DORLAND'S ILLUSTRATED

Medical Dictionary

Twenty-sixth Edition

DORLAND'S ILLUSTRATED

Medical Dictionary

Twenty-sixth Edition

W. B. SAUNDERS COMPANY Philadelphia London Toronto
Mexico City Sydney Tokyo

Preface

Each day, through the efforts of workers in the scientific community, including the many specialties and subspecialties of medicine and related fields, new concepts are formed and old theories are discarded, answers to hitherto seemingly unanswerable questions are found, and new techniques evolve. The results of these efforts must be made known to all who are concerned with or interested in what is current in the language of science. This places strenuous demands on those who have the obligation of recording and defining these developments in a manner that may be comprehended readily not only by specialists in a particular field but also by those who, for various reasons, seek to learn more about an unfamiliar subject.

As in all previous twenty-five editions of Dorland's Illustrated Medical Dictionary, the compilers of this, the twenty-sixth, edition have endeavored to meet the challenges presented by the ever-expanding terminology of all the sciences.

The use of computer technology for composition of the twenty-fifth edition of the Dictionary served us well in preparing the present edition. The coded master file on which the entire contents of the Dictionary had been transcribed and stored enabled us to sort and retrieve all entries relating to a particular discipline, thereby allowing us and our consultants to review the entire lexicon of each discipline. Also, the system of computer coding enabled us to integrate new terms and to revise others without disturbing already existing material — that is, only new portions of the vocabulary or those that needed emendation were phototypeset. The time saved in typography and the flexibility of this method made it possible for us to continue updating our material even after the phototypesetting process had begun and to utilize the latest data gathered from our reference sources during the final stages of manuscript preparation. Such methods helped to ensure that the vocabulary recorded here is as current as the increasingly rapid expansion of the terminology of science allows at any given time.

While making full use of such new tools and procedures, however, we have adhered to the fundamental concepts that have guided our efforts throughout the history of the Dictionary. These concepts have been stated in previous editions:

All learning in science is based on education in vocabulary, for the imagery of words and symbols is the only means to expression of scientific data and concepts. For the continuing successful interchange of ideas, the words and ideographs of science must have precise and specific meanings and these must be recorded in a carefully arranged repository of such information. Accuracy, comprehensiveness, ease of understanding, and typographic legibility are obvious standards of usefulness in such a work. The occasional assembly of related data in tables and illustrations serves the additional purpose of grouping information under broad headings of reference or educative value.

Codification of knowledge is made increasingly difficult by the steadily broadening scope and mounting complexity of contemporary medical science. In this situation we believe that writers and editors constitute the first line of defense, particularly against erosion and adulteration of the language. We believe that editors should not be unmindful of the advisability of safeguarding the faithful transmission of ideas, by insuring the integrity of the words in which they are expressed. In furtherance of this purpose, we believe that the exercise of judgment is a legitimate activity of the compiler of a dictionary of scientific terms: to lend support to words properly compounded and to favor such terms over words which may bear the taint of ambiguity.

The function of a dictionary must then be something more than that of a record of usage. It is our belief that maintenance of certain standards of etymological propriety and of selection is also a responsibility of the lexicographer — no less in the language of science than in that of imaginative or creative writing. Validity of formation of a word supplies its best assurance of intact passage across language barriers that are fast disappearing in medicine, as in other sciences. And the extensive usage of this Dictionary outside the United States makes us all the more aware of this responsibility.

In exercising this belief, it is not our intention to assume an unyielding attitude toward words that, although imprecisely coined, enjoy a ready, almost universal acceptance within the biomedical sciences. Rather, we attempt to lend our influence to the preference of etymologically sound and unambiguous terms to communicate new concepts. In most instances, this preference is indicated within the Dictionary by assigning the definition to the "term of choice" and cross-referring synonyms to that term.

Certain questions that arise in writing or editing, as those regarding the use of diphthongs or the hyphenation of compound words, may be entirely a matter of style, and their answers are not primarily to be established by recourse to a dictionary. It would be impossible, except in unabridged volumes, to present every variation on such themes that might be completely acceptable and proper.

ACKNOWLEDGMENTS

As in the preceding edition, the definitions of the various anatomical structures are placed on the NA terms, that is, on the terms as they appear in the *Nomina Anatomica* as approved by the Sixth International Congress of Anatomists held in Paris in 1955, and revised by the Seventh and Eighth Congresses held respectively in New York in 1960 and in Wiesbaden in 1965.

In enzyme nomenclature, we have relied heavily on the Recommendations of the International Union of Pure and Applied Chemistry and the International Union of Biochemistry on the Nomenclature and Classification of Enzymes.

For psychiatric terms, we have been guided in many instances by *A Psychiatric Glossary*, edited by the Subcommittee on Public Information and published by the American Psychiatric Association.

In pharmacology, as noted on the copyright page, we have made use of portions of the text of the *United States Pharmacopeia,* the *National Formulary,* and *USAN and the USP Dictionary of Drug Names,* all publications of the United States Pharmacopeial Convention, Inc.

In acknowledging our indebtedness to the compilers, editors, and publishers of the aforementioned publications, we emphasize that any inaccuracies that may have arisen from our transcription or interpretation of this material are our sole responsibility.

In addition to the contributions from these publications, hundreds of persons have made valuable suggestions for this book of words. To them, we gratefully acknowledge our great debt for help beyond measure, help that can be repaid only insofar as we have succeeded in combining these separate threads into a fabric useful and authoritative to all.

The more than 50 new illustrations were drawn by Susan Shapiro Brenman. Her fine drawings with their precise attention to detail and structure not only enhance the pages of the Dictionary but also provide at a glance information that is sometimes difficult to convey in words.

We would also like especially to thank Dr. I. Eban of London, England, for all the useful advice and suggestions that he has given us over so many years.

Lastly and most importantly, we must express our overwhelming debt and enduring gratitude to our Consultants, whom we take great pleasure in listing on the following page. Without their dedication, forbearance, and expert knowledge, the massive and intricate task of compiling this twenty-sixth edition of the Dictionary could never have been completed.

JOHN P. FRIEL

Dictionary Editor for the Publisher

Consultants

FRANK J. BIA, M.D., M.P.H.
Assistant Professor of Medicine and Laboratory Medicine, Yale University School of Medicine

JOHN PAUL BRADY, M.D.
Kenneth E. Appel Professor of Psychiatry and Chairman of the Department, University of Pennsylvania; Consulting Psychiatrist, Veterans Administration Hospital, Philadelphia, Institute of the Pennsylvania Hospital, Philadelphia, and Philadelphia Psychiatric Center; and Visiting Professor of Psychiatry, Trinity College, Dublin, Ireland

LUTHER W. BRADY, M.D.
Hylda Cohn/American Cancer Society Professor of Clinical Oncology and Chairman of the Department of Radiation and Nuclear Medicine, Hahnemann Medical College

NICHOLAS P. CHRISTY, M.D.
Chief of Staff, Veterans Administration, Brooklyn, New York; Professor of Medicine, Downstate Medical Center, State University of New York, Brooklyn; and Lecturer in Medicine, College of Physicians and Surgeons, Columbia University

JULIUS M. CRUSE, D.MICROBIOL., M.D., PH.D., F.A.A.M., F.R.S.H.
Professor of Pathology, Director of Immunopathology Section and Tissue Typing Laboratories, Director of Graduate Studies in Pathology, and Associate Professor of Microbiology, The University of Mississippi Medical Center

JOHN BERNARD HENRY, B.A., M.D.
Dean and Professor of Pathology, Georgetown University School of Medicine

ROBERT E. LEWIS, JR., B.A., M.S., PH.D., M.B.S.H.
Assistant Professor of Anesthesiology, Assistant Professor of Pathology, Co-Director of Clinical Immunopathology Laboratory and of the Tissue Typing Laboratory, The University of Mississippi Medical Center

MILTON MARKOWITZ, M.D.
Professor and Head, Department of Pediatrics, University of Connecticut School of Medicine; and Director of Pediatric Services, John Dempsy Hospital

RONAN O'RAHILLY, M.D.
Director, Carnegie Laboratories of Embryology and Professor of Human Anatomy and Neurology, University of California, Davis

STEVEN J. PHILLIPS, M.D.
Professor of Anatomy, Temple University School of Medicine

GEORGE C. POPPENSIEK, M.S., V.M.D.
The James Law Professor of Comparative Medicine, College of Veterinary Medicine, Cornell University

STANLEY G. SCHADE, M.D.
Professor of Medicine, University of Illinois at the Medical Center, Chicago; Chief, Section of Hematology, University of Illinois Hospital; and Staff Member, Westside Veterans Administration Hospital

JAMES SNOW, JR., M.D.
Professor and Chairman, Department of Otorhinolaryngology and Human Communication, University of Pennsylvania School of Medicine

JOHN B. WEST, M.D., PH.D., D.SC., M.R.C.P. (LOND.)
Professor of Medicine and Physiology, School of Medicine, University of California, San Diego; and Physician, University of California, San Diego Medical Center

DOROTHY WHITCOMB, B.A., M. LIB. SCI.
Historical Librarian, University of Wisconsin Health Science Center Libraries and William S. Middleton Library, University of Wisconsin

Contents

Index to Tables

Index to Plates

Notes on Use
of This Dictionary

The new user of this Dictionary, we believe, will profit from an understanding of the policies that have been followed in its actual construction. This section is therefore presented to explain some of the mechanics which were involved in the compilation of the material.

It is our hope that a corollary of the conventional use of this Dictionary, to discover the spelling, meaning, and derivation of specific terms, will be assistance in the reverse direction — to aid in the creation of words desired to express new concepts. To this end individual elements — prefixes, suffixes, and stems — may be found both in the vocabulary portion and in the section entitled Fundamentals of Medical Etymology. An understanding of the elements of a term encountered for the first time, if the term is too new to be in any dictionary, will aid one in arriving at an approximation if not an exact distillation of its meaning. Similarly, knowledge of these elements and of the conventions governing their combination will be of help to a person seeking to construct a new word. We believe the serious user of the Dictionary will find familiarity with these features highly rewarding.

ARRANGEMENT OF ENTRIES

Quick simple usefulness continues to be one of the principal objectives of this work. Words appearing as main entries are recognizable at a glance, not being distorted by accents or other indication of syllabication. Accents and syllables are shown in the phonetic respelling immediately following the bold face entry. Subentries — terms consisting of two words which are ordinarily defined under the second (or principal) word, the *noun* — are immediately apparent as subentries, run on in the same paragraph, and set in the same bold face type as the word constituting the main entry. For example, acetic acid, acetrizoic acid, iopanoic acid, neuraminic acid, shikimic acid, and the like, are included as subentries under acid, regardless of the pH of the specific compounds. Absorption bands, Büngner's bands, Lane's band, Parham band are defined under band; Heinz-Ehrlich bodies, Howell-Jolly bodies, Leishman-Donovan bodies are defined under body.

The space-imposed practice of defining a term only once accounts for the cross references necessitated on eponymic terms where biographical information is given. Thus you will find such entries as "Apgar score . . . See under *score*" and "Budin's joint, rule . . . See under *joint* and *rule*." An exception to this policy of arrangement occurs in the case of specific chemical terms embodying the name of the element: aluminum acetate, aluminum hydroxide, aluminum sulfate, and the like are defined under aluminum; calcium carbonate, calcium oxide, calcium sulfate under calcium.

If biographical information is not given for an individual named in an eponymic term, such as Kortzeborn's operation, the definition should be sought directly under the noun, in this case under operation. For certain phrases, because of prevalent multiplicity of terminology, it may be necessary to look in more than one place. For example, what one person may speak of as a disease may originally have been called a syndrome; if the desired term does not appear under one, it should be sought under the alternative term. Similarly for phenomenon and sign, and numerous other entities.

SEQUENCE OF ENTRIES

Entries will be found alphabetized on the sequence of the letters, regardless of space or hyphens which may occur between them. Thus sequences such as

bloodless,	or	formboard,
blood plasma,		form-class,
blood pressure,		forme,
bloodroot		form-family

appear in that order. An exception to this occurs in the case of compound eponymic terms: Bard-Pic's syndrome precedes Bardach's test. In eponymic terms, the apostrophe s ('s) is ignored in determining the alphabetical sequence, thus *Addison's planes* precedes *addisonian*, *Sabouraud's agar* precedes *Sabouraudia*, and *Förster's operation* precedes *Förster-Penfield operation*, both as a main entry and under operation. Similarly umlauts (ö, ü) are ignored in alphabetizing the entries, and *Löwenthal's tract, Lower's rings, Löwitt's bodies, Lowman balance board,* and *Lowry's test* appear in that sequence. Proper names beginning with "Mc" or "Mac" are alphabetized as though spelled "mac" in every instance, the sequence being determined by the letters immediately following the *c*.

Proper names (or capitalized entries) commonly appear before a common noun (or lower case entry) with the identical spelling. Thus *Diplococcus* precedes *diplococcus*, *Micrococcus* precedes *micrococcus*.

INDICATION OF PRONUNCIATION

As in the twenty-five preceding editions, phonetic respelling of a term appears in parentheses immediately following the main bold face entry. As a rule only the most commonly heard pronunciation is given, with no effort to represent any variants. Such phonetic respelling is presented in the simplest possible manner, with a minimum of diacritical markings. The basic rule is this: An unmarked vowel ending a syllable is long; an unmarked vowel in a syllable ending with a consonant is short. By this same token, a long vowel in a syllable which must end with a consonant is indicated by a macron (ā, ē, ī, ō, ū, and o͞o): for example ah-bāt′, lēd, la′bīl, mi′o-fōn, mol′e-kūl, to͞oth. A short vowel ending or alone constituting a syllable is usually indicated by use of the breve (ĕ, ĭ, ŏ, ŭ, o͝o): for example ĕ-fish′ent, ĭ-mu′nĭ-te, ŏ-kloo′zhun.

The use of the syllable *ah* for the sound of *a* in open, unaccented syllables (ah-bāt′, ah-lu′mĭ-num, ah-pof′ĭ-sis, ah-tak′se-ah) has been continued; *ah* is also used in syllables ending with a consonant, to indicate a broader *a* sound (fahr′mah-se, in contrast to am-ne′se-ah). No effort has been made to complicate the system by introduction of additional diacritical marks showing the finer gradations of sound, such as the circumflex (â, ô), diaeresis (ä, ü), tilde (ē). The primary (′) and secondary (″) accents are indicated in polysyllabic words (as pol″e-sĭ-lab′ik); an unstressed syllable is followed by a hyphen.

To recapitulate, unmarked vowels not followed by a consonant have the long sound:

> ba, da, ka, la, ma, na, etc., are all pronounced to rhyme with *fay*
>   (bāt, kām, mān, etc., have the same vowel sound).
> be, de, le, re, te, we, etc., are all pronounced to rhyme with *fee*
>   (bēm, dēp, rēt, etc., have the same vowel sound).
> bi, di, ni, pi, ti, zi, etc., are all pronounced to rhyme with *sigh*
>   (bīd, pīnt, tīm, etc., have the same vowel sound).
> bo, do, lo, mo, to, wo, etc., are all pronounced to rhyme with *go*
>   (bōd, lōm, tōt, etc., have the same vowel sound).
> bu, du, hu, mu, nu, su, etc., are all pronounced to rhyme with *few*
>   (kūt, mūt, etc., have the same vowel sound).

Short vowels terminating syllables are affected by the value or the consonantal sounds of the adjoining syllables. For example, as usually pronounced, the sound of *i* in the second syllable more closely approaches that of long *e* in mult*i*articular than it does in mult*i*gravida, although in either word it may show any gradation between the long *e* and an indeterminate vowel sound. Combinations of vowels are also indicated: *oi* as in oil; *ou* as in out; *aw* as in paw.

It has been impossible, within the framework of this simplified system, to represent the exact pronunciation of many foreign words and proper names which have entered the medical vocabulary. They have been represented as well as possible by an English approximation.

The important key to remember in interpreting the phonetic respelling is that an unmarked vowel not followed by a consonant has the long value; one followed by a consonant has the short. A long vowel which must perforce be followed by a consonant is indicated by use of the macron; a short vowel ending its respective syllable is indicated by use of the breve.

PRESENTATION OF PLURAL FORMS

The plural of a word which is irregularly formed or of a foreign word is given following the phonetic respelling and often, but not invariably, is given a separate bold face listing in proper alphabetical order. Alternate plurals (e.g., exanthemas, exanthemata) are frequently shown. Subentries appear in proper alphabetical order, determined by the subsequent, modifying word or phrases, regardless of whether they are singular or plural. For example, under *ligamentum,* the entries

> l. annulare baseos stapedis
> ligamenta annularia digitorum manus
> ligamenta annularia digitorum pedis
> l. annulare radii
> ligamenta annularia (trachealia)

appear in that order.

ETYMOLOGY

Information on the derivation of a word appears in square brackets following the phonetic respelling, or following the plural form of the word, when that is given. Greek characters are no longer used in presentation of the etymological information in the vocabulary portion of this book,* being transliterated into the English alphabet as shown in the following tabulation:

	α	= a		λ	= l	
initial	$\dot{\alpha}$	= a		μ	= m	
"	$\dot{\alpha}$	= ha		ν	= n	
diphthong	$\alpha\iota$	= ai		ξ	= x	
initial	$\alpha\iota$	= ai		o	= o	
"	$\alpha\iota$	= hai	initial	$\dot{o}$	= o	
diphthong	$\alpha\upsilon$	= au	"	$\dot{o}$	= ho	
initial	$\alpha\dot{\upsilon}$	= au	diphthong	$o\iota$	= oi	
"	$\alpha\dot{\upsilon}$	= hau	initial	$o\iota$	= oi	
	β	= b	"	$o\iota$	= hoi	
	γ	= g	diphthong	$o\upsilon$	= ou	
	$\gamma\gamma$	= ng [as in "angeion"]	initial	$o\dot{\upsilon}$	= ou	
	$\gamma\kappa$	= nk [as in "ankyle"]	"	$o\dot{\upsilon}$	= hou	
	$\gamma\xi$	= nx [as in "salpinx"]		π	= p	
	$\gamma\chi$	= nch [as in "anchousa"]		ρ	= r	
	δ	= d	initial	ρ	= rh	
	ϵ	= e		$\rho\rho$	= rrh	[used in compounds, although the root has only initial rh, e.g. diarrhoia—(English) diarrhea]
initial	$\dot{\epsilon}$	= e				
"	$\dot{\epsilon}$	= he				
diphthong	$\epsilon\iota$	= ei				
initial	$\epsilon\iota$	= ei				
"	$\epsilon\iota$	= hei		σ, s	= s	
diphthong	$\epsilon\upsilon$	= eu		τ	= t	
initial	$\epsilon\dot{\upsilon}$	= eu		υ	= y	
"	$\epsilon\dot{\upsilon}$	= heu	[initial	υ	does not occur]	
	ζ	= z	"	$\dot{\upsilon}$	= hy	
	η	= $\bar{e}$	diphthong	$\upsilon\iota$	= ui	
initial	$\dot{\eta}$	= $\bar{e}$	initial	$\upsilon\iota$	= hui	
"	$\dot{\eta}$	= h$\bar{e}$		ϕ	= ph	
	θ	= th		χ	= ch	
	ι	= i		ψ	= ps	
initial	ι	= i		ω	= $\bar{o}$	
"	ι	= hi	initial	$\dot{\omega}$	= $\bar{o}$	
	κ	= k	"	$\dot{\omega}$	= h$\bar{o}$	

*The Greek characters do appear, however, in the section entitled Fundamentals of Medical Etymology (pp. xvii–xxix).

The original words from which the terms presented in this Dictionary are derived are reproduced in italic, the language of their origin being indicated by the appropriate abbreviation (see Abbreviations Used in This Dictionary).

As a guide to related vocabulary, especially on anatomical terms, the main entry may be followed in brackets by its Latin and/or Greek equivalent, such as "liver [L. *jecur;* Gr. *hepar*]" and "kidney [L. *ren;* Gr. *nephros*]."

SYNONYMS AND THE PLACEMENT OF DEFINITIONS

With few exceptions in this Dictionary, a definition (as opposed to a cross-reference) is given at only one place for two or more synonymous terms. Thus, for example, definitions of most anatomical terms appear on the terms official in the *Nomina Anatomica,* and the common names are cross-referred to the official names. The reader, then, will find on the anglicized common names of anatomical structures, as those under artery, ligament, muscle, nerve, and vein, a cross-reference to the official name of the specific structure. The complete descriptions, in these particular instances, are given in the tables of arteriae, ligamenta, musculi, nervi, and venae.

Such cross-references are also given for synonyms of terms listed in other official publications, including the *United States Pharmacopeia* and the *National Formulary,* the full descriptions again being given on the official names.

This practice of cross-referring is also followed for earlier terms that have been supplanted in the vocabulary as well as for terms which are currently used with the same meaning as the term on which a full description is given. In most such instances, the term on which the definition appears is the currently preferred term for the entity. In others, the shade of preference may be slight, or even denied by some persons. In the latter cases, the practice has been adhered to as a means of keeping down the size of the Dictionary by avoiding duplication of definitions.

ABBREVIATIONS USED IN THIS DICTIONARY

a.	artery (L. *arteria*); agar	l.	ligament (L. *ligamentum*); left
aa.	arteries (L. *arteriae*)	lat.	lateral
ant.	anterior	lev.	levator
Ar.	Arabic	m.	muscle (L. *musculus*); medium
A.S.	Anglo-Saxon	med.	medial, median
b.	broth	Mex.	Mexican
bas.	basal	n.	nerve (L. *nervus*)
br.	branch	NA	Nomina Anatomica
C.	cervical	neg.	negative
c.	about (L. *circa*); culture medium	NF	National Formulary
cf.	compare (L. *confer*)	obs.	obsolete
Coc.	coccygeal	Peruv.	Peruvian
Dan.	Danish	pl.	plural
def.	definition	Port.	Portuguese
dim.	diminutive	post.	posterior
e.g.	for example (L. *exempli gratia*)	priv.	privative
Fin.	Finnish	q.v.	which see (L. *quod vide*)
Fr.	French	r.	right
gen.	genitive	Russ.	Russian
Ger.	German	S.	sacral
Gr.	Greek	sing.	singular
Hind.	Hindu	Sp.	Spanish
i.e.	that is (L. *id est*)	sup.	superior
inf.	inferior	T.	thoracic
It.	Italian	USP	United States Pharmacopeia
Jap.	Japanese	v.	vein (L. *vena*)
L.	Latin; lumbar		

Fundamentals of Medical Etymology

By Lloyd W. Daly, A.M., Ph.D., Litt.D.

Allen Memorial Professor of Greek, University of Pennsylvania

The very size of current medical dictionaries is evidence of the massive proportions which the medical, scientific, and technical vocabulary has attained within the English language. As this vocabulary grows, its mastery by each succeeding generation becomes increasingly difficult. It is popularly believed that the study of Latin at least, if not also of Greek, is prerequisite for the study of medicine. Although this is no longer literally true, the composition of the medical vocabulary makes it evident why such study was formerly considered necessary. At least fifty per cent of the general English vocabulary is of Greek and Latin derivation, and it is a conservative estimate that as much as seventy-five per cent of the scientific element is of such origin.

Some familiarity with these two languages which contribute so largely to the terminology must obviously simplify the task of learning a basic vocabulary and of comprehending new words as they are encountered. Experience shows that it does. However, since it no longer seems economical to learn to read the two languages for this purpose, some short cut to the necessary information is needed, and again experience has shown that certain fundamentals of vocabulary and linguistic principle can easily be mastered and are of great assistance. The purpose of the present introduction is to present those fundamentals in as practical and concise a form as possible; any statements in the following pages which are contrary to historical linguistic fact are made deliberately, in keeping with this purpose.

GREEK

Alphabet and transcription
The Latin alphabet as we use it is derived, with slight modifications, from the Greek alphabet, which is almost completely phonetic. The table (p. xviii) shows as nearly as possible the sound equivalent of each letter in terms of our own alphabet, the names of the letters, and their transcribed equivalents in English. The first syllable of the name of each letter, properly pronounced, also gives its sound equivalent.

Greek words are written with an accent ($\theta\acute{\epsilon}\sigma\iota\varsigma$, $\varphi\hat{v}\lambda o\nu$); for present purposes, the two kinds of accent mark may be regarded simply as indicating the syllable on which the stress of accent is placed. Words beginning with a vowel, diphthong, or *rho* (ρ) are written with a breathing mark over the initial vowel or *rho*, or over the second vowel of the diphthong ($\ddot{\alpha}\lambda\lambda o\varsigma$, $\dot{\rho}v\theta\mu\acute{o}\varsigma$, $a\dot{v}\tau\acute{o}\varsigma$). The so-called rough breathing mark (') indicates that the syllable over which it is placed should be initiated in pronunciation with an *h* sound, and words beginning with such a sound are usually transcribed into English with an initial *h*. Rarely they may appear with or without the *h*.* The smooth breathing mark (') has no effect on pronunciation.

---

*For example, in the Analytical Word List, following, compare -em- and hem(at)-, -aph- and hapt-, -elc- and helc-; such forms without the *h* rarely appear as the initial element of a compound.

Capital	Small Letter	Sound	Name	Transcription
Α	α	*aha*	alpha	a
Β	β	*bet*	beta	b
Γ	γ	*get*	gamma	g
Δ	δ	*do*	delta	d
Ε	ε	*egg*	epsilon	e
Ζ	ζ	*adze*	zeta	z
Η	η	*fête*	eta	ē
Θ	θ	*thin*	theta	th
Ι	ι	*it* / ma*chi*ne	iota	i
Κ	κ	*key*	kappa	k
Λ	λ	*let*	lambda	l
Μ	μ	*met*	mu	m
Ν	ν	*net*	nu	n
Ξ	ξ	*hex*	xi	x
Ο	ο	*oho*	omicron	o
Π	π	*pet*	pi	p
Ρ	ρ	*r* (trilled)	rho	r
Σ	σ, ς*	*set*	sigma	s
Τ	τ	*tell*	tau	t
Υ	υ	*ü* (German)	upsilon	y
Φ	φ	*photo*	phi	ph
Χ	χ	a*ch* (German)	chi	ch
Ψ	ψ	*tips*	psi	ps
Ω	ω	*oho*	omega	ō

* Sigma is written σ at the beginning or in the middle of a word and ς at the end of a word. E.g., σύνδεσις.

The vowels are α, ε, η, ι, ο, υ, and ω, which may be combined to give the diphthongs shown in the listing below. The letter *iota* (ι) may also be written as a subscript (ᾳ, ῃ, ῳ), but as such it has no effect on pronunciation.

Diphthong	Sound	Transcription
αι	*aisle*	ae, e, or ai
αυ	*out*	au
ει	*eight*	i, e, or ei
ευ	*eh-oo*	eu
οι	*oil*	oe or e
ου	*ghoul*	ou or u
υι	*quit*	ui

Words are transcribed from Greek into our own alphabet as indicated in the foregoing tables, with the following exceptions: *Gamma* (γ) before *gamma* (γ), *kappa* (κ), *chi* (χ), or *xi* (ξ) is nasal and so is transcribed as *n*. Initial *rho* (ῥ) is transcribed as *rh*, and double *rho* (ρρ) as *rrh*. *Upsilon* (υ) is transcribed as *y* except in diphthongs, where it is reproduced by *u*, as indicated in the table.

Many Greek words have come into English through Latin, in which they have undergone some change (Greek στέονον, Latin *sternum*), or through a second intermediary language, such as French, with still further change (Greek χειρουργία, Latin *chirurgia*, French *cirurgerie*, English *surgery*). Such evolution explains many of the apparent peculiarities of Greek words in English. Other changes are accounted for by our tendency to drop inflectional terminations which indicate grammatical function in Greek but have no function in English (σπέρμα, sperm), or to simplify the termination (γονοφόρος, gonophore).

Combining forms The most constant change, however, in the transition of Greek words to English, is the loss of termination which produces what we may call the *combining form*. This combining form, which is used when the word enters into a compound with another word, may differ markedly from the *lexical form*, under which the word would be located in a dictionary of the Greek language.

For most nouns (those ending in -η, -α, -ος, -ον), the combining form may be derived by dropping the termination from the lexical form. For another large class the combining form must be derived from a secondary form of the word (indicated in parentheses in the following table) by dropping the ending -ος. For most words ending in -ις only ς need be dropped. In some instances, as in terms derived from the words for blood (hemat-) and body (somat-), different combining forms are used, derived from either the lexical or the secondary form. Adjectives are similar in formation to nouns. For those ending in -υς only the ς need be dropped.

LEXICAL FORM	COMBINING FORM	ENGLISH
ἀρχή	ἀρχ-	*arch*enteron
ἰδέα	ἰδε-	*ide*ology
τόπος	τοπ-	*top*esthesia
ὀστέον	ὀστε-	*oste*otome
βάσις	βασι-	*basi*cranial
μῦς (μυός)	μυ-	*my*ectomy
αἷμα (αἵματος)	αἱμ-, αἱματ-	*hem*angioma, *hemat*ophyte
παῖς (παιδός)	παιδ-	*paed*iatrics

For verbs the combining form may be derived from several of the six principal parts, which may show a variable vowel just as English verbs do (sing, sang, sung). Thus the verb meaning to *stretch* has the forms τείνω and τέτακα, and English words may be derived from either, e.g., *tein*oscope, *ectasis*. In most cases, however, the combining form may be derived from the lexical form ending in -ω, -μαι, or -μι, or from the infinitive form ending in -ειν, -αν, -ουν, -σθαι, or -ναι, the latter being the form often cited in the etymology given in dictionaries. The commonest vowel variation is from ε to ο, as in the verb τρέφω, which frequently shows the combining form τροφ-, as in a*troph*y.

Compounds   Most derivatives are composed not of single Greek words but of a combination of two or more words or word elements. Thus the word *osteotome* is composed of the noun ὀστέον (oste) plus τέμνω (tom). When the second member of the compound begins with a consonant, as in this instance, a connective *o* is usually inserted between the two members to facilitate pronunciation.

Prefixes   Many compounds consist of a word preceded by a prefix, commonly a preposition. As shown in the table, most of these prepositions have a final vowel, which is dropped when the word to which it is affixed begins with a vowel, the prefix περί (peri-) being an exception. A final consonant may also be changed as indicated, to accommodate it to a succeeding initial consonant. The negative prefix ἀν- before a vowel (*an*omaly) must not be confused with the preposition ἀνά with the final vowel dropped (*an*ode).

PREPOSITION	COMBINING FORMS	ENGLISH
ἀμφί	ἀμφι-	*amphi*crania
	ἀμφ-	*amph*eclexis
ἀνά	ἀνα-	*ana*bolism
	ἀν-	*an*ode
ἀντί	ἀντι-	*anti*gen
	ἀντ-	*ant*helminthic
ἀπό	ἀπο-	*apo*physis
	ἀπ-	*ap*andria
διά	δια-	*dia*thermy
	δι-	*di*uretic
ἐκ	ἐκ-	*ec*topia
ἐξ	ἐξ-	*ex*osmosis
ἐν	ἐν-	*en*ostosis
	ἐμ-	*em*bolus
ἐπί	ἐπι-	*epi*nephrin
	ἐπ-	*ep*arterial
κατά	κατα-	*cata*lepsy
	κατ-	*cat*ion
μετά	μετα-	*meta*morphosis
	μετ-	*met*encephalon
παρά	παρα-	*para*mastoid
	παρ-	*par*otid
περί	περι-	*peri*toneum
πρό	προ-	*pro*gnosis
σύν	συν-	*syn*thesis
	συμ-	*sym*physis
	συλ-	*syl*lepsis
	συ-	*sy*stole
ὑπέρ	ὑπερ-	*hyper*trophy
ὑπό	ὑπο-	*hypo*dermic
	ὑπ-	*hyp*axial

Suffixes Suffixes, which constitute a third element in the formation of compounds, are added directly to the combining forms of words without insertion of a connective *o*, but when the result would be a combination of consonants difficult to pronounce, certain euphonic changes are made in the final consonant of the combining form. The combinations shown

Consonant Changes	English
β or $\varphi + \tau = \pi\tau$	epile*ptic*
γ or $\chi + \tau = \kappa\tau$	ta*ctic*
δ or $\theta + \tau = \sigma\tau$	schi*st*
π, β or $\varphi + \mu = \mu\mu$	le*mma*
κ, γ or $\chi + \mu = \gamma\mu$	paradi*gm*
τ, δ or $\theta + \mu = \sigma\mu$	pla*sma*
π, β or $\varphi + \sigma = \psi$	auto*psy*
κ, γ or $\chi + \sigma = \xi$	cache*xia*
τ, δ or $\theta + \sigma = \sigma$	do*se*

in the table represent the results of the addition of those suffixes which are the commonest in the vocabulary. The suffixes -$\tau\eta s$ (-*t*), -$\tau\eta\rho$ (-*ter*), -$\sigma\iota s$ (-*sis*), -$\sigma\iota\alpha$ (-*sia* or -*sy*), -μos (-*m*), -$\mu\alpha$ (-*ma* or -*m*) are usually added to verbal combining forms to produce nouns; -τos (-*t*, -*te*) and -$\tau\iota\kappa os$ (-*tic*) are added to verbal combining forms to produce adjectives or nouns; -$\iota\zeta\omega$ (-*ize*) is added to noun or adjective combining forms to produce verbs; -$\iota\alpha$ (-*ia* or -*y*) is added to noun or verb combining forms to produce nouns; -$\iota\tau\iota s$ (-*itis*) and -κos or -$\iota\kappa os$ (-*c* or -*ic*) are added to noun combining forms to produce nouns or adjectives. The following examples illustrate such compounding and indicate some of the possibilities of adding one suffix to another. It should be noted that nouns ending with the suffix -$\mu\alpha$ have a combining form ending in -$\mu\alpha\tau$- and that verbs ending with the suffix -$\iota\zeta\omega$ have a combining form ending in -$\iota\delta$-.

Greek Components	English
$\dot{o}\sigma\tau\acute{e}ov + \kappa\lambda\acute{a}\omega + -\tau\eta s$	osteo*clast*
$\sigma\varphi\acute{\iota}\gamma\gamma\omega + -\tau\eta\rho$	sphin*cter*
$\dot{\epsilon}\mu\acute{e}\omega + -\sigma\iota s$	eme*sis*
$\kappa\iota\nu\acute{e}\omega + -\sigma\iota\alpha$	cine*sia*
$\dot{\epsilon}\pi\acute{\iota} + \lambda\alpha\mu\beta\acute{a}\nu\omega + -\sigma\iota\alpha$	epile*psy*
$\sigma\pi\acute{a}\omega + -\mu os$	spa*sm*
$\kappa\alpha\rho\kappa\iota\nu\acute{o}\omega + -\mu\alpha$	carcino*ma*
$\dot{o}\rho\acute{a}\omega + -\tau os + \mu\acute{e}\tau\rho ov$	opto*meter*
$\zeta\upsilon\gamma\acute{o}\omega + -\tau os$	zyg*ote*
$\ddot{\iota}\sigma\tau\eta\mu\iota + -\tau\iota\kappa os$	sta*tic*
$\kappa\rho\acute{\upsilon}\sigma\tau\alpha\lambda\lambda os + -\iota\zeta\omega$	crystal*lize*
$\mu\alpha\acute{\iota}\nu\omega + -\iota\alpha$	man*ia*
$\nu\epsilon\hat{\upsilon}\rho ov + \gamma\rho\acute{a}\varphi\omega + -\iota\alpha$	neuro*graphy*
$o\hat{\upsilon}s + -\iota\tau\iota s$	ot*itis*
$\kappa\acute{o}\lambda ov + -\iota\kappa os$	col*ic*
$\varphi\acute{\upsilon}\sigma\iota s + -\kappa os$	physi*c*
$\ddot{\alpha}\rho\theta\rho ov + -\iota\tau\iota s + -\kappa os$	arth*ritic*
$\sigma\upsilon\mu\pi\acute{\iota}\pi\tau\omega + -\mu\alpha + -\iota\kappa os$	sympto*matic*
$\kappa\rho\acute{e}as + \varphi\alpha\gamma\epsilon\hat{\iota}\nu + -\iota\zeta\omega + -\mu os$	creopha*gism*
$\varphi\acute{\upsilon}\omega + -\sigma\iota s + -\kappa os + -\iota\zeta\omega + -\tau\eta s$	phy*sicist*

In the formation of compounds English follows natural tendencies of the Greek language but often goes far beyond the actual Greek vocabulary. For example, there is no such Greek verb as $\varphi\upsilon\sigma\iota\kappa\acute{\iota}\zeta\omega$ nor even such an English verb as *physicize*, yet the word physicist is formed as though there were, on the analogy of such verbs as *stigmatize*, which actually have Greek counterparts. In a similar manner, the need for new terms is met by coining new words composed of prefixes, combining forms, and suffixes, on the basis of analogy.

LATIN

A high percentage of medical terms is of Latin origin, but a good proportion of this element, being in the form of anatomical nomenclature, is original Latin and not derivative. The purpose of this introduction is to explain derivatives, words which have undergone some change in the transfer to English. For original Latin words the reader may refer to the body of the Dictionary.

Alphabet The Latin alphabet is a modification of the Greek which has been adopted for English with the addition of the characters *J*, *U*, and *W*, which were developed during the Middle Ages. The ease with which the Romans adapted the Greek alphabet is evidence of the close relationship of the two languages.

The inflectional terminations of Latin words, as of Greek, tend to be modified or to be dropped in English. Thus *nervus* becomes nerve, *spina* becomes spine, *penicillum* becomes pencil, and *oleum* appears usually as -ol. However, Latin terminations are more frequently tolerated than those of Greek, and are adopted into English, as occurred with the terms *fetus, rectum, pelvis,* and *vagina.*

Combining forms   Combining forms of Latin words, as of Greek, are derived by dropping an inflectional termination. Thus for most nouns ending in *-a, -us,* or *-um,* this ending must be dropped from the lexical form, whereas for others *-is* must be dropped from a secondary form (indicated in parentheses in the table).

LEXICAL FORM	COMBINING FORM	ENGLISH
retina	*retin-*	*retin*opapillitis
bulbus	*bulb-*	*bulb*iform
ovum	*ov-*	*ov*iduct
frons (frontis)	*front-*	*front*oparietal
cortex (corticis)	*cortic-*	*cortic*ipetal

Adjectives follow these same patterns. The comparative form, ending in *-ior,* frequently appears in English without change, as in *inferior.*

The lexical forms of all regular Latin verbs end in either *-o* or *-or,* but the forms most commonly used in English derivatives are the participles, or verbal adjectives, present and past. Whereas the English present participle ends in *-ing,* the combining form of the Latin ends in *-nt* preceded by a vowel, either *a* or *e.* Whereas the English past participle usually ends in *-ed* or *-en,* the combining form of the Latin regularly ends in *-t* or *-s,* which may be preceded by a vowel, either *a* or *i.* The *-us* termination of these past participles is regularly modified to an *e,* thus producing the common English ending *-ate.*

LEXICAL FORM	ENGLISH	
	(From Pres. Part.)	(From Past Part.)
consulto	*consultant*	*consulta*tion
aperio	*aperient*	*aper*ture
nutrio	*nutrient*	*nutri*tive
sentio	*sentient*	*sens*ory

Use of the past participial form ending in *-atus* is greatly extended in English by the formation of numerous derivatives, including not only such verbs as rotate, from the Latin verb *roto* but also, by analogy, such verbs as aerate, although there is no such Latin verb as *aero.*

Compounds   In the formation of compound derivatives from Latin words a combining form is linked to the following element by what may be called, regardless of its origin, a connective vowel. This vowel is most commonly either *o* (lumb*o*costal, genit*o*urinary) or *i* (nerv*i*motor, bil*i*rubin), or less frequently *u* (gran*u*lation).

Prefixes   As in Greek, most of the prefixes in Latin are prepositions. Most of these may be added to other words without change, but some of those which end in a consonant assimilate this consonant to the initial sound of the word to which it is affixed.

CONSONANT CHANGES			ENGLISH
ad-	before *c* becomes *ac-*		*ac*celerate
ad-	before *f* becomes *af-*		*af*finity
ad-	before *g* becomes *ag-*		*ag*glutinant
ad-	before *p* becomes *ap-*		*ap*pendix
ad-	before *s* becomes *as-*		*as*similate
ad-	before *t* becomes *at-*		*at*trition
ex-	before *f* becomes *ef-*		*ef*fusion
in-	before *l* becomes *il-*		*il*linition
in-	before *m* becomes *im-*		*im*mersion
in-	before *r* becomes *ir-*		*ir*radiation
ob-	before *c* becomes *oc-*		*oc*clusion
sub-	before *f* becomes *suf-*		*suf*focate
sub-	before *p* becomes *sup-*		*sup*pository
trans-	before *s* becomes *tran-*		*tran*spiration

The addition of a prefix may also affect the following word by changing its characteristic vowel; thus *ob* + *caput* becomes *occiput*, and *in* + *iactus* becomes *inject*.

Suffixes   The commonest Latin suffixes used in forming nouns are: *-arium, -orium* (-ary, -ory), *-io* (-ion added to past participles), *-or* (-or added to past participles), and *-tas* (-ty). Those used in forming adjectives are: *-abilis, -ibilis* (-able, -ible), *-alis, -ilis* (-al, -ile), *-aris* (-ar), *-arius, -orius* (-ary, -ory), *-atus* (-ate), *-idus* (-id), *-ivus* (-ive), and *-osus* (-ous or -ose).

Latin Components	English
avis + *-arium*	avi*ary*
dormio (*dormitus*) + *-orium*	dormit*ory*
nutrio (*nutritus*) + *-io*	nutrit*ion*
moveo (*motus*) + *-or*	mot*or*
porosus + *-tas*	porosi*ty*
frio + *-abilis*	fri*able*
edo + *-ibilis*	ed*ible*
corpus (*corporis*) + *-alis*	corpor*al*
febris + *-ilis*	febr*ile*
oculus + *-aris*	ocul*ar*
cilium + *-arius*	cili*ary*
sensus + *-orius*	sens*ory*
reticulum + *-atus*	reticul*ate*
morbus + *-idus*	morb*id*
aborior (*abortus*) + *-ivus*	abort*ive*
squama + *-osus*	squam*ous*
adeps (*adipis*) + *-osus*	adip*ose*
prae + *caveo* (*cautus*) + *-io* + *-arius*	precaut*ionary*

HYBRID TERMS

The examples hitherto cited have been purely Greek or purely Latin, but elements from the two languages are often combined in one compound word, which is called a hybrid. A prefix from one language may be added to a word from the other (*de* + ὕδωρ + *-atus* = dehydrate), or a Greek and a Latin word may be combined (δόλιχος + *facialis* = dolichofacial). However, the most productive source of such hybrids is the addition of a Latin suffix to a Greek word (κρανίον + *-alis* = cranial) or vice versa (*cerebellum* + *-ιτις* = cerebellitis).

ANALYTICAL WORD LIST

The following list includes those Greek and Latin words which an actual count* shows occur most frequently in the vocabulary of this dictionary, arranged alphabetically under their English combining forms as rubrics. The dash appended to a combining form indicates that it is not a complete word and, if the dash precedes the combining form, that it commonly appears as the terminal element of a compound. Infrequently a combining form is both preceded and followed by a dash, showing that it usually appears between two other elements. Closely related forms are shown in one entry by the use of parentheses: thus carbo(n)-, showing it may be either carbo-, as in *carbo*hydrate, or carbon-, as in *carbon*uria.

Following each combining form the first item of information is the Greek or Latin word from which it is derived. Those words which are not printed in Greek characters are Latin. Occasionally both a Greek and a Latin word are given. Presence of a dash before or after such an element indicates that it does not occur as an independent word in the original language. Information necessary to the understanding of the form appears next in parentheses. Then the meaning or meanings of the word are given, followed where appropriate by reference to a synonymous combining form in the other language, that is, on a combining form of Latin derivation, to the synonymous form of Greek derivation, and vice versa. Finally, an example is given to illustrate use of the combining form in a compound English derivative.

If this list is used in close conjunction with the etymological information given in the body of the Dictionary, no confusion should be caused by the similarity of elements in such words as *mel*algia, *mel*ancholia, and *mel*icera, where the similarity is only apparent and the derivation of each word is different.

---

*For the count upon which the selection was based, thanks are due to my wife, Bernadine A. Daly, whose expert work will, I am sure, greatly increase the practical usefulness of the list.

a-   a- (n is added before words beginning with a vowel) negative prefix. Cf. in-³. ametria

ab-   ab away from. Cf. apo-. abducent

abdomin-   abdomen, abdominis. abdominoscopy

ac-   See ad-. accretion

acet-   acetum vinegar. acetometer

acid-   acidus sour. aciduric

acou-   ἀκούω hear. acouesthesia. (Also spelled acu-)

acr-   ἄκρον extremity, peak. acromegaly

act-   ago, actus do, drive, act. reaction

actin-   ἀκτίς, ἀκτῖνος ray, radius. Cf. radi-. actinogenesis

acu-   See acou-. osteoacusis

ad-   ad (d changes to c, f, g, p, s, or t before words beginning with those consonants) to. adrenal

aden-   ἀδήν gland. Cf. gland-. adenoma

adip-   adeps, adipis fat. Cf. lip- and stear-. adipocellular

aer-   ἀήρ air. anaerobiosis

aesthe-   See esthe-. aesthesioneurosis

af-   See ad-. afferent

ag-   See ad-. agglutinant

-agogue   ἀγωγός leading, inducing. galactagogue

-agra   ἄγρα catching, seizure. podagra

alb-   albus white. Cf. leuk-. albocinereous

alg-   ἄλγος pain. neuralgia

all-   ἄλλος other, different. allergy

alve-   alveus trough, channel, cavity. alveolar

amph-   See amphi-. ampheclexis

amphi-   ἀμφί (i is dropped before words beginning with a vowel) both, doubly. amphicelous

amyl-   ἄμυλον starch. amylosynthesis

an-¹   See ana-. anagogic

an-²   See a-. anomalous

ana-   ἀνά (final a is dropped before words beginning with a vowel) up, positive. anaphoresis

ancyl-   See ankyl-. ancylostomiasis

andr-   ἀνήρ, ἀνδρός man. gynandroid

angi-   ἀγγεῖον vessel. Cf. vas-. angiemphraxis

ankyl-   ἀγκύλος crooked, looped. ankylodactylia. (Also spelled ancyl-)

ant-   See anti-. antophthalmic

ante-   ante before. anteflexion

anti-   ἀντί (i is dropped before words beginning with a vowel) against, counter. Cf. contra-. antipyogenic

antr-   ἄντρον cavern. antrodynia

ap-¹   See apo-. apheter

ap-²   See ad-. append

-aph   ἅπτω, ἀφ- touch. dysaphia. (See also hapt-)

apo-   ἀπό (o is dropped before words beginning with a vowel) away from, detached. Cf. ab-. apophysis

arachn-   ἀράχνη spider. arachnodactyly

arch-   ἀρχή beginning, origin. archenteron

arter(i)-   ἀρτηρία elevator (?), artery. arteriosclerosis, periarteritis

arthr-   ἄρθρον joint. Cf. articul-. synarthrosis

articul-   articulus joint. Cf. arthr-. disarticulation

as-   See ad-. assimilation

at-   See ad-. attrition

aur-   auris ear. Cf. ot-. aurinasal

aux-   αὔξω increase. enterauxe

ax-   ἄξων or axis axis. axofugal

axon-   ἄξων axis. axonometer

ba-   βαίνω, βα- go, walk, stand. hypnobatia

bacill-   bacillus small staff, rod. Cf. bacter-. actinobacillosis

bacter-   βακτήριον small staff, rod. Cf. bacill-. bacteriophage

ball-   βάλλω, βολ- throw. ballistics. (See also bol-)

barb-   βάρος weight. pedobarometer

bi-¹   βίος life. Cf. vit-. aerobic

bi-²   bi- two (see also di-¹). bilobate

bil-   bilis bile. Cf. chol-. biliary

blast-   βλαστός bud, child, a growing thing in its early stages. Cf. germ-. blastoma, zygotoblast.

blep-   βλέπω look, see. hemiablepsia

blephar-   βλέφαρον (from βλέπω; see blep-) eyelid. Cf. cili-. blepharoncus

bol-   See ball-. embolism

brachi-   βραχίων arm. brachiocephalic

brachy-   βραχύς short. brachycephalic

brady-   βραδύς slow. bradycardia

brom-   βρῶμος stench. podobromidrosis

bronch-   βρόγχος windpipe. bronchoscopy

bry-   βρύω be full of life. embryonic

bucc-   bucca cheek. distobuccal

cac-   κακός bad, abnormal. Cf. mal-. cacodontia, arthrocace. (See also dys-)

calc-¹   calx, calcis stone (cf. lith-), limestone, lime. calcipexy

calc-²   calx, calcis heel. calcaneotibial

calor-   calor heat. Cf. therm-. calorimeter

cancr-   cancer, cancri crab, cancer. Cf. carcin-. cancrology. (Also spelled chancr-)

capit-   caput, capitis head. Cf. cephal-. decapitator

caps-   capsa (from capio; see cept-) container. encapsulation

carbo(n)-   carbo, carbonis coal, charcoal. carbohydrate, carbonuria

carcin-   καρκίνος crab, cancer. Cf. cancr-. carcinoma

cardi-   καρδία heart. lipocardiac

cary-   See kary-. caryokinesis

cat-   See cata-. cathode

cata-   κατά (final a is dropped before words beginning with a vowel) down, negative. catabatic

caud-   cauda tail. caudad

cav-   cavus hollow. Cf. coel-. concave

cec-   caecus blind. Cf. typhl-. cecopexy

cel-¹   See coel-. amphicelous

cel-²   See -cele. celectome

-cele   κήλη tumor, hernia. gastrocele

cell-   cella room, cell. Cf. cyt-. celliferous

cen-   κοινός common. cenesthesia

cent- — *centum* hundred. Cf. hect-. Indicates fraction in metric system. [This exemplifies the custom in the metric system of identifying fractions of units by stems from the Latin, as centimeter, decimeter, millimeter, and multiples of units by the similar stems from the Greek, as hectometer, decameter, and kilometer.] *centi*meter, *centi*pede

cente- — κεντέω puncture. Cf. punct-. entero*cente*sis

centr- — κέντρον or *cenrum* point, center. neuro*centr*al

cephal- — κεφαλή head. Cf. capit-. en*cephal*itis

cept- — *capio, -cipientis, -ceptus* take, receive. re*cept*or

cer- — κηρός or *cera* wax. *cer*oplasty, *cer*omel

cerat- — See kerat-. a*cerat*osis

cerebr- — *cerebrum. cerebr*ospinal

cervic- — *cervix, cervicis* neck. Cf. trachel-. *cervic*itis

chancr- — See cancr-. *chancr*iform

cheil- — χεῖλος lip. Cf. labi-. *cheil*oschisis

cheir- — χείρ hand. Cf. man-. macro*cheir*ia. (Also spelled chir-)

chir- — See cheir-. *chir*omegaly

chlor- — χλωρός green. a*chlor*opsia

chol- — χολή bile. Cf. bil-. hepato*chol*angeitis

chondr- — χόνδρος cartilage. *chondr*omalacia

chord- — χορδή string, cord. peri*chord*al

chori- — χόριον protective fetal membrane. endo*chori*on

chro- — χρώς color. poly*chro*matic

chron- — χρόνος time. syn*chron*ous

chy- — χέω, χυ- pour. ec*chy*mosis

-cid(e) — *caedo, -cisus* cut, kill. infanti*cide*, germi*cid*al

cili- — *cilium* eyelid. Cf. blephar-. super*cili*ary

cine- — See kine-. auto*cine*sis

-cipient — See cept-. in*cipient*

circum- — *circum* around. Cf. peri-. *circum*ferential

-cis- — *caedo, -cisus* cut, kill. ex*cis*ion

clas- — κλάω, κλασ- break. cranio*clas*t

clin- — κλίνω bend, incline, make lie down. *clin*ometer

clus- — *claudo, -clusus* shut. Maloc*clus*ion

co- — See con-. *co*hesion

cocc- — κόκκος seed, pill. gono*cocc*us

coel- — κοῖλος hollow. Cf. cav-. *coel*enteron. (Also spelled cel-)

col-¹ — See colon-. *col*ic

col-² — See con-. *col*lapse

colon- — κόλον lower intestine. *colon*ic

colp- — κόλπος hollow, vagina. Cf. sin-. endo*colp*itis

com- — See con-. *com*masculation

con- — *con-* (becomes co- before vowels or *h*; col- before *l*; com- before *b, m,* or *p*; cor- before *r*) with, together. Cf. syn-. *con*traction

contra- — *contra* against, counter. Cf. anti-. *contra*indication

copr- — κόπρος dung. Cf. sterco-. *copr*oma

cor-¹ — κόρη doll, little image, pupil. iso*cor*ia

cor-² — See con-. *cor*rugator

corpor- — *corpus, corporis* body. Cf. somat-. intra*corpor*al

cortic- — *cortex, corticis* bark, rind. *cortic*osterone

cost- — *costa* rib. Cf. pleur-. inter*cost*al

crani- — κρανίον or *cranium* skull. peri*crani*um

creat- — κρέας, κρεατ- meat, flesh. *creat*orrhea

-crescent — *cresco, crescentis, cretus* grow. ex*crescent*

cret-¹ — *cerno, cretus* distinguish, separate off. Cf. crin-. dis*cret*e

cret-² — See -crescent. ac*cret*ion

crin- — κρίνω distinguish, separate off. Cf. cret-¹. endo*crin*ology

crur- — *crus, cruris* shin, leg. brachio*crur*al

cry- — κρύος cold. *cry*esthesia

crypt- — κρύπτω hide, conceal. *crypt*orchism

cult- — *colo, cultus* tend, cultivate. *cult*ure

cune- — *cuneus* wedge. Cf. sphen-. *cune*iform

cut- — *cutis* skin. Cf. derm(at)-. sub*cut*aneous

cyan- — κύανος blue. antho*cyan*in

cycl- — κύκλος circle, cycle. *cycl*ophoria

cyst- — κύστις bladder. Cf. vesic-. nephro*cyst*itis

cyt- — κύτος cell. Cf. cell-. plasmo*cyt*oma

dacry- — δάκρυ tear. *dacry*ocyst

dactyl- — δάκτυλος finger, toe. Cf. digit-. hexa*dactyl*ism

de- — *de* down from. *de*composition

dec-¹ — δέκα ten. Indicates multiple in metric system. Cf. dec-². *deca*gram

dec-² — *decem* ten. Indicates fraction in metric system. Cf. dec-¹. *deci*para, *deci*meter

dendr- — δένδρον tree. neuro*dendr*ite

dent- — *dens, dentis* tooth. Cf. odont-. inter*dent*al

derm(at)- — δέρμα, δέρματος skin. Cf. cut-. endo*derm*, *dermat*itis

desm- — δεσμός band, ligament. syn*desm*opexy

dextr- — *dexter, dextr-* right-hand. ambi*dextr*ous

di-¹ — *di-* two. *di*morphic. (See also bi-²)

di-² — See dia-. *di*uresis.

di-³ — See dis-. *di*vergent.

dia- — διά (*a* is dropped before words beginning with a vowel) through, apart. Cf. per-. *dia*gnosis

didym- — δίδυμος twin. Cf. gemin-. epi*didym*al

digit- — *digitus* finger, toe. Cf. dactyl-. *digit*igrade

diplo- — διπλόος double. *diplo*myelia

dis- — *dis-* (*s* may be dropped before a word beginning with a consonant) apart, away from. *dis*location

disc- — δίσκος or *discus* disk. *disc*oplacenta

dors- — *dorsum* back. ventro*dors*al

drom- — δρόμος course. hemo*drom*ometer

-ducent — See duct-. ad*ducent*

duct- — *duco, ducentis, ductus* lead, conduct. ovi*duct*

dur-   *durus* hard. Cf. scler-. in*dura*tion

dynam(i)-   δύναμις power. *dynam*oneure, neuro*dynam*ic

dys-   δυσ- bad, improper. Cf. mal-. *dys*trophic. (See also cac-)

e-   *e* out from. Cf. ec- and ex-. *e*mission

ec-   ἐκ out of. Cf. e- *ec*centric

-ech-   ἔχω have, hold, be. syn*ech*otomy

ect-   ἐκτός outside. Cf. extra-. *ecto*plasm

ede-   οἰδέω swell. *ede*matous

ef-   See ex-. *ef*florescent

-elc-   ἕλκος sore, ulcer. enter*elc*osis. (See also helc-)

electr-   ἤλεκτρον amber. *electr*otherapy

em-   See en-. *em*bolism, *em*pathy, *em*phlysis

-em-   αἷμα blood. an*em*ia. (See also hem(at)-)

en-   ἐν (*n* changes to *m* before *b, p,* or *ph*) in, on. Cf. in-². *en*celitis

end-   ἔνδον inside. Cf. intra-. *end*angium.

enter-   ἔντερον intestine. dys*enter*y

ep-   See epi-. *ep*axial

epi-   ἐπί (*i* is dropped before words beginning with a vowel) upon, after, in addition. *epi*glottis

erg-   ἔργον work, deed. en*erg*y

erythr-   ἐρυθρός red. Cf. rub(r)-. *erythr*ochromia

eso-   ἔσω inside. Cf. intra-. *eso*phylactic

esthe-   αἰσθάνομαι, αἰσθη- perceive, feel. Cf. sens-. an*esthe*sia

eu-   εὖ good, normal. *eu*pepsia

ex-   ἐξ or *ex* out of. Cf. e-. *ex*cretion

exo-   ἔξω outside. Cf. extra-. *exo*pathic

extra-   *extra* outside of, beyond. Cf. ect- and exo-. *extra*cellular

faci-   *facies* face. Cf. prosop-. brachio*faci*olingual

-facient   *facio, facientis, factus, -fectus* make. Cf. poie-. cale*facient*

-fact-   See facient-. arte*fact*

fasci-   *fascia* band. *fasci*orrhaphy

febr-   *febris* fever. Cf. pyr-. *febr*icide

-fect-   See -facient. de*fect*ive

-ferent   *fero, ferentis, latus* bear, carry. Cf. phor-. ef*ferent*

ferr-   *ferrum* iron. *ferr*oprotein

fibr-   *fibra* fibre. Cf. in-¹. chondro*fibr*oma

fil-   *filum* thread. *fil*iform

fiss-   *findo, fissus* split. Cf. schis-. *fiss*ion

flagell-   *flagellum* whip. *flagell*ation

flav-   *flavus* yellow. Cf. xanth-. ribo*flav*in

-flect-   *flecto, flexus* bend, divert. de*flect*ion

-flex-   See -flect-. re*flex*ometer

flu-   *fluo, fluxus* flow. Cf. rhe-. *flu*id

flux-   See flu-. af*flux*ion

for-   *foris* door, opening. per*for*ated

-form   *forma* shape. Cf. -oid. ossi*form*

fract-   *frango, fractus* break. re*fract*ive

front-   *frons, frontis* forehead, front. naso*front*al

-fug(e)   *fugio* flee, avoid. vermi*fuge*, centri*fug*al

funct-   *fungor, functus* perform, serve, function. mal*funct*ion

fund-   *fundo, fusus* pour. in*fund*ibulum

fus-   See fund-. dif*fus*ible

galact-   γάλα, γάλακτος milk. Cf. lact-. dys*galact*ia

gam-   γάμος marriage, reproductive union. a*gam*ont

gangli-   γάγγλιον swelling, plexus. neuro*gangli*itis

gastr-   γαστήρ, γαστρός stomach. cholangio*gastr*ostomy

gelat-   *gelo, gelatus* freeze, congeal. *gela*tin

gemin-   *geminus* twin, double. Cf. didym-. quadri*gemin*al

gen-   γίγνομαι, γεν-, γον- become, be produced, originate, or γεννάω produce, originate. cyto*gen*ic

germ-   *germen, germinis* bud, a growing thing in its early stages. Cf. blast-. *germ*inal, ovi*germ*

gest-   *gero, gerentis, gestus* bear, carry. con*gest*ion

gland-   *glans, glandis* acorn. Cf. aden-. intra*gland*ular

-glia   γλία glue. neuro*glia*

gloss-   γλῶσσα tongue. Cf. lingu-. tricho*gloss*ia

glott-   γλῶττα tongue, language. *glott*ic

gluc-   See glyc(y)-. *gluc*ophenetidin

glutin-   *gluten, glutinis* glue. ag*glutin*ation

glyc(y)-   γλυκύς sweet. *glyc*emia, *glycy*rrhizin. (Also spelled gluc-)

gnath-   γνάθος jaw. ortho*gnath*ous

gno-   γιγνώσκω, γνω- know, discern. dia*gno*sis

gon-   See gen-. amphi*gon*y

grad-   *gradior* walk, take steps. retro*grad*e

-gram   γράφω, γραφ- + -μα scratch, write, record. cardio*gram*

gran-   *granum* grain, particle. lipo*gran*uloma

graph-   γράφω scratch, write, record. histo*graph*y

grav-   *gravis* heavy. multi*grav*ida

gyn(ec)-   γυνή, γυναικός woman, wife. andro*gyn*y, *gynec*ologic

gyr-   γῦρος ring, circle. *gyr*ospasm

haem(at)-   See hem(at)-. *haem*orrhagia, *haemat*oxylon

hapt-   ἅπτω touch. *hapt*ometer

hect-   ἑκτ- hundred. Cf. cent-. Indicates multiple in metric system. *hect*ometer

helc-   ἕλκος sore, ulcer. *helc*osis

hem(at)-   αἷμα, αἵματος blood. Cf. sanguin-. *hem*angioma, *hemat*ocyturia. (See also -em-)

hemi-   ἡμι- half. Cf. semi-. *hemi*ageusia

hen-   εἷς, ἑνός one. Cf. un-. *hen*ogenesis

hepat-   ἧπαρ, ἥπατος liver. gastro*hepat*ic

hept(a)-   ἑπτά seven. Cf. sept-². *hept*atomic, *hepta*valent

hered-   *heres, heredis* heir. *hered*oimmunity

hex-¹   ἕξ six. Cf. sex-. *hex*yl-. An *a* is added in some combinations.

hex-²   ἔχω, ἐχ- (added to σ becomes ἐξ-) have, hold, be. cach*ex*y

hexa-   See hex-¹. *hexa*chromic

hidr-   ἱδρώς sweat. hyper*hidr*osis

hist-   ἱστός web, tissue. *hist*odialysis

hod-   ὁδός road, path. *hod*oneuromere.
            (See also od- and -ode[1])

hom-   ὁμός common, same. *homo*morphic

horm-   ὁρμή impetus, impulse. *horm*one

hydat-   ὕδωρ, ὕδατος water. *hydat*ism

hydr-   ὕδωρ, ὑδρ- water. Cf. lymph-. achlor*hydr*ia

hyp-   See hypo-. *hyp*axial

hyper-   ὑπέρ above, beyond, extreme. Cf. super-. *hyper*trophy

hypn-   ὕπνος sleep. *hypn*otic

hypo-   ὑπό (o is dropped before words beginning with a vowel) under, below. Cf. sub-. *hypo*metabolism

hyster-   ὑστέρα womb. colpo*hyster*opexy

iatr-   ἰατρός physician. ped*iatr*ics

idi-   ἴδιος peculiar, separate, distinct. *idi*osyncrasy

il-   See in-[2, 3]. *il*linition (in, on), *il*legible (negative prefix)

ile-   See ili- [ile- is commonly used to refer to the portion of the intestines known as the ileum]. *ile*ostomy

ili-   *ilium (ileum)* lower abdomen, intestines [ili- is commonly used to refer to the flaring part of the hip bone known as the ilium]. *ili*osacral

im-   See in-[2, 3]. *im*mersion (in, on), *im*perforation (negative prefix)

in-[1]   ἴς, ἰνός fiber. Cf. fibr-. *in*osteatoma

in-[2]   *in* (n changes to *l*, *m*, or *r* before words beginning with those consonants) in, on. Cf. en-. *in*sertion

in-[3]   *in*- (n changes to *l*, *m*, or *r* before words beginning with those consonants) negative prefix. Cf. a-. *in*valid

infra-   *infra* beneath. *infra*orbital

insul-   *insula* island. *insul*in

inter-   *inter* among, between. *inter*carpal

intra-   *intra* inside. Cf. end- and eso-. *intra*venous

ir-   See in-[2, 3]. *ir*radiation (in, on), *ir*reducible (negative prefix)

irid-   ἴρις, ἴριδος rainbow, colored circle. kerato*irid*ocyclitis

is-   ἴσος equal. *is*otope

ischi-   ἰσχιον hip, haunch. *ischi*opubic

jact-   *iacio, iactus* throw. *jact*itation

ject-   *iacio, -iectus* throw. in*ject*ion

jejun-   *ieiunus* hungry, not partaking of food. gastro*jejun*ostomy

jug-   *iugum* yoke. con*jug*ation

junct-   *iungo, iunctus* yoke, join. con*junct*iva

kary-   κάρυον nut, kernel, nucleus. Cf. nucle-. mega*kary*ocyte. (Also spelled cary-)

kerat-   κέρας, κέρατος horn. *kerat*olysis. (Also spelled cerat-)

kil-   χίλιοι one thousand. Cf. mill-. Indicates multiple in metric system. *kil*ogram

kine-   κινέω move. *kine*matograph. (Also spelled cine-)

labi-   *labium* lip. Cf. cheil-. gingivo*labi*al

lact-   *lac, lactis* milk. Cf. galact-. gluco*lact*one

lal-   λαλέω talk, babble. glosso*lal*ia

lapar-   λαπάρα flank. *lapar*otomy

laryng-   λάρυγξ, λάρυγγος windpipe. *laryng*endoscope

lat-   *fero, latus* bear, carry. See -ferent. trans*lat*ion

later-   *latus, lateris* side. ventro*later*al

lent-   *lens, lentis* lentil. Cf. phac-. *lent*iconus

lep-   λαμβάνω, ληπ- take, seize. cata*lep*tic

leuc-   See leuk-. *leuc*inuria

leuk-   λευκός white. Cf. alb-. *leuk*orrhea. (Also spelled leuc-)

lien-   *lien* spleen. Cf. splen-. *lien*ocele

lig-   *ligo* tie, bind. *lig*ate

lingu-   *lingua* tongue. Cf. gloss-. sub*lingu*al

lip-   λίπος fat. Cf. adip-. glyco*lip*in

lith-   λίθος stone. Cf. calc-[1]. nephro*lith*otomy

loc-   *locus* place. Cf. top-. *loc*omotion

log-   λέγω, λογ- speak, give an account. *log*orrhea, embry*olog*y

lumb-   *lumbus* loin. dorso*lumb*ar

lute-   *luteus* yellow. Cf. xanth-. *lute*oma

ly-   λύω loose, dissolve. Cf. solut-. kerato*ly*sis

lymph-   *lympha* water. Cf. hydr-. *lymph*adenosis

macr-   μακρός long, large. *macr*omyeloblast

mal-   *malus* bad, abnormal. Cf. cac- and dys-. *mal*function

malac-   μαλακός soft. osteo*malac*ia

mamm-   *mamma* breast. Cf. mast-. sub*mamm*ary

man-   *manus* hand. Cf. cheir-. *man*iphalanx

mani-   μανία mental aberration. *mani*graphy, klepto*mani*a

mast-   μαστός breast. Cf. mamm-. hyper*mast*ia

medi-   *medius* middle. Cf. mes-. *medi*frontal

mega-   μέγας great, large. Also indicates multiple (1,000,000) in metric system. *mega*colon, *mega*dyne. (See also megal-)

megal-   μέγας, μεγάλου great, large. acro*megal*y

mel-   μέλος limb, member. sym*mel*ia

melan-   μέλας, μέλανος black. hippo*melan*in

men-   μήν month. dys*men*orrhea

mening-   μῆνιγξ, μήνιγγος membrane. encephalo*mening*itis

ment-   *mens, mentis* mind. Cf. phren-, psych- and thym-. de*ment*ia

mer-   μέρος part. poly*mer*ic

mes-   μέσος middle. Cf. medi-. *mes*oderm

met-   See meta-. *met*allergy

meta-   μετά (a is dropped before words beginning with a vowel) after, beyond, accompanying. *meta*carpal

metr-[1]   μέτρον measure. stereo*metr*y

metr-[2]   μήτρα womb. endo*metr*itis

micr-   μικρός small. photo*micr*ograph

mill-   *mille* one thousand. Cf. kil-. Indicates fraction in metric system. *mill*igram, *mill*ipede

miss-   See -mittent. intro*miss*ion

-mittent	*mitto, mittentis, missus* send. inter*mittent*	par-[1]	*pario* bear, give birth to. primi*parous*
mne-	μιμνήσκω, μνη- remember. pseudo*mnesia*	par-[2]	See para-. *parepigastric*
mon-	μόνος only, sole. *mono*plegia	para-	παρά (final *a* is dropped before words beginning with a vowel) beside, beyond. *para*mastoid
morph-	μορφή form, shape. poly*morpho*nuclear		
mot-	*moveo, motus* move. vaso*motor*	part-	*pario, partus* bear, give birth to. *part*urition
my-	μῦς, μυός muscle. inoleio*myoma*		
-myces	μύκης, μύκητος fungus. myelo*myces*	path-	πάθος that which one undergoes, sickness. psycho*pathic*
myc(et)-	See -myces. asco*mycetes*, strepto*mycin*	pec-	πήγνυμι, πηγ- (πηκ- before τ) fix, make fast. sym*pecto*thiene. (See also pex-)
myel-	μυελός marrow. polio*myelitis*		
myx-	μύξα mucus. *myx*edema	ped-	παῖς, παιδός child. ortho*ped*ic
narc-	νάρκη numbness. topo*narc*osis	pell-	*pellis* skin, hide. *pell*agra
nas-	*nasus* nose. Cf. rhin-. palato*nasal*	-pellent	*pello, pellentis, pulsus* drive. re*pellent*
ne-	νέος new, young. *ne*ocyte	pen-	πένομαι need, lack. erythrocyto*penia*
necr-	νεκρός corpse. *necr*ocytosis		
nephr-	νεφρός kidney. Cf. ren-. para*nephr*ic	pend-	*pendeo* hang down. ap*pend*ix
		pent(a)-	πέντε five. Cf. quinque-. *pent*ose, *penta*ploid
neur-	νεῦρον nerve. esthesio*neure*		
nod-	*nodus* knot. *nod*osity	peps-	πέπτω, πεψ- (before σ) digest brady*peps*ia
nom-	νόμος (from νέμω deal out, distribute) law, custom. tax*onomy*	pept-	πέπτω digest. dys*pept*ic
		per-	*per* through. Cf. dia-. *per*nasal
non-	*nona* nine. *non*acosane	peri-	περί around. Cf. circum-. *peri*phery
nos-	νόσος disease. *nos*ology		
nucle-	*nucleus* (from *nux, nucis* nut) kernel. Cf. kary-. *nucle*ide	pet-	*peto* seek, tend toward. centri*pet*al
nutri-	*nutrio* nourish. mal*nutri*tion	pex-	πήγνυμι, πηγ- (added to σ becomes πηξ-) fix, make fast. hepato*pexy*
ob-	*ob* (b changes to c before words beginning with that consonant) against, toward, etc. *ob*tuse		
		pha-	φημί, φα- say, speak. dys*pha*sia
oc-	See ob-. *oc*clude.	phac-	φακός lentil, lens. Cf. lent-. *phac*osclerosis. (Also spelled phak-)
ocul-	*oculus* eye. Cf. ophthalm-. *oculo*motor		
-od-	See -ode[1]. peri*od*ic	phag-	φαγεῖν eat. lipo*phag*ic
-ode[1]	ὁδός road, path. cath*ode*. (See also hod-)	phak-	See phac-. *phak*itis
		phan-	See phen-. dia*phan*oscopy
-ode[2]	See -oid. nemat*ode*	pharmac-	φάρμακον drug. *pharmac*ognosy
odont-	ὀδούς, ὀδόντος tooth. Cf. dent-. ortho*dont*ia	pharyng-	φάρυγξ, φαρυγγ- throat. glosso*pharyng*eal
-odyn-	ὀδύνη pain, distress. gastro*dyn*ia		
-oid	εἶδος form. Cf. -form. hy*oid*	phen-	φαίνω, φαν- show, be seen. phos*phen*e
-ol	See ole-. cholester*ol*	pher-	φέρω, φορ- bear, support. peri*pher*y
ole-	*oleum* oil. *ole*oresin		
olig-	ὀλίγος few, small. *olig*ospermia	phil-	φιλέω like, have affinity for. eosino*phil*ia
omphal-	ὀμφαλός navel. peri*omphal*ic		
onc-	ὄγκος bulk, mass. hemat*onc*ometry	phleb-	φλέψ, φλεβός vein. peri*phleb*itis
onych-	ὄνυξ, ὄνυχος claw, nail. an*onych*ia	phleg-	φλέγω, φλογ- burn, inflame. adeno*phleg*mon
oo-	ᾠόν egg. Cf. ov-. peri*oo*thecitis	phlog-	See phleg-. anti*phlog*istic
op-	ὁράω, ὀπ- see. erythr*op*sia	phob-	φόβος fear, dread. claustro*phob*ia
ophthalm-	ὀφθαλμός eye. Cf. ocul-. ex*ophthalm*ic		
		phon-	φωνή sound. echo*phon*y
or-	*os, oris* mouth. Cf. stom(at)-. intra*or*al	phor-	See pher-. Cf. -ferent. exo*phor*ia
orb-	*orbis* circle. sub*orb*ital	phos-	See phot-. *phos*phorus
orchi-	ὄρχις testicle. Cf. test-. *orchi*opathy	phot-	φῶς, φωτός light. *phot*erythrous
organ-	ὄργανον implement, instrument. *organ*oleptic	phrag-	φράσσω, φραγ- fence, wall off, stop up. Cf. sept-[1]. dia*phrag*m
orth-	ὀρθός straight, right, normal. *orth*opedics		
oss-	*os, ossis* bone. Cf. ost(e)-. *oss*iphone	phrax-	φράσσω, φραγ- (added to σ becomes φραξ-) fence, wall off, stop up. em*phrax*is
ost(e)-	ὀστέον bone. Cf. oss-. en*ost*osis, *oste*anaphysis		
		phren-	φρήν mind, midriff. Cf. ment-. meta*phren*ia, meta*phren*on
ot-	οὖς, ὠτός ear. Cf. aur-. par*ot*id		
ov-	*ovum* egg. Cf. oo-. syn*ov*ia	phthi-	φθίνω decay, waste away. ophthalmo*phthi*sis
oxy-	ὀξύς sharp. *oxy*cephalic	phy-	φύω beget, bring forth, produce, be by nature. noso*phy*te
pachy(n)-	παχύνω thicken. *pachy*derma, myo*pachyn*sis		
		phyl-	φῦλον tribe, kind. *phyl*ogeny
pag-	πήγνυμι, παγ- fix, make fast. thoraco*pag*us	-phyll	φύλλον leaf. xantho*phyll*
		phylac-	φύλαξ guard. pro*phylac*tic

phys(a)- φυσάω blow, inflate. *physocele, physalis*

physe- φυσάω, φυση- blow, inflate. em*physema*

pil- *pilus* hair. e*pilation*

pituit- *pituita* phlegm, rheum. *pituitous*

placent- *placenta* (from πλακοῦς) cake. extra*placental*

plas- πλάσσω mold, shape. cine*plasty*

platy- πλατύς broad, flat. *platyrrhine*

pleg- πλήσσω, πληγ- strike. di*plegia*

plet- *pleo, -pletus* fill. de*pletion*

pleur- πλευρά rib, side. Cf. cost-. peri*pleural*

plex- πλήσσω, πληγ- (added to σ becomes πληξ-) strike. apo*plexy*

plic- *plico* fold. com*plication*

pne- πνοιά breathing. traumato*pnea*

pneum(at)- πνεῦμα, πνεύματος breath, air. *pneumodynamics, pneumatothorax*

pneumo(n)- πνεύμων lung. Cf. pulmo(n)-. *pneumocentesis, pneumonotomy*

pod- πούς, ποδός foot. *podiatry*

poie- ποιέω make, produce. Cf. -facient. sarco*poietic*

pol- πόλος axis of a sphere. peri*polar*

poly- πολύς much, many. *polyspermia*

pont- *pons, pontis* bridge. *ponto-cerebellar*

por-¹ πόρος passage. myelo*pore*

por-² πῶρος callus. *porocele*

posit- *pono, positus* put, place. re*positor*

post- *post* after, behind in time or place. *postnatal, postoral*

pre- *prae* before in time or place. *prenatal, prevesical*

press- *premo, pressus* press. *pressoreceptive*

pro- πρό or *pro* before in time or place. *progamous, procheilon, prolapse*

proct- πρωκτός anus. entero*proctia*

prosop- πρόσωπον face. Cf. faci-. di*prosopus*

pseud- ψευδής false. *pseudoparaplegia*

psych- ψυχή soul, mind. Cf. ment-. *psychosomatic*

pto- πίπτω, πτω- fall. nephro*ptosis*

pub- *pubes* & *puber, puberis* adult. ischio*pubic*. (See also puber-)

puber- *puber* adult. *puberty*

pulmo(n)- *pulmo, pulmonis* lung. Cf. pneumo(n)-. *pulmolith, cardiopulmonary*

puls- *pello, pellentis, pulsus* drive. pro*pulsion*

punct- *pungo, punctus* prick, pierce. Cf. cente-. *punctiform*

pur- *pus, puris* pus. Cf. py-. sup*puration*

py- πύον pus. Cf. pur-. nephro*pyosis*

pyel- πύελος trough, basin, pelvis. nephro*pyelitis*

pyl- πύλη door, orifice. *pylephlebitis*

pyr- πῦρ fire. Cf. febr-. galacto*pyra*

quadr- *quadr-* four. Cf. tetra-. *quadrigeminal*

quinque- *quinque* five. Cf. pent(a)-. *quinquecuspid*

rachi- ῥάχις spine. Cf. spin-. encephalo*rachidian*

radi- *radius* ray. Cf. actin-. ir*radiation*

re- *re-* back, again. *retraction*

ren- *renes* kidneys. Cf. nephr-. ad*renal*

ret- *rete* net. *retothelium*

retro- *retro* backwards. *retrodeviation*

rhag- ῥήγνυμι, ῥαγ- break, burst. hemor*rhagic*

rhaph- ῥαφή suture. gastror*rhaphy*

rhe- ῥέω flow. Cf. flu-. diar*rheal*

rhex- ῥήγνυμι, ῥηγ- (added to σ becomes ῥηξ-) break, burst. metror*rhexis*

rhin- ῥίς, ῥινός nose. Cf. nas-. basi*rhinal*

rot- *rota* wheel. *rotator*

rub(r)- *ruber, rubri* red. Cf. erythr-. bili*rubin, rubrospinal*

salping- σάλπιγξ, σάλπιγγος tube, trumpet. *salpingitis*

sanguin- *sanguis, sanguinis* blood. Cf. hem(at)-. *sanguineous*

sarc- σάρξ, σαρκός flesh. *sarcoma*

schis- σχίζω, σχιδ- (before τ or added to σ becomes σχισ-) split. Cf. fiss-. *schistorachis, rachischisis*

scler- σκληρός hard. Cf. dur-. *sclerosis*

scop- σκοπέω look at, observe. endo*scope*

sect- *seco, sectus* cut. Cf. tom-. *sectile*

semi- *semi-* half. Cf. hemi-. *semiflexion*

sens- *sentio, sensus* perceive, feel. Cf. esthe-. *sensory*

sep- σήπω rot, decay. *sepsis*

sept-¹ *saepio, saeptus* fence, wall off, stop up. Cf. phrag-. naso*septal*

sept-² *septem* seven. Cf. hept(a)-. *septan*

ser- *serum* whey, watery substance. *serosynovitis*

sex- *sex* six. Cf. hex-¹. *sexdigitate*

sial- σίαλον saliva. poly*sialia*

sin- *sinus* hollow, fold. Cf. colp-. *sinobronchitis*

sit- σῖτος food. para*sitic*

solut- *solvo, solventis, solutus* loose, dissolve, set free. Cf. ly-. dis*solution*

-solvent See solut-. dis*solvent*

somat- σῶμα, σώματος body. Cf. corpor-. psycho*somatic*

-some See somat-. dictyo*some*

spas- σπάω, σπασ- draw, pull. *spasm, spastic*

spectr- *spectrum* appearance, what is seen. micro*spectroscope*

sperm(at)- σπέρμα, σπέρματος seed. *spermacrasia, spermatozoon*

spers- *spargo, -spersus* scatter. dis*persion*

sphen- σφήν wedge. Cf. cune-. *sphenoid*

spher- σφαῖρα ball. hemi*sphere*

sphygm- σφυγμός pulsation. *sphygmomanometer*

spin- *spina* spine. Cf. rachi-. cerebro*spinal*

spirat- *spiro, spiratus* breathe. in*spiratory*

splanchn- σπλάγχνα entrails, viscera. neuro*splanchnic*

splen- σπλήν spleen. Cf. lien-. *splenomegaly*

spor- σπόρος seed. *sporophyte, zygospore*

squam-   *squama* scale. de*squam*ation

sta-   ἵστημι, στα- make stand, stop. genesi*stasis*

stal-   στέλλω, σταλ- send. peri*stal*sis. (See also stol-)

staphyl-   σταφυλή bunch of grapes, uvula. *staphylo*coccus, *staphylec*tomy

stear-   στέαρ, στέατος fat. Cf. adip-. *stear*odermia

steat-   See stear-. *steat*opygous

sten-   στενός narrow, compressed. *steno*cardia

ster-   στερεός solid. chole*ster*ol

sterc-   *stercus* dung. Cf. copr-. *sterco*porphyrin

sthen-   σθένος strength. a*sthen*ia

stol-   στέλλω, στολ- send. dia*stol*e

stom(at)-   στόμα, στόματος mouth, orifice. Cf. or-. ana*stom*osis, *stomato*gastric

strep(h)-   στρέφω, στρεπ- (before τ) twist. Cf. tors-. *streph*osymbolia, *strep*tomycin. (See also stroph-)

strict-   *stringo, stringentis, strictus* draw tight, compress, cause pain. con*strict*ion

-stringent   See strict-. a*stringent*

stroph-   στρέφω, στροφ- twist. ana*stroph*ic. (See also strep(h)-)

struct-   *struo, structus* pile up (against). ob*struct*ion

sub-   *sub* (b changes to f or p before words beginning with those consonants) under, below. Cf. hypo-. *sub*lumbar

suf-   See sub-. *suf*fusion

sup-   See sub-. *sup*pository

super-   *super* above, beyond, extreme. Cf. hyper-. *super*motility

sy-   See syn-. *sy*stole

syl-   See syn-. *syl*lepsiology

sym-   See syn-. *sym*biosis, *sym*metry, *sym*pathetic, *sym*physis

syn-   σύν (n disappears before s, changes to l before l, and changes to m before b, m, p, and ph) with, together. Cf. con-. myo*syn*izesis

ta-   See ton-. ec*ta*sis

tac-   τάσσω, ταγ- (τακ- before τ) order, arrange. a*tac*tic

tact-   *tango, tactus* touch. con*tact*

tax-   τάσσω, ταγ- (added to σ becomes ταξ-) order, arrange. a*tax*ia

tect-   See teg-. pro*tect*ive

teg-   *tego, tectus* cover. in*teg*ument

tel-   τέλος end. *tel*osynapsis

tele-   τῆλε at a distance. *tele*ceptor

tempor-   *tempus, temporis* time, timely or fatal spot, temple. *tempo*romalar

ten(ont)-   τένων, τένοντος (from τείνω stretch) tight stretched band. *teno*dynia, *teno*nitis, *tenon*tagra

tens-   *tendo, tensus* stretch. Cf. ton-. ex*tens*or

test-   *testis* testicle. Cf. orchi-. *test*itis

tetra-   τετρα- four. Cf. quadr-. *tetrag*enous

the-   τίθημι, θη- put, place. syn*the*sis

thec-   θήκη repository, case. *theco*stegnosis

thel-   θηλή teat, nipple. *thel*erethism

therap-   θεραπεία treatment. hydro*therapy*

therm-   θέρμη heat. Cf. calor-. dia*therm*y

thi-   θεῖον sulfur. *thi*ogenic

thorac-   θώραξ, θώρακος chest. *thoraco*plasty

thromb-   θρόμβος lump, clot. *thrombo*penia

thym-   θυμός spirit. Cf. ment-. dys*thym*ia

thyr-   θυρεός shield (shaped like a door θύρα). *thyr*oid

tme-   τέμνω, τμη- cut. axono*tme*sis

toc-   τόκος childbirth. dys*toc*ia

tom-   τέμνω, τομ- cut. Cf. sect-. ap pend*ec*tomy

ton-   τείνω, τον- stretch, put under tension. Cf. tens-. peri*ton*eum

top-   τόπος place. Cf. loc-. *top*esthesia

tors-   *torqueo, torsus* twist. Cf. strep-. ex*tors*ion

tox-   τοξικόν (from τόξον bow) arrow poison, poison. *tox*emia

trache-   τραχεῖα windpipe. *trache*otomy

trachel-   τράχηλος neck. Cf. cervic-. *trachel*opexy

tract-   *traho, tractus* draw, drag. pro*tract*ion

traumat-   τραῦμα, τραύματος wound. *traumat*ic

tri-   τρεῖς, τρία or *tri-* three. *tri*gonid

trich-   θρίξ, τριχός hair. *trich*oid

trip-   τρίβω rub. en*trip*sis

trop-   τρέπω, τροπ- turn, react. sito*trop*ism

troph-   τρέφω, τροφ- nurture. a*troph*y

tuber-   *tuber* swelling, node. *tuber*cle

typ-   τύπος (from τύπτω strike) type. a*typ*ical

typh-   τῦφος fog, stupor. adeno*typh*us

typhl-   τυφλός blind. Cf. cec-. *typhl*ectasis

un-   *unus* one. Cf. hen-. *un*ioval

ur-   οὖρον urine. poly*ur*ia

vacc-   *vacca* cow. *vacc*ine

vagin-   *vagina* sheath. in*vagin*ated

vas-   *vas* vessel. Cf. angi-. *vas*cular

vers-   See vert-. in*vers*ion

vert-   *verto, versus* turn. di*vert*iculum

vesic-   *vesica* bladder. Cf. cyst-. *vesico*vaginal

vit-   *vita* life. Cf. bi-¹. de*vit*alize

vuls-   *vello, vulsus* pull, twitch. con*vuls*ion

xanth-   ξανθός yellow, blond. Cf. flav- and lute-. *xanth*ophyll

-yl-   ὕλη substance. cacod*yl*

zo-   ζωή life, ζῷον animal. micro*zo*aria

zyg-   ζυγόν yoke, union. *zyg*odactyly

zym-   ζύμη ferment. en*zym*e

DORLAND'S ILLUSTRATED
Medical Dictionary

A or **Å**   symbol for *Angström unit* or *angstrom*.

A   symbol for *mass number*.

A.   absorbance, accommodation, acetum, anode, anterior, arteria, atomic weight, and axial. See also *point A,* under *point*.

A₂   aortic second sound.

a   symbol for *thermodynamic activity*.

a.   accommodation, ampere, anode, anterior, aqua, and arteria.

a-   1. [Gr.] an inseparable prefix signifying want or absence; appears as *an* before stems beginning with a vowel or with *h.*   2. [L.] a prefix signifying separation, or away from.

α   the first letter of the Greek alphabet; see *alpha*.

A.A.   achievement age; Alcoholics Anonymous.

aa.   abbreviation for L. *arteriae*.

AA, aa   [Gr. *ana* of each]   an abbreviation used in prescription writing, following the names of two or more ingredients and signifying "of each"; also written *ana*.

AAA   acute anxiety attack.

aaa.   amalgama, an obsolete variant of *amalgam*.

A.A.A.   American Academy of Allergy; American Association of Anatomists.

AA-AMP   amino acid adenylate.

A.A.A.S.   American Association for the Advancement of Science.

A.A.B.B.   American Association of Blood Banks.

A.A.C.P.   American Academy of Cerebral Palsy.

A.A.D.P.   American Academy of Denture Prosthetics.

A.A.D.R.   American Academy of Dental Radiology.

A.A.D.S.   American Association of Dental Schools.

A.A.E.   American Association of Endodontists.

A.A.F.P.   American Academy of Family Physicians.

A.A.G.P.   American Academy of General Practice.

A.A.I.   American Association of Immunologists.

A.A.I.D.   American Academy of Implant Dentures.

A.A.I.N.   American Association of Industrial Nurses.

A.A.M.A.   American Association of Medical Assistants.

A.A.M.C.   American Association of Medical Colleges.

A.A.M.R.L.   American Association of Medical Record Librarians.

A.A.O.   American Association of Orthodontists; American Academy of Otolaryngology.

A.A.O.P.   American Academy of Oral Pathology.

A.A.P.   American Academy of Pediatrics; American Academy of Pedodontics; American Academy of Periodontology; American Association of Pathologists.

A.A.P.A.   American Academy of Physician Assistants.

A.A.P.B.   American Association of Pathologists and Bacteriologists.

A.A.P.M.R.   American Academy of Physical Medicine and Rehabilitation.

A.A.P.S.   American Association of Plastic Surgeons.

Aarane (ār'ān)   trademark for a preparation of cromolyn sodium.

Aaron of Alexandria (ār'on) (7th century A.D.)   a physician who wrote medical works in the Syriac language, all of which are lost except fragments (e.g., on smallpox) preserved by Rhazes.

Aaron's sign (ār'onz) [Charles Dettie *Aaron*, American physician, 1866–1951]   see under *sign*.

aasmus (a-as'mus) [Gr. *aasmos* breathing]   (*obs.*) asthma.

AAV   adeno-associated virus.

A.B.   abbreviation for L. *Artium Baccalaureus,* Bachelor of Arts.

Ab   abbreviation for antibody.

ab   Latin preposition meaning from.

ab- [L. *ab* of, off]   prefix signifying from, off, away from.

abacterial (a"bak-te're-al)   free from bacteria.

abactio (ah-bak'she-o) [L.]   (*obs.*) induced abortion.

abactus venter (ah-bak'tus ven'ter) [L.]   (*obs.*) induced abortion.

Abadie's sign (ah-bah-dēz') [1. Charles *Abadie,* ophthalmologist in Paris, 1842–1932.   2. Jean *Abadie,* Bordeaux neurologist, 1873–1946]   see under *sign*.

abaissement (ah-bās-maw') [Fr.]   1. a lowering or a depressing.   2. couching.

abalienated (ab-āl'yen-āt"ed)   (*obs.*) mentally deranged.

abalienatio (ab-āl"yen-a'she-o) [L. "made alien," "deprived"]   abalienation.   **a. men'tis,** former term for mental derangement.

abalienation (ab-āl"yen-a'shun) [L. *abalienatio*]   former term for mental derangement.

Abano (ah-ba'no), **Pietro d'**   see *Peter of Abano*.

abaptiston (ah"bap-tis'ton), pl. *abaptis'ta* [*a* neg. + Gr. *baptein* to dip]   a trephine so shaped that it will not penetrate the brain.

abarognosis (a"bar-og-no'sis) [*a* neg. + Gr. *baros* weight + *gnōsis* knowledge]   loss of weight sense; baragnosis.

abarthrosis (ab"ar-thro'sis) [*ab-* + L. *arthrosis*]   diarthrosis.

abarticular (ab"ar-tik'u-lar)   1. not affecting a joint.   2. remote from a joint.

abarticulation (ab"ar-tik"u-la'shun) [*ab-* + L. *articulatio* joint]   1. a dislocation of a joint.   2. junctura synovialis.

abasia (ah-ba'zhe-ah) [*a* neg. + Gr. *basis* step + *-ia*]   inability to walk.   **a. asta'sia,** astasia-abasia.   **a. atac'tica,** abasia characterized by uncertainty of movement, due to a defect of coordination.   **choreic a.,** a form due to chorea of the legs.   **paralytic a.,** a form due to paralysis of the leg muscles.   **paroxysmal trepidant a.,** astasia-abasia caused by spastic stiffening of the legs on attempting to stand; called also *spastic a.*   **spastic a.,** paroxysmal trepidant a.   **trembling a., a. trep'idans,** abasia due to trembling of the legs.

abasic (ah-ba'sik)   pertaining to abasia.

abatardissement (ah-bah"tar-dēs-maw') [Fr.]   deterioration of a race or breed.

abate (ah-bāt')   to lessen or decrease.

abatement (ah-bāt'ment)   a decrease in the severity of a pain or a symptom.

abatic (ah-bat'ik)   abasic.

abbau (ab'ow) [Ger.]   catabolic products.

Abbé's condenser (ah-bāz') [Ernst Karl *Abbé,* German physicist, 1840–1905]   see under *condenser*.

Abbe's operation, string method (ab'ez) [Robert *Abbe,* New York surgeon, 1851–1928]   see under *operation, ring,* and *treatment*.

Abbé-Zeiss counting cell, counting chamber [E. K. *Abbé;* Carl *Zeiss,* German optician, 1816–1888]   see *Thoma-Zeiss counting chamber,* under *chamber*.

Abbocillin-DC (ab"bo-sil'lin)   trademark for preparations of penicillin G procaine.

Abbott's method (ab'ots) [Edville Gerhardt *Abbott,* surgeon in Portland, Maine, 1870–1938]   see under *method*.

Abbott-Miller tube (ab'ot-mil'er) [William Osler *Abbott,* American physician, 1902–1943; T. Grier *Miller,* Philadelphia physician, born 1886]   see *Miller-Abbott tube,* under *tube*.

Abbott-Rawson tube (ab'ot-raw'son) [William Osler *Abbott;* Arthur J. *Rawson,* American medical physicist]   see under *tube*.

ABC   aspiration biopsy cytology.

Abderhalden's reaction (dialysis, test) (ahb'der-hal"denz) [Emil *Abderhalden,* Swiss physiologist, 1877–1950]   see under *reaction*.

Abdollatif (ab″dol-lat′if) (1162–1231) an Arabian physician and traveler who criticized Galen's anatomical observations.

abdomen (ab-do′men) [L., possibly from *abdere* to hide] that portion of the body which lies between the thorax and the pelvis; called also *venter*. It contains a cavity (*abdominal cavity*) separated by the diaphragm from the thoracic cavity, and lined with a serous membrane, the peritoneum. This cavity contains the viscera (see Plate accompanying *viscera*) and is enclosed by a wall (*abdominal wall* or *parietes*) formed by the abdominal muscles, vertebral column, and the ilia. It is divided into nine regions by four

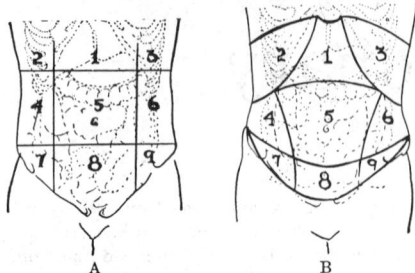

Regions of abdomen bounded according to (A) the standard and (B) a variant system: 1, epigastric; 2, right hypochondriac; 3, left hypochondriac; 4, right lateral (or lumbar); 5, umbilical; 6, left lateral (or lumbar); 7, right inguinal (or iliac); 8, pubic (hypogastric); 9, left inguinal (or iliac).

imaginary lines, of which two pass horizontally around the body (the upper at the level of the cartilages of the ninth ribs, the lower at the tops of the crests of the ilia), and two extend vertically on each side of the body from the cartilage of the eighth rib to the center of the inguinal ligament, as in A above. The regions are: three upper—right hypochondriac, epigastric, left hypochondriac; three middle—right lateral, umbilical, left lateral; and three lower—right inguinal, pubic, left inguinal. Called also *belly*. **acute a.,** an abdominal condition of abrupt onset usually associated with abdominal pain due to inflammation, perforation, obstruction, infarction, or rupture of intra-abdominal organs. Emergency surgical intervention is usually required. Examples are acute cholecystitis or appendicitis, perforated peptic ulcer, strangulated hernia, superior mesenteric artery thrombosis, and splenic rupture. Called also *surgical a.* **boat-shaped a.,** scaphoid a. **carinate a.,** scaphoid a. **navicular a.,** scaphoid a. **a. obsti′pum,** congenital shortness of the rectus abdominis muscle. **pendulous a.,** a relaxed condition of the abdominal wall, so that the anterior abdominal wall hangs over the pubis; called also *venter propendens*. **scaphoid a.,** an abdomen whose anterior wall is hollowed out; seen in children with cerebral disease. Called also *boat-shaped a., carinate a.,* and *navicular a.* **surgical a.,** acute a.

abdominal (ab-dom′ĭ-nal) [L. *abdominalis*] pertaining to the abdomen.

abdomino- [L. *abdomen* the belly] a combining form denoting relationship to the abdomen.

abdominoanterior (ab-dom″ĭ-no-an-te′re-or) (*obs.*) with the abdomen forward (denoting a position of the fetus in utero).

abdominocentesis (ab-dom″ĭ-no-sen-te′sis) [*abdomino-* + Gr. *kentēsis* puncture] surgical puncture (paracentesis) of the abdominal cavity.

abdominocystic (ab-dom″ĭ-no-sis′tik) pertaining to the abdomen and gallbladder.

abdominogenital (ab-dom″ĭ-no-jen′ĭ-tal) pertaining to the abdomen and the reproductive organs.

abdominohysterectomy (ab-dom″ĭ-no-his″ter-ek′to-me) hysterectomy performed through an abdominal incision.

abdominohysterotomy (ab-dom″ĭ-no-his″ter-ot′o-me) hysterotomy performed through an abdominal incision; called also *abdominouterotomy*.

abdominoposterior (ab-dom″ĭ-no-pos-te′re-or) (*obs.*) having the abdomen turned backward (denoting a position of the fetus in utero).

abdominoscopy (ab-dom″ĭ-nos′ko-pe) [*abdomino-* + Gr. *skopein* to inspect] inspection or examination of the abdominal cavity, particularly direct examination of the abdominal organs by endoscopy; peritoneoscopy.

abdominoscrotal (ab-dom″ĭ-no-skro′tal) pertaining to the abdomen and scrotum.

abdominothoracic (ab-dom″ĭ-no-tho-ras′ik) pertaining to the abdomen and thorax.

abdominouterotomy (ab-dom″ĭ-no-u″ter-ot′o-me) abdominohysterotomy.

abdominovaginal (ab-dom″ĭ-no-vaj′ĭ-nal) pertaining to the abdomen and the vagina.

abdominovesical (ab-dom″ĭ-no-ves′ĭ-k'l) pertaining to the abdomen and urinary bladder.

abducens (ab-du′senz) [L. "drawing away"] Latin adjective

used in names of structures (e.g., nervus abducens) which serve to abduct a part.

abducent (ab-du′sent) [L. *abducens*] abducting, or effecting a separation, as an abducent nerve.

abduct (ab-dukt′) [*ab-* + L. *ducere* to draw] to draw away from the median plane or (in the digits) from the axial line of a limb.

abduction (ab-duk′shun) the act of abducting or state of being abducted.

abductor (ab-duk′tor) [L.] that which abducts; see *Table of Musculi.*

Abegg's rule (ab′egz) [Richard *Abegg,* Danish chemist, 1869–1910] see under *rule.*

Abelin's reaction (test) (ab′e-linz) [Isaak *Abelin,* Swiss physiologist, born 1883] see under *reaction.*

abembryonic (ab″em-bre-on′ik) [*ab-* + Gr. *embryon* embryo] away from the embryo.

abepithymia (ab″ep-ĭ-thi′me-ah) [*ab-* + Gr. *epithymia* desire] paralysis of the solar plexus.

A.B.E.P.P. American Board of Examiners in Professional Psychology.

abequose (ab′ĕ-kwōs) an unusual sugar found to be a polysaccharide somatic antigen of *Salmonella* species.

Abercrombie's degeneration (syndrome) (ab′er-krom″bēz) [John *Abercrombie,* Scottish physician, 1780–1844] see *amyloid degeneration,* under *degeneration.*

Abernethy's fascia, sarcoma (ab′er-ne″thēz) [John *Abernethy,* British surgeon and anatomist, 1764–1831] see *fascia iliaca,* under *fascia,* and see under *sarcoma.*

aberrant (ab-er′ant) [L. *aberrans, ab* from + *errare* to wander] wandering or deviating from the usual or normal course.

aberratio (ab″er-a′she-o) [L.] aberration. **a. tes′tis,** situation of the testis in a part distant from the path which it takes in normal descent.

aberration (ab″er-a′shun) [*ab-* + L. *errare* to wander] 1. deviation from the usual course or condition. 2. unequal refraction or focalization of light rays by a lens, resulting in degradation of the image they produce. **chromatic a.,** unequal deviation of light rays of different wavelengths passing through a refractive medium, resulting in fringes of color around the image produced; called also *newtonian a.* **chromatic a., lateral,** difference in magnification due to differences in position of the principal points for light of different wavelength; also a difference of focal length. **chromatic a., longitudinal,** difference in position along the axis for the focal points of light, produced by unequal deviation of light rays of different wavelengths by a lens. **chromosome a.,** an irregularity in the number or constitution of chromosomes that may alter the course of development of the embryo, usually in the form of a gain (duplication), loss (deletion), exchange (translocation), or alteration in sequence (inversion) of genetic material. **dioptric a.,** spherical a. **distantial a.,** a blurring of vision for distant objects. **heterosomal a.,** one affecting more than one chromosome; a translocation. **homosomal a.,** one affecting a single chromosome. **mental a.,** unsoundness of mind of mild degree, not including disorders of intelligence; usually limited to a circumscribed deviation in an otherwise adapted individual. **meridional a.,** unequal refraction of light rays as a result of variation of refractive power in different portions of the same meridian of a lens. **newtonian a.,** chromatic a. **penta-X chromosomal a.,** one in which there are five X chromosomes in a female. **spherical a.,** zonal aberration in relation to an axial point; see *spherical a., negative,* and *spherical a., positive.* Called also *dioptric a.* **spherical a., negative,** unequal refraction of light rays by a lens, those passing through the outer zones of the lens being focused farther from the lens than those passing through the central zones. **spherical a., positive,** unequal refraction of light rays by a lens, those passing through the outer zones of the lens being focused closer to the lens than those passing through the central zones. **tetra-X chromosomal a.,** one in which there are four X chromosomes in a female. **triple-X chromosomal a.,** one in which there are three X chromosomes in a female. **zonal a.,** unequal refraction of light rays by a lens, the rays passing through different zones being focused at different distances from the lens.

aberrometer (ab″er-om′ĕ-ter) [*aberration* + Gr. *metron* measure] an instrument for measuring errors in delicate experiments or observations.

abesterase (ab-es′ter-ās) a simple esterase that hydrolyzes short-chain aliphatic esters.

abetalipoproteinemia (a-ba″tah-lip″o-pro-te″in-e′me-ah) a hereditary syndrome, transmitted as an autosomal recessive trait, characterized by a lack of β-lipoproteins in the blood, acanthocytosis, hypocholesterolemia, progressive ataxic neuropathy, atypical retinitis pigmentosa with involvement of the macula, and malabsorption. Called also *Bassen-Kornzweig syndrome.*

abeyance (ah-ba′ans) a suspension of function or of action; a state of suspended activity.

abiatrophy (ah″bi-at′ro-fe) premature and endogenous loss of vitality or tissue substance. See also *abiotrophy*.

abient (ab′e-ent) avoiding the source of stimulation; said of a response to a stimulus. Cf. *adient*.

abietate (ab′e-ĕ-tāt) a salt of abietic acid.

abiogenesis (ab″e-o-jen′ĕ-sis) [*a* neg. + Gr. *bios* life + Gr. *genesis* generation] the spontaneous generation of life; the origin of living things from things inanimate. Cf. *biogenesis*.

abiogenetic (ab″e-o-jĕ-net′ik) pertaining to or marked by spontaneous generation.

abiogenous (ab″e-oj′ĕ-nus) abiogenetic.

abiologic, abiological (ab″bi-o-loj′ik, a″bi-o-loj′e-k′l) (*obs.*) pertaining to abiology.

abiology (a″bi-ol′o-je) [*a* neg. + Gr. *bios* life + *-logy*] (*obs.*) the study of nonliving things; anorganology.

abionergy (ab″e-on′er-je) [*a* neg. + Gr. *bios* life + *ergon* work] abiotrophy.

abiophysiology (ab″e-o-fiz″e-ol′o-je) [*a* neg. + Gr. *bios* life + *physiology*] the study of inorganic processes in living organisms.

abiosis (ab″e-o′sis) [*a* neg. + Gr. *bios* life + *-osis*] 1. absence or deficiency of life. 2. abiotrophy.

abiotic (ab″e-ot′ik) pertaining to or characterized by absence of life; incapable of living; antagonistic to life.

abiotrophia (ab″e-o-tro′fe-ah) abiotrophy.

abiotrophic (ab″e-o-trof′ik) pertaining to or characterized by abiotrophy.

abiotrophy (ab″e-ot′ro-fe) [*a* neg. + Gr. *bios* life + *trophē* nutrition] progressive loss of vitality of certain tissues or organs leading to disorders or loss of function; applied especially to degenerative hereditary diseases of late onset, e.g., Huntington's chorea. **retinal a.,** a general term for a group of degenerative diseases of the retina, such as retinitis pigmentosa and amaurotic familial idiocy.

abirritant (ab-ir′rĭ-tant) [*ab*- + L. *irritans* irritating] 1. diminishing or relieving irritation; soothing. 2. an agent that relieves irritation.

abirritation (ab″ir-rĭ-ta′shun) 1. diminished responsiveness to stimulation. 2. atony.

abirritative (ab-ir′rĭ-ta″tiv) reducing irritability; soothing.

abiuret (ah-bi′u-ret) [*a* neg. + *biuret*] not giving a positive reaction to the biuret test.

abiuretic (ah-bi″u-ret′ik) not responsive to the biuret test.

ablactation (ab″lak-ta′shun) [L. *ablactatio*, from *ab* from + *lactare* to give milk] the weaning of a child or the cessation of milk secretion.

ablastemic (a-blas-tem′ik) [*a* neg. + Gr. *blastēma* a shoot] not concerned with germination.

ablastin (ah-blas′tin) an antibody that prevents the multiplication of invading microorganisms.

ablate (ab-lāt′) [L. *ablatus* removed] to remove, especially by cutting; to extirpate.

ablatio (ab-la′she-o) [L.] ablation. **a. placen′tae,** premature detachment of a placenta. **a. ret′inae** (*obs.*), detachment of the retina.

ablation (ab-la′shun) [L. *ablatio*] 1. separation or detachment; extirpation; eradication. 2. removal of a part, especially by cutting.

ablepharia (ah″blef-a′re-ah) [*a* neg. + Gr. *blepharon* eyelid + *-ia*] congenital reduction or absence of the eyelids.

ablepharon (ah-blef′ah-ron) ablepharia.

ablepharous (ah-blef′ah-rus) 1. lacking eyelids. 2. pertaining to ablepharia.

ablephary (ah-blef′ah-re) ablepharia.

ablepsia (ah-blep′se-ah) [*a* neg. + Gr. *blepsis* sight + *-ia*] lack or loss of sight; blindness.

ablepsy (ah-blep′se) ablepsia.

abluent (ab′lu-ent) [*ab*- + L. *luens* washing] 1. detergent. 2. a cleansing agent.

ablution (ab-lu′shun) [L. *ablutio* a washing] the act of washing or cleansing; the application of water by the hand, which may be covered with a bath mitt or towel.

ablutomania (ab-lu″to-ma′ne-ah) [L. *ablutio* a washing + *mania*] abnormal interest in washing or bathing.

abmortal (ab-mor′tal) situated or directed away from a dead or injured part; applied especially to electric currents set up in injured tissue.

abneural (ab-nu′ral) [L. *ab*- + Gr. *neuron* nerve] (*obs.*) 1. distant from the central nervous system. 2. abneural.

abnormal (ab-nor′mal) [*ab*- + L. *norma* rule] not normal; contrary to the usual structure, position, condition, behavior, or rule.

abnormality (ab″nor-mal′ĭ-te) 1. the quality or fact of being abnormal. 2. a malformation or deformity; see also *abnormity* and *anomaly*.

abnormity (ab-nor′mĭ-te) 1. abnormality; deformity. 2. monstrosity.

abocclusion (ab″o-kloo′zhun) (*obs.*) open bite.

abomasitis (ab″o-mah-si′tis) inflammation of the abomasum.

abomasum (ab″o-ma′sum) [*ab*- + L. *omasum* paunch] the fourth stomach of a ruminant animal.

aborad (ab-o′rad) directed away from the mouth.

aboral (ab-o′ral) opposite to, away from, or remote from the mouth.

aboriginal (ab-ŏ-rij′ĭ-nal) native to the place inhabited.

abort (ah-bort′) [L. *aboriri* to miscarry] 1. to check the usual course of a disease. 2. to miscarry before the fetus is viable. 3. an abortion. 4. to become checked in development.

aborticide (ah-bor′tĭ-sīd) [L. *aboriri* to miscarry + *caedere* to kill] abortifacient.

abortient (ah-bor′shent) abortifacient.

abortifacient (ah-bor″tĭ-fa′shent) [L. *abortio* abortion + *facere* to make] 1. causing abortion. 2. an agent which causes abortion; called also *abortient* and *aborticide*.

abortin (ah-bor′tin) a glycerin extract of the *Brucella abortus*, prepared and used as is tuberculin, but in the diagnosis of brucellosis in man.

abortion (ah-bor′shun) [L. *abortio*] 1. the premature explusion from the uterus of the products of conception—of the embryo, or of a nonviable fetus. The four classic symptoms, usually present in each type of abortion, are uterine contractions, uterine hemorrhage, softening and dilatation of the cervix, and presentation or expulsion of all or part of the products of conception. 2. premature stoppage of a natural or a morbid process. **accidental a.,** an abortion which is due to an accident. **afebrile a.,** abortion in which the temperature is not elevated above 100.4° F. **ampullar a.,** a variety of tubal abortion occurring from the ampulla of the oviduct. **artificial a.,** induced abortion; an abortion which is brought on purposely. **cervical a.,** abortion in which the ovum is retained in the cervix uteri because the external os fails to dilate. **complete a.,** abortion in which all of the products of conception have been expelled from the uterus and identified. **contagious a.,** in cattle, infectious a., def. 1. **contagious equine a.,** infectious a., def. 2. **criminal a.,** an abortion that is produced illegally. **enzootic of cattle,** an infectious abortion caused by organisms of the genus *Chlamydia*; also known as *foothill abortion* in western United States. **enzootic a. of ewes,** abortion in ewes, usually late in the gestation period, caused by *Chlamydia psittaci*. **equine epizootic a.,** an infectious abortion of horses, caused by the virus of equine rhinopneumonitis. **equine virus a.,** see under *rhinopneumonitis*. **foothill a.,** enzootic a. of cattle. **habitual a.,** the spontaneous expulsion of a dead or nonviable fetus in three or more consecutive pregnancies, at about the same period of development. **idiopathic a.,** abortion for which no recognized organic cause can be found. **imminent a.,** impending abortion in which the bleeding is profuse, the cervix softened and dilated, and the uterine contractions approach the character of labor pains. **incomplete a.,** abortion in which the uterus is not entirely rid of its contents. **induced a.,** abortion brought on intentionally; called also *artificial* or *therapeutic a.* **inevitable a.,** a condition in which vaginal bleeding has been profuse or prolonged and the cervix has become effaced or dilated, and abortion will proceed naturally. **infected a.,** abortion associated with infection of the genital tract. **infectious a.,** 1. an infectious disease of cattle caused by *Brucella abortus*, marked by inflammatory changes in the uterine mucosa and fetal membranes, resulting in premature expulsion of the fetus. 2. an infectious disease of horses due to *Salmonella abortusequi* and of sheep due to *S. abortusovis*. Called also (in horses) *contagious equine a.* **justifiable a.,** therapeutic a. **missed a.,** retention in the uterus of an abortus that has been dead for at least four weeks, indicated either by cessation of growth and hardening of the uterus or by actual diminution of its size; absence of fetal heart tones after they have been heard is also definitive; more accurate information of fetal death is obtainable by fetal electrocardiography and sonar. **a. in progress,** a condition marked by profuse hemorrhage from the uterus and pains resembling those of labor, with softening and dilatation of the cervix, going on to expulsion of the products of conception. **recurrent a.,** habitual a. **septic a.,** abortion associated with serious infection of the uterus, leading to generalized infection; more common after criminal abortion. **spontaneous a.,** abortion occurring naturally. **therapeutic a.,** abortion induced to save the life or health (physical or mental) of a pregnant woman; sometimes performed after rape or incest. Called also *justifiable a.* **threatened a.,** a condition in which there is bloody discharge from the uterus but the loss of blood is less than in inevitable abortion and there is no dilatation of the cervix; it may proceed to actual abortion or the symptoms may subside and the pregnancy go to full term. **tubal a.,** extrusion of the conceptus through the open end of the uterine tube into the abdominal cavity, occurring in tubal (ectopic) pregnancy. **vibrio a.,** an infectious abortion of cattle, sheep, and goats, caused by *Campylobacter* (*Vibrio*) *fetus*.

abortionist (ah-bor′shun-ist)   one who makes a business of inducing criminal abortions.

abortive (ah-bor′tiv) [L. *abortivus*]   1. incompletely developed. 2. effecting an abortion; abortifacient.   3. cutting short the course of a disease.

abortus (ah-bor′tus) [L.]   a fetus weighing less than 500 gm. (17 oz.) at time of expulsion from the uterus, having no chance of survival.

abouchement (ah-bōōsh-maw′) [Fr.]   the termination of a vessel in a larger one.

ab-oukine   the native name in Gabun for yaws (q.v.).

aboulia (ah-boo′le-ah)   abulia.

aboulomania (ah-boo″lo-ma′ne-ah)   abulomania.

ABP   arterial blood pressure.

abrachia (ah-bra′ke-ah) [*a* neg. + Gr. *brachiōn* arm + -*ia*]   congenital absence of the arms.

abrachiatism (ah-bra′ke-ah-tizm″)   abrachia.

abrachiocephalia (ah-bra″ke-o-sĕ-fa′le-ah) [*a* neg. + Gr. *brachiōn* arm + *kephalē* head + -*ia*]   congenital absence of the arms and head.

abrachiocephalus (ah-bra″ke-o-sef′ah-lus)   a monster exhibiting abrachiocephalia.

abrachius (ah-bra′ke-us)   an individual exhibiting abrachia.

abradant (ah-bra′dant)   abrasive.

abrade (ah-brād′)   to rub away the external covering or layer of a part; see also *planing*.

Abrahams' sign (a′brah-hamz) [Robert *Abrahams*, New York physician, 1861–1935]   see under *sign*.

Abrami's disease (ah-brahm′ēz) [Pierre *Abrami*, French physician, 1879–1943]   hemolytic anemia.

Abrams' (heart) reflex (a′bramz) [Albert *Abrams*, physician in San Francisco, 1863–1924]   see under *reflex*.

abrasio (ah-bra′se-o) [L.]   abrasion.   **a. cor′neae,** a rubbing off of the superficial layers of the cornea.

abrasion (ah-bra′zhun) [L. *abrasio*]   1. the wearing away of a substance or structure (such as the skin or the teeth) through some unusual or abnormal mechanical process; see also *planing*.   2. an area of body surface denuded of skin or mucous membrane by some unusual or abnormal mechanical process.   **dental a.,** abrasion of the teeth.

abrasive (ah-bra′siv)   1. causing abrasion. 2. a substance used for abrading, grinding, or polishing.

abrasor (ah-bra′zor)   an instrument used for abrasion.

abreaction (ab″re-ak′shun) [*ab-* + *reaction*]   the reliving of an experience in such a way that previously repressed emotions associated with it are released.   **motor a.,** an abreaction achieved through motor or muscular expression.

abreuography (ab″roo-og′rah-fe) [Manoel de *Abreu*, Brazilian physician, 1892–1962]   (*obs.*) photofluorography.

Abrikosov's (Abrikossoff's) tumor (ab″rĭ-kos′ofs) [Aleksei Ivanovich *Abrikosov*, Moscow pathologist, 1875–1955]   myoblastoma.

abrin (a′brin)   a powerful phytotoxin or toxalbumin present in the seeds of *Abrus precatorius* L., Leguminosae; once used topically in certain chronic eye disorders. The plant is also known as jequirity or precatory bean, and rosary pea.

abrism (a′brizm)   poisoning by jequirity; see *abrin*.

abrosia (ah-bro′ze-ah) [Gr. *abrōsia* fasting]   lack of food.

abruptio (ab-rup′she-o) [L.]   a rending asunder.   **a. placen′tae,** premature detachment of a placenta, often attended by maternal systemic reactions in the form of shock, oliguria, and fibrinogenopenia.

Abrus precatorius L. (Leguminosae) (a′brus pre-kah-to′re-us)   a species of tree native to tropical Asia, also found in Central America and Florida. Its seeds, called rosary beads, crab eyes, or jequirity beans, contain a toxalbumin (abrin) that is extremely irritant to mucous membranes. Used for jewelry and rosary beads.

abs-   a prefix signifying away, from.

abscess (ab′ses) [L. *abscessus*, from *ab* away + *cedere* to go]   a localized collection of pus in a cavity formed by the disintegration of tissues.   **acute a.,** one which runs a relatively short course, producing some fever and a painful local inflammation.   **acute dentoalveolar a.,** alveolar a.   **alveolar a.,** a collection of pus at the alveolar border, resulting .from infection of the periodontal ligament and the bony tissues surrounding the root of a tooth; called also *acute dentoalveolar a.*   **amebic a., amoebic a.,** an abscess cavity of the liver resulting from liquefaction necrosis due to entrance of *Entamoeba histolytica* into the portal circulation in amebiasis; amebic abscesses may also effect the lungs, brain, and spleen.   **anorectal a.,** one in the celluloadipose tissue near the anus.   **apical a.,** one situated at the apex of an organ.   **apical periodontal a., acute,** a localized infection of short duration, arising at or near the apex of a tooth root, resulting in pain, swelling, and a collection of pus; called also *periapical a.* and *dentoalveolar a.*   **apical periodontal a., chronic,** a localized collection of inflammatory

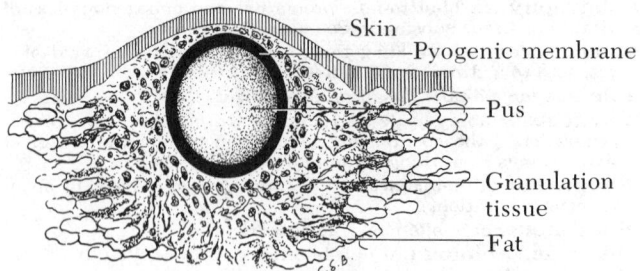

Diagram of cross-section of abscess.

tissue and occasionally a little pus in the alveolar bone at or near the apex of a tooth root, usually resulting from infection or the presence of pulpal degradation products within the root canal; the process may result in dental granuloma.   **appendiceal a., appendicular a.,** abscess resulting from perforation of an acutely inflamed appendix.   **arthrifluent a.,** a wandering abscess which has its point of origin in a diseased joint.   **axillary a.,** an abscess, usually multiple, in the axilla.   **bartholinian a.,** abscess of the excretory duct of Bartholin's gland.   **Bezold's a.,** an abscess deep in the neck resulting from a complication of acute mastoiditis in which pus tracts deep to the superior portion of the sternocleidomastoid muscle.   **bicameral a.,** one which has two chambers or pockets; see *shirt-stud a.*   **bile duct a.,** cholangitic a.   **bilharziasis a.,** one in the wall of the intestine caused by *Schistosoma* (*Bilharzia*) *mansoni*.   **biliary a.,** abscess of the gallbladder or some part of the biliary tract.   **bone a.,** osteomyelitis; suppurative periostitis.   **brain a.,** one affecting the brain as a result of extension of an infection (e.g., otitis media) from an adjacent area or through bloodborne infection.   **broad ligament a.,** an abscess between the folds of the broad ligament of the uterus; called also *parametric* or *parametrial a.*   **Brodie's a.,** a roughly spherical region of bone destruction, filled with pus or connective tissue, usually found in the metaphyseal region of long bones and caused by *Staphylococcus aureus* or *albus*.   **bursal a.,** one occurring in a bursa.   **canalicular a.,** a mammary abscess communicating with a milk duct.   **carniform a.** (*obs.*), a hard sarcoma of a joint.   **caseous a.,** one that contains cheesy matter; called also *cheesy a.*   **cerebral a.,** one in the brain substance.   **cheesy a.,** caseous a.   **cholangitic a.,** intrahepatic abscess complicating bacterial cholangitis; called also *bile duct a.*   **chronic a.,** cold a.   **circumscribed a.,** an abscess limited by a layer of fibroblasts.   **circumtonsillar a.,** peritonsillar a.   **cold a.,** an abscess of comparatively slow development with little evidence of inflammation; it is usually tuberculous. Called also *chronic a.* and *scrofulous a.*   **collar-button a.,** shirt-stud a.   **deep a.,** one occurring below the deep fascia.   **Delpech's a.,** a rapidly developing abscess accompanied by great prostration but little fever.   **dental a.** (*obs.*), an abscess in or about a tooth.   **dentoalveolar a.,** apical periodontal a., acute.   **diffuse a.,** an abscess the pus of which, or a part of it, is widely diffused in the surrounding tissues.   **Douglas' a.,** an abscess in the rectouterine pouch.   **dry a.,** one that disappears without pointing or breaking.   **Dubois' a.,** abscess of the thymus in congenital syphilis; called also *thymus a.*   **emphysematous a.,** gas a.   **encysted a.,** one in which pus is circumscribed in a serous cavity.   **endamebic a., entamebic a.,** amebic a.   **epidural a.,** extradural a.   **epiploic a.,** an abscess in the omentum.   **extradural a.,** an abscess of the brain situated between the dura and the cranial bone; called also *epidural a.*   **fecal a.,** an abscess, usually pericolic or perirectal, resulting from lower bowel perforation and containing pus and fecal matter; extension to the skin or mucosa leads to a fecal fistula.   **filarial a.,** an abscess caused by filaria.   **fixation a., Fochier's a.** (*obs.*), an abscess produced artificially (as by injection of turpentine) for the purpose of attracting and fixing at the site of the abscess the bacteria of an acute infection.   **follicular a.,** one developing in a follicle.   **frontal a.,** one in the frontal lobe of the brain.   **fungal a.,** one caused by a fungus, such as *Nocardia*.   **gangrenous a.,** one attended with gangrene of the surrounding parts.   **gas a.,** a localized collection of seropurulent material containing gas, caused by gas-forming bacteria such as *Clostridium perfringens*. Called also *tympanitic a.* and *Welch's a.*   **gastric a.,** phlegmonous gastritis.   **gingival a.,** one situated in the oral gingival tissues arising from the periodontal pocket.   **glandular a.,** one formed around a lymph gland.   **gravitation a., gravity a.,** one in which the pus migrates or gravitates to a lower or deeper portion of the body.   **helminthic a.,** one caused by a worm, such as filaria.   **hemorrhagic a.,** one which contains blood.   **hepatic a.,** an abscess of the liver.   **hot a.,** an acute abscess with symptoms of local inflammation.   **hypostatic a.,** wandering a.   **idiopathic a.,** one due to unknown causes.   **iliac a.,** one in the iliac region.   **intradural a.,** one within the layers of the dura mater.   **intramammary a.,** one in the substance of the mammary gland.   **intramastoid a.,** an abscess of the mastoid process of the temporal bone.   **intratonsillar**

a., tonsillar a. **ischiorectal a.,** one located in the ischiorectal fossa. **kidney a.,** renal a. **lacrimal a.,** one in or around the lacrimal sac. **lacunar a.,** one in the lacunae of the urethra. **lateral a., lateral alveolar a.,** periodontal a. **lumbar a.,** one in the lumbar region. **lymphatic a.,** an abscess of a lymph node. **mammary a.,** abscess of the mam-

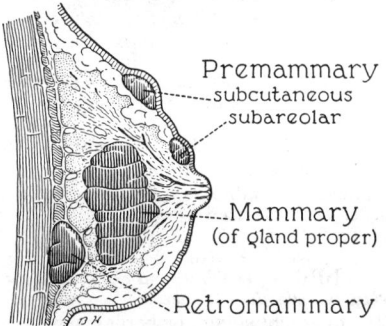

Premammary
---subcutaneous
---subareolar

---Mammary
(of gland proper)

---Retromammary

Abscesses of breast.

mary gland. **marginal a.,** one near the orifice of the anus. **mastoid a.,** suppuration within the cells of the mastoid portion of the temporal bone. **mediastinal a.,** suppuration in the mediastinum. **metastatic a.,** a secondary abscess, usually of embolic origin, in which organisms are carried by the circulation to a point distant from the primary lesion. **migrating a.,** wandering a. **miliary a.,** one of a set of small multiple abscesses. **milk a.,** an abscess of the mammary gland during lactation. **Monro's a's,** minute intraepidermal accumulations of cellular debris in the upper part of the epidermis; seen in psoriasis. **mother a.,** a primary abscess from which other abscesses arise. **multiple a.,** one of a set of many abscesses usually accompanying pyemia. **mural a.,** one in the abdominal wall. **nocardial a.,** one caused by a species of *Nocardia*. **orbital a.,** suppuration in the orbit. **ossifluent a.,** an abscess dependent on a breaking down of bone tissue. **Paget's a.,** one recurring about the residue of a former abscess. **palatal a.,** a periapical or periodontal abscess of a maxillary tooth which erupts or extends toward the palate. **palmar a.,** a purulent effusion into the tissues of the palm of the hand. **pancreatic a.,** an abscess formed following secondary bacterial contamination of necrotic pancreatic debris and hemorrhagic exudate; it is a serious complication of severe acute pancreatitis and of postoperative pancreatitis. **parafrenal a.,** abscess of the preputial gland. **parametrial a., parametric a.,** broad ligament a. **paranephric a.,** one in the tissues around the kidney. **parapancreatic a.,** one in the tissues around the pancreas. **parietal a.,** periodontal a. **parotid a.,** an abscess of the parotid gland. **Pautrier's a.,** focal collections of reticular cells in the epidermis. **pelvic a.,** abscess of the pelvic peritoneum, usually of the rectouterine pouch. **pelvirectal a.,** one lying immediately above the levator ani muscle, in close relation to the wall of the rectum. **perianal a.,** one located immediately beneath the skin adjacent to the anal canal. **periapical a.,** acute apical periodontal a. **pericemental a.** (*obs.*), periodontal a. **pericoronal a.,** an abscess around the crown of a partially erupted tooth. **peridental a.,** periodontal a. **perinephric a.,** one in the tissues immediately around the kidney. **periodontal a.,** a localized purulent inflammation situated in the periodontal tissues; called also *lateral a., lateral alveolar a., parietal a.,* and *peridental a.* **peripleuritic a.,** an abscess between the parietal pleura and the chest wall. **perirectal a.,** one in the areolar tissue around the rectum. **perisinus a., perisinuous a.,** an abscess around a venous sinus, usually the lateral sinus. **peritoneal a.,** a confined collection of inflammatory exudate in peritonitis. **peritonsillar a.,** an abscess in the peritonsillar tissue extending into the tonsil capsule, resulting from suppuration of the tonsil; called also *quinsy*. **periureteral a.,** one around the ureter. **periurethral a.,** one formed around the urethra. **perivesical a.,** one in the tissues around the bladder. **phlegmonous a.,** one associated with acute inflammation of the subcutaneous connective tissues. **postanal a.,** one located posterior to the anal canal, between the coccygeal attachments of the superficial part of the external sphincter and the levator ani muscle. **postcecal a.,** one occurring posterior to the cecum, usually of appendiceal origin; called also *retrocecal a.* **Pott's a.,** one associated with tuberculosis of the spine. **premammary a.,** a small cutaneous abscess of the mammary gland. **primary a.,** one formed at the seat of the infection. **protozoan a.,** one caused by a protozoon. **psoas a.,** one which arises from disease of the lumbar or lower dorsal vertebrae, the pus descending in the sheath of the psoas muscle. **pulmonary a.,** an abscess of the lungs. **pulp a.,** 1. a cavity that discharges pus formed in the pulp tissue of a tooth. 2. an abscess of the tissues of the pulp of a finger; see also *felon*. **pyemic a.,** a constitutional abscess due to pyemia. **renal a.,** a localized renal parenchy-

mal suppuration consequent to bacterial infection. **residual a.,** one seated near the residue of a former inflammation. **retrocecal a.,** postcecal a. **retromammary a.,** one situated between the mammary gland and the chest wall. **retroperitoneal a.,** subperitoneal a. **retropharyngeal a.,** a suppurative inflammation of the lymph nodes in the posterior and lateral walls of the pharynx; called also *hippocratic angina*. **retrotonsillar a.,** an abscess behind a tonsil caused by any of the common pyogenic bacteria, usually occurring with or closely following acute tonsillitis or pharyngitis. **ring a.,** a ring-shaped purulent infiltration at the periphery of the cornea. **root a.,** a chronic or acute pustular condition affecting the supporting tissues of the root of a tooth; when it is of endodontic origin, it is called *periapical abscess* (q.v.); when it is periodontal in origin, it is called *periodontal abscess* (q.v.). **sacrococcygeal a.,** one over the sacrum and coccyx. **satellite a.,** a secondary abscess arising from a primary one and situated near the latter. **scrofulous a.,** tuberculous a. **secondary a.,** one occurring as the result of another process. **septal a.** (*obs.*), one at the proximal surface of the root of a tooth. **septicemic a.,** one resulting from septicemia. **serous a.,** periostitis albuminosa. **shirt-stud a.,** a superficial abscess connected with a deeper one by a passage; called also *collar-button a.* **spermatic a.,** one in the seminiferous tubules. **spirillar a.,** one containing spirilla. **splenic a.,** an abscess of the spleen. **stercoraceous a., stercoral a.,** fecal a. **sterile a.,** one which contains no microorganisms. **stitch a.,** one which develops adjacent to a stitch or suture. **streptococcal a.,** one caused by streptococci. **strumous a.,** tuberculous a. **subaponeurotic a.,** one beneath an aponeurosis or fascia. **subareolar a.,** a subcutaneous abscess of the areola of the nipple. **subdiaphragmatic a.,** one beneath the diaphragm. **subdural a.,** a brain abscess situated just under the dura mater. **subfascial a.,** one beneath a fascia. **subgaleal a.,** one under the galea aponeurotica. **subhepatic a.,** one situated beneath the liver. **submammary a.,** one beneath the mammary gland. **subpectoral a.,** one beneath the pectoral muscles. **subperiosteal a.,** a bone abscess situated just below the periosteum. **subperitoneal a.,** one between the parietal peritoneum and the abdominal wall. **subphrenic a.,** one beneath the diaphragm. **subscapular a.,** one between the serratus anterior and the posterior thoracic wall. **sudoriparous a.,** an abscess arising in a sweat gland. **superficial a.,** one occurring near the surface. **suprahepatic a.,** one situated in the suspensory ligament between the liver and the diaphragm. **sympathetic a.,** one arising some distance from the exciting cause. **syphilitic a.,** one occurring in the bones during tertiary syphilis. **thecal a.,** one arising in an enveloping sheath, such as a tendon sheath. **Thornwaldt (Tornwaldt) a.,** an abscess of the adenoids, usually associated with adenoid hyperplasia. **thymus a.,** Dubois' a. **tonsillar a.,** acute suppurative tonsillitis. **tooth a.** (*obs.*), dental a. **traumatic a.,** one provoked by injury. **tropical a.,** amebic a. **tuberculous a.,** one due to infection with tubercle bacilli (*Mycobacterium tuberculosis*); called also *cold a., scrofulous a.,* and *strumous a.* **tubo-ovarian a.,** abscess of the uterine tube and ovary resulting from extension of infection along the tube. **tympanitic a.,** gas a. **tympanocervical a.,** one arising in the tympanum and extending to the neck. **tympanomastoid a.,** a combined abscess of the tympanum and the mastoid. **urethral a.,** an abscess of the urethra. **urinary a.,** one caused by extravasation of infected urine. **urinous a.** (*obs.*), one which contains pus mixed with urine. **verminous a.,** one which contains insect larvae or other animal parasites. **vitreous a.,** abscess of the vitreous humor of the eye due to infection, trauma, or foreign body. **von Bezold's a.,** Bezold's a. **wandering a.,** one that burrows in the tissues and finally points at a distance from the site of origin; called also *hypostatic a.* and *migrating a.* **web-space a.,** one in the loose connective tissue and fat between the bases of the fingers. **Welch's a.,** gas a. **worm a.,** one caused by or containing worms.

abscessus (ab-ses′us) [L.] abscess. **a. sic′cus cor′neae,** keratitis disciformis.

abscise (ab-sīz′) to cut off or remove.

abscissa (ab-sis′ah) [L. *ab* from + *scindere* to cut] one of two coordinates, the other of which is called ordinate, used as a frame of reference. The abscissa is usually horizontal and the ordinate vertical and, when suitable values have been assigned to them, corresponding data can be plotted.

abscission (ab-sish′un) [L. *ab* from + *scindere* to cut] removal by cutting. **corneal a.,** excision of the prominence of the cornea in staphyloma.

absconsio (ab-skon′se-o), pl. *absconsio′nes* [L.] the cavity of a bone receiving and concealing the head of another bone.

abscopal (ab-sko′p'l) pertaining to the effect on nonirradiated tissue resulting from irradiation of other tissue of the organism.

absence (ab′sens) temporary loss of consciousness, as may occur in some forms of epilepsy.

absentia (ab-sen′she-ah) [L.] absence. **a. epilep′tica,** temporary loss of consciousness in mild epilepsy.

abs. feb. abbreviation for L. *absen'te feb're,* while fever is absent. Cf. *adst. feb.*

Absidia (ab-sid'e-ah) a genus of fungi of the family Mucoraceae, order Mucorales. *A. corymbifera* (*Mucor rhizopodiformis*) and several other species are pathogenic for laboratory animals and may cause localized or generalized mycosis in man. *A. ramosa* (*Mucor ramosa*) is a pathogenic species that grows on bread and decaying vegetation, and causes otomycosis and sometimes mucormycosis. Formerly called *Leptomitus* and *Lichthemimia.* See also *mucormycosis.*

absinthe (ab'sinth) an extract of absinthium and other bitter herbs, containing 60 per cent alcohol; prolonged ingestion causes nervousness, convulsions, trismus, amblyopia, optic neuritis, and mental deterioration.

absinthin (ab-sin'thin) a crystalline compound, $C_{30}H_{40}O_6$, the chief bitter principle of wormwood (*Artemisia absinthium* L.), used as a flavoring in alcoholic beverages; formerly used as an anthelmintic and bitter tonic.

absinthium (ab-sinth'e-um) wormwood; the dead leaves and flowering tops of *Artemisia absinthium* L. (Compositae).

absolute (ab'so-lūt) [L. *absolutus,* from *absolvere* to set loose] free from limitations; unlimited; uncombined.

absorb (ab-sorb') [L. *absorbēre*] to take in or assimilate, as to take up substances into or across tissues, e.g., the skin, intestine, or kidney tubules, or to react with radiation energy so as to attenuate it.

absorbance (ab-sor'bans) in radiology, a measure of the ability of a medium to absorb radiation, expressed as the logarithm of the quotient of the intensity of the radiation entering the medium divided by that leaving it.

absorbefacient (ab-sor''be-fa'shent) [L. *absorbere* to absorb + *facere* to make] 1. causing or promoting absorption. 2. a medicine or an agent that promotes absorption.

absorben (ab-sor'ben) an antigen used to adsorb homologous antibodies from antiserum.

absorbency (ab-sor'ben-se) absorbance.

absorbent (ab-sor'bent) [L. *absorbens,* from *ab* away + *sorbere* to suck] 1. able to take in, or suck up and incorporate. 2. a tissue structure involved in absorption. 3. a substance that absorbs or acts as an absorbefacient.

absorptiometer (ab-sorp''she-om'ĕ-ter) [*absorption* + Gr. *metron* measure] 1. an instrument for measuring the solubility of gas in a liquid. 2. a device for measuring the layer of liquid absorbed between two glass plates; used as a hematoscope.

absorption (ab-sorp'shun) [L. *absorptio*] 1. the uptake of substances into or across tissues, e.g., skin, intestine, and kidney tubules. 2. in psychology, devotion of thought to one object or activity, with inattention to others. 3. in radiology, the taking up of energy by matter with which the radiation interacts. Cf. *attenuation,* def. 3. **agglutinin a.,** the removal of antibody from an immune serum by treatment with particulate antigen (usually bacteria) homologous to that antibody, followed by centrifugation and separation of the antigen-antibody complex. **cutaneous a.,** absorption through the skin. **disjunctive a.** (*obs.*), the process by which a slough separates from healthy tissue by the absorption of the thin layer of the latter which is in direct contact with the necrosed portion. **enteral a.,** internal a. **excrementitial a.,** pathologic a. **external a.,** the absorption of foods, poisons, or other agents through the skin or mucous membrane. **internal a.,** the normal absorption of foods, water, etc., in digestion. **interstitial a.,** removal of waste matter by the absorbent system. **intestinal a.,** the uptake from the intestinal lumen of fluids, solutes, proteins, fats, and other nutrients into the intestinal epithelial cells, blood, lymph, or interstitial fluids of the intestine. **net a.,** the difference between uptake and efflux from a tissue or cell. **parenteral a.,** absorption otherwise than through the digestive tract. **pathologic a., pathological a.,** the absorption into the blood of any bodily excretion or morbid product, such as bile or pus.

absorptive (ab-sorp'tiv) capable of absorbing; absorbent; pertaining to absorption.

abst., abstr. abstract.

abstergent (ab-ster'jent) [L. *abstergere* to cleanse] 1. cleansing or purifying. 2. a cleansing application or medicine.

abstinence (ab'stĭ-nens) a refraining from the use of or indulgence in food, stimulants, or sexual intercourse. **alimentary a.,** fasting, hunger, or starvation.

abstr. abstract.

abstract (ab'strakt) [L. *abstractum,* from *abstrahere* to draw off] 1. a summary or epitome of a book, paper, or case history. 2. (*obs.*) a powder made from a drug or its fluidextract with lactose, and brought to twice the strength of the original drug or extract.

abstraction (ab-strak'shun) [L. *abstractio*] 1. the withdrawal of any ingredient from a compound. 2. (*obs.*) the letting of blood. 3. in dentistry and anthropology, malocclusion in which the occlusal plane is further than normal from the eye-ear plane; it causes lengthening of the face. Cf. *attraction,* def. 2.

abterminal (ab-ter'mĭ-nal) [*ab-* + L. *terminus* end] moving from the terminus toward the center; said of electric currents in muscular substance.

abtorsion (ab-tor'shun) disclination.

abtropfung (ahb-trop-foong) [Ger. "a trickling or dropping down"] the proliferative transition of collections of nevus cells (theques) from the epidermis down into the dermis.

Abulcasis (ah''bool-kas'is) Albucasis.

abulia (ah-bu'le-ah) [*a* neg. + Gr. *boulē* will + *-ia*] loss or deficiency of will power, initiative, or drive. **cyclic a.,** abulia occurring periodically. **social a.,** social inactivity resulting from inability to select a course of action, although a wish to participate may be present.

abulic (ah-bu'lik) affected with or pertaining to abulia.

Abulkasim (ah''bool-kas'im) Albucasis.

abulomania (ah-bu''lo-ma'ne-ah) [*abulia* + Gr. *mania* madness] mental disorder characterized by weakness of the will or indecision of character.

abuse (ah-būs') misuse or wrong use, particularly excessive use of anything. **child a.,** see *battered-child syndrome,* under *syndrome.* **drug a.,** see *dependence.*

abut (ah-but') to touch, adjoin, or border upon.

abutment (ah-but'ment) a supporting structure to sustain lateral or horizontal pressure; applied in dentistry to any tooth to which either a fixed or a removable partial denture is attached. **auxiliary a.,** secondary a. **intermediate a.,** a natural tooth, without other natural teeth in proximal contact, used for the support or anchorage of a fixed or removable partial denture. Sometimes called *pier* or *isolated a.* **isolated a.,** an intermediate abutment, particularly one used to support a removable partial denture. **multiple a.,** one resulting from the fixed splinting of two or more adjacent natural teeth to serve as a unit in the support and retention of a fixed or removable partial denture. **primary a.,** a natural tooth providing both retention and support for a removable partial denture; sometimes used in reference to a terminal abutment for a fixed partial denture. **secondary a.,** a natural tooth used in addition to the primary abutments to provide support or indirect retention for a removable partial denture; called also *auxiliary a.* **terminal a.,** a natural tooth located at an extremity of a fixed partial denture and used for the support and retention of the prosthesis.

abwehrfermente (ahb-vair'fer-men''te) [Ger.] protective ferments.

A.C. air conduction; alternating current; aortic closure; anodal closure; axiocervical; acromioclavicular.

Ac chemical symbol for *actinium.*

a.c. abbreviation for L. *an'te ci'bum,* before meals.

A.C.A. American College of Angiology; American College of Apothecaries.

Acacia (ah-ka'she-ah) [L.; Gr. *akakia*] a genus of leguminous shrubs or trees containing several economically and medically important species; e.g., *A. senegal* yields acacia (gum arabic). **A. cat'echu** Willd. (Leguminosae), a small tree native to India and Burma, which is a source of catechu. **A. georgi'nae** F. M. Bail. (Leguminosae), a tree in northern Australia; the fluoroacetate content of its leaves is fatal to sheep and cattle.

acacia (ah-ka'shah) [NF] the dried, gummy exudate from the stems and branches of *Acacia senegal* and other African species of *Acacia,* prepared as a mucilage or syrup; formerly used intravenously in the treatment of shock and now employed as a suspending agent, emollient, and demulcent for pharmaceutical preparations. Called also *gum arabic* and *gum senegal.*

acalcerosis (ah-kal''ser-o'sis) a deficiency of calcium in the system.

acalcicosis (ah-kal''sĭ-ko'sis) a condition caused by a deficiency of calcium in the diet.

acalculia (ah''kal-ku'le-ah) [*a* neg. + L. *calculare* to reckon + *-ia*] inability to do simple arithmetical calculations.

acampsia (ah-kamp'se-ah) [*a* neg. + Gr. *kamptein* to bend + *-ia*] rigidity or inflexibility of a part or of a joint.

acantha (ah-kan'thah) [Gr. *akantha* thorn] 1. the spine. 2. the spinous process of a vertebra.

acanthaceous (ak''an-tha'shus) bearing prickles or spines.

acanthamebiasis (ah-kan''thah-me-bi'ah-sis) infection with *Acanthamoeba castellani.*

Acanthamoeba (ah-kan''thah-me'bah) a genus of amebas of the order Amoebida. **A. castella'ni,** a free-living ameba which ordinarily inhabits moist soil or water, but has been found as an opportunistic parasite of man, causing a fatal meningoencephalitis. The infection seems to be acquired by bathing in fresh-water lakes inhabited by the ameba.

acanthesthesia (ah-kan''thes-the'ze-ah) [*acantho-* + Gr. *aisthēsis* sensation + *-ia*] perverted sensibility with a feeling as of pressure of a sharp point.

Acanthia lectularia (ah-kan'the-ah lek''tu-la're-ah) *Cimex lectularius.*

acanthion (ah-kan'the-on) [Gr. *akanthion* little thorn] a point at the base of the anterior nasal spine.

acantho- [Gr. *akantha* a thorn or prickle] a combining form meaning thorny or spiny, or denoting a relationship to a sharp spine or thorn.

Acanthobdellidea (ah-kan″tho-del-lid′e-ah) an order of leeches of the class Hirudinea, characterized by the presence of spines on the surface of the body.

Acanthocephala (ah-kan″tho-sef′ah-lah) [*acantho-* + Gr. *kephalē* head] a phylum of animal parasites, the thorny-headed or spiny-head worms, so called because of the proboscis which projects anteriorly, and is covered with thornlike recurved spines for attachment to the digestive tract of the host. In some systems of classification, they are considered to be a class of the phylum Nemathelminthes.

acanthocephalan (ah-kan″tho-sef′ah-lan) any individual of the phylum Acanthocephala.

acanthocephaliasis (ah-kan″tho-sef″ah-li′ah-sis) infestation with any species of the phylum Acanthocephala.

acanthocephalous (ah-kan″tho-sef′ah-lus) pertaining to or caused by worms of the phylum Acanthocephala.

Acanthocephalus (ah-kan″tho-sef′ah-lus) a genus of parasitic worms of the phylum Acanthocephala.

Acanthocheilonema (ah-kan″tho-ki″lo-ne′mah) a genus of filarial nematodes. **A. per′stans,** *Dipetalonema perstans.* **A. streptocer′ca,** *Dipetalonema streptocerca.*

acanthocheilonemiasis (ah-kan″tho-ki″lo-ne-mi′ah-sis) dipetalonemiasis.

acanthocyte (ah-kan′tho-sīt) [*acantho-* + Gr. *kytos* cell] a distorted erythrocyte characterized by protoplasmic projections of varying sizes and shapes, irregularly spaced, which give the cell a "thorny" appearance; seen in abetalipoproteinemia.

acanthocytosis (ah-kan″tho-si-to′sis) the presence in the blood of acanthocytes, characteristically occurring in abetalipoproteinemia.

acanthoid (ah-kan′thoid) [*acantho-* + Gr. *eidos* form] resembling a spine; spinous.

acanthokeratodermia (ah-kan″tho-ker″ah-to-der′me-ah) [*acantho-* + Gr. *keras* horn + *derma* skin + *-ia*] (*obs.*) hyperkeratosis.

acantholysis (ak″an-thol′ĭ-sis) [*acantho-* + Gr. *lysis* a loosening] dissolution of the intercellular bridges in the prickle-cell layer of the epidermis; it is the mechanism of formation of the intraepidermal vesicles in pemphigus vulgaris. Cf. *acanthorrhexis* and *epidermolysis.* **a. bullo′sa** (*obs.*), epidermolysis bullosa.

acantholytic (ah-kan″tho-lit′ik) pertaining or relating to acantholysis.

acanthoma (ak″an-tho′mah, a″kan-tho′mah), pl. *acantho′mas* or *acantho′mata* [*acantho-* + *-oma*] a tumor composed of epidermal or squamous cells. **a. adenoi′des cys′ticum,** trichoepithelioma. **basal cell a.,** seborrheic keratosis. **a. verruco′sa seborrhe′ica,** seborrheic keratosis.

acanthopelvis (ah-kan″tho-pel′vis) [*acantho-* + Gr. *pelyx* bowl] a pelvis with a very sharp and prominent pubic crest; called also *acanthopelyx.*

acanthopelyx (ah-kan″tho-pel′iks) acanthopelvis.

Acanthophacetus (ah-kan″tho-fah-se′tus) a genus of small fish. **A. reticula′tus,** *Lebistes reticulatus.*

Acanthophis (ah-kan′tho-fis) a genus of elapid snakes; see table accompanying *snake.* **A. antarc′tica,** a widespread, live-bearing elapid snake of Australia and New Guinea, remarkable for its viper-like form; next to the tiger snake it is the most feared snake in Australia. Called also *death adder.*

Acanthopterygii (ah-kan″tho-tĕ-rij′e-i) a superorder of spiny-finned teleosts.

acanthorrhexis (ah-kan″tho-rek′sis) rupture (as opposed to dissolution, or acantholysis) of the intercellular bridges of the prickle-cell layer of the epidermis, as in blisters caused by severe edema of the skin.

acanthosis (ak″an-tho′sis) [*acantho-* + *-osis*] diffuse hyperplasia and thickening of the prickle-cell layer of the epidermis, as in psoriasis. Also used in the clinical sense to denote diffuse "thorniness" without such hyperplasia. Cf. *acanthosis nigricans.* **a. ni′gricans,** diffuse velvety acanthosis with gray, brown, or black pigmentation, chiefly in axillae and other body folds, occurring in an adult form, often associated with an internal carcinoma (called *malignant acanthosis nigricans*), and in a benign, nevoid form, more or less generalized. A benign juvenile form associated with obesity, which is sometimes due to endocrine disturbance, is called *pseudoacanthosis nigricans.* **a. seborrhe′ica, a. verruco′sa,** seborrheic keratosis.

acanthotic (ak″an-thot′ik) marked by acanthosis.

acanthrocyte (ah-kan′thro-sīt) acanthocyte.

acanthrocytosis (ah-kan″thro-si-to′sis) acanthocytosis.

a cap′ite ad cal′cem (ah kap′ĭ-te ad kal′sēm) [L.] from head to heel, the classic order for describing symptoms.

acapnia (ah-kap′ne-ah) [*a* neg. + Gr. *kapnos* smoke + *-ia*] a condition of diminished carbon dioxide in blood; hypocapnia.

acapnial (ah-kap′ne-al) acapnic.

acapnic (ah-kap′nik) pertaining to or characterized by acapnia.

Acarapis (a-kar′ah-pis) a genus of mites, including *A. woodi,* the tracheal mite of the honeybee, which causes Isle of Wight disease.

acarbia (ah-kar′be-ah) a condition in which the blood bicarbonate is lowered.

acardia (a-kar′de-ah) [*a* neg. + Gr. *kardia* heart] congenital absence of the heart.

acardiac (a-kar′de-ak) having no heart.

acardiacus (ah″kar-di′ah-kus) acardius.

acardiotrophia (ah-kar″de-o-tro′fe-ah) [*a* neg. + Gr. *kardia* heart + *trophē* nutrition + *-ia*] (*obs.*) atrophy of the heart.

acardius (a-kar′de-us) [*a* neg. + Gr. *kardia* heart] an imperfectly formed free twin fetus, lacking a heart and invariably lacking other body parts as well; called also *fetus a.* **a. aceph′alus,** holoacardius acephalus. **a. acor′mus,** holoacardius acormus. **a. amor′phus,** holoacardius amorphus. **a. an′ceps,** hemiacardius.

acari (ak′ah-ri) [L.] plural of *acarus,* a mite.

acarian (ah-ka′re-an) pertaining to the acarids or mites.

acariasis (ak″ah-ri′ah-sis) [Gr. *akari* mite + *-iasis*] an infestation with mites; called also *acarinosis.* **chorioptic a.,** see *Chorioptes.* **demodectic a.,** infestation of the hair follicles with the mite *Demodex folliculorum*; it affects man, dogs, horses, cattle, and sheep. In animals it is called *demodectic* or *follicular mange.* **psoroptic a.,** infestation with mites which deposit their eggs on the skin of the host and produce scabs, e.g., *Psoroptes.* **pulmonary a.,** a disease of monkeys produced by mites which live in the lungs of the host. **sarcoptic a.,** an infestation with mites of species which burrow into the skin, producing channels in which their eggs are deposited, e.g., *Sarcoptes.* See also *scabies.*

acaricide (ah-kar′ĭ-sīd) [L. *acarus* mite + *caedere* to slay] 1. destructive to mites. 2. an agent that destroys mites.

acarid (ak′ah-rid) a mite or tick of the order Acarina, or a mite of the family Acaridae.

Acaridae (ah-kar′ĭ-de) a family of small mites of the order Acarina; several species cause skin rashes, such as grocers' itch, copra itch, and vanillism.

acaridan (ah-kar′ĭ-dan) acarid.

acaridiasis (ah-kar″ĭ-di′ah-sis) acariasis.

Acarina (ak″ah-ri′nah) an order of the class Arachnida, including the ticks and mites.

acarine (ak′ah-rīn) any member of the order Acarina.

acarinosis (ah-kar″ĭ-no′sis) any disease caused by mites; acariasis.

acariosis (ah-kar″e-o′sis) acariasis.

acaro- [Gr. *akari;* L. *acarus,* a mite] a combining form denoting relationship to mites.

acarodermatitis (ak″ah-ro-der″mah-ti′tis) any skin inflammation caused by mites. **a. urticarioi′des,** grain itch.

acaroid (ak′ah-roid) [Gr. *akari* a mite + *eidos* form] resembling a mite.

acarologist (ak″ah-rol′o-jist) a specialist in acarology.

acarology (ak″ah-rol′o-je) [*acaro-* + *-logy*] the scientific study of mites and ticks.

acarophobia (ak″ah-ro-fo′be-ah) [*acaro-* + *phobia*] morbid dread of mites (*acarus*), or of small objects.

acarotoxic (ak″ah-ro-tok′sik) destructive to mites.

Acartomyia (ah-kar″to-mi′yah) a genus of culicine mosquitoes.

Acarus (ak′ah-rus) [L.; Gr. *akari* a mite] a genus of small mites, often ectoparasitic; they cause itch, mange, and other skin diseases. **A. folliculo′rum,** *Demodex folliculorum.* **A. galli′nae,** *Dermanyssus gallinae.* **A. hor′dei,** the barley bug, a mite which burrows under the skin of man. **A. rhyzoglyp′ticus hyacin′thi,** the onion mite which occurs on decaying onions and produces a dermatitis (onion-mite dermatitis) on persons who handle them. **A. scabie′i,** *Sarcoptes scabiei.* **A. si′ro,** a mite that causes vanillism in vanilla pod handlers; called also *Tyrophagus siro* and *Tyroglyphus siro.* **A. trit′ici,** former name for *Pyemotes ventricosus.*

acarus (ak′ah-rus), pl. *ac′ari* [L.] a mite.

acaryote (a-kār′e-ōt) [*a* neg. + Gr. *karyon* kernel] akaryote.

acatalasemia (a″kat-ah-la-se′me-ah) [*a* neg. + *catalase* + Gr. *haima* blood] deficiency of catalase in the blood; now called *acatalasia* (q.v.).

acatalasia (a″kat-ah-la′ze-ah) a rare disease characterized by congenital absence of the enzyme catalase, due to homozygosity for a mendelian gene occurring mostly in Japanese persons. Only about half the patients have symptoms, which consist of recurrent infections of the gingiva and associated oral structures. Originally called *acatalasemia* because the absence of catalase was first detected in the red blood cells. Called also *anenzymia catalasea.*

acatalepsia (ah-kat″ah-lep′se-ah) [*a* neg. + Gr. *katalepsis* comprehension] (*obs.*) 1. lack of understanding. 2. uncertainty of diagnosis.

acatalepsy (ah-kat′ah-lep″se)   acatalepsia.

acataleptic (ah-kat″ah-lep′tik)   1. mentally deficient. 2. doubtful or uncertain.

acatamathesia (a-kat″ah-mah-the′ze-ah) [*a* neg. + Gr. *katamathēsis* understanding + *-ia*]   1. loss or impairment of the power to understand speech. 2. impairment of any one of the perceptive faculties, due to a central lesion.

acataphasia (a-kat″ah-fa′ze-ah) [*a* neg. + Gr. *kataphasis* orderly utterance + *-ia*]   inability to express one's thoughts in a connected manner, due to a central lesion.

acataposis (a-kat″ah-po′sis) [*a* neg. + Gr. *kata* down + *posis* drinking]   (*obs.*) dysphagia.

acatastasia (ak″ah-tas-ta′ze-ah) [*a* neg. + Gr. *katastasis* stability + *-ia*]   irregularity; variation from the normal.

acatastatic (ak″ah-tas-tat′ik)   irregular; varying from the normal.

acathectic (ak″ah-thek′tik) [*a* neg. + Gr. *kathexis* a retention]   pertaining to or characterized by acathexia.

acathexia (ak″ah-thek′se-ah)   inability to retain bodily secretions.

acathexis (ah″kah-thek′sis)   a mental disturbance in which certain things, such as objects, ideas, and memories, that ordinarily have great significance to an individual arouse no emotional response.

acathisia (ak″ah-the′ze-ah)   akathisia.

acaudal (a-kaw′dal)   acaudate.

acaudate (a-kaw′dāt) [*a* neg. + L. *cauda* tail]   lacking a tail.

acauline (a-kaw′lin) [*a* neg. + L. *caulis* stem]   (*obs.*) having no stem, as certain fungi.

acaulinosis (a-kaw″lĭ-no′sis)   infection with a fungus of the genus *Acaulium* (*Scopulariopsis*); scopulariopsosis.

Acaulium (ah-kaw′le-um)   former name for *Scopulariopsis.*

ACC   anodal closure contraction.

Acc.   accommodation.

accelerans (ak-sel′er-anz) [L. "hastening"]   (*obs.*) an autonomic nerve, stimulation of which hastens the heart's action.

accelerant (ak-sel′er-ant)   a catalyst.

acceleration (ak-sel″er-a′shun) [L. *acceleratio,* from *ad* intensification + *celerare* to quicken]   a quickening, as of the pulse rate or respiration. **negative a.,** a slowing.

accelerator (ak-sel′er-a″tor) [L. "hastener"]   1. an agent or apparatus that is used to increase the rate at which an object proceeds or a substance acts, or at which some reaction occurs. 2. any nerve or muscle which hastens the performance of a function. 3. any of a group of chemicals used in the vulcanization of rubber or other polymerizations; they frequently cause dermatitis in workers. **linear a.,** an apparatus for the acceleration of subatomic particles, using alternating hollow electrodes in a straight vacuum tube, so arranged that when their high frequency potentials are properly varied the particles traveling through them receive successive increases in energy. **serum prothrombin conversion a. (SPCA),** Factor VII; see *coagulation factors,* under *factor.* **serum thrombotic a.,** a factor in serum which possesses procoagulant properties and the ability, when infused experimentally into locally arrested flow systems, to induce blood coagulation; its precise nature and role in normal blood coagulation has not been delineated and hence it has not been assigned a number in the conventional scheme of blood coagulation factors. **a. uri′nae,** musculus bulbospongiosus; see *Table of Musculi.*

accelerin (ak-sel′er-in)   Factor VI; see *coagulation factors,* under *factor.*

accelerometer (ak-sel′er-om′ĕ-ter)   an instrument for measuring the acceleration (rate of change of velocity) of an object.

accentuation (ak-sen″chu-a′shun) [L. *accentus* accent]   increased loudness or distinctness; intensification.

acceptor (ak-sep′tor)   a substance which unites with another substance; specifically a substance which unites with hydrogen or oxygen in an oxidoreduction reaction and so enables the reaction to proceed. Cf. *donor.* **hydrogen a.,** the substance that is reduced in the oxidation and reduction occurring anaerobically in the body tissues. **oxygen a.,** a substance that is oxidized.

accès pernicieux (ak-sa′ păr-nis-yuh′) [Fr. "pernicious attack"]   a sudden and severe paroxysm in falciparum malaria.

accessiflexor (ak-ses′ĕ-flek″sor)   any accessory flexor muscle.

accessorius (ak″ses-o′re-us) [L. "supplementary"]   accessory; used in naming certain structures thought to serve a supplementary function.

accessory (ak-ses′o-re) [L. *accessorius*]   supplementary or affording aid to another similar and generally more important thing; complementary; concomitant.

accident (ak′sĭ-dent)   an unforeseen occurrence, especially one of an injurious character; an unexpected complicating occurrence in the regular course of a disease. **cerebrovascular a.,** stroke syndrome.

accidentalism (ak″sĭ-den′tal-izm)   the theory of medicine that attends only the symptoms of disease, ignoring the etiology and pathology.

accident prone (ak′sĭ-dent prŏn)   specially susceptible to accidents owing to psychological factors.

accipiter (ak-sip′ĭ-ter) [L. "hawk"]   a facial bandage with tails like the talons of a hawk.

ACCl   anodal closure clonus.

acclimatation (ah-kli″mah-ta′shun)   acclimation.

acclimation (ak″li-ma′shun)   the process of becoming accustomed to a new environment.

acclimatization (ah-kli″mah-ti-za′shun)   acclimation.

accolé   see *appliqué form,* under *form.*

accommodation (ah-kom″o-da′shun) [L. *accommodere* to fit to]   adjustment, especially that of the eye for various distances (see illustration). **absolute a.,** the accommodation of either eye

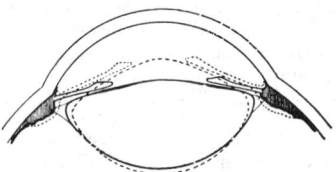

Changes during accommodation: Contraction of ciliary muscle; approximation of ciliary muscle to lens; relaxation of suspensory ligament; increased curvature of anterior surface of lens. (Helmholtz.)

separately. **binocular a.,** accommodation in both eyes in coordination with convergence. **excessive a.,** accommodation of the eye which is persistently above the normal. **histologic a.,** a group of changes in the morphology and function of cells following changed conditions. **negative a.,** adjustment of the eye for long distances by relaxation of the ciliary muscle. **nerve a.,** the rise in the threshold during the passage of a constant, direct electric current because of which only the make and break of the current stimulates the nerve. **positive a.,** adjustment of the eye for short distances by contraction of the ciliary muscle. **relative a.,** the change in accommodation that is possible with a fixed amount of convergence. **subnormal a.,** insufficient power of accommodation of the eye.

accommodative (ah-kom′o-da″tiv)   pertaining to, of the nature of, or affecting accommodation.

accommodometer (ah-kom″o-dom′ĕ-ter)   a device for measuring the accommodative capacity of the eye.

accomplice (ak-om-plēs′) [Fr.]   a bacterium which accompanies the chief infecting agent in a mixed infection and which influences the virulence of the chief organism.

accouchement (ah-kōōsh-maw′) [Fr.]   labor. **a. forcé** (ah-kōōsh-maw′ for-sa′), rapid forcible delivery from below by any one of several methods; originally applied to rapid dilatation of the cervix with the hands, followed immediately by version and extraction of the fetus.

accoucheur (ah-kōōsh-er′) [Fr.]   one skilled in obstetrics; an obstetrician.

accoucheuse (ah-kōōsh-ez′) [Fr.]   a midwife.

accrementition (ak″re-men-tish′un) [L. *ad* to + *crementum* increase]   growth or increase by the addition of similar tissue.

accretio (ah-kre′she-o) [L.]   abnormal adhesion of parts normally separate. **a. cor′dis, a. pericar′dii,** a form of adhesive pericarditis in which adhesions extend from the pericardium to the pleurae, diaphragm, and chest wall.

accretion (ah-kre′shun) [L. *ad* to + *crescere* to grow]   1. growth by addition of material. 2. accumulation. 3. adherence of parts normally separated.

A.C.D.   acid citrate dextrose (see under *solution*).

ACE   adrenocortical extract.

acebutolol (ah″se-bu′to-lŏl)   chemical name: (+)-*N*-[3-acetyl-4-[2-hydroxy-3-[(1-methylethyl)amino]propoxy]pheynl]butanamide; a beta-adrenergic blocking agent, $C_{18}H_{28}N_2O_4$.

acecainide hydrochloride (as″ĕ-ka′nīd)   chemical name: 4-(acetylamino)-*N*-[2-(diethylamino)ethyl]benzamide monohydrochloride; an antiarrhythmic cardiac depressant, $C_{15}H_{23}N_3O_2 \cdot HCl$.

aceclidine (as-sek′lĭ-dēn)   chemical name: 3-quinuclidinol acetate ester; a cholinergic, $C_9H_{15}NO_2$.

acedapsone (as-ĕ-dap′sŏn)   chemical name: 4′,4‴-sulfonylbis[acetanilide]. The diacetyl derivative of dapsone, $C_{16}H_{16}N_2O_4S$, having actions similar to those of the parent compound; used as a leprostatic and antimalarial. Called also *diacetyl diaminodiphenylsulfone* (*DADDS*).

acedia (ah-se′de-ah) [*a* neg. + Gr. *kēdos* care + *-ia*]   a mental disorder characterized by apathy and melancholy.

acellular (a-sel′u-lar)   not made up of or containing cells.

acelomate (a-se′lo-māt)   not having a coelom or body cavity.

acelous (a-se′lus) [*a* neg. + Gr. *koilos* hollow]   not concave on either surface; said of the vertebrae of certain animals. Cf. *opisthocelous* and *procelous.*

acenesthesia (ah-sen″es-the′ze-ah) [*a* neg. + *cenesthesia*] abolition of the sense of well being, seen in melancholia and hypochondriasis.

acenocoumarin (ah-se″no-koo′mah-rin) acenoumarol.

acenocoumarol (ah-se″no-koo′mah-rol) chemical name: 2*H*-1-benzopyran-2-one-4-hydroxy-3-[1-4(4-nitrophenyl)-3-oxobutyl]-3-α-acetonyl-*p*-nitrobenzyl)-4-hydroxycoumarin. One of the synthetic coumarin anticoagulants, $C_{19}H_{15}NO_6$, occurring as an off-white to light tan powder, having a rapid onset, intermediate duration of action, and little cumulative effect; administered orally.

acentric (ah-sen′trik) [Gr. *akentrikos* not centric] 1. not central; not located in the center. 2. lacking a centromere, so that the chromosome will not survive subsequent cell divisions.

ACEP American College of Emergency Physicians.

acephalia (ah″sĕ-fa′le-ah) [*a* neg. + Gr. *kephalē* head] congenital absence of the head.

acephalism (ah-sef′ah-lizm) acephalia.

acephalobrachia (ah-sef″ah-lo-bra′ke-ah) [*a* neg. + Gr. *kephalē* head + *brachiōn* arm + *-ia*] congenital absence of the head and arms.

acephalobrachius (ah-sef″ah-lo-bra′ke-us) a monster exhibiting acephalobrachia.

acephalocardia (ah-sef″ah-lo-kar′de-ah) [*a* neg. + Gr. *kephalē* head + *kardia* heart + *-ia*] congenital absence of the head and heart.

acephalocardius (ah-sef″ah-lo-kar′de-us) a monster exhibiting acephalocardia.

acephalochiria (ah-sef″ah-lo-ki′re-ah) [*a* neg. + Gr. *kephalē* head + *cheir* hand + *-ia*] congenital absence of the head and hands.

acephalochirus (ah-sef″ah-lo-ki′rus) a monster exhibiting acephalochiria.

acephalocyst (ah-sef″ah-lo′sist) [*a* neg. + Gr. *kephalē* head + *kystis* bladder] sterile cyst.

acephalocystis racemosa (ah-sef″ah-lo-sis′tis ra-se-mo′sah) (*obs.*) a hydatid mole of the uterus.

acephalogaster (ah-sef″ah-lo-gas′ter) [*a* neg. + Gr. *kephalē* head + *gastēr* belly] a monster exhibiting acephalogastria.

acephalogastria (ah-sef″ah-lo-gas′tre-ah) congenital absence of the head, chest, and upper part of the abdomen.

acephalopodia (ah-sef″ah-lo-po′de-ah) [*a* neg. + Gr. *kephalē* head + *pous* foot + *-ia*] congenital absence of the head and feet.

acephalopodius (ah-sef″ah-lo-po′de-us) a monster exhibiting acephalopodia.

acephalorhachia (ah-sef″ah-lo-ra′ke-ah) [*a* neg. + Gr. *kephalē* head + *rhachis* spine + *-ia*] congenital absence of the head and vertebral column.

acephalostomia (ah-sef″ah-lo-sto′me-ah) [*a* neg. + Gr. *kephalē* head + *stoma* mouth + *-ia*] congenital absence of the head, yet with a kind of mouth on the superior aspect.

acephalostomus (ah-sef″ah-los′to-mus) a monster exhibiting acephalostomia.

acephalothoracia (ah-sef″ah-lo-tho-ra′se-ah) [*a* neg. + Gr. *kephalē* head + *thōrax* chest *-ia*] congenital absence of the head and chest.

acephalothorus (ah-sef″ah-lo-tho′rus) a monster exhibiting acephalothoracia.

acephalous (ah-sef′ah-lus) headless.

acephalus (ah-sef′ah-lus), pl. *aceph′ali* [*a* neg. + Gr. *kephalē* head] a headless monster. **a. dibra′chius,** an acephalus with both upper limbs more or less undeveloped. **a. di′pus,** an acephalus with both lower limbs more or less undeveloped. **a. monobra′chius,** an acephalus with only one upper limb. **a. mon′opus,** an acephalus with only one foot or lower limb. **a. paraceph′alus,** a monster with a partially formed skull but no brain. **a. sym′pus,** an acephalus with the two lower limbs fused into one.

acephaly (ah-sef′ah-le) acephalia.

acepromazine maleate (ah″se-pro′mah-zēn) 1-[10-[3-(dimethylamino)propyl]-10*H*-phenothiazin-2-yl]ethanone (*Z*)-2-butenedioate(1:1). A tranquilizer, $C_{19}H_{22}N_2OS·C_4H_4O_4$; used in veterinary medicine to immobilize large animals.

Aceraria (as″ĕ-ra′re-ah) a genus of nematode parasites. **A. spira′lis,** a nematode parasite occurring in growths in the esophagus of fowls.

acerin (ah′ser-in) an extract from the dried fruit of the Norway maple, *Acer plantanoides* L. (Aceraceae); effective against *Escherichia coli* and the vaccinia virus.

acerola (ah-sĕ-ro′lah) the West Indian cherry fruit (*Malpighia punicifolia* L., Malpighiaceae), thought to be the richest natural source of vitamin C (about 1690 mg. per 100 grams of pitted fruit). It is given in the diet of individuals allergic to citrus fruits.

acervuli (ah-ser′vu-li) [L.] plural of *acervulus.*

acervuline (ah-ser′vu-lin) [L. *acervulus* little heap] aggregated; said of certain glands.

acervuloma (ah-ser″vu-lo′mah) [L. *acervulus* little heap + *-oma*] (*obs.*) a meningioma containing psammoma bodies.

acervulus (ah-ser′vu-lus), pl. *acer′vuli* [L., dim. of *acervus* a heap] the mass of gritty matter which lies in or near the pineal body, the choroid plexus, and other parts of the brain; called also *acervulus cerebri, brain sand,* and *sand bodies.*

acescence (ah-ses′ens) [L. *acescere* to become sour] 1. sourness. 2. the process of becoming sour.

acescent (ah-ses′ent) somewhat or slightly acid.

acesodyne (ah-ses′o-dīn) [Gr. *akesis* cure + *odynē* pain] anodyne; allaying pain.

acestoma (ah″ses-to′mah) [Gr. *akesis* cure + *-oma*] (*obs.*) a mass of granulations.

acetabular (as″ĕ-tab′u-lar) pertaining to the acetabulum.

Acetabularia (as″ĕ-tab″u-la′re-ah) a genus of large single-celled green algae having a foot, a stalk, and a cap. *A. mediterra′nea* and *A. crenula′ta* have been used in genetic experiments.

acetabulectomy (as″ĕ-tab″u-lek′to-me) [*acetabulum* + Gr. *ektomē* excision] excision of the acetabulum.

acetabuloplasty (as″ĕ-tab′u-lo-plas″te) [*acetabulum* + Gr. *plassein* to form] plastic reconstruction of the acetabulum.

acetabulum (as″ĕ-tab′u-lum), pl. *acetab′ula* [L. "vinegar-cruet," from *acetum* vinegar] [NA] the large cup-shaped cavity on the lateral surface of the os coxae in which the head of the femur articulates; called also *acetabular bone, cotyloid cavity,* and *os acetabulum.* **sunken a.,** Otto pelvis.

acetal (as′ĕ-tal) an organic compound formed by a combination of an aldehyde with an alcohol.

acetaldehydase (as″et-al′dĕ-hi″dās) an enzyme that catalyzes the oxidation of acetic aldehyde to acetic acid.

acetaldehyde (as″et-al′dĕ-hīd″) a colorless flammable liquid, CH_3CHO, with a pungent odor, used in the manufacture of acetic acid, perfumes, and flavors. It is also an intermediate in the metabolism of alcohol. Acetaldehyde may cause irritation of mucous membranes, lacrimation, photophobia, conjunctivitis, corneal injury, rhinitis, anosmia, bronchitis, pneumonia, pleurisy, headache, and unconsciousness. Called also *acetic aldehyde, ethanal,* and *ethylaldehyde.*

acetamide (as″et-am′īd) a white crystalline substance, CH_3-$CONH_2$, used in organic synthesis and as a general solvent when melted.

acetamidine (as″et-am′ĭ-dīn) chemical name: α-amino-α-iminoethane. The imine, $CH_3CH(NH)NH_2$, of acetamide, used in the synthesis of imidazoles and pyrimidines.

***p*-acetamidobenzene sulfonamide** (as″et-am″ĭ-do-ben′zēn sul-fon′ah-mīd) one of the conjugated forms in which benzene sulfonamide is excreted in the urine.

acetaminophen (as″et-am′ĭ-no-fen) [USP] chemical name: *N*-(4-hydroxyphenyl)acetamide. An analgesic and antipyretic, C_8H_9-NO_2, occurring as a white, crystalline powder; administered orally.

acetanilid (as″ĕ-tan′ĭ-lid) [*acetic* + *aniline*] chemical name: *N*-phenylacetamide; it is a white, crystalline, sublimable solid, $C_6H_5NH·OC·CH_3$, produced by combining glacial acetic acid with aniline. It is analgesic and antipyretic and is used in neuralgia and rheumatism. Called also *acetylaminobenzene, acetylaniline,* and *antifebrin.*

acetannin (as″ĕ-tan′in) acetyltannic acid.

acetarsol (as″et-ar′sol) acetarsone.

acetarsone (as″et-ar′sōn) chemical name: 3-acetamido-hydroxyphenyl arsonic acid. A pentavalent arsenical, $C_8H_{10}AsNO_5$, occurring as a white, crystalline powder. It is used orally in the treatment of intestinal amebiasis, orally and topically in necrotizing ulcerative gingivitis, and topically in trichomonas vaginitis. Called also *acetphenarsine.*

acetas (ah-se′tas) [L.] acetate.

acetate (as′ĕ-tāt) any salt of acetic acid.

acetazolamide (as″et-ah-zol′ah-mīd) [USP] chemical name: *N*-[5-(aminosulfonyl)-1,3,4-thiadiazol-2-yl]acetamide. A white to faintly yellowish white crystalline powder, $C_4H_6N_4O_3S_2$, it is a diuretic of the carbonic anhydrase inhibitor type, useful in treatment of carbon dioxide retention in chronic lung disease, to reduce intraocular pressure in glaucoma, and formerly in management of edema associated with heart disease. **sodium a., sterile** [USP], a preparation suitable for parenteral use, prepared from acetazolamide with the aid of sodium hydroxide, $C_4H_5N_4Na$-O_3S_2, and containing between 95 and 110 per cent of the labeled amount of acetazolamide.

acetenyl (ah-se′tĕ-nil) ethynyl.

Acetest (ah′sĕ-test) trademark for reagent tablets containing sodium nitroprusside, aminoacetic acid, disodium phosphate, and lactose. A drop of urine is placed on a tablet on a sheet of white paper; if significant quantities of acetone are present the tablet changes from a purple tint (1+), to lavender (2+), to moderate purple (3+), or deep purple (4+).

aceteugenol (as″et-u′jĕ-nol) an essential oil from oil of cloves: 1-ethyl, 3-methoxy, 4-acetoxy benzene.

acetic (ah-se′tik, ah-set′ik) pertaining to vinegar or its acid; sour.

aceticoceptor (ah-se″te-ko-sep′tor) a ceptor or side chain having specific affinity for the acetic acid radical.

acetify (ah-set′ĭ-fi) to turn into acetic acid or vinegar.

acetimeter (as″ĕ-tim′ĕ-ter) [L. *acetum* vinegar + Gr. *metron* measure] an apparatus for determining the amount of acetic acid present in a solution.

acetin (as′ĕ-tin) a glyceryl acetate; it may contain one, two, or three acetyl groups.

Acetobacter (ah-se″to-bak′ter) [L. *acetum* vinegar + *bactrum* (Gr. *baktērion*) little rod] a genus of schizomycetes of the family Pseudomonadaceae, order Pseudomonadales, occurring as ellipsoidal to rod-shaped cells, singly, or in pairs or short or long chains, important for their role in completion of the carbon cycle and in production of vinegar. It includes seven species, *A. ace′ti, A. melano′genus, A. ox′ydans, A. ran′cens, A. ro′seus, A. subox′ydans,* and *A. xy′linum; A. kuetzingia′nus* and *A. pasteuria′nus* are considered varieties of *A. rancens.*

acetoform (ah-se′to-form) methenamine.

acetohexamide (as″ĕ-to-heks′ah-mīd) [USP] chemical name: 4-acetyl-*N*-[[cyclohexylamino]carbonyl]benzenesulfonamide. An oral hypoglycemic agent, $C_{15}H_{20}O_4S$, occurring as a white, crystalline powder.

acetoin (ah-set′o-in) 3-hydroxy-2-butanone: a liquid ketone product of carbohydrate fermentation.

acetokinase (as″ĕ-to-ki′nās) acetate kinase.

acetolase (ah-set′o-lās) an enzyme that catalyzes the conversion of alcohol into acetic acid.

acetolysis (as″ĕ-tol′ĭ-sis) combined hydrolysis and acetylation.

acetomeroctol (as″ĕ-to-mer-ok′tol) chemical name: 2-acetoxymercuri-4(1,1,3,3-tetramethylbutyl) phenol; a crystalline substance, $C_{16}H_{24}HgO_3$, formerly used as a topical antiseptic.

acetometer (as″ĕ-tom′ĕ-ter) acetimeter.

acetomorphine (as″ĕ-to-mor′fēn) diacetylmorphine.

acetonaphthone (as″e-to-naf′thōn) an acetyl derivative of naphthalene, $C_{10}H_7COCH_3$, occurring in two isomeric forms. The 2-acetonaphthone isomer is a mosquito repellent; derivatives are used as bactericides and as an antitubercular agent.

acetonasthma (as″ĕ-tōn-az′mah) (*obs.*) air hunger due to acidosis.

acetonation (as″ĕ-to-na′shun) combination with acetone.

acetone (as′ĕ-tōn) [*acetic* + *ketone*] 1. dimethyl ketone, CH_3-CO·CH_3, a colorless liquid with a pleasant ethereal odor, found in small quantities in normal urine and in larger amounts in diabetic urine. It is acrid and inflammable, and is used as a solvent for fats, resins, rubber, and plastic and to cleanse the skin before injections and vaccinations. The USP preparation contains not less than 99 percent of acetone on the anhydrous basis. 2. any member of the series to which the normal or typical acetone belongs. See also *ketone bodies,* under *body.* **a. diethyl-sulfone,** sulfonmethane.

acetonemia (as″ĕ-to-ne′me-ah) [*acetone* + Gr. *haima* blood + *-ia*] an excess of acetone bodies in the blood; now called *ketonemia.*

acetonemic (as″ĕ-to-ne′mik) pertaining to or marked by acetonemia.

acetonglycosuria (as″ĕ-tōn″gli-ko-su′re-ah) glycosuria due to acetone poisoning.

acetonitrile (as″ĕ-to-ni′tril) a poisonous colorless liquid, CH_3-CN, with an ether-like odor; see also *Hunt's reaction,* under *reaction.*

acetonum (as″ĕ-to′num) [L.] acetone.

acetonumerator (as″ĕ-to-nu′mer-a″tor) an instrument for estimating the amount of acetone in the urine.

acetonuria (as″ĕ-to-nu′re-ah) an excess of acetone bodies in the urine; it occurs in diabetes, fever, starvation, carcinoma, and digestive disorders. Now called *ketonuria.*

aceto-orcein (as″ĕ-to-or′se-in) orcein dissolved in acetic acid, used in making squash preparations of polytene chromosomes.

acetophenazine maleate (as″ĕ-to-fen′ah-zēn) [USP] chemical name: 10-[3-[4-(2-hydroxyethyl)-1-piperazinyl]propyl]phenothiazin-2-yl methyl ketone maleate. A fine, yellow powder, $C_{23}H_{29}N_3O_2S·2C_4H_4O_4$, used as a major tranquilizer.

acetophenetidin (as″ĕ-to-fĕ-net′ĭ-din) phenacetin.

acetosal (ah-se′to-sal) acetylsalicylic acid.

acetosoluble (as″ĕ-to-sol′u-b′l) soluble in acetic acid.

acetosulfone sodium (as″ĕ-to-sul′fōn) chemical name: *N*-[[5-amino-2-[(4-aminophenyl)sulfonyl]phenyl]sulfonyl]acetamide monosodium salt. An antibacterial derivative of dapsone, $C_{14}N_{14}N_3$-NaO_5S_2, having actions similar to those of the parent compound, occurring as a white to pinkish-white crystalline powder; used as

a leprostatic in lepromatous and tuberculoid leprosy and as a dermatitis herpetiformis suppressant, administered orally.

acetous (as′ĕ-tus) [L. *acetosus*] pertaining to, producing, or resembling acetic acid.

acetphenarsine (as″et-fen-ar′sēn) acetarsone.

acetphenetidin (as″et-fĕ-net′ĭ-din) phenacetin.

acetpyrogall (as″et-pi′ro-gal) chemical name: pyrogall triacetate. A white crystalline compound, $C_6H_3(CH_3CO_2)_3$, used as a topical caustic and keratolytic.

acetract (as′ĕ-trakt) (*obs.*) an extract of a drug made with a menstruum containing acetic acid.

acetum (ah-se′tum), pl. *ace′ta* [L.] 1. vinegar. 2. a medicinal solution of a drug in dilute acetic acid. **a. plum′bi, a. satur′ni,** lead subacetate solution.

aceturate (ah-set′u-rāt) USAN contraction for *N*-acetylglycinate.

acetyl (as′ĕ-til) [L. *acetum* vinegar + Gr. *hylē* matter] the monovalent radical, CH_3CO. **a. chloride,** a colorless liquid, CH_3·CO·Cl, used as a reagent for forming acetate esters of alcohols. **a. peroxide,** diacetyl peroxide. **a. sulfisoxazole,** chemical name: N^1-acetyl-N^1-(3,4-dimethyl-5-isoxazolyl)-sulfanilamide. Tasteless crystals, $C_{13}H_{15}N_3O_4S$, used as an antimicrobial.

acetylaminobenzene sulfonate (as″ĕ-til-am″ĭ-no-ben′zēn) a compound, CH_3·CO·NH·C_6H_4·SO_2·NH_2, the form in which sulfanilamide is excreted.

acetylaminobenzene (as″ĕ-til-am″ĭ-no-ben′zēn) acetanilid.

acetylaminofluorene (as″ĕ-til-am″ĭ-no-floo′o-rēn) a compound, $C_6H_4CH_2C_6H_3NH·CO·CH_3$, which is carcinogenic when ingested.

acetylaniline (as″ĕ-til-an′ĭ-lin) acetanilid.

acetylation (ah-set″ĭ-la′shun) the introduction of an acetyl group into the molecule of an organic compound.

acetylator (ah-set″ĭ-la′tor) an organism capable of metabolic acetylation; in man, acetylator status (fast or slow) is determined by the rate of acetylation of sulfamethazine.

acetyl-beta-methylcholine chloride (as″ĕ-til-ba″tah-meth″il-ko′lin) methacholine chloride.

acetylcholine (as″ĕ-til-ko′lēn) a reversible acetic acid ester of choline, CH_3·CO·O·CH_2·CH_2·N(CH_3)₃·OH, normally present in many parts of the body and having important physiological functions, such as serving as a neurotransmitter at the myoneural junction, in sympathetic and parasympathetic ganglia, and at parasympathetic nerve endings; used also in medicine as a parasympathomimetic agent. Abbreviated ACh. **a. chloride,** a miotic administered by instillation into the anterior chamber of the eye.

acetylcholinesterase (as″ĕ-til-ko″lin-es′ter-ās) an enzyme present in nervous tissue, muscle, and red cells that catalyzes the hydrolysis of acetylcholine to choline and acetic acid; called also *true cholinesterase.* Abbreviated AChE.

acetyl-CoA acetylcoenzyme A.

acetylcoenzyme A (as″ĕ-til-ko-en′zīm) acetyl-CoA, an important intermediate in the citric acid (Krebs') cycle and the chief precursor of lipids; it is formed by the attachment to coenzyme A of an acetyl group during the oxidation of pyruvate, fatty acids, or amino acids.

acetylcysteine (as″ĕ-til-sis′te-in) [USP] chemical name: *N*-acetyl-L-cysteine. A white, crystalline powder, $C_5H_9NO_3S$, used as a mucolytic agent for adjunct therapy in bronchopulmonary disorders to reduce the viscosity of mucus and facilitate its removal. Administered by instillation or nebulization.

acetyldigitoxin (as″ĕ-til-dij″ĭ-tok′sin) chemical name: (3,β,5,β)-3-[(*O*-2,6-dideoxy-β-D-*ribo*-hexopyranosyl-(1 → 4)-*O*-2,6-dideoxy-β-D-*ribo*-hexopyranosyl)-1(1 → 4)-2,6-dideoxy-β-D-*ribo*-hexopyranosyl)oxy]-14-hydroxy-card-20(22)-enolide monoacetate. A derivative of digitalis, $C_{43}H_{66}O_{14}$, obtained from lantoside A, composed of the aglycone digitoxigenin and three molecules of digitoxose, to one of which an acetyl group is attached; used as a cardiotonic.

acetylene (ah-set′ĭ-lēn) a colorless, volatile, explosive gas, C_2-H_4; it is the simplest of a class of unsaturated (triple-bonded) hydrocarbons, the alkynes.

acetylization (ah-set″il-i-za′shun) acetylation.

acetylmethadol (as″ĕ-til-meth′ah-dol) methadyl acetate.

acetylphenylhydrazine (as″ĕ-til-fen″il-hi-dra′zēn) chemical name: β-acetylphenylhydrazine. A compound, $C_8H_{10}N_2O$, that has been used as an oral erythrocyte depressant in the treatment of polycythemia vera and was once used as an antipyretic. Called also *hydracetin.*

acetylphosphatase (as″ĕ-til-fos′fah-tās) an enzyme in muscle which catalyzes the splitting of acetylphosphate.

acetylstrophanthidin (as″ĕ-til-stro-fan′thĭ-din) a synthetic fast-acting digitalis-like preparation.

acetylsulfadiazine (as″ĕ-til-sul″fah-di′ah-zēn) the form in which sulfadiazine is excreted in the urine, often occurring in dark green crystalline spheres.

acetylsulfaguanidine (as″ĕ-til-sul″fah-gwan′ĭ-dēn) the form in which sulfaguanidine is excreted in the urine, often occurring in thin oblong crystalline plates.

acetylsulfanilamide (as″ĕ-til-sul″fah-nil′ah-mīd) 1. N^1-acetylsulfanilamide (see *sulfacetamide*). 2. N^4-acetylsulfanilamide, $C_8H_{10}O_3S$, the acetylated (unconjugated) sulfanilamide as it appears in the body after administration.

acetylsulfathiazole (as″ĕ-til-sul″fah-thi′ah-zōl) the form in which sulfathiazole is excreted in the urine, often occurring in the form of sheaves-of-wheat crystals.

acetyltannin (as″ĕ-til-tan′in) acetyltannic acid.

acetyltransferase (as″ĕ-til-trans′fer-ās) any of a group of enzymes that catalyze the transfer of an acetyl group from one substance to another; called also *transacetylase*. **acetyl-CoA a.,** acetyl-CoA:acetyl-CoA *C*-acetyltransferase: an enzyme occurring in the liver and heart that catalyzes the transfer of the acetyl group from one molecule of acetylcoenzyme A to another, releasing free coenzyme A; called also *acetoacetyl thiolase*. **phosphate a.,** an enzyme that catalyzes the transfer of an acetyl group between acetylphosphate and acetylcoenzyme A; called also *phosphotransacetylase*.

A.C.G. American College of Gastroenterology; angiocardiography.

AcG accelerator globulin (coagulation Factor V; see under *factor*).

ACH (*obs.*) adrenocortical hormone.

ACh acetylcholine.

A.C.H.A. American College of Hospital Administrators.

achalasia (ak″ah-la′ze-ah) [*a* neg + Gr. *chalasis* relaxation + *-ia*] failure to relax of the smooth muscle fibers of the gastrointestinal tract at any point of junction of one part with another. Especially the failure of the esophagogastric sphincter to relax with swallowing, due to degeneration of ganglion cells in the wall of the organ. The thoracic esophagus also loses its normal peristaltic activity and becomes dilated (megaesophagus). Called also *cardiospasm*. **pelvirectal a.,** congenital absence of ganglion cells in a distal segment of the large bowel; the resultant loss of normal motor function in this segment causes hypertrophic dilatation of the normal proximal colon. Called also *Hirschsprung's disease*. **sphincteral a.,** failure of any sphincter of a tubular organ to relax in response to a normal physiological stimulus.

Achard-Castaigne method, test (ash-ar′ kas-tān′) [Émile Charles *Achard*, Paris physician, 1860–1941; Joseph *Castaigne*, French physician, 1871–1951] see *methylene blue test* (def. 1), under *test*.

Achard-Thiers syndrome (ash-ar′ tērz′) [Émile Charles *Achard*; Joseph *Thiers*] see under *syndrome*.

Achatina (ak″ah-ti′nah) a genus of very large land snails. **A. fuli′ca,** a giant land snail that serves as an intermediate host of the rat lungworm, *Angiostrongylus cantonensis*, the causative agent of eosinophilic meningitis.

AChE acetylcholinesterase.

ache (āk) 1. to suffer a continuous pain. 2. a continuous, fixed pain, as distinguished from twinges.

acheilia (ah-ki′le-ah) [*a* neg. + Gr. *cheilos* lip + *-ia*] congenital absence of one or both lips.

acheilous (ah-ki′lus) lacking lips; exhibiting acheilia.

acheiria (ah-ki′re-ah) [*a* neg. + Gr. *cheir* hand + *-ia*] congenital absence of one or both hands.

acheiropodia (ah-ki″ro-po′de-ah) [*a* neg. + Gr. *cheir* hand + *pous* foot + *-ia*] congenital absence of hands and feet.

acheirus (ah-ki′rus) [L.] an individual exhibiting acheiria.

Achillea (ak″ĭ-le′ah) [L.; Gr. *achilleia*] a genus of composite-flowered plants. *A. millefolium*, milfoil, has been used as a bitter and stimulant tonic; it contains an essential oil and a bitter alkaloid, achilleine;

Achilles bursa, jerk (reflex), tendon (ah-kil′ēz) [Gr. *Achilleus* Greek hero, whose mother held him by the ankle to dip him in the Styx] see *bursa tendinis calcanei* [*Achillis*], *triceps surae jerk*, under *jerk*, and *tendo calcaneus*.

Achillini (ak″ĭ-le′ne) Alessandro (1463–1512) a celebrated Bolognese physician and philosopher who left several works on anatomy.

achillobursitis (ah-kil″o-bur-si′tis) [*Achilles* + Gr. *byrsa* bursa + *-itis*] inflammation and thickening of the bursae about the Achilles tendon, especially of the bursa in front of it; called also *achillodynia*.

achillodynia (ak″ĭ-lo-din′e-ah) [*Achilles* (tendon) + Gr. *odynē* pain + *-ia*] pain in the Achilles tendon or in its bursa; achillobursitis.

achillorrhaphy (ak″ĭ-lor′ah-fe) [*Achilles* (tendon) + Gr. *rhaphē* suture] the operation of suturing the Achilles tendon.

achillotenotomy (ah-kil″o-ten-ot′o-me) [*Achilles* + Gr. *tenōn* tendon + *tomē* cut] surgical division of the Achilles tendon. **plastic a.,** elongation of the Achilles tendon by plastic operation.

achillotomy (ak″ĭ-lot′o-me) achillotenotomy.

achiria (ah-ki′re-ah) acheiria.

achirus (ah-ki′rus) acheirus.

achlorhydria (ah″klor-hi′dre-ah) [*a* neg. + *chlorhydria*] absence of hydrochloric acid from maximally stimulated gastric secretions; a result of gastric mucosal atrophy. Called also *gastric anacidity*. **a. apep′sia** (*obs.*), absence of pepsinogens in secretions of the stomach.

achlorhydric (ah″klor-hi′drik) characterized by achlorhydria.

achloroblepsia (ah-klo″ro-blep′se-ah) achloropsia.

achloropsia (ah″klo-rop′se-ah) [*a* neg. + Gr. *chlōros* green + *opsis* vision + *-ia*] inability to distinguish green tints, as in deuteranopia.

Achlya (ak′le-ah) a genus of phycomycetous fungi of the order Saprolegniales, subclass Oomycetes, which form molds on certain fish and insects.

achlys (ak′lis) [Gr. *achlys* darkness] (*obs.*) a mild corneal opacity (Himly).

acholia (ah-ko′le-ah) [*a* neg. + Gr. *cholē* bile + *-ia*] lack or absence of the secretion of bile.

acholic (ah-kol′ik) free from bile.

acholuria (ah-ko-lu′re-ah) [*a* neg. + Gr. *cholē* bile + *ouron* urine + *-ia*] lack of bile pigment in the urine.

acholuric (ah-ko-lu′rik) pertaining to or characterized by acholuria, as acholuric jaundice.

achondrogenesis (ah-kon″dro-jen′ĕ-sis) a hereditary disorder characterized by hypoplasia of bone, resulting in markedly shortened limbs; the head and trunk are normal.

achondroplasia (ah-kon″dro-pla′ze-ah) [*a* neg. + Gr. *chondros* cartilage + *plassein* to form + *-ia*] a hereditary, congenital disturbance of epiphyseal chondroblastic growth and maturation, causing inadequate enchondral bone formation and resulting in a peculiar form of dwarfism with short limbs, normal trunk, small face, normal vault, lordosis, and trident hand. It may be accompanied by other anomalies. Called also *chondrodystrophia fetalis*. See also *achondroplastic dwarf*, under *dwarf*.

achondroplastic (ah-kon″dro-plas′tik) pertaining to, or affected with, achondroplasia.

achondroplasty (ah-kon′dro-plas″te) achondroplasia.

achor (a′kor) [Gr. *achōr* dandruff] (*obs.*) 1. an eruption of small papules on the hairy parts. 2. a scaly or scabby eruption on the face and scalp in infants. 3. an acuminate pustule.

achordal (a-kor′dal) achordate.

achordate (a-kor′dāt) without a notochord; used with reference to animals which are not chordates.

achoresis (ak″o-re′sis) [*a* neg. + Gr. *chōrein* to hold] (*obs.*) diminution of the capacity of a hollow organ.

Achorion (ah-ko′re-on) *Trichophyton*.

achrestic (ah-kres′tik) [Gr. *achrēstia* the nonusance of a thing] pertaining to the lack of use of a principle which is present in the body, as in achrestic anemia, a condition in which the body is unable to use the antianemic principle.

achroacytosis (ah-kro″ah-si-to′sis) [*a* neg. + Gr. *chroa* color + *kytos* hollow vessel + *-osis*] a term once used to designate pathologically excessive numbers of lymphocytes in organs, as in Mikulicz's disease.

achroma (ah-kro′mah) [*a* neg. + Gr. *chrōma* color] (*obs.*) absence of color or of normal pigmentation.

achromachia (ah″kro-mak′e-ah) (*obs.*) grayness or whiteness of the hair; now called *canities*.

achromasia (ak″ro-ma′se-ah) [*a* neg. + Gr. *chrōma* color + *-ia*] 1. lack of normal pigmentation of the skin. 2. absence of the usual staining reaction in a tissue or cell.

achromat (ak′ro-mat) [*a* neg. + *chromatic*] 1. an achromatic objective. 2. monochromat.

achromate (ah-kro′māt) monochromat.

Achromatiaceae (ak″ro-ma″she-a′se-e) a family of schizomycetes (order Beggiatoales), made up of cells which are spherical to ovoid, or short cylinders with hemispherical ends, not possessing photosynthetic pigments. It includes a single genus, *Achromatium*.

achromatic (ak″ro-mat′ik) [*a* neg. + Gr. *chrōmatikos* pertaining to color] 1. producing no discoloration. 2. staining with difficulty. 3. containing achromatin. 4. refracting light without decomposing it into its component colors. 5. monochromatic, def. 2.

achromatin (ah-kro′mah-tin) [*a* neg. + Gr. *chrōma* color] the faintly staining substance forming the karyolymph, linin, and nuclear membrane of the nucleus of a cell.

achromatinic (ah-kro″mah-tin′ik) pertaining to or containing achromatin.

achromatism (ah-kro′mah-tizm″) 1. the quality or condition of being achromatic. 2. monochromatism.

Achromatium (ak″ro-ma′she-um) a genus of schizomycetes of the family Achromatiaceae.

achromatize (ah-kro′mah-tīz) to render achromatic.

achromatolysis (ah-kro″mah-tol′ĭ-sis) [*achromatin* + Gr. *lysis* dissolution] disorganization of the achromatin of a cell.

achromatophil (ah″kro-mat′o-fil) [*a* neg. + Gr. *chrōma* color + *philein* to love] 1. having no affinity for stains. 2. an organism or tissue element that does not stain easily.

achromatophilia (ah-kro″mah-to-fil′e-ah) the property of resisting the coloring action of stains.

achromatopia (ah″kro-mah-to′pe-ah) [*a* neg. + Gr. *chrōma* color + *ōpē* vision + *-ia*] monochromatism.

achromatopic (ah″kro-mah-top′ik) monochromatic, def. 2.

achromatopsia (ah-kro″mah-top′se-ah) monochromatism.

achromatosis (ah-kro″mah-to′sis) [*a* neg. + Gr. *chrōma* color + *-osis*] 1. deficiency of pigmentation in the tissues, as in the skin and the iris. 2. lack of staining power in a cell or tissue.

achromatous (ah-kro′mah-tus) having no color; colorless.

achromaturia (ah-kro″mah-tu′re-ah) [*a* neg. + Gr. *chrōma* color + *ouron* urine + *-ia*] the excretion of colorless urine.

achromia (ah-kro′me-ah) [*a* neg. + Gr. *chrōma* color + *-ia*] the lack or absence of normal color or pigmentation, as of the skin. **congenital a.**, albinism. **cortical a.**, a condition in which an area of the cerebral cortex shows disappearance of ganglion cells. **a. parasit′ica**, a name applied to the nonpigmented or whitish variety of macular patches occurring in tinea versicolor. **a. un′guium** (*obs.*), leukonychia.

achromic (ah-kro′mik) pertaining to or characterized by achromia.

achromin (ah-kro′min) achromatin.

Achromobacter (ah-kro″mo-bak′ter) [*a* neg. + Gr. *chrōma* color + *baktērion* little rod] a genus of schizomycetes of the family Achromobacteraceae, order Eubacteriales, made up of nonpigment-forming gram-negative rod-shaped bacteria occurring in soil or in fresh or salt water. Fifteen species have been described.

Achromobacteraceae (ah-kro″mo-bak″tĕ-ra′se-e) a family of schizomycetes (order Eubacteriales), made up of motile or nonmotile small to medium-sized rods, generally in soil or in fresh or salt water. Some are parasitic or pathogenic. It includes five genera, *Achromobacter, Agarbacterium, Alcaligenes, Berneckea,* and *Flavobacterium.*

achromocyte (ah-kro′mo-sīt) a red cell artifact in the shape of a quarter moon which stains more faintly than intact red cells; called also *selenoid* or *crescent body.*

achromoderma (ah-kro″mo-der′mah) [*a* neg. + Gr. *chrōma* color + *derma* skin] (*obs.*) leukoderma.

achromophil (ah-kro′mo-fil) [*a* neg. + Gr. *chrōma* color + *philein* to love] achromatophil.

achromophilous (ah″kro-mof′ĭ-lus) having no affinity for stains.

Achromycin (ak′ro-mi″sin) trademark for preparations of tetracycline.

achrooamyloid (a-kro″o-am′ĭ-loid) [Gr. *achroos* uncolored + *amyloid*] amyloid in its early nonstainable stage.

achroocytosis (ah-kro″o-si-to′sis) achroacytosis.

achroodextrin (ah-kro″o-dek′strin) [Gr. *achroos* uncolored + *dextrin*] a kind of lower-molecular-weight dextrin not colored by iodine.

Achucárro's stain (ach″oo-kah′roz) [Nicolás *Achucárro,* Spanish histologist, 1881–1918] see *Table of Stains.*

achylia (ah-ki′le-ah) [Gr. *achylos* juiceless + *-ia*] absence of hydrochloric acid and pepsinogens (pepsin) in the gastric juice (*a. gas′trica*). **a. gas′trica hemorrha′gica** (*obs.*), absence of hydrochloric acid from, and presence of occult blood in, the stomach. **a. pancreat′ica** (*obs.*), absence of exocrine pancreatic secretion, occurring in pancreatic ductal obstruction, pancreatic atrophy, or chronic pancreatitis with pancreatic insufficiency.

achylous (ah-ki′lus) [Gr. *achylos* juiceless] (*obs.*) deficient in chyle.

achymia (ah-ki′me-ah) imperfect, insufficient, or absence of formation of chyme.

achymosis (ak″ĭ-mo′sis) achymia.

acicular (ah-sik′u-lar) [L. *acicularis*] shaped like a needle or needle point.

aciculum (ah-sik′u-lum) a bent, finger-like spine or bristle found in certain flagellates.

acid (as′id) 1. [L. *acidus,* from *acere* to be sour] sour; having properties opposed to those of the alkalis. 2. [L. *acidum*] any compound of an electronegative element with one or more hydrogen atoms that are readily replaceable by electropositive atoms; a compound which, in aqueous solution, undergoes dissociation with the formation of hydrogen ions (protons) a substance whose molecule or ion can give up a proton (to a base); a substance capable of accepting a pair of electrons to form a coordinate covalent bond. Acids have a sour taste, turn blue litmus red, and unite with bases to form salts. Acids are distinguished as *binary* or *hydracids,* and *ternary* or *oxacids:* the former contain no oxygen; in the latter the hydrogen is united to the electronegative element by oxygen. The hydracids are distinguished by the prefix *hydro-.* The names of acids end in "ic," except in the case in which there are two degrees of oxygenation. The acid containing the

greater amount of oxygen has the termination *-ic,* the one having the lesser amount, the termination *-ous.* Acids ending in *-ic* form the salts with the termination *-ate;* those ending in *-ous* form the salts ending in *-ite.* The salts of hydracids end in *-ide.* Acids are called *monobasic, dibasic, tribasic,* and *tetrabasic,* respectively, when they contain one, two, three, or four replaceable hydrogen atoms. **abietic a., abietinic a.,** an acid resin, $C_{20}H_{30}O_2$, forming about 83 per cent of American rosin; its esters are used in lacquers and varnishes. **abscissic a.,** a growth-inhibiting plant hormone, which promotes abscission of plant parts, such as leaves and petals, and is associated with the onset and maintenance of dormancy. **acetic a.** [NF], a saturated fatty acid, CH_3COOH, the characteristic component of vinegar. It may be obtained by destructive distillation of wood, by oxidative bacterial fermentation of ethyl alcohol, and by oxidation of acetylaldehyde via interaction of acetylene and water; in the form of acetyl-CoA, acetic acid is the precursor of fatty acids, cholesterol, steroids, prostaglandins, and other compounds. It is used in solutions of various strengths, as *dilute acetic a.* (6 per cent) and *glacial acetic a.* (99.4 per cent). Called also *ethanoic a.* **acetic a., diluted** [NF], a clear, colorless liquid containing, in each 100 ml., between 5.7 and 6.3 g. of the pure acid; used as a solvent. **acetic a., glacial** [USP], a clear, colorless liquid with a pungent characteristic odor, containing not less than 99.4 per cent by weight of acetic acid; used as an acidifying agent in pharmaceutical preparations and in solution to irrigate the bladder. **acetoacetic a.,** a colorless syrupy compound, $CH_3 \cdot CO \cdot CH_2 \cdot COOH$, one of the ketone bodies, occurring in trace amounts in normal urine and in elevated amounts in the urine of diabetes mellitus (especially in ketoacidosis) and in starvation due to incomplete fatty acid oxidation; called also *beta-ketobutyric a.* and *diacetic a.* **acetrizoic a.,** chemical name: 3-acetamido-2,4,6-triiodobenzoic acid. An odorless white powder, $C_9H_8I_3NO_3$, soluble in alcohol and slightly soluble in water, ether, and chloroform; its sodium salt is used as an x-ray contrast medium. **acetylaminobenzoic a.,** $CH_3 \cdot CO \cdot NH \cdot C_6H_4 \cdot COOH$, the form in which aminobenzoic acid is detoxicated by acetylation and eliminated. **acetylenic a.,** an unsaturated fatty acid having the general formula $C_nH_{2n-3}COOH$, commonly found in microorganisms. **acetylpropionic a.,** levulinic a. **acetylsalicylic a.,** aspirin. **acetyltannic a.,** a diacetic ester of tannic acid, a grayish or white powder, insoluble in water, soluble in alcohol, and having astringent properties; formerly used as an antiperistaltic in the treatment of diarrhea. Called also *diacetyltannic a.* **acrylic a.,** an olefinic acid, $CH_2:CH \cdot COOH$, found in animal and vegetable tissues. **adenosine triphosphoric a.,** a normal constituent of most cells, $C_5H_4N_5 \cdot C_5H_8O_4 \cdot PO_3H_2 \cdot P_2O_3(OH)_4$, which participates in metabolic energy transformations; abbreviated ATP. **adenylic a.,** a mononucleotide, $NH_2 \cdot C_5H_3N_4 \cdot C_4H_3O(OH)_2 \cdot CH_2OH \cdot PO_2(OH)_2$, made up of adenine, ribose, and phosphoric acid. It is one of the decomposition products of ribonucleic acid and occurs in muscle, blood corpuscles, yeast, and other nuclear material. *Yeast adenylic a.* is adenosine 3′-phosphate; *muscle adenylic a.* is adenosine 5′-phosphate. Called also *adenine nucleotide* and *adenosine monophosphate (AMP).* **adipic a.,** a crystalline acid, $COOH(CH_2)_4COOH$, obtained by oxidizing certain fats with nitric acid; made commercially by oxidation of cyclohexanol and used in the manufacture of resins and nylon. **agaric a., agaricic a.,** a resinous acid, $C_{19}H_{36} \cdot (OH)(COOH)_3 \cdot 1\frac{1}{2}H_2O$, from the fungus *Polyporus officinalis,* or white agaric; formerly used as an anhidrotic. **ailantic a.,** a bitter acid from *Ailantus excelsa.* **aldobionic a.,** $C_{11}H_{19}O_{10} \cdot COOH$, a disaccharide containing a uronic acid as one of its component sugars and occurring in various plant gums and certain pathogenic organisms; it can be formed by the hydrolysis of the specific polysaccharide of Type III pneumococcus. **alepric a.,** a homologue of chaulmoogric acid. **aleprylic a.,** a homologue of chaulmoogric acid. **alginic a.,** an organic acid from various species of algae; called also *algin.* **aliphatic a.,** an organic acid with an open carbon chain. **allanic a., allanturic a.,** an acid, glyoxalyl urea, $NH_2CO \cdot N:CH \cdot COOH$, formed along with urea by the action of nitric acid on allantoin. **allonic a.,** one of the isomeric forms of pentahydroxycaproic acid, $CH_2OH(CHOH)_4COOH$, formed by the gentle oxidation of allose. **allophanic a.,** an acid, urea carbonic acid, $NH_2CO \cdot NH \cdot COOH$, not known in the free state. Its amide is biuret. Formerly combined with various substances to make them less disagreeable to take. **alloxanic a.,** a crystalline acid, $NH_2 \cdot CO \cdot NH \cdot CO \cdot COOH$, obtainable from alloxan. **alloxyproteic a.,** a sulfur compound sometimes found in the urine. **alluranic a.,** an acid, $C_5H_4N_4O_4$, derived from alloxan and urea. **alpha-aminobetahydroxypropionic a.,** serine. **alpha-aminodeltaguanidovaleric a.,** arginine. **alpha-aminoisocaproic a.,** leucine. **alpha-hydroxypropionic a.,** lactic a. **alpha-oxynaphthoic a.,** a crystalline acid, $OH \cdot C_{10}H_6COOH$, formerly used as an antiseptic and deodorant. **alpharsonic a.,** an arsonic acid containing an alphyl radical. **alphatoluic a.,** phenylacetic a. **altronic a.,** one of the isomeric forms of penta-hydroxycaproic acid, $CH_3OH(CHOH)_4COOH$, formed by the gentle oxidation of altrose. **amalic a.,** a crystalline acid, $C_8(CH_3)_4N_4O_7$, formed by the reduction of dimethyl alloxan with hydrogen disulfide. **ambrettolic a.,** an unsaturated hydroxy acid, 16-hydroxy-7-hexadecenoic acid, CH_2-

NATURALLY OCCURRING AMINO ACIDS

The substances listed below have been found either free as components of plant or animal tissues or as products of the hydrolysis of proteins. The year refers to the earliest occasion upon which the substance was characterized. As found in nature, all belong to the L family, being configurationally related to L-glyceraldehyde. However, in recent years, the D-enantiomorphs of a few of these substances have been detected in complex polypeptides produced by bacterial metabolism.

YEAR	COMMON NAME	SYSTEMATIC NAME	DISCOVERER
1806	Asparagine	2-amino-4-succinamic acid	Vauquelin and Robiquet
1810	Cystine	3,3'-dithiobis-(2-aminopropionic acid)	Wollaston
1819	Leucine	2-aminoisocaproic acid	Proust
1820	Glycine	aminoacetic acid	Braconnot
1846	Tyrosine	2-amino-3-(4-hydroxyphenyl)-propionic acid	Liebig
1856	Valine	2-aminoisovaleric acid	von Gorup-Besanez
1865	Serine	2-amino-3-hydroxypropionic acid	Cramer
1866	Glutamic acid	2-aminoglutaric acid	Ritthausen
1869	Aspartic acid[1]	2-aminosuccinic acid	Ritthausen
1879	Phenylalanine	2-amino-3-phenylpropionic acid	Schulze
1883	Glutamine	2-amino-5-glutaramic acid	Schulze and Bosshard
1884	Cysteine	2-amino-3-mercaptopropionic acid	Baumann
1886	Arginine	2-amino-5-guanidinovaleric acid	Schulze
1888	Alanine[2]	2-aminopropionic acid	Weyl
1889	Lysine	2,6-diaminohexanoic acid	Drechsel
1896	3,5-Diiodotyrosine (Iodogorgoic acid)	2-amino-3-(3,5-diiodo-4-hydroxyphenyl)-propionic acid	Drechsel
1896	Histidine	2-amino-3-(5-imidazolyl)-propionic acid	Hedin: Kossel
1898	Ornithine[3]	2,5-diaminovaleric acid	Schulze and Winterstein
1901	Proline[4]	2-pyrrolidinecarboxylic acid	Fischer
1901	Tryptophan	2-amino-3-(3-indo yl)-propionic acid	Hopkins and Cole
1902	Hydroxyproline	4 hydroxy-2-pyrrolidinecarboxylic acid	Fischer
1903	Isoleucine	2-amino-3-methylvaleric acid	Ehrlich
1913	3,5-Dibromotyrosine[5]	2-amino-3-(3,5-dibromo-4-hydroxyphenyl)-propionic acid	Morner
1913	3,4-Dihydroxyphenylalanine	2-amino-3-3,4-(dihydroxyphenyl)-propionic acid	Guggenheim
1915	Thyroxine	2-amino-3[(3,5-diiodo-4-hydroxyphenoxy)-3,5-diiodophenyl]-propionic acid	Kendall
1922	Methionine	2-amino-4-methylmercaptobutyric acid	Mueller
1929	Canavanine	2-amino-4-guanidinoöxy-butyric acid	Kitagawa and Tomita
1930	Citrulline[6]	2-amino-5-ureidovaleric acid	Wada
1935	Djenkolic acid	3,3'-methylenedithiobis-(2-aminopropionic acid)	van Veen and Hyman
1936	Threonine	2-amino-3-hydroxybutyric acid	Meyer and Rose
1938	Hydroxylysine[7]	2,6-diamino-5-hydroxyhexanoic acid	Van Slyke, Hiller, Dillon, and MacFadyen
1948	α,γ-Diaminobutyric acid	2,4-diaminobutyric acid	Catch, Jones, and Wilkenson
1950	α,ε-Diaminopimelic acid	2,6-diaminopimelic acid	Work

[1] Aspartic acid was prepared from asparagine by Plisson in 1827.
[2] Synthesized by Strecker, 1850.
[3] Ornithuric acid, the dibenzoyl derivative of ornithine, was discovered by Jaffé in 1877. The base was first characterized as a decomposition product of arginine by Schulze and Winterstein in 1898 and in 1943 was shown to be a product of the hydrolysis of tyrocidine by Gordon, Martin, and Synge.
[4] Synthesized by Willstätter, 1900.
[5] 3,5-Dibromotyrosine was synthesized from tyrosine by von Gorup-Besanez in 1863.
[6] Isolated but not characterized by Koga and Odake in 1914.
[7] Van Slyke and Hiller announced the probable presence of a new basic amino acid in gelatin in 1921. It was identified as an hydroxylysine in 1938.

$OH(CH_2)_7CH{:}CH(CH_2)_5COOH$, that occurs as a lactone in ambrette-seed oil. **amfonelic a.,** chemical name: 1-ethyl-1,4-dihydro-4-oxo-7-(phenylmethyl)-1,8-naphthyridine-3-carboxylic acid; a central nervous system stimulant, $C_{18}H_{16}N_2O_3$. **amino a.,** any of a class of organic compounds containing the amino (NH_2) group and the carboxyl (COOH) group. The amino acids form the chief structure of proteins, and several are essential in human nutrition. (See table listing names of amino acids occurring in nature, referred to as *natural amino a's.*) **amino a., essential,** one that is essential for optimal growth in a young animal or for nitrogen equilibrium in an adult. Those essential for nitrogen equilibrium in man are isoleucine, leucine, lysine, methionine, phenylalanine, threonine, tryptophan, and valine; histidine, in addition to these eight, is required by infants. **aminoacetic a.,** a nonessential amino acid, NH_2CH_2COOH, occurring as a constituent of many proteins. It has been synthetized, and is used as a gastric antacid, dietary supplement, and in the treatment of various myopathies and peripheral vascular insufficiencies. A solution [USP] is used as an irrigating fluid. Its hydrochloride salt is used as a source of hydrochloric acid in the treatment of achlorhydria gastrica. Called also *aminoethanoic a.* **aminobenzoic a.,** an acid, $C_7H_7NO_2$, widely distributed in plant and animal tissues, and considered to be associated with, or a member of, the group of B vitamins. It is a growth factor for rats, chicks, and yeast, and an essential constituent of bacterial culture media. It nullifies the clot-lysing properties of plasmin, and synthetic preparations [USP] are used for this purpose (as a hemostatic). **ε-aminocaproic a.,** chemical name: 6-aminohexanoic acid. A synthetic amino acid that is an inhibitor of plasminogen activator and plasmin, and indirectly of fibrinolysis. **aminoethanoic a.,** aminoacetic a. **aminoglutaric a.,** glutamic a. **2-amino-5-guanidinovaleric a.,** arginine. **aminohippuric a.** [USP], chemical name: N-(4-aminobenzoyl)glycine. The N-acetic acid of aminobenzoic acid, $C_9H_{10}N_2O_3$. Its sodium salt (aminohippurate sodium) is used to measure the effective renal plasma flow and to determine the functional capacity of the tubular excretory mechanism. Called also *para-aminohippuric a.,* and *PAH* or *PAHA.* **aminohydroxybenzoic a.,** a group of chemotherapeutic agents used in the treatment of infections with acid-fast bacilli. **2-amino-3-p-hydroxyphenylpropionic a.,** tyrosine. **2-amino-3-indole propionic a.,** tryptophan. **aminoisocaproic a.,** leucine. **2-aminoisovaleric a.,** valine. **δ-aminolevulinic a., 5-aminolevulinic a.,** an acid, $NH_2CH_2COCH_2CH_2COOH$, biosynthesized from succinyl coenzyme A and glycine; two molecules of it then condense to form porphobilinogen. **2-aminopropionic a.,** alanine. **aminopteroylglutamic a.,** aminopterin. **aminosalicylic a.** [USP], chemical name: 4-amino-2-hydroxybenzoic acid. An antibacterial, $C_7H_7NO_3$, occurring as a white, or nearly white, bulky powder; used orally as a tuberculostatic. Called also *para-aminosalicylic* acid (*PAS* or *PASA*). **aminosuccinic a.,** aspartic a. **2-amino-3-thiopropionic a.,** cysteine. **2-aminovaleric a.,** an amino acid, $CH_3 \cdot CH_2 \cdot CH_2 \cdot CH(NH_2) \cdot COOH$, reported to occur rarely in protein. **amygdalic a.,** mandelic a. **anacardic a.,** a crystalline principle, normal pentadecylene salicylic acid, $C_{15}H_{27} \cdot C_6H_3 \cdot (OH) \cdot COOH$, from *Anacardium occidentale;* formerly used as an anthelmintic. **angelic a.,** an unsaturated fatty acid, $CH_3 \cdot CH{:}C(CH_3) \cdot COOH$, from the roots of *Angelica archangelica,* formerly used as a sedative. **anilinparasulfonic a.,** sulfanilic acid. **anisic a.,** a crystalline acid, $CH_3O \cdot C_6H_4 \cdot CO_2H$, from anise and fennel, forming anisates; it was once used as a local antiseptic and antirheumatic. Called also *draconic a.* **anisuric a.,** an acid, $C_{10}H_{11}NO_2$, in leafy crystals, obtainable from urine after the ingestion of anisic acid. **anthranilic a.,** a crystalline acid, O-aminobenzoic acid, $NH_2C_6H_4 \cdot COOH$; its cadmium salt is used as an ascaricide in swine. **anthropodeoxycholic a.,** chenodeoxycholic a. **anticyclic a.,** a fragrant powdery acid that was used as an antipyretic. **anti-**

monic a., antimony pentoxide. **antoxyproteic a.**, an organic acid obtained from urine. **aposorbic a.**, a crystalline acid, $C_5H_8O_7$, obtained by oxidizing sorbose with HNO_3. **arabic a.**, arabin. **arabonic a.**, one of the forms of tetrahydroxy-normal valeric acid, $CH_2OH(CHOH)_3COOH$, formed by the action of bromine water on arabinose. **arachic a.**, **arachidic a.**, a fatty acid, $CH_3(CH_2)_{18}COOH$, from the oil of the peanut, *Arachis hypogaea.* **arachidonic a.**, a polyunsaturated essential fatty acid, $CH_3(CH_2)_4(CH{:}CH{:}CH_2)_4(CH_2)_2COOH$, a constituent of lecithin and a biosynthetic source of some prostaglandins. **argininosuccinic a.**, an amino acid, one of the key intermediates in the ornithine cycle; large amounts are excreted in the urine in an inborn error of metabolism manifested by mental retardation. **aristolochic a.**, an acid, 8-methoxy-6-nitrophenanthro[3,4-*d*]-1,3-dioxole-5-carboxylic acid, $C_{17}H_{11}NO_7$, the major aromatic bitter principle of herbs of the genus *Aristolochia* and related species; called also *aristolochine.* **aromatic a.**, any of a group of acids containing a carboxylic acid function attached to the benzene or other aromatic ring. **arsanilic a.**, chemical name: *p*-aminobenzenearisonic acid. An acid, $NH_2{\cdot}C_6H_4{\cdot}A_sO(OH)_2$, used in tne manufacture of medicinal arsenicals and to control dysentery in swine. **arsenic a.**, the acid, H_3AsO_4, some of whose salts, called arsenates, are used as medicines. **arsenous a.**, 1. a monobasic acid, $HAsO_2$, forming arsenites. 2. arsenic trioxide, As_2O_3, or arsenous anhydride. **arsinic a.**, an organic compound containing the group —As-$(OH)_2$. **arsinosalicylic a.**, a colorless crystalline substance formerly used in African sleeping sickness. **arsonic a.**, an organic compound containing the group —A_sO_2OH. **arylarsonic a.**, arsonic acid combined with an aryl radical. **ascorbic a.**, a water-soluble vitamin, $C_6H_8O_6$, present in citrus fruits, and in tomatoes, strawberries, and many other fruits and vegetables; it is also made synthetically. Deficiency of this substance produces scurvy and poor wound repair. Pharmaceutical preparations [USP] are used parenterally and orally as antiscorbutic vitamins in vitamin C deficiency. Called also *vitamin C, antiscorbutic vitamin, cevitamic a.,* and *hexuronic a.* **aseptic a.**, mixture of boric acid, water, hydrogen dioxide, and salicylic acid, formerly used as an antiseptic. **aspartic a.**, a nonessential, natural dibasic amino acid, $COOH{\cdot}CH(NH_2){\cdot}CH_2{\cdot}COOH$, widely distributed in proteins; called also *aminosuccinic a.* **aspergillic a.**, chemical name: 1-hydroxy-6-(1-methylpropyl)-3-(2-methylpropyl)-2(1*H*)pyrazinone. An antibiotic substance, $C_{12}H_{20}N_2O_2$, isolated from cultures of *Aspergillus flavus.* **atractylic a.**, a poisonous glycoside, $C_{30}H_{25}O_{18}S_2$, from *Atractylis gummifer.* **auric a.**, 1. the acid, H_3AuO_3, forming salts called aurates. 2. auric anhydride. **azelaic a.**, an acid of widespread occurrence, $COOH{\cdot}(CH_2)_7COOH$, formed by oxidation of oleic acid. **barbituric a.**, chemical name: 2,4,6,-trioxohexahydropyrimidine. A crystalline substance, $CO(NHCO)_2CH_2$, known in medicine chiefly because of its derivatives, such as barbital and phenobarbital, and from which the term applied to the class of drugs, barbiturates, is derived. Called also *malonyl urea.* **basic amino a's**, amino acids (e.g., lysine and arginine) having, in addition to the alpha amino group, another amino, a guanido, or an imidazole group; as a result they bear a net positive charge at neutral pH. **behenic a.**, a fatty acid, $CH_3(CH_2)_{20}COOH$, present in oil of black mustard and other plant-seed oils. **benzoic a.** [USP], an acid, $C_6H_5{\cdot}COOH$, in the form of white crystals, scales, or needles from benzoin and other resins and from coal tar, used as an antifungal agent in pharmacopeial preparations and in combination with salicylic acid as a topical antifungal agent. Called also *flores benzoini* and *flowers of benzoin.* **benzoylaminoacetic a.**, hippuric a. **benzoylglucuronic a.**, a conjugate of benzoic acid and glucuronic acid, by which the former is detoxicated and eliminated. **beta-acetylpropionic a.**, levulinic a. **beta-aminobutyric a.**, an acid, $CH_3CH(NH_2)$-CH_2COOH, which causes profound narcotism and symptoms resembling coma. **beta-hydroxybutyric a.**, beta-oxybutyric a. **beta-ketobutyric a.**, acetoacetic a. **beta-ketopalmitic a.**, an oxidized form of palmitic acid, $CH_3(CH_2)_{12}CO{\cdot}CH_2{\cdot}COOH$. **beta-naphtholsulfonic a.**, white pearly scales tinged with red, $OH{\cdot}C_{10}H_6SO_2{\cdot}OH$, used as a test for albumin in the urine; a toxic drug which causes profound narcotism and symptoms resembling diabetic coma, not used as a medication. **beta-oxybutyric a.**, an acid, $CH_3CHOH{\cdot}CH_2$-$COOH$, one of the ketone bodies, occurring in the urine in diabetic ketoacidosis and in starvation due to incomplete fatty acid oxidation; called also *beta-hydroxybutyric a.* **beta-phenylpropionic a.**, hydrocinnamic a. **bichloracetic a.**, dichloracetic a. **bile a.**, a steroid acid of the bile, usually occurring in conjugate form, e.g., glycocholic acid, metabolically derived from cholesterol. **bilianic a.**, an acid, $C_{24}H_{34}O_8$, formed by oxidizing dehydrocholic acid. **bilic a.**, a crystalline acid, $C_{16}H_{22}O_6$, formed by oxidizing cholic acid with chromic acid. **bilirubinic a.**, bilirubin. **biliverdinic a.**, biliverdine. **binary a.**, an acid which contains only two elements, e.g., HCl; called also *hydracid.* **bionic a.**, **biotic a.**, a compound composed of a mixture of substances that stimulates growth of yeast cells; its active ingredient is probably biotin. **bismuthic a.**, the monobasic acid, $HBiO_3$. **blattic a.**, a substance derived from cockroaches that has diuretic properties. See *Blatta.* **boracic a.**, boric a. **boric a.** [NF], colorless odorless scales, crystals, or crystalline powder, H_3BO_3, used as a buffer. It was formerly used as a local anti-infective and in solution as an ophthalmic irrigant; rarely used now because of the occurrence of fatal poisoning due to absorption from damaged skin. Called also *boracic a.* and *orthoboric a.* **borocitric a.**, a white crystalline combination of boric and citric acids, employed as a solvent for urates and phosphates. **borophenylic a.**, a white aromatic powder, $C_6H_5{\cdot}OB(OH)_2$, formerly used as an antiseptic agent. **borosalicylic a.**, a white powder, $BOH(OC_6H_4COOH)_2$, prepared by evaporating a mixture of aqueous solution of boric acid and alcoholic solution of salicylic acid; formerly used as an antiseptic. **botulinic a.**, an acid found in putrid sausages, believed to consist of allantotoxicon mixed with other substances. **brassic a.**, **brassidic a.**, $CH_3{\cdot}(CH_2)_7{\cdot}CH{:}CH{\cdot}(CH_2)_{11}{\cdot}COOH$, the transisomer of erucic acid produced by treating erucic acid with nitric acid; called also *isoerucic a.* **brassilic a.**, a dibasic acid, $COOH(CH_2)_{11}COOH$, obtained by the oxidation of erucic acid. **brenz-catechin sulfuric a.**, pyrocatechin sulfuric acid, $OH{\cdot}C_6H_4{\cdot}O{\cdot}SO_2OH$, found in the urine after the administration of salicin, hydroquinone, etc. **bromauric a.**, a brownish crystalline acid, $HAuBr_4 + 5H_2O$, used as a readily soluble form of gold and as a source of colloidal gold (by reduction). **bromphenylmercapturic a.**, a compound, bromphenylacetylcysteine, C_6H_4-$Br{\cdot}S{\cdot}CH_2{\cdot}CH(NH{\cdot}CO{\cdot}CH_3)COOH$, found conjugated with glycuronic acid in the urine of dogs fed bromobenzene; called also *bromphenylacetylcysteine* and *phenylmercapturic a.* See also *mercapturic a.* **bursic a.**, **bursinic a.**, a pale yellow substance derived from *Capsella bursa-pastoris,* a species of weeds; once used as an astringent. **butylcarboxylic a.**, valeric a. **butylethylbarbituric a.**, butethal. **butyric a.**, a rancid sticky acid, $CH_3CH_2CH_2COOH$, found in butter, sweat, feces, and urine, and in traces in the spleen and in blood. **cacodylic a.**, a crystalline deliquescent solid, dimethylarsinic acid, $(CH_3)_2{\cdot}AsO{\cdot}OH$, used as a herbicide; formerly used in treatment of various skin conditions. **caffeic a.**, a crytalline solid, dihydroxycinnamic acid, $(OH)_2C_6H_3CH{:}CH{\cdot}COOH$, obtained from coffee. **caffetannic a.**, a glucoside, $C_{15}H_{18}O_8$, found in coffee; it is resolvable into dextrose and caffeic acid. **caffuric a.**, a crystalline acid, $C_6H_9N_3O_4$, formed by the oxidation of caffeine. **camphoglycuronic a.**, $C_{16}H_{24}O_8$, a combination of glycuronic acid and camphor, found in the urine after the ingestion or injection of camphor. **campholic a.**, a compound, $C_{10}H_{18}O_2$, formed by distilling camphor with alcoholic potash. **camphoric a.**, a colorless crystalline substance, $C_8H_{14}(COOH)_2$, from the oxidation of camphor; it may stimulate the respiratory center. **cantharic a.**, a crystalline acid, $C_{10}H_{12}O_4$, derivable from its isomer cantharidin. **cantharidic a.**, a dibasic acid, $C_{10}H_{14}O_5$, formed by the combination of cantharidin with water. **capobenic a.**, chemical name: 6-(3,4,5-trimethoxybenzamido)hexanoic acid; a cardiac depressant, $C_{16}H_{23}NO_6$. **capric a.**, a crystalline, rancid-smelling fatty acid, $CH_3(CH_2)_8COOH$, from butter; called also *decanoic a.* **caproic a.**, a fatty acid, CH_3-$(CH_2)_4COOH$, occurring in milk fat and some plant oils, used in the manufacture of artificial flavors; called also *hexanoic a.* **caproleic a.**, see *decenoic a.* **caprylic a.**, a fatty acid, CH_3-$(CH_2)_6COOH$, from goat and cow milk fat and some seed oils, used in manufacture of perfumes; called also *octanoic a.* **capsic a.**, an irritating principle existing in *Pimenta.* **carbamic a.**, a monobasic acid, the monoamide of carbonic acid (aminoformic acid), $NH_2CO{\cdot}OH$; it is not known in the free state. Its ethyl ester is urethan. **carbaminocarboxylic a.**, an acid, $COOH{\cdot}NH{\cdot}CH_2{\cdot}COOH$, formed by CO_2 in the presence of the amino acid glycine and alkali. **carbolic a.**, phenol. **carbonaphthoic a.**, hydroxynaphthoic a. **carbonic a.**, 1. an acidulous unstable liquid, H_2CO_3, made by dissolving carbon dioxide in water; it forms carbonates. 2. carbon dioxide. **γ-carboxyglutamic a.**, an amino acid occurring in biologically active prothrombin and formed in the liver in the presence of vitamin K by carboxylation of glutamic acid residues in prothrombin precursor molecules. **carboxylic a's**, a group of organic acids containing the carboxyl group, —COOH, in the molecule, and widely distributed in nature, especially in foodstuffs. **carminic a.**, a red anthraquinonoid dye, $C_{22}H_{20}O_{13}$, the essential component of carmine and cochineal. **carnaubic a.**, an acid, $CH_3(CH_2)_{22}COOH$, from carnauba wax or from wool fat. **carolic a.**, a C_9 acid that is a metabolic product of *Penicillium charlesii.* **carthamic a.**, a red dye, $C_{21}H_{22}O_{10}$, obtained by alkaline extraction of safflower petals. **caryophyllic a.**, eugenol. **catechuic a.**, catechin. **catechutannic a.**, the tannin of catechu, a powerfully astringent extract of *Acacia catechu.* **cathartic a.**, **cathartinic a.**, a laxative principle from senna. **cellulosic a.**, oxidized cellulose. **cerebronic a.**, a fatty acid, $C_{24}H_{48}O_3$, derived from sphingomyelin; the principal hydroxy saturated fatty acid from the brain. **cerotic a.**, **cerotinic a.**, a fatty acid, $CH_3(CH_2)_{24}{\cdot}COOH$, from beeswax and other insect and plant waxes; called also *hexacosanoic a.* **cevitamic a.**, ascorbic a. **chaulmoogric a.**, chemical name: (*S*)-2-cyclopentene-1-tridecanoic acid. An unsaturated fatty acid, $C_{18}H_{32}O_2$, from chaulmoogra oil. See also *ethyl chaulmoograte.* **chenic a.**, chenodeoxycholic a. **chenodeoxycholic a.**, an acid, 3,7-dihydroxycholanic acid, the third most abundant acid of human bile; it was first found in the bile of geese [Gr. *chēn* goose]. It has gallstone-dissolving properties, probably because it suppresses synthesis of cholesterol by the liver, and is administered for this purpose. Called also *anthropodeoxycholic a.* and *chenic a.* **chenotaurocholic a.,** a crystalline compound, $C_{29}H_{49}NSO_6$, a bile acid formed by the conjugation of chenodeoxycholic acid and taurine, and occurring in the bile of geese. **chinovic a.,** quinovic a. **chitonic a.,** an acid, trihydroxymethyl-tetrahydrofurfurane-carboxylic acid, $CH_2OH \cdot CHO(CHOH)_2 \cdot CH \cdot COOH$, formed by the oxidation of chitose. **chloracetic a.,** an acid in which the three hydrogen atoms of acetic acid are wholly or partly replaced by chlorine; it occurs, therefore, in three forms, called respectively monochloracetic, dichloracetic, and trichloracetic acid, all being strongly acidic: the more chlorine, the more acidic the acid. **chloranilic a.,** chemical name: 2,5-dichloro-3,6-dihydroxy-*p*-benzoquinone. Red crystals, $C_6H_2Cl_2O_4$, used in spectrophotometry for several chemical measurements that yield a colored product. **chlorauric a.,** yellow hygroscopic crystals of gold chloride, $AuCl_3 \cdot HCl \cdot 4H_2O$ (or $HAuCl_4 + 4H_2O$), which contain 48 per cent of gold. **chlorhydric a.,** hydrochloric a. **chlorogenic a.,** a simple phenolic compound of low molecular weight isolated from raw coffee bean, castor bean, and oranges. **chloroplatinic a.,** $H_2PtCl_6 \cdot 6H_2O$, made by dissolving metallic platinum in nitrohydrochloric acid (aqua regia). Soluble source of platinum for reduction (mirrors, photography) and for preparation of other compounds of platinum. **chlorosulfonic a.,** an irritant war gas and lacrimator, HSO_3Cl, used widely as an intermediate in chemical synthesis. **chlorous a.,** a feebly acid compound, $HClO_2$, forming salts called chlorites. **cholanic a.,** the product, $C_{24}H_{40}O_2$, of the reduction of cholic acid or other bile acids. **choleic a's,** complexes of fatty acids with deoxycholeic acid. **cholic a.,** an acid, 3,7,12-trihydroxycholanic acid, $C_{24}H_{40}O_5$, from bile. **choloidanic a.,** an acid, $C_{24}H_{36}O_{10}$, formed by oxidative splitting of deoxycholic acid. **chondroitic a., chondroitin-sulfuric a.,** a mucopolysaccharide occurring in cartilage. **chondrosaminic a.,** an oxidation product of chondrosamine. **chromic a.,** 1. a dibasic acid, H_2CrO_4; its salts are called chromates. 2. brilliant red crystals, flakes, or granular powder, CrO_3, formerly used in solutions as an astringent, topical antiseptic, and corrosive; called also *chromic anhydride* and *chromium trioxide.* **chromonucleic a.,** deoxyribonucleic a. **chrysenic a.,** a crystalline compound, $C_{17}H_{12}O_2$. **chrysophanic a.,** chemical name: 1,8-dihydroxy-3-methylanthraquinone. A yellow crystalline acid, dioxymethyl-anthraquinone, $CH_3(OH) \cdot C_6H_2(CO)_2C_6H_3OH$, from a glycoside in senna, certain lichens, and various species of rhubarb, and from chrysarobin, whose therapeutic properties it shares. Called also *rheic a.* **cinchomeronic a.,** pyridine-dicarboxylic acid, $C_5H_3N(COOH)_2$, formed from cinchonine by oxidation. **cinchonic a.,** quinolin-carboxylic acid, $C_9H_6N(COOH)$, formed from cinchonine by oxidation. **cinchoninic a.,** an acid, $C_{10}H_7O_2N$, produced in the oxidation of cinchonine. **cinnamic a.,** a white crystalline acid, phenyl acrylic acid, $C_6H_5(CH)_2COOH$, from cinnamon, storax, the balsams, and other aromatic resins. **citraconic a.,** a crystalline compound, $COOH \cdot C \cdot (CH_3){:}CH \cdot COOH$, formed by distilling citric acid; called also *methylmaleic a.* and *pyrocitric a.* **citric a.,** chemical name: 2-hydroxy-1,2,3-propanetricarboxylic acid. A tribasic acid in the form of crystals or crystalline powder, $CH_2(COOH)C(OH)(COOH)CH_2COOH$, from lemons, limes, etc., that forms citrates and is antiscorbutic, refrigerant, and diuretic; it is used as an ingredient of anticoagulant citrate dextrose solution, anticoagulant citrate phosphate dextrose solution, and citric acid syrup. Citric acid is an intermediate in the tricarboxylic acid (Krebs') cycle, formed by acetylation of oxaloacetic acid and itself converted to isocitric acid. **clodronic a.,** chemical name: (dichloromethylene)bisphosphoric acid; a bone calcium regulator, $CH_4Cl_2O_6P_2$. **clofenamic a.,** chemical name: *N*-(2,3-dichlorophenyl)anthranilic acid; an anti-inflammatory agent, $C_{13}H_9ClNO_2$. **clorazepic a.,** chemical name: 7-chloro-2,3-dihydro-2-oxy-5-phenyl-1*H*-1,4-benzodiazepine-3-carboxylic acid. A derivative of benzodiazepine, $C_{16}H_{13}ClN_2O$, whose dipotassium and monopotassium salts are used as minor tranquilizers. **clupanodonic a.,** an unsaturated fatty acid, $C_{22}H_{34}O_2$, derived from sardine oil and oils of other fish; called also *docosapentaenoic a.* **cocatannic a.,** a compound found in the leaves of *Erythroxylon coca.* **cojic a.,** kojic a. **colchicinic a.,** an acid, $C_{16}H_{15}O_5$, formed from colchicine by heating it with hydrochloric acid. **comanic a.,** an acid, $C_6H_4O_4$, derived from succinic acid. **comenic a.,** a crystalline acid, oxypyrone-carboxylic acid, $OH \cdot C_5H_2O_2 \cdot COOH$, from opium. **copaibic a.,** an acid nearly identical with the resin of copaiba. **coumaric a.,** an acid, $OH \cdot C_6H_4 \cdot (CH)_2 \cdot COOH$, from coumarin, readily convertible into salicylic acid. **coumarilic a.,** a crystalline acid, $C_9H_6O_3$, from coumarin. **cresolsulfuric a.,** a substance, $CH_3C_6H_4SO_2 \cdot OH$, found in small quantities in the urine. **cresotic a., cresotinic a.,** an acid, $CH_3C_6H_3(OH) \cdot COOH$, occurring in three modified forms, ortho-, meta-, and para-; its sodium salt is antipyretic but is not used in medicine. Called also *oxytoluic a.* **cresylic a.,** cresol. **croconic a.,** chemical name: 4,5-dihydroxy-4-cyclopentene-1,2,3-trione. A yellow crystalline acid, $C_5H_2O_5$, used as a diuretic and to enhance the deodorizing action of chlorophyll. **cromoglycic a.,** chemical name: 5,5′-[(2-hydroxy-1,3-propanediyl)bis(oxy)]bis[4-oxo-4*H*-benzopyran-2-carboxylic acid]. An acid, $C_{23}H_{16}O_{11}$, the disodium salt of which (*cromolyn sodium*) is used in the prophylaxis of allergic asthma and allergic rhinitis. Called also *cromolyn.* **crotonic a.,** an unsaturated fatty acid, $CH_3 \cdot CH{:}CH \cdot COOH$, found in croton oil. **cryptophanic a.,** an amorphous acid, $C_{10}H_{18}O_{10}N_2$, said to be found in the urine. **cubebic a.,** a principle, $C_{13}H_{14}O_7$, from cubeb (q.v.); it has diuretic actions but is not used in medicine. **cumic a., cuminic a.,** chemical name: *p*-isopropylbenzoic acid. An acid, $C_6H_4(C_3H_7)COOH$, formed by the oxidation of cumic aldehyde. **cuminuric a.,** the excretion product of cumic acid and aminoacetic acid, $(CH_3)_2 \cdot CH \cdot C_6H_4 \cdot CO \cdot NH \cdot CH_2 \cdot COOH$. **cyanhydric a.,** hydrocyanic a. **cyanic a.,** an acid, $H \cdot CNO$, with vesicant actions; not used in medicine. **cyanuric a.,** a white crystalline compound, formed by heating urea. **cyclamic a.,** chemical name: cyclohexanesulfamic acid. An acid, $C_6H_{13}NO_3S$, whose calcium and sodium salts were once used widely as non-nutritive sweeteners, but were banned as food additives in 1969 in the United States because of an association with bladder tumors in animals. **cyclohexanesulfamic a.,** cyclamic a. **cysteic a.,** $SO_2OH \cdot CH_2CH \cdot (NH_2)COOH$, an intermediate product in the metabolism of cysteine. **cytidylic a.,** a pyrimidine nucleotide constituent of ribonucleic acid. **damalic a.,** C_7H_8O, said to occur in urine. **damaluric a.,** $C_7H_{12}O_2$, found in human urine and in that of cows. **decenoic a.,** an unsaturated fatty acid, $C_{10}H_{20}O_2$; 4-decenoic acid (common name *obtusilic a.*) is found in a spice bush, and 9-decenoic acid (common name *caproleic a.*) is found in butter fat. **decoic a.,** capric a. **dehydroascorbic a.,** an acid resulting from the oxidation of ascorbic acid. **dehydrocholalic a.,** dehydrocholic a. **dehydrocholic a.** [USP], a white bitter powder, $C_{24}H_{34}O_5$, formed by the oxidation of cholic acid and derived from natural bile acids; used as a choleretic. **deoxyadenylic a.,** a purine nucleotide constituent of deoxyribonucleic acid. **deoxycholeic a.,** one of the bile acids; see also *choleic a's.* **deoxycholic a.,** one of the bile acids, capable of forming soluble, diffusible complexes with fatty acids. **deoxycytidylic a.,** a pyrimidine nucleotide constituent of deoxyribonucleic acid. **deoxyguanylic a.,** a purine nucleotide constituent of deoxyribonucleic acid. **deoxypentosenucleic a.,** deoxyribonucleic a. **deoxyribonucleic a.,** a nucleic acid originally isolated from fish sperm and thymus gland, but later found in all living cells; on hydrolysis it yields adenine, guanine, cytosine, thymine, deoxyribose, and phosphoric acid. It is the carrier of genetic information for all organisms except the RNA viruses. See also *Watson-Crick helix* (and illustration), under *helix.* Abbreviated DNA. **desoxyribonucleic a., desoxyribose nucleic a.,** deoxyribonucleic a. **dextrotartaric a.,** ordinary tartaric acid, which turns the plane of polarization to the right. **diacetic a.,** acetoacetic a. **diacetyltannic a.,** acetyltannic a. **diallylbarbituric a.,** former name for allobarbital. **dialuric a.,** a crystalline acid, $CO(NH \cdot CO)_2CH \cdot OH$, obtainable from alloxan. **diamino a.,** one containing two amino, or NH_2, groups. **diaminoacetic a.,** an acid, $CH(NH_2)_2COOH$, formed by heating casein in sealed tubes with concentrated hydrochloric acid. **α,γ-diaminobutyric a.,** a naturally occurring amino acid discovered in 1948. **α,ϵ-diaminocaproic a.,** lysine. **α,ϵ-diaminopimelic a.,** a naturally occurring amino acid discovered in 1950. **α,δ-diaminovaleric a.,** ornithine. **diatrizoic a.** [USP], chemical name: 3,5-bis(acetylamino)-2,4,6-triiodobenzoic acid. A white powder, $C_{11}H_9I_3N_2O_4$, used in the preparation of certain radiopaque media (see *diatrizoate meglumine* and *diatrizoate sodium*). **diazobenzenesulfonic a.,** chemical name: *p*-sulfobenzenediazonium hydroxide inner salt. White or slightly red crystals, $C_6H_4N_2O_3S$, prepared by the diazotization of sulfanilic acid and used in Ehrlich's diazo reaction. **dichloroacetic a.,** $CHCl_2 \cdot COOH$, a caustic acid formed from acetic acid by substitution and used as a topical keratolytic, topical astringent, and escharotic. **2,4-dichlorophenoxyacetic a.,** a phytohormone with herbicidal properties. **diethylbarbituric a.,** barbital. **digallic a.,** an incorrect term for tannic a. **3,6-dihydroxycholanic a.,** hyodeoxycholic a. **2,5-dihydroxyphenylacetic a.,** homogentisic a. **4,8-dihydroxyquinaldic a.,** xanthurenic a. **dihydroxystearic a.,** an acid, $CH_3(CH_2)_7(CHOH)_2(CH_2)_7COOH$, obtained by oxidizing oleic acid and found in castor oil. **diiodosalicylic a.,** chemical name: 3,5-diiodosalicylic acid. A yellowish white crystalline powder, $OH \cdot C_6H_2I_2 \cdot COOH$, used as an iodine source in feeds for cattle, hogs, and poultry. **dimethylarsinic a.,** cacodylic a. **dimethylcolchicinic a.,** an acid, $C_{18}H_{19}O_5N$, formed from colchicine by heating it with hydrochloric acid. **dithiochloralsalicylic a.,** a reddish yellow powder, $S_2C_6H \cdot Cl \cdot OH \cdot COOH$, formerly used as an antiseptic. **djenkolic a.,** an alpha-diamino acid, $CH_2(S \cdot CH_2 \cdot CH(NH_2)COOH)_2$, obtained by hydrolyzing djenkol nuts. **docosapentaenoic a.,** clupanodonic a. **draconic a.,** anisic a. **durylic a.,** a crystalline compound, trimethylbenzoic acid, $(CH_3)_3C_6H_2 \cdot COOH$. **edetic a.** [NF], chemical name: *N,N′*-1,2-ethanediylbis[*N*-(carboxymethyl)glycin]. An acid, $C_{10}H_{16}N_2O_8$, occurring as a white, crystalline powder, which is an organic chelating agent and is used as a pharmaceutic aid. A number of its salts are available as chelating agents (see *edetate*). Called also *ethylenediamine-tetraacetic acid* (*EDTA*). **elaidic a.,** an unsaturated fatty acid, $CH_3(CH_2)_7 \cdot$

CH:CH(CH₂)₇·COOH, isomeric with oleic acid and formed by treating the latter with nitrous acid. **enanthic a., enanthylic a.,** a saturated fatty acid, $C_7H_{14}O_2$, not known definitely to occur naturally, but may be produced by certain oxidations of fats; called also *heptanoic a.* and *heptylic a.* **epicladosporic a.,** a mycotoxin produced by *Cladosporium epiphyllum.* **ergotinic a.,** an acid from ergot that is toxic if injected. **erucic a.,** an unsaturated fatty acid, cis-13-docosenoic acid, CH₃(CH₂)₇-CH:CH(CH₂)₁₁COOH, the cis-isomer of brassidic acid; it exists as a glyceride in oil of rape seed and of mustard. **ethacrynic a.** [USP], chemical name: [2,3-dichloro-4-(2-methylene-1-oxobutyl)-phenoxy]acetic acid. A powerful, rapid-acting diuretic of short duration, $C_{13}H_{12}Cl_2O_4$, occurring as a white or almost white, crystalline powder, used orally or, in the form of the sodium salt, intravenously. **ethanal a.,** glyoxylic a. **ethanoic a.,** acetic a. **ethylamine sulfonic a.,** taurine (def. 1). **ethylenediamine tetra-acetic a. (EDTA),** edetic a. **ethylene lactic a., ethylidene lactic a.,** see under *lactic a.* **5-ethyl-5-isoamylbarbituric a.,** amobarbital. **ethylsulfonic a.,** an acid, CH₃·CH₂·SO₂·OH, found in the urine after administration of sulfonmethane. **etidronic a.,** chemical name: (1-hydroxyethylidene)diphosphoric acid; a bone calcium regulator, $C_2H_8O_7P_2$. **etodolic a.,** chemical name: 1,8-diethyl-1,3,4,9-tetrahydropyrano[3,4-*b*]indole-1-acetic acid; an anti-inflammatory, $C_{17}H_{21}NO_3$. **eugenic a.,** eugenol. **excretoleic a., excretolic a.,** a fatty acid derived from feces. **fagicladosporic a.,** a mycotoxin produced by *Cladosporium epiphyllum.* **fatty a.,** any monobasic aliphatic acid containing only carbon, hydrogen, and oxygen and made up of an alkyl radical attached to the carboxyl group. The saturated fatty acids have the general formula $C_nH_{2n}O_2$. There are also several series of unsaturated fatty acids having one or more double bonds, and a few instances of cyclic acids. **fatty a., essential,** an unsaturated fatty acid that cannot be formed in the body and therefore must be provided by the diet; the most important are linoleic acid, linolenic acid, and arachidonic acid. **filicic a.,** a tasteless white amorphous powder, (CH₃)₂C₆HO(OH)₂, from filix mas (male fern); in veterinary medicine, it has limited use in the treatment of helminthiasis of cattle, sheep, and goats. **filixic a.,** a principle from filix mas (male fern). **flavaspidic a.,** a compound from the root of aspidium. **flufenamic a.,** chemical name: 2-[[3-(trifluoromethyl)phenyl]amino]benzoic acid; an anti-inflammatory and analgesic agent, $C_{14}H_{10}F_3NO_2$. **fluohydric a.,** hydrofluoric a. **fluoroacetic a.,** a metabolic poison from *Chailletia cymosa,* a tree of South Africa, that blocks the tricarboxylic acid cycle, causing convulsions and ventricular fibrillation. **fluorosilicic a.,** fluosilicic a. **fluosilicic a.,** an acid, H_2SiF_6, whose salts are fluorosilicates; its sodium salt, Na_2SiF_6, is used as an insecticide. Fluorosilicates are toxic because they release fluoride ion in solution, disturbing the calcium balance in the blood. Called also *fluorosilicic* or *hydrofluosilicic a.* **folic a.,** chemical name: *N*-{*p*|[(2-amino-4-hydroxy-6-pteridinyl)methyl]-amino}benzoyl} glutamic acid. A widely distributed water-soluble vitamin, $C_{19}H_{19}$-N_7O_6, existing in a number of natural products in free form or in various conjugates, which have been designated by various names, including *pteroylglutamic acid,* fermentation *Lactobacillus casei factor,* liver *L. casei factor, Norit eluate factor, factor R, Streptococcus lactis R* (or *SLR*) *factor, factor U,* yeast *L. casei factor, vitamin B₂, vitamin B₂ conjugate,* and *vitamin M.* It is an essential growth factor for many animals and microorganisms. Folic acid serves as a coenzyme in the transfer of one-carbon units, and its deficiency in man inhibits the synthesis of DNA, which first becomes obvious clinically in hematopoietic cells, resulting in certain types of macrocytic anemias. Synthetic folic acid is pteroylglutamic acid, COOH·(CH₂)₂·CH·(COOH)·NH·CO·C₆-HN₄·(NH₃)·OH. **folinic a.,** chemical name: 5-formyl-5,6,7,8-tetrahydropteroyl-L-glutamic acid. A derivative of folic acid, $C_{20}H_{23}N_7O_7$, necessary for the growth of *Leuconostoc citrovorum;* the calcium salt (*leucovorin calcium* [USP]) is used as an antidote for folic acid antagonists when there is need to reverse the toxic effects of the latter and in the treatment of megaloblastic anemias due to folic acid deficiency. Called also *citrovorum factor* and *leucovorin.* **formic a.,** a colorless pungent liquid, HCOOH, from nettles and ants and other insects; derivable from oxalic acid and from glycerin and from the oxidation of formaldehyde, it is a vesicant, but is not now used in medicine. **formiminoglutamic a.,** an intermediate product in the metabolism of histidine which accumulates in the urine of humans and rats deficient in folic acid. An increased urinary excretion, although not completely specific, may be employed clinically as a test for folic acid deficiency. Abbreviated *FIGLU.* **fulminic a.,** an unstable acid, carbyloxime, C:N·OH, isomeric with cyanic acid; it has the odor of hydrocyanic acid and is equally poisonous. **fumaric a.,** an unsaturated dibasic acid, HO₂C·CH:CH·CO₂H, the *trans*-isomer of maleic acid; it is an intermediate in the tricarboxylic acid (Krebs') cycle, formed from succinic acid and itself converted to malic acid. An NF preparation is used as an acidifier. **fusidic a.,** chemical name: 3α,11α,16β-trihydroxy-29-nor-8α,-9β,13α,14β-dammara-17(20),24-dien-21-oic acid 16-acetate. A fermentation product of *Fusidium coccineum,* $C_{31}H_{48}O_6$, used as an antibiotic. **gadelaidic a.,** the trans-isomer of gadoleic acid. **gadoleic a.,** an unsaturated fatty acid, $C_{20}H_{38}O_2$, from cod liver

oil. **gaidic a.,** a fatty acid crystalline compound, hexadecenoic acid, $C_{16}H_{30}O_2$, from hypogeic acid. **galactonic a.,** lactonic a. **galacturonic a.,** an acid isomeric with glucuronic acid, being an oxidized form of galactose, COH·(CHOH)₄COOH; it is the principal constituent of pectin. **galic a.,** chemical name: 3,4,5-trihydroxybenzoic acid. A white crystalline acid, (OH)₃C₆H₂·COOH·-H₂O, obtained by hydrolysis of the tannins from nutgalls or by hydrolysis of broths from *Penicillium glaucum* or *Aspergillus niger;* formerly used internally as an astringent. In veterinary medicine, it is sometimes used in the treatment of diarrhea. Called also *trihydroxybenzoic a.* **gallotannic a.,** tannic a. **gambogic a.,** a resin, $C_{29}H_{23}O_4$, obtainable in large quantities from cambogia. **gamma-aminobutyric a. (GABA),** an amino acid occurring in the brain, bacteria, green plants, and yeast. It functions as a neurotransmitter in the brain, inhibiting neural excitation. Called also *γ-aminobutyric* and *4-aminobutyric a.* **gentiotannic a.,** a variety of tannic acid, $C_{14}H_{10}O_5$, from gentian; once used as astringent on skin, especially in burns, but now discarded because of danger of liver damage. **gentisic a.,** dihydroxybenzoic acid, (OH)₂C₆H₃·COOH, obtained by melting gentianin with potassium hydroxide. **gigantic a.,** an antibiotic substance, $C_{14}H_{22}O_9N_2S$, isolated from *Aspergillus giganteus.* **glucic a.,** a colorless soluble acid formed from cane sugar by the action of potassium hydroxide. **glucoascorbic a.,** an analogue of ascorbic acid, which competitively inhibits the activity of the latter. **α-glucoheptonic a.,** a heptahydroxy acid, CH₂-OH(CHOH)₅COOH. **gluconic a.,** one of the isomeric forms of pentahydroxycaproic acid, CH₂OH(CHOH)₄COOH; it is made by the gentle oxidation of dextrose, cane sugar, etc. **glucothionic a.,** a sulfuric acid ester of an unknown carbohydrate isolated from the mammary gland. **glucuronic a.,** a uronic acid formed by oxidation in animal metabolism. It is a tetrahydroxy-aldehyde acid, CHO(CHOH)₄COOH, with the configuration of glucose and is found in the urine combined with camphor, chloroform, chloral, and other aromatic bodies in the form of glucuronides. D-Glucuronic acid is a precursor of L-gulonic acid in the biosynthesis of ascorbic acid. **glutamic a.,** chemical name: 2-aminoglutaric acid. A crystalline dibasic amino acid, COOH·(CH₂)₂·CH(NH₂)·COOH, widely distributed in proteins; it is thought to be a neurotransmitter, inhibiting neural excitation in the central nervous system. Called also *aminoglutaric a.* **glutamic a. hydrochloride,** a white crystalline powder, C₅-H₉NO₄HCl, used as a gastric acidifier; formerly used in the treatment of achlorhydria and hypochlorhydria, and as an antiepileptic. **glutaric a.,** an acid, COOH(CH₂)₃COOH obtained from cyclopentanone. **glyceric a.,** a dihydroxymonobasic acid formed by the oxidation of glycerol; it is 2,3-dihydroxypropanoic acid, CH₂OH·CHOH·COOH. **glycerophosphoric a.,** a clear syrupy liquid, CH₂OH·CHOH·CH₂·O·PO(OH)₂, used in the manufacture of certain glycerophosphates. **glycocholic a.,** a conjugated form of one of the bile acids that yields glycine and cholic acid on hydrolysis. **glycolic a.,** an acid, CH₂OH·-COOH, formed by electrolytic reduction of oxalic acid or by the action of sodium hydroxide on monochloroacetic acid and used in pH control; also produced in the body as an intermediate product in the conversion of serine to glycine. Called also *hydroxyacetic a., hydroxyethanoic a.,* and *oxyacetic a.* **glycoluric a.,** a crystalline acid, a ureid of glycolic acid, NH₂CO·NH·CH₂·COOH, formed by heating urea with aminoacetic acid. Called also *hydantoic a.* and *uraminoacetic a.* **glycosuric a.,** an acid found in the urine in certain conditions; it causes the urine to turn black on exposure to the air. **glycuronic a.,** glucuronic a. **glycyrrhizic a.,** glycyrrhizin. **glyoxylic a.,** a crystalline acid, dihydroxyacetic acid, (O:HC·COOH)₂, used in Hopkins-Cole test for protein; called also *ethanal a.* **gorlic a.,** a dehydrochaulmoogric acid, C₅H₇(CH₂)₆CH:CH(CH₂)₄·COOH, from *Corpotroche brasiliensis* and *Oncoba echinata* (gorli seed). **granatotannic a.,** the tannic acid, $C_{20}H_{16}O_{13}$, of pomegranate bark, a greenish yellow, amorphous powder. **guanidinoacetic a.,** a nitroge-
$$H$$
$$|$$
nous compound, H₂N—C(=NH)—N—CH₂·COOH, formed enzymatically in human liver, pancreas, and kidney by a transamidination reaction between arginine and glycine, and *N*-methylated in the liver by *S*-adenosylmethionine to form creatine. **guanidinosuccinic a.,** a metabolite first found in the urine of uremic patients, which at high levels inhibits platelet aggregation. **guanylic a.,** a mononucleotide made up of guanine, phosphoric acid, and a pentose. **gulonic a.,** one of the isomeric forms of pentahydroxycaproic acid, CH₃OH(CHOH)₄COOH, formed by the gentle oxidation of gulose or the reduction of D-glucuronic acid; L-gulonic acid is a precursor of gulonolactone in the biosynthesis of ascorbic acid. **gymnemic a.,** a yellow to brown, bitter powder, $C_{32}H_{55}O_{12}$, from leaves of *Gymnema sylvestre,* a southern Asiatic shrub; placed in the mouth, it temporarily abolishes the sense of taste for sweet and bitter, but not for pungent, sour, or astringent substances; not used in medicine. **gynocardic a.,** an oily acid, $C_{18}H_{34}O_2$, from the seeds of *Gynocardia odorata.* **haloid a.,** an acid which contains no oxygen in the molecule, but is composed of hydrogen and a halogen element; called also *hydracid* and *hydrohalogen a.* **helvellic a.,** a cytotoxic thermolabile hemolysin that is an active constituent of the fungus *Helvella infula* (*Gyromitra esculenta*). **helvolic a.,** an antibi-

otic acid, $C_{32}H_{42}O_8$, from cultures of *Aspergillus fumigatus* and *A. fumigatus* var. *helvola;* used as an antimicrobial. Called also *fumigacin.* **hemipinic a.,** an acid, $(CH_3O)_2C_6H_2(COOH)$, obtained by oxidizing noscapine. **heptaiodic a.,** a periodic acid, made by dissolving iodine in aqueous hydriodic acid. **heptanoic a.,** enanthic a. **heptylic a.,** enanthic a. **heterocyclic amino a's,** the amino acids proline, hydroxyproline, tryptophan, histidine, and pyroglutamic acid (or 5-oxoproline), all of which contain a ring which includes a noncarbon atom. **hexanoic a.,** caproic a. **hexonic a.,** any of several isomeric forms of gluconic acid. **hexosediphosphoric a.,** a normal intermediate of the glycolytic pathway that may accumulate in the products of fermentation of sugars by yeasts in the presence of phosphates. **hexuronic a.,** ascorbic a. **hidrolic a., hidrotic a.,** sudoric a. **hippuric a.,** a crystallizable acid, $C_6H_5·CO·NH·CH_2·COOH$, from the urine of domestic animals; more rarely found in human urine. Called also *benzoylaminoacetic a., benzoylglycine,* and *urobenzoic a.* **hircic a.,** an acid with a peculiar odor, found in goat's milk. **hirsutic a.,** a group of acidic materials, $C_{15}H_{20}O_4$, obtained from *Stereum hirsutum,* which show antibiotic activity. **homogentisic a.,** an intermediate product of the catabolism of tyrosine and phenylalanine, which is ultimately metabolized to acetone; called also *2,5-dihydroxyphenylacetic a.* and *hydroquinone-acetic a.* See also *alkapton bodies,* under *body.* **homophthalic a.,** a crystalline acid, $COOH·C_6H_4·CH_2·COOH$, formed by fusing cambogia with potassium hydroxide. **homopiperidinic a.,** an amino acid, $NH_2-(CH_2)_4·COOH$, found in decomposing meat. **homovanillic a.,** a major terminal urinary metabolite, converted from dopa, dopamine, and norepinephrine. **humic a.,** polymeric materials from peat, soil, certain waters, etc.; called also *humin.* **hyaluronic a.,** a mucopolysaccharide which is a polymer of acetylglucosamine and glucuronic acid; it is highly viscous in aqueous solution and occurs in the intercellular substance of various tissues, especially the skin, and has also been isolated from the vitreous humor, the umbilical cord, and the fluids of the synovial, pleural, pericardial, and peritoneal spaces. **hydantoic a.,** glycoluric a. **hydnocarpic a.,** chemical name: 11-(2-cyclopenten-1-yl)undecanoic acid. An unsaturated fatty acid, $C_{16}H_{28}O_2$, obtained from chaulmoogra (hydnocarpus) oil. See also *ethyl chaulmoograte.* **hydracrylic a.,** an isomer of lactic acid, $HOCH_2CH_2COOH$, that decomposes to acrylic acid when heated. **hydrazoic a.,** triazoic a. **hydriodic a.,** a gaseous haloid acid, HI; its aqueous solution and its syrup have been used as alteratives, but have no material advantage over the alkali iodides. **hydrobromic a.,** a gaseous haloid acid, HBr; its 10 per cent aqueous solution was once used like the bromides. **hydrocaffeic a.,** chemical name: β-(3,4-dihydroxyphenyl) propionic acid. An acid, $(OH)_2·C_6H_3·CH_2·CH_2·COOH$, formed by treating caffeic acid with sodium amalgam. **hydrochloric a.,** 1. a normal constituent of the gastric juice in man and other mammals, HCl. 2. a colorless, fuming liquid with a pungent odor that ceases to fume on the addition of water, containing 35–38 per cent, by weight, of HCl. It is used medicinally only in the dilute form (*diluted hydrochloric a.* [NF]), which contains 9.5–10.5 gm. of HCl in 100 ml.; used as an acidifying agent. Called also *chlorhydric a.* **hydrochloroplatinic a.,** chloroplatinic a. **hydrocinnamic a.,** chemical name: β-phenylpropionic acid. A white crystalline powder, $C_6H_5·CH_2·CH_2·COOH$, prepared by reduction of cinnamic acid. Called also *phenylpropionic a.* **hydrocumaric a.,** an acid, β-p-hydroxyphenylpropionic acid, $OH·C_6H_4-(CH_2)_2·COOH$, sometimes found in the urine and derived from the putrefaction of protein; called also *parahydroxyhydratropic a.* and *phloretic a.* **hydrocyanic a.,** hydrogen cyanide. **hydrofluoric a.,** a gaseous haloid acid, HF, extremely poisonous and corrosive; called also *fluoric a., fluohydric a.,* and *hydrogen fluoride.* **hydrofluosilicic a.,** fluosilicic a. **hydrohalogen a.,** haloid a. **hydroparacumaric a.,** an isomer of hydrocumaric acid, sometimes found in the urine of dogs. **hydroquinone-acetic a.,** homogentisic a. **hydrosulfuric a.,** hydrogen sulfide. **hydrosulfurous a.,** an unstable acid, $H_2S_2O_4$, known only in the form of its organic esters. **hydroxyacetic a.,** glycolic a. **p-hydroxybenzoic a.,** an acid isomeric with salicylic acid and used as an intermediate in dye manufacture and fungicides. **hydroxybutyric a.,** a poisonous acid, $CH_3CHOHCH_2COOH$, sometimes occurring in the urine in diabetes (ketoacidosis) and sometimes in the blood; it frequently occurs in several isomeric forms. Called also *oxybutyric a.* See also *beta-oxybutyric a.* **hydroxy-n-decanoic a.,** a saturated, monohydroxy fatty acid, $CH_3(CH_2)_7(CHOH)COOH$, found in brain phospholipids. **hydroxyethanoic a.,** glycolic a. **hydroxyformobenzoylic a.,** a crystalline compound, parahydroxyphenylglycolic acid, $OH·C_6H_4·CHOH·COOH$, sometimes occurring in the urine in acute yellow atrophy of the liver; called also *oxyamygdalic a., oxyformobenzoylic a.,* and *oxymandelic a.* **hydroxyglutamic a.,** a non-natural amino acid, $COOH·CH_2-CHOH·CH(NH_2)·COOH$. **5-hydroxyindoleacetic a.,** a product of serotonin metabolism present in cerebrospinal fluid and in increased amount in the urine in carcinoid. **hydroxymandelic a.,** parahydroxyphenylglycolic a. **hydroxynaphthoic a.,** chemical name: 1-naphthol-2-carboxylic acid. An acid, $OH·C_{10}H_6·COOH$, a naphthalene homologue of salicylic acid;

called also *carbonaphthoic a.* and *oxynaphthoic a.* **hydroxyphenylaminopropionic a.,** tyrosine. **2-hydroxypropionic a.,** lactic a. **hydroxystearic a.,** one of several monohydroxylated stearic acids, $C_{18}H_{36}O_3$, present in wool fat, rose wax, and castor oil. **hydroxytetracosanic a.,** cerebronic a. **hydrurilic a.,** an acid, $C_8H_7N_4O_6·2H_2O$, obtained as the ammonium salt on boiling alloxantin (uroxin) with dilute sulfuric acid. **hyodeoxycholic a.,** a major bile acid, $C_{24}H_{40}O_4$, of the hog; called also *3,6-dihydroxycholanic a.* **hyoglycocholic a.,** an acid, $C_{26}H_{43}NO_5$, from the conjugation of glycine with hyocholic acid, found in hog bile. **hyotaurocholic a.,** an acid, $C_{26}H_{45}NSO_6$, from the conjugation of taurine with hyocholic acid, occurring in hog bile. **hypobromous a.,** the acid, HBrO, forming hypobromites, which are used in testing for urea. **hypochlorous a.,** an unstable compound, HClO, a disinfectant and bleaching agent; its salts (hypochlorites) are used as medicinal agents, particularly as surgical solution of chlorinated soda. See *sodium hypochlorite solution* (*diluted*), under *solution.* **hypogeic a.,** an unsaturated fatty acid, 2-hexadecenoic acid, $CH_3(CH_2)_7·CH:CH(CH_2)_5COOH$, found in the oil of the peanut, *Arachis hypogaea.* **hyponitrous a.,** an unstable acid of the composition HO—N=N—OH, formed by the action of nitrous acid on hydroxylamine. The pure acid and its salts explode on heating; its organic esters release N_2 at room temperature. **hypophosphoric a.,** an acid, $H_4P_2O_6$, of phosphorus, forming salts called hypophosphates; it is formed on sticks of white phosphorus when they are exposed to air. **hypophosphorous a.,** the acid, H_3PO_2, forming hypophosphites; it is a toxic, monobasic acid with strong reducing properties, used in 30 to 32 per cent and 50 per cent solutions. **hypoxanthylic a.,** inosinic a. **ichthyolsulfonic a.,** an ichthammol derivative; called also *sulfichthyolic a.* **idonic a.,** an acid, $CH_2OH-(CHOH)_4COOH$, produced by the catalytic reduction of ascorbic acid. **indoleacetic a., 5-OH-indoleacetic a.,** a major end-product of tryptophan metabolism, occurring in minute amounts in normal urine and in elevated amounts when carcinoid tumors are present. **indopropionic a.,** a decomposition product of tryptophan. **indoxylic a.,** an acid, $C_9H_7NO_3$, formed by fusing its ethyl ester with sodium hydroxide. **indoxylsulfonic a.,** one of the ethereal sulfates found in the urine. **infectious nucleic a.,** viral nucleic acid capable of infecting a cell and inducing the production of viruses. **inorganic a.,** one containing no carbon atoms. **inosinic a.,** a mononucleotide made up of hypoxanthine, ribose, and phosphoric acid; it is a precursor of purine nucleotides (AMP and GMP), components of nucleic acids, and is also found in muscle tissue. Called also *hypoxanthylic a.* and *inosine monophosphate.* **inositol hexaphosphoric a.,** phytic a. **iobenzamic a.,** chemical name: N-(3-amino-2,4,6-triiodobenzoyl)-N-phenyl-β-alanine; a diagnostic radiopaque medium (cholecystography), $C_{13}H_{13}I_3N_2O_3$. **iocarmic a.,** chemical name: 3,3'-[(1,6-dioxo-1,6-hexanediyl)diimino]bis[2,4,6-triiodo-5-[(methylamino)carbonyl]benzoic acid; a radiopaque medium, $C_{24}H_{20}N_4O_8$. See *iocarmate meglumine.* **iocetamic a.** [USP], chemical name: 3-[acetyl-(3-amino-2,4,6-triiodophenyl)amino]-2-methylpropanoic acid; a radiopaque medium, $C_{12}H_{13}I_3N_2O_3$. **iodic a.,** a monobasic acid, HIO_3, formed by the oxidation of iodine with nitric acid or chlorates. The sodium salt occurs in Chile saltpeter, and is the chief source of iodine. It is a strong acid and a strong oxidizing agent. **iodipamic a.,** iodipamide. **iodoacetic a.,** $CH_2-ICOOH$, whose sodium salt is used in physiological study of muscle contraction. **iodoalphionic a.,** chemical name: 4-hydroxy-3,5-diiodo-α-phenylbenzenepropanoic acid; a radiopaque medium used in cholecystography, $C_{15}H_{12}I_2O_3$. **iodogorgoric a.,** 3,5-diiodotyrosine. **iodopanoic a.,** iopanoic a. **p-iodophenylarsenic a.,** a colorless crystalline compound, $C_6H_4I·AsO(OH)_2$. **iodosalicylic a.,** an antipyretic, analgesic, and antiseptic compound, $OH·C_6H_3I·COOH$, not now used in medicine. **iodosobenzoic a.,** a compound, $C_6H_4(IO)COOH$, formerly used as an antiseptic. **iodoxamic a.,** chemical name: 3,3'-[(1,16-dioxo-4,7,10,13-tetraoxohexadecane-1,16-diyl)diimino]bis[2,4,6-triiodobenzoic acid]; a radiopaque medium, $C_{26}H_{26}I_6N_2O_{10}$, used in cholecystography. **iodoxybenzoic a.,** a compound, $C_6H_4(IO_2)COOH$; the salts of ortho-iodoxybenzoic acid, once used in arthritis. **ioglicic a.,** chemical name: 3-(acetylamino)-2,4,6-triiodo-5-[[[2-(methylamino)-2-oxoethyl]amino]carbonyl] benzoic acid; a radiopaque medium, $C_{13}H_{12}I_3N_3O_5$. **ioglycamic a.,** chemical name: 3,3'-[oxobis(1-oxo-2,1-ethanediyl)]bis[2,4,6-triiodobenzoic acid]. An acid, $C_{18}H_{10}I_6N_2O_7$, the meglumine and sodium salts of which are used as diagnostic radiopaque media in cholecystography. **iopanoic a.** [USP], chemical name: 3-amino-α-ethyl-2,4,6-triiodobenzenepropanoic acid. A tasteless cream-colored powder, $C_{11}H_{12}I_3NO_2$, with a characteristic odor; used as a radiopaque medium in cholecystography. **iophenoxic a.,** chemical name: α-ethyl-3-hydroxy-2,4,6-triiodobenzenepropanoic acid. A compound, $C_{11}H_{11}I_3O_3$, used as a radiopaque medium in cholecystography. Called also *triiodoethionic a.* **iopronic a.,** chemical name: (±)-2-[[2-[3-(acetylamino)-2,4,6-triiodophenoxy]ethoxy]methyl]butanoic acid; a radiopaque medium for use in cholecystography, $C_{15}H_{18}I_3NO_5$. **iosefamic a.,** chemical name: 3,3'-[(1,10-dioxo-1,10-decanediyl)diimino]bis-[2,4,6-triiodo-5-[(methylamino)carbonyl]benzoic acid; a radiopaque medium, $C_{28}H_{28}I_6N_4O_8$. **ioseric a.,** chemical name: 3-[[[1-(hydroxymethyl)-2-(methylamino)-2-oxoethyl]amino]carbonyl]-2,4,6-triiodo-5-[(methoxyacetyl) amino]benzoic acid; a radiopaque medium, $C_{15}H_{16}I_3N_3O_7$. **iosumetic a.,** chemical name: 4-[ethyl-[2,4,6-triiodo-3-(methylamino)-phenyl]amino]-4-oxobutanoic acid; a radiopaque medium, $C_{13}H_{15}I_3N_2O_3$. **iotetric a.,** chemical name: benzoic acid, 3,3′-[(1,14-dioxo-3,6,9,12-tetraoxatetradecane-1,14-diyl)diimino]bis[2,4,6-triiodobenzoic acid]; a radiopaque medium, $C_{24}H_{22}I_6N_2O_{10}$. **iothalamic a.** [USP], chemical name: 3-(acetylamino)-2,4-6-triiodo-5-[(methylamino)carbonyl]-benzoic acid. A white powder, $C_{11}H_9I_3N_2O_4$, used in the preparation of certain radiopaque media (see *iodothalamate meglumine* and *iodothalamate sodium*). **iotroxic a.,** chemical name: 3,3′-[oxybis[2,1-ethanediyloxy-(1-oxo-2,1-ethanediyl)imino]]bis[2,-4,6-triiodobenzoic acid]; a radiopague medium, $C_{22}H_{18}I_6N_2O_9$. **iridic a.,** an acid, $C_{10}H_{12}O_5$, from orris. **isanic a.,** a crystalline acid, $C_{14}H_{20}O_2$, from isano oil, a violent purgative; it is not now used in medicine. **isethionic a.,** a thick liquid, hydroxyethylsulfonic acid, $CH_2(OH)\cdot CH_2\cdot SO_2\cdot OH$, isomeric with ethylsulfuric acid; formed by the action of nitrous acid on taurine. **isoamylethylbarbituric a.,** amobarbital. **isobilianic a.,** an acid, $C_{24}H_{34}O_8$, derived along with bilianic acid by the oxidation of dehydrocholalic acid. **isobutylallylbarbituric a.,** former name for butalbital. **isobutylaminoacetic a.,** leucine. **isobutyric a.,** an acid, $(CH_3)_2CH\cdot COOH$, a product of putrefaction of protein, found in the urine. **isocitric a.,** an intermediate in the tricarboxylic acid cycle, formed from oxaloacetic acid and itself converted to ketoglutaric acid. **isoerucic a.,** brassidic a. **isolysergic a.,** $C_{16}H_{16}N_2O_2$, one of the main cleavage products of the alkaline hydrolysis of the alkaloids characteristic of ergot, and the parent compound of the ergotinine group of alkaloids. **isopentoic a.,** isovalerianic a. **isopropylacetic a.,** isovalerianic a. **isopropylaminoacetic a.,** valine. **isosaccharic a.,** an acid, $COOH\cdot CH(O)\cdot (CHOH)_2\cdot CH\cdot COOH$, resulting from the oxidation of glucosamine with nitric acid. **isosulfocyanic a., isothiocyanic a.,** an acid, HNCS, whose salts are isosulfocyanates or isothiocyanates. **isouric a.,** an acid, $NC\cdot NH\cdot CH\cdot (CO\cdot NH)_2CO$, formed by the combination of cyanamide and alloxantin and which yields uric acid when boiled with hydrochloric acid. **isovalerianic a., isovaleric a.,** an acid, $(CH_3)_2CHCH_2COOH$, of unpleasant odor, found in cheese, in the sweat of the feet, in the urine in smallpox, in typhus, and in acute yellow atrophy of the liver. Called also *isopentoic a.* and *isopropylacetic a.* **jervic a.,** an acid, $C_{14}H_{10}O_{12}\cdot 2H_2O$, from *Veratrum album.* **juglandic a.,** an acid from the bark of *Juglans cinerea;* one of the constituents of juglone. Called also *nucin.* **kermisic a.,** a red dye similar to carminic acid, from kermes insects. **keto a.,** a chemical compound containing the group CO and COOH. **ketocholanic a.,** an oxidized form of cholanic acid. **α-ketoglutaric a.,** 2-oxopentanedioic acid, an intermediate in the tricarboxylic acid (Krebs') cycle, formed by oxidation of isocitric acid and itself oxidized to form succinyl-CoA; it is also formed in transamination involving the α-amino group of amino acids. **ketostearic a.,** an oxidized form of stearic acid, $CH_3(CH_2)_{11}CO(CH_2)_4COOH$, found in mushrooms; called also *lactaric a.* **kinic a.,** quinic acid. **kinotannic a.,** the tannic acid of kino. **kojic a.,** a pyrone, formed from sugars by certain molds and aerobic bacteria; it has a toxic action on animals. **krameric a.,** the tannic acid derived from *Krameria;* called also *ratanhiatannic a.* **kynurenic a.,** a crystalline acid, C_9H_5N-(OH)COOH (4-hydroxyquinaldic acid), a metabolite of tryptophan found in microorganisms and in the urine of normal mammals. **lactaric a.,** ketostearic a. **lactic a.,** 1. a monobasic acid, hydroxypropionic acid, $C_3H_6O_3$, alpha-hydroxypropionic acid known in three stereoisomeric forms: (*a*) a dextrorotatory form, L-lactic acid (paralactic acid) is produced by anaerobic glycolysis in muscle during heavy muscular exertion, and can be converted into glucose by the liver; called also sarcolactic acid because it occurs in flesh; it can be obtained conveniently from beef extract; (*b*) a levorotatory form, D-lactic acid, is produced by the fermentation of dextrose by *Micrococcus acidi levolactici;* (*c*) DL-lactic acid, the inactive, ethylidene, racemic, or fermentation lactic acid, the ordinary kind found in sour milk, in the stomach, and in certain fermented foods, such as sauerkraut and in silage. Beta-hydroxypropionic acid, $CHOH\cdot CH_2\cdot COOH$, called also ethylene lactic acid, is not found in the body. 2. [USP] a colorless or yellowish syrupy liquid consisting of a mixture of lactic acid and lactic acid lactate, obtained by lactic fermentation of sugars or produced synthetically; use in the preparation of sodium lactate (def. 2). **lactonic a.,** a crystallizable monobasic acid, $CH_2OH\cdot (CHOH)_4\cdot$-COOH, produced by the oxidation of milk sugar, gum arabic, or galactose. **lanoceric a.,** a saturated dihydroxy fatty acid present in wool fat, $CH_3(CH_2)_{26}(CHOH)_2COOH$. **lanopalmic a.,** a saturated monohydroxy fatty acid present in wool fat, CH_3-$(CH_2)_{13}(CHOH)COOH$. **laricic a.,** agaricic a. **laricinolic a.,** an acid resin, $C_{20}H_{30}O_2$, found in Venice turpentine. **lauric a., laurostearic a.,** a saturated fatty acid, dodecanoic acid, $C_{12}H_{24}O_2$, from laurel seed oil, coconut oil, and milk fat. **leuconic a.,** a crystalline acid, pentoketocyclopentane, obtained by oxidizing croconic acid. **levo-tartaric a.,** a form of tartaric acid which turns the plane of polarized light to the left. **levulinic a.,** an acid $CH_3COCH_2CH_2COOH$, formed by action of heat and acid on carbohydrates; it occurs in the form of hygroscopical scales. Called also *acetylpropionic a.* and *beta-acetylpropionic a.* **lignoceric a.,** a saturated fatty acid, $CH_3(CH_2)_{22}\cdot$-COOH, obtained from kerasin and sphingomyelin by hydrolysis. **linoleic a.,** a doubly unsaturated essential fatty acid, $C_{18}H_{32}O_2$, the most abundant such acid in various vegetable oils. **linolenic a.,** a triply unsaturated essential fatty acid, $C_{18}H_{30}O_2$, from linseed and other vegetable oils. **linolic a.,** linoleic a. **lipoic a.,** 6,8-dithio-octanoic acid: a bacterial growth factor present in the water-soluble fraction of liver and yeast. It is necessary for the oxidative decarboxylation of pyruvic acid by *Streptococcus fecalis* and for the growth of *Tetrahymena gelii,* and replaces acetate for the growth of *Lactobacillus casei.* It has been variously known as *acetate replacing factor, protogen A,* and *pyruvate oxidation factor.* **lithic a.,** uric a. **lithocholic a.,** an acid, 3-d-hydroxycholanic acid, from ox, human, and rabbit bile. **luteic a.,** a highly mucilaginous polysaccharide acid produced by the growth of *Penicillium luteum* on liquid media that contain sugar; it seems to be a malonyl ester of luteose, and on acid hydrolysis yields glucose. **lysergic a.,** a constituent of the ergot alkaloids, $C_6H_4\cdot NH\cdot C_5H_2N(CH_3)(CH{:}CH\cdot CH_3)\cdot COOH$, obtained by hydrolysis. **lysergic a. diethylamide,** lysergide. **lysuric a.,** a crystalline dibenzoyl lysine, $C_6H_5\cdot CO\cdot NH(CH_2)_4\cdot$-$CH(COOH)\cdot NH\cdot CO\cdot C_6H_5$, obtained from lysine. **lyxonic a.,** one of the isomeric forms of tetrahydroxy valeric acid, CH_2OH-$(CHOH)_3COOH$, formed by the gentle oxidation of lyxose. **maleic a.,** an unsaturated dibasic acid, $(CH\cdot COOH)_2$; fumaric acid is the trans form of its cis configuration. **malic a.,** hydroxysuccinic acid, $COOH\cdot CH_2CH(OH)\cdot COOH$, an intermediate in the tricarboxylic acid (Krebs') cycle, formed from fumaric acid and itself oxidized to form oxaloacetic acid; found in unripe and sour apples and in many other fruits. It has been prescribed for scurvy, and its iron salt, ferric malate, was once employed in medicine. **malonic a.,** a crystalline dibasic acid, $COOH\cdot CH_2COOH$, formed by oxidizing malic acid with chromium trioxide and used in the manufacture of barbiturates. **mandelic a.,** chemical name: α-hydroxybenzeneacetic acid. A crystalline acid, $C_8H_8O_3$, with active bacteriostatic properties, used in urinary tract infections, usually in the form of one of its salts. Called also *amygdalic a.* and *phenylglycolic a.* **manganic a.,** a green acid, H_2MnO_4, formed by fusing manganese dioxide with potassium or sodium hydroxide (in air) and then acidifying; it is readily oxidized to deep red permanganic acid, $HMnO_4$. **mannitic a.,** a compound, $CH_2OH(CHOH)_4\cdot COOH$, derived from mannitol by the action of platinum black. **mannonic a.,** a compound, CH_2OH-$(CHOH)_4\cdot COOH$, formed by oxidizing mannose. **mannosaccharic a.,** a dicarboxylic acid, $COOH(CHOH)_4COOH$. **margaric a.,** 1. an artificial fatty acid, $CH_3(CH_2)_{15}\cdot COOH$. 2. the incorrect name of a mixture of stearic and palmitic acids. **meclofenamic a.,** chemical name: 2-[(2,6-dichloro-3-methylphenyl)amino]benzoic acid; an anti-inflammatory, $C_{14}H_{11}Cl_2NO_2$. **meconic a.,** chemical name: 3-hydroxy-4-oxo-4H-pyran-2,6-dicarboxylic acid. A white crystalline acid, $C_7H_4O_7$, derived from opium. **mefenamic a.,** chemical name: 2-[(2,3-dimethylphenyl)amino]benzoic acid. A white to off-white, crystalline powder, $C_{15}H_{15}NO_2$, having analgesic, anti-inflammatory, and antipyretic properties; used orally chiefly in the relief of mild to moderate pain. **melassic a.,** a dark colored insoluble acid formed from cane sugar by the action of potassium hydroxide. **melilotic a.,** phenolpropionic acid, $OH\cdot C_6H_4(CH_2)_2\cdot COOH$, derived from coumarin. **melissic a.,** a crystalline fatty acid, $CH_3(CH_2)_{29}COOH$, from beeswax. **mellitic a.,** benzenehexacarboxylic acid, $C_6(COOH)_6$, prepared by oxidation of carbonaceous material. **mercapturic a.,** one of a series of acids formed in the body on the introduction of a halogen derivative of benzol; they are formed by combination with cysteine. See also *bromphenylmercapturic a.* **mesitylenic a.,** $C_6H_3(CH_3)_2COOH$, an oxidized form of mesitylene. **mesityluric a.,** the form in which mesitylene is excreted in the urine combined with acetoacetic acid, $C_6H_3(CH_3)_2CO\cdot NH\cdot CH_2\cdot COOH$. **meso-tartaric a.,** an optically inactive form of tartaric acid by internal compensation, $COOH(CHOH)_2COOH$. **mesoxalic a.,** $(OH)_2C(COOH)_2$, an oxidation product of glycerin. **metaphosphoric a.,** a glassy solid substance, HPO_3, soluble in water; used as a reagent for chemical analysis and as a test for albumin in the urine. Called also *glacial phosphoric a.* **metarsenic a.,** the acid, $HAsO_3$, which forms metarsenates; a dehydrated form of arsenic acid, H_3AsO_4. **metasaccharic a.,** a dibasic tetrahydroxy acid formed by the oxidation of mannitol; it is $COOH(CHOH)_4COOH$, and in the free state passes into a double lactone. **metastannic a's,** two acids from the oxidation of tin: the alpha-acid is $H_4SnO_4[Sn(OH)_4]$; the beta-acid is $H_2SnO_3[SnO(OH)_2]$. **metavanadic a.,** vanadic a. **methionic a.,** an acid, $CH_2(SO_2$-$OH)_2$, used in the preparation of ether. **3-methoxy-4-hydroxymandelic a.,** vanillylmandelic a. **methylarsinic a.,** a white crystalline compound, $CH_3\cdot AsO(OH)_2$, an organic derivative of arsenic. **methylguanidinoacetic a.,** creatine. **methylhydantoic a.,** an acid, glycoluric acid, $NH_2CO\cdot N$-$(CH_3)\cdot CH_2\cdot COOH$, obtained by boiling creatine with barium hydroxide. **methylmaleic a.,** citraconic acid. **methylmalonic a.,** a structural isomer of succinic acid. **methylprotocatechuic a.,** vanillic a. **methylsuccinic a.,** pyrotartaric

a. ***N*⁵-methyltetrahydrofolic a.**, a derivative of folic acid which seems to be the most important type of folic acid found in human blood serum. **mevalonic a.**, a dihydroxy acid; see *mevalonate.* **molybdenic a., molybdic a.**, the acid, H_2MoO_4; used in homeopathic medicine. **monamino a.**, an organic acid which contains an NH_2 group. **monoaminodicarboxylic a.**, an acid containing one amino group and two carboxyl groups in the molecule, e.g., glutamic acid. **monoaminomonocarboxylic a.**, an acid having one amino group and one carboxyl group in the molecule, e.g., alanine. **monobasic a.**, an acid having but one replaceable hydrogen atom and therefore yielding only one series of salts, e.g., HCl. **monochloracetic a.**, $CH_2Cl{\cdot}COOH$; see *chloracetic a.* **moritannic a.**, the tannic acid, $C_{13}H_{10}O_6$, of fustic, the wood of *Morus tinctoria,* $C_{13}H_{10}O_6$. **morphoxylacetic a.**, a narcotic, $C_{17}H_{18}NO_3{\cdot}CH_2{\cdot}COOH$, not used in medicine. **mucic a.**, a tetrahydroxy dibasic acid, $COOH(CHOH)_4COOH$, produced by oxidizing galactose or any carbohydrate containing galactose, such as milk sugar, agar, galactitol, or the galactans. **mucoitin-sulfuric a.**, a mucopolysaccharide occurring in gastric mucus and in the cornea of the eye; it is isomeric with chondroitin sulfuric acid but contains glucosamine in place of galactosamine. **muconic a.**, a dibasic acid, $COOH{\cdot}(CH)_4{\cdot}COOH$, found in the urine of dogs that have been given benzene. **muramic a.**, a condensation product of glucosamine and lactic acid; it is found in the cell wall of certain bacteria. **muriatic a.**, hydrochloric a. **muscle adenosine phosphoric a.**, a substance obtained from striated muscle, adenosine-5′-monophosphate. **mycolic a's**, acid-fast hydroxy acids of high molecular weight, which are specific components of mycobacteria. **mycophenolic a.**, a crystalline antibiotic substance, $C_{17}H_{20}O_6$, from cultures of *Penicillium brevi-compactum* and related species, which is both bacteriostatic and fungistatic. **myristic a.**, a widely occurring saturated fatty acid, $CH_3{\cdot}(CH_2)_{12}{\cdot}COOH$, found in spermaceti, nutmeg butter, and other fats under the form of myristin. **myronic a.**, a glycoside, $C_{10}H_{19}NS_2O_{10}$, found in black mustard; this acid, by the myrosin present, is changed into allyl mustard oil, glucose, and potassium sulfate on the addition of water. **nalidixic a.** [USP], chemical name: 1-ethyl-1,4-dihydro-7-methyl-4-oxo-1,8-naphthyridine-3-carboxylic acid. A synthetic antibacterial agent, $C_{12}H_{12}N_2O_3$, occurring as a white to slightly yellow crystalline powder; used orally in the treatment of urinary infections caused by gram-negative organisms, especially those caused by *Proteus* species. **naphtholcarboxylic a.**, a white crystalline substance, $C_{10}H_6(CH)CO_2H$, not now used in medicine. **naphtholdisulfonic a.**, any of several isomeric substances derived from naphthol and used in the preparation of azo dyes. **naphtholsulfonic a.**, any of the isomeric sulfonic acids, $C_{10}H_6(OH)SO_2OH$, derived from naphthol. **naphthylmercapturic a.**, a compound found in the urine of rabbits to which naphthalene has been administered. **nastinic a.**, a fatty acid of high molecular weight found in nastin. **nervonic a.**, an unsaturated fatty acid, $CH_3(CH_2)_7{\cdot}CH{:}CH(CH_2)_{13}{:}COOH$, occurring in sphingomyelin. **neuraminic a.**, a widely distributed 9-carbon aminosugar acid, one of the sialic acids. **nicotinic a.**, niacin. **nicotinuric a.**, a urinary metabolite of nicotine, $(C_5H_4N)CONHCH_2COOH$. **nitric a.**, a colorless liquid, HNO_3, with a characteristic choking odor; it is extremely caustic and escharotic, decomposing most organic substances, and combining with bases to form nitrates. Nitric acid is occasionally used as a cauterizing agent for warts, etc. *Fuming nitric acid* is a yellow to brownish red corrosive liquid giving off a suffocating vapor and containing some dissolved nitrogen peroxide; called also *nitrosonitric a.* **nitroferrocyanic a.**, a complex cyano-acid, $H_2[Fe(NO)Cy_5]$, formed by the action of nitric acid on potassium ferrocyanide; it is used as a salt in several tests. Called also *nitroprussic a.* **nitrohydrochloric a.**, a yellowish mixture of concentrated nitric acid and hydrochloric acid; it gives off chlorine continuously, and dissolves gold and platinum. Called also *nitromuriatic a.* and *aqua regia.* **nitromuriatic a.**, nitrohydrochloric a. **nitroprussic a.**, nitroferrocyanic a. **nitrosonitric a.**, fuming nitric acid. **nitrous a.**, an unstable weak acid, HNO_2, with which free amino groups react to form hydroxyl groups and liberate gaseous nitrogen; it is used in the determination of urea, the liberated N_2 being collected and measured. **nitroxanthic a.**, trinitrophenol. **noncarbonic a's**, all acids other than carbonic acid; called also *fixed* (*nonvolatile*) *acids.* **nonesterified fatty a.**, a fatty acid fraction of blood plasma; usually abbreviated NEFA. **normal fatty a.**, a fatty acid that has a straight carbon chain, or at least one that is not branched. **norpinic a.**, a dicarboxylic acid, $C_8H_{12}O_4$, that results from the oxidation of pinene. **nucleic a's**, high-molecular-weight polymeric substances composed of nucleotides, which constitute the acidic groups of the nucleoproteins and contain phosphoric acid, sugars, and purine and pyrimidine bases. Two types, ribonucleic a. and deoxyribonucleic a., are distinguished on the basis of the contained sugar and a difference in the pyrimidine bases. **nucleinic a.**, nucleic a. **nucleothymimic a.**, a patented yellowish white powder prepared from the pancreas of the calf or from nucleic acid; no longer used in medicine. **obtusilic a.**, 4-decenoic a. **octanoic a.**, caprylic a. **oenanthylic a.**, absolute forms of heptanoic acid. **olefinic a.**, an unsaturated fatty acid having the general formula $C_nH_{2n-1}COOH$. **oleic a.** [NF], chemical name: (*Z*)-9-octadenenoic acid. A colorless to pale yellow, unsaturated oily liquid that darkens on exposure to air, $CH_3(CH_2)_7CH{:}CH(CH_2)_7COOH$, obtained from tallow and other fats; used as an emulsion adjunct in pharmaceutical preparations. **opianic a.**, a compound, $CHO{\cdot}C_6H_2(CH_3O)_2{\cdot}COOH$, obtained from noscapine. **organic a.**, any acid the radical of which is a carbon derivative; a compound in which a hydrocarbon radical is united to COOH (a carboxylic acid) or to SO_3H (a sulfonic acid). **ornithuric a.**, an acid, $C_6H_5{\cdot}CO{\cdot}NH{\cdot}(CH_2)_3{\cdot}CH{\cdot}NH{\cdot}CO{\cdot}C_6H_5$, or dibenzoylornithin, occurring in the urine of birds fed on benzoic acid. **orotic a.**, chemical name: 1,2,3,6-tetrahydro-2,6-dioxo-4-pyrimidinecarboxylic acid. An intermediate in the biosynthesis of pyrimidine nucleotides, $C_5H_4N_2O_4$. It is also found in milk. **orsellinic a.**, a crystalline acid, $C_8H_8O_4$, from certain lichens. **orthoarsenic a.**, arsenic a. **orthoboric a.**, boric a. **orthohydroxybenzoic a.**, salicylic a. **ortho-oxybenzoic a.**, salicylic a. **orthophosphoric a.**, phosphoric a. **oshaic a.**, a principle resembling angelic acid and found in osha. **osmic a.**, 1. a dibasic acid, H_2OsO_4, forming salts called osmates. 2. osmium tetroxide. **oxalic a.**, a white crystalline dibasic acid, $(COOH)_2 + 2H_2O$, occurring in certain foods and formed in the body by enzymatic cleavage of glyoxalate. Its calcium salt (calcium oxalate), when formed in high concentrations in the urine, may lead to formation of urinary calculi. It is used as a disinfectant for the skin and as a chemical reagent. **oxaloacetic a.**, oxobutanedioic acid, $HOOC{\cdot}COCH_2{\cdot}COOH$, an intermediate in the tricarboxylic acid (Krebs') cycle, formed by oxidation of malic acid and itself acetylated to form citric acid; it is also formed in transamination reactions of aspartic acid. **oxaluric a.**, an acid, $NH_2{\cdot}CO{\cdot}NH{\cdot}CO{\cdot}COOH$, found in healthy urine. **oxamic a.**, the monoamide of oxalic acid; a monobasic crystalline acid, $NH_2{\cdot}CO{\cdot}COOH$. **oxolinic a.**, chemical name: 5-ethyl-5,8-dihydro-8-oxo-1,3-dioxolo[4,5-*g*]quinoline-7-carboxylic acid. A synthetic antibacterial, $C_{13}H_{11}NO_5$, used orally in urinary tract infections caused by susceptible gram-negative organisms. **oxyacetic a.**, glycolic a. **oxyamygdalic a.**, hydroxyformobenzoylic a. **oxybenzoic a.**, salicylic a. **oxybutyric a.**, hydroxybutyric a. **oxyformobenzoylic a.**, hydroxyformobenzoylic a. **oxygen a.**, an acid that contains oxygen; an oxyacid. **oxymandelic a.**, hydroxyformobenzoylic a. **oxynaphthoic a.**, any of the isomeric hydroxynaphthoic acids. **oxynervonic a.**, an unsaturated hydroxy lignoceric acid, $C_{24}H_{46}O_3$; it is one of the components of the cerebroside, oxynervone. **oxyphenylacetic a.**, parahydroxyphenylacetic a. **oxypropionic a.**, see under *lactic a.* **oxyproteic a.**, a nitrogenous substance of unknown constitution, perhaps a peptide, sometimes found in urine. **oxyproteinic a.**, a compound occurring in normal urine. **oxytoluic a.**, cresotic a. **palmitic a.**, a saturated fatty acid, $CH_3(CH_2)_{14}COOH$, found in most of the common fats and oils. **palmitoleic a.**, an unsaturated fatty acid, hexadecenoic acid, $CH_3(CH_2)_5{\cdot}CH{:}CH(CH_2)_7COOH$, found in marine animal, reptilian, avian, amphibian, and, to a lesser extent, mammalian fats; called also *physetoleic a.* **pangamic a.**, a substance originally defined as an ester of gluconic acid and dimethylglycine hydrochloride, said to be isolated from apricot kernels, but the term has been applied to several different substances and mixtures. **pantothenic a.**, an amide, $C_9H_{17}NO_5$, of α,γ-dihydroxy-β,β-dimethyl butyric acid (pantoic acid) and β-alanine, the antidermatitis factor of chicks essential for the normal development of rats and chicks. It is widely distributed in foods and tissues, and stimulates the growth of yeast. It is a vitamin of the B complex and occurs in bound form in coenzyme A. **para-aminobenzoic a.**, aminobenzoic a. **para-aminohippuric a.**, aminohippuric a. **para-aminosalicylic a.**, aminosalicylic a. Often abbreviated PAS or PASA. **parabanic a.**, a solid acid, $CO(NH{\cdot}CO)_2$, derivable from uric acid by oxidation. **parahydroxyhydratropic a.**, hydrocumaric a. **parahydroxyphenylacetic a.**, an acid, $OH{\cdot}C_6H_4{\cdot}CH_2{\cdot}COOH$, derived from tyrosine by putrefactive changes in the intestines and sometimes found in the urine. **parahydroxyphenylglycolic a.**, an acid, $OH{\cdot}C_6H_4{\cdot}CHOH{\cdot}COOH$, derived from tyrosine by deaminization and oxidation; it is found in the urine at times especially in cases of acute yellow atrophy of the liver. Called also *hydroxymandelic a.* **parahydroxyphenylpropionic a.**, an acid, $OH{\cdot}C_6H_4(CH_2)_2COOH$, sometimes found in the urine. **paralactic a.**, see under *lactic a.* **pararosolic a.**, aurin. **paratartaric a.**, see under *tartaric a.* **pectic a.**, a complex polysaccharide present in pectin, composed of four mols of galacturonic acid, one of arabinose, one of galactose, two of acetic acid, and two of methyl alcohol. **pelargonic a.**, a normal fatty acid, nonoic acid, $CH_3(CH_2)_7COOH$, found in oil of the garden geranium (pelargonium) and other plants. **penicillic a.**, chemical name: 3-methoxy-5-methyl-4-oxo-2,5-hexadienoic acid. An antibiotic substance, $C_8H_{10}O_4$, isolated from cultures of various species of *Penicillium* and *Aspergillus.* **pentacosanic a.**, an acid, $C_{25}H_{50}O_2$, from phrenosin. **pentanoic a.**, normal valeric a. **pentetic a.**, chemical name: *N,N*-bis[2-[bis(carboxymethyl)amino]ethyl]glycine; a chelating agent, $C_{14}H_{23}N_3O_{10}$. See also *pentetate calcium trisodium.* **pentosenucleic a.**, ribonucleic a. **peptohydrochloric a.**, the acid supposed to be formed by the combination of pepsin and dilute hydrochloric acid. **peracetic a.,** an acid, $C_2H_4O_3$, which explodes on heating to 110° C.; called also *peroxyacetic a.* **perchloric a.,** a volatile colorless fuming liquid, $HClO_4$, strongly resembling sulfuric acid in its properties. The pure acid alone is quite stable, but in the presence of organic matter or anything reducible, powerful explosions can result. **periodic a.,** a series of acids formed by the union of different amounts of water with periodic anhydride (I_2O_7) varying from HIO_4 to H_7IO_7. Sodium periodate occurs in small amounts in Chile saltpeter. **permanganic a.,** a monobasic acid, $HMnO_4$, with a persistent deep red color. Its salts are permanganates: see *potassium permanganate.* **perosmic a.,** a yellow crystalline acid anhydride, OsO_4, with suffocating odor, used as a stain in pathology; it is toxic and can cause blindness because its vapors are readily reduced to a film of osmium directly on the eyeball. **peroxyacetic a.,** peracetic a. **peroxydisulfuric a.,** persulfuric a. **peroxymonosulfuric a.,** persulfuric a. **persulfuric a.,** an oxidized form of sulfuric acid which can be either peroxymonosulfuric acid, H_2SO_5, or peroxydisulfuric acid, $H_2S_2O_8$. **petroselinic a.,** an unsaturated acid, $CH_3(CH_2)_{10}CH:CH(CH_2)_4COOH$, the principal constituent of the fatty oil from seeds of the *Umbelliferae,* e.g., fennel, carrot, parsley, and coriander. **phenaceturic a.,** an alpha amino acid, $C_6H_5CH_2·CO·NH·CH_2·COOH$, found in horse and dog urine. **phenic a.,** phenol. **phenylacetic a.,** a decarboxylation product, $C_6H_5·CH·COOH$, of phenylpyruvic acid, formed in the metabolism of phenylalanine in the body; it is conjugated with glutamine and excreted in the urine. Called also *alphatoluic a.* **β-phenyl-α-aminopropionic a.,** phenylalanine. **phenylcinchoninic a.,** cinchophen. **phenylethylbarbituric a.,** phenobarbital. **phenylglycolic a.,** mandelic a. **phenylglycuronic a.,** a compound of phenol and glucuronic acid, $C_6H_5·O·CO·(CHOH)_4·CHO$, found in the urine after the ingestion of phenol. **phenylic a.,** phenol. **phenyllactic a.,** an acid excreted in the urine in phenylketonuria. **phenylmercapturic a.,** bromphenylmercapturic a. **phenyloboric a.,** a white powder, $C_6H_5·B(OH)_2$, used as a germicide. **phenylpropionic a.,** hydrocinnamic a. **phenylpyruvic a.,** an intermediary product, $C_6H_5CH_2·COCOOH$, in the metabolism of phenylalanine. **phenylsalicylic a.,** a white powder, $C_6H_3(OH)(C_6H_5)COOH$, used as an antiseptic dusting powder. **phloretic a.,** hydrocumaric a. **phocenic a.,** isovaleric a.; see under *valeric a.* **phosphatidic a.,** a compound formed by the esterification of the three hydroxyl groups of glycerol with two fatty acid groups and one phosphoric acid group; characteristic group of the phosphatides, occurring widely in animals and plants. **phosphocarnic a.,** an acid consisting of carnic acid united with phosphorus, found in muscle, blood, and milk. **2-phosphoglyceric a.,** $CH_2OH—CH[OPO(OH)_2]—COOH$, an intermediate in the metabolic formation of pyruvate. **phosphomolybdic a.,** an acid, $H_3PO_4·12MoO_3 + H_2O$, important as a precipitant for all the alkaloids. **phosphoric a.,** 1. a crystalline acid, H_3PO_4, formed by the oxidation of phosphorus. 2. [NF] a colorless liquid of syrupy consistency, containing in each ml., between 85 and 88 per cent phosphoric acid; used as a solvent having many laboratory and industrial uses. Called also *orthophosphoric a.* **phosphoric a., diluted** [NF], a preparation of phosphoric acid in purified water, containing in each milliliter between 9.5 and 10.5 gm. of phosphoric acid; used as a solvent in pharmaceutical preparations. It is also used orally as a gastric acidifier. **phosphoric a., glacial,** metaphosphoric a. **phosphorous a.,** a dibasic reducing acid, H_3PO_3, whose salts are called phosphites. **phosphotungstic a.,** a white crystalline powder, approximately $24WO_3·P_2O_5·51H_2O$, used in preparing histologic stains, in testing for ptomaines, and as a reagent. **phrenosinic a.,** cerebronic a. **phthalic a.,** a crystalline dibasic acid, benzene dicarboxylic acid, $C_6H_4(COOH)_2$, formed by oxidizing naphthalene. **phthioic a.,** an optically active fraction of the phosphatide portion of the tubercle bacillus. **physetoleic a.,** palmitoleic a. **phytic a.,** an acid, $6CHOPO(OH)_2$, occurring in the leaves of plants; called also *inositol hexaphosphoric a.* **picramic a.,** dinitroaminophenol. **picric a.,** trinitrophenol. **picronitric a.,** trinitrophenol. **picrosulfuric a.,** a mixture used as a fixing agent in histologic work. **pimaric a.,** an acid resin, $C_{20}H_{30}O_2$, soluble in sodium hydroxide solution and forming 8 to 10 per cent of European turpentine. **pimelic a.,** a dibasic acid, $COOH(CH_2)_5COOH$, homologous with adipic acid. **pipecolic a.,** a heterocyclic intermediate in the catabolism of lysine. **piperic a., piperidic a.,** chemical name: 5-(3,4-methylenedioxyphenyl)-2,4-pentadienoic acid. A crystalline unsaturated acid, $CH_2O_2·C_6H_3·(CH)_4·COOH$, formed when piperine is boiled with alcoholic potassium hydroxide. **pivalic a.,** see under *valeric a.* **plasminic a.,** an acid obtained by splitting up nucleic acids; it may be decomposed into phosphoric acid and nucleic bases. **plasmonucleic a.,** ribonucleic a. **platinochloric a.,** chloroplatinic a. **plumbodithio-pyridine carboxylic a.,** a yellow powder, soluble in water, containing 42.4 per cent of lead; once used in the treatment of cancer. **podophyllinic a. 2-ethylhydrazide,** an acid, $C_{24}H_{30}N_2O_8$, obtained from podophyllum, which has antineoplastic properties. **polybasic a.,** an acid which contains two or more hydrogen atoms which may be neutralized by alkalies and replaced by organic radicals. **polygalic a.,** a saponin found, along with senegenin, in senega. **polyglycolic a.,** chemical name: poly(oxycarbonylmethylene); a surgical suture material, $(C_2H_2O_2)_n$. **polyunsaturated fatty a's,** acids with abundant unsaturated bonds; in large amounts in diets, they tend to lower plasma cholesterol levels. **prodolic a.,** chemical name: 1,3,4,9-tetrahydro-1-propylpyrano[3,4-b]indole-1-acetic acid; an anti-inflammatory, $C_{16}H_{19}NO_3$. **propargylic a.,** propiolic a. **propiolic a.,** an acetylenic unsaturated fatty acid, $CH·C·COOH$; called also *propargylic a.* **propionic a.,** an acid, $CH_3CH_2·COOH$, found in chyme and in sweat, and one of the products of bacterial fermentation of wood pulp waste; its salts (calcium and sodium propionate) are used as antifungal agents. **propionylsalicylic a.,** the salicylic ester of propionic acid, $CH_3·CH_2·CO·O·C_6H_4·COOH$. **protocatechuic a.,** dioxybenzoic acid, $(OH)_2C_6H_3·COOH$, sometimes found in the urine. **prussic a.,** hydrocyanic a. **pteroic a.,** folic acid with glutamic acid removed. **pteroyldiglutamic a.,** chemical name: pteroyl-α-glutamylglutamic acid. A compound that has been tried and discarded as an antineoplastic agent. **pteroylglutamic a.,** folic acid (q.v.) found in nature and produced synthetically; abbreviated P.G.A. **pteroylmonoglutamic a.,** folic a. **pteroyltriglutamic a.,** chemical name: N-[N-(N-pteroyl-γ-glutamyl)-γ-glutamyl]glutamic acid. A compound $C_{29}H_{33}N_9O_{12}·H_2O$, formerly used in the treatment of neoplastic disease. **puberulic a.,** chemical name: 3,4,6-trihydroxy-5-oxo-1,3,6-cycloheptatriene-1-carboxylic acid. An antibiotic substance, $C_8H_6O_6$, isolated from cultures of *Penicillium,* bacteriostatic for gram-positive bacteria. **puberulonic a.,** chemical name: 5,6,7-trihydroxy-1H-cyclohepta[c]furan-1,3,4-trione. An antibiotic substance, $C_9H_4O_7$, isolated from cultures of *Penicillium,* bacteriostatic for gram-positive bacteria. **punicotannic a.,** the tannic acid of pomegranate root. **purpuric a.,** an imino-condensation product of alloxan, $CO(NH·CO)_2C·NH·C(NH·CO)_2CO$, found in Weidel's test for uric acid. See also *murexide,* and see *Weidel's test* (1), under *tests.* **pyolipic a.,** an antibiotic substance isolated from *Pseudomonas aeruginosa.* **pyridoxic a.,** a pyridine compound sometimes occurring in the urine, the chief metabolic product of pyridoxine, pyridoxal, and pyridoxamine. **pyroarsenic a.,** the condensed acid, $H_4As_2O_7$, forming pyroarsenates. **pyroboric a.,** a condensed dibasic acid, $H_2B_4O_7$, obtained by heating boric acid; borax, $Na_2B_4O_7$, is the most common salt. Called also *tetraboric a.* **pyrocechatuic a.,** an acid formerly thought to be concerned in the reaction of alkapton urine. **pyrocinchonic a.,** an acid, dimethylmaleic acid, $(CH_3·C·COOH)_2$, known as an anhydride, which is formed when cinchonic acid is heated. **pyrocitric a.,** citraconic acid. **pyroglutamic a.,** 5-oxoproline. **pyroligneous a.,** the dark brown volatile fraction obtained when wood is heated without access of air; its acid constituent is mainly acetic acid. **pyrophosphoric a.,** a condensed crystalline acid, $H_4P_2O_7$; its salts are pyrophosphates; see also *phosphoric acid.* **pyrosulfuric a.,** see *sulfuric a., fuming.* **pyrotartaric a.,** an acid, $COOH·CH_2CH_2(CH_3)COOH$, produced in the dry distillation of tartaric acid; called also *methylsuccinic a.* **pyrrolidinecarboxylic a.,** proline. **pyruvic a.,** an acid, $CH_3CO·CO_2H$, that is an intermediate in carbohydrate metabolism (see *pyruvate*); it may be prepared by dry distillation of racemic or tartaric acid. Called also *pyroracemic a.* **quercitannic a.,** the tannic acid of oak bark, $C_{17}H_{16}O_9$, differing in its properties slightly from ordinary tannic acid. **quillaic a.,** an acid, $C_{30}H_{46}O_5$, from a saponin in quillaia, the bark of the rosaceous tree *Quillaja saponaria* Molina. **quinaldinic a.,** a crystalline acid, $C_9H_5N(CO_2H)$. **quinic a.,** an acid, $CH_2·(CHOH)_3CH_2·C(OH)·COOH$, found in cinchona bark, coffee, cranberries, and in many other plants; in man, largely transformed into benzoic acid and excreted as hippuric acid; called also *kinic a.* **quininic a.,** a crystalline acid, $CH_3O·C_9H_5N·COOH$, formed by oxidizing quinine and quinidine. **quinotannic a.,** a variety of tannic acid from cinchona bark. **quinovic a.,** an acid, $C_{30}H_{46}O_5$, from a cinchona glucoside. **ratanhiatannic a.,** krameric a. **Reinecke's a.,** tetrathiocyanodiaminochromic acid, $(SCN)_4Cr(NH_3)_2·NH_4$, used as a reagent for the isolation of proline and other basic substances. **retinoic a.,** an acid, $C_{20}H_{28}O_2$, obtained by oxidizing the alcohol group of vitamin A (retinol) to an aldehyde and then to carboxyl. The term is used to designate the all-*trans* stereoisomer (*tretinoin* [q.v.]), which is used as a topical keratolytic. A synthetic isomer, 13-*cis*-retinoic acid (isotretinoin), given orally, has been reported effective in clearing cystic and conglobate acne. Called also *vitamin A a.* **rheic a.,** chrysophanic a. **rhodanic a.,** rhodanine. **ribonic a.,** an acid, $CH_2OH(CHOH)_3COOH$, which results from oxidation of ribose. **ribonucleic a.,** a nucleic acid originally isolated from yeast, but later found in all living cells; on hydrolysis it yields adenine, guanine, cytosine, uracil, ribose, and phosphoric acid. Abbreviated RNA. *Messenger RNA* is an RNA fraction of intermediate molecular weight, with a base ratio corresponding to the DNA of the same organism, which transmits information from DNA to the protein-forming system of the cell. In bacteria it turns over rapidly. *Ribosomal RNA* comprises about half of the substance of ribosomes, which presumably perform a nonspecific function in polypeptide synthesis. *Soluble RNA.* See *transfer RNA. Transfer RNA* is an RNA fraction of low molecular weight (S = 4), existing in 20 species, each of which combines with one amino acid species, transferring it from activating enzyme to ribosome. **ribose nucleic a.,** ribonucleic a. **ricinoleic a., ricinolic a.,** an unsaturated hydroxyacid, $CH_3(CH_2)_5 \cdot CHOH \cdot CH_2 \cdot CH{:}CH(CH_2)_7 \cdot COOH$, found as a glyceride in castor oil. **rosacic a.,** purpurin (def. 2). **rosolic a.,** aurin. **ruberythric a.,** a glycoside found in madder root which on hydrolysis yields alizarin. **rufigallic a.,** a brownish crystalline acid, $C_{14}H_8O_8$, derived from anthracene, used to analytically detect Zr and Hf. **saccharic a.,** 1. a dibasic acid, $COOH \cdot (CHOH)_4CO \cdot OH$, formed by the action of nitric acid on dextrose or carbohydrates containing dextrose. 2. a monobasic acid, $C_6H_{12}O_6$, or tetraoxycaproic acid, not existing in the free state. **saccharonic a.,** an acid, methyltrihydroxyglutaric acid, $CH_3 \cdot C(OH)(COOH)(CHOH)_2COOH$, formed by the oxidation of saccharin (2) with nitric acid. **salicylacetic a.,** salicyloacetic acid. **salicylic a.** [USP], chemical name: 2-hydroxybenzoic acid. A white crystalline powder or white crystals, $OH \cdot C_6H_4 \cdot COOH$, obtained from several sources, notably wintergreen leaves and bark of white birch but usually prepared synthetically; it is used as a topical keratolytic. Its salts are the salicylates. **salicyloacetic a.,** a compound, $C_9H_8O_5$, formerly used as an antiseptic. **salicylsalicylic a.,** salsalate. **salicylsulfonic a.,** sulfosalicylic a. **salicyluric a.,** an acid, $CH_2 \cdot NH_2 \cdot CO \cdot O \cdot C_6H_4 \cdot COOH$, found in urine after the exhibition of salicylic acid. **santenic a.,** chemical name: 1,2-dimethyl-1,3-cyclopentane dicarboxylic acid. A crystalline compound from santene in oil of sandalwood, $C_9H_{12}O_4$, produced by oxidation with solution of potassium permanganate. **santonic a.,** the acid, $C_{15}H_{20}O_4$, from santonica. **santoninic a.,** santonin. **sarcolactic a.,** see *lactic a.* **Scheele's a.,** hydrocyanic acid 4 per cent. **sclerotic a., sclerotinic a.,** an acid found in ergot, of which it is one of the active principles. **sebacic a.,** a crystalline dibasic acid, decanedioic acid, $COOH \cdot (CH_2)_8 \cdot COOH$, derivable from olein and various fixed oils. **selenic a.,** a clear liquid, H_2SeO_4, resembling sulfuric acid but less stable and much more easily reduced. **selenous a.,** 1. an acid, H_2SeO_3, forming selenites. 2. less correctly, selenium oxide, SeO_2. **shikimic a.,** chemical name: 3,4,5-trihydroxycyclohexene-1-carboxylic acid. It is found in the fruit of the Japanese star anise, *Illicium verum,* and is a precursor in the biosynthesis of several aromatic compounds, including phenylalanine and tyrosine. **sialic a's,** a group of acetylated derivatives of neuraminic acid which occur in a number of mucopolysaccharides and glycolipids. **silicic a.,** 1. an acid of which silicon is the base, forming silicates. It is of several kinds, as orthosilicic acid, H_4SiO_4; metasilicic acid, H_2SiO_3; and parasilicic acid, H_6SiO_6. 2. less correctly, silica, SiO_2, or silicic anhydride. **silicotungstic a.,** an acid, $12WO_3SiO_2 + 2H_2O$, in white or yellow crystals, used as a reagent for alkaloids. **sinapinic a.,** an aromatic acid, $(CH_3O)_2C_6H_2 \cdot OH \cdot CH{:}CH \cdot CO_2H$, from the seeds of black mustard. **skatol carboxylic a.,** a compound, $C_8H_5(CH_3)N \cdot COOH$, formed during the putrefaction of proteins. **skatoxylglycuronic a.,** a detoxicated form of skatoxyl produced by conjugation with glucuronic acid. **skatoxylsulfuric a.,** one of the ethereal sulfates, $C_9H_8N \cdot O \cdot SO_3OH$, found in the urine in the form of its potassium salt. **sorbic a.,** 1. chemical name: 2,4-hexadienoic acid. An acid $CH_3(CH)_4COOH$, found in berries of mountain ash, *Sorbus aucuparia.* 2. [NF] a preparation occurring as a free-flowing, white, crystalline powder, containing 99 to 101 per cent of the labeled amount of sorbic acid; used as an antimicrobial preservative. **spermanucleic a.,** nucleic acid from the spermatozoa of various animals. **sphacelinic a.,** a poisonous substance from ergot. **stannic a.,** a colloidal or gelatinous compound, $Sn(OH)_4$, formed by the addition of alkalies to tin salts. It is amphoteric, forming tin salts with strong acids and alkali stannates with strong bases. **stearic a.,** 1. chemical name: octadecanoic acid. A saturated fatty acid, $CH_3(CH_2)_{16}COOH$, widely distributed in plant and animal fats. 2. [NF] a mixture of solid acids, mainly stearic acid and palmitic acid, obtained from edible tallow, containing not less than 40 per cent each of stearic and palmitic acids, the sum of the two not less than 90 per cent; used as an emulsion adjunct and tablet lubricant. Also available as *purified stearic a.,* in which the amount of stearic acid and palmitic acid together constitute not less than 98 per cent of the total content; the content of stearic acid being not less than 90 per cent of the total. **stearolic a.,** an acetylenic fatty acid, $CH_3(CH_2)_7 \cdot C{:}C(CH_2)_7COOH$, from oleic or elaidic acids. **stibanilic a.,** a white powder, $NH_2C_6H_5SbO(OH)_2$, formerly used in leishmaniasis. **suberic a.,** a dibasic acid, $COOH(CH_2)_6COOH$, obtained from castor oil by heating it with nitric acid. **succinic a.,** 1,4-butanedioic acid, $COOH(CH_2)_2COOH$, an intermediate in the tricarboxylic acid (Krebs') cycle; it is formed from succinyl-CoA and is itself oxidized to form fumaric acid. It was once used in the treatment of diabetic ketosis and, combined with salicylates, in the treatment of rheumatic fever and arthritis. **sudoric a.,** an acid, $C_5H_9O_7N$, said to exist in sweat; called also *hidrolic a.* and *hidrotic a.* **sulfacetic a.,** acetylsalicylic acid. **sulfaminic a.,** an aminosulfonic acid, $NH_2 \cdot SO_2OH$, once used in the treatment of cholera. **sulfanilic a.,** chemical name: *p*-aminobenzenesulfonic acid. A white crystalline compound, $NH_2 \cdot C_6H_4 \cdot SO_2 \cdot OH \cdot 2H_2O$; the diazotized form (diazobenzenesufonic acid) is used in Ehrlich's diazo reaction. Called also *anilinparasulfonic a.* **sulfhydric a.,** hydrogen sulfide. **sulfichthyolic a.,** ichthyolsulfonic a. **sulfinic a.,** an organic compound containing the group —SO·OH. **sulfo-a.,** an acid in which oxygen or carbon is replaced by sulfur. **sulfoconjugate a.,** the arylsulfuric acid formed as a metabolite of phenolic compounds. **sulfocyanic a.,** thiocyanic acid. **sulfoichthyolic a.,** ichthyolsulfonic acid. **sulfonic a.,** a compound of SO_2OH with another radical, especially a hydrocarbon. **sulforicinic a.,** an acid derived from castor oil by the action of sulfuric acid. **sulforicinoleic a.,** an acid formed by treating castor oil with sulfuric acid. **sulfosalicylic a.,** chemical name: 3-carboxy-4-hydroxybenzenesulfonic acid. A compound, $C_6H_3COOH(OH)(SO_3H)$-1,2,5·$2H_2O$, occurring as white or slightly pinkish needle-like crystals, or crystalline powder, soluble in water and alcohol; used as a reagent for protein and as a colorimetric reagent for ferric ion. Called also *salicylsulfonic a.* **α-sulfostearic a.,** an acid, $CH_3(CH_2)_{15} \cdot CH(SO_2OH) \cdot COOH$, formed by the action of liquid sulfur trioxide on stearic acid. **sulfovinic a.,** ethylsulfuric acid, $C_2H_5 \cdot HSO_4$, formed by the action of sulfuric acid in alcohol. **sulfuric a.,** an oily, highly caustic, and poisonous acid, H_2SO_4, used widely in chemistry, industry, and the arts, and formerly used as a topical caustic and in serous diarrhea and gastric hypoacidity. The concentrated acid, formerly called oil of vitriol, causes severe skin burns by dehydration; explosive spattering occurs when water is added. **sulfuric a., fuming,** a heavy, colorless, oily liquid compounded of sulfuric acid, H_2SO_4, and sulfur trioxide, SO_3, which gives off suffocating fumes; it is widely used in industry for sulfonations and nitrations. Called also *pyrosulfuric a.* **sulfurous a.,** 1. a dibasic acid, H_2SO_3, produced by combining sulfur dioxide, a gas, SO_2, with water to form a clear colorless solution used as a reagent; its salts are called sulfites. 2. sulfur dioxide. **talonic a.,** one of the isomeric forms of pentahydroxycaproic acid $CH_2OH(CHOH)_4 \cdot CO_2H$, formed by the gentle oxidation of talose. **tannic a.,** a yellowish white to light brown powder, $(OH)_3C_6H_2 \cdot CO \cdot O \cdot C_6H_2(OH)_2 \cdot COOH$, usually obtained from nutgalls and used as an astringent; it is no longer used in the treatment of burns because of the possibility of severe liver damage. Called also *gallotannic a., tannin,* and, erroneously, *digallic a.* **tariric a.,** a complex organic acid, $C_{17}H_{31}COOH$, found in the seeds of *Picramnia,* a species of tropical American shrubs. **tartaric a.,** a white powder from the lees of wine and from various plants, 2,3-dihydroxysuccinic acid, $COOH(CHOH)_2COOH$. It is known in four forms: (*a*) ordinary or dextrotartaric acid; (*b*) levotartaric acid (these two are so called because their solutions rotate the plane of polarized light to the right and the left respectively); (*c*) paratartaric acid, a mixture of (*a*) and (*b*) hence optically inactive; and (*d*) mesotartaric acid, optically inactive from internal compensation. It is used in baking and tanning, and as a chemical reagent. **tartronic a.,** a dibasic acid, hydroxymalonic acid, $COOH \cdot CHOH \cdot COOH$, produced by the oxidation of glycerin or the ozonization of malonic acid. **taurocarbamic a.,** the form in which taurine when fed is excreted in the urine; it is taurine paired with carbamic acid, $NH_2 \cdot CO \cdot NH(CH_2)_2 \cdot SO_2OH$. **taurocholic a.,** one of the bile acids, $C_{26}H_{45}NSO_7$, formed by the conjugation of taurine and cholic acid. **taurylic a.,** a compound, $C_7H_{14}O$, found in urine. **teichoic a's,** antigenic polymers of glycerol or ribitol phosphates found attached to the cell walls or in intracellular association with membranes of gram-positive bacteria; they determine group specificity of some species, e.g., the staphylococci. **telluric a.,** an unstable dibasic and toxic acid, H_2TeO_4, readily reduced to tellurium; it is liberated in some smelting operations and may poison surrounding plant and animal life. **terebic a.,** a monobasic acid, $C_7H_{10}O_4$, from oxidizing turpentine. **ternary a.,** an acid which contains three distinct radicals; called also *oxacid.* **terrestric a.,** a tetronic acid, $C_{11}H_{14}O_4$, which is a metabolic product of *Penicillium terrestre.* **testicular nucleic a.,** an acid derivable from testicular nuclein. **tetraboric a.,** pyroboric a. **tetracosanic a.,** an acid, $C_{24}H_{48}O_2$, from phrenosin. **tetradeconic a.,** an acid occurring in small amounts in milk. **tetrahydrofolic a.,** the coenzyme of folic acid, being a reduced folic acid with four hydrogen atoms attached; in dissociated form, called *tetrahydrofolate.* **tetramethyluric a.,** a methylated purine found in tea, $C_9H_{12}N_4O_3$. **tetrodonic a.,** a poisonous acid from various fishes of the genus *Tetraodon.* **thapsic a.,** an acid said to occur in *Thapsia garganica.* **thebolactic a.,** the lactic acid found in opium. **thioacetic a.,** a colorless or yellowish liquid, CH_3COSH; called also *thiuretic a.* **β-thio-α-aminopropionic a.,** cysteine. **thiobarbituric a.,** a condensation of malonic acid and thiourea, $C_4H_4N_2O_2S$, differing from barbituric acid only by the presence of a sulfur atom instead of an oxygen atom at the number 2 carbon; it is the parent compound of a class of drugs, thiobarbiturates. Thiobarbiturates and barbiturates are analogous in their effects. **thioctic a.,** a naturally occurring acid used in growing bacterial cultures, and reported to be an antidote to mushroom (*Amanita*) poisoning; also prepared synthetically. **thiocyanic a.,** an unstable acid, HCNS; it forms salts called thiocyanates or sulfocyanides, which give a blood-red color with ferric salts. Called also *sulfocyanic a.* **thiolactic a.,** an acid, $CH_3CH(SH)COOH$, derived from keratin. **thionic a.,** any of a series of acids composed of hydrogen, sulfur, and oxygen. **thiopanic a.,** a compound, (dihydroxy dimethyl butyryl) taurine, $CH_2OH \cdot C(CH_3)_2 \cdot CHOH \cdot CO \cdot NH \cdot CH_2 \cdot CH_2 \cdot SO_2OH$, which inhibits bacterial growth in competition with pantothenic acid. **thiopyruvic a.,** one of the intermediary products in the metabolism of cysteines. **thiosalicylic a.,** chemical name: 2-mercaptobenzoic acid. A compound, $C_7H_6O_2S$, used in the manufacture of dyes and as a reagent for the determination of iron. **thiosulfuric a.,** a very unstable acid, $H_2S_2O_3$, not known in the free state, but which forms salts called thiosulfates; the sodium salt is the photographer's "hypo," which forms soluble complexes with silver halides and is a standard reducing agent in chemical analysis. **thiuretic a.,** thioacetic a. **thymic a.,** the residue left after partial acid hydrolysis of nucleic acid; it is a combination of phosphoric acid, carbohydrate, and pyrimidine bases. **thymidylic a.,** a mononucleotide with a thymine base, occurring in deoxyribonucleic acid, but not in ribonucleic acid. **thyminic a.,** an acid formed by the splitting up of deoxyribonucleic acid. **thymonucleic a., thymus nucleic a.,** deoxyribonucleic a. **tibric a.,** chemical name: 2-chloro-5-[(3,5-dimethyl-1-piperidinyl)sulfonyl]benzoic acid; an antihyperlipidemic, $C_{14}H_{18}ClNO_4S$. **tienilic a.,** ticrynafen. **tiglic a.,** an unsaturated acid, methyl crotonic acid, $CH_3 \cdot CH:C(CH_3) \cdot COOH$, the cis-isomer of angelic acid, found in croton oil. **toluic a.,** $CH_3 \cdot C_6H_4 \cdot COOH$, produced by the oxidation of xylene. **toluric a.,** the form in which toluic acid, paired with glycine, is excreted in the urine. **toxicodendric a.,** a volatile acid from *Rhus toxicodendron*, supposed to be poisonous. **tranexamic a.,** chemical name: *trans*-4-(aminomethyl)cyclohexanecarboxylic acid. An acid, $C_8H_{15}NO_2$, which acts as an antifibrinolytic agent by competitively inhibiting plasminogen; used as a hemostatic in the treatment of severe hemorrhage associated with excessive fibrinolysis. **traumatic a.,** chemical name: 2-dodecenedioic acid. An acid, $HOOC(CH_2)_8CH{=}CHCOOH$, which functions as a plant-wound hormone, stimulating the production of wound periderm. **triazoic a.,** a strong monobasic acid, HN_3, a colorless liquid with an unpleasant odor; it is explosive and forms salts called hydrazoates, azides, or trinitrides; its heavy-metal salts are used in detonators. Called also *hydrazoic a.* **tribasic a.,** an acid that has three replaceable hydrogen atoms. **trichlorethylglucuronic a.,** $CHCl_2 \cdot CHCl \cdot C_6H_9O_7$, the conjugated form of chloral hydrate, the form in which it is excreted in the urine. **trichloroacetic a.** [USP], a poisonous, extremely caustic acid, $C_2HCl_3O_2$, occurring as colorless, deliquescent crystals; used as a topical caustic for local destruction of lesions and for treatment of dermatological diseases. **tricyanic a.,** a crystalline acid, $C_3N_3(OH)_3$, formed when urea is heated dry. **trihydroxybenzoic a.,** gallic a. **triiodoethionic a.,** iophenoxic a. **trimethylaminoacetic a.,** methylated aminoacetic acid, $OH(CH_3)_3 \cdot N \cdot CH_2 \cdot COOH$; its anhydride is betaine. **triticonucleic a.,** the nucleic acid of the wheat embryo. **tropic a.,** a crystalline acid, alphaphenyl betahydroxy propionic acid, $C_6H_5 \cdot CH(CH_2OH) \cdot COOH$, obtained from atropine by digesting it with baryta water. **tuberculostearic a.,** an acid, $CH_3(CH_2)_7 \cdot CH(CH_3) \cdot (CH_2)_8 \cdot COOH$, isolated from the acetone-soluble lipid of tubercle bacilli. **tungstic a.,** a yellow crystalline compound, H_2WO_4, used as a source of metallic tungsten and as precipitant for many nitrogenous organic substances. **undecenoic a.,** undecylenic a. **undecylenic a.,** 1. chemical name: 10-undecenoic acid. A normal constituent of sweat, $C_{11}H_{20}O_2$, which may be prepared by heating castor oil. 2. [USP] a pharmaceutical preparation, occurring as a clear, colorless to pale yellow liquid, used in combination with zinc undecylenate or alone as a topical antifungal. **uramilic a.,** an acid, $C_8H_9N_5O_2$, obtained by treating uramil with sulfuric acid. **uraminoacetic a.,** glycoluric a. **uraminobenzoic a.,** an acid found in the urine after the ingestion of aminobenzoic acid; the latter is paired with carbamic acid, giving $NH_2 \cdot CO \cdot NH \cdot C_6H_4 \cdot COOH$. **uraminotauric a.,** a compound occurring in the urine after the administration of taurine. **uric a.,** a crystallizable acid, 2,6,8-trioxypurine, $C_5H_4N_4O_3$, from the urine of man and animals, being one of the products of nuclein metabolism and the end-product of purine metabolism in man. It is nearly insoluble in water, alcohol, and ether, but soluble in solutions of alkaline salts. In the form of its sodium salt (monosodium urate), it forms a large portion of certain calculi, and in the blood it causes morbid symptoms, among which are those of gout. Called also *lithic a.* **uridylic a.,** a pyrimidine nucleotide constituent of ribonucleic acid. **urobenzoic a.,** hippuric a. **urocanic a.,** an intermediate metabolite, $C_6H_6N_2O_2$, of histamine, convertible normally to glutamic acid. **urochloralic a., urochloric a.,** an acid, $C_{14}H_{12}Cl_2O_{12} \cdot [C_7H_{12}Cl_2O_6]$, found in the urine after the exhibition of chloral. **uroferric a.,** a substance found in urine. **uroleucic a.,** **uroleucinic a.,** a crystalline acid, $C_9H_{10}O_5$, found in the urine in alkaptonuria. **uronic a.,** any of certain aldehyde acids derived from simple sugars by oxidation of the alcohol end of the chain; see *glucuronic a.* and *galacturonic a.* **ursodeoxycholic a.,** a bile acid (an isomer of chenodeoxycholic acid) normally present only in small amounts in man; first isolated from the bile of bears [L. *ursus* bear], it is administered to dissolve cholesterol gallstones. **ursolic a.,** ursone. **usnic a.,** a complex organic acid occurring in the lichen, *Usnea barbata*. **uvitic a.,** a crystalline acid, methylisophthalic acid, $CH_3 \cdot C_6H_3 \cdot$

$(COOH)_2$, obtained by oxidizing mesitylene. **vaccenic a.,** an unsaturated fatty acid, $CH_3(CH_2)_5CH{:}CH(CH_2)_9 \cdot COOH$, isomeric with oleic acid; found in butterfat. **valerianic a.,** normal valeric a.; see under *valeric a.* **valeric a.,** an organic acid found in the roots of *Valeriana officinalis* and *Angelica archangelica*, and which may be synthesized in various ways. Called also *butyrcarboxylic a.* and *phoenic a.* There are four valeric acids: (*a*) normal valeric acid (valeric acid, pentanoic acid), $CH_3(CH_2)_3COOH$, (*b*) isovaleric acid, $(CH_3)_2CH \cdot CH_2 \cdot COOH$, (*c*) β-methylbutyric acid, $CH_3(C_2H_5) \cdot CH \cdot COOH$, and (*d*) trimethylacetic acid (pivalic acid), $(CH_3)_3 \cdot C \cdot COOH$. The salts were once considered medicinal. **valproic a.,** 2-propylpentanoic acid, $C_8H_{16}O_2$. A simple eight-carbon branched-chain fatty acid, it is used as an antiepileptic, especially for control of absence seizures. Its salt, valproate sodium, is used for the same purpose. **vanadic a.,** an acid, HVO_3, formed by the oxidation of vanadium; it may cause chronic poisoning. Called also *metavanadic a.* **vanillic a.,** an acid, $CH_3 \cdot O \cdot C_6H_3(OH)COOH$, obtained by the oxidation of vanillin; called also *methylprotocatechuic a.* **vanillic a. diethylamide,** ethamivan. **vanillylmandelic a.,** chemical name: 3-methoxy-4-hydroxymandelic acid; an excretory product of the catecholamines, used as a test for epinephrine metabolism. Abbreviated VMA. **veratric a.,** a white crystalline acid, 3,4-dimethoxybenzoic acid, $(CH_3 \cdot O)_2C_6H_3 \cdot COOH$, found in sabadilla seeds. **viburnic a.,** acid from the bark of *Viburnum prunifolium*, identical with valeric a. **violuric a.,** a barbituric acid compound, 5-isonitrosobarbituric acid, $OHN{:}C(CO \cdot NH)_2CO$. **vitamin A a.,** 1. retinoic a. 2. tretinoin. **vulpic a., vulpinic a.,** a yellow crystalline acid, $C_{19}H_{14}O_5$, from the lichen, *Cetraria vulpina*; called also *pulvinic a. methyl ester.* **xanthic a.,** an oily liquid, $C_2H_5O \cdot CS \cdot SH$, with a penetrating odor; called also *xanthogenic a.* **xanthogenic a.,** xanthic a. **xanthoproteic a.,** a yellow compound obtained by treating protein with nitric acid. **xanthurenic a.,** chemical name: 4,8-dihydroxyquinaldic acid. A metabolite, $C_9H_5N(OH)_2COOH_2$, of L-tryptophan, present in normal urine and found in increased amounts in vitamin B_6 deficiency; L-kynurenine is a precursor. **xanthylic a.,** one of the nucleic acids. **xanthylicnucleic a.,** a nucleic acid which may be made to afford xanthine. **xylic a.,** a crystalline acid, dimethylbenzoic acid, $(CH_3)_2C_6H_3 \cdot COOH$. **xylidic a.,** a dibasic acid, methylisophthalic acid, $CH_3 \cdot C_6H_3 \cdot (COOH)_2$. **xylonic a.,** one of the isomeric forms of tetrahydroxyvaleric acid, $CH_2OH(CHOH)_3COOH$, formed by the gentle oxidation of xylose. **yeast nucleic a.,** ribonucleic a.

acidalbumin (as″id-al′bu-min) a protein that dissolves in acids and shows an acid reaction.

acidaminuria (as″id-am″ĭ-nu′re-ah) aminoaciduria.

acidemia (as″ĭ-de′me-ah) [*acid* + Gr. *haima* blood + *-ia*] a decreased pH (increased hydrogen ion concentration) of the blood. **argininosuccinic a.,** argininosuccinicaciduria. **isovaleric a.,** an inborn error of leucine metabolism characterized by high levels of isovaleric acid in the blood, periodic acidosis with coma, objectionable body odor, and psychomotor retardation. **methylmalonic a.,** an inborn error of metabolism characterized by excretion of excessive amounts of methylmalonic acid in the urine, recurrent vomiting, failure to thrive, developmental retardation, hepatomegaly, intermittent neutropenia, and thrombocytopenia, and often by severe metabolic acidosis. It is due to an inability to convert D- to L-methylmalonyl CoA or of the latter to succinyl CoA or to a defect in the metabolism of vitamin B_{12}. **propionic a.,** an excess of propionic acid in the blood, due to failure of activity of propionyl-CoA carboxylase and characterized by ketosis, acidosis, and hyperglycinemia and, in the absence of dietary controls, by developmental retardation, ECG abnormalities, and osteoporosis.

acid-fast (as′id-fast) not readily decolorized by acids when stained, a characteristic of mycobacteria stained by the Ziehl-Neelsen procedure.

acidic (ah-sid′ik) of or pertaining to an acid; acid-forming.

acidifiable (ah-sid′ĭ-fi″ah-b′l) susceptible of being made acid.

acidifier (ah-sid″ĭ-fi′er) an agent that causes acidity; a substance used to increase gastric acidity.

acidify (ah-sid′ĭ-fi) 1. to render acid, as by addition of a strong acid. 2. to become acid.

acidimeter (as″ĭ-dim′ĕ-ter) [L. *acidum* acid + Gr. *metron* measure] an instrument used in performing acidimetry.

acidimetry (as-ĭ-dim′ĕ-tre) the determination of the amount of free acid in a solution.

acidism (as′ĭ-dizm) a condition due to introduction into the body of acids from outside; called also *acidismus*.

acidismus (as″ĭ-diz′mus) acidism.

acidity (ah-sid′ĭ-te) [L. *aciditas*] the quality of being acid or sour; containing acid (hydrogen ions).

acidocyte (as′ĭ-do-sīt″) (*obs.*) 1. an acidophilic cell. 2. eosinophil.

acidogenic (as″ĭ-do-jen′ik) producing acid or acidity, especially acidity of the urine.

Acidol (a′sĭ-dol) trademark for a preparation of betaine hydrochloride.

acidology (as″ĭ-dol′o-je) [Gr. *akis* bandage + *-logy*] the science of surgical appliances.

acidophil (as′id-o-fil″) [L. *acidum* acid + Gr. *philein* to love] 1. a structure, cell, or other histologic element staining readily with acid dyes. 2. an alpha cell of the adenohypophysis; see also *carminophil* and *orangeophil*. 3. an organism that grows well in highly acid media. 4. acidophilic. **alpha a.,** orangeophil, def. 3. **epsilon a.,** carminophil, def. 3.

acidophile (as′id-o-fīl″) acidophil.

acidophilic (as″ĭ-do-fil′ik) 1. readily stained with acid dyes. 2. growing in highly acid media; said of microorganisms.

acidophilism (as″ĭ-dof′ĭ-lizm) the condition produced by acidophilic adenoma of the pituitary, resulting in acromegaly.

acidosic (as″ĭ-do′sik) acidotic.

acidosis (as″ĭ-do′sis) a pathologic condition resulting from accumulation of acid or depletion of the alkaline reserve (bicarbonate content) in the blood and body tissues, and characterized by an increase in hydrogen ion concentration (decrease in pH). Cf. *alkalosis*. **compensated a.,** a condition in which the compensatory mechanisms have returned the pH toward normal; see *metabolic a., compensated,* and *respiratory a., compensated*. **diabetic a.,** a variety of metabolic acidosis produced by accumulation of ketone bodies resulting from uncontrolled diabetes mellitus. **hypercapnic a.,** respiratory a. **hyperchloremic a.,** metabolic acidosis accompanied by elevated plasma chloride. **metabolic a.,** a disturbance in which the acid-base status of the body shifts toward the acid side because of loss of base or retention of noncarbonic, or fixed (nonvolatile), acids; called also *nonrespiratory a*. **metabolic a., compensated,** a state of metabolic acidosis in which the pH of the blood has been returned toward normal by respiratory compensatory mechanisms. **nonrespiratory a.,** metabolic a. **renal hyperchloremia a.,** renal tubular a. **renal tubular a.,** a variety of metabolic acidosis resulting from impairment of renal function. **respiratory a.,** a state due to excess retention of carbon dioxide in the body; called also *hypercapnic a*. **respiratory a., compensated,** respiratory acidosis in which the pH of the blood has been returned toward normal by renal compensatory mechanisms. **starvation a.,** a variety of metabolic acidosis produced by accumulation of ketone bodies which may accompany a caloric deficit. **uremic a.,** the condition in chronic renal disease in which the ability to excrete acid is decreased, causing acidosis.

acidosteophyte (as″ĭ-dos′te-o-fīt″) [Gr. *akis* point + *osteon* bone + *phyton* plant] a sharp-pointed osteophyte.

acidotic (as″ĭ-dot′ik) pertaining to or characterized by acidosis.

acidulated (ah-sid′u-lāt″ed) rendered acid in reaction.

Acidulin (ah-sid′u-lin) trademark for a preparation of glutamic acid hydrochloride.

acidulous (ah-sid′u-lus) somewhat acid.

acidum (as′ĭ-dum) [L.] acid (def. 2).

aciduria (as″ĭ-du′re-ah) the presence of acid in the urine. **acetoacetic a.,** diaceturia. **beta-aminoisobutyric a.,** excessive excretion of β-aminoisobutyric acid in the urine; it occurs as a benign genetic metabolic variant and in certain illnesses. **methylmalonic a.,** excretion of excessive amounts of methylmalonic acid in the urine; a characteristic symptom of methylmalonic acidemia. **orotic a.,** a hereditary disorder, transmitted as an autosomal recessive trait, in which a defect in the metabolism of pyrimidines is associated with excessive excretion of orotic acid in the urine, characterized by megaloblastic anemia, crystalluria, and frequently physical and mental retardation. **pyroglutamic a.,** 5-oxoprolinuria.

aciduric (as″ĭ-du′rik) [L. *acidum* acid + *durare* to endure] acid-tolerant; said of bacteria which are able to withstand a degree of acidity usually fatal to nonsporulating bacteria.

acidyl (as′ĭ-dil) any acid radical.

acidylation (ah-sid″ĭ-la′shun) acylation.

acies (a′se-ēz) [L.] edge, margin, or border. **a. thal′ami op′tici** (*obs.*), stria medullaris thalami.

acinar (as′ĭ-nar) pertaining to or affecting an acinus or acini.

acinesia (as″ĭ-ne′ze-ah) akinesia.

acinetic (as″ĭ-net′ik) akinetic (def. 1).

Acinetobacter (as″ĭ-net″o-bak′ter) [*a* neg. + Gr. *kinētos* movable + *bactērion* rod] a genus of nonmotile, paired, gram-negative bacilli widely distributed in nature. **A. anitra′tus,** *Herellea vaginicola*. **A. lwof′fi,** *Mima polymorpha*.

acini (as′ĭ-ni) [L.] plural of *acinus*.

acinic (ah-sin′ik) pertaining to an acinus.

aciniform (ah-sin′ĭ-form) [L. *acinus* grape + *forma* form] shaped like an acinus, or grape.

acinitis (as″ĭ-ni′tis) inflammation of the acini of a gland.

acinitrazole (as″ĭ-ni′tro-zōl) aminitrozole.

acinose (as′ĭ-nōs) [L. *acinosus* grape-like] 1. made up of acini. 2. acinar.

acinotubular (as″ĭ-no-tu′bu-lar) composed of tubular acini or of tubules ending in acini.

acinous (as′ĭ-nus) 1. resembling a grape. 2. acinar.

acinus (as′ĭ-nus), pl. *ac′ini* [L. "grape"] a general term used in anatomical nomenclature to designate a small saclike dilatation, particularly one found in various glands; see also *alveolus*. **a. liena′lis, a. lie′nis,** folliculi lymphatici lienales. **liver a.,** a functional unit of the liver, smaller than a portal lobule, being a diamond-shaped mass of liver parenchyma that is supplied by a terminal branch of the portal vein and of the hepatic artery and drained by a terminal branch of the bile duct. **a. rena′lis [malpig′hii],** corpuscula renis. **a. re′nis [malpig′hii],** corpuscula renis.

acipenserin (as″ĭ-pen′ser-in) a toxic substance from the gonads of the sturgeon, *Acipenser*.

ackee (ah′ke) akee.

acladiosis (ak-lad″e-o′sis) an ulcerative dermatomycosis caused by *Acladium castellani*, occurring in Ceylon, the Malay States, and Macedonia, and marked by the formation of roundish or oval ulcers with sharply defined edges and a granulating fundus.

Acladium (ah-kla′de-um) a genus of imperfect fungi of the family Moniliaceae, order Moniliales, sometimes found in human infection; possibly identical with *Olpitrichum* or *Oidium*.

aclasia (ah-kla′ze-ah) aclasis.

aclasis (ah′klah-sis) [*a* neg. + Gr. *klasis* a breaking] pathologic continuity of structure, as in dyschondroplasia. **diaphyseal a.,** enchondromatosis. **tarsoepiphyseal a.,** dysplasia epiphysealis hemimelica.

aclastic (a-klas′tik) [*a* neg. + Gr. *klan* to break] 1. pertaining to or characterized by aclasis. 2. not refracting.

acleistocardia (ah-klīs″to-kar′de-ah) [*a* neg. + Gr. *kleistos* closed + *kardia* heart] an open condition of the foramen ovale cordis.

aclusion (ah-klu′zhun) [*a* neg. + *occlusion*] (*obs.*) open bite.

acmastic (ak-mas′tik) (*obs.*) pertaining to acme; having a period of increase (*epacmastic*) followed by a period of decline (*paracmastic*).

acme (ak′me) [Gr. *akmē* point] the crisis or critical stage of a disease.

acmesthesia (ak″mes-the′ze-ah) [Gr. *akmē* + *aisthēsis* perception + *-ia*] a sensation of a sharp point touching the skin.

acne (ak′ne) [possibly a corruption of Greek *akmē* a point or of *achnē* chaff] an inflammatory disease of the pilosebaceous unit, the specific type usually being indicated by a modifying term; frequently used alone to designate common acne, or *acne vulgaris*. **a. agmina′ta** (*obs.*), papulonecrotic tuberculid. **a. al′bida** (*obs.*), milium. **a. atroph′ica,** acne in which, after the disappearance of small papular lesions, there is left a stippling of tiny atrophic pits and scars. **beatle a.,** seborrheic dermatitis. **bromide a.,** an acneiform eruption without comedones, one of the most constant symptoms of brominism. **a. cachectico′rum** (Hebra), a form of acne which may accompany wasting diseases or rapid growth; the pustular lesions are soft, scarcely infiltrated, and almost lacking in inflammatory reaction. **chlorine a.,** chloracne. **common a.,** a. vulgaris. **a. conglobu′ta,** a form of acne characterized by the presence of numerous comedones, marked suppuration, the formation of cysts and sinuses, and severe scarring. **contagious a.,** a contagious skin disease of horses caused by *Corynebacterium* or *Staphylococcus* and characterized by the formation of pustules which when ruptured release a sticky pus that rapidly dries and leaves a yellow crust. **cystic a.,** acne with the formation of cysts enclosing a mixture of keratin and sebum in varying proportions. **a. erythemato′sa,** rosacea. **a. excoriée des jeunes filles,** Brocq's name for a superficial acne of the face of girls caused chiefly by the patient's picking at and squeezing out small blackheads. **a. fronta′lis,** a. varioliformis. **a. ful′minans,** a rare form affecting teenage males, marked by sudden onset of fever and eruption of highly inflammatory, tender, ulcerative, and crusted lesions on the back, chest, and face. **halogen a.,** acne caused by the use of or exposure to halogens (such as chlorine, bromine, or iodine, or their salts) or chloronaphthalene. **halowax a.,** chloracne. **a. hordeola′ris** (*obs.*), acne in which the tubercles are hard, tough, and arranged in rows. **a. indura′ta,** a progression of papular acne, with deep-seated and destructive lesions that may produce severe scarring. **iodide a.,** an eruption caused by the use of iodine compounds. **a. keloid,** keloidal folliculitis. **a. kerato′sa,** acne characterized by horny conical plugs, typically at the angles of the mouth, which become inflamed. **a. necrot′ica milia′ris,** a rare and chronic form of folliculitis of the scalp, occurring principally in adults, with formation of tiny superficial pustules which are destroyed by scratching. See also *a. varioliformis*. **a. neonato′rum,** a condition found in newborn infants with oily skins, characterized by comedones, papules, and pustules on nose, cheeks, and forehead. **a. papulo′sa,** acne vulgaris in which the lesions are papular. **petroleum a.,** acne-like lesions sometimes seen in petroleum workers. **a. picea′lis,** a form of acne caused by contact with tar or exposure to its vapors. **premenstrual a.,** acne of a cyclic nature, appearing shortly before (rarely after) the onset of menses. **a. pustulo′sa,** acne in which the lesions show central suppuration. **a. rosa′cea,** rosacea. **a. scorbu′tica** (*obs.*), a papular eruption in scurvy.

a. scrofuloso′rum (Bazin), papulonecrotic tuberculid. **a. syphilit′ica** (*obs.*), an acuminated pustular syphiloderm. **tropical a., a. tropica′lis,** a severe and extensive form of acne occurring in hot, humid climates, characterized by nodular, cystic, and pustular lesions chiefly on the back, buttocks, and thighs. Conglobate abscesses frequently form, especially on the back. **a. urtica′ta,** an acneiform eruption characterized by edematous papular wheals, resembling acne papules. **a. variolifor′mis,** a rare condition, with persistent brown papulopustules, usually localized to the brow and scalp; probably a deep variant of acne necrotica miliaris. Called also *a. frontalis* and *folliculitis varioliformis.* **a. vulga′ris,** a chronic inflammatory disease of the pilosebaceous apparatus, the lesions occurring most frequently on the face, chest, and back. The inflamed glands may form small pink papules, which sometimes surround comedones so that they have black centers, or form pustules or cysts; the cause is unknown, but it has been suggested that many factors, including certain foods, stress, hereditary factors, hormones, drugs, and bacteria, especially *Corynebacterium acnes, Staphylococcus albus,* and *Pityrosporon ovale,* play an etiologic role. Called also *common a.*

acneform (ak′ne-form) acneiforⁿn.

acnegen (ak′ne-jen) a substance that causes acne.

acnegenic (ak″ne-jen′ik) [*acne* + Gr. *gennan* to produce] causing or capable of producing acne.

acneiform (ak-ne′ĭ-form″) resembling acne.

acnemia (ak-ne′me-ah) [*a* neg. + Gr. *knēmē* leg] atrophy of the calves of the legs.

acnitis (ak-ni′tis) papulonecrotic tuberculid.

acnitrazole (ak-ni′trah-zōl) aminitrozole.

A.C.N.M. American College of Nurse-Midwives; see *nurse-midwife* and *nurse-midwifery.*

acoasma (a″ko-as′mah) acousma.

Acocanthera (ak″o-kan-the′rah) [Gr. *akōkē* a point, edge + *anthēros* blooming] a genus of apocynaceous plants of African origin whose members yield a juice from stems and leaves which is used by natives to prepare arrow poison. *A. schimperi* (A.D.C.) Schwf. and other species yield the toxic glycoside ouabain (acocantherin).

acocantherin (ak″o-kan′ther-in) ouabain.

Acoela (ah-se′lah) an order of the class Turbellaria, made up of minute marine flatworms with no intestines that receive food into a porous mass of endodermal tissue.

acoelomate (ah-sēl′o-māt) 1. lacking a body cavity. 2. an animal lacking a body cavity, as the platyhelminths.

acoenesthesia (ah-sen″es-the′ze-ah) acenesthesia.

A.C.O.G. American College of Obstetricians and Gynecologists.

acognosia (ak″og-no′se-ah) [Gr. *akos* cure + *gnōsis* knowledge] knowledge of or study of remedies.

acognosy (ah-kog′no-se) acognosia.

A.C.O.H.A. American College of Osteopathic Hospital Administrators.

Acokanthera (ak″o-kan-the′rah) *Acocanthera.*

acology (ah-kol′o-je) [Gr. *akos* cure + *-logy*] the science of remedies; therapeutics, def. 1.

acomia (ah-ko′me-ah) [*a* neg. + Gr. *komē* hair + *-ia*] (*obs.*) baldness.

Acon (a′kon) trademark for a preparation of vitamin A.

aconative (ah-kon′ah-tiv) without conation; not involving desire or volition.

aconine (ak′o-nin) an alkaloid, $C_{25}H_{41}NO_9$, from aconitine, much less toxic than aconitine.

aconitase (ah-kon′ĭ-tās) an enzyme that catalyzes the transformation of citric acid into cisaconitic acid and l-isocitric acid.

aconite (ak′o-nīt) [L *aconitum;* Gr. *akoniton*] a poisonous drug, from the dried tuberous root of *Aconitum napellus,* which contains several closely related alkaloids, the major one being aconitine. It was once given internally as a febrifuge and gastric anesthetic. Called also *monkshood* and *wolfsbane.*

aconitine (ah-kon′ĭ-tin) [L. *aconitina, aconitia*] a poisonous white crystalline alkaloid, $C_{34}H_{47}O_{11}N$, the active principle of aconite.

Aconitum (ak-o-ni′tum), gen. *aconi′ti* [L.] a genus of poisonous ranunculaceous herbs; *A. napellus* is the source of aconite.

aconuresis (ak″on-u-re′sis) [Gr. *akōn* unwilling + *ourēsis* urination] the involuntary passage of urine.

A.C.O.O.G. American College of Osteopathic Obstetricians and Gynecologists.

acoprosis (ak″o-pro′sis) [*a* neg. + Gr. *kopros* excrement] absence of fecal matter from the intestine.

acoprous (ah-kop′rus) having no fecal matter in the intestine.

acor (a′kor) [L.] 1. acidity. 2. acrimony or bitterness.

acorea (ah″ko-re′ah) [*a* neg. + Gr. *korē* pupil] absence of the pupil of the eye.

acoria (ah-ko′re-ah) [*a* neg. + Gr. *koros* satiety + *-ia*] a form of polyphagia due to loss of the sensation of satiety, a condition in which the patient never feels that he has enough, although the appetite may not be large.

acorin (ak′o-rin) a bitter glycoside, $C_{36}H_{60}O_6$, from calamus; it splits into oil of calamus and sugar.

acortan (a-kor′tan) corticotropin.

Acorus (ak′o-rus) [L.; Gr. *akoros*] a genus of araceous plants; see *calamus,* def. 2.

A.C.O.S. American College of Osteopathic Surgeons.

acosmia (a-koz′me-ah) [*a* neg. + Gr. *kosmos* order + *-ia*] (*obs.*) ill health.

Acosta′s disease (ah-kos′tas) [José d′Acosta, 1539–1600, a Jesuit priest who first described it after his travels in Peru in 1590] acute mountain sickness.

acou- [Gr. *akouein* to hear] a combining form denoting relationship to hearing.

acouasm (ah-koo′azm) acousma.

acousma (ah-kōōs′mah), pl. *acous′mata* [Gr. *akousma* a thing heard] (*obs.*) an auditory hallucination or imaginary sound.

acousmatamnesia (ah-kōōs″mat-am-ne′ze-ah) [Gr. *akousma* hearing + *amnēsia* forgetfulness] failure of the memory to call up the images of sounds.

acoustic (ah-kōōs′tik) [Gr. *akoustikos*] pertaining to sound.

Acousticon (ah-koo′stĕ-kon) trademark for an apparatus for a hearing aid.

acousticophobia (ah-koos″tĕ-ko-fo′be-ah) [Gr. *akoustos* heard + *phobia*] morbid fear of sounds.

acoustics (ah-kōōs′tiks) the science of sounds.

acoustigram (ah-koos′tĭ-gram) acoustogram.

acoustogram (ah-koos′to-gram) the graphic tracing of the curves, delineated in frequencies per second and decibel levels, of sounds produced by motion of a joint. Applied to the knee joint, an acoustogram will show the sound of the moving semilunar cartilages, the moving contact between the articular surfaces of the femur and tibia, and the circulation of the synovia.

A.C.P. American College of Pathologists.

acquired (ah-kwīrd′) [L. *acquirere* to obtain] not genetic, but produced by influences originating outside the organism.

acquisition (ah″kwĭ-zĭ′shun) in psychology, the period in learning during which progressive increments in response strength can be measured. Also the process involved in such learning.

acquisitus (ah-kwis′ĕ-tus) [L.] acquired.

A.C.R. American College of Radiology.

acragnosis (ak″rag-no′sis) acroagnosis.

acral (ak′ral) [Gr. *akron* extremity] pertaining to an extremity or apex; affecting the extremities.

acrania (ah-kra′ne-ah) [*a* neg. + Gr. *kranion* skull + *-ia*] a developmental anomaly characterized by partial or complete absence of the cranium, or skull.

acranial (ah-kra′ne-al) having no cranium.

Acraniata (ah-kra″ne-a′tah) a subphylum of Chordata comprising species without a true skull.

acranius (ah-kra′ne-us) a monster exhibiting acrania.

acrasia (ah-kra′ze-ah) (*obs.*) lack of self-control; intemperance.

acratia (ah-kra′she-ah) [*a* neg. + Gr. *kratos* power + *-ia*] (*obs.*) loss of power or strength.

acraturesis (ah-krat″u-re′sis) [Gr. *akratēs* feeble + *ourēsis* urination] difficult urination due to atony of the bladder or to obstruction of the urethra, as in prostatism.

Acree-Rosenheim reagent, test (reaction) (ak′re-ro′zen-hīm) [Solomon Farley *Acree,* American chemist, born 1875; Otto *Rosenheim,* London scientist] see under *reagent* and *tests.*

Acrel′s ganglion (ak′relz) [Olof (or Olaf) *Acrel,* Swedish surgeon, 1717–1806] see under *ganglion.*

Acremoniella (ak″rĕ-mo-ne-el′ah) a genus of dematiacious imperfect fungi of the order Moniliales, resembling *Acremonium;* reportedly isolated from lesions of the lung.

acremoniosis (ak″rĕ-mo-ne-o′sis) infection with the fungus *Acremonium,* producing a state marked by fever and the formation of gumma-like swellings.

Acremonium (ak″rĕ-mo′ne-um) a genus of imperfect fungi of the family Moniliaceae, order Moniliales, rarely isolated from human infection. **A. kilien′se,** an etiologic agent of white mycetoma in South and Central America; called also *Cephalosporium falciforme.*

acribometer (ak″rĭ-bom′ĕ-ter) [Gr. *akribēs* exact + *metron* measure] an instrument for measuring minute objects.

acrid (ak′rid) [L. *acer, acris* sharp] pungent; producing an irritation.

acridine (ak′rĭ-din) a dibenzopyridine, $CH:(C_6H_4)_2:N$, used in the synthesis of dyes and drugs; its derivatives are mostly fluorescent yellow dyes (acridine dyes), and those used in medicine (as antiseptic agents) are acriflavine hydrochloride, acriflavine base, and proflavine. **a. orange,** tetramethyl acridine, CH-

[N(CH₃)₂C₆H₃]₂N, a fluorescent basic dye; sometimes used for vital staining.

acriflavine (ak″rĭ-fla′vin) a mixture of 3,6-diamino-10-methyl-acridinium chloride and 3,6-diaminoacridine, occurring as a deep orange granular powder; used in solution as a topical antiseptic for the skin and mucous membranes, and has been used orally as a urinary antiseptic. Called also *chromoflavine, euflavine, neutral acriflavine,* and *neutroflavine.* **a. hydrochloride,** a mixture of the hydrochloride salts of 3,6-diamino-10-methylacridinium chloride and 3,6-diaminoacridine, occurring as a brownish red, crystalline powder; used like the base. This substance was originally prepared by Benda in 1911 for use in trypanosomiasis, and was by him given the name of *trypaflavine.* It has also been called *flavine.* Its use is rapidly diminishing in modern medicine. **neutral a.,** acriflavine.

acrimony (ak′rĭ-mo″ne) [L. *acrimonia*] an acrid quality, property, or condition; called also *acor.*

acrinyl sulfocyanate (ak-ri′nil sul″fo-si′ah-nāt) an acrid vesicating principle found in white mustard.

acrisia (ah-kri′se-ah) (*obs.*) uncertainty about the diagnosis and, especially, about the prognosis of a disease.

acrisorcin (ak-rĭ-sor′sin) [USP] chemical name: 4-hexyl-1,3-benzenediol compound with 9-acridinamine. A salt of aminacrine and hexylresorcinol, C₁₂H₁₈O₂·C₁₃H₁₀N₂, occurring as a yellow powder; used as a local antifungal, applied topically in the treatment of tinea versicolor.

acritical (ah-krit′ĭ-kal) [*a* neg. + Gr. *krisis* a crisis] having no crisis, said especially of febrile diseases ending by lysis.

acritochromacy (ah-krit″o-kro′mah-se) [*a* neg. + Gr. *krinein* to judge + *chrōma* color] defective perception of color.

acro- (ak′ro) [Gr. *akron* extremity; *akros* extreme] a combining form denoting relation to an extremity, top, or summit, or to an extreme.

acroagnosis (ak″ro-ag-no′sis) [*acro-* + *a* neg. + Gr. *gnōsis* knowledge] lack of sensory recognition of a limb; lack of acrognosis. Called also *acragnosis.*

acroanesthesia (ak″ro-an″es-the′ze-ah) [*acro-* + *anesthesia*] loss of sensation in the extremities.

acroarthritis (ak″ro-ar-thri′tis) [*acro-* + *arthritis*] arthritis affecting the extremities.

acroasphyxia (ak″ro-as-fik′se-ah) [*acro-* + *asphyxia*] (*obs.*) acrocyanosis.

acroblast (ak′ro-blast) [*acro-* + Gr. *blastos* germ] Golgi material in the spermatid from which arises the acrosome.

acrobrachycephaly (ak″ro-brak″ĕ-sef′ah-le) [*acro-* + Gr. *brachys* short + *kephalē* head] a condition resulting from fusion of the coronal suture, causing abnormal shortening of the anteroposterior diameter of the skull.

acrobystiolith (ak″ro-bis′te-o-lith) [Gr. *akrobystia* prepuce + *lithos* stone] postholith.

acrobystitis (ak″ro-bis-ti′tis) [Gr. *akrobystia* prepuce + *-itis*] inflammation of the prepuce.

acrocentric (ak″ro-sen′trik) [*acro-* + Gr. *kentron,* L. *centrum* center] having the centromere near one end of the replicating chromosome, so that one arm is much longer than the other. Cf. *metacentric* and *submetacentric.*

acrocephalia (ak″ro-sĕ-fa′le-ah) [Gr. *akra* point + *kephalē* head + *-ia*] oxycephaly.

acrocephalic (ak″ro-sĕ-fal′ik) oxycephalic.

acrocephalopolysyndactyly (ak″ro-sef″ah-lo-pol″e-sin-dak′-tĭ-le) [*acrocephaly* + *polysyndactyly*] acrocephalosyndactyly (Apert's syndrome) with polydactyly as an additional feature. Two types are known: *type I,* the typical form (Noack's syndrome) is transmitted as an autosomal dominant trait, and *type II* (see *Carpenter's syndrome,* under *syndrome*) is transmitted as an autosomal recessive trait.

acrocephalosyndactylia (ak″ro-sef″ah-lo-sin″dak-til′e-ah) acrocephalosyndactyly.

acrocephalosyndactylism (ak″ro-sef″ah-lo-sin-dak′tĭ-lizm) acrocephalosyndactyly.

acrocephalosyndactyly (ak″ro-sef″ah-lo-sin-dak′tĭ-le) [*acrocephaly* + *syndactyly*] craniostenosis characterized by acrocephaly associated with syndactyly. Called also *acrocephalosyndactyly type I* and *Apert's disease* or *syndrome.* It also occurs in combination with a variety of other anomalies, which have been designated: *Apert-Crouzon disease* (type II), *Chotzen's syndrome* (type III), *Waardenburg's syndrome,* def. 2 (type IV), and *Pfeiffer's syndrome* (type V). See also *acrocephalopolysyndactyly.*

acrocephalous (ak″ro-sef′ah-lus) oxycephalic.

acrocephaly (ak″ro-sef′ah-le) oxycephaly. **a.-syndactyly,** acrocephalosyndactyly.

acrochordon (ak″ro-kor′don) [*acro-* + Gr. *chordē* string] a soft pendulous growth, usually occurring on the neck, eyelids, or axillary or intercrural areas, consisting of a pedunculated excrescence of normal epidermis and dermis.

acrocinesis (ak″ro-si-ne′sis) [*acro-* + Gr. *kinēsis* motion] excessive motility; abnormal freedom of movement. Called also *acrokinesia.*

acrocinetic (ak″ro-si-net′ik) affected with acrocinesis.

acrocontracture (ak″ro-kon-trak′chūr) [*acro-* + *contracture*] contracture of an extremity; contracture of muscles of the hand or foot.

acrocyanosis (ak″ro-si″ah-no′sis) [*acro-* + *cyanosis*] a condition marked by symmetrical cyanosis of the extremities, with persistent, uneven, mottled blue or red discoloration of the skin of the digits, wrists, and ankles and with profuse sweating and coldness of the digits. Called also *Raynaud's sign.*

acrodermatitis (ak″ro-der″mah-ti′tis) [*acro-* + *dermatitis*] inflammation of the skin of the hands or feet. **a. chron′ica atroph′icans,** a diffuse idiopathic atrophy of the skin, usually confined to the extremities and occurring in two phases: the early, erythematous, edematous phase, and the more characteristic later, atrophic phase. **a. contin′ua,** a chronic inflammation of the skin of the extremities, in some cases becoming more generalized; regarded by many as a variant of inverse or flexural (volar) psoriasis. Called also *Hallopeau's a., a. perstans,* and *dermatitis repens.* **a. enteropath′ica,** a severe gastrointestinal and cutaneous disease of early childhood, due to an autosomal recessive disorder of zinc uptake and characterized by a vesiculo-pustulous dermatitis, preferentially located around the body orifices and on the head, hands, and feet, with diarrhea, true steatorrhea, and loss of hair. **Hallopeau's a.,** a. continua. **infantile lichenoid a., infantile papular a.,** Gianotti-Crosti syndrome. **a. papulo′sa infan′tum,** Gianotti-Crosti syndrome. **a. per′stans,** a. continua.

acrodermatoses (ak″ro-der″mah-to′sēz) plural of *acrodermatosis.*

acrodermatosis (ak″ro-der″mah-to′sis), pl. *acrodermato′ses* [*acro-* + *dermatosis*] any disease of the skin of the hands or feet.

acrodolichomelia (ak″ro-dol″ĕ-ko-me′le-ah) [*acro-* + Gr. *dolichos* long + *melos* limb + *-ia*] abnormal or disproportionate length of hands and feet.

acrodont (ak′ro-dont) [*acro-* + Gr. *odous* tooth] having the teeth attached to the upper surface of the jaw rather than encased in a socket, a condition seen in many lizards.

acrodynia (ak″ro-din′e-ah) [*acro-* + Gr. *odynē* pain + *-ia*] a disease of infancy and early childhood characterized by pain and swelling in, and pink coloration of, the fingers and toes, and by listlessness, irritability, failure to thrive, generalized inconstant rashes, profuse perspiration, photophobia, loss of teeth, and sometimes scarlet coloration of cheeks and tip of nose; repeated ingestion of or contact with mercury is a possible cause, and individual sensitivity may also be a factor. Called also *erythredema polyneuropathy* and *pink disease.* **rat a.,** a condition in rats, dogs, and pigs due to deficiency of pyridoxine, and marked by swelling and necrosis of the paws, the tips of ears and nose, and the lips.

acrodysplasia (ak″ro-dis-pla′se-ah) acrocephalosyndactyly.

acroedema (ak″ro-ĕ-de′mah) [*acro-* + *edema*] (*obs.*) permanent edema of the hand or foot.

acroesthesia (ak″ro-es-the′ze-ah) [*acro-* + Gr. *aisthēsis* sensation + *-ia*] 1. increased sensitiveness. 2. pain in the extremities.

acrognosis (ak″rog-no′sis) [*acro-* + Gr. *gnōsis* knowledge] sensory recognition of the limbs and of the different portions of each limb in relation to each other; limb knowledge.

acrohypothermy (ak″ro-hi″po-ther′me) [*acro-* + Gr. *hypo* under + *thermē* heat] abnormal coldness of the hands and feet.

acrohysterosalpingectomy (ak″ro-his″ter-o-sal″pin-jek′to-me) [*acro-* + Gr. *hystera* uterus + *salpinx* tube + *ektomē* excision] excision of both fallopian tubes and part of the fundus uteri; formerly done for pelvic inflammatory disease.

acrokeratosis (ak″ro-ker″ah-to′sis) a condition involving the skin of the extremities, with the appearance of horny growths. **a. verrucifor′mis,** a condition resembling epidermodysplasia verruciformis, but with the lesions appearing chiefly on the palms and soles, and not on the face.

acrokinesia (ak″ro-ki-ne′ze-ah) acrocinesis.

acrolein (ak-ro′le-in) [L. *acer* acrid + *oleum* oil] a volatile acrid liquid, CH₂:CHCHO, from the decomposition of glycerin; called also *acrylic aldehyde, acryaldehyde,* and *allyl aldehyde.*

acromacria (ak″ro-mak′re-ah) [*acro-* + Gr. *makros* long] arachnodactyly.

acromania (ak″ro-ma′ne-ah) [*acro-* + Gr. *mania* madness] mania marked by great motor activity.

acromastitis (ak″ro-mas-ti′tis) [*acro-* + Gr. *mastos* mamma + *-itis*] inflammation of the nipple.

acromegalia (ak″ro-mĕ-ga′le-ah) acromegaly.

acromegalic (ak″ro-mĕ-gal′ik) pertaining to or characterized by acromegaly.

acromegalogigantism (ak″ro-meg″ah-lo-ji′gan-tizm) gigantism and acromegaly due to hypersecretion of the pituitary growth hormone beginning before puberty and continuing into maturity.

acromegaloidism (ak"ro-meg'ah-loid-izm) a bodily condition resembling acromegaly but not due to pituitary disorder.

acromegaly (ak"ro-meg'ah-le) [*acro-* + Gr. *megalē* great] a condition caused by hypersecretion of the pituitary growth hormone after maturity and characterized by enlargement of the extremities of the skeleton—the nose, jaws, fingers, and toes; the converse of acromicria. Called also *Marie's disease.*

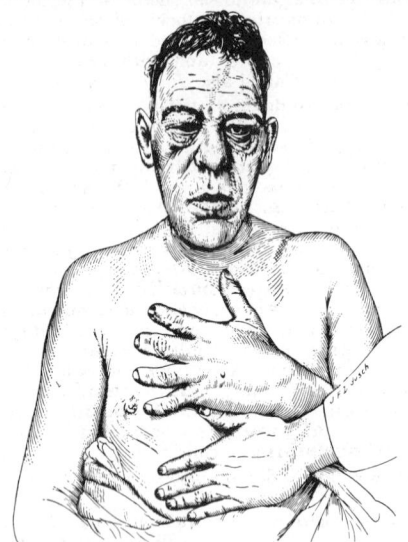

Acromegaly (Dunphy and Botsford).

acromelalgia (ak"ro-mĕ-lal'je-ah) erythromelalgia.

acromelic (ak"ro-me'lik) [*acro-* + Gr. *melos* limb] pertaining to or affecting the end of a limb.

acrometagenesis (ak"ro-met"ah-jen'ĕ-sis) [*acro-* + Gr. *meta* beyond + *genesis* production] undue growth of the extremities.

acromial (ah-kro'me-al) pertaining to the acromion.

acromicria (ak"ro-mik're-ah) [*acro-* + Gr. *mikros* small + *-ia*] a condition characterized by hypoplasia of the extremities of the skeleton—the nose, jaws, fingers, and toes; the converse of acromegaly. **congenital a.,** Down's syndrome.

acromikria (ak"ro-mik're-ah) acromicria.

acromioclavicular (ah-kro"me-o-klah-vik'u-lar) pertaining to the acromion and clavicle, especially to the articulation between the acromion and clavicle. See also *articulatio acromioclavicularis.*

acromiocoracoid (ah-kro"me-o-kor'ah-koid) pertaining to the acromion and the coracoid process; called also *coracoacromial.*

acromiohumeral (ah-kro"me-o-hu'mer-al) pertaining to the acromion and humerus.

acromion (ah-kro'me-on) [*acro-* + Gr. *ōmos* shoulder] [NA] the lateral extension of the spine of the scapula, projecting over the shoulder joint and forming the highest point of the shoulder; called also *acromial process* and *acromion scapulae.*

acromionectomy (ah-kro"me-on-ek'to-me) resection of the distal end of the acromion, done in the treatment of acromioclavicular arthritis.

acromioscapular (ah-kro"me-o-skap'u-lar) pertaining to the acromion and scapula.

acromiothoracic (ah-kro"me-o-tho-ras'ik) pertaining to the acromion and thorax.

acromphalus (ah-krom'fah-lus) [*acro-* + Gr. *omphalos* navel] 1. undue prominence of the navel; sometimes a sign of umbilical hernia. 2. the center of the navel.

acromycosis (ak"ro-mi-ko'sis) (*obs.*) mycosis of the limbs.

acromyotonia (ak"ro-mi-o-to'ne-ah) [*acro-* + Gr. *mys* muscle + *tonos* contraction + *-ia*] contracture of the hand or foot resulting in spastic deformity (Sicard, 1915).

acromyotonus (ak"ro-mi-ot'o-nus) acromyotonia.

acronarcotic (ak"ro-nar-kot'ik) both acrid and narcotic.

acroneurosis (ak"ro-nu-ro'sis) [*acro-* + *neurosis*] any neuropathy of the extremities.

acronine (a'kro-nēn) chemical name: 3,12-dihydro-6- methoxy-3,3,12- trimethyl -7*H*- pyrano[2,3 - *c*]acridin -7- one; an antineoplastic agent, $C_{20}H_{19}NO_3$.

acronym (ak'ro-nim) [*acro-* + Gr. *onoma* name] a word formed by the initial letters of the principal components of a compound term, as laser or maser.

acro-osteolysis (ak"ro-os"te-ol'ĭ-sis) osteolysis involving the distal phalanges of the fingers and toes.

acropachy (ak'ro-pak"e) [*acro-* + Gr. *pachys* thick] clubbing of the fingers and toes, with distal periosteal bone changes and swelling of the overlying soft tissues.

acropachyderma (ak"ro-pak"e-der'mah) [*acro-* + Gr. *pachys* thick + *derma* skin] a condition marked by thickening of the skin over the face, scalp, and extremities, clubbing of the extremities, and deformities of the long bones; usually associated with acromegaly. Called also *pachyacria.*

acroparalysis (ak"ro-pah-ral'ĭ-sis) [*acro-* + *paralysis*] paralysis of the extremities.

acroparesthesia (ak"ro-par"es-the'ze-ah) [*acro-* + *paresthesia*] 1. paresthesia of the tips of the extremities due to nerve compression at any of several levels, or polyneuritis. 2. a disease marked by attacks of tingling, numbness, and stiffness in the extremities, chiefly the fingers, hands, and forearms, sometimes with pain, pallor of the skin, or slight cyanosis. Two forms have been described—the simple form (Schultze's type), which tends to end in acrocyanosis, and the vasomotor or angiospastic form (Nothnagel's type), which may end in recovery or go on to gangrene.

acropathology (ak"ro-pah-thol'o-je) [*acro-* + *pathology*] the pathology of diseases affecting the extremities.

acropathy (ah-krop'ah-the) [*acro-* + Gr. *pathos* disorder] any disease of the extremities.

acropeptide (ak"ro-pep'tīd) a protein fraction obtained by heating protein to above 140° C. in nonaqueous solvents.

acropetal (ah-krop'e-tal) [*acro-* + L. *petere* to seek] rising toward the summit.

acrophobia (ak"ro-fo'be-ah) morbid dread of high places.

acroposthitis (ak"ro-pos-thi'tis) [Gr. *acroposthia* prepuce + *-itis*] inflammation of the prepuce.

acropurpura (ak"ro-pur'pu-rah) purpura affecting the extremities, especially the digits.

acroscleroderma (ak"ro-skle"ro-der'mah) acrosclerosis.

acrosclerosis (ak"ro-skle-ro'sis) [*acro-* + *sclerosis*] a condition combining the features of Raynaud's disease with scleroderma of the distal parts of the extremities, especially of the digits (sclerodactyly), and of the neck and the face, particularly the nose; called also *acroscleroderma.* It is generally regarded as a form of systemic or generalized scleroderma.

acrosome (ak'ro-sōm) [*acro-* + Gr. *sōma* body] the caplike, membrane-bound structure derived from Golgi elements found at the anterior portion of the nucleus of a spermatozoon; it contains lysosomal enzymes and a proteolytic enzyme, which are believed to facilitate entry of spermatozoa into ova. Called also *acrosomal cap* and *anterior head cap.* See also *acrosome reaction,* under *reaction.*

acrosphenosyndactylia (ak"ro-sfe"no-sin"dak-til'e-ah) acrocephalosyndactylia.

acrostealgia (ak"ros-te-al'je-ah) [*acro-* + Gr. *osteon* bone + *algos* pain + *-ia*] a painful apophysitis of the bones of the extremities.

acrosyndactyly (ak"ro-sin-dak'tĭ-le) [*acro-* + Gr. *syn* with + *daktylos* finger] fusion of the terminal portion of two or more digits, with clefts or sinuses present between their proximal phalanges.

acroteric (ak"ro-ter'ik) pertaining to the tips or outermost parts.

Acrotheca pedrosoi (ak"ro-the'kah pĕ-dro'soi) *Fonsecaea pedrosoi.*

Acrothesium floccosum (ak"ro-the'se-um flok-ko'sum) *Epidermophyton floccosum.*

acrotic (ah-krot'ik) 1. [Gr. *akros* extreme] affecting the surface. 2. [*a* neg. + Gr. *krotos* beat] pertaining to absence or weakness of the pulse.

acrotism (ak'ro-tizm) [*a* neg. + Gr. *krotos* beat + *-ism*] absence or imperceptibility of the pulse.

acrotrophodynia (ak"ro-trof"o-din'e-ah) [*acro-* + Gr. *trophē* nutrition + *odynē* pain + *-ia*] a trophic disorder with neuritis and paresthesia from exposure of extremities to cold and moisture.

acrotrophoneurosis (ak"ro-trof"o-nu-ro'sis) trophoneurotic disturbance of the extremities.

acrylaldehyde (ak"ril-al'de-hīd) acrolein.

acrylamide (ah-kril'ah-mīd) the crystalline amide of acrylic acid, $CH_2CHCONH_2$.

acrylic (ah-kril'ik) an acrylic resin; see under *resin.*

acrylonitrile (ak"rĭ-lo-ni'tril) chemical name: 2-propenenitrile. A compound, $CH_2:CH\cdot CN$, used in the making of plastics and as a pesticide; its vapors are irritant to the respiratory tract and eyes, and may cause systemic poisoning.

A.C.S. American Chemical Society; antireticular cytotoxic serum.

A.C.S.M. American College of Sports Medicine.

act (akt) a doing, or a thing done; a performance involving motor activity. **compulsive a.,** a ritualistic and repetitive act, such as touching the slats in a fence, or handwashing, carried out by an individual contrary to his wishes and standards, being a feature of the obsessive-compulsive personality. Failure to perform the act leads to increasing anxiety and tension. **Harrison antinarcotic a.,** see under *H.* **imperious a.,** compulsive a. **impulsive a.,** a sudden unpremeditated act likely to be regretted after its performance but momentarily in synchrony with the emotional needs of the individual; such acts are characteristic of persons with poor behavior controls and low inhibition. **reflex a.,** a relatively fixed action or pattern of response performed as a result of the triggering of a reflex arc and usually without involvement of the higher centers.

Actaea (ak-te′ah) [L.; Gr. *aktē* elder-tree] a genus of ranunculaceous plants. **A. odora′ta,** bitter weed, a plant that causes heavy losses of sheep and goats in the Southwest. **A. richardso′ni,** rubber weed which is poisonous to sheep. **A. spica′ta,** red cohosh.

actaplanin (ak″tah-pla′nin) a glycopeptide antibiotic of unknown structure derived from a species of *Actinoplanes*, containing a chlorophenyl group, glucose, mannose rhamnose, and several unknown amino acids; a veterinary growth stimulant.

ACTe anodal closure tetanus.

ACTH adrenocorticotropic hormone; see *corticotropin.*

Acthar (ak′thar) trademark for preparations of corticotropin.

ACTH-RF corticotropin (adrenocorticotropic hormone) releasing factor.

Actidil (ak′tĭ-dil) trademark for a preparation of triprolidine hydrochloride.

Actidione (ak″tĭ-di′ōn) trademark for a preparation of cycloheximide.

actin (ak′tin) a protein of the myofibril, localized in the I band; acting along with myosin particles it is responsible for the contraction and relaxation of muscle. In the absence of salt, it becomes globular (*G-actin*), and in the presence of potassium chloride and adenosine triphosphate it polymerizes, forming long fibers (F-actin). Cf. *actomyosin* and *myosin.*

acting out (ak′ting owt) the behavioral expression of hidden emotional conflicts, such as hostile feelings, in various kinds of neurotic behavior, as a defense pattern analogous to somatic conversion.

actinic (ak-tin′ik) [Gr. *aktis* ray] pertaining to those rays of light beyond the violet end of the spectrum that produce chemical effects.

actinicity (ak″tĭ-nis′ĭ-te) actinism.

actiniform (ak-tin′ĭ-form) [Gr. *aktis* ray] formed like a ray; radiate.

actinine (ak′tĭ-nin) a base occurring in the sea anemone *Actinia equina.*

actinism (ak′tĭ-nizm) [Gr. *aktis* ray] that property of radiant energy which produces chemical changes, as in photography or heliotherapy; called also *actinicity.*

actinium (ak-tin′e-um) [Gr. *aktis* ray] a rare metallic chemical element occurring in the ores of uranium and having radioactive properties; its atomic number is 89, its atomic weight 227, and its symbol Ac.

actino- (ak′tĭ-no) [Gr. *aktis, aktinos* a ray] a combining form denoting relation to a ray, as ray-shaped, or pertaining to some form of radiation.

actinobacillosis (ak″tĭ-no-bas″ĭ-lo′sis) a disease of domestic animals resembling actinomycosis and caused by *Actinobacillus lignieresii,* sometimes seen in man; the bacillus forms radiating structures in the tissues.

Actinobacillus (ak″tĭ-no-bah-sil′lus) a genus of schizomycetes of the family Brucellaceae, order Eubacteriales. **A. actinoi′des,** an organism isolated from chronic pneumonias in calves and rats and of uncertain relation to the disease. **A. actinomycetemcom′itans,** a microorganism found in the actinomycotic granules in bovine actinomycosis and of doubtful relation to the disease. **A. equu′li,** the causative agent of equulosis of foals. **A. ligniere′sii,** the causative agent of actinomycosis-like disease of cattle and other domestic animals. **A. mal′lei,** *Pseudomonas mallei.* **A. pseudomal′lei,** *Pseudomonas pseudomallei.* **A. whitmor′i,** *Pseudomonas pseudomallei.*

actinobolin (ak″tĭ-nob′o-lin) a broad-spectrum antibiotic elaborated by *Streptomyces griseoviridus* var. *atrofaciens,* $C_{13}H_{20}N_2O_6$, which exhibits activity against a wide range of bacteria and against various neoplasms, and inhibits cariogenic microorganisms in rats; it is being studied for use in the control of caries in humans.

actinochemistry (ak″tĭ-no-kem′is-tre) [*actino-* + *chemistry*] chemistry dealing with action of rays of light; photochemistry.

actinocongestin (ak″tĭ-no-kon-jĕs′tin) congestin.

actinocutitis (ak″tĭ-no-ku-ti′tis) [*actino-* + *cutitis*] radiodermatitis.

actinodaphnine (ak″tĭ-no-daf′nin) a crystalline alkaloid, $C_{18}H_{17}O_4N$, from the bark of *Actinodaphne hookeri.*

actinodermatitis (ak″tĭ-no-der″mah-ti′tis) radiodermatitis.

actinodiastase (ak″tĭ-no-di′as-tās) an enzyme found in the

body of coelenterate animals which performs the intracellular digestion characteristic of these animals.

actinoerythrin (ak″tĭ-no-er′ĭ-thrin) an ester of violerythrin, which gives the color to sea anemones.

actinogen (ak-tin′o-jen) a substance which produces radiation.

actinogenesis (ak″tĭ-no-jen′ĕ-sis) [*actino-* + Gr. *genesis* production] the production of rays; radiogenesis.

actinogenic (ak″tĭ-no-jen′ik) producing or forming rays; radiogenic.

actinogenics (ak″tĭ-no-jen′iks) the science or study of radiation.

actinogram (ak-tin′o-gram) (*obs.*) roentgenogram.

actinograph (ak-tin′o-graf) [*actino-* + Gr. *graphein* to write] 1. (*obs.*) roentgenogram. 2. an instrument for recording variations in the actinic effect of the sun's rays.

actinography (ak″tĭ-nog′rah-fe) (*obs.*) roentgenography.

actinohematin (ak″tĭ-no-hem′ah-tin) a red respiratory pigment occurring in certain sea anemones.

actinokymography (ak″tĭ-no-ki-mog′rah-fe) [*actino-* + Gr. *kyma* wave + *graphein* to write] (*obs.*) motion picture radiography.

actinolite (ak-tin′o-līt) any substance that is markedly changed by light.

actinology (ak″tĭ-nol′ŏ-je) [*actino-* + *-logy*] 1. the science of photochemistry; the science of the chemical effects of light. 2. the study of radiant energy.

Actinomadura (ak″tĭ-no-mad′ŭ-rah) a genus of microorganisms of the family Actinomycetaceae, order Actinomycetales. **A. madu′rae,** a species distributed worldwide in soil, and a common cause of maduromycosis in which the granules in the discharged pus are white; called also *Nocardia madurae.* **A. pelletier′ii,** a species commonly found in north central Africa and the Sudan; it is the cause of maduromycosis in which the granules discharged in the pus are red.

actinometer (ak″tĭ-nom′ĕ-ter) [*actino-* + Gr. *metron* measure] 1. an instrument for measuring the intensity of actinic effects. 2. an apparatus for measuring the penetrating power of actinic rays.

actinometry (ak″tĭ-nom′ĕ-tre) the measurement of the photochemical power of light.

actinomycelial (ak″tĭ-no-mi-se′le-al) 1. pertaining to the mycelium of an actinomyces. 2. actinomycetic.

Actinomyces (ak″tĭ-no-mi′sēz) [*actino-* + Gr. *mykēs* fungus] a genus of microorganisms of the family Actinomycetaceae, order Actinomycetales, made up of three pathogenic species; called also *ray fungus.* **A. actinoi′des,** *Actinobacillus actinoides.* **A. baudet′ii,** an etiologic agent of actinomycosis in cats and dogs. **A. bo′vis,** a non–acid-fast anaerobic or microaerophilic microorganism;

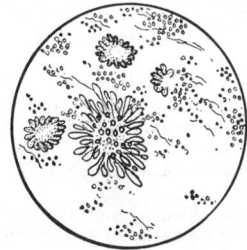

Actinomyces bovis (de Rivas)

the specific etiologic agent of actinomycosis in cattle. **A. erikson′ii,** an etiologic agent of pulmonary actinomycosis in which there is no granule formation. **A. israe′lii,** a non–acid-fast anaerobic actinomyces parasitic in the mouth, proliferating in necrotic tissue, and occurring as the etiologic agent in some cases of human actinomycosis. **A. mur′is,** **A. mur′is-rat′ti,** *Streptobacillus moniliformis.* **A. necroph′orus,** *Fusobacterium necrophorum.* **A. rhusiopath′iae,** *Erysipelothrix insidosa.* **A. vina′ceus,** a species that produces viomycin.

actinomyces (ak″tĭ-no-mi′sēz), pl. *actinomyce′tes.* An organism of the genus *Actinomyces.*

Actinomycetaceae (ak″tĭ-no-mi″sĕ-ta′se-e) a family of Schizomycetes, order Actinomycetales, divided into three genera, the anaerobic or microaerophilic *Actinomyces,* and two aerobic genera, *Nocardia* and *Actinomadura.*

Actinomycetales (ak″tĭ-no-mi″sĕ-ta′lēz) an order of Schizomycetes made up of elongated cells which have a definite tendency to branch; it includes four families, Actinomycetaceae, Actinoplanaceae, Mycobacteriaceae, and Streptomycetaceae.

actinomycete (ak″tĭ-no-mi′sēt) any organism of the order Actinomycetales.

actinomycetes (ak″tĭ-no-mi-se′tēz) plural of *actinomyces* and *actinomycete.*

actinomycetic (ak″tĭ-no-mi-set′ik) of or caused by actinomyces; of or pertaining to organisms of the order Actinomycetales or diseases caused by such organisms.

actinomycetin (ak″tĭ-no-mi-se′tin) a substance derived from cultures of the actinomycete *Streptomyces albus;* it lyses dead bacteria.

actinomycin (ak″tĭ-no-mi′sin) a large, complex family of antibiotics obtained from cultures of various species of *Streptomyces,* which have antibacterial, antifungal, and cytotoxic properties. Some, especially actinomycins C (cactinomycin) and D (dactinomycin), are used as antineoplastic agents.

actinomycoma (ak″tĭ-no-mi-ko′mah) [*actinomyces* + *-oma*] a tumor-like reactive lesion due to actinomycetes.

actinomycosis (ak″tĭ-no-mi-ko′sis) [*actino-* + Gr. *mykēs* fungus] an infectious disease caused by *Actinomyces israelii* in man and by *A. bovis* in cattle. It is characterized by indolent inflammatory lesions of the lymph nodes draining the mouth (*cervicofacial area*), by intraperitoneal abscesses, including liver abscess, or by lung abscess due to aspiration, in that order of frequency. The lymphadenitis is characterized by slow, relatively painless enlargement of the lymph nodes (lumpy jaw), with reddening of the overlying skin. Infection of the peritoneal cavity or lung is associated with gradually increasing fever and loss of weight, but few localizing signs. Pus drained from a suppurative lesion sometimes contains dense mycelial clusters in the form of yellowish granules (sulfur granules).

actinomycotic (ak″tĭ-no-mi-kot′ik) pertaining to or affected with actinomycosis.

actinomycotin (ak″tĭ-no-mi′ko-tin) a therapeutic preparation of cultures of *Actinomyces,* used in treating actinomycosis.

actinon (ak′tĭ-non) radon-219.

actinoneuritis (ak″tĭ-no-nu-ri′tis) [*actino-* + *neuritis*] radioneuritis.

actinophage (ak-tin′o-fāj) a virus that causes the lysis of actinomycetes.

actinophytosis (ak″tĭ-no-fi-to′sis) infection with *Actinomyces* or *Nocardia.*

Actinoplanaceae (ak″tĭ-no-plah-na′se-e) a family of schizomycetes, order Actinomycetales.

Actinoplanes (ak″tĭ-no-pla′nēz) [*actino-* + Gr. *planēs* one who wanders] a genus of schizomycetes of the family Actinoplanaceae, order Actinomycetales, made up of saprophytic forms found in soil and water.

actinopraxis (ak″tĭ-no-prak′sis) [*actino-* + Gr. *praxis* doing] (*obs.*) the diagnostic and therapeutic use of the rays of radioactive substances; radiopraxis.

actinoquinol sodium (ak-tin′o-kwĭ-nōl) chemical name: 8-ethoxy-5-quinolinesulfonic acid sodium salt; an ultraviolet screen, $C_{11}H_{10}NNaO_4S$.

actinoscopy (ak″tĭ-nos′ko-pe) [*actino-* + Gr. *skopein* to view] (*obs.*) examination by means of the roentgen ray.

actinostereoscopy (ak″tĭ-no-ste″re-os′ko-pe) (*obs.*) actinoscopy.

actinotherapeutics (ak″tĭ-no-ther″ah-pu′tiks) actinotherapy.

actinotherapy (ak″tĭ-no-ther′ah-pe) [*actino-* + Gr. *therapeia* treatment] treatment of disease with ultraviolet or actinic rays.

actinotoxemia (ak″tĭ-no-tok-se′me-ah) [*actino-* + *toxemia*] radiation sickness.

actinotoxin (ak″tĭ-no-tok′sin) a crude poison derived from alcoholic extracts of the tentacles of sea anemones.

action (ak′shun) [L. *actio*] any performance of function or movement either of any part or organ or of the whole body. **ball-valve a.,** the intermittent obstruction caused by a free or partially attached foreign body in a tubular or cavitary structure, as by a foreign body in a bronchus, a stone in a bile duct, or a tumor in the cardiac atrium. **buffer a.,** an action that tends to stabilize an inanimate system or a body function or state, such as pH, blood pressure, [Ca^{++}], etc.; most commonly used to denote the stabilization of pH by acid-base buffers (tampon a.). **calorigenic a.,** 1. specific dynamic action. 2. the total energy released in the body by a food or food constituent. **capillary a.,** the transport of a fluid in a tube, caused by adhesion of the fluid to the tube wall. **contact a.,** contact catalysis. **cumulative a.,** action of increased intensity, as may be evidenced after administration of several doses of a drug due to the accumulation of the drug in the body so that the biological effect is greater than after the first dose. Called also *cumulative effect.* **diastasic a., diastatic a.,** the action of diastase in converting starch into glucose. **opsonic a.,** the effect that opsonins exert on bacteria and other cells, increasing their susceptibility to phagocytosis. **reflex a.,** a response resulting from the passage of excitation potential from a receptor to a muscle or gland, over a system of neurons without the necessity of volition. **specific a.,** the action of a drug which is exerted on a certain definite pathogenic organism. **specific dynamic a.,** the increase in metabolism over the basal rate brought about by the ingestion and assimilation of food, varying from 4 to 6 per cent for fats and carbohydrates

to 30 per cent for protein. **tampon a.,** buffer a. **thermogenic a.,** the action of a food or drug in increasing the production of heat or the temperature of the body. **trigger a.,** an action that releases energy whose character has no relation to the process which released it. **vitaminoid a.,** an action resembling the action of vitamins.

activate (ak′tĭ-vāt) to render active.

activation (ak″tĭ-va′shun) the act or process of rendering active, as (*a*) in the transformation of pre-enzyme into an active enzyme by the action of a kinase or another pre-enzyme, or gain in the purifying of sewage by means of activated sludge; (*b*) the process by which the central nervous system is stimulated into activity through the mediation of the reticular activating system; (*c*) the deliberate induction of a pattern of electrical activity in the brain, as in the electrocardiographic diagnosis of epilepsy. **lymphocyte a.,** the biochemical interactions that initiate activation of lymphocytes and release of biologically active mediators. This process may be initiated either by antigens or by plant mitogens. **ovum a.,** initiation of ovum development by a spermatozoon or an artificial substitute. **plasma a.,** the stimulation of the cellular metabolism produced by the successful application of nonspecific agents, such as the injection of foreign proteins or of colloidal metals.

activator (ak′tĭ-va″tor) 1. a substance that renders some other substance active, especially a substance that combines with an inactive enzyme to render it capable of effecting its proper action. Cf. *coenzyme.* 2. a substance that stimulates the development of a particular structure in the embryo. Cf. *inductor* and *organizer.* **monobloc a.,** a removable orthodontic appliance utilizing muscle forces to achieve therapeutic correction; called also *Andresen appliance* and *functional a.* **plasminogen a.,** a substance that has the ability to activate plasminogen and convert it into plasmin, its active form. **tissue a.,** fibrinokinase.

active (ak′tiv) characterized by action; not passive; not expectant. **optically a.,** capable of rotating the plane of polarization of a light wave.

activity (ak-tiv′i-te) the quality or process of exerting energy or of accomplishing an effect. In physical chemistry, the ratio of the fugacity of a substance in a particular experimental state to the fugacity in its standard state at the same temperature. **displacement a.,** irrelevant activity produced by an excess of one of two conflicting drives in an organism. **enzyme a.,** the catalytic effect exerted by an enzyme, expressed as units per milligram of enzyme (specific activity) or as molecules of substrate transformed per minute per molecule of enzyme (molecular activity). **leukemia-associated inhibitory a. (LIA),** the inhibition of normal marrow cells of donors from forming colonies of granulocytes and macrophages, induced *in vitro* by the presence of cell extracts, or of culture media conditioned by cells, from the bone marrow, spleen, or blood of patients with acute leukemia. **optical a.,** the ability of a chemical compound to rotate the plane of polarization of plane-polarized light. **specific a.,** the ratio of radioactive to nonradioactive atoms or molecules of the same kind.

actodigin (ak″to-dij′in) chemical name: 3β-(β-D-glucopyranosyloxy)-14,23-dihydroxy-24-nor-5β,14β-chol-20(22)-en-21-oic acid γ-lactone; a cardiotonic, $C_{29}H_{44}O_9$.

actometer (ak-tom′ĕ-ter) a device for measuring activity, as in hyperkinesis, as reflected in locomotion in the horizontal plane.

actomyosin (ak″to-mi′o-sin) a complex of the proteins actin and myosin occurring in muscle. Cf. *actin* and *myosin.*

Actonia (ak-to′ne-ah) a genus of ascomycetous fungi of the order Endomycetales, described as producing creamy patches in the throat resembling diphtheria; it is probably not a valid genus.

ACTP adrenocorticotropic polypeptide, a hydrolysate of ACTH (corticotropin).

actual (ak′chu-al) [L. *actualis*] real rather than potential.

actuary (ak′chu-a″re) a person whose business is the calculation of premiums and risks in insurance.

acu- (ak′u) [L *acus* needle] a combining form denoting relationship to a needle.

Acuaria spiralis (ak″u-a′re-ah spi-ra′lis) a filarioid parasite in the proventriculus and esophagus of fowls.

acuclosure (ak″u-klo′zhur) arrest of hemorrhage by means of a needle.

acufilopressure (ak″u-fi′lo-presh″er) [*acu-* + L. *filum* thread + *pressura* pressure] a combination of acupressure and ligation.

acuity (ah-ku′ĭ-te) [L. *acuitas* sharpness] clarity or clearness, especially of the vision. **Vernier a.,** displacement threshold; see under *threshold.*

aculeate (ah-ku′le-āt) [L. *aculeatus* thorny] covered with sharp points; pointed.

acuminate (ah-ku′mĭ-nāt) [L. *acuminatus*] sharp pointed.

acupoint (ak′u-point) a specific site of needle insertion along a body meridian in acupuncture.

acupression (ak″u-presh′un) acupressure.

acupressure (ak′u-presh″er) [*acu-* + L. *pressio* or *pressura* pressure] compression of a bleeding vessel by inserting needles into adjacent tissue.

acupuncture (ak″u-pungk′chūr) [*acu-* + L. *punctura* a prick] the Chinese practice of piercing specific peripheral nerves with needles to relieve the discomfort associated with painful disorders, to induce surgical anesthesia, and for therapeutic purposes.

acus (a′kus) [L.]   a needle or needle-like process.

acusection (ak″ı-sek′shun)   cutting by means of the electrosurgical needle.

acusector (aı″u-sek′tor) [*acu-* + L. *sectere* to cut]   an electric needle used like a scalpel for incising tissues.

acute (ah-kūt′) [L. *acutus* sharp]   1. sharp; poignant.   2. having a short and relatively severe course.

acutorsion (ak″u-tor′shun) [*acu-* + L. *torsio* a twisting]   the twisting of a blood vessel with a needle for the control of hemorrhage.

acyanoblepsia (ah-si″ah-no-blep′se-ah) [*a* neg. + Gr. *kyanos* blue + *blepsia* vision]   inability to distinguish blue tints.

acyanopsia (ah-si″ah-nop′se-ah)   acyanoblepsia.

acyanotic (ah-si″ah-not′ik)   characterized by absence of cyanosis.

acyclia (ah-si′kle-ah)   arrest of circulation of body fluids.

acyclic (a-si′klik)   1. in chemistry, having an open-chain structure; aliphatic.   2. occurring independently of a cycle, as of the menstrual cycle.

acyesis (ah″si-e′sis) [*a* neg. + Gr. *kyēsis* pregnancy]   1. sterility in women.   2. absence of pregnancy.

acyl (as′il)   an organic radical derived from an organic acid by removal of the hydroxyl group.

Acylanid (as″il-an′id)   trademark for a preparation of acetyldigitoxin.

acylase (as′ĭ-lās)   any enzyme that catalyzes the hydrolysis of acylated amino acids.

acylation (as″ĕ-la′shun)   the introduction of an acid radical into the molecule of a chemical compound.

acylmutase (as″il-mu′tās)   an enzyme of the isomerase class that catalyzes the intermolecular transfer of acyl groups. **lysolecithin a.,** an enzyme that catalyzes the conversion of 2- to 3-lysolecithin.

acylphosphatase (as″il-fos′fah-tās)   acylphosphate hydrolase: an enzyme occurring in muscle, liver, and kidney that catalyzes the hydrolysis of an acyl phosphate to an anion and an orthophosphate.

acyltransferase (as″il-trans′fer-ās)   any of a group of enzymes that catalyze the transfer of an acyl group from one substance to another.

acystia (ah-sis′te-ah) [*a* neg. + Gr. *kystis* bladder]   congenital absence of the bladder.

acystinervia (ah-sis″tĕ-ner′ve-ah) [*a* neg. + Gr. *kystis* bladder + L. *nervus* nerve + *-ia*]   defective nervous tone in the bladder.

acystineuria (ah-sis″te-nu′re-ah)   acystinervia.

Acystosporidia (ah-sis″to-spo-rid′e-ah) [*a* neg. + Gr. *kystis* bladder + *sporidia*]   *Haemosporidia.*

AD   diphenylchlorarsine; anodal duration.

A.D.   abbreviation for L. *au′ris dex′tra,* right ear.

ad [L. *ad* to]   used in writing prescriptions to indicate that a substance (usually a diluent) be added up to a certain amount.

ad- [L. *ad* to]   a prefix expressing to or toward, addition to, nearness, or intensification.

-ad   1. [L. *ad* to] adverbial suffix expressing toward, as in cephalad, caudad.   2. [Gr.] suffix indicating a numerical group, as in triad, or derivation from or connection with.

A.D.A.   American Dental Association; American Diabetic Association; American Dietetic Association.

adactylia (ah″dak-til′e-ah)   adactyly.

adactylism (a-dak′tĭ-lizm)   adactyly.

adactylous (a-dak′tĭ-lus)   pertaining to adactyly; lacking digits on the hand or foot.

adactyly (a-dak′tĭ-le) [*a* neg. + Gr. *daktylos* finger]   a developmental anomaly characterized by the absence of digits on the hand or foot.

adamantine (ad″ah-man′tin)   pertaining to the enamel of the teeth.

adamantinocarcinoma (ad″ah-man″tĭ-no-kar″-sĭ-no′mah) (*obs.*)   ameloblastic sarcoma.

adamantinoma (ad″ah-man″tĭ-no′mah)   ameloblastoma. **pituitary a.,** craniopharyngioma. **a. polycys′ticum,** an adamantinoma (ameloblastoma) that has undergone cystic degeneration.

adamantoblast (ad″ah-man′to-blast) [Gr. *adamas* a hard substance + *blastos* germ]   ameloblast.

adamantoblastoma (ad″ah-man″to-blas-to′mah)   ameloblastoma.

adamantoma (ad″ah-man-to′mah)   ameloblastoma.

adamas (ad′ah-mas) [Gr. "unconquerable"]   anything fixed or unalterable.   **a. den′tis,** the enamel of the teeth.

Adami's theory (ad-am′ēz) [John George *Adami,* Canadian pathologist, 1862–1926]   see under *theory.*

Adamkiewicz's demilunes, test (reaction) (ah-dam-ke′viks) [Albert *Adamkiewicz,* Polish pathologist, 1850–1921]   see under *demilune* and *test.*

Adams' operation, saw (ad′amz)   1. [William *Adams,* English surgeon, 1810–1900] see under *operation,* defs. 1, 2, and 3, and under *saw.*   2. [Sir William *Adams,* British surgeon, 1783–1827] see under *operation,* def. 5.

Adams-Stokes disease (syncope, syndrome) [Robert *Adams,* Irish physician, 1791–1875; William *Stokes,* Irish physician, 1804–1878]   see under *disease.*

adamsite (ad′amz-īt)   diphenylaminearsine chloride.

Adansonia (ad″an-so′ne-ah) [after Michel *Adanson,* French naturalist, 1727–1806]   a genus of trees in the Bombacaceae family. *A. digita′ta* is the baobab, a huge tree of Africa, found also in India. In Africa, the young leaves and seeds are eaten as food and the pulp is widely used for its diaphoretic properties.

adansonian (ad″an-son′ne-an)   named for Michel *Adanson;* see *numerical taxonomy,* under *taxonomy.*

adaptation (ad″ap-ta′shun) [L. *adaptare* to fit]   1. the adjustment of an organism to its environment, or the process by which it enhances such fitness.   2. immunization.   3. the normal ability of the eye to adjust itself to variations in the intensity of light; the adjustment to such variations.   4. the decline in the frequency of firing of a neuron, particularly of a receptor, under conditions of constant stimulation.   5. in dentistry, (*a*) the proper fitting of a denture, (*b*) the degree of proximity and interlocking of restorative material to a tooth preparation, (*c*) the exact adjustment of bands to teeth.   6. in microbiology, the adjustment of bacterial physiology to a new environment; see *genetic a.* and *phenotypic a.*   **color a.,**   1. fading of hue and dulling of brightness of visual perceptions with prolonged stimulation.   2. adjustment of vision to degree of brightness or color tone of illumination indoors or out; includes *dark a.* **dark a.,** the adaptation of the eye to vision in the dark or in reduced illumination (night vision), with build-up of rhodopsin in the retinal rods; called also *scotoptic a.*   **enzymatic a.,** inducible enzyme synthesis; see under *synthesis.*   **genetic a.,** the natural selection of the progeny of a mutant better adapted to a new environment; especially seen in the development of microbes resistant to chemotherapeutic agents or to other inhibitors of growth (drug resistance).   **light a.,** adaptation of the eye to vision in the sunlight or in bright illumination (photopia), with reduction in the concentration of the photosensitive pigments of the eye; called also *photopic a.*   **phenotypic a.,** a change in the properties of an organism, without any change in genotype, in response to a change in the environment. In microbiology, especially the formation of specific enzymes required for the utilization of new foodstuffs (induced enzyme formation), or a change in cell size and composition with variation in growth rate. Called also *physiological a.*   **photopic a.,** light a.   **retinal a.,** the adjustment of the photoreceptor cell of the eye to the surrounding illumination.   **scotopic a.,** dark a.

adapter (ah-dap′ter)   a device by which different parts of an apparatus or instrument are connected.

adaptometer (ad″ap-tom′ĕ-ter) [*adaptation* + Gr. *metron* measure]   an instrument for measuring the time required for retinal adaptation: i.e., for regeneration of the visual purple. It is used to help detect night blindness, vitamin A deficiency, and retinitis pigmentosa.   **color a.,** an instrument using colored and neutral filters and control of illuminant to demonstrate adaptation of eye to color or light.

adaxial (ad-ak′se-al)   located alongside of, or directed toward, the axis.

ADC   anodal duration contraction; axiodistocervical.

add.   abbreviation for L. *ad′de* add, or *adde′tur* let there be added; used in writing prescriptions.

adde (ad′e) [L.]   add.

Ad def. an.   abbreviation for L. *ad defectio′nem an′imi,* to the point of fainting.

Ad deliq.   abbreviation for L. *ad deli′quium,* to fainting.

adder (ad′er)   1. *Vipera berus.*   2. any of many venomous snakes of the family Viperidae, such as the puff adder and the European viper. See table accompanying *snake.*   **death a.,** an extremely venomous elapid snake, *Acanthophis antarcticus* of Australia and New Guinea, with a short, stout body and a tail with a spine at the tip.   **puff a.,** an extremely venomous, brightly colored, viperine snake, *Bitis arientans,* of Africa and Arabia; when annoyed it inflates its stubby body and hisses loudly.

addict (ad′ikt)   a person who cannot resist a habit, especially the use of drugs or alcohol, for physiological or psychological reasons.

addiction (ah-dik′shun)   the state of being given up to some habit, especially strong dependence on a drug.   **alcohol a.,** alcoholism.   **drug a.,** a state of periodic or chronic intoxication produced by the repeated consumption of a drug, characterized by (1) an overwhelming desire or need (compulsion) to continue use of the drug and to obtain it by any means, (2) a tendency to increase the dosage, (3) a psychological and usually a physical dependence on its effects, and (4) a detrimental effect on the individual and on society. Cf. *habituation,* def. 3. **opium a.,** the habitual misuse of opium or the consequences of such misuse; see also *drug a.* **polysurgical a.,** habitual seeking of surgical treatment.

addiment (ad′ĭ-ment) complement.

Addis count (method, test) [Thomas *Addis,* San Francisco physician, 1881–1949] see under *count.*

addisin (ad′ĭ-sin) a substance present in the gastric juice that has stimulating power on bone-marrow formation; such an extract from the gastric juice of the hog is used in pernicious anemia.

Addison's anemia, disease, keloid (ad′-ĭ-sonz) [Thomas *Addison,* English physician, 1793–1860; he was a colleague of Bright at Guy's Hospital] see *pernicious anemia,* under *anemia;* see *circumscribed scleroderma,* under *scleroderma;* and see under *disease.*

Addison's planes, point (ad′ĭ-sonz) [Christopher *Addison,* English anatomist, 1869–1951] see under *plane* and *point.*

addisonian (ad″dĭ-so′ne-an) named for Thomas *Addison;* see pernicious *anemia,* under *anemia,* and see under *disease.*

addisonism (ad′ĭ-son-izm″) a group of symptoms associated with tuberculosis, consisting of pigmentation and debility, resembling those of Addison's disease.

additive (ad′ĭ-tiv) characterized by addition; see also under *effect.* 2. a substance, as a flavoring agent, preservative, or vitamin, added to another substance to improve its appearance, increase its nutritional value, etc.

adducent (ah-du′sent) performing adduction.

adduct (ah-dukt′) [L. *adducere* to draw toward] 1. to draw toward the median plane or (in the digits) toward the axial line of a limb. 2. a chemical addition product.

adduction (ah-duk′shun) the act of adducting or the state of being adducted.

adductor (ah-duk′tor) [L.] that which adducts; see *Table of Musculi.*

Adelmann's method, operation (ad′el-manz) [Georg Franz Blasius *Adelmann,* German surgeon, 1811–1888] see under *method* and *operation.*

adelomorphic (ah-del″o-mor′fik) adelomorphous.

adelomorphous (ah-del″o-mor′fus) [Gr. *adēlos* not evident + *morphē* form] not having a clearly defined form; see under *cell.*

aden- see *adeno-.*

adenalgia (ad″ĕ-nal′je-ah) [*aden-* + Gr. *algos* pain + *-ia*] pain in a gland; called also *adenodynia.*

adenase (ad′ĕ-nās) [*aden-* + *-ase*] a deaminizing enzyme that catalyzes the conversion of adenine into hypoxanthine and ammonia.

adenasthenia (ad″en-as-the′ne-ah) [*aden-* + *a* neg. + Gr. *sthenos* strength + *-ia*] deficient glandular activity.

adendric (ah-den′drik) adendritic.

adendritic (ah″den-drit′ik) [*a* neg. + Gr. *dendron* tree] lacking dendrites.

adenectomy (ad″ĕ-nek′to-me) [*aden-* + Gr. *ektomē* excision] surgical removal of a gland.

adenectopia (ad″ĕ-nek-to′pe-ah) [*aden-* + Gr. *ektopos* displaced + *-ia*] malposition or displacement of a gland.

adenemphraxis (ad″ĕ-nem-frak′sis) [*aden-* + Gr. *emphraxis* stoppage] (*obs.*) glandular obstruction.

adenia (ah-de′ne-ah) chronic great enlargement of the lymphatic glands; see also *lymphoma* and *pseudoleukemia.*

adenic (ah-de′nik) pertaining to or resembling a gland.

adeniform (ah-den′ĭ-form) [*aden-* + L. *forma* shape] resembling a gland, especially in shape.

adenine (ad′ĕ-nin) a white crystalline base, 6-aminopurine, $C_5H_5N_5$, found in various animal and vegetable tissues as one of the purine base constituents of DNA and RNA. It is one of the decomposition products of nuclein and may be found in the urine. Adenine is nonpoisonous, and occurs in the form of pearly crystals. **a. arabinoside,** vidarabine. **a. hypoxanthine,** a leukomaine, $C_5H_5N_5 + C_4H_4N_4O$, a compound of adenine and hypoxanthine. **a. nucleotide,** adenylic a. **a. sulfate,** white crystals, $(C_5H_5N_5)_2 \cdot H_2SO_4$, formerly used in nucleotide therapy in agranulocytosis.

adenitis (ad″ĕ-ni′tis) inflammation of a gland. Cf. *acinitis.* **acute epidemic infectious a.** (*obs.*), infectious mononucleosis. **acute salivary a.,** Pirera's name for an epidemic disease in Naples and vicinity, marked by inflammation of the parotid and other salivary glands, enlargement of the spleen, and pain in the axillary glands. **cervical a.,** a condition characterized by enlarged, inflamed, and tender lymph nodes of the neck; seen in certain infectious diseases of children, such as acute infections of the throat. **mesenteric a.,** mesenteric lymphadenitis. **phlegmonous a.,** inflammation of a gland and the surrounding connective tissue; called also *adenophlegmon.* **a. tropica′lis,** venereal lymphogranuloma.

Adenium (ah-de′ne-um) a genus of African plants of the family Aponcynaceae which are used for arrow poisons; they contain cardioactive glycosides (e.g., somalin) which are close in structure and action to the digitalis glycosides.

adenization (ad″ĕ-ni-za′shun) the assumption by other tissue of an abnormal glandlike appearance; adenoid change.

adeno-, aden- (ad′ĕ-no, ad′en) [Gr. *adēn, adenos* gland] a combining form denoting relationship to a gland or glands.

adenoacanthoma (ad″ĕ-no-ak″an-tho′mah) an adenocarcinoma in which some or the majority of the cells exhibit squamous differentiation; called also *adenocancroid.*

adenoameloblastoma (ad″ĕ-no-ah-mel″o-blas-to′mah) an odontogenic tumor characterized by the formation of ductlike structures in place of or in addition to a typical ameloblastic pattern.

adenoangiosarcoma (ad″ĕ-no-an″je-o-sar-ko′mah) (*obs.*) an angiosarcoma involving gland structures.

adenoblast (ad′ĕ-no-blast″) [*adeno-* + Gr. *blastos* germ] an embryonic cell that gives rise to glandular tissue.

adenocancroid (ad″ĕ-no-kang′kroid) adenoacanthoma.

adenocarcinoma (ad″ĕ-no-kar″sĭ-no′mah) carcinoma derived from glandular tissue or in which the tumor cells form recognizable glandular structures; adenocarcinomas may be classified according to the predominant pattern of cell arrangement, as papillary, alveolar, etc., or according to a particular product of the cells, as mucinous adenocarcinoma. **acinar a., acinous a.,** alveolar a. **alveolar a.,** adenocarcinoma composed of cells arranged in the form of alveoli. **follicular a.,** one in which the cells are arranged in the form of follicles, usually of thyroid origin. **a. of kidney,** renal cell carcinoma. **mucinous a.,** mucinous carcinoma. **papillary a., polypoid a.,** an adenocarcinoma in which the tumor elements are arranged as finger-like processes or as a solid spherical nodule projecting from an epithelial surface.

adenocele (ad′ĕ-no-sēl′) [*adeno-* + Gr. *kēlē* tumor] an adenomatous cystic tumor.

adenocellulitis (ad″ĕ-no-sel″u-li′tis) inflammation of a gland and the tissue around it.

adenochirapsology (ad″ĕ-no-ki″rap-sol′o-je) [*adeno-* + Gr. *cheir* hand + *hapsis* touch + *-logy*] see *royal touch,* under *touch.*

adenochondroma (ad″ĕ-no-kon-dro′mah) a tumor containing both adenomatous and chondromatous elements, as in the mixed tumor of salivary gland; called also *chondroadenoma.*

adenochondrosarcoma (ad″ĕ-no-kon″dro-sar-ko′mah) (*obs.*) a tumor containing the elements of adenoma, chondroma, and sarcoma.

adenocyst (ad′ĕ-no-sist″) [*adeno-* + Gr. *kystis* bladder] adenocystoma.

adenocystoma (ad″ĕ-no-sis-to′mah) an adenoma in which there is cyst formation. **papillary a. lymphomato′sum,** a rare cystic tumor containing epithelial and lymphoid tissues found in the regions of the submaxillary and parotid glands; called also *Warthin's tumor* and *adenolymphoma.*

adenocyte (ad′ĕ-no-sīt″) [*adeno-* + Gr. *kytos* hollow vessel] a mature secretory cell of a gland.

adenodynia (ad″ĕ-no-din′e-ah) [*adeno-* + Gr. *odynē* pain + *-ia*] pain in a gland.

adenoepithelioma (ad″ĕ-no-ep″ĭ-the′le-o′mah) a tumor composed of glandular and epithelial elements.

adenofibroma (ad″ĕ-no-fi-bro′mah) a tumor composed of connective tissue containing glandular structures. **a. edemato′des,** a tumor composed of glandular and connective tissue elements in which there is marked edema of the stroma, as in nasal polyp.

adenofibrosis (ad″ĕ-no-fi-bro′sis) fibroid change in a gland.

adenogenous (ad″ĕ-noj′ĕ-nus) [*adeno-* + Gr. *gennan* to produce] originating from glandular tissue.

adenographic (ad″ĕ-no-graf′ik) pertaining to adenography.

adenography (ad″ĕ-nog′rah-fe) [*adeno-* + Gr. *graphein* to write] roentgenography of a gland or glands.

adenohypersthenia (ad″ĕ-no-hi″per-sthe′ne-ah) [*adeno-* + Gr. *hyper* over + *sthenos* strength + *-ia*] (*obs.*) excessive glandular activity.

adenohypophyseal (ad″ĕ-no-hi″po-fiz′e-al) pertaining to the adenohypophysis.

adenohypophysectomy (ad″ĕ-no-hi-pof″ĭ-sek′to-me) excision of the glandular portion (the adenohypophysis) of the hypophysis.

adenohypophysial (ad″ĕ-no-hi″po-fiz′e-al) adenohypophyseal.

adenohypophysis (ad″ĕ-no-hi-pof′ĭ-sis) [*adeno-* + *hypophysis*] [NA alternative] the anterior (or glandular) lobe of the pituitary gland (hypophysis), as distinguished from the posterior lobe, or neurohypophysis. See *pituitary gland,* under *gland.*

adenoid (ad′ĕ-noid) [*aden-* + Gr. *eidos* form] 1. resembling a gland. 2. in the plural, lymphoid tissue that normally exists in the nasopharynx of children and is known as the pharyngeal tonsil. Also, a popular term for hypertrophy of this tissue. 3. pertaining to adenoids.

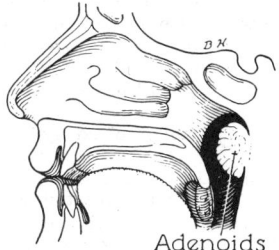

Adenoids

adenoidectomy (ad″ĕ-noid-ek′to-me) [*adenoid* + Gr. *ektomē* excision] excision of the adenoids.

adenoidism (ad′ĕ-noid-izm) the symptom-complex which results from the presence of greatly enlarged adenoids.

adenoiditis (ad″ĕ-noid-i′tis) inflammation of the adenoid tissue of the nasopharynx.

adenoleiomyofibroma (ad″ĕ-no-li″o-mi″o-fi-bro′mah) a leiomyofibroma containing adenomatous elements.

adenolipoma (ad″ĕ-no-lĭ-po′mah) a tumor composed of both glandular and fatty tissue elements.

adenolipomatosis (ad″ĕ-no-lip″o-mah-to′sis) a condition characterized by the development of multiple adenolipomas.

adenologaditis (ad″ĕ-no-log″ah-di′tis) [*adeno-* + Gr. *logades* whites of the eyes + *-itis*] 1. ophthalmia neonatorum. 2. inflammation of the glands of the conjunctiva.

adenology (ad″ĕ-nol′o-je) [*adeno-* + *-logy*] the scientific study of or the body of knowledge relating to glands.

adenolymphitis (ad″ĕ-no-lim-fi′tis) lymphadenitis.

adenolymphocele (ad″ĕ-no-lim′fo-sēl) [*adeno-* + *lymphocele*] lymphadenocele.

adenolymphoma (ad″ĕ-no-lim-fo′mah) papillary adenocystoma lymphomatosum (Warthin's tumor) of salivary glands.

adenoma (ad″ĕ-no′mah) [*adeno-* + *-oma*] a benign epithelial tumor in which the cells form recognizable glandular structures or in which the cells are clearly derived from glandular epithelium. **acidophilic a.,** a tumor, usually found in the anterior lobe of the pituitary gland, whose cells stain with acid dyes; such pituitary tumors may give rise to excessive secretion of growth hormone, resulting in gigantism or acromegaly. **a. adamantiʹnum,** ameloblastoma. **a. alveolaʹre,** an adenoma whose cells are arranged like those of an alveolar gland. **basophil a., basophilic a.,** a tumor of the anterior lobe of the pituitary gland whose cells stain with basic dyes and may give rise to excessive secretion of adrenocorticotropic hormone (ACTH), resulting in Cushing's syndrome. **bronchial a's,** adenomas situated in the submucosal tissues of large bronchi; they have a glandular structure and are thought to be derived from the mucous glands of the bronchi or from the ducts of those glands. Sometimes composed of well differentiated cells and usually circumscribed, these tumors have two histologic forms: carcinoid and cylindroma. Although termed "adenomas," these tumors are now recognized as being of low grade malignancy. **carcinoid a. of bronchus,** carcinoid tumor of bronchus; see under *tumor.* **chief-cell a.,** adenoma of the parathyroid composed of solid masses of small chief cells similar to those seen in the normal gland. **chromophobe a., chromophobic a.,** a tumor of the anterior lobe of the pituitary gland whose cells do not stain readily with either acid or basic dyes and whose presence may be associated with hypopituitarism; although classically these adenomas have been said to be composed of sparsely granulated or degranulated (nonfunctioning) cells, some contain functioning cells and may be associated with a hyperpituitary state. **cortical a's,** minute adenomas in the cortex of the kidney, arising from the renal tubules. **a. desʹtruens** (*obs.*), an invasive, destructive adenocarcinoma of the stomach. **a. endometrioiʹdes ovaʹrii,** ovarian endometriosis. **eosinophil a.,** a tumor of eosinophilic cells of the anterior lobe of the pituitary gland whose presence is associated with acromegaly and gigantism. **a. fibroʹsum,** fibroadenoma. **follicular a.,** adenoma of the thyroid in which the cells are arranged in the form of follicles. **a. gelatinoʹsum,** colloid goiter. **Getsowa's a.** (*obs.*), Hürthle cell tumor; see under *tumor.* **a. hidradenoiʹdes,** hidradenoma. **Hürthle cell a.,** see under *tumor.* **islet a., langerhansian a.,** an islet cell adenoma of the pancreas. **a's of kidney,** cortical a's. **malignant a.,** adenocarcinoma. **mucinous a.,** an epithelial tumor whose cells produce mucin. **a. ovaʹrii testiculaʹre,** a Sertoli cell tumor of the ovary, now generally regarded as a variant of arrhenoblastoma. **oxyphilic granular cell a.,** a benign adenoma of salivary glands composed of acidophilic granular cells; called also *oncocytoma* and *pyknocytoma.* **papillary cystic a.,** a form of adenoma in which the alveoli are distended by fluid or by outgrowths of tissue. **pituitary a.,** a benign neoplasm of the pituitary gland; see *acidophilic a., basophilic a.,* and *chromophobe a.* **pleomorphic a.,** a benign mixed tumor of adult glandular epithelium, commonly of the parotid gland. **racemose a.,** an adenoma whose structure resembles that of a racemose gland. **sebaceous a.,** hypertrophy or benign hyperplasia of a sebaceous gland. **a. sebaʹceum,** nevoid hyperplasia of sebaceous glands, forming multiple yellow papules or nodules of the face (Balzer type); a cutaneous malformation or hamartoma of the face involving blood vessels and connective tissue associated with the tuberous sclerosis complex (Pringle type). In the Pringle type the term adenoma sebaceum is a misnomer since the sebaceous glands are rarely involved. Called also *Pringle's disease.* **a. simʹplex** (*obs.*), simple hyperplasia of a gland. **a. sudoripʹarum,** adenoma of the sweat glands; called also *spiradenoma* and *hidradenoma.* **tubular a.,** a Sertoli cell tumor. **a. tubulaʹre testiculaʹre ovaʹrii,** a Sertoli cell tumor of the ovary, now generally recognized as a variant of arrhenoblastoma; called also *adenoma ovarii testiculare.* **villous a.,** a large soft papillary polyp on the mucosa of the large intestine.

adenomalacia (ad″ĕ-no-mah-la′she-ah) [*adeno-* + Gr. *malakia* softness] abnormal softening of a gland.

adenomatoid (ad″ĕ-no′mah-toid) resembling adenoma.

adenomatosis (ad″ĕ-no-mah-to′sis) a condition characterized by development of numerous adenomatous growths. **multiple endocrine a.,** polyendocrine a. **a. oʹris,** enlargement of the mucous glands of the lip without secretion or inflammation. **pluriglandular a.,** polyendocrine a. **polyendocrine a.,** a rare syndrome in which there are adenomas or hyperplasia of more than one endocrine tissue; common sites are the anterior pituitary gland, the islets of Langerhans, and the parathyroid. The Zollinger-Ellison syndrome may occur in affected families. Called also *multiple endocrine a., pluriglandular a., polyendocrinoma,* and *Wermer's syndrome.* **pulmonary a.,** 1. alveolar cell carcinoma. 2. a chronic progressive pneumonia of sheep, probably of viral origin, with adenomatous proliferation in the alveoli and small bronchioles. Called also *jaagsiekte* and *lunger disease.*

adenomatous (ad″ĕ-nom′ah-tus) pertaining to adenoma or to nodular hyperplasia of a gland.

adenomegaly (ad″ĕ-no-meg′ah-le) enlargement of the glands.

adenomere (ad′ĕ-no-mēr″) [*adeno-* + Gr. *meros* part] the blind terminal portion of a developing gland, becoming the functional portion of the organ.

adenomyoepithelioma (ad″ĕ-no-mi″o-ep″ĭ-the-le-o′mah) adenoid cystic carcinoma. **a. of stomach,** malformation of the gastric glands or Brunner's glands.

adenomyofibroma (ad″ĕ-no-mi″o-fi-bro′mah) a fibroma containing adenomatous and myomatous tissue.

adenomyoma (ad″ĕ-no-mi-o′mah) [*adeno-* + Gr. *mys* muscle + *-oma*] see *adenomyosis.* **a. psammopapillaʹre,** a multiple papillary tumor in the broad ligament, described by Pick.

adenomyomatosis (ad″ĕ-no-mi″o-mah-to′sis) the formation of multiple adenomyomatous nodules in the parauterine tissues or in the uterus.

adenomyomatous (ad″ĕ-no-mi-o′mah-tus) pertaining to or resembling adenomyoma.

adenomyometritis (ad″ĕ-no-mi″o-mĕ-tri′tis) adenomyosis.

adenomyosarcoma (ad″ĕ-no-mi″o-sar-ko′mah) a mixed mesodermal tumor in which striated muscle cells are one component. **embryonal a.,** Wilms' tumor.

adenomyosis (ad″ĕ-no-mi-o′sis) a benign condition characterized by ingrowth of the endometrium into the uterine musculature, sometimes associated with an overgrowth of the latter. If the lesion forms a circumscribed tumor-like nodule, it is called *adenomyoma.* Called also *endometriosis interna* or *uterina, adenomyosis uteri,* and *adenomyometritis.* **a. exterʹna,** endometriosis. **stromal a.,** stromatosis. **a. subbasaʹlis,** a bandlike, usually diffuse and superficial invasion of the myometrium by epithelial elements, accompanied by small clusters of endometrial stromal cells. **a. tuʹbae,** 1. an old term for salpingitis isthmica nodosa. 2. the growth of the endometrium into the lumen of the uterine tube from the uterus, replacing the endosalpinx. **a. uʹteri,** adenomyosis.

adenomyxoma (ad″ĕ-no-mik-so′mah) (*obs.*) a tumor composed of both glandular and mucous elements.

adenomyxosarcoma (ad″ĕ-no-mik″so-sar-ko′mah) (*obs.*) a sarcoma containing both glandular and mucous elements.

adenoncus (ad″ĕ-nong′kus) [*adeno-* + Gr. *onkos* weight] enlargement of a gland.

adenoneural (ad″ĕ-no-nu′ral) pertaining to a gland and a nerve.

adenopathy (ad″ĕ-nop′ah-the) [*adeno-* + Gr. *pathos* disease] enlargement of the glands, especially of the lymphatic glands.

adenopharyngitis (ad″ĕ-no-far″in-ji′tis) [*adeno-* + Gr. *pharynx* pharynx + *-itis*] inflammation of the adenoids and pharynx, usually involving the tonsils.

adenophlegmon (ad″ĕ-no-fleg′mon) [*adeno-* + *phlegmon*] phlegmonous adenitis.

adenophthalmia (ad″ĕ-nof-thal′me-ah) [*adeno-* + Gr. *ophthalmos* eye + *-ia*] inflammation of the meibomian glands.

adenopituicyte (ad″ĕ-no-pĭ-tu′ĭ-sīt) see *pituicyte.*

adenosarcoma (ad″ĕ-no-sar-ko′mah) a mixed tumor composed of sarcomatous and glandular elements, as Wilms' tumor. **embryonal a.,** Wilms' tumor.

adenosclerosis (ad″ĕ-no-skle-ro′sis) [adeno- + Gr. sklērōsis hardening] the hardening of a gland.

adenosinase (ad-ĕ-no′sin-ās) an enzyme that splits adenosine hydrolytically.

adenosine (ah-den′o-sēn) a nucleoside, adenine-D-ribose, $C_5H_5\cdot N_5\cdot CH(CHOH)_2\cdot CH\cdot CH_2OH$, derived from nucleic acid. **a. 3′:5′-cyclic phosphate,** a cyclic nucleotide participating in the activities of many hormones, including catecholamines, ACTH, vasopressin, etc. Because this compound is formed from ATP by the action of adenyl cyclase which in turn is stimulated by the interaction of the aforementioned hormones with the plasma membrane of target cells, it has been called the "second messenger" in a mechanism of hormone action. Called also cyclic AMP. **a. deaminase,** an enzyme that converts adenosine into inosine. **a. diphosphate (ADP),** a product, along with organic phosphate, of the hydrolysis of adenosine triphosphate (ATP), with the release of free energy; ADP is then readily rephosphorylated to ATP. **a. hydrolase,** an enzyme that converts adenosine into adenine and pentose. **a. monophosphate (AMP),** adenylic acid. **a. phosphate,** any of the three interconvertible compounds in which adenosine is attached through its ribose group to one (a. monophosphate), two (a. diphosphate), or three (a. triphosphate) phosphoric acid molecules. **a. 3′-phosphate,** see adenylic acid, under acid. **a. 5′-phosphate,** see adenylic acid, under acid. **a. triphosphate (ATP),** a nucleotide compound occurring in all cells, where it represents energy storage in the form of high-energy phosphate bonds; free energy is released when it is hydrolyzed to ADP and a phosphate group.

adenosinetriphosphatase (ah-den″o-sin-tri-fos′fah-tās) any enzyme that catalyzes the splitting of adenosine triphosphate, with liberation of inorganic phosphate and release of free energy; abbreviated ATPase. These enzymes are activated by Ca^{++} and/or Mg^{++} or by Na^+ and K^+ and are associated with formed elements, such as intracellular structures and cell membranes. Thus myosin ATPase is concerned in muscle contraction, mitochondrial ATPase in securing energy from biological oxidations, etc.

adenosis (ad″ĕ-no′sis) 1. any disease of the glands. 2. the abnormal development or formation of gland tissue. **blunt duct a.,** a form of mammary dysplasia characterized by dominance of the proliferation of the epithelial parenchyma; it is often accompanied by fibrosis and cystic disease of the breast. **a. vagi′nae,** the presence in the vagina of multiple ectopic areas of folded endocervical mucosa.

S-adenosylmethionine (ah-den″o-sil-mĕ-thi′o-nēn) a reaction product of ATP and methionine in which the S atom of methionine is bound to the ribose of adenosine; it serves as a methyl donor in transmethylation reactions.

adenotome (ad′ĕ-no-tōm″) [adeno- + Gr. tomē cutting] an instrument for excision of the adenoids.

adenotonsillectomy (ad″ĕ-no-ton″sil-lek′to-me) removal of the adenoids and tonsils.

adenous (ad′ĕ-nus) pertaining to a gland.

adenoviral (ad″ĕ-no-vi′ral) pertaining to or caused by adenoviruses.

adenovirus (ad″ĕ-no-vi′rus) one of a group of viruses found in all parts of the world, causing disease of the upper respiratory tract and conjunctivae, and also present in latent infections in normal persons. Some 31 differentiable serotypes have been described and given numbers. Types 1, 2, and 5 have been recovered from tonsils and adenoids of persons not ill with respiratory disease, as well as from patients with febrile respiratory infections; types 3, 4, 7, 14, and 21 have been isolated from patients with acute respiratory disease. Adenovirus type 3 is the specific etiologic agent of pharyngoconjunctival fever, and adenovirus type 8 is thought to be the specific cause of epidemic keratoconjunctivitis. In addition to the human adenovirus types, there are simian, bovine, avian, canine, and murine types. Many adenoviruses induce malignancy in certain species.

adenyl (ad′ĕ-nil) a chemical radical resulting from the formal loss of an OH group attached to phosphorus from adenosine-5′-monophosphoric acid (5′-AMP). **a. cyclase,** an enzyme found in the liver and muscle cell membranes, which catalyzes the conversion of adenosine triphosphate (ATP) to cyclic adenosine monophosphate (AMP) (see adenosine 3′:5′cyclic phosphate) plus pyrophosphate, and is activated by many hormones. Called also adenylate cyclase.

adenylate (ah-den′ĭ-lāt) adenylic acid, or a salt of adenylic acid. **a. cyclase,** see under adenyl. **a. kinase,** ATP:AMP phosphotransferase. An enzyme occurring in muscle, heart, brain, and liver that converts AMP and ATP to two molecules of ADP. Called also myokinase.

adenylcyclase (ad″ĕ-nil-si′klās) adenyl cyclase.

adenylosuccinase (ad″ĕ-nil-o-suk′sĭ-nās) adenylosuccinate lyase.

adenylosuccinate (ad″ĕ-nil-o-suk′sĭ-nāt) a derivative of ade-

nylic and succinic acids, which is cleaved to form adenylic acid plus fumaric acid. **a. lyase,** adenylosuccinate AMP-lyase: an enzyme occurring in the liver that catalyzes the conversion of adenylosuccinate to adenylic acid and fumarate.

adenylpyrophosphate (ad″ĕ-nil-pi″ro-fos′fāt) adenosine triphosphate.

adenylyl (ad′ĕ-nĭ-lil) the radical of adenylic acid with one H ion removed.

adephagia (ad″ĕ-fa′ji-ah) [Gr. adēn enough + phagein to eat + -ia] obsolete term for gluttony and insatiable hunger (bulimia).

adeps (ad′eps), gen. ad′ipis [L.] lard; the purified omental fat of the hog, used in the preparation of ointments. **a. anseri′nus,** goose grease. **a. benzoina′tus,** benzoinated lard. **a. la′nae,** anhydrous lanolin. **a. la′nae hydro′sus,** lanolin. **a. ovil′lus,** sheep lard, or tallow. **a. por′ci,** hog lard. **a. re′nis,** the fatty capsule of the kidney. **a. suil′lus,** hog lard.

adequacy (ad′ĕ-kwah-se) the state of being sufficient for a specific purpose. **velopharyngeal a.,** sufficient functional closure of the velum against the postpharyngeal wall so that air and hence sound cannot enter the nasopharyngeal and nasal cavities.

adermia (ah-der′me-ah) [a neg. + Gr. derma skin + -ia] congenital defect or absence of the skin.

adermine (ah-der′min) pyridoxine; vitamin B_6.

adermogenesis (ah-der″mo-jen′ĕ-sis) [a neg. + Gr. derma skin + genesis production] imperfect development of the skin.

Ad grat. acid abbreviation for L. ad gra′tum acidita′tem, to an agreeable sourness, an obsolete instruction in pharmacy.

ADH antidiuretic hormone; see vasopressin.

Adhatoda (ad-hat′o-dah) a plant genus of the Acanthaceae family. A. vasica, known as the Malabar nut tree, is used in India for its antispasmodic and expectorant properties.

adhere (ad-hēr′) to cling together; to become fastened.

adherence (ad-hēr′ens) the act or quality of sticking to something. **immune a.,** a complement-dependent phenomenon in which antigen-antibody complexes or particulate antigens coated with antibody (e.g., antibody-coated bacteria) adhere to red blood cells when complement component C3 is bound. It is a sensitive detector of complement-fixing antibody.

adhesio (ad-he′ze-o), pl. adhesio′nes [L. "clinging together"] a connecting band or structure. **a. interthalam′ica** [NA], a mass of gray matter connecting the thalami across the midline of the third ventricle; it develops as a secondary adhesion and is often absent. Called also intermediate mass and massa intermedia.

adhesion (ad-he′zhun) [L. adhaesio, from adhaerere to stick to] 1. the property of remaining in close proximity, as that resulting from the physical attraction of molecules to a substance, or the molecular attraction existing between the surfaces of contacting bodies. 2. the stable joining of parts to each other, which may occur abnormally. 3. a fibrous band or structure by which parts abnormally adhere. **amniotic a's,** fibrous adhesions from the amnion to the fetus. **attic a's** (obs.), adhesions about the gallbladder and pyloric region. **primary a.,** healing by first intention. **secondary a.,** healing by second intention. **serological a.,** a phenomenon in which nonspecific particulate material tends to adhere to particulate antigen in the presence of antibody and complement. **sublabial a.,** abnormal union of the sublabial mucosa of the upper lip to the alveolar process; usually present in a unilateral or bilateral cleft of the lip. **traumatic uterine a's,** adhesions of the uterus, most often in the cervical canal, frequently in the uterine cavity, and sometimes in both the cervix and the corpus, which are usually caused by curettage; cervical adhesions cause amenorrhea (see Asherman's syndrome, under syndrome), whereas corporeal adhesions usually are asymptomatic.

adhesiotomy (ad-he″ze-ot′o-me) the cutting or division of adhesions.

adhesive (ad-he′siv) 1. sticky; tenacious. 2. a substance that causes close adherence of adjoining surfaces. **denture a.,** a compound of natural or artificial gums used to stabilize denture bases.

adhesiveness (ad-he′siv-nes) the property of remaining adherent. **platelet a.,** the physical property of platelets by which they stick to a variety of materials in vivo and in vitro, but more specifically this phenomenon as it occurs in the initial formation of a clot and in the maintenance of hemostasis.

Adhib. abbreviation for L. adhiben′dus, to be administered.

adiabatic (ah-di″ah-bat′ik) conducted without the evolution or absorption of heat.

adiactinic (ah-di″ak-tin′ik) [a neg. + Gr. dia through + aktis ray] not permitting the passage of actinic rays.

adiadochocinesia (ah-di″ah-do″ko-si-ne′se-ah) adiadochokinesia.

adiadochocinesis (ah-di″ah-do″ko-si-ne′sis) adiadochokinesia.

adiadochokinesia (ah-di″ah-do″ko-ki-ne′se-ah) [a neg. + Gr. diadochos succeeding + kinesis motion + -ia] inability to perform rapid alternating movements. Cf. diadochokinesia.

adiadochokinesis (ah-di″ah-do″ko-ki-ne′sis) adiadochokine-sia.

adiadokokinesia (ah-di″ah-do″ko-ki-ne′se-ah) adiadochokine-sia.

adiadokokinesis (ah-di″ah-do″ko-ki-ne′sis) adiadochokinesia.

Adiantum (ad″e-an′tum) [*a* neg. + Gr. *dianein* to moisten] a genus of ferns of the family Polypodiaceae, popularly called maidenhair. *A. pedatum* (North America, eastern Asia) has been used as an expectorant and demulcent.

adiaphoria (ah-di″ah-fo′re-ah) [Gr. "indifference"] nonresponse to stimuli as a result of previous exposure to similar stimuli; see also *refractory period*, under *period*.

adiaspiromycosis (ad″ĭ-ah-spi″ro-mi-ko′sis) a pulmonary disease of many species of rodents throughout the world and rarely of man. It is caused by the inhalation of spores produced by the saprophytic soil fungus *Emmonsia parva* or *E. crescens*, and marked by the presence of huge spherules (adiaspores) without endospores in the lungs. The condition is often confused with the tissue phase of *Coccidioides immitis*. Called also *haplomycosis*.

adiaspore (ad′ĭ-ah-spōr) a spore produced by the soil fungi *Emmonsia parva* and *E. crescens*, which, after inhalation into the lungs, enlarges to form a huge spherule without endospores.

adiathermance (ah-di″ah-ther′mans) adiathermancy.

adiathermancy (ah-di″ah-ther′man-se) [*a* neg. + Gr. *dia* through + *thermansis* heating] the condition of being impervious to heat waves.

adicillin (ad″ĭ-sil′in) chemical name: (4-amino-4-carboxybutyl)-penicillin. A cephalosporin that is less active against gram-positive bacteria than penicillin G but more active against gram-negative organisms and is highly active against *Neisseria;* it has been used in the treatment of typhoid fever and gonorrhea. Called also *cephalosporin N* and *penicillin N*.

Adie's pupil, syndrome (a′dēz) [William John *Adie*, British neurologist, 1886–1935] see *tonic pupil*, under *pupil*, and see under *syndrome*.

adiemorrhysis (ah-di″ĕ-mor′ĭ-sis) [*a* neg. + Gr. *dia* through + *haima* blood + *rhysis* flow] stoppage of circulation of blood.

adient (ad′e-ent) tending toward the source of stimulation; positive. Cf. *abient*.

Adinida (ah-din′ĭ-dah) a suborder of dinoflagellate protozoa marked by the flagella being free and not enclosed in furrows.

adipectomy (ad″ĭ-pek′to-me) [L. *adeps* + Gr. *ektomē* excision] lipectomy.

adiphenine hydrochloride (ad″ĭ-fen′ēn) chemical name; α-phenyl-2-(diethylamino)ethyl ester hydrochloride. An antispasmodic anticholinergic, $C_{20}H_{25}NO_2 \cdot HCl$, used orally as a smooth muscle relaxant in the treatment of hypermotility and spasm of the genitourinary and gastrointestinal tracts.

adipic (ah-dip′ik) [L. *adeps* fat] adipose.

adipo- (ad′ĭ-po) [L. *adeps, adipis* fat] a combining form denoting relationship to fat.

adipocele (ad′ĭ-po-sēl″) [*adipo-* + Gr. *kēlē* hernia] a hernia containing fat or fatty tissue, as an epiplocele.

adipocellular (ad″ĭ-po-sel′u-lar) composed of connective tissue and fat.

adipoceratous (ad″ĭ-po-ser′ah-tus) pertaining to or resembling adipocere.

adipocere (ad′ĭ-po-sēr″) [*adipo-* + L. *cera* wax] a peculiar waxy substance formed during the decomposition of animal bodies, and seen especially in human bodies buried in moist places; it consists principally of insoluble salts of fatty acids. Called also *grave wax* and *corpse* or *grave fat*.

adipocyte (ad′ĭ-po-sīt″) a fat cell; see under *cell*.

adipofibroma (ad″ĭ-po-fi-bro′mah), pl. *adipofibro′mas*. A lipoma containing fibrous tissue component.

adipogenesis (ad″ĭ-po-jen′ĕ-sis) the formation of fat.

adipogenic (ad″ĭ-po-jen′ik) [*adipo-* + Gr. *gennan* to produce] producing fat or fatness.

adipogenous (ad″ĭ-poj′ĕ-nus) adipogenic.

adipohepatic (ad″ĭ-po-hĕ-pat′ik) pertaining to or marked by fatty degeneration of the liver.

adipoid (ad′ĭ-poid) [*adipo-* + Gr. *eidos* form] lipoid, def. 1.

adipokinesis (ad″ĭ-po-ki-ne′sis) the mobilization of fat in the body, often with the liberation of free fatty acids into the blood plasma; see also *lipolytic hormones*, under *hormone*.

adipokinetic (ad″ĭ-po-ki-net′ik) pertaining to, characterized by, or promoting adipokinesis.

adipokinin (ad″ĭ-po-ki′nin) a theoretical lipolytic hormone of the anterior lobe of the pituitary gland.

adipolysis (ad″ĭ-pol′ĭ-sis) [*adipo-* + Gr. *lysis* dissolution] lipolysis.

adipolytic (ad″ĭ-po-lit′ik) lipolytic.

adipoma (ad″ĭ-po′mah) (*obs.*) lipoma.

adipometer (ad″ĭ-pom′ĕ-ter) an instrument for measuring the

thickness of the skin fold, as a means of determining the presence of obesity.

adiponecrosis (ad″ĭ-po-nĕ-kro′sis) necrosis of fatty tissue in the body. **a. subcuta′nea neonato′rum,** subcutaneous fat induration in newborn and young infants; called also *subcutaneous fat necrosis* and *pseudosclerema*.

adipopectic (ad″ĭ-po-pek′tik) pertaining to, characterized by, or promoting adipopexis.

adipopexia (ad″ĭ-po-pek′se-ah) adipopexis.

adipopexic (ad″ĭ-po-pek′sik) adipopectic.

adipopexis (ad″ĭ-po-pek′sis) [*adipo-* + Gr. *pēxis* fixation] the fixation or storing of fats.

adiposalgia (ad″ĭ-pōs-al′je-ah) [*adipo-* + Gr. *algos* pain + *-ia*] a neuropathic state in which there are painful areas of subcutaneous fat.

adipose (ad″ĭ-pōs) [L. *adiposus* fatty] 1. of a fatty nature; fatty; fat. 2. the fat present in the cells of adipose tissue.

adiposis (ad″ĭ-po′sis) [L. *adeps* fat + *-osis*] 1. obesity or corpulence; an excessive accumulation of fat in the body. 2. fatty change of an organ or tissue. **a. cerebra′lis,** cerebral adiposity. **a. doloro′sa,** a disease accompanied by painful localized fatty swellings and by various nerve lesions. The disease is usually seen in women, and may cause death from pulmonary complica-

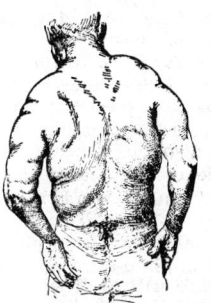

Adiposis dolorosa (Homans).

tions. Called also *Dercum's disease.* **a. hepat′ica,** fatty change of the liver. **a. tubero′sa sim′plex,** a disorder resembling adiposis dolorosa, marked by development in the subcutaneous tissue of fatty masses which are sometimes painful to pressure; called also *Anders' disease.* **a. universa′lis,** a deposit of fat generally throughout the body, including the internal organs.

adipositas (ad″ĭ-pos′ĭ-tas) [L.] fatness. **a. abdom′inis,** hyperadiposity of the abdominal wall. **a. cerebra′lis,** cerebral adiposity. **a. cor′dis,** fat heart, def. 2. **a. ex vac′uo,** fatty atrophy.

adipositis (ad″ĭ-po-si′tis) panniculitis.

adiposity (ad″ĭ-pos′ĭ-te) the state of being fat; fatness; obesity. See *adiposogenital dystrophy*, under *dystrophy*. **cerebral a.,** fatness due to cerebral disease, especially disease of the hypothalamus, as in adiposogenital dystrophy. **pituitary a.,** obesity due to pituitary insufficiency.

adiposuria (ad″ĭ-po-su′re-ah) [*adipo-* + Gr. *ouron* urine + *-ia*] the occurrence of fat in the urine; lipuria, or lipiduria.

adipsa (ah-dip′sah) remedies to allay thirst; foods which do not produce thirst.

adipsia (ah-dip′se-ah) [*a* neg. + Gr. *dipsa* thirst + *-ia*] absence of thirst, or abnormal avoidance of drinking.

adipsous (ah-dip′sus) quenching thirst, as certain fruits.

adipsy (ah-dip′se) adipsia.

aditus (ad′ĭ-tus), pl. *ad′itus* [L.] [NA] a general term for the entrance or approach to an organ or part. **a. ad an′trum** [NA], an opening between the epitympanum and the mastoid antrum. **a. ad aquaeduc′tum cer′ebri** (*obs.*), the posterior portion of the third ventricle where it passes over into the aqueductus cerebri. **a. ad pel′vis,** the pelvic inlet. **a. ad sac′cum peritonae′i mino′rem,** epiploic foramen. **a. laryn′gis** [NA], the aperture by which the pharynx communicates with the larynx; called also *aperture of larynx*. **a. or′bitae** [NA], the opening to the orbit in the cranium; called also *orbital aperture, orbital opening*, and *anterior opening of orbital cavity*. **a. vagi′nae,** ostium vaginae.

adjection (ad-jek′shun) addition; specifically, the principle that as many microbes can be added to the living microbes in the body as will form in combination with the latter the proper dose to immunize the patient.

adjunct (ad′junkt) an accessory or auxiliary agent or measure.

adjunctive (ad-junk′tiv) assisting or aiding.

adjustment (ad-just′ment) 1. a rearrangement of physical parts made in response to changing conditions. 2. in psychology, the relative state of harmony of personality; the relative degree of resolution of emotional conflicts. 3. in chiropractic, manipulation of the spine, said to restore normal nerve function and cure disease.　4. the mechanism for raising and lowering the tube of a microscope, for bringing the object being examined into proper focus.　5. a modification made in a denture after its completion and insertion in the mouth.　**occlusal a.,** modification of the occluding surfaces of teeth to develop more harmonious relationships between these surfaces, usually by grinding away interferences.

adjuvant (ad′ju-vant) [L. *adjuvans* aiding]　1. assisting, or aiding.　2. a substance which aids another, such as an auxiliary remedy; in immunology, nonspecific stimulator (e.g., BCG vaccine) of the immune response.　**Freund's a.,** a water-in-oil emulsion incorporating antigen, in the aqueous phase, into light-weight paraffin oil with the aid of an emulsifying agent. On injection, this mixture (*Freund's incomplete a.*) induces strong persistent antibody formation. The addition of killed, dried mycobacteria, e.g., *Mycobacterium butyricum,* to the oil phase (*Freund's complete a.*) elicits cell-mediated immunity (delayed hypersensitivity), as well as humoral antibody formation.　**mycobacterial a.,** Freund's complete a.; see *Freund's a.*

adjuvanticity (ad″ju-van-tĭ′sĭ-te)　the ability to modify the immune response.

Adler's test (ad′lerz) [Oscar *Adler,* German physician, 1879–1932, and his brother Rudolph, 1882–1952]　benzidine test; see *Table of Tests.*

Adler's theory (ad′lerz) [Alfred *Adler,* Vienna psychiatrist, 1870–1937]　see under *theory.*

ad lib.　abbreviation for L. *ad lib′itum,* at pleasure.

adlumidine (ad-loo′mi-din)　a crystalline alkaloid, $C_{19}H_{16}O_6N$, from *Adlumia fungosa,* a species of herbaceous ferns.

adlumine (ad-loo′min)　a crystalline alkaloid, $C_{21}H_{21}NO_6$, from *Adlu′mia fungosa,* a species of herbaceous ferns.

admedial (ad-me′de-al)　situated near the median plane.

admedian (ad-me′de-an)　toward the median plane, or midline of the body.

adminicula (ad″mĭ-nik′u-lah) [L.]　plural of *adminiculum.*

adminiculum (ad″mĭ-nik′u-lum), pl. *adminic′ula* [L.]　a prop or support.　**a. lin′eae al′bae** [NA], the expansion of fibers extending from the superior pubic ligament to the posterior surface of the linea alba.

admov.　abbreviation for L. *ad′move, admovea′tur,* add, let there be added.

ad nauseam (ad-naw′se-am) [L.]　to the extent of producing nausea.

adnerval (ad-ner′val)　1. situated near a nerve.　2. toward a nerve, said of an electric current which passes through muscle toward the entrance point of a nerve.

adneural (ad-nu′ral) [*ad-* + Gr. *neuron* nerve]　adnerval.

adnexa (ad-nek′sah) [L., pl]　appendages or adjunct parts; see also *appendage.*　**a. oc′uli,** the eyelids, lacrimal apparatus, and other appendages of the eye.　**a. u′teri,** the uterine appendages: the ovaries, uterine tubes, and ligaments of the uterus.

adnexal (ad-nek′sal)　pertaining to adnexa, especially the adnexa uteri.

adnexectomy (ad″nek-sek′to-me) [*adnexa* + Gr. *ektomē* excision]　excision or removal of the adnexa.

adnexitis (ad″nek-si′tis)　inflammation of the adnexa uteri.

adnexogenesis (ad-nek″so-jen′ĕ-sis) [L. *adnexa* + Gr. *genesis* production]　embryonic development of the adnexa or accessory structures.

adnexopexy (ad-nek′so-pek″se) [L. *adnexa* + Gr. *pēxis* fixation] (*obs.*) ovariopexy.

adnexorganogenic (ad-neks″or-gah-no-jen′ik)　giving rise to or originating in the adnexa uteri.

adolescence (ad″o-les′ens) [L. *adolescentia*]　the period of life beginning with the appearance of secondary sex characters and terminating with the cessation of somatic growth, roughly from 11 to 19 years of age; cf. *puberty.*

adolescent (ad″o-les′ent)　1. pertaining to adolescence.　2. an individual during the period of adolescence.

adonidin (ah-don′i-din)　a poisonous glycoside, $C_{24}H_{42}O_9$, from *Adonis vernalis,* not unlike digitalin in its effects; formerly used as a cardiac stimulant.

adonin (ah-do′nin)　a glucoside, $C_{20}H_{40}O_9$, from *Adonis amurensis,* a plant of Asia.

Adonis (ah-do′nis) [L.]　a genus of poisonous ranunculaceous plants, native to Europe, Asia, and Africa. *A. aestiva′lis* and *A. verna′lis* were formerly used as cardiac stimulants.

adonite (ad′o-nit)　adonitol.

adonitol (ah-don′i-tol)　a pentahydric alcohol found in *Adonis vernalis;* by oxidation it yields ribose.

adoral (ad-o′ral) [L. *ad* near + *os, oris* mouth]　toward or near the mouth.

ADP　adenosine diphosphate.

Ad pond. om.　abbreviation for L. *ad pon′dus om′nium,* to the weight of the whole.

adrenal (ah-dre′nal) [L. *ad* near + *ren* kidney]　1. situated near the kidney.　2. an adrenal gland.　**Marchand's a's,** accessory adrenal bodies in the broad ligament.

adrenalectomize (ah-dre″nal-ek′to-mīz)　to extirpate one or both adrenal glands by surgical means.

adrenalectomy (ah-dre″nal-ek′to-me) [*adrenal* + Gr. *ektomē* excision]　excision of one or both adrenal glands; suprarenalectomy.

Adrenalin (ah-dren′ah-lin)　trademark for preparations of epinephrine; in Great Britain, a generic name.

adrenaline (ah-dren′ah-lēn)　the official British Pharmacopoeia name for epinephrine.　**a. acid tartrate,** epinephrine bitartrate.

adrenalinemia (ah-dren″ah-lin-e′me-ah) [*adrenalin* + Gr. *haima* blood + *-ia*]　the presence of epinephrine in the blood.

adrenalinogenesis (ah-dren″ah-lin-o-jen′ĕ-sis)　the formation of epinephrine.

adrenalinuria (ah-dren″ah-lin-u′re-ah)　the presence of epinephrine in the urine.

adrenalism (ah-dren′al-izm)　ill health due to adrenal dysfunction. Cf. *dysadrenalism.*

adrenalitis (ah-dre″nal-i′tis)　inflammation of the adrenal glands.

adrenalone (ah-dren′ah-lōn)　chemical name: 1-(3,4-dihydroxyphenyl)-2-(methylamino)ethanone. An adrenergic, $C_9H_{11}NO_3$, obtained by oxidation of an epinephrine derivative; it has vasoconstrictor activity.

adrenalopathy (ah-dre″nal-op′ah-the) [*adrenal* + Gr. *pathos* disease]　any disease of the adrenal glands.

adrenalotropic (ah-dren″ah-lo-trop′ik) [*adrenal* + Gr. *tropos* a turning]　having a special affinity for the adrenal glands.

adrenarche (ad″ren-ar′ke) [*adrenal* + Gr. *archē* beginning]　augmentation of adrenal cortex function, involving especially androgens, a physiologic change that occurs at approximately the age of eight years.

adrenergic (ad″ren-er′jik)　1. activated by, characteristic of, or secreting epinephrine or substances with similar activity; the term is applied to those nerve fibers that liberate norepinephrine at a synapse when a nerve impulse passes, i.e., the sympathetic fibers. See also under *receptor.*　2. an agent that produces such an effect. Called also *sympathomimetic.* Cf. *cholinergic.*

adrenic (ah-dren′ik)　pertaining to the adrenal glands.

adrenin (ah-dre′nin)　epinephrine.

adrenine (ah-dre′nin)　epinephrine.

adrenitis (ad″re-ni′tis)　adrenalitis.

adreno- [L. *ad* near + *ren* kidney]　a combining form denoting relationship to the adrenal gland.

adrenoceptive (ah-dre″no-sep′tiv)　pertaining to the sites on effector organs that are acted upon by adrenergic transmitters.

adrenoceptor (ah-dre″no-sep′tor)　adrenergic receptor; see under *receptor.*

adrenochrome (ad-re′no-krōm″)　chemical name: 2,3-dihydro-3-hydroxy-1-methyl-1*H*-indole-5,6-dione. A red oxidation product of epinephrine, $C_9H_9NO_3$, which possesses hemostatic properties due to its effect on capillary permeability, and has been used as an experimental psychomimetic. It is used in the form of its stable derivative *carbazochrome salicylate.*

adrenocortical (ad-re″no-kor′te-kal)　pertaining to or arising from the cortex of the adrenal gland.

adrenocorticohyperplasia (ah-dre″no-kor″tĭ-ko-hi″per-pla′ze-ah)　adrenal cortical hyperplasia.

adrenocorticomimetic (ad-re″no-kor″te-ko-mi-met′ik)　producing effects similar to those of hormones of the cortex of the adrenal glands.

adrenocorticotrophic (ad-re″no-kor″te-ko-trof′ik)　corticotropic.

adrenocorticotrophin (ad-re″no-kor″te-ko-trof′in)　corticotropin.

adrenocorticotropic (ad-re″no-kor″te-ko-trop′ik)　corticotropic.

adrenocorticotropin (ad-re″no-kor″te-ko-trop′in)　corticotropin.

adrenodontia (ad-ren″o-don′she-ah) [*adreno-* + Gr. *odous* tooth]　tooth form once thought to be indicative of adrenal predominance: the canines are large and sharp, and the occlusal surfaces of the teeth have a brownish coloration.

adrenodoxin (ad-dre″no-dok′sin)　an iron-sulfide protein of the adrenal cortex that serves as an electron carrier in the biosynthesis of adrenal steroids.

adrenogenous (ad″ren-oj′ĕ-nus) [*adreno-* + Gr. *gennan* to produce]　produced or arising in the adrenals.

adrenoglomerulotropin (ah-dre″no-glo-mer″u-lo-tro′pin)　a hormone alleged to stimulate the production of aldosterone by the adrenal cortex.

adrenogram (ad-ren′o-gram)　a roentgenogram of the adrenal glands.

adrenokinetic (ad-re″no-kǐ-net′ik) [adreno- + Gr. kinētikos moving] stimulating the adrenal gland.

adrenoleukodystrophy (ah-dre″no-loo″ko-dis′tro-fe) a hereditary disease of childhood marked by diffuse abnormality of the cerebral white matter and adrenal atrophy. It is marked by mental deterioration progressing to dementia and by aphasia, apraxia, dysarthria, and loss of vision. Clinical adrenal insufficiency occurs in about a third of the patients, but almost all show abnormal adrenal functioning when tested. It is transmitted as a sex-linked recessive trait.

adrenolutin (ah-dre″no-lu′tin) chemical name: 1-methyl-1H-indole-3,5,6-triol; degradation product of epinephrine, $C_9H_9NO_3$.

adrenolytic (ad″ren-o-lit′ik) [adreno- + Gr. lysis a loosening] inhibiting the action of adrenergic nerves; inhibiting the response to epinephrine.

adrenomedullotropic (ad-re″no-med″u-lo-trop′ik) having a hormonal influence on the adrenal medulla.

adrenomegaly (ad-ren″o-meg′ah-le) [adreno- + Gr. megaleia bigness] enlargement of one or both of the adrenal glands.

adrenomimetic (ah-dre″no-mi-met′ik) having actions similar to those of adrenergic compounds; sympathomimetic.

adrenopathy (ad″ren-op′ah-the) [adreno- + Gr. pathos disease] adrenalopathy.

adrenopause (ad-ren′o-pawz) cessation or suppression of function of the adrenal glands.

adrenoprival (ad-ren′o-pri″val) pertaining to or characterized by deprivation of the adrenal glands, as a result of their removal or suppression of their function.

adrenoreceptor (ah-dre″no-re-sep′tor) adrenergic receptor; see under receptor.

Adrenosem (ah-dren′o-sem) trademark for preparations of carbazochrome salicylate.

adrenostatic (ad-re″no-stat′ik) 1. inhibiting the activity of the adrenal glands. 2. an agent that inhibits the activity of the adrenal glands.

adrenosterone (ad″re-no′ster-ōn″) androst-4-ene-3,11,77-trione, a crystalline androgenic steroid, $C_{19}H_{24}O_3$, isolated from the adrenal cortex.

adrenotoxin (ad-ren″o-tok′sin) any substance that is toxic to the adrenals.

adrenotrophic (ad-ren″o-trof′ik) [adreno- + Gr. trophē nutrition] adrenotropic.

adrenotrophin (ad-ren″o-trof′in) corticotropin.

adrenotropic (ad-ren″o-trop′ik) [adreno- + Gr. tropos a turning] having specific affinity for or influence on the adrenal glands; suprarenotropic.

adrenotropin (ad-ren″o-trop′in) corticotropin.

adrenoxidase (ad″ren-ok′sǐ-dās) an oxygenized adrenal secretion presumed to be distributed by the blood plasma and to act catalytically.

Adriamycin (a″dre-ah-mi′sin) [from "Adriatic" + mycin] trademark for preparations of doxorubicin hydrochloride.

Adrian (a′dre-an), Edgar Douglas. An English physiologist, born 1889; co-winner, with Sir Charles Scott Sherrington, of the Nobel prize for medicine and physiology in 1932, for their work on the neuron.

adromia (ah-dro′me-ah) [a neg. + Gr. dromos a running + -ia] absence of conduction in nerve of muscle.

Adroyd (ad′roid) trademark for a preparation of oxymetholone.

adrue (ad-ru′a) the Cyperus articulatus, a grasslike plant of the West Indies, with an aromatic tonic, antiemetic, and anthelmintic root.

ADS antidiuretic substance; see vasopressin.

adsorb (ad-sorb′) to attract and retain other material on the surface.

adsorbate (ad-sor′bāt) a substance taken up on a surface by adsorption.

adsorbent (ad-sor′bent) 1. pertaining to or characterized by adsorption. 2. an agent that attracts other materials or particles to its surface.

adsorption (ad-sorp′shun) [L. ad to + sorbere to suck] 1. the attachment of one substance to the surface of another; the concentration of a gas or a substance in solution in a liquid on a surface in contact with the gas or liquid, resulting in a relatively high concentration of the gas or solution at the surface. Cf. absorption. 2. in spectroscopy, the uptake of light energy by a substance. **agglutinin a.**, the taking up by bacteria suspended in diluted antiserum of those agglutinins specific for that microorganism.

adsternal (ad-ster′nal) toward or near the sternum.

adst. feb. abbreviation for L. adstan′te feb′re, while fever is present; cf. abs. feb.

ADTe symbol for tetanic contraction, produced by an application of the positive pole with the circuit closed.

adterminal (ad-ter′mǐ-nal) passing toward the end of a muscle; said of an electric current.

adtorsion (ad-tor′shun) conclination.

Ad 2 vic. abbreviation of L. ad du′as vi′ces, at two times, for two doses.

adult (ah-dult′) [L. adultus grown up] 1. having attained full growth or maturity. 2. a living organism which has attained full growth or maturity.

adulterant (ah-dul′ter-ant″) a substance used as an addition to another substance for sophistication or adulteration.

adulteration (ah-dul″ter-a′shun) addition of an impure, cheap, or unnecessary ingredient to cheat, cheapen, or falsify a preparation; in legal terminology, incorrect labeling, including dosage not in accordance with the label.

adumbration (ah″dum-bra′shun) a geometric lack of sharpness; an inherent property of the focal spot which causes the production of double images. In radiology, the giving forth of a shadow.

Adv. abbreviation for L. adver′sum, against.

advance (ad-vans′) to perform the operation of advancement.

advancement (ad-vans′ment) surgical detachment, as of a muscle or tendon, followed by reattachment at an advanced point; chiefly an operation for strabismus. The round ligaments of the uterus have sometimes been advanced for retrodisplacement. **capsular a.**, the artificial attachment of a part of a vaginae bulbi (Tenon's capsule) in such a way as to draw forward the insertion of an ocular muscle. **tendon a.**, advancement applied to a tendon.

adventitia (ad″ven-tish′e-ah) [L. adventicious from without] outermost; denoting the layer of loose connective tissue forming the outermost coating of an organ. See tunica adventitia.

adventitial (ad″ven-tish′al) pertaining to the tunica adventitia.

adventitious (ad″ven-tish′us) [L. ad to + venire to come] 1. accidental or acquired; not natural or hereditary. 2. found out of the normal or usual place.

adynamia (ah″di-na′me-ah) [a neg. + Gr. dynamis might + -ia] lack or loss of the normal or vital powers; asthenia. **a. episod′ica heredita′ria**, a hereditary form of periodic paralysis.

adynamic (ad″i-nam′ik) characterized by adynamia; asthenic.

A.E. abbreviation for Ger. antitoxineinheit (antitoxic unit).

ae- for words beginning thus, see also those beginning e-.

Aeby's muscle, plane (a′bēz) [Christopher Theodore Aeby, Swiss anatomist, 1835–1885] see musculus depressor labii inferioris, and see under plane.

aec- for words beginning thus, see words beginning ec-.

aeciospore (e′se-o-spōr″) [Gr. aikia injury + sporas seed] a yellow, thin-walled, single-celled, binucleate spore of the wheat rust fungus formed in chainlike series within an aecium, produced in the spring on the leaves of barberry plants.

aecium (e′se-um), pl. ae′cia [Gr. aikia injury] 1. a cuplike structure formed on certain plants by wheat rust fungi, containing aeciospores. 2. a fruiting body of a fungus that bursts through the epidermis of the host.

Aedes (a-e′dēz) [Gr. aēdēs unpleasant] a genus of culicine mosquitoes with broad appressed scales on the head and scutellum. The palpi in the female are short and sparsely tufted and have three segments of equal length; in the male, the palpi are long and tufted. In addition to the vectors listed below, the following species are annoying because of their bites: A. aldrichi, A. communis, A. excrucians, A. punctor, A. stimulans, and A. vexans. Also Aëdes. See mosquito. **A. aegyp′ti**, the tiger mosquito, which breeds near houses and transmits urban yellow fever and dengue; it may also transmit filariasis and encephalitis. **A. africa′nus**, an arboreal mosquito that attacks monkeys and is a carrier of the yellow fever virus over much of Central Africa. It also carries the Zika virus. **A. albopic′tus**, a species that transmits yellow fever, equine encephalomyelitis, and dengue. **A. cine′reus**, a species occurring in certain parts of the United States which transmits equine encephalomyelitis. **A. flaves′cens**, a species of the Pacific Islands which transmits filariasis. **A. in-gram′i**, a species found in the pool from which Uganda S virus was isolated in 1947. **A. leucocelae′nus**, a South American species that transmits jungle yellow fever. **A. polynesien′sis**, a species of the South Pacific islands which is a vector of filaria and dengue. **A. pseudoscutella′ris**, a species of the Pacific Islands which is a vector of filaria. **A. scapula′ris**, a vector of the Cache Valley virus in Trinidad. **A. simp′soni**, a vector of jungle yellow fever in Africa. **A. sollic′itans**, the common salt-marsh mosquito of the Atlantic and Gulf coasts; it may transmit equine encephalomyelitis. **A. spenc′erii**, a species of mosquito found on the Saskatchewan prairies. **A. taeniorhyn′chus**, a species which transmits dengue in Florida. **A. to′goi**, a species of Japan that serves as a vector of Brugia malayi, which causes filariasis malayi. **A. varipal′pus**, a species found along the Pacific coast.

aedoeocephalus (ed″e-o-sef′ah-lus) [Gr. aidoia genitals + kephalē head] a monster with no mouth, a nose like a penis, and but one orbit.

Aeg. abbreviation for L. aeger, aegra, the patient.

Aegyptianella pullorum (e-jip″she-ah-nel′ah pul-lo′rum)   a sporozoan parasite of the family Babesiidae, order Haemosporidia, found in the blood of fowls; called also *Balfour's bodies.*

aelurophobia (e-loo″ro-fo′be-ah) [Gr. *ailouros* cat + *phobia*] ailurophobia.

aeluropsis (e″loo-rop′sis) [Gr. *ailouros* cat + *opsis* vision]   a slanting palpebral fissure like that of a cat.

aequator (e-kwa′tor) [L. "equalizer"]   equator.

aequum (e′kwum) [L. "equal"]   Pirquet's term for the amount of food required to maintain weight under a given condition of activity.

aer (a′er) [Gr. *aēr*]   atmos.

aer-   see *aero-.*

aerase (a′er-ās) [*aer-* + *-ase*]   a hypothetical substance once believed to be the respiratory enzyme of aerobic bacteria; cf. *anaerase.*

aerasthenia (a″er-as-the′ne-ah) [*aer-* + *asthenia*]   aeroneurosis.

aerated (a′er-āt″ed) [L. *aeratus*]   1. charged with air.   2. charged with carbon dioxide.   3. oxygenated.

aeration (a″er-a′shun)   1. the exchange of carbon dioxide for oxygen by the blood in the lungs.   2. the charging of a liquid with air or gas.

aeremia (a″er-e′me-ah) [*aer-* + Gr. *haima* blood + *-ia*]   aeroembolism; decompression sickness (bends).

aerendocardia (a″er-en″do-kar′de-ah) [*aer-* + Gr. *endon* in + *kardia* heart]   (obs.) the presence of gas or air within the heart.

aerenterectasia (a″er-en″ter-ek-ta′ze-ah) [*aer-* + Gr. *enteron* intestine + *ektasis* distention + *-ia*]   (obs.) distention of the intestines with air or gas.

aerial (a-e′re-al)   pertaining to the air.

aeriferous (a″er-if′er-us) [*aer-* + L. *ferre* to bear]   conveying air, as the bronchi.

aeriform (a-er′ĭ-form) [*aer-* + L. *forma* form]   like the air; gaseous.

aero-, aer- (a′er-o, a′er) [Gr. *aēr;* L. *aer* air or gas]   a combining form denoting relationship to air or gas.

aeroasthenia (a″er-o-as-the′ne-ah)   aeroneurosis.

Aerobacter (a″er-o-bak′ter) [*aero-* + Gr. *baktērion* little rod]   a genus of bacteria of the tribe Escherichieae, family Enterobacteriaceae, order Eubacteriales, made up of short, motile or nonmotile, gram-negative rods, which ferment glucose and lactose to produce acid and gas. It includes two species, *A.* (*Bacterium*) *aero′genes* and *A.* (*Bacterium*) *cloa′cae.*

aerobe (a′er-ōb) [*aero-* + Gr. *bios* life]   a microorganism that can live and grow in the presence of free oxygen.   **facultative a's,** microorganisms that are able to live under either aerobic or anaerobic conditions.   **obligate a's,** microorganisms that require molecular oxygen for growth.

aerobic (a-er-o′bik)   1. having molecular oxygen present.   2. growing, living, or occurring in the presence of molecular oxygen.   3. requiring oxygen for respiration.

aerobiology (a″er-o-bi-ol′o-je) [*aero-* + *biology*]   that branch of biology which deals with the distribution of living organisms by the air, either the exterior or outdoor air (extramural a.) or the indoor air (intramural a.).

aerobiosis (a″er-o-bi-o′sis) [*aero-* + Gr. *biosis* way of life]   life in the presence of molecular oxygen.

aerobiotic (a″er-o-bi-ot′ik)   pertaining to aerobiosis.

aerobullosis (a″er-o-bu-lo′sis)   decompression sickness.

aerocele (a′er-o-sēl″) [*aero-* + Gr. *kēlē* tumor]   a tumor formed by air filling an adventitious pouch, such as laryngocele and tracheocele.   **epidural a.,** a collection of air between the dura mater and the wall of the spinal column.   **intracranial a.,** traumatic pneumocephalus.

Aerococcus (a″er-o-kok′us)   in some systems of classification, a genus of aerobic, gram-positive cocci of the family Streptococcaceae.   **A. vir′idans,** a species indistinguishable from *Gaffkya homari,* which may be pathogenic for lobsters, and has been found in infections of the urinary tract and in endocarditis in humans.

aerocolpos (a″e-ro-kol′pos) [*aero-* + Gr. *kolpos* bosom or fold]   distention of the vagina with gas.

aerocystography (a″er-o-sis-tog′rah-fe)   roentgenography of the bladder after it has been injected with air; called also *pneumocystography.*

aerocystoscope (a″er-o-sis′to-skōp)   aerourethroscope.

aerocystoscopy (a″er-o-sis-tos′ko-pe) [*aero-* + Gr. *kystis* bladder + *skopein* to inspect]   examination of the bladder with the aerourethroscope.

aerodermectasia (a″er-o-der″mek-ta′ze-ah) [*aero-* + Gr. *derma* skin + *ektasis* extension + *-ia*]   subcutaneous emphysema; it may be spontaneous, traumatic, or surgical in origin.

aerodontalgia (a″er-o-don-tal′je-ah)   pain experienced in the teeth at lowered atmospheric pressures, as in aircraft flight or ascent of high mountains; sometimes simulated by pain arising

from maxillary aerosinusitis which occurs during recompression. Called also *aero- odontodynia* and *barodontalgia.*

aerodontia (a″er-o-don′she-ah)   aerodontics.

aerodontics (a″er-o-don′tiks)   that branch of dentistry which is concerned with effects on the teeth of high altitude flying.

aerodromophobia (a″er-o-dro″mo-fo′be-ah) [*aero* + Gr. *dromos* quick movement + *phobos* fear + *-ia*]   (obs.) morbid fear of traveling by air.

aerodynamics (a″er-o-di-nam′iks) [*aero-* + Gr. *dynamis* might]   the science of air and gases in motion.

aeroembolism (a″er-o-em′bo-lizm)   embolism due to air; it may occur in surgery of head, neck, and heart, induced abortion, and severe decompression sickness.

aeroemphysema (a″er-o-em″fĭ-ze′mah)   pulmonary emphysema and edema with collection of nitrogen bubbles in the tissues of the lung; due to excessively rapid atmospheric decompression.

aerogastria (a″er-o-gas′tre-ah)   the presence of gas in the stomach; stomach bubble. See also *magenblase.*   **blocked a.,** retention of air in the stomach due to spasm of the esophagus.

aerogel (a′er-o-jel″)   a solid formed by replacing the liquid of a gel with a gas.

aerogen (a′er-o-jen″)   an aerogenic, or gas-producing, bacterium.

aerogenesis (a″er-o-jen′ĕ-sis) [*aero-* + Gr. *genesis* production]   gas production.

aerogenic (a″er-o-jen′ik)   producing gas; said of bacteria that liberate free gaseous products.

aerogenous (a″er-oj′ĕ-nus)   aerogenic.

aerogram (a′er-o-gram″) [*aero-* + Gr. *gramma* mark]   a roentgenogram of an organ after it has been injected with air; called also *pneumogram.*

aerohydrotherapy (a″er-o-hi″dro-ther′ah-pe) [*aero-* + Gr. *hydōr* water + *therapeia* treatment]   (obs.) the therapeutic use of air and water.

aeroionotherapy (a″er-o-i″o-no-ther′ah-pe) [*aero-* + *ionotherapy*]   treatment of respiratory conditions by the inhalation of air with altered electrical charges.

aeromedicine (a″er-o-med′ĕ-sin)   aviation medicine.

aerometer (a″er-om′ĕ-ter) [*aero-* + Gr. *metron* measure]   an instrument for weighing air or for estimating the density of air.

Aeromonas (a″er-o-mo′nas)   a genus of bacteria of the family Pseudomonadaceae, suborder Pseudomonadineae, order Pseudomonadales, occurring as small rod-shaped cells and usually found in water, some being pathogenic for fish and amphibians. It includes four species: *A. hydro′phila, A. liquefa′ciens, A. puncta′ta,* and *A. salmoni′cida.*

aeroneurosis (a″er-o-nu-ro′sis) [*aero-* + *neurosis*]   a functional nervous disorder occurring in pilots, characterized by gastric distress, nervous irritability, insomnia, emotional instability, and increased motor activity. Called also *aeroasthenia* and *flying sickness.*

aero-odontalgia (a″er-o-o″don-tal′je-ah)   aerodontalgia.

aero-odontodynia (a″er-o-o-don″to-din′e-ah)   aerodontalgia.

aero-otitis (a″er-o-o-ti′tis) [*aero-* + *otitis*]   barotitis.

aeropathy (a″er-op′ah-the) [*aero-* + Gr. *pathos* disease]   any disease due to change in atmospheric pressure, such as decompression sickness or air sickness.

aeropause (a′er-o-paws″)   the region between the stratosphere and outer space, where to all practical purposes the atmosphere does not exist.

aeroperitoneum (a″er-o-per′ĭ-to-ne′um) [*aero-* + *peritoneum*]   pneumoperitoneum.

aeroperitonia (a″er-o-per′ĭ-to′ne-ah)   pneumoperitoneum.

aerophagia (a″er-o-fa′je-ah) [*aero-* + Gr. *phagein* to eat]   spasmodic swallowing of air followed by eructations, often seen in conjunction with functional gastrointestinal disturbances; called also *gastrospiry.*

aerophagy (a″er-of′ah-je)   aerophagia.

aerophil (a′er-o-fil″) [*aero-* + Gr. *philein* to love]   an aerophilic organism.

aerophilic (a″er-o-fil′ik)   requiring air for proper growth.

aerophilous (a″er-of′ĭ-lus)   aerophilic.

aerophobia (a″er-o-fo′be-ah) [*aero-* + *phobia*]   1. morbid dread of air, drafts of air, airborne influences, or bad air (body odor).   2. morbid dread of being up in the air; acrophobia.

aerophyte (a′er-o-fit″) [*aero-* + Gr. *phyton* plant]   an air plant; any microbe or other plant organism that derives its sustenance from the air.

aeropiesotherapy (a″er-o-pi-e″so-ther′ah-pe) [*aero-* + Gr. *piesis* pressure + *therapy*]   the therapeutic use of compressed or rarefied air.

aeroplankton (a″er-o-plank′ton)   the organisms (bacteria, pollen, etc.) present in the air.

Aeroplast (ār′o-plast″)   trademark for a preparation of vibesate.

aeroplethysmograph (a″er-o-plĕ-thiz′mo-graf) [*aero-* + Gr. *plēthysmos* enlargement + *graphein* to record] an apparatus for measuring respiratory volumes by recording changes in body volume; see also *plethysmograph.*

aeroporotomy (a″er-o-po-rot′o-me) [*aero-* + Gr. *poros* passage + *tomē* cutting] the operation of letting air into the air passages, as by intubation or tracheotomy.

aerosialophagy (a″er-o-si″ah-lof′ah-je) sialoaerophagy.

aerosinusitis (a″er-o-si″nus-i′tis) barosinusitis.

aerosis (a″er-o′sis) the production of gas in the tissues or organs of the body.

aerosol (a′er-o-sol″) 1. a colloid system in which the continuous phase (dispersion medium) is a gas, e.g., fog. 2. a bactericidal solution which can be finely atomized for the purpose of sterilizing the air of a room. 3. a solution of a drug which can be atomized into a fine mist for inhalation therapy.

aerosolization (a″er-o-sol″ĭ-za′shun) the process of dispersing in a fine mist.

aerosolology (a″er-o-sol-ol′o-je) the scientific study of aerosol therapy.

aerosome (a′er-o-sōm″) [*aero-* + Gr. *sōma* body] one of the hypothetical bodies once thought to be in the air of tropical climates and to affect the acclimatization of Europeans.

Aerosporin (a″er-o-spo′rin) trademark for a preparation of polymyxin B sulfate.

aerostatics (a″er-o-stat′iks) [*aero-* + Gr. *statikos* causing to stand] the science of gases in equilibrium.

aerotaxis (a″er-o-tak′sis) [*aero-* + Gr. *taxis* arrangement] a movement of an organism in reaction to the presence of molecular oxygen.

aerotherapeutics (a″er-o-ther″ah-pu′tiks) [*aero-* + Gr. *therapeia* treatment] (*obs.*) the use of air in treating diseases.

aerotherapy (a″er-o-ther′ah-pe) (*obs.*) aerotherapeutics.

aerothermotherapy (a″er-o-ther″mo-ther′ah-pe) [*aero-* + Gr. *thermē* heat + *therapeia* treatment] (*obs.*) treatment with currents of hot air.

aerotitis (a″er-o-ti′tis) barotitis.

aerotolerant (a″er-o-tol′er-ant) surviving and growing in small amounts of air; said of anaerobic microorganisms.

aerotonometer (a″er-o-to-nom′ĕ-ter) [*aero-* + Gr. *tonos* tension + *metron* measure] an instrument for measuring the partial pressure of the gases in the blood.

aerotropism (a″er-ot′ro-pizm) [*aero-* + Gr. *tropos* a turning] movement of an organism toward (*positive a.*) or away from (*negative a.*) a supply of air.

aerotympanal (a″er-o-tim′pah-nal) [*aero-* + L. *tympanum* drum] pertaining to atmospheric pressure (air) and the middle ear.

aerourethroscope (a″er-o-u-re′thro-skōp″) [*aero-* + *urethroscope*] a urethroscope by which the urethra is dilated with air before inspection; called also *aerocystoscope.*

aerourethroscopy (a″er-o-u″re-thros′ko-pe) the use of the aerourethroscope.

A.E.S. American Encephalographic Society; American Epidermological Society.

aes-, aet- for words beginning thus, see also those beginning *es-, et-.*

aesculapian (es″ku-la′pe-an) 1. pertaining to Aesculapius, the god of medicine, or to the art of medicine. 2. a physician.

Aesculapius (es″ku-la′pe-us) [Gr. *Asklēpios*] the mythical god of healing, son of Apollo and the nymph Coronis; called also *Asclepios.* See also *Asclepiad, asclepion, Hygeia,* and *Panacea,* and under *staff.*

aesculin (es′ku-lin) esculin.

Aesculus (es′ku-lus) a genus of trees, species of which contain a coumarin type of glycoside, esculin, which has been held responsible for their veterinary toxicity. The bark and seeds of *A. hippocastanum,* the horse chestnut, were formerly used in treatment of rheumatism and malaria and as an anticoagulant. *A. glabrus* is popularly known as *buckeye* (q.v.).

aesthesio- for words beginning thus, see those beginning *esthesio-.*

aesthetic (es-thet′ik) esthetic.

aesthetics (es-thet′iks) esthetics.

aet. abbreviation for L. *aétas,* age.

Aethusa (e-thoo′sah) a genus of umbelliferous plants, one species of which, *A. cynapium* L. (fool's parsley), has a reputation for human toxicity. The fruit contains a volatile alkaloid, cynapine, purported to be related to coniine.

aethylenum (eth″ĭ-le′num) [L.] ethylene. **a. pro narco′si,** ethylene used for producing surgical anesthesia.

Aëtius (a-e′she-us) (or **Aetios**) **of Amida** (or **Antiochenus**) (6th century A.D.) a Byzantine Greek writer, whose *Tetrabiblion* gives details of the works of Rufus (of Ephesus), Leonides, Soranus, and Philumenus, and good accounts of diseases of the eye, ear, nose, and throat, and also of technical procedures (e.g., tonsillectomy, urethrotomy, and the treatment of hemorrhoids).

A.F. albumose-free; see under *tuberculin.*

afebrile (a-feb′ril) without fever.

afetal (ah-fe′tal) without a fetus.

affect (af′fekt) a freudian term for the feeling of pleasantness or unpleasantness evoked by a stimulus; also the emotional complex associated with a mental state; the feeling experienced in connection with an emotion.

affection (ah-fek′shun) 1. a state of emotion or feeling. 2. a morbid condition or diseased state. **celiac a.,** the infant form of nontropical sprue (q.v.).

affective (ah-fek′tiv) pertaining to a feeling or mental state.

affectivity (af″ek-tiv′ĭ-te) the affective faculty. In psychology, the feeling tone; the basal tone or tendency of the feeling life.

affectomotor (ah-fek″to-mo′tor) combining emotional disturbance with muscular activity.

affektepilepsie (af″fekt-ep″ĭ-lep′se) Bratz's name for a psychogenic convulsion occurring in psychasthenia and obsessive states.

affenspalte (af″en-spahl″te) [Ger. "ape fissure"] Reidinger's term for sulcus lunatus.

afferent (af′er-ent) [L. *ad* to + *ferre* to carry] centripetal; esodic; conveying toward a center, as an afferent nerve.

afferentia (af″er-en′she-ah) [L.] 1. any afferent vessels, whether blood or lymph vessels. 2. the lymph vessels in general.

affinin (af′ĭ-nin) a lipid amide obtained from *Heliopsis longipes* (A. Gray) Blake, Compositae. It has insecticidal and local anesthetic properties. The plant is used in Mexico as a dental analgesic.

affinity (ah-fin′ĭ-te) [L. *affinitas* relationship] 1. inherent likeness or relationship. 2. a special attraction for a specific element, organ, or structure. 3. a driving force (thermodynamics). **chemical a.,** 1. the force that unites atoms into molecules. 2. the tendency of substances to undergo reaction with one another. **elective a.,** that force by which a substance chooses or elects to unite with one substance rather than with another. **residual a.,** the force which enables molecules to combine into larger aggregates.

affirmation (af″er-ma′shun) one of the stages in autosuggestion by which is secured a positive reactive tendency.

afflux (af′luks) [L. *affluxus, affluxio*] the rush of blood or liquid to a part.

affluxion (ah-fluk′shun) afflux.

affusion (ah-fu′zhun) [L. *affusio*] the pouring of water upon a part or upon the body for reducing fever; now rarely done. See *ablution.*

afibrinogenemia (ah-fi″brin-o-jĕ-ne′me-ah) deficiency or, more literally, absence of fibrinogen (coagulation factor I) in the blood. **congenital a.,** an uncommon hemorrhagic coagulation disorder, probably transmitted by an autosomal recessive gene, and characterized by complete incoagulability of the blood.

aflatoxicosis (af″lah-tok″sĭ-ko′sis) a form of mycotoxicosis affecting turkeys and other farm animals fed on ground nut meal contaminated with the molds *Aspergillus flavus* and related species, which produce aflatoxin; widespread epidemics with high mortality rates have been reported from all parts of the world. Called also *x disease.*

aflatoxin (af″lah-tok′sin) a toxic factor, $C_{17}H_{12}O_6$, produced by *Aspergillus flavus* and *A. parasiticus,* molds contaminating ground nut seedlings. It is responsible for deaths of fowl and other farm animals (aflatoxicosis) fed on infected ground nut meal. In experimental animals, aflatoxin causes liver necrosis, bile duct proliferation, and cirrhosis and, on prolonged administration, leads to hepatocellular carcinoma and cholangiocarcinoma. It has also been implicated as a cause of human hepatic carcinoma.

Afrin (af′rin) trademark for a preparation of oxymetazoline hydrochloride.

afteraction (af″ter-ak′shun) an effect occurring after cessation of the causative stimulus, such as the negative variation of the electric current continuing for a short time in a tetanized muscle.

afterbirth (af′ter-berth″) the placenta and membranes, delivered from the uterus after the birth of the child.

afterbrain (af′ter-brān″) metencephalon.

aftercare (af′ter-kār) the care and treatment of a convalescent patient, especially one who has undergone surgery; called also *aftertreatment.*

aftercataract, after-cataract (af″ter-kat′ah-rakt) see under *cataract.*

aftercurrent (af″ter-kur′ent) a current produced in a muscle and nerve after cessation of an electric current that has been flowing through it.

afterdischarge (af″ter-dis′charj) the portion of the response to stimulation in a sensory nerve which persists after the stimulus has ceased.

aftergilding (af″ter-gild′ing) the histologic application of gold salts to nerve tissue after fixation and hardening.

afterimage (af′ter-im″ij) a visual impression persisting briefly after cessation of the stimuli causing the original image. A *positive* afterimage is one in which the bright parts of the appearance remain bright, the dark parts dark. In a *negative* afterimage, the bright parts appear dark and the dark parts bright; called also *accidental* or *negative image.*

afterimpression (af″ter-im-presh′un) aftersensation.

aftermovement (af″ter-moov′ment) spontaneous elevation of the arm by idiomuscular contraction after benumbing it by powerful pressure against a rigid object; called also *Kohnstamm's phenomenon.*

afterpains (af′ter-pānz″) the cramplike pains felt after the birth of the child, due to the contractions of the uterus.

afterperception (af″ter-per-sep′shun) the perception of a sensation after the stimulus producing it has ceased.

afterpotential (af″ter-po-ten′shal) see under *potential.*

aftersensation (af″ter-sen-sa′shun) a sensation lasting after the stimulus that produced it has been removed; called also *afterimpression.*

afterstain (af′ter-stān″) (obs.) counterstain.

aftertaste (af′ter-tāst″) a taste continuing after the substance producing it has been removed.

aftertreatment (af″ter-trēt′ment) aftercare.

aftervision (af″ter-vizh′un) persistence of visual sensation after cessation of the stimuli producing it.

aftosa (af-to′sah) [Sp.] foot-and-mouth disease.

afunction (a-funk′shun) loss of function.

AG atrial gallop.

Ag chemical symbol for *silver* (L. *argentum*); abbreviation for *antigen.*

A.G.A. American Geriatrics Association.

agalactia (ah″gah-lak′she-ah) [*a* neg. + Gr. *gala* milk + *-ia*] absence or failure of the secretion of milk; called also *agalactosis.* **contagious a.,** a contagious disease of goats and sometimes of sheep, caused by mycoplasma, a pleuropneumonia-like organism. The disease occurs principally in parts of southern Europe and North Africa, affecting both females and males; it is marked by lesions of the eyes and joints and in the mammary glands of females.

agalactosis (ah-gal″ak-to′sis) agalactia.

agalactosuria (ah-gal″ak-to-su′re-ah) [*a* neg. + *galactose* + Gr. *ouron* urine + *-ia*] absence of galactose from the urine.

agalactous (ah″gah-lak′tus) 1. suppressing the secretion of milk. 2. not nursed; artificially fed.

agalorrhea (ah-gal″o-re′ah) [*a* neg. + Gr. *gala* milk + *rhoia* flow] absence or arrest of the flow of milk.

agamete (ag′ah-mēt) [*a* neg. + Gr. *gamos* marriage] the product of asexual multiple fission in protozoa.

agametic (a″gah-met′ik) devoid of germ cells; not possessing gametes.

agamic (ah-gam′ik) [*a* neg. + Gr. *gamos* marriage] (obs.) 1. asexual. 2. reproducing without impregnation.

agammaglobulinemia (a-gam″ah-glob″u-lĭ-ne′me-ah) [*a* neg. + *gamma globulin* + Gr. *haima* blood + *-ia*] an immunological deficiency state characterized by an extremely low level of generally all classes of gamma globulin in the blood, resulting in heightened susceptibility to those infectious diseases vulnerable to immunoglobulin-associated defense mechanisms. Called also *hypogammaglobulinemia* (q.v.). Cf. *dysgammaglobulinemia.* **Swiss type a.,** a lethal combined immunity deficiency syndrome associated with thymic aplasia, alymphocytosis, absence of the ability to develop delayed or cell-mediated immunities, and variable capacity to produce humoral immunity.

agamobium (ag″ah-mo′be-um) [*a* neg. + Gr. *gamos* marriage + *bios* life] (obs.) the asexual stage in the alternation of generations; cf. *gamobium.*

agamocytogeny (ah-gam″o-si-toj′ĕ-ne) schizogony.

Agamodistomum (ag″ah-mo-dis′to-mum) a genus of immature trematodes whose sexual organs are undeveloped and whose relationship to adult types has not been determined. **A. ophthalmo′bium,** an immature trematode parasite reported to have been found in the crystalline lens of the human eye.

Agamofilaria (ah-gam″o-fi-la′re-ah) a name given to filarial worms which are known only in immature stages and which cannot be assigned to any known genus or species.

agamogenesis (ag″ah-mo-jen′ĕ-sis) [*a* neg. + Gr. *gamos* marriage + *genesis* production] schizogony.

agamogenetic (ag″ah-mo-jĕ-net′ik) reproducing asexually.

agamogony (ag″ah-mog′o-ne) [*a* neg. + Gr. *gamos* marriage + *gonos* offspring] schizogony.

Agamomermis culicis (ag″ah-mo-mer′mis ku′lĭ-sis) a mermithid nematode parasitic in the mosquito.

Agamonema (ag″ah-mo-ne′mah) a genus of immature and unidentified nematodes, whose relationship to adult types has not yet been determined.

Agamonematodum migrans (ag″ah-mo-ne″mah-to′dum mi′grans) a name once applied to the nematode larva which

causes creeping eruption in the southern United States. See *Ancylostoma.*

agamont (ag′ah-mont) [*a* neg. + Gr. *gamos* marriage + *on* being] schizont.

agamous (ag′ah-mus) 1. asexual. 2. having no recognizable sexual organs.

aganglionic (a-gang″gle-on′ik) pertaining to or characterized by the absence of ganglion cells.

aganglionosis (ah-gang″gle-on-o′sis) congenital absence of parasympathetic ganglion cells, as in congenital megacolon.

agar (ahg′ar) [NF] a dried mucilaginous substance extracted from *Gelidium cartilagineum, Gracilaria confervoides,* and related red algae, having the property of melting at 100° C. and solidifying into a gel at 40° C. It is not digested by most bacteria and is used as a gel in the preparation of solid culture media for microorganisms, as a bulk laxative, in making emulsions, and as a supporting medium for immunodiffusion and immunoelectrophoresis. See *Table of Culture Media* for specific agars.

agar-agar (ag″ar-ag′ar) [Singhalese] agar.

Agarbacterium (ag″ar-bak-te′re-um) a genus of bacteria of the family Achromobacteraceae, order Eubacteriales, made up of short to medium-sized, motile or nonmotile, rod-shaped bacteria which characteristically digest agar; found primarily on decomposing seaweed and in sea water, they also occur in soil and fresh water. There are twelve species.

agaric (ah-gar′ik) [Gr. *agarikon* a sort of tree fungus] 1. any mushroom, more especially any species of *Agaricus.* 2. the tinder or punk prepared from dried mushrooms. **fly a.,** a poisonous species, *Amanita muscaria.* **larch a., purging a.,** a preparation obtained from *Polyporus officinalis,* a spongy mass growing on several species of trees; formerly used as an anhidrotic. **surgeons' a.,** a preparation obtained from *Polyporus officinalis,* which grows on several species of trees; used as a hemostatic. **white a.,** larch a.

Agaricales (ah-gar″ĭ-ka′lēz) an order of basidiomycetous fungi of the series Hymenomycetes, subclass Homobasidiomycetidae, made up of the mushrooms, including the genera *Agaricus* and *Amanita.*

Agaricus (ah-gar′ĭ-kus) a genus of mushrooms. See also *agaric,* and *agaric acid,* under *acid.* **A. campes′tris,** the common edible, or field, mushroom. **A. musca′rius,** *Amanita muscaria.*

agastria (ah-gas′tre-ah) absence of the stomach.

agastric (ah-gas′trik) [*a* neg. + Gr. *gastēr* stomach] having no alimentary canal.

Agathinus (ag″ah-thi′nus) **of Sparta** (1st century A.D.) a Greek physician who was a pupil of Athenaeus and, like his master, a Pneumatist.

Agave (ah-ga′ve) [L.; Gr. *agauē* noble] a genus of amaryllidaceous plants with many species possessing spiny-margined leaves and tall candelabra-shaped inflorescences. Some species serve as a source of an alcoholic beverage. The fresh juice of *A. americana* L. is purgative and diuretic, and has been used as an abortifacient. Several species contain saponins.

AGCT Army General Classification Test, an intelligence test whose results have been used for purposes of placement in the military situation.

age (āj) 1. the duration of individual existence measured in units of time. 2. the measure of some individual attribute in terms of the chronological age of an average normal individual showing the same degree of proficiency, e.g., achievement age. 3. to undergo change as the result of the passage of time. **achievement a.,** proficiency in study expressed in terms of the chronological age of an average child showing the same degree of attainment. **anatomical a.,** age expressed in terms of the chronological age of the average individual showing the same body development. **Binet a.,** mental age as determined by the Binet tests. **bone a.,** osseous development shown roentgenographically, stated in terms of the chronological age at which the development is ordinarily attained. **chronological a.,** the age of a person expressed in terms of the period elapsed from the time of birth. **coital a.,** the age of a conceptus defined by the time elapsed since the coitus that led to fertilization. **developmental a.,** age estimated from the degree of anatomical development. In psychology, the age of an individual as determined by the degree of his emotional, mental, anatomical, and physiologic maturation. **emotional a.,** the age of an individual expressed in terms of the chronological age of an average normal individual showing the same degree of emotional maturity. **fertilization a.,** conceptus age defined by the time elapsed since fertilization. **functional a.,** the combined expression of the chronological, emotional, mental, and physiological ages of an individual. **gestational a.,** age of conceptus or pregnancy. In human clinical practice, pregnancy is timed from onset of the last normal menstruation. Elsewhere the onset may be timed from estrus, coitus, artificial insemination, vaginal plug formation, fertilization, or implantation. **menstrual a.,** conceptus age defined by the time elapsed since the onset of the mother's last normal menstruation. **mental a.,** the score achieved by a person in an intelligence test, expressed in terms of the chronological age of an average normal individual showing the same degree of attainment. **physical a., physiological a.,** the age of an individual expressed in terms of the chronological age of a normal individual showing the same degree of anatomical and physiological development. **postovulatory a.,** conceptus age defined by the time elapsed since release of the oocyte from the ovary.

agenesia (ah″jĕ-ne′se-ah) agenesis. **a. cortica′lis,** congenital failure of development of the cortical cells, especially the pyramidal cells, of the brain, resulting in infantile cerebral paralysis and idiocy.

agenesis (ah-jen′ĕ-sis) [*a* neg. + Gr. *genesis* production] 1. absence of an organ; frequently used to designate such absence resulting from failure of appearance of the primordium of an organ in embryonic development. Cf. *aplasia.* 2. sterility or impotence. **callosal a.,** defect of the callosal structures of the brain. **gonadal a.,** complete failure of gonadal development; see *Turner's syndrome,* under *syndrome.* **nuclear a.,** Möbius' syndrome. **ovarian a.,** failure of development of the ovaries; see *Turner's syndrome,* under *syndrome.*

agenitalism (ah-jen′ĭ-tal-izm) a condition due to lack of the internal secretion of the testes or ovaries.

agenized (a′jĕn-izd″) treated with nitrogen trichloride for bleaching purposes, as flour.

agenosomia (ah-jen″o-so′me-ah) congenital absence or rudimentary development of the genitals and eventration of the lower part of the abdomen.

agenosomus (ah-jen″o-so′mus) [*a* neg. + Gr. *gennan* to beget + *sōma* body] a monster exhibiting agenosomia.

agent (a′jent) [L. *agens* acting] any power, principle, or substance capable of producing an effect, whether physical, chemical, or biological. **activating a.,** one of two factors present in adult tissues which, when administered to embryos, interact to induce regional development; when administered alone, this factor induces archencephalic development. Called also *dorsalizing* or *neuralizing a.* Cf. *caudalizing a.* **adrenergic blocking a.,** a compound that selectively inhibits response to sympathetic impulses and to catecholamines and other adrenergic amines. See *alpha-adrenergic blocking a., beta-adrenergic blocking a.,* and *adrenergic neuron blocking a.* **adrenergic neuron blocking a.,** one that inhibits the release of norepinephrine from postganglionic adrenergic nerve endings. **alkylating a.,** any synthetic compound containing two or more end (alkyl) groups that combine readily with other molecules. They react with many cellular components and have a toxic reaction on many types of cells, normal as well as malignant. The exact mechanism of action is not completely understood, but their major biological effect seems to be caused by interaction with the nuclear deoxyribonucleic acid, resulting in inhibition of cell division and the production of mutations, and also inhibition of antibody formation. Although they do not damage malignant cells selectively, they are used in chemotherapy of many types of malignancies, the most widely used being the nitrogen mustards (see under *mustard*). **alpha-adrenergic blocking a.,** one that blocks the alpha receptor sites of effector organs to the effects of catecholamines. **beta-adrenergic blocking a.,** an agent that blocks the beta receptor sites of effector organs to the effects of catecholamines. **Bittner a.,** mouse mammary tumor virus. **blocking a.,** an agent that inhibits the response of effector organs to neural impulses of the autonomic nervous system; it may be an adrenergic or cholinergic blocking agent. **caudalizing a.,** one of two factors present in adult tissues which, when administered to embryos, interact to induce regional development; when administered alone, this factor induces only mesodermal development. Called also *mesodermalizing* or *transforming a.* Cf. *activating a.* **chelating a.,** 1. a compound that combines with metal ions by means of two or more coordinating positions to form stable ring structures, e.g., heme. 2. a substance used to reduce the concentration of free metal ion in solution by complexing it. Called also *metal complexing a.* **chimpanzee coryza a.,** respiratory syncytial virus. **cholinergic blocking a.,** one that blocks or inactivates acetylcholine. **clearing a.,** an agent used in staining technique for fixed cells, which has the same refractive index as that of protein particles. **dorsalizing a.,** activating a. **Eaton a.,** *Mycoplasma pneumoniae.* **fixing a's,** agents, such as formalin, alcohol, acids, salts of heavy metals, or mixtures of these, that precipitate the proteins of cells or tissues and render them insoluble. **ganglionic blocking a.,** one that blocks nerve impulses at autonomic ganglionic synapses. **Gordon a.,** a substance present in certain human and animal tissues which produces characteristic clinical symptoms and pathological changes on intracerebral injection into rabbits and guinea pigs. **levigating a.,** a material used for moistening a solid before reducing it to a powder. **mammary tumor a., mouse mammary tumor a.,** mouse mammary tumor virus. **Marcy a.,** a virus causing afebrile diarrhea in man. **mesodermalizing a.,** caudalizing a. **metal complexing a.,** chelating a. **milk a.,** mouse mammary tumor virus. **Norwalk a.,** the causative agent, probably a virus, of an acute infectious gastroenteritis. **A. Orange,** a herbicide containing 2,4,5-trichlorophenoxyacetic acid and 2,4-dichlorophenoxyacetic acid and

used to kill broadleaf plants by overstimulating their phototropic response; it also contains the contaminant dioxin. The compound is suspected of having oncogenic and teratogenic properties. **progestational a's,** a group of hormones secreted by the corpus luteum and placenta and, in small amounts, by the adrenal cortex, including progesterone, Δ⁴-3-ketopregnene-20(α)-ol, and Δ⁴-3-ketopregnene-20(β)-ol. Agents having progestational activity are also produced synthetically. Called also *gestogens, progestins, progestational hormones,* and *progestogens.* **reducing a.,** a substance capable of donating electrons to another substance, thereby reducing the second substance and itself becoming oxidized. **transforming a.,** any substance that produces transformation in a cell, e.g., a substance, shown to be a form of DNA, isolated from pneumococci and certain other bacteria, which on introduction into bacteria of that type of bacteria produces a permanent, inherited change; see also *bacterial transformation,* under *transformation.* **vacuolating a.,** see under *virus.* **virus inactivating a.,** an agent present in the serous secretion of the nose which inactivates the influenza and certain other viruses. Abbreviated VIA. **wetting a's,** substances that lower the surface tension of water and promote wetting.

ageotropic (ah-je″o-tro′pik) [*a* neg. + Gr. *gē* earth + *tropikos* turning] not responding to gravity; said of certain plant roots.

agerasia (ah″jer-a′zee-ah) [*a* neg. + Gr. *gēras* old age] an unusually youthful appearance in a person of advanced years.

ageusia (ah-gu′ze-ah) [*a* neg. + Gr. *geusis* taste] lack or impairment of the sense of taste.

ageusic (ah-gu′sik) pertaining to ageusia.

ageustia (ah-goōs′te-ah) ageusia.

agger (aj′er), pl. *ag′geres* [L.] an eminence; [NA] a general term for such a structure. **a. na′si** [L. "ridge of the nose"] [NA], a ridgelike elevation midway between the anterior extremity of the middle nasal concha and the inner surface of the dorsum of the nose; called also *ridge of nose* and *nasoturbinal concha.* **a. perpendicula′ris,** eminentia fossae triangularis auriculae. **a. val′vae ve′nae,** an elevation of the wall of a vein over the site of a valve.

aggeres (aj′er-ēz) [L.] plural of *agger.*

agglomerated (ah-glom′er-āt″ed) [L. *agglomeratus,* from *ad* together + *glomus* mass] crowded into a mass.

agglutinable (ah-gloo′tĭ-nah-bl) capable of agglutination.

agglutinant (ah-gloo′tĭ-nant) [L. *agglutinans* gluing] 1. promoting union by adhesion. 2. a tenacious or gluey substance which holds parts together during the process of healing.

agglutination (ah-gloo″tĭ-na′shun) [L. *agglutinatio*] 1. the action of an agglutinant substance. 2. the process of union in the healing of a wound. 3. the clumping together in suspension of antigen-bearing cells, microorganisms, or particles in the presence of specific antibodies (agglutinins). Called also *clumping.* **acid**

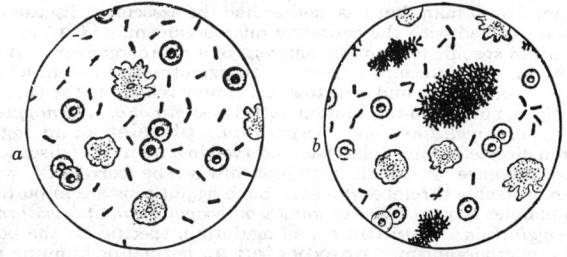

Agglutination: *a,* bacilli unagglutinated; *b,* bacilli agglutinated.

a., the nonspecific agglutination of microorganisms at relatively low hydrogen ion concentration; it occurs without participation of antibody. **bacteriogenic a.,** clumping of cells due to bacterial action, as in the *Huebener-Thomsen-Friedenreich phenomenon;* called also *T-agglutination.* **chief a.,** see *chief agglutinin,* under *agglutinin.* **cold a.,** agglutination of red cells in the presence of cold agglutinins. **cross a.,** the agglutination of particulate antigen by antibody raised against a different but related antigen; see also *group a.* **group a.,** agglutination—usually to a lower titer—of various members of a group of biologically related organisms or corpuscles by an agglutinin specific for one of that group. For instance, the specific agglutinin of typhoid bacilli may agglutinate other members of the colon-typhoid group, such as *Escherichia coli* and *Salmonella enteritidis.* **H a.,** the agglutination of motile bacteria in the presence of antibody to the heat-labile flagellar antigens. **intravascular a.,** clumping of particulate elements within the blood vessels; used conventionally to denote red blood cell aggregation. **macroscopic a.,** agglutination in which the product of the reaction, the agglutinate, can be observed with the unaided eye. **microscopic a.,** agglutination so done, usually by means of a hanging drop, that the clumping of the microorganisms or corpuscles can be observed with the microscope. **minor a.,** see *partial agglutinin,* under *agglutinin.* **O a.,** the agglutination of bacteria in the presence of antibody to the heat-stable somatic antigen. **part a.**, see *partial agglutinin*, under *agglutinin*. **passive a.**, agglutination in antiserum of particles upon which specific soluble antigen has been adsorbed. **platelet a.**, the clumping together of platelets; sometimes used interchangeably with aggregation (q.v.), but probably better reserved for immunological or analogous phenomena. **salt a.**, agglutination that occurs in concentrations of certain salts. **spontaneous a.**, the agglutination of bacteria or other cells in physiologic salt solution due to the lack of sufficient surface polar groups to give stable suspensions in the presence of electrolytes. **T-a.**, bacteriogenic a. **Vi a.**, agglutination of bacteria containing Vi antigen on their surface, in the presence of specific agglutinin.

agglutinative (ah-gloo″tĭ-na″tiv) promoting adhesion or agglutination.

agglutinator (ah-gloo′tĭ-na″tor) something which agglutinates; an agglutinin.

agglutinin (ah-gloo′tĭ-nin) antibody which aggregates a particulate antigen, e.g., bacteria, following combination with the homologous antigen in vivo or in vitro. Also, any substance other than antibody, e.g., lectin, that is capable of agglutinating particles. **anti-Rh a.**, an agglutinin not normally present in human plasma but which may be produced in Rh– mothers carrying an Rh+ fetus or after transfusion of Rh+ blood into an Rh– patient. See *blood type*. **chief a.**, the specific immune agglutinin in the blood of an animal immunized against an infectious disease agent; it is active at a higher dilution of the blood serum than are the partial agglutinins. Called also *haupt-agglutinin* and *major agglutinin*. **cold a.**, an agglutinin that acts only at relatively low temperatures (ranging from 0° to 20° C.) Cf. *autoagglutinin*. **complete a's**, agglutinins, e.g., IgM hemagglutinins, demonstrable by simple direct tests. **cross a.**, an agglutinin which, although formed in response to one particulate antigen, also has specific action on a different but related antigen. **expected a's**, normal human agglutinins directed against erythrocytic antigens of blood group A and/or B. **flagellar a.**, an agglutinin specific for the flagella of a microorganism. **group a.**, an agglutinin which has a specific action on certain organisms or cells, but which will agglutinate other closely related species as well. **H a.**, an agglutinin specific for flagellar antigens of the motile strain of a microorganism. **haupt-a.**, chief a. **immune a.**, a specific agglutinin found in the blood as a result of recovering from the disease or of having been injected with the microorganism causing the disease. **incomplete a.**, an agglutinin which at appropriate concentrations fails to agglutinate the homologous antigen. **leukocyte a.**, a type of agglutinin, directed against neutrophilic and other leukocytes, found in a variety of disorders, the presence of which may not necessarily be related to the manifestations of a particular clinical entity or to the pathogenesis of the manifest leukopenic state. Called also *leukoagglutinin*. **major a.**, chief a. **MG a.**, a specific agglutinin developed against *Streptococcus MG*. **minor a.**, partial a. **normal a.**, a specific agglutinin found in the blood of an animal or of man that has neither had the associated disease nor been injected with the causative microorganism. **O a.**, an agglutinin specific for somatic antigens of a microorganism. **partial a.**, an agglutinin present in an agglutinative serum which acts on organisms and cells that are closely related to the specific antigen, but in a lower dilution; called also *minor a.*, *nebenagglutinin*, *para-agglutinin*, and *coagglutinin*. **platelet a.**, an agglutinin directed against platelets, observed in a number of disorders, the presence of which may not always be correlated with demonstrable thrombocytopenia. Such agglutinins are important in platelet typing. See also *autothromboagglutinin* and *isothromboagglutinin*. **somatic a.**, an agglutinin specific for the body of a microorganism. **unexpected a.**, normal or immune agglutinin directed against erythrocytic antigens other than those of blood groups A and B. **warm a.**, an antibody (IgG) that reacts best at 37° C., usually without producing agglutination, although the immune reaction occasionally fixes small amounts of complement.

agglutinogen (ag″loo-tin′o-jen) 1. any substance which, acting as an antigen, stimulates the production of agglutinin. 2. the particulate antigen used in conducting agglutination tests.

agglutinogenic (ah-gloo″tĭ-no-jen′ik) pertaining to the production of agglutinin; producing agglutinin.

agglutinophilic (ah-gloo″tĭ-no-fil′ik) agglutinating readily.

agglutinoscope (ah-gloo″tĭ-no-skōp″) [*agglutinin* + Gr. *skopein* to view] an apparatus for examining test tubes to ascertain the degree of agglutination in the agglutination reaction.

agglutogenic (ah-gloo″to-jen′ik) agglutinogenic.

agglutometer (ag″loo-tom′ĕ-ter) an apparatus for performing the test for Gruber's reaction without the use of a microscope.

aggred. feb. abbreviation for L. *aggredien′te feb′re*, while the fever is coming on.

aggregate (ag′re-gāt) [L. *aggregatus*, from *ad* to + *grex* flock] 1. to crowd or cluster together. 2. crowded or clustered together. 3. a mass or assemblage.

aggregation (ag″re-ga′shun) 1. massing of materials together as in clumping. 2. a clumped mass of material. **familial a.**, a concentration of cases of a disease in families; the occurrence of

more cases of a given disorder in close relatives of a person with the disorder than in control families. **platelet a.**, a clumping together of platelets induced in vitro and, probably in vivo, by a number of agents, such as ADP, thrombin, and collagen, as part of a sequential mechanism leading to the initiation and formation of a thrombus or hemostatic plug.

aggregon (ag′rĕ-jen) [L. *aggregare* to collect together + Gk. *gennan* to produce] an organized mass of mammalian cells growing in agitated culture, resembling an aggregate in having a continuous layer of peripheral cells forming a smooth surface, but differing from it in having the capacity to fragment to form daughter aggregons.

aggregometer (ag″grĕ-gom′ĕ-ter) an instrument that detects changes in optical density of plasma (or solution) caused by platelet (or particle) clustering.

aggregometry (ag″grĕ-gom′ĕ-tre) the measurement of platelet aggregation by means of an aggregometer.

aggressin (ah-gres′in) any of a postulated group of nontoxic substances produced by pathogenic bacteria that inhibit the mechanisms of host resistance.

aggression (ah-gresh′un) [L. *aggressus*, from *ad* to + *gradi* to step] a form of behavior which leads to self-assertion; it may arise from innate drives and/or a response to frustration; it may be manifested by destructive and attacking behavior, by covert attitudes of hostility and obstructionism, or by a healthy self-expressive drive to mastery.

AgI chemical symbol for *silver iodide*.

aging (āj′ing) the gradual changes in the structure of any organism that occur with the passage of time, that do not result from disease or other gross accidents, and that eventually lead to the increased probability of death as the individual grows older. Cf. *senescence*.

agitated (aj′e-tāt″ed) marked by restlessness and increased activity intermingled with anxiety, fear, and tension.

agitation (aj″e-ta′shun) 1. exceeding restlessness associated with mental distress. 2. a shaking.

agitographia (aj″e-to-graf′e-ah) [L. *agitare* to hurry + Gr. *graphein* to write + *-ia*] excessive rapidity of writing with unconscious omission of words or parts of words; it is usually associated with agitophasia.

agitolalia (aj″e-to-la′le-ah) agitophasia.

agitophasia (aj″e-to-fa′ze-ah) [L. *agitare* to hurry + Gr. *phasis* speech + *-ia*] excessive rapidity of speech in which words or syllables are unconsciously omitted or imperfectly uttered; called also *agitolalia*.

Agit. vas. abbreviation for L. *agita′to va′se*, the vial being shaken.

Agkistrodon (ag-kis′tro-don) [Gr. *agkistron* fishhook + *odous* tooth] a genus of venomous serpents of the family Crotalidae. *A. contor′trix* is the copperhead and *A. pisciv′orus*, the water moccasin of North America. Called also *Ancistrodon*. See table accompanying *snake*.

aglaucopsia (ah″glaw-kop′se-ah) [*a* neg. + Gr. *glaukos* green + *opsis* vision + *-ia*] deuteranopia.

aglaukopsia (ah″glaw-kop′se-ah) deuteranopia.

aglomerular (ah″glo-mer′u-lar) having no glomeruli; said of a kidney in which the glomeruli have been absorbed or in which they have never formed (as in some fishes).

aglossia (ah-glos′e-ah) [*a* neg. + Gr. *glōssa* tongue + *-ia*] congenital absence of the tongue.

aglossostomia (ah″glos-o-sto′me-ah) [*a* neg. + Gr. *glōssa* tongue + *stoma* mouth + *-ia*] a developmental anomaly characterized by absence of the tongue and mouth opening.

aglucone (ah-gloo′kōn) aglycone.

aglutition (ag-loo-tish′un) inability to swallow.

aglycemia (ah″gli-se′me-ah) [*a* neg. + Gr. *glykys* sweet + *haima* blood + *-ia*] absence of sugar from the blood. Cf. *hyperglycemia* and *hypoglycemia*.

aglycone (ah-gli′kōn) [*a* neg. + Gr. *glykys* sweet + *ōn* being] the noncarbohydrate group of a glycoside molecule; called also *genin*.

aglycosuric (ah-gli″ko-su′rik) free from glycosuria.

agmatology (ag″mah-tol′o-je) [Gr. *agmos* fracture + *-logy*] the sum of what is known regarding fractures.

agminated (ag′min-āt″ed) [L. *agmen* a group] clustered.

agnate (ag′nāt) in Scotch law, the nearest relative on the father's side of one adjudged insane, and appointed guardian of the same.

Agnatha (ăg′na-tha) [*a* neg. + Gr. *gnathos* jaw] the jawless fishes; a class of vertebrates including lampreys, hagfishes, and many extinct forms.

agnathia (ag-na′the-ah) [*a* neg. + Gr. *gnathos* jaw + *-ia*] a developmental anomaly characterized by total or virtual absence of the lower jaw.

agnathus (ag-na′thus) a fetus exhibiting agnathia.

agnea (ag-ne′ah) a condition in which objects are not recognized.

Agnew's splint (ag′nūz) [David Hayes *Agnew*, Philadelphia surgeon, 1818–1892] see under *splint.*

AgNO₃ chemical symbol for *silver nitrate.*

agnogenic (ag″no-jen′ik) [Gr. *agnōs* unknown, obscure + *genesis* origin] of unknown origin or etiology.

agnosia (ag-no′ze-ah) [*a* neg. + Gr. *gnōsis* perception] loss of the power to recognize the import of sensory stimuli; the varieties correspond with the several senses and are distinguished as *auditory, visual, olfactory, gustatory,* and *tactile.* **acoustic a., auditory a.,** inability to recognize the significance of sounds. **body-image a.,** autotopagnosia. **finger a.,** loss of ability to indicate one's own or another's fingers. **ideational a.,** loss of the special associations which make up the idea of an object from its component ideas. **tactile a.,** inability to recognize familiar objects by touch or feel. **time a.,** loss of comprehension of the succession and duration of events. **visual a.,** inability to recognize familiar objects by sight.

agnosterol (ag-nos′ter-ol″) polyunsaturated sterol, $C_{30}H_{48}O$, present in wool fat.

agnus castus (ag′nus kas′tus) [L. "chaste lamb"] the chaste-tree, *Vi′tex ag′nus-cas′tus;* the herb and fruit were used for centuries as an anaphrodisiac and symbol of chastity.

Ag₂O chemical symbol for *silver oxide.*

agofollin (ah-gof′o-lin) estradiol.

-agogue [Gr. *agōgos* leading, inducing] a word termination meaning an agent which leads or induces.

agomphiasis (ag″om-fi′ah-sis) [*a* neg. + Gr. *gomphios* molar + *-ia*] absence of the teeth.

agomphious (ah-gom′fe-us) without teeth.

agonad (ah-go′nad) [*a* neg. + *gonad*] an individual without gonads.

agonadal (ah-gon′ah-dal) having no sex glands; due to absence of sex glands.

agonadism (ah-go′nah-dizm) the condition of being without sex glands.

agonal (ag′o-nal) 1. pertaining to the death agony; occurring at the moment of or just before death. 2. pertaining to terminal infection.

agoniadin (ag″o-ni′ah-din) a glycoside from *Plume′ria suc′cuba,* a genus of tropical American shrubs.

agonist (ag′o-nist) a prime mover; a muscle opposed in action by another muscle, called the antagonist. In pharmacology, a drug that has affinity for and stimulates physiologic activity at cell receptors normally stimulated by naturally occurring substances.

agony (ag′o-ne) [Gr. *agōnia*] 1. severe pain or extreme suffering. 2. the death struggle.

agoraphilia (ag″ŏ-rah-fil′e-ah) [Gr. *agora* marketplace + *philein* to love] an unusual or morbid attraction to large open spaces.

agoraphobia (ag″o-rah-fo′be-ah) [Gr. *agora* marketplace + *phobia*] fear of being in a large open space; overwhelming and incapacitating anxiety on traveling away from the safety of home or on being in crowded places.

Agostini's test (reaction) (ag-os-te′nēz) see under *tests.*

agouti (ah-goo′te) 1. a rodent of the genus *Dasyprocta,* about the size of a rabbit, found in tropical America. 2. a term used in genetics to indicate the natural wild color pattern of the hair of certain mammals.

-agra (ag′rah) [Gr. *agra* a catching, seizure] a word termination meaning a seizure of acute pain.

agraffe (ah-graf′) [Fr.] a clamplike instrument for maintaining the edges of a wound in apposition.

agrammatica (ag″rah-mat′e-kah) agrammatism.

agrammatism (ah-gram′ah-tizm″) [Gr. *agrammatos* unlettered] inability to speak grammatically because of brain injury or disease.

agrammatologia (ah-gram″ah-to-lo′je-ah) agrammatism.

agranulocyte (ah-gran′u-lo-sīt″) a nongranular leukocyte.

agranulocytosis (ah-gran″u-lo-si-to′sis) a symptom complex characterized by marked decrease in the number of granulocytes and by lesions of the throat and other mucous membranes, of the gastrointestinal tract, and of the skin; called also *granulocytopenia* and *Schultz's disease.* **infectious feline a.,** panleukopenia.

agranuloplastic (ah-gran″u-lo-plas′tik) [*a* neg. + *granule* + Gr. *plassein* to form] forming nongranular cells only; not forming granular cells.

agraphia (ah-graf′e-ah) [*a* neg. + Gr. *graphein* to write + *-ia*] inability to express thoughts in writing, due to a lesion of the cerebral cortex. **absolute a.,** loss of the power to write even single letters. **acoustic a.,** loss of the power of writing from dictation. **a. amnemon′ica,** agraphia in which letters and words can be written, but not so arranged as to express any idea. **a. atac′tica,** absolute a. **cerebral a.,** mental a. **jargon a.,** agraphia in which the patient can write, but forms only senseless combinations of letters. **literal a.,** inability to write let-

ters of the alphabet. **mental a.,** agraphia due to inability to put thought into phrases. **motor a.,** inability to write because of lack of motor coordination. **musical a.,** loss of the power to write musical symbols. **optic a.,** inability to copy written or printed words, but with ability to write from dictation. **verbal a.,** ability to write single letters, with loss of ability to combine them into words.

agraphic (ah-graf′ik) pertaining to, affected with, or of the nature of agraphia.

agremia (ah-gre′me-ah) [Gr. *agra* seizure + *haima* blood + *-ia*] (*obs.*) that condition of the blood which characterizes gout.

agria (ag′re-ah) [L.; Gr. *agrios* wild] an obstinate pustular eruption.

Agriolimax (ag″re-o-li′maks″) a genus of slugs. **A. lae′vis,** a species that serves as an intermediate host of *Angiostrongylus cantonensis,* which transmits eosinophilic meningitis.

agriothymia (ag″re-o-thim′e-ah) [Gr. *agrios* wild + *thymos* spirit + *-ia*] (*obs.*) insane ferocity.

agrius (a′gre-us) [L. "wild"] very severe; said of skin eruptions.

Agrobacterium (ag″ro-bak-te′re-um) [Gr. *agros* field + *bacterium*] a genus of bacteria of the family Rhizobiaceae, order Eubacteriales, made up of small, short, flagellated rods, found in soil or in the roots or stems of plants; seven species have been named, the type species being *A. tumefa′ciens.*

agromania (ag″ro-ma′ne-ah) [Gr. *agros* field + *mania* madness] morbid passion for solitude or for wandering in the fields.

Agropyron (ag″ro-pi′ron) a genus of grasses, including *A. repens* (L.) Beauv. (Gramineae), couch grass; see *triticum.*

Agropyrum (ag″ro-pi′rum) triticum.

Agrostemma githa′go (ag″ro-stem′ah gith-a′go) corn cockle, *Lychnis githago,* a plant whose seeds may cause poisoning (githagism).

agrypnia (ah-grip′ne-ah) [Gr. *agrypnos* sleepless + *-ia*] former term for sleeplessness, or insomnia.

agrypnocoma (ah-grip″no-ko′mah) wakeful coma; lethargy with wakefulness and muttering delirium.

agrypnode (ah-grip′nōd) agrypnotic.

agrypnotic (ah″grip-not′ik) [Gr. *agrypnotikos*] promoting wakefulness.

Ag₂SO₄ chemical symbol for *silver sulfate.*

AGTH adrenoglomerulotropin.

aguamiel (ag″wah-me-el′) the sap from which pulque is made.

ague (a′gu) [Fr. *aigu* sharp] 1. malarial fever, or any other severe recurrent symptom of malarial origin. 2. a chill. **brass-founders' a.,** a disease of brass-founders, caused by inhalation of zinc fumes. **dumb a.,** ague without well-marked chill, and with only a slight periodicity. **quartan a.,** that in which paroxysms are seventy-two hours apart. **quintan a.,** that in which the paroxysms are ninety-six hours apart. **quotidian a.,** that in which there is a twenty-four hour interval between the paroxysms. **shaking a.,** a severe form of malarial paroxysm, beginning with a marked chill. **tertian a.,** that in which the paroxysms are forty-eight hours apart.

A.G.V. aniline gentian violet.

agyria (ah-ji′re-ah) [*a* neg. + Gr. *gyros* ring + *-ia*] a malformation in which the convolutions of the cerebral cortex are not normally developed and the brain is usually small; called also *lissencephaly.*

agyric (ah-ji′rik) 1. pertaining to or characterized by agyria. 2. having no gyri.

ah symbol for *hyperopic astigmatism.*

A.H.A. American Heart Association; American Hospital Association.

ahaptoglobinemia (a-hap″to-glo″bĭ-ne′me-ah) the presence of little or no haptoglobin in the blood serum.

AHF antihemophilic factor (blood coagulation Factor VIII, see under *factor*).

AHG antihemophilic globulin (blood coagulation Factor VIII, see under *factor*).

ahistidasia (ah-his″tĭ-da′ze-ah) absence of histidase activity; see *histidinemia.*

A.H.P. Assistant House Physician.

A.H.S. Assistant House Surgeon.

A.I. aortic incompetence; aortic insufficiency; apical impulse; artificial insemination.

A.I.C. Association des Infirmières Canadiennes.

aichmophobia (āk″mo-fo′be-ah) [Gr. *aichmē* spearpoint + *phobos* fear + *-ia*] abnormal fear of sharp-pointed objects.

aid (ād) help or assistance; by extension, applied to any device by which a function can be improved or augmented, as a hearing aid. **first a.,** emergency assistance and treatment furnished in cases of accident, injury, or illness pending regular surgical or medical therapy. **hearing a.,** a device which amplifies sound to help persons with hearing loss; audiphone; otophone. **pharmaceutic a., pharmaceutical a.,** see under *necessity.* **speech a.,** an appliance used to improve an individual's speech, or therapy which is designed to promote the improvement of speech. **speech a., prosthetic,** an appliance which is used to close a cleft in the hard or soft palate, or both, or to restore other tissue necessary to the production of vocal sounds.

A.I.D. donor insemination.

aidoiomania (a″doy-o-ma′ne-ah) [Gr. *aidoia* genitals + *mania* madness] (*obs.*) abnormal sexual desire.

A.I.H. American Institute of Homeopathy; homologous insemination.

A.I.H.A. American Industrial Hygiene Association.

Ailanthus (a-lan′thus) [L. from Malacca name] a genus of simarubaceous trees; the bark of *A. glandulosa* (tree of heaven) is purgative, tonic, and anthelmintic, and contains a bitter principle (ailanthin), glycosides, and a saponin.

Ailantus (a-lan′tus) *Ailanthus.*

ailment (āl′ment) any disease or affection of the body, usually referring to slight or mild disorder.

ailurophilia (i-lu″ro-fil′e-ah) [Gr. *ailouros* cat + *philein* to love] a morbid or inordinate fondness for cats.

ailurophobia (i-lu″ro-fo′be-ah) [Gr. *ailouros* cat + *phobia*] pathologic fear of cats (Weir Mitchell).

ainhum (ān′hum, i′num, or [Portuguese] īn-yoom′) [African] a condition occurring chiefly in Negroes in tropical countries, marked by linear constriction of a toe, especially the little one, which by its contraction gradually amputates the toe.

air (ār) [L. *aer;* Gr. *aēr*] the gaseous mixture which makes up the earth's atmosphere; it is an odorless, colorless gas, consisting of about 1 part by volume of oxygen and 4 parts of nitrogen, the proportion varying somewhat according to conditions. It also contains a small amount of carbon dioxide, ammonia, argon, nitrites, and organic matter. **alkaline a.** (*obs.*), free ammonia. **alveolar a.,** see under *gas.* **complemental a., complementary a.** (*obs.*), inspiratory capacity. **factitious a.,** nitrous oxide. **functional residual a.** (*obs.*), functional residual capacity; see under *capacity.* **liquid a.,** air liquefied by great pressure; on evaporation it produces intense cold. Liquid air has been used to produce local anesthesia and in the treatment of neuralgia and herpes zoster, and as a source of oxygen for medical use. **reserve a.** (*obs.*), see *expiratory* and *inspiratory reserve volume,* under *volume.* **residual a.,** see under *volume.* **stationary a.** (*obs.*), functional residual capacity. **supplemental a.** (*obs.*), expiratory reserve volume; see under *volume.* **tidal a.,** see under *volume.* **venous alveolar a.,** alveolar air in CO₂ equilibrium with mixed venous blood.

Airbrasive (ār′bra-siv) trademark for (*a*) an instrument for preparing a cavity in a tooth or removing deposits from teeth by application of a mixture of sand and aluminum oxide by air blast; (*b*) the abrasive cutting powder used with the instrument.

Airdent (ār′dent) trademark for a dental unit which utilizes abrasive particles applied by air blast for the preparation of dental cavities.

airway (ār′wa) 1. the route for passage of air into and out of the lungs. 2. a tubular device for securing unobstructed passage of air into and out of the lungs during general anesthesia or on occasions when the patient is not ventilating properly. **oropharyngeal a.,** a hollow tube inserted into the mouth and back of the throat to prevent the tongue from blocking off passage of air in unconscious persons.

Ajellomyces (ah″jĕ-lo-mi′sēz) a genus of ascomycetous perfect fungi of the family Gymnoascaceae, order Eurotiales. *A. dermatitidis,* the perfect stage of *Blastomyces dermatitidis,* is the etiologic agent of North American blastomycosis.

ak- for words beginning thus, see also words beginning *ac-.*

akaryocyte (ah-kar′e-o-sit″) [*a* neg. + Gr. *karyon* kernel + *kytos* hollow vessel] a non-nucleated cell, e.g., an erythrocyte.

akaryota (ah-kar″e-o′tah) akaryocyte.

akaryote (ah-kar′e-ōt) [*a* neg. + Gr. *karyon* kernel] akaryocyte.

akatama (ak″ah-tam′ah) a form of chronic peripheral neuritis once observed in West Africa; it is marked by swelling, erythema, prickling sensations, burning, numbness, and sometimes excessive sweating.

akatamathesia (ah-kat″ah-mah-the′zhe-ah) [*a* neg. + Gr. *katamathēsis* understanding] inability to understand.

akatanoesis (ah-kat″ah-no′ĕ-sis) [*a* neg. + Gr. *katanoein* to understand] inability to understand oneself (Heveroch, 1914).

akathisia (ak″ah-the′ze-ah) [*a* neg. + Gr. *kathisis* a sitting down + *-ia*] a condition of motor restlessness, ranging from a feeling of inner disquiet to inability to sit or lie quietly or to sleep; seen in toxic reactions to the phenothiazines. Called also *acathisia* and *kathisophobia.*

akee (ah′ke) native Jamaican name for the fruit of the tree *Blighia sapida,* Kon. Sapindaceae. The seeds contain the toxic principles hypoglycine A and B, and the aril of the unripe fruit contains hypoglycine A. The whitish, ripe aril is cooked and consumed as a delicacy. Ingestion of unripe fruit causes Jamaican vomiting sickness.

akembe (ah-kem′be) onyalai.

Åkerlund deformity (ek′er-loond) [Åke Olof Åkerlund, Swedish roentgenologist, 1885–1958] see under *deformity.*

akidogalvanocautery (ak″i-do-gal″vah-no-kaw′ter-e) cauterization by means of a needle electrode.

akinesia (ah″ki-ne′ze-ah) [*a* neg. + Gr. *kinēsis* motion + *-ia*] 1. absence or poverty of movements. 2. the temporary paralysis of a muscle by the injection of procaine. **a. al′gera,** Möbius' syndrome. **O'Brien a.,** paralysis of the orbicularis oculi muscle produced by injection of an anesthetic solution directly over the orbital branch of the seventh nerve as it emerges from behind the ear and extends toward the orbital region along the ramus of the jaw, permitting better exposure of the bulb of the eye. **reflex a.,** loss of reflex movement.

akinesis (ah″ki-ne′sis) akinesia.

akinesthesia (ah-kin″es-the′zhe-ah) absence of kinesthesia; absence of the movement sense.

akinetic (ah″ki-net′ik) 1. pertaining to, characterized by, or causing akinesia. 2. amitotic.

Akineton (a″ki-ne′ton) trademark for preparations of biperiden.

akiyami (ah″ke-yah′me) nanukayami.

aklomide (ak′lo-mīd) chemical name: 2-chloro-4-nitrobenzamide. A substance, C₇H₅ClN₂O₃, used as a coccidiostatic agent in poultry.

aknephascopia (ak″nef-ah-sko′pe-ah) [*a* neg. + Gr. *knephas* twilight + *skopein* to view] twilight blindness; reduced visual acuity in weak daylight, such as twilight, or in inadequate artificial illumination. Cf. *nyctalopia.*

Akokanthera (ak″o-kan-the′rah) *Acocanthera.*

akoria (ah-ko′re-ah) acoria.

Akrinol (ak′rin-ol) trademark for a preparation of acrisorcin.

Akureyri disease (ah-ku′ra-re) [*Akureyri,* a town in northern Iceland] benign myalgic encephalomyelitis.

Al chemical symbol for *aluminum.*

-al a suffix used in forming the names of chemical compounds, indicating presence of the aldehyde group, —CHO, as *chloral;* also used to form adjectives (usu*al*) and nouns (tri*al*).

A.L.A. American Laryngological Association.

Ala alanine.

ala (a′lah), pl. *a′lae* [L. "wing"] [NA] a general term for a winglike structure or process; called also *wing.* **a. al′ba media′lis,** area vestibularis. **a. au′ris,** auricula. **a. cerebel′li,** a. lobuli centralis. **a. cine′rea,** trigonum nervi vagi. **a. cris′tae gal′li** [NA], a small winglike process on the anterior part of the crista galli of the ethmoid bone; called also *frontal hamulus, hamulus frontalis,* and *processus alaris ossis ethmoidalis.* **a. il′ii,** a. ossis illi. **a′lae lin′gulae cerebel′li,** vincula lingulae cerebelli. **a. lob′uli centra′lis cerebel′li** [NA], the hemispheric extensions of the central lobule of the vermis of the cerebellum; called also *a. cerebelli.* **a. mag′na os′sis sphenoida′lis, a. ma′jor os′sis sphenoida′lis** [NA], great (major) wing of sphenoid bone: a large wing-shaped process arising from either side of the body of the sphenoid bone; its cerebral surface forms the anterior part of the floor of the middle cranial fossa, and its orbital surface forms the chief part of the lateral wall of the orbit. Called also *a. temporalis ossis sphenoidalis, lateral wing of sphenoid bone,* and *alisphenoid bone.* **a. mi′nor os′sis sphenoida′lis** [NA], small wing of sphenoid bone: the thin triangular plate of bone that extends horizontally and laterally from either side of the anterior part of the body of the sphenoid bone; it articulates with the frontal bone and helps form the roof of the orbit and the floor of the anterior cranial fossa. **a. na′si** [NA], wing of nose: the flaring cartilaginous expansion forming the outer side of each naris. **a. os′sis il′ii** [NA], **a. os′sis il′ium,** the expanded superior portion of the ilium which forms the lateral boundary of the greater pelvis. **a. par′va os′sis sphenoida′lis,** a. minor ossis sphenoidalis. **a. pon′tis,** tenia ventriculi quarti. **a. sacra′lis, a. sa′cri, a. of the sacrum,** pars lateralis ossis sacri. **a. tempora′lis os′sis sphenoida′lis,** a. major ossis sphenoidalis. **a. vespertilio′nis** ["bat's wing"], mesosalpinx. **a. of vomer, a. vo′meris** [NA], wing of vomer: one of the two lateral expansions on the superior border of the vomer, coming into contact with the sphenoidal process of the palatine bone and the vaginal process of the medial pterygoid plate.

alacrima (a-lak′rĭ-mah) [*a* neg. + L. *lacrima* tear] marked deficiency or absence of secretion of tears.

alactasia (ah-lak-ta′se-ah) malabsorption of lactose due to deficiency of lactase; it is a genetically determined condition in which lactose is not absorbed from the intestine, but is degraded in the large intestine and excreted in the feces as lactic acid, glucose, and galactose. It is very rare in infants of any race, but is common in nonwhite adults.

alae (a′le) [L.] plural of *ala.*

alalia (ah-la′le-ah) [*a* neg. + Gr. *lalein* to speak + *-ia*] lack of ability to talk; see also *aphasia.* **a. coph′ica,** deaf-mutism.

a. organ'ica, alalia due to organic disease. **a. physiolo'gica,** deaf-mutism. **a. prolonga'ta,** delayed speech.

alalic (ah-lal'ik) pertaining to, affected with, or of the nature of alalia.

alamecin (al-ah-me'sin) an antibiotic substance produced by *Trichoderma viride.*

alangine (ah-lan'jin) a yellowish amorphous alkaloid from *Alangium lamarckii.*

Alangium lamarckii (ah-lan'je-um lah-mark'e-e) an East Indian plant whose root is emetic, antipyretic, diuretic, and purgative. *A. salviifolium* is much used in Indian medicine as an emetic substitute for ipecac.

alanine (al'ah-nēn) a natural amino acid occurring in two forms: alpha-alanine, $CH_3CH(NH_2)\cdot COOH$, 2-aminopropionic acid, and beta-alanine, $CH_2NH_2\cdot CH_2COOH$, 3-aminopropionic acid. **a. mercury,** mercury aminopropionate, $[CH_3\cdot CH(NH_2)\text{-}COO]_2Hg.$

Alanson's amputation [Edward *Alanson,* British surgeon, 1747–1823] see under *amputation.*

alantin (ah-lan'tin) inulin.

alanyl-leucine (al''ah-nil-loo'sin) a dipeptide, $CH_3\cdot CH(NH_2)\cdot\text{-}CO\cdot NH(COOH)\cdot CH\cdot CH_2\cdot CH(CH_3)_2.$

alar (a'lar) [L. *alaris*] pertaining to an ala, or wing.

alastrim (ah-las'trim) variola minor.

alastrimic (al''as-trim'ik) pertaining to variola minor (alastrim).

alastrinic (al''as-trin'ik) alastrimic.

alate (a'lāt) [L. *alatus* winged] having wings; winged.

alba (al'bah) [L.] white; used as an adjective in names of certain anatomical tissues or structures, as substantia alba, and of certain diseases, as pityriasis alba.

Albalon (al'bah-lon) trademark for preparations of naphazoline hydrochloride.

Albamycin (al'bah-mi''sin) trademark for preparations of novobiocin.

Albarrán's disease, gland, test, tubules (al''bar-anz') [Joaquin *Albarrán* y Domínguez, Cuban surgeon in Paris, 1860–1912] see *colibacilluria,* and under *gland, test,* and *tubule.*

albedo (al-be'do) [L.] whiteness. **a. ret'inae,** edema of the retina.

Albee's operation (awl'bēz) [Fred. Houdlett *Albee,* New York surgeon, 1876–1945] see under *operation.*

albendazole (al-ben'dah-zōl) chemical name: [5-(propylthio)-1*H*-benzimidazol-2-yl] carbamic acid methyl ester; an anthelmintic, $C_{12}H_{15}N_3O_2S.$

Albers-Schönberg disease [Heinrich Ernst *Albers-Schönberg,* Hamburg roentgenologist, 1865–1921] osteopetrosis.

Albert's diphtheria stain (al'bertz) [Henry *Albert,* American physician, 1878–1930] see *Table of Stains.*

Albert's operation, suture [Eduard *Albert,* Austrian surgeon, 1841–1900] see under *operation* and *suture.*

Albertini's treatment (al-ber-tēn'ēz) [Ippolito Francesco *Albertini,* Italian physician, 1662–1738] see under *treatment.*

albicans (al'bĭ-kanz), pl. *albican'tia* [L.] white; see *corpus albicans.*

albiduria (al''bĭ-du're-ah) [L. *albidus* whitish + Gr. *ouron* urine + *-ia*] the discharge of white or pale urine.

albidus (al'bĭ-dus) [L.] whitish.

Albini's nodules (al-be'nēz) [Giuseppe *Albini,* Italian physiologist, 1827–1911] see under *nodule.*

albinism (al'bĭ-nizm) [L. *albus* white + *-ism*] congenital absence of pigment in the skin, hair, and eyes, due to absence or defect of tyrosinase, an enzyme that catalyzes the oxidation of tyrosine, a precursor of melanin. It is accompanied by photophobia and astigmatism. **localized a.,** partial a. **ocular a.,** absence of pigmentation in the tissues of the eye. **partial a.,** absence of pigment in local areas only; called also *localized a.* and *piebaldism.* **total a.,** complete absence of pigment in the eyes and in the skin and its appendages, often attended with astigmatism, photophobia, and nystagmus; called also *albinismus totalis* and *albinismus universalis.*

albinismus (al''bĭ-niz'mus) [L.] albinism. **a. circumscrip'tus,** partial albinism manifested as piebaldism, white forelock (a. circumscriptus pilorum), or circumscribed areas of depigmentation of the skin. See *piebaldism.* **a. tota'lis, a. universa'lis,** total albinism.

albino (al-bi'no) an individual affected with albinism.

albinoidism (al-bi-noid'izm) deficiency of pigment in the hair, skin, and eyes, but not to the degree seen in albinism.

albinoism (al-bi'no-izm) (*obs.*) albinism.

albinotic (al''bĭ-not'ik) pertaining to or characterized by albinism.

albinuria (al''bĭ-nu're-ah) albiduria.

Albinus' muscle (al-bi'nus) [Bernard Siegfried *Albinus,* anato-

mist and surgeon in Leyden, 1697–1770] 1. musculus risorius. 2. musculus scalenus medius.

albocinereous (al''bo-sĭ-ne're-us) [L. *albus* white + *cinereus* gray] (*obs.*) containing both white and gray matter.

Albrecht's bone (al'brektz) [Karl Martin Paul *Albrecht,* German anatomist, 1851–1894] basiotic bone.

Albright's syndrome (awl'brīts) [Fuller *Albright,* Boston physician, born 1900] see under *syndrome.*

Albucasis (al''boo-kas'is) [936–1013] the most famous Arabic writer on surgery; the surgical part of his encyclopedic *Altrasrif* greatly influenced medieval European medicine. Known also as *Abulcasis* and *Abulkasim.*

albuginea (al''bu-jin'e-ah) [L. from *albus* white] a tough whitish layer of fibrous tissue investing a part, especially a dense white membrane forming the immediate covering of the testicle; called also *tunica albuginea testis* [NA]. **a. oc'uli,** the sclera. **a. ova'rii,** the outer layer, or tunica, of the ovary. **a. pe'nis,** the outer envelope of the corpora cavernosa.

albugineotomy (al''bu-jin''e-ot'o-me) [*albuginea* + Gr. *tomē* a cutting] incision of the tunica albuginea of the testis.

albugineous (al''bu-jin'e-us) [L. *albugineus*] pertaining to or resembling a tough whitish layer of fibrous tissue (tunica albuginea testis).

albuginitis (al''bu-jĭ-ni'tis) inflammation of any one of the albugineous tissues or tunics.

albugo (al-bu'go) [L. from *albus* white] a white corneal opacity.

albukalin (al''bu-ka'lin) a substance, $C_8H_{16}N_2O_6$, found in leukemic blood.

albumen (al-bu'men) [L., from *albus* white] albumin.

albumimeter (al''bu-mim'ĕ-ter) albuminimeter.

albumin (al-bu'min) a protein found in nearly every animal and in many vegetable tissues, and characterized by being soluble in water and coagulable by heat; it contains carbon, hydrogen, nitrogen, oxygen, and sulfur. The formula for crystallized albumin has been given as $C_{720}H_{1134}N_{218}S_5O_{248}.$ **a. A,** a certain constituent of the blood serum which in cancer patients is reduced in amount but which gathers abundantly in cancer cells; see *Kahn test* (def. 2), under *tests.* **acid a.,** albumin altered by the action of an acid. **alkali a.,** any albumin which has been treated with an alkali. **blood a.,** serum a. **circulating a.,** that which is found in the fluids of the body. **coagulated a.,** albumin altered by heat or chemical action so as to be insoluble in water, neutral salt solutions, or dilute acid and alkaline solutions. **derived a.,** any albumin denatured by chemical action, as albuminate. **egg a.,** a glycoprotein that constitutes 20 per cent of the white of hens' eggs; called also *ovalbumin.* **hematin a.,** a preparation of ox blood rich in iron. **human a.,** normal human serum a. **iodinated I 125 serum a.,** iodinated I 125 albumin injection; see under *injection.* **iodinated I 131 serum a.,** iodinated I 131 albumin injection; see under *injection.* **Mayer's a.,** white of egg 50 ml., glycerol 50 ml., sodium salicylate 1 gm. **muscle a.,** a variety found in muscle juice. **native a.,** any albumin normally present in the body. **normal human serum a.** [USP], a sterile preparation of serum albumin obtained by fractionating blood from healthy, human donors, not less than 96 per cent of its total volume being albumin; used as a blood-volume supporter in the treatment of shock, hypoproteinemia, hyperbilirubinemia, and erythroblastosis fetalis. Administered intravenously. **organ a.,** any albumin normally present in a particular organ. **radioiodinated (^{125}I) serum a. (human),** iodinated I 125 albumin injection; see under *injection.* **radioiodinated (^{131}I) serum a. (human),** iodinated I 131 albumin injection; see under *injection.* **serum a.,** a major protein of human blood plasma. **soap a.,** a combination of soap and albumin which is supposed to constitute the intracellular granules of soap. **a. tannate,** a yellowish white astringent powder containing about 50 per cent tannic acid combined with protein; used in diarrhea. **technetium Tc 99m aggregated a.,** see under *technetium.* **vegetable a.,** any albumin of vegetable origin.

albuminate (al-bu'mĭ-nāt'') albumin denatured by a base or an acid, characterized by solubility in dilute acids or alkalis and by being insoluble in dilute salt solutions, water, or alcohol; called also *derived albumin* and *derived protein.*

albuminaturia (al-bu''mĭ-na-tu're-ah) [*albuminate* + *urine*] proteinuria in which there is an excess of albuminates in the urine.

albuminemia (al-bu''mĭ-ne'me-ah) [*albumin* + Gr. *haima* blood + *-ia*] the presence of albumin in the blood plasma or serum; proteinemia.

albuminimeter (al-bu''mĭ-nim'ĕ-ter) [*albumin* + *meter*] an instrument used in determining the proportion of albumin present, as in the urine.

albuminimetry (al-bu''mĭ-nim'ĕ-tre) the determination of the proportion of albumin present.

albuminocholia (al-bu''mĭ-no-ko'le-ah) [*albumin* + Gr. *cholē* bile + *-ia*] the presence of albumin in the bile.

albuminocytological (al-bu''mĭ-no-si''to-loj'ĭ-k'l) pertaining to the level of protein as albumin in relation to number of cells present in cerebrospinal fluid.

albuminoid (al-bu′mĭ-noid″) [*albumin* + Gr. *eidos* form] 1. resembling albumin. 2. fibrous protein. 3. a scleroprotein.

albuminolysin (al″bu-mĭ-nol′ĭ-sin) [*albumin* + *lysin*] 1. a lysin that disintegrates albumins. 2. anaphylactin.

albuminolysis (al-bu″mĭ-nol′ĭ-sis) the splitting up of albumins.

albuminometer (al-bu″mĭ-nom′ĕ-ter) albuminimeter.

albuminoptysis (al″bu-mĭ-nop′tĭ-sis) [*albumin* + Gr. *ptyein* to spit] presence of albumin in the sputum.

albuminoreaction (al-bu″mĭ-no-re-ak′shun) the reaction of the sputum to tests for albumin; the presence of albumin (positive reaction) is indicative of pulmonary inflammation.

albuminorrhea (al-bu″mi-no-re′ah) [*albumin* + Gr. *rhoia* flow] excessive excretion of albumins.

albuminous (al-bu′mĭ-nus) containing, charged with, or of the nature of an albumin.

albuminuretic (al-bu″mĭ-nu-ret′ik) [*albumin* + Gr. *ourētikos* diuretic] 1. pertaining to, characterized by, or promoting albuminuria. 2. an agent that promotes albuminuria.

albuminuria (al″bu-mĭ-nu′re-ah) [*albumin* + Gr. *ouron* urine + *-ia*] the presence in the urine of serum albumin; see *proteinuria*. **Bamberger's hematogenic a.,** that which occurs during the latter periods of severe anemia.

albuminuric (al″bu-mĭ-nu′rik) proteinuric.

albuminurophobia (al-bu″min-u″ro-fo′be-ah) [*albuminuria* + *phobia*] 1. an exaggerated fear of acquiring albuminuria. 2. overemphasis on the significance of albumin in the urine.

Albumisol (al-bu′mĭ-sol) trademark for a preparation of albumin human.

albumoscope (al-bu′mo-skōp″) [*albumin* + Gr. *skopein* to view] an instrument for determining the presence and amount of albumin in the urine.

albuterol (al-bu′ter-ōl) chemical name: α¹-[(*tert*-butylamino)-methyl]-4-hydroxy-*m*-xylene-α,α′-diol; a β-adrenergic stimulant, $C_{13}H_{21}NO_3$, used as a bronchodilator. Called also *salbutamol*. **a. sulfate,** the sulfate salt of albuterol, $(C_{13}H_{21}NO_3)\cdot H_2SO_4$, having the same actions and uses as the base.

Alcaine (al′kān) trademark for a preparation of proparacaine hydrochloride.

Alcaligenes (al″kah-lij′ĕ-nēz) a genus of microorganisms of the family Achromobacteraceae, order Eubacteriales, made up of gram-negative rod-shaped bacteria generally found in the intestinal tracts of vertebrates or in dairy products. It includes six species, *A. boo′keri, A. faeca′lis* (*Bacillus faecalis alcaligenes*), *A. marshal′lii, A. metalcalig′enes, A. rec′ti,* and *A. viscolac′tis.*

alcapton (al-kap′ton) alkapton body; see under *body*.

alcaptonuria (al-kap″to-nu′re-ah) alkaptonuria.

alcaptonuric (al-kap″to-nu′rik) alkaptonuric.

alchemy (al′kĕ-me) the supposed art of transmutation of baser metals into gold; also chemical magic.

alclofenac (al-klo′fen-ak) chemical name: 3-chloro-4-(2-propenyloxy)benzene-acetic acid; an analgesic, antipyretic, and anti-inflammatory, $C_{11}H_{11}ClO_3$.

Alcmaeon (alk-me′on) **of Crotona** (c. 500 B.C.) a famous physician, supposedly a pupil of Pythagoras, and the reputed discoverer of the optic nerve and the auditory tube.

Alcock's canal (al′koks) [Benjamin *Alcock,* Professor of Anatomy, Queen's College, Cork, from 1849 to 1855; born 1801, date of death in America unknown] canalis pudendalis.

alcohol (al′ko-hol) [Arabic *al-koh′l* something subtle] 1. chemical name: ethanol. A transparent, colorless, mobile, volatile liquid, C_2H_5OH, miscible with water, ether, and chloroform, obtained by fermentation of carbohydrates with yeast. Called also *ethyl alcohol.* 2. [USP] a preparation containing not less than 92.3 per cent and not more than 93.8 per cent by weight, corresponding to not less than 94.9 per cent and not more than 96.0 per cent by volume, at 15.56° C., of C_2H_5OH; used as a topical anti-infective and solvent. 3. any of a class of organic compounds formed from the hydrocarbons by the substitution of one or more hydroxyl groups for an equal number of hydrogen atoms; the term is extended to various substitution products which are neutral in reaction and which contain one or more of the alcohol groups. They are distinguished as *monohydric, dihydric, trihydric,* etc., depending on the number of hydroxyl groups present. Alcohols may be classified as *primary, secondary,* or *tertiary* according to whether the hydroxyl group is attached to a carbon atom that is covalently bonded to one, two, or three other carbon atoms. **absolute a.,** dehydrated a. **amyl a.,** a colorless oily liquid, $C_5H_{11}OH$, with characteristic odor; miscible with alcohol, ether, and chloroform and slightly soluble in water. **amyl a., tertiary,** amylene hydrate. **anisyl a.,** an alcohol, *p*-methoxybenzyl alcohol, $CH_3O\cdot C_6H_4\cdot OH$, in pungent shining prisms. **aromatic a.,** any of the phenols. **azeotropic isopropyl a.** [USP], a preparation containing 91 to 93 per cent of isopropyl alcohol by volume, and the remainder consisting of water.

batyl a., the monooctadecyl ether of glycerol, CH_2-OHCHOHCH$_2$O(CH$_2$)$_{17}$CH$_3$; 3-(octadecyloxy)-1,2-propanediol. An isolate from shark liver oils and from yellow bone marrow, now synthesized. Has been reported for bracken fern (*Pteridium aquilinum* (L.) Kuhn; Polypodiaceae) poisoning in cattle. **benzyl a.** [NF], a clear colorless oily liquid, $C_6H_5\cdot CH_2\cdot OH$, occurring in balsam of Peru, tolu balsam, and styrax; used as a bacteriostatic in solutions for injection. It is also applied topically as a local anesthetic. Called also *phenylcarbinol* and *phenylmethanol.* **bornyl a.,** Borneo camphor. **butyl a.,** a clear liquid, C_4H_9OH, from the molasses of beets; four isomeric forms are known. **camphyl a.,** borneol. **carnaubyl a.,** a constituent, $CH_3(CH_2)_{23}OH$, of carnauba wax and of wool fat. **ceryl a.,** a fatty alcohol, CH_3-$(CH_2)_{24}CH_2OH$, from Chinese wool; called also *cerotin.* **cetyl a.** [NF], a fatty alcohol, $CH_3(CH_2)_{14}CH_2OH$, from spermaceti; used as an emulsifying and stiffening agent. Called also *ethal.* **cinnamyl a.,** chemical name: 3-phenyl-2-propen-1-ol. It is obtained from storax and balsam of Peru. **dehydrated a.** [USP], an extremely hygroscopic, transparent, colorless, volatile liquid with characteristic odor and burning taste, containing not less than 99.5 per cent by volume of C_2H_5OH; called also *absolute a.* **denatured a.,** alcohol which has been rendered unfit for beverage or medicinal purposes by addition of methanol or acetone, but which may still be used for industrial purposes or as a solvent. **deodorized a.,** one that contains 92.5 per cent of absolute alcohol and is free from fusel oil (amyl alcohol) and organic impurities. **dihydric a.,** an alcohol containing two hydroxyl groups. **diluted a.** [NF], a mixture of alcohol and water containing 41 to 42 per cent by weight, or 48.4 to 49.5 per cent by volume, at 15.56° C., of C_2H_5OH; used as a solvent. **ethyl a.,** alcohol. **fatty a.,** any hydroxide of a hydrocarbon derived from the paraffin series. **glyceryl a., glycyl a.,** glycerin. **isoamyl a.,** amyl a. **isobutyl a.,** chemical name: (2-methyl-1-propanol). A clear colorless liquid, $(CH_3)_2CHCH_2OH$, with a characteristic odor; miscible with alcohol and with ether; called also *isobutanol.* **isopropyl a.** [USP], chemical name: 2-propanol. A clear colorless liquid, CH_3-CH(OH)CH$_3$, an isomer of propyl alcohol and a homologue of ethyl alcohol. It is miscible with water, alcohol, ether, and chloroform; used as a solvent and as a basis for isopropyl rubbing alcohol (q.v.). Called also *avantin* and *dimethyl carbinol,* and *isopropanol.* **isopropyl rubbing a.** [USP], a preparation containing between 68 and 72 per cent isopropyl alcohol in water, used as a rubefacient. Formerly called *isopropyl alcohol rubbing compound.* **ketone a.,** an alcohol which contains the ketone (carbonyl) group. **lanolin a's** [NF], a mixture of aliphatic alcohols, triterpenoid alcohols, and sterols, obtained by hydrolysis of lanolin and containing not less than 30 per cent cholesterol. **methyl a.,** methanol. **monohydric a.,** an alcohol containing only one hydroxyl group. **nicotinyl a.,** chemical name: 3-pyridinemethanol. An alcohol, C_6H_7NO, used as a peripheral vasodilator in vasospastic conditions. **palmityl a.,** cetyl a. **pantothenyl a.,** 1. panthenol. 2. dexpanthenol. **phenylethyl a.** [USP], chemical name: 2-phenylethanol. A colorless liquid, $C_8H_{10}O$, with a roselike odor and a sharp, burning taste; used as a bacteriostatic for drug solutions. Called also *benzyl carbonol.* **phenylic a.,** phenol. **polyglucosic a.,** an alcohol having the formula $C_{6n}H_{10n}$ + $2O_{5n}$. **polyvinyl a.** [USP], a water-soluble synthetic resin, represented by the formula $(C_2H_4O)_n$, in which *n* varies between 500 and 5000; used as a viscosity-increasing agent in pharmaceutical preparations and as a pharmaceutic necessity for ophthalmic solution dosage forms. **primary a.,** an alcohol containing the monovalent carbinol group, —CH_2OH. **n-propyl a.,** chemical name: 1-propanol. A clear colorless liquid with an alcohol-like odor, $CH_3\cdot CH_2\cdot CH_2OH$, miscible with water and most organic solvents; used as a solvent for resins. **rubbing a.** [USP], a preparation of acetone, methyl isobutyl ketone, and 68.5 to 71.5 per cent ethyl alcohol; used as a rubefacient. **secondary a.,** an alcohol containing the divalent group ═CHOH. **stearyl a.,** a solid alcohol [$CH_3(CH_2)_{16}CH_2OH$], prepared from stearic acid by catalytic hydrogenation; a pharmacological preparation [NF], containing not less than 90 per cent of stearyl alcohol, the remainder consisting chiefly of cetyl alcohol, is used as an ingredient of hydrophilic ointment, hydrophilic petrolatum, and polethylene glycol ointment. **sugar a's,** alcohols that result from the reduction of the functional group (aldehyde or ketone) of sugars. **tertiary a.,** an alcohol containing the trivalent group, ≡COH. **tribromoethyl a.,** tribromoethanol. **trihydric a.,** an alcohol containing three hydroxyl groups. **unsaturated a.,** alcohol that is derived from unsaturated hydrocarbons (alkenes, or olefins). **wood a.,** methanol.

alcoholase (al′ko-hol-ās″) a hypothetical substance once believed to be responsible for the conversion of lactic acid into alcohol.

alcoholemia (al″ko-hol-e′me-ah) [*alcohol* + Gr. *haima* blood + *-ia*] the presence of alcohol in the blood.

alcoholic (al″ko-hol′ik) [L. *alcoholicus*] 1. pertaining to or containing alcohol. 2. a person suffering from alcoholism (q.v.).

alcoholism (al′ko-hol-izm) a chronic behavioral disorder manifested by repeated drinking of alcoholic beverages in excess of the dietary and social uses of the community and to an extent that interferes with the drinker's health or his social or economic functioning; some degree of habituation, dependence, or addiction is implied. **acute a.,** simple drunkenness due to excessive intake of ethyl alcohol, resulting in depression of the centers of the nervous system. **chronic a.,** long-continued, excessive intake of ethyl alcohol characterized by various conditions, including anorexia, diarrhea, weight loss, mental deterioration, personality changes, peripheral neuropathy, and fatty deterioration of the liver.

alcoholization (al″ko-hol″i-za′shun) treatment by application or injection of alcohol.

alcoholize (al′ko-hol-īz″) 1. to treat with alcohol. 2. to transform into alcohol.

alcoholometer (al″ko-hol-om′ĕ-ter) [alcohol + Gr. metron measure] an instrument used in determining the percentage of alcohol in a solution.

alcoholuria (al″ko-hol-u′re-ah) the presence of alcohol in the urine.

alcoholysis (al″ko-hol′ĭ-sis) [alcohol + Gr. lysis dissolution] a process analogous to hydrolysis, but in which alcohol takes the place of water.

alcuronium chloride (al-kūr-o′nĭ-um) chemical name: N,N′-diallylnortoxiferinium dichloride; a skeletal muscle relaxant, $C_{44}H_{50}Cl_2N_4O_2$.

Aldactazide (al-dak′tah-zīd) trademark for a preparation of spironolactone with hydrochlorothiazide.

Aldactone (al-dak′tōn) trademark for a preparation of spironolactone.

aldehydase (al″de-hi′dās) an enzyme that oxidizes an aldehyde into its corresponding acid; it may also refer to anaerobic conversion to the corresponding acid and alcohol.

aldehyde (al′dĕ-hīd) [alcohol + L. de away from + hydrogen] 1. any one of a large class of organic compounds containing the group —CHO, that is, with the carbonyl group, C=O, occurring at the end of the carbon chain. 2. acetaldehyde. **acetic a.,** acetaldehyde. **acrylic a.,** acrolein. **amylic a.,** n-valeraldehyde. **anisic a.,** a volatile oil, p-methoxybenzaldehyde, CH_3·O·C_6H_4·CHO, obtainable from oil of anise and other volatile oils. **benzoic a.,** benzaldehyde. **butylic a.,** a substance, isobutyraldehyde, $(CH_3)_2CH$·CHO. **cinnamic a.,** a colorless aldehyde, $C_6H_5(CH)_2$CHO, obtained from oil of cinnamon, and used in flavors and perfumes. **cumic a.,** an aromatic volatile oil, para-isopropylbenzaldehyde, C_3H_7·C_6H_4·CHO, from several essential oils. **glyceric a., glycerin a.,** one of the allomeric forms of triose; it is CH_2OH·CHOH·CHO, a reference substance for the stereochemical classification of the simple sugars. **glycolic a.,** see diose. **keto a.,** an aldehyde that contains the keto group CO and CHO. **salicylic a.,** a fragrant colorless liquid, C_6H_4OH·CHO, soluble in water, from volatile oil of shrubs of the genus Spiraea; called also salicylaldehyde. **trichloracetic a.,** chloral. **valeric a.,** n-valeraldehyde.

aldehyde-lyase (al′dĕ-hīd-li′ās) a group of lyases that catalyze the removal of an aldehyde group, as from 4-hydroxy-2-oxobutyrate to form pyruvate and formaldehyde, or from L-threonine to form glycine and acetaldehyde. It includes the aldolases.

aldin (al′din) an aldehyde base.

Aldinamide (al-din′ah-mīd) trademark for preparations of pyrazinamide.

aldohexose (al″do-hek′sōs) a hexose that is an aldehyde derivative; any of a class of sugars that contain six carbon atoms and an aldehyde group, as glucose or mannose.

aldolase (al′do-lās) an enzyme in muscle extract that acts as a catalyst in the production of dihydroxyacetone phosphate and glyceraldehyde phosphate from fructose 1,6-diphosphate.

Aldomet (al′do-met) trademark for a preparation of methyldopa.

aldopentose (al″do-pen′tōs) any of a class of sugars that contain five carbon atoms and an aldehyde group, as arabinose.

aldose (al′dōs) a sugar containing an aldehyde group, —CHO.

aldoside (al′do-sīd) a glycoside that on hydrolysis yields an aldose sugar.

aldosterone (al′do-ster-ōn″, al-dos′ter-ōn) the main mineralocorticoid hormone secreted by the adrenal cortex, the principal biological activity of which is the regulation of electrolyte and water balance by promoting the retention of sodium (and therefore of water) and the excretion of potassium; the retention of water induces an increase in plasma volume and an increase in blood pressure. The secretion of aldosterone is stimulated by angiotensin II.

aldosteronism (al″do-ster′ōn-izm″) an abnormality of electrolyte metabolism caused by excessive secretion of aldosterone; called also hyperaldosteronism. **primary a.,** that arising from oversecretion of aldosterone by an adrenal adenoma, characterized typically by hypokalemia, alkalosis, muscular weakness, polyuria, polydipsia, and hypertension. Called also Conn's syndrome. **pseudoprimary a.,** that caused by bilateral adrenal hyperplasia and having the same signs and symptoms as primary aldosteronism. **secondary a.,** that due to extra-adrenal stimulation of aldosterone secretion; it is commonly associated with

edematous states, as in nephrotic syndrome, hepatic cirrhosis, heart failure, and accelerated phase hypertension.

aldosteronogenesis (al″do-ster-o-no-jen′e-sis) the production of aldosterone by the adrenal glands.

aldosteronoma (al″do-ster″on-o′mah) an aldosterone-secreting tumor of the adrenal cortex.

aldosteronopenia (al″do-ster-o-no-pe′ne-ah) hypoaldosteronism.

aldosteronuria (al″do-ster″ōn-u′re-ah) the presence of aldosterone in the urine.

aldotetrose (al″do-tet′rōs) an aldehyde sugar containing four atoms of carbon.

aldoxime (al-dok′sīm) a compound formed by the union of an aldehyde with hydroxylamine.

Aldrich mixture (awl′drich) [Robert Henry Aldrich, American surgeon, born 1902] see under mixture.

Aldrich syndrome (awl′drich) [Robert A. Aldrich, American pediatrician, born 1917] Wiskott-Aldrich syndrome.

Aldrich-McClure test (awl′drich-mah-kloor′) [Charles Anderson Aldrich, American pediatrician, 1888–1949; William Bradbury McClure, 1884–1936, American physician] McClure-Aldrich test.

aldrin (al′drin) chemical name: 1,2,3,4,10,10-hexachloro-1,4,4a,5,8,8a-hexahydro-1,4:8-dimethanonaphthalene. A chlorinated naphthalene derivative, $C_{12}H_8Cl_6$, used as an insecticide.

alecithal (ah-les′ĭ-thal) [a neg. + Gr. lekithos yolk] without yolk; applied to eggs with very little yolk. See under ovum.

Alectorobius talaje the tick Ornithodoros talaje.

alembic (ah-lem′bik) [Arabic al-imbīq, the still, from Gr. ambix cup] a retort with a removable cap formerly used by chemists.

alembroth (ah-lem′broth) a compound, $(NH_4Cl)_2HgCl_2$ + $2H_2O$, of mercuric and ammonium chlorides, formerly used as an antiseptic dressing.

alemmal (ah-lem′al) [a neg. + Gr. lemma husk] (obs.) having no neurilemma; said of a nerve fiber.

alethia (ah-le′the-ah) [a neg. + Gr. lēthē forgetfulness] (obs.) the inability to forget.

aletocyte (ah-le′to-sīt″) [Gr. alētēs wanderer + kytos hollow vessel] a wandering cell.

Aletris farinosa L. (Liliaceae) (al′ĕ-tris fah-rĭ-nōs′ah) a perennial herb indigenous to eastern North America, used medicinally by the Catawba Indians. The dried roots (colic root, or unicorn root) are used as a diuretic and uterine tonic; cold-water leaf infusion is used for colic and stomach ailments. It contains starch and diosgenin.

aleukemia (ah″lu-ke′me-ah) [a neg. + Gr. leukos white + haima blood + -ia] 1. absence or deficiency of leukocytes in the blood. 2. aleukemic leukemia.

aleukemic (ah″lu-ke′mik) marked by aleukemia; see under leukemia.

aleukia (ah-lu′ke-ah) [a neg. + Gr. leukos white + -ia] absence of leukocytes from the blood; leukopenia. **alimentary toxic a.,** a form of mycotoxicosis associated with the ingestion of grain that has overwintered in the field; causative agents include members of the genera Fusarium, Cladosporium, Alternaria, Penicillium, Mucor, Piptocephalis, Trichoderma, Rhizopus, Trichothecium, Thammidium, Verticillium, and Actinomyces. Abbreviated ATA. **a. hemorrha′gica,** an accessory or auxiliary term which actually refers to the condition of aplastic anemia (see under anemia).

aleukocytic (ah-lu″ko-sit′ik) showing no leukocytes.

aleukocytosis (ah-lu″ko-si-to′sis) [a neg. + leukocyte + -osis] deficiency in the proportion of white cells in the blood; leukopenia.

aleuriospore (ah-lu′re-o-spōr) [Gr. aleuron flour + spore] a terminal or lateral, asexual spore similar to a conidium except that it is not shed (not deciduous), being released only by dissolution of its attachment to the mycelium.

Aleurisma (al″u-riz′mah) Chrysosporium.

Aleurobius farinae (ah-lu-ro′bĭ-us fah-ri′ne) Tyroglyphus farinae.

Aleuronat (ah-lu′ro-nat″) trademark for a brand of wheat flour from which most of the starch has been removed; used by diabetics.

aleurone (ah-loor′ōn″, al′yah-rōn″) 1. the protein granule of globulins and peptones found in ripe seeds. 2. the outer layer of the endosperm in gluten-rich cereal grains.

aleuronoid (ah-lu′ro-noid″) resembling flour.

Alexander (al″ek-san′der) **of Tralles** (c. 525–605 A.D.) a Byzantine Greek physician and compiler who practiced latterly in Rome; his writings were mainly on pathology and the treatment of internal diseases, his descriptions of parasites being outstanding. He is also known as Alexander Trallianus.

Alexander's operation (al″ek-zan′derz) 1. [Samuel Alexander, New York surgeon, 1858–1910] see under operation (def. 3). 2. [William Alexander, Liverpool surgeon, 1844–1919] see under operation (defs. 1 and 2).

Alexander-Adams operation (al″ek-zan′der-ad′amz) [William *Alexander* 1844–1919; James Alexander *Adams*, gynecologist in Glasgow, 1857–1930] see *Alexander's operation* (def. 1), under *operation*.

alexeteric (ah-lek″sĕ-ter′ik) [Gr. *alexētēr* defender] effective against infection or poison.

alexia (ah-lek′se-ah) [*a* neg. + Gr. *lexis* word + *-ia*] a form of receptive aphasia in which there is loss of the ability to understand written language as a result of a cerebral lesion; called also *aphemesthesia, optical alexia, visual amnesia, visual aphasia,* and *word blindness.* **cortical a.,** a form of sensory aphasia due to lesions of the left gyrus angularis. **motor a.,** alexia in which the patient understands what he sees written or printed, but cannot read it aloud. **musical a.,** loss of the ability to read music; music blindness. **optical a.,** alexia. **subcortical a.,** a form due to interruption of the connection between the optic center and the gyrus angularis.

alexic (ah-lek′sik) 1. having the properties of an alexin. 2. pertaining to alexia.

alexidine (ah-leks′ĭ-dēn) chemical name: N,N″-bis(2-ethylhexyl)-3,12-diimino-2,4,11,13-tetraazatetradecanediimidamide; an antibacterial, $C_{26}H_{56}N_{10}$.

alexin (ah-lek′sin) [Gr. *alexein* to ward off] a nonspecific thermolabile substance which in the presence of specific sensitizer exerts a lytic action on bacteria and other cells. It is not increased by immunization and is present in plasma and serum. See *complement* and *cytase,* def. 1. **leukocytic a.,** see *leukin,* def. 1.

alexinic (ah″ek-sin′ik) pertaining to or having the properties of an alexin.

alexipharmac (ah-lek″se-far′mak) [Gr. *alexein* to ward off + *pharmakon* poison] 1. warding off the ill effects of a poison. 2. an antidote or remedy for poisoning.

alexipyretic (ah-lek″sĭ-pi-ret′ik) [Gr. *alexein* to ward off + *pyretos* fever] (*obs.*) dispelling or preventing fever.

alexocyte (ah-lek′so-sit″) [Gr. *alexein* to ward off + *kytos* hollow vessel] a cell of the animal organism secreting alexins; the term was formerly applied to eosinophil cells.

aleydigism (ah-li′dig-izm″) absence of androgen secretion of the interstitial cells of Leydig.

Alflorone (al′flo-rōn) trademark for preparations of fludrocortisone.

A.L.G. antilymphocyte globulin.

alga (al′gah) any individual organism of the algae.

algae (al′je) [L., pl., "seaweeds"] a group of cryptogamous plants, in which the body is unicellular or consists of a thallus; it includes the seaweed and many unicellular fresh-water plants, most of which contain chlorophyll. Algae account for about 90 per cent of the earth's photosynthetic activity.

algal (al′gal) of, pertaining to, or caused by algae.

alganesthesia (al-gan″es-the′ze-ah) [Gr. *algos* pain + *anesthesia*] analgesia.

algaroba (al″gah-ro′bah) the finely pulverized meal of the dried ripe fruit (St. John's bread, or carob fruit) of *Ceratonia siliqua* L., Leguminosae. It contains albuminous proteins, carbohydrates, and small amounts of fat and crude fiber, and is used in pharmaceutical formulations as an adsorbent and demulcent in treatment of diarrhea.

alge- see *algesi-*.

algedonic (al″je-don′ik) [*alge-* + Gr. *hēdonē* pleasure] characterized by or relating to pain.

algefacient (al″je-fa′shent) [L. *algere* to be cold + *faciens* making] cooling; refrigerant.

algeldrate (al-jel′drāt) nonreactive, powdered, hydrated aluminum hydroxide; an antacid, $AlH_3O_3 \cdot xH_2O$.

algeoscopy (al″je-os′ko-pe) [Gr. *algos* pain + *skopein* to view] physical examination by pressure, to ascertain whether such pressure produces pain, often used in neurological examinations and in ascertaining depth of coma.

algesi-, alge-, algio-, algo- (al-je′ze, al′je, al′je-o, al′go) [Gr. *algos* pain] combining form denoting relationship to pain.

algesia (al-je′ze-ah) sensitiveness to pain; hyperesthesia.

algesic (al-je′zik) painful.

algesichronometer (al-je″ze-kro-nom′ĕ-ter) [*algesi-* + Gr. *chronos* time + *metron* measure] an instrument for recording the time required to produce a painful impression.

algesimeter (al″je-sim′ĕ-ter) [*algesi* + Gr. *metron* measure] an instrument used in measuring the sensitiveness to pain as produced by pricking with a sharp point. **Björnström's a.,** an apparatus for determining the sensitiveness of the skin. **Boas' a.,** an instrument for determining the sensitiveness over the epigastrium.

algesimetry (al″jĕ-sim′ĕ-tre) the measurement of sensitiveness to pain; called also *algesiometry*.

algesiogenic (al-je″ze-o-jen′ik) [*algesi-* + Gr. *gennan* to produce] producing pain.

algesiometer (al-je″ze-om′ĕ-ter) algesimeter.

algesthesia (al″jes-the′ze-ah) pain sensibility; algesthesis.

algesthesis (al″jes-the′sis) [*algesi-* + Gr. *aisthēsis* perception] the perception of pain; any painful sensation.

algestone acetophenide (al-jes′tōn) chemical name: 16α,17-dihydroxypregn-4-ene-3,20-dione cyclic acetal with acetophenone; a progestin, $C_{29}H_{36}O_4$.

algetic (al-jet′ik) painful.

-algia (al′je-ah) [Gr. *algos* pain + *-ia* condition] a word termination indicating a painful condition.

algicide (al′jĭ-sīd) [*algae* + L. *caedere* to kill] a substance which is destructive to algae.

algid (al′jid) [L. *algidus*] chilly or cold, def. 1.

algin (al′jin) sodium alginate, a purified carbohydrate (sodium mannuronate) extracted from brown algae species and used as a stabilizing colloid in numerous pharmaceuticals, cosmetics, and foods.

alginate (al′jĭ-nāt) a salt of alginic acid, which is extracted from marine kelp. Calcium, sodium, and ammonium alginates have been used as foam, clot, or gauze for absorbable surgical dressings. Soluble alginates, such as sodium, potassium, and magnesium alginates, form a viscous sol which can be changed into a gel by a chemical reaction with compounds such as calcium sulfate, a property which makes them useful as materials for taking dental impressions.

Alginobacter (al″jĭ-no-bak′ter) a genus of microorganisms of the tribe Escherichieae, family Enterobacteriaceae, order Eubacteriales, made up of short motile rods, found in the soil. The type species is *A. acidofa′ciens.*

Alginomonas (al″jĭ-no-mo′nas) a genus of microorganisms of the family Pseudomonadaceae, suborder Pseudomonadineae, order Pseudomonadales, occurring as motile coccoid rods, found on algae and in sea water and soil. It includes five species, *A. algi′nica, A. algino′vora, A. fuci′cola, A. nonfermen′tans, A. terrestralgi′nica.*

alginuresis (al″jin-u-re′sis) [Gr. *algos* pain + *ourēsis* urination] painful urination.

algio- see *algesi-*.

algioglandular (al″je-o-glan′du-lar) pertaining to glandular action resulting from painful stimulation.

algiometabolic (al″je-o-met″ah-bol′ik) pertaining to metabolic changes resulting from painful stimulation.

algiomotor (al″je-o-mo′tor) producing painful movements, such as spasm or dysperistalsis.

algiomuscular (al″je-o-mus′ku-lar) causing painful muscular movements.

algiovascular (al″je-o-vas′ku-lar) pertaining to vascular action resulting from painful stimulation.

algo- see *algesi-*.

algodystrophy (al″go-dis′tro-fe) [*algo-* + *dystrophy*] a combination of pain and dystrophic changes in bone, as in Sudeck's atrophy.

algogenesia (al″go-jĕ-ne′ze-ah) [*algo-* + Gr. *gennan* to produce] the production of pain.

algogenesis (al″go-jen′ĕ-sis) algogenesia.

algogenic (al-go-jen′ik) 1. [*algo-* + Gr. *gennan* to produce] causing pain. 2. [L. *algor* cold + Gr. *gennan* to produce] producing cold.

algolagnia (al″go-lag′ne-ah) [*algo-* + Gr. *lagneia* lust] abnormal sexual impulse toward persons of opposite sex with a desire for experiencing or causing pain. **active a.,** sadism. **passive a.,** masochism.

algologist (al-gol′o-jist) 1. one who specializes in algology. 2. phycologist.

algology (al-gol′o-je) 1. [*algo-* + *-logy*] the discipline that deals with the study of pain. 2. [*alga* + *-logy*] phycology.

algomenorrhea (al″go-men-o-re′ah) [*algo-* + *menorrhea*] (*obs.*) dysmenorrhea.

algometer (al-gom′ĕ-ter) [*algo-* + Gr. *metron* measure] an instrument for testing sensitivity to painful stimuli. **pressure a.,** an instrument for measuring sensitivity to pressure.

algometry (al-gom′ĕ-tre) the measurement of sensitivity to painful stimuli, as with an algometer.

algophilia (al″go-fil′e-ah) (*obs.*) masochism.

algophily (al-gof′ĭ-le) [*algo-* + Gr. *philein* to love] (*obs.*) sexual perversion marked by a desire for experiencing pain; masochism.

algophobia (al″go-fo′be-ah) [*algo-* + *phobia*] morbid dread of experiencing or of witnessing pain.

algopsychalia (al″go-si-ka′le-ah) [*algo-* + Gr. *psychē* soul] (*obs.*) a condition of melancholia with perverted imaginary perceptions of sounds and sights which cause dread, despair, and inclination to suicide.

algor (al′gor) [L.] (*obs.*) a chill or rigor; coldness. **a. mor′tis** ["chill of death"], the gradual decrease of temperature of the body after death.

algoscopy (al-gos'ko-pe) [L. *algor* cold + Gr. *skopein* to view] (*obs.*) cryoscopy.

algosis (al-go'sis) the presence of algae or fungi in a part of the body.

algospasm (al'go-spazm) [*algo-* + *spasm*] painful spasm or cramp.

algovascular (al"go-vas'ku-lar) algiovascular.

Ali Abbas (ah'le ab'bas) (10th century A.D.) a celebrated Persian physician who wrote *Al-Maliki* (the "Royal Book"), a comprehensive treatise on medicine.

Ali ben Iza (ah'le ben i'zah) [11th century A.D.] a noted Arabic ophthalmologist, who wrote *Tadhkirat* (or *risala*) *al-kah-halin* (the "Book of Memoranda for Eye-doctors"); known also as *Jesu Haly*.

Alibert's disease, keloid (al-e-berz') [Jean Louis Marc *Alibert*, French dermatologist, 1768–1837] see *mycosis fungoides*, and under *keloid*.

alible (al'ĭ-b'l) [L. *alibilis*] nutritive; assimilable as a food.

alices (al'ĭ-sēz) [pl.] the red spots that appear before the pustules in smallpox.

alicyclic (al"ĭ-sik'lik) having the properties of both aliphatic and cyclic substances.

Alidase (al'ĭ-dās) trademark for a preparation of hyaluronidase for injection.

alienation (āl"yen-a'shun) [L. *alienatio*] 1. a feeling of disconnection or isolation from the standards and values of society. 2. former term for mental derangement.

alienia (ah"li-e'ne-ah) [*a* neg. + L. *lien* spleen] absence of the spleen.

alienism (āl'yen-izm) [L. *alienus* alien] 1. mental disorder. 2. the practice of forensic psychiatry.

alienist (āl'yen-ist) 1. former term for psychiatrist. 2. a forensic psychiatrist.

aliflurane (al"ĭ-floo'rān) chemical name: 1-chloro-1,2,2,3-tetra-fluoro-3-methoxy-cyclopropane; an inhalation anesthetic, $C_4H_3ClF_4O$.

aliform (al'ĭ-form) [L. *ala* wing + *forma* shape] shaped like a wing.

alignment (ah-līn'ment) [Fr. *aligner* to put in a straight line] the act of arranging in a line; the state of being arranged in a line. In dentistry, the bringing of natural teeth into normal articulation, or the arranging of artificial teeth in normal articulation and appearance.

aliment (al'ĕ-ment) [L. *alimentum*] food or nutritive material.

alimentary (al"ĕ-men'tar-e) pertaining to food or nutritive material, or to the organs of digestion.

alimentation (al"ĕ-men-ta'shun) the act of giving or receiving nutriment. **artificial a.,** the giving of food or nourishment to persons who cannot take it in the usual way. **forced a.,** 1. the feeding of a person against his will. 2. the giving of more food to a person than his appetite calls for. **rectal a.,** the administration of concentrated nourishment by instillation into the rectum. **total parenteral a.,** parenteral hyperalimentation.

alimentology (al"ĕ-men-tol'o-je) the science of nutrition.

alimentotherapy (al"ĕ-men"to-ther'ah-pe) [*aliment* + Gr. *therapeia* treatment] dietetic treatment; treatment by systematic feeding.

alinasal (al"e-na'sal) pertaining to the ala nasi.

alinement (ah-līn'ment) alignment.

alinjection (al"in-jek'shun) (*obs.*) repeated injection of alcohol for preserving anatomic specimens.

alipamide (ah-lip'ah-mīd) chemical name: 3-(aminosulfonyl)-4-chloro-2,2-dimethylhydrazine benzoic acid; a diuretic and antihypertensive, $C_9H_{12}ClN_3O_3S$.

aliphatic (al"ĕ-fat'ik) [Gr. *aleiphar, aleiphatos* oil] pertaining to an oil; a term applied to the "open-chain" or fatty series of hydrocarbons.

alipogenic (a-lip"o-jen'ik) not lipogenic; not forming fat.

alipoidic (a"lip-oi'dik) free from lipoids.

alipotropic (al"lip-o-trop'ik) having no influence on the metabolism of fat.

aliquot (al'ĕ-kwot) the part of a number which will divide it without a remainder; e.g., 2 is an aliquot of 6. By extension, any portion that bears a known quantitative relationship to a whole or to other portions of the same whole, as an aliquot portion of a solution; a sample of a whole taken to determine the quantitative composition of the whole.

alismin (ah-lis'min) an extractive from *Alisma plantago*, or water plantain.

alisphenoid (al-e-sfe'noid) [*ala* + *sphenoid*] 1. pertaining to the greater wing of the sphenoid. 2. a cartilage of the fetal chondrocranium on either side of the basisphenoid; later in development it forms the greater part of the greater wing of the sphenoid.

alizarin (ah-liz'ah-rin) [Arabic *ala sara* extract] a red crystalline dye, 1,2-dihydroxyanthraquinone, $C_6H_4(CO)_2C_6H_2(OH)_2$ pre-pared synthetically or obtained from madder; its compounds are used as indicators. **a. monosulfonate,** a. red; see under *red*. **a. No. 6,** purpurin (def. 2). **a. red,** see under *red*. **a. yellow, a. yellow g.,** see under *yellow*.

alizarinopurpurin (al"ĭ-zar"ĭ-no-pur'pu-rin) purpurin (def. 2).

alkalemia (al"kah-le'me-ah) [*alkali* + Gr. *haima* blood + *-ia*] increased pH or decreased hydrogen ion concentration of the blood.

alkalescence (al"kah-les'ens) slight or incipient alkalinity.

alkalescent (al"kah-les'ent) having a tendency to alkalinity.

alkali (al'kah-li) [Arabic *al-qalīy* potash] any of a class of compounds which form soluble soaps with fatty acids, turn red litmus blue, and form soluble carbonates. Essentially the hydroxides of cesium, lithium, potassium, rubidium, and sodium, they include also the carbonates of these metals and of ammonia. **caustic a.,** any solid hydroxide of a fixed alkali. **fixed a.,** any of the alkalis except ammonium. **volatile a.,** ammonia, NH_3; also ammonium hydroxide.

alkalify (al-kal'e-fi) to make alkaline.

Alkaligenes (al"kah-lij'e-nēz) *Alcaligenes*.

alkaligenous (al"kah-lij'ĕ-nus) yielding an alkali.

alkalimeter (al"kah-lim'ĕ-ter) [*alkali* + *meter*] an instrument for measuring the alkali contained in any mixture.

alkalimetry (al"kah-lim'ĕ-tre) the measurement of the alkalis present in any substance. **Engel's a.,** a method of determining the alkalinity of the blood by titrating a diluted specimen with normal tartaric acid solution until it reddens litmus paper; the amount of tartaric solution necessary to produce the result indicates the degree of alkalinity of the blood.

alkaline (al'kah-lin) [L. *alkalinus*] having the reactions of an alkali.

alkalinity (al"kah-lin'ĭ-te) the fact or quality of being alkaline.

alkalinization (al"kah-lin"ĭ-za'shun) alkalization.

alkalinize (al'kah-lin-iz") alkalize.

alkalinuria (al"kah-lin-u're-ah) [*alkaline* + *urine*] an alkaline condition of the urine.

alkalitherapy (al"kah-li-ther'ah-pe) treatment by alkalis; the administration of large amounts of alkali in the treatment of peptic ulcer and hyperchlorhydria.

alkalization (al"kah-li-za'shun) the act of making alkaline.

alkalize (al'kah-līz) to render alkaline.

alkalizer (al"kah-līz'er) an agent that neutralizes acids or causes alkalinization.

alkalogenic (al"kah-lo-jen'ik) producing alkalinity.

alkaloid (al'kah-loid") [*alkali* + Gr. *eidos* form] one of a large group of nitrogenous basic substances found in plants. They are usually very bitter and many are pharmacologically active. Examples are atropine, caffeine, coniine, morphine, nicotine, quinine, strychnine. The term is also applied to synthetic substances (*artificial a's*) which have structures similar to plant alkaloids, such as procaine. **animal a.,** 1. a ptomaine. 2. a leukomaine. **artificial a.,** an alkaloid that is made by synthetic chemical processes.

alkalometry (al"kah-lom'ĕ-tre) [*alkaloid* + Gr. *metron* measure] the dosimetric administration of alkaloids.

alkalosis (al"kah-lo'sis) a pathologic condition resulting from accumulation of base, or from loss of acid without comparable loss of base in the body fluids, and characterized by decrease in hydrogen ion concentration (increase in pH). Cf. *acidosis*. **altitude a.,** increased alkalinity in blood and tissues due to exposure to high altitudes. **compensated a.,** a condition in which compensatory mechanisms have returned the pH toward normal; see *metabolic a., conpensated*, and *respiratory a., compensated*. **hypokalemic a.,** a variety of metabolic alkalosis associated with a low serum potassium level; retention of alkali or loss of acid occurs in the extracellular (but not intracellular) fluid compartment, although the pH of the intracellular fluid may be below normal. It may be caused by hypertrophy and hypoplasia of the juxtaglomerular cells, as in Bartter's syndrome. **metabolic a.,** a disturbance in which the acid-base status of the body shifts toward the alkaline side because of retention of base or loss of noncarbonic, or fixed (nonvolatile), acids. **metabolic a., compensated,** a state of alkalosis in which the pH of the blood has been returned toward normal by respiratory compensation. **respiratory a.,** a state due to excess loss of carbon dioxide from the body. **respiratory a., compensated,** a respiratory alkalosis in which the pH of the blood has been returned toward normal through retention of acid or excretion of base by renal mechanisms.

alkalotherapy (al"kah-lo-ther'ah-pe) alkalitherapy.

alkalotic (al"kah-lot'ik) pertaining to or characterized by alkalosis.

alkaluria (al"kah-lu're-ah) the presence of an alkali in the urine.

alkamine (al'kah-min) an alcohol which contains an amine group.

alkane (al'kān) a saturated hydrocarbon of the methane series, one in which all carbon atoms are joined by single bonds; called also *paraffin.*

alkanet (al′kă-net) the reddish dye-containing root of *Alkanna tinctoria* Tausch, Boraginaceae; formerly used as an astringent, but now mainly as a colorant for candies, cosmetics, and wines. It contains alkannin (the dye principle) and tannin.

alkapton (al-kap′tōn) [*alk*ali + Gr. *haptō* to fasten or bind to] see *alkapton bodies,* under *body.*

alkaptonuria (al″kap-to-nu′re-ah) [*alkaptone* + Gr. *ouron* urine + *-ia*] excretion in the urine of alkapton bodies (most commonly homogentisic acid), which causes the urine to turn dark on standing, or on addition of alkali. It may occur without other symptoms, or it may in long-standing cases be associated with ochronosis and arthritic symptoms. **spontaneous a.,** a hereditary and congenital anomaly of the metabolism of tyrosine with excretion in the urine of homogentisic acid.

alkaptonuric (al-kap″to-nu′rik) pertaining to, characterized by, or causing alkaptonuria; by extension, sometimes used as a noun to designate an individual with alkaptonuria.

alkatriene (al″kah-tri′ēn) an unsaturated aliphatic hydrocarbon containing three double bonds.

alkavervir (al″kah-ver′vir) a yellow powdery mixture of alkaloids obtained from selective extraction of *Veratrum viride;* it is used orally as a vasodilator in the treatment of hypertension.

alkene (al′kēn) an unsaturated aliphatic hydrocarbon containing one double bond; olefin.

Alkeran (al-ker′an) trademark for a preparation of melphalan.

alkyl (al′kil) the radical which results when an aliphatic hydrocarbon loses one hydrogen atom.

alkylamine (al″kil-ah′mēn) an amine containing an alkyl radical.

alkylate (al′kĭ-lāt) to treat with an alkylating agent.

alkylation (al″kĭ-la′shun) the substitution of an alkyl group for an active hydrogen atom in an organic compound.

alkylogen (al-kil′o-jen) an alkyl ester of any of the halogen acids, e.g., ethyl chloride.

alkyne (al′kīn) an unsaturated hydrocarbon containing a triple bond between two carbon atoms; the alkynes are members of the acetylene series.

allachesthesia (al″ah-kes-the′ze-ah) [Gr. *allachē* elsewhere + *aisthēsis* perception + *-ia*] allesthesia. **optical a.,** visual allesthesia.

allantiasis (al″an-ti′ah-sis) [*allanto-* + *-iasis*] sausage poisoning; poisoning from sausages containing the toxins of *Clostridium botulinum.* See *botulism.*

allanto- (ah-lan′to) [Gr. *allas, allantos* sausage] a combining form denoting relationship to a sausage or to the allantois.

allantochorion (ah-lan″to-ko′re-on) a compound membrane formed by fusion of the allantois and chorion.

allantogenesis (al″an-to-jen′ĕ-sis) the formation and development of the allantois.

allantoic (al″an-to′ik) pertaining to the allantois.

allantoicase (al″an-to′i-kās) an enzyme that converts the allantoic acid formed by allantoinase from allantoin, producing glyoxylic acid and urea.

allantoid (ah-lan′toid) [*allanto-* + Gr. *eidos* form] 1. resembling the allantois. 2. sausage shaped.

allantoidean (al″an-toi′de-an) 1. pertaining to the allantois. 2. any animal with an allantois during its embryonic development; in the plural, *amniotes* is the more usual term.

allantoidoangiopagous (al″an-toi″do-an″je-op′ah-gus) [*allanto-* + Gr. *angeion* vessel + *pagos* thing fixed] joined by the vessels of the umbilical cord; see under *twin.*

allantoidoangiopagus (al″an-toi″do-an″je-op′ah-gus) twin fetuses joined by the vessels of the umbilical cord; allantoidoangiopagous twins. Called also *omphaloangiopagus.*

allantoin (ah-lan′to-in) chemical name: 5-ureidohydantoin. A white crystallizable substance, $C_4H_6N_4O_3$, the diureide of glyoxylic acid, found in allantoic fluid, fetal urine, and many plants, and as a urinary excretion product of purine metabolism in most mammals but not in man or the higher apes. It is produced synthetically by the oxidation of uric acid, and was once used to encourage epithelial formation in wounds and ulcers and in osteomyelitis. It is the active substance in maggot treatment, being secreted by the maggots as a product of purine metabolism.

allantoinase (al″an-to′ĭ-nās) an enzyme that catalyzes the conversion of allantoin into allantoic acid.

allantoinuria (ah-lan″to-in-u′re-ah) the presence of allantoin in the urine.

allantois (ah-lan′to-is) [Gr. *allantos* sausage + *eidos* form] an initially tubular ventral diverticulum of the hindgut of embryos of reptiles, birds, and mammals. In reptiles and birds, it expands to a large sac for storing urine and, after fusing with the chorion which lines the shell, provides for gas exchange. The allantois is prominent in some mammals (carnivores, ungulates); in others, including man, it is vestigial except that its blood vessels give rise to those of the umbilical cord. See illustration under *amnion.*

allantotoxicon (ah-lan″to-tok′se-kon) [*allanto-* + Gr. *toxikon* poison] a hypothetical poison formerly supposed to cause allantiasis.

allassotherapy (ah-las″o-ther′ah-pe) [Gr. *allassein* to alter + *therapy.*] treatment based on producing a change in the general biologic conditions of the organism.

allaxis (ah-lak′sis) [Gr. "exchange"] transformation.

allel (ah-lēl′) allele.

allele (ah-lēl′) [Gr. *allēlōn* of one another] 1. one of two or more alternative forms of a gene occupying corresponding sites (loci) on homologous chromosomes, any two of which may be carried by a given individual and which determine alternative characters in inheritance. The existence of more than two alleles at a single locus is known as multiple allelism. See also *Mendel's law,* under *law.* 2. one of two or more contrasting characters transmitted by alternative genes. **multiple a's,** alleles of which there are more than two alternative forms possible at any one locus. **silent a.,** one which has no detectable expression.

allelic (ah-le′lik) pertaining to alleles; produced by alternative genes.

allelism (al′e-lizm) the existence of alleles, or their relationship to one another.

allelo- (ah-le′lo) [Gr. *allēlōn* of one another] a combining form denoting relationship to another.

allelocatalysis (ah-le″lo-kah-tal′ĭ-sis) [*allelo-* + *catalysis*] the once held theory of mutual stimulation of cells to growth, or stimulation of growth in a bacterial culture by the addition to it of other cells of the same type.

allelocatalytic (ah-le″lo-kat-ah-lit′ik) catalyzing each other; causing or marked by allelocatalysis.

allelochemics (al-le″lo-kem′iks) chemical interactions between species, involving release of active chemical substances, such as scents, pheromones, and toxins.

allelomorph (ah-le′lo-morf) [*allelo-* + Gr. *morphē* form] allele.

allelomorphic (ah-le″lo-mor′fik) allelic.

allelomorphism (ah-le″lo-mor′fizm) allelism.

allelotaxis (ah-le″lo-tak′sis) [*allelo-* + Gr. *taxis* arrangement] the development of an organ from several embryonic structures.

allelotaxy (ah-le′lo-tak″se) allelotaxis.

Allen's fossa [Harrison *Allen,* Philadelphia anatomist, 1841–1897] see under *fossa.*

Allen's paradoxic law, treatment [Frederick Madison *Allen,* American physician, 1879–1964] see under *law* and *treatment.*

Allen's test (al′lenz) 1. [Alfred Henry *Allen,* American chemist, 1846–1904] see under *tests* (1) and (2). 2. [Charles Warren *Allen,* American physician, 1854– 1906], see under *tests* (4); 3. [Edgar V. *Allen,* American physician, born 1900] see under *tests* (5).

Allen-Doisy test, unit (al′en doi′se) [Edgar V. *Allen,* American anatomist, 1892–1943; Edward Adelbert *Doisy,* American biochemist, born 1893] see under *test,* and see *mouse unit* and *rat unit,* under *unit.*

allenthesis (ah-len′thĕ-sis) (*obs.*) introduction into the body of a foreign substance.

allergen (al′er-jen) [*allergy* + Gr. *gennan* to produce] 1. a substance capable of inducing allergy or specific hypersensitivity; such a substance may be a protein or a nonprotein. 2. any of the extracts of certain foods, bacteria, or pollen, for example, the proteins of milk, egg, or wheat; they are used in the treatment of or testing for hypersensitivity to specific substances. **pollen a.,** see *pollen antigen,* under *antigen.*

allergenic (al″er-jen′ik) acting as an allergen; inducing allergy.

allergic (ah-ler′jik) pertaining to, caused by, affected with, or of the nature of allergy.

allergid (al′er-jid) a papular or nodular allergic skin reaction.

allergie (al′er-je) variant of allergy.

allergin (al′er-jin) 1. the antibody responsible for anaphylaxis. 2. allergen.

allergist (al′er-jist) a physician who specializes in the diagnosis and treatment of allergic conditions.

allergization (al″er-jĭ-za′shun) active sensitization or the introduction of allergens into the body.

allergize (al′er-jīz) to subject to sensitization; to make allergic.

allergological (al″er-go-loj′ĭ-kal) pertaining to allergology.

allergologist (al″er-gol′o-jist) one who specializes in allergology.

allergology (al″er-gol′o-je) the branch of medicine devoted to the study of allergy, its etiology, diagnosis, and treatment.

allergosis (al″er-go′sis), pl. *allergo′ses.* Any allergic disease.

allergy (al′er-je) [Gr. *allos* other + *ergon* work] a hypersensitive state acquired through exposure to a particular allergen, reexposure bringing to light an altered capacity to react. Originally, the term denoted any altered reactivity, whether decreased or increased, but is now usually used to denote a hypersensitive state. Allergies may be classified as immediate and delayed, and include atopy, serum sickness, allergic drug reactions, contact dermatitis, and anaphylactic shock. The allergies are principally manifested in the gastrointestinal tract, the skin, and the respiratory tract. Cf. *anaphylaxis* and *hypersensitivity*. **atopic a.,** atopy. **bacterial a.,** specific hypersensitiveness to a particular bacterial antigen, e.g., *Mycobacterium tuberculosis;* it is dependent on previous infection with the specific organism and shows no circulating antibodies. **bronchial a.,** see *asthma.* **cold a.,** a condition manifested by local and systemic reactions, mediated by histamine, which is released from mast cells and basophils as a result of exposure to cold. **contact a.,** hypersensitiveness marked by an eczematous reaction to contact between the epidermis and the allergen. **delayed a.,** see under *hypersensitivity.* **drug a.,** an allergic reaction occurring as the result of unusual sensitivity to a drug. **endocrine a.,** allergy to an endogenous hormone. **food a., gastrointestinal a.,** allergy in which the ingested antigens include food as well as drugs; strawberries, milk, and eggs are the most common offenders. The organ affected is usually the skin. **hereditary a.,** atopy. **immediate a.,** see under *hypersensitivity.* **induced a.,** allergy resulting from the injection of an antigen, contact with an antigen, or infection with a microorganism, as contrasted with hereditary allergy; called also *normal a.* and *physiologic a.* **latent a.,** allergy which is not manifested by symptoms but which may be detected by tests. **nonatopic a.,** one of two general groups of clinical allergies, which includes contact dermatitis and some food and drug allergies. Cf. *atopy.* **normal a.,** induced a. **pathologic a.,** hereditary a. **physical a.,** a condition in which the patient is sensitive to the effects of physical agents, such as heat, cold, light, etc. **physiologic a.,** induced a. **pollen a.,** hay fever. **polyvalent a.,** see *pathergy,* def. 2. **spontaneous a.,** atopy.

Allescheria (al″es-ke′re-ah) a genus of ascomycetous fungi of the family Eurotiaceae, order Eurotiales, representing the perfect (sexual) stage of *Monosporium.* **A. boy′dii,** a species of fungi, commonly isolated from maduromycosis and other human infection; its imperfect (asexual) stage is *Monosporium apiospermum.*

allesthesia (al″es-the′ze-ah) [Gr. *allos* other + *aisthēsis* perception + *-ia*] a condition in which a sensation, as of pain or touch, is experienced at a point remote from that at which the stimulus is applied or occurs, as in allochiria. **visual a.,** a condition in which visual images are transposed from one half of the visual field to the other, either vertically or horizontally; called also *optical allachesthesia.*

allethrin (al′ĕ-thrin) a viscous fluid, $C_{19}H_{26}O_3$, insoluble in water, used as an insecticide.

alliaceous (al″e-a′shus) pertaining to or resembling the smell of garlic; pertaining to the genus *Allium.*

alligation (al″ĭ-ga′shun) the process of finding the cost of a mixture of known quantities of ingredients, each of known value, or of determining the quantities of solutions of various strengths to be used to form a mixture of a particular strength.

alligator boy (al′ĭ-ga″tor boi) a child with severe ichthyosis.

Allingham's operation [Herbert William *Allingham,* English surgeon, 1862–1904] see under *operation,* def. 1.

Allingham's operation, ulcer [William *Allingham,* English surgeon, 1829–1908] see under *operation,* def. 2, and under *ulcer.*

Allis's inhaler, sign (al′is-iz) [Oscar Huntington *Allis,* Philadelphia surgeon, 1833–1921] see under *inhaler* and *sign.*

alliteration (ah-lit″er-a′shun) [L. *ad* to + *litera* letter] a dysphrasia in which the patient uses words containing the same consonant sounds.

allithiamine (al″ĭ-thi′ah min) any of several analogues of thiamine that are easily absorbed from the intestinal tract.

Allium (al′e-um) [L. "garlic"] a genus of liliaceous plants, including the garlic and onion. Garlic contains a sulfur ester derivative known as allicin, which has antimicrobial activity. It is a common home remedy among various European ethnic groups as an antitussive, antiseptic, rubefacient, diaphoretic, toothache and earache remedy, vermifuge, and as an aid in nervous conditions.

allo- (al′o) [Gr. *allos* other] a combining form denoting a condition differing from the normal, or reversal, or referring to another.

alloantibody (al″o-an′-tĭ-bod″e) isoantibody.

alloantigen (al″o-an′tĭ-jen) isoantigen.

alloantiserum (al″o-an″tĭ-se′rum) antiserum against antigens of another strain of animal of the same species.

allobar (al′o-bar) [*allo-* + Gr. *baros* weight] a form of a chemical element having an atomic weight different from that of the naturally occurring form.

allobarbital (al″o-bar′bĭ-tal) chemical name: 5,5-di-2-propenyl-2,4,6(1*H*,3*H*,5*H*)pyrimidinetrione. An intermediate to long-acting barbiturate, $C_{10}H_{12}N_2O_3$, occurring as a white, crystalline powder; used orally as a sedative and hypnotic, and orally in combination with acetaminophen or with acetaminophen and codeine as an analgesic. Formerly called *diallylbarbituric acid.*

allobiosis (al″o-bi-o′sis) [*allo-* + Gr. *bios* life] the condition of altered reactivity which an organism manifests under changed environmental or physiologic conditions.

allocentric (al″o-sen′trik) having all of one's ideas centered on others. Cf. *egocentric.*

allocheiria (al″o-ki′re-ah) allochiria.

allochesthesia (al″o-kes-the′ze-ah) allesthesia.

allochezia (al″o-ke′ze-ah) [*allo-* + Gr. *chezein* to defecate] (obs.) 1. the discharge of nonfecal matter by the anus. 2. the discharge of feces by an abnormal passage.

allochiral (al″o-ki′ral) [*allo-* + Gr. *cheir* hand] pertaining to allochiria.

allochiria (al″o-ki′re-ah) [*allo-* + Gr. *cheir* hand + *-ia*] a condition in which, if one extremity is stimulated, the sensation is referred to the opposite side (Obersteiner).

allochroic (al″o-kro′ik) changeable in color, a term generally applied to minerals.

allochroism (al″o-kro′izm) [*allo-* + Gr. *chroa* color + *-ism*] change or variation in color, as in certain minerals.

allochromacy (al″o-kro′mah-se) the formation of other coloring agents from a dye that is unstable in solution.

allochromasia (al″o-kro-ma′ze-ah) change in color of the hair or skin.

allocinesia (al″o-si-ne′ze-ah) [*allo-* + Gr. *kinēsis* motion + *-ia*] a condition in which the patient performs a movement on the side of the body opposite to that directed.

allocolloid (al″o-kol′oid) [*allo-* + *colloid*] a colloid in which a single element in its allotropic forms makes up the colloid system.

allocortex (al″o-kor′teks) [*allo-* + L. *cortex* bark or outer layer] archipallium.

allocrine (al′o-krin) [*allo-* + Gr. *krinein* to separate] heterocrine.

allocytophilic (al″o-si″to-fil′ik) [*allo-* + Gr. *kytos* hollow vessel + *philein* to love] having an affinity for cells derived from the same species.

Allodermanyssus (al″o-der″mah-nis′sus) a genus of bloodsucking mites. **A. sanguin′eus,** a species that parasitizes mice and is a vector of *Rickettsia akari,* the causative agent of rickettsialpox.

allodesmism (al″o-des′mizm) [*allo-* + Gr. *desmos* bond] allomerism based on a difference in the bonds uniting the atoms.

allodiploid (al″o-dip′loid) [*allo-* + *diploid*] 1. having two sets of chromosomes derived from different parental species, as in hybrids. 2. an individual or cell having two such sets of chromosomes.

allodiploidy (al″o-dip′loi-de) the state of having two sets of chromosomes derived from different parental species, as in hybrids; see also *alloploidy* and *allopolyploidy.*

allodynia (al″o-din′e-ah) [*allo-* + Gr. *odynē* pain] pain resulting from a non-noxious stimulus to normal skin.

alloeosis (al″e-o′sis) (obs.) change in the character of a disease.

alloeroticism (al″o-e-rot′ĭ-izm) sexuality directed to another, in contrast to autoeroticism.

alloerotism (al″o-er′o-tizm) [*allo-* + *erotism*] alloeroticism.

alloesthesia (al″o-es-the′ze-ah) allesthesia.

allogamy (al-log′ah-me) [*allo-* + Gr. *gamos* marriage] cross fertilization.

allogeneic (al″o-jĕ-ne′ik) 1. having cell types that are antigenically distinct. 2. in transplantation biology, denoting individuals (or tissues) that are of the same species but antigenically distinct. Called also *homologous.* NOTE: In contrast, *syngeneic* (or *isogeneic*) refers to individuals having identical genotypes, and *xenogeneic* to individuals of different species, which by definition have different genotypes.

allogenic (al″o-jen′ik) allogeneic.

allogotrophia (al″o-go-tro′fe-ah) nourishment of one part of the body at the expense of another part.

allograft (al′o-graft) a graft of tissue between individuals of the same species but of disparate genotype; called also *allogeneic graft* and *homograft.*

alloimmune (al″o-im-mūn′) specifically immune to an allogeneic antigen.

alloimmunization (al″o-im″u-ni-za′shun) isoimmunization; the development of an immune response to alloantigens (isoantigens), as during pregnancy or in blood transfusions or organ transplantations.

alloisomerism (al″o-i-som′er-izm) isomerism which does not appear in the formula.

allokeratoplasty (al″o-ker′ah-to-plas″te) [*allo-* + *keratoplasty*] repair of the cornea by the use of foreign material.

allokinesis (al″o-ki-ne′sis) movement that is not performed voluntarily but is produced passively or occurs reflexly.

allokinetic (al″o-ki-net′ik) [*allo-* + Gr. *kinēsis* movement] pertaining to or characterized by allokinesis.

allolactose (al″o-lak′tōs) a disaccharide, isomeric with lactose, occurring in milk.

allolalia (al″o-la′le-ah) [*allo-* + Gr. *lalein* to speak + *-ia*] any defect of speech of central origin.

allomerism (ah-lom′er-izm) [*allo-* + Gr. *meros* part] change of chemical constitution without change in the crystalline form. Cf. *allomorphism.*

allometric (al′o-met′rik) [*allo-* + Gr. *metron* measure] denoting the disproportionate growth of organs or parts of an organism; pertaining to allometry.

allometron (al″o-met′ron) [*allo-* + Gr. *metron* measure] an evolutionary change in bodily form or proportion as expressed in measurements and indices.

allometry (al-lom′ĕ-tre) the measurement of changing shape of an organism with increase in size, i.e., the determination of the relationship of two varying dimensions, usually linear.

allomorphism (al″o-mor′fizm) [*allo-* + Gr. *morphē* form] change of crystalline form without change in chemical constitution. Cf. *allomerism.*

allongement (al-onzh-mon′) [Fr.] elongation; especially any procedure for elongating a uterine tumor after it has been severed from its connections, so as to admit of its extraction. Usually done by making a spiral incision into its substance while it is being pulled down.

allonomous (al-lon′o-mus) [*allo-* + Gr. *nomos* law] regulated by stimuli from the outside.

allopath (al′o-path) a term sometimes applied to a practitioner of allopathy.

allopathic (al′o-path′ik) pertaining to or characteristic of allopathy.

allopathist (al-lop′ah-thist) allopath.

allopathy (al-lop′ah-the) [*allo-* + Gr. *pathos* disease] a term applied to that system of therapeutics in which diseases are treated by producing a condition incompatible with or antagonistic to the condition to be cured or alleviated. Called also *heteropathy.* Cf. *homeopathy.*

allophanamide (al-o-fan-am′id) biuret.

allophanate (al′o-fan′āt) a salt of allophanic acid.

allophasis (al-lof′ah-sis) [*allo-* + Gr. *phasis* speech] incoherent speech; delirium.

allophenic (al″o-fe′nik) [*allo-* + Gr. *phainein* to show] of or relating to single individuals originating from more than one conceptus; having orderly coexistence of cells with different phenotypes ascribable to known allelic genotypic differences; mosaic.

allophore (al′o-fōr) erythrophore.

allophthalmia (al″of-thal′me-ah) heterophthalmia.

alloplasia (al″o-pla′ze-ah) [*allo-* + Gr. *plasis* formation + *-ia*] heteroplasia.

alloplasmatic (al″o-plaz-mat′ik) [*allo-* + Gr. *plassein* to form] formed by differentiation from the cytoplasm.

alloplast (al′o-plast) an inert foreign body used for implantation into tissue.

alloplastic (al″o-plas′tik) [*allo-* + Gr. *plassein* to form] pertaining to or characterized by alloplasty; pertaining to an alloplast.

alloplasty (al′o-plas-te) [*allo-* + Gr. *plassein* to form] the developmental direction of the libido away from self to other people or objects, resulting in the direct and unmodified expression of impulses, as seen in certain antisocial individuals. Cf. *autoplasty.*

alloploid (al′o-ploid) [*allo-* + *-ploid*] 1. having any number (two or many) of chromosome sets derived from different ancestral species. 2. an individual or cell having any number (two or many) of chromosome sets derived from different ancestral species.

alloploidy (al″o-ploi′de) the state of having any number (two or many) of chromosome sets derived from different ancestral species; see also *allodiploidy* and *allopolyploidy.*

allopolyploid (al″lo-pol′e-ploid″) [*allo-* + *polyploid*] 1. having more than two chromosome sets derived from different ancestral species. 2. an individual or cell having more than two chromosome sets derived from different ancestral species.

allopolyploidy (al″lo-pol′e-ploi-de) the state of having more than two chromosome sets derived from different ancestral species; see also *allodiploidy* and *alloploidy.*

allopregnandiol (al″o-preg-nan′de-ol) an isomer of pregnandiol occurring in female urine.

allopregnane (al″o-preg′nān) see *pregnane.*

allopregnenolone (al″o-preg-nen′o-lōn) a chemical compound which can be transformed into progesterone, testosterone, or other steroid hormones.

allopsychic (al″o-si′kik) [*allo-* + Gr. *psychē* soul] pertaining to mind in its relation to the external world.

allopsychosis (al″o-si-ko′sis) a psychosis marked by disorganization of the perceptive powers for the outer world (hallucinations and illusions), but without disorder of motor powers such as speech and action (Wernicke).

allopurinol (al″o-pu′rin-ol) [USP] chemical name: 1*H*-[3,4-*d*]-pyrimidin-4-ol. An isomer of hypoxanthine, $C_5H_4N_4O$, capable of inhibiting xanthine oxidase and thus of reducing serum and urinary levels of uric acid; it occurs as a fluffy white to off-white powder and is used orally in the treatment of gout.

allorhythmia (al″o-rith′me-ah) [*allo-* + Gr. *rhythmos* rhythm + *-ia*] irregularity in the rhythm of the heart beat or pulse that recurs in a regular fashion.

allorhythmic (al″o-rith′mik) affected with or of the nature of allorhythmia.

all or none the fact, discovered by Bowditch (1871), that the heart muscle, under whatever stimulus, will contract to the fullest extent or not at all. In the heart, stimulation of any single atrial or ventricular muscle fiber causes the action potential to travel over the entire atrial or ventricular mass, or not to travel at all. In other muscles and in nerves, this principle is limited to individual fibers; i.e., stimulation of a fiber causes an action potential to travel over the entire fiber, or not to travel at all. Called also *all-or-none law.*

allorphine (al′lor-fēn) nalorphine.

allose (al′ōs) a sugar, $C_6H_{12}O_6$, isomeric with glucose.

allosensitization (al″o-sen″sĭ-ti-za′shun) sensitization to alloantigens (isoantigens), as to Rh antigens during pregnancy (see *Rh isoimmunization*). Called also *isosensitization.*

allosome (al′o-sōm) [*allo-* + Gr. *sōma* body] 1. (*obs.*) a sex chromosome; see under *chromosome.* 2. a foreign constituent of the cytoplasm of a cell which has entered from the outside. **paired a.,** a diplosome. **unpaired a.,** a monosome, def. 1.

allosteric (al″o-ster′ik) [*allo-* + Gr. *stereos* solid] denoting a macromolecule (an enzyme) whose reactivity with another molecule is altered by combination with a third molecule that is not a substrate; also, denoting the enzyme inhibition exercised by such alteration. See also under *effector* and *site.*

allotetraploid (al″o-tet′rah-ploid) an individual having two sets of chromosomes derived from different ancestral species.

allotherm (al′o-therm″) [*allo-* + Gr. *thermē* heat] 1. poikilotherm. 2. heterotherm.

allotope (al′o-tōp) a site on the constant or nonvarying portion of an antibody molecule that can be recognized by a combining site of other antibodies. Cf. *idiotype.*

allotopia (al″o-to′pe-ah) dystopia.

allotopic (al″o-top′ik) dystopic.

allotoxin (al″o-tok′sin) [*allo-* + *toxin*] any substance formed by tissue change within the body which serves as a defense against toxins by neutralizing their poisonous properties.

allotransplantation (al″o-trans″plan-ta′shun) [*allo-* + *transplantation*] transplantation of tissue from one individual into the body of another member of the same species but of a different genotype from the donor.

allotrio- (ah-lot′re-o) [Gr. *allotrios* strange] a combining form meaning strange or foreign.

allotriodontia (ah-lot″re-o-don′she-ah) [*allotrio-* + Gr. *odous* tooth + *-ia*] 1. the transplantation of teeth. 2. the existence of teeth in abnormal places, as in tumors.

allotriogeustia (ah-lot″re-o-gu′ste-ah) [*allotrio-* + Gr. *geusis* taste + *-ia*] a perverted condition of the sense of taste.

allotriolith (al″o-tri′o-lith) [*allotrio-* + Gr. *lithos* stone] a calculus in an abnormal situation, or one composed of unusual materials.

allotriophagia (ah-lot″re-o-fa′je-ah) allotriophagy.

allotriophagy (ah-lot″re-of′ah-je) [*allotrio-* + Gr. *phagein* to eat] former term for pica.

allotriosmia (al″o-tri-os′me-ah) heterosmia.

allotriuria (ah-lot″re-u′re-ah) [*allotrio-* + Gr. *ouron* urine + *-ia*] a strange or perverted condition of the urine.

allotrope (al′o-trōp) an allotropic form.

allotrophic (al″o-trof′ik) rendered non-nutritious by the process of digestion.

allotropic (al″o-trop′ik) 1. exhibiting allotropism. 2. concerned with others; said of a type of personality which is inclined to be preoccupied by others rather than oneself; not self-centered.

allotropism (ah-lot′ro-pizm) [*allo-* + Gr. *tropos* a turning] 1. the existence of a substance in two or more distinct forms (allotropic forms) with distinct physical properties, e.g., graphite and diamond, allotropic forms of carbon. 2. a tropism between different structures, e.g., between spermatozoa and ova (Roux).

allotropy (ah-lot′ro-pe) allotropism.

allotrylic (al″o-tril′ik) [*allotrio-* + Gr. *hylē* matter] produced by the presence of a foreign body or principle.

allotype (al′o-tīp) any of the alternative characters controlled by allelic genes; see also *allotypy.* **Inv a.,** Km antigen. **Km a.,** an allotypic antigenic marker on the kappa chain of human immunoglobulins. **Oz a.,** an allotypic antigenic marker on the lambda chain of human immunoglobulins, equivalent to the Km allotypes on kappa light chains.

allotypic (al″o-tip′ik) characterized by allotypes.

allotypy (al″o-ti′pe) [*allo-* + Gr. *typos* type] the genetically controlled property, in proteins, of existing in antigenically distinguishable forms in different members of the same species, i.e., as serum protein isoantigens (not yet distinguishable by chemical or physiochemical means); the condition of being an allotype.

alloxan (al′ok-san) a reddish, crystalline substance, mesoxalyl urea, CO·NH·CO:NH·CO, an oxidized product of uric acid. It

   └──CO──┘

tends to destroy the islet cells of the pancreas, thus producing diabetes. It has been obtained from the mucus of the intestine in diarrhea and has been used in nutrition experiments and as an antineoplastic agent.

alloxantin (al″ok-san′tin) a crystalline derivative of alloxan and dialuric acid, [CO(NH·CO)₂C(OH)—]₂, obtained by reduction.

alloxazine (ah-lok′sah-zēn) a heterocyclic compound, $C_{10}H_6N_4O_2$, an isomer of isoalloxazine, which is the basic structure of riboflavin.

alloxuremia (al″ok-su-re′me-ah) [*alloxur* + Gr. *haima* blood + *-ia*] the presence of purine bases in the blood, causing a form of intoxication.

alloxuria (al″ok-su′re-ah) [*alloxur* + Gr. *ouron* urine + *-ia*] the presence of purine bases in the urine.

alloxuric (al″ok-su′rik) pertaining to or characterized by alloxuria.

alloy (al′loi) [Fr. *aloyer* to mix metals] a solid mixture of two or more metals or metalloids that are mutually soluble in the molten condition; distinguished as binary, ternary, quaternary, etc., depending on the number of metals in the mixture. An alloy may also be classified on the basis of its behavior when solidified. **amalgam a.,** a metal in the form of filings or spheres which is to be blended with mercury to form an amalgam. **Newton's a.,** Melotte's metal.

alloyage (ah-loi′ij) the combining of metals into alloys.

allspice (awl′spīs) pimenta.

all-*trans* retinal see *retinal* (def. 2).

allyl (al′il) [L. *allium* garlic + Gr. *hylē* matter] a univalent organic group, CH₂:CH·CH₂. **a. aldehyde,** acrolein. **a. isothiocyanate,** chemical name: 3-isothiocyanato-1-propene. Volatile oil of mustard, C_3H_5NCS, used as a counterirritant in ointments and plasters and in the preparation of flavors; it is also used in the manufacture of war gas. **a. sulfide,** a synthetically prepared compound, $(C_3H_5)S$, formerly used in cholera and subcutaneously in tuberculosis; called also *diallyl sulfide* and *thiollylic ether*. **a. sulfocarbamide, a. thiocarbamide, a. thiourea,** thiosinamine. **a. tribromide,** a colorless or yellowish liquid, $C_3H_5Br_3$, formerly used as an antispasmodic and anodyne.

allylamine (al″il-am′in) a caustic liquid with an ammoniacal odor, 3-aminopropylene, CH₂:CH·CH₂·NH₂, used in the manufacture of mercurial diuretics.

allylguaiacol (al″lil-gwi′ah-kol) eugenol.

allylnormorphine hydrochloride (al″il-nor-mor′fēn) nalorphine hydrochloride.

almadrate sulfate (al′mah-drāt) aluminum magnesium hydroxide oxide sulfate hydrate; an antacid, $Al_4H_6Mg_2O_{14}S·xH_2O$.

Almeida's disease (al-ma-ēd′ahz) [Floriano Paulo de *Almeida*, Brazilian physician born 1898] paracoccidioidomycosis.

Almén's reagent, test (al-mānz′) [August Teodor *Almén*, Swedish physiologist, 1833–1903] see under *reagent* and *tests*.

almond (ah′mund) [Fr. *amande*, from L. *amygdala* almond] the fruit of *Prunus amygdalus* Batsch. (*P. communis* L.), almond tree, seeds of the sweet variety (var. *dulcis*) being edible. **bitter a.,** the fruit of *P. amygdalus* var. *amara*, whose seeds are inedible but which contains a volatile oil and amygdalin. On maceration and distillation, the seeds yield bitter almond oil, which contains about 80 per cent benzaldehyde and 2–4 per cent hydrocyanic acid. Used in low doses in various cough mixtures, in liqueurs, and in perfumery. **sweet a.,** the fruit of *P. amygdalus* var. *dulcis*.

almoner (al′mo-ner) a person who dispenses alms. **hospital a.,** *Brit.*, a person trained in dispensing the social service funds of a hospital, and in administering social service work.

Al₂O₃ aluminum oxide.

alochia (ah-lo′ke-ah) [L.; *a* neg. + Gr. *lochia* lochia] absence of the lochia.

Aloe (al′o) [L. *alöe*; Gr. *aloē*] a large genus of succulent South African plants of the Liliaceae family. The dried juice of several species (e.g., *A. barbadensis, A. ferox, A. perryi*) contains purgative principles. Aloe may also refer to the fragrant wood of *Aquilaria agallocha* (East Indian tree) of the family Thymelaeaceae.

aloe (al′o) [USP] the dried juice of the leaves of various species of liliaceous plants of the genus *Aloe*, which has purgative properties; it is now used only as an ingredient of *compound benzoin tincture*.

aloe-emodin (al′o-em′o-din) chemical name: 1,8-dihydroxy-3-(hydroxymethyl)-9,10-antracenedione. A compound having cathartic principles, occurring in the free state and as a glycoside in rhubarb, senna leaves, and in various species of *Aloe*.

aloetic (al″o-et′ik) [L. *aloeticus*] pertaining to or containing aloe.

alogia (ah-lo′je-ah) [*a* neg. + Gr. *logos* word + *-ia*] inability to speak, due to a central lesion.

Al(OH)₃ aluminum hydroxide.

aloin (al′o-in) chemical name: 10-glucopyranosyl-1,8-dihydroxy-3-(hydroxymethyl)-9(10H)-anthracenone. A mixture of active principles, chiefly barbaloin, $C_{21}H_{22}O_9$, extracted from aloes; used as a purgative to relieve temporary constipation and/or atonic chronic constipation.

alonimid (ah-lon′ĭ-mid) chemical name: 2,3-dihydrospiro[naphthalene-1(4H),3′-piperidine]-2′,4,6′-trione; a sedative and hypnotic, $C_{14}H_{13}NO_3$.

alopecia (al″o-pe′she-ah) [Gr. *alōpekia* a disease in which the hair falls out] baldness; absence of the hair from skin areas where it normally is present. **a. adna′ta,** congenital a. **a. area′ta,** a microscopically inflammatory, usually reversible, patchy loss of hair, occurring in sharply defined areas and usually involving the beard or scalp; called also *a. circumscripta* and *area celsi*. **a. cap′itis tota′lis,** complete loss of hair from the scalp. **a. cel′si,** a. areata. **cicatricial a., a. cicatrisa′ta,** an irreversible loss of hair associated with scarring, usually occurring on the scalp; called also *alopecia orbicularis*. **a. circumscrip′ta,** a. areata. **congenital a., a. congenita′lis,** congenital absence of hair, usually from the scalp. **drug a.,** a medicamentosa. **a. generalisa′ta,** 1. a. universalis. 2. a. totalis. **a. limina′ris,** loss of hair along the front and back margins of the scalp, occurring as the result of trauma or pressure; see *ophiasis*. Called also *a. marginalis* or *marginal a*. **male pattern a.,** a progressive, diffuse, symmetrical loss of scalp hair, beginning with characteristic frontal recession and leaving ultimately only a sparse peripheral rim of scalp hair (the hippocratic wreath); the condition is androgen-dependent and is caused by an autosomal dominant gene of variable expressivity. Called also *common male baldness* and *hereditary a*. **marginal a., a. margina′lis,** a. liminaris. **marginal traumatic a.,** baldness occurring above and anterior to the ears. **a. medicamento′sa,** loss of hair caused by the ingestion of a drug, such as heparin, thallium, or one of the radiomimetic drugs; called also *drug a*. **a. mucino′sa,** a patchy loss of hair associated with follicular mucinosis. **a. orbicula′ris,** a. cicatrisata. **physiologic a.,** the normal shedding of hair at the end of telogen. **a. pityroi′des,** loss of scalp hair associated with, and presumably at least partially due to, dandruff or seborrheic dermatitis of the scalp. **postpartum a.,** a common, diffuse, temporary loss of resting scalp hair (telogen effluvium), beginning soon after parturition. **a. prematu′ra, a. preseni′lis,** early, rapidly progressive male pattern alopecia. **pressure a.,** loss of hair from a body area subjected to prolonged pressure. **radiation a.,** loss of hair after exposure to ionizing radiation, the extent and permanence of which are dependent on the skin field, quality of radiation beam, time-dose relationship, and probably other factors. **roentgen a.,** x-ray a. **a. seborrhe′ica,** loss of scalp hair associated with chronic disorder of the scalp, marked by itching, hyperemia, and dandruff. **senile a., a. seni′lis,** loss of hair accompanying old age. **symptomatic a., a. symptomat′ica,** loss of hair occurring after fever or childbirth, as a result of systemic or psychogenic causes, or after some other stress of which the effluvium is symptomatic. **syphilitic a., a. syphilit′ica,** loss of hair resulting from either secondary or tertiary syphilis. **a. tota′lis,** complete loss of hair from the entire scalp, resulting from progression of alopecia areata. **traction a.,** baldness as a consequence of continuous or prolonged traction on the roots of the hair, as applied in certain styles of dressing the hair or in the habit of twisting the hair. **traumatic a., a. traumat′ica,** loss of hair occurring as the result of injury, as in alopecia liminaris or traction alopecia. **a. universa′lis,** loss of hair over the entire body, resulting from progression of alopecia areata. **x-ray a.,** loss of hair after exposure to roentgen radiation, the extent and permanence of which are dependent on the field and dosage; called also *roentgen a*.

alopecic (al″o-pe′sik) pertaining to or characterized by alopecia.

alopécie (al-ŏ-pa-se′) [Fr.] alopecia. **a. du chignon,** baldness developing at the site on which the chignon, or bun of hair, rests on the scalp. **a. marginale traumatique,** marginal traumatic alopecia.

aloxanthin (al″ok-san′thin) a yellow principle, $C_{15}H_{10}O_6$, derivable from aloes by the action of potassium dichromate.

aloxiprin (al-ok′sĭ-prin) chemical name: 2-(acetyloxy)benzoic acid polymer with aluminum hydroxide. A polymeric condensation product of aluminum hydroxide and aspirin, $Al_3O_2[C_6H_4(OOCCH_3)COO]_5$, used as an analgesic.

alpenstich (ahl′pen-stikh″) [Ger. "alpine stab"] epidemic pneumonia in Alpine valleys.

alpertine (al-per′tēn) chemical name: 5,6-dimethoxy-3-[2-4(4-phenyl-1-piperazinyl)ethyl]-1H-indole-2-carboxylic acid ethyl ester; a tranquilizer, $C_{25}H_{31}N_3O_4$.

alpha (al′fah) the first letter of the Greek alphabet, α or *a*; used as a part of a chemical name to denote the first of a series of isomeric compounds, or the carbon atom next to the carboxyl group. The succeeding letters of the Greek alphabet, beta (β), gamma (γ), delta (δ), etc., are used to name, in order, succeeding compounds or carbon atoms.

alpha-amylose (al″fah-am′ĭ-lōs) the linear component of starch, usually amylose.

alpha₁-antitrypsin (al″fa-an″te-trip′sin) a plasma protein (an α_1-globulin, molecular weight 45000) produced in the liver, which inhibits the activity of trypsin and other proteolytic enzymes. Deficiency of this protein is associated with development of emphysema. Also written α_1-antitrysin.

Alpha Chymar (al′fah ki′mar) trademark for a preparation of chymotrypsin.

alpha-dinitrophenol (al″fah-di-ni″tro-fe′nol) see under *dinitrophenol.*

alphadione (al″fah-di′ōn) a steroid anesthetic, a combination of two steroids (3α-hydroxy-5α-pregnane-11,20-dione and 21-acetoxy-3α-hydroxy-5α-pregnane-11,20-dione) which are structurally similar to progesterone. It has a wide margin of safety between anesthetic dose and lethal dose.

Alphadrol (al′fah-drol) trademark for a preparation of fluprednisolone.

alpha-estradiol (al″fah-es″trah-di′ol) see *estradiol.*

alpha-hypophamine (al″fah-hi-pof′ah-min) oxytocin.

alpha-lobeline (al″fah-lob′e-lin) see *lobeline.*

alphalytic (al″fah-lit′ik) blocking the α-adrenergic receptors of the sympathetic nervous system; also, an agent that so acts.

alphamimetic (al″fah-mi-met′ik) stimulating or mimicking the stimulation of the α-adrenergic receptors of the sympathetic nervous system; also, an agent that so acts.

alphanaphthol (al″fah-naf′thol) a form of naphthol occurring as a white or pinkish crystalline compound, soluble in alcohol, ether, and hot water and slightly soluble in cold water; used in the manufacture of dyes, intermediates, and perfumes, and in microscopy.

alphaprodine hydrochloride (al″fah-pro′dēn) [USP] chemical name: *cis*-(+)-13-dimethyl-4-phenyl-4-piperidinol propanoate (ester) hydrochloride. A white, crystalline powder, $C_{16}H_{23}NO_2$·HCl, used intravenously or subcutaneously as a narcotic analgesic in conditions requiring rapid and brief analgesia.

alpha-tocopherol (al″fah-to-kof′er-ol) see under *tocopherol.*

alpha-tropeine (al″fah-tro′pe-in) a substance derivable from scopolamine and hyoscine.

alphelasma (al″fel-as′mah) (*obs.*) leukoplakia.

alphitomorphous (al″fit-o-mor′fus) [Gr. *alphiton* barley-meal + *morphē* form] having a mealy appearance; said of certain fungous parasites of plants.

alphodermia (al″fo-der′me-ah) (*obs.*) absence of pigmentation of the skin.

alphonsin (al-fon′sin) [named for *Alphonse* Ferri, Italian surgeon, 1515–1595] a bullet-forceps having three prongs.

alphos (al′fos) [L.; Gr. *alphos*] a nummular variety of psoriasis.

alprazolam (al-pra′zo-lam) chemical name: 8-chloro-1-methyl-6-phenyl-4*H*-[1,2,4]triazolo[4,3-α][1,4]benzodiapine; a tranquilizer, $C_{17}H_{13}ClN_4$.

alprenolol hydrochloride (al-pren′o-lol) chemical name: 1-[(1-methylethyl)amino]-3-[2-(2-propenyl)phenyl]-2-propanol hydrochloride; a beta-adrenergic blocking agent, $C_{15}H_{23}NO_2HCl$, having the same actions as propranolol (q.v.).

alprostadil (al-pros′tah-dil) chemical name: 11α,15S-dihydroxy-9-oxo-prost-13-en-1-oic acid; a vasodilator, $C_{20}H_{34}O_5$. Called also *prostaglandin* E₁.

alrestatin sodium (al′rĕ-stat″in) chemical name: 1,3-dioxo-1*H*-benz[*de*]isoquinoline-2(3*H*)acetic acid sodium salt; an aldose reductase inhibitor, $C_{14}H_8NNaO_4$.

A.L.R.O.S. American Laryngological, Rhinological, and Otological Society.

ALS antilymphocytic serum.

alseroxylon (al″ser-ok′sĭ-lon) a purified extract of *Rauwolfia serpentina*, containing reserpine and other amorphous alkaloids, occurring as a reddish brown amorphous powder; used orally as an antihypertensive and sedative.

alstonine (al′stŏ-nēn) an alkaloid obtained from several apocynaceous plants, e.g., *Alstonia constricta* F. Muell., *Rauwolfia* species, *Catharanthus roseus* G. Don, etc. The bark of several species of *Alstonia* has been used for its tonic, astringent, antiperiodic, and antipyretic properties.

Alström's syndrome (al′strumz) [Carl Henry *Alström*, Swedish geneticist] see under *syndrome.*

Alt. dieb. abbreviation for L. *alter′nis die′bus,* every other day.

alter (awl′ter) to castrate, as housepets or livestock.

alterant (awl′ter-ant) alterative.

alterative (awl′ter-a″tiv) [L. *alterare* to change] an obsolete term originally used for drugs said to re-establish healthy functions of the system.

alteregoism (awl″ter-e′go-izm) interest and sympathy only for persons who are in the same situation as one's self.

alternans (awl-ter′nanz) [L.] alternating or alternation, as in pulsus alternans (alternating strength of the pulse). **electrical a.,** alternating variations in the amplitude of electrocardiographic waves. **a. of the heart,** alternating strength in the heart beat or pulse. **pulsus a.,** the presence of alteration of intensity of heat sounds, indicating left ventricular failure.

Alternaria (awl″ter-na′re-ah) a genus of dematiacious Fungi Imperfecti of the order Moniliales, having dark-colored conidia somewhat resembling *Trichophyton;* it causes several diseases of plants and has been reported in diseases of the lungs and in skin infection in man, and is also a common allergen in human bronchial asthma.

alternariatoxicosis (awl″ter-nar″ĭ-ah-tok-sĭ-ko′sis) a form of mycotoxicosis caused by members of the genus *Alternaria.*

alternating (awl′ter-nāt″ing) occurring in regular succession; alternately direct and reversed.

alternation (awl″ter-na′shun) [L. *alternatio*] interrupted occurrence, being interspersed with different or opposite events. **cardiac a.,** a condition in which, during sphygmoscopy, every other beat is weak at 2 to 10 mm. Hg below the systolic level. **a. of generations,** alternate occurrence in regular sequence of asexual and sexual methods of reproduction in the same species; metagenesis.

Althaea (al-the′ah) [L.] a genus of malvaceous plants; the root and leaves of *A. officinalis* (marshmallow) contain sugar, pectin, and mucilage and are used as a demulcent and poultice.

Althausen test (awlt′how-zen) [Theodore L. *Althausen,* American physician, born 1897] see under *tests.*

althea (al-the′ah) the dried root of *Althaea officinalis,* or marshmallow root; a decoction was once used as a demulcent, and the boiled root as a poultice.

althiazide (al-thi′ah-zīd) chemical name: 3-[(allylthio)methyl]-6-chloro-3,4-dihydro-2*H*-1,2,4-benzothiadiazine-7-sulfonamide 1,-1-dioxide; an antihypertensive agent, $C_{11}H_{14}ClN_3O_4S_3$.

Alt. hor. abbreviation for L. *alter′nis ho′ris,* every other hour.

Altmann's fluid, granule, theory (ahlt′manz) [Richard *Altmann,* German histologist, 1852–1900] see under *fluid* and *theory,* and see *mitochondrion.*

Altmann-Gersh method (ahlt′man gersh) [Richard *Altmann;* Isidore *Gersh,* American anatomist, born 1907] see under *method.*

altofrequent (al″to-fre′quent) [L. *altus* high + *frequent*] marked by high frequency; see *high-frequency current,* under *current.*

altricious (al-trish′us) requiring a long period of nursing care.

altrose (al′trōs) a sugar, $C_6H_{12}O_6$, isomeric with glucose.

Alu-Cap (al′u-kap) trademark for a preparation of dried aluminum hydroxide gel.

Aludrine (ah-lu′drin) trademark for a preparation of isoproterenol.

Aludrox (al-u′droks) trademark for a preparation of alumina and magnesia.

alum (al′um) [L. *alumen*] 1. [USP] an odorless, colorless, crystalline substance, with local astringent and styptic properties and sweetish taste, and soluble in water, but insoluble in alcohol; it is either potassium alum, $AlK(SO_4)_2 + 12H_2O$, or ammonium alum, $AlNH_4(SO_4)_2 + 12H_2O$. Used as a topical application. 2. a generic term for any member of a class of double sulfates formed on the type of the foregoing compounds. 3. any member of a class of double aluminum-containing compounds. **ammonioferric a.,** a powerfully styptic alum, sulfate of iron, and ammonium; no longer used in medicine. **ammonium a.,** see *alum,* def. 1. **burnt a.,** exsiccated a. **chrome a.,** chromium and potassium sulfate; a violet pigment. **concentrated a.,** aluminum sulfate, incorrectly called an alum. **dried a.,** exsiccated a. **exsiccated a.,** a white odorless powder, with a sweetish, astringent taste, either exsiccated ammonium alum, $AlNH_4(SO_4)_2$, or exsiccated potassium alum, $AlK(SO_4)_2$, and containing at least 96.5 per cent of the labeled product. Called also *burnt* or *dried a.,* and *alumen exsiccatum.* **iron a.,** iron and potassium sulfate. **potassium a.,** see *alum,* def. 1. **sodium a.,** aluminum and sodium sulfate.

alumen (ah-loo′men), gen. *alu′minis* [L.] alum. **a. exsicca′tum,** exsiccated alum.

alumina (ah-loo′mi-nah) aluminum oxide, Al_2O_3; it occurs in sapphire and ruby, and is extracted from clay and bauxite as raw material for aluminum production. **a. and magnesia** [USP], a preparation containing 90 to 110 per cent of the labeled amounts of aluminum hydroxide and magnesium hydroxide; used as an antacid in tablet form.

aluminated (ah-loo′mi-nāt″ed) charged with alum.

aluminium (al″u-min′e-um) [L.] aluminum.

Aluminoid (ah-loo′mĭ-noid) trademark for preparations of aluminum hydroxide gel for use in gastric ulcers and hyperacidity.

aluminosis (ah-loo″mĭ-no′sis) a form of pneumoconiosis due to the presence of aluminum-bearing dust in the lungs; called also *a. pulmonum.*

aluminum (ah-loo'mĭ-num) an extremely light, whitish, lustrous, metallic element, obtainable from bauxite or clay: specific gravity, 2.699; atomic weight, 26.982; atomic number, 13; symbol, Al. It is very malleable and ductile, and is used for the manufacture of instruments and as a base for artificial dentures. The aluminum of the pharmacopeia is a fine, free-flowing, silvery powder, free from gritty or discolored particles. Aluminum compounds are used chiefly for their antacid and astringent properties. **a. acetate,** a compound, $C_6H_9AlO_6$, used in solution as an astringent and antiseptic; called also *eston.* **a. aminoacetate,** dihydroxyaluminum aminoacetate. **a. ammonium sulfate,** ammonium alum. **a. carbonate, basic,** an aluminum hydroxide–aluminum carbonate complex, available only in the form of *basic aluminum carbonate gel* (see under *gel*). **a. chloride** [USP], a white or yellowish white, deliquescent powder, $AlCl_3 \cdot 6H_2O$, used as a local astringent in a 10 to 25 per cent solution applied topically to the skin. It is also used as a topical antiseptic and in many deodorant preparations to diminish sweating. **a. chlorhydrex,** a topical astringent, reportedly consisting of a coordination complex of basic aluminum chloride and propylene glycol or polyethylene glycol in which the water molecules normally coordinated to the aluminum in aluminum chlorohydrate have been displaced by the glycol, resulting in a relatively less polar complex of low water content. **a. glycinate,** dihydroxyaluminum aminoacetate. **a. hydrate,** a. hydroxide. **a. hydroxide,** a white, bulky, amorphous powder, $Al(OH)_3$, used as a gastric antacid in the form of *aluminum hydroxide gel* or *dried aluminum hydroxide gel* (see under *gel*). **a. hydroxide, colloidal,** aluminum hydroxide gel. **a. monostearate** [NF], a combination of aluminum with variable proportions of stearic acid and palmitic acid; used in preparation of a suspension of procaine penicillin G. **a. nicotinate,** chemical name: 3-pyridinecarboxylic acid aluminum salt. A complex consisting of aluminum nicotinate, aluminum hydroxide, and nicotinic acid; used chiefly as an anticholesterolemic, antilipoproteinemic, and peripheral vasodilator, administered orally. **a. oxide,** a pure compound, Al_2O_3, produced in various grain sizes and used as an abrasive agent in dentistry; called also *alumina* or *alumina corundum.* **a. penicillin,** see under *penicillin.* **a. phosphate,** a white infusible powder, $AlPO_4$, used with calcium sulfate and sodium silicate in dental cements, and as a gastric antacid in the form of aluminum phosphate gel (see under *gel*). **a. potassium sulfate,** potassium alum. **a. subacetate** [USP], a yellow liquid prepared by the interaction of aluminum sulfate, acetic acid, and precipitated calcium carbonate, and used as an astringent wash when diluted with 20 to 40 volumes of water. **a. sulfate,** an odorless white, crystalline powder, with a sweet taste, $Al_2(SO_4)_3 + 18H_2O$, that is astringent and antiperspirant. Incorrectly called *concentrated alum.*

alundum (ah-lun'dum) electrically fused alumina, used in making laboratory appliances which are to be subjected to intense heat.

Alupent (al'u-pent) trademark for preparations of metaproterenol sulfate.

Alurate (al'ūr-āt) trademark for a preparation of aprobarbital.

Alv. adst. abbreviation for L. *al'vo adstric'ta,* when the bowels are constipated.

Alv. deject. abbreviation for L. *al'vi dejectio'nes,* alvine dejections.

alvei (al've-i) [L.] plural of *alveus.*

alveobronchiolitis (al″ve-o-brong″ke-o-li'tis) inflammation of the bronchioles and alveoli of the lungs.

alveolalgia (al″ve-o-lal'je-ah) [*alveolus* + *-algia*] pain occurring in a dental alveolus.

alveolar (al-ve'o-lar) [L. *alveolaris*] pertaining to an alveolus.

alveolate (al-ve'o-lāt) marked by honeycomb-like pits; called also *faveolate.*

alveolectomy (al″ve-o-lek'to-me) [*alveolus* + Gr. *ektomē* excision] excision of a portion of the alveolar process to aid in the removal of teeth, in the restoration of the normal contour following the removal of teeth, and in the preparation of the mouth for dentures.

alveoli (al-ve'o-li) plural of *alveolus.*

alveolitis (al″ve-o-li'tis) inflammation of an alveolus. **allergic a., extrinsic allergic a.,** hypersensitivity pneumonitis; a respiratory hypersensitivity reaction to repeated inspiration of organic particles, most often in an occupational setting, with onset about 4 to 8 hours after exposure to the allergen. There is fever, fatigue, chills, unproductive cough, tachycardia, and tachypnea. In the chronic form there is interstitial fibrosis with collagenous thickening of the alveolar septa. The disorder includes farmer's lung, bagassosis, pigeon breeder's lung, etc. **fibrosing a.,** diffuse interstitial pulmonary fibrosis. **a. sic'ca doloro'sa,** dry socket.

alveolo- (al-ve'o-lo) [L. *alveolus*] a combining form denoting relationship to an alveolus, probably most often used in reference to a dental alveolus.

alveolocapillary (al″o-lo-kap'ĭ-lār″e) pertaining to the pulmonary alveoli and capillaries.

alveoloclasia (al-ve″o-lo-kla'ze-ah) [*alveolo-* + Gr. *klasis* breaking] disintegration or resorption of the inner wall of a tooth alveolus, causing looseness of the teeth.

alveolodental (al-ve″o-lo-den'tal) pertaining to a tooth and its alveolus.

alveololabial (al-ve″o-lo-la'be-al) pertaining to the alveolar processes and the lips.

alveololabialis (al-ve″o-lo-la″be-a'lis) musculus buccinator.

alveololingual (al-ve″o-lo-ling'gwal) pertaining to the alveolar processes and the tongue.

alveolomerotomy (al-ve″o-lo″mĕ-rot'o-me) [*alveolus* + Gr. *meros* part + *tomē* a cutting] alveolectomy.

alveolonasal (al-ve″o-lo-na'sal) pertaining to the alveolar point and the nasion.

alveolopalatal (al-ve″o-lo-pal'ah-tal) pertaining to the alveolar process and palate.

alveoloplasty (al-ve'o-lo-plas″te) [*alveolo-* + Gr. *plassein* to form] the surgical alteration of the shape and condition of the alveolar process, in preparation for immediate or future denture construction. **interradicular a.,** the surgical removal of the interradicular bone and the collapsing of the cortical plates to a more desirable contour. **intraseptal a.,** interradicular a.

alveolotomy (al″ve-o-lot'o-me) [*alveolo-* + Gr. *tomē* a cutting] incision into a dental alveolus; see also *alveolectomy.*

alveolus (al-ve'o-lus), pl. *alve'oli* [L., dim. of *alveus* hollow] a general term used in anatomical nomenclature to designate a small saclike dilatation; see also *acinus.* **dental alveoli,** the bony cavities or sockets in the mandible or maxilla in which the roots of the teeth are attached. See *alveoli dentales mandibulae* and *alveoli dentales maxillae.* **alve'oli denta'les mandib'-ulae** [NA], dental alveoli of the mandible: the cavities or sockets in the alveolar process of the mandible in which the roots of the teeth are held by the periodontal ligament; called also *alveolar cavities.* **alve'oli denta'les maxil'lae** [NA], dental alveoli of the maxilla: the cavities or sockets in the alveolar process of the maxilla in which the roots of the teeth are held by the periodontal ligament; called also *alveolar cavities.* **alve'oli pulmo'nis** [NA], small polyhedral outpouchings along the walls of the alveolar sacs and alveolar ducts through the walls of which gas exchange takes place between alveolar gas and pulmonary capillary blood; called also *pulmonary alveoli, a. pulmonum, Malpighi's vesicles, vesiculae pulmonales,* and *pulmonary vesicles.* **alveoli pulmo'num,** alveoli pulmonis.

alveoplasty (al-ve″o-plas'te) alveoloplasty.

alverine citrate (al've-rēn) [NF] chemical name: *N*-ethyl-3,3′-diphenyldipropylamine citrate. An anticholinergic, $C_{20}H_{27}N \cdot C_6H_8O_7$, occurring as a white to off-white powder with a sweet odor and slightly bitter taste; used as a smooth muscle relaxant and antispasmodic.

alveus (al've-us), pl. *al'vei* [L.] a trough or a canal. **a. commu'nis,** utriculus, def. 2. **a. hippocam'pi** [NA], **a. of hippocampus,** the thin layer of white matter that covers the ventricular surface of the hippocampus.

alvine (al'vin) [L. *alvinus*] (*obs.*) pertaining to the abdomen or intestines.

alvinolith (al'vi-no-lith″) [L. *alvus* abdomen + Gr. *lithos* stone] (*obs.*) enterolith.

Alvodine (al'vo-din) trademark for preparations of piminodine esylate.

alvus (al'vus) [L.] the abdomen with its contained viscera.

alymphia (ah-lim'fe-ah) [*a* neg. + L. *lympha* lymph] deficiency or absence of the lymph.

alymphocytosis (ah-lim″fo-si-to'sis) complete or nearly complete absence of lymphocytes from the blood; lymphopenia.

alymphoplasia (ah″lim-fo-pla'ze-ah) failure of development of lymphoid tissue. **thymic a.,** a type of congenital agammaglobulinemia in which there is thymic hypoplasia, sparsity of lymphocytes in the thymus, spleen, lymph nodes, and intestines, absence of plasma cells, and absence of Hassall's corpuscles.

alymphopotent (ah-lim″fo-po'tent) [*a* neg. + *lymphoid* + L. *potens* able] incapable of producing lymphocytes or lymphoid cells.

Alzheimer's basket cells, dementia (disease, sclerosis), stain (altz'hi-merz) [Alois *Alzheimer,* German neurologist, 1864–1915] see *presenile dementia,* under *dementia,* and see under *basket* (def. 2), *cell,* and *stain.*

A.M. abbreviation for L. *artium magister,* Master of Arts.

Am chemical symbol for *americium.*

am symbol for *myopic astigmatism, meterangle,* and *ametropia.*

A.M.A. American Medical Association; Australian Medical Association.

ama (a'mah), pl. *a'mae* [L.] an enlargement of a semicircular canal of the internal ear at the end opposite the ampulla.

amaas (ah'mahs) variola minor.

amacratic (am″ah-krat′ik) [Gr. *hama* together + *kratos* strength] amasthenic.

amacrinal (am″ah-kri′nal) of the nature of amacrines.

amacrine (am′ah-krin) [*a* neg. + Gr. *makros* long + *is, inos* fiber] 1. having no long processes. 2. any of a group of branched retinal structures regarded as modified nerve cells.

Amadil (am′ah-dil) trademark for a preparation of acetaminophen.

amadinone acetate (ah-mad′ĭ-nōn) chemical name: 17-(acetyloxy)-6-chloronorpregna-4,6-diene-3,20-dione acetate; a progestin, $C_{22}H_{27}ClO_4$.

amadou (am′ah-doo) [Fr.] touchwood or punk; the fungus *Polyporus fomentarius*, which grows on old trees; formerly used as a wound dressing and a hemostatic.

amakrine (am′ah-krin) amacrine.

AMAL Aero-Medical Acceleration Laboratory.

amalgam (ah-mal′gam) [Gr. *malagma* poultice or soft mass] an alloy of two or more metals, one of which is mercury. **dental a.,** an amalgam of silver, tin, and mercury ($Ag_3Sn + Hg$) with low concentrations of copper and sometimes zinc; used for filling cavities in teeth. **emotional a.,** an unconscious attempt to bind, neutralize, deny, or counteract anxiety. **emotional-object a.,** the union of emotion or emotional significance with a person, event, object, or circumstance, as in phobias, in which anxiety becomes associated with an unconsciously selected phobic object. **retrograde a.,** see under *filling.*

amalgamable (ah-mal′gah-mah-b'l) capable of forming an amalgam with mercury.

amalgamate (ah-mal′gah-māt″) to unite a metal in an alloy with mercury; to form an amalgam.

amalgamation (ah-mal″gah-ma′shun) 1. the formation of an amalgam. 2. trituration.

amalgamator (ah-mal′gah-ma″tor) triturator.

amandin (am′an-din) a globulin from the almond nut.

Amanita (am″ah-ni′tah) [Gr. *amanitai* a sort of fungus] a genus of mushrooms of the family Agaricaceae, several species of which are poisonous. *A. phalloi′des* (destroying angel, death cup) contains a hemolysin and a mixture of peptide toxins (e.g., phalloidin) which are protoplasmic poisons. These cause irreversible damage in cardiac musculature, liver, and kidney cells after 24 hours. Mortality ranges from 50 to 90 per cent. *A. musca′ria* (fly agaric) contains muscarine and ibotenic acid. The latter is psychotropic. Ingestion of this species causes intoxication (drunkenness) and ultimate loss of consciousness. Other species are also toxic; some are edible.

amanitine (ah-mă-ni′tin) a poisonous alkaloid from fly agaric; also a poisonous glycoside from the various mushrooms, especially from *Amanita phalloides.*

amanitotoxin (ah-man″ĭ-to-tok′sin) *Amanita* toxin.

Amann's test (ah-manz′) [Jules *Amann*, Swiss physician] see under *tests.*

amantadine hydrochloride (ah-man′tah-dēn) [USP] chemical name: tricyclo[3.3.1.1³,⁷]decan-1-amine hydrochloride. An antiviral compound, $C_{10}H_{17}N \cdot HCl$, occurring as a white or nearly white crystalline powder; used in the prophylaxis and management of type A influenza and, because it augments the release of dopamine, as an antidyskinetic in the treatment of parkinsonism.

amara (ah-ma′rah) [L., pl.] (*obs.*) bitters, def. 2

Amaranth (am′ah-ranth) a genus of herbs of the family Amarantaceae, several species of which have various medical and food uses. Some species of the western United States are a problem in causing hay fevers. A source of the dye called amaranth, now prepared synthetically.

amaranth (am′ah-ranth) a dark, red-brown powder, $C_{10}H_6$-$(SO_2 \cdot ONa) \cdot N:N \cdot C_{10}H_4(SO_2 \cdot ONa)_2 \cdot OH$, once used as a coloring agent in food, cosmetics, and drugs.

amaril (am′ah-ril) [Sp. *amarillo*] yellow; a name formerly given to a hypothetical poison that was considered at that time to be a cause of yellow fever. **virus a.,** yellow fever.

amarillic (am″ah-ril′ik) pertaining to amaril.

amarine (am′ah-rin) [L. *amarus* bitter] a poisonous crystalline base, $C_6H_5 \cdot CH \cdot NH \cdot C:(C_6H_5)N \cdot CH \cdot C_6H_5$, triphenyl dihydroglyoxaline, from oil of bitter almonds, and also prepared artificially.

amaroid (am′ah-roid) a bitter principle.

amaroidal (am-ah-roi′dal) somewhat bitter; also resembling a bitter in properties.

amarthritis (am″ar-thri′tis) [Gr. *hama* together + *arthron* joint + *-itis*] inflammation of several joints at the same time; polyarthritis.

amasesis (am″ah-se′sis) [*a* neg. + Gr. *masēsis* chewing] inability to chew food.

amasthenic (am″as-then′ik) [Gr. *hama* together + *sthenos* strength] bringing the rays of light into one focus; said of a lens.

amastia (ah-mas′te-ah) [*a* neg. + Gr. *mastos* breast] congenital absence of the mammae; sometimes applied to masculine breast characteristics in an adult female. Called also *amazia.*

amastigote (ah-mas′tĭ-gōt) [*a* neg. + Gr. *mastix* whip] the nonflagellate, intracellular, morphologic stage in the development of certain hemoflagellates, resembling the typical adult form of *Leishmania;* called also *leishmanial stage* or *form.* Cf. *epimastigote, promastigote,* and *trypomastigote.*

amathophobia (ah-math″o-fo′be-ah) [Gr. *amathos* sand + *phobia*] morbid dread of dust.

amativeness (am′ah-tiv′nes) [L. *amare* to love] inclination to love.

amatol (am′ah-tol) a war explosive, being a mixture of trinitrotoluene and ammonium nitrate.

amaurosis (am″aw-ro′sis) [L. from Gr. *amaurōsis* darkening] blindness (Hippocrates), especially blindness occurring without apparent lesion of the eye, as from disease of the optic nerve, spine, or brain. Cf. *amblyopia.* **albuminuric a.,** that which is due to renal disease. **Burns's a.** (*obs.*), postmarital amblyopia. **cat's eye a.,** blindness of one eye, with bright reflection from the pupil, as from the tapetum of a cat (Beer). **central a., a. centra′lis,** amaurosis due to disease of the central nervous system. **cerebral a.,** that which is due to cerebral or brain disease. **a. congen′ita of Leber, Leber's congenital a.,** a characteristic and rare type of blindness transmitted as an autosomal recessive trait, occurring at or shortly after birth and associated with an atypical form of diffuse pigmentation and commonly with optic atrophy and attenuation of the retinal vessels. **congenital a.,** that which exists from birth. **diabetic a.,** that which is associated with diabetes. **a. fu′gax,** a transient episode of monocular blindness, or partial blindness, lasting ten minutes or less. **hysteric a.,** that which is associated with hysteria. **intoxication a.,** amaurosis caused by some systemic poison, as alcohol or tobacco. **a. partia′lis fu′-gax,** sudden transitory partial blindness. **reflex a.,** that which is caused by the reflex action of a remote irritation. **saburral a.,** that which occurs in an attack of acute gastritis. **uremic a.,** an amaurotic condition due to uremia; sometimes attendant on nephritis.

amaurotic (am″aw-rot′ik) pertaining to, or of the nature of, amaurosis.

amaxophobia (ah-mak″so-fo′be-ah) [Gr. *hamaxa* carriage + *phobia*] (*obs.*) morbid dread of vehicles.

amazia (ah-ma′ze-ah) [*a* neg. + Gr. *mazos* breast + *-ia*] amastia.

amb- see *ambi-.*

Ambard's formula (coefficient, constant, equation), laws (ahm-barz′) [Léon *Ambard*, physiologist in Strassburg, born 1876] see under *formula* and *law.*

ambenonium chloride (am″be-no′ne-um) [USP] chemical name: *N,N′*-[(1,2-dioxo-1,2-ethanediyl)bis-(imino-2,1-ethanediyl)]-bis[2-chloro-*N,N*-diethylbenzenemethanaminium] dichloride. A cholinergic, $C_{28}H_{42}Cl_4N_4O_2$, occurring as a white powder; used in the treatment of myasthenia gravis to treat the symptoms of muscular weakness and fatigue, administered orally.

amber (am′ber) a yellowish fossil resin, the gum of several species of coniferous trees, found in the alluvial deposits of northeastern Germany.

Amberg's line (am′bergz) [Emil *Amberg*, Detroit otologist, 1868–1948] see under *line.*

ambergris (am′ber-gris) [L. *ambra grisea* gray amber] a grayish waxy mass of material ejected from the intestinal tract of the sperm whale, *Physeter catodon,* and made up of cholesterol and varying amounts of fatty oil, benzoic acid, ambrein, and other materials. Used as a fixative in perfumery.

ambi- [L.] an inseparable prefix signifying on both sides; appears as *amb* before stems beginning with a vowel.

ambidexterity (am″bĭ-dek-ster′ĭ-te) the ability to perform acts requiring manual skill with either hand, some ordinarily being performed with one and some with the other.

ambidextrality (am″bĭ-dek-stral′ĭ-te) ambidexterity.

ambidextrism (am″bĭ-deks′trizm) ambidexterity.

ambidextrous (am″bĭ-dek′strus) pertaining to or characterized by ambidexterity.

ambient (am′be-ent) [L. *ambire* to surround] surrounding; encompassing; prevailing.

ambilateral (am″bĭ-lat′er-al) [*ambi-* + L. *latus* side] pertaining to or affecting both the right and the left side.

ambilevosity (am″bĭ-lĕ-vos′ĭ-te) the inability to perform acts requiring manual skill with either hand.

ambilevous (am″bĭ-le′vus) [*ambi-* + L. *laevus* left-handed] pertaining to or characterized by ambilevosity.

ambiopia (am″be-o′pe-ah) [L.] diplopia.

ambisexual (am″bĭ-seks′u-al) denoting sexual characteristics common to both sexes, e.g., pubic hair. Cf. *bisexual.*

ambisinister (am″bĭ-sin′is-ter) [*ambi-* + L. *sinister* left] ambilevous.

ambisinistrous (am″bĭ-sĭ-nis′trus) ambilevous.

ambivalence (am-biv′ah-lens) [ambi- + L. *valentia* strength, power] the simultaneous existence of conflicting attitudes, as of love and hate, toward the same object.

ambivalent (am-biv′ah-lent) 1. characterized by or pertaining to ambivalence. 2. having equal power in two opposite directions.

ambiversion (am″bĭ-ver′zhun) a personality state intermediate between introversion and extroversion.

ambivert (am′bĭ-vert) a person who is intermediate between an extrovert and an introvert.

ambly- (am′ble) [Gr. *amblys* dull] a combining form denoting dullness.

amblyaphia (am-ble-a′fe-ah) [ambly- + Gr. *haphe* touch + -ia] bluntness or dullness of the sense of touch.

amblychromasia (am″ble-kro-ma′ze-ah) the condition of staining faintly or of having little chromatin.

amblychromatic (am″ble-kro-mat′ik) [ambly- + Gr. *chrōma* color] feebly staining.

amblygeustia (am″ble-gu′ste-ah) [ambly- + Gr. *geusis* taste + -ia] dullness of the sense of taste.

Amblyomma (am″ble-om′ah) [ambly- + Gr. *omma* eye] a genus of ticks. **A. america′num,** the Lone Star tick of the southern United States, particularly Texas and Louisiana; it is a vector of Rocky Mountain spotted fever. **A. cajennen′se,** a particularly obnoxious species of tropical America; it transmits Rocky Mountain spotted fever. **A. hebrae′um,** the bont tick, an African species which transmits the rickettsial disease of sheep, goats, and cattle known as "heartwater" as well as South African tick-bite fever of man. **A. macula′tum,** a species found on the Gulf Coast. **A. ova′le,** a tropical tick of dogs and tapirs. **A. tubercula′tum,** a species found in Florida. **A. variega′tum,** a species which, like *A. hebraeum*, transmits heartwater; it also transmits the virus causing Nairobi sheep disease.

amblyope (am′blĕ-ōp) a person with amblyopia.

amblyopia (am″ble-o′pe-ah) [ambly- + Gr. *ōps* eye + -ia] dimness of vision without detectable organic lesion of the eye. Cf. *amaurosis.* **a. alcohol′ica,** impairment of the vision as a result of alcohol poisoning; called also *a. crapulosa.* **arsenic a.,** disturbance of vision due to the use of arsenic. **color a.,** impairment of color vision, caused by toxic or other influences. **a. crapulo′sa,** a. alcoholica. **crossed a., a. crucia′ta,** that which affects one eye, with hemianesthesia of the opposite side. **a. ex anop′sia,** that which results from long disuse. **hysteric a.,** that which is associated with hysteria. **nocturnal a.,** abnormal dimness of vision at night. **postmarital a.,** that which was once thought to be caused by sexual excess. **quinine a.,** amblyopia following large doses of quinine; thought to be due to anemia of the retina. **reflex a.,** that which results from peripheral irritation. **strabismic a.,** amblyopia resulting from suppression of vision in one eye to avoid diplopia. **tobacco a.,** a visual disturbance affecting tobacco users, marked by cecocentral scotoma and visual field defect. **toxic a.,** amblyopia due to poisoning, as from tobacco or alcohol. **traumatic a.,** amblyopia due to injury. **uremic a.,** loss of vision sometimes seen during a uremic attack.

amblyopiatrics (am″ble-o″pe-at′riks) [amblyopia + Gr. *iatreia* healing] the therapeutics or treatment of amblyopia.

amblyoscope (am′ble-o-skōp″) [amblyopia + Gr. *skopein* to view] an instrument for training an amblyopic eye to take part in vision and for measuring and increasing fusion of the eyes.

Amblystoma (am-blis′to-mah) *ambystoma.*

ambo (am′bo) ambon.

ambo- [L. *ambo* both] a combining form signifying both, or on both sides.

amboceptor (am″bo-sep′tor) [ambo- + L. *capere* to take] Ehrlich's term for hemolysin, particularly for its double receptors, the one combining with the blood cell, the other with complement. **bacteriolytic a.,** an amboceptor that takes part in bacteriolysis. **Bordet's a.,** an alexin-fixing amboceptor. **hemolytic a.,** a hemolysin; an amboceptor which takes part in hemolysis.

amboceptorgen (am″bo-sep′tor-jen) an antigen giving rise to amboceptors.

Ambodryl (am′bo-dril) trademark for preparations of bromodiphenhydramine hydrochloride.

ambomycin (am″bo-mi′sin) an antibiotic substance with antineoplastic properties produced by *Streptomyces ambofaciens;* formerly called *duazomycin C.*

ambon (am′bon) the ring of fibrocartilage forming the edge of the sockets in which the heads of long bones are lodged.

ambosexual (am″bo-seks′u-al) [ambo- + *sexual*] ambisexual.

ambrain (am-bra′in) ambrein.

ambrein (am-bre′in) ambrin.

ambrin (am′brin) a white crystalline tricyclic terpenoid, $C_{30}H_{49}O_2$, resembling cholesterol, found in ambergris and derived metabolically from squalene.

Ambrine (am′brēn) trademark for preparations of paraffin, rosin, and wax; formerly used as a dressing in the treatment of extensive burns and in rheumatic disorders, introduced by Barthe de Sandfort (1913).

Ambrosia (am-bro′zhe-ah) [L. and Gr., from Gr. *ambrotos* immortal] a genus of annual weeds which produce quantities of windborne pollen and so cause much hay fever. *A. artemisiaefo′lia* is the common or small ragweed; *A. trif′ida* is the giant ragweed.

ambrosin (am-bro′sin) (*obs.*) a substance contained in the pollen of ragweed (*Ambrosia*).

ambrosterol (am-bros′tĕ-rol) a phytosterol, $C_{20}H_{34}O$ with a melting point of 147° to 149° C. found in the pollen of ragweed (*Ambrosia*).

ambruticin (am″broo-ti′sin) chemical name: 6-[2-[2-[5-(6-ethyl-3,6-dihydro-5-methyl-2H-pyran-2-yl]-3-methyl-1,4-hexadienyl]-3-methycyclopropyl]ethenyl]tetrahydro-4,5-dihydroxy-2H-pyran-2-acetic acid; an antifungal antibiotic derived from *Polyangium cellulosum* subspecies *fulvum*, $C_{28}H_{42}O_6$.

ambulance (am′bu-lans) [Fr.] a vehicle for conveying the sick or injured, and equipped with apparatus for rendering emergency treatment.

ambulant (am′bu-lant) [L. *ambulans* walking] walking or able to walk.

ambulation (am″bu-la′shun) the act of walking.

ambulatory (am′bu-lah-to″re) ambulant.

ambuphylline (am-bu′fĭ-lēn) chemical name: theophylline compound with 2-amino-2-methyl-1-propanol; a diuretic and smooth muscle relaxant, $C_7H_8N_4O_2 \cdot C_4H_{11}NO$.

ambustion (am-bust′yun) a burn or scald.

ambutoxate hydrochloride (am-bu-toks′āt) chemical name: 2-(diethylamino)ethyl 4-amino-2-butoxybenzoate hydrochloride; a spinal anesthetic. Called also *ambucaine.*

Ambystoma (am-bis′to-mah) a genus of salamanders used for experimental purposes; called also *amblystoma.* See *axolotl.*

amcinafal (am-sin′ah-fal) chemical name: 9-fluoro-11β,21-dihydroxy-16α,17-[(1-ethylpropylidene)bis(oxy)]pregna-1,4-diene-2,-3-dione; an anti-inflammatory, $C_{26}H_{35}FO_6$.

amcinafide (am-sin′ah-fīd) chemical name: (R)-9-fluoro-11β,21-dihydroxy-16α,17-[(1-phenylethylidine)bis(oxy)]pregna-1,-4-diene-3,20-dione; an anti-inflammatory, $C_{26}H_{35}FO_6$.

amcinonide (am-sin′o-nīd) chemical name: 21-(acetyloxy)-16α,17-[cyclopentylidenebis(oxy)]-9-fluoro-11β-hydroxy-pregna-1,-4-diene-3,20-dione; a glucocorticoid, $C_{28}H_{35}FO_7$.

A.M.D.S. Association of Military Dental Surgeons.

ameba (ah-me′bah), pl. *amebae* or *amebas* [L., from Gr. *amoibē* change] a minute protozoon of the subphylum Sarcodina. It is a single-celled nucleated mass of protoplasm which changes shape by extending cytoplasmic processes, called pseudopodia, by means of which it moves about and absorbs nourishment. The majority of amebae are free-living in soil or water, but the following are parasitic in man: *Entamoeba coli, E. hartmanni, E. histolytica, E. gingivalis, Dientamoeba fragilis, Endolimax mana,* and *Iodamoeba bütschlii.* **artificial a.,** combinations of chemicals which behave somewhat like living amebae; for example, a drop of mercury will move toward a crystal of potassium dichromate if they are close together in dilute nitric acid. **coprozoic a.,** free-living amebae, sometimes found in human feces and characterized by the fact that they grow readily on artificial media. There are four genera: *Hartmanella, Naegleria, Sappinia,* and *Vahlkampfia.*

amebacidal (ah-me″bah-si′dal) amebicidal.

amebacide (ah-me′bah-sīd) amebicide.

amebadiastase (ah-me″bah-di′as-tās) an intracellular enzyme found in amebae which catalyzes the digestion of material engulfed by them.

amebaism (ah-me′bah-izm) the power or property of ameboid motion.

ameban (ah-me′ban) carbarsone.

amebiasis (am″e-bi′ah-sis) the state of being infected with amebae, especially with *Entamoeba histolytica.* **a. cu′tis,** a form of amebiasis in which there is invasion of the skin, with formation of indolent ulcers. **hepatic a.,** amebic hepatitis. **intestinal a.,** amebic dysentery. **pulmonary a.,** amebic infection in the thoracic space, secondary to intestinal amebiasis and usually associated with amebic liver abscesses; it may affect the pleura, the diaphragm, the lung, and/or the bronchi.

amebic (ah-me′bik) pertaining to or of the nature of an ameba.

amebicidal (ah-me″bĭ-si′dal) destructive to amebae.

amebicide (ah-me′bĭ-sīd) [ameba + L. *caedere* to kill] an agent which is destructive to amebae.

amebiform (ah-me′bĭ-form) shaped like or resembling an ameba.

amebiosis (am″e-bi-o′sis) amebiasis.

amebism (am′e-bizm) 1. ameboid movement. 2. invasion of the system with amebae.

amebocyte (ah-me′bo-sīt″) [ameba + Gr. *kytos* hollow vessel] an ameba-like cell found in coelomic fluid, blood (leukocytes), or other tissues of almost all animals.

amebodiastase (ah-me″bo-di′as-tās) amebadiastase.

ameboid (ah-me′boid) [ameba + Gr. eidos form] resembling an ameba in form or in movements.

ameboididity (am″e-boi-did′ĭ-te) (obs.) ameboidism.

ameboidism (ah-me′boid-izm) a type of motility characteristic of amebae and certain other cells, occurring as a result of protrusion of pseudopods.

ameboma (am″e-bo′mah) a tumor-like mass produced by localized inflammation due to amebiasis.

amebosis (am″ĕ-bo′sis) amebiasis.

amebula (ah-me′bu-lah) [dim. of L. amoeba] 1. one of the small amebae formed by division of the multinucleate mass (metacyst) produced by excystation of Entamoeba histolytica or other parasitic amebae. 2. the motile ameboid stage of the spores of certain sporozoan parasites; called also pseudopodiospore.

ameburia (am″ĕ-bu′re-ah) [ameba + Gr. ouron urine + -ia] the discharge or presence of amebae in the urine.

amedalin hydrochloride (ah-me′dah-lin) chemical name: 1,3-dihydro-3-methyl-3-[3-(methylamino)-propyl]-1-phenyl-2H-indol-2-one monohydrochloride; an antidepressant, $C_{19}H_{22}N_2O$·HCl.

ameiosis (a″mi-o′sis) aberrant meiosis in which only an equational division occurs, as in parthenogenesis.

AMEL Aero-Medical Equipment Laboratory.

amelanotic (ah″mel-ah-not′ik) containing no melanin; unpigmented.

amelia (ah-me′le-ah) [a neg. + Gr. melos limb + -ia] congenital absence of a limb or limbs; cf. phocomelia.

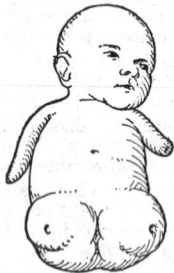

Amelia in legs; hemimelia in arms (Arey).

amelification (ah-mel″ĭ-fi-ka′shun) [Old Fr. amel enamel + L. facere to make] the development of enamel cells into enamel.

amelioration (ah-mēl″yo-ra′shun) [L. ad to + melior better] improvement, as of the condition of a patient.

ameloblast (ah-mel′o-blast″) [Old Fr. amel enamel + Gr. blastos germ] a cylindrical epithelial cell in the innermost layer of the enamel organ which takes part in the elaboration of the enamel prism. The ameloblasts cover the dental papilla. Called also adamantoblast, ganoblast, enamel builder, and enameloblast.

ameloblastoma (ah-mel″o-blas-to′mah) a true neoplasm of tissue of the type characteristic of the enamel organ, but which does not undergo differentiation to the point of enamel formation; called also adamantinoma. **melanotic a.,** melanotic neuroectodermal tumor. **pigmented a.,** melanotic neuroectodermal tumor. **pituitary a.,** craniopharyngioma.

amelodentinal (am″ĕ-lo-den′tĭ-nal) pertaining to the enamel and dentin of a tooth.

amelogenesis (am″ĕ-lo-jen′ĕ-sis) the formation of enamel. **a. imperfec′ta,** a hereditary condition resulting in defective development of enamel of the teeth, caused by improper differentiation of the ameloblasts and characterized by a brown color of the teeth. The condition takes three forms: agenesis, in which there is complete absence of enamel; enamel hypoplasia, in which the enamel is hard but deficient in quantity; and enamel hypocalcification, in which the enamel is soft but normal in quantity. Called also hereditary brown enamel and hereditary enamel hypoplasia.

amelogenic (am″ĕ-lo-jen′ik) forming enamel.

amelogenin (am″ĕ-lo-jen′in) any of several proteins secreted by ameloblasts and forming the organic matrix of tooth enamel.

amelus (am′ĕ-lus) an individual exhibiting amelia.

amenia (ah-me′ne-ah) [a neg. + menses + -ia] amenorrhea.

amenomania (am″ĕ-no-ma′ne-ah) [L. amoenus pleasant + mania] (obs.) psychosis with agreeable hallucinations.

amenorrhea (ah-men″o-re′ah) [a neg. + Gr. mēn month + rhoia flow] absence or abnormal stoppage of the menses; called also amenia. **dietary a.,** cessation of menstruation accompanying loss of weight due to dietary restriction, the loss of weight and of appetite being less extreme than in anorexia nervosa and unassociated with psychological problems. Called also nutritional a.

dysponderal a., amenorrhea associated with disorder of weight, such as obesity or extreme underweight. **hypothalamic a.,** amenorrhea associated with disorders of the hypothalamus. **lactation a.,** absence of the menses incidental to lactation. **nutritional a.,** dietary a. **ovarian a.,** amenorrhea resulting from deficiency of ovarian (estrus-producing) hormone. **physiologic a.,** absence of menses not due to organic disorder, usually occurring in pregnancy. **pituitary a.,** absence of the menses owing to pituitary deficiency. **premenopausal a.,** physiologic decrease of menstruation during establishment of the climacterium. **primary a.,** failure of menstruation to occur at puberty. **relative a.,** menstrual flow which is less than normal for the individual; called also oligomenorrhea. **secondary a.,** cessation of menstruation after it has once been established at puberty. **traumatic a.,** amenorrhea due to blockage of the cervical canal by adhesions, most often a result of curettage, as in Asherman's syndrome.

amenorrheal (ah-men-o-re′al) pertaining to amenorrhea.

amensalism (a-men′sal-izm) symbiosis in which one population (or individual) is adversely affected and the other is unaffected.

ament (a′ment) [L. a away + mens mind] an idiot; a person with profound mental deficiency. Used in contrast with dement.

amentia (ah-men′she-ah) [L. a away + mens mind + -ia] 1. congenital mental retardation of varying extent. 2. a mental disorder characterized by marked mental confusion, sometimes so severe as to approach stupor; called also confusion and confusional insanity. **a. agita′ta** (obs.), amentia attended by great excitement and continuous hallucinations. **a. atton′ita** (obs.), amentia marked by stupor, immobility, and indifference. **nevoid a.,** Sturge-Weber syndrome. **a. occul′ta** (obs.), mild melancholia with sudden violent actions. **a. paranoi′des** (obs.), amentia with mild symptoms. **phenylpyruvic a.,** idiocy attended by the excretion of phenylpyruvic acid in the urine; now called phenylketonuria (q.v.). **Stearns' alcoholic a.,** a form of temporary alcoholic insanity marked by less emotional disturbance than delirium tremens, but of longer duration and characterized by greater mental clouding and amnesia.

amential (ah-men′she-al) pertaining to or characterized by amentia.

Americaine (ah-mer′ĭ-kān″) trademark for preparations of benzocaine.

americium (am″ĕ-ris′e-um) the chemical element of atomic number 95, atomic weight 243, symbol Am, obtained by cyclotron bombardment of uranium and plutonium.

amerism (am′er-izm) [a neg. + Gr. meros part] the quality of not splitting into segments or fragments.

ameristic (am″er-is′tik) [a neg. + Gr. meristos divided] not split into segments.

ametabolon (ah″mĕ-tab′o-lon) an animal that develops without undergoing metamorphosis.

ametabolous (ā″mĕ-tab′o-lus) not undergoing metamorphosis.

ametachromophil (ah″met-ah-kro′mo-fil) orthochromophil.

ametamorphosis (ah-met″ah-mor′fo-sis) (obs.) undue activity of thought leading to a condition of mental absorption and abstraction.

ametaneutrophil (ah-met-ah-nu′tro-fil) orthochromophil.

amethocaine hydrochloride (ah-meth′o-kān) tetracaine hydrochloride.

amethopterin (ah-meth-op′ter-in) methotrexate.

ametria (ah-me′tre-ah) [a neg. + Gr. mētra uterus] congenital absence of the uterus.

ametrometer (am″ĕ-trom′ĕ-ter) [ametropia + Gr. metron measure] an instrument for measuring the degree of ametropia.

ametropia (am″ĕ-tro′pe-ah) [Gr. ametros disproportionate + ōps eye + -ia] discrepancy between the size and refractive powers of the eye, such that images are not brought to a proper focus on the retina; consequently hypermetropia, myopia, or astigmatism are produced. See illustration. **axial a.,** ametropia due to lengthening of the eyeball along the optic axis. **curvature a.,** ametropia due to variations in the curvature of the surface of the eye. **index a.,** ametropia due to alterations in the refractive index media of the eye. **position a.,** ametropia due to faulty position of the crystalline lens. **refractive a.,** ametropia due to fault in the dioptric system of the eye.

ametropic (am″ĕ-trop′ik) affected with or pertaining to ametropia.

amfenac sodium (am′fĕ-nak) chemical name: 2-amino-3-benzoylbenzeneacetic acid sodium salt monohydrate; an anti-inflammatory, $C_{15}H_{12}NNaO_3H_2O$.

Amh mixed astigmatism with myopia predominating.

AMI acute myocardial infarction.

amianthoid (am″e-an′thoid) [Gr. amianthos asbestos + eidos form] having the appearance of asbestos; a term applied to certain fibers seen in degenerated costal and laryngeal cartilage.

amianthosis (am″e-an-tho′sis) [Gr. amianthos asbestos + -osis] (obs.) asbestosis.

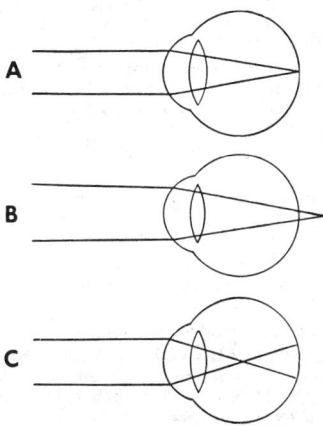

Refraction by the eye in (*A*) emmetropia; (*B*) hyperopia, and (*C*) myopia (Scheie and Albert).

amibiarson (am″ĭ-bĭ-ar′sŏn) carbarsone.

Amicar (am′ĭ-kar) trademark for a preparation of aminocaproic acid.

amichloral (am″ĭ-klor′ah) chemical name: 6-*O*-[2,2,2-trichloro-1-hydroxyethyl]-α-D-glucopyranose polymer with α-D-glucopyranose; a food additive for use in veterinary medicine, $(C_8H_{11}Cl_3O_6)_x(C_8H_{10}O_5)_y$.

Amici's disk, line, striae (ah-me′chēz) [Giovanni Battista *Amici*, Italian physicist, 1784–1863] see *Z band*, under *band*, and see under *stria*.

amicine (am′ĭ-sin) a substance in the posterior lobe of the pituitary gland which inhibits the growth of both plants and animals.

amicrobic (ah″mi-kro′bik) [*a* neg. + *microbe*] not caused by microbes.

amicroscopic (ah-mi″kro-skop′ik) too small to be observed by use of the microscope.

amiculum (ah-mik′u-lum) a dense surrounding coat of white fibers, as the sheath of the inferior olive and of the dentate nucleus.

amidapsone (ah″me-dap′sŏn) chemical name: [4-[(4-aminophenyl)sulfonyl]phenyl]urea; an antiviral for use in poultry, $C_{13}H_{13}N_3O_3S$.

amidase (am′ĭ-dās) a deamidizing enzyme.

amide (am′īd) [*ammonia* + *-ide*] an organic compound derived from ammonia by substituting an acyl radical for hydrogen, or from an acid by replacing the —OH group by —NH₂. **niacin a., nicotinic acid a.,** niacinamide.

amidin (am′ĭ-din) [Fr. *amidon* starch] amylose, def. 2.

amidine (am′ĭ-din) any compound containing the monovalent group ·C(:NH)·NH₂. **insoluble a., tegumentary a.,** amylopectin.

amidine-lyase (am′ĭ-dēn-li′ās) an enzyme that catalyzes the removal of an amindino group, as from L-argininosuccinate to form fumarate and L-arginine.

amidinotransferase (ah″mĭ-din″o-trans′fer-ās) transamidinase.

amido- a prefix indicating the presence of the radical NH₂ along with the radical CO.

amidoazotoluene (am″ĭ-do-a″zo-tol′u-ēn) a reddish brown powder, $CH_3·C_6H_4·N_2·C_6H_3·CH_2·NH_2$, derived from scarlet red; used in an 8 per cent ointment to stimulate the growth of epithelium.

amidobenzene (am″ĕ-do-ben′zēn) aniline.

amidogen (am′ĕ-do-jen″) the hypothetic radical, NH₂, found in amido compounds.

amidohexose (am″ĕ-do-hek′sōs) a hexose combined with the amido group NH₂.

amido-ligase (am′ĭ-do-li′gās) any enzyme that catalyzes the coupling of two molecules, with glutamine acting as an ammonia donor.

amidopyrine (am″ĭ-do-pi′rēn) aminopyrine.

Amidostomum (am″ĭ-dos′to-mum) a genus of roundworms. **A. an′seris,** a roundworm parasitic in the mucous membrane of the intestinal tract of ducks and geese.

amidoxime (am-ĭ-dok′sīm) any of a class of compounds formed from the amidines by substituting hydroxyl for a hydrogen atom of the amido group.

amidulin (am-mid′u-lin) the granulose of starch freed from its envelope of amylose by the action of hydrochloric acid; called also *soluble starch*.

Amigen (am′ĭ-jen) trademark for a protein hydrolysate preparation for intravenous injection.

amikacin sulfate (am″ĭ-ka′sin) [USP] chemical name: (*S*)-*O*-3-amino-3-deoxy-α-D-glucopyranosyl-(1 → 6)-*O*-[6-amino-6-deoxy-α-D-glucopyranosyl(1 → 4)]-*N*¹-(4-amino-2-hydroxy-1-oxobutyl)-2-deoxy-D-streptamine sulfate (1:1) salt. A semisynthetic aminoglycoside antibiotic derived from kanamycin, $C_{22}H_{43}N_5O_{13}·2H_2SO_4$, effective against gram-negative bacteria including *Pseudomonas, Providencia, Klebsiella-Enterobacter-Serratia, Acinetobacter,* and *Proteus* species, and *Escherichia coli* and *Citrobacter freundii,* and some gram-positive organisms, including penicillinase- and nonpenicillinase-producing staphylococci; used in the treatment of a wide range of infections due to susceptible organisms, administered intramuscularly and intravenously.

Amikin (am′ĭ-kin) trademark for a preparation of amikacin sulfate.

amimia (ah-mim′e-ah) [*a* neg. + Gr. *mimos* mimic + *-ia*] loss of the power of expression by the use of signs or gestures. **amnesic a.,** a condition in which gestures can be made, but their meaning cannot be remembered.

aminacrine hydrochloride (am-in-ak′rin) chemical name: 9-aminoacridine monohydrochloride. An antiseptic dye, $C_{13}H_{10}N_2·HCl$, occurring as a pale yellow, crystalline powder, which is effective against many gram-negative and gram-positive bacteria; used as a topical anti-infective, mainly in the treatment of infected wounds. Called also *aminoacridine hydrochloride*.

aminarsone (am-in-ar′sŏn) carbarsone.

amine (ah-mēn′; am′in) an organic compound containing nitrogen; any member of a group of chemical compounds formed from ammonia by replacement of one or more of the hydrogen atoms by organic (hydrocarbon) radicals. The amines are distinguished as *primary, secondary,* and *tertiary,* according to whether one, two, or three hydrogen atoms are replaced. The amines include allylamine, amylamine, ethylamine, methylamine, phenylamine, propylamine, and many other compounds. **biogenic a's,** amines arising by biosynthesis that play a role in neural functioning, e.g., norepinephrine, serotonin, dopamine, and acetycholine; called also *bioamines*. **catechol a.,** catecholamine. **methyl dimethoxy methyl phenyl a.,** a long-acting hallucinogenic substance. Abbreviated DMP. **vasoactive a.,** amines that cause vasodilation and increase small vessel permeability, e.g., histamine and serotonin.

aminitrozole (am″ĭ-ni′tro-zōl) chemical name: 2-acetamido-5-nitrothiazole. A compound, $C_5H_5N_3O_3S$, formerly used in treatment of trichomoniasis. In veterinary medicine, it is used in treatment of blackhead in turkeys. Called also *acnitrazole*.

amino (ah-me′no, am′ĭ-no) the monovalent chemical group —NH₂. As a prefix (amino-) it indicates the presence in a compound of the group —NH₂.

aminoacidemia (ah-me″no-, am″ĭ-no-as″ĭ-de′me-ah) [*amino acid* + Gr. *haima* blood + *-ia*] an excess of amino acids in the blood.

aminoacidopathy (am″ĭ-no-as″ĭ-dop′ah-the) any of a group of disorders due to a defect in an enzymatic step in the metabolic pathway of one or more amino acids or in a protein mediator necessary for transport of certain amino acids into or out of cells.

aminoaciduria (ah-me″no-, am″ĭ-no-as″ĭ-du′re-ah) [*amino acid* + Gr. *ouron* urine + *-ia*] an excess of amino acids in the urine; called also *acidaminuria*.

aminoacridine hydrochloride (am′ĭ-no-ak′rĭ-din) aminacrine hydrochloride.

aminoacylase (am″ĭ-no-as″ĭ-lās) *N*-acylamino-acid amidohydrolase: an enzyme occurring in the kidney that catalyzes the hydrolysis of hippuric acid to benzoic acid and glycine; called also *dehydropeptidase* and *hippuricase*. **a. II,** aspartoacylase.

***o*-aminoazotoluene** (ah-me″no-, am″ĭ-no-az″o-tol′u-ēn) chemical name: methyl-4-[(2-methylphenyl)azo]benzeneamine; a red crystalline solid, $CH_3·C_6H_4·N_2·C_6H_3(CH_3)NH_2$, that is actively carcinogenic.

aminobenzene (ah-me″no-, am″ĭ-no-ben′zēn) aniline.

γ-aminobutyrate (ah-me″no-, am″ĭ-no-bu″tĭ-rāt) a salt or dissociated form of gamma-aminobutyric acid; see under *acid*.

aminodinitrophenol (am″ĭ-no-di-ni″tro-fe′nol) dinitroaminophenol.

2-aminoethanol (am″ĭ-no-eth′ah-nol) ethanolamine.

aminoform (ah-min′o-form) methenamine.

aminoglutethimide (ah-me″no-, am″ĭ-no-gloo-teth′ĭ-mīd) chemical name: 3-(4-aminophenyl)-3-ethyl-2,6-piperididedione. A glutethimide derivative, $C_{13}H_{16}N_2O_2$, occurring as a white, crystalline powder; formerly used as an anticonvulsant in epilepsy. It inhibits adrenal cortical secretion, and has been used experimentally in the treatment of secondary hyperaldosteronism and edema.

aminoglycoside (am″ĭ-no-gli-ko′sīd) any of a group of antibacterial antibiotics (e.g., streptomycin and gentamicin), derived from various species of *Streptomyces*, which interfere with the function of bacterial ribosomes. These compounds contain an inositol substituted with two amino or guanidino groups and with one or more sugars and aminosugars.

aminogram (am-i′no-gram) a graphic representation of the pattern of amino acids present in a substance as determined quantitatively.

aminoheterocyclic (am″ĭ-no-het″er-o-sik′lik) having a closed chain or ring formation which includes the —NH₂ group.

aminohippurate (am″ĭ-no-hip′u-rāt) a salt of aminohippuric acid. **a. sodium** [USP], the sodium salt of aminohippuric acid, $C_9H_9N_2NaO_3$, which is injected intravenously for the measurement of effective renal plasma flow and determination of the functional capacity of the tubular excretory mechanism.

aminolevulinate (ah-me″no-lev″u-lin′āt) a salt or dissociated form of 5-aminolevulinic acid (see under *acid*).

aminolipid (ah-me″no-, am″ĭ-no-lip′id) any of a class of fatty substances containing amino nitrogen and fatty acids.

aminolipin (ah-me″no-, am″ĭ-no-li′pin) aminolipid.

aminolysis (am″ĭ-nol′ĭ-sis) [*amine* + Gr. *lysis* dissolution] reaction with an amine, resulting in the addition of (or substitution by) an imino group, —NH—.

aminometradine (ah-me″no-, am″ĭ-no-met′rah-dēn) chemical name: 6-amino-3-ethyl-1-(2-propenyl)-2,4(1*H*,3*H*)-pyrimidinedione; a nonmercurial diuretic for oral administration, $C_9H_{13}N_3O_2$.

aminometramide (ah-me″no-, am″ĭ-no-met′rah-mĭd) aminometradine.

aminonitrogen (ah-me″no-, am″ĭ-no-ni′tro-jen) see under *nitrogen*.

aminonitrothiazole (am″ĭ-no-ni″tro-thi′ah-zōl) chemical name: 2-amino-5-nitrothiazole. A greenish-yellow to orange-yellow fluffy powder, $C_3H_3N_3O_2S$, used in the treatment and prevention of blackhead in turkeys.

aminopentamide sulfate (ah-me″no-, am″ĭ-no-pen′tah-mīd) chemical name: α-[2-(dimethylamino)propyl]-α-phenylbenzeneacetamide sulfate; an anticholinergic, $C_{19}H_{24}N_2OH_2SO_4$, with atropine-like action.

aminopeptidase (ah-me″no-, am″ĭ-no-pep′ti-dās) an exopeptidase that acts on the peptide bond of terminal amino acids possessing a free amino group. **leucine a.,** an enzyme that acts preferentially on peptides in which the free amino group is that of an L-leucine residue; found in all human tissues analyzed, with high activity in the duodenum, liver, and kidney.

aminophenazone (am″ĭ-no-phen′ah-zōn) aminopyrine.

aminopherase (am″ĭ-nof′er-ās) transaminase.

aminophylline (ah-me″no-fil′in) [USP] chemical name: 3,7-dihydro-1,3-dimethyl-1*H*-purine-2,6-dione compound with 1,2-ethanediamine. A salt of theophylline, $C_{16}H_{24}N_{10}O_4$, occurring as white or slightly yellowish granules or powder. Aminophylline is a smooth muscle relaxant and is used chiefly for its bronchodilator effect in such diseases as asthma, bronchitis, and emphysema; administered orally, rectally, or intravenously. It also may be used for its myocardial stimulant and coronary vasodilator actions, diuretic action, and respiratory center stimulant effect. Called also *theophylline ethylenediamide*.

aminopolypeptidase (ah-me″no-, am″ĭ-no-pol″e-pep′tĭ-dās) an enzyme that hydrolyzes polypeptides by cleaving the peptide linkage adjacent to a free amino group.

aminopterin (am″ĭ-nop′ter-in) chemical name: *N*-{p-{[(2,4-diamino-6-pteridinyl)methyl]amino}benzoyl}glutamic acid. An antimetabolite that functions as a folic acid antagonist, $C_{19}H_{20}N_8O_5$, which has been used as an antineoplastic in the treatment of acute leukemia; it also is used as a rodenticide. Called also *aminopteroylglutamic acid*. **a. sodium,** the sodium salt of aminopterin, having the same actions and uses as the base.

aminopurine (ah-me″no-, am″ĭ-no-pu′rin) a purine that is a component of nucleic acid and the nucleotides; the aminopurines include adenine and guanine.

aminopyrine (ah-me″no-, am″ĭ-no-pi′rin) chemical name: 4-(dimethylamino)-1,2-dihydro-1,5-dimethyl-2-phenyl-3*H*-pyrazol-3-one. A pyrazole derivative, $C_{13}H_{17}N_3O$, occurring as a white, bulky powder, which darkens on exposure to light and air. It is an effective analgesic and antipyretic, but is seldom used because it has been associated with cases of fatal agranulocytosis. Called also *amidopyrine* and *aminophenazone*.

aminorex (ah-min′o-reks) chemical name: 4,5-dihydro-5-phenyl-2-oxazoline; a sympathomimetic anorexic, $C_9H_{10}N_2O$.

aminosaccharide (ah-me″no-, am″ĭ-no-sak′ah-rīd) a sugar in which the OH group has been replaced by an amino group, —NH₂.

aminosalicylate (am″ĭ-no-sal″ĭ-sil′-āt) any salt of aminosalicylic acid. The USP preparations, *Aminosalicylate calcium, aminosalicylate potassium,* and *aminosalicylate sodium,* are used as tuberculostatic antibacterials.

aminosidine sulfate (am″ĭ-no-si′din) paromomycin sulfate.

aminosis (am″ĭ-no′sis) the pathologic production of amino acids in the body.

Aminosol (ah-me′no-sol) trademark for an amino acid preparation for intravenous injection.

aminostiburia (ah-me″no-, am″ĭ-no-sti-bu′re-ah) the glycoside of urea stibamine.

aminosuria (ah-me″no-, am″ĭ-no-su′re-ah) [*amine* + Gr. *ouron* urine + *-ia*] an excess of amines in the urine.

Aminosyn (ah-me′no-sin) trademark for a crystalline amino acid solution for intravenous administration; it contains a mixture of essential and nonessential amino acids but no peptides.

aminothiazole (ah-me″no-, am″ĭ-no-thi′ah-zol) chemical name: 2-thiazylamine. A sulfonamide compound, $NH_2 \cdot C$:$N \cdot CH:CH \cdot S$, that has been used in the treatment of hyperthyroidism.

aminotransferase (ah-me″no-, am″ĭ-no-trans′fer-ās) transaminase.

aminotrate (am″ĭ-no-trāt″) the generic name for compounds composed of proteins and vitamins, used as a dietary food supplement. **a. phosphate,** trolnitrate phosphate.

aminuria (am″ĭ-nu′re-ah) an excess of amines in the urine.

amiodarone (ah-me′o-dah-rōn″) a cardiac vasodilator and antiarrhythmic agent.

Amipaque (am′ĭ-pāk) trademark for metrizamide.

amiphenazole hydrochloride (am″ĭ-fen′ah-zōl) chemical name: 2,4-diamino-5-phenylthiazole monohydrochloride; a respiratory stimulant, $C_9H_9N_3S \cdot HCl$, which acts as an antagonist to morphine and other narcotics.

amiquinsin hydrochloride (am″ĭ-kwin′sin) chemical name: 4-amino-6,7-dimethoxyquinoline hydrochloride monohydrate; an antihypertensive agent, $C_{11}H_{12}N_2O_2 \cdot HCl \cdot H_2O$.

amisometradine (am-i″so-met′rah-dēn) chemical name: 6-amino-3-methyl-1-(2-methyl-2-propenyl)-2,4(1*H*,3*H*)-pyrimidinedione. A white crystalline powder, $C_9H_{13}N_3O_2$, used as an oral diuretic.

amithiozone (am″ĭ-thi″ŏ-zōn) thiacetazone.

amitosis (am″ĭ-to′sis) [*a* neg. + Gr. *mitos* thread + *-osis*] direct cell division; cell division by simple cleavage of the nucleus without the formation of spireme (mitotic) spindle figure or chromosomes. Called also *holoschisis.*

amitotic (am″ĭ-tot′ik) of the nature of amitosis; not occurring by mitosis; called also *akinetic.*

amitriptyline hydrochloride (am″ĭ-trip′tĭ-lēn) [USP] chemical name: 3-(10,11-dihydro-5*H*-dibenzo[*a*,*d*]cyclohepten-5-ylidene)-*N*,*N*-dimethyl-1-propanamine hydrochloride. An antidepressant, $C_{20}H_{23}N \cdot HCl$, occurring as a white or practically white, crystalline powder; administered orally or intramuscularly.

ammeter (am′me-ter) [*ampere* + Gr. *metron* measure] an instrument calibrated to read in amperes or subdivisions of amperes the strength of a current flowing in a circuit.

Ammi (am′me) a genus of umbelliferous plants. *A. visna'ga* grows in Mediterranean countries and has been used in the treatment of urethral spasm and renal colic. Fruits of this species contain khellin. **A. ma'jus** (L.) Lam. Khella. (Umbelliferae), a species found in Mediterranean countries that is a source of methoxsalen.

ammoaciduria (am″o-as″ĭ-du′re-ah) an excess of ammonia and amino acids in the urine.

Ammon's filaments, fissure, operation (am′unz) [Friedrich August von *Ammon,* ophthalmologist and pathologist in Dresden, 1799–1861] see under the nouns.

Ammon's horn (am′unz) [*Ammon,* a ram-headed god of the Egyptians] hippocampus.

ammonemia (ah″mo-ne′me-ah) [*ammonia* + Gr. *haima* blood + *-ia*] hyperammonemia.

ammonia (ah-mo′ne-ah) [named from Jupiter *Ammon,* near whose temple in Libya it was formerly obtained] a colorless alkaline gas, NH_3, of a penetrating odor and soluble in water, forming ammonia water; called also *volatile alkali.* **a. hemate,** a compound of ammonia and hematein, used as a violet-black stain for microscopic specimens.

ammoniac (ah-mo′ne-ak) [L. *ammoniacum*] a fetid gum-resin, stimulant and expectorant, from a Persian umbelliferous plant, *Dorema ammoniacum,* used in bronchitis and asthma. Ammoniac plaster and plaster of ammoniac and mercury are used as counterirritants in pleurisy and rheumatism.

ammoniacal (am″o-ni′ah-kal) containing ammonia or treated with excess ammonia.

ammonia-lyase (ah-mo′ne-ah-li′ās) any of a group of lyases that catalyze the removal of ammonia by cleaving a C—N bond. **β-alanyl-CoA a.,** one that catalyzes the conversion of β-alanyl-CoA to acrylyl-CoA and ammonia. **aspartate a.,** an enzyme that catalyzes the conversion of L-aspartate to fumarate and ammonia; called also *aspartase.* **histadine a.,** one that catalyzes the conversion of L-histidine to urocanate and ammonia; called also *histidase.* **methylaspartate a.,** one that catalyzes the conversion of methylaspartate to mesaconate and ammonia. **phenylalanine a.,** one that catalyzes the conversion of L-phenylalanine to *trans*-cinnamate and ammonia.

ammoniate (ah-mo′ne-āt) 1. to treat or to combine with ammonia. 2. the product of combination with ammonia.

ammoniemia (ah-mo″ne-e′me-ah) hyperammonemia.

ammonification (ah-mo″nĭ-fi-ka′shun) the formation of ammonia by the action of bacteria on proteins.

ammonirrhea (am″o-nĭ-re′ah) [*ammonia* + Gr. *rhoia* flow] the excretion of ammonia in the urine or sweat.

ammonium (ah-mo′ne-um) the hypothetical radical, NH₄; it forms salts analogous to those of the alkaline metals. **a. acetate,** a crystal compound with an acetous odor, NH₄C₂H₃O₂, formerly used as a diaphoretic; in veterinary medicine it is used as a diuretic, diaphoretic, antipyretic, and as a vehicle. **a. alum,** see *alum,* def. 1. **a. benzoate,** a white crystalline salt, C₆H₅·CO·ONH₄, stimulant and diuretic. **a. bromide,** a sedative, NH₄Br, occurring as colorless crystals or a yellowish white crystalline powder; used occasionally in treatment of grand mal seizures. See also *bromides.* **a. carbonate,** 1. a white powder, or hard white or translucent masses, with a strong odor of ammonia and a sharp ammoniacal taste. 2. [NF] a compound, (NH₂COONH₄), consisting of ammonium bicarbonate and ammonium carbamate in varying amounts, and yielding between 30 and 34 per cent ammonia; used as a source of ammonia. It is also used as an ingredient of aromatic ammonia spirit and of smelling salts. Called also *sal volatile* or *volatilis.* **a. chloride** [USP], a hygroscopic compound, NH₄Cl, occurring as colorless crystals or as a fine or coarse, white crystalline powder, with a cool saline taste; used as a systemic acidifier. Called also *a. muriate.* **ferric a. citrate, brown,** a preparation containing 16.5 to 18.5 per cent iron, about 9 per cent ammonia, and about 65 per cent hydrated citric acid; formerly used in treatment of iron deficiency anemia. Called also *iron and ammonium citrate.* **ferric a. citrate, green,** a preparation containing 14.5 to 16 per cent iron, about 7.5 per cent ammonia, and about 75 per cent hydrated citric acid; formerly used in treatment of iron deficiency anemia. **a. ferric sulfate, ferric a. sulfate,** pale violet crystals, FeNH₄(SO₄)₂·12H₂O, very soluble in water, used as a reagent. It has also been used as an astringent, styptic, and an *in vitro* diagnostic aid in phenylketonuria. **a. ferric tartrate, ferric a. tartrate,** reddish brown transparent scales used as a hematinic in iron deficiency anemia; called also *iron and ammonium tartrate.* **a. ferrous sulfate, ferrous a. sulfate,** pale bluish green crystals or granules, (NH₄)₂(SO₄)₂·6H₂O, soluble in water, used as a reagent. **a. hypophosphite,** white powder or colorless crystals, NH₄H₂PO₂, formerly used as an expectorant. **a. ichthyolate,** a reddish brown viscous fluid used like ichthammol. **a. ichthyosulfonate,** ichthammol. **a. iodide,** an odorless compound, NH₄I, occurring as minute, colorless, cubic crystals or as a white granular powder, with a sharp salty taste; formerly used as an expectorant. **a. mandelate,** the ammonium salt of mandelic acid, C₈H₁₁NO₃, used orally as a urinary anti-infective. **a. muriate,** a. chloride. **a. nitrate,** a colorless crystalline or white granular compound, NH₄NO₃, readily soluble in water and soluble in 20 parts of alcohol. Used in making nitrous oxide gas; formerly used as a diuretic and urine acidifier. **a. oxalate,** (NH₄)₂C₂O₄ + H₂O; used as a test solution. **a. persulfate,** a colorless crystalline substance, (NH₄)₂S₂O₈; formerly used as a deodorant and disinfectant. **a. phosphate,** a compound occurring in colorless translucent prisms, (NH₄)₂HPO₄ and NH₄H₂PO₄; formerly used in gout and rheumatism. **a. purpurate,** murexide. **a. rhodanilate,** a reagent for proline; it is NH₄[Cr(CNS)₄(C₆H₄·NH₂)₂]. **a. salicylate,** an odorless compound, C₇H₅NH₄O₃, occurring as colorless lustrous prisms or plates, or as a faintly pink crystalline powder; formerly used as an analgesic. **a. sulfoichthyolate,** ichthammol. **a. valerate,** a sedative, CH₃(CH₂)₃COONH₄.

ammoniuria (ah-mo″ne-u′re-ah) [*ammonia* + Gr. *ouron* urine + *-ia*] an excess of ammonia in the urine.

Ammonius (ah-mo′ne-us) (3rd century B.C.) an Alexandrian surgeon who, according to Celsus, devised a lithotrite.

ammonolysis (am″o-nol′ĭ-sis) a process analogous to hydrolysis, but in which ammonia takes the place of water, resulting in attachment of (or replacement by) an amino group, NH₂.

ammonotelic (ah-mo″no-tel′ik) [*ammonia* + Gr. *telikos* belonging to the completion, or end] having ammonia as the chief excretory product of nitrogen metabolism, as in fresh-water fishes.

Ammospermophilus (am″mo-sper-mof′ĭ-lus) a genus (or subgenus) of desert ground squirrels of western North America. **a. leucu′rus,** the desert antelope ground squirrel, which is a natural host of the plague-transmitting flea, *Thrassis francisi.*

ammotherapy (am″o-ther′ah-pe) [Gr. *ammos* sand + *therapeia* healing] (*obs.*) treatment of disease by the sand bath.

amnalgesia (am″nal-je′ze-ah) [*amnesia* + *algesia*] a technique by which all pain and memory of a potentially painful procedure are abolished, involving the use of drugs or, for minor procedures, hypnosis.

amnemonic (am″ne-mon′ik) [*a* neg. + Gr. *mnēmē* a remembrance, record] (*obs.*) pertaining to, characterized by, or causing loss of memory.

amnesia (am-ne′ze-ah) [Gr. *amnēsia* forgetfulness] lack or loss of memory, especially inability to remember past experiences. **anterograde a.,** amnesia for events occurring after the trauma or disease which caused the condition. **auditory a.,** word deafness. **Broca's a.,** inability to remember spoken words. **circumscribed a.,** amnesia with sharply delineated limits in time or with respect to events. **emotional a.,** amnesia which is primarily emotional in origin, as in certain hysterical or dissociative states following intolerable emotional stress. **episodic a.,** amnesia for a particular episode or a small area of experience. **immunologic a.,** the failure of the anamnestic immunologic response to antigens. **infantile a.,** the usual inability to recall the events of the first five or six years of life. **lacunar a.,** loss of memory for certain isolated events only; called also *patchy.* **localized a.,** amnesia for events connected with a certain place, time, or incident. **olfactory a.,** loss of memory for smell. **organic a.,** amnesia secondary to organic defects, damage, or disease. **patchy a.,** lacunar a. **post-hypnotic a.,** a directed forgetfulness of the subject for experiences undergone while he was in the hypnotic state. **retroactive a., retrograde a.,** amnesia for events which occurred before the trauma or disease causing the condition. **tactile a.,** astereognosis. **transient global a.,** an episode of short-term memory loss, usually nonrecurrent, and lasting a few hours, without other signs or symptoms of neurological impairment; the cause is unknown but may involve an ischemic or epileptic attack. **traumatic a.,** amnesia following physical injury; it most often occurs following a blow to the head (concussion). **tropic a., tropical a.,** loss of memory affecting white men in the tropics; a condition once very prevalent on the west coast of Africa, where it was called *coast memory.* **verbal a.,** loss of memory for words. **visual a.,** alexia.

amnesiac (am-ne′se-ak) a person affected with amnesia.

amnesic (am-ne′sik) affected with or characterized by amnesia.

amnésie (am-naze′) [Fr.] amnesia. **a. memoration,** a defect in memorizing.

amnestic (am-nes′tik) 1. amnesic. 2. causing amnesia.

Amnestrogen (am-nes′tro-jen) trademark for a preparation of esterified estrogens.

amnio- [Gr. *amnion* bowl; membrane enveloping the fetus] a combining form denoting relationship to the amnion.

amniocele (am′ne-o-sēl) omphalocele.

amniocentesis (am″ne-o-sen-te′sis) surgical transabdominal perforation of the uterus, to obtain amniotic fluid.

amniochorial (am″ne-o-ko′re-al) pertaining to the amnion and chorion.

Amniocolidae (am″ne-o-kol′ĭ-de) Hydrobiidae.

amniogenesis (am″ne-o-jen′ĕ-sis) [*amnio-* + Gr. *genesis* formation] the development of the amnion.

amniography (am″ne-og′rah-fe) [*amnio-* + Gr. *graphein* to record] roentgenography of the gravid uterus after injection of opaque media into the amniotic fluid, outlining the amniotic cavity and fetus.

amnioma (am″ne-o′mah) [*amnio-* + *-oma*] (*obs.*) a tumor formed from the amnion.

amnion (am′ne-on) [Gr. "bowl"; "membrane enveloping the fetus"] the thin but tough extraembryonic membrane of reptiles, birds, and mammals that lines the chorion and contains the fetus and the amniotic fluid around it; in mammals it is derived from trophoblast by folding or splitting. **a. nodo′sum,** multiple fo-

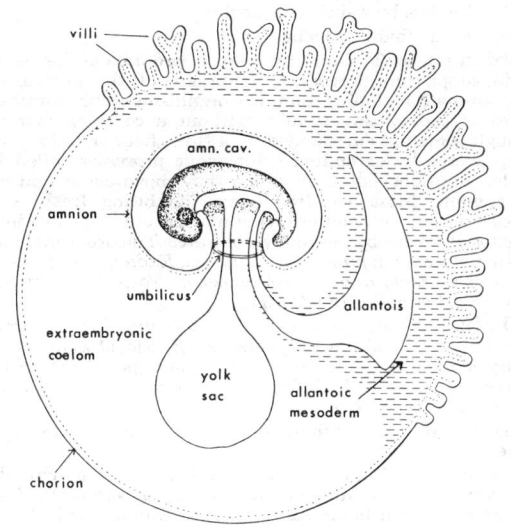

Amnion, chorion, and other embryonic membranes surrounding the embryo of a placental mammal; *amn. cav.* = amniotic cavity. (Balinsky.)

cal lesions of the amnion, consisting of masses of adherent amniotic squamae partially invaded by amniotic mesoderm; a nodular condition of the fetal surface of the amniotic membrane.

amnionic (am″ne-on′ik) amniotic.

amnionitis (am″ne-o-ni′tis) inflammation of the amnion.

Amnioplastin (am-ne-o-plas′tin) trademark for the dried and sterilized amnionic membrane applied to prevent adhesions after craniotomy.

amniorrhea (am″ne-o-re′ah) [*amnion* + Gr. *rhoia* flow] the escape of the amniotic fluid, or liquor amnii.

amniorrhexis (am″ne-o-rek′sis) [*amnion* + Gr. *rhēxis* rupture] rupture of the amnion.

amnioscope (am′ne-o-skōp″) an endoscope that, by passage through the maternal abdominal wall into the amnionic cavity, permits direct visualization of the fetus and the amniotic fluid.

amnioscopy (am″ne-os′ko-pe) direct observation of the fetus and the color and amount of the amniotic fluid by means of a specially designed endoscope inserted through the uterine cervix.

Amniota (am-ne-o′tah) a major group of vertebrates comprising those which develop an amnion, including reptiles, birds, and mammals; opposed to Anamniota.

amniote (am′ne-ōt) any animal or group belonging to the Amniota.

amniotic (am″ne-ot′ik) pertaining to or developing an amnion.

Amniotin (am-ni′o-tin) trademark for estrogens derived from the urine of pregnant mares.

amniotome (am′ne-o-tōm″) [*amnion* + Gr. *tomē* a cutting] an instrument for cutting the fetal membranes.

amniotomy (am″ne-ot′o-me) [*amnion* + Gr. *tomē* a cutting] deliberate rupture of the fetal membranes to induce labor.

amobarbital (am″o-bar′bǐ-tal) [USP] chemical name: 5-ethyl-5-(methylbutyl)-2,4,6(1H,3H,5H)-pyrimidinetrione. An intermediate-acting barbiturate, $C_{11}H_{18}N_2O_3$, occurring as a white, crystalline powder; used orally as a sedative and hypnotic. Called also amylobarbitone and *isoamylethylbarbituric acid*. **a. sodium** [USP], the monosodium salt of ammobarbital, $C_{11}H_{17}N_2NaO_3$, occurring as a white, friable, granular powder; administered orally, intravenously, and intramuscularly as a hypnotic and sedative.

amodiaquine hydrochloride (am″o-di′ah-kwin) [USP] chemical name: 4-[(7-chloro-4-quinolinyl)amino]-2-[(diethylamino)-methyl]-phenol dihydrochloride dihydrate. An antimalarial, $C_{20}H_{22}ClN_3O \cdot 2HCl \cdot 2H_2O$, occurring as a yellow, crystalline powder, whose activity is limited to the asexual erythrocytic forms of plasmodia; administered orally.

Amoeba (ah-me′bah) a genus of amebae of the order Amoebida, class Rhizopoda, including many free-living species found in fresh, salt, and brackish water, and characterized by an extremely flexible membrane covering the body and a vesicular nucleus. Many species once included in this genus are now assigned to other taxonomic catagories. **A. bucca′lis,** *Entamoeba gingivalis.* **A. co′li,** *Entamoeba coli.* **A. denta′lis,** *Entamoeba gingivalis.* **A. dysente′riae** (*obs.*), *Entamoeba histolytica.* **A. histolyt′ica** (*obs.*), *Entamoeba histolytica.* **A. li′max,** *Endolimax nana.* **A. meleag′ridis,** *Histomonas meleagridis.* **A. pro′teus,** a species found in fresh water and widely studied in the laboratory. **A. uri′nae granula′ta,** an ameba-like cell found in the urine in cases of infective jaundice with proteinuria. **A. verruco′sa,** an ameba-like cell having a large knobby nucleus and a deeply staining nucleolus.

amoeba (ah-me′bah) ameba.

Amoebida (ah-me′bǐ-dah) an order of protozoa of the class Rhizopoda, subphylum Sarcodina, comprising all the amebae symbiotic in animals, including man. The organisms occur as unicellular masses of protoplasm, usually without a covering membrane, although some are surrounded by a thin shell, or testa. Amebae change shape by extending cytoplasmic processes called lobose pseudopodia (lobopodia), by which they move about and absorb nourishment. Most are free-living, inhabiting fresh, salt, or brackish water, soil, and decaying matter, but some are internal parasites of invertebrates and vertebrates. The order includes the genera Amoeba, Sappinia, Vahlkampfia, Endamoeba, Entamoeba, Iodamoeba, Endolimax, Dientamoeba, Naegleria, Trimastigamoeba, Hartmanella, and Craigia.

Amoebobacter (ah-me″bo-bak′ter) a genus of microorganisms of the family Thiorhodaceae, suborder Rhodobacteriineae, order Pseudomonadales, made up of cells usually occurring without a common capsule. It includes three species, *A. bacillo′sus*, *A. gran′ula*, and *A. ro′seus.*

Amoebotaenia (ah-me″bo-te′ne-ah) a tapeworm parasitic in chickens.

amok (ah-mok′) [Malay "impulse to murder"] a psychic disturbance seen chiefly in Malaya, the Philippines, and parts of Africa, marked by sudden homicidal mania, screaming, and attacks on people and inanimate objects, tending to result in social retribution and leading to death of the individual.

Amomum (ah-mo′mum) [L.; Gr. *amōmon*] a genus of perennial herbs of the ginger family native to tropical Asia; its seeds are used as a substitute for cardamom (q.v.).

amopyroquin hydrochloride (am-o-pi′ro-kwin) chemical name: 4-[(7-chloro-4-quinolyl)amino]-α-1-pyrrolidinyl-*o*-cresol dihydrochloride; an antimalarial drug.

amor (a′mor) [L.] love. **a. les′bicus** (*obs.*), lesbianism.

amorph (ah′morf) a gene that has no effect on its substrate; an inactive gene.

amorpha (ah-mor′fah) [*a* neg. + Gr. *morphē* form] diseases that evince no definite structural changes.

amorphia (ah-mor′fe-ah) [*a* neg. + Gr. *morphē* form + *-ia*] the fact or quality of being amorphous.

amorphic (ah-mor′fik) amorphous; in genetics, almost completely inactive, as an amorph.

amorphinism (ah-mor′fǐ-nizm) the state produced by depriving a morphine addict of his drug.

amorphism (ah-mor′fizm) amorphia.

amorphous (ah-mor′fus) [*a* neg. + Gr. *morphē* form] having no definite form; shapeless; having no specific orientation of atoms; in pharmacy, not crystallized.

amorphus (ah-mor′fus) [*a* neg. + Gr. *morphē* form] a shapeless monster.

Amoss′ sign (a′mos) [Harold Lindsay *Amoss*, American physician, 1886–1956] see under *sign*.

amotio (ah-mo′she-o) [L.] a removing. **a. ret′inae,** detachment of the retina.

amoxapine (ah-moks′ah-pēn) chemical name: 2-chloro-11-(1-piperazinyl)dibenz[*b,f*][1,4]oxazepine; an antidepressant, $C_{17}H_{16}ClN_3O$.

amoxicillin (ah-moks″ǐ-sil′in) [USP] chemical name: 6-[[amino(4-hydroxyphenyl)acetyl]amino]-3,3-dimethyl-7-oxo-4-thia-1-azabicyclo[3.2.0]heptane-2-carboxylic acid. A semisynthetic derivative of ampicillin, $C_{16}H_{19}N_3O_5S$, effective against a broad spectrum of gram-positive and gram-negative bacteria; used especially in the treatment of infections due to susceptible strains of *Hemophilus influenzae, Escherichia coli, Proteus mirbilis, Neisseria gonorrhoeae,* streptococci (including *S. faecalis* and *S. pneumoniae*), and nonpenicillinase-producing staphylococci. It is administered orally.

Amoxil (ah-moks′il) trademark for a preparation of amoxicillin.

AMP adenosine monophosphate. **cyclic AMP,** adenosine 3′:5′-cyclic phosphate.

amp. ampere.

ampelotherapy (am″pě-lo-ther′ah-pe) [Gr. *ampelos* grape + *therapy*] the therapeutic use of grape products.

amperage (am′per-ij) the strength of an electric current expressed in amperes or milliamperes.

ampere (am′pēr) [André M. *Ampère,* 1775–1836] the unit of electric current in the M.K.S. system of measurement, being the current produced by one volt acting through a resistance of one ohm. The international ampere is the unvarying electrical current which, when passed through a solution of silver nitrate in accordance with certain specifications, deposits silver at the rate of 0.001118 gm. per second. Abbreviated a. or amp.

amphamphoterodiplopia (am″fam-fo″ter-o-dǐ-plo′pe-ah) [Gr. *amphi* on both sides + *amphoteros* both together + *diplopia*] double vision with both eyes together, or with either eye separately.

ampheclexis (am″fě-klek′sis) [Gr. *amphi* on both sides + *eklexis* selection] sexual selection on the part of both male and female.

Amphedroxyn (am″fě-drok′sin) trademark for a preparation of methamphetamine.

amphemerous (am-fem′er-us) (*obs.*) quotidian; occurring daily, as a fever.

amphetamine (am-fet′ah-min) 1. chemical name: (±)-α-methylbenzeneethannine. Racemic amphetamine; a sympathomimetic amine, $C_9H_{13}N$, occurring as a colorless mobile liquid, has a stimulating effect on both the central and peripheral nervous systems. It relaxes both systolic and diastolic blood pressure and bronchial muscle, contracts the sphincter of the urinary bladder, and depresses the appetite. Abuse of this drug and its salts may lead to dependence, characterized by strong psychic dependence, to marked tolerance, and to mild physical dependence associated with tachycardia, increased blood pressure, restlessness, irritability, insomnia, personality changes, and in the severe form of chronic intoxication, psychosis similar to schizophrenia. Abrupt withdrawal can cause severe fatigue, mental depression, and abnormalities in the electroencephalogram. 2. [pl.] a group of closely related compounds having similar actions, including both racemic amphetamine and its salts, dextroamphetamine, and methamphetamine. **a. phosphate,** a white, crystalline powder, $C_9H_{16}NO_4P$, having the same actions and uses as the sulfate salt; administered orally and parenterally. **a. sulfate** [USP], a white, crystalline powder, $C_{18}N_{28}N_2H_2O_4S$, having the same actions as the base, used chiefly for its central stimulant effects in the treatment of mental depression, psychopathic states, narcolepsy, hyperkinetic behavior disorders in children, and exogenous obesity; administered orally. **a. sulfate, dextro,** dextroamphetamine.

amphi- (am′fe) [Gr. *amphi* on both sides] a prefix signifying on both sides; around or about; double.

amphiarkyochrome (am″fe-ar′ke-o-krōm″) [*amphi-* + Gr. *arkys* net + *chrōma* color] a nerve cell, the stainable portion of whose body is a pale network, of which the nodal points are joined by a readily and intensely stainable network.

amphiarthrodial (am″fe-ar-thro′de-al) pertaining to amphiarthrosis.

amphiarthrosis (am″fe-ar-thro′sis) [amphi- + Gr. arthrōsis joint] a form of articulation permitting little motion, the apposed surfaces of bone being connected by fibrocartilage; called also junctura cartilaginea [NA].

amphiaster (am′fe-as″ter) [amphi- + Gr. astēr star] the figure of achromatin fibers formed in karyokinesis, consisting of two asters joined by a spindle; called also diaster.

Amphibia (am-fib′e-ah) [amphi- + Gr. bios life] a class of vertebrate animals that breathe by means of gills in the larval state, but after metamorphosis generally breathe by means of lungs; it includes frogs, toads, newts, and salamanders.

amphibious (am-fib′e-us) [see Amphibia] capable of living both on land and in water.

amphiblastic (am″fe-blas′tik) [amphi- + Gr. blastos germ] denoting the complete but unequal cleavage of a telolecithal egg.

amphiblastula (am″fe-blas′tu-lah) [amphi- + blastula] a blastula with unequal blastomeres.

amphiblestritis (am″fe-bles-tri′tis) [Gr. amphiblēstron net + -itis] retinitis.

amphibolia (am″fe-bo′le-ah) [Gr. amphibolia uncertainty] a term once used to describe the course of an untreatable febrile disease at a stage before its outcome was clear.

amphibolic (am″fe-bol′ik) 1. uncertain; vacillating; of doubtful prognosis. 2. having both a catabolic and an anabolic function.

amphibolous (am-fib′o-lus) [Gr. amphibolos] amphibolic.

amphicarcinogenic (am″fe-kar″sĭ-no-jen′ik) tending, optionally, to increase or to decrease carcinogenic activity.

amphicelous (am″fe-se′lus) [amphi- + Gr. koilos hollow] concave at both ends; a term usually applied to the hollow-ended vertebral centra of certain cold-blooded vertebrates.

amphicentric (am″fe-sen′trik) [amphi- + Gr. kentron center] beginning and ending in the same vessel, as a branch of a rete mirabile.

amphichroic (am″fe-kro′ik) [amphi- + Gr. chrōma color] exhibiting two colors; affecting both red and blue litmus.

amphichromatic (am″fe-kro-mat′ik) amphichroic.

amphicreatine (am″fe-kre′ah-tin) [amphi- + creatine] a leukomaine, $C_9H_{19}N_7O_4$, from muscle, occurring in the form of opaque yellowish white crystals.

amphicreatinine (am″fe-kre-at′ĭ-nin) [amphi- + creatinine] a poisonous leukomaine, $C_9H_{19}N_7O_4$, from muscle.

amphicroic (am″fe-kro′ik) [amphi- + Gr. krouein to test] amphichroic.

amphicyte (am′fe-sīt) [amphi- + Gr. kytos hollow vessel] a satellite cell, def. 1.

amphicytula (am″fe-sit′u-lah) [amphi- + cytula] a fertilized telolecithal ovum.

amphidiarthrosis (am″fe-di″ar-thro′sis) [amphi- + diarthrosis] a joint having the nature of both a ginglymus and arthrodia, as the articulation of the lower jaw.

amphidiploid (am″fe-dip′loid) allotetraploid.

amphigastrula (am″fe-gas′tru-lah) [amphi- + gastrula] a gastrula composed of cells unequal in size in its upper and lower hemispheres.

amphigenetic (am″fe-jĕ-net′ik) produced by means of both sexes, as amphigenetic reproduction.

amphigonadism (am″fe-gon′ah-dizm) possession of both ovarian and testicular tissue; true hermaphroditism.

amphigonium (am″fe-go′ne-um) [amphi- + Gr. gonos generation] (obs.) that stage of the life of a malaria parasite which is passed in the mosquito.

amphigony (am-fig′o-ne) sexual reproduction.

amphikaryon (am″fe-kar′e-on) [amphi- + Gr. karyon kernel] a diploid nucleus.

Amphileptus (am″fe-lep′tus) a genus of ciliate protozoa, most species of which are free-living. **A. branchia′rum,** a ciliate parasite on the gills of frog tadpoles.

amphileukemic (am″fe-lu-ke′mik) [amphi- + leukemic] showing leukemic changes which vary in degree with the changes in the organ.

Amphimerus (am-fim′er-us) a genus of trematodes. A. nover′ca is a biliary-duct parasite of dogs and foxes and occasionally of hogs and man. A. pseudofelin′eus infects cats and coyotes in the central United States.

amphimicrobian (am″fe-mi-kro′be-an) [amphi- + microbe] (obs.) see facultative aerobes, under aerobe.

amphimorula (am″fe-mor′u-lah) [amphi- + morula] the morula resulting from unequal cleavage, the cells of the two hemispheres being of unequal size.

amphinucleus (am″fe-nu′kle-us) [amphi- + nucleus] a nucleus that consists of a single body made of spindle fibers and centrosome, around which the chromatin is massed; it is the ordinary form of protozoan nucleus. Called also centronucleus.

Amphioxus (am″fe-ok′sus) a primitive fishlike marine chordate, considered similar to the ancestor of the vertebrates.

amphipath (am′fe-path) a molecule showing amphipathic properties.

amphipathic (am″fe-path′ik) of or relating to molecules containing groups with characteristically different properties, e.g., both hydrophilic and hydrophobic properties.

amphipyrenin (am″fe-pi′re-nin) [amphi- + Gr. pyrēn stone of a fruit] the substance of the nuclear membrane of a cell.

Amphistoma, Amphistomum (am-fis′to-mah, am-fis′to-mum) [amphi- + Gr. stoma mouth] a genus of parasitic trematode worms, many species of which have been reassigned to other genera. **A. con′icum,** Paramphistomum cervi. **A. hom′inis,** Gastrodiscoides hominis. **A. watso′ni,** Watsonius watsoni.

amphistome (am-fis′tōm) a fluke having the ventral sucker near the posterior end, usually found in the rumen or intestine of herbivorous mammals. The genera Paramphistomum and Watsonius include most of the medically important amphistomes.

amphistomiasis (am″fe-sto-mi′ah-sis) the condition of being infected with trematodes of the genus Amphistoma or of the family Paramphistomidae.

amphitene (am′fĕ-tēn) zygotene.

amphitheater (am″fe-the′ah-ter) an operating room or lecture room with seats arranged in tiers for students or spectators.

amphithymia (am″fe-thi′me-ah) [amphi- + Gr. thymos spirit + -ia] (obs.) a mental state characterized by both depression and elation.

amphitrichous (am-fit′rĕ-kus) [amphi- + Gr. thrix hair] having a single flagellum, or a single tuft of flagella, at each end; said of a bacterial cell. See flagellum.

amphitypy (am-fit′ĭ-pe) the condition of showing both types.

ampho- (am′fo) [Gr. amphō both] a prefix signifying both.

amphochromatophil (am″fo-kro-mat′o-fil) 1. amphophil. 2. amphophilic.

amphochromophil (am″fo-kro′mo-fil) [ampho- + Gr. chrōma color + philein to love] 1. amphophil. 2. amphophilic.

amphocyte (am′fo-sīt) an amphophilic cell.

amphodiplopia (am″fo-dĭ-plo′pe-ah) [ampho- + diplopia] double vision in both eyes.

amphogenic (am″fo-jen′ik) [ampho- + Gr. gennan to produce] producing offspring of both sexes.

Amphojel (am′fo-jel) trademark for a preparation of aluminum hydroxide gel.

ampholyte (am′fo-līt) [ampho- + electrolyte] an amphoteric electrolyte.

amphomycin (am-fo-mi′sin) an antibiotic substance produced by Streptomyces canus.

amphophil (am′fo-fil) 1. a cell that stains readily with acid or basic dyes; an amphophilic cell. Called also amphochromatophil and amphochromophil. 2. amphophilic.

amphophile (am′fo-fīl″) denoting cells of the adenohypophysis that are thought to be actively secreting: the lightly granulated acidophils and basophils.

amphophilic (am-fo-fil′ik) [ampho- + Gr. philein to love] stainable with either acid or basic dyes. **a.-basophil,** staining with both acid and basic stains, but having a greater affinity for basic ones. **gram-a.,** tending to stain both positive and negative with Gram stain. **a.-oxyphil,** staining with both acid and basic dyes, but having a greater affinity for the acid ones.

amphophilous (am-fof′i-lus) amphophilic.

amphoric (am-for′ik) [L. amphoricus, from L. amphora, Gr. amphoreus jar] pertaining to a bottle; resembling the sound made by blowing across the mouth of a bottle, particularly such a sound resulting from percussion or a breath sound heard over a cavity in the lung.

amphoricity (am″fo-ris′ĭ-te) the condition of giving off amphoric sounds on percussion or auscultation.

amphoriloquy (am″fo-ril′o-kwe) [L. amphora jar + loqui to speak] the production of amphoric sounds in speaking.

amphorophony (am″fo-rof′o-ne) [Gr. amphoreus jar + phonē voice] an amphoric sound of the voice.

amphoteric (am-fo-ter′ik) [Gr. amphoteros pertaining to both] having opposite characters; capable of acting either as an acid or as a base; combining with both acids and bases; affecting both red and blue litmus.

amphotericin B (am″fo-ter′ĭ-sin) [USP] one of two antifungal antibiotics, the other designated amphotericin A (not used clinically), derived from a strain of Streptomyces nodosus, $C_{47}H_{73}NO_{17}$; administered by intravenous infusion in the treatment of systemic fungal infections, such as aspergillosis, histoplasmosis, cryptococcosis, coccidioidomycosis, etc. It may also be applied topically to the skin in lotion or cream in the treatment of candidiasis and related infections.

amphotericity (am″fo-ter-is′ĭ-te) amphoterism.

amphoterism (am-fo′ter-izm) the condition or quality of possessing both basic and acid properties.

amphoterodiplopia (am-fot″er-o-dĭ-plo′pe-ah) [Gr. *amphoteros* pertaining to both + *diplopia*] amphodiplopia.

amphoterous (am-fot′er-us) amphoteric.

amphotony (am-fot′o-ne) [*ampho-* + Gr. *tonos* tension] a condition in which both sympathicotonia and vagotony is said to exist; hypertonia of the entire sympathetic nervous system.

ampicillin (amp″ĭ-sil′in) [USP] chemical name: [2S-[2α,5α-6β(S*)]][(aminophenylacetyl)amino]-3,3-dimethyl-7-oxo-4-thia-1-azabicyclo[3.2.0]heptane-2-carboxylic acid. A semisynthetic, acid-resistant penicillin, $C_{16}H_{19}N_3O_4S$, occurring as a white, crystalline powder, effective orally against many gram-negative and gram-positive bacteria; used mainly in the treatment of infections of the urinary tract and urinary system, and in chronic bronchial infections, especially those due to susceptible strains of *Shigella, Salmonella, Escherichia coli, Hemophilus influenzae, Proteus mirabilis,* and *Neisseria gonorrhoeae.* **a. sodium** [USP], **sodium a.,** the monosodium salt of ampicillin, $C_{16}H_{18}N_3$-NaO_4S, having the same actions and uses as the base; administered intramuscularly or intravenously.

amplexation (am″plek-sa′shun) [L. *amplexus* embrace] treatment of fractured clavicle by an apparatus which fixes the shoulder and embraces the chest and neck.

amplexus (am-plek′sus) [L.] an embrace, as in the sexual clasping of the female by the male frog; see *pseudocopulation.*

amplification (am″plĭ-fĭ-ka′shun) [L. *amplifica′tio*] the process of making larger, as the increase of an auditory or visual stimulus, as a means of improving its perception. **image a.,** amplification of an image by means of an electron-image or electron multiplier tube.

amplifier (am′plĕ-fi″er) an electronic device that increases the strength of an input signal, or an apparatus for increasing the magnification of a microscope.

amplitude (am′plĕ-tūd) [L. *amplitudo*] largeness or fullness; wideness or breadth of range or extent. **a. of accommodation,** the total amount of accommodative power of the eye; the difference in refractive power of the eye when adjusted for farthest vision and that when adjusted for nearest vision. **a. of convergence,** the difference in the power required to turn the eyes from their far point to their near point of convergence.

ampoule (am′pūl) ampule.

amprotropine phosphate (am″pro-tro′pēn) chemical name: α-(hydroxymethyl)benzeneacetic acid 3-(diethylamino)-2,2-dimethylpropyl ester phosphate. An anticholinergic, $C_{18}N_{32}NO_7$, occurring as a white, crystalline powder, which has been used as a spasmolytic to depress gastrointestinal motility.

ampul (am′pūl) ampule.

ampule (am′pūl) [Fr. *ampoule*] a small glass or plastic container capable of being sealed so as to preserve its contents in a sterile condition; used principally for containing sterile parenteral solutions.

ampulla (am-pul′lah), pl. *ampul′lae* [L. "a jug"] a general term used in anatomical nomenclature to designate a flasklike dilatation of a tubular structure. **anterior membranaceous a.,** a. membranacea anterior. **a. canalic′uli lacrima′lis** [NA], ampulla of lacrimal canaliculus: a dilatation of a lacrimal canaliculus just before it opens into the lacrimal sac; called also *a. ductus lacrimalis.* **a. chy′li,** cisterna chyli. **a. duc′tus deferen′tis** [NA], the enlarged and tortuous distal end of the ductus deferens; called also *Henle's a.* and *a. of vas deferens.* **a. duct′us lacrima′lis,** a. canaliculi lacrimalis. **Henle's a.,** a. ductus deferentis. **hepatopancreatic a., a. hepatopancreat′ica** [NA], the dilatation formed by junction of the common bile and the pancreatic duct proximal to their opening into the lumen of the duodenum; called also *a. of Vater.* **a. of lacrimal canaliculis,** a. canaliculi lacrimalis. **ampul′lae lactif′erae,** sinus lactiferi. **lateral membranaceous a.,** a. membranacea lateralis. **Lieberkühn's a.,** the termination of a lacteal in an intestinal villus. **ampul′lae membrana′ceae** [NA], membranaceous ampullae: the dilatations at one end of each of the three membranous semicircular ducts, each named according to the duct of which it forms a part. **a. membrana′cea ante′rior** [NA], anterior membranaceous ampulla: the dilatation at the end of the anterior membranous semicircular duct. **a. membrana′cea latera′lis** [NA], lateral membranaceous ampulla: the dilatation at the end of the lateral membranous semicircular duct. **a. membrana′cea poste′rior** [NA], posterior membranaceous ampulla: the dilatation at the end of the posterior membranous semicircular duct. **ampul′lae os′seae** [NA], osseous ampullae: the dilatations at one of the ends of the bony semicircular canals, each named according to the canal of which it forms a part, and lodging the correspondingly named ampulla of a semicircular duct. **a. os′sea ante′rior** [NA], the dilatation at one end of the anterior semicircular canal; see *ampullae osseae.* **a. os′sea latera′lis** [NA], the dilatation at one end of the lateral semicircular canal; see *ampullae osseae.* **a. os′sea poste′rior** [NA], the dilatation at one end of the posterior semicircular canal; see *ampullae osseae.* **phrenic a.,** the dilatation at the lower end of the

esophagus. **posterior membranaceous a.,** a. membranacea posterior. **rectal a., a. rec′ti** [NA], the dilated portion of the rectum just proximal to the anal canal. **a. of Thoma,** one of the small terminal expansions of an interlobar artery in the pulp of the spleen. **a. tu′bae uteri′nae** [NA], a. of uterine tube: the thin-walled, almost muscle-free, midregion of the uterine tube; its mucosa is greatly plicated. **a. of uterine tube,** a. tubae uterinae. **a. of vas deferens,** a. ductus deferentis. **a. of Vater,** a. hepatopancreatica.

ampullae (am-pul′le) [L.] plural of *ampulla.*

ampullar (am-pul′ar) pertaining to an ampulla, especially to the ampulla hepatopancreatica.

ampullary (am′pu-la″re) ampullar.

ampullate (am-pul′āt) flask shaped.

ampullitis (am″pul-li′tis) inflammation of an ampulla, especially of the ampulla ductus deferentis.

ampullula (am-pul′u-lah) [L.] any minute ampulla, like many of those of the lymphatic and lacteal vessels.

amputation (am″pu-ta′shun) [L. *amputare* to cut off, or to prune] the removal of a limb or other appendage or outgrowth of the body; called also *apocope.* **Alanson's a.,** circular amputation, the stump being shaped like a hollow cone. **Alouette's a.,** amputation at the hip, with a semicircular outer flap to the great trochanter and a large internal flap from within outward; called also *Alouette's operation.* **amniotic a.,** the alleged amputation of a fetal limb by a band of amnion. **aperiosteal a.,** amputation with complete removal of the periosteum from the end of the stump of the bone; called also *Bunge's a.* **Béclard's a.,** amputation at the hip joint by cutting the posterior flap first. **Bier's a.,** osteoplastic amputation of the leg with a bone flap cut out of the tibia and fibula above the stump; called also *Bier's operation.* **Bunge's a.,** aperiosteal a. **Callander's a.,** a tendoplastic amputation at the knee joint with long anterior and posterior flaps, the patella being removed to leave a fossa for the end of the divided femur. **Carden's a.,** a single-flap operation, cutting through the femur just above the knee. **central a.,** one in which the scar is situated at or near the center of the stump. **chop a.,** amputation by a circular cut through the parts without the formation of a flap. **Chopart's a.,** amputation of the foot, with the calcaneus, talus, and other parts of the tarsus being retained; called also *mediotarsal a.* **cinematic a., cineplastic a.,** kineplasty. **circular a.,** one performed by means of a single flap and by a circular cut in a direction vertical to the long axis of a limb. **closed a.,** one in which flaps are made from the skin and subcutaneous tissue and sutured over the end of the bone; called also *flap a.* **coat-sleeve a.,** a circular amputation, with a single skin flap made very long, the end being closed with a tape. **complete a.,** amputation in which the entire limb or segment of the limb is removed. **congenital a.,** the alleged amputation of a fetal limb *in utero* by a constricting band; called also *intrauterine a.* and *natural a.* **consecutive a.,** amputation performed during or after the period of suppuration. **a. in contiguity,** an amputation at a joint. **a. in continuity,** an amputation elsewhere than at a joint. **cutaneous a.,** amputation in which the flaps are composed entirely of skin. **diaclastic a.,** an amputation in which the bone is broken by the osteoclast and the soft tissues divided by the écraseur. **Dieffenbach's a.,** see under *operation,* def. 1. **double-flap a.,** one in which two flaps are formed. **Dupuytren's a.,** amputation of the arm at the shoulder joint; called also *Lisfranc's a.* **eccentric a.,** one in which the scar is not at the center of the stump. **elliptic a.,** one in which the cut has an elliptic outline on account of the oblique direction of the incision. **Farabeuf's a.,** amputation of the leg at the "place of choice," with a large external flap. **flap a.,** closed a. **flapless a.,** guillotine a. **Forbe's a.,** a foot amputation which retains the calcaneus, astragalus, scaphoid, and a part of the cuboid bones. **forequarter a.,** interscapulothoracic a. **galvanocaustic a.,** one in which the soft parts are divided with the galvanocautery. **Gritti's a.,** amputation of the leg through the knee, using the patella as an osteoplastic flap over the end of the femur. **Gritti-Stokes a.,** a modification of Gritti's amputation, using an oval anterior flap; called also *Stoke's a.* or *operation.* **guillotine a.,** rapid amputation of a limb by a circular sweep of the knife and a cut of the saw, the entire cross-section being left open for dressing; done when primary closure of the stump is contraindicated, owing to the possibility of recurrent or developing infection. Called also *flapless a.* and *open a.* **Guyon's a.,** amputation above the malleoli. **Hancock's a.,** a modification of Pirogoff's amputation, a part of the astragalus (talus) being retained in the flap, the lower surface being sawed off, and the cut surface of the calcaneus being brought into contact with it; called also *Hancock's operation.* **Hey's a.,** disarticulation of the metatarsus from the tarsus, with removal of a part of the medial cuneiform bone; called also *Hey's operation.* **hindquarter a.,** interilioabdominal a. **immediate a.,** one performed within hours after the injury which made it necessary. **interilioabdominal a., interinnominoabdominal a.,** amputation of an entire lower limb, including the whole or part of the hip bone; called also *hindquarter a.* **intermediary a., intermediate a.,** one done during the period of reaction and before suppuration;

called also *intrapyretic a.* and *mediate a.* **interpelviabdominal a.,** amputation of the thigh with excision of the lateral half of the pelvis; called also *Jaboulay's a.* or *operation.* **interscapulothoracic a.,** amputation of the upper extremity, including the scapula and the clavicle; called also *forequarter a.* **intrapyretic a.,** intermediary a. **intrauterine a.,** congenital a. **Jaboulay's a.,** interpelviabdominal a. **kineplastic a.,** kineplasty. **Kirk's a.,** a tendoplastic amputation just above the femoral condyles, the tendon of the quadriceps femoris muscle being sutured over the end of the divided femur. **Langenbeck's a.,** amputation in which the flaps are cut from without inward. **Larrey's a.,** a method of disarticulation of the humerus at the shoulder joint by an incision extending from the acromion about three inches down the arm, splitting the deltoid muscle, and from this point going around the arm to the center of the axilla; called also *Larrey's operation.* **Le Fort's a.,** a modification of Pirogoff's amputation in which the calcaneus is sawed through horizontally instead of vertically. **linear a.,** amputation by a simple straight division of all the tissues. **Lisfranc's a.,** Dupuytren's a. 2. a division of the foot between the tarsus and the metatarsus. **MacKenzie's a.,** amputation like that of Syme except that the flap is taken from the inner side of the ankle. **Maisonneuve's a.,** amputation by breaking the bone, followed by cutting of the soft parts. **major a.,** amputation of a leg above the ankle or of an arm above the wrist. **Malgaigne's a.,** subastragalar a. **mediate a.,** intermediary a. **mediotarsal a.,** Chopart's a. **minor a.,** amputation of a small part, as of a finger or toe. **mixed a.,** that which is performed by a combination of the circular and flap methods. **multiple a.,** amputation of two or more parts at the same time. **musculocutaneous a.,** one in which the flap consists of muscle and skin. **natural a.,** congenital a. **oblique a.,** oval a. **open a.,** guillotine a. **operative a.,** removal of a part by surgery. **osteoplastic a.,** one in which the two severed surfaces of bone are brought into contact so as to unite. **oval a.,** one in which the incision consists of two reversed spirals; called also *oblique a.* and *loxotomy.* **partial a.,** amputation of only a portion or segment of a limb. **pathological a.,** amputation of a part because of its diseased condition. **periosteoplastic a.,** subperiosteal a. **phalangophalangeal a.,** amputation of a digit at a phalangeal joint. **Pirogoff's a.,** amputation of the foot at the ankle, part of the calcaneus being left in the lower end of the stump. **primary a.,** one performed after the period of shock and before the development of inflammation. **pulp a.,** pulpotomy. **quadruple a.,** amputation of all four extremities. **racket a.,** one in which there is a single longitudinal incision continuous below with a spiral incision on each side of the limb. **rectangular a.,** one with a long and a short rectangular skin flap, as in Teale's amputation. **Ricard's a.,** intertibiocalcaneal disarticulation, astragalectomy, and the placing of the calcaneus in the tibiofibular mortise. **root a.,** the removal of one or more roots from a multirooted tooth, leaving at least one root to support the crown; when only the apical portion of a root is involved, it is called *apicoectomy.* **secondary a.,** one performed during the period of healing of a granulative surface. **spontaneous a.,** loss of a part which occurs without surgical intervention, as in leprosy, diabetes mellitus, and Buerger's disease. **Stokes's a.,** Gritti-Stokes a. **subastragalar a.,** amputation of the foot, leaving the astragalus (talus) in the lower end of the stump; called also *Malgaigne's a.* **subperiosteal a.,** one in which the cut end of the bone is covered with a flap of periosteum; called also *periosteoplastic a.* **Syme's a.,** amputation of the foot at the ankle joint with removal of both malleoli; called also *Syme's operation.* **synchronous a.,** multiple amputation, especially multiple amputation in which two or more parts are removed simultaneously by different operators. **Teale's a.,** amputation with preservation of a long rectangular flap of muscle and integument on one side of the limb and a short rectangular flap on the other. **tertiary a.,** amputation done after the secondary stage of inflammatory reaction has subsided. **a. by transfixion,** one performed by thrusting a long knife through the limb and cutting the flaps from within outward. **traumatic a.,** amputation of a part by accidental injury. **Tripier's a.,** one like Chopart's, except that a part of the tarsus is removed. **triple a.,** amputation of three extremities. **Vladimiroff-Mikulicz a.,** osteoplastic resection of the foot with incision of the calcaneus and talus.

amputee (am″pu-te′) a person who has one or more of his limbs amputated.

amrinone (am′rĭ-nōn) chemical name: 5-amino-[3,4′-bipyridin]-6(1*H*)-one; an oral cardiotonic, $C_{10}H_9N_3O$.

A.M.R.L. Aerospace Medical Research Laboratories.

A.M.S. American Meteorological Society.

ams. *amount of a substance.*

Amsler's marker (am′slerz) a form of caliper compass used for marking with a dot of India ink the point for the application of the cautery in the Gonin operation.

Amsustain (am′sus-tān) trademark for a preparation of dextroamphetamine.

amu atomic mass unit.

amuck (ah-muk′) amok.

amusia (ah-mu′ze-ah) [Gr. *amousia* want of harmony] inability to produce (*motor a.*) or to comprehend (*sensory a., tone deafness*) musical sounds (Knoblunch). **instrumental a.,** that in which the patient has lost the power of playing a musical instrument. **vocal motor a.,** that in which the patient cannot sing in tune.

Amussat's operation, probe, valve (am″oo-sahz′) [Jean Zuléma *Amussat,* French surgeon, 1796–1856] see under *operation* and *probe.*

A.M.W.A. American Medical Women's Association; American Medical Writers' Association.

amyasthenia (ah-mi″as-the′ne-ah) amyosthenia.

amyasthenic (ah-mi″as-then′ik) amyosthenic.

amychophobia (ah-mi″ko-fo′be-ah) [Gr. *amychē* a scratch + *phobia*] morbid fear of being scratched, as by the claws of a cat.

amyctic (ah-mik′tik) caustic or irritating.

amyelencephalia (ah-mi″el-en-seh-fa′le-ah) [*a* neg. + Gr. *myelos* marrow + *enkephalos* brain + *-ia*] congenital absence of both brain and spinal cord.

amyelencephalus (ah-mi″el-en-sef′ah-lus) a monster exhibiting amyelencephalia.

amyelia (ah″mi-e′le-ah) [*a* neg. + Gr. *myelos* marrow + *-ia*] congenital absence of spinal cord.

amyelic (ah″mi-el′ik) having no spinal cord.

amyelinic (ah-mi″ĕ-lin′ik) without myelin; having no medullary sheath.

amyelonic (ah-mi″ĕ-lon′ik) [*a* neg. + Gr. *myelos* marrow] 1. having no spinal cord. 2. having no bone marrow.

amyelotrophy (ah-mi″ĕ-lot′ro-fe) [*a* neg. + Gr. *myelos* marrow + *trophē* nourishment] atrophy of the spinal cord.

amyelus (ah-mi′e-lus) [*a* neg. + Gr. *myelos* marrow] a monster exhibiting amyelia.

amygdala (ah-mig′dah-lah) [Gr. *amygdalē* almond] a term used in anatomical nomenclature to designate an almond-shaped structure; often used alone to refer to the corpus amygdaloideum (see under *corpus*). **a. accesso′ria, accessory a.,** tonsilla lingualis. **a. ama′ra,** the bitter almond; see *almond.* **a. of cerebellum,** tonsilla cerebelli. **a. dul′cis,** the sweet almond of many varieties; see *almond.*

amygdalase (ah-mig′dah-lās) an enzyme that splits amygdalose.

amygdalin (ah-mig′dah-lin) chemical name: (*R*)-α-[(6-*O*-β-glucopyranosyl-β-D-glucopyranosyl)oxy]benzeneacetonitrile. A cyanogenic glycoside, $C_6H_5CH(CN)\cdot O\cdot C_{12}H_{21}O_{10}$, characteristically found in seeds and other plant parts of members of the Rosaceae family, e.g., almonds. It is split by the enzyme emulsin into glucose, benzaldehyde, and hydrocyanic acid. The term is sometimes used interchangeably with *Laetrile.*

amygdaline (ah-mig′dah-lin″) [L. *amygdalinus*] 1. like an almond. 2. pertaining to a tonsil; tonsillar.

amygdalo- (ah-mig′dah-lo) [Gr. *amygdalē* almond] a combining form denoting relationship to an almond-shaped structure or to the tonsil.

amygdaloid (ah-mig′dah-loid) [*amygdalo-* + Gr. *eidos* form] resembling an almond, or tonsil.

amygdalophenin (ah-mig″dah-lof′ĕ-nin) salicyl phenetidin, $C_6H_4(OC_2H_5)NH\cdot OC\cdot CH(OH)C_6H_5$.

amygdalose (ah-mig′dah-los) a disaccharide from amygdalin; it splits into two molecules of dextrose.

amyl (am′il) [Gr. *amylon* starch] the univalent radical, C_5H_{11}. **a. acetate,** a colorless limpid liquid, the acetic acid ester of amyl alcohol, $CH_3\cdot CO\cdot OC_5H_{11}$; it has the odor of bananas and is called *banana oil.* **a. chloride,** the colorless liquid, $C_5H_{11}Cl$, used as a solvent; formerly used as an anesthetic. **a. nitrite** [USP], a flammable, clear, yellowish liquid, $C_5H_{11}NO_2$, with a peculiar, ethereal, fruity odor, which is volatile at low temperatures; it is a vasodilator, administered by inhalation to relieve pain of anginal syndrome (angina pectoris, angina of effort) and of biliary colic, to relieve asthmatic paroxysms, to control convulsions, and in cyanide poisoning. Called also *isoamyl nitrite.* **a. salicylate,** a compound, $C_5H_{11}\cdot O_2C\cdot C_6H_4\cdot OH$, formerly used locally as an analgesic.

amylaceous (am″ĭ-la′she-us) [L. *amylaceus*] starchy; containing starch; of the nature of starch.

amylase (am′ĭ-lās) [*amyl* + *-ase*] an enzyme that catalyzes the hydrolysis of starch into smaller molecules. The α-amylases are found in animals and include salivary amylase and pancreatic amylase; the β-amylases are found in higher plants. α-Amylases act in a random manner in catalyzing the hydrolysis of α-1,4-glucan links in polysaccharides. **pancreatic a.,** the α-amylase of the pancreas. **salivary a.,** α-amylase occurring in the saliva.

amylasuria (am″ĭ-lās-u′re-ah) an excess of amylase in the urine, a sign of pancreatitis.

amylatic (am-ĭ-lat′ik) characterized by conversion of starch into sugar.

Amylcaine Hydrochloride (am″il-kān hi″dro-klo′rīd) trademark for a preparation of naepaine.

amylemia (am″ĭ-le′me-ah) [Gr. *amylon* starch + *haima* blood + *-ia*] an excess of starch in the blood.

amylene (am′ĭ-lēn) chemical name: 2-methyl-2-butene. A flammable liquid hydrocarbon of five isomeric forms, C_5H_{10}, practically insoluble in water and miscible with alcohol and ether. It is an unsafe anesthetic. **a. chloral,** an oily colorless liquid, composed of chloral and amylene hydrate; formerly used as a hypnotic. **a. hydrate** [NF], chemical name: 2-methyl-2-butanol. A clear colorless liquid, with camphoraceous odor, $C_2H_5 \cdot C(CH_3)_2OH$; miscible with alcohol, chloroform, ether, and glycerin, it is used as a solvent in pharmaceutical preparations and also as an ingredient of *tribromoethanol solution* and as a hypnotic. Called also *a. alcohol.*

amylenization (am″ĭ-len-i-za′shun) anesthesia produced by amylene.

amylic (ah-mil′ik) [L. *amylicus*] pertaining to amyl.

amylin (am′ĭ-lin) amylopectin.

amylism (am′ĭ-lizm) poisoning by amylene hydrate.

amylo- (am′ĭ-lo) [Gr. *amylon* starch] a combining form denoting relationship to starch.

amylobarbitone (am″ĭ-lo-bar′bĭ-tōn) amobarbital.

amylocellulose (am″ĭ-lo-sel′u-lōs) amylose, def. 2.

amyloclast (am′ĭ-lo-klast″) a starch-splitting enzyme.

amyloclastic (am″ĭ-lo-klas′tik) [*amylo-* + Gr. *klastikos* breaking up] digesting or splitting up starch.

amylocoagulase (am″ĭ-lo-ko-ag′u-lās) a ferment occurring in cereals which coagulates soluble starch.

amylodextrin (am″ĭ-lo-deks′trin) a compound colored yellow by iodine, formed during the change of starch into sugar.

amylodyspepsia (am″ĭ-lo-dis-pep′se-ah) [*amylo-* + *dyspepsia*] inability to digest starch-containing foods.

amylogen (ah-mil′o-jen) amylose, def. 2.

amylogenesis (am″ĭ-lo-jen′ĕ-sis) [*amylo-* + Gr. *gennan* to produce] the formation of starch.

amylogenic (am″ĭ-lo-jen′ik) producing starch.

amylo-1,6-glucosidase (am″ĭ-lo-glu-ko′sĭ-dās) dextrin-1,6-glucosidase.

amylohemicellulose (am″ĭ-lo-hem″e-sel′u-lōs) a polysaccharide found in the cell wall of plants; it is much like the amylose of starch in that it is insoluble in water and stains blue with iodine.

amylohydrolysis (am″ĭ-lo-hi-drol′ĭ-sis) hydrolysis of starch; amylolysis.

amyloid (am′ĭ-loid) [*amylo-* + Gr. *eidos* form] 1. resembling starch; characterized by a starchlike formation. 2. an abnormal complex material, most probably a glycoprotein, the exact biochemical composition of which has not been defined. Its protein component may be related to the immunoglobulins (gamma globulins), and it bears only a superficial resemblance to starch. 3. a substance produced by the action of sulfuric acid on cellulose; it gives a blue color when treated with iodine.

amyloidemia (am″ĭ-loi-de′me-ah) the presence of amyloid in the blood.

amyloidosis (am″ĭ-loi-do′sis) the accumulation of amyloid in various body tissues, which, when advanced, engulfs and obliterates parenchymal cells and thus injures the affected organ. The disorder is divided, mainly for descriptive purposes, into the following categories: (1) primary, (2) secondary, (3) familial, (4) associated with multiple myeloma, and (5) associated with familial Mediterranean fever. **a., Andrade type,** see *hereditary neuropathic a.* **cutaneous a., a. cu′tis,** amyloid degeneration of the skin characterized by an eruption of papules, nodules, plaques, or pigmentation, usually associated with itching. Called also *gammaloidosis.* See also *lichen amyloidosus.* **hereditary neuropathic a.,** hereditary amyloidosis affecting the peripheral nerves, characterized by paresthesias, sharp pains, and diminished sensitivity to pain. In the Andrade or Portuguese form, the manifestations are predominantly in the legs, but vitreous opacities are frequent. In the Indiana form, they are predominantly in the upper limbs, with carpal tunnel syndrome the characteristic feature. Both forms are autosomal dominant traits. **a., Indiana type,** see *hereditary neuropathic a.* **lichenoid a.,** lichen amyloidosus. **pericollagen a.,** amyloidosis in which the amyloid is originally deposited along collagen fibers. **perireticulin a.,** amyloidosis in which the amyloid is originally deposited along reticular fibers. **a., Portuguese type,** see *hereditary neuropathic a.* **primary a.,** that with no antecedent or coexisting disease, producing depositions chiefly in mesodermal tissue, including the cardiovascular system. **secondary a.,** that following some chronic destructive disease such as tuberculosis, osteomyelitis, etc., and producing depositions in parenchymal organs (kidney, spleen, liver, etc.) **senile a.,** amyloidosis of the elderly, most frequently affecting the heart.

amylolysis (am″ĭ-lol′ĭ-sis) [*amylo-* + Gr. *lysis* solution] the digestion and disintegration of starch, or its conversion into sugar; called also *amylohydrolysis.*

amylolytic (am″ĭ-lo-lit′ik) pertaining to, characterized by, or promoting amylolysis.

amylopectin (am″ĭ-lo-pek′tin) the insoluble constituent of starch; it stains violet red with iodine and forms a paste with hot water. The soluble constituent of starch is amylose. Called also *alpha-amylose, amylin, insoluble* or *tegumentary amidine,* and *starch cellulose.*

amylopectinosis (am″ĭ-lo-pek″tĭ-no′sis) glycogen storage disease, type IV; see under *disease.*

amylophagia (am″ĭ-lo-fa′je-ah) [*amylo-* + Gr. *phagein* to eat + *-ia*] starch eating; an abnormal craving for starch.

amyloplast (ah-mil′o-plast″) [*amylo-* + Gr. *plassein* to form] a starch-forming vegetable leuko-plastid.

amyloplastic (am″ĭ-lo-plas′tik) forming starch.

amylopsin (am″ĭ-lop′sin) [*amylo-* + *trypsin*] α-amylase occurring in the pancreas.

amylorrhea (am″ĭ-lo-re′ah) [*amylo-* + Gr. *rhoia* flow] the presence of an abnormal amount of starch in the stools.

amylorrhexis (am″ĭ-lo-rek′sis) [*amylo-* + Gr. *rhēxis* a breaking] the enzymatic hydrolysis of starch.

amylose (am′ĭ-lōs) 1. any carbohydrate of the starch group; a polysaccharide. 2. the soluble constituent of starch; it stains blue with iodine and does not form a paste with hot water. The other constituent is amylopectin. Called also *amidin, amylocellulose, amylogen,* and *granulose.* **alpha-a.** amylopectin. **crystalline a's,** crystalline compounds, produced by the growth of *Bacillus macerans* in a solution of starch or glycogen; the degree of polymerization may vary from 4 to 8 residues.

amylosis (am″ĭ-lo′sis) amyloidosis.

amylosuria (am″ĭ-lo-su′re-ah) the presence of amylose in the urine.

amylosynthesis (am″ĭ-lo-sin′the-sis) the synthesis of starch from sugar.

Amylsine Hydrochloride (am′il-sin hi″dro-klo′-rīd) trademark for a preparation of naepaine.

amylum (am′ĭ-lum) [L.; Gr. *amylon*] starch. **a. ioda′tum,** iodized starch.

amyluria (am″ĭ-lu′re-ah) [*amylo-* + Gr. *ouron* urine + *-ia*] an excess of starch in the urine.

amyoesthesis (ah-mi″o-es-the′sis) [*a* neg. + Gr. *mys* muscle + *aisthēsis* sensation] the lack of muscle sense.

amyoplasia (ah-mi″o-pla′ze-ah) [*a* neg. + Gr. *mys* muscle + *plassein* to form] lack of muscle formation. **a. congen′ita,** a generalized lack of muscular development and growth, with contracture and deformity at most of the joints; called *congenital multiple arthrogryposis* and *arthrogryposis multiplex congenita.*

amyostasia (ah-mi″o-sta′ze-ah) [*a* neg. + Gr. *mys* muscle + *stasis* a standing still] a tremor of the muscles, seen especially in locomotor ataxia.

amyostatic (ah-mi″o-stat′ik) marked by amyostasia or muscular tremors.

amyosthenia (ah-mi″os-the′ne-ah) [*a* neg. + Gr. *mys* muscle + *sthenos* strength] deficient muscular power, especially a feeling of weakness in the arms and legs, often seen in hysteria.

amyosthenic (ah-mi″os-then′ik) pertaining to, characterized by, or causing amyosthenia.

amyotaxia (ah-mi″o-tak′se-ah) ataxia.

amyotaxy (ah-mi′o-tak″se) [*a* neg. + Gr. *mys* muscle + *tassein* to arrange] ataxia.

amyotonia (a″mi-o-to′ne-ah; ah-mi″o-to′ne-ah) [*a* neg. + Gr. *mys* muscle + *tonos* tension + *-ia*] atonic condition of the musculature of the body; called also *myatonia* and *myatony.* **a. congen′ita** (Oppenheim, 1900), a vague term denoting any of several rare congenital diseases of children marked by general hypotonia of the muscles; called also *congenital atonic pseudoparalysis, myatonia congenita,* and *Oppenheim's disease.*

amyotrophia (ah-mi″o-tro′fe-ah) [*a* neg. + Gr. *mys* muscle + *trophē* nourishment + *-ia*] amyotrophy. **neuralgic a.,** neuralgic amyotrophy. **a. spina′lis progressi′va,** progressive muscular atrophy.

amyotrophic (ah-mi″o-trof′ik) pertaining to or characterized by amyotrophy.

amyotrophy (ah″mi-ot′ro-fe) atrophy of muscle tissue. **diabetic a.,** progressive weakening and wasting of muscles accompanied by an aching or stabbing pain, usually limited to the muscles of the pelvic girdle and thigh, and associated with diabetes. **neuralgic a.,** a condition characterized by pain across the shoulder and upper arm, with atrophy and paralysis of the muscles of the shoulder girdle.

amyous (am′e-us) [*a* neg. + Gr. *mys* muscle] deficient in muscular tissue.

amyrol (am′ĭ-rol) two isomeric principles, $C_5H_{26}O$, from sandalwood oil.

Amytal (am′ĭ-tal) trademark for amobarbital.

amyxia (ah-mik′se-ah) [*a* neg. + Gr. *myxa* mucus + *-ia*] absence of mucus.

amyxorrhea (ah-mik″so-re′ah) [*a* neg. + Gr. *myxa* mucus + *rhoia* flow] absence of mucus secretion. **a. gas′trica,** deficiency of mucus in the gastric secretion.

An chemical symbol for *actinon*.

An. anode; anodal; anisometropia.

an- 1. see *a* (def. 1). 2. see *ana-*.

A.N.A. American Nurses' Association; American Neurological Association.

ana (an′ah) [Gr.] so much of each; usually written āā.

ana-, an- (an′ah, an) [Gr. *ana* up, back, again] a prefix indicating upward, backward, excessive, or again.

anabasine (ah-nab′ah-sin) an alkaloid, $C_5H_4N \cdot C_5H_{10}N$, from the plant, *Anabasis aphylla,* which closely resembles nicotine; it is used as an insecticide.

anabasis (ah-nab′ah-sis) [Gr. "ascent"] the stage of increase in a disease.

anabatic (an″ah-bat′ik) [Gr. *anabatikos*] 1. increasing or growing more intense. 2. pertaining to or characterized by anabasis.

Anabena (ah-nab′ĕ-nah) a genus of blue-green algae which sometimes impart an objectionable odor to a water supply.

anabiosis (an″ah-bi-o′sis) [Gr. *anabiōsis* a reviving] restoration of vital processes after their apparent cessation.

anabiotic (an″ah-bi-ot′ik) apparently lifeless, but still capable of living.

anabolergy (an″ah-bol′er-je) [Gr. *anabolē* a throwing up + *ergon* work] energy expended in anabolism or in anabolic processes.

anabolic (an″ah-bol′ik) [Gr. *anabolikos*] pertaining to or promoting anabolism.

anabolin (ah-nab′o-lin) anabolite.

anabolism (ah-nab′o-lizm″) [Gr. *anabolē* a throwing up] any constructive process by which simple substances are converted by living cells into more complex compounds, especially into living matter.

anabolistic (ah-nab″o-lis′tik) pertaining to anabolism.

anabolite (ah-nab′o-līt″) any product of anabolism or of a constructive metabolic process.

anacamptic (an″ah-kamp′tik) pertaining to reflection, as of sound or light.

anacamptometer (an″ah-kamp-tom′ĕ-ter) [Gr. *anakampsis* reflection + *metron* measure] an instrument for measuring the reflexes (Duprat, 1886).

Anacardium (an″ah-kar′de-um) [L.; *ana-* + Gr. *kardia* heart] a genus of tropical trees with a poisonous juice. *A. occidentale,* the cashew tree, affords the cashew nut and a useful gum, as well as anacardic acid.

anacardol (an″ah-kar′dol) a constituent, 3-pentadecadienyl-phenol, $C_{15}H_{27} \cdot C_6H_4OH$, of cashew nut shell liquid; it causes reactions in persons sensitive to poison ivy.

anacatadidymus (an″ah-kat″ah-did′ĭ-mus) anakatadidymus.

anacatesthesia (an″ah-kat″es-the′ze-ah) anakatesthesia.

anachoresis (an″ah-ko-re′sis) [Gr. *anachōrēsis* a retreating] the preferential collection or deposits of particles at a certain site, as of bacteria or of metals which have localized out of the blood stream in areas of inflammation; called also *anachoretic effect*.

anachoretic (an″ah-ko-ret′ik) pertaining to, characterized by, or resulting from anachoresis.

anachoric (an″ah-ko′rik) anachoretic.

anachronobiology (an″ah-kron″o-bi-ol′o-je) a term suggested to denote the study of the constructive effects (growth, development, and maturation) of time on a living system. Cf. *catachronobiology*.

anacidity (an″ah-sid′ĭ-te) [*an* neg. + *acidity*] lack of normal acidity. **gastric a.,** achlorhydria.

anaclasimeter (an″ah-klah-sim′ĕ-ter) [Gr. *anaklasis* reflection + *metron* measure] an instrument for measuring eye refraction.

anaclasis (ah-nak′lah-sis) [Gr. *anaklasis* reflection] 1. reflection or refraction of light. 2. reflex action. 3. refracture. 4. forcible flexion of a limb; the breaking up of an ankylosis.

anaclisis (an″ah-kli′sis) the state of being anaclitic.

anaclitic (an″ah-klit′ik) [*ana-* + Gr. *klinein* to lean] leaning against or depending on something; in psychoanalysis, the development of the infant's love for his mother from his original dependence on her for care.

anacmesis (an-ak′me-sis) anakmesis.

anacobra (an″ah-ko′brah) cobra venom treated with formaldehyde and heat.

anacousia (an″ah-ku′ze-ah) anakusis.

anacrotic (an″ah-krot′ik) pertaining to or characterized by anacrotism.

anacrotism (ah-nak′ro-tizm) [*ana-* + Gr. *krotos* beat + *-ism*] an anomaly of the pulse evidenced by the presence of a prominent notch on the ascending limb of the pulse tracing.

anacusis (an″ah-ku′sis) anakusis.

anadenia (an″ah-de′ne-ah) [*an* neg. + Gr. *adēn* gland + *-ia*] (*obs.*) 1. absence of glands. 2. insufficiency of glandular function. **a. ventric′uli,** absence or destruction of the glands of the stomach.

anadidymus (an″ah-did′ĭ-mus) [*ana-* + Gr. *didymos* twin] a twin monster, divided below but single toward the cephalic pole (monstra duplicia anadidyma—Förster); called also *duplicitas inferior* and *duplicitas posterior*.

anadipsia (an″ah-dip′se-ah) [*ana-* + Gr. *dipsa* thirst + *-ia*] intense thirst.

anadrenalism (an″ah-dre′nal-izm) absence or failure of adrenal functioning.

anadrenia (an″ah-dre′ne-ah) anadrenalism.

Anadrol (an′ah-drol) trademark for a preparation of oxymetholone.

anaerase (an-a′er-ās″) [*an* neg. + Gr. *aēr* air + *-ase*] a hypothetical substance once believed to be the respiratory enzyme of anaerobic bacteria; cf. *aerase*.

anaerobe (an-a′er-ōb) [*an* neg. + Gr. *aēr* air + *bios* life] a microorganism that lives and grows in the complete, or almost complete, absence of molecular oxygen. **facultative a's,** microorganisms which are able to grow under either anaerobic or aerobic conditions. **obligate a's,** microorganisms that can grow only in the complete absence of molecular oxygen; some are killed by oxygen. **spore-forming a.,** *Clostridium*.

anaerobia (an″a-er-o′be-ah) plural of anaerobion.

anaerobian (an″a-er-o′be-an) (*obs.*) 1. living without air. 2. an anaerobe.

anaerobiase (an-a″er-o-bi′ās) a hypothetical substance from *Clostridium welchii* and other anaerobes which was thought to be fully active under anaerobic conditions.

anaerobic (an″a-er-o′bik) 1. lacking molecular oxygen. 2. growing in the absence of molecular oxygen.

anaerobion (an″a-er-o′be-on), pl. *anaero′bia*. Former term for anaerobe.

anaerobiosis (an-a″er-o-bi-o′sis) [*an* neg. + Gr. *aēr* air + *biosis* way of life] life only in the absence of molecular oxygen; called also *anoxybiosis*.

anaerobiotic (an-a″er-o-bi-ot′ik) (*obs.*) anaerobic.

anaerobism (an-a′er-o-bizm″) (*obs.*) the ability to live without oxygen.

anaerogenic (an-a″er-o-jen′ik) [*an* neg. + Gr. *aēr* air + *gennan* to produce] 1. producing little or no gas. 2. suppressing the formation of gas by the gas-producing bacteria.

anaeroplasty (an-a′er-o-plas″te) [*an* neg. + Gr. *aēr* air + *plassein* to form] exclusion of the air from wounds, as by applying water.

anaerosis (an″a-er-o′sis) [*an* neg. + Gr. *aēr* air + *-osis*] interruption of the respiratory function, especially in the newborn.

anagen (an′ah-jen) the phase of the hair cycle during which synthesis of hair takes place.

anagenesis (an″ah-jen′ĕ-sis) [*ana-* + Gr. *genesis* production] (*obs.*) reproduction or regeneration of tissue.

anagenetic (an″ah-jĕ-net′ik) pertaining to or producing anagenesis.

anagnosasthenia (an-ag″nos-as-the′ne-ah) [Gr. *anagnōsis* reading + *asthenia*] (*obs.*) neurasthenia with distress at any attempt to read.

Anagnostakis' operation (ah-nag″nos-ta′kis) [Andreas *Anagnostakis,* Greek ophthalmologist, 1826–1897] see under *operation*.

anagocytic (an-ag″o-si′tik) retarding or inhibiting the growth of cells.

anagoge (an″ah-go′je) anagogy.

anagogic (an″ah-goj′ik) [*ana-* + Gr. *agogē* leading] pertaining to the moral, uplifting, progressive strivings of the unconscious.

anagogy (an″ah-go′je) psychic material that has an idealistic quality.

anagotoxic (an-ag″o-tok′sik) acting antagonistically to toxin; counteracting toxic action.

anahormone (an″ah-hor′mōn) a substance capable of inducing antibody formation and of suppressing the secretion of protein hormones.

anakatadidymus (an″ah-kat″ah-did′ĭ-mus) [*ana-* + Gr. *kata* down + *didymos* twin] a twin monster separate above and below, but united in the middle (monstra duplicia anakatadidyma—Förster).

anakatesthesia (an″ah-kat″es-the′ze-ah) [*ana-* + Gr. *kata* down + *aisthēsis* perception + *-ia*] a hovering feeling or sensation.

anakhre (an-ak′er) goundou.

anakmesis (an-ak′me-sis) [*an* neg. + Gr. *akmēnos* full grown] arrest of maturation; specifically, increase of early granular cells (stem cells) in the marrow with lack of further maturation, as observed in the marrow in agranulocytosis.

anakusis (an″ah-koo′sis) [*an* neg. + Gr. *akouein* to hear] total deafness.

anal (a′nal) [L. *analis*]   pertaining to the anus.

analbuminemia (an″al-bu″mǐ-ne′me-ah)   a state characterized by deficiency or absence of albumins in the blood serum.

analeptic (an″ah-lep′tik) [Gr. *analepsis* a repairing]   a drug which acts as a restorative, such as caffeine, amphetamine, pentylenetetrazol, etc.

analgesia (an″al-je′ze-ah) [*an* neg. + Gr. *algēsis* pain + *-ia*] absence of sensibility to pain; absence of pain on noxious stimulation; designating particularly the relief of pain without loss of consciousness; called also *alganesthesia*. **a. al′gera,** spontaneous pain in a denervated part; pain in an area or region which is anesthetic; called also *a. dolorosa*. **audio a.,** audioanalgesia. **continuous caudal a.,** the relief of the pain of labor and childbirth by the continuous bathing of the sacral and lumbar plexuses within the epidural space by the injection of an anesthetic solution. This method is used also in general surgery to block the pain pathways below the navel. Called also *continuous caudal anesthesia*. **a. doloro′sa,** a. algera. **epidural a.,** analgesia induced by introduction of the analgesic agent into the epidural space of the vertebral canal. **infiltration a.,** paralysis of the nerve endings at the site of operation by subcutaneous injection of an anesthetic. **narcolocal a.,** local analgesia preceded by premedication. **paretic a.,** loss of the sense of pain accompanied by partial paralysis. **permeation a.,** surface a. **relative a.,** in dental anesthesia, a maintained level of conscious-sedation, short of general anesthesia, in which the pain threshold is elevated, usually induced in inhalation of nitrous oxide and oxygen. **surface a.,** local analgesia produced by an anesthetic applied to the surface of such mucous membranes as those of the eye, nose, throat, larynx, and urethra; called also *permeation a.*

analgesic (an″al-je′zik)   1. relieving pain. 2. not sensitive as to pain. 3. an agent that alleviates pain without causing loss of consciousness.

Analgesine (an″al-je′sin)   trademark for a preparation of antipyrine.

analgetic (an″al-jet′ik)   analgesic.

analgia (an-al′je-ah) [*an* neg. + Gr. *algos* pain + *-ia*]   absence of pain.

analgic (an-al′jik)   insensible to pain.

anallergic (an″ah-ler′jik)   not allergic; not causing anaphylaxis or hypersensitivity.

analogous (ah-nal′o-gus) [Gr. *analogos* according to a due ratio, conformable, proportionate]   resembling or similar in some respects, as in function or appearance, but not in origin or development; cf. *homologous*, def. 1.

analogue (an′ah-log)   1. a part or organ having the same function as another, but of a different evolutionary origin; cf. *homologue* (def. 1). 2. a chemical compound with a structure similar to that of another but differing from it in respect to a certain component; it may have a similar or opposite action metabolically. Cf. *homologue* (def. 2). **base a.,** an analogue of a purine or pyrimidine base, as aminopurine. **homologous a.,** a part that is similar to another in both function and structure. **metabolic a.,** a closely similar compound which tends to replace an essential metabolite. **substrate a.,** a substance with a structure similar to the natural substrate of an enzyme and which, because of this similarity, inhibits the action of the enzyme, as in competitive inhibition.

analogy (ah-nal′o-je) [Gr. *analogia* equality of ratios, proportion] the quality of being analogous; resemblance or similarity in function or appearance, but not in origin or development.

analphalipoproteinemia (an-al″fah-lip″o-pro″te-in-e′me-ah) Tangier disease.

analysand (ah-nal′ǐ-sand)   one who is being psychoanalyzed.

analysis (ah-nal′ǐ-sis), pl. *anal′yses* [*ana-* + Gr. *lysis* dissolution] 1. separation into component parts or elements; the act of determining the component parts of a substance. 2. psychoanalysis. **activation a.,** a quantitative determination of the presence of certain types of nuclei in a sample by transmuting them into radioactive nuclei and analyzing the emanating radiation. **antigenic a.,** the determination of the components of the antigenic mosaic of a bacterial species. **bite a.,** occlusal a. **blood gas a.,** the determination of oxygen and carbon dioxide concentrations and the pH of the blood by laboratory tests; the following measurements may be made: Po_2, partial pressure of oxygen in arterial blood; Pco_2, partial pressure of carbon dioxide in arterial blood; So_2, percent saturation of hemoglobin with oxygen in arterial blood; the total CO_2 content of (venous) plasma; and the pH. **bradycinetic a.,** cineradiographic study of motor activity. **cephalometric a.,** a study or analysis of the skeletal and dental relationships used in orthodontic case analysis, as seen in cephalograms. **character a.,** the systematic psychotherapeutic investigation or analysis of the personality traits or defenses of an individual. **chromatographic a.,** chromatography. **colorimetric a.,** analysis by means of the various color tests. **densimetric a.,** analysis by ascertaining the specific gravity of a solution and estimating the amount of matter dissolved. **distributive a.,** psychobiologic treatment by the

directed study and interpretation of the patient's present and past behavior. **Downs' a.,** a series of cephalometric criteria developed by Downs as an aid in orthodontic diagnosis. **ego a.,** the intensive therapeutic study and analysis of the ways in which the ego resolves or attempts to deal with intrapsychic conflicts. **end-group a.,** evaluation of the degree of linearity and branching of polysaccharide by determination of the number of end groups; determination of the amino- and carboxyl-terminal amino acids of a protein permitting an evaluation of the number of peptide chains per molecule as well as the state of purity of the protein. **existential a.,** existential psychoanalysis. **gasometric a.,** the measurement of the different components of a gaseous mixture. **gravimetric a.,** quantitative a. **group a.,** intensive psychotherapeutic analysis in which two or more patients actively participate. **occlusal a.,** a study of the relations of the occlusal surfaces of opposing teeth, and of the relations of the teeth in one jaw to those in the opposite jaw as units; called also *bite a.* **organic a.,** the analysis of animal and vegetable tissues. **polariscopic a.,** analysis by means of the polariscope. **proximate a.,** the determination of the simpler constituents of a substance. **qualitative a., qualitive a.,** the determination of the nature of the constituents of a compound or a mixture of compounds. **quantitative a., quantitive a.,** the determination of the proportionate quantities of the constituents of a compound. **radiochemical a.,** direct or indirect identification or determination of the content of specific elements in a substance through measurement of the disintegration rates of radionuclides. **spectroscopic a., spectrum a.,** analysis by means of determining the wave length(s) at which electromagnetic energy is absorbed by a sample. **tetrad a.,** the analysis of crossing over by studying all the tetrads arising from the meiotic divisions of a single primary gametocyte. **transactional a.,** a type of psychotherapy involving an understanding of the interpersonal interchanges between the components of the personalities of the participants (individuals or members of a group). **ultimate a.,** the determination of the ultimate elements of a compound. **vector a.,** analysis of a moving force to determine both its magnitude and its direction, e.g., analysis of the scalar electrocardiogram to determine the magnitude and direction of the electromotive force for one complete cycle of the heart. **volumetric a.,** quantitative analysis by measuring volumes of liquids.

analysor (an′ah-li″zor)   analyzer.

analyte (an′ah-līt)   a substance undergoing analysis.

analytic (an″ah-lit′ik)   pertaining to analysis.

analyzer (an′ah-li″zer)   1. a Nicol prism attached to a polarizing apparatus which extinguishes the ray of light polarized by the polarizer. 2. Pavlov's name for a specialized part of the nervous system which controls the reactions of the organism to changing external conditions. 3. a nervous receptor together with its central connections, by means of which sensitivity to stimulations is differentiated. **amino acid a.,** an analytical instrument that separates, identifies, and measures quantities of amino acids and related compounds. **amino acid sequence a.,** an instrument for determining protein components in plasma, useful in blood-lipid evaluation. **blood gas a.,** an instrument for measuring partial pressures of oxygen, carbon dioxide, carbon monoxide, and nitrogen in blood. **breath a.,** an instrument for determining the volume and composition of respired gases; some types are specifically designed for detecting alcohol in the breath. **image a.,** an instrument that counts, measures and classifies cells and images viewed on microscopes, photographs, transparencies, etc. **oxygen gas a.,** an instrument for measuring the oxygen content of a gaseous mixture, or dissolved oxygen in a liquid, or saturation of blood hemoglobin with O_2 or partial pressure of O_2 in blood. **voice a.,** an electronic instrument for printing out waveforms corresponding to vocal characteristics, as an aid in identifying voice and speech problems or a particular speaker.

Aname (an′ah-me)   a genus comprising the venomous "bird spiders" of the family Theraphosidae.

Anamirta cocculus   L. Wight & Arn. (Menispermaceae) (an″-ah-mer′tah kok′u-lus) a species of East Indian woody vines whose dried berries or fruit, cocculus indicus, yield picrotoxin. Called also *A. paniculata*.

anamirtin (an″ah-mer′tin)   an oily glyceride, $C_{19}H_{24}O_{10}$, from the dried berries or fruit of *Anamirta cocculus*.

anamnesis (an″am-ne′sis) [Gr. *anamnēsis* a recalling]   1. the faculty of memory. 2. the collected data concerning a patient, his family, previous environment, and experiences, including any abnormal sensations, moods, or acts observed by the patient himself or by others, with the dates of their appearance and duration, as well as any results of treatment. 3. in immunology, the faculty of immunological memory as exemplified by events in the secondary or anamnestic immune response.

anamnestic (an″am-nes′tik)   pertaining to anamnesis. See also under *response*.

Anamniota (an″am-ne-o′tah) [*an* priv. + Gr. *amnion*]   a major group of vertebrates comprising those which develop no amnion, including fishes and amphibians; opposed to Amniota.

anamniote (an-am′ne-ōt″) any animal or group belonging to the Anamniota.

anamniotic (an″am-ne-ot′ik) [*an* neg. + *amnion*] having no amnion.

anamorphosis (an″ah-mor-fo′sis) [*ana-* + Gr. *morphē* form] an ascending progression or change of form in the evolution of a group of animals or plants.

ananabasia (an-an″ah-ba′se-ah) [*an* neg. + Gr. *anabasis* ascent + *-ia*] (*obs.*) inability to ascend high places.

ananabolic (an″an-ah-bol′ik) [*an* neg. + *anabolic*] characterized by absence of anabolism.

ananaphylaxis (an-an″ah-fĭ-lak′sis) antianaphylaxis.

Ananase (an′ah-nās) trademark for a preparation of bromelains.

ananastasia (an-an″as-ta′se-ah) [*an* neg. + Gr. *anastasis* a standing up + *-ia*] inability to stand up or to rise from a sitting posture.

anancastic (an″an-kas′tik) [Gr. *anankastos* forced] obsessive-compulsive.

anandia (an-an′de-ah) aphemia.

anandria (an-an′dre-ah) [*an* neg. + Gr. *anēr* man] (*obs.*) the loss of masculinity or virility.

anangioid (an-an′je-oid) [*an* neg. + Gr. *angeion* vessel + *eidos* form] seemingly without blood vessels.

anapepsia (an″ah-pep′se-ah) complete absence of pepsin from the stomach secretion.

anaphalantiasis (an-af″ah-lan-ti′ah-sis) [Gr. "forehead-baldness"] absence of the eyebrows. Cf. *madarosis*.

anaphase (an′ah-fāz) [*ana-* + Gr. *phasis* phase] that stage in meiosis and mitosis, following the metaphase, in which the centromeres split and the chromatids lined up on the spindle begin to move apart toward the poles of the spindle to form the daughter chromosomes. See also *meiosis* and *mitosis*. **flabby a.,** a mitotic phase in which the gel is disoriented and separation of the doubled chromosomes fails to occur, owing to interference with spindle formation caused by cell poisoning.

anaphia (an-a′fe-ah) [*an* neg. + Gr. *haphē* touch + *-ia*] lack or loss of the sense of touch.

anaphoresis (an″ah-fo-re′sis) 1. the passage of charged particles toward the positive pole (anode) in electrophoresis. 2. (*obs.*) diminution in the activity of the sweat glands.

anaphoria (an″ah-fo′re-ah) [*ana-* + Gr. *pherein* to bear + *-ia*] a tendency for the visual axes of both eyes to divert above the horizontal plane.

anaphrodisia (an″af-ro-diz′e-ah) [*an* neg. + Gr. *Aphroditē* Venus + *-ia*] absence or loss of sexual desire; called also *sexual anesthesia*.

anaphrodisiac (an″af-ro-diz′e-ak) 1. repressing sexual desire. 2. a drug or medicine that allays sexual desire.

anaphylactic (an″ah-fĭ-lak′tik) decreasing immunity instead of increasing it; pertaining to anaphylaxis; possessing anaphylaxis.

anaphylactin (an″ah-fĭ-lak′tin) the antibody in anaphylaxis; it is formed after the first injection of the foreign protein (antigen) and interacts with it on the second injection. Called also *sensibilisin*. Cf. *anaphylactic antibody*.

anaphylactogen (an″ah-fĭ-lak′to-jen) a substance which is capable of inducing a condition of anaphylaxis; see also *allergen,* def. 1., *anaphylactic antibody,* under *antibody,* and *sensitinogen*.

anaphylactogenesis (an″ah-fĭ-lak″to-jen′ĕ-sis) the production of anaphylaxis.

anaphylactogenic (an″ah-fĭ-lak″to-jen′ik) producing anaphylaxis.

anaphylactoid (an″ah-fĭ-lak′toid) resembling anaphylaxis.

anaphylactotoxin (an″ah-fĭ-lak″to-tok′sin) anaphylatoxin.

anaphylatoxin (an″ah-fĭ″lah-tok′sin) a substance produced in blood serum during complement fixation which serves as a mediator of inflammation by inducing mast cell degranulation and histamine release (thereby indirectly increasing vascular permeability). Its injection into animals results in the development of signs and symptoms consistent with those of systemic anaphylaxis. Anaphylatoxin activity is a property of low-molecular-weight complement fragments C3a and C5a.

anaphylaxin (an″ah-fĭ-lak′sin) anaphylactin.

anaphylaxis (an″ah-fĭ-lak′sis) [*ana-* + Gr. *phylaxis* protection] an unusual or exaggerated allergic reaction of an organism to foreign protein or other substances. Use of the term was originally restricted to a condition of sensitization in laboratory animals produced by the injection of foreign matter, such as horse serum, but has since been extended to human reactions. Such an injection renders the individual hypersusceptible to a subsequent injection. This is termed *active a.* Anaphylaxis produced in an animal by injecting the blood serum of a sensitized animal is termed *passive a.* The reaction results from the release of histamine, serotonin, and other vasoactive substances when antigen combines with antibody on cell surfaces. Cf. *allergy* and *hypersensitivity*. Called also *hypersensitization, Theobald Smith phenomenon, hypersus-*

ceptibility, and *protein sensitization.* **acquired a.,** anaphylaxis in which sensitization is known to have been produced by the administration of a foreign immunogen. **active a.,** the anaphylactic state produced in an individual by the injection of a foreign immunogen; distinguished from passive anaphylaxis. **aggregate a.,** an anaphylactic reaction caused by pharmacological mediators whose release is effected by large amounts of soluble antigen-antibody complexes; it occurs within minutes after antigen is injected. **antiserum a.,** passive anaphylaxis. **cutaneous a., active,** localized anaphylaxis in the form of the wheal and flare reaction on injection of antigen into the skin of a sensitized subject; used as a test for allergy to pollen. **cutaneous a., passive (PCA),** localized anaphylaxis passively transferred by intradermal injection of an antibody and, after a latent period (about 24 to 72 hours), intravenous injection of the homologous antigen and Evans blue dye. Blueing of the skin at the site of the intradermal injection is evidence of the permeability reaction. Used in studies of antibodies causing immediate hypersensitivity reactions. **cytotoxic a.,** anaphylaxis following the injection of antibodies specific for natural antigenic constituents of the body cell surfaces. **cytotropic a.,** that induced by antigen reacting with antibody that has become fixed to mediator cells (mast cells, basophilic leukocytes) which release mediators of anaphylaxis when reacting with allergens. **heterologous a.,** a passive anaphylaxis induced by the transference of serum from a donor animal of a species different from that of the recipient. **homologous a.,** a passive anaphylaxis induced by the transference of serum from one animal to another of the same species. **indirect a.,** anaphylaxis induced by an animal's own antigen modified in some way. **inverse a.,** 1. anaphylaxis in which the shocking agent is antibody (anaphylactin) rather than antigen (anaphylactogen). 2. anaphylactic shock produced by a single intravenous injection into guinea pigs of Forssman antibody which interacts with Forssman antigen in their tissues. Called also *reverse anaphylaxis*. **local a.,** anaphylaxis confined to a limited area, e.g., cutaneous anaphylaxis. **passive a.,** anaphylaxis occurring in a normal individual as a result of the injection of the serum of a previously sensitized individual; called also *antiserum a.* **reverse a.,** anaphylaxis following the injection of antigen succeeded by the injection of antiserum; also local reactions from the union of circulating antibodies with antigen fixed by tissue cells. **systemic a.,** that in which many tissues are involved, in contrast to local anaphylaxis. Target tissues or organs vary from one species to another, e.g., terminal bronchiole smooth muscle in the guinea pig and portal vascular system in the dog.

anaphylodiagnosis (an″ah-fī″lo-di″ag-no′sis) diagnosis of disease by means of anaphylactic reactions.

anaphylotoxin (an″ah-fī″lo-tok′sin) anaphylatoxin.

anaplasia (an″ah-pla′ze-ah) [Gr. *ana* backward + *plassein* to form] a loss of differentiation of cells (dedifferentiation) and of their orientation to one another and to their axial framework and blood vessels, a characteristic of tumor tissue. **monophasic a.,** reversion of a cell form to embryonic type, as in cancer formation. **polyphasic a.,** change of a cell into a cell of more complex character.

Anaplasma (an″ah-plaz′mah) [Gr. *anaplasma* something formed] a genus of microorganisms of the family Anaplasmataceae (q.v.), including three species, *A. centra′le, A. margina′le* (the causative agent of anaplasmosis), and *A. ovis*.

Anaplasmataceae (an″ah-plaz″mah-ta′se-e) a family of the order Rickettsiales, made up of microorganisms parasitic in red blood cells, in which they appear as spherical granules staining a deep reddish violet; naturally parasitic in ruminants and transmitted by arthropods. It includes a single genus, *Anaplasma*.

anaplasmodastat (an″ah-plaz-mo′dah-stat″) any of a group of chemical agents for control of anaplasmosis in animals.

anaplasmosis (an″ah-plaz-mo′sis) a disease of cattle and related ruminants marked by high temperature, anemia, and icterus, and caused by *Anaplasma marginale,* which is transmitted by ticks and other blood-sucking arthropods. Called also *gallsickness*.

anaplastia (an″ah-plas′te-ah) anaplasia.

anaplastic (an″ah-plas′tik) [*ana-* + Gr. *plassein* to form] 1. restoring a lost or absent part. 2. characterized by anaplasia or reversed development; said of cells.

anaplasty (an′ah-plas″te) [*ana-* + Gr. *plassein* to form] (*obs.*) restorative or plastic surgery.

anaplerosis (an″ah-ple-ro′sis) (*obs.*) the repair or replacement of lost or defective parts.

anaplerotic (an″ah-plĕ-rot′ik) 1. pertaining to anaplerosis. 2. relating to a sequence of enzymatic actions in central metabolic cycles (e.g., the tricarboxylic acid cycle) by which intermediates are produced from catabolic products of a substrate needed for the growth of an organism; the mechanism thus serves to replenish an intermediate depleted during growth.

anapnograph (an-ap′no-graf) [Gr. *anapnoē* respiration + *graphein* to record] (*obs.*) a device once used to register the speed and pressure of the respired air current; replaced by the pneumotachygraph.

anapnometer (an″ap-nom′ĕ-ter) [Gr. *anapnoē* respiration + *metron* measure] (*obs.*) a spirometer.

anapnotherapy (an″ap-no-ther′ah-pe) [Gr. *anapnein* to inhale + *therapeia* treatment] treatment by inhalation of gas, as in resuscitation.

anapophysis (an″ah-pof′ĭ-sis) [*ana-* + Gr. *apophysis* process of a bone] an accessory vertebral process, especially an accessory process of a thoracic or lumbar vertebra.

anaptic (an-ap′tik) [*an* neg. + Gr. *haphē* touch] marked by anaphia.

anarchic (an-ar′kik) of the nature of anarchy; against rule; different from the usual.

anaric (ah-na′rik) [*a* neg. + L. *naris* nose] having no nose.

anarithmia (an″ah-rith′me-ah) [*an* neg. + Gr. *arithmos* number] inability to count, due to a central lesion.

anarrhexis (an″ah-rek′sis) [*ana-* + Gr. *rhēxis* fracture] the operation of refracturing a bone.

anarthria (an-ar′thre-ah) [*an* neg. + Gr. *arthroun* to articulate + *-ia*] severe dysarthria resulting in speechlessness. **a. litera′lis,** stuttering.

anasarca (an″ah-sar′kah) [*ana-* + Gr. *sarx* flesh] generalized massive edema.

anasarcous (an″ah-sar′kus) affected with or of the nature of anasarca.

anascitic (an″ah-sit′ik) without ascites.

anastalsis (an″ah-stal′sis) [*ana-* + Gr. *stalsis* contraction] reversed peristalsis.

anastaltic (an″ah-stal′tik) [Gr. *anastaltikos* contracting] 1. astringent 2. a styptic medicine.

anastate (an′ah-stāt″) [Gr. *anastatos* raised up] an anabolite.

anastigmatic (an″ah-stig-mat′ik) not astigmatic; corrected for astigmatism.

anastole (ah-nas′to-le) [Gr. *anastolē*] retraction, as of the edges of a wound.

anastomose (ah-nas′to-mōs) 1. to communicate with one another by anastomosis, as arteries and veins. 2. to create a communication between two formerly separate structures.

anastomosis (ah-nas″to-mo′sis), pl. *anastomo′ses* [Gr. *anastomōsis* opening, outlet] 1. a communication between two vessels by collateral channels. 2. an opening created by surgical, traumatic, or pathological means between two normally distinct spaces or organs. **antiperistaltic a.,** enterostomy in which the in-

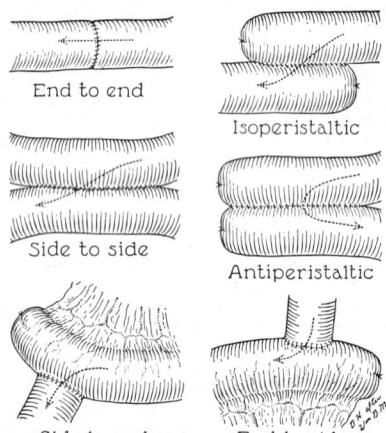

End to end
Isoperistaltic
Side to side
Antiperistaltic
Side to end
End to side

Methods of intestinal anastomosis (Babcock).

testinal segments are so joined that the directions of the peristaltic waves in the two conjoined portions are opposed. See illustration. **a. arterioveno′sa** [NA], a vessel that directly interconnects an artery and a vein and that acts as a shunt to bypass the capillary bed. **arteriovenous a.,** 1. anastomosis arteriovenosa [NA]. 2. a communication surgically created between an artery and a vein. **Braun's a.,** formation of an anastomosis between the afferent and efferent intestinal loops just distal to a gastroenteric stoma to prevent vicious cycling of gastric and duodenal contents. **Clado's a.,** the anastomosis between the appendicular and ovarian arteries in the appendiculo-ovarian ligament. **crucial a.,** an arterial anastomosis in the proximal part of the thigh, formed by the anastomotic branch of the sciatic, the internal circumflex, the first perforating, and the transverse portion of the external circumflex. **Galen's a.,** the anastomosis between the superior and inferior laryngeal nerves; called also *Galen's nerve.* **heterocladic a.,** an anastomosis between branches of different arteries. **homocladic a.,** an anastomosis between branches of the same artery. **Hyrtl's a.,** see *Hyrtl's loop,* under *loop.* **ileorectal a.,** surgical anastomosis of the ileum and rectum after total colectomy, as is sometimes done in ulcerative colitis. **in-**

testinal a., the establishment of a communication between two portions of the intestinal tract; see illustration. **isoperistaltic a.,** enterostomy in which the intestinal segments are so joined that the peristaltic waves in the two conjoined portions progress in the same direction; see illustration. **Jacobson's a.** (*obs.*), the anastomosing part of the tympanic plexus. **portosystemic a.,** anastomosis between the portal and systemic venous circulation. **postcostal a.,** a longitudinal linkage of the seven highest intersegmental arteries in the embryo that gives rise to the vertebral artery. **precapillary a.,** anastomosis between small arteries just before they become capillaries. **precostal a.,** a longitudinal anastomosis of intersegmental arteries in the embryo that gives rise to the thyrocervical and costocervical trunks. **pyeloileocutaneous a.,** direct connection of the renal pelvis to an isolated loop of the ileum, which is then anchored to the abdominal wall at the stoma, to drain exteriorly. **a. of Riolan,** anastomosis of the superior and inferior mesenteric arteries. **Roux-en-Y a.,** any Y-shaped anastomosis in which the small intestine is included. **stirrup a.,** an arterial branch joining the dorsalis pedis with the external plantar artery. **Sucquet-Hoyer a.,** regulatory connections between small peripheral arteries and veins, especially in the hands and feet; called also *Sucquet-Hoyer canal.* **terminoterminal a.,** surgical anastomosis between the peripheral end of an artery and the central end of the corresponding vein and between the central end of the artery and the terminal end of the vein. **transureteroureteral a.,** the operation of transplanting one ureter into the ureter on the opposite side. **ureteroileocutaneous a.,** connection of the transected ureter to an isolated loop of the ileum, which is then anchored to the abdominal wall at the stoma, to drain exteriorly. **ureterotubal a.,** an anastomosis between the ureter and fallopian tube. **ureteroureteral a.,** the operation of joining portions of the same ureter.

anastomotic (ah-nas″to-mot′ik) pertaining to or of the nature of an anastomosis.

anastral (an-as′tral) [*an* neg. + Gr. *astēr* star] lacking, or pertaining to the lack of, an aster; used in reference to a mitotic figure.

anastrophic (an″ah-strof′ik) [Gr. *anastrophē* a turning back, reversal] capable of being inactivated and then reactivated; said of certain proteinases.

anat. anatomy; anatomical.

anatherapeusis (an″ah-ther″ah-pu′sis) [Gr. *ana* upward + *therapeusis*] treatment by increasing doses.

anatomic (an″ah-tom′ik) anatomical.

anatomical (an″ah-tom′ĭ-kal) pertaining to anatomy, or to the structure of the organism.

anatomicomedical (an-ah-tom″e-ko-med′ĭ-kal) pertaining to anatomy and medicine or to medical anatomy.

anatomicopathological (an″ah-tom″e-ko-path″o-loj′ĭ-kal) pertaining to pathological anatomy.

anatomicophysiological (an-ah-tom″e-ko-fiz″e-o-loj′ĭ-kal) pertaining to anatomy and physiology.

anatomicosurgical (an-ah-tom″e-ko-ser′jĭ-kal) pertaining to anatomy and surgery.

anatomist (ah-nat′o-mist) a person skilled or learned in anatomy; a specialist in the field of anatomy.

anatomist's snuff-box the hollow at the back of the hand and the base of the thumb, between the tendons of the extensor pollicis longus and extensor pollicis brevis muscles.

anatomopathology (an″ah-to-mo-pah-thol′o-je) the anatomical aspects of pathology.

anatomy (ah-nat′o-me) [*ana-* + Gr. *temnein* to cut] 1. the science of the structure of the animal body and the relation of its parts; it is largely based on dissection, from which it obtains its name. 2. dissection of an organized body. **applied a.,** anatomy as applied to diagnosis and treatment. **artificial a.,** the study of anatomical structure by use of models or other artificial means. **artistic a.,** the study of anatomy as applied to painting and sculpture. **clastic a.,** anatomy studied by the aid of models in which various layers can be removed to show the position of organs and parts underneath. **comparative a.,** a comparison of the structure of different animals and plants, one with another. **corrosion a.,** anatomy studied by means of corrosive agents that remove the tissues not intended to be observed. **dental a.,** the study of the structure of the teeth and their correlated parts. **descriptive a.,** the study or description of individual parts of the body; called also *systematic a.* **developmental a.,** the field of embryology concerned with the changes that cells, tissues, organs, and the body as a whole undergo from a germ cell of each parent to the resulting, adult offspring. **general a.,** the study of the structure and composition of the body, and its tissues and fluids in general. **gross a.,** that which deals with structures that can be distinguished with the naked eye; called also *macroscopic a.* **histologic a.,** histology. **homologic a.,** the study of the correlated parts of the body in different animals. **macroscopic a.,** gross a. **medical a.,** anatomy concerned with the study of points connected with the diagnosis and situation of internal diseases. **microscopic a., minute a.,** histology. **morbid a., pathologi-**

cal a., the anatomy of diseased tissues. **physiognomonic a.,** the study of the external expression of the body surface, especially of the face. **physiological a.,** the study of the organs with respect to their normal functions. **plastic a.,** the study of anatomy by the aid of models and manikins, especially those that can be taken apart. **practical a.,** anatomy studied by means of demonstration and dissection. **radiological a.,** the study of the anatomy of organs and tissues based on their visualization on x-ray films. **regional a.,** the study of limited portions or regions of the body, and the relationships of their parts. **special a.,** the study of particular organs or parts. **surface a.,** the study of the form and markings of the surface of the body, especially in relation to deeper parts. **surgical a.,** the study of limited portions or regions of the body, with a view to the diagnosis and treatment of surgical conditions. **systematic a.,** descriptive a. **topographic a.,** the study of parts in their relation to surrounding parts. **transcendental a.,** the study of the general design and morphology of the body and the analogies and homologies of its parts. **veterinary a.,** the anatomy of domestic animals. **x-ray a.,** radiological a.

anatopism (ah-nat′o-pizm) [ana- + Gr. topos place + -ism] (obs.) a mental condition in which the patient fails to conform to the customs of the social group to which he belongs; called also ectopism.

anatoxic (an″ah-tok′sik) pertaining to anatoxin.

anatoxin (an″ah-tok′sin) [ana- + toxin] toxoid. **diphtheria a., a.-Ramon,** diphtheria toxoid.

anatoxireaction (an″ah-tok″se-re-ak′shun) Moloney's test; see under tests.

anatripsis (an″ah-trip′sis) [Gr. "rubbing"] (obs.) therapeutic rubbing or friction massage.

anatriptic (an″ah-trip′tik) [Gr. anatriptos rubbed up] 1. pertaining to anatripsis. 2. a medication applied by rubbing.

anatrophic (an″ah-trof′ik) 1. correcting or preventing atrophy. 2. a remedy that prevents waste of the tissues.

anatropia (an″ah-tro′pe-ah) [ana- + Gr. trepein to turn] upward deviation of the visual axis of one eye when the other eye is fixing.

anatropic (an″ah-trop′ik) pertaining to anatropia; deviating upward.

anavenin (an″ah-ven′in) a venom which has become inactivated by the addition of formaldehyde but which retains its antigenic properties.

anaxon (an-ak′son) [an neg. + Gr. axōn axis] a term formerly used to describe a nerve cell which appears to lack an axon.

anazolene sodium (an-az′o-lēn) chemical name: 4-[(4-anilino-5-sulfo-1-naphthyl)azo]-5-hydroxy-2, 7-naphthalenedisulfonic acid trisodium salt. A reddish black powder, $C_{26}H_{16}N_3Na_3O_{10}S_3$, used as a diagnostic aid in the determination of blood volume and cardiac output; called also anoxynaphthonate sodium.

Ancef (an′sef) trademark for a preparation of cefazolin sodium.

anchone (ang-ko′ne) (obs.) spasmodic constriction of the throat in hysteria.

anchor (ang′ker) a means by which something is held securely.

anchorage (ang′ker-ij) fixation, such as the surgical fixation of a displaced viscus. In operative dentistry, the fixation of fillings or of artificial crowns or bridges; in orthodontics, the support used for a regulating apparatus, which may be intramaxillary, by means of teeth located in the same arch; intermaxillary, by means of both maxillary and mandibular teeth; or extramaxillary (extraoral), by means of a device that is located outside the mouth. **cervical a.,** anchorage in which the back of the neck is used for resistance through means of a cervical headgear. **extraoral a.,** anchorage in which the resistance unit is outside the oral cavity, as in cranial, occipital, or cervical anchorage. **intraoral a.,** anchorage in which the resistance units are all located within the oral cavity. **multiple a.,** anchorage in which more than one type of resistance unit is utilized. **occipital a.,** anchorage in which the top and back of the head are used for resistance through means of a headgear. **reciprocal a.,** anchorage in which the movement of one or more dental units is balanced against the movement of one or more opposing dental units. Cf. reciprocal force. **reinforced a.,** multiple a. **simple a.,** dental anchorage in which the resistance to the movement of one or more dental units comes solely from resistance to the tipping movement of the anchorage unit. **stationary a.,** dental anchorage in which the resistance to the movement of one or more dental units comes from the resistance to bodily movement of the anchorage unit. A questionable concept of anchorage implying that selected teeth remain stable.

anchylo- for words beginning thus, see those beginning ankylo-.

ancillary (an′sil-lār″e) [L. ancillaris relating to a maid servant] assisting in the performance of a service or the achievement of a result.

ancipital (an-sip′ĭ-tal) [L. an′ceps two headed] having two heads or two edges.

Ancistrodon (an-sis′tro-don) Agkistrodon.

ancistroid (an-sis′troid) [Gr. ankistron fishhook + eidos form] hook shaped.

Ancobon (an′ko-bon) trademark for a preparation of flucytosine.

anconad (ang′ko-nad) [Gr. ankōn elbow + L. ad toward] toward the elbow or olecranon.

anconagra (ang″kon-ag′rah) [Gr. ankōn elbow + agra seizure] gout of the elbow.

anconal (ang′ko-nal) anconeal.

anconeal (ang-ko′ne-al) pertaining to the elbow.

anconitis (ang″ko-ni′tis) inflammation of the elbow joint.

anconoid (ang′ko-noid) resembling the elbow.

ancrod (an′krod) a proteinase obtained from the venom of the Malayan pit viper Agkistrodon rhodostoma, acting specifically on fibrinogen; used as an anticoagulant in the treatment of retinal vein occlusion and deep vein thrombosis and to prevent postoperative rethrombosis.

ancylo- for words beginning thus, see also words beginning ankylo-.

Ancylostoma (an″kĭ-los′to-mah, an″sĭ-los′to-mah) [Gr. ankylos crooked + stoma mouth] a genus of nematode parasites of the family Ancylostomidae, the Old World hookworms. **A. america′num,** Necator americanus. **A. brazilien′se,** a species found in cats and dogs in the southeastern United States, Brazil, and other tropical countries; its larvae may cause creeping eruption in man. **A. cani′num,** the common hookworm of dogs and cats; the larvae of which may cause creeping eruption in man. **A. ceylon′icum,** A. braziliense. **A. duodena′le,** the common European or Old World hookworm, a nematode worm, the male being 10 to 12 mm. ($\frac{1}{3}$ to $\frac{1}{2}$ inch) long and 0.4 mm. ($\frac{1}{60}$ inch) broad, the female somewhat larger; the mature parasites inhabit the small intestine, producing the condition known as ancylostomiasis. Called also Uncinaria duodenale.

ancylostomatic (an″kĭ-lo-sto-mat′ik, an″sĭ-lo-sto-mat′ik) caused by Ancylostoma.

ancylostome (an-kil′o-stōm, an-sil′o-stōm) 1. an individual of the genus Ancylostoma. 2. an individual of the family Ancylostomidae; a hookworm.

ancylostomiasis (an″kĭ-los″to-mi′ah-sis, an″sĭ-los″to-mi′ah-sis) hookworm disease; see under disease. **a. brazilien′sis,** larva migrans.

Ancylostomidae (an″kĭ-lo-sto′mĭ-de, an″sĭ-lo-sto′mĭ-de) a family of phasmid nematodes of the superfamily Strongyloidea, comprising all the hookworms, including the genera Ancylostoma, Bunostomum, Necator, and Uncinaria.

Ancylostomum (an″kĭ-los-to′mum, an″sĭ-los-to′mum) Ancylostoma.

ancyroid (an′sĭ-roid) [Gr. ankyra anchor + eidos form] shaped like an anchor or hook.

Anda (an′dah) [Brazilian] a genus of euphorbiaceous trees. A. as′su and A. gome′sii, of Brazil, afford purgative oils.

Andernach's ossicles (ahn′der-nahks) [Johann Winther von Andernach, German physician, 1487–1574] ossa suturarum.

Anders' disease (an′ders) [James Meschter Anders, Philadelphia physician, 1854–1936] adiposis tuberosa simplex.

Andersch's ganglion, nerve (an′dersh-ez) [Carolus Samuel Andersch, German anatomist of the 18th Century] see ganglion inferius nervi glossopharyngei and nervus tympanicus.

Andersen's disease, syndrome (triad) (an′der-sonz) [Dorothy Hansine Andersen, New York pathologist, born 1901] see under disease and syndrome.

Anderson splint (an′der-son) [Roger Anderson, Seattle orthopedic surgeon, born 1891] see under splint.

Anderson-Goldberger test (an′der-son-gōld′ber-ger) [John F. Anderson, American Physician, born 1873; Joseph Goldberger, American physician, 1874–1929] see under tests.

Andira (an-di′rah) a genus of tropical leguminous trees. Goa powder (q.v.) and chrysarobin (q.v.) are derived from A. araro′ba, of Brazil. Many species afford poisons, and several are anthelmintic.

andirine (an-di′rin) surinamine.

andr- see andro-.

Andrade's indicator (an-drah′dēz) [Eduardo Penny Andrade, American bacteriologist, 1872–1906] see under indicator.

Andral's decubitus (sign) (an-dralz′) [Gabriel Andral, French physician, 1797–1876] see under decubitus.

andreioma (an″dre-o′mah) [andr- + -oma] arrhenoblastoma.

andreoblastoma (an″dre-o-blas-to′mah) arrhenoblastoma.

Andrewes' test (an′drōōz) [Sir Christopher Howard Andrewes, British physician, born 1896] see under tests.

Andrews' disease [George Clinton Andrews, New York dermatologist, born 1891] pustular bacterid.

andriatrics, andriatry (an″dre-at′riks; an-dri′ah-tre) [Gr. anēr man + iatrikos healing] (obs.) that branch of medicine which deals with diseases of men and their treatment.

andrin (an'drin) [Gr. *anēr* man] a general term for the androgens of the testis, namely testosterone, androsterone, and dehydroandrosterone.

andro-, andr- (an'dro) [Gr. *anēr, andros* man] a combining form denoting relationship to man or to the male.

androblastoma (an″dro-blas-to'mah) 1. a rare, benign tumor of the testis that histologically resembles the fetal testis; there are three varieties: diffuse stromal, mixed (stromal and epithelial), and tubular (epithelial). The epithelial elements contain Sertoli cells, which may produce estrogen and thus cause feminization. Called also *Sertoli cell tumor.* 2. arrhenoblastoma.

androcyte (an'dro-sīt) [*andro-* + Gr. *kytos* hollow vessel] male sex cell, especially an immature stage.

androdedotoxin (an″dro-de'do-tok'sin) a poisonous principle from the leaves of rhododendrons.

androecium (an″dro-e'she-um) stamen.

androgalactozemia (an″dro-gah-lak″to-ze'me-ah) [*andro-* + Gr. *gala* milk + *zēmia* loss] the secretion or escape of milk from the male breast.

androgamone (an″dro-gam'ōn) a gamone released by spermatozoa.

androgen (an'dro-jen) [*andro-* + Gr. *gennan* to produce] any substance that possesses masculinizing activities, such as the testicular hormone; see *androsterone* and *testosterone.*

androgenesis (an″dro-jen'ĕ-sis) [*andro-* + Gr. *genesis* production] development of an egg which contains only paternal chromosomes.

androgenic (an″dro-jen'ik) producing masculine characteristics.

androgenicity (an″dro-jĕ-nis'ĭ-te) the quality of exerting a masculinizing effect.

androgenization (an″dro-jen-ĭ-za'shun) the state of producing an excess of androgens in the female.

androgenized (an-droj'ĕ-nizd) subjected to the production or presence of an excess of androgen in the female.

androgenous (an-droj'ĕ-nus) [*andro-* + Gr. *gennan* to beget] pertaining or tending to the production of male rather than female offspring.

androglossia (an″dro-glos'e-ah) [*andro-* + Gr. *glōssa* tongue] a quality of maleness in a woman's voice.

androgone (an'dro-gōn) [*andro-* + Gr. *gonos* seed] a spermatogenic cell.

androgyne (an'dro-jīn) a female pseudohermaphrodite.

androgyneity (an″dro-jĭ-ne'ĭ-te) female pseudohermaphroditism.

androgynism (an-droj'ĭ-nizm) female pseudohermaphroditism.

androgynoid (an-droj'ĭ-noid) 1. a pseudohermaphrodite. 2. pertaining to female pseudohermaphroditism.

androgynous (an-droj'ĭ-nus) pertaining to or characterized by female pseudohermaphroditism.

androgynus (an-droj'ĭ-nus) [*andro-* + Gr. *gynē* woman] a female pseudohermaphrodite.

androgyny (an-droj'ĭ-ne) female pseudohermaphroditism.

android (an'droid) [*andro-* + Gr. *eidos* shape] resembling a man; manlike.

androidal (an-droi'dal) android.

androkinin (an″dro-kin'in) [*andro-* + Gr. *kinein* to move] a general term for androgenic substances; no longer in good usage.

andrology (an-drol'o-je) [*andro-* + *-logy*] scientific study of the masculine constitution and of the diseases of the male sex; especially the study of diseases of the male organs of generation. Cf. *andriatrics.*

androma (an-dro'mah) [*andr-* + *-oma*] arrhenoblastoma.

Andromachus (an-drom'ah-kus) (1st century A.D.) known as Andromachus the Elder, of Crete, he was body physician to the Emperor Nero and supposedly the originator of a famous universal remedy, theriaca andromachi.

andromania (an″dro-ma'ne-ah) [*andro-* + Gr. *mania* madness] (*obs.*) nymphomania.

Andromeda (an-drom'ĕ-dah) [L.] a genus of ericaceous shrubs and trees, some of which afford a poisonous narcotic principle. *A. maria'na, A. nit'ida,* and *A. polifo'lia* are among the poisonous species.

andromedotoxin (an-drom″ĕ-do-tok'sin) [*Andromeda* + *toxin*] a poisonous crystalline principle, $C_{22}H_{36}O_7$, from various ericaceous plants, such as *Kalmia latifolia* (mountain laurel) and related species; it is toxic to sheep and other livestock that graze on the plants, causing salivation, nasal discharge, emesis, paralysis, coma, and death.

andromerogon (an″dro-mer'o-gon) [*andro-* + Gr. *meros* part + *gonē* seed] an organism developed from an ovum containing the male pronucleus only, the cells, as a result, containing only the paternal set of chromosomes.

andromerogone (an″dro-mer'o-gon) andromerogon.

andromerogony (an″dro-mĕ-rog'o-ne) [*andro-* + Gr. *meros* a part + *gonos* procreation] development of a portion of an ovum containing the male pronucleus only, the nucleus of the ovum having been removed before fusion of the male and female pronuclei occurred. Cf. *gynomerogony* and *merogony.*

andromimetic (an″dro-mĭ-met'ik) [*andro-* + Gr. *mimētikos* imitating] producing male characteristics; having a masculinizing effect; simulating the action of androgen.

andromorphous (an″dro-mor'fus) [*andro-* + Gr. *morphē* form] having a masculine appearance.

andropathy (an-drop'ah-the) [*andro-* + Gr. *pathos* disease] any disease peculiar to males.

androphile (an'dro-fīl) anthropophilic.

androphilous (an-drof'ĭ-lus) anthropophilic.

androphobia (an″dro-fo'be-ah) [*andro-* + Gr. *phobein* to be affrighted by + *-ia*] morbid dislike of the male sex.

Andropogon (an″dro-po'gon) a genus of grasses. *A. sor'ghum* includes broom corn, kafir corn, and sorghum.

androstane (an'dro-stān) the tetracyclic hydrocarbon nucleus ($C_{19}H_{32}$) from which the androgens are derived.

androstanediol (an″dro-stān'de-ol) an androgen, $C_{19}H_{32}O_2$.

androstanedione (an″dro-stān'de-ōn) an androgen, $C_{19}H_{28}O_2$, (3,17-diketo androstane), formed in the testes.

androstanolone (an″dro-stan'o-lōn) an androgen, $C_{19}H_{30}O_2$, occurring in two isomeric forms; see *androsterone.*

androstene (an'dro-stēn) a cyclic hydrocarbon, $C_{19}H_{30}$, with one double bond; a steroid occurring in two isomeric forms forming the nucleus of testosterone and some other androgens.

androstenediol (an″dro-stēn'de-ol) an androgen, $C_{19}H_{30}O_2$, occurring in two isomeric forms, 3-trans, 17-dihydroxy Δ⁵-androstene and 3-cis, 17-dihydroxy Δ⁵-androstene.

androstenedione (an″dro-stēn'de-ōn) an androgen, $C_{19}H_{26}O_2$, 3,17-diketo Δ⁴-androstene; less potent than testosterone, it is secreted by the testis, adrenal cortex, and ovary.

androsterone (an-dros'ter-ōn) an androgen excreted in the urine of both men and women. It is 3α-hydroxy-5α-androstan-17-one, $C_{19}H_{30}O_2$. When injected intramuscularly it counteracts the effects of castration.

androtin (an'dro-tin) a generic term for androgenic substances; no longer in good usage.

-ane a word termination denoting (1) a saturated open-chain hydrocarbon, C_nH_{2n+2}; (2) an organic compound in which hydrogen has replaced the hydroxyl group.

anecdotal (an″ek-do'tal) [Gr. *anekdotos* not published] based on descriptions of unmatched individual cases rather than on controlled studies.

anecdysis (an-ek'dĭ-sis) [*an* neg. + Gr. *ekdysis* a way out] a long period during the molting cycle of arthropods when there are no signs of either recovery from a molt or preparations for the next molt.

anechoic (an-ĕ-ko'ik) without echoes; quiet; said of a chamber for measuring the effects of sound.

anectasin (an-ek'tah-sin) [*an* neg. + Gr. *ektasis* distention] a hypothetical substance once thought to be produced by bacteria and to have an effect on the vasomotor nerves opposite to that of ectasin.

anectasis (an-ek'tah-sis) [*an* neg. + Gr. *ektasis* distention] congenital atelectasis due to developmental immaturity.

Anectine (an-ek'tin) trademark for preparations of succinylcholine chloride.

Anel's operation, probe, syringe [Dominique *Anel*, French surgeon, 1679–1730] see under *operation, probe,* and *syringe.*

anelectrotonic (an″e-lek-tro-ton'ik) pertaining to anelectrotonus.

anelectrotonus (an″e-lek-trot'o-nus) [Gr. *ana* up + *electrotonus*] lessened irritability of a nerve in the region of the positive pole or anode during the passage of an electric current.

anemia (ah-ne'me-ah) [Gr. *an* neg. + *haima* blood + *-ia*] a reduction below normal in the number of erythrocytes per cu. mm., in the quantity of hemoglobin, or in the volume of packed red cells per 100 ml. of blood which occurs when the equilibrium between blood loss (through bleeding or destruction) and blood production is disturbed. **achrestic a.,** megaloblastic anemia morphologically resembling pernicious anemia, but with multiple other causes. **achylic a., a. achy'lica,** hypochromic a., idiopathic. **acute a.,** a nonspecific term indicating anemia of relatively short duration, as acute hemorrhagic anemia. **acquired sideroachrestic a.,** refractory sideroblastic a. **Addison's a., Addison-Biermer a., addisonian a.** (*obs.*), pernicious a. **anhematopoietic a., anhemopoietic a.,** anemia due to defective formation of erythrocytes. **aplastic a.,** a form of anemia generally unresponsive to specific antianemia therapy, often accompanied by granulocytopenia and thrombocytopenia, in which the bone marrow may not necessarily be acellular or hypoplastic but fails to produce adequate numbers of peripheral blood elements. The term actually is all-inclusive and most probably encompasses several clinical syndromes. Called also *aregenerative a.* and *refractory a.* **aregenerative a.,** aplastic a. **aregenerative a., chronic congenital,** hypoplastic a., congenital. **Bagdad Spring a.** (*obs.*) a type of hemolytic anemia most probably due to erythrocyte deficiency of glucose-6-phosphate dehydrogenase. **Bartonella a.,** Oroya fever in man; also occurring in a number of animals, e.g., the dog, as well as in the rat, in which the anemia is latent until splenectomy. **Biermer's a., Biermer-Ehrlich a.** (*obs.*), pernicious a. **a. of Blackfan and Diamond** (*obs.*), hypoplastic a., congenital. **cameloid a.,** elliptocytosis. **cattle a.,** a condition caused by infection with *Theileria parva;* East Coast fever. **chlorotic a.,** chlorosis. **congenital hypoplastic a.,** see *hypoplastic a., congenital.* **congenital a. of newborn,** erythroblastosis fetalis. **congenital nonspherocytic hemolytic a.,** see *hemolytic a., congenital nonspherocytic.* **Cooley's a.,** see *β-thalassemia,* under *thalassemia.* **cow's milk a.,** anemia in infants due to lack of iron in a cow's milk diet. **cytogenic a.** (*obs.*), progressive pernicious a. **deficiency a.,** anemia caused by a lack of a specific substance required for normal hemoglobin synthesis and erythrocytic maturation arising by several means, such as malabsorption or poor dietary intake; called also *nutritional a.* **dilution a.,** a condition in which the anemia is more apparent than real, being due to an increased plasma volume rather than to a decreased total circulating red cell mass. **dimorphic a.,** a condition characterized by a dual erythrocyte population, as defined by a double peak of the diameter frequency curve, observed when combined deficiencies of vitamin B_{12} (or analogous substance) and iron exist concurrently in the same patient. It may also occur in persons receiving blood transfusions. **drepanocytic a.** (*obs.*), sickle cell a. **Edelmann's a.** (*obs.*), a type of chronic infectious anemia. **elliptocytary a., elliptocytotic a.,** elliptocytosis. **equine infectious a.,** a viral disease of equines marked by recurring attacks of malaise with abrupt rises of temperature, and spread through the blood by inoculation, especially by blood-sucking insects. Called also *infectious a. of horses, Vallee's disease,* and *swamp fever.* **erythroblastic a. of childhood,** erythroblastic a., familial; see *β-thalassemia,* under *thalassemia.* **erythronormoblastic a.** (*obs.*), hypochromic a. **essential a.,** primary a. **familial erythroblastic a.,** see *thalassemia.* **Fanconi's a.,** see under *syndrome* (def. 1). **folic acid deficiency a.,** macrocytic anemia due to deficiency of folic acid. **globe cell a.** (*obs.*), hereditary spherocytosis. **glucose-6-phosphate dehydrogenase deficiency a.,** a genetically determined hemolytic anemia caused by a deficiency of this enzyme in erythrocytes which results in hemolysis of the erythrocyte by drugs of certain groups (such as antimalarials, sulfonamides, nitrofurans, antipyretics and analgesics, and sulfones), fava beans, and other agents. Recent studies imply that this predisposition to hemolysis may be expressed in varying degrees and that other biochemical defects, in addition to that involving glucose-6-phosphate dehydrogenase, may also be present in the erythrocytes. **goat's milk a.,** a macrocytic anemia, observed particularly in Germany and Italy, occurring in infants fed exclusively on goat's milk, associated with a megaloblastic bone marrow, thrombocytopenia, leukopenia, hyperbilirubinemia, and hyperferremia. **ground itch a.,** hookworm disease. **Heinz-body a's,** a group of hemolytic syndromes of diverse etiology with the common morphologic characteristic of having one or more Heinz bodies within affected erythrocytes. **hemolytic a.,** anemia due to shortened *in vivo* survival of mature red blood cells and inability of the bone marrow to compensate completely for their decreased life span. **hemolytic a., acquired,** that due to causes other than hereditary factors, including infectious agents, poisons, and physical agents, in which there is premature destruction of red blood cells. **hemolytic a., acute,** a condition characterized by sudden destruction of erythrocytes by hemolysis. **hemolytic a., autoimmune,** acquired hemolytic anemia in which serum antibodies, usually of the IgG class, react with erythrocytes and the Coombs test is positive. It occurs in several autoimmune diseases, including systemic lupus erythematosus. The antibodies may be of the cold or warm type. **hemolytic a., congenital,** a general term for anemia, present at birth, in which the lifespan of red blood cells is diminished. **hemolytic a., congenital nonspherocytic,** a heterogeneous group of nonspherocytic hereditary anemias in which shortened red cell survival is associated with erythrocyte membrane defects, multiple intracellular deficiencies, or unstable hemoglobins. **hemolytic a., hereditary nonspherocytic,** a heterogeneous group of congenital hemolytic anemias characterized by absence of spherocytosis, negative antiglobulin tests, and absence of a detectable abnormal hemoglobin. **hemolytic a., infectious,** that due to an incompletely compensated decrease in red blood cell survival secondary to infectious agents, including protozoa (e.g., *Plasmodium* in malaria), bacteria, and certain viruses. **hemolytic a., microangiopathic,** hemolytic anemia due to intravascular fragmentation of red blood cells. **hemolytic a., toxic,** that due to toxic agents, including drugs and animal and vegetable poisons. **hemorrhagic a.,** anemia caused by the sudden and acute loss of blood; called also *acute posthemorrhagic a.* **hookworm a.,** hypochromic microcytic anemia resulting from infection with *Ancylostoma* or *Necator.* **hypochromic a.,** a condition characterized by a disproportionate reduction of red cell hemoglobin and an increased area of central pallor in the red cells. **hypo-**

chromic a., idiopathic, iron deficiency a. **hypochromic microcytic a.,** hypochromic anemia in which the red cells are reduced in size and in hemoglobin content. **a. hypochro′mica siderochres′tica heredita′ria,** a hereditary, chronic, refractory sideroblastic anemia affecting males; called also *hereditary sideroachrestic a.* **hypoferric a.** (*obs.*), iron deficiency a. **hypoplastic a.,** a general term indicating a form of anemia due to varying degrees of erythrocytic hypoplasia without leukopenia or thrombocytopenia. **hypoplastic a., congenital,** 1. a progressive anemia of unknown etiology encountered in the first year of life, unaccompanied by leukopenia and thrombocytopenia, unresponsive to hematinics, and often requiring multiple blood transfusions to sustain life; called also *chronic congenital aregenerative anemia, erythrogenesis imperfecta,* and *anemia of Blackfan and Diamond.* 2. Fanconi's syndrome, def. 1. **icterohemolytic a.** (*obs.*), hemolytic anemia with jaundice. **idiopathic a.,** primary a. **infectious a. of horses,** equine infectious a. **intertropical a.,** hookworm disease. **iron deficiency a.,** anemia characterized by low or absent iron stores, low serum iron concentration, low transferrin saturation, elevated transferrin, low serum ferritin, low hemoglobin concentration or hematocrit, and hypochromic microcytic red blood cells. Symptoms may include pallor, angular stomatitis and other oral lesions, gastrointestinal complaints, and thinning and brittleness of the nails, occasionally leading to spoon nails (koilonychia). **kennel a.,** a disease of dogs caused by *Ancylostoma caninum.* **Lederer's a.** (*obs.*), an acute hemolytic anemia of short duration and unknown etiology, possibly autoimmune, which, when originally described, further helped to establish the concept of acquired hemolytic anemia as distinct from the congenital spherocytic type. **Leishman's a.** (*obs.*), kala-azar. **leukoerythroblastic a.,** leukoerythroblastosis. **macrocytic a.,** a name applied to a category of anemias, of varying etiologies, characterized by larger than normal red cells, absence of the customary central area of pallor, and an increased mean corpuscular volume and mean corpuscular hemoglobin. **macrocytic a., nutritional,** folic acid deficiency a. **macrocytic a., tropical,** a type of nutritional macrocytic anemia occurring in India, China, and the African west coast, resembling pernicious anemia in many respects but without achlorhydria and only erratically responsive to vitamin B_{12}. Folic acid produces marked improvement in most cases. **Mediterranean a.,** see *β-thalassemia,* under *thalassemia.* **megaloblastic a.,** anemia characterized by the presence of megaloblasts in the bone marrow. **megaloblastic a., familial,** a rare familial form of anemia observed in Norwegian and Finnish children, characterized by selective intestinal malabsorption of vitamin B_{12} uninfluenced by intrinsic factor, and associated with proteinuria, and structural genitourinary tract anomalies. **megalocytic a.,** macrocytic a. **microangiopathic a.,** hemolytic a., microangiopathic. **microcytic a.,** anemia characterized by erythrocytes the majority of which are smaller than normal. **milk a.,** cow's milk a. **miners' a.,** hookworm disease. **mountain a.,** a form of mountain sickness. **myelopathic a., myelophthisic a.,** leukoerythroblastosis. **a. neonato′rum,** the mildest form of erythroblastosis fetalis in which anemia is the chief manifestation; now replaced by the term erythroblastosis qualified by an adjective indicating the degree of severity. **normochromic a.,** anemia in which the hemoglobin content of the red cells as measured by the MCHC is in the normal range. **normocytic a.,** anemia characterized by a proportionate decrease in the hemoglobin content, the packed red cell volume, and the number of erythrocytes per cubic millimeter of blood. **nutritional a.,** deficiency a. **osteosclerotic a.,** a form of myelophthisis occurring in association with osteosclerosis, as a result of the effect on bone marrow of changes in the bones. **pernicious a.,** a megaloblastic anemia occurring in children but more commonly in later life, characterized by histamine-fast achlorhydria, in which the laboratory and clinical manifestations are based on malabsorption of vitamin B_{12} due to a failure of the gastric mucosa to secrete adequate and potent intrinsic factor. Called also *Addison's* or *addisonian a., Addison-Biermer a., cytogenic a.,* and *malignant a.* **pernicious a., juvenile,** megaloblastic anemia occurring in infancy, childhood, or adolescence, resembling the adult form in its response to vitamin B_{12} but distinguished from it by inconstant histamine-fast achlorhydria. **phenylhydrazine a.,** a hemolytic anemia resulting from ingestion of phenylhydrazine, which most probably is converted to a compound that, by acting as an oxidant, transforms oxyhemoglobin to methemoglobin, and then sulfhemoglobin, and finally produces Heinz-Ehrlich bodies. In certain instances, due to an intracellular deficiency of reduced glutathione, and enzymes such as glucose-6-phosphate dehydrogenase, erythrocytes may be particularly sensitive to this agent. **physiologic a.,** the normocytic, normochromic anemia that occurs in infants at the age of two or three months, owing to normal depression of erythropoiesis and hemoglobin synthesis, probably resulting as an adjustment to the change-over from placental to pulmonary oxygenation. **polar a.,** an anemic condition that occurs during exposure to low temperature; initially microcytic, but subsequently becoming normocytic. The basic mechanism is not defined precisely, but it may be due to loss of circulating erythrocytes secondary to trauma or capillary wall diapedesis, in addition to failure of compensatory bone marrow response. Called also *arctic a.* **posthemorrhagic a., acute,** hemorrhagic a. **posthemorrhagic a. of newborn,** anemia of the newborn due to hemorrhage into the placenta or from umbilical vessels; it may range from mild to severe. **primaquine-sensitive a.,** glucose-6-phosphate dehydrogenase a. **primary a.,** an outmoded concept, since all the anemias are regarded as symptoms, and are therefore "secondary." **a. pseudoleuke′mica infan′tum,** a condition originally described as a specific entity in children under age three, with anisocytosis, poikilocytosis, peripheral red blood cell immaturity, leukocytosis, lymphadenopathy, and hepatosplenomegaly; now considered to be a syndrome produced by many factors such as malnutrition, chronic infection, malabsorption, and hemoglobinopathies. **pure red cell a.,** anemia characterized by absence of red cell precursors in the bone marrow. **pyridoxine-responsive a.,** a form of sideroblastic anemia in which there is a therapeutic response to pyridoxine; it affects predominately young or middle-aged males. **refractory a.,** anemia unresponsive to hematinics. **a. refracto′ria sideroblas′tica, refractory sideroblastic a.,** sideroblastic anemia characterized by failure to respond to hematinics; called also *acquired sideroachrestic a.* **Runeberg's a.** (*obs.*), a remittent form of pernicious anemia; called also *Runeberg's disease* or *type.* **scorbutic a.,** anemia due to deficiency of ascorbic acid (vitamin C); in naturally occurring human scurvy the anemia is generally normocytic, although in experimentally induced vitamin C deficiency the anemia is of the megaloblastic type. **secondary a.,** a term originally used to distinguish anemia due to antecedent or associated disease from anemia thought to be a fundamental disease of the hematopoietic system (primary anemia); the distinction is obsolete since anemia is now recognized as a symptom and thus is always "secondary." **sickle cell a.,** a hereditary, genetically determined hemolytic anemia, one of the hemoglobinopathies, occurring almost exclusively in Negroes, characterized by arthralgia, acute attacks of abdominal pain, ulcerations of the lower extremities, sickle-shaped erythrocytes in the blood, and, for full clinical expression, the homozygous presence of S hemoglobin in the red blood cells, as defined by hemoglobin electrophoresis. Called also *sicklemia,* and *Herrick's a.* See also *sickle cell-thalassemia disease,* under *disease.* **sideroachrestic a.,** sideroblastic a. **sideroblastic a.,** a heterogeneous group of anemias with diverse clinical manifestations and with multiple causes each involving a derangement in the final pathway of heme synthesis, in which iron stores of the reticuloendothelial tissues are almost always increased and bone marrow normoblasts contain iron (sideroblasts). Called also *sideroachrestic a.* **sideropenic a.,** a group of anemias characterized by low levels of iron in the plasma; it includes iron deficiency anemia and the anemias of chronic disorders. **simple achlorhydric a.,** (*obs.*), iron deficiency a. **slaty a.,** a term applied to a grayish color of the face in poisoning by acetanilid or silver. **spherocytic a.,** hereditary spherocytosis. **splenic a., a. splenet′ica,** congestive splenomegaly; Banti's disease. **spur-cell a.,** anemia in which the red cells have a bizarre spiculated shape and are destroyed prematurely, primarily in the spleen; it is an acquired form occurring in severe liver disease and represents an abnormality in the cholesterol content of the red-cell membrane. **tropical a.,** hookworm disease. **Von Jaksch's a.,** a. pseudoleukemic infantum.

anemic (ah-ne′mik) pertaining to or characterized by anemia.

anemo- [Gr. *anemos* wind] a combining form denoting relationship to wind.

anemometer (an″ĕ-mom′ĕ-ter) [*anemo-* + Gr. *metron* measure] an instrument for measuring the velocity of air or gas flow.

Anemone (ah-nem′o-ne) a large genus of plants of the family Ranuculaceae, with divided leaves and conspicuous flowers of sepals. They generally contain ranunculin, which converts enzymatically to toxic protoanemonin, a principle held responsible for animal poisoning. Protoanemonin ultimately converts to anemonin, a substituted diacrylic acid dilactone, which has been used as a sedative and antispasmodic. Anemonin is present in *A. pulsatilla* and other species. Several species have been used medicinally.

anemonin (ah-nem′o-nin) the active principle of *Anemone pulsatilla,* a colorless crystalline substance, $C_{10}H_8O_4$, or pulsatilla camphor.

anemonism (ah-nem′o-nizm) poisoning by plants of the genus *Anemone.*

anemonol (ah-nem′o-nol) an exceedingly poisonous volatile oil from various species of *Anemone* and from other ranunculaceous plants.

anemophilous (an″ĕ-mof′ĭ-lus) [*anemo-* + Gr. *philein* to love] pollinated by the wind; said of certain flowers.

anemophobia (an″ĕ-mo-fo′be-ah) [*anemo-* + Gr. *phobein* to be affrighted by + *ia*] morbid fear of wind or of drafts.

anemotaxis (an″ĕ-mo-tak′sis) [*anemo-* + Gr. *taxis* arrangement] adjustment with reference to the wind.

anemotrophy (an″ĕ-mot′ro-fe) [*an* neg. + Gr. *haima* blood + *trophē* nourishment] deficiency of blood nourishment.

anemotropism (an″ĕ-mot′ro-pism) [*anemo-* + Gr. *tropos* a turning] a turning toward or away from the wind.

anencephalia (an″en-sĕ-fa′le-ah) anencephaly.

anencephalic (an″en-sĕ-fal′ik) exhibiting anencephaly; having no brain.

anencephalous (an″en-sef′ah-lus) having no brain.

anencephalus (an″en-sef′ah-lus) a monster exhibiting anencephaly.

anencephaly (an″en-sef′ah-le) [*an* neg. + Gr. *enkephalos* brain] congenital absence of the cranial vault, with cerebral hemispheres completely missing or reduced to small masses attached to the base of the skull.

anenterous (an-en′ter-us) [*an* neg. + Gr. *enteron* intestine] lacking intestines.

anenzymia (an″en-zi′me-ah) a morbid condition resulting from absence of an enzyme normally present in the body. **a. cata·la′sea,** acatalasia.

anephric (a-nef′rik) being without kidneys.

anephrogenesis (a″nef-ro-jen′ĕ-sis) [*a* neg. + Gr. *nephros* kidney + *genesis*] congenital absence of kidney tissue.

anepiploic (an-ep″e-plo′ik) devoid of omentum.

anepithymia (an-ep″ĕ-thim′e-ah) loss of any natural appetite.

anerethisia (an-er″ĕ-thiz′e-ah) [*an* neg. + Gr. *erethizein* to excite + *-ia*] deficient irritability.

aneretic (an″e-ret′ik) [Gr. *anairetikos*] destructive.

anergasia (an″er-ga′ze-ah) [*an* neg. + Gr. *ergasia* work] lack of functional activity; Meyer's term for a psychosis associated with a structural lesion of the central nervous system.

anergastic (an″er-gas′tik) Meyer's term for psychic disorders from structural loss of brain function (loss of memory and judgment, fits, contractures, palsies, etc.).

anergia (an-er′je-ah) anergy.

anergic (an-er′jik) [*an* neg. + Gr. *ergon* work] 1. characterized by abnormal inactivity; inactive. 2. marked by asthenia or lack of energy. 3. pertaining to anergy.

anergy (an′er-je) diminished reactivity to specific antigen(s); it may take the form of diminished immediate hypersensitivity or diminished delayed hypersensitivity, or both. **absolute a.,** transient reduction or complete lack of reactivity to antigen (or allergen), e.g., tuberculin allergens, in a sensitized individual, occurring as a result of intervening events, such as cachexia. **cachectic a.,** transient lessened reactivity to allergens in a sensitized individual, occurring as a result of debilitation. **negative a.,** transient reduction in reactivity to allergens in a sensitized individual, occurring as a result of intervening events, such as cachexia. **positive a.,** reduction in reactivity to allergens in a sensitized individual, owing to alterations in the immune response in the course of disease, as in tuberculosis.

aneroid (an′er-oid) [*a* neg. + Gr. *nēros* liquid + *eidos* form] not containing liquid.

anerythroblepsia (an″ĕ-rith″ro-blep′se-ah) anerythropsia.

anerythroplasia (an″ĕ-rith″ro-pla′ze-ah) [*an* neg. + Gr. *erythros* red + *plassein* to form + *-ia*] absence of erythrocyte formation.

anerythroplastic (an″ĕ-rith″ro-plas′tik) pertaining to or characterized by anerythroplasia.

anerythropoiesis (an″ĕ-rith″ro-poi-e′sis) [*an* neg. + *erythropoiesis*] deficient production of erythrocytes.

anerythropsia (an″er-ĭ-throp′se-ah) [*an* neg. + Gr. *erythros* red + *opsis* sight + *-ia*] impaired perception of red tints.

anerythroregenerative (an″ĕ-rith″ro-re-jen′er-a″tiv) see *aregenerative.*

anesthecinesia (an-es″the-sĭ-ne′ze-ah) [*an* neg. + Gr. *aisthēsis* perception + *kinēsis* movement + *-ia*] loss of sensibility and motor power.

anesthekinesia (an-es″the-kĭ-ne′ze-ah) anesthecinesia.

anesthesia (an″es-the′ze-ah) [*an* neg. + Gr. *aisthēsis* sensation] loss of feeling or sensation. Although the term is used for loss of tactile sensibility, or of any of the other senses, it is applied especially to loss of the sensation of pain, as it is induced to permit performance of surgery or other painful procedures. **angiospastic a.,** loss of sensibility dependent on spasm of the blood vessels. **balanced a.,** anesthesia which utilizes a combination of drugs, each in an amount sufficient to produce its major or desired effect to the optimum degree and keep its undesirable or unnecessary effects to a minimum. **basal a.,** anesthesia which acts as a basis for further and deeper anesthesia; a state of narcosis produced by preliminary medication so profound that the added inhalation anesthetic necessary to produce surgical anesthesia is greatly reduced. **Bier's local a.,** local anesthesia produced by injection of a 0.5 per cent solution of procaine in the veins of a limb that has been rendered bloodless by elevation and constriction; called also *vein a.* **block a.,** see *regional a.* and *block.* **bulbar a.,** lack of sensation caused by a lesion of the pons. **caudal a.,** anesthesia produced by injection of a local anesthetic into the caudal or sacral canal. **central a.,** lack of sensation caused by disease of the nerve centers. **cerebral a.,**

lack of sensation caused by a cerebral lesion. **closed a.,** inhalational anesthesia maintained by the continuous rebreathing of a relatively small amount of the anesthetic gas, normally used with an absorption apparatus for the removal of carbon dioxide. **colonic a.,** anesthesia induced by injection of the anesthetic agent into the rectum and lower colon. **compression a.,** loss of sensation resulting from pressure on a nerve. **conduction a.,** regional a. **continuous caudal a.,** see under *analgesia*. **Corning's a.,** see *spinal a.,* def. 1. **crossed a.,** hemianesthesia cruciata. **dissociated a., dissociation a.,** loss of certain sensations while others remain intact. **doll's head a.,** loss of sensation affecting the head, neck, and upper part of the thorax. **a. doloro′sa,** pain in an area or region that is anesthetic. **electric a.,** anesthesia induced by passage of an electric current. **endobronchial a.,** anesthesia produced by introduction of a gaseous mixture through a slender tube placed in a large bronchus. **endotracheal a.,** anesthesia produced by introduction of a gaseous mixture through a wide-bore tube inserted into the trachea. **epidural a.,** anesthesia produced by injection of the anesthetic agent between the vertebral spines and beneath the ligamentum flavum into the extradural space; called also *peridural a.* **facial a.,** loss of sensation caused by a lesion of the facial nerve. **frost a.,** abolition of feeling or sensation as a result of topical refrigeration produced by a jet of highly volatile liquid. **gauntlet a.,** loss of sensation in the hand and wrist; called also *glove a.* **general a.,** a state of unconsciousness, produced by anesthetic agents, with absence of pain sensation over the entire body and a greater or lesser degree of muscular relaxation; the drugs producing this state can be administered by inhalation, intravenously, intramuscularly, rectally, or via the gastrointestinal tract. **girdle a.,** loss of sensation in a zone encircling the hips. **glove a.,** gauntlet a. **gustatory a.,** loss of the sense of taste. **Gwathmey's oilether a.,** anesthesia produced by introduction into the rectum of a mixture of liquid ether and olive oil. **high pressure a.,** anesthesia produced by controlled application of pressure to a nerve trunk or its branches. **hypnosis a.,** production of insensibility to pain during surgical procedures by means of hypnotism. **hypotensive a.,** anesthesia accompanied by the deliberate lowering of the blood pressure, a procedure said to reduce blood loss. **hypothermic a.,** anesthesia accompanied by the deliberate lowering of the body temperature. **hysterical a.,** loss of sensation occurring in hysteria, characterized by its failure to conform to anatomical nerve distributions, as in *gauntlet a.* **infiltration a.,** the production of local anesthesia by deposition of a local anesthesia solution in the area of small, terminal nerve endings. **inhalation a.,** anesthesia produced by the inhalation of vapors of a volatile liquid or gaseous anesthetic agent. **insufflation a.,** anesthesia produced by blowing a mixture of gases or vapors through a tube introduced into the respiratory tract. **intercostal a.,** anesthesia produced by blocking intercostal nerves with a local anesthetic. **intranasal a.,** local anesthesia produced by insertion into the nasal fossae of pledgets soaked in a solution of an anesthetic agent which is effective after topical application, or by insufflation of a mixture of anesthetic gases or vapors through a tube introduced into the nose. **intraoral a.,** anesthesia produced within the oral cavity by injection, spray, pressure, etc. **intraosseous a.,** a local anesthetic effect produced by the administration of an anesthetic agent directly into the cancellous portion of bone. **intrapulpal a.,** a local anesthetic effect produced by the administration of an anesthetic agent directly into the dental pulp. **intraspinal a.,** spinal a., def. 1. **intravenous a.,** anesthesia produced by introduction of an anesthetic agent into a vein. **Kulenkampff's a.,** anesthesia of the upper extremity produced by injection of a local anesthetic around the brachial plexus. **local a.,** anesthesia confined to one part of the body. **lumbar epidural a.,** anesthesia produced by injection of the anesthetic agent into the epidural space at the second or third lumbar interspace. **Meltzer's a.,** see under *method*. **mental a.,** loss of ability to recognize or identify sensory stimulations. **mixed a.,** anesthesia which is produced by administration of more than one anesthetic agent; see also *balanced a.* **muscular a.,** loss of the muscular sense. **nausea a.,** loss of the sensation of nausea, usually stimulated by noxious and disgusting substances. **nerve blocking a.,** regional a. **olfactory a.,** anosmia. **open a.,** general inhalation anesthesia utilizing a cone; there is no significant rebreathing of expired gases. **paraneural a.,** anesthesia produced by injection of the anesthetic agent around a nerve; called also *paraneural infiltration*. **parasacral a.,** regional anesthesia produced by injection of a local anesthetic around the sacral nerves as they emerge from the sacral foramina. **paravertebral a.,** regional anesthesia produced by injection of a local anesthetic around the spinal nerves at their exit from the spinal column, and outside the spinal dura. **partial a.,** anesthesia with retention of some degree of sensibility. **peridural a.,** epidural a. **perineural a.,** regional anesthesia produced by injection of the anesthetic agent close to the nerve. **peripheral a.,** loss of sensation which is due to changes in the peripheral nerves. **permeation a.,** analgesia of a body surface produced by the application of a local anesthetic, most commonly to mucous membranes; called also *surface a.*

plexus a., anesthesia produced by the injection of a local anesthetic around a nerve plexus. **pressure a.,** anesthesia produced by a local anesthetic forced into the tissues by pressure. **rectal a.,** anesthesia induced by introduction of an anesthetic agent into the rectum. **refrigeration a.,** local anesthesia produced by applying a tourniquet and chilling the part to near freezing temperature; called also *crymoanesthesia*. **regional a.,** the production of insensibility of a part by interrupting the sensory nerve conductivity from that region of the body. It may be produced by (1) *field block*, that is, the creation of walls of anesthesia encircling the operative field by means of injections of a local anesthetic; or (2) *nerve block*, that is, injection of the anesthetic agent close to the nerves whose conductivity is to be cut off. Called also *blocking a., conduction a.,* and *block*. **sacral a.,** anesthesia produced by injection of a local anesthetic into the extradural space of the sacral canal. **saddle block a.,** the production of anesthesia in a region corresponding roughly with the areas of the buttocks, perineum, and inner aspects of the thighs which impinge on the saddle in riding, by introducing the anesthetic agent low in the dural sac. **segmental a.,** loss of sensation caused by lesions of nerve roots. **semiclosed a.,** general inhalation anesthesia in which there is partial rebreathing of the expired gases, with a carbon dioxide absorber in the circuit. **semiopen a.,** general inhalation anesthesia administered by use of an open cone or a partially open circuit; there is partial rebreathing of the expired gases without a carbon dioxide absorber in the circuit. **sexual a.,** anaphrodisia. **spinal a.,** 1. anesthesia produced by injection of a local anesthetic into the subarachnoid space around the spinal cord; called also *Corning's a.* or *method, intraspinal a.,* and *subarachnoid a.* 2. loss of sensation due to a spinal lesion. **splanchnic a.,** anesthesia produced by injection of a local anesthetic around the semilunar ganglia. **subarachnoid a.,** spinal a., def. 1. **surface a.,** permeation a. **surgical a.,** that degree of anesthesia at which surgery may safely be performed; ordinarily used to designate such depth of general anesthesia. **tactile a.,** loss or impairment of the sense of touch. **thalamic hyperesthetic a.,** see *thalamic syndrome,* under *syndrome*. **thermal a., thermic a.,** loss of the temperature sense. **topical a.,** anesthesia produced by application of a local anesthetic directly to the area involved, as to the oral mucosa or the cornea. **total a.,** loss of all sensibility in the affected part. **transsacral a.,** spinal anesthesia produced by injection of the anesthetic agent into the sacral canal and about the sacral nerves through each of the posterior sacral foramina. **traumatic a.,** loss of sensation caused by injury to a nerve. **twilight a.,** twilight sleep. **unilateral a.,** hemianesthesia. **vein a.,** Bier's local a. **visceral a.,** loss of visceral sensations.

anesthesimeter (an-es″thĕ-sim′ĕ-ter) [*anesthesia* + Gr. *metron* measure] 1. an instrument to regulate the amount of an anesthetic administered. 2. an instrument for taking the degree of insensitiveness.

Anesthesin (ah-nes′thĕ-sin) trademark for a preparation of benzocaine.

anesthesiologist (an″es-the″ze-ol′o-jist) a physician specializing in anesthesiology. Cf. *anesthetist*.

anesthesiology (an″es-the″ze-ol′o-je) [*anesthesia* + *-logy*] that branch of medicine which studies anesthesia and anesthetics.

anesthesiophore (an″es-the′ze-o-fōr″) [*anesthesia* + Gr. *phoros* bearing] 1. conveying the anesthetic action. 2. the portion of the molecule of a chemical compound which is responsible for its anesthetic action.

anesthetic (an″es-thet′ik) 1. pertaining to, characterized by, or producing anesthesia. 2. a drug or agent that is used to abolish the sensation of pain. **general a.,** an agent that produces general anesthesia. **local a.,** an agent whose anesthetic action is limited to an area of the body determined by the site of its application; it produces its effect by blocking nerve conduction. **topical a.,** a local anesthetic applied directly to the area to be anesthetized, usually the mucous membranes or the skin.

anesthetist (ah-nes′thĕ-tist) a person, such as a nurse or technician, trained in the administration of anesthetics. Cf. *anesthesiologist*.

anesthetization (ah-nes″thĕ-tĭ-za′shun) the production of insensibility to pain.

anesthetize (ah-nes′thĕ-tīz) to put under the influence of anesthetics.

anesthetometer (an″es-thĕ-tom′ĕ-ter) an apparatus for measuring and mixing anesthetic vapors and gases.

anesthetospasm (an″es-thet′o-spazm) spasm with anesthesia.

anestrum (an-es′trum) anestrus.

anestrus (an-es′trus) a period of sexual inactivity intervening between two estrous cycles.

anethene (an′e-thēn) a hydrocarbon, $C_{10}H_{16}$, from oil of dill.

anethole (an′ĕ-thōl) [NF] chemical name: (*E*)-1-methoxy-4-(1-propenyl)benzene. A colorless or faintly yellow liquid, $C_{10}H_{12}O$, obtained from anise and fennel oils and other sources, or prepared synthetically; used as a flavoring agent for drugs, and formerly as a carminative and expectorant. Called also *anise camphor*.

Anethum (ah-ne′thum) [L.; Gr. *anēthon*] a genus of plants, including fennel and dill, the source of oil of dill and a source of carvone. The fruit of *A. graveolens* (*Peucedanum graveolens*), or dill, is carminative and stimulant.

anetic (ah-net′ik) relaxing or soothing.

anetiological (an-e″te-o-loj′e-kal) [*an* neg. + *etiologic*] not conforming to etiologic principles.

anetoderma (an″ĕ-to-der′mah) [Gr. *anetos* slack + *derma* skin] atrophy and looseness of the skin; primary macular atrophy. There are two forms: that of Schweninger and Buzzi, in which the skin becomes loosened, gray, thickened, and stiff and contains multiple new growths; that of Jadassohn in which erythematous lesions develop which become baglike protrusions. Called also *atrophia maculosa cutis*.

aneugamy (an-u′gah-me) [*an-* neg. + Gr. *eu* well + *gamos* marriage] union of gametes in one or both of which the chromosomes have not been reduced to the normal haploid number, resulting in an abnormal number of chromosomes (aneuploidy) in the zygote.

aneuploid (an′u-ploid) [*an-* + *euploid*] 1. having more or less than the normal diploid number of chromosomes. 2. an individual or cell having more or less than the normal diploid number of chromosomes.

aneuploidy (an″u-ploi′de) any deviation from an exact multiple of the haploid number of chromosomes, whether fewer (hypoploidy, as in Turner's syndrome) or more (hyperploidy, as in Down's syndrome). Individuals exhibiting aneuploidy are usually abnormal physiologically and morphologically, and animals especially, seldom survive. Cf. *euploidy* and *polyploidy*.

aneurin (ah-nu′rin) [*an* neg. + Gr. *neuron* nerve] thiamine hydrochloride (vitamin B₁).

aneurine hydrochloride (an′u-rin) thiamine hydrochloride.

aneurogenic (a″nu-ro-jen′ik) pertaining to or characterized by absence of formation of nerve fibers.

aneurysm (an′u-rizm) [Gr. *aneurysma* a widening] a sac formed by the dilatation of the wall of an artery, a vein, or the heart. The chief signs of arterial aneurysm are the formation of a pulsating tumor, and often a bruit (*aneurysmal bruit*) heard over the swelling. Sometimes there are symptoms from pressure on contiguous parts. **abdominal a.,** an aneurysm of the abdominal aorta. **ampullary a.,** sacculated a. **a. by anastomosis, a. anastomot′ica** (obs.), a dilatation of several arteries which forms a pulsating tumor under the skin. **aortic a.,** aneurysm of the aorta. **aortic sinusal a.,** aneurysm arising in the aortic sinuses of Valsalva; these rare lesions may be either developmental or syphilitic. **arteriovenous a.** (William Hunter, 1761), a communication, sometimes congenital, often traumatic, between an artery and a vein in which the blood flows directly into a neighboring vein (*aneurysmal varix*) or else is carried into such a vein by a connecting sac (*varicose aneurysm*). **arteriovenous pulmonary a.,** arteriovenous fistula. **atherosclerotic a.,** an aneurysm arising as a result of weakening of the media in severe atherosclerosis. **axillary a.,** aneurysm of the axillary artery. **bacterial a.,** infected a. **berry a.,** a small saccular aneurysm of a cerebral artery, usually at the junction of vessels in the circle of Willis, having a narrow opening into the artery; such aneurysms frequently rupture, causing subarachnoid hemorrhage. **brain a.,** berry a. **cardiac a.,** thinning and dilatation of a portion of the wall of the left ventricle, usually consequent to myocardial infarction but rare forms have been described. **cerebral a.,** berry a. **cirsoid a.,** racemose a. **compound a.,** one in which some of the coats are ruptured and others merely dilated; called also *mixed a.* **congenital cerebral a.,** berry a. **Crisp's a.** (obs.), aneurysm of the splenic artery. **cylindroid a.,** the uniform dilatation of a considerable part of an artery; called also *tubular a.* **cystogenic a.** (obs.), one formed by the rupture of a cyst into an artery. **dissecting a.,** one resulting from hemorrhage that causes longitudinal splitting of the arterial wall, producing a tear in the intima and establishing communication with the lumen; it usually affects the thoracic aorta. Called also *aortic dissection, Laennec's disease,* and *Shekelton's a.* **ectatic a.,** one formed by distention of a section of an artery without rupture of any of its coats. **embolic a.,** the most common form of mycotic aneurysm. **embolomycotic a.** (obs.), aneurysm due to embolism from some vegetative condition in the heart. **false a.,** one in which the entire wall is injured and the blood is contained by the surrounding tissues, with eventual formation of a sac communicating with the artery (or heart); called also *aneurysmal hematoma, pulsatile hematoma,* and *spurious a.* **fusiform a.,** a spindle-shaped arterial aneurysm in which the stretching process affects the entire circumference of the artery; called also *Richet's a.* Cf. *saccular a.* **hernial a.,** one in which the sac is formed by an inner coat projecting through the outer. **infected a.,** aneurysm produced by growth of microorganisms in the vessel wall, or infection arising within a preexisting arteriosclerotic aneurysm. Called also *bacterial a.* and *mycotic a.* **innominate a.,** aneurysm of the innominate artery (brachiocephalic trunk). **intracranial a.,** any aneurysm situated within the cranium. **lateral a.,** one that projects from one side of an artery. **miliary a.,** aneu-

rysm of a minute artery, chiefly intracranial or retinal. **mixed a.** (obs.), compound a. **mural a.** (obs.), aneurysm of the heart wall. **mycotic a.,** infected a. **orbital a.,** one situated within the orbit of the eye. **Park's a.,** an arteriovenous aneurysm occurring at the elbow and establishing communication between the brachial artery and the brachial and median basilic veins. **pelvic a.,** one situated within the pelvis. **Pott's a.,** an aneurysmal varix. **racemose a.,** a condition in which the blood vessels become dilated, lengthened, and tortuous; called also *cirsoid a.* and *diffuse arterial ectasia.* **Rasmussen's a.,** dila-

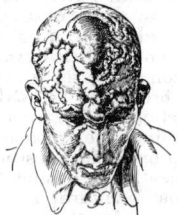

Racemose aneurysm (Homans).

tation of an artery in a tuberculous cavity; its rupture produces hemorrhage. **renal a.,** an aneurysm within the kidney. **Richet's a.,** fusiform a. **Rodrigues' a.,** a varicose aneurysm with the sac lying contiguous to the artery. **saccular a., sacculated a.,** an eccentric localized distended sac affecting only a part of the circumference of the arterial wall. Cf. *fusiform a.* **serpentine a.,** an elongated and varicose senile condition of certain arteries, such as the splenic, iliac, and temporal. **Shekelton's a.,** dissecting a. **spurious a.,** false a. **suprasellar a.,** aneurysm of the internal carotid artery above the sella turcica. **syphilitic a.,** aortic aneurysm occurring in cases of cardiovascular syphilis. **thoracic a.,** one situated within the thorax. **traumatic a.,** an aneurysm due to injury. **true a.,** an aneurysm in which the sac is formed by the arterial walls one of which, at least, is unbroken. **tubular a.,** cylindroid a. **varicose a.,** an aneurysm in which the artery communicates with contiguous veins by means of an intervening sac. **venous a.,** aneurysm of a vein. **ventricular a.,** an aneurysmal dilatation of a portion of the wall of the left ventricle or, rarely, a saccular protrusion through it (*false a. of the heart*). **verminous a.,** aneurysm of equines caused by strongylid worms; called also *worm a.* **worm a.,** verminous a.

aneurysmal (an″u-riz′mal) pertaining to or resembling an aneurysm.

aneurysmatic (an″u-riz-mat′ik) aneurysmal.

aneurysmectomy (an″u-riz-mek′to-me) [*aneurysm* + Gr. *ektomē* excision] extirpation of an aneurysm by removal of the sac.

aneurysmoplasty (an″u-riz′mo-plas″te) [*aneurysm* + Gr. *plassein* to form] plastic restoration of the artery in the treatment of aneurysm.

aneurysmorrhaphy (an″u-riz-mor′ah-fe) [*aneurysm* + Gr. *rhaphē* suture] the operation of suturing an aneurysm.

aneurysmotomy (an″u-riz-mot′o-me) [*aneurysm* + Gr. *tomē* cut] the operation of incising the sac of an aneurysm.

ANF antinuclear factor.

anfractuosity (an-frak″tu-os′ĭ-te) [L. *anfractus* a bending] (obs.) a cerebral sulcus.

anfractuous (an-frak′tu-us) (obs.) convoluted, sinuous, or tortuous.

angei- for words beginning thus, see those beginning *angi-*.

Angelica (an-jel′e-kah) [L., from Gr. *angelikos* angelic] a genus of umbelliferous plants; the roots and fruit of *A. archangelica* (garden angelica) afford volatile oils, angelic acid (formerly a sedative), and several acids. The plant has carminative, diaphoretic, and diuretic properties.

angeline (an′jĕ-lin) surinamine.

Angelucci's syndrome (an″jĕ-loo′chēz) [Arnaldo *Angelucci,* Naples ophthalmologist, 1854–1933] see under *syndrome.*

Anghelescu's sign (ahn-jĕ-les′kōoz) [Constantin *Anghelescu,* Roumanian surgeon, 1869–1948] see under *sign.*

angi- see *angio-.*

angialgia (an″je-al′je-ah) [*angi-* + Gr. *algos* pain + *-ia*] pain in a blood vessel; called also *angiodynia.*

angiasthenia (an″je-as-the′ne-ah) [*angi-* + *a* neg. + Gr. *sthenos* strength + *-ia*] loss of tone in the vascular system; vascular instability.

angiectasis (an″je-ek′tah-sis) [*angi-* + Gr. *ektasis* dilatation] gross dilatation and often lengthening of a blood vessel.

angiectatic (an″je-ek-tat′ik) pertaining to or characterized by angiectasis.

angiectomy (an″je-ek′to-me) [*angi-* + Gr. *ektomē* excision] the excision or resection of a vessel.

angiectopia (an″je-ek-to′pe-ah) [*angi-* + Gr. *ek* out + Gr. *topos* place + *-ia*] abnormal position or course of a vessel.

angiemphraxis (an″je-em-frak′sis) [*angi-* + Gr. *emphraxis* stoppage] (*obs.*) the stopping up of a vessel, as by an embolus.

angiitis (an″je-i′tis), pl. *angii′tides* [*angi-* + *-itis*] inflammation of a vessel, chiefly of a blood or a lymph vessel; called also *vasculitis.* **allergic cutaneous a.,** angiitis due to allergic reaction, marked by such cutaneous lesions as papules, macules, vesicles, urticarial wheals, purpura, and small ulcers, and accompanied by itching and usually by a slight fever and malaise; called also *allergic cutaneous vasculitis* and *nodular vasculitis.* **consecutive a.,** inflammation of a vessel caused by extension of the inflammation from the neighboring tissues. **necrotizing a.,** any condition in which vascular inflammation leads to fibrinoid necrosis of the vessel walls (arteries or veins, or both). **necrotizing a. with granulomata,** allergic granulomatosis. **nodular cutaneous a.,** angiitis in which small muscular-walled arteries are involved, along with cutaneous lesions. **visceral a.,** a term proposed for a group of disorders marked by peculiar lesions of the small arteries, such as periarteritis nodosa, allergic angiitis, and lupus erythematosus disseminatus.

angina (an-ji′nah, an′ji-nah) [L.] spasmodic, choking, or suffocative pain; now used almost exclusively to denote angina pectoris. **abdominal a., a. abdomina′lis, a. abdom′inis,** intestinal a. **a. acu′ta,** simple sore throat. **agranulocytic a.,** agranulocytosis. **benign croupous a.,** pharyngitis herpetica. **Bretonneau's a.,** diphtheria. **a. cap′itis,** headache, especially that due to refractive errors. **a. catarrha′lis,** acute pharyngitis. **a. cor′dis,** a. pectoris. **a. croupo′sa** (*obs.*), pseudomembranous or croupous sore throat. **a. cru′ris,** intermittent claudication. **a. decu′bitus,** cardiac pain occurring in a recumbent position. **a. diphtherit′ica,** diphtheritic pharyngitis or laryngitis. **a. dyspep′tica,** a condition resembling angina pectoris but due to distention of the stomach with gas. **a. epiglottide′a,** inflammation of the epiglottis. **exudative a.,** croup. **a. follicula′ris,** follicular tonsillitis. **fusospirochetal a.** (*obs.*), necrotizing ulcerative gingivitis. **a. gangreno′sa,** gangrenous inflammation of the fauces. **hippocratic a.,** retropharyngeal abscess. **hysteric a.,** pain simulating angina in a hysterical patient. **intestinal a.,** cramping postprandial abdominal pain caused by ischemia of the smooth muscle of the bowel in patients with mesenteric vascular insufficiency. **a. inver′sa,** a variant form of angina pectoris in which there is elevation, rather than depression, of the RS-T interval of the electrocardiogram. **lacunar a.,** tonsillitis. **a. laryn′gea,** laryngitis. **a. ludovi′ci, a. ludwig′ii, Ludwig's a.,** diffuse purulent inflammation of the floor of the mouth, its fascial spaces, muscles, and glands, and spreading to the soft tissues of the upper neck; edema may cause airway obstruction. Called also *Gensoul's disease.* **malignant a.,** a. gangrenosa. **a. membrana′cea,** croup. **monocytic a.** (*obs.*), infectious mononucleosis. **neutropenic a.,** agranulocytosis. **a. nosoco′mii,** pharyngitis ulcerosa. **a. parotid′ea,** mumps. **a. pec′toris,** a paroxysmal thoracic pain, with a feeling of suffocation and impending death, due, most often, to anoxia of the myocardium and precipitated by effort or excitement; has been called *a. cordis, angor pectoris, Elsner's asthma, Heberden's asthma* or *disease, Rougnon-Heberden disease,* and *stenocardia.* **a. pec′toris vasomoto′ria,** a condition marked by precordial pain due to vasomotor disturbance and showing no organic disease of the heart; called also *vasomotor a.* **a. phlegmono′sa,** peritonsillar abscess. **Plaut's a., pseudomembranous a.,** necrotizing ulcerative gingivitis. **preinfarction a.,** status anginosus. **Prinzmetal's a.,** a variant of angina pectoris in which the attacks occur during rest, exercise capacity is well preserved, and attacks are associated electrocardiographically with elevation of the ST-segment. Called also *variant a. pectoris.* **a. rheumat′ica,** pharyngitis associated with rheumatic diathesis. **a. scarlatino′sa,** pharyngitis associated with scarlet fever. **Schultz's a.,** agranulocytosis. **a. sim′plex,** simple sore throat. **a. sine dolo′re,** an episode of coronary insufficiency in which no pain is experienced. **streptococcal a.,** angina due to a streptococcus. **a. tonsilla′ris,** peritonsillar abscess. **a. trachea′lis,** croup. **ulceromembranous a.** (*obs.*), necrotizing ulcerative gingivitis. **a. ulcero′sa,** pharyngitis ulcerosa. **variant a. pectoris,** Prinzmetal's a. **vasomotor a.,** a. pectoris vasomotoria. **Vincent's a.,** necrotizing ulcerative gingivitis.

anginal (an-ji′nal, an′ji-nal) pertaining to or characteristic of angina.

anginiform (an-jin′i-form) resembling angina.

anginoid (an′ji-noid) resembling angina.

anginophobia (an″jin-o-fo′be-ah) [*angina* + Gr. *phobein* to be affrighted by + *-ia*] morbid dread of angina pectoris.

anginose (an′ji-nōs) [L. *anginosus*] pertaining to or affected with angina, especially angina pectoris.

anginosis (an″ji-no′sis) a general term for anginal conditions; angina; often used to denote continuing pain; status anginosus.

anginous (an′ji-nus) anginose.

angio-, angi- (an′je-o, an′je) [Gr. *angeion* vessel] a combining form denoting relationship to a vessel, usually a blood vessel.

angioasthenia (an″je-o-as-the′ne-ah) angiasthenia.

angioataxia (an″je-o-ah-tak′se-ah) [*angio-* + *ataxia*] irregular tension of the blood vessels.

angioblast (an′je-o-blast″) [*angio-* + Gr. *blastos* germ] 1. the mesenchymal tissue of the embryo from which the blood cells and blood vessels differentiate; called also *angioderm.* 2. an individual vessel-forming cell.

angioblastic (an″je-o-blas′tik) pertaining to angioblast.

angioblastoma (an″je-o-blas-to′mah) a term applied to certain blood-vessel tumors of the brain: those arising in the cerebellum (cerebellar angioblastoma) may be cystic and associated with Von Hippel-Lindau's disease; also, a blood-vessel tumor arising from the meninges of the brain or spinal cord (angioblastic meningioma).

angiocardiogram (an″je-o-kar′de-o-gram) the film produced by angiocardiography.

angiocardiography (an″je-o-kar″de-og′rah-fe) [*angio-* + Gr. *kardia* heart + *graphein* to write] roentgenography of the heart and great vessels after introduction of contrast material into a blood vessel or one of the cardiac chambers.

angiocardiokinetic (an″je-o-kar″de-o-ki-net′ik) [*angio-* + Gr. *kardia* heart + *kinēsis* motion] 1. affecting the motions or movements of the heart and blood vessels. 2. any agent that affects the movements of the heart and vessels.

angiocardiopathy (an″je-o-kar″de-op′ah-the) any disease of the heart and blood vessels.

angiocarditis (an″je-o-kar-di′tis) [*angio-* + Gr. *kardia* heart + *-itis*] inflammation of the heart and great blood vessels.

angiocavernous (an″je-o-kav′er-nus) of the nature of angioma and cavernoma.

angioceratoma (an″je-o-ser″ah-to′mah) angiokeratoma.

angiocheiloscope (an″je-o-ki′lo-skōp″) [*angio-* + Gr. *cheilos* lip + *skopein* to view] an instrument for observing blood circulation of the lips under magnification.

angiochondroma (an″je-o-kon-dro′mah) a chondroma about which there is an excessive development of blood vessels.

angioclast (an′je-o-klast″) [*angio-* + Gr. *klastos* broken] former name for hemostat.

Angiococcus (an″je-o-kok′us) [Gr. *angeion* vessel + *kokkos* berry] a genus of microorganisms of the family Myxococcaceae, with two species, *A. cellulosum* and *A. discoformis.*

Angio-CONRAY (an″je-o-kon′ra) trademark for a preparation of sodium iothalamate.

angiocrine (an′je-o-krīn) [*angio-* + *endocrine*] denoting vasomotor disorders of endocrine origin.

angiocrinosis (an″je-o-kri-no′sis) a vasomotor disorder of endocrine origin.

angiocyst (an′je-o-sist″) [*angio-* + *cyst*] angioblastic cyst.

angioderm (an′je-o-derm) angioblast, def. 1.

angiodermatitis (an″je-o-der-mah-ti′tis) (*obs.*) inflammation of the vessels of the skin.

angiodiascopy (an″je-o-di-as′ko-pe) [*angio-* + Gr. *dia* through + *skopein* to view] direct visual inspection of blood vessels of the extremities, a light being held behind the part.

angiodiathermy (an″je-o-di′ah-ther″me) [*angio-* + *diathermy*] coagulation by diathermy of the long posterior ciliary arteries in treatment of glaucoma; now rarely done.

angiodynia (an″je-o-din′e-ah) [*angio-* + Gr. *odynē* pain + *-ia*] angialgia.

angiodysplasia (an″je-o-dis-pla′ze-ah) small vascular abnormalities, especially of the intestinal tract.

angiodystrophia (an″je-o-dis-tro′fe-ah) [*angio-* + *dystrophy*] defective nutrition of blood vessels. **a. ova′rii,** angiodystrophia of the blood vessels of the ovary.

angiodystrophy (an″je-o-dis′tro-fe) angiodystrophia.

angioectatic (an″je-o-ek-tat′ik) angiectatic.

angioedema (an″je-o-e-de′mah) angioneurotic edema.

angioelephantiasis (an″je-o-el″ĕ-fan-ti′ah-sis) extensive angiomatous condition of the subcutaneous tissues.

angioendothelioma (an″je-o-en″do-the″le-o′mah) hemangioendothelioma.

angiofibroma (an″je-o-fi-bro′mah) an angioma containing fibrous tissue; called also *telangiectatic fibroma.* **a. contagio′sum trop′icum,** a skin disease of Brazil characterized by an eruption of red papules which develop into bluish nodules. **juvenile a.,** nasopharyngeal a. **nasopharyngeal a.,** a tumor of the nasopharynx composed of fibrous connective tissue with abundant endothelium-lined vascular spaces, usually occurring during puberty, most commonly in boys. It is characterized by nasal obstruction which may become total, hyponasality, discomfort in swallowing, auditory tube obstruction and massive epistaxis. Called also *juvenile a.* and *nasopharyngeal fibroangioma.*

angiofollicular (an″je-o-fol-lik′u-lar) pertaining to a lymphoid follicle and its blood vessels.

angiogenesis (an″je-o-jen′ĕ-sis) [*angio-* + *genesis*] the development of the vessels. **tumor a.,** the induction of the growth of blood vessels from surrounding tissue into a solid tumor by a diffusible chemical factor released by the tumor cells.

angiogenic (an″je-o-jen′ik) 1. arising in the vascular system. 2. developing into blood vessels.

angioglioma (an″je-o-gli-o′mah) a very vascular form of glioma.

angiogliomatosis (an″je-o-gli″o-mah-to′sis) a condition marked by the formation of multiple vascular gliomas.

angiogliosis (an″je-o-gli-o′sis) (*obs.*) a condition marked by the development of angiogliomas.

angiogram (an′je-o-gram″) a roentgenogram of blood vessels filled with a contrast medium.

angiograph (an′je-o-graf″) [*angio-* + Gr. *graphein* to record] angiogram.

angiography (an″je-og′rah-fe) [*angio-* + Gr. *graphein* to record] 1. the roentgenographic visualization of blood vessels following introduction of contrast material; used as a diagnostic aid in such conditions as cerebrovascular attacks (strokes) and myocardial infarctions. 2. a treatise on the vessels; the study of the vessels. **cerebral a.**, radiography of the vascular system of the brain after injection of contrast material into the arterial blood stream. **coronary a.**, radiographic visualization of the coronary arteries after the introduction of contrast material.

angiohemophilia (an″je-o-he″mo-fil′e-ah) von Willebrand's disease.

angiohyalinosis (an″je-o-hi″ah-lĭ-no′sis) [*angio-* + *hyalinosis*] hyaline degeneration of the walls of blood vessels. **a. hemorrhag′ica**, a variety characterized by congenital hemorrhage.

angioid (an′je-oid) [*angio-* + Gr. *eidos* form] resembling a blood vessel.

angioinvasive (an″je-o-in-va′siv) tending to invade the walls of blood vessels.

angiokeratoma (an″je-o-ker″ah-to′mah) [*angio-* + Gr. *keras* horn + *-oma*] a disease of the skin characterized by telangiectases or warty growths, in groups, together with thickening of the epidermis (Mibelli); the dorsal aspect of the fingers and toes, and the scrotum are sites of predilection. Called also *angiokeratosis*. **a. circumscrip′tum**, a rare form characterized by discrete papules and nodules usually localized to a small area on the leg or trunk. **a. cor′poris diffu′sum**, Fabry's disease.

angiokeratosis (an″je-o-ker″ah-to′sis) angiokeratoma.

angiokinesis (an″je-o-kĭ-ne′sis) [*angio-* + Gr. *kinēsis* movement] vascular activity.

angiokinetic (an″je-o-kĭ-net′ik) pertaining to vascular activity; vasomotor.

angioleucitis (an″je-o-lu-si′tis) [*angio-* + Gr. *leukos* white + *-itis*] lymphangitis.

angioleukitis (an″je-o-lu-ki′tis) lymphangitis.

angiolipoleiomyoma (an″je-o-lip″o-li-o-mi-o′mah) see *angiomyolipoma*.

angiolipoma (an″je-o-lĭ-po′mah) a tumor composed of a mixture of adipose tissue and blood vessels.

angiologia (an″je-o-lo′je-ah) angiology; in NA terminology *angiologia* encompasses the nomenclature relating to the heart, arteries, veins, lymphatic system, and spleen.

angiology (an″je-ol′o-je) [*angio-* + Gr. *logos* treatise] the scientific study of the vessels of the body; applied also to the sum of knowledge relating to the blood vessels and lymph vessels.

angiolupoid (an″je-o-lu′poid) a granuloma consisting of small red oval infiltrated plaques with telangiectases over the surface and occurring chiefly on the sides of the nose.

angiolymphangioma (an″je-o-lim-fan″je-o′mah) a mixed angioma in which lymph vessels and blood vessels are involved.

angiolymphitis (an″je-o-lim-fi′tis) lymphangitis.

angiolymphoma (an″je-o-lim-fo′mah) (*obs.*) a tumor made up of lymph vessels.

angiolysis (an″je-ol′ĭ-sis) [*angio-* + Gr. *lysis* dissolution] retrogression or obliteration of blood vessels, such as occurs during embryonic development.

angioma (an″je-o′mah) [*angio-* + *-oma*] a tumor whose cells tend to form blood vessels (*hemangioma*) or lymph vessels (*lymphangioma*); a tumor made up of blood vessels or lymph vessels. **a. arteria′le racemo′sum**, a dilatation and complex intertwining of many new-formed and altered vessels of small caliber with subsequent involvement of normal vessels. **arteriovenous a. of brain**, congenital angioma of the brain composed of arterial and venous channels with many arteriovenous shunts, and characterized by frequent focal epileptic seizures and progressive impairment of the blood supply, which gives rise to increasing hemiparesis. It is distinguished by an intracranial bruit. **capillary a's**, cherry a's. **a. caverno′sum, cavernous a.**, cavernous hemangioma. **cherry a's**, bright red, circumscribed, round or oval angiomas, 2 to 6 mm. in diameter, containing many vascular loops, caused by a telangiectatic vascular disturbance; they are usually seen on the trunk but may appear on other areas of the body, as in angioma serpiginosum, and occur in well over 85 per cent of the middle-aged and elderly.

Called also *capillary a's, De Morgan's spots*, and *senile a's*. **a. cu′tis**, a kind of nevus made up of a network of dilated blood vessels. **fissural a.**, angioma occurring in embryonal fissures of the face, neck, or lips. **hereditary hemorrhagic a.**, hereditary hemorrhagic telangiectasia. **hypertrophic a.**, hemangioendothelioma. **infective a.** (*obs.*), a. serpiginosum. **a. lymphat′icum**, lymphangioma. **a. pigmento′sum atroph′icum** (*obs.*), xeroderma pigmentosum. **plexiform a.**, ordinary angioma made up of dilated and tortuous capillaries usually located in the skin. **senile a's**, cherry a's. **a. serpigino′sum**, a skin disease characterized by minute vascular points, looking like grains of cayenne pepper, arranged in rings on the skin; called also *Hutchinson's disease*. **simple a.**, a nevus or telangiectasis; a tumor composed of a network of small vessels or of distended capillaries bound together by connective tissue. **spider a.**, vascular spider. **strawberry a.**, cavernous angioma resembling a strawberry in size and color, occurring in the newborn and infants. **telangiectatic a.**, an angioma made up of dilated blood vessels. **a. veno′sum racemo′sum**, the swellings caused by severe varicosity of superficial veins. **venous a. of brain**, congenital angioma of the brain composed of abnormal venous arteries and characterized by frequent focal epileptic seizures and progressive hemiparesis.

angiomatosis (an″je-o-mah-to′sis) a diseased state of the vessels with the formation of multiple angiomas. **cerebroretinal a.**, von Hippel-Lindau disease. **encephalofacial a., encephalotrigeminal a.**, Sturge-Weber syndrome. **hemorrhagic familial a.**, hereditary hemorrhagic telangiectasia. **hepatic a.**, peliosis hepatis. **a. of retina**, von Hippel's disease. **retinocerebral a.**, von Hippel-Lindau disease.

angiomatous (an″je-om′ah-tus) of the nature of angioma.

angiomegaly (an″je-o-meg′ah-le) [*angio-* + Gr. *megas* large] enlargement of blood vessels; especially a condition of the eyelid marked by great increase in its volume.

angiometer (an″je-om′ĕ-ter) [*angio-* + Gr. *metron* measure] an instrument once used for measuring the diameter or caliber and the tension of the blood vessels.

angiomyolipoma (an″je-o-mi″o-lĭ-po′mah) a benign tumor containing vascular, adipose, and muscle elements; it occurs most often in the kidney with smooth muscle elements (angiolipoleiomyoma) in association with tuberous sclerosis, and is considered to be a hamartoma.

angiomyoma (an″je-o-mi-o′mah) a hamartoma composed of blood vessels and smooth muscle. **a. cu′tis**, a variety of leiomyoma cutis arising from the tunica media of blood vessels and embryonic muscle rests, usually on the lower leg.

angiomyoneuroma (an″je-o-mi″o-nu-ro′mah) glomangioma.

angiomyosarcoma (an″je-o-mi″o-sar-ko′mah) a tumor made up of elements of angioma, myoma, and sarcoma.

angiomyxoma (an″je-o-mik-so′mah) a chorioangioma in which capillary-like blood vessels are very evident; it may extend into the umbilical cord and often contains myxomatous tissue resembling that in the normal cord.

angionecrosis (an″je-o-nĕ-kro′sis) [*angio-* + Gr. *nekros* dead + *-osis*] necrosis of the walls of blood vessels.

angioneoplasm (an″je-o-ne′o-plazm) [*angio-* + *neoplasm*] a tumor or neoplasm of blood vessels.

angioneuralgia (an″je-o-nu-ral′jĕ-ah) [*angio-* + *neuralgia*] a condition marked by burning pain in an extremity attended by edema and redness of the part; thought to be an early stage of Raynaud's disease.

angioneurectomy (an″je-o-nu-rek′to-me) [*angio-* + Gr. *neuron* nerve + *ektomē* excision] excision of vessels and nerves.

angioneuroedema (an″je-o-nu″ro-e-de′mah) [*angio-* + Gr. *neuron* nerve + *oidēma* swelling] (*obs.*) angioneurotic edema.

angioneuroma (an″je-o-nu-ro′mah) glomangioma.

angioneuromyoma (an″je-o-nu″ro-mi-o′mah) glomangioma.

angioneuropathic (an″je-o-nu″ro-path′ik) pertaining to or of the nature of an angioneuropathy.

angioneuropathy (an″je-o-nu-rop′ah-the) [*angio-* + *neuropathy*] any neuropathy affecting primarily the blood vessels; a disorder of the vasomotor system, as angiospasm, angioparalysis, or vasomotor paralysis.

angioneurotic (an″je-o-nu-rot′ik) denoting a neuropathy affecting the vascular system; see under *edema*.

angioneurotomy (an″je-o-nu-rot′o-me) [*angio-* + Gr. *neuron* nerve + *tomē* cutting] the operation of cutting vessels and nerves.

angionoma (an″je-o-no′mah) [*angio-* + Gr. *nomē* ulcer] ulceration of a blood vessel.

angiopancreatitis (an″je-o-pan″kre-ah-ti′tis) (*obs.*) inflammation of the pancreatic vessels or of the vascular tissue of the pancreas.

angioparalysis (an″je-o-pah-ral′ĭ-sis) [*angio-* + *paralysis*] vasomotor paralysis.

angioparesis (an″je-o-par′e-sis) [*angio-* + *paresis*] vasomotor paralysis.

angiopathology (an″je-o-pah-thol′o-je) the pathology of, or the changes seen in, diseases of the blood vessels.

angiopathy (an-je-op′ah-the) [*angio-* + Gr. *pathos* disease] any disease of the vessels.

angiophakomatosis (an″je-o-fak″o-mah-to′sis) [*angio-* + Gr. *phakos* lens + -*oma*] von Hippel-Lindau disease.

angioplasty (an′je-o-plas″te) [*angio-* + Gr. *plassein* to form] surgical reconstruction of blood vessels. **percutaneous transluminal a.,** dilatation of a blood vessel by means of a balloon catheter inserted through the skin and into the chosen vessel and then passed through the lumen of the vessel to the site of the lesion, where the balloon is inflated to flatten plaque against the artery wall.

angiopoiesis (an″je-o-poi-e′sis) [*angio-* + Gr. *poiein* to make] the process of vessel formation.

angiopoietic (an″je-o-poi-et′ik) pertaining to or causing angiopoiesis.

angiopressure (an′je-o-presh″ur) the application of pressure to a blood vessel to control hemorrhage.

angioreticuloendothelioma (an″je-o-rĕ-tik″u-lo-en″do-the-le-o′mah) Kaposi's sarcoma.

angioreticuloma (an″je-o-re-tik″u-lo′mah) a hemangioma, especially one of the brain.

angiorrhaphy (an″je-or′ah-fe) [*angio-* + Gr. *rhaphē* suture] suture of a vessel or vessels. **arteriovenous a.,** the suturing of an artery to a vein, so as to divert the arterial current into the vein.

angiosarcoma (an″je-o-sar-ko′mah) [*angio-* + *sarcoma*] a hemangiosarcoma. **a. myxomato′des** (*obs.*), an angiosarcoma in which the walls of the vessels are affected with mucous degeneration.

angiosclerosis (an″je-o-skle-ro′sis) [*angio-* + *sclerosis*] a nonspecific term indicating hardening of the walls of the blood vessels.

angiosclerotic (an″je-o-skle-rot′ik) pertaining to or marked by angiosclerosis.

angioscope (an′je-o-skōp″) [*angio-* + Gr. *skopein* to view] a microscope for observing capillary blood vessels.

angioscotoma (an″je-o-sko-to′mah) a scotoma, or defect in the visual field, caused by shadows of the retinal blood vessels.

angioscotometry (an″je-o-sko-tom′ĕ-tre) [*angio-* + *scotoma* + Gr. *metron* measure] the plotting or mapping of the scotoma caused by the shadow of retinal blood vessels; used particularly in the diagnosis of glaucoma.

angiospasm (an′je-o-spazm″) [*angio-* + Gr. *spasmos* spasm] spasmodic contraction of the blood vessels.

angiospastic (an″je-o-spas′tik) of the nature of angiospasm; causing contraction of the blood vessels.

angiosperm (an′je-o-sperm″) [*angio-* + Gr. *sperma* seed] a true flowering plant; a plant having its seeds in an enclosed ovary.

angiospermin (an″je-o-sper′min) a substance derived from flowering plants and said to have hormone-like properties.

angiostaxis (an″je-o-stak′sis) [*angio-* + Gr. *staxis* hemorrhage] (*obs.*) hemorrhagic diathesis.

angiostenosis (an″je-o-ste-no′sis) [*angio-* + *stenosis*] narrowing of the caliber of a vessel.

angiosteosis (an″je-os″te-o′sis) [*angio-* + Gr. *osteon* bone] ossification or calcification of a vessel.

angiosthenia (an″je-os-the′ne-ah) [*angio-* + Gr. *sthenos* strength + -*ia*] arterial tension.

angiostomy (an″je-os′to-me) [*angio-* + Gr. *stomoun* to provide with an opening, or mouth] the operation of making an opening into a blood vessel and inserting a cannula therein.

angiostrongyliasis (an″je-o-stron″jĭ-li′ah-sis) infection with *Angiostrongylus cantonensis.*

Angiostrongylus (an″je-o-stron′jĭ-lus) [Gr. *angeion* vessel + *strongylos* round] a genus of parasitic nematodes of the family Metastrongylidae. **A. cantonen′sis,** the lungworm that parasitizes the domestic rat in Australia and many of the Pacific islands, including Hawaii. Larval development occurs in snails, slugs, and planarians; in rats, the adult worms are found in the bronchioles. Human infection, which is thought usually to be due to ingestion of larvae in paratenic hosts, such as prawns or freshwater crabs, results in migration of the larval worms to the central nervous system, where they provoke eosinophilic meningoencephalitis. **A. vaso′rum,** a species parasitic in the pulmonary arteries of dogs.

angiostrophe (an″je-os′tro-fe) [*angio-* + Gr. *strophē* a twist] the twisting of a vessel to arrest hemorrhage.

angiostrophy (an″je-os′tro-fe) angiostrophe.

angiotelectasis (an″je-o-tĕ-lek′tah-sis), pl. *angiotelectases* [*angio-* + Gr. *telos* end + *ektasis* dilatation] dilatation of the minute arteries and veins.

angiotensin (an″je-o-ten′sin) a polypeptide present in the blood and formed by the catalytic action of renin on angiotensinogen in the blood plasma. The decapeptide angiotensin I, the inactive form, is in turn acted upon by a peptidase (converting enzyme), chiefly in the lungs, to form the octapeptide hormone angiotensin II, a powerful vasopressor and a stimulator of aldosterone secretion by the adrenal cortex. By its vasopressor action, it raises blood pressure and diminishes fluid loss in the kidney by restricting flow. Angiotensin II is hydrolyzed to form the heptapeptide angiotensin III, which has lesser vasopressor activity but is more active on the adrenal cortex. **a. amide,** chemical name: 1-L-asparagine-5-L-valineangiotensin II. An amide derivative of angiotensin, $C_{49}H_{70}N_{14}O_{11}$, occurring as a white to slightly off-white, amorphous powder, which is a powerful vasoconstrictor and vasopressor, and is used in the treatment of certain hypotensive states; usually administered by slow intravenous infusion, and sometimes intramuscularly or subcutaneously.

angiotensinase (an″je-o-ten′sĭ-nās) any of a group of peptidases in plasma and tissues that inactivate angiotensin.

angiotensinogen (an″je-o-ten′sin-o-jen) a serum α_2-globulin secreted in the liver which, on hydrolysis by renin, gives rise to angiotensin; formerly called *hypertensinogen.*

angiotome (an′je-o-tōm″) [*angio-* + Gr. *tomē* a cutting] any one of the segments of the vascular system of the embryo; called also *vascular segment* and *intersegment.*

angiotomy (an″je-ot′o-me) [*angio-* + Gr. *tomē* a cutting] the cutting or severing of a blood or lymph vessel.

angiotonase (an″je-o-to′nās) an enzyme formed by the kidneys which inactivates angiotensin.

angiotonia (an″je-o-to′ne-ah) vasotonia.

angiotonic (an″je-o-ton′ik) [*angio-* + Gr. *tonos* tension] increasing the vascular tension.

angiotonin (an″je-o-to′nin) angiotensin.

angiotribe (an′je-o-trib″) [*angio-* + Gr. *tribein* to crush] an exceedingly strong forceps in which pressure is applied by means of a screw; the instrument is used to crush tissue containing an artery in order to check hemorrhage from the vessel. Called also *vasotribe.*

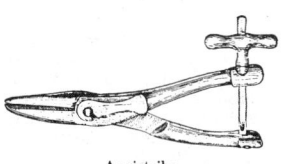

Angiotribe.

angiotripsy (an′je-o-trip″se) production of hemostasis by use of the angiotribe; called also *vasotripsy.*

angiotrophic (an″je-o-trof′ik) [*angio-* + Gr. *trophē* nutrition] pertaining to vascular nutrition.

angitis (an-ji′tis) angiitis.

angle (ang′g'l) [L. *angulus*] 1. the area or point of junction of two intersecting borders or surfaces; see *angulus.* 2. the degree of divergence of two intersecting lines or planes. **a. of aberration,** a. of deviation. **acromial a.,** angulus acromialis. **acromial a. of scapula,** angulus lateralis scapulae. **alpha a.,** that formed by the intersection of the visual line with the optic axis at the nodal point. It is *positive* when the visual axis crosses the cornea on the nasal side of the optic axis, as in most individuals; *negative* when the visual axis crosses the cornea on the temporal side of the optic axis; and *nil* when the visual axis and the optic axis coincide. **Alsberg's a.,** see Alsberg's triangle, under *triangle.* **alveolar a.,** the angle between a line running through a point beneath the nasal spine and the most prominent point of the lower border of the alveolar process of the superior maxilla and the cephalic horizontal. **anterior a. of petrous portion of temporal bone,** angulus anterior pyramidis ossis temporalis. **a. of aperture,** the angle between two lines from the focus of a lens to the ends of its diameter. **auriculo-occipital a.,** the angle between lines from the auricular point to the lambda and opisthion. **axial a.,** any angle the formation of which is partially dependent on the axial wall of a tooth cavity. **axial line a.,** any line angle which is parallel with the long axis of a tooth. For names of various angles see the table of *Cavity Angles* and illustration of *Tooth Angles.* **Bennett a.,** the angle formed by the sagittal plane and the path of the advancing condyle during lateral movement of the mandible, as viewed in the horizontal plane. **beta a.,** the angle between the radius fixus and a line joining the bregma and hormion. **biorbital a.,** the angle formed by intersection of a posterior extension of the axes of the two orbits. **Broca's a.,** ophryospinal a. **buccal a's,** the angles formed between the buccal surface and the other surfaces of a posterior tooth, or between the buccal wall of a tooth cavity and other walls, named according to the surfaces which participate in their formation. See the table of *Cavity Angles* and illustration of *Tooth Angles.* **cardiodiaphragmatic a.,** the angle formed by the junction of the shadows of the heart and diaphragm in posteroanterior roentgenograms of the chest; called also *cardiophrenic a.* **cardiohepatic a.,** the angle formed by the horizontal limit of hepatic dullness with the upright line of cardiac dullness in the fifth right intercostal space, close to the sternal border; called also *Ebstein's a.* **cardio-**

phrenic a., cardiodiaphragmatic a. **carrying a.,** angle formed by the axes of the arm and forearm when the forearm is extended in the anatomical position. **cavity a's,** the angles formed by the junction of two or more walls of a tooth cavity, named according to the walls participating in their formation. See table of *Cavity Angles.* **cavosurface a.,** the angle formed by

CAVITY ANGLES
Line Angles
(Formed by the junction of two walls)

axiodistal	gingivoaxial
axiogingival	labiogingival
axioincisal	linguoaxial
axiolabial	linguodistal
axiolingual	linguogingival
axiomesial	linguomesial
axio-occlusal	linguopulpal
axiopulpal	mesiobuccal
buccoaxial	mesiogingival
buccodistal	mesiolabial
buccogingival	mesiolingual
buccomesial	mesio-occlusal
buccopulpal	mesiopulpal
distobuccal	pulpoaxial
distogingival	pulpodistal
distolabial	pulpolabial
distolingual	pu'polingual
disto-occlusal	pulpomesial
distopulpal	

Point Angles
(Formed by the junction of three walls)

axiodistogingival	distopulpolingual
axiodisto-occlusal	gingivobuccoaxial
axiolabiogingival	gingivolinguoaxial
axiolinguogingival	mesiobuccopulpal
axiomesiogingival	mesiolinguopulpal
axiomesio-occlusal	mesiopulpolabial
distobuccopulpal	mesiopulpolingual
distolinguopulpal	pulpobuccoaxial
distopulpolabial	pulpolinguoaxial

the junction of a wall of a cavity and a surface of the crown of the tooth. **cephalic a.,** various angles of the skull or face. **cephalic-medullary a.,** the angle at which the brain stem meets the base of the brain. **cephalometric a.,** measurement of intersecting anthropometric lines on tracings made of oriented head films in radiologic orthodontic diagnosis. **cerebellopontile a.,** that between the cerebellum and the pons. **chi a.,** the angle between two lines from the hormion to the staphylion and to the basion, respectively. **collodiaphyseal a.,** the angle formed by the intersection of the long axes of the neck and shaft of the femur. **condylar a.,** the angle between the planes of the basilar clivus and the foramen magnum. **a. of convergence,** that between the visual axis and the median line when an object is looked at. **a. of convexity,** a cephalometric measurement formed by connecting the nasion, point A, and pogonion (NAP), which reflects the convexity or concavity of the facial profile. **coronary a.,** angulus frontalis ossis parietalis. **costal a.,** angulus costae. **costophrenic a.,** the angle formed at the junction of the costal and diaphragmatic pleurae. **costovertebral a.,** the angle formed on either side of the vertebral column, between the last rib and the lumbar vertebrae. **craniofacial a.,** the angle between the basifacial and basicranial axes at the middle of the ethmoidosphenoid suture. **critical a.,** the angle of incidence at which a ray of light passing from one medium to another of different density changes from refraction to total reflection; called also *limiting a.* **cusp a.,** 1. the angle made by the slopes of a cusp of a tooth with the plane that passes through the tip of the cusp and that is perpendicular to a line bisecting the cusp, measured mesiodistally or buccolingually. 2. the angle made by the slopes of a cusp with a perpendicular line bisecting the cusp, measured mesiodistally or buccolingually. 3. one half of the included angle between the buccal and lingual or mesial and distal cusp inclines. **cusp plane a.,** the incline of the cusp plane in relation to the plane of occlusion. **Daubenton's a.,** an angle formed by junction of the opisthiobasal and opisthionasial lines; called also *occipital a.* **a. of declination,** Mikulicz's a. **a. of deviation,** the angle between a refracted ray and the incident ray prolonged; called also *a. of aberration.* **a. of direction,** the angle through which the eye must move to bring the image onto the fovea. **distal a's,** the angles formed between the distal surface and other surfaces of a tooth, or between the distal wall of a tooth cavity and other walls; named according to the surfaces which participate in their formation. See table of *Cavity Angles* and illustration of *Tooth Angles.* **Ebstein's a.,** cardiohepatic a. **elevation a.,** 1. the angle made by the visual plane when moved upward or downward with its normal position. 2. see *Alsberg's triangle,* under *triangle.* **epigastric a.,** the angle made by the xiphoid process with the body of the sternum. **ethmocranial a.,** the angle formed by the plane of the cribriform plate of the ethmoid bone prolonged to meet the basicranial axis; called also *ethmoid angle.* **ethmoid a.,** ethmocranial a. **external a. of border of tibia,** margo interosseus tibiae. **external a. of scapula,** angulus lateralis scapulae. **facial a.,** an expression of the degree of recession or protrusion of the chin, determined by a line drawn from the nasion to the pogonion as it intersects

with the eye-ear (Frankfort) plane; a cephalometric diagnostic measurement. **filtration a.,** angulus iridocornealis. **frontal a. of parietal bone,** angulus frontalis ossis parietalis. **gamma a.,** the angle formed by junction of the line of fixation and the optic axis at the center of rotation of the eye. **gonial a.,** the angle formed by the intersection of the body of the mandible and the ascending mandibular ramus; an important consideration in prognathic procedures. Called also *angulus mandibulae* [NA]. **horizontal a.,** in dental radiology the angle, measured within a horizontal plane, at which the central ray of the useful beam is projected relative to a vertical plane of reference. **impedance a.,** the ratio between the resistance of the body to an electric current and its condenser function; cf. *impedance.* **a. of incidence,** the angle made with the perpendicular by a ray of light which strikes a denser or a rarer medium; see *refraction.* **incisal a.,** one of the angles formed by the junction of the incisal and the mesial or distal surface of an anterior tooth; called the *mesial* and the *distal incisal angle,* respectively. **incisal guide a.,** the angle formed with the horizontal plane by drawing a line in the sagittal plane between incisal edges of the maxillary and mandibular central incisors when the teeth are in centric occlusion. **incisal mandibular plane a.,** one of the three angles composing the Tweed triangle, designating the axial inclination of the lower incisor to the mandibular plane in the lateral cephalometric radiograph. **a. of inclination,** inclinatio pelvis. **inferior a. of duodenum,** flexura duodeni inferior. **inferior a. of parietal bone, anterior,** angulus sphenoidalis ossis parietalis. **inferior a. of parietal bone, posterior,** angulus mastoideus ossis parietalis. **inferior a. of scapula,** angulus inferior scapulae. **infrasternal a. of thorax,** angulus infrasternalis thoracis. **inner a. of humerus,** margo medialis humeri. **internal a. of tibia,** margo medialis tibiae. **iridial a., iridocorneal a., a. of iris,** angulus iridocornealis. **Jacquart's a.,** ophryospinal a. **a. of jaw,** angulus mandibulae. **kappa a.,** the angle between the pupillary axes. **kyphotic a.,** the superior angle formed by intersection of two lines drawn on the lateral chest roentgenogram, tangential to the anterior borders of the second and eleventh intervertebral spaces, an index of the degree of deformity in thoracic kyphosis. **labial a's,** the angles formed between the labial surface and other surfaces of an anterior tooth, or between the labial wall of a tooth cavity and other walls; named according to the surfaces participating in their formation. See tables of *Cavity Angles* and *Tooth Angles.* **lambda a.,** the angle between the pupillary axis and the line of sight. **lateral a. of border of tibia,** margo interosseus tibiae. **lateral a. of eye,** angulus oculi lateralis. **lateral a. of humerus,** margo lateralis humeri. **lateral a. of scapula,** angulus lateralis scapulae. **limiting a.,** critical a. **line a.,** an angle formed by junction of two planes. Used in dentistry to designate the junction of two surfaces of a tooth, or of two walls of a tooth cavity; named according to the tooth surfaces or the cavity walls which participate in its formation. See tables of *Cavity Angles* and *Tooth Angles.* **lingual a's,** the angles formed between the lingual and other surfaces of a tooth, or between the lingual wall of a tooth cavity and other walls; named according to the surfaces which participate in their formation. See tables of *Cavity Angles* and *Tooth Angles.* **Louis' a., Ludwig's a.,** angulus sterni. **lumbosacral a.,** sacrovertebral a. **a. of mandible, mandibular a.,** angulus mandibulae. **mastoid a. of parietal bone,** angulus mastoideus ossis parietalis. **maxillary a.,** the angle between two lines extending from the point of contact of the upper and lower central incisors to the ophryon and the most prominent point of the lower jaw. **medial a. of eye,** angulus oculi medialis. **medial a. of humerus,** margo medialis humeri. **medial a. of scapula,** angulus superior scapulae. **medial a. of tibia,** margo medialis tibiae. **mesial a's,** the angles formed between the mesial surface and other surfaces of a tooth, or between the mesial wall of a tooth cavity and other walls, named according to the surfaces participating with the mesial in their formation. See tables of *Cavity Angles* and *Tooth Angles.* **metafacial a.,** the angle between the base of the skull and the pterygoid process; called also *Serres' a.* **meter a.,** a unit of convergence of the eye: that amount of convergence required for binocular fixation of an object at 1 meter and using 1 diopter of accommodation. **Mikulicz's a.,** an angle formed by two planes, one passing through the long axis of the epiphysis of the femur and the other through the long axis of the diaphysis; it is normally 130 degrees. Called also *a. of declination.* **minimum visual a.,** the angle which the minimum separabile subtends at the eye; 60 seconds of arc is usually taken as standard for a normal eye. **a. of mouth,** angulus oris. **a. of Mulder,** the angle formed by the intersection of the facial line of Camper and a line from the root of the nose to the spheno-occipital suture. **nu a.,** the angle between the radius fixus and a line joining the hormion and nasion. **occipital a.,** Daubenton's a. **occipital a. of parietal bone,** angulus occipitalis ossis parietalis. **ocular a's,** see *angulus oculi lateralis* and *angulus oculi medialis.* **olfactive a.,** the angle formed by the line of the olfactory fossa and the os planum of the sphenoid bone; called also *olfactory a.* **olfactory a.,** olfactive a. **ophryospinal a.,** the angle at the anterior nasal spine between lines from the auricular point

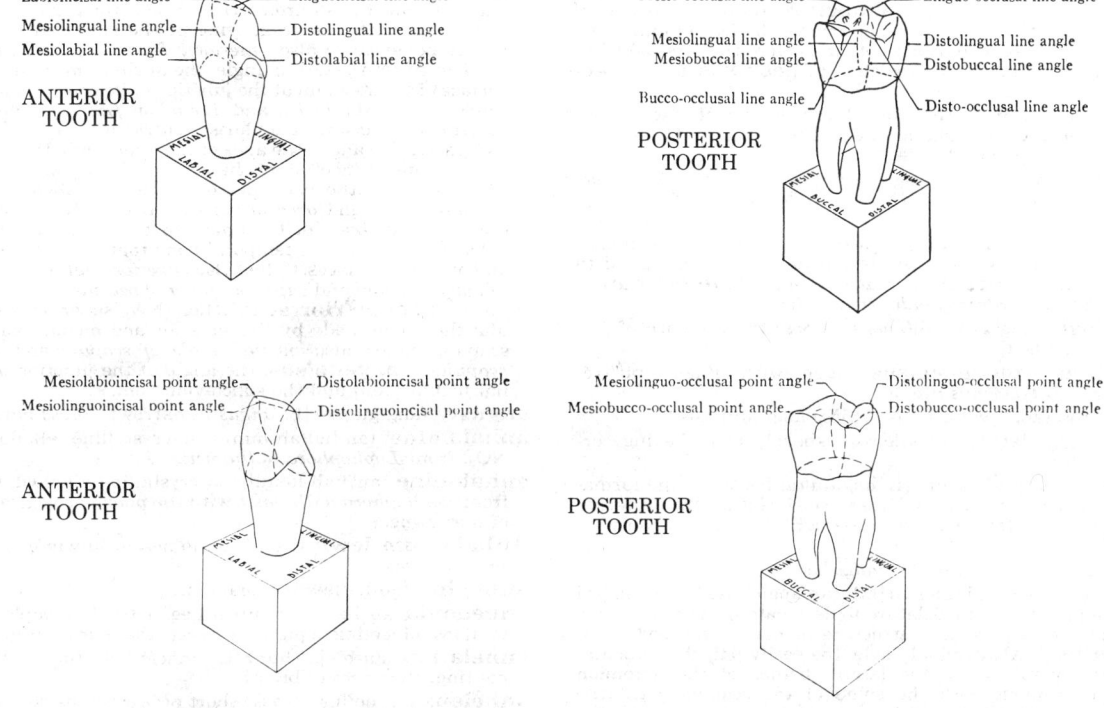

Tooth angles: *Top*, line angles; *Bottom*, point angles (Wheeler).

and the glabella; called also *Jacquart's a.*, *Topinard's a.*, and *Broca's a.* **optic a.**, visual a. **orifacial a.**, in cephalometrics, the angle formed by the junction of the Frankfort horizontal plane (eye-ear plane) with the facial plane (nasion-pogonion). **parietal a.**, the angle formed by junction of lines passing through the extremities of the transverse bizygomatic diameter and the maximum transverse frontal diameter; called also *Quatrefage's a.* **parietal a. of sphenoid bone**, margo parietalis alae majoris. **a. of pelvis**, inclinatio pelvis. **pelvivertebral a.**, inclinatio pelvis. **phrenopericardial a.**, the space or angle between the pericardium and the diaphragm. **Pirogoff's a.**, venous a. **point a.**, in dentistry, the junction of three surfaces of a tooth, or of three walls of a tooth cavity, named according to the tooth surfaces or the cavity walls participating in its formation. See tables of *Cavity Angles* and *Tooth Angles.* **a. of polarization**, the angle at which light is most completely polarized. **posterior a. of petrous portion of temporal bone**, angulus posterior pyramidis ossis temporalis. **principal a.**, refracting a. **a. of pubis**, angulus subpubicus. **Quatrefage's a.**, parietal a. **Ranke's a.**, the angle between the horizontal plane of the skull and a line through the center of the maxillary alveolar margin and the center of the nasofrontal suture. **a. of reflection**, that which a reflected ray makes with a line perpendicular to the reflecting surface. **refracting a.**, that between the two refracting faces of a prism; called also *principal a.* **a. of refraction**, the angle between a refracted ray and a line perpendicular to the refracting surface; see *refraction.* **a. of rib**, angulus costae. **rolandic a.**, **a. of Rolando**, the angle formed by junction of the median plane and the central sulcus (fissure of Rolando). **sacrovertebral a.**, the angle formed at the junction of the sacrum with the lowest lumbar vertebra; called also *lumbosacral a.* **Serres' a.**, metafacial a. **sigma a.**, the angle between the radius fixus and a line from the staphylion to the hormion. **somatosplanchnic a.**, the angle formed by junction of the somatic and splanchnic layers of the mesoblast in the embryo. **sphenoid a.**, **sphenoidal a.**, 1. an angle at the top of the sella turcica between lines from the nasal point and from the tip of the rostrum of the sphenoid. 2. the anterior inferior angle of the parietal bone; called also *Welcher's a.* **sphenoidal a. of parietal bone**, angulus sphenoidalis ossis parietalis. **squint a.**, the angle by which the visual line of the squinting eye deviates from a line drawn to the object which should be fixed; called also *squint deviation.* **sternal a.**, angulus sterni. **sternoclavicular a.**, the angle formed by junction of the sternum and clavicle. **a. of sternum**, angulus sterni. **subcostal a.**, angulus infrasternalis thoracis. **subpubic a.**, angulus subpubicus. **subscapular a.**, a transverse depression on the costal or ventral surface of the scapula, where the bone appears bent on itself perpendicular to and passing through the glenoid cavity. **substernal a.**, angulus infrasternalis thoracis. **superior a. of**

duodenum, flexura duodeni superior. **superior a. of parietal bone, anterior**, angulus frontalis ossis parietalis. **superior a. of parietal bone, posterior**, angulus occipitalis ossis parietalis. **superior a. of petrous portion of temporal bone**, angulus superior pyramidis ossis temporalis. **superior a. of scapula**, angulus superior scapulae. **a. of Sylvius**, the angle formed by junction of the lateral sulcus (fissure of Sylvius) and a line perpendicular to the horizontal plane tangential to the highest point of the hemisphere. **tentorial a.**, the angle between the basicranial axis and the plane of the tentorium. **tooth a's**, the angles formed by the junction of two or more surfaces of a tooth, named according to the surfaces participating in their formation (see illustration). **Topinard's a.**, ophryospinal a. **a. of torsion**, the angle between the axes of any two different portions of long bones. **tuber a.**, the angle formed by junction of two lines, one parallel with the superior surface of the tuber calcanei and the other joining the anterior and posterior articular facets; normally about 30 degrees. **venous a.**, the angle formed by junction of the internal jugular and subclavian veins; called also *Pirogoff's a.* **vertical a.**, in dental radiology the angle, measured within a vertical plane, at which the central ray of the useful beam is projected relative to a horizontal plane of reference. **vesicourethral a.**, the angle formed by junction of the bladder wall and the urethra. **vesicourethral a., anterior**, the angle formed by junction of the anterior wall of the bladder and the urethra. **vesicourethral a., posterior**, the angle formed by junction of the posterior wall of the bladder and the urethra. **a. of Virchow**, the angle between the nasobasilar line and the nasosubnasal line. **visual a.**, the angle formed between two lines extending from the nodal point of the eye to the extremities of the object seen; called also *optic a.* **Vogt's a.**, the angle between the nasobasilar and alveolonasal lines. **Weisbach's a.**, the angle at the alveolar point between lines passing from the basion and from the middle of the frontonasal suture. **Welcher's a.**, sphenoid a. **xiphoid a's**, the angles formed by the borders of the xiphoid notch. **Y a.**, the angle between the radius fixus and line joining the lambda and the inion.

Angle's classification, splint (ang'elz) [Edward Hartley *Angle*, American orthodontist, 1855–1930] see under *malocclusion* and *splint.*

Anglesey leg (ang'g'l-se) [Marquis of *Anglesey*, 1768–1854, for whom the leg was made] see under *leg.*

anglicus sudor (ang'le-kus su'dor) the English sweating fever; a deadly pestilential fever which has several times ravaged England.

angophrasia (ang"go-fra'zhe-ah) [Gr. *anchein* to choke + *phrasis* utterance + *-ia*] a drawling and broken form of speech occurring in dementia (Kussmaul).

angor (ang′gŏr) [L. "a strangling"] angina. **a. an′imi**, a feeling of impending dissolution. **a. noctur′nus** (*obs.*), pavor nocturnus. **a. ocula′ris**, a condition marked by fear of imminent blindness and by sudden attacks of mist before the eyes, possibly due to angiospasm of ocular vessels. **a. pec′toris**, angina pectoris.

angstrom (ang′strem) the unit of wavelength of electromagnetic and corpuscular radiations, equal to 10^{-7} mm. Called also *Angström unit.* Symbol A or Å.

Angström's law, unit (awng′strem) [Anders Jonas *Angström*, Swedish physicist, 1814–1874] see under *law*, and see *angstrom*.

Anguillula (ang-gwil′u-lah) [L. "little eel"] a genus of nematode parasites, many species of which have been reassigned to other genera. **A. ace′ti,** *Turbatrix aceti.* **A. intestina′lis,** **A. stercora′lis,** *Strongyloides stercoralis.*

anguilluliasis (ang″gwil-u-li′ah-sis) (*obs.*) the presence of *Anguillula* in the body.

Anguilluli′na putrefa′ciens (ang-gwil″u-li′nah pu″trě-fa″she-enz) *Ditylenchus dipsaci.*

anguillulosis (ang″gwil-u-lo′sis) (*obs.*) anguilluliasis.

angular (ang′gu-lar) [L. *angula′ris*] sharply bent; having corners or angles.

angulation (ang″gu-la′shun) [L. *angula′tus* bent] 1. the formation of a sharp obstructive angle, as in the intestine, the ureter, or similar tubes. 2. deviation from a straight line, as in a badly set bone.

anguli (ang′gu-li) [L.] plural of *angulus*.

angulus (ang′gu-lus), pl. *an′guli* [L.] an angle; used as a general term in anatomical nomenclature to designate a triangular area or the angle of a particular structure or part of the body. **a. acromia′lis** [NA], acromial angle: the easily palpable subcutaneous bony point where the lateral border of the acromion becomes continuous with the spine of the scapula. **a. ante′rior pyram′idis os′sis tempora′lis**, a short area on the petrous part of the temporal bone consisting of two parts: one, adjoined to the squamous part of the bone at the petrosquamous suture; the other, a free part articulating with the great wing of the sphenoid; called also *anterior angle of petrous portion of temporal bone.* **a. cos′tae** [NA], costal angle: a prominent line on the external surface of a rib, a little in front of the tubercle, where the rib is bent in two directions and at the same time twisted on its long axis; called also *angle of rib.* **a. fronta′lis os′sis parieta′lis** [NA], frontal angle of parietal bone: the anterosuperior angle of the parietal bone, which is membranous at birth and forms part of the anterior fontanelle; called also *anterior superior angle of parietal bone* and *coronary angle.* **a. infecti′o′sus**, perlèche. **a. infe′rior scap′ulae** [NA], inferior angle of scapula: the angle formed by the junction of the medial and lateral borders of the scapula. **a. infrasterna′lis thora′cis** [NA], infrasternal angle of thorax: the angle on the anteroinferior surface of the thorax, the apex of which is the sternoxiphoid junction, and the sides of which are the seventh, eighth, and ninth costal cartilages; it partially delimits two sides of the triangular epigastric region on the ventral body surface; called also *subcostal* or *substernal angle.* **a. i′ridis**, a. iridocornealis. **a. iridocornea′lis** [NA], iridocorneal angle: a narrow recess between the sclerocorneal junction and the attached margin of the iris, marking the periphery of the anterior chamber of the eye; it is the principal exit site for the aqueous fluid. Called also *filtration angle, iridial angle, angle of iris,* and *angulus iridis.* **a. latera′lis scap′ulae** [NA], lateral angle of scapula: the head of the scapula, which bears the glenoid cavity and articulates with the head of the humerus; called also *acromial* or *external angle of scapula,* and *condyle of scapula.* **a. latera′lis tib′iae**, margo interosseus tibiae. **a. Ludovi′ci**, a. sterni. **a. mandib′ulae** [NA], angle of mandible: the angle created at the junction of the posterior edge of the ramus and the lower edge of the mandible; called also *angle of jaw, gonial angle,* and *mandibular angle.* **a. mastoi′deus os′sis parieta′lis** [NA], mastoid angle of parietal bone: the posteroinferior angle of the parietal bone, which articulates with the posterior part of the temporal bone and the occipital bone; called also *posterior inferior angle of parietal bone.* **a. media′lis scap′ulae**, a. superior scapulae. **a. media′lis tib′iae**, margo medialis tibiae. **a. occipita′lis os′sis parieta′lis** [NA], occipital angle of parietal bone: the posterosuperior angle of the parietal bone, which during fetal life participates in the formation of the posterior fontanelle; called also *posterior superior angle of parietal bone.* **a. oc′uli latera′lis** [NA], lateral angle of eye: the angle formed by the lateral junction of the superior and inferior eyelids. **a. oc′uli media′lis** [NA], medial angle of eye: the angle formed by the medial junction of the superior and inferior eyelids. **a. o′ris** [NA], angle of mouth: the angle formed at either side of the mouth by junction of the upper and the lower lip. **a. parieta′lis os′sis sphenoida′lis**, margo parietalis alae majoris. **a. poste′rior pyram′idis os′sis tempora′lis**, the angle on the petrous portion of the temporal bone that separates the posterior from the inferior surface; called also *posterior angle* or *border of petrous portion of temporal bone.* **a. pubis**, a. subpubicus.

a. sphenoida′lis os′sis parieta′lis [NA], sphenoid angle of parietal bone: the anteroinferior angle of the parietal bone, which articulates with the great wing of the sphenoid bone and the frontal bone; called also *anterior inferior angle of sphenoid bone.* **a. ster′ni** [NA], sternal angle: the angle formed on the anterior surface of the sternum at the junction of its body and manubrium; called also *a. Ludovici,* and *Louis'* or *Ludwig's angle.* **a. of stomach**, incisura angularis ventriculi. **a. subpu′bicus** [NA], subpubic angle: the apex of the pubic arch; the angle formed at the point of meeting of the conjoined rami of the ischial and pubic bones of the two sides of the body. Called also *a. pubis, subpubic arch,* and *arch of pelvis.* **a. supe′rior pyram′idis os′sis tempora′lis**, the angle on the internal surface of the petrous portion of the temporal bone that separates its posterior and anterior surfaces. Called also *superior angle of petrous portion of temporal bone* and *superior border of petrous portion of temporal bone.* **a. supe′rior scap′ulae** [NA], superior angle of scapula: the angle made by the superior and medial borders of the scapula; called also *medial angle of scapula* and *a. medialis scapulae.* **a. veno′sus,** the angle at the junction of the internal jugular vein and the subclavian vein.

angusty (ang-gus′te) [L. *angustus* narrow] (*obs.*) narrowness.

anhalamine (an-hal′ah-min) a crystalline alkaloid, $C_{11}H_{15}$-NO_3, from *Lophophora williamsii.*

anhalonine (an″hah-lo′nin) a crystalline alkaloid, $C_{12}H_{15}NO_3$, from *Lophophora williamsii,* with the pharmacological properties of mescaline.

Anhalonium lewinii (an″hah-lo′ne-um lu-win′e-e) *Lophophora williamsii.*

anhaphia (an-ha′fe-ah) anaphia.

anhedonia (an″he-do′ne-ah) [*an* neg. + Gr. *hēdonē* pleasure + *-ia*] total loss of feeling of pleasure in acts that normally give pleasure.

anhelation (an-hě-la′shun) [L. *anhela′tio*] (*obs.*) dyspnea, with panting; shortness of breath.

anhelous (an-he′lus) (*obs.*) short of breath; marked by dyspnea.

anhidrosis (an″hĭ-dro′sis) [*an* neg. + Gr. *hidrōs* sweat + *-osis*] an abnormal deficiency of sweat. **thermogenic a.,** tropical anhidrotic asthenia.

anhidrotic (an″hĭ-drot′ik) 1. checking the secretion of sweat. 2. an agent that checks the secretion of sweat.

anhydrase (an-hi′drās) an enzyme that catalyzes the removal of water from a compound. **carbonic a.,** a zinc-containing enzyme that catalyzes the decomposition of carbonic acid into carbon dioxide and water and thus facilitates the transfer of carbon dioxide from tissues to blood and to alveolar air.

anhydration (an″hi-dra′shun) dehydration.

anhydremia (an″hi-dre′me-ah) [*an* neg. + Gr. *hydōr* water + *haima* blood + *-ia*] deficiency of water in the blood.

anhydride (an-hi′drīd) [*an* neg. + Gr. *hydōr* water] a chemical compound derived from a substance, especially an acid, by the abstraction of a molecule of water. The anhydrides of bases are oxides; those of alcohols are ethers. **abietic acid a.,** a resinous substance, $C_{44}H_{62}O_4$, found in rosin. **acetic a.,** a colorless mobile liquid of a pungent acetic odor, the anhydride of acetic acid $(CH_3CO)_2O$. **arsenous a.,** arsenic trioxide. **carbonic a.,** carbon dioxide. **chromic a.,** chromic acid. **perosmic a.,** osmium tetroxide. **silicic a.,** silica. **sorbitol a.,** sorbitan. **sulfurous a.,** sulfur dioxide.

anhydrochloric (an″hi-dro-klo′rik) achlorhydric.

anhydrohydroxyprogesterone (an-hi″dro-hi-drok″se-projes′ter-ōn) ethisterone.

anhydromuscarine (an″hi-dro-mus′kah-rin) a synthetic alkaloid, $OH(CH_3)_3N\cdot CH_2,CHO$, that has been used in experimental medicine.

Anhydron (an-hi′dron) trademark for a preparation of cyclothiazide.

anhydrosugar (an″hi-dro-shug′ar) a substance produced from cane sugar by heating it under diminished pressure to about 170° C. It does not ferment nor reduce copper solutions, and it has been used as a food in diabetes.

anhydrous (an-hi′drus) [*an* neg. + Gr. *hydōr* water] deprived or destitute of water.

anhypnia, anhypnosis (an-hip′ne-ah; an″hip-no′sis) [*an* neg. + Gr. *hypnos* sleep + *-ia*] (*obs.*) insomnia.

aniacinamidosis (ah-ni″ah-sin-am″ĭ-do′sis) any disorder due to nicotinamide deficiency.

aniacinosis (ah-ni″ah-sĭ-no′sis) nicotinic acid (niacin) deficiency.

anianthinopsy (an″e-an′thĭ-nop″se) [*an* neg. + Gr. *ianthinos* violet + *opsis* vision] inability to distinguish violet tints.

Anichkov's (Anitschkow's) myocyte (cell) (ah-nich′kofs) [Nikolai Nikolaevich *Anichkov,* Russian pathologist, born 1885] see under *myocyte.*

anicteric (an″ik-ter′ik) without icterus; not associated with jaundice.

anidean (ah-nid′e-an) pertaining to anideus.

anideus (ah-nid′e-us) [*an* neg. + Gr. *idea* form] holoacardius amorphous. **embryonic a.,** a blastoderm in which no embryonic axis develops.

anidoxime (an″ĭ-doks′ēm) chemical name: 3-(diphenylamino)-1-phenyl-1-propanone O-[[(4-methylphenyl)amino]carbonyl]oxime; an analgesic, $C_{21}H_{27}N_3O_3$.

anidrosis (an-ĭ-dro′sis) anhidrosis.

anidrotic (an″ĭ-drot′ik) anhidrotic.

anile (a′nīl) [L. *anus*, old woman] 1. like an old woman. 2. imbecilic.

anileridine (an″ĭ-ler′ĭ-dēn) [USP] chemical name: 1-[2-(4-aminophenyl)ethyl]-4-phenyl-4-piperidinecarboxylic acid. A synthetic narcotic analgesic, $C_{22}H_{28}N_2O_2$, occurring as a white, crystalline powder, used as the phosphate salt for premedication for general anesthesia in surgery, as a postoperative sedative, and obstetric analgesic; administered subcutaneously or intramuscularly. Abuse of this drug may lead to dependence. **a. hydrochloride** [USP], a white or nearly white, crystalline powder, $C_{22}H_{28}N_2O_2 \cdot 2HCl$, having the same actions and uses as the base; administered orally.

anilid (an′ĭ-lid) anilide.

anilide (an′ĭ-lid) any compound formed from aromatic amines by substitution of an acyl group for the hydrogen of NH_2.

anilinction (a″nĭ-link′shun) [L. *anus* + *lingere, linctum* to lick] application of the mouth to, or licking of, the anus.

anilinctus (a″nĭ-link′tus) anilinction.

aniline (an′ĭ-lin) [Arabic *an′nil* indigo, *nīl* blue; L. *nil* indigo] a colorless oily liquid, $C_6H_5NH_2$, from coal tar and from indigo, made commercially by reducing nitrobenzene. It is slightly soluble in water; freely so in ether and alcohol. Combined with other substances, especially chlorine and the chlorates, it forms the aniline colors or dyes that are derived from coal tar. It is an important cause of serious industrial poisoning associated with bone-marrow depression as well as methemoglobinemia. Called also *amidobenzene* and *aminobenzene*. See also *anilinism*. **a. sulfate,** a white crystalline substance, $(C_6H_5NH_2)_2H_2SO_4$.

anilingus (a″nĭ-lin′gus) an individual who practices anilinction.

anilinism (an′ĭ-lin-izm) a condition produced by exposure to aniline, and marked by methemoglobinemia and aplastic anemia, vertigo, muscular weakness, cyanosis, and digestive derangement.

anilinophil (an-ĭ-lin′o-fil) [*aniline* + Gr. *philein* to love] (obs.) an anilinophilous element or structure.

anilinophile (an″ĭ-lin′o-fīl) (obs.) 1. anilinophilous. 2. anilinophil.

anilinophilous (an″ĭ-lin-of′ĭ-lus) (obs.) staining readily with aniline dyes.

anilism (an′ĭ-lizm) anilinism.

anility (ah-nil′ĭ-te) [L. *anus*, old woman] 1. the state of being like an old woman. 2. imbecility.

anilopam hydrochloride (an′ĭl-o-pam″) chemical name: 4-[2-(1,2,4,5-tetrahydro-8-methoxy-2-methyl-3H-3-benzazepin-3-yl)-ethyl]benzeneamine dihydrochloride; an analgesic, $C_{20}H_{26}N_2O \cdot 2HCl$.

anil-quinoline (an″il-kwin′o-lin) synthetic quinoline prepared from aniline.

anima (an′ĭ-mah) [L. "air"] 1. the soul. 2. the active principle of a drug. 3. Jung's term for the unconscious, or inner being, of the individual, as opposed to the personality he presents to the world (persona). In Jungian psychoanalysis, the more feminine soul or feminine component of a man's personality; cf. *animus*.

animal (an′ĭ-mal) [L. *animalis*, from *anima* life, breath] 1. a living organism having sensation and the power of voluntary movement and requiring for its existence oxygen and organic food. 2. pertaining to such an organism. **control a.,** see *control,* def. 2. **conventional a.,** an experimental animal that has not been reared under gnotobiotic conditions. **decerebrate a.,** an experimental animal that has been subjected to decerebration; such an animal exhibits rigid extension of the legs, with strong tonic contraction of the extensor muscles and to some extent the flexor muscles. See also *decerebrate,* and see *decerebrate rigidity,* under *rigidity.* **experimental a.,** an animal which is used as a subject of experimental procedures in the laboratory. **Houssay a.,** an experimental animal deprived of both pituitary gland and pancreas. **hyperphagic a.,** an experimental animal in which the cells of the ventromedial nucleus of the hypothalamus have been destroyed, abolishing its awareness of the point at which it should stop eating; excessive eating and savageness characterize such an animal. **Long-Lukens a.,** an experimental animal which has been deprived of the pancreas and adrenal glands. **nuclein a.,** an animal into which a certain amount of nuclein has been injected. **slime a.,** a protozoon of the order Mycetozoida; slime mold. **spinal a.,** an animal whose spinal cord has been severed, thus cutting off communication with the brain. **thalamic a.,** an animal in which the brain stem has been transected just above the thalamus.

animalcule (an″ĭ-mal′kūl) [L. *animalculum*] any minute or microscopic animal organism.

animalculist (an″ĭ-mal′ku-list) a believer in the theory that the undeveloped embryo exists preformed in the spermatozoon; cf. *ovist.*

animality (an″ĭ-mal′ĭ-te) the distinguishing characteristics of animals.

animation (an″ĭ-ma′shun) 1. the state of being alive. 2. liveliness of spirits. **suspended a.,** a temporary state of apparent death.

animism (an′ĭ-mizm) [L. *anima* soul] 1. the obsolete doctrine that the soul is the source of all organic development. 2. the belief that nonliving objects and phenomena (such as clouds) are inhabited and motivated by a nonphysical agent; it is a characteristic of the thinking of early childhood. 3. the theory that behavior is controlled by an immaterial mind or soul.

animus (an′ĭ-mus) in Jungian psychoanalysis, the more male soul or masculine component of a woman's personality; cf. *anima,* def. 3.

anincretinosis (an-in″kre-tĭ-no′sis) [*an* neg. + *incretion*] (obs.) a disorder due to defect or lack of some internal secretion.

anion (an′ĭ-on) [Gr. *ana* up + *iōn* going] an ion carrying a negative charge owing to the gain of one or more electrons. Hence, because unlike forms of electricity attract each other, it is attracted by, and travels to, the anode or positive pole. See *ion.* The anions include all the nonmetals, the acid radicals, and the hydroxyl ion. They are indicated by a minus sign, as Cl^- (formerly by an accent mark, as Cl′).

anionic (an″i-on′ik) pertaining to or containing an anion.

anionotropy (an″e-on-ot′ro-pe) [*anion* + Gr. *tropos* a turning] a type of tautomerism in which the migrating group is a negative ion rather than the more usual hydrogen ion. Cf. *prototropy.*

aniridia (an″ĭ-rid′e-ah) [*an* neg. + *iris*] absence of the iris; a rare, usually bilateral, hereditary anomaly that is rarely complete, a rudimentary stump usually being visible on gonioscopy.

anisakiasis (an″is-sa-ki′ah-sis) infection with the roundworm *Anisakis marina.* Human infection is caused by third-stage larvae eaten in undercooked infected marine fish (e.g., herring); the larvae then burrow into the stomach wall, producing an eosinophilic granulomatous mass. Called also *eosinophilic granuloma.*

Anisakis (an″ĭ-sa′kis) a genus of nematodes that parasitize the stomachs of marine mammals and birds, where they reach the adult stage; the infective third-stage larvae occur in various marine fishes. See also *anisakiasis.* **A. ma′rina,** a species causing anisakiasis.

anisate (an′ĭ-sāt) a salt of anisic acid.

anischuria (an″is-ku′re-ah) [*an* neg. + Gr. *ischouria* retention of the urine] (obs.) incontinence of urine; enuresis.

anise (an′is) [L. *anisum*] the fruit of *Pimpinella anisum,* an umbelliferous plant; it is used as a carminative and expectorant. **Chinese a., Indian a.,** the dried ripe fruit of *Illicium verum,* an Asian tree. It yields anise oil and is used as a stimulant and carminative. **star a.,** the fruit of *Illicium religiosum* (*I. japonicum; I. anisatum*), the Japanese star anise (shikimmi); it is very poisonous due to content of hananomin.

aniseikonia (an″ĭ-si-ko′ne-ah) [Gr. *anisos* unequal + *eikōn* image + *-ia*] a condition in which the ocular image of an object as seen by one eye differs in size and shape from that seen by the other.

aniseikonic (an″ĭ-si-kon′ik) pertaining to or correcting aniseikonia.

anisindione (an″is-in-di′ōn) [NF] chemical name: 2-(4-methoxyphenyl)-1H-indene-1,3(2H)-dione. One of the indanedione anticoagulants, $C_{16}H_{12}O_3$, occurring as a white to creamy white powder; administered orally.

anisine (an′ĭ-sin) a crystalline alkaloid, $C_{22}H_{24}N_2O_3$, from anise; used as a bactericide and wood fungicide.

aniso- (an-i′so) [Gr. *anisos* unequal, uneven] a combining form denoting unequal or dissimilar.

anisoaccommodation (an-i″so-ah-kom″mo-da′shun) a difference in the accommodative capacity of the two eyes.

anisochromasia (an-i″so-kro-ma′ze-ah) [*aniso-* + Gr. *chrōma* color] a condition in which only the peripheral zone of an erythrocyte is colored.

anisochromatic (an-i″so-kro-mat′ik) [*aniso-* + Gr. *chrōma* color] not of the same color throughout; applied to solutions used for testing color blindness, containing two pigments which are distinguished by both the normal and the color blind eye. Cf. *pseudoisochromatic.*

anisochromia (an″ĭ-so-kro′me-ah) [*aniso-* + Gr. *chrōma* color + *-ia*] variation in the color of the erythrocytes due to unequal hemoglobin content.

anisocoria (an″ĭ-so-ko′re-ah) [*aniso-* + Gr. *korē* pupil + *-ia*] inequality of the pupils in diameter.

anisocytosis (an-i″so-si-to′sis) [*aniso-* + Gr. *kytos* hollow vessel + *-osis*] presence in the blood of erythrocytes showing excessive variation in size.

anisodactylous (an-i-so-dak′tĭ-lus) [*aniso-* + Gr. *daktylos* finger] having corresponding digits of unequal length.

anisodactyly (an-i-so-dak'tĭ-le) a condition characterized by having corresponding digits of unequal length.

anisodiametric (an-i″so-di″ah-met'rik) characterized by different dimensions in different diameters.

anisodont (an-i'so-dont) [aniso- + Gr. odous tooth] having teeth of unequal size or length.

anisogamete (an″ĭ-so-gam'ĕt) a gamete of different size and structure than the one with which it unites.

anisogametic (an″ĭ-so-gah-met'ik) characterized by the production of gametes of different size and structure.

anisogamous (an″ĭ-sog'ah-mus) having conjugating elements (gametes) that differ in size and structure.

anisogamy (an″i-sog'ah-me) [aniso- + Gr. gamos marriage] sexual conjugation in which the gametes differ in structure and size, as in the malarial parasites.

anisoic (an″ĭ-so'ik) pertaining to anise.

anisoiconia (an-i″so-i-ko'ne-ah) aniseikonia.

anisokaryosis (an-i″so-kar'e-o'sis) [aniso- + Gr. karyon nucleus + -osis] inequality in the size of the nuclei of cells.

Anisolobis (an-i″so-lo'bis) a genus of beetles, the earwigs. Nymphs and adults of A. euborellia (Lucas) are intermediate hosts of helminth parasites of man and animals.

anisomastia (an-i″so-mas'te-ah) [aniso- + Gr. mastos breast + -ia] inequality in the size of the breasts.

anisomelia (an-i″so-me'le-ah) [aniso- + Gr. melos limb + -ia] inequality between paired limbs.

anisomeric (an-i″so-mer'ik) not isomeric.

anisometrope (an-i″so-met'rōp) a person affected with anisometropia.

anisometropia (an-i″so-mĕ-tro'pe-ah) [aniso- + Gr. metron measure + ōps eye + -ia] a difference in the refractive power of the two eyes.

anisometropic (an-i″so-mĕ-trop'ik) pertaining to or characterized by anisometropia.

Anisomorpha (an-i″so-mor'fah) a genus of insects. **A. bu-prestoi′des,** the walking stick; a species of orthopterous insects capable of discharging an irritating fluid.

anisophoria (an″i-so-fo're-ah) [aniso- + phoria] a condition in which the balance of the vertical muscles of one eye differs from that of the other eye, so that the visual lines do not lie in the same horizontal plane.

anisopia (an″i-so'pe-ah) [aniso- + Gr. ōps eye + -ia] inequality of vision in the two eyes.

anisopiesis (an-i″so-pi-e'sis) [aniso- + Gr. piesis pressure] variation or inequality in the blood pressure as registered in different parts of the body.

anisopoikilocytosis (an-i″so-poi″kĭ-lo-si-to'sis) the presence in the blood of erythrocytes of varying sizes and abnormal shapes.

anisorhythmia (an-i″so-rith'me-ah) [aniso- + Gr. rhythmos rhythm + -ia] (obs.) irregular heart action marked by lack of synchronism in the rhythm of atria and ventricles.

anisosmotic (an″ĭ-sos-mot'ik) not having the same osmotic pressure or not containing the same effective concentration of osmotically active components.

anisospore (an-i'so-spōr″) [aniso- + Gr. sporos spore] 1. an anisogamete of organisms that reproduce by spores. 2. an asexual spore produced by a heterosporous organism. See isospore.

anisosporous (an-i″sos'po-rus) having anisospores.

anisosthenic (an-i″sos-then'ik) [aniso- + Gr. sthenos strength] not having equal strength; said of paired muscles.

anisotonic (an-i″so-ton'ik) 1. showing a variation in tonicity or tension. 2. having an osmotic pressure differing from that of a solution with which it is compared.

anisotropal (an″i-sot'ro-pal) anisotropic.

anisotropic (an-i″so-trop'ik) [aniso- + Gr. tropos a turning] 1. having unlike properties in different directions, as in any unit lacking spherical symmetry. 2. doubly refracting or having a double polarizing power.

anisotropine methylbromide (an-is″o-tro'pēn) chemical name: endo-8,8-dimethyl-3-[(1-oxo-2-propylpentyl)oxy]-8-azonia-bicyclo[3.2.1]octane bromide. An anticholinergic, $C_{17}H_{32}BrNO_2$, occurring as a white, crystalline powder or plates, which produces relaxation of visceral smooth muscle, and is used as a spasmolytic in various gastrointestinal disorders; administered orally.

anisotropy (an″i-sot'ro-pe) the quality or condition of being anisotropic.

anisum (an-i'sum), gen. ani'si [L.] anise.

anisuria (an″i-su're-ah) [aniso- + Gr. ouron urine + -ia] a condition marked by alternating oliguria and polyuria.

anitrogenous (ah″ni-troj'ĕ-nus) not nitrogenous.

Anitschkow Anichkov.

ankle (ang'k'l) 1. the part of the leg just above the foot. 2. the joint between the foot and the leg; ankle joint (articulatio talocruralis [NA]. **cocked a.,** a partial anterior flexion of the fetlock joint of a horse. **deck a's,** edema of the ankles ob-

served on troop ships. **tailors′ a.,** an abnormal bursa over the lower end of the fibula in tailors, from pressure caused by sitting on the floor with the legs crossed in front.

ankylo- (ang'kĭ-lo) [Gr. ankylos bent or crooked] a combining form meaning bent, or in the form of a noose or loop.

ankyloblepharon (ang″kĭ-lo-blef'ah-ron) [ankylo- + Gr. blepharon eyelid] the adhesion of the ciliary edges of the eyelid to each other. **a. filifor′me adna′tum,** congenital adhesion of the margins of the upper and lower lids by filamentous bands. **a. tota′le,** cryptophthalmos.

ankylocheilia (ang″kĭ-lo-ki'le-ah) [ankylo- + Gr. cheilos lip + -ia] adhesion of the lips to each other.

ankylocolpos (ang-kĭ-lo-kol'pos) [ankylo- + Gr. kolpos vagina] atresia or imperforation of the vagina.

ankylodactyly (ang″kĭ-lo-dak'tĭ-le) [ankylo- + Gr. daktylos finger] fusion or adhesion of fingers or toes to one another.

ankyloglossia (ang″kĭ-lo-glos'e-ah) [ankylo- + Gr. glōssa tongue + -ia] tongue-tie. **a. supe′rior,** an unusual association of an extensive adhesion of the tongue to the palate, with deformities of the extremities.

ankylophobia (ang″kĭ-lo-fo'be-ah) [ankylo- + Gr. phobein to be affrighted by + -ia] morbid fear of ankylosis in cases of fracture or joint affection.

ankylopoietic (ang″kĭ-lo-poi-et'ik) [ankylo- + Gr. poiein to make] producing or characterized by ankylosis.

ankyloproctia (ang″kĭ-lo-prok'she-ah) [ankylo- + Gr. prōktos anus + -ia] (obs.) a stricture of the anus.

Ankyloproglypha (ang″kĭ-lo-pro-glif'ah) Proteroglypha.

ankylosed (ang'kĭ-lōsd) fused or obliterated, as a joint.

ankyloses (ang″kĭ-lo'sēz) plural of ankylosis.

ankylosis (ang″kĭ-lo'sis, pl. ankylo'ses [Gr. ankylōsis] immobility and consolidation of a joint due to disease, injury, or surgical procedure. **artificial a.,** arthrodesis. **bony a.,** the union of the bones of a joint by proliferation of bone cells, resulting in complete immobility; called also true a. **cricoarytenoid joint a.,** complete fixation of the cricoarytenoid joint of the larynx due to inflammation and characterized by hoarseness, cough, and difficulty in expectoration. **dental a.,** solid fixation of a tooth, resulting from fusion of the cementum and alveolar bone, with obliteration of the periodontal membrane. **extracapsular a.,** ankylosis due to rigidity of structures exterior to the joint capsule. **false a.,** fibrous a. **fibrous a.,** reduced mobility of a joint due to proliferation of fibrous tissue; called also false a. and spurious a. **intracapsular a.,** obliteration of joint motion due to disease, injury, or surgical procedure within the joint capsule. **spurious a.,** fibrous a. **stapedial a.,** fixation of the footplate of the stapes in otosclerosis, causing a conductive hearing loss. **true a.,** bony a.

Ankylostoma (ang″kĭ-los'to-mah) Ancylostoma.

ankylostomiasis (ang″kĭ-lo-sto-mi'ah-sis) hookworm disease.

ankylotic (ang″kĭ-lot'ik) pertaining to or marked by ankylosis.

ankylotomy (ang″kĭ-lot'o-me) [ankylo- + Gr. tomē cut] the surgical procedure for relieving tonguetie; frenectomy.

ankylurethria (ang″kil-u-re'thre-ah) [ankylo- + urethra + -ia] stricture of the urethra.

ankyroid (ang'kĭ-roid) [Gr. ankyra hook + eidos form] hook-shaped.

anlage (ahn'lah-geh, or an'lāj), pl. anla'gen [Ger. "a laying on"] primordium.

Annandale′s operation (an'an-dālz) [Thomas Annandale, Scottish surgeon, 1838–1907] see under operation.

anneal (ah-nēl') to soften a material, such as a metal, by controlled heating and cooling, making it less brittle and more easily adapted, bent, or swaged.

annectent (ah-nek'tent) [L. annectens] connecting or joining.

annelid (ah'nel-id) any member of Annelida.

Annelida (ah-nel'ĭ-dah) a phylum of metazoan invertebrates, the segmented worms; it contains only one class of medical interest, Hirudinea, the leeches.

Annona (ah-no'nah) a genus of trees and shrubs of tropical America; the bark, fruit, and leaves of various species are used in native medicine, and the seeds are poisonous for fish and insects and have emetic properties. A. muricata L. is the soursop, a popular tropical American edible fruit.

annotto (ah-not'o) a red color or stain from the fruit of Bixa orellana, a South American tree, used for coloring butter, cheese, margarine, and other foods; called also arnotto.

annoyer (ah-noi'er) a stimulus which arouses an unpleasant feeling reaction.

annular (an'u-lar) [L. annularis] shaped like a ring.

annuli (an'u-li) [L.] plural of annulus.

annuloplasty (an'u-lo-plas'te) plastic repair of a cardiac valve.

annulorrhaphy (an'u-lor'ah-fe) [L. annulus ring + Gr. rhaphē suture] closure of a hernial ring or defect by sutures.

annulus (an'u-lus), pl. an'nuli [L. "a ring"; dim. of annus a year, originally a circuit] a ring, or ringlike or circular structure. This word has been replaced by *anulus* in NA terminology. For official names which were otherwise unchanged, see under *anulus*. **a. abdomina′lis,** see *anulus inguinalis profundus* and *anulus inguinalis superficialis.* **a. abdomina′lis abdom′inis,** anulus inguinalis profundus. **a. cilia′ris,** orbiculus ciliaris. **a. haemorrhoida′lis,** zona hemorrhoidalis. **a. inguina′lis abdomina′lis,** anulus inguinalis profundus. **a. inguina′lis subcuta′neus,** anulus inguinalis superficialis. **a. mi′grans,** a disease marked by formation on the tongue of raised red patches with a yellow border, which spread in eccentric circles over the upper and under surfaces; cf. *geographic tongue,* under *tongue.* **a. of nuclear pore,** a filamentous, circular structure at the edge of the nuclear pore of a cell nucleus and extending into the pore as a lining layer; the pore and its annulus together form the pore complex. **a. ova′lis,** limbus of recessus ellipticus vestibuli. **a. of spermatozoon,** the so-called ring centriole (see under *centriole*). **a. tendin′eus commu′nis [Zinni],** anulus tendineus communis. **a. tra′cheae,** any of the rings of the trachea. **tympanic a.,** anulus tympanicus. **a. urethra′lis,** a thickening around the urethral opening of the bladder formed by a thickening of the middle muscular coat. **Vieussens' a.,** 1. limbus of the recessus ellipticus vestibuli. 2. ansa subclavia. **a. zin′nii,** anulus tendineus communis.

Anocentor (a″no-sen′tor) a genus of ticks of the family Ixodidae. **A. ni′tans,** a species of yellow-brown ticks parasitizing horses and related animals, originally described in Jamaica and Santo Domingo, and later found in the United States in southern Texas, Florida, and Georgia. It transmits *Babesia caballi,* an etiologic agent of biliary fever of horses. Called also *Dermacentor nitans* and *Otocentor nitans.*

anochlesia (an″o-kle′ze-ah) (*obs.*) 1. tranquillity. 2. catalepsy.

anochromasia (an″o-kro-ma′se-ah) 1. absence of the usual staining reaction from a tissue or cell. 2. a condition in which the erythrocytes show a piling up of hemoglobin at the periphery so that the center is pale.

anociassociation (ah-no″se-ah-so″se-a′shun) [*a* neg. + L. *nocere* to injure + *association*] the blunting of harmful association impulses; a method of anesthesia designed to minimize the effect of surgical shock. [The mind of the patient is calmed by an injection of scopolamine and morphine one hour before the operation. The general anesthetic employed is usually nitrous oxide and oxygen.] The field of operation is blocked by infiltration with procaine and every division of sensitive tissue during the operation is preceded by the injection of procaine. Sharp dissection and gentle manipulations are employed. [To minimize postoperative discomfort in serious cases, quinine and urea hydrochloride solution is injected at some distance from the wound] (Crile). Called also *anocithesia.*

anociated (ah-no′se-āt″ed) in a condition of anociassociation.

anociation (ah-no″se-a′shun) anociassociation.

anocithesia (ah-no″se-the′ze-ah) anociassociation.

anococcygeal (a″no-kok-sij′e-al) pertaining to the anus and coccyx.

anodal (an-o′dal) pertaining to the anode.

anode (an′ōd) [Gr. *ana* up + *hodos* way] the positive electrode or pole to which negative ions are attracted. In x-ray tubes, it is usually made of solid copper equipped with a tungsten insert which serves as a target. **hooded a.,** in radiology, an anode incorporating a copper shield to overcome problems of secondary x-ray emission. **rotating a.,** in radiology, an anode on which the tungsten target area is constantly rotated in relation to the electron stream.

anoderm (a′no-derm) the epithelial lining of the anal canal.

anodmia (an-od′me-ah) [*an* neg. + Gr. *odmē* smell + -*ia*] anosomia.

anodontia (an″o-don′she-ah) [*an* neg. + Gr. *odous* tooth + -*ia*] congenital absence of the teeth; it may involve all (*total a.*) or only some of the teeth (*partial a., hypodontia*), and both the deciduous and the permanent dentition, or only teeth of the permanent dentition. **partial a., a. partia′lis,** congenital absence of some of the teeth; called also *hypodontia.* **total a., a tota′lis,** congenital absence of all of the teeth. **a. ve′ra,** total failure of development of the teeth, usually associated with other anomalies, such as absence of sebaceous glands and deficiency of the sweat, lacrimal, pharyngeal, conjunctival, and salivary glands, and other congenital defects.

anodontism (an″o-don′tizm) anodontia.

anodyne (an′o-dīn) [*an* neg. + Gr. *odynē* pain] 1. relieving pain. 2. a medicine that relieves pain; the anodynes include opium, morphine, codeine, aspirin, and others. Called also *acesodyne.* **Hoffmann's a.,** compound ether spirit.

anodynia (an″o-din′e-ah) [*an* neg. + Gr. *odynē* pain + -*ia*] freedom from pain.

anoia (ah-noi′ah) [Gr. *anoia*] idiocy; amentia.

anol (a′nol) a compound, *p*-hydroxy propenyl benzene, which is readily polymerized to form active carcinogenic and estrogenic substances.

anomalad (ah-nom′ah-lad) [*anomaly* + Gr. -*ad* connected with] a term proposed to designate a single, localized anomaly occurring during morphogenesis, together with the pattern of subsequent morphologic defects that stem from it.

anomalo- (ah-nom′ah-lo) [Gr. *anōmalos* irregular, *anōmalia* irregularity, unevenness; from *an* neg. + Gr. *homalos* even] a combining form meaning irregular or uneven.

anomalopia (ah-nom″ah-lo′pe-ah) [*anomalo-* + Gr. *ōpe* vision + -*ia*] a slight anomaly of visual perception. **color a.,** a minor deviation of color vision, without loss of ability to distinguish the four primary colors; see *deuteranomalopia* and *protanomalopia.*

anomaloscope (ah-nom′ah-lo-skōp″) [*anomalo-* + Gr. *skopein* to view] an instrument used in testing for anomalies of color vision by having the subject match mixed spectral lines.

anomalotrophy (ah-nom″al-ot′ro-fe) [*anomalo-* + Gr. *trophē* nutrition] abnormality of nutrition.

anomalous (ah-nom′ah-lus) [Gr. *anōmalos*] irregular; marked by deviation from the natural order. Applied particularly to congenital and hereditary defects.

anomaly (ah-nom′ah-le) [Gr. *anōmalia*] marked deviation from the normal standard, especially as a result of congenital or hereditary defects. **Alder's a., Alder's constitutional granulation a., Alder-Reilly a.,** a hereditary, clinically unimportant condition in which all leukocytes, but mainly those of the myelocytic series, contain coarse azurophilic granules. **Aristotle's a.,** if the first and second fingers are crossed and a pencil is placed between them, the person feels two pencils. **Axenfeld's a.,** see under *syndrome.* **Chédiak-Higashi a., Chédiak-Steinbrinck-Higashi a.,** see under *syndrome.* **developmental a.,** a defect which is the result of imperfect development of the embryo. **Ebstein's a.,** a malformation of the tricuspid valve, the septal and posterior leaflets being attached to the wall of the right ventricle to a varying degree, and the anterior leaflet being normally attached to the anulus fibrosis; usually associated with an atrial septal defect. Called also *Ebstein's disease.* **Freund's a.,** stenosis of the upper thoracic aperture from shortening of the first rib, resulting in deficient expansion of the apex of the lung. **May-Hegglin a.,** a rare dominantly inherited disorder of blood cell morphology, characterized by the presence of blue, RNA-containing cytoplasmic inclusions similar to Döhle bodies in most granulocytes (neutrophils, eosinophils, basophils, and monocytes), accompanied by abnormally large, poorly granulated platelets and, at times, thrombocytopenia, usually without associated distinguishing features. **Pelger's nuclear a., Pelger-Huët nuclear a.,** Pelger-Huët nuclear a., def. 1. **Pelger-Huët nuclear a.,** 1. an inherited defect interfering with normal nuclear lobulation of neutrophils and eosinophils so that the nuclei appear rodlike, spherical, or dumbbell-shaped. The nuclear structure is coarse and lumpy. Called also *Pelger's nuclear a.* and *Pelger-Huët a.* 2. an acquired condition with changes similar to those observed in the genetically determined abnormality, occurring in certain types of anemia and leukemia. **Poland's a.,** see under *syndrome.* **Rieger's a.,** see under *syndrome.* **Uhl's a.,** congenital hypoplasia of the myocardium of the right ventricle, resulting in decreased output of the right side of the heart. **Undritz a.,** hereditary hypersegmentation of neutrophils; see under *hypersegmentation.*

anomer (an′o-mer) [Gr. *ana* up + *meros* part] the α or β form of a sugar produced when the possibility of steroisomerism is available to the reducing carbon atom by the formation of an oxygen-containing ring.

anomeric (an″o-mer′ik) pertaining to an anomer; denoting the reducing carbon atom in an anomer.

anomia (ah-no′me-ah) [*an* neg. + Gr. *anoma* name + -*ia*] loss of the power of naming objects or of recognizing and recalling their names; cf. *nominal aphasia* and *dysnomia.*

anonacein (an″o-na′se-in) an alkaloid of *Hylopia aethiopica* used in Africa as an aphrodisiac.

anonaine (an″o-na′in) an alkaloid, $C_{17}H_{17}O_2N$, from *Annona reticulata.*

anonychia (an″o-nik′e-ah) [*an* neg. + Gr. *onyx* nail + -*ia*] congenital absence of a nail or nails.

anonymous (ah-non′ĭ-mus) nameless; innominate.

anoopsia (an″o-op′se-ah) hypertropia.

anoperineal (a″no-per-ĭ-ne′al) pertaining to the anus and perineum.

Anopheles (ah-nof′ĕ-lēz) [Gr. *anōphelēs* hurtful] a genus of mosquitoes characterized by long slender palpi, nearly as long as the proboscis, and by holding the body at an angle with the surface on which it rests while the head and proboscis are in line with the body. Many species are vectors of malaria, and some are vectors of *Wuchereria bancrofti;* called also *Cellia.* See table on following page.

anophelicide (ah-nof′ĕ-lĭ-sīd″) [*anopheles* + L. *caedere* to kill] destructive to anopheline mosquitoes.

anophelifuge (ah-nof′ĕ-lĭ-fūj) [*anopheles* + L. *fugare* to put to flight] preventing the bite or attack of anopheline mosquitoes.

anopheline (ah-nof′ĭ-lĭn) pertaining to or caused by mosquitoes of the tribe Anophelini.

CHIEF MALARIA-CARRYING ANOPHELES SPECIES OF THE WORLD

Modified from Russell et al., *Practical Malariology.*

A. aconitus	A. maculatus maculatus
A. albimanus	A. maculipennis
A. albitarsis	A. mangyanus
A. amictus	A. messeae
A. annularis	A. minimus
A. annulipes annulipes	A. minimus flavirostris
A. aquasalis	A. moucheti moucheti
A. atroparvus	A. moucheti nigeriensis
A. bancroftii	A. multicolor
A. barbirostris barbirostris	A. nili
A. bellator	A. pattoni
A. claviger	A. pharoensis
A. culicifacies	A. philippinensis
A. darlingi	A. pretoriensis
A. farauti	A. pseudopunctipennis
A. fluviatilis	pseudopunctipennis
A. freeborni	A. punctimacula
A. funestus	A. punctulatus
A. gambiae	punctulatus
A. hancocki	A. quadrimaculatus
A. hargreavesi	A. sacharovi
A. hyrcanus nigerrimus	A. sergentii
A. hyrcanus sinensis	A. stephensi stephensi
A. jeyporiensis candidiensis	A. subpictus subpictus
A. jeyporiensis jeyporiensis	A. sundaicus
A. kochi	A. superpictus
A. labranchiae atroparvus	A. umbrosus
A. labranchiae labranchiae	A. varuna
A. leucosphyrus leucosphyrus	A. walkeri
A. lungae	

Anophelini (ah-nof″ĭ-li′ni) a tribe of mosquitoes of the subfamily Culicinae, family Culicidae. It includes the genera *Anopheles, Chagasia,* and *Nyssorhynchus,* and the subgenus *Stethomyia.* Members of the genus *Anopheles* act as carriers of the malarial parasite.

anophelism (ah-nof′ĕ-lizm) infestation of a district with anopheline mosquitoes.

anophoria (an-o-fo′re-ah) [Gr. *anō* upward + Gr. *pherein* to bear] hyperphoria.

anophthalmia (an″of-thal′me-ah) [*an* neg. + Gr. *ophthalmos* eye] a developmental defect characterized by complete absence of the eyes (rare) or by the presence of vestigial eyes.

anophthalmos (an″of-thal′mos) anophthalmia.

anophthalmus (an″of-thal′mus) an individual exhibiting anophthalmia.

anopia (an-o′pe-ah) [*an* neg. + Gr. *ōpē* sight + *-ia*] 1. absence or rudimentary condition of the eye. 2. anopsia (def. 1). 3. hypertropia.

anoplasty (a′no-plas″te) [L. *anus* anus + Gr. *plassein* to form] a plastic or restorative operation on the anus.

Anoplocephala (an″op-lo-sef′ah-lah) [Gr. *anoplos* unarmed + Gr. *kephalē* head] a genus of tapeworms of the family Anoplocephalidae, found in horses.

Anoplocephalidae (an″o-plo-sĕ-fal′ĭ-de) a family of medium-sized or large tapeworms of the order Cyclophyllidea, subclass Cestoda, commonly parasitic in various herbivorous animals and man. Genera of medical and veterinary importance are *Anoplocephala, Moniezia, Bertiella,* and *Thysanosoma.*

Anoplura (an″o-plu′rah) [Gr. *anoplos* unarmed + *oura* tail] an order of insects, the sucking lice, characterized by the absence of wings; it includes only two genera of medical interest, *Pediculus* and *Phthirus.* Cf. *Mallophaga.*

anopsia (an-op′se-ah) [*an* neg. + Gr. *opsis* vision + *-ia*] 1. nonuse or suppression of vision in one eye, as in heterotropia. 2. hypertropia.

anorchia (an-or′ke-ah) anorchism.

anorchid (an-or′kid) [*an* neg. + Gr. *orchis* testis] an individual with no testes in the scrotum.

anorchidic (an″or-kid′ik) pertaining to anorchism; having no testes in the scrotum.

anorchidism (an-or′kĭ-dizm″) anorchism.

anorchis (an-or′kis) anorchid.

anorchism (an-or′kizm) congenital absence of the testis, which may occur unilaterally or bilaterally.

anorectal (a″no-rek′tal) pertaining to the anus and rectum or to the junction region between the two.

anorectic (an″o-rek′tik) [Gr. *anorektos* without appetite for] 1. pertaining to anorexia; having no appetite. 2. a substance that diminishes the appetite.

anorectitis (a″no-rek-ti′tis) inflammation of the anorectum.

anorectocolonic (a″no-rek″to-ko-lon′ik) pertaining to the anus, rectum, and colon.

anorectum (a″no-rek′tum) [*anus* + *rectum*] the anus and rectum considered together as a single unit.

anoretic (an″o-ret′ik) anorectic.

anorexia (an″o-rek′se-ah) [Gr. "want of appetite"] lack or loss of the appetite for food. **a. nervo′sa,** a psychophysiologic condition, usually seen in girls and young women, characterized by severe and prolonged inability or refusal to eat, sometimes accompanied by spontaneous or induced vomiting, extreme emaciation, amenorrhea (impotence in males), and other biological changes.

anorexiant (an″o-rek′se-ant) anorexigenic.

anorexic (an″o-rek′sik) anorectic.

anorexigenic (an″o-rek″sĭ-jen′ik) [*anorexia* + Gr. *gennan* to produce] 1. producing anorexia, or diminishing the appetite. 2. an agent that produces anorexia, or controls the appetite. Called also *anorexiant.*

anorganic (an″or-gan′ik) denoting tissue (e.g., bone) from which the organic material has been removed.

anorganology (an″or-gan-ol′o-je) the study of nonliving things; abiology.

anorgasmy (an-or-gaz′me) [*an* neg. + *orgasm*] failure to experience orgasm in coitus.

anorthography (an″or-thog′rah-fe) [*an* neg. + Gr. *orthos* straight + *graphein* to write] loss of the power of writing correctly.

anorthopia (an″or-tho′pe-ah) [*an* neg. + Gr. *orthos* straight + *opsis* vision + *-ia*] distorted vision.

anorthoscope (an-or′tho-skōp) [*an* neg. + Gr. *orthos* straight + *skopein* to examine] an instrument for combining two disconnected pictures in one perfect visual image.

anorthosis (an″or-tho′sis) [*an* neg. + Gr. *orthos* straight + *-osis*] absence of penile erectility, a form of impotence.

anoscope (a′no-skōp) [*anus* + Gr. *skopein* to examine] a speculum for examining the anus and lower rectum.

anoscopy (ah-nos′ko-pe) examination of the anus and lower rectum by means of an anoscope.

anosigmoidoscopic (a″no-sig-moi″do-skop′ik) pertaining to anosigmoidoscopy.

anosigmoidoscopy (a″no-sig″moi-dos′ko-pe) [*anus* + *sigmoid* + Gr. *skopein* to examine] endoscopic examination of the anus, rectum, and sigmoid colon.

anosmatic (an″oz-mat′ik) [*an* neg. + Gr. *osmasthai* to smell] having no sense of smell, or only an imperfect sense of smell. Cf. *osmatic,* def. 2.

anosmia (an-oz′me-ah) [*an* neg. + Gr. *osmē* smell + *-ia*] absence of the sense of smell; called also *anosphrasia* and *olfactory anesthesia.* **a. gustato′ria,** the loss of the power to smell foods. **preferential a.,** lack of ability to sense certain odors only. **a. respirato′ria,** loss of smell due to nasal obstruction.

anosmic (an-oz′mik) 1. pertaining to or characterized by anosmia. 2. odorless. Called also *aosmic.*

anosodiaphoria (an-o″so-di-ah-fo′re-ah) [*a* neg. + Gr. *nosos* disease + *diaphoria* difference] (*obs.*) indifference to the existence of disease.

anosognosia (an-o″so-no′zhe-ah) [*a* neg. + Gr. *nosos* disease + *gnosis* knowledge + *-ia*] loss of ability to recognize or to acknowledge bodily defect; it is usually associated with lesions of the nondominant hemisphere and nondominant left hemiparesis, but it may also occur with other brain lesions.

anosphrasia (an″os-fra′ze-ah) [*an* neg. + Gr. *osphrasis* sense of smell] anosmia.

anospinal (a″no-spi′nal) pertaining to the anus and the spinal cord.

anosteoplasia (an-os″te-o-pla′se-ah) [*an* neg. + Gr. *osteon* bone + *plasis* formation + *-ia*] defective bone formation.

anostosis (an″os-to′sis) [*an* neg. + Gr. *osteon* bone + *-osis*] defective development of bone.

anotia (an-o′she-ah) [*an* neg. + Gr. *ous* ear + *-ia*] congenital absence of the external ear(s).

anotropia (an″o-tro′pe-ah) [Gr. *anō* upward + *trepein* to turn] a condition in which the visual axes tend to rise above the object looked at.

anotus (an-o′tus) [*an* neg. + Gr. *ous* ear] an earless fetus.

anovaginal (a″no-vaj′ĭ-nal) pertaining to the anus and vagina, or communicating with the anal canal and vagina, as an anovaginal fistula.

anovaria (an″o-va′re-ah) anovarism.

anovarism (an-o′var-izm) [*an* neg. + *ovary*] absence of the ovaries.

anovesical (a″no-ves′ĭ-kal) [L. *anus* fundament + *vesica* bladder] pertaining to the anus and urinary bladder.

anovular (an-ov′u-lar) not accompanied with the discharge of an ovum.

anovulation (an″ov-u-la′shun) absence of ovulation.

anovulatory (an-ov′u-lah-to″re) anovular.

anovulia (an″ov-u′le-ah) (*obs.*) anovulation.

anovulomenorrhea (an-ov″u-lo-men″o-re′ah) anovular menstruation.

anoxemia (an″ok-se′me-ah) [*an* neg. + *oxygen* + Gr. *haima* blood + *-ia*] reduction of oxygen content of the blood below physiologic levels.

anoxemic (an″ok-se′mik) characterized by or due to a lack of the normal proportion of oxygen in the blood.

anoxia (ah-nok′se-ah) absence of oxygen supply to tissue despite adequate perfusion of the tissue by blood; the term is often used interchangeably with *hypoxia*, to indicate a reduced oxygen supply. **altitude a.,** high-altitude sickness. **anemic a.,** anoxia resulting from a decrease in amount of hemoglobin or number of erythrocytes in the blood. **anoxic a.,** anoxia resulting from interference with the source of oxygen. **fulminating a.,** a rapid fall in the oxygen content of the blood. **histotoxic a.,** anoxia resulting from disturbance in the tissues that impairs utilization of oxygen. **myocardial a.,** failure of coronary blood flow to keep up with myocardial needs. **a. neonato′-rum,** anoxia of the newborn. **stagnant a.,** anoxia resulting from inadequate blood flow through the capillaries with resultant abnormal oxygen extraction and low tissue oxygen tension.

anoxiate (ah-nok′se-āt) to put into a state of anoxia.

anoxic (ah-nok′sik) pertaining to or charcterized by anoxia.

anoxybiontic (an-ok″se-bi-on′tik) (*obs.*) anaerobic.

anoxybiosis (an-ok″se-bi-o′sis) [*an* neg. + *oxygen* + Gr. *bios* life] (*obs.*) anaerobiosis.

ANS 1. anterior nasal spine, a cephalometric landmark; the tip of the anterior nasal spine as seen on the x-ray film in norma lateralis. 2. autonomic nervous system.

ansa (an′sah), pl. *an′sae* [L. "handle"] a general term used in anatomical nomenclature to designate a looplike structure; called also *loop*. **a. cervica′lis** [NA], a nerve loop in the neck that supplies the infrahyoid muscles and that presents a superior root, which connects with the hypoglossal nerve (and actually consists of fibers of the second or first cervical nerve), and an inferior root (nervus descendens cervicalis), which connects with the second and third cervical nerves. Called also *a. hypoglossi*. **a. hypo-glos′si,** a. cervicalis. **a. lenticula′ris** [NA], a small fiber tract arising in the globus pallidus of the lenticular nucleus and extending around the medial border of the internal capsule to reach the anterior portion of the ventral thalamic nucleus. **an′sae nervo′rum spina′lium** [NA], loops of nerve fibers joining the ventral roots of the spinal nerves. **a. peduncula′ris** [NA], a complex grouping of fibers connecting the amygdaloid nucleus, the piriform area, and the anterior part of the hypothalamus, and various thalamic nuclei. The fiber bundles pass below the internal capsule, a principal bundle being the inferior peduncle of the thalamus. **a. subcla′via** [NA], nerve filaments that pass anterior and posterior to the subclavian artery to form a loop interconnecting the middle and inferior cervical ganglia; called also *a. of Vieussens* and *annulus of Vieussens*. **a. of Vieussens,** a. subclavia. **a. vitelli′na,** an embryonic vein from the yolk sac to the umbilical vein.

ansae (an′se) [L.] plural of *ansa*.

ansate (an′sāt) [L. *ansatus,* from *ansa* handle] having a handle; loop-shaped.

Ansbacher unit (ahns′bahk-er) [Stefan *Ansbacher,* German-American biologist, born 1905] see under *unit*.

anseriform (an′ser-ĭ-form″) of or belonging to the Anseriformes.

Anseriformes (an″ser-i-form′ēz) the order including ducks, geese, and swans.

anserine (an′ser-in) [L. *anserinus*] 1. pertaining to or like a goose. 2. a basic substance, beta-alanylmethylhistidine, first found in goose muscle, and subsequently in the muscle of many animals, not including man.

ansiform (an′sĭ-form) loop-shaped.

Ansolysen (an″so-li′sen) trademark for preparations of pentolinium tartrate.

Anspor (an′spōr) trademark for a preparation of cephradine.

Anstie's limit, reagent, rule (limit), test (an′stēz) [Francis Edmund *Anstie,* English physician, 1833–1874] see under *reagent, rule,* and *tests*.

ant. anterior.

ant- see *anti-*.

Antabuse (an′tah-būs″) trademark for a preparation of disulfiram.

antacid (ant-as′id) [*ant-* + L. *acidus* sour] 1. counteracting acidity. 2. a substance that counteracts or neutralizes acidity, usually of the stomach.

antagonism (an-tag′o-nizm″) [Gr. *antagōnisma* struggle] opposition or contrariety between similar things, as between muscles, medicines, or organisms; cf. *antibiosis*. **bacterial a.,** the antagonistic (inhibiting) effect of one bacterial organism on another by reason of its production of an antibiotic (antibiosis) or by its superior competitive ability to absorb nutrients. **induced bacterial a.,** the interaction between two bacteria, induced by close association, which results in antagonism between them. **metabolic a.,** interference with the metabolism or function of a given chemical compound by another bearing a close structural resemblance, the similarity in structure being the basis of the interference. For the various forms of such antagonism, see under

inhibition. **salt a.,** the antagonistic action of different salts in maintaining normal permeability of the plasma membrane.

antagonist (an-tag′o-nist) [Gr. *antagōnistēs* an opponent] 1. a muscle that acts in opposition to the action of another muscle, its agonist. 2. a substance that tends to nullify the action of another, as a drug that binds to a cell receptor without eliciting a biological response. 3. a tooth in one jaw that articulates with a tooth in the other jaw. **associated a's,** muscles that act on different parts, and by their combined actions move the parts in parallel directions. **competitive a.,** a substance that competes with a substrate or with an enzyme which ordinarily attacks the substrate, thus interfering with usual metabolic activity. The antagonist is usually a substrate analogue. See *antimetabolite*. **direct a's,** muscles that act on the same part, and by their combined actions keep the part at rest. **enzyme a.,** an antimetabolite that interferes with the normal action of an enzyme. See *enzyme inhibition,* under *inhibition*. **insulin a.,** any of a number of factors which block the action of insulin, including epinephrine, somatotropin, glucocorticoids, and glucagon (all of which counteract the metabolic effects of insulin), and the more direct-acting factors associated with plasma protein fractions. **metabolic a.,** an antimetabolite that interferes with the utilization of a substance essential in metabolism. **narcotic a.,** an agent that opposes the action of narcotics on the nervous system. **sulfonamide a.,** para-aminobenzoic acid.

antalgesic (ant-al-je′zik) antalgic.

antalgic (ant-al′jik) 1. counteracting or avoiding pain, as a posture or gait assumed so as to lessen pain. 2. analgesic.

antalkaline (ant-al′kah-līn″) [*ant-* + *alkali*] 1. neutralizing alkalinity. 2. an agent that neutralizes alkalis.

antaphrodisiac (ant″af-ro-diz′e-ak) 1. abrogating the sexual instinct. 2. an agent that allays sexual impulses; called also *anterotic*.

antapoplectic (ant″ap-o-plek′tik) [*ant-* + Gr. *apoplēxia* apoplexy] an agent for alleviating stroke.

antarthritic (ant″ar-thrit′ik) [*ant-* + Gr. *arthritikos* gouty] 1. alleviating arthritis. 2. an agent that alleviates arthritis.

antasthenic (ant″as-then′ik) [*ant-* + Gr. *astheneia* weakness] 1. alleviating weakness, or restoring strength. 2. an agent that alleviates weakness and restores strength.

antasthmatic (ant″az-mat′ik) [*ant-* + Gr. *asthma* asthma] 1. affording relief in asthma. 2. an agent that relieves the spasm of asthma.

antatrophic (ant″ah-trof′ik) correcting or opposing the progress of atrophy.

antazoline (an-taz′o-lēn) chemical name: 4,5-dihydro-*N*-phenyl-*N*-(phenylmethyl)-1*H*-imidazole-2-methanamine. An antihistaminic, $C_{17}H_{19}N_3$. Called also *imidamine*. **a. hydrochloride,** a white or almost white, crystalline powder, $C_{17}H_{20}ClN_3$, used to relieve allergic symptoms and to treat allergic manifestations; administered orally. **a. phosphate** [USP], a white to off-white crystalline powder, $C_{17}H_{19}N_3 \cdot H_2PO_4$, used in a 0.5 per cent solution, applied topically to the eyes in the treatment of allergic conjunctivitis.

ante- (an′te) [L. *ante* before] a prefix signifying "before" in time or place.

antebrachium (an″te-bra′ke-um) [*ante-* + L. *brachium* arm] [NA] the part of the upper member of the body, between the elbow and the wrist; called also *antibrachium* and *forearm*.

antecardium (an-te-kar′de-um) epigastrium.

antecedent (an″te-se′dent) [L. *antecedere* to go before, precede] a precursor. **plasma thromboplastin a. (PTA),** Factor XI; see *coagulation factors,* under *factor*.

ante cibum (an′te si′bum) [L.] before meals, usually abbreviated *a.c.* in prescriptions, etc.

antecornu (an″te-kor′nu) (*obs.*) cornu anterius ventriculi lateralis.

antecubital (an″te-ku′bĭ-tal) situated in front of the cubitus, or elbow.

antecurvature (an″te-kur′vah-chur″) [*ante-* + L. *curvatura* bend] a slight anteflexion.

antefebrile (an″te-feb′ril) [*ante-* + L. *febris* fever] before the onset of fever.

anteflect (an′te-flekt) to bend forward.

anteflexed (an′te-flekst) in a condition of anteflexion.

anteflexio (an″te-flek′se-o) [L.] anteflexion. **a. u′teri,** anteflexion, def. 2.

anteflexion (an-te-flek′shun) [*ante-* + L. *flexio* bend] 1. an abnormal forward curvature of an organ or part. 2. the normal forward curvature of the uterus (anteflexio uteri).

antegrade (an′te-grād) anterograde.

antelocation (an″te-lo-ka′shun) [*ante-* + L. *locatio* placement] the forward displacement of an organ.

antemetic (ant″e-met′ik) antiemetic.

ante mortem (an′te mor′tem) [L.] before death.

antenatal (an″te-na′tal) [*ante-* + L. *natus* born] occurring or formed before birth; prenatal. Cf. *antepartal*.

antenna (an-ten′ah), pl. *anten′nae*. a feeler of an arthropod; one of the two lateral appendages on the anterior segment of the head of arthropods.

Antepar (an′te-par) trademark for a preparation of piperazine citrate and piperazine phosphate.

antepartal (an″te-par′tal) occurring before parturition, or childbirth, with reference to the mother. Cf. *antenatal.*

ante partum (an′te par′tum) [L.] in obstetrics, before the onset of labor, with reference to the mother.

antepartum (an″te-par′tum) [L.] antepartal.

antephase (an′te-fāz) the portion of interphase immediately preceding mitosis (or meiosis) when energy is being produced and stored for mitosis (or meiosis) and chromosome reproduction is taking place.

antephialtic (ant″ef-e-al′tik) [*ant-* + Gr. *ephialtēs* nightmare] alleviating or preventing nightmare.

anteposition (an″te-po-zish′un) forward displacement, as of the uterus.

anteprostate (an″te-pros′tāt) [*ante-* + *prostate*] glandula bulbourethralis.

anteprostatitis (an″te-pros-tah-ti′tis) inflammation of glandula bulbourethralis.

antepyretic (an″te-pi-ret′ik) [*ante-* + *pyretic*] occurring before the stage of fever.

Antergan (ant′er-gan) trademark for a preparation of phenbenzamine.

antergia (ant-er′je-ah) [*ant-* + Gr. *ergon* work] antagonism; resistance.

antergic (ant-er′jik) working in opposite directions; a term applied to antagonistic muscles.

antergy (ant′er-je) antergia.

anteriad (an-te′re-ad) toward the anterior surface of the body.

anterior (an-ter′e-or) [L. "before"; neut. *anterius*] situated in front of or in the forward part of an organ, toward the head end of the body; [NA] a term used in reference to the ventral or belly surface of the body.

antero- [L. *anterior* before] a prefix signifying before.

anteroclusion (an″ter-o-kloo′zhun) mesioclusion.

anteroexternal (an″ter-o-eks-ter′nal) situated on the front and to the outer side.

anterograde (an′ter-o-grād″) [*antero-* + L. *gredi* to go] moving or extending forward; called also *antegrade.*

anteroinferior (an″ter-o-in-fer′e-or) situated in front and below.

anterointernal (an″ter-o-in-ter′nal) situated on the front and to the inner side.

anterolateral (an″ter-o-lat′er-al) situated in front and to one side.

anteromedian (an″ter-o-me′de-an) situated in front and toward the median plane.

anteroposterior (an″ter-o-pos-ter′e-or) from front to back of the body; in roentgenology it denotes such direction of the beam.

anteroseptal (an″ter-o-sep′tal) situated in front of the atrioventricular septum.

anterosuperior (an″ter-o-su-per′e-or) situated in front and above.

anterotic (ant″e-rot′ik) antaphrodisiac.

anteroventral (an″ter-o-ven′tral) situated in front and toward the ventral surface.

anteversion (an″te-ver′zhun) [*ante-* + L. *versio* a turning] the forward tipping or tilting of an organ; displacement in which the organ is tipped forward, but is not bent at an angle, as occurs in anteflexion.

antexed (an-tekst′) bent forward.

antexion (an-tek′shun) an abnormal forward bending, as of the spine.

anthelix (ant′he-liks) [*ant-* + Gr. *helix* coil] [NA] the prominent semicircular ridge seen on the lateral aspect of the auricle of the external ear, anteroinferior to the helix; called also *antihelix.*

anthelminthic (ant″hel-min′thik) anthelmintic.

anthelmintic (ant″hel-min′tik) [*ant-* + Gr. *helmins* worm] 1. destructive to worms. 2. an agent that is destructive to worms.

anthelmycin (an-thel-mi′sin) an antibiotic substance produced by *Streptomyces longissimus,* which has anthelmintic activity.

anthelone (ant-he′lōn) [*ant-* + Gr. *helkos* ulcer] a substance obtained from the small intestine (anthelone E; see *enterogastrone*) or from the urine (anthelone U; see *urogastrone*).

anthelotic (ant″he-lot′ik) [*ant-* + Gr. *hēlos* nail] 1. effective against corns. 2. a remedy for corns.

anthema (an′the-mah) (*obs.*) an exanthem; a skin eruption.

Anthemis (an′the-mis) [L.; Gr. *anthemis*] 1. a genus of composite-flowered plants. 2. the flower heads of *A. nobilis,* or common camomile, formerly used for coughs, in spasmodic conditions in infants, and as a stomachic tonic.

anthemorrhagic (ant″hem-o-raj′ik) [*ant-* + *hemorrhage*] antihemorrhagic.

anther (an′ther) [Gr. *anthēros* blooming] the portion of the stamen of flowering plants containing the microsporangia (pollen sacs) in which haploid microspores (pollen grains) are formed.

antheridium (an″ther-id′e-im), pl. *antherid′ia* [L. *anthera* medicine made from flowers + Gr. *idion* a diminutive ending] male organ of a cryptogamic plant in which microgametes are produced. Cf. *archegonium.*

antherozoid (an′ther-o-zoid″) the motile fertilizing cell of certain fungi.

antherpetic (ant″her-pet′ik) curing or preventing herpes.

anthiolimine (an-thi-o′li-mēn) antimony lithium thiomalate.

Anthiomaline (an″thi-o-mal′in) trademark for antimony lithium thiomalate.

anthocyanidin (an″tho-si-an′i-din) a pigment obtained by hydrolysis of anthocyanin.

anthocyanin (an″tho-si′ah-nin) [Gr. *anthos* flower + *kyanos* blue] any of a class of pigments of blue, red, and violet flowers; they are glycosides, yielding anthocyanidin and a sugar on hydrolysis.

anthocyaninemia (an″tho-si″ah-nin-e′me-ah) the presence of anthocyanin in the blood.

anthocyaninuria (an″tho-si″ah-nin-u′re-ah) the presence of anthocyanin in the urine.

Anthomyia (an″tho-mi′yah) a genus of small black houseflies. Two species of medical importance were formerly assigned to this genus. See *Fannia canicularis* and *F. scalaris.*

Anthomyiidae (an″tho-mi′i-de) [Gr. *anthos* flower + *myia* fly] in some systems of classification, a family of the order Diptera; the only genus of medical importance is *Fannia,* the larvae of which may cause both urinary and intestinal myiasis in man.

anthophobia (an″tho-fo′be-ah) [Gr. *anthos* flower + *phobein* to be affrighted by + *ia*] (*obs.*) a morbid dislike or dread of flowers.

anthorisma (an″tho-riz′mah) [*ant-* + Gr. *horisma* boundary] (*obs.*) a diffuse swelling.

Anthozoa (an″tho-zo′ah) [Gr. *anthos* flower + *zoia* animal] a class of coelenterates with large polyps and no medusa stage; it includes corals.

anthracene (an′thrah-sēn) 1. a colorless crystalline hydrocarbon, $C_6H_4(CH)_2C_6H_4$, from coal tar, used in the manufacture of anthracene dyes. 2. a ptomaine obtained from cultures of the anthrax bacillus, *Bacillus anthracis.*

anthracic (an-thras′ik) pertaining to or resembling anthrax.

anthracidal (an″thrah-si′dal) (*obs.*) destructive to *Bacillus anthracis.*

anthraco- [Gr. *anthrax* coal] a combining form denoting relationship to coal or to a carbuncle; also to carbon dioxide.

anthracoid (an′thrah-koid) [*anthraco-* + Gr. *eidos* form] resembling anthrax or a carbuncle.

anthracometer (an″thrah-kom′ĕ-ter) [*anthraco-* + Gr. *metron* measure] an instrument for measuring the carbon dioxide of the air.

anthracomucin (an″thrah-ko-mu′sin) a protective substance against anthrax existing in the tissues.

anthraconecrosis (an″thrah-ko-nĕ-kro′sis) [*anthraco-* + Gr. *nekrōsis* death] necrotic transformation of a tissue into a black dry mass.

anthracosilicosis (an″thrah-ko-sil″ĭ-ko′sis) [*anthraco-* + *silicon*] a mixed condition of anthracosis and silicosis.

anthracosis (an-thrah-ko′sis) [*anthraco-* + *-osis*] a usually asymptomatic form of pneumoconiosis caused by deposition of coal dust in the lungs; it is present in most urban dwellers. When the coal dust accumulates in large amounts, it may result in pneumoconiosis of coal workers. **a. lin′guae,** black tongue.

anthracotherapy (an″thrah-ko-ther′ah-pe) [Gr. *anthrax* coal + *therapy*] treatment with charcoal.

anthracotic (an″thrah-kot′ik) pertaining to or affected with anthracosis.

anthracycline (an″thrah-si′klēn) a class of fermentation products of the fungus *Streptomyces peucetius;* it includes doxorubicin and daunomycin, both used as antineoplastic agents.

Anthra-Derm (an′thrah-derm) trademark for a preparation of anthralin.

anthragallol (an″thrah-gal′ol) chemical name: 1,2,3-trihydrox-9,10-anthracenedione. A product of the interaction of gallic, benzoic, and sulfuric acids, $C_{14}H_8O_5$.

anthralin (an′thrah-lin) [USP] chemical name: 1,8,9-anthracenetriol. A synthetic compound, $C_{14}H_{10}O_3$, occurring as a yellowish brown, crystalline powder; applied topically to the skin in the treatment of dermatophytoses, chronic eczema, alopecia areata, and other skin diseases. Called also *dithranol.*

anthramucin (an″thrah-mu′sin) (*obs.*) anthrax capsule.

anthramycin (an″thrah-mi′sin) (*E*)-3-(5,10,11,11a-tetrahydro-9,11-dihydroxy-8-methyl-5-oxo-1*H*-pyrrolo[2,1-*c*] [1,4]benzodiazepin-2-yl)-2-propenamide. An antineoplastic antibiotic, $C_{16}H_{17}N_3$-O_4, produced by *Streptomyces refuineus* var. *thermotolerans.*

anthraquinone (an″thrah-kwin′ōn)   chemical name: 9,10-anthracenedione. A derivative of anthracene, $C_{14}H_8O_2$; its derivatives, which are found in aloes, cascara sagrada, senna, and rhubarb, have cathartic properties.

anthrarobin (an″thrah-ro′bin) [*anthracene* + *araroba*] chemical name: 1,2,10-anthracenetriol. A yellowish white powder from alizarin, C_6H_4:C(OH)·CH:C_6H_2(OH)$_2$; it is useful in psoriasis and various skin diseases in 10 to 20 per cent ointment, and as a parasiticide.

anthrax (an′thraks) [Gr. "coal", "carbuncle"] an infectious disease of ruminants resulting from the ingestion of spores of *Bacillus anthracis* in the soil, often leading to sudden death due to bacteremia (*malignant a.*). It is transmissible to man by direct inoculation from contaminated wool or other animal products, by ingestion of raw meat, or by inhalation of airborne spores from such products, and is characterized by a papule, often with one or more satellite lesions, that enlarges, ulcerates, and becomes crusted with an adherent, dense black eschar. The reddened or red (erythematous) underlying skin is elevated by subcutaneous edema. The lesion persists for two weeks or longer unless treated at its inception. Spread of the bacilli to regional lymph nodes may result in systemic disease marked by widespread edema and hemorrhage. Called also *charbon* and *splenic fever*. **acute a.,**

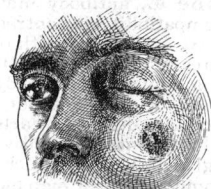

Anthrax: showing the malignant pustule (Homans).

a usually rapidly fatal form with high fever, death occurring in a day or two. **apoplectic a.,** fulminant anthrax, so called because the symptoms resemble those of cerebral apoplexy. **cerebral a.,** anthrax in which the bacilli invade the brain. **chronic a.,** a persistent form with local lesions confined to the tongue and throat. **cutaneous a.,** anthrax due to inoculation of *Bacillus anthracis* into superficial wounds or abrasions of the skin, producing a black crusted pustule surmounting a broad zone of edema. **industrial a.,** anthrax in man due to contact with wool, hair, hides, or other material from infected animals. **intestinal a.,** a severe form of anthrax in which the intestine is affected. **localized a.,** cutaneous anthrax. **malignant a.,** anthrax. **pulmonary a.,** anthrax of the lungs due to the inhalation of dust or animal hair containing anthrax spores; it is an occupational disease, usually affecting those who handle and sort wools and fleeces. Called also *a. pneumonia* and *woolsorter's disease* or *pneumonia*. **symptomatic a.,** blackleg.

anthropo- (an′thro-po) [Gr. *anthrōpos* man] a combining form denoting a relationship to man, or to a human being.

anthropobiology (an″thro-po-bi-ol′o-je) the biological study of man and the anthropoid apes.

anthropocentric (an″thro-po-sen′trik) [*anthropo-* + Gr. *kentrikos* of or from the center] with a human bias; considering man the center of the universe.

anthropocracy (an″thro-pok′rah-se) [*anthropo-* + Gr. *kratein* to rule] (*obs.*) the tendency in therapeutics to actively interfere in the course of disease; cf. *physiocracy*.

anthropogeny (an″thro-poj′ĕ-ne) [*anthropo-* + Gr. *gennan* to produce] the evolution and development of man.

anthropography (an″thro-pog′rah-fe) [*anthropo-* + Gr. *graphein* to write] that branch of anthropology which deals with the distribution of the varieties of man, as distinguished by physical character, institutions, customs, etc.; cf. *ethnography*.

anthropoid (an′thro-poid) [*anthropo-* + Gr. *eidos* form] resembling man. The anthropoid apes are the tailless apes, including the chimpanzee, gibbon, gorilla, and orang-utan.

Anthropoidea (an″thro-poi′de-ah) a suborder of Primates including the monkeys, apes, and man.

anthropokinetics (an″thro-po-ki-net′iks) [*anthropo-* + Gr. *kinētikos* for putting in motion] the study of the total human being in action, with integrated applications from the special fields of the biological and physical sciences, psychology, and sociology.

anthropology (an″thro-pol′o-je) [*anthropo-* + *-ology*] the science that treats of man, his origins, historical and cultural development, and races. **criminal a.,** that branch of anthropology which treats of criminals and crimes. **cultural a.,** that branch of anthropology which treats of man in relation to his fellows and to his environment. **physical a.,** that branch of anthropology which treats of the physical characteristics of man.

anthropometer (an″thro-pom′ĕ-ter) an instrument especially designed for measuring various dimensions of the body.

anthropometric (an″thro-po-met′rik) pertaining to or connected with anthropometry.

anthropometrist (an″thro-pom′ĕ-trist) a person skilled in anthropometry.

anthropometry (an″thro-pom′ĕ-tre) [*anthropo-* + Gr. *metron* measure] the science which deals with the measurement of the size, weight, and proportions of the human body.

anthropomorphism (an″thro-po-mor′fizm) [*anthropo-* + Gr. *morphē* form] the attribution of human form or character to nonhuman objects.

anthroponomy (an″thro-pon′o-me) [*anthropo-* + Gr. *nomos* law] the science that deals with the laws of human development in relation to environment and to other organisms.

anthropopathy (an″thro-pop′ah-the) [*anthropo-* + Gr. *pathos* suffering] the ascription of human emotions to nonhuman subjects.

anthropophagy (an″thro-pof′ah-je) [*anthropo-* + Gr. *phagein* to eat] 1. cannibalism. 2. a sexual perversion with cannibalistic tendencies.

anthropophilic (an″thro-po-fil′ik) [*anthropo-* + Gr. *philein* to love] preferring human beings to other animals; said of certain mosquitoes. Cf. *anthropozoophilic* and *zoophilic*.

anthropophobia (an″thro-po-fo′be-ah) [*anthropo-* + Gr. *phobein* to be affrighted by + *-ia*] (*obs.*) morbid dread of human society.

anthroposcopy (an″thro-pos′ko-pe) [*anthropo-* + Gr. *skopein* to examine] the judging of the type of body build by inspection rather than by anthropometry.

anthroposophy (an″thro-pos′o-fe) [*anthropo-* + Gr. *sophos* wise] knowledge of the nature of man.

anthropozoonosis (an″thro-po-zo″o-no′sis), pl. *anthropozoonoses* [*anthropo-* + *zoonosis*] a disease of either animals or man that may be transmitted from one species to the other.

anthropozoophilic (an″thro-po-zo″o-fil′ik) [*anthropo-* + Gr. *zōon* animal + *philein* to love] attracted to both human beings and animals; said of certain mosquitoes. Cf. *anthropophilic* and *zoophilic*.

anthypnotic (ant″hip-not′ik) (*obs.*) antihypnotic.

anthysteric (ant″his-ter′ik) antihysteric.

anti-, ant- (Gr. *anti* against) a prefix signifying counteracting, effective against, or opposing.

antiabortifacient (an″tĭ-ah-bor″tĭ-fa′shent) an agent that prevents abortion or promotes successful gestation.

antiabortus (an″tĭ-ah-bor′tus) (*obs.*) neutralizing or destructive to *Brucella abortus*.

antiadrenergic (an″tĭ-ah-dren-er′jik) 1. opposing the effects of impulses conveyed by adrenergic postganglionic fibers of the sympathetic nervous system. 2. an agent that so acts. Called also *sympatholytic*. Cf. *anticholinergic*.

antiagglutinating (an″tĭ-ah-gloo′tĭ-nāt″ing) preventing agglutination.

antiagglutinin (an″tĭ-ah-gloo′tĭ-nin) a substance that opposes the action of an agglutinin.

antiaggressin (an″tĭ-ah-gres′in) a substance once thought to be formed in the body by repeated injection of an aggressin, and tending to oppose the action of the aggressin.

antialbumin (an″tĭ-al-bu′min) a precipitin for albumin.

antialexic (an″tĭ-ah-lek′sik) opposing or counteracting an alexin.

antialexin (an″tĭ-ah-lek′sin) a substance which opposes the action of alexin.

antiamboceptor (an″tĭ-am′bo-sep″tor) a substance which opposes the action of an amboceptor. Called also *anti-immune body*.

antiamebic (an″tĭ-ah-me′bik) 1. destroying or suppressing the growth of amebas. 2. an agent that destroys or suppresses the growth of amebas.

antiamylase (an″tĭ-am′ĭ-lās) a substance counteracting the action of amylase.

antianaphylactin (an″tĭ-an-ah-fi-lak′tin) an antibody which counteracts an anaphylactin.

antianaphylaxis (an″tĭ-an-ah-fi-lak′sis) a condition in which the anaphylaxis reaction is not obtained because of the presence of free antibodies in the blood; the state of desensitization to antigens.

antiandrogen (an″tĭ-an′dro-jen) any substance capable of inhibiting the biological effects of androgenic hormones.

antianemic (an″tĭ-ah-ne′mik) 1. counteracting or preventing anemia. 2. an agent that counteracts or prevents anemia.

antianopheline (an″tĭ-ah-nof′ĕ-lin) directed against anopheline mosquitoes or their larvae.

antiantibody (an″tĭ-an′tĭ-bod″e) an immunoglobulin which is formed in the body following the administration of antibody acting as an immunogen, and which interacts with the latter.

antiantidote (an″tĭ-an′tĭ-dōt″) a substance that counteracts the action of an antidote.

antiantitoxin (an″tĭ-an′tĭ-tok′sin) an antibody, formed in immunization with an antitoxin, which counteracts the effect of the latter.

antianxiety (an″te-ang-zi′ĕ-te)   dispelling anxiety; relating to an anxiolytic.

antiapoplectic (an″tĭ-ap″o-plek′tik)   affording relief in or preventing stroke (apoplexy).

antiarachnolysin (an″tĭ-ar″ak-nol′ĭ-sin)   a substance counteracting spider toxin.

antiarin (an-te′ar-in)   a poisonous principle, $C_{14}H_{20}O_5 + 2H_2O$, from the upas tree, *Antiaris toxicaria;* formerly used as a heart depressant.

Antiaris (an″tĭ-a′ris) [Javanese *antiar*]   a genus of artocarpous trees. *A. toxicaria* (*Bohun upas*), the upas tree of Java, yields a latex used as an arrow poison. The major toxic principle is a digitalis-like cardioactive glycoside, α-antiarin.

antiarrhythmic (an″tĭ-ah-rith′mik)   1. preventing or alleviating cardiac arrhythmia. 2. an agent that prevents or alleviates cardiac arrhythmia.

antiarsenin (an″tĭ-ar′sĕ-nin)   a nonarsenical substance believed to be developed in the body by immunizing doses of arsenous acid.

antiarthritic (an″tĭ-ar-thrit′ik)   antarthritic.

antiasthmatic (an″tĭ-az-mat′ik)   antasthmatic.

antiatherogenic (an″tĭ-ath″er-o-jen′ik)   combating the formation of atheromatous lesions in arterial walls.

antiautolysin (an″tĭ-aw-tol′ĭ-sin)   a substance which opposes the action of autolysin.

antibacterial (an″tĭ-bak-te′re-al)   1. destroying or suppressing the growth or reproduction of bacteria. 2. a substance that destroys bacteria or suppresses their growth or reproduction.

antibechic (an″tĭ-bek′ik) [*anti-* + Gr. *bēchikos* suffering from cough]   1. relieving a cough. 2. an agent that relieves cough.

antibiosis (an″tĭ-bi-o′sis) [*anti-* + Gr. *bios* life]   an association between two organisms that is detrimental to one of them, or between one organism and an antibiotic produced by another.

antibiotic (an″tĭ-bi-ot′ik) [*anti-* + Gr. *bios* life]   1. destructive of life.   2. a chemical substance produced by a microorganism which has the capacity, in dilute solutions, to inhibit the growth of or to kill other microorganisms. Antibiotics that are sufficiently nontoxic to the host are used as chemotherapeutic agents in the treatment of infectious diseases of man, animals, and plants. **bactericidal a.,** one that kills bacteria. **bacteriostatic a.,** one that suppresses the growth or reproduction of bacteria. **broad-spectrum a.,** one that is effective against a wide range of bacteria. **macrolide a.,** an antibiotic characterized by a lactone ring, a ketone function, commonly an α-β unsaturated system, and a deoxyamino sugar containing a dimethylamino group. **oral a.,** one that is effective when administered orally. **polyene a.,** an antibiotic having the general structure (CH=CH)ₙ, and containing large lactone rings; active against a variety of fungi.

antibiotin (an″tĭ-bi′o-tin)   a compound that is antagonistic to biotin; avidin.

antiblastic (an″tĭ-blas′tik) [*anti-* + Gr. *blastos* germ]   retarding growth or multiplication, as of tumor or bacterial cells.

antiblennorrhagic (an″tĭ-blen-o-raj′ik)   1. preventing or relieving gonorrhea. 2. an agent that prevents or relieves gonorrhea.

antibody (an″tĭ-bod″e)   an immunoglobulin molecule that has a specific amino acid sequence by virtue of which it interacts only with the antigen that induced its synthesis in cells of the lymphoid series (especially plasma cells), or with antigen closely related to it. Antibodies are classified according to their mode of action as agglutinins, bacteriolysins, hemolysins, opsonins, precipitins, etc. See *immunoglobulin.* **allocytophilic a.,** see *cytotropic a.* **anaphylactic a.,** a substance formed as a result of the first injection of a foreign anaphylactogen and responsible for the anaphylactic symptoms following the second injection of the same anaphylactogen. Cf. *anaphylactin.* **anti-D a.,** an antibody active against Rh-D-antigen–positive erythrocytes. **antinuclear a's,** autoantibodies directed against components of the cell nucleus, e.g., DNA, RNA, histone, etc.; they may be detected by immunofluorescence and are present in systemic lupus erythematosus and sometimes in rheumatoid arthritis and in other collagen-vascular diseases with autoimmune manifestations. **autologous a.,** self-derived antibody; autoantibody. **blocking a.,** 1. an antibody which possesses the same specificity as one from another source and interferes with the reactivity of the other by combining with available epitopes of homologous specificity, thereby preventing undesirable sequelae of antigen-antibody reactions *in vivo.* 2. incomplete a. (def. 2). **cell-bound a., cell-fixed a.,** any antibody bound to the cell surface, such as saline inagglutinable antibody or cytotropic antibody. **complete a.,** Wiener's term for the Rh antibody that is capable of directly agglutinating Rh-positive erythrocytes in physiologic saline and implying that the antibody is mulitvalent, that is, possesses two or more reactive groups. The definition may be extended to include a number of other globulins with similar agglutinating, but not necessarily type-specific, features. **cross-reacting a.,** one that combines with an antigen other than the one that induced its production. **cytophilic a.,** cytotropic a. **cytotoxic a.,** any specific antibody directed against

cellular antigens, which when bound to the antigen, activates the complement pathway or activates killer cells, resulting in cell lysis. **cytotropic a.,** any of a class of antibodies that attach to tissue cells (such as mast cells and basophils) through their Fc segments to induce the release of histamine and other vasoconstrictive amines important in immediate hypersensitivity reactions. In man this antibody, also known as *reagin,* is primarily of the immunoglobulin class IgE. Called also *cytophilic a.* Cytotropic antibodies derived from the same species are called *homocytotropins,* or *homocytotropic* or *allocytophilic a's;* those from different species, *heterocytotropins,* or *heterocytotropic* or *xenocytophilic a's.* **despeciated a.,** an antibody that has been deprived of its species characteristics.   **Forssman a.,** an antibody produced by injecting rabbits with sheep erythrocytes, saline solutions containing guinea pig kidney, or other tissues that contain Forssman antigen.   **heterocytotropic a.,** see *cytotropic a.* **heterogenetic a.,** an antibody capable of reacting with antigens phylogenetically unrelated to the antigen that stimulated its production as well as with the homologous antigen.   **heterophile a.,** an accessory antibody produced by the injection of a heterogenetic or heterophilic antigen.   **homocytotropic a.,** see *cytotropic a.* **horse-type a.,** antibody from any species which, like that from the horse, forms highly soluble antigen-antibody complexes in both antibody excess and in antigen excess, so that precipitation occurs with sharp peaks.   **immune a.,** antibody induced by immunization or by transfusion incompatibility, in contrast to the natural antibodies.   **incomplete a.,** 1. antibody with only one antigen-binding site or with two sites so close together that the antibody behaves functionally as a univalent antibody. Such antibodies coat antigen-bearing cells or particles but do not agglutinate them. 2. a gamma globulin, described earlier as a univalent antibody combining specifically with Rh-positive erythrocytes without causing visible agglutination but which, in the presence of antihuman globulin (Coombs) serum or high molecular weight media, e.g., albumin, will cause red cell clumping. Other red cell coating proteins, not group specific, may demonstrate similar properties.   **inhibiting a.,** blocking a.   **isophil a.,** antibodies against red blood cell antigens produced in members of the species from which the red cells originated.   **lipoidotropic a.,** the substance in the blood serum of syphilitics which combines with the (lipoidal) antigen to produce a positive Wassermann test.   **maternal a's,** antibodies (e.g., of the IgG class) produced in the body of the mother and transferred to the fetal circulation.   **natural a's,** serum proteins present in low titer with the structural properties of immunoglobulins, which can react specifically with their antigens, even though the individuals in which they are formed have had no known previous exposure to those antigens. They may result from unknown exposure to naturally occurring antigens, e.g., food or bacterial flora.   **neutralizing a.,** antibody that, on mixture with the homologous toxin or infectious agent, detoxifies or reduces the infectious titer; components of the antigen-antibody complex can be dissociated and recovered in their original forms; reversibility of the association often decreases with time; the host cell influences effectiveness of interaction—e.g., a virus that is neutralized for one kind of host cell may be infectious for another.   **P-K a's,** Prausnitz-Küstner a's.   **Prausnitz-Küstner a's,** homocytotropic antibodies of the immunoglobulin class IgE that are responsible for cutaneous anaphylaxis. Abbreviated P-K a's. See *reagin.* **protective a.,** antibody responsible for immunity to an infectious agent observed in passive immunity.   **reaginic a.,** reagin.   **Rh a's,** those directed against Rh antigen(s) of human erythrocytes. Not normally present, but may be produced when Rh-negative persons receive Rh-positive blood by transfusion or when an Rh-negative person is pregnant with an Rh-positive fetus. **saline a.,** complete a.   **sensitizing a.,** a loosely used term, applied to antibodies that are attached to body cells and that "sensitize" the cells or render them susceptible to destruction by body defenses.   **Vi a.,** an antibody produced by immunizing rabbits with cultures of highly virulent typhoid bacilli; it will agglutinate the virulent strain which is resistant to ordinary O antibodies.   **warm a.,** antibody that reacts more strongly at temperatures of 37° C. or higher, than at lower temperatures. **xenocytophilic a.,** see *cytotropic a.* **7S a's,** antibodies with a sedimentation coefficient of 7S, including all those of immunoglobulin classes IgG and IgD and some of class IgA.

antibrachium (an″tĭ-bra′ke-um)   antebrachium.

antibromic (an″tĭ-bro′mik) [*anti-* + Gr. *brōmos* smell]   deodorant.

antibubonic (an″tĭ-bu-bon′ik)   effective against bubonic plague.

anticachectic (an″tĭ-kah-kek′tik)   1. preventing or relieving cachexia.   2. an agent that prevents or relieves cachexia.

anticalculous (an″tĭ-kal′ku-lus)   preventing or alleviating calculus.

anticarcinogen (an″tĭ-kar-sin′o-jen)   an agent that counteracts the effect of a carcinogen.

anticarcinogenic (an″tĭ-kar-sin″o-jen′ik)   inhibiting or preventing the development of carcinoma.

anticardium (an″tĭ-kar′de-um) [*anti-* + Gr. *kardia* heart]   antecardium (epigastrium).

anticariogenic (an″tĭ-kār″e-o-jen′ik) effective in suppressing caries production.

anticarious (an″tĭ-ka′re-us) anticariogenic.

anticatalyst (an″tĭ-kat′ah-list) a substance that retards the action of a catalyzer by acting on the catalyzer itself.

anticatalyzer (an″tĭ-kat′ah-līz″er) anticatalyst.

anticataphylactic (an″tĭ-kat″ah-fĭ-lak′tik) 1. pertaining to, characterized by, or causing anticataphylaxis. 2. an agent that inhibits cataphylaxis.

anticataphylaxis (an″tĭ-kat″ah-fĭ-lak′sis) inhibition of cataphylaxis.

anticathexis (an″tĭ-kah-thek′sis) [anti- + cathexis] expression of an emotional impulse as an emotion of opposite character; called also counterinvestment.

anticathode (an″tĭ-kath′ōd) the part of a vacuum tube opposite the cathode; the target.

anti-Cellano (an″tĭ-seh-lan′o) see Cellano.

anticephalalgic (an″tĭ-sef-ah-lal′jik) curing or preventing headache.

anticheirotonus (an″tĭ-ki-rot′o-nus) [Gr. anticheir thumb + tonos tension] spasmodic flexion of the thumb.

antichlorotic (an″tĭ-klo-rot′ik) effective against chlorosis.

anticholelithogenic (an″tĭ-ko″lĭ-lith″o-jen′ik) 1. serving to prevent the formation of gallstones. 2. an agent that so acts.

anticholerin (an″tĭ-kol′er-in) [anti- + cholera] a substance from cultures of the cholera vibrio, used against cholera.

anticholesteremic (an″tĭ-ko-les″ter-e′mik) 1. promoting a reduction of cholesterol levels in the blood. 2. any agent that promotes a reduction of blood cholesterol levels, e.g., the sitosterols and clofibrate. Called also anticholesterolemic.

anticholesterolemic (an″tĭ-ko-les″tĕ-ro-le′mik) anticholesteremic.

anticholinergic (an″tĭ-ko″lin-er′jik) [anti- + cholinergic] 1. blocking the passage of impulses through the parasympathetic nerves. 2. an agent that blocks the parasympathetic nerves. Called also parasympatholytic. Cf. antiadrenergic.

anticholinesterase (an″tĭ-ko-lin-es′ter-ās) [anti- + cholinesterase] a drug that prevents the hydrolysis of acetylcholine by the enzyme acetylcholinesterase, thereby permitting high levels of acetylcholine to accumulate at reactive sites.

antichymosin (an″tĭ-ki′mo-sin) an antibody that prevents the action of rennin on milk.

anticipate (an-tis′ĭ-pāt) [ante- + L. capere to take] to occur or recur before the regular time; said of a disease or of symptoms. See anticipation.

anticipation (an-tis″ĭ-pa′shun) the apparent occurrence of a hereditary disease at a progressively earlier age in successive generations; now considered by most authorities to be an artifact arising from the ease of identification of succeeding cases.

anticlinal (an″tĭ-kli′nal) [anti- + Gr. klinein to slope] sloping in opposite directions, as opposite sides of triangular structures.

anticnemion (an″tik-ne′me-on) [anti- + Gr. kēmē leg] the shin.

anticoagulant (an″tĭ-ko-ag′u-lant) 1. serving to prevent the coagulation of blood. 2. any substance that, in vivo or in vitro, suppresses, delays, or nullifies coagulation of the blood. **circulating a.,** a substance present in the blood which inhibits normal blood clotting and thus may cause a hemorrhagic syndrome; it may be directed against a specific coagulation factor and may accompany various hematologic and nonhematologic diseases.

anticoagulative (an″tĭ-ko-ag′u-la″tiv) preventing or opposing coagulation.

anticoagulin (an″tĭ-ko-ag′u-lin) a substance that suppresses, delays, or nullifies the coagulation of blood.

anticodon (an″tĭ-ko′don) a triplet of nucleotides in transfer RNA that is complementary to the codon in messenger RNA which specifies the amino acid.

anticollagenase (an″tĭ-ko-laj′ĭ-nās) an antienzyme that neutralizes the activity of collagenase.

anticomplement (an″tĭ-kom′ple-ment) a substance that opposes or counteracts the action of a complement.

anticomplementary (an″tĭ-kom″plĕ-men′ta-re) capable of reducing or destroying the power of a complement.

anticonceptive (an″tĭ-kon-sep′tiv) contraceptive.

anticoncipiens (an″tĭ-kon-sip′e-enz) a contraceptive agent.

anticonvulsant (an″tĭ-kon-vul′sant) 1. preventing or relieving convulsions. 2. an agent that prevents or relieves convulsions.

anticonvulsive (an″tĭ-kon-vul′siv) anticonvulsant.

anticrotin (an″tĭ-kro′tin) the antitoxin of crotin.

anticurare (an″tĭ-koo-rah′re) an agent that counteracts the action of curare on skeletal muscle.

anticus (an-ti′kus) [L.] anterior.

anticutin (an″tĭ-ku′tin) [anti- + cutaneous reaction] an antibody in the blood of certain tuberculous persons which, when added to tuberculin, neutralizes the latter so that it will not produce the cutaneous reaction.

anticytolysin (an″tĭ-si-tol′ĭ-sin) a substance opposing the action of cytolysin.

anticytotoxin (an″tĭ-si″to-tok′sin) a substance that opposes the action of a cytotoxin.

anti-D the antibody against the principal D-antigen of the Rh blood groups. IgG antibody formed by the mother against D-positive fetal red cells may lead to hemolytic disease of the newborn. Commercial preparation of anti-D, such as RhoGam, may be administered following parturition to prevent maternal alloimmunization against the D-antigen.

antidepressant (an″tĭ-de-pres′sant) 1. preventing or relieving depression. 2. an agent that stimulates the mood of a depressed patient. **tricyclic a's,** a group of antidepressant drugs that contain three fused rings in their chemical structure and that potentiate the action of catecholamines; they include imipramine, amitriptyline, nortriptyline, protriptyline, desipramine, and doxepin.

antidiabetic (an″tĭ-di″ah-bet′ik) 1. preventing or alleviating diabetes. 2. an agent that prevents or alleviates diabetes.

antidiabetogenic (an″tĭ-di-ah-be″to-jen′ik) 1. preventing the development of diabetes. 2. an agent that prevents the development of diabetes.

antidiarrheal (an″tĭ-di″ah-re′al) 1. counteracting diarrhea. 2. an agent that is effective in combating diarrhea.

antidiarrheic (an″tĭ-di″ah-re′ik) antidiarrheal.

antidiastase (an″tĭ-di′as-tās) a substance formed in the blood serum on the injection of a diastase, which opposes the action of the diastase.

antidinic (an″tĭ-din′ik) [anti- + Gr. dinos whirl] effective against vertigo.

antidipsetic (an″tĭ-dip-set′ik) pertaining to or causing the suppression of thirst.

antidipsia (an″tĭ-dip′se-ah) [anti- + Gr. dipsa thirst + -ia] (obs.) aversion to the ingestion of fluids; hydrophobia.

antidipticum (an″tĭ-dip′te-kum) an agent that lessens thirst.

antidiuresis (an″tĭ-di″u-re′sis) suppression of urinary secretion.

antidiuretic (an″tĭ-di″u-ret′ik) 1. suppressing the rate of urine formation. 2. an agent that suppresses urine formation.

antidiuretin (an″tĭ-di-u-re′tin) vasopressin.

antidotal (an″tĭ-do′tal) serving as an antidote.

antidote (an′tĭ-dōt) [L. antidotum, from Gr. anti against + didonai to give] a remedy for counteracting a poison. **a. against arsenic,** dimercaprol; hydrated oxide of iron with magnesia was once used. **Bibron's a.,** an antidote once used against snake bite: potassium iodide 0.24, mercury bichloride 0.12, bromine 20. **chemical a.,** an antidote that reacts chemically with a poison to form a harmless compound. **Fantus' a.,** an antidote once used for mercury poisoning, consisting of calcium sulfide solution; given by intravenous injection. **Hall a.,** a solution of 7.35 parts potassium iodide and 4 parts quinine hydrochloride in 480 parts water; once used as an antidote for mercuric chloride poisoning. **mechanical a.,** an antidote that prevents the absorption of a poison. **physiologic a.,** an antidote that counteracts the effects of a poison by producing opposing physiologic effects. **universal a.,** a mixture of 2 parts activated charcoal, 1 part magnesium oxide, and 1 part tannic acid, given as ½ ounce in a half glass of warm water, to be followed, except after ingestion of a corrosive substance, by gastric lavage or an emetic; considered by some to be useful in poisoning by acids, alkaloids, glycosides, and heavy metals.

antidotic (an″tĭ-dot′ik) antidotal.

antidromic (an″tĭ-drom′ik) [Gr. antidromein to run in a contrary direction] conducting impulses in a direction opposite to the normal; said of neurons in the posterior roots of the spinal cord. Evidence suggests, however, that this phenomenon results from ephaptic transmission rather than backward transmission. Cf. orthodromic.

antidysenteric (an″tĭ-dis″en-ter′ik) 1. preventing, alleviating, or curing dysentery. 2. an agent that prevents, alleviates, or cures dysentery.

antidysentericum (an″tĭ-dis″en-ter′e-kum) a preparation of myrobalan, pelletierin, extract of rose, extract of pomegranate, and gum arabic.

antieczematic (an″tĭ-ek-zĕ-mat′ik) 1. effective against eczema. 2. an agent that is effective against eczema.

antieczematous (an″tĭ-ek-zem′ah-tus) effective against eczema; antieczematic.

antiedematous (an″tĭ-e-dem′ah-tus) antiedemic.

antiedemic (an″tĭ-e-dem′ik) 1. preventing or alleviating edema. 2. an agent that prevents or alleviates edema.

antiemetic (an″tĭ-e-met′ik) [anti- + Gr. emetikos inclined to vomit] 1. preventing or alleviating nausea and vomiting. 2. an agent that prevents or alleviates nausea and vomiting.

antiemulsin (an″tĭ-e-mul′sin) an immune serum counteracting emulsin.

antiendotoxic (an″tĭ-en″do-tok′sik) counteracting the effect of endotoxins.

antiendotoxin (an″tĭ-en″do-tok′sin) an antibody that counteracts the effect of endotoxin.

antienzyme (an″tĭ-en′zīm) [*anti-* + *enzyme*] an agent that prevents or retards the action of an enzyme.

antiepileptic (an″tĭ-ep″ĕ-lep′tik) 1. combating epilepsy. 2. an agent that combats epilepsy.

antiepithelial (an″tĭ-ep″ĕ-the′le-al) destructive to epithelial cells.

antierotica (an″tĭ-e-rot′e-kah) drugs which have an anaphrodisiac effect.

antiesterase (an″tĭ-es′ter-ās) an agent that inhibits or counteracts the activity of ester-hydrolyzing enzymes.

antiestrogen (an″te-es-tro′jen) 1. blocking the action of estrogens. 2. an agent that so acts.

antiestrogenic (an″tĭ-es″tro-jen′ik) counteracting or suppressing estrogenic activity.

antifebrile (an″tĭ-feb′ril) antipyretic.

antifebrin (an″tĭ-feb′rin) acetanilid.

antifertilizin (an″tĭ-fer′tĭ-li″zin) a substance with which fertilizin reacts in agglutinating spermatozoa of certain marine invertebrates.

antifibrillatory (an″tĭ-fib′rĭ-lah-tor″e) 1. preventing or stopping fibrillation of the heart. 2. an agent that prevents or stops fibrillation of the heart.

antifibrinolysin (an″tĭ-fi″brĭ-nol′ĭ-sin) an inhibitor of fibrinolysin.

antifibrinolytic (an″tĭ-fi″brĭ-no-lit′ik) inhibiting fibrinolysis.

antifilarial (an″tĭ-fĭ-la′re-al) 1. effective against filaria. 2. an agent that is effective against filaria.

antiflatulent (an″tĭ-flat′u-lent) 1. relieving or preventing flatulence. 2. an agent that relieves or prevents flatulence.

antiflux (an′tĭ-fluks) a substance that prevents the attachment of solder.

Antiformin (an″tĭ-for′min) trademark for a preparation of alkaline sodium hypochlorite solution.

antifungal (an″tĭ-fung′gal) 1. destructive to fungi, or suppressing their reproduction or growth; effective against fungal infections. 2. an agent that is destructive to fungi, suppresses the growth or reproduction of fungi, or is effective against fungal infections.

antigalactic (an″tĭ-gah-lak′tik) [*anti-* + Gr. *gala* milk] 1. diminishing the secretion of milk. 2. an agent that tends to suppress milk secretion.

antigametocyte (an″tĭ-gah-me′to-sīt) effective against the gametocytes of malaria.

antigelatinase (an″tĭ-jeh-lat′ĭ-nās) a substance in the serum of animals infected with bacteria which prevents the digestion of gelatin.

antigen (an′tĭ-jen) [*antibody* + Gr. *gennan* to produce] any substance which is capable, under appropriate conditions, of inducing a specific immune response and of reacting with the products of that response, that is, with specific antibody or specifically sensitized T-lymphocytes, or both. Antigens may be soluble substances, such as toxins and foreign proteins, or particulate, such as bacteria and tissue cells; however, only the portion of the protein or polysaccharide molecule known as the antigenic determinant (q.v.) combines with antibody or a specific receptor on a lymphocyte. Abbreviated Ag. **acetone-insoluble a.,** an antigen for the Wassermann reaction consisting of the acetone-insoluble constituents of an alcoholic extract of beef heart. **allergic a.,** allergen. **allogeneic a.,** one occurring in some but not all individuals of the same species, e.g., histocompatibility antigens and human blood group antigens; isoantigen. **Au a., Australia a.,** hepatitis B surface a. **B a.,** an antigenic component of the K antigen complex. **beef heart a.,** an antigen for the Wassermann reaction made by extracting fresh normal beef heart tissue with absolute alcohol; the fresh normal hearts of guinea pigs, rabbits, and human beings are also used. **blood-group a's,** secreted soluble mucopolysaccharides possessing the H, A, and B haptenic structures that are characteristic of erythrocytes and some other tissues of the body; see specific *soluble blood group substances,* under *substance.* **capsular a.,** specific capsular substance. **carbohydrate a's,** numerous polysaccharides isolated from bacteria, other cells, and natural substances, which function as specific haptens or as complete antigens. **carcinoembryonic a.,** oncofetal antigen; a cancer-specific glycoprotein antigen of colon carcinoma, also present in many adenocarcinomas of endodermal origin and in normal gastrointestinal tissues of human embryos. **chick embryo a.,** see *Frei a.* **cholesterinized a.,** beef heart antigen to which has been added 0.4 per cent of cholesterol. **common a.,** an antigenic determinant group (epitope) that is present in two or more different antigen molecules and frequently leads to cross-reactions among them. **complete a.,** an antigen which

both stimulates the immune response and reacts with the products (e.g., antibody) of that response. **conjugated a.,** antigen produced by coupling a hapten to a protein carrier molecule through covalent bonds; when it induces immunization, the resultant immune response is directed against both the hapten and the carrier. **cross-reacting a.,** 1. one that combines with antibody produced in response to a different but related antigen, owing to similarity of antigenic determinants. 2. identical antigens in two bacterial strains, so that antibody produced against one strain will react with the other. **D a.,** a red cell antigen of the Rh blood group system, important in the development of isoimmunization in Rh-negative persons exposed to the blood of Rh-positive persons. **E a.,** a red cell antigen of the Rh blood group system. **e a.,** an antigen contained on the outer lipoprotein coat of the hepatitis B virus (Dane particle); also designated HB$_e$Ag. **envelope a's,** K a's. **F a.,** 1. a fast-migrating tumor-associated antigen first found in association with Hodgkin's disease and identified as a ferritin compound. 2. Forssman a. **febrile a's,** proprietary preparations consisting of suspensions of members of the typhoid-paratyphoid group for the performance of agglutination tests for enteric infections. **fetal a's,** antigens demonstrable during fetal life but not normally in adults; their reappearance in adults is attributed to reactivation of genes associated with cellular transformation to the malignant state. See also *fetoprotein.* **flagellar a.,** H antigen. **Forssman a.,** a heterogenetic antigen inducing the production of antisheep hemolysin, occurring in various unrelated animals, mainly in the organs but not in the erythrocytes (guinea pig, horse), but sometimes only in the erythrocytes (sheep), and occasionally in both (chicken). In the original and strict sense, the antigen is typified by that found in the guinea pig kidney and characterized by heat stability and solubility in alcohol; the antigenic determinant is polysaccharide in nature. Its antibody is absorbed by tissues containing the antigen, contains no lysin for bovine cells and little or no agglutinin for sheep cells. The term is also used loosely to refer to any antigen producing sheep hemolysin, but antibodies to it are not identical, as they are in the case of the true Forssman (or F) antigen. **Frei a.,** sterile pus from an unruptured bubo of suspected venereal lymphogranuloma for use in the intradermal Frei test. The virus of the disease is now propagated by inoculating it into the yolk sac of developing chick embryos (*yolk sac antigen, chick embryo antigen*), or by inoculating it into the brain tissue of mice (*mouse brain a.*). **Gm group a.,** one of more than twenty allotypic markers on human γ heavy chains usually located on the Fc or the Fd portion of the chain. **H a.** (Ger. *Hauch,* film), 1. the antigen of the flagella of motile bacteria; called also *flagellar a.* Cf. *O a.* 2. H substance. **heat-aggregated protein a.,** a protein antigen, which on modest heating, for example, to 63° C., undergoes partial denaturation, which lessens the solubility of the molecule and causes it to express new antigenic determinants. **hepatitis a., hepatitis-associated a. (HAA),** hepatitis B surface a. **hepatitis B core a. (HB$_c$Ag),** the antigen of the DNA-containing core of the Dane particle, produced in the nuclei of hepatocytes in viral hepatitis type B. **hepatitis B surface a. (HB$_s$Ag),** an antigen present in the serum of those infected with viral hepatitis type B, consisting of the outer lipoprotein coat (surface) of the Dane particle. Originally called *Australia (Au) antigen* because it was first found in an Australian aborigine, it is also known as *hepatitis-associated* a. (HAA) and *serum-hepatitis (SH)* a. **heterogeneic a.,** xenogeneic a. **heterogenetic a., heterologous a.,** an antigen common to more than one species whose species distribution is unrelated to its phylogenetic distribution (viz., Forssman's antigen, lens protein, certain caseins, etc.). Called also *heterophile a.* **heterophile a.,** heterogenetic a. **Hikojima a.,** one of the three serological types of cholera vibrio, the other two being the Inaba antigen and the Ogawa antigen. **histocompatibility a's,** genetically determined isoantigens present on the lipoprotein membranes of nucleated cells of most tissues, which incite an immune response when grafted onto a genetically disparate individual and thus determine the compatibility of tissues in transplantation. **Hitchens and Hansen's a.,** one from cultures of meningococcus that are grown on salt-free agar, suspended in water, precipitated with alcohol then with ether, dried, and rubbed up in a mortar with physiologic sodium chloride solution for use. **HLA a's** (*h*uman *l*eukocyte *a*ntigen) histocompatibility antigens (glycoproteins) on the surface of nucleated cells (including circulating and tissue cells) determined by a region on chromosome 6 bearing several genetic loci, each having multiple alleles and designated HLA-A, HLA-B, HLA-C, HLA-D, and HLA-DR, according to the locus at which the allele appears. Specific antigens are further designated by a numeral (e.g., HLA-B5), and provisionally identified antigens are labeled with the letter "w" (e.g., HLA-Bw22). They are important in cross-matching procedures, and are partially responsible for the rejection of transplanted tissues when donor and recipient HLA antigens do not match. A statistical association has been shown between certain HLA antigens and a number of diseases, e.g., HLA-B27 and ankylosing spondylitis. **homologous a.,** isoantigen. **H-Y a.,** a histocompatibility antigen of the cell membrane, dependent on the Y chromosome; it is the mediator of testicular organization (hence, sexual differentiation) in the male.

Ia a's, histocompatibility antigens governed by the I region of the major histocompatibility complex (MHC), located principally on B cells, although T cells, skin and certain macrophages may also contain Ia antigens. **Inaba a.,** one of the three serological types of cholera vibrio, the other two being the Hikojima antigen and the Ogawa antigen. **Inv group a.,** Km a. **isogeneic a.,** an antigen carried by an individual which is capable of eliciting an immune response in genetically different individuals of the same species, but not in an individual bearing it. **isophile a.,** allogeneic a. **K a's,** antigens that function as blocking antigens in that their presence interferes with agglutination with O antisera; called also *somatic surface a's* and *envelope a's.* **Km a.,** one of three alloantigens found in the constant region of the κ light chains in human immunoglobulins. Called also *Inv group a.* and *Inv allotype.* **Kveim a.,** an antigen prepared from human sarcoid tissue, usually lymph node or spleen; see under *tests.* **lens a's,** a series of proteins produced during development of the lens of the eye. **Ly a's,** antigenic cell-surface markers of subpopulations of T-lymphocytes, classified as Ly 1, 2, and 3; they are associated with helper and suppressor activities of T-lymphocytes. **lymphogranuloma venereum a.** [USP], a sterile suspension of inactivated *Chlamydia trachomatis* prepared by growing the organism in embryonic tissue of the domestic fowl (*Gallus domesticus*). It is used as a dermal reactivity indicator in the diagnosis of lymphogranuloma venereum. **M a.,** a type-specific antigen that appears to be located primarily in the cell wall and is associated with virulence of *Streptococcus pyogenes.* **Mitsuda a.,** lepromin. **mouse brain a.,** see *Frei a.* **mumps skin test a.,** [USP], a sterile suspension of formaldehyde-inactivated mumps virus–infected chick embryo, concentrated and purified by differential centrifugation, and diluted with isotonic sodium chloride solution so that each milliliter contains not less than 20 complement-fixing units; used as a dermal reactivity indicator. **Nègre a.,** an antigen prepared from dead, dried, and triturated tubercle bacilli by means of acetone and methyl alcohol; used in serum tests for tuberculosis. **NP a.,** a nucleoprotein antigen present in the pox group of viruses. **nuclear a's,** the components of cell nuclei with which antinuclear antibodies (see under *antibody*) react. **O a.** (Ger. *ohne Hauch,* without film), the antigen that occurs in the lipopolysaccharide layer of the wall of gram-negative bacteria; called also *somatic a.* Cf. *H a.* **Ogawa a.,** one of the three serological types of cholera vibrio, the other two being the Hikojima antigen and the Inaba antigen. **oncofetal a.,** carcinoembryonic a. **organ-specific a.,** any antigen that occurs exclusively in a particular organ and serves to distinguish it from other organs. Two types of organ specificity have been proposed: (1) first-order or tissue specificity is attributed to the presence of an antigen characteristic of a particular organ in a single species; (2) second-order organ specificity is attributed to an antigen characteristic of the same organ in many, even unrelated species. **partial a.,** hapten. **pollen a.,** the essential polypeptides of the pollen of plants extracted with a suitable menstruum; used in diagnosis, prophylaxis, and desensitization in hay fever. Called also *pollen allergen.* **private a's,** antigens of the low frequency blood groups, so called because they are found only in members of a single kindred, probably differing from ordinary blood group systems only in their incidence. **public a's,** antigens of the high frequency blood groups, so called because they are found in almost all persons tested. **R a.,** a type-specific antigen similar to M antigen except that it is resistant to tryptic digestion. **recall a.,** an antigen to which an individual has previously been sensitized and which is subsequently administered as a challenging dose to elicit a hypersensitivity reaction. **residue a's,** naturally occurring haptens split from the antigenic complex by autolysis or methods of preparation of purified antigen. **S a.,** a heat-stable, soluble viral antigen that is nucleoprotein in nature; it is found in influenza and mumps viruses. **Sachs's a.,** an antigen consisting of a cholesterinized alcoholic extract of beef heart. **self-a.,** self-antigen. **sequestered a's,** the cellular constituents of tissue (e.g., lens of the eye, thyroid, etc.) sequestered anatomically from the lymphoreticular system during embryonic development and thus thought not to be recognized as "self." Should such tissue be exposed to the lymphoreticular system during adult life, an autoimmune response would be elicited. **serum hepatitis a., SH a.,** hepatitis B surface a. **shock a.,** the specific antigen which is capable of eliciting the characteristic immunological reaction (e.g., anaphylaxis) in a sensitized animal. **somatic a.,** O a. **somatic surface a's,** K a's. **species-specific a's,** specific antigens that are restricted to a single species but occur in all members of that species. **Stein's a.,** an antigen for the serologic diagnosis of relapsing fever. **T a.,** a nonstructural, complement-fixing viral antigen synthesized in the early stage of the infectious cycle; it persists in cells that have been modified by oncogenic adenoviruses. **therapeutic a.,** any substance which, on injection into the body, stimulates the formation of protective antibodies. **Thy 1 a., theta (θ) a.,** a surface antigenic determinant of mice, present on thymus-dependent lymphocytes (T-lymphocytes) in the peripheral lymphoid tissues, in the central nervous system, and on the skin and fibroblasts in small amounts. It occurs in two allelic forms: Thy 1.1 and Thy 1.2. **TL a.,** a surface antigenic determinant on thymic lymphocytes of

mice. **tumor-specific a.,** cell-surface antigens of tumors that elicit a specific immune response in the host; abbreviated TSA. **tumor-specific transplantation a.,** any of the cell surface histocompatibility antigens of any given tumor, that evoke a specific immune response on transplantation to a syngeneic host; abbreviated TSTA. **V a., Vi a.,** an antigen contained in the capsule of a bacterium, as the typhoid bacillus, and thought to contribute to its virulence. **VDRL a.,** an alcohol solution containing 0.03 per cent cardiolipin, 0.99 per cent cholesterol, and enough lecithin to produce standard reactivity. **virulence a's,** V a. **W a.,** an antigen which appears to be invariably associated with virulence of the plague bacillus. **xenogeneic a.,** an antigen common to members of one species but not to members of other species; called also *heterogeneic a.* **yolk sac a.,** see *Frei a.*

antigenemia (an″tǐ-jě-ne″me-ah) [*antigen* + *-emia*] the presence of antigen (e.g., hepatitis B antigen) in the blood.

antigenemic (an″tǐ-jen-e′mik) exhibiting antigenemia.

antigenic (an-tǐ-jen′ik) having the properties of an antigen.

antigenicity (an″tǐ-jě-nis′ǐ-te) the capacity to react with the antibodies induced in an immune response.

antigenophil (an″tǐ-jen′o-fil) antigentophil.

antigenotherapy (an″tǐ-jen″o-ther′ah-pe) the treatment of disease by the injection of an antigen to stimulate antibody formation.

antigentophil (an″tǐ-jen′to-fil) [*antigen* + Gr. *philein* to love] having an affinity for the antigen, a property of the antigen-binding sites of immunoglobulin (antibody) molecules.

antigentotherapy (an″tǐ-jen″to-ther′ah-pe) antigenotherapy.

antiglobulin (an″tǐ-glob′u-lin) an antibody directed against gamma globulin, as used in the Coombs' test.

antiglyoxalase (an″tǐ-gli-ok″sah-lās) a pancreatic substance that inhibits the action of glyoxalase.

antigoitrogenic (an″tǐ-goi″tro-jen′ik) [*anti-* + *goiter* + Gr. *gennan* to produce] preventing or inhibiting the development of goiter.

antigonadotropic (an″tǐ-go″nad-o-tro′pik) inhibiting the gonadotropic hormones.

antigonorrheic (an″tǐ-gon″o-re′ik) effective against gonorrhea.

antigrowth (an″tǐ-grōth) counteracting the growth hormone.

antihallucinatory (an″tǐ-hah-lu″sǐ-nah-to″re) counteracting hallucinogenesis; suppressing hallucinations.

anti-HB_c antibody to hepatitis B core antigen (HB$_c$Ag).

anti-HB_s antibody to hepatitis B surface antigen (HB$_s$Ag).

antihelix (an″tǐ-he′liks) anthelix.

antihelmintic (an″tǐ-hel-min′tik) anthelmintic.

antihemagglutinin (an″tǐ-hem-ah-gloo″tǐ-nin) a substance whose action is antagonistic to hemagglutinin.

antihemolysin (an″tǐ-he-mol′ǐ-sin) any agent that opposes the action of a hemolysin.

antihemolytic (an″tǐ-he″mo-lit′ik) preventing hemolysis; hemosozic.

antihemophilic (an″tǐ-he″mo-fil′ik) see *coagulation Factor VIII,* under *factor.*

antihemorrhagic (an″tǐ-hem″o-raj′ik) 1. stopping hemorrhage. 2. an agent that prevents or stops hemorrhage.

antiheterolysin (an″tǐ-het″er-ol′ǐ-sin) a substance that counteracts heterolysin.

antihidrotic (an″tǐ-hi-drot′ik) anhidrotic.

antihistamine (an″tǐ-his′tah-mēn) a drug that counteracts the action of histamine. The antihistamines are of two types. The conventional ones, as those used in allergies, block the H$_1$ histamine receptors, whereas the others block the H$_2$ receptors. See *histamine.* Called also *antihistaminic.*

antihistaminic (an″tǐ-his-tah-min′ik) 1. counteracting the effect of histamine. 2. antihistamine.

antihormone (an″tǐ-hor′mōn) chalone.

antihyaluronidase (an″tǐ-hi-ah-lu-ron′ǐ-dās) an antienzyme that opposes the action of hyaluronidase.

antihydrophobic (an″tǐ-hi-dro-fo′bik) counteracting the development of hydrophobia (rabies).

antihypercholesterolemic (an″tǐ-hi″per-ko-les″ter-ol-e′mik) effective in decreasing or preventing an excessively high level of cholesterol in the blood. By extension, sometimes used to designate an agent that exerts such an effect.

antihyperglycemic (an″tǐ-hi″per-gli-se′mik) 1. counteracting high levels of glucose in the blood. 2. an agent that counteracts high levels of glucose in the blood.

antihyperlipoproteinemic (an″tǐ-hi″per-lip″o-pro″te-in-e′mik) 1. promoting a reduction of lipoprotein levels in the blood. 2. an agent that so acts.

antihypertensive (an″tǐ-hi″per-ten′siv) 1. counteracting high blood pressure. 2. an agent that reduces high blood pressure.

antihypnotic (an″tĭ-hip-not′ik) 1. preventing or hindering sleep. 2. an agent that prevents or hinders sleep.

antihypotensive (an″tĭ-hi″po-ten′siv) 1. counteracting low blood pressure. 2. an agent that so acts.

antihysteric (an″tĭ-his-ter′ik) 1. preventing or relieving hysteria. 2. an agent that counteracts hysteria.

anti-icteric (an″tĭ-ik-ter′ik) relieving icterus or jaundice.

anti-immune (an″tĭ-im-mūn′) acting so as to prevent immunity.

anti-infectious (an″tĭ-in-fek′shus) counteracting infection.

anti-infective (an″tĭ-in-fek′tiv) 1. counteracting infection. 2. an agent that counteracts infection.

anti-inflammatory (an″tĭ-in-flam′ah-to″re) 1. counteracting or suppressing inflammation. 2. an agent that counteracts or suppresses the inflammatory process.

anti-insulin (an″tĭ-in′su-lin) a substance that counteracts the action of insulin.

anti-invasin (an″tĭ-in-va′sin) an enzyme that antagonizes hyaluronidase. **a. I,** an enzyme present in normal blood plasma which antagonizes hyaluronidase. **a. II,** an enzyme present in normal blood plasma which antagonizes proinvasin I.

anti-isolysin (an″tĭ-i-sol′ĭ-sin) a substance that counteracts an isolysin.

antikataphylactic (an″tĭ-kat″ah-fi-lak′tik) interfering with kataphylaxis.

antikenotoxin (an″tĭ-ke″no-tok′sin) a substance that inhibits the action of kenotoxin.

antiketogen (an″tĭ-ke′to-jen) a substance that inhibits the formation of ketone bodies.

antiketogenesis (an″tĭ-ke″to-jen′ĕ-sis) inhibition of the formation of ketone bodies.

antiketogenetic (an″tĭ-ke″to-jĕ-net′ik) antiketogenic.

antiketogenic (an″tĭ-ke″to-jen′ik) preventing or inhibiting the formation of ketone bodies.

antiketoplastic (an″tĭ-ke″to-plas′tik) antiketogenic.

antikinase (an″tĭ-ki′nās) an antibody thought to inhibit the action of kinase.

antikinesis (an″tĭ-ki-ne′sis) [anti- + Gr. kinēsis movement] the tendency of organisms to resist and lean in an opposite direction to a dragging rotary force, e.g., on a slowly revolving plane (Dubois, 1898).

antilactase (an″tĭ-lak′tās) an antienzyme that counteracts lactase.

antilactoserum (an″tĭ-lak″to-se′rum) a substance that inhibits the action of lactoserum.

antileishmanial (an″tĭ-lesh-ma′ne-al) 1. effective against leishmania. 2. an agent that is effective against leishmania.

antilemic (an″tĭ-le′mik) [anti- + Gr. loimos plague] (obs.) effective against the plague.

antileprotic (an″tĭ-lep-rot′ik) 1. therapeutically effective against leprosy. 2. an agent that is therapeutically effective against leprosy.

antilethargic (an″tĭ-lĕ-thar′jik) 1. overcoming a tendency toward lethargy. 2. an agent that counteracts a tendency toward lethargy.

antileukocidin (an″tĭ-lu-ko′si-din) a substance that counteracts leukocidin; called also antileukotoxin.

antileukocytic (an″tĭ-lu″ko-sit′ik) destructive to white blood corpuscles (leukocytes).

antileukoprotease (an″tĭ-lu″ko-pro′te-ās) an antienzyme of the blood plasma that inhibits the digestion of protein by leukoprotease.

antileukotoxin (an″tĭ-lu″ko-tok′sin) antileukocidin.

antilewisite (an″tĭ-lu′ĭ-sīt) dimercaprol; also called British antilewisite, or BAL.

antilipase (an″tĭ-lip′ās) a substance that counteracts a lipase.

antilipemic (an″tĭ-li-pe′mik) 1. counteracting high levels of lipids in the blood. 2. an agent that counteracts high levels of lipids in the blood.

antilipoid (an″tĭ-lip′oid) an antibody having the power of reacting with a lipid.

antilipotropic (an″tĭ-lip″o-trop′ik) interfering with the mobilization of fat in the liver.

antilipotropism (an″tĭ-lip-ot′ro-pizm) interference with the mobilization of fat in the liver.

Antilirium (an″tĕ-lir′e-um) trademark for a preparation of physostigmine salicylate.

antilithic (an″tĭ-lith′ik) [anti- + Gr. lithos stone] 1. preventing the formation of stone or calculus. 2. an agent that prevents the formation of stone or calculus.

antiluetic (an″tĭ-lu-et′ik) antisyphilitic.

antilysin (an″tĭ-li′sin) [anti- + lysin] a substance that opposes the action of a lysin.

antilysis (an″tĭ-li′sis) the inhibition or suppression of lysis.

antilyssic (an″tĭ-lis′ik) [anti- + Gr. lyssa rabies] (obs.) antirabic.

antilytic (an″tĭ-lit′ik) pertaining to antilysis; inhibiting or suppressing lysis.

antimalarial (an″tĭ-mah-la′re-al) 1. therapeutically effective against malaria. 2. an agent that is therapeutically effective against malaria. Called also antipaludian.

antimaniacal (an″tĭ-mah-ni′ah-kal) 1. preventing or diminishing mania. 2. an agent that prevents or diminishes mania.

antimephitic (an″tĭ-mĕ-fit′ik) preventing or neutralizing mephitic substances.

antimere (an′tĭ-mēr) [anti- + Gr. meros a part] one of the opposite corresponding parts of an organism which are symmetrical with respect to the longitudinal axis of its body; cf. metamere.

antimeristem (an″tĭ-me-ris′tem) a preparation of a fungus, Mucor racemus (var. malignus), isolated from malignant tumors of animals; a supposed antitoxin used against the microorganisms that caused the tumors.

antimesenteric (an″tĭ-mes′en-ter″ik) designating that part of the intestine which is opposite to the site of attachment of the mesentery.

antimetabolite (an″tĭ-mĕ-tab′o-līt) a substance bearing a close structural resemblance to one required for normal physiological functioning, and exerting its effect by interfering with the utilization of the essential metabolite. For various ways in which antimetabolites inhibit metabolic processes, see under inhibition.

antimethemoglobinemic (an″tĭ-met″he-mo-glo″bĭ-ne′mik) 1. promoting reduction of methemoglobin levels in the blood. 2. an agent that so acts.

antimetropia (an″tĭ-mĕ-tro′pe-ah) [anti- + Gr. metron measure + ōps eye + -ia] hyperopia in one eye with myopia in the other; heterometropia.

antimiasmatic (an″tĭ-mi″az-mat′ik) [anti- + Gr. miasma pollution] effective against noxious emanations or exhalations.

antimicrobial (an″tĭ-mi-kro′be-al) 1. killing microorganisms, or suppressing their multiplication or growth. 2. an agent that kills microorganisms or suppresses their multiplication or growth.

antimicrobic (an″tĭ-mi-kro′bik) (obs.) antimicrobial.

antimineralocorticoid (an″tĭ-min″er-al-o-kor′tĭ-koid) a substance that suppresses the action of mineralocorticoids.

Antiminth (an′tĭ-minth) trademark for a preparation of pyrantel pamoate.

antimitotic (an″tĭ-mi-tot′ik) inhibiting or preventing mitosis.

antimongoloid (an″tĭ-mon′go-loid) denoting a feature opposite to one characteristic of mongolism, as antimongoloid slant of the palpebral fissures.

antimongolism (an″te-mon′go-lizm) a term applied to clinical signs opposite to those of Down's syndrome (mongolism), as the syndromes associated with group G (21 and 22) chromosome deletions or chromosome 21 monosomy, characterized by antimongoloid obliquity of the palpebral fissures, hypertonia, high-arched palate, micrognathia, and microcephaly, and by mental and growth retardation.

antimonial (an″tĭ-mo′ne-al) pertaining to or containing antimony.

antimonic (an″tĭ-mon′ik) containing antimony in its pentad valency.

antimonid (an″tĭ-mo′nīd) any binary compound of antimony.

antimonious (an″tĭ-mo′ne-us) containing antimony in its triad valency.

antimonium (an″tĭ-mo′ne-um), gen. antimo′nii [L.] antimony.

antimony (an′tĭ-mo″ne) [L. antimonium or stibium] a crystalline metallic element with a bluish luster, symbol Sb, atomic number 51, atomic weight 121.75, forming various medicinal and poisonous salts. **a. chloride,** a. trichloride. **a. dimercaptosuccinate,** stibocaptate. **a. lithium thiomalate,** a compound, $Li_6C_{12}H_9O_{12}SbS_3 \cdot 9H_2O$, which has been used for the same purposes as antimony potassium tartrate, especially in the treatment of schistosomiasis; administered intramuscularly. Called also anthiolimine. **a. pentoxide,** a white or yellowish powder, Sb_2O_5, used in preparation of antimony compounds; called also antimonic acid. **a. potassium tartrate** [USP], a trivalent antimony compound, $C_8H_4K_2Sb_2O_{12} \cdot 3H_2O$, used as an antischistosomal, especially in Schistosoma japonicum infections; administered intravenously. It has been used in various tropical infections, such as leishmaniasis, trypanosomiasis, and granuloma inguinale, and rarely as a nauseant expectorant. Called also tartar emetic and potassium antimonyltartrate. **a. sodium dimercaptosuccinate,** stibocaptate. **a. sodium gluconate,** 1. a pentavalent antimony compound, $C_6H_9Na_2O_9Sb$, used as an antileishmanial, administered intravenously and intramuscularly. 2. a trivalent antimony compound, $C_6H_8NaO_7Sb$, used as an antischistosomal, administered intravenously. Called also sodium stibogluconate, stibogluconate sodium, and sodium antimony gluconate. **a. sodium tartrate,** a trivalent antimony compound, $C_4H_4NaO_7Sb$, having the same actions and uses as the potassium tartrate but more water-soluble and less irritant when injected. Called also Plimmer's a. and sodium antimonyltartrate. **a. so-**

dium thioglycollate, a trivalent antimony compound, C_4H_4-NaO_4S_2Sb, which has been used as an antileishmanial and antischistosomal. Called also *sodium antimonylthioglycollate.*
tartrated a., a. potassium tartrate. **a. thioglycollamide,** an organic antimony compound, $Sb(S·CH_2·CO·NH_2)_3$, the triamide of antimony thioglycollic acid; used in the treatment of granuloma inguinale, kala-azar, and filariasis. **a. trichloride,** very deliquescent, colorless, transparent crystals or crystalline mass, $SbCl_3$, highly soluble in water. **a. trioxide,** a white odorless crystalline powder, Sb_2O_3, used in the preparation of tartar emetic (antimony potassium tartrate).

antimonyl (an-tim′o-nil″) the univalent radical SbO—.

antimorph (an′tĭ-morf) a mutant gene that acts to antagonize or inhibit the influence of its allele.

antimorphic (an″tĭ-mor′fik) in genetics, antagonizing or inhibiting normal activity; of or pertaining to an antimorph.

antimuscarinic (an″tĭ-mus′kah-rin′ik) effective against the poisonous activity of muscarine.

antimutagen (an″tĭ-mu′tah-jen) a substance that antagonizes the mutagenic effects of other substances.

antimyasthenic (an″tĭ-mi″as-then′ik) 1. counteracting or relieving muscular weakness in myasthenia gravis. 2. an agent that counteracts or relieves muscular weakness in myasthenia gravis.

antimycobacterial (an″tĭ-mi″ko-bak-te′re-al) active against mycobacteria.

antimycotic (an″tĭ-mi-kot′ik) suppressing the growth of fungi.

antinarcotic (an″tĭ-nar-kot′ik) counteracting narcotic depression.

antinatriuresis (an″tĭ-nā″tre-u-re′sis) inhibition of the excretion of sodium in the urine.

antinauseant (an″tĭ-naw′ze-ant) 1. preventing or relieving nausea. 2. an agent that prevents or relieves nausea.

antineoplastic (an″tĭ-ne″o-plas′tik) 1. inhibiting or preventing the development of neoplasms; checking the maturation and proliferation of malignant cells. 2. an agent having such properties.

antineoplaston (an″te-ne″o-plas′ton) any of a number of peptides isolated from human urine that inhibit cell division in certain cancer cells but not in normal cells.

antinephritic (an″tĭ-nĕ-frit′ik) counteracting inflammation of the kidneys.

antineuralgic (an″tĭ-nu-ral′jik) counteracting neuralgia.

antineuritic (an″tĭ-nu-rit′ik) counteracting neuritis.

antineurotoxin (an″tĭ-nu″ro-tok′sin) a substance that counteracts a neurotoxin.

antineutrino (an″tĭ-nu-tre′no) the antiparticle of the neutrino.

antineutron (an″tĭ-nu′tron) an elementary particle without a charge and with a mass and spin equal to that of a neutron, but with magnetic moment opposite to that of a neutron; the antiparticle of a neutron.

antiniad (an-tin′e-ad) toward the antinion.

antinial (an-tin′e-al) pertaining to the antinion.

antinion (an-tin′e-on) [*anti-* + Gr. *inion* occiput] the frontal pole of the head; the median frontal point farthest from the inion.

antinuclear (an″tĭ-nu′kle-ar) destructive to or reactive with components of the cell nucleus, as antinuclear antibody.

antiodontalgic (an″tĭ-o″don-tal′jik) relieving toothache.

antioncotic (an″t-ong-kot′ik) [*anti-* + Gr. *onkos* bulk, mass] 1. tending to reduce swelling and effective against tumors. 2. an agent that reduces swelling or suppresses growth of tumors.

antiophidica (an″tĭ-o-fid′i-kah) [*anti-* + Gr. *ophis* snake] remedies that combat the effects of snake bite.

antiophthalmic (an″tĭ-of-thal′mik) counteracting ophthalmia.

antiopsonin (an″te-op′so-nin) a substance that has an inhibitory influence on opsonins; antitropin.

antiovulatory (an″tĭ-ov′u-lah-to″re) suppressing ovulation.

antioxidant (an″tĭ-ok′sĭ-dant) one of many widely used synthetic or natural substances added to a product to prevent or delay its deterioration by action of oxygen in the air. Rubber, paints, vegetable oils, and prepared foods commonly contain antioxidants.

antioxidase (an″tĭ-ok′sĭ-dās) a substance that impairs oxidase activity.

antioxidation (an″tĭ-ok-sĭ-da′shun) the prevention of oxidation.

antioxygen (an″tĭ-ok′sĭ-jen) antioxidant.

antipaludian (an″tĭ-pah-lu′de-an) antimalarial.

antiparalytic (an″tĭ-par″ah-lit′ik) [*anti-* + *paralysis*] relieving paralysis.

antiparasitic (an″tĭ-par″ah-sit′ik) 1. destructive to parasites. 2. an agent destructive to parasites.

antiparastata (an″tĭ-pah-ras′tah-tah) [*anti-* + Gr. *parastatēs* testis] bulbourethral gland (glandula bulbourethralis [NA]).

antiparastatitis (an″tĭ-par″ah-stah-ti′tis) inflammation of the glandula bulbourethralis.

antiparasympathomimetic (an″tĭ-par″ah-sim″pah-tho-mĭ-met′ik) producing effects that resemble those of interruption of the parasympathetic nerve supply.

antiparkinsonian (an″tĭ-par″kin-so′ne-an) 1. effective in the treatment of parkinsonism. 2. an agent effective in the treatment of parkinsonism.

antiparticle (an′tĭ-par″tĭ-k′l) either of two particles, one of matter and one of antimatter, that annihilate each other upon collison, as an electron and a positron.

antipathic (an″tĭ-path′ik) [*anti-* + Gr. *pathos* feeling] of diverse nature; antagonistic; marked by antipathy.

antipathogen (an″tĭ-path′o-jen) any substance that acts against a pathogen.

antipathy (an-tip′ah-the) [*anti-* + Gr. *pathos* feeling] an opposing quality or property; a feeling or attitude of strong aversion.

antipedicular (an″tĭ-pĕ-dik′u-lar) effective against *Pediculus* (sucking lice), or in the treatment of pediculosis; antipediculotic.

antipediculotic (an″tĭ-pĕ-dik″u-lot′ik) 1. effective against lice. 2. an agent effective against lice.

antipepsin (an″tĭ-pep′sin) an antienzyme that inhibits the action of pepsin.

antiperiodic (an″tĭ-pe″re-od′ik) preventing periodic recurrence of symptoms, as in malaria.

antiperistalsis (an″tĭ-per″ĭ-stal′sis) reversed peristalsis.

antiperistaltic (an″tĭ-per″ĭ-stal′tik) 1. pertaining to or causing antiperistalsis. 2. diminishing peristaltic action. 3. an agent that diminishes peristaltic action.

antiperspirant (an″tĭ-per′spĭ-rant″) 1. inhibiting or preventing perspiration. 2. an agent that inhibits or prevents perspiration.

antiphagin (an″tĭ-fa′jin) a hypothetical substance once thought to be the specific component of virulent bacteria which renders them resistant to phagocytosis.

antiphagocytic (an″tĭ-fag-o-sit′ik) counteracting or opposing phagocytosis.

antiphlogistic (an″tĭ-flo-jis′tik) 1. counteracting inflammation and fever. 2. an agent that counteracts inflammation and fever.

antiphrynolysin (an″tĭ-frĭ-nol′ĭ-sin) the antivenin for the toxin of toad venom.

antiphthiriac (an″tĭ-ther′e-ak) effective against lice.

antiphthisic (an″tĭ-tiz′ik) checking or relieving pulmonary tuberculosis (phthisis).

antiplasmin (an″tĭ-plaz′min) a substance in the blood that inhibits plasmin.

antiplasmodial (an″tĭ-plaz-mo′de-al) having a destructive action on plasmodia.

antiplastic (an″tĭ-plas′tik) [*anti-* + Gr. *plassein* to form] 1. unfavorable to the healing process. 2. an agent that suppresses formation of the blood or other cells.

antiplatelet (an″tĭ-plāt′let) directed against or destructive to blood platelets.

antipneumococcic (an″tĭ-nu″mo-kok′sik) destroying pneumococci.

antipodagric (an″tĭ-po-dag′rik) effective against gout.

antipodal (an″tip′ŏ-dal) occupying opposite positions; diametrically opposed; pertaining to an antipode.

antipode (an′tĭ-pōd) something occupying a directly opposed position. In chemistry, a molecule whose atoms are arranged in a directly opposite manner.

antipolycythemic (an″tĭ-pol″e-si-the′mik) 1. effective against polycythemia. 2. an agent effective against polycythemia.

antiport (an′tĭ-port) a mechanism of coupling the transport of two compounds across a membrane in opposite directions.

antiposia (an″tĭ-po′se-ah) antipathy to drinking.

antiprecipitin (an″tĭ-pre-sip′ĭ-tin) a substance antagonistic in its action to precipitin.

antiprostate (an″tĭ-pros′tāt) the bulbourethral gland (glandula bulbourethralis [NA]).

antiprostatitis (an″tĭ-pros″tah-ti′tis) inflammation of the glandula bulbourethralis.

antiprotease (an″tĭ-pro′te-ās) a substance that checks the proteolytic action of enzymes, as antitryptase.

antiprothrombin (an″tĭ-pro-throm′bin) directed against prothrombin; a general term indicating a type of anticoagulant that acts by retarding the conversion of prothrombin to thrombin, without actually designating the specific means by which this occurs.

antiprotozoal (an″tĭ-pro-to-zo′al) 1. destroying protozoa, or checking their growth or reproduction. 2. an agent that destroys protozoa, or checks their growth or reproduction.

antiprotozoan (an″tĭ-pro″to-zo′an) antiprotozoal.

antipruritic (an″tĭ-proo-rit′ik) 1. relieving or preventing itching. 2. an agent, usually a topical application, that relieves or prevents itching.

antipsoriatic (an″tĭ-so″re-at′ik) 1. effective against psoriasis. 2. an agent effective against psoriasis.

antipsychomotor (an″tĭ-si′ko-mo′tor) suppressing or inhibiting the motor effects of cerebral or psychic activity.

antipsychotic (an″tĭ-si-kot′ik) neuroleptic.

antiputrefactive (an″tĭ-pu″tre-fak′tiv) counteracting putrefaction.

antipyogenic (an″tĭ-pi″o-jen′ik) [anti- + Gr. pyon pus + gennan to produce] preventing or hindering the development of pus.

antipyresis (an″tĭ-pi-re′sis) [anti- + Gr. pyressein to have a fever] the therapeutic use of antipyretics.

antipyretic (an″tĭ-pi-ret′ik) [anti- + Gr. pyretos fever] 1. relieving or reducing fever. 2. an agent that relieves or reduces fever. Called also antifebrile, antithermic, and febrifuge.

antipyrine (an″tĭ-pi′rin) [anti- + Gr. pyr fire] [USP] chemical name: 1,2-dihydro-1,5-dimethyl-2-phenyl-3H-pyrazol-3-one. A pyrazole derivative, $C_{11}H_{12}N_2O$, occuring as colorless crystals or white, crystalline powder. An effective analgesic, it is seldom used because of an association with cases of fatal agranulocytoses. A solution of antipyrine and benzocaine in dehydrated glycerine is used in the treatment of acute otitis media. It was formerly used as an antipyretic and anti-inflammatory. Called also phenazone and phenyldimethylpyrazolon. **a. camphorate,** an antipyretic compound formerly used in night sweats. **a. mandelate,** a salt, $C_{19}H_{20}N_2O_4$, prepared by fusing antipyrine and mandelic acid.

antipyrotic (an″tĭ-pi-rot′ik) [anti- + Gr. pyrōsis a burning] 1. therapeutically effective against burns. 2. an agent that is effective in the treatment of burns.

antirabic (an″tĭ-ra′bik) directed against or effective in preventing the development of rabies; antilyssic.

antirachitic (an″tĭ-rah-kit′ik) therapeutically effective against rickets.

antiradiation (an″tĭ-ra″de-a′shun) capable of counteracting the effects of radiation; effective against radiation injury.

antirennin (an″tĭ-ren′in) an antienzyme formed in the blood serum of animals injected with rennin; it counteracts the rennitic coagulation of milk.

antirheumatic (an″tĭ-ru-mat′ik) [anti- + rheumatic] 1. relieving or preventing rheumatism. 2. an agent that relieves or prevents rheumatism.

antiricin (an″tĭ-ri′sin) a substance that opposes the action of ricin (e.g., antitoxin produced following the introduction of ricin into the animal body).

antirickettsial (an″tĭ-rĭ-ket′se-al) 1. effective against rickettsiae. 2. an agent that is effective against rickettsiae.

antirobin (an″tĭ-ro′bin) the antitoxin of robin, a poison of the locust tree.

antisaluresis (an″tĭ-sal″u-re′sis) antinatriuresis.

antiscabietic (an″tĭ-ska″be-et′ik) 1. effective against scabies. 2. an agent effective against scabies.

antiscabious (an″tĭ-ska′be-us) [anti- + L. scabies itch] antiscabietic.

antiscarlatinal (an″tĭ-skar-lah-ti′nal) effective against scarlatina.

antischistosomal (an″tĭ-shis″to-so′mal) 1. effective against schistosomes. 2. an agent that is destructive to schistosomes.

antiscorbutic (an″tĭ-skor-bu′tik) [anti- + scorbutus] effective in the prevention or relief of scurvy.

antiseborrheic (an″tĭ-seb″o-re′ik) 1. effective against seborrhea. 2. an agent effective against seborrhea.

antisecretory (an″tĭ-se-kre′to-re) 1. inhibiting or diminishing secretion; secretoinhibitory. 2. an agent that so acts, as certain drugs that inhibit or diminish gastric secretions.

antisensibilisin (an″tĭ-sen-sĭ-bil′ĭ-zin) antianaphylactin.

antisensitizer (an″tĭ-sen′sĭ-tīz″er) a substance that opposes the action of a sensitizer (e.g., antiantibody or antiamboceptor).

antisepsis (an″tĭ-sep′sis) [anti- + Gr. sēpsis putrefaction] the prevention of sepsis by the inhibition or destruction of the causative organism. **physiologic a.,** the combination of methods by which the body excludes germs; called also autoantisepsis.

antiseptic (an″tĭ-sep′tik) 1. preventing decay or putrefaction. 2. a substance that will inhibit the growth and development of microorganisms without necessarily destroying them. Cf. disinfectant. **Credé's a.,** silver citrate. **Dakin's a.,** see diluted sodium hypochlorite solution, under solution. **Lister's a.,** mercury-zinc cyanide.

antisepticism (an″tĭ-sep′tĭ-sizm) the systematic employment of antiseptic agents.

antisepticize (an″tĭ-sep′tĭ-sīz) to render antiseptic.

antiserum (an″tĭ-se′rum) a serum that contains antibody or antibodies; it may be obtained from an animal that has been immunized either by injection of antigen into the body or by infection with microorganisms containing the antigen. **Reenstierna a.,** a serum once used in the treatment of leprosy, prepared by inoculating sheep with glycerin bouillon cultures of an organism then thought to be the mycobacterium of leprosy. **Rh a.,** serum that contains antibodies against antigenic determinants shared by some humans and all Rhesus monkeys.

antisialagogue (an″tĭ-si-al′ah-gog) 1. counteracting the formation of saliva. 2. an agent that counteracts any influence that promotes the flow of saliva.

antisialic (an″tĭ-si-al′ik) [anti- + Gr. sialon saliva] 1. checking the flow of saliva. 2. an agent that checks the secretion of saliva.

antisideric (an″tĭ-sĭ-der′ik) [anti- + Gr. sidēros iron] incompatible with iron.

antisocial (an″tĭ-so′shal) denoting a personality disorder marked by a basic lack of socialization and repeated conflict with society. Called also psychopathic and sociopathic. See antisocial personality, under personality.

antisocialism (an″tĭ-so′shal-izm″) the manifestation of antisocial personality.

antispasmodic (an″tĭ-spaz-mod′ik) 1. relieving spasm, usually of smooth muscle, as in arteries, bronchi, intestine, bile duct, ureters or sphincters, but also of voluntary muscle. Cf. antispastic. 2. an agent that relieves spasm. **biliary a.,** an agent that relieves spasm of the biliary duct and sphincter. **bronchial a.,** an agent that relieves bronchial spasm.

antispastic (an″tĭ-spas′tik) antispasmodic with specific reference to skeletal muscle.

antispermotoxin (an″tĭ-sper″mo-tok′sin) a substance that opposes the action of a spermotoxin.

antistaphylococcic (an″tĭ-staf″ĭ-lo-kok′sik) killing or suppressing staphylococci.

antistaphylohemolysin (an″tĭ-staf″ĭ-lo-he-mol′ĭ-sin) antistaphylolysin.

antistaphylolysin (an″tĭ-staf-ĭ-lol′ĭ-sin) a substance that opposes the action of staphylolysin.

antisteapsin (an″tĭ-ste-ap′sin) an antibody that counteracts steapsin.

antisterility (an″tĭ-ste-ril′ĭ-te) combating sterility.

Antistine (an-tis′tin) trademark for preparations of antazoline.

antistreptococcic (an″tĭ-strep″to-kok′sik) antagonistic to streptococci.

antistreptokinase (an″tĭ-strep-to′kĭ-nās) an antibody that inhibits streptokinase.

antistreptolysin (an″tĭ-strep-tol′ĭ-sin) an antibody that inhibits streptolysin.

antisubstance (an″tĭ-sub′stans) antibody.

antisudoral (an″tĭ-su′dor-al) antisudorific.

antisudorific (an″tĭ-su″dor-if′ik) [anti- + L. sudor sweat] 1. inhibiting perspiration. 2. an agent that inhibits perspiration.

antisympathetic (an″tĭ-sim″pah-thet′ik) 1. producing effects that resemble those of interruption of the sympathetic nerve supply. 2. an agent that produces effects resembling those of interruption of the sympathetic nerve supply.

antisyphilitic (an″tĭ-sif″ĭ-lit′ik) [anti- + syphilitic] 1. effective against syphilis. 2. a remedy for syphilis. Called also antiluetic.

antitemplate (an″tĭ-tem′plāt) a hypothetical substance said to inhibit mitosis of normal cells and, on injury to cells, to diffuse out of the cells to initiate mitosis.

antitetanic (an″tĭ-tĕ-tan′ik) preventing or curing tetanus.

antitetanolysin (an″tĭ-tet-ah-nol′ĭ-sin) the antibody to tetanolysin.

antithenar (an″tĭ-the′nar) [anti- + Gr. thenar palm, sole] situated opposite to the palm or the sole.

antithermic (an″tĭ-ther′mik) [anti- + Gr. thermē heat] antipyretic.

antithrombin (an″tĭ-throm′bin) [anti- + thrombin] a general term for a naturally occurring or therapeutically administered substance (e.g., heparin) that neutralizes the action of thrombin and thus limits or restricts blood coagulation. Six naturally occurring antithrombins have been designated by Roman numerals (I to VI); of these, antithrombins I and III appear to be of major importance. **a. I,** a term referring to the capacity of fibrin to adsorb large amounts of thrombin and thus neutralize (but not inactivate) it. **a. III,** a protein (an α_2-globulin molecular weight 64,000) of normal plasma and extravascular sites that inactivates thrombin in a time-dependent irreversible reaction and serves as a cofactor of heparin in its anticoagulant activities. Antithrombin III also inhibits certain coagulation factors.

antithromboplastin (an″tĭ-throm″bo-plas′tin) any agent or substance that prevents or interferes with the interaction of the blood coagulation factors as they generate prothrombinase (prothrombin converting principle).

antithrombotic (an″tĭ-throm-bot′ik) preventing or interfering with the formation of thrombi; an agent that so acts.

antithyroid (an″tĭ-thi′roid) counteracting the functioning of the thyroid, especially in its synthesis of thyroid hormone.

antithyrotoxic (an″tĭ-thi″ro-tok′sik) counteracting the toxic effect of thyroid and thyroid products.

antithyrotropic (an″tĭ-thi″ro-trop′ik) inhibiting the action of the thyrotropic hormone.

antitonic (an″tĭ-ton′ik) reducing tone or tonicity.

antitoxic (an″tĭ-tok′sik) effective against a poison; pertaining to antitoxin.

antitoxigen (an″tĭ-tok′sĭ-jen) [antitoxin + Gr. gennan to produce] any substance that induces the formation of antitoxin in the animal body; antitoxinogen.

antitoxin (an″tĭ-tok′sin) [anti- + Gr. toxicon poison] antibody to the toxin of a microorganism (usually the bacterial exotoxins), to a zootoxin (e.g., spider or bee venom), or to a phytotoxin (e.g., ricin of the castor bean), which combines specifically with the toxin, in vivo and in vitro, with neutralization of toxicity. **botulinal a., botulinum a., botulinus a.**, botulism a. **botulism a.** [USP], a sterile solution of antitoxic substances (antibodies) from the blood serum or plasma of healthy horses immunized against the toxins of Clostridium botulinum, used as a passive immunizing agent. It is available in bivalent (types A and B), trivalent (types A, B, and E), and monovalent (type E) forms. Called also botulinum a. and botulinus a. **bovine a.**, antitoxin containing antibodies derived from the cow instead of from the horse, for use on persons who are hypersensitive to horse serum. **diphtheria a.** [USP], a sterile solution of refined and concentrated antibody globulins derived from the blood serum or plasma of a healthy animal, usually the horse, immunized against diphtheria toxins; used as a passive immunizing agent, administered intramuscularly or intravenously. **gas gangrene a.**, a sterile solution of antibody globulins from the blood of horses immunized against the toxins of certain species of pathogenic clostridia. Bivalent antitoxin contains antibodies against Clostridium perfringens and Cl. septicum; trivalent contains these plus antibodies against Cl. novyi. Antibodies against Cl. histolyticum and Cl. bifermentans are added to these in polyvalent antitoxins. **normal a.**, antitoxin capable of neutralizing an equal quantity of normal toxin solution. **scarlet fever streptococcus a.**, a sterile solution of antitoxic substances (i.e., immunoglobulins) from blood serum of healthy animals immunized against toxin from the streptococci causing scarlet fever. **tetanus a.** [USP], a sterile solution of refined and concentrated antibody globulins obtained from the blood serum or plasma of a healthy animal, usually the horse, immunized against tetanus toxin or toxoid; used as a passive immunizing agent, administered intramuscularly, subcutaneously, or intravenously. **tetanus and gas gangrene a's**, a sterile solution of antitoxic substances (immunoglobulins) obtained from the blood of healthy animals immunized against the toxins of Clostridium tetani, C. perfringens, and C. septicum; used for prophylactic immunization against tetanus.

antitoxinogen (an″tĭ-tok-sin′o-jen) [antitoxin + Gr. gennan to produce] an antigen that stimulates the production of antitoxin.

antitoxinum (an″tĭ-tok-si′num) [L.] antitoxin.

antitragicus (an″tĭ-traj′e-kus) see Table of Musculi.

antitragus (an″tĭ-tra′gus) [anti- + tragus] [NA] a projection opposite the tragus, bounding the cavum conchae posteroinferiorly and continuous above with the anthelix.

antitreponemal (an″tĭ-trep″o-ne′mal) 1. effective against Treponema. 2. an agent that is effective against Treponema.

antitrichomonal (an″tĭ-trich″o-mo′nal) 1. effective against Trichomonas. 2. an agent that is destructive to Trichomonas.

antitrismus (an″tĭ-triz′mus) a spasm that prevents the closure of the mouth.

antitrope (an′tĭ-trōp) [anti- + Gr. trepein to turn] 1. any organ that forms a symmetrical pair with another. 2. antibody.

antitropic (an″tĭ-tro′pic) corresponding, but oppositely oriented, as a right and a left glove.

antitropin (an″tĭ-tro′pin) any substance that opposes the action of tropin; antiopsonin.

antitrypanosomal (an″tĭ-trĭ-pan″o-so′mal) 1. effective against trypanosomes. 2. a drug for combating trypanosomiasis.

antitrypsic (an″tĭ-trip′sik) antitryptic.

α₁-antitrypsin (an″tĭ-trip′sin) alpha₁-antitrypsin.

antitryptase (an″tĭ-trip′tās) a substance that inhibits or counteracts the action of tryptase.

antitryptic (an″tĭ-trip′tik) [anti- + tryptic] counteracting the activity of trypsin.

antituberculin (an″tĭ-tu-ber′ku-lin) an antibody developed following the injection of tuberculin into the animal body.

antituberculotic (an″tĭ-tu-ber″ku-lot′ik) 1. therapeutically effective against tuberculosis. 2. an agent that is therapeutically effective against tuberculosis.

antituberculous (an″tĭ-tu-ber′ku-lus) therapeutically effective against tuberculosis.

antitubulin (an″tĭ-too′bu-lin) an agent that prevents the polymerization of tubulin, and thus the formation of microtubules in a cell.

antitumorigenic (an″tĭ-tu″mor-ĭ-jen′ik) counteracting tumor formation.

antitussive (an″tĭ-tus′iv) 1. relieving or preventing cough. 2. an agent that relieves or prevents cough.

antityphoid (an″tĭ-ti′foid) counteracting or preventing typhoid.

antityrosinase (an″tĭ-ti-ro′sĭ-nās) an antienzyme that counteracts tyrosinase.

antiulcerative (an″tĭ-ul′ser-a″tiv) 1. preventing or promoting the healing of ulcers. 2. an agent that so acts.

antiuratic (an″tĭ-u-rat′ik) preventing the deposit of urates.

antiurease (an″tĭ-u′re-ās) an antibody that inhibits the activity of urease.

antiurokinase (an″tĭ-u″ro-ki′nās) a naturally occurring substance that inhibits clot dissolution by inhibiting the action of urokinase.

antivaccinationist (an″tĭ-vak″sĭ-na′shun-ist) a person who is opposed to vaccination.

antivenene (an″tĭ-vĕ-nēn′) [anti- + L. venenum poison] antivenin.

antivenereal (an″tĭ-vĕ-ne′re-al) effective against venereal diseases.

antivenin (an″tĭ-ven′in) [anti- + L. venenum poison] a proteinaceous material used in the treatment of poisoning by animal venom. See also antivenomous serum, under serum. **black widow spider a.**, Latrodectus mactans a. **Latrodectus mactans a.**, an antitoxic serum specific in the treatment of black widow spider (L. mactans) bites, prepared by immunizing horses against venom of the black widow spider; called also black widow spider a. **a. (Micrurus fulvius)** [USP], a sterile, nonpyrogenic preparation derived by drying a frozen solution of specific venom-neutralizing globulins obtained from serum of horses immunized against the venom of Eastern coral snakes (Micrurus fulvius). **a. (Crotalidae) polyvalent** [USP], polyvalent crotaline a., a sterile serum containing specific venom-neutralizing globulins, produced by hyperimmunization of horses with the venoms of the fer-de-lance and the Florida, Texas, and tropical rattlesnakes; used as a passive immunizing agent for the treatment of envenomation by most pit vipers throughout the world.

antivenom (an″tĭ-ven′om) antivenin.

antivenomous (an″tĭ-ven′o-mus) counteracting venom.

antiviral (an″tĭ-vi′ral) 1. destroying viruses or suppressing their replication. 2. an agent that destroys viruses or suppresses their replication.

antivirotic (an″tĭ-vi-rot′ik) 1. antiviral. 2. an agent that destroys viruses or checks their growth or multiplication.

antivirulin (an″tĭ-vir′u-lin) any substance that opposes the action of virulin; the substance in animals immunized against rabies, which neutralizes or inactivates the virus of rabies.

antivirus (an″tĭ-vi′rus) Besredka's name for the filtered and heated broth cultures of bacteria used by him to produce local immunity.

antivitamer (an″tĭ-vi′tah-mer) a substance that inactivates a vitamer.

antivitamin (an″tĭ-vi′tah-min) a substance that inactivates a vitamin.

antivivisection (an″tĭ-viv″ĭ-sek′shun) opposition to vivisection.

antivivisectionist (an″tĭ-viv″ĭ-sek′shun-ist) an individual opposed to vivisection.

antixenic (an″tĭ-ze′nik) [anti- + Gr. xenos strange or foreign] pertaining to the reaction of living tissue to any foreign substance.

antixerophthalmic (an″tĭ-ze″rof-thal′mik) counteracting xerophthalmia.

antixerotic (an″tĭ-ze-rot′ik) counteracting or preventing xerosis.

antizyme (an″tĭ-zīm) a protein whose synthesis is induced by a product of an enzyme reaction and which combines with and inhibits the action of that enzyme.

antizymohexase (an″tĭ-zi″mo-hek′sās) an antienzyme that counteracts zymohexase.

antizymotic (an″tĭ-zĭ-mot′ik) inhibiting or suppressing the action of enzymes.

antodontalgic (an″to-don-tal′jik) antiodontalgic.

Anton's symptom (syndrome) (an′tonz) [Gabriel Anton, German neuropsychiatrist, 1858–1933] see under symptom.

antophthalmic (ant″of-thal′mik) relieving ophthalmia.

antorphine (an-tor′fēn) nalorphine.

antra (an′trah) [L.] plural of antrum.

antracele (an′trah-sēl) antrocele.

antral (an′tral) of or pertaining to an antrum.

antrectomy (an-trek′to-me) [antrum + Gr. ektomē excision] surgical excision of an antrum, as resection of the pyloric antrum of the stomach.

Antrenyl (an′trĕ-nil) trademark for a preparation of oxyphenonium.

Antricola (an-trik′ŏ-lah) a genus of soft ticks that infest birds; several species feed on bats.

antritis (an-tri′tis) inflammation of an antrum, chiefly the maxillary antrum.

antro- (an′tro) [L. *antrum;* Gr. *antron* cave] a combining form denoting relationship to an antrum, or sinus; often used with specific reference to the maxillary antrum, or sinus.

antroatticotomy (an″tro-at″ĭ-kot′o-me) atticoantrotomy.

antrobuccal (an″tro-buk′kal) pertaining to or communicating with the maxillary antrum (sinus) and (oral) buccal cavity, as an antrobuccal fistula.

antrocele (an′tro-sēl) [*antro-* + Gr. *kēlē* tumor] a cystic accumulation of fluid in the maxillary antrum (sinus).

antroduodenectomy (an″tro-du″o-de-nek′to-me) surgical removal of the pyloric antrum and adjacent portion of the duodenum, formerly done in the treatment of duodenal ulcer.

antrodynia (an″tro-din′e-ah) [*antro-* + Gr. *odynē* pain] pain in an antrum.

antronalgia (an″tro-nal′je-ah) [*antro-* + *-algia*] pain in the maxillary antrum.

antronasal (an″tro-na′zal) pertaining to the maxillary antrum and the nose.

antroneurolysis (an″tro-nu-rol′ĭ-sis) denervation of the entire gastric antrum by submucosal dissection.

antrophore (an′tro-fōr) [*antro-* + Gr. *pherein* to bear] a form of soluble medicated bougie.

antrophose (an′tro-fōz) [*antro-* + *phose*] a phose originating in the central ocular mechanism.

antropyloric (an″tro-pǐ-lor′ik) pertaining to or affecting the pyloric part of the stomach, including its antrum.

antroscope (an′tro-skōp″) [*antro-* + Gr. *skopein* to examine] an instrument for illuminating and examining the maxillary antrum.

antroscopy (an-tros′ko-pe) the use of the antroscope; inspection of an antrum.

antrostomy (an-tros′to-me) [*antro-* + Gr. *stomoun* to provide with an opening, or mouth] the operation of making an opening into an antrum for purposes of drainage.

antrotome (an′tro-tōm) an instrument for performing antrotomy.

antrotomy (an-trot′o-me) [*antro-* + Gr. *tomē* cut] the cutting open of an antrum.

antrotympanic (an″tro-tim-pan′ik) pertaining to the mastoid antrum and the tympanic cavity.

antrotympanitis (an″tro-tim″pah-ni′tis) [*antro-* + *tympanitis*] inflammation of the mastoid antrum and of the middle ear.

antrum (an′trum), pl. *an′trums* or *an′tra* [L.; Gr. *antron* cave] a cavity or chamber; used as a general term in anatomical nomenclature, especially to designate a cavity or chamber within a bone. **a. au′ris,** meatus acusticus externus. **cardiac a., a. cardi′acum,** the short conical portion of the esophagus below the diaphragm, its base being continuous with the cardiac orifice of the stomach. **ethmoid a., a. ethmoida′le,** bulla ethmoidalis cavi nasi. **frontal a.,** sinus frontalis. **gastric a.,** a. pylori. **a. of Highmore, a. highmo′ri,** sinus maxillaris. **Malacarne's a.** (obs.), substantia perforata posterior. **mastoid a., a. mastoi′deum** [NA], an air space in the mastoid portion of the temporal bone, communicating with the tympanic cavity and the mastoid cells; called also *a. tympanicum, tympanic a.,* and *mastoid cavity.* **a. maxilla′re, maxillary a.,** sinus maxillaris. **a. pylo′ri, pyloric a., a. pylor′icum** [NA], the dilated portion of the pyloric part of the stomach, between the body of the stomach and the pyloric canal; called also *a. of Willis* and *gastric a.* **tympanic a., a. tympan′icum,** a. mastoideum. **a. of Willis,** a. pyloricum.

Antrypol (an′trĭ-pol) trademark for a preparation of suramin sodium.

ANTU a powerful rodenticide, alphanaphthyl thiourea, that produces massive pulmonary edema and pleural effusion in rats.

antuitarism (an-tu′ĭ-tah-rizm) [*ante-* + *pituitarism*] (obs.) hyperpituitarism.

Anturane (an′choo-rān) trademark for a preparation of sulfinpyrazone.

Antyllus (an-til′lus) (2nd century A.D.) a noted Greek surgeon of antiquity, a Pneumatist, whose treatment of aneurysms by ligation above and below remained standard practice until the time of John Hunter (18th century). He also made contributions to plastic surgery, ophthalmology, and public health. His writings remain only in fragments, and in the works of others (particularly Oribasius).

anuclear (ah-nu′kle-ar) having no nuclei; said of cells, such as erythrocytes, which have lost their nuclei.

anucleated (a-nu′kle-āt″ed) denucleated.

anulus (an′u-lus), pl. *an′uli* [L. dim. of *anus*] [NA] a term used to designate a ringlike anatomical structure; called also *annulus.* **a. of conjunctiva, a. conjuncti′vae** [NA], a ring at the junction of the conjunctiva and cornea. **a. femora′lis** [NA], femoral ring: the abdominal opening of the femoral canal,

normally closed by the crural septum and peritoneum; called also *crural fossa, inferior digital fossa, crural fovea, femoral fovea, femoral fossa,* and *hiatus femoralis.* **a. fibrocartilagin′eus membra′nae tym′pani** [NA], fibrocartilaginous ring of tympanic membrane: the margin of the pars tensa of the tympanic membrane, which attaches to the sulcus tympanicus. **an′uli fibro′si cor′dis** [NA], fibrous rings of the heart: dense fibrous rings, one of which surrounds each of the four major cardiac orifices: the right and left atrioventricular, the aortic, and the pulmonary trunk orifices. To these four rings, either directly or indirectly, are attached the atrial and ventricular muscle fibers. Called also *Lower's rings.* **a. fibro′sus dis′ci interverte-bra′lis** [NA], the circumferential ringlike portion of an intervertebral disk, composed of fibrocartilage and fibrous tissue; called also *annulus fibrosus fibrocartilaginis intervertebralis* and *fibrous ring of intervertebral disk.* **a. inguina′lis profun′dus** [NA], deep inguinal ring: an aperture in the fascia transversalis for the spermatic cord or for the round ligament; called also *annulus abdominalis abdominis, annulus inguinalis abdominalis, deep* or *internal abdominal ring,* and *internal inguinal ring.* **a. inguina′lis superficia′lis** [NA], superficial abdominal ring: an opening in the aponeurosis of the external oblique muscle for the spermatic cord or for the round ligament; called also *annulus inguinalis subcutaneus, external abdominal ring,* and *superficial* or *external inguinal ring.* **a. i′ridis ma′jor** [NA], greater ring of iris: the less coarsely striated outer concentric circle on the anterior surface of the iris; called also *greater circle of iris.* **a. i′ridis mi′nor** [NA], lesser ring of iris: the more coarsely striated inner concentric circle on the anterior surface of the iris; called also *lesser circle of iris.* **a. tendin′eus commu′nis** [NA], common tendinous ring: the anular ligament of origin common to the recti muscles of the eye, attached to the edge of the optic canal and the inner part of the superior orbital fissure; called also *annulus tendineus communis* [Zinni], *annulus zinii,* and *Zinn's ring* or *ligament.* **a. tympan′icus** [NA], tympanic ring: the bony ring forming part of the temporal bone at the time of birth and developing into the pars tympanica of the bone; called also *tympanic annulus.* **a. umbilica′lis** [NA], umbilical ring: the aperture in the abdominal wall through which the umbilical cord communicates with the fetus. After birth it is felt for some time as a distinct fibrous ring surrounding the umbilicus; these fibers later shrink progressively. Called also *umbilical canal.*

Anura (ah-nu′rah) the order of frogs and toads.

anuran (ah-nu′ran) any member of Anura.

anuresis (an″u-re′sis) 1. retention of urine in the bladder. 2. anuria.

anuretic (an-u-ret′ik) pertaining to or characterized by anuresis.

anuria (ah-nu′re-ah) [*an* neg. + Gr. *ouron* urine + *-ia*] complete suppression of urinary secretion by the kidneys; called also *anuresis.* **angioneurotic a.,** anuria occurring in cortical necrosis of the kidney. **calculous a.,** anuria caused by a renal calculus. **obstructive a.,** failure of urinary excretion due to a blockage, as by a calculus, in the urinary passages. **postrenal a.,** anuria resulting from obstruction of the ureters. **prerenal a.,** cessation of renal secretion of urine resulting from fall of blood pressure below the level necessary to maintain adequate filtration pressure in the glomeruli. **renal a.,** failure of urinary secretion by the kidney in the presence of adequate filtration pressure in the glomeruli and patency of the ureters. **suppressive a.,** failure of secretion of urine in the kidneys.

anuric (ah-nu′rik) pertaining to or characterized by anuria.

anurous (ah-nu′rus) [*an* neg. + Gr. *oura* tail] without a tail.

anus (a′nus), pl. *anus,* gen. *a′ni* [L.; said originally to have been derived from an Anglo-Saxon word meaning to sit] the distal or terminal orifice of the alimentary canal. **artificial a.,** an opening from the bowel formed by the operation of colostomy. **ectopic a.,** imperforate a. **imperforate a.,** persistence of the anal membrane, so that the anus is closed. The defect is not always complete; sometimes a narrow opening permits the passage of the bowel contents. When completely imperforate, the anus is seen as a dimple (the proctodeal pit) in the skin of the perineum. The latter condition is often associated with atresia of the lower rectum. **preternatural a.,** an anus situated at some unusual or abnormal place. **a. of Rusconi,** the blastopore. **a. vesica′lis,** anomalous opening of the rectum into the bladder, the anus being imperforate. **a. vestibula′ris,** anomalous opening of the rectum on the vulva, the anus being imperforate. **vulvovaginal a.,** a. vestibularis.

anusitis (a-nus-i′tis) inflammation of the anus.

anvil (an′vil) incus.

anxietas (ang-zi′ĕ-tas) [L.] a nervous restlessness; anxiety. **a. preseni′lis,** a state of extreme anxiety preceding senility.

anxiety (ang-zi′ĕ-te) a feeling of apprehension, uncertainty, and fear without apparent stimulus, and associated with physiological changes (tachycardia, sweating, tremor, etc.). **castration a.,** castration complex. **free-floating a.,** fear in the absence of known cause for anxiety. **neurotic a.,** that in which the apprehension is objectively out of proportion to any apparent cause. **separation a.,** apprehension due to removal of significant persons or familiar surroundings; common in infants 6 to 10 months old. **situation a.,** a feeling of apprehension coming on with the starting of some undertaking.

anxiolytic (ang″zi-o-lit′ik) 1. dispelling anxiety. 2. any sedative or hypnotic, e.g., diazepam and chlorodiazepoxide, used in the psychoneuroses and anxiety states to reduce anxiety, agitation, or tension; called also *minor tranquilizer.*

anydremia (an″ĭ-dre′me-ah) [*an* neg. + Gr. *hydōr* water + *haima* blood + *-ia*] anhydremia.

AO anodal opening; opening of the atrioventricular valves.

A.O.A. American Optometric Association; American Orthopaedic Association; American Orthopsychiatric Association; American Osteopathic Association.

AOC anodal opening contraction.

AOCl anodal opening clonus.

AOO anodal opening odor.

AOP anodal opening picture.

A.O.P.A. American Orthotics and Prosthetics Association.

aorta (a-or′tah), pl. *aor′tas, aor′tae* [L.; Gr. *aortē*] the main trunk from which the systemic arterial system proceeds [NA]. It arises from the left ventricle of the heart; passes upward (*a. ascen′dens*), bends over (*arcus aortae*), passes down through the thorax (*a. thoraca′lis*) and through the abdomen to about the level of the fourth lumbar vertebra (*a. abdomina′lis*), where it divides into the two common iliac arteries. Called also *arteria a.* and *arteria maxima Galeni.* See *Table of Arteriae.* **abdominal a., a. abdomina′lis** [NA], the continuation of the thoracic aorta, which gives rise to the inferior phrenic, lumbar, median sacral, superior mesenteric, inferior mesenteric, middle suprarenal, renal, and testicular or ovarian arteries, and the celiac trunk. **a. ascen′dens** [NA], **ascending a.,** the proximal portion of the aorta, arising from the left ventricle, and giving origin to the right and left coronary arteries before continuing as the arch of the aorta. **a. descen′dens** [NA], **descending a.,** the continuation of the aorta from the arch of the aorta, in the thorax, to the point of its division into the common iliac arteries, in the abdomen. See also *a. abdominalis* and *a. thoracica.* **dextrapositioned a.,** a congenital anomaly resulting from increased rotation of the lower end of the bulbar septum, bringing the aorta farther to the right. It is seen in tetralogy of Fallot. **overriding a.,** a congenital anomaly occurring in tetralogy of Fallot, in which the aorta is displaced to the right so that it appears to arise from both ventricles and straddles the ventricular septal defect. **palpable a.,** one which, on account of a thin retracted abdominal wall, is easily palpable. **primitive a.,** either of two main vascular trunks before fusion into a single aorta in the early embryo. **a. sacrococcyg′ea,** arteria sacralis mediana. **a. thoraca′lis,** a. thoracica. **thoracic a., a. thorac′ica** [NA], the proximal portion of the descending aorta, proceeding from the arch of the aorta, and giving rise to the bronchial, esophageal, pericardiac, and mediastinal branches, and the superior phrenic, posterior intercostal III to XI, and subcostal arteries; it is continuous through the diaphragm with the abdominal aorta. **ventral a.,** a single short vascular segment that, in fishes, in some amphibians, and in the embryo of higher vertebrates, connects the heart with the aortic arches. In mammalian development, it becomes continuous with the aortic arch.

aortae (a-or′te) [L.] plural and genitive of *aorta.*

aortal (a-or′tal) aortic.

aortalgia (a″or-tal′je-ah) [*aorta* + Gr. *algos* pain] pain in the region of the aorta.

aortectomy (a″or-tek′to-me) [*aorta* + Gr. *ektomē* excision] excision of part of the aorta.

aortic (a-or′tik) of or pertaining to the aorta.

aorticopulmonary (a-or″tĭ-ko-pul′mo-ner″e) pertaining to or lying between the aorta and pulmonary artery.

aorticorenal (a-or″te-ko-re′nal) pertaining to the aorta and the kidneys.

aortitis (a″or-ti′tis) [*aorta* + *-itis*] inflammation of the aorta. **Döhle-Heller a.,** syphilitic a. **luetic a.,** syphilitic a. **nummular a.,** aortitis with white circular patches on the inner coat of the vessel. **rheumatic a.,** inflammation of the aorta due to rheumatism, which may progress to patchy fibrosis. **syphilitic a., a. syphilit′ica,** aortitis caused by syphilis; its complications include insufficiency of the aortic valve, stenosis of occlusion of the coronary orifices, and aortic aneurysm. Called also *Döhle-Heller a., Heller-Döhle disease,* and *luetic a.*

aortocoronary (a-or″to-kor′o-na-re) pertaining to or communicating with the aorta and coronary arteries.

aortogram (a-or′to-gram″) the roentgenographic record resulting from aortography.

aortography (a″or-tog′rah-fe) [*aorta* + Gr. *graphein* to write] roentgenography of the aorta after the intravascular injection of an opaque medium. **retrograde a.,** roentgenography of the aorta after passage of a catheter through a peripheral artery to the aorta and the rapid injection of a radiopaque substance. **translumbar a.,** roentgenography of the aorta after injection of

a radiopaque medium into it through a needle inserted into the lumbar area at about the level of the 12th thoracic vertebra.

aortopathy (a″or-top′ah-the) [*aorta* + Gr. *pathos* disease] any disease of the aorta.

aortorrhaphy (a″or-tor′ah-fe) [*aorta* + Gr. *rhaphē* suture] suture of the aorta.

aortosclerosis (a-or″to-skle-ro′sis) sclerosis of the aorta.

aortotomy (a″or-tot′o-me) [*aorta* + Gr. *tomē* a cutting] incision of the aorta.

AOS anodal opening sound.

A.O.S. American Otological Society.

aosmic (a-oz′mik) anosmic.

A.O.T.A. American Occupational Therapy Association.

AOTe anodal opening tetanus.

AP anterior pituitary (gland); angina pectoris; anteroposterior; arterial pressure.

ap- see *apo-.*

APA antipernicious anemia factor; see *cyanocobalamin.*

A.P.A. American Pharmaceutical Association; American Podiatric Association; American Psychiatric Association; American Psychoanalytic Association; American Psychological Association; American Psychopathological Association.

apaconitine (ap″ah-kon′ĭ-tin) [*ap-* + *aconitine*] a poisonous base derived from aconitine.

apallesthesia (ah-pal″es-the′ze-ah) pallanesthesia.

Apamide (ap′ah-mīd) trademark for a preparation of acetaminophen.

apancrea (ah-pan′kre-ah) absence of the pancreas.

apancreatic (ah-pan″kre-at′ik) due to absence of the pancreas.

apandria (ap-an′dre-ah) [*ap-* + Gr. *anēr* man] (*obs.*) morbid aversion to the male sex.

apanthropia (ap-an-thro′pe-ah) [*ap-* + Gr. *anthrōpos* man + *-ia*] (*obs.*) 1. morbid fear of human companionship. 2. apandria.

apanthropy (ap-an′thro-pe) (*obs.*) apanthropia.

aparalytic (ah-par″ah-lit′ik) without paralysis.

aparathyreosis (ah-par″ah-thi-re-o′sis) aparathyrosis.

aparathyroidism (ah-par″ah-thi′roid-izm) aparathyrosis.

aparathyrosis (ah-par″ah-thi-ro′sis) absence or deficiency of the parathyroid glands.

apareunia (ah″par-u′ne-ah) abstinence from or inability to perform coitus.

aparthrosis (ap″ar-thro′sis) [Gr. *aparthrōsis*] junctura synovialis.

apastia (ah-pas′te-ah) [Gr. "fasting"] abstention from food, as a neurologic symptom.

apastic (ah-pas′tik) pertaining to or characterized by apastia.

apathetic (ap″ah-thet′ik) indifferent; undemonstrative.

apathic (ah-path′ik) without sensation or feeling.

apathism (ap′ah-thizm) the state of being slow in responding to stimuli.

apathy (ap′ah-the) [Gr. *apatheia*] lack of feeling or emotion; indifference.

apatite (ap′ah-tīt) a calcium phosphate of the composition $Ca_5(PO_4)_3OH$, one of the two mineral constituents of bones and teeth (the other being $CaCO_3$). Apatite is soluble in acids of soft drinks and in carbohydrate fermentation, but its OH^- ion is readily exchanged for F^- ion from some fluorides, and the resulting fluoroapatite is not susceptible to acid decay.

apazone (ap′ah-zōn) chemical name: 5-(dimethylamino)-9-methyl-2-propyl-1*H*-pyrazolo[1,2-*a*][1,2,4]benzotriazine-1,3-(2*H*)-dione; an anti-inflammatory agent, $C_{16}H_{20}N_4O_2$, which has been used in the treatment of rheumatoid disorders. Called also *azapropazone.*

APC 1. abbreviation for *acetylsalicylic acid, phenacetin,* and *caffeine,* available in capsule or tablet form; antipyretic and analgesic. 2. atrial premature contraction.

APE anterior pituitary extract.

apeidosis (ap″i-do′sis) [*ap-* + Gr. *eidos* form] progressive disappearance of characteristic form in either the histologic or clinical aspect of a disease.

apellous (a-pel′us) [*a* neg. + L. *pellis* skin] 1. skinless; not covered with skin; not cicatrized (said of a wound). 2. having no prepuce.

apepsia (ah-pep′se-ah) [*a* neg. + Gr. *peptein* to digest] (*obs.*) cessation or failure of the digestive functions.

apepsinia (ah″pep-sin′e-ah) (*obs.*) total absence or lack of secretion of pepsinogen by the stomach.

aperient (ah-pe′re-ent) [L. *aperiens* opening] a mild or gentle purgative; called also *aperitive* and *laxative.*

aperiodic (ah″pe-rĭ-od′ik) having no definite period; said of membranes that have no definite periods of vibration of their own, but are free to take up any vibrations imparted to them.

aperistalsis (ah″per-ĭ-stal′sis) [*a* neg. + *peristalsis*] absence of peristaltic action.

aperitive (ah-per′ĭ-tiv) 1. stimulating the appetite. 2. aperient.

Apert's disease (syndrome) (ah-parz′) [Eugène *Apert*, French pediatrician, 1868–1940] acrocephalosyndactylia.

Apert-Crouzon disease (ah-par′kroo-zon′) [Eugène *Apert*; Octave *Crouzon*, French neurologist, 1874–1938] see under *disease.*

apertognathia (ah-per″tog-na′the-ah) open bite.

apertometer (ap″er-tom′ĕ-ter) an apparatus for measuring the angle of aperture of microscopical objectives.

apertura (ap″er-tu′rah), pl. *apertu′rae* [L.] a general term used in anatomical nomenclature to designate an opening. **a. exter′na aqueduc′tus vestib′uli** [NA], external aperture of aqueduct of vestibule: the external opening for the aqueduct of the vestibule, located on the posterior surface of the petrous part of the temporal bone, lateral to the opening for the internal acoustic meatus; called also *fissure of aqueduct of vestibule.* **a. exter′na canalic′uli coch′leae** [NA], external aperture of canaliculus of cochlea: the external opening of the cochlear canaliculus on the margin of the jugular foramen in the temporal bone. **a. infe′rior canalic′uli tympan′ici,** inferior aperture of tympanic canaliculus: the lower opening of the tympanic canaliculus on the inferior surface of the petrous portion of the temporal bone; called also *external aperture of tympanic canaliculus.* **a. latera′lis ventric′uli quar′ti** [NA], an opening at the end of each lateral recess of the fourth ventricle by which the ventricular cavity communicates with the subarachnoid space; called also *lateral aperture of fourth ventricle, foramen of Luschka,* and *foramen of Key and Retzius.* **a. media′lis ventric′uli quar′ti,** a. mediana ventriculi quarti. **a. media′na ventric′uli quar′ti** [NA], a deficiency in the lower portion of the roof of the fourth ventricle through which the ventricular cavity communicates with the subarachnoid space; called also *a. medialis ventriculi quarti, median aperture of fourth ventricle,* and *foramen of Magendie.* **a. pel′vis infe′rior** [NA], **a. pel′vis [mino′ris] infe′rior,** the inferior, very irregular aperture of the minor pelvis, bounded by the coccyx, the sacrotuberous ligaments, part of the ischium, the sides of the pubic arch, and the pubic symphysis; called also *exitus pelvis* and *inferior aperture of minor pelvis.* **a. pel′vis supe′rior** [NA], **a. pel′vis [mino′ris] supe′rior,** the superior aperture of the minor pelvis, bounded by the crest and pecten of the pubic bones, the arcuate lines of the ilia, and the anterior margin of the base of the sacrum; called also *superior aperture of minor pelvis.* **a. pirifor′mis** [NA], piriform aperture: the anterior nasal opening in the skull; called also *bony anterior nasal aperture.* **a. si′nus fronta′lis** [NA], aperture of frontal sinus: the external opening of the frontal sinus into the nasal cavity. **a. si′nus sphenoida′lis** [NA], aperture of sphenoid sinus: a round opening just above the superior nasal concha, interconnecting the sphenoid sinus and nasal cavity; called also *sphenoidal ostium.* **a. supe′rior canalic′uli tympan′ici,** superior aperture of tympanic canaliculus: the upper opening of the tympanic canaliculus in the temporal bone, leading to the tympanum; called also *internal aperture of tympanic canaliculus.* **a. thora′cis infe′rior** [NA], inferior aperture of thorax: the irregular opening at the inferior part of the thorax bounded by the twelfth thoracic vertebra, the twelfth ribs, and the curving edge of the costal cartilages as they meet the sternum; called also *inferior thoracic aperture.* **a. thora′cis supe′rior** [NA], superior aperture of thorax: the elliptical opening at the summit of the thorax, bounded by the first thoracic vertebra, the first ribs, and the upper margin of the manubrium sterni; called also *superior thoracic aperture.* **a. tympan′ica canalic′uli chor′dae tym′pani** [NA], tympanic aperture of canaliculus of chorda tympani: the opening through which the chorda tympani enters the tympanic cavity.

aperturae (ap″er-tu′re) [L.] plural of *apertura.*

aperture (ap′er-chūr) [L. *apertura*] an opening, or orifice; see also *apertura.* **angle of a., angular a.,** the angle formed at a luminous point between the most divergent rays that are capable of passing through the objective of a microscope; called also *a. of lens.* **external a. of aqueduct of vestibule,** apertura externa aqueductus vestibuli. **external a. of canaliculus of cochlea,** apertura externa canaliculi cochleae. **external a. of tympanic canaliculus,** apertura inferior canaliculi tympanici. **a. of frontal sinus,** apertura sinus frontalis. **a. of glottis,** rima glottidis. **inferior a. of minor pelvis,** apertura pelvis inferior. **inferior a. of thorax,** apertura thoracis inferior. **inferior a. of tympanic canaliculus,** apertura inferior canaliculi tympanici. **internal a. of tympanic canaliculus,** apertura superior canaliculi tympanici. **a. of larynx,** aditus laryngis. **lateral a. of fourth ventricle,** apertura lateralis ventriculi quarti. **a. of lens,** angle of a. **median a. of fourth ventricle,** apertura mediana ventriculi quarti. **nasal a., bony anterior,** apertura piriformis. **numerical a.,** a measure of the efficiency of a microscope objective, being the product of the sine of one-half the angle of the aperture times the lowest refractive index of any medium between the objective and specimen; usually abbreviated N.A. **orbital a.,** aditus orbitae. **piriform a.,** apertura piriformis. **a. of sphenoid sinus,** apertura sinus sphenoidalis. **spinal a.,** foramen vertebrale. **spurious a. of facial canal,** hiatus canalis nervi petrosi majoris. **spurious a. of fallopian canal,** hiatus canalis nervi petrosi majoris. **superior a. of minor pelvis,** apertura pelvis superior. **superior a. of thorax,** apertura thoracis superior. **superior a. of tympanic canaliculus,** apertura superior canaliculi tympanici. **thoracic a., inferior,** apertura thoracis inferior. **thoracic a., superior,** apertura thoracis superior. **tympanic a. of canaliculus of chorda tympani,** apertura tympanica canaliculi chordae tympani.

apex (a′peks), pl. *apexes* or *a′pices* [L.] 1. a general term used in anatomical nomenclature to designate the top of a body, organ, or part, or the pointed extremity of a conical structure; called also *tip.* 2. the point of greatest activity, or the point of greatest response to any type of stimulation, such as electrical stimulation of a muscle. **a. of arytenoid cartilage,** a. cartilaginis arytenoideae. **a. auric′ulae** [NA], a pointed protrusion sometimes observed on the upper border of the ear; called also *darwinian a.* **a. of bladder,** a. vesicae urinariae. **a. cap′itis fib′ulae** [NA], a process pointing upward on the posterior surface of the head of the fibula, giving attachment to the arcuate popliteal ligament of the knee joint and part of the biceps tendon; called also *a. capituli fibulae* and *a. of head of fibula.* **a. capit′uli fib′ulae,** a. capitis fibulae. **a. cartilag′inis arytenoi′deae** [NA], apex of arytenoid cartilage: the upper part of the arytenoid cartilage, which bends posteriorly and medially and connects with the corniculate cartilage. **a. colum′nae posterio′ris medul′lae spina′lis,** a. cornus posterioris medullae spinalis. **a. cor′dis** [NA], apex of the heart: the blunt rounded extremity of the heart formed by the left ventricle; it is directed ventrally, inferiorly, and to the left. **a. cor′nus posterio′ris medul′lae spina′lis** [NA], a rim of large neurons just dorsal to the substantia gelatinosa of the spinal cord; sometimes used to refer to the gelatinous substance. Called also *a. columnae posterioris medullae spinalis* and *a. of posterior horn of spinal cord.* **a. cus′pidis** [NA], the apex of the cusp of a tooth. **darwinian a.,** a. auriculae. **a. of head of fibula,** a. capitis fibulae. **a. of heart,** a. cordis. **a. lin′guae** [NA], the most distal portion of the tongue; called also *a. of tongue.* **a. of lung,** a. pulmonis. **a. na′si** [NA], the most distal portion of the nose. **a. os′sis sa′cri** [NA], apex of the sacrum: the caudal end of the body of the fifth sacral vertebra, which articulates with the coccyx. **a. par′tis petro′sae os′sis tempora′lis** [NA], apex of petrous portion of temporal bone: the truncated portion of the petrous part of the temporal bone that is directed anteriorly and medially and ends at the medial opening of the carotid canal; called also *a. pyramidis ossis temporalis.* **a. of patella, a. patel′lae** [NA], the inferiorly directed blunt point of the patella, to which the patellar ligament is attached. **a. of petrous portion of temporal bone,** a. partis petrosae ossis temporalis. **a. of posterior horn of spinal cord,** a. cornus posterioris medullae spinalis. **a. prosta′tae** [NA], **a. of prostate gland,** the lower portion of the prostate, located just above the urogenital diaphragm. **a. pulmo′nis** [NA], apex of the lung: the rounded upper extremity of either lung, extending upward as high as the first thoracic vertebra. **a. pyram′idis os′sis tempora′lis,** a. partis petrosae ossis temporalis. **a. rad′icis den′tis** [NA], the terminal end of the root of a tooth. **root a.,** the terminal end of the root of the tooth. **a. of sacrum,** a. ossis sacri. **a. suprarena′lis [gl. dex′trae],** the apex of the right suprarenal (adrenal) gland. **a. of tongue,** a. linguae. **a. vesi′cae urina′riae** [NA], apex of bladder: the site of junction of the superior and inferolateral surfaces of the urinary bladder, from which the middle umbilical ligament (urachus) extends to the umbilicus; called also *fundus of bladder, vertex vesicae urinariae,* and *fundus* or *vertex of urinary bladder.*

apexcardiogram (a″peks-kar′de-o-gram) the graphic record obtained by apexcardiography.

apexcardiography (a″peks-kar″de-og′rah-fe) a method of graphically recording the pulsations of the precordium in the region of the cardiac apex.

A.P.F. animal protein factor; anabolism-promoting factor.

Apgar score (scale) (ap′gar) [Virginia *Apgar*, American anesthesiologist, 1909–1974] see under *score.*

APH anterior pituitary hormone.

A.P.H.A. American Public Health Association; American Protestant Hospital Association.

A.Ph.A. American Pharmaceutical Association.

aphacia (ah-fa′se-ah) aphakia.

aphacic (ah-fa′sik) aphakic.

aphagia (ah-fa′je-ah) [*a* neg. + Gr. *phagein* to eat + *-ia*] abstention from eating. **a. al′gera,** refusal of a person to take food because it causes pain.

aphagopraxia (ah-fa″go-prak′se-ah) loss of the ability to swallow.

aphakia (ah-fa′ke-ah) [*a* neg. + Gr. *phakos* lentil + *-ia*] absence of the lens of the eye; it may occur congenitally or from trauma, but is most commonly caused by extraction of a cataract.

aphakic (ah-fa′kik) pertaining to aphakia; having no lens in the eye.

aphalangia (ah″fah-lan′je-ah) a developmental anomaly characterized by absence of a digit or of one or more phalanges of a finger or toe.

Aphanozoa (af″ah-no-zo′ah) [Gr. *aphanēs* invisible + *zōon* animal] ultramicroscopic organisms.

aphantobiont (ah-fan″to-bi′ont) [Gr. *aphantos* invisible + *bioun* a living being] obsolete term for virion.

aphasia (ah-fa′ze-ah) [*a* neg. + Gr. *phasis* speech] defect or loss of the power of expression by speech, writing, or signs, or of comprehending spoken or written language, due to injury or disease of the brain centers. For types of aphasia not given below, see *agrammatism, anomia, paragrammatism,* and *paraphasia.* **acoustic a.,** auditory a. **ageusic a.,** loss of power to express words relating to the sense of taste. **amnemonic a.,** forgetfulness of words, with consequent aphasia; called also *a. lethica.* **amnesic a., amnestic a.,** anomic a. **anomic a.,** fluent aphasia in which comprehension and repetition are both preserved; called also *amnestic a.* **anosmic a.,** inability to express in words sensations of smell. **associative a.,** aphasia due to a disturbance of connection between the parts comprising the central structure. **ataxic a.,** expressive a. **auditory a.,** aphasia due to disease of the hearing center of the brain; word deafness. **Broca's a.,** expressive a. **central a.,** global a. **combined a.,** aphasia of two or more forms occurring concomitantly in the same person. **commissural a.,** aphasia due to a lesion in the insula interrupting the path between the motor and sensory speech centers; called also *frontolenticular a.* and *lenticular a.* **complete a.,** aphasia due to lesion of all the speech centers, producing inability to communicate with others in any way. **conduction a.,** fluent aphasia in which there is normal comprehension of spoken language but words are repeated incorrectly. **cortical a.,** global a. **expressive a.,** aphasia in which there is impairment of the ability to speak and write, due to a lesion of the cortical center. The patient understands written and spoken words, and knows what he wants to say, but cannot utter the words. Called also *ataxic a., Broca's a., motor a., frontocortical a.,* and *verbal a.* **expressive-receptive a.,** global a. **fluent a.,** aphasia in which speech is well articulated and grammatically correct but is lacking in content. **frontocortical a.,** expressive a. **frontolenticular a.,** commissural a. **functional a.,** aphasia resulting from hysteria or severe hysterical disorder. **gibberish a.,** jargon a. **global a.,** aphasia which involves all the functions which go to make up speech or communication; called also *central a., cortical a., expressive-receptive a.,* and *pictorial a.* **graphomotor a.,** aphasia in which the person cannot express himself in writing. **Grashey's a.,** aphasia due to lessened duration of sensory impressions, causing disturbance of perception and association, without lack of function of the centers or conductivity of the tracts; it is seen in acute diseases and concussion of the brain. **impressive a.,** sensory a. **intellectual a.,** true a. **jargon a.,** a form of receptive aphasia with utterance of meaningless phrases; called also *gibberish a.* **Kussmaul's a.,** voluntary refraining from speech, as in the insane. **lenticular a.,** commissural a. **a. leth′ica,** amnemonic a. **Lichtheim's a.,** a form of aphasia in which spontaneous speech is lost but the ability to repeat words is retained. **mixed a.,** global a. **motor a.,** expressive a. **nominal a.,** aphasia marked by the defective use of names of objects; cf. *anomia* and *dysnomia.* **nonfluent a.,** aphasia in which little speech is produced, and is uttered slowly, with great effort and poor articulation; it is due to a lesion in Broca's area. **optic a.,** inability to name objects seen, due to interruption of the connection between the speech and visual centers. **parieto-occipital a.,** combined alexia and apraxia. **pathematic a.,** aphasia due to passion or fright. **pictorial a.,** global a. **psychosensory a.,** receptive a. **receptive a.,** inability to understand written, spoken, or tactile speech symbols, due to disease of the auditory and visual word centers, as in word blindness; called also *impression a., sensory a., temporoparietal a.,* and *Wernicke's a.* **semantic a.,** aphasia characterized by a lack of recognition of the full significance of words and phrases or by loss of memory for words. **sensory a.,** receptive a. **subcortical a.,** aphasia due to a lesion interrupting impulses toward the afferent tracts that proceed to the auditory speech center. **syntactical a.,** aphasia characterized by inability to arrange words properly, so that the patient talks jargon. **tactile a.,** inability to name objects which are felt. **temporoparietal a.,** receptive a. **total a.,** global a. **transcortical a.,** aphasia caused by a lesion of a pathway between the speech center and other cortical centers. **true a.,** aphasia due to lesion of any one of the speech centers; called also *intellectual a.* **verbal a.,** expressive a. **visual a.,** alexia. **Wernicke's a.,** receptive a.

aphasiac (ah-fa′ze-ak) aphasic, def. 2.

aphasic (ah-fa′zik) 1. pertaining to or affected with aphasia. 2. a person affected with aphasia.

aphasiologist (ah-fa″ze-ol′o-jist) one who specializes in aphasiology, as a neurologist or psychologist.

aphasiology (a-fa″ze-ol′o-je) the scientific study of aphasia and the specific neurologic lesions producing it.

aphasmid (a-faz′mid) [*a* neg. + phasmid] a nematode belonging to the subclass Aphasmidia. Cf. *phasmid.*

Aphasmidia (a-faz-mid′e-ah) a subclass of Nematoda comprising those organisms which do not possess phasmids, and including the superfamilies Trichuroidea, Mermithoidea, and Dioctophymoidea.

apheliotropism (ap″he-le-ot′ro-pizm) negative heliotropism.

aphemesthesia (ah″fe-mes-the′ze-ah) [*a* neg. + Gr. *phēmē* voice + *aisthēsis* perception] alexia.

aphemia (ah-fe′me-ah) [*a* neg. + Gr. *phēmē* voice] loss of the power of speech, due to a central lesion; see *expressive aphasia,* under *aphasia.* Called also *anandia.*

aphemic (ah-fem′ik) pertaining to or characterized by aphemia.

aphephobia (af″e-fo′be-ah) [Gr. *haphē* touch + *phobein* to be affrighted by + *-ia*] (*obs.*) a morbid dread of touching or of being touched.

apheresis (ah-fer′ĕ-sis) [Gr. *aphairesis* removal] any procedure in which blood is withdrawn from a donor, a portion (plasma, leukocytes, platelets, etc.) is separated and retained, and the remainder is retransfused into the donor. It includes leukapheresis, thrombocytapheresis, etc. Called also *pheresis.*

apheter (af′ĕ-ter) [Gr. *aphienai* to dissolve] a supposed material that gives to inogen the stimulus that decomposes it, and thus causes muscular contraction.

aphilopony (ah″fil-op′ŏ-ne) [*a* neg. + Gr. *philein* to love + *ponos* bodily exertion] (*obs.*) fear of or disinclination to work.

Aphiochae′ta ferrugin′ea *Megaselia scalaris.*

aphonia (ah-fo′ne-ah) [*a* neg. + Gr. *phōnē* voice] loss of voice. **a. clerico′rum,** see under *dysphonia.* **hysteric a.,** loss of speech due to hysteria. **a. paralyt′ica,** aphonia due to paralysis or disease of the laryngeal nerves. **a. parano′ica,** stubborn and willful silence. **spastic a.,** interference with the voice caused by muscular spasm.

aphonic (ah-fon′ik) 1. pertaining to or affected with aphonia. 2. without audible voice.

aphonogelia (ah″fo-no-je′le-ah) [*a* neg. + Gr. *phōnē* voice + *gelōs* laughter] inability to laugh aloud.

aphose (ah-fōz′) [*a* neg. + Gr. *phōs* light] any phose or subjective visual sensation due to absence or interruption of light.

aphosphagenic (ah-fos″fah-jen′ik) due to deficiency of phosphorus.

aphosphorosis (ah-fos″fo-ro′sis) a morbid condition caused by a deficiency of phosphorus in the diet.

aphotesthesia (a″fot-es-the′ze-ah) [*a* neg. + Gr. *phōs* light + *aisthēsis* perception] reduced sensitivity of the retina to light resulting from excessive exposure to rays of the sun.

aphotic (ah-fot′ik) without light; totally dark.

aphrasia (ah-fra′ze-ah) [*a* neg. + Gr. *phrasis* utterance] inability to speak or to understand words arranged as phrases. **a. parano′ica** (*obs.*), voluntary abstention from speech in the mentally ill.

aphrenia (ah-fre′ne-ah) [*a* neg. + Gr. *phrēn* mind] dementia.

aphrodisia (af″ro-diz′e-ah) [Gr. *aphrodisia* sexual pleasures] 1. sexual excitement, especially if morbid or excessive. 2. coitus or sexual congress.

aphrodisiac (af″ro-diz′e-ak) 1. exciting the libido. 2. any drug that arouses the sexual instinct.

aphrodisiomania (af″ro-diz″e-o-ma′ne-ah) (*obs.*) erotomania.

aphronesia (af″ro-ne′ze-ah) [*a* neg. + Gr. *phronēsis* good sense] (*obs.*) dementia.

aphronia (ah-fro′ne-ah) [*a* neg. + Gr. *phronein* to understand] (*obs.*) deficiency in mental discernment; defect in cerebration.

aphtha (af′thah), pl. *aph′thae* [L.; Gr. *aphtha*] [usually plural] a small ulcer, especially the reddish or whitish spots in the mouth that characterize aphthous stomatitis. **Bednar's a.,** an infected traumatic ulcer on the posterior portion of the hard palate in infants. **chronic intermittent recurrent aphthae,** periadenitis mucosa necrotica recurrens. **contagious aphthae, epizootic aphthae,** foot-and-mouth disease of cattle. **epizootic aphthae,** foot-and-mouth disease. **malignant aphthae** (*obs.*), foot-and-mouth disease of cattle. **Mikulicz's aphthae,** periadenitis mucosa necrotica recurrens. **recurrent scarring aphthae,** periadenitis mucosa necrotica recurrens. **aphthae resisten′tiae,** periadenitis mucosa necrotica recurrens.

aphthae (af′the) [L.] plural of *aphtha.*

aphthoid (af′thoid) [Gr. *aphtha* thrush + *eidos* form] 1. resembling thrush; thrushlike. 2. an exanthema resembling that of thrush.

aphthongia (af-thon′je-ah) [*a* neg. + Gr. *phthongos* sound] aphasia due to spasm of the speech muscles.

aphthosis (af-tho′sis) any condition marked by aphthae.

aphthous (af′thus) pertaining to, characterized by, or affected with aphthae.

aphylactic (a″fi-lak′tik) pertaining to or characterized by aphylaxis.

aphylaxis (a″fi-lak′sis) absence of phylaxis.

apical (ap′e-kal) pertaining to or located at the apex.

apicectomy (a″pĭ-sek′to-me) 1. excision of the apex of the petrous portion of the temporal bone. 2. (obs.) apicoectomy.

apices (ap′ĭ-sēz) [L.] plural of apex.

apicitis (a″pe-si′tis) inflammation of an apex, as the apex of a tooth, the apex of the lung, or the apex of the petrous portion of the temporal bone (petrositis).

apicoectomy (a″pĕ-ko-ek′to-me) [apex + Gr. ektomē excision] excision of the apical portion of a tooth root through an opening made in the overlying labial, buccal, or palatal alveolar bone; see also root amputation.

apicolysis (a″pĕ-kol′ĭ-sis) [apex + Gr. lysis dissolution] the operation of causing the apex of the lung to collapse, for the purpose of obliterating an apical cavity.

apicostomy (a″pĕ-kos′to-me) [apex + Gr. stomoun to provide with an opening, or mouth] surgical formation of an opening through the gum and bone to the apical end of a tooth; called also dental trephination.

apicotomy (a″pe-kot′o-me) puncture of the apex of the petrous portion of the temporal bone.

apii (a′pe-i) genitive of apium. **a. fruc′tus,** see under Apium.

A.P.I.M. abbreviation for Association Professionnelle Internationale des Médecins, an international body which deals with the conduct of medical practice from the economic point of view.

apinealism (ah-pin′e-al-izm) the effects allegedly produced by removal of the pineal body.

apinoid (ap′ĭ-noid) [a neg. + Gr. pinos dirt + eidos form] clean; free from filth.

apiotherapy (a″pe-o-ther′ah-pe) treatment with bee venom.

apiphobia (a″pĕ-fo′be-ah) [L. apis bee + phobia] (obs.) morbid dread of bees and their sting.

apisination (a″pis-ĭ-na′shun) [L. apis bee] poisoning by the sting of bees.

apitoxin (a″pĕ-tok′sin) the toxic protein constituent of bee venom.

apituitarism (ah″pĭ-tu′ĭ-tar-izm″) hypopituitarism.

Apium (a′pe-um) [L.] a genus of umbelliferous plants, including celery; celery seed (apii fructus), the ripe fruit of A. graveolens; has been used as a diuretic and antispasmodic.

A.P.L. trademark for a preparation of human chorionic gonadotropin.

aplacental (a″plah-sen′tal) [a neg. + placenta] having no placenta.

aplanatic (ap″lah-nat′ik) [a neg. + Gr. planan to wander] pertaining to an optical system in which, for every position of a light source, all the light rays converge to a corresponding image point without aberrations.

aplanatism (ah-plan′ah-tizm) freedom from spherical aberration.

aplasia (ah-pla′zhe-ah) [a neg. + Gr. plassein to form] lack of development of an organ or tissue, or of the cellular products from an organ or tissue. Cf. agenesis and hypoplasia. **a. axia′lis extracortica′lis congen′ita,** familial centrolobar sclerosis. **a. cu′tis congen′ita,** localized failure of development of skin, most commonly of the scalp, less frequently of the trunk and limbs. The defects are usually covered by a thin translucent membrane or scar tissue, or may be raw, ulcerated, or covered by granulation tissue. **dental a.,** lack of formation or development of a tooth or teeth. **germinal a.,** gonadal a. **gonadal a.,** complete failure of gonad development; see Turner's syndrome, under syndrome. **nuclear a.,** Möbius' syndrome. **a. of ovary,** gonadal dysgenesis. **retinal a.,** failure of the retina to develop into functioning tissue, with subsequent secondary degenerative changes. **thymic a.,** absence of the thymus gland, as in DiGeorge's syndrome. **thymic-parathyroid a.,** DiGeorge's syndrome.

aplasmic (ah-plaz′mik) containing no protoplasm or sarcoplasm.

aplastic (ah-plas′tik) [a neg. + Gr. plassein to form] pertaining to or characterized by aplasia; anatomically undeveloped from the primordium or from the stem cell.

Aplectana (ah-plek′tah-nah) a genus of nematodes parasitic in the intestinal tract of amphibians and reptiles.

apleuria (ah-plu′re-ah) absence of ribs.

A.P.M. Academy of Physical Medicine; Academy of Psychosomatic Medicine.

apnea (ap-ne′ah) [a neg. + Gr. pnoia breath] 1. cessation of breathing. 2. asphyxia. **deglutition a.,** a temporary arrest of the activity of the respiratory nerve center during an act of swallowing. **initial a.,** a condition in which an infant fails to establish sustained respiration within two minutes of delivery. **late a.,** cessation of respiration in an infant for more than 60 seconds after spontaneous breathing has been established and sustained. **a. neonato′rum,** failure of the newborn infant to initiate pulmonary ventilation. **sleep a.,** transient attacks of failure of automatic control of respiration, resulting in alveolar hypoventilation, which becomes more pronounced during sleep. It may result in acidosis and in vasoconstriction of pulmonary arterioles, producing pulmonary arterial hypertension. **traumatic a.,** cessation of pulmonary ventilation following physical injury.

apneic (ap′ne ik) pertaining or relating to apnea or affected with apnea.

apneumatic (ap″nu-mat′ik) 1. free from air. 2. done with the exclusion of air.

apneumatosis (ap″nu-mah-to′sis) [a neg. + Gr. pneumatōsis inflation] congenital atelectasis of the lungs.

apneumia (ap-nu′me-ah) [a neg. + Gr. pneumōn lung] congenital absence of the lungs.

apneusis (ap-nu′sis) a condition marked by maintained inspiratory activity unrelieved by expiration, each inspiration being long and cramplike; it follows excision of the upper portion of the pons (pneumotaxic center).

apneustic (ap-nu′stik) pertaining to or characterized by apneusis.

apo-, ap- [Gr. apo from] a prefix implying separation or derivation from.

apoatropine (ap″o-ah′tro-pēn) chemical name: endo-α-methylenebenzeneacetic acid 8-methyl-8-azabicyclo[3.2.1]oct-3-yl ester. An antispasmodic alkaloid, $C_{17}H_{21}NO_2$, derived from belladonna.

apocamnosis (ap″o-kam-mo′sis) apokamnosis.

apocenosis (ap″o-sĕ-no′sis) an increased flow of blood or other body fluid.

apochromat (ap″o-kro-mat′) [apo- + chromatic aberration] an apochromatic objective; see under objective.

apochromatic (ap″o-kro-mat′ik) free from chromatic and spherical aberration; see under objective.

apocope (ah-pok′o-pe) [Gr. apokopē a cutting off; amputation.

apocoptic (ap″o-kop′tik) resulting from or pertaining to an amputation.

apocrine (ap′o-krin) [Gr. apokrinesthai to be secreted] denoting that type of glandular secretion in which the free end or apical portion of the secreting cell is cast off along with the secretory products that have accumulated therein.

apocrinitis (ap″o-krin-i′tis) bacterial infection of isolated single apocrine sweat glands.

apocrustic (ap″o-krus′tik) 1. astringent and repellent. 2. an astringent and repellent agent.

apocynin (ah-pos′ĕ-nin) see Apocynum.

Apocynum (ah-pos′ĕ-num) a genus of poisonous North American apocynaceous plants noted for their digitalis-like cardioactive principles, e.g., A. androsaemifolium L. (dogbane, wild or milk ipecac, rheumatism weed) and A. cannabinum L. (Canadian hemp, black Indian hemp). Both contain apocynin, formerly used like digitalis.

apodal (ah-po′dal) having no feet.

apodemialgia (ap″o-de″me-al′je-ah) [Gr. apodēmia journey + algos pain + -ia] (obs.) a morbid longing to go away from home.

Apodemus (ap″o-de′mus) a genus of Old World field mice. **A. sylvat′icus,** the wood mouse, a species that serves as a reservoir of Leptospira grippotyphosa.

apodia (ah-po′de-ah) [a neg. + Gr. pous foot + -ia] a developmental anomaly characterized by absence of one or both of the feet.

apoenzyme (ap″o-en′zīm) the protein component of an enzyme that is separable from the prosthetic group (or coenzyme) but that requires the presence of the prosthetic group to form the functioning compound (holoenzyme).

apoferment (ap-o-fer′ment) apoenzyme.

apoferritin (ap″o-fer′ĭ-tin) a colorless protein, with a molecular weight of 460,000, occurring in the mucosal cells of the small intestine, forming a compound with iron called ferritin, which has been implicated in the regulation of iron absorption in the gastrointestinal tract.

apogamia, apogamy (ap″o-gam′e-ah; ah-pog′ah-me) [apo- + Gr. gamein to wed] 1. reproduction without conjugation of gametes and usually without meiosis, as in certain seed plants. 2. parthenogenesis.

apogee (ap′o-je) the state of greatest severity of a disease.

apokamnosis (ap″o-kam-no′sis) abnormal liability to fatigue in myasthenia; a feeling of tiredness, numbness, and heaviness in a limb motion.

apolar (ah-po′lar) [a neg. + Gr. polos pole] not having poles or processes.

apolegamic (ap″o-leh-gam′ik) [Gr. apolegein to pick out + gamos marriage] pertaining to selection, especially sexual selection.

apolegamy (ap″o-leg′ah-me) selection, especially sexual selection in breeding.

apolepsis (ap″o-lep′sis) the suppression of a natural secretion.

apolipoprotein (ah″po-lip′o-pro′te-in) the protein moiety (moieties) of plasma lipoproteins which binds the lipid moiety to form the holoprotein.

Apollonia (ap″o-lo′ne-ah) the patron saint of dentistry; a Christian martyr who was first persecuted by having her teeth knocked out and then burned alive in A.D. 249. Her feast is observed February 9.

Apollonius (ap″o-lo′ne-us) the name by which several physicians of classical antiquity were known. For example, (1) a Greek physician, also called "the Empiric," who lived c. 200 B.C.; (2) a physician of Citium in Cyprus, who lived in the first century B.C. and who wrote a commentary on Hippocrates' treatise on articulations.

apomixia, apomixis (ap″o-mik′se-ah; ap″o-mik′sis) [apo- + Gr. mixis a mingling] 1. asexual reproduction in a species normally reproducing sexually, as in certain seed plants. 2. apogamia.

apomorphine (ap″o-mor′fin) [apo- + morphine] a crystalline alkaloid, $C_{17}H_{17}NO_2$, derived from morphine by the abstraction of a molecule of water; it is administered intravenously to induce instantaneous vomiting and was formerly used as an expectorant. **a. hydrochloride** [USP], a grayish crystalline compound, C_{17}-$H_{17}NO_2 \cdot HCl \cdot \frac{1}{2}H_2O$, a potent and prompt emetic.

aponeurectomy (ap″o-nu-rek′to-me) [aponeurosis + Gr. ektomē excision] excision of the aponeurosis of a muscle.

aponeurology (ap″o-nu-rol′o-je) [aponeurosis + -logy] the sum of knowledge regarding aponeuroses and fasciae.

aponeurorrhaphy (ap″o-nu-ror′ah-fe) [aponeurosis + Gr. rhaphē suture] suture of an aponeurosis; fasciorrhaphy.

aponeuroses (ap″o-nu-ro′sēz) plural of aponeurosis.

aponeurosis (ap″o-nu-ro′sis), pl. aponeuro′ses [Gr. aponeurōsis] [NA] 1. a white, flattened or ribbon-like tendinous expansion, serving mainly to connect a muscle with the parts that it moves. 2. a term formerly applied to certain fasciae. **abdominal a.,** the conjoined tendons of the oblique and transverse muscles on the abdomen. **bicipital a.,** a. musculi bicipitis brachii. **clavicoracoaxillary a.,** fascia clavipectoralis. **crural a.,** fascia cruris. **Denonvilliers' a.,** septum rectovesicale. **epicranial a.,** galea aponeurotica. **falciform a. of rectus abdominis muscle,** falx inguinalis. **femoral a.,** fascia lata femoris. **a. of insertion,** the connection of a muscle with the part or parts that it moves. **interchondral aponeuroses, internal** (obs.), see membrana intercostalis interna. **intercostal aponeuroses, external,** see membrana intercostalis externa. **intercostal aponeuroses, internal,** see membrana intercostalis interna. **a. of investment** (obs.), the fascial investment of a muscle. **ischioprostatic a.** (obs.), fascia diaphragmatis urogenitalis inferior. **ischiorectal a.** (obs.), fascia diaphragmatis pelvis inferior. **a. lin′guae** [NA], **lingual a.,** the connective tissue framework of the tongue, supporting and giving attachment to the intrinsic and extrinsic muscles; composed of the connective tissue layer of the tunica mucosa, the lingual septum, and the posterior transverse expansion of the septum which attaches to the hyoid bone. **a. mus′culi bicip′itis bra′chii** [NA], an expansion of the tendon of the biceps brachii muscle by which it is attached to the fascia of the forearm and to the ulna; called also bicipital a. or fascia, and lacertus fibrosus, semilunar fascia, and fibrous fasciculus of biceps muscle. **a. of occipitofrontal muscle,** galea aponeurotica. **palatine a.,** a fibrous sheet in the anterior part of the soft palate, derived mainly from the tendons of the two tensor muscles, giving attachment to the musculus uvulae and to the palatopharyngeus and levator veli palatini muscles. **palmar a., a. palma′ris** [NA], bundles of fibrous tissue radiating toward the bases of the fingers from the tendon of the palmaris longus muscle; called also volar fascia. **perineal a.,** fascia diaphragmatis urogenitalis inferior. **perineal a., superficial,** fascia diaphragmatis pelvis inferior. **perineal a., superior,** fascia diaphragmatis pelvis superior. **pharyngeal a., a. pharyn′gis, pharyngobasilar a., a. pharyngobasila′ris,** fascia pharyngobasilaris. **plantar a., a. planta′ris** [NA], bands of fibrous tissue radiating toward the bases of the toes from the medial process of the tuber calcanei; called also plantar fascia. **prostatic a., lateral** (obs.), fascia diaphragmatis urogenitalis superior. **Sibson's a.,** membrana suprapleuralis. **subscapular a.,** a fascia attached to the circumference of the subscapular fossa. **a. of superior surface of levator ani muscle,** fascia diaphragmatis pelvis superior. **supraspinous a.,** a dense fascia that partly envelops the supraspinous muscle. **temporal a.,** fascia temporalis. **vertebral a.,** fascia thoracolumbalis. **a. of Zinn,** see fibrae zonulares.

aponeurositis (ap″o-nu-ro-si′tis) [aponeurosis + -itis] inflammation of an aponeurosis.

aponeurotic (ap″o-nu-rot′ik) pertaining to or of the nature of an aponeurosis.

aponeurotome (ap″o-nu′ro-tōm) a knife for cutting aponeuroses.

aponeurotomy (ap″o-nu-rot′o-me) [aponeurosis + Gr. tomē a cut] surgical cutting of an aponeurosis.

aponia (ah-po′ne-ah) [Gr.] (obs.) freedom from pain.

aponic (ah-po′nik) relieving pain or fatigue.

aponoia (ap″o-noi′ah) [apo- + Gr. nous mind] (obs.) amentia.

Aponomma (ap″o-nom′ah) a genus of ticks infesting tropical reptiles of the Old World.

apopathetic (ap″o-pah-thet′ik) (obs.) a term applied to behavior in which the individual adapts his actions to the presence of other persons.

apophlegmatic (ap″o-fleg-mat′ik) causing a discharge of mucus; expectorant.

apophylactic (ap″o-fi-lak′tik) pertaining to or marked by apophylaxis.

apophylaxis (ap″o-fi-lak′sis) [apo- + phylaxis] decrease of the phylactic power of the blood, as seen in the negative phase of vaccine therapy.

apophysary (ah-pof′ĭ-za-re) apophyseal.

apophyseal (ap″o-fiz′e-al) pertaining to or of the nature of an apophysis.

apophyseopathy (ap″o-fiz-e-op′ah-the) [apophysis + Gr. pathos disease] disease of an apophysis, particularly Osgood-Schlatter disease.

apophyses (ah-pof′ĭ-sēz) plural of apophysis.

apophysial (ap″o-fiz′e-al) apophyseal.

apophysiary (ap″o-fiz′e-a″re) apophyseal.

apophysis (ah-pof′ĭ-sis), pl. apoph′yses [Gr. "an offshoot"] [NA] any outgrowth or swelling, especially a bony outgrowth that has never been entirely separated from the bone of which it forms a part, such as a process, tubercle, or tuberosity. **basilar a.,** pars basilaris ossis occipitalis. **cerebral a., a. cer′ebri,** pineal body. **genial a.,** spina mentalis. **a. of Ingrassias,** ala minor ossis sphenoidalis. **a. lenticula′ris in′cudis,** processus lenticularis incudis. **odontoid a., a. os′sium,** epiphysis. **a. raviana, a. raw′ii,** processus anterior mallei.

apophysitis (ah-pof″ĭ-zi′tis) inflammation of an apophysis, especially a disorder of the foot caused by disease of the epiphysis of the calcaneus. **a. tibia′lis adolescen′tium,** Osgood-Schlatter disease.

apoplasmatic (ap″o-plaz-mat′ik) pertaining to substances that are produced by cells and form a constituent part of the tissues of an organism, such as fibers of connective tissue or the matrix of bone and cartilage.

apoplectic (ap″o-plek′tik) [Gr. apoplēktikos] pertaining to, caused by, or affected with apoplexy.

apoplectiform (ap-o-plek′tĕ-form) resembling apoplexy.

apoplectoid (ap″o-plek′toid) resembling apoplexy.

apoplexia (ap″o-plek′se-ah) [L.] apoplexy. **a. u′teri,** sudden uterine hemorrhage, due to arterial degeneration or hemorrhagic infarct.

apoplexy (ap′o-plek″se) [Gr. apoplēxia] 1. an apoplectic stroke; sudden neurologic impairment due to a cerebrovascular disorder, limited by some to intracranial hemorrhage, extended by others to include occlusive cerebrovascular lesions. See stroke syndrome, under syndrome. 2. copious extravasation of blood within any organ. **abdominal a.,** spontaneous intraperitoneal hemorrhage due to rupture of an intra-abdominal blood vessel, independent of any trauma to the abdomen. **adrenal a.,** a morbid condition resulting from massive hemorrhage into the adrenal glands, occurring in Waterhouse-Friderichsen syndrome. **asthenic a.,** stroke syndrome resulting from debility. **bulbar a.,** hemorrhage into the substance of the pons; called also pontile a. or pontine a. **capillary a.,** stroke syndrome resulting from the rupture of capillary vessels. **cerebellar a.,** hemorrhage into the cerebellum. **cerebral a.,** cerebral hemorrhage. **delayed a.,** cerebral hemorrhage which comes on several days after the receipt of the injury. **embolic a.,** stroke syndrome due to stopping of a cerebral artery by an embolus. **fulminating a.,** cerebral hemorrhage in which the patient suddenly falls and quickly becomes unconscious. **heat a.,** heat stroke. **ingravescent a.,** progressive paralysis due to the slow leakage of blood from a ruptured vessel. **neonatal a.,** stroke syndrome in newborn infants. **ovarian a.,** extensive extravasation of blood into the ovary. **pancreatic a.,** extensive hemorrhage of the pancreas; seen in cardiac failure and portal hypertension. **parturient a.,** milk fever, def. 3. **pituitary a.,** sudden massive degeneration with hemorrhagic necrosis of the pituitary gland, associated with pituitary tumor, signaled by abrupt headache, followed by loss of sight, diplopia, drowsiness, and confusion, or coma. **placental a.,** hemorrhage into a separated placenta with formation of a hematoma between the placenta and uterine wall. **pontile a., pontine a.,** bulbar a. **Raymond's a.,** a type of ingravescent apoplexy marked by paresthesia of the hand on the side which later becomes paralyzed; called also Raymond's type of a. **renal a.,** a morbid condition resulting from rupture of an intrarenal blood vessel. **spinal a.,** bleeding or hemorrhage into the substance of the spinal cord. **thrombotic a.,** stroke syndrome due to thrombosis of a cerebral artery. **trau-**

matic late a., cerebral hemorrhage following trauma and appearing several days or weeks after the accident. **uteroplacental a.,** Couvelaire's term for a severe uterine condition seen in some cases of separation of the placenta, in which the uterine musculature is disrupted and infiltrated with blood.

apoprotein (ap″o-pro′te-in) the protein moiety of a compound, as of a lipoprotein. **a. CII,** an apoprotein of high-density and very-low-density lipoproteins, which functions to activate the enzyme lipoprotein lipase.

aporepressor (ap″o-re-pres′or) in genetic theory, a product of regulator genes, of unknown structure, which combines with low-molecular weight corepressor to form the complete repressor, which specifically represses the activity of certain structural genes.

aporioneurosis (ap-o″re-o″nu-ro′sis) [Gr. *aporia* doubt + *neurosis*] (*obs.*) anxiety neurosis.

aposia (ah-po′ze-ah) [*a* neg. + Gr. *posis* drinking + *-ia*] (*obs.*) absence of drinking, or reluctance to ingest fluids.

apositia (ap″o-sish′e-ah) [*apo-* + Gr. *sitos* food + *-ia*] (*obs.*) aversion to food.

apositic (ap″o-sit′ik) (*obs.*) pertaining to, characterized by, or causing apositia.

aposome (ap′o-sōm) [*apo-* + Gr. *sōma* body] an inclusion within the cytoplasm that has been made by the activity of the cell itself.

apostasis (ah-pos′tah-sis) [Gr.] 1. an abscess. 2. the end or crisis of an attack of disease.

apostem (ap′os-tem) (*obs.*) an abscess.

apostema (ap″os-te′mah) [Gr. *apostēma*] (*obs.*) an abscess.

aposthia (ah-pos′the-ah) [*a* neg. + Gr. *posthē* foreskin + *-ia*] congenital absence of the prepuce.

apothanasia (ap″o-thah-na′ze-ah) [*apo-* + Gr. *thanatos* death] the postponing of death; the prolongation of life.

apothecary (ah-poth′ĕ-ka″re) [Gr. *apothēke* storehouse] pharmacist. **surgeon a.,** in Great Britain, a practitioner who has passed the examinations required of a surgeon and of an apothecary.

apothecium (ap″o-the′se-um) an open or expanded fruiting body whose asci are contained on its exposed surface. Cf. *cleistothecium, gymnothecium,* and *perithecium.*

apothem (ap′o-them) [*apo-* + Gr. *thema* deposit] a dark deposit that sometimes appears in vegetable infusions and decoctions exposed to the air.

apotheme (ap′o-thēm) apothem.

apotoxin (ap′o-tok′sin) Richet's term for the poison that produces the symptoms of anaphylaxis.

apotripsis (ap″o-trip′sis) [Gr. *apotribein* to abrade] removal of a corneal opacity (Hirschberg).

apotropaic (ap″o-tro-pa′ik) [Gr. *apotropaios* averting evil] prophylactic, in the sense of averting evil influence (in Greek medicine).

apoxemena (ap″ok-sem′ĕ-nah) the material removed from a periodontal pocket in treatment of periodontitis.

apoxesis (ap″ok-se′sis) [Gr. *apoxein* to scrape off] the removal of detritus from a periodontal pocket.

apozem, apozema, apozeme (ap′o-zem, ap-oz′e-mah, ap′o-zēm) [Gr. *apozema* decoction, from *apo-* away + *zein* to boil] a medicinal or medicated decoction.

apozymase (ap″o-zi′mās) the portion of a zymase that requires the presence of a cozymase to become a complete or holozymase.

apparatus (ap″ah-ra′tus), pl. *apparatus* or *apparatuses* [L., from *ad* to + *parare* to make ready] an arrangement of a number of parts acting together in the performance of some special function; used in anatomical nomenclature to designate a number of structures or organs which act together in serving some particular function. **Abbe-Zeiss a.,** Thoma-Zeiss counting chamber. **absorption a.,** an apparatus used in gas analysis by means of which the sample to be examined is absorbed and its quantity thus estimated. **Barcroft's a.,** a differential manometer for studying small samples of blood or other tissues. **Beckmann's a.,** an apparatus for determining the molecular weight of a substance by dissolving the substance in a pure liquid and observing either the depression of the freezing point or the elevation of the boiling point of the liquid produced by the dissolved substance. **biliary a.,** the parts concerned in the formation, conduction, and storage of bile, including the secreting cells of the liver, bile ducts, and gallbladder. **central a.,** the dynamic organ of the cell that participates in mitosis; it consists of a centrosome, a centrosphere, and an astrosphere. **chromidial a.,** the chromatin staining material of the cytoplasm of a cell, occurring in the form of granules, rods, strands, and networks. **ciliary a.,** corpus ciliare. **a. derivato′rius,** the direct opening of small arteries into small veins without intervention of capillaries, as in phalanges and erectile tissues. **Desault's a.,** Desault's bandage. **digestive a., a. digesto′rius** [NA], the organs associated with the ingestion and digestion of food, including the mouth and associated structures, pharynx, and components of the digestive tube, as well as the associated organs and glands; called also *systema digestorius* [NA alternative]. **Fell-O'Dwyer a.,** a de-

vice used in performing artificial respiration and for preventing collapse of the lung in thoracic operations. **Finsen's a.,** Finsen's lamp; see under *lamp.* **genitourinary a.,** a. urogenitalis. **Golgi a.,** see under *complex.* **a. of Golgi-Rezzonico** (*obs.*), spiral filaments seen in the incisures of the myelin sheath, probably artifacts. **a. of Goormaghtigh,** juxtaglomerular cells. **Haldane a.,** see under *chamber.* **Hodgen's a.,** see under *splint.* **Jaquet's a.,** a recording apparatus for venous and cardiac impulses. **Junker a.,** see under *inhaler.* **juxtaglomerular a.,** a collective term for the juxtaglomerular cells in a nephron; see under *cell.* **Kirschner's a.,** an apparatus consisting of a wire and stirrup for applying skeletal traction in fractures of the limbs. **lacrimal a., a. lacrima′lis** [NA], the system concerned with the secretion and circulation of the tears and the normal fluid of the conjunctival sac; it consists of the lacrimal gland and ducts, and associated structures. See Plate accompanying *eye.* **a. ligamento′sus col′li,** membrana tectoria. **masticatory a.,** see under *system.* **mental a.,** the hypothetical aspects or parts of the mind or psyche, i.e., the id, the ego, and the superego. **a. of Perroncito,** a mass of fibrils in the form of spirals and networks with newly formed axons which develop in the cut stump of a nerve during regeneration; called also *Perroncito's spirals.* **pilosebaceous a.,** the complex consisting of a hair follicle and its sebaceous gland, and the erector pili muscle. **Potain's a.,** an apparatus used for aspiration. **a. respirato′rius** [NA], **respiratory a.,** the tubular and cavernous organs and structures by means of which pulmonary ventilation and gas exchange between ambient air and the blood are brought about. The chief organs involved are the nose, larynx, trachea, bronchi, bronchioles, and lungs. See Plate XLIX. Called also *respiratory system* and *systema respiratorium.* **Sayre's a.,** an apparatus for suspending a patient during the application of a plaster-of-Paris jacket. **Soxhlet's a.,** an apparatus by which fatty or lipid constituents can be extracted from solid matter by repeated treatment with distilled solvent. **spindle a.,** see *spindle,* def. 1. **steadiness a.,** ataxiagraph. **subneural a.,** evenly spaced, ribbon-like lamellae, formed by infolding of the sarcolemma lining the primary synaptic cleft, and projecting into the underlying sarcoplasm of muscle; the clefts between the lamellae are known as *secondary synaptic clefts.* **sucker a.,** sucker foot; see under *foot.* **a. suspenso′rius len′tis,** zonula ciliaris. **Taylor's a.,** see under *splint.* **a. of Timofeew,** a terminal nervous globular network within a lamellar corpuscle. **Tiselius a.,** an apparatus for the electrophoretic separation of the proteins of blood serum, plasma, and other body fluids. **urogenital a., a. urogenita′lis** [NA], the organs concerned in the production and excretion of urine, together with the organs of reproduction; see Plate L, under *system.* Called also *genitourinary a., genitourinary* or *urogenital system,* and *systema urogenitale.* **vasomotor a.,** the neuromuscular mechanism controlling the constriction and dilation of blood vessels and thus the amount of blood supplied to a part. **Waldenberg's a.,** an apparatus for exhausting or compressing air which is inhaled by the patient or into which the patient exhales. **Wangensteen's a.,** see under *tube.* **Warburg a.,** a device for measuring the quantity of gas liberated or consumed by respiring tissue slices enclosed in a chamber which is attached to a manometer and immersed in water at constant temperature. **Zander a.,** a group of machines designed for exercise of various parts of the body; rarely employed today.

appearance (ah-pēr′ans) [L. *apparere* to be visible] the visible manifestation of the characteristics of an object or entity.

appendage (ah-pen′dij) a thing or part appended; see also *adnexa* and *appendix.* **atrial a., auricular a.,** auricula atrii. **cecal a.,** appendix vermiformis. **a. of epididymis,** appendix epididymidis. **epiploic a's,** appendices epiploicae. **a's of the eye,** the lids, eyebrows, lacrimal apparatus, and conjunctiva; called also *adnexa oculi.* **a's of the fetus,** the trophoblast derivatives or extraembryonic membranes, including the umbilical cord, amnion, and chorion (placenta). **fibrous a. of liver,** appendix fibrosa hepatis. **ovarian a.,** the parovarium. **a's of the skin,** the hair, nails, sebaceous glands, sweat glands, and mammary glands. **testicular a., a. of the testis,** appendix testis. **uterine a's,** the ligaments of the uterus, and the oviducts and the ovaries; called also *adnexa uteri.* **a. of ventricle of larynx,** sacculus laryngis. **vermicular a.,** appendix vermiformis. **vesicular a's of epoophoron of Morgagni** (*obs.*), appendices vesiculosi epoophori.

appendagitis (ah-pen″dah-ji′tis) inflammation of an appendage, particularly of the epiploic appendages. **epiploic a.,** inflammation of one or more of the epiploic appendages of the colon, characterized by pain and tenderness over the affected area.

appendectomy (ap″en-dek′to-me) surgical removal of the vermiform appendix. **auricular a.,** excision of the auricular appendage (auricle) of the heart.

appendical (ah-pen′de-kal) appendiceal.

appendiceal (ap-en-dis′e-al) pertaining to an appendix.

appendicectomy (ah-pen″dĭ-sek′to-me) [*appendix* + Gr. *ektomē* excision] appendectomy.

appendices (ah-pen′dĭ-sēz) [L.] plural of *appendix.*

appendicitis (ah-pen″dĭ-si′tis) inflammation of the vermiform appendix. **actinomycotic a.,** that caused by *Actinomyces israeli.* **acute a.,** appendicitis of acute onset requiring surgical intervention and usually characterized by pain in the right lower abdominal quadrant with local and referred rebound tenderness, overlying muscle spasm, and cutaneous hyperesthesia. Periumbilical, colicky pain at the onset may be due to obstruction of the appendix by a fecalith. Fever and polymorphonuclear leukocytosis result from the localized infection. Symptoms and signs may be modified by the location of the appendix, by adhesive bands, or by kinking. **amebic a.,** appendicitis caused by infection with *Entamoeba histolytica.* **chronic a.,** 1. appendicitis characterized by fibrotic thickening of the wall of the organ due to previous acute inflammation. 2. a term formerly applied to chronic or recurrent pain in the appendiceal area in the absence of evidence of acute inflammation. **a. by contiguity,** appendicitis caused by infection from neighboring tissues. **foreign-body a.,** appendicitis, usually obstructive, due to a foreign body in the lumen. **fulminating a.,** appendicitis marked by sudden onset and rapid, fatal termination. **gangrenous a.,** appendicitis complicated by gangrene of the organ, owing to interference with the blood supply. **a. granulo′sa,** appendicitis developing on a disease of the mucous membrane which is marked by formation of granulation tissue between the gland tubules (Riedel). **helminthic a.,** verminous appendicitis. **left-sided a.,** 1. diverticulitis; so called because the symptoms resemble those of appendicitis, and the descending (or left) colon is the usual site of involvement. 2. left-sided appendicitis associated with situs inversus. **lumbar a.,** a type of appendicitis in which the appendix is posterior, lying against the peritoneum behind or below the cecum. **a. oblit′erans,** appendicitis with sclerosis and shrinking of the submucous tissue and plastic peritonitis, causing obliteration of the lumen of the appendix; called also *protective a.* **obstructive a.,** a common form of appendicitis attended by obstruction of the lumen of the appendix, usually by a fecalith. **perforating a., perforative a.,** appendicitis with perforation of the organ. **protective a.,** a. obliterans. **purulent a.,** suppurative a. **recurrent a.,** that characterized by recurrent attacks of acute appendicitis. **relapsing a.,** recurrence of appendiceal inflammation after improvement; recurrent appendicitis. **segmental a.,** inflammation confined to a segment of the appendix; it may be proximal, central, or distal. **skip a.,** appendicitis in which two or more areas of focal inflammation are separated by normal appendiceal tissue. **stercoral a.,** appendicitis in which a fecal concretion is the assumed cause. **subperitoneal a.,** appendicitis in which the appendix is buried under the peritoneum instead of being free in the peritoneal cavity. **suppurative a.,** purulent infiltration of the walls of the appendix; called also *purulent a.* **traumatic a.,** appendicitis caused by external trauma. **verminous a.,** appendicitis due to the presence of a worm in the appendix.

appendicocecostomy (ah-pen″dĭ-ko-se-kos′to-me) the formation of an abnormal opening between the appendix and cecum, usually by surgical means; also, the orifice so established.

appendicocele (ah-pen′dĭ-ko-sēl″) hernia containing the vermiform appendix.

appendicoenterostomy (ah-pen″dĭ-ko″en-ter-os′to-me) the formation of an anastomosis between the vermiform appendix and the intestine.

appendicolithiasis (ah-pen″dĭ-ko″lĭ-thi′ah-sis) [*appendix* + *lithiasis*] a condition marked by concretions in the vermiform appendix.

appendicolysis (ah-pen″dĭ-ko-li′sis) [*appendix* + Gr. *lysis* dissolution] the surgical division of adhesions about the appendix.

appendicopathia (ah-pen″dĭ-ko-path′e-ah) (*obs.*) appendicopathy. **a. oxyu′rica,** disease of the vermiform appendix caused by *Oxyuris.*

appendicopathy (ah-pen″dĭ-kop′ah-the) [*appendix* + Gr. *pathos* disease] any diseased condition of the vermiform appendix.

appendicostomy (ah-pen″dĭ-kos′to-me) [*appendix* + Gr. *stomoun* to provide with an opening, or mouth] surgical creation of an opening from the surface of the abdominal wall into the vermiform appendix for the purpose of irrigating or draining the large bowel; called also *Weir's operation.*

appendicular (ap″en-dik′u-lar) 1. pertaining to the vermiform appendix. 2. pertaining to an appendage.

appendix (ah-pen′diks), pl. *appendixes, appen′dices* [L. from *appendere* to hang upon] a general term used in anatomical nomenclature to designate a supplementary, accessory, or dependent part attached to a main structure; called also *appendage.* Frequently used alone to refer to the *appendix vermiformis* [NA], or *vermiform appendix.* **auricular a.,** auricula atrii. **cecal a.,** a. vermiformis. **ensiform a.,** processus xiphoideus. **a. epidid′ymidis** [NA], **a. of epididymis,** a remnant of the mesonephros sometimes situated on the head of the epididymis; called also *appendage of epididymis.* **epiploic appendices, appen′dices epiplo′icae** [NA], peritoneum-covered tabs of fat, 2 to 10 cm. long, attached in rows along the tenia of the colon. **a. fibro′sa hep′atis** [NA], **fibrous a. of liver,** a fibrous band at the left extremity of the liver, being the atrophied remnant of

formerly more extensive liver tissue. **a. morgagn′ii,** see *appendix testis* and *appendices vesiculosi epoophori.* **a. tes′tis** [NA], the remnant of the müllerian duct (ductus paramesonephricus) on the upper end of the testis; called also *a. morgagnii, testicular appendage, hydatid of Morgagni,* and *sessile hydatid.* **a. of ventricle of larynx, a. ventriculilaryn′gis,** sacculus laryngis. **a. vermic′ularis, vermiform a.,** a vermiformis. **a. vermifor′mis** [NA], vermiform appendix; a wormlike diverticulum of the cecum, varying in length from 3 to 6 inches, and measuring about 1/3 inch in diameter. **appen′dices vesiculo′si epooph′ori** [NA], small pedunculated structures attached to the uterine tubes near their fimbriated end, being remnants of the mesonephric ducts; called also *a. morgagnii, vesicular appendages of epoophoron,* and *hydatids of Morgagni.* **xiphoid a.,** processus xiphoideus.

appendolithiasis (ah-pen″do-lĭ-thi′ah-sis) appendicolithiasis.

apperception (ap″er-sep′shun) [L. *ad* to + *percipere* to perceive] conscious perception and appreciation; the power of receiving, appreciating, and interpreting sensory impressions.

apperceptive (ap″er-sep′tiv) pertaining to apperception.

appersonification (ap″er-son″ĭ-fi-ka′shun) the identification of one's self with another person.

appestat (ap′pĕ-stat) [appetite + Gr. *statoe* standing] the brain center (probably in the hypothalamus) concerned with controlling the amount of food intake.

appet (ap′et) Dunlap's term for that which in connection with anticipatory thinking constitutes a desire.

appetite (ap′ĕ-tīt) [L. *appetere* to desire] a natural longing or desire, especially the natural and recurring desire for food. **excessive a.,** bulimia. **perverted a.,** the longing for unnatural and indigestible things as articles of food; pica.

appetition (ap″ĕ-tish′un) [L. *ad* toward + *petere* to seek] the directing of desire toward a definite purpose or object.

appetitive (ap-pet′ĭ-tiv″) characterized by approach, or exciting approach behavior; said of stimuli or behavior. Cf. *aversive.*

applanation (ap″lah-na′shun) [L. *applanatio*] undue flatness, as of the cornea.

applanometer (ap″lah-nom′ĕ-ter) an instrument for determining intraocular pressure in the detection of glaucoma; it may be mechanical or electronic. See *tonometer.*

apple (ap′'l) the edible fruit of the rosaceous tree, *Pyrus malus* L. (= *Malus sylvestrus* Mill); also the tree itself. Apple seeds are known to be cyanogenetic, and ingestion of large quantities (cupful) have proven fatal to man. Dried apples in powdered form are used as an antidiarrheal. **Adam's a.,** prominentia laryngea. **bitter a.,** colocynth. **Indian a., May a.,** podophyllum. **thorn a.,** stramonium.

appliance (ah-pli′ans) a device used for performing or for facilitating the performance of a particular function. In orthodontics, a device used in the mouth to produce or prevent movement of teeth, so that malopposed teeth and jaws may be brought into proper alignment and occlusion. **Andresen a.,** monobloc activator. **Begg a.,** a fixed, multibanded orthodontic appliance incorporating a concept of differential light forces and using a modified ribbon-arch attachment. **Bimler a.,** a removable orthodontic appliance. **craniofacial a.,** a device used to immobilize and/or reduce mandibular or midfacial fractures. **Crozat a.,** a removable wrought-wire orthodontic appliance, used to align the teeth and correct malocclusion. **extraoral a.,** an appliance that utilizes the top and back of the head and/or neck for anchorage or a resistance unit, such as a headgear, cervical gear, etc. **fixed a.,** an appliance that is cemented to the teeth or attached by means of an adhesive material. **Frankel a.,** function corrector. **functional a.,** monobloc a. **Johnson twin wire a.,** a light wire orthodontic appliance; see *twin wire,* under *wire.* **orthodontic a.,** a mechanism for the application of force to the teeth and their supporting tissues to produce changes in the relationship of the teeth and related osseous structures. **prosthetic a.,** a device affixed to or implanted in the body, designed to take the place, or perform the function, of a missing body part, such as an artificial arm or leg, or a complete or partial denture. **removable a.,** any orthodontic appliance that the patient is able to insert and remove from the mouth. **thumb-sucking a.,** an appliance designed to discourage a deforming thumb-sucking habit. **universal a.,** an orthodontic device incorporating the edgewise and ribbon arch techniques, affording precise control of individual teeth in all planes of space.

applicator (ap′lĭ-ka″tor) an instrument for making local applications. **sonic a.,** an electromechanical transducer used in the local application of sound for therapeutic purposes, as in the treatment of muscular ailments.

appliqué (ap″lĭ-ka′) see under *form.*

Apponus, Petrus see *Peter of Abano.*

apposition (ap″o-zish′un) [L. *appositio*] the placing of things in juxtaposition or proximity; specifically, the deposition of successive layers upon those already present, as in cell walls. Called also *juxtaposition.*

apprehension (ap″re-hen′shun) 1. perception and understanding. 2. anticipatory fear or anxiety.

approach (ah-prōch′) 1. in surgery, the specific procedures by which an organ or part is exposed. 2. in psychiatry, the manner in which personal conflicts are dealt with. **Risdon a.,** a surgical method of exposing the ascending ramus of the mandible by means of an incision made below and behind the angle of the mandible, for treatment of fractures, e.g., condylar fractures, or for reconstructive surgery.

approximal (ah-prok′sĭ-mal) situated close together.

approximate (ah-prok′sĭ-māt″) 1. to bring close together, or into apposition. 2. approximal.

approximation (ah-prok″sĭ-ma′shun) the act or process of bringing closer together or into apposition. **successive a.,** shaping.

apractic (ah-prak′tik) pertaining to or characterized by apraxia.

apramycin (ap″rah-mi′sin) an antibacterial antibiotic, $C_{21}H_{41}$-N_5O_{11}, produced by *Streptomyces tenebrarius.*

apraxia (ah-prak′se-ah) [Gr. "a not acting," "want of success"] loss of ability to carry out familiar, purposeful movements in the absense of paralysis or other motor or sensory impairment, especially inability to make proper use of an object. **akinetic a.,** loss of ability to carry out spontaneous movement. **amnestic a.,** loss of ability to carry out a movement on command as a result of inability to remember the command, although ability to perform the movement is present. **Bruns' a. of gait,** apraxia in which the patient walks with a broad-based gait, taking short steps with the feet placed flat on the ground and with a tendency to retropulsion. **classic a.,** ideokinetic a. **constructional a.,** a type of motor incapacity characterized by lack of ability to copy simple drawings or to reproduce patterns created with building blocks or matchsticks. **cortical a.,** motor a. **ideational a.,** sensory a. **ideokinetic a., ideomotor a.,** a form due to an interruption between the ideation center and the center for the limb; in it, simple movements can be performed but not complicated ones. Called also *limb-kinetic a.* and *transcortical a.* **innervation a.,** motor a. **Liepmann's a.,** inability to perform coordinated movements of the limbs, without actual paralysis. **limb-kinetic a.,** ideokinetic a. **motor a.,** loss of ability to make proper use of an object, although its proper nature is recognized; called also *cortical* or *innervation a.* **sensory a.,** loss of ability to make proper use of an object, due to lack of perception of its proper nature and purpose; called also *ideational a.* **transcortical a.,** ideokinetic a.

apraxic (ah-prak′sik) apractic.

Apresoline (ah-pres′o-lēn) trademark for preparations of hydralazine.

aprindine (ah-prin′dēn) chemical name: *N*-(2,3-dihydro-1*H*-inden-2-yl)-*N*′,*N*′-diethyl-*N*-phenyl-1,3-propandiamine; a cardiac depressant, $C_{22}H_{30}N_2$, which has been used as an antirrhythmic. **a. hydrochloride,** the monohydrochloride salt of aprindine, $C_{22}H_{30}N_2 \cdot HCl$, having the same actions and uses as the base.

aprobarbital (ap″ro-bar′bĭ-tal) chemical name: 5-(1-methylethyl)-5-(2-propenyl)-2,4,6(1*H*,3*H*,5*H*)-pyrimidinetrione. An intermediate-acting barbiturate, $C_{10}H_{14}N_2O_3$, occurring as a fine, white, crystalline powder; used as a sedative and hypnotic, administered orally. Abuse of this drug may lead to dependence.

Aprocta (ah-prok′tah) a genus of filarial organisms. *A. microanalis* and *A. semenova* infest the orbital and nasal cavities of birds.

aproctia (ah-prok′she-ah) [*a* neg. + Gr. *prōktos* anus] congenital absence or imperforation of the anus.

apron (a′prun) a piece of clothing worn as a protection for the body in front. **Hottentot a., pudendal a.,** artificially or abnormally elongated nymphae.

aprosexia (ap″ro-sek′se-ah) [*a* neg. + Gr. *prosechein* to heed] (*obs.*) a condition in which there is inability to fix the attention; inattention due to mental weakness or to defective hearing, and often seen in chronic catarrh of the nose or of the nasopharynx (*aprosexia nasalis*).

aprosody (a-pros′o-de) absence of the normal variations in stress, pitch, and rhythm of speech.

aprosopia (ap″ro-so′pe-ah) [*a* neg. + Gr. *prosōpon* face] partial or complete congenital absence of structures of the face.

aprosopus (ah-pro′so-pus) a monster exhibiting aprosopia.

aprotic (a-pro′tik) denoting a substance that does not possess dissociable protons.

aprotinin (ah-pro-ti′nin) a polypeptide, obtained from animal organs, which inhibits proteinase and kallikrein; it has been used in the treatment of pancreatitis.

A.P.S. American Pediatric Society; American Physiological Society; American Proctologic Society; American Psychological Society; American Psychosomatic Society.

apselaphesia (ap″sel-ah-fe′ze-ah) [*a* neg. + Gr. *psēlaphēsis* touch] diminution of the sense of touch.

apsithyria (ap″sĭ-thi′re-ah) [*a* neg. + Gr. *psithyros* whispering + *ia*] (*obs.*) hysterical loss of speech and even of the ability to whisper.

apsychia (ah-si′ke-ah) [*a* neg. + Gr. *psychē* soul + *-ia*] 1. loss or lack of consciousness. 2. a faint or swoon.

apsychical (ah-si′ke-kal) not psychical or mental.

apsychosis (ah″si-ko′sis) [*a* neg. + Gr. *psychē* soul + *-osis*] (*obs.*) absence or loss of the function of thought.

A.P.T. alum-precipitated toxoid.

A.P.T.A. American Physical Therapy Association.

apterous (ap′ter-us) [*a* neg. + Gr. *pteron* wing] wingless.

Apterygiformes (ap″tĕ-rij″ĭ-form′ēz) the order of kiwis, flightless birds with vestigial wings.

aptitude (ap′tĭ-tūd) natural ability and skill in certain lines of endeavor.

aptyalia, aptyalism (ap″ti-a′le-ah, ap-ti′ah-lizm) [*a* neg. + Gr. *ptyalizein* to spit] deficiency or absence of the saliva; xerostomia; asialia.

APUD [*amine precursor uptake (and) decarboxylation*] an acronym for a group of apparently unrelated endocrine cells which share a number of cytochemical and ultrastructural characteristics and that produce polypeptide hormones and neurotransmitters. See *amine precursor uptake and decarboxylation cells,* under *cell.*

apudoma (ah″pud-o′mah) any tumor composed of APUD cells.

apulmonism (ah-pul′mo-nizm) [*a* neg. + L. *pulmo* lung] a developmental anomaly characterized by partial or complete absence of a lung.

apus (a′pus) [*a* neg. + Gr. *pous* foot] an individual exhibiting apodia.

apyetous (ah-pi′ĕ-tus) [*a* neg. + Gr. *pyon* pus] showing no pus; not suppurating.

apyknomorphous (ah-pik″no-mor′fus) [*a* neg. + Gr. *pyknos* compact + *morphē* form] not pyknomorphous; not having the stainable cell elements compactly placed—said of certain nerve cells.

apyogenous (ah″pi-oj′ĕ-nus) not caused by pus.

apyous (ah-pi′us) [*a* neg. + Gr. *pyon* pus] having no pus; nonpurulent.

apyrene (ah′pi-rēn) [*a* neg. + Gr. *pyrēn* fruit stone, nucleus] having no nucleus or nuclear material.

apyretic (ah″pi-ret′ik) [*a* neg. + *pyretic*] having no fever; afebrile.

apyrexia (ah″pi-rek′se-ah) [*a* neg. + *pyrexia*] the absence or intermission of fever.

apyrexial (ah″pi-rek′se-al) pertaining to apyrexia, or to the stage of intermission of a fever.

apyrogenic (ah-pi″ro-jen′ik) [*a* neg. + Gr. *pyr* fever + *gennan* to produce] not producing fever.

A.Q. achievement quotient.

Aq. Abbreviation for L. *a′qua,* water. **Aq. dest.,** L. *a′qua destilla′ta,* distilled water. **Aq. pur.,** L. *a′qua pu′ra,* pure water. **Aq. tep.** L. *a′qua tep′ida,* tepid water.

aqua (ah′kwah, ak′wah), gen. and pl. *a′quae* [L.] water. See also *aromatic water* and various other forms listed under *water.* **a. am′nii,** amniotic fluid. **a. ani′si,** anise water. **a. aromat′ica,** aromatic water. **a. astric′ta,** frozen water. **a. bul′liens,** boiling water. **a. cal′cis,** calcium hydroxide solution. **a. cam′phorae,** camphor water. **a. chlorofor′mi,** chloroform water. **a. cinnamo′mi,** cinnamon water. **a. commu′nis,** ordinary water. **a. destilla′ta,** distilled water. **a. destilla′ta steril′is,** sterile distilled water. **a. fer′vens,** hot water. **a. foenic′uli,** fennel water. **a. for′tis,** a solution of nitric acid. **a. gaulthe′ria,** wintergreen water. **a. hamamel′idis,** hamamelis water. **a. labyrin′thi** (*obs.*), the clear fluid in the labyrinth of the ear. **a. men′thae piperi′tae,** peppermint water. **a. men′thae vir′idis,** spearmint water. **a. oc′uli,** the aqueous humor or fluid of the eye. **a. pericar′dii,** the pericardial fluid. **a. pro injectio′ne,** water for injection. **a. pu′ra,** pure water. **a. re′gia,** nitrohydrochloric acid. **a. ro′sae,** rose water. **a. ro′sae for′tior,** stronger rose water. **a. sterilisa′ta,** sterilized water. **a. tep′ida,** warm water. **a. vi′tae,** brandy.

Aquacare (ah′kwah-kār) trademark for preparations of urea.

aquae (ak′we, ah′kwe) [L.] plural of *aqua.*

aquaeductus (ak″we-duk′tus), pl. *aquaeduc′tus* [L.] aqueductus.

AquaMEPHYTON (ak″wah-mef′ĭ-ton) trademark for a preparation of phytonadione.

aquaphobia (ak″wah-fo′be-ah) morbid fear of water.

aquapuncture (ak″wah-pungk′tūr) [L. *aqua* water + *puncture*] the subcutaneous injection of water.

Aquatag (ah′kwah-tag) trademark for a preparation of benzthiazide.

Aquatensen (ak″wah-ten′sen) trademark for a preparation of methyclothiazide.

aquatic (ah-kwat′tik) inhabiting or frequenting water.

aqueduct (ak′we-dukt″) a passage or channel in a body structure or organ; see also *aqueductus.* **cerebral a.,** aqueductus cerebri. **a. of cochlea,** 1. ductus perilymphatici. 2. canaliculus cochleae. **a. of Cotunnius,** 1. aqueductus vestibuli. 2. canaliculus cochleae. **fallopian a., a. of Fallopius,** canalis facialis. **a. of midbrain,** aqueductus cerebri. **a. of Sylvius,** aqueductus cerebri. **ventricular a.,** aqueductus cerebri. **a. of the vestibule,** aqueductus vestibuli.

aqueductus (ak″we-duk′tus) [L., from *aqua* water + *ductus* canal] [NA] a passage or channel in a body structure or organ, especially a channel for the conduction of fluid; called also *aqueduct* and *aquaeductus.* **a. cer′ebri** [NA], cerebral aqueduct: the narrow channel in the midbrain, about 1 cm. long, that connects the third and fourth ventricles; called also *aqueduct* or *iter of Sylvius,* and *mesocele.* **a. cochle′ae,** 1. NA alternative for *ductus perilymphatici.* 2. canaliculus cochleae. **a. endolymphat′icus,** ductus endolymphaticus. **a. vestib′uli** [NA], aqueduct of vestibule: 1. a small canal extending from the vestibule of the inner ear to open onto the posterior surface of the petrous part of the temporal bone. It lodges the endolymphatic duct and an arteriole and a venule. Called also *aqueduct of Cotunnius.* 2. NA alternative for ductus endolymphaticus.

aqueous (a′kwe-us) [L. *aqua* water] 1. watery; prepared with water. 2. the aqueous humor of the eye; see under *humor.*

Aquex trademark for a preparation of clopamide.

aquiparous (ak-wip′ah-rus) [L. *aqua* water + *parere* to produce] producing water or a watery secretion.

aquocapsulitis (a″kwo-kap″su-li′tis) [L. *aqua* water + *capsulitis*] serous iritis.

aquula (ak′woo-lah) [L.] a little stream. **a. auditi′va exter′na** (*obs.*), perilymph. **a. auditi′va inter′na** (*obs.*), endolymph. **a. cotun′nii, a. labyrin′thi exter′na** (*obs.*), perilymph. **a. labyrin′thi inter′na** (*obs.*), **a. labyrin′thi membrana′cei** (*obs.*), endolymph.

AR alarm reaction; aortic regurgitation; artificial respiration.

Ar chemical symbol for *argon.*

A.R.A. American Rheumatism Association.

ara-A adenine arabinoside; see *vidarabine.*

araban (ar′ah-ban) a pentosan, $(C_5H_{10}O_5)_n$, found in various gums and pectins, consisting of a mixture of anhydrides of l-arabinose.

arabanase (ah-rab′ĭ-nās) an enzyme that catalyzes the hydrolysis of araban to arabinose.

arabate (ar′ah-bāt) a salt of arabic acid.

arabin (ar′ah-bin) an amorphous carbohydrate, $(C_5H_{10}O_5)_2 + H_2O$, from gum arabic, soluble in water; called also *arabic acid.*

arabinose (ah-rab′ĭ-nōs) gum sugar; a crystalline aldo-pentose, $CH_2OH(CHOH)_3CHO$, obtained from vegetable gums by acid hydrolysis and sometimes found in urine. d-Arabinose is a constituent of aloin; l-arabinose is the gum sugar.

arabinosis (ah-rab″ĭ-no′sis) poisoning by arabinose, which may produce nephrosis.

arabinosuria (ah-rab″ĭ-no-su′re-ah) the presence of arabinose in the urine.

arabinosylcytosine (ah-rab″ĭ-no-sil-si′to-sēn) cytarabine.

arabinulose (ar″ah-bin′u-lōs) a ketopentose.

arabite (ar′ah-bīt) a sweet crystalline principle, $C_5H_{12}O_5$, derivable from arabinose by the action of sodium amalgam.

arabitol (ah-rab′ĭ-tol) an alcohol, $CH_2OH(CHOH)_3CH_2OH$, formed by the reduction of arabinose.

arabopyranose (ar″ah-bo-pi′rah-nōs) arabinose.

ara-C cytosine arabinoside; see *cytarabine.*

arachidate (ah-rak′ĭ-dāt) eicosanoate: the ionic form of arachidic acid, $C_{20}H_{40}O_2$, a naturally occurring fatty acid.

arachidic (ar″ah-kid′ik) [L. *arachis* peanut] caused by peanut kernels, as arachidic bronchitis following accidental inhalation of a peanut.

arachnephobia (ah-rak″ne-fo′be-ah) arachnophobia.

arachnid (ah-rak′nid) any member of the class Arachnida.

Arachnida (ah-rak′nĭ-dah) [Gr. *arachnē* spider] a class of the Arthropoda, including the spiders, ticks, mites, and scorpions.

arachnidism (ah-rak′nĭ-dizm) the condition produced by the bite of a venomous spider; spider envenomation. Called also *araneism.*

arachnitis (ar″ak-ni′tis) [*arachno-* + *-itis*] arachnoiditis.

arachno- (ah-rak′no) [Gr. *arachnē* spider] a combining form denoting relationship to the arachnoid membrane or to a spider.

arachnodactylia (ah-rak″no-dak-til′e-ah) arachnodactyly.

arachnodactyly (ah-rak″no-dak′tĭ-le) [*arachno-* + Gr. *daktylos* finger] a condition characterized by abnormal length and slenderness of the fingers and toes; called also *acromacria, dolichostenomelia,* and *spider finger.* Sometimes used in the past as a synonym for *Marfan's syndrome.*

arachnogastria (ah-rak″no-gas′tre-ah) [*arachno-* + Gr. *gastēr* stomach + *-ia*] the prominent network of veins on the protuberant abdomen caused by ascites, especially in hepatic cirrhosis.

arachnoid (ah-rak′noid) 1. resembling a spider's web. 2.

arachnoidea. **a. of brain, cranial a.,** arachnoidea encephali. **spinal a., a. of spinal cord,** arachnoidea spinalis.

arachnoidal (ar″ak-noi′dal) or of pertaining to the arachnoid.

arachnoidea (ar″ak-noi′de-ah), pl. *arachnoi′deae* [Gr. *arachnoeidēs* like a cobweb] [NA] a delicate membrane interposed between the dura mater and the pia mater, being separated from the pia mater by the subarachnoid space. **a. enceph′ali** [NA], the arachnoidea covering the brain; called also *arachnoid of brain* and *cranial arachnoid.* **a. spina′lis** [NA], spinal arachnoid: the arachnoidea covering the spinal cord; called also *arachnoid of spinal cord.*

arachnoideae (ar″ak-noi′de-e) plural of *arachnoidea.*

arachnoidism (ah-rak′noi-dizm″) the condition produced by the bite of venomous spiders.

arachnoiditis (ah-rak″noid-i′tis) [*arachnoid* + *-itis*] inflammation of the arachnoidea; called also *arachnitis.* **chronic adhesive a.,** thickening and adhesions of the leptomeninges in the brain or spinal cord, resulting from previous meningitis, other disease processes, or trauma; the signs and symptoms vary with extent and location.

arachnolysin (ar″ak-nol′ĭ-sin) [*arachno-* + *lysin*] the active hemolytic principle of spider venom.

arachnophobia (ah-rak″no-fo′be-ah) [*arachno-* + Gr. *phobos* fear + *-ia*] morbid fear of spiders.

arachnopia (ar″ak-no′pe-ah) [*arachno-* + *pia*] (*obs.*) the pia-arachnoid.

arachnorhinitis (ah-rak″no-ri-ni′tis) [*arachno-* + *rhinitis*] disease of the nasal passages caused by the presence of a spider.

arack (ah-rak′) arrack.

Aradidae (ah-rad′ĭ-de) a family of broad flat bugs which inhabit crevices under bark and similar sites; some species bite man, but are of no medical importance.

Aralen (ār′ah-len) trademark for a preparation of chloroquine.

Aralia (ah-ra′le-ah) [L.] a genus of aromatic and diaphoretic plants, including spikenard or pettymorrel (*A. racemosa*), dwarf elder (*A. hispida*), and other plants used in domestic medicine. Volatile oil appears to be the active constituent. It is one of the ingredients of compound white pine syrup. Called also *spice berry.*

aralia (ah-ra′le-ah) the dried rhizome and roots of *Aralia racemosa;* an ingredient of compound white pine syrup.

aralkyl (ah-ral′kil) an aryl derived from an alkyl radical.

Aramine (ār′ah-min) trademark for a preparation of metaraminol.

Aran's law (ar-ahnz′) [François Amilcar *Aran,* French physician, 1817–1861] see under *law.*

Aran-Duchenne muscular atrophy (disease) (ar-ahn′doo-shen′) [François Amilcar *Aran;* Guillaume Benjamin Amand *Duchenne,* French neurologist, 1806–1875] muscular atrophy; see under *atrophy.*

Araneae (ah-rän′e-e) an order of the Arachnida comprising the spiders; it is divided into the suborders Labidognatha and Orthognatha.

Araneida (ar″ah-ne′ĭ-dah) Araneae.

araneism (ah-ra′ne-izm) spider envenomation.

araneous (ah-ra′ne-us) [L. *araneum* cobweb] like a cobweb.

Arantius' bodies, etc. (ah-ran′she-us) [Julius Caesar *Arantius* (Italian *Aranzi*), an Italian anatomist and physician, 1530–1589] see under *body, canal, duct, ligament, nodule,* and *ventricle.*

Aranzi see *Arantius.*

araphia (ah-ra′fe-ah) [*a* neg. + Gr. *rhaphē* seam] dysraphia.

araroba (ar″ah-ro′bah) [Brazilian] 1. *Andira.* 2. Goa powder.

arbaprostil (ar″bah-prost′il) chemical name: (5Z,11α,13E,-15R)-11,15-dihydroxy-15-methyl-9-oxo-prosta-5,13-diene-1-oic acid; a synthetic 15-methyl analogue of dinoprostone, a prostaglandin of the E type, $C_{21}H_{34}O_5$; its esters have been used orally to reduce gastric secretion in the treatment of gastric ulcer and intramuscularly for termination of pregnancy.

arbor (ar′bor), pl. *arbo′res* [L.] a treelike structure or part; a structure or system resembling a tree with its branches. **a. medulla′ris ver′mis,** a. vitae cerebelli. **a. vi′tae,** *Thuja occidentalis,* or white cedar, a tree of the family Cupressaceae, native to eastern North America. Oil from the leaves is used as an expectorant, antirheumatic, and emmenagogue, and externally as a counterirritant and for dermatological diseases. **a. vi′tae cerebel′li** [NA], the treelike outline of white substance seen in a median section of the cerebellum; called also *a. medullaris vermis, a. vitae of vermis, medullary body of vermis, corpus medullare vermis,* and *arborescent white substance of cerebellum.* **a. vi′tae u′teri,** plicae palmatae. **a. vitae of vermis,** a. vitae cerebelli.

arboreal (ar-bo′re-al) pertaining to trees; inhabiting or attached to trees.

arbores (ar′bo-rēz) [L.] plural of *arbor.*

arborescent (ar″bo-res′ent) [L. *arborescens*] branching like a tree.

arborization (ar″bor-ĭ-za′shun) 1. the branching termination of certain nerve cell processes. 2. a form of the termination of a nerve fiber when in contact with a muscle fiber. 3. the treelike appearance of capillary vessels in inflamed conditions.

arboroid (ar′bo-roid) [L. *arbor* a tree] branching like a tree.

arborvirus (ar″bor-vi′rus) former term for *arbovirus*.

arboviral (ar″bo-vi′ral) pertaining to or caused by arboviruses.

arbovirus (ar″bo-vi′rus) [from *arthropod-borne* + virus] any of a group of viruses, including the causative agents of yellow fever, viral encephalitides, and certain febrile infections, which are transmitted to man by various mosquitoes and ticks; those transmitted by ticks are often considered in a separate category (tickborne viruses).

arbutin (ar′bu-tin) [L. *Arbutus*] see *Arbutus*.

Arbutus (ar′bu-tus) [L.] a genus of ericaceous trees and shrubs which contain arbutin, a hydroquinone glycoside that has been used for its diuretic and urinary antiseptic properties. **A. u′va-ur′si**, *Arctostaphylos uva-ursi*.

A.R.C. American Red Cross; anomalous retinal correspondence.

arc (ark) [L. *arcus* bow] a structure or projected path having a curved or bowlike outline; by extension, a visible electrical discharge generally taking the outline of an arc. In neurophysiology, the pathway of neural reactions. **auricular a., binauricular a.,** a measurement from the center of one auditory meatus to that of the other. **bregmatolambdoid a.,** the arc extending along the course of the sagittal suture from the bregma to the lambda. **carbon a.,** an electrical discharge between carbon electrodes that gives off an intense white light. **mercury a.,** an electric discharge between electrodes in mercury vapor in a vacuum tube which gives off light rich in ultraviolet rays. **nasobregmatic a.,** the arc extending from the nasion to the bregma. **naso-occipital a.,** the arc extending from the nasion to the most inferior part of the external occipital protuberance. **neural a.,** a series of two or more neurons connecting certain receptors and effectors, and constituting the pathway for neural reactions and reflexes; called also *sensorimotor a.* **nuclear a.,** vortex lentis. **reflex a.,** the neural arc utilized in a reflex action; an impulse travels centrally over afferent fibers to

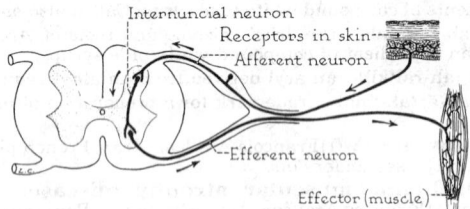

Three-neuron reflex arc (King and Showers).

a nerve center, and the response outward to an effector organ or part over efferent fibers. **sensorimotor a.,** neural a. **tungsten a.,** see under *lamp*.

arcade (ar-kād′) an anatomical structure composed of a series of arches. **arterial a's,** a series of anastomosing arterial arches as in the intestinal branches of the superior mesenteric artery. **Flint's a.,** an arteriovenous arch at the base of the renal pyramids.

arcanum (ar-ka′num) [L. "secret"] a secret medicine or nostrum.

arcate (ar′kāt) arcuate.

arch (arch) [L. *arcus* bow] a structure with a curved or bowlike outline; see also *arcus*. **abdominothoracic a.,** the lower boundary of the front of the thorax. **alveolar a.,** see *arcus alveolaris mandibulae* and *arcus alveolaris maxillae*. **anterior a. of atlas,** arcus anterior atlantis. **a. of aorta,** arcus aortae. **aortic a's,** paired vessels arching from the ventral to the dorsal aorta through the branchial arches of fishes and amniote embryos. In mammalian development, arches 1 and 2 disappear; arch 3 joins the common to the internal carotid; the left arch 4 remains as the arch of the definitive aorta while the right arch 4 joins the aorta to the subclavian artery; arch 5 disappears; and the ventral halves of arch 6 form the pulmonary arteries while the connections to the dorsal aorta are lost, although the left half, or ductus arteriosus, serves until birth. **arterial a's of kidney,** arteriae arcuatae renis. **axillary a.,** a muscular slip occasionally arising from the cranial border of the latissimus dorsi muscle, crossing the axilla ventral to the axillary vessels and nerves, and joining the under surface of the tendon of the pectoralis major, the coracobrachialis, or the fascia of the biceps brachii muscle. **basal a.,** apical base. **branchial a's,** paired arched columns that bear the gills in lower aquatic vertebrates and that, in the embryos of higher vertebrates, appear in comparable form before subsequent modification into structures of the ear and neck. Each arch contains a cartilaginous bar, consisting of right and left halves. The first arch (*mandibular a.*) differentiates into the sphenomandibular and anterior malleolar ligaments, malleus, and incus, the second (*hyoid a.*) into the styloid process, stylohyoid ligament, lesser cornu of the hyoid bone, and

cranial part of the hyoid body, the third into the greater cornu of the hyoid bone and the caudal part of its body, and the fourth and fifth into certain laryngeal cartilages. Called also *pharyngeal a's* and *visceral a's*. **carpal a., anterior,** an arch formed by anastomosis of the anterior carpal branches of the radial and ulnar arteries. **carpal a., dorsal, carpal a., posterior,** rete carpi dorsale. **a's of Corti,** a series of arches in the organ of Corti formed by inner and outer pillar cells. **costal a.,** arcus costalis. **a. of cricoid cartilage,** arcus cartilaginis cricoideae. **crural a.,** ligamentum inguinale. **crural a., deep,** a thickened band of fibers derived from the transversalis fascia, which arches over the external iliac vessels as they pass under the inguinal ligament; called also *iliopubic tract*. **dental a.,** the curving structure formed by the teeth in their normal position; called also *arcus dentalis*. The *inferior dental arch* (*arcus dentalis inferior* or *arch of the mandible*) is formed by the mandibular teeth, and the *superior dental arch* (*arcus dentalis superior* or *maxillary arch*) is formed by the maxillary teeth. **dental a., inferior,** see under *dental a.* **dental a., superior,** see under *dental a.* **diaphragmatic a., external,** ligamentum arcuatum laterale. **diaphragmatic a., internal,** ligamentum arcuatum mediale. **digital venous a's,** arcus venosi digitales. **dorsal venous a. of foot,** arcus venosus dorsalis pedis. **double aortic a.,** a congenital anomaly in which the aorta divides into two branches which embrace the trachea and esophagus and reunite to form the descending aorta. **epiphyseal a.,** the embryonic structure in the roof of the third ventricle from which the pineal body develops. **expansion a.,** a wire appliance made to conform to the arch of the jaw, used in orthodontic work to produce movement of the teeth into a larger arc and to eliminate space deficiency and irregularities. **femoral a., superficial,** ligamentum inguinale. **fibrous a. of soleus muscle,** arcus tendineus musculi solei. **a's of foot,** see *arcus pedis longitudinalis* and *arcus pedis transversalis*. **glossopalatine a.,** arcus palatoglossus. **Gothic a.,** a tracing made by the excursions to left and right and the protrusive movement of the mandible, to provide a graphic record of the range of mandibular movement in the occlusal plane. **Haller's a's,** see *ligamentum arcuatum laterale* and *ligamentum arcuatum mediale*. **hemal a.,** the arch formed by the body, pedicles, and transverse processes of a vertebra, a pair of ribs and their costal cartilages, and the sternum; the sum of all such arches forming the thoracic cage. **high labial a.,** a labial arch placed gingival to the anterior tooth crowns, with springs extending downward to maintain pressure on the teeth to be moved. **hyoid a.,** the second branchial arch; see *branchial a's*. **jugular venous a.,** arcus venosus juguli. **labial a.,** a wire appliance made to conform to the outside perimeter of the dental arch; used to promote or to prevent movement of the teeth in orthodontic therapy. **Langer's axillary a.,** axillary a. **lingual a.,** a wire appliance made to conform to the lingual aspect of the dental arch; used to promote or to prevent movement of the teeth in orthodontic work. **longitudinal a. of foot,** arcus pedis longitudinalis. **lumbocostal a., external, of diaphragm,** ligamentum arcuatum laterale. **lumbocostal a., internal, of diaphragm,** ligamentum arcuatum mediale. **lumbocostal a., lateral, of Haller,** ligamentum arcuatum laterale. **lumbocostal a., medial, of Haller,** ligamentum arcuatum mediale. **malar a.,** arcus zygomaticus. **mandibular a.,** 1. the first branchial arch; see *branchial a's*. 2. the inferior dental arch; see under *dental a.* **maxillary a.,** 1. the palatal arch. 2. the superior dental arch; also the residual dental arch. See under *dental a.* **nasal a.,** the arch formed by the nasal bones and by the nasal processes of the maxilla. **neural a. of vertebra,** arcus vertebrae. **open pubic a.,** a congenital anomaly in which the pubic arch is not fused, the bodies of the pubic bones being spread apart. **oral a.,** see palatal a. **orbital a. of frontal bone,** margo supraorbitalis ossis frontalis. **palatal a.,** the arch formed by the roof of the mouth from the teeth on one side of the maxilla to the teeth on the other or, if the teeth are missing, from the residual dental arch on one side to that on the other. Called also *maxillary a., palatomaxillary a.,* and *oral a.* **palatine a., anterior,** arcus palatoglossus. **palatine a., posterior,** arcus palatopharyngeus. **palatoglossal a.,** arcus palatoglossus. **palatomaxillary a.,** palatal a. **palatopharyngeal a.,** arcus palatopharyngeus. **palmar arterial a., deep,** arcus palmaris profundus. **palmar arterial a., superficial,** arcus palmaris superficialis. **palmar venous a., deep,** arcus venosus palmaris profundus. **palmar venous a., superficial,** arcus venosus palmaris superficialis. **palpebral a., inferior,** arcus palpebralis inferior. **palpebral a., superior,** arcus palpebralis superior. **paraphyseal a.,** the embryonic structure in the roof of the third ventricle of vertebrates from which the paraphysis develops. **passive lingual a.,** an orthodontic appliance for maintaining space and preserving arch length when bilateral primary molars are prematurely lost. **a. of pelvis,** angulus subpubicus. **pharyngeal a's,** branchial a's. **pharyngoepiglottic a.,** arcus palatopharyngeus. **pharyngopalatine a.,** arcus palatopharyngeus. **plantar arterial a.,** arcus plantaris. **plantar venous a.,** arcus venosus plantaris. **popliteal a.,** ligamentum popliteum arcuatum. **postaural a's,** branchial a's. **poste-**

rior a. of atlas, arcus posterior atlantis. **pubic a., a. of pubis,** arcus pubis. **pulmonary a's,** the most caudal of the aortic arches, which become the pulmonary arteries. **residual dental a.,** the curved contour of the ridge remaining after tooth removal. **ribbon a.,** an appliance of flattened wire made to conform to the arch of the jaw and used in producing bodily movement of the teeth in orthodontic work. **a. of ribs,** arcus costalis. **right aortic a.,** a congenital anomaly in which the aorta is displaced to the right and passes behind the esophagus, thus forming a vascular ring that may cause compression of the trachea and esophagus. **Riolan's a.,** the arch formed by the mesentery of the transverse colon. **saddle a., saddle-shaped a.,** a palatal arch in which the lateral parts are contrasted. **Salus' a.,** the arching of a vein where it crosses an artery in the retina, seen in arteriosclerosis. **Shenton's a.,** Shenton's line. **stationary lingual a.,** a lingual arch soldered to the anchor bands. **subpubic a.,** angulus subpubicus. **superciliary a.,** arcus superciliaris. **supraorbital a. of frontal bone,** margo supraorbitalis ossis frontalis. **tarsal a's,** see *arcus palpebralis inferior* and *arcus palpebralis superior.* **tendinous a.,** arcus tendineus. **tendinous a. of diaphragm, external,** ligamentum arcuatum laterale. **tendinous a. of diaphragm, internal,** ligamentum arcuatum mediale. **tendinous a. of levator ani muscle,** arcus tendineus musculi levatoris ani. **tendinous a. of lumbodorsal fascia,** ligamentum lumbocostale. **tendinous a. of pelvic fascia,** arcus tendineus fasciae pelvis. **tendinous a. of soleus muscle,** arcus tendineus musculi solei. **thyrohyoid a.,** the third pharyngeal arch, which becomes represented by the greater cornu of the hyoid bone. **transverse a. of foot,** arcus pedis transversalis. **Treitz's a.,** an arch composed of the left superior colic artery and the inferior mesenteric vein; it lies between the ascending portion of the duodenum and the inner edge of the left kidney. **venous a's of kidney,** venae arcuatae renis. **a. of vertebra, vertebral a.,** arcus vertebrae. **visceral a's,** branchial a's. **volar venous a., deep,** arcus venosus palmaris profundus. **volar venous a., superficial,** arcus venosus palmaris superficialis. **V-shaped a.,** a dental arch which narrows and comes to a point at the lingual junction of the maxillary central incisors. **wire a.,** an arch or splint of wire adjusted to the dental arch, used in orthodontic work to produce movement of the teeth and achieve a normal contour of the dental arch. **Zimmermann's a.,** an inconstant, rudimentary arch of the embryo, supposed to explain the origin of certain occasionally occurring vessels between the fourth aortic and the pulmonary arch. **zygomatic a.,** arcus zygomaticus.

arch- See *archi-.*

archaeus (ar-ke'us) Paracelsus' term for the vital principle, the living force in the body or the animate universe.

Archagathus (ark-ag'ah-thus) the first Greek physician to practice in Rome (219 B.C.), according to Pliny. At first known as "the wound-curer" (*Vulnerarius*), because of his surgical exploits he was later termed "the executioner" (*Carnifex*).

archaic (ar-ka'ik) [Gr. *archaios* ancient] very ancient; pertaining to early evolutionary stages.

archamphiaster (ark-am''fe-as''ter) [arch- + Gr. *amphi* around + *astēr* star] the primitive amphiaster associated with the formation of polar bodies.

Archangelica (ar''kan-jel'e-kah) [L. from Gr. *archangelikos* archangelic] a genus of umbelliferous plants. See *angelica.*

Archangiaceae (ark-an''je-a'se-e) a systematic family of schizomycetes, order Myxobacterales, and made up of two genera (*Archangium* and *Stelangium*) of soil microorganisms.

Archangium (ark-an''je-um) a genus of schizomycetes of the family Archangiaceae, order Myxobacterales.

arche- see *archi-.*

archebiosis (ar''ke-bi-o'sis) [arche- + Gr. *biōsis* way of life] the spontaneous generation of organisms, a concept proved to be false; called also *archegenesis, archigenesis,* or *archegony.*

archecentric (ar''kĕ-sen'trik) [arche- + *centric*] denoting a primitive type of structure from which the other types in the members of the group are derived.

archegenesis (ar''kĕ-jen'ĕ-sis) [arche- + Gr. *genesis* reproduction] archebiosis.

archegonium (ar''kĕ-go'ne-um) [arche- + Gr. *gonos* offspring] the female organ of a cryptogamic plant taking part in the formation of sexually produced spores; cf. *antheridium.*

archegony (ar-keg'o-ne) [arche- + Gr. *gonē* seed] archebiosis.

archencephalon (ar''ken-sef'ah-lon) [arche- + Gr. *enkephalos* brain] the primitive brain, anterior to the end of the notochord, from which the midbrain and the forebrain are developed.

archenteron (ar-ken'ter-on) [arche- + Gr. *enteron* intestine] the primitive digestive cavity of those embryonic forms whose blastula becomes a gastrula by invagination; called also *archigaster, coelenteron, gastrocoele,* and *primitive gut.*

archeocinetic (ar''ke-o-si-net'ik) archeokinetic.

archeocyte (ar'ke-o-sit'') [Gr. *archaios* ancient + *kytos* hollow vessel] any free or wandering ameboid cell.

archeokinetic (ar''ke-o-ki-net'ik) [Gr. *archaios* ancient + *kinēsis* motion] a term applied to the primitive type of motor nerve mechanism, as seen in the peripheral and ganglionic nervous systems; cf. *neokinetic* and *paleokinetic.*

archepyon (ar-kep'e-on) [arche- + Gr. *pyon* pus] (*obs.*) very thick, cheesy pus.

archespore (ar'kĕ-spōr) [arche- + Gr. *sporos* seed] the mass of cells that give rise to spore mother cells; called also *archesporium* and *archispore.*

archesporium (ar''kĕ-spo're-um) archespore.

archetype (ar''kĕ-tīp) [arche- + Gr. *typos* type] an ideal, original, or standard type or form.

archi-, arch-, arche- [Gr. *archē* beginning] a combining form denoting first, beginning, or original.

archiblast (ar'kĭ-blast) [archi- + Gr. *blastos* germ] 1. the components of an ovum that actively form the embryo, as distinguished from the yolk. 2. His' term for the fundamental part of the blastodermic layers as distinguished from the parablast or peripheral portion of the mesoderm.

archiblastic (ar''kĭ-blas'tik) derived from or pertaining to the archiblast.

archicarp (ar'kĭ-karp) the group of cells, including the ascogonium, that give rise to the fruiting body of ascomycetous fungi. Cf. *ascocarp.* See also *ascogonium.*

archicenter (ar''kĭ-sen'ter) [archi- + Gr. *kentron* sharp point] an archetype; an organ or organism that is the primitive form from which another organ or organism is descended.

archicentric (ar-kĭ-sen'trik) pertaining to an archicenter.

archicerebellum (ar''kĭ-ser''ĕ-bel'um) [archi- + *cerebellum*] a term sometimes applied to the phylogenetically old part of the cerebellum, viz., the flocculonodular lobe, which is predominantly supplied by vestibulocerebellar fibers and dominated by vestibular functions.

archicortex (ar''kĭ-kor'teks) archipallium.

archicyte (ar'kĭ-sīt) [archi- + Gr. *kytos* hollow vessel] zygote.

archicytula (ar''kĭ-sit'u-lah) [archi- + Gr. *kytos* hollow vessel] a fertilized ovum in the stage in which the nucleus is first discernible.

archigaster (ar'kĭ-gas''ter) [archi- + Gr. *gastēr* belly] archenteron.

archigastrula (ar''kĭ-gas'troo-lah) [archi- + *gastrula*] the gastrula in its most primitive form of development.

Archigenes (ar-kij'ĕ-nēz) **of Apamea** (1st century A.D.) a celebrated Greek physician, a pupil of Agathinus (and a Pneumatist). He practiced in Rome and wrote several works, some portions of which are preserved; his surgical observations (e.g., on amputation and ligation) are noteworthy.

archigenesis (ar-kĭ-jen'ĕ-sis) archebiosis.

archikaryon (ar''kĭ-kar'e-on) [archi- + Gr. *karyon* kernel] the nucleus of a fertilized ovum.

archil (ar'kil) the lichen *Roccella tinctoria;* also, a violet coloring matter from this and other lichens, employed as an indicator dye for litmus paper: alkalies give a blue color, and acids a red color.

archimorula (ar-kĭ-mor'u-lah) [archi- + *morula*] a mass of cells arising from the division of the archicytula and preceding the archigastrula.

archinephron (ar''kĭ-nef'ron) [archi- + Gr. *nephros* kidney] a unit of the pronephros.

archineuron (ar''kĭ-nu'ron) [archi- + Gr. *neuron* nerve] the neuron at which an efferent impulse starts (Waldeyer).

archipallial (ar''kĭ-pal'e-al) pertaining to the archipallium.

archipallium (ar''kĭ-pal'e-um) [archi- + L. *pallium* cloak] that portion of the pallium (cerebral cortex) which, with the paleopallium, develops in association with the olfactory system and which is phylogenetically older than the neopallium and lacks its layered structure. The embryonic archipallium corresponds to the cortex of the dentate gyrus and hippocampus in mature mammals. Called also *allocortex, archicortex, heterotypical cortex,* and *olfactory cortex.*

archiplasm (ar'kĭ-plazm'') [archi- + Gr. *plasma* something formed] (*obs.*) Boveri's name for the material of the spindle fibers and astral rays. This material was thought to exist during the entire cell cycle but to become visible after aggregation at mitosis.

archispore (ar'kĭ-spōr) archespore.

archistome (ar'kĭ-stōm) [archi- + Gr. *stoma* mouth] blastopore.

archistriatum (ar''ke-stri-a'tum) [archi- + *striatum*] the primitive corpus striatum, represented in man by the corpus amygdaloideum.

architectonic (ar''ke-tek-ton'ik) 1. pertaining to architectural pattern. 2. the structure or construction of, as architectonic structure of the brain.

archo- [Gr. *archos* rectum, from *archē* beginning, the rectum having been considered the first part of the bowel] a combining form once used to denote relationship to the rectum or anus.

archocele (ar'ko-sēl) [*archo-* + Gr. *kēlē* hernia] (*obs.*) rectocele.

archocystocolposyrinx (ar″ko-sis″to-kol″po-sir'inks) [*archo-* + Gr. *kystis* bladder + *kolpos* vagina + *syrinx* pipe] (*obs.*) fistula of the anus, vagina, and bladder.

archocystosyrinx (ar″ko-sis″to-sir'inks) [*archo-* + Gr. *kystis* bladder + *syrinx* pipe] fistula of the anus and bladder.

archoptoma (ar″ko-to'mah) [*archo-* + Gr. *ptōma* fall] (*obs.*) a prolapsed portion of the rectum.

archoptosis (ar″ko-to'sis) [*archo-* + Gr. *ptōsis* fall] (*obs.*) prolapse of the lower rectum through the anal canal.

archorrhagia (ar″ko-ra'je-ah) [*archo-* + Gr. *rhēgnynai* to burst forth + *-ia*] (*obs.*) hemorrhage from the rectum.

archorrhea (ar″ko-re'ah) [*archo-* + Gr. *rhoia* flow] (*obs.*) a liquid discharge from the rectum.

archostenosis (ar″ko-ste-no'sis) [*archo-* + Gr. *stenōsis* stricture] (*obs.*) stricture of the rectum.

archosyrinx (ar″ko-sir'inks) [*archo-* + Gr. *syrinx* pipe] (*obs.*) 1. fistula in ano. 2. a rectal syringe.

archusia (ar-ku'se-ah) a hypothetical substance once thought to be necessary for cell growth.

arciform (ar'sĭ-form) [L. *arcus* bow + *forma* shape] bow-shaped; arcuate.

arctation (ark-ta'shun) [L. *arctatio*] contracture or narrowing of any canal or opening.

Arctostaphylos uva-ursi (ark″to-staf'ĭ-los u'vah-ur'si) the bearberry shrub of the family Ericaceae. The fruits are edible, and the leaves are used medicinally as an astringent, diuretic tea. It contains arbutin (see *Arbutus*). Called also *Arbutus uva-ursi* L.

arcual (ar'ku-al) [L. *arcualis*] pertaining to an arch.

arcualia (ar″ku-a'le-ah) nodules of cartilage in the continuous mesenchymal sheath in close apposition to the external surface of the notochord in vertebrate embryos.

arcuate (ar'ku-āt) [L. *arcuatus* bow shaped] shaped like an arc; arranged in arches.

arcuation (ark-u-a'shun) [L. *arcuatio*] curvature; especially an abnormal curvature.

arcus (ar'kus), pl. *ar'cus* [L. "a bow"] an arch; a general term used in anatomical nomenclature to designate any structure having a curved or bowlike outline. **a. adipo'sus**, a. senilis. **a. alveola'ris mandib'ulae** [NA], alveolar arch of mandible: the superior free border of the alveolar process of the mandible. Called also *alveolar border* or *alveolar limbus of mandible*, and *limbus alveolaris mandibulae*. **a. alveola'ris maxil'lae** [NA], alveolar arch of maxilla: the inferior free border of the alveolar process of the maxilla; called also *alveolar border* or *alveolar limbus of maxilla*, and *limbus alveolaris maxillae*. **a. ante'rior atlan'tis**, anterior arch of atlas: the more slender portion joining the lateral masses of the atlas ventrally, constituting about one-fifth of its entire circumference. **a. aor'tae** [NA], arch of the aorta: the continuation of the ascending aorta, giving rise to the brachiocephalic trunk, and the left common carotid and left subclavian arteries; it continues as the thoracic aorta (aorta thoracica). **a. cartilag'inis cricoi'deae** [NA], arch of cricoid cartilage: the slender anterior portion of the cricoid cartilage. **a. costa'lis** [NA], **a. costa'rum**, costal arch: the anterior portion of the apertura thoracis inferior, consisting of the costal cartilages of ribs 7 to 10, inclusive; called also *arch of ribs*. **a. denta'lis** [NA], the curving structure formed by the crowns of the teeth in their normal position in the jaw; see *dental arch*, under *arch*. **a. denta'lis infe'rior** [NA], the curving structure formed by the teeth of the mandible; see *dental arch*, under *arch*. **a. denta'lis supe'rior** [NA], the curving structure formed by the teeth of the maxilla; see *dental arch*, under *arch*. **a. dorsa'lis pe'dis**, arteria arcuata pedis. **a. glossopalati'nus**, a. palatoglossus. **a. iliopectin'eus** [NA], the fascial partition that separates the lacuna musculorum and the lacuna vasorum; called also *fascia iliopectinea*. **a. juveni'lis**, a condition identical to arcus senilis, except that it occurs congenitally or before or during middle life, and may be due to early degeneration of the cornea, corneal irritation, interstitial keratitis, or familial hypercholesterolemia; called also *anterior embryotoxon*. **a. lipoi'des cor'neae**, a crescentic deposit of fat and cholesterol crystals in the cornea. **a. lipoi'des myr-in'gis**, a ring of degeneration in the tympanic membrane of the aged. **a. lumbocosta'lis latera'lis**, ligamentum arcuatum laterale. **a. lumbocosta'lis media'lis**, ligamentum arcuatum mediale. **a. palati'ni**, see *a. palatoglossus* and *a. palatopharyngeus*. **a. palatoglos'sus** [NA], palatoglossal arch: the anterior of the two folds of mucous membrane on either side of the oropharynx, connected with the soft palate and enclosing the palatoglossal muscle; called also *a. glossopalatinus, glossopalatine arch, anterior palatine arch*, and *anterior column* or *pillar of fauces*. **a. palatopharyn'geus** [NA], palatopharyngeal arch: the posterior of the two folds of mucous membrane on each side of the oropharynx, connected with the soft palate and enclosing the palatopharyngeal muscle; called also *a. pharyngopalatinus, pharyngopalatine* or *pharyngoepiglottic arch, posterior palatine arch*, and *posterior column* or *pillar of fauces*. **a. pal-ma'ris profun'dus**, deep palmar arterial arch: an arch formed by the terminal part of the radial artery and its anastomosis with the deep branch of the ulnar, and extending from the base of the metacarpal bone of the little finger to the proximal end of the first interosseous space; it gives off palmar metacarpal arteries and perforating branches. Called also *a. volaris profundus*. **a. palma'ris superficia'lis** [NA], superficial palmar arterial arch: an arch formed by the terminal part of the ulnar artery and its anastomosis with the superficial palmar branch of the radial, giving rise to the palmar digital arteries and supplying blood to the palmar aspect of the hands and fingers. Called also *a. volaris superficialis*. **a. palpebra'les**, see *a. palpebralis inferior* and *a. palpebralis superior*. **a. palpebra'lis infe'rior** [NA], inferior palpebral arch: an arch derived from the medial palpebral artery, supplying the lower lid of the eye; called also *a. tarseus inferior*. **a. palpebra'lis supe'rior** [NA], superior palpebral arch: an arch derived from the medial palpebral artery, supplying the upper lid of the eye; called also *a. tarseus superior*. **a. parieto-occipita'lis**, the curved convolution formed by the backward continuation into the occipital lobe of the superior postcentral sulcus. **a. pe'dis longitudina'lis** [NA], the longitudinal arch of the foot, comprising the pars medialis and the pars lateralis. **a. pe'dis transversa'lis** [NA], transverse arch of foot: the metatarsal arch of the foot, formed by the navicular, cuneiform, cuboid, and the five metatarsal bones. **a. pharyngopalati'nus**, a. palatopharyngeus. **a. planta'ris** [NA], plantar arterial arch: the deep arterial arch in the foot, formed by the anastomosis of the lateral plantar artery with the deep plantar branch of the dorsal artery of the foot, and giving off the plantar metatarsal arteries. **a. poste'rior atlan'tis** [NA], posterior arch of atlas: the slender portion joining the lateral masses of the atlas dorsally, constituting about two-fifths of its entire circumference. **a. pu'bis** [NA], pubic arch: the arch formed by the conjoined rami of the ischial and pubic bones of the two sides of the body. **a. senil'is**, a gray opaque ring surrounding the margin of the cornea, but separated from the margin by an area of clear cornea, usually occurring bilaterally in persons of 50 years or older as a result of lipoid degeneration; called also *gerontoxon*. Cf. *a. juvenilis*. **a. supercilia'ris** [NA], superciliary arch: a smooth elevation arching upward and laterally from the glabella, a little above the margin of the orbit. **a. tar'seus infe'rior**, a palpebralis inferior. **a. tar'seus supe'rior**, a palpebralis superior. **a. tendin'eus** [NA], tendinous arch: a linear thickening of fascia over some part of a muscle, such as that over the soleus or the obturator internus. **a. tendin'eus fas'ciae pel'vis** [NA], tendinous arch of pelvic fascia: a thickening of the superior fascia, extending from the ischial spine to the posterior part of the body of the pubis. **a. tendin'eus mus'culi levato'ris a'ni** [NA], tendinous arch of levator ani muscle: a linear thickening of the fascia over the levator ani muscle. **a. tendin'eus mus'culi so'lei** [NA], tendinous arch of soleus muscle: an aponeurotic band in the front part of the soleus muscle, extending from a tubercle on the neck of the fibula to the soleal line of the tibia. **a. veno'si digi-ta'les**, digital venous arches: communicating branches of veins across the backs of the fingers at their bases. **a. veno'sus dorsa'lis pe'dis** [NA], dorsal venous arch of foot: a transverse venous arch across the dorsum of the foot near the bases of the metatarsal bones. **a. veno'sus jug'uli** [NA], jugular venous arch: a transverse connecting trunk between the anterior jugular veins of either side. **a. veno'sus palma'ris profun'dus** [NA], deep palmar venous arch: a venous arch accompanying the deep palmar arterial arch; called also *a. volaris venosus profundus*. **a. veno'sus palma'ris superficia'lis** [NA], superficial palmar venous arch: a venous arch accompanying the superficial palmar arterial arch; called also *a. volaris venosus superficialis*. **a. veno'sus planta'ris** [NA], plantar venous arch: the deep venous arch that accompanies the arterial plantar arch. **a. ver'tebrae** [NA], vertebral arch: the bony arch composed of the laminae and pedicles of a vertebra; called also *arch of vertebra* and *neural arch of vertebra*. **a. vola'ris profun'dus**, a. palmaris profundus. **a. vola'ris superficia'lis**, a. palmaris superficialis. **a. vola'ris veno'sus profun'dus**, a. venosus palmaris profundus. **a. vola'ris veno'sus superficia'lis**, a. venosus palmaris superficialis. **a. zygomat'icus** [NA], zygomatic arch: the arch formed by the articulation of the broad temporal process of the zygomatic bone and the slender zygomatic process of the temporal bone, giving attachment to the masseter muscle and serving as a line of demarcation between the temporal and infratemporal fossae; called also *malar arch*.

ARD acute respiratory disease (of any undefined form).

ardanesthesia (ar″dan-es-the'ze-ah) [L. *ardor* heat + *anesthesia*] thermanesthesia.

ardent (ar'dent) [L. *ardere* to glow] 1. hot or feverish. 2. characterized by eager desire.

ardor (ar'dor) [L.] 1. intense heat. 2. eager desire. **a. uri'-nae**, a scalding sensation during the passage of urine. **a. ven-tric'uli** (*obs.*), pyrosis or heartburn.

Arduen'na (ar″du-en'nah) *Ascarops*.

area (a're-ah), pl. *a'reae* or *areas* [L.] a limited space; a general term used in anatomical nomenclature to designate a specific surface or functional region. See also *region*. **acoustic a., a.**

acus′tica, a. vestibularis. **alisphenoid a.,** the surface of the great wing of the sphenoid bone. **aortic a.,** the area on the chest over the inner end of the right second costal cartilage. **apical a.,** the area about the apex of the root of a tooth. **association a′s,** areas of the cerebral cortex (excluding the primary areas) that are connected with each other and with the neothalamus by numerous fibers passing through the corpus callosum and the white matter of the hemispheres; these areas are responsible for the higher mental and emotional processes, including memory, learning, etc. **auditory a.,** a. vestibularis. **axial a.,** an area on a limb in which there is a hiatus in the numerical sequence of the spinal nerves in their cutaneous distribution. **Bamberger′s a.,** an area of cardiac dullness in the left intercostal region, suggestive of pericardial effusion. **bare a. of liver,** a. nuda hepatis. **basal seat a.,** that portion of the structures of the mouth that is available to support a denture. **Betz cell a.,** motor a. **Broca′s motor speech a.,** an area comprising parts of the opercular and triangular portions of the inferior frontal gyrus; injury to this area may result in motor aphasia. **Broca′s parolfactory a.,** a. subcallosa. **Brodmann′s a′s,** areas of the cerebral cortex distinguished by differences in the arrangement of their six cellular layers and identified by numbering each area. **a. cel′si,** alopecia areata. **a. centra′lis,** a circular area of cells around the foveola in the ganglion cell layer of the retina. **cingulate a.,** the area comprising cingulate gyrus and isthmus. **a. coch′leae** [NA], the anterior part of the inferior portion of the fundus of the internal acoustic meatus, near the base of the cochlea; called also *cochlear a. of internal acoustic meatus.* **cochlear a. of internal acoustic meatus,** a. cochleae. **Cohnheim′s a′s,** dark, polygonal areas of myofibrils seen on cross-section of a poorly fixed muscle fiber. **contact a.,** the area at which two bodies or materials touch. In dentistry, the site on the proximal surfaces at which two adjacent teeth touch. **cribriform a. of renal papilla,** a. cribrosa papillae renalis. **a. cribro′sa me′dia,** a. vestibularis inferior. **a. cribro′sa papil′lae rena′lis** [NA], cribriform area of renal papilla: the tip of a pyramid of a kidney, which is perforated by 10–25 openings for the papillary ducts. **a. cribro′sa supe′rior,** a. vestibularis superior. **a. of critical definition,** that part of an optic image within which the detail is clear. **denture-bearing a.,** that portion of the basal seat area that, in occlusion, supports the complete or partial denture base; called also *denture foundation a.* or *denture-supporting a.* **denture foundation a.,** denture-bearing a. **denture-supporting a.,** denture-bearing a. **dermatomic a.,** dermatome. **embryonic a.,** embryonic disk. **excitable a.,** a motor area in the cerebral cortex. **excitomotor a.,** motor a. **eye a.,** the area comprising the frontal eye fields of the cortex in the frontal lobe, which are concerned with the control of eye movements. **a. of facial nerve,** a. nervi facialis. **Flechsig′s a′s** (*obs.*), three areas—anterior, lateral, and posterior—on each lateral half of the sections of the medulla oblongata, marked out by the fibers of the vagus and hypoglossal nerves. **gastric a′s, a′reae gas′tricae,** the several areas on organs adjacent to the stomach by which the organs make contact with the stomach. **genital a′s,** areas on the inferior nasal concha and upper part of the nasal septum that may become engorged during menstruation. **germinal a., a. germinati′va,** embryonic disk. **glove a.,** that area—fingers, hand, and wrist—ordinarily covered by a glove, which sometimes coincides with the distribution of anesthesia in cases of polyneuropathy. **a. hypoglos′si,** the portion of the mouth beneath the tongue. **impression a.,** the surface of the oral structures recorded in an impression. **insular a.,** the cortex of the insula. **intercondylar a′s of tibia,** see *a. intercondylaris anterior tibiae* and *a. intercondylaris posterior tibiae.* **a. intercondyla′ris ante′rior tib′iae** [NA], the broad area between the superior articular surfaces of the tibia; called also *anterior intercondylar a., fossa intercondyloidea anterior tibiae, anterior intercondylar fossa of tibia* and *patellar fossa of tibia.* **a. intercondyla′ris poste′rior tib′iae** [NA], a deep notch separating the condyles on the posterior surface of the tibia; called also *posterior intercondylar a., fossa intercondyloidea posterior tibiae, posterior intercondylar fossa of tibia,* and *popliteal fossa of tibia.* **interglobular a′s,** the areas of dentin lying between the calcoglobules. **Kiesselbach′s a.,** an area on the anterior part of the nasal septum above the intermaxillary bone, which is richly supplied with blood vessels and is a common site of nosebleed; called also *Little′s a.* **Krönig′s a.** (*obs.*), Krönig′s field. **Laimer-Haeckerman a.,** the region of the lower pharynx and upper esophagus, where diverticula most frequently develop. **language a.,** any center of the cortex, usually in the dominant hemisphere, controlling the understanding or use of language. **Little′s a.,** Kiesselbach′s a. **a. luna′ta** (*obs.*), the posterior semilunar lobule of the cerebellar hemisphere situated rostral to the postlunate (postclival) fissure. **a. martegia′ni,** a slightly enlarged space at the optic disk, marking the beginning of the hyaloid canal. **a. medullovasculo′sa,** a median elongated area of vascular granulation-like tissue in rachischisis. **mesobranchial a.,** the pharyngeal floor, between the pharyngeal arches and pouches of each side. **mirror a.,** the reflecting surface of the cornea and lens when illuminated through the slit lamp. **motor a.,** that area of the

cerebral cortex which, upon application of brief electrical stimuli, shows the lowest threshold and shortest latency for the production of muscle movement. Called also *Betz cell a., excitomotor a., precentral a., psychomotor a.,* and *rolandic a.* **a. ner′vi facia′lis** [NA], area of facial nerve: the part of the fundus of the internal acoustic meatus where the facial nerve enters the facial canal. **a. nu′da hep′atis** [NA], bare area of liver: the superior surface of the liver, adjacent to the diaphragm, that lacks a peritoneal covering; its boundaries are formed by the hepatic coronary ligament proper and the triangular ligaments. **Obersteiner-Redlich a.** (*obs.*), the constricted area at the point where a posterior nerve root enters the spinal cord. **olfactory a.,** a general area, including the olfactory bulb, tract, and trigone, the anterior portion of the gyrus cinguli, and the uncus. **a. opa′ca,** the outer part of the embryonic disk, as seen in the bird egg: **Panum′s a′s,** fusional areas on the retina. **a. parolfacto′ria [Brocae], parolfactory a. of Broca,** a. subcallosa. **a. pellu′cida,** the central clear part of the embryonic disk, as seen in the bird egg. **a. perfora′ta,** substantia perforata (perforated space). **peristriate a.,** an area of the occipital cortex nearly surrounding the striate (visual) cortex. **piriform a.,** an area in the rhinencephalon comprising the lateral olfactory process or gyrus, the limen insulae, the uncus, and at least part of the parahippocampal gyrus; in some species it is pear-shaped. Called also *piriform lobe.* **postcentral a.,** the sensory area just posterior to the central sulcus of the cerebral hemisphere, the primary receptive area for general sensations; called also *postrolandic a.* and *somesthetic cortex.* **post dam a.,** posterior palatal seal a. **posterior hypothalamic a.,** see *hypothalamic a′s.* **posterior palatal seal a.,** the soft tissues along the junction of the hard and soft palates on which pressure can be applied by a denture to aid in its retention; called also *post dam a.* **a. postpterygoi′dea** (*obs.*), the part of the ansiform lobule of the cerebellar hemisphere immediately behind the postclival fissure. **a. postre′ma,** an area on the floor of the fourth ventricle immediately lateral to the trigonum nervi vagi and separated from it by the sulcus limitans. **postrolandic a.,** postcentral a. **precentral a.,** motor a. **prefrontal a.,** the cortex of the frontal lobe immediately in front of the premotor cortex, concerned chiefly with associative functions. **premotor a.,** the motor cortex of the frontal lobe immediately in front of the precentral gyrus. **preoptic a.,** several groups of cells in the median plane immediately below the anterior commissure which are functionally related to the hypothalamus. **pressure a.,** an area which is subjected to excessive pressure, with consequent displacement of tissue. **primary a′s,** areas of the cerebral cortex comprising the motor and sensory regions. Cf. *association a′s.* **primary receptive a.,** the area of cerebral cortex which receives the thalamic projections of the primary sensory modalities, such as vision, hearing, touch, etc. **projection a′s,** those areas of the cerebral cortex that receive the most direct projection of the sensory systems of the body. **psychomotor a.,** motor a. **a. pterygoi′dea** (*obs.*), the part of the ansiform lobule of the cerebellar hemisphere immediately behind the great horizontal (postpterygoid) fissure. **pyriform a.,** piriform a. **receptive a.,** primary receptive a. **relief a.,** that portion of the surface of oral structures upon which pressures exerted by a denture are reduced or eliminated. **rest a.,** that portion of a tooth or of a restoration in a tooth prepared to receive the incisal, lingual, or occlusal rest of a removable partial denture. **rolandic a.,** motor a. **rugae a.,** the portion of the mouth in which rugae are found; called also *rugae zone.* **saddle a.,** the edentulous portion of the dental arch upon which a fixed or removable prosthesis rests. **sensorimotor a.,** the cortex of the pre- and postcentral gyri—the motor area and the primary receptive area for general sensations, respectively. **sensory a.,** primary receptive a. **septal a.,** the area on either cerebral hemisphere comprising the parolfactory area of Broca (area subcallosa) and the corresponding half of the septum pellucidum; the area has olfactory, hypothalamic, and hippocampal connections. **silent a.,** an area of the brain in which pathologic conditions may occur without producing symptoms. **somatic sensory a., somatosensory a.,** the cortical projection area in the postcentral gyrus for information initiated by stimulation of receptors in the skin, joints, muscles, and viscera; it is involved in conscious perception of somatic sensation. Called also *somesthetic a.* **somesthetic a.,** somatosensory a. **stress-bearing a.,** 1. the portion of the mouth capable of providing support for a denture. 2. surfaces of oral structures which resist forces, strains, or pressures brought upon them during function. **a. stria′ta,** striate cortex. **strip a.,** a strip of cortex between the motor and premotor areas thought to be suppressor in function. **a. subcallo′sa** [NA], **subcallosal a.,** a small area of cortex on the medial surface of each cerebral hemisphere, immediately in front of the gyrus subcallosus; called also *a. parolfactoria* [Brocae], *parolfactory a. of Broca,* and *gyrus olfactorius medialis* (*of Retzius*). **supporting a.,** 1. the surface of the mouth available for support of a denture. 2. those areas of the maxillary and mandibular edentulous ridges which are considered best suited to carry the forces of mastication when the dentures are in function. **supplementary a′s,** small motor and sensory areas of the cerebral cortex in addition to the primary areas.

suppressor a's, cortical areas whose activation suppresses or prevents movement. **temporal a.,** an area above the temporal fossa, reaching to the outer canthus of the eye. **thymus-dependent a's,** those areas of the peripheral lymphoid organs populated by thymus-dependent lymphocytes, e.g., the pericortical areas of the lymph nodes, the centers of the malpighian corpuscle of the spleen, and the internodular zone of Peyer's patches. See also *T-lymphocytes*, under *lymphocyte*. **thymus-independent a's,** those areas of the peripheral lymphoid organs populated by thymus-independent lymphocytes, e.g., the medullary and outer cortical regions of the lymph node; see also *B-lymphocytes*, under *lymphocyte*. **trigger a.,** an area the stimulation of which may cause physiologic or pathologic changes in another area. **vagus a.,** the area on the floor of the fourth ventricle in which the vagus nerve has its origin (trigonum nervi vagi [NA]). **a. vasculo'sa,** that part of the area opaca where the blood vessels are first seen, as in the bird egg. **vestibular a.,** a. vestibularis. **vestibular a., inferior, of internal acoustic meatus,** a. vestibularis inferior. **vestibular a., superior, of internal acoustic meatus,** a. vestibularis superior. **a. vestibula'ris** [NA], the triangular lateral and median part of the floor of the fourth ventricle over which pass the striae medullares of the fourth ventricle; called also *a. acustica, acoustic a., auditory a.,* and *ala alba medialis.* **a. vestibula'ris infe'rior** [NA], the lower portion of the fundus of the internal acoustic meatus; called also *inferior vestibular a. of internal acoustic meatus* and *a. cribrosa media.* **a. vestibula'ris supe'rior** [NA], the upper portion of the fundus of the internal acoustic meatus; called also *superior vestibular a. of internal acoustic meatus* and *a. cribrosa superior.* **visual a.,** the striate and peristriate cortex of the occipital lobe. **visuopsychic a.,** the area of the cerebral cortex concerned in the interpretation of visual sensations. **visuosensory a.,** cortical projection area for information initiated by stimulation of the retina surrounding the calcarine fissure; the area involved in conscious perception of visual information. **a. vitelli'na,** the yolk area beyond the area vasculosa in meroblastic eggs. **vocal a.,** the part of the glottis between the vocal cords. **Wernicke's a.,** originally a term denoting a speech center on the posterior part of the superior temporal gyrus, now used to include the supramarginal and angular gyri as well; called also *Wernicke's center, field,* or *zone.*

areata, areatus (ar″e-a'tah; ar″e-a'tus) occurring in patches, as alopecia areata.

Areca (ar'ĕ-kah) [L.; East Indian] a genus of palm trees, chiefly Asiatic. *A. catechu* L., Palmaceae affords betel nut and an inferior catechu (see *areca*).

areca (ar'e-kah) the dried ripe seed of *Areca catechu* L., Palmaceae, a palm native to the East Indies. It is a common masticatory throughout Asia and India, and contains the alkaloid arecoline and astringent tannins; it has parasympathomimetic and anthelmintic properties. Called also *betel nut* and *pinang.*

arecoline (ah-rek'o-lin) chemical name: 1,2,5,6-tetrahydro-1-methyl-3-pyridinecarboxylic acid methyl ester. An alkaloid obtained from areca (betel nut), $C_8H_{13}NO_2$. **a. hydrobromide,** a cholinergic, $C_8H_3NO_2 \cdot HBr$, occurring as a white, crystalline powder, having actions similar to those of pilocarpine; it was formerly used in the treatment of glaucoma. Now used as a cathartic and anthelmintic in veterinary medicine.

areflexia (ah″re-flek'se-ah) [*a* neg. + *reflex* + *-ia*] absence of the reflexes.

aregenerative (ah″re-jen'er-a″tiv) characterized by absence of regeneration; applied especially to blood cells in aplastic anemia.

arenaceous (ar″ĕ-na'se-us) sandy; gritty.

arenation (ar″ĕ-na'shun) [L. *arena* sand] (*obs.*) ammotherapy.

Arenaviridae (ah″re-nah-vi'ri-de) a family of viruses comprising the arenaviruses (genus *Arenavirus*).

arenavirus (ah″re-nah-vi'rus) [L. *arenaceus* sandy + *virus*] any of a group of viruses made up of pleomorphic virions, from 50 to 300 nm. in diameter, having four large and one to three small segments of single-stranded RNA and having ribosomes within the virions that give a sandy appearance. It includes the lymphocytic choriomenigitis virus, the American hemorrhagic fever viruses (Amapari, Junin, Latino, Machupo, Parana, Pichinde, Tacaribe, and Tamiami viruses), and the Lassa fever virus. Rodents are the common hosts of these viruses. The term (*Arenavirus*) is also used as the genus name (of the family Arenaviridae) of the group.

arenoid (ar'ĕ-noid) [L. *arena* sand + Gr. *eidos* form] resembling sand.

areola (ah-re'o-lah), pl. *are'olae* [L., dim. of *area* space] 1. any minute space or interstice in a tissue. 2. a circular area of a different color, surrounding a central point, as such an area surrounding a pustule or vesicle, or the part of the iris surrounding the pupil of the eye, or surrounding the nipple of the breast. **Chaussier's a.,** the areola of induration of a malignant pustule. **a. mam'mae** [NA], **a. of mammary gland,** the darkened ring surrounding the nipple of a breast. **a. of nipple,** a. mammae. **a. papilla'ris,** a. mammae. **second a.,** a ring which, during pregnancy, surrounds the areola mammae. **um-**

bilical a., a pigmented patch that sometimes surrounds the navel. **vaccinal a.,** the ring of redness that surrounds a vaccinia pustule.

areolae (ah-re'o-le) [L.] plural of *areola.*

areolar (ah-re'o-lar) pertaining to or containing areolae; containing minute interspaces.

areolitis (ar″e-o-li'tis) inflammation of the areola of the breast.

areometer (ar″e-om'ĕ-ter) [Gr. *araios* thin + *metron* measure] a hydrometer.

areometric (ar″e-o-met'rik) pertaining to hydrometry.

areometry (ar″e-om'ĕ-tre) hydrometry.

Aretaeus (ar-ĕ-te'us) **of Cappadocia** (2nd century A.D.) a famous Greek Pneumatist who wrote works on acute and chronic diseases. His clinical descriptions (e.g., of diabetes, pleurisy, tetanus) are outstanding, and in the best Hippocratic tradition.

Arey's rule (ār'ēz) [Leslie Brainerd *Arey*, American anatomist, born 1891] see under *rule.*

Arfonad (ar'fon-ad) trademark for a preparation of trimethaphan camsylate.

Arg arginine.

arg. abbreviation for L. *argen'tum*, silver.

argamblyopia (ar″gam-ble-o'pe-ah) [Gr. *argos* idle + *amblyopia*] amblyopia due to long disuse of the eye.

Argand burner [Aimé *Argand*, Swiss physicist, 1755–1803] see under *burner.*

Argas (ar'gas) a genus of ticks. **A. america'nus,** *A. persicus.* **A. brump'ti,** a species found in Africa whose bite causes local inflammation in man. **A. minia'tus,** *A. persicus.* **A. per'sicus,** a cosmopolitan tick, the tampan or tampan tick, one of the most important parasites of poultry, which sucks the blood of fowls, producing a weak condition of flocks, with great economic losses. In Iran, Egypt, India, Australia, and Brazil, it acts as the carrier of fowl spirochetosis. Called also *A. americanus* and *A. minatus,* and *miana bug.* **A. reflex'us,** an ectoparasite of pi-

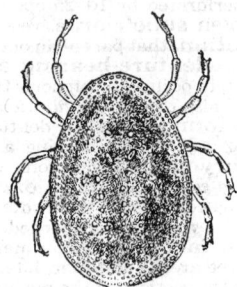

Argas persicus (after Braun).

geons and other roosting birds, which frequently attacks man and may cause a cutaneous inflammatory lesion.

Argasidae (ar-gas'ĭ-de) a family of the superfamily Ixodoidea, comprising the soft ticks, distinguished from the hard-bodied ticks (Ixodidae) by absence of the scutum. The genera are *Argas, Otobius, Antricola,* and *Ornithodoros.*

argema (ar'je-mah) a white ulcer of the cornea.

argentaffin (ar-jen'tah-fin) [L. *argentum* silver + *affinis* having affinity for] having an affinity for silver and chromium salts; said of tissues. See also under *cell.*

argentaffinoma (ar″jen-taf″ĭ-no'mah) carcinoid; a tumor of the gastroenteric tract formed from the argentaffin cells (Kultschitzky's cells) found in the enteric canal; such tumors elaborate a variety of catecholamines that produce the symptom complex called carcinoid syndrome. Cf. *enterochromaffin gland.* **a. of bronchus,** carcinoid tumor of the bronchus, highly vascular tumors of the bronchus similar to argentaffinoma of the gastrointestinal tract.

argentation (ar″jen-ta'shun) [L. *argentum* silver] staining with a silver salt.

argenti (ar-jen'ti) genitive of *argentum.* **a. io'didum colloida'le,** colloidal silver iodide. **a. ni'tras,** silver nitrate.

argentic (ar-jen'tik) containing silver.

argentoproteinum (ar-jen″to-pro″te-i'num) silver protein; see under *silver.*

argentum (ar-jen'tum), gen. *argen'ti* [L.] silver. **a. protein'icum for'te,** strong silver protein; see under *silver.* **a. protein'icum mi'te,** mild silver protein; see under *silver.*

argilla (ar-jil'lah) kaolin.

argillaceous (ar″jĭ-la'shus) composed of clay.

arginase (ar'jĭ-nās) an enzyme existing primarily in the liver, but also in the mammary gland, testis, and kidney, which splits arginine into urea and ornithine.

arginine (ar'jĭ-nin) chemical name: 2-amino-5-guanidovaleric acid. An amino acid, $C_6H_{14}N_4O_2$, produced by the hydrolysis or digestion of proteins. It is one of the hexone bases (Schulze and

Steiger, 1886), and it supplies the amidine group for the synthesis of creatine. Arginine is also formed by the transfer of a nitrogen atom from aspartate to citrulline in the urea cycle. It then gives off urea, to form ornithine. **a. glutamate,** the L(+)-arginine salt, $C_{11}H_{23}N_5O_6$, of L(+)-glutamic acid, used intravenously as an adjunct in the management of ammonia intoxication due to hepatic failure; called also *glutargin.* **a. hydrochloride** [USP], the L(+)-arginine salt of hydrochloric acid, used intravenously as an adjunct in the management of conditions in which there is an excess of ammonia in the blood. **a. monohydrochloride,** a salt of arginine sometimes used in place of ammonium chloride to potentiate mercurial diuretics in refractory heart failure. **suberyl a.,** a compound that functions in the bufotoxins as glucose does in the glucosides; it is $COOH(CH_2)_6CONHCO:NH(CH_2)_3CH(NH_2)COOH$.

argininosuccinate (ar″jĭ-nĭ-no-suk′sĭ-nāt) a compound formed by the condensation of aspartic acid and citrulline, which is an intermediate in the urea cycle. **a. lyase,** L-argininosuccinate arginine-lyase: an enzyme occurring in the liver that converts argininosuccinate to arginine and fumarate.

argininosuccinicacidemia (ar″jĭ-nĭ″no-suk-sin″ik-as″ĭ-de′me-ah) the presence in the blood of argininosuccinic acid.

argininosuccinicaciduria (ar″jĭ-nĭ″no-suk-sin″ik-as″ĭ-du′re-ah) presence in the urine of argininosuccinic acid, characteristic of a condition resulting from an inborn error of metabolism and accompanied by mental retardation.

argipressin (ar″jĕ-pres′in) chemical name: 8-α-arginine vasopressin. Vasopressin containing arginine, as that from most mammals, including man. See also *lypressin.*

argon (ar′gon) [Gr. *argos* inert] a chemical element, atomic number 18, discovered in the atmosphere in 1895. One of the inert gases, its symbol is Ar and its atomic weight 39.948.

Argyll Robertson pupil (sign) (ar-gīl′ rob′ert-son) [Douglas Moray Cooper Lamb *Argyll Robertson,* Scottish physician, 1837–1909] see under *pupil.*

argyremia (ar″jĭ-re′me-ah) [Gr. *argyros* silver + *haima* blood + *-ia*] the presence of silver or silver salts in the blood.

argyria (ar-jir′e-ah) a permanent ashen-gray discoloration of the skin, conjunctiva, and internal organs that results from long-continued use of silver salts. Called also *argyrosis.* **a. nasa′lis,** argyric discoloration of the nasal mucosa.

argyriasis (ar″jĭ-ri′ah-sis) argyria.

argyric (ar-ji′rik) pertaining to or caused by silver; pertaining to argyria.

argyrism (ar′jĭ-rizm) argyria.

Argyrol (ar′jĭ-rol) trademark for mild silver protein; see under *silver.*

argyrophil (ar-ji′ro-fil) [Gr. *argyros* silver + *philein* to love] capable of binding silver salts, which may subsequently be reduced by light or by a reducing agent to give a black deposit of silver; said of tissues.

argyrosis (ar″jĭ-ro′sis) [Gr. *argyros* silver] argyria.

arhigosis (ah″rĭ-go′sis) [*a* neg. + Gr. *rhigos* cold] inability to perceive cold; absence of the cold sense.

arhinencephalia (ah″rin-en″se-fa′le-ah) [*a* neg. + *rhinencephalon*] congenital absence of the rhinencephalon.

arhinia (ah-rin′e-ah) [*a* neg. + Gr. *rhis* nose + *-ia*] congenital absence of the nose.

arhythmia (ah-rith′me-ah) arrhythmia.

Arias-Stella reaction [Javier *Arias-Stella,* Peruvian pathologist, born 1920] see under *reaction.*

ariboflavinosis (a-ri″bo-fla″vĭ-no′sis) deficiency of riboflavin in the diet, a condition marked by lesions in the angles of the mouth, on the lips, and around nose and eyes, by corneal or other eye changes, and by seborrheic dermatitis.

aril (ar′il) [L. *arillus* dried grape] an accessory covering or appendage of seeds.

arildone (ar′il-dōn) chemical name: 4-[6-(2-chloro-4-methoxyphenoxy)hexyl]-3,5-heptanedione; an antiviral agent, $C_{20}H_{29}ClO_4$.

arillode (ar′ĭ-lōd) an appendage of certain seeds attached to the micropyle or raphe.

aristin (ah-ris′tin) a crystalline principle from various species of *Aristolochia.*

Aristocort (ah-ris′to-cort) trademark for preparations of triamcinolone and its derivatives.

Aristogel (ah-ris′to-jel) trademark for a preparation of triamcinolone acetonide.

aristogenesis (ah-ris″to-jen′ĕ-sis) [Gr. *aristos* best + *genesis* generation] the gradual continuous adaptive genoplastic origin of new and better organic mechanisms.

aristogenics (ah-ris″to-jen′iks) [Gr. *aristos* best + *gennan* to produce] improvement of the race through promotion of optimal mating between individuals possessing superior characteristics.

Aristolochia (ah-ris″to-lo′ke-ah) [L.; Gr. *aristos* best + *lochia* lochia] a genus of shrubs and herbs of many species, often actively medicinal; see *serpentaria. A. reticulata* Nutt. (Texas snakeroot) and *A. serpentaria* L. (Virginia snakeroot) are the

source (dried rhizome and roots) of serpentaria, an aromatic bitter. The plants contain aristolochic acid, a phenanthrene-carboxylic acid derivative, the major aromatic bitter principle. It is toxic to experimental animals in sufficient dosage, causing cardiac and respiratory arrest.

aristolochine (ah-ris-tol′o-chēn) aristolochic acid.

Aristospan (ah-ris′to-span) trademark for preparations of triamcinolone hexacetonide.

Aristotle's anomaly (ar′ĭ-stot-elz) [A Greek philosopher, 384–322 B.C.] see under *anomaly.*

arithmomania (ah-rith″mo-ma′ne-ah) [Gr. *arithmos* number + *mania* madness] (*obs.*) a morbid impulse to count, with worriment about numbers.

arkyochrome (ar′ke-o-krōm) [Gr. *arkys* net + *chrōma* color] any nerve cell in which the chromatic substance arranges itself in the form of a network. Cf. *gyrochrome, perichrome,* and *stichochrome.*

arkyostichochrome (ar″ke-o-stik′o-krōm) [Gr. *arkys* net + *stichos* row + *chrōma* color] any nerve cell that is both an arkyochrome and a stichochrome.

Arlidin (ar′lĭ-din) trademark for preparations of nylidrin hydrochloride.

Arloing-Courmont test (ahr-lyahn′koor′mont) [Saturnin *Arloing,* French pathologist, 1846–1911; *Courmont,* Paul] see under *test.*

Arlt's operation, recessus, sinus, trachoma (arltz) [Carl Ferdinand Ritter von *Arlt,* ophthalmologist in Vienna, 1812–1887] see under *operation, recess,* and *trachoma,* and see *sinus of Maier.*

arm (arm) [L. *armus*] 1. the part of the upper extremity between the shoulder and elbow, as distinguished from the forearm; popularly the upper extremity from shoulder to hand. See also *brachium.* 2. an armlike appendage or extension. In dentistry, the portion of the clasp by which a removable partial denture is retained in position in the mouth. In genetics, one of the portions of a mitotic chromosome on either side of the centromere. **bar clasp a.,** an extension originating in the base or major connector of a denture, and consisting of the arm that traverses but does not contact the gingival structures, and a terminal end that approaches its contact with the tooth in a gingivo-occlusal direction. **bird a.,** a wasted condition of the forearm due to atrophy of the muscles. **circumferential clasp a.,** an extension originating in a minor connector of a removable partial denture, which follows the contour of the tooth approximately in a plane perpendicular to the path of insertion of the denture. **glass a.,** a painful condition of the upper arm due to an injury to the long tendon of the biceps muscle or to the tendon of the supraspinatus muscle, at times resulting in subdeltoid bursitis. **golf a.,** a form of neuritis seen in golf players after excessive exercise. **Krukenberg's a.,** see under *hand.* **lawn tennis a.,** tennis elbow. **reciprocal a.,** the arm of the clasp of a removable partial denture which stabilizes against lateral movement of the appliance and resists force transmitted by the retentive arm, during seating and removal of the prosthesis; called also *stabilizing a.* **retention a., retentive a.,** the arm of the clasp of a removable partial denture which aids in resistance to displacement of the appliance in an occlusal direction and stabilizes against lateral forces. **stabilizing a.,** reciprocal a.

armadillo (ar″mah-dil′o) one of a group of burrowing mammals belonging to the order Edentata and possessing horny shields on the dorsal surface of the body; one species in South America is a reservoir for *Trypanosoma cruzi.*

armamentarium (ar″mah-men-tā′re-um) [L.] the equipment of a practitioner or institution, including books, instruments, medicines, and surgical appliances.

Armanni-Ebstein cells [Luciano *Armanni,* Italian pathologist, 1839–1903; Wilhelm *Ebstein,* German internist, 1836–1912] see under *cell.*

armarium (ar-ma′re-um) [L.] armamentarium.

armature (ar′mah-chūr) [L. *armatura* a defensive apparatus] 1. the iron bar or keeper across the open end of a horseshoe magnet. 2. a protective organ or structure.

A.R.M.H. Academy of Religion and Mental Health.

Armigeres (ar-mij′er-ēz) a genus of mosquitoes. **A. obtur′bans,** a mosquito which transmits dengue in Japan.

Armillifer (ar-mil′lĭ-fer) a genus of endoparasitic animals of the family Porocephalidae, order Porocephalida. **A. armilla′tus,** a species whose adult members are found in the lungs and trachea of the python (*Python sebae* and *P. regius*) and whose larvae occur in the internal organs of monkeys and lions and occasionally of man in Africa. Called also *Porocephalus armillatus* and *P. constrictus.* **A. monilifor′mis,** a species whose larvae are parasitic in man in China, the Philippines, and other Asian islands.

armpit (arm′pit) 1. fossa axillaris. 2. axilla.

Arnaldus de Villanova see *Arnold of Villanova.*

Arndt's law, Arndt-Schulz law [Rudolf *Arndt,* German psychiatrist, 1835–1900; Hugo *Schulz,* German pharmacologist, 1853–1932] see under *law.*

Arneth's formula (classification, count, index) (ar-nāts′) [Joseph *Arneth,* German physician, 1873– 1955] see under *formula.*

Arnica (ar′nĕ-kah) [L.] a genus of composite-flowered plants, known also as *leopard's bane, wolf's bane,* and *mountain tobacco.* The dried flowerheads of *A. montana* contain a volatile oil, arnicin, arnisterol, and anthoxanthine, tannin, and resin. Used topically as a tincture for contusions, sprains, and superficial wounds, and as a counterirritant.

arnica (ar′nĭ-kah) the dried flowerheads of *Arnica montana.* Called also *wolf's bane* and *leopard's bane.*

A.R.N.M.D. Association for Research in Nervous and Mental Disease.

Arnold (ar′nold) **of Villanova,** or **Arnaldus de Villanova** (c. 1235 to c. 1312) a celebrated Catalan physician who wrote extensively on medicine, alchemy, and religion and who translated Avicenna's writings on the heart from Arabic into Latin.

Arnold's bodies [Julius *Arnold,* German pathologist, 1835–1915] see under *body.*

Arnold's canal, etc. [Philipp Friedrich *Arnold,* German anatomist, 1803–1890] see under *canal, fold, ganglion, ligament, nerve, substance,* and *syndrome.*

Arnold's test [Vincenz *Arnold,* Austrian physician, born 1864] see under *tests.*

Arnold-Chiari deformity (malformation, syndrome) [Julius *Arnold;* Hans *Chiari,* German pathologist, 1851–1916] see under *deformity.*

Arnott's bed (ar′nots) [Neil *Arnott,* Scottish physician, 1788–1874] see under *bed.*

arnotto (ar-not′o) annotto.

A.R.O. Association for Research in Ophthalmology.

aroma (ah-ro′mah) [Gr. *arōma* spice] fragrance or odor, especially that of a spice or medicine or of articles of food or drink.

aromatase (ah-ro′mah-tās) an enzyme that catalyzes the aromatization of its substrate, as in the conversion of testosterone to estradiol.

aromatic (ar″o-mat′ik) [L. *aromaticus;* Gr. *arōmatikos*] 1. having a spicy odor. 2. (in chemistry) denoting a compound characterized by the benzene ring.

aromatization (ah-ro″mah-tĭ-za′shun) chemical conversion to an aromatic form.

aromine (ah-ro′min) a fragrant alkaloid from urine containing benzene derivatives.

Aron's test (ar′onz) [Hans *Aron,* German pediatrician, born 1881] see under *test.*

arousal (ah-row′sal) a state of responsiveness to sensory stimulation; called also *activation, vigilance,* and *wakefulness.*

arprinocid (ar-pri′no-sid) chemical name: 9-[(2-chloro-6-fluorophenyl)methyl]-9*H*-purin-6-amine; a coccidiostat, $C_{12}H_9ClFN_5$.

arrachement (ar″ash-mahw′) [Fr. "extraction"] extraction of a membranous cataract by pulling out the capsule through a corneal incision.

arrack (ar′rak) an alcoholic liquor distilled from fermented dates, rice, the sap of palms, mahua flowers, etc.

arrangement (ah-rānj′ment) the disposal or positioning of parts. **anterior tooth a.,** the arrangement of anterior teeth for esthetic or phonetic effects. **tooth a.,** 1. the positioning of teeth on a denture for specific purposes. 2. the setting of teeth on temporary bases.

arrector (ah-rek′tor), pl. *arrecto′res* [L.] raising, or that which raises. **a. pi′li,** pl. **arrecto′res pilo′rum** [L. "raisers of the hair"], minute smooth muscles of the skin, attached to the connective tissue sheath of the hair follicles, the contraction of which causes the hair to stand erect and produces the appearance called cutis anserina, or goose flesh.

arrectores (ar″rek-to′rez) [L.] plural of *arrector.*

arrest (ah-rest) stoppage; the act of stopping. **cardiac a.,** sudden cessation of cardiac function, with disappearance of arterial blood pressure, connoting either ventricular fibrillation or ventricular standstill. **deep transverse a.,** the condition during delivery in which the occiput of the fetus turns and stops in the transverse diameter of the pelvis. **developmental a.,** a temporary or permanent cessation of the process of development. **epiphyseal a.,** interruption of growth at the epiphysis of a bone by diaphyseal-epiphyseal fusion. **heart a.,** cardiac a. **maturation a.,** interruption of the process of development before it is complete; applied especially to failure of maturation of granulocytes, with myeloblasts and promyelocytes constituting the dominant bone marrow elements. **sinus a.,** a pause in cardiac rhythm due to a momentary failure of the sinus node to initiate an impulse; called also *sinus standstill.*

arrested (ah-rest′ed) detained; stopped. In obstetrics, the head of the child is said to be arrested when it is *detained,* but not *impacted,* in the pelvic cavity.

arrhaphia (ah-ra′fe-ah) status dysrhaphia.

Arrhenius' equation, formula, theory (doctrine) (ah-re′ne-us) [Svante August *Arrhenius,* Swedish chemist, 1859–1927] see under *equation, formula,* and *theory.*

arrheno- (ah-re′no) [Gr. *arrhēn* male] a combining form meaning male.

arrhenoblastoma (ah-re″no-blas-to′mah) [*arrheno-* + Gr. *blastos* germ + *-oma*] a neoplasm of the ovary, arising from the ovarian stroma, mimicking to a greater or lesser extent derivatives of the sex cord mesenchyme of the testis, and sometimes causing defeminization and virilization. Called also *andreioma, andreoblastoma, androma, arrhenoma,* and *Sertoli-Leydig cell tumor.*

arrhenogenic (ar″ĕ-no-jen′ik) [*arrheno* + Gr. *gennan* to produce] producing only male offspring.

arrhenokaryon (ar″ĕ-no-kar′e-on) an organism that is produced by androgenesis.

arrhenoma (ar″ĕ-no′mah) arrhenoblastoma.

arrhenoplasm (ah-re′no-plazm) [*arrheno-* + *plasm*] the male element of idioplasm.

arrhenotocia (ar″ĕ-no-to′se-a) arrhenotoky.

arrhenotoky (ar″ĕ-not′o-ke) [*arrheno-* + Gr. *tokos* birth] the production of males only by a virgin mother, as in the unfertilized queen bee.

arrhigosis (ah″rĭ-go′sis) arhigosis.

arrhinencephalia (ah″rin-en″se-fa′le-ah) arhinencephalia.

arrhinia (ah-rin′e-ah) arhinia.

arrhythmia (ah-rith′me-ah) [*a* neg. + Gr. *rhythmos* rhythm] any variation from the normal rhythm of the heart beat, including sinus arrhythmia, premature beat, heart block, atrial fibrillation, atrial flutter, pulsus alternans, and paroxysmal tachycardia. **continuous a.,** irregularity in the force, quality, and sequence of the pulse beat, continuing as a permanent phenomenon; called also *perpetual a.* **juvenile a.,** sinus arrhythmia occuring in children. **nodal a.,** nodal rhythm; see under *rhythm.* **perpetual a.,** continuous a. **phasic a.,** sinus a. **respiratory a.,** sinus a. **sinus a.,** the physiologic cyclic variation in heart rate related to vagal impulses to the sinoatrial node; it occurs commonly in children (juvenile a.) and in the aged, and requires no treatment. Called also *phasic a.* and *respiratory a.*

arrhythmic (ah-rith′mik) [*a* neg. + Gr. *rhythmos* rhythm] characterized by absence of rhythm.

arrhythmogenic (ah-rith″mo-jen′ik) [*a* neg. + Gr. *rhythmos* rhythm + *gennan* to produce] producing or promoting arrhythmia.

arrhythmokinesis (ah-rith″mo-kĭ-ne′sis) [*a* neg. + Gr. *rhythmos* rhythm + *kinēsis* movement] defective ability to perform voluntary successive movement of a definite rhythm.

arrow (ar′o) a sharply pointed instrument or tool. **caustic a.,** a sharply pointed bit of nitrate of silver or other caustic substance.

arrowroot (ar′o-root) a starch prepared from the rhizome of *Maranta arundinacea* L., Marantaceae, a plant native to northern South America and the West Indies and now extensively cultivated in almost all tropical countries. It is a prominent constituent of infant, geriatric, and convalescent diets.

Arroyo's sign (ar-ro′yōz) [Carlos F. *Arroyo,* American physician, 1892–1928] asthenocoria.

A.R.R.S. American Roentgen Ray Society.

A.R.S. American Radium Society.

arsambide (ar-sam′bīd) carbarsone.

arsenate (ar′sĕ-nāt) any salt of arsenic acid. **ferric a.,** a brownish yellow powder, $4Fe_2O_3 \cdot 5H_2O$, used in anemia; called also *iron arsenate.* **ferrous a.,** a green amorphous powder, $Fe_3(AsO_4)_2 \cdot 6H_2O$, insoluble in water; formerly used in chronic skin conditions and now employed as an insecticide. Called also *iron arsenate.*

arseniasis (ar″sĕ-ni′ah-sis) chronic arsenical poisoning.

arsenic[1] (ar′sĕ-nik) [L. *arsenicum, arsenium,* or *arsenum;* from Gr. *arsēn* strong] 1. a medicinal and poisonous element; it is a brittle, lustrous, grayish solid, with a garlicky odor. Symbol, As; atomic number, 33; atomic weight, 74.922; specific gravity, 5.73. See also under *poisoning.* 2. arsenic trioxide. **a. chloride,** a. trichloride. **a. disulfide,** a poisonous compound, As_2S_2, used as a pigment, in fireworks, in shot manufacture, and in the leather industry; called also *red arsenic sulfide* and *realgar.* **fuming liquid a.,** a. trichloride. **a. iodide,** a red crystalline compound, AsI_3, once used in coryza and skin diseases. **red a. sulfide,** a. disulfide. **a. trichloride,** a very poisonous fuming liquid, $AsCl_3$, which readily liberates highly irritant hydrochloric acid; it is used in war gas and as an intermediate for organic chemicals. **a. trioxide,** white arsenic, a white or glassy compound, As_2O_3, with a sweetish taste and erythropoietic effect; taken in repeated small doses in Alpine countries to increase hemoglobin, resulting in increased working capacity and a ruddy complexion. Formerly used in treatment of skin and hematologic disorders. Called also *arsenous acid, arsenous anhydride,* and *flowers of arsenic.* **a. trisulfide,** a poisonous substance, As_2S_3, occurring in nature as the mineral orpiment; used as a pigment and sometimes as a medicine. Called also *a. yellow* and *auripigment.* **white a.,** a. trioxide. **a. yellow,** a. trisulfide.

arsenic² (ar-sen′ik) pertaining to or containing arsenic in a pentavalent state.

arsenical (ar-sen′ĭ-kal) [L. *arsenicalis*] 1. pertaining to or containing arsenic. 2. a drug containing arsenic.

arsenicalism (ar-sen′ĕ-kal″izm) chronic arsenical poisoning.

arsenicophagy (ar″sen-ĭ-kof′ah-je) [*arsenic* Gr. *phagein* to eat] the eating of arsenic.

arsenicum (ar-sen′ĕ-kum) [L.] arsenic.

arsenide (ar′sĕ-nīd) any compound of arsenic with another element, in which arsenic is the negative element.

arsenious (ar-sen′e-us) arsenous; pertaining to arsenic in a trivalent state.

arsenism (ar′sen-izm) chronic arsenic poisoning.

arsenite (ar′sĕ-nīt) any salt of arsenous acid.

arsenium (ar-se′ne-um) [L.] the element arsenic.

arsenization (ar″sen-ĭ-za′shun) treatment with arsenic.

arseno- (ar′sĕ-no) a prefix indicating the chemical group —As: As—.

arsenoactivation (ar″sĕ-no-ak″tĭ-va′shun) increase in the manifestations of syphilis under treatment by arsenicals.

arsenoautohemotherapy (ar″sĕ-no-aw″to-he″mo-ther′ah-pe) treatment of syphilis by injection of arsenical drug mixed with some of the patient's own blood.

arsenobenzene (ar″sĕ-no-ben′zēn) a general term for the various arsphenamine compounds used in the treatment of spirochetal diseases.

arsenoblast (ar-sen′o-blast) [Gr. *arsēn* male + *blastos* germ] the male element of a zygote; a male pronucleus.

arsenoceptor (ar-sen′o-sep″tor) a supposed receptor in cells for arsenic.

arsenolysis (ar″sen-ol′ĭ-sis) the enzyme-induced, reversible combination and separation of sugar and arsenic acid.

arsenophagy (ar″sĕ-nof′ah-je) arsenicophagy.

arsenorelapsing (ar-sen″o-re-laps′ing) relapsing after apparent cure by arsenical treatment; said of certain cases of syphilis.

arsenoresistant (ar-sen″o-re-zis′tant) resistant to arsenicals such as arsphenamine; said of certain cases of syphilis.

arsenotherapy (ar″sĕ-no-ther′ah-pe) [*arsenic* + Gr. *therapeia* treatment] treatment of disease by the use of arsenic and arsenical preparations.

arsenous (ar′sĕ-nus) containing arsenic in its lower or triad valency.

arsenoxide (ar″sen-ok′sīd) oxophenarsine.

arsenum (ar-se′num) [L.] arsenic.

arsine (ar′sin) any member of a peculiar group of volatile arsenical bases, formed when arsenous acid is brought in contact with albuminous substances. The typical arsine is AsH_3, arsenous hydride or arseniuretted hydrogen, a very poisonous gas, and some of its compounds have been used in warfare. It causes hemolysis, jaundice, gastroenteritis, and nephritis.

arsonium (ar-so′ne-um) the univalent radical or ion, AsH_4, which acts in combination like the ammonium ion, NH_4.

arsonvalization (ar″son-val″i-za′shun) d'arsonvalism.

arsphenamine (ars-fen′ah-min) chemical name: 4,4′-(1,2-diarsenediyl)bis[2-aminophenol]dihydrochloride. A yellow hygroscopic powder, $[OH \cdot C_6H_3(NH_2 \cdot HCl) \cdot As]_2$, introduced as the first specific for the treatment of syphilis, yaws, and other spirillum infections but later virtually replaced in medicine, first by arsenoxide and then by penicillin. It rapidly oxidizes on exposure to air, and is, therefore, put up in hermetically sealed capsules. The substance is converted, immediately before injection, into an unstable sodium salt by the addition of sodium hydroxide solution. Called also *salvarsan* (Germany), *arsenobenzol* (France), *diarsenol* (Canada), *arsaminol* (Japan), *606*, *Ehrlich-Hata* or *Hata's preparation*, and *magic bullet.* **silver a.,** sodium salt of silver diaminodihydroxyarsenobenzene; it contains about 19 per cent arsenic and 12 to 14 per cent silver; formerly used in the treatment of the neurologic complications in syphilis. Called also *argentum arsphenamina* and *silver salvarsan.* **sodium a.,** a bright yellow powder, the sodium salt of arsphenamine, $C_{12}H_{10}As_2N_2Na_2O_2$, unstable in air and freely soluble in water; formerly used in the treatment of syphilis. Called also *sodiarsphenamine.* **a. sulfoxylate,** a condensation product of arsphenamine and sodium formaldehyde bisulfite, $[NaO \cdot SO_2 \cdot CH \cdot NH(OH)C_6H_4As]_2$.

arsthinol (ars′thĭ-nol) chemical name: *N*-[2-hydroxy-5-[4-(hydroxymethyl)-1,3,2-dithiarsolan-2-yl]phenyl]acetamide. An antiprotozoal agent, $C_{11}H_{14}AsNO_3S_2$, effective in amebiasis and yaws; administered orally.

A.R.T. Accredited Record Technicians.

Artane (ar′tān) trademark for preparations of trihexyphenidyl.

artarine (ar′tah-rin) an alkaloid, $C_{21}H_{23}NO_4$, from the root of *Xanthoxylum senegalense.*

artefact (ar′te-fakt) artifact.

Artemisia (ar″tĕ-mis′e-ah) [L.; Gr. *artemisia* from *Artemis* Diana] a genus of composite-flowered plants, including *A. abrot′anum* (southernwood), *A. absin′thium* (wormwood), and *A. marit′ima* (*A. pauciflora*), from which santonin is derived. The oil of *A. absinthium* was formerly used in the preparation of the alcoholic beverage, absinthe, but because it contains neurotoxic agents (1-thujone and d-isothujone), its use has been discontinued. Absinthin is the active bitter principle.

arteralgia (ar″ter-al′je-ah) pain emanating from an artery, such as headache from an inflamed temporal artery.

arterectomy (ar″tĕ-rek′to-me) arteriectomy.

arterenol (ar″tĕ-re′nol) norepinephrine.

arteria (ar-te′re-ah) pl. *arte′riae* [L.; Gr. *artēria*] a general term used in anatomical nomenclature to designate any vessel carrying blood away from the heart. For names and description of specific vessels, see *Table of Arteriae.* See also *artery.* **a. luso′ria,** an abnormally situated retroesophageal vessel, usually the subclavian artery from the aortic arch, which may cause symptoms by compression of the esophagus, the trachea, or a nerve.

arteriae (ar-te′re-e) [L.] plural of *arteria.*

TABLE OF ARTERIAE

Description of vessels are given on NA terms, and include anglicized names of specific arteries. Although each artery is identified by its origin, branches, and distribution, it should be borne in mind that there are variations in the point of origin, that only named branches are listed, and that only the more noteworthy structures are given in the distribution.

a. aceta′buli, ramus acetabularis arteriae obturatoriae.

a. alveola′ris infe′rior [NA], inferior alveolar artery: *origin,* maxillary artery; *branches,* dental, mylohyoid rami, mental artery; *distribution,* lower jaw, lower lip, and chin. Called also *inferior dental artery* and *mandibular artery.*

arte′riae alveola′res superio′res anterio′res [NA], anterior superior alveolar arteries: *origin,* infraorbital artery; *branches,* dental; *distribution,* incisors and canine regions of upper jaw, maxillary sinus. Called also *anterior dental arteries.*

a. alveola′ris supe′rior poste′rior [NA], posterior superior alveolar artery: *origin,* maxillary artery; *branches,* dental; *distribution* molar and premolar regions of upper jaw, maxillary sinus. Called also *superior dental artery.*

a. angula′ris [NA], angular artery: *origin,* facial artery; *branches,* none; *distribution,* lacrimal sac, lower eyelid, nose.

a. anon′yma, truncus brachiocephalicus.

a. aor′ta, aorta.

a. appendicula′ris [NA], appendicular artery: *origin,* ileocolic artery; *branches,* none; *distribution,* vermiform appendix. Called also *vermiform artery.*

arte′riae arcifor′mes re′nis, arteriae arcuatae renis.

a. arcua′ta pe′dis [NA], arcuate artery of foot: *origin,* dorsal artery of foot; *branches,* deep plantar branch and dorsal metatarsal artery; *distribution,* foot, toes. Called also *arcus dorsalis pedis.*

arte′riae arcua′tae re′nis [NA], arcuate arteries of kidney: *origin,* interlobar artery; *branches,* interlobular artery and arteriolae rectae; *distribution,* parenchyma of kidney. Called also *arteriae arciformes renis* and *arterial arches of kidney.*

a. ascen′dens ileocol′ica [NA], *origin,* ileocecal; *branches,* none; *distribution,* ascending colon.

a. auditi′va inter′na, a. labyrinthi.

arte′riae auricula′res anterio′res, rami auriculares anteriores arteriae temporalis superficialis.

a. auricula′ris poste′rior [NA], posterior auricular artery: *origin,* external carotid; *branches,* auricular and occipital rami, stylomastoid artery; *distribution,* middle ear, mastoid cells, auricle, parotid gland, digastric and other muscles.

a. auricula′ris profun′da [NA], deep auricular artery: *origin,* maxillary artery; *branches,* none; *distribution,* skin of auditory canal, tympanic membrane, temporomandibular joint.

a. axilla′ris [NA], axillary artery: *origin,* continuation of subclavian artery; *branches,* subscapular rami, and supreme thoracic, thoracoacromial, lateral thoracic, subscapular, and anterior and posterior circumflex humeral arteries; *distribution,* upper limb, axilla, chest, shoulder.

a. basila′ris [NA], basilar artery: *origin,* from junction of right and left vertebral arteries; *branches,* pontine branches, and anterior inferior cerebellar, labyrinthine, superior cerebellar, and posterior cerebral arteries; *distribution,* brain stem, internal ear, cerebellum, posterior cerebrum.

a. brachia′lis [NA], brachial artery: *origin,* continuation of axillary artery; *branches,* superficial brachial, deep brachial, nutrient of humerus, superior ulnar collateral, inferior ulnar collateral, radial, and ulnar arteries; *distribution*, shoulder, arm, forearm, hand.

a. brachia′lis superficia′lis [NA], superficial brachial artery: a name given to a vessel that arises from high bifurcation of the brachial artery and assumes a more superficial course than usual.

arte′riae bronchia′les, rami bronchiales aortae thoracicae.

a. bucca′lis [NA], buccal artery: *origin*, maxillary artery; *branches*, none; *distribution*, buccinator muscle, mucous membrane of mouth. Called also *a. buccinatoria* and *buccinator artery*.

a. buccinato′ria, a. buccalis.

a. bul′bi pe′nis [NA], artery of bulb of penis: *origin*, internal pudendal artery; *branches*, none; *distribution*, bulbourethral gland, bulb of penis. Called also *a. bulbi urethrae* and *bulbourethral artery*.

a. bul′bi ure′thrae, a. bulbi penis.

a. bul′bi vestib′uli vagi′nae [NA], artery of bulb of vestibule of vagina: *origin*, internal pudendal artery; *branches*, none; *distribution*, vestibular bulb, greater vestibular glands.

a. cana′lis pterygoi′dei [NA], artery of pterygoid canal: *origin*, maxillary artery; *branches*, none; *distribution*, roof of pharynx, auditory tube. Called also *vidian artery*.

a. carot′is commu′nis [NA], common carotid artery: *origin*, brachiocephalic trunk (right), aortic arch (left); *branches*, external and internal carotids; *distribution*, see *a. carotis externa* and *a. carotis interna*. Called also *cephalic artery*.

a. carot′is exter′na [NA], external carotid artery: *origin*, common carotid; *branches*, superior thyroid, ascending pharyngeal, lingual, facial, sternocleidomastoid, occipital, posterior auricular, superficial temporal, maxillary; *distribution*, neck, face, skull. Called also *facial artery*.

a. carot′is inter′na [NA], internal carotid artery: *origin*, common carotid; *branches*, caroticotympanic rami, and ophthalmic, posterior communicating, anterior choroid, anterior cerebral, and middle cerebral arteries; *distribution*, middle ear, brain, pituitary gland, orbit, choroid plexus.

a. cau′dae pancre′atis [NA], *origin*, splenic; *branches and distribution*, supplies branches to tail of pancreas, and accessory spleen (if present).

a. ceca′lis ante′rior [NA], anterior cecal artery: *origin*, ileocecal; *branches*, none; *distribution*, cecum.

a. ceca′lis poste′rior [NA], posterior cecal artery: *origin*, ileocecal; *branches*, none; *distribution*, cecum.

a. centra′lis ret′inae [NA], central artery of retina: *origin*, ophthalmic artery; *branches*, none; *distribution*, retina. Called also *Zinn's artery*.

a. cerebel′li infe′rior ante′rior [NA], anterior inferior cerebellar artery: *origin*, basilar artery; *branches*, labyrinthine artery; *distribution*, anteroinferior part of cerebellum, inner ear.

a. cerebel′li infe′rior poste′rior [NA], posterior inferior cerebellar artery: *origin*, vertebral artery; *branches*, none; *distribution*, lower cerebellum, medulla, choroid plexus of fourth ventricle.

a. cerebel′li supe′rior [NA], superior cerebellar artery: *origin*, basilar artery; *branches*, none; *distribution*, upper cerebellum, midbrain, pineal body, choroid plexus of third ventricle.

arte′riae cer′ebri [NA], cerebral arteries: the arteries supplying the cerebral cortex, including *a. cerebri anterior*, *a cerebri media*, and *a. cerebri posterior*.

a. cer′ebri ante′rior [NA], anterior cerebral artery: *origin*, internal carotid; *branches*, cortical (orbital, frontal, parietal), anterior choroidal, and central branches (including the medial striate artery), and anterior communicating artery; *distribution*, orbital, frontal, and parietal cortex, corpus callosum, diencephalon, corpus striatum, internal capsule, choroid plexus of lateral ventricle.

a. cer′ebri me′dia [NA], middle cerebral artery: *origin*, internal carotid; *branches*, cortical (orbital, frontal, parietal, temporal) and central (striate) branches; *distribution*, orbital, frontal, parietal, and temporal cortex, corpus striatum, internal capsule. Called also *sylvian artery*.

a. cer′ebri poste′rior [NA], posterior cerebral artery: *origin*, terminal bifurcation of basilar artery; *branches*, cortical (temporal, occipital, parietooccipital), central, and choroid branches; *distribution*, occipital and temporal cortex, diencephalon, midbrain, choroid plexus of lateral and third ventricles.

a. cervica′lis ascen′dens [NA], ascending cervical artery: *origin*, inferior thyroid artery; *branches*, spinal rami; *distribution*, muscles of neck, vertebrae, vertebral canal.

a. cervica′lis profun′da [NA], deep cervical artery: *origin*, costocervical trunk; *branches*, none; *distribution*, deep neck muscles.

a. cervica′lis superficia′lis, NA alternative for *ramus superficialis arteriae transversae colli*.

arte′riae cervicovagi′nales, several large branches of the uterine artery given off at the side of the uterus at the level of the cervix, to supply the vagina.

a. chorioi′dea, a. choroidea anterior.

a. choroi′dea ante′rior [NA], anterior choroidal artery: *origin*, internal carotid or middle cerebral artery; *branches*, none; *distribution*, choroid plexus of lateral ventricle and adjacent parts. Called also *a. chorioidea*.

arte′riae cilia′res anterio′res [NA], anterior ciliary arteries: *origin*, ophthalmic and lacrimal arteries; *branches*, episcleral and anterior conjunctival arteries; *distribution*, iris, conjunctiva.

arte′riae cilia′res posterio′res bre′ves [NA], short (poste-

rior) ciliary arteries: *origin*, ophthalmic artery; *branches*, none; *distribution*, choroid coat of eye.

arte′riae cilia′res posterio′res lon′gae [NA], long (posterior) ciliary arteries: *origin*, ophthalmic artery; *branches*, none; *distribution*, iris, ciliary process.

a. circumflex′a fem′oris latera′lis [NA], lateral circumflex femoral artery: *origin*, deep femoral artery; *branches*, ascending, descending, and transverse branches; *distribution*, hip joint, thigh muscles.

a. circumflex′a fem′oris media′lis [NA], medial circumflex femoral artery: *origin*, deep femoral artery; *branches*, deep, ascending, transverse, and acetabular branches; *distribution*, hip joint, thigh muscles.

a. circumflex′a hu′meri ante′rior [NA], anterior circumflex humeral artery: *origin*, axillary artery; *branches*, none; *distribution*, shoulder joint and head of humerus, long tendon of biceps, tendon of pectoralis major muscle.

a. circumflex′a hu′meri poste′rior [NA], posterior circumflex humeral artery: *origin*, axillary artery; *branches*, none; *distribution*, deltoideus, shoulder joint, teres minor and triceps muscles.

a. circumflex′a il′ium profun′da [NA], deep circumflex iliac artery: *origin*, external iliac artery; *branches*, ascending branches; *distribution*, iliac region, abdominal wall, groin. Called also *external epigastric artery*.

a. circumflex′a il′ium superficia′lis [NA], superficial circumflex iliac artery: *origin*, femoral artery; *branches*, none; *distribution*, groin, abdominal wall.

a. circumflex′a scap′ulae [NA], circumflex artery of scapula: *origin*, subscapular artery; *branches*, none; *distribution*, inferolateral muscles of the scapula.

a. clitor′idis, artery of clitoris.

a. coelia′ca, truncus celiacus.

a. col′ica dex′tra [NA], right colic artery: *origin*, superior mesenteric artery; *branches*, none; *distribution*, ascending colon.

a. col′ica me′dia [NA], middle colic artery: *origin*, superior mesenteric artery; *branches*, none; *distribution*, transverse colon. Called also *accessory superior colic artery*.

a. col′ica sinis′tra [NA], left colic artery: *origin*, inferior mesenteric; *branches*, none; *distribution*, descending colon.

a. collatera′lis me′dia [NA], middle collateral artery: *origin*, deep brachial artery; *branches*, none; *distribution*, triceps muscle, elbow joint.

a. collatera′lis radia′lis [NA], radial collateral artery: *origin*, deep brachial artery; *branches*, none; *distribution*, brachioradialis and brachialis muscles.

a. collatera′lis ulna′ris infe′rior [NA], inferior ulnar collateral artery: *origin*, brachial artery; *branches*, none; *distribution*, arm muscles at back of elbow.

a. collatera′lis ulna′ris supe′rior [NA], superior ulnar collateral artery: *origin*, brachial artery; *branches*, none; *distribution*, elbow joint, triceps muscle.

a. comitans′ ner′vi ischia′dici [NA], sciatic artery: *origin*, inferior gluteal artery; *branches*, none; *distribution*, accompanies sciatic nerve. Called also *accompanying artery of ischiatic nerve*.

a. commu′nicans ante′rior cer′ebri [NA], anterior communicating artery of cerebrum: *origin*, anterior cerebral artery; *branches*, none; *distribution*, establishes connection between the anterior cerebral arteries.

a. commu′nicans poste′rior cer′ebri [NA], posterior communicating artery of cerebrum: establishes connection between internal carotid and posterior cerebral arteries; *branches*, none.

arte′riae conjunctiva′les anterio′res [NA], anterior conjunctival arteries: *origin*, anterior ciliary; *branches*, none; *distribution*, conjunctiva.

arte′riae conjunctiva′les posterio′res [NA], posterior conjunctival arteries: *origin*, medial palpebral artery; *branches*, none; *distribution*, caruncula lacrimalis, conjunctiva.

a. corona′ria [cor′dis] dex′tra, a. coronaria dextra.

a. corona′ria dex′tra [NA], right coronary artery of heart: *origin*, right aortic sinus; *branches*, posterior interventricular; *distribution*, right ventricle, right atrium. Formerly called *right auricular artery*.

a. corona′ria [cor′dis] sinis′tra, a. coronaria sinistra.

a. corona′ria sinis′tra [NA], left coronary artery of heart: *origin*, left aortic sinus; *branches*, anterior interventricular and circumflex rami; *distribution*, left ventricle, left atrium. Formerly called *left auricular artery*.

a. cremaster′ica [NA], cremasteric artery: *origin*, inferior epigastric; *branches*, none; *distribution*, cremaster muscle, coverings of spermatic cord. Called also *a. spermatica externa* and *external spermatic artery*.

a. cys′tica [NA], cystic artery: *origin*, right branch of proper hepatic artery; *branches*, none; *distribution*, gallbladder.

a. deferentia′lis, a. ductus deferentis.

arte′riae digita′les dorsa′les ma′nus [NA], dorsal digital arteries of hand: *origin*, dorsal metacarpal arteries; *branches*, none; *distribution*, dorsum of fingers.

arte′riae digita′les dorsa′les pe′dis [NA], dorsal digital arteries of foot: *origin*, dorsal metatarsal arteries; *branches*, none; *distribution*, dorsum of toes.

arte′riae digita′les palma′res commu′nes [NA], common palmar digital arteries: *origin*, superficial volar arch; *branches*,

Plate I   arteries

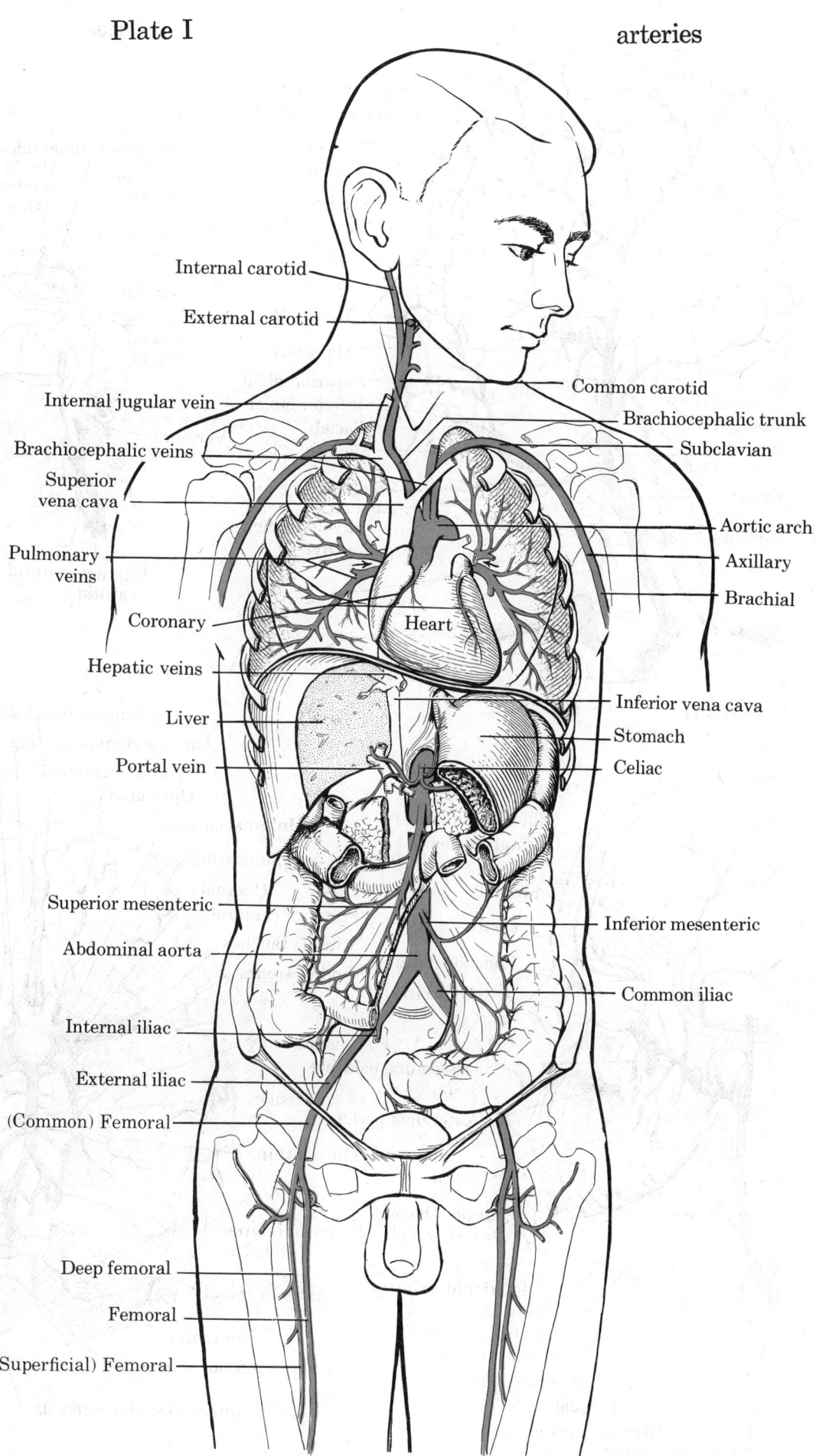

Internal carotid

External carotid

Common carotid

Brachiocephalic trunk

Internal jugular vein

Subclavian

Brachiocephalic veins

Superior
vena cava

Aortic arch

Pulmonary
veins

Axillary

Brachial

Coronary

Heart

Hepatic veins

Inferior vena cava

Liver

Stomach

Portal vein

Celiac

Superior mesenteric

Inferior mesenteric

Abdominal aorta

Common iliac

Internal iliac

External iliac

(Common) Femoral

Deep femoral

Femoral

(Superficial) Femoral

PRINCIPAL ARTERIES OF THE BODY AND PULMONARY VEINS

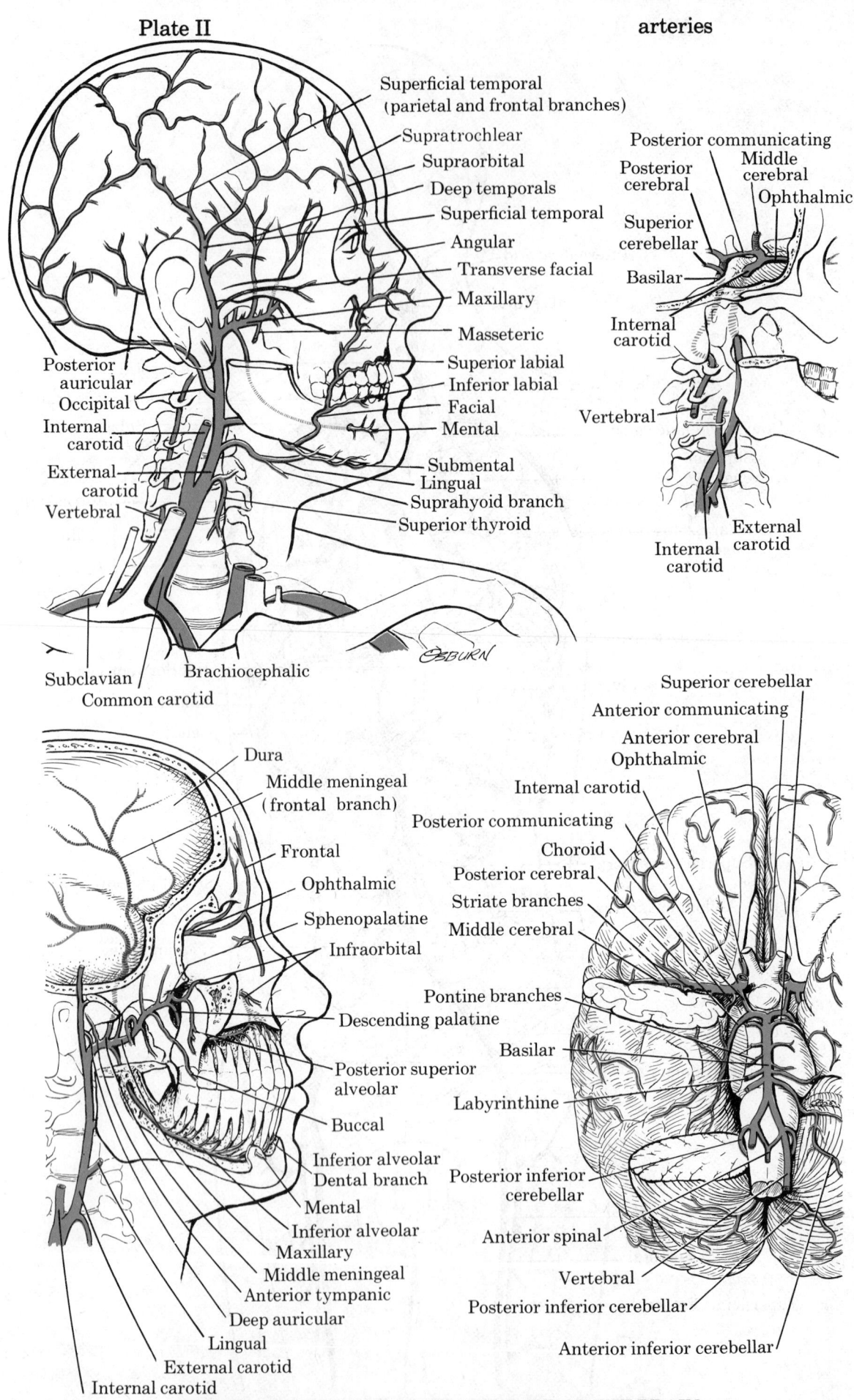

Plate II

arteries

Superficial temporal
(parietal and frontal branches)

Supratrochlear

Supraorbital

Deep temporals

Superficial temporal

Angular

Transverse facial

Maxillary

Masseteric

Superior labial

Inferior labial

Facial

Mental

Submental

Lingual

Suprahyoid branch

Superior thyroid

Posterior
auricular

Occipital

Internal
carotid

External
carotid

Vertebral

Subclavian

Brachiocephalic

Common carotid

Posterior communicating

Posterior
cerebral

Middle
cerebral

Ophthalmic

Superior
cerebellar

Basilar

Internal
carotid

Vertebral

External
carotid

Internal
carotid

Dura

Middle meningeal
(frontal branch)

Frontal

Ophthalmic

Sphenopalatine

Infraorbital

Descending palatine

Posterior superior
alveolar

Buccal

Inferior alveolar

Dental branch

Mental

Inferior alveolar

Maxillary

Middle meningeal

Anterior tympanic

Deep auricular

Lingual

External carotid

Internal carotid

Superior cerebellar

Anterior communicating

Anterior cerebral

Ophthalmic

Internal carotid

Posterior communicating

Choroid

Posterior cerebral

Striate branches

Middle cerebral

Pontine branches

Basilar

Labyrinthine

Posterior inferior
cerebellar

Anterior spinal

Vertebral

Posterior inferior cerebellar

Anterior inferior cerebellar

ARTERIES OF THE HEAD, NECK, AND BASE OF THE BRAIN

Plate III   arteries

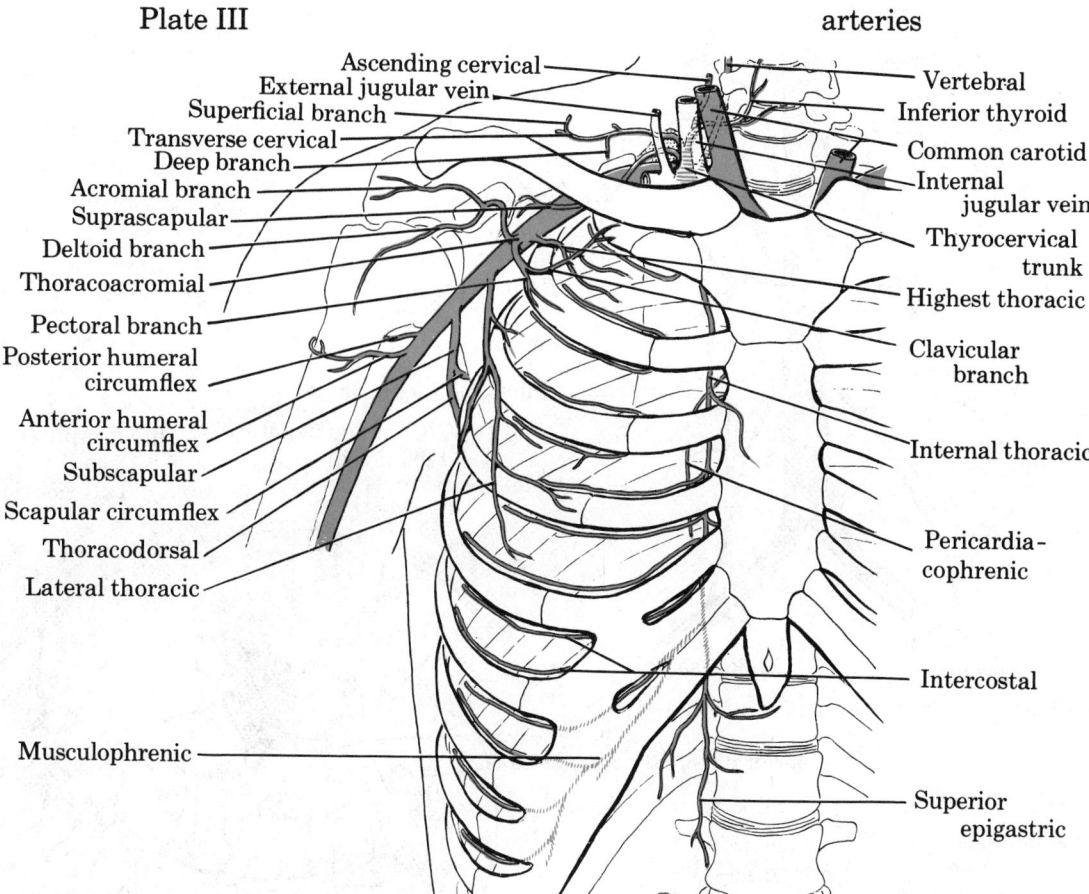

Ascending cervical
External jugular vein
Superficial branch
Transverse cervical
Deep branch
Acromial branch
Suprascapular
Deltoid branch
Thoracoacromial
Pectoral branch
Posterior humeral circumflex
Anterior humeral circumflex
Subscapular
Scapular circumflex
Thoracodorsal
Lateral thoracic
Musculophrenic

Vertebral
Inferior thyroid
Common carotid
Internal jugular vein
Thyrocervical trunk
Highest thoracic
Clavicular branch
Internal thoracic
Pericardia-cophrenic
Intercostal
Superior epigastric

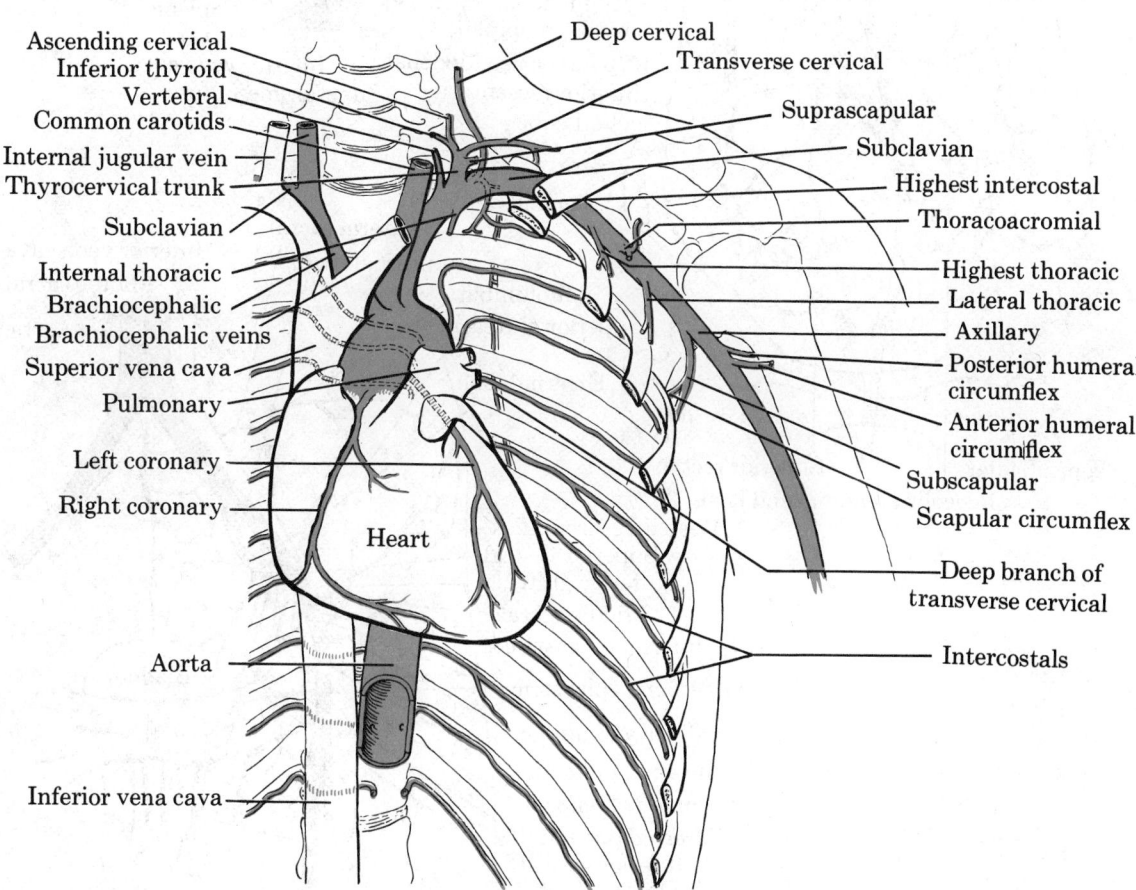

Ascending cervical
Inferior thyroid
Vertebral
Common carotids
Internal jugular vein
Thyrocervical trunk
Subclavian
Internal thoracic
Brachiocephalic
Brachiocephalic veins
Superior vena cava
Pulmonary
Left coronary
Right coronary
Heart
Aorta
Inferior vena cava

Deep cervical
Transverse cervical
Suprascapular
Subclavian
Highest intercostal
Thoracoacromial
Highest thoracic
Lateral thoracic
Axillary
Posterior humeral circumflex
Anterior humeral circumflex
Subscapular
Scapular circumflex
Deep branch of transverse cervical
Intercostals

ARTERIES OF THE THORAX AND AXILLA

Plate IV

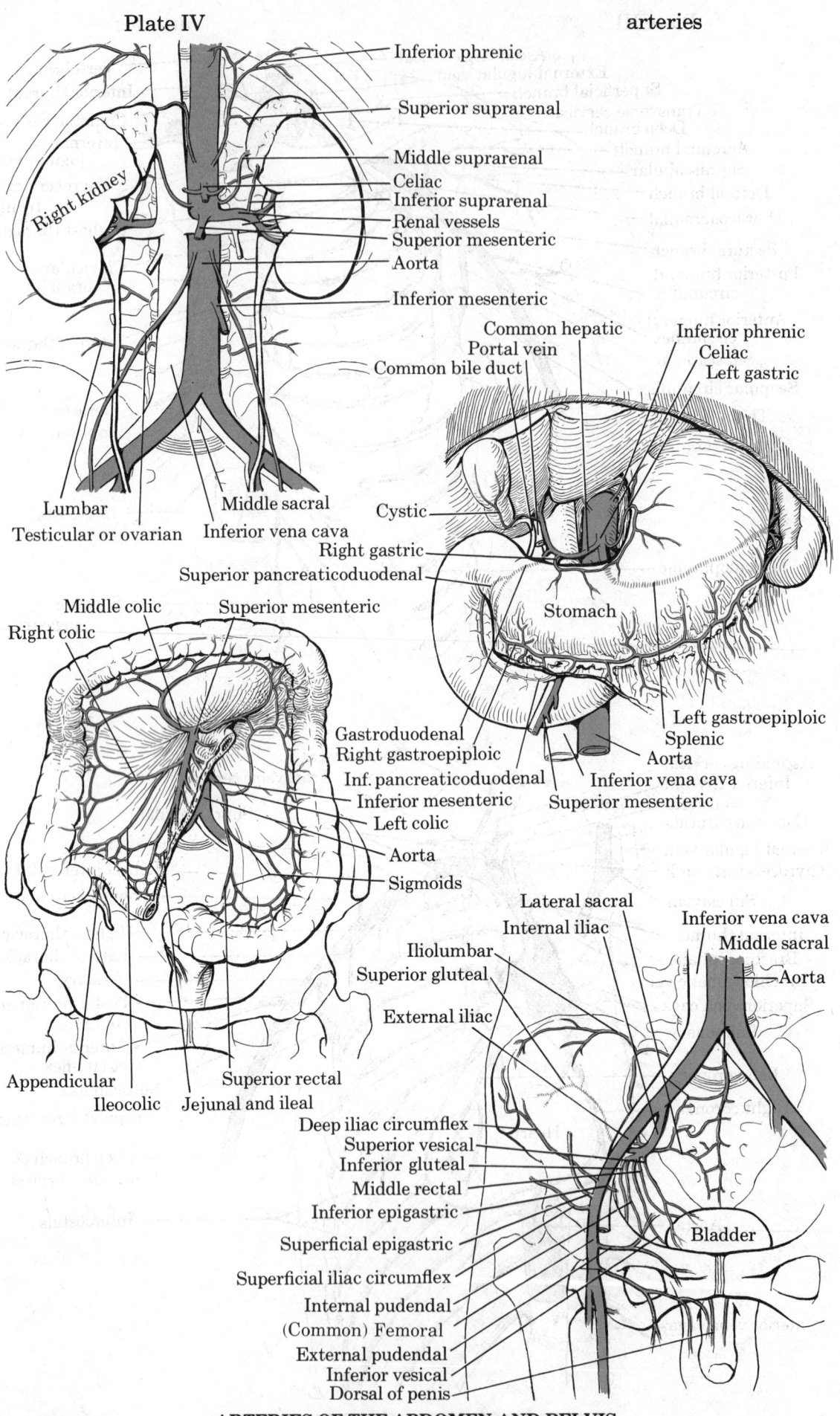

Inferior phrenic

Superior suprarenal

Middle suprarenal
Celiac
Inferior suprarenal
Renal vessels
Superior mesenteric
Aorta

Inferior mesenteric

Right kidney

Lumbar
Testicular or ovarian

Middle sacral
Inferior vena cava

Common hepatic
Portal vein
Common bile duct

Inferior phrenic
Celiac
Left gastric

Cystic

Right gastric

Superior pancreaticoduodenal

Stomach

Left gastroepiploic
Splenic
Aorta
Inferior vena cava
Superior mesenteric

Middle colic   Superior mesenteric
Right colic

Gastroduodenal
Right gastroepiploic
Inf. pancreaticoduodenal
Inferior mesenteric
Left colic
Aorta
Sigmoids

Appendicular   Superior rectal
Ileocolic   Jejunal and ileal

Lateral sacral
Internal iliac
Iliolumbar
Superior gluteal
External iliac

Inferior vena cava
Middle sacral
Aorta

Deep iliac circumflex
Superior vesical
Inferior gluteal
Middle rectal
Inferior epigastric

Superficial epigastric

Superficial iliac circumflex

Internal pudendal
(Common) Femoral
External pudendal
Inferior vesical
Dorsal of penis

Bladder

ARTERIES OF THE ABDOMEN AND PELVIS

Plate V   arteries

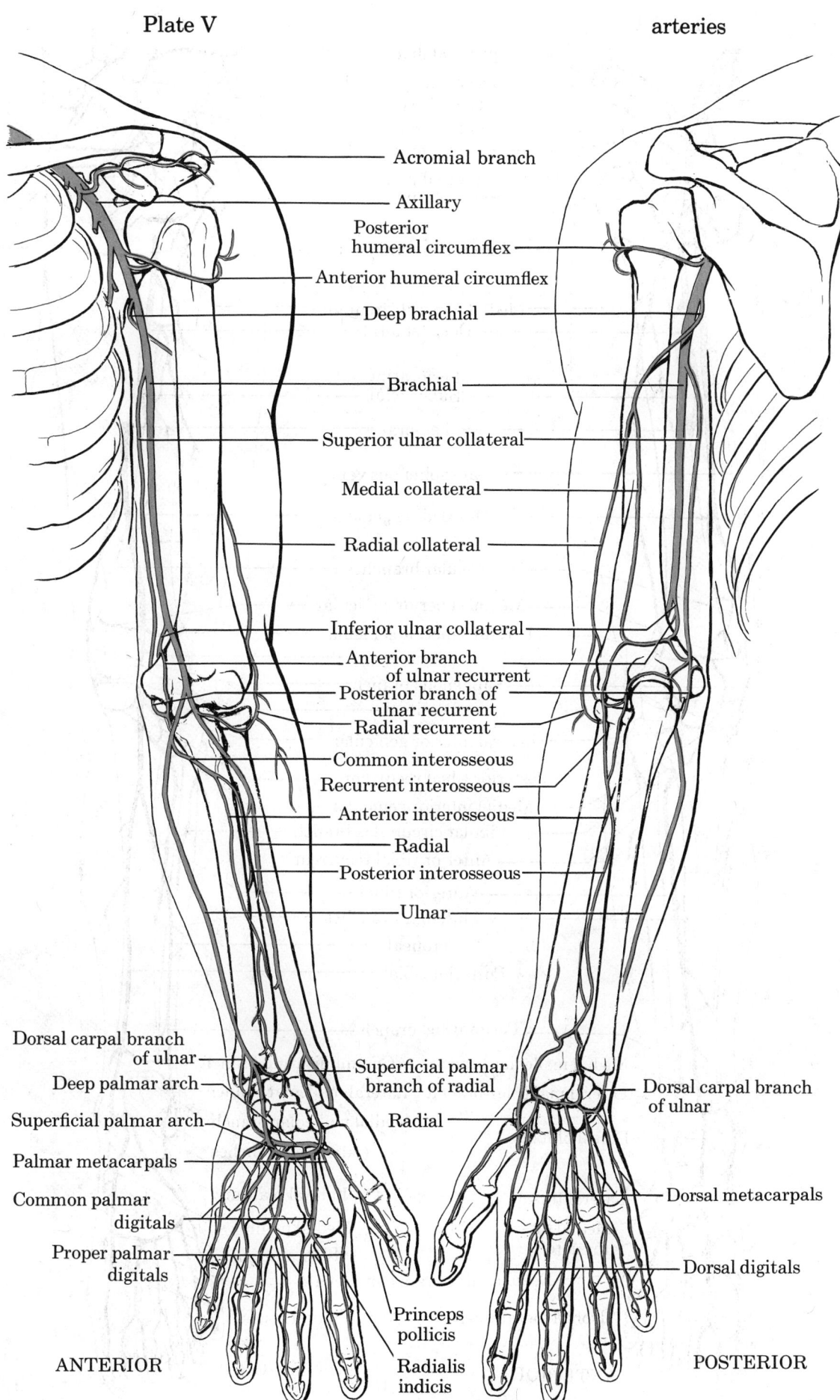

Acromial branch

Axillary

Posterior
humeral circumflex

Anterior humeral circumflex

Deep brachial

Brachial

Superior ulnar collateral

Medial collateral

Radial collateral

Inferior ulnar collateral

Anterior branch
of ulnar recurrent

Posterior branch of
ulnar recurrent

Radial recurrent

Common interosseous

Recurrent interosseous

Anterior interosseous

Radial

Posterior interosseous

Ulnar

Dorsal carpal branch
of ulnar

Deep palmar arch

Superficial palmar arch

Palmar metacarpals

Common palmar
digitals

Proper palmar
digitals

Superficial palmar
branch of radial

Radial

Princeps
pollicis

Radialis
indicis

Dorsal carpal branch
of ulnar

Dorsal metacarpals

Dorsal digitals

ANTERIOR

POSTERIOR

ARTERIES OF THE UPPER EXTREMITY

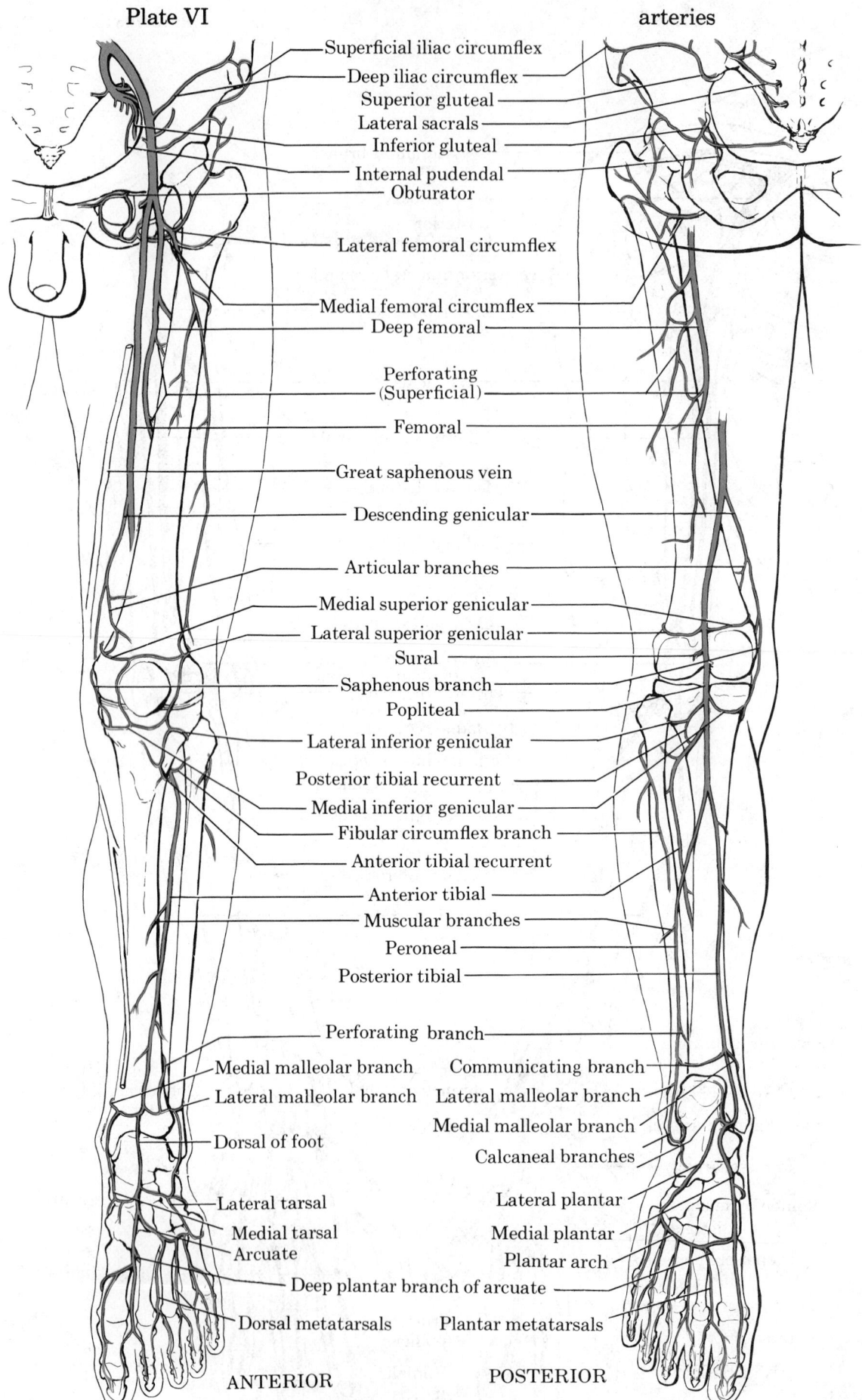

Plate VI   arteries

Superficial iliac circumflex
Deep iliac circumflex
Superior gluteal
Lateral sacrals
Inferior gluteal
Internal pudendal
Obturator

Lateral femoral circumflex

Medial femoral circumflex
Deep femoral

Perforating
(Superficial)

Femoral

Great saphenous vein

Descending genicular

Articular branches
Medial superior genicular
Lateral superior genicular
Sural
Saphenous branch
Popliteal
Lateral inferior genicular
Posterior tibial recurrent
Medial inferior genicular
Fibular circumflex branch
Anterior tibial recurrent

Anterior tibial
Muscular branches
Peroneal
Posterior tibial

Perforating branch
Medial malleolar branch   Communicating branch
Lateral malleolar branch   Lateral malleolar branch
                                 Medial malleolar branch
Dorsal of foot   Calcaneal branches

Lateral tarsal   Lateral plantar
Medial tarsal   Medial plantar
Arcuate   Plantar arch
Deep plantar branch of arcuate
Dorsal metatarsals   Plantar metatarsals

ANTERIOR   POSTERIOR

ARTERIES OF THE LOWER EXTREMITY

proper palmar digital arteries; *distribution*, fingers. Called also *arteriae digitales volares communis, common volar digital arteries,* and *ulnar metacarpal arteries.*

arte′riae digita′les palma′res pro′priae [NA], proper palmar digital arteries: *origin*, common palmar digital arteries; *branches*, none; *distribution*, fingers. Called also *arteriae digitales volares propriae, collateral digital arteries,* and *proper volar digital arteries.*

arte′riae digita′les planta′res commu′nes [NA], common plantar digital arteries: *origin*, plantar metatarsal arteries; *branches*, proper plantar digital arteries; *distribution*, toes.

arte′riae digita′les planta′res pro′priae [NA], proper plantar digital arteries: *origin*, common plantar digital arteries; *branches*, none; *distribution*, toes.

arte′riae digita′les vola′res commu′nes, arteriae digitales palmares communes.

arte′riae digita′les vola′res pro′priae, arteriae digitales palmares propriae.

a. dorsa′lis clitor′idis [NA], dorsal artery of clitoris: *origin*, internal pudendal artery; *branches*, none; *distribution*, clitoris.

a. dorsa′lis na′si [NA], dorsal artery of nose: *origin*, ophthalmic artery; *branches*, lacrimal; *distribution*, dorsum of nose.

a. dorsa′lis pe′dis [NA], dorsal artery of foot: *origin*, continuation of anterior tibial; *branches*, lateral and medial tarsal and arcuate arteries; *distribution*, foot, toes.

a. dorsa′lis pe′nis [NA], dorsal artery of penis: *origin*, internal pudendal artery; *branches*, none; *distribution*, glans, corona, prepuce of penis.

a. duc′tus deferen′tis [NA], artery of ductus deferens, deferential artery: *origin*, umbilical artery; *branches*, ureteral artery; *distribution*, ureter, ductus deferens, seminal vesicles, testes. Called also *a. deferentialis.*

a. epigas′trica infe′rior [NA], inferior epigastric artery: *origin*, external iliac; *branches*, pubic branch, cremasteric artery, a. of round ligament of uterus; *distribution*, abdominal wall.

a. epigas′trica superficia′lis [NA], superficial epigastric artery: *origin*, femoral; *branches*, none; *distribution*, abdominal wall, groin.

a. epigas′trica supe′rior [NA], superior epigastric artery: *origin*, internal thoracic artery; *branches*, none; *distribution*, abdominal wall, diaphragm.

arte′riae episcle′rales [NA], episcleral arteries: *origin*, anterior ciliary artery; *branches*, none; *distribution*, iris, ciliary process.

a. ethmoida′lis ante′rior [NA], anterior ethmoidal artery: *origin*, ophthalmic artery; *branches*, anterior meningeal; *distribution*, dura mater, nose, frontal sinus, anterior ethmoidal cells.

a. ethmoida′lis poste′rior [NA], posterior ethmoidal artery: *origin*, opthalmic artery; *branches*, none; *distribution*, posterior ethmoidal cells, dura mater, nose.

a. facia′lis [NA], facial artery: *origin*, external carotid; *branches*, ascending palatine, tonsillar, submental, inferior labial, superior labial, angular, glandular; *distribution*, face, tonsil, palate, submandibular gland. Called also *a. maxillaris externa* or *external maxillary artery.*

a. femora′lis [NA], femoral artery: *origin*, continuation of external iliac; *branches*, superficial epigastric, superficial circumflex iliac, external pudendal, deep femoral, descending geniculate; *distribution*, lower abdominal wall, external genitalia, lower extremity. NOTE: Vascular surgeons refer to the portion of the femoral artery proximal to the branching of the deep femoral as the *common femoral a.,* and to its continuation as the *superficial femoral a.* In this classification, the descending geniculate artery is a branch of the superficial femoral artery.

a. fibula′ris, NA alternative for *a. peronea.*

a. fronta′lis, a. supratrochlearis.

arte′riae gas′tricae bre′ves [NA], short gastric arteries: *origin*, splenic; *branches*, none; *distribution*, upper part of stomach.

a. gas′trica dex′tra [NA], right gastric artery: *origin*, common hepatic artery; *branches*, none; *distribution*, lesser curvature of stomach. Called also *right coronary artery of stomach* and *pyloric artery.*

a. gas′trica sinis′tra [NA], left gastric artery: *origin*, celiac; *branches*, espohageal; *distribution*, esophagus, lesser curvature of stomach. Called also *left coronary artery of stomach.*

a. gastroduodena′lis [NA], gastroduodenal artery: *origin*, common hepatic artery; *branches*, superior pancreaticoduodenal, right gastroepiploic; *distribution*, stomach, duodenum, pancreas, greater omentum.

a. gastroepiplo′ica dex′tra [NA], right gastroepiploic artery: *origin*, gastroduodenal artery; *branches*, epiploic branches; *distribution*, stomach, greater omentum. Called also *right inferior gastric artery.*

a. gastroepiplo′ica sinis′tra [NA], left gastroepiploic artery: *origin*, splenic artery; *branches*, epiploic branches; *distribution*, stomach, greater omentum. Called also *left inferior gastric artery.*

a. ge′nu infe′rior latera′lis, a. genus inferior lateralis.

a. ge′nu infe′rior media′lis, a. genus inferior medialis.

a. ge′nu me′dia, a. genus media.

a. ge′nu supe′rior latera′lis, a. genus superior lateralis.

a. ge′nu supe′rior media′lis, a. genus superior medialis.

a. ge′nu supre′ma, a. genus descendens.

a. ge′nus descen′dens [NA], descending geniculate artery: ori-

gin, femoral artery; *branches*, saphenous, articular; *distribution*, knee joint, upper and medial part of leg. Called also *a. genu suprema.*

a. ge′nus infe′rior latera′lis [NA], lateral inferior genicular artery: *origin*, popliteal artery; *branches*, none; *distribution*, knee joint. Called also *a. genu inferior lateralis.*

a. ge′nus infe′rior media′lis [NA], medial inferior genicular artery: *origin*, popliteal artery; *branches*, none; *distribution*, knee joint. Called also *a. genu inferior medialis.*

a. ge′nus me′dia [NA], middle genicular artery: *origin*, popliteal artery; *branches*, none; *distribution*, knee joint, cruciate ligaments, patellar synovial and alar folds. Called also *a. genu media.*

a. ge′nus supe′rior latera′lis [NA], lateral superior genicular artery: *origin*, popliteal artery; *branches*, none; *distribution*, knee joint, femur, patella, contiguous muscles. Called also *a. genu superior lateralis.*

a. ge′nus supe′rior media′lis [NA], medial superior genicular artery: *origin*, popliteal artery; *branches*, none; *distribution*, knee joint, femur, patella, contiguous muscles. Called also *a. genu superior medialis.*

a. glu′taea infe′rior, a. glutea inferior.

a. glu′taea supe′rior, a. glutea superior.

a. glu′tea infe′rior [NA], inferior gluteal artery: *origin*, internal iliac; *branches*, sciatic; *distribution*, buttock, back of thigh. Called also *a. glutaea inferior.*

a. glu′tea supe′rior [NA], superior gluteal artery: *origin*, internal iliac artery; *branches*, superficial and deep branches; *distribution*, buttocks. Called also *a. glutaea superior.*

a. haemorrhoida′lis infe′rior, a. rectalis inferior.

a. haemorrhoida′lis me′dia, a. rectalis media.

a. haemorrhoida′lis supe′rior, a. rectalis superior.

arte′riae helici′nae pe′nis [NA], helicine arteries of penis: helicine arteries arising from the vessels of the penis, whose engorgement causes erection of the organ. Called also *arteries of Mueller.*

a. hepat′ica, a. hepatica communis.

a. hepat′ica commu′nis [NA], common hepatic artery: *origin*, celiac trunk; *branches*, right gastric, gastroduodenal, hepatic proper; *distribution*, stomach, pancreas, duodenum, liver, gallbladder, greater omentum. Called also *a. hepatica.*

a. hepat′ica pro′pria [NA], proper hepatic artery: *origin*, common hepatic artery; *branches*, right and left branches; *distribution*, liver, gallbladder. Called also *hepatic funiculus of Rauber.*

a. hyaloi′dea [NA], hyaloid artery: a fetal vessel that continues forward from the central retinal artery through the vitreous body to supply the lens; it normally is not present after birth.

a. hypogas′trica, a. iliaca interna.

arte′riae il′eae, arteriae ilei.

arte′riae il′ei [NA], ileal arteries: *origin*, superior mesenteric; *branches*, none; *distribution*, ileum. Called also *a. ileae.*

a. ileoco′lica [NA], ileocolic artery: *origin*, superior mesenteric; *branches*, ascending, anterior, and posterior cecal, appendicular; *distribution*, ileum, cecum, vermiform appendix, ascending colon. Called also *inferior right colic artery.*

a. ili′aca commu′nis [NA], common iliac artery: *origin*, abdominal aorta; *branches*, internal and external iliac; *distribution*, pelvis, abdominal wall, lower limb.

a. ili′aca exter′na [NA], external iliac artery: *origin*, common iliac; *branches*, inferior epigastric, deep circumflex iliac; *distribution*, abdominal wall, external genitalia, lower limb. Called also *anterior iliac artery.*

a. ili′aca inter′na [NA], internal iliac artery: *origin*, continuation of common iliac; *branches*, iliolumbar, obturator, superior gluteal, inferior gluteal, umbilical, inferior vesical, uterine, middle rectal, and internal pudendal arteries; *distribution*, wall and viscera of pelvis, buttock, reproductive organs, medial aspect of thigh. Called also *a. hypogastrica, hypogastric artery,* and *posterior pelvic artery.*

a. iliolumba′lis [NA], iliolumbar artery: *origin*, internal iliac; *branches*, iliac and lumbar branches, lateral sacral arteries; *distribution*, pelvic muscles and bones, fifth lumbar segment, sacrum. Called also *small iliac artery.*

a. infraorbita′lis [NA], infraorbital artery: *origin*, maxillary artery; *branches*, anterior superior alveolar; *distribution*, maxilla, maxillary sinus, upper teeth, lower lid, cheek, nose.

a. innomina′ta, truncus brachiocephalicus.

arte′riae intercosta′les, see *arteriae intercostales posteriores I et II, III–XI.*

arte′riae intercosta′les posterio′res I et II [NA], posterior intercostal arteries I and II: *origin*, highest intercostal artery; *branches*, dorsal and spinal rami; *distribution*, upper thoracic wall.

arte′riae intercosta′les posterio′res III–XI [NA], posterior intercostal arteries III–XI: *origin*, thoracic aorta; *branches*, dorsal, lateral, and lateral cutaneous; *distribution*, thoracic wall.

a. intercosta′lis supre′ma [NA], highest intercostal artery: *origin*, costocervical trunk; *branches*, posterior intercostal arteries I and II; *distribution*, upper thoracic wall.

arte′riae interlobula′res hep′atis [NA], interlobular arteries of liver: arteries originating from the right or left branch of the proper hepatic artery, and passing between the lobules of the liver.

arte′riae interlobula′res re′nis [NA], interlobular arteries of kidney: arteries originating from the arcuate arteries of the kidney and distributed to the renal glomeruli. Called also *radiate arteries of kidney.*

a. interos'sea ante'rior [NA], anterior interosseous artery: *origin*, posterior or common interosseous artery; *branches*, median artery; *distribution*, deep parts of front of forearm. Called also *a. interossea volaris* or *volar interosseous artery.*

a. interos'sea commu'nis [NA], common interosseous artery: *origin*, ulnar artery; *branches*, anterior and posterior interosseous arteries; *distribution*, antecubital fossa.

a. interos'sea dorsa'lis, a. interossea posterior.

a. interos'sea poste'rior [NA], posterior interosseous artery: *origin*, common interosseous artery; *branches*, recurrent interosseous; *distribution*, deep parts of back of forearm. Called also *a. interossea dorsalis,* and *dorsal* or *posterior interosseous artery of forearm.*

a. interos'sea recur'rens [NA], recurrent interosseous artery: *origin*, posterior interosseous or common interosseous artery; *branches*, none; *distribution*, back of elbow joint.

a. interos'sea vola'ris, a. interossea anterior.

arte'riae intestina'les, intestinal arteries: the arteries arising from the superior mesenteric, and supplying the intestines, including the pancreaticoduodenal, jejunal, ileal, ileocolic, and colic arteries.

arte'riae jejuna'les [NA], jejunal arteries: *origin*, superior mesenteric; *branches*, none; *distribution*, jejunum.

arte'riae labia'les anterio'res vul'vae, rami labiales anteriores arteriae femoralis.

a. labia'lis infe'rior [NA], inferior labial artery: *origin*, facial artery; *branches*, none; *distribution*, lower lip.

arte'riae labia'les posterio'res vul'vae, rami labiales posteriores arteriae pudendae internae.

a. labia'lis supe'rior [NA], superior labial artery: *origin*, facial artery, *branches*, septal and alar; *distribution*, upper lip, nose.

a. labyrin'thi [NA], artery of labyrinth, labyrinthine artery: *origin*, basilar or anterior inferior cerebellar artery; *branches*, vestibular and cochlear rami; *distribution*, internal ear. Called also *a. auditiva interna* and *internal auditory artery.*

a. lacrima'lis [NA], lacrimal artery: *origin*, ophthalmic artery; *branches*, lateral palpebral artery; *distribution*, lacrimal gland, upper and lower eyelids, conjunctiva.

a. laryn'gea infe'rior [NA], inferior laryngeal artery: *origin*, inferior thyroid artery; *branches*, none; *distribution*, larynx, trachea, esophagus.

a. laryn'gea supe'rior [NA], superior laryngeal artery: *origin*, superior thyroid; *branches*, none; *distribution*, larynx.

a. liena'lis [NA], splenic artery: *origin*, celiac trunk; *branches*, pancreatic and splenic branches, left gastroepiploic, and short gastric arteries; *distribution*, spleen, pancreas, stomach, greater omentum.

a. ligamen'ti ter'etis u'teri [NA], artery of round ligament of uterus: *origin*, inferior epigastric artery; *branches*, none; *distribution*, round ligament of uterus.

a. lingua'lis [NA], lingual artery: *origin*, external carotid; *branches*, suprahyoid, sublingual, dorsal lingual, deep lingual; *distribution*, tongue, sublingual gland, tonsil, epiglottis.

a. lo'bi cauda'ti [NA], either of two branches, one from the right and one from the left hepatic artery, supplying twigs to the caudate lobe of the liver.

arte'riae lumba'les [NA], lumbar arteries: *origin*, abdominal aorta; *branches*, dorsal and spinal branches; *distribution*, posterior abdominal wall, renal capsule.

a. lumba'lis i'ma [NA], lowest lumbar artery: *origin*, middle sacral; *branches*, none; *distribution*, sacrum, gluteus maximus muscle. Called also *fifth lumbar artery.*

a. malleola'ris ante'rior latera'lis [NA], lateral anterior malleolar artery: *origin*, anterior tibial artery; *branches*, none; *distribution*, ankle joint.

a. malleola'ris ante'rior media'lis [NA], medial anterior malleolar artery: *origin*, anterior tibial artery; *branches*, none; *distribution*, ankle joint.

a. malleola'ris poste'rior latera'lis, see *rami malleolares laterales arteriae peroneae.*

a. malleola'ris poste'rior media'lis, see *rami malleolares mediales arteriae tibialis posterioris.*

a. mammar'ia inter'na, a. thoracica interna.

a. masseter'ica [NA], masseteric artery: *origin*, maxillary artery; *branches*, none; *distribution*, masseter muscle.

a. maxilla'ris [NA], maxillary artery: *origin*, external carotid artery; *branches*, pterygoid rami, and deep auricular, anterior tympanic, inferior alveolar, middle meningeal, masseteric, deep temporal, buccal, posterior superior alveolar, infraorbital, descending palatine, sphenopalatine, and the artery of the pterygoid canal; *distribution*, both jaws, teeth, muscles of mastication, ear, meninges, nose, nasal sinus, palate. Called also *a. maxillaris interna, internal maxillary artery,* and *deep facial artery.*

a. maxilla'ris exter'na, a. facialis.

a. maxilla'ris inter'na, a. maxillaris.

a. max'ima Gale'ni, aorta.

a. media'na [NA], median artery: *origin*, anterior interosseous artery; *branches*, none; *distribution*, median nerve, muscles of front forearm.

arte'riae mediastina'les anterio'res, rami mediastinales arteriae thoracicae internae.

a. menin'gea ante'rior [NA], anterior meningeal artery: *ori-gin*, anterior ethmoidal artery; *branches*, none; *distribution*, dura mater of anterior cranial fossa.

a. menin'gea me'dia [NA], middle meningeal artery: *origin*, maxillary artery; *branches*, frontal, parietal, and lacrimal anastomotic, accessory meningeal, and petrosal rami, and the superior tympanic artery; *distribution*, cranial bones, dura mater.

a. menin'gea poste'rior [NA], posterior meningeal artery: *origin*, ascending pharyngeal; *branches*, none; *distribution*, bones, dura mater of posterior cranial fossa.

a. menta'lis [NA], mental artery: *origin*, inferior alveolar; *branches*, none; *distribution*, chin.

a. mesenter'ica infe'rior [NA], inferior mesenteric artery: *origin*, abdominal aorta; *branches*, left colic, sigmoid, and superior rectal arteries; *distribution*, descending colon, rectum.

a. mesenter'ica supe'rior [NA], superior mesenteric artery: *origin*, abdominal aorta; *branches*, inferior pancreaticoduodenal, jejunal, ileal, ileocolic, right colic, and middle colic arteries; *distribution*, small intestine, proximal half of colon.

arte'riae metacar'peae dorsa'les [NA], dorsal metacarpal arteries: *origin*, dorsal carpal rete and radial artery; *branches*, dorsal digital arteries; *distribution*, dorsum of fingers.

arte'riae metacar'peae palma'res [NA], palmar metacarpal arteries: *origin*, deep palmar arch; *branches*, none; *distribution*, deep parts of metatarsus. Called also *arteriae metacarpeae volares, volar metacarpal arteries,* and *palmar intermetacarpal arteries.*

arte'riae metacar'peae vola'res, arteriae metacarpeae palmares.

arte'riae metatar'seae dorsa'les [NA], dorsal metatarsal arteries: *origin*, arcuate artery of foot; *branches*, dorsal digital arteries; *distribution*, foot, toes.

arte'riae metatar'seae planta'res [NA], plantar metatarsal arteries: *origin*, plantar arch; *branches*, perforating branches, common and proper plantar digital arteries; *distribution*, toes. Called also *common digital arteries of foot.*

a. musculophren'ica [NA], musculophrenic artery: *origin*, internal thoracic artery; *branches*, none; *distribution*, diaphragm, abdominal and thoracic walls.

arte'riae nasa'les posterio'res, latera'les et sep'ti [NA], lateral and septal posterior nasal arteries: *origin*, sphenopalatine artery; *branches*, none; *distribution*, nasal cavity, nasal septum, adjacent sinuses.

arte'riae nutri'ciae hu'meri [NA], nutrient arteries of humerus: *origin*, brachial and deep brachial arteries; *branches*, none; *distribution*, humerus.

a. obturato'ria [NA], obturator artery: *origin*, internal iliac; *branches*, pubic, acetabular, anterior, and posterior branches; *distribution*, pelvic muscles, hip joint.

a. obturato'ria accesso'ria [NA], accessory obturator artery, a name given to the obturator artery when it arises from the inferior epigastric instead of the internal iliac artery.

a. occipita'lis [NA], occipital artery: *origin*, external carotid; *branches*, auricular, meningeal, mastoid, descending, occipital, and sternocleidomastoid rami; *distribution*, muscles of neck and scalp, meninges, mastoid cells.

arte'riae oesoph'ageae, rami esophagei aortae thoracicae.

a. ophthal'mica [NA], ophthalmic artery: *origin*, internal carotid; *branches*, lacrimal, supraorbital, central artery of retina, ciliary, posterior and anterior ethmoidal, palpebral, supratrochlear, dorsal nasal; *distribution*, eye, orbit, adjacent facial structures.

a. ova'rica [NA], ovarian artery: *origin*, abdominal aorta; *branches*, ureteral branch; *distribution*, ureter, ovary, uterine tube. Called also *tubo-ovarian artery* or *aortic uterine artery.*

a. palati'na ascen'dens [NA], ascending palatine artery: *origin*, facial artery; *branches*, none; *distribution*, soft palate, wall of pharynx, tonsil, auditory tube.

a. palati'na descen'dens [NA], descending palatine artery: *origin*, maxillary artery; *branches*, greater and lesser palatine arteries; *distribution*, soft palate, hard palate, tonsil.

a. palati'na ma'jor [NA], greater palatine artery: *origin*, descending palatine; *branches*, none; *distribution*, hard palate.

arte'riae palati'nae mino'res [NA], lesser palatine arteries: *origin*, descending palatine; *branches*, none; *distribution*, soft palate, tonsil.

arte'riae palpebra'les latera'les [NA], lateral palpebral arteries: *origin*, lacrimal artery; *branches*, none; *distribution*, eyelids, conjunctiva.

arte'riae palpebra'les media'les [NA], medial palpebral arteries: *origin*, ophthalmic artery; *branches*, posterior conjunctival; *distribution*, eyelids.

a. pancreat'ica dorsa'lis [NA], dorsal pancreatic artery: *origin*, splenic; *branches*, inferior pancreatic; *distribution*, neck and body of pancreas.

a. pancreat'ica infe'rior [NA], inferior pancreatic artery: *origin*, dorsal pancreatic; *branches*, none; *distribution*, body and tail of pancreas.

a. pancreat'ica mag'na [NA], great pancreatic artery: *origin*, splenic artery; *branches and distribution*, right and left branches anastomose with other pancreatic arteries.

arteriae pancreaticoduodena'les infe'riores [NA], inferior pancreaticoduodenal arteries: *origin*, superior mesenteric artery; *branches*, none; *distribution*, pancreas, duodenum. Called also *duodenal arteries.*

a. pancreaticoduodena′lis supe′rior, superior pancreaticoduodenal artery: *origin,* gastroduodenal artery; *branches,* none; *distribution,* pancreas, duodenum.

arte′riae perforan′tes [NA], perforating arteries: *origin,* deep femoral artery; *branches,* none; *distribution,* adductor, hamstring, and gluteal muscles, and femur. Called also *a. perforans prima femoris, a. perforans secunda femoris,* and *a. perforans tertia femoris.*

a. per′forans pri′ma fem′oris, see *arteriae perforantes.*

a. per′forans secun′da fem′oris, see *arteriae perforantes.*

a. per′forans ter′tia fem′oris, see *arteriae perforantes.*

a. pericardiacophren′ica [NA], pericardiacophrenic artery: *origin,* internal thoracic artery; *branches,* none; *distribution,* pericardium, diaphragm, pleura. Called also *superior phrenic artery.*

a. perinea′lis [NA], perineal artery: *origin,* internal pudendal artery; *branches,* none; *distribution,* perineum, skin of external genitalia. Called also *a. perinei.*

a. perine′i, *a.* perinealis.

a. pero′nea [NA], peroneal artery: *origin,* posterior tibial artery; *branches,* perforating, communicating, calcaneal, and lateral and medial malleolar branches, and the calcaneal rete; *distribution,* outside and back of ankle. Called also *a. fibularis* [NA alternative] and *fibular artery.*

a. pharyn′gea ascen′dens [NA], ascending pharyngeal artery: *origin,* external carotid; *branches,* posterior meningeal, pharyngeal, and inferior tympanic; *distribution,* pharynx, soft palate, ear, meninges.

arteriae phren′icae infe′riores [NA], inferior phrenic arteries: *origin,* abdominal aorta; *branches,* superior suprarenal; *distribution,* diaphragm, suprarenal gland. Called also *great phrenic arteries* and *diaphragmatic arteries.*

arte′riae phren′icae superio′res [NA], superior phrenic arteries: *origin,* thoracic aorta; *branches,* none; *distribution,* upper surface of vertebral portion of diaphragm. Called also *superior diaphragmatic arteries.*

a. planta′ris latera′lis [NA], lateral plantar artery: *origin,* posterior tibial artery; *branches,* plantar arch, and plantar metatarsal arteries; *distribution,* sole of foot and toes. Called also *external plantar artery.*

a. planta′ris media′lis [NA], medial plantar artery: *origin,* posterior tibial artery; *branches,* deep and superficial branches; *distribution,* sole of the foot and toes.

a. poplit′ea [NA], popliteal artery: *origin,* continuation of femoral artery; *branches,* lateral and medial superior genicular, middle genicular, sural, lateral and medial inferior genicular, anterior and posterior tibial arteries, and the genicular articular and the patellar rete; *distribution,* knee, calf.

a. prin′ceps pol′licis [NA], principal artery of thumb: *origin,* radial artery; *branches,* radial of index finger; *distribution,* each side and palmar aspect of thumb.

a. profun′da bra′chii [NA], deep brachial artery: *origin,* brachial artery; *branches,* deltoid ramus, nutrient artery, medial and radial collateral arteries; *distribution,* humerus, muscles and skin of arm.

a. profun′da clitor′idis [NA], deep artery of clitoris: *origin,* internal pudendal artery; *branches,* none; *distribution,* clitoris.

a. profun′da fem′oris [NA], deep femoral artery: *origin,* femoral artery; *branches,* medial and lateral circumflex arteries of thigh, perforating arteries; *distribution,* thigh muscles, hip joint, gluteal muscles, femur.

a. profun′da lin′guae [NA], deep lingual artery: *origin,* lingual artery; *branches,* none; *distribution,* tongue. Called also *ranine artery.*

a. profun′da pe′nis [NA], deep artery of penis: *origin,* internal pudendal artery; *branches,* none; *distribution,* corpus cavernosum penis.

arte′riae puden′dae exter′nae [NA], external pudendal arteries: *origin,* femoral artery; *branches,* anterior scrotal or anterior labial and inguinal branches; *distribution,* external genitalia, upper medial thigh.

a. puden′da inter′na [NA], internal pudendal artery: *origin,* internal iliac artery; *branches,* posterior scrotal or posterior labial branches and inferior rectal, perineal, urethral arteries, artery of bulb of penis or vestibule, deep artery of penis or clitoris, dorsal artery of penis or clitoris; *distribution,* external genitalia, anal canal, perineum.

a. pulmona′lis, truncus pulmonalis.

a. pulmona′lis dex′tra [NA], right pulmonary artery: *origin,* pulmonary trunk; *branches,* numerous branches named according to the part of the lung to which they distribute unaerated blood; *distribution,* right lung.

a. pulmona′lis sinis′tra [NA], left pulmonary artery: *origin,* pulmonary trunk; *branches,* numerous branches named according to the part of the lung to which they distribute unaerated blood; *distribution,* left lung.

a. radia′lis [NA], radial artery: *origin,* brachial artery; *branches,* palmar carpal, superficial palmar and dorsal carpal rami, recurrent radial artery, principal artery of thumb, deep palmar arch; *distribution,* forearm, wrist, hand.

a. radia′lis in′dicis [NA], radial artery of index finger: *origin,* principal artery of thumb; *branches,* none; *distribution,* index finger. Called also *a. volaris indicis radialis* and *volar radial artery of index finger.*

a. recta′lis infe′rior [NA], inferior rectal artery: *origin,* internal pudendal artery; *branches,* none; *distribution,* rectum, anal canal. Called also *a. haemorrhoidalis inferior* and *inferior hemorrhoidal artery.*

a. recta′lis me′dia [NA], middle rectal artery: *origin,* internal iliac artery; *branches,* none; *distribution,* rectum. Called also *a. haemorrhoidalis media* and *middle hemorrhoidal artery.*

a. recta′lis supe′rior [NA], superior rectal artery: *origin,* inferior mesenteric artery; *branches,* none; *distribution,* rectum. Called also *a. haemorrhoidalis superior* and *superior hemorrhoidal artery.*

a. recur′rens radia′lis [NA], radial recurrent artery: *origin,* radial artery; *branches,* none; *distribution,* brachioradialis, brachialis, elbow region.

a. recur′rens tibia′lis ante′rior [NA], anterior tibial recurrent artery: *origin,* anterior tibial artery; *branches,* none; *distribution,* tibialis anterior, extensor digitorum longus, knee joint, contiguous fascia and skin.

a. recur′rens tibia′lis poste′rior [NA], posterior tibial recurrent artery: *origin,* anterior tibial artery; *branches,* none; *distribution,* knee.

a. recur′rens ulna′ris [NA], ulnar recurrent artery: *origin,* ulnar artery; *branches,* anterior and posterior; *distribution,* elbow joint region.

arte′riae recurren′tes ulna′res, see *a. recurrens ulnaris.*

a. rena′lis [NA], renal artery: *origin,* abdominal aorta; *branches,* ureteral branches, inferior suprarenal artery; *distribution,* kidney, suprarenal gland, ureter. Called also *emulgent artery.*

arte′riae re′nis [NA], renal arteries: the arteries of the kidney, including the interlobar, arcuate, and interlobular arteries, and arteriolae rectae.

arte′riae retroduodena′les [NA], retroduodenal arteries: *origin,* first branch of gastroduodenal; *branches,* none; *distribution,* bile duct, duodenum, head of pancreas.

a. sacra′lis latera′lis, see *rami spinales arteriarum sacralium lateralium.*

arte′riae sacra′les latera′les [NA], lateral sacral arteries: *origin,* iliolumbar artery; *branches,* spinal branches; *distribution,* structures about coccyx and sacrum.

a. sacra′lis me′dia, a. sacralis mediana.

a. sacra′lis media′na [NA], median sacral artery: *origin,* continuation of abdominal aorta; *branches,* lowest lumbar artery; *distribution,* sacrum, coccyx, rectum. Called also *a. sacralis media, aorta sacrococcygea,* and *caudal, coccygeal,* or *sacrococcygeal artery.*

a. scapula′ris descen′dens [dorsa′lis], NA alternative for *ramus profundus arteriae transversae colli.*

arte′riae scrota′les anterio′res, rami scrotales anteriores arteriae femoralis.

arte′riae scrota′les posterio′res, rami scrotales posteriores arteriae pudendae internae.

a. segmen′ti anterio′ris [NA], anterior segmental artery: *origin,* right hepatic; *branches,* none; *distribution,* anterior segment of right lobe of liver.

a. segmen′ti anterio′ris inferio′ris [NA], anterior inferior segmental artery: *origin,* anterior branch of renal artery; *branches,* none; *distribution,* anterior inferior segment of kidney.

a. segmen′ti anterio′ris superio′ris [NA], anterior superior segmental artery: *origin,* anterior branch of renal artery; *branches,* none; *distribution,* anterior superior segment of kidney.

a. segmen′ti inferio′ris [NA], inferior segmental artery: *origin,* anterior branch of renal artery; *branches,* none; *distribution,* inferior segment of kidney.

a. segmen′ti latera′lis [NA], lateral segmental artery: *origin,* left branch of common hepatic artery; *branches,* none; *distribution,* lateral segment of left lobe of liver.

a. segmen′ti media′lis [NA], medial segmental artery: *origin,* left branch of common hepatic artery; *branches,* none; *distribution,* medial segment of left lobe of liver.

a. segmen′ti posterio′ris [NA], posterior segmental artery: 1. *origin,* right hepatic; *branches,* none; *distribution,* posterior segment of right lobe of liver. 2. *origin,* posterior branch of renal artery; *branches,* none; *distribution,* posterior segment of kidney.

a. segmen′ti superio′ris [NA], superior segmental artery: *origin,* anterior branch of renal artery; *branches,* none; *distribution,* superior segment of kidney.

arte′riae sigmoi′deae [NA], sigmoid arteries: *origin,* inferior mesenteric artery; *branches,* none; *distribution,* sigmoid colon.

a. spermat′ica exter′na, a. cremasterica.

a. sphenopalati′na [NA], sphenopalatine artery: *origin,* maxillary artery; *branches,* lateral and septal posterior nasal arteries; *distribution,* structures adjoining nasal cavity, the nasopharynx. Called also *nasopalatine artery.*

a. spina′lis ante′rior [NA], anterior spinal artery: *origin,* vertebral artery; *branches,* none; *distribution,* spinal cord.

a. spina′lis poste′rior [NA], posterior spinal artery: *origin,* vertebral artery; *branches,* none, *distribution,* spinal cord.

a. sternocleidomastoi′dea, see *rami sternocleidomastoidei arteriae occipitalis.*

a. stylomastoi′dea [NA], stylomastoid artery: *origin,* posterior auricular; *branches,* mastoid and stapedial rami, posterior tympanic artery; *distribution,* tympanic cavity walls, mastoid cells, stapedius muscle.

a. subcla′via [NA], subclavian artery: *origin,* brachiocephalic trunk (right), arch of aorta (left); *branches*, vertebral, internal thoracic arteries, thyrocervical and costocervical trunks; *distribution*, neck, thoracic wall, spinal cord, brain, meninges, upper limb.

a. subcosta′lis [NA], subcostal artery: *origin*, thoracic aorta; *branches*, dorsal and spinal branches; *distribution*, upper posterior abdominal wall.

a. sublingua′lis [NA], sublingual artery: *origin*, lingual artery; *branches*, none; *distribution*, sublingual gland.

a. submenta′lis [NA], submental artery: *origin*, facial artery; *branches*, none; *distribution*, tissues under chin.

a. subscapula′ris [NA], subscapular artery: *origin*, axillary artery; *branches*, thoracodorsal and circumflex scapular arteries; *distribution*, scapular and shoulder region.

arte′riae supraduodena′les superio′res [NA], superior supraduodenal arteries: *origin*, gastroduodenal; *branches*, pancreatic and duodenal; *distribution*, pancreas, duodenum.

a. supraorbita′lis [NA], supraorbital artery: *origin*, ophthalmic artery; *branches*, none; *distribution*, forehead, upper muscles of orbit, upper eyelid, frontal sinus.

a. suprarena′lis infe′rior [NA], inferior suprarenal artery: *origin*, renal artery; *branches*, none; *distribution*, suprarenal gland. Called also *inferior capsular artery.*

a. suprarena′lis me′dia [NA], middle suprarenal artery: *origin*, abdominal aorta; *branches*, none; *distribution*, suprarenal gland. Called also *middle capsular artery* and *aortic suprarenal artery.*

arte′riae suprarena′les superio′res [NA], superior suprarenal arteries: *origin*, inferior phrenic artery; *branches*, none; *distribution*, suprarenal gland.

a. suprascapula′ris [NA], suprascapular artery: *origin*, thyrocervical trunk; *branches*, acromial branch; *distribution*, clavicular, deltoid, and scapular regions. Called also *a. transversa scapulae* and *transverse scapular artery.*

a. supratrochlea′ris [NA], supratrochlear artery: *origin*, ophthalmic artery; *branches*, none; *distribution*, anterior scalp. Called also *a. frontalis* and *frontal artery.*

arte′riae sura′les [NA], sural arteries: *origin*, popliteal artery; *branches*, none; *distribution*, popliteal space, calf.

a. tar′sea latera′lis [NA], lateral tarsal artery: *origin*, dorsal artery of foot; *branches*, none; *distribution*, tarsus.

arte′riae tar′seae media′les [NA], medial tarsal arteries: *origin*, dorsal artery of foot; *branches*, none; *distribution*, side of foot.

a. tempora′lis me′dia [NA], middle temporal artery: *origin*, superficial temporal artery; *branches*, none; *distribution*, temporal region.

arte′riae tempora′les profun′dae [NA], deep temporal arteries: *origin*, maxillary artery; *branches*, none; *distribution*, deep parts of temporal region.

a. tempora′lis profun′da ante′rior, see *arteriae temporales profundae.*

a. tempora′lis profun′da poste′rior, see *arteriae temporales profundae.*

a. tempora′lis superficia′lis [NA], superficial temporal artery: *origin*, external carotid; *branches*, parotid, anterior auricular, frontal, and parietal rami, transverse facial, zygomaticoorbital, and middle temporal arteries; *distribution*, parotid and temporal regions.

a. testicula′ris [NA], testicular artery: *origin*, abdominal aorta; *branches*, ureteral branches; *distribution*, ureter, epididymis, testis. Called also *funicular artery.*

a. thoraca′lis latera′lis, a. thoracica lateralis.

a. thoraca′lis supre′ma, a. thoracica suprema.

a. thora′cica inter′na [NA], internal thoracic artery: *origin*, subclavian artery; *branches*, mediastinal, thymic, bronchial, sternal, perforating, lateral costal, and anterior intercostal branches, pericardiacophrenic, musculophrenic, and superior epigastric arteries; *distribution*, anterior thoracic wall, mediastinal structures, diaphragm. Called also *a. mammaria interna* and *internal mammary artery.*

a. thora′cica latera′lis [NA], lateral thoracic artery: *origin*, axillary artery; *branches*, mammary branches; *distribution*, pectoral muscles, mammary gland. Called also *a. thoracalis lateralis* and *external mammary artery.*

a. thora′cica supre′ma [NA], highest thoracic artery: *origin*, axillary artery; *branches*, none; *distribution*, axillary aspect of chest wall. Called also *a. thoracalis suprema.*

a. thoracoacromia′lis [NA], thoracoacromial artery: *origin*, axillary artery; *branches*, clavicular, pectoral, deltoid, acromial rami; *distribution*, deltoid, clavicular, and thoracic regions. Called also *thoracic axis.*

a. thoracodorsa′lis [NA], thoracodorsal artery: *origin*, subscapular artery; *branches*, none; *distribution*, subscapular and teretes muscles.

arte′riae thy′micae, rami thymici arteriae thoracicae internae.

a. thyreoi′dea i′ma, a. thyroidea ima.

a. thyreoi′dea infe′rior, a. thyroidea inferior.

a. thyreoi′dea supe′rior, a. thyroidea superior.

a. thyroi′dea i′ma [NA], lowest thyroid artery: *origin*, arch of aorta, brachiocephalic trunk or right common carotid; *branches*, none; *distribution*, thyroid gland. Called also *a. thyreoidea ima* and *Neubauer's artery.*

a. thyroi′dea infe′rior [NA], inferior thyroid artery: *origin*, thyrocervical trunk; *branches*, pharyngeal, esophageal, and tracheal rami, inferior laryngeal and ascending cervical arteries; *distribution*, thyroid gland and adjacent structures. Called also *a. thyreoidea inferior.*

a. thyroi′dea supe′rior [NA], superior thyroid artery: *origin*, external carotid artery; *branches*, hyoid, sternocleidomastoid, superior laryngeal, cricothyroid, muscular, and glandular branches; *distribution*, thyroid gland and adjacent structures. Called also *a. thyreoidea superior.*

a. tibia′lis ante′rior [NA], anterior tibial artery: *origin*, popliteal artery; *branches*, posterior and anterior tibial recurrent, and lateral and medial anterior malleolar arteries, lateral and medial malleolar retes; *distribution*, leg, ankle, foot.

a. tibia′lis poste′rior [NA], posterior tibial artery: *origin*, popliteal artery; *branches*, fibular circumflex branch, peroneal, medial plantar, and lateral plantar arteries; *distribution*, leg, foot.

a. transver′sa col′li [NA], transverse cervical artery: *origin*, subclavian artery; *branches*, deep and superficial rami; *distribution*, root of neck, muscles of scapula.

a. transver′sa facie′i [NA], transverse facial artery: *origin*, superficial temporal artery; *branches*, none; *distribution*, parotid region.

a. transver′sa scap′ulae, a. suprascapularis.

a. tympan′ica ante′rior [NA], anterior tympanic artery: *origin*, maxillary artery; *branches*, none; *distribution*, tympanic cavity.

a. tympan′ica infe′rior [NA], inferior tympanic artery: *origin*, ascending pharyngeal; *branches*, none; *distribution*, tympanic cavity.

a. tympan′ica poste′rior [NA], posterior tympanic artery: *origin*, stylomastoid artery; *branches*, none; *distribution*, tympanic cavity.

a. tympan′ica supe′rior [NA], superior tympanic artery: *origin*, middle meningeal artery; *branches*, none; *distribution*, tympanic cavity.

a. ulna′ris [NA], ulnar artery: *origin*, brachial artery; *branches*, palmar carpal, dorsal carpal, and deep palmar rami, ulnar recurrent and common interosseous arteries, superficial palmar arch; *distribution*, forearm, wrist, hand.

a. umbilica′lis [NA], umbilical artery: *origin*, internal iliac artery; *branches*, deferential, superior vesical arteries; *distribution*, ductus deferens, seminal vesicles, testes, urinary bladder, ureter.

a. urethra′lis [NA], urethral artery: *origin*, internal pudendal artery; *branches*, none; *distribution*, urethra.

a. uteri′na [NA], uterine artery: *origin*, internal iliac artery; *branches*, ovarian and tubal rami, vaginal artery; *distribution*, uterus, vagina, round ligament of uterus, uterine tube, ovary. Called also *fallopian artery.*

a. vagina′lis [NA], vaginal artery: *origin*, uterine artery; *branches*, none; *distribution*, vagina, fundus of bladder.

a. vertebra′lis [NA], vertebral artery: *origin*, subclavian artery; *branches*, spinal and meningeal branches, posterior inferior cerebellar, basilar, and anterior and posterior spinal arteries; *distribution*, muscles of neck, vertebrae, spinal cord, cerebellum, interior of cerebrum.

a. vesica′lis infe′rior [NA], inferior vesical artery: *origin*, internal iliac; *branches*, none; *distribution*, bladder, prostate, seminal vesicles.

arte′riae vesica′les superio′res [NA], superior vesical arteries: *origin*, umbilical artery; *branches*, none; *distribution*, bladder, urachus, ureter.

a. vola′ris in′dicis radia′lis, a. radialis indicis.

a. zygomaticoorbita′lis [NA], zygomaticoorbital artery: *origin*, superficial temporal; *branches*, none; *distribution*, lateral side of orbit.

---

arterial (ar-te′re-al)   pertaining to an artery or to the arteries.

arterialization (ar-te″re-al-i-za′shun)   (*obs.*) the change of venous into arterial blood; the provision or supplying of oxygenated instead of venous blood.

arteriarctia (ar″tĕ-re-ark′she-ah) [*artery* + L. *arctare* to contract] (*obs.*) contraction of an artery; narrowing of the caliber of an artery.

arteriectasia (ar″tĕ-re-ek-ta′ze-ah)   arteriectasis.

arteriectasis (ar″tĕ-re-ek′tah-sis) [*artery* + Gr. *ektasis* dilatation] dilatation and, usually, lengthening of an artery.

arteriectomy (ar″tĕ-re-ek′to-me) [*artery* + Gr. *ektome* excision] excision of a portion of an artery.

arteriectopia (ar″tĕ-re-ek-to′pe-ah) [*artery* + Gr. *ektopos* out of place] displacement of an artery from its normal location.

arterio- (ar-te′re-o) [L. *arteria*, Gr. *artēria*] a combining form denoting relationship to an artery or arteries.

arteriocapillary (ar-te″re-o-kap′ĭ-la″re)   pertaining to the arteries and the capillaries.

arteriodilating (ar-te″re-o-di′lāt-ing) increasing the caliber of the arteries, particularly of arterioles.

arteriogenesis (ar-te″re-o-jen′ĕ-sis) [*artery* + Gr. *genesis* production] the formation of arteries.

arteriogram (ar-te′re-o-gram″) [*artery* + Gr. *gramma* a writing] 1. a roentgenogram of an artery after injection of a radiopaque medium. 2. (*obs.*) a sphygmographic tracing of the arterial pulse.

arteriograph (ar-te′re-o-graf) a film produced by arteriography.

arteriography (ar″te-re-og′rah-fe) [*artery* + Gr. *graphein* to write] roentgenography of arteries after injection of radiopaque material into the blood stream. **catheter a.,** radiography of vessels after introduction of contrast material through a catheter inserted into an artery. **selective a.,** radiography of a specific vessel which is opacified by a medium introduced directly into it, usually via a catheter.

arteriola (ar-te″re-o′lah), pl. *arterio′lae* [L., dim. of *arteria*] arteriole: a minute arterial branch, especially [NA] one just proximal to a capillary. **a. macula′ris infe′rior** [NA], inferior macular arteriole: the inferior arteriole supplying the macula retinae. **a. macula′ris supe′rior** [NA], superior macular arteriole: the superior arteriole supplying the macula retinae. **a. media′lis ret′inae** [NA], medial arteriole of retina: the small branch supplying blood to the central region of the retina. **a. nasa′lis ret′inae infe′rior** [NA], inferior nasal arteriole of retina: a small branch of the central artery of the retina supplying the inferior nasal region of the retina. **a. nasa′lis ret′inae supe′rior** [NA], superior nasal arteriole of retina: a small branch of the central artery of the retina, supplying the superior nasal region of the retina. **arterio′lae rec′tae re′nis** [NA], branches of the arcuate arteries of the kidney arising from the efferent glomerular arterioles, and passing down to the renal pyramids; called also *straight arteries*, or *arterioles, of the kidney* and *vasa recta.* Also sometimes called *arteriolae rectae spuriae* or *false straight arterioles* of the kidney to distinguish them from straight direct branches from the arcuate and interlobular arteries that are called *arteriolae rectae vera* or *true straight arterioles* of the kidney. **arterio′lae rec′tae spu′riae,** see *arteriolae rectae renis.* **arterio′lae rec′tae ve′ra,** see *arteriolae rectae renis.* **a. tempora′lis ret′inae infe′rior** [NA], inferior temporal arteriole of retina: a branch of the central artery of the retina, supplying the inferior temporal region of the retina. **a. tempora′lis ret′inae supe′rior** [NA], superior temporal arteriole of retina: a branch of the central artery of the retina, supplying the superior temporal region of the retina.

arteriolae (ar-te″re-o′le) [L.] plural of arteriola.

arteriolar (ar″te-re′o-lar) pertaining to or resembling arterioles.

arteriole (ar-te′re-ōl) [L. *arteriola*] a minute arterial branch, especially one just proximal to a capillary; called also *arteriola* [NA]. **ellipsoid a's,** sheathed arteries. **glomerular a., afferent,** a branch of an interlobular artery that goes to a renal glomerulus; called also *vas afferens glomeruli* [NA]. **glomerular a., efferent,** an arteriole that arises from a renal glomerulus, breaking up into capillaries to supply renal tubules; called also *vas efferens glomeruli* [NA]. **Isaacs-Ludwig a.,** an arteriolar twig that sometimes branches from the afferent glomerular arteriole of the kidney to communicate directly with the tubular capillary plexus. **macular a., inferior,** arteriola macularis inferior. **macular a., superior,** arteriola macularis superior. **medial a. of retina,** arteriola medialis retinae. **nasal a. of retina, inferior,** arteriola nasalis retinae inferior. **nasal a. of retina, superior,** arteriola nasalis retinae superior. **postglomerular a.,** efferent glomerular a. **precapillary a's,** arterial capillaries. **preglomerular a.,** afferent glomerular a. **sheathed a's,** see under *artery.* **straight a's of kidney,** arteriolae rectae renis. **straight a's of kidney, false,** see *arteriolae rectae renis.* **straight a's of kidney, true,** see *arteriolae rectae renis.* **temporal a. of retina, inferior,** arteriola temporalis retinae inferior. **temporal a. of retina, superior,** arteriola temporalis retinae superior.

arteriolith (ar-te′re-o-lith″) [*artery* + Gr. *lithos* stone] a chalky concretion in an artery.

arteriolitis (ar-tēr″ĭ-o-li′tis) inflammation of the arterioles.

arteriology (ar-te″re-ol′o-je) [*artery* + *-logy*] the sum of what is known regarding the arteries; the science or study of the arteries.

arteriolonecrosis (ar-te″re-o″lo-ne-kro′sis) necrosis of arterioles, as may be seen in nephrosclerosis; called also *arteriolar necrosis.*

arteriolosclerosis (ar-te″re-o″lo-sklĕ-ro′sis) sclerosis and thickening of the walls of the smaller arteries (arterioles). *Hyaline arteriolosclerosis,* in which there is homogeneous pink hyaline thickening of the arteriolar walls, is associated with benign nephrosclerosis. *Hyperplastic arteriolosclerosis,* in which there is a concentric thickening with progressive narrowing of the lumina, may be associated with malignant hypertension, nephrosclerosis, and scleroderma.

arteriolosclerotic (ar-te″re-o″lo-skle-rot′ik) pertaining to or characterized by arteriolosclerosis.

arteriomalacia (ar-te″re-o-mah-la′she-ah) [*artery* + Gr. *malakia* softness] (*obs.*) abnormal softness of the arterial coats.

arteriometer (ar″te-re-om′ĕ-ter) [*artery* + Gr. *metron* measure] (*obs.*) an apparatus used for measuring any changes in the caliber of a pulsating artery.

arteriomotor (ar-te″re-o-mo′tor) pertaining to or causing change in the caliber of an artery.

arteriomyomatosis (ar-te″re-o-mi″o-mah-to′sis) a growth of irregular muscular fibers in the walls of an artery causing thickening of the walls.

arterionecrosis (ar-te″re-o-ne-kro′sis) necrosis of an artery or of arteries.

arteriopalmus (ar-te″re-o-pal′mus) (*obs.*) palpitation or throbbing of an artery.

arteriopathy (ar″te-re-op′ah-the) [*artery* + Gr. *pathos* disease] any arterial disease. **hypertensive a.,** widespread involvement, chiefly of arterioles and small arteries, associated with arterial hypertension and characterized primarily by hypertrophy and thickening of the media.

arterioperissia (ar-te″re-o-pĕ-ris′e-ah) [*artery* + Gr. *perissos* excessive] (*obs.*) excessive arterial development.

arterioplania (ar-te″re-o-pla′ne-ah) [*artery* + Gr. *planan* to wander + *-ia*] (*obs.*) the condition in which an artery takes an unusual course.

arterioplasty (ar-te″re-o-plas′te) [*artery* + Gr. *plassein* to form] surgical repair or reconstruction of an artery; applied to Matas' operation (endoaneurysmorraphy) for aneurysm, restoring the continuity of the parent artery by making a new channel out of the sac walls.

arteriopressor (ar-te″re-o-pres′or) producing increased blood pressure in the arteries.

arteriorenal (ar-te″re-o-re′nal) pertaining to the arteries of the kidney.

arteriorrhagia (ar-te″re-o-ra′je-ah) (*obs.*) arterial hemorrhage.

arteriorrhaphy (ar-te″re-or′ah-fe) [*artery* + Gr. *rhaphē* suture] suture of an artery.

arteriorrhexis (ar-te″re-o-rek′sis) [*artery* + Gr. *rhēxis* rupture] rupture of an artery.

arteriosclerosis (ar-te″re-o-sklĕ-ro′sis) [*artery* + Gr. *sklēros* hard] a group of diseases characterized by thickening and loss of elasticity of arterial walls; it comprises three distinct forms: atherosclerosis, Mönckeberg's arteriosclerosis, and arteriolosclerosis. **cerebral a.,** arteriosclerosis of the arteries of the brain. **coronary a.,** arteriosclerosis (atherosclerosis) of the coronary arteries. **hyaline a.,** a homogeneous hyaline thickening of the walls of arterioles with consequent narrowing of the lumina. **hypertensive a.,** arteriosclerosis intensified by hypertension. **infantile a.,** see *infantile arteritis,* under *arteritis.* **intimal a.,** arteriosclerosis in which the major changes affect the intima of the arteries. **medial a.,** a condition of large and medium-sized arteries, with primary destruction of the muscle and elastic fibers of the medial coat, which are replaced by fibrous tissue; sometimes there are deposits of calcium (akin to Mönckeberg's arteriosclerosis). **Mönckeberg's a.,** medial arteriosclerosis with extensive deposits of calcium in the media of the artery; called also *Mönckeberg's calcification, degeneration, sclerosis,* or *medial calcific sclerosis.* **nodose a., nodular a.** (*obs.*), disease of the arteries marked by the formation of fibrous nodes or plaques in the lining membrane of the arteries. **a. oblit′erans,** arteriosclerosis in which proliferation of the intima of small vessels has caused complete obliteration of the lumen of the artery. **peripheral a.,** arteriosclerosis of the extremities. **presenile a.,** physiological arteriosclerosis occurring at an unusually early age and without apparent cause. **senile a.,** arteriosclerosis that accompanies old age, but is not specifically age related.

arteriosclerotic (ar-te″re-o-sklĕ-rot′ik) pertaining to or affected with arteriosclerosis.

arteriosity (ar-te″re-os′ĭ-te) the condition or quality of being arterial.

arteriospasm (ar-te′re-o-spazm″) spasm of an artery.

arteriospastic (ar-te″re-o-spas′tik) pertaining to, characterized by, or causing arteriospasm.

arteriostenosis (ar-te″re-o-ste-no′sis) [*artery* + Gr. *stenos* narrow] the narrowing or diminution of the caliber of an artery.

arteriosteogenesis (ar-te″re-os″te-o-jen′ĕ-sis) [*artery* + Gr. *osteon* bone + *gennan* to produce] calcification of an artery.

arteriostosis (ar-te″re-os-to′sis) [*artery* + Gr. *osteon* bone + *-osis*] ossification of an artery.

arteriostrepsis (ar-te″re-o-strep′sis) [*artery* + Gr. *streptos* twisted] the twisting of an artery for the arrest of hemorrhage.

arteriosympathectomy (ar-te″re-o-sim″pah-thek′to-me) periarterial sympathectomy; see under *sympathectomy.*

arteriotomy (ar″te-re-ot′o-me) [*artery* + Gr. *tomē* cut] incision of an artery.

arteriotony (ar-te″re-ot′o-ne) [*artery* + Gr. *tonos* tension] the intra-arterial tension of the blood; blood pressure.

arteriotrepsis (ar-te″re-o-trep′sis) arteriostrepsis.

arterious (ar-te′re-us) pertaining to the arteries; arterial.

arteriovenous (ar-te″re-o-ve′nus) both arterial and venous; pertaining to or affecting an artery and a vein.

arteritides (ar″tĕ-rit′ĭ-dēz) plural of *arteritis*.

arteritis (ar″tĕ-ri′tis), pl. *arterit′ides* [*artery* + *-itis*] inflammation of an artery; cf. *endarteritis* and *periarteritis*. **brachiocephalic a., a. brachiocephal′ica,** pulseless disease. **coronary a.,** inflammation of the coronary arteries. **cranial a.,** temporal a. **a. defor′mans** (*obs.*), chronic endarteritis with calcareous infiltration. **equine viral a.,** a frequently fatal viral disease of horses affecting especially the smaller arteries, with hemorrhagic enteritis, abdominal pain and diarrhea, and pulmonary edema. Abortion is common in affected mares. **giant cell a.,** temporal a. **Horton′s a.,** temporal a. **a. hyperplas′tica** (*obs.*), arteritis with the formation of new connective tissue. **infantile a.,** diffuse arteritis in infants and children, rarely with atherosclerotic processes. **localized visceral a.,** allergic vasculitis. **a. nodo′sa,** periarteritis (polyarteritis) nodosa. **a. oblit′erans,** endarteritis obliterans. **rheumatic a.,** generalized inflammation of arterioles and arterial capillaries occurring in rheumatic fever. **syphilitic a.,** a late manifestation of syphilis characterized by intimal proliferation and degeneration of the medial coat, usually involving the ascending aorta, aortic arch, and pulmonary artery, which may lead to aneurysm. **Takayasu′s a.,** pulseless disease. **temporal a.,** a chronic vascular disease of unknown origin, largely confined to the carotid arterial system, characterized by proliferative inflammation, often with giant cells and granulomas, and by headache, difficulty in chewing, weakness, weight loss, fever, and symptoms of sepsis, with a markedly increased erythrocyte sedimentation rate and leukocytosis. Ocular involvement, ranging from diplopia to complete blindness, occurs in about half the subjects. The disease occurs exclusively in older persons, and is often associated with polymyalgia rheumatica. Called also *cranial a., giant cell a.,* and *Horton′s arteritis, disease,* or *syndrome.* **tuberculous a.,** endarteritis obliterans in those arteries intimately involved in a tubercular focus. **a. umbilica′lis,** septic inflammation of the umbilical artery in newborn infants. **a. verruco′sa** (*obs.*), arteritis marked by finger-like projections from the wall into the lumen of the blood vessel.

artery (ar′ter-e) [L. *arteria;* Gr. *artēria,* from *aēr* air + *tērein* to keep, because the arteries were supposed by the ancients to contain air, or from Gr. *aeirein* to lift or attach] a vessel through which the blood passes away from the heart to the various parts of the body; called also *arteria* [NA]. The wall of an artery consists typically of an outer coat (tunica adventitia), a middle coat (tunica media), and an inner coat (tunica intima). **accompa-**

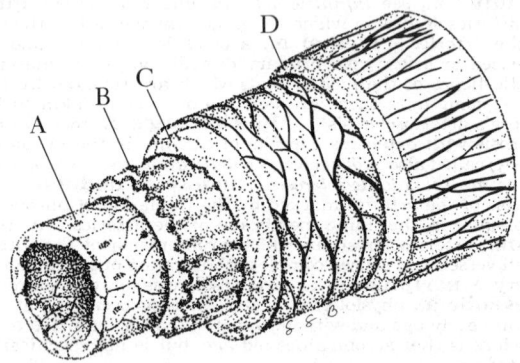

Artery; representation of arterial coats; *A,* tunica intima; *B,* internal elastic lamina; *C,* tunica media; *D,* tunica adventitia.

nying a. of ischiadic nerve, arteria comitans nervi ischiadici. **acetabular a.,** 1. ramus acetabularis arteriae circumflexae femoris medialis. 2. ramus acetabularis arteriae obturatoriae. **adipose a′s of kidney,** rami capsulares arteriae renis. **afferent a. of glomerulus,** vas afferens glomeruli. **alveolar a., inferior,** arteria alveolaris inferior. **alveolar a′s, superior, anterior,** arteriae alveolares superiores anteriores. **alveolar a., superior, posterior,** arteria alveolaris superior posterior. **angular a.,** arteria angularis. **appendicular a.,** arteria appendicularis. **arcuate a. of foot,** arteria arcuata pedis. **arcuate a′s of kidney,** arteriae arcuatae renis. **articular a., proper, of little head of fibula,** ramus circumflexus fibulae arteriae tibialis posterioris. **auditory a., internal,** arteria labyrinthi. **auricular a′s, anterior,** rami auriculares anteriores arteriae temporalis superficialis. **auricular a., deep,** arteria auricularis profunda. **auricular a., left,** arteria coronaria sinistra. **auricular a., posterior,** arteria auricularis posterior. **auricular a., right,** arteria coronaria dextra. **axillary a.,** arteria axillaris. **basilar a.,** arteria basilaris. **brachial a.,** arteria brachialis.

brachial a., deep, arteria profunda brachii. **brachial a., superficial,** arteria brachialis superficialis. **brachiocephalic a.,** truncus brachiocephalicus. **bronchial a′s, anterior,** rami bronchiales aortae thoracicae. **bronchial a′s, anterior,** rami bronchiales arteriae thoracicae internae. **buccal a.,** arteria buccalis. **buccinator a.,** arteria buccalis. **bulbourethral a.,** arteria bulbi penis. **a. of bulb of penis,** arteria bulbi penis. **a. of bulb of vestibule of vagina,** arteria bulbi vestibuli vaginae. **capsular a., inferior,** arteria suprarenalis inferior. **capsular a., middle,** arteria suprarenalis media. **caroticotympanic a.,** see *rami caroticotympanici.* **carotid a., common,** arteria carotis communis. **carotid a., external,** arteria carotis externa. **carotid a., internal,** arteria carotis interna. **caudal a.,** arteria sacralis mediana. **celiac a.,** truncus celiacus. **cecal a., anterior,** arteria cecalis anterior. **cecal a., posterior,** arteria cecalis posterior. **central a. of retina,** arteria centralis retinae. **central a′s of spleen,** branches of the splenic artery after they leave the trabeculae; their tunica adventitia is replaced by a cylindrical lymphoid sheath and they pass through the aggregations of lymphatic nodules and branch out to terminate as splenic penicilli. **cephalic a.,** arteria carotis communis. **cerebellar a., inferior, anterior,** arteria cerebelli inferior anterior. **cerebellar a., inferior, posterior,** arteria cerebelli inferior posterior. **cerebellar a., superior,** arteria cerebelli superior. **cerebral a′s,** arteriae cerebri. **cerebral a., anterior,** arteria cerebri anterior. **a. of cerebral hemorrhage,** lenticulostriate a. **cerebral a., middle,** arteria cerebri media. **cerebral a., posterior,** arteria cerebri posterior. **a′s of cerebrum,** arteriae cerebri. **cervical a., ascending,** arteria cervicalis ascendens. **cervical a., deep,** a. cervicalis profunda. **cervical a., descending, deep,** see *rami occipitales arteriae occipitalis.* **cervical a., superficial,** ramus superficialis arteriae transversae colli. **cervical a., transverse,** arteria transversa colli. **choroidal a., anterior,** arteria choroidea anterior. **ciliary a′s, anterior,** arteriae ciliares anteriores. **ciliary a′s, long,** arteriae ciliares posteriores longae. **ciliary a′s, posterior, long,** arteriae ciliares posteriores longae. **ciliary a′s, posterior, short,** arteriae ciliares posteriores breves. **ciliary a′s, short,** arteriae ciliares posteriores breves. **circumflex a., deep, internal,** ramus profundus arteriae circumflexae femoris medialis. **circumflex a., femoral, lateral,** arteria circumflexa femoris lateralis. **circumflex a., femoral, medial,** arteria circumflexa femoris medialis. **circumflex a., humeral, anterior,** arteria circumflexa humeri anterior. **circumflex a., humeral, posterior,** arteria circumflexa humeri posterior. **circumflex a., iliac, deep,** arteria circumflexa ilium profunda. **circumflex a., iliac, superficial,** arteria circumflexa ilium superficialis. **circumflex a. of scapula,** arteria circumflexa scapulae. **a. of clitoris, deep,** arteria profunda clitoridis. **a. of clitoris, dorsal,** arteria dorsalis clitoridis. **coccygeal a.,** arteria sacralis mediana. **cochlear a.,** ramus cochlearis arteriae labyrinthi. **Cohnheim′s a.,** terminal a. **colic a., left,** arteria colica sinistra. **colic a., middle,** arteria colica media. **colic a., right,** arteria colica dextra. **colic a., right, inferior,** arteria ileocolica. **colic a., superior, accessory,** arteria colica media. **collateral a., middle,** arteria collateralis media. **collateral a., radial,** arteria collateralis radialis. **collateral a., ulnar, inferior,** arteria collateralis ulnaris inferior. **collateral a., ulnar, superior,** arteria collateralis ulnaris superior. **communicating a., anterior, of cerebrum,** arteria communicans anterior cerebri. **communicating a., posterior, of cerebrum,** arteria communicans posterior cerebri. **conducting a′s,** large arterial trunks, characterized by their large size and elasticity, such as the aorta, subclavian, and common carotid, and the brachiocephalic and pulmonary trunks. **conjunctival a′s, anterior,** arteriae conjunctivales anteriores. **conjunctival a′s, posterior,** arteriae conjunctivales posteriores. **copper-wire a′s,** retinal arteries on which the bright line of reflex is exaggerated; seen in arteriosclerosis. **corkscrew a′s,** small arteries in the macular region of the eye that appear markedly tortuous. **coronary a., descending, posterior,** ramus interventricularis posterior. **coronary a., left, of heart,** arteria coronaria sinistra. **coronary a., left, of stomach,** arteria gastrica sinistra. **coronary a., right, of heart,** arteria coronaria dextra. **coronary a., right, of stomach,** arteria gastrica dextra. **cremasteric a.,** arteria cremasterica. **cricothyroid a.,** ramus cricothyroideus arteriae thyroideae superioris. **cystic a.,** arteria cystica. **deferential a.,** arteria ductus deferentis. **deltoid a.,** ramus deltoideus arteriae thoracoacromialis. **dental a′s, anterior,** arteriae alveolares superiores anteriores. **dental a., inferior,** arteria alveolaris inferior. **dental a., posterior,** arteria alveolaris superior posterior. **diaphragmatic a′s,** arteriae phrenicae inferiores. **diaphragmatic a′s, superior,** arteriae phrenicae superiores. **digital a′s, collateral,** arteriae digitales palmares propriae. **digital a′s of foot, common,** arteriae metatarseae plantares. **digital a′s of foot, dorsal,** arteriae digitales dorsales pedis. **digital a′s of hand, dorsal,** arteriae digitales dorsales manus. **digital a′s, palmar,**

common, arteriae digitales palmares communes. **digital a's, palmar, proper,** arteriae digitales palmares propriae. **digital a's, plantar, common,** arteriae digitales plantares communes. **digital a's, plantar, proper,** arteriae digitales plantares propriae. **digital a's, volar, common,** arteriae digitales palmares communes. **digital a's, volar, proper,** arteriae digitales palmares propriae. **distributing a's,** most of the arteries except the conducting arteries; of muscular type, they extend from the large vessels to the arterioles. **dorsal a. of clitoris,** arteria dorsalis clitoridis. **dorsal a. of foot,** arteria dorsalis pedis. **dorsal a. of nose,** arteria dorsalis nasi. **dorsal a. of penis,** arteria dorsalis penis. **a. of ductus deferens,** arteria ductus deferentis. **duodenal a's,** arteriae pancreaticoduodenales inferiores. **efferent a. of glomerulus,** vas efferens glomeruli. **elastic a's,** conducting a's. **emulgent a.,** arteria renalis. **end a.,** one which undergoes progressive branching without development of channels connecting with other arteries, so that if occluded it cannot supply sufficient blood to the tissue depending on it. **epigastric a., external,** arteria circumflexa ilium profunda. **epigastric a., inferior,** arteria epigastrica inferior. **epigastric a., superficial,** arteria epigastrica superficialis. **epigastric a., superior,** arteria epigastrica superior. **episcleral a's,** arteriae episclerales. **esophageal a's,** rami esophagei aortae thoracicae. **esophageal a's, inferior,** rami esophagei arteriae gastricae sinistrae. **ethmoidal a., anterior,** arteria ethmoidalis anterior. **ethmoidal a., posterior,** arteria ethmoidalis posterior. **facial a.,** 1. arteria facialis. 2. arteria carotis externa. **facial a., deep,** arteria maxillaris. **facial a., transverse,** arteria transversa faciei. **fallopian a.,** arteria uterina. **femoral a.,** arteria femoralis. **femoral a., common,** see *arteria femoralis.* **femoral a., deep,** arteria profunda femoris. **femoral a., superficial,** see *arteria femoralis.* **fibular a.,** arteria peronea. **a. of foot, dorsal,** arteria dorsalis pedis. **frontal a.,** arteria supratrochlearis. **funicular a.,** arteria testicularis. **gastric a., left,** arteria gastrica sinistra. **gastric a., left inferior,** arteria gastroepiploica sinistra. **gastric a., right,** arteria gastrica dextra. **gastric a., right inferior,** arteria gastroepiploica dextra. **gastric a's, short,** arteriae gastricae breves. **gastroduodenal a.,** arteria gastroduodenalis. **gastroepiploic a., left,** arteria gastroepiploica sinistra. **gastroepiploic a., right,** arteria gastroepiploica dextra. **genicular a., descending,** arteria genus descendens. **genicular a., inferior, lateral,** arteria genus inferior lateralis. **genicular a., inferior, medial,** arteria genus inferior mediales. **genicular a., middle,** arteria genus media. **genicular a., superior, lateral,** arteria genus superior lateralis. **genicular a., superior, medial,** arteria genus superior medialis. **a. of glomerulus,** vas afferens glomeruli. **gluteal a., inferior,** arteria glutea inferior. **gluteal a., superior,** arteria glutea superior. **hardening of a's,** arteriosclerosis. **helicine a's,** small arteries that possess on one side, throughout their length, a band of thickened intima in which longitudinal muscle fibers are embedded. They follow a convoluted or curled course and open directly into cavernous sinuses instead of capillaries; they play a dominant role in erection of erectile tissue. **helicine a's of penis,** arteriae helicinae penis. **hemorrhoidal a., inferior,** arteria rectalis inferior. **hemorrhoidal a., middle,** arteria rectalis media. **hemorrhoidal a., superior,** arteria rectalis superior. **hepatic a., common,** arteria hepatica communis. **hepatic a., proper,** arteria hepatica propria. **hyaloid a.,** arteria hyaloidea. **a's of hybrid type,** a term denoting the short transitional regions where arteries of mixed or elastic (conducting) type pass into arteries of the muscular (distributing) type. **hyoid a.,** ramus suprahyoideus arteriae lingualis. **hypogastric a.,** arteria iliaca interna. **hypogastric a., obliterated,** ligamentum umbilicale mediale. **hypophyseal a.,** any of a series of minute branches of the internal carotid artery that supply the pituitary gland. **ileal a's,** arteriae ilei. **ileocolic a.,** arteria ileocolica. **iliac a., anterior,** arteria iliaca externa. **iliac a., common,** arteria iliaca communis. **iliac a., external,** arteria iliaca externa. **iliac a., internal,** arteria iliaca interna. **iliac a., small,** arteria iliolumbalis. **iliolumbar a.,** arteria iliolumbalis. **infracostal a.,** ramus costalis lateralis arteriae thoracicae internae. **infraorbital a.,** arteria infraorbitalis. **inguinal a's,** rami inguinales arteriae femoralis. **innominate a.,** truncus brachiocephalicus. **intercostal a's, anterior,** rami intercostales anteriores arteriae thoracicae internae. **intercostal a., highest,** arteria intercostalis suprema. **intercostal a's, posterior, I and II,** arteriae intercostales posteriores I et II. **intercostal a's, posterior, III–XI,** arteriae intercostales posteriores III–XI. **interlobar a's of kidney,** arteriae interlobares renis. **interlobular a's of kidney,** arteriae interlobulares renis. **interlobular a's of liver,** arteriae interlobulares hepatis. **intermetacarpal a's, palmar,** arteriae metacarpeae palmares. **interosseous a., anterior,** arteria interossea anterior. **interosseous a., common,** arteria interossea communis. **interosseous a., dorsal, of forearm,** arteria interossea posterior. **interosseous a., posterior (of forearm),** arteria interossea posterior. **interosse-**

ous a., recurrent, arteria interossea recurrens. **interosseous a., volar,** arteria interossea anterior. **intersegmental a's,** paired dorsal branches of the embryonic aorta, originally going to the spinal cord but later mainly to the neck, back, and body wall. **interventricular a., anterior,** ramus interventricularis anterior. **intestinal a's,** arteriae intestinales. **jejunal a's,** arteriae jejunales. **labial a's, anterior, of vulva,** rami labiales anteriores arteriae femoralis. **labial a., inferior,** arteria labialis inferior. **labial a's, posterior, of vulva,** rami labiales posteriores arteriae pudendae internae. **labial a., superior,** arteria labialis superior. **a. of labyrinth, labyrinthine a.,** arteria labyrinthi. **lacrimal a.,** arteria lacrimalis. **laryngeal a., inferior,** arteria laryngea inferior. **laryngeal a., superior,** arteria laryngea superior. **lenticulostriate a.,** one of the central branches (lateral striate arteries) of the middle cerebral artery; it supplies the lenticular (lentiform) nucleus, internal capsule, and caudate nucleus (which together form the corpus striatum) and is a common site of cerebral hemorrhage. Called also *a. of cerebral hemorrhage.* **lingual a.,** arteria lingualis. **lingual a., deep,** arteria profunda linguae. **lumbar a's,** arteriae lumbales. **lumbar a., fifth, lumbar a., lowest,** arteria lumbalis ima. **malleolar a., anterior, lateral,** arteria malleolaris anterior lateralis. **malleolar a., anterior, medial,** arteria malleolaris anterior medialis. **malleolar a., posterior, lateral,** see *rami malleolares laterales arteriae peroneae.* **malleolar a., posterior, medial,** see *rami malleolares mediales arteriae peroneae.* **mammary a., external,** 1. arteria thoracica lateralis. 2. see *rami mammarii laterales arteriae thoracicae lateralis.* **mammary a., internal,** arteria thoracica interna. **mandibular a.,** arteria alveolaris inferior. **marginal a. (of Drummond),** a long channel running parallel to the large intestine, from the cecum to the sigmoid colon, formed by branches from the superior and inferior mesenteric arteries and giving rise to straight arteries that supply the intestinal wall. **masseteric a.,** arteria masseterica. **mastoid a's,** rami mastoidei arteriae auricularis posterioris. **maxillary a.,** arteria maxillaris. **maxillary a., external,** arteria facialis. **maxillary a., internal,** arteria maxillaris. **medial a. of foot, superficial,** ramus superficialis arteriae plantaris medialis. **median a.,** arteria mediana. **mediastinal a's, anterior,** rami mediastinales arteriae thoracicae internae. **mediastinal a's, posterior,** rami mediastinales aortae thoracicae. **medullary a.,** nutrient a. **meningeal a., accessory,** ramus meningeus accessorius arteriae meningeae mediae. **meningeal a., anterior,** arteria meningea anterior. **meningeal a., middle,** arteria meningea media. **meningeal a., posterior,** 1. arteria meningea posteria. 2. ramus meningeus arteriae vertebralis. **mental a.,** arteria mentalis. **mesenteric a., inferior,** arteria mesenterica inferior. **mesenteric a., superior,** arteria mesenterica superior. **metacarpal a's, dorsal,** 1. arteriae metacarpeae dorsales. 2. see *ramus carpeus dorsalis arteriae ulnaris.* **metacarpal a's, palmar,** arteriae metacarpeae palmares. **metacarpal a's, ulnar,** arteriae digitales palmares communes. **metacarpal a's, volar,** arteriae metacarpeae palmares. **metacarpal a., volar, deep,** ramus palmaris profundus arteriae ulnaris. **metatarsal a's, dorsal,** arteriae metatarseae dorsales. **metatarsal a's, plantar,** arteriae metatarseae plantares. **a's of mixed type,** arteries having elastic (conducting) and muscular (distributing) elements. **a's of Mueller,** arteriae helicinae penis. **muscular a's,** distributing a's. **musculophrenic a.,** arteria musculophrenica. **mylohyoid a.,** ramus mylohyoideus arteriae alveolaris inferioris. **myomastoid a.,** ramus occipitalis arteriae auricularis posterioris. **nasal a's, posterior, lateral and septal,** arteriae nasales posteriores, laterale et septi. **nasopalatine a.,** arteria sphenopalatina. **Neubauer's a.,** arteria thyroidea ima. **a. of nose, dorsal,** arteria dorsalis nasi. **nutrient a.,** any artery that supplies the marrow or medulla of bone; called also *medullary a.* **nutrient a's of humerus,** arteriae nutriciae humeri. **nutrient a's of kidney,** rami capsulares arteriae renis. **obturator a.,** arteria obturatoria. **obturator a., accessory,** arteria obturatoria accessoria. **occipital a.,** arteria occipitalis. **ophthalmic a.,** arteria ophthalmica. **ovarian a.,** arteria ovarica. **palatine a., ascending,** arteria palatina ascendens. **palatine a., descending,** arteria palatina descendens. **palatine a., greater,** arteria palatina major. **palatine a's, lesser,** arteriae palatinae minores. **palpebral a's, lateral,** arteriae palpebrales laterales. **palpebral a's, medial,** arteriae palpebrales mediales. **pancreatic a., dorsal,** arteria pancreatica dorsalis. **pancreatic a., great,** arteria pancreatica magna. **pancreatic a., inferior,** arteria pancreatica inferior. **pancreaticoduodenal a's, inferior,** arteriae pancreaticoduodenales inferiores. **pancreaticoduodenal a., superior,** arteria pancreaticoduodenalis superior. **pelvic a., posterior,** arteria iliaca interna. **a. of penis, deep,** arteria profunda penis. **a. of penis, dorsal,** arteria dorsalis penis. **perforating a's,** arteriae perforantes. **pericardiac a's, posterior,** rami pericardiaci aortae thoracicae. **pericardiacophrenic a.,** arteria pericardiacophrenica. **perineal a.,** arteria perinealis. **peroneal a.,** arteria peronea.

peroneal a., perforating, ramus perforans arteriae peroneae. **pharyngeal a., ascending,** arteria pharyngea ascendens. **phrenic a's, great,** arteriae phrenicae inferiores. **phrenic a's, inferior,** arteriae phrenicae inferiores. **phrenic a., superior,** arteria pericardiacophrenica. 2. see *arteriae phrenicae superiores.* **plantar a., external,** arteria plantaris lateralis. **plantar a., lateral,** arteria plantaris lateralis. **plantar a., medial,** arteria plantaris medialis. **popliteal a.,** arteria poplitea. **principal a. of thumb,** arteria princeps pollicis. **pterygoid a's,** rami pterygoidei. **a. of pterygoid canal,** arteria canalis pterygoidei. **pubic a.,** ramus pubicus arteriae epigastricae inferioris. **pudendal a's, external,** arteriae pudendae externae. **pudendal a., internal,** arteria pudenda interna. **pulmonary a.,** truncus pulmonalis. **pulmonary a., left,** arteria pulmonalis sinistra. **pulmonary a., right,** arteria pulmonalis dextra. **a. of the pulp,** a name given the first portion of a brushlike group of blood vessels in the spleen. **pyloric a.,** arteria gastrica dextra. **quadriceps a. of femur,** ramus descendens arteriae circumflexae femoris lateralis. **radial a.,** arteria radialis. **radial a., collateral,** arteria collateralis radialis. **radial a. of index finger,** arteria radialis indicis. **radial a., volar, of index finger,** arteria radialis indicis. **radiate a's of kidney,** arteriae interlobulares renis. **radicular a's,** a name applied to arteries that enter the spinal canal along the anterior and posterior nerve roots. **ranine a.,** arteria profunda linguae. **rectal a., inferior,** arteria rectalis inferior. **rectal a., middle,** arteria rectalis media. **rectal a., superior,** arteria rectalis superior. **recurrent a., radial,** arteria recurrens radialis. **recurrent a., tibial, anterior,** arteria recurrens tibialis anterior. **recurrent a., tibial, posterior,** arteria recurrens tibialis posterior. **recurrent a., ulnar,** arteria recurrens ulnaris. **renal a.,** arteria renalis. **renal a's,** arteriae renis. **retrocostal a.,** ramus costalis lateralis arteriae thoracicae internae. **retroduodenal a's,** arteriae retroduodenales. **revehent a.,** vas efferens glomeruli. **a. of round ligament of uterus,** arteria ligamenti teretis uteri. **sacral a's, lateral,** arteriae sacrales laterales. **sacral a., median,** arteria sacralis mediana. **sacrococcygeal a.,** arteria sacralis mediana. **scapular a., dorsal,** ramus profundus arteriae transversae colli. **scapular a., posterior,** ramus profundus arteriae transversae colli. **scapular a., transverse,** arteria suprascapularis. **sciatic a.,** arteria comitans nervi ischiadici. **scrotal a's, anterior,** rami scrotales anteriores arteriae femoralis. **scrotal a's, posterior,** rami scrotales posteriores arteriae pudendae internae. **segmental a., anterior,** arteria segmenti anterioris. **segmental a., anterior inferior,** arteria segmenti anterioris inferioris. **segmental a., anterior superior,** arteria segmenti anterioris superioris. **segmental a., inferior,** arteria segmenti inferioris. **segmental a., lateral,** arteria segmenti lateralis. **segmental a., medial,** arteria segmenti medialis. **segmental a., posterior,** arteria segmenti posterioris. **segmental a., superior,** arteria segmenti superioris. **sheathed a's,** arterial branches having spindle-shaped thickenings in their walls (Schweigger-Seidel sheaths) and forming the penicilli of the spleen; called also *ellipsoid* or *sheathed arterioles.* **sigmoid a's,** arteriae sigmoideae. **spermatic a., external,** arteria cremasterica. **spermatic a., internal,** arteria testicularis. **sphenopalatine a.,** arteria sphenopalatina. **spinal a's,** rami spinales arteriae vertebralis. **spinal a., anterior,** arteria spinalis anterior. **spinal a., posterior,** arteria spinalis posterior. **splenic a.,** arteria lienalis. **sternal a's, posterior,** rami sternales arteriae thoracicae internae. **sternocleidomastoid a.,** see *rami sternocleidomastoidei arteriae occipitalis.* **sternocleidomastoid a., superior,** ramus sternocleidomastoideus arteriae thyroideae superioris. **straight a's of kidney,** arteriolae rectae renis. **striate a's,** rami striati arteriae cerebri mediae. **striate a., medial,** a branch of the anterior medial artery; it supplies the lower anterior portion of the basal ganglia. **stylomastoid a.,** arteria stylomastoidea. **subclavian a.,** arteria subclavia. **subcostal a.,** 1. arteria subcostalis. 2. ramus costalis lateralis arteriae thoracicae internae. **sublingual a.,** arteria sublingualis. **submental a.,** arteria submentalis. **subscapular a.,** arteria subscapularis. **supraduodenal a's, superior,** arteriae supraduodenales superiores. **supraorbital a.,** arteria supraorbitalis. **suprarenal a., aortic,** arteria suprarenalis media. **suprarenal a., inferior,** arteria suprarenalis inferior. **suprarenal a., middle,** arteria suprarenalis media. **suprarenal a's, superior,** arteriae suprarenales superiores. **suprascapular a.,** arteria suprascapularis. **supratrochlear a.,** arteria supratrochlearis. **sural a's,** arteriae surales. **sylvian a.,** arteria cerebri media. **tarsal a., lateral,** arteria tarsea lateralis. **tarsal a's, medial,** arteriae tarseae mediales. **temporal a's, deep,** arteriae temporales profundae. **temporal a., deep, anterior,** see *arteriae temporales profundae.* **temporal a., deep, posterior,** see *arteriae temporales profundae.* **temporal a., middle,** arteria temporalis media. **temporal a., superficial,** arteria temporalis superficialis. **terminal a.,** an artery that does not divide into branches, but is directly continuous with capillaries; called also *Cohnheim's a.* **testicular a.,** arteria

testicularis. **thoracic a., highest,** arteria thoracica suprema. **thoracic a., internal,** arteria thoracica interna. **thoracic a., lateral,** arteria thoracica lateralis. **thoracicoacromial a.,** arteria thoracoacromialis. **thoracodorsal a.,** arteria thoracodorsalis. **thymic a's,** rami thymici arteriae thoracicae internae. **thyroid a., inferior,** arteria thyroidea. **thyroid a., inferior, of Cruveilhier,** ramus cricothyroideus arteriae thyroideae superioris. **thyroid a., lowest,** arteria thyroidea ima. **thyroid a., superior,** arteria thyroidea superior. **tibial a., anterior,** arteria tibialis anterior. **tibial a., posterior,** arteria tibialis posterior. **a. of tongue, dorsal,** see *rami dorsales linguae arteriae lingualis.* **tonsillar a.,** ramus tonsillaris arteriae facialis. **transverse a. of face,** arteria transversa faciei. **transverse a. of neck,** ramus superficialis arteriae transversae colli. **tubo-ovarian a.,** arteria ovarica. **tympanic a., anterior,** arteria tympanica anterior. **tympanic a., inferior,** arteria tympanica inferior. **tympanic a., posterior,** arteria tympanica posterior. **tympanic a., superior,** arteria tympanica superior. **ulnar a.,** arteria ulnaris. **ulnar collateral a., inferior,** arteria collateralis ulnaris inferior. **ulnar collateral a., superior,** arteria collateralis ulnaris superior. **umbilical a.,** arteria umbilicilis. **urethral a.,** arteria urethralis. **uterine a.,** arteria uterina. **uterine a., aortic,** arteria ovarica. **vaginal a.,** arteria vaginalis. **venous a's,** venae pulmonales. **vermiform a.,** arteria appendicularis. **vertebral a.,** arteria vertebralis. **vesical a., inferior,** arteria vesicalis inferior. **vesical a's, superior,** arteriae vesicales superiores. **vestibular a's,** rami vestibulares arteriae labyrinthi. **vidian a.,** arteria canalis pterygoidei. **a. of Zinn,** arteria centralis retinae. **zygomaticoorbital a.,** arteria zygomaticoorbitalis.

arthr- see *arthro-.*

arthragra (ar-thrag'rah) [*arthr-* + Gr. *agra* seizure] a gouty seizure in a joint or in the joints.

arthral (ar'thral) pertaining to a joint.

arthralgia (ar-thral'je-ah) [*arthr-* + *-algia*] pain in a joint. **a. saturni'na,** arthralgia of lead poisoning.

arthralgic (ar-thral'jik) pertaining to arthralgia; affected with arthralgia.

arthrectomy (ar-threk'to-me) [*arthr-* + Gr. *ektomē* excision] the excision of a joint; called also *erasion of joint.*

arthrempyesis (ar"threm-pi-e'sis) [*arthr-* + Gr. *empyēsis* suppuration] suppuration in a joint.

arthresthesia (ar"thres-the'ze-ah) [*arthr-* + Gr. *aisthēsis* perception] joint sensibility; the perception of joint motions.

arthrifuge (ar'thrĭ-fūj) [*arthritis* + L. *fugare* to put to flight] a cure for gout.

arthritic (ar-thrit'ik) 1. pertaining to or affected with gout or arthritis. 2. a person affected with arthritis.

arthritide (ar'thrĭ-tīd) any skin eruption of arthritic or gouty origin.

arthritides (ar-thrit'ĭ-dēz) plural of *arthritis.*

arthritis (ar-thri'tis), pl. *arthrit'ides* [Gr. *arthron* joint + *-itis*] rheumatism in which the inflammatory lesions are confined to the joints. **acute a.,** arthritis marked by pain, heat, redness, and swelling, due to inflammation, infection, or trauma. **acute gouty a.,** acute arthritis associated with gout. **acute rheumatic a.,** rheumatic fever. **acute suppurative a.,** pyarthrosis. **atrophic a.,** rheumatoid a. **Bekhterev's a.,** rheumatoid spondylitis. **blennorrhagic a.,** gonococcal a. **chronic inflammatory a.,** rheumatoid a. **chronic villous a.,** a form of rheumatoid arthritis due to villous outgrowths from the synovial membranes, which cause impairment of function and crepitation; called also *dry joint.* **climactic a.,** menopausal a. **cricoarytenoid a.,** inflammation of the cricoarytenoid joint in rheumatoid arthritis; causing laryngeal stridor. **a. defor'mans,** rheumatoid a. **degenerative a.,** osteoarthritis. **dysenteric a.,** arthritis with joint effusion and redness of overlying skin following *Shigella* dysentery or, less frequently, *Salmonella* enteritis; possibly the result of antigen-antibody reaction. **exudative a.,** arthritis with exudate into or about the joint. **a. fungo'sa,** abnormal changes within a joint secondary to mycotic disease, most commonly blastomycosis. It resembles and is sometimes indistinguishable from tuberculous arthritis. **gonococcal a., gonorrheal a.,** acute arthritis due to gonococcus; called also *blennorrhagic a.* and *urethral a.* **gouty a.,** arthritis due to gout; called also *uratic a.* **hemophilic a.,** bleeding into the joint cavities. **a. hiema'lis,** special forms of arthritis occurring in winter. **hypertrophic a.,** osteoarthritis. **infectional a.,** arthritis due to infection (gonococcal, tuberculous, etc.). **Lyme a.,** a recurrent form of migratory arthritis affecting a few large joints, especially the knees, shoulders, and elbows, and associated with erythema chronicum migrans, malaise, and myalgia. First reported in Old Lyme, Connecticut, it is transmitted by a tick. **menopausal a.,** a condition sometimes seen in women at the menopause, due to ovarian hormonal deficiency and marked by pain in the small joints, shoulders, elbows, or knees; called also *arthropathia ovaripriva* and *climactic a.* **a. mu'tilans,** a severe deforming polyarthritis with gross bone and cartilage destruction, usually an atypical variant of rheumatoid arthritis. **navicular a.,** inflammation of the navicular bursa and the cartilage covering the navicular bone of the foot of a horse. **neuropathic a.,** neuropathic arthropathy. **a. nodo′sa,** 1. rheumatoid a. 2. gout. **a. pau′perum,** 1. rheumatoid a. 2. poor man's gout. **proliferative a.,** rheumatoid a. **psoriatic a.,** arthritis associated with severe psoriasis, classically affecting the terminal interphalangeal joints. **rheumatoid a.,** a chronic systemic disease primarily of the joints, usually polyarticular, marked by inflammatory changes in the synovial membranes and articular structures and by atrophy and rarefaction of the bones. In late stages deformity and ankylosis develop. The cause is unknown, but autoimmune mechanisms and virus infection have been postulated. Called also *atrophic a., a. deformans, a. nodosa, a. pauperum, chronic inflammatory a., proliferative a., arthronosos deformans, arthrosis deformans,* and *rheumatic gout.* **rheumatoid a., juvenile,** rheumatoid arthritis of children, with swelling, tenderness, and pain involving one or more joints, leading to impaired growth and development, limitation of movement, and ankylosis and flexion contractures of the joints. It is frequently accompanied by systemic manifestations which may include spiking fever, transient rash on the trunk and extremities, hepatosplenomegaly, generalized lymphadenopathy, and anemia. Called also *Still's disease.* **rheumatoid a. of spine,** rheumatoid spondylitis. **a. sic′ca,** arthritis without exudation into a joint cavity. **suppurative a.,** a form marked by purulent joint infiltration, chiefly due to bacterial infection but also seen in Reiter's syndrome. **syphilitic a.,** a form associated with or due to syphilis. **tuberculous a.,** arthritis due to tuberculous infection; it usually affects a single joint and is characterized by chronic inflammation with effusion and destruction of contiguous bone. **uratic a.,** gouty a. **urethral a.,** gonococcal a. **a. urethrit′ica,** Reiter's syndrome. **venereal a.,** Reiter's syndrome. **vertebral a.,** inflammation involving the intervertebral disks, secondary to joint involvement.

arthritism (ar′thrĭ-tizm) [*arthritis* + -*ism*] the gouty diathesis; the peculiar diathesis or disposition of body that predisposes to joint disease.

arthro-, arthr- [Gr. *arthron* joint] a combining form denoting some relationship to a joint or joints.

Arthrobacter (ar″thro-bak′ter) [Gr. *arthron* a joint + *baktron* a rod] a genus of microorganisms of the family Corynebacteriaceae, order Eubacteriales, consisting of pleomorphic, gram-variable soil bacteria.

arthrobacterium (ar″thro-bak-te′re-um) [*arthro-* + *bacterium*] a bacterium that reproduces by separation into joints or arthrospores.

Arthrobotrys (ar″thro-bo′tris) a genus of imperfect fungi of the family Moniliaceae, order Moniliales, some of which infect and destroy nematodes.

arthrocace (ar-throk′ah-se) [*arthro-* + Gr. *kakōs* bad] caries of a joint.

arthrocele (ar′thro-sel) [*arthro-* + Gr. *kēlē* tumor] a swollen joint.

arthrocentesis (ar″thro-sen-te′sis) puncture and aspiration of a joint.

arthrochalasis (ar″thro-kal′ah-sis) [*arthro-* + Gr. *chalasis* relaxation] abnormal relaxation or flaccidity of a joint. **a. mul′tiplex congen′ita,** overflaccidity of multiple joints, not associated with hyperelasticity of the skin.

arthrochondritis (ar″thro-kon-dri′tis) [*arthro-* + *chrondritis*] inflammation of the cartilage of a joint.

arthroclasia (ar″thro-kla′ze-ah) [*arthro-* + Gr. *klaein* to break] the surgical breaking down of an ankylosis in order to secure free movement in a joint.

arthroclisis (ar″thro-kli′sis) arthrokleisis.

Arthroderma (ar″thro-der′mah) a genus of ascomycetous fungi (family Gymnoascaceae, order Eurotiales) in which the hyphae around the gymnothecium are dichotomously branched, with deep constrictions of the cells to give a dumbbell shape. It contains the perfect (sexual) stages of imperfect fungi of the genus *Trichophyton.*

arthrodesia (ar″thro-de′se-ah) arthrodesis.

arthrodesis (ar″thro-de′sis) [*arthro-* + Gr. *desis* binding] the surgical fixation of a joint by a procedure designed to accomplish fusion of the joint surfaces by promoting the proliferation of bone cells; called also *artificial ankylosis.* **Moberg a.,** fusion of a finger joint with a small squared bone peg.

arthrodia (ar-thro′de-ah) [Gr. *arthrōdia* a particular kind of articulation] articulatio plana [NA].

arthrodial (ar-thro′de-al) of the nature of an arthrodia.

arthrodynia (ar″thro-din′e-ah) [*arthro-* + *odynē* pain] pain in a joint.

arthrodysplasia (ar″thro-dis-pla′ze-ah) [*arthro-* + *dysplasia*] a hereditary condition marked by deformity of various joints.

arthroempyesis (ar″thro-em″pi-e′sis) [*arthro-* + Gr. *empyēsis* suppuration] suppuration within a joint.

arthroendoscopy (ar″thro-en-dos′ko-pe) arthroscopy.

arthroereisis (ar″thro-ĕ-ri′sis) [*arthro-* + Gr. *ereisis* a raising up] operative limiting of the motion in a joint that is abnormally mobile from paralysis.

arthrogenous (ar-throj′ĕ-nus) [*arthro-* + Gr. *gennan* to produce] formed as a separate joint, as arthrogenous spore.

arthrogram (ar′thro-gram) a roentgenographic record after introduction of opaque contrast material into a joint.

Arthrographis (ar-throg′rah-fis) a genus of imperfect fungi of uncertain classification, tentatively placed in the family Dermaticeae, order Moniliales. **A. langero′ni,** a species of fungi reported to produce an onychomycosis in man and a benign dermatomycosis in animals. The term is no longer considered valid.

arthrography (ar-throg′rah-fe) [*arthro-* + Gr. *graphein* to write] roentgenography of a joint after injection of opaque contrast material. **air a.,** pneumoarthrography.

arthrogryposis (ar″thro-grĭ-po′sis) [*arthro-* + Gr. *grypōsis* a crooking] 1. persistent flexure or contracture of a joint. 2. tetanoid spasm. **congenital multiple a., a. mul′tiplex congen′ita,** amyoplasia congenita.

arthrokatadysis (ar″thro-kah-tad′ĭ-sis) [*arthro-* + Gr. *katadysis* a falling down] a sinking in or subsidence of the floor of the acetabulum with protrusion of the femoral head through it (intrapelvic protrusion) resulting in limitation of movement of the hip joint; called also *Otto's disease.*

arthrokleisis (ar″thro-kli′sis) [*arthro-* + Gr. *kleisis* closure] ankylosis of a joint, or the production of such ankylosis.

arthrolith (ar′thro-lith) [*arthro-* + Gr. *lithos* stone] a calculous deposit in a joint; cf. *arthrophyte* and *joint mouse.*

arthrolithiasis (ar″thro-lĭ-thi′ah-sis) gout.

arthrology (ar-throl′o-je) [*arthro-* + -*logy*] the sum of what is known regarding the joints.

arthrolysis (ar-throl′ĭ-sis) [*arthro-* + Gr. *lysis* dissolution] the operative loosening of adhesions in an ankylosed joint.

arthromeningitis (ar″thro-men″in-ji′tis) [*arthro-* + Gr. *mēninx* membrane + -*itis*] synovitis.

arthrometer (ar-throm′ĕ-ter) [*arthro-* + Gr. *metron* measure] an instrument for measuring the angles of movements of joints.

arthrometry (ar-throm′ĕ-tre) the measurement of the range of mobility of joints.

Arthromitaceae (ar″thro-mi-ta′se-e) a family of Schizomycetes (order Caryophanales), made up of parasitic microorganisms found in the intestinal tracts of insects and crustaceans; it includes two genera, *Arthromitus* and *Coleomitus.*

Arthromitus (ar-throm′ĭ-tus) a genus of bacteria, species of which occur in the intestinal walls of insects, tadpoles, and crustaceans.

arthroncus (ar-throng′kus) [*arthro-* + Gr. *onkos* mass] swelling of a joint.

arthroneuralgia (ar″thro-nu-ral′je-ah) [*arthro-* + *neuralgia*] pain arising in or around a joint.

arthronosos (ar″thro-no′sos) [*arthro-* + Gr. *nosos* disease] a disease of the joints. **a. defor′mans,** rheumatoid arthritis.

arthro-onychodysplasia (ar″thro-on″ĕ-ko-dis-pla′ze-ah) [*arthro-* + Gr. *onyx* nail + *dysplasia*] a hereditary syndrome with involvement of the head of the radius, hypoplasia or absence of the patellae, posterior iliac spurs, and dystrophy of the nails; called also *nail-patella syndrome.*

arthro-ophthalmopathy (ar″thro-of-thal-mop′ah-the) an association of degenerative joint disease and eye disease. **hereditary progressive a.,** a hereditary disorder consisting of myopia, progressing to retinal detachment and blindness, and premature degenerative changes in the joints; it is transmitted as an autosomal dominant trait.

Arthropan (ar′thro-pan) trademark for a preparation of choline salicylate.

arthropathia (ar″thro-path′e-ah) [L.] arthropathy. **a. ovaripri′va,** menopausal arthritis. **a. psoriat′ica,** a disease of the joints seen in persons suffering from psoriasis; it resembles rheumatoid arthritis.

arthropathic (ar″thro-path′ik) pertaining to or characterized by arthropathy.

arthropathology (ar″thro-pah-thol′o-je) [*arthro-* + *pathology*] the study of the structural and functional changes produced in the joints by disease.

arthropathy (ar-throp′ah-the) [*arthro-* + Gr. *pathos* disease] any joint disease. **Charcot's a.,** neuropathic a. **chondrocalcific a.,** progressive polyarthritis with joint swelling and bony enlargement, most commonly in the small joints of the hand but also affecting other joints, characterized roentgenographically by narrowing of the joint space with subchondral erosions and sclerosis and frequently chondrocalcinosis. **inflammatory a.,** a disease of a joint of inflammatory origin. **neurogenic a.,** neuropathic a. **neuropathic a.,** chronic progressive degeneration of the stress-bearing portion of a joint, with bizarre hypertrophic changes at the periphery. It is probably a complication of a variety of neurologic disorders, particularly tabes dorsalis, involving loss of sensation, which leads to relaxation of supporting structures and chronic instability of the joint. Called also *Charcot's a.*, *neurogenic a.*, *Charcot's disease* or *joint*, and *neuropathic arthritis*. **osteopulmonary a.**, clubbing of the fingers and toes, enlargement and swelling of the ends of the long bones associated with cardiac and pulmonary disease. **psoriatic a.**, see under *arthritis*. **static a.**, a disturbance in a joint of the extremity secondary to a disturbance in some other joint of the same extremity, as one in the knee joint secondary to one in the hip joint. **syphilitic a.**, see under *arthritis*. **tabetic a.**, neuropathic arthropathy (q.v.) occurring in patients with tabes dorsalis.

arthrophyma (ar″thro-fi′mah) [*arthro-* + Gr. *phyma* swelling] the swelling of a joint.

arthrophyte (ar′thro-fīt) [*arthro-* + Gr. *phyton* plant] an abnormal growth in a joint cavity; cf. *arthrolith* and *joint mouse*.

arthroplastic (ar″thro-plas′tik) pertaining to arthroplasty.

arthroplasty (ar′thro-plas″te) [*arthro-* + Gr. *plassein* to form] plastic surgery of a joint or of joints; the formation of movable joints. **gap a.**, surgical correction of dental ankylosis by creating a space between the ankylosed part and the portion to be made moveable. **interposition a.**, surgical correction of ankylosis of the temporomandibular joint by separating the immobile fragment from the mobilized fragment and interposing a substance, such as fascia, cartilage, metal, or plastic, between them. **intracapsular temporomandibular joint a.**, operative recontouring of the articular surface of the mandibular condyle without the removal of the articular disk.

arthropneumography (ar″thro-nu-mog′rah-fe) arthropneumoroentgenography.

arthropneumoroentgenography (ar″thro-nu″mo-rent-gen-og′rah-fe) [*arthro-* + Gr. *pneuma* air + *roentgenography*] roentgenography of a joint after injection into it of air, oxygen, or carbon dioxide.

arthropod (ar′thro-pod) an animal belonging to the Arthropoda.

Arthropoda (ar-throp′o-dah) [*arthro-* + Gr. *pous* foot] a phylum of the animal kingdom composed of organisms having a hard, jointed exoskeleton and paired, jointed legs, and including, among other classes, the Arachnida and Insecta, many species of which are important medically as parasites or as vectors of organisms capable of causing disease in man.

arthropodan (ar′thro-po″dan) arthropodous.

arthropodic (ar″thro-po′dic) arthropodous.

arthropodous (ar-throp′o-dus) pertaining to or caused by arthropods.

arthropyosis (ar″thro-pi-o′sis) [*arthro-* + Gr. *pyōsis* suppuration] the formation of pus in a joint cavity.

arthrorheumatism (ar″thro-roo′mah-tizm) [*arthro-* + *rheumatism*] inflammation within a joint.

arthrorisis (ar″thro-ri′sis) arthroereisis.

arthroscintigram (ar″thro-sin′tĭ-gram) a scintiscan of a joint.

arthroscintigraphy (ar″thro-sin-tig′rah-fe) scintigraphy of a joint.

arthrosclerosis (ar″thro-skle-ro′sis) [*arthro-* + *sklērōsis* hardening] stiffening or hardening of the joints.

arthroscope (ar′thro-skōp) [*arthro-* + Gr. *skopein* to examine] an endoscope for examining the interior of a joint and for carrying out diagnostic and therapeutic procedures within the joint.

arthroscopy (ar-thros′ko-pe) examination of the interior of a joint with an arthroscope.

arthrosis (ar-thro′sis) 1. [Gr. *arthrōsis* a jointing] a joint or articulation. 2. [*arthro-* + *-osis*] a disease of a joint. **a. defor′mans**, rheumatoid arthritis.

arthrospore (ar′thro-spōr) [*arthro-* + Gr. *sporos* seed] a type of spore formed in a close sequence in the hyphae of certain fungi, and leading to hyphal fragmentation.

arthrosteitis (ar″thros-te-i′tis) [*arthro-* + Gr. *osteon* bone + *-itis*] inflammation of the bony structures of a joint.

arthrostomy (ar-thros′to-me) [*arthro-* + Gr. *stomoun* to provide with a mouth, or opening] surgical creation of an opening into a joint, as for the purpose of drainage.

arthrosynovitis (ar″thro-sin″o-vi′tis) [*arthro-* + *synovitis*] inflammation of the synovial membrane of a joint.

arthrotome (ar′thro-tōm) [*arthro-* + Gr. *tomē* cut] a knife for incising a joint.

arthrotomy (ar-throt′o-me) [*arthro-* + Gr. *tomē* cut] surgical incision of a joint.

arthrotropic (ar″thro-trop′ik) [*arthro-* + Gr. *tropos* a turning] having an affinity for or tending to settle in the joints.

arthrotyphoid (ar″thro-ti′foid) [*arthro-* + *typhoid*] typhoid fever beginning with symptoms resembling those of rheumatic fever.

arthroxerosis (ar″thro-ze-ro′sis) [*arthro-* + Gr. *xeros* dry + *-osis*] chronic osteoarthritis.

arthroxesis (ar-throk′sĕ-sis) [*arthro-* + Gr. *xesis* scraping] the scraping of an articular surface.

Arthus's reaction (phenomenon) (ar-toos′ez) [Nicolas-Maurice *Arthus*, French physiologist, 1862–1945] see under *reaction*.

article (ar′te-kl) [L. *articulus* a little joint] an interarticular segment; one of the portions or segments forming a jointed series.

articular (ar-tik′u-lar) [L. *articularis*] of or pertaining to a joint.

articulare (ar-tik″u-la′re) a cephalometric landmark, being the point of intersection of the dorsal contours of the articular process of the mandible and the temporal bone.

articulate (ar-tik′u-lāt) [L. *articulatus* jointed] 1. divided into or united by joints. 2. enunciated in words and sentences. 3. to divide into or to unite so as to form a joint. 4. in dentistry, to adjust or place the teeth in their proper relation to each other in making an artificial denture.

articulated (ar-tik′u-lāt″ed) connected by movable joints; consisting of separate segments so joined as to be movable on each other.

articulatio (ar-tik″u-la′she-o), pl. *articulatio′nes* [L.] an articulation: a place of junction between two discrete objects; used in anatomical nomenclature to designate the place of union or junction between two or more bones of the skeleton, indicated by the modifying term. Also used in the plural as a general term to indicate such joints. Called also *joint*, *junctura ossium* [NA alternative], and *osseous junction*. **a. acromioclavicula′ris** [NA], acromioclavicular articulation: the joint formed by the acromion of the scapula and the acromial extremity of the clavicle; called also *scapuloclavicular articulation* or *joint*. **a. atlantoaxia′lis latera′lis** [NA], lateral atlantoaxial articulation: one of a pair of joints, one on either side of the body, formed by the inferior articular surface of the atlas and the superior surface of the axis. **a. atlantoaxia′lis media′na** [NA], medial atlantoaxial articulation: a single joint formed by the two articular facets of the dens of the axis, one in relation with the articular facet on the anterior arch of the atlas, the other in relation with the transverse ligament of the atlas. **a. atlantoepistroph′ica**, see *a. atlantoaxialis lateralis* and *a. atlantoaxialis mediana*. **a. atlantooccipita′lis** [NA], atlanto-occipital articulation: one of two joints, each formed by a superior articular pit of the atlas and a condyle of the occipital bone; called also *craniovertebral, occipital,* or *occipitoatlantal articulation,* and *Cruveilhier's joint*. **a. bicondyla′ris**, a condylar joint with a meniscus between the articular surfaces, as in the temporomandibular joint. **a. calcaneocuboi′dea** [NA], calcaneocuboid articulation: one formed between the cuboidal articular surface of the calcaneus and the cuboid bone. **a. cap′itis cos′tae** [NA], one of the two types of articulations between ribs and vertebrae: the articulation of the head of the rib with the bodies of two vertebrae. Called also *articulation of head of rib, articulationes capitulorum costarum,* and *capitular* or *costocentral articulation*. Cf. *a. costotransversaria*. **articulatio′nes capitulo′rum costa′rum**, see *a. capitis costae*. **articulatio′nes carpometacar′peae** [NA], carpometacarpal articulations: joints formed by the trapezial, trapezoid, capitate, and hamate bones together with the bases of the four medial metacarpal bones; called also *metacarpocarpal articulations*. **a. carpometacar′pea pol′licis** [NA], the joint formed by the first metacarpal and the trapezial bones; called also *carpometacarpal articulation of thumb* and *first carpometacarpal articulation*. **a. cochlea′ris**, a form of hinge joint that permits of some lateral motion. **a. compos′ita** [NA], composite articulation: a type of synovial joint in which more than two bones are involved; called also *compound articulation* and *compound* or *composite joint*. **a. condyla′ris** [NA], condylar articulation: a modification of the ball-and-socket type of synovial joint in which, due to the arrangement of the muscles and ligaments around the joint, all movements are permitted except rotation about a vertical axis. Three types have been recognized: a. bicondylaris, a. ellipsoidea, and a. sellaris. Called also *condyloid joint*. **a. condyla′ris inver′sus**, a. sellaris. **a. costotransversa′ria** [NA], costotransverse articulation: one of the two types of articulations between ribs and vertebrae: the articulation of the tubercle of the rib with the transverse process of a vertebra. This is lacking for the eleventh and twelfth ribs. Called also *articulation of tubercle of rib*. Cf. *a. capitis costae*. **articulatio′nes costovertebra′les** [NA], costovertebral articulations: the articulations between the ribs and vertebrae, of which there are two types: a. capitis costae and a. costotransversaria. **a. cotyl′ica**, NA alternative for *a. spheroidea*. **a. cox′ae** [NA], articulation of hip: the joint formed between the head of the femur and the acetabulum of the hip bone; called also *coxofemoral articulation of Buisson, femoral articulation,* and *hip joint*; loosely called *hip*. **a. cricoarytenoi′dea** [NA], cricoarytenoid articulation: the synovial joint between the upper border of the cricoid cartilage and the base of the arytenoid cartilage. **a. cricothyroi′dea** [NA], the articulation between the lateral aspect of the cricoid cartilage and the inferior horn of the thyroid cartilage. **a. cu′biti** [NA], cubital articulation: the joint between the arm and forearm, comprising the humeroulnar, humeroradial, and proximal radioulnar articulations; called also *cubital articulation, articulation of elbow,* and *elbow joint.* **a. cuneonavicula′ris** [NA], cuneonavicular articulation: the joint between the anterior surface of the navicular bone and the proximal ends of the three cuneiform bones. **articulatio′nes digito′rum ma′nus,** articulations interphalangeae manus. **articulatio′nes digito′rum pe′dis,** articulationes interphalangeae pedis. **a. ellipsoi′dea** [NA], ellipsoidal articulation: a modification of the spheroidal form of synovial joint in which the articular surfaces are ellipsoid rather than spheroid, as in the radiocarpal joint. Called also *ellipsoidal joint* and *condylarthrosis.* **a. ge′nu, a. ge′nus** [NA], articulation of knee: the compound joint formed between the articular surface of the patella, the condyles and patellar surface of the femur, and the superior articular surface of the tibia; called also *knee joint.* **a. hu′meri** [NA], articulation of shoulder: the joint formed by the head of the humerus and the glenoid cavity of the scapula; called also *articulation of humerus,* and *shoulder joint.* **a. humeroradia′lis** [NA], humeroradial articulation: the joint between the humerus and the radius; called also *brachioradial articulation.* **a. humeroulna′ris** [NA], humeroulnar articulation: the joint between the humerus and the ulna; called also *brachioulnar articulation.* **a. incudomallea′ris** [NA], incudomalleolar articulation: the junction of the incus and the malleus. **a. incudomalleola′ris,** a. incudomallearis. **a. incudostape′dia** [NA], incudostapedial articulation: the junction of the incus and the stapes. **articulatio′nes intercar′peae** [NA], intercarpal articulations: articulations between the various carpal bones themselves; called also *intercarpal joints.* **articulatio′nes interchondra′les** [NA], the unions, on either side, between the costal cartilages of the upper false ribs, usually ribs seven through ten; called also *articulationes interchondrales costarum, intercostal articulations,* and *interchondral articulations of ribs.* **articulatio′nes interchondra′les costa′rum,** articulationes interchondrales. **articulatio′nes intermetacar′peae** [NA], intermetacarpal articulations: the joints formed between the adjoining bases of the second, third, fourth, and fifth metacarpal bones; called also *articulations of metacarpal bones.* **articulatio′nes intermetatar′seae** [NA], intermetatarsal articulations: the joints formed between the adjoining bases of the five metatarsal bones; called also *articulations of metatarsal bones.* **articulatio′nes interphalan′geae ma′nus** [NA], interphalangeal articulations of hand: the joints between the phalanges of the fingers; called also *articulationes digitorum manus, interphalangeal articulations of fingers, articulations of digits of hand,* and *articulations of fingers.* **articulatio′nes interphalan′geae pe′dis** [NA], interphalangeal articulations of foot: the joints between the phalanges of the toes; called also *articulationes digitorum pedis* and *interphalangeal articulations of toes, articulations of digits of foot,* and *articulations of toes.* **articulatio′nes intertar′seae** [NA], intertarsal articulations: the articulations between the various tarsal bones. **a. mandibula′ris,** a. temporomandibularis. **articulatio′nes ma′nus** [NA], articulations of hand: the joints of the hand. **a. mediocar′pea** [NA], metacarpal articula- tion: the joint between the two rows of carpal bones; called also *mediocarpal joint.* **articulatio′nes metacarpophalan′geae** [NA], metacarpophalangeal articulations: joints formed between the heads of the five metacarpal bones and the bases of the corresponding proximal phalanges. **articulatio′nes metatarsophalan′geae** [NA], metatarsophalangeal articulations: the joints formed between the heads of the five metatarsal bones and the bases of the corresponding proximal phalanges. **articulatio′nes ossiculo′rum audi′tus** [NA], articulations of auditory ossicles, including *a. incudomallearis* and *a. incudostapedia.* **a. os′sis pisifor′mis** [NA], articulation of pisiform bone: the joint formed by the pisiform and triquetral bones. **articulatio′nes pe′dis** [NA], articulations of foot: the joints of the foot, including those of the ankle, the tarsus, the metatarsus, and the phalanges. **a. pla′na** [NA], plane articulation: a type of synovial joint in which the opposed surfaces are flat or only slightly curved; it permits only simple gliding movement, in any direction, within narrow limits imposed by ligaments. Called also *arthrodia, gliding articulation, plane* or *gliding joint,* and *arthrodial joint.* **a. radiocar′pea** [NA], radiocarpal articulation: a condylar joint formed by the radius and the articular disk with the scaphoid, lunate, and triquetral bones; called also *brachiocarpal articulation.* **a. radioulna′ris dista′lis** [NA], distal radioulnar articulation: the joint formed by the head of the ulna and the ulnar notch of the radius; called also *inferior radioulnar* (or *cubitoradial*) *articulation.* **a. radioulna′ris proxima′lis** [NA], proximal radioulnar articulation: the proximal of the two joints between the radius and the ulna; it enters into pronation and supination of the forearm. Called also *superior radioulnar* (or *cubitoradial*) *articulation.* **a. sacroili′aca** [NA], sacroiliac articulation: the joint formed between the auricular surfaces of the sacrum and the ilium; called also *sacroiliac symphysis,* and *ileosacral articulation.* **a. sella′ris** [NA], a type of synovial joint in which the articular surface of one bone is concave in one direction and convex in the direction at right angles to the first (concavoconvex), and the articular surface of the second bone is reciprocally convexoconcave; movement is permitted along two main axes at right angles to each other.

Called also *a. condylaris inversus, saddle articulation,* and *saddle* or *sellar joint.* **a. sim′plex** [NA], simple articulation: a type of synovial joint in which only two bones are involved; called also *simple joint.* **a. sphaeroi′dea,** a. spheroidea. **a. spheroi′dea** [NA], spheroidal articulation: a type of synovial joint in which a spheroidal surface on one bone ("ball") moves within a concavity ("socket") on the other bone; it is the most moveable type of joint. Called also *a. cotylica, a. sphaeroidea, ball-and-socket articulation* or *joint, spheroidal joint, multiapial* or *polyaxial joint,* and *enarthrodial joint.* **a. sternoclavicula′ris** [NA], sternoclavicular articulation: the joint formed by the sternal extremity of the clavicle, the clavicular notch of the manubrium of the sternum, and the first costal cartilage. **articulatio′nes sternocosta′les** [NA], sternocostal articulations: the joints between the costal notches of the sternum and the medial ends of the costal cartilages of the upper seven ribs; called also *costosternal* or *chondrosternal articulations.* **a. subtala′ris** [NA], subtalar articulation: the joint formed between the posterior calcaneal articular surface of the talus and the posterior articular surface of the calcaneus; called also *a. talocalcanea.* **a. talocalca′nea,** a. subtalaris. **a. talocalcaneonavicula′ris** [NA], talocalcaneonavicular articulation: a joint formed by the head of the talus, the anterior articular surface of the calcaneus, the plantar calcaneonavicular ligament, and the posterior surface of the navicular bone. **a. talocrura′lis** [NA], talocrural articulation: the ankle joint, formed by the inferior articular and malleolar articular surfaces of the tibia, the malleolar articular surface of the fibula, and the medial malleolar, lateral malleolar, and superior surfaces of the talus; called also *talocrural ankle,* and *talotibiofibular joint.* **a. talonavicula′ris,** talonavicular articulation: the junction between the talus and navicular bone. **a. tar′si transver′sa** [NA], transverse tarsal articulation: a joint comprising the articulation of the calcaneus and the cuboid bone and the articulation of the talus and the navicular bone. Called also *a. tarsi transversa* [*Choparti*], *transverse tarsal joint,* and *Chopart's articulation* or *joint.* **articulatio′nes tarsometatar′seae** [NA], tarsometatarsal articulations: joints formed by the cuneiform and cuboid bones together with the bases of the metatarsal bones; called also *Lisfranc's joint.* **a. temporomandibula′ris** [NA], temporomandibular articulation: a bicondylar joint formed by the head of the mandible and the mandibular fossa, and the articular tubercle of the temporal bone; called also *a. mandibularis, temporomaxillary articulation,* and *mandibular articulation.* **a. tibiofibula′ris** [NA], 1. the joint formed at the proximal end of the tibia and fibula between the articular surface of the head of the fibula and the fibular articular surface of the tibia; called also *tibiofibular articulation.* 2. NA alternative for *syndesmosis tibiofibularis* when it contains a prolongation of the cavity of the talocrural articulation. **a. trochoi′dea** [NA], trochoidal articulation: a type of synovial joint that allows a rotary motion in but one plane; a pivot-like process turns within a ring, or a ring turns on a pivot. Called also *pivot articulation* or *joint.*

articulation (ar-tik″u-la′shun) [L. *articulatio*] 1. the place of union or junction between two or more bones of the skeleton; see also *articulatio, junctura,* and *joint.* 2. the enunciation of words and sentences. 3. in dentistry: (*a*) the contact relationship of the occlusal surfaces of the teeth while in action; (*b*) the arrangement of artificial teeth so as to accommodate the various positions of the mouth and to serve the purpose of the natural teeth which they are to replace. **acromioclavicular a.,** articulatio acromioclavicularis. **articulator a.,** in dentistry, the use of a mechanical device by which movements of the temporomandibular joint or mandible can be simulated, to facilitate the arrangement of teeth in complete or removable partial dentures so that they articulate properly. **atlantoaxial a., lateral,** articulatio atlantoaxialis lateralis. **atlantoaxial a., medial,** articulatio atlantoaxialis mediana. **atlantoepistrophic a.,** see *articulatio atlantoaxialis lateralis* and *articulatio atlantoaxialis mediana.* **atlantooccipital a.,** articulatio atlantooccipitalis. **a's of auditory ossicles,** articulationes ossiculorum auditus. **balanced a.,** in dentistry, a continuous change from one balanced occlusion into another for all occluded mandibular excursions. **ball-and-socket a.,** articulatio spheroidea. **brachiocarpal a.,** articulatio radiocarpea. **brachioradial a.,** articulatio humeroradialis. **brachioulnar a.,** articulatio humeroulnaris. **calcaneocuboid a.,** articulatio calcaneocuboidea. **capitular a.,** articulatio capitis costae. **carpal a's,** the junctions between the various carpal bones and between them and the bones of the forearm and hand. **carpometacarpal a's,** articulationes carpometacarpeae. **carpometacarpal a., first,** articulatio carpometacarpea pollicis. **carpometacarpal a. of thumb,** articulatio carpometacarpea pollicis. **chondrosternal a's,** articulationes sternocostales. **Chopart's a.,** articulatio tarsi transversa. **composite a.,** articulatio composita. **compound a.,** articulatio composita. **condylar a.,** articulatio condylaris. **confluent a.,** a manner of speaking in which the syllables are run together. **costocentral a.,** articulatio capitis costae. **costosternal a's,** articulationes sternocostales. **costotransverse a.,** articulatio costotransversaria. **costovertebral a's,** articulationes costovertebrales. **coxofemoral a. of Buisson,** articulatio coxae.

craniovertebral a., articulatio atlantooccipitalis. **cricoarytenoid a.,** articulatio cricoarytenoidea. **cricothyroid a.,** articulatio cricothyroidea. **cubital a.,** articulatio cubiti. **cubitoradial a., inferior,** articulatio radioulnaris distalis. **cubitoradial a., superior,** articulatio radioulnaris proximalis. **cuneonavicular a.,** articulatio cuneonavicularis. **a's of digits of foot,** articulationes interphalangeae pedis. **a's of digits of hand,** articulationes interphalangeae manus. **a. of elbow,** articulatio cubiti. **ellipsoidal a.,** articulatio ellipsoidea. **femoral a.,** articulatio coxae. **a's of fingers,** articulationes interphalangeae manus. **a's of foot,** articulationes pedis. **gliding a.,** articulatio plana. **a's of hand,** articulationes manus. **a. of head of rib,** articulatio capitis costae. **a. of hip,** articulatio coxae. **humeroradial a.,** articulatio humeroradialis. **humeroulnar a.,** articulatio humeroulnaris. **a. of humerus,** articulatio humeri. **iliosacral a.,** articulatio sacroiliaca. **incudomalleolar a.,** articulatio incudomallearis. **incudostapedial a.,** articulatio incudostapedia. **intercarpal a's,** articulationes intercarpeae. **interchondral a's of ribs,** articulationes interchondrales. **intercostal a's,** articulationes interchondrales. **intermetacarpal a's,** articulationes intermetacarpeae. **intermetatarsal a's,** articulationes intermetatarseae. **interphalangeal a's of fingers,** articulationes interphalangeae manus. **interphalangeal a's of foot,** articulationes interphalangeae pedis. **interphalangeal a's of hand,** articulationes interphalangeae manus. **interphalangeal a's of toes,** articulationes interphalangeae pedis. **intertarsal a's,** articulationes intertarseae. **a. of knee,** articulatio genus. **mandibular a.,** articulatio temporomandibularis. **maxillary a.,** articulatio temporomandibularis. **mediocarpal a.,** articulatio mediocarpea. **a's of metacarpal bones,** articulationes intermetacarpeae. **metacarpocarpal a's,** articulationes carpometacarpeae. **metacarpophalangeal a's,** articulationes metacarpophalangeae. **a's of metatarsal bones,** articulationes intermetatarseae. **metatarsophalangeal a's,** articulationes metatarsophalangeae. **occipital a.,** articulatio atlantooccipitalis. **occipitoatlantal a.,** articulatio atlantooccipitalis. **petrooccipital a.,** synchondrosis petrooccipitalis. **phalangeal a's,** see *articulationes interphalangeae manus* and *articulationes interphalangeae pedis.* **a. of pisiform bone,** articulatio ossis pisiformis. **pisocuneiform a.,** articulatio ossis pisiformis. **pivot a.,** articulatio trochoidea. **plane a.,** articulatio plana. **a. of pubis,** symphysis pubica. **radiocarpal a.,** articulatio radiocarpea. **radioulnar a., distal, radioulnar a., inferior,** articulatio radioulnaris distalis. **radioulnar a., proximal, radioulnar a., superior,** articulatio radioulnaris proximalis. **sacrococcygeal a.,** junctura sacrococcygea. **sacroiliac a.,** articulatio sacroiliaca. **saddle a.,** articulatio sellaris. **scapuloclavicular a.,** articulatio acromioclavicularis. **a. of shoulder,** articulatio humeri. **simple a.,** articulatio simplex. **spheroidal a.,** articulatio spheroidea. **sternoclavicular a.,** articulatio sternoclavicularis. **sternocostal a's,** articulationes sternocostales. **subtalar a.,** articulatio subtalaris. **talocalcaneonavicular a.,** articulatio talocalcaneonavicularis. **talocrural a.,** articulatio talocruralis. **talonavicular a.,** articulatio talonavicularis. **tarsometatarsal a's,** articulationes tarsometatarseae. **temporomandibular a.,** articulatio temporomandibularis. **temporomaxillary a.,** articulatio temporomandibularis. **tibiofibular a.,** 1. articulatio tibiofibularis. 2. syndesmosis tibiofibularis. **a's of toes,** articulationes interphalangeae pedis. **transverse tarsal a.,** articulatio tarsi transversa. **trochoidal a.,** articulatio trochoidea. **a. of tubercle of rib,** articulatio costotransversaria.

articulationes (ar-tik″u-la″she-o′nēz) [L.] plural of *articulatio.*

articulator (ar-tik′u-la″tor) a device for effecting a jointlike union; see also *dental articulator.* **adjustable a.,** 1. a dental articulator which may be adjusted to permit movement of the casts into recorded eccentric relationships. 2. a dental articulator capable of adjustment to more than one eccentric position. **dental a.,** a mechanical device by which movements of the temporomandibular joints or mandible can be simulated; used in matching upper and lower dentures and for mounting artificial teeth in order to obtain proper relations of occlusion and articulation. **hinge a., plain-line a.,** a dental articulator with only a hinge joint, permitting no lateral or gliding motion. **semiadjustable a.,** a dental articulator that may be adjusted so that at least one movement conforms with a mandibular movement of the patient.

articulatory (ar-tik′u-la″to-re) pertaining to utterance.

articulo (ar-tik′u-lo) [L.] moment; crisis. **a. mor′tis,** at the moment or point of death.

articulus (ar-tik′u-lus), pl. *articuli* [L.] a joint.

artifact (ar′tĭ-fakt) [L. *ars* art + *factum* made] any artificial product. In histology or microscopy, any structure or feature that has been introduced by processing a tissue. In radiology, a substance or structure not naturally present in living tissue, but of which an authentic image appears in a radiograph.

artifactitious (ar′tĭ-fak-tish′us) having the character of an artifact.

artificial (ar″tĭ-fish′al) [L. *ars* art + *facere* to make] made by art; not natural or pathological.

Artiodactyla (ar″te-o-dak′tĭ-lah) [Gr. *artios* even + *daktylos* finger] an order of ungulates, having an even number of toes, including ruminants, pigs, deer, and antelopes. Cf. *Perissodactyla.*

artiodactylous (ar″te-o-dak′tĭ-lus) having an even number of digits on a hand or foot; pertaining to Artiodactyla.

Artyfechinostomum (ar″te-fek″ĭ-nos′to-mum) *Paryphostomum.* **A. sufrar′tyfex,** *Paryphostomum sufrartyfex.*

arucase (ah′ru-kās) an extract of *Calea pinnatifida* (R. Br.) Less. (aruca plant) of the family Compositae; it has been used in the management of intestinal amebiasis.

Arum (a′rum) a genus of plants. *A. dracontium* is highly poisonous; *A. maculatum* furnishes sago.

Arvin (ar′vin) a purified fraction of the venom of the Malayan pit viper, used as an anticoagulant in thromboembolic disorders.

aryepiglottic (ar″e-ep″ĭ-glot′ik) arytenoepiglottic.

aryepiglotticus (ar″e-ep″ĭ-glot′ĭ-kus) see *Table of Musculi.*

aryepiglottidean (ar″e-ep″ĭ-glo-tid′e-an) arytenoepiglottic.

aryl- (ar′il) a chemical prefix indicating a radical belonging to the aromatic series.

arylamine (ar″il-ah-mēn′, ar″il-am′in) any of a group of amines in which one or more of the hydrogen atoms are replaced by aromatic groups.

arytenoepiglottic (ar-it″ĕ-no-ep″ĭ-glot′ik) [Gr. *arytaina* ladle + *epiglottis*] pertaining to the arytenoid cartilage and to the epiglottis.

arytenoid (ar″ĕ-te′noid) [Gr. *arytaina* ladle + *eidos* form] shaped like a jug or pitcher, as arytenoid cartilage.

arytenoidectomy (ar″ĕ-te″noid-ek′to-me) [*arytenoid* + Gr. *ektomē* excision] surgical removal of an arytenoid cartilage.

arytenoideus (ar″ĕ-te-noi′de-us) [L.] see *musculus arytenoideus obliquus* and *transversus.*

arytenoiditis (ar-it″ĕ-noi-di′tis) inflammation of the arytenoid cartilage or muscles.

arytenoidopexy (ar″ĭ-tĕ-noi′do-pek″se) [*arytenoid* + Gr. *pēxis* fixation] surgical fixation of arytenoid cartilage or muscle; called also *Kelly's operation.*

Arzberger's pear (arz′ber-gerz) [Friedrich *Arzberger,* Austrian physicist, 1833–1905] a pear-shaped vessel or container for insertion into the rectum, which may be cooled by passing water through the instrument.

As chemical symbol for *arsenic.*

As. astigmatism.

AS aortic stenosis; arteriosclerosis.

A.S. abbreviation for L. *au′ris sinis′tra,* left ear.

ASA argininosuccinic acid.

A.S.A. 1. American Society of Anesthesiologists; American Standards Association; American Stomatological Association; American Surgical Association. 2. trademark for a preparation of aspirin.

asacria (ah-sa′kre-ah) congenital absence of the sacrum.

asafetida (as″ah-fet′ĭ-dah) the oleo-gum-resin obtained from the roots of *Ferula asafoetida* L. and other related species of Umbelliferae. The main odorous principle is isobutylpropanyldisulfide. Used in India, Iran, etc., as a condiment and food flavoring, and has been used as an animal repellent in veterinary medicine to prevent bandage chewing, and as a carminative, expectorant, and antispasmodic both in humans and animals.

A.S.A.I.O. American Society for Artificial Internal Organs.

asaphia (ah-sa′fe-ah) [Gr. *asapheia*] indistinctness of utterance.

asaron (as′ah-ron) see *Asarum.*

Asarum (as′ah-rum) [Gr. *asaron*] a genus of the family Aristolochiaceae. *A. europaeum* L. yields a camphor-like aromatic principle known as asaron. *A. canadense* L. (Indian ginger, Canadian snakeroot, wild ginger) yields from its dried roots and rhizomes an acrid resin, methyl eugenol, and an aromatic volatile oil. Both species have been used as aromatics.

A.S.B. American Society of Bacteriologists.

asbestiform (as-bes′tĭ-form) having a fibrous structure like asbestos.

asbestos (as-bes′tos) [Gr. *asbestos* unquenchable] a fibrous, incombustible, magnesium and calcium silicate, used as thermal insulation; its dust causes asbestosis.

asbestosis (as″bĕ-sto′sis) [*asbestos* + *-osis*] a form of lung disease (pneumoconiosis) caused by inhaling fibers of asbestos and marked by interstitial fibrosis of the lung varying in extent from minor involvement of the basal areas to extensive scarring; it is associated with pleural mesothelioma and bronchogenic carcinoma. Called also *amianthosis.*

A-scan see *scan,* def. 2.

ascariasis (as″kah-ri′ah-sis) [*ascaris* + *-iasis*] infection by the roundworm *Ascaris lumbricoides,* which is found in the small intestine, causing colicky pains and diarrhea, especially in children. On ingestion, the larvae migrate from the intestine to the lungs, where they cause a pneumonitis, and then to the trachea, esophagus, and intestine, where they mature. If adult worms are present in sufficient number they may cause intestinal obstruction. **sarcoptic a.,** scabies.

ascaricidal (as-kar″ĭ-si′dal) destructive to intestinal parasites of the genus *Ascaris*.

ascaricide (as-kar′ĭ-sid) [Gr. *askaris* ascaris + L. *caedere* to kill] an agent that destroys worms of the genus *Ascaris*.

ascarid (as′kah-rid) any member of the superfamily Ascaridoidea.

ascarides (as-kar′ĭ-dēz) plural of *ascaris*.

Ascaridia (as″kah-rid′e-ah) a genus of nematode parasites of the superfamily Ascaridoidea. **A. gal′li,** a species parasitic in the large intestine of chickens. **A. linea′ta,** a nematode parasite in the small intestine of fowls, the common roundworm of chickens in the United States.

ascaridiasis (as″kar-ĭ-di′ah-sis) ascariasis.

Ascaridoidea (as″kah-rĭ-doi′de-ah) a superfamily of phasmid nematodes, including the genera *Ascaridia, Ascaris, Toxocara,* and *Toxascaris.*

ascaridole (ah-skar′ĭ-dōl″) chemical name: 1,4-peroxido-*p*-menthene-2. The major constituent of oil of chenopodium or American wormseed (*Chenopodium ambrosioides* L., Chenopodiaceae). The oil was once used as an anthelmintic.

ascaridosis (as-kar-ĭ-do′sis) ascariasis.

ascariosis (as-kar-e-o′sis) ascariasis.

Ascaris (as′kah-ris) [L.; Gr. *askaris*] a genus of large intestinal nematode parasites of the superfamily Ascaridoidea. **A. ala′ta, A. ca′nis,** see *Toxocara canis.* **A. e′qui, A. equo′rum,** *Parascaris equorum.* **A. lumbricoi′des,** the eelworm or roundworm, a common worm resembling the earthworm; it is found in the small intestine, causing colicky pains and diarrhea, especially in children (see *ascariasis*). **A. margina′ta,** see

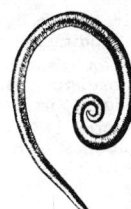

Ascaris lumbricoides (after Brumpt).

Toxocara canis. **A. megaloceph′ala,** *A. equorum.* **A. mys′tax,** *Toxocara cati.* **A. o′vis,** a name given to immature specimens of *A. lumbricoides,* occasionally found in sheep and cattle. **A. su′is, A. suil′la, A. su′um,** a name given to *A. lumbricoides* found in swine. **A. vermicula′ris,** see *Enterobius vermicularis.* **A. vitulo′rum,** a species found in cattle and the Indian buffalo.

ascaris (as-kah-ris), pl. *ascar′ides.* a worm of the genus *Ascaris.*

Ascarops (as′kah-rops) a genus of parasitic nematodes; formerly called *Arduenna.* **A. strongyli′na,** a small red blood-sucking species found in the stomach of pigs.

ascending (ah-send′ing) having an upward course.

ascensus (ah-sen′sus) [L.] a going up; ascent. **a. u′teri,** an abnormally high position of the uterus.

ascertainment (ah″ser-tān″ment) in genetic studies, the method by which persons with a trait or disease are selected or found by an investigator. **complete a.,** the method in which every sibship in the population that has at least one affected member is enumerated. **single a.,** the method in which only a sample of the affected sibships is included in the series. **truncate a.,** ascertainment in which only sibships that include at least one affected child are enumerated.

A.S.C.H. American Society of Clinical Hypnosis.

Asch's operation, splint [Morris Joseph *Asch,* American laryngologist, 1833–1902] see under *operation* and *splint.*

aschelminth (ask′hel-minth) any worm of the phylum Aschelminthes.

Aschelminthes (ask″hel-minth′ēz) a phylum of unsegmented, bilaterally symmetrical, pseudocoelomate, mostly vermiform animals whose bodies are almost entirely covered with a cuticle, and possess a complete digestive tract lacking definite muscular walls. It includes the classes Gastrotricha, Kinorhyncha, Nematoda, Nematomorpha, and Rotifera.

Ascher's glass-rod phenomenon, syndrome [Karl Wolfgang *Ascher,* Cincinnati ophthalmologist, born in Prague, 1887] see *aqueous-influx phenomenon,* under *phenomenon,* and under *syndrome.*

Ascherson's membrane, vesicles (ash′er-sunz) [Ferdinand Moritz *Ascherson,* German physician, 1798–1879] see under *membrane* and *vesicle.*

Aschheim-Zondek hormone, test (ash′him-tson′dek) [Selmar *Aschheim,* German gynecologist, 1878–1965; Bernhardt *Zondek,*

German gynecologist, born 1891] see *luteinizing hormone,* under *hormone,* and see under *test.*

aschistodactylia (ah-skis″to-dak-til′e-ah) [*a* neg. + Gr. *schistos* cleft + *daktylos* finger + *-ia*] syndactyly.

Aschner's phenomenon (test), reflex, sign (ash′nerz) [Bernhard *Aschner,* Austrian gynecologist, 1883–1960] see under *phenomenon,* and see *oculocardiac reflex,* under *reflex.*

Aschoff's bodies (nodules), cell, node (ash′ofs) [Karl Albert Ludwig *Aschoff,* German pathologist, 1866–1942] see under *body* and *cell,* and see *nodus atrioventricularis.*

Aschoff-Tawara node [Karl Albert Ludwig *Aschoff ;* Sunao *Tawara,* Japanese pathologist, born 1873] nodus atrioventricularis.

A.S.C.I. American Society for Clinical Investigation.

asci (as′i) plural of *ascus.*

ascia (as′e-ah) [L. "ax," from the shape of its folds] a form of spiral bandage.

ascites (ah-si′tēz) [L.; Gr. *askitēs,* from *askos* bag] effusion and accumulation of serous fluid in the abdominal cavity; called also *abdominal* or *peritoneal dropsy, hydroperitonia,* and *hydrops abdominis.* **a. adipo′sus,** a variety characterized by a milky appearance of the contained fluid, due to the presence of cells that have undergone fatty degeneration; called also *fatty* or *milky a.* **bile a.,** choleperitoneum. **bloody a.,** hemorrhagic a. **chyliform a., a. chylo′sus, chylous a.,** the presence of chyle in the peritoneal cavity as a result of anomalies, injuries, or obstruction of the thoracic duct. **exudative a.,** ascites in which the fluid in the peritoneal cavity is an exudate. **fatty a.,** a. adiposus. **hemorrhagic a.,** that in which the fluid is mixed with blood. **hydremic a.,** that which is associated with, or due to, a watery state of the blood, as in severe malnutrition. **milky a.,** a. adiposus. **a. prae′cox,** ascites that develops prior to edema in constrictive pericarditis. **preagonal a.,** a flow of serum into the peritoneal cavity just before death. **pseudochylous a.,** ascites in which the contained fluid resembles chyle in appearance, but does not contain fatty matter. **transudative a.,** ascites in which the fluid in the peritoneal cavity is a transudate.

ascitic (ah-sit′ik) pertaining to or characterized by ascites.

ascitogenous (as″ĭ-toj′ĕ-nus) causing ascites.

asclepia (as-kle′pe-ah) plural of *asclepion.*

Asclepiad (as-kle′pe-ad) [Gr. *Asklēpiadēs*] a member of an organized guild of physicians, followers of Æsculapius, who were the priests in the early Greek temples of healing (see *asclepion*). The name is also applied to any devoted, high-minded physician.

Asclepiades (as″kle-pi′ah-dēz) born in Bithynia (Asia Minor), in 124 B.C., this celebrated physician studied in Alexandria, and later popularized Greek medicine in Rome. Opposed to Hippocratic humoralism, he taught that disease resulted from a mechanical disturbance of the passage of atoms through the pores of the body. His followers, the Methodists, further simplified this concept.

Asclepias (as-kle′pe-as) [L.] the milkweeds or swallow-worts, a genus of herbs most species of which are generally recognized as poisonous to animals, while some have medicinal qualities; e.g., *A. tuberosa* L. (pleurisy root) has been used as an emetic, diaphoretic, laxative, and expectorant. They contain asclepiadin, volatile oils, and toxic resins.

asclepion (as-kle′pe-on), pl. *asclepia* [Gr. *Asklēpieion* temple of Asklepios (Æsculapius)] one of the early Greek temples of healing, the most celebrated of which were at Cos, Epidaurus, Cnidus, and Pergamos. Greek temple medicine flourished during the time of Hippocrates (late 5th century B.C.), but was quite independent of his school. See also *Æsculapius* and *Asclepiad.*

Asclepios (as-klep′e-os) Æsculapius.

A.S.C.L.T. American Society of Clinical Laboratory Technicians.

Ascobolus (as-kob′ŏ-lus) a genus of ascomycetous fungi (family Pezizaceae, order Pezizales) used in genetic studies of crossing over.

ascocarp (as′ko-karp) [Gr. *askos* bag + *karpos* fruit] the developed sporophore (fruiting body) in ascomycetous fungi, including the asci and ascospores. Cf. *archicarp.*

Ascocotyle (as″ko-ko′tĭ-le) a genus of nematode parasites. **A. pithecophagic′ola,** a nematode parasite in the monkey-eating eagle in the Philippines.

ascogonium (as″ko-go′ne-um) the receiving (female) organ in ascomycetous fungi which, after fertilization, gives rise to ascogenous hyphae and later to asci and ascospores. Called also *carpogonium* and, in British usage, *archicarp.*

Ascoli's reaction, test (as-ko′lēz) [Maurizio *Ascoli,* Italian pathologist, 1876–1958] miostagmin reaction.

Ascoli's test, treatment (as-ko′lēz) [Alberto *Ascoli,* Italian serologist, 1877–1957] see under *test* (def. 1) and under *treatment.*

Ascomycetae (as″ko-mi-sē′te) Ascomycetes.

ascomycete (as-ko′mi-sēt) any individual fungus of the Ascomycetes.

Ascomycetes (as″ko-mi-se′tēz) [Gr. *askos* bag + *mykēs* fungus] a class of perfect fungi of the division Eumycetes, the individual members of which form ascospores. The class consists of the yeasts, mildews, and cheese, jelly, and fruit molds, and includes the subclasses Hemiascomycetidae, Euascomycetidae, and Loculoascomycetidae. Called also *Ascomycetae* and *sac fungus.*

ascomycetous (as″ko-mi-se′tus) of or pertaining to the Ascomycetes.

ascorbate (as-kor′bāt) a compound or derivative of ascorbic acid.

ascorbemia (as″kor-be′me-ah) the presence of ascorbic acid in the blood.

ascorburia (as-kor-bu′re-ah) the presence of ascorbic acid in the urine.

ascorbyl palmitate (as-kor′bil) [NF] chemical name: 6-hexadecanoate L-ascorbic acid. An antioxidant, $C_{22}H_{38}O_7$, occurring as a white to yellowish white powder; used as a preservative in pharmaceutical preparations.

ascospore (as′ko-spōr) [Gr. *askos* bag + *sporos* seed] a sexual spore formed within a special sac, or ascus, as in ascomycetous fungi. See *spore.*

A.S.C.P. American Society of Clinical Pathologists.

ascus (as′kus), pl. *as′ci* [Gr. *askos* a bag] the sporangium or spore case of certain lichens and fungi, consisting of a single terminal cell. See *spore.*

-ase (ās) a word termination used in forming the names of enzymes, ordinarily affixed to a stem that indicates the general nature of the substrate, the actual name of the substrate, the type of reaction catalyzed, or a combination of these factors.

asecretory (ah-se′kre-to″re) without secretion.

Aselli's pancreas (glands) (ah-sel′ēz) [Gasparo *Aselli* (or Gaspare Asellio, or Gaspar Asellius), Italian anatomist, 1581–1626] see under *pancreas.*

Asellio, Asellius see *Aselli.*

asemantic (a-sĕ-man′tik) [*a* neg. + Gr. *sēmantikos* significant] being or pertaining to a molecule that is not produced by an organism and so is not influenced by the presence in the organism of semantides (q.v.).

asemasia (as″ĕ-ma′ze-ah) [*a* neg. + Gr. *sēmasia* the giving of a signal] aphasia in which there is lack or loss of the power of communication by words or by signals.

asemia (ah-se′me-ah) [*a* neg. + Gr. *sēma* sign + *-ia*] aphasia with inability to employ or to understand either speech or signs, due to a central lesion. **a. graph′ica,** inability either to write (agraphia) or to understand (dyslexia) writing, due to a central lesion. **a. mim′ica,** inability to understand or to perform any action expressive of thought or emotion. **a. verba′lis,** inability to make use of or to understand words.

asepsis (a-sep′sis) [*a* neg. + Gr. *sēpesthai* to decay] 1. freedom from infection. 2. the prevention of contact with microorganisms. **integral a.,** an aseptic technique in which not only the instruments, the drapes, and the gloved hands of the surgical team are sterile, but also the entire operating room and the air are free of viable microorganisms.

aseptic (a-sep′tik) [*a* neg. + Gr. *sēpsis* decay] free from infection or septic material; sterile. **a.-antiseptic,** both aseptic and antiseptic.

asepticism (a-sep′tĭ-sizm) the principles and practices of aseptic surgery.

asetake (as″e-tak′e) a poisonous Japanese fungus of the genus *Hebeloma.*

asexual (a-seks′u-al) having no sex; not sexual; not pertaining to sex. Called also *agamic* or *agamous.*

asexuality (a″seks-u-al′ĭ-te) the state of being asexual; absence of sexual interests.

asexualization (a-seks″u-al-ĭ-za′shun) sterilization of an individual, as by castration or vasectomy.

ASF a synthetic resin composed of aniline, formaldehyde, and sulfur, used for mounting microscopic objects.

A.S.G. American Society for Genetics.

A.S.H. American Society for Hematology.

As. H. hypermetropic astigmatism.

ash (ash) 1. the incombustible residue remaining after any process of incineration. 2. any tree or species of the genus *Fraxinus.* *F. ornus* and others afford mannitol. The bark of many species is astringent and antiperiodic.

A.S.H.A. American School Health Association; American Speech and Hearing Association.

Ashby's agar (culture medium) (ash′bēz) [Sir Eric *Ashby,* English botanist, born 1904] see under *culture medium.*

Ashhurst's splint (ash′hursts) [John *Ashhurst,* Philadelphia surgeon, 1839–1900] see under *splint.*

A.S.H.I. Association for the Study of Human Infertility.

A.S.H.P. American Society of Hospital Pharmacists.

asialia (ah″si-a′le-ah) [*a* neg. + Gr. *scialon* spittle] absence or deficiency of the secretion of the saliva; aptyalism; xerostomia.

asialo (a-si′ah-lo) [*a* neg. + *sialo*] lacking a sialic acid group, as do certain sphingolipids.

asiaticoside (a″zhe-at′ĭ-ko-sīd″) a steroidal glycoside of a trisaccharide and asiatic acid, which is the active principle of the umbelliferous plant *Centella asiatica* L. The compound has been used for various dermatological conditions, including wounds and burns.

asiderosis (ah″sid-er-o′sis) [*a* neg. + Gr. *sidēros* iron] abnormal decrease of the iron reserve of the body.

A.S.I.I. American Science Information Institute.

A.S.I.M. American Society of Internal Medicine.

Asimina (ah-sim′ĭ-nah) [L., from its Algonkian name] a genus of North American trees and shrubs of the family Annonaceae. *A. triloba* (L.) Dunal is the papaw or pawpaw; see *papaw,* def. 2. *A. reticulata* is used to make Seminole tea, used by Seminole Indians in Florida for kidney problems.

asiminine (ah-sim′ĭ-nin) an alkaloid from the seeds of *Asimina triloba.*

-asis a word termination denoting state or condition; see *-sis.*

asitia (ah-sish′e-ah) [*a* neg. + Gr. *sitos* food] a loathing for food.

asjike (ahs-ji′ke) beriberi.

Asklepios (as-klep′e-os) [Gr. *Asklēpios* son of Apollo and Coronis, tutelary god of medicine] see *Æsculapius.*

ASL antistreptolysin.

Aslanvitol (as-lan-vi′tol) [named for Anna *Asland,* Romanian physiologist, who discovered it] a drug containing procaine hydrochloride, purported to increase longevity by restoring chemical balances in the brain so that its regulatory functions, such as those governing glandular activities, are made more effective.

As.M. myopic astigmatism.

Asn asparagine.

As₂O₃ arsenic trioxide.

ASO arteriosclerosis obliterans.

asoma (a-so′mah), pl. *aso′mata* [*a* neg. + Gr. *sōma* body] a monster with an imperfect head and the merest rudiments of a trunk.

asomatophyte (a-so′mah-to-fīt″) [*a* neg. + Gr. *sōma* body + *phyton* plant] a plant in which there is no distinction between body and reproductive cells; bacteria belong to this class.

Asopia (a-so′pe-ah) a genus of pyralid moths. *A. farinalis,* the meal moth, or worm, acts as the intermediate host of *Hymenolepis diminuta.*

A.S.P. American Society of Parasitologists.

Asp aspartic acid.

aspalasoma (as″pal-ah-so′mah) [Gr. *aspalax* the mole + *sōma* body] a monster with lateral or median abdominal eventration and other deformities.

asparaginase (as-par′ah-jin-ās″) chemical name: L-asparaginase. An enzyme that catalyzes the hydrolysis of asparagine to aspartic acid and ammonia. Asparaginase has antineoplastic activity, and a preparation derived from *Escherichia coli, Erwinia* species, or obtained from other sources has been used in the treatment of acute lymphocytic leukemia. Called also *colaspase.*

asparagine (as-par′ah-jēn, as-par′ah-jin) [Gr. *asparagos* asparagus] chemical name: α-aminosuccinic acid. A nonessential amino acid, $C_4H_8N_2O_3$, which is the β-amide of aspartic acid. It is found in most plants, and has diuretic properties. It is used as a culture medium for certain bacteria.

Asparagus (ah-spar′ah-gus) [L.; Gr. *asparagos*] a genus of liliaceous plants; the root of *A. officinalis* is a mild diuretic. It is claimed by some that methylmercaptan is excreted in urine after ingestion of the vegetable. Others feel that the odoriferous material is asparagine-aminosuccinic acid monoamide.

aspartame (ah-spar′tām) chemical name: N-L-α-aspartyl-L-phenylalanine methyl ester. An artificial sweetener, $C_{14}H_{18}N_2O_5$, which is about 200 times as sweet as sucrose and has potential as a low-calorie sweetener.

aspartase (as′par-tās) an enzyme that splits aspartic acid into fumaric acid and ammonia.

aspartate (ah-spahr′tāt) a salt of aspartic acid, or aspartic acid in dissociated form.

asparthione (as-par′thi-ōn″) a tripeptide analogous to glutathione but containing aspartic acid in place of glutamic acid.

aspartoacylase (ah-spahr″to-as′ĭ-lās) N-acylaspartate amidohyrolase: an enzyme occurring in the kidney that catalyzes the hydrolysis of N-acylaspartate to aspartate and a fatty acid ion; called also *aminoacylase II.*

aspartocin (ah-spar′to-sin) an antibacterial substance produced by *Streptomyces griseus.*

aspartokinase (ah-spar″to-ki′nās) aspartate kinase.

aspecific (ah″spĕ-sif′ik) nonspecific; not caused by a specific organism.

aspect (as′pekt) [L. *aspectus,* from *aspicere* to look toward] 1. that part of a surface facing in any designated direction. 2. the look or appearance. **dorsal a.,** the surface of a body as viewed from the back (human anatomy) or from above (veterinary anatomy). **ventral a.,** the surface of a body as viewed from the front (human anatomy) or from below (veterinary anatomy).

aspergillar (as″per-jil′ar) pertaining to or caused by *Aspergillus*.

aspergilli (as″per-jil′i) plural of *aspergillus*.

aspergillin (as″per-jil′in) a black antibiotic substance, from the spore of various species of *Aspergillus;* formerly called *vegetable hematin*.

aspergilloma (as″per-jil-o′mah) a tumor-like granulomatous mass formed by colonization of the fungus *Aspergillus* in a bronchus or pulmonary cavity; the organism may disseminate through the blood stream to the brain, heart, and kidneys. Called also *fungus ball*.

aspergillomycosis (as″per-jil″o-mi-ko′sis) aspergillosis.

aspergillosis (as″per-jil-o′sis) a diseased condition caused by species of *Aspergillus* and marked by inflammatory granulomatous lesions in the skin, ear, orbit, nasal sinuses, lungs, and sometimes in the bones and meninges; called also *aspergillomycosis*. **aural a.,** see *otomycosis*. **bronchopneumonic a.,** infection of the bronchi and lungs by *Aspergillus;* see *aspergilloma*. **pulmonary a.,** infection of the lungs with *Aspergillus*.

aspergillotoxicosis (as″per-jil″o-tok″sĭ-ko′sis) aspergillustoxicosis.

Aspergillus (as″per-jil′us) [L. *aspergere* to scatter] a genus of imperfect fungi of the family Moniliaceae. When found, the perfect, or sexual, stage is classified with the ascomycetous fungi in the family Eurotiaceae, order Eurotiales. It includes several of the common molds and some that are opportunistic pathogens. It is characterized by elongated conidiophores thickly set with chains of basipetally formed conidia. See Plate under *mold*. **A.**

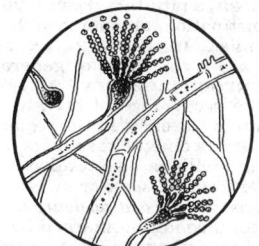

Aspergillus (de Rivas).

auricula′ris, a mold of uncertain classification, found in the cerumen of the ear. **A. bar′bae,** a species of uncertain classification that has been found in mycosis of the beard. **A. clava′tus,** a species occurring in soils and manure; its cultures produce the antibacterial substance patulin. **A. concen′tricus,** a species formerly considered to be the cause of tinea imbricata, now known to be caused by *Trichophyton concentricum*. **A. cook′ei,** *A. mucoroides*. **A. fisher′ii,** a thermophilic soil fungus. **A. fla′vus,** a mold found on corn, peanuts, and grain; it produces aflatoxin (q.v.). **A. fumiga′tus,** a thermotolerant fungus growing in soils and manure. It has been found in infections of the ear, nose, lungs, and other organs of humans and animals, and is considered to be a primary pathogen of birds. Its cultures produce various antibiotics, such as fumagillin and helvolic acid. Formerly called *A. gliocladium* and *Eurotium malignum*. **A. gigan′teus,** a species from which gigantic acid is obtained. **A. glau′cus,** a group of species of bluish molds common on dry and decaying vegetation and rarely occurring in otomycosis or other human infectious processes. **A. gliocla′dium,** former name for the species that furnishes the antibiotic gliotoxin; now called *A. fumigatus*. **A. mucoroi′des,** a species of uncertain classification, probably of the *A. glaucus* group, reported in lung tissue; called also *A. cookei*. **A. nid′ulans,** a species common in soil and occasionally isolated from onychomycosis and rarely from maduromycosis and other disease processes. **A. ni′ger,** a species common in soil and often isolated from otomycosis; it may produce a severe and very persistent infection. **A. ochra′ceus,** the species that ferments the coffee berry and produces the characteristic and desirable odor. **A. parasit′icus,** a mold found on ground nut seedlings that elaborates aflatoxin (q.v.). **A. pic′tor,** a formerly recognized species, probably identical with *A. versicolor*, once thought to cause pinta, a treponeme disease. **A. re′pens,** a species found in the external auditory canal, where it may produce a false membrane. Its perfect stage is *Eurotium repens*. **A. ter′reus,** a species occasionally associated with infection of the bronchi and lungs; see *aspergilloma*. **A. versic′olor,** a species of common soil saprophytes often isolated from dried salted beef; see also *A. pictor*.

aspergillus (as″per-jil′us), pl. *aspergil′li*. An individual of the genus *Aspergillus*.

aspergillustoxicosis (as″per-jil″us-tok″sĭ-ko′sis) a form of mycotoxicosis caused by a member of the genus *Aspergillus*.

asperkinase (ah-sper-ki′nās) a proteolytic enzyme elaborated by *Aspergillus oryzae*.

aspermatism (ah-sper′mah-tizm) aspermia.

aspermatogenesis (ah-sper″mah-to-jen′ĕ-sis) absence of development of spermatozoa.

aspermia (ah-sper′me-ah) [*a* neg. + Gr. *sperma* seed + *-ia*] failure of formation or emission of semen.

asphalgesia (as″fal-je′ze-ah) [Gr. *asphe-* self + *algos* pain] a sensation of burning felt on touching certain articles, occurring during hypnosis.

asphyctic (as-fik′tik) pertaining to, or affected with, asphyxia.

asphyctous (as-fik′tus) asphyctic.

asphygmia (as-fig′me-ah) temporary disappearance of the pulse.

asphyxia (as-fik′se-ah) [Gr. "a stopping of the pulse"] a condition due to lack of oxygen in respired air, resulting in impending or actual cessation of apparent life. **blue a.,** a. livida. **a. carbon′ica,** suffocation from the inhalation of coal gas, water gas, or carbon monoxide. **a. cyanot′ica,** a. livida. **fetal a.,** asphyxia in utero due to anoxia caused by premature placental separation (abruptio placentae), injudicious use of anesthetics, etc. **a. liv′ida,** asphyxia in which the skin is cyanotic from the lack of oxygen in the blood; called also *blue a.* and *a. cyanotica*. **local a.,** Raynaud's disease (def. 2); see under *disease*. **a. neonato′rum,** respiratory failure in the newborn; see also *respiratory distress syndrome*, under *syndrome*. **a. pal′lida,** asphyxia attended with paleness of the skin; called also *white a.* **a. reticula′ris,** livedo reticularis. **secondary a.,** asphyxia recurring after apparent recovery from suffocation. **traumatic a.,** asphyxia occurring as a result of sudden or severe compression of the thorax or upper abdomen, or both; called also *traumatic apnea*. **white a.,** a. pallida.

asphyxial (as-fik′se-al) characterized by or pertaining to asphyxia.

asphyxiant (as-fik′se-ant) a substance capable of producing asphyxia.

asphyxiate (as-fik′se-āt) to put into a state of asphyxia.

asphyxiation (as-fik″se-a′shun) suffocation.

Aspidium (as-pid′e-um) [L.; Gr. *aspidion* little shield] a group of ferns called male shield ferns and male ferns which yield an oleoresin (see under *oleoresin*).

aspidium (as-pid′e-um) the rhizome and stipes of filix mas (male fern), yielding not less than 1.5 per cent of crude filicin. It is a violent poison and is highly irritant to the gastrointestinal tract when taken internally. See also *aspidium oleoresin*, under *oleoresin*.

aspidosperma (as″pĭ-do-sper′mah) the dried bark of *Aspidosperma quebracho-blanco* Schlecht., a tree of the family Apocynaceae. It contains several alkaloids, the main one being aspidospermine. It has been used to control parasitic worms in soil. Medically, it has been used in asthma and dyspnea as a respiratory stimulant.

aspidospermine (as″pĭ-do-sper′mēn) an alkaloid, $C_{22}H_{30}N_2O_2$, from aspidosperma (q.v.).

aspirate (as′pĭ-rāt) 1. to treat by aspiration. 2. the substance or material obtained by aspiration. 3. a consonantal sound in which some part of the respiratory tract is constricted, the nasal cavity shut off, and the breath makes a whistling noise.

aspiration (as″pĭ-ra′shun) [L. *ad* to + *spirare* to breathe] 1. the act of inhaling. 2. the removal of fluids or gases from a cavity by the application of suction. **meconium a.,** aspiration of meconium by the fetus or newborn, which may result in atelectasis, emphysema, or pneumonia. **vacuum a.,** removal of the uterine contents by application of a vacuum through a hollow curet or a cannula introduced into the uterus. Called also *vacuum extraction*.

aspirator (as″pĭ-ra′tor) an apparatus used for removal by suction of fluids or gases contained within a cavity. **Dieulafoy's a.,** an apparatus that consists of a glass cylinder containing a piston and having two openings, one for a trocar and cannula, the other for a discharge tube.

aspirin (as′pĭ-rin) chemical name: 2-(acetyloxy) benzoic acid. A compound, $C_9H_8O_4$, occurring as white crystals that are commonly tabular or needle-like, or as a white, crystalline powder; used as an analgesic, antipyretic, and antirheumatic. Called also *acetylsalicylic acid*. **aluminum a.,** chemical name: hydroxybis-(salicylato)aluminum diacetate. A combination of aspirin and aluminum oxide used as an analgesic and antipyretic.

asplenia (a-sple′ne-ah) absence of the spleen. **functional a.,** impaired reticuloendothelial function of the spleen, as in children with sickle-cell anemia.

asplenic (a-splen′ik) pertaining to asplenia; caused by absence of the spleen.

asporogenic (as″po-ro-jen′ik) [*a* neg. + *sporogenic*] not producing spores; not reproduced by spores.

asporogenous (as″po-roj′ĕ-nus) asporogenic.

asporous (ah-spo′rus) [*a* neg. + Gr. *sporos* seed] having no true spores; applied to microorganisms.

A.S.R.T. American Society of Radiologic Technologists.

A.S.S. anterior superior spine.

assanation (as"ah-na′shun) [L. *ad* to + *sanus* sound]   sanitation; the improvement of sanitary conditions.

assay (as-sa′)   determination of the amount of a particular constituent of a mixture, or of the biological or pharmacological potency of a drug.   **biological a.,** bioassay.   **four-point a.,** an assay based on a mixture of two doses of test material and two doses of standard material.   **immune a.,** immunoassay.   **microbiological a.,** assay by the use of microorganisms.   **stem cell a.,** a test for determining the effectiveness of particular drugs against human cancer, in which human tumor cell suspensions are first incubated with various drugs and then suspended in agar and plated over a layer of agar at the bottom of the plate. Effectiveness of the drugs is determined by counting the number of colonies that grow in comparison with the number of colonies on control plates.

Assézat's triangle (ah-se-zahz′) [Jules *Assézat,* French anthropologist, 1832–1876]   facial triangle.

assident (as′ĭ-dent)   generally but not always accompanying a disease.

assimilable (ah-sim′ĭ-lah-bl)   susceptible of being assimilated.

assimilation (ah-sim″ĭ-la′shun) [L. *assimilatio,* from *ad* to + *similare* to make like]   1. the transformation of food into living tissue; anabolism.   2. in psychology, the absorption of new experiences into the existing psychological make-up.

assistant (ah-sis′tant)   one who aids or helps another; an auxiliary.   **physician a.,** see under *physician.*

Assmann's focus (tuberculous infiltrate) [Herbert *Assmann,* German internist, 1882–1950]   see under *focus.*

association (ah-so″se-a′shun) [L. *associatio,* from *ad* to + *socius* a fellow]   the coordination of the functions of similar parts. In neurology, correlation involving a high degree of modifiability and also consciousness; see *association areas,* under *area.* In genetics, the occurrence together of two characteristics at a frequency greater than would be predicted on the basis of chance, i.e., at a frequency greater than the product of the frequency of each. An example is the association of blood group O and peptic ulcers.   **clang a.,** association of disconnected ideas resulting only from the similarity of the sounds of words, called also *klang a.*   **controlled a's,** ideas called up into the consciousness in response to words spoken by the examiner.   **dream a's,** emotions or thoughts associated with previous dreams, as developed by the patient in psychoanalysis.   **free a.,** a psychoanalytical method in which the patient is encouraged to describe the association of thoughts and emotions as they arise spontaneously during the analysis.   **klang a.,** clang a.

assonance (as′o-nans)   a morbid tendency to alliteration in speaking.

assortment (ah-sort′ment)   the random distribution of nonhomologous chromosomes to daughter cells in metaphase of the first meiotic division.   **independent a.,** the phenomenon that during meiosis members of different pairs of genes are distributed to the gametes independently of one another.

assurin (as′u-rin)   a diaminodiphosphatide, $C_{46}H_{94}N_2P_2O_9$, said to occur in the brain substance.

Ast.   astigmatism.

astacene (as′tah-sēn)   astacin.

astacin (as′tah-sin)   a carotenoid pigment, $C_{40}H_{48}O_4$, obtained from the shells of various crustaceans, where it occurs partly protein-bound and partly esterified.

astasia (as-ta′zhe-ah) [*a* neg. + Gr. *stasis* stand]   motor incoordination with inability to stand.   **a.-abasia,** inability to stand or to walk although the legs are otherwise under control; called also *abasia astasia.*

astatic (as-tat′ik)   pertaining to astasia.

astatine (as′tah-tin) [Gr. *astatos* unstable]   the radioactive element of atomic number 85, atomic weight 210, symbol At. It is prepared by alpha particle bombardment of bismuth on the cyclotron. It has a half-life of 75 hours and may be of use in the treatment of hyperthyroidism.

astaxanthin (as″tah-zan′thin)   a red carotenoid pigment, $C_{40}H_{52}O_4$, constituent of the green chromoprotein from the eggs of crayfish.

asteatodes (as″te-ah-to′dēz)   asteatosis.

asteatosis (as″te-ah-to′sis) [*a* neg. + Gr. *stear* tallow + *-osis*]   any disease characterized by such persistent fine dry scaling of the skin surface as to suggest scantiness or absence of the sebaceous secretion.   **a. cu′tis,** a dry, scaly, or fissured state of the skin, attended with a deficient secretion of sebaceous matter; called also *xerosis cutis.*

aster (as′ter) [L.; Gr. *astēr* star]   a structure seen in a cell during the prophase of mitosis, composed of a system of microtubules arranged in astral rays around the centrosome; called also *astrosphere, cytaster,* and *kinosphere.*   **sperm a.,** the centriole, with astral rays, that precedes the male pronucleus during fertilization.

astereocognosy (ah-ste″re-o-kog′nŏ-se)   astereognosis.

astereognosis (ah-ster″e-og-no′sis) [*a* neg. + Gr. *stereos* solid + *gnōsis* recognition]   loss of power to recognize objects or to ap-

preciate their form by touching or feeling them; called also *tactile amnesia.*

asterion (as-te′re-on), pl. *aste′ria* [Gr. "starred"]   the point on the surface of the skull where the lambdoid, parietomastoid, and occipitomastoid sutures meet.

asterixis (as″ter-ik′sis) [*a* neg. + Gr. *stērixis* a fixed position]   a motor disturbance marked by intermittent lapse of an assumed posture, as a result of intermittency of the sustained contraction of groups of muscles, a characteristic of hepatic coma but observed also in numerous other conditions; called also *liver flap* and *flapping tremor.*

asternal (a-ster′nal)   1. not joined to the sternum.   2. pertaining to asternia; lacking a sternum.

asternia (ah-ster′ne-ah) [*a* neg. + Gr. *sternon* sternum + *-ia*]   congenital absence of the sternum.

Asterococcus (as″ter-o-kok′us)   a genus of bacteria resembling filtrable viruses, which cause pleuropneumonia (def. 2) and other diseases; called also *Coccobacillus.*   **A. ca′nis,** pleuropneumonia-like microorganisms found in the purulent nasal discharge of dogs with distemper.   **A. mycoi′des,** *Mycoplasma myocides.*

asteroid (as′ter-oid) [Gr. *astēr* star + *eidos* form]   star-shaped; resembling the aster.

Asterol (as′ter-ol)   trademark for preparations of diamthazole dihydrochloride.

asterubin (as″te-roo′bin)   a basic substance, NH:C(NH·CH₂·· SO₂OH)·N(CH₃)₂, that has been isolated from the starfish.

Asth.   asthenopia.

asthenia (as-the′ne-ah) [Gr. *asthenēs* without strength + *-ia*]   lack or loss of strength and energy; weakness.   **a. gra′vis hypophyseogen′ea,** a pituitary dysfunction marked by emaciation, anorexia, constipation, amenorrhea, hypothermia, hypotonia, and hypoglycemia.   **myalgic a.,** a condition in which the general symptoms are a sensation of general fatigue and muscular pains.   **neurocirculatory a.,** a symptom-complex characterized by the occurrence of breathlessness, giddiness, a sense of fatigue, pain in the chest in the region of the precordium, and palpitation. It occurs chiefly in soldiers in active war service, though it is seen in civilians also. Called also *effort syndrome, cardiac neurosis, DaCosta's disease* or *syndrome, anxiety neurosis, neurasthenia, cardiasthenia, cardiac neurasthenia,* and *cardioneurosis.*   **periodic a.,** a condition marked by periodically returning attacks of marked asthenia.   **a. pigmento′sa,** Addison's disease; see under *disease.*   **tropical anhidrotic a.,** a condition resulting from generalized, sometimes almost complete, anhidrosis in conditions of high temperature, characterized by a tendency to overfatigability, irritability, anorexia, inability to concentrate, and drowsiness, with headache and vertigo. Called also *anhidrotic heat exhaustion, sweat retention syndrome, type II heat exhaustion,* and *thermogenic anhidrosis.*

asthenic (as-then′ik)   pertaining to or characterized by asthenia.

asthenobiosis (as-the″no-bi-o′sis) [*asthenia* + Gr. *bios* life + *-osis*]   a condition of reduced biologic activity resembling hibernation or estivation but not directly related to or dependent on temperature or humidity.

asthenocoria (as-the″no-ko′re-ah) [*asthenia* + Gr. *korē* pupil + *-ia*]   a condition in which the pupillary light reflex is sluggish; seen in hypoadrenalism. Called also *Arroyo's sign.*

asthenometer (as″thĕ-nom′ĕ-ter) [*asthenia* + Gr. *metron* measure]   an instrument for measuring the degree of muscular asthenia or of asthenopia.

asthenope (as′then-ōp)   a person affected with asthenopia.

asthenophobia (as″thĕ-no-fo′be-ah) [*asthenia* + *phobia*]   (obs.) morbid fear of being weak.

asthenopia (as″thĕ-no′pe-ah) [*asthenia* + Gr. *ōpē* sight + *-ia*]   weakness or easy fatigue of the visual organs, attended by pain in the eyes, headache, dimness of vision, etc. Previously a diagnostic term; now used mainly as a descriptive term.   **accommodative a.,** asthenopia due to strain of the ciliary muscle.   **muscular a.,** that which is due to weakness of the external ocular muscles.   **nervous a.,** asthenopia occurring as one of the symptoms of neurosis and marked by fatigue and contraction of the visual field; called also *retinal a.* and *asthenia of the retina.*   **retinal a.,** that which is due to retinal disease.   **tarsal a.,** asthenopia due to irregular astigmatism produced by the pressure of the lids on the cornea.

asthenopic (as″thĕ-nop′ik)   characterized by asthenopia.

asthenospermia (as″thĕ-no-sper′me-ah) [*asthenia* + Gr. *sperma* seed + *-ia*]   reduction in the vitality of spermatozoa.

asthenoxia (as″then-ok′se-ah) [*asthenia* + *oxygen*]   lack of power to oxidize waste products.

asthma (az′mah) [Gr. *asthma* panting]   a condition marked by recurrent attacks of paroxysmal dyspnea, with wheezing due to spasmodic contraction of the bronchi. Some cases of asthma are allergic manifestations in sensitized persons (*bronchial allergy*); others are provoked by a variety of factors, including vigorous exercise, irritant particles, psychologic stresses, etc.   **abdominal a.,** asthma due to upward pressure on the diaphragm.   **al-**

lergic a., bronchial asthma due to allergy; called also *atopic a.* **alveolar a.,** that which is characterized by dilatation of the alveoli of the lungs. **atopic a.,** allergic asthma. **bacterial a.,** asthma due to bacterial infection. **bronchial a.,** see *asthma.* **bronchitic a.,** asthmatic disorder accompanying bronchitis. **cardiac a.,** paroxysmal dyspnea that occurs in association with heart disease, such as left ventricular failure; called also *cardiasthma.* **cat a.,** asthma brought on by inhalation of cat dander by a sensitized person. **catarrhal a.,** bronchitic a. **a. convulsi′vum,** bronchial a. **cotton-dust a.,** byssinosis. **cutaneous a.,** reflex asthma believed to be caused by some irritation of the skin. **diisocyanate a.,** isocyante a. **dust a.,** asthma caused by inhalation of dust. **Elsner's a.,** angina pectoris. **emphysematous a.,** emphysema of the lungs attended with asthmatic paroxysms. **essential a.,** asthma of unknown or inapparent cause; called also *true a.* **extrinsic a.,** asthma caused by some factor in the environment, usually allergic asthma. **food a.,** asthma brought on by ingestion of certain foods to which the person is allergic. **grinders' a.,** asthmatic symptoms related to the inhalation of fine particles set free in the grinding of metals. **Heberden's a.,** angina pectoris. **horse a.,** a form of allergic asthma in which the attacks are brought on by the presence of horses or of horse products. **humid a.,** asthma with profuse expectoration. **infective a.,** asthma due to infection. **intrinsic a.,** asthma attributed to pathophysiologic disturbances and not to environmental factors. **isocyanate a.,** bronchial asthma caused by allergy to toluene diisocyanate and similiar materials. **Kopp's a.,** laryngismus stridulus. **Millar's a.,** laryngismus stridulus. **millers' a.,** a condition of the lungs found in millers, caused by the inhalation of cereal dusts. **miners' a.,** asthma associated with anthracosis. **nasal a.,** asthma caused by a disease of the nose. **nervous a.,** essential asthma, usually associated with emotional disturbances. **pollen a.,** hay fever. **potters' a.,** asthmatic symptoms associated with the pneumoconiosis of workers in the ceramic industries. **reflex a.,** asthma attributed to some reflex action. **Rostan's a.,** cardiac a. **sexual a.,** asthma resulting from sexual intercourse. **spasmodic a.,** bronchial a. **steam-fitters' a.,** asthmatic symptoms associated with asbestosis. **stone a.,** asthmatic symptoms due to broncholithiasis. **stripper's a.,** asthmatic symptoms associated with byssinosis. **symptomatic a.,** asthma that is secondary to some other physical condition. **thymic a.,** an alleged condition occurring usually in children, associated with enlargement of the thymus, paroxysmal attacks of asthma, and a tendency to sudden death. **true a.,** essential asthma. **Wichmann's a.,** laryngismus stridulus.

asthmatic (az-mat′ik) [L. *asthmaticus*] pertaining to or affected with asthma.

asthmatiform (az-mat′ĭ-form) resembling asthma.

asthmogenic (az″mo-jen′ik) 1. causing asthma. 2. a substance capable of causing asthma.

astigmagraph (ah-stig′mah-graf) an instrument for demonstrating astigmatism.

astigmatic (as″tig-mat′ik) pertaining to or affected with astigmatism.

astigmatism (ah-stig′mah-tizm) [*a* neg. + Gr. *stigma* point] unequal curvature of the refractive surfaces of the eye as a result of which a ray of light is not sharply focused on the retina but is spread over a more or less diffuse area. This results from the radius of curvature in one plane being longer or shorter than that of the radius at right angles to it (Airy, 1827). **acquired a.,**

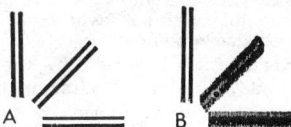

Astigmatism: the appearance of lines as seen by (*a*) the normal eye and (*b*) the astigmatic eye.

that due to some disease or injury of the eye. **a. against the rule,** that in which the meridian along which the greatest refraction takes place is horizontal; called also *inverse a.* **compound a.,** that which is complicated with hypermetropia in all meridians or with myopia in all meridians. **congenital a.,** that which exists at birth. **corneal a.,** that due to irregularity in the curvature or refracting power of the cornea. **direct a.,** a. with the rule. **hypermetropic a., hyperopic a.,** that which complicates hyperopia. **hyperopic a., simple,** astigmatism in which one meridian, usually the vertical, is emmetropic and the horizontal meridian is hyperopic. The focus of the vertical meridian is not in the retina; that of the horizontal is behind the retina: horizontal lines appear distinct. **inverse a.,** a. against the rule. **irregular a.,** astigmatism in which the curvature in different parts of the same meridian of the eye varies or in which successive meridians differ irregularly in refraction, the image produced being an irregular area. **lenticular a.,** that which is due to some irregularity or abnormality

of the lens. **mixed a.,** that in which one principal meridian is myopic and the other hyperopic. **myopic a.,** that which complicates myopia. **myopic a., compound,** astigmatism in which all meridians are myopic, both principal meridians having their foci in front of the retina; vertical lines are usually more distinct. **myopic a., simple,** astigmatism in which the focus of one meridian is situated on the retina, while that of the other lies in front of the retina; vertical lines appear distinct. **oblique a.,** astigmatism in which the direction of the principal meridians approaches 45° and 135°. **physiological a.,** the slight astigmatism possessed by nearly all eyes and causing the twinkling sensation when distant points of light are viewed. **regular a.,** astigmatism in which the refractive power of the eye shows a uniform increase or decrease from one meridian to the other, being practically constant in each meridian; the image produced is regular in shape, either a line, an oval, or a circle. See also *Sturm's conoid,* under *conoid.* **a. with the rule,** that wherein the meridian in which the greatest refraction takes place is vertical or nearly so; called also *direct a.*

astigmatometer (as″tig-mah-tom′ĕ-ter) [*astigmatism* + Gr. *metron* measure] an instrument used in measuring astigmatism.

astigmatoscope (as″tig-mat′o-skōp) [*astigmatism* + Gr. *skopein* to inspect] an instrument for discovering and measuring astigmatism.

astigmatoscopy (ah-stig″mah-tos′ko-pe) the use of the astigmatoscope.

astigmia (ah-stig′me-ah) [*a*- neg. + Gr. *stigma* a mathematical point + *ia*] astigmatism.

astigmic (ah-stig′mik) astigmatic.

astigmometer (as″tig-mom′ĕ-ter) astigmatometer.

astigmometry (as″tig-mom′ĕ-tre) [*astigmatism* + Gr. *metron* measure] the measurement of astigmatism, the use of the astigmatometer.

astigmoscope (as-tig′mo-skōp) astigmatoscope.

A.S.T.M.H. American Society of Tropical Medicine and Hygiene.

astomatous (as-tom′ah-tus) [*a* neg. + Gr. *stoma* mouth] having no mouth, as certain ciliates.

astomia (ah-sto′me-ah) [*a* neg. + Gr. *stoma* mouth] congenital absence of the mouth.

astomus (ah-sto′mus) a fetus without a mouth opening.

Astrafer (as′trah-fer) trademark for a preparation of dextriferron.

astragalar (as-trag′ah-lar) pertaining to the astragalus (talus).

astragalectomy (as″trag-ah-lek′to-me) [*astragalus* + Gr. *ektomē* excision] excision of the astragalus (talus).

astragalocalcanean (as-trag″ah-lo-kal-ka′ne-an) pertaining to the astragalus (talus) and the calcaneus.

astragalocrural (as-trag″ah-lo-kroo′ral) relating to the astragalus (talus) and the leg.

astragaloscaphoid (as-trag″ah-lo-skaf′oid) pertaining to the astragalus (talus) and the scaphoid (navicular) bone.

astragalotibial (as-trag″ah-lo-tib′e-al) pertaining to the astragalus (talus) and the tibia.

Astragalus (ah-strag′ah-lus) a genus of leguminous plants or many species. *A. gummifer* and other oriental species afford tragacanth; others are poisonous. *A. mollissimus,* of the United States (one of the plants called loco), is poisonous, and its active principle is mydriatic.

astragalus (ah-strag′ah-lus) [L.; Gr. *astragalos* ball of the ankle joint or dice] the talus, def. 1.

astral (as′tral) of or relating to an aster.

astraphobia (as″tra-fo′be-ah) (*obs.*) morbid fear of thunder and lightning.

astrapophobia (as″trah-po-fo′be-ah) [Gr. *astrapē* lightning + *phobia*] (*obs.*) astraphobia.

astriction (ah-strik′shun) [L. *astringere* to constrict] 1. the action of an astringent. 2. (*obs.*) constipation.

astringe (ah-strinj′) to act as an astringent.

astringent (ah-strin′jent) [L. *astringens,* from *ad* to + *stringere* to bind] 1. causing contraction, usually locally after topical application. 2. an agent which has an astringent action.

astro- (as′tro) [Gr. *astron* star] a combining form indicating some relation to a star, as star-shaped.

astroblast (as′tro-blast) [*astro-* + Gr. *blastos* germ] a cell that develops into an astrocyte.

astroblastoma (as″tro-blas-to′mah) an astrocytoma of Grade II, composed of cells with abundant cytoplasm and two or three nuclei.

astrocele (as′tro-sēl) astrocoele.

astrocinetic (as″tro-si-net′ik) astrokinetic.

astrocoele (as′tro-sēl) [*astro-* + Gr. *koilos* hollow] the clear space within the astrosphere of a cell in which the centrosome lies.

astrocyte (as′tro-sīt) [*astro-* + Gr. *kytos* hollow vessel] a neuroglial cell of ectodermal origin, characterized by fibrous, protoplasmic, or plasmatofibrous processes. Collectively, such cells are called *astroglia*. **fibrous a's,** astrocytes found mainly in the white matter of the brain, having long, thin, infrequently branched cytoplasmic processes containing numerous fibrillar structures. **gemistocytic a.,** gemistocyte. **plasmatofibrous a's,** astrocytes found at the junction of the gray and white matter of the brain; the cytoplasmic processes extending into the white matter are fibrous and those extending into the gray matter are protoplasmic. **protoplasmic a's,** astrocytes found mainly in the gray matter of the brain, having many branching, thick cytoplasmic processes.

astrocytin (as″tro-si′tin) an antigen present on the cell membrane of astrocytes, found in the serum of patients with malignant glial tumors.

astrocytoma (as″tro-si-to′mah) a tumor composed of astrocytes; such tumors have been classified in order of increasing malignancy as: *Grade I*, consisting of fibrillary or protoplasmic astrocytes; *Grade II* (see *astroblastoma*); and *Grades III* and *IV* (see *glioblastoma multiforme*). **anaplastic a.,** glioblastoma multiforme. **a. fibrilla′re,** an astrocytoma composed of astrocytes which produce fibrillary or neuroglial fibers. **gemistocytic a.,** an astrocytoma in which the cytoplasm of the tumor cells is swollen, homogeneously hyaline, and acidophilic in appearance. **pilocytic a.,** a variant of the fibrillary type of astrocytoma in which the fibrils are arranged in parallel rows. **a. protoplasmat′icum,** a tumor composed of protoplasmic astrocytes.

astrocytosis (as″tro-si-to′sis) the proliferation of astrocytes owing to the destruction of nearby neurons during a hypoxic or hypoglycemic episode.

astroglia (as-trog′le-ah) [*astro-* + *neuroglia*] the astrocytes considered as tissue; see *macroglia*.

astroid (as′troid) [*astro-* + Gr. *eidos* form] 1. star-shaped. 2. (*obs.*) a structure of the neuroglia formed by a felted mass of fibers.

astrokinetic (as″tro-ki-net′ik) [*astro-* + Gr. *kinēsis* motion] pertaining to the movements of the centrosome.

astroma (as-tro′mah) (*obs.*) astrocytoma.

astrophobia (as″tro-fo′be-ah) [*astro-* + *phobia*] (*obs.*) fear of the stars and celestial space.

astrophorous (as-trof′o-rus) [*astro-* + Gr. *phoros* bearing] having star-shaped processes.

astroplankton (as″tro-plank′ton) [Gr. *astron* star + *planktos* wandering] hypothetical living material drifting in outer space.

astrosphere (as′tro-sfēr) [*astro-* + Gr. *sphaira* sphere] 1. the central mass of an aster, exclusive of the rays. 2. aster.

astrostatic (as″tro-stat′ik) [*astro-* + Gr. *statikos* standing] pertaining to the centrosome in its resting condition.

astyclinic (as″tĕ-klin′ik) [Gr. *asty* city + *klinē* bed] a city or municipal hospital, dispensary, or clinic.

asuerotherapy (as″oo-ār′o-ther″ah-pe) a system of healing exploited in 1929 by Fernando Asuero, a Spanish physician, and consisting of cauterization of the sphenopalatine ganglion combined with suggestion.

asulfurosis (ah-sul-fu-ro′sis) a condition due to lack of sulfur in the body.

asyllabia (ah″sil-la′be-ah) a condition in which letters are recognized by the patient, but he is unable to form them into syllables.

asylum (ah-si′lum) [L.] a place of refuge and shelter, as an institution of the past for the support and care of helpless and deprived individuals, such as the mentally deficient, emotionally disturbed, or the blind.

asymbolia (ah-sim-bo′le-ah) [*a* neg. + Gr. *symbolon* symbol + *-ia*] loss of power to comprehend symbolic things, as words, figures, gestures, signs, etc. (Wernicke). **pain a.,** absence of psychic reaction to pain sensations; it may be congenital or result from brain lesion, particularly of the supramarginal gyrus of the dominant parietal lobe.

asymboly (ah-sim′bo-le) asymbolia.

asymmetrical (a″sim-met′rĭ-kal) characterized by or pertaining to asymmetry.

asymmetry (a-sim′ĕ-tre) [*a* neg. + Gr. *symmetria* symmetry] lack or absence of symmetry; dissimilarity in corresponding parts or organs on opposite sides of the body which are normally alike. In chemistry, lack of symmetry in the special arrangements of the atoms and radicals within the molecule or crystal. **chromatic a.,** difference in color in the irides of the two eyes. **encephalic a.,** a condition in which the two sides of the brain are not the same size.

asymphytous (ah-sim′fĭ-tus) separate or distinct; not grown together.

asymptomatic (a″simp″to-mat′ik) showing or causing no symptoms.

asynapsis (ah-sĭ-nap′sis) [*a* neg. + Gr. *synapsis* conjunction] the failure of homologous chromosomes from the male and female to pair during meiosis.

asynchronism (a-sin′kro-nizm) [*a* neg. + *synchronism*] the occurrence at distinct times of events normally synchronous; disturbance of coordination.

asynchrony (a-sin′kro-ne) asynchronism.

asynclitism (ah-sin′klĭ-tizm) [*a* neg. + *synclitism*] 1. oblique presentation of the fetal head in labor. 2. asynchronous maturation of the nucleus and cytoplasm of blood cells. **anterior a.,** Nägele's obliquity. **posterior a.,** Litzmann's obliquity.

asyndesis (ah-sin′dĕ-sis) [*a* neg. + Gr. *syn* together + *desis* binding] a disorder of language in which related elements of a sentence cannot be welded together as a whole; observed in schizophrenia and organic brain syndromes.

asynechia (ah″sĭ-nek′e-ah) [*a* neg. + Gr. *synecheia* continuity] absence of continuity of structure.

asynergia (a″sin-er′je-ah) asynergy.

asynergic (a″sin-er′jik) marked by asynergy.

asynergy (a-sin′er-je) [*a* neg. + Gr. *synergia* cooperation] lack of coordination among parts or organs normally acting in harmony. In neurology, disturbance of that proper association in the contraction of muscles which assures that the different components of an act follow in proper sequence, at the proper moment, and are of the proper degree, so that the act is executed accurately. **truncal a.,** see under *ataxia*.

asynodia (ah″sĭ-no′de-ah) [*a* neg. + Gr. *synodia* a journeying together] sexual impotence.

asynovia (a′h-sĭ-no″ve-ah) deficiency of the synovial secretion.

asyntaxia (ah″sin-tak′se-ah) [Gr. "want of arrangement"] lack of proper and orderly embryonic development. **a. dorsa′lis,** failure of the neural groove to close in the developing embryo.

asystole (a-sis′to-le) [*a* neg. + *systole*] cardiac standstill or arrest—absence of a heartbeat; called also *Beau's syndrome*.

asystolia (ah″sis-to′le-ah) asystole.

asystolic (ah″sis-tol′ik) characterized by asystole.

A. T. German abbreviation for *old tuberculin* (Alt Tuberculin).

A. T. 10 dihydrotachysterol.

At chemical symbol for *astatine*.

ATA alimentary toxic aleukia; see under *aleukia*.

Atabrine (ah′tah-brin) trademark for a preparation of quinacrine hydrochloride.

atactic (ah-tak′tik) [Gr. *ataktos* irregular] lacking coordination; irregular; pertaining to or characterized by ataxia.

atactiform (ah-tak′tĭ-form) resembling ataxia.

ataractic (at″ah-rak′tik) [Gr. *ataraktos* without disturbance; quiet] 1. pertaining to or capable of producing ataraxia. 2. an agent capable of inducing ataraxia; a tranquilizer.

ataralgesia (at″ar-al-je′ze-ah) [Gr. *ataraktos* without trouble + *-algesia*] a method of combined sedation and analgesia designed to abolish the mental distress and pain attendant on surgical procedures, with the patient remaining conscious and alert.

Atarax (ah′tah-raks) trademark for preparations of hydroxyzine hydrochloride.

ataraxia (at″ah-rak′se-ah) [Gr. "impassiveness," "calmness"] perfect peace or calmness of mind: used especially to designate a detached serenity without depression of mental faculties or clouding of consciousness.

ataraxic (at″ah-rak′sik) ataractic.

ataraxy (at″ah-rak′se) ataraxia.

atavic (at′ah-vik) atavistic.

atavism (at′ah-vizm) [L. *atavus* grandfather] the apparent inheritance of a characteristic from remote rather than from immediate ancestors, due to a chance recombination of genes or to unusual environmental conditions favorable to their expression in the embryo. Called also *reversion*.

atavistic (at-ah-vis′tik) characterized by atavism.

ataxaphasia (ah-tak″sah-fa′ze-ah) ataxiaphasia.

ataxia (ah-tak′se-ah) [Gr., from *a* negative + *taxis* order] failure of muscular coordination; irregularity of muscular action. **acute a.,** ataxia of sudden onset. **acute cerebellar a.,** cerebellar ataxia, usually unilateral, associated with infectious disease, tumor, or trauma, resulting in marked hypotonia of muscles on the affected side, asynergy, and assumption of a characteristic posture. **alcoholic a.,** a condition resembling tabes dorsalis, due to loss of proprioception in chronic alcoholism. **autonomic a.,** defective coordination between the sympathetic and parasympathetic nervous systems. **Briquet's a.,** a hysteric condition with anesthesia of the skin and leg muscles. **Broca's a.,** hysteric a. **central a.,** ataxia due to lesion of the centers controlling coordination. **cerebellar a.,** ataxia due to disease of the cerebellum. **cerebral a.,** ataxia due to disease of the cerebrum. **a. cor′dis** (*obs.*), atrial fibrillation. **enzootic a.,** congenital locomotor ataxia of lambs, thought to be associated with copper deficiency; called also *swayback*. **family a.,** Friedreich's a. **Fergusson and Critchley's a.,** a hereditary ataxia resembling multiple sclerosis found in only a few families and appearing between the ages of 30 and 45. **Friedreich's a.,** Friedreich's disease: an inherited disease, usually beginning in childhood or youth, with sclerosis of the dorsal and lateral columns of the spinal cord. It is attended by ataxia, speech impairment, lateral curvature of the spinal column, and peculiar swaying and irregular movements, with paralysis of the muscles, especially of the lower extremities (Friedreich 1863–76). It is often associated with hypertrophic cardiomyopathy. Called also *hereditary a., family a.,* and *Friedreich's tabes.* **frontal a.,** disturbance of equilibrium occurring in tumor of the frontal lobe. **hereditary a.,** Friedreich's a. **hereditary cerebellar a.,** a disease of early adult life, due to atrophy of the cerebellum, and marked by ataxia, increased knee jerk, speech defects, and nystagmus; called also *cerebellar syndrome, Marie's a.,* and *Nonne's syndrome.* **hysteric a.,** hysteria simulating ataxia; called also *Broca's a.* **intrapsychic a.,** an apparent lack of unity of ideation and emotional reaction, as in a patient who weeps at a funny occurrence or laughs outright at the death of a close relative. **kinetic a.,** motor a. **labyrinthic a.,** vestibular a. **Leyden's a.,** pseudotabes. **locomotor a.,** tabes dorsalis. **Marie's a.,** hereditary cerebellar a. **motor a.,** inability to control the coordinate movements of the muscles; called also *kinetic a.* **ocular a.,** nystagmus. **professional a.,** occupation neurosis. **Sanger-Brown's a.,** spinocerebellar a. **sensory a.,** ataxia due to loss of proprioception (joint position sensation) between the motor cortex and peripheral nerves, resulting in poorly judged movements, the incoordination becoming aggravated when the eyes are closed. **spinal a.,** that which is due to disease of the spinal cord. **spinocerebellar a.,** hereditary cerebellar ataxia marked by degeneration of the spinocerebellar tracts; called also *Sanger-Brown's a.* **a.-telangiectasia,** severe progressive cerebellar ataxia, associated with oculocutaneous telangiectasia, sinopulmonary disease with frequent respiratory infections, and abnormal eye movements; it is a hereditary disorder transmitted as an autosomal recessive trait, usually appearing when the child attempts to learn to walk. It is also associated with immunodeficiency (IgA and IgE) and sometimes with cell-mediated dysfunction. Called also *Louis-Bar syndrome.* **thermal a.,** a condition characterized by great and paradoxic fluctuations of the temperature of the body. **trunkal a.,** ataxia affecting the muscles of the trunk. **vasomotor a.** (*obs.*), paralysis or spasm of blood vessels due to some derangement of vasomotor nerves or centers. **vestibular a.,** incoordination due to vestibular disease; called also *labyrinthine a.*

ataxiadynamia (ah-tak″se-ah-di-na′me-ah) ataxoadynamia.

ataxiagram (ah-tak′se-ah-gram″) [*ataxia* + Gr. *gramma* a writing] a tracing drawn by an ataxic patient; also the record made by an ataxiagraph.

ataxiagraph (ah-tak′se-ah-graf″) [*ataxia* + Gr. *graphein* to write] an apparatus used in ascertaining the extent of ataxia by measuring the amount of swaying of the body when standing erect and with the eyes closed.

ataxiameter (ah-tak″se-am′ĕ-ter) [*ataxia* + Gr. *metron* measure] an apparatus for measuring ataxia.

ataxiamnesic (ah-tak″se-am-ne′sik) characterized by both ataxia and amnesia.

ataxiaphasia (ah-tak″se-ah-fa′ze-ah) [*ataxia* + Gr. *aphasia*] a condition characterized by inability to arrange words into sentences.

ataxic (ah-tak′sik) atactic.

ataxiophemia (ah-tak″se-o-fe′me-ah) ataxophemia.

ataxiophobia (ah-tak″se-o-fo′be-ah) ataxophobia.

ataxoadynamia (ah-tak″so-ad″ĕ-na′me-ah) (*obs.*) ataxia associated with marked weakness.

ataxophemia (ah-tak″so-fe′me-ah) [Gr. *ataxia* disorder + *phēmē* speech] lack of coordination of the speech muscles.

ataxophobia (ah-tak″so-fo′be-ah) [Gr. *ataxia* disorder + *phobia*] (*obs.*) morbid or insane dread of disorder.

ataxy (ah-tak′se) ataxia.

-ate (āt) a word termination forming a participial noun, as the object of the process indicated by the root to which it is affixed, e.g., *hemolysate,* something hemolyzed; *homogenate,* something homogenized; *injectate,* something injected. Also forming adjectives, signifying possession of the quality indicated by the root, e.g., *dentate* and *corticate;* and verbs, signifying performance of the action indicated by the root, e.g., *decussate* and *pulsate.* In organic chemistry, this suffix replaces the *-ic* ending in names of acids (as in glycerate for glyceric acid), indicating that the acid involved is in dissociated form or combined in an ester.

atelectasis (at″e-lek′tah-sis) [Gr. *atelēs* imperfect + *ektasis* expansion] 1. incomplete expansion of a lung or a portion of a lung, occurring congenitally as a primary or secondary condition, or as an acquired condition. 2. airlessness of a lung that had once been expanded. 3. collapse of a lung. **absorption a., acquired a.,** that produced by any factor, e.g., secretions, foreign body, tumor, abnormal external pressure, etc., which completely obstructs the airway, preventing intake of air into the alveolar sacs and permitting absorption of air into the bloodstream. Called also *obstructive a., reabsorption a.,* and *secondary a.* **compression a.,** acquired atelectasis due to abnormal external pressure on the lung. **congenital a.,** that present at birth or shortly thereafter; it may occur as a primary condition (see *primary a.*) or secondary to some other congenital disorder (see *secondary a.*).

initial a., primary a. **lobar a.,** that affecting only a lobe of the lung; called also *segmental a.* **lobular a.,** that affecting a lobule of the lung; called also *patchy a.* **obstructive a.,** absorption a. **patchy a.,** lobular a. **primary a.,** congenital atelectasis, common among premature infants, in which there is failure of initial alveolar expansion, due to pulmonary immaturity or to inadequacy of respiratory effort that may be a result of weakness of respiratory muscles, severe illness, softness of thoracic cage, brain damage with injury to the respiratory center, or oversedation. Called also *initial a.* **relaxation a.,** absorption atelectasis due to bronchial collapse resulting from large amounts of air or fluid in the pleural cavity, as in pneumothorax or pleural effusion. **resorption a.,** absorption a. **secondary a.,** 1. absorption atelectasis occurring at birth or in the newborn period, in which the pulmonary alveoli collapse after initial expansion by air; it is due to obstruction of the airway which prevents further entrance of air or to prevention of air from remaining in the alveoli by increased surfaces forces, occurring as a result of inhalation of amniotic debris or mucous plugs, deficiency of pulmonary surfactant, obstruction by congenital abnormalities, or abnormal external pressure upon the lung. 2. absorption a. **segmental a.,** lobar a.

atelectatic (at″ĕ-lek-tat′ik) pertaining to or characterized by atelectasis.

ateleiosis (ah-te″le-o′sis) [*a* neg. + Gr. *teleios* complete] hypophyseal infantilism.

atelencephalia (ah-tel″en-sĕ-fa′le-ah) [Gr. *ateleia* incompleteness + *enkephalos* brain + *-ia*] congenital imperfect development of the brain.

atelia (ah-te′le-ah) [Gr. *ateleia* incompleteness] imperfect or incomplete development.

ateliosis (ah-te″le-o′sis) hypophyseal infantilism.

ateliotic (ah-te″le-ot′ik) pertaining to or characterized by atelia.

atelo- (at′ĕ-lo) [Gr. *atelēs* incomplete] a combining form meaning imperfect or incomplete.

atelocardia (at″ĕ-lo-kar′de-ah) [*atelo-* + Gr. *kardia* heart] congenitally incomplete development of the heart.

atelocephalous (at″ĕ-lo-sef′ah-lus) [*atelo-* + Gr. *kephalē* head] having an incomplete head.

atelocephaly (at″ĕ-lo-sef′ah-le) imperfect development of the skull.

atelocheilia (at″ĕ-lo-ki′le-ah) [*atelo-* + Gr. *cheilos* lip + *-ia*] a congenitally incomplete development of a lip.

atelocheiria (at″ĕ-lo-ki′re-ah) [*atelo-* + Gr. *cheir* hand + *-ia*] congenitally incomplete development of the hand.

ateloencephalia (at″ĕ-lo-en″sĕ-fa′le-ah) atelencephalia.

ateloglossia (at″ĕ-lo-glos′e-ah) [*atelo-* + Gr. *glōssa* tongue + *-ia*] congenitally incomplete development of the tongue.

atelognathia (at″ĕ-log-na′the-ah) [*atelo-* + Gr. *gnathos* jaw + *-ia*] congenitally incomplete development of the jaw.

atelomyelia (at″ĕ-lo-mi-e′le-ah) [*atelo-* + Gr. *myelos* marrow + *-ia*] congenitally incomplete development of the spinal cord.

atelopidtoxin (a-tel-op″id-tok′sin) a potent dialyzable toxin derived from the skin of frogs of the genus *Atelopus,* of Central and South America. The LD$_{50}$ in mice is 16 μg/kg. Its chemical and pharmacological nature has not been fully defined.

atelopodia (at″ĕ-lo-po′de-ah) [*atelo-* + Gr. *pous* foot + *-ia*] congenitally incomplete development of the foot.

ateloprosopia (at″ĕ-lo-pro-so′pe-ah) [*atelo-* + Gr. *prosōpon* face + *-ia*] congenitally incomplete development of the face.

atelorachidia (at″ĕ-lo-rah-kid′e-ah) [*atelo-* + Gr. *rhachis* spine + *-ia*] congenitally incomplete development of the vertebral column.

Atelosaccharomyces (at″ĕ-lo-sak″ah-ro-mi′sēz) former name for *Cryptococcus.*

atelostomia (at″ĕ-lo-sto′me-ah) [*atelo-* + Gr. *stoma* mouth + *-ia*] congenitally incomplete development of the mouth.

atenolol (ah-ten′o-lōl) chemical name: 4-[2-hydroxy-3-[(1-methyethyl)amino]propoxyl]benzeneacetamide; an antiadrenergic (β-receptor), $C_{14}H_{22}N_2O_3$.

athalposis (ah″thal-po′sis) [*a* neg. + Gr. *thalpos* warmth + *-osis*] inability to perceive warmth.

athelia (ah-the′le-ah) [*a* neg. + Gr. *thēlē* nipple + *-ia*] congenital absence of the nipple(s).

Athenaeus (ath″ĕ-ne′us) **of Attalia** (1st century A.D.) a celebrated physician, latterly of Rome, and founder of the Pneumatist school of medicine. Only fragments of his many writings remain.

athermal (ah-ther′mal) [*a* neg. + Gr. *thermē* heat] not warm; said of springs the water of which is below 15° C.

athermancy (ah-ther′man-se) the state of being athermanous.

athermanous (ah-ther′mah-nus) [*a* neg. + Gr. *thermē* heat] absorbing heat rays and not permitting them to pass.

athermic (ah-ther′mik) [*a* neg. + Gr. *thermē* heat] without fever or rise of temperature; apyretic; afebrile.

athermosystaltic (ah-ther″mo-sis-tal′tik) [*a* neg. + Gr. *thermē* heat + Gr. *systaltikos* drawing together] not contracting under the action of cold or heat; said of skeletal muscle.

atheroembolism (ath″er-o-em′bo-lizm) embolism due to blockage of a blood vessel by an atheroembolus.

atheroembolus (ath″er-o-em′bo-lus), pl. *atheroem′boli*. An embolus composed of cholesterol or its esters (typically lodging in small arteries) or of fragments of atheromatous plaques.

atherogenesis (ath″er-o-jen′ĕ-sis) the formation of atheromatous lesions in the arterial intima.

atherogenic (ath″er-o-jen′ik) conducive to or causing atherogenesis.

atheroma (ath″er-o′mah) [Gr. *athērē* gruel + *-oma*] a mass of plaque of degenerated, thickened arterial intima occurring in atherosclerosis. **a. cu′tis,** sebaceous cyst.

atheromatosis (ath″er-o″mah-to′sis) a diffuse atheromatous disease of the arteries.

atheromatous (ath″er-o′mah-tus) affected with or of the nature of atheroma.

atheronecrosis (ath″er-o″ne-kro′sis) (*obs.*) the necrosis or degeneration accompanying atherosclerosis.

atherosclerosis (ath″er-o″skle-ro′sis) an extremely common form of arteriosclerosis in which deposits of yellowish plaques (atheromas) containing cholesterol, lipoid material, and lipophages are formed within the intima and inner media of large and medium-sized arteries. **a. oblit′erans,** arteriosclerosis obliterans.

atherosis (ath″er-o′sis) (*obs.*) atherosclerosis.

athetoid (ath′ĕ-toid) [Gr. *athetos* not fixed + *eidos* form] resembling or affected with athetosis.

athetosic (ath″ĕ-to′sik) athetotic.

athetosis (ath″ĕ-to′sis) [Gr. *athetos* not fixed + *-osis*] a derangement marked by ceaseless occurrence of slow, sinuous, writhing movements, especially severe in the hands, and performed involuntarily; it may occur after hemiplegia, and is then known as *posthemiplegic chorea.* Called also *mobile spasm.*

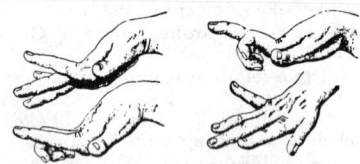

Position of fingers in movements of athetosis.

double a., double congenital a., congenital bilateral athetosis due to birth trauma, which may occur in association with spastic paraplegia, as in *Vogt's syndrome* and *Little's disease.* **pupillary a.,** hippus.

athetotic (ath″e-tot′ik) pertaining to athetosis.

athiaminosis (ah-thi″ah-mĭ-no′sis) thiamine deficiency.

Athiorhodaceae (a″thi-o-ro-da′se-e) a family of Schizomycetes (order Pseudomonadales, suborder Rhodobacteriineae), made up of non–sulfur photosynthetic microorganisms that characteristically produce a pigment composed of bacteriochlorophyll and one or more carotenoids. It includes two genera, *Rhodopseudomonas* and *Rhodospirillum.*

athomin (ath′o-min) a bactericidal principle isolated from the root bark of the "horseradish" tree, *Moringa pterygosperma* Gaertn., Moringaceae, used in India as an antiemetic and in the clinical management of cholera. Called also *GL 54.*

athrepsia (ah-threp′se-ah) [*a* neg. + Gr. *threpsis* nutrition] 1. marasmus. 2. Ehrlich's term for immunity to tumor inoculation due to a supposed lack of the special nutritive material necessary for tumor growth.

athrepsy (ath′rep-se) athrepsia.

athreptic (ah-threp′tik) pertaining to or characterized by athrepsia.

athrocytosis (ath″ro-si-to′sis) absorption of macromolecules from the lumen of the renal tubules by renal tubular cells by means of a process similar to phagocytosis.

athrophagocytosis (ath″ro-fag″o-si-to′sis) non-nutritive phagocytosis; phagocytosis of inert particles, as the removal of injected carbon particles from the body by phagocytes in the carbon clearance test.

athymia (ah-thim′e-ah) [*a* neg. + Gr. *thymos* mind] 1. dementia. 2. loss of consciousness. 3. absence of the thymus gland.

athymism (ah-thi′mizm) absence of the thymus or the condition induced by absence or removal of the thymus.

athymismus (ah″thi-mis′mus) athymism.

athyrea (ah-thi′re-ah) hypothyroidism.

athyreosis (ah-thi″re-o′sis) [*a* neg. + *thyreoid* thyroid + *-osis*] hypothyroidism.

athyria (ah-thi′re-ah) 1. a condition resulting from absence of the thyroid gland. 2. hypothyroidism.

athyroidation (ah-thi″roi-da′shun) hypothyroidism.

athyroidemia (ah-thi″roi-de′me-ah) [*a* neg. + *thyroid* + Gr. *haima* blood + *-ia*] absence of thyroid hormone from the blood.

athyroidism (ah-thi′roid-izm) hypothyroidism.

athyroidosis (ah-thi″roi-do′sis) hypothyroidism.

athyrosis (ah″thi-ro′sis) hypothyroidism.

athyrotic (ah″thi-rot′ik) pertaining to or characterized by hypothyroidism.

Athysanus (ah-this′ah-nus) a genus of blood-sucking flies of Algeria.

atite (at′īt) a substance in milk that reduces nitrate to nitrite.

atlantad (at-lan′tad) toward the atlas.

atlantal (at-lan′tal) pertaining to the atlas.

atlantoaxial (at-lan″to-ak′se-al) pertaining to the atlas and the axis.

atlantodidymus (at-lan″to-did′ĭ-mus) a monster with one body and two heads.

atlantomastoid (at-lan″to-mas′toid) pertaining to the atlas and the mastoid process.

atlanto-odontoid (at-lan″to-o-don′toid) pertaining to the atlas and the odontoid process of the axis.

atlas (at′las) [Gr. *Atlas* the Greek god who bears up the pillars of Heaven] 1. [NA], the first cervical vertebra, which articulates above with the occipital bone and below with the axis. 2. a collection of illustrations on one subject, such as anatomy, blood and bone marrow, brain, cardiac disease.

atloaxoid (at″lo-ak′soid) pertaining to the atlas and the axis.

atlodidymus (at″lo-did′ĭ-mus) [*atlas* + Gr. *didymos* twin] atlantodidymus.

atloido-occipital (at-loi″do-ok-sip′ĭ-tal) pertaining to the atlas and the occiput.

atmiatrics (at″me-at′riks) [*atmo-* + Gr. *iatrikos* healing] treatment by medicated vapors (P. Niemeyer).

atmiatry (at-mi′ah-tre) atmiatrics.

atm. atmosphere.

atmo- (at′mo) [Gr. *atmos* steam or vapor] a combining form denoting relationship to steam or vapor.

atmocausis (at″mo-kaw′sis) [*atmo-* + Gr. *kausis* burning] (*obs.*) treatment by the direct application of superheated steam; used chiefly in nonmalignant uterine affections and to arrest bleeding (*a. u′teri*).

atmocautery (at″mo-kaw′ter-e) (*obs.*) an instrument for performing atmocausis.

atmograph (at′mo-graf) [*atmo-* + Gr. *graphein* to record] an instrument for recording respiratory movements.

atmolysis (at-mol′ĭ-sis) [*atmo-* + Gr. *lysis* loosing] 1. the separation of mixed gases by passing through a porous plate, the more diffusible passing through first. 2. the disintegration of organic tissue by the fumes of volatile fluids, such as benzine, ether, alcohol, etc.

atmometer (at-mom′ĕ-ter) [*atmo-* + Gr. *metron* measure] an instrument for measuring exhaled vapors, or the amount of water exhaled by evaporation in a given time, in order to ascertain the humidity of the atmosphere.

atmos (at′mos) [Gr. "steam" or "vapor"] a unit of air pressure, being a pressure of one degree per square centimeter; called also *aer.*

atmosphere (at′mos-fēr) [*atmo-* + Gr. *sphaira* sphere] 1. the entire gaseous envelope surrounding the earth, including the troposphere, tropopause, and stratosphere. 2. the unit of pressure of the air upon the earth at sea level, about 14.7 pounds to the square inch.

atmospheric (at″mos-fer′ik) of or pertaining to the atmosphere.

atmotherapy (at″mo-ther′ah-pe) [*atmo-* + Gr. *therapeia* treatment] 1. treatment by medicated vapors. 2. treatment by methodic reduction of respiration.

at. no. atomic number.

atocia (ah-to′se-ah) [*a* neg. + Gr. *tokos* birth] sterility in the female.

atolide (ah′to-līd) chemical name: 2-amino-4′-(diethylamino)-o-benzotoluidide; an anticonvulsant, $C_{18}H_{23}N_3O$.

atom (at′om) [Gr. *atomos* indivisible; *a-* + *tomos* from *temnein* to cut] any one of the ultimate particles of a molecule or of any matter. An atom is the smallest particle of an element that is capable of entering into a chemical reaction. The atom consists of a minute central nucleus, in which practically all of the mass of the atom is concentrated, and of surrounding electrons. The nucleus is positively charged; the amount of the charge corresponds to the atomic number of the atom. See *Table of Elements,* under *element.* In a neutral atom the surrounding negative electrons are equal in number to the positive charges on the nucleus. The number and arrangement of these electrons determine all the properties of the atom except its atomic weight and its radioactivity. **activated a.,** 1. an ionized atom. 2. an atom in which some of the orbital electrons have been driven out into larger and less stable orbits; the atom is thus prepared to release its stored energy as these electrons return to their normal and stable orbits. Called also *excited a.* **Bohr a.,** the conception of a nulcear atom in which the orbital electrons are able to occupy only certain orbits, these orbits being determined by quantum limitations. **excited a.,** activated atom. **ionized a.,** an atom from which one or more of the outer or valence electrons have been removed, or to which one or more electrons have been added (hence positive and negative ions). **nuclear a.,** the conception or theory of the atom as composed of a small central nucleus surrounded by orbital electrons; called also *Rutherford a.* For table of the atoms see under *element.* **recoil a., rest a.,** the portion of an atom from which an alpha particle or other subatomic particle has been given off; this remaining part recoils with a velocity inversely proportional to its mass. **Rutherford a.,** nuclear a. **stripped a.,** an atom from which the orbital electrons have been more or less completely removed. **tagged a.,** one which has been made radioactive, so that its course in the body may be checked; see *radioactive tracer,* under *tracer.*

atomic (ah-tom′ik) of or pertaining to an atom.

atomism (at′om-izm) the hypothesis that the universe is composed of atoms.

atomization (at″om-ĭ-za′shun) the act or process of breaking a liquid up into spray.

atomizer (at′om-iz″er) an instrument for throwing a jet of spray.

atonia (ah-to′ne-ah) atony. **choreatic a.,** deficient muscular tonicity often seen in chorea.

atonic (ah-ton′ik) lacking normal tone or strength; pertaining to or characterized by atony.

atonicity (at″o-nis′ĭ-te) the quality or condition of being without normal tone or strength.

atony (at′o-ne) [L. *atonia,* from *a* neg. + Gr. *tonos* tension] lack of normal tone or strength. **primary ureteral a.,** megaloureter.

atopen (at′o-pen) the antigen responsible for atopy; cf. *reagin.*

atopic (ah-top′ik, a-top′ik) [*a* neg. + Gr. *topos* place] 1. ectopic. 2. pertaining to an atopen or to atopy; allergic.

atopognosia (ah-top″og-no′ze-ah) [*a* neg. + Gr. *topos* place + *gnōsis* knowledge + *-ia*] loss of power of correctly locating a sensation.

atopognosis (ah-top″og-no′sis) atopognosia.

atopomenorrhea (at″ŏ-po-men-o-re′ah) [*a* neg. + Gr. *topos* place + *men* month + *rhoia* flow] (*obs.*) vicarious menstruation.

atopy (at′o-pe) a clinical hypersensitivity state, or allergy, with a hereditary predisposition; that is, the tendency to develop some form of allergy is inherited, but the specific clinical form, e.g., hay fever, asthma, eczema, is not. An unusual type of antibody, termed reagin, which is in the immunoglobulin E (IgE) class, is involved. Called also *hereditary* or *spontaneous allergy.*

atoxic (ah-tok′sik) [*a* neg. + Gr. *toxikon* poison] not poisonous; not due to a poison.

atoxigenic (a-tok″sĭ-jen′ik) not producing or elaborating toxins.

ATP adenosine triphosphate.

ATPase adenosinetriphosphatase.

atrabiliary (at″rah-bil′e-ă-re) [L. *atra* black + *bilis* bile] pertaining to black bile, one of the four humors, according to the humoral theory; by extension, characterized by melancholy or gloom; melancholic or gloomy.

Atractaspis (ah-trak-tas′pis) a genus of African vipers whose bite is toxic to man.

atransferrinemia (a-trans″fer-ĭ-ne′me-ah) absence from the circulating blood of iron-binding protein (transferrin).

atraumatic (a″traw-mat′ik) [*a* neg. + Gr. *traumatikos* of or for wounds] not inflicting or causing damage or injury.

Atrax (a′traks) a genus of tarantula-like spiders (funnel-web spiders) of Australia belonging to the family Dipluridae. The venom of *A. robustus, A. formidabilis*(tree funnel-web spider), and six other species is harmful to man; *A. robustus* has caused several deaths.

atremia (ah-tre′me-ah) [*a* neg. + Gr. *tremein* to tremble] 1. absence of tremor. 2. hysterical inability to walk.

atrepsy (at′rep-se) [*a* neg. + Gr. *threpsis* nutrition] athrepsia (def. 1).

atreptic (ah-trep′tik) athreptic.

atresia (ah-tre′ze-ah) [*a* neg. + Gr. *trēsis* a hold + *-ia*] congenital absence or closure of a normal body orifice or tubular organ; as esophageal and pulmonary atrial a.; called also *clausura.* **anal a., a. a′ni,** imperforate anus. **aortic a.,** absence or closure of the aortic root orifice, a rare congenital anomaly in which the left ventricle is hypoplastic or nonfunctioning, oxygenated blood passing from the left into the right atrium through a septal defect, and the mixed venous and arterial blood passing from the pulmonary artery to the aorta by way of a patent ductus. **aural a.,** absence or closure of the external auditory canal. **bili-**

ary a., obliteration or hypoplasia of one or more components of the bile ducts due to arrested fetal development, resulting in persistent jaundice and liver damage ranging from biliary stasis to biliary cirrhosis, with splenomegaly as portal hypertension progresses. **choanal a.,** congenital bony or membranous occlusion of one or both choanae, due to failure of the embryonic bucconasal membrane to rupture. **duodenal a.,** congenital absence or occlusion of a portion of the duodenum, characterized by vomiting a few hours after birth, cessation of bowel movements after one to three days, and usually distention of the epigastrium. It is often associated with Down's syndrome. **esophageal a.,** congenital lack of continuity of the esophagus, commonly associated with tracheoesophageal fistula and characterized by excessive salivation, gagging, vomiting when fed, cyanosis, and dyspnea. **folliclar a., a. follic′uli,** the degeneration and resorption of an ovarian follicle before it reaches maturity and ruptures. **intestinal a.,** congenital obstruction of the intestine at any level, most commonly of the ileum, due to lack of continuity of the lumen; symptoms vary with the site of obstruction. **a. i′ridis,** closure of the pupillary opening. **mitral a.,** congenital obliteration of the mitral valve orifice; it is associated with hyperplastic left-heart syndrome or transposition of the great vessels. **prepyloric a.,** congenital membranous obstruction of the gastric outlet, characterized by vomiting of gastric contents only. **pulmonary a.,** congenital severe narrowing of the opening between the pulmonary artery and the right ventricle, characterized by cardiomegaly, reduced pulmonary vascularity, and right ventricular atrophy. It is usually associated with tetralogy of Fallot, transposition of the great vessels, or other cardiovascular anomalies. **tricuspid a.,** absence of the orifice between the right atrium and ventricle, circulation being made possible by the presence of an atrial septal defect, blood passing from the right to the left atrium and thence to the left ventricle and aorta. Classification by type is made according to the presence or absence of transposition of the great vessels and of pulmonary stenosis.

atresic (ah-tre′zik) atretic.

atretic (ah-tret′ik) [Gr. *atrētos* not perforated] without an opening; pertaining to or characterized by atresia.

atreto- (ah-tre′to) [Gr. *atrētos* not perforated] a combining form denoting absence of a normal opening; imperforate, or closed.

atretoblepharia (ah-tre″to-blĕ-fa′re-ah) [*atreto-* + Gr. *blepharon* eyelid + *-ia*] symblepharon.

atretocephalus (ah-tre″to-sef′ah-lus) [*atreto-* + Gr. *kephalē* head] a monster lacking the orifices normally present in the head.

atretocormus (ah-tre″to-kor′mus) [*atreto-* + Gr. *kormos* trunk] a fetus or infant having one of the body openings imperforate.

atretocystia (ah-tre″to-sis′te-ah) [*atreto-* + Gr. *kystis* bladder + *-ia*] lack of the normal opening from the bladder.

atretogastria (ah-tre″to-gas′tre-ah) [*atreto-* + Gr. *gastēr* stomach + *-ia*] lack of the normal opening into the stomach.

atretolemia (ah-tre″to-le′me-ah) [*atreto-* + Gr. *laimos* gullet + *-ia*] lack of the normal opening into the larynx or the esophagus.

atretometria (ah-tre″to-me′tre-ah) [*atretro-* + Gr. *mētra* uterus + *-ia*] lack of the normal opening into the uterus.

atretopsia (ah″tre-top′se-ah) [*atreto-* + Gr. *ōps* eye + *-ia*] lack of the normal opening in the iris of the eye.

atretorrhinia (ah-tre″to-rin′e-ah) [*atreto-* + Gr. *rhis* nose + *-ia*] absence of the normal opening into the nose.

atretostomia (ah-tre″to-sto′me-ah) [*atreto-* + Gr. *stoma* mouth + *-ia*] lack of the normal opening into the oral cavity.

atreturethria (ah-tre″tu-re′thre-ah) [*atreto-* + Gr. *ourēthra* urethra + *-ia*] lack of the normal urethral opening.

atria (a′tre-ah) [L.] plural of *atrium.*

atrial (a′tre-al) pertaining to an atrium.

atrichia (ah-trik′e-ah) [*a* neg. + Gr. *thrix* hair + *-ia*] 1. absence of the hair; alopecia. 2. absence of flagella or cilia. **universal congenital a.,** congenital universal alopecia.

atrichosis (at″rĭ-ko′sis) (*obs.*) alopecia.

atrichous (ah-trik′us) [*a* neg. + Gr. *thrix* hair] 1. having no flagella; said of bacteria. 2. having no hair.

atrio- (a′tre-o) [L. *atrium* hall] a combining form denoting relationship to an atrium of the heart.

atriocommissuropexy (a″tre-o-kom″ĭ-su′ro-pek″se) [*atrio-* + *commissure* + *-pexy*] fixation of the mitral valve with sutures passed from the ventricle through the valve leaflets and the atrial wall, for correction of mitral insufficiency.

atriomegaly (a″tre-o-meg′ah-le) [*atrio-* + Gr. *megaleios* magnitude] abnormal dilatation or enlargement of an atrium of the heart.

atrionector (at″re-o-nek′tor) [*atrio-* + L. *nector* connector] the sinoatrial node.

atrioseptopexy (a″tre-o-sep″to-pek′se) [*atrio-* + *septum* + Gr. *pēxis* a fixing, putting together] surgical repair of a defect in the interatrial septum.

atrioseptoplasty (a″tre-o-sep″to-plas′te) plastic repair of the interatrial septum.

atriotomy (a″tre-ot′o-me) [*atrio-* + Gr. *tomē* a cutting] surgical incision of an atrium of the heart.

atrioventricular (a″tre-o-ven-trik′u-lar) pertaining to an atrium of the heart and to a ventricle.

atrioventricularis communis (a″tre-o-ven-trik″u-la′ris kŏ-mu′nis) a congenital cardiac anomaly in which the endocardial cushions fail to fuse, the ostium primum persists, the atrioventricular canal is undivided, a single atrioventricular valve has anterior and posterior cusps, and there is a defect of the membranous interventricular septum. Called also *persistent common atrioventricular canal.*

atriplicism (ah-trip′lĭ-sizm) poisoning produced by eating a kind of spinach, *Atriplex littoralis.*

atrium (a′tre-um), pl. *a′tria* [L.; Gr. *atrion* hall] a chamber; used in anatomical nomenclature to designate a chamber affording entrance to another structure or organ. Usually used alone to designate an atrium of the heart (a. cordis). **common a.,** the single atrium found in a form of three-chambered heart. **a. cor′dis** [NA], one of the pair of smaller cavities of the heart, with thin muscular walls, from which the blood passes to the ventricles; see *a. dextrum* and *a. sinistrum.* **a. dex′trum** [NA], right atrium: the atrium of the right side of the heart; it receives blood from the superior and the inferior vena cava, and delivers it to the right ventricle. **a. glot′tidis, a. of glottis,** vestibulum laryngis. **a. laryn′gis, a. of larynx,** vestibulum laryngis. **left a.,** a. sinistrum. **a. mea′tus me′dii** [NA], a. of middle meatus of nose: a depression in front of the middle nasal meatus, between the agger nasi and the middle nasal concha. **a. pulmona′le, pulmonary a.,** 1. atrium sinistrum. 2. respiratory atrium. **respiratory a.** (*obs.*), the expanded cavity at the end of an alveolar duct, into which the alveolar sacs open; called also *a. pulmonale* or *pulmonary a.* **right a.,** a. dextrum. **a. sinis′trum** [NA], left atrium: the atrium of the left side of the heart; it receives blood from the pulmonary veins, and delivers it to the left ventricle. Called also *a. pulmonale* and *pulmonary a.* **a. vagi′nae,** vestibulum vaginae.

Atromid-S (at′ro-mid) trademark for a preparation of clofibrate.

Atropa (at′ro-pah) [Gr. *Atropos* "undeviating," one of the Fates] a genus of solanaceous plants, from which various alkaloids are derived, including atropine, hyoscyamine, and scopolamine, which generally possess anticholinergic properties. The genus includes *A. belladonna* and *A. belladonna* var. *acuminata.* See *belladonna.*

atrophedema (ah-trof″ĕ-de′mah) [*atrophy* + *edema*] a chronic hereditary disease probably of angioneurotic origin.

atrophia (ah-tro′fe-ah) [L.; Gr., from *a* neg. + Gr. *trophē* nourishment] atrophy. **a. bul′bi,** atrophy and fibrosis of all components of the globe of the eye resulting from uveitis. **a. bulbo′rum heredita′ria,** Norrie's disease. **a. cer′ebri seni′lis sim′plex,** senile dementia in which there is marked atrophy of the brain associated with conspicuous loss of neurons and abundant lipochrome in those that survive. **a. choroi′deae et ret′inae,** atrophy of the choroid and retina, formerly associated with night blindness. **a. cu′tis, a. cu′tis idiopath′ica,** atrophoderma. **a. cu′tis seni′lis,** senile atrophy of the skin. **a. doloro′sa,** atrophy of the eyeball accompanied by violent attacks of pain. **a. infan′tum** (*obs.*), tabes mesenterica. **a. maculo′sa cu′tis** (Jadassohn), anetoderma. **a. mesenter′ica** (*obs.*), tabes mesenterica. **a. musculo′rum lipomato′sa,** pseudohypertrophic muscular dystrophy. **a. pilo′rum pro′pria,** atrophy of the hair. **a. seni′lis,** atrophy accompanying old age. **a. stria′ta et maculo′sa,** cutaneous atrophy occurring in white, shining, depressed lines or spots. **a. testic′uli,** wasting of the testis. **a. un′guium,** atrophy of the nails.

atrophic (ah-trof′ik) pertaining to or characterized by atrophy.

atrophie (at″ro-fe) [Fr.] atrophy. **a. blanche** (blahnsh) [Fr. "white atrophy"], a condition marked by areas of atrophy, sometimes with painful and tender ulceration, and vesicular, bullous, or hemorrhagic lesions, eventuating in characteristic whitened plaques, usually on legs and ankles, of middle-aged or older women, with varicosities and associated cutaneous changes. **a. noir** (nwahr) [Fr. "black atrophy"], a condition characterized by ulcers surrounded by areas of blue-black pigmentation on the ankles, the pigmentation occurring after recurrent attacks of dermatitis with ulceration.

atrophied (at′ro-fēd) marked by atrophy; shrunken.

atrophoderma (at″ro-fo-der′mah) [Gr. *atrophia* want of nourishment + *derma* skin] atrophy of the skin or of any part of it; called also *atrophia cutis.* **a. biotrip′ticum,** senile atrophy of the skin. **a. diffu′sum** (*obs.*), acrodermatitis chronica atrophicans. **idiopathic a. of Pasini and Pierini,** a condition observed in youths and young adults, affecting chiefly the trunk and back, with variously sized pale, bluish, violaceous, or brownish blue depressions, histologically there is edema of collagen bundles of the deep part of the cutis, with loss of elastic tissue in this area. **a. macula′tum,** a condition characterized by atrophic changes in the skin and the formation of macules which gradually fade, leaving shiny white depressed spots; it may occur as a primary condition or be secondary to other diseases. **a.**

neurit′icum, a painful condition of the skin resulting from injury to the nerves, characterized by profuse perspiration and smooth, glossy, pink, ruddy, or blotched appearance. **a. pigmento′sum** (*obs.*), xeroderma pigmentosum. **a. reticula′tum symmet′ricum facie′i** (*obs.*), folliculitis ulerythematosa reticulata. **a. seni′le** (*obs.*), a weatherbeaten condition of the skin common in the aged, with dyspigmentation, telangiectasia, loss of elasticity, and dryness with fine scaling. **a. vermicula′re** (*obs.*), folliculitis ulerythematosa reticulata.

atrophodermatosis (at-ro″fo-der-mah-to′sis) any skin disease having cutaneous atrophy as a prominent symptom.

atrophy (at′ro-fe) [L., Gr. *atrophia*] 1. a wasting away; a diminution in the size of a cell, tissue, organ, or part. See also *atrophia* and *atrophie.* 2. to undergo atrophy, or to cause atrophy. **acute yellow a.,** a pathological term describing the shrunken, yellow liver of patients who have suffered from fulminant hepatitis with massive necrosis of the liver. It is an uncommon, usually fatal complication of viral hepatitis, or it may be due to toxic hepatitis, as that resulting from ingestion of carbon tetrachloride, fluorinated hydrocarbons, or *Amanita phalloides.* Called also *acute parenchymatous hepatitis, Budd's jaundice, malignant jaundice, massive hepatic necrosis,* and *Rokitansky's disease.* See also *postnecrotic cirrhosis,* under *cirrhosis* and *fulminant hepatitis,* under *hepatitis.* **Aran-Duchenne muscular a.,** spinal muscular a. **arthritic a.,** wasting of the muscles and bone that surround a joint, due to injury or to constitutional disease. **black a.,** atrophie noir. **blue a.,** a blue pigmentation that sometimes follows self-injection of drugs by individuals addicted to their use. **bone a.,** resorption of bone evident both in external form and in internal density. Cf. *osteoporosis.* **brown a.,** atrophy in which the affected viscus assumes a brownish hue, due to intracellular accumulation of lipofuscin; it is seen chiefly in the heart, liver, and spleen of the aged. **Buchwald's a.** (*obs.*), progressive atrophy of the skin. **Charcot-Marie a., Charcot-Marie-Tooth a.,** a progressive neuropathic (peroneal) muscular a. **circumscribed a. of brain,** lobar a. **compensatory a.,** atrophy, particularly of an endocrine organ, following excessive exogenous supply of its normal secretion or excessive secretion by its paired organ. **compression a.,** atrophy of a part due to constant pressure. **concentric a.,** atrophy of a hollow organ in which its cavity is contracted. **convolutional a.,** lobar a. **correlated a.,** the wasting of a part following the destruction or removal of a correlated part. **corticostriatospinal a.,** Creutzfeldt-Jakob syndrome. **Cruveilhier's a.,** spinal muscular atrophy. **degenerative a.,** the wasting of a part due to a degeneration of its cells. **Dejerine-Sottas type of a.,** progressive hypertrophic interstitial neuropathy. **Dejerine-Thomas a.,** olivopontocerebellar a. **denervated muscle a.,** muscular atrophy resulting from severance of the motor nerve supplying the muscle. **dental a.** (*obs.*), erosion of the teeth. **a. of disuse,** wasting caused by lack of normal exercise of a part. **Duchenne-Aran muscular a.,** spinal muscular a. **eccentric a.,** atrophy of a hollow organ in which the size of the cavity is increased. **Eichhorst's a.,** the femorotibial form of progressive muscular atrophy with contraction of the toes; called also *Eichhorst's type.* **endocrine a.,** atrophy in organs that are dependent upon endocrine stimulation for the maintenance of their normal structure, occurring when their tropic hormone stimulation diminishes or is absent. **endometrial a.,** atrophy of the endometrium occurring physiologically at menopause or pathologically before menopause, and accompanied by absence of menstrual flow and shrinkage of the uterus. **Erb's a.,** pseudohypertrophic muscular dystrophy. **exhaustion a.,** atrophy of an endocrine organ caused by prolonged overwork of that organ. **facial a.,** progressive unilateral facial a. **facioscapulohumeral muscular a.,** Landouzy-Dejerine dystrophy. **familial spinal muscular a.,** Werdnig-Hoffmann paralysis. **fat replacement a.,** the destruction of subcutaneous fat and its replacement by inflammatory cells, as in erythema induratum; called also *wucher a.* **fatty a.,** fatty infiltration following atrophy of the tissue elements of a part; called also *adipositas ex vacuo.* **Fazio-Londe a.,** progressive bulbar paralysis in children; see *bulbar paralysis,* under *paralysis.* **Fuchs' a.,** peripheral atrophy of the optic nerve. **gastric a.,** a condition in which the thickness of the mucosa of the stomach is greatly reduced, with complete or almost complete disappearance of the gastric and pyloric glands and their replacement by simple mucus-secreting epithelium and by extensive intestinal metaplasia. **granular a. of kidney,** chronic interstitial inflammation of the kidney producing compression and atrophy of the parenchyma. **gray a.,** secondary optic a. **gyrate a. of choroid and retina,** a rare, hereditary, slowly progressive atrophy of the choroid and pigment epithelium of the retina marked by ring-shaped areas of thinning in the periphery of the fundus which enlarge and become confluent, resulting in tunnel vision; night blindness and other disturbances of vision follow. It is inherited as an autosomal recessive trait. **healed yellow a.,** postnecrotic cirrhosis. **hemifacial a.,** atrophy of one side of the face. **hemilingual a.,** atrophy of one side of the tongue. **Hoffmann's a.,** Werdnig-Hoffmann paralysis. **Hunt's a.,** neuropathic atrophy of the small muscles of the hand unattended by sensory disturbance. **idiopathic muscular a.,** progressive muscular dystrophy. **infantile a.,** marasmus. **inflammatory a.,** atrophy of the functioning part of an organ caused by overgrowth of the fibrous elements from inflammation. **interstitial a.,** absorption of the mineral matter of bones, so that only the reticulated portion remains. **a. of iris, essential,** a progressive disease of unknown etiology, marked by patchy degeneration and disappearance of the iris stroma followed by loss of epithelium and formation of holes in the iris; it is associated with severe glaucoma. **ischemic muscular a.,** Volkmann's contracture. **Jadassohn's macular a.,** see *anetoderma.* **juvenile muscular a.,** pseudohypertrophic muscular dystrophy. **lactation a.,** hyperinvolution of the uterus which may follow prolonged lactation. **Landouzy-Dejerine a.,** Landouzy-Dejerine dystrophy. **leaping a.,** progressive muscular atrophy beginning in the hand and extending to the shoulder without affecting the muscles of the arm. **Leber's optic a.,** a hereditary disorder of males characterized by bilateral progressive optic atrophy, with onset usually at about the age of twenty. It is thought to be an X-linked trait. **linear a.,** atrophy of the papillary layer of the skin, causing the appearance of blue and white lines. **lobar a.,** progressive atrophy of the cerebral convolutions in a limited area (lobe) of the brain, marked by progressive degeneration of the higher faculties and by the gradual development of aphasia; called also *circumscribed a. of brain* and (*Pick's*) *convolutional a.* **macular a.,** anetoderma. **muscular a.,** a wasting of muscle tissue; there are many kinds and causes. See also *spinal muscular a.* **myelopathic muscular a.,** muscular atrophy due to lesion of the spinal cord, as in spinal muscular atrophy. **myopathic a.,** muscular atrophy due to disease of the muscle tissue. **neural a.,** neuropathic a. **neuritic muscular a.,** neuropathic a. **neuropathic a.,** atrophy of muscular tissue due to disease of the peripheral nervous system; called also *neural a.* **neurotic a.,** neuropathic a. **neurotrophic a.,** atrophy attributed to destruction of the peripheral neurons that maintain the nutrition of a tissue. **numeric a.,** atrophy due to diminution in the number of the constituent elements of a tissue, as well as skrinkage of those that remain. **olivopontocerebellar a.,** atrophy affecting the cerebellar cortex, the middle peduncles, and the inferior olivary bodies. **optic a.,** atrophy of the optic disk resulting from degeneration of the nerve fibers of the optic nerve and optic tract. **optic a., primary,** a form in which the optic disk is characterized by sharp margins, enlarged physiologic cup, enhanced visibility of the lamina cribrosa, and a white color. **optic a., secondary,** a form in which the optic disk is characterized by blurred margins, poor visibility of the lamina cribrosa, filling-in of the physiologic cup, and gray-white glial tissue on its surface and along its blood vessels; called also *gray a.* **pallidal a.,** juvenile paralysis agitans (of Hunt); see under *paralysis.* **Parrot's a. of the newborn,** primary infantile atrophy or marasmus. **pathologic a.,** a decrease in the size of tissues or organs beyond the range of normal variability. **peroneal a.,** progressive neuropathic (peroneal) muscular a. **physiologic a.,** atrophy which affects certain organs in all individuals as part of the normal aging process. **Pick's convolutional a.,** lobar sclerosis. **pigmentary a.,** wasting marked by the deposit of pigment in the atrophied cells. **postmenopausal a.,** atrophy of various tissues, such as the genital mucosa, occurring after menopause. **post-traumatic a. of bone,** post-traumatic osteoporosis. **pressure a.,** decrease in the size of a tissue cell caused by excessive pressure. **progressive choroidal a.,** choroideremia. **progressive muscular a.,** spinal muscular a. **progressive neural muscular a., progressive neuromuscular a.,** progressive neuropathic (peroneal) muscular a. **progressive neuropathic (peroneal) muscular a.,** a hereditary form of muscular atrophy, beginning in the muscles supplied by the peroneal nerves, progressing slowly to involve the muscles of the hands and arms. Called also *peroneal a., Charcot-Marie-Tooth a.* or *disease, Charcot-Marie type, Tooth type,* and *progressive neural muscular (neuromuscular) a.* **progressive spinal muscular a.,** spinal muscular a. **progressive unilateral facial a.,** an affection attended by progressive wasting of the skin, tissues, and bone, often of the muscles of one side of the face. **pseudohypertrophic muscular a.,** pseudohypertrophic muscular dystrophy. **pulp a.,** a degenerative state of the dental pulp characterized by a decrease of cellular elements. **receptoric a.,** a condition assumed to be due to atrophy of the cell receptors; animals kept immune by repeated injections of an antigen sometimes cease to respond by the formation of antibodies. **red a.,** atrophy, mainly of the liver, due to chronic congestion from valvular heart disease. **reversionary a.,** anaplasia. **rheumatic a.,** atrophy of muscles after an attack of rheumatism. **Schweninger-Buzzi macular a.,** see *anetoderma.* **senile a.,** the normal atrophy of old age. **serous a.,** atrophy with the effusion of a serous fluid into the wasted tissues; wasting of fat. **simple a.,** atrophy due to a shrinkage in size of individual cells. **spinal muscular a.,** a progressive degenerative disease of the motor cells of spinal cord. Beginning usually in the small muscles of the hands, but in some cases (scapulohumeral type) in those of the upper arm and shoulder, the atrophy progresses slowly to the muscles of the lower extremity. Called

also *Aran-Duchenne muscular a., Aran-Duchenne disease, Duchenne-Aran muscular a., Duchenne-Aran disease, Cruveilhier's disease, Duchenne's disease,* and *progressive spinal muscular a.* **subacute yellow a.,** submassive necrosis of the liver associated with broad zones of necrosis, due to viral, toxic, or drug-induced hepatitis; it may have an acute course with death occurring after several weeks of liver failure, or clinical recovery may be associated with regeneration of the parenchymal cells. **Sudeck's a.,** posttraumatic osteoporosis. **Tooth's a.,** progressive neuropathic (peroneal) muscular atrophy. **toxic a.,** atrophy of an organ in the course of infectious diseases. **trophoneurotic a.,** atrophy due to disease of the nerves or of a center supplying a part. **unilateral facial a.,** progressive unilateral facial a. **vascular a.,** progressive loss of substance in cells and organs when the blood supply to that organ or tissue becomes reduced below a critical level. **von Leber's a.,** Leber's optic a. **Vulpian's a.,** scapulohumeral type of spinal muscular atrophy. **Werdnig-Hoffmann a.,** see under *paralysis.* **white a.,** 1. atrophy of a nerve, leaving only white connective tissue. 2. atrophie blanche. **wucher a.,** fat replacement a. **yellow a.,** acute yellow a. **Zimmerlin's a.,** a hereditary form of progressive muscular atrophy, beginning in the upper part of the body; called also *Zimmerlin's type.*

atropine (at′ro-pēn) [USP] chemical name: *endo*-(+)-α-(hydroxymethyl)benzeneacetic acid 8-methyl-8-azabicyclo[3.2.1]oct-3-yl ester. An alkaloid, $C_{17}H_{23}NO_3$, derived from species of belladonna, hyoscyamus, or strammonium, or produced synthetically, and occurring as white crystals, usually needle-like, or as a white, crystalline powder. Atropine is an anticholinergic and is used chiefly as an antispasmodic to relax smooth muscles; to relieve the tremor and rigidity of parkinsonism; to increase the heart rate by blocking the vagus nerve; as an antidote for various toxic and anticholinesterase agents; and as an antisecretory, mydriatic, and cycloplegic. **a. methonitrate, a. methylnitrate,** methylatropine nitrate. **a. oxide hydrochloride,** a salt of atropine, having the same actions as atropine. **a. sulfate** [USP], colorless crystals or white, crystalline powder, $(C_{17}H_{23}NO_3)_2 \cdot H_2SO_4 \cdot H_2O$, having the same actions as the base; administered parenterally and orally as an anticholinergic, intravenously as a cholinesterase inhibitor, and applied topically to the conjunctiva as a cycloplegic and mydriatic.

atropinic (at″ro-pin′ik) having actions similar to atropine, that is, antagonizing the muscarinic effects of acetylcholine.

atropinism (at′ro-pin-izm) poisoning caused by ingestion of atropine or belladonna or parts or preparations of any of the plants from which the drugs are derived; the symptoms include excessive dryness of the mouth and throat, dilation of the pupils, fever, rapid pulse, flushing of the face, confusion, mania, and hallucinations, and sometimes a skin rash.

atropinization (at-ro″pin-i-za′shun) subjection to the influence of atropine.

atropism (at′ro-pizm) atropinism.

Atropisol (at′ro-pĭ-sol) trademark for preparations of atropine sulfate.

A.T.S antitetanic serum (tetanus antitoxin); anxiety tension state.

attachment (ah-tach′ment) 1. the state of being fixed or attached. 2. the means or device by which something is fixed or stabilized. In dentistry, anything, as a clasp, retainer, or artificial crown, that is used to stabilize or to attach a partial denture to a natural tooth in the mouth. **epithelial a. (of Gottlieb),** the attachment of the oral epithelium (a continuation of the gingiva) to the tooth, forming a peripheral seal around the part of the tooth exposed to the oral cavity. **frictional a., internal a., key-and-keyway a., parallel a.,** precision a. **precision a.,** an attachment used in fixed and removable partial dentures, consisting of closely fitting male and female parts, the latter usually inserted in the crown of the abutment tooth; the denture is maintained precisely because of the friction or resistance between the parallel surfaces of the two parts forming the attachment. Called also *frictional a., internal a., key-and-keyway a., parallel a.,* and *slotted a.* **slotted a.,** precision a.

attack (ah-tak′) an episode or onset of illness. **transient ischemic a's,** brief attacks (from a few minutes to hours) of cerebral dysfunction of vascular origin, with no persistent neurological deficit; they are most commonly associated with occlusive vascular disease, especially in the distribution of the carotid and vertebral-basilar systems. **vagal a.,** vasovagal a. **vasovagal a.,** a transient vascular and neurogenic reaction marked by pallor, nausea, sweating, bradycardia, and rapid fall in arterial blood pressure which, when below a critical level, results in loss of consciousness and characteristic electroencephalographic changes. It is most often evoked by emotional stress associated with fear or pain. Called also *vasovagal* or *vasodepressor syncope,* and *Gower's syndrome.*

attar (at′ar) [Persian "essence"] any essential or volatile oil of vegetable origin. **a. of roses,** rose oil.

attention (ah-ten′shun) 1. selective awareness of a part or aspect of the environment. 2. selective responsiveness to one class of stimuli.

attenuant (ah-ten'u-ant) 1. causing thinness, as of the blood. 2. a medicine that thins the blood.

attenuate (ah-ten'u-āt) [L. *attenuare* to thin] 1. to render thin. 2. to render less virulent; see *attenuation*, def. 2.

attenuation (ah-ten''u-a'shun) [L. *attenuatio*, from *ad* to + *tenuis* thin] 1. the act of thinning or weakening. 2. the alteration of the virulence of a pathogenic microorganism by passage through another host species, decreasing the virulence of the organism for the native host and increasing it for the new host. 3. the process by which a beam of radiation is reduced in energy when passed through tissue or other material. Cf. *absorption*, def. 3.

Attenuvac (ah-ten'u-vak) trademark for a preparation of live attenuated measles virus vaccine.

attic (at'ik) [L. *atticus*] the superior part of the tympanic cavity, above the level of the tympanic membrane; called also *recessus epitympanicus* [NA], *epitympanum*, and *attic of middle ear*.

atticitis (at''i-ki'tis) inflammation of the attic.

atticoantrotomy (at''i-ko-an-trot'o-me) the operation of opening the mastoid antrum and the attic of the middle ear; called also *antroatticotomy*.

atticomastoid (at''i-ko-mas'toid) pertaining to the attic and the mastoid process of the temporal bone.

atticotomy (at''i-kot'o-me) [*attic* + Gr. *temnein* to cut] the surgical opening of the attic. **transmeatal a.,** removal through the external auditory meatus of the outer wall of the attic.

attitude (at'i-tūd) [L. *attitudo* posture] 1. a posture or position of the body. In obstetrics, the relation of the various parts of the fetal body to one another, the normal attitude being one of moderate flexion of all the joints, with the back curved forward, the head slightly bent on the chest, and the arms and legs free to move in all natural directions (habitus). 2. a tendency to respond positively or negatively to other individuals, institutions, or programs of activity. **a. of combat** [Fr. *attitude de combat*], the stiff defensive position of the corpse of one burned to death in a conflagration. **crucifixion a.,** rigidity of the body, with the arms extended at right angles; seen in hysteroepilepsy and in catatonia. **deflexion a.,** the condition early in labor in which the fetal head lies over the pelvic inlet, the large fontanel is lower than the small one or is even with the root of the nose, and the eyes are palpable. **Devergie's a.,** the posture of a dead body marked by flexed elbows and knees and with closed fingers and extended ankles. **discobolus a.,** a position resembling that of a discus thrower, caused by stimulation of the semicircular canals. **forced a.,** an abnormal position or attitude due to some disease, such as is seen in meningitis or as the result of contractures. **illogical a's,** the strange and grotesque attitudes assumed by those suffering from hysteroepilepsy. **a. passionnelle, passionate a.,** the dramatic or theatrical expression or gesture often assumed by hysterical patients. **stereotyped a.,** an attitude assumed and maintained for a long time, a phenomenon often seen in mental disease.

atto- [Danish *atten* eighteen] a prefix signifying one quintillionth, or 10^{-18}.

attollens (ah-tol'enz) [L.] lifting up. **a. au'rem** (*obs.*), musculus auricularis superior.

attractant (ah-trak'tant) [L. *attrahere* to draw toward] a substance that exerts an attracting influence, such as one used to attract insect or animal pests to traps or to poisons.

attraction (ah-trak'shun) [L. *attractio*] 1. the force, act, or process that draws one body toward another. 2. in dentistry and anthropology, malocclusion in which the occlusal plane is closer than normal to the eye-ear plane; it causes shortening of the face. Cf. *abstraction*, def. 3. **a. of affinity,** chemical a. **capillary a.,** the force that attracts the particles of a fluid into and along the caliber of a tube. **chemical a.,** the tendency of atoms of one element to unite with those of another; called also *a. of affinity*. **electric a.,** the tendency of bodies bearing opposite electric charges to move toward each other. **magnetic a.,** the tendency of bodies possessing circulating electric currents to move toward each other.

attrahens (at'rah-henz) [L.] drawing toward. **a. au'rem** (*obs.*), musculus auricularis anterior.

attraxin (ah-trak'sin) Fischer's name for supposed specific bodies existing in solutions which, when the solution is injected into the tissues, exert a chemotactic influence on the epithelial cells.

attrition (ah-trish'un) [L. *attritio* a rubbing against] the physiologic wearing away of a substance or structure (such as the teeth) in the course of normal use.

at. vol. atomic volume.

At. wt. atomic weight.

atypia (a-tip'e-ah) the condition of being irregular or not conforming to type.

atypical (a-tip'i-kal) [*a* neg. + Gr. *typos* type or model] irregular; not conformable to the type; in microbiology, applied specifically to strains of unusual type.

atypism (a-tip'izm) atypia.

A. U. Angström unit; aures unitas (both ears together) or auris uterque (each ear).

Au chemical symbol for *gold* (L. *au'rum*); abbreviation for Australian antigen (see under *antigen*).

Au-antigenemia (an''ti-je-ne''me-ah) the presence of Australian antigen in the blood.

Aub-Dubois table (awb-doo-bois') [Joseph Charles *Aub*, Boston physician, born 1890; Eugene Floyd *Dubois*, New York physician, 1882–1953] see under *table*.

Aubert's phenomenon (o-bārz') [Hermann *Aubert*, German physiologist, 1826–1892] see under *phenomenon*.

Auchmeromyia (awk''mer-o-mi'yah) a genus of flies of the family Calliphoridae. **A. lute'ola,** a fly of the Congo and Nigeria having a blood-sucking larva known as the Congo floor maggot; called also *Musca luteola*.

audile (aw'dil) pertaining to hearing; a term applied to that type of mentality which recalls most easily that which has been heard.

audioanalgesia (aw''de-o-an''al-je'ze-ah) alleged reduction or abolition of pain accomplished by listening, through a stereophonic head set, to recorded music to which may be added a background sound, so-called "white noise."

audiogenic (aw''de-o-jen'ik) produced by sound.

audiogram (aw'de-o-gram'') [L. *audire* to hear + Gr. *gramma* a writing] a record of the thresholds of hearing of an individual for various sound frequencies. **cortical a.,** a graphic representation of the result of cortical audiometry.

audiologist (aw''de-ol'o-jist) a person skilled in audiology, including the rehabilitation of those whose impaired hearing cannot be improved by medical or surgical means.

audiology (aw''de-ol'o-je) [L. *audire* to hear + *-logy*] the science of hearing, particularly the study of impaired hearing that cannot be improved by medication or surgical therapy.

audiometer (aw''de-om'ĕ-ter) [L. *audire* to hear + Gr. *metron* measure] an electronic device that produces acoustic stimuli of known frequency and intensity for the measurement of hearing. **evoked response a.,** an instrument that detects response to sound stimuli by changes in the electroencephalogram.

audiometric (aw''de-o-met'rik) pertaining to the measurement of hearing, as by means of an audiometer.

audiometrician (aw''de-o-mĕ-trish'an) a technician specializing in the measurement of hearing ability (audiometry).

audiometry (aw''de-om'ĕ-tre) measurement of hearing, as by means of an audiometer. **Békésy a.,** audiometry in which the patient, by pressing a signal button, traces his monaural thresholds for pure tones: the intensity of the tone decreases as long as the button is depressed and increases when it is released. Both continuous and interrupted tones are used. **cortical a.,** an objective method of determining auditory acuity by recording and averaging electric potentials evoked from the cortex of the brain in response to stimulation by pure tones. **electrocochleographic a.,** measurement of electrical potentials from the middle ear or external auditory canal (cochlear microphonics and eighth nerve action potentials) in response to acoustic stimuli. **electrodermal a.,** audiometry in which the subject is conditioned by harmless electric shock to pure tones; thereafter he anticipates a shock when he hears a pure tone, the anticipation resulting in a brief electrodermal response, which is recorded. The lowest intensity at which the response is elicited is taken to be his hearing threshold. **localization a.,** a technique for measuring the capacity to locate the source of a pure tone received binaurally in a sound field. **pure tone a.,** audiometry utilizing pure tones that are relatively free of noise and overtones. **speech a.,** that in which the threshold of speech perception (speech reception threshold) in decibels and the ability to understand speech (speech discrimination) are measured.

audiovisual (aw''de-o-vizh'u-al) simultaneously stimulating, or pertaining to simultaneous stimulation of, the senses of both hearing and sight.

audition (aw-dish'un) [L. *auditio*] the act of hearing; ability to hear. **chromatic a., a. colorée,** a sensation of color produced by sound; a variety of chromesthesia. **gustatory a.,** a condition in which certain sounds call up a sensation of taste.

auditive (aw'di-tiv) a person in whom the prime sense is hearing.

auditognosis (aw''di-tog-no'sis) [L. *auditio* hearing + Gr. *gnōsis* knowledge] the sense by which sounds are understood and interpreted.

auditory (aw'di-to''re) [L. *auditorius*] pertaining to the sense of hearing.

Audouin's microsporon (ow-doo-anz') [Jean-Victor *Audouin*, Parisian physician, 1797–1841] *Microsporum audouini*.

Auenbrugger's sign (ow-en-broog'erz) [Leopold Elder von *Auenbrugger*, Austrian physician, 1722–1809] see under *sign*.

Auer's bodies (ow'erz) [John *Auer*, American physician, 1875–1948] see under *body*.

Auerbach's ganglion, plexus (ow'er-bahks) [Leopold *Auerbach*, German anatomist, 1828–1897] see under *ganglion*, and see *plexus myentericus*.

Aufrecht's sign (owf′rekhts) [Emanual *Aufrecht*, German physician, 1844–1933] see under *sign*.

augmentor (awg-men′tor) 1. increasing; a term applied to nerves or nerve cells concerned in increasing the size and force of heart contractions. 2. a substance supposed to increase the action of an auxetic.

augnathus (awg-na′thus) [Gr. *au* again + *gnathos* jaw] a monster with a double lower jaw.

Aujeszky's disease (aw-jes′kēz) [Aladár *Aujeszky*, Hungarian physician, 1869–1933] pseudorabies.

aula (aw′lah) [L.; Gr. *aulē* hall] 1. (*obs.*) the anterior end of the third ventricle of the cerebrum. 2. the red erythematous areola formed about the periphery of the vesicle of the vaccination lesion.

auliplexus (aw-lĕ-plek′sus) [*aula* + *plexus*] (*obs.*) a part of the choroid plexus within the aula (def. 1).

aulix (aw′liks) [L. "furrow"] (*obs.*) sulcus hypothalamicus.

aura (aw′rah), pl. *au′rae* [L. "breath"] a subjective sensation or motor phenomenon that precedes and marks the onset of a paroxysmal attack, such as an epileptic attack (Galen). **a. asthmat′ica,** premonitory symptoms preceding an attack of bronchial asthma. **auditory a.,** an auditory sensation that sometimes precedes an attack of epilepsy. **electric a.,** a breezy sensation experienced on the receipt of a discharge of static electricity. **epigastric a.,** an uncomfortable sensation in the epigastrium that sometimes precedes an epileptic attack. **epileptic a.,** a sensation that sometimes gives warning of an approaching attack of epilepsy. **a. hyster′ica,** an aura like that preceding an epileptic attack sometimes experienced by hysterical patients. **intellectual a.,** a dreamy condition that sometimes precedes an attack of epilepsy; called also *reminiscent a.* **kinesthetic a.,** a sensation of movement of some part of the body, with or without such actual movement. **motor a.,** movement that precedes an epileptic attack. **a. procursi′va,** a spell of running that precedes an epileptic attack. **reminiscent a.,** intellectual a. **a. vertigino′sa,** a sudden attack of vertigo.

aural (aw′ral) [L. *auralis*] 1. pertaining to or perceived by the ear, as an aural stimulus. 2. pertaining to or of the nature of an aura.

auranofin (aw-rān′o-fin) chemical name: (2,3,4,6-tetra-*O*-acetyl-1-thio-β-D-glucopyranosato-*S*)(triethylphosphine)gold; an antirheumatic, $C_{20}H_{34}AuO_9PS$.

aurantia (aw-ran′she-ah) an orange coal tar stain, the ammonium salt of hexanitrodiphenylamine, $C_6H_2(NO_2)_3 \cdot N:C_6H_2(NO_2)_2 \cdot N \cdot O \cdot O \cdot NH_4$; used in staining mitochondria.

aurantiamarin (aw-ran″te-am′ah-rin) a glycoside from orange peel.

aurantiasis (aw″ran-ti′ah-sis) [L. *aurantium* orange + *-iasis*] carotenemia.

Aurelia (aw-rel′ĭ-ah) a genus of large discophorous jellyfish found in Atlantic, Indian, and Pacific waters; nematocysts of many of the larger forms can penetrate the human skin and produce intense pain.

Aureobasidium (aw-re″o-bah-sid′ĭ-um) a genus of imperfect fungi of the family Dematiaceae, order Moniliales, which produce black yeastlike cells; called also *Pullularia*. **A. pul′lulans,** a common soil organism and contaminant; called also *Pullularia pullans*.

aureolin (aw-re′o-lin) a yellow dye.

Aureomycin (aw″re-o-mi′sin) trademark for preparations of crystalline chlortetracycline hydrochloride.

aures (aw′rēz) [L.] plural of *auris*.

auriasis (aw-ri′ah-sis) chrysiasis.

auric (aw′rik) pertaining to or containing gold.

auricle (aw′rĕ-kl) [L. *auricula* a little ear] 1. the portion of the external ear not contained within the head; the pinna, or flap of the ear. Called also *auricula*. 2. auricula atrii. The term *auricle* was formerly used to designate an atrium of the heart. **cervical a.,** a flap of skin and yellow cartilage sometimes seen on the side of the neck at the external opening of a persistent branchial cleft. **left a. of heart,** auricula atrii sinistri. **right a. of heart,** auricula atrii dextri.

auricula (aw-rik′u-lah), pl. *auric′ulae* [L., dim. of *auris*] a little ear; the NA term for the portion of the external ear not contained within the head; the pinna, or flap of the ear. Called also *ala auris* and *auricle*. Applied also to the ear-shaped appendage of either atrium of the heart (*auricula atrii*), and formerly used as a synonym for the atrium (*atrium cordis*). **a. a′trii** [NA], the ear-shaped appendage of either atrium of the heart; called also *atrial appendage*. **a. a′trii dex′tri** [NA], the ear-shaped appendage of the right atrium of the heart. **a. a′trii sinis′tri** [NA], the ear-shaped appendage of the left atrium of the heart. **a. cor′dis,** a. atrii. **a. dex′tra cor′dis,** a. atrii dextri. **a. sinis′tra cor′dis,** a. atrii sinistri.

auriculae (aw-rik′u-le) [L.] plural of *auricula*.

auricular (aw-rik′u-lar) [L. *auricularis*] pertaining to an auricle or to the ear, and, formerly, to an atrium of the heart.

auriculare (aw-rik″u-la′re) [L. *auricularis* pertaining to the ear] a craniometric point at the top of the opening of the external auditory meatus.

auricularis (aw″rik-u-la′ris) [L.] pertaining to the ear; auricular.

auriculocranial (aw-rik″u-lo-kra′ne-al) pertaining to an ear and the cranium.

auriculotemporal (aw-rik″u-lo-tem′pŏ-ral) pertaining to an ear and the temporal region.

auriculoventricular (aw-rik″u-lo-ven-trik′u-lar) a former term for atrioventricular.

aurid (aw′rid) [L. *aurum* gold] a skin eruption produced by the systemic administration of gold salts.

auriform (aw′rĭ-form) ear-shaped.

aurin (aw′rin) chemical name: 4-[bis(*p*-hydroxyphenyl)methylene]-2,5-cyclohexdien-1-one. A triphenylmethane derivative, $C_{19}H_{14}O_3$, occurring as deep red masses with a greenish metallic luster; used as an indicator and dye intermediate. Called also *pararosolic acid, rosolic acid,* and *corallin.*

aurinarium (aw″ri-na′re-um) a medicated suppository for insertion onto the external auditory meatus.

aurinasal (aw″rĭ-na′zal) pertaining to the ear and the nose.

auriphone (aw′rĭ-fōn) [L. *auris* ear + Gr. *phonē* voice] a form of ear trumpet in which the sound conveyed is amplified.

auripigment (aw″rĭ-pig′ment) arsenic trisulfide.

auris (aw′ris), pl. *au′res* [L.] [NA] the ear; the organ of hearing. See Plate XVI. **a. exter′na** [NA], external ear: the portion of the auditory organ comprising the auricle and the external acoustic meatus. **a. inter′na** [NA], internal ear: the labyrinth, comprising the vestibule, cochlea, and semicircular canals; called also *inner ear.* **a. me′dia** [NA], middle ear: it includes the space medial to the tympanic membrane (mesotympanum), the epitympanum, and the hypotympanum, and it contains the auditory ossicles and connects with the mastoid cells and auditory tube. Called also *cavum tympani* [NA alternative], *eardrum, tympanic cavity,* and *tympanum.*

auriscalpium (aw″rĭ-skal′pe-um) [L. *auris* ear + *scalpere* to scrape] an instrument for scooping or scraping foreign matter from the ear.

auriscope (aw′rĭ-skōp) [L. *auris* ear + Gr. *skopein* to examine] a form of otoscope.

aurist (aw′rist) a specialist in ear diseases.

auristics (aw-ris′tiks) [L. *auris* ear] the art of treating diseases of the ear.

aurochromoderma (aw″ro-kro″mo-der′mah) [L. *aurum* gold + Gr. *chrōma* color + Gr. *derma* skin] a permanent greenish-blue staining of the skin due to injection of certain gold compounds.

aurotherapy (aw″ro-ther′ah-pe) [L. *aurum* gold + *therapy*] the use of gold in the treatment of disease; chrysotherapy.

aurothioglucose (aw″ro-thi″o-gloo′kōs) [USP] chemical name: (1-thio-D-glucopyranosato)gold. A gold preparation, $C_6H_{11}AuO_5S$, occurring as a yellow powder, used in the treatment of rheumatoid arthritis; it is also used in nondisseminated lupus erythematosus. Administered intramuscularly. Called also *gold thioglucose.*

aurothiomalate disodium (aw″ro-thi″o-ma′lāt) gold sodium thiomalate.

aurum (aw′rum) [L.] gold.

auscult (aws-kult′) auscultate.

auscultate (aws′kul-tāt) [L. *auscultare* to listen to] to examine by listening, usually to the sounds of the thoracic or abdominal viscera, with or without a stethoscope.

auscultation (aws″kul-ta′shun) the act of listening for sounds within the body, chiefly for ascertaining the condition of the lungs, heart, pleura, abdomen and other organs, and for the detection of pregnancy. **direct a., immediate a.,** auscultation performed without the stethoscope. **Korányi's a.,** auscultatory percussion done by tapping with one forefinger the second joint of the other forefinger applied perpendicularly to the part; called also *Korányi's percussion.* **mediate a.** (Laennec, 1819), auscultation performed by the aid of an instrument (stethoscope) interposed between the ear and the part being examined. **obstetric a.,** auscultation in pregnancy for the study of the sounds of the fetal heart.

auscultatory (aws-kul′tah-to″re) of or pertaining to auscultation.

auscultoplectrum (aws-kul″to-plek′trum) an instrument for use both in auscultation and percussion.

auscultoscope (aws-kul′to-skōp) phonendoscope.

Austin Flint murmur, respiration (aws′tin flint) [*Austin Flint*, American physiologist, 1812–1886] see *Flint's murmur,* under *murmur,* and *cavernous respiration,* under *respiration.*

Australorbis (aws″trah-lor′bis) *Biomphalaria.*

aut- see *auto-.*

autacoid (aw′tah-koid) [*aut-* + Gr. *akos* remedy] a term once proposed to replace the term *hormone* and recently suggested as a general term for various physiologically active, endogenous substances (histamine, serotonin, angiotensin, prostaglandins, etc.) that do not yet fit into existing functional classifications.

autesthetic (awt″es-thet′ik) [*auto-* + *esthetic*] pertaining to an activity (e.g., play or pair-ritual) that rewards the performer as much as other individuals.

autacoid (aw′tah-koid) [*aut-* + Gr. *akos* remedy] an organic substance formed by the cells of one organ and carried through the circulatory fluid to other organs upon which the substance acts. **chalonic a.,** a chalone. **duodenal a.,** secretin. **excitatory a.,** a hormone. **hormonic a.,** a hormone. **inhibitory a., restraining a.,** a chalone.

autarcesiology (awt″ar-se″se-ol′o-je) [*autarcesis* + *-logy*] the branch of immunology that has to do with autarcesis.

autarcesis (awt-ar-se′sis) [*aut-* + Gr. *arkein* to ward off] the power to resist infection by the normal activity of the body cells as distinguished from immunity of the antibody type.

autarcetic (awt-ar-set′ik) pertaining to autarcesis.

autechoscope (aw-tek′o-skōp) [*aut-* + Gr. *ēchos* sound + Gr. *skopein* to examine] an instrument for auscultating one's own body.

autecic (aw-te′sik) autoecious.

autecious (aw-te′shus) autoecious.

autecology (aw″te-kol′o-je) [*aut-* + *ecology*] the ecology of an organism as an individual; cf. *synecology.*

autemesia (aw″tĕ-me′se-ah) [*aut-* + Gr. *emesis* vomiting] functional or idiopathic vomiting.

autism (aw′tizm) [Gr. *autos* self + *-ism*] the condition of being dominated by subjective, self-centered trends of thought or behavior; it may occur in adults or children (see *early infantile a.*). Called also *autistic thinking.* **akinetic a.,** coma vigil. **early infantile a., infantile a.,** a severe disorder of communication and behavior, usually beginning at birth, invariably present by age three; it is characterized by self-absorption, profound withdrawal from contact with people, including the mother figure, a desire for sameness, preoccupation with inanimate objects, and developmental language disorders. Called also *Kanner's syndrome.*

autistic (aw-tis′tik) self-centered; sufficient unto itself.

auto-, aut- [Gr. *autos* self] a prefix denoting relationship to self.

autoactivation (aw″to-ak″te-va′shun) the activation of a gland by its own secretion.

autoagglutination (aw″to-ah-gloo″tĭ-na′shun) 1. clumping or agglutination of an individual's cells by his own serum, as in autohemagglutination. Autoagglutination occurring at low temperatures is called cold agglutination (see under *agglutination*). 2. agglutination of particulate antigens, e.g., bacteria, in the absence of specific antigens.

autoagglutinin (aw″to-ah-gloo″tĭ-nin) an autologous serum factor with the property of agglutinating the individual's own cellular elements: e.g., the red cells (autoagglutinin) and platelets (platelet autoagglutinin). An autoagglutinin that functions at low temperatures is called a cold agglutinin (see under *agglutinin*).

autoallergic (aw′to-ah-ler′jik) pertaining to or characterized by autoallergy.

autoallergy (aw″to-al′er-je) autoimmunity.

autoamputation (aw″to-am″pu-ta′shun) the spontaneous detachment from the body and elimination of an appendage or of an abnormal growth, such as a polyp.

autoanalysis (aw″to-ah-nal′ĭ-sis) the analysis and interpretation, on the part of a neurotic patient, of the state of mind underlying his disorder; employed as a means of treatment.

autoanamnesis (aw″to-an″am-ne′sis) a history obtained from the patient himself.

autoanaphylaxis (aw″to-an″ah-fĭ-lak′sis) anaphylaxis from reactions within the body independent of the introduction of substances from without and induced by substances derived from the individual himself; anaphylaxis induced by serum or other substances from the individual himself.

autoantibody (aw″to-an′tĭ-bod″e) an antibody (immunoglobulin) formed in response to, and reacting against, one of the individual's own normal antigenic endogenous body constituents.

autoanticomplement (aw″to-an″tĭ-kom′ple-ment) an anticomplement formed in the body against its own complement.

autoantigen (aw″to-an′tĭ-jen) a tissue constituent that is immunogenic in the animal in which it occurs; it stimulates the production of autoantibody in the tissues of the organism in which it occurs.

autoantisepsis (aw″to-an″tĭ-sep′sis) physiological antisepsis.

autoantitoxin (aw″to-an″tĭ-tok′sin) [*auto-* + *antitoxin*] antitoxin produced by the tissues of the body to protect it from injury by the homologous toxin.

autoaudible (aw″to-aw′dĭ-bl) audible to one's self; said of heart sounds.

autobacteriophage (aw″to-bak-te′re-o-fāj) bacteriophage derived from the patient under treatment.

autobiotic (aw″to-bi-ot′ik) any of a group of substances produced by cells and controlling the behavior of the producing cells.

autoblast (aw″to-blast) an independent solitary bioblast; a microorganism.

autocatalysis (aw″to-kah-tal′ĭ-sis) a catalytic reaction that gradually accelerates in velocity because some of the products of the reaction themselves act as catalytic agents.

autocatalyst (aw″to-kat′ah-list) an element participating in autocatalysis.

autocatalytic (aw″to-kat-ah-lit′ik) pertaining to, characterized by, or producing autocatalysis.

autocatharsis (aw″to-kah-thar′sis) psychiatric treatment by encouraging the patient to write out his troubles and thus rid himself of his mental complexes.

autocatheterism (aw″to-kath′ĕ-ter-izm) [*auto-* + *catheterism*] the passage of the catheter by the patient himself.

autocerebrospinal (aw″to-ser″ĕ-bro-spi′nal) the patient's own cerebrospinal fluid used in treating epidemic meningitis.

autocholecystectomy (aw″to-ko″le-sis-tek′to-me) [*auto-* + *cholecystectomy*] invagination of the gallbladder into the intestine, with final separation and expulsion of the organ.

autochthonous (aw-tok′tho-nus) [Gr. *autochthōn* sprung from the land itself] 1. found in the place of formation; not removed to a new site. 2. denoting a tissue graft to a new site on the same individual. Cf. *heterochthonous.*

autocinesis (aw″to-si-ne′sis) [*auto-* + Gr. *kinēsis* motion] autokinesis.

autoclasia (aw″to-kla′ze-ah) [*auto-* + Gr. *klasis* breaking] a self-perpetuating destructive process in which an autoimmune reaction causes breakdown of tissue, liberating more antigen, which in turn elicits the formation of more autoantibody, and so on.

autoclasis (aw-tok′lah-sis) [*auto-* + Gr. *klasis* breaking] destruction of a part by influences developed within itself.

autoclave (aw′to-klāv) [*auto-* + L. *clavis* key] an apparatus for effecting sterilization by steam under pressure; it is fitted with a gauge that automatically regulates the pressure, and therefore the degree of heat to which the contents are subjected.

Autoclip (aw″to-klip′) trademark for a stainless steel surgical clip inserted by means of a mechanical applier that automatically feeds a series of clips for wound closing.

autocondensation (aw″to-kon-den-sa′shun) (*obs.*) application of high-frequency currents to the entire body for therapeutic purposes in which the patient constitutes one plate of a condenser. Rarely employed today.

autoconduction (aw″to-kon-duk′shun) a method of applying high-frequency currents by electromagnetic induction in which the patient placed inside a large solenoid constitutes the secondary of a transformer. Though not employed in this country, this procedure is still used in treatment of psychoses in the U.S.S.R.

autocystoplasty (aw″to-sis′to-plas″te) a plastic operation on the bladder with grafts from the patient's body.

autocytolysin (aw″to-si-tol′ĭ-sin) autolysin.

autocytolysis (aw″to-si-tol′ĭ-sis) autolysis.

autocytolytic (aw″to-si″to-lit′ik) autolytic.

autocytotoxin (aw″to-si″to-tok′sin) a cytotoxin for the cells of the body in which it is formed.

autodermic (aw″to-der′mik) [*auto-* + Gr. *derma* skin] of the patient's own skin; a term applied to skin grafts. See *dermatoautoplasty* and *autograft.*

autodestruction (aw″to-de-struk′shun) self-destruction, specifically that which certain enzymes undergo in solution.

autodigestion (aw″to-di-jes′chun) self-digestion; autolysis; applied especially to the digestion of the walls of the stomach and contiguous structures after death.

autodiploid (aw″to-dip′loid) [*auto-* + *diploid*] 1. having two sets of chromosomes as a result of redoubling of the chromosomes of a haploid individual or cell. 2. an individual or cell having two sets of chromosomes as a result of redoubling of the haploid set.

autodiploidy (aw″to-dip′loi-de) the state of having two sets of chromosomes as a result of redoubling of the haploid set.

autodrainage (aw″to-drān′ij) drainage of an abscess or cavity by diversion of the fluid into a different channel or viscus within the patient's own body; this may be accomplished by surgery or may occur spontaneously.

autoecholalia (aw″to-ek″o-la′le-ah) [*auto-* + *echolalia*] repetition of one's own words.

autoecic (aw-te′sik) [*auto-* + Gr. *oikos* house] autoecious.

autoecious (aw-to-e′shus) [*auto-* + Gr. *oikos* house] pertaining to or denoting parasitic fungi that pass through their entire developmental cycle upon the same host. Cf. *heteroecious.*

autoeczematization (aw″to-ek-zem″ah-tĭ-za′shun) the spread, at first locally, and later more generally, of lesions from an originally circumscribed focus of eczema.

autoerotic (aw″to-e-rot′ik) marked by autoerotism.

autoeroticism (aw″to-ĕ-rot′ĭ-sizm) erotic behavior directed toward oneself; cf. *heteroerotism*.

autoerotism (aw″to-er′o-tizm) autoeroticism.

autoerythrophagocytosis (aw″to-ĕ-rith″ro-fag″o-si-to′sis) [*auto + erythrocyte + phagocytosis*] phagocytosis of erythrocytes by autologous phagocytic cells (e.g., neutrophils, monocytes).

autofluorescence (aw″to-floo″o-res′ens) fluorescence in tissues produced by substances normally present in the tissues. Cf. *secondary fluorescence*, under *fluorescence*.

autofluoroscope (aw″to-floo′o-ro-skōp″) a type of scintillation camera that utilizes in its detector sodium iodide crystals packed in an array especially suited to the study of small tumors in large organs.

autofundoscope (aw″to-fun′do-skōp) an instrument that makes use of the fact that by observing an illuminated blank space through a pin-perforated card one can see faint images of the retinal vessels of his own eyes.

autofundoscopy (aw″to-fun-dos′ko-pe) examination with the autofundoscope.

autogamous (aw-tog′ah-mus) characterized by self-fertilization.

autogamy (aw-tog′ah-me) [*auto-* + Gr. *gamos* marriage] 1. self-fertilization; fertilization within a cell itself by union of two chromatin masses derived from the same primary nucleus; called also *automixis* and *syngamic nuclear union.* Cf. *endogamy* (def. 1) and *exogamy* (def. 1). 2. a special case of syngamy in which the gametes are sister cells, resulting from the division of a single mother cell.

autogeneic (aw″to-jen-e′ik) autogenous; pertaining to an autograft.

autogenesis (aw″to-jen′ĕ-sis) [*auto-* + Gr. *genesis* production] self-generation; origination within the organism.

autogenetic (aw″to-jĕ-net′ik) pertaining to autogenesis.

autogenous (aw-toj′ĕ-nus) [*auto-* + *genesis*] self-generated; originated within the body. As applied to bacterial vaccines, the term denotes those vaccines which are made from the patient's own bacteria, as opposed to stock vaccines which are made from standard cultures. In transplantation immunology, denoting tissue arising, transferred, or transplanted within an individual.

autognosis (aw″tog-no′sis) [*auto-* + Gr. *gnōsis* knowledge] (*obs.*) self-diagnosis; a form of psychoanalysis consisting of giving the patient self-knowledge by revealing to him through his own confessions the course of mental change leading to his symptoms.

autognostic (aw″tog-nos′tik) characterized by self-diagnosis; a term applied to the psychoanalytical method.

autograft (aw′to-graft) a graft of tissue derived from another site in or on the body of the organism receiving it; called also *autologous* or *autochthonous graft,* and *autoplast.*

autografting (aw″to-graft′ing) autotransplantation.

autogram (aw′to-gram) [*auto-* + Gr. *gramma* mark] a mark forming on the skin following pressure by a blunt instrument.

autographism (aw-tog′rah-fizm) [*auto-* + Gr. *graphein* to write] (*obs.*) dermatographism.

autohemagglutination (aw″to-hem″ah-gloo″tĭ-na′shun) agglutination of autologous erythrocytes.

autohemagglutinin (aw″to-hem-ah-gloo′tĭ-nin) a hemagglutinin that causes the clumping or agglutination of autologous erythrocytes.

autohemic (aw″to-he′mik) [*auto-* + Gr. *haima* blood] done with the patient's own blood.

autohemolysin (aw″to-he-mol′ĭ-sin) a type of autoantibody or related factor having the ability to lyse autologous erythrocytes.

autohemolysis (aw″to-he-mol′ĭ-sis) hemolysis of the blood cells of a person by his own serum.

autohemolytic (aw″to-he″mo-lit′ik) pertaining to autohemolysis.

autohemopsonin (aw″to-hem″op-so′nin) an opsonin that renders the red cells susceptible to destruction by the other cells of the patient's body.

autohemotherapy (aw″to-he″mo-ther′ah-pe) [*auto-* + Gr. *haima* blood + *therapeia* treatment] treatment by reinjection of the individual's own blood.

autohemotransfusion (aw″to-he″mo-trans-fu′zhun) the withdrawal of a small amount of venous blood and reinjection directly into the same individual.

autohistoradiograph (aw″to-his″to-ra′de-o-graf) autoradiograph.

autohormonoclasis (aw″to-hor″mōn-ok′lah-sis) [*auto-* + *hormone* + Gr. *klasis* destruction] the inactivation of the hormone of a given gland in the presence of activity of the gland.

autohypnosis (aw″to-hip-no′sis) the act or process of hypnotizing oneself.

autohypnotic (aw″to-hip-not′ik) (*obs.*) 1. pertaining to self-induced hypnotism. 2. one who can put himself into a hypnotic state.

autoimmune (aw″to-im-mūn′) directed against the body's own tissue; see under *disease* and *response.*

autoimmunity (aw″to-im-mu′nĭ-te) a condition characterized by a specific humoral or cell-mediated immune response against the constituents of the body's own tissues (autoantigens); it may result in hypersensitivity reactions or, if severe, in autoimmune disease. Called also *autoallergy.*

autoimmunization (aw″to-im″u-ni-za′shun) the induction in an individual of an immune response to its own tissue constituents, which may lead to pathological sequelae, *i.e.,* to autoimmune disease. Called also *autosensitization.* See also *autoantibody.*

autoinfection (aw″to-in-fek′shun) [*auto-* + *infection*] infection by an agent already present in the body or transferred from one part of the body to another.

autoinfusion (aw″to-in-fu′zhun) [*auto-* + *infusion*] the forcing of the blood toward the heart by bandaging the extremities, compression of the abdominal aorta, etc.

autoinoculable (aw″to-in-ok′u-lah-bl) [*auto-* + *inoculable*] susceptible of being inoculated with microorganisms from one's own body.

autoinoculation (aw″to-in-ok′u-la″shun) [*auto-* + *inoculation*] inoculation with microorganisms from one's own body.

autointerference (aw″to-in″ter-fer′ens) interference with the replication of a virus by an intact, attenuated, or inactivated virus of the same kind.

autointoxicant (aw″to-in-tok′sĭ-kant) a poison generated within the system.

autointoxication (aw″to-in-tok″sĭ-ka′shun) [*auto-* + *intoxication*] intoxication by some poison generated within the body. **intestinal a.,** a disordered state due to the accumulation of intestinal poisons in the blood; called also *alimentary toxemia* and *intestinal intoxication.*

autoisolysin (aw″to-i-sol′ĭ-sin) a lysin that destroys cells (e.g., blood cells) of the subject from which it was obtained, as well as those of other animals of the same species.

autokeratoplasty (aw″to-ker′ah-to-plas″te) [*auto-* + *keratoplasty*] corneal grafting with tissue from the patient's other eye.

autokinesis (aw″to-ki-ne′sis) [*auto-* + Gr. *kinēsis* motion] voluntary motion. **visible light a.,** see *autokinetic visible light phenomenon,* under *phenomenon.*

autokinetic (aw″to-ki-net′ik) having the power of voluntary motion.

autolaryngoscopy (aw″to-lar″in-gos′ko-pe) observation of one's own larynx.

autolavage (aw″to-lah-vahzh′) [*auto-* + *lavage*] lavage performed on one's self or on one's own stomach.

autolesion (aw′to-le″zhun) a self-inflicted injury.

autoleukoagglutinin (aw″to-lu″ko-ah-gloo′tĭ-nin) see *leukoagglutinin.*

autoleukocytotherapy (aw″to-lu″ko-si″to-ther′ah-pe) treatment by administration of the patient's own, previously withdrawn leukocytes.

autologous (aw-tol′o-gus) [*auto-* + Gr. *logos* relation] 1. related to self; designating products or components of the same individual organism. 2. autogenous.

autology (aw-tol′o-je) the science of one's own self.

autolysate (aw-tol′ĭ-sāt) a substance or substances produced by autolysis; autolysates of cancer tissue have been used subcutaneously in the treatment of cancer.

autolysin (aw-tol′ĭ-sin) a lysin present in an organism and capable of destroying the cells or tissues of that organism; called also *autocytolysin.*

autolysis (aw-tol′ĭ-sis) [*auto-* + Gr. *lysis* dissolution] 1. the spontaneous disintegration of tissues or of cells by the action of their own autogenous enzymes, such as occurs after death and in some pathological conditions; called also *autodigestion, self-digestion,* and *autoproteolysis.* 2. the destruction of cells of the body by its own serum; called also *autocytolysis.* **postmortem a.,** enzymatic self-digestion of cells or tissues after death.

autolysosome (aw″to-li′so-sōm) a vacuolar element of the lysosome system of cells to which hydrolases have been added by fusion with lysosomes.

autolytic (aw-to-lit′ik) pertaining to or causing autolysis; autocytolytic.

autolyze (aw′to-līz) to undergo or to cause to undergo autolysis.

automatic (aw″to-mat′ik) [Gr. *automatos* self-acting] 1. spontaneous or involuntary; done by no act of the will. 2. self-moving; self-regulating.

automatin (aw-tom′ah-tin) an extract of bovine heart muscle formerly used in circulatory disorders.

automatism (aw-tom′ah-tizm) [Gr. *automatismos* self-action] 1. the performance of nonreflex acts without conscious volition; called also *automatic behavior.* 2. the doctrine that the brain causes, manufactures, or calls into action mental processes and that all mental processes are dependent on brain activity. Cf. *parallelism.* **ambulatory a.,** a condition in which the patient walks about and performs acts mechanically and without consciousness of what he is doing. Cf. *poriomania*. **command a.,** an abnormal responsiveness to commands, the subject performing suggested acts without exercising any critical judgment, as observed in hypnosis and certain mental states.

automatograph (aw″to-mat′o-graf) [Gr. *automatismos* self-action + *graphein* to write] an instrument for recording involuntary movements.

Autom′eris i′o the io moth that produces dermatitis (io-moth dermatitis) by means of irritant hairs on its larva.

automixis (aw″to-mik′sis) [*auto-* + Gr. *mixis* mixture] autogamy, def. 1.

automnesia (aw″tom-ne′ze-ah) [*auto-* + Gr. *mnēsis* memory] spontaneous recall to memory of past conditions of one's life.

automysophobia (aw″to-mi″so-fo′be-ah) [*auto-* + *mysophobia*] (*obs.*) abnormally exaggerated dread of personal uncleanness.

autonarcosis (aw″to-nar-ko′sis) insensibility due to autosuggestion.

autonephrectomy (aw″to-nĕ-frek′to-me) [*auto-* + Gr. *nephros* kidney + Gr. *ektomē* excision] obliteration of a kidney as the result of disease.

autonephrotoxin (aw″to-nef″ro-tok′sin) a substance toxic to the cells of the kidney of the body in which it is formed.

autonomic (aw″to-nom′ik) self-controlling; functionally independent. See *autonomic nervous system*, under *system*.

autonomotropic (aw″to-nom-o-trop′ik) [*autonomic* + Gr. *tropos* a turning] having an affinity for the autonomic nervous system.

autonomous (aw-ton′o-mus) pertaining to or characterized by autonomy.

autonomy (aw-ton′o-me) [*auto-* + Gr. *nomos* law] the state of functioning independently, without extraneous influence.

auto-ophthalmoscope (aw″to-of-thal′mo-skōp) [*auto-* + *ophthalmoscope*] an ophthalmoscope for examining one's own eyes.

auto-ophthalmoscopy (aw″to-of-thal-mos′ko-pe) the use of the auto-ophthalmoscope.

auto-oxidation (aw″to-ok″sĭ-da′shun) the phenomenon of combining directly with oxygen at ordinary temperatures, without catalysis.

autopath (aw′to-path) a person who has allergic symptoms because of a sensitive autonomic nervous system.

autopathography (aw″to-pah-thog′rah-fe) [*auto-* + Gr. *pathos* disease + *graphein* to write] a written description of one's own disease.

autopathy (aw-top′ah-the) [*auto-* + Gr. *pathos* disease] a disease without apparent external causation; idiopathic disease.

autopepsia (aw″to-pep′se-ah) [*auto-* + Gr. *peptein* to digest] (*obs.*) autolysis, def. 1.

autophagia (aw″to-fa′je-ah) [*auto-* + Gr. *phagein* to eat + *-ia*] 1. the eating of one's own flesh. 2. nutrition of the body by the consumption of its own tissues. 3. autophagy.

autophagosome (aw″to-fag′o-sōm) [*auto-* + *phagosome*] an intracytoplasmic vacuole containing elements of the cell's own cytoplasm; it fuses with a lysosome, subjecting its contents to enzymatic digestion. Called also *autophagic vesicle, autosome*, and *cytolysosome*.

autophagy (aw-tof′ah-je) 1. the segregation of part of the cell's own cytoplasmic material within a membrane and its digestion after fusion of the segregated vacuole with a lysosome. Cf. *heterophagy*. 2. autophagia.

autopharmacologic (aw″to-fahr″mah-ko-loj′ik) pertaining to substances (e.g., hormones) produced in the body that have pharmacologic activities.

autopharmacology (aw″to-far″mah-kol′o-je) the chemical regulation of bodily function by the natural constituents of the body tissues.

autophil (aw′to-fil) a person with a tendency to allergic manifestations because of a sensitive autonomic nervous system.

autophilia (aw″to-fil′e-ah) [*auto-* + Gr. *philein* to love] pathological self-esteem; narcissism.

autophobia (aw″to-fo′be-ah) [*auto-* + Gr. *phobos* fear] (*obs.*) abnormal dread of being alone.

autophonomania (aw″to-fo″no-ma′ne-ah) [*auto-* + Gr. *phonos* murder + *mania* madness] (*obs.*) suicidal mania.

autophonometry (aw″to-fo-nom′ĕ-tre) [*auto-* + Gr. *phōne* voice + *metron* measure] the application of a vibrating tuning fork to the body of a patient for the purpose of having him describe the sensations that it produces.

autophthalmoscope (aw″tof-thal′mo-skōp) auto-ophthalmoscope.

autophyte (aw′to-fīt) [*auto-* + Gr. *phyton* plant] a plant that does not depend on organized food material, but derives its nourishment directly from inorganic matter. Cf. *saprophyte*.

autoplasmotherapy (aw″to-plaz″mo-ther′ah-pe) [*auto-* + L. *plasma* + Gr. *therapeia* treatment] treatment of disease by injections of the patient's own blood plasma.

autoplast (aw′to-plast) an autograft.

autoplastic (aw″to-plas′tik) pertaining to autoplasty.

autoplasty (aw″to-plas′te) [*auto-* + Gr. *plassein* to form] 1. the replacement or reconstruction of diseased or injured parts by tissue taken from another part of the patient's own body. 2. in psychoanalysis, instinctive modification within the psychic systems in adaptation to reality. **peritoneal a.,** peritonization.

autoploid (aw′to-ploid) [*auto-* + *-ploid*] autopolyploid.

autoploidy (aw′to-ploi′de) autopolyploidy.

autopodium (aw″to-po′de-um) see *limb* (def. 1).

autopoisonous (aw″to-poi′zun-us) poisonous to the organism by which it is formed.

autopolymer (aw″to-pol′ĭ-mer) a material that polymerizes without the use of heat, but on the addition of an activator and a catalyst.

autopolymerization (aw″to-pol″ĭ-mer″i-za′shun) polymerization occurring without the use of heat but as a chemical reaction following the addition of an activator and a catalyst.

autopolyploid (aw″to-pol″ĭ-ploid) [*auto-* + *polyploid*] 1. having more than two chromosome sets as a result of redoubling of the chromosomes of a haploid individual or cell. 2. an individual or cell having more than two chromosome sets as a result of redoubling of the haploid set.

autopolyploidy (aw″to-pol″ĭ-ploi″de) the state of having more than two chromosome sets as a result of redoubling of the haploid set.

autoprecipitin (aw″to-pre-sip′ĭ-tin) an autoantibody with the characteristics of a precipitin.

autoprotection (aw″to-pro-tek′shun) self-protection, e.g., the protection of the body from disease by the formation of autoantitoxins.

autoproteolysis (aw″to-pro-te-ol′ĭ-sis) autolysis, def. 1.

autoprothrombin (aw″to-pro-throm′bin) Seegers' term for an activation product of prothrombin. **a. I,** Factor VII; see *coagulation factors*, under *factor*. **a. II,** Factor IX; see *coagulation factors*, under *factor*. **a. C,** Factor X; see under *coagulation factors*, under *factor*.

autoprotolysis (aw″to-pro-tol′ĭ-sis) self-ionization involving proton transfer.

autopsia (aw-top′se-ah) autopsy.

autopsy (aw′top-se) [*auto-* + Gr. *opsis* view] the postmortem examination of a body, including the internal organs and structures after dissection, so as to determine the cause of death or the nature of pathological changes. Called also *necropsy*.

autopsychic (aw″to-si′kik) [*auto-* + Gr. *psychē* soul] pertaining to self-consciousness.

autopsychorhythmia (aw″to-si-ko-rith′me-ah) [*auto-* + Gr. *psychē* soul + Gr. *rhythmos* rhythm] pathological rhythmic activity of the brain.

autopsychosis (aw″to-si-ko′sis) (*obs.*) a psychosis or mental disease marked by derangement of ideas relating to the patient's self.

autopsychotherapy (aw″to-si″ko-ther′ah-pe) psychotherapy administered by a patient on himself, such as by the exercise of self-control and will power.

autoradiogram (aw″to-ra′de-o-gram) an autoradiograph.

autoradiograph (aw″to-ra′de-o-graf) a radiograph of an object or tissue made by recording the radiation emitted by radioactive material within it, especially after the purposeful introduction of radioactive material.

autoradiography (aw″to-ra″de-og′rah-fe) the making of a radiograph of an object or tissue by recording on a photographic plate the radiation emitted by weakly emitting radioactive material within the object; the technique has been used widely for studying DNA synthesis and location within cells, with tritium-labeled precursors (like thymidine) as the radioactive marker.

autoreactive (aw″to-re-ak′tiv) directed against the body's own tissues, as an autoreactive immune response.

autoregulation (aw″to-reg″u-la′shun) the control of certain phenomena by factors inherent in a situation, usually restricted to circulatory physiology; specifically (1) the intrinsic tendency of an organ or tissue to maintain constant blood flow despite changes in arterial pressure, (2) the adjustment of blood flow through an organ in order to provide for its metabolic needs, and (3) (*obs.*) the factors tending to maintain a constant blood pressure. **heterometric a.,** those intrinsic mechanisms controlling the strength of ventricular contractions that depend on the length of myocardial fibers at the end of diastole. **homeometric a.,** those intrinsic mechanisms controlling the strength of ventricular contractions that are independent of the length of myocardial fibers at the end of diastole.

autoreinfusion (aw″to-re″in-fu′zhun) intravenous infusion of a patient's own blood or serum which has escaped into the pleural or peritoneal cavities, usually because of trauma or spontaneous rupture of a major vessel.

autorrhaphy (aw-tor′ah-fe) [*auto-* + Gr. *rhaphē* suture] (*obs.*)

closure of a wound by the use of strands of tissue taken from the flaps of the wound.

autosensitization (aw″to-sen″sĭ-ti-za′shun) sensitization toward one's own tissues; see *autoimmunization.* **erythrocyte a.,** autoerythrocyte sensitization; see under *syndrome.*

autosensitized (aw″to-sen′sĭ-tīzd) rendered hypersensitive to one's own serum or tissues; see *autoimmunization.*

autosepticemia (aw″to-sep″tĭ-se′me-ah) septicemia due to poisons developed within the body.

autoserodiagnosis (aw″to-se″ro-di-ag-no′sis) diagnostic use of a serum from the patient's own blood.

autoserosalvarsan (aw″to-se-ro-sal′var-san) Swift-Ellis treatment; see under *treatment.*

autoserous (aw″to-se′rus) accomplished by means of one's own serum.

autoserum (aw″to-se′rum) [*auto-* + *serum*] a serum administered to the patient from whom it was derived.

autosexing (aw″to-seks′ing) in avian genetics, the deliberate breeding of an early-appearing sex-linked phenotype to distinguish male from female chicks.

autosite (aw′to-sīt) [*auto-* + Gr. *sitos* food] the larger, more nearly normal component of asymmetrical conjoined twins, to which the parasite is attached as a dependent growth.

autositic (aw″to-sit′ik) pertaining to or of the nature of an autosite.

autosmia (aw-tos′me-ah) [*auto-* + Gr. *osmē* smell] the smelling of one's own bodily odor.

autosomal (aw″to-so′mal) pertaining to an autosome.

autosomatognosis (aw″to-so″mah-tog-no′sis) [*auto-* + Gr. *sōma* body + *gnosis* recognition] the feeling that a part of the body that has been removed, as by amputation, is still present. See *phantom limb,* under *limb.*

autosomatognostic (aw″to-so″mah-tog-nos′tik) pertaining to autosomatognosis.

autosome (aw′to-sōm) [*auto-* + Gr. *sōma* body] 1. any ordinary paired chromosome as distinguished from a sex chromosome; in man there are 22 pairs of autosomes. 2. autophagosome.

autospermotoxin (aw″to-sper″mo-tok′sin) a substance capable of agglutinating the spermatozoa of the animal in which they are formed.

autosplenectomy (aw″to-sple-nek′to-me) the almost complete disappearance of the spleen through progressive fibrosis and shrinkage, such as may occur in sickle cell anemia.

autospray (aw′to-spra) an apparatus for spraying, to be used by the patient himself.

autosterilization (aw″to-ster″ĭ-li-za′shun) a supposed tendency of certain viruses (e.g., poliovirus) to disappear from the tissues after a short time; a concept found to be erroneous.

autostimulation (aw″to-stim″u-la′shun) stimulation of an animal with antigenic material originating from its own tissues.

autosuggestibility (aw″to-sug-jes″tĭ-bil′ĭ-te) a peculiar mental state with loss of will, in which suggestion becomes easy.

autosuggestion (aw″to-sug-jes′chun) [*auto-* + *suggestion*] the spontaneous occurrence to the mind of ideas produced in the individual himself. Also the peculiar mental state often occurring after accidents, in which suggestions are easily received, so that the slightest injury to a part induces an hysterical paralysis or other disability. Cf. *ectosuggestion.*

autosynnoia (aw″to-sin-noi′ah) [*auto-* + Gr. *synnoia* meditation] (*obs.*) a mental condition in which the patient is so concentrated in his thoughts and hallucinations that he loses all interest in the outside world.

autosynthesis (aw″to-sin′thĕ-sis) self-reproduction.

autotemnous (aw″to-tem′nus) [*auto-* + Gr. *temnein* to cut] capable of spontaneous division.

autotherapy (aw″to-ther′ah-pe) [*auto-* + Gr. *therapeia* treatment] 1. the spontaneous cure of disease. 2. self-cure. 3. treatment of disease by filtrates from the patient's own secretions.

autotomographic (aw″to-tom″o-graf′ik) pertaining to autotomography.

autotomography (aw″to-to-mog′rah-fe) a method of body-section roentgenography involving movement of the patient instead of the x-ray tube.

autotomy (aw-tot′o-me) [*auto-* + Gr. *tomē* cut] 1. self-division; fission. 2. the spontaneous shedding of an appendage, as in some invertebrates.

autotopagnosia (aw″to-top″ag-no′se-ah) [*auto-* + Gr. *topos* place + *a* neg. + *gnōsis* knowledge] inability to localize or orient correctly different parts of the body; body-image agnosia.

autotoxemia (aw″to-tok-se′me-ah) autotoxicosis.

autotoxic (aw″to-tok′sik) [*auto-* + Gr. *toxikon* poison] pertaining to autointoxication.

autotoxicosis (aw″to-tok″sĭ-ko′sis) [*auto-* + Gr. *toxikon* poison + *-osis*] poisoning by material generated within the body; called also *autotoxemia.*

autotoxin (aw″to-tok′sin) any pathogenic principle developed within the body from tissue metamorphosis.

autotoxis (aw″to-tok′sis) autotoxicosis.

autotransfusion (aw″to-trans-fu′zhun) reinfusion of the patient's own blood.

autotransplant (aw″to-trans′plant) autograft.

autotransplantation (aw″to-trans″plan-ta′shun) the operation of taking a piece of tissue from one part of a subject and inserting it in another part of the same individual; called also *autografting.*

autotrepanation (aw″to-trep″ah-na′shun) erosion of the skull by a brain tumor.

autotroph (aw′to-trōf) an autotrophic organism. **facultative a.,** a microorganism which can live as a chemoautotroph or as a chemoheterotroph; an organism with a flexible requirement for oxidizable substrate. **obligate a.,** a microorganism that can exist only by autotrophic means.

autotrophic (aw″to-trof′ik) [*auto-* + Gr. *trophē* nutrition] self-nourishing; said of organisms that can build their organic constituents from carbon dioxide and inorganic salts. Cf. *heterotrophic.*

autotrophy (aw-tot′ro-fe) the state of being autotrophic; autotrophic nutrition.

autotuberculin (aw″to-tu-ber″ku-lin) tuberculin made from cultures obtained from a patient's own sputum.

autotuberculinization (aw″to-tu-ber″ku-lin-i-za′shun) absorption of tuberculin or similar products from a patient's own foci of disease.

autovaccination (aw″to-vak″sĭ-na′shun) 1. treatment of a patient with autovaccine. 2. treatment of a patient by causing liberation of antigenic products from some invading microorganism or diseased tissue and thus bringing about the formation of antibodies.

autovaccine (aw″to-vak′sēn) a bacterial vaccine prepared from cultures of organisms isolated from the patient's own secretions or tissues.

autovaccinotherapy (aw″to-vak″sĭ-no-ther′ah-pe) autovaccination.

autoxemia (aw″tok-se′me-ah) autotoxicosis.

autoxidation (aw″tok-sĭ-da′shun) spontaneous oxidation of a substance that is in direct contact with oxygen.

autoxidizable (aw-tok″sĭ-dīz′ah-bl) spontaneously oxidizable.

autozygous (aw″to-zi′gus) homozygous by virtue of parental descent from a common ancestor.

auxanogram (awks-an′o-gram) the plate culture in auxanography.

auxanographic (awks″an-o-graf′ik) pertaining to auxanography.

auxanography (awks″an-og′rah-fe) [Gr. *auxanein* to increase + *graphein* to write] determination of the most suitable medium for a microbe by placing drops of various solutions on a plate containing a poor medium; the microbe will develop the strongest colonies on the spot that contains the best medium.

auxanology (awks″an-ol′o-je) [Gr. *auxanein* to increase + *-logy*] (*obs.*) the science of growth; applied especially to the study or science of the growth of microorganisms.

auxesis (awk-se′sis) [Gr. *auxēsis*] increase in the size of an organism; often used specifically to designate increase in volume of an organism as a result of growth of its individual cells, without increase in their number.

auxetic (awk-set′ik) [Gr. *auxētikos* growing] 1. pertaining to auxesis. 2. a substance that stimulates auxesis.

auxiliary (awk-sil′e-a″re) [L. *auxiliaris*] 1. affording aid. 2. that which affords aid. **torquing a.,** an accessory arch wire used to apply torsion on a tooth in any of the three planes of space.

auxiliomotor (awk-sil″e-o-mo′tor) aiding or stimulating motion.

auxilytic (awk-sĭ-lit′ik) [Gr. *auxein* to increase + *lysis*] increasing the lytic or destructive power.

auximone (awk′sĭ-mōn) [Gr. *auxein* to increase + *hormone*] a hypothetical substance, akin to vitamin, that favors growth in plants.

auxin (awk′sin) [Gr. *auxē* increase] a phytohormone (plant hormone) from sprouts of plants and from human urine that promotes growth in plant cells and tissues by elongation rather than by multiplication of cells; there are two forms, *auxin A,* a cyclopentene derivative of trihydroxy valeric acid, $C_{18}H_{32}O_5$, and *auxin B,* which is heteroauxin.

auxiometer (awk″se-om′ĕ-ter) [Gr. *auxein* to increase + *metron* measure] 1. an apparatus for measuring the magnifying powers of lenses; called also *auxometer.* 2. a dynamometer.

auxo- [Gr. *auxē* increase] a combining form denoting relationship to growth, or to stimulation or to acceleration.

auxoaction (awk″so-ak′shun) the accelerating or stimulating action of a substance.

auxoamylase (awk″so-am′ĭ-lās) a substance that accelerates the action of amylase.

auxocardia (awk″so-kar′de-ah) [auxo- + Gr. kardia heart] (obs.) 1. diastole. 2. enlargement of the heart.

auxochrome (awk′so-krōm) [auxo- + Gr. chrōma color] a chemical group which, if introduced into a chromogen, will convert the latter into a dye.

auxochromous (awk″so-kro′mus) pertaining to an auxochrome.

auxocyte (awk′so-sīt) [auxo- + Gr. kytos hollow vessel] an oocyte, spermatocyte, or sporocyte in the early stages of its development; called also gonotokont.

auxodrome (awk′so-drōm) [Gr. auxé growth + dromos a course] the course of growth as plotted on a Wetzel grid.

auxoflore (awk′so-flōr) a substance that increases the intensity of fluorescence of a compound. Cf. bathoflore.

auxoflur (awk′so-floor) auxoflore.

auxogluc (awk′so-glook) [auxo- + Gr. glykys sweet] a tasteless atom with which a glucophore combines to form a compound that has a sweet taste.

auxohormone (awk″so-hor′mōn) [auxo- + hormone] a vitamin.

auxology (awk-sol′o-je) (obs.) auxanology.

auxometer (awks-om′ĕ-ter) auxiometer, def. 1.

auxometric (awks″o-met′rik) pertaining or relating to auxometry.

auxometry (awks-om′ĕ-tre) [Gr. auxein to increase + to measure metron] measurement of rate of growth.

auxoneurotropic (awk″so-nu″ro-trop′ik) [auxo- + neurotropic] increasing or strengthening the neurotropic properties of any substance.

auxospireme (awk″so-spi′rēm) the spireme of an auxocyte during the growth cycle.

auxospore (awk′so-spōr) a rejuvenescent cell of certain diatoms formed in response to a diminution in the size of the organism as a result of repeated cell divisions; it sheds the cell walls, enlarges, and then forms new, larger walls.

auxotherapy (awk″so-ther′ah-pe) [auxo- + therapy] substitution therapy, as by hormonotherapy or organotherapy.

auxotonic (awk″so-ton′ik) [auxo- + Gr. tonos tension] contracting against increasing resistance.

auxotox (awk′so-toks) a chemical group that causes a compound to be toxic.

auxotroph (awk′so-trōf) an auxotrophic organism.

auxotrophic (awk″so-trof′ik) [auxo- + Gr. trophē nutrition] 1. requiring a growth factor that is not required by the parental or prototype strain; said of microbial mutants. 2. requiring specific organic growth factors in addition to the carbon source present in a minimal medium.

AV, A-V, atrioventricular; arteriovenous.

Av. average; avoirdupois.

avalvular (ah-val′vu-lar) having no valves.

avantin (av′an-tin) isopropyl alcohol.

avascular (ah-vas′ku-lar) [a neg. + vascular] not supplied with blood vessels.

avascularization (ah-vas″ku-lar-i-za′shun) the diversion of blood from tissues; it may be accomplished by ligating vessels or by applying tight elastic bandages.

Aveling's repositor (av′el-ingz) [James Hobson Aveling, British obstetrician, 1828–1892] see under repositor.

Avellis's syndrome (paralysis) (av-el′ēz) [Georg Avellis, German laryngologist, 1864–1916] see under syndrome.

Avena (ah-ve′nah) [L.] a genus of grasses. The grains of A. sativa constitute the oats of commerce, a nutritive and edible cereal.

avenin (ah-ve′nin) an albuminoid obtained from Avena sativa, or oats, said to be identical with gluten casein; called also plant casein and legumin.

avenolith (ah-ve′no-lith) [L. avena oats + Gr. lithos stone] an intestinal calculus or enterolith formed around a grain of oats.

Aventyl (ah-ven′til) trademark for a preparation of nortriptyline hydrochloride.

Avenzoar (av″en-zo′ar) (1113–1162) a renowned Islamic physician, born in Seville, Spain, whose principal writing was a compendium of practice, al-Teïsir, which contains many interesting clinical reports. Also in his writings he described the itch-mite (Acarus scabiei), and did not hesitate to criticize Galen. He is also known as Ibn Zuhr.

Averroes (av-er′ro-ēz) (1126–1198) a distinguished Spanish-Islamic philosopher and physician, born at Cordova. Better known as a philosopher, his chief philosophical work is his commentary on Aristotle; his chief medical work is the Colliget, a predominantly philosophical approach to a system of medicine. Known also as Ibn Rushd.

aversive (ah-ver′siv) characterized by or giving rise to avoidance; noxious. Cf. appetitive.

Avertin (ah-ver′tin) trademark for a preparation of tribromoethanol.

avian (a′ve-an) [L. avis bird] of or pertaining to birds.

Avicenna (av″ĭ-sen′nah) (980–1037) a celebrated Persian physician and philosopher, surnamed the "Prince of Physicians." His great encyclopedia, the Canon, written in Arabic, influenced medical thought and teaching for hundreds of years, its dogmatic, pontifical style having particular appeal for the medieval physician. Known also as Ibn Sinā.

avidin (av′ĭ-din) a specific protein in egg albumin that interacts with biotin to render it unavailable to an animal, thus producing the syndrome known as biotin deficiency. See also biotin.

avidity (ah-vid′ĭ-te) 1. the strength of an acid or base. 2. in immunology, a measure of the quantity of antigen-antibody complexes formed with respect to time (kinetically derived quantity). It differs from affinity, a thermodynamically derived quantity measuring the strength of binding. By contrast, avidity is a relatively imprecise term.

avifauna (a″vĭ-faw′nah) the bird life present in or characteristic of a given region or locality.

avirulence (a-vir′u-lens) lack of virulence; lack of competence of an infectious agent to produce pathologic effects.

avirulent (a-vir′u-lent) not virulent.

avitaminosis (a-vi″tah-mĭ-no′sis) hypovitaminosis.

avitaminotic (a-vi″tah-mĭ-not′ik) pertaining to or characterized by avitaminosis.

avivement (ah-vēv-mon′) [Fr.] the refreshing of the edges of a wound by surgical procedure.

Avlosulfon (av-lo-sul′fon) trademark for a preparation of dapsone.

Avogadro's law, number (constant) (av-o-gad′rōz) [Amedeo Avogadro, Italian physicist, 1776–1856] see under law and number.

avogram (av′o-gram) one septillionth (10^{-24}) of a gram, or one picopicogram (ppg); so named from Avogadro's number, 6.03×10^{23}. The mass of a molecule in avograms is therefore 1.66 times its conventional molecular weight.

avoidance (ah-void′ans) a conscious or unconscious defensive reaction intended to escape anxiety, conflict, danger, fear, or pain.

avoirdupois (av″er-dŭ-poiz′) see under weight, and see Table of Weights and Measures.

avoparcin (av-o-par′sin) a glycopeptide antibiotic derived from Streptomyces candidus; an antibacterial.

avulsion (ah-vul′shun) [L. avulsio, from a- away + vellere to pull] the tearing away of a part of structure. **nerve a.,** the operation of tearing a nerve by traction. **phrenic a.,** extraction of a piece of the phrenic nerve through an incision at the base of the neck; done in pulmonary tuberculosis to paralyze the corresponding side of the diaphragm in order to secure rest of the lung.

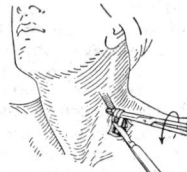

Avulsion of a phrenic nerve.

awu atomic weight unit; see atomic mass unit, under unit.

ax. axis.

axanthopsia (ak″san-thop′se-ah) [a neg. + Gr. xanthos yellow + opsis vision + -ia] yellow blindness.

Axenfeld's syndrome (anomaly) (ak′sen-feltz″) [Theodor Axenfeld, German ophthalmologist, 1867–1930] see under syndrome.

Axenfeld's test (ak′sen-feltz) [David Axenfeld, German physiologist, 1848–1912] see under tests.

Axenfeld-Morax see Morax-Axenfeld.

axenic (a-zen′ik) [a neg. + Gr. xenos a guestfriend, stranger] not contaminated by or associated with any foreign organisms; used in reference to pure cultures of microorganisms or to germ-free animals. Cf. gnotobiotic.

axes (ak′sēz) [L.] plural of axis.

axial (ak′se-al) of or pertaining to the axis of a structure or part. In dentistry, pertaining to the long axis of a tooth.

axiation (ak″se-a′shun) the establishment of an axis, or the development of polarity, in an ovum, embryo, organ, or other body structure.

axifugal (ak-sif′u-gal) [L. axis axis + fugere to flee] directed away from an axon or axis.

axilemma (ak″si-lem′ah) [axis + Gr. lemma husk] axolemma.

axilla (ak-sil′ah), pl. *axil′lae* [L.] [NA] a small pyramidal space between the upper lateral part of the chest and the medial side of the arm, and including, in addition to the armpit, axillary vessels, the brachial plexus of nerves, a large number of lymph nodes, and fat and loose areolar tissue; called also *armpit, fossa axillaris,* and *axillary space.*

axillae (ak-sil′e) [L.] plural of *axilla.*

axillary (ak′sĭ-lar″e) pertaining to the axilla.

axio- (ak′se-o) [L. *axis;* Gr. *axōn* axle] a combining form denoting relationship to an axis. In dentistry, it is used in special reference to the long axis of a tooth, as in the names of cavity angles. See specific terms.

axiobuccal (ak″se-o-buk″kal) pertaining to or formed by the axial and buccal walls of a tooth cavity.

axiobuccocervical (ak-se-o-buk″ko-ser″vĭ-kal) pertaining to or formed by the axial, buccal, and cervical walls of a tooth cavity.

axiobuccogingival (ak″se-o-buk″ko-jin′jĭ-val) pertaining to or formed by the axial, buccal, and gingival walls of a tooth cavity.

axiobuccolingual (ak″se-o-buk″ko-ling′gwal) pertaining to the long axis and the buccal and lingual surfaces of a posterior tooth.

axiocervical (ak″se-o-ser′vĭ-kal) pertaining to or formed by the axial and cervical walls of a tooth cavity.

axiodistal (ak″se-o-dis′tal) pertaining to or formed by the axial and distal walls of a tooth cavity.

axiodistocervical (ak″se-o-dis″to-ser′vĭ-kal) pertaining to or formed by the axial, distal, and cervical walls of a tooth cavity.

axiodistogingival (ak″se-o-dis″to-jin′jĭ-val) pertaining to or formed by the axial, distal, and gingival walls of a tooth cavity.

axiodistoincisal (ak″se-o-dis″to-in-si′zal) pertaining to or formed by the axial, distal, and incisal walls of a tooth cavity.

axiodisto-occlusal (ak″se-o-dis″to-ŏ-kloo′zal) pertaining to or formed by the axial, distal, and occlusal walls of a tooth cavity.

axiogingival (ak″se-o-jin′jĭ-val) pertaining to or formed by the axial and gingival walls of a tooth cavity.

axioincisal (ak″se-o-in-si′zal) pertaining to or formed by the axial and incisal walls of a tooth cavity.

axiolabial (ak″se-o-la′be-al) pertaining to or formed by the axial and labial walls of a tooth cavity.

axiolabiogingival (ak″se-o-la″be-o-jin′jĭ-val) pertaining to or formed by the axial, labial, and gingival walls of a tooth cavity.

axiolabiolingual (ak″se-o-la″be-o-ling′gwal) pertaining to the long axis and the labial and lingual surfaces of an anterior tooth.

axiolingual (ak″se-o-ling′gwal) pertaining to or formed by the axial and lingual walls of a tooth cavity.

axiolinguocervical (ak″se-o-ling″gwo-ser′vĭ-kal) pertaining to or formed by the axial, lingual, and cervical walls of a tooth cavity.

axiolinguogingival (ak″se-o-ling″gwo-jin′jĭ-val) pertaining to or formed by the axial, lingual, and gingival walls of a tooth cavity.

axiolinguo-occlusal (ak″se-o-ling″gwo-ŏ-kloo′sal) pertaining to or formed by the axial, lingual, and occlusal walls of a tooth cavity.

axiomesial (ak″se-o-me′ze-al) pertaining to or formed by the axial and mesial walls of a tooth cavity.

axiomesiocervical (ak″se-o-me″ze-o-ser′vĭ-kal) pertaining to or formed by the axial, mesial, and cervical walls of a tooth cavity.

axiomesiodistal (ak″se-o-me″ze-o-dis′tal) pertaining to the long axis and the mesial and distal surfaces of a tooth.

axiomesiogingival (ak″se-o-me″ze-o-jin′jĭ-val) pertaining to or formed by the axial, mesial, and gingival walls of a tooth cavity.

axiomesioincisal (ak″se-o-me″ze-o-in-si′zal) pertaining to or formed by the axial, mesial, and incisal walls of a tooth cavity.

axiomesio-occlusal (ak″se-o-me″ze-o-ŏ-kloo′zal) pertaining to or formed by the axial, mesial, and occlusal walls of a tooth cavity.

axion (ak-se′on) (*obs.*) the brain and spinal cord.

axio-occlusal (ak″se-o-ŏ-kloo′zal) pertaining to or formed by the axial and occlusal walls of a tooth cavity.

axiopodium (ak″se-o-po′de-um) axopodium.

axiopulpal (ak″se-o-pul′pal) pertaining to or formed by the axial and pulpal walls of a tooth cavity.

axipetal (ak-sip′ĕ-tal) [L. *axis* axis + *petere* to seek] directed toward an axon or axis.

axis (ak′sis), pl. *ax′es* [L.; Gr. *axōn* axle] 1. a line about which a revolving body turns or about which a structure would turn if it did revolve; a line around which specified parts of the body are arranged. Used as a general term in NA terminology. 2. [NA] the second cervical vertebra; called also *epistropheus, odontoid vertebra,* and *vertebra dentata.* **arterial a., costocervical,** truncus costocervicalis. **basibregmatic a.,** a vertical line from the basion to the bregma; the maximum height of the cranium. **basicranial a.,** a line from the basion to the gonion. **basifacial a.,** a line joining the gonion and the subnasal point; called also *facial a.* **binauricular a.,** a line joining the two auricular points. **brain a.** (*obs.*), brain stem; see under B. **a. bul′bi exter′nus** [NA], an imaginary line that passes from the anterior to the posterior pole of the eyeball; called also *external axis of eye* and *axis oculi externa.* **a. bul′bi inter′nus** [NA], an imaginary line in the eyeball, passing from the anterior pole to a point on the anterior surface of the retina just deep to the posterior pole; called also *internal axis of eye* and *axis oculi interna.* **celiac a.,** truncus celiacus. **cell a.,** a line connecting the proximal and distal sides of a cell or passing through the centrosome and nucleus of a cell. **cephalocaudal a.,** the long axis of the body. **cerebrospinal a.** (*obs.*), the central nervous system. **condylar a.,** a line through the two mandibular condyles around which the mandible may rotate during a part of the opening movement of the jaw; called also *condyle chord.* **conjugate a.** (*obs.*), the conjugate diameter of the pelvis; see under *diameter.* **craniofacial a.,** the axis of the bones at the base of the skull, including the mesethmoid, presphenoid, basisphenoid, and basioccipital. **dorsoventral a.,** any line in the median plane at right angles to the long axis of the body. **electrical a. of heart,** the resultant of the electromotive forces within the heart at any instant. **embryonic a.,** an imaginary line from the head end to the tail end of an embryo or, before that, the line of elongation of the primitive streak and groove. **encephalomyelonic a., encephalospinal a.** (*obs.*), the central nervous system. **external a. of eye,** a. bulbi externus. **facial a.,** basifacial a. **frontal a.,** an imaginary line running from right to left through the center of the eyeball. **a. of heart,** a line passing through the center of the base of the heart and the apex. **hinge a.,** the imaginary line connecting the mandibular condyles around which the mandible can rotate without translatory movement; called also *mandibular a.* **internal a. of eye,** a. bulbi internus. **a. of lens, a. len′tis** [NA], an imaginary line joining the anterior and posterior poles of the lens of the eye. **long a. of body,** the imaginary straight line through the neck, thorax, abdomen, and pelvis about which the weights of the torso are most symmetrically distributed. **mandibular a.,** hinge a. **neural a.,** the central nervous system. **a. oc′uli exter′na,** a. bulbi externus. **a. oc′uli inter′na,** a. bulbi internus. **opening a.,** an imaginary line around which the condyles may rotate during opening and closing movements of the mandible. **optic a.,** 1. axis opticus. 2. optical axis. 3. the hypothetical straight line that passes through the centers of curvature of the front and back surfaces of a simple lens; a light ray coinciding with this line will pass through the lens undeviated. **a. op′tica,** a. opticus. **optical a.,** the line formed by the coinciding principal axes of elements composing an optical system, being the continuous line passing through the centers of curvature of the optical surfaces of those elements; called also *principal a.* **a. op′ticus** [NA], optic axis: an imaginary line passing from the midpoint of the visual field to the fovea centralis of the macula; called also *a. optica, sagittal a. of eye,* and *visual a.* **a. pel′vis** [NA], **a. of pelvis,** an imaginary curved line drawn through the minor pelvis at right angles to the planes of the superior aperture, of the cavity, and of the inferior aperture at their central points. **a. of preparation,** the path taken by a dental restoration as it slides on or off the preparation. **principal a.,** optical a. **pupillary a.,** the line perpendicular to the cornea that passes through the center of the pupil of entrance. **renal a.,** an imaginary straight line extending through the upper and lower poles of the kidney or, radiographically, through the most inferior and superior calices of the kidney; when projected superiorly, it intersects the thoracic spine. **sagittal a. of eye,** a. opticus. **secondary a.,** an imaginary line passing through the optical center of a lens. **thoracic a.,** arteria thoracoacromialis. **thyroid a.,** truncus thyrocervicalis. **vertical a. of eye,** an imaginary line connecting the extreme upper and lower points of the eyeball. **visual a.,** a. opticus. **Y a.,** the angle of a line connecting the sella turcica and the gnathion related to a horizontal plane; it is an indicator of downward and forward growth of the mandible.

axis cylinder (ak″sis-sil′in-der) [*axis* + *cylinder*] axon, def. 2.

axite (ak′sīt) (*obs.*) terminal filaments of an axon.

axoaxonic (ak″so-ak-son′ik) referring to a synapse between the axon of one neuron and the axon of another.

axodendritic (ak″so-den-drit′ik) [*axo-* + Gr. *dendron* tree] referring to a synapse between the axon of one neuron and dendrites of another; see *synapse.*

axofugal (ak-sof′u-gal) axifugal.

axograph (ak′so-graf) an apparatus for recording axes in kymographic tracings.

axoid (ak′soid) pertaining to the axis or second cervical vertebra.

axoidean (ak-soi′de-an) axoid.

axolemma (ak″so-lem′ah) [*axon* + Gr. *eilēma* sheath] the surface membrane of an axon; called also *Mauthner's membrane* or *sheath.*

axolotl (ak′so-lot″l) a larval salamander of the genus *Ambystoma;* used in experiments with thyroid feeding.

axolysis (ak-sol′ĭ-sis) [*axon* + Gr. *lysis* dissolution] degeneration and breaking up of the axon of a nerve cell.

axometer (ak-som′ĕ-ter) [*axis* + Gr. *metron* measure] an instrument for measuring an axis, especially an instrument for adjusting a pair of spectacles with respect to the optic axes of the eyes.

axon (ak'son) [Gr. *axōn* axle, axis] 1. the axis of the body; the vertebral column (columna vertebralis [NA]). 2. that process of a neuron by which impulses travel away from the cell body; at the terminal arborization of the axon, the impulses are transmitted to other nerve cells or to effector organs. In the peripheral nervous system, the larger (myelinated) axons are surrounded by a myelin sheath, formed by concentric layers of plasma membrane of the Schwann cell, individual Schwann cells being separated by gaps called nodes of Ranvier. In the central nervous system, the function of the Schwann cell is supplied by oligodendrocytes. Called also *axis cylinder*. **giant a.,** an axon of certain invertebrates, e.g., the squid, whose size (500 to 700 microns) has facilitated physiological studies of cell membrane excitation. **naked a.,** an axon which has no myelin sheath. **unmyelinated a.,** naked a.

axonal (ak'so-nal) pertaining to or affecting an axon.

axonapraxia (ak"son-ah-prak'se-ah) neurapraxia.

axone (ak'sōn) axon.

axoneme (ak'so-nēm) [*axon* + Gr. *nēma* thread] 1. the axial thread of the chromosome in which is located the axial combination of genes. 2. the central core of a cilium or flagellum, consisting of a central pair of filaments surrounded by nine other pairs; called also *axial filament*.

axoneuron (ak"so-nu'ron) [*axis* + Gr. *neuron* nerve] (*obs.*) a neuron of the central nervous system.

axonometer (ak"so-nom'ĕ-ter) [*axon* + Gr. *metron* measure] an apparatus for the rapid determination of the cylindrical axis of a lens.

axonotmesis (ak"son-ot-me'sis) [*axon* + Gr. *tmēsis* a cutting apart] nerve injury characterized by disruption of the axon and myelin sheath but with preservation of the connective tissue fragments, resulting in degeneration of the axon distal to the injury site; regeneration of the axon is spontaneous and of good quality. Cf. *neurapraxia* and *neurotmesis*.

axopetal (ak-sop'ĕ-tal) axipetal.

axophage (ak'so-fāj) a neuroglial cell occurring in excavations in the myelin in myelitis.

axoplasm (ak'so-plazm) [*axon* + Gr. *plasma* plasma] the cytoplasm of an axon.

axoplasmic (ak"so-plas'mik) pertaining to the axoplasm.

axopodium (ak-so-po'de-um) [*axon* + Gr. *pous* foot] a more or less permanent type of pseudopodium, long and needle-like, characterized by an axial rod, composed of a bundle of fibrils inserted near the center of the body of the cell. Cf. *filopodium, lobopodium,* and *rhizopodium*.

axosomatic (ak'so-so-mat'ik) [*axo-* + Gr. *sōma* body] referring to a synapse between the axon of one neuron and the cell body of another.

axospongium (ak"so-spun'je-um) [*axon* + Gr. *spongos* sponge] the meshwork structure making up the substance of the axon of a nerve cell.

axostyle (ak'so-stīl) 1. the central supporting structure of an axiopodium. 2. a supporting rod running through the body of a trichomonad and protruding posteriorly.

Ayala's quotient (equation, index) [A. G. *Ayala*, Italian neurologist, 1878–1943] see under *quotient*.

ayapana (ah"yah-pah'nah) the leaves of *Eupato'rium tripliner've*, a plant growing in many tropical countries; used as an aromatic, stomachic, diaphoretic, and stimulant, and as a household remedy for many conditions in various hot regions.

Ayer's test (ārz) [James Bourne *Ayer*, Boston neurologist, born 1882] see under *test*.

Ayer-Tobey test (a'er-to'be) [James Bourne *Ayer*, Boston neurologist, born 1882; George L. *Tobey*, Jr., Boston otolaryngologist, 1881–1947] Tobey-Ayer test.

Ayerza's disease, syndrome (ah-yer'thaz) [Abel *Ayerza*, Buenos Aires physician, 1861–1918] see under *disease* and *syndrome*.

ayurvedism (ah"yoor-va'dism) Asiatic Indian treatment by means of plants and drugs indiginous to India.

Az. azote, French for nitrogen.

azabon (a'zah-bon) chemical name: 4-(3-azobicyclo[3.2.2]non-3-ylsulfonyl)benzenamine; a central nervous system stimulant, $C_{14}H_{20}N_2O_2S$.

azaclorzine hydrochloride (a"zah-klor'zēn) chemical name: 2-chloro-10-[3-(hexahydropyrrolo[1,2-*a*]pyrazin-2-(1*H*)-yl)-1-oxopropyl]-10*H*-phenothiazine dihydrochloride; a coronary vasodilator, $C_{22}H_{24}ClN_3OS \cdot 2HCl$.

azacosterol hydrochloride (ah"zah-kos'ter-ōl) chemical name: 17β-[[3-(diethylamino)-propyl]methylamino]androst-5-en-3β-ol dihydrochloride; a hypocholesterolemic agent and avian chemosterilant, $C_{25}H_{44}N_2O \cdot 2HCl$.

azacyclonol (a"zah-si'klo-nol) chemical name: α,α-diphenyl-4-piperidinemethanol. The gamma isomer of pipradol, $C_{18}H_{21}NO$, occurring as small white odorless crystals; used in the hydrochlo-

ride form as a tranquilizer in the treatment of schizophrenia. Called also *gamma-pipradol*.

azacytidine (ah"zah-si'tĭ-dēn) chemical name: 5-azacytidine-4-amino-1-ribofuranosyl-1,3,5-triazin-2(1*H*)-one. An antineoplastic, $C_8H_{12}N_4O_5$, which has been used in the treatment of acute myelogenous and lymphocytic leukemia.

azaguanine (az"ah-gwan'in) a mitotic poison, which resembles the purine guanine, but is actually incorporated into nucleic acids and acts to block nucleic acid synthesis by competitive inhibition.

azamethonium bromide (a"zah-mĕ-tho'ne-um) chemical name: 2,2'-(methylimino)bis[*N*-ethyl-*N,N*-dimethylethanaminium]dibromide. A ganglionic blocking agent, $C_{13}H_{33}Br_2N_3$, which has been used as an antihypertensive agent.

azanator maleate (a'zah-na"tor) chemical name: 5-(1-methyl-4-piperidinylidene)-5*H*-[1]benzopyrano[2,3-*b*]pyridine (*Z*)-2-butenedioate(1:1); a bronchodilator, $C_{18}H_{18}N_2O \cdot C_4H_4O_4$.

azanidazole (a"zah-nid'ah-zōl) chemical name: (*E*)-4-[2-(1-methyl-5-nitro-1*H*-imidazol-2-yl)ethenyl]-2-pyrimidinamine; an antiprotozoal, $C_{10}H_{10}N_6O_2$.

azapetine phosphate (a"zah-pet'ēn) chemical name: 6,7-dihydro-6,7-dihydro-6-(2-propenyl)-5*H*-dibenz[*c,e*]azepine phosphate. An α-adrenergic blocking agent, $C_{17}H_{20}NO_4P$, occurring as white crystalline powder; used as a vasodilator in peripheral vascular disease in which vasospasm is prominent, administered orally.

azapropazone (ah"zah-pro'pah-zōn) apazone.

azaserine (a"zah-ser'ēn) chemical name: L-serine diazoacetate (ester). An antifungal antibiotic, $C_5H_7N_3O_4$, produced by *Streptomyces* species or by synthesis; it is a glutamine antagonist, inhibiting the synthesis of purine, and has been used as an antineoplastic agent.

azastene (a'zah-stēn) chemical name: 4,4,17-trimethylandrosta-2,5-dieno[2,3-*d*]isoxazol-17β-ol; a contraceptive, $C_{23}H_{33}NO_2$.

azatadine maleate (ah-zat'ah-dēn) chemical name: 6,11-dihydro-11-(1-methyl-4-piperidylidene)-5*H*-benzol[5,6]cyclohepta-[1,2-*b*]pyridine maleate (1:2); an antihistaminic, $C_{20}H_{22}N_2 \cdot 2C_4H_4O_4$, used in the treatment of perennial and seasonal allergic rhinitis and chronic urticaria, administered orally.

azathioprine (a"zah-thi'o-prēn) [USP] chemical name: 6-[(1-methyl-4-nitro-1*H*-imidazol-5-yl)thio]-1*H*-purine. A purine antagonist that interferes with DNA synthesis, it is an imidazole derivative of mercaptopurine, $C_9H_7N_7O_2S$, occurring as a pale yellow powder; used as an immunosuppressive agent in tissue transplantation and in autoimmune diseases, administered orally. **a. sodium,** the sodium salt of azathioprine, suitable for injection; used for the same purposes as the base.

6-azauridine (a"zah-u'rĭ-dēn) chemical name: 2-β-D-ribofuranoxyl-1,2,4-triazine-3,5(2*H*,4*H*)-dione; an antimetabolite, the triazine analogue of uridine, $C_8H_{11}N_3O_6$, which particularly affects neoplastic cells; it has been used in the treatment of acute leukemias.

azedarach (ah-zed'ă-rak") a common name for *Melia azedarach* L. (Meliaceae) (the chinaberry tree; umbrella tree; pride of China). Its seeds are used for beads and rosaries, and the bark of roots for its anthelmintic properties. Leaf juice is used as a diuretic and emmenagogue. In the United States, it is considered a poisonous plant for humans and animals, the toxicity being felt to reside in the resinous fraction of fruit pulp. Its pharmacological actions include severe local irritation, nervous symptoms, cardioactivity, and dyspnea.

azeotropic (a"ze-o-trop'ik) pertaining to or characterized by azeotropy.

azeotropy (a"ze-ot'ro-pe) [*a* neg. + Gr. *zein* to boil + *tropē* a turn, or turning] the absence of any change in the composition of a mixture of substances when it is boiled under a given pressure.

azepindole (a"zĕ-pin'dōl) chemical name: 2,3,4,5-tetrahydro-1*H*-[1,4]diazepino[1,2-*a*]indole; an antidepressant, $C_{12}H_{14}N_2$.

azerin (az'er-in) an enzyme from *Drosera, Nepenthes,* and various other insectivorous plants.

azid, azide (az'id) a compound that contains the group N_3.

azipramine (ah-zip'rah-mēn) chemical name: 6,7-dihydro-*N*-methyl-*N*-(phenylmethyl)-indolo[1,7-*ab*][1]benzazepine-1-ethanamine monohydrochloride; an antidepressant, $C_{26}H_{26}N_2 \cdot HCl$.

azlocillin (az"lo-sil'in) an antibiotic derivative of penicillin, $C_{20}H_{23}N_5O_6S$.

azo- a prefix indicating the presence of the group —N:N—, as in azobenzene.

azoamyly (a-zo-am'ĭ-le) [*a* neg. + Gr. *zōon* animal + *amylon* starch] inability of the hepatic cells to store up a normal amount of glycogen.

Azobacter (a-zo-bak'ter) (*obs.*) azotobacter.

azobenzene (az"o-ben'zēn) [*azote* + *benzene*] an orange-red crystalline product, $C_6H_5N:N \cdot C_6H_5$, of the reduction of nitrobenzene, soluble in alcohol and ether, but only sparingly so in water; it is the parent substance of azo dyes and some pH indicators.

azocarmine (az″o-kar′min) either azocarmine G or azocarmine B, red basic dyes used in certain staining procedures.

azoic (ah-zo′ik) [*a* neg. + Gr. *zōe* life] destitute of living organisms.

azoimide (az″o-im′īd) 1. the group:

$$—N{\displaystyle <}^{\substack{N\\ \|\\ N}}$$

2. a protoplasmic poison, hydrazoic acid, N_3H, resembling hydrocyanic acid in its action, made by heating hydrogen chloride with sodium nitrate. It is highly explosive. Called also *triazoic acid* and *hydronitric acid.*

azole (az′ōl) 1. a derivative of a five-membered ring containing nitrogen and either oxygen, sulfur, or an additional nitrogen atom, as well as carbon atoms. 2. pyrrole.

Azolid (az′o-lid) trademark for preparations of phenylbutazone.

azolimine (ah-zo′li-mēn) chemical name: 2-imino-3-methyl-1-phenyl-4-imidazolidinone; a potassium-sparing diuretic, $C_{10}H_{11}N_3O$.

azolitmin (az″o-lit′min) a coloring principle, $C_7H_7NO_4$, from litmus; it is used as a pH indicator, being red at a pH of 4.5 and blue at 8.3.

azomycin (a″zo-mi′sin) chemical name: 2-nitroimidazole. An antibiotic, $C_3H_3N_3O_2$, produced by a species of *Streptomyces.*

azoospermatism (a-zo″o-sper′mah-tizm) azoospermia.

azoospermia (a-zo″o-sper′me-ah) [*a* neg. + *zoosperm*] absence of spermatozoa in the semen, or failure of formation of spermatozoa.

azopigment (a″zo-pig′ment) a purple derivative of bile pigment containing an azo (—N=N—) linkage; formed by reacting bile pigments with diazotizing agents.

azoprotein (az″o-pro′te-in) a protein some constituents of which have been diazotized.

azosulfamide (az″o-sul′fah-mīd) chemical name: 6-(acetylamino)-3-[[4-(aminosufonyl)phenyl]azo]-4-hydroxy-2, 7-naphthalenedisulfonic acid. An antibacterial compound, $C_{18}H_{14}N_4Na_2O_{10}S$, occurring as a reddish-brown powder; it was one of the forerunners of the sulfonamide drugs.

azote (az′ōt) [*a* neg. + Gr. *zōe* life] nitrogen.

azotemia (az″o-te′me-ah) [*azote* + Gr. *haima* blood + *-ia*] an excess of urea or other nitrogenous bodies in the blood. **chloropenic a.,** hypochloremic a. **extrarenal a.,** excess of non-protein nitrogen in the blood in the absence of renal disease sufficient to account for it; called also *prerenal a.* **hypochloremic a.,** a condition characterized by deficiency of sodium chloride, fixation of chlorine in the tissues, and azoturia; called also *chloropenic a.* **prerenal a.,** extrarenal a.

azotemic (az″o-te′mik) pertaining to or characterized by azotemia.

azotenesis (az″o-te-ne′sis) any disease due to an excess of nitrogenous substances in the system.

azothermia (az″o-ther′me-ah) [*azote* + Gr. *thermē* heat] temperature increase produced by nitrogenous matter in the blood.

azotification (az-o″ti-fi-ka′shun) the fixation of atmospheric nitrogen.

azotize (az′o-tīz) to combine or charge with nitrogen.

Azotobacter (ah-zo′to-bak″ter) a genus of microorganisms of the family Azotobacteraceae, order Eubacteriales; it includes three species, *A. a′gilis, A. chroococ′cum,* and *A. in′dicus.* Sometimes called *Azobacter.*

Azotobacteraceae (ah-zo″to-bak″tĕ-ra′se-e) a family of Schizomycetes, order Eubacteriales, occurring as relatively large rods and even cocci. They are free-living nitrogen-fixing bacteria widely distributed in soil, which are capable of fixing atmospheric nitrogen in the presence of carbohydrate or other source of energy, and grow best on media deficient in nitrogen. The family includes a single genus, *Azotobacter.*

azotometer (az″o-tom′ĕ-ter) [*azote* + Gr. *metron* measure] an instrument for measuring the proportion of nitrogen compounds in a solution.

Azotomonas (ah-zo″to-mo′nas) a genus of microorganisms of the family Pseudomonadaceae, suborder Pseudomonadineae, order Pseudomonadales, occurring as rod-shaped to coccoid cells

found in the soil and active in fixation of atmospheric nitrogen. It includes two species, *A. fluores′cens* and *A. inso′lita.*

azotomycin (ah-zo″to-mi′sin) an antibiotic substance with antineoplastic properties produced by *Streptomyces ambofaciens;* formerly called *duazomycin B.*

azotorrhea (az″o-to-re′ah) [*azote* + Gr. *rhoia* flow] excessive loss of nitrogen in the feces.

azoturia (az″o-tu′re-ah) [*azote* + Gr. *ouron* urine] 1. an excess of urea or other nitrogen compounds in the urine. 2. a disease of horses marked by a sudden attack of perspiration and paralysis of the hind quarters and by the passing of light red to dark brown urine. It occurs in horses that, after being engaged in continuous work, are rested and well fed for a few days and then returned to work.

azoturic (az″o-tu′rik) pertaining to azoturia or the urinary excretion of nitrogen.

azoxybenzene (az″ok-se-ben-zēn′) a pale yellow product, $C_6H_5 \cdot N \cdot (\cdot O)N \cdot C_6H_5$, of the reduction of nitrobenzene.

azoxy compound (az-ok′se) a compound which contains the group

$$O{\displaystyle <}^{\substack{N—\\ \|\\ N—}}$$

AZT Aschheim-Zondek test.

Aztec idiocy, type (az′tek) [*Aztec,* a tribe of aboriginal Mexicans] microcephalic idiocy.

azul (az′ool) pinta.

azulene (az′u-lēn) a blue crystalline hydrocarbon, $C_{10}H_8$, with an odor similar to that of naphthalene, obtained from certain volatile oils, such as oil of cubebs.

Azulfidine (a-zul′fi-dēn) trademark for a preparation of sulfasalazine.

azure (azh′-ūr) any of the partially methylated homologues of the series of basic dyes extending from thionine to methylene blue, or to certain mixtures of members of this series. They are metachromatic, and are used in many important staining procedures. **a. A,** asymmetrical dimethylthionine, $(CH_3)_2N \cdot C_6H_3 \cdot (SN)C_6H_3 \cdot NH_2 \cdot Cl.$ **a. B,** trimethylthionin, $(CH_3)_2N \cdot C_6H_3(SN) \cdot C_6H_3 \cdot N(CH_3) \cdot Cl.$ **a. C,** monomethylthionine chloride, $(CH_3) \cdot N \cdot C_6H_3(SN)C_6H_3NH_2 \cdot Cl.$ **a. I,** azure B. **a. II,** a mixture of equal parts of azure I and methylene blue. **methylene a.,** azure B.

azuresin (azh″u-rez′in) a complex combination of azure A dye and carbacrylic cationic exchange resin, used as a diagnostic aid in detection of gastric secretion.

azurophil (azh-u′ro-fil) [*azure* + Gr. *philein* to love] an element or cell that stains well with blue aniline dyes.

azurophile (azh′u-ro-fīl) 1. azurophil. 2. azurophilic.

azurophilia (azh″u-ro-fil′e-ah) a condition in which the blood contains cells having azurophil granulations.

azurophilic (azh″u-ro-fil′ik) staining well with blue aniline dyes; pertaining to or characterized by azurophilia.

azygogram (az′i-go-gram) the roentgenographic record obtained by azygography.

azygography (az″i-gog′rah-fe) roentgenography of the azygous venous system following its opacification with radiographic contrast material; usually employed for evaluation of abnormal tumor masses in the mediastinum, as evidenced by extrinsic pressure upon, or complete obstruction of, the visualized azygous vein.

azygos (az′i-gos) [*a* neg. + Gr. *zygon* yoke or pair] 1. unpaired. 2. any unpaired part, such as the azygos vein.

azygosperm (ah-zi′go-sperm″) [*a* neg. + Gr. *zygon* yoke or pair + *sperma* seed] azygospore.

azygospore (ah-zi′go-spōr″) [*a* neg. + Gr. *zygon* yoke or pair + *sporos* seed] a spore developed directly from a gamete without conjugation; called also *azygosperm.*

azygous (az′i-gus) having no fellow; unpaired.

azymia (ah-zim′e-ah) [*a* neg. + Gr. *zymē* ferment] absence of an enzyme.

azymic (ah-zim′ik) (*obs.*) not causing fermentation; not arising from fermentation.

azymous (ah-zi′mus) (*obs.*) azymic.

B

B   chemical symbol for *boron;* in physics the symbol for magnetic flux density measured in *gauss.*

B.   bacillus; [L.] *bal'neum* (bath); Baumé scale; Benoist scale; boils at; buccal. See also *point B,* under *point.*

β   the second letter of the Greek alphabet; see *beta-.*

Ba   chemical symbol for *barium.*

B.A.   abbreviation for L. *bal'neum are'nae* (sand bath); Bachelor of Arts.

Babbitt metal (bab'it) [Isaac *Babbitt,* American inventor, 1799–1862]   see under *metal.*

Babcock's operation (bab'koks) [William Wayne *Babcock,* Philadelphia surgeon, 1872–1963]   see under *operation.*

Babcock's test (bab'koks) [Stephen Moulton *Babcock,* American agricultural chemist, 1843–1931]   see under *tests.*

Babès' treatment, tubercles (bah'bāz) [Victor *Babès,* Roumanian bacteriologist, 1854–1926]   see under *treatment* and *tubercle.*

Babès-Ernst granules (bodies) (bah'bāz-ernst) [Victor *Babès;* Paul *Ernst,* German pathologist, 1859–1937]   metachromatic granules.

Babesia (bah-be'ze-ah) [Victor *Babès*]   a genus of sporozoa of the family Babesiidae, order Haemosporidia, found in red blood cells of various animals, including cattle, dogs, sheep, goats, swine, and horses, and transmitted by ticks; formerly called *Babesiella* and *Piroplasma.* **B. bigem'ina,** the causative organism of Texas fever; transmitted by the genus *Boophilus,* primarily by *B. annulatus.* **B. bo'vis,** the cause of hemoglobinuria, fever, and anemia in cattle in Europe; transmitted by *Ixodes ricinus.* **B. cabal'li,** a species causing biliary fever of horses in Africa, Siberia, and Russia, transmitted by ticks of the genera *Anocentor, Dermacentor, Hyalomma,* and *Rhipicephalus.* **B. ca'nis,** the cause of malignant jaundice in dogs; transmitted by *Haemaphysalis leachi, Rhipicephalus sanguineus, Ixodes ricinus,* and *Dermacentor reticulatus.* **B. e'qui,** a species causing biliary fever of horses in the eastern part of the Soviet Union, Italy, Africa, India, and Brazil, transmitted by ticks of the genera *Dermacentor, Rhipicephalus,* and *Hyalomma;* called also *Nuttallia equi.* **B. gibso'ni,** a species found in dogs; called also *Nuttallia gibsoni.* **B. mota'si,** a species infecting sheep and goats in Europe and Africa. **B. o'vis,** the etiologic agent of carceag and icterohematuria of sheep.

babesiasis, babesiosis (bah-bě-si'ah-sis, bah-be''ze-o'sis)   infection with *Babesia;* called also *piroplasmosis.*

Babesiella (bah-be''ze-el'ah)   *Babesia.*

Babesiidae (bah-be-ze'ĭ-de)   a family of protozoa of the order Haemosporidia, subphylum Sporozoa, comprising intraerythrocytic parasites of various vertebrates, usually mammals, reptiles, and amphibians. It includes the genera *Aegyptianella, Babesia,* and *Theileria.*

Babinski's law, etc. (bah-bin'skēz) [Joseph François Felix *Babinski,* physician in Paris, 1857–1932]   see under *law, phenomenon, reflex, sign,* and *syndrome.*

Babinski-Fröhlich syndrome (bah-bin'ske-fra'lik) [J.F.F. *Babinski;* Alfred *Fröhlich,* Vienna neurologist, 1871–1953]   adiposogenital dystrophy.

Babinski-Nageotte syndrome (bah-bin'ske-nazh-yot') [J.F.F. *Babinski;* Jean *Nageotte,* Paris pathologist, 1866–1948]   see under *syndrome.*

Babinski-Vaquez syndrome (bah-bin'ske-vak-a') [J.F.F. *Babinski;* Louis Henri *Vaquez,* French physician, 1860–1936]   Babinski syndrome.

baby (ba'be)   an infant; a child not yet able to walk. **blue b.,** an infant born with cyanosis due to a congenital heart lesion or to congenital atelectasis. **collodion b.,** an infant born completely covered by a collodion- or parchment-like membrane; see *lamellar exfoliation of the newborn,* under *exfoliation.*

bacampicillin hydrochloride (bah-kam''pĭ-sil'in)   chemical name: 6-[(aminophenylacetyl)amino]-3,3-dimethyl-7-oxo-4-thia-1-azabicyclo[3.2.0]heptane-2-carboxylic acid 1-[(ethoxycarbonyl)oxy]ethyl ester monohydrochloride; an antibacterial, $C_{21}H_{27}N_3O_7 \cdot HCl.$

bacca (bak'ah), pl. *bac'cae* [L.]   a berry.

baccate (bak'āt)   resembling a berry.

Baccelli's mixture, sign (bak-chel'ēz) [Guido *Baccelli,* Italian physician, 1832–1916]   see under *mixture,* and see *aphonic pectoriloquy,* under *pectoriloquy.*

bacciform (bak'sĭ-form) [L. *bacca* berry + *forma* shape]   berry-shaped.

Bachman test (reaction) [George William *Bachman,* American parasitologist, born 1890]   see under *tests.*

Bachmann's bundle [Jean George *Bachmann,* American physiologist, born 1877]   see under *bundle.*

Baciguent (bas'ĭ-gwent)   trademark for preparations of bacitracin.

Bacillaceae (bas''il-la'se-e)   a family of Schizomycetes, order Eubacteriales, made up of rod-shaped cells capable of producing cylindrical, ellipsoidal, or spherical endospores which are located terminally, subterminally, or centrally. They are mostly saprophytic, commonly found in the soil, but a few are parasitic on insects or animals, and may produce disease. It includes two genera, *Bacillus* and *Clostridium,* the former aerobic, and the latter obligate anaerobes.

bacillary (bas'ĭ-la''re)   pertaining to bacilli or to rodlike forms.

bacillemia (bas''ĭ-le'me-ah) [*bacillus* + Gr. *haima* blood]   the presence of bacilli in the blood.

bacilli (bah-sil'i) [L.]   plural of *bacillus.*

bacilliculture (bah-sil'ĭ-kul-chur)   the artificial propagation of bacilli.

bacilliferous (bah''sil-lif'er-us)   bearing or carrying bacilli.

bacilliform (bah-sil'ĭ-form) [*bacillus* + L. *forma* form]   having the appearance of a bacillus.

bacilligenic (bah-sil'ĭ-jen'ik)   bacillogenic.

bacillin (bah-sil'in)   an antibiotic substance isolated from strains of *Bacillus subtilis,* highly active on both gram-positive and gram-negative bacteria.

bacilliparous (bas''ĭ-lip'ah-rus) [*bacillus* + L. *parere* to produce]   producing bacilli.

bacillogenic (bah-sil''o-jen'ik)   1. caused by bacilli. 2. producing bacilli.

bacillogenous (bas''ĭ-loj'ě-nus)   caused by bacilli.

bacilluria (bas''ĭ-lu're-ah) [*bacillus* + Gr. *ouron* urine + *-ia*]   the presence of bacilli in the urine.

Bacillus (bah-sil'lus) [L. "little rod"]   a genus of microorganisms of the family Bacillaceae, order Eubacteriales, including large gram-positive, aerobic, spore-forming bacteria separated into 33 species, of which three are pathogenic, or potentially pathogenic, and the remainder are saprophytic soil forms. Many organisms historically called *Bacillus* are now classified in other genera. **B. abor'tus,** the microorganism responsible for contagious abortion in cattle (Bang's disease). **B. aerog'enes capsula'tus,** *Clostridium perfringens.* **B. al'vei,** the etiologic agent of European foulbrood of honeybees. **B. an'thracis,** the causative agent of anthrax in lower animals and man. **B. botuli'nus,**

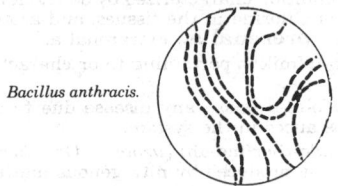

Bacillus anthracis.

Clostridium botulinum. **B. bre'vis,** an organism that is the source of the antibiotics gramicidin and tyrocidin. **B. bronchisep'ticus,** *Brucella bronchiseptica.* **B. cer'eus,** a saprophytic, usually motile, aerobic, spore-forming bacillus that has been implicated in several outbreaks of food poisoning. **B. co'li,** *Escherichia coli.* **B. cras'sus,** a normally nonpathogenic species sometimes found in vaginal cultures; it has been implicated as the cause of ulcus vulvae acutum. **B. dysente'riae,** *Shigella dysenteriae.* **B. enterit'idis,** *Salmonella enteritidis.* **B. faeca'lis alcalig'enes,** *Alcaligenes faecalis.* **B. frag'ilis,** *Bacteroides fragilis.* **B. fusifor'mis,** *Fusobacterium plauti-vincenti.* **B. lar'vae,** the specific etiologic agent of American foulbrood of honeybees, not pathogenic for man. **B. lep'rae,** *Mycobacterium leprae.* **B. mal'lei,** *Pseudomonas mallei.* **B. megathe'rium,** a widely distributed saprophytic soil form, commonly occurring as a laboratory contaminant. **B. necroph'orus,** *Fusobacterium necrophorum.* **B. oedemat'iens,** *Clostridium novyi.* **B. oedem'atis malig'ni No. II,** *Clostridium novyi.* **B. parabotuli'nus,** *Clostridium botulinum* type Cβ. **B. pneumo'niae,** *Klebsiella pneumoniae.* **B. polymyx'a,** a saprophytic soil and water microorganism that produces the antibiotic polymyxin. **B. pseudomal'lei,** *Pseudomonas pseudomallei.* **B. pyocya'neus,** *Pseudomonas aeruginosa.* **B. sub'tilis,** a common saprophytic soil and water form, often occurring as a laboratory contaminant, and in rare instances found in apparently causal relation to pathologic processes, such as conjunctivitis. **B. tet'ani,** *Clostridium tetani.* **B. trop'icus,** an aerobic sporulating bacillus found in Australia as a natural parasite of the rat and bandicoot. **B. ty'phi, B. typho'sus,** *Salmonella ty-*

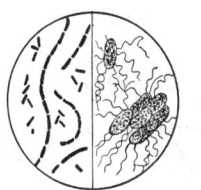

Bacillus subtilis.

phosa. **B. welchi'ii,** *Clostridium perfringens.* **B. whit'-mori,** *Pseudomonas pseudomallei.*

bacillus (bah-sil'us), pl. *bacil'li* [L.] 1. an organism of the genus *Bacillus.* 2. in general, any rod-shaped bacterium; any spore-forming, rod-shaped microorganism of the order Eubacteriales. **b. aborti'vus equi'nus,** *Salmonella abortus equi.* **Bang's b.,** *Brucella abortus.* **Battey bacilli,** unclassified mycobacteria of Group III (nonphotochromogens), which may produce tuberculosis-like disease in man. **Boas-Oppler b.,** an organism first found in the gastric juice of patients with stomach carcinoma, similar to if not identical with *Lactobacillus bulgaricus;* called also *lactobacillus of Boas-Oppler.* **Bordet-Gengou b.,** *Bordetella pertussis.* **butter b.,** *Mycobacterium butyricum.* **Calmette-Guerin b.,** an organism of the strain *Mycobacterium bovis,* rendered completely avirulent by cultivation for many years on bile-glycero-potato medium. **Chauveau's b.,** *Clostridium chauvoei.* **colon b.,** *Escherichia coli.* **diphtheria b.,** *Corynebacterium diphtheriae.* **Döderlein's b.,** a large gram-positive microorganism commonly found in the vagina, said to be identical with *Lactobacillus acidophilus.* **Ducrey's b.,** *Hemophilus ducreyi.* **dysentery bacilli,** gram-negative, non-spore-forming rods related to other enteric bacteria, and causing dysentery in man; see *Shigella.* **Escherich's b.,** *Escherichia coli.* **Fick's b.,** *Proteus vulgaris.* **Flexner's b.,** *Shigella flexneri.* **Friedländer's b.,** *Klebsiella pneumoniae.* **fusiform b.,** a rod-shaped bacterium in which the cell is thicker in the center and tapers towards the ends. **Gärtner's b.,** *Salmonella enteritidis.* **Ghon-Sachs b.,** *Clostridium septicum.* **glanders b.,** *Pseudomonas mallei.* **Hansen's b.,** *Mycobacterium leprae.* **hay b.,** *Bacillus subtilis.* **Hofmann's b.,** *Corynebacterium pseudodiphtheriticum.* **hog cholera b.,** *Salmonella choleraesuis.* **Johne's b.,** *Mycobacterium paratuberculosis.* **Klebs-Löffler b.,** *Corynebacterium diphtheriae.* **Koch-Weeks b.,** *Hemophilus aegyptius.* **lepra b., leprosy b.,** *Mycobacterium leprae.* **Morax-Axenfeld b.,** *Hemophilus duplex.* **Morgan's b.,** *Proteus morgani.* **Newcastle-Manchester b.,** *Shigella flexneri* type 6, Boyd 88. **Nocard's b.,** *Salmonella typhimurium.* **paracolon bacilli,** microorganisms commonly found in the intestinal flora, distinguished by delayed (5–21 days) fermentation of lactose. See *Paracolobactrum.* **Pfeiffer's b.,** *Hemophilus influenzae.* **Preisz-Nocard b.,** *Corynebacterium pseudotuberculosis.* **rhinoscleroma b.,** a microorganism closely resembling *Klebsiella pneumoniae,* isolated from granulomatous lesions in rhinoscleroma. **Schmitz's b.,** *Shigella dysenteriae* type 2. **Schmorl's b.,** *Fusobacterium necrophorum.* **Shiga b.,** *Shigella dysenteriae* type 1. **smegma b.,** *Mycobacterium smegmatis.* **Sonne-Duval b.,** *Shigella sonnei.* **Stanley b.,** a serotype of *Salmonella* isolated from patients with food poisoning in Stanley, England. **Strong's b.,** *Shigella flexneri.* **swine rotlauf b.,** *Erysipelothrix rhusiopathiae.* **tetanus b.,** *Clostridium tetani.* **timothy b.,** *Mycobacterium phlei.* **tubercle b.,** *Mycobacterium tuberculosis.* **typhoid b.,** *Salmonella typhosa.* **vole b.,** *Mycobacterium microti.* **Weeks' b.,** *Hemophilus aegyptius.* **Welch's b.,** *Clostridium perfringens.* **Whitmore's b.,** *Pseudomonas pseudomallei.*

bacitracin (bas"ĭ-tra'sin) [USP] an antibacterial polypeptide produced by the growth of a gram-positive, spore-forming organism belonging to the *licheniformis* group of *Bacillus subtilis,* occurring as a white to pale buff powder. It is effective against many gram-positive bacteria, such as staphylococci, streptococci, and pneumococci, and some gram-negative bacteria, such as gonococci and meningococci. It is applied topically to the skin or conjunctiva or administered by intramuscular injection in the treatment of infections caused by susceptible organisms. **b. zinc** [USP], the zinc salt of bacitracin, occurring as a white to pale tan powder; used for topical application to the skin.

back (bak) the posterior part of the trunk from the neck to the pelvis; called also *dorsum* [NA]. **flat b.,** a back that appears flat as a result of a decrease of normal lumbar lordosis and normal thoracic kyphosis. **functional b.,** a condition of fatigue and defective balance marked by more or less continuous lumbar or dorsal pain. **hollow b.,** see *lordosis.* **hump b., hunch b.,** kyphosis. **poker b.,** rheumatoid spondylitis. **saddle b.,** see *lordosis.*

backalgia (bak-al'je-ah) back pain not explained on the basis of structural abnormality or disease process.

backbone (back'bōn) the vertebral column, forming a continuous, comparatively rigid structure in the midline of the back; see *columna vertebralis* [NA].

back-cross (bak'kros) in experimental genetics, a mating between a heterozygote and a homozygote (as between an F_1 hybrid and an individual of a genotype identical to one of the two parental strains [P_1]). **double b.,** the mating between a double heterozygote and a homozygote; it is the mating most informative for analysis of the linkage of various genes.

backflow (bak'flo) the flowing of a current in a direction the reverse of that normally taken; regurgitation. **pyelovenous b.,** the drainage of fluid from the pelvis of the kidney into the venous system under certain conditions of back pressure.

backing (bak'ing) in dentistry, the piece of metal that supports the porcelain facing, and to which the pins of the artificial tooth are soldered. **alloy b.,** one made of an alloy instead of pure platinum or gold.

backknee (bak'ne) genu recurvatum.

back-raking (bak-rāk'ing) extraction of impacted feces from the rectum of an animal.

backscatter (bak'skat-er) in radiology, radiation deflected by scattering processes at angles greater than 90 degrees to the original direction of the beam of radiation; see also *scatter radiation,* under *radiation.*

BaCl₂ barium chloride.

baclofen (bak'lo-fen) chemical name: 4-amino-3-(4-chlorophenyl)butanoic acid. A muscle relaxant, $C_{10}H_{12}ClNO_2$, which is an analogue of gamma-aminobutyric acid; administered orally in the treatment of spasticity in multiple sclerosis and other disorders of the spinal cord.

Bacon's anoscope (ba'kunz) [Harry Ellicott *Bacon,* Philadelphia proctologist, born 1900] see under *anoscope.*

Bact. *Bacterium.*

bacteremia (bak"ter-e'me-ah) [Gr. *baktērion* little rod + *haima* blood] the presence of bacteria in the blood.

Bacteria (bak-te're-ah) in some systems of classification, a division of the kingdom Procaryotae, including all prokaryotic organisms that are not blue-green algae (see *Cyanophyceae*). In other systems, prokaryotic organisms without a true cell wall are considered to be unrelated to the Bacteria and are placed in a separate class—the Mollicutes.

bacteria (bak-te're-ah) [L.] plural of *bacterium.*

Bacteriaceae (bak"te-re-a'se-e) a name formerly given a family of Schizomycetes.

bacterial (bak-te're-al) pertaining to or caused by bacteria.

bactericidal (bak-tēr"ĭ-si'dal) [*bacterium* + L. *caedere* to kill] destructive to bacteria.

bactericide (bak-tēr'ĭ-sīd) an agent that destroys bacteria. **specific b.,** bacteriolysin.

bactericidin (bak"ter-rĭ-si'din) a substance that leads to the death of bacteria; such substances include both antibody and nonantibody components in the blood.

bacterid (bak'ter-id) a skin eruption caused by a bacterial infection elsewhere in the body; usually pustular bacterid (q.v.). **pustular b.,** a grouped eruption of sterile intraepidermal pustules on the palms or soles, believed by some to be due to bacterial infection elsewhere in the body; called also *pustular b. of Andrews.*

bacteride (bak"ter-īd) (obs.) bacterid.

bacteridium (bak"ter-id'e-um), pl. *bacterid'ia.* A former generic name for certain bacilli.

Bacterieae (bak-te're-e-e) a name formerly given a tribe of Schizomycetes.

bacteriemia (bak-tēr"e-e'me-ah) bacteremia.

bacteriform (bak-tēr'ē-form) resembling a bacterium in form.

bacterin (bak'ter-in) a bacterial vaccine; a suspension of bacteria for stimulating the production of antibodies in humans and animals for prophylactic or therapeutic purposes, or for the production of antisera. Cf. *vaccine.*

bacterinia (bak-tĕ-rin'e-ah) the condition of unfavorable action which sometimes follows inoculation with bacterial vaccines.

bacterioagglutinin (bak-te"re-o-ah-gloo'tĭ-nin) an agglutinin that causes the clumping of bacteria.

bacteriochlorophyll (bak-te"re-o-klo'ro-fil) a form of chlorophyll occurring in certain bacteria and capable of carrying out photosynthesis. It is designated bacteriochlorophyll a, b, c, or d, according to its absorption spectrum.

bacteriocidin (bak-te"re-o-si'din) an antibacterial antibody that causes death of bacteria. Originally used to define a specific antibody though actually referring to only one of several activities, such as agglutination and precipitation.

bacteriocin (bak-te"rĭ-o-sin) any of a group of substances, e.g., colicin, released by certain bacteria that kill but do not lyse other strains of bacteria. Specific bacteriocins attach to specific receptors on cell walls and induce specific metabolic block, e.g., cessation of nucleic acid or protein synthesis or of oxidative phosphorylation.

bacteriocinogenic (bak-te"re-o-sin"o-jen'ik) giving rise to bacteriocin; denoting bacterial plasmids that synthesize bacteriocin.

bacterioclasis (bak-te"re-ok'lah-sis) [*bacteria* + Gr. *klasis* breaking] bacteriolysis.

bacterioerythrin (bak-te"re-o-er'ĭ-thrin) a red pigment obtained from bacteriopurpurin.

bacteriofluorescein (bak-te"re-o-floo-o-res'e-in) a fluorescent coloring matter produced by bacteria.

bacteriogenic (bak-te"re-o-jen'ik) 1. bacterial in origin. 2. producing bacteria.

bacteriogenous (bak-te"re-oj'ĕ-nus) bacteriogenic.

bacteriohemagglutinin (bak-te"re-o-hem"ah-gloo'tĭ-nin) a hemagglutinin formed by body tissues in response to bacterial antigens.

bacteriohemolysin (bak-te"re-o-he-mol'ĭ-sin) a hemolysin formed in the body in response to bacterial antigens.

bacterioid (bak-te're-oid) [Fr. *baktērion* little rod + *eidos* form] 1. resembling the bacteria. 2. a structure resembling a bacterium.

bacteriologic, bacteriological (bak-te"re-o-loj'ik, bak-te"-re-o-loj'ĭ-k'l) pertaining to bacteriology.

bacteriologist (bak-te"re-ol'o-jist) an expert in bacteriology.

bacteriology (bak-te"re-ol'o-je) [*bacteria* + *-logy*] the science that treats of bacteria. Cf. *microbiology.* **hygienic b.,** sanitary b. **medical b.,** that branch of bacteriology which treats of the microorganisms that cause disease in the animal body. **pathological b.,** that branch of bacteriology which treats chiefly of the effects produced upon the animal body by the presence of bacteria and their toxins. **sanitary b.,** bacteriology which deals chiefly with methods of disease prevention based upon the knowledge of the organisms causing disease and the manner in which they spread; called also *hygienic b.* **systematic b.,** that branch of bacteriology which studies the classification and relationship of bacteria.

bacteriolysant (bak-te"re-ol'ĭ-sant) an agent that causes bacteriolysis.

bacteriolysin (bak-te"re-ol'ĭ-sin) an antibacterial antibody that produces lysis of bacterial cells.

bacteriolysis (bak-te"re-ol'ĭ-sis) [*bacteria* + Gr. *lysis* dissolution] disruption of the structural integrity of a bacterial cell resulting in release of the cell contents.

bacteriolytic (bak-te"re-o-lit'ik) pertaining to, characterized by, or promoting the dissolution or destruction of bacteria.

bacteriolyze (bak-te're-o-līz") to produce or cause bacteriolysis.

bacterio-opsonin (bak-te"re-o-op-so'nin) an opsonin that acts on bacteria.

bacteriopexia (bak-te"re-o-pek'se-ah) bacteriopexy.

bacteriopexy (bak-te"re-o-pek'se) [*bacteria* + Gr. *pēxis* fixation] the fixing of bacteria by histiocytes.

bacteriophage (bak-te're-o-fāj") [*bacteria* + Gr. *phagein* to eat] a virus that lyses bacteria; see *bacterial virus,* under *virus.* **temperate b.,** a bacteriophage whose genetic material (prophage) becomes an intimate part of the bacterial cell, persisting through many cell division cycles. The affected bacterial cell is known as a *lysogenic bacterium* (q.v.).

bacteriophagia (bak-te"re-o-fa'je-ah) the destruction of bacteria by a lytic agent; bacteriolysis.

bacteriophagic (bak-te"re-o-faj'ik) [*bacteria* + Gr. *phagein* to eat] pertaining to, characterized by, or producing bacteriophagia.

bacteriophagology (bak-te"re-o-fah-gol'o-je) the study of bacteriophage.

bacterioph'agum intestina'le (bak-te"re-of'ah-gum in-tes"tĭ-na'le) (*obs.*) bacteriophage.

bacteriophagy (bak-te"re-of'ah-je) bacteriophagia.

bacteriophytoma (bak-te"re-o-fi-to'mah) a tumor-like, reactive lesion caused by bacteria.

bacterioplasmin (bak-te"re-o-plaz'min) any one of a class of unchanged albuminous poisons existing in the expressed juice of certain bacteria.

bacterioprecipitin (bak-te"re-o-pre-sip'ĭ-tin) a precipitin formed in the body in response to bacterial antigens.

bacterioprotein (bak-te"re-o-pro'te-in) any one of a class of poisonous albuminous (protein) bodies, unaltered by heat, derivable from certain bacteria; the bacterioproteins produce fever, inflammation, and suppuration, but are not thought to be specific.

bacteriopsonic (bak-te"re-op-son'ik) exerting an opsonic effect on bacteria.

bacteriopsonin (bak-te"re-op'so-nin) an antibody that interacts with bacteria to render them more susceptible to ingestion by phagocytic cells than they otherwise would be.

bacteriopurpurin (bak-te"re-o-pur'pu-rin) [*bacteria* + L. *purpur* purple] a light purple pigment produced by certain bacteria.

bacteriorhodopsin (bak-te"re-o-ro-dop'sin) [*bacteria* + Gr. *rhodon* rose + *opsis* vision] a purple pigment, similar to rhodopsin, occurring in the cell membrane of bacteria of the genus

Halobacterium, which converts sunlight directly into electrochemical energy.

bacteriosis (bak-te"re-o'sis) any bacterial disease.

bacteriospermia (bak-te"re-o-sper'me-ah) the presence of bacteria in the semen.

bacteriostasis (bak-te"re-os'tah-sis) [*bacteria* + Gr. *stasis* stoppage] the inhibition of growth, but not the killing, of bacteria by chemicals or biologic materials.

bacteriostat (bak-te're-o-stat") an agent that inhibits the growth of bacteria.

bacteriostatic (bak-te"re-o-stat'ik) 1. inhibiting the growth or multiplication of bacteria. 2. an agent that inhibits the growth or multiplication of bacteria.

bacteriotherapy (bak-te"re-o-ther'ah-pe) [*bacteria* + *therapy*] treatment of disease by the introduction of bacteria into the system.

bacteriotoxemia (bak-te"re-o-tok-se'me-ah) the presence of bacterial toxins in the blood.

bacteriotoxic (bak-te"re-o-tok'sik) 1. toxic to bacteria. 2. caused by bacterial toxins.

bacteriotoxin (bak-te"re-o-tok'sin) [*bacteria* + *toxin*] any toxin produced by or toxic to bacteria.

bacteriotropic (bak-te"re-o-trop'ik) [*bacteria* + Gr. *tropos* a turning] turning toward or changing bacteria; opsonic.

bacteriotropin (bak-te"re-ot'ro-pin) immune opsonin.

bacteriotrypsin (bak-te"re-o-trip'sin) a proteolytic.

bacteritic (bak"ter-it'ik) caused by or characterized by bacteria.

Bacterium (bak-te're-um) [L.; Gr. *baktērion* little rod] a name formerly given a genus of bacteria, order Eubacteriales, made up of non–spore-forming, rod-shaped bacteria, not necessarily closely related, that were not fitted into other formally defined genera. **B. aci'di propion'ici,** a species formerly including all the propionic acid bacteria; it is now divided into a number of species under the generic name *Propionibacterium.* **B. aerog'enes,** *Aerobacter aerogenes.* **B. aerugino'sum,** *Pseudomonas aeruginosa.* **B. chol'erae su'is,** *Salmonella choleraesuis.* **B. cloa'cae,** *Aerobacter cloacae.* **B. co'li, B. co'li commu'ne,** *Escherichia coli.* **B. dysente'riae,** *Shigella dysenteriae.* **B. faeca'lis alcalig'enes,** *Alcaligenes faecalis.* **B. pes'tis bubon'icae,** *Pasteurella pestis.* **B. son'nei,** *Shigella sonnei.* **B. tularen'se,** *Francisella tularensis.* **B. typho'sum,** *Salmonella typhosa.*

bacterium (bak-te're-um), pl. *bacte'ria* [L.; Gr. *baktērion* little rod] in general, any of the unicellular prokaryotic microorganisms that commonly multiply by cell division (fission) and whose cell is typically contained within a cell wall. They may be aerobic or anaerobic, motile or nonmotile, and may be free-living, saprophytic, parasitic, or even pathogenic, the last causing disease in plants or animals. See also *Bacteria.* **acid-fast b.,** one that retains aniline stains so tenaciously that it is not decolorized by 5 per cent mineral acids. **autotrophic b.,** one that has no organic nutritional requirements; none are pathogenic. **beaded b.,** one having deeply staining granules equally spaced along the rod. **bifid b.,** *Lactobacillus bifidus.* **blue-green b.,** see *Cyanophyceae.* **Chauveau's b.,** *Clostridium chauvoei.* **chemoautotrophic b.,** an autotrophic microorganism that obtains energy by the oxidation of inorganic compounds of iron, nitrogen, sulfur, or hydrogen; none are pathogenic. **chemoheterotrophic b.,** a heterotrophic microorganism that obtains energy through the oxidation of organic compounds by mechanisms closely similar to those existing in higher animals. **chromo b., chromogenic b.,** a microorganism that produces pigment. **coliform bacteria,** see *Escherichia, Aerobacter,* and *Paracolobactrum.* **Dar es Salaam b.,** a microorganism identified as a *Salmonella* serotype. **denitrifying b.,** a microorganism that is able to reduce nitrates to nitrites and even to ammonia and nitrogen gas. **gram-negative b.,** see under *G.* **gram-postive b.,** see under *G.* **hemophilic bacteria,** microorganisms of the genera *Hemophilus* and *Bordetella,* which have a nutritional affinity for constituents of fresh blood or whose growth is significantly stimulated on blood-containing media. **heterotrophic b.,** a microorganism that requires organic compounds of carbon and nitrogen as sources of energy or as essential parts of the cell. **higher bacteria,** microorganisms, mostly filamentous in form, which seem to be intermediate between Schizomycetes and the fungi (Hyphomycetes). **hydrogen b.,** a facultative autotrophic microorganism that respires by the oxidation of hydrogen to end-products such as H_2O, H_2S, and CH_4 (*Hydrogenomonas, Sporovibrio, Methanobacterium*). **iron b.,** an autotrophic microorganism that oxidizes iron from the ferrous to the ferric state (*Gallionella, Leptothrix*). **lysogenic b.,** a bacterial cell that harbors in its genome the genetic material (prophage) of a temperate bacteriophage and thus reproduces the bacteriophage in cell division; occasionally the prophage develops into the mature form, replicates, lyses the bacterial cell, and is free to infect other cells. **mantle b.,** see *Chlamydia.* **mesophilic b.,** a microorganism whose optimum temperature for growth is about the same as the temperature of the human body.

Plate VII

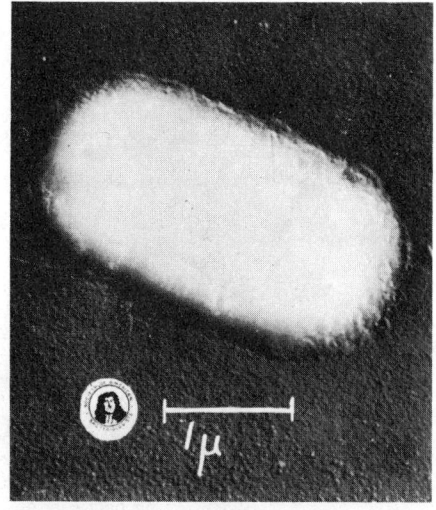

Escherichia coli. (Hedén and Wyckoff, S.A.B. LS-290.)

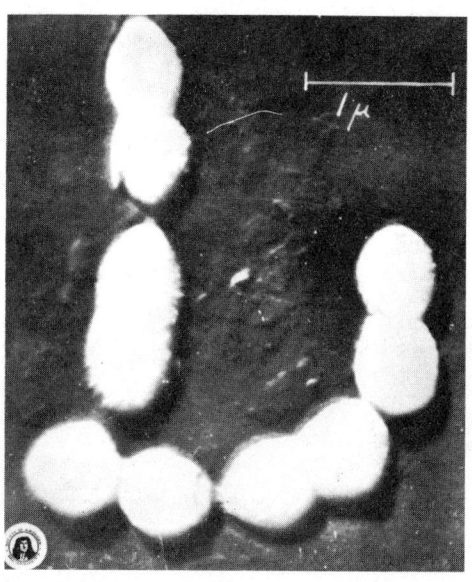

Streptococcus pneumoniae, type 2. (Williams, S.A.B. LS-162.)

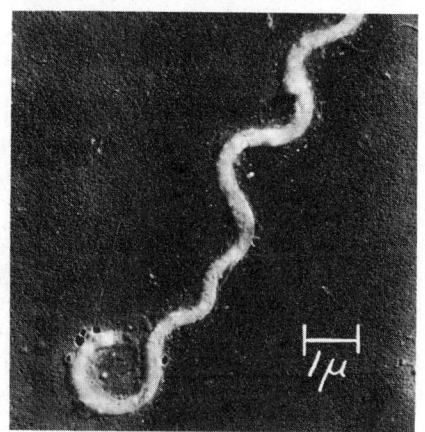

Borrelia vincentii. (Hampp, Scott, and Wyckoff, S.A.B. LS-248.)

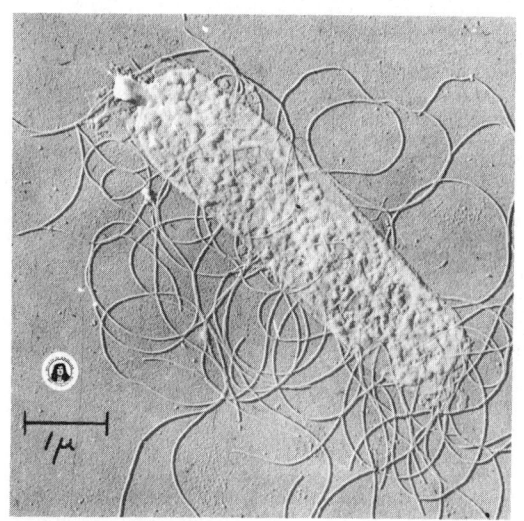

Proteus vulgaris. (Robinow and van Iterson, S.A.B. LS-260.)

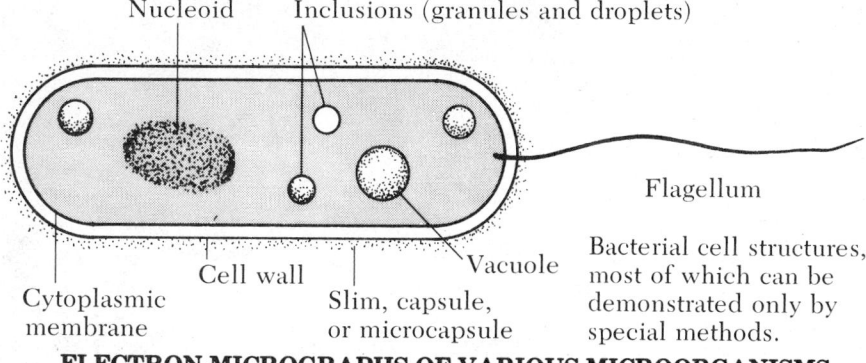

Nucleoid   Inclusions (granules and droplets)

Flagellum

Bacterial cell structures, most of which can be demonstrated only by special methods.

Vacuole

Cell wall

Cytoplasmic membrane

Slim, capsule, or microcapsule

ELECTRON MICROGRAPHS OF VARIOUS MICROORGANISMS, AND DIAGRAM SHOWING VARIOUS STRUCTURES OF TYPICAL BACTERIAL CELL

nitrifying b., a microorganism in the soil that oxidizes ammonia to nitrite (*Nitrosomonas, Nitrosococcus*), and nitrite to nitrate (*Nitrobacter*). **nodule bacteria,** bacteria which by their growth in specific nodules on the roots of plants (legumes) tend to bring about fixation of atmospheric nitrogen. **parasitic b.,** a microorganism that is dependent on a living host for its nutrition. **pathogenic b.,** a microorganism capable of causing disease. **photoautotrophic b.,** an autotrophic microorganism capable of deriving energy from light. **photoheterotrophic b.,** a heterotrophic microorganism capable of deriving energy from light. **photosynthetic b.,** any of the anaerobic bacteria that contain bacteriochlorophyll and carotenoid pigments and that carry out photosynthesis and assimilate carbon dioxide without the production of oxygen; the process depends on the presence of oxidizable electron donors other than water, such as reduced sulfur compounds. **psychrophilic b.,** a microorganism whose optimum temperature for growth is 15° to 20° C. **pyogenic b.,** a microorganism, infection with which produces suppuration. **pyrogenetic b.,** a microorganism, infection with which produces fever. **rough b.,** a variant form of a bacterium that grows in rough colonies in solid media. **saprophytic b.,** a microorganism that lives in decaying organic matter. **sulfur b.,** an obligate and facultative chemoautotrophic microorganism that respires by the oxidation of sulfur and its compounds, belonging predominantly to the genera *Beggiatoa* and *Thiobacillus*. **sulfur b., purple,** a photosynthetic anaerobic microorganism whose photoreduction of CO_2 and oxidation of H_2S is catalyzed by the pigment bacteriochlorin (*Thiorhodaceae*). **thermophilic b.,** a microorganism that grows best at high temperatures. **toxigenic b., toxinogenic b.,** a microorganism that produces a toxin.

bacteriuria (bak-te″re-u′re-ah) [*bacteria* + Gr. *ouron* urine + -*ia*] the presence of bacteria in the urine.

bacteriuric (bak-te″re-u′rik) pertaining to bacteriuria.

bacteroid (bak′tĕ-roid) [*bacteria* + Gr. *eidos* form] 1. resembling a bacterium. 2. a structurally modified bacterium.

Bacteroidaceae (bak″tĕ-roi-da′se-e) [Gr. *baktērion* rod + *eidos* form] a family of Schizomycetes, order Eubacteriales, occurring as nonsporulating obligate anaerobic rods with rounded or pointed ends, and varying in size from minute filtrable forms to long, branching, filamentous forms; it includes five genera.

Bacteroideae (bak″tĕ-roi′de-e) a name formerly given a tribe of Schizomycetes.

Bacteroides (bak″tĕ-roi′dēz) a genus of nonsporulating obligate anaerobic filamentous bacteria occurring as normal flora in the mouth and large bowel; often found in necrotic tissue, probably as secondary invaders. Thirty species have been described. **B. frag′ilis,** a species found in appendicitis, in septicemia with metastatic abscesses, in urinary tract infections, and in abscesses of the liver, pelvis, and lungs; called also *Bacillus fragilis*. **B. fundulifor′mis,** *Fusobacterium necrophorum*. **B. fusifor′mis,** *Fusobacterium plautivincenti*. **B. melaninogen′icus,** a species found in sepsis occurring after childbirth, in wounds of the abdomen that have become infected, in kidney infections, in the feces of patients affected with chronic amebic dysentery, and in the mouth and tonsils. Called also *Ristella melaninogenica*. **B. nodo′sus,** the causative agent of foot rot in sheep. **B. ochra′ceus,** a species isolated from the gingival crevices, closely resembling *Capnocytophaga* (q.v.). **B. pneumosin′tes,** *Dialister pneumosintes*. **B. ramo′sus,** a gram-positive species found in the pus of appendicitis and in gangrene of the lungs, and which causes abscesses in rabbits and guinea pigs on subcutaneous injection and fatal infections when inoculated intravenously. Called also *Ramibacterium ramosum*.

bacteroides (bak″tĕ-roi′dēz) 1. a general term for highly pleomorphic rod-shaped bacteria. 2. a microorganism of the genus *Bacteroides*.

bacteroidosis (bak″te-roi-do′sis) infection with organisms of the genus *Bacteroides*.

bacteruria (bak″te-ru′re-ah) bacteriuria.

Bactocill (bak′to-sil) trademark for a preparation of oxacillin sodium.

Bactoscilla (bak″tos-sil′ah) a genus of schizomycetes of the family Vitreoscillaceae.

baculovirus (bak″u-lo-vi′rus) any of a group of morphologically similar, ether- and heat-labile DNA viruses, which infect various insects, producing granular inclusion capsules in the cells; called also *granulosis virus*.

baculum (bak′u-lum) [L. "a stick, staff"] a heterotopic bone developed in the fibrous septum between the corpora cavernosa and above the urethra, forming the skeleton of the penis in all insectivores, bats, rodents, carnivores, and pinnipeds, and in primates except man; called also *os penis* and *os priapi*.

Badal's operation (bah-dahlz′) [Antoine Jules *Badal*, French ophthalmologist, 1840–1929] see under *operation*.

badge (baj) see *film badge*.

Baelz's disease (bāltz′es) [Erwin von *Baelz*, German physician, 1849–1913] see *cheilitis glandularis*.

Baer's cavity, law, vesicle (bārz) [Karl Ernst von *Baer* (Ber),

Russian anatomist, 1792–1876] see under *cavity, law,* and *vesicle*.

Baer's method (bārz) [William Stevenson *Baer*, American orthopedic surgeon, 1872–1931] see under *method*.

Baerensprung's erythrasma (bār′en-sproongs) [Friedrich Wilhelm Felix von *Baerensprung*, German physician, 1822–1864] see under *erythrasma*.

Baeyer's test (ba′erz) [Adolf von *Baeyer*, German chemist, 1835–1917] see under *test*.

bag (bag) a sac or pouch. **Barnes' b.,** a water-filled rubber bag for dilating the cervix uteri; called also *Barnes' dilator*. **Bunyan b.,** a bag of light waterproof material for covering wet dressings. **Champetier de Ribes' b.,** a conic water-filled bag of silk or rubber for dilating the cervix uteri. **colostomy b.,** a receptacle worn over the stoma to receive the fecal discharge from a colostomy. **Douglas b.,** a receptacle for the collection of expired air, permitting measurement of respiratory gases. **Hagner b.,** an inflatable rubber bag to be used by traction through the urethra to prevent hemorrhage following prostatectomy. **ice-b.,** a bag filled with ice, for applying cold to the body. **ileostomy b.,** any of various plastic or latex bags for the collection of urine or fecal material following ileostomy or the establishment of an ileal bladder; a flange or similar device fits closely about the ileal stoma and the bag is cemented to the skin or strapped to the body. **Lyster b.,** a rubber-lined bag with faucets and with straps for slinging; used for the water supply in temporary camps. **micturition b.,** a receptacle for urine used by ambulatory patients with urinary incontinence. **nuclear b.,** the central portion of the central or equatorial segment of intrafusal fibers of muscle; it is usually devoid of obvious cross striations and contains an accumulation of 40 to 50 spherical nuclei, which completely fill and often slightly distend the fiber. **Perry b.,** an ileostomy bag with a small latex cuff reinforced by a plastic disk which fits snugly around a protruding stoma; the cuff is held down by a large plastic ring to which a belt is attached. **Petersen's b.,** an inflatable rubber bag inserted into the rectum so as to elevate the bladder in the operation of suprapubic cystotomy. **Pilcher b.,** a modification of the Hagner bag which provides urethral drainage as well as hemostasis. **Politzer's b.,** a soft bag of rubber for inflating the middle ear. **testicular b.,** scrotum. **Voorhees' b.,** a rubber bag that can be inflated with water; used for dilating the cervix uteri. **b. of waters,** the membranes that enclose the amniotic fluid of the fetus. **Whitmore b.,** an ileostomy bag with a malleable flange and a valvular device for urine drainage at the lower end of the bag.

bagasscosis (bag″as-ko′sis) bagassosis.

bagassosis (bag″ah-so′sis) a respiratory disorder due to the inhalation of the dust of bagasse, the waste of sugar cane after the sugar has been extracted.

Baillarger's lines (bands, layer, striae, striation, stripes), sign (bi-yar-zhāz′) [Jules Gabriel François *Baillarger*, French psychiatrist, 1809–1890] see under *line* and *sign*.

Bainbridge reflex (bān′brij) [Francis Arthur *Bainbridge*, English physiologist, 1874–1921] see under *reflex*.

bake (bāk) to expose to high temperature at low humidity, as in the hardening of porcelain.

Baker's cyst (ba′kerz) [William Morrant *Baker*, British surgeon, 1839–1896] see under *cyst*.

Baker's velum (ba′kerz) [Henry A. *Baker*, Boston surgeon] see under *velum*.

bakkola (bak′o-lah) a fungus obtained from birch trees in Finland, used in folk medicine in the form of a decoction containing a chrysarobin-like principle or chrysophanic acid, in the treatment of cancer.

BAL [*British anti-lewisite*] dimercaprol.

balance (bal′ans) [L. *bilanx*] 1. an instrument for weighing. 2. the harmonious adjustment of parts; the harmonious performance of functions. **acid-base b.,** a condition in which the net rate of acid or alkali production by the body is balanced by the net rate of acid or alkali excretion from the body, resulting in a stable concentration of H^+ (hydrogen ions) in the body fluids. **analytical b.,** a laboratory balance sensitive to variations of the order of 0.05 to 0.1 mg. **calcium b.,** the balance between the calcium intake and its output through the body excretions. **enzyme b.** (in bacteria), a once-postulated steady state in relative enzyme and substrate concentrations in a bacterial culture that is altered in a different environment, thus accounting for bacterial adaptation. **fluid b.,** the state of the body in relation to ingestion and excretion of water and electrolytes; called also *water b.* **genic b.,** the ratio of male- to female-sex producers in the chromosome assortment as the determiner of sex. **inhibition-action b.,** the balance maintained in every person between emotional feelings and response to them. **microchemical b.,** a laboratory balance sensitive to variations of the order of 0.001 mg. **nitrogen b.,** the state of the body in regard to ingestion and excretion of nitrogen. In *negative nitrogen balance* the amount of nitrogen excreted is greater than the quantity ingested; in *positive nitrogen balance* the amount excreted is smaller than the amount ingested. **occlusal b.,** see *balanced occlusion*, under *occlu-*

sion. **semimicro b.,** a balance sensitive to variations of 0.01 mg. **torsion b.,** 1. a weighing balance in which the scale beam is supported by metallic ribbons that act by torsion. 2. an electrometer that acts by the twisting of a single fiber of the web of a silkworm. **water b.,** fluid b.

balanic (bah-lan′ik) pertaining to the glans penis or glans clitoridis.

balanism (bal′ah-nizm) [L. *balanismus*] (*obs.*) treatment with pessaries or suppositories.

balanitis (bal″ah-ni′tis) [*balano-* + *-itis*] inflammation of the glans penis; it is usually associated with phimosis. **amebic b.,** a variety caused by *Entamoeba histolytica*. **b. circina′ta,** a variety attributed to the presence of spirochetes. **b. diabet′ica,** a variety caused by the irritation of the urine in diabetes. **Follmann's b.,** a serous balanitis and posthitis without induration. **b. gangraeno′sa, gangrenous b.,** a rapidly destructive infection producing erosion of the glans penis and often destruction of the entire external genitals; the infection is believed to be due to a spirochete. Called also *balanoposthomycosis* and *Corbus' disease*. **phagedenic b.,** gangrenous b. **plasma cell b.,** Zoon's erythroplasia. **b. plasmocellula′re,** Zoon's erythroplasia. **b. xerot′ica oblit′erans,** atrophy of the glans penis resulting in stricture of the urethral meatus, usually representing lichen sclerosus et atrophicus of the male genitalia, but sometimes resulting from chronic irritation or benign mucosal pemphigoid.

balano- (bal′ah-no) [Gr. *balanos* an acorn] a combining form indicating relationship to the glans penis or to the glans clitoridis.

balanoblennorrhea (bal″ah-no-blen″o-re′ah) [*balano-* + Gr. *blennos* mucus + *rhoia* flow] gonorrheal inflammation of the glans penis.

balanocele (bal′ah-no-sēl″) [*balano-* + Gr. *kēlē* hernia] protrusion of the glans penis through a rupture of the prepuce.

balanochlamyditis (bal″ah-no-klam″e-di′tis) [*balano-* + Gr. *chlamys* hood + *-itis*] (*obs.*) inflammation of the glans clitoridis and hood.

balanoplasty (bal′ah-no-plas″te) [*balano-* + Gr. *plassein* to form] plastic surgery of the glans penis.

balanoposthitis (bal″ah-no-pos-thi′tis) [*balano-* + Gr. *posthē* prepuce + *-itis*] inflammation of the glans penis and prepuce. **enzootic b.,** disease of uncertain etiology, affecting sheep in Australia and New Zealand, marked by spreading ulceration of the glans penis and prepuce and severe swelling and distention of the sheath; called also *pizzle rot* and *sheath rot*. **specific gangrenous and ulcerative b.,** an acute inflammatory disease of the glans penis and opposed surface of the prepuce, marked by ulcerations and sometimes by gangrene, with a flow of odorous pus, and caused by a spirochete; called also *fourth venereal disease*.

balanoposthomycosis (bal″ah-no-pos″tho-mi-ko′sis) gangrenous balanitis.

balanopreputial (bal″ah-no-pre-pu′she-al) pertaining to the glans penis and the prepuce.

balanorrhagia (bal″ah-no-ra′je-ah) [*balano-* + Gr. *rhēgnynai* to break] balanitis with free discharge of pus.

balantidiasis (bal″an-tĭ-di′ah-sis) infection by protozoan parasites of the genus *Balantidium;* in man, *B. coli* may cause diarrhea and dysentery, with ulceration of the colon mucosa.

balantidicidal (bal-an″tĭ-dĭ-si′dal) [*Balantidium* + L. *caedere* to kill] destructive to *Balantidium*.

balantidiosis (bal″an-tid-e-o′sis) balantidiasis.

Balantidium (bal″an-tid′e-um) [Gr. *balantidion* little bag] a genus of ciliated protozoa of the subclass Euciliatia, including many species found in the intestine of vertebrates and invertebrates. **B. co′li** (Malmsten, 1857), the largest protozoan parasite of man, being 50 to 100μ in length and 40 to 70μ in width. It is commonly found in the intestines of swine, has been found in orangutans and monkeys, and is rarely found in man (see *balantidiasis*). It is oval in form, actively motile, and may be found free in the contents of the cecum if they are fluid, or may form ulcers in the walls. It has been called *Holophrya coli, Leukophrya coli*, and *Paramecium coli*. **B. su′is,** a species occurring in pigs, often considered identical to *B. coli*.

balantidosis (bal″an-tĭ-do′sis) balantidiasis.

balanus (bal′ah-nus) the glans penis.

balata (bal′ah-tah) the inspissated juice or latex of *Mimusops globosa*, a tree of tropical America; used much like gutta-percha.

Balbiani's body, nucleus (bahl-be-ah′nēz) [Edouard Gérard *Balbiani*, French embryologist, 1823–1899] yolk nucleus.

balbuties (bal-bu′she-ēz) [L.] (*obs.*) stuttering.

baldness (bawld′nes) alopecia, especially absence of hair from the scalp. **common male b.,** male pattern alopecia; thinning or absence of hair from around the vertex of the scalp, and recession of the frontal scalp margin on each side of the forehead, forming the so-called "professor angles."

Baldwin's operation (bawld′winz) [James Fairchild *Baldwin*, American gynecologist, 1850–1936] see under *operation*.

Baldy's operation (bawl′dēz) [John Montgomery *Baldy*, American gynecologist, 1860–1934] Webster's operation.

Baldy-Webster operation (bawl′de-web′ster) [John Montgomery *Baldy;* John Clarence *Webster*, American gynecologist, 1863–1950] Webster's operation.

baleri (bah-le′ri) a local name for nagana in the French Sudan.

Balfour's infective granule (bal′forz) [Sir Andrew *Balfour*, physician in Khartoum, 1873–1931] see under *granule*.

Balkan frame, splint (bawl′kan) see under *frame* and *splint*.

ball (bawl) a more or less spherical mass. **chondrin b.,** one of the ball-like masses in hyaline cartilage, consisting of cells surrounded by a capsule of basophilic matrix. **fatty b. of Bichat,** sucking pad (corpus adiposum buccae [NA]). **food b.,** phytobezoar. **fungus b.,** aspergilloma. **hair b.,** trichobezoar. **Marchi b's,** ellipsoid or ovoid segments of myelin produced by degeneration, staining brown by Marchi methods. **oat hair b.,** a trichobezoar formed in the stomach of the horse from the fine hairs within the outer husk of the oat grain and other materials. **pleural fibrin b's,** fibrin bodies in the pleural space. **wool b's,** a trichobezoar containing wool fibers and other substances.

Ball's valve (bawlz) [Sir Charles Bent *Ball*, Irish surgeon, 1851–1916] see *valvula anales*.

Ballance's sign (bal′an-siz) [Sir Charles Alfred *Ballance*, British surgeon, 1856–1936] see under *sign*.

Ballet's sign (bal-āz′) [Gilbert *Ballet*, French neurologist, 1853–1916] see under *sign*.

Ballingall's disease (bal′ing-gawlz) [Sir George *Ballingall*, British surgeon, 1780–1855] maduromycosis.

ballism (bal′izm) ballismus.

ballismus (bah-liz′mus) [Gr. *ballismos* a jumping about, dancing] violent flinging movements caused by contractions of the proximal limb muscles as a result of destruction of the subthalamic nucleus of Luysii or its fiber connections, sometimes affecting only one side of the body (hemiballismus). Called also *ballism*.

ballistic (bah-lis′tik) 1. jerking or twitching; pertaining to or characterized by ballismus. 2. pertaining to or caused by projectiles.

ballistics (bah-lis′tiks) [Gr. *ballein* to throw] the scientific study of the motion of projectiles in flight. **wound b.,** the scientific study of the speed and direction of missiles (bullets and other projectiles) in relation to the injuries they produce.

ballistocardiogram (bah-lis″to-kar′de-o-gram″) the tracing made by a ballistocardiograph; abbreviated BCG.

ballistocardiograph (bah-lis″to-kar′de-o-graf″) an apparatus for recording the movements of the body caused by the heartbeat, used to determine the degree of elasticity or atheroma of the aorta, and, more rarely, to calculate cardiac output.

ballistocardiography (bah-lis″to-kar″de-og′rah-fe) the graphic recording, by means of a ballistocardiograph, of the recoil movements of an animal body which result from motion of its heart and blood.

balloon (bah-lōōn′) 1. a sac that can be inserted into a body cavity or tube and distended with air or gas. 2. to distend with air or gas; to inflate. **Shea-Anthony antral b.,** sinus b. **sinus b.,** a hollow rubber structure, expandable with either liquid or air, used to support depressed fractures of the walls of the maxillary sinus; called also *Shea-Anthony antral balloon*. The balloon of a Foley catheter is frequently used for this purpose.

ballooning (bah-lōōn′ing) distending any cavity of the body with air or gas for therapeutic purposes.

ballotable (bah-lot′ah-bl) capable of showing ballottement.

ballottement (bah-lot′ment) [Fr. "a tossing about"] a palpatory maneuver to test for a floating object. The term is applied especially to a maneuver for detecting the existence of pregnancy by pushing up the head or breech of a fetus by fingers inserted into the vagina, so as to cause the fetus to rise and fall again like a heavy body in water. **abdominal b., indirect b.,** that

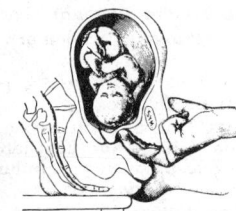

Ballottement (Jewett).

which is effected by the finger applied to the abdominal wall. **renal b.,** palpation of the kidney by pressing one hand into the abdominal wall while the other hand makes quick thrusts forward from behind so as to throw the kidney against the anterior hand.

balm (bahm) [Fr. *baume*] 1. a healing or soothing medicine. 2. a plant of the genus *Melis′sa*, especially *M. officina′lis;* it is carminative and aromatic. 3. b. of Gilead. 4. balsam. **blue b.,** *Melissa*. **b. of Gilead,** 1. a liquid oleoresin from *Abies balsamea* (L.) Mill., the balsam fir of North America, which was once used in the treatment of diseases of the urinary tract. 2.

the buds of the poplar tree *Populus candicans* Aiton (Salicaceae), which contain volatile oils and resins; used as a stimulating expectorant in cough syrups. 3. Mecca balsam. Called also *balsam of Gilead*. **lemon b.,** *Melissa.* **mountain b.,** *Eriodictyon.* **sweet b.,** *Melissa.*

Balme's cough (bahlmz) [Paul Jean *Balme*, French physician, born 1857] see under *cough.*

balneology (bal″ne-ol′o-je) [L. *balneum* bath + *-logy*] the science of baths and their therapeutic uses.

balneotherapeutics (bal″ne-o-ther-ah-pu′tiks) balneotherapy.

balneotherapy (bal″ne-o-ther′ah-pe) [L. *balneum* bath + Gr. *therapeia* treatment] the treatment of disease by baths.

balneum (bal′ne-um), pl. *bal′nea* [L.] a bath, def. 1. **b. are′nae,** a sand bath; also *ammotherapy.* **b. lac′teum,** milk bath. **b. pneumat′icum,** air bath.

Balopticon (bal-op′te-kon) [Gr. *ballein* to throw + *optikos* pertaining to sight] trademark for a projection apparatus for throwing an enlarged image on a screen.

balsam (bawl′sam) [L. *balsamum;* Gr. *balsamon*] 1. a semifluid, resinous, and fragrant liquid of vegetable origin, usually trees, which is often composed chiefly of resins, volatile oils, and various esters. 2. balm. **Canada b.,** a liquid oleoresin from *Abies balsamea* (L.) Mill. (Pinaceae), the balsam fir of North America, containing volatile oils, chiefly *l*-pinene, and over 70 per cent resins; a microscopic medium. **b. of copaiba,** copaiba. **friars' b.,** compound benzoin tincture. **b. of Gilead,** see under *balm.* **gurjun b.,** an oleoresin from *Dipterocarpus alatus* Roxb. (Dipterocarpaceae) and other species of *Dipterocarpus* growing in East India; an adulterant of copaiba. **Holland b.,** juniper tar. **Mecca b.,** a light-colored, mobile to viscid liquid with an aromatic odor; it is the resinous juice of *Commiphora opobalsamum,* a small evergreen of the Red Sea region. It is still used as a medicine and cosmetic in eastern countries. **b. of Peru,** peruvian b. **peruvian b.** [NF], a dark brown viscid liquid obtained from *Myroxylon pereirae* Klotzsch (Leguminosae) used as a local protectant and as a rubefacient, applied topically to the skin in ointment or alcohol solution. Called also *b. of Peru.* **St. Thomas' b.,** a resinous juice obtained from the tree, *Santiriopsis balsamifera,* grown on the island of St. Thomas. **silver b.,** juniper tar. **b. of sulfur,** a preparation made by boiling sulfur in linseed or olive oil. **tolu b.** [USP], a balsam obtained from *Myroxylon balsamum,* used as an ingredient of compound benzoin tincture and as an expectorant. **Turlington's b.,** **Wade's b.,** compound benzoin tincture.

balsamo (bal′sah-mo) [Sp.] balsam. **b. de tolu′,** tolu balsam. **b. del Peru′,** peruvian balsam.

Balsamodendron (bal″sah-mo-den′dron) [L.; Gr. *balsamon* balsam + *dendron* tree] a genus of old world amyridaceous trees of many species, producing bdellium and other balsamic drugs.

balsamum (bal′sah-mum) [L.] balsam. **b. peruvia′num,** peruvian balsam.

Balser's fatty necrosis (bahl′zerz) [W. *Balser,* German physician] see under *necrosis.*

balteum (bal′te-um) [L.] belt or girdle. **b. vene′reum,** Venus' girdle.

Baltimore (bal′tĭ-mor) David. American biologist, born 1938; co-winner, with Renato Dulbecco and Howard Temin, of the Nobel prize in medicine and physiology for 1975, for discoveries concerning the interaction between tumor viruses and the genetic material of host cells and the role of reverse transcriptase.

Bamberger's albuminuria, etc. (bahm′ber-gerz) [Heinrich von *Bamberger,* Austrian physician, 1822–1888] see under *albuminuria, disease,* and *sign.*

Bamberger-Marie disease [Eugen *Bamberger,* Austrian physician, 1858–1921; Pierre *Marie,* French physician, 1853–1940] hypertrophic pulmonary osteoarthropathy.

bambermycins (bam″ber-mi′sinz) an antibacterial antibiotic complex containing mainly moenomycin A and C, produced by *Streptomyces bambergiensis, S. ederensis, S. geysiriensis,* and *S. ghansensis,* and related strains, or the same substance produced by other means; used as a feed additive in foodstuffs for pigs, poultry, and calves and in veterinary supplements.

bamboo brier (bam-boo′ bri′er) the root of species of *Smilax,* of the United States, used as a food by Indians.

bamnidazole (bam-nid′ah-zōl) chemical name: 2-methyl-5-nitro-1*H*-imidazol-1-ethanol carbamate (ester); an antiprotozoal effective against *Trichomonas,* $C_7H_{10}N_4O_4$.

Bancroft's filariasis (ban′krofts) [Joseph *Bancroft,* English physician in Australia, 1836–1894] see under *filariasis.*

bancroftosis (ban″krof-to′sis) infection with *Wuchereria bancrofti.*

band (band) 1. a part, structure, or appliance that binds. 2. in dentistry, a thin strip of band formed to encircle horizontally the crown of a natural tooth or its root. 3. in cytogenetics, a part of a chromosome which, after staining, is clearly distinguishable from its adjacent segment by appearing darker or lighter, brighter or duller; bands are named, according to the procedure used,

C-bands, F-bands, G-bands, etc. 4. see *band cells,* under *cell.* **A b.,** the dark-staining zone of a sarcomere, whose center is traversed by the paler H band, which in turn contains the darker M band; called also *A disk, Q disk, anisotropic disk,* and *transverse disk.* **absorption b's,** dark bands in the spectrum due to absorption of light by the medium (a solid, a liquid, or a gas) through which the light has passed. Cf. *absorption lines,* under *line.* **amniotic b.,** a fibrous band passing from fetus to amnion. **anchor b.,** a band applied to a tooth to secure anchorage in order to influence the movement of other teeth in the mouth. **Angle b.,** a clamp band tightened by a threaded screw on the lingual side; once used in orthodontics. **anogenital b.,** a fetal fillet that is the rudiment of the perineum. **anterior b. of colon,** tenia libera. **atrioventricular b.,** bundle of His. **auriculoventricular b.,** atrioventricular b. **axis b.,** the primitive streak. **Baillarger's b's,** see under *line.* **belly b.,** a strip of flannel worn around the abdomen, usually by infants or young children. **b. of Broca,** a part of the primordial rhinencephalon close to the anterior perforated substance. **Büngner's b's,** bands of syncytium formed by the union of sheath cells during the regeneration of peripheral nerves; called also *Ledbänder.* **C-b.,** a band produced on a chromosome by the centric heterochromatin method; see *Table of Stains and Staining Methods,* under *stain.* **Clado's b.,** the suspensory ligament of the ovary covered with peritoneum. **clamp b.,** an anchor band held in place with a screw nut. **coagulation b.,** the band formed in Weltmann's coagulation test. **b's of colon, longitudinal,** teniae coli. **contoured b.,** a dental band shaped to the contour of the tooth. **coronary b.,** a band of vascular tissue at the upper edge of the wall of the hoof which is concerned in the secretion of the wall; called also *coronary cusion, coronary ring, cutidure,* or *cutiduris.* **dentate b.,** gyrus dentatus, def. 1. **F-b.,** a band produced on a chromosome by the F-staining method; see *Table of Stains and Staining Methods,* under *stain.* **free b. of colon,** tenia libera. **G-b.,** a band produced on a chromosome by the Giemsa method; see *Table of Stains and Staining Methods,* under *stain.* **Gennari's b.,** see *Baillarger's lines,* under *line.* **Giacomini's b.,** the grayish band constituting the anterior extension of the gyrus dentatus of the hippocampus over the inferior surface of the uncus. **H b.,** a relatively pale zone sometimes seen traversing the center of the A band of fibrils of striated muscle; called also *Hensen's* or *Engelmann's disk.* **Hall b.,** an intrauterine contraceptive device of surgical stainless steel, measuring $\frac{13}{16}$ inch in diameter and consisting of three flat circular members $\frac{1}{16}$ inch wide and $\frac{1}{1000}$ inch thick, located within the lumen of an open coiled spring. **Harris' b.,** anomalous peritoneal folds which extend from the gallbladder to the inferior surface of the liver to the proximal duodenum, sometimes traversing the mesocolon near the hepatic flexure. **Henle's b.,** fibers from the anterior aponeurosis of the transversus abdominis muscle extending behind the rectus below the arcuate line. **His' b.,** see under *bundle.* **horny b.** (obs.), the band or disk of the stria terminalis; called also *b. of Tarinus.* **b's of Hunter-Schreger,** a series of bands visible by reflected light in the enamel of longitudinal sections of human teeth. **I b.,** the band or disk within a striated muscle fibril that appears as a light region under the light microscope and as a dark region under polarized light; it contains the proteins actin, troponin, and tropomyosin. Called also *isotropic disk* and *J disk.* **iliotibial b.,** tractus iliotibialis. **Lane's b's,** adhesions between tight loops of the terminal ileum which may extend as ligamentous bands to the right iliac fossa. See also *Lane's kink,* under *kink.* **Leonardo's b.,** a term proposed by Sudhoff for the band of Reil, first delineated by Leonardo da Vinci. **limbic b's,** a superior and an inferior muscular band developed in the right atrium of the fetal heart that become the basis of Lower's tubercle and the sinus septum. **M b.,** the narrow dark band in the center of the H band of the sarcomere; called also *M disk, Hensen's line,* and *mesophragma.* Cf. *Z band.* **Maissiat's b.,** tractus iliotibialis. **Matas' b.,** an aluminum band for temporarily occluding large blood vessels in order to test the condition of the collateral circulation. **matrix b.,** a thin piece of metal that is fitted around a tooth to supply a missing wall of a multisurface cavity in order to allow adequate condensation of amalgam into the cavity. **Meckel's b.,** a part of the anterior ligament fastening the malleus to the wall of the tympanum. **mesocolic b.,** tenia mesocolica. **moderator b.,** trabecula septomarginalis. **molar b.,** a plain anchor band used in orthodontics. **N-b.,** a band produced on a chromosome by the N-staining method; see *Table of Stains and Staining Methods,* under *stain.* **omental b.,** tenia omentalis. **orthodontic b.,** a thin strip of metal closely encircling the crown of a tooth mesiodistally and buccolabiolingually; an integral part of a fixed orthodontic appliance. **Parham b.,** a metallic ribbon used to fix a fractured long bone by encircling the bone at the site of the fracture. **periopic b.,** the band of secretor cells at the upper border of the hoof of animals; it secretes the periople. **periosteal b.,** see under *collar.* **phonatory b's,** the vocal cords, or an artificial substitute for them. **Q b.,** A b. **Q-b.,** any of the light and dark transverse bands on chromosomes visible on fluorescence microscopy after staining by quinacrine mustard (or related substance). **R-b.,** a band produced on a chromosome by the reverse Giemsa method; see *Table of Stains and*

Staining Methods, under *stain*. **b. of Reil**, 1. a muscular fillet extending across the right ventricle of the heart, now regarded as forming one of the terminal parts of the moderator band; see *bundle of His*. 2. (obs.) see under *ribbon*. **b. of Remak**, axon. **retention b.**, musculus suspensorius duodeni. **b's of Schreger**, b's of Hunter-Schreger. **Sebileau's b's** (obs.), three thickenings in the membrana suprapleuralis. **Simonart's b's**, Simonart's threads; see under *thread*. **Soret's b.**, a band in the violet end of the spectrum of hemoglobin. **T-b.**, a band produced on a chromosome by the T-staining method; see *Table of Stains and Staining Methods*, under *stain*. **b. of Tarinus**, horny b. **Vicq d'Azyr's b.**, a thin stripe of fine myelinated fibers in Brodmann's external granular layer; sometimes called stripe of Kaes, and often incorrectly defined as the outer line of Baillarger. **Z b.**, a thin membrane seen on longitudinal section as a dark line in the center of the I band; the distance between successive Z bands serves to delimit the sarcomeres of striated muscle. Called also *Z disk* or *line*, *Amici's disk*, *Dobie's line* or *layer*, *intermediate disk*, *Krause's membrane*, *telophragma*, and *thin disk*. See *inophragma* and cf. *M b.* **zinc b.**, Z b. **zonular b.**, zona orbicularis articulationis coxae.

bandage (ban'dij) 1. a strip or roll of gauze or other material for wrapping or binding any part of the body. 2. to cover by wrapping with a strip of gauze or other material. See also *dressing* and *strapping*. **abdominal b.**, a wide support worn around the abdomen after an abdominal operation, often during pregnancy, and for obesity. **Ace b.**, trademark for a bandage of woven elastic material. **A-S-E b.**, the third roller of Desault's bandage, which forms a triangle, the angles of which are located at the axilla, shoulder, and elbow. **Barton's b.**, a figure-of-8 bandage supporting the lower jaw below and in front. **Baynton's b.**, a binding of adhesive plaster applied to the leg in the treatment of indolent ulcer. **binocle b.**, a bandage covering both eyes. **Borsch's b.**, an eye bandage covering both the diseased and the healthy eye. **Buller's b.**, see under *shield*. **capeline b.**, a bandage applied like a cap or hood to the head or shoulder or to an amputation stump; called also *Hippocrates' b.* **circular b.**, a bandage applied in circular turns, usually about a limb. **compression b.**, a bandage by which pressure is applied to a limb to prevent edema. **crucial b.**, T bandage. **demigauntlet b.**, a bandage that covers the hand but leaves the fingers exposed. **Desault's b.**, a bandage binding the elbow to the side, with a pad in the axilla, for fractured clavicle; called also *Desault's apparatus*. **elastic b.**, a bandage of India rubber applied to an area to exert continuous pressure upon it. **Esmarch's b.**, an India rubber bandage applied upward around (from the distal part to the proximal) a part in order to expel blood from it; the limb is often elevated as the elastic pressure is applied. **figure-of-8 b.**, a bandage in which the turns cross each other like the figure eight (8). **Fricke's b.**, strapping of the scrotum for orchitis and epididymitis. **Galen's b.**, a bandage with each end split into three pieces: the middle section is placed on the crown of the head; the two anterior strips are fastened at the back of the neck; the two posterior ones, on the forehead; and the two middle ones are tied under the chin. **Garretson's b.**, a bandage for the lower jaw, running above the forehead and back again, crossing under the occiput, and ending under the chin. **gauntlet b.**, a bandage that covers the hand and fingers like a glove. **gauze b.**, a continuous strip of tightly rolled absorbent gauze in various widths and lengths. **Genga's b.**, Theden's b. **Gibney b.**, strips of ½-inch adhesive overlapped along the sides and back of the foot and leg to hold the foot in slight varus position and leave the dorsum of the foot and anterior aspect of the leg exposed; called also *Gibney's strapping*. **Hamilton's b.**, a compound bandage for the lower jaw, composed of a leather string with straps of linen webbing. **hammock b.**, a bandage for retaining dressings on the head; it consists of a broad strip placed over the dressing, brought down over the ears, and held in place by a circular bandage around the head. **Heliodorus' b.**, a T bandage. **Hippocrates' b.**, capeline b. **Hueter's b.**, a perineal bandage applied as a spica bandage. **immobilizing b.**, a bandage for partially immobilizing a part. **Kiwisch's b.**, a modified figure-of-8 bandage applied to both breasts to support and firmly compress them. **Maisonneuve's b.**, a plaster-of-Paris bandage made of folded cloth held in place by other bandages. **many-tailed b.**, a wide bandage with each end cut into several strips of equal width which may be overlapped as the bandage is applied, usually to the abdomen or chest. See *scultetus b.* **Martin's b.**, a roller bandage of thin elastic rubber. **oblique b.**, a bandage applied obliquely up a limb without reverses. Cf. *reversed b.* **plaster b.**, a bandage stiffened with a paste of plaster of Paris, which sets and becomes very hard. **pressure b.**, a bandage for applying pressure. **protective b.**, a bandage for covering underlying injured tissue or dressings. **reversed b.**, one applied to a limb in such a way that the roll is inverted or half-turned at each revolution, so as to make it fit smoothly the varying dimensions of the limb. **Ribble's b.**, a spica bandage applied to the instep. **Richet's b.**, a bandage of plaster of Paris to which a little gelatin has been added. **roller b.**, a tightly rolled, circular bandage of varying widths and materials, often commercially prepared. **Sayre's b.**, an adhesive plaster bandage used in cases of fracture of the clavicle.

scultetus b., a many-tailed bandage applied with the tails overlapping each other and held in position by safety pins; see illustration. **Seutin's b.**, a starch and plaster bandage. **spica b.**, a figure-of-8 bandage with turns that cross one another regularly like the letter V, usually applied to anatomical areas of quite different dimensions, as the pelvis and thigh or the thorax and arm. See illustration. **spiral b.**, a roller bandage applied spirally around a limb. **spiral reverse b.**, a spiral bandage applied with reverse turns in order to fit more snugly the varying contours and dimensions of a limb. **starch b.**, a bandage that has been impregnated with a solution of starch which hardens after the bandage is applied. **suspensory b.**, a bandage for supporting the scrotum. **T b.**, a bandage shaped like the letter T; called also *crucial b.* and *Heliodorus' b.* **Theden's b.**, a roller bandage applied from below upward over a graduated compress to control hemorrhage; called also *Genga's b.* **triangular b.**, a triangle of cloth used as a sling. **Velpeau's b.**, a bandage to support the arm and provide immobilization of the elbow and shoulder; it is useful in supporting the upper extremity in severe injuries involving the shoulder girdle and upper end of humerus. **Y b.**, a bandage shaped like the letter Y.

bandicoot (ban'de-koot) an Indian rodent, *Nesokia bengalensis*, which is a reservoir of *Spirillum minus*, the causative organism of rat-bite fever; it also harbors *Coxiella burneti*, which may be transmitted by the bandicoot tick, *Haemaphysalis humerosa*.

banding (band'ing) 1. the act of encircling and binding with a thin strip of material. 2. in genetics, any of several techniques of staining chromosomes so that a characteristic pattern of transverse dark and light bands becomes visible, permitting identification of individual chromosome pairs. **chromosome b.**, any staining procedure resulting in a banding pattern of light and dark or bright and dull regions on a chromosome; known as C-banding, G-banding, etc., according to the staining technique used. **pulmonary artery (PA) b.**, an operation performed to control pulmonary blood flow in children with certain congenital cardiac defects.

Bandl's ring (ban'dl) [Ludwig *Bandl*, German obstetrician, 1842–1892] *pathologic retraction ring*; see *retraction ring*, under *ring*.

bane (bān) a poison. **leopard's b., wolf's b.**, see *arnica*.

banewort (bān'wort) belladonna leaf.

bang (bang) bhang.

Bang's bacillus, disease, test (bangz) [Bernhard Laurits Frederik *Bang*, Danish physician, 1848–1932] see *Brucella abortus*, and under *disease* and *tests*.

Bang's method (bangz) [Ivar Christian *Bang*, Swedish physiological chemist, 1869–1918] see under *method*.

banian (ban'yan) the *Ficus bengalensis* (L.), an East Indian fig tree; its seeds and bark are tonic, antifebrile, and diuretic.

banisterine (ban-is'ter-in) an alkaloid from *Banisteria caapi*, a woody vine of South America; it has hallucinogenic properties.

bank (bangk) a stored supply of human material or tissues for future use by other individuals, as *blood b.*, *bone b.*, *eye b.*, *human-milk b.*, *skin b.*, etc.

Bannister's disease (ban'nis-terz) [Henry Martyn *Bannister*, Chicago physician, 1844–1920] angioneurotic edema.

Banthine (ban'thīn) trademark for preparations of methantheline bromide.

Banti's disease, syndrome (ban'tēz) [Guido *Banti*, Italian pathologist, 1852–1925] see under *disease*, and see *congestive splenomegaly*, under *splenomegaly*.

Banting (ban'ting) Sir Frederick Grant. A Canadian physician, 1891–1941; co-discoverer of insulin, in 1922, with Charles Herbert Best and John James Rickard Macleod; co-winner, with Macleod, of the Nobel prize for medicine in 1923.

Banting's treatment (cure, diet) (ban'tingz) [William *Banting*, English coffin-maker, 1787–1878] see under *treatment*.

bantingism (ban'ting-izm) [William *Banting*, English coffin-maker, 1797–1878, who devised the method in 1863] Banting treatment.

Baptisia (bap-tiz'e-ah) [L.; Gr. *baptizein* to dip in or under water] a genus of leguminous plants. **B. leucan'tha** Torr. and Gray, a species, known as wild indigo, which contains quinolizidine alkaloids and has caused poisoning in horses and cows. **B. tincto'ria** R. Br., a species of herbs of North America, which contains cytisine; used as a dye. The dried root has been used as a cathartic and emetic.

baptisin (bap'tĭ-zin) a glycoside from *Baptisia tinctoria*, a brownish powder, soluble in alcohol.

baptitoxine (bap-tĭ-tok'sin) cytisine.

bar (bahr) 1. the upper part of the gums of a horse, between the grinders and the tusks, which bears no teeth. 2. that portion of the wall of a horse's hoof which is reflected posteriorly at an acute angle. 3. a unit of pressure, being a pressure by one megadyne per square centimeter; called also *barye*. 4. in orthodontics, a connector which may consist of a heavy wire or a wrought or cast metal segment, longer than it is wide, which connects different parts of a removable partial denture. **arch b.**, a heavy wire

Plate VIII

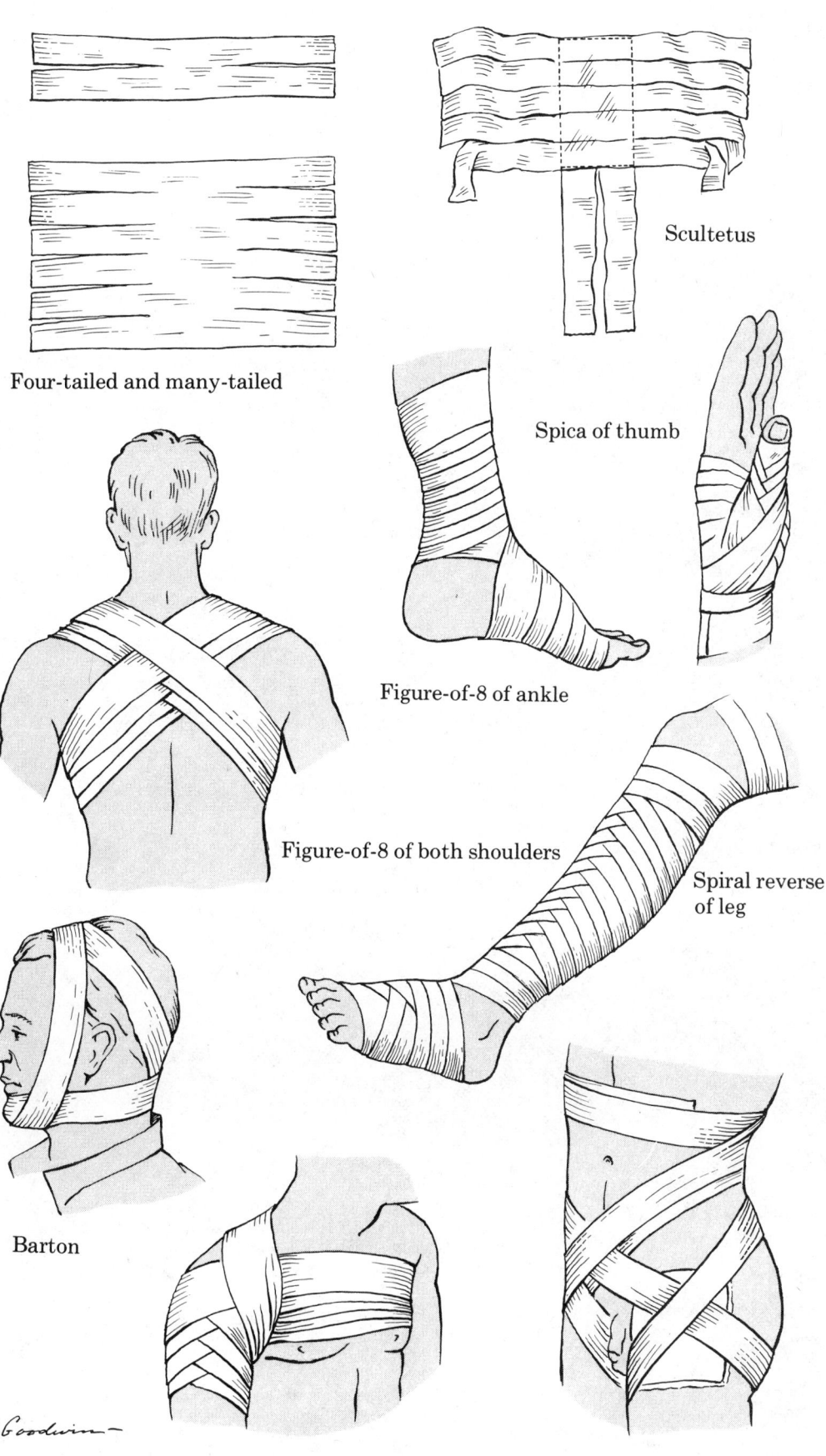

bandage

Scultetus

Four-tailed and many-tailed

Spica of thumb

Figure-of-8 of ankle

Figure-of-8 of both shoulders

Spiral reverse of leg

Barton

Spica of shoulder

Spica of groin

H. Goodwin

VARIOUS TYPES OF BANDAGE

shaped to the outer circumference of the dental arch and extending from one side to the other so that intervening teeth may be attached to it; usually used for fixation in jaw fractures. **b. of bladder,** interureteric ridge (plica interureterica [NA]). **chromatoidal b.,** chromatoid body, def. 1. **connector b.,** a minor connector; see under *connector.* **Erich arch b.,** an arch bar made of soft, readily contoured metal, used for intermaxillary fixation. **hyoid b's,** a pair of cartilaginous plates forming the second visceral arch, from which a part of the hyoid bone is developed. **Kazanjian T b.,** an appliance useful in reconstruction of the lip and jaw; it is fixed with an acrylic prosthesis to provide soft tissue support during reconstruction. **Kennedy b.,** a secondary lingual bar, usually placed on the cingula of incisor teeth, used as an indirect retainer and may be used to stabilize poorly supported anterior teeth; called also *continuous bar retainer.* **labial b.,** a major connector located labial to the dental arch, and joining two or more bilateral parts of a mandibular removable partial denture. **lingual b.,** 1. a heavy wrought or cast structure, usually of gold, cobalt-chromium alloy, or stainless steel, placed along the gums on the lingual surface of the teeth of the lower jaw. 2. a major connector located lingual to the dental arch, and joining two or more bilateral parts of a mandibular removable partial denture. **median b.,** a fibrotic formation across the neck of the prostate gland, causing obstruction of the urethra. **Mercier's b.,** interureteric ridge (*plica interureterica* [NA]). **occlusal rest b.,** a minor connector used to attach an occlusal rest to a major part of a removable partial denture. **palatal b.,** a major connector that extends across the palate and joins two or more parts of a maxillary removable partial denture. **Passavant's b.,** a horizontal ridge that appears on the posterior wall of the pharynx during swallowing, produced by contraction of the palatopharyngeal sphincter; it also occurs during speech in persons with cleft palate. Called also *pharyngeal ridge* and *Passavant's cushion, pad,* or *ridge.* **sternal b.,** one of the paired cartilaginous bars in the embryo that unite to form the sternum. **terminal b's,** zones where epithelial cells contact one another, once thought to represent an accumulation of dense cementing substance, but with the electron microscope shown to be a junctional complex (see under *complex*).

Bar's incision (bahrz) [Paul *Bar,* French obstetrician, 1853–1945] see under *incision.*

Barach's index (bar′aks) [Alvan Leroy *Barach,* New York physician, born 1895] see under *index.*

baragnosis (bar″-ag-no′sis) [Gr. *baros* weight + *a* neg. + *gnōsis* knowledge] absence of the power to recognize weight.

Bárány's symptom (sign, test), pointing test (bah′rah-nēz) [Robert *Bárány,* Austrian otologist, 1876–1936; winner of the Nobel prize for medicine in 1914] see under *symptom* and *tests.*

barba (bar′bah) [L. "the beard"] [NA] the beard.

barbaloin (bar′bah-loin) an anthraquinone pentoside that occurs in various species of *Aloe* and is mainly responsible for their purgative properties.

barbaralalia (bar″bar-ah-la′le-ah) a form of dyslalia that is shown when speaking a foreign language.

barbasco (bar-bas′ko) tropical plants, *Jacquinia paramensis* and *Paullinia pinnata;* used as fish poisons.

barbeiro (bar-ba′ro) [Port.] Brazilian name for *Panstrongylus megistus.*

barberry (bar′ber-e) the shrub *Berberis vulgaris* and its fruit, which is the source of a yellow dye. The chief constituents are resins and the alkaloid berberine. Its berries are used as preservatives, and the bark of the stems and roots is used as a bitter tonic.

barbital (bar′bĭ-tal) chemical name: 5,5-diethyl-2,4,6(1H,3H,-5H)-pyrimidinetrione. A long-acting barbiturate, $C_8H_{12}N_2O_3$, the first of the barbiturate series; used as a hypnotic and sedative, administered orally. **b. sodium, b. soluble,** the soluble monosodium salt of barbital, $C_8H_{11}N_2NaO_3$, having the same actions and uses as the base.

barbitalism (bar′bĭ-tal-izm) (*obs.*) Barbituism.

barbitone (bar′bĭ-tōn) a British name for barbital.

barbituism (bar-bit′u-izm) (*obs.*) a condition caused by the use of barbital or its derivatives and marked by chill, headache, fever, and cutaneous eruptions.

barbiturate (bar-bit′u-rāt) a salt or derivative of barbituric acid.

barbiturism (bar-bit′u-rizm) (*obs.*) barbituism.

barbotage (bar″bo-tahzh′) [Fr. *barboter* to dabble] repeated injection and withdrawal of fluid, as in gastric lavage, or the administration of an anesthetic into the subarachnoid space by alternate injection of a small amount of the anesthetic and withdrawal of a small quantity of cerebrospinal fluid into the syringe, until the anesthetic is completely administered.

barbula (bar′bu-lah) [L.] a little beard. **b. hir′ci,** 1. axillary hair (hirci [NA]). 2. tufts of hair in the ears.

Barcoo disease, rot (bar-koo′) [*Barcoo,* a river in South Australia] see *desert sore,* under *sore.*

Barcroft's apparatus (bar′krofts) [Sir Joseph *Barcroft,* British physiologist, 1872–1947] see under *apparatus.*

Bard's sign (bardz′) [Louis *Bard,* French physician, 1857–1930] see under *sign.*

Bard-Pic syndrome [Louis *Bard;* Adrien *Pic,* French physician, 1862–1944] see under *syndrome.*

Bardach's test (bar′dakz) [Bruno *Bardach,* Vienna chemist] see under *tests.*

Bardenheuer's extension (bar′den-hoi-erz) [Bernhard *Bardenheuer,* Cologne surgeon, 1839–1913] see under *extension.*

Bardet-Biedl syndrome (bar-da′ be′del) [Georges *Bardet,* French physician, born 1885] Laurence-Biedl syndrome.

baresthesia (bar″es-the′ze-ah) [Gr. *baros* weight + *aisthēsis* perception + *-ia*] sensibility for weight or pressure; pressure sense.

baresthesiometer (bar″es-the″ze-om′ĕ-ter) [Gr. *baros* weight + *aisthēsis* perception + *metron* measure] an instrument for determining sensitiveness as to weight or pressure.

Baréty's method (bar″a-tēz′) [Jean Paul *Baréty,* French surgeon, 1887–1912] see under *method.*

Barfoed's reagent, test (bahr′fedz) [Christen Thomsen *Barfoed,* Swedish physician, 1815–1899] see under *tests.*

Bargen's serum, streptococcus, (bar′genz) [J. Arnold *Bargen,* California physician, born 1894] see under *serum* and see *Streptococcus bovis.*

bariatrics (bar″e-at′riks) [Gr. *baros* weight + *iatrikē* medicine, surgery] a field of medicine encompassing the study of overweight, its causes, prevention, and treatment.

baritosis (bar-ĭ-to′sis) pneumoconiosis due to inhalation of barite or barium dust.

barium (ba′re-um), gen. *ba′rii* [L.; Gr. *baros* weight] a pale yellowish, metallic element belonging to the alkaline earths, whose acid-soluble salts are poisonous; its atomic number is 56; atomic weight 137.34; symbol, Ba. **b. arsenate,** a salt, $Ba_3(AsO_4)_2$, formerly used in tuberculosis and in skin diseases. **b. bromide,** a compound, $BaBr_2 + 2H_2O$, formerly used as a heart tonic and in aneurysm and scrofula. **b. carbonate,** a poisonous salt, $BaCO_3$, formerly used in medicine; now employed in preparing the chloride, etc. **b. chloride,** a compound, $BaCl_2 + 2H_2O$, a cardiac stimulant; formerly used in sclerosis of the nervous tissues and in heart block and aneurysm. **b. cyanoplatinate,** a substance, $BaPt(CN)_4 \cdot 4H_2O$, used for coating the screen of the fluoroscope; called also *b. platinocyanide.* **b. hydrate, b. hydroxide,** $Ba-(OH)_2$, a crystalline soluble base employed as a test for sulfates. **b. oxide,** white to yellowish white powder, BaO, used for drying gases; called also *baryta.* **b. platinocyanide,** b. cyanoplatinate. **b. sulfate,** a bulky, fine, white powder without odor or taste, and free from grittiness, $BaSO_4$; used as a contrast medium in roentgenography of the digestive tract. Called also *synthetic baryta.* **b. sulfide,** a heavy, grayish white or pale yellow, poisonous powder, BaS, sometimes used in veterinary medicine as a depilatory for preoperative preparation.

bariumize (bār′e-um-īz) (*obs.*) to treat with barium.

bark (bark) [L. *cortex*] the rind or outer cortical cover of the woody parts of a plant, tree, or shrub; called also *cascara.* **bearberry b.,** cascara sagrada. **bitter b.,** the dried bark of *Alstonia constricta,* a tree of New South Wales and Queensland. **buck-thorn b.,** the dried bark of *Rhamnus frangula.* **butternut b.,** the dried inner bark of the root of *Juglans cinerea.* **calisaya b.,** cinchona. **casca b.,** the bark of *Erythrophloeum guineense;* called also *Mancona b.* **chittem b.,** cascara sagrada. **cinchona b.,** cinchona. **cotton root b.,** the air dried bark of roots of various species of *Gossypium;* formerly used as an oxytocic. Called also *gossypii radicis cortex.* **cramp b.,** the dried bark of *Viburnum opulus.* **cuprea b.,** the bark of *Remijia purdieana* or *R. pedunculata.* **dita b.,** the dried bark of *Alstonia scholaris,* a tree of India and the Philippines. **dogwood b.,** 1. cascara sagrada. 2. see *Cornus.* **elm b.,** the dried inner bark of *Ulmus fulva.* **Jesuits' b.,** cinchona. **Mancona b.,** casca b. **Persian b.,** cascara sagrada. **Peruvian b.,** cinchona. **Purshiana b.,** cascara sagrada. **quebracho b.,** bark derived from a large evergreen tree of the genus *Aspidosperma,* indigenous to various parts of South America. **quillay b.,** quillaia. **sacred b.,** cascara sagrada. **seven b's,** *Hydrangea.* **soap b., soap tree b.,** quillaia. **white oak b.,** the dried inner bark of *Quercus alba.* **wild black cherry b.,** wild cherry; see under *cherry.*

Barkan's operation (bar′kanz) [Otto *Barkan,* San Francisco ophthalmologist, born 1887] goniotomy.

barley (bar′le) the annual grasses, *Hordeum vulgare, H. distichon,* etc.; also their seed, a cereal grain. Used for malting and distillation and to some extent as a food substance. Boiled barley water has demulcent properties and has been used as a home remedy in the management of infant diarrhea. **pearl b.,** decorticated polished barley grain.

Barlow's disease (bar′lōz) [Sir Thomas *Barlow,* physician in London, 1845–1945] infantile scurvy.

barn (barn) a unit of nuclear cross-section, being 10^{-24} square centimeter.

Barnes's bag (dilator), curve (barn'zes) [Robert *Barnes*, English obstetrician, 1817–1907] see under *bag* and *curve*.

baro- [Gr. *baros* weight] a combining form denoting relationship to weight or pressure.

baroagnosis (bar″o-ag-no′sis) baragnosis.

baroceptor (bar″o-sep′tor) baroreceptor.

barodontalgia (bar″o-don-tal′je-ah) aerodontalgia.

baroelectroesthesiometer (bar″o-e-lek″tro-es-the″ze-om′ĕ-ter) [*baro-* + *electric* + Gr. *aisthēsis* perception + *metron* measure] an instrument to measure the amount of pressure at the time electric sensibility to tingling or pain is felt.

barognosis (bar″og-no′sis) [*baro-* + Gr. *gnōsis* knowledge] conscious perception of weight; the faculty by which weight is recognized; weight knowledge.

baromacrometer (bar″o-mah-krom′ĕ-ter) [*baro-* + Gr. *makros* long + *metron* measure] an instrument for measuring and weighing newborn infants.

baro-otitis (bar″o-o-ti′tis) barotitis. **b. me′dia,** barotitis media.

baropacer (bar″o-pās′er) an electronic unit implanted in the necks of dogs for continuous stimulation of the carotid sinuses.

barophilic (bar″o-fil′ik) [*baro-* + Gr. *philein* to love] growing best under high atmospheric pressure; said of bacterial cells.

baroreceptor (bar″o-re-sep′tor) a sensory nerve ending that is stimulated by changes in pressure, as those in the walls of blood vessels; called also *baroceptor.*

baroscope (bar′ŏ-skōp) [*baro-* + Gr. *skopein* to examine] an instrument used in the quantitative determination of urea.

barosinusitis (bar″o-si″nu-si′tis) inflammation of one or more paranasal sinuses (usually the frontal sinus) due to difference in pressure between the surrounding atmosphere and the air within the sinus cavity; severe localized pain is the predominant symptom. It occurs on ascent or descent in an aircraft to or from high altitude, in the absence of free communication between the sinus and the atmosphere. Called also *aerosinusitis* and *sinus barotrauma.*

barospirator (bar″o-spi′ra-tor) [*baro-* + L. *spirare* to breathe] a machine for producing artificial respiration by means of variations in the air pressure in a closed chamber.

barotaxis (bar″o-tak′sis) [*baro-* + Gr. *taxis* arrangement] stimulation of living matter by change of the pressure relations under which it exists; see also *barotropism.*

barotitis (bar″o-ti′tis) a morbid condition of the ear produced by exposure to differing atmospheric pressures. **b. me′dia,** traumatic inflammation of the middle ear caused by a difference in pressure between the surrounding atmosphere and air in the middle ear space, marked by otalgia, tinnitus, hearing loss, and, occasionally, vertigo. It occurs in descent of aircraft from high altitude. Called also *aerotitis media* and *otitic barotrauma.*

barotrauma (bar″o-traw′mah) [*baro-* + Gr. *trauma* wound] injury caused by pressure: specifically injury of the cartilaginous walls of the eustachian tube and the ear drum due to the difference between atmospheric and intratympanic pressures. **odontalgia b.,** aerodontalgia. **otitic b.,** barotitis media. **sinus b.,** barosinusitis.

barotropism (bar-ot′ro-prizm) [*baro-* + Gr. *tropos* a turning] a relatively stereotyped response, often a movement, in response to pressure stimuli.

Barr body (bahr) [Murray Llewellyn *Barr*, Canadian anatomist, born 1908] sex chromatin.

Barraquer's disease (bar-rak-erz′) [Roviralta José Antonio *Barraquer*, Spanish physician] lipodystrophia progressiva.

Barraquer's method, operation (bar-rak-erz′) [Ignacio *Barraquer*, Spanish ophthalmologist, 1884–1965] phacoerysis.

Barré-Guillain syndrome (bar-ra′ ge-yan′) acute febrile polyneuritis.

barren (bar′en) sterile; unfruitful.

barrier (bār′e-er) an obstruction. **blood-air b., blood-gas b.,** alveolocapillary membrane. **blood-aqueous b.,** the physiologic mechanism that prevents exchange of materials between the chambers of the eye and the blood. **blood-brain b., blood-cerebral b.,** the barrier separating the blood from the parenchyma of the central nervous system. Presumably it consists of the walls of the capillaries of the central nervous system and the surrounding glial membranes (glial end-feet). Abbreviated BBB. **blood-cerebrospinal fluid b.,** blood-brain b. **blood-testis b.,** a barrier separating the blood from the seminiferous tubules, consisting of special junctional complexes between adjacent Sertoli cells near the base of the seminiferous epithelium. **blood-thymus b.,** a barrier in the thymus which excludes certain substances, possibly constituted by the interposition of a sheet of epithelial cell processes around the periphery of the lobules and between the lymphocytes and the perivascular connective tissue. **filtration b.,** the structures separating the blood in the glomerular capillaries and capsular space of the renal corpuscle, consisting of the fenestrated epithelium, the basal lamina, and the slit pores between the pedicels of the podocytes. **gastric mucosal b.,** a physiological property of the gastric mucosa rendering the epithelium relatively impermeable to ions. Its function is impaired by aspirin, organic acids, and bile salts, and in patients subjected to severe trauma or shock. Back diffusion of acid from the gastric lumen may cause mucosal erosion or ulceration. **hematoencephalic b.,** blood-brain b. **histohematic connective tissue b.,** the barrier between the blood and the dependent parenchymal tissue through which diffusion of nutrients and gases takes place. **placental b.,** the placental separation of fetal from maternal blood and bloodborne materials of greater than molecular size. **protective b.,** an intervening shield of radiation-absorbing material such as lead, concrete, or plastic whose atomic number and thickness are specifically sufficient to give adequate body protection against ionizing radiation of various types. **protective b's, primary,** barriers sufficient to reduce a primary beam of radiation to a permissible exposure rate. **protective b's, secondary,** barriers sufficient to reduce stray or scattered radiation to a permissible exposure rate. **radiation b.,** protective b. **stimulus b.,** the mechanisms, consisting of a combination of neurophysiological properties of the nervous system and mental processes, by which the organism is protected from overwhelming and destructive stimulation, both from internal and external sources.

barsati (bar-sat-e′) cutaneous habronemiasis.

Barth's hernia (barths) [Jean Baptiste Philippe *Barth*, German physician, 1806–1877] see under *hernia.*

Barthélemy's disease (bar-tāl′mez) [P. Toussaint *Barthélemy*, French dermatologist, 1850–1906] tuberculosis papulonecrotica.

Bartholin's anus (bar′to-linz) [Thomas *Bartholin*, Danish anatomist, 1616–1680] see under *anus.*

Bartholin's duct, gland (bar′to-linz) [Caspar Thomèson *Bartholin*, Jr., Danish anatomist, 1655–1738] see *ductus sublingualis major* and *glandula vestibularis major.*

bartholinitis (bar″to-lin-i′tis) inflammation of Bartholin's ducts.

Barton's bandage, fracture, operation (bar′tunz) [John Rhea *Barton*, Philadelphia surgeon, 1794–1871] see under *bandage, fracture,* and *operation.*

Bartonella (bar″to-nel′lah) [A. L. *Barton*, Peruvian physician, who described the organisms in 1909] a genus of the family Bartonellaceae, order Rickettsiales, occurring as a single species. **B. bacillifor′mis,** the etiologic agent of Carrión's disease (bartonellosis); called also *Bartonia bodies.*

Bartonellaceae (bar″to-nel-la′se-e) a family of the order Rickettsiales, made up of small rod-shaped, coccoid, or ring- or disk-shaped, filamentous and beaded organisms, usually measuring less than 3μ, occurring as pathogenic parasites in the erythrocytes of man and other animals. It includes four genera, *Bartonella, Eperythrozoon, Grahamella,* and *Haemobartonella.*

bartonellemia (bar″to-nel-e′me-ah) presence in the blood of organisms of the genus *Bartonella.*

bartonelliasis (bar″to-nel-li′ah-sis) Carrión's disease.

bartonellosis (bar″to-nel-lo′sis) Carrión's disease.

Baruch's law, sign (bar′ooks) [Simon *Baruch*, physician in New York, 1840–1921] see under *law* and *sign.*

baruria (bah-roo′re-ah) [Gr. *baros* weight + *ouron* urine + *-ia*] the passage of urine of a high specific gravity.

Barwell's operation (bar′welz) [Richard *Barwell*, London surgeon, 1826–1916] see under *operation.*

bary- [Gr. *barys* heavy] a combining form meaning heavy or difficult.

barye (bar′e) bar, def. 3.

baryencephalia (bar″ĭ-en-se-fa′le-ah) [*bary-* + Gr. *enkephalos* brain] dullness of the intellect.

baryesthesia (bar″ĭ-esthe′ze-ah) baresthesia.

baryglossia (bar″ĭ-glos′e-ah) [*bary-* + Gr. *glōssa* tongue + *-ia*] thick, slow utterance of speech.

barylalia (bar″ĭ-la′le-ah) [*bary-* + Gr. *lalia* speech] thick, indistinct speech due to imperfect articulation.

baryphonia (bar″ĭ-fo′ne-ah) [*bary-* + Gr. *phōnē* voice + *-ia*] a thick, heavy quality of voice.

baryta (bah-ri′tah) any of several compounds of barium, including calcinated baryta (barium oxide) and caustic baryta (barium hydroxide). **synthetic b.,** barium sulfate.

barytosis (bar″ĭ-to′sis) baritosis.

barytron (bar′ĭ-tron) [*bary-* + *electron*] an electrical particle lighter than a proton but heavier than an electron, and charged both positively and negatively; called also *yukon.*

basad (ba′sad) toward a base or basal aspect.

basal (ba′sal) pertaining to or situated near a base.

Basaljel (ba′sal-jel) trademark for basic aluminum carbonate gel.

basaloid (ba′sah-loid) resembling basal cells of the skin; see under *carcinoma.*

basaloma (ba″sah-lo′mah) basal cell carcinoma.

basculation (bas″ku-la′shun) [Fr. *basculer* to swing] (*obs.*) replacement of a retroverted uterus by simultaneously elevating the corpus and depressing the cervix.

base (bās) [L., Gr., *basis*] 1. the lowest part or foundation of anything; see also *basis*. 2. the main ingredient of a compound. 3. in chemistry, the nonacid part of a salt; a substance that combines with acids to form salts; a substance that dissociates to give hydroxide ions in aqueous solutions; a substance whose molecule or ion can combine with a proton (hydrogen ion); a substance capable of donating a pair of electrons (to an acid) for the formation of a coordinate covalent bond. **acidifiable b.**, a chemical substance that will unite with water to form an acid. **acrylic resin b.**, a denture base made of an acrylic resin. **alloxur b's, alloxuric b's,** purine b's. **animal b.**, a ptomaine or leukomaine. **apical b.**, that portion of the jaws giving support to the teeth; called also *basal arch.* **cement b.**, a layer of insulated, sometimes medicated dental cement placed in the deep portions of a cavity preparation to protect the pulp, reduce the bulk of the metallic restoration, or eliminate undercuts in tapered preparation. **cheoplastic b.**, a denture base produced by casting molten metal in a mold. **cranial b.**, the endochondral bony support for the brain, separating the cranial from the facial region. **denture b.**, the material in which the teeth of a denture are set and which rests on the supporting tissues when the denture is in place in the mouth. **extension b.**, a unit of a removable prosthesis that extends anteriorly or posteriorly, terminating in a free end. **film b.**, a thin, flexible, transparent sheet of cellulose acetate or similar material which carries the radiation- and light-sensitive emulsion of x-ray or photographic films. **b. of heart,** basis cordis. **hexone b's,** diaminomonocarboxylic acids formed by the hydrolysis of proteins, and containing six atoms of carbon; they include arginine, lysine, and histidine. Called also *histone b's* and *diaminoacids.* **histone b's,** hexone b's. **Lewis b.**, an electron-pair donor, e.g., ammonia and halide ion. **b. of lung,** basis pulmonis. **metal b.**, a metallic portion of a denture base forming a part or all of the basal surface of the denture, which serves as the attachment for the plastic (resin) part of the denture. **nitrogenous b.**, an aromatic, nitrogen-containing molecule that serves as a proton acceptor, e.g., purine or pyrimidine. **nuclein b's, nucleinic b's,** purine b's. **ointment b.**, a vehicle for medicinal substances intended for external application to the body. **plastic b.**, a denture or baseplate, made of a plastic material. **b. of prostate,** basis prostatae. **purine b's,** a group of chemical compounds of which purine is the base, including 6-oxypurine (hypoxanthine); 2,6-dioxypurine (xanthine); 6-aminopurine (adenine); 2-amino-6-oxypurine (guanine); 2,6,8-trioxypurine (uric acid); 3,7-dimethyl xanthine (theobromine). Called also *nuclein* or *nucleinic b's*, and *xanthine b's.* **pyrimidine b's,** a group of chemical compounds of which pyrimidine is the base, including 2,4-dioxy-pyrimidine (uracil), 2,4-dioxy-5-methylpyrimidine (thymine), and 2-oxy-4-aminopyrimidine (cytosine), which are common constituents of nucleic acids. **record b.**, baseplate. **Schreiner's b.**, spermine. **shellac b's,** resinous materials adapted to maxillary or mandibular casts to form baseplates. **b. of stapes,** footplate. **temporary b.**, baseplate. **tinted denture b.**, a denture base which simulates the coloring and shading of natural oral tissues. **tooth-borne b.**, the base of a partial denture which is supported by the abutment teeth and not by the tissues beneath it. **trial b.**, baseplate. **xanthine b's,** purine b's.

basedoid (bas′ĕ-doid) a condition resembling Basedow's (Graves') disease, but without thyrotoxicosis.

Basedow's disease, triad (bas′e-dōz) [Carl Adolph von *Basedow*, German physician, 1799–1854] see *Graves' disease,* under *disease,* and *Merseburg triad,* under *triad.*

basedowian (bas″e-do′e-an) a person affected with Basedow's (Graves') disease.

basedowiform (bas″e-do′ĭ-form) resembling Basedow's (Graves') disease.

baseline (bās′līn) a known value or quantity used to measure or assess an unknown, as a baseline urine sample.

baseplate (bās′plāt) 1. a sheet of wax, gutta-percha, or other plastic material used as a temporary base in the construction and fitting of artificial dentures; called also *record base, temporary base,* and *trial base.* 2. Hutch's term for the tissue circumferential to and somewhat eccentric to the urethral orifice which, it is postulated, may act as a floor during the filling of the bladder and assume a cone-shape during micturition to allow the proximal urethra to fill. **stabilized b.**, a baseplate lined with a plastic material to improve its fit and stability in the mouth.

bases (ba′sēz) [L.] plural of *basis.*

bas-fond (bah-fon′) [Fr.] a fundus, especially that of the urinary bladder.

Basham's mixture (Bash′amz) [William Richard *Basham*, English physician, 1804–1877] iron and ammonium acetate solution; see under *solution.*

basi-, basio- (ba′se, ba′se-o) [L., Gr. *basis*] a combining form denoting relationship to a base or foundation.

basial (ba′se-al) pertaining to the basion.

basialis (ba″se-a′lis) [L.] basial; used in the NA terminology as denoting relationship to a base or to the basion.

basialveolar (ba″se-al-ve′o-lar) extending from the basion to the alveolar point.

basiarachnitis (ba″se-ar″ak-ni′tis) inflammation of the basal part of the arachnoid; called also *basiarachnoiditis.*

basiarachnoiditis (ba″se-ah-rak″noi-di′tis) basiarachnitis.

basic (ba′sik) 1. pertaining to or having the properties of a base. 2. capable of neutralizing acids.

basicaryoplastin (ba″se-kar″e-o-plas′tin) [*basi-* + Gr. *karyon* kernel + *plassein* to form] the basophil paraplastin of the cell nucleus.

basichromatin (ba″se-kro′mah-tin) the basophil portion of the chromatin of the cell nucleus.

basichromiole (ba″se-kro′me-ōl) [*basophil* + *chromiole*] one of the basophil particles forming the chromatin of the cell nucleus.

basicity (bah-sis′ĭ-te) 1. the quality of being a base, or basic. 2. the combining power of an acid; it is measured by the number of hydrogen atoms replaceable by a base.

basicranial (ba″se-kra′ne-al) [*basi-* + Gr. *kranion* cranium] pertaining to the base of the skull.

basicytoparaplastin (ba″se-si″to-par″ah-plas′tin) the basophil paraplastin of the cytoplasm.

basidia (bah-sid′e-ah) plural of *basidium.*

Basidiobolus (bah-sid″ĭ-ob′o-lus) a genus of phycomycetous fungi of the family Entomophthoraceae, order Entomophthorales. **B. haptospo′rus,** the etiologic agent of subcutaneous phycomycosis; called also *B. meristosporus.* **B. meristospo′rus,** *B. haptosporus.*

basidiocarp (bah-sid′ĕ-o-karp″) the basidium-producing large fruiting body, the mushroom, composed of masses of intertwined hyphal elements, which is characteristic of the majority of the Basidiomycetes.

Basidiomycetes (bah-sid″e-o-mi-se′tēz) a class of perfect fungi of the division Eumycetes, the club fungi, in which the spores are borne on club-shaped organs (basidia); it includes the subclasses Heterobasidiomycetidae and Homobasidiomycetidae.

basidiomycetous (ba″sid-ĭ-o-mi-se′tus) of or pertaining to fungi of the class Basidiomycetes.

basidiospore (bah-sid′e-o-spōr) a spore formed on a basidium. See *Basidiomycetes* and *spore.*

basidium (bah-sid′e-um), pl. *basid′ia* [Gr. *basis* base] the club-like organ of the fungal class Basidiomycetes which, following karyogamy and meiosis, bears the basidiospore. See *spore.*

basifacial (ba-se-fa′shal) [L. *basis* base + *facies* face] pertaining to the lower part of the face.

basigenous (bah-sij′ĕ-nus) capable of forming a chemical base.

basihyal (ba″se-hi′al) basihyoid.

basihyoid (ba″se-hi′oid) the body of the hyoid bone; in certain of the lower animals, either of the two lateral bones that are its homologues; called also *basihyal,* and *corpus ossis hyoidei.*

basil (ba′sil) any aromatic plant of the genus *Osimum,* especially *O. basilicum;* a condiment with carminative properties. Called also *sweet b.*

basilad (bas′ĭ-lad) toward the basilar aspect.

basilar (bas′ĭ-lar) [L. *basilaris,* from *basis* base] pertaining to a base or basal part.

basilaris (bas′ĭ-la′ris) [L.] situated at the base. **b. cra′nii,** a composite of the numerous bones which serve the brain as a supportive floor and form the axis of the whole skull.

basilateral (ba″se-lat′er-al) both basilar and lateral.

basilemma (ba″se-lem′ah) [*basi-* + Gr. *lemma* husk] basement membrane.

basilic (bah-sil′ik) [L. *basilicus;* Gr. *basilikos* royal] important or prominent.

basilicon (bah-sil′ĭ-kon) [Gr. *basilikos* royal] a once popular name for various ointments, and especially for resin cerate.

basiloma (bas-ĕ-lo′mah) basal cell carcinoma. **b. tere′brans,** an invasive basal-cell epithelioma.

basilysis (bah-sil′ĭ-sis) [*basi-* + Gr. *lysis* dissolution] (*obs.*) craniotomy, def. 2.

basilyst (bas′ĭ-list) (*obs.*) cranioclast.

basin (ba′sn) the pelvis.

basinasial (ba″se-na′ze-al) pertaining to the basion and the nasion.

basio- see *basi-.*

basioccipital (ba″se-ok-sip′ĭ-tal) pertaining to the basilar process of the occipital bone.

basioglossus (ba″se-o-glos′us) [*basio-* + Gr. *glōssa* tongue] the part of the hyoglossus muscle that is attached to the base of the hyoid bone.

basion (ba′se-on) [Gr. *basis* base] the midpoint of the anterior border of the foramen magnum.

basiotic (ba″se-ot′ik) [basi- + Gr. ous ear]   see under bone.

basiotribe (ba′se-o-trib″) [basio- + Gr. tribein to crush]   (obs.) cranioclast.

basiotripsy (ba′se-o-trip″se)   (obs.) craniotomy, def. 2.

basiotriptor (ba′se-o-trip″ter)   (obs.) cranioclast.

basiparachromatin (ba″se-par″ah-kro′mah-tin)   basicaryoplastin.

basiparaplastin (ba″se-par″ah-plas′tin)   the basophil portion of the paraplastin.

basipetal (ba-sip′ĕ-tal) [basi- + L. petere to seek]   descending toward the base; developing in the direction of the base, as a spore.

basiphilic (ba″se-fil′ik)   basophilic.

basirhinal (ba″se-ri′nal) [basi- + Gr. rhis nose]   pertaining to the base of the brain and to the nose.

basis (ba′sis), pl. bases [L.; Gr.]   the lower, basic, or fundamental part of an object; [NA] a general term designating the base of a structure or organ, or the part opposite to or distinguished from the apex.   **b. cartilag′inis arytenoi′deae** [NA], base of arytenoid cartilage: the triangular inferior part of the arytenoid cartilage, which bears the articular surface.   **b. cer′ebri**, facies inferior cerebri.   **b. coch′leae** [NA], base of cochlea: the posterior of the cochlea, which rests upon the internal acoustic meatus.   **b. cor′dis** [NA], base of heart: a poorly delimited region of the heart, formed, in general, by the atria and the area occupied by the roots of the great vessels. It lies opposite the middle thoracic vertebrae, its exact position varying with heart action, and is directed superiorly, posteriorly, and to the right.   **b. cra′nii exter′na** [NA], external base of cranium: the outer surface of the inferior region of the skull.   **b. cra′nii inter′na** [NA], internal base of cranium: the inner surface of the inferior region of the skull, constituting the floor of the cranial cavity.   **b. enceph′ali**, facies inferior cerebri.   **b. glan′dulae suprarena′lis**, facies renalis glandulae suprarenalis.   **b. mandib′ulae** [NA], base of mandible: the lower margin of the body of the mandible; called also inferior border of mandible.   **b. modi′oli** [NA], base of modiolus: the broad part of the modiolus situated near the lateral part of the internal acoustic meatus.   **b. na′si**, the portion of the nose opposite to the apex.   **b. os′sis metacarpa′lis** [NA], base of metacarpal bone: the proximal end of a metacarpal bone, that articulates with bone(s) of the carpus and with adjacent metacarpal bones.   **b. os′sis metatarsa′lis** [NA], base of metatarsal bone: the wedge-shaped proximal end of a metatarsal bone, which articulates with bone(s) of the tarsus and with adjacent metatarsal bones.   **b. os′sis sa′cri** [NA], base of the sacral bone: the cranial surface of the sacrum; its lateral portions consist of the alae of the sacrum, and its middle portion is the upper surface of the body of the first sacral vertebra that articulates with the fifth lumbar vertebra. Called also base of the sacrum.   **b. patel′lae** [NA], base of patella: the superior border of the patella, to which the tendon of the quadriceps femoris muscle is attached; called also superior border of patella.   **b. pedun′culi cer′ebri**, crus cerebri.   **b. phalan′gis digito′rum ma′nus** [NA], base of phalanx of fingers: the proximal end of each phalanx of the fingers; called also proximal extremity of phalanx of finger.   **b. phalan′gis digito′rum pe′dis** [NA], base of phalanx of toes: the proximal end of each phalanx of the toes; called also proximal extremity of phalanx of toe.   **b. prosta′tae** [NA], base of prostate: the broad upper part of the prostate, in contact with the lower surface of the urinary bladder.   **b. pulmo′nis** [NA], base of lung: the portion of each lung that is directed toward the diaphragm.   **b. pyram′idis rena′lis** [NA], base of renal pyramid: the part of a renal pyramid that is directed away from the renal sinus.   **b. scap′ulae**, a name applied to both the vertebral and the axillary borders of the scapula (margo medialis and margo lateralis).   **b. sta′pedis** [NA], base of stapes: the oval plate of bone on the stapes that fits into the fenestra vestibuli.

basisphenoid (ba″se-sfe′noid)   an embryonic bone that becomes the back part of the body of the sphenoid.

basisylvian (ba″se-sil′ve-an) [basi- + sylvian]   (obs.) pertaining to the basilar part of the sylvian fissure (sulcus lateralis).

basitemporal (ba″se-tem′po-ral) [basi- + temporal]   pertaining to the lower part of the temporal bone.

basivertebral (ba″se-ver′te-bral) [basi- + L. vertebra joint]   pertaining to the body of a vertebra.

basket (bas′ket)   1. basket cell, the inferior stellate cell of the cerebellar cortex.   2. one of the condensations of intracellular neurofibrils in senile dementia; called also Alzheimer's neurofibrillary degeneration and, less commonly, Alzheimer's b.   **fiber b's**, fine fibers extending from the external limiting membrane of the retina to surround the adjacent portions of the rods and cones.

Basle Nomina Anatomica (bah′zl no′mĭ-nah an-ah-tom′ĭ-kah)   the official body of anatomical nomenclature prepared by a group of German anatomists with some help from anatomists in other countries, and presented for final criticism at the annual meeting of the German Anatomic Society held in Basle, Switzerland in 1895. Abbreviated BNA. It has been superseded by Nomina Anatomica.

BaSO₄   barium sulfate.

basocyte (ba′so-sīt)   (obs.) a basophilic cell or leukocyte.

basocytopenia (ba″so-si″to-pe′ne-ah) [basocyte + Gr. penia poverty]   (obs.) basophilic leukopenia.

basocytosis (ba″so-si-to′sis)   (obs.)   1. basophilic leukocytosis.   2. basophilia, def. 1.

basoerythrocyte (ba″so-ĕ-rith′ro-sīt)   (obs.) an erythrocyte containing basophilic granules.

basoerythrocytosis (ba″so-ĕ-rith″ro-si-to′sis)   (obs.) basophilia, def. 1.

basograph (ba′so-graf) [Gr. basis a walking + graphein to write]   an instrument for recording abnormalities of gait.

basometachromophil (ba″so-met″ah-kro′mo-fil) [basic + Gr. meta beyond + chrōma color + philein to love]   staining with basic dyes to a color different from that of surrounding substances.

Basommatophora (ba-som″mah-tof′o-rah)   a suborder of mostly freshwater snails (order Pulmonata, subclass Euthyneura, class Gastropoda); two families of medical importance are Planorbidae and Lymnaeidae.

basopenia (ba″so-pe′ne-ah)   (obs.) basophilic leukopenia.

basophil (ba′so-fil) [Gr. basis base + philein to love]   1. a structure, cell, or other histologic element staining readily with basic dyes.   2. a granular leukocyte with an irregularly shaped, relatively pale-staining nucleus that is partially constricted into two lobes, and with cytoplasm that contains coarse bluish black granules of variable size. Basophils contain vasoactive amines, e.g., histamine and serotonin, which are released on appropriate stimulation. Called also basophilic leukocytes.   3. a beta cell of the adenohypophysis; see also gonadotrope (def. 3) and thyrotrope (def. 2).   4. basophilic.   **beta b.**, thyrotrope, def. 2.   **Crooke-Russell b's**, the basophils in Crooke's hyaline degeneration; see under degeneration.   **delta b.**, gonadotrope, def. 3.

basophile (ba′so-fīl)   basophilic.

basophilia (ba″so-fil′e-ah)   1. the reaction of relatively immature erythrocytes to basic dyes whereby the stained cells appear blue, gray, or grayish-blue (diffuse basophilia), or bluish granules appear (punctate basophilia or stippling).   2. an abnormal increase in the blood of basophilic erythrocytes; called also basocytosis and basoerythrocytosis.   3. basophilic leukocytosis.

basophilic (ba-so-fil′ik)   staining readily with basic dyes.

basophilism (ba-sof′ĭ-lizm)   abnormal increase of basophil cells.   **Cushing's b., pituitary b.**, Cushing's syndrome (def. 1); see under syndrome.

basophilous (ba-sof′ĭ-lus)   basophilic.

basoplasm (ba′so-plazm″)   cytoplasm that stains with basic dyes.

Bass-Watkins test (bas-wot′kinz) [Charles Cassedy Bass, American physician, born 1875; J. A. Watkins]   see under tests.

Basset's operation (bas-sāz′) [Antoine Basset, French surgeon, 1882–1951]   see under operation.

Bassini's operation (bah-se′nēz) [Edoardo Bassini, surgeon in Padua, 1844–1924]   see under operation.

bassorin (bas′o-rin)   a principal constituent of tragacanth gum, made up of a complex of polymethoxylated acids (bassoric acid) which swell in water to form an irreversible gel; used as pharmaceutical adjuvant.

basswood (bas′wood)   the wood of the Linden tree, Tilia americana L. (Tiliaceae). Long used in American folk medicine as a decoction of the wood, bark, or flowers for bile and liver disorders.

bast (bast)   a strong woody fiber obtained chiefly from the phloem of higher plants; used to a very limited extent in surgery.

bastard (bas′tard) [Old Fr.]   1. an illegitimate person; one born out of wedlock.   2. illegitimate.   3. of inferior quality; not genuine.

Bastedo's rule (bas-te′dōz) [Walter Arthur Bastedo, physician in New York, 1873–1952]   see under rule.

Bastian-Bruns law (sign) (bas′chan-broonz′) [Henry Charlton Bastian, British neurologist, 1837–1915; Ludwig Bruns, neurologist in Hanover, 1856–1916]   see under law.

basylous (bas′ĭ-lus)   acting as a base in chemical composition.

Bateman's disease (bāt′manz) [Thomas Bateman, English physician, 1778–1821]   molluscum contagiosum.

Bates' operation (bātz′) [William Horatio Bates, American surgeon]   see under operation.

bath (bath)   1. a conductive or convective medium, as water, vapor, sand, or mud, with which the body is laved or in which the body is wholly or partly immersed for therapeutic or cleansing purposes; called also balneum.   2. the application of a conductive or convective medium to the body for therapeutic or cleansing purposes.   3. a piece of equipment or scientific apparatus in which a body or object may be immersed.   **acid b.**, one of water medicated with a mineral acid.   **air b.**, the therapeutic exposure of the body to air, which is usually warm; called also balneum pneumaticum.   **alcohol b.**, the laving of the body with dilute alcohol; it is defervescent and stimulant.   **alkaline b.**, the washing of a patient in a weak solution of an alkaline carbonate; useful in skin diseases.   **alum b.**, the use of alum water as a bathing medium.   **antipyretic b.**, a bath given to reduce fever. **antiseptic b.,** a bath containing an antiseptic. **aromatic b.,** a medicated bath in which the water is scented with a decoction of aromatic plants or volatile oils. **astringent b.,** a bath in a liquid containing tannic acid, alum, or other astringent. **borax b.,** one in water medicated with glycerin and borax. **bran b.,** an emollient bath of water in which bran has been boiled. **Brand b.** (1861), a cold bath of short duration in which the water is at 68° F., and during which the patient is gently massaged. **bubble b.,** a bath in which the water has been filled with bubbles produced by mechanical or chemical means. **cabinet b.,** a hot-air bath or a radiant heat bath in which the patient is inclosed in a special cabinet. **camphor b.,** a bath given in an atmosphere containing the vapor of camphor. **carbon dioxide b.,** a water bath impregnated with carbon dioxide, such as the Nauheim bath. **Charcot's b.** (*obs.*), a bath taken by standing in ankle-deep hot water and sponging the body locally with cold water. **cold b.,** one in which cold water is used at a temperature of less than 65° F. **colloid b.,** a bath containing gelatin, bran, starch, or similar substances. **continuous b.,** a bath of flowing water. **contrast b.,** immersion of a part of the body alternately in hot and in cold water. **cool b.,** one in water from 65° to 75° F. **creosote b.,** a bath containing creosote and glycerin; used in scaly skin diseases. **douche b.,** the application of water to the body from a jet spray. **drip-sheet b.,** see *drip sheet*, under *sheet*. **earth b.,** the placing of a patient in a mass of earth or of sand, usually warmed. **emollient b.,** a bath in an emollient liquid, like a decoction of bran. **Finnish b.,** a sweat bath given in an enclosed, steamy room. Hyperemia of the skin is increased by beating with twigs, and the bath is followed by a cold plunge. **Finsen b.,** a general irradiation of the patient's body with ultraviolet rays. **foam b.,** a bath of foam produced by blowing air or oxygen through the water to which a foam-forming substance (saponin) has been added. **full b.,** one in which the patient's body is fully immersed in the water. **gas-bubble b.,** a bath of water containing gases in such quantities that gas bubbles are set free and ascend to the surface of the water, as in carbon dioxide and oxygen baths. **gelatin b.,** an emollient bath in a thin warm solution of gelatin. **glycerin b.,** a warm emollient bath in water containing glycerin and gum acacia. **graduated b.,** one in which the temperature of the water is gradually modified. **grease b.,** a scrubbing of the body with some greasy preparation (petrolatum, lanolin). **Greville b.** (*obs.*), an electric hot-air bath. **half b.,** a bath of the hips and lower part of the body. **herb b.,** one which contains a decoction of aromatic herbs. **hip b.,** sitz b. **hot b.,** one in water from 98° to 104° F. **hot-air b.,** one in air or vapor from 100° to 130° F. **hyperthermal b.,** a hot bath in which the water is above 104° F. **immersion b.,** one in which the body of the patient is immersed. **iron b.,** one in water which contains iron sulfate. **kineto-therapeutic b.,** a bath providing facilities for underwater exercise. **light b.,** exposure of all or part of the body to light rays, either of the sun or from an apparatus. **linseed b.,** a bath to which has been added the mucilage extracted from linseed. **lukewarm b.,** a neutral bath in which the water is between 92° and 97° F. **medicated b.,** a bath variously charged with medicinal substances. **milk b.,** one taken in milk; called also *balneum lacteum*. **moor b.,** a mud bath containing earth from a moor or waste land. **mud b.,** application of wet sticky earth to the body, or immersion of the body in such material. **Nauheim b.,** a bath in which the patient is immersed in warm carbonated water. **needle b.,** a shower bath in which the water is projected in a fine, needle-like spray. **oil b.,** one taken in warm olive oil, sometimes variously medicated. **oxygen b.,** a bath impregnated with oxygen. See *gas-bubble b.* **pack b.,** see *pack.* **paraffin b.,** wax b. **peat b.,** a mud bath utilizing partially carbonized vegetable matter. **sand b.,** 1. the immersion of the body in dry, heated sand. 2. the covering of the body with the damp sand of the seashore. Called also *balneum arenae.* **sauna b.,** a sweat bath given in an enclosed, steamy room, usually followed by a cold shower. See *Finnish b.* **Schott b.,** see *Schott's treatment*, under *treatment.* **sea b.,** **sea-water b.,** a bath in water from the sea; usually warm. **sedative b.,** a warm bath in which the patient's body is immersed, usually for several hours, to reduce agitated behavior. **sheet b.,** the applications of wet sheets to the body. **sitz b.,** a bath in which the patient sits in the tub, the hips and buttocks being immersed; called also *hip b.* **sponge b.,** one in which the patient's body is not immersed in water but is rubbed with a wet cloth or sponge. **stimulating b.,** a bath containing tonic, astringent, or aromatic substances. **sweat b.,** any bath given to promote sweating. **tepid b.,** one in water from 75° to 92° F. **vapor b.,** exposure of the body to steam. **warm b.,** one taken in water from 92° to 97° F. **water b.,** a vessel containing water for immersing bodies or for immersing liquid-containing vessels that are to be heated or cooled, or are to be held at a given temperature. **wax b.,** the application of heated liquid wax to a part of the body, the wax being permitted to solidify; also the immersion of a part of the body in heated liquid wax maintained at a constant temperature. Called also *paraffin b.* **whirlpool b.,** a variously sized tank in which the body or an extremity can be submerged as the heated water is mechanically agitated.

bathesthesia (bath″es-the′ze-ah) bathyesthesia.

bathmotropic (bath″mo-trop′ik) [Gr. *bathmos* threshold + *tropos* a turning] influencing the response of tissue to stimuli. **negatively b.,** lessening response to stimuli. **positively b.,** increasing response to stimuli.

bathmotropism (bath-mot′ro-pizm) influence on the excitability of muscular tissue.

batho- see *bathy-*.

bathochrome (bath′o-krōm) an atom or group whose introduction into a compound shifts the compound's absorption peak to a longer wavelength; cf. *hypsochrome*.

bathochromy (bath″o-kro′me) a shift of the absorption band toward lower frequencies (longer wavelengths) with deepening of color from yellow to red to black.

bathoflore (bath′o-flōr) [*batho-* + *fluorescence*] a substance that decreases the intensity of fluorescence of a parent compound; cf. *auxoflore*.

bathomorphic (bath″o-mor′fik) [*batho-* + Gr. *morphē* form] having a deep or myopic eye.

bathrocephaly (bath′ro-sef′ah-le) [Gr. *bathron* a step + *kephalē* head] a developmental anomaly characterized by a steplike posterior projection of the skull, caused by excessive bone formation at the lambdoid suture.

bathy-, batho- (bath′e, bath′o) [Gr. *bathys* deep, *bathos* depth] a combining form meaning deep, or denoting relationship to depth.

bathyanesthesia (bath″e-an″es-the′ze-ah) [*bathy-* + *anesthesia*] loss of deep sensibility.

bathycardia (bath″e-kar′de-ah) [*bathy-* + Gr. *kardia* heart] a low position of the heart due to anatomical conditions and not to disease.

bathyesthesia (bath″e-es-the′ze-ah) [*bathy-* + Gr. *aisthēsis* perception] deep sensibility; the sensibility in the parts of the body beneath the surface, such as muscle sensibility and joint sensibility.

bathyhyperesthesia (bath″e-hi″per-es-the′ze-ah) [*bathy-* + *hyperesthesia*] increased sensitiveness of deep structures of the body.

bathyhypesthesia (bath″e-hip″es-the′za-ah) [*bathy-* + *hypesthesia*] decreased sensitiveness of the deep structures of the body.

bathypnea (bath″e-ne′ah) [*bathy-* + Gr. *pnoia* breath] deep breathing.

batonet (ba-to-net′) pseudochromosome.

batrachoplasty (bat′rah-ko-plas″te) [Gr. *batrachos* frog + *plassein* to form] a surgical operation for the cure of ranula.

battarism (bat′ah-rizm) stuttering.

battarismus (bat′ah-riz-mus) [Gr. *battarizein* to stammer] stuttering.

battery (bat′er-e) 1. a set or series of cells which afford an electric current. 2. any set, series, or grouping of similar things, as a battery of tests.

Battey bacilli (bat′e) [*Battey*, a tuberculosis hospital in Rome, Georgia, where many strains of these mycobacteria were first recognized] see under *bacillus.*

batteyin (bat′e-in) [*Battey* bacillus] a product prepared from Battey bacilli (Group III of the unclassified mycobacteria), comparable to tuberculin, used in a cutaneous test of hypersensitivity.

Battle's operation, sign (bat′t'lz) [William Henry *Battle*, London Surgeon, 1855–1936] see under *operation* and *sign.*

Battley's sedative (bat′lēz) [Richard *Battley*, English chemist, 1770–1856] see under *sedative.*

Baudelocque's diameter (line) (bo-dloks′) [Jean Louis *Baudelocque*, French obstetrician, 1746–1810] see under *diameter.*

Bauhin's gland, valve (bo′anz) [Gaspard (Caspar) *Bauhin*, Swiss anatomist, 1560–1624] see *glandulae linguales anteriores* and *valva ileocecalis.*

Baumé's scale (bo-māz′) [Antoine *Baumé*, French chemist, 1728–1804] see under *scale.*

Baumès' law (bo-mez′) [Pierre Prosper François *Baumès*, French physician, 1791–1871] see *Colles' law*, under *law.*

Baumès' symptom (bo-mez′) [Jean Baptiste Timothée *Baumès*, French physician, 1756–1828] see under *sign.*

baunscheidtism (bown′shīd-tizm) [from Karl *Baunscheidt*, the inventor] (*obs.*) treatment of chronic rheumatism, etc., by acupuncture with the révulseur, an instrument furnished with many fine needle points, which are dipped into an irritant liquid, as oil of mustard.

bay (ba) a recess or inlet. **lacrimal b.,** the depression at the inner canthus of the eye in which the lacrimal canaliculi lie.

bayberry (ba′ber-e) 1. the fruit of *Laurus nobilis*, the European laurel. 2. the wax myrtle, *Myrica cerifera*, and its berry. 3. the tree, *Pimenta afficinalis*, and its fruit.

Bayer 205 (ba′er) suramin sodium.

Bayle's disease (bālz) [Antoine Laurent Jesse *Bayle*, French physician, 1799–1858] see under *disease.*

Bayle's granulations (bālz) [Gaspard Laurent *Bayle*, French physician, 1774–1816]　see under *granulation*.

Baynton's bandage (bān'tonz) [Thomas *Baynton*, English surgeon, 1761–1820]　see under *bandage*.

Bayrac's test (bi-rakz') [Henri Pierre *Bayrac*, French physician]　see under *tests*.

Bazillenemulsion [Ger.]　bacillary emulsion.

Bazin's disease (bah-zaz') [Antoine Pierre Ernest *Bazin*, French dermatologist, 1807–1878]　erythema induratum.

B.B.B.　blood-brain barrier; see under *barrier*.

BBT　basal body temperature.

BCG　bacille Calmette Guérin (see *BCG vaccine*, under *vaccine*); bicolor guaiac test (see under *tests*); ballistocardiogram.

BCNU　carmustine.

b.d.　abbreviation for L. *bis di'e*, twice a day.

B.D.A.　British Dental Association.

Bdella (del'ah) [Gr. "leech"]　a genus of mites.　**B. cardina'-lis,** a species that is parasitic on other insects.

bdellepithecium (del"ĕ-pĭ-the'se-um) [Gr. *bdella* leech + *epithesis* application]　a kind of artificial leech, as a tube used in leeching.

bdellium (del'le-um) [L.; Gr. *bdellion*]　the fragrant gum-resin of several species of *Commiphora* trees; used as an adulterant of myrrh because of its similar appearance and aromatic properties.

bdellometer (del-lom'ĕ-ter)　a mechanical substitute for a leech.

bdellotomy (del-lot'ŏ-me) [Gr. *bdella* leech + *tomē* cutting]　incision into a sucking leech to increase the amount of blood it will take.

Bdellovibrio (del"o-vib're-o)　a genus of small, rod-shaped or curved, actively motile bacteria that are obligate parasites on certain gram-negative bacteria, including *Pseudomonas*, *Salmonella*, and coliform bacteria; they replicate between the cell wall and plasma membrane of the host bacterium and are considered to be related to the vibrios.

bdellovibrio (del"o-vib're-o)　any microorganism of the genus *Bdellovibrio*.

B.D.S.　Bachelor of Dental Surgery.

B.D.Sc.　Bachelor of Dental Science.

B.E.　Bacillen emulsion; see under *tuberculin*.

Be　chemical symbol for *beryllium*.

bead (bēd)　a small spherical structure or mass.　**rachitic b's,** a series of palpable or visible prominences at the points where the ribs join their cartilages; seen in certain cases of rickets.

beaded (bēd'ed)　having the appearance of a string of beads.

Beadle (be'd'l), George Wells.　United States biochemist, born 1903; co-winner, with Edward Lawrie Tatum and Joshua Lederberg, of the Nobel prize in medicine and physiology for 1958, for the discovery that genes act by regulating specific chemical processes.

beaker (bēk'er)　a form of glass cup, usually with a lip for pouring, used by chemists and pharmacists.

Beale's ganglion cells (bēlz) [Lionel Smith *Beale*, British physician, 1828–1906]　see under *cell*.

beam (bēm)　1. a unidirectional or approximately unidirectional emission of electromagnetic radiation or particles.　2. a dental bar whose curvature changes under load.　**cantilever b.,** a beam that is supported by one fixed support at only one of its ends.　**continuous b.,** a beam that continues over three or more supports; those supports not at the beam ends being equally free supports.　**restrained b.,** one that has two or more supports; at least one of which permits some freedom of rotation to the point of support.　**simple b.,** a straight beam that has two supports, one at either end.　**useful b.,** in radiology, that part of the primary radiation which is permitted to emerge from the tubehead assembly of an x-ray machine, as limited by the tubehead aperture or port and accessory collimating devices.

beamtherapy (bēm-ther'ah-pe)　see *beam therapy*, under *therapy*, and *chromotherapy*, def. 2.

bean (bēn)　any of the seeds contained in pods of various leguminous plants.　**broad b.,** *Vicia faba*.　**Calabar b.,** the poisonous seed of the tropical West African leguminous plant *Physostigma venenosum*; it is the source of physostigmine and has been used by natives in ordeal trials. Called also *ordeal b.*　**castor b.,** the seed of the castor oil plant, *Ricinus communis*, which affords castor oil.　**ordeal b.,** Calabar b.　**St. Ignatius' b.,** the poisonous seed of the tropical tree *Strychnos ignatii*; it contains strychnine and brucine.

beard (bērd)　the heavy hair growing on the lower part of a man's face, normally appearing after puberty as a secondary sex characteristic; called also *barba* [NA].

Beard's disease (bērdz) [George Miller *Beard*, American psychiatrist, 1839–1883]　neurasthenia.

bearing (bār'ing)　a supporting surface or point.　**central b.,** application of forces between the maxillae and mandible at a single point as near as possible to the center of the supporting areas of the upper and lower jaws, for the purpose of distributing closing forces evenly throughout the areas of the supporting structures during the registration and recording of maxillomandibular (jaw) relations and during the correction of occlusal errors.

bearing down (bār'ing down)　1. a feeling of weight in the pelvis occurring in certain diseases.　2. the expulsive effort of a woman in labor.

bearwood (bār'wood)　cascara sagrada.

beat (bēt)　a throb or pulsation, as of the heart or of an artery; see also *pulse*.　**apex b.,** the pulsation of the heart felt over its apex normally in the fifth left intercostal space, 8 or 9 cm. from the midline.　**capture b's,** occasional ventricular responses to a sinus impulse that reaches the atrioventricular node in a nonrefractory phase.　**ciliary b.,** the rhythmic, coordinated contraction of cilia of cells in a two-step process involving intraciliary excitation followed by interciliary conduction.　**dropped b.,** absence of a single ventricular contraction.　**ectopic b.,** a heart beat originating at some point other than the sinus node.　**escaped b's,** heart beats that follow an abnormally long pause.　**forced b.,** an extrasystole produced by artificial stimulation of the heart.　**fusion b.,** in electrocardiography, the complex resulting when an ectopic ventricular beat coincides with normal conduction to the ventricle; the complex has features of both the normal and the ectopic beat.　**premature b.,** extrasystole.　**reciprocal b's,** an additional ventricular contraction induced when the ventricle is activated significantly before the sinus impulse reaches the atria, so that the impulse, after effecting an atrial contraction, may retrace its path to induce another ventricular contraction.

Beatson's operation (bēt'sonz) [George Thomas *Beatson*, Glasgow surgeon, 1848–1933]　see under *operation*.

Beau's disease, lines, syndrome (bōz) [Joseph Honoré Simon *Beau*, French physician, 1806–1865]　see *cardiac insufficiency*, under *insufficiency*; see under *line*, and see *asystole*.

Beauvaria (bo-var'e-ah)　a genus of imperfect fungi of the family Moniliaceae, order Moniliales.　*B. bassia'na* causes muscardine in silkworms, and *B. tenel'la* causes a disease of the larvae of beetles; formerly called *Botrytis bassiana* and *Botrytis tenella*, respectively.

bebeerine (be-be'rēn)　an alkaloid, $C_{36}H_{38}N_2O_6$, obtained from the bark of *Nectandra rodioei* Hook (Lauraceae), the root of *Chondodendron microphyllum* (Eichl.) Moldenke (menispermaceae), and related species; it has been used as a tonic in malaria. Called also *chondodendrine* and *pelosine*.

bebeeru (be-be'roo)　the greenheart tree, *Nectandra rodioei* Hook (Lauraceae), of tropical America; its bark, which contains bebeerine, has been used as a tonic in malaria.

becanthone hydrochloride (bĕ-kan'thōn)　chemical name: 1-[[2-[ethyl(2-hydroxy-2-methylpropyl)amino]ethyl]amino]-4-methylthioxanthen-9-one monohydrochloride; an antischistosomal agent, $C_{22}H_{28}N_2O_2S \cdot HCl$.

Beccari process (bĕ-kah're) [Giuseppe *Beccari*, physician in Florence]　see under *process*.

bechic (bek'ik) [L. *bechicus*, from Gr. *bēx* cough]　pertaining to cough.

Bechterew　see *Bekhterev*.

Beck's gastrostomy (beks) [Carl *Beck*, American surgeon, 1856–1911]　see under *gastrostomy*.

Beck's triad (beks) [Claude Schaeffer *Beck*, Cleveland surgeon, born 1894]　see under *triad*.

Becker's phenomenon (sign), test (bek'erz) [Otto Heinrich Enoch *Becker*, German oculist, 1828–1890]　see under *phenomenon* and *tests*.

Beckmann's apparatus (bek'manz) [Ernst Otto *Beckmann*, Berlin chemist, 1853–1923]　see under *apparatus*.

Béclard's amputation, etc. (ba-klahrz') [Pierre Augustin *Béclard*, French anatomist, 1785–1825]　see under *amputation*, *hernia*, *nucleus*, and *triangle*.

beclomethasone dipropionate (bek"lo-meth'ah-sōn) [USP]　chemical name: 9-chloro-11β-hydroxy-16β-methylpregna-1,4-diene-3,20-dione. A glucocorticoid, $C_{28}H_{37}ClO_7$, administered by aerosol inhalation to patients who require chronic treatment with corticosteroids for control of bronchial asthma symptoms. It has also been used topically in the treatment of glucocorticoid-responsive skin diseases.

Becquerel's rays (bek-relz') [Antoine Henri *Becquerel*, French physicist, 1852–1908; co-winner, with M. S. Curie and P. Curie, of the Nobel prize in physics for 1903, for studies on spontaneous radioactivity]　see under *ray*, and see *becquerel*.

becquerel (bek-rel') [Antoine Henri *Becquerel*]　a proposed unit of radioactivity, defined as that of quantity of a radioactive nuclide whose rate of spontaneous nuclear transformation in one second to the minus one power (s⁻¹) is 2.703 × 10¹¹; it is the reciprocal of the curie. Abbreviated Bq.

bed (bed)　1. a supporting structure or tissue.　2. a couch or support for the body during sleep.　**air b.,** an airtight, inflatable mattress.　**Arnott's b.,** water bed.　**Bandeloux's b.,** an air bed with a vessel beneath for the collection of urine, the whole being surmounted by a cradle covered with gauze. **capillary b.,** the total combined mass of capillaries forming a large reservoir which may be more or less completely filled with blood. **Circoelectric b.,** trademark for a revolving circular bed which induces constant pressure alteration. **ether b.,** a bed made up to facilitate the transfer of an unconscious patient from an operating table or stretcher to the bed. **fracture b.,** a bed for the use of patients with broken bones. **Gatch b.,** a bed fitted with joints beneath the hips and knees of the patient, allowing him to be raised to a half-sitting position and be so maintained by elevating his knees to prevent his sliding toward the footboard. **hydrostatic b.,** a water bed. **Klondike b.,** a bed arranged for outdoor sleeping so that the patient is protected from draughts. **metabolic b.,** a bed so arranged that all the feces and urine of the patient are saved; the amount of excreta compared with the intake gives an indication of the metabolism in the body. **nail b.,** the modified area of epidermis beneath the nail, over which the nail plate slides forward as it grows; called also *matrix unguis* [NA]. **Sanders b.,** a powered, rocking bed, used in the treatment of chronic occlusive arterial disease to improve circulation. **sawdust b.,** a bed made from sawdust which is used to prevent bed sores. **Vickers hyperbaric b.,** a small portable unit for administering hyperbaric oxygen therapy, particularly in myocardial infarction; its maximum pressure is 2 atmospheres. **water b.,** a rubber mattress filled with water; used to prevent bed sores by evenly distributing the patient's weight; called also *Arnott's b.*

bedbug (bed′bug) a bug of the family Cimicidae, genus *Cimex. C. lectularius,* of temperate regions, and *C. rotundatus* (*hempterus*), of the tropics, are flattened, oval, reddish insects which inhabit houses, furniture and neglected beds and feed on man, usually at night.

bedfast (bed′fast) unable to leave the bed.

bedlam (bed′lam) [*Bedlam,* the Bethlehem Royal Hospital, London, a mental hospital established in 1402] 1. an institution for patients with mental illness. 2. bedlamism.

bedlamism (bed′lam-izm) a state of wild tumult; bedlam.

Bednar's aphtha (bed′narz) [Alois *Bednar,* physician in Vienna, 1816–1888] see under *aphtha.*

bedpan (bed′pan) a vessel for receiving the urinary and fecal discharges of a patient unable to leave his bed.

Bedsonia (bed-so′ne-ah) *Chlamydia.*

bedsore (bed-sor) decubitus ulcer.

beef (bēf) the meat of an adult bull, steer, ox, or cow. **b., iron, and wine,** a preparation of beef extract, ferric ammonium citrate, and other ingredients in sherry wine; formerly used as a hematinic agent.

beer (bēr) the fermented infusion of malted barley and hops.

Beer's collyrium, knife, operation (ba′erz) [Georg Joseph *Beer,* German ophthalmologist, 1763–1821] see under *collyrium, knife,* and *operation.*

beerwort (bēr′wert) an infusion of malt in water intended to be converted into beer; it is sometimes used for the cultivation of yeasts and molds.

beeswax (bēz′waks) wax derived from the honeycomb of *Apis mellifera;* see *yellow wax,* under *wax.* **bleached b.,** see *white wax,* under *wax.* **unbleached b.,** see *yellow wax,* under *wax.*

Beevor's sign (be′vorz) [Charles Edward *Beevor,* British neurologist, 1854–1908] see under *sign.*

Begbie's disease (beg′bēz) [James *Begbie,* Scottish physician, 1798–1869] Graves' disease.

Beggiatoa (bej″je-ah-to′ah) [named for F. S. *Beggiato*] a genus of microorganisms, order Beggiatoales, family Beggiatoaceae.

Beggiatoaceae (bej″je-ah-to-a′se-e) a family of Schizomycetes (order Beggiatoales), made up of cells which are generally not visible without staining, arranged in chains within trichomes which show flexing motion and also show gliding movements when in contact with a substrate. It includes four genera, *Beggiatoa, Thioploca, Thiospirillopsis,* and *Thiothrix.* These are free-living sulfur bacteria, often found in association with blue-green algae.

Beggiatoales (bej″je-ah-to-a′lēz) a taxonomic order of class Schizomycetes, made up of cells which occur singly, or in motile or nonmotile trichomes, and which multiply by transverse fission. They are found in fresh or salt water, and in soil and decomposing organic material, especially algae. It includes four families, Achromatiaceae, Beggiatoaceae, Leukotrichaceae, and Vitreoscillaceae.

begma (beg′mah) [Gr. *begma* phlegm] 1. a cough. 2. the material evacuated from the lungs by coughing (sputum).

behavior (be-hāv′yor) deportment or conduct; any or all of a person's total activity, especially that which can be externally observed. **automatic b.,** automatism, def. 1. **invariable b.,** activity whose character is determined by innate structure, such as reflex action. **operant b.,** see under *conditioning.* **protean b.,** an irregular, unpredictable sequence of movements by prey when pursued by predators. **respondent b.,** see *conditioning.* **variable b.,** behavior that is modifiable by individual experience.

behaviorism (be-hāv′yor-izm) a school of psychology based upon a purely objective observation and analysis of human and animal behavior without reference to the testimony of consciousness.

behaviorist (be-hāv′yor-ist) a psychologist who is a disciple of behaviorism.

Behçet's syndrome (disease) (ba′sets) [Hulusi *Behçet,* dermatologist, Istanbul, Turkey, 1889–1948] see under *syndrome.*

Béhier-Hardy sign (symptom) (ba′he-a har′de) [Louis Jules *Béhier,* French physician, 1813–1876; Louis Phillipe Alfred *Hardy,* French physician, 1811–1893] see under *sign.*

Behla's bodies (ba′lahs) [Robert Franz *Behla,* German physician, 1850–1921] Plimmer's bodies.

Behring's law, tuberculin (ba′ringz) [Emil Adolph von *Behring,* German bacteriologist, 1854–1917; winner of the Nobel prize for medicine in 1901] see under *law,* and see *tuberculose* and *tulose.*

BEI butanol-extractable iodine.

Beigel's disease (bi′gelz) [Hermann *Beigel,* German physician, 1830–1879] piedra.

beikost (bi′kōst) [Ger.] solid and semisolid baby foods, i.e., those other than milk or formula feedings.

bejel (bej′el) nonvenereal syphilis (q.v.) occurring in Africa, the Middle East, the Balkans, Central Asia, and Africa.

Békésy (bek′ĕ-se), Georg von. Hungarian-born physicist, born 1899; winner of the Nobel prize in medicine and physiology for 1961, for his discoveries concerning the physical mechanisms of stimulation within the cochlea.

Bekhterev's (Bechterew's) arthritis, etc. (bek- ter′yevs) [Vladimir Mikhailovich *Bekhterev,* Russian neurologist, 1857–1927] see under *arthritis, disease, layer, nucleus, reaction, reflex, symptom,* and *tests.*

Bekhterev-Mendel reflex (bek-ter′yev-men′del) [V. M. *Bekhterev;* Kurt *Mendel,* German neurologist, 1857–1927] Mendel-Bekhterev reflex.

bel (bel) the common logarithm of the ratio of two powers, usually electric or acoustic powers; such ratios are usually expressed in decibels (q.v.). An increase of one bel in intensity approximately doubles the loudness of most sounds.

Belascaris (bĕ-las″kah-ris) *Toxocara.* **B. ca′ti,** *Toxocara cati.* **B. margina′ta,** *Toxocara canis.* **B. mys′tax,** *Toxocara cati.*

belching (belch′ing) eructation; the noisy voiding of gas from the stomach through the mouth.

belemnoid (be-lem′noid) [Gr. *belemnon* dart + *eidos* form] 1. dart-shaped. 2. the styloid process of the ulna or of the temporal bone.

Belfield's operation (bel′fēldz) [William Thomas *Belfield,* surgeon in Chicago, 1856–1929] vasotomy.

Bell's law, nerve, palsy (paralysis), phenomenon [Sir Charles *Bell,* Scottish physiologist in London, 1774–1842] see *nervus thoracicus longus,* and see under *law, palsy,* and *phenomenon.*

Bell's mania (disease) [Luther Vose *Bell,* American physician, 1806–1862] see under *mania.*

Bell's muscle [John *Bell,* Scottish surgeon and anatomist, 1763–1820] see under *muscle.*

Bell's treatment [William Blair *Bell,* British gynecologist, 1871–1936] see under *treatment.*

Bell-Magendie law (bel′ma-jen′de) [Sir Charles *Bell;* François *Magendie,* French physiologist, 1783–1855] Bell's law.

belladonna (bel″ah-don′ah) [Ital. "fair lady"] the *Atropa belladonna* L. (Solanaceae), or deadly nightshade, a perennial plant indigenous to central and southern Europe and cultivated in North America, containing various anticholinergic alkaloids (e.g., atropine, hyoscyamine, belladonnine, scopolamine, etc.), some of which are produced during the extraction process. Called also *banewort, death's herb,* and *dwale. Belladonna leaf* [USP], consisting of the dried leaves and fruiting tops of *A. belladonna* or *A. belladonna* var. *acuminata,* is used in the preparation of standardized dosage forms; see under *extract* and *tincture.* The root has also been used.

belladonnine (bel″ah-don′nēn) chemical name: 1,2,3,4-tetrahydro-1-phenyl-1,4-naphthalenedicarboxylic acid bis(8-methyl-8-azobicyclo[3.2.1]oct-3-yl)ester. An alkaloid, $C_{34}H_{42}N_2O_4$, derived from belladonna and related solanaceous plants, produced during the process of extraction.

bellaradine (bel-ar′ah-din) cuscohygrine.

bell-crowned (bel-krownd′) having a crown somewhat bell-shaped; said of a tooth that is larger than usual at the occlusal measurement and that tapers toward the neck, or cervix.

Bellini's ducts (tubules), ligament (bel-e′nēz) [Lorenzo *Bellini,* Italian anatomist, 1643–1704] see *tubuli renales recti,* and see under *ligament.*

Bellocq's cannula (sound, tube) (bel-oks′) [Jean Jacques *Bellocq,* French surgeon, 1732–1807] see under *cannula.*

belly (bel′e) 1. the abdomen. 2. the fleshy, contractile part of a muscle; called also *venter musculi* [NA]. **anterior b. of di-**

gastric muscle, venter anterior musculi digastrici. **delhi b.,** a dysenteric infection occurring in tropical countries, manifested as an acute diarrheal disease. **drum b.,** tympanitic abdomen. **frontal b. of occipitofrontal muscle,** venter occipitalis musculi occipitofrontalis. **occipital b. of occipitofrontal muscle,** venter occipitalis musculi occipitofrontalis. **posterior b. of digastric muscle,** venter posterior musculi digastrici. **prune b.,** see under *syndrome.* **swollen b.,** tympanites in animals. **wooden b.,** abdominal rigidity.

belonoid (bel′o-noid) [Gr. *belonē* needle + *eidos* form] needle-shaped; styloid.

belonoskiascopy (bel″o-no-ski-as′ko-pe) [Gr. *belonē* needle + *skia* shadow + *skopein* to examine] a method of retinoscopy.

beloxamide (bel-oks′ah-mīd) chemical name: *N*-(benzyloxy)-*N*-(3-phenylpropyl)acetamide; an anticholesteremic agent, $C_{18}H_{21}NO_2$.

belt (belt) an encircling band worn about the waist or abdomen; called also *balteum.* Cf. *girdle.*

bemegride (bem′ĕ-grīd) chemical name: 4-ethyl-4-methyl-2,6-piperidinedione. An analeptic drug, $C_8H_{13}NO_2$, which has been used in the treatment of barbiturate poisoning.

bemidone (bem′ĭ-dōn) chemical name: ethyl 4-(*m*-hydroxyphenyl)-1-methylisonipecotate. A crystal compound, $C_{15}H_2NO_3$, soluble in water; formerly used as a narcotic and analgesic.

benactyzine hydrochloride (ben-ak′tĭ-zēn) chemical name: α-hydroxy-α-phenylbenzeneacetic acid 2-(diethylamino)ethyl ester hydrochloride. An anticholinergic, $C_{20}H_{26}ClNO_3$, occurring as a white, crystalline powder, which has the ability to increase the emotional threshold of outside influences and to block the thought processes; used as a tranquilizer, administered orally.

Benadryl (ben′ah-dril) trademark for preparations of diphenhydramine hydrochloride.

benapryzine hydrochloride (ben-ah-pri′zēn) chemical name: 2(ethylpropylamino)ethyl benzilate hydrochloride; an anticholinergic, $C_{21}H_{27}NO_3 \cdot HCl$.

Bence Jones protein, etc. [Henry *Bence Jones,* English physician, 1814–1873] see under *cylinder, protein, proteinuria,* and *reaction.*

bend (bend) a flexure or curve; a flexed or curved part. **first order b′s,** adjustments made in a labial arch wire, incorporating offsets in the horizontal plane, which are usually made in the areas of the cuspids and premolar and molar teeth, accommodating differences in thickness in the labiolingual or buccolingual diameters of the teeth. **head b.,** cephalic flexure. **neck b.,** cervical flexure. **second order b′s,** bends in the vertical plane of an arch wire. **third order b′s,** bends in an arch wire to maintain or produce torsion of a tooth. **V b′s,** V-shaped bends incorporated in an arch wire, usually placed mesial or distal to the cuspids to improve the axial relationship of teeth. **varolian b.,** the third cerebral flexure in the developing fetus.

bendazac (ben′dah-zak) chemical name: [(1-benzyl-1*H*-indazol-3-yl)oxy]acetic acid; an anti-inflammatory agent, $C_{16}H_{14}N_2O_3$.

Bendectin (ben-dek′tin) trademark for tablets containing a combination of doxylamine succinate and pyridoxine hydrochloride; used in management of nausea and vomiting during pregnancy.

bendrofluazide (ben″dro-floo′ah-zīd) bendroflumethiazide.

bendroflumethiazide (ben″dro-floo″mĕ-thi′ah-zīd) [USP] chemical name: 3,-dihydro-3-(phenylmethyl)-6-(trifluoromethyl)-2*H*-1,2,4-benzothiadiazine-7-sulfonamide 1,1-dioxide. A white to cream-colored crystalline powder, $C_{15}H_{14}F_3N_3O_4S_2$, used as an oral diuretic and antihypertensive.

bends (bendz) pain in the limbs and abdomen occurring as a result of rapid reduction of air pressure; see *decompression sickness,* under *sickness.*

Bendylate (ben′dĭ-lāt) trademark for preparations of diphenhydramine hydrochloride.

bene (be′ne) [L.] well.

beneceptor (ben′e-sep-tor) [L. *bene* well + *ceptor*] a rarely used term for a receptor that transmits stimuli of a beneficial character. Cf. *nociceptor* and *ceptor,* def. 2.

Beneckea (be-nek′e-ah) a genus of microorganisms of the family Achromobacteraceae, order Eubacteriales, made up of small to medium-sized rods, found in salt and fresh water and soil, which may or may not be chromogenic. It includes six species, *B. chitino′vora, B. hyperop′tica, B. indolthe′tica, B. la′bra, B. lipo′phaga,* and *B. ureaso′phora.*

Benedict's test (ben′e-dikts) [Stanley Rossiter *Benedict,* American physiological chemist, 1884–1936] see under *tests.*

Benedict-Hopkins-Cole reagent (ben′ĕ-dikt-hop′kinz-kōl) [Stanley Rossiter *Benedict;* Sir Frederick Gowland *Hopkins,* English biologist, 1861–1947; Sidney William *Cole,* English physiologist, born 1877] see under *reagent.*

Benedikt's syndrome (ben′e-dikts) [Moritz *Benedikt,* Austrian physician, 1835–1920] see under *syndrome.*

Benemid (ben′ĕ-mid) trademark for probenecid.

benign (be-nīn′) [L. *benignus*] not malignant; not recurrent; favorable for recovery.

benignant (be-nig′nant) benign.

Béniqué's sound (ba-ne-kāz′) [Pierre Jules *Béniqué,* French physician, 1806–1851] see under *sound.*

Benisone (ben′ĭ-sōn) trademark for preparations of betamethasone benzoate.

benjamin (ben′jah-min) benzoin, def. 1.

Bennet's corpuscles (ben′ets) [James Henry *Bennet,* English obstetrician, 1816–1891] see *Nunn's gorged corpuscles* and *Drysdale's corpuscles,* under *corpuscle.*

Bennett's disease (ben′ets) [John Hughes *Bennett,* English physician, 1812–1875] leukemia.

Bennett's fracture, operation (ben′ets) [Edward Hallaran *Bennett,* Irish surgeon, 1837–1907] see under *fracture* and *operation.*

Benoquin (ben′o-kwin) trademark for preparations of monobenzone.

benorterone (bĕ-nor′ter-ōn) chemical name: 17β-17-hydroxy-17-methyl-*B*-norandrost-4-en-3-one; an antiandrogen, $C_{19}H_{28}O_2$.

benoxaprofen (ben-oks″ah-pro′fen) chemical name: 2-(4-chlorophenyl)-α-methyl-5-benzoxazoleacetic acid; an anti-inflammatory and analgesic, $C_{16}H_{12}ClNO_3$.

benoxinate hydrochloride (ben-ok′sĭ-nāt) [USP] chemical name: 4-amino-3-butoxybenzoic acid 2-(diethylamino)ethyl ester monohydrochloride. A local anesthetic, $C_{17}H_{28}N_2O_3 \cdot HCl$, occurring as white crystals or as a white, crystalline powder; used in ophthalmology, applied topically to the conjunctiva.

Benoxyl (ben-ok′sil) trademark for preparations of benzoyl peroxide.

benserazide (ben-ser′ah-zīd) chemical name: 2-[(2,3,4-trihydroxyphenyl)-methyl]hydrazide DL serine; a decarboxylase inhibitor, $C_{10}H_{15}N_3O_5$.

Benson's disease (ben′sunz) [Alfred Hugh *Benson,* Irish ophthalmologist, 1852–1912] asteroid hyalosis.

bentazepam (ben-taz′ĕ-pam) chemical name: 1,3,6,7,8,9-hexahydro-5-phenyl-2*H*-[1]benzothieno[2,3-*e*]-1,4-diazepin-2-one; a tranquilizer, $C_{17}H_{16}N_2OS$.

benthos (ben′thos) [Gr. *benthos* bottom of the sea] the flora and fauna of the bottom of oceans.

bentonite (ben′ton-īt) [NF] a native, colloidal, hydrated aluminum silicate, which on the addition of water swells to produce a slippery paste; its chief pharmaceutical use is as a suspending agent, and it has also been used as a bulk laxative.

Bentyl (ben′til) trademark for preparations of dicyclomine hydrochloride.

benzaldehyde (ben-zal′dĕ-hīd) [NF] artificial essential oil of almond; used as a flavoring agent in orally administered medicaments.

benzalin (ben′zah-lin) nigrosin.

benzalkonium chloride (ben″zal-ko′ne-um) [NF] a mixture of alkylbenzyl dimethylammonium chlorides of the general formula, $[C_6H_5CH_2N(CH_3)_2R]Cl$. A rapidly acting surface disinfectant and detergent, occurring as a white or yellowish white, thick gel or gelatinous pieces, which is active against both gram-negative and gram-positive bacteria and certain viruses, fungi, yeasts, and protozoa; applied topically to the skin and mucous membranes. It is also used as an antimicrobial preservative in ophthalmic solution.

benzamidase (ben-zam′i-dās) an enzyme that catalyzes the change of benzoic acid into benzamide.

benzamine (ben′zah-mēn) eucaine.

benzanthracene (ben-zan′thrah-sēn) one of a group of hydrocarbons some of which have carcinogenic properties.

benzazoline hydrochloride (benz-az′o-lēn) tolazoline hydrochloride.

benzbromarone (benz-bro′mah-rōn) chemical name: (3,5-dibromo-4-hydroxyphenyl)-(2-ethyl-3-benzofuranyl)methanone; a uricosuric drug, $C_{17}H_{12}Br_2O_3$.

benzcurine iodide (benz′ku-rēn) gallamine triethiodide.

Benzedrex (ben′zĕ-dreks) trademark for a propylhexedrine inhaler.

Benzedrine (ben′zĕ-drēn) trademark for preparations of amphetamine sulfate.

benzene (ben′zēn) a colorless volatile liquid hydrocarbon, C_6H_6, obtained mainly as a by-product in the destructive distillation of coal, along with coal tar, etc. It has an aromatic odor, and burns with a light-giving flame. It dissolves sulfur, phosphorus, iodine, and organic compounds. The fumes may cause fatal poisoning. It was formerly used as a pulmonary antiseptic in influenza, etc., as a teniacide, externally as a parasiticide, and has been suggested in leukemias. Called also *benzol.* **dimethyl b.,** xylene. **b. hexachloride,** chemical name: 1,2,3,4,5,6-hexachlorocyclohexane. A compound, $C_6H_6Cl_6$, prepared by chlorination of benzene in actinic light, consisting of five isomers, the gamma isomer being a powerful insecticide; see also *gamma benzene hexachloride.* Called also *hexachlorocyclohexane.* **methyl b.,** toluene.

benzenoid (ben'zĕ-noid) a compound having a structure related to benzene or other compounds of aromatic character.

benzestrofol (ben-zes'tro-fōl) estradiol benzoate.

benzestrol (ben-zes'trol) [USP] chemical name: 4,4'-(1,2-diethyl-3-methyl-1,3-propanediyl)bisphenol. A synthetic estrogen, $C_{20}H_{26}O_2$, occurring as a white, crystalline powder; administered orally. Called also *octoxollin.*

benzethonium chloride (ben''zĕ-tho'ne-um) [USP] chemical name: N,N-dimethyl-N-[2-[2-[4-(1,1,3,3-tetra-methylbutyl)phenoxy]ethoxy]ethyl]benzene-methanaminium chloride. A synthetic quarternary ammonium compound, $C_{27}H_{42}ClNO_2$, occurring as white crystals; used as a local anti-infective applied topically as a solution, and as a preservative in pharmaceutical preparations. It is also used in various concentrations for cleaning eating and cooking utensils, as a disinfectant in laundering, to control algal growth in swimming pools, and as an environmental deodorant.

benzhexol hydrochloride (benz-hek'sol) trihexyphenidyl hydrochloride.

benzhydramine hydrochloride (benz-hi'drah-mēn) diphenhydramine hydrochloride.

benzidine (ben'zĭ-din) a colorless, crystalline compound, para-diaminodiphenyl, $(NH_2 \cdot C_6H_4 \cdot C_6H_4 \cdot NH_2)$, formed by the action of acids on hydrazobenzene; used as a test for blood.

benzilonium bromide (benz''il-o'ne-um) chemical name: 1,1-diethyl-3-[(hydroxydiphenylacetyl)oxy] pyrrolidinium bromide; an anticholinergic, $C_{22}H_{28}BrNO_3$, used in the treatment of peptic ulcer and functional gastrointestinal disorders.

benzimidazole (ben''zim-ĭ-da'zōl) a compound, $C_7H_6N_2$, which is toxic to yeast and animals in the absence of its homologous compounds, adenine and guanine. It is also a naturally occurring analog of vitamin B_{12}.

benzin, benzine (ben'zin) [L. *benzinum*] petroleum benzin. **petroleum b., purified b.,** a purified distillate from petroleum consisting of hydrocarbons chiefly of the methane series (mainly pentanes and hexanes), which occurs as a clear, colorless, volatile liquid with a strong ethereal odor; it is highly flammable and may be explosive if the vapors mix with air and are ignited. It is used as a solvent for organic compounds. Called also *benzin* or *benzine, petroleum ether,* and *naphtha.*

benzoate (ben'zo-āt) a salt of benzoic acid.

benzoated (ben'zo-āt-ed) containing or combined with benzoic acid.

benzocaine (ben'zo-kān) [USP] chemical name: 4-aminobenzoic acid ethyl ester. A local anesthetic, $C_9H_{11}NO_2$, occurring as small, white crystals or as a white crystalline powder; applied topically to the skin and mucous membranes.

benzodepa (ben''zo-dep'ah) chemical name: [bis(1-aziridinyl)-phosphenyl]carbamic acid phenylmethyl ester. An antineoplastic, $C_{12}H_{16}N_3O_3P$.

benzodiazepine (ben''zo-di-az'ĕ-pēn) any of a group of minor tranquilizers, including chlordiazepoxide, clorazepate, diazepam, flurazepam, oxazepam, etc., having a common molecular structure and similar pharmacological activities, such as antianxiety, muscle relaxing, and sedative and hypnotic effects.

benzodioxan (ben''zo-di-oks'an) a class of α-adrenergic blocking agents, the most important member of which is piperoxan.

benzogynestryl (ben''zo-gi-nes'tril) estradiol benzoate.

benzoin (ben'zoin) 1. [USP] a balsamic resin with an aromatic odor and taste, which is obtained from *Styrax benzoin* or *S. paralleloneurus* (known as Sumatra b.), or from *S. tonkinensis* or other species of *Styrax* (known as Siam b.); the former is composed of reddish brown, reddish gray, or grayish brown masses, and the latter of yellowish brown to rusty brown masses. It is used as a topical protectant, and as a topical antiseptic, irritant expectorant, and as an inhalant in respiratory tract inflammation. Called also *benjamin, gum benjamin,* and *gum b.* 2. chemical name: α-hydroxy-α-phenylacetophenone. A white crystalline compound, $C_{14}H_{12}O_2$, prepared by condensation of benzaldehyde in potassium cyanide solution; called also *benzoylphenylcarbinol.*

benzol (ben'zol) benzene.

benzolism (ben'zo-lizm) poisoning by benzene or its vapor.

benzomethamine (ben''zo-meth'ah-mēn) chemical name: N-diethylaminoethyl-N'-methylbenzilamide; formerly used to produce parasympathetic blockade and to reduce the secretion of hydrochloric acid in the stomach.

benzonatate (ben-zo'nah-tāt) [USP] chemical name: 2,5,-8,11,14,17,20,23,26-nonaoxaoctacos-28-yl ester benzoic acid. An antitussive, $C_{30}H_{53}NO_{11}$, occurring as a clear, pale yellow, viscous liquid, administered orally.

benzononatine (ben-zo''no-na'tin) benzonatate.

Benzopropyl (ben''zo-pro'pil) trademark for a preparation of amydricaine.

benzopurpurine (ben''zo-pur'pu-rin) any one of a series of azo-dyes of a scarlet color, used especially as a contrast stain with

hematoxylin and other blue stains. **b. B,** an indicator with a pH range of 2.0 to 4.0.

1,2-benzopyran (ben''zo-pir'an) 1,2-chromene.

benzopyrronium bromide (ben''zo-pēr-o'ne-um) chemical name: 3-hydroxy-1,1-dimethylpyrrolidinium bromide benzilate; an anticholinergic, $C_{20}H_{24}BrNO_3$.

benzotherapy (ben''zo-ther'ah-pe) treatment with benzoates, especially the treatment of pulmonary abscess by intravenous injection of sodium benzoate.

benzothiadiazide, benzothiadiazine (ben''zo-thi''ah-di'ah-zīd; ben''zo-thi''ah-di'ah-zēn) thiazide.

benzoxiquine (ben-zoks'ĭ-kwin') chemical name: 8-quinolinol benzoate (ester); a disinfectant, $C_{16}H_{11}NO_2$.

benzoyl (ben'zo-il) the radical, $C_6H_5 \cdot CO$, of benzoic acid and of an extensive series of compounds. **b. peroxide, b. peroxide, hydrous** [USP], a crystalline substance formed by the action of sodium peroxide on benzoyl chloride, used to initiate free radical reactions and to induce skin peeling so as to promote evacuation of comedones in acne vulgaris.

benzoylglycine (ben''zol-gli'sin) hippuric acid.

benzoylpas calcium (ben''zo-il'paz) [USP] chemical name: 4-(benzoylamino)-2-hydroxybenzoic acid calcium salt (2:1) pentahydrate. An antibacterial, $C_{28}H_{20}CaN_2O_8 \cdot 5H_2O$, occurring as a white to cream-colored powder; used as an oral tuberculostatic.

benzoylphenylcarbinol (ben''zol-fen''il-kar'bĭ-nol) benzoin, def. 2.

benzphetamine hydrochloride (benz-fet'ah-mēn) chemical name: N,α-dimethyl-N-(phenylmethyl)benzeneethanamine hydrochloride. A sympathomimetic amine, $C_{17}H_{21}N \cdot HCl$, related to amphetamine, occurring as an odorless, white to off-white, crystalline powder; used as an oral anorexiant in the control of exogenous obesity.

benzpiperylon (benz''pĭ-per'ĭ-lōn) chemical name: 4-benzyl-1-(1-methyl-4-piperidyl)-3-phenyl-3-pyrazolin-5-one. A substance, $C_{22}H_{25}N_3O$, used in the treatment of connective tissue disorders.

benzpyrene (benz-pi'rēn) a carcinogenic polycyclic hydrocarbon, $C_{20}H_{12}$.

benzpyrinium bromide (benz''pi-rin'e-um) chemical name: 3-[(dimethylamino)-carbonyl]oxy]-1-(phenylmethyl) pyridinium bromide. A cholinergic, $C_{15}H_{17}BrN_2O_3$, having anticholinesterase actions similar to those of neostigmine.

benzpyrrole (benz-pir'ol) indole.

benzquinamide (benz-kwin'ah-mīd) chemical name: 2-(acetyloxy)-N,N-diethyl-1,3,4,6,7,11b-hexahydro-9,10-dimethoxy-2H-benzo[a]quinolizine-3-carboxamide. A compound, $C_{22}H_{32}N_2O_5$, used intramuscularly or intravenously as an antiemetic; it also has antihistaminic and mild anticholinergic and sedative action.

benzthiazide (benz-thi'ah-zīd) [USP] chemical name: 6-chloro-3-[[(phenyl-methyl)thio]methyl]-2H-1,2,4-benzothiadiazine-7-sulfonamide 1,1-dioxide. An orally effective diuretic and antihypertensive agent, $C_{15}H_{14}ClN_3O_4S_3$, occurring as a white, crystalline powder.

benztropine mesylate (benz'tro-pēn) [USP] chemical name: endo-3-(diphenylmethoxy)-8-azabicyclo[3.2.1]octane methanesulfonate. A drug, $C_{21}H_{25}NO \cdot CH_4O_3S$, occurring as a white, crystalline powder, having anticholinergic, antihistaminic, and local anesthetic actions; used as an antiparkinsonian agent, administered intramuscularly, intravenously, and orally.

benzurestat (ben-zur'ĕ-stat) chemical name: 4-chloro-N-[2-(hydroxyamino)-2-oxoethyl]benzamide; an enzyme (urease) inhibitor, $C_9H_9ClN_2O_3$.

benzydroflumethiazide (ben-zid''ro-floo-mĕ-thi'ah-zīd) bendroflumethiazide.

benzyl (ben'zil) the hydrocarbon radical, C_7H_7 or $C_6H_5 \cdot CH_2$, of benzyl alcohol and various other bodies. **b. benzoate** [USP], a clear, colorless oily liquid, $C_{14}H_{12}O_2$; used as a pharmaceutic necessity in the preparation of dimercaprol for injection and applied topically to the skin as a scabicide. **b. bromide,** a war gas, $C_6H_5CH_2Br$, causing lacrimation and irritation of the skin; called also *cylite.* **b. carbinol,** phenyl ethyl alcohol, a constituent of oil of rose, possessing anesthetic properties. **b. fumarate,** a white crystalline substance, $C_6H_5CH_2 \cdot OOC \cdot CH:CH:COO \cdot CH_2C_6H_5$, containing 63.6 per cent of benzyl. **b. mandelate,** the benzyl ester of mandelic acid; formerly used as an antispasmodic on smooth muscle fiber, as in high blood pressure. **b. succinate,** the dibenzyl ester of succinic acid, $(C_6H_5 \cdot CH_2 \cdot O \cdot CO \cdot CH_2)_2$; formerly used as an antispasmodic to nonstriated muscle.

benzylidene (ben-zil'ĭ-dēn) a hydrocarbon radical, C_6H_5CH:.

p-benzyloxyphenol (ben''zil-ok''se-fe'nol) monobenzone.

benzylpenicillin (ben''zil-pen-ĭ-sil'in) penicillin G; see under *penicillin.* **b. potassium,** penicillin G potassium; see under *penicillin.* **b. procaine,** penicillin G procaine; see under *penicillin.* **b. sodium,** penicillin G sodium; see under *penicillin.*

bephenium (bĕ-fen'ĭ-um) a substance whose salts, e.g., *b. embonate* and *b. hydroxynaphthoate,* are used in veterinary medicine as anthelmintic agents.

Béraneck's tuberculin (ba-ran-eks′) [Edmund *Béraneck*, Swiss bacteriologist, 1859–1920] see under *tuberculin.*

Bérard's aneurysm, ligament (ba-rarz′) [Auguste *Bérard*, French surgeon, 1802–1846] see under *aneurysm* and *ligament.*

Béraud's valve (ba-rōz′) [Bruno Jean Jacques *Béraud*, French surgeon, 1825–1865] see under *valve.*

berberine (ber′ber-ēn) an alkaloid obtained from *Hydrastis canadensis* L. (Berberidaceae), *Berberis* species, and other members of this family; used variously as an antimalarial, carminative, and febrifuge, and externally in dressings for indolent ulcers.

Berberis (ber′ber-is) [L.] a genus of berberidaceous shrubs, the barberries, which contain berberine.

bergamot (ber′gah-mot) [L. *bergamium*] 1. the tree, *Citrus bergamia;* also its orange-like fruit, whose rind affords the fragrant oil of bergamot. 2. a popular name for various fragrant labiate plants, such as *Mentha citrata* and *Monarda fistulosa.*

Bergenhem's operation (ber′gen-hemz) [Bengt *Bergenhem*, Swedish surgeon, born 1898] see under *operation.*

Berger's method, operation (bār-zhāz′) [Paul *Berger*, French surgeon, 1845–1908] see under *method* and *operation.*

Berger's paresthesia (ber′gerz) [Oskar *Berger*, neurologist in Breslau, 1845–1908] see under *paresthesia.*

Berger rhythm (ber′ger) [Hans *Berger*, Jena neurologist, 1873–1941] alpha rhythm; see under *rhythm.*

Berger's sign (symptom) (ber′gerz) [Émile *Berger*, Austrian ophthalmologist, 1855–1926] see under *sign.*

Bergeron's chorea (disease) (berzh′ronz) [Étienne Jules *Bergeron*, French physician, 1817–1900] see under *chorea.*

Bergmann's cells, cords, fibers (berg′manz) [Gottlieb Heinrich *Bergmann*, German physician, died 1861] see *striae acusticae,* and see under *cell* and *fiber.*

Bergmann's incision (berg′manz) [Ernst von *Bergmann*, German surgeon, 1836–1907] see under *incision.*

Bergonié treatment (method) (bār-go-nya′) [Jean Alban *Bergonié*, French physician, 1857–1925] see under *treatment.*

Bergonié-Tribondeau law (bār-go-nya′tre-bon-do′) [J. A. *Bergonié;* Louis *Tribondeau*, French naval physician, 1872–1918] see under *law.*

beriberi (ber″e-ber′e) [Singhalese, "I cannot," signifying that the person is too ill to do anything] a disease caused by a deficiency of thiamine (vitamin B₁) and characterized by polyneuritis, cardiac pathology, and edema. The epidemic form is found primarily in areas in which white (polished) rice is the staple food, as in Japan, China, the Philippines, India, and other countries of Southeast Asia. **atrophic b.,** dry b. **dry b.,** a form of beriberi in which flaccid paralysis, muscular atrophy, and areflexia are the prominent signs; cardiac enlargement and tachycardia may be present. Called also *atrophic b.* and *paralytic b.* **infantile b.,** a disease of breast-fed infants whose mothers have thiamine deficiency; it is characterized by diminished urine secretion, progressive edema, and often by acute cardiac failure, which may terminate in sudden death. Vomiting, aphonia, opisthotonos, and convulsions may occur. **paralytic b.,** dry b. **ship b.,** a disease resembling tropical beriberi, seen on Norwegian ships, but with edema a more prominent symptom than neuritis. **wet b.,** a form marked by cardiac failure and edema, but without extensive nervous system involvement.

beriberic (ber″e-ber′ik) pertaining to or of the nature of beriberi.

Berkefeld filter (ber′ke-feld) [Wilhelm *Berkefeld*, manufacturer, 1836–1897] see under *filter.*

berkelium (berk′le-um) [named for *Berkeley*, California, where it was produced] an element of atomic number 97, atomic weight 247, symbol Bk, produced by bombardment of the isotope of americium of atomic weight 241 by helium ions; half-life 4½ hours.

Berlin's disease, edema (ber′linz) [Rudolf *Berlin*, German oculist, 1833–1897] commotio retinae.

berlock, berloque (ber-lok′) [Fr. *breloque,* Ger. *Berlocke* a charm (especially on a chain)] see under *dermatitis.*

Bernard's canal, etc. (ber-narz′) [Claude *Bernard*, French physiologist, 1813–1878] see under *canal, duct, layer, puncture,* and *syndrome.*

Bernard-Horner syndrome (ber-nar′hor′ner) [Claude *Bernard;* Johann Friedrich *Horner*, Swiss ophthalmologist, 1831–1886] Horner's syndrome.

Bernays' sponge (ber′nāz) [Augustus Charles *Bernays*, American surgeon, 1854–1907] see under *sponge.*

Bernhardt's disease, paresthesia (bern′harts) [Martin *Bernhardt*, German neurologist, 1844–1915] meralgia paresthetica.

Bernhardt-Rot disease, syndrome [Martin *Bernhardt;* Vladimir K. *Rot*, Russian neurologist, 1848–1916] meralgia paresthetica.

Bernheimer's fibers (bern′hi-merz) [Stefan *Bernheimer*, Austrian ophthalmologist, 1861–1918] see under *fiber.*

berry (ber′e) a small fruit with a succulent pericarp. **bear b.,** *Uva ursi.* **buckthorn b.,** *Rhamnus cathartica.* **elder b.,** *Sambucus.* **fish b.,** cocculus indicus. **horse nettle b.,** *Sola-*

num. **Indian b.,** cocculus indicus. **juniper b.,** juniper. **saw palmetto b.,** *Serenoa.* **spice b.,** aralia.

Berry's ligament (ber′ēz) [Sir James *Berry*, Canadian surgeon, 1860–1946] ligamentum thyroideum.

Bertiella (ber″te-el′lah) a genus of tapeworms of the family Anoplocephalidae. **B. sat′yri, B. stu′deri,** a tapeworm found occasionally in man and in the higher apes in Mauritius, India, Africa, Borneo, the West Indies, and the Philippines.

bertielliasis (ber″te-el-li′ah-sis) infection with *Bertiella.*

Bertin's bones (ossicles), column, ligament (ber′tinz) [Exupère Joseph *Bertin*, French anatomist, 1712–1781] see *concha sphenoidalis, columnae renales,* and *ligamentum iliofemorale.*

Bertrand's method, reagent, test (bār-trahnz′) [Gabriel *Bertrand*, Paris biological chemist, born 1867] see under *method, reagent,* and *tests.*

Berubigen (be-roo′bĭ-jen) trademark for preparations of cyanocobalamin.

berylliosis (ber″il-le-o′sis) beryllium poisoning, a morbid condition, usually of the lungs, more rarely of the skin, subcutaneous tissue, lymph nodes, liver, and other structures, characterized by formation of granulomas. Fumes of beryllium salts or finely divided dust may be inhaled or the substance may be accidentally implanted in the skin or subcutaneous tissue by laceration or puncture.

beryllium (ber-il′le-um) [Gr. *bēryllos* beryl] a metallic element of atomic number 4, atomic weight 9.012, symbol Be.

berythromycin (bĕ-rith″ro-mi′sin) chemical name: 12-deoxyerythromycin; an antiamebic and antibacterial, $C_{37}H_{67}NO_{12}$. Called also *erythromycin B.*

Berzelius' test (bār-za′le-us) [Jöns Jacob *Berzelius*, Swedish chemist, 1779–1848] see under *tests.*

besiclometer (bes″ĭ-klom′ĕ-ter) an instrument for measuring the forehead to ascertain the proper width of spectacle frames.

Besnier's prurigo [Ernest *Besnier*, Paris dermatologist, 1831–1909] see under *prurigo.*

Besnier-Boeck disease [Ernest *Besnier;* Caesar P. M. *Boeck,* Norwegian dermatologist and syphilologist in Christiana, 1845–1917] sarcoidosis.

Besnoitia (bes-noi′te-ah) a genus of sporozoa; formerly called *Globidium.* **B. bennet′ti,** a species causing besnoitiosis in horses. **B. besnoi′ti,** a species causing besnoitiosis in cattle; viscerotropic strains have been found in the impala and blue wildebeest. **B. darlin′gi,** a species found in lizards. **B. jelliso′ni,** a species found in rodents and opossums. **B. taran′di,** a species found in reindeer.

besnoitiosis (bes-noi″te-o′sis) a disease of cattle, horses, sheep, goats, and other herbivorous animals, due to sporozoan parasites of the genus *Besnoitia,* transmitted mechanically by certain biting flies. The organisms localize in the skin, blood vessels, mucous membranes of the upper respiratory tract, and subcutaneous and other tissues, where they eventually form characteristic thick-walled cysts. Other symptoms include fever, anasarca, loss of appetite, photophobia, rhinitis, sclerodermatitis, and alopecia of varying severity. Formerly called *globidiosis.*

Besredka's antivirus, reaction (bes-red′kahz) [Alexandre *Besredka*, Russian pathologist at Pasteur Institute, Paris, 1870–1940] see under *antivirus* and *reaction.*

Best (best), Charles Herbert. A Canadian physiologist, born in Maine 1899; discovered histaminase and was associated with Sir Frederick Banting and John James Macleod in the discovery of insulin in 1922.

bestiality (bes-te-al′ĭ-te) [L. *bestia* beast] sexual connection with an animal.

besylate (bes′ĭ-lāt) USAN contraction for benzenesulfonate.

Beta (be′tah) [L.] a genus of plants to which the beet belongs. *B. vulga′ris* L. is the sugar beet, a commercial source of sugar (sucrose).

beta (ba′tah) the second letter of the Greek alphabet, β; used as part of a chemical name to distinguish one of two or more isomers or to indicate the position of substituting atoms or groups in certain compounds. Cf. *alpha.*

Betabacterium (ba″tah-bak-te′re-um) a subgenus of *Lactobacillus.*

Beta-Chlor (ba′tah-klōr) trademark for a preparation of chloral betaine.

beta-cholestanol (ba″tah-ko-les′tah-nol) see under *cholestanol.*

betacism (ba′tah-sizm) [Gr. *bēta* the second letter of the Greek alphabet] the excessive use of the *b* sound in speaking.

Betadine (ba′tah-dīn) trademark for preparations of povidone-iodine.

beta-estradiol (ba″tah-es″trah-di′ol) see *estradiol.*

betaglobulin (ba″tah-glob′u-lin) see under *globulin.* **pregnancy-specific b.,** a beta globulin secreted by the placenta; its function is unknown.

betahistine hydrochloride (ba″tah-his′tēn) chemical name: *N*-methyl-2-pyridineethanamine dihydrochloride. A compound,

$C_8H_{12}N_2 \cdot 2HCl$, occurring as a white or creamy white, crystalline powder, which has histamine-like action; used orally as a vasodilator to reduce the frequency of the episodes of vertigo in some patients with Meniere's disease, especially those having a high frequency of such episodes.

beta-hypophamine (ba″tah-hi-pof′ah-min) vasopressin.

betaine (be′tah-in, be′tah-ēn, bēt′ān) chemical name: 1-carboxy-N,N,N-trimethylmethanaminium hydroxide inner salt. An oxidation product of choline, $C_5H_{11}NO_2$, which is a transmethylating intermediate in metabolism, and has been shown to have lipotropic activity. Betaine was first found in the sugar beet and was later shown to be present in many other plants and in animals. It is produced synthetically, and has been used in the treatment of muscular weakness and degeneration. The term has also been used to designate any of a class of trimethyl derivatives of amino acids, e.g., carnitine, or, more generally, the internal salts of quarternary ammonium bases. Called also *lycine* and *oxyneurine*. **b. hydrochloride,** the hydrochloride salt of betaine, $C_5H_{12}ClNO$, which on hydrolysis yields hydrochloric acid; used as a gastric acidifier. It has been used as a lipotropic agent in the treatment of fatty infiltration of the liver.

beta-lactose (ba″tah-lak′tōs) a disaccharide isomeric with lactose, obtained by allowing a solution of lactose to crystallize above 93° C.; it is more soluble and sweeter than lactose.

Betalin (ba′tah-lin) trademark for preparations containing components of the vitamin B complex. *Betalin Complex* is a sterile solution of synthetic B complex factors in sterile distilled water. *Betalin Complex F.C.* consists of synthetic vitamin B factors and synthetic ascorbic acid in sterile distilled water. *Betalin S* is a synthetic preparation of thiamine hydrochloride. *Betalin 12 crystalline* is a sterile isotonic solution of crystalline cyanocobalamin.

betalysin (ba-tal′ĭ-sin) a relatively thermostable lysin for gram-positive bacteria (Patterson).

betamethasone (ba″tah-meth′ah-sōn) [NF] chemical name: 9-fluoro-11β,17,21-trihydroxy-16β-methylpregna-1,4-diene-3,20-dione. A synthetic glucocorticoid, occuring as a white to creamy white, crystalline powder, which is the most active of the anti-inflammatory steroids; administered orally or applied to the skin. **b. acetate** [USP], an ester of betamethasone, $C_{24}H_{31}$-FO_6, occurring as a white to creamy white powder, having the same actions as the base; used in combination with betamethasone sodium phosphate for intramuscular, intra-articular, intrasynovial, or intralesional injection. **b. benzoate** [USP], the 17-benzoate ester of betamethasone, $C_{29}H_{33}FO_6$, having the same actions as the base; applied topically to the skin. **b. dipropionate** [USP], the 17,21-dipropionate ester of betamethasone, C_{28}-$H_{37}FO_7$, having the same uses as the base; applied topically to the skin. **b. sodium phosphate** [USP], the disodium salt of the 21-phosphate ester of betamethasone, $C_{22}H_{28}FNa_2O_8P$, occurring as a white to almost white powder, having the same actions as the base; used in combination with betamethasone acetate for intramuscular, intra-articular, intrasynovial, or intralesional injection. **b. valerate** [USP], the 17-valerate ester of betamethasone, C_{27}-$H_{37}FO_6$, occurring as a white or almost white powder, having the same actions as the base; applied topically to the skin.

betamicin sulfate (ba″tah-mi′sin) chemical name: O-6-amino-6-deoxy-α-D-glucopyranosyl-(1→4)-O-[3-deoxy-4-C-methyl-3-(methylamino)β-L-arabinopyranosyl-(1→6)]-2-deoxy-D-streptamine sulfate; an antibacterial, $C_{19}H_{38}N_4O_{10} \cdot xH_2SO_4$.

betanaphthol (ba″tah-naf′thol) a form of naphthol, $C_{10}H_8O$, occurring as a colorless or pale-buff crystalline compound having the odor of carbolic acid. Formerly used locally as a counterirritant in alopecia and as an anthelmintic; now used as a topical antiseptic, especially in fungal infections. Called also *isonaphthol*.

betanaphthyl (ba″tah-naf′thil) the combining group, $C_{10}H_8$, of betanaphthol. **b. benzoate,** betanaphthol benzoate. **b. salicylate,** betanaphthol salicylate.

betanin (be′tah-nin) the red pigment of the root of the beet.

beta-oxybutyria (ba″tah-ok″se-bu-ti′re-ah) the presence of beta-oxybutyric acid in the urine. Cf. *ketonuria*.

Betapar (ba′tah par) trademark for a preparation of meprednisone.

Betapen-VK (ba′tah-pen) trademark for a preparation of penicillin V potassium.

Betaprone (ba′tah-prōn) trademark for a preparation of propiolactone.

betapropiolactone (ba″tah-pro″pe-o-lak′tōn) propiolactone.

betaquinine (ba″tah-kwin′in) quinidine.

betatron (ba′tah-tron) an apparatus for accelerating electrons to millions of electron volts by means of magnetic induction.

Betaxin (be-tak′sin) trademark for preparations of thiamine hydrochloride.

betazole hydrochloride (ba′tah-zōl) [USP] chemical name: 1H-pyrazole-3-ethanamine dihydrochloride. A histamine analogue, $C_5H_9N_3 \cdot 2HCl$, occurring as a white crystalline powder, which stimulates gastric secretion of hydrochloric acid; used in diagnostic tests of gastric secretion, administered intramuscularly or subcutaneously. Called also *gastramine hydrochloride*.

bête (bet) [Fr.] beast. **b. rouge** (bet-rōōzh′) [Fr. "red beast"], chigger.

betel (be′t'l) [Tamil *vettilei*] an East Indian masticatory, consisting of a piece of betel nut rolled up with lime in a betel leaf; it is tonic, astringent, and stimulant. **b. leaf,** the leaf of *Piper betle;* formerly used as a masticatory and topically as a counterirritant. The oil was used internally for cough and for diphtheria. **b. nut,** the dried ripe seed of *Areca catechu*, a palm tree of South Asia; formerly used as an anthelmintic in veterinary medicine. Called also *areca*.

bethanechol chloride (bĕ-tha′nĕ-kol) [USP] chemical name: 2-[(aminocarbonyl)oxy]-N,N,N-trimethyl-1-propanaminium chloride. A cholinergic, $C_7H_{17}ClN_2O_2$, occurring as colorless or white crystals or as a white crystalline powder; used in the treatment of gastric retention following vagotomy, postoperative urinary retention, postoperative abdominal distention, and in other conditions in which stimulation of the parasympathetic nervous system is desirable; it is administered orally or subcutaneously.

bethanidine sulfate (be-than′ĭ-dēn) chemical name: N,N-dimethyl-N-(phenylmethyl)guanidine sulfate (2:1). An adrenergic neuron-blocking agent, $C_{10}H_{15}N_3 \cdot \frac{1}{2}H_2SO_4$, used in the treatment of essential hypertension, particularly in the malignant phase.

Bethea's sign (method) (bĕ-tha′ez) [Oscar Walter *Bethea*, New Orleans physician, 1878–1963] see under *sign*.

Betonica (be-ton′ĭ-kah) [L.] a genus of labiate plants. *B. officinalis*, wood betony, was formerly used in medicine: the tops are astringent and aromatic; the root, emetic and cathartic.

Bettendorff's test (bet′en-dorf) [Anton Joseph Hubert Maria *Bettendorff*, German chemist, 1839–1902] see under *tests*.

Betula (bet′u-lah) [L.] a genus of trees: the birches. **B. al′ba** (white birch), the source of a bark from which rectified birch tar oil is derived; used as an expectorant in various cough syrup formulations, and formerly in certain skin diseases. **B. len′ta** (black birch), a tree whose bark is an important commercial source of methyl salicylate. Now used mainly as a flavoring oil for confections and soda beverages.

betweenbrain (be-twēn′brān) diencephalon (interbrain).

Betz's cells, cell area (bet′zes) [Vladimir Aleksandrovich *Betz*, Russian anatomist, 1834–1894] see under *cell*, and see *psychomotor area*, under *area*.

Bev Abbreviation for *billion electron volts;* the equivalent of 3.82×10^{-11} gram calorie, or 1.6×10^{-3} erg.

Bevan's incision, operation (bev′anz) [Arthur Dean *Bevan*, American surgeon, 1861–1943] see under *incision* and *operation*.

Bevan Lewis cells (bev′an loo′is) [William *Bevan Lewis*, English physiologist, 1847–1929] see under *cell*.

bevel (bev′el) 1. a slanting edge. 2. to produce a slanting of the enamel margins of a tooth cavity.

Bevidox (bev′ĭ-doks) trademark for a solution of vitamin B_{12}; see *cyanocobalamin*.

beziehungswahn (ba-ze′hoongz-vahn″) [Ger.] a form of guilt psychosis marked by morbid ideas of reference.

bezoar (be′zōr) [Persian] a concretion of various character sometimes found in the stomach or intestines of man or other animals. They may belong to one of three types: trichobezoar (hair), phytobezoar (fruit and vegetable fibers), or trichophytobezoar (a mixture of hair, and fruit and vegetable fibers).

Bezold's abscess, etc. (ba′zoltz) [Friedrich *Bezold*, otologist in Munich, 1842–1908] see under *abscess, mastoiditis, perforation, sign,* and *triad*.

Bezold's ganglion (ba′zoltz) [Albert von *Bezold*, German physiologist, 1836–1868] see under *ganglion*.

BF blastogenic factor; see *lymphocyte transforming factor*, under *factor*.

BFP abbreviation for *biologically false positivity* (*biologic false positive* reaction), the presence of positive findings in serologic tests for syphilis when syphilis is known not to exist.

BFU-E burst-forming unit—erythroid, the earliest red cell precursor presently detectable in *in-vitro* culture, where it has a high requirement for erythropoietin; so named because its growth is composed of subcolonies which give the appearance of a burst.

bhang (bang) [Hindi] the Asian Indian name for a mixture of the dried leaves and young stems of uncultivated *Cannabis sativa* L. (Cannabaceae), usually ingested as a decoction with milk, sugar, and water, or sometimes smoked or chewed. See *cannabis*.

Bi chemical symbol for *bismuth*.

bi- [L. *bi* two] 1. a prefix meaning two or twice. 2. see *bio-*.

Bial's reagent, test (be′alz) [Manfred *Bial*, German physician, 1869–1908] see under *reagent* and *tests*.

bialamicol hydrochloride (bi″ah-lam′ĭ-kōl) chemical name: 3,3′-bis[(diethylamino)methyl]-5,5′-di-2-propenyl-1,1′-biphenyl]-4-4′-diol dihydrochloride. An antiamebic agent, $C_{28}H_{40}N_2O_2 \cdot 2HCl$, administered orally. Formerly called *biallylamicol*.

biallylamicol (bi-al″il-am′ĭ-kol) former name for bialamicol hydrochloride.

Bianchi's nodules, valve (be-ang′kēz) [Giovanni Battista *Bian-*

chi, Italian anatomist, 1681–1761] see *noduli valvularum aortae*, and under *valve*.

Bianchi's syndrome (be-ang′kēz) [Leonardo *Bianchi*, Italian psychiatrist, 1848–1927] see under *syndrome*.

biarticular (bi″ar-tik′u-lar) pertaining to two joints.

biarticulate (bi″ar-tik′u-lāt) having two joints.

biasteric (bi″as-ter′ik) pertaining to the two asteria, especially to the shortest distance between them (biasteric width).

biauricular (bi″aw-rik′u-lar) pertaining to the two auricles of the ears.

Bib. abbreviation for L. *bi′be*, drink.

bib (bib) the remaining fragment of an erythrocyte in which the crescentic gametocyte of *Plasmodium falciparum* is developing in malaria.

bibasic (bi-ba′sik) doubly basic; having two hydrogen atoms that may react with bases; Cf. *dibasic*.

bibeveled (bi′bev-eld) having a slanting surface on two sides, as some dental instruments; hatchet-edged.

Bibliofilm (bib′le-o-film) a negative microfilm of material for a library. It is a trademark registered by Science Service with the idea that it would be applied only to the product of Bibliofilm Services, Incorporated, under the proposed Documentation Institute.

bibliomania (bib″le-o-ma′ne-ah) [Gr. *biblion* book + *mania* madness] abnormally intense desire to collect books.

bibliotherapy (bib″le-o-ther′ah-pe) [Gr. *biblion* book + *therapeia* treatment] the employment of books and the reading of them in the treatment of nervous disorders.

Bibron's antidote (bib′ronz) [Gabriel *Bibron*, French naturalist, 1806–1848] see under *antidote*.

bibulous (bib′u-lus) [L. *bibulus*, from *bibere* to drink] 1. absorbent or spongy. 2. having the property of absorbing moisture. Cf. *hygroscopic*.

bicameral (bi-kam′er-al) [*bi-* + L. *camera* chamber] having two chambers.

bicapsular (bi-kap′su-lar) [*bi-* two + L. *capsula* a capsule] having two capsules, as an articular capsule.

bicarbonate (bi-kar′bo-nāt) any salt containing the HCO_3^- anion. **blood b.,** the bicarbonate of the blood, an index of the alkali reserve. **plasma b.,** blood b. **b. of soda,** sodium bicarbonate.

bicarbonatemia (bi-kar″bo-nāt-e′me-ah) hyperbicarbonatemia.

bicardiogram (bi-kar′de-o-gram″) (*obs.*) a curve in an electrocardiogram indicating the composite effect of the right and left atria.

bicaudal (bi-kaw′dal) [*bi-* + L. *cauda* tail] having two tails.

bicaudate (bi-kaw′dāt) bicaudal.

bicellular (bi-sel′u-lar) made up of two cells, or having two cells.

bicephalus (bi-sef′ah-lus) dicephalus.

biceps (bi′seps) [*bi-* + L. *caput* head] a muscle having two heads. **b. bra′chii, b. fem′oris,** see *Table of Musculi*.

Bichat's canal, etc. (be-shaz′) [Marie François Xavier *Bichat*, an eminent French anatomist and physiologist, 1771–1802, founder of scientific histology and pathological anatomy] see under *canal, fissure, foramen, ligament, membrane,* and *tunic*.

bichloride (bi-klo′rīd) any chloride that contains two equivalents of chlorine.

bichromate (bi-kro′māt) dichromate.

Bicillin (bi′sĭ-lin) trademark for a preparation of penicillin G benzathine.

bicipital (bi-sip′ĭ-tal) 1. having two heads. 2. pertaining to a biceps muscle.

biconcave (bi-kon′kāv) [*bi-* + L. *concavus* hollow] having two concave surfaces, as the opposite sides of a structure.

biconvex (bi-kon′veks) having two convex surfaces, as the opposite sides of a structure.

bicornate (bi-kor′nāt) bicornuate.

bicornuate (bi-kor′nu-āt) [*bi-* + L. *cornutus* horned] having two horns or having horn-shaped branches, as the uterus of most mammals.

bicoronial (bi″ko-ro′ne-al) pertaining to the two coronas, one radiating from each internal capsule of the brain.

bicorporate (bi-kor′pŏ-rāt) [*bi-* + L. *corpus* body] having two bodies.

bicuspid (bi-kus′pid) [*bi-* + L. *cuspis* point] 1. having two cusps or points. 2. a bicuspid valve. 3. a term used mainly in the United States for a premolar tooth.

bicuspidal (bi-kus′pĭ-dal) 1. pertaining to a bicuspid tooth. 2. having two cusps.

bicuspidate (bi-kus′pĭ-dāt) having two cusps.

bicuspoid (bi-kus′poid) a figure in space resembling a bicuspid tooth and representing the space traversed in all its movements by a point in one jaw in relation to the other jaw.

b.i.d. abbreviation for L. *bis in di′e*, twice a day.

Bidder's ganglia, organ [Heinrich Friedrich *Bidder*, German anatomist, 1810–1894] see under *ganglion* and *organ*.

bidental (bi-den′tal) [*bi-* + L. *dens* tooth] having, pertaining to, or affecting two teeth.

bidentate (bi-den′tāt) having two teeth.

bidermoma (bi″der-mo′mah) [*bi-* + Gr. *derma* skin + *-oma*] a variety of teratoma composed of cells and tissues derived from two germ layers.

biduotertian (bid″u-o-ter′shun) denoting malaria caused by *Plasmodium vivax*, in which two broods of parasites are segmenting on alternate days, so that febrile paraoxysms occur daily.

biduous (bid′u-us) lasting for two days, as a fever.

Biederman's sign (be′der-manz) [Joseph Bear *Biederman*, Cincinnati physician, born 1907] see under *sign*.

Biedert's cream mixture (be′derts) [Philipp *Biedert*, pediatrist in Strasburg, 1847–1916] see under *mixture*.

Biedl's disease, syndrome (be′dlz) [Artur *Biedl*, Austrian physician, 1869–1933] Laurence-Moon-Biedl syndrome.

Bielschowsky's method (be″el-show′skēz) [Max *Bielschowsky*, German neuropathologist, 1869–1940] see *Table of Stains and Staining Methods*.

Bielschowsky-Jansky disease (be″el-show′ske- yan′ske) late infantile form of amaurotic family idiocy; see under *idiocy*.

Bier's amputation, etc. (bērz) [August Karl Gustav *Bier*, surgeon in Berlin, 1861–1949] see under *amputation, anesthesia, hyperemia,* and *treatment*.

Biermer's anemia (disease), sign (bēr′merz) [Anton *Biermer*, German physician, 1827–1892] see *pernicious anemia*, under *anemia*, and see under *sign*.

Biernacki's sign (byēr-naht′skēz) [Edmund *Biernacki*, Polish physician, 1866–1911] see under *sign*.

Biesiadecki's fossa (bya-syah-det′skēz) [Alfred von *Biesiadecki*, Polish physician, 1839–1888] iliacosubfascial fossa.

Biett's disease (be-ets′) [Laurent Théodore *Biett*, Parisian dermatologist, 1781–1840] discoid lupus erythematosus.

bifid, bifidus (bi′fid, bif′ĭ-dus) [L.] cleft into two parts or branches.

Bifidobacterium (bi″fid-o-bak-te′re-um) a genus of obligate anaerobic lactobacilli commonly occurring in the feces.

bifocal (bi-fo′kal) 1. having two foci. 2. pertaining to the compound spectacle, which contains a smaller lens for near vision placed below the center of the larger lens, which is for distant vision. 3. (pl.) bifocal glasses.

biforate (bi-fo′rāt) [*bi-* + L. *fora* opening] having two foramina or openings.

biformyl (bi-for′mil) glyoxal.

bifurcate (bi-fur′kāt) [L. *bifurcatus*, from *bi-* + *furca* fork] forked; divided into two branches.

bifurcatio (bi″fur-ka′she-o), pl. *bifurcatio′nes* [L.] the site of division of a single structure into two. **b. tra′cheae** [NA], bifurcation of trachea: the site of division of the trachea into the right and left main bronchi.

bifurcation (bi″fur-ka′shun) [L. *bifurcatio*, from *bi-* + *furca* fork] 1. division into two branches. 2. the site where a single structure divides into two. **b. of trachea,** bifurcatio tracheae.

bifurcationes (bi″fur-ka″she-o′nēz) [L.] plural of *bifurcatio*.

Bigelow's ligament, litholapaxy, operation, septum (big′ĕ-lōz) [Henry Jacob *Bigelow*, Boston surgeon, 1818–1890] see *ligamenta iliofemorale*, and see under *litholapaxy, operation,* and *septum*.

bigemina (bi-jem′ĭ-nah) 1. plural of *begeminum*. 2. a bigeminal pulse.

bigeminal (bi-jem′ĭ-nal) occurring in twos; twin.

bigeminum (bi-jem′ĭ-num), pl. *bigem′ina* [L. "twin"] either one of the corpora bigemina of the fetus or of a bird; the fetal bigemina become the corpora quadrigemina (colliculi).

bigeminy (bi-jem′ĭ-ne) the condition of occurring in pairs; especially the occurrence of two beats of the pulse in rapid succession; see *bigeminal pulse*, under *pulse*. **nodal b.,** a form of arrhythmia consisting of nodal extrasystoles followed by nodal automatic beats.

bigerminal (bi-jer′mĭ-nal) pertaining to two germs or ova.

bighead (big′hed) 1. bulging of the skull bones of an animal, due to osteomalacia. 2. an acute infectious disease of young rams due to *Clostridium novyi*, which enters the tissues through head wounds acquired in fighting; it is characterized by intense edematous swelling of the head, face, and neck; called also *swelled head*. 3. photosensitivity in white-faced sheep, occurring after the ingestion of certain plants, characterized by thickening and pendulous swelling of the face and ears. 4. hydrocephalus in mink.

bigjaw (big′jaw) actinomycosis in cattle.

bigleg (big′leg) lymphangitis of a horse's leg.

bigonial (bi-go′ne-al) connecting the two gonions.

bilabe (bi'lāb) [*bi-* + L. *labium* lip] an instrument for taking small calculi from the bladder through the urethra.

bilaminar (bi-lam'ĭ-nar) [*bi-* + L. *lamina* layer] having or pertaining to two layers, as the basement membrane that comprises the basal lamina and the reticular lamina.

bilateral (bi-lat'er-al) [*bi-* + L. *latus* side] having two sides, or pertaining to both sides.

bilateralism (bi-lat'er-al-izm) bilateral symmetry.

bile (bīl) [L. *bilis*] a fluid secreted by the liver and poured into the small intestine via the bile ducts. Important constituents are conjugated bile salts, cholesterol, phospholipid, bilirubin diglucuronide, and electrolytes. Bile is alkaline due to its bicarbonate content, golden brown to greenish yellow in color, and has a bitter taste. Hepatic bile (see *A b.*) secreted by the liver, is concentrated in the gallbladder. Its formation depends on active secretion by liver cells into the bile canaliculi. Excretion of bile salts by liver cells and secretion of bicarbonate rich fluid by ductular cells in response to secretin are the major factors which normally determine the volume of secretion. Conjugated bile salts and phospholipid normally dissolve cholesterol in a mixed micellar solution. In the upper small intestine, bile is in part responsible for alkalinizing the intestinal content, and conjugated bile salts play an essential role in fat absorption by dissolving the products of fat digestion (fatty acids and monoglyceride) in water soluble micelles. Called also *gall*. **A b.**, bile from the common bile duct; samples are obtained by use of a duodenal tube before gallbladder stimulation. It usually contains 20–200 mg. of bilirubin per 100 ml. **B b.**, bile from the gallbladder; samples are obtained by use of a duodenal tube after gallbladder contraction stimulation, usually with magnesium sulfate. It may occur despite absence of the gallbladder and contains up to 1 gram of bilirubin per 100 ml. **C b.**, heptatic bile; it is obtained from a duodenal drainage tube after the gallbladder has been emptied. **cystic b., gallbladder b.,** the bile that is held for some time in the gallbladder before moving into the intestine. **limy b.,** bile containing an increased amount of calcium, usually as the carbonate but sometimes as the phosphate or bilirubinate. It varies in consistency from a thick, milky fluid to a putty, gel, or solid. It is usually suspended in a thin, more watery bile. Called also *milk of calcium b.* **milk of calcium b.,** limy b. **ox b.,** the fresh bile of the ox, a brownish green to dark green viscous fluid; the extract is used as a choleretic. Called also *fel bovis* and *oxgall*. **Platner's crystallized b.,** a crystalline substance obtained by the action of ether in an alcoholic extract of bile. **white b.,** the colorless liquid containing mucoproteins and calcium salts sometimes found in the gallbladder in obstructions above the entrance of the cystic duct. Its accumulation in the distended biliary tract is called *hydrops*.

Bilharzia (bil-har'ze-ah) [Theodor Maximilian *Bilharz*, German physician, 1825–1862] *Schistosoma*.

bilharzial (bil-har'ze-al) pertaining to or caused by *Schistosoma* (*Bilharzia*).

bilharziasis (bil'har-zi'ah-sis) schistosomiasis.

bilharzic (bil-har'zik) bilharzial.

bilharzioma (bil-har''ze-o'mah) a tumor in the skin or mucous membrane caused by a schistosome.

bilharziosis (bil-har''ze-o'sis) schistosomiasis.

bili- [L. *bilis* bile] a combining form denoting relationship to the bile.

biliary (bil'e-a-re) pertaining to the bile, to the bile ducts, or to the gallbladder.

biliation (bil''e-a'shun) the secretion of bile.

bilicyanin (bil''ĭ-si'ah-nin) [*bili-* + L. *cyaneus* blue] a blue pigment derivable from biliverdin by oxidation; called also *cholecyanin* and *cholocyanin*.

bilidigestive (bil''e-di-jes'tiv) pertaining to the gallbladder and digestive tract.

biliflavin (bil''ĭ-fla'vin) [*bili-* + L. *flavus* yellow] a yellow pigment obtainable from biliverdin.

bilifulvin (bil''ĭ-ful'vin) [*bili-* + L. *fulvus* tawny] an impure bilirubin of a tawny color; also a tawny pigment from extract of ox bile; not normally found in healthy human bile.

bilifuscin (bil''ĭ-fus'in) [*bili-* + L. *fuscus* brown] a pigment from human bile and gallstones.

biligenesis (bil''ĭ-jen'ĕ-sis) the production or formation of bile.

biligenetic (bil''ĭ-jĕ-net'ik) 1. pertaining to biligenesis. 2. biligenic.

biligenic (bil''ĭ-jen'ik) [*bili-* + Gr. *gennan* to produce] producing bile.

biligulate (bi-lig'u-lāt) [*bi-* + L. *ligula* little tongue] having two tonguelike structures.

bilihumin (bil''ĭ-hu'min) [*bili-* + L. *humus* earth] an insoluble ingredient of gallstones.

bilin (bi'lin) [L. *bilis* bile] collective name for yellow bile pigments including i-urobilin, stercobilin, and d-urobilin, formed by spontaneous oxidation of the central methyene group of corresponding bilinogen; they are generated in the final steps of bilirubin catabolism.

bilious (bil'yus) [L. *biliosus*] characterized by bile, by excess of bile, or by biliousness.

biliousness (bil'yus-nes) a symptom complex comprising nausea, abdominal discomfort, headache, and constipation, formerly attributed to excessive secretion of bile.

biliprasin (bil'ĭ-pra'sin) [*bili-* + Gr. *prasinos* green] a green pigment from gallstones.

bilipurpurin (bil''ĭ-pur'pu-rin) [*bili-* + L. *purpur* purple] a purple pigment, $C_{34}H_{36}O_8N_4$, occurring in the bile of ruminants; derived from chlorophyll.

bilirachia (bil''ĭ-ra'ke-ah) the presence of bile pigments in the spinal fluid.

bilirhachia (bil''ĭ-ra'ke-ah) [*bili-* + Gr. *rhachis* spine + *-ia*] the presence of bile pigments in the spinal fluid.

bilirubin (bil''ĭ-roo'bin) [*bili-* + L. *ruber* red] a bile pigment; it is a breakdown product of heme mainly formed from the degradation of erythrocyte hemoglobin in reticuloendothelial cells, but also formed by breakdown of other heme pigments, e.g., cytochromes. Bilirubin normally circulates in plasma as a complex with albumin, and is taken up by the liver cells and conjugated to form bilirubin diglucuronide, which is the water-soluble pigment excreted in bile. In patients with cholestasis conjugated bilirubin (bilirubin diglucuronide) accumulates in the blood and tissues and is excreted in the urine; unconjugated bilirubin is not excreted in the urine. High concentrations of bilirubin may result in jaundice. **direct b., conjugated b.,** bilirubin that has been taken up by the liver cells and conjugated to form the water-soluble bilirubin diglucuronide. **indirect b.,** unconjugated bilirubin. **unconjugated b.,** the lipid-soluble form of bilirubin that circulates in loose association with the plasma proteins; called also *indirect b.*

bilirubinate (bil''ĭ-roo'bĭ-nāt) a salt of bilirubin.

bilirubinemia (bil''ĭ-roo-bĭ-ne'me-ah) [*bilirubin* + Gr. *haima* blood + *-ia*] the presence of bilirubin in the blood; see *hyperbilirubinemia*.

bilirubinic (bil''ĭ-roo-bin'ik) pertaining to bilirubin.

bilirubinuria (bil''ĭ-roo-bĭ-nu're-ah) presence of bilirubin in the urine.

bilis (bi'lis) [L.] bile. **b. bovi'na, b. buba'ta,** ox bile extract; see under *extract*.

bilitherapy (bil''ĭ-ther'ah-pe) (*obs.*) treatment with bile or bile salts.

biliuria (bil''ĭ-u're-ah) [*bili-* + Gr. *ouron* urine + *-ia*] the presence of bile pigments in the urine.

biliverdin (bil''ĭ-ver'din) [*bili-* + L. *viridis* green] a green pigment, $C_{33}H_{34}O_6N_4$, the initial bile pigment from catabolism of hemoglobin, converted to bilirubin by reduction of a methene bridge; it may arise from air oxidation of bilirubin. Called also *biliverdinic acid* and *dehydrobilirubin*.

biliverdinate (bil''ĭ-ver'dĭ-nāt) a salt of biliverdin.

bilixanthin, bilixanthine (bil''ĭ-zan'thin) [*bili-* + Gr. *xanthos* yellow] choletelin.

Billroth's cords, disease, etc. (bil'rōts) [Christian Albert Theodor *Billroth*, surgeon in Vienna, 1829–1894] see under *cord*, *disease*, *operation*, and *strand*.

bilobate (bi-lo'bāt) [*bi-* + L. *lobus* lobe] having two lobes.

bilobular (bi-lob'u-lar) having two lobules.

bilobulate (bi-lob'u-lāt) bilobular.

bilocular (bi-lok'u-lar) [*bi-* + L. *loculus* cell] having two compartments.

biloculate (bi-lok'u-lāt) bilocular.

biloma (bi'lo-mah) an encapsulated collection of bile in the peritoneal cavity.

Bilopaque (bil'o-pāk) trademark for a preparation of tyropanoate sodium.

bilophodont (bi-lof'ŏ-dont) [*bi-* + Gr. *lophos* ridge + *odous* tooth] having molariform teeth with two ridges on them; applied to certain mammals, e.g., the kangaroo.

Bimana (bim'ah-nah) [*bi-* + L. *manus* hand] a name sometimes applied to a category of mammals distinguished by possessing hands of character differing from that of the feet, and made up of man alone.

bimanual (bi-man'u-al) [*bi-* + L. *manualis* of the hand] with both hands; performed by both hands.

bimastoid (bi-mas'toid) pertaining to both mastoid processes.

bimaxillary (bi-mak'sĭ-ler''e) pertaining to or affecting both jaws.

bimeter (bīm'ĕ-ter) see under *gnathodynamometer*.

bimethoxycaine lactate (bi''mĕ-thoks'ĭ-kān) lactic acid compound with 2,2'-dimethoxy-α-α'-dimethyldiphenethylamine (1:1); a local anesthetic.

bimodal (bi-mo'dal) having two modes or peaks; said of a graphic curve.

bimolecular (bi''mo-lek'u-lar) relating to or formed from two molecules.

binangle (bin'ang-g'l) having two angles; Black's term for a dental instrument having two angulations in the shank connecting the handle, or shaft, with the working portion of the instrument, known as the blade, or nib.

binary (bi′na-re) [L. *binarius* of two] made up of two elements or of two equal parts; denoting a number system with a base of two.

binaural (bi-naw′ral, bin-aw′ral) [L. *bini* two + *auris* ear] pertaining to both ears.

binauricular (bin″aw-rik′u-lar) [L. *bini* two + *auricula* little ear] pertaining to both auricles of the ears.

binder (bīnd′er) an abdominal girdle or bandage, chiefly for women in labor who have pendulous abdomens (obstetric b.). **abdominal b.,** a binder applied to the abdomen after childbirth to support the relaxed abdominal walls.

binegative (bi-neg′ah-tiv) having two negative charges, especially in ions such as SO_4^{--}.

Binet's test (be-nāz′) [Alfred *Binet*, French physiologist, 1857–1911] see under *tests*.

Binet-Simon test (be-na′ se-mon′) [Alfred *Binet;* Theodore *Simon,* French physician, born 1873] Binet's test.

Bing's test (bingz) [Albert *Bing*, German otologist, 1844–1922] see under *tests*.

biniramycin (bin-ēr-ah-mi′sin) an antibacterial substance produced by a variant of *Streptomyces bikiniensis*.

binocular (bin-ok′u-lar) [L. *bini* two + *oculus* eye] 1. pertaining to both eyes. 2. having two eyepieces, as in a microscope.

binoculus (bin-ok′u-lus) the two eyes considered as one organ.

binomial (bi-no′me-al) [*bi-* + L. *nomen* name] composed of two terms, as the names of organisms formed by the combination of genus and species names.

binophthalmoscope (bin″of-thal′mo-skōp) an ophthalmoscope for examining both fundi of the patient at one time.

binoscope (bin′o-skōp) [L. *bini* two + Gr. *skopein* to examine] an instrument for inducing binocular vision in squint by presenting one object in the central part of the field of vision, the peripheral parts of the field being screened out.

binotic (bin-ot′ik) [L. *bini* two + Gr. *ous* ear] pertaining to both ears.

binovular (bin-ov′u-lar) [L. *bini* two + *ovum* an egg] pertaining to or derived from two distinct ova.

Binswanger's dementia (encephalitis) (bins′wang-er) [Otto *Binswanger,* German neurologist, 1852–1929] see under *dementia*.

binuclear (bi-nu′kle-ar) [*bi-* + L. *nucleus* nut] having two nuclei.

binucleate (bi-nu′kle-āt) binuclear.

binucleation (bi″nu-kle-a′shun) the formation of two nuclei within a cell through division of the nucleus without division of the cytoplasm.

binucleolate (bi-nu-kle′o-lāt) [*bi-* + L. *nucleolus*] having two nucleoli.

Binz's test (bints′ez) [Karl *Binz*, German pharmacologist, 1832–1913] see under *tests*.

bio-, bi- [Gr. *bios* life] combining form denoting relationship to life.

bioacoustics (bi″o-ah-koo′stiks) the science dealing with the communicating sounds made by animals.

bioactive (bi″o-ak′tiv) having an effect on or eliciting a response from living tissue.

bioaeration (bi″o-a″er-a′shun) a modification of the activated sludge method of purifying sewage.

bioamine (bi″o-am′ēn) biogenic amine.

bioaminergic (bi″o-am″in-er′jik) of or pertaining to neurons that secrete biogenic amines.

bioassay (bi″o-as-sa′) [*bio-* + *assay*] determination of the active power of a sample of a drug by noting its effect on a live animal or an isolated organ preparation, as compared with the effect of a standard preparation; called also *biological assay*.

bioastronautics (bi″o-as′tro-naw-tiks) the science concerned with study of the effects of space and interplanetary travel on living organisms.

bioavailability (bi″o-ah-vāl″ah-bil′ĭ-te) the degree to which a drug or other substance becomes available to the target tissue after administration.

bioblast (bi′o-blast) [*bio-* + Gr. *blastos* germ] 1. mitochondrion. 2. elementary unit of protoplasmic structure; Altmann's granule.

biocatalyst (bi″o-kat′ah-list) [*bio-* + *catalyst*] a name once suggested by Bayliss for enzyme.

biocenosis (bi″o-se-no′sis) [*bio-* + Gr. *koinos* common] the relation of diverse organisms that live in association.

biocenotic (bi″o-se-not′ik) characterized by biocenosis.

biochemistry (bi″o-kem′is-tre) [*bio-* + *chemistry*] the chemistry of living organisms and of vital processes; physiological chemistry.

biochemorphic (bi″o-ke-mor′fik) pertaining to biochemorphology.

biochemorphology (bi″o-ke-mor-fol′o-je) the study of the relationship between chemical constitution and biological action.

biocidal (bi″o-si′dal) pertaining to that which kills living organisms.

bioclimatics (bi″o-kli-mat′iks) bioclimatology.

bioclimatologist (bi″o-kli″mah-tol′ŏ-jist) an individual skilled in bioclimatology.

bioclimatology (bi″o-kli″mah-tol′ŏ-je) [*bio-* + *climatology*] the science devoted to the study of effects on living organisms of conditions of the natural environment (rainfall, daylight, temperature, humidity, air movement) prevailing in specific regions of the earth. See also *biometeorology*.

$(BiO)_2CO_2$ subcarbonate of bismuth.

biocoenosis (bi″o-se-no′sis) biocenosis.

biocolloid (bi″o-kol′oid) [*bio-* + *colloid*] a colloid from animal, plant, or microbial tissue.

biocompatible (bi″o-kom-pat′ĭ-b'l) being harmonious with life; not having toxic or injurious effects on biological function.

biocompatibility (bi″o-kom-pat″ĭ-bil′ĭ-te) the quality of being biocompatible.

biocybernetics (bi″o-si″ber-net′iks) the science of communications and control in animals.

biocycle (bi″o-si′k'l) [*bio-* + Gr. *kyklos* cycle] the rhythmic repetition of certain phenomena observed in living organisms.

biodegradable (bi″-o-de-grād′ah-b'l) susceptible of degradation by biological processes, as by bacterial or other enzymatic action.

biodegradation (bi″o-deg″rah-da′shun) the series of processes by which living systems render chemicals less noxious to the environment.

Bio-des (bi′o-des) trademark for a preparation of diethylstilbestrol.

biodetritus (bi″o-de-tri′tus) detritus derived from the disintegration and decomposition of once-living organisms; further designated as phytodetritus or zoodetritus, depending on whether the original organism was vegetal or animal.

biodynamics (bi″o-di-nam′iks) [*bio-* + Gr. *dynamis* might] the scientific study of the nature and determinants of all organismic (including human) behavior.

bioelectricity (bi″o-e″lek-tris′ĭ-te) the electrical phenomena that appear in living tissues, as that generated by muscle and nerve tissue.

bioelectronics (bi″o-e″lek-tron′iks) the study of the role of intermolecular transfer of electrons in biological regulation and defense.

bioelement (bi″o-el′e-ment) any chemical element that is a component of living tissue.

bioenergetics (bi″o-en″er-jet′iks) the study of the energy transformations in living organisms.

bioequivalence (bi″o-e-kwiv′ah-lens) the quality of being bioequivalent.

bioequivalent (bi″o-e-kwiv′ah-lent) having the same strength and similar bioavailability in the same dosage form as another specimen of a given drug substance.

biofeedback (bi″o-fēd′bak) the process of furnishing an individual information, usually in an auditory or visual mode, on the state of one or more physiological variables such as heart rate, blood pressure, or skin temperature; such a procedure often enables the individual to gain some voluntary control over the physiologic variable being sampled. **alpha b.,** a procedure in which a person is presented with continuous information, usually auditory, on the state of his brain-wave pattern, with the intent of increasing the percentage of alpha activity; this is done with the expectation that it will be associated with a state of relaxation and peaceful wakefulness. Called also *alpha feedback*.

bioflavonoid (bi″o-fla′vo-noid) a generic term for a group of compounds that are widely distributed in plants and that are concerned with maintenance of a normal state of walls of small blood vessels. See *flavonoid*.

biogen (bi′o-jen) [*bio-* + Gr. *gennan* to produce] one of several labile proteins supposedly representing the ultimate molecular basis of life.

biogenesis (bi″o-jen′ē-sis) [*bio-* + Gr. *genesis* origin] 1. the origin of life, or of living organisms. 2. the theory that living organisms can originate only from other organisms already living. Cf. *abiogenesis*.

biogenetic (bi″o-jĕ-net′ik) pertaining to biogenesis.

biogenic (bi″o-jen′ik) having origins in biological processes, as a biogenic amine.

biogenous (bi-oj′ĕ-nus) originating from life or producing life.

biogeochemistry (bi″o-je″o-kem′is-tre) [*bio-* + Gr. *gē* earth + *chemistry*] the study of interactions between the biosphere and its mineral environment, e.g., the study of the effect of living organisms on the weathering of rocks, of the concentration of elements by living systems, etc.

biogeography (bi″o-je-og′rah-fe) the scientific study of geographic distribution of living organisms.

biograph (bi′o-graf) 1. an instrument for analyzing and rendering visible the movements of animals; used in diagnosis of certain nervous diseases. 2. spirograph.

biohydraulic (bi″o-hī-draw′lik) [*bio-* + Gr. *hydōr* water] pertaining to the action of water and solutions in living tissue.

bioimplant (bi″o-im′plant) denoting a prosthesis made of biosynthetic material.

biokinetics (bi″o-ki-net′iks) [*bio-* + Gr. *kinētikos* of or for putting in motion] the science of the movements within developing organisms.

biologic, biological (bi-o-loj′ik; bi-o-loj′ĕ-kal) pertaining to biology.

biologicals (bi-o-loj′ĕ-kalz) medicinal preparations made from living organisms and their products, including serums, vaccines, antigens, antitoxins, etc.

biologist (bi-ol′ŏ-jist) an expert in biology.

biologos (bi-ol′ŏ-gos) [*bio-* + Gr. *logos* reason] the intelligent power displayed in organic activities.

biology (bi-ol′ŏ-je) [*bio-* + *-logy*] the science that deals with the phenomena of life and living organisms in general. **molecular b.,** the study of molecular structures and events underlying biological processes, including the relation between genes and the functional characteristics they determine. **radiation b.,** the scientific study of effects of ionizing radiation on living organisms.

bioluminescence (bi″o-loo″mĭ-nes′ens) chemoluminescence occurring in living cells, especially the emission of light as a result of cellular oxidation of a heat-stable substrate (luciferin) in the presence of a heat-sensitive enzyme (luciferase).

biolysis (bi-ol′ĭ-sis) chemical decomposition of organic matter by the action of living organisms.

biolytic (bi-o-lit′ik) [*bio-* + Gr. *lytikos* loosening] 1. pertaining to or characterized by biolysis. 2. destructive to life.

biomass (bi′o-mass) the entire assemblage of living organisms, both animal and vegetable, of a particular region, considered collectively.

biomaterial (bi″o-mah-te′re-al) a synthetic dressing with selective barrier properties, used in treatment of burns; it consists of a liquid solvent (polyethylene glycol-400) and a powdered polymer.

biomathematics (bi″o-math″ĕ-mat′iks) [*bio-* + *mathematics*] mathematics as applied to the phenomena of living things.

biome (bi′ōm) [Gr. *bios* life + *-ome* (-oma) mass] the recognizable community unit of a given region, produced by interaction of climatic factors, biota, and substrate, usually designated according to the characteristic adult or climax vegetation, as tundra, coniferous forest or taiga, deciduous forest, grassland, and the like.

biomechanics (bi″o-mĕ-kan′iks) [*bio-* + *mechanics*] the application of mechanical laws to living structures, specifically to the locomotor system of the human body. **dental b.,** the relationship between the biologic behavior of oral structures and the physical influence of a dental restoration.

biomedical (bi″o-med′ĭ-kal) biological and medical; pertaining to the application of the natural sciences (biology, biochemistry, biophysics, etc.) to the study of medicine.

biomedicine (bi″o-med′ĭ-sin) clinical medicine based on the principles of the natural sciences (biology, biochemistry, biophysics, etc.).

biomembrane (bi″o-mem′brān) any membrane, e.g., cell membrane, of an organism.

biomembranous (bi″o-mem′brah-nus) of or pertaining to a biomembrane.

biometeorologist (bi″o-me″te-or-ol′ŏ-jist) an individual skilled in biometeorology.

biometeorology (bi″o-me″te-or-ol′ŏ-je) [*bio-* + Gr. *meteōros* raised from off the ground + *logos* treatise] that branch of ecology which deals with the effects on living organisms of the extraorganic aspects of the physical environment (such as temperature, humidity, barometric pressure, rate of air flow, and air ionization). It considers not only the natural atmosphere but also artificially created atmospheres such as those to be found in buildings and shelters, and in closed ecological systems, such as satellites and submarines.

biometer (bi-om′ĕ-ter) [*bio-* + Gr. *metron* measure] an apparatus by which extremely minute quantities of carbon dioxide can be measured; used in measuring the carbon dioxide given off from functioning tissue.

biometrician (bi″o-mĕ-trish′an) an individual skilled in biometry.

biometrics (bi-o-met′riks) biometry.

biometry (bi-om′ĕ-tre) [*bio-* + Gr. *metron* measure] 1. the science of the application of statistical methods to biological facts; mathematical analysis of biological data. 2. in life insurance, the calculation of the expectation of life.

biomicroscope (bi″o-mi′krŏ-skōp) a microscope for examining living tissue in the body. **slit-lamp b.,** Gullstrand's slit lamp.

biomicroscopy (bi″o-mi-kros′ko-pe) 1. microscopic examination of living tissue in the body. 2. examination of the cornea or the lens by a combination of slit lamp and corneal microscope.

biomolecule (bi″o-mol′ĕ-kūl) a molecule produced by a living cell, as a protein, carbohydrate, or lipid.

biomotor (bi″o-mo′tor) an apparatus for producing artificial respiration.

Biomphalaria (bi-om″fah-la′re-ah) a genus of planorbid snails, species of which are intermediate hosts of *Schistosoma mansoni;* called also *Australorbis.*

bion (bi′on) [Gr. *bioun* a living being] an individual living organism.

bionecrosis (bi″o-ne-kro′sis) necrobiosis.

bionergy (bi-on′er-je) [*bion* + Gr. *ergon* work] life force; the force exercised in the living organism.

bionics (bi-on′iks) the science concerned with study of the functions, characteristics, and phenomena found in the living world and application of the knowledge gained to new devices and techniques in the world of machines.

bionomics (bi″o-nom′iks) [*bio-* + Gr. *nomos* law] the study of the relations of organisms to their environment; ecology.

bionomy (bi-on′ŏ-me) [*bio-* + Gr. *nomos* law] the sum of knowledge regarding the laws of life.

bionosis (bi-o-no′sis) [*bio-* + Gr. *nosos* disease] any disease caused by living agencies, as by bacteria or parasites.

bionucleonics (bi″o-nu″kle-on′iks) the study of the biological applications of radioactive and rare stable isotopes.

bio-osmotic (bi″o-oz-mot′ik) [*bio-* + *osmotic*] a term applied to osmotic pressure phenomena in living organisms.

biophagism (bi-of′ah-jizm) [*bio-* + Gr. *phagein* to eat] the eating or absorption of living matter.

biophagous (bi-of′ah-gus) feeding on living matter.

biophagy (bi-of′ah-je) biophagism.

biophore (bi′o-fōr) [*bio-* + Gr. *phoros* bearing] one of the hypothetical vital units which, according to Weismann, are aggregated into groups called *determinants,* these groups being gathered into larger ones called *ids,* which are the visible chromatin granules, and these in turn into larger groups called *idants,* which are the chromosomes. Called also *idioblast* and *plastidule.*

biophoric (bi-o-for′ik) relating to biophores.

biophotometer (bi″o-fo-tom′ĕ-ter) [*bio-* + Gr. *phōs* light + *metron* measure] an instrument for measuring the dark adaptation of the eye as an indication of vitamin A deficiency.

biophysical (bi-o-fiz′ĭ-kal) pertaining to biophysics.

biophysics (bi-o-fiz′iks) [*bio-* + *physics*] the science dealing with the application of physical methods and theories to biological problems. **dental b.,** the relationship between the biologic behavior of oral structures and the physical influence of a dental restoration.

biophysiography (bi″o-fiz-e-og′rah-fe) [*bio-* + *physiography*] structural or descriptive biology.

biophysiology (bi″o-fiz-e-ol′ŏ-je) [*bio-* + Gr. *physis* nature + *-logy*] that part of biology which includes organogeny, morphology, and physiology.

bioplasia (bi-o-pla′ze-ah) [*bio-* + Gr. *plassein* to form] the storing up of food energy in the form of growth.

bioplasm (bi′o-plazm) [*bio-* + Gr. *plasma* anything molded] 1. protoplasm. 2. the more essential or vital part of cytoplasm, contrasted with the *hyaloplasm.* Called also *plasmogen.*

bioplasmic (bi-o-plaz′mik) of or pertaining to bioplasm.

bioplast (bi′o-plast) 1. an independently existing mass of living matter. 2. an ameboid cell.

biopoiesis (bi″o-poi-e′sis) [*bio-* + Gr. *poiein* to make] the origin of life from inorganic matter.

biopolymer (bi″o-pol′ĭ-mer) a polymer formed in a living organism, as a polypeptide formed from amino acids (monomers).

biopsy (bi′op-se) [*bio-* + Gr. *opsis* vision] the removal and examination, usually microscopic, of tissue from the living body, performed to establish precise diagnosis. **aspiration b.,** biopsy in which the tissue is obtained by the application of suction through a needle attached to a syringe. **bite b.,** the instrumental removal of a fragment of tissue. **brush b.,** biopsy in which cells or tissue is obtained by manipulating tiny brushes against the tissue or lesion in question (e.g., through a bronchoscope) at the desired site. **cone b.,** biopsy in which an inverted cone of tissue is excised, as from the uterine cervix. **cytological b.,** a procedure in which cells are obtained by various methods for pathological examinations, as by irrigation of hollow viscera. **endoscopic b.,** removal of tissue by appropriate instruments introduced through an endoscope. **excisional b.,** biopsy of tissue removed by excision; biopsy of an entire lesion, including a significant margin of contiguous normal-appearing tissue. **exploratory b.,** exploration combined with biopsy to determine the type and extent of neoplasms, both deep and superficial. **incisional b.,** biopsy of a selected portion of a lesion and, if possible, of adjacent normal-appearing tissue. **needle b.,** biopsy in which tissue is obtained by the puncture of a tumor, the tissue within the lumen of the needle being detached by rotation and withdrawal of the needle. See also *aspiration b.* **punch b.,** biopsy in which tissue is obtained by a punch. **sternal b.,** biopsy of bone marrow of the sternum; done by puncture or trephining. **surface b.,** biopsy of cells scraped from the surface of suspicious or obvious lesions, most commonly employed in examination for cancer of the cervix. **surgical b.,** biopsy of tissue obtained by surgical excision. **total b.,** biopsy of an entire growth, a procedure of both therapeutic and diagnostic value.

biopsychic (bi″o-si′kik) pertaining to psychical phenomena in their relation to the living organism.

biopsychical (bi″o-si′kĭ-kal) biopsychic.

biopsychology (bi″o-si-kol′o-je) psychobiology.

biopterin (bi-op′ter-in) a naturally occurring pteridine, 2-amino-4-hydroxy-6-(1,2-dihydroxypropyl) pteridine.

bioptic (bi-op′tik) pertaining to or dependent on biopsy.

bioptome (bíop-tōm″) a cutting instrument for taking biopsy specimens.

biopyoculture (bi″o-pi′o-kul″tūr) [*bio-* + Gr. *pyon* pus + *culture*] a culture made from pus whose cells are alive.

biorbital (bi-or′bĭ-tal) [*bi-* + L. *orbita* orbit] pertaining to both orbits.

bioreversible (bi″o-re-ver′sĭ-b'l) capable of being changed back to the original biologically active chemical form by processes within the organism; said of drugs.

biorgan (bi′or-gan) a physiological organ, as distinguished from a morphological organ, or *idorgan.*

biorheology (bi″o-re-ol′o-je) the study of the deformation and flow of matter in living systems and in materials directly derived from them.

biorhythm (bi′o-rithm) the cyclic occurrence of physiological events, as a circadian rhythm.

bioroentgenography (bi″o-rent″gen-og′rah-fe) [*bio-* + *roentgenography*] the making of kinematographic x-ray pictures.

bios (bi′os) [Gr. "life"] any one of a group of growth factors for single-celled organisms such as yeast. Bios occurs in yeast, leaves of plants, bran, and the outer covering of seeds, and is probably a mixture of B vitamins and pantothenic acid. **b. I,** inositol. **b. II,** biotin.

bioscience (bi″o-si′ens) the study of biology wherein all the applicable sciences (physics, chemistry, etc.) are applied.

bioscopy (bi-os′ko-pe) [*bio-* + Gr. *skopein* to examine] the examination of the body to determine whether the patient is living or dead.

biose (bi′ōs) a sugar containing two carbon atoms.

biosis (bi-o′sis) [Gr. *bios* life] vitality, or life.

biosmosis (bi″os-mo′sis) osmosis through a living membrane.

biospectrometry (bi″o-spek-trom′ĕ-tre) measurement by a spectroscope of the quantity of a substance in living tissue.

biospectroscopy (bi″o-spek-tros′ko-pe) examination of living tissue with the spectroscope.

biosphere (bi′ŏ-sfēr) 1. that part of the universe in which living organisms are known to exist, comprising the atmosphere, hydrosphere, and lithosphere. 2. the sphere of action between an organism and its environment.

biostatics (bi″ŏ-stat′iks) [*bio-* + Gr. *statikos* causing to stand] the science of the structure of organisms in relation to their function.

biostatistics (bi″o-stah-tis′tiks) vital statistics; see under *statistics.*

biostereometrics (bi″o-ste″re-o-met′riks) analysis of the spatial and spatial-temporal characteristics of biological form and function by means of three-dimensional mapping of the body.

biosynthesis (bi″o-sin′thĕ-sis) the building up of a chemical compound in the physiologic processes of a living organism.

biosynthetic (bi″o-sin-thet′ik) pertaining to or characterized by biosynthesis.

Biot's respiration (breathing, sign) (be-ōz′) [Camille *Biot,* French physician of 19th century] see under *respiration.*

biota (bi-o′tah) [Gr. *bios* life] all the living organisms of a particular area; the combined flora and fauna of a region.

biotaxis (bi″o-tak′sis) [*bio-* + Gr. *taxis* arrangement] the selecting and arranging powers of living cells.

biotaxy (bi″o-tak′se) 1. biotaxis. 2. taxonomy.

biotelemetry (bi″o-tel-em′ĕ-tre) the recording and measuring of certain vital phenomena of living organisms that are situated at a distance from the measuring device.

biothesiometer (bi″o-the″se-om′ĕ-ter) an instrument for measuring the vibratory-perception threshold.

biotic (bi-ot′ik) 1. pertaining to life or living matter. 2. pertaining to the biota.

biotics (bi-ot′iks) [Gr. *biōtikos* living] the functions and qualities peculiar to living organisms, or the sum of knowledge regarding these qualities.

biotin (bi′o-tin) a colorless crystalline compound, 2′-keto-3,4-imidazolido-2-tetrahydrothiophene-δ-n-valeric acid, $CH_2 \cdot CH \cdot NH \cdot CO \cdot NH \cdot CH \cdot (CH_2)_4 \cdot COOH$, identical with vitamin H and coenzyme R; it is a ubiquitous member of the vitamin B complex required by or occurring in all forms of life tested. Deficiency of biotin has been produced in men and experimental animals fed uncooked egg white, such deficiency being due to the avidin present in the egg white, which renders the biotin of the diet unavailable. Manifestations of biotin deficiency in experimental animals include paralysis, usually of the hindquarters (cows, dogs, rats), dermatitis (rats, pigs, fowl), alopecia (mice, pigs, monkeys), and graying of brown and black fur (mice, monkeys). *Alpha b.* is the product isolated from egg yolk; *beta b.* is that isolated from liver. Called also *bios II.* Cf. *avidin.*

biotomy (bi-ot′ŏ-me) [*bio-* + Gr. *tomē* a cutting] 1. the study of animal and plant structure by dissection. 2. vivisection.

biotoxication (bi″o-tok″sĭ-ka′shun) an intoxication resulting from a plant or animal poison (biotoxin).

biotoxicology (bi″o-tok″sĭ-kol′o-je) [*bio-* + Gr. *toxikon* poison + *-logy*] the science of poisons produced by living things, their cause, detection, and their effects, and of the treatment of conditions produced by them.

biotoxin (bi″o-tok′sin) any poisonous substance produced by and derived from a living organism, either plant or animal.

biotransformation (bi″o-trans″for-ma′shun) the series of chemical alterations of a compound (e.g., a drug) which occur within the body, as by enzymatic activity.

biotrepy (bi-ot′rĕ-pe) the study of the body by means of its reactions to chemical substances.

biotype (bi′o-tīp) 1. a group of individuals possessing the same genotype. 2. any one of a number of strains of a species of microorganisms that have differentiable physiologic characteristics.

biotypology (bi″o-ti-pol′o-je) the study of anthropological types with their constitutional variations, inadequacies, etc.

biovular (bi-ov′u-lar) binovular.

B.I.P. bismuth iodoform paraffin; see *Morison's method,* under *method.*

biparasitic (bi″par-ah-sit′ik) living parasitically upon a parasite; hyperparasitic.

biparental (bi″pah-ren′tal) derived from two parents, male and female.

biparietal (bi″pah-ri′ĕ-tal) pertaining to the two parietal eminences or bones.

biparous (bip′ah-rus) [*bi-* + L. *parere* to produce] producing two ova or offspring at one time.

bipartite (bi-par′tīt) [L. *bipartitus*] having two parts or divisions, as the uterus of most mammals.

biped (bi′ped) [*bi-* + L. *pes* foot] 1. having two feet. 2. an animal with two feet.

bipedal (bip′ĕ-dal) [*bi-* + L. *pes* foot] having or pertaining to both feet.

bipenniform (bi-pen′ĭ-form) doubly feather-shaped; said of muscles whose fibers are arranged on each side of a tendon, like the barbs on the shaft of a feather.

biperforate (bi-per′fŏ-rāt) [*bi-* + L. *perforatus* bored through] having two perforations.

biperiden (bi-per′ĭ-den) [USP] chemical name: α-bicyclo-[2.2.1]hept-5-en-2-yl-α-phenyl-1-piperidenepropanol. A synthetic anticholinergic, $C_{21}H_{29}NO$, occurring as a white, crystalline powder, having antisecretory, spasmolytic, and mydriatric actions. It is used, in the form of the hydrochloride or lactate salts, as an antiparkinsonian agent, and is also useful in the treatment of drug-induced extrapyramidal reactions. **b. hydrochloride** [USP], the hydrochloride of biperiden, $C_{21}H_{29}NO \cdot HCl$, administered orally. **b. lactate** [NF], the lactate of biperiden, $C_{21}H_{29}NO \cdot C_3H_6O_3$, administered intramuscularly and intravenously.

biphenamine hydrochloride (bi-fen′ah-mēn) chemical name: 2-(diethylamino)ethyl 2-hydroxy-3-biphenylcarboxylate hydrochloride; an antibacterial, antifungal, and topical anesthetic, $C_{19}H_{23}NO_3 \cdot HCl$.

biphenyl (bi-fe′nil) diphenyl. **polychlorinated b. (PCB),** any of a group of substances in which chlorine replaces hydrogen in biphenyl and which are toxic and accumulate in animal tissues; it is used as a heat-transfer agent and as an insulator in electrical equipment.

bipolar (bi-po′lar) 1. having two poles; having processes at both poles. 2. pertaining to both poles; denoting electrotherapeutic treatments in which two poles are used; also bacterial staining confined to the poles (ends) of the organism. 3. a two-poled nerve cell. **cone b.,** any one of those bipolar nerve cells of the inner nuclear layer of the retina that are related to the terminations of the cone visual cells. **giant b's,** those cone bipolars that lie beneath the external plexiform layer of the retina. **rod b.,** any one of those bipolar nerve cells that are related to the terminations of the rod visual cells.

bipositive (bi-poz′ĭ-tiv) having two positive charges, as in Ca^{++}.

bipotential (bi″po-ten′shal)   pertaining to or characterized by bipotentiality.

bipotentiality (bi″po-ten″she-al′ĭ-te) [*bi-* + L. *potentia* power]   possession of the power of developing or acting in either of two possible ways.   **b. of the gonad,** the capability of an undifferentiated gonad to develop into either an ovary or a testis.

bipp   a vernacular term in the British Isles for bismuth iodoform paraffin paste; see *Morison's method,* under *method.*

biramous (bi-ra′mus) [*bi-* + L. *ramus* branch]   consisting of or possessing two branches.

Bird's formula, treatment (birdz) [Golding *Bird,* English physician, 1814–1854]   see under *formula* and *treatment.*

Bird's sign (birdz) [Samuel Dougan *Bird,* Australian physician, 1832–1904]   see under *sign.*

bird-arm (bird′arm)   a forearm that is greatly reduced in size as the result of atrophy of the muscles.

bird-face (bird′fās)   a form of dyscephaly in which the skull is small and the facial bones are large, giving a birdlike appearance. The appearance of the face in microcephaly, the skull being small and the facial bones large.

bird-leg (bird′leg)   a leg that is greatly reduced in size as the result of atrophy of the muscles.

bird-lime (bird′līm) [*bird* + L. *limus* slime]   a viscous or gummy substance of various origin, used for catching small birds; some kinds were used formerly in dressing wounds and sores.

birefractive (bi″re-frak′tiv)   doubly refractive.

birefringence (bi″re-frin′jens)   the quality of transmitting light unequally in different directions; double refraction. In biological materials, it indicates an ordering of the molecules, e.g., they may be oriented to one another much as in a crystal.   **crystalline b.,** birefringence occurring in systems in which the bonds between molecules or ions have a regular asymmetrical arrangement; it is independent of the refractive index of the medium.   **flow b.,** that exhibited only when the substance is in solution and flowing; e.g., it is seen in solutions of long thin molecules, such as nucleoproteins.   **form b.,** that produced by regular orientation of submicroscopic asymmetrical particles in a substance or object, differing in refractive index from the surrounding medium; it is the most common form occurring in organisms.   **intrinsic b.,** crystalline b.   **strain b.,** birefringence observed occasionally in isotropic structures when subjected to tension or pressure; it occurs in muscle and in embryonic tissues.   **streaming b.,** flow b.

birefringent (bi″re-frin′jent) [*bi-* + L. *refringere* to break up]   doubly refractive.

Birkett's hernia (ber′kets) [John *Birkett,* English surgeon, 1815–1904]   synovial hernia.

Birkhaug's test (birk′hawg) [Konrad Elias *Birkhaug,* Norwegian bacteriologist in America, born 1892]   see under *tests.*

Birnberg bow (bern′berg) [Charles H. *Birnberg,* American obstetrician and gynecologist, born 1900]   see under *bow.*

birth (birth)   the act or process of being born.   **complete b.,** the complete separation of the infant from the maternal body (after cutting of the umbilical cord).   **cross b.,** labor with the fetus lying transversely in the uterus.   **dead b.,** birth of a fetus which, during or before birth, has lost all signs of antenatal life, heart beat, pulsation, movement.   **head b.,** a birth in which the head presents.   **multiple b.,** the birth of two or more offspring produced in the same gestation period, the frequency of birth of viable offspring after such multiple pregnancy having been computed as follows: twins, 1 in 80; triplets, 1 in 6400 (80 × 80); quadruplets, 1 in 512,000 (80 × 80 × 80); etc. (Hellin's law).   **post-term b.,** birth of a post-mature, or over-term, infant.   **premature b.,** birth of a premature infant.

birthmark (birth′mark)   nevus; a circumscribed new growth of congenital origin, as a vascular nevus (hemangioma) or a mole.   **physiologic b.,** one so common as to be considered normal; a term once applied to nevus flammeus in the suboccipital region.

bis-   a prefix signifying two or twice.

bisacodyl (bis-ak′o-dil; bis″ah-ko′dil) [USP]   chemical name: 4,4′-(2-pyridinylmethylene)bisphenol diacetate (ester). A cathartic, $C_{22}H_{19}NO_4$, occurring as a white to off-white, crystalline powder; administered orally or by rectal suppository.   **b. tannex,** a water-soluble complex of bisacodyl and tannic acid; a cathartic.

bisacromial (bis″ah-kro′me-al)   pertaining to the two acromial processes.

bisalbuminemia (bis″al-bu″mĭ-ne′me-ah)   a congenital abnormality characterized by the presence of two distinct serum albumins which differ in their electrophoretic mobility.

bisaxillary (bis-ak′sĭ-lar″e)   pertaining to both axillae.

Bischoff's test (bish′ofs) [Carl Adam *Bischoff,* German chemist, 1855–1908]   see under *tests.*

biscuit (bis′ket)   in dentistry, porcelain that has undergone the first baking, before it is subjected to the glazing or enameling; called also *bisque.*   **hard b.,** biscuit after shrinking but before

vitrification has begun.   **soft b.,** biscuit during the process of stiffening, before shrinkage has begun.

biscuiting (bis′ket-ing)   the first baking of porcelain paste, by which biscuit is formed.

bisection (bi-sek′shun) [*bi-* + L. *sectio* a cut]   a division into two parts by cutting; called also *hemisection.*

biseptate (bi-sep′tāt) [*bi-* + L. *septum* partition]   divided into two parts by a septum.

bisexual (bi-seks′u-al) [*bi-* + L. *sexus* sex]   1. having gonads of both sexes. Cf. *ambisexual.* 2. hermaphrodite. 3. having both active and passive sexual interests or characteristics. 4. capable of the function of both sexes; cf. *unisexual.* 5. both heterosexual and homosexual. 6. an individual who is both heterosexual and homosexual. 7. of, relating to, or involving both sexes, as bisexual reproduction; see *sexual reproduction,* under *reproduction.*

bisexuality (bi-seks″u-al′ĭ-te)   1. the condition of being bisexual or of being a bisexual. 2. hermaphroditism.

bisferious (bis-fe′re-us) [L. *bis* twice + *ferire* to beat]   having two beats; usually refers to a widely notched arterial pulse, sometimes palpable.

Bishop's sphygmoscope (bish′ups) [Louis Faugères *Bishop,* American physician, 1864–1941]   see under *sphygmoscope.*

bishydroxycoumarin (bis″hi-drok″se-koo′mah-rin) [USP]   dicumarol.

bisiliac (bi-sil′e-ak) [L. *bis* twice + *iliac*]   pertaining to both iliac bones or to any two corresponding points on the two iliac bones.

bis in die (bis in de′a) [L.]   twice a day; abbreviated b.d. or b.i.d.

bismuth (biz′muth) [L. *bismuthum*]   a silver-white metal; atomic number 83; atomic weight 208.980; symbol Bi: its salts have been used in inflammatory diseases of the stomach and intestine, and in the treatment of syphilis. Since the introduction of antibiotics, treatment with bismuth has declined.   **b. albuminate,** a white or grayish insoluble powder formerly used for intestinal and gastric cramps.   **b. and ammonium citrate,** a white crystalline compound formerly used as an astringent in intestinal irritation.   **b. arsanilate,** a compound, $NH_2C_6H_4\cdot\cdot AsO$, formerly used in the treatment of syphilis.   **b. benzoate,** a whitish tasteless powder, $Bi(C_6H_5CO_2)_3Bi(OH)_3$, formerly used as an external and internal antiseptic.   **b. betanaphthol,** a light brown insoluble aromatic powder, $(C_{10}H_7\cdot O)_3\cdot Bi\cdot 3H_2O$, formerly used as an intestinal astringent and antiseptic.   **b. borophenate,** a compound formerly used as an antiseptic dusting powder.   **b. carbonate, basic,** b. subcarbonate.   **b. cerium salicylate,** a bismuth salt in the form of a pinkish, insoluble powder, formerly used in enteritis, diarrhea, etc.   **b. chrysophanate,** an amorphous yellow powder, $(C_{15}H_9O_4)_3Bi_2O_3$, resulting from the mixture of chrysarobin and bismuth hydroxide; formerly used in skin diseases.   **b. citrate,** an amorphous powder, $BiC_6H_5O_7$, used in pharmacy and in the preparation of other bismuth remedies.   **b. ethyl camphorate,** a bismuth preparation, $(C_{12}H_{19}O_4)_3Bi$, containing 23.5 per cent of bismuth; formerly used as an antisyphilitic.   **b. glycollylarsanilate,** glycobiarsol.   **b. magma,** milk of bismuth.   **b. nitrate,** $Bi(NO_3)_3\cdot 5H_2O$, formerly used in diarrhea.   **b. oxybromide,** an impalpable yellowish powder, $BiOBr$, to be given in a tragacanth emulsion; formerly used in nervous dyspepsia.   **b. oxychloride,** a white powder, sometimes known as pearl white, $BiOCl$, formerly used as a local antiseptic.   **b. oxyiodide,** a brownish-red powder, $BiOI$, formerly used as a local antiseptic.   **b. oxyiodopyrogallate,** a fine, yellowish-red powder, $C_6H_2(OH)_2\cdot O\cdot Bi(OH)I$, formerly used as a surgical antiseptic powder.   **b. permanganate,** a black bulky powder, $Bi(MnO_4)_3$, formerly used as an antiseptic dusting powder.   **b. phosphate,** a white odorless powder, $BiPO_4$, formerly used as an intestinal antiseptic.   **b. and potassium tartrate,** a white odorless powder, $C_4H_2O_9\cdot Bi_3K\cdot 4H_2O$, formerly used intramuscularly in syphilis.   **b. pyrogallate,** a yellow powder, $C_6H_3\cdot OH\cdot O\cdot O\cdot BiOH$, formerly used as an internal and external antiseptic.   **b. salicylate,** a white, tasteless, and insoluble powder formerly used as an intestinal antiseptic.   **b. sodium tartrate,** a compound, $BiNa(C_4H_4O_6)_2$, formerly used in the treatment of syphilis.   **b. sodium triglycollamate,** double salt of sodium bismuthyl triglycollamate and disodium triglycollamate; formerly used for lupus erythematosus and chronic syphilis.   **b. subcarbonate,** a white to yellowish white powder, $(BiO)_2CO_3\cdot H_2O$, yielding at least 90 per cent Bi_2O_3; it is used as a topical protectant to relieve skin irritations, and it has been used internally as an antacid and astringent. Called also *basic bismuth carbonate.*   **b. subgallate,** a basic salt, $Bi(OH)_2\cdot C_7H_5O_5$, which on drying yields 52 to 57 per cent of bismuth trioxide; formerly used as an astringent and protective in the treatment of ulcerative colitis, dysentery, and diarrhea.   **b. subnitrate** [USP], a basic salt, $BiO\cdot NO_3\cdot H_2O$, which on ignition yields not less than 71 per cent of bismuth trioxide, occurring as a white, slightly hygroscopic powder; used as a pharmaceutic necessity, and formerly as an antacid, antiseptic, and radiopaque medium. Called also *b. white* and *Spanish water.*   **b. subsalicylate,** a basic salt, $C_7H_5BiO_4$, which on ignition yields 62 to 66 per cent bismuth trioxide; it has been given orally in the treatment of enteritis and intramuscularly in the treatment of syphilis, lupus erythematosus, and necrotizing ulcerative gingivitis. **b. tannate,** a compound formed by the action of tannic acid on bismuth hydroxide; formerly used as an astringent in diarrhea. **b. tribromphenate,** a yellow powder, $C_{18}H_6BiBr_9$-O_3, formerly used as a topical antiseptic. **b. white,** b. subnitrate.

bismuthia (biz-mu′the-ah) blue discoloration of the skin and mucous membranes as the result of the administration of bismuth compounds.

bismuthism (biz′muth-izm) bismuthosis.

bismuthosis (biz″mu-tho′sis) chronic bismuth poisoning, characterized by anuria, stomatitis, dermatitis, and diarrhea.

bisobrin lactate (bis′o-brin) chemical name: *meso*-1,1′-tetramethylenebis[1,2,3,4-tetrahydro-6,7-dimethoxyisoquinoline] dilactate; a fibrinolytic agent, $C_{26}H_{36}N_2O_4 \cdot 2C_3H_6O_3$.

2,3-bisphosphoglycerate (bis-fos″fo-glis′er-āt) a salt or ester of bisphosphoglyceric acid; it is contained in red blood cells, where it plays a role in liberating oxygen from hemoglobin in the peripheral circulation. It is also an intermediate in the conversion of 3-phosphoglycerate to 2-phosphoglycerate. Called also *2,3-diphosphoglycerate.*

bispore (bi′spōr) one of two asexual spores produced by the red algae.

bisque (bisk) [Fr.] biscuit. **hard b., soft b.,** see under *biscuit.*

bistephanic (bi″ste-fan′ik) pertaining to the two stephanions, especially to the shortest distance between them (bistephanic width).

Biston betularia (bis′ton be-tu-la′re-ah) the peppered moth, used in the study of industrial melanism.

bistort (bis′tort) [L. *bis* twice + *tortus* twisted] the plant, *Polygonum bistorta;* its root [L. *bistortae radix*] contains tannins and has mild astringent and tonic properties.

bistoury (bis′too-re) [Fr. *bistouri*] a long narrow surgical knife, straight or curved, used for incising abscesses and enlarging sinuses, fistulas, etc.

bistratal (bi-stra′tal) [*bi-* + L. *stratum* layer] disposed in two layers.

bisulfate (bi-sul′fāt) an acid sulfate (not to be confused with *disulfate*).

bisulfide (bi-sul′fīd) disulfide.

bisulfite (bi-sul′fīt) an acid sulfite.

bitartrate (bi-tar′trāt) any salt containing the anion $C_4H_5O_6^-$ derived from the diacid tartaric acid ($C_4H_6O_6$).

bite (bīt) 1. seizure with the teeth. 2. a wound or puncture made by the teeth or other mouth parts of a living organism. 3. an impression made by closure of the teeth upon a thin sheet of some malleable material, e.g., wax. 4. occlusion, def. 3. **balanced b.,** balanced occlusion. **check b.,** a thin sheet of wax or paraffin placed between the teeth in the mouth and used as a check upon the teeth in the dental articulator. **closed b.,** dental malocclusion in which the mandible protrudes; that is, the incisal edges of the mandibular anterior teeth extend lingually past the incisal edges of the maxillary, approaching the lingual gingival margin, when the jaws are in habitual occlusion. See also *retrusion.* **cross b.,** crossbite. **edge-to-edge b., end-to-end b.,** occlusion in which the incisors of both jaws meet along the incisal edges when the jaws are in centric or habitual occlusion. **open b.,** a condition marked by failure of certain opposing teeth to establish occlusal contact when the jaws are closed, usually confined to the anterior teeth; called also *apertognathia.* **over b.,** overbite. **stork b's,** 1. capillary flames. 2. nevi flammeus. **underhung b.,** a characteristic of mandibular prognathism in which the incisal edges of the mandibular anterior teeth extend labially to the incisal edges of the maxillary anterior teeth when the jaws are in habitual occlusion. **wax b.,** an impression, made simultaneously, of both the upper and the lower jaw, by having the subject bite on a double layer of soft baseplate wax. **X-b.,** crossbite.

bite-block (bīt′blok) occlusion rim; see under *rim.*

bitegage (bīt′gāj) a device used in prosthetic dentistry as an aid in securing proper occlusion of the maxillary and mandibular teeth.

bitelock (bīt′lok) a device used in dentistry for retaining the occlusion rims in the same relation outside of the mouth which they occupied in the mouth.

bitemporal (bi-tem′po-ral) pertaining to both temples or temporal bones.

biteplate (bīt′plāt) a tooth- and tissue-borne appliance, usually fabricated of plastic and wire and worn in the palate; used as a diagnostic or therapeutic adjunct in orthodontics or prosthodontics. Sometimes used for temporomandibular joint disorders, or as a diagnostic splint in full mouth restorations.

biterminal (bi-ter′min-al) performed by using two terminals of an alternating current.

bite-wing (bīt′wing) a wing or fin attached along the center of the tooth side of a dental x-ray film and bitten on by the patient; used for making radiographic projections showing simultaneously

the corona of the teeth in both dental arches and their contiguous periodontal tissues.

bithionol (bĭthi′o-nol) chemical name: 2,2′-thiobis(4,6-dichlorophenol). A bacteriostatic agent, $C_{12}H_6Cl_4O_2S$, especially effective against gram-positive cocci; formerly used in the formulation of surgical soap compositions. Called also *TBP.*

Bithynia (bĭ-thin′ĕ-ah) a genus of snails, species of which are the intermediate hosts of *Opisthorchis.* **B. longicor′nus,** *Alocimna longicornis.*

Bitis (bi′tis) a genus of venomous, brightly colored, thick-bodied, viperine snakes, possessing heart-shaped heads; it includes the puff adder (*B. arientans*), Gaboon viper (*B. gabonica*), and rhinoceros viper (*B. nasicornis*). See table accompanying *snake.*

bitolterol (bi-tōl′ter-ōl) chemical name: 4-methylbenzoic acid 4-[2-[(1,1-dimethylethyl)amino]-1-hydroxyethyl]-1,2-phenylene ester; a bronchodilator, $C_{28}H_{31}NO_5$.

Bitot's spots (patches) (be′tōz) [Pierre A. *Bitot,* Bordeaux physician, 1822–1888] see under *spot.*

bitrochanteric (bi″tro-kan-ter′ik) pertaining to both trochanters on one femur or to both greater trochanters.

bitter (bit′er) 1. having an austere and unpalatable taste, like that of quinine. 2. [pl.] a medicinal agent that has a bitter taste; used as a tonic, alterative, or appetizer. Called also *amara.* **aromatic b's,** bitter vegetable drugs that have an aromatic quality. **simple b's,** any drug with a bitter taste that has no general influence upon the system except through its action upon the stomach or intestine. **styptic b's,** bitter drugs with a markedly astringent quality. **Swedish b's,** compound tincture of aloes.

bitterling (bit′er-ling) see *bitterling test,* under *tests.*

bitters (bit′erz) a popular name for various alcoholic medicines and drinks; see under *bitter.*

Bittorf's reaction (bit′orfs) [Alexander *Bittorf,* German physician, 1876–1949] see under *reaction.*

bitumen (bĭ-tu′men) [L.] any one of various natural and artificial dry petroleum products. **sulfonated b.,** ichthammol.

bituminosis (bi″tu-mĭ-no′sis) a form of pneumoconiosis due to the dust from soft coal.

biurate (bi′u-rāt) an acid urate; a monobasic salt of uric acid.

biuret (bi′u-ret) [L. *bis* twice + *urea*] a derivative of urea, H_2-$NCO \cdot NH \cdot CO \cdot NH_2$, equivalent to two molecules of urea less one of ammonia; called also *allophanamide.* See also under *tests.*

bivalence (biv′ah-lens) [*bi-* + L. *valens* powerful] the property of an atom of certain chemical elements of forming chemical bonds with two other atoms or groups.

bivalent (bi-va′lent, biv′ah-lent) 1. having a valence of two; characterized by bivalence. 2. denoting homologous chromosomes associated in pairs, during the zygotene stage of the first meiotic prophase, each of which splits (pachytene stage) into two sister chromatids to form a tetrad. Called also *divalent.*

bivalve (bi′valv) [*bi-* + L. *valva* valve] having two valves, as the shells of such mollusks as clams.

Bivalvia (bi-val′ve-ah) [*bi-* + L. *valva* valve + *-ia*] Pelecypoda.

biventer (bi′ven-ter) [*bi-* + L. *venter* belly] a part or organ (as a muscle) with two bellies. **b. cer′vicis,** musculus spinalis capitis.

biventral (bi-ven′tral) 1. having two bellies. 2. musculus digastricus.

biventricular (bi″ven-trik′u-lar) pertaining to or affecting both ventricles of the heart.

bivitelline (bi″vi-tel′in) having two yolks.

bixin (bik′sin) [L. *Bixa* a plant genus] an orange-red color or stain, $C_{25}H_{30}O_4$, from annotto.

bizygomatic (bi″zi-go-mat′ik) [*bi-* + Gr. *zygōma* zygoma] pertaining to the two most prominent points on the two zygomatic arches. See also *bizygomatic breadth,* under *breadth.*

Bizzozero's cells, corpuscles, platelets (bit-sot′ ser-ōz) [Giulio *Bizzozero,* Italian physician, 1846–1901] platelets.

Bjerrum's scotoma (sign) (byer′oomz) [Jannik Petersen *Bjerrum,* Danish ophthalmologist, 1851–1920] see under *scotoma.*

Bjerrum's screen (byer′oomz) [J. *Bjerrum,* Danish ophthalmologist, 1827–1892] tangent screen.

Bk chemical symbol for *berkelium.*

black (blak) reflecting no light or true color; of the darkest hue. **animal b., bone-b.,** animal charcoal. **indulin b.,** nigrosin. **ivory b.,** animal charcoal. **lamp b.,** finely divided carbon deposited from the smoky flame of burning oils, rosin, etc. **Paris b.,** animal charcoal.

Black's formula (blaks) [J. A. *Black,* English army surgeon] see under *formula.*

Black's test (blaks) [Otis Fischer *Black,* American chemist, 1867–1933] see under *tests.*

Blackberg and Wanger's test (blak′berg, wang′gerz) [Solon Nathaniel *Blackberg,* Chicago physician, 1897–1962; J. O. *Wanger*] see under *tests.*

black haw (blak haw) see *Viburnum prunifolium* L. (Caprifoliaceae), a North American medicinal plant.

blackhead (blak′hed) 1. a comedo. 2. a disease of turkeys; see *histomoniasis of turkeys*.

blackleg (blak′leg) an acute anaerobic bacterial disease of cattle and sheep producing crepitant swelling in the musculature, caused by *Clostridium chauvoei*. Called also *symptomatic anthrax*, *blackquarter*, and *quarter evil*.

blackout (blak′owt) a condition characterized by failure of vision and momentary unconsciousness, due to diminished circulation to the brain.

blackquarter (blak kwor′ter) blackleg.

blacksnake (blak′snāk) usually *Pseudechis porphyriacus*, a large, semiaquatic, venomous, elapid snake of Australia, whose body is black on top and red underneath. See table accompanying *snake*. Also, *Coluber constrictor*, the American blacksnake or black racer.

blacktongue (blak-tung′) pellagra in dogs.

bladder (blad′der) [L. *vesica, cystis*; Gr. *kystis*] a membranous sac, such as one serving as receptacle for a secretion; often used alone to designate the urinary bladder. Called also *vesica*. **allantoic b.,** a membranous sac formed in amphibians as an outgrowth of the cloaca for the storage of urine. **atonic b.,** a condition marked by a dilated, poorly contracting urinary bladder without evidence of a lesion of the central nervous system. **atonic neurogenic b.,** neurogenic bladder due to destruction of the sensory nerve fibers from the bladder to the spinal cord, marked by the absence of control of bladder functions and of the desire to void, overdistention of the bladder, and an abnormal amount of residual urine; it is most frequently associated with tabes dorsalis (*tabetic b.*) and pernicious anemia, but may be seen in association with other diseases. Called also *paralytic b.* and *sensory paralytic b.* **automatic b.,** neurogenic bladder due to complete transection of the spinal cord above the sacral segments, marked by complete loss of micturition reflexes and bladder sensation, violent involuntary voiding, and an abnormal amount of residual urine. Called also *cord b., reflex b.,* and *spastic b.* **autonomic b.,** autonomous b. **autonomous b.,** neurogenic bladder due to a lesion in the sacral portion of the spinal cord that interrupts the reflex arc which controls the bladder. The lesion may be in the cauda equina, conus medullaris, sacral roots, or pelvic nerve. It is marked by loss of normal bladder sensation and reflex activity, inability to initiate urination normally, and incontinence. Called also *denervated b.* and *nonreflex b.* **chyle b.,** cisterna chyli. **cord b.,** automatic b. **denervated b.,** autonomous b. **double b.,** reduplication of the bladder. **fasciculated b.,** a bladder which, from hypertrophy of the muscular coat, is ridged on its inner surface. **gall b.,** see *gallbladder*. **irritable b.,** a state of the bladder marked by increased frequency of contraction with associated desire to urinate. **motor paralytic b.,** neurogenic bladder due to impairment of the motor neurons or nerves controlling the bladder. The *acute* form is marked by painful distention and inability to initiate micturition, the *chronic* form by difficulty in initiating micturition, straining, decrease in size and force of stream, interrupted stream, and recurrent infection of the urinary tract. **nervous b.,** a colloquial term for a functional condition characterized by a constant desire to urinate without the power to do so completely. **neurogenic b.,** any condition of dysfunction of the urinary bladder caused by a lesion of the central or peripheral nervous system, as *atonic neurogenic b., automatic b., autonomous b., motor paralytic b.,* and *uninhibited neurogenic b.* **nonreflex b.,** autonomous b. **paralytic b.,** atonic neurogenic b. **reflex b.,** automatic b. **sacculated b.,** a bladder with pouches between the hypertrophied muscular fibers. **sensory paralytic b.,** atonic neurogenic b. **spastic b.,** automatic b. **string b.,** a term sometimes erroneously used as a synonym for cord bladder; see *automatic b.* **tabetic b.,** see *atonic neurogenic b.* **uninhibited neurogenic b.,** neurogenic bladder due to a lesion in the region of the upper motor neurons with subtotal interruption of the corticospinal pathways, marked by urgency, frequent involuntary voiding, and small-volume threshold of activity. **urinary b.,** the musculomembranous sac, situated in the anterior part of the pelvic cavity, that serves as a reservoir for urine, which it receives through the ureters and discharges through the urethra. Called also *vesica urinaria* [NA].

Blainville's ear (blah′vēlz) [Henri Marie Ducrotay de *Blainville*, French zoologist, 1777–1850] see under *ear*.

Blake's disks (blākz) [Clarence John *Blake*, Boston otologist, 1843–1919] see under *disk*.

Blalock-Taussig operation (bla′lok taw′sig) [Alfred *Blalock*, American surgeon, 1899–1964; Helen Brooke *Taussig*, American pediatrician, born 1898] see under *operation*.

blanc (blaw) [Fr.] white. **b. fixe,** barium sulfate.

Blanchard's method, treatment (blanch′ardz) [Wallace *Blanchard*, American surgeon, 1848–1922] see under *treatment*.

Blancophor (blank′o-fŏr) trademark for optical whitening agents (blankophores) chemically related to the sulfonamides, which produce brightness by absorbing invisible ultraviolet light and reflecting it as visible blue light. They are added to detergents,

paper, and textiles, and may produce phototoxic effects, e.g., phototoxic dermatitis; they may also produce allergic contact sensitization.

bland (bland) [L. *blandus*] mild or soothing.

Blandin's glands (blah-daz′) [Philippe Frédéric *Blandin*, French surgeon, 1798–1849] see *glandulae linguales anteriores* and *ganglion submandibulares*.

Blandlube (bland′lūb) trademark for a preparation of mineral oil.

blankophore (blank′o-fōr) see *Blancophor*.

Blasius' duct (blah′se-ooz) [Gerhard *Blasius* (Blaes), Dutch anatomist of the 17th century] ductus parotideus.

blast (blast) [Gr. *blastos* germ] 1. an immature stage in cellular development before appearance of the definitive characteristics of the cell; used also as a word termination, as in adamantoblast, hematoblast, neuroblast, etc. See *blasto-*. 2. one of the small filamentous spindles formed by the splitting up of meres. See under *mere*. 3. [Anglo-Saxon *blœst* a puff of wind] the wave of air pressure (*air concussion*) produced by the detonation of a high-explosive bomb, shell or other explosion. A wave of high-pressure velocity (shock wave) is created and this is followed by one of negative decreased velocity, exerting a suction-like action. Blast causes pulmonary concussion and hemorrhage (*lung blast, blast chest*), laceration of other thoracic and abdominal viscera, ruptured ear drums, and minor effects in the central nervous system. **immersion b.,** internal injury to seamen in the water caused by explosion of a depth bomb near them.

blastation (blas-ta′shun) any variation of the germ plasm that is inheritable.

blastema (blas-te′mah) [Gr. *blastēma* shoot] 1. the primitive substance from which cells are formed. 2. a group of cells that give rise to a new individual, in asexual reproduction, or to an organ or part, in either normal development or in regeneration.

blastemic (blas-tem′ik) pertaining to the blastema.

blastid (blas′tid) the site indicative of an organizing nucleus in a fertilized ovum.

blastide (blas′tīd) blastid.

blastin (blas′tin) a substance that stimulates or increases cell proliferation; a substance providing alimentation for cells.

blasto- (blas′to) [Gr. *blastos* germ] a combining form denoting relationship to a bud or budding, particularly to an early embryonic stage, as to a primitive or formative element, cell, or layer.

Blastocaulis (blas″to-kaw′lis) a genus of microorganisms of the family Pasteuriaceae, order Hyphomicrobiales, made up of pear-shaped or globular cells with long slender stalks, attached to a firm substrate in fresh-water environments. The type species is *B. sphaerica*.

blastocele (blas′to-sēl) blastocoele.

blastocelic (blas″to-se′lik) blastocoelic.

blastochyle (blas′to-kīl) [*blasto-* + Gr. *chylos* juice] the fluid contained in the blastocoele.

blastocoele (blas′to-sēl) [*blasto-* + Gr. *koilos* hollow] the fluid-filled cavity of the mass of cells (blastula) produced by cleavage of a fertilized ovum; see illustration under *blastula*. Sometimes spelled *blastocoel*. Called also *cleavage, segmentation,* or *subgerminal cavity*.

blastocoelic (blas″to-se′lik) pertaining to the blastocoele.

blastocyst (blas′to-sist) [*blasto-* + Gr. *kystis* bladder] the mammalian conceptus in the post-morula stage; it is like a blastula in having a fluid-filled cavity, unlike it in having the surface layer not exclusively embryoblast but mainly or entirely trophoblast, in having an eccentric embryoblast, and in not being limited to one germ layer.

Blastocystis (blas″to-sis′tis) a genus of yeasts of uncertain classification. **B. hom′inis,** microorganism appearing as a spherical cystic structure, 5 to 15μ in diameter, frequently found in human feces.

blastocyte (blas′to-sīt) [*blasto-* + Gr. *kytos* hollow vessel] an embryonic cell that has not yet become differentiated.

blastocytoma (blas″to-si-to′mah) blastoma.

Blastodendrion (blas″to-den′dre-on) (obs.) *Candida*.

blastodendriosis (blas″to-den″dre-o′sis) candidiasis.

blastoderm (blas′to-derm) [*blasto-* + Gr. *derma* skin] collectively, the mass of cells produced by cleavage of a fertilized ovum, forming the hollow sphere of the blastula, or the cellular cap above a floor of segmented yolk in the discoblastula of telolecithal eggs; see illustration under *blastula*. Called also *germinal membrane*, or *membrana germinativa*. **bilaminar b.,** the stage of development in which the embryo is represented by two primary layers: the ectoderm and the entoderm. See *gastrula*. **embryonic b.,** the region of the blastoderm forming the embryo proper. **extraembryonic b.,** the region of the blastoderm forming membranes rather than the embryo proper. **trilaminar b.,** the stage of development in which the embryo is represented by the three primary layers: the ectoderm, the mesoderm, and the entoderm.

blastodermal (blas″to-der′mal)   pertaining to or derived from the blastoderm.

blastodermic (blas″to-der′mik)   blastodermal.

blastodisc (blas′to-disk) [*blasto-* + Gr. *diskos* disk]   the convex structure formed by the blastomeres at the animal pole of an ovum undergoing incomplete cleavage.

blastogenesis (blas″to-jen′ĕ-sis)   1. the development of an individual from a blastema, that is, by asexual reproduction.   2. transmission of inherited characters by the germ plasm.   3. the morphological transformation of small lymphocytes into larger cells resembling blast cells, occurring on exposure to phytohemagglutin or to antigens to which the donor is immunized.

blastogenetic (blas″to-jĕ-net′ik)   blastogenic.

blastogenic (blas″to-jen′ik)   originating in the germ or germ cell; pertaining to or characterized by blastogenesis.

blastogeny (blas-toj′ĕ-ne) [*blasto-* + Gr. *genesis* production]   the germ history of an organism or species.

blastokinin (blas″to-ki′nin)   a globulin found in the uterine lumen of some mammals near the time of blastocyst implantation; called also *uteroglobulin.*

blastolysis (blas-tol′ĭ-sis) [*blasto-* + Gr. *lysis* dissolution]   destruction or splitting up of germ substance.

blastolytic (blas″to-lit′ik)   pertaining to, characterized by, or producing blastolysis.

blastoma (blas-to′mah), pl. *blasto′mas* or *blasto′mata* [*blasto-* + *-oma*]   a neoplasm composed of embryonic cells derived from the blastema of an organ or tissue; called also *blastocytoma.*   **pluricentric b.,** a blastoma that arises from a number of scattered cells or groups of cells.   **unicentric b.,** a blastoma arising from one cell or from a single group of cells.

blastomatoid (blas-to′mah-toid) [*blastoma* + Gr. *eidos* form]   resembling blastomas.

blastomatosis (blas″to-mah-to′sis)   the formation of blastomas; tumor formation.

blastomatous (blas-to′mah-tus)   pertaining to or of the nature of blastoma.

blastomere (blas′to-mēr) [*blasto-* + Gr. *meros* a part]   one of the cells produced by cleavage of a fertilized ovum, forming the blastoderm; called also *segmentation sphere* and *cleavage cell.*

blastomerotomy (blas″to-mēr-ot′o-me) [*blastomere* + Gr. *tomē* a cut]   destruction of a blastomere or of blastomeres; called also *blastotomy.*

blastomogenic (blas″to-mo-jen′ik)   producing or tending to produce new growths or tumors.

blastomogenous (blas″to-moj′ĕ-nus)   blastomogenic.

Blastomyces (blas″to-mi′sēz) [*blasto-* + Gr. *mykēs* fungus]   a genus of thermal dimorphic imperfect fungi of the family Moniliaceae, order Moniliales, which grow as mycelial forms at room temperature and as yeastlike forms at body temperature. The term is applied to the yeasts pathogenic for man and animals.   **B. brasilien′sis,** *Paracoccidioides brasiliensis.*   **B. coccidioi′des,** former name for *Coccidioides immitis.*   **B. dermatit′idis,** the etiologic agent of North American blastomycosis; its perfect, or sexual, stage is known as *Ajellomyces dermatitidis.* Formerly called *Cryptococcus gilchristi* and *Endomyces capsulatus, E. epidermatidis,* and *E. epidermidis.*   **B. farcimino′sus,** former name for *Histoplasma farciminosus.*

blastomyces (blas″to-mi′sēz), pl. *blastomyce′tes.*   A fungus of the genus *Blastomyces.*

blastomycete (blas″to-mi′sēt)   any organism of the genus *Blastomyces;* also, any yeastlike organism.

blastomycetes (blas″to-mi-se′tēz)   plural of *blastomyces* and *blastomycete.*

blastomycin (blas″to-mi′sin)   a sterile broth filtrate of a culture of *Blastomyces dermatitidis;* it is injected intracutaneously as a test for blastomycosis.

Blastomycoides immitis (blas″to-mi-koi′dēz im-mi′tis)   former name for *Coccidioides immitis.*

blastomycosis (blas″to-mi-ko′sis)   1. infection caused by organisms of the genus *Blastomyces.*   2. a general term for any infection caused by a yeastlike organism.   **Brazilian b.,** paracoccidioidomycosis.   **cutaneous b.,** see *North American b.*   **European b.,** infection caused by *Cryptococcus neoformans,* especially the cutaneous form of cryptococcosis (q.v.).   **keloidal b.,** an infection caused by *Loboa loboi,* characterized by the appearance of red, smooth, hard cutaneous nodules which, histologically, have the appearance of a keloid. Called also *Lobo's disease.*   **North American b.,** an infection usually acquired through the pulmonary route, caused by *Blastomyces dermatitidis,* and marked by suppurating tumors in the skin (*cutaneous b.*) or by lesions in the lungs, bones, subcutaneous tissues, liver, spleen, and kidneys (*systemic b.*). Called also *Gilchrist's disease* and *Chicago disease.*   **South American b.,** paracoccidioidomycosis.   **systemic b.,** see *North American b.*

blastoneuropore (blas″to-nu′ro-pōr) [*blasto-* + Gr. *neuron* nerve + *poros* opening]   in certain embryos, a temporary aperture formed by the coalescence of the blastopore and neuropore.

blastophthoria (blas″tof-tho′re-ah) [*blasto-* + Gr. *phthora* corruption]   degeneration of the germ cells.

blastophthoric (blas″tof-tho′rik)   pertaining to, characterized by, or producing blastophthoria.

blastophyllum (blas″to-fil′um) [*blasto-* + Gr. *phyllon* leaf]   a primitive germ layer.

blastophyly (blas-tof′ĭ-le) [*blasto-* + Gr. *phylē* tribe]   the tribal history, or arrangement, of organisms.

blastopore (blas′to-pōr) [*blasto-* + Gr. *poros* opening]   the opening of the archenteron to the exterior of the embryo, at the gastrula stage; called also *archistome, protostoma,* and *anus of Rusconi.*

blastosphere (blas′to-sfēr) [*blasto-* + Gr. *sphaira* sphere]   blastula.

blastospore (blas′to-spōr) [*blasto-* + *spore*]   a spore formed by budding, as in yeast.

blastostroma (blas″to-stro′mah)   that part of the egg which takes an active part in the formation of the blastoderm.

blastotomy (blas-tot′o-me)   blastomerotomy.

blastozooid (blas″to-zo′oid) [*blasto-* + Gr. *zōo-eidēs* like an animal]   an individual developed as a result of asexual reproduction. Cf. *oozooid.*

blastula (blas′tu-lah), pl. *blas′tulae* [L.]   the usually spherical structure produced by cleavage of a fertilized ovum, consisting of a single layer of cells (blastoderm) surrounding a fluid-filled cavity (blastocoele); called also *blastosphere.* See also *discoblastula.*

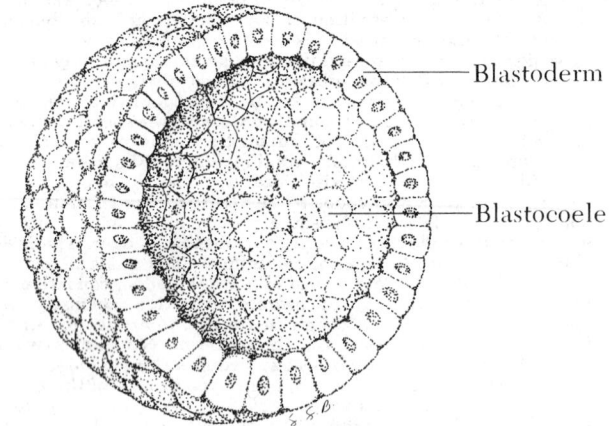

Blastoderm

Blastocoele

Section of a blastula.

blastulae (blas′tu-le) [L.]   plural of *blastula.*

blastular (blas′tu-lar)   pertaining to the blastula.

blastulation (blas″tu-la′shun)   conversion of morula to blastula by development of a central cavity (blastocoele or cleavage cavity).

Blatta (blat′ah) [L.]   a genus of insects—the cockroaches. The dried insects exert diuretic action, but are no longer used in medicine. They may act as the intermediate host of *Raillietina madagascariensis* and *Gongylonema scutatum. B. (Blatella) germanica,* the German roach, now widely distributed, is called the Croton bug. It is light brown in color and small in size. *B. orientalis,* the black beetle, a common European species.

Blaud's pills (blōz) [Pierre *Blaud,* French physician, 1774–1858]   ferrous carbonate pills; see under *pill.*

blaze (blāz)   an abnormal streak or spot of white in the hair of the scalp; called also *leucismus pilorum.*

bleaching (blēch′ing)   the act or process of removing stains or color by chemical means.   **coronal b.,** the use of a chemical agent, usually but not necessarily in combination with heat, to remove discolorations from the crown of a pulpless tooth.

bleb (bleb)   a large flaccid vesicle, usually at least 1 cm. in diameter.

bleeder (blēd′er)   1. one who bleeds freely or is subject to hemorrhagic diathesis.   2. any large blood vessel cut during a surgical procedure.   3. one who lets blood; a phlebotomist.

bleeding (blēd′ing)   1. the escape of blood from an injured vessel.   2. the letting of blood, phlebotomy.   **functional b.,** bleeding from the uterus when no organic lesions are present.   **implantation b.,** bleeding occurring at the time of implantation of the fertilized ovum in the decidua, being due to leakage of blood into the uterine lumen from disrupted blood vessels about the implantation site. Cf. *placentation b.*   **occult b.,** escape of such a small amount of blood that it can be detected only by chemical test or by examination with the microscope or spectroscope.   **placentation b.,** bleeding occurring from the uterus during the early weeks of pregnancy, when the maternal blood vessels are being eroded. Cf. *implantation b.*   **summer b.,** dermatorrhagia parasitica.

blenn-   see *blenno-.*

blennadenitis (blen″ad-ĕ-ni′tis) [*blenn-* + Gr. *adēn* gland + *-itis*] inflammation of mucous glands.

blennaphrosin (blen-af′ro-sin) a preparation of a double salt of potassium nitrate and methenamine with extract of kava-kava; formerly used in gonorrhea and cystitis.

blennemesis (blen-em′ĕ-sis) [*blenn-* + Gr. *emesis* vomiting] the vomiting of mucus.

blenno-, blenn- (blen′no, blen′) [Gr. *blennos* mucus] a combining form denoting relationship to mucus.

blennogenic (blen″no-jen′ik) [*blenno-* + Gr. *gennan* to produce] producing mucus.

blennogenous (blen-noj′ĕ-nus) blennogenic.

blennoid (blen′noid) [*blenn-* + Gr. *eidos* form] resembling mucus.

blennorrhagia (blen″no-ra′je-ah) [*blenno-* + Gr. *rhēgnynai* to break forth] 1. any excessive discharge of mucus; blennorrhea. 2. gonorrhea.

blennorrhagic (blen″no-raj′ik) pertaining to or of the nature of blennorrhagia.

blennorrhea (blen″no-re′ah) [*blenno-* + Gr. *rhoia* flow] a free discharge from the mucous surfaces, especially a gonorrheal discharge from the urethra or vagina; gonorrhea. **b. adulto′rum,** gonorrheal ophthalmia. **inclusion b.,** inclusion conjunctivitis. **b. neonato′rum,** ophthalmia neonatorum. **Stoerk's b.,** blennorrhea with profuse chronic suppuration producing hypertrophy of the mucosa of the nose, pharynx, and larynx.

blennorrheal (blen″no-re′al) pertaining to or of the nature of blennorrhea.

blennostasis (blen-nos′tah-sis) [*blenno-* + Gr. *stasis* standing] the suppression of an abnormal mucous discharge, or the correction of an excessive one.

blennostatic (blen″no-stat′ik) [*blenno-* + Gr. *histanai* to halt] correcting of excessive mucous secretion.

blennothorax (blen″no-tho′raks) [*blenno-* + Gr. *thōrax* chest] an accumulation of mucus in the chest.

blennuria (blen-nu′re-ah) [*blenn-* + Gr. *ouron* urine] the existence of mucus in the urine.

Blenoxane (blen-oks′ān) trademark for a preparation of bleomycin sulfate.

bleomycin (ble-o-mi′sin) a polypeptide antibiotic mixture having antineoplastic properties, obtained from cultures of *Streptomyces verticellus*, or the same substance obtained by other means; it is separable into 13 fractions, including bleomycins A and B and their components. Evidence indicates that bleomycin inhibits cell division, thymidine incorporation into DNA, and DNA synthesis. **b. sulfate,** a mixture of the sulfate salts of the components of bleomycin, especially that of bleomycin A₂. Sterile *bleomycin sulfate* [USP] is used alone or in conjunction with other chemotherapeutic agents in the palliative treatment of squamous cell carcinoma of the head and neck, Hodgkin's disease and other lymphomas, and testicular tumors; administered intravenously, intramuscularly, intra-arterially, or subcutaneously.

Bleph (blef) trademark for preparations of sulfacetamide sodium.

blephar- see *blepharo-*.

blepharadenitis (blef″ar-ad″ĕ-ni′tis) [*blephar-* + Gr. *adēn* gland + *-itis*] inflammation of the meibomian glands; called also *blepharoadenitis*.

blepharal (blef′ah-ral) pertaining to the eyelids.

blepharectomy (blef″ah-rek′to-me) [*blephar-* + Gr. *ektomē* excision] excision of a lesion of the eyelids.

blepharelosis (blef″ah-rel-o′sis) [*blephar-* + Gr. *eilein* to roll] entropion.

blepharism (blef′ah-rizm) [L. *blepharismus*: Gr. *blepharizein* to wink] spasm of the eyelids; continuous blinking.

blepharitis (blef″ah-ri′tis) [*blephar-* + *-itis*] inflammation of the eyelids. **b. angula′ris,** blepharitis ulcerosa affecting the medial commissure (angle) and blocking the punctum lacrimalis. **b. cilia′ris, b. margina′lis,** a chronic inflammation of the hair follicles and sebaceous gland openings of the margins of the eyelids; called also *blear eye, lippa,* and *lippitude.* **nonulcerative b.,** blepharitis often associated with seborrhea of the scalp, brows, and skin behind the ears, marked by greasy scaling of the margins of the lids, scales around the lashes, hyperemia, and thickening; called also *seborrheic b.* and *squamous seborrheic b.* **seborrheic b.,** nonulcerative b. **b. squamo′sa,** a marginal blepharitis in which the edges of the lids are covered with scales. **squamous seborrheic b.,** nonulcerative b. **b. ulcero′sa,** an ulcerous form of marginal blepharitis.

blepharo-, blephar- (blef′ah-ro, blef′ahr) [Gr. *blepharon* eyelid] a combining form denoting relationship to an eyelid or eyelash.

blepharoadenitis (blef″ah-ro-ad″ĕ-ni′tis) blepharadenitis.

blepharoadenoma (blef″ah-ro-ad″ĕ-no′mah) adenoma of the eyelid.

blepharoatheroma (blef″ah-ro-ath″er-o′mah) an encysted tumor or sebaceous cyst of an eyelid.

blepharochalasis (blef″ah-ro-kal′ah-sis) [*blepharo-* + Gr. *chalasis* relaxation] relaxation of the skin of the eyelid, due to atrophy of the intercellular tissue; called also *dermatolysis palpebrarum.*

blepharochromidrosis (blef″ah-ro-kro-mĭ-dro′sis) [*blepharo-* + Gr. *chrōma* color + Gr. *hidrōs* sweat + *-osis*] excretion of a sweat containing pigment from the eyelids, usually of a bluish shade.

blepharoclonus (blef″ah-rok′lo-nus) [*blepharo-* + *clonus*] clonic spasm of the orbicularis oculi muscle, appearing as an increased winking of the eye.

blepharoconjunctivitis (blef″ah-ro-kon-junk″tĭ-vi′tis) inflammation of the eyelids and conjunctiva.

blepharodiastasis (blef″ah-ro-di-as′tah-sis) [*blepharo-* + Gr. *diastasis* separation] excessive separation of the eyelids, causing the fissure to be very wide.

blepharoncus (blef″ah-rong′kus) [*blepharo-* + Gr. *onkos* bulk, mass] a tumor on the eyelid.

blepharopachynsis (blef″ah-ro-pak-in′sis) [*blepharo-* + Gr. *pachynsis* thickening] abnormal thickening of an eyelid.

blepharophimosis (blef″ah-ro-fĭ-mo′sis) [*blepharo-* + Gr. *phimōsis* a muzzling] abnormal narrowness of the palpebral fissures in the horizontal direction, caused by lateral displacement of the inner canthi.

blepharoplast (blef′ah-ro-plast″) [*blepharo-* + Gr. *plassein* to form] basal body.

blepharoplasty (blef′ah-ro-plas″te) plastic surgery of the eyelids.

blepharoplegia (blef″ah-ro-ple′je-ah) [*blepharo-* + Gr. *plēgē* stroke] paralysis of an eyelid (Desmarres); paralysis of both muscles of the eyelid (Graefe-Saemisch).

blepharoptosis (blef″ah-ro-to′sis) [*blepharo-* + Gr. *ptōsis* a fall] drooping of an upper eyelid due to paralysis; ptosis.

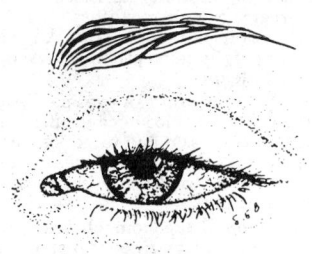

Blepharoptosis.

blepharopyorrhea (blef″ah-ro-pi-ŏ-re′ah) [*blepharo-* + Gr. *pyon* pus + *rhoia* flow] purulent ophthalmia.

blepharorrhaphy (blef″ah-ror′ah-fe) [*blepharo-* + Gr. *rhaphē* suture] the operation of suturing the eyelids together; tarsorrhaphy.

blepharospasm (blef′ah-ro-spazm″) [*blepharo-* + Gr. *spasmos* spasm] tonic spasm of the orbicularis oculi muscle, producing more or less complete closure of the eyelids. **essential b.,** blepharospasm that is present when there is no abnormality of the eye, or trigeminal (fifth cranial) nerve. **symptomatic b.,** blepharospasm occurring in association with a lesion of the eye or of the trigeminal (fifth cranial) nerve.

blepharosphincterectomy (blef″ah-ro-sfingk″ter-ek′to-me) [*blepharo-* + Gr. *sphinktēr* sphincter + *ektomē* excision] excision of some of the fibers of the orbicularis muscle, together with overlying skin, to relieve pressure of the eyelid on the cornea in blepharospasm.

blepharostat (blef′ah-ro-stat″) [*blepharo-* + Gr. *histanai* to cause to stand] an instrument for holding the eyelids and keeping them apart during surgical operations on the eye.

blepharostenosis (blef″ah-ro-stĕ-no′sis) [*blepharo-* + Gr. *stenōsis* a narrowing] an abnormal narrowing of the palpebral slit.

blepharosynechia (blef″ah-ro-sĭ-ne′ke-ah) [*blepharo-* + Gr. *synecheia* a holding together] the growing together or adhesion of the eyelids.

blepharotomy (blef″ah-rot′o-me) [*blepharo-* + Gr. *tomē* a cut] surgical incision of an eyelid; tarsotomy.

blepharoxysis (blef″ah-ro-zi′sis) [*blepharo-* + Gr. *xysis* a polishing] Hippocrates' treatment for trachoma, consisting of rubbing the inner surface of the lid with wool wound round a core of wood, followed by cauterization and instillation of copper peroxide.

Blessig's cysts (spaces), (lacunae), groove (bles′sigz) [Robert *Blessig*, German physician, 1830–1878] see under *cyst* and *groove.*

blight (blīt) any fungal disease of plants.

blind (blīnd) not having the sense of sight; see *blindness.*

blindgut (blīnd′gut) the cecum, def. 1.

blindness (blīnd′nes) lack or loss of ability to see; lack of perception of visual stimuli, due to disorder of the organs of sight or to lesions in certain areas of the brain; see also *amaurosis.* **amnesic color b.,** inability to recognize or to name a hue, although it is correctly perceived. **blue b.,** imperfect perception of the blue spectrum; see *tritanopia.* **blue-yellow b.,** imperfect perception of blue and yellow tints; see *tetartanopia,* def. 2. **Bright's b.,** former term for dimness or complete loss of sight occurring in uremia, without lesion of the retina or optic disk. **color b.,** a term colloquially and incorrectly applied to any deviation from normal perception of hues; see *deuteranopia, protanopia,* etc. **concussion b.,** functional blindness due to violent explosions, as by high explosive shells, bombs, etc. **cortical b.,** blindness due to a lesion of the cortical visual center. **cortical psychic b.,** loss of optic memory image and of spatial orientation due to lesion of the optic lobe. **day b.,** hemeralopia. **epidemic b.,** a form of avian leukosis with blindness and misshapen pupil or irregular depigmentation of the iris in one or both eyes. **flight b.,** amaurosis fugax caused by high centrifugal forces encountered in aviation. **functional b.,** inability to see, occurring without disorder of the organs of sight. **green b.,** imperfect perception of green tints; see *deuteranopia.* **legal b.,** blindness as defined by law; in most states of the United States, maximal visual acuity of the better eye, after correction, of 20/200 or less, with a total diameter of the visual field in that eye of 20 degrees or less. **letter b.,** inability to recognize individual letters. **mind b.,** psychic b. **moon b.,** periodic ophthalmia. **night b.,** nyctalopia, def. 1. **note b.,** inability to read musical notes, due to a lesion of the central nervous system. **object b.,** inability to recognize the nature and purpose of objects seen. **psychic b.,** inability to recognize the nature of the source of visual stimuli, because of some lesion of the brain; called also *mind b.* and *soul b.* **red b.,** imperfect perception of red tints; see *protanopia.* **red-green b.,** imperfect perception of red and green tints. **river b.,** onchocerciasis caused by *Onchocerca volvulus* (q.v.). **snow b.,** dimness of vision, usually temporary, due to the glare of the sun upon snow. **soul b.,** psychic b. **syllabic b.,** inability to recognize syllables. **taste b.,** inability to perceive certain gustatory stimuli, some substances producing no sensation of taste. **text b.,** alexia. **total b.,** complete absence of light perception. **twilight b.,** aknephascopia. **word b.,** alexia.

blister (blis′ter) [L. *vesicula*] a vesicle, especially a bulla. **blood b.,** a vesicle having bloody contents; it may be caused by a pinch or bruise, but is often due to persistent friction. **fever b.,** herpes simplex, usually of the face. **Marochetti's b's,** small blisters seen under the tongue in rabies. **water b.,** one with clear watery contents.

bloat (blōt) 1. tympany of the stomach or cecum. 2. enteritis in young rabbits, accompanied by gaseous distention of the abdomen.

Bloch (blok), Konrad. German biochemist in the United States, born 1912; co-winner, with Feodor Lynen, of the Nobel prize for medicine and physiology in 1964, for investigations in biosynthesis of cholesterol and fatty acids.

Bloch's scale (bloks) [Marcel *Bloch,* French pathologist, 1885–1925] see under *scale.*

Bloch-Sulzberger syndrome (blok-sulz-berg′er) [Bruno *Bloch,* Swiss dermatologist, 1878–1933; Marion Baldur *Sulzberger,* American dermatologist, born 1895] incontinentia pigmenti.

block (blok) 1. an obstruction or stoppage. 2. a term introduced by Romanes to express the obstruction of the passage of muscular or nervous impulses. 3. regional anesthesia; see under *anesthesia.* **adrengeric b.,** see under *blockade.* **air b.,** interference with the normal inflation and deflation of the lungs and with the pulmonary blood flow, produced by the leakage of air from the pulmonary alveoli into the interstitial tissue of the lung (interstitial emphysema) and into the mediastinum (mediastinal emphysema). **alveolar-capillary b.,** interference in the normal diffusion of gases across the membrane between the alveolar spaces and the pulmonary capillaries. **arborization b.,** a gross intraventricular conduction defect in the distal ramifications of the bundle branches. **bundle-branch b.,** see under *heart block.* **caudal b.,** anesthesia produced by injection of a local anesthetic into the caudal or sacral canal. **comparator b.,** see *comparator.* **cryogenic b.,** local cooling of tissue. **dynamic b.,** spinal subarachnoid b. **ear b.,** trauma of the middle ear and the resulting inflammation and pain in compressed-air workers in which the eustachian tube is not patulous; called also *tubal b.* **epidural b.,** anesthesia produced by injection of the anesthetic agent between the vertebral spines and beneath the ligamentum flavum into the extradural space. **field b.,** regional anesthesia obtained by blocking conduction in nerves with chemical or physical agents. **heart b.,** see *heart block,* under *H.* **intercostal b., intercostal nerve b.,** anesthesia produced by blocking intercostal nerves with a local anesthetic. **intranasal b.,** local anesthesia produced by insertion into the nasal fossae of pledgets soaked in a solution of an anesthetic agent that is effective after topical application, or by insufflation of a mixture of anesthetic gases or vapors through a tube introduced into the nose. **intraspinal b.,** subarachnoid b. **mental b.,** obstruction to thought or memory, particularly that produced by emotional factors. **methadone b.,** see *nar-*

cotic blockade, under *blockade.* **Mobitz b.,** dropped beat. **nerve b.,** regional anesthesia secured by making extraneural or paraneural injections of anesthetics in close proximity to the nerve whose conductivity is to be cut off. **paracervical b.,** anesthesia of the inferior hypogastric plexus and ganglia produced by injection of the local anesthetic into the lateral fornices of the vagina; called also *uterosacral b.* **paraneural b.,** anesthesia produced by injection of the anesthetic agent around a nerve. **parasacral b.,** regional anesthesia produced by injection of a local anesthetic around the sacral nerves as they emerge from the sacral foramina. **paravertebral b.,** infiltration of the cervicothoracic (stellate) ganglion with procaine hydrochloride; done for stroke, tachycardia, etc. **peri-infarction b.,** the association of myocardial infarction with surrounding intraventricular conduction disturbance other than left or right bundle-branch block. **perineural b.,** regional anesthesia produced by injection of the anesthetic agent close to the nerve. **presacral b.,** anesthesia produced by injection of the local anesthetic into the sacral nerves on the anterior aspect of the sacrum. **pudendal b.,** anesthesia produced by blocking the pudendal nerves, accomplished by injection of the local anesthetic into the tuberosity of the ischium. **sacral b.,** anesthesia produced by injection of a local anesthetic into the extradural space of the spinal canal. **saddle b.,** the production of anesthesia in a region corresponding roughly with the areas of the buttocks, perineum, and inner aspects of the thighs which impinge on the saddle in riding, by introducing the anesthetic agent low in the dural sac. **sinoatrial b., sinoauricular b.,** a disturbance in which the atrial response is delayed or omitted because of partial or complete interference with the propagation of impulses from the sinoatrial node to the atria. **sinus b.,** 1. pain in the paranasal sinuses due to air being trapped in them in decompression sickness. 2. sinoatrial b. **spinal b.,** subarachnoid b. **spinal subarachnoid b.,** a condition in which the flow of cerebrospinal fluid is interfered with by an obstruction in the spinal canal; called also *dynamic b.* **splanchnic b.,** anesthesia produced by blocking the splanchnic nerves and the celiac ganglia; it is accomplished by injection of the anesthetic agent into the retroperitoneal tissues in the immediate vicinity of the celiac or solar plexuses. **stellate b.,** the analgesic blocking of the stellate (cervicothoracic) ganglion. **subarachnoid b.,** anesthesia produced by the injection of a local anesthetic into the subarachnoid space around the spinal cord; called also *intraspinal b.* and *spinal b.* **sympathetic b.,** blocking of the sympathetic trunk by paravertebral infiltration with an anesthetic agent. **transsacral b.,** anesthesia produced by injection of the anesthetic agent into the sacral canal and about the sacral nerves through each of the posterior sacral foramina. **tubal b.,** ear b. **uterosacral b.,** paracervical b. **vagal b., vagus nerve b.,** blocking of vagal impulses obtained by injection of a solution of local anesthetic into the vagus nerve at its exit from the skull. **ventricular b.,** obstruction to the flow of cerebrospinal fluid within the ventricular system or through the exit foramina (foramina of Magendie and Luschka) by which the ventricles communicate with the subarachnoid space; it results in obstructive hydrocephalus. **Wenckebach b.,** partial heart block in which the ventricular rhythm is irregular, partly because of the changing P-R interval and partly because of dropped beats.

blockade (blok-ād′) 1. the rendering of the reticuloendothelial cells of the body less capable of phagocytosis by the intravenous injection of harmless material, such as carmine, lampblack, etc. 2. the prevention by drugs of certain physiologic or enzymatic actions. 3. the prevention of the effects of certain drugs by an agent, as the effect of nalorphine on heroin action. **adrenergic b.,** selective inhibition of the response to sympathetic impulses and to catecholamines and other adrenergic amines at either the alpha or beta receptor sites of the effector organ or at the postganglionic adrenergic neuron. **adrenergic neuron b.,** see *adrenergic b.* **alpha-adrenergic b., alpha-b.,** see *adrenergic b.* **beta-adrenergic b., beta-b.,** see *adrenergic b.* **cholinergic b.,** selective inhibition of cholinergic nerve impulses at autonomic ganglionic synapses, at postganglionic parasympathetic effectors, or the neuromuscular junction. **narcotic b.,** inhibition of the euphoric effects of narcotic drugs by the use of other drugs, such as methadone, in the treatment of addiction. **renal b.,** obstructive uropathy with involvement of the genitourinary system distal to the collecting tubules; blockade of individual nephrons or nephron groups and the resultant anuria. **virus b.,** interference by a virus with the action of another virus; attenuated virus of a disease has been used to inhibit the multiplication of an active virus. Called also *virus interference* and *cell blockade.*

blockage (blok′ij) the process of blocking or obstructing; the condition of being blocked or obstructed. **tendon b.,** fixation of tendon by a Kirschner wire to bone or tendon sheath to relieve tension and prevent retraction.

Blockain (blok′ān) trademark for a preparation of propoxycaine hydrochloride.

blocker (blok′er) something that blocks or obstructs passage, activity, etc. **α-b.,** a drug that induces adrenergic blockade at α-adrenergic receptors. **β-b.,** a drug that induces adrenergic blockade at either β_1- or β_2-adrenergic receptors or at both.

blocking (blok′ing) 1. the cutting off of an afferent nerve path, as by the injection of cocaine (*cocaine b.*). 2. the inhibition of an intracellular biosynthetic process, as by the injection of dactinomycin (actinomycin D). 3. the freudian term for a sudden stop in an association produced when a complex is touched. 4. the fastening of a histological specimen impregnated with celloidin to a block of wood or other suitable material which may be clamped in the microtome. **adrenergic b.,** see under *blockade.* **b. of thought,** a mental condition in which the patient expresses himself with difficulty, because, as he claims, "the avenues of thought are obstructed"; seen in schizophrenia.

Blocq's disease (bloks) [Paul Oscar *Blocq*, French physician, 1860–1896] astasia-abasia.

Blondlot rays (blond-lo′) [Prosper René *Blondlot*, French physicist, 1849–1930] n rays.

blood (blud) [L. *sanguis, cruor*; Gr. *haima*] the fluid that circulates through the heart, arteries, capillaries, and veins, carrying nutriment and oxygen to the body cells; called also *sangius* [NA]. It consists of a pale yellow liquid, the *plasma*, containing the microscopically visible formed elements of the blood: the erythrocytes, or red blood corpuscles; the leukocytes, or white blood corpuscles; and the thrombocytes, or blood platelets. **aerated b.,** that which carries oxygen to the tissues through the systemic arteries. **anticoagulated b.,** blood that remains fluid due to presence of an anticoagulant. **arterial b.,** aerated b. **central b.,** blood obtained from the pulmonary venous system; some-

times used to designate splanchnic blood, or blood obtained from chambers of the heart or from bone marrow. **cord b.,** blood contained within the umbilical vessels at the time of delivery of the infant. **defibrinated b.,** whole blood from which fibrin was separated during the clotting process. **laky b.,** blood containing at least some lysed erythrocytes. **occult b.,** blood present in such small quantities that it can be detected only by chemical tests of suspected material, or by microscopic or spectroscopic examination. **peripheral b.,** blood obtained from acral areas, or from the circulation remote from the heart, as from earlobe, fingertip, or heel pad (in a child), or from the antecubital vein; the blood in the systemic circulation. **sludged b.,** blood in which the red cells have become aggregated into masses; it occurs particularly in the smaller blood vessels, where the velocity of blood flow is diminished. **splanchnic b.,** a general term applied to blood in the thoracic, abdominal, and pelvic viscera; further distinguished, in the case of blood from a specific organ, by the appropriate modifier, e.g., pulmonary, hepatic, or splenic blood. **venous b.,** blood that has given up its oxygen to the tissues and carries carbon dioxide back through the systemic veins for gas-exchange in the lungs. **whole b.,** blood from which none of the elements have been removed. *Whole blood* [USP] or *whole human blood* is blood that has been drawn from a selected donor under strict aseptic conditions, containing citrate ion or heparin as an anticoagulant, and used as a blood replenisher.

blood bank (blud bangk) see *bank.*

HUMAN BLOOD GROUP SYSTEMS AND ERYTHROCYTIC ANTIGENIC DETERMINANTS

Antigenic determinants are systematized according to observed and assumed independent assortment of their responsible genes. Within many systems, alleles are responsible for differing combinations of antigenic determinants.

BLOOD GROUP SYSTEM	ANTIGENIC DETERMINANTS*
ABO	A, A_1, B
H	H
I	I, i, I^T, I^D, I^F
MN	M, N, S, s, U, Clᵃ, Far, He, Hill, Hu, Mᴬ, Mᶜ, Mᵉ, Mᵍ, M₁, Miᵃ, Mtᵃ, Mur, Mᵛ, Nyᵃ, Riᵃ, Sᴮ, Sj, Stᵃ, Sul, Tm, Uᴮ, Vr, Vw, Nᴬ, Z
P	P1, P2 (Tjᵃ), P3 (Pᴷ)
Rh	Rh1 (D, Rh₀), Rh2 (C, rh′), Rh3 (E, rh″), Rh4 (c, hr′), Rh5 (e, hr″), Rh6 (f, ce, hr), Rh7 (Ce, rhᵢ), Rh8 (Cᵂ, rhᵂ¹), Rh9 (Cˣ, rhˣ), Rh10 (V, ceˢ, hrᵛ), Rh11 (Eᵂ, rhᵂᶻ), Rh12 (G, rhᴳ), Rh13 (Rhᴬ), Rh14 (Rhᴮ), Rh15 (Rhᶜ), Rh16 (Rhᴰ), Rh17 (Hr₀), Rh18 (Hr), Rh19 (hrˢ), Rh20 (VS, eˢ), Rh21 (Cᴳ), Rh22 (CE), Rh23 (Dᵂ), Rh24 (Eᵀ), Rh26, Rh27 (cE), Rh28 (hrᴴ), Rh29 (RH), Rh30 (Goᵃ), Rh31 (hrᴮ), Rh32, Rh33
Lutheran	Luᵃ (Lu1), Luᵇ (Lu2), Luᵃᵇ (Lu3), Lu4, Lu5, Lu6, Lu7, Lu8, Lu9, Lu10, Lu11, Lu12, Lu13, Lu14 (Swᵃ)
Kell	K1 (K), K2 (k), K3 (Kpᵃ), K4 (Kpᵇ), K5 (Ku), K6 (Jsᵃ), K7 (Jsᵇ), K8 (kw), K9 (KL), K10 (U1ᵃ), K11, K12, K13, K14, K15, K16
Lewis	Leᵃ (Le1), Leᵇ (Le2), Leˣ (Leᵃᵇ, Le3), Mag (Le4), Leᶜ (Le5), Leᵈ
Duffy	Fyᵃ (Fy1), Fyᵇ (Fy2), Fyᵃᵇ (Fy3), Fy4
Kidd	Jkᵃ (Jk1), Jkᵇ (Jk2), Jkᵃᵇ (Jk3)
Cartwright	Ytᵃ, Ytᵇ
Xg	Xgᵃ
Dombrock	Doᵃ, Doᵇ
Auberger	Auᵃ
Cost-Sterling	Csᵃ, Ykᵃ
Wright	Wrᵃ, Wrᵇ
Diego	Diᵃ, Diᵇ
Vel	Vel 1, Vel 2
Sciana	Sm, Buᵃ
Bg	Bgᵃ, Bgᵇ, Bgᶜ, Ho, Ho-like, Ot, Sto, DBG (similar to HL-A7 of lymphocytes)
Gerbich	Ge1, Ge2, Ge3 (anti-Gel = M.Y.; anti-Ge1,2 = Ge; anti-Ge1,2,3 = Yus)
Coltan	Coᵃ, Coᵇ
Stoltzfus	Sfᵃ

Low-incidence antigenic determinants not thus far associated with a blood group system:

Beᵃ, Bec, Bi, Big Charles, Bpᵃ, Bxᵃ, By, Cad, Chrᵃ, Coates, Craig, Dahl, Donaviesky, Driver, Duch, Evans, Evelyn, Fin, Fuerhart, Gfᵃ, Gilbraith, Good, Green, Hands, Heibel, Hil, Htᵃ, Jeᵃ, Jnᵃ, Job, Kam, Ken, Kosis, Lev, Lwᵃ, McCall, Man, Mar, Moᵃ, Nij, Orr, Ptᵃ, Rdᵃ, Reid, Rm, Skjelbred, Thᵃ, Toᵃ, Trᵃ, Ven, Wb, Weeks, Wu, Yhᵃ, Za, 754

High-incidence antigenic determinants not thus far associated with a blood group system:

Anᵃ, Atᵃ, Bou, Bra, Car, Chido (Gursha), Cip, Dp, El, Enᵃ, Fuj, Gnᵃ Goᵇ, Gyᵃ, Hen, Hy, Joᵃ, Jr, Kelly, Knops, Lan, MZ443, Ola, Pea Savior, Sch, Sdᵃ, Simon, Ters, Todd, Vennera, Wil, Winbourne

Antigenic determinants that depend on gene interactions:

ABO/I	IH, IA, IB, iH
P/I	IP1, IP2(ITⱼᵃ), IᵀP1, iP1
Lewis/I	ILeᵇʰ
Lewis/ABO	A₁Leᵇ
P/ABO	Luke
Xor/Duffy	Fy5
Rh/LW	Rh25 (LW)

*Symbols within parentheses are those of alternative nomenclatures.
(Compiled by Dr. Fred H. Allen, Jr.)

Bloodgood's disease (blud′goodz) [Joseph Colt *Bloodgood*, Baltimore surgeon, 1866–1935] cystic disease of the breast; see under *disease*.

blood group (blud′ groop) 1. an erythrocytic allotype (or phenotype) defined by one or more cellular antigenic structural groupings under the control of allelic genes. Erythrocytic antigenic determinants irregularly incite allotypic and sometimes xenotypic immune responses. Blood groups, especially for man, are identified by agglutination supported by specific human or animal antisera and by lectins extracted from certain plants. Bovine blood group reactions, however, are usually lytic. An abbreviated classification of human blood groups is given in the accompanying table. 2. any characteristic, function, or trait of a cellular or fluid component of blood, considered as the expression (phenotype or allotype) of the actions and interactions of dominant genes, and useful in medicolegal and other studies of human inheritance. Such characteristics include the antigenic groupings of erythrocytes, leukocytes, platelets, and plasma proteins. Called also *blood type*. **ABO b. g.,** the major human blood type system, which depends on the presence or absence of two antigenic structures, A and B. The gene for A is responsible for synthesis *N*-acetyl-α-D-galactosaminyl transferase, whereas that for B is responsible for α-D-galactosyl transferase. Either A or B is created when one of these hexasaccharides is positioned by a specific transferase in $1 \rightarrow 3$ linkage to the β-D-galactose of an H-active oligosaccharide. Type O occurs when neither transferase is present or, very rarely (Bombay type), when H does not exist. When both transferases are present, type AB results. Differences in degree of transferase activity are determined at the same locus: weak transferase give rise to weak antigens (A_2, A_3 A_x, B_3 B_x). Similar oligosaccharides, especially in bacterial cell walls, immunize persons lacking A or B so that their serum contains anti-A or anti-B activity. A and B antigens are on the mucopolysaccharides of secretors; persons with dominant genes have H-active mucoids. A and B are largely glycolipids in the red cell membrane. **Auberger b. g.,** Au^a, related to the Lutheran blood group. **Cartwright b. g.,** erythrocytic antigens Yt^a and Yt^b. **Diego b. g.,** the blood group antigens Di^a and Di^b, determined by allelic genes. Di^a is most frequent in South American Indians, Japanese, and Chinese. **Dombrock b. g.,** an erythrocytic antigen commonest in whites (65 per cent) but not rare elsewhere. **Duffy b. g.,** a blood group consisting principally of the antigens Fy^a and Fy^b, determined by allelic genes. Amorphic genes are common in Negroes. **high frequency b. g.,** erythrocytic antigens found over 99 per cent of individuals; hence, also known as *public antigens*. **I b. g.,** that involving receptors of most cold reactive hemagglutinins; it is best expressed on cells of almost all normal adults, but is strongest on cord blood cells. **Kell b. g.,** multiple red cell antigens, especially three pairs of alternates, determined by complex genes at one locus, including an amorph; also regulated by the X chromosome, it is associated with sex-linked chronic granulomatous disease. One antigen, K6, is more frequent in Negroes. **Kidd b. g.,** a group consisting principally of Jk^a and Jk^b antigens, determined by allelic genes; amorphic genes are commonest in Orientals. **Lewis b. g.,** a blood group determined by plasma glycolipids which adhere to erythrocytic surfaces. It is based on dominant independent *Le* genes, but interacts with the H precursor oligosaccharides of A and B. Whereas *le/le* provides the "double negative" blood type Le (a–b–), *Le* without H gives rise to Le^a, i.e., blood type Le (a+b–) and with H gives rise to Le^bH, i.e., blood type Le(a–b+). **low frequency b. g.,** erythrocytic antigens found in fewer than 1 per cent of individuals; also known as *private antigens*. **Lutheran b. g.,** a complex system somewhat resembling the Kell group in having pairs of alternative antigens and amorphic genes, but also subject to a dominant independently segregating repressor. **MN b. g.,** a complex system (MNSs) consisting principally of two pairs of antigens determined by closely linked genes (crossovers have been observed, but rarely). M and N, determined by allelic genes, depend on sialic (neuraminic) acid residues. S and s are also determined by allelic genes, and an amorphic gene is common in Negroes when another antigen (U) is missing. The system also includes numerous low frequency antigens. **P b. g.,** a system originally consisting of only P (now P1) but found to include P2 (Tj^a), a very high frequency antigen, and P3 (P^K), a very low frequency antigen. P1 is most common in Negroes (90 per cent), less common in Caucasians (75 per cent) and least common in Orientals (30 per cent). **Rh b. g.,** the most complex of all human blood groups because the genes differ by determining a different number of the 33 antigens thus far described, and do so with remarkably different quality. Negroes show the greatest degree of diversity, Orientals the least. The major antigen, Rh1 (Rh_o,D), is highly immunogenic and, before the development of passive immunization prophylaxis, was responsible for serious hemolytic disease of the newborn. Two other pairs of alternative antigens are inherited with or without Rh1; these are Rh21 (rh^G, C^G) and Rh4 (hr′, c), and Rh3 (rh″, E) and Rh5 (hr″, e). The commonest groups of antigens are $R^{1,-3,-21}$ (in Caucasians), $R^{1,-3,-21}$ (in Negroes), $R^{1,-3,21}$ (in Orientals and Caucasians), and $R^{1,3,-21}$ (in Orientals and Caucasians). Another antigen Rh10 (hr^v, V) is common in Negroes.

bloodless (blud′les) 1. deprived of blood; anemic or exsanguinate. 2. performed with little or no loss of blood.

blood plasma (blud plaz′mah) the liquid portion of the blood in which the particulate components are suspended; see *blood*.

blood pressure (blud presh′ur) see under *pressure*.

bloodroot (blud′root) sanguinaria.

blood serum (blud se′rum) the clear liquid that separates from the blood when it is allowed to clot completely. It is therefore blood plasma from which fibrinogen has been removed in the process of clotting. **alkaline b. s.,** blood serum to which sodium hydroxide has been added, consisting mostly of alkali albuminate. **coagulated b. s.,** plain blood serum from the horse, cow, sheep, dog, or other animal, coagulated and sterilized at a temperature not above 80° C. **Councilman and Mallory's b. s.,** blood serum coagulated in a hot-air sterilizer and sterilized with steam. **glycerin b. s.,** blood serum containing glycerin; called also *glycerin culture medium*. **inspissated b. s.,** blood serum heated to coagulation, usually in test tubes and in an inclined position. **Löffler's b. s.,** nutrient bouillon containing dextrose and blood serum, mixed, and heat-coagulated in an inclined position; called also *Löffler's serum* or *culture medium*. **Lorrain Smith's b. s.,** blood serum containing sodium hydroxide.

blood type (blud′ tīp) see *blood group*.

Bloor's method test [Walter Ray *Bloor*, American biochemist, born 1877] see under *method* and *test*.

blotch (bloch) a blemish or spot.

blowpipe (blo′pīp) a tube through which a current of air or other gas is forced upon a flame to concentrate and intensify the heat.

B.L.R.O.A. British Laryngological, Rhinological, and Otological Association.

blue (bloo) 1. one of the principal colors of the spectrum, the color of the sky. 2. having the color of the clear sky. 3. a dye that is blue in color. **alcian b.,** a copper-containing dye for staining acid mucopolysaccharides; it may be combined with periodic acid–Schiff reagent. **alizarin b.,** a blue dyestuff derived from anthracene. **alkali b.,** a dye, sodium triphenyl-rosaniline monosulfate; called also *isamine b*. **aniline b.,** a mixture of the trisulfonates of triphenyl rosaniline and diphenyl rosaniline; also known variously as *anthracene b., China b., marine b., soluble b.* (3*M* or 2*R*), and *water b*. **aniline b., W. S.,** a mixture of the sulfonation products of mixtures of phenylated rosaniline and pararosaniline, soluble in water. **anthracene b.,** alizarin b. **azidine b., 3 B.,** trypan b. **benzamine b., 3 B.,** trypan b. **benzo b.,** trypan b. **Berlin b.,** Prussian b. **Borrel's b.,** a silver oxide stain for spirochetes. **brilliant b., C.,** brilliant cresyl b. **brilliant cresyl b.,** an oxazin dye, usually $C_{15}H_{16}N_3OCl$, used in staining blood; called also *C. brilliant b.* and *cresyl b. 2R. N* or *B. B. S.* **bromchlorphenol b.,** an indicator, dibrom-dichlor-phenol-sulfonphthalein, $(C_6H_2ClBrOH)_2 \cdot C_6H_4 \cdot SO_2ONa$. **bromophenol b.,** a dye, tetrabromophenolsulfonphthalein, used as an indicator in determining hydrogen ion concentration, being yellow at pH 3 and blue at pH 4.6. **bromothymol b.,** a dye, dibromothymolsulfonphthalein, used as an indicator in determining hydrogen ion concentration; it has a pH range of 6.0 to 7.6, being yellow at 6.0 and blue at 7.6. **china b.,** aniline b. **chlorazol b., 3 B.,** trypan b. **Congo b., 3 B.,** trypan b. **cresyl b., 2 R. N.** or **B. B. S.,** brilliant cresyl b. **cyanol b.,** a bright blue acid coal tar color related to triphenylmethane. **diamine b.,** trypan b. **dianil b., H. 3 G.,** trypan b. **Evans b.,** a green, bluish green, or brown odorless powder, $C_{34}H_{24}N_6Na_4O_{14}S_4$, injected intravenously in determining blood volume; called also *T-1824*. **Helvetia b.,** methyl b. **indigo b.,** indigotin. **indigo b., soluble,** indigotin disulfonate sodium. **indophenol b.,** the blue pigment produced in the Nadi reaction and in the indophenol test; it is $(CH_3)_2N \cdot C_6H_4 \cdot N:C_{10}H_6:O$. **isamine b.,** alkali b. **Kühne's methylene b.,** a mixture of methylene blue and dehydrated alcohol in phenol solution. **Löffler's methylene b.,** a mixture of methylene blue and alcohol in aqueous solution of potassium hydroxide. **marine b.,** aniline b. **methyl b.,** a dark blue powder, sodium triphenyl-para-rosaniline sulfonate, formerly used as an antiseptic. Called also *Helvetia b*. **methylene b.** [USP], 3,7-bis(dimethylamino)phenazothionium chloride. Dark green crystals or crystalline powder having a bronze-like luster, $C_{16}H_{18}ClN_3S \cdot 3H_2O$, used as a stain and as an indicator; also used as an antidote in cyanide poisoning, and in treatment of methemoglobinemia. Called also *Swiss b.* and *methylthionine chloride*. **methylene b., N. N.,** new methylene blue, N. **methylene b., O.,** toluidine blue, O. **naphthamine b., 3 B. X.,** trypan b. **new methylene b., N.,** $C_2H_5 \cdot NH(CH_3)C_6-H_2(SN)C_6H_2(CH_3)N(C_2H_5)HCl$. Called also *methylene blue, N. N.* **Niagara b., 3 B.,** trypan b. **Nile b., A.,** Nile b. sulfate, an oxazin dye which stains fatty acids blue; it is $(C_2H_5)_2N \cdot C_6H_3-(ON)C_{10}H_5 \cdot NH_2 \cdot (SO_4)_{\frac{1}{2}}$. **polychrome methylene b.,** a mixture of methylene green, methylene azure, methylene violet, and methylene blue. **Prussian b.,** an amorphous blue powder, $Fe_4[Fe(CN)_6]_3$; called also *Berlin b*. **pyrrole b.,** $C_4H_4N \cdot C-[C_6H_4 \cdot N(CH_3)_2]_2$. **quinaldine b.,** chemical name: 1-ethyl-2-[3-(1-ethyl-2(1*H*)quinolylidene)propenyl]quinolinium chloride. A bright blue-green stain, $C_{25}H_{25}ClN_2$, used in the cytodiagnosis of ruptured fetal membranes. **soluble b., 3 M.** or **2 R.,** aniline

b. **spirit b.,** a mixture of diphenylrosaniline, $C_6H_5 \cdot NHCl \cdot C_6H_4 \cdot C[C_6H_3(CH_3)NH_2]C_6H_4 \cdot NH \cdot C_6H_5$, and triphenylrosaniline, $C_6H_5 \cdot NHCl \cdot C_6H_4C$ $[C_6H_4(CH_3)NH \cdot C_6H_5]$ $C_6H_4 \cdot NH \cdot C_6H_5$. **Swiss b.,** methylene b. **thymol b.,** an indicator, thymolsulfonphthalein, with an acid pH range of 1.2 to 2.8, being red at 1.2 and yellow at 2.8, and an alkaline pH range of 8.0 to 9.6, being yellow at 8.0 and blue at 9.6. **toluidine b., toluidine b., O,** the chloride salt or zinc chloride double salt of aminodimethylaminotoluphenazthionium chloride; useful as a stain for demonstrating basophilic and metachromatic substances. Called also *methylene blue, O.* **trypan b.,** an acid, azo dye that has been used in vital staining and as a remedy in protozoan infections; it is the sodium salt of toluidin-diazo-diamino-naphthol-disulfonic acid, $[CH_3 \cdot C_6H_3 \cdot N:N \cdot C_{10}H_3(NH_2)(SO_2 \cdot ONa)_2 \cdot OH]_2$. Variously known as *azidine b., 3 B; benzamine b., 3 B; benzo b.; chlorazol b.; Congo b., 3 B; diamine b.; dianil b., H. 3G.; naphthamine b., 3 B. X.;* and *Niagara b., 3 B. X.* **Victoria b.,** a triphenylmethane dye with bacteriostatic properties; it is a phenyltetramethyltriaminotriphenylmethane chloride, $C_6H_5 \cdot NH(Cl)C_6H_4:C$ $[C_6H_4 \cdot N(CH_3)_2]_2Cl$. **b. vitriol,** cupric sulfate. **water b.,** aniline blue.

bluensomycin (blu″en-so-mi′sin) an antibiotic substance obtained from cultures of *Streptomyces bluensis*, or the same substance produced by other means.

bluestone (blu′stōn) cupric sulfate.

Blum's reagent, test (bloomz) [Léon *Blum*, German physician, 1878–1930] see under *tests*.

Blum's syndrome (bloomz) [Paul *Blum*, Strasbourg physician, 1878–1933] hypochloremic azotemia.

Blumberg's sign (blum′bergz) [Jacob Moritz *Blumberg*, surgeon and gynecologist in Berlin, and later in London, 1873–1955] see under *sign*.

Blumenau's nucleus (bloo′men-owz) [Leonid Wassiljewitsch *Blumenau*, Russian neurologist, 1862–1931] see under *nucleus*.

Blumenbach's clivus, plane, process (bloo′men-bahks) [Johann Friederich *Blumenbach*, German physiologist, 1752–1840] see *clivus* and *processus uncinatus ossis ethmoidalis*, and see under *plane*.

Blumenthal's disease (bloo′men-tahlz) [Ferdinand *Blumenthal*, German physician, born 1870] erythroleukemia.

blunthook (blunt′hook) an instrument used mainly in embryotomy.

blush (blush) sudden, brief erythema of the face and neck, resulting from vascular dilatation due to emotion or heat.

Blutene (bloo′tēn) trademark for a preparation of tolonium.

Blyth's test [Alexander Wynter *Blyth*, English physician, 1844–1921] see under *tests*.

B.M. abbreviation for L. *bal′neum ma′ris* (seawater bath); Bachelor of Medicine.

B.M.A. British Medical Association.

B.M.R. basal metabolic rate.

B.M.S. Bachelor of Medical Science.

BNA abbreviation for *Basle Nomina Anatomica*, the anatomical terminology accepted at Basel, Switzerland, in 1895; superseded by *Nomina Anatomica*.

B.O.A. British Orthopaedic Association.

board (bord) 1. a long flat piece of wood or other material. 2. a group of administrators or experts serving a special function. **angle b.,** in dental radiology, a device used to facilitate the establishment of reproducible angular relationships between a patient's head and the plane of an x-ray film.

Boas' algesimeter, etc. (bo′az) [Ismar Isidor *Boas*, physician in Berlin, 1858–1938] see under *algesimeter, point, test,* and *test meal*.

Boas-Oppler bacillus (lactobacillus) (bo′az op′ler) [Ismar Isidor *Boas*; Bruno *Oppler*, German physician] see under *bacillus*.

Bobroff's operation (bob′rofs) [V. F. *Bobroff*, Russian surgeon, born 1858] see under *operation*.

Bochdalek's foramen (gap, sinus), ganglion (pseudoganglion), hernia, valve (bok′dal-eks) [Vincent Alexander *Bochdalek*, anatomist in Prague, 1801–1883] see *hiatus pleuroperitonealis* and *plexus dentalis superior*, and see under *hernia* and *valve*.

Bock's ganglion, nerve (boks) [August Carl *Bock*, German anatomist, 1782–1833] see *carotid ganglion*, under *ganglion*, and see *rami pharyngei nervi vagi*, under *ramus*.

Bockhart's impetigo (bok′harts) [Max *Bockhart*, German physician of the nineteenth century] see under *impetigo*.

Bodansky unit (bo-dan′ske) [Aaron *Bodansky*, American biochemist, 1887–1961] see under *unit*.

bodenplatte (bo″den-plaht′tĕ) [Ger.] floor plate.

Bodo (bo′do) a genus of small, ovoid, plastic, biflagellate protozoa of the family Bodonidae, order Protomastigida; called also *Cystomonas* and *Prowazekia*. **B. cauda′tus,** a common coprozoic flagellate with a highly flattened body that usually tapers at the posterior end; found in stagnant water and in human feces.

B. sal′tans, the "springing monad" that has been found in ulcers. **B. urina′ria,** a species found in urine.

Bodonidae (bo-don′ĭ-de) a family of probably nonpathogenic flagellate protozoa of the order Protomastigida, class Zoomastigophora, characterized by the presence of two flagella, one projecting forward and the other trailing backward, and by the absence of an undulating membrane; it is commonly found in stagnant water, as well as in both fresh and salt water, in sewage, and in the digestive tract and feces of various animals, including man. It includes the genera *Bodo, Pleuromons, Proteromonas,* and *Retortamonas.*

body (bod′e) 1. the trunk, or animal frame, with its organs. 2. a cadaver or corpse. 3. the largest and most important part of any organ; see also *corpus* and *soma.* 4. any mass or collection of material. **acetone b's,** ketone b's. **adipose b. of cheek,** corpus adiposum buccae. **adipose b. of ischiorectal fossa,** corpus adiposum fossae ischiorectalis. **adipose b. of orbit,** corpus adiposum orbitae. **adrenal b.,** adrenal gland. **alkapton b's,** a class of substances with an affinity for alkali, found in the urine and causing the condition known as alkaptonuria; the compound commonly found, and most commonly referred to by the term, is homogentisic acid. **Amato b's,** irregular, pale-staining, blue cytoplasmic clumps, occurring in neutrophils of patients with various infectious diseases, such as diphtheria, scarlet fever, and pneumonia, and probably identical with Döhle bodies. **amygdaloid b.,** corpus amygdaloideum. **amylaceous b's, amyloid b's,** corpora amylacea. **anaphylactic reaction b.,** anaphylactin. **anococcygeal b.,** ligamentum anococcygeum. **anti-immune b., anti-intermediary b.,** antiantibody. **aortic b's,** small neurovascular structures on either side of the aorta in the region of the aortic arch; they contain chemoreceptors that play a role in reflex regulation of respiration by responding to changes in oxygen, carbon dioxide, and hydrogen ion concentration in the blood. Called also *glomera aortica.* **apical b.,** acrosome. **b's of Arantius,** nodules of aortic valve; see *noduli valvularum semilunarium.* **Arnold's b's** (*obs.*), small pieces of erythrocytes in the blood, or red cell shadows. **asbestos b's, asbestosis b's,** golden yellow bodies of various shapes formed by the deposition of calcium and iron salts and proteins on a spicule of asbestos, occurring in the sputum, lung secretion, and feces of patients with asbestosis. Cf. *ferruginous b's.* **Aschoff b's,** submiliary collections of cells and leukocytes in the interstitial tissues of the heart in rheumatic myocarditis; called also *Aschoff's nodules.* **asteroid b.,** an irregularly star-shaped inclusion body found in the giant cells in sarcoidosis and also found in numerous other diseases. **Auer b's,** finely granular, lamellar bodies having acid-phosphatase activity, found in the cytoplasm of myeloblasts, myelocytes, monoblasts, and granular histiocytes, rarely in plasma cells, absent in lymphoblasts or lymphocytes, and virtually pathognomonic of leukemia. **Babès-Ernst b's,** metachromatic granules. **Balbiani's b.,** yolk nucleus. **Balfour b's,** *Aegyptianella pullorum.* **bamboo b's,** asbestos b's. **Barr b.,** sex chromatin. **Bartonia b's,** *Bartonella bacilliformis.* **basal b.,** a small cylindrical thickening at the base of each cilium and flagellum, consisting of nine triplets of microtubules around the edge of the cylinder from which extend the cilium and flagellum; basal bodies originate from centrioles which replicate and migrate to the plasma membrane. Called also *basal corpuscle, basal granule,* and *blepharoplast.* **Behla's b's,** Plimmer's b's. **Bence Jones b's,** Bence Jones protein; see under *protein.* **bigeminal b's** (*obs.*), superior and inferior colliculi. **Bollinger's b's,** inclusion bodies found in all tissue cells in fowlpox; called also *Bollinger's granules.* Cf. *Borrel b's.* **Borrel b's,** minute granules composing the Bollinger bodies of fowlpox. **Bracht-Wächter b's,** nonspecific inflammatory foci of lymphocytic and mononuclear cells in the myocardium, observed in bacterial endocarditis. **brassy b.,** a dark, shrunken blood corpuscle seen in malaria. **Buchner's b's,** defensive proteins. **Cabot's ring b's,** lines in the form of loops or figures of eight, seen in stained erythrocytes in severe anemias; they are stained red with the Wright-Leishman stain and blue with eosinate of methylthionine chlorides. **Call-Exner b's,** the accumulations of densely staining material that appear among granulosa cells in maturing ovarian follicles and that may be intracellular precursors of follicular fluid. **cancer b's,** see *Plimmer's b's,* and *Russell b's.* **carotid b.,** a small neurovascular structure lying in the bifurcation of the right and left carotid arteries; it contains chemoreceptors that monitor the oxygen content of the blood and help to regulate respiration. Called also *glomus caroticum.* **cavernous b. of clitoris,** corpus cavernosum clitoridis. **cavernous b. of penis,** corpus cavernosum penis. **cell b.,** that portion of a cell which contains the nucleus independent of any such projections as an axon or dendrites which the cell may have. **central b.,** the structures at the center of the aster during mitosis. **chromaffin b.,** paraganglion. **chromatin b's,** chromatinic b's. **chromatinic b's,** aggregates of deoxyribonucleic acid found in bacterial cells, and demonstrable by staining with Giemsa following hydrolysis of cytoplasmic ribonucleic acid and osmic acid fixation. They are tentatively regarded as representing a morphologically discrete bacterial nucleus. **chromatoid b.,** 1. one of the deeply staining rodlike bodies with rounded extremities found in the cysts of certain amebas; called also *chromatoidal bar.* 2. a dense chromatoid mass near the distal centriole of a spermatozoon, from which the so-called ring centriole seemingly arises. **chromophilous b's,** Nissl b's. **ciliary b.,** corpus ciliare. **coccoid x b's,** minute bodies found in the blood in psittacosis. **coccygeal b.,** glomus coccygeum. **colostrum b's,** colostrum corpuscles. **Councilman b's,** acidophilic round bodies of hepatocellular origin seen in viral hepatitis, yellow fever, and other hepatic diseases; called also *Councilman's lesions.* **crystalloid b.,** a body seen near the nuclei of the cells of the seminiferous tubules. **cytoid b's,** globular, shiny white structures resembling cell nuclei in size and shape, appearing in degenerated retinal nerve fibers; seen histologically in cotton-wool spots. **Deetjen's b's,** blood platelets. **demilune b.,** achromocyte. **dense b's,** small regions of increased density in the sarcoplasm of skeletal muscles to which myofilaments seem to attach; cf. *attachment plaques,* under *plaque.* **dentate b. of cerebellum** (*obs.*), nucleus dentatus. **dentate b. of medulla oblongata** (*obs.*), nucleus olivaris. **denticulate b.** (*obs.*), gyrus dentatus. **Döhle's b's, Döhle's inclusion b's,** discrete, round or oval, blue-staining inclusions seen in the periphery of the cytoplasm of neutrophils, consisting mainly of RNA derived from rough endoplasmic reticulum, found in association with many infections, burns, aplastic anemia, uncomplicated pregnancy, and after administration of toxic agents. Similar structures, which are often larger and more prominent, are present in granulocytes other than neutrophils in the May-Hegglin anomaly. Called also *leukocyte inclusions.* **Donné's b's,** colostrum corpuscles. **Donovan's b's,** *Calymmatobacterium granulomatis.* **Ehrlich's hemoglobinemic b's** (*obs.*), dark bodies, occurring in the center of degenerated red cells but which do not represent true red cell inclusions. **elementary b.,** 1. a blood platelet. 2. an inclusion body. **Elschnig b's,** clear grapelike clusters formed by proliferation of epithelial cells after extracapsular extraction of a cataractous lens; called also *Elschnig's pearls.* **Elzholz's b's,** bodies described by Elzholz in degenerated medullated nerve fibers. **end b.,** see *complement.* **epithelial b.,** parathyroid gland. **falciform b.,** sporozoite. **ferruginous b's,** structures similar to asbestos bodies, composed of a central mineral filament coated with a protein-iron complex. **fibrin b's of pleura,** movable or adherent, round, homogeneous, sharply demarcated opacities near the base of the pleural cavity, which may occur secondary to pleural effusion, pneumothorax, or hemopneumothorax; called also *pleural fibrin balls.* **filling b's,** fullkörper. **flagellated b.,** the male gametocyte of the malarial parasite, *Plasmodium.* **foreign b.,** a mass or particle of material that is not normal to the place where it is found. **b. of fornix,** corpus fornicis. **fruiting b.,** a specialized structure, as an apothecium, which produces spores; see Plate accompanying *mold.* **fuchsin b's,** Russell's b's. **gamma-Favre b's,** small intracytoplasmic inclusion bodies found in lymphogranuloma venereum. **geniculate b.,** see *corpus geniculatum laterale* and *corpus geniculatum mediale.* **Giannuzzi's b's,** crescents of Giannuzzi. **glomus b's,** glandulae glomiformes. **Golgi b.,** see under *complex.* **Gordon's elementary b.,** a particle originally thought to be the viral cause of Hodgkin's disease, but later shown to be obtainable from any tissue containing eosinophils or involved with this neoplasm; called also *Gordon's encephalopathic agent.* **Guarnieri's b's,** inclusion bodies in the cells of the affected tissues in smallpox and vaccinia, regarded as caused by the reaction of the cell to the virus of the disease; called also *Guarnieri's corpuscles.* **habenular b.,** habenula, def. 2. **Halberstaedter-Prowazek b's,** trachoma b's. **Harting b's,** deposits of calcium (calcospherites) in the cerebral capillaries. **Hassall's b's,** Hassall's corpuscles. **Hassall-Henle b's,** see under *wart.* **Heinz b's, Heinz-Ehrlich b's,** coccoid inclusion bodies resulting from oxidative injury to and precipitation of hemoglobin, seen in the presence of certain abnormal hemoglobins (HHb H, Köln, etc.) and erythrocytes with enzyme deficiencies. Refractile in fresh blood smears, they are not visible when stained with Romanowsky dyes but may be stained supravitally. Called also *Heinz granules.* See also *Heinz-body anemia.* **Hensen's b.,** a rounded modified Golgi net under the cuticle of an outer hair cell of the organum spirale. **Herring b's,** hyaline or colloid masses scattered throughout the pars nervosa of the pituitary gland. **b. of Highmore,** mediastinum testis. **Howell's b's,** Howell-Jolly b's. **Howell-Jolly b's,** smooth, round remnants of nuclear chromatin seen in erythrocytes in megaloblastic anemia, hemolytic anemia, and after splenectomy. Called also *Howell's b's* and *Jolly's b's.* **hyaline b's,** drusen. **hyaloid b.,** vitreous body (corpus vitreum [NA]). **immune b.,** antibody. **inclusion b.,** round, oval, or irregular shaped bodies occurring in the cytoplasm and nuclei of cells of the body, as in disease caused by filtrable virus infection such as rabies, smallpox, herpes, etc.; called also *elementary b's* and *intranuclear inclusions.* **infrapatellar fatty b.,** corpus adiposum infrapatellare. **infundibular b.,** posterior lobe of the pituitary gland (lobus posterior hypophyseos [NA]). **inner b's,** round bodies seen in erythrocytes after certain stainings, such as Ehrlich's hemoglobinemic bodies, Heinz-Ehrlich bodies, and Schmauch's bodies. **intercarotid b.,** glomus caroticum. **in-**

termediary b., see *amboceptor.* **intermediate b. of Flemming,** a small bridge of acidophil material connecting the two daughter cells for a time at the end of mitosis. **interrenal b.,** an elongated organ that lies between the kidneys in elasmobranch fishes and that corresponds to the adrenal medulla in mammals. **intravertebral b.,** corpus vertebrae. **Jaworski b's,** see under *corpuscle.* **Joest's b's,** intranuclear inclusion bodies found in the brain of animals with Borna disease. **Jolly's b's,** Howell-Jolly b's. **juxtarestiform b.,** a structure connecting the lateral vestibular nucleus with the nucleus fastigii and conveying vestibular impulses. **ketone b's,** the substances acetone, acetoacetic acid, and β-hydroxybutyric acid. Except for acetone (which may arise spontaneously from acetoacetic acid), they are normal metabolic products of lipid (and pyruvate) metabolism via acetyl-CoA within the liver, and are oxidized by the muscles. Acetoacetic acid is convertible to fatty acids and to steroids. Excessive production leads to urinary excretion of these bodies, as in diabetes mellitus. Called also *acetone b's.* **Kurloff's b's,** bodies seen in the large mononuclear leukocytes of guinea pigs and related rodents. Observations with the electron microscope indicate that they probably result from intracellular secretion or from a sequestering and concentration of a serum molecular component. **L b's,** amorphous bodies of various size formed from granules of bacteria. **Lafora's b's,** intracytoplasmic inclusions consisting of a complex of glycoprotein and acid mucopolysaccharide; widespread deposits of these bodies are found in myoclonus epilepsy. **Lallemand's b's, Lallemand-Trousseau b's,** Bence Jones cylinders. **Landolt's b's,** small elongate bodies between the rods and cones on the outer nuclear layer of the retina. **Laveran's b's,** former name for the malarial parasite; see *Plasmodium.* **L.C.L. b's,** minute coccoid bodies found in tissue infected with psittacosis; called also *Levinthal-Coles-Lillie b's.* **Leishman-Donovan b's,** small round or oval bodies found in the reticuloendothelial cells, especially those of the spleen and liver, of patients suffering with kala-azar; they are the nonflagellate intracellular forms of the protozoan *Leishmania donovani,* the parasite causing the disease. Also used to designate similar forms of *L. tropica* found in macrophages in the lesions of cutaneous leishmaniasis. **lenticular b.** (*obs.*), nucleus lentiformis. **Levinthal-Coles-Lillie b's,** L.C.L. b's. **Lewy b's,** concentrically laminated, round bodies found in vacuoles in the cytoplasm of some of the neurons of the midbrain in paralysis agitans. **Lieutaud's b.,** trigonum vesicae. **Lindner's initial b's,** bodies resembling inclusion bodies found in epithelial cells in trachoma. **Lipschütz b's,** intranuclear inclusion bodies found in the lesions of herpes simplex, both in the epithelial cells of the primary skin lesion (skin or cornea) and in the affected nerve cells. **Lostorfer's b's,** Lostorfer's corpuscles. **Luschka's b.,** glomus coccygeum. **Luys' b.,** nucleus subthalamicus. **lyssa b's,** red staining masses somewhat resembling Negri bodies but less sharply defined and with less internal structure. **Mallory's b's,** 1. hyaline endoplasmic reticulum within hepatocytes in nutritional cirrhosis. 2. bodies in the lymph spaces and epidermal cells in scarlet fever. **malpighian b's of kidney,** corpuscula renis. **malpighian b's of spleen,** folliculi lymphatici lienales. **mamillary b., mammillary b.,** corpus mamillare. **Marchal b's,** cell inclusion bodies observed in ectromelia. **Masson b's,** the cellular components that fill the pulmonary alveoli and alveolar ducts in rheumatic pneumonia; they are possibly the equivalent of modified Aschoff bodies. **medullary b. of cerebellum,** corpus medullare cerebelli. **medullary b. of vermis,** arbor vitae cerebelli. **melon-seed b.,** any of a class of small fibrous masses sometimes occurring in the joints and in cysts of the tendon sheaths. **metachromatic b's,** metachromatic granules. **Michaelis-Gutmann b's,** bodies found in the lesion of malacoplakia of the bladder. **mitochondrial b.,** a fused colony of mitochondria found in the spermatids of insects. **molluscous b's** (*obs.*), molluscum b's. **molluscum b's,** peculiar round or oval eosinophilic bodies occupying the central crater of the papular lesions of molluscum contagiosum; formerly called *Patterson's corpuscles* or *nodules.* **Mooser b's,** bodies resembling rickettsiae, seen in the epithelial cells of the tunica vaginalis exudate in some forms of typhus. **Mörner's b.,** nucleoalbumin. **Mott b's,** clear globules present in the cytoplasm of plasma cells in multiple myeloma. **multilamellar b.,** any of the osmiophilic, lipid-rich, layered bodies found in the type II alveolar cells of the lung; called also *cytosome.* **multivesicular b.,** a secondary lysosome manifested as a spherical, membrane-bound vacuole, containing numerous small vesicles in a matrix that exhibits acid phosphatase activity. **Negri b's,** oval or round inclusion bodies, seen in the cytoplasm and sometimes in the processes of nerve cells of rabid animals after death; their presence is considered conclusive proof of rabies. Called also *Neurorrhyctes hydrophobiae* and *Encephalocytozoon rabiei.* **Neill-Mooser b.,** large mononuclear cells filled with rickettsiae, seen in the inflammatory exudate of the scrotal swelling of laboratory animals infected with murine typhus. See also under *reaction.* **nigroid b.,** granula iridica of the equine or bovine iris. **Nissl b's,** large granular basophilic bodies found in the cytoplasm of neurons, composed of rough endoplasmic reticulum and free polyribosomes; called also *chromophilous b's*, *trigoid b's*, *chromophil corpuscles* or *substance*, and *chromatic granules*. **Nothnagel's b's**, oval or round bodies, plain or striated, from 15 to 60 μ in diameter, sometimes found in the stools of persons who eat meat. **no-threshold b's**, no-threshold substances. **Oken's b.**, mesonephros. **olivary b.**, oliva. **onion b's**, epithelial pearls. **oryzoid b's**, rice b's. **pacchionian b's**, granulationes arachnoideales. **pampiniform b.**, epoophoron. **Pappenheimer b's**, basophilic iron-containing granules observed in various types of erythrocytes. **para-aortic b's**, corpora paraaortica; see also *paraganglion*. **parabasal b.**, an oval or rodlike body in the kinetoplast, larger than the blepharoplast, and connected therewith by a delicate fibril. **paranuclear b.**, centrosome. **paraphyseal b.**, paraphysis (def. 1). **paraterminal b.**, gyrus paraterminalis. **parathyroid b.**, a parathyroid gland. **parietal b.**, epiphyseal eye. **parolivary b's**, accessory olivary nuclei; see *nucleus olivaris accessorius dorsalis* and *medialis*. **Paschen's b's**, inclusion bodies in the cells of the tissues in variola and vaccinia; they are infective but whether they are the infective agents or mechanical carriers of the invisible virus is not known. Called also *Paschen's corpuscles* or *granules*. **pearly b's**, epithelial pearls. **perineal b.**, centrum tendineum perinei. **pheochrome b.**, paraganglion. **pineal b.**, 1. a small, somewhat flattened, cone-shaped body in the epithalamus, lying above the superior colliculi and below the splenium of the corpus callosum. Arising embryologically from the ependyma of the third ventricle of the brain and consisting of cords of pinealocytes supported by interstitial cells, it is the site of synthesis of melatonin, which inhibits gonad development and influences estrus in mammals and produces marked lightening of the dermal pigmentation in amphibians by stimulating the aggregation of melanosomes into melanophores. Melatonin secretion is diminished during exposure to environmental light; the pineal body synthesizes and releases melatonin in response to norepinephrine, whose rate of release, in turn, declines when light activates retinal photoreceptors. Called also *corpus pineale* [NA], *conarium*, *epiphysis cerebri*, and *pineal gland*. 2. the posterior eyelike structure arising from the median of the dorsal wall of the thalamus in some lower vertebrates. See also *epiphyseal eye*, under *eye*. **pituitary b.**, pituitary gland. **Plimmer's b's**, small round capsulated bodies found in cancer, and thought by the discoverer to be the parasite causing the disease; called also *Behla's b's* and *cancer b's*. **polar b's**, 1. the small abortive cells with a haploid chromosome complement, consisting of a tiny piece of cytoplasm and a nucleus, resulting from unequal division of the primary oocyte (*first polar b.*) and, if fertilization occurs, of the secondary oocyte (*second polar b.*); the polar body appears as a speck at the animal pole of the egg. 2. metachromatic granules located at the ends of bacteria. **postbranchial b's**, ultimobranchial b's. **presegmenting b's**, malarial parasites (*Plasmodium*) before they undergo segmentation. **Prowazek's b's**, 1. trachoma bodies. 2. extremely small inclusion bodies found in the material from smallpox pustules and in cowpox vaccine and regarded by Prowazek as the cause of the disease. **Prowazek-Greeff b's**, trachoma b's. **psammoma b.**, a spherical, concentrically laminated mass of calcareous material, usually of microscopic size; such bodies occur in both benign and malignant epithelial and connective-tissue tumors, and are sometimes associated with chronic inflammation. **pseudolutein b.**, corpus atreticum. **purine b's**, purine bases. **pyknotic b's**, bodies in the mucus of stools in amebiasis; they are the nuclear remains of tissue cells and leukocytes. **quadrigeminal b's**, corpora quadrigemina. **Reilly b's**, large, coarse granulations found in the leukocytes in Hurler's syndrome. **Renaut's b's**, pale granules in the degenerating nerve fibers in muscular dystrophy. **residual b.**, 1. a secondary lysosome that has completed its digestive processes but retains indigestible or very slowly digestible material. 2. the mass of protoplasm left after the completion of schizogony, as in *Plasmodium;* called also *sporal residuum* and *sporenrest*. **residual b. of Regnaud**, an anucleate mass consisting of fine granules, lipid droplets, and degenerating organelles, cast off after the completion of regional differentiation of the tail during spermiogenesis. **restiform b.**, see *pedunculus cerebellaris inferior*. **restiform b. of Clark** (*obs.*), fasciculus cuneatus medullae oblongatae. **b. of Retzius**, a protoplasmic mass containing pigment granules at the lower end of a hair cell of the organum spirale. **rice b's**, small bodies resembling grains of rice which form in the tendons of joints and in the fluid of hygroma; called also *oryzoid b's*, and *corpora oryzoidea*. **Rosenmüller's b.**, epoophoron. **Ross's b's**, spherical copper-colored bodies showing dark granulations and sometimes having ameboid movements; seen in the blood and tissue fluids in syphilis. **Russell b's**, globular plasma cell inclusions, mucoprotein in nature, containing surface gamma globulin, and representing aggregates of immunoglobulins synthesized by the cell; called also *cancer b's* and *fuchsin b's*. **sand b's**, acervulus. **Sandström's b's**, parathyroid glands. **Schaumann's b's**, the red or brown, nodular, shell-like lesions of sarcoidosis. **Schmorl b.**, a portion of the nucleus pulposus that has protruded into an adjoining vertebra. **Seidelin b's**, a name once applied to structures observed in the red cells in yellow fever,

believed by the discoverer to be the cause of the disease. **semilunar b's**, crescents of Giannuzzi. **Spengler's immune b's**, a preparation extracted from the blood cells of animals immunized against both human and bovine tubercle bacilli, based on the concept that the immunizing substances in tuberculosis are in the blood cells and not in the serum; used at one time in the management of tuberculosis. Called also *I.K.* (*Immunkörper*). **spherical b.** (*obs.*), the first stage of the sexual cycle of the malarial parasite (*Plasmodium*), developing later into the gametocyte. **spongy b. of male urethra**, corpus spongiosum penis. **spongy b. of penis**, corpus cavernosum penis. **striate b.**, corpus striatum. **supracardial b's**, aortic paraganglia. **suprarenal b.**, adrenal gland. **Symington's b.**, ligamentum anococcygeum. **telobranchial b's**, ultimobranchial b's. **thermostabile b.**, in immunology, the term usually refers to antibodies that remain stable in serum heated to 56° C., which inactivates complement. **threshold b's**, threshold substances. **thyroid b.**, thyroid gland (glandula thyroidea [NA]). **tigroid b's**, Nissl b's. **Todd b's**, eosinophilic structures formed in the cytoplasm of the red cells of certain amphibians. **Torres-Teixeira b's**, inclusion bodies found in the cells in variola minor. **trachoma b's**, inclusion bodies found in clusters in the cytoplasm of the epithelial cells from the conjunctiva of trachomatous eye; called also *Halberstaedter-Prowazek b's*, *Prowazek's b's*, and *Prowazek-Greeff b's*. **trapezoid b.**, corpus trapezoideum. **Trousseau-Lallemand b's**, Bence Jones cylinders. **ultimobranchial b's**, embryonic derivatives of the fifth pharyngeal pouches, which migrate along with the parathyroid glands and are incorporated in the thyroid gland; in submammalian vertebrates they remain as discrete masses in the neck or mediastinum throughout adult life. The parafollicular cells of these bodies produce calcitonin. Called also *postbranchial b's* and *telobranchial b's*. **vermiform b's**, peculiar sinuous invaginations of the plasma membrane of Kupffer cells of the liver, having a central linear density between parallel membranes and a faint transverse striation; similar structures are seen in macrophages of certain organs and in the Langerhans cells of the epidermis. **Verocay b's**, small groups of fibrils surrounded by rows of palisaded nuclei, seen in schwannomas. **vitelline b.**, yolk nucleus. **vitreous b.**, the transparent gel that fills the inner portion of the eyeball between the lens and the retina; called also *corpus vitreum* [NA], *hyaloid b.*, *humor cristallinus*, and *crystalline* or *vitreous humor*. **Winkler's b.**, spherical bodies seen in the lesions of syphilis. **wolffian b.**, mesonephros. **xanthine b's**, purine bases. **yellow b. of ovary**, corpus luteum. **zebra b.**, concentric, laminated, figure-like, cytoplasmic inclusions of Schwann cells, occurring singly or in clusters as a result of degeneration phenomena. **Zuckerkandl's b's**, paraganglia found along the course of the aorta near its bifurcation.

body rocking (bod′e rok′ing) a rhythmic backward and forward motion in a sitting position.

body snatching (bod′e snach′ing) the illegal procural of dead bodies, especially the robbing of a grave of a recently buried corpse.

Boeck's disease, sarcoid (beks) [Caesar P. M. *Boeck*, Norwegian dermatologist and syphilologist, 1845–1913] sarcoidosis.

Boedeker's test (ba′dek-erz) [Carl Heinrich Detlef *Boedeker*, German chemist, 1815–1895] see under *tests*.

Boerhaave's glands, syndrome (boor′hahv-ēz) [Hermann *Boerhaave*, Dutch physician, 1668–1738] the sweat glands (glandulae sudoriferae); see under *syndrome*.

Boettcher (bet′sher) see *Böttcher*.

Boettger see *Böttger*.

Bogomolets' serum [Aleksandr Alexsandrovich *Bogomolets*, Russian physiopathologist, 1881–1946] antireticular cytotoxic serum.

Bogros' space (bŏg-rōz′) [Annet Jean *Bogros*, French anatomist, 1786–1823] see under *space*.

Böhler splint (bāl′er) [Lorenz *Böhler*, Vienna surgeon, born 1885] see under *splint*.

Bohr effect (bor) [Christian *Bohr*, Scandinavian physiologist, 1855–1911] see under *effect*.

Bohun upas (bo′hun u′pas) the poison tree of Java, *Antiaris toxicaria*.

boil (boil) furuncle. **Aleppo b.**, **Bagdad b.**, **Biskra b.**, cutaneous leishmaniasis. **blind b.**, a boil that does not develop a white or yellow "head" at its apex through which pus may be discharged; an abscess. **Bulama b.** [from *Bulama*, an island of West Africa], a chronic sore of West Africa, said to be due to a burrowing insect larva. **Delhi b.**, cutaneous leishmaniasis. **Gafsa b.** [from *Gafsa*, in Tunis], a variety of cutaneous leishmaniasis. **godovnik b.**, cutaneous leishmaniasis. **gum b.**, parulis. **Jerico b.**, cutaneous leishmaniasis. **Natal b.**, **oriental b.**, **Penjdeh b.**, cutaneous leishmaniasis. **shoe b.**, capped elbow in the horse. **tropical b.**, cutaneous leishmaniasis.

Bol. abbreviation for L. *bo′lus*, pill.

bolasterone (bōl-ah′ster-ōn)   chemical name: 17β-hydroxy-7α,17-dimethylandrost-4-en-3-one; an anabolic agent, $C_{21}H_{32}O_2$.

boldenone undecylenate (bōl′dĕ-nōn)   chemical name: 17β-hydroxyandrosta-1,4-dien-3-one 10-undecenoate; an anabolic agent, $C_{30}H_{44}O_3$.

boldine (bol-dēn′)   an alkaloid from *Peumus* (*Boldu*) *boldus* Molina (Monimiaceae), which possesses diuretic properties.

boldo (bol′do) [L. *boldus*, *boldoa*]   the leaves and stems of *Peumus* (*Boldu*) *boldus* Molina (Monimiaceae), a Chilean evergreen shrub. Once official in the U.S. National Formulary (1936) and still common in numerous over-the-counter remedies in Canada and other countries, it contains over 15 alkaloids and is used variously as a choleretic, diuretic, stomachic, sedative, and anthelmintic.

boldoa (bol′do-ah) [L.]   boldo.

boldoin (bōl′do-in)   a glycoside obtainable from boldo.

bolenol (bōl′ĕ-nōl)   chemical name: 19-nor-17α-pregn-5-en-17-ol; an anabolic agent, $C_{20}H_{32}O$.

Boletus (bo-le′tus) [L.; Gr. *bōlitēs*]   a genus of basidiomycetous Hymenomycetes, some of which are edible and others poisonous. **B. sata′nas**, a species that causes mycetismus gastrointestinalis.

Bolk's retardation theory [Louis *Bolk*, Dutch anatomist, 1866–1930]   see under *theory*.

Bollinger's bodies, granules (bol′in-gerz) [Otto von *Bollinger*, German pathologist, 1843–1909]   see under *body* and *granule*.

bolometer (bo-lom′ĕ-ter) [Gr. *bolē* a throw, a ray + *metron* measure]   1. an instrument for measuring the force of the heart beat.   2. an instrument for measuring minute changes in heat radiated by an object, such as a portion of the human body.

boloscope (bo′lŏ-skōp) [Gr. *bolē* a ray + *skopein* to examine]   an apparatus for detecting and locating metallic foreign bodies in tissues.

Boltz test (reaction) [Oswald Hermann *Boltz*, American neurologist, born 1895]   see under *tests*.

bolus (bo′lus) [L.; Gr. *bolos* lump]   1. a rounded mass of food or a pharmaceutical preparation ready to swallow, or such a mass passing through the gastrointestinal tract.   2. a concentrated mass of pharmaceutical preparation given intravenously for diagnostic purposes, e.g., an opaque contrast medium or radioactive isotope.   3. a mass of scattering material, such as wax, paraffin, bags of water, or a rice-flour mixture, placed between the radiation source and the skin so as to achieve precalculated isodose pattern in the tissue irradiated. **b. al′ba**, kaolin. **alimentary b.**, the mass of food in the oropharynx or the esophagus, comprising one swallow.

bomb (bom)   a heavy metal-shielded apparatus containing a quantity of radium or other radioactive element for use in clinical teleradiation therapy.

bombard (bom-bard′)   to expose the whole body or a specific tissue target to the action of ionizing radiation.

bombesin (bom′bĕ-sin)   a tetradecapeptide first isolated from the skin of certain frogs; on infusion into dogs, it stimulates gastric acid secretion, gallbladder contraction, pancreatic secretion, and relaxation of the choledochoduodenal junction; a pressor substance, it is present in the brain tissue and gut of man and is classified as a neuropeptide.

bombicesterol (bom″be-ses′ter-ol)   a sterol obtained from the chrysalis of the silkworm and from sponges.

bombykol (bom′bĭ-kol)   a pheromone secreted by silkworms that serves as a sex attractant; it is a 16-carbon alcohol with two double bonds.

Bombyx mori (bom′biks mor′i)   the commercial silkworm, used extensively in experimental genetics.

bond (bond)   1. the linkage between two atoms or radicals of a chemical compound.   2. a mark used to indicate the number and attachment of the valencies of an atom in constitutional formulas; it is represented by a pair of dots or a line between the atoms, e.g., H—O—H, H—C≡C—H or H:O:H, H:C:::C:H. **coordinate covalent b.**, a covalent bond in which one of the bonded atoms furnishes both of the shared electrons. **covalent b.**, a chemical bond between two atoms or radicals formed by the sharing of a pair (single bond), 2 pairs (double bond), or 3 pairs of electrons (triple bond). **disulfide b.**, a strong covalent bond, —S—S—, important in linking polypeptide chains in proteins, the linkage arising as a result of the oxidation of the sulfhydryl (SH) groups of two molecules of cysteine; called also *disulfide bridge*. **energy-rich b.**, high-energy b. **glycosidic b's**, the bonds between the monosaccharide components of a polysaccharide. **high-energy b.**, a chemical bond the hydrolysis of which yields high levels of free energy; such bonds involve phosphate (high-energy phosphate b.) or sulfur (high-energy sulfur b.) or other mixed anhydride types of chemical structure. **high-energy phosphate b.**, an energy-rich phosphate linkage present in adenosine triphosphate, phosphocreatine, and certain other intermediates of carbohydrate metabolism. On hydrolysis at pH 7 it yields about 8000 calories per mole, in contrast to the 3000 calories of the ester phosphate bond. This energy can be transferred, stored, or used in metabolic processes, such as the synthesis of glycogen from

glucose, or in the supply of energy for muscle activity. **high-energy sulfur b.**, an energy-rich sulfur linkage, the most important of which occurs in the acetyl-CoA molecule, the main source of energy for fatty acid biosynthesis. **hydrogen b.**, a weak, primarily electrostatic, bond between a hydrogen atom bound to a highly electronegative element (such as oxygen or nitrogen) in a given molecule, or part of a molecule, and a second highly electronegative atom in another molecule or in a different part of the same molecule. The hydrogen bond is generally represented by three dots, e.g., X—H···Y, where X and Y are electronegative atoms. **hydrophobic b.**, a linkage resulting from the tendency of nonpolar molecules (or their side chains) to aggregate in an aqueous environment because of their mutual repulsion of solvent. **ionic b.**, a chemical bond in which electrons are transferred from one atom (e.g., sodium) to another (e.g., chlorine) so that one bears a positive and the other a negative charge, the attraction between these opposite charges forming the bond. **pair b.**, in ethology, the more or less permanent relationship between a male and a female for the purposes of mating and rearing the young. **peptide b.**, the ·CO·NH· bond formed between the carboxyl group of one amino acid and the amino group of another; it is an amide linkage joining amino acids to form peptides. **Van der Waals b.**, a weak chemical bond arising from a nonspecific attractive force originating when two atoms are close to one another; this weak binding is only effective when several atoms of one molecule are bound to several atoms in another molecule.

Bond's splint [Thomas *Bond*, Philadelphia physician and surgeon, 1712–1784]   see under *splint*.

bone (bōn) [L. *os*; Gr. *osteon*]   1. the hard form of connective tissue that constitutes the majority of the skeleton of most vertebrates; it consists of an organic component (the cells and matrix) and an inorganic, or mineral, component; the matrix contains a framework of collagenous fibers and is impregnated with the mineral component, chiefly calcium phosphate (85 per cent) and calcium carbonate (10 per cent), which imparts the quality of rigidity to bone. Called also *osseous tissue*.   2. any distinct piece of the osseous framework, or skeleton, of the body; called also *os*. See Plate accompanying *skeleton*. **accessory b.**, an occasionally occurring bone or ossicle adjoining one of the bones of the carpus or of the tarsus; recognized in the roentgenogram. **acetabular b.**, acetabulum. **acromial b.**, acromion. **alar b.**, os sphenoidale. **Albers-Schönberg marble b's**, osteopetrosis. **Albrecht's b.**, basiotic b. **alisphenoid b.**, ala major ossis sphenoidalis. **alveolar b.**, the thin layer of bone making up the bony processes of the maxilla and mandible, and surrounding and containing the teeth; it is pierced by many small openings through which blood vessels, lymphatics, and nerve fibers pass. **ankle b.**, talus, def. 1. **astragaloid b.**, talus, def. 1. **astragaloscaphoid b.**, Pirie's b. **back b.**, see *backbone*. **basal b.**, the relatively fixed and unchangeable framework of the mandible and maxilla, which limits the extent to which teeth can be moved in the alveolar or supporting bone if the occlusion is to remain stable. **basihyal b.**, the body of the hyoid bone. **basilar b.**, basioccipital b. **basioccipital b.**, a bone developing from a separate ossification center in the fetus, which becomes the basilar part of the occipital bone; called also *basilar b*. **basiotic b.**, a small bone of the fetus between the basisphenoid and the basioccipital bones; called also *Albrecht's b*. **basisphenoid b.**, an embryonic bone that becomes the back part of the body of the sphenoid. **Bertin's b.**, concha sphenoidalis. **breast b.**, sternum. **bregmatic b.**, parietal b. **brittle b's**, osteogenesis imperfecta. **bundle b.**, one of the two types of bone comprising the alveolar bone, so called because of the continuation into it of the principal fibers of the periodontal membrane. Cf. *lamellated b.* **calcaneal b.**, calcaneus. **calf b.**, fibula. **cancellated b.**, cancellous b., substantia spongiosa ossium. **cannon b.**, a bone in the limb of hoofed animals, extending from the fetlock to the knee or hock joint. **capitate b.**, os capitatum. **carpal b's**, the eight bones of the wrist; see *ossa carpi*. [NA]. **carpal b., central**, os centrale. **carpal b., first**, os trapezium. **carpal b., fourth**, os hamatum. **carpal b., great**, os capitatum. **carpal b., intermediate**, os lunatum. **carpal b., radial**, os scaphoideum. **carpal b., second**, os trapezoideum. **carpal b., third**, os capitatum. **carpal b., ulnar**, os triquetrum. **cartilage b.**, any bone that develops within cartilage, in contrast to membrane bone, ossification taking place within a cartilage model; called also *endochondral b.*, *replacement b.*, and *substitution b.* **cavalry b.**, rider's b. **central b.**, os centrale. **chalky b's**, osteopetrosis. **cheek b.**, os zygomaticum. **chevron b.**, the V-shaped hemal arches of the third, fourth, and fifth coccygeal vertebrae of a dog. **coccygeal b.**, coccyx (os coccygis [NA]). **coffin b.**, the third or distal phalanx of the foot of a horse; called also *pedal b.* and *os pedis*. **collar b.**, clavicula. **compact b.**, substantia compacta ossium. **coronary b.**, the small pastern bone of the horse. **cortical b.**, the compact bone of the shaft of a bone that surrounds the medullary cavity. **costal b.**, os costale. **cranial b's, b's of cranium**, the bones that constitute the cranial part of the skull, including the occipital, sphenoid, temporal, parietal, frontal, ethmoid, lacrimal and nasal bones, the inferior nasal concha, and vomer; called also *ossa cranii.* [NA]. See also *facial b's.* **cribriform b.,** os ethmoidale. **cuboid b.,** os cuboideum. **cuckoo b.,** os coccygis. **cuneiform b. of carpus,** os triquetrum. **cuneiform b., external,** os cuneiforme laterale. **cuneiform b., first,** os cuneiforme mediale. **cuneiform b., intermediate,** os cuneiforme intermedium. **cuneiform b., internal,** os cuneiforme mediale. **cuneiform b., lateral,** os cuneiforme laterale. **cuneiform b., medial,** os cuneiforme mediale. **cuneiform b., middle, cuneiform b., second,** os cuneiforme intermedium. **cuneiform b., third,** os cuneiforme laterale. **dermal b.,** a bone developed by ossification in the skin. **ear b's,** auditory ossicles. **ectethmoid b's,** the lateral masses of the ethmoid bone. **ectocuneiform b.,** os cuneiforme laterale. **endochondral b.,** cartilage b. **entocuneiform b.,** os cuneiforme mediale. **epactal b's,** ossa suturarum. **epactal b., proper,** os interparietale. **ethmoid b.,** os ethmoidale. **exercise b.,** a bone developed in a muscle, tendon, or fascia, as a result of excessive exercise. **exoccipital b.,** one of the two lateral portions of the occipital bone, developing, from separate centers of ossification, into the portions that bear the condyles. **b's of face, facial b's,** the bones that constitute the facial part of the skull, including the hyoid, palatine, and zygomatic bones, the mandible, and the maxilla; called also *ossa faciei* [NA]. The facial bones are considered by many to include the lacrimal and nasal bones, the inferior nasal concha, and the vomer, but not the hyoid bone. **femoral b.,** femur, def. 1. **fibular b.,** fibula. **b's of fingers,** ossa digitorum manus. **flank b.,** ilium (os ilium [NA]). **flat b.,** one whose thickness is slight, sometimes consisting of only a thin layer of compact bone, or of two layers with intervening spongy bone and marrow; usually bent or curved, rather than flat. Called also *os planum* [NA]. **frontal b.,** os frontale. **funny b.,** the region of the median condyle of the humerus where it is crossed by the ulnar nerve. **hamate b.,** os hamatum. **haunch b.,** os coxae. **heel b.,** calcaneus. **hip b.,** os coxae. **humeral b.,** humerus. **hyoid b.,** a horseshoe-shaped bone situated at the base of the tongue, just above the thyroid cartilage; called also *os hyoideum* [NA], *lingual b.,* and *tongue b.* **iliac b.,** ilium (os ilium [NA]). **incarial b.,** os interparietale. **incisive b.,** os incisivum. **innominate b.,** os coxae. **intermediate b.,** os lunatum. **interparietal b.,** os interparietale. **intrachondrial b.,** osseous tissue occurring in cartilage matrix which has undergone calcification; consistently found in patches within the middle layer of the otic capsule. **ischial b.,** ischium (os ischii [NA]). **ivory b's,** osteopetrosis. **jaw b., lower,** mandibula. **jaw b., upper,** maxilla. **jugal b.,** os zygomaticum. **lacrimal b.,** a thin scalelike bone at the anterior part of the medial wall of the orbit, articulating with the frontal and ethmoidal bones and the maxilla and inferior nasal concha; called also *os lacrimale* [NA] and *os unguis.* **lamellated b.,** one of the two types of bone comprising the alveolar bone, with some lamellae roughly parallel with the marrow spaces and others forming haversian systems. Cf. *bundle b.* **lenticular b. of hand, lentiform b.,** os pisiforme. **lingual b.,** hyoid b. (os hyoideum [NA]). **long b.,** a bone that has a longitudinal axis of considerable length, consisting of a shaft (the diaphysis) and an expanded portion (the epiphysis) at each end that is usually articular; any of the long bones of the limbs. Called also *os longum* [NA]. **lunate b.,** os lunatum. **malar b.,** os zygomaticum. **marble b's,** osteopetrosis. **mastoid b.,** pars mastoidea ossis temporalis. **maxillary b.,** maxilla. **maxillary b., inferior,** mandibula. **maxillary b., superior,** maxilla. **maxilloturbinal b.,** concha nasalis inferior. **membrane b.,** any bone that develops within a connective tissue membrane, in contrast to cartilage bone. **mesocuneiform b.,** os cuneiforme intermedium. **metacarpal b's,** the five cylindrical bones of the hand; see *ossa metacarpalia I–V.* **metatarsal b's,** the five bones extending from the tarsus to the phalanges of the toes, forming the skeleton of the metatarsus; called also *ossa metatarsalia I–V* [NA]. **multangular b., accessory,** os centrale. **multangular b., larger,** os trapezium. **multangular b., smaller,** os trapezoideum. **nasal b.,** either of the two small oblong bones that together form the bridge of the nose; called also *os nasale* [NA]. **navicular b. of foot,** os naviculare. **navicular b. of hand,** os scaphoideum. **nonlamellated b.,** woven b. **occipital b.,** a single trapezoidal-shaped bone situated at the posterior and inferior part of the cranium; see *os occipitale* [NA]. **odontoid b.,** dens axis. **orbital b.,** os zygomaticum. **orbitosphenoidal b.,** ala minor ossis sphenoidalis. **palate b.,** palatine b. **palatine b.,** one of the two irregularly shaped bones forming the posterior part of the hard palate, the lateral wall of the nasal fossa between the medial pterygoid plate and the maxilla, and the posterior part of the floor of the orbit. Called also *os palatinum* [NA] and *palate b.* **parietal b.,** one of the two quadrilateral bones forming part of the superior and lateral surfaces of the skull, and joining each other in the midline at the sagittal suture; called also *os parietale* [NA] and *bregmatic b.* **pastern b.,** either of two bones of the horse's foot: *large pastern b.,* the first phalanx of a horse's foot; *small pastern b.,* the second phalanx of a horse's foot. **pedal b.,** coffin b. **pelvic b.,** os coxae. **periosteal b.,** bone that is developed directly from and beneath the periosteum. **petro-**

sal b., petrous b., pars petrosa ossis temporalis. **phalangeal b's of foot,** ossa digitorum pedis. **phalangeal b's of hand,** ossa digitorum manus. **Pirie's b.,** an occasionally occurring ossicle found above the head of the talus; called also *astragaloscaphoid b.* **pisiform b.,** os pisiforme. **pneumatic b.,** one that contains air-filled cavities or sinuses; called also *os pneumaticum* [NA]. **postsphenoidal b.,** the posterior portion of the sphenoid bone. **postulnar b.,** os pisiforme. **prefrontal b.,** pars nasalis ossis frontalis. **prefrontal b. of von Bardeleben,** processus frontalis maxillae. **preinterparietal b.,** a wormian bone sometimes observed, detached from the anterior part of the interparietal bone. **premaxillary b.,** premaxilla. **presphenoidal b.,** the anterior portion of the sphenoid bone that develops separately and unites with the posterior portion (postsphenoidal bone) between the seventh and eighth months of intrauterine life. **primitive b.,** woven b. **pterygoid b.,** processus pterygoideus ossis sphenoidalis. **pubic b.,** the anterior inferior part of the hip bone (os coxae) on either side; see *os pubis* [NA]. **pyramidal b.,** os triquetrum. **radial b.,** radius, def. 2. **replacement b.,** cartilage b. **resurrection b.,** sacrum (os sacrum [NA]). **rider's b.,** a localized ossification of the inner aspect of the lower end of the tendon of the adductor muscle of the thigh (adductor tubercle), sometimes seen in horseback riders; called also *cavalry b.* **Riolan's b's,** small bones resembling wormian bones, sometimes found in the suture between the occipital bone and the petrous portion of the temporal bone. **rudimentary b.,** a bone that has only partially developed. **sacral b.,** os sacrum. **scaphoid b.,** os scaphoideum. **scaphoid b. of foot,** os naviculare. **scaphoid b. of hand,** os scaphoideum. **scapular b.,** scapula. **semilunar b.,** os lunatum. **sesamoid b's,** a type of short bone occurring mainly in the hands and feet, and found embedded in tendons or joint capsules; called also *ossa sesamoidea* [NA]. **sesamoid b's of foot,** ossa sesamoidea pedis. **sesamoid b's of hand,** ossa sesamoidea manus. **shin b.,** tibia. **short b.,** one whose main dimensions are approximately equal, e.g., one of the bones of the carpus or tarsus; called also *os breve* [NA]. **b's of skull,** ossa cranii. **solid b.,** substantia compacta ossium. **sphenoid b.,** a single, irregular, wedge-shaped bone at the base of the skull, which forms a part of the floor of the anterior, middle, and posterior cranial fossae; called also *os sphenoidale* [NA] and *alar b.* **sphenoturbinal b.,** concha sphenoidalis. **splint b's,** the reduced second and fourth metacarpal and metatarsal bones of the Equidae. **spoke b.,** radius, def. 2. **spongy b.,** substantia spongiosa ossium. **spongy b., inferior,** concha nasalis inferior. **spongy b., superior,** concha nasalis superior. **squamo-occipital b.,** the squamous portion of the fetal occipital bone, including the supraoccipital and interparietal bones. **squamous b.,** pars squamosa ossis temporalis. **stifle b.,** the patella of the horse. **stirrup b.,** stapes. **substitution b.,** cartilage b. **supernumerary b.,** a bone occurring in addition to the normal one, as a vertebra or a rib (cervical rib). **suprainterparietal b.,** a wormian bone sometimes occurring at the posterior part of the sagittal suture. **supraoccipital b.,** a bone developing from a separate ossification center in the fetus, which becomes the squamous part of the occipital bone below the superior nuchal line. **suprapharyngeal b.,** os sphenoidale. **suprasternal b's,** ossa suprasternalia. **sutural b's,** ossa suturarum. **tarsal b's,** the seven bones of the ankle; see *ossa tarsi.* **tarsal b., first,** os cuneiforme mediale. **tarsal b., second,** os cuneiforme intermedium. **tarsal b., third,** os cuneiforme laterale. **temporal b.,** one of the two irregular bones forming part of the lateral surfaces and base of the skull, and containing the organs of hearing; called also *os temporale* [NA]. **thigh b.,** femur, def. 1. **b's of toes,** ossa digitorum pedis. **tongue b.,** os hyoideum. **trapezium b.,** os trapezium. **trapezium b., lesser,** os trapezoideum. **trapezium b. of Lyser,** os trapezoideum. **trapezoid b.,** os trapezoideum. **trapezoid b. of Henle,** processus pterygoideus ossis sphenoidalis. **trapezoid b. of Lyser,** os trapezium. **triangular b.,** os triquetrum. **triangular b. of tarsus,** os trigonum tarsi. **triquetral b.,** os triquetrum. **turbinate b., highest,** concha nasalis suprema. **turbinate b., inferior,** concha nasalis inferior. **turbinate b., middle,** concha nasalis media. **turbinate b., superior,** concha nasalis superior. **turbinate b., supreme,** concha nasalis suprema. **tympanic b.,** pars tympanica ossis temporalis. **ulnar b.,** ulna. **unciform b.,** os hamatum. **uncinate b.,** os hamatum. **vesalian b.,** os vesalianum pedis. **vomer b.,** vomer. **whettle b's,** vertebrae thoracicae. **whirl b.,** 1. the patella. 2. the head of the femur. **wormian b's,** ossa suturarum. **woven b.,** bony tissue found in the embryo and young children and in various pathologic conditions in adults, in which the bone fails to show the oriented arrangement of collagen fibers characteristic of lamellated bone; called also *nonlamellated b.* and *primitive b.* **xiphoid b.,** sternum. **zygomatic b.,** the triangular bone of the cheek; see *os zygomaticum.*

bonelet (bōn′let) a small bone, or ossicle.

Bonhoeffer's symptom (bon′hef-erz) [Karl *Bonhoeffer,* psychiatrist in Berlin, 1868–1948] see under *symptom.*

Bonine (bo′nēn) trademark for preparations of meclizine hydrochloride.

Bonnaire's method (bon-ārz′) [Érasme *Bonnaire*, French obstetrician, 1858–1918] see under *method*.

Bonnet's capsule, sign (bo-nāz′) [Amédée *Bonnet*, French surgeon, 1809–1858] the capsule enclosing the posterior part of the eyeball. See *vagina bulbi*, and under *sign*.

Bonnier's syndrome (bon-e-āz′) [Pierre *Bonnier*, French physician, 1861–1918] see under *syndrome*.

Bonwill triangle (bon′wil) [William Gibson Arlington *Bonwill*, American dentist, 1833–1899] see under *triangle*.

boomslang (boom′slang) a venomous, colubrid, arboreal snake, *Dispholidus typus*, of South Africa. See table accompanying *snake*.

Boophilus (bo-of′ĭ-lus) [Gr. *bous* ox + *philein* to love] a genus of cattle ticks. **B. annula′tus, B. bo′vis,** the southern cattle tick, which transmits *Babesia bigemina*, the causative agent of Texas fever. Called also *Margaropus annulatus*. **B. decolora′tus,** a tick of South Africa that serves as the means of transmitting *Anaplasma marginale*, the causative agent of gallsickness in cattle. **B. microplus,** the common cattle tick in Panama; it transmits Texas fever.

Booponus (bo-op′o-nus) [Gr. *bous* ox + *ponos* pain] a fly of the Philippines whose larvae (foot maggots) cause lameness in cattle and goats.

booster (boost′er) see under *dose*. **patch b.,** a permanent artificial heart pump composed of silicone rubber and Dacron attached to a helium-powered driving unit and compressed air tank worn on a belt about the waist.

boot (boot) an encasement for the foot; a protective casing or sheath. **Gibney's b.,** an adhesive tape support used in treatment of sprains and other painful conditions of the ankle, the tape being applied in a basketweave fashion with strips placed alternately under the sole of the foot and around the back of the leg. **Junod's b.,** an air-tight boot to which is fitted an air pump. A partial vacuum causes a flow of blood to the parts enclosed in the boot, producing the effect of bloodletting by causing a fainting spell. **Unna's paste b.,** a dressing for varicose ulcers, consisting of a paste made from gelatin, zinc oxide, and glycerin, which is applied to the entire leg, then covered with a spiral bandage, this in turn being given a coat of the paste; the process is repeated until satisfactory rigidity is attained.

borate (bo′rāt) any salt of boric acid.

borated (bo′rāt-ed) combined with or containing borax or boric acid.

borax (bo′raks), gen. *bora′cis* [L. from Arabic; Persian *būrah*] sodium borate.

borborygmus (bor″bo-rig′mus), pl. *borboryg′mi* [L.] a rumbling noise caused by the propulsion of gas through the intestines.

Borchardt's test (bor′chartz) [Leo *Borchardt*, German chemist, born 1879] see under *tests*.

border (bor′der) a bounding line, edge, or surface. For names of borders of various anatomical structures not included here, see entries under *margo*. **b. of acetabulum,** labrum acetabulare. **alveolar b. of mandible,** arcus alveolaris mandibulae. **alveolar b. of maxilla,** arcus alveolaris maxillae. **brush b.,** a specialization of the free surface of a cell, consisting of minute cylindrical processes (microvilli) that greatly increase the surface area; noted especially on the cells of the proximal convolution in a renal tubule and on the intestinal epithelium of vertebrates. Called also *striated b.* **denture b.,** 1. the limit, boundary, or circumferential margin of a denture base. 2. the margin of the denture base at the junction of the polished surface with the impression (tissue) surface. 3. the extreme edges of a denture base at the buccolabial, lingual, and posterior limits. 4. the extreme margins of a denture base. Called also *denture edge.* **external b. of tibia,** facies lateralis tibiae. **inferior b. of mandible,** basis mandibulae. **orbital b. of sphenoid bone,** facies orbitalis alae majoris. **b. of oval fossa,** limbus fossae ovalis. **posterior b. of petrous portion of temporal bone,** angulus posterior pyramidis ossis temporalis. **posterointernal b. of fibula,** crista medialis fibulae. **striated b.,** brush b. **superior b. of patella,** basis patellae. **superior b. of petrous portion of temporal bone,** angulus superior pyramidis ossis temporalis. **vermilion b.,** the exposed red portion of the upper or lower lip.

Bordet's phenomenon, test (bor-dāz′) [Jules Jean Baptiste Vincent *Bordet*, Belgian bacteriologist, 1870–1961; winner of Nobel prize in medicine and physiology for 1919] see *serum test*, under *tests*.

Bordet-Gengou agar (culture medium), bacillus, phenomenon (reaction) (bor-da′-zhaw-goo′) [Jules Jean Baptiste Vincent *Bordet;* Octave *Gengou*, French bacteriologist, 1875–1957] see *Table of Culture Media*, and see *Hemophilus pertussis* and *fixation of the complement*.

Bordetella (bor″dĕ-tel′lah) [Jules Jean Baptiste Vincent *Bordet*] in some systems of classifications, a genus of microorganisms of the family Brucellaceae, order Eubacteriales, made up of minute motile or nonmotile gram-negative coccobacilli that are parasitic and produce a dermonecrotic toxin. **B. bronchisep′tica,** the causative agent of bronchopneumonia in guinea pigs and other rodents, swine, dogs, and lower primates. Formerly called *Bacillus bronchisepticus, Brucella bronchiseptica,* and *Hemophilus bronchisepticus.* **B. parapertus′sis,** a species occasionally found in whooping cough in man; called also *Hemophilus parapertussis.* **B. pertus′sis,** the causative agent of whooping cough in man; called also *Hemophilus pertussis.*

borism (bo′rizm) poisoning by a boron compound.

borjom (bor′jom) a natural mineral water from Caucasia.

Borna disease [*Borna*, a district in Saxony where an epidemic occurred] see under *disease*.

borneol (bor′ne-ol) chemical name: *endo*-1,7,7-trimethylbicyclo-[2.2.1]heptan-2-ol. A terpene alcohol, $C_{10}H_{18}O$, found in the Borneo camphor tree (*Dryobalanops aromatica*) and many other plants, or prepared synthetically, and used, chiefly in the form of its esters, in the manufacture of perfume and incense. Called also *Borneo camphor, bornyl alcohol,* and *camphyl alcohol.* **b. acetate,** see under *bornyl*.

Bornholm disease (born′hōm) [named from the Danish island, *Bornholm*] epidemic pleurodynia.

bornyl (bor′nil) a univalent radical of borneol. **b. acetate,** an ester of borneol found in the oil of *Rosmarinus officinalis* and many other oils, and used as a flavoring agent and in the manufacture of perfume; called also *borneol acetate.* **b. alcohol,** borneol. **b. chloride,** chemical name: *endo*-2-chlorol-7,7-trimethylbicyclo[2.2.1]heptane. A compound, $C_{10}H_{17}Cl$, prepared from pinene, the chief constituent of turpentine oil, by the action of hydrochloric acid, in the process of producing synthetic camphor. Called also *artificial camphor, pinene hydrochloride,* and *turpentine camphor.*

boroglyceride (bo″ro-glis′er-īd) boroglycerin.

boroglycerin (bo″ro-glis′er-in) a compound $(C_3H_5BO_3)$ prepared by heating 2 parts of boric acid and 3 parts of glycerin; formerly used as an antiseptic. **b. glycerite,** a preparation of boric acid and glycerin, containing between 47.5 and 52.5 per cent of boroglycerin; formerly used as an antibacterial. Called also *glyceritum boroglycerini* and *glycerol boroglycerite.*

boroglycerol (bo″ro-glis′er-ol) boroglycerin.

boron (bo′ron) [L. *borium*] a nonmetallic element occurring in the form of crystals and as a powder. It is the base of borax and boric acid: symbol B, atomic number 5, specific gravity 2.54, atomic weight 10.811. **b. carbide,** a substance, B_4C, obtained by heating boron at an extremely high temperature to effect its union with carbon, used in dentistry as an abrasive agent.

Borrelia (bŏ-rel′e ah) [after Amédée *Borrel*, French bacteriologist in Strasbourg, 1867–1936] a genus of microorganisms of the family Treponemataceae, order Spirochaetales, made up of cells 8 to 16μ long, with coarse, shallow, irregular spirals, generally tapering into fine filaments at the ends; parasitic in many animals, some of them causing relapsing fever in birds and in man and other mammals. Twenty-eight different species have been described. **B. aegyp′tica,** an etiologic agent of relapsing fever in the Sudan. **B. anseri′na,** the etiologic agent of fowl spirochetosis, transmitted by the tick *Argas persicus,* nonpathogenic for man. **B. ber′bera,** the causative agent of relapsing fever in North Africa, thought to be transmitted by the human body louse. **B. bucca′lis,** a parasite of the human oral cavity that has slight pathogenicity. **B. car′teri,** the etiologic agent of Indian relapsing fever, transmitted by the human body louse. **B. caucas′ica,** an etiologic agent of relapsing fever in the Caucasus, transmitted by the tick *Ornithodoros verrucosus* from a reservoir of infection in field mice. **B. dutto′nii,** an etiologic agent of relapsing fever in central and south Africa, transmitted by the tick *Ornithodoros moubata;* called also *Dutton's spirochete.* **B. herm′sii,** an etiologic agent of relapsing fever in western North America, transmitted by the tick *Ornithodoros hermsi* but not by other species of ticks. **B. hispan′ica,** the etiologic agent of relapsing fever in the Iberian peninsula and northwest Africa, transmitted by ticks of the genus *Ornithodoros.* **B. ko′chii,** an etiologic agent of African relapsing fever, considered to be identical with *B. duttonii.* **B. neotropica′lis,** an etiologic agent of relapsing fever in South America. **B. no′vyi,** an etiologic agent of relapsing fever in North America. **B. par′keri,** an etiologic agent of relapsing fever in western United States, transmitted by the tick *Ornithodoros parkeri* but not by other species of *Ornithodoros.* **B. per′sica,** an etiologic agent of relapsing fever in Iran, transmitted by the tick *Ornithodoros tholozani.* **B. recurren′tis,** the causative agent of relapsing fever transmitted by the human body louse; considered by some to include all relapsing fever spirochetes, other named species being regarded as serotypes or serological variants of a single species of organisms. **B. theile′ri,** a microorganism associated with a benign affection of cattle of South Africa and regarded as the transmitter of tickborne relapsing fever; *Rhipicephalus decoloratus* is regarded as the vector. **B. turica′tae,** an etiologic agent of relapsing fever in southwestern United States, transmitted by the tick *Ornithodoros turicata* but not by other species of *Ornithodoros.* **B. venezuelen′sis,** an etiologic agent of relapsing fever in northern South America and Central America, transmitted by the tick *Ornithodoros rudis.* **B. vincen′tii,** a parasite of the human oral cavity, occurring in large numbers with a fusiform bacillus (*Fusobacterium plauti-vincenti*) in necrotizing ulcerative gingivitis and in necrotizing ulcerative gingivostomatitis; called also *spirillium of Vincent.*

borreliosis (bŏ-rel″e-o′sis) infection with *Borrelia;* see *relapsing fever,* under *fever.*

Borsieri's sign (line) (bor″se-er′ēz) [Giovanni Battista *Borsieri* de Kanilfeld, French physician, 1725–1785] see under *line.*

Borthen's operation (bor′tenz) [Johan *Borthen,* Norwegian ophthalmologist] iridotasis.

Bose's hooks, operation (bo′sez) [Heinrich *Bose,* German surgeon, 1840–1900] see under *hook* and *operation.*

boss (bos) a rounded eminence, as on the surface of a bone or tumor. **parietal b's,** sharp prominences on each side of the parietal bones.

bosselated (bos′ĕ-lāt-ed) [Fr. *bosseler*] marked or covered with bosses.

bosselation (bos″ĕ-la′shun) 1. a small eminence; one of a set of bosses. 2. the condition or fact of being bosselated; the process of becoming bosselated.

Bossi's dilator (bos′ēz) [Luigi Maria *Bossi,* gynecologist in Genoa, 1859–1919] see under *dilator.*

Bostock's catarrh (disease) (bos′toks) [John *Bostock,* English physician, 1773–1846] hay fever.

Boston's sign (bos′tonz) [L. Napoleon *Boston,* American physician, 1871–1931] see under *sign.*

bot (bot) the larva of botflies, which may be parasitic in the stomach of animals and sometimes in that of man. **sheep nose b.,** the larva of *Oestrus ovis,* which is frequently found in the nasal passages of sheep.

Botallo's duct, foramen, ligament [Leonardo *Botallo,* Italian surgeon in Paris, born 1530] see *ductus arteriosus, foramen ovale cordis,* and *ligamentum arteriosum.*

botanic (bo-tan′ik) 1. pertaining to or derived from plants; of the vegetable kingdom. 2. pertaining to botany.

botany (bot′ah-ne) [L. *botanica* from Gr. *botanē* herb] the science of plants or of the vegetable kingdom. **medical b.,** the botany of plants used in medicine.

Botelho's test (bo-tel′yōz) [Dr. *Botelho,* physician in Paris] see under *tests.*

botfly (bot′fli) an insect of the order Diptera, family Oestridae, whose larvae are parasitic in animals, especially horses and sheep. The genera include *Oestrus, Gasterophilus, Dermatobia,* and *Cuterebra.*

bothridium (both-rid′e-um) one of the four leaf-like suckers symmetrically placed around the anterior end of the scolex of a tetraphyllidean cestode; called also *phyllidea.*

bothriocephaliasis (both″re-o-sef″ah-li′ah-sis) diphyllobothriasis.

Bothriocephalus (both″re-o-sef′ah-lus) [Gr. *bothrion* pit + *kephalē* head] diphyllobothrium.

bothrium (both′re-um) [Gr. *bothrion* pit] a sucker in the form of a groove such as is seen on either side of the head of *Diphyllobothrium latum.*

bothropik (both-rop′ik) pertaining to, characteristic of, or derived from snakes of the genus *Bothrops.*

Bothrops (both-rops) [Gr. *bothros* pit + *ōps* eye] a genus of South American serpents. *B. atrox* is the fer-de-lance and *B. jararaca* is the jararaca (q.v.). See table accompanying *snake.*

botogenin (bot-o-je′nin) a steroid sapogenin, $C_{27}H_{40}O_4$, derived from *Dioscorea mexicana,* which is a precursor in a patented process for the partial synthesis of steroid hormones.

botryoid (bot′re-oid) [Gr. *botrys* bunch of grapes + *eidos* form] resembling a bunch of grapes.

botryomycoma (bot″re-o-mi-ko′mah) one of the lesions of botryomycosis.

botryomycosis (bot″re-o-mi-ko′sis) a purulent infection of domestic animals, such as horses and cattle, resembling maduromycosis and marked by the formation of granulomatous masses in the skin and sometimes the viscera. It is caused by *Staphylococcus aureus* and other bacteria and is associated especially with castration or other wounds or injuries. Formerly thought to be caused by a fungus. **b. hom′inis** (*obs.*), granuloma pyogenicum.

botryomycotic (bot″re-o-mi-kot′ik) pertaining to or affected with botryomycosis.

botryotherapy (bot-re-o-ther′ah-pe) [Gr. *botrys* cluster of grapes + *therapeia* therapy] the grape cure.

botrytimycosis (bo-tri″te-mi-ko′sis) infection with fungi of the genus *Botrytis.*

Botrytis (bo-tri′tis) a genus of fungi of the family Moniliaceae, order Moniliales, including the common gray mold and some plant pathogens, which causes onion rot, peony blight, and turnip fire. **B. bassia′na,** *Beauvaria bassiana.* **B. tenel′la,** *Beauvaria tenella.*

bots (bots) a name given the diseased condition in horses and

other animals, attributed to the presence of larvae of botflies of various genera.

Böttcher's cells, crystals (bet′sherz) [Arthur *Böttcher,* German anatomist, 1831–1889] see under *cell* and *crystals.*

Böttger's test (bet′gerz) 1. [Rudolf *Böttger,* German chemist, 1806–1881] see under *tests* (def. 1). 2. [Wilhelm Carl *Böttger,* German chemist, 1871–1949] see under *tests* (def. 2).

Bottini's operation (bo-te′nēz) [Enrico *Bottini,* Italian surgeon, 1837–1903] see under *operation.*

bottle (bot′l) a hollow narrow-necked vessel of glass or other material, used in laboratory procedures or for other purposes. **Junker b.,** see under *inhaler.* **Spritz b.,** a wash bottle for laboratory use. **wash b.,** 1. a flexible squeeze-bottle with delivery tube, or a bottle having two tubes through the cork, so arranged that blowing into one will force a stream of liquid from the other; used in washing chemical materials. 2. a bottle containing some washing fluid, through which gases are passed for the purpose of freeing them from impurities. **Woulfe's b.,** a three-necked bottle used for washing gases or for saturating liquids with a gas.

botuliform (boch′oo-li-form) [L. *botulus* sausage + *forma* shape] sausage-shaped.

botulin (boch′oo-lin) [L. *botulus* sausage] a highly active neurotoxin sometimes found in imperfectly preserved or canned meats and vegetables; it is produced by *Clostridium botulinum* and is peculiar in that it resists the action of the gastric juice. The toxin occurs in six antigenically distinct forms, A, B, C, D, E, and F. Called also *botulinum toxin.* See *botulism.*

botulinal (boh″oo-li′nal) pertaining to *Clostridium botulinum* or to its toxin (botulin).

botulinogenic (boch′oo-lin″o-jen′ik) [*botulin* + Gr. *gennan* to produce] producing or containing botulin.

botulism (boch′oo-lizm) [L. *botulus* sausage] a type of food poisoning caused by a neurotoxin (botulin) produced by the growth of *Clostridium botulinum* in improperly canned or preserved foods. It is characterized by vomiting, abdominal pain, difficulty of vision, nervous symptoms of central origin, disturbances of secretion, motor disturbances, dryness of the mouth and pharynx, dyspepsia, a barking cough, mydriasis, ptosis, etc. *Botulism* is the broader term; *allantiasis* refers only to sausage poisoning. **infant b.,** that affecting infants, typically 4 to 26 weeks of age, marked by constipation, lethargy, hypotonia, and feeding difficulty; it may lead to respiratory insufficiency. It is thought to result from toxin produced in the gut by ingested organisms, rather than from preformed toxins. **wound b.,** botulism resulting from infection of a wound with *Clostridium botulinum;* it is marked by the same symptoms as the foodborne form except for the absence of gastrointestinal symptoms.

botulismotoxin (boch′oo-liz″mo-tok′sin) botulin.

bouba (boo′bah) yaws. **b. braziliana,** mucocutaneous leishmaniasis.

Bouchard's coefficient, disease, nodes (nodules), sign (boo-sharz′) [Charles Jacques *Bouchard,* French physician, 1837–1915] see under *coefficient, disease, node,* and *sign.*

Bouchardat's test, treatment (boo-shar-dahz′) [Apollinaire *Bouchardat,* French chemist, 1806–1886] see under *tests* and *treatment.*

bouche (boosh′) [Fr.] mouth. **b. de tapir** (de tah-pēr′), tapir mouth.

Bouchut's respiration, tubes (boo-shooz′) [Jean Antoine Eugène *Bouchut,* French physician, 1818–1891] see under *respiration* and *tube.*

Boudin's law (boo-dahz′) [Jean Christian Marc François Joseph *Boudin,* French physician, 1806–1867] see under *law.*

bougie (boo-zhe′) [Fr. "wax candle"] a slender, flexible, hollow or solid, cylindrical instrument for introduction into the urethra or other tubular organ, usually for the purpose of calibrating or dilating constricted areas. **b. à boule** (ah-bool′) [Fr.], bulbous

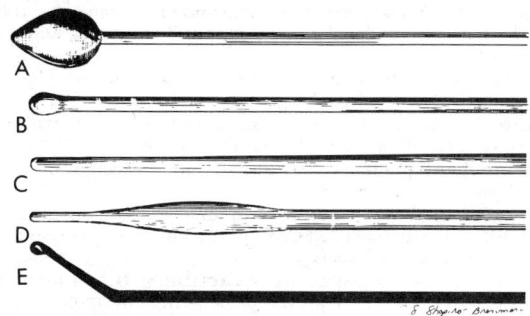

Bougies: *A,* Otis bougie à boule; *B,* olive-tipped bougie; *C,* Garceau bougie; *D,* Braasch bulbous bougie; *E,* filiform bougie.

b. **acorn-tipped b.,** a bulbous bougie with a tip shaped like an acorn. **bulbous b.,** one with a bulb-shaped tip; called also *bougie à boule.* **caustic b.,** one that has a piece of silver nitrate or other caustic agent attached to its end; used as a portcaustic. **conic b.,** one with a cone-shaped tip. **cylindrical b.,** one with a round or circular section. **dilating b.,** a bougie whose diameter can be increased by turning a screw; commonly used for dilating a stricture of the urethra. **ear b.,** one for use in aural surgery. **elastic b.,** one made of India rubber or other elastic material. **elbowed b.,** one with an elbow or sharp, beaklike bend, near the tip. **filiform b.,** one of very slender caliber; often used for the gentle exploration of strictures or sinus tracts of small diameter with multiple false passages. **fusiform b.,** one with a belly or expansion in its shaft. **Gruber's b's** (*obs.*), bougies of medicated gelatin for insertion into the auditory meatus. **Hurst's b's,** a series of mercury-filled tubes of graded diameter for dilating the cardioesophageal region. **Maloney b's,** a series similar to Hurst's bougies but having cone-shaped tips. **medicated b.,** one that is charged with a medicinal substance. **olive-tipped b.,** a bulbous bougie with a tip shaped like an olive. **rosary b.,** a beaded bougie for use in a strictured urethra. **soluble b.,** one composed of a material that will melt or dissolve in situ. **wax b.,** one made of linen, gauze, or silk dipped in melted wax and then rolled. **wax-tipped b.,** a long, slender, flexible bougie with a wax tip for passage into the ureter through the cystoscope to confirm the diagnosis of ureteral calculus. **whip b.,** one with a filiform point and a stem of gradually increasing caliber.

bougienage (boo-zhe-nahzh′) the passage of a bougie through a tubular structure or organ, to increase its caliber, as in the treatment of stricture of the esophagus.

bouginage (boo-zhe-nahzh′) bougienage.

Bouillaud's disease, sign, syndrome, (boo-e-yōz′) [Jean Baptiste *Bouillaud,* French physician, 1796–1881] see *rheumatic endocarditis,* under *endocarditis,* and see under *sign* and *syndrome.*

bouillon (boo-e-yaw′) [Fr.] a broth or soup prepared from the flesh of animals; used in food preparations and as a bacteriological culture medium. In the latter use, it is generally called *broth;* see Table of Culture Media for specific broths.

Bouin's fluid (solution) (bwahz′) [Paul *Bouin,* French anatomist, 1870–1962] see under *fluid.*

boulimia (boo-lim′e-ah) bulimia.

bound (bownd) 1. restrained or confined; not free. 2. held in chemical combination.

bouquet (boo-ka′) [Fr.] a structure suggesting resemblance to a bunch of flowers, as a cluster of vessels, nerves, or fibers, or the polarized stage of synapsis at the start of meiosis.

bourdonnement (boor-don-maw′) [Fr.] (*obs.*) an abnormal humming or buzzing sound in the ears; tinnitus.

Bourgery's ligament (boor′jer-ēz) [Marc Jean *Bourgery,* French anatomist and surgeon, 1797–1849] ligamentum popliteum obliquum.

Bourget's test (boor-zhāz′) [Louis *Bourget,* Swiss physician, 1856–1913] see under *tests.*

Bourneville's disease (boor′ne-vēz) [Désiré-Magloire *Bourneville,* French neurologist, 1840–1909] sclerosis tuberosa.

bout (bout) an attack or episode of illness.

bouton (boo-taw′) [Fr.] button. **b. de Biskra, b. d'o′rient,** cutaneous leishmaniasis. **b's terminaux′,** synaptic end-feet.

boutonneuse (boo-ton-ez′) boutonneuse fever.

boutonnière (boo-ton-yār′) an incision made into the urethra in order to extract an impacted calculus.

Bouveret's disease (syndrome), ulcer (boo-ver-āz′) [Léon *Bouveret,* French physician, 1850–1929] see *paroxysmal tachycardia,* under *tachycardia,* and see under *ulcer.*

Boveri's test (bo′va-rēz) [Piero *Boveri,* Italian neurologist, 1879–1932] see under *tests.*

Bovet (bo′vet), Daniel. Swiss pharmacologist in Italy, born 1907; winner of the Nobel prize in medicine and physiology for 1957, for work that led to development of antihistamines and muscle relaxants.

Bovimyces pleuropneumoniae (bo″vě-mi′sēz ploor″o-numo′ne-e) *Mycoplasma mycoides.*

bovine (bo′vīn) [L. *bos, bovis* ox, bullock, cow] pertaining to, characteristic of, or derived from the ox (cattle).

bovovaccination (bo″vo-vak″sĭ-na′shun) vaccination with bovovaccine.

bovovaccine (bo″vo-vak″sēn) an attenuated and ground human tubercle bacillus used by von Behring for protective inoculation against bovine tuberculosis.

bow (bo) a bow-shaped device. **Birnberg b.,** an intrauterine contraceptive device consisting of polyethylene molded in a rod and shaped in the outline of two isosceles triangles of equal size placed apex to apex, one containing a nylon tail to facilitate removal of the appliance. **Logan b.,** an appliance used to prevent tension on sutures after surgical repair of cleft lip.

Bowditch's law (bow′dich-ez) [Henry Pickering *Bowditch,* Bos-

ton physiologist, 1840–1911] see *all-or-none,* under A; see under *law;* and see *treppe.*

bowel (bow′el) [Fr. *boyau*] the intestine.

bowenoid (bo′en-oid) anaplastic; said of the neoplastic cells derived from the epidermis, which constitute lesions of intraepidermal squamous cell carcinoma (Bowen's disease).

Bowen's disease (precancerous dermatosis) (bo′enz) [John Templeton *Bowen,* American dermatologist, 1857–1941] see under *disease.*

bowie (bo′e) a disease resembling rickets, which affects unweaned lambs in New Zealand.

bowleg (bo′leg) an outward curvature of one or both legs near the knee; genu varum. **nonrachitic b.,** osteochondrosis deformans tibiae.

Bowman's capsule, etc. (bo′manz) [Sir William *Bowman,* an English physician, 1816–1892] see under *capsule, lamina, muscle, probe, theory,* and *tube.*

box (boks) a rectangular structure. **fracture b.,** a long box without cover or ends, to support a broken limb. **Skinner b.,** an experimental enclosure for testing animal conditioning, in which the subject animal performs (e.g., presses a bar or lever) to obtain a reward. **Yerkes discrimination b.,** a maze with a series of doors, used in the laboratory in studies of visual discrimination in animals; opening of the proper door produces a reward, but opening of the wrong door produces an electric stimulus.

boxing (boks′ing) in dentistry, the building up of vertical walls, usually in wax, around the impression to produce the desired size and form of the base of the cast, and to preserve certain landmarks of the impression.

box-note (boks′nōt) a hollow sound heard in percussing the chest in emphysema.

Boyer's bursa, cyst (bwah-yāz′) [Alexis, Baron, *de Boyer,* French surgeon, 1757–1833] see under *bursa* and *cyst.*

Boyle's law (boilz) [Robert *Boyle,* British physicist, 1627–1691] see under *law.*

Bozeman's catheter, operation, position speculum (boz′manz) [Nathan *Bozeman,* American surgeon, 1825–1905] see under *catheter, position,* and *speculum,* and see *hysterocytocleisis.*

Bozeman-Fritsch catheter (boz′man-fritsh) [Nathan *Bozeman;* Heinrich *Fritsch,* German gynecologist, 1844–1915] Bozeman's catheter.

Bozzolo's sign (bot′tso-lōz) [Camillo *Bozzolo,* Italian physician, 1845–1920] see under *sign.*

B.P. 1. blood pressure. 2. British Pharmacopoeia, a publication of the General Medical Council, describing and establishing standards for medicines, preparations, materials, and articles used in the practice of medicine, surgery, or midwifery.

b.p. *boiling point.*

B.P.A. British Paediatric Association.

B. Ph. British Pharmacopoeia.

Bq abbreviation for *becquerel.*

Br chemical symbol for *bromine.*

brace (brās) an orthopedic appliance or apparatus (an orthosis) used to support, align, or hold parts of the body in correct position; also, usually in the plural, an orthodontic appliance for the correction of malaligned teeth.

bracelet (brās′let) a small encircling band, denoting, in the plural, transverse markings across the palmar surface of the skin of the wrists. **Nageotte's b's,** bands covered with circular spines on the axons at the level of the nodes of Ranvier.

brachia (bra′ke-ah) [L.] plural of *brachium.*

brachial (bra′ke-al) [L. *brachialis,* from *brachium* arm] pertaining to the arm.

brachialgia (bra″ke-al′je-ah) [Gr. *brachiōn* arm + *-algia*] pain in the arm or arms. **b. stat′ica paresthet′ica,** painful paresthesias in the arm and hand during sleep due to compression of the blood vessels; called also *Wartenberg's disease.*

brachiation (bra″ke-a′shun) [L. *brachium* + *-ation* suffix implying action] locomotion in a position of suspension by means of the hands and arms, as exhibited by monkeys when swinging from branch to branch.

brachiocephalic (brak″e-o-sĕ-fal′ik) [Gr. *brachiōn* arm + *kephalē* head] pertaining to the arm and head.

brachiocrural (brak″e-o-kroo′ral) [L. *brachium* arm + *crus* leg] pertaining to the arm and leg.

brachiocubital (brak″e-o-ku′bĭ-tal) [L. *brachium* arm + *cubitus* elbow] pertaining to the arm and elbow or forearm.

brachiocyllosis (brak″e-o-sĭ-lo′sis) [Gr. *brachiōn* arm + *kyllōsis* a crooking] brachiocyrtosis.

brachiocyrtosis (brak″e-o-ser-to′sis) [Gr. *brachiōn* arm + *kyrtos* bent] crookedness of the arm.

brachiofaciolingual (brak″e-o-fa″she-o-ling′gwal) pertaining to or affecting the arm, the face, and the tongue.

brachiogram (brak′e-o-gram) (*obs.*) a tracing of the pulse beat at the brachial artery.

brachiotomy (bra″ke-ot′o-me) [Gr. *brachiōn* arm + *tomē* a cut] (*obs.*) the surgical or obstetrical cutting or removal of an arm.

brachium (bra′ke-um), pl. *bra′chia* [L.; Gr. *brachiōn*] [NA] 1. the arm; specifically the arm from shoulder to elbow. 2. a general term used to designate an armlike process or structure. **b. collic′uli inferio′ris** [NA], fibers from the lateral lemniscus that pass deep to the inferior colliculus and run forward to terminate in the medial geniculate body; called also *b. quadrigeminum inferius, b. conjunctivum posterius, b. of inferior colliculus, inferior b. of mesencephalon,* and *posterior conjunctival b.* **b. collic′uli superio′ris** [NA], fibers from the optic tract that pass dorsal to the superior colliculus to enter the superior colliculus; called also *b. quadrigeminum superius, anterior conjunctival b., b. conjunctivum anterius, b. of superior colliculus,* and *superior b. of mesencephalon.* **conjunctival b., anterior** (*obs.*), b. colliculi superioris. **conjunctival b., posterior** (*obs.*), b. colliculi inferioris. **b. conjuncti′vum ante′rius** (*obs.*), b. colliculi superioris. **b. conjuncti′vum [cerebel′li]**, pedunculus cerebellaris superior. **b. conjuncti′vum poste′rius** (*obs.*), b. colliculi inferioris. **b. of inferior colliculus,** b. colliculi inferioris. **b. of mesencephalon, inferior** (*obs.*), b. colliculi inferioris. **b. of mesencephalon, superior** (*obs.*), b. colliculi superioris. **b. op′ticum,** one of the processes extending from the corpora quadrigemina to the optic thalamus. **b. pon′tis,** pedunculus cerebellaris medius. **b. quadrigem′inum infe′rius,** b. colliculi inferioris. **b. quadrigem′inum supe′rius,** b. colliculi superioris. **b. of superior colliculus,** b. colliculi superioris.

brachy- (brak′e) [Gr. *brachys* short] a combining form meaning short.

brachybasia (brak″e-ba′se-ah) [*brachy-* + Gr. *basis* walking] a slow, shuffling, short-stepped gait, as seen in double hemiplegia.

brachycardia (brak″e-kar′de-ah) bradycardia.

brachycephalia (brak″e-se-fa′le-ah) brachycephaly.

brachycephalic (brak″e-se-fal′ik) [*brachy-* + Gr. *kephalē* head] having a short wide head, with a cephalic index of 81.0 to 85.4.

brachycephalism (brak″e-sef′ah-lizm) brachycephaly.

brachycephalous (brak″e-sef′ah-lus) brachycephalic.

brachycephaly (brak″e-sef′ah-le) the fact or quality of having a short head, with a cephalic index of 81.0 to 85.4.

brachycheilia (brak″e-ki′le-ah) [*brachy-* + Gr. *cheilos* lip + *-ia*] shortness of the lip.

brachychily (brak-ik′ĭ-le) brachycheilia.

brachychronic (brak″e-kron′ik) [Gr. *brachychronios* of short duration] acute; said of a disease (Rabagliati).

brachycranic (brak″e-kra′nik) having a short head, with a cephalic index of 80.0 to 84.9.

brachydactyly (brak″e-dak′tĭ-le) [*brachy-* + Gr. *daktylos* finger] abnormal shortness of the fingers and toes.

brachyesophagus (brak″e-ĕ-sof′ah-gus) [*brachy-* + *esophagus*] abnormal shortness of the esophagus.

brachyfacial (brak″e-fa′shal) having a low broad face, with a facial index of 90 or less.

brachygnathia (brak-ig-na′the-ah) [*brachy-* + Gr. *gnathos* jaw + *-ia*] abnormal shortness of the lower jaw.

brachygnathous (brah-kig′nah-thus) [*brachy-* + Gr. *gnathos* jaw] having an unusually short lower jaw.

brachykerkic (brak″e-ker′kik) [*brachy-* + Gr. *kerkis* the radius of the arm] having a short radius, with a radiohumeral index less than 75.

brachyknemic (brak″e-ne′mik) having a short leg, with a tibiofemoral index of 82 or less.

brachymetacarpalism (brak″e-met″ah-kar′pal-izm) brachymetacarpia.

brachymetacarpia (brak″e-met″ah-kar′pe-ah) abnormal shortness of the metacarpal bones.

brachymetapody (brak″e-mĕ-tap′o-de) abnormal shortness of some of the metacarpal or metatarsal bones.

brachymetatarsia (brak″e-met″ah-tar′se-ah) abnormal shortness of the metatarsal bones.

brachymetropia (brak″e-mĕtro′pe-ah) [*brachy-* + Gr. *metron* measure + *opsis* sight] myopia, or nearsightedness.

brachymetropic (brak″e-mĕ-trop′ik) nearsighted, or myopic.

brachymorphic (brak″e-mor′fik) [*brachy-* + Gr. *morphe* form] built along lines that are shorter and broader than those of the normal figure; called also *brachytypical* and *brevilineal*.

brachyphalangia (brak″e-fah-lan′je-ah) [*brachy-* + *phalanx*] abnormal shortness of one or more of the phalanges of a finger or toe.

brachyskelous (brak″e-ske′lus) having short legs.

brachystaphyline (brak″e-staf′ĭ-lin) [*brachy-* + Gr. *staphylē* uvula] having a short palate, with palatal index of 85.0 or more.

brachystasis (brah-kis′tah-sis) [*brachy-* + *stasis*] a state in which a muscle fiber is relatively decreased in length, and resists stretch; it contracts and relaxes, manifesting the same tension after contraction as before.

brachytherapy (brak″e-ther′ah-pe) in radiotherapy, treatment with ionizing radiation whose source is applied to the surface of the body or is located a short distance from the body area being treated; cf. *teletherapy.*

brachytypical (brak″e-tip′e-k′l) brachymorphic.

brachyuranic (brak″e-u-ran′ik) having a narrow maxilla, with a maxilloalveolar index of 115.0 or more.

bracing (bra′sing) resistance to the horizontal components of masticatory force.

bracken (brak′en) a fern, *Pteridium aquilinum* (L.) Kuhn (Polypodiaceae), of worldwide distribution noted as a poisonous plant in veterinary medicine. In monogastric animals, the plant produces severe intoxication due to enzymatic destruction of thiamine by a thiaminase present in the plant. In ruminants, the poisoning is apparently due to a dialyzable, small molecule which causes bone-marrow hypoplasia, leading to death.

bract (brakt) a small modified leaf in a flower cluster.

Bradford frame (brad′ford) [Edward Hickling *Bradford*, Boston orthopedic surgeon, 1848–1926] see under *frame.*

bradshot (brad′shot) braxy.

bradsot (brad′sot) braxy.

brady- (brad′e) [Gr. *bradys* slow] a combining form meaning slow.

bradyacusia (brad″e-ah-ku′se-ah) [*brady-* + Gr. *akouein* to hear] dullness of hearing.

bradyarrhythmia (brad″e-ah-rith′me-ah) [*brady-* + *a* neg. + Gr. *rhythmos* rhythm] bradycardia associated with an irregularity in the heart rhythm.

bradyarthria (brad″e-ar′thre-ah) [*brady-* + Gr. *arthroun* to utter distinctly] bradylalia.

bradyauxesis (brad″e-awk-se′sis) [*brady-* + Gr. *auxēsis* increase] a form of heterauxesis in which the part grows more slowly than the whole.

Bradybaena (brad″e-be′nah) a genus of snails that serve as hosts to *Dicrocoelium dentriticum.*

bradycardia (brad″e-kar′de-ah) [*brady-* + Gr. *kardia* heart] slowness of the heart beat, as evidenced by slowing of the pulse rate to less than 60. **Branham's b.,** see under *sign.* **cardiomuscular b.** (*obs.*), that caused by disease of the muscle of the heart. **central b.,** bradycardia dependent on disease of the central nervous system. **essential b.,** bradycardia occurring without discoverable cause. **nodal b.,** bradycardia in which the stimulus of the heart's contraction arises in the atrioventricular node or main bundle. **postinfective b.,** bradycardia occurring after infectious disease. **sinoatrial b.,** sinus b. **sinus b.,** a slow sinus rhythm, with a heart rate less than 60. **vagal b.,** bradycardia due to increased vagal tone.

bradycardiac (brad″e-kar′de-ak) 1. pertaining to, characterized by, or causing bradycardia. 2. an agent that acts to slow the pulse.

bradycardic (brad″e-kar′dik) bradycardiac.

bradycinesia (brad″e-sĭ-ne′ze-ah) bradykinesia.

bradycrotic (brad″e-krot′ik) [*brady-* + Gr. *krotos* pulsation] pertaining to, characterized by, or inducing slowness of pulse.

bradydiastalsis (brad″e-di″ah-stal′sis) (*obs.*) slow or delayed bowel movement.

bradydiastole (brad″e-di-as′to-le) [*brady-* + *diastole*] abnormal prolongation of the diastole.

bradyecoia (brad″e-e-koi′ah) [Gr. *bradyēkoos* slow of hearing] partial deafness.

bradyesthesia (brad″e-es-the′ze-ah) [*brady-* + Gr. *aisthēsis* perception] slowness or dullness of perception.

bradygenesis (brad″e-jen′ĕ-sis) [*brady-* + *genesis*] the lengthening of certain stages in embryonic development.

bradyglossia (brad″e-glos′e-ah) [Gr. *bradyglōssos* slow of speech] abnormal slowness of utterance.

bradykinesia (brad″e-kĭ-ne′se-ah) [*brady-* + Gr. *kinēsis* movement] abnormal slowness of movement; sluggishness of physical and mental responses.

bradykinetic (brad″e-kĭ-net′ik) [*brady-* + Gr. *kinēsis* motion] 1. characterized by or performed by slow movement. 2. denoting a method of showing the details of motor action by motion pictures taken very rapidly and shown very slowly.

bradykinin (brad″e-ki′nin) [*brady-* + Gr. *kinein* to move] a kinin composed of a chain of nine amino acids (arginine, proline, proline, glycine, phenylalanine, serine, proline, phenylalanine, and arginine), formed from kallidin II by the action of kallikrein; it is a very powerful vasodilator and causes increased capillary permeability. In addition, it constricts smooth muscle and stimulates pain receptors.

bradylalia (brad″e-la′le-ah) [*brady-* + Gr. *lalein* to talk] abnormally slow utterance of words due to a brain lesion; called also *bradyarthria* and *bradyphasia.*

bradylexia (brad″e-lek′se-ah) [*brady-* + Gr. *lexis* word] abnormal slowness in reading, due neither to defect of intelligence or of vision nor to ignorance of the alphabet.

bradylogia (brad″e-lo′je-ah) [Gr.] abnormal slowness of speech due to slowness of thinking, as in a mental disorder.

bradymenorrhea (brad″e-men″o-re′ah) [*brady-* + *menorrhea*] menstruation marked by long duration.

bradyphagia (brad″e-fa′je-ah) [*brady-* + Gr. *phagein* to eat] abnormal slowness in eating.

bradyphasia (brad″e-fa′ze-ah) [*brady-* + Gr. *phasis* speech] bradylalia.

bradyphemia (brad″e-fe′me-ah) [*brady-* + Gr. *phēmē* speech] slowness of speech.

bradyphrasia (brad″e-fra′ze-ah) [*brady-* + Gr. *phrasis* utterance] slowness of speech due to mental disorder.

bradyphrenia (brad″e-fre′ne-ah) [*brady-* + Gr. *phrēn* mind] a condition marked by extreme fatigability of initiative, interest, and psychomotor activity resulting from epidemic encephalitis.

bradypnea (brad″e-ne′ah) [*brady-* + Gr. *pnoia* breath] abnormal slowness of breathing.

bradypragia (brad″e-pra′je-ah) [*brady-* + Gr. *prattein* to act] slowness of action.

bradyrhythmia (brad″e-rith′me-ah) [*brady-* + Gr. *rhythmos* rhythm] bradycardia.

bradyspermatism (brad″e-sper′mah-tizm) [*brady-* + Gr. *sperma* semen] abnormally slow ejaculation of semen.

bradysphygmia (brad″e-sfig′me-ah) [*brady-* + Gr. *sphygmos* pulse] bradycardia.

bradystalsis (brad″e-stal′sis) [*brady-* + (*peri*)-*stalsis*] abnormal slowness of peristalsis.

bradytachycardia (brad″e-tak″e-kar′de-ah) [*brady-* + Gr. *tachys* swift + *kardia* heart] alternating attacks of bradycardia and tachycardia, as may occur in sick sinus syndrome.

bradyteleocinesia (brad″e-tel″e-o-si-ne′ze-ah) bradyteleokinesis.

bradyteleokinesis (brad″e-tel″e-o-ki̇̆-ne′sis) [*brady-* + Gr. *telein* to complete + *kinēsis* movement] a defect of motor coordination in which a movement is slowed or stopped prior to reaching its goal.

bradytocia (brad″e-to′se-ah) [*brady-* + Gr. *tokos* birth] lingering or slow parturition.

bradytrophia (brad″e-tro′fe-ah) a condition characterized by slow-acting nutritive processes.

bradytrophic (brad″e-trof′ik) [*brady-* + Gr. *trophē* nutrition] having slow-acting nutritive processes.

bradyuria (brad″e-u′re-ah) [*brady-* + Gr. *ouron* urine] abnormally slow passage of urine.

braidism (brād′izm) [after James *Braid*] hypnotism.

Braid's strabismus (brādz) [James *Braid*, English surgeon 1795–1860] see under *strabismus*.

Brailey's operation (bra′lēz) [William Arthur *Brailey*, English ophthalmologist, 1845–1915] see under *operation*.

braille (brāl) [Louis *Braille*, a French teacher of the blind, 1809–1852] a system of writing and printing for the blind by means of tangible points or dots.

brain (brān) [Anglo-Saxon *braegen*] that part of the central nervous system contained within the cranium, comprising the prosencephalon, mesencephalon, and rhombencephalon; it is derived (developed) from the anterior part of the embryonic neural tube. Called also *encephalon*. See also *cerebrum*. **new b.,** neencephalon (neoencephalon). **old b.,** paleencephalon (paleoencephalon). **olfactory b.,** smell b., rhinencephalon, def. 1. **respirator b.,** the brain after clinical brain death but while vital functions are being artificially maintained; it is characterized by marked autolysis and necrosis. **'tween b.,** diencephalon (interbrain). **water b.,** gid. **wet b.,** an edematous condition of the brain; see *brain edema*, under *edema*.

Brain's reflex (brānz) [Walter Russell *Brain*, British neurologist, 1895–1966] see under *reflex*.

brain stem (brān′stem) the stemlike portion of the brain connecting the cerebral hemispheres with the spinal cord and comprising the pons, medulla oblongata, and mesencephalon; the diencephalon is considered part of the brain stem by some.

brainwashing (brān′wash-ing) systematic emotional and mental conditioning of an individual or a group of individuals designed to instill attitudes and beliefs conformable to the wishes of those administering the conditioning, accomplished by means of propaganda, torture, drugs, conditioning procedures, or by other means. Called also *menticide*.

brake (brāk) a mechanism for arresting or inhibiting an activity. **duodenal b.,** a mechanism lodged largely in the duodenum that inhibits gastric secretion and motility.

bran (bran) the meal derived from the epidermis or outer covering of a cereal grain.

branch (branch) a division or offshoot from a main stem, especially of blood vessels, nerves, or lymphatics; for specific anatomical structures, see under *ramus*.

branchia (brang′ke-ah) [Gr. *branchia* gills] the gills of fishes and of others of the lower vertebrates; represented in the human fetus by the branchial arches, separated by clefts.

branchial (brang′ke-al) pertaining to or resembling the gills of a fish or the derivatives of homologous parts in higher forms.

branchiogenic (brang″ke-o-jen′ik) gill-forming; forming a branchial arch.

branchiogenous (brang″ke-oj′e̅-nus) [*branchia* + Gr. *gennan* to produce] formed from a branchial cleft or arch.

branchioma (brang″ke-o′mah) a tumor derived from branchial epithelium or branchial rests.

branchiomere (brang′ke-o-mēr″) a segment of the splanchnic mesoderm from which the branchial arches are developed.

branchiomeric (brang″ke-o-mer′ik) pertaining to the branchiomeres or visceral arches.

branchiomerism (brang″ke-om′er-izm) [*branchia-* + Gr. *meros* part] metamerism based on the serial repetition of the branchial arches.

Branchiostoma (brang″ke-o-sto′mah) [*branchia* + Gr. *stoma* mouth] *Amphioxus*.

Brand bath (brahnt) [Ernst *Brand*, German physician, 1827–1897] see under *bath*.

Brande's test (brands) [William Thomas *Brande*, English chemist, 1788–1866] see under *tests*.

Brandt's method (treatment) (brahnts) [Thure *Brandt*, Swedish physician, 1819–1895] see under *method*.

brandy (bran′de) the potable alcoholic distillate of fermented juices of various fruits, e.g., grapes, apples, cherries, peaches, etc., containing 48 to 54 per cent ethanol; used medically as a stomachic, tonic, peripheral vasodilator, and sedative.

Branham's sign (bradycardia) (bran′hamz) [H. H. *Branham*, American surgeon of 19th century] see under *sign*.

Branhamella (bran″hah-mel′ah) a genus of aerobic, nonmotile, non–spore-forming cocci. The type species, *B. catarrha′lis*, is a normal inhabitant of the nasopharynx but occasionally causes disease; called also *Neisseria catarrhalis*.

brash (brash) heartburn. **water b.,** heartburn with regurgitation of sour fluid or almost tasteless saliva into the mouth. **weaning b.,** diarrhea in an infant when put on food other than its mother's milk.

Brassica (bras′e-kah) [L.] a genus of cruciferous plants to which the cabbage, turnip, mustard, and related species belong. *B. al′ba* (L.) Rabenh. (*Sinapis alba* L.) is white mustard, and *B. ni′gra* (L.) Koch. is black mustard. When the seeds of these plants are crushed and moistened, volatile oils are liberated. See *mustard* and *oil of mustard*.

Braun's anastomosis (brawnz) [Heinrich *Braun*, German surgeon, 1847–1911] see under *anastomosis*.

Braun's canal (brawnz) [Carl von *Braun*, Viennese obstetrician, 1822–1891] neurenteric canal; see under *canal*.

Braun's hook (brawnz) [Gustav *Braun*, Austrian gynecologist, 1829–1911] see under *hook*.

Braun's test (brawnz) [Christopher Heinrich *Braun*, German physician, born 1847] see under *tests*.

Braun-Husler test (reaction) (brawn hoos′ler) [Ludwig *Braun*, German physician, born 1881] see under *tests*.

Braune's canal (brawn′ez) [Christian Wilhelm *Braune*, German anatomist, 1831–1892] see under *canal*.

Braxton Hicks' sign (braks′ton hiks) [John *Braxton Hicks*, English gynecologist, 1823–1897] see *Hicks sign*, under *sign*.

braxy (brak′se) a disease of sheep caused by *Clostridium septicum*, and marked by hemorrhagic abomasitis, with hemorrhage into the peritoneal cavity, by abdominal pain, and, usually, by diarrhea and high fever.

brayera (bra-ye′rah) the dried panicles of the pistillate flowers of *Hagenia abyssinica* J. F. Gmel., having medical and veterinary use as a vermifuge and teniacide, respectively.

brazilin (brah-zil′in) a yellow crystalline substance obtained from the bark of *Biancea sappan* and other redwood trees; it is very similar to hematoxylin and oxidizes to a bright red dye, brazilein.

breadth (bredth) the distance measured horizontally from side to side; see also under *diameter*. **b. of accommodation,** range of accommodation. **bizygomatic b.,** the distance between the most laterally situated points (zygia) on the zygomatic arches.

break (brāk) 1. to interrupt the continuity, or an interruption in the continuity of a structure, especially a bone. See *fracture*. 2. the interruption of an electric circuit, as distinguished from the make. **chromatid b.,** interruption of the continuity of a chromatid, the portions immediately proximal and distal to the site being out of alignment.

breast (brest) the anterior aspect of the chest, often applied especially to the modified cutaneous glandular structure it bears; see *mamma* [NA]. **caked b.,** stagnation mastitis. **chicken b.,** pigeon b. **Cooper's irritable b.,** neuralgia of the breast. **funnel b.,** funnel chest. **hysterical b.,** painful swelling of the breast due to hysteria. **irritable b.,** Cooper's irritable b.

Plate IX

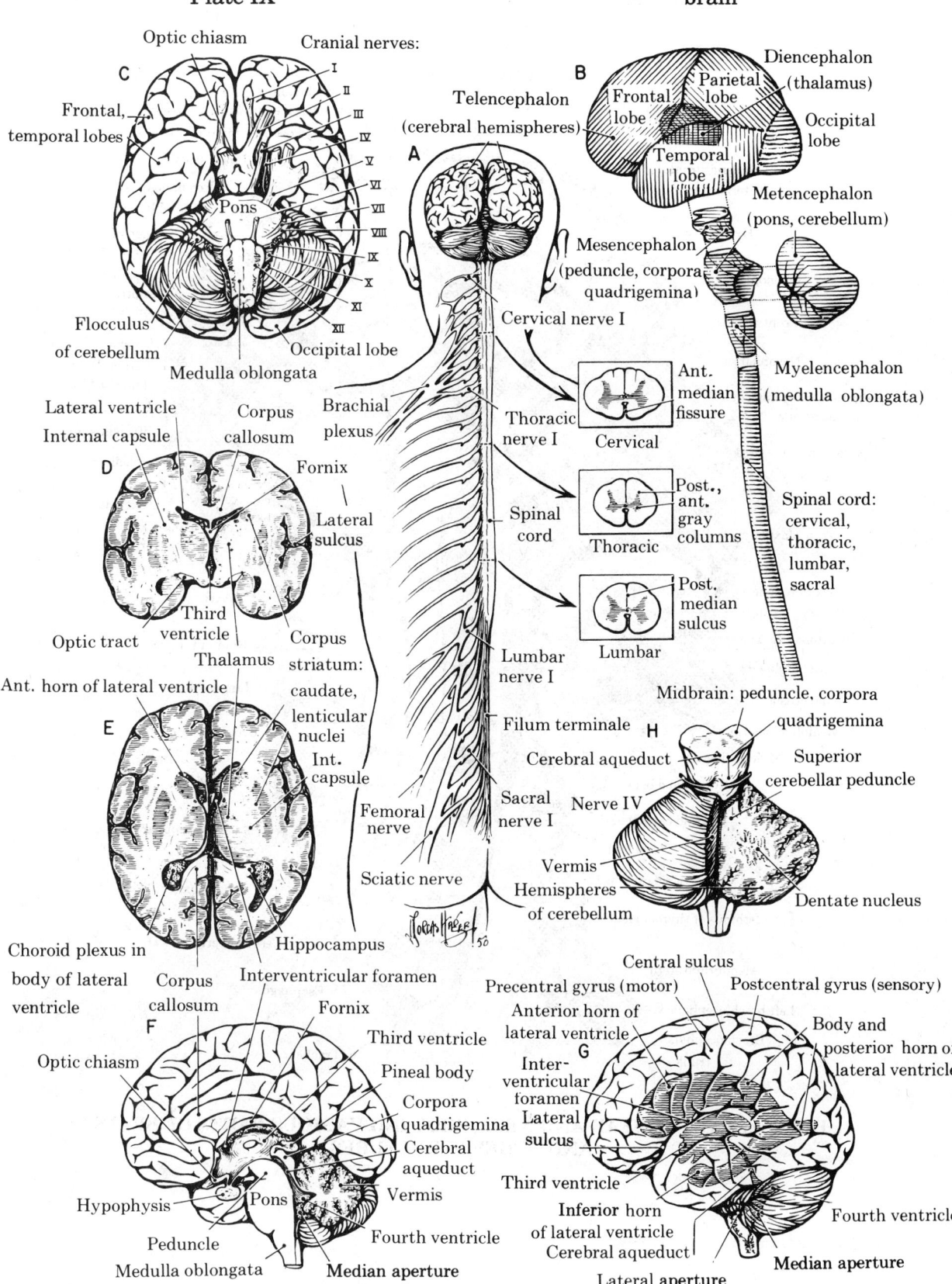

Optic chiasm Cranial nerves:

C I
II
Frontal, III
temporal lobes IV
V
VI
VII
Pons VIII
IX
X
Flocculus XI
of cerebellum XII **Occipital lobe**
Medulla oblongata

B Diencephalon
(thalamus)
Frontal Parietal
lobe lobe Occipital
lobe
Temporal
lobe Metencephalon
(pons, cerebellum)

Telencephalon
(cerebral hemispheres) Mesencephalon
(peduncle, corpora
quadrigemina)

A Myelencephalon
(medulla oblongata)

Cervical nerve I

Lateral ventricle Corpus
Internal capsule callosum
Ant.
D median
Fornix fissure
Cervical
Lateral
sulcus Post.,
ant.
Third gray
Optic tract ventricle Corpus columns
striatum: Thoracic
Thalamus caudate,
Ant. horn of lateral ventricle lenticular Post.
nuclei median
Int. sulcus
E capsule Lumbar

Thoracic
nerve I

Spinal
cord

Lumbar
nerve I

Spinal cord:
cervical,
thoracic,
lumbar,
sacral

Midbrain: peduncle, corpora
quadrigemina
Filum terminale H
Cerebral aqueduct Superior
cerebellar peduncle
Nerve IV
Sacral
nerve I
Choroid plexus in Vermis
body of lateral Corpus Femoral Hemispheres Dentate nucleus
ventricle callosum nerve of cerebellum
Interventricular foramen Hippocampus
Sciatic nerve

Central sulcus
Precentral gyrus (motor) Postcentral gyrus (sensory)
F Anterior horn of
Fornix lateral ventricle Body and
Third ventricle Inter- G posterior horn of
Optic chiasm Pineal body ventricular lateral ventricle
foramen
Corpora Lateral
quadrigemina sulcus
Cerebral
aqueduct Third ventricle
Hypophysis Vermis
Pons Inferior horn Fourth ventricle
Peduncle Fourth ventricle of lateral ventricle
Medulla oblongata **Median aperture** Cerebral aqueduct **Median aperture**
Lateral **aperture**

VARIOUS ASPECTS AND SECTIONS OF BRAIN AND SPINAL CORD

Plate X   brain

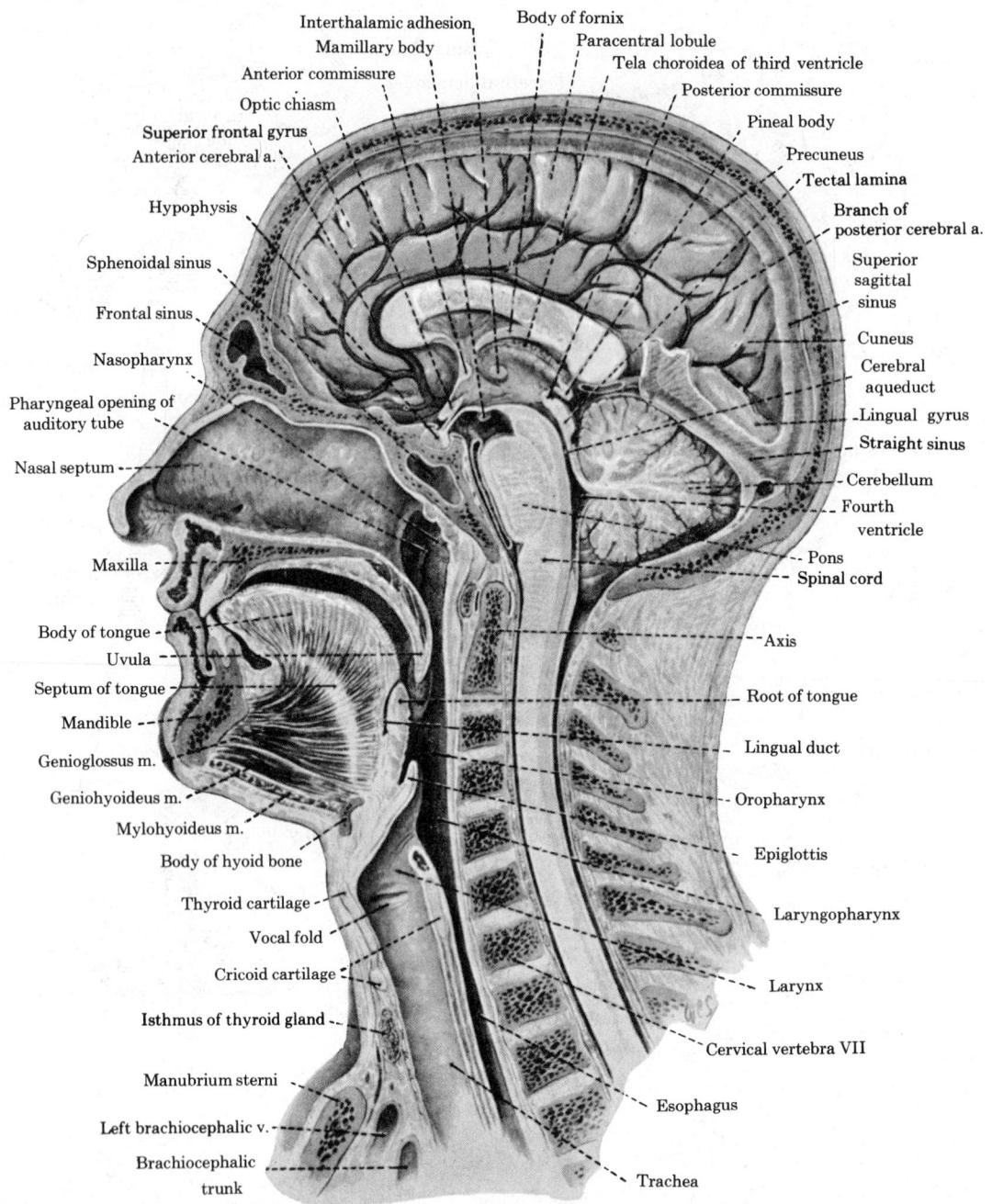

Interthalamic adhesion
Mamillary body
Anterior commissure
Optic chiasm
Superior frontal gyrus
Anterior cerebral a.
Hypophysis
Sphenoidal sinus
Frontal sinus
Nasopharynx
Pharyngeal opening of auditory tube
Nasal septum
Maxilla
Body of tongue
Uvula
Septum of tongue
Mandible
Genioglossus m.
Geniohyoideus m.
Mylohyoideus m.
Body of hyoid bone
Thyroid cartilage
Vocal fold
Cricoid cartilage
Isthmus of thyroid gland
Manubrium sterni
Left brachiocephalic v.
Brachiocephalic trunk

Body of fornix
Paracentral lobule
Tela choroidea of third ventricle
Posterior commissure
Pineal body
Precuneus
Tectal lamina
Branch of posterior cerebral a.
Superior sagittal sinus
Cuneus
Cerebral aqueduct
Lingual gyrus
Straight sinus
Cerebellum
Fourth ventricle
Pons
Spinal cord
Axis
Root of tongue
Lingual duct
Oropharynx
Epiglottis
Laryngopharynx
Larynx
Cervical vertebra VII
Esophagus
Trachea

HEMISECTION OF HEAD AND NECK, SHOWING VARIOUS PARTS OF BRAIN AND OTHER STRUCTURES

(Anson)

pigeon b., a condition of the chest in which the sternum is prominent, due to obstruction to infantile respiration or to rickets; called also *chicken b., keeled chest, pectus carinatum,* and *pectus gallinatum.* **proemial b.,** that condition of the female breast which is a prelude to pathologic changes. **shoe-makers' b.,** sinking in of the sternum in shoe-makers, produced by the pressure of tools against the lower part of the sternum and the xiphoid cartilage. **shotty b.,** cystic disease of the breast; see under *disease.* **thrush b.,** the speckled appearance of the myocardium under the endocardium in fatty degeneration of the heart.

breast-feeding (brest′ fēd′ing) the nursing of an infant at the mother's breast.

breath (breth) [L. *spiritus halitus*] the air taken in and expelled by the expansion and contraction of the thorax. **lead b.,** the metallic odor of the breath in lead poisoning; called also *halitus saturninus.* **liver b.,** fetor hepaticus (hepatic fetor).

breathing (brēth′ing) the alternate inspiration and expiration of air into and out of the lungs; see *respiration.* **Biot's b.,** see under *respiration.* **bronchial b.,** vesicular breath sounds. **frog b., glossopharyngeal b.,** respiration unaided by the primary or ordinary accessory muscles of respiration, the air being "swallowed" rapidly into the lungs by use of the tongue and muscles of the pharynx; used by patients with chronic muscle paralysis to augment their breathing. **intermittent positive pressure b.,** the active inflation of the lungs during inspiration under positive pressure from a cycling valve; abbreviated IPPB. **periodic b.,** Cheyne-Stokes respiration.

Breda's disease (bra′dahz) [Achille *Breda,* Italian dermatologist, 1850–1933] yaws.

bredouillement (bra-dwe-maw′) a speech defect in which only part of the word is pronounced, due to extreme rapidity of utterance.

breech (brēch) buttocks (nates [NA]). **frank b.,** see under *presentation.*

bregma (breg′mah) [L.; Gr.] the point on the surface of the skull at the junction of the coronal and sagittal sutures.

bregmatic (breg-mat′ik) pertaining to the bregma.

bregmatodymia (breg″mah-to-dim′e-ah) [*bregma* + Gr. *didymos* twin + *-ia*] the state of conjoined twins fused at the bregmas.

Brehmer's treatment (method) (bra′merz) [Hermann *Brehmer,* German physician, 1826–1889] see under *treatment.*

brei (bri) [Ger. "pulp"] tissue that has been ground to a pulp; a homogenate.

Breisky's disease (bri′skēz) [August *Breisky,* German gynecologist, 1832–1889] kraurosis vulvae.

Bremer's test (brem′erz) [Ludwig *Bremer,* St. Louis physician, 1844–1914] see under *tests.*

bremsstrahlung (brem′strah-lung) [Ger. "braking radiation"] the electromagnetic radiation produced by the sudden deflection of a fast-charged particle (usually an electron) by another charged particle (usually a nucleus), the spectral distribution being continuous.

Brennemann's syndrome (bren′e-manz) [Joseph *Brennemann,* Chicago pediatrician, 1872–1944] see under *syndrome.*

Brenner's formula (test) (bren′erz) [Rudolf *Brenner,* German physician, 1821–1884] see under *formula.*

Brenner operation [Alexander *Brenner,* Austrian surgeon, 1859–1936] see under *operation.*

Brenner tumor [Fritz *Brenner,* German pathologist, born 1877] see under *tumor.*

brenz- (brents) a pure German prefix, meaning burnt; for words beginning thus, see those beginning *pyro-.*

brephic (bref′ik) [Gr. *brephos* embryo] pertaining to an early stage of development.

brepho- (bref′o) [Gr. *brephos* embryo or newborn infant] a combining form denoting relationship to the embryo or fetus, or to the newborn infant.

brephoplastic (bref″o-plas′tik) [*brepho-* + Gr. *plassein* to form] formed from embryonic tissue or during embryonic life.

brephopolysarcia (bref″o-pol″e-sar′se-ah) [*brepho-* + *polysarcia*] (obs.) excessive fleshiness in an infant.

brephotrophic (bref″o-trof′ik) [*brepho-* + Gr. *trophē* nutrition] pertaining to the nourishment of infants.

Breschet's canals, hiatus, sinus, veins (brĕ-shaz′) [Gilbert *Breschet,* French anatomist, 1784-1845] see *canales diploici, helicotrema, sinus sphenoparietalis,* and *venae diploicae.*

Brethine (breth′ēn) trademark for preparations of terbutaline sulfate.

Bretonneau's diphtheria (angina, disease) (bret-o-nōz′) [Pierre Fidèle *Bretonneau,* French physician, 1778–1862] diphtheria.

bretylium tosylate (brĕ-til′e-um) chemical name: 2-bromo-*N*-ethyl-*N,N*-dimethylbenzenemethanaminium 4-methylbenzenesulfonate. An adrenergic blocking agent, $C_{18}H_{24}BrNO_3S$, occurring as a white, crystalline powder; originally used as an antihy-

pertensive agent, it is now used as an antiarrhythmic in certain cases of ventricular tachycardia or fibrillation.

Breus mole (broys) [Carl *Breus,* Austrian obstetrician, 1852–1914] see under *mole.*

brevi- (brev′e) [L. *brevis* short] a combining form meaning short.

Brevibacteriaceae (brev″e-bak-te″re-a′se-e) a family of Schizomycetes (order Eubacteriales), occurring as motile or nonmotile cells without endospores. It includes two genera, *Brevibacterium* and *Kurthia.*

Brevibacterium (brev″e-bak-te′re-um) a genus of microorganisms of the family Brevibacteriaceae, order Eubacteriales, made up of generally nonmotile, short, unbranched rods. Found in soil, salt and fresh water, dairy products, and decomposing material of many types. It includes 23 species.

brevicollis (brev″ĕ-kol′is) [*brevi-* + L. *collum* neck] shortness of the neck; see *dystrophia brevicollis.*

breviductor (brev″ĕ-duk′tor) [*brevi-* + L. *ductor* leader] (obs.) musculus adductor brevis.

breviflexor (brev″ĕ-flek′sor) [*brevi-* + L. *flexor* bender] a short flexor muscle.

brevilineal (brev″ĕ-lin′e-al) brachymorphic.

breviradiate (brev″ĕ-ra′de-āt) having short processes; a term applied to one type of neuroglia cells.

Brevital (brev′ĭ-tal) trademark for a preparation of methohexital sodium.

brevium (bre′ve-um) a name formerly given to a supposed isotope of tantalum now known to be the element protactinium.

Brewer's infarcts, point (broo′erz) [George Emerson *Brewer,* New York surgeon, 1861–1939] see under *infarct* and *point.*

Bricanyl (brik′ah-nil) trademark for preparations of terbutaline sulfate.

Brickner's sign (brik′nerz) [Richard Max *Brickner,* New York neurologist, born 1896] see under *sign.*

brickpox (brik′poks) a form of swine erysipelas (Ger. *Backsteinblattern*) caused by *Erysipelothrix insidiosa.*

bridge (brij) 1. a form of dental prosthesis that replaces one or more lost or missing teeth, being supported and held in position by attachments to adjacent teeth; see *partial denture,* under *denture.* 2. see *pons.* 3. a protoplasmic structure that unites adjacent elements of a cell, similar in plants and animals. **arteriolovenular b.,** the main and largest capillary connecting an arteriole and a venule; it retains some muscle elements and is rarely completely collapsed. **cantilever b.,** a fixed partial denture that is attached at one end to one or more natural teeth or roots, the other end not being rigidly attached. **cell b's,** see *intercellular b.* and *protoplasmic b.* **cytoplasmic b.,** 1. protoplasmic b. 2. intercellular b. **dentin b.,** a scarlike deposit of reparative dentin or other calcific substance which reseals exposed pulp or which forms across the excised surface of pulp after pulpotomy. **disulfide b.,** see under *bond.* **extension b.,** one having an artificial tooth attached beyond the point of anchorage of the tooth; sometimes called *cantilever b.* **fixed b.,** a fixed partial denture. **Gaskell's b.,** bundle of His. **intercellular b.,** a structure seen especially in the prickle cell layer of the epidermis, formed by the meeting of short cytoplasmic projections from the cell surface of adjacent cells. The structure was formerly thought to constitute a bridge for cytoplasmic continuity between cells, but it has been demonstrated that the processes make contact at a desmosome (q.v.); hence each cell is independent. Called also *cytoplasmic b.* **b. of the nose,** the upper portion of the external nose formed by the junction of the nasal bones. **protoplasmic b.,** a strand of protoplasm connecting two secondary spermatocytes, occurring as a result of incomplete cytokinesis; called also *cytoplasmic b.* **removable b.,** a removable partial denture. **salt b.,** 1. an inverted-U–shaped tube filled with a gel, usually composed of agar, water, and potassium chloride, used to separate two chemically incompatible solutions in an electrochemical cell. 2. a chemical bond between a nitrogen atom, carrying a positive charge, and an oxygen atom, carrying a negative charge. **stationary b.,** a fixed partial denture. **ureteric b.,** Bell's muscle. **b. of Varolius,** pons, def. 2.

bridgework (brij′werk) a partial denture retained by attachments other than clasps. **fixed b.,** a partial denture retained by crowns or inlays cemented to the natural teeth. **removable b.,** a partial denture retained by attachments which permit its removal.

bridle (bri′d'l) 1. a frenum. 2. a loop or filament that crosses the lumen of a passage or the surface of an ulcer.

bridou (bre-doo′) perlèche.

Brieger's cachexia reaction, test (bre′gerz) [Ludwig *Brieger,* physician in Berlin, 1849–1919] see *cachexia reaction,* under *reaction,* and see under *tests.*

Bright's blindness, disease, eye (brīts) [Richard *Bright,* English physician, 1789–1858] see under *blindness, disease,* and *eye.*

brightic (bri′tik) 1. affected with glomerulonephritis (Bright's disease). 2. a person with glomerulonephritis.

brightism (brīt′izm) acute or chronic nephritis.

Brill's disease (brilz) [Nathan Edwin *Brill*, American physician, 1860–1925] see under *disease*.

Brill-Symmers disease [Nathan Edwin *Brill*; Douglas *Symmers*, American physician, 1879–1952] giant follicular lymphoma.

Brill-Zinsser disease (bril′zin′ser) [Nathan E. *Brill*; Hans *Zinsser*, American bacteriologist, 1878–1940] Brill's disease.

brim (brim) the edge of the superior strait of the true pelvis; apertura pelvis superior.

Brinell hardness number (brin-el′) [Johann August *Brinell*, Swedish engineer, 1849–1925] see under *number*.

brinolase (bri′no-lās) a fibrinolytic enzyme produced by the fungus *Aspergillus oryzae*.

Brinton's disease (brin′tonz) [William *Brinton*, English physician, 1823–1867] linitis plastica.

Brion-Kayser disease (bre-on′ ki′zer) [Albert *Brion*, physician in Strasburg; Heinrich *Kayser*, German physician] paratyphoid, def. 2.

Briquet's ataxia, syndrome (bre-kāz′) [Paul *Briquet*, French physician, 1796–1881] see under *ataxia* and *syndrome*.

brisement (brēz-maw′) [Fr. "crushing"] the breaking up or tearing of anything, as of an ankylosis. **b. forcé**, the forcible breaking up or tearing of a bony ankylosis.

brise-pierre (brēs-pe-ār′) [Fr. "stone-breaker"] a form of lithotrite.

Brissaud's dwarf, infantilism, reflex, scoliosis (bre-sōz′) [Edouard *Brissaud*, French physician, 1852–1909] see under *dwarf*; see *infantile myxedema*, under *myxedema*; see under *reflex*; and see *sciatic scoliosis*, under *scoliosis*.

Brissaud-Sicard syndrome (bre-so′-se-kar′) [Edouard *Brissaud*; Jean Athanase *Sicard*, Paris neurologist, 1872–1929] see under *syndrome*.

Bristacycline (bris″tah-si′klēn) trademark for a preparation of tetracycline hydrochloride.

Bristamin (bris′tah-min) trademark for a preparation of phenyltoloxamine.

broach (brōch) a fine instrument used by dentists for assisting in the instrumental cleansing of a root canal or for extirpating the pulp. **barbed b.**, one whose surface is covered with barbs. **root-canal b.**, a broach for use in removing the contents of a root canal of a tooth. **smooth b.**, one without barbs, used for exploring fine and tortuous root canals.

Broadbent's sign (brod′bentz) [Sir William Henry *Broadbent*, English physician, 1835–1907] see under *sign*.

Broca's amnesia, etc. (bro′kahz) [Pierre Paul *Broca*, celebrated French anatomist, anthropologist, and surgeon, 1824–1880] see under *amnesia*, *aphasia*, *area*, *ataxia*, *band*, *center*, *convolution*, *fissure*, *formula*, *gyrus*, *plane*, *point*, *pouch*, and *region*.

Brock's syndrome (brok) [Russell Claude *Brock*, British surgeon, born 1903] middle lobe syndrome.

Brödel's white line (brü′del) [Max *Brödel*, Baltimore physician, 1870–1941] see under *line*.

Broders' index (classification) (bro′derz) [Albert Compton *Broders*, American pathologist, 1885–1964] see under *index*.

Brodie's abscess, disease, knee (bro′dēz) [Sir Benjamin Collins *Brodie*, English surgeon, 1783–1862] see under *abscess*, *disease*, and *knee*.

Brodie's ligament (bro′dēz) [J. Gordon *Brodie*, Edinburgh anatomist, 1786–1818] transverse humeral ligament.

Brodmann's area [Korbinian *Brodmann*, German neurologist, 1868–1918] see under *area*.

Broesike's fossa (bre′ze-kēz) [Gustav *Broesike*, German anatomist, born 1853] see *parajejunal fossa*, under *fossa*.

brofoxine (bro-foks′ēn) chemical name: 6-bromo-1,4-dihydro-4,4-dimethyl-2*H*-3,1-benzoxazin-2-one; a tranquilizer, $C_{10}H_{10}BrNO_2$.

broken wind (bro′ken wind) heaves.

brom-, bromo- (brōm, bro′mo) [Gr. *brōmos* stink] a combining form indicating the presence of bromine.

bromated (bro′māt-ed) brominated.

bromatherapy (bro″mah-ther′ah-pe) bromatotherapy.

bromatology (bro″mah-tol′o-je) [Gr. *brōma* food + *-logy*] the science of foods and dietetics.

bromatotherapy (bro″mah-to-ther′ah-pe) [Gr. *brōma* food + *therapeia* treatment] the use of food in treating disease; called also **bromatherapy**.

bromatotoxin, bromatotoxismus (bro″mah-to- tok′sin; bro″-mah-to-tok-sis′mus) [Gr. *brōma* food + *toxin*] the poison formed in food by fermentation, etc.

bromatoxism (bro-mah-tok′sizm) [Gr. *brōma* food + *toxikon* poison] food poisoning.

bromazepam (bro-mah′zĕ-pam) chemical name: 7-bromo-1,3-dihydro-5-(2-pyridyl)-2*H*-1,4-benzodiazepin- 2-one; a minor tranquilizer, $C_{14}H_{10}BrN_3O$.

bromelain (bro′mĕ-lān) a proteolytic and milk-clotting enzyme derived from the pineapple plant, *Ananas sativus*; called also *bromelin*. In the plural, a concentrate of these enzymes, used as an anti-inflammatory agent. Also used in tenderizing meat, preparing protein hydrolysates, and chill-proofing beer.

bromelin (bro-mel′in) [L. *bromelia* pineapple] bromelain.

bromethol (bro-meth′ol) tribromoethanol solution.

bromhexine hydrochloride (brom-heks′ēn) chemical name: 2-amino-3,5-dibromo-*N*-cyclohexyl-*N*-methylbenzenemethanamine monohydrochloride; an expectorant and mucolytic, $C_{14}H_{20}$-$Br_2N_2 \cdot HCl$.

bromhidrosis (bro″mĭ-dro′sis) [Gr. *brōmos* stench + *hidrōs* sweat] axillary (apocrine) sweat which has become foul-smelling as a result of its bacterial decomposition.

bromic (bro′mik) pertaining to or containing pentavalent bromine, as in bromic acid, $HBrO_3$.

bromide (bro′mīd) any binary compound of bromine in which the bromine carries a negative charge (Br^-); specifically a salt (or organic ester) of hydrobromic acid (H^+Br^-). Bromides produce depression of the central nervous system, and were once widely used for their sedative effect. Because overdosage causes serious mental disturbances they are now used seldomly, except occasionally in grand mal seizures. See also *bromism*.

bromidrosis (bro″mĭ-dro′sis) bromhidrosis.

brominated (bro″mĭ-nāt′ed) combined with or containing bromine; bromated; brominized.

bromine (bro′mēn; bro′min) [L. *bromium, brominium, bromum*; Gr. *brōmos* stench] a reddish-brown liquid element, symbol Br, giving off suffocating vapors. Its atomic number is 35; atomic weight, 79.909. See also *bromide* and *bromism*.

brominism (bro′min-izm) a condition of poisoning produced by the excessive use of bromine or a bromine compound; it is marked by such neurological symptoms as mental dullness, deficient memory, slurred speech, drowsiness, and unsteady gait, and by skin eruptions of various forms and fetor of breath. Called also *bromism*.

brominized (bro′min-īzd) brominated.

bromism (bro′mizm) brominism.

bromisovalum (brōm″i-so-val′um) chemical name: *N*-(aminocarbonyl)-2-bromo-3-methylbutanamide. A sedative and hypnotic, $C_6H_{11}BrN_2O_2$, occurring as white, needle-shaped or scale-like crystals; administered orally.

bromization (bro″mi-za′shun) impregnation with bromides or bromine; the administration of large doses of bromides.

bromized (bro′mīzd) under the influence of bromides.

bromobenzene (bro″mo-ben′zēn) a colorless liquid, C_6H_5Br, with a pleasant, characteristic odor, obtained by bromination of benzene in the presence of iron.

bromochlorotrifluoroethane (bro″mo-klo″ro-tri-floo-o″ro-eth′ān) halothane.

bromocriptine (bro″mo-krip′tēn) 2-bromo-α-ergocryptine, a dopamine agonist, an ergot alkaloid used to suppress prolactin secretion and thereby to inhibit lactation and stimulate ovulation in galactorrhea-amenorrhea syndrome and hypogonadism. It raises serum growth hormone levels in normal persons, but lowers them in those with acromegaly.

5-bromodeoxyuridine (bro″mo-de-ok-se-u′rĭ-din) a thymidine analogue causing breakage in chromosomal regions rich in heterochromatin.

bromoderma (bro″mo-der′mah) [*bromine* + Gr. *derma* skin] a skin eruption due to the use of bromides.

bromodiphenhydramine hydrochloride (bro″mo-di″fen-hi′drah-mēn) [USP] chemical name: 2-[(4-bromophenyl)phenylmethoxy]-*N,N*-dimethylethanamine hydrochloride. An antihistaminic, $C_{17}H_{20}BrNO \cdot HCl$, occurring as a white to pale buff, crystalline powder; administered orally.

bromoiodism (bro″mo-i′o-dizm) poisoning with bromine and iodine or their compounds.

bromomania (bro″mo-ma′ne-ah) [*bromin* + *mania*] mental disorder induced by the injudicious use of the bromine compounds.

bromomenorrhea (bro″mo-men-o-re′ah) [Gr. *brōmos* stench + *mēn* month + *rhoia* flow] the discharge of menses characterized by an offensive odor.

bromopnea (brōm″op-ne′ah) [Gr. *brōmos* stench + *pnoia* breath] halitosis.

5-bromouracil (bro″mo-u′rah-sil) a pyrimidine analogue with mutagenic properties.

bromoxanide (bro-moks′ah-nīd) chemical name: *N*-[4-bromo-2-(trifluoromethyl)phenyl]-3-(1,1-dimethylethyl)-2-hydroxy-6-methyl-5-nitrobenzamide; an anthelmintic, $C_{19}H_{18}BrF_3N_2O_4$.

bromperidol (brom-per′ĭ-dōl) chemical name: 4-[4-(4-bromophenyl)-4-hydroxy-1-piperidinyl]-1-butanone; a tranquilizer, C_{21}-$H_{23}BrFNO_2$.

brompheniramine (brōm″fen-ir′ah-mēn) chemical name: γ-(4-bromophenyl)-*N,N*-dimethyl-2-pyridinepropanamine. The bromine analogue of chlorpheniramine, $C_{16}H_{19}BrN_2$, an antihistaminic drug. **b. maleate** [USP], the maleate salt of brompheniramine, $C_{16}H_{19}BrN_2 \cdot C_4H_4O_4$, occurring as white crystalline powder; administered orally or by intramuscular, subcutaneous, or intravenous injection for therapy and prophylaxis of conditions in which antihistamines may be effective.

bromphenol (brŏm-fe′nol) one of a series of brominized phenols, sometimes found in the precipitates of tested urine.

bromphenylacetylcysteine (brŏm-fen″il-as″e-til-sis′te-in) bromphenylmercapturic acid.

Bromsulphalein (brom-sul′fah-lin) trademark for a preparation of sulfobromophthalein sodium. Abbreviated BSP.

bromum (brō′mum) [L.] bromine.

Bromural (brŏm-u′ral) trademark for preparations of bromisovalum.

bromurated (brŏm′u-rāt″ed) containing bromine or bromine salts; brominated.

bromuret (brŏm′u-ret) a bromide.

bronchadenitis (brong″kad-ĕ-ni′tis) [Gr. *bronchia* bronchia + *adēn* gland + *-itis*] inflammation of the bronchial glands.

bronchi (brong′ki) [L.] plural of *bronchus*.

bronchia (brong′ke-ah) [L.; Gr.] plural of *bronchium*.

bronchial (brong′ke-al) [L. *bronchialis*] pertaining to one or more bronchi.

bronchiarctia (brong″ke-ark′she-ah) [*bronchus* + L. *arctare* to constrict] bronchostenosis.

bronchiectasia (brong″ke-ek-ta′ze-ah) bronchiectasis.

bronchiectasic (brong″ke-ek-ta′zik) bronchiectatic.

bronchiectasis (brong″ke-ek′tah-sis) [*bronchus* + Gr. *ektasis* dilatation] chronic dilatation of the bronchi marked by fetid breath and paroxysmal coughing, with the expectoration of mucopurulent matter. It may affect the tube uniformly (*cylindric b.*), or occur in irregular pockets (*sacculated b.*), or the dilated tubes may have terminal bulbous enlargements (*fusiform b.*). **capillary b.,** dilatation of the bronchioles. **cystic b.,** bronchiectasis in which the dilatations of the bronchi are spherical. **dry b.,** that in which the infection is episodic and may be attended by hemoptysis, the cough being nonproductive during quiescent periods. **follicular b.,** bronchiectasis in which the lymphoid tissue in the affected regions becomes greatly enlarged and, by projecting into the bronchial lumen, may seriously distort and partially obstruct the bronchus.

bronchiectatic (brong″ke-ek-tat′ik) pertaining to or characterized by bronchiectasis.

bronchiloquy (brong-kil′o-kwe) [*bronchus* + L. *loqui* to speak] a high-pitched pectoriloquy due to a consolidated lung.

bronchiocele (brong′ke-o-sēl) [*bronchiole* + Gr. *kēlē* tumor] a dilatation or swelling of a branch smaller than a bronchus.

bronchiocrisis (brong″ke-o-kri′sis) bronchial crisis; see under *crisis*.

bronchiogenic (brong″ke-o-jen′ik) bronchogenic.

bronchiole (brong′ke-ōl) [L. *bronchiolus*] one of the finer (1 mm. or less) subdivisions of the branched bronchial tree, differing from the bronchi in having no cartilage plates and having cuboidal epithelial cells. Called also *bronchiolus*. **alveolar b.,** respiratory b. **lobular b.,** terminal b. **respiratory b.,** the final branch of a bronchiole; a subdivision of a terminal bronchiole, it has alveolar outcroppings and itself divides into several alveolar ducts. Called also *alveolar b.* **terminal b.,** the last portion of a bronchiole whose sole function is gas conduction; it subdivides into respiratory bronchioles. Called also *lobular b.*

bronchiolectasis (brong″ke-o-lek′tah-sis) [*bronchiole* + Gr. *ektasis* dilatation] dilatation of the bronchioles.

bronchioli (brong-ki′o-li) [L.] plural of *bronchiolus*.

bronchiolitis (brong″ke-o-li′tis) bronchopneumonia. **acute obliterating b.,** cirrhosis of the lung due to induration of the walls of the bronchioles. **b. exudati′va** (Curschmann), inflammation of the bronchioles, with exudation of Curschmann's spirals and spiral, tenacious sputum; often associated with asthma. **b. fibro′sa oblit′erans,** bronchiolitis marked by ingrowth of connective tissue from the wall of the terminal bronchi with occlusion of their lumina. **vesicular b.,** bronchopneumonia.

bronchiolus (brong-ki′o-lus), pl. *bronchi′oli* [L.] [NA] bronchiole: one of the finer subdivisions of the branched bronchial tree; see *bronchiole*. **bronchi′oli respirato′rii** [NA], respiratory bronchioles: the final branches of the bronchioles, into which the alveolar ducts open; see *respiratory bronchiole*, under *bronchiole*.

bronchiospasm (brong′ke-o-spazm″) bronchospasm.

bronchiostenosis (brong″ke-o-stĕ-no′sis) bronchostenosis.

bronchisepticin (brong″ke-sep′tĭ-sin) an antigen prepared from *Brucella bronchiseptica*; used in the skin test for canine distemper.

bronchismus (brong-kis′mus) bronchospasm.

bronchitic (brong-kit′ik) [L. *bronchiticus*] pertaining to, affected with, or of the nature of bronchitis.

bronchitis (brong-ki′tis) [*bronchus* + *-itis*] inflammation of one or more bronchi. **acute b.,** a bronchitic attack with a short and more severe course. It is due to exposure to cold, to the

breathing of irritant substances, and to acute infection. It is marked by fever, pain in the chest, especially on coughing, dyspnea, and cough. **acute laryngotracheal b.,** a form of nondiphtheritic croup, clinically resembling diphtheria, except that there is no membrane; it mainly affects boys during the first year of life, usually in the winter. **arachidic b.,** bronchitis caused by the presence of a peanut kernel in a bronchus. **capillary b.,** bronchopneumonia. **Castellani's b.,** bronchospirochetosis. **catarrhal b.,** a form of acute bronchitis with a profuse mucopurulent discharge. **cheesy b.,** a form accompanying some cases of tuberculosis of the lung, in which the alveoli are filled with cells that undergo a cheesy degeneration (caseous necrosis). **chronic b.,** a long-continued form, often with a more or less marked tendency to recurrence after stages of quiescence. It is due to repeated attacks of acute bronchitis or to chronic general diseases; characterized by attacks of coughing, by expectoration, either scanty or profuse, and secondary changes in the lung tissue. **croupous b.,** bronchitis characterized by violent cough and paroxysms of dyspnea, in which casts of the bronchial tubes are expectorated with Charcot-Leyden crystals and eosinophil cells. Variously known as *exudative, fibrinous, membranous, plastic,* and *pseudomembranous bronchitis*. **dry b.,** a form with a scanty secretion of tough sputum. **epidemic b.,** influenza. **epidemic capillary b.,** bronchiolitis due to measles virus, respiratory syncytial virus, or other respiratory pathogens. **ether b.,** that due to the irritation of ether. **exudative b.,** croupous b. **fibrinous b.,** croupous b. **hemorrhagic b.,** bronchospirochetosis. **infectious asthmatic b.,** a syndrome marked by the development of symptoms of bronchospasm following respiratory tract infections in persons with asthma; also, asthma of bacterial origin. **infectious avian b.,** an acute, highly contagious, respiratory viral disease of chickens characterized by tracheal rales, coughing, sneezing, nasal discharge, and a drop in egg production. **mechanic b.,** a variety caused by the inhalation of dust or of solid particles. **membranous b.,** croupous b. **b. obliterans,** a form in which the smaller bronchi become filled with nodules made up of fibrinous exudate. **parasitic b.,** hoose. **phthinoid b.,** tuberculous bronchitis with purulent expectoration. **plastic b.,** croupous b. **productive b.,** bronchitis associated with a productive cough. **pseudomembranous b.,** croupous b. **putrid b.,** a form of chronic bronchitis in which the sputum is very offensive. **secondary b.,** that which occurs either as a complication of some acute disease, such as a local expression of some constitutional disorder. **staphylococcus b.,** bronchitis caused by staphylococci. **streptococcal b.,** bronchitis caused by streptococci. **suffocative b.,** suffocation produced by excessive secreting and exudates in acute bronchopneumonia. **verminous b.,** hoose. **vesicular b.,** that in which the inflammation extends into the alveoli, which are sometimes visible under the pleura as whitish-yellow granulations like millet seeds.

bronchium (brong′ke-um), pl. *bron′chia* [L.] one of the subdivisions of a bronchus, smaller than the bronchus and larger than the bronchioles.

bronchoadenitis (brong″ko-ad″e-ni′tis) bronchadenitis.

bronchoalveolar (brong″ko-al-ve′o-lar) pertaining to a bronchus and alveoli; called also *bronchovesicular*.

bronchoalveolitis (brong″ko-al″ve-o-li′tis) bronchopneumonia.

bronchoaspergillosis (brong″ko-as″per-jil-lo′sis) bronchial disease resulting from infection with *Aspergillus*.

bronchoblastomycosis (brong″ko-blas″to-mi-ko′sis) North American blastomycosis of the pulmonary type; see under *blastomycosis*.

bronchoblennorrhea (brong″ko-blen″o-re′ah) chronic bronchitis in which the sputum is copious, thin, and mucopurulent.

bronchocandidiasis (brong″ko-kan″dĭ-di′ah-sis) candidiasis of the respiratory tract. It has been reported in two forms: an afebrile *mild form* manifested as chronic bronchitis with dyspnea and cough, and a usually fatal *severe form* that resembles tuberculosis. Called also *bronchomoniliasis* and *broncho-oidiosis*.

bronchocavernous (brong″ko-kav′er-nus) both bronchial and cavitary.

bronchocele (brong′ko-sēl) [*bronchus* + Gr. *kēlē* tumor] a localized dilatation of a bronchus.

bronchocephalitis (brong″ko-sef″ah-li′tis) (*obs.*) whooping cough.

bronchoconstriction (brong″ko-kon-strik′shun) the act or process of decreasing the caliber of a bronchus; bronchostenosis.

bronchoconstrictor (brong″ko-kon-strik′tor) 1. constricting or narrowing the lumina of the air passages of the lungs. 2. an agent that causes narrowing of the lumina of the air passages of the lungs.

bronchodilatation (brong″ko-dil-ah-ta′shun) a dilated state of a bronchus, or the site at which a bronchus is dilated.

bronchodilation (brong″ko-di-la′shun) the act or process of increasing the caliber of a bronchus.

bronchodilator (brong″ko-di-la′tor) 1. dilating or expanding the lumina of air passages of the lungs. 2. an agent that causes expansion of the lumina of the air passages of the lungs.

bronchoegophony (brong″ko-e-gof′o-ne) egobronchophony.

bronchoesophageal (brong″ko-ĕ-sof″ah-je′al) pertaining to or communicating with a bronchus and the esophagus, as a bronchoesophageal fistula.

bronchoesophagology (brong″ko-ĕ-sof-ah-gol′o-je) that branch of medicine which deals with the tracheobronchial tree and the esophagus.

bronchoesophagoscopy (brong″ko-ĕ-sof-ah-gos′ko-pe) the instrumental examination of the bronchi and esophagus.

bronchofiberscope (brong″ko-fi′ber-skōp) a flexible bronchoscope utilizing fiberoptics.

bronchofibroscopy (brong″ko-fi-bros′ko-pe) examination of the bronchi through a bronchofiberscope.

bronchogenic (brong-ko-jen′ik) originating in a bronchus.

bronchogram (brong′ko-gram) the roentgenogram obtained by bronchography.

bronchographic (brong″ko-graf′ik) pertaining to or obtained by bronchography.

bronchography (brong-kog′rah-fe) [*bronchus* + Gr. *graphein* to write] roentgenography of the lung after the instillation of an opaque medium in a bronchus.

broncholith (brong′ko-lith) [*bronchus* + Gr. *lithos* stone] lung calculus.

broncholithiasis (brong″ko-lĭ-thi′ah-sis) a condition in which calculi (broncholiths) are present within the lumen of the tracheobronchial tree.

bronchologic (brong″ko-loj′ik) pertaining to bronchology.

bronchology (brong-kol′o-je) the study and treatment of diseases of the tracheobronchial tree.

bronchomalacia (brong″ko-mah-la′she-ah) a deficiency in the cartilaginous wall of the trachea or a bronchus that may lead to atelectasis or obstructive emphysema; it may be congenital or acquired.

bronchomoniliasis (brong″ko-mo-nĭ-li′ah-sis) bronchocandidiasis.

bronchomotor (brong″ko-mo′tor) affecting the caliber of the bronchi.

bronchomucotropic (brong″ko-mu″ko-trop′ik) augmenting secretion by the respiratory mucosa.

bronchomycosis (brong″ko-mi-ko′sis) [*bronchus* + Gr. *mykēs* fungus] any bronchial disorder due to fungi, particularly infection of the lungs caused by *Candida albicans*.

bronchonocardiosis (brong″ko-no-kar″de-o′sis) nocardial infection of the bronchi.

broncho-oidiosis (brong″ko-o-id″e-o′sis) bronchocandidiasis.

bronchopancreatic (brong″ko-pan″kre-at′ik) communicating with a bronchus and the pancreas, as a bronchopancreatic fistula.

bronchopathy (brong-kop′ah-the) [*bronchus* + Gr. *pathos* disease] any disease of the air passages of the lungs.

bronchophony (brong-kof′o-ne) [*bronchus* + Gr. *phōnē* voice] the sound of the voice as heard through the stethoscope applied over a healthy large bronchus. Heard elsewhere, it indicates solidification of the lung tissue. **pectoriloquous b.,** a bronchophony with an accompaniment of pectoriloquy. **sniffling b.,** that which is accompanied with a sniffing sound, as of air drawn through the nose. **whispered b.,** that which is heard while the patient is whispering.

bronchoplasty (brong′ko-plas″te) [*bronchus* + Gr. *plassein* to mold] plastic surgery of the bronchus; surgical closure of a fistula in the bronchus.

bronchoplegia (brong″ko-ple′je-ah) paralysis of the muscles of the walls of the bronchial tubes.

bronchopleural (brong″ko-ploor′al) pertaining to a bronchus and the pleura, or communicating with a bronchus and the pleural cavity, as a bronchopleural fistula.

bronchopleuropneumonia (brong″ko-plu″ro-nu-mo′ne-ah) pneumonia complicated by bronchitis and pleurisy.

bronchopneumonia (brong″ko-nu-mo′ne-ah) [*bronchus* + *pneumonia*] a name given to an inflammation of the lungs which usually begins in the terminal bronchioles. These become clogged with a mucopurulent exudate forming consolidated patches in adjacent lobules. The disease is frequently secondary in character, following infections of the upper respiratory tract, specific infectious fevers, and debilitating diseases. In infants and debilitated persons of any age it may occur as a primary affection. Called also *bronchial pneumonia, bronchiolitis, bronchoalveolitis, bronchopneumonitis, catarrhal pneumonia, lobular pneumonia, capillary bronchitis* and *vesicular bronchiolitis.* **postoperative b.,** bronchopneumonia following surgical operations, particularly those on the abdomen. The cause is related to the inhalation of irritant vapors during anesthesia and the inhalation of infected material from the mouth or nose during the temporary depression of the cough reflex. **subacute b.,** bronchopneumonia that is more indolent than usual. **virus b.,** pneumonia caused by viral infection.

bronchopneumonic (brong″ko-nu-mon′ik) pertaining to, affected with, or caused by bronchopneumonia.

bronchopneumonitis (brong″ko-nu″mo-ni′tis) bronchopneumonia.

bronchopneumopathy (brong″ko-nu-mop′ah-the) disease of the bronchi and lung tissue.

bronchopulmonary (brong″ko-pul′mo-ner″e) pertaining to the lungs and their air passages; both bronchial and pulmonary.

bronchoradiography (brong″ko-ra-de-og′rah-fe) radiographic visualization of the bronchial tree.

bronchorrhagia (brong″ko-ra′je-ah) [*bronchus* + Gr. *rhēgnynai* to burst forth] hemorrhage from the bronchi.

bronchorrhaphy (brong-kor′ah-fe) [*bronchus* + Gr. *rhaphē* suture] the repair of an incised or wounded bronchus.

bronchorrhea (brong-ko-re′ah) [*bronchus* + Gr. *rhoia* flow] excessive discharge of mucus from the air passages of the lungs.

bronchoscope (brong′ko-skōp) an instrument for inspecting the interior of the tracheobronchial tree and carrying out endobronchial diagnostic and therapeutic maneuvers, such as taking specimens for culture and biopsy and removing foreign bodies. **fiberoptic b.,** bronchofiberscope.

bronchoscopic (brong″ko-skop′ik) pertaining to bronchoscopy or to the bronchoscope.

bronchoscopy (brong-kos′ko-pe) [*bronchus* + Gr. *skopein* to examine] examination of the bronchi through a bronchoscope. **fiberoptic b.,** bronchofibroscopy.

bronchosinusitis (brong″ko-si″nus-i′tis) coexisting infection of the paranasal sinuses and the lower respiratory passages.

bronchospasm (brong′ko-spazm) spasmodic contraction of the smooth muscle of the bronchi, as occurs in asthma.

bronchospirochetosis (brong″ko-spi″ro-ke-to′sis) an infectious disease caused by the presence in the bronchi of the *Spirochaeta bronchialis* and marked by chronic bronchitis attended by the spitting of blood; called also *Castellani's bronchitis* or *disease,* and *hemorrhagic bronchitis.*

bronchospirography (brong″ko-spi-rog′rah-fe) the recording of bronchospirometry results.

bronchospirometer (brong″ko-spi-rom′ĕ-ter) an instrument used in bronchospirometry.

bronchospirometry (brong″ko-spi-rom′ĕ-tre) determination of the vital capacity, oxygen intake, and carbon dioxide excretion of a single lung, or simultaneous measurements of the function of each lung seperately. **differential b.,** measurement of the function of each lung separately.

bronchostaxis (brong″ko-stak′sis) bleeding from the bronchial wall.

bronchostenosis (brong″ko-ste-no′sis) [*bronchus* + Gr. *stenōsis* a narrowing] stricture or cicatricial diminution of the caliber of a bronchial tube; called also *bronchiarctia* and *bronchoconstriction.*

bronchostomy (brong-kos′to-me) [*bronchus* + Gr. *stomoun* to provide with a mouth, or opening] the surgical creation of an opening into a bronchus.

bronchotome (brong′ko-tōm) a cutting instrument used in performing bronchotomy.

bronchotomy (brong-kot′o-me) [*bronchus* + Gr. *tomē* a cutting] surgical incision of a bronchus.

bronchotracheal (brong″ko-tra′ke-al) pertaining to the bronchi and trachea; tracheobronchial.

bronchotyphoid (brong″ko-ti′foid) typhoid fever beginning with severe bronchitis.

bronchotyphus (brong″ko-ti′fus) typhus complicated with acute bronchitis.

bronchovesicular (brong″ko-ve-sik′u-lar) bronchoalveolar.

bronchus (brong′kus), pl. *bron′chi* [L.; Gr. *bronchos* windpipe] any of the larger air passages of the lungs, having an outer fibrous coat with irregularly placed plates of hyaline cartilage, an interlacing network of smooth muscle, and a mucous membrane of columnar ciliated epithelial cells. **apical b.,** b. segmentalis apicalis. **cardiac b.,** b. segmentalis basalis medialis. **eparterial b.,** ramus bronchialis eparterialis. **hyparterial bronchi,** rami bronchiales hyparteriales. **lingular b., inferior,** b. lingularis inferior. **lingular b., superior,** b. lingularis superior. **b. lingula′ris infe′rior** [NA], inferior lingular bronchus: the branch of the left upper lobar bronchus that supplies the inferior lingular bronchopulmonary segment. **b. lingula′ris supe′rior** [NA], superior lingular bronchus: the branch of the left upper lobar bronchus that supplies the superior lingular bronchopulmonary segment. **lobar bronchi, bron′chi loba′res** [NA], passages arising from the primary bronchi and passing to the lobes of the right and left lungs, being the *right upper, middle,* and *right lower,* and the *left upper* and *left lower lobar bronchi.* **primary b., b. principa′lis** [NA], either of the two main branches, right (*dex′ter*) and left (*sinis′ter*) bronchi, into which the trachea divides, each passing to the respective lung. **secondary bronchi,** subdivisions of the primary bronchi, including the lobar and segmental bronchi.

segmental b., anterior, b. segmentalis anterior. **segmental b., anterior basal**, b. segmentalis basalis anterior. **segmental b., apical**, b. segmentalis apicalis. **segmental b., apicoposterior**, b. segmentalis apicoposterior. **segmental bronchi, bronchi segmenta′les** [NA], air passages arising from the lobar bronchi and passing to the different segments of the two lungs, where they further subdivide into smaller and smaller passages (bronchioles). **segmental b., cardiac**, b. segmentalis basalis medialis [cardiacus]. **segmental b., lateral**, b. segmentalis lateralis. **segmental b., lateral basal**, b. segmentalis basalis lateralis. **segmental b., medial**, b. segmentalis medialis. **segmental b., medial basal**, b. segmentalis basalis medialis [cardiacus]. **segmental b., posterior**, b. segmentalis posterior. **segmental b., posterior basal**, b. segmentalis basalis posterior. **segmental b., superior**, b. segmentalis superior. **b. segmenta′lis ante′rior** [NA], anterior segmental bronchus: the branch of the right upper or of the left upper lobar bronchus that supplies the anterior bronchopulmonary segment. **b. segmenta′lis apica′lis** [NA], apical segmental bronchus: the branch of the upper right lobar bronchus that supplies the apical bronchopulmonary segment. The term is also used for corresponding branches in the right lower or left lower lobar bronchus; see *b. segmentalis superior*. **b. segmenta′lis apicoposte′rior** [NA], apicoposterior segmental bronchus: the branch of the left upper lobar bronchus that supplies the apicoposterior bronchopulmonary segment. **b. segmenta′lis basa′lis ante′rior** [NA], anterior basal segmental bronchus: the branch of the right lower or left lower lobar bronchus that supplies the anterior basal bronchopulmonary segment. **b. segmenta′lis basa′lis latera′lis** [NA], lateral basal segmental bronchus: the branch of the right lower or left lower lobar bronchus that supplies the lateral basal bronchopulmonary segment. **b. segmenta′lis basa′lis media′lis [cardi′acus]** [NA], medial basal segmental bronchus: the branch of the lower right or of the lower left segmental bronchus that supplies the medial basal bronchopulmonary segment; called also *cardiac segmental b.* **b. segmenta′lis basa′lis poste′rior** [NA], posterior basal segmental bronchus: the branch of the right lower or of the left lower lobar bronchus that supplies the posterior basal bronchopulmonary segment. **b. segmenta′lis latera′lis** [NA], lateral segmental bronchus: the branch of the right middle lobar bronchus that supplies the lateral bronchopulmonary segment. **b. segmenta′lis media′lis** [NA], medial segmental bronchus: the branch of the right middle lobar bronchus that supplies the medial bronchopulmonary segment. **b. segmenta′lis poste′rior** [NA], posterior segmental bronchus: the branch of the upper right lobar bronchus that supplies the posterior bronchopulmonary segment. **b. segmenta′lis supe′rior** [NA], superior segmental bronchus: the branch of the right lower or left lower lobar bronchus that supplies the superior bronchopulmonary segment; called also *b. segmentalis apicalis* or *apical segmental b.* **stem b.**, the continuation of the primary bronchus of the embryo, from which branches are given off to the lobes of the lungs. **tracheal b.**, an ectopic or supernumerary bronchus, extending directly from the trachea to the apical segment of the upper lobe of the right lung, occurring normally in some animals but as a congenital anomaly in man.

Brooke's disease, tumor (brooks) [Henry Ambrose Grundy *Brooke*, English (Manchester) dermatologist, 1854–1919] see *adenoid basal cell carcinoma*, under *carcinoma*, see *keratosis follicularis contagiosa*, and see *trichoepithelioma*.

Brophy's operation (bro′fēz) [Truman William *Brophy*, American oral surgeon, 1848–1928] see under *operation*.

broth (broth) 1. a thin soup prepared by boiling meat or vegetables. 2. a liquid culture medium for the cultivation of microorganisms; see *Table of Culture Media* for specific broths.

broussaisism (broo-sa′izm) [after François Joseph Victor *Broussais*, French physician, 1772–1838] the obsolete opinion taught by Broussais, that irritability of the mucous membrane of the alimentary canal was a point of primary importance in the causation of disease.

brow (brow) the forehead, or either lateral half of it. **olympic b.**, the overdeveloped forehead seen in congenital syphilis.

brown (brown) a dusky, reddish yellow color. **aniline b., Bismarck b.**, a basic aniline dye, phenylene-diazo-metaphenylene-diamine, $C_6H_4[N_2C_6H_3(NH)_2]_2$, much used as a stain and counterstain in histology; called also *Manchester b.* and *phenylene b.* **Manchester b., phenylene b.**, aniline b.

Brown's test (reaction) [Thomas Kenneth *Brown*, American gynecologist, 1898–1951] see under *tests*.

Brown-Séquard's injection, etc. (brown′ sa-karz′) [Charles Edouard *Brown-Séquard*, French physiologist, 1817–1894] see under *injection, paralysis, syndrome*, and *treatment*.

brownian movement (brow′ne-an) [Robert *Brown*, English botanist, 1773–1858] see under *movement*.

Browning's vein (brown′ingz) [William *Browning*, Brooklyn anatomist, 1855–1941] see under *vein*.

brownism (brown′izm) brunonianism.

Broxolin (brok′so-lin) trademark for a preparation of glycobiarsol.

B.R.S. British Roentgen Society.

Bruce's septicemia (broos′ez) [Sir David *Bruce*, surgeon in British army, 1855–1931] brucellosis.

Bruce's tract (broos′ez) [Alexander *Bruce*, Edinburgh anatomist, 1854–1911] the septomarginal tract; see under *tract*.

Brucella (broo-sel′lah) [Sir David *Bruce*] a genus of microorganisms of the family Brucellaceae, order Eubacteriales, made up of nonmotile short, rod-shaped to coccoid, gram-negative encapsulated cells. It includes three species which may be differentiated on the basis of (1) the relative content of two antigens, A and M, (2) sensitivity to thionine and basic fuchsin, (3) production of hydrogen sulfide, and (4) the requirement for carbon dioxide on primary isolation. **B. abor′tus**, the commonest cause of brucellosis (undulant fever) in man; it is the causative agent of infectious abortion of cattle, which constitutes the animal reservoir of infection; called also *Bang's bacillus*. **B. bronchisep′tica**, the causative agent of bronchopneumonia in guinea pigs and other rodents; formerly called *Bacillus bronchosepticus, Bordetella bronchiseptica*, and *Hemophilus bronchisepticus*. **B. ca′nis**, a species causing epidemic abortion in beagles. **B. meliten′sis**, the causative agent of brucellosis (undulant fever), occurring primarily, although not exclusively, in goats as the reservoir of infection. **B. o′vis**, the causative agent of an infectious disease in sheep. **B. rangif′eri taran′di**, a species found in Eskimos in Canada and Alaska and in reindeer in northern Russia. **B. su′is**, a species found primarily in swine, and which is capable of producing severe disease in man. **B. tularen′sis**, British name for *Pasteurella tularensis*.

brucella (broo-sel′ah) an individual organism of the genus *Brucella*.

Brucellaceae (broo″sel-la′se-e) a family of Schizomycetes, order Eubacteriales, occurring as small coccoid to rod-shaped cells, singly or in pairs, chains, or groups. It includes eight genera, *Actinobacillus, Bordetella, Brucella, Calymmatobacterium, Haemophilus, Moraxella, Noguchia*, and *Pasteurella*, some of which are parasitic on and pathogenic for warm-blooded animals, including man and birds.

brucellar (broo-sel′ar) pertaining to or caused by *Brucella*.

Brucellergen (broo-sel′er-jin) trademark for a suspensoid of nucleoproteins derived from *Brucella* (melitin from *B. melitensis* and abortin from *B. abortus*); used in a skin test for brucellosis.

brucelliasis (broo″sel-li′ah-sis) brucellosis.

brucellin (broo-sel′in) a preparation from pooled cultures of the three species of *Brucella*, used in the diagnosis of brucellosis.

brucellosis (broo″sel-lo′sis) a generalized infection of man involving primarily the reticuloendothelial system, caused by species of *Brucella*, namely, *B. melitensis, B. abortus, B. suis*, and *B. canis*, derived from contact respectively with goats, cattle, pigs, and dogs. Its incubation is an average of three weeks, and symptoms include fever of varying pattern, malaise, and headache. It has been variously called *undulant fever, abortus fever, Malta* or *Maltese fever, Mediterranean fever* or *phthisis, Cyprus fever, goat fever, goat's milk fever, Gibraltar fever, mountain fever, Neapolitan fever, rock fever, febris melitensis, febris sudoralis, febris undulans, fièvre caprine, Bruce's septicemia, brucellemia, brucelliasis, melitensis septicemia*, and *melitensis*.

Bruch's glands, membrane (layer) (brooks) [Karl Wilhelm Ludwig *Bruch*, German anatomist, 1819–1884] see under *gland*, and see *lamina basalis choroideae*.

brucine (broo′sin) [from *Brucea*, a genus of shrubs named for J. *Bruce*, 1730–1794] chemical name: 2,3-dimethoxystrychnidin. A poisonous alkaloid, $C_{23}H_{26}N_2O_4$, from *Strychnos ignatii* and *S. nux-vomica*, which resembles strychnine in its action, but is less poisonous. One of the principal constituents of nux vomica and ignatia, it was formerly used in the same manner as strychnine (q.v.).

Bruck's disease (brooks) [Alfred *Bruck*, German physician, born 1865] see under *disease*.

Bruck's reaction, test (brooks) [Carl *Bruck*, German dermatologist, 1879–1944] see under *reaction* and *tests*.

Brücke's lines, etc. (bre′kez) [Ernst Wilhelm von *Brücke*, Austrian physiologist, 1819–1892] see under *line, muscle, reagent, test*, and *tunic*.

Brudzinski's sign (reflex) (brood-zin′skēz) [Józef *Brudzinski*, Polish physician, 1874–1917] see under *sign*.

Brugia (bruj′ĕ-ah) a genus of filarial worms once considered to be members of the genus *Wuchereria*. **B. ma′layi**, a species causing human filariasis and elephantiasis throughout Southeast Asia, the China Sea, and eastern India; it is similar to, and often found in association with, *Wuchereria bancrofti*. Called also *Wuchereria malayi* and *Brug's filaria*. **B. pahan′gi**, a species found in man, cats, tigers, and other wild and domestic animals in Malaya; in man, it may produce the symptoms of tropical eosinophilia.

bruise (brooz) a superficial injury produced by impact without laceration; a contusion. **stone b.**, a painful bruise, especially of the bare feet of children.

bruissement (brwĕs-maw′) [Fr.] a purring tremor; see under *tremor*.

bruit (brwe, broot) [Fr.] a sound or murmur heard in auscultation, especially an abnormal one. **aneurysmal b.,** a blowing sound heard over an aneurysm. **b. d'airain** (brwe da-ră′) [Fr. "sound of brass"], a clear ringing musical note sometimes heard on percussion over a pneumothorax cavity. **b. de bois** (brwe duh bwah′) [Fr. "sound of wood"], a dull wooden nonmusical note sometimes heard on percussion over a pneumothorax cavity. **b. de canon** (brwe duh kah-naw′) [Fr. "sound of cannon"], an abnormally loud first heart sound, heard intermittently in complete heart block. **b. de choc** (brwe duh shawk′) [Fr. "sound of impact"], the second cardiac sound, accompanied by a sound of impact, such as is heard over an aneurysm of the aorta. **b. de clapotement** (brwe duh klah-pŏt-maw′) [Fr. "sound of rippling"], a splashing sound indicative of dilatation of the stomach when pressure is made on the wall of the abdomen. **b. de claquement** (brwe duh klak′maw) [Fr. "sound of clapping"], a snapping sound caused by the sudden contact of parts. **b. de craquement** (brwe duh krak-maw′) [Fr. "a sound of crackling"], a crackling pericardial or pleural bruit. **b. de cuir neuf** (brwe duh kwēr nuf) [Fr. "sound of new leather"], a creaking noise; usually a sign of pericarditis or pleurisy. **b. de diable** (brwe duh de-ahbl′) [Fr. "humming top"], a buzzing venous murmur in anemia; see *venous hum,* under *hum*. **b. de drapeau** (brwe duh drah-po′) [Fr. "sound of a flag"], a flapping rustle heard in croup and laryngitis, and sometimes in nasal polyp. **b. de froissement** (brwe duh frwahs-maw′) [Fr. "sound of clashing"], a clashing noise of various origin. **b. de frolement** (brwe duh frol-maw′) [Fr. "sound of rustling"], a rustling murmur from pericardial or pleural friction. **b. de frottement** (brwe duh frot-maw′) [Fr. "sound of friction"], a rubbing sound of various origin. **b. de galop** (brwe duh gah-lo′) [Fr. "sound of galloping"], triple heart sounds in gallop cadence. **b. de grelot** (brwe duh gruh-lo′) [Fr. "sound of a rattle"], a rattling sound usually caused by the presence of a foreign body in the respiratory passages. **b. de Leudet** (brwe duh led-a′), Leudet's tinnitus. **b. de lime** (brwe duh lēm) [Fr. "sound of a file"], a filing cardiac sound. **b. de moulin** (brwe duh moo-lă′) [Fr. "sound of a mill"], a splashing or waterwheel sound synchronous with systole, sometimes audible at some distance from the patient, variously attributed to cardiac, pericardiac, or mediastinal causes. **b. de parchemin** (brwe duh parsh-maw′) [Fr. "sound of parchment"], a sound as of two pieces of parchment rubbed together, of valvular cardiac origin. **b. de piaulement** (brwe duh pyŏl-maw′) [Fr. "sound of whining"], a cardiac murmur like the mewing of a cat. **b. de pot fêlé** (brwe duh po fĕ-la′) [Fr. "cracked-pot sound"], a sound heard in percussion over cavities of the chest. **b. de rape** (brwe duh rahp) [Fr. "sound of a grater"], a rasping, cardiac, valvular murmur. **b. de rappel** (brwe duh rah-pel′) [Fr. "sound of drum beating to arms"], a sound as of a drum; a delayed mitral murmur. **b. de Roger** (brwe duh ro-zha′), a loud long systolic murmur heard in the third interspace to the left of the sternum, characteristic of a small ventricular septal defect. Called also *Roger's bruit* or *murmur*. **b. de scie** (brwe duh se) [Fr. "sound of a saw"], a cardiac murmur resembling the sound of a saw. **b. de soufflet** (brwe duh soo-fla′) [Fr. "sound of a bellows"] see *souffle*. **b. de tabourka** (brwe duh tah-bŏŏr′kah), timbre métallique. **b. de tambour** (brwe duh tahm-bor′) [Fr. "sound of drum"], a ringing sound heard in syphilitic aortic regurgitation. **false b.,** one due to pressure by the stethoscope, or derived from the circulation in the ear of the auscultator. **Leudet's b.,** see under *tinnitus*. **b. placentaire** (brwe pla″-sawn-tār′) [Fr. "placental sound"], placental souffle. **Roger's b.,** b. de Roger. **b. skodique** (brwe skaw-dēk′), skodaic resonance. **systolic b.,** a noise (heard on auscultation) occurring with the systole of the heart. **Verstraeten's b.,** an abnormal sound heard in auscultation over the lower border of the liver in cachectic patients.

Brunn's membrane, epithelial nests (brōōnz) [Albert von *Brunn,* German anatomist, 1849–1895] see under *membrane* and *nest*.

Brunner's glands (brun′erz) [Johann Conrad *Brunner,* Swiss anatomist, 1653–1727] glandulae duodenales.

Brünninghausen's method (brin′ing-how″senz) [Herrmann J. *Brünninghausen,* German physician, 1761–1834] see under *method*.

brunonianism (broo-no′ne-an-izm″) [John *Brown,* Scottish physician, 1735–1788] the obsolete doctrine that all disease is due to either excess (sthenia) or lack (asthenia) of stimulus; called also *brownism*.

Bruns' disease (brunz′ez) [John Dickson *Bruns,* New Orleans physician, 1836–1883] pneumopaludism.

Bruns' syndrome (sign) (brōōnz) [Ludwig *Bruns,* neurologist in Hanover, 1858–1916] see under *syndrome*.

Brunschwig's operation (brōōn′swigz) [Alexander *Brunschwig,* American surgeon, 1901–1969] pancreatoduodenectomy.

brush (brush) tufts of bristles, hair, or other flexible materials set into a handle. **Haidinger's b.,** two conical brushlike images with apexes touching, seen on looking through a Nicol prism; used in determining visual function. **b's of Ruffini,** a form

of nerve ending occurring in the papillae of the skin in the form of densely interlaced branches; called also *terminal cylinders* and *organ of Ruffini*. **stomach b.,** a brush used to cleanse and stimulate the mucous lining of the stomach.

bruxism (bruk′sizm) [Gr. *brychein* to gnash the teeth] rhythmic or spasmodic grinding of the teeth in other than chewing movements of the mandible, especially such movements performed during sleep. Dental malocclusion and tension-release factors are the usual inciting causes. Cf. *bruxomania* and *clenching*.

bruxomania (bruk″so-ma′ne-ah) grinding of the teeth occurring as a tension-release habit in the waking state; called also *brychomania*. Cf. *bruxism*.

Bryant's line (bri′ants) [Thomas *Bryant,* English surgeon, 1828–1914] see under *line*.

Bryce's test (bris′ez) [James *Bryce,* Scottish physician of the 19th century] see under *tests*.

Bryce-Teacher ovum [Thomas Hastie *Bryce,* Scottish anatomist, 1862–1946; John Hammond *Teacher,* Scottish pathologist, 1869–1930] see under *ovum*.

brychomania (bri″ko-ma′ne-ah) [Gr. *brychē* a gnashing of teeth + *mania*] bruxomania.

Bryobia (bri-o′be-a) a genus of spider mites. **B. praetio′sa,** the clover, or spinning, mite; a spider mite found on clover, which may greatly annoy man.

bryonia (bri-o′ne-ah) [L.; Gr. *bryōnia*] the air-dried root of *Bryonia alba* L. or other related species (Cucurbitaceae). It contains several glycosides, including bryonin and bryonidin. Formerly used both medically and in veterinary practice as a drastic and irritant purgative.

Bryson's sign (bri′sonz) [Alexander *Bryson,* English physician, 1802–1869] see under *sign*.

B.S. Bachelor of Surgery; Bachelor of Science; breath sounds; blood sugar.

BSA body surface area.

B-scan see *scan,* def. 2.

BSP Bromsulphalein.

B.T.U., B.Th.U British thermal unit.

buba (boo′bah) a native name in South American countries for mucocutaneous leishmaniasis.

bubo (bu′bo) [L. from Gr. *boubōn* groin] an enlarged and inflamed lymph node, particularly in the axilla or groin, due to such infections as plague, syphilis, gonorrhea, lymphogranuloma venereum, and tuberculosis. **bullet b.,** the characteristic hard bubo of primary syphilis. **chancroidal b.,** a suppurating form accompanying or following chancroid; called also *virulent b.* **climatic b.,** lymphogranuloma venereum. **Frei's b.** (obs.), lymphogranuloma venereum. **gonorrheal b.,** a bubo following or accompanying gonorrhea. **indolent b.,** one that is hard and nearly painless, and shows little tendency to suppurate. **malignant b.,** the bubo of bubonic plague. **nonvenereal b.,** that associated with lymphogranuloma venereum. **pestilential b.,** that which is associated with plague. **primary b.,** a bubo which is due to venereal exposure but which is not preceded by any visible lesion; called also *bubon d'emblée*. **strumous b.,** lymphogranuloma venereum. **sympathetic b.,** one due to friction or injury. **syphilitic b.,** an indolent bubo following a hard chancre. **tropical b.,** lymphogranuloma venereum. **venereal b.,** one due to venereal disease. **virulent b.,** chancroidal b.

bubon (bu-baw′) [Fr.] bubo. **b. d'emblée** (bu-baw″dah-bla′) [Fr. "at the first onset"], primary bubo.

bubonalgia (bu″bo-nal′je-ah) [Gr. *boubōn* groin + *-algia*] pain in the groin.

bubonic (bu-bon′ik) [L. *bubonicus*] characterized by or pertaining to buboes; see also under *plague*.

bubonocele (bu-bon′o-sēl) [Gr. *boubōn* groin + *kēlē* tumor] inguinal or femoral hernia forming a swelling in the groin.

bubonulus (bu-bon′u-lus) [L. "a small bubo"] a nodule or abscess along a lymphatic vessel, especially one on the dorsum of the penis (Nisbet's chancre).

bucainide maleate (bu-ka′nīd) chemical name: 1-hexyl-4-[[(methylpropyl) imino] phenylmethyl]-piperazine (Z)-2-butenedioate (1:2); a cardiac depressant with antiarrhythmic action, $C_{21}H_{35}N_3 \cdot 2C_4H_4O_4$.

bucardia (bu-kar′de-ah) [Gr. *bous* ox + *kardia* heart] cor bovinum.

bucca (buk′ah) [L.] [NA] the fleshy portion of the side of the face; the cheek. Called also *mala* [NA alternative]. **b. ca′vi o′ris** [NA], the fleshy portion of the side of the oral cavity, which is continuous with the commissure of the lips.

buccal (buk′al) [L. *buccalis,* from *bucca* cheek] pertaining to or directed toward the cheek.

buccally (buk′al-le) toward the cheek.

buccinator (buk′sĭ-na″tor) [L. "trumpeter"] see *Table of Musculi*.

bucco- (buk′ko) [L. *bucca* cheek] a combining form denoting relationship to the cheek.

buccoaxial (buk-ak′se-al) pertaining to or formed by the buccal and axial walls of a tooth cavity.

buccoaxiocervical (buk″ko-ak″se-o-ser′vĭ-kal) buccoaxiogingival.

buccoaxiogingival (buk″ko-ak″se-o-jin′jĭ-val) pertaining to or formed by the buccal, axial, and gingival walls of a tooth cavity; called also *buccoaxiocervical*.

buccocervical (buk″ko-ser′vĭ-kal) 1. pertaining to the cheek and neck. 2. pertaining to the buccal surface of the neck of a posterior tooth. 3. buccogingival.

buccoclination (buk″ko-kli-na′shun) (*obs.*) buccoversion.

buccoclusal (buk″ko-kloo′sal) 1. pertaining to buccoclusion. 2. bucco-occlusal.

buccoclusion (buk″ko-kloo′zhun) malocclusion in which the dental arch or a quadrant or group of teeth is buccal to the normal.

buccodistal (buk″ko-dis′tal) pertaining to or formed by the buccal and distal surfaces of a tooth, or the buccal and distal walls of a tooth cavity.

buccogingival (buk″ko-jin′jĭ-val) 1. pertaining to the cheek and gingiva. 2. pertaining to or formed by the buccal and gingival walls of a tooth cavity.

buccoglossopharyngitis (buk″ko-glos′o-far″in-ji′tis) inflammation involving the cheek, tongue, and pharynx. **b. sic′ca,** inflammation and dryness of the buccal mucosa, tongue, and pharynx. Cf. *Sjögren's syndrome,* under *syndrome.*

buccolabial (buk″ko-la′be-al) pertaining to the cheek and lip.

buccolingual (buk″ko-ling′gwal) 1. pertaining to the cheek and tongue. 2. pertaining to the buccal and lingual surfaces of a posterior tooth.

buccolingually (buk″ko-ling′gwal-le) from the cheek toward the tongue.

buccomaxillary (buk″ko-mak′sĭ-ler″e) 1. pertaining to the cheek and maxilla. 2. communicating with the buccal cavity and the maxillary sinus, as a buccomaxillary fistula.

buccomesial (buk″ko-me′ze-al) pertaining to or formed by the buccal and mesial surfaces of a tooth, or the buccal and mesial walls of a tooth cavity.

bucco-occlusal (buk″ko-ŏ-kloo′zal) pertaining to or formed by the buccal and occlusal surfaces of a tooth.

buccopharyngeal (buk″ko-fah-rin′je-al) pertaining to the mouth and pharynx.

buccoplacement (buk′ko-plās″ment) displacement of a tooth toward the cheek.

buccopulpal (buk″ko-pul′pal) pertaining to or formed by the buccal and pulpal walls of a tooth cavity.

buccostomy (buk-kos″to-me) the surgical creation of permanent buccal fistulae to prevent wind-sucking in horses.

buccoversion (buk″ko-ver′zhun) the position of a tooth which lies buccally to the line of occlusion.

buccula (buk′ŭ-lah) [L. "a little cheek"] (*obs.*) a redundant fold under the chin, commonly called a double chin.

Bucephalus (bu-sef′ah-lus) a genus of trematodes. **B. papillo′sus,** a trematode parasitic in the stomach and intestines of fresh-water fish.

Buchner's bodies (book′nerz) [Hans *Buchner,* German bacteriologist, 1850–1902] see *defensive protein,* under *protein.*

buchu (bu′ku) the name of several species of *Barosma* (Rutaceae), which contain urinary antiseptic and diuretic volatile oils.

Buck's extension, fascia, operation (buks) [Gurdon *Buck,* American surgeon, 1807–1877] see under *extension, fascia,* and *operation.*

buckeye (buk′i) a popular designation for *Aesculus glabra* and other trees and shrubs of the same genus. The fruit of trees in this genus are toxic to livestock due to a glycoside, esculin.

buckling (buk′ling) the process or an instance of becoming crumpled or warped. **scleral b.,** a technique for repair of detachment of the retina, in which indentations or infoldings of the sclera are made over the tears in the retina so as to promote adherence of the retina to the choroid.

Bucky diaphragm, rays (buk′e) [Gustav P. *Bucky,* German roentgenologist in America, 1880–1963] see under *diaphragm,* and see *grenz rays,* under *ray.*

buclizine hydrochloride (bu′klĭ-zēn) chemical name: 1-[(4-chlorophenyl)phenylmethyl]-4-[[4-(1,1-dimethylethyl)phenyl]-methyl]piperazine dihydrochloride. An antihistamine, $C_{28}H_{33}Cl-N_2 \cdot 2HCl$, used mainly as an antinauseant in the management of motion sickness; administered orally.

bucnemia (buk-ne′me-ah) [L., from Gr. *bous* ox + *knēmē* leg] a diffuse, tense, and inflammatory swelling of the leg.

bucrylate (bu′krĭ-lāt) chemical name: isobutyl 2-cyanoacrylate; a tissue adhesive, $C_8H_{11}NO_2$.

bud (bud) any small part of the embryo or adult metazoon more or less resembling the bud of a plant and presumed to have potential for growth and differentiation. **bronchial b.,** an outgrowth from the stem bronchus giving rise to the air passages of its respective pulmonary lobe. **end b.,** the remnant of the primitive knot, from which arises the caudal portion of the trunk; called also *tail b.* **gustatory b.,** taste b. **limb b.,** a swelling on the trunk of the embryo that becomes a limb. **liver b.,** a diverticulum from the foregut that gives rise to the liver and its ducts. **lung b.,** an outgrowth from the foregut that gives rise to the trachea, bronchi, and all the branchings that form a tracheobronchial tree. **metanephric b.,** ureteric b. **periosteal b.,** vascular connective tissue from the periosteum growing through apertures in the periosteal bone collar into the cartilaginous matrix of the primary center of ossification. **tail b.,** 1. the primordium of the caudal appendage. 2. end bud. **taste b.,** one of the minute terminal organs of the gustatory nerve that contain the receptor surfaces for the sense of taste. See also *caliculus gustatorius* [NA]. **tooth b.,** the knoblike primordium of a tooth. **ureteric b.,** an outgrowth of the mesonephric duct that gives rise to all but the nephrons of the permanent kidney; called also *metanephric b.* **b. of urethra,** bulbus penis. **vascular b.,** an outgrowth of an existing vessel from which a new blood vessel arises. **wing b.,** a swelling on the trunk of an avian embryo that gives rise to a wing.

Budd's cirrhosis (disease), jaundice (budz) [George *Budd,* London physician, 1808–1882] see under *cirrhosis* and see *acute yellow atrophy of liver,* under *atrophy.*

Budd-Chiari syndrome (disease) (bud′ke-ar′e) [George *Budd;* Hans *Chiari,* Austrian pathologist, 1851–1916] see under *syndrome.*

buddeized milk (boo′de-īzd) [E. *Budde,* Danish sanitary engineer] see under *milk.*

budding (bud′ing) 1. gemmation; a form of asexual reproduction in which the body divides into two unequal parts, the larger part being considered the parent and the smaller one the bud. 2. the process by which a new blood vessel arises from a preexisting vessel.

Budge's center (bood′gēz) [Julius Ludwig *Budge,* German physiologist, 1811–1888] 1. the ciliospinal center. 2. the genital center.

budgerigar, budgie (buj′er-e-gar″; buj′e) [Australian name] a species of parakeet, *Melopsittacus undulatus,* used for experimental work in psittacosis, and also popular as cage pets; called also *shell parakeet.*

Budin's joint, rule (boo-daz′) [Pierre-Constant *Budin,* Paris gynecologist, 1846–1907] see under *joint* and *rule.*

BUDR 5-bromodeoxyuridine.

Buerger's disease, symptom (ber′gerz) [Leo *Buerger,* physician in New York, 1879–1943] see under *disease* and *symptom.*

Buergi's theory (ber′gēz) [Emil *Buergi,* Swiss pharmacologist, born 1872] see under *theory.*

büffelseuche (bif′el-zoi″kĕ) [Ger.] pasteurellosis of the buffalo.

buffer (buf′er) 1. a chemical system that prevents change in the concentration of another chemical substance, e.g., proton donor and acceptor systems serve as buffers preventing marked changes in hydrogen ion concentration (pH). 2. a physical or physiological system that tends to maintain constancy, e.g., reflexes regulating blood pressure. **bicarbonate b.,** a buffer system composed of bicarbonate ions and dissolved carbon dioxide; in the body, this system is an important factor in determining the pH of the blood as the concentration of bicarbonate ions is regulated by the kidneys and of carbon dioxide by the respiratory system. **cacodylate b.,** one containing an organic arsenical salt, used in preparing fixatives for electron microscopy. **phosphate b.,** a buffer system composed of acid phosphate and sodium or potassium salts, e.g., monosodium and disodium acid phosphate; in the body, it is important in regulating the pH of the renal tubular fluids. **protein b.,** a buffer system involving proton donor and proton acceptor groups of the amino acid residues of proteins. **TRIS b.,** see *tromethamine.* **veronal b.,** a barbital buffer commonly used in the preparation of fixatives for electron microscopy.

buffering (buf′er-ing) the action produced by a buffer.

bufilcon A (bu-fil′kon) chemical name: 2-hydroxyethyl methacrylate polymer with N-(1,1-dimethyl-3-oxobutyl)acrylamide and 2-ethyl-2-(hydroxymethyl)-1,3-propanediol trimethacrylate; a contact lens material (hydrophilic), $(C_6H_{10}O_3)_x(C_9H_{15}NO_2)_y(C_{18}-H_{26}O_6)_z$.

bufin (bu′fin) a white secretion obtained by stimulating the parotid gland of certain species of toads by electricity; it has a physiologic action similar to that of digitalis but is not used in Western medicine.

Bufo (bu′fo) [L. "toad"] a genus of toads, species of which have been extensively studied by population geneticists.

buformin (bu-for′min) chemical name: N-butylimidocarbonimidic diamide; an oral hypoglycemic agent, $C_6H_{15}N_5$.

bufotalin (bu-fo-tal′in) a poisonous principal, $C_{26}H_{36}O_6$, present in the skin and saliva of the common European toad, *Bufo vulgaris.*

bufotenin (bu-fo′tĕ-nin) a specific basic pressor principle, 5-hydroxy indole ethyl dimethyl amine, $OH \cdot C_8H_5N \cdot CH_2 \cdot CH_2 \cdot N$-

$(CH_3)_2$, prepared from the skin glands of the toad, *Bufo bufo bufo*. It is used as a hallucinogenic in experimental medicine.

bufotherapy (bu''fo-ther'ah-pe) [L. *bufo* toad + *therapy*] the use of toad toxins in the treatment of disease.

bufotoxin (bu''fo-tok'sin) any toxin derived from the skin of toads.

bug (bug) an insect of the order Hemiptera. **assassin b.,** see *Reduviidae*. **barley b.,** *Acarus hordei*. **blister b.,** *Lytta vesicatoria*. **blue b.,** *Argas persicus*. **cone-nose b.,** see *Reduviidae*. **croton b.,** *Blatta (Blatella) germanica*. **harvest b.,** chigger. **hematophagous b.,** a bug that lives on blood, such as the bedbug. **kissing b.,** see *Reduviidae*. **Malay b.,** see *Reduviidae*. **miana b., Mianeh b.,** *Argas persicus*. **red b.,** chigger. **wheat b.,** *Pyemotes*.

Buhl's disease, desquamative pneumonia (būlz) [Ludwig von *Buhl*, German pathologist, 1816–1880] see under *disease* and *pneumonia*.

Buhl-Dittrich law (būl-dit-rik) [Ludwig von *Buhl*; Franz *Dittrich*, German pathologist, 1815–1859] see under *law*.

buiatrics [Gr. *bous* ox, cow + *iatrikos* surgery, medicine] the treatment of diseases of cattle.

Buist's method (būsts) [Robert C. *Buist*, Scotch obstetrician, 1860–1939] see *artificial respiration*, under *respiration*.

bulb (bulb) [L. *bul'bus*; Gr. *bolbos*] 1. a rounded mass, or enlargement. 2. (*obs.*) medulla oblongata. **b. of aorta,** bulbus aortae. **auditory b.,** the membranous labyrinth and cochlea. **b. of corpus cavernosum,** bulbus penis. **duodenal b.,** pars superior duodeni. **end b.,** 1. an ovoid or spheroid body located at the termination of a nerve fiber, and dispersed in the skin, mucous membranes, muscles, joints, and connective tissue of the internal organs. End-bulbs show a wide diversity, from simple end knobs to complex sensory end organs with connective tissue sheaths. For descriptions of specific types, see under *corpusculum*. 2. one of the end-feet. **end b's of Krause,** corpuscula bulboidea; see under *corpusculum*. **b. of eye,** bulbus oculi. **gustatory b.,** taste bud (caliculus gustatorius). **b. of hair,** the bulbous expansion at the proximal end of a hair in which the hair shaft is generated; called also *bulbus pili* [NA]. **b. of heart,** bulbus cordis. **b. of jugular vein, inferior,** bulbus venae jugularis inferior. **b. of jugular vein, superior,** bulbus venae jugularis superior. **b's of Krause,** corpuscula bulboidea; see under *corpusculum*. **olfactory b.,** bulbus olfactorius. **b. of ovary,** a bulb formed by the interweaving of veins with the bundles of involuntary muscle within the mesovarium; called also *Rouget's b.* **b. of penis,** bulbus penis. **b. of posterior horn,** bulbus cornus posterioris. **Rouget's b.,** b. of ovary. **sinovaginal b.,** one of paired sacculations of the urogenital sinus, forming the lowermost part of the vagina. **taste b.,** taste bud (caliculus gustatorius). **terminal b's of Krause,** corpuscula bulboidea; see under *corpusculum*. **b. of urethra,** bulbus penis. **vaginal b.,** 1. a solid end of a paramesonephric duct in the embryo. 2. bulbus vestibuli vaginae. **b. of vestibule of vagina, vestibulovaginal b.,** bulbus vestibuli vaginae.

bulbar (bul'bar) pertaining to a bulb; pertaining to or involving the medulla oblongata, as bulbar paralysis.

bulbi (bul'bi) [L.] plural of *bulbus*.

bulbiform (bul'bĭ-form) bulb-shaped.

bulbitis (bul-bi'tis) inflammation of the bulb of the penis.

bulboatrial (bul''bo-a'tre-al) pertaining to the bulbus cordis and atrium.

bulbocapnine (bul''bo-kap'nin) an alkaloid, $C_{19}H_{19}NO_4$, derived from the roots of *Corydalis bulbosa* DC. or *C. cava* (L.) Schweigg. & Korte (Fumariaceae) (*Capnoides cavum*). It has an inhibitory effect on the reflex and motor activities of striated muscle, and has been used in the treatment of muscular tremors and vestibular nystagmus. See also under *experiment*.

bulbocavernosus (bul''bo-kav''er-no'sus) musculus bulbospongiosus.

bulbogastrone (bul''bo-gas'trōn) a polypeptide secreted by the duodenal bulb when the bulb is acidified; it inhibits gastric acid secretion in dogs.

bulboid (bul'boid) bulb-shaped.

bulbonuclear (bul''bo-nu'kle-ar) (*obs.*) pertaining to the medulla oblongata and its nerve nuclei.

bulbopontine (bul''bo-pon'tin) a term once applied to that portion of the brain made up of the pons and the region of the medulla oblongata situated dorsad to it.

bulbospongiosus (bul''bo-spon''je-o'sus) see Table of *Musculi*.

bulbourethral (bul''bo-u-re'thral) pertaining to the bulb of the urethra (bulbus penis [NA]).

bulbous (bul'bus) having the form or nature of a bulb; bearing or arising from a bulb.

bulbus (bul'bus), pl. *bul'bi* [L.] a rounded mass, or enlargement. **b. aor'tae** [NA], bulb of aorta: the enlargement of the aorta at its point of origin from the heart, where the bulges of the aortic sinuses occur. **b. arterio'sus,** b. cordis. **b. carot'icus,** carotid sinus. **b. cor'dis,** the foremost of the three parts of the

primitive heart of the embryo; called also *bulb of heart* and *bulbus arteriosus*. **b. cor'nu posterio'ris ventric'uli latera'lis,** b. cornus posterioris. **b. cor'nus posterio'ris** [NA], bulb of posterior horn: an eminence produced in the posterior horn of the lateral ventricle by the splenial fibers of the corpus callosum as they pass posteriorly into the occipital lobe; called also *b. cornu posterioris ventriculi lateralis*. **b. oc'uli** [NA], the bulb, or globe, of the eye; called also *eyeball* and *bulb of eye*. See under *eye*. **b. olfacto'rius** [NA], olfactory bulb; the bulblike expansion of the olfactory tract on the under surface of the frontal lobe of each cerebral hemisphere; the olfactory nerves enter it. Called also *Morgagni's tubercle*. **b. pe'nis** [NA], bulb of penis: the enlarged proximal part of the corpus spongiosum found between the two crura of the penis. Called also *b. urethrae, bulb of corpus cavernosum*, and *bulb of urethra*. **b. pi'li** [NA], bulb of hair: the bulbous expansion at the proximal end of a hair, in which the hair shaft is generated. **b. ure'thrae,** b. penis. **b. ve'nae jugula'ris infe'rior** [NA], inferior bulb of jugular vein: a dilatation of the internal jugular vein just before it joins the brachiocephalic vein. **b. ve'nae jugula'ris supe'rior** [NA], superior bulb of jugular vein: a dilatation at the beginning of the internal jugular vein; called also *Heister's diverticulum*. **b. vestib'uli vagi'nae** [NA], bulb of vestibule of vagina: a body consisting of paired elongated masses of erectile tissue, one on either side of the vaginal opening, united anteriorly in a thin strand that passes along the lower surface of the clitoris.

bulesis (bu-le'sis) [Gr. *boulēsis*] the will, or an act of the will.

bulimia (bu-lim'e-ah) [L.; Gr. *bous* ox + *limos* hunger] abnormal increase in the sensation of hunger; cynorexia. Cf. *polyphagia*.

bulimiac (bu-lim'e-ak) bulimic.

bulimic (bu-lim'ik) pertaining to or affected with bulimia.

Buliminae (bu-lim'ĭ-ne) a subfamily of snails (family Hydrobiidae, order Mesogastropoda) that includes the medically important genera *Bulimus, Alocinma,* and *Parafossarulus*.

Bulimus (bu-li'mus) a genus of small fresh-water snails. **B. fuchsia'nus,** the chief intermediate host of the human liver flukes *Clonorchis* and *Opisthorchis;* it is commonly found in southern China. **B. leach'ii,** a species found in northern Europe and the northwestern United States, which ingests the eggs of *Opisthorchis felineus* and in whose body the eggs hatch.

Bulinus (bu-li'nus) a genus of snails, several species of which are the intermediate hosts of *Schistosoma haematobium* and *Opisthorchis*.

bulkage (bulk'ij) material that will increase the bulk of the intestinal contents and consequently stimulate peristalsis.

Bull. abbreviation for L. *bul'liat,* let it boil.

bulla (bul'ah), pl. *bul'lae* [L.] a large vesicle, usually 2 cm. or more in diameter. **emphysematous b.,** any space of more than 1 centimeter in diameter in distended areas of the emphysematous lung. **ethmoid b.,** see *b. ethmoidalis cavi nasi* and *b. ethmoidalis ossis ethmoidalis*. **b. ethmoida'lis ca'vi na'si** [NA], ethmoidal bulla of nasal cavity: the large ethmoid air cell lodged in the bulla ethmoidalis ossis ethmoidalis. **b. ethmoida'lis os'sis ethmoida'lis** [NA], ethmoidal bulla of ethmoidal bone: a rounded projection of the ethmoid bone into the lateral wall of the middle nasal meatus just below the middle nasal concha, enclosing a large ethmoid air cell; called also *antrum ethmoidale* and *ethmoid antrum*. **b. for'nicis, b. of fornix,** corpus mamillare. **b. mastoi'dea,** a large air cell in the mastoid of lower animals. **b. os'sea,** the dilated part of the bony external meatus of the ear.

bullae (bul'e) plural of *bulla*.

bullate (bul'āt) [L. *bullatus*] 1. characterized by the presence of bullae. 2. inflated.

bullation (bul-la'shun) [L. *bullatio*] 1. the condition characterized by the presence of bullae. 2. the state of being inflated.

Buller's shield (bandage) (bul'erz) [Frank *Buller*, Canadian ophthalmologic surgeon, 1844–1905] see under *shield*.

bullosis (bul-lo'sis) the production of, or a condition characterized by, bullous lesions. **b. diabetico'rum,** a condition in which bullae appear spontaneously, usually on the ankles and feet, in some uncontrolled diabetics.

bullous (bul'us) pertaining to or characterized by bullae.

bumblefoot (bum'bel-foot) inflammation of the ball of the foot of fowls, usually caused by staphylococcus.

bumetanide (bu-met'ah-nīd) chemical name: 3-(aminosulfonyl)-5-(butylamino)-phenoxybenzoic acid; a rapid-acting, potent diuretic, $C_{17}H_{20}N_2O_5S$.

Bumke's pupil (boom'kez) [Oswald Conrad Edward *Bumke*, German neurologist, 1877–1950] see under *pupil*.

bumps (bumpz) a symptom of the primary form of coccidioidomycosis (q.v.); called also *desert* or *valley bumps*.

BUN blood urea nitrogen; see *urea nitrogen*.

bunamidine hydrochloride (bu-nah'mĭ-dēn) chemical name: *N,N*-dibutyl-4-(hexyloxy)-1-naphthamidine monohydrochloride; an anthelmintic, $C_{25}H_{38}N_2O \cdot HCl$.

bunamiodyl (bu''nah-mi'o-dil) chemical name: 2-[[2,4,6-triiodo-3-[(1-oxobutyl)amino]phenyl]methylene]butanoic acid monosodium salt. A radiopaque medium, $C_{15}H_{16}I_3NO_3$, used in roentgenography of the biliary tract. Called also *buniodyl*.

bundle (bun'd'l) a collection of fibers or strands, as of muscle fibers, or a fasciculus or band of nerve fibers. **aberrant b's,** collections of pyramidal fibers leaving the corticonuclear tract at successive levels of the brain stem, and giving off fibers to the motor nuclei of the cranial nerves. **atrioventricular b., a-v. b.,** b. of His. **Bachmann's b.,** a transverse band of muscle fibers extending between the bases of the right and left auricles of the heart in dogs. **basis b's,** fasciculi proprii; see under *fasciculus*. **Bruce's b.,** cornucommissural b. **cornucommissural b.,** a name once given the fasciculus proprius on the surface of the posterior column and posterior commissure of the spinal cord. **forebrain b., medial,** a complex group of fibers arising from the basal olfactory regions, the periamygdaloid region, and the septal nuclei, and passing to the lateral hypothalamus; some fibers continue into the midbrain tegmentum and are relayed to the autonomic and visceral nuclei of the brain stem. **fundamental b's, ground b's,** fasciculi proprii; see under *fasciculus*. **b. of Helweg,** olivospinal tract. **b. of His,** a small band of atypical cardiac muscle fibers that originates in the atrioventricular node in the interatrial septum, passes through the atrioventricular junction, and then runs beneath the endocardium of the right ventricle on the membranous part of the interventricular septum. It divides at the upper end of the muscular part of the interventricular septum into right and left branches which descend in the septal wall of the right and left ventricle, respectively, to be distributed to those two chambers. This bundle propagates the atrial contraction rhythm to the ventricles, and its interruption produces heart block. Called also *fasciculus atrioventricularis* [NA], atrioventricular or *a-v b., Kent-His b.,* b. of Stanley Kent, His' band, Gaskell's bridge, and *ventriculonector*. **Keith's b.,** a bundle of fibers in the wall of the right atrium, between the openings of the venae cavae; called also *sinoatrial b.* **Kent's b.,** a muscular bundle in the heart of several mammalian species (sometimes in man), forming a direct connection between the atrial and ventricular walls. **Kent-His b.,** b. of His. **longitudinal medial b.,** fasciculus longitudinalis medialis. **main b.,** the portion of the bundle of His between the atrioventricular node and the division into right and left branches; see *b. of His.* **medial forebrain b.,** a group of nerve fibers in the lateral area of the hypothalamus, connecting the midbrain tegmentum and elements of the limbic system. **Meynert's b.,** fasciculus retroflexus. **Monakow's b.,** tractus rubrospinalis. **muscle b.,** one of the primary longitudinal subdivisions of a muscle, made up of muscle fibers and separated from other bundles by fascial septa or perimysium. **olivocochlear b. of Rasmussen,** a bundle of fibers originating in the superior olivary complex and usually terminating in the cochlea of the opposite side; called also *b. of Oort* and *b. of Rasmussen.* **b. of Oort,** olivocochlear b. of Rasmussen. **posterior longitudinal b.,** fasciculus longitudinalis medialis. **predorsal b.** (*obs.*), tectospinal tract. **b. of Rasmussen,** olivocochlear b. of Rasmussen. **Schultze's b.,** interfascicular fasciculus. **Schutz's b.,** fasciculus longitudinalis dorsalis. **sinoatrial b.,** Keith's b. **solitary b.,** tractus solitarius medullae oblongatae. **b. of Stanley Kent,** b. of His. **thalamomamillary b.,** fasciculus mamillothalamicus. **Thorel's b.,** a bundle of muscle fibers in the human heart, connecting the sinoatrial and atrioventricular nodes, and passing around the mouth of the inferior vena cava. **transverse b's of palmar aponeurosis,** fasciculi transversi aponeurosis palmaris; see under *fasciculus*. **Türck's b.,** tractus temporopontinus. **b. of Vicq d'Azyr,** fasciculus mamillothalamicus. **Weissmann's b.,** the bundle of striated muscle fibers of a neuromuscular spindle.

bundle branch (bun'd'l branch) a branch of the bundle of His.

bungarotoxin (bung″gah-ro-tok'sin) a strong neurotoxin from the venom of kraits (*Bungarus*); three electrophoretic fractions, α-, β-, and γ-bungarotoxin, have been identified. α-Bungarotoxin, the chief fraction, binds irreversibly with acetylcholine receptors, producing neuromuscular block.

Bungarus (bung'gah-rus) a genus of venomous elapid snakes found in India; the krait. See table accompanying *snake*.

Bunge's amputation (boong'gez) [Richard *Bunge*, German surgeon, born 1870] aperiosteal amputation.

Bunge's law (boong'gez) [Gustav von *Bunge*, physiologist at Basel, 1844–1920] see under *law*.

Bunge's spoon (boong'gez) [Paul *Bunge*, German ophthalmologist, 1853–1926] see under *spoon*.

bungeye (bung'i) a condition caused by infestation of the eye of horses with *Habronema*, and marked by small worm-containing granulomas in the conjunctiva; called also *blue-eye*.

Büngner's bands (cell cordons) (bing'nerz) [Otto von *Büngner*, German neurologist, 1858–1905] see under *band*.

bungpagga (bung-pag'gah) tropical pyomyositis.

buninoid (boo'ne-noid) [Gr. *bounos* hill + *eidos* form] having a rounded form; said of tumors.

buniodyl (bu-ni'o-dil) bunamiodyl.

bunion (bun'yun) [L. *bunio*; Gr. *bounion* turnip] abnormal prominence of the inner aspect of the first metatarsal head,

accompanied by bursal formation and resulting in a lateral or valgus displacement of the great toe. **tailor's b.,** bunionette.

bunionectomy (bun-yun-ek'to-me) [*bunion* + Gr. *ektomē* excision] excision of an abnormal prominence on the mesial aspect of the first metatarsal head.

bunionette (bun-yun-et') enlargement of the lateral aspect of the fifth metatarsal head; called also *tailor's bunion*.

bunodont (bu'no-dont) [Gr. *bounos* hill + *odous* tooth] having cheek teeth with low rounded cusps on the occlusal surface of the crown, as in mammals with mixed diet, such as swine, many rodents, and man.

bunolol hydrochloride (bu'no-lōl) chemical name: 5-[3-[(1,1-dimethylethyl)amino]-2-hydroxypropoxy]-3-4-dihydro-1(2*H*)-naphthalenone hydrochloride; a beta-adrenergic blocking agent, $C_{17}H_{25}NO_3 \cdot HCl$, having the same actions as propranolol (q.v.).

bunolophodont (bu″no-lo'fo-dont) [Gr. *bounos* hill + *lophos* ridge + *odous* tooth] having cheek teeth with both rounded cusps and transverse ridges on the occlusal surface of the crown, as in some kangaroos.

bunoselenodont (bu″no-sĕ-le'no-dont) [Gr. *bounos* hill + *selēnē* moon + *odous* tooth] having cheek teeth with both rounded cusps and crescentic ridges on the occlusal surface of the crown.

Bunostomum (bu″no-sto'mum) a genus of hookworms of the family Ancylostomidae that parasitize cattle, sheep, and other ruminants; called also *Monodontus*.

Bunsen burner, coefficient (bun'sen) [Robert Wilhelm Eberhard von *Bunsen*, German chemist, 1811–1899] see under *burner*, and see *absorption coefficient* (def. 2.), under *coefficient*.

buphthalmia (būf-thal'me-ah) buphthalmos; hydrophthalmos.

buphthalmos (buf-thal'mos) [Gr. *bous* ox + *ophthalmos* eye] enlargement and distention of the fibrous coats of the eye; hydrophthalmos; infantile glaucoma. Called also *cornea globosa* and *megophthalmos*.

buphthalmus (būf-thal'mus) buphthalmos; hydrophthalmos.

bupicomide (bu-pik'o-mīd) chemical name: 5-butyl-2-pyridinecarboxamide; an antihypertensive, $C_{10}H_{14}N_2O$.

bupivacaine hydrochloride (bu-piv'ah-kān) chemical name: *dl*-1-butyl-2'-6'-pipecoloxylidide hydrochloride. A local anesthetic, $C_{18}H_{28}N_2O \cdot HCl$, occurring as a white crystalline powder; used for peripheral nerve block, infiltration, and sympathetic, caudal, or epidural block.

buprenorphine hydrochloride (bu″pre-nor'fēn) chemical name: 17-(cyclopropylmethyl)-α-(1,1-dimethylethyl)-4,5α-epoxy-18,19-dihydro-3-hydroxy-6-methoxy-α-methyl-6,14-ethenomorphinan-7α(*S*)-methanol hydrochloride; a synthetic derivative of thebaine, $C_{29}H_{41}NO_4 \cdot HCl$, used as an analgesic.

bupropion hydrochloride (bu-pro'pe-on) chemical name: (±)-1-(3-chlorophenyl)-2-[(1,1-dimethylethyl) amino]-1-propanone hydrochloride; an antidepressant, $C_{13}H_{18}ClNO \cdot HCl$.

bur (ber) a form of drill used for creating openings in bone or similar hard substances. Such an instrument is used in dentistry, in the hand piece of a dental engine, for opening and preparing tooth cavities; called also *bur drill*. **carbide b.,** one in which the steel is alloyed with tungsten carbide to increase its hardness and cutting ability.

Burdach's columns, etc. (boor'daks) [Karl Friedrich *Burdach*, German physiologist, 1776–1847] see under *columns, fasciculus, fiber, fissure, nucleus*, and *tract*.

buret, burette (bu-ret') a graduated glass tube used in volumetric chemistry to deliver a measured amount of liquid.

Burghart's symptom (sign) (boorg'harts) [Hans Gerny *Burghart*, German physician, 1862–1932] see under *symptom*.

burimamide (bu-rim'ah-mīd) an antagonist to histamine, competing for the histamine$_2$ receptor site on cells.

burn (bern) a lesion caused by the contact of heat or fire. Burns of the first degree show redness; of the second degree, vesication; of the third degree, necrosis through the entire skin. Burns of the first and second degree are known as partial thickness burns, those of the third degree as full-thickness burns. **brush b.,** a wound caused by violent rubbing or friction, as by a rope pulled through the hands; called also *friction b.* **cement b., concrete b.,** a corrosive destruction of tissue caused by contact with cement or concrete. **chemical b.,** see *primary irritant dermatitis*, under *dermatitis*. **contact b.,** an electric burn produced by contact with electric current. **electric b., electrical b.,** see *flash b.* and *contact b.* **flash b.,** a thermal lesion produced by a very brief exposure to radiant heat of high intensity, as in an explosion or a sudden discharge of electricity. **friction b.,** brush b. **Kangri b.,** a burn on the abdomen caused by the portable stove (Kangri) carried by natives of Kashmir; such a burn may be followed by cancer. **radiation b.,** a burn caused by exposure to x-ray, radium, sunlight, atomic, or any other type of radiant energy. **sun b.,** sunburn. **thermal b.,** injury due to contact with flame, hot objects, or hot liquids, as distinguished from chemical and electric burns. **x-ray b.,** a lesion caused by exposure to x-rays.

Burnam's test (bur'namz) [Curtis Field *Burnam*, Baltimore surgeon, 1877–1947] see under *tests*.

burner (ber′ner) the part of a lamp, stove, or furnace from which the flame issues. **Argand b.,** a burner for oil or gas, with an inner tube for supplying air to the flame. **Bunsen b.,** a gas burner in which the gas is mixed with air before ignition, in order to give complete oxidation.

Burnet (bur-net′), Sir Frank Macfarlane. Australian physician-virologist, born 1899; co-winner, with Peter B. Medawar, of the Nobel prize in medicine and physiology for 1960, for the theoretical solution to the problem of transplanting tissues and vital organs from one animal to another.

Burnett's disinfecting fluid, (solution) (bur′nets) [Sir William *Burnett,* English surgeon, 1779–1861] see under *fluid.*

burnisher (ber′nish-er) a smooth, rounded dental instrument for adapting, finishing and polishing metal dental restorations and dentures.

burnishing (ber′nish-ing) a dental procedure somewhat related to polishing and abrading.

Burns' amaurosis (bernz) [John *Burns,* Scottish physician, 1774–1850] postmarital amblyopia.

Burns' ligament, space (bernz) [Allan *Burns,* Scottish anatomist, 1781–1813] see *margo falciformis hiatus saphenus* and *fossa jugularis,* def. 1.

Burow's operation, solution, vein (bōōr′ovz) [Karl August *Burow,* surgeon in Königsberg, 1809–1874] see under *operation* and *vein,* and see *aluminum acetate solution,* under *solution.*

burquism (burk′izm) [V. B. *Burg,* French neurologist, 1823–1884] a system of metallotherapy.

burr (bur) bur.

bursa (ber′sah), pl. *bur′sae* [L.; Gr. "a wine skin"] a sac or saclike cavity filled with a viscid fluid and situated at places in the tissues at which friction would otherwise develop. **b. of Achilles (tendon),** b. tendinis calcanei. **acromial b.,** b. subdeltoidea. **adventitious b.,** an abnormal cyst due to friction or some other mechanical cause, and containing synovial fluid; called also *supernumerary b.* **anconeal b.,** b. subcutanea olecrani. **anconeal b. of triceps muscle,** b. subtendinea musculi tricipitis brachii. **b. anseri′na** [NA], **anserine b.,** a bursa between the tendons of the sartorius, gracilis, and semitendinosus muscles, and the tibial collateral ligament; called also *anterior genual b.* **bicipital b., bicipitofibular b.,** b. subtendinea musculi bicipitis femoris inferior. **bicipitoradial b., b. bicipitoradia′lis** [NA], a bursa between the radial tuberosity and the biceps tendon; called also *b. mucosa radialis.* **Boyer's b.,** one situated beneath the hyoid bone. **Brodie's b.,** b. subtendindea musculi gastrocnemii lateralis. **calcaneal b.,** b. tendinis calcanei. **calcaneal b., subcutaneous,** b. subcutanea calcanea. **b. of calcaneal tendon,** b. tendinis calcanei. **Calori's b.,** a bursa situated between the trachea and the arch of the aorta. **b. copula′trix,** an appendage at the posterior end of the male of certain nematodes. **coracobrachial b.,** b. musculi coracobrachialis. **coracoid b.,** b. subtendinea musculi subscapularis. **b. cubita′lis interos′sea** [NA], **cubitoradial b.,** a bursa between the ulna, the biceps tendon, and nearby muscles; called also *interosseous cubital b.* and *ulnoradial b.* **deltoid b.,** b. subacromialis. **b.-equivalent,** requiring interaction with human tissue analogous to the bursa of Fabricius in birds (*bursal equivalent tissue*). See *B-lymphocytes,* under *lymphocyte.* **b. of Fabricius,** an epithelial outgrowth of the cloaca in chick embryos, which develops in a manner similar to that of the thymus in mammals, atrophying after 5 or 6 months and persisting as a fibrous remnant in sexually mature birds. It contains lymphoid follicles, and before involution is a site of formation of lymphocytes associated with humoral immunity. See also *b.-equivalent,* and *bursal equivalent tissue,* under *tissue.* **fibular b.,** b. subtendinea musculi bicipitis femoris inferior. **Fleischmann's b.,** one beneath the tongue. **b. of flexor carpi radialis muscle,** vagina synovialis tendinis musculi flexoris carpi radialis. **gastrocnemiosemimembranous b.,** b. musculi semimembranosi. **genual b., anterior,** b. anserina. **genual b., external inferior,** b. subtendinea musculi bicipitis femoris inferior. **genual bursae, internal superior,** bursae subtendineae musculi sartorii. **genual b., posterior,** b. musculi semimembranosi. **bur′sae glutaeofemora′les** bursae intermusculares musculorum gluteorum. **gluteal b.,** one situated beneath the gluteus maximus muscle. **gluteal intermuscular bursae,** bursae intermusculares musculorum gluteorum. **gluteofascial bursae,** bursae intermusculares musculorum gluteorum. **gluteofemoral bursae,** bursae intermusculares musculorum gluteorum. **gluteotuberosal b.,** b. ischiadica musculi glutei maximi. **His's b.,** the dilatation at the end of the archenteron. **humeral b.,** 1. b. subacromialis. 2. b. subtendinea musculi gastrocnemii lateralis. **hyoid b.,** b. subcutanea prominentiae laryngeae. **iliac b., subtendinous, b. ili′aca subtendin′ea,** b. subtendinea iliaca. **b. iliopectine′a** [NA], **iliopectineal b.,** a bursa between the iliopsoas tendon and the iliopectineal eminence; called also *subiliac b.* and *ileopubic vesicular b.* **b. of iliopsoas muscle,** b. subtendinea iliaca. **inferior b. of biceps femoris muscle,** b. subtendinea musculi bicipitis femoris inferior. **infracardiac b.,** the cranial

end of a celomic recess of the embryo, extending upward between the esophagus and right lung bud; frequently persisting in the adult. **infracondyloid b., external,** recessus subpopliteus. **infragenual b.,** infrapatellaris profunda. **infrahyoid b., b. infrahyoi′dea** [NA], a bursa sometimes present below the hyoid bone at the attachment of the sternohyoid muscle. **infrapatellar b.,** b. subtendinea prepatellaris. **infrapatellar b., deep,** b. infrapatellaris profunda. **infrapatellar b., subcutaneous,** b. subcutanea infrapatellaris. **infrapatellar b., superficial inferior,** b. subcutanea tuberositatis tibiae. **b. infrapatella′ris profun′da** [NA], a bursa between the patellar ligament and the tibia. Called also *deep infrapatellar b., infragenual b., subpatellar b., subligamentous b.,* and *subpatellar mucous b.* **b. infrapatella′ris subcuta′nea,** b. subcutanea infrapatellaris. **bur′sae intermuscula′res musculo′rum gluteo′rum** [NA], intermuscular gluteal bursae: several sacs that surround the tendon attaching the gluteus maximus to the femur; called also *bursae glutaeofemorales, gluteofascial bursae,* and *gluteofemoral bursae.* **interosseous cubital b.,** cubitalis interossea. **intertubercular b.,** vagina synovialis intertubercularis. **b. intratendin′ea olecra′ni** [NA], intratendinous bursa of olecranon: a bursa within the triceps tendon near its insertion; called also *intratendinous supra-anconeal b.* and *Monro's b.* **ischiadic b.,** b. ischiadica musculi obturatoris interni. **b. ischiad′ica mus′culi glu′tei max′imi** [NA], ischial bursa of gluteus maximus muscle: a bursa between the ischial tuberosity and the gluteus maximus; called also *gluteotuberosal b.* **b. ischiad′ica musculi obturato′rii inter′ni** [NA], ischial bursa of internal obturator muscle: a bursa between the tendon of the obturator internus muscle and the lesser sciatic notch; called also *ischiadic b., b. musculi obturatoris interni, sciatic b. of obturator internus muscle,* and *tuberoischiadic b.* **ischial b. of gluteus maximus muscle,** b. ischiadica musculi glutei maximi. **ischial b. of internal obturator muscle,** b. ischiadica musculi obturatorii interni. **lateral b. of gastrocnemius muscle,** b. subtendinea musculi gastrocnemii lateralis. **b. of latissimus dorsi muscle,** subtendinea musculi latissimi dorsi. **Luschka's b.,** b. pharyngea. **medial b. of gastrocnemius muscle,** b. subtendinea musculi gastrocnemii medialis. **Monro's b.,** b. intratendinea olecrani. **b. muco′sa,** b. synovialis. **b. muco′sa patella′ris profun′da,** b. subtendinea prepatellaris. **b. muco′sa radia′lis,** b. bicipitoradialis. **b. muco′sa radia′lis inter′ni,** vagina synovialis tendinis musculi flexoris carpi radialis. **b. muco′sa subcuta′nea,** b. synovialis subcutanea. **b. muco′sa subfascia′lis,** b. synovialis subfascialis. **b. muco′sa submuscula′ris,** b. synovialis submuscularis. **b. muco′sa subtendin′ea,** b. synovialis subtendinea. **b. muco′sa superficia′lis ge′nu,** Loder, b. subtendinea prepatellaris. **mucous b.,** b. synovialis. **mucous b., subpatellar,** b. infrapatellaris profunda. **mucous b., supracondyloid, medial,** b. subtendinea musculi gastrocnemii medialis. **mucous b. of knee, superficial,** b. subtendinea prepatellaris. **multilocular b.,** one which is subdivided into several compartments. **b. mus′culi bicip′itis fem′oris infe′rior,** b. subtendinea musculi bicipitis femoris inferior. **b. mus′culi bicip′itis fem′oris supe′rior** [NA], superior bursa of biceps femoris muscle: a bursa between the long head of the biceps, the semitendinosus, the tendon of the semimembranosus, and the ischial tuberosity; called also *subtendinous b.* **b. mus′culi coracobrachia′lis** [NA], a bursa between the coracobrachialis and subscapularus muscles and the coracoid process; called also *coracobrachial b.* and *subcoracoid b.* **b. mus′culi extenso′ris car′pi radia′lis bre′vis** [NA], a bursa between the tendon and the base of the third metacarpal bone. **b. mus′culi flexo′ris car′pi radia′lis,** vagina synovialis tendinis musculi flexoris carpi radialis. **b. mus′culi gastrocne′mii latera′lis,** b. subtendinea musculi gastrocnemii lateralis. **b. mus′culi gastrocne′mii media′lis,** b. subtendinea musculi gastrocnemii medialis. **b. mus′culi infraspina′ti,** b. subtendinea musculi infraspinati. **b. mus′culi latis′simi dor′si,** b. subtendinea musculi latissimi dorsi. **b. mus′culi obturato′ris inter′ni,** see *b. ischiadica musculi obturatorii interni* and *b. subtendinea musculi obturatorii interni.* **b. mus′culi pirifor′mis** [NA], bursa of piriform muscle: a bursa between the piriformis tendon, the superior gemellus muscle, and the femur; called also *piriform b.* **b. mus′culi poplite′i,** recessus subpopliteus. **b. mus′culi sarto′rii pro′pria** see *bursae subtendineae musculi sartorii.* **b. mus′culi semimembrano′si** [NA], bursa of semimembranosus muscle: a bursa between the semimembranosus muscle and the medial head of the gastrocnemius. Called also *gastrocnemiosemimembranous b., posterior genual b., retrocondyloid b., semimembranosagastrocnemial b.,* and *semimembranous b.* **b. mus′culi sternohyoi′dei,** see *b. intrahyoidea* and *b. retrohyoidea.* **b. mus′culi subscapula′ris,** b. subtendinea musculi subscapularis. **b. mus′culi tenso′ris ve′li palati′ni** [NA], bursa of tensor veli palatini muscle: a bursa between the hamular process of the sphenoid bone and the tendon of the tensor veli palatini. **b. mus′culi tere′tis majo′ris,** b. subtendinea musculi teretis majoris. **b. mus′culi thyreohyoi′dei,** a bursa under the thyrohyoid muscle. **b. mus′culi trochlea′ris,** vagina synovialis musculi obliqui superioris. **b. of olecranon,** b. subcutanea olecrani. **omental b., b. omenta'lis** [NA], a serous peritoneal cavity situated behind the stomach, the lesser omentum, and part of the liver and in front of the pancreas and duodenum. It communicates with the general peritoneal cavity (greater sac) through the epiploic foramen and sometimes is continuous with the cavity of the greater omentum. Called also *lesser peritoneal cavity*. **ovarian b., b. ova'rica,** the peritoneal fossa in which the ovary is situated. **patellar b., deep,** b. subtendinea prepatellaris. **patellar b., middle,** b. subfascialis prepatellaris. **patellar b., prespinous,** b. subcutanea tuberositatis tibiae. **patellar b., subcutaneous,** b. subcutanea prepatellaris. **peroneal b., common,** vagina synovialis musculorum peroneorum communis. **b. pharyn'gea** [NA], **pharyngeal b.,** an inconstant blind sac located above the pharyngeal tonsil in the midline of the posterior wall of the nasopharynx; it represents persistence of an embryonic communication between the anterior tip of the notochord and the roof of the pharynx. Called also *Luschka's b., Tornwaldt's b.* and *Tornwaldt's cyst*. **b. of piriform muscle,** b. musculi piriformis. **popliteal b., b. of popliteal muscle,** recessus subpopliteus. **postcalcaneal b.,** b. subcutanea calcanea. **postcalcaneal b., deep,** b. tendinis calcanei. **postgenual b., external,** b. subtendinea musculi gastrocnemii lateralis. **b. praepatella'ris subcuta'nea,** b. subcutanea prepatellaris. **b. praepatella'ris subfascia'lis,** b. subfascialis prepatellaris. **b. praepatella'ris subtendin'ea,** b. subtendinea prepatellaris. **prepatellar b., middle,** b. subfascialis prepatellaris. **prepatellar b., subcutaneous,** b. subcutanea prepatellaris. **prepatellar b., subfascial,** b. subfascialis prepatellaris. **prepatellar b., subtendinous,** b. subtendinea prepatellaris. **bur'sae prepatella'res,** see *b. subcutanea prepatellaris, b. subfascialis prepatellaris,* and *b. subtendinea prepatellaris*. **b. prepatella'ris profun'da, b. prepatella'ris subaponeurot'ica,** b. subtendinea prepatellaris. **pretibial b.,** b. subcutanea tuberositatis tibiae. **bur'sae pro'priae mus'culi sarto'rii,** bursae subtendineae musculi sartorii. **pyriform b.,** b. musculi piriformis. **b. of quadratus femoris muscle,** b. subtendinea iliaca. **retrocondyloid b.,** b. musculi semimembranosi. **retroepicondyloid b., lateral, deep,** b. subtendinea musculi gastrocnemii lateralis. **retrohyoid b., b. retrohyoi'dea** [NA], a bursa sometimes present behind the hyoid bone at the attachment of the sternohyoid muscle. **retromammary b.,** a well defined loose areolar tissue between the deep layer of superficial fascia on the posterior aspect of the breast, and the deep fascia covering the pectoralis major and other muscles of the chest wall. **sciatic b. of obturator internus muscle,** b. ischiadica musculi obturatorii interni. **semimembranosogastrocnemial b., semimembranous b.,** b. of semimembranosus muscle. **semitendinous b.,** b. musculi bicipitis femoris superior. **sternohyoid b., b. sternohyoi'dea,** see *b. infrahyoidea* and *b. retrohyoidea*. **subachilleal b.,** b. tendinis calcanei. **subacromial b., b. subacromia'lis** [NA], one between the acromion and the insertion of the supraspinatus muscle, extending between the deltoid and the greater tubercle of the humerus; called also *deltoid b.* and *humeral b.* **subcalcaneal b., b. subcutanea calcanea. subclavian b.,** an inconstant bursa between the fibers of the rhomboid ligament. **subcoracoid b.,** 1. bursa musculi coracobrachialis. 2. bursa subtendinea musculi subscapularis. **subcrural b.,** b. suprapatellaris. **b. subcuta'nea acromia'lis** [NA], a bursa between the acromion and the overlying skin; called also *subcutaneous acromial b.* **b. subcuta'nea calca'nea** [NA], subcutaneous calcaneal bursa: a bursa between the calcaneus and the skin on the sole of the foot; called also *postcalcaneal b.,* and *subcalcaneal b.* **b. subcuta'nea infrapatella'ris** [NA], subcutaneous intrapatellar bursa: a bursa between the upper end of the patellar ligament and the skin; called also *b. infrapatellaris subcutanea, subpatellar b.,* and *superficial b. of knee*. **b. subcuta'nea malle'oli latera'lis** [NA], subcutaneous bursa of lateral malleolus: a bursa between the lateral malleolus and the skin. **b. subcuta'nea malle'oli media'lis** [NA], subcutaneous bursa of medial malleolus: a bursa between the medial malleolus and the skin. **b. subcuta'nea olecra'ni** [NA], subcutaneous bursa of olecranon: a bursa between the olecranon process and the skin; called also *anconeal b.* and *superficial b. of olecranon*. **b. subcuta'nea prepatella'ris** [NA], subcutaneous prepatellar bursa: a bursa between the patella and the skin; called also *b. prepatellaris subcutanea*. **b. subcuta'nea prominen'tiae laryn'geae** [NA], subcutaneous bursa of prominence of larynx: a bursa over the anterior prominence of the thyroid cartilage of the larynx, under the skin; called also *hyoid b., subhyoid b.,* and *thyrohyoid b*. **b. subcuta'nea tuberosita'tis tib'iae** [NA], subcutaneous bursa of tuberosity of tibia: a bursa between the tibial tuberosity and the skin; called also *patellar b., prespinous b., pretibial b.,* and *superficial inferior infrapatellar b.* **subcutaneous acromial b.,** b. subcutanea acromialis. **subcutaneous b. of lateral malleolus,** b. subcutanea malleoli lateralis. **subcutaneous b. of medial malleolus,** b. subcutanea malleoli medialis. **subcutaneous b. of olecranon,** b. subcutanea olecrani. **subcutaneous b. of prominence of**

larynx, b. subcutanea prominentiae laryngeae. **subcutaneous b. of tuberosity of tibia,** b. subcutanea tuberositatis tibiae. **subdeltoid b., b. subdeltoi'dea** [NA], a bursa between the deltoid and the shoulder joint capsule, usually connected to the subacromial bursa; called also *acromial b.* **b. subfascia'lis prepatella'ris** [NA], subfascial prepatellar bursa: a bursa between the front of the patella and the investing fascia of the knee; called also *b. praepatellaris subfascialis, middle patellar* (or *prepatellar*) *b.* **subhyoid b.,** b. subcutanea prominentiae laryngeae. **subiliac b.,** 1. b. iliopectinea. 2. b. subtendinea iliaca. **subligamentous b.,** b. infrapatellaris profunda. **subpatellar b.,** 1. b. infrapatellaris profunda. 2. b. subcutanea infrapatellaris. **b. subtendin'ea ili'aca** [NA], subtendinous iliac bursa: a bursa between the iliopsoas tendon and the lesser trochanter; called also *b. iliaca subtendinea, b. of quadratus femoris muscle, b. of iliopsoas muscle,* and *subiliac b.* **b. subtendin'ea mus'culi bicip'itis fem'oris infe'rior** [NA], inferior subtendinous bursa of bicipitis femoris muscle: a bursa between the tendon of the biceps femoris muscle and the fibular collateral ligament of the knee joint; called also *bicipital b., biciptofibular b., fibular b., external inferior genual b.,* and *b. musculi bicipitus femoris inferior*. **b. subtendin'ea mus'culi gastrocne'mii latera'lis** [NA], a bursa between the tendon of the lateral head of the gastrocnemius muscle and the joint capsule; called also *b. musculi gastrocnemii lateralis, subtendinous b. of lateral head of gastrocnemius muscle, Brodie's b., humeral b., lateral b. of gastrocnemius muscle, external postgenual b.,* and *deep lateral retroepicondyloid b.* **b. subtendin'ea mus'culi gastrocne'mii media'lis** [NA], a bursa between the tendon of the medial head of the gastrocnemius, the condyle of the femur, and the joint capsule; called also *b. musculi gastrocnemii medialis, subtendinous b. of medial head of gastrocnemius muscle, internal supracondyloid b., medial b. of gastrocnemius muscle,* and *medial supracondyloid* (*mucous*) *b.* **b. subtendin'ea mus'culi infraspina'ti** [NA], subtendinous bursa of infraspinatus muscle: a bursa between the tendon of the infraspinatus and the joint capsule or the greater tubercle; called also *b. musculi infraspinati*. **b. subtendin'ea mus'culi latis'simi dor'si** [NA], a bursa between the tendons of the latissimus dorsi and teres major muscles; called also *b. musculi latissimi dorsi* and *b. of latissimus dorsi muscle*. **b. subtendin'ea mus'culi obturato'rii inter'ni** [NA], subtendinous bursa of internal obturator muscle: a bursa beneath the tendon of the obturator internus muscle; called also *b. musculi obturatoris interni*. **bur'sae subtendin'eae mus'culi sarto'rii** [NA], subtendinous bursa of sartorius muscle: bursae between the tendons of the sartorius, semitendinosus, and gracilis muscles; called also *internal superior genual bursae, b. musculi sartorii propria,* and *bursae propriae musculi sartorii*. **b. subtendin'ea mus'culi subscapula'ris** [NA], subtendinous bursa of subscapularis muscle: a bursa between the tendon of the subscapularis muscle and the glenoid border of the scapula; called also *b. musculi subscapularis, coracoid b.,* and *subcoracoid b.* **b. subtendin'ea mus'culi tere'tis majo'ris** [NA], subtendinous bursa of teres major muscle: a bursa deep to the tendon of insertion of the teres major muscle; called also *b. musculi teretis majoris*. **b. subtendin'ea mus'culi tibia'lis anterio'ris** [NA], subtendinous bursa of anterior tibial muscle: a bursa between the tibialis anterior and the medial surface of the medial cuneiform bone. **b. subtendin'ea mus'culi tibia'lis posterio'ris** [NA], subtendinous bursa of posterior tibial muscle: a bursa between the tibialis posterior and the navicular bone. **b. subtendin'ea mus'culi trape'zii** [NA], a bursa between the trapezius and the medial end of the spine of the scapula. **b. subtendin'ea mus'culi tricip'itis bra'chii, b. subtendin'ea olecra'ni,** an inconstant sac between the triceps tendon, the olecranon, and the dorsal ligament of the elbow; called also *anconeal b. of triceps muscle*. **b. subtendin'ea prepatella'ris** [NA], subtendinous prepatellar bursa: a bursa sometimes present between the quadriceps tendon and the patellar periosteum; called also *b. prepatellaris subtendinea, deep patellar b., infrapatellar b., mucosa superficialis* (*Loder*) *b., mucosa patellaris profunda, b. prepatellaris profunda* or *subaponeurotica, subcutaneous patellar b.,* and *superficial mucous b. of knee*. **subtendinous b. of anterior tibial muscle,** b. subtendinea musculi tibialis anterioris. **subtendinous b. of biceps femoris muscle, inferior,** b. subtendinea musculi bicipitis femoris inferior. **subtendinous b. of infraspinatus muscle,** b. subtendinea musculi infraspinati. **subtendinous b. of internal obturator muscle,** b. subtendinea musculi obturatorii interni. **subtendinous b. of lateral head of gastrocnemius muscle,** b. subtendinea musculi gastrocnemii lateralis. **subtendinous b. of medial head of gastrocnemius muscle,** b. subtendinea musculi gastrocnemii medialis. **subtendinous b. of obturator internus muscle,** b. subtendinea musculi obturatorii interni. **subtendinous b. of posterior tibial muscle,** b. subtendinea musculi tibialis posterioris. **subtendinous bursae of sartorius muscle,** bursae subtendineae musculi sartorii. **subtendinous b. of subscapularis muscle,** b. subtendinea musculi subscapularis. **subtendinous b. of teres major muscle,** b. subtendinea musculi teretis majoris. **superficial b. of knee,** b. subcutanea infrapatellaris. **superficial b. of olecranon,** b. subcutanea olecrani. **superior b. of biceps femoris muscle,** b. musculi bicipitis femoris superior. **supernumerary b.,** adventitious b. **supra-anconeal b., intratendinous,** b. intratendinea olecrani. **supracondyloid b., internal, supracondyloid b., medial,** b. subtendinea musculi gastrocnemii medialis. **supragenual b., suprapatellar b.,** b. suprapatellaris. **b. suprapatella'ris** [NA], suprapatellar bursa: a bursa between the distal end of the femur and the quadriceps tendon; called also *supragenual b.* and *subcrural b.* **synovial b.,** b. synovialis. **synovial b., subcutaneous,** b. synovialis subcutanea. **synovial b. of trochlea,** b. synovialis trochlearis. **b. synovia'lis** [NA], synovial bursa: a closed synovial sac interposed between surfaces which glide upon each other; it may be simple or multilocular in structure, and subcutaneous, submuscular, subfascial, or subtendinous in location; called also *b. mucosa* and *mucous b.* **b. synovia'lis subcuta'nea** [NA], subcutaneous synovial bursa: a synovial sac found beneath the skin; called also *b. mucosa subcutanea.* **b. synovia'lis subfascia'lis** [NA], a synovial sac found beneath a fascial layer; called also *b. mucosa subfascialis.* **b. synovia'lis submuscula'ris** [NA], a synovial sac found beneath a muscle; called also *b. mucosa submuscularis.* **b. synovia'lis subtendin'ea** [NA], a synovial sac found beneath a tendon; called also *b. mucosa subtendinea.* **b. synovia'lis trochlea'ris** [NA], synovial bursa of trochlea: the synovial bursa that encloses the tendon of the superior oblique muscle as it passes through the trochlea. **b. ten'dinis Achil'lis,** NA alternative for b. tendinis calcanei. **b. ten'dinis calca'nei** [NA], bursa of calcaneal tendon: a bursa between the calcaneal tendon and the back of the calcaneus; called also *b. of Achilles* (*tendon*), *calcaneal b., deep postcalcaneal b., subachilleal b.,* and *b. tendinis Achillis* [NA alternative]. **b. of tendon of Achilles,** b. tendinis calcanei. **b. of tensor veli palatini muscle,** b. musculi tensoris veli palatini. **b. of testes,** scrotum. **thyrohyoid b.,** b. subcutanea prominentiae laryngeae. **thyrohyoid b., anterior,** see *b. infrahyoidea* and *b. retrohyoidea.* **Tornwaldt's b.,** b. pharyngea. **trochanteric b., subcutaneous,** b. trochanterica subcutanea. **trochanteric b. of gluteus maximus muscle,** b. trochanterica musculi glutei maximi. **trochanteric bursae of gluteus medius muscle,** bursae trochantericae musculi glutei medii. **trochanteric b. of gluteus minimus muscle,** b. trochanterica musculi glutei minimi. **b. trochanter'ica mus'culi glu'taei me'dii ante'rior,** see *bursae trochantericae musculi glutei medii.* **b. trochanter'ica mus'culi glu'taei me'dii poste'rior,** see *bursae trochantericae musculi glutei medii.* **b. trochanter'ica mus'culi glu'tei max'imi** [NA], trochanteric bursa of gluteus maximus muscle: a bursa between the fascial tendon of the gluteus maximus, the posterolateral surface of the greater trochanter, and the vastus lateralis muscle. **bur'sae trochanter'icae mus'culi glu'tei me'dii** [NA], trochanteric bursae of gluteus medius muscle: bursae between the gluteus medius and the lateral surface of the greater trochanter, and sometimes between the tendons of the gluteus medius and the piriformis. **b. trochanter'ica mus'culi glu'tei min'imi** [NA], trochanteric bursa of gluteus minimus muscle: a bursa between the edge of the gluteus minimus and the greater trochanter. **b. trochanter'ica subcuta'nea** [NA], subcutaneous trochanteric bursa: a bursa between the greater trochanter of the femur and the skin. **tuberoischiadic b.,** b. ischiadica musculi obturatorii interni. **ulnoradial b.,** b. cubitalis interossea. **vesicular b., ileopubic,** b. iliopectinea. **vesicular b. of sternohyoideus muscle,** see *b. infrahyoidea* and *b. retrohyoidea.*

bursae (ber'se) [L.] plural of *bursa.*

bursal (ber'sal) [L. *bursalis*] of or pertaining to a bursa.

bursalogy (ber-sal'o-je) [*bursa* + *-logy*] the sum of knowledge regarding the bursae.

Bursata (ber-sa'tah) a term sometimes used to designate those Nematoda which have a bursa copulatrix.

bursatti, bursautee (ber-sat'e, ber-sawt'e) cutaneous habronemiasis.

bursectomy (ber-sek'to-me) [*bursa* + Gr. *ektomē* excision] excision of a bursa.

bursicon (bur'sĭ-kon) an insect hormone appearing in the blood after molting, which is required for the tanning and hardening of new cuticle.

bursitis (ber-si'tis) inflammation of a bursa, occasionally accompanied by a calcific deposit in the underlying supraspinatus tendon; the most common site is the subdeltoid bursa. **Achilles b.,** achillobursitis. **adhesive b.,** see under *capsulitis.* **calcific b.,** see under *tendinitis.* **Duplay's b.** (*obs.*), inflammation of the subacromial or subdeltoid bursa; see *calcific tendinitis,* under *tendinitis.* **ischiogluteal b.,** inflammation of the bursa over the ischial tuberosity, characterized by sudden onset of excruciating pain over the center of the buttock and down the back of the leg. **olecranon b.,** inflammation and enlargement of the bursa over the olecranon; called also *miners' elbow.* **omental b.,** peritonitis localized to the omental bursa (lesser sac). **pharyngeal b.,** Tornwaldt's b. **popliteal b.,** a swelling behind the knee, caused by escape of synovial fluid

which then becomes enclosed in a sac or membrane; called also *Baker's cyst* and *synovial cyst of the popliteal space.* **prepatellar b.,** inflammation of the bursa in front of the patella, with fluid accumulating within it; called also *housemaid's knee.* **radiohumeral b.,** tennis elbow. **retrocalcaneal b.,** achillodynia. **scapulohumeral b.,** calcific tendinitis. **subacromial b.,** see *calcific tendinitis,* under *tendinitis.* **subdeltoid b.,** see *calcific tendinitis,* under *tendinitis.* **superficial calcaneal b.,** achillobursitis. **Thornwaldt's b., Tornwaldt's b.,** chronic inflammation of the pharyngeal bursa, attended with formation of a pus-containing cyst, and nasopharyngeal stenosis; called also *pharyngeal b.,* and *Tornwaldt's disease.*

bursolith (ber'so-lith) [*bursa* + Gr. *lithos* stone] a calculus or concretion in a bursa.

bursopathy (ber-sop'ah-the) [*bursa* + Gr. *pathos* disease] any disease of a bursa.

bursotomy (ber-sot'o-me) [*bursa* + Gr. *tomē* a cutting] incision of a bursa.

burst (berst) a sudden, intense increase or outbreak. **respiratory b.,** a sharply increased consumption of oxygen and production of superoxides and peroxide occurring in actively phagocytizing leukocytes.

bursula (ber'su-lah) [L.] a small bag or pouch.

Burton's line (sign) (ber'tunz) [Henry *Burton,* British physician, 1799–1849] see *lead line,* under *line.*

Bury's disease [Judson Sykes *Bury,* English physician, 1852–1944] erythema elevatum diutinum.

Buscaino's test (reaction) (bus-ki'nōz) [Vito Maria *Buscaino,* Italian neurologist, born 1887] see under *tests.*

Buschke's disease, scleredema (boōsh'kez) [Abraham *Buschke,* German dermatologist, 1868–1943] see *cryptococcosis* and *scleredema.*

Buschke-Löwenstein's tumor (boōsh'kēz-la'ven-stīnz) [Abraham *Buschke;* Ludwig W. *Löwenstein*] see under *tumor.*

bushmaster (bush'mas-ter) a large venomous pit viper, *Lachesis muta,* of the Amazon region of South America. See table accompanying *snake.*

buspirone hydrochloride (bu-spi'rōn) chemical name: 8-[4-[4-(2-pyrimidinyl)-1-piperazinyl]butyl]-8-azaspiro[4,5]decane-7,9-dione; a tranquilizer, $C_{21}H_{31}N_5O_2 \cdot HCl$.

Busquet's disease (boōs-kāz') [P. *Busquet,* French physician] see under *disease.*

Busse-Buschke disease [Otto *Busse,* German physician, 1867–1922; Abraham *Buschke,* German dermatologist, 1868–1943] cryptococcosis.

busulfan (bu-sul'fan) [USP] chemical name: 1,4-butanediol dimethanesulfonate. An alkylating agent, $C_6H_{14}O_6S_2$, occurring as a white, crystalline powder; used as an antineoplastic, chiefly in the treatment of granulocytic (myelocytic) leukemia, administered orally.

But. abbreviation for L. *bu'tyrum,* butter.

butabarbital sodium (bu-tah-bar'bĭ-tal) [USP] chemical name: 5-ethyl-5-(1-methylpropyl)-2,4-6(1*H*,3*H*,5*H*)pyrimidinetrione monosodium salt. A barbituric acid derivative, $C_{10}H_{15}N_2NaO_3$, occurring as a white powder; used as a sedative and hypnotic, administered orally.

butacaine sulfate (bu''tah-kān' sul'fāt) [USP] chemical name: 3-(dibutylamino)-1-propanol 4-aminobenzoate sulfate. A local anesthetic, $(C_{18}H_{30}N_2O_2)_2 \cdot H_2SO_4$, occurring as a white to practically white, crystalline powder; used to produce topical anesthesia in the eye or in the mouth.

butaclamol hydrochloride (bu''tah-kla'mōl) chemical name: (+)-3α-(1,1-dimethylethyl)-2,3,4,4aα,8,9,13bβ,14-octahydro-1*H*-benzo[6,7]cyclohepta[1,2,3-de]pyrido[2,1-*a*]isoquinolin hydrochloride; a tranquilizer, $C_{25}H_{31}NO \cdot HCl$.

butadiazamide (bu''tah-di-az'ah-mīd) chemical name: *N*-(5-butyl-1,3,4-thiadiazol-2-yl)-*p*-chlorobenzenesulfonamide; a hypoglycemic agent, $C_{12}H_{14}ClN_3O_2S_2$.

butalbital (bu-tal'bĭ-tal) [USP] chemical name: 5-(2-methylpropyl)-5-(2-propenyl)-2,4,6(1*H*,3*H*,5*H*)-pyrimidinetrione. An intermediate-acting barbiturate, occurring as a white, crystalline powder, $C_{11}H_{16}N_2O_3$; administered orally.

butallylonal (bu-tah-lil'o-nal) chemical name: 5-(2-bromo-2-propenyl)-5-(1-methylpropyl)-2,4,6(1*H*,3*H*,5*H*) pyrimidinetrione. An intermediate-acting barbiturate, $C_{11}H_{15}BrN_2O_3$, used as a hypnotic.

butamben (bu-tam'ben) [USP] chemical name: 4-aminobenzoic acid butyl ester. A local anesthetic, $C_{11}H_{15}NO_2$, occurring as a white, crystalline powder; applied topically in the treatment of painful skin conditions and pain associated with hemorrhoids or anal fissure. Called also *butyl aminobenzoate.*

butamirate citrate (bu''tah-mi'rāt) chemical name: α-ethyl-2-[2-(diethylamino)ethoxy]ethyl ester benzeneacetic acid 2-hydroxy-1,2,3-propanetricarboxylate (1:1); an antitussive, $C_{18}H_{29}NO_3 \cdot C_6H_8O_7$.

butamisole hydrochloride (bu-tam'ĭ-sōl) chemical name: (−)-2-methyl-*N*-[3-(2,3,5,6-tetrahydroimidazo[2,1-*b*]thiazol-6-yl)-

phenyl]propanamide monohydrochloride; a veterinary anthelmintic, $C_{15}H_{19}N_3OS \cdot HCl$.

butamoxane hydrochloride (bu-tah-moks'an) chemical name: N-butyl-1,4-benzodioxan-2-methylamine hydrochloride; a tranquilizer, $C_{13}H_{19}NO_2 \cdot HCl$.

butane (bu'tān) n-butane; an aliphatic hydrocarbon of the methane series, C_4H_{10}, from petroleum, occurring as a colorless flammable gas with a characteristic odor. **normal b.,** CH_3—$(CH_2)_2CH_3$.

butaperazine (bu-tah-per'ah-zēn) chemical name: 1-[10-[3-(4-methyl-1-piperazinyl)propyl]10H-phenothiazin-2-yl]-1-butanone. A phenothiazide derivative, $C_{24}H_{31}N_3OS$, used as an antipsychotic drug in the treatment of acute and chronic schizophrenia; administered orally. **b. maleate,** the maleate ester of butaperazine, $C_{24}H_{31}N_3OS \cdot 2C_4H_4O_4$, having the same actions and uses as the base.

Butazolidin (bu″tah-zol'ĭ-din) trademark for preparations of phenylbutazone.

Butcher's saw (booch'erz) [Richard George Herbert *Butcher*, Irish surgeon, 1819–1891] see under *saw*.

Butesin (bu-te'sin) trademark for a preparation of butyl aminobenzoate.

butethal (bu'tĕ-thal) chemical name: 5-butyl-5-ethyl-2,4,6-(1H,3H,5H)pyrimidinetrione. An intermediate-acting barbiturate, $C_{10}H_{16}N_2O_3$, used as a sedative; administered orally.

butethamine hydrochloride (bu-teth'ah-mēn) chemical name: 2-[(2-methylpropyl)amino]ethanol 4-aminobenzoate (ester) hydrochloride. A local anesthetic, $C_{13}H_{20}N_2O_2 \cdot HCl$, occurring as small, white crystals or white, crystalline powder; used for nerve block anesthesia in dentistry.

Buthus (bu'thus) a genus of scorpions. **B. carolinia'nus,** a species occurring in the southern United States. **B. quinquestria'tus,** a dangerous species occurring in Egypt.

butirosin sulfate (bu-tēr'o-sin) an aminoglycoside antibiotic complex, $C_{21}H_{41}N_5O_{12} \cdot 2H_2SO_4 \cdot 2H_2O$, obtained from certain strains of *Bacillus circulans*, consisting of butirosins A and B; an antibacterial.

Butisol sodium (bu'tĭ-sol) trademark for preparations of sodium butabarbital.

butonate (bu'to-nāt) chemical name: butanoic acid 2,2,2-trichloro-1-(dimethoxyphosphinyl)ethyl ester; an insecticide and anthelminthic that is a potent cholinesterase inhibitor, $C_8H_{14}Cl_3O_5P$.

butoprozine hydrochloride (bu″to-pro'zēn) chemical name: [4-[3-(dibutylamino)propoxy]phenyl](2-ethyl-3-indolizinyl)methanone monohydrochloride; an antiarrhythmic cardiac depressant and antianginal, $C_{28}H_{38}N_2O_2 \cdot HCl$.

butopyronoxyl (bu″to-pi″ro-nok'sil) chemical name: 3,4-dihydro-2,2-dimethyl-4-oxo-2H-pyran carboxylic acid butyl ester. An insect repellent effective against ticks, $C_{12}H_{18}O_4$, occurring as a yellow to pale reddish brown liquid.

butorphanol (bu-tor'fah-nōl) chemical name: 17-(cyclobutyl-methyl)morphinan-3,14-diol; a synthetic opioid, $C_{21}H_{29}NO_2$, having analgesic and antitussive properties. **b. tartrate,** the tartrate salt of butorphanol, $C_{21}H_{29}NO_2 \cdot C_4H_6O_6$, administered intramuscularly as an analgesic.

butoxamine hydrochloride (bu-toks'ah-mēn) chemical name: α-[1-[(1,1-dimethylethyl)amino]ethyl]-2,5-dimethoxybenzenemethanol. A beta-adrenergic blocking agent, $C_{15}H_{25}NO_3 \cdot HCl$.

butriptyline hydrochloride (bu-trip'tĭ-lēn) chemical name: (±)-10,11-dihydro-N,N,β-trimethyl-5H-dibenzo[a,d]cyclohep-tene-5-propylamine hydrochloride; an antidepressant, $C_{21}H_{27}N \cdot HCl$.

Bütschli's nuclear spindle (bitsh'lēz) [Otto *Bütschli*, German zoologist, 1848–1920] see *spindle*, def. 1.

Bütschlia (bitsh'le-ah) a genus of ciliates, species of which have been found in the stomachs of cattle.

butt (but) to bring the surfaces of two distinct objects squarely or directly into contact with each other.

butter (but'er) [L. *butyrum*; Gr. *boutyron*] the oily mass procured by churning cream. **b. of antimony,** antimony trichloride. **b. of arsenic,** arsenic trichloride. **cacoa b., cocoa b.,** [NF] the fat obtained from the roasted seed of *Theobroma cacao*; used as a suppository base, and has been used for its emollient properties in cosmetics and is sometimes used to soften and protect the skin. Called also *theobroma oil*. **b. of tin,** stannic chloride. **b. of zinc,** zinc chloride.

butterfly (but'er-fli) 1. a mass of absorbent cotton with wing-shaped appendages, used mainly in uterine surgery. 2. a form of doubly wing-shaped skin flaps. 3. a small piece of adhesive tape with broad, wing-shaped ends by means of which the edges of a superficial wound may be approximated. 4. a pattern formed by a skin eruption across the nose and adjacent areas of the cheeks, as in systemic lupus erythematosus, seborrheic dermatitis, and rosacea.

buttock (but'ok) one of the gluteal prominences; called also *clunis* or *breech* and, in the plural, *nates*.

button (but'n) 1. a knoblike elevation or structure. 2. a small appliance shaped like a spool or disk and used in surgery for the construction of intestinal anastomosis. **Aleppo b.,** cutaneous leishmaniasis. **Bagdad b., Biskra b.,** cutaneous leishmaniasis. **Boari b.,** a device analogous to the Murphy button for use in ureterocystostomy. **bromide b.,** a verrucous cutaneous lesion occurring as a result of sensitivity to bromides. **Chlumsky's b.,** a button for intestinal suture made of pure magnesium on the pattern of the Murphy button. **dog b.,** nux vomica. **iodide b.,** a verrucous cutaneous lesion occurring as a result of sensitivity to iodides. **Jaboulay b.,** a device for performing lateral intestinal anastomosis without the aid of sutures, consisting of two button-like cylinders of metal that are fitted together on the screw and key-ring principle through a small intestinal opening. **Lardennois's b.,** a modified form of Murphy button for intestinal anastomosis. **mescal b's,** transverse slices of the flowering heads of the Mexican dumpling cactus, *Lophophora williamsii* or mescal, whose major active principle is mescaline; used in divinatory and religious ceremonies by North American Indians. **Murphy's b.,** a device for joining the ends of a divided intestine so that union may take place. It consists of two short metal cylinders of different diameter, each having a collar at one end; the collars are sutured to the divided ends, and the narrower cylinder is locked into its mate. **oriental b.,** cutaneous leishmaniasis. **peritoneal b.,** a short flanged glass tube for insertion between the peritoneal cavity and a subcutaneous pocket through which peritoneal transudate may be drained. **quaker b.,** nux vomica. **terminal b's,** see *end-feet*. **Villard's b.,** a modified Murphy button.

buttonhole (but'n-hōl) a short straight incision into a cavity or organ; an abnormal narrowing of the caliber of a structure. **mitral b.,** an advanced state of stenosis of the mitral orifice of the heart, adhesion and shortening of the cusps having produced a narrow slit-like orifice.

butyl (bu'til) a hydrocarbon radical, C_4H_9 or $CH_3 \cdot CH_2 \cdot CH_2 \cdot CH_2$. **b. acetate,** a liquid compound, $C_6H_{12}O_2$, used in the manufacture of lacquer, artificial leather, photographic film, plastics, and safety glass; it is an irritant which may cause conjunctivitis, and is narcotic in high concentrations. **b. aminobenzoate** [NF], chemical name, n-butyl p-aminobenzoate. A white, odorless, tasteless crystalline powder, $C_{11}H_{15}NO_2$, soluble in dilute acids, alcohol, ether, and chloroform; used as a local anesthetic. Called also *butamben*. **b. chloride,** chemical name: 1-chlorobutane. A clear colorless volatile liquid, C_4H_9Cl, miscible with dehydrated alcohol and with ether; used as a veterinary anthelmintic. **b. formate,** an industrial solvent, $CH_3(CH_2)_3COOH$, the vapors of which are powerfully lacrimatory and suffocating. **b. hydride,** a hydrocarbon, C_4H_{10}, from petroleum; its vapor is an unsafe anesthetic.

butylene (bu'ti-lēn) a gaseous hydrocarbon, C_4H_8.

butylmercaptan (bu″til-mer-kap'tan) a thioalcohol, thiobutyl alcohol, $CH_3 \cdot CH_2 \cdot CH_2CH_2SH$, the active principle of the odoriferous secretion of the skunk.

butylparaben (bu-til-par'ah-ben) [NF] chemical name: 4-hydroxybenzoic acid butyl ester. An antifungal agent, $C_{11}H_{14}O_3$, occurring as small, colorless crystals or white powder, used as a pharmaceutic preservative.

Butyn (bu'tin) trademark for a preparation of butacaine sulfate.

butyr- (bu'tir) [L. *butyrum*; Gr. *boutyron* butter] a combining form denoting a relationship to butter.

butyraceous (bu″tĭ-ra'she-us) of a buttery consistency.

butyrase (bu'tĭ-rās) butyrinase.

butyrate (bu'tĭ-rāt) a salt of butyric acid.

Butyribacterium (bu-ti″re-bak-te're-um) [Gr. *boutyron* butter + *baktērion* little rod] a genus of microorganisms of the family Propionibacteriaceae, order Eubacteriales, made up of non-spore-forming, anaerobic or microaerophilic gram-positive bacilli, nonpathogenic but occurring as parasites in the intestinal tract.

butyric (bu-tir'ik) derived from butter, as butyric acid.

butyrin (bu'tĭ-rin) a triglyceride of butyric acid existing in butter, $C_3H_5(C_4H_7O_2)_3$, a liquid fat with an acrid, bitter taste; called also *tributyrin*.

butyrinase (bu'tĭ-rin-ās) an enzyme of the blood serum that is capable of catalyzing the hydrolysis of butyrin; called also *butyrase*.

butyrine (bu'tĭ-rin) an amino acid derivative of butyric acid; it is α-amino butyric acid.

butyroid (bu'tĭ-roid) [butyr- + Gr. *eidos* form] resembling or having the consistency of butter.

butyromel (bu-tir'o-mel) fresh, unsalted butter, 2 parts, and honey, 1 part: a substitute for cod liver oil.

butyrometer (bu″tĭ-rom'ĕ-ter) [butyr- + Gr. *metron* measure] an apparatus for estimating the proportion of butter fat in milk; called also *butyroscope*.

butyrophenone (bu″tĭ-ro-fe'nōn) a chemical class of major tranquilizers especially useful in the treatment of manic and moderate to severe agitated states and in the control of vocal utterances and tics of Gilles de la Tourette's syndrome.

butyroscope (bu-ti′ro-skōp) [butyr- + Gr. skopein to examine] butyrometer.

butyrous (bu′tĭ-rus) like butter; having a butter-like appearance.

bypass (bi′pas) an auxiliary flow; a shunt. **aortocoronary b.**, a section of saphenous vein or suitable substitute grafted between the aorta and a coronary artery distal to an obstructive lesion in the latter. Called also coronary artery b. **aortoiliac b.**, insertion of a vascular prosthesis from the abdominal aorta to the femoral artery to bypass intervening atherosclerotic segments. **aortorenal b.**, insertion of a section of saphenous vein, hypogastric artery, or suitable substitute between the aorta and renal artery to bypass occluded segments. **cardiopulmonary b.**, diversion of the flow of blood from the entrance of the right atrium directly to the aorta, usually via a pump oxygenator, avoiding both the heart and the lungs; a form of extracorporeal circulation used in heart surgery. **coronary b., coronary artery b.**, aortocoronary b. **femoropopliteal b.**, insertion of a vascular prosthesis from the femoral to the popliteal artery to bypass occluded segments. **gastric b.**, gastrojejunostomy in which the stomach is transected high on the body, the proximal remnant being joined to a loop of jejunum in end-to-side anastomosis. **intestinal b.**, resection of the intestine, with anastomosis of the proximal to the distal portion, as in jejunoileostomy. **jejunal b., jejunoileal b.**, surgical anastomosis of the proximal part of the jejunum to the distal part of the ileum so as to bypass much of the small intestine and reduce intestinal absorption. **left heart b.**, diversion of the flow of blood from the pulmonary veins directly to the aorta, avoiding the left atrium and the left ventricle. **partial b.**, the deviation of only a portion of blood flowing through an artery. **right heart b.**, diversion of the flow of blood from the entrance of the right atrium directly to the pulmonary arteries, avoiding the right atrium and right ventricle.

by-product (bi-prod′ukt) a secondary product obtained during the manufacture of a primary product.

byssaceous (bis-sa′she-us) [Gr. byssos flax] composed of fine flaxlike threads.

byssinosis (bis″ĭ-no′sis) [Gr. byssos flax + -osis] a pulmonary disease occurring among cotton textile workers and preparers of flax and soft hemp, due to inhalation of textile dust. The acute form is marked by tightness of the chest, wheezing, and cough on return to work after a brief absence (Monday dyspnea). The chronic form, occurring after years of exposure, is marked by permanent dyspnea. It is probably due to smooth muscle contraction resulting from histamine release induced by chemicals in the dust. Called also brown lung, cotton-dust or stripper's asthma, cotton-mill fever, and Monday fever.

byssinotic (bis″ĭ-not′ik) 1. pertaining to byssinosis. 2. one affected with byssinosis.

byssocausis (bis″o-kaw′sis) [Gr. byssos flax + kausis burning] moxibustion; counterirritation produced by igniting a cone or cylinder of moxa placed on the skin.

byssoid (bis′oid) [Gr. byssos flax + eidos form] made up of a fringe, the filaments of which are unequal in length.

byssophthisis (bis″o-thi′sis) [Gr. byssos flax + phthisis consumption] (obs.) byssinosis.

byssus (bis′us) [L.; Gr. byssos] lint, charpie, or cotton.

Bythnia (bith′ne-ah) Bithynia.

bythus (bith′us) [Gr. bythos depth] (obs.) the lower portion of the abdomen.

C

C 1. chemical symbol for carbon. 2. in the electrocardiogram, C stands for chest (precordial) lead, CR for chest and right arm, CL for chest and left arm, CF for chest and left leg; see precordial leads, under lead². 3. symbol for complement.

C. cathode (or cathodal); Celsius or centigrade; congius (gallon); closure; contraction; color sense; cylinder; cervical (in vertebral formulas); clonus; clearance (in kidney function tests).

c. contact; curie.

C′ former symbol for complement; replaced by C.

c′ symbol for coefficient of partage.

C$_{alb}$ albumin clearance; see clearance.

C$_{cr}$ creatinine clearance; see clearance.

C$_{in}$ inulin clearance; see clearance.

C$_{T-1824}$ clearance of Evans blue, or T–1824.

CA chronological age; Croup-associated (virus); cardiac arrest; coronary artery.

Ca 1. chemical symbol for calcium. 2. abbreviation for cathode, cathodal, cancer.

ca. abbreviation for L. circa about.

cabinet (kab′ĭ-net) a small closet, or place of enclosure. **Sauerbruch's c.** (obs.), a cabinet within which the air pressure can be increased or diminished; formerly used in operations on the chest, the patient's head being outside the cabinet, and his body and the surgeon within it.

Cabot's ring bodies (kab′ots) [Richard Clarke Cabot, Boston physician, 1868–1939] see under body.

Cabot's splint (kab′ots) [Arthur Tracy Cabot, Boston surgeon, 1852–1912] see under splint.

cabufocon A (kab″u-fo′kon) chemical name: cellulose acetate butanoate; a contact lens material (hydrophobic).

cac- see caco-.

cacaerometer (kak″a-er-om′ĕ-ter) [cac- + Gr. aēr air + metron measure] an instrument for measuring the impurity of air.

cacanthrax (kak-an′thraks) anthrax.

cacao (kah-ka′o) 1. cocoa. 2. Theobroma cacao. 3. the seeds of T. cacao.

cacation (kak-a′shun) defecation.

cacatory (kak′ah-to″re) marked by severe diarrhea.

cacergasia (kak″er-gas′e-ah) [cac- + Gr. ergon work] (obs.) poor functioning, either bodily or mental.

cacesthenic (kak″es-then′ik) having defective sense organs.

cacesthesia (kak″es-the′ze-ah) [cac- + Gr. aisthēsis perception] any morbid sensation or any disorder of sensibility.

cachectic (kah-kek′tik) pertaining to or characterized by cachexia.

cachet (kah-sha′) [Fr.] a disk-shaped wafer or capsule for enclosing a dose of medicine.

cachexia (kah-kek′se-ah) [cac- + Gr. hexis habit + -ia] a profound and marked state of constitutional disorder; general ill health and malnutrition. **cancerous c.**, the weak, emaciated condition seen in cases of malignant tumor. **c. exophthal′mica**, Graves' disease. **fluoric c.**, that seen in fluorosis. **hypophyseal c.**, see panhypopituitarism. **c. hypophysiopri′va**, the train of symptoms resulting from total deprivation of function of the pituitary gland, including loss of sexual function, bradycardia, hypothermia, apathy, and coma. **lymphatic c.**, pseudoleukemia. **malarial c.**, a group of physical signs of a chronic nature that result from antecedent attacks of severe malaria; the principal signs are anemia, sallow skin, yellow sclera, splenomegaly, hepatomegaly, and, in children, retardation of body growth and puberty. **c. mercuria′lis**, that seen in chronic mercurial poisoning. **pachydermic c.**, myxedema. **pituitary c.**, see panhypopituitarism. **saturnine c.**, that seen in chronic lead poisoning. **c. strumipri′va**, myxedema resulting from deprivation of the function of the thyroid gland by surgery or irradiation; called also c. thyreoidectomica and c. thyreopriva. **c. suprarena′lis**, Addison's disease. **c. thymopri′va**, cachexia due to loss of the thymus gland. **c. thyreoidectom′ica, c. thyreopri′va**, c. strumipriva. **thyroid c.**, Graves' disease. **tropical c.**, a general condition of ill health affecting residents in the tropics, frequently associated with disease of the liver or spleen. **uremic c.**, cachexia associated with other systemic symptoms of advanced renal failure. **verminous c.** (obs.), the condition of anemia and debility which accompanies infection with worms, especially Ancylostoma.

cachexy (kah-kek′se) cachexia.

cachinnation (kak″ĭ-na′shun) [L. cachinnare to laugh aloud] excessive, hysterical laughter.

CaCl$_2$ calcium chloride.

CaCl(OCl) chlorinated lime.

CaCO$_3$ calcium carbonate.

CaC$_2$O$_4$ calcium oxalate.

caco-, cac- [Gr. kakos bad] a combining form meaning bad, or ill.

cacodemonomania (kak″o-de″mon-o-ma′ne-ah) a condition marked by delusions of being possessed by evil spirits.

cacodontia (kak″o-don′she-ah) [cac- + Gr. odous tooth] an obsolete term for unsound teeth.

cacodyl (kak′o-dil) [caco- + Gr. ozein to smell + hylē matter] tetramethylbiarsine, a colorless liquid, (CH$_3$)$_2$As—As(CH$_3$)$_2$, with an offensive odor; it gives off a poisonous vapor and is inflammable when exposed to air. **c. cyanide**, a white powder, (CH$_3$)$_2$As-CN, which, when exposed to the air, gives off an extremely poisonous vapor. **c. hydride**, a colorless liquid, (CH$_3$)$_2$AsH, with a strong, garlicky odor; on exposure to air, it gives off a poisonous vapor and ignites spontaneously. Symptoms of poisoning are the same as those of arsenic poisoning.

cacodylate (kak′o-dil-āt) a salt of cacodylic acid; the cacodylates were once used in skin diseases, tuberculosis, malaria, and other conditions.

cacoethes (kak″o-e′thēz) [Gr. *kakoēthēs* an ill habit or itch for doing a thing] (*obs.*) a bad habit.

cacoethic (kak″o-e′thik) ill-conditioned; malignant.

cacogenesis (kak″o-jen′ĕ-sis) [*caco-* + Gr. *genesis* production] defective development.

cacogenic (kak″o-jen′ik) 1. having a tendency toward racial deterioration through bad sexual selection. 2. pertaining to cacogenesis.

cacogenics (kak″o-jen′iks) [*caco-* + Gr. *gennan* to generate] deterioration of the physical and moral properties of a race resulting from the mating and propagation of inferior individuals.

cacogeusia (kak″o-ju′se-ah) [*caco-* + Gr. *geusis* taste] a bad taste; it may be a complaint in idiopathic epilepsy (uncinate fit) and of patients receiving neuroleptic agents or lithium, and a somatic delusion in psychoses.

cacomelia (kak″o-me′le-ah) [*caco-* + Gr. *melos* limb] congenital deformity of a limb.

cacomorphosis (kak″o-mor-fo′sis) [*caco-* + Gr. *morphē* form] malformation.

cacoplastic (kak″o-plas′tik) [*caco-* + Gr. *plastikos* forming] susceptible of only an imperfect formation.

cacorhythmic (kak″o-rith′mik) [*caco-* + Gr. *rhythmos* rhythm] marked by irregularity of rhythm.

cacosmia (kak-oz′me-ah) [*caco-* + Gr. *osmē* smell] a bad odor; stench.

cacostomia (kak″o-sto′me-ah) [*caco-* + Gr. *stoma* mouth] (*obs.*) a foul or gangrenous state of the mouth.

cacothenic (kak″o-then′ik) pertaining to cacothenics.

cacothenics (kak″o-then′iks) [Gr. *kakothēneein* to be in a bad state] deterioration of a race resulting from deleterious influences in the environment.

cacothymia (kak″o-thi′me-ah) a morbid condition caused by derangement of the thymus gland.

cacotrophy (kak-ot′ro-fe) [*caco-* + Gr. *trophē* nourishment] malnutrition; impaired or disordered nourishment.

cactinomycin (kak″tin-o-mi′sin) a highly toxic antibiotic of the actinomycin group, actinomycin C, produced by *Streptomyces chrysomallus*, consisting of a mixture of actinomycins C_2 and C_3 and dactinomycin (actinomycin D); formerly used as an antineoplastic.

cacumen (kak-u′men), pl. *cacu′mina* [L. "summit"] (*obs.*) 1. the top or apex of an organ. 2. the top and uppermost branchlets of a plant. 3. culmen.

cacuminal (kak-u′mĭ-nal) pertaining to the cacumen.

cadaver (kah-dav′er) [L., from *cadere*, to fall, to perish] a dead body; generally applied to a human body preserved for anatomical study.

cadaveric (kah-dav′er-ik) of or pertaining to a cadaver.

cadaverine (kah-dav′er-in) [L. *cadaver* corpse] a nitrogenous base, pentamethylenediamine, $NH_2 \cdot CH_2(CH_2)_3CH_2 \cdot NH_2$, produced by decarboxylation of lysine. It is sometimes one of the products of *Vibrio proteus* and of *Vibrio cholerae* and occasionally occurs in the urine in cystinuria.

cadaverous (kah-dav′er-us) resembling a cadaver.

caddis (kad′is) see under *fly*.

caderas (kad-e′ras) mal de caderas.

cadmiosis (kad″me-o′sis) pneumoconiosis due to inhalation of and tissue reaction to cadmium dust.

cadmium (kad′me-um) [Gr. *kadmia* earth] a bivalent metal, not unlike tin in appearance and properties; symbol, Cd; atomic number, 48; atomic weight, 112.40. Its salts are poisonous. **c. anthranilate,** a salt of anthranilic acid (o-aminobenzoic acid) used as an ascaricide in swine. **c. bromide,** a poisonous substance, $CdBr_2$, used in photography, process engraving, and lithography; when swallowed it causes increased salivation, choking, abdominal pain, diarrhea, and tenesmus. **c. iodide,** a compound, CdI_2, formerly used as a nematocide. **c. oleate,** a preparation formerly used in various skin diseases. **c. salicylate,** a salt, $(C_6H_4(OH)CO_2)_2Cd + H_2O$, in fine, white, tabular crystals, or in an amorphous powder, formerly used as an antiseptic. **c. sulfate,** a salt, $CdSO_4$, weak solutions of which were formerly used as astringents in eye, ear, and urethral inflammations. **c. sulfide,** a light yellow or orange powder, CdS, used in 1 per cent suspension in treatment of seborrheic dermatitis of the scalp.

caduca (kah-du′kah) the decidua (membranae deciduae [NA]).

caduceus (kah-du′se-us) the wand of Hermes or Mercury, the messenger of the gods. Used as a medical symbol and as the emblem of the Medical Corps, U.S. Army. The official symbol of the medical profession is the staff of Æsculapius.

caducous (kah-du′kus) [L. *cadere* to fall] falling off; deciduous.

cae- for words beginning thus, see also those beginning *ce-*.

caecitas (ses′ĭ-tas) [L.] blindness.

caecum (se′kum) [L.] cecum.

caecus (se′kus) [L.] a blind pouch. **c. mi′nor ventric′uli,** the cardiac part of the stomach (pars cardiaca ventriculi [NA]).

Caelius Aurelianus (se′le-us aw-re″le-a′nus) (5th century A.D.) an outstanding physician and medical writer, whose most famous work, *De morbis acutis et chronicis,* although clearly influenced by Soranus, contains much fresh material and "conforms to the modern standard of what a medical work should be" (Major).

caelotherapy (se″lo-ther′ah-pe) [L. *caelum* heaven + *therapy*] the use of religion and religious symbols for therapeutic purposes.

caeno- see *ceno-*.

caesarean (se-za′re-an) see *cesarean section,* under *section.*

caesium (se′ze-um) cesium.

CaF₂ calcium fluoride.

cafard (kah-far′) [Fr.] a severe form of mental depression.

caffea (kaf′e-ah) [L.] coffee.

caffeine (kaf-fēn′, kaf′fe-in) [L. *caffeina*] [USP] chemical name: 1,3,7-trimethyl-3,7-dihydro-1*H*-purine-2,6-dione. An odorless, bitter, white powder, $C_8H_{10}N_4O_2$, one of the xanthines (q.v.), soluble in water and alcohol, and obtainable from coffee, tea, guarana, and maté. Caffeine stimulates the central nervous system, mainly affecting the cerebrum; has a diuretic effect on the kidneys; stimulates striated muscle; has a group of effects on the cardiovascular system. It is used as a central and respiratory stimulant and for the relief of headache; administered orally. A combination of caffeine and sodium benzoate in water for injection is administered parenterally. Called also *guaranine* and *methyltheobromine.* See also *caffeinism.* **c. borocitrate,** a white soluble powder having sedative and antiseptic effects; no longer used in medicine. **c. chloral,** a soluble crystalline combination of caffeine and chloral, $C_8H_{10}N_4O_2$—CCl_3COH, formerly used as an analgesic. **c. citrate, citrated c.,** a preparation of equal parts of caffeine and citric acid, used for the same purposes as caffeine; administered orally. **c. hydrobromide,** colorless, efflorescent crystals, formerly used as a diuretic. **c. nitrate,** a salt in yellowish, needle-like crystals. **c. phthalate,** a sedative and antiseptic; no longer used in medicine. **c. and sodium benzoate,** see *caffeine.* **c. triiodide,** a compound in dark-green prisms, $(C_8H_{10}N_4O_2I_2 \cdot HI)_2 + 3H_2O$, formerly used as an iodine substitute. **c. valerianate,** a former remedy for whooping cough and hysteric vomiting.

caffeinism (kaf′en-izm, kaf′e-in-izm″) a morbid condition resulting from ingestion of excessive amounts of caffeine. The manifestations include insomnia, restlessness, excitement, tachycardia, tremors, and diuresis.

Caffey's disease (kaf′fēz) [John *Caffey,* American pediatrician, 1895–1966] infantile cortical hyperostosis.

cage (kāj) a box or enclosure. **population c.,** an enclosure in which populations of *Drosophilia* can be isolated through many generations. **thoracic c.,** the bony structure enclosing the thorax, consisting of the ribs, vertebral column, and sternum.

CaH₂O₂ calcium hydroxide.

Cain complex (cān) see under *complex.*

caino- see *ceno-*.

Cajal's cells, interstitial nucleus, stain (ka-halz′) [Santiago Ramón y *Cajal,* Spanish histologist, 1852–1934; co-winner, with Camillo Golgi, of the Nobel prize in medicine for 1906] see under *cell,* see *nucleus interstitialis,* under *nucleus,* and see *Table of Stains.*

cajeputol (kaj′e-pu-tol) eucalyptol.

Cal. large calorie.

cal. small calorie.

calage (kah-lahzh′) [Fr.] propping with pillows to immobilize the viscera and thus relieve seasickness.

calamine (kal′ah-mīn) [USP] a mild astringent and protectant, consisting of zinc oxide with a small proportion of ferric oxide, and occurring as a fine, pink powder; applied topically in the treatment of skin diseases.

calamus (kal′ah-mus) [L.] 1. a reedlike structure. 2. the plant *Acorus calamus* L. (Araceae), and its aromatic rhizome; it is used as a flavoring agent and insect repellent, and was formerly used as a carminative and vermifuge. **c. scripto′rius,** the lowest portion of the floor of the fourth ventricle, shaped like a pen and situated between the restiform bodies.

calcaneal (kal-ka′ne-al) pertaining to the calcaneus.

calcanean (kal-ka′ne-an) calcaneal.

calcaneitis (kal-ka″ne-i′tis) inflammation of the calcaneus.

calcaneoapophysitis (kal-ka′ne-o-ah-pof″ĕ-zi′tis) an affection of the posterior part of the calcaneus marked by pain at the point of insertion of the Achilles tendon, with swelling of the soft parts.

calcaneoastragaloid (kal-ka″ne-o-ah-strag′ah-loid) pertaining to the calcaneus and astragalus.

calcaneocavus (kal-ka″ne-o-ka′vus) clubfoot in which talipes calcaneus is combined with talipes cavus.

calcaneocuboid (kal-ka″ne-o-ku′boid) pertaining to the calcaneus and cuboid bone.

calcaneodynia (kal-ka″ne-o-din′e-ah) pain in the heel, or calcaneus.

calcaneofibular (kal-ka″ne-o-fib′u-lar) pertaining to the calcaneus and the fibula.

calcaneonavicular (kal-ka″ne-o-nah-vik′u-lar) pertaining to the calcaneus and navicular bone.

calcaneoplantar (kal-ka″ne-o-plan′tar) pertaining to the calcaneus and the sole of the foot.

calcaneoscaphoid (kal-ka″ne-o-ska′foid) calcaneonavicular.

calcaneotibial (kal-ka″ne-o-tib′e-al) pertaining to the calcaneus and the tibia.

calcaneovalgocavus (kal-ka″ne-o-val″go-ka′vus) clubfoot in which talipes calcaneus, talipes valgus, and talipes cavus are combined.

calcaneum (kal-ka′ne-um), pl. *calca′nea* [L.] calcaneus.

calcaneus (kal-ka′ne-us), pl. *calca′nei* [L.] 1. [NA] the irregular quadrangular bone at the back of the tarsus; called also *calcaneal bone, calcaneum, heel bone, os calcis,* and *os tarsi fibulare.* 2. *talipes calcaneus.*

calcanodynia (kal″kah-no-din′e-ah) calcaneodynia.

calcar (kal′kar) [L. "spur"] a spur, or a structure resembling a spur. **c. a′vis** [NA], the lower of two medial elevations in the posterior horn of the lateral cerebral ventricle, produced by the lateral extension of the calcarine sulcus. **c. femora′le,** the plate of strong tissue which strengthens the neck of the femur. **c. pe′dis,** the heel.

calcarea (kal-ka′re-ah) [L.] calcium oxide or hydroxide. **c. chlora′ta,** chlorinated lime, a disinfectant and bleaching agent. **c. hy′drica,** a solution of calcium hydroxide; liquor calcis, or lime water. **c. phosphor′ica,** precipitated calcium phosphate. **c. us′ta,** quicklime or caustic lime; calcium oxide or unslaked lime.

calcareous (kal-ka′re-us) [L. *calcarius*] pertaining to or containing lime or calcium; chalky.

calcarine (kal′kar-in) [L. *calcarinus* spur-shaped] 1. spur-shaped. 2. pertaining to the calcar.

calcariuria (kal-ka″re-u′re-ah) [L *calcarius* containing lime + Gr. *ouron* urine + *-ia*] the presence of lime salts in the urine.

calcaroid (kal′kar-oid) resembling calcium; a term given to certain deposits in cerebral tissue which resemble calcification but do not give a specific reaction for calcium.

calcemia (kal-se′me-ah) [*calcium* + Gr. *haima* blood + *-ia*] hypercalcemia.

calcibilia (kal″sĭ-bil′e-ah) the presence of calcium in the bile.

calcic (kal′sik) of or pertaining to lime or to calcium.

calcicosilicosis (kal″sĭ-ko-sil″ĭ-ko′sis) a variety of pneumoconiosis due to the inhalation of mineral dust containing silica and lime.

calcicosis (kal″sĭ-ko′sis) [L. *calx* lime] a morbid condition of the lung resulting from the inhalation of marble dust.

calcidiol (kal″sĭ-di′ol) 25-hydroxycholecalciferol.

calcifames (kal-sif′ah-mēz) calcium hunger; see under *hunger.*

calcifediol (kal″sif-ĕ-di′ōl) 25-hydroxycholecalciferol.

calciferol (kal-sif′er-ol) 1. see *vitamin D,* under *vitamin.* 2. ergocalciferol.

calcific (kal-sif′ik) forming lime.

calcification (kal″sĭ-fĭ-ka′shun) [*calcium* + L. *facere* to make] the process by which organic tissue becomes hardened by a deposit of calcium salts within its substance. **dystrophic c.,** the deposition of calcium in abnormal tissue, such as scar tissue or atherosclerotic plaques, but without abnormalities of blood calcium. **metastatic c.,** the deposition of calcium in tissues as a result of abnormalities in calcium and phosphate levels in the blood and tissue fluids. **Mönckeberg's c.,** see under *arteriosclerosis.*

calcigerous (kal-sij′er-us) [*calcium* + L. *gerere* to bear] producing or carrying calcium salts.

Calcimar (kal′sĭ-mar) trademark for a preparation of salmon calcitonin, available for clinical use.

calcimeter (kal-sim′ĕ-ter) [*calcium* + Gr. *metron* measure] an instrument for estimating the amount of calcium present, as in the blood.

calcination (kal″sĭ-na′shun) [L. *calcinare* to char] the process of reducing to a dry powder by heat.

calcine (kal′sin) to reduce to a dry powder by heat.

calcinosis (kal″sĭ-no′sis) a condition marked by the deposition of calcium salts in various tissues of the body; called also *exudative calcifying fasciitis* and *calcium gout.* **c. circumscrip′ta,** localized deposition of calcium in small nodules in subcutaneous tissues or muscle, usually in systemic scleroderma or dermatomyositis. **c. cu′tis,** a condition marked by deposits of calcium salts in the skin in the form of nodules or plaques. **c. interstitia′lis,** a disorder of calcium metabolism marked by abnormal deposits of calcium in the connective tissues. **c. intervertebra′lis,**

deposit of calcium in one or more intervertebral disks; called also *chondritis intervertebralis calcanea* and *Verse's disease.* **tumoral c.,** development of large periarticular masses about the shoulder, elbow, and hip, marked by symptoms such as sciatica due to pressure on adjacent nerves. It is of unknown etiology, with onset usually in the first or second decade of life. **c. universa′lis,** widespread deposition of calcium salts in the dermis, panniculus, and muscles, in the form of nodules or plaques, most often in children, principally girls, with dermatomyositis.

calciokinesis (kal″se-o-ki-ne′sis) mobilization of calcium stored in the body.

calciokinetic (kal″se-o-ki-net′ik) pertaining to or causing calciokinesis.

calciorrhachia (kal″se-o-ra′ke-ah) [*calcium* + Gr. *rhachis* spine + *-ia*] the presence of calcium in the spinal fluid.

calciotropism (kal″se-ot′ro-pizm) an exaggerated reaction of cells to the administration of calcium.

calcipectic (kal″sĭ-pek′tik) pertaining to, characterized by, or causing calcipexy.

calcipenia (kal″sĭ-pe′ne-ah) [*calcium* + Gr. *penia* poverty] deficiency of calcium.

calcipenic (kal″sĭ-pe′nik) pertaining to or characterized by calcipenia.

calcipexic (kal″sĭ-pek′sik) calcipectic.

calcipexis (kal″sĭ-pek′sis) calcipexy.

calcipexy (kal′sĭ-pek″se) [*calcium* + Gr. *pēxis* fixation] fixation of calcium in the tissues of the organism.

calciphilia (kal″sĭ-fil′e-ah) [*calcium* + Gr. *philein* to love] a tendency to absorb lime salts from the blood and thus to become calcified.

calciphylactic (kal″sĭ-fi-lak′tik) pertaining to or characterized by calciphylaxis.

calciphylaxis (kal″sĭ-fi-lak′sis) the formation of calcified tissue in response to administration of a challenging agent subsequent to induction of a hypersensitive state. **systemic c.,** the generalized appearance of calcifications in internal organs or tissues, occurring in response to intravenous or intraperitoneal injection of the challenging agent. **topical s.,** the formation of a circumscribed area of calcification in response to subcutaneous injection of the challenging agent.

calciprivia (kal″sĭ-priv′e-ah) [*calcium* + L. *privus* without + *-ia*] deprivation or loss of calcium.

calciprivic (kal″sĭ-priv′ik) pertaining to or characterized by calciprivia.

calcipyelitis (kal″sĭ-pi-ĕ-li′tis) calculous pyelitis.

calcitonin (kal″sĭ-to′nin) a polypeptide hormone elaborated by the parafollicular cells of the thyroid gland in response to hypercalcemia; it lowers plasma calcium and phosphate levels, inhibits bone resorption, and serves as an antagonist to parathyroid hormone. It is secreted in lower vertebrates by the ultimobranchial glands. It is used in the treatment of severe hypercalcemia and Paget's disease of bone. Called also *thyrocalcitonin.*

calcitriol (kal″sĭ-tri′ol) 1,25-dihydroxycholecalciferol.

calcium (kal′se-um), gen. *cal′cii* [L. *calx* lime] a silvery yellow metal, the basic element of lime. Symbol, Ca; atomic number, 20; atomic weight, 40.08. It is found in nearly all organized tissues, being the most abundant mineral in the body. In combination with phosphorus it forms calcium phosphate, the dense, hard material of the teeth and bones. It is an essential dietary element, a constant blood calcium level being essential for the maintenance of the normal heartbeat, and for the normal functioning of nerves and muscles. It also plays a role in multiple phases of blood coagulation (in which it is called *coagulation factor IV*) and in many enzymatic processes. **c. acetate,** a resolvent, $Ca(C_2H_3O_2)_2$. **c. benzamidosalicylate,** benzoylpas calcium. **c. benzoate,** a compound, $Ca(C_6H_5CO_2)_2 + 3H_2O$, formerly used in nephritis. **c. bromide,** an odorless white deliquescent granular salt, $CaBr_2$, formerly used as a sedative and anticonvulsant. **c. carbide,** grayish black lumps or crystals, CaC_2, which yields acetylene on decomposition by water. **c. carbimide,** 1. c. cyanamide. 2. c. carbimide, citrated. **c. carbimide, citrated,** a mixture containing calcium cyanamide and citric acid; an antialcoholic. See also *c. cyanamide.* **c. carbonate,** a compound, $CaCO_3$, occurring naturally in bones, shells, etc. It is used chiefly as an antacid in its native form, in a prepared form (see *prepared chalk,* under *chalk*), and in a precipitated form (see *c. carbonate, precipitated*). **c. carbonate, precipitated** [USP], an odorless, tasteless, fine white crystalline powder, $CaCO_3$, used as an antacid; called also *precipitated chalk.* **c. caseinate,** a nutrient preparation of casein and calcium. **c. chloride** [USP], a salt, $CaCl_2 \cdot 2H_2O$, occurring as white, hard fragments or granules. It is used as a calcium replenisher, administered intravenously, and has been used as an acid-producing diuretic and urinary acidifier and to control bleeding in such conditions as purpura, intestinal bleeding, and small multiple hemorrhages. It is also a specific antidote for magnesium poisoning, administered intravenously. **c. creosotate,** a mixture of the calcium constituents of creosote, formerly used as a disinfectant and antiseptic. **c. cyanamide,** a compound, $CaCN_2$, obtained by the interaction of nitrogen and calcium carbide in an electric furnace, which inhibits one or more of the enzymes required for oxidation of acetaldehyde formed from alcohol; used as a fertilizer, defoliant, herbicide, pesticide, and anthelmintic for swine. Because the drinking of alcohol after inhalation or ingestion of calcium cyanamide produces very unpleasant symptoms (see *mal rouge*) it has been considered as a basis for treating alcholism; a mixture of calcium cyanamide and citric acid (*citrated c. carbamide*) has been used for this purpose. Called also *c. carbimide* and, sometimes, *cyanamide*. **c. cyclamate,** cyclamate calcium. **c. disodium edathamil, c. disodium edetate,** edetate calcium disodium. **c. Disodium Versenate,** trademark for edetate calcium disodium. **c. EDTA,** edetate calcium disodium. **c. fluoride,** a compound, CaF_2, occurring in the bones and teeth. **c. glubionate,** chemical name: (4-O-β-D-galactopyranosyl-D-gluconato-O^1) (D-gluconato-O^1)calcium monohydrate. A calcium replenisher, $C_{18}H_{32}CaO_{19}H_2O$, administered orally. **c. gluconate,** a calcium salt of gluconic acid, $C_{12}H_{22}CaO_{14}$, occurring as odorless, tasteless, white crystalline granules or powder. It is used as a calcium replenisher, administered intravenously or orally, and has been used to decrease capillary permeability in various conditions. It is an oral antidote for fluoride or oxalic acid poisoning. **c. glycerophosphate,** the calcium salt of glycerophosphoric acid, $C_3H_7CaO_6P$; it has been used as a calcium and phosphorus dietary supplement and as a pharmaceutic necessity. **c. hydroxide** [USP], a salt, $Ca(OH)_2$, occurring as a white powder; used in solution as a topical astringent. **c. hypophosphite,** an odorless bitter compound, $Ca(PH_2O_2)_2$, occurring in colorless, transparent, monoclinic prisms, as small lustrous scales, or as a white crystalline powder; formerly used in conditions of impaired nutrition or vigor. **c. iodate,** a compound, $Ca(IO_3)_2$ + $6H_2O$, formerly used as an antiseptic. **c. iodide,** a hygroscopic compound, CaI_2, formerly used as an expectorant. **c. iodobehenate,** a white or yellowish powder, $(C_{21}H_{42}ICOO)_2Ca$, containing at least 23.5 per cent of iodine; formerly used as an antigoitrogenic. **c. iodostearate,** a cream-colored odorless powder, $C_{36}H_{68}CaIO_4$, formerly used in the treatment of colloid goiter. **c. ipodate** [NF], chemical name: calcium 3-[[(dimethylamino) methylene] amino]-2,4,6-triiodohydrocinnamate. A white to off-white, odorless, fine crystalline powder, $C_{24}H_{24}CaI_6N_4O_4$, used as a diagnostic radiopaque medium in cholangiography and cholecystography. **c. lactate** [USP], chemical name: 2-hydroxypropanoic acid calcium salt. A calcium replenisher, $C_6H_{10}CaO_6 \cdot xH_2O$, occurring as white granules or powder; administered orally in the treatment of calcium deficiency. **c. levulinate** [USP], chemical name: 4-oxo-pentanoic acid calcium salt. A calcium replenisher, $C_{10}H_{14}CaO_6 \cdot 2H_2O$, occurring as a white, crystalline or amorphous powder; administered parenterally in the treatment of calcium deficiency. **c. mandelate,** the calcium salt of mandelic acid, $C_{16}H_{14}CaO_6$, used orally as a urinary anti-infective. **c. oxalate,** a typical compound, CaC_2O_4, occurring in the urine as crystals and in certain calculi. **c. oxide,** a corrosively alkaline and caustic earth, CaO, used for absorbing carbon dioxide from air, and industrially as a cheap alkali and as a base for mortar; called also *calcarea usta, calx, lime,* and *quicklime*. **c. pantothenate** [USP], chemical name: N-(2,4,-dihydroxy-3,3-dimethyl-1-oxobutyl)-β-alanine calcium salt. The calcium salt of the dextrorotatory isomer of pantothenic acid, $C_{18}H_{32}CaN_2O_{10}$, the B-complex vitamin, occurring as a white powder; used, usually in combination with other B vitamins, as a nutritional supplement. See also *racemic c. pantothenate*. **c. pantothenate, racemic** [USP], a mixture of the calcium salts of the dextrorotatory and levorotatory isomers of pantothenic acid, with a physiological activity about half that of calcium pantothenate. **c. permanganate,** a crystalline salt, $Ca(MnO_4)_2$ + $5H_2O$, formerly used as an antiseptic. **c. phenolsulfonate,** c. sulfocarbolate. **c. phosphate,** any of three salts containing calcium and the phosphate radical (PO_4); see *c. phosphate, dibasic, monobasic,* and *tribasic*. **c. phosphate, dibasic** [USP], an odorless, tasteless, white powder, $CaHPO_4 \cdot 2H_2O$, used as a calcium supplement and as a base in preparation of tablets; called also *dicalcium phosphate*. **c. phosphate, monobasic,** colorless shining scales or powder, $CaH_4(PO_4)_2$, used in fertilizers, baking powders, and wheat flours, and as a mineral supplement in foods and feeds. Called also *c. superphosphate*. **c. phosphate, tribasic** [NF], an odorless, tasteless, white powder, $Ca_3(PO_4)_2$, used as a calcium supplement; it is also used as an antacid and as a laxative. **c. polycarbophil,** a calcium salt of a loosely cross-linked, hydrophilic resin of the polycarboxylic type; a cathartic. **c. propionate,** the calcium salt of propionic acid, $C_6H_{10}CaO_4$, which has antifungal properties; used alone or in combination with sodium propionate or other agents as a preservative to inhibit mold production in bakery and milk products, other foods, tobacco, and pharmaceuticals and as a topical antifungal in the treatment of various mycoses. **radioactive c.,** radiocalcium. **c. stearate** [NF], chemical name: octadecanoic acid calcium salt. A compound of calcium with organic acids obtained from fats, $C_{36}H_{70}CaO_4$, occurring as a fine, white to yellow white, bulky powder; used as a tablet lubricant. **c. sulfate** [NF], an abundant natural product, CaO_4S, found in nature as anhydrite, and occurring in a hydrated form known as gypsum; when gypsum is calcined it forms *plaster of Paris*. Dried

calcium sulfate dihydrate is used as a tablet diluent. **c. sulfhydrate,** a preparation of sulfuretted calcium, once used as a depilatory. **c. sulfide,** a compound, CaS. **c. sulfite,** a compound, $CaSO_3$, resulting from the extraction of sulfur dioxide, by calcium hydroxide, from air or flue gas. **c. sulfocarbolate,** a white crystalline substance, $Ca(C_6H_5SO_4)_2$ + $6H_2O$, soluble in water. **c. superphosphate,** monobasic c. phosphate. **c. trisodium pentetate,** pentetate calcium trisodium.

calciumedetate sodium (kal″se-um-ed′ĕ-tāt) edetate calcium disodium.

calciuria (kal″sĭ-u′re-ah) the presence of calcium in the urine.

calcoglobule (kal″ko-glob′ūl) one of the irregular shaped globules of calcium salts deposited in developing dentin and constituting the spherical type of calcification. See also *calcospherite*.

calcoglobulin (kal″ko-glob′u-lin) the form of globulin that occurs in calcifying tissue.

calcospherite (kal″ko-sfēr′it) one of the small globular bodies formed during the process of calcification, by chemical union between the calcium particles and the albuminous organic matter of the intercellular substance. These particles coalesce to form calcoglobulin.

calculary (kal′ku-la-re) pertaining to a calculus.

calculi (kal′ku-li) plural of *calculus*.

calculifragous (kal″ku-lif′rah-gus) [*claculus* + L. *frangere* to break] the crushing of a bladder stone; lithotriptic.

calculogenesis (kal″ku-lo-jen′ĕ-sis) the formation of calculi.

calculosis (kal″ku-lo′sis) lithiasis.

calculous (kal′ku-lus) pertaining to, of the nature of, or affected with calculus.

calculus (kal′ku-lus), pl. *cal′culi* [L. "pebble"] an abnormal concretion occurring within the animal body and usually composed of mineral salts. **alternating c.,** a urinary calculus made up of successive layers of different composition; called also *combination c.* **alvine c.,** a concretion in the intestine formed by hardening of portions of the fecal contents. **articular c.,** a deposit in a joint; it is usually composed of sodium urate, sometimes of calcium urate. Called also *joint c., calculous conretion,* and *chalk stone.* **biliary calculi,** gallstones (cholelithiasis) composed almost entirely of the excessive blood pigment liberated by hemolysis, with calcium deposits in some. **bronchial c.,** lung c. **calcium oxalate c.,** a hard, rough calculus composed of calcium oxalate. **cardiac c.** (*obs.*), cardiolith. **cholesterol c.,** a calculus formed of cholesterol; called also *metabolic c.* and *metabolic stone.* **combination c.,** alternating c. **cystine c.,** a soft variety of urinary calculus composed of cystine. **decubitus c.,** a calculus formed in the urinary tract as a result of long immobilization. **dental c.,** calcium phosphate and carbonate, with organic matter, deposited upon the surfaces of the teeth; see *subgingival c.* and *supragingival c.* **encysted c.,** a urinary calculus enclosed in a sac developed from the wall of the bladder; called also *pocketed c.* **fibrin c.,** urinary calculi formed largely from fibrinogen in blood. **fusible c.,** a calculus formed of a mixture of calcium phosphate and triple phosphates which fuses to a black, enamel-like mass when tested under the blowpipe. **gastric c.,** gastrolith. **gonecystic c.,** calculus of a seminal vesicle. **hematogenic c.,** subgingival c. **hemic c.,** a calculus developed from a blood clot. **hemp seed c.,** a small, smooth, pale urinary calculus of calcium oxalate of the size and shape of a hemp seed. **hepatic c.,** a gallstone formed in the intrahepatic bile ducts. **indigo c.,** calculus formed by oxidation of the indican of the urine. **intestinal c.,** enterolith. **joint c.,** articular c. **lacrimal c.,** one in a lacrimal gland or duct; dacryolith. **lacteal c.,** mammary c. **lung c.,** a concretion formed in the bronchi by accretion about an inorganic nucleus, or from calcified portions of lung tissue or adjacent lymph nodes; called also *lung stone* and *broncholith.* **mammary c.,** a concretion in one of the lactiferous ducts; called also *lacteal c.* **matrix c.,** a yellowish white to light tan urinary calculus with the consistency of putty, containing calcium salts but composed chiefly of an organic matrix consisting of a mucoprotein and a sulfated mucopolysaccharide. **metabolic c.,** cholesterol c. **mulberry c.,** a hard, smooth urinary calculus of calcium oxalate, so called from its shape. **nasal c.,** rhinolith. **nephritic c.,** renal c. **ovarian c.** (*obs.*), an enlarged and calcified corpus luteum. **oxalate c.,** a hard urinary calculus of calcium oxalate. Some are covered with minute sharp spines that may abrade the renal pelvic epithelium; others are smooth (see *mulberry c.*). **pancreatic c.,** a concretion formed in the pancreatic duct from calcium carbonate with other salts and organic materials. **phosphate c., phosphatic c.,** a renal calculus composed of calcium oxalate and ammonium urate; it may be hard, soft, or friable, and so large that it may fill the pelvis and calices. **pocketed c.,** encysted c. **preputial c.,** postholith. **prostatic c.,** a concretion formed in the prostate, chiefly of calcium carbonate and phosphate. **renal c.,** a calculus occurring in the kidney; called also *nephritic c.* **renal c., primary,** one formed in an apparently healthy urinary tract, usually composed of oxalates or urates. **renal c., secondary,** one associated with infection and obstruction, usually composed of ammonium magnesium phosphate. **salivary c.,** 1. a concretion occurring in a salivary gland or duct; called also *salivary stone*. See *sialolithiasis*. 2. supragingival c. **serumal c.,** subgingival c., so called because it is supposed to result from exudation of serum. **shellac c.,** a gastrolith caused by drinking shellac varnish. **spermatic c.,** a concretion in a seminal vesicle. **staghorn c.,** a calculus of the renal pelvis usually extending into multiple calices. **stomachic c.,** a bezoar or other concretion in the stomach; a gastrolith. **struvite c.,** a urinary calculus composed of very pure ammoniomagnesium phosphate, forming the hard crystals known to mineralogists as struvite. **subgingival c.,** a calculus on the concealed surface of a tooth, that is, apical to the crest of the gingival margin; called also *hematogenic c.* and *serumal c.* **submorphous c.,** a calculus made up of molecules of a crystalline salt, together with molecules of the colloid matter in which the salt is contained. **supragingival c.,** a dental calculus on the exposed surface of a tooth, that is, coronal to the crest of the gingival margin; called also *salivary c.* **tonsillar c.,** a calcareous concretion in a tonsil. **urate c.,** a calculus composed of urates, usually smooth, round, and yellow-brown, occurring chiefly in newborn or young infants. **urethral c.,** calculus of the urethra with symptoms varying according to sex and the site of lodgment. **uric acid c.,** hard, yellow or reddish-yellow calculi formed from uric acid. **urinary c.,** a calculus in any part of the urinary tract; it is *vesical* when lodged in the bladder (stone, gravel), and *renal* when in the pelvis of the kidney. **urostealith c.,** a urinary calculus formed of fatty matter. **uterine c.,** an intrauterine concretion formed mainly by the calcification of a tumor; called also *womb stone*. **vesical c.,** a form found in the urinary bladder; called also *bladder stone* and *cystolith*. **vesicoprostatic c.,** a prostatic calculus extending into the bladder. **xanthic c.,** a urinary calculus composed mainly of xanthine.

Caldani's ligament (kal-dah′nēz) [Leopoldo Marcantonio *Caldani*, Italian anatomist, 1725–1813] see under *ligament*.

Caldwell-Luc operation (kald′wel-luk′) [George W. *Caldwell*, American physician, 1834–1918; Henry *Luc*, French laryngologist, 1855–1925] see under *operation*.

Caldwell-Moloy classification [William Edgar *Caldwell*, American obstetrician, 1880–1943; Howard Carman *Moloy*, American obstetrician, 1903–1953] classification of female pelves as gynecoid, android, anthropoid, and platypelloid; see under *classification*.

Calef. abbreviation for L. *calefactus*, warmed, or for L. *calefac*, make warm.

calefacient (kal″e-fa′shent) [L. *calidus* warm + *facere* to make] 1. warming; causing a sensation of warmth. 2. an agent that causes a sensation of warmth.

Calendula (kah-len′du-lah) [L.] a genus of composite-flowered plants. The dried florets of *C. officinalis*, pot marigold, are stimulant and resolvent, and were once used externally for inflammatory lesions of the skin and mucous membranes.

calentura (kal-en-too′rah) [Sp. "fever"] a name applied to various tropical fevers; sunstroke.

calenture (kal′en-tūr) [Sp. *calentura*] sunstroke, or thermic fever; the name is applied also to various tropical fevers.

calf (kaf) [L. *sura*] the fleshy mass formed chiefly by the gastrocnemius muscle at the back of the leg (below the knee). Called also *sura* [NA].

caliber (kal′ĭ-ber) [Fr. *calibre* the bore of a gun] the diameter of a canal or tube.

calibration (kal″ĭ-bra′shun) determination of the accuracy of an instrument, usually by measurement of its variation from a standard, to ascertain necessary correction factors.

calibrator (kal′ĭ-bra-tor) an instrument for dilating a tubular structure, such as the urethra, or for determining the inner or outer diameter of such a passage.

caliceal (kal″ĭ-se′al) pertaining to or affecting a calix.

calicectasis (kal″ĭ-sek′tah-sis) dilatation of a calix of a kidney.

calicectomy (kal″ĭ-sek′to-me) excision of a calix of a kidney.

calices (kal′ĭ-sēz) plural of *calix*.

calicine (kal′ĭ-sēn) related to or resembling a calix.

calicivirus (kal′ĭ-sĭ-vi′rus) a subgroup of picornaviruses, including the virus of vesicular exanthem.

caliculi (kah-lik′u-li) plural of *caliculus*.

caliculus (kah-lik′u-lus), pl. *calic′uli* [L., dim. of *calix*] a small cup or cup-shaped structure. **c. gustato′rius** [NA], one of the minute, barrel-shaped terminal organs of the gustatory nerve, situated around the bases of the circumvallate papillae of the tongue, each consisting of a group of spindle-shaped cells made up of outer supporting cells and inner sense cells. Called also *taste bud* or *bulb*, *gustatory bud* or *bulb*, and *Schwalbe's corpuscle*. **c. ophthal′micus** [NA], an indentation of the distal wall of the optic vesicle, brought about by rapid marginal growth and producing a double-layered cup, attached to the diencephalon by a tubular stalk. Called also *ocular cup*, *ophthalmic cup*, and *optic cup*.

caliectasis (ka″lĭ-ek′tah-sis) [*calix* + Gr. *ektasis* dilatation] caliectasis.

caliectomy (ka″lĭ-ek′to-me) [*calix* + Gr. *ektomē* excision] calicectomy.

californium (kal′ĭ-for′ne-um) [named from *California* (University and state), where it was first produced] chemical element of atomic number 98, atomic weight 249, symbol Cf, produced by irradiation of the isotope of curium of atomic weight 242 with helium ions; half-life 45 minutes.

caligation (kal″ĭ-ga′shun) caligo.

caligo (kah-li′go) [L. "fog"] dimness of vision. **c. cor′neae**, obscurity of vision due to an opacity of the cornea. **c. len′tis**, obscurity of vision due to cataract. **c. pupil′lae**, dimness of vision due to contraction of the pupil.

calipers (kal′ĭ-perz) [from *caliber*] compasses with bent or curved legs used for measuring the thickness or diameter of a solid. **skinfold c.,** an instrument designed for measuring the thickness of folds of skin gathered at various areas of the body; used in studies of nutritional status and of physical constitution.

calisthenics (kal″is-then′iks) [Gr. *kalos* beautiful + *sthenos* strength] a system of light gymnastics for promoting strength and grace of carriage.

calix (ka′liks), pl. *cal′ices* [L.] a cup-shaped organ or cavity. **renal calices**, calices renales. **renal calices, greater,** calices renales majores. **renal calices, major,** calices renalis majores. **renal calices, minor,** calices renales minores. **cal′ices rena′les** [NA], renal calices: any one of the recesses of the pelvis of the kidney which enclose the pyramids; called also *calyces renales* and *infundibula of kidney*. **cal′ices rena′les majo′res** [NA], major renal calices: the two or more larger subdivisions of the renal pelvis, into which the minor calices open; called also *calyces renales majores* and *greater renal calices*. **cal′ices rena′les mino′res** [NA], minor renal calices: a varying number of smaller subdivisions of the renal pelvis which enclose the pyramids, and open into the major calices; called also *calyces renales minores*.

Callander's amputation (kal′an-derz) [C. Latimer *Callander*, San Francisco surgeon, 1892–1947] see under *amputation*.

Callaway's test (kal′ah-wāz) [Thomas *Callaway*, English physician, 1791–1848] see under *tests*.

Calleja's islets (islands) (kal-ya′hahz) [Camilo *Calleja* y Sanchez, Spanish anatomist, died 1913] see under *islet*.

callicrein (kal″ik-re′in) kallikrein.

Callimastix (kal″ĭ-mas′tiks) a genus of parasitic protozoa (order Polymastigida, class Zoomastigophora), characterized by the presence of 12 to 15 anterior flagella. *C. cy′clops* is found in the body cavity of species of *Cyclops*, *C. fronta′lis* in the rumen of the cow, sheep, and goat, and *C. e′qui* in the colon and cecum of the horse.

Calliphora (kah-lif′o-rah) [Gr. *kallos* beauty + *phoros* bearing] a genus of scavenger flies of the family Calliphoridae, the blow flies or bluebottle flies, which deposit their eggs in decaying matter, on wounds, or in the openings of the body. **C. vomi-**

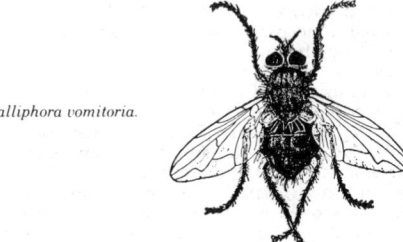

Calliphora vomitoria.

to′ria, the common blow fly or bluebottle fly, whose larvae may invade the nasal fossae or produce intestinal myiasis. Other species are *C. azurea*, *C. erythrocephala*, and *C. lionensis*.

Calliphoridae (kal″lĭ-for′ĭ-de) a family of medium-sized to large flies of the order Diptera, including the genera *Auchmeromyia*, *Calliphora* (type genus), *Cordylobia*, *Cochliomyia*, *Chrysomyia*, *Lucilia*, *Phaenicia*, and *Phormia*; all species may serve as vectors of pathogens and may also produce myiasis in man.

Callison's fluid (kal′ĭ-sunz) [James S. *Callison*, American physician, born 1873] see under *fluid*.

Callitroga (kal″lĭ-tro′gah) *Cochliomyia*.

callomania (kal″o-ma′ne-ah) [Gr. *kallos* beauty + *mania* madness] a condition marked by delusions of personal beauty; cf. *narcissism*.

callosal (kah-lo′sal) pertaining to the corpus callosum.

callositas (kah-los′ĭ-tas) [L.] a callus.

callosity (kah-los′ĭ-te) [L. *callositas*, from *callus*] a callus.

callosomarginal (kah-lo″so-mar′jĭ-nal) pertaining to the callosal and marginal gyri.

callosum (kah-lo′sum) corpus callosum.

callous (kal′us) hard; like callus.

callus (kal′us) [L.] 1. localized hyperplasia of the horny layer of the epidermis due to pressure or friction; called also *callosity*. 2. an unorganized meshwork of woven bone developed on the pattern of the original fibrin clot, which is formed following fracture of a bone and is normally ultimately replaced by hard adult bone; called also *bony c.* 3. a mass of plant tissue formed over a wound or at the base of a cutting. **bony c.,** see callus (def. 2). **central c.,** a provisional callus formed within the medullary cavity of a fractured bone; it arises from the cells covering the endosteal and trabecular surfaces near the fracture. Called also *inner c., medullary c.,* and *myelogenous c.* **definitive c.,** the exudate formed between the fractured ends of the bone, which is permanent and becomes changed into true bone; called also *intermediate c.* and *permanent c.* **ensheathing c.,** provisional callus forming a sheath about the ends of the fragments of a fractured bone. **external c.,** the collar of callus formed by the periosteum in a long bone. **inner c.,** central c. **intermediate c.,** definitive c. **internal c., medullary c., myelogenous c.,** central c. **permanent c.,** definitive c. **provisional c.,** callus formed within the medullary cavity and about the ends of a broken bone, and which is absorbed as the repair is completed. **temporary c.,** provisional c.

calmative (kal′mah-tiv, kahm′ah-tiv) 1. sedative; allaying excitement. 2. an agent that allays excitement or has a sedative effect.

Calmette's reaction (ophthalmoreaction, test), serum, tuberculin, vaccine (kal-metz′) [Albert Léon Charles *Calmette,* French bacteriologist, 1863–1933] see *ophthalmic reaction,* under *reaction; antivenomous serum,* under *serum;* and *BCG vaccine,* under *vaccine;* and see under *tuberculin.*

Calobata (kah-lo′bah-tah) a genus of South American flies whose larvae sometimes occur in the human intestine.

calomel (kal′o-mel) [L. *calomelas;* Gr. *kalos* fair + *melas* black] chemical name: mercurous chloride. A heavy, white, odorless, impalpable powder, HgCl, insoluble in water, alcohol, ether, and cold dilute acids; rarely used today as a cathartic. **vegetable c.,** podophyllum.

calor (ka′lor) [L.] heat; one of the cardinal signs of inflammation. **c. febri′lis,** the heat of fever. **c. fer′vens,** an intense heat. **c. inna′tus,** the normal or natural heat of the body. **c. inter′nus,** the heat of the interior of the body. **c. mor′dax, c. mor′dicans,** 1. biting or stinging heat. 2. the hot, burning, reddish-colored skin occurring in scarlet fever.

caloradiance (kal″o-ra′de-ans) the radiation or rays which lie between 250 and 55,000 millimicrons, such as the rays from the sun, carbon arcs, incandescent rods and filaments, and hot black bodies.

calorescence (kal″o-res′ens) the conversion of nonluminous into luminous heat rays.

Calori's bursa (kah-lo′rēz) [Luigi *Calori,* Italian anatomist, 1807–1896] see under *bursa.*

caloric (kah-lo′rik) pertaining to heat or to calories.

caloricity (kal″o-ris′ĭ-te) the power of the animal body of developing and maintaining heat.

calorie (kal′o-re) [Fr.; L. *calor* heat] a unit of heat. The term is commonly used alone to designate the *small calorie* (abbreviated cal.). The calorie used in the study of metabolism is the *large calorie,* or *kilocalorie* (abbreviated Cal.). **gram c.,** small c. **I.T. c., International Table c.,** a unit of heat, equivalent to 4.1868 joules. **large c.,** the calorie used in metabolic studies, being the amount of heat required to raise the temperature of 1 kilogram of water 1 degree Celsius (centigrade), specifically from 14.5° to 15.5° C. at a pressure of 1 atmosphere; abbreviated kg.-cal. Called also *kilocalorie.* Also used to express the fuel or energy value of food. **mean c.,** one one-hundredth of the amount of heat required to raise the temperature of 1 gram of water from 0 to 100° C. **small c.,** the amount of heat required to raise the temperature of 1 gram of water 1 degree Celsius (centigrade), specifically from 14.5° to 15.5° C. at a pressure of 1 atomosphere; abbreviated g.-cal. Called also *gram c.* and *standard c.* **standard c.,** small c. **thermochemical c.,** a unit of heat, equivalent to 4.184 joules.

calorifacient (kah-lor″ĭ-fa′shent) [L. *calor* heat + *facere* to make] producing heat; said of certain foods.

calorific (kal″o-rif′ik) [L. *calor* heat + *facere* to make] producing heat.

calorigenetic (kah-lor″ĭ-jĕ-net′ik) calorigenic.

calorigenic (kah-lor″ĭ-jen′ik) [L. *calor* heat + Gr. *gennan* to produce] producing heat or energy; increasing heat or energy production; increasing the consumption of oxygen.

calorimeter (kal″o-rim′ĕ-ter) [L. *calor* heat + Gr. *metron* measure] an instrument for measuring the amount of heat exchanged in any system. In physiology, an apparatus for measuring the amount of heat produced by an individual. **bomb c.,** an apparatus for measuring the potential energy of food, a weighed amount of the food being placed on a platinum dish inside a hollow steel container (bomb) filled with pure oxygen. The heat produced by its combustion is absorbed by a known quantity of water in which the container is immersed, permitting its measurement. **compensating c.,** an apparatus in which the object to be tested,

such as a developing chick in an egg, is placed at one junction of a thermocouple and an electrical resistance at the other. From the amount of current that must pass through the resistance to keep both junctions at the same temperature (as shown by lack of current in the thermocouple circuit), it is possible to calculate the amount of heat generated in the object being tested. **respiration c.,** an apparatus for the measurement of the gaseous exchange between a living organism and the atmosphere surrounding it and the simultaneous measurement of the amount of heat produced by that organism.

calorimetric (kah-lor″ĭ-met′rik) pertaining to or performed by calorimetry.

calorimetry (kal″o-rim′ĕ-tre) [L. *calor* heat + Gr. *metron* measure] measurement of the amounts of heat absorbed or given out. **direct c.,** measurement of the amount of heat produced by a subject enclosed within a small chamber. **indirect c.,** measurement of the amount of heat produced by a subject by determination of the amount of oxygen consumed and the quantity of nitrogen and carbon dioxide eliminated.

caloripuncture (kal″o-rĭ-punk′tūr) [L. *calor* heat + *puncture*] puncture by the use of heat.

caloriscope (kah-lor′ĭ-skōp) an instrument for showing the caloric values of mixtures for infant feedings.

caloritropic (kah-lor″ĭ-trop′ik) [L. *calor* heat + Gr. *tropos* a turning] thermotropic.

calory (kal′o-re), pl. *calories.* Calorie.

Calot's operation, treatment, triangle (kah-ōz′) [Jean-François *Calot,* French surgeon, 1861–1944] see under *operation, treatment,* and *triangle.*

calotte (kah-lot′) [Fr. "cap"] a part shaped like a skull cap. In ophthalmology, a cap-shaped specimen removed from the eyeball for histopathologic examination.

calsequestrin (kal″sĕ-kwes′trin) [*calcium* + *sequester* + *-in* chemical suffix] a calcium-binding protein rich in carboxylate side chains, occurring on the inner membrane surface of the sarcoplasmic reticulum; it serves to chelate and store calcium ions.

Calurin (kal″u-rin) trademark for a preparation of carbaspirin calcium.

calusterone (kal-u′ster-ōn) chemical name: (7β-17β)-17-hydroxy-7,17-dimethylandrost-4-en-3-one; an antineoplastic agent, $C_{21}H_{32}O_2$, used for palliation of inoperable or metastatic breast carcinoma in postmenopausal women.

calutron (kal′u-tron) an apparatus for separating the isotopes of uranium.

calvacin (kal′vah-sin) an antineoplastic substance derived from the fungus *Calvatia gigantea.*

calvaria (kal-va′re-ah) [L.] [NA] the domelike superior portion of the cranium, composed of the superior portions of the frontal, parietal, and occipital bones; called also *calvarium, concha of cranium,* and *skullcap.*

calvarial (kal-va′re-al) pertaining to the calvaria.

calvarium (kal-va′re-um) the calvaria.

Calvatia (kal-va′she-ah) a genus of basidiomycetous fungi of the order Lycoperdales, series Gasteromycetes. **C. gigan′tea,** the giant puffball, the source of calvacin.

Calvé-Perthes disease (kal-va′per-tās) [Jacques *Calvé,* French orthopedist, 1875–1954; Georg Clemens *Perthes,* German surgeon, 1869–1927] osteochondrosis of the capitular epiphysis of the femur; see under *osteochondrosis.*

Calvert's test (kal′vertz) [E. G. B. *Calvert,* British physician] see under *tests.*

Calvin cycle (kal′vin) [Melvin *Calvin,* American chemist, born 1911; winner of the Nobel prize in chemistry for 1961 for development of techniques to determine the chemical reactions of plant carbon dioxide assimilation] see under *cycle.*

calvities (kal-vish′e-ēz) [L.] baldness; see *alopecia.*

calx (kalks) [L.] 1. lime or chalk. 2. [NA] the hindmost part of the foot; the heel. 3. any residue obtained by calcination. 4. lime or calcium oxide, CaO; quicklime: alkaline, caustic, and escharotic. **c. chlora′ta, c. chlorina′ta,** chlorinated lime. **c. sulfura′ta,** a mixture of at least 60 per cent of calcium sulfide with a variable proportion of calcium sulfate and carbon. It is used in skin and pustular diseases, and as a depilatory. Called also *sulfurated lime.*

calyceal (kal″ĭ-se′al) caliceal.

calycectasis (kal″ĭ-sek′tah-sis) calicectasis.

calycectomy (kal″ĭ-sek′to-me) calicectomy.

calyces (kal′ĭ-sēz) plural of *calyx.*

calycine (kal′ĭ-sin) calicine.

calycle (kal′ĭ-kl) a caliculus.

calyculi (kah-lik′u-li) [L.] caliculi.

calyculus (kah-lik′u-lus), pl. *calyc′uli* [L. "a little cup," from Gr. *kalyx* cup of a flower] caliculus. **c. gustato′rius,** caliculus gustatorius. **c. ophthal′micus,** caliculus ophthalmicus.

Calymmatobacterium (kah-lim″mah-to-bak-te′re-um) [Gr. *kalymma* a hood or veil + *baktērion* a little staff] a genus of microorganisms of the family Brucellaceae, order Eubacteriales, made up of pleomorphic nonmotile, gram-negative rods, which may or may not be encapsulated. **C. granulo′matis,** a gram-negative, pleomorphic, rod-shaped microorganism that is not cultivable on non-viable media but grows in the yolk, yolk sac, and amniotic fluid of the chick embryo. It is serologically related to *Klebsiella pneumoniae* and coliform bacilli, and is grouped with *Pasteurella, Malleomyces,* and *Actinobacillus* by some workers. It is the causative agent of granuloma inguinale in man. Called also *Donovania granulomatis* and *Donovan body.*

calyx (ka′liks), pl. *cal′yces* [Gr. *kalyx* cup of a flower]   calix. **cal′yces rena′les,** calices renales; see under *calix.* **cal′- yces rena′les majo′res,** calices renales majores; see under *calix.* **cal′yces rena′les mino′res,** calices renales minores; see under *calix.*

Camallanus (kam″ah-la′nus)   a genus of nematodes of the order Spiraroidea, species of which are parasites in the intestines of fishes, reptiles, and amphibians.

Cambaroides (kam″bah-roi′dēz)   a genus of crayfish which harbor the metacercariae of *Paragonimus.*

cambendazole (kam-ben′dah-zōl)   chemical name: [2-(4-thia- zolyl)-1*H*-benzimidazol-5-yl]cambaʳnic acid; an antihelmintic, C_{14}- $H_{14}N_4O_2S$.

cambium (kam′be-um) [L. "exchange"]   1. the loose cellular in- ner layer of the periosteal tissue in the intramembranous ossifica- tion of bone.   2. a layer of cells beneath the bark of woody plants.

cambogia (kam-bo′je-ah) [L.]   gamboge.

cameloid (kam′ĕ-loid)   possessing characteristics similar to those observed in a camel.

camelpox (kam′el-poks)   an eruptive disease of camels due to a poxvirus.

camera (kam′er-ah), pl. *cameras* or *cam′erae* [L. "chamber"]   1. a box, chamber, or compartment.   2. any enclosed space or ventri- cle.   **c. ante′rior bul′bi** [NA], anterior chamber of eye: that portion of the aqueous-containing space between the cornea and the lens which is bounded in front by the cornea and part of the sclera, and behind by the iris, part of the ciliary body, and that part of the lens which presents through the pupil. Called also *c. oculi anterior.*   **c. lu′cida,** an optical device utilizing a prism or mir- rors so arranged as to throw the reflected image of an object upon paper, thus permitting its outlines to be traced with a pencil. **c. obscu′ra,** a combined box, lens, and screen, used for viewing, tracing, or making photographs.   **c. oc′uli,** either one of the chambers of the eye.   **c. oc′uli ante′rior,** c. anterior bulbi. **c. oc′uli poste′rior,** c. posterior bulbi.   **c. poste′rior bul′bi** [NA], posterior chamber of the eye: that portion of the aqueous-containing space between the cornea and the lens which is bounded in front by the iris, and behind by the lens and suspensory ligament; called also *c. oculi posterior.*   **c. pul′pi,** the pulp cavity of a tooth.   **recording c.,** photokymograph. **scintillation c.,** an electronic instrument that produces photo- graphs or cathode-ray tube images of the gamma ray or positron emissions from organs containing tracer compounds.   **c. sep′ti pellu′cidi** (*obs.*), cavum septi pellucidi.   **c. vi′trea bul′bi** [NA], vitreous chamber.

camerae (kam′er-e) [L.]   plural of *camera.*

Camerer's law (kam′er-erz) [Johann Friedrich Wilhelm *Camerer,* German pediatrician, 1842–1910]   see under *law.*

camisole (kam′ĭ-sōl) [Fr.]   straitjacket.

Cammann's stethoscope (kam′anz) [George Philip *Cammann,* American physician, 1804–1863]   a binaural stethoscope.

Cammidge reaction (test) (kam′ij) [Percy John *Cammidge,* En- glish physician born 1872]   see *pancreatic reaction,* under *reac- tion.*

Camoquin (kam′o-kwin)   trademark for a preparation of amo- diaquine hydrochloride.

campanula (kam-pan′u-lah) [L. *campana* a bell]   a bell-shaped organ or part.   **c. hal′leri,** the swollen end of the falciform process in the eye of fish.

Campbell's ligament (kam′belz) [William Francis *Campbell,* American surgeon, 1867–1926]   the suspensory ligament of the axilla.

campeachy, campechy (kam-pe′che)   *Haematoxylon.*

Camper's angle, fascia, ligament, line (kam′perz) [Pieter *Camper,* Dutch physician, 1722–1789]   see *facial angle* and *maxillary angle,* under *angle;* see *diaphragma urogenitale;* and see under *fascia* and *line.*

campesterol (kam-pes′ter-ol)   a sterol, $C_{28}H_{48}O$, from rape seed oil, soy bean oil, and wheat germ oil; it is isomeric with ergastanol.

camphene (kam-fēn′)   chemical name: 2,2-dimethyl-3-me- thylenebicyclo[2.2.1]heptane. A terpene, $C_{10}H_{16}$, found in many essential oils or prepared synthetically from pinene in the process of producing synthetic camphor.

camphol (kam′fol)   Borneo camphor.

camphor (kam′for, kam′fer) [L. *camphora;* Gr. *kamphora*]   1. [USP] chemical name: 1,7,7-trimethylbicyclo[2.2.1]heptane-2-one. A ketone, $C_{10}H_{16}O$, obtained from the wood of *Cinnamomum*

camphora, an evergreen tree native to eastern Asia, or produced synthetically (see *synthetic c.*), and occurring as colorless or white crystals, granules, or crystalline masses or as colorless to white, translucent, tough masses, with a penetrating characteristic odor and a pungent, aromatic taste. It is applied topically to the skin as an antipruritic and anti-infective and is used as a pharmaceutic necessity in certain pharmaceutic preparations. Called also *gum c.* 2. any compound having characteristics similar to those of camphor.   **anise c.,** anethole.   **artificial c.,** bornyl chloride. **Borneo c.,** 1. the dextrorotatory form of borneol.   2. borneol. **monobromated c.,** that in which one hydrogen atom has been replaced by one bromine atom; formerly used as a sedative. **peppermint c.,** natural menthol.   **synthetic c.,** a camphor produced from pinene, the principal constituent of turpentine. **thyme c.,** thymol.   **turpentine c.,** bornyl chloride.

camphora (kam-fo′rah) [L.]   camphor.

camphoraceous (kam″fo-ra′shus)   having characteristics re- sembling those of camphor.

camphorated (kam′fo-rāt″ed) [L. *camphoratus*]   containing or tinctured with camphor.

camphorism (kam′for-izm)   poisoning by camphor; the condi- tion is marked by convulsions, coma, and gastritis.

campimeter (kam-pim′ĕ-ter) [L. *campus* field + *metrum* measure] an apparatus for mapping the central portion of the visual field on a flat surface.

campimetry (kam-pim′ĕ-tre)   the determination of the pres- ence of defects in the central portion of the visual field by use of the campimeter.

campospasm (kam′po-spazm) [Gr. *kampē* a bending + *spasm*] camptocormia.

campotomy (kam-pot′o-me) [L. *campi* fields (of Forel) + Gr. *tomē* a cutting]   the stereotaxic surgical technique of producing a le- sion in Forel's fields, beneath the thalamus, for correction of tremor in Parkinson's disease.

camptocormia (kamp″to-kor′me-ah) [Gr. *kamptos* bent + *kormos* trunk + *-ia*]   a static deformity consisting of forward flexion of the trunk; called also *camptospasm.*

camptocormy (kamp″to-kor′me)   camptocormia.

camptodactylia (kamp″to-dak-til′e-ah)   camptodactyly.

camptodactylism (kamp″to-dak′til-izm)   camptodactyly.

camptodactyly (kamp″to-dak′tĭ-le) [Gr. *kamptos* bent + *daktylos* finger]   permanent and irreducible flexion of one or more fin- gers (Landouzy).

camptomelia (kamp″to-me′le-ah) [Gr. *kamptos* bent + *melos* limb + *-ia*]   bending of the limbs, producing permanent bowing or curving of the affected part; see also *camptomelic syndrome,* under *syndrome.*

camptomelic (kamp″to-me′lik)   pertaining to camptomelia; see also under *syndrome.*

camptospasm (kamp′to-spazm)   camptocormia.

Campylobacter (kam′pĭ-lo-bak′ter) [Gr. *kampylos* curved + *baktērion* little rod]   a genus of bacteria, family Spirillaceae, made up of gram-negative, non–spore-forming, motile, spirally curved rods, which are microaerophilic to anaerobic. The type species is *C. fetus.*   **c. fe′tus,** the microaerophilic type species, occurring as three subspecies: *C. fetus* subspecies *fe′tus* causes abortion and infertility in cattle; *C. fetus* subspecies *intestina′lis* causes abortion in sheep and sporadic abortion in cattle, as well as human infection; *C. fetus* subspecies *jeju′ni* causes an acute gastroenteritis of man. Called also *Vibrio fetus.*

campylognathia (kam″pĭ-lo-na′the-ah) [Gr. *kampylos* curved + *gnathos* jaw + *-ia*]   harelip.

camsylate (kam′sĭ-lāt)   USAN contraction for camphorsulfon- ate.

Canada-Cronkhite syndrome (kan′ah-dah-krong′kīt) [Wilma Jeanne *Canada,* American radiologist; Leonard W. *Cronkhite,* Jr., American internist, born 1919]   see under *syndrome.*

canal (kah-nal′)   a relatively narrow tubular passage or channel; see also *canalis.*   **abdominal c.,** canalis inguinalis.   **acces- sory palatine c's,** canales palatini minores.   **adductor c.,** canalis adductorius.   **Alcock's c.,** canalis pudendalis.   **ali- mentary c.,** that part of the digestive tract formed by the esoph- agus, stomach, and small and large intestines (canalis alimenta- rius [NA]).   **alisphenoid c.,** a canal in the alisphenoid bone which in many animals transmits the internal carotid artery. **alveolar c's,** see *canalis mandibulae* and *canales alveolares maxillae.*   **alveolar c., anterior; alveolar c. of maxilla; alveolar c., posterior,** see *canales alveolares maxillae.* **anal c.,** the terminal portion of the alimentary canal, extending from the rectum to its distal opening; called also *canalis analis* [NA].   **arachnoid c.** (*obs.*), cisterna venae magnae cerebri. **c. of Arantius,** ductus venosus.   **archenteric c.,** neuren- teric c.   **archinephric c.,** pronephric duct.   **Arnold's c.,** a channel in the petrous portion of the temporal bone for passage of the auricular branch of the vagus nerve.   **arterial c.,** ductus arteriosus.   **atrioventricular c.,** the common canal connect- ing the primitive atrium and ventricle. It sometimes persists as a congenital anomaly, as a result of failure of closure of the gap between the interatrial and interventricular septa due to arrest in development of the endocardial cushions. **auditory c., external,** meatus acusticus externus. **auditory c., internal,** meatus acusticus internus. **basipharyngeal c.,** canalis vomerovaginalis. **Bichat's c.,** cisterna venae magnae cerebri. **biliary c's, interlobular,** ductuli interlobulares. **biliary c's, intralobular,** small passages for conducting the bile within the substance of the lobules of the liver (ductuli biliferi [NA]). **birth c.,** the canal through which the fetus passes in birth, comprising the cervix uteri, vagina, and vulva; called also *obstetric c.* and *parturient c.* **blastoporic c.,** neurenteric c. **blunderbuss c.,** a descriptive term used to denote an incompletely formed tooth root in which the apical third of the root canal possesses a wider diameter than the coronal two thirds. **bony c's of ear,** see entries beginning *canalis semicircularis.* **branching c.,** collateral pulp c. **Braun's c.,** neurenteric c. **Braune's c.** (*obs.*), the uterine cavity and vagina, after complete dilation of the os of the cervix in labor. **Breschet's c's,** canales diploici. **bullular c's,** spatia zonularia. **calciferous c's,** canals containing lime salts in cartilage that is undergoing calcification. **caroticotympanic c's,** canaliculi caroticotympanici. **carotid c.,** canalis caroticus. **carpal c.,** canalis carpi. **c's of cartilage,** canals in an ossifying cartilage during its stage of vascularization. **central c. of modiolus,** see *canales longitudinales modioli.* **central c. of spinal cord,** canalis centralis medullae spinalis. **central c. of Stilling, central c. of vitreous,** canalis hyaloideus. **cerebrospinal c.,** the primitive cavity of the brain and spinal cord. **cervical c. of uterus,** canalis cervicis uteri. **chordal c.,** notochordal c. **c. of chorda tympani,** canaliculus chordae tympani. **ciliary c's,** spatia anguli iridocornealis. **Civinini's c.,** canaliculus chordae tympani. **Cloquet's c.,** canalis hyaloideus. **cochlear c.,** ductus cochlearis. **collateral pulp c.,** a branch of a dental pulp canal that emerges from the root at a place other than the apex; called also *branching c.* **condylar c., condyloid c.,** canalis condylaris. **condyloid c., anterior,** canalis hypoglossi. **connecting c.,** the arched or coiled part of a uriniferous tubule, joining it to a collecting tubule. **c. of Corti,** inner tunnel. **c. of Cotunnius,** the aqueductus vestibuli and canaliculus cochleae considered as a continuous passage. **craniopharyngeal c.,** an occasional passage through the sphenoid bone, opening into the sella turcica. **crural c.,** canalis femoralis. **crural c. of Henle,** canalis adductorius. **c. of Cuvier,** ductus venosus. **dental c., inferior,** canalis mandibulae. **dental c's, posterior,** 1. see *canales alveolares maxillae.* 2. foramina alveolaria maxillae. **dentinal c's,** canaliculi dentales. **digestive c.,** canalis alimentarius. **diploic c's,** canales diploici. **Dorello's c.,** an opening sometimes found in the temporal bone through which the abducens nerve and inferior petrosal sinus together enter the cavernous sinus. **entodermal c.,** the primitive gut or alimentary canal (canalis alimentarius [NA]). **c. of epididymis,** ductus epididymidis. **ethmoid c., anterior,** a passage in the frontal and ethmoid bones for the nasal branch of the ophthalmic nerve and anterior ethmoid vessels. **ethmoid c., posterior,** foramen ethmoidale posterius. **eustachian c.,** tuba auditiva. **eustachian c., osseous,** canalis musculotubarius. **facial c., c. for facial nerve,** canalis facialis. **fallopian c.,** canalis facialis. **femoral c.,** canalis femoralis. **Ferrein's c.,** a canal said to be formed by the edges of the closed eyelids, which conducts the tears during sleep to the puncta lacrimale. **flexor c.,** canalis carpi. **ganglionic c.,** canalis spiralis modioli. **Gartner's c.,** ductus epoophori longitudinalis. **genital c.,** any canal for the passage of ova or for copulatory use; called also *genital duct.* **gubernacular c's,** four small openings in young crania, one behind each incisor tooth. **c. of Guidi,** canalis pterygoideus. **gynecophoral c., gynecophorous c.,** the ventral slot in which the male schistosome carries the female. **hair c.,** an epidermal canal through which a hair grows in order to erupt. **Hannover's c.,** a potential space existing between the anterior and posterior portions of the suspensory ligament of the lens. **haversian c.,** one of the freely anastomosing channels of the haversian system in compact bone. Called also *canalis nutricius ossis* [NA], *haversian space, nutrient c. of bone,* and *plasmatic c.* **hemal c.,** the space within the hemal arch. **Henle's c's,** Henle's loops. **Hensen's c.,** ductus reuniens. **c's of Hering,** openings through which the bile canaliculi communicate with the terminal branches of the bile duct system, the cholangioles; distinguished by their walls, which consist of parenchymal liver cells on one side and cells of the ductules (cholangioles) on the other. **hernial c.,** the passage which transmits a hernia. **Hirschfeld's c's,** interdental c's. **His's c.,** ductus thyroglossus. **Holmgren-Golgi c's,** minute canals in the cytoplasm of cells, particularly of nerve cells, forming a complex apparatus throughout the cytoplasm; called also *intracytoplasmic c's.* **c. of Hovius,** one of a series of connections between the venae vorticosae in certain mammals. **Huguier's c.,** iter chordae anterius. **Hunter's c.,** canalis adductorius. **Huschke's c.,** a passage formed by union of the tubercles of the tympanic ring (anulus tympanicus); it commonly disappears during the years of childhood. **hyaloid c.,** canalis hyaloideus. **hypoglossal c.,** canalis hypoglossi. **iliac c.,** lacuna muscu-

lorum. **incisive c.,** canalis incisivus. **infraorbital c.,** canalis infraorbitalis. **inguinal c.,** canalis inguinalis. **intercellular c's,** interfacial c's. **interdental c's,** channels in the alveolar process of the mandible, between the roots of the medial and lateral incisors, for the passage of anastomosing blood vessels between the sublingual and inferior dental arteries; called also *Hirschfeld's c's.* **interfacial c's.,** a labyrinthine system of expanded intercellular spaces between desmosomes; called also *intercellular c's.* **intersacral c's,** foramina intervertebralia ossis sacri. **intestinal c.,** the intestine; that part of the alimentary canal which lies between the pylorus and the anus. **intracytoplasmic c's,** Holmgren-Golgi c's. **Jacobson's c., c. for Jacobson's nerve,** canaliculus tympani. **Kovalevsky's c.,** neurenteric c. **lacrimal c.,** 1. canalis nasolacrimalis. 2. any passage for transmission of the secretion of the lacrimal glands. **lateral c.,** a lateral extension of the major root canal. **Laurer's c.,** a passage in trematode worms extending from the ovarian duct to the dorsal surface of the body. **longitudinal c's of modiolus,** canales longitudinales modioli. **Löwenberg's c.,** the part of the ductus cochlearis above the membrane of Corti. **mandibular c.,** canalis mandibulae. **maxillary c., superior,** foramen rotundum ossis sphenoidalis. **medullary c.,** 1. canalis vertebralis. 2. cavum medullare ossium. **c's of modiolus,** see *canalis spiralis modioli* and *canales longitudinales modioli.* **Müller's c.,** ductus paramesonephricus. **musculotubal c.,** canalis musculotubarius. **nasal c.,** canalis nasolacrimalis. **nasolacrimal c.,** canalis nasolacrimalis. **nasopalatine c.,** canalis incisivus. **neural c.,** canalis vertebralis. **neurenteric c. (of Kovalevsky),** a passage, in the embryo, from the posterior part of the neural tube into the archenteron; called also *Braun's c., archenteric c.,* and *blastoporic c.* **notochordal c.,** a tunnel extending from the primitive pit into the notochordal process of the embryo; called also *chordal c.* **c. of Nuck,** processus vaginalis peritonei. **nutrient c. of bone,** haversian c., or canalis nutricius ossis. **obstetric c.,** birth c. **obturator c.,** canalis obturatorius. **obturator c. of pubic bone,** sulcus obturatorius ossis pubis. **c. of Oken,** ductus mesonephricus. **olfactory c.,** the nasal fossae at an early stage of their embryonic development. **omphalomesenteric c.,** yolk stalk. **optic c.,** canalis opticus. **orbital c's,** foramina ethmoidalia. **orbital c., anterior internal,** foramen ethmoidale anterius. **orbital c., posterior internal,** foramen ethmoidale posterius. **palatine c's, accessory,** canales palatini minores. **palatine c., anterior,** 1. canalis incisivus. 2. foramen incisivum. **palatine c's, lesser, palatine c's, posterior,** canales palatini minores. **palatomaxillary c.,** 1. canalis palatinus major. 2. see *foramen palatinum majus.* **palatovaginal c.,** canalis palatovaginalis. **parturient c.,** birth c. **pelvic c.,** the passage from the superior to the inferior strait of the pelvis. **perivascular c.,** a lymph space about a blood vessel. **persistent common atrioventricular c.,** atrioventricularis communis. **Petit's c.,** see *spatia zonularia.* **pharyngeal c.,** canalis palatovaginalis. **plasmatic c.,** haversian c. **pleural c's,** a pair of passages in the embryo, connecting the primitive pericardial and peritoneal cavities. **portal c.,** a space within the capsule of Glisson and liver substance, containing branches of the portal vein, of the hepatic artery, and of the hepatic duct. **pterygoid c.,** canalis pterygoideus. **pterygopalatine c.,** 1. canalis palatinus major. 2. canalis palatovaginalis. **pudendal c.,** canalis pudendalis. **pulmoaortic c.,** ductus arteriosus. **pulp c.,** root c. **pyloric c.,** canalis pyloricus. **c's of Recklinghausen,** small lymph spaces in the connective tissue. **recurrent c.,** canalis pterygoideus. **Reichert's c.,** ductus reuniens. **c's of Rivinus,** ductus sublinguales minores. **root c. (of tooth),** that portion of the pulp cavity in the root of a tooth extending from the pulp chamber to the apical foramen; more than one canal may be present in a root, two commonly being present in the mesial root of the mandibular first molar. Called also *canalis radicis dentis* [NA] and *pulp c.* **root c., accessory,** a lateral branching of the main root canal, usually occurring in the apical third of the root. **Rosenthal's c.,** canalis spiralis modioli. **ruffed c.,** see *spatia zonularia.* **sacculocochlear c.,** a passage connecting the sacculus and the cochlea. **sacculoutricular c.,** ductus utriculosaccularis. **sacral c.,** canalis sacralis. **Santorini's c.,** ductus pancreaticus accessorius. **Schlemm's c.,** a branching, circumferential vessel lying in the internal scleral sulcus, a major component of the drainage pathway for aqueous humor; called also *sinus venosus sclerae*[NA]. **scleral c., scleroticochoroidal c.,** the channel in the choroid and sclera of the eye through which the optic nerve passes; see also *lamina cribrosa sclerae.* **semicircular c's,** three long canals of the bony labyrinth of the ear. See *canales semicirculares ossei* [NA]. **semicircular c., anterior,** canalis semicircularis anterior. **semicircular c., horizontal,** canalis semicircularis lateralis. **semicircular c., lateral,** canalis semicircularis lateralis. **semicircular c's, membranous,** see *ductus semicircularis anterior, ductus semicircularis lateralis,* and *ductus semicircularis posterior.* **semicircular c., posterior,** canalis semicircularis posterior. **seminal c.,** a passage for the transmission of semen, or of spermatozoa. **serous c.,** a minute lymph space. **sheathing c.,** the passage from the peritoneal cavity to the tunica vaginalis testis. **Sondermann's c's,** conical extensions of the lumen of Schlemm's canal sometimes observed in the inner wall of the canal. **spermatic c.,** the canalis inguinalis in the male, providing for passage of the spermatic cord. **sphenopalatine c.,** 1. canalis palatovaginalis. 2. canalis palatinus major. **sphenopharyngeal c.,** canalis palatovaginalis. **spinal c.,** canalis vertebralis. **spinal medullary c.** (*obs.*), canalis centralis medullae spinalis. **spiral c. of cochlea,** canalis spiralis cochleae. **spiral c. of modiolus,** canalis spiralis modioli. **spiroid c.,** canalis facialis. **c. of Steno, Stensen's c.,** parotid duct (ductus parotideus [NA]). **c. of Stilling,** canalis hyaloideus. **subsartorial c.,** canalis adductorius. **Sucquet-Hoyer c.,** Sucquet-Hoyer anastomosis. **supraciliary c.,** a small opening sometimes present near the supraorbital notch, which transmits a nutrient artery and a branch of the supraorbital nerve to the frontal sinus. **supraoptic c.,** a minute canal which is the anterior continuation of the optic recess above the optic chiasma. **supraorbital c.,** incisura frontalis. **tarsal c.,** sinus tarsi. **c. for tensor tympani muscle,** semicanalis musculi tensoris tympani. **Theile's c.,** a space formed by reflection of the pericardium on the aorta and the pulmonary artery. **Tourtual's c.,** canalis palatinus major. **tubal c.,** semicanalis tubae auditivae. **tubotympanic c.,** the inner division of the first branchial cleft in the fetus, from which the auditory tube and middle ear cavity are derived. **tympanic c. of cochlea,** scala tympani. **umbilical c.,** anulus umbilicalis. **urogenital c's,** that portion of the urogenital sinus used jointly by the müllerian and mesonephric ducts. **uterine c.,** the cavity of the uterus. **uterocervical c.,** canalis cervicis uteri. **utriculosaccular c.,** ductus utriculosaccularis. **vaginal c.,** the space within the vagina; called also *vulvouterine c.* **Van Hoorne's c.,** thoracic duct (ductus thoracicus [NA]). **vector c.** (*obs.*), a channel for the passage of ova; an oviduct, def. 1. **ventricular c.,** canalis ventriculi. **Verneuil's c's,** collateral vessels of a venous trunk. **vertebral c.,** canalis vertebralis. **vestibular c.,** scala vestibuli. **vidian c.,** canalis pterygoideus. **Volkmann's c's,** passages other than haversian canals, for the passage of blood vessels through bone. **vomerine c.,** canalis vomerovaginalis. **vomerobasilar c., lateral inferior,** canalis palatovaginalis. **vomerobasilar c., lateral superior,** canalis vomerovaginalis. **vomerovaginal c.,** canalis vomerovaginalis. **vulvar c.,** vestibulum vaginae. **vulvouterine c.,** vaginal c. **c. of Wirsung,** ductus pancreaticus. **zygomaticofacial c.,** foramen zygomaticofaciale. **zygomaticotemporal c.,** foramen zygomaticotemporale.

canales (kah-na'lēz) [L.] plural of *canalis.*

canalicular (kan″ah-lik'u-lar) resembling or pertaining to a canaliculus.

canaliculi (kan″ah-lik'u-li) [L.] plural of *canaliculus.*

canaliculization (kan″ah-lik″u-li-za'shun) the development of canaliculi, as in bone.

canaliculodacryocystostomy (kan″ah-lik″u-lo-dak″re-o-sis-tos′to-me) correction of a congenitally blocked tear duct by excision of the blocked portion and anastomosis of the patent portion to the lacrimal sac.

canaliculorhinostomy (kan″ah-lik″u-lo-ri-nos′to-me) dacryocystorhinostomy.

canaliculus (kan″ah-lik'u-lus), pl. *canalic'uli* [L. dim. of *canalis*] [NA] an extremely narrow tubular passage or channel; used as a general term in anatomical nomenclature for various small channels. **apical c.,** any of the numerous tubular invaginations arising from the clefts between the microvilli of the proximal convoluted tubule of the kidney and extending downward into the apical cytoplasm. **bile canaliculi, biliary canaliculi,** fine tubular canals running between liver cells, throughout the parenchyma, usually occurring singly between each adjacent pair of cells, and forming a three-dimensional network of polyhedral meshes, with a single cell in each mesh. Called also *bile capillaries.* **bone canaliculi,** branching tubular passages radiating like wheel spokes from each bone lacuna to connect with the canaliculi of adjacent lacunae, and with the haversian canal. **caroticotympanic canaliculi, canalic'uli caroticotympan'ici** [NA], caroticotympanic canals: tiny passages in the temporal bone interconnecting the carotid canal and the tympanic cavity, and carrying communicating twigs between the internal carotid and tympanic plexuses; called also *caroticotympanic foramina.* **c. of chorda tympani, c. chor'dae tym'pani** [NA], a small canal that opens off the facial canal just before its termination, transmitting the chorda tympani nerve into the tympanic cavity; called also *canal of chorda tympani, canalis chordae tympani,* and *Civinini's canal.* **c. of cochlea, c. coch'leae** [NA], a small canal in the petrous part of the temporal bone that interconnects the scala tympani of the inner ear with the subarachnoid cavity; it lodges the perilymphatic duct and a small vein. Called also *aqueduct of cochlea* and *aqueduct of Cotunnius.* **dental canaliculi, canalic'uli denta'les** [NA], dentinal canals: minute channels in dentin, extending from the pulp cavity to the cementum and enamel. Called also *dental* or *dentinal tubules.* **haversian c.,** any one of a system of minute channels in compact bone connected with each haversian canal. **incisor c.,**

ductus incisivus. **innominate c., c. innomina'tus,** sulcus nervi petrosi minoris. **intercellular c.,** one located between adjacent cells, such as one of the secretory capillaries, or canaliculi, of the gastric parietal cells. **intracellular canaliculi of parietal cells,** a system of canaliculi that seem to be intracellular, but are formed by deep invaginations of the surface of the gastric parietal cells rather than extending into the cytoplasm of the cell. **c. lacrima'lis** [NA], the short passage in an eyelid, beginning at the punctum, that leads from the lacrimal lake to the lacrimal sac; called also *lacrimal duct* and *ductus lacrimalis.* **c. laqueifor'mis,** Henle's loops. **mastoid c., mastoid c. for Arnold's nerve,** c. mastoideus. **c. mastoi'deus** [NA], a minute passage beginning in the lateral wall of the jugular fossa of the temporal bone and passing into the temporal bone. The tympanic branch of the vagus nerve passes through it to exit via the tympanomastoid fissure. Called also *mastoid c.* (*for Arnold's nerve*). **c. petro'sus, petrous c.,** sulcus nervi petrosi minoris. **pseudobile c.,** one of the dark-staining columns of cells from the bile ducts seen in the portal area of the liver in cirrhosis. **secretory c.,** see under *capillary.* **Thiersch's c.,** one of the small channels in newly formed repair tissue through which the nutritive fluids circulate. **tympanic c., tympanic c. for Jacobson's nerve,** c. tympanicus. **c. tympan'icus** [NA], a small opening on the inferior surface of the petrous part of the temporal bone in the floor of the petrosal fossa; it transmits the tympanic branch of the glossopharyngeal nerve and a small artery. Called also *Jacobson's canal, canal for Jacobson's nerve,* and *tympanic canaliculus* (*for Jacobson's nerve*).

canalis (kah-na'lis), pl. *cana'les* [L.] [NA] a general term for a relatively narrow tubular passage or channel; called also *canal.* **c. adducto'rius** [NA], adductor canal: an intramuscular interval on the medial aspect of the middle third of the thigh, which contains the femoral vessels and the saphenous nerve. The lateral wall is formed by the vastus medialis, the posterior wall by the adductor longus and adductor magnus, the roof by a layer of fascia, and it is covered by the sartorius. Called also *crural canal of Henle, Hunter's canal, subsartorial canal,* and *canalis subsartorialis.* **c. alimenta'rius** [NA], alimentary canal: that part of the digestive tract formed by the esophagus, stomach, and small and large intestines; called also *alimentary tract, digestive canal, tract,* or *tube,* and *tubus digestorius.* **cana'les alveola'res,** see *canales alveolares maxillae* and *c. mandibulae.* **cana'les alveola'res maxil'lae** [NA], alveolar canals of maxilla: several canals in the maxilla for the passage of the posterior superior alveolar vessels and nerves, each canal beginning on the infratemporal surface of the maxilla at an alveolar foramen; called also *posterior dental canals.* **c. ana'lis** [NA], anal canal: the terminal portion of the alimentary canal, extending from the rectum to the anus; called also *pars analis recti.* **c. basipharyn'geus,** canalis vomerovaginalis. **c. carot'icus** [NA], carotid canal: a passage in the petrous portion of the temporal bone, beginning on the inferior surface just anterior to the jugular foramen, and running anteromedially for about 2 cm.; it is seen interiorly in the floor of the middle cranial fossa, where it meets the carotid sulcus on the body of the sphenoid bone. It lodges the internal carotid artery. **c. car'pi** [NA], carpal canal: an osseofibrous tunnel for passage of the tendons of the flexor muscles of the hand and digits, formed by the flexor retinaculum as it roofs over the concavity of the carpus on the palmar surface; called also *carpal tunnel* and *flexor canal.* **c. centra'lis medul'lae spina'lis** [NA], central canal of spinal cord: a small canal extending throughout the length of the spinal cord, lined by ependymal cells. Above, it continues into the medulla oblongata, where it opens into the fourth ventricle. **c. cerv'icis u'teri** [NA], cervical canal of uterus: the part of the uterine cavity that lies within the cervix. **c. chor'dae tym'pani,** canaliculus chordae tympani. **c. condyla'ris** [NA], condylar canal: an opening sometimes present in the floor of the condylar fossa for the transmission of a vein from the transverse sinus; called also *c. condyloideus, condyloid canal,* and *posterior condyloid foramen.* **c. condyloi'deus,** canalis condylaris. **cana'les diplo'ici** [NA], diploic canals: bony canals in the cranial bones, located in the spongy bone between the compact tables and providing for passage of the veins of the diploë; called also *canales diploici* [*Brescheti*] and *Breschet's canals.* **c. facia'lis** [NA], **c. fascia'lis** [*Fallo'pii*], facial canal: a canal in the temporal bone for the facial nerve, beginning in the internal acoustic meatus and passing anterolaterally dorsal to the vestibule of the inner ear for about 2 mm. Turning sharply backward at the genu of the facial canal, it runs along the medial wall of the tympanic cavity, then turns inferiorly and reaches the exterior of the petrous part of the bone at the stylomastoid foramen. Called also *canal for facial nerve, fallopian aqueduct* or *canal, aqueduct of Fallopius,* and *spiroid canal.* **c. femora'lis** [NA], femoral canal: the cone-shaped medial part of the femoral sheath lateral to the base of the lacunar ligament; called also *crural canal.* **c. hyaloi'deus** [NA], hyaloid canal: a passage running from in front of the optic disk to the lens of the eye; in the fetus it transmits the hyaloid artery. Called also *central canal of Stilling, central canal of vitreous,* and *Cloquet's canal.* **c. hypoglos'si** [NA], hypoglossal canal: an opening in the lateral part of the occipital bone at the base of the condyle, which transmits the hypoglossal nerve and a branch of the posterior meningeal artery; called also *anterior condyloid canal*, and *anterior condyloid foramen*. **c. incisi′vus** [NA], incisive canal: one of the small canals opening into the incisive fossa of the hard palate, and transmitting small vessels and nerves from the floor of the nose into the front part of the roof of the mouth; called also *anterior palatine canal*, or *groove, nasopalatine canal*, and *foramen of Stensen*. **c. infraorbita′lis** [NA], infraorbital canal: a passage beneath the orbital surface of the maxilla, continuous posteriorly with the infraorbital sulcus, and opening anteriorly on the anterior surface of the body of the maxilla in the infraorbital foramen. It contains the infraorbital vessels and nerve. **c. inguina′lis** [NA], inguinal canal: the passage superficial to the deep inguinal ring for transmission of the spermatic cord in the male and the round ligament in the female; called also *abdominal canal*. **cana′les longitudina′les modi′oli** [NA], longitudinal canals of modiolus: short tunnels in the modiolus that transmit blood vessels and nerves. **c. mandib′ulae** [NA], mandibular canal: a canal that traverses the ramus and body of the mandible between the mandibular and mental foramina, transmitting the inferior alveolar vessels and nerve; called also *inferior dental canal*. **c. musculotuba′rius** [NA], musculotubal canal: the combined canals of the auditory tube and the tensor tympani muscle in the temporal bone; called also *osseous eustachian canal*. **c. nasolacrima′lis** [NA], nasolacrimal canal: a canal formed by the lacrimal sulcus of the maxilla, lacrimal bone, and inferior nasal concha; it contains the nasolacrimal duct. Called also *lacrimal canal*, and *nasal canal*. **c. nutri′cius os′sis** [NA], one of the freely anastomosing channels of the haversian system of compact bone, which contain blood vessels, lymph vessels, and nerves; called also *haversian canal* and *haversian space*. **c. obturato′rius** [NA], obturator canal: an opening within the obturator membrane for the passage of the obturator vessels and nerve; its boundaries are the edge of the obturator membrane, together with the obturator groove of the pubic bone. **c. op′ticus** [NA], optic canal: one of the paired openings in the sphenoid bone where the small wings are attached to the body of the bone at the apex of the orbit; each canal transmits one of the optic nerves and the ophthalmic artery of that side. Called also *foramen opticum ossis sphenoidalis* and *optic foramen of sphenoid bone*. **cana′les palati′ni**, canales palatini minores. **c. palati′nus ma′jor** [NA], great palatine canal: a passage in the sphenoid and palatine bones for the greater palatine vessels and nerve; called also *c. pterygopalatinus, palatomaxillary canal, pterygopalatine canal, sphenopalatine canal*, and *Tourtual's canal*. **cana′les palati′ni mino′res** [NA], lesser palatine canals: openings in the palatine bone that branch off the great palatine canal to carry the lesser and middle palatine nerves and vessels to the roof of the mouth. Called also *canales palatini*, and *accessory or posterior palatine canals*. **c. palatovagina′lis** [NA], palatovaginal canal: a narrow canal located in the roof of the nasal cavity between the inferior surface of the body of the sphenoid bone and the sphenoidal process of the palatine bone; it opens posteriorly into the nasal cavity and anteriorly into the pterygopalatine fossa. Called also *c. pharyngeus, pharyngeal canal, pterygopalatine canal, sphenopalatine canal, sphenopharyngeal canal*, and *lateral inferior vomerobasilar canal*. **c. pharyn′geus**, canalis palatovaginalis. **c. pterygoi′deus** [NA], pterygoid canal: a horizontally running canal that passes forward through the base of the medial pterygoid plate of the sphenoid bone to open into the posterior wall of the ptergopalatine fossa just medial and inferior to the foramen rotundum; it transmits the pterygoid vessels and nerves. Called also *c. pterygoideus [Vidii], canal of Guidi, recurrent canal*, and *vidian canal*. **c. pterygopalati′nus**, c. palatinus major. **c. pudenda′lis** [NA], pudendal canal: the tunnel in the special fascial sheath through which the pudendal vessels and nerve pass; it is intimately related to the obturator fascia. Called also *Alcock's canal*. **c. pylor′icus** [NA], pyloric canal: the short narrow part of the stomach extending from the gastroduodenal junction to the pyloric antrum. **c. rad′icis den′tis** [NA], that portion of the pulp cavity in the root of a tooth, extending from the pulp chamber to the apical foramen; called also *root canal (of tooth)* and *pulp canal*. **c. reu′niens**, ductus reuniens. **c. sacra′lis** [NA], sacral canal: the continuation of the vertebral canal through the sacrum. **c. semicircula′ris ante′rior** [NA], anterior semicircular canal: the anterior of the osseous semicircular canals, lodging the ductus semicircularis anterior. Called also *c. semicircularis superior*. See *canales semicirculares ossei*. **c. semicircula′ris latera′lis** [NA], lateral semicircular canal: the lateral of the semicircular canals, lodging the ductus semicircularis lateralis; called also *horizontal semicircular canal*. See *canales semicirculares ossei*. **cana′les semicircular′es os′sei** [NA], three long canals of the bony labyrinth of the ear (lateral, anterior, and posterior), forming loops and opening into the vestibule by five openings. They lodge the semicircular ducts (ductus semicirculares [NA]) of the membranous labyrinth. Called also *semicircular canals*. **c. semicircula′ris poste′rior** [NA], posterior semicircular canal: the posterior of the semicircular canals, lodging the ductus semicircularis posterior; see *canales semicirculares ossei*. **c. semicircula′ris supe′rior**, c. semicircularis anterior. **c. spina′lis**, c. vertebralis. **c. spira′lis**

coch′leae [NA], spiral canal of cochlea: a winding tube that makes two and one-half turns about the modiolus of the cochlea; it is divided into two compartments, scala tympani and scala vestibuli, by the lamina spiralis. Called also *cochlear duct*. **c. spira′lis modio′li** [NA], spiral canal of modiolus: a canal following the course of the bony spiral lamina of the cochlea and containing the spiral ganglion of the cochlear division of the vestibulocochlear nerve. Called also *ganglionic canal* and *Rosenthal's canal*. **c. subsartoria′lis**, c. adductorius. **c. ventric′uli** [NA], ventricular canal: the longitudinal grooved channel formed by the more or less regular ridges along the lesser curvature of the stomach; called also *magenstrasse*. **c. vertebra′lis** [NA], vertebral canal: the canal formed by the foramina in the successive vertebrae, which encloses the spinal cord and meninges; called also *c. spinalis, medullary canal, neural canal*, and *spinal canal*. **c. vomerovagina′lis** [NA], vomerovaginal canal: an inconstant opening formed by the articulating margins of the ala of the vomer and the body of the sphenoid bone; called also *c. basipharyngeus, basipharyngeal canal, lateral superior vomerobasilar canal*, and *vomerine canal*.

canalization (kan″al-i-za′shun) 1. the formation of canals, natural or morbid. 2. the surgical establishment of canals for drainage. 3. the formation of new canals or paths, especially blood vessels, through an obstruction, such as a clot. 4. in psychology, the formation in the central nervous system of new pathways by the repeated passage of nerve impulses.

canaloplasty (kah-nal′o-plas″te) plastic reconstruction of a passage, as of the external auditory meatus.

canarypox (kah-na′re-poks) an eruptive disease of canaries due to a poxvirus.

Canavalia (kan″ah-val′i-ah) a genus of leguminous plants, the Jack bean, native to the West Indies but widely cultivated as a source of food for humans and livestock. *C. ensifor′mis* D.C. and other species are the source of canavalin and concanavallin.

canavalin (kan″ah-val′in) an antibacterial substance isolated from the meal of the Jack bean (*Canavalia ensiformis* D.C., and other species of *Canavalia*).

canavanase (kan-av′ah-nās) an enzyme from human liver that catalyzes the hydrolysis of canavanine into caveline and urea.

canavanine (kan-av′ĭ-nin) 2-amino-4-(guanidino-oxy)-butyric acid isolated from soy bean meal; it is $NH_2 \cdot C(:NH) \cdot NH \cdot O \cdot CH_2 \cdot CH_2 \cdot CH(NH_2) \cdot COOH$.

cancellated (kan′sel-lāt-ed) having a lattice-like structure.

cancelli (kan-sel′i) [L.] plural of *cancellus*.

cancellous (kan′sĕ-lus) of a reticular, spongy, or lattice-like structure; said mainly of bony tissue.

cancellus (kan-sel′us), pl. *cancel′li* [L. "a lattice"] [NA] any structure arranged like a lattice.

cancer (kan′ser) [L. "crab"] a cellular tumor the natural course of which is fatal. Cancer cells, unlike benign tumor cells, exhibit the properties of invasion and metastasis and are highly anaplastic. Cancers are divided into two broad categories of carcinoma and sarcoma. **acinar c., acinous c.,** alveolar adenocarcinoma. **adenoid c.,** a malignant tumor made up of or containing cylindrical tubes lined with epithelium. **c. à deux** [Fr. "cancer in two"], cancer attacking simultaneously or consecutively two persons who live together. **alveolar c.,** see under *adenocarcinoma*. **aniline c.,** cancer due to aniline dyes, occurring among those who work in dye factories and dyeing establishments. **apinoid c.,** scirrhous c. **c. aquat′icus** (*obs.*), gangrenous stomatitis. **areolar c.** (*obs.*), mucinous carcinoma. **c. atroph′icans,** scirrhous cancer surrounded by sclerosed and atrophied tissue. **betel c.,** buyo cheek c. **black c.,** malignant melanoma. **boring c.,** epithelioma of the skin of the face. **branchiogenous c.,** cancer originating in the superior cervical triangle, and supposed to be derived from a relic of an embryonal branchial cleft. **Butter's c.,** carcinoma of the hepatic flexure of the colon. **buyo cheek c.,** cancer of the cheek seen in natives of the Philippine Islands from chewing buyo leaf or betel; called also *betel c.* **cellular c.,** medullary carcinoma. **cerebriform c.,** medullary carcinoma. **chimney-sweeps' c.,** carcinoma of the scrotum due to soot poisoning; called also *soot c.* **chondroid c.,** scirrhous carcinoma with a cartilage-like texture. **claypipe c.,** carcinoma of the lip due to irritation caused by a pipe stem. **colloid c.,** mucinous carcinoma. **contact c.,** cancer developing in a part of the body in contact with a previously existing cancer. **corset c.,** cancer en cuirasse. **cystic c.,** carcinoma that has undergone cystic degeneration. **dendritic c.,** papillary carcinoma. **dermoid c.** (*obs.*), squamous cell carcinoma. **duct c.,** carcinoma arising from the epithelium of a duct. **dye workers' c.,** carcinoma of the urinary bladder frequently observed among workers in aniline dyes. **c. en cuirasse,** a carcinoma about the skin of the thorax; called also *corset c.* and *jacket c.* **endothelial c.,** endothelioma. **epidermal c.,** malignant epithelioma of the skin. **epithelial c.,** carcinoma. **fungous c.** (*obs.*), fungus haematodes. **glandular c.,** adenocarcinoma. **green c.,** chloroma. **hard c.,** scirrhous carcinoma. **hematoid c.** (*obs.*), fungus haematodes. **c. in si′tu,** carcinoma in situ. **jacket c.,** c. en cuirasse.

kang c., kangri c., epithelioma in the thigh or abdomen affecting Indian and Chinese natives, and attributed to irritation from the kang (heated brick oven) or from the kangri (fire basket). **latent c.,** microscopic carcinomas of the prostate discovered, in the absence of any clinical manifestations, in the course of histological examination. **medullary c.,** see under *carcinoma.* **melanotic c.,** malignant melanoma. **mule-spinners' c.,** a form of epithelioma affecting mule spinners in the cotton-spinning industry. **occult c.,** a small prostatic carcinoma that gives rise to clinically evident distant metastases before it is itself clinically detectable. **paraffin c.,** a malignant growth occurring in those who work in paraffin. **pitchworkers' c.,** epithelioma of the face, neck, and scrotum seen in those who work in pitch. **retrograde c.,** a dormant atrophied malignant growth. **rodent c.,** rodent ulcer. **roentgenologist's c.,** cancer affecting the hands of those who work with roentgen rays. **scirrhous c.,** see under *carcinoma.* **soft c.,** medullary carcinoma. **solanoid c.,** (*obs.*), scirrhous carcinoma. **soot c.,** chimney-sweeps' c. **spindle cell c.,** a rare type of carcinoma affecting older persons, in which spindle-cell growth predominates, often associated with giant-cell cancer. These tumors may arise from any epithelial surface, but are most often found in sites that usually produce squamous or transitional cell carcinomas. **tar c.,** carcinoma caused by inflammatory irritation of fumes of tar or by the irritating effect of tar on the skin. **tubular c.,** an adenocarcinoma in which the cells are arranged in the form of tubules. **villous duct c.,** carcinoma with a villous growth pattern arising from the wall of a cyst. **water c.** (*obs.*), gangrenous stomatitis. **withering c.** (*obs.*), scirrhous carcinoma.

canceration (kan-ser-a'shun)   (*obs.*) malignant or carcinomatous degeneration.

canceremia (kan″ser-e'me-ah)   the presence of cancer cells in the blood.

cancericidal (kan″ser-ĭ-si'dal) [*cancer* + L. *caedere* to kill]   destructive to cancer or malignant cells.

cancerigenic (kan″ser-ĭ-jen'ik)   giving rise to a malignant tumor.

cancerin (kan'ser-in)   a white crystalline ptomaine, $C_8H_5NO_3$, from the urine in carcinoma.

cancerism (kan'ser-izm)   the cancerous diathesis, i.e., the tendency to the development of malignant disease.

cancerization (kan″ser-ĭ-za'shun)   canceration.

cancerocidal (kan″ser-o-si'dal)   cancericidal.

cancerogenic (kan″ser-o-jen'ik)   cancerigenic.

cancerology (kan″ser-ol'o-je)   (*obs.*) oncology.

cancerophobia (kan″ser-o-fo'be-ah)   cancerphobia.

cancerous (kan'ser-us)   of the nature of or pertaining to cancer.

cancerphobia (kan″ser-fo'be-ah)   1. morbid dread of becoming affected with cancer. 2. delusion of being affected with cancer. Called also *carcinophobia.*

cancer-ulcer (kan'ser-ul'ser)   carcinomatous ulceration.

cancriform (kang'krĭ-form)   resembling a cancer.

cancroid (kang'kroid) [*cancer* + Gr. *eidos* form]   1. resembling cancer. 2. a skin cancer of a moderate degree of malignancy.

cancrology (kang-krol'o-je) [*cancer* + *-logy*]   (*obs.*) oncology.

cancrum (kang'krum) [L.]   canker. **c. na′si,** gangrenous rhinitis of children. **c. o′ris,** gangrenous stomatitis. **c. puden′di,** see *noma.*

candela (kan-del'ah) [L. *candēla* candle]   the SI unit of luminous intensity equal to one-sixtieth of the luminous intensity per square centimeter of a blackbody radiating at the temperature of the freezing point of platinum. Called also *candle, new candle,* and *standard candle.* Abbreviated cd.

Candeptin (kan-dep'tin)   trademark for preparations of candicidin.

candicidin (kan″dĭ-si'din) [USP]   an antifungal antibiotic produced by a strain of *Streptomyces griseus;* it is especially effective against *Candida albicans,* and is administered intravaginally in the treatment of vaginal candidiasis.

Candida (kan'dĭ-dah) [L. *candidus* glowing white]   a genus of yeastlike imperfect fungi of the family Cryptococcaceae, order Moniliales, characterized by producing yeast cells, mycelia, pseudomycelia, and blastospores. It is commonly part of the normal flora of the skin, mouth, intestinal tract, and vagina, but can cause a variety of infections, including candidiasis, onychomycosis, tinea corporis, tinea pedis, vaginitis, and thrush. *C. albicans* is the usual pathogen, but *C. tropicalis* may also cause infection. Other species are *C. guilliermondi* and *C. krusei.* Called also *Monilia* and *Oidium,* and, formerly, *Blastodendrion,* and *Castellania.* **C. al′bicans,** the most frequent agent of candidiasis. **C. mesenter′ica,** a species which causes fermentation in fruit acids; called also *Saccharomyces mesentericus.* **C. parapsilo′sis,** a species of limited pathogenicity but particularly associated with endocarditis, paronychia, and otitis externa. **C. tropica′lis,** a species that is an occasional cause of candidiasis. **C. vin′i,** a species from fermenting liquors and diabetic urine, in which it produces a slight fermentation seen as cylindrical, oval,

or elliptical cells, forming branched chains; called also *Saccharomyces mycoderma.*

candidal (kan'dĭ-dal)   pertaining to or caused by *Candida.*

candidemia (kan″dĭ-de'me-ah)   the presence in the blood of fungi of the genus *Candida,* usually resulting from candidal endocarditis or systemic candidiasis.

candidiasis (kan″dĭ-di'ah-sis)   infection with a fungus of the genus *Candida.* It is usually a superficial infection of the moist cutaneous areas of the body, and is generally caused by *C. albicans;* it most commonly involves the skin (dermatocandidiasis), oral mucous membranes (thrush, def. 1), respiratory tract (bronchocandidiasis), and vagina (vaginitis). Rarely there is a systemic infection or endocarditis. Called also *moniliasis, candidosis, oidomycosis,* and, formerly, *blastodendriosis.* **cutaneous c.,** candidiasis of the skin, which may be manifested as eczema-like lesions of the interdigital spaces, perlèche, or chronic paronychia; called also *dermatocandidiasis.* **endocardial c.,** mycotic endocarditis caused by various species of *Candida.*

candidid (kan'dĭ-did)   a secondary skin eruption that is the expression of hypersensitivity to infection with *Candida* elsewhere on the body; called also *moniliid.*

candidin (kan'dĭ-din)   a skin test antigen derived from *Candida albicans,* used in testing for the development of delayed-type hypersensitivity to constituents of the microorganism.

candidosis (kan-dĭ-do'sis)   candidiasis.

candiduria (kan″did-u're-ah)   the presence of *Candida* organisms in the urine.

candiru (kan-dĭ-roo′)   any of certain small catfishes of the Amazon River which are said to enter the urethra of men and the vulva of women who bathe in the river.

candle (kan'd'l)   1. a mass of wax or similar substance, usually cylindrical in shape, with a wick for burning, to furnish illumination or heat. 2. a cylindrical mass of material used as a filter in microbiology. 3. candela. **foot c.,** see under *F.* **meter c.,** see *lux.* **new c., standard c.,** candela.

candlefish (kan'd'l fish)   a marine fish, *Thaleichthys pacificus,* of the smelt family, yielding a fixed oil with properties similar to those of cod liver oil.

candol (kan'dol)   a dry malt extract.

cane (kān)   a wooden stick or metal rod used for support in walking. **adjustable c.,** a cane whose length can be easily altered. **English c.,** a supporting device consisting of a single upright with a hand rest at right angles to it; an extension piece above the hand rest, attached at an angle of about 125 degrees to the upright and bent away from the body, has a holder at the top which fits around the forearm, permitting the weight of the body to be supported on the hand and back of the forearms. **quadripod c.,** one adapted for increased stability by forking to provide a four-legged rectangular base of support. **tripod c.,** one similar to a quadripod cane except that it forks to provide a three-legged, triangular base of support.

canescent (kah-nes'ent) [L. *canus* gray]   1. becoming white or grayish. 2. in biology, having grayish or whitish hairs or down; hoary.

canine (ka'nīn) [L. *canis* a dog, hound]   1. of, pertaining to, or like that which belongs to a dog. 2. a canine tooth; see under *tooth.*

caniniform (ka-nīn'ĭ-form)   resembling a canine tooth.

caninus (ka-ni'nus)   musculus levator anguli oris.

canities (kah-nish'e-ēz) [L.]   grayness or whiteness of the scalp hair.

canker (kang'ker)   1. ulceration, chiefly of the mouth and lips; see *aphthous stomatitis,* under *stomatitis.* 2. disease of the keratogenous membrane in horses, beginning at the frog and extending to the sole and wall, marked by a loss of function of the horn-secreting cells and the discharge of a serous exudate in place of normal horn. 3. inflammation of the lining of the external ear in dogs and cats. Called also *cancrum.*

canna (kan'ah) [L.]   a reed, or cane. **c. ma′jor,** the tibia. **c. mi′nor,** the fibula.

cannabidiol (kan″ah-bĭ-di'ōl)   a nonpsychoactive diphenol, $C_{21}H_{30}O_2$, isolated from cannabis.

cannabinoid (kan-ab'ĭ-noid)   any of the principles of *Cannabis,* including tetrahydrocannabinol, cannabinol, and cannabidiol.

cannabinol (kah-nab'ĭ-nol)   a nonpsychoactive constituent, $C_{21}H_{26}O_2$, of resinous exudates of *Cannabis sativa* L.; its tetrahydro derivatives are active principles.

cannabis (kan'ah-bis) [Gr. *kannabis* hemp]   the dried flowering tops of hemp plants, *Cannabis sativa* L. (Cannabaceae), which contains the euphoric principles Δ^1-3,4-*trans* and Δ^6-3,4-*trans* tetrahydrocannabinol, as well as cannabinol and cannabidiol. It is classified as a hallucinogenic and is prepared as bhang, ganja, hashish, and marihuana. See also *cannabism.*

cannabism (kan'ah-bizm)   a morbid state produced by misuse of cannabis; it is usually responsive to simple reassurance in its acute stage. The occurrence of a chronic brain syndrome as a result of frequent and prolonged use is unsubstantiated.

cannibalism (kan'ĭ-bal-izm)   phagocytosis of one malignant cell by another.

Cannizzaro's reaction (kan"e-zah'rōz) [Stanislao *Cannizzaro*, chemist in Rome, 1826–1910]   see under *reaction*.

Cannon's ring (point) (kan'unz) [Walter Bradford *Cannon*, Boston physiologist, 1871–1945, the first to adapt x-ray techniques to the study of digestive function]   see under *ring*.

cannula (kan'u-lah) [L. dim. of *canna* "reed"]   a tube for insertion into a duct or cavity; during insertion its lumen is usually occupied by a trocar.   **Bellocq's c.,** a curved cannula containing a stylet to which is attached a watch spring; used for plugging the posterior nares to control nosebleed. Called also *Bellocq's sound*.   **Lindemann's c.,** a special needle for use with a syringe in the transfusion of unmodified blood.   **perfusion c.,** a double tube for running a continuous flow of liquid into and out of an organ.   **Strauss' c.,** see *Strauss needle*, under *needle*.   **Trendelenburg's c.,** a cannula covered with a dilatable rubber bag, used for closing the trachea to prevent the entrance of blood after tracheotomy.   **washout c.,** a cannula attached to a manometer and inserted into a blood vessel so that the connection between the artery and the manometer can be washed out in long observations.

cannulate (kan'u-lāt)   to introduce a cannula, which may be left in place.

cannulation (kan"u-la'shun)   the insertion of a cannula.

cannulization (kan"u-li-za'shun)   cannulation.

Canomyces (ka"no-mi'sēz)   a microorganism of the pleuropneumonia group found in dog distemper.

canon (kan'un) [L. "rule"]   a working rule or formula for use in scientific procedure.

canrenoate potassium (kan-ren'o-āt)   chemical name: 17-hydroxy-3-oxo-17α-pregna-4,6-diene-21-carboxylic acid monopotassium salt; an aldosterone antagonist, $C_{22}H_{29}KO_4$.

canrenone (kan-ren'ōn)   chemical name: 17-hydroxy-3-oxo-17α-pregna-4,6-diene-21-carboxylic acid γ-lactone. An aldosterone antagonist, $C_{22}H_{28}O_3$; called also *phanurane*.

cant (kant)   an inclination or slope.   **c. of mandible,** the angle formed by the intersection of the mandibular (gonion-gnathion) plane with the sella-nasion or Frankfort plane.

Cantani's treatment (kahn-tah'nēz) [Arnaldo *Cantani*, Italian physician, 1837–1893]   see under *treatment*.

canthal (kan'thal)   pertaining to a canthus.

canthariasis (kan"thah-ri'ah-sis) [Gr. *kantharos* beetle]   infection by beetles as endoparasites in the body of a mammal, following ingestion of larval or adult forms.

cantharidal (kan-thar'ĭ-dal)   containing or pertaining to cantharides.

cantharidate (kan-thar'ĭ-dāt)   any salt of cantharidic acid.

cantharides (kan-thar'ĭ-dēz) [L.]   the dried Spanish fly, *Lytta* (*Cantharis*) *vesicatoria*, sometimes called "blister bug." Cantharides were once applied externally as a powerful rubefacient and blistering agent and given internally as a diuretic and aphrodisiac.

cantharidin (kan-thar'ĭ-din)   the most important active principle of cantharides; it is the lactone of cantharidic acid, $C_{10}H_{12}O_4$, occurs in crystalline form, has a bitter taste, and produces blistering of the skin.

cantharidism (kan-thar'ĭ-dizm)   a morbid condition resulting from the misuse of cantharides.

Cantharis (kan'thah-ris) [L.; Gr. *kantharos* beetle]   *Lytta.*   **C. vesicato'ria,** *Lytta vesicatoria*.

canthectomy (kan-thek'to-me) [Gr. *kanthos* canthus + *ektomē* excision]   surgical removal of a canthus.

canthi (kan'thi) [L.]   plural of *canthus*.

canthitis (kan-thi'tis)   inflammation of a canthus or of the canthi.

cantho- (kan'tho) [Gr. *kanthos*]   a combining form denoting relationship to the canthus.

cantholysis (kan-thol'ĭ-sis) [*cantho-* + *lysis* dissolution]   surgical division of the canthus of an eye or of a canthal ligament.

canthoplasty (kan'tho-plas"te) [*cantho-* + Gr. *plassein* to form]   plastic surgery of the medial and/or lateral canthus, especially section of the lateral canthus to lengthen the palpebral fissure; also the surgical restoration of a defective canthus.   **provisional c.,** canthotomy performed as a temporary measure to enlarge the palpebral aperture.

canthorrhaphy (kan-thor'ah-fe) [*cantho-* + Gr. *rhaphē* suture]   the suturing of the palpebral fissure at either canthus.

canthotomy (kan-thot'o-me) [*cantho-* + Gr. *temnein* to cut]   surgical division of the outer canthus.

canthus (kan'thus), pl. *can'thi* [L.; Gr. *kanthos*]   the angle at either end of the fissure between the eyelids; the canthi are distinguished as outer or temporal, inner or nasal.

Cantil (kan'til)   trademark for a preparation of mepenzolate bromide.

Cantlie's foot tetter [Sir James *Cantlie*, British physician, 1851–1926]   see under *tetter*.

Cantor tube (kan'tor) [Meyer D. *Cantor*, American physician, born 1907]   see under *tube*.

cantus galli (kan'tus gal'li) [L. "cock-crowing"]   laryngismus stridulus.

canula (kan'u-lah)   cannula.

CaO   calcium oxide.

Ca(OH)₂   calcium hydroxide.

caoutchouc (koo'chŏŏk) [Fr.]   gum-elastic or India rubber; the concrete juice of various trees and plants, such as *Siphonia elastica*. It is a hydrocarbon, $C_{20}H_{32}$, soluble in chloroform, ether, and carbon disulfide. Called also *elastica*.

C.A.P.   College of American Pathologists.

Cap.   abbreviation for L. *ca'piat*, let him take.

cap (kap)   a protective covering for the head or for a similar structure.   **acrosomal c.,** acrosome.   **bishop's c.,** pars superior duodeni.   **cradle c.,** crusta lactea.   **duodenal c.,** pars superior duodeni.   **dutch c.,** a contraceptive cervical diaphragm.   **enamel c.,** the enamel organ after it covers the top of the growing tooth papilla.   **head c.,** the double-layed cap-like structure over the upper two-thirds of the acrosome of a spermatozoon, consisting of the collapsed acrosomal vesicle.   **head c., anterior,** acrosome.   **knee c.,** patella.   **metanephric c's,** masses of metanephric blastema that adhere to the primordial pelvis of the kidney and to its ampullary dilatations.   **phrygian c.,** the cholecystographic appearance of the gallbladder showing kinking between the body and the fundus, in which the fundus is fixed and folded.   **postnuclear c.,** a broad band encircling the postacrosomal region of the nucleus of a spermatozoon.   **pyloric c.,** pars superior duodeni.   **root c.,** a thimble-shaped group of cells forming a protective covering over the apical meristem in the tip of a plant root.   **skull c.,** calvaria.   **c. of Zinn,** a prominence of the pulmonary arc in the left upper portion of the cardiac silhouette, usually seen in posteroanterior roentgenograms in cases of patent ductus arteriosus, and representing the dilated pulmonary artery.

capacitance (kah-pas'ĭ-tans)   1. the property of being able to store an electric charge.   2. the ratio of charge to potential in a conductor.   **membrane c.,** the electrical capacitance of a cell membrane, as of an axon or muscle fiber.

capacitation (kah-pas"ĭ-ta'shun)   the process by which spermatozoa become capable of fertilizing an ovum after it reaches the ampullary portion of the uterine tube.

capacitor (kah-pas'ĭ-tor)   a device for holding and storing charges of electricity.

capacity (kah-pas'ĭ-te) [L. *capacitas*, from *capere* to take]   1. power or ability to hold, retain, or contain, or the ability to absorb.   2. an expression of the measurement of material that may be held or contained.   3. in electricity, the property by which a given body will take and hold an electric charge.   4. mental ability to receive, accomplish, endure, or understand.   **cranial c.,** an expression of the amount of space within the cranium.   **functional residual c.,** the amount of air remaining at the end of normal quiet respiration; abbreviated FRC. See accompanying illustration.   **heat c.,** thermal c.   **inspiratory c.,** the volume of gas that can be taken into the lungs on a full inspiration, starting from the resting inspiratory position; it is equal to the tidal volume plus the inspiratory reserve volume. Abbreviated IC. See accompanying illustration.   **maximal breathing c.,** the greatest volume of gas that can be breathed per minute by voluntary effort; abbreviated MBC.   **maximal tubular excretory c.,** see *tubular maximum*, under *maximum*.   **respiratory c.,** the ability of the blood to absorb oxygen from the lungs and carbon dioxide from the tissues.   **thermal c.,** the amount of heat absorbed by a body in being raised from 15° to 16° C. in temperature; called also *heat c.*   **total lung c.,** the volume of gas contained in the lungs at the end of a maximal inspiration; abbreviated TLC. See accompanying illustration.   **virus neutralizing c.,** the ability of a serum to inhibit the infectivity of a virus.   **vital c.,** the volume of gas that can be expelled from the lungs from a position of full inspiration, with no limit to the duration of expiration; it is equal to the inspiratory capacity plus the expiratory reserve volume. See diagram on following page.

Capastat (kap'ah-stat)   trademark for a preparation of capreomycin sulfate.

capelet (kap'e-let) [L. *capelletum*]   a swelling on the point of a horse's hock or on its elbow; called also *capulet*.

capeline (kap'ĕ-lin) [Fr.]   a cap-shaped bandage for the head or for the stump of an amputated limb.

capiat (ka'pe-at) [L. "let it take"]   (obs.) an instrument for removing foreign bodies from a cavity, as from the uterus.

capillarectasia (kap"ĭ-lār"ek-ta'se-ah) [*capillary* + Gr. *ektasis* distention]   dilatation of capillaries.

Capillaria (kap"ĭ-la're-ah)   a genus of nematodes of the superfamily Trichuroidea; called also *Hepaticola* and *Trichosoma*.   **C. contor'ta,** a roundworm parasitic in domestic fowls; called also *Trichosoma contortum*.   **C. hepat'ica,** a species parasitic in the liver tissue of rats and of a wide variety of other mammals; a few human infections have been reported.   **C. philip-**

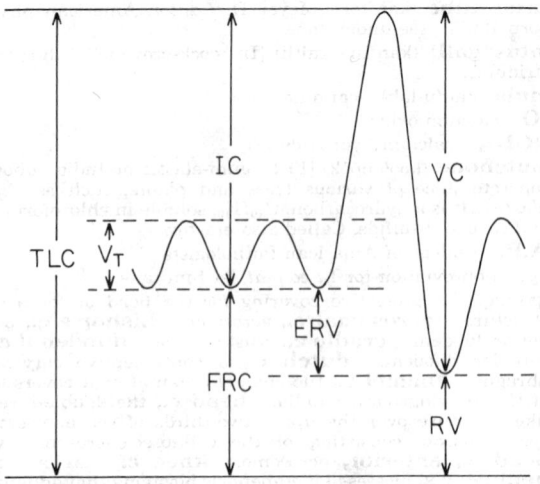

Subdivisions of total lung capacity: *TLC* = total lung capacity; *V_T* = tidal volume; *IC* = inspiratory capacity; *FRC* = functional residual capacity; *ERV* = expiratory reserve volume; *VC* = vital capacity; *RV* = residual volume. (Bates, Macklem, and Christie.)

pinen′sis, a parasite of the human intestine in Luzon, causing severe diarrhea, malabsorption, and high mortality.

capillariasis (kap″ĭ-lah-ri′ah-sis) infection with nematodes of the genus *Capillaria*, especially *C. philippinensis*.

capillariomotor (kap″ĭ-lār″e-o-mo′tor) pertaining to the functional activity of the capillaries.

capillarioscopy (kap″ĭ-lār″e-os′ko-pe) capillaroscopy.

capillaritis (kap″ĭ-lār-i′tis) inflammation of the capillaries.

capillarity (kap″ĭ-lār′ĭ-te) the action by which the surface of a liquid where it is in contact with a solid, as in capillary tubes, is elevated or depressed.

capillaropathy (kap″ĭ-lār-op′ah-the) [*capillary* + Gr. *pathos* disease] any disease of the capillaries.

capillaroscopy (kap″ĭ-lār-os′ko-pe) [*capillary* + Gr. *skopein* to examine] diagnostic examination of the capillaries with the microscope.

capillary (kap′ĭ-lar″e) [L. *capillaris* hair-like] 1. pertaining to or resembling a hair. 2. any one of the minute vessels that connect the arterioles and venules, forming a network in nearly all parts of the body. Their walls act as semipermeable membranes for the interchange of various substances, including fluids, between the blood and tissue fluid; called also *vas capillare* [NA]. **arterial c's,** minute vessels lacking a continuous mus-

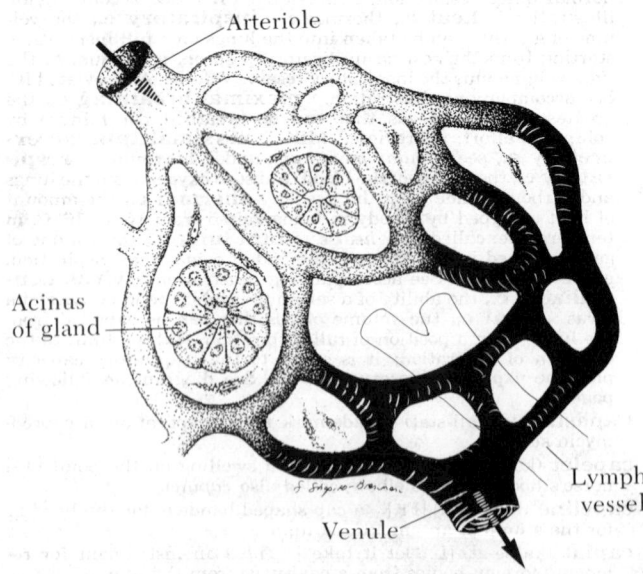

Capillary bed: lighter areas indicate oxygenated blood.

cular coat, intermediate in structure and location between arterioles and capillaries; called also *precapillaries, precapillary arterioles,* and *metarterioles.* **bile c's,** 1. bile canaliculi. 2. a term sometimes used to designate the cholangioles. **continuous c's,** one of the two major types of capillaries found in muscle, skin, lung, central nervous system, and other tissues, characterized by the presence of an uninterrupted endothelium and a continuous

basal lamina, and by fine filaments and numerous pinocytotic vesicles. Cf. *fenestrated c's.* **erythrocytic c's,** capillaries of the bone marrow of early life which seem to produce erythrocytes. **fenestrated c's,** one of the two major types of capillaries, found in the intestinal mucosa, renal glomeruli, pancreas, endocrine glands, and other tissues, and characterized by the presence of circular fenestrae or pores that penetrate the endothelium; these pores may be closed by a very thin diaphragm. Cf. *continuous c's.* **glomerular c.,** any of the capillaries of a renal glomerulus. **lymph c., lymphatic c.,** one of the most minute vessels of the lymphatic system, having a caliber slightly greater than that of a capillary of the blood circulatory system. **Meigs' c's,** capillaries in the myocardium. **secretory c's,** any of the extremely fine intercellular canaliculi situated between adjacent gland cells, such as the gastric parietal cells, being formed by the apposition of grooves in the surfaces of the cells, and opening into the gland's lumen. **sheathed c's,** see under *artery.* **sinusoidal c's,** sinusoid, def. 2. **venous c's,** minute vessels lacking a muscular coat, intermediate in structure and location between venules and capillaries; called also *postcapillaries* and *postcapillary venules.*

capilli (kah-pil′li) [L.] plural of *capillus.*

capillitium (kap″ĭ-lish′e-um) [L. "head of hair"] the interlacing, filamentous structure which, with the spores, fills the spore case of Myxobacteriales.

capillomotor (kap″ĭ-lo-mo′tor) capillariomotor.

capillus (kah-pil′lus), pl. *capil′li* [L.] a hair; used in the plural, in anatomical terminology, especially to designate the aggregate of hair on the scalp.

capistration (kap″ĭ-stra′shun) [L. *capistratus* masked] phimosis.

capita (kap′ĭ-tah) [L.] plural of *caput.*

capital (kap′ĭ-tal) 1. of the highest importance; involving danger to life. 2. of or pertaining to the head of the femur.

capitate (kap′ĭ-tāt) [L. *caput* head] head-shaped.

capitation (kap″ĭ-ta′shun) the annual fee paid to a physician or group of physicians by each participant in a health plan.

capitatum (kap″ĭ-ta′tum) [L. "having a head"] the capitate bone, or os capitatum [NA].

capitellum (kap″ĭ-tel′um) [L. dim. of *caput* head] capitulum humeri.

capitonnage (kap″ĭ-to-nahzh′) [Fr.] the surgical closure of a cyst cavity by applying sutures in such a way as to cause approximation of the opposing surfaces.

capitopedal (kap″ĭ-to-ped′al) pertaining to the head and foot.

Capitrol (kap′ĭ-trol) trademark for a preparation of chloroxine.

capitula (kah-pit′u-lah) [L.] plural of *capitulum.*

capitular (kah-pit′u-lar) pertaining to a capitulum or head of a bone.

capitulum (kah-pit′u-lum), pl. *capit′ula* [L. dim. of *caput*] a general term for a little head, or a small eminence on a bone by which it articulates with another bone; in NA applied only to the distal end of the humerus, since that bone already possesses a head (caput). **c. cos′tae,** caput costae. **c. fib′ulae,** caput fibulae. **c. hu′meri** [NA], **c. of humerus,** an eminence on the distal end of the lateral epicondyle of the humerus for articulation with the head of the radius; called also *capitellum* and *little* or *radial head of humerus.* **c. mal′lei,** caput mallei. **c. os′sis metacarpa′lis,** caput ossis metacarpalis. **c. os′sis metatarsa′lis,** caput ossis metatarsalis. **c. [proces′sus condyloi′dei] mandib′ulae,** caput mandibulae. **c. ra′dii,** caput radii. **c. sta′pedis,** caput stapedis. **c. ul′nae,** caput ulnae.

Capla (kap′lah) trademark for a preparation of mebutamate.

capno- [Gr. *kapnos* smoke] a combining form signifying a sooty or smoky appearance.

Capnocytophaga (kap″no-si-tof′ah-gah) [*capno-* + Gr. *kytos* cell + *phagein* to eat] a genus of anaerobic, gram-negative, rod-shaped bacteria that are implicated in the pathogenesis of periodontal disease; they closely resemble *Bacteroides ochraceus.*

capnohepatography (kap″no-hep″ah-tog′rah-fe) radiography of the liver after intravenous injection of carbon dioxide gas.

capnophilic (kap-no-fil′ik) [Gr. *kapnos* smoke + *philein* to love] growing best in the presence of carbon dioxide; said of bacteria.

Ca₃(PO₄)₂ tribasic calcium phosphate.

capobenate sodium (kap-o-ben′āt) chemical name: 6-[(3,4,5-trimethoxybenzoyl) amino]hexanoic acid monosodium salt. The monosodium salt of capobenic acid, $C_{16}H_{22}NNaO_6$, having cardiac depressant activity; used as an antiarrhythmic.

capon (ka′pon) a castrated domestic fowl.

caponize (ka′pon-īz) to castrate, especially male domestic fowl.

capotement (kah-pōt-maw′) [Fr.] a splashing sound heard in the dilated stomach.

cappie (kap′e) a disease of young sheep characterized by thinning of the bones of the scalp, possibly due to phosphorus-deficient diet.

capping (kap′ing) 1. the provision of a protective or obstructive covering. 2. the formation of a polar cap on the surface of a lymphoid cell concerned with immunologic responses, occurring as a result of movement of components on the cell surface into clusters or patches that coalesce to form the cap. The cap later undergoes endocytosis and disappears. The process is produced by reaction of antibody with the cell membrane, and appears to involve cross-linking of antigenic determinants. It is seen also in various other cells such as protozoa. **direct pulp c.**, a procedure in which an antiseptic, anodyne, or protective material is placed directly over the pulp at the site of exposure. **indirect pulp c.**, a procedure in which an antiseptic, anodyne, or protective material is placed over a thin partition of dentin at a site in which the pulp is nearly exposed. **pulp c.**, the covering of an exposed or nearly exposed dental pulp with some material, medicated or nonmedicated, to provide protection against external influences and to encourage healing.

caprate (kap′rāt)   any salt of capric acid.

capreolary (kap′re-o-la″re)   capreolate.

capreolate (kap′re-o-lāt)   tendril shaped, like the spermatic vessels.

capreomycin (kap″re-o-mi′sin)   a polypeptide antibiotic produced by Streptomyces capreolus, which is active against human strains of Mycobacterium tuberculosis and has four microbiologically active components. **c. sul′ate, sterile** [USP], the disulfate salt of capreomycin, occurring as a white to practically white, amorphous powder; used as a tuberculostatic, administered intramuscularly.

caprillic (kah-pril′ik) [L. caper goat]   goatlike; said of sounds resembling the bleating of a goat.

capriloquism (kah-pril′o-kwizm) [L. caper goat + loqui to speak]   egophony.

caprin (kap′rin)   any one of the caprates of glycerin (glycerol) especially the glyceryl tricaprate, or tricaprin, $C_3H_5[CH_3(CH_2)_8$-$COO]_3$, from ordinary butter.

caprine (kap′rin) [L. caper goat]   1. pertaining to or derived from a goat.   2. norleucine.

caprizant (kap′rĭ-zant) [L. caprizans, from caper a goat]   leaping or bounding (like a goat); said of the pulse.

caproate (kap′ro-āt)   1. any salt of caproic acid.   2. USAN contraction for hexanoate.

caproin (kah-pro′in)   any caproate of glycerin (glycerol) especially the tricaproate, $C_3H_5(C_6H_{13}O_2)_3$; it occurs in butter.

caprone (kap′rōn)   a volatile oil, di-n-amylketone 6-undecanone, $CH_3(CH_2)_4\cdot CO(CH_2)_4\cdot CH_3$, from butter.

caproyl (kap-ro′il)   the hydrocarbon radical, C_6H_{13}; hexyl.

caproylamine (kap″ro-il-am′in)   n-hexylamine.

caprylate (kap′rĭ-lāt)   any salt of caprylic acid.

caprylin (kap′rĭ-lin)   any caprylate of glycerin (glycerol) especially the tricaprylate, $C_3H_5(C_7H_{15}CO_2)_3$.

Capsebon (kap′se-bon)   trademark for a suspension of cadmium sulfide.

Capsicum (kap′sĭ-kum) [L.]   a genus of solanaceous plants of various species, including the cayenne or red pepper.

capsicum (kap′sĭ-kum)   the dried fruit of various species of Capsicum, used as an irritant and carminative. It is known in commerce as African chillies (C. frutescens), tabasco pepper (C. annum var. conoidis), Louisiana long pepper (C. annum var. longum), and Louisiana sport pepper (a hybrid).

capsid (kap′sid) [L. capsa a box]   the shell of protein that protects the nucleic acid of a virus; it may have helical or cubic symmetry and is composed of structural units, or capsomers. According to the number of subunits possessed by capsomers, they are called dimers (2), trimers (3), pentamers (5), or hexamers (6).

capsitis (kap-si′tis)   inflammation of the capsule of the crystalline lens.

capsomer (kap′so-mer) [L. capsa a box + Gr. meros part]   the morphological unit of the capsid of a virus.

capsomere (kap′so-mēr)   capsomer.

capsotomy (kap-sot′o-me)   capsulotomy.

Capsul.   abbreviation for L. cap′sula, capsule.

capsula (kap′su-lah), pl. cap′sulae [L. "a small box"] [NA]   a general term for a cartilaginous, fatty, fibrous, or membranous structure enveloping another structure, organ, or part; called also capsule. **c. adipo′sa**, a capsule consisting principally of fat. **c. adipo′sa re′nis** [NA], adipose capsule of kidney: the investment of perirenal fat surrounding the fibrous capsule of the kidney and continuous at the hilus with the fat in the renal sinus; called also fatty capsule of kidney. **articula′ris** [NA], articular capsule: the sac-like envelope which encloses the cavity of a synovial joint by attaching to the circumference of the articular end of each involved bone; it consists of a fibrous membrane and a synovial membrane. Called also joint or synovial capsule. **c. articula′ris acromioclavicula′ris** [NA], acromioclavicular articular capsule: a ligamentous sac surrounding the acromioclavicular joint. **c. articula′ris articulatio′nis tar′si transver′sae** [NA], a ligamentous sac surrounding the transverse tarsal joint. **c. articula′ris articulatio′nis temporomandibula′ris** [NA], a ligamentous sac surrounding the temporomandibular joint; called also c. articularis mandibulae and capsule

of temporomandibular joint. **c. articula′ris articulatio′num vertebra′rum** [NA], capsule of vertebral articulations: one of the bands of tissue, partly white fibrous and partly yellow elastic, that unite the articular processes of adjacent vertebrae. **c. articula′ris atlantoaxia′lis latera′lis** [NA], atlantoaxial articular capsule: a ligamentous sac surrounding the lateral atlantoaxial joint; called also (pl.) capsulae articulares atlantoepistrophicae. **cap′sulae articula′res atlantoepistro′phicae**, see c. articularis atlantoaxialis lateralis. **c. articula′ris atlantooccipita′lis** [NA], capsule of atlantooccipital articulation: one of a pair of distinct ligamentous bands, each of which is attached at one end to the lateral mass of the atlas and at the other end to the margins of an occipital condyle. **c. articula′ris calcaneocuboi′dea** [NA], capsule of calcaneocuboidal joint: a ligamentous sac surrounding the calcaneocuboidal joint. **c. articula′ris capi′tis cos′tae** [NA], articular capsule of head of rib: a ligamentous sac surrounding the articulation of the head of a rib; called also capsulae articulares capituli costae. **cap′sulae articula′res capit′uli cos′tae**, see c. articularis capitis costae. **cap′sulae articula′res carpometacar′peae** [NA], capsules of carpometacarpal joints: ligamentous sacs surrounding the carpometacarpal joints; they are continuous with the capsules of the intercarpal joints. **c. articula′ris carpometacar′pea pol′licis** [NA], capsule of carpometacarpal articulation of thumb: a ligamentous sac surrounding the carpometacarpal joint of the thumb. **c. articula′ris costotransversa′ria** [NA], capsule of costotransverse joint: a ligamentous sac surrounding the costotransverse articulation. **c. articula′ris cox′ae** [NA], capsule of hip joint: a large, strong ligamentous sac surrounding the hip joint. **c. articula′ris cricoarytenoi′dea** [NA], cricoarytenoid articular capsule: the fibrous and synovial layers enclosing the cricoarytenoid joint; called also c. articularis cricoarytaenoidea. **c. articula′ris cricothyroi′dea** [NA], the capsule of the cricothyroid joint; called also c. articularis cricothyreoidea. **c. articula′ris cu′biti** [NA], articular capsule of elbow: the capsule formed around the cubital articulation by its various ligaments. **cap′sulae articula′res digito′rum man′us**, capsulae articulares interphalangearum manus. **cap′sulae articula′res digito′rum pe′dis**, capsulae articulares interphalangearum pedis. **c. articula′ris ge′nus** [NA], capsule of knee joint: the loose, thin, but strong sac enclosing the knee joint; called also c. articularis genu. **c. articula′ris hu′meri** [NA], articular capsule of humerus: a ligamentous sac surrounding the shoulder joint. **cap′sulae articula′res intermetacar′peae** [NA], capsules of intermetacarpal joints: ligamentous sacs that surround the intermetacarpal joints; they are continuous with the capsules of the carpometacarpal joints. **cap′sulae articula′res intermetatar′seae** [NA], capsules of intermetatarsal joints: the capsules around the four joints between the bases of the metatarsal bones. **cap′sulae articula′res interphalangea′rum man′us** [NA], capsules of interphalangeal joints of hand: incomplete ligamentous sacs surrounding the interphalangeal joints of the hand; called also capsulae articulares digitorum manus. **cap′sulae articula′res interphalangea′rum pe′dis** [NA], capsules of interphalangeal joints of foot: the capsules surrounding the interphalangeal articulations of the toes; called also capsulae articulares digitorum pedis. **c. articula′ris mandib′ulae**, c. articularis articulationis temporomandibularis. **c. articula′ris man′us** [NA], a loose ligamentous sac surrounding the radiocarpal joint and the intercarpal joints together; called also capsule of radiocarpal joint. **cap′sulae articula′res metacarpophalan′geae** [NA], capsules of metacarpophalangeal joints: ligamentous sacs that surround the metacarpophalangeal joints. **cap′sulae articula′res metatarsophalan′geae** [NA], capsules of metatarsophalangeal joints: the five capsules surrounding the metatarsophalangeal articulations. **c. articula′ris os′sis pisifor′mis** [NA], articular capsule of pisiform bone: a thin, loose ligamentous sac surrounding the joint of the pisiform bone. **c. articula′ris radioulna′ris dista′lis** [NA], distal radioulnar articular capsule: a loose ligamentous sac surrounding the distal radioulnar joint. **c. articula′ris sternoclavicula′ris** [NA], capsule of sternoclavicular joint: a ligamentous sac surrounding the sternoclavicular joint. **c. articula′ris sternocosta′lis** [NA], sternocostal articular capsule: the ligamentous sac that surrounds a sternocostal joint. **c. articula′ris talocalca′nea** [NA], a loose ligamentous sac surrounding the subtalar joint; called also capsule of subtalar joint. **c. articula′ris talocrura′lis** [NA], a thin ligamentous sac surrounding the ankle joint; called also capsule of ankle joint. **c. articula′ris talonavicula′ris**, a capsule surrounding the talonavicular joint. **cap′sulae articula′res tarsometatar′seae** [NA], capsules of tarsometatarsal joints: the three capsules that surround the joints between the metatarsal and cuneiform bones. **c. articula′ris tibiofibula′ris** [NA], capsule of tibiofibular joint: a fibrous sac enclosing the tibiofibular articulation. **c. bul′bi**, see vagina bulbi. **c. cor′dis**, pericardium. **c. exter′na** [NA], the layer of white fibers which lies between the putamen and the claustrum; called also c. externa nuclei lentiformis, and external capsule. **c. exter′na nu′clei lentifor′mis**, c. externa. **c. extre′ma**, the

white matter between the claustrum and the cortex of the insula.
c. fibro′sa, a capsule consisting largely of fibrous elements.
c. fibro′sa glan′dulae thyroi′deae [NA], fibrous capsule of thyroid gland: a connective tissue coat intimately adherent to the underlying gland; called also *c. glandulae thyroideae.* **c. fibro′sa [Glisso′ni], c. fibro′sa hep′atis,** c. fibrosa perivascularis. **c. fibro′sa perivascula′ris** [NA], perivascular fibrous capsule: the connective tissue sheath that accompanies the vessels and ducts through the hepatic portal. It is continuous with the fibrous coat. Called also *c. fibrosa hepatis, fibrous capsule of liver, Glisson's capsule, hepatobiliary capsule,* and *c. fibrosa [Glissoni].* **c. fibro′sa re′nis** [NA], fibrous capsule of kidney: the connective tissue investment of the kidney, which continues through the hilus to line the renal sinus; called also *tunica fibrosa renis.* **c. glan′dulae thyroi′deae,** c. fibrosa glandulae thyroideae. **c. glomer′uli** [NA], capsule of glomerulus: the double-walled globular dilatation that forms the beginning of a uriniferous tubule of the kidney and surrounds the glomerulus; it consists of an inner, or visceral, layer (*capsular epithelium*) and an outer, or parietal, layer (*glomerular epithelium*); called also *Bowman's, glomerular, malpighian,* and *müllerian capsule.* **c. inter′na** [NA], internal capsule: a fanlike mass of white fibers that separates the lentiform nucleus laterally from the head of the caudate nucleus, the dorsal thalamus, and the tail of the caudate nucleus medially; it consists of an anterior limb, a genu, a posterior limb, and retrolentiform and sublentiform parts, and carries both afferent and efferent fibers of the cerebral cortex. Called also *c. interna nuclei lentiformis.* **c. inter′na nu′clei lentifor′mis,** c. interna. **c. len′tis** [NA], capsule of lens: the elastic envelope covering the lens of the eye and fusing with the fibers of the ciliary zonule; called also *crystalline capsule.* **c. lien′is,** folliculi lymphatici lienales. **c. nu′clei denta′ti,** a layer formed by fibers passing to and from the dentate nucleus. **cap′sulae nu′clei lentifor′mis,** see *c. externa* and *c. interna.* **cap′sulae re′nis,** see *c. adiposa renis* and *c. fibrosa renis.* **c. sero′sa lie′nis,** tunica serosa lienis.

capsulae (kap′su-le) [L.] plural of *capsula.*

capsular (kap′su-lar) pertaining to a capsule.

capsulation (kap″su-la′shun) the enclosure of a medicine in a capsule.

capsule (kap′sūl) [L. *capsula* a little box] 1. a structure in which something is enclosed, such as a hard or a soft, soluble container of a suitable substance, for enclosing a dose of medicine. 2. an anatomical structure enclosing an organ or body part; see *capsula.* **adherent c.,** an investing structure that is not readily separated from the organ or substance contained within it. **adipose c.,** one consisting largely of fat. **adrenal c.,** adrenal gland (glandula suprarenalis [NA]). **adrenal c's, accessory,** accessory adrenal glands (glandulae suprarenales accessoriae [NA]). **anthrax c.,** the capsule of *Bacillus anthracis,* which is capable of neutralizing the anthracidal substance of the host. **articular c.,** the sac-like envelope which encloses the cavity of a synovial joint; see *capsula articularis,* and for names of capsules of particular joints see other entries beginning *capsula articularis,* under *capsula.* Called also *joint c.* and *synovial c.* **articular c., fibrous,** membrana fibrosa capsulae articularis. **auditory c.,** the cartilaginous capsule of the embryo that develops into the bony labyrinth of the inner ear. **bacterial c.,** an envelope of gel surrounding a bacterial cell, usually polysaccharide but sometimes polypeptide in nature, which is associated with the virulence of pathogenic bacteria. **biopsy c.,** a device which may be passed into the intestine for the purpose of securing specimens of the mucosa for examination under the microscope. **Bonnet's c.,** see *vagina bulbi.* **Bowman's c.,** capsula glomeruli. **c's of the brain,** layers of white matter in the cerebrum; see *capsula externa* and *capsula interna.* **brood c's,** capsular projections from the internal membrane of hydatid cysts, from which the scoleces arise. **cartilage c.,** a basophilic zone of cartilage matrix bordering on a lacuna and its enclosed cartilage cell. **Crosby c.,** an instrument used to obtain intestinal material for biopsy, consisting of a cylindrical capsule containing a knife which is spring-activated and triggered by suction. **crystalline c.,** capsula lentis. **decavitamin c.** [USP], a capsule containing not less than 1.2 mg. of vitamin A, 10 μg. of vitamin D, 70 mg. of ascorbic acid, 10 mg. of calcium pantothenate, 1 μg. of cyanocobalamin, 50 μg. of folic acid, 20 mg. of niacinamide, 2 mg. of pyridoxine hydrochloride, 2 mg. of riboflavin, 2 mg. of thiamine hydrochloride or its equivalent as thiamine mononitrate, and a suitable form of alpha tocopherol. It is used as a dietary supplement. **dental c.,** periodontium. **external c.,** capsula externa. **extreme c.,** capsula extrema. **fatty c. of kidney,** capsula adiposa renis. **fibrous c.,** one composed chiefly of fibrous elements. **fibrous c. of corpora cavernosa of penis,** tunica albuginea corporum cavernosorum penis. **fibrous c. of graafian follicle,** theca externa thecae folliculi. **fibrous c. of kidney,** capsula fibrosa renis. **fibrous c. of liver,** capsula fibrosa perivascularis. **fibrous c. of spleen,** tunica fibrosa lienis. **fibrous c. of testis,** tunica albuginea testis. **fibrous c. of thyroid gland,** capsula fibrosa glandulae thyroideae. **Gerota's c.,** the fascia surrounding the kidney. **Glisson's c.,** capsula fibrosa perivascularis. **glomerular c., c. of glomerulus,** capsula glomeruli. **Hearson's**

c. (*obs.*), a thermostatic chamber for regulating the temperature in incubators. **c. of heart,** pericardium. **hepatobiliary c.,** capsula fibrosa perivascularis. **hexavitamin c.** [NF], a capsule containing not less than 1.5 mg. of vitamin A, 10 μg. of vitamin D, 75 mg. of ascorbic acid, 2 mg. of thiamine hydrochloride or an equivalent amount of thiamine mononitrate, 3 mg. of riboflavine, and 20 mg. of niacinamide; used as a dietary supplement. **internal c.,** capsula interna. **joint c.,** articular c.; see also under *capsula articularis.* **c. of lens,** capsula lentis. **malpighian c.,** capsula glomeruli. **Müller c., müllerian c.,** capsula glomeruli. **ocular c.,** see *vagina bulbi.* **optic c.,** the embryonic structure from which the sclera is developed. **otic c.,** the skeletal element enclosing the inner ear mechanism. In the human embryo, it develops as cartilage at various ossification centers and becomes completely bony and unified at about the twenty-third week of fetal life. **pelvioprostatic c.,** fascia prostatae. **perinephric c.,** see *capsula adiposa renis* and *capsula fibrosa renis.* **periotic c.,** the tissue surrounding the otic sac in the embryo. **radiotelemetering c.,** telemetering c. **renal c.,** see *capsula adiposa renis* and *capsula fibrosa renis.* **serous c. of spleen,** tunica serosa lienis. **sodium iodide ^{131}I c's,** capsules containing radioactive iodine as sodium iodide, used in tests of thyroid disease and in the suppression of thyroid function. **suprarenal c.,** adrenal gland (glandula suprarenalis [NA]). **synovial c.,** articular c. (capsula articularis [NA]). **telemetering c.,** a small radio transmitter encased in a capsule the size of an ordinary drug capsule that can be swallowed or otherwise inserted in the body to give information about conditions (pressure, temperature, pH, etc.) within an organ; called also *radio pill.* **Tenon's c.,** see *vagina bulbi.* **triasyn B c's,** capsules containing thiamine, riboflavin, and nicotinamide, used as a vitamin supplement.

capsulectomy (kap″su-lek′to-me) [L. *capsula* capsule + Gr. *ektomē* excision] excision of a capsule, especially a joint capsule or the capsule of the lens. **renal c.,** excision of the capsule of the kidney.

capsulitis (kap″su-li′tis) the inflammation of a capsule, as that of the lens. **adhesive c.,** adhesive inflammation between the joint capsule and the peripheral articular cartilage of the shoulder with obliteration of the subdeltoid bursa, characterized by painful shoulder of gradual onset, with increasing pain, stiffness, and limitation of motion. Called also *adhesive bursitis, peritendinitis,* or *tendinitis, frozen shoulder,* and *periarthritis of shoulder.* **hepatic c.,** perihepatitis.

capsulolenticular (kap″su-lo-len-tik′u-lar) pertaining to the lens of the eye and its capsule.

capsuloma (kap″su-lo′mah) a capsular or subcapsular tumor of the kidney.

capsuloplasty (kap′su-lo-plas″te) [*capsule* + Gr. *plassein* to form] a plastic operation on a joint capsule.

capsulorrhaphy (kap″su-lor′ah-fe) [*capsule* + Gr. *raphē* suture] suturing of a capsule, especially a joint capsule.

capsulotome (kap-su′lo-tōm) a cutting instrument used for incising the capsules of the lens.

capsulotomy (kap″su-lot′o-me) [*capsule* + Gr. *temnein* to cut] the incision of a capsule, especially of that of the eye, as in cataract operation; or that of a joint. **renal c.,** incision of a renal capsule.

captamine hydrochloride (kap′tah-mēn) chemical name: 2-(dimethylamino)ethanethiol hydrochloride; a depigmenting agent, $C_4H_{11}NS \cdot HCl$.

captation (kap-ta′shun) [L. *captatio* seizure] (*obs.*) the first stage of hypnotism.

captodiame hydrochloride (kap-to-di′am) captodiamine hydrochloride.

captodiamine hydrochloride (kap″to-di′ah-mēn) chemical name: 2[[[4-(butylthio)phenyl]phenylmethyl]thio]-*N,N*-dimethylethamine hydrochloride. A tranquilizer and muscle relaxant, $C_{21}H_{29}NS_2HCl$, used as a sedative. Called also *captodiame hydrochloride.*

captopril (kap′to-pril)) a drug that inhibits the activity of angiotensin-converting enzymes, thus preventing the conversion of angiotensin I to the active form, angiotensin II.

capulet (kap′u-let) capelet.

capuride (kap′ur-īd) chemical name: *N*-(aminocarbonyl)-2-ethylmethylpentamide; a hypnotic, $C_9H_{18}N_2O_2$.

Capuron's points [Joseph *Capuron,* French physician, 1767–1850] see under *point.*

caput (kap′ut), pl. *cap′ita* [L. "head"] [NA] 1. the superior extremity of the body, comprising the cranium and face, and containing the brain, the organs of special sense, and the first organs of the digestive system; the head. 2. a general term applied to the expanded or chief extremity of an organ or part. **c. angula′re mus′culi quadra′ti la′bii superio′ris,** musculus levator labii superioris alaeque nasi. **c. bre′ve mus′culi bicip′itis bra′chii** [NA], the short head of the biceps brachii muscle, arising from the apex of the coracoid process; called also *medial head of biceps brachii muscle, short head of coracoradialis muscle,* and *coracoradialis.* **c. bre′ve**

mus′culi bicip′itis fem′oris [NA], the short head of the biceps femoris muscle, arising from the linea aspera femoris. **c. co′li**, cecum, def. 1. **c. cos′tae** [NA], head of rib: the posterior end of a rib, which articulates with the body of a vertebra; called also *capitulum costae*. **c. distor′tum**, torticollis. **c. epididym′idis** [NA], head of epididymis: the upper part of the epididymis, in which are found the straight and coiled portions of the efferent ductules of the testis; called also *globus major epididymidis*. **c. fem′oris** [NA], head of femur: the proximal end of the femur, articulating with the hip bone. **c. fib′ulae** [NA], head of fibula: the proximal extremity of the fibula; called also *capitulum fibulae*. **c. gallinag′inis** [L. "woodcock's head"], colliculus seminalis. **c. humera′le mus′culi flex-o′ris car′pi ulna′ris** [NA], the humeral head of the flexor carpi ulnaris muscle, arising from the medial epicondyle of the humerus. **c. humera′le mus′culi flexo′rum digito′rum subli′mis**, c. humeroulnare musculi flexoris digitorum superficialis. **c. humera′le mus′culi pronato′ris tere′tis** [NA], the humeral head of the pronator teres muscle arising from the medial epicondyle of the humerus. **c. humera′lis**, c. humeri. **c. hu′meri** [NA], head of humerus: the proximal end of the humerus, which articulates with the glenoid cavity of the scapula; called also *c. humeralis*. **c. humeroulna′re mus′culi flex-o′ris digito′rum superficia′lis**, the humeroulnar head of the flexor digitorum superficialis muscle, arising from the medial epicondyle of the humerus and coronoid process of ulna; called also *c. humerale musculi flexoris digitorum sublimis* and *humeral head of flexor digitorum sublimis muscle*. **c. in-cunea′tum** (*obs.*), impaction of the fetal head during labor. **c. infraorbita′le mus′culi quadra′ti la′bii superio′ris**, musculus levator labii superioris. **c. latera′le mus′culi gastrocne′mii** [NA], the lateral head of the gastrocnemius muscle, arising from the lateral condyle and posterior surface of the femur, and the capsule of the knee joint; called also *lateral gastrocnemius muscle*. **c. latera′le mus′culi tricip′itis bra′chii** [NA], the lateral head of the triceps brachii muscle, arising from the posterior surface of the humerus, the lateral border of the humerus, and the lateral intermuscular septum; called also *great* or *second head of triceps brachii muscle*, and *lateral* or *short anconeus muscle*. **c. lie′nis**, extremitas posterior lienis. **c. lon′gum mus′culi bicip′itis bra′chii** [NA], the long head of the biceps brachii muscle, arising from the upper border of the glenoid cavity; called also *interarticular ligament of articulation of humerus*. **c. lon′gum mus′culi bicip′itis fem′oris**, the long head of the biceps femoris muscle, arising from the ischial tuberosity. **c. lon′gum mus-culi tricip′itis bra′chii** [NA], the long head of the triceps brachii muscle, arising from the infraglenoid tubercle of the scapula; called also *first, middle,* or *scapular head of triceps brachii muscle*. **c. mal′lei** [NA], head of malleus: the upper portion of the malleus, which articulates with the incus; called also *capitulum mallei*. **c. mandib′ulae** [NA], head of mandible: the articular surface of the condyloid process of the mandible; called also *capitulum[processus condyloidei] mandibulae* and *head of condyloid process of mandible*. **c. media′le mus′culi gastrocne′mii** [NA], the medial head of the gastrocnemius muscle, arising from the medial condyle of the femur and the capsule of the knee joint; called also *medial gastrocnemius muscle*. **c. media′le mus′culi tricip′itis bra′chii** [NA], the medial head of the triceps brachii muscle, arising from the posterior surface of the humerus below the radial groove, the medial border of the humerus, and the medial intermuscular septum; called also *medial anconeus muscle* and *deep* or *short head of triceps brachii muscle*. **c. medu′sae**, Medusa's head: dilated cutaneous veins around the umbilicus, seen mainly in the newborn and in patients suffering with cirrhosis of the liver; so called because the veins resemble the head of the snake-haired Gorgon, Medusa. Called also *cirsomphalos*. **c. mus′culi** [NA], head of muscle: the end of a muscle at the site of its attachment to a bone or other fixed structure (origin). **c. natifor′me**, a head in rickets in which the eminences of the frontal and parietal bones form elevations separated by depressions which mark the lines of the cranial sutures; called also *hot cross bun head*. **c. nu′clei cauda′ti** [NA], head of caudate nucleus: the largest and most anterior part of the caudate nucleus, which bulges into the anterior horn of the lateral ventricle. **c. obli′quum mus′culi adducto′ris hal′lucis** [NA], the oblique head of the adductor hallucis muscle, originating from the bases of the second, third, and fourth metatarsal bones, and the sheath of the peroneus longus muscle; called also *great* or *long head of adductor hallucis muscle*. **c. obli′quum mus′culi adducto′ris pol′licis** [NA], the oblique head of the adductor pollicis muscle, arising from the capitate and trapezoid bones and the base of the second metacarpals. **c. os′sis metacarpa′lis** [NA], head of metacarpal bone: the distal extremity of each metacarpal bone, which articulates with the base of a proximal phalanx; called also *capitulum ossis metacarpalis* and *condyle of metacarpal bone*. **c. os′sis metatarsa′lis** [NA], head of metatarsal bone: the distal part of each metatarsal bone, which articulates with the base of a proximal phalanx; called also *capitulum ossis metatarsalis* and *little head of metatarsal bone*. **c. pancre′atis** [NA], head of pancreas: the discoidal mass forming the enlarged right

extremity of the pancreas, lying in a flexure of the duodenum. **c. pe′nis**, glans penis. **c. phalan′gis digito′rum ma′nus** [NA], head of phalanx of fingers: the distal articular surface of each of the proximal and middle phalanges of the fingers; called also *trochlea phalangis digitorum manus*. **c. phalan′gis digito′rum pe′dis** [NA], head of phalanx of toes: the distal articular extremity of each of the proximal and middle phalanges of the toes; called also *trochlea phalangis digitorum pedis*. **c. pla′num**, a flattened head occurring with osteochondrosis deformans juvenilis. **c. proge′neum**, forward projection of the jaw (prognathism). **c. quadra′tum**, an abnormally shaped head, sometimes occurring with rickets. **c. radia′le mus′culi flexo′ris digito′rum superficia′lis** [NA], the radial head of the flexor digitorum superficialis muscle, arising from the oblique line and anterior border of the radius. **c. ra′dii** [NA], head of radius: the disk on the proximal end of the radius that articulates with the capitulum of the humerus and the radial notch of the ulna; called also *capitulum radii*. **c. stape′dis** [NA], the head of the stapes, which articulates with the incus; called also *capitulum stapedis*. **c. succeda′neum**, edema occurring in and under the fetal scalp during labor. **c. ta′li** [NA], head of talus: the rounded anterior end of the talus; called also *head of astragalus*. **c. transver′sum mus′culi adducto′ris hal′lucis** [NA], the transverse head of the adductor hallucis muscle, arising from the capsules of the metatarso-phalangeal joints of the third, fourth, and fifth toes. **c. transver′sum mus′culi adducto′ris pol′licis** [NA], the transverse head of the adductor pollicis muscle arising from the lower two thirds of the anterior surface of the third metacarpal. **c. ul′nae** [NA], head of ulna: the articular surface of the distal extremity of the ulna; called also *capitulum ulnae*. **c. ulna′re mus′culi flexo′ris car′pi ulna′ris** [NA], the ulnar head of the flexor carpi ulnaris muscle, arising from the olecranon, and the adjacent part of the ulna. **c. ulna′re mus′culi pronato′ris ter′etis** [NA], the ulnar head of the pronator teres muscle, arising from the coronoid process of the ulna; called also *coronoid head of pronator teres muscle*. **c. zygomat′icum mus′culi quadra′ti la′bii superio′ris**, musculus zygomaticus minor.

C.A.R. Canadian Association of Radiologists.

caraate (kah″rah-ah′ta)   pinta.

Carabelli cusp (sign, tubercle) (kah-rah-bel′e) [Georg C. *Carabelli*, dentist in Vienna, 1787–1842]   see under *cusp*.

caramel (kar′ah-mel, kahr′mel) [NF]   a concentrated solution of the product obtained by heating sugar or glucose until the sweet taste is destroyed and a uniform dark brown mass results; used as a coloring agent for pharmaceuticals and foods.

caramiphen (kah-ram′ĭ-fen)   chemical name: 1-phenylcyclopentanecarboxylic acid 2-(dimethylamino)ethyl; an anticholinergic with actions similar to but weaker than those of atropine (q.v.). **c. edisylate, c. ethanedisulfonate**, an ester of caramiphen, $C_{38}H_{60}N_2O_{10}S_2$, with the anticholingeric effects of the base; used as an antitussive, administered orally. **c. hydrochloride**, an ester of caramiphen, $C_{18}H_{28}ClNO_2$, with the anticholinergic effects of the base; used mainly in the treatment of Parkinson's disease and parkinsonism, administered orally.

Carassini's spool (kar-ah-se′nēz)   see under *spool*.

carat (kar′at)   1. a measure of the fineness of gold, pure gold being 24 carats. 2. a unit of weight of precious stones, being 205.5 milligrams or $3\frac{1}{6}$ grains troy.

carate (kah-rah′ta)   pinta.

caraway (kar′ah-wa) [NF]   the dried ripe fruit of the umbelliferous plant *Carum carvi* of Europe and central and western Asia; its brown mericarps have an aromatic odor and taste and are used as a flavoring agent for pharmaceuticals.

carbachol (kar′bah-kol) [USP]   chemical name: 2-[(aminocarbonyl)oxy]-*N,N,N*-trimethylethanaminium chloride. A cholinergic, $C_6H_{15}ClN_2O_2$, occurring as white or faintly yellow crystals or crystalline powder; applied topically to the conjunctiva in the treatment of glaucoma. Called also *carbamylcholine chloride* and *carbocholine*.

carbadox (kar′bah-doks)   chemical name: 2-(2-quinoxalinylmethylene)hydrazine carboxylic acid methyl ester N^1,N^4-dioxide; an antibacterial, $C_{11}H_{10}N_4O_4$, used in veterinary medicine.

carbamate (kar′bah-māt)   any ester of carbamic acid. **ethyl c.**, urethan.

carbamazepine (kar-bah-maz′ĕ-pēn)   chemical name: 5*H*-dibenz[*b,f*]azepin-5-carboxamide. An anticonvulsant and analgesic, $C_{15}H_{12}N_2O$, occurring as a white to off-white powder; used in the treatment of pain associated with trigeminal neuralgia and in epilepsy manifested by certain types of seizures, administered orally.

carbamide (kar-bam′ĭd)   urea in anhydrous, lyophilized, sterile powder form; it is injected intravenously in dextrose or invert sugar solution to induce diuresis.

carbaminohemoglobin (kar-bam″ĭ-no-he″mo-glo′bin)   a chemical combination of carbon dioxide with hemoglobin, CO_2-HHb, being one of the forms in which carbon dioxide exists in the blood.

carbamoyl (kar′bah-moil) the radical NH₂—CO—; see *carbamoyltransferase.* Called also *carbamyl.*

carbamoyltransferase (kar″bah-moil-trans′fer-ās) an enzyme that catalyzes the transfer of carbamoyl, as from carbamoylphosphate to L-ornithine to form orthophosphate and citrulline in the synthesis of urea; called also *transcarbamoylase.*

carbamyl (kar′bah-mil) carbamoyl.

carbamylcholine chloride (kar″bah-mil-ko′lēn klo′rīd) carbachol.

carbantel lauryl sulfate (kar′ban-tel) chemical name: *N*-[[(4-chlorophenyl)amino]carbonyl]pentanimidamide compound with dodecyl hydrogen sulfate (1:1); an anthelmintic, $C_{12}H_{16}ClN_3O \cdot C_{12}H_{26}O_4S$.

carbaril (kar′bah-ril) chemical name: 1-naphthalenol methylcarbamate; an insecticide and parasiticide, $C_{12}H_{11}NO_2$. Called also *carbaryl.*

carbarsone (kar′bar-sōn) [USP] chemical name: [4-[(aminocarbonyl)amino]phenyl]arsonic acid. A pentavalent organic arsenical, $C_7H_9AsN_2O_4$, occurring as a white powder; used as an antiamebic, administered orally or in a retention enema. It is also administered orally in the treatment of balantiasis and intravaginally in vaginitis due to *Trichomonas vaginalis.*

carbaryl (kar′bah-ril) carbaril.

carbaspirin calcium (kar-kas′pĭ-rin) chemical name: 2-(acetyloxy)benzoic acid calcium salt compound with urea (1:1); an analgesic, $C_{19}H_{18}CaN_2O_9$, which also has antipyretic properties, and has been used like aspirin.

carbasus (kar′bah-sus) [L.; Gr. *karpasos* cotton] an old name for lint, charpie, or cotton.

carbazide (kar′bah-zīd) a urea derivative, carbodiazide, CO-(N₃)₂, in which both the amide groups of urea have been replaced by hydrazine residues.

carbazochrome salicylate (kar-baz′o-krōm) chemical name: 2-hydroxybenzoic acid monosodium salt compound with 2-(1,-2,3,5-tetrahydro-3-hydroxy-1-methyl-5-oxo-6*H*-indol-6-ylidene)-hydrazinecarboxamide (1:1). A complex of adrenochrome monosemicarbazone with sodium salicylate, $C_{17}H_{17}N_4NaO_6$, occurring as an orange-red crystallized powder; used as a hemostatic to control capillary bleeding and to prevent capillary permeability, administered orally or intramuscularly.

carbazocine (kar-bah′zo-sēn) chemical name: *cis*-14-(cyclopropylmethyl)-1,2,3,4,4a,5,6,11-octahydro-5,11b-iminoethano-11b-*H*-benzo[*a*]carbazole; an analgesic, $C_{22}H_{28}N_2$.

carbazotate (kar-baz′o-tāt) any salt of picric acid; a picrate.

carbenicillin (kar″ben-ĭ-sil′in) chemical name: *N*-(2-carboxy-3,3-dimethyl-7-oxo-4-thia-1-azabicyclo[3·2·0]hept-6-yl)-2-phenylmalonamic acid. A semisynthetic penicillin, $C_{17}H_{18}N_2O_6S$, effective against gram-negative bacteria, such as susceptible strains of *Pseudomonas aeruginosa,* indole-positive *Proteus* species, certain strains of *Escherichia coli,* and *Hemophilus influenzae;* it also inhibits the growth of some gram-positive pathogens. Called also *carfecillin.* **c. disodium,** the disodium salt of carbenicillin, $C_{17}H_{16}N_2Na_2O_6S$, occurring as a white to off-white, crystalline powder, and having the same actions as the base; administered intramuscularly or intravenously in severe systemic infections and septicemia, urinary and genitourinary tract infections, acute and chronic respiratory infections, and soft-tissue infections. A sterile preparation is prepared in conformance with USP standards. Called also *c. sodium.* **c. indanyl sodium** [USP], the sodium salt of the indanyl ester of carbenicillin disodium, $C_{26}H_{25}N_2NaO_6S$, having the same actions as the base; administered orally in the treatment of upper and lower urinary tract infections due to susceptible strains of *Pseudomonas* species, *Proteus* species, *Escherichia coli, Enterobacter,* and enterococci. Called also *carindacillin sodium.* **c. phenyl sodium,** the sodium salt of the phenyl ester of carbenicillin disodium, $C_{23}H_2N_2NaO_6S$, which has been used for the same purposes as carbenicillin indanyl sodium. Called also *carfecillin sodium.* **c. potassium,** the potassium salt of carbenicillin, $C_{17}H_{17}KN_2O_6S$. **c. sodium,** c. disodium.

carbenoxolone sodium (kar″ben-oks′o-lōn) chemical name: 3-(3-carboxy-1-oxopropoxy)-11-oxo-olean-12-en-29-oic acid disodium salt. A derivative of glycyrrhizin, $C_{34}H_{48}Na_2O_7$, having marked anti-inflammatory actions and aldosterone-like activity; used in the treatment of gastric ulcer.

carbetapentane citrate (kar-ba″tah-pen′tān) chemical name: 1-phenylcyclopentanecarboxylic acid 2-(2-diethylaminoethoxy)ethyl citrate. An antitussive agent, $C_{20}H_{31}NO_3 \cdot C_6H_8O_7$, with mild atropine-like antisecretory activity; used in the treatment of cough associated with upper respiratory infections, administered orally.

carbethyl salicylate (kar-beth′il) chemical name: salicylic ethyl ester carbonate. It is used as an analgesic and antiarthritic.

carbhemoglobin (karb″he-mo-glo′bin) carbaminohemoglobin.

carbide (kar′bīd) a compound of carbon with an element or radical. **metallic c.,** a compound of carbon with a transition metal, as in Fe_3C (as distinguished from a salt-like carbide, such as CaC_2).

carbidopa (kar″bĭ-do′pah) [USP] chemical name: (*S*)-α-hy-

drazino-3,4-dihydroxy-α-methylomonohydrate benezene propranoic acid. An inhibitor, $C_{10}H_{14}N_2O_4 \cdot H_2O$, of the decarboxylation of peripheral levodopa to dopamine, which does not penetrate the central nervous system. When given with levodopa, carbidopa produces higher brain concentrations of dopamine with lower doses of levodopa, thus lessening the side effects seen with higher doses. It is used orally, in combination with levodopa, as an antiparkinsonian agent, and has been used in the treatment of Lesch-Nyhan syndrome and Gilles de la Tourette syndrome.

carbimazole (kar-bi′mah-zōl) chemical name: carbonothioic acid *O*-ethyl *S*-(1-methyl-1 *H*-imidazol-2-yl) ester. An inhibitor of thyroid hormone synthesis occurring as a white or creamy white, crystalline powder; administered orally in the treatment of hyperthyroidism.

carbinol (kar′bĭ-nol) 1. methanol. 2. any aromatic or fatty alcohol formed by substituting one, two, or three hydrocarbon groups for hydrogen in methanol. **acetylmethyl c.,** a keto-isomer of aldol, $CH_3 \cdot CHOH \cdot CO \cdot CH_3$, which is formed from glucose by certain bacteria and which is detected in a broth culture of bacteria by the Voges-Proskauer reaction. **dimethyl c.,** isopropyl alcohol.

carbinoxamine maleate (kar″bin-ok′sah-mēn) [USP] chemical name: 2-[(4-chlorophenyl)-2-pyridinylmethoxy-*N*,*N*-dimethylethanamine (*Z*)-2-butenedioate. A potent antihistaminic, $C_{16}H_{19}ClN_2O \cdot C_4H_4O_4$, occurring as a white, crystalline powder; used in the treatment of allergic disorders, administered orally.

carbo (kar′bo) [L.] charcoal. **c. activa′tus,** activated charcoal. **c. anima′lis,** a variety prepared from bones and other animal matter; a decolorizing agent. **c. anima′lis purifica′tus,** purified animal charcoal. **c. lig′ni,** wood charcoal, a deodorant, adsorbent, and disinfectant.

Carbocaine (kar′bo-kān) trademark for preparations of mepivacaine hydrochloride.

carbocholine (kar″bo-ko′lēn) carbachol.

carbocromen hydrochloride (kar″bo-kro′mēn) chromonar hydrochloride.

carbocyclic (kar″bo-si′klik) having or pertaining to a closed chain or ring formation which includes only carbon atoms; said of chemical compounds.

carbocysteine (kar″bo-sis-te′in) chemical name: *S*-(carboxymethyl)cysteine; a mucolytic, $C_5H_9NO_4S$.

carbodiimide (kar″bo-di-im′id) a derivative of urea, NH:C:NH.

carbogaseous (kar″bo-gas′e-us) charged with carbon dioxide gas.

carbogen (kar′bo-jen) a mixture of oxygen with 5 per cent carbon dioxide.

carbohemia (kar″bo-he′me-ah) [*carbon* dioxide + Gr. *haima* blood + -*ia*] the presence of carbon dioxide in the blood.

carbohemoglobin (kar″bo-he-mo-glo′bin) carbaminohemoglobin.

carbohydrase (kar″bo-hi′drās) any of a group of enzymes that catalyze the hydrolysis of higher carbohydrates to lower forms, each enzyme being usually specific for one substrate only.

carbohydrate (kar″bo-hi′drāt) an aldehyde or ketone derivative of a polyhydric alcohol, particularly of the pentahydric and hexahydric alcohols. They are so named because the hydrogen and oxygen are usually in the proportion to form water, $(CH_2O)_n$. The most important carbohydrates are the starches, sugars, celluloses, and gums. They are classified into mono-, di-, tri-, poly- and heterosaccharides. **reserve c's,** carbohydrates that can be stored in the plant or animal in the form of high molecular weight, hydrolyzable compounds such as starch or glycogen.

carbohydraturia (kar″bo-hi″drah-tu′re-ah) excess of carbohydrates in the urine.

carbohydrogenic (kar″bo-hi″dro-jen′ik) producing carbohydrates.

carbolate (kar′bo-lāt) 1. phenolate. 2. to charge with carbolic acid.

carbolfuchsin (kar″bol-fōōk′sin) see *Table of Stains,* and see under *solution.*

carboligase (kar″bol-i′gās) an enzyme found in both plant and animal tissues that catalyzes the linking up of carbon atoms and thus changes pyruvic acid to acetyl-methyl-carbinol.

carbolism (kar′bol-izm) phenol poisoning.

carbolize (kar′bol-īz) to treat with phenol.

carboluria (kar″bo-lu′re-ah) [*carbolic* + Gr. *ouron* urine + -*ia*] the presence of phenol in the urine.

carbolxylene (kar″bol-zi′lēn) a mixture of 1 part carbolic acid and 3 parts xylene, used for clearing microscopical sections.

carbomer, carbomer 934 P (kar′bo-mer) [NF] a polymer of acrylic acid, cross-linked with a polyfunctional agent; used as an emulsifying agent and as a suspending agent in pharmaceutical preparations.

carbometer (kar-bom′ĕ-ter) (*obs.*) carbonometer.

carbometry (kar-bom′ĕ-tre) (*obs.*) carbonometry.

carbomycin (kar″bo-mi′sin) a crystalline monobasic antibiotic isolated from the elaborated products of *Streptomyces halstedii* or produced by other means; it is bacteriostatic for gram-positive organisms.

carbon (kar'bon) [L. *carbo*, coal, charcoal] 1. a nonmetallic tetrad element, found nearly pure in the diamond, and approximatley pure in charcoal, graphite, and anthracite; symbol, C; atomic number, 6; atomic weight, 12.011. 2. an electrode made of carbon shell in which medicaments may be enclosed. **¹³C**, a natural isotope of carbon, of atomic mass 13, used as a tracer in chemical reactions in living tissue. **¹⁴C**, a radioactive isotope of carbon, of atomic mass 14, used in cancer and metabolic research. **c. dioxide,** an odorless, colorless gas, CO_2, resulting from the oxidation of carbon. It is formed in the tissues and eliminated by the lungs. CO_2 and the carbonates assist in maintaining the neutrality of the tissues and fluids of the body. Inhalations of carbon dioxide, containing not less than 99 percent by volume of CO_2 [USP], mixed with air or oxygen, are used to stimulate respiration. Solid carbon dioxide (*Dry Ice* or *carbon dioxide snow*) has been used as an escharotic to destroy certain skin lesions. **c. disulfide,** a colorless, flammable, poisonous liquid, CS_2, used as a solvent; it is a counterirritant and has local anesthetic properties but is not used as such. **c. monoxide,** a colorless poisonous gas, CO, formed by burning carbon or organic fuels with a scanty supply of oxygen; it causes asphyxiation by combining irreversibly with the blood hemoglobin. **c. oxysulfide,** a colorless gas, COS, uniting with air to form an explosive mixture. **radioactive c.,** radiocarbon. **c. tetrachloride** [NF], a clear, colorless, volatile liquid, CCl_4, used as a solvent in pharmaceutical preparations. Inhalation of its vapors can depress central nervous system activity and cause degeneration of the liver and kidneys. Called also *perchlormethane* and *tetrachlormethane*. **c. trichloride,** a white solid, hexachlorethane, C_2Cl_6; it is a stimulant and has local anesthetic properties but is not used as such.

carbonate (kar'bon-āt) any salt of carbonic acid. **ferrous c.,** a compound, $FeCO_3$, used in iron deficiency anemia; called also *iron carbonate*.

carbonemia (kar″bon-e'me-ah) carbohemia.

carbonize (kar'bo-nīz) to char or to convert into charcoal.

carbonometer (kar″bo-nom'ĕ-ter) (*obs.*) an apparatus for performing carbonometry.

carbonometry (kar″bo-nom'ĕ-tre) [*carbon* + Gr. *metron* measure] (*obs.*) measurement of the amount of carbon dioxide exhaled with the breath.

carbonuria (kar″bo-nu're-ah) [*carbon* + Gr. *ouron* urine + *-ia*] the presence of carbon dioxide or other carbon compounds in the urine. **dysoxidative c.,** pathologic increase of carbon compounds in the urine due to deficient oxidation.

carbonyl (kar'bo-nil) [*carbon* + Gr. *hylē* matter] the organic radical, C:O, occurring in compounds such as aldehydes, ketones, carboxylic acids, and esters. **c. chloride,** phosgene.

carbophilic (kar-bo-fil'ik) capnophilic.

carboprost (kar'bo-prost) chemical name: (5z)-9α,11α,15-trihydroxy-15S-methyl-prosta-5,13E-dien-1-oic acid. A synthetic 15-methyl analogue of dinoprost, a prostaglandin in the F type, $C_{21}H_{36}O_5$; it has been used as an oxytocic for termination of pregnancy and missed abortion, administered intramuscularly. **c. methyl,** the methyl ester of carboprost, $C_{22}H_{38}O_5$, having the same actions and similar uses as the base; administered in vaginal suppositories or in an intravaginal device. **c. tromethamine,** an oxytocic compound of carboprost and 2-amino-2-(hydroxymethyl)-1,3-propanediol (1:1), $C_{21}H_{36}O_5 \cdot C_4H_{11}NO_3$.

Carborundum (kar″bo-run'dum) trademark for a compound of carbon and silicon, silicon carbide, SiC, a substance which ranks next to the diamond in hardness; used as an abrasive and as a refractory.

Carbowax (kar'bo-waks) trademark for a series of polyethylene glycols; used in compounding water-soluble ointment vehicles.

carboxydismutase (kar-bok″se-dis'mu-tās) an enzyme employed in autotrophic fixation of carbon dioxide; it catalyzes the reaction in which CO_2 is fixed to ribulose-1,5-diphosphate with the formation of two molecules of 3-phosphoglyceric acid.

Carboxydomonas (kar-bok″se-do-mo'nas) a genus of microorganisms of the family Methanomonadaceae, suborder Pseudomonadineae, order Pseudomonadales, occurring as chemoautotrophic rod-shaped cells capable of securing growth energy by oxidizing CO to CO_2. The type species is *C. oligocarb'ophila*.

γ-carboxyglutamate (kar-bok″se-gloo'tah-māt) a salt or dissociated form of carboxyglutamic acid; see under *acid*.

carboxyhemoglobin (kar-bok″se-he″mo-glo'bin) hemoglobin combined with carbon monoxide, which occupies the sites on the hemoglobin molecule that normally bind with oxygen and which is not readily displaced from the molecule; exposure to carbon monoxide thus results in cellular anoxia.

carboxyhemoglobinemia (kar-bok″se-he″mo-glo″bin-e′me-ah) the presence of carboxyhemoglobin in the blood.

carboxyl (kar-bok'sil) the monovalent radical, —COOH, occurring in those organic acids termed carboxylic acids.

carboxylase (kar-bok'sĭ-lās) an enzyme that catalyzes the removal of carbon dioxide from the carboxyl group of alpha keto

acids. Decarboxylation of pyruvic acid is the essential step in alcoholic fermentation by which pyruvic acid is converted into acetaldehyde and carbon dioxide. **acetyl-CoA c.,** an enzyme that catalyzes the conversion of ATP, acetyl-CoA, CO_2, and water to ADP, orthophosphate, and malonyl-CoA. **amino acid c.,** an enzyme in many bacteria that catalyzes the removal of CO_2 from amino acids, thus producing amines. **methylcrotonoyl CoA c.,** an enzyme that catalyzes the conversion of ATP, 3-methylcrotonoyl-CoA, CO_2, and water to ADP, orthophosphate, and 3-methylglutaconyl-CoA. **phosphopyruvate c.,** an enzyme of the lyase class that catalyzes the conversion of GTP and oxaloacetate to phosphoenolpyruvate, CO_2, and GDP. **propionyl-CoA c.,** an enzyme that catalyzes the conversion of ATP, propionyl-CoA, CO_2, and water to ADP, orthophosphate, and methylmalonyl-CoA. **pyruvate c.,** an enzyme (biotin protein) that catalyzes the conversion of pyruvic acid to acetaldehyde and carbon dioxide.

carboxylation (kar-bok″sĭ-la'shun) the addition of a carboxyl group, as to pyruvate to form oxaloacetate.

carboxylesterase (kar-bok″sil-es′ter-ās) carboxylic-ester hydrolase: an enzyme that catalyzes the hydrolysis of the esters of carboxylic acids.

carboxyltransferase (kar-bok″sil-trans'fer-ās) an enzyme that catalyzes the transfer of a carboxyl group, as in the carboxylation of pyruvate to form oxaloacetate; called also *transcarboxylase*.

carboxy-lyase (kar-bok'se-li′ās) any of a group of lyases that catalyzes the removal of a carboxyl group; it includes the carboxylases and decarboxylases.

carboxymethylcellulose sodium (kar-bok″se-meth″il-sel′u-lōs) [USP] the sodium salt of a polycarboxymethyl ether of cellulose; used as a suspending agent, tablet excipient, and viscosity-increasing agent in pharmaceutical preparations, and administered orally as a cathartic.

carboxymyoglobin (kar-bok″se-mi″o-glo'bin) a compound formed from myoglobin on exposure to carbon monoxide, with formation of a covalent bond with oxygen and without change of the charge of the ferrous state.

carboxypeptidase (kar-bok″se-pep'tĭ-dās) an exopeptidase that acts on the peptide bond of terminal amino acids possessing a free carboxyl group. Carboxypeptidase A (peptidyl-L-amino-acid hydrolase) and B (peptidyl-L-lysine hydrolase) are zinc-proteins that occur in the pancreas. Yeast carboxypeptidase is peptidyl-glycine hydrolase.

carboxypolypeptidase (kar-bok″se-pol″e-pep'tĭ-dās) an exopeptidase that, in a polypeptide, attacks the peptide linkage of a terminal amino acid possessing a free carboxyl group, releasing a free amino acid.

carbromal (kar-bro'mal) chemical name: *N*-(aminocarbonyl)-2-bromo-2-ethylbutaneamide. A sedative with weak hypnotic activity, $C_7H_{13}BrN_2O$, occurring as a white, crystalline powder; administered orally.

carbuncle (kar'bung-kl) [L. *carbunculus* little coal] a necrotizing infection of skin and subcutaneous tissue composed of a cluster of boils (furuncles), usually due to *Staphylococcus aureus*, with multiple formed or incipient drainage sinuses. **malignant c.,** anthrax in man. **renal c.,** a massive localized parenchymal suppuration consequent to bacterial metastasis, following localized vascular thrombosis or infarction of the kidney.

carbuncular (kar-bung'ku-lar) resembling or of the nature of a carbuncle.

carbunculoid (kar-bung'ku-loid) resembling a carbuncle.

carbunculosis (kar-bung″ku-lo'sis) a condition marked by the development of carbuncles.

carbutamide (kar-bu'tah-mīd) chemical name: 1-butyl-3-sulfanilylurea; a hypoglycemic agent, $C_{11}H_{17}N_3O_3S$.

carbuterol hydrochloride (kar-bu'ter-ōl) chemical name: [5-[2-(1,1-dimethylethyl)amino]-1-hydroxyethyl]-2-hydroxyphenyl]urea monohydrochloride. An adrenergic, $C_{13}H_{21}N_3O_3 \cdot HCl$, which has been used as a bronchodilator, administered by inhalation.

carcass (kar'kas) [Fr. *carcasse*] a dead body; generally applied to other than a human body.

Carcassonne's ligament, perineal ligament (kar-kah-sonz′) [Bernard Gauderic *Carcassonne*, French surgeon, born 1728] see *ligamentum puboprostaticum* and *ligamentum transversum perinei*.

carceag (kar'se-ag) a disease of sheep in the Balkan States caused by *Babesia* (*Piroplasma*) *ovis* and transmitted by the tick *Rhipicephalus bursa*.

carciag (kar'se-ag) carceag.

carcinectomy (kar″sin-ek'tŏ-me) [*carcinoma* + Gr. *ektomē* excision] excision of carcinoma.

carcinelcosis (kar″sin-el-ko'sis) [Gr. *karkinos* cancer + *helkōsis* ulceration] (*obs.*) malignant ulceration.

carcinemia (kar″sin-e'me-ah) [*carcinoma* + Gr. *haima* blood + *-ia*] cancerous cachexia.

carcino- [Gk. *karkinos* a crab] a combining form meaning relationship to carcinoma.

carcinoembryonic (kar″sin-o-em″bre-on′ik) oncofetal; relating to carcinoma and to the embryonic state; see under *antigen*.

carcinogen (kar-sin′o-jen) any cancer-producing substance.

carcinogenesis (kar″sĭ-no-jen′ĕ-sis) [Gr. *karkinos* cancer + *genesis* production] the production of carcinoma.

carcinogenic (kar″sĭ-no-jen′ik) producing carcinoma.

carcinogenicity (kar″sĭ-no-jĕ-nis′ĭ-te) the power, ability, or tendency to produce carcinoma.

carcinoid (kar′sĭ-noid) a yellow circumscribed tumor occurring in the small intestine, appendix, stomach, or colon; argentaffinoma (q.v.). See also under *syndrome*.

carcinology (kar″sĭ-nol′o-je) (*obs.*) oncology.

carcinolysin (kar″sĭ-nol′ĭ-sĭn) [*carcinoma* + Gr. *lysis* dissolution] a ferment derived from a Chinese variety of pine called "haisung." It has been given subcutaneously or intramuscularly for cancer.

carcinolysis (kar″sĭ-nol′ĭ-sis) destruction of carcinoma cells, as by perfusion of an antineoplastic agent through the vessels of the body segment in which the growth occurs.

carcinolytic (kar″sĭ-no-lit′ik) [*carcinoma* + Gr. *lytikos* destroying] pertaining to, characterized by, or causing carcinolysis.

carcinoma (kar″sĭ-no′mah), pl. **carcinomas** or **carcino′mata** [Gr. *karkinōma* from *karkinos* crab, cancer] a malignant new growth made up of epithelial cells tending to infiltrate the surrounding tissues and give rise to metastases. **acinar c., acinous c.,** alveolar adenocarcinoma. **adenocystic c.,** adenoid cystic c. **adenoid cystic c.,** carcinoma characterized by bands or cylinders of hyalinized or mucinous stroma separating or surrounded by nests or cords of small epithelial cells. When the cylinders occur within masses of epithelial cells, they give the tissue a perforated, sievelike, or cribriform appearance. Such tumors occur in the mammary glands, the mucous glands of the upper and lower respiratory tract, and the salivary glands. They are malignant but slow-growing, and tend to spread locally via the nerves. Called also *adenocystic c., adenomyoepithelioma, cribriform c.,* and *cylindroma.* NOTE: Certain unrelated tumors may have a cylindromatous or adenoid cystic pattern, e.g., cutaneous cylindroma, ameloblastoma, and a type of basal cell carcinoma of the skin. **c. adenomato′sum,** adenocarcinoma. **c. of adrenal cortex,** malignant tumors of adrenal cortical cells that may cause endocrine disorders such as Cushing's syndrome and adrenogenital syndrome. **alveolar c.,** alveolar adenocarcinoma. **alveolar cell c.,** carcinoma of the lung marked clinically by severe cough with voluminous expectoration and histologically by distinctive, tall, columnar to cuboidal epithelial cells that line up along the alveolar septa, project into the alveolar spaces in numerous branching papillary formations, and may contain mucinous secretion; called also *bronchiolar c., alveolar cell tumor,* and *pulmonary adenomatosis.* **basal cell c., c. basocellula′re,** an epithelial tumor that seldom metastasizes but has potentialities for local invasion and destruction. Clinically, it is divided into types: nodular, cicatricial, morphaic, and erythematoid (pagetoid). Called also *basaloma* or *basiloma,* and *hair matrix c.* **basaloid c.,** a rare transitional-cell carcinoma of the anus, resembling basal cell carcinoma of the skin. **basosquamous cell c.,** carcinoma that histologically exhibits both basal and squamous elements. **bronchioalveolar c., bronchiolar c.,** alveolar cell c. **bronchiolar c.,** alveolar cell c. **bronchogenic c.,** carcinoma of the lung, so called because it arises from the epithelium of the bronchial tree. **cerebriform c.,** medullary c. **cholangiocellular c.,** primary carcinoma of the liver originating in bile duct cells, called also *cholangioma* and *cholangiocarcinoma.* **chorionic c.,** choriocarcinoma. **colloid c.,** mucinous c. **comedo c.,** comedocarcinoma. **corpus c.,** carcinoma of the body of the uterus. **cribriform c.,** adenoid cystic c. **c. en cuirasse,** a rare carcinoma infiltrating the entire skin of the anterior chest wall and frequently breaking it down. **c. cuta′neum,** malignant epithelioma of the skin. **cylindrical c., cylindrical cell c.,** carcinoma in which the cells are cylindrical or nearly so. **duct c.,** carcinoma of any duct. **c. du′rum** (*obs.*), scirrhous c. **embryonal c.,** 1. a highly malignant, primitive form of carcinoma, probably of germinal cell or teratomatous derivation, usually arising in a gonad and rarely in other sites. 2. (*obs.*) seminoma. **encephaloid c.** (*obs.*), medullary c. **epibulbar c.,** carcinoma that starts at the edge of the cornea and spreads over the cornea and conjunctiva. **epidermoid c.,** carcinoma in which the cells tend to differentiate in the same way that the cells of the epidermis do; that is, they tend to form prickle cells and undergo cornification. **c. epithelia′le adenoi′des,** adenoid basal cell c. **exophytic c.,** a malignant epithelial neoplasm with marked outward growth like a wart or papilloma. **c. ex ul′cere** (*obs.*), carcinomatous degeneration of a benign ulcer. **c. fibro′sum,** scirrhous c. **gelatiniform c.,** mucinous c. **gelatinous c.,** colloid c. **giant cell c.,** carcinoma containing many giant cells. **c. gigantocellula′re,** carcinoma containing many giant cells. **glandular c.,** adenocarcinoma. **granulosa cell c.,** see under *tumor.* **hair-matrix c.,** basal cell c. **hematoid c.** (*obs.*), a highly vascular carcinoma.

hepatocellular c., primary carcinoma of the liver cells; called also *hepatoma, malignant hepatoma,* and *hepatocarcinoma.* **Hürthle cell c.,** see under *tumor.* **hyaline c.** (*obs.*), mucinous c. **hypernephroid c.,** renal cell c. **infantile embryonal c.,** mesonephroma (type 2). **c. in si′tu,** a neoplastic entity wherein the tumor cells are confined to the epithelium of origin, without invasion of the basement membrane; popularly applied to such cells in the uterine cervix. Called also *cancer in situ* and *preinvasive c.* **intraepidermal c.,** carcinoma confined within the epidermis, the basal layer of the epidermis not being penetrated by the proliferating cells; Bowen's disease. **intraepithelial c.,** c. in situ. **Krompecher's c.,** rodent ulcer. **Kulchitzky-cell c.,** carcinoid tumor of the small or large intestine. **large-cell c.,** a bronchogenic tumor of undifferentiated (anaplastic) cells of large size. **lenticular c., c. lenticula′re,** scirrhous carcinoma of the skin with the formation of flattened papules and nodules which run together, forming fungoid masses. **lipomatous c.,** (*obs.*), carcinoma with fatty degeneration. **lymphoepithelial c.,** lymphoepithelioma. **c. mastitoi′des** (*obs.*), medullary carcinoma of the breast. **c. medulla′re, medullary c.,** carcinoma composed mainly of epithelial elements with little or no stroma. **c. melano′des, melanotic c.** (*obs.*), malignant melanoma. **c. mol′le,** medullary c. **mucinous c.,** adenocarcinoma producing mucin in significant amounts; sometimes erroneously called *colloid* or *gelatinous colloma.* **c. mucip′arum,** mucinous c. **c. mucocellula′re,** Krukenberg's tumor. **mucoepidermoid c.,** a malignant epithelial tumor of glandular tissue, especially the salivary glands, characterized by acini with mucus-producing cells and by the presence of malignant squamous elements. **c. muco′sum, mucous c.,** mucinous c. **c. myxomato′des,** carcinoma in which the stroma has undergone myxomatous degeneration. **nasopharyngeal c.,** a malignant tumor arising in the epithelial lining of the space behind the nose (the nasopharynx) and occurring at high frequency in southern China. The Epstein-Barr virus has been implicated as a causative agent. **c. ni′grum** (*obs.*), malignant melanoma. **oat cell c.,** a small-cell c. **c. ossif′icans, osteoid c.,** carcinoma in which there is osteoid or osseous metaplasia of the stroma. **papillary c.,** carcinoma in which there are papillary excrescences. **periportal c.,** carcinoma of the liver, extending along and around the portal vessels. **preinvasive c.,** c. in situ. **prickle cell c.,** squamous cell c. **pultaceous c.** (*obs.*), comedocarcinoma. **renal cell c. of kidney,** carcinoma of the renal parenchyma usually occurring in middle age or later and composed of tubular cells in varying arrangements; symptoms depend on extent of invasion. Called also *adenocarcinoma of kidney* and *hypernephroid carcinoma.* **reserve cell c.,** oat cell c. **c. sarcomato′des** (*obs.*), spindle cell c. **schneiderian c.,** a neoplasm of the mucosa of the nose and the paranasal sinuses. **scirrhous c.,** carcinoma with a hard structure owing to the formation of dense connective tissue in the stroma. **c. scro′ti,** carcinoma of the scrotum. **signet-ring cell c.,** a highly malignant, mucus-secreting tumor in which the mucus-secreting cells are anaplastic and appear rounded, with the nucleus displaced to one side by a globule of mucus in the cytoplasm. **c. sim′plex,** an undifferentiated carcinoma. **small-cell c.,** a radiosensitive tumor composed of small, oval, undifferentiated cells that are intensely hematoxyphilic and typically bronchogenic. Called also *oat-cell c.* **solanoid c.** (*obs.*), scirrhous c. **spheroidal cell c.,** c. simplex. **spindle cell c.,** squamous cell carcinoma marked by fusiform development of rapidly proliferating cells. **c. spongio′sum,** medullary c. **squamous c., squamous cell c.,** carcinoma developed from squamous epithelium, and having cuboid cells. **string c.,** a carcinoma of the large intestine, most commonly the ascending or transverse colon, giving it the appearance of being bound tightly by a string. **c. telangiectat′icum, c. telangiecto′des,** carcinoma involving the cutaneous capillaries and producing telangiectatic changes. **transitional cell c.,** a malignant tumor arising from a transitional type of stratified epithelium, usually affecting the urinary bladder. **c. tubero′sum, tuberous c.,** scirrhous carcinoma of the skin with the formation of nodular projections. **verrucous c.,** a variety of epidermoid carcinoma that has a predilection for the buccal mucosa but also affects other oral soft tissue, the larynx, and the genitals. It is a slow-growing, somewhat invasive, exophytic neoplasm, either papillary or verrucous in appearance. **c. villo′sum,** carcinoma in which the cells are arranged in a villous pattern.

carcinomata (kar″sĭ-no′mah-tah) plural of *carcinoma.*

carcinomatoid (kar″sĭ-nom′ah-toid) resembling carcinoma.

carcinomatophobia (kar″sĭ-no″mah-to-fo′be-ah) cancerphobia.

carcinomatosis (kar″sĭ-no-mah-to′sis) the condition of widespread dissemination of cancer throughout the body; called also *carcinosis.*

carcinomatous (kar″sĭ-nom′ah-tus) pertaining to or of the nature of cancer; malignant.

carcinomectomy (kar″sĭ-no-mek′to-me) carcinectomy.

carcinomelcosis (kar″sĭ-no-mel-ko′sis) [*carcinoma* + Gr. *helkōsis* ulceration] (*obs.*) an ulcerated carcinoma.

carcinophilia (kar″sĭ-no-fil′e-ah) [*carcinoma* + Gr. *philein* to love] special affinity for cancerous tissue.

carcinophilic (kar″sĭ-no-fil′ik) having an affinity for cancerous tissue.

carcinophobia (kar″sĭ-no-fo′be-ah) [*carcinoma* + *phobia*] cancerphobia.

carcinosarcoma (kar″sĭ-no-sar-ko′mah) a malignant tumor composed of carcinomatous and sarcomatous tissues. **embryonal c.**, Wilms' tumor.

carcinosis (kar″sĭ-no′sis) carcinomatosis. **miliary c.**, carcinomatosis marked by development of numerous nodules resembling miliary tubercles. **c. pleu′rae**, secondary cancer of the pleura in which the membrane is studded with nodules. **pulmonary c.**, alveolar cell carcinoma.

carcinostatic (kar″sĭ-no-stat′ik) tending to check the growth of carcinoma.

carcinous (kar′sĭ-nus) carcinomatous.

card- see *cardio-*.

cardamom (kar′dah-mom) [L. *cardamomum;* Gr. *kardamōmon*] the fruit of *Elettaria cardamomum* of the ginger family, a perennial herb native to tropical Asia; its seed is used as a flavoring agent, and has been used as a carminative. Also, the fruit of herbs of the same family, e.g., that of *Amomum*.

Cardarelli's sign (symptom) (kar-dar-el′ēz) [Antonio *Cardarelli*, Italian physician, 1831–1927] see under *sign.*

cardelmycin (kar-del-mi′sin) novobiocin.

Carden's amputation (kar′denz) [Henry Douglas *Carden*, English surgeon, 19th century] see under *amputation.*

cardia (kar′de-ah) [Gr. *kardia* heart] 1. ostium cardiacum. 2. that part of the stomach surrounding the esophagogastric junction which contains cardiac glands but lacks acid (parietal) and pepsin (chief) cells. **c. of stomach, c. ventric′uli**, ostium cardiacum [NA].

cardiac (kar′de-ak) [L. *cardiacus,* from Gr. *kardiakos*] 1. pertaining to the heart. 2. a cordial, or restorative medicine. 3. a person with a heart disorder. 4. pertaining to the portion of the stomach close to the esophagus; see also *cardiac glands,* under *gland.*

cardiagra (kar-de-ag′rah) [*cardia-* + Gr. *agra* seizure] (*obs.*) gout or pain of the heart.

cardialgia (kar″de-al′je-ah) [*cardia-* + *-algia*] 1. (*obs.*) an uneasy or painful sensation in the anterior chest or upper abdomen; heartburn. 2. cardiodynia.

cardianesthesia (kar″de-an″es-the′ze-ah) [*cardia-* + *anesthesia*] (*obs.*) absence of sensation in the heart.

cardianeuria (kar″de-ah-nu′re-ah) [*cardia-* + Gr. *aneuros* without nerves + *-ia*] (*obs.*) deficiency of tone in the heart.

cardiant (kar′de-ant) a drug or agent stimulating the heart.

cardiasthenia (kar″de-as-the′ne-ah) [*cardia-* + Gr. *astheneia* weakness] neurocirculatory asthenia.

cardiasthma (kar-de-as′mah) cardiac asthma.

cardiataxia (kar″de-ah-tak′se-ah) [*cardia-* + *ataxia*] (*obs.*) incoordination in the movements of the heart.

cardiectasis (kar″de-ek′tah-sis) [*cardia-* + Gr. *ektasis* dilatation] dilatation of the heart.

cardiectomized (kar″de-ek′tŏ-mīzd) having the heart removed, as a cardiectomized animal.

cardiectomy (kar″de-ek′tŏ-me) [*cardia-* + Gr. *ektomē* excision] excision of the cardiac portion of the stomach.

Cardilate (kar′dĭ-lāt) trademark for a preparation of erythrityl tetranitrate.

cardinal (kar′dĭ-nal) [L. *cardinalis,* from *cardo* a hinge] of primary or preeminent importance.

cardio-, card- [Gr. *kardia* heart] a combining form denoting relationship to the heart or to the cardiac orifice or portion of the stomach.

cardioaccelerator (kar″de-o-ak-sel′er-a-tor) 1. quickening the heart action. 2. an agent that accelerates the heart action.

cardioactive (kar″de-o-ak′tiv) having an effect upon the heart.

cardioangiography (kar″de-o-an″je-og′rah-fe) angiocardiography.

cardioangiology (kar″de-o-an″je-ol′o-je) [*cardio-* + Gr. *angeion* vessel + *-logy*] the medical specialty which deals with the heart and blood vessels.

cardioaortic (kar″de-o-a-or′tik) pertaining to the heart and the aorta.

cardioarterial (kar″de-o-ar-te′re-al) pertaining to the heart and the arteries.

cardiocairograph (kar″de-o-ki′ro-graf) [*cardio-* + Gr. *kairos* time + *graphein* to write.] a technique by means of which roentgenograms of the heart can be made at any chosen phase of its cycle.

cardiocele (kar′de-o-sēl″) [*cardio-* + Gr. *kēlē* tumor] protrusion of the heart through a fissure of the diaphragm or through a wound.

cardiocentesis (kar″de-o-sen-te′sis) [*cardio-* + Gr. *kentēsis* puncture] surgical puncture or incision of the heart; called also *cardiopuncture.*

cardiochalasia (kar″de-o-kah-la′ze-ah) [*cardio-* + Gr. *chalasis* relaxation + *-ia*] relaxation or incompetence of sphincter action of the cardiac orifice of the stomach.

cardiocinetic (kar″de-o-sĭ-net′ik) cardiokinetic.

cardiocirculatory (kar″de-o-ser′ku-lah-tor′e) pertaining to blood flow through the heart and vascular system.

cardiocirrhosis (kar″de-o-sir-ro′sis) [*cardio-* + *cirrhosis*] cirrhosis of the liver complicating heart disease with recurrent intractable congestive heart failure; cardiac cirrhosis. See *Hutinel's disease,* under *disease.*

cardioclasis (kar″de-ok′lah-sis) [*cardio-* + Gr. *klasis* break] (*obs.*) rupture of the heart.

cardiodiaphragmatic (kar″de-o-di″ah-frag-mat′ik) pertaining to the heart and diaphragm.

cardiodilator (kar″de-o-di′la-tor) an instrument for dilating the cardia in cardiospasm or stricture.

cardiodiosis (kar″de-o-di-o′sis) the dilatation of the cardiac end of the stomach.

cardiodynamics (kar″de-o-di-nam′iks) [*cardio-* + *dynamics*] the science of the motions and forces involved in the heart's action.

cardiodynia (kar″de-o-din′e-ah) [*cardio-* + Gr. *odynē* pain] pain in the heart.

cardioesophageal (kar″de-o-ĕ-sof″ah-je′al) pertaining to the cardia of the stomach and the esophagus, as the cardioesophageal junction or sphincter.

cardiogenesis (kar″de-o-jen′ĕ-sis) [*cardio-* + Gr. *gennan* to produce] the development of the heart in the embryo.

cardiogenic (kar″de-o-jen′ik) [*cardio-* + Gr. *gennan* to produce] 1. originating in the heart; caused by abnormal function of the heart. 2. pertaining to cardiogenesis.

Cardiografin (kar″de-o-gra′fin) trademark for meglumine diatrizoate injection.

cardiogram (kar′de-o-gram″) [*cardio-* + Gr. *gramma* a writing] a tracing of a cardiac event made by means of the cardiograph. **apex c.**, a graphic record, in the form of a simple displacement curve, of the thrust of the apex of the heart as manifested on the surface of the body. **esophageal c.**, a tracing of the contractions of the left atrium made by registering the pulsations in the esophagus. **negative c.**, a cardiogram in which the curve falls below the abscissa instead of rising above it. **precordial c.**, kinetocardiogram. **vector c.**, vectorcardiogram.

cardiograph (kar′de-o-graf″) [*cardio-* + Gr. *graphein* to write] an instrument designed to record some element of the heartbeat.

cardiographic (kar″de-o-graf′ik) pertaining to cardiography.

cardiography (kar″de-og′rah-fe) the technique of graphically recording some physical or functional aspects of the heart. See also *ballistocardiography, echocardiography, electrocardiography, electrokymography, kinetocardiography, phonocardiography, roentgen kymography, vibrocardiography,* etc. **apex c.**, the graphic recording of low-frequency pulsations at the anterior chest wall over the apex of the heart. **ultrasonic c.**, echocardiography. **vector c.**, vectorcardiography.

Cardio-Green (kar′de-o-grēn) trademark for a preparation of indocyanine green.

cardiohepatic (kar″de-o-hĕ-pat′ik) pertaining to the heart and the liver.

cardiohepatomegaly (kar″de-o-hep′ah-to-meg′ah-le) enlargement of the heart and liver.

cardioid (kar′de-oid) heartlike; resembling a heart.

cardioinhibitor (kar″de-o-in-hib′ĭ-ter) an agent which restrains the heart's action.

cardioinhibitory (kar″de-o-in-hib′ĭ-to-re) restraining or inhibiting the movements of the heart.

cardiokinetic (kar″de-o-ki-net′ik) 1. stimulating the action of the heart. 2. an agent that stimulates action of the heart.

cardiokymographic (kar″de-o-ki″mo-graf′ik) pertaining to cardiokymography.

cardiokymography (kar″de-o-ki-mog′rah-fe) the recording of the motion of the heart by means of the electrokymograph.

cardiolipin (kar″de-o-lip′in) [*cardio-* + Gr. *lipos* fat] 1,3-diphosphatidylglycerol, a phospholipid synthesized in mitochondria and also abundant in bacterial cell membranes; it has immunologic properties and, when combined with lecithin and cholesterol, forms an antigen for use in flocculation and precipitation tests for syphilis. It combines with Wassermann antibody but not with the antibody responsible for treponema immobilization.

cardiolith (kar′de-o-lith″) [*cardio-* + Gr. *lithos* stone] (*obs.*) a concretion or calculus within the heart.

cardiologist (kar-de-ol′o-jist) a physician skilled in the diagnosis and treatment of heart disease.

cardiology (kar-de-ol′o-je) [*cardio-* + *-logy*]   the study of the heart and its functions.

cardiolysin (kar″de-ol′ĭ-sin)   a lysin that acts on heart muscle.

cardiolysis (kar″de-ol′ĭ-sis) [*cardio-* + Gr. *lysis* loosening]   an operation of freeing the heart and its adherent pericardium from its adhesion to the sternal periosteum in adhesive mediastinopericarditis; it is done by resecting the ribs and the sternum over the pericardium. See also *Brauer's operation,* under *operation.*

cardiomalacia (kar″de-o-mah-la′she-ah) [*cardio-* + Gr. *malakia* softness]   morbid softening of the muscular substance of the heart.

cardiomegalia (kar″de-o-mĕ-ga′le-ah)   cardiomegaly.   **c. glycogen′ica circumscrip′ta,** glycogenic cardiomegaly. **c. glycogen′ica diffu′sa,** glycogen storage disease, type II; see under *disease.*

cardiomegaly (kar″de-o-meg′ah-le) [*cardio-* + Gr. *megas* large]   cardiac hypertrophy.   **glycogenic c.,** a morbid condition characterized by enlargement of the heart, with localized deposits of glycogen in the heart muscle; called also *cardiomegalia glycogenica circumscripta.*

cardiomelanosis (kar″de-o-mel″ah-no′sis)   melanosis of the heart.

cardiometer (kar″de-om′ĕ-ter) [*cardio-* + Gr. *metron* measure]   an instrument used in estimating the power of the heart's action.

cardiometry (kar″de-om′ĕ-tre)   the estimation of the force of the heart's action.

cardiomotility (kar″de-o-mo-til′ĭ-te)   the movements of the heart; the motility of the heart.

cardiomyoliposis (kar″de-o-mi″o-li-po′sis) [*cardio-* + Gr. *mys* muscle + *lipos* fat]   fatty degeneration of the heart muscle.

cardiomyopathy (kar″de-o-mi-op′ah-the) [*cardio-* + Gr. *mys* muscle + *pathos* disease]   a general diagnostic term designating primary myocardial disease, often of obscure or unknown etiology.   **alcoholic c.,** a congestive cardiomyopathy resulting in cardiac enlargement and low cardiac output, occurring in chronic alcoholics; the heart disease in beriberi (thiamine deficiency) is also associated with alcoholism.   **congestive c.,** a syndrome characterized by cardiac enlargement, especially of the left ventricle, myocardial dysfunction, and congestive heart failure.   **infiltrative c.,** myocardial disease resulting from deposition in the heart tissue of abnormal substances, as may occur in amyloidosis, hemochromatosis, etc.   **peripartum c.,** cardiac enlargement and congestive heart failure of unknown cause beginning in the last month of gestation or the first few months after delivery.   **postpartum c.,** cardiac enlargement and congestive heart failure of unknown cause occurring in a mother during the first few months after delivery of a child.   **primary c.,** that in which the basic pathological process involves the myocardium itself and not other cardiac structures and in which the cause is unknown and not part of a disease affecting other organs.   **restrictive c.,** a form in which the ventricular walls are excessively rigid, impeding ventricular filling; it is marked by abnormal diastolic function but by normal or nearly normal systolic function.   **secondary c.,** any form that is due to another cardiovascular disorder (e.g., hypertension) or is a manifestation of systemic disease (e.g., sarcoidosis).

cardiomyopexy (kar″de-o-mi′o-pek″se) [*cardio-* + Gr. *mys* muscle + *pēxis* fixation]   surgical removal of the epicardium and application of a pedicled flap of adjacent muscle to the denuded myocardium and pericardium, as a means of supplying collateral circulation to the heart.

cardiomyotomy (kar″de-o-mi-ot′ŏ-me) [*cardio-* + Gr. *mys* muscle + *tomē* a cutting]   esophagogastromyotomy.

cardionecrosis (kar″de-o-nĕ-kro′sis)   necrosis or gangrene of the heart.

cardionector (kar″de-o-nek′ter) [*cardio-* + L. *nector* joiner]   the structures that regulate the heart beat, comprising the sinoatrial node (atrionector), the bundle of His (ventriculonector), and the atrioventricular node.

cardionephric (kar″de-o-nef′rik)   pertaining to the heart and the kidney.

cardioneural (kar″de-o-nu′ral)   pertaining to the heart and nervous system.

cardioneurosis (kar″de-o-nu-ro′sis) [*cardio-* + *neurosis*]   neurocirculatory asthenia.

cardio-omentopexy (kar″de-o-o-men′to-pek″se)   the operation of suturing a portion of the omentum to the heart, the omentum having been drawn through an incision in the diaphragm.

cardiopalmus (kar″de-o-pal′mus) [*cardio-* + Gr. *palmos* palpitation]   (*obs.*) palpitation of the heart.

cardiopaludism (kar″de-o-pal′u-dizm)   heart disease due to malaria, marked by gallop rhythm in the tricuspid area, intermittent heart action, dilatation of the right heart, and reduplication of the diastolic sound.

cardiopath (kar′de-o-path)   a person with heart disease.

cardiopathia (kar″de-o-path′e-ah)   cardiopathy.

cardiopathic (kar″de-o-path′ik)   pertaining to or marked by disease of the heart.

cardiopathy (kar″de-op′ah-the) [*cardio-* + Gr. *pathos* disease]   any disorder or disease of the heart. In addition to heart disease of inflammatory origin, there are *arteriosclerotic cardiopathy,* due to arteriosclerosis; *fatty cardiopathy,* due to growth of fatty tissue; *hypertensive cardiopathy,* due to high blood pressure; *nephropathic cardiopathy,* due to kidney disease; *thyrotoxic cardiopathy,* due to thyroid intoxication; *toxic cardiopathy,* due to the effect of some toxin; *valvular cardiopathy,* due to faulty valve action.   **infarctoid c.,** a heart condition with symptoms resembling those of myocardial infarction.

cardiopericardiopexy (kar″de-o-per″ĭ-kar′de-o-pek-se) [*cardio-* + *pericardium* + Gr. *pēxis* fixation]   the operative establishment of adhesive pericarditis, for the relief of coronary disease.

cardiopericarditis (kar″de-o-per″ĭ-kar-di′tis) [*cardio-* + *pericarditis*]   inflammation of both the heart and the pericardium.

cardiophobia (kar″de-o-fo′be-ah) [*cardio-* + Gr. *phobein* to be affrighted by + *-ia*]   morbid dread of heart disease.

cardiophone (kar′de-o-fōn″) [*cardio-* + Gr. *phōnē* voice]   (*obs.*) an instrument for recording the heart sounds.

cardiophrenia (kar″de-o-fre′ne-ah)   (*obs.*) neurocirculatory asthenia.

cardioplasty (kar′de-o-plas″te) [*cardio-* + Gr. *plassein* to form]   esophagogastroplasty.

cardioplegia (kar″de-o-ple′je-ah) [*cardio-* + Gr. *plēgē* stroke + *-ia*]   arrest of contraction of the myocardium, as may be induced by the use of chemical compounds or of cold (cryocardioplegia) in the performance of surgery upon the heart.

cardioplegic (kar″de-o-plej′ik)   pertaining to cardioplegia.

cardiopneumatic (kar″de-o-nu-mat′ik) [*cardio-* + Gr. *pneuma* breath]   of or pertaining to the heart and respiration.

cardiopneumograph (kar″de-o-nu′mo-graf) [*cardio-* + Gr. *pneuma* breath + *graphein* to record]   an apparatus that registers cardiopneumatic movements.

cardiopneumonopexy (kar″de-o-nu-mon′o-pek″se)   an operation designed to provide collateral blood supply to the heart muscle by various methods of connecting the heart with the left lung, including production of vascular adhesions through the use of mechanical abrasion or chemical irritants.

cardioptosia (kar″de-o-to′se-ah)   cardioptosis.

cardioptosis (kar″de-op′tŏ-sis) [*cardio-* + Gr. *ptōsis* falling]   downward displacement of the heart; called also *Rummo's disease* and *Wenckebach's disease.*

cardiopulmonary (kar″de-o-pul′mo-ner-e)   pertaining to the heart and lungs.

cardiopuncture (kar″de-o-punk′cher)   cardiocentesis.

cardiopyloric (kar″de-o-pi-lor′ik)   pertaining to the cardia (ostium cardiacum [NA]) and the pylorus.

Cardioquin (kar′de-o-kwin″)   trademark for a preparation of quinidine polygalacturonate.

cardiorenal (kar″de-o-re′nal)   pertaining to the heart and the kidney.

cardiorrhaphy (kar″de-or′ah-fe) [*cardio-* + Gr. *raphē* suture]   the operation of suturing the heart muscle.

cardiorrhexis (kar″de-o-rek′sis) [*cardio-* + Gr. *rhēxis* rupture]   rupture of the heart.

cardiosclerosis (kar″de-o-skle-ro′sis) [*cardio-* + Gr. *sklēros* hard]   fibrous induration of the heart.

cardioscope (kar′de-o-skōp″) [*cardio-* + Gr. *skopein* to examine]   an instrument once used for inspecting the interior of the heart and for manipulation within the heart.

cardioselective (kar″de-o-sĕ-lek′tiv)   having greater activity on heart tissue than on other tissue.

cardiospasm (kar′de-o-spazm″)   achalasia of the esophagus; see under *achalasia.*   **tropical c.,** entalação.

cardiosphygmogram (kar″de-o-sfig′mŏ-gram)   a tracing made by the cardiosphygmograph.

cardiosphygmograph (kar″de-o-sfig′mŏ-graf)   a combination of the cardiograph and sphygmograph for recording the movements of the heart and an arterial pulse.

cardiosplenopexy (kar″de-o-splen′o-pek″se)   suture of splenic parenchyma to the denuded surface of the heart, as a method of revascularization of the myocardium.

cardiosymphysis (kar″de-o-sim′fĭ-sis) [*cardio-* + Gr. *symphysis* growing together]   (*obs.*) a condition in which the heart has become fixed to the chest by combined adhesion of the visceral and parietal pericardia to each other and by adhesion of the parietal pericardium to the mediastinal structures.

cardiotachometer (kar″de-o-tah-kom′ĕ-ter) [*cardio-* + Gr. *tachos* speed + *metron* measure]   the instrument used in cardiotachometry.

cardiotachometry (kar″de-o-tah-kom′ĕ-tre)   continuous recording of the heart rate for long periods of time.

cardiotherapy (kar″de-o-ther′ah-pe) [*cardio-* + Gr. *therapeia* treatment]   the treatment of heart diseases.

cardiothyrotoxicosis (kar″de-o-thi″ro-tok″se-ko′sis)   hyperthyroidism with cardiac involvement.

cardiotocograph (kar″de-o-to′ko-graf) the instrument used in cardiotocography.

cardiotocography (kar″de-o-to-kog′rah-fe) [*cardio-* + Gr. *tokos* childbirth + *graphein* to write] the monitoring of the fetal heart rate and uterine contractions, as during delivery. Also spelled *cardiotokography*.

cardiotokography (kar″de-o-to-kog′rah-fe) cardiotocography.

cardiotomy (kar″de-ot′ŏ-me) [*cardio-* + Gr. *tomē* a cutting] 1. surgical incision of the heart for repair of cardiac defects. 2. incision into the cardiac end of the stomach or the cardiac orifice.

cardiotonic (kar″de-o-ton′ik) 1. having a tonic effect on the heart. 2. an agent that has a tonic effect on the heart.

cardiotopometry (kar″de-o-to-pom′ĕ-tre) [*cardio-* + Gr. *topos* place + *metron* measure] measurement of the area of cardiac dullness.

cardiotoxic (kar″de-o-tok′sik) having a poisonous or deleterious effect upon the heart.

cardiovalvular (kar″de-o-val′vu-lar) pertaining to the valves of the heart.

cardiovalvulitis (kar″de-o-val″vu-li′tis) inflammation of the valves of the heart.

cardiovalvulotome (kar″de-o-val′vu-lo-tōm″) [*cardio-* + L. *valvula* valve + Gr. *tomē* cut] an instrument for performing cardiovalvulotomy.

cardiovalvulotomy (kar″de-o-val″vu-lot′o-me) [*cardio-* + L. *valvula* valve + Gr. *tomē* a cutting] the operation of incising a cardiac valve, or of excising a portion of it, done for the relief of stenosis.

cardiovascular (kar″de-o-vas′ku-lar) pertaining to the heart and blood vessels.

cardiovascular-renal (kar″de-o-vas′ku-lar-re′nal) pertaining to the heart, blood vessels, and kidney.

cardiovasology (kar″de-o-vas-ol′o-je) cardioangiology.

cardioversion (kar′de-o-ver″zhun) the restoration of normal rhythm of the heart by electrical shock.

cardioverter (kar′-de-o-ver″ter) an energy-storage capacitor-discharge type of condenser which is discharged with an inductance; it delivers a direct-current shock which restores normal rhythm of the heart.

carditis (kar-di′tis) [*cardio-* + *-itis*] inflammation of the heart. **rheumatic c.,** cardiac involvement in rheumatic fever, which when severe may be manifested by congestive heart failure, progressive cardiac enlargement, pericarditis, and significant murmurs. **streptococcal c.,** carditis occurring as a result of streptococcal sore throat. **verrucous c.,** a nonbacterial endocarditis marked by a continuous chain of wartlike vegetations near the line of closure of the cusps of the mitral and tricuspid valves; seen in lupus erythematosus and occasionally in scleroderma, thrombotic purpura, and other collagen diseases.

Cardrase (kar′drās) trademark for a preparation of ethoxzolamide.

carfecillin sodium (kar″fĕ-sil′in) carbenicillin phenyl sodium.

carfentanil citrate (kar-fen′tah-nil) chemical name: 4-[(1-oxopropyl) phenyl amino]-1-(2-phenylethyl)-4-piperidine carboxylic acid methyl ester 2-hydroxy 1,2,3-propanetricarboxylate (1:1); an analgesic and narcotic, $C_{24}H_{30}N_2O_3 \cdot C_6H_8O_7$.

caricous (kar′ĭ-kus) [L. *carica* fig] shaped like or resembling a fig.

caries (ka′re-ēz, kar′ēz) [L. "rottenness"] 1. the molecular decay or death of a bone, in which it becomes softened, discolored, and porous. It produces a chronic inflammation of the periosteum and surrounding tissues, and forms a cold abscess filled with a cheesy, fetid, puslike liquid, which generally burrows through the soft parts until it opens externally by a sinus or fistula. 2. dental c. **backward c.,** dental caries that progresses backward from the dentinoenamel junction into the enamel; called also *internal c.* **cemental c.,** dental caries that involves the cementum of a tooth. **central c.,** a chronic abscess in the interior of a bone. **dental c.,** a disease of the calcified tissues of the teeth resulting from the action of microorganisms on carbohydrates, characterized by decalcification of the inorganic portions of the tooth and accompanied or followed by disintegration of the organic portion. Formerly classified by degree of severity: *c. of first degree* (enamel alone decalcified); *c. of second degree* (enamel and dentin affected); *c. of third degree* (pulp exposed); *c. of fourth degree* (putrefactive decomposition of pulp). Now classified as *enamel c.* (q.v.). See also *cavity.* **dentinal c.,** dental caries that involves the dentin of a tooth. **dry c.,** a form of tuberculous caries of the joints and ends of bones; called also *c. sicca.* **enamel c.,** dental caries that involves the enamel of a tooth. **c. fungo′sa,** a form of tuberculosis of a bone. **internal c.,** backward c. **lateral c.,** dental caries that extends laterally at the dentinoenamel junction. **necrotic c.,** a disease in which pieces of bone lie in a suppurating cavity. **primary c.,** dental caries that attacks either the pits and fissures, or the smooth surfaces of a previously uninvolved area of a tooth. **secondary c.,** dental caries recurring around or beneath a previously placed dental restoration. **c. sic′ca,**

dry c. **spinal c.,** tuberculotic osteitis of the vertebrae and of the intervertebral cartilages.

carina (kah-ri′nah), pl. *cari′nae* [L. "keel"] a ridgelike structure. **c. for′nicis,** a ridge on the under surface of the fornix. **c. of trachea, c. tra′cheae** [NA], a projection of the lowest tracheal cartilage, forming a prominent semilunar ridge running anteroposteriorly between the orifices of the two bronchi. **urethral c. of vagina, c. urethra′lis vagi′nae** [NA], the column of rugae in the lower part of the anterior wall of the vagina, immediately beneath the urethra.

carinae (kah-ri′ne) [L.] plural of *carina*.

carinate (kar′ĭ-nāt) [L. *carina* a keel] keel shaped; having a keel-like process.

carination (kar″ĭ-na′shun) a ridged condition of a part.

carindacillin sodium (kar″in-dah-sil′in) carbenicillin indanyl sodium.

cariogenesis (kār″e-o-jen′ĕ-sis) development of caries.

cariogenic (kār″e-o-jen′ik) [*caries* + Gr. *gennan* to produce] conducive to caries.

cariogenicity (kār″e-o-jĕ-nis′ĭ-te) the quality of being conducive to the production of caries.

cariology (kar″e-ol′o-je) 1. the study of the cell nucleus and of chromosomal activity within it. 2. the study of caries formation and prevention.

cariosity (kar″e-os′ĭ-te) the quality of being carious.

carious (ka′re-us) [L. *cariosus*] affected with or of the nature of caries.

carisoprodol (kar″i-so-pro′dol) chemical name: (1-methylethyl)carbamic acid-2-[[aminocarbonyl)oxy]methyl]-2-methylpentyl ester. A centrally acting skeletal muscle relaxant, $C_{12}H_{24}N_2O_4$, occurring as a white, crystalline powder; used for the symptomatic management of acute, painful musculoskeletal disorders, administered orally. Called also *isopropyl meprobamate*.

Carleton's spots (karl′tonz) [Bukk G. *Carleton*, American physician, 1856–1914] see under *spot*.

carmalum (kar-mal′um) a stain composed of carmine, alum, and water.

carmantadine (kar-man′tah-dēn) chemical name: 1-tricyclo-[3.3.1.1³,⁷]dec-1-yl-azetidinecarboxylic acid; an antiparkinsonian agent, $C_{14}H_{21}NO_2$.

Carmichael's crown (kar′mi-kel) [J. P. *Carmichael*, American dentist, 1856–1946] partial veneer crown; see under *crown*.

carminative (kar-min′ah-tiv) [L. *carminare* to card, to cleanse, from *carmen*, a card for wool] 1. relieving flatulence. 2. a medicine that relieves flatulence and assuages pain.

carmine (kar′min) a red coloring matter derived from cochineal by the addition of alum and used as a histologic stain; called also *carminum* and *coccinellin*. **alizarin c.,** alizarin red. **indigo c.,** indigotin disulfonate sodium. **lithium c.,** vital stain for macrophages. **Schneider's c.,** a saturated solution of carmine in concentrated acetic acid.

carminophil (kar-min′o-fil) [*carmine* + Gr. *philein* to love] 1. easily stainable with carmine. 2. a cell or other element that readily takes a stain from carmine. 3. one of the acidophils, or alpha cells (*mammotropes*), of the adenohypophysis staining readily with azocarmine; called also *epsilon acidophil*.

carminum (kar-mi′num) carmine.

carmustine (kar-mus′tēn) chemical name: *N,N′*-bis(2-chloroethyl)-*N*-nitrosourea (BCNU); a nitrosourea, $C_5H_9Cl_2N_3O_2$, used as an antineoplastic agent.

carneous (kar′ne-us) [L. *carneus*, from *caro* flesh] fleshy.

carnidazole (kar-nid′ah-zōl) chemical name: [2-(2-methyl-5-nitro-1*H*-imidazol-1-yl)ethyl]carbamothioic acid *O*-methyl ester; an antiprotozoal, $C_8H_{12}N_4O_3S$.

carnification (kar″nĭ-fĭ-ka′shun) [L. *caro* flesh + *facere* to make] the change of tissue, such as that of the lungs, into a substance resembling flesh.

carnitine (kar′nĭ-tin) a naturally occurring amino acid, $C_7H_{15}NO_3$, required for mitochondrial oxidation of long-chain fatty acids; it is a betaine derivative found in skeletal muscle and liver, which acts as a carrier of acyl groups (fatty acids) across the mitochondrial membrane to the matrix, where they combine with coenzyme A to form acyl CoA. It has been used as an investigational antithyroid and antiangina agent.

Carnivora (kar-niv′ŏ-rah) [L. *caro* flesh + *vorare* to devour] an order of mammals that are primarily carnivorous, with teeth adapted for flesh eating, a simple stomach, and a short intestine.

carnivore (kar′nĭ-vōr) an animal that eats flesh, especially members of the order Carnivora.

carnivorous (kar-niv′o-rus) eating or subsisting on flesh.

Carnochan's operation (kar′nok-anz) [John Murray *Carnochan*, American surgeon, 1817–1887] see under *operation*.

carnosinase (kar′no-sĭ-nās) an enzyme that hydrolyzes carnosine (amino-acyl-L-histidine) and other dipeptides containing L-histidine into their constituent amino acids.

carnosine (kar′no-sin) chemical name: β-alanylhistidine. A dipeptide, $C_9H_{14}N_4O_2$, composed of beta-alanine and histidine, found in skeletal muscle of vertebrates.

carnosinemia (kar″no-sĭ-ne′me-ah) excessive amounts of carnosine in the blood; it has been associated with a progressive neurologic disease characterized by severe mental defect and myoclonic seizures, and is probably due to a genetic deficiency of carnosinase in the serum.

carnosinuria (kar″no-sĭ-nu′re-ah) an aminoaciduria characterized by excess of carnosine in the urine; occurs in carnosinemia or may be dietary in origin, especially in young children.

carnosity (kar-nos′ĭ-te) [L. *carnositas* fleshiness] any abnormal fleshy excrescence.

Carnot's test (kar′nōz) [Paul *Carnot*, French physician, 1869–1957] see under *tests*.

carnutine (kar-nu′tin) a ptomaine found in muscle tissue.

caro (ka′ro), pl. *car′nes* [L.] flesh or muscular tissue. **c. quadra′ta ma′nus,** musculus palmaris brevis. **c. quadra′ta syl′vii,** musculus quadratus plantae.

carota (kah-ro′tah), pl. *caro′tae* [L.] carrot.

carotenase (kar-ot′ĕ-nās) an enzyme capable of converting carotene into vitamin A; called also *carotinase*.

carotene (kar′o-tēn) a yellow or red pigment found in carrots, sweet potatoes, leafy vegetables, milk fat, body fat, egg yolk, etc. It is a chromolipoid hydrocarbon and exists in several forms; alpha, beta, and gamma carotene are pro-vitamins and may be converted into vitamin A in the body. Called also *carotin*. **beta c.,** chemical name: β,β-carotene; an ultraviolet screen, $C_{40}H_{56}$.

carotenemia (kar″o-te-ne′me-ah) [*carotene* + Gr. *haima* blood + *-ia*] presence of excessive carotene in the blood; it sometimes occurs in sufficient quantities to produce yellowing of the skin resembling jaundice (carotenodermia).

carotenoderma (kar-ot″en-o-der′mah) carotenodermia.

carotenodermia (kar-rot″ĕ-no-der′me-ah) yellowness of the skin due to carotenemia.

carotenoid (kah-rot′ĕ-noid) 1. any member of a group of red, orange, or yellow pigmented polyisoprenoid lipids found in carrots, sweet potatoes, green leaves, and some animal tissues; examples are the carotenes, lycopene, and xanthophyll. In plants, blue-green algae, and photosynthetic bacteria, carotenoids absorb energy from light and transfer it to chlorophyll. 2. marked by yellow color. 3. lipochrome.

carotenosis (kar″o-te-no′sis) carotenemia.

carotic (kah-rot′ik) [Gr. *karos* deep sleep] pertaining to or of the nature of carus, or stupor.

caroticotympanic (kah-rot″ĭ-ko-tim-pan′ik) pertaining to the carotid canal and the tympanum.

carotid (kah-rot′id) [Gr. *karōtis* from *karos* deep sleep] relating to the principal artery of the neck (arteria carotis communis); see also under *body, sinus,* etc.

carotidynia (kah-rot″ĭ-din′e-ah) carotodynia.

carotin (kar′o-tin) carotene.

carotinase (kar′o-tĭ-nās) carotenase.

carotinemia (kar″o-tin-e′me-ah) carotenemia.

carotinosis (kar″o-tĭ-no′sis) carotenemia.

carotodynia (kah-rot″o-din′e-ah) [*carotid* + Gr. *odynē* pain] tenderness along the course of the common carotid artery.

caroxazone (kah-roks′ah-zōn) chemical name: 2-oxo-2*H*-1,3-benzoxazine-3(4*H*)-acetamide; an antidepressant, $C_{10}H_{10}N_2O_3$.

carp (karp) a fruiting body of a fungus.

carpal (kar′pal) [L. *carpalis*] of or pertaining to the carpus, or wrist.

carpale (kar-pa′le) a carpal bone.

carpectomy (kar-pek′to-me) [*carpus* + Gr. *ektomē* excision] excision of a carpal bone.

carpel (kar′pel) a one-celled pistil, or one of the members composing a compound pistil or seed vessel.

carphenazine maleate (kar-fen′ah-zēn) [USP] chemical name: 1-[10-[3-[4-(2-hydroxyethyl)1-piperazinyl]propyl]-10*H*-phenothiazin-2-yl]-1-propanone(*Z*)-2-butenedioate (1:2). A phenothiazine antipsychotic agent, $C_{24}H_{31}N_3O_2S·2C_4H_4O_4$, occurring as a yellow, finely divided powder; used in the treatment of acute or chronic schizophrenic reactions in hospitalized patients, administered orally.

carphologia (kar″fo-lo′je-ah) carphology.

carphology (kar-fol′o-je) [Gr. *karphologein* to pick bits of wool off a person's coat] the involuntary picking at the bedclothes seen in grave fevers and in conditions of great exhaustion; called also *carphologia* and *crocidismus*.

carpitis (kar-pi′tis) inflammation of the synovial membranes of the bones of the carpal joint of domestic animals, producing swelling, pain, and lameness.

carpocarpal (kar″po-kar′pal) pertaining to two parts of the carpus, especially to the articulations between carpal bones.

Carpoglyphus (kar″po-gli′fus) a genus of mites. **C. pas-**

sula′rum, a tyroglyphid mite that infests dried fruit, causing dermatitis in those who handle the infested fruit.

carpogonium (kar″po-go′ne-um) ascogonium; more specifically the female sex organ in members of the order Erysiphales, class Ascomycetes.

carpometacarpal (kar″po-met″ah-kar′pal) pertaining to the carpus and metacarpus.

carpopedal (kar″po-pe′dal) [*carpus* + L. *pes, pedalis* foot] pertaining to or affecting the carpus and the foot, as carpopedal spasm.

carpophalangeal (kar″po-fah-lan′je-al) pertaining to the carpus and the phalanges.

carpoptosis (kar″pop-to′sis) [*carpus* + *ptosis*] wristdrop.

carpospore (kar′po-spōr) a diploid spore in the red algae which, by germination, produces tetraspores.

carprofen (kar-pro′fen) chemical name: (±)-6-chloro-α-methyl-carbazole-2-acetic acid; an anti-inflammatory, $C_{15}H_{12}ClNO_2$.

Carpue's operation, rhinoplasty (kar′pūz) [Joseph Constantine *Carpue*, English surgeon, 1764–1846] Indian rhinoplasty.

Carpule (kar′pūl) trademark for a glass, rubber-stoppered cartridge containing local anesthetic solutions, fitted in a special syringe for hypodermic injection.

carpus (kar′pus) [L.; Gr. *karpos*] [NA] the joint between the arm and hand, the wrist, made up of eight bones; see *ossa carpi,* and names of specific bones. Also, the part of the hand between the forearm and metacarpus. The term is also applied to the corresponding forelimb joint in quadrupeds. **c. cur′vus,** Madelung's deformity.

Carr-Price test [Francis Howard *Carr*, British chemist, born 1874; E. A. *Price*] see under *tests*.

carrageen, carragheen (kar′ah-gēn) the dried and bleached plant *Chondrus crispus* (L.) Stackhouse, or *Gigartina mammillosa* (Goodenough and Woodward) J. Aghardt (Gigartinaceae). It contains a valuable polysaccharide widely used as a gel, thickening agent, and emulsifier. It also has demulcent properties.

carrageenan, carragheenin (kar″ah-ge′nan) a colloidal extractive derived from various species of red marine algae (*Chondrus, Eucheuma, Gigartina,* etc.), composed of a mixture of sodium, potassium, calcium, and magnesium salts of an acid sulfate of a galactose-containing polysaccharide. Used chiefly as a suspending agent in foods, pharmaceuticals, cosmetics, etc.

carreau (kar-ro′) [Fr.] (*obs.*) enlargement and hardening of the abdomen caused by disease of the peritoneum and abdominal walls.

carrefour (kahr″uh-foōr′) [Fr.] crossway; decussation.

Carrel's method, treatment, tube (kar-elz′) [Alexis *Carrel,* French surgeon who spent many years in the United States, 1873–1944; winner of the Nobel prize for physiology and medicine in 1912] see under *method, treatment, and tube*.

Carrel-Dakin fluid, treatment [Alexis *Carrel;* Henry Drysdale *Dakin,* American chemist, 1880–1952] see *diluted sodium hypochorite solution,* under *solution,* and see under *treatment*.

carrier (kar′e-er) 1. an individual who harbors in his body the specific organisms of a disease without manifest symptoms and thus acts as a carrier or distributor of the infection; the condition of such an individual is known as *carrier state.* 2. a substance in a cell which can accept one or two electrons and so be reduced and can then be re-oxidized. 3. an instrument or apparatus for carrying or transporting something. 4. a heterozygote, i.e., one who carries a recessive gene, either autosomal or sex-linked, together with its normal allele. 5. in radiology, a substance in appreciable amount, which when associated with a trace of another substance, will carry the trace through a chemical or physical process, especially a precipitation process. 6. a molecule to which a substance may be reversibly attached for transport, as across an intracellular membrane. 7. a macromolecular immunogen which when chemically coupled to a hapten may facilitate an immune response to the hapten. **amalgam c.,** a dental instrument for transporting portions of mixed amalgam, used as a restorative material, to a prepared tooth cavity. **electron c.,** see *carrier,* def. 2. **female c.,** a woman who is heterozygous for a recessive X-linked gene; half of the sons of a female carrier show the recessive X-chromosomal feature. **foil c.,** a dental instrument for transporting foil, used as a restorative material, from the annealor to a prepared tooth cavity. **gametocyte c.,** in malaria, a person who has gametocytes in his blood stream and so can infect *Anopheles* mosquitoes that feed on him. **hemophilia c.,** the female transmitter of classical sex-linked, recessive hemophilia who generally, but not always, demonstrates no overt manifestations of a hemorrhagic diathesis but in whom a coagulation factor deficiency may be detected by quantitative assay.

carrier-free (kar′e-er-fre) a term denoting a radioisotope of an element in pure form, i.e., essentially undiluted with a stable isotope carrier.

Carrión's disease (kar-e-onz′) [Daniel A. *Carrión,* (1850–1885), a student in Peru who inoculated himself and died of the disease] see under *disease*.

carrot (kar′ut) [L. *carota*] the umbelliferous plant, *Daucus carota;* its seed is diuretic and stimulant.

carrotene (kar′o-tēn) carotene.

cart (kart) a wheeled vehicle for conveying patients or equipment and supplies in a hospital. **crash c.,** resuscitation c. **dressing c.,** one containing all the supplies and equipment that may be necessary for changing dressings of surgical or injured patients. **resuscitation c.,** one containing all the equipment necessary for initiating emergency resuscitation.

cartazolate (kar-taz′o-lāt) chemical name: 4-(butylamino)-1-ethyl-1*H*-pyrazolo[3,4-*b*]pyridine-5-carboxylic acid ethyl ester; an antidepressant, $C_{15}H_{22}N_4O_2$.

carteolol hydrochloride (kar′te-o-lōl) chemical name: 5-[3-[(1,1-dimethylethyl)amino]-2-hydroxypropoxy]-3,4-dihydro-2(1*H*)-quinolinone monohydrochloride; an antiadrenergic (β-receptor), $C_{16}H_{24}N_2O_3 \cdot HCl$.

Carter's operation, intranasal splint (kar′terz) [William Wesley *Carter*, New York rhinologist, born 1869] see under *operation* (2d def.) and *splint.*

cartilage (kar′tĭ-lij) [L. *cartilago*] a specialized, fibrous connective tissue, forming most of the temporary skeleton of the embryo, providing a model in which most of the bones develop, and constituting an important part of the growth mechanism of the organism. It exists in several types, the most important of which are hyaline cartilage, elastic cartilage, and fibrocartilage. Also used as a general term to designate a mass of such tissue in a particular site in the body. See *cartilago.* **accessory c's of nose,** cartilagines alares minores. **c. of acoustic meatus,** cartilago meatus acustici. **alar c., greater,** cartilago alaris major. **alar c's, lesser,** cartilagines alares minores. **annular c.,** cartilago cricoidea. **aortic c.,** the second costal cartilage on the right side. **arthrodial c.,** articular c. **articular c.,** a thin layer of cartilage, usually hyaline, on the articular surface of bones in synovial joints. Called also *cartilago articularis* [NA], *arthrodial c., diarthrodial c., investing c.,* and *obducent c.* **arytenoid c.,** cartilago arytenoidea. **c. of auditory tube,** cartilago tubae auditivae. **c. of auricle, auricular c.,** cartilago auriculae. **branchial c.,** one of the rods of cartilage in the branchial arches of the embryo. **calcified c.,** cartilage in which granules of calcium phosphate and calcium carbonate have been deposited in the interstitial substance. **cariniform c.,** the cartilaginous prolongation at the anterior end of the sternum of a horse. **cellular c.,** a variety composed almost entirely of cells, with little interstitial substance; called also *parenchymatous c.* **central c.,** former term for an opacity in the center of the crystalline lens. **ciliary c's,** see *tarsus inferior palpebrae* and *tarsus superior palpebrae.* **circumferential c.,** labrum glenoidale. **conchal c.,** cartilago auriculae. **connecting c.,** cartilage connecting the surfaces of an immovable joint; called also *interosseous c.* **corniculate c.,** cartilago corniculata. **costal c.,** cartilago costalis. **costal c., interarticular,** ligamentum sternocostale intraarticulare. **cricoid c.,** cartilago cricoidea. **cuneiform c.,** cartilago cuneiformis. **dentinal c.,** the substance remaining after the lime salts of dentin have been dissolved in an acid. **diarthrodial c.,** articular c. **elastic c.,** a substance that is more opaque, flexible, and elastic than hyaline cartilage, and is further distinguished by its yellow color. The interstitial substance is penetrated in all directions by frequently branching fibers which give all the reactions for elastin. Called also *reticular c.* and *yellow c.* **ensiform c.,** processus xiphoideus. **epactal c's,** cartilagines nasales accessoriae. **epiglottic c.,** cartilago epiglottica. **epiphyseal c.,** cartilago epiphysialis. **eustachian c.,** cartilago tubae auditivae. **falciform c's,** see *meniscus lateralis articulationis genus* and *meniscus medialis articulationis genus.* **floating c.,** a detached piece of cartilage, usually from the articular surface of the medial condyle and femur, but also from the patella or lateral condyle of the femur. **gingival c.,** the tissue covering the loculus which contains an unerupted tooth. **guttural c.,** cartilago arytenoidea. **hyaline c.,** a flexible, somewhat elastic, semitransparent substance with an opalescent bluish tint, composed of a basophilic, fibril-containing interstitial substance with cavities in which the chondrocytes occur; called also *chondroid.* **inferior c. of nose,** cartilago alaris major. **innominate c.,** cartilago cricoidea. **interarticular c.,** 1. ligamentum longitudinale posterius. 2. an interarticular disk. **interarticular c. of little head of rib,** ligamentum capitis costae intraarticulare. **interosseous c.,** connecting c. **intervertebral c's,** disci intervertebrales. **intrathyroid c.,** a cartilage connecting the alae of the thyroid cartilage in early life. **investing c.,** articular c. **Jacobson's c.,** cartilago vomeronasalis. **laryngeal c's,** cartilagines laryngis. **laryngeal c. of Luschka,** cartilago sesamoidea ligamenti vocalis. **lateral c's,** in the horse, the cartilages from the end of the third phalanx to the heel of the hoof. **lateral c. of nose,** cartilago nasi lateralis. **Luschka's c.,** cartilago sesamoidea ligamenti vocalis. **mandibular c.,** Meckel's c. **meatal c.,** cartilago meatus acustici. **Meckel's c.,** the cartilaginous bar (in the embryo) into which the mesenchymal core of the mandibular process of the first mandibular arch is converted; from it or its sheath, the sphenomandibular ligament, the anterior malleolar ligament, the

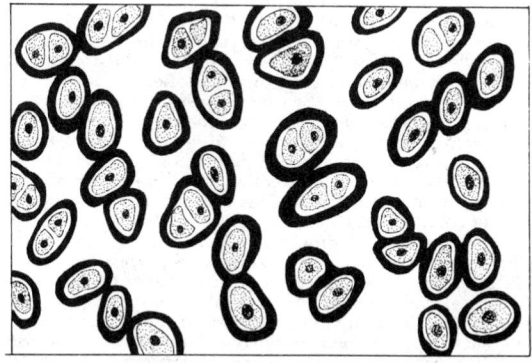

Hyaline cartilage: chondrocytes embedded in a gel-like matrix.

malleus, and the incus develop. Called also *mandibular c., tympanomandibular c.,* and *Meckel's rod.* **minor c's,** cartilagines nasales accessoriae. **mucronate c.,** processus xiphoideus. **nasal c's,** cartilagines nasi. **nasal c's, accessory,** cartilagines nasales accessoriae. **nasal c., lateral,** cartilago nasi lateralis. **c. of nasal septum,** cartilago septi nasi. **c's of nose,** cartilagines nasi. **obducent c.,** articular c. **ossifying c.,** temporary c. **palpebral c's,** see *tarsus inferior palpebrae* and *tarsus superior palpebrae.* **parachordal c's,** the two cartilages at the sides of the occipital part of the notochord of the embryo. **parenchymatous c.,** cellular c. **periotic c.,** an oval mass on the upper surface of the fetal chondrocranium investing the inner ear. **permanent c.,** cartilage that does not normally become ossified. **posterior cricoarytenoid c.,** ligamenta cricoarytenoideum posterius. **precursory c.,** temporary c. **pulmonary c.,** the third costal cartilage on the left side. **pyramidal c.,** cartilago arytenoidea. **Reichert's c's,** cartilaginous bars in the lateral side of the embryonic tympanum from which develop the styloid processes, the stylohyoid ligaments, and the lesser cornua of the hyoid bone. **reticular c.,** elastic c. **Santorini's c.,** cartilago corniculata. **scutiform c.,** cartilago thyroidea. **semilunar c. of knee joint, external,** meniscus lateralis articulationis genus. **semilunar c. of knee joint, internal,** meniscus medialis articulationis genus. **septal c. of nose,** cartilago septi nasi. **sesamoid c. of larynx,** cartilago triticea. **sesamoid c's of nose,** cartilagines nasales accessoriae. **sesamoid c. of vocal ligament,** cartilago sesamoidea ligamenti vocalis. **sigmoid c's,** see *meniscus lateralis articulationis genus* and *meniscus medialis articulationis genus.* **slipping rib c.,** loosening and deformity of the costal cartilages, causing painful symptoms. **sternal c.,** cartilago costalis. **stratified c.,** fibrocartilage. **subvomerine c's,** cartilago vomeronasalis. **supra-arytenoid c.,** cartilago corniculata. **tarsal c's,** see *tarsus inferior palpebrae* and *tarsus superior palpebrae.* **temporary c.,** any cartilage that is being replaced by bone or that is normally destined to be replaced by bone; called also *ossifying c.* and *precursory c.* **tendon c.,** a form of embryonic cartilage by which tendons and bones are united. **thyroid c.,** cartilago thyroidea. **tracheal c's,** cartilagines tracheales. **triangular c. of nose,** cartilago nasi lateralis. **triquetral c., triquetrous c.,** 1. cartilago arytenoidea. 2. discus articularis articulationis radioulnaris distalis. **triticeal c., triticeous c.,** cartilago triticea. **tubal c.,** cartilago tubae auditivae. **tympanomandibular c.,** Meckel's c. **vomeronasal c.,** cartilago vomeronasalis. **Weitbrecht's c.,** discus articularis articulationis acromioclavicularis. **Wrisberg's c.,** cartilago cuneiformis. **xiphoid c.,** processus xiphoideus. **Y c.,** a Y-shaped cartilage in the acetabulum, joining the ilium, ischium, and pubes. **yellow c.,** elastic c.

cartilagin (kar′tĭ-laj″in) a protein found in cartilage, which is changed by boiling into chondrin; called also *chondrigen.*

cartilagines (kar″tĭ-laj′ĭ-nēz) [L.] plural of *cartilago.*

cartilaginification (kar″tĭ-lah-jin″ĭ-fĭ-ka′shun) conversion into cartilage.

cartilaginiform (kar″tĭ-lah-jin′ĭ-form) resembling cartilage; called also *cartilaginoid.*

cartilaginoid (kar″tĭ-laj′ĭ-noid) cartilaginiform.

cartilaginous (kar″tĭ-laj′ĭ-nus) consisting of or of the nature of cartilage.

cartilago (kar-tĭ-lah′go), pl. *cartilag′ines* [L.] a specialized, fibrous connective tissue; see *cartilage.* Used in anatomical nomenclature to designate a mass of such tissue in a particular site in the body. **c. ala′ris ma′jor** [NA], greater alar cartilage: either of two thin, curved cartilages, one on either side at the apex of the nose, each of which possesses a lateral and a medial crus; called also *inferior cartilage of nose.* **cartilag′ines ala′res mino′res** [NA], lesser alar cartilages: various small cartilages located in the fibrous tissue of the alae nasi; called also *accessory* *cartilages of nose.* **c. articula′ris** [NA], articular cartilage: a thin layer of cartilage, usually hyaline, on the articular surface of bones in synovial joints; called also *arthrodial, diarthrodial, investing,* and *obducent cartilage.* **c. arytenoi′dea** [NA], arytenoid cartilage: one of the paired, pitcher-shaped cartilages of the back of the larynx at the upper border of the cricoid cartilage; called also *c. arytaenoidea* and *c. triquetra,* and *guttural, pyramidal, triquetral,* and *triquetrous cartilage.* **c. auric′ulae** [NA], cartilage of auricle: the internal plate of elastic cartilage which is found in the external ear; called also *auricular* and *conchal cartilage.* **c. cornicula′ta** [NA], corniculate cartilage: a small nodule of cartilage at the apex of each arytenoid cartilage; called also *c. corniculata* [*Santorini*], *c. santorini, Santorini's* and *supra-arytenoid cartilage, corniculum,* and *corpus santoriana.* **c. cornicula′ta [Santori′ni],** c. corniculata. **c. costa′lis** [NA], costal cartilage: a bar of hyaline cartilage by which the ventral extremity of a rib is attached to the sternum in the case of the true ribs, or to the superiorly adjacent ribs in the case of the upper false ribs; called also *sternal cartilage.* **c. cricoi′dea** [NA], cricoid cartilage: a ringlike cartilage forming the lower and back part of the larynx; called also *annular* or *innominate cartilage.* **c. cuneifor′mis** [NA], cuneiform cartilage: either of the paired cartilages, one on either side in the aryepiglottic fold; called also *c. cuneiformis* [*Wrisbergi*], *c. wrisbergi,* and *Wrisberg's cartilage.* **c. cuneifor′mis [Wrisber′gi],** c. cuneiformis. **c. ensifor′mis,** processus xiphoideus. **c. epiglot′tica** [NA], epiglottic cartilage: the plate of cartilage that constitutes the central part of the epiglottis. **c. epiphysia′lis** [NA], epiphyseal cartilage: cartilage interposed between the epiphysis and the shaft of the bone during the period of growth; by its growth the bone increases in length. Called also *epiphyseal synchondroses,* and *synchondrosis epiphyseos.* **cartilag′ines falca′tae,** see *meniscus lateralis articulationis genus* and *meniscus medialis articulationis genus.* **c. jacobso′ni,** c. vomeronasalis. **cartilag′ines laryn′gis** [NA], laryngeal cartilages: cartilages of the larynx, including the cricoid, thyroid, and epiglottic, and two each of arytenoid, corniculate, and cuneiform cartilages. **c. mea′tus acus′tici** [NA], cartilage of acoustic meatus: the trough-shaped cartilage of the cartilaginous part of the external acoustic meatus; called also *meatal cartilage.* **cartilag′ines nasa′les accesso′riae** [NA], accessory nasal cartilages: one or more small cartilages on either side of the nose between the greater alar and lateral nasal cartilages; called also *cartilagines sesamoideae nasi, epactal* or *minor cartilages,* and *sesamoid cartilages of nose.* **cartilag′ines na′si** [NA], nasal cartilages: the cartilages of the nose, including the lateral nasal, greater and lesser alar, nasal septal, vomeronasal, and the accessory nasal cartilages. **c. na′si latera′lis** [NA], lateral nasal cartilage: a lateral expansion of the septal cartilage on either side of the nose just inferior to the nasal bone; called also *lateral* or *triangular cartilage of nose.* **c. santori′ni,** c. corniculata. **c. sep′ti na′si** [NA], cartilage of nasal septum: the hyaline cartilage forming the framework of the cartilaginous part of the nasal septum, and including the lateral nasal cartilages; called also *septal cartilage of nose.* **c. sesamoi′dea laryn′gis, Luschka,** c. sesamoidea ligamenti vocalis. **c. sesamoi′dea ligamen′ti voca′lis** [NA], sesamoid cartilage of vocal ligament: a small cartilage occasionally found within the vocal ligaments; called also *laryngeal cartilage of Luschka,* and *Luschka's cartilage.* **cartilag′ines sesamoi′deae na′si,** cartilagines nasales accessoriae. **c. thyroi′dea** [NA], thyroid cartilage: the largest cartilage of the larynx, with two broad, posteriorly diverging laminae and two pairs of horns, superior and inferior, that extend from the posterior borders of the laminae; called also *c. thyreoidea* and *scutiform cartilage.* **cartilag′ines trachea′les** [NA], tracheal cartilages: the 16 to 20 incomplete rings which, held together and enclosed by a strong, elastic, fibrous membrane, constitute the wall of the trachea. **c. triquet′ra,** 1. cartilago arytenoidea. 2. discus articularis articulationis radioulnaris distalis. **c. tritic′ea** [NA], triticeal cartilage: a small cartilage in the thyrohyoid ligament. Called also *sesamoid cartilage, corpusculum triticeum,* and *corpus triticeum.* **c. tu′bae auditi′vae** [NA], cartilage of auditory tube: the cartilage on the inferomedial surface of the temporal bone that supports the walls of the cartilaginous portion of the auditory tube; called also *tubal* or *eustachian cartilage.* **c. vomeronasa′lis** [NA], vomeronasal cartilage: either of the two narrow, longitudinal strips of cartilage, one lying on either side of the anterior portion of the lower margin of the septal cartilage; called also *c. vomeronasalis* [*Jacobsoni*], *c. jacobsoni,* and *Jacobson's* or *subvomerine cartilage.* **c. vomeronasa′lis [Jacobso′ni],** c. vomeronasalis. **c. wrisbergi,** c. cuneiformis.

cartilagotropic (kar″tĭ-lag-o-trop′ik) [L. *cartilago* cartilage + Gr. *tropos* a turning] having affinity for cartilage.

caruncle (kar′ung-kl) a small fleshy eminence, whether normal or abnormal; called also *caruncula* [NA]. **amniotic c's,** small epithelial amniotic growths occasionally found at the placental insertion of the umbilical cord, the fold of amnion, or Schultze's fold, carrying the vitelline duct. **hymenal c's,** caruncula hymenales. **lacrimal c.,** caruncula lacrimalis. **major c. of Santorini,** papilla duodeni major. **Morgagni's c., morgagnian c.,** lobus medius prostatae. **myrti-**

form c's, carunculae hymenales. **sublingual c.,** caruncula sublingualis. **urethral c.,** a small, polypoid, deep red growth on the mucous membrane of the urinary meatus in women.

caruncula (kah-rung′ku-lah), pl. *carun′culae* [L. dim. of *caro* flesh] [NA] a small fleshy eminence; called also *caruncle.* **carun′culae hymena′les** [NA], hymenal caruncles: small elevations of the mucous membrane encircling the vaginal orifice, being relics of the torn hymen; called also *carunculae myrtiformis.* **c. lacrima′lis** [NA], lacrimal caruncle: the red eminence at the medial angle of the eye. **c. mammilla′ris** (*obs.*), trigonum olfactorium. **carun′culae myrtifor′mes,** carunculae hymenales. **c. saliva′ris,** c. sublingualis. **c. sublingua′lis** [NA], an eminence on each side of the frenulum of the tongue, at the apex of which are the openings of the major sublingual duct and the submandibular duct. Called also *c. salivaris* and *sublingual caruncle.*

carunculae (kah-rung′ku-le) [L.] plural of *caruncula.*

Carus' curve (circle) (kah′rus) [Karl Gustav *Carus,* German obstetrician, 1789–1869] see under *curve.*

carver (kar′ver) an instrument for producing and perfecting anatomical forms in artificial teeth and dental restorations.

carvone (kar′vōn) chemical name: *p*-mentha-6,8-dien-2-one. A terpene ketone, $C_3H_5 \cdot C_6H_6O_6 \cdot CH_3$, found in many volatile oils, such as caraway oil, oil of dill, and spearmint oil.

caryo- (kar′e-o) [Gr. *karyon* nucleus, or nut] a combining form denoting relationship to a nucleus; see also words beginning *karyo-.*

Caryococcus (kar″e-o-kok′kus) [*caryo-* + Gr. *kokkos* berry] a genus of bacteria parasitic on protozoa.

Caryophanaceae (kar″e-o-fah-na′se-e) a family of the class Schizomycetes (order Caryophanales), made up of large motile or nonmotile trichomes and bacillary structures which do not form spores. It includes three genera, *Caryophanon, Lineola,* and *Simonsiella,* comprising nonpathogenic parasitic forms found in the oral cavity and in the intestinal content of ruminants.

Caryophanales (kar″e-o-fah-na′lēz) an order of the class Schizomycetes, made up of microorganisms that occur as cylindrical or discoidal cells enclosed in a continuous wall, forming long filaments or shorter structures which function as hormogonia; found in water and in decomposing organic materials, and in the intestines of arthropods and vertebrates. It includes three families, Arthromitaceae, Caryophanaceae, and Oscillospiraceae.

Caryophanon (ka″re-o′fah-non) a genus of Schizomycetes of the order Caryophanales, family Caryophenaceae.

caryophil (kar′e-o-fil) staining easily with thiazinammonium stains.

Carysomyia (kar″ĭ-so-mi′yah) *Chrysomyia.*

carzenide (kar′zĕ-nīd) chemical name: *p*-sulfamoylbenzoic acid; a carbonic anhydrase inhibitor, $C_7H_7NO_4S.$

Casal's necklace (kah-salz′) [Gaspar *Casal,* Spanish physician, 1679–1759] see under *necklace.*

casanthranol (kah-san′thrah-nōl) a purified mixture of the anthranol glycosides derived from *Cascara sagrada;* a cathartic.

cascade (kas-kād′) a series of steps or stages (as of a physiological process) which, once initiated continues to the final step by virtue of each step being triggered by the preceding one, sometimes with cumulative effect. **electron c.,** the passage of electrons during oxidative phosphorylation from a large negative (reducing) potential through a series of cytochromes to a positive (oxidizing) potential.

cascara (kas-kār′ah) [Sp.] bark. **c. amar′ga** [Sp. "bitter bark"], the bark of *Sweetia panamensis* Benth. (Leguminosae), a tree of tropical America; it is alterative and tonic. **c. sagra′da** [Sp. "sacred bark"] [USP], the dried bark of *Rhamnus purshiana* DC. (Rhamnaceae), a shrub of the Pacific states of the United States, used as a cathartic; called also *bearberry bark, chittem bark, dogwood bark, Persian bark,* and *Purshiana bark.* Its laxative principles are glycosidal anthraquinones, e.g., emodin and barbaloin.

case (kās) 1. a particular instance of disease, as a *case* of leukemia; sometimes used incorrectly to designate the patient with the disease. 2. a term sometimes used incorrectly in dentistry to designate a flask, denture, casting, or the like. **borderline c.,** an instance of a disease in which the symptoms resemble those of a recognized condition but are not typical of it. **custodial c.,** the case of an individual who requires supervision or removal from society because of mental disease, chronic illness, etc.; an offensive term which is to be avoided because it implies hopelessness and may result in the abandonment of rehabilitative or ameliorative measures. **index c.,** the case of the original patient (propositus or proband), which provides the stimulus for study of other members of the family, to ascertain a possible genetic factor in causation of the presenting condition. In epidemiology of contagious disease, the first case of a disease, as opposed to subsequent cases. **trial c.,** a box containing convex and concave spherical, and convex and concave cylindrical lenses, arranged in pairs, a trial spectacle frame, and various other devices used in testing vision.

casease (ka′se-ās) [L. *caseus* cheese] a protease derived from bacterial cultures, capable of dissolving albumin and the casein of milk and cheese.

caseation (ka″se-a′shun) [L. *caseus* cheese] 1. the precipitation of casein. 2. a form of necrosis in which the tissue is changed into a dry, amorphous mass resembling cheese.

casebook (kās-book) a book in which a physician enters the records of his cases.

case history (kās his-to′re) the collected data concerning an individual, his family, and environment, including his medical history and any other information that may be useful in analyzing and diagnosing his condition or for instructional purposes.

casein (ka′se-in, ka′sēn, ka-sēn′) [L. *caseus* cheese] a phosphoprotein, the principal protein of milk, the basis of curd and of cheese. It is precipitated from milk as a white amorphous substance by dilute acids, and redissolves on the addition of alkalis or of excess acid. Rennin (and other milk-clotting enzymes) influence the hydrolysis of casein to soluble paracasein, which in the presence of calcium (Ca^{++}) is converted to an insoluble curd (insoluble paracasein or calcium paracaseinate). Casein, usually in the form of its calcium, potassium, or sodium salts, is added to other ingredients of the diet to increase its protein content. NOTE: In British nomenclature, casein is called *caseinogen*, and paracasein is called *casein*. **c.-calcium,** calcium caseinate. **gluten c.,** a casein-like substance in the seeds of various cereal plants; glutin. **Panum's c.,** paraglobulin. **serum c.,** paraglobulin. **c.-sodium,** a nutrient preparation of casein and sodium hydroxide. **vegetable c.,** a protein resembling casein, e.g., wheat gluten.

caseinate (ka′se-ah-nāt″, ka-se′nāt) 1. any salt of casein. 2. a combination of casein and a metal.

caseinogen (ka″se-in′o-jen) [*casein* + Gr. *gennan* to produce] the British term for casein.

caseinogenate (ka″se-in′o-jĕ-nāt) a salt of caseinogen.

caseogenous (ka″se-oj′ĕ-nus) producing caseation; conversion into cheese (casein).

caseoserum (ka″se-o-se′rum) an antiserum produced by immunization with casein.

caseous (ka′se-us) resembling cheese or curd; cheesy.

caseum (ka′se-um) [L. "cheese"] cellular debris of a cheeselike consistency, produced as a result of caseation.

caseworm (kās′werm) echinococcus.

CaSO₄ calcium sulfate.

Casoni's intradermal test (reaction) (kah-so′nēz) [Tommaso *Casoni*, Italian physician, 1880–1933] see under *tests.*

cassava (kah-sah′vah) [Sp. *casabe*] a shrub of the genus *Manihot*, especially *M. esculenta* Crantz (Euphorbiaceae), and their starchy root products. The roots contain hydrogen cyanide, which is removed during processing to obtain starch. The starch is used in foods (soups, breads, tapioca) and glues.

Casselberry's position (kas′el-ber-e) [William Evans *Casselberry*, American laryngologist, 1859–1916] see under *position.*

Casser's (Casserio's, Casserius') fontanelle, etc. (kah′serz) [Giulio *Casserio*, Italian anatomist, 1556– 1616] see under *fontanelle, ligament,* and *muscle.*

casserian (kah-se′re-an) named for Giulio Casserio, as casserian fontanelle.

cassette (kah-set′) [Fr. "a little box"] 1. a lightproof housing for x-ray film, containing front and back intensifying screens between which the film is placed. 2. a magazine for film or magnetic tape.

Cassia (kash′e-ah) [L.; Gr. *kasia*] a genus of leguminous trees, shrubs, and herbs, found in the warmer regions of the world. *C. acutifo′lia* Del., native to Africa and cultivated in India, and *C. angustifo′lia* Vahl., native to Arabia, afford Alexandria senna and Tinnevelly senna, respectively.

cast (kast) 1. a positive copy or likeness of an object, such as a mold of a hollow organ (a renal tubule, bronchiole, etc.), formed of effused plastic matter and extruded from the body, as a urinary cast. 2. a positive reproduction of the form of the tissues of the upper or lower jaw, which is made in an impression, and over which denture bases or other dental restorations may be fabricated. 3. to form an object in a mold. 4. a stiff dressing or casing made of bandage impregnated with plaster of Paris or other hardening material, used for immobilization of various parts of the body, in cases of fractures, dislocations, and infected wounds. 5. strabismus. **bacterial c.,** a urinary cast made up of bacteria or containing a large number of bacteria. **blood c.,** a urinary cast that bears blood cells on its surface. **coma c.,** a urinary cast containing strongly refracting granules; said to indicate oncoming coma in diabetes. Called also *Külz's c.* or *cylinder.* **decidual c.,** the mass of degenerating or necrotic decidua discharged from the uterus at the time of rupture of an ectopic pregnancy. **dental c.,** the facsimile of oral structures obtained by pouring plaster into an impression made of the mouth; see cast, def. 2. **diagnostic c.,** a facsimile of oral structures made for the specific purpose of study as a means of determining the proper method of treatment, usually made of plaster of Paris;

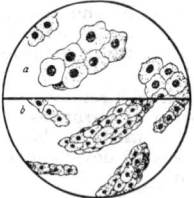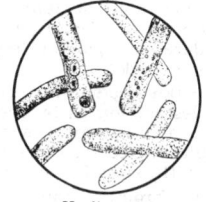

a, Squamous epithelium from urine; *b,* epithelial casts.   Hyaline casts.

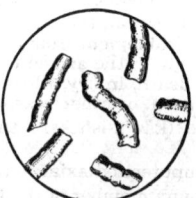

Granular casts.   Waxy casts.

called also *preoperative c.* and *study c.* **epithelial c.,** a urinary cast made up of columnar renal epithelium or of round cells. **false c.,** pseudocast. **fatty c.,** any cast made up of material loaded with fat globules. **fibrinous c.,** a cast resembling a waxy cast, but having a distinctly yellow color like beeswax, often seen in acute nephritis. **gnathostatic c.,** a cast of the teeth trimmed so that the occlusal plane is in its normal position in the mouth when the cast is set on a plane surface; used in orthodontic diagnosis. **granular c.,** a dark colored urinary cast of granular or cell-like substance, it being a degenerated form of a hyaline or waxy cast. **hair c.,** 1. trichobezoar. 2. (usually pl.) discrete, white, shiny, freely movable tubular accretions 2 to 7 mm. long that encircle the hair shafts of the scalp and which may be mistaken for nits; called also *peripilar keratin c's* and *pseudonits.* **hanging c.,** one applied to the arm in fracture of the shaft of the humerus and suspended by a sling looped around the neck. **hemoglobin c.,** an irregular, dark, granular cast composed of disintegrated red blood corpuscles. **hyaline c.,** a nearly transparent urinary cast made up of homogeneous protein, but slightly refractive. **investment c.,** refractory c. **Külz's c.,** coma c. **leukocyte c.,** a hyaline cast in which leukocytes are incorporated; called also *pus c.* **master c.,** a facsimile of oral structures, including the prepared tooth surfaces, residual ridge areas, and/or other parts of the dental arch, reproduced from an impression. **mucous c.,** cylindroid, def. 2. **peripilar keratin c.,** hair c., def. 2. **preextraction c.,** preoperative c., diagnostic c. **pus c.,** leukocyte cast. **quarter c.,** a cut in the quarter of a horse's hoof. **red cell c.,** hyaline cast in which red cells are incorporated. **refractory c.,** one made of material that will not disintegrate at the high temperatures used in casting and/or soldering; called also *investment c.* **renal c.,** urinary c. **spiral c.,** a urinary cast having a spiral or twisted shape. **spurious c., spurious tube c.,** cylindroid, def. 2. **study c.,** diagnostic c. **tube c.,** urinary c. **urate c.,** an agglomeration of urates on a shred of fibrin or other substance. **urinary c.,** a cast formed from gelled protein precipitated in the renal tubules and molded to the tubular lumen; pieces of these casts break off and are washed out with the urine. Urinary casts may be classified as granular, hyaline, epithelial, etc. Called also *renal c., tube c.,* and *urinary cylinder.* **waxy c.,** a urinary cast made up of a highly refractive, translucent, amyloid substance.

Castanea (kas-ta′ne-ah) [L.; Gr. *kastanea*] a genus of trees, the chestnuts. *C. dentata* (Marsh.) Borkh. (Fagaceae) is the American chestnut. Its wood and leaves contain 6–11 per cent tannin. It has been used as an astringent and in pertussis. The leaves and buds may be poisonous to livestock if consumed in sufficient quantities. The nut is edible.

Castellanella (kas″tel-ah-nel′ah) [Aldo *Castellani*] *Trypanosoma.* **C. castellan′i,** *Trypanosoma rhodesiense.* **C. gambien′se,** *Trypanosoma gambiense.*

Castellani's bronchitis (disease), mixture, paint, test (kas-tel-ah′nēz) [Sir Aldo *Castellani,* Italian physician 1877–1971] see *bronchospirochetosis,* and see under *mixture, paint,* and *tests.*

Castellani-Low symptom [Aldo *Castellani;* George Carmichael *Low,* English physician, 1872–1952] see under *symptom.*

Castellania (kas-tel-a′ne-ah) [Aldo *Castellani*] (obs.) *Candida.*

casting (kast′ing) an object formed by the solidification of plastic material, such as molten metal or gypsum product, poured into an impression or mold, or the act of formation of such an object. **vacuum c.,** the pouring of plastic material into an impression or mold, under conditions of lowered atmospheric pressure.

Castle's factors (kas′elz) [William Bosworth *Castle,* American physician, born 1897] 1. intrinsic factor. 2. cyanocobalamin (extrinsic factor).

castrate (kas′trāt) 1. to deprive of the gonads, rendering the individual incapable of reproduction. In the male, to geld or emasculate; in the female, to spay. 2. an individual that has been rendered incapable of reproduction by removal or destruction of the gonads.

castration (kas-tra′shun) [L. *castratio*] removal of the gonads, or their destruction as by radiation or parasites. **female c.,** bilateral oophorectomy, or spaying. **male c.,** bilateral orchiectomy. **parasitic c.,** defective sexual development due to infestation with parasites in early life.

castroid (kas′troid) eunuchoid.

casual (kaz′u-al) [L. *casualis*] 1. pertaining to accidental injuries or to accidents. 2. an occupant of a casual bed in a hospital.

casualty (kaz′u-al-te) 1. an accident; an accidental wound; death or disablement from an accident; also the person so injured or killed. 2. in the armed forces, one missing from his unit as a result of death, injury, illness, capture, because his whereabouts are unknown, or other reasons.

casuistics (kaz″u-is′tiks) the recording and study of cases of disease.

CAT computerized axial tomography.

cat (kat) any member of the family Felidae (lions, leopards, wildcats, etc.), especially the domesticated cat, *Felis catus*. **calico c.,** a cat with fur of three colors: black, white, and orange. Most are female; affected males are sterile, having extra X chromosomes (XXY, XXXY, etc.). **tortoise-shell c.,** calico c.

cata- [Gr. *kata* down] a prefix signifying down, lower, under, against, along with, very; see also words beginning *kata-*.

catabasial (kat-ah-ba′ze-al) [*cata-* + *basion*] having the basion lower than the opisthion; said of certain skulls.

catabasis (kah-tab′ah-sis) [*cata-* + Gr. *bainein* to go] the stage of decline of a disease.

catabatic (kat-ah-bat′ik) pertaining to the decline of a disease; abating.

catabiosis (kat″ah-bi-o′sis) [Gr. *katabiōsis* a passing life] the normal senescence of cells.

catabiotic (kat″ah-bi-ot′ik) 1. pertaining to or characterized by catabiosis. 2. dissipated or used up in the performance of function; said of the energy obtained from food.

catabolergy (kat″ah-bol′er-je) [*catabolic* + Gr. *ergon* work] the energy consumed in a catabolic process.

catabolic (kat″ah-bol′ik) pertaining to or of the nature of catabolism; retrograde or destructive.

catabolin (kah-tab′o-lin) catabolite.

catabolism (kah-tab′o-lizm) [Gr. *katabole* a throwing down] any destructive process by which complex substances are converted by living cells into more simple compounds. **antibody c.,** the rapid degradation (shortened half-life) of foreign gamma globulin in the body.

catabolite (kah-tab′o-līt) any product of catabolism, or of a destructive metabolic process.

catabolize (kah-tab′ŏ-liz) to subject to catabolism; to undergo catabolism.

catachronobiology (kat″ah-kron″o-bi-ol′o-je) a term suggested to denote the study of the deleterious effects of time on a living system. Cf. *anachronobiology*.

catacrotic (kat″ah-krot′ik) pertaining to or characterized by catacrotism.

catacrotism (kah-tak′ro-tizm) [*cata-* + Gr. *krotos* beat] an anomaly of the pulse evidenced by appearance of a small additional wave or notch in the descending limb of the pulse tracing.

catadicrotic (kat″ah-di-krot′ik) pertaining to or characterized by catadicrotism.

catadicrotism (kat″ah-di′kro-tizm) [*cata-* + Gr. *dis* twice + *krotos* beat] an anomaly of the pulse evidenced by appearance of two small additional waves or notches in the descending limb of the pulse tracing.

catadidymus (kat″ah-did′ĭ-mus) katadidymus.

catadioptric (kat″ah-di-op′trik) deflecting and reflecting light at the same time.

catagen (kat′ah-jen) the brief portion of the hair growth cycle in which growth (anagen) stops and resting (telogen) starts.

catagenesis (kat″ah-jen′ĕ-sis) [*cata-* + Gr. *genesis* production] involution or retrogression.

catagenetic (kat″ah-jĕ-net′ik) pertaining to catagenesis.

catagmatic (kat″ag-mat′ik) [Gr. *katagma* fracture] having the power of consolidating a broken bone.

catalase (kat′ah-lās) hydrogen-peroxide:hydrogenperoxide oxidoreductase. A crystalline enzyme that specifically catalyzes the decomposition of hydrogen peroxide and that is found in practically all cells except certain anaerobic bacteria.

catalatic (kat″ah-lat′ik) pertaining to catalase.

catalepsy (kat′ah-lep″se) [Gr. *katalēpsis*] a condition of diminished responsiveness usually characterized by trancelike states and by a waxy rigidity of the muscles (flexibilitas cerea) so that the patient tends to remain in any position in which he is placed; it

occurs in organic and psychological disorders and under hypnosis. Called also *anochlesia*.

cataleptic (kat″ah-lep′tik) 1. pertaining to, characterized by, or inducing catalepsy. 2. a person affected with catalepsy.

cataleptiform (kat″ah-lep′tĭ-form) resembling catalepsy.

cataleptoid (kat″ah-lep′toid) cataleptiform.

catalogia (kat″ah-lo′je-ah) verbigeration.

Catalpa (kah-tal′pah) a genus of bignoniaceous trees. *C. bignonioides* Walt. and *C. speciosa* Warder., of the United States, afford seeds formerly used in asthma.

catalysis (kah-tal′ĭ-sis) [Gr. *katalysis* dissolution] increase in the velocity of a chemical reaction or process produced by the presence of a substance that is not consumed in the net chemical reaction or process; *negative catalysis* denotes the slowing down or inhibition of a reaction or process by the presence of such a substance. **contact c., heterogeneous c.,** catalysis produced by the adsorbing power of contact surfaces; e.g., catalysis caused by colloidal platinum. **surface c.,** catalysis in which the reacting substances are adsorbed onto the surface of the catalyst and there react. Cf. *contact c.*

catalyst (kat′ah-list) any substance that brings about catalysis; called also *accelerant*. **negative c.,** a catalyst that retards the velocity of a reaction.

catalytic (kat″ah-lit′ik) [Gr. *katalyein* to dissolve] 1. causing or pertaining to an alterative effect; causing catalysis. 2. an alterative or specific medicine.

catalyzator (kat″ah-lĭ-za′tor) catalyst.

catalyze (kat′ah-līz) to cause or produce catalysis.

catalyzer (kat′ah-līz″er) catalyst.

catamenia (kat″ah-me′ne-ah) [Gr. *katamēnia*] the monthly uterine discharge; menstruation, or the menses.

catamenial (kat″ah-me′ne-al) pertaining to the menses or to menstruation.

catamenogenic (kat″ah-men″o-jen′ik) inducing menstruation.

catamite (kat′ah-mīt) in psychiatric terminology, a boy who submits to pederasty.

catamnesis (kat″am-ne′sis) the follow-up history of a patient after he is discharged from treatment or a hospital.

catamnestic (kat″am-nes′tik) pertaining to catamnesis.

catapasm (kat′ah-pazm) [Gr. *katapasma*] a dusting powder applied to an injured surface.

cataphasia (kat″ah-fa′ze-ah) [*cata-* + Gr. *phasis* speech] a speech disorder in which the patient constantly or repeatedly utters the same word or phrase.

cataphora (kah-taf′o-rah) [Gr. *kataphora*] lethargy with intervals of imperfect waking; called also *coma somnolentium*.

cataphoresis (kat″ah-fo-re′sis) [*cata-* + Gr. *phorēsis* bearing] the passage of charged particles toward the negative pole (cathode) in electrophoresis.

cataphoretic (kat″ah-fo-ret′ik) of, or pertaining to, cataphoresis.

cataphoria (kat″ah-fo′re-ah) [*cata-* + Gr. *pherein* to bear] a permanent downward turning of the visual axes of both eyes after the visual fusional stimuli have been eliminated; double hypophoria.

cataphoric (kat″ah-for′ik) pertaining to cataphoresis or to cataphora.

cataphrenia (kat″ah-fre′ne-ah) [*cata-* + Gr. *phrēn* mind] a state of mental debility of the dementia type that tends to eventuate in recovery.

cataphylaxis (kat″ah-fĭ-lak′sis) [*cata-* + Gr. *phylaxis* a guarding] 1. the movement of leukocytes and antibodies to the locality of an infection (Wright). 2. a breaking down of the body's natural defense to infection (Bullock and Cranmer).

cataplasia (kat″ah-pla′se-ah) [*cata-* + Gr. *plassein* to form] retrograde metamorphosis, a form of atrophy in which the tissues revert to earlier and more embryonic conditions.

cataplasis (kat-ap′lah-sis) cataplasia.

cataplasm (kat′ah-plazm) [L. *cataplasma*; Gr. *kataplasma*] a poultice or soft external application, often medicated. **kaolin c.,** a poultice prepared with kaolin, boric acid, and glycerin; called also *cataplasma kaolini*.

cataplasma (kat″ah-plaz′mah) [L.; Gr. *kataplasma*] cataplasm. **c. fermen′ti,** a poultice containing yeast. **c. kaoli′ni,** kaolin cataplasm.

cataplectic (kat″ah-plek′tik) 1. pertaining to or characterized by cataplexy. 2. coming on suddenly and overwhelmingly.

cataplexie (kat′ah-plek″se) [Fr.] cataplexy. **c. du réveil,** awakening of the psyche occurring before physical awakening.

cataplexis (kat′ah-plek″sis) [Gr.] cataplexy.

cataplexy (kat′ah-plek-se) a condition in which there are abrupt attacks of muscular weakness and hypotonia triggered by an emotional stimulus such as mirth, anger, fear, or surprise. It is often associated with narcolepsy.

catapophysis (kat″ah-pof′ĭ-sis) a process, or projection, of bone or of brain matter.

Catapres (kat″ah-pres) trademark for a preparation of clonidine hydrochloride.

cataract (kat′ah-rakt) [L. *cataracta*, from Gr. *katarrhēgnynai* to break down] an opacity of the crystalline lens of the eye. **adherent c.**, a cataract with adhesions between the iris and the lens capsule. **adolescent c.**, cataract developing during puberty. **after-c.**, a recurrent capsular cataract; any membrane in the pupillary area after performance of a procedure for extraction or absorption of the lens. **anterior pyramidal c.**, an anterior capsular opacity projecting forward into the aqueous humor. **arborescent c.**, one in which the opacity has a branched appearance. **aridosiliculose c., aridosiliquate c.**, siliculose c. **atopic c.**, cataract occurring, most often in the second to third decade, in those with longstanding atopic dermatitis. **axial c., nuclear c. axiliary c.**, spindle c. **black c.**, a nuclear cataract with a dark colored opacity; called also *cataracta brunescens* and *cataracta nigra*. **blood c.**, blocking of the lens by a blood clot. **blue c., blue dot c.**, a condition characterized by the presence of small blue punctate opacities scattered throughout the nucleus and cortex of the lens; vision is usually not interfered with, nor does the condition usually progress. Called also *cerulean c.* and *cataracta cerulea*. **bony c.**, cataracta ossea. **bottlemakers' c.**, glassblowers' c. **brown c., brunescent c.**, senile cataract appearing as a brown opacity. **calcareous c.**, one containing a chalky calcific deposit. **capsular c.**, one that consists of an opacity in the capsule. **capsulolenticular c.**, one that is seated partly in the capsule and partly in the lens. **central c.**, opacity of the center of the eye lens. **cerulean c.**, blue c. **choroidal c.**, a brownish diffuse opacity of the lens nucleus associated with chronic choroidal disease. **complete c.**, one that involves the whole lens. **complicated c.**, cataract due to disease of other parts of the eye; called also *secondary c.* and *cataracta complicata*. **congenital c.**, one that originates before birth. **contusion c.**, one due to shock or to injury of the eyeball. **coralliform c.**, a cataract having the shape of coral. **coronary c.**, a congenital condition in which club-shaped opacities are arranged in a ring or crown around the lens, the center of the lens and the extreme periphery remaining clear. **cortical c.**, a stellate opacity in the cortical layers of the lens; called also *stellate c.* **cupuliform c.**, a senile cataract of the capsule and subcapsular cortical fibers at the posterior pole of the lens. **cystic c.**, a cataract showing cystic degeneration. **diabetic c.**, one that occurs as a complication of diabetes. **dry-shelled c.**, siliculose c. **electric c.**, cataract attributed to the light formed in electric welding or to a flash of lightning; called also *cataracta electrica*. **embryonal nuclear c.**, an opacity confined to the embryonal nucleus of the lens. **fibroid c.**, a variety of capsular cataract that does not affect the lens. **floriform c.**, a cataract having the form of a rayed flower (sunflower). **fluid c.**, a hypermature cataract in which the lens has become a milky fluid; called also *lacteal* or *milky c.* **fusiform c.**, spindle c. **general c.**, a cataract in which the opacity affects both the cortex and nucleus of the lens; called also *mixed c.* **glassblowers' c.**, cataract in glassblowers, due to exposure to infrared heat and characterized by exfoliation of the lens capsule; called also *bottlemaker's c.* **glaucomatous c.**, an opacity that results from one or more attacks of glaucoma. **gray c.**, senile cortical cataract. **green c.**, a greenish opacity, sometimes glaucomatous and sometimes due to a slight lack of transparency in the mediums. **hard c.**, one with a hard nucleus. **heat-ray c.**, cataract due to long-continued exposure to high temperatures, e.g., glassblowers' c. **hedger's c.**, perforation of the cornea by a thorn, occurring in persons who trim hedges. **heterochromic c.**, cataract associated with heterochromia of the iris. **hypermature c.**, one in which the lens capsule is wrinkled and the contents have become either solid and shrunken or soft and liquid; called also *overripe c.* **immature c.**, an early opacity, or any cataract that affects only a part of the lens or capsule. **incipient c.**, any cataract in its early stages, or one that has sectors of opacity with clear spaces intervening. **infantile c.**, a lamellar cataract of early childhood, commonly associated with rickets or convulsions. **intumescent c.**, one in which the lens is swollen and opaque. **irradiation c.**, cataract caused by large doses of roentgen rays, radium, or similar energy. **juvenile c.**, a soft cataract in a young person. **lacteal c.**, fluid c. **lamellar c.**, an opacity that affects certain layers only between the cortex and nucleus of the lens; called also *zonular c.* **lenticular c.**, opacity of the lens not affecting the capsule. **lightning c.**, cataract caused by a stroke of lightning passing through the body. **mature c.**, one in which the lens is completely opaque; called also *ripe c.* **membranous c.**, a condition in which the lens substance has shrunk, leaving remnants of the capsule and fibrous tissue formation. **milky c.**, fluid c. **mixed c.**, general c. **morgagnian c.**, a hypermature cataract in which the cortex has become completely liquefied and the nucleus settles at the bottom of the lens. **naphthalinic c.**, cataract caused by the injection of naphthalene. **nuclear c.**, one in which the opacity is seated in the central nucleus of the lens; called also *axial c.* **overripe c.**, hypermature c. **partial c.**, any cataract that affects only a

part of the lens; it may be central or peripheral. **perinuclear c.**, a disklike opacity around the nucleus of the lens. **peripheral c.**, a cataract in the periphery of the lens. **polar c., anterior**, one seated at the center of the anterior capsule of the lens. **polar c., posterior**, one seated at the center of the posterior capsule of the lens. **primary c.**, a cataract developing independently of any other disease. **progressive c.**, one in which the opacification advances and finally becomes total. **puddler's c.**, cataract in iron puddlers due to intense radiation from open-hearth furnaces. **punctate c.**, one made up of a collection of dotlike opacities. **pyramidal c.**, a conoid anterior polar cataract with its apex pointing forward. **reduplication c.**, a series of similar opacities situated at various levels in the lens, usually connected by opaque lines. **ripe c.**, mature cataract. **sanguineous c.**, former term for a blood clot in the prepupillary opening. **secondary c.**, 1. a cataract that forms after most of the opaque lens has been removed surgically. 2. complicated cataract. **sedimentary c.**, a soft cataract in which the denser parts have gravitated downward. **senile c.**, a hard opacity of the nucleus of the lens of the eye, occurring in the aged. **siliculose c., siliquose c.**, a cataract in which there is absorption of the lens, with calcareous deposit in the capsule, so that the atrophied lens resembles a silique; called also *dry-shelled c., aridosiliculose c., aridosiliquate c.*, and *cataracta aridosiliquata*. **snowflake c., snowstorm c.**, a cataract that has the appearance of numerous grayish or bluish-white flaky opacities, frequently seen in young diabetics. **Soemmering's ring c.**, see under *ring*. **soft c.**, one with no hard nucleus. **spindle c.**, a cataract characterized by a spindle-shaped opacity reaching through the capsule in an anteroposterior direction; called also *axiliary c.* and *fusiform c.* **stationary c.**, an opacity of the lens that does not increase in extent. **stellate c.**, cortical c. **subcapsular c.**, an opacity situated beneath the anterior or posterior capsule of the lens. **sunflower c.**, a sunflower-shaped cataract caused by the presence of copper in the eye, as in Wilson's disease. Called also *chalcosis lentis*. **sutural c.**, a congenital opacity of the lens affecting the Y-shaped sutures of the fetal membrane. **total c.**, an opacity of all the fibers of the lens. **toxic c.**, that due to exposure to a toxic drug, e.g., naphthalene. **traumatic c.**, cataract following an injury. **tremulous c.**, one attended by a tremulous movement of the pupil and iris. **zonular c.**, 1. lamellar cataract. 2. one that involves the zonula.

cataracta (kat″ah-rak′tah) [L.] cataract. **c. accre′ta**, a condition in which the lens and the iris are fastened together as a result of iritis. **c. aridosiliqua′ta**, siliculose cataract. **c. brunes′cens**, brown cataract. **c. ceru′lea**, blue cataract. **c. complica′ta**, complicated cataract. **c. congen′ita membrana′cea**, congenital membranaceous cataract. **c. corona′ria**, a crown-shaped cataract. **c. elec′trica**, electric cataract. **c. membrana′cea accre′ta**, an after-cataract due to adhesions of the remains of the anterior capsule to the posterior capsule. **c. neurodermat′ica**, a type of cataract occurring as a complication of generalized dermatitis. **c. ni′gra**, black cataract. **c. os′sea**, bony cataract: a condition in which lens tissue has become ossified. **c. syndermot′ica**, cataract occurring as an accompaniment of a skin disease.

cataractogenic (kat″ah-rak″to-jen′ik) tending to induce the formation of cataracts.

cataractopiesis (kat″ah-rak″to-pi-e′sis) couching.

cataractous (kat″ah-rak″tus) of the nature of or affected with cataract.

cataria (kah-ta′re-ah) [L. "catnip"] the leaves and tops of *Nepeta cataria* L. (Labi.), or catnip, a labiate plant; used as a carminative and mild nerve stimulant. Feline species are attracted to and fondle the plant because of its aromatic oils, which contain nepetalactone.

catarrh (kah-tahr′) [L. *catarrhus*, from Gr. *katarrhein* to flow down] inflammation of a mucous membrane, with a free discharge (Hippocrates); especially such inflammation of the air passages of the head and throat. **atrophic c.**, chronic rhinitis with wasting of mucous and submucous tissues. **autumnal c.**, hay fever. **Bostock's c.**, hay fever. **epidemic c.**, influenza or grip. **Fruehjahr c.**, vernal conjunctivitis. **hypertrophic c.**, chronic catarrh that results in irregular, and sometimes papillary, thickening of the mucous and the submucous tissues. **Laennec's c.**, a kind of asthmatic bronchitis, with viscous, pearly expectoration. **malignant c. of cattle**, a virus disease of cattle characterized by exudative inflammation of the mucous membranes, corneal opacities, and enlargement of the lymphatic glands. **postnasal c.**, chronic rhinopharyngitis. **Russian c.**, influenza. **sinus c.**, a disorder of the lymph nodes characterized by dilatation of the sinuses accompanied by some proliferation of the littoral cells, which become swollen and detach themselves from the wall of the sinuses to lie free in the lumen. **spring c.**, vernal conjunctivitis. **suffocative c.**, asthma. **vernal c.**, allergic rhinitis and conjunctivitis attributed to spring pollens.

catarrhal (kah-tahr′al) of the nature of or pertaining to catarrh.

Catarrhina (kat″ah-ri′nah) [cata- + Gr. rhis nose] Cercopithecoidea.

catarrhine (kat′ah-rīn) 1. pertaining to the superfamily Catarrhina. 2. characterized by nostrils that are close together and directed downward.

catastalsis (kat″ah-stal′sis) [cata- + Gr. stalsis contraction] (obs.) a downward moving wave of contraction without a preceding wave of inhibition occurring in the digestive tube.

catastaltic (kat″ah-stal′tik) [Gr. katastaltikos] 1. inhibitory; restraining. 2. an agent that tends to restrain or check any process.

catastate (kat′ah-stāt) [cata- + Gr. histanai to stand] a result of catabolism; any substance or condition resulting from a catabolic process.

catastatic (kat″ah-stat′ik) of the nature of or pertaining to a catastate.

catatasis (kah-tat′ah-sis) [Gr. katatasis a stretching] extension of a limb or part, applied for the reduction of a dislocation or fracture.

catathermometer (kat″ah-ther-mom′ĕ-ter) katathermometer.

catathymic (kat″ah-thi′mik) H. W. Maier's term for psychic disorders marked by perseveration, in the course of which a single depressive topic tends to be complex-determined.

catatonia (kat-ah-to′ne-ah) [cata- + Gr. tonos tension + -ia] catatonic schizophrenia.

catatoniac (kat″ah-to′ne-ak) catatonic.

catatonic (kat″ah-ton′ik) 1. see under schizophrenia. 2. an individual affected with catatonic schizophrenia.

catatony (kah-tat′o-ne) catatonia.

catatricrotic (kat″ah-tri-krot′ik) pertaining to or characterized by catatricrotism.

catatricrotism (kat″ah-tri′kro-tizm) [cata- + Gr. treis three + krotos beat] an anomaly of the pulse evidenced by appearance of three small additional waves or notches in the descending limb of the pulse tracing.

catatropia (kat″ah-tro′pe-ah) [cata- + Gr. trepein to turn] a downward turning of the visual axis of both eyes in the presence of the visual fusional stimuli.

cataxia (kah-tak′se-ah) [Gr. katagnymai to break in pieces] (obs.) the separation or breaking up of bacterial associations; especially in those cases in which the association is pathogenic, but individual bacterial species are not.

catechin (kat′ĕ-kin) chemical name: trans-2-(3,4-dihydroxyphenyl)-3,4-dihydro-2H-1-benzopyran-3,5,7-triol. A crystalline astringent principle, $C_{15}H_{14}O_6·4H_2O$, from catechu (e.g., Acacia catechu Willd., Leguminosae and gambier, Uncaria gambier [Hunter] Roxb., Rubiaceae). Called also catechol and catechuic acid.

catechol (kat′ĕ-kol) 1. catechin. 2. pyrocatechol.

catecholamine (kat″ĕ-kol′ah-mēn, kat″ĕ-kol′ah-min) one of a group of similar compounds having a sympathomimetic action, the aromatic portion of whose molecule is catechol, and the aliphatic portion an amine. Such compounds include dopamine, norepinephrine, and epinephrine.

catecholaminergic (kat″e-kol-am″in-er′jik) activated by or secreting catecholamines.

catechu (kat′ĕ-ku) 1. a powerfully astringent extract from the heartwood of Acacia catechu Willd., Leguminosae, the chief constituents of which are catechin, quercetin, and catechutannic acid; formerly used as an antidiarrheal agent. Called also black c. 2. gambir. **pale c.,** gambir.

catelectrotonus (kat″e-lek-trot′o-nus) [cata- + electrotonus] increase of irritability of a nerve or muscle near the cathode during passage of an electric current.

Catenabacterium (kat″ĕ-nah-bak-te′re-um) [L. catena chain + bacterium] a genus of microorganisms of the tribe Lactobacilleae, family Lactobacillaceae, order Eubacteriales, made up of nonsporulating, anaerobic, gram-positive bacilli, found in the intestinal tract and occasionally associated with purulent infections.

catenating (kat′e-nāt″ing) [L. catena a chain] forming part of a chain or complex of symptoms.

catenoid (kat′e-noid) [L. catena chain] arranged like a chain or resembling a chain.

catenulate (kah-ten′u-lāt) catenoid.

catgut (kat′gut) an absorbable sterile strand obtained from collagen derived from healthy mammals, originally prepared from the submucous layer of the intestines of sheep; used as a surgical ligature. **chromic c., chromicized c.,** catgut sterilized and impregnated with chromium trioxide to prolong its tensile strength in tissues. **formaldehyde c.,** catgut impregnated with a solution of formaldehyde by boiling in an alcohol-formaldehyde solution. **I.K.I. c.,** catgut treated with a solution of 1 part of iodine in 100 parts of a potassium iodide solution; called also iodine c. **iodine c.,** I.K.I. c. **iodochromic c.,** catgut treated with a solution of iodine, potassium, iodide, and potassium

dichromate. **silverized c.,** catgut impregnated with silver to give it increased strength and resisting qualities.

Cath. abbreviation for L. cathar′ticus, cathartic.

Catha (kath′ah) a genus of plants. **C. ed′ulis** Forsk. (Celastraceae), a shrub or tree native to tropical East Africa, whose leaves are chewed or brewed into a tea and consumed for its central nervous system stimulating properties. The active principle is D-norpseudoephedrine.

cathaeresis (kah-thēr′ĕ-sis) catheresis.

catharma (kah-thar′mah) [Gr. katharma] the refuse of sacrifice, used as remedies in Greek medicine.

catharmos (kah-thar′mos) [Gr. katharmos a cleansing] incantations (hymns) against disease.

catharometer (kath″ah-rom′ĕ-ter) an instrument for measuring the thermal conductivity of air by the rate of heat loss from a heated platinum wire.

catharsis (kah-thar′sis) [Gr. katharsis a cleansing] 1. a cleansing or purgation. 2. in psychiatry, the expression and discharge of repressed emotions and ideas; called also psychocatharsis and Freud's cathartic method.

cathartic (kah-thar′tik) [Gr. kathartikos] 1. causing evacuation of the bowels. 2. an agent that causes evacuation of the bowels by increasing bulk, stimulating peristaltic action, etc. Called also purgative (q.v.), coprogogue, and eccoprotic. 3. producing catharsis. **bulk c.,** one that stimulates evacuation of the bowel by increasing the bulk of the feces. **lubricant c.,** one that acts by softening the feces and reducing friction between them and the intestinal wall. **saline c.,** one that increases fluidity of the intestinal contents by retention of water by osmotic forces, and indirectly increases motor activity. **stimulant c.,** one that directly increases motor activity of the intestinal tract.

cathectic (kah-thek′tik) pertaining to cathexis.

Cathelin's method, segregator (kat-laz′) [Fernand Cathelin, Paris urologist, born 1873] see under method and segregator.

cathemoglobin (kath″em-o-glo′bin) a substance produced by oxidizing hemochromogen; it consists of oxidized heme and denatured globin.

cathepsin (kah-thep′sin) an endopeptidase found in most cells, which takes part in cell autolysis and in the self-digestion of tissues.

catheresis (kah-thēr′ĕ-sis) [Gr. kathairesis a reduction] 1. weakness caused by medicine. 2. a mild action.

catheretic (kath″ĕ-ret′ik) 1. mildly caustic. 2. weakening or prostrating.

catheter (kath′ĕ-ter) [Gr. kathetēr] a tubular, flexible, surgical instrument for withdrawing fluids from (or introducing fluids into) a cavity of the body, especially one for introduction into the bladder through the urethra for the withdrawal of urine. **acorn-tipped c.,** one used in ureteropyelography to occlude the ureteral orifice and prevent backflow from the ureter during and following the injection of an opaque medium. **angiographic c.,** a catheter through which a contrast medium is injected for visualization of the vascular system of an organ. Such catheters may have pre-formed ends to facilitate selective locating (as in a renal or coronary vessel) from a remote entry site. They may be named according to the site of entry and destination, as femoral-renal, brachial-coronary, etc. **bicoudate c., c. bicoudé,** a twice-bent Mercier catheter. **Bozeman's c., Bozeman-Fritsch c.,** a double-current uterine catheter; called also Fritsch's c. **Braasch bulb c.,** a bulb-tipped catheter used for dilatation and calibration. **cardiac c.,** a long, fine catheter especially designed for passage, usually through a peripheral blood vessel, into the chambers of the heart under roentgenologic control. **central venous c.,** a long, fine catheter introduced into a large (jugular, subclavian, etc.) vein for the purposes of administering parenteral fluids (as in hyperalimentation) or medications or for measurement of central venous pressure. **conical c.,** a catheter with a cone-shaped tip designed to dilate the ureter. **c. coudé,** an elbowed c. **c. à demeure,** a catheter that is held in position in the urethra. **de Pezzer c.,** a self-retaining catheter having a bulbous extremity. **double-current c.,** a catheter having two channels; one for injection and one for removal of fluid. **Drew-Smythe c.,** an instrument used for the artificial rupture of the amniotic membranes to induce labor. **elbowed c.,** one with a sharp bend near the beak; used principally in cases of enlarged prostate. Called also c. coudé. **eustachian c.,** an instrument for inflating the eustachian tube, used in treating some diseases of the middle ear. **faucial c.,** a eustachian catheter to be used through the fauces. **female c.,** a short catheter for passage through the female urethra. **filiform-tipped c's,** catheters used to dilate tight ureteral strictures and to bypass obstructions due to angulations or calculi in the ureter. **flexible c.,** Nélaton's c. **Foley c.,** an indwelling catheter retained in the bladder by a balloon which may be inflated with air or liquid. **Fritsch's c.,** Bozeman-Fritsch c. **Garceau c.,** conical c. **Gouley's c.,** a solid, curved steel instrument, grooved on its inferior surface so that it can be passed over a guide through a urethral stricture. **indwelling c.,** a catheter that is held in position in the urethra.

Itard's c., a variety of eustachian catheter. **lobster-tail c.,** one with three joints at the tip. **Malecot c.,** a two- or four-winged catheter for use in the female bladder. **Mercier's c.,** a flexible catheter elbowed at the end; used in hypertrophied prostate. **Nélaton's c.,** a catheter of soft India rubber; called also *flexible c.* and *soft c.* **Odman-Ledin c.,** a polyethylene thermoplastic radiopaque catheter used for percutaneous insertion in cardiac catheterization. **olive-tip c.,** a ureteral catheter with an olive-shaped end, used to dilate a constricted ureteral orifice; larger sizes are also utilized for dilating urethral strictures or for calibrating the diameter of such strictures. **Pezzer's c.,** see *de Pezzer c.* **Phillips' c.,** a urethral catheter with a woven filiform guide. **prostatic c.,** a catheter having a short angular tip for passing an enlarged prostate. **railway c.,** a straight elastic catheter with an open end to be introduced with a filiform guide in cases of stricture. **Robinson c.,** a straight catheter with two to six openings to allow drainage, especially useful in the presence of blood clots which may occlude one or more openings. **Schrötter's c.,** a hard-rubber catheter of varying caliber, used for dilating laryngeal strictures. **self-retaining c.,** a catheter so constructed as to be retained at will and effect a drainage of the bladder. **Skene's c.,** a srong, self-retaining glass catheter for the female bladder. **soft c.,** Nélaton's c. **spiral-tip c.,** a catheter with an off-center filiform tip. **Squire's c.,** a vertebrated catheter. **Swan-Ganz c.,** a soft, flow-directed catheter with a balloon at the tip for measuring pulmonary arterial pressures; it is introduced into the basilic vein and is guided by blood flow into the subclavian vein, the superior vena cava, through the right atrium and ventricle, into the pulmonary artery. **tracheal c.,** an instrument for removing mucus from the trachea by application of suction. **two-way c.,** a form used in irrigation. **vertebrated c.,** a catheter made in small sections fitted together so as to be flexible; called also *Squire's c.* **whistle-tip c.,** a catheter with a terminal opening as well as a lateral one. **winged c.,** a catheter with two projections on the end to retain it in the bladder.

catheterization (kath″ĕ-ter-i-za′shun) the employment or passage of a catheter. **cardiac c.,** passage of a small catheter through a vein in an arm or leg or the neck and into the heart, permitting the securing of blood samples, determination of intracardiac pressure, and detection of cardiac anomalies. **hepatic vein c.,** passage of a cardiac catheter through an arm vein, right atrium, inferior vena cava, and hepatic vein, into a small hepatic venule, for recording of intrahepatic venous pressures. **laryngeal c.,** insertion of a catheter into the larynx, for the evacuation of secretions or introduction of a gas. **retrourethral c.,** passage through the urethra of a catheter first introduced through an incision into the bladder, and then passed through the internal urethral orifice.

catheterize (kath′ĕ-ter-īz) to introduce a catheter within a body cavity; usually used to designate the passage of a catheter into the bladder for the withdrawal of urine.

catheterostat (kath-e′ter-o-stat) a holder for containing and sterilizing catheters.

cathetometer (kath″ĕ-tom′ĕ-ter) an instrument for aiding in the reading of thermometers, burets, etc.

cathexis (kah-thek′sis) [Gr. *kathexis*] the charge or attachment of mental or emotional energy upon an idea or object.

cathisophobia (kath″ĭ-so-fo′be-ah) [Gr. *kathizein* to sit down + *phobein* to be affrighted by + *ia*] akathisia.

cathode (kath′ōd) [Gr. *kata* down + *hodos* way] 1. the negative electrode from which electrons are emitted and to which positive ions are attracted. 2. the electrode through which a current leaves a nerve or other substance. Cf. *anode.*

cathodic (kah-thod′ik) pertaining to or emanating from a cathode.

catholicon (kah-thol′ĭ-kon) [Gr. *katholikos* general] a panacea or universal medicine.

catholyte (kath′o-līt) that portion of an electrolyte that adjoins the cathode.

Cathomycin (kath′o-mi″sin) trademark for preparations of novobiocin.

cation (kat′i-on) [Gr. *kata* down + *iōn* going] an ion having a positive charge owing to the loss of one or more electrons, and hence being attracted to and traveling to the cathode, or negative pole, under the influence of an applied electric field.

cationic (kat″ĭ-on′ik) pertaining to or containing a cation.

cationogen (kat″ĭ-on′o-jen) a compound that may become or may liberate a cation in the body.

cativi (kah-te′ve) pinta.

catlin (kat′lin) a long, straight, sharp-pointed, double-edged knife used in amputations.

catling (kat′ling) catlin.

catoptric (kah-top′trik) [Gr. *katoptrikos* in a mirror] pertaining to a reflected image, or to reflected light.

catoptrics (kah-top′triks) that branch of physics which treats of reflected light.

catoptroscope (kah-top′tro-skōp) [Gr. *katoptron* mirror + *sko-pein* to examine] an instrument for examining objects by reflected light.

catotropia (kat″o-tro′pe-ah) cataphoria.

Cattani's serum (kah-tan′ez) [Giuseppina *Cattani,* Italian pathologist, 1859–1915] see under *serum.*

cauda (kaw′dah), pl. *cau′dae* [L.] [NA] a tail, or tail-like appendage; in anatomical nomenclature, a general term for a structure resembling such an appendage. **c. cerebel′li,** vermis cerebelli. **c. cor′poris stria′ti,** c. nuclei caudati. **c. epididym′idis** [NA], tail of epididymus: the lower part of the epididymis, where the ductus epididymidis is continuous with the ductus deferens; called also *globus minor epididymidis.* **c. equi′na** [NA], the collection of spinal roots that descend from the lower part of the spinal cord and occupy the vertebral canal below the cord; their appearance resembles the tail of a horse. **c. he′licis** [NA], the termination of the posterior margin of the cartilage of the helix. **c. lie′nis,** extremitas anterior lienis. **c. nu′clei cauda′ti** [NA], tail of caudate nucleus: the part of the caudate nucleus that tapers off from the body, curves around in the roof of the inferior horn of the lateral ventricle, and extends rostrally as far as the amygdaloid nucleus; called also *c. corporis striati.* **c. pancre′atis** [NA], tail of pancreas: the left extremity of the pancreas, usually in contact with the medial aspect of the spleen and the junction of the transverse and descending colon.

caudad (kaw′dad) directed toward the tail; opposite to craniad or cephalad.

caudae (kaw′de) [L.] plural of *cauda.*

caudal (kaw′dal) 1. pertaining to a cauda. 2. denoting a position more toward the cauda, or tail, than some specified point of reference; same as inferior, in human anatomy. See *caudalis.*

caudalis (kaw-da′lis) pertaining to the cauda (tail), or to the inferior end of the body; [NA] a term used to denote relationship to the caudal or inferior extremity of an organ or part.

caudalward (kaw′dal-ward) toward the caudal end; in a direction away from the head.

caudamoeba sinen′sis (kaw″dah-me′bah sin-en′sis) *Entamoeba histolytica.*

caudate (kaw′dāt) [L. *caudatus*] having a tail.

caudatolenticular (kaw-da″to-len-tik′u-lar) pertaining to the caudate and lenticular nuclei of the striatum.

caudatum (kaw-da′tum) [L.] the nucleus caudatus.

caudectomy (kaw-dek′to-me) the surgical removal of all or part of the tail, as of a dog.

caudex (kaw′deks), pl. *cau′dices* or *caudexes* [L.] (*obs.*) a stem or stemlike part. **c. cer′ebri** (*obs.*), pedunculus cerebri.

caudocephalad (kaw-do-sef′ah-lad) [L. *cauda* tail + Gr. *kephalē* head + L. *ad* toward] 1. proceeding in a direction from the tail toward the head. 2. in both a caudal and a cephalic direction.

caul (kawl) 1. a piece of amnion that sometimes envelops a child's head at birth; pileus. Called also *cowl.* 2. the omentum, usually used to designate the greater omentum.

Caulk's punch [John Roberts *Caulk,* St. Louis urologist, 1881–1938] see under *punch.*

Caulobacter (kaw″lo-bak′ter) [Gr. *kaulos* stalk + *baktron* a staff] a genus of microorganisms of the family Caulobacteraceae, suborder Pseudomonadineae, order Pseudomonadales, occurring as stalked, curved, rod-shaped cells, the long axis of the cell coinciding with the long axis of the stalk. The type species is *C. vibrioi′des.*

Caulobacteraceae (kaw″lo-bak″ter-a′se-e) a family of Schizomycetes (order Pseudomonadales, suborder Pseudomonadineae), occurring as nonfilamentous rod-shaped bacteria singly or in pairs or short chains, in fresh or salt water. It includes five genera, *Caulobacter, Gallionella, Nevskia,* and *Siderophacus.*

Caulobacteriineae (kaw″lo-bak-te-re-in′e-e) a name formerly given a suborder of microorganisms now considered to constitute a family (Caulobacteraceae) of the suborder Pseudomonadineae, order Pseudomonadales.

caumesthesia (kaw″mes-the′ze-ah) [Gr. *kauma* burn + *aisthēsis* perception] a condition in which, with a low temperature, the patient experiences a sense of burning heat.

causal (kaw′zal) pertaining to a cause; directed against a cause.

causalgia (kaw-zal′je-ah) [Gr. *kausos* heat + *-algia*] a burning pain, often accompanied by trophic skin changes, due to injury of a peripheral nerve.

causative (kawz′ah-tiv) effective or responsible as a cause or agent.

cause (kawz) [L. *causa*] that which brings about any condition or produces any effect. **constitutional c.,** one acting within the body that is not restricted to a specific site, but is systemic or has a genetic basis. **exciting c.,** one that leads directly to a specific condition. **immediate c.,** a cause that is operative at the beginning of the specific effect; called also *precipitating c.* **local c.,** one that is not general or constitutional, but is confined to the site where the effect is produced. **precipitating c.,** immediate c. **predisposing c.,** anything that renders a person more liable to a specific condition without actually producing it. **primary c.,** the principal factor contributing to the production of a specific result. **proximate c.,** that which immediately precedes and produces an effect. **remote c.,** any cause that does not immediately precede and produce a specific condition; a predisposing, secondary, or ultimate cause. **secondary c.,** one that is supplemental to the primary cause. **specific c.,** one that produces a special or specific effect. **ultimate c.,** the earliest factor, in point of time, that has contributed to production of a specific result.

caustic (kaws'tik) [L. *causticus;* Gr. *kaustikos*] 1. burning or corrosive; destructive to living tissues. 2. having a burning taste. 3. an escharotic or corrosive agent. Called also *cauterant*. **Churchill's iodine c.,** a caustic solution of iodine and potassium iodide in water. **Filhos's c.,** 5 parts of potassium hydroxide and 1 part of calcium oxide. **Landolfi's c.,** a compound containing chlorides of antimony, bromine, gold, and zinc. **Lugol's c.,** 1 part each of iodine and potassium iodide dissolved in 2 parts of water. **lunar c.,** toughened silver nitrate. **mitigated c.,** silver nitrate diluted with potassium nitrate. **Plunket's c.,** a caustic paste made of 60 parts of arsenic, 100 of sulfur, and 480 each of *Ranunculus acris* and *R. flammula*. **Rousselot's c.,** a caustic containing red mercuric sulfide, burnt sponge, and arsenic trioxide. **Vienna c.,** caustic potash with lime. **zinc c.,** a mixture of 1 part of zinc chloride and 3 parts of flour.

causticize (kaws'tĭ-sīz) to render caustic.

cauter (kaw'ter) [Gr. *kauter*] (*obs.*) a cautery iron.

cauterant (kaw'ter-ant) 1. any caustic material or application. 2. caustic.

cauterization (kaw"ter-i-za'shun) the destruction of tissue with a hot instrument, an electric current, or a caustic substance.

cautery (kaw'ter-e) [L. *cauterium;* Gr. *kauterion*] 1. the application of a caustic substance, a hot instrument, an electric current, or other agent to destroy tissue. 2. a caustic substance or hot instrument used in cauterization. **actual c.,** 1. a red-hot iron used as a cauterizing agent. 2. the application of an agent that actually burns tissue. **button c.,** an iron disk with a handle, used as a cautery. **chemical c.,** chemocautery. **cold c.,** cautery produced by the application of carbon dioxide; called also *cryocautery*. **Corrigan's c.,** a form of button cautery. **electric c., galvanic c.,** see *galvanocautery*. **gas c.,** cauterization by means of a specially controlled jet of burning gas. **Paquelin's c.,** a platinum point for use in cauterization; it is hollow and filled with platinum sponge through which a heated hydrocarbon vapor is blown. **potential c.,** cauterization by an escharotic without applying heat; called also *virtual c*. **solar c.,** cauterization by using heat produced by concentrating the rays of the sun with a lens or mirror; called also *sun c*. **Souttar's c.,** a steam-heated cautery producing a constant temperature of about 100° C. **steam c.** (*obs.*), atmocausis. **sun c.,** solar c. **virtual c.,** potential c. **Ziegler c.,** a method of treating minor degrees of senile ectropion.

cava (ka'vah) [L.] 1. plural of *cavum*. 2. a vena cava.

caval (ka'val) pertaining to a vena cava.

cavascope (kav'ah-skōp) [L. *cavum* hollow + Gr. *skopein* to examine] an instrument for illuminating and examining a cavity.

cave (kāv) [L. *cavum*] a small enclosed space within the body or an organ; see under *cavity* and *cavum*.

caveola (ka-ve-o'lah), pl. *caveo'lae* [L.] a small pit, depression, or invagination, such as any of the minute pits or incuppings of the cell membrane formed during pinocytosis, which close and then pinch off to form small, free, fluid-filled vesicles (pinosomes) in the cytoplasm. Called also *c. intracellularis* and *plasmalemmal vesicle*.

cavern (kav'ern) a pathologic cavity, such as occurs in the lung in tuberculosis. **c's of corpora cavernosa of penis,** cavernae corporum cavernosorum penis. **c's of corpus spongiosum,** cavernae corporis spongiosi. **Schnabel's c's,** pathologic spaces in the optic nerve in glaucoma.

caverna (ka-ver'nah), pl. *caver'nae* [L.] [NA] a general term used to designate a cavity. **caver'nae cor'poris spongio'si** [NA], caverns of corpus spongiosum: the dilatable spaces within the corpus spongiosum of the penis, which fill with blood and become distended with erection. **caver'nae corpo'rum cavernoso'rum pe'nis** [NA], caverns of corpora cavernosa of penis: the dilatable spaces within the corpora cavernosa of the penis, which fill with blood and become distended with erection.

caverniloquy (kav"er-nil'o-kwe) [L. *caverna* cavity + *loqui* to speak] the low-pitched pectoriloquy indicative of a pulmonary cavity.

cavernitis (kav"er-ni'tis) inflammation of the corpora cavernosa or corpus spongiosum of the penis. **fibrous c.,** Peyronie's disease.

cavernoma (kav"er-no'mah), pl. *caverno'mas, cavernoma'ta*. Hemangioma cavernosum. **c. lymphat'icum,** lymphangioma cavernosum.

cavernoscope (kav'er-no-skōp") an instrument for viewing pulmonary cavities; it is pushed through an intercostal space and on into the cavity.

cavernoscopy (kav"er-nos'ko-pe) the inspection of pulmonary cavities by the aid of a cavernoscope.

cavernositis (kav"er-no-si'tis) cavernitis.

cavernostomy (kav"er-nos'to-me) operative drainage of a pulmonary abscess cavity.

cavernous (kav'er-nus) [L. *cavernosus*] containing caverns or hollow spaces.

Cavia (ka've-ah) a genus of small South American rodents. **C. coba'ya,** the guinea pig.

cavilla (kah-vil'ah) os sphenoidale.

cavitary (kav'ĭ-ta"re) 1. characterized by the presence of a cavity or cavities. 2. any entozoon with a body space or alimentary canal.

cavitas (kav'ĭ-tas), pl. *cavita'tes* [L. from *cavus* hollow] a hollow space or depression; called also *cavity*. See also *cavum*. **c. den'tis,** pulp cavity (cavum dentis [NA]). **c. glenoida'lis** [NA], glenoid cavity: a depression in the lateral angle of the scapula for articulation with the humerus; called also *glenoid fossa of scapula*.

cavitates (kav"ĭ-ta'tēz) [L.] plural of *cavitas*.

cavitation (kav"ĭ-ta'shun) the formation of cavities, as in pulmonary tuberculosis. Also, a cavity.

Cavite fever (kah-ve'tah) [*Cavite*, a province and city in the Philippine Islands] see under *fever*.

cavitis (ka-vi'tis) inflammation of a vena cava.

cavity (kav'ĭ-te) [L. *cavitas*] 1. a hollow place or space, or a potential space, within the body or in one of its organs; it may be normal or pathological. See also *cavitas* and *cavum*. 2. in dentistry, the lesion, or area of destruction in a tooth, produced by dental caries; classified as simple, compound, or complex, according to the number of surfaces involved. Also classified by Greene

BLACK'S CLASSIFICATION OF TOOTH CAVITIES

Class I. Cavities beginning as structural defects in pits and fissures.
Class II. Cavities in the proximal surfaces of bicuspids and molars.
Class III. Cavities in the proximal surfaces of incisors and cuspids not requiring the removal of the incisal angle.
Class IV. Cavities in the proximal surfaces of incisors and cuspids which require the removal of the incisal angle.
Class V. Cavities in the gingival third of the labial, or lingual, or buccal surfaces.
[Class VI. Cavities in the incisal edge or occlusal cusps due to either abrasion, erosion, attrition, or developmental defect.]

Vardiman Black into five groups on the basis of similarity of treatment required. (See table for Black's Classification of Tooth Cavities, to which a sixth group is sometimes added.) **abdominal c.,** the cavity of the body, located between the diaphragm above and the pelvis below, which contains all the abdominal organs; called also *cavum abdominis* [NA]. See also *abdomen*. **absorption c's,** cavities in developing compact bone due to osteoclastic erosion, usually occurring in the areas laid down first. **alveolar c's,** see *alveoli dentales mandibulae* and *alveoli dentales maxillae*. **amniotic c.,** the closed sac between the embryo and the amnion, containing the amniotic fluid. **articular c.,** cavum articulare. **Baer's c.,** the cleavage cavity beneath the blastoderm. **body c.,** a visceral cavity, such as the thoracic, abdominal, or pelvic cavity. **bony c. of nose,** cavum nasi osseum. **buccal c.,** 1. that portion of the oral cavity bounded on one side by the teeth and gingivae (or the residual alveolar ridges), and on the other by the cheeks. 2. a carious lesion beginning on the buccal surface of a posterior tooth. **cleavage c.,** the cavity of the blastula; blastocoele. **complex c.,** a carious lesion that involves three or more surfaces of a tooth in its prepared state. **compound c.,** a carious lesion that involves two surfaces of a tooth in its prepared state. **c. of concha,** cavum conchae. **cotyloid c.,** acetabulum. **cranial c.,** the space enclosed by the bones of the cranium. **dental c.,** the defect (lesion) produced by destruction of enamel and dentin in a tooth affected by caries. **distal c.,** a carious lesion beginning on the distal surface of a tooth. **epidural c.,** cavum epidurale. **faucial c.,** cavum pharyngis. **fibrotic c's,** cavities of the lung in tuberculosis composed of tuberculous granulation tissue surrounded by scar tissue, often the source from which the disease spreads to other pulmonary segments. **fissure c.,** a carious lesion beginning in a fissure of a tooth. **gastrovascular c.,** the body cavity of a coelenterate, which opens to the outside at one end to form a mouth; called also *coelenteron*. **glandular c.,** a hollow sac formed by invagination of the epithelial sheath in the developing multicellular gland. **glenoid c.,** cavitas glenoidalis. **head c.,** modified somites that in lower vertebrates give rise to the extrinsic eye muscles. **hemal c.,** hemocoelom. **incisal c.,** a carious lesion beginning on the incisal surface of an anterior tooth. **infraglottic c.,** cavum infraglotticum. **ischiorectal c.,** fossa ischiorectalis. **labial c.,** a carious lesion beginning on the labial surface of an anterior tooth. **laryngeal c.,** cavum laryngis. **laryngopharyngeal c.,** the laryngopharynx (pars laryngea pharyngis [NA]).

lingual c., a carious lesion beginning on the lingual surface of a tooth. **lymph c's,** the larger lymph spaces and cisterns of the body. **marrow c.,** cavum medullare ossium. **mastoid c.,** antrum mastoideum. **Meckel's c.,** cavum trigeminale. **mediastinal c., anterior,** mediastinum anterius. **mediastinal c., posterior,** mediastinum posterius. **medullary c. of bones,** cavum medullare ossium. **mesial c.,** a carious lesion beginning on the mesial surface of a tooth. **nasal c.,** cavum nasi. **nasal c., bony,** cavum nasi osseum. **nerve c.,** pulp c. (cavum dentis [NA]). **occlusal c.,** a carious lesion beginning on the occlusal surface of a posterior tooth. **oral c.,** the cavity of the mouth; see *cavum oris* [NA]. **oral c., external,** vestibulum oris. **oral c., proper,** cavum oris proprium. **orbital c.,** orbita. **pectoral c.,** thoracic c. (cavum thoracis [NA]). **pelvic c.,** the space within the walls of the pelvis; called also *cavum pelvis*. **pericardial c.,** cavum pericardii. **peritoneal c., peritoneal c., greater,** cavum peritonei. **peritoneal c., lesser,** bursa omentalis. **pharyngeal c.,** cavum pharyngis. **pharyngolaryngeal c.,** the laryngopharynx (pars laryngea pharyngis [NA]). **pharyngonasal c.,** the nasopharynx (pars nasalis pharyngis [NA]). **pharyngo-oral c.,** the oropharynx (pars oralis pharyngis [NA]). **c. of pharynx,** cavum pharyngis. **pit c.,** a carious lesion beginning in a pit of a tooth. **pleural c.,** cavum pleurae. **pleuroperitoneal c.,** the temporarily continuous coelomic cavity in the embryo that will later be partitioned by the developing diaphragm. **popliteal c.,** fossa poplitea. **prepared c.,** one that is produced in a tooth to support and retain the filling material and protect the tooth structure remaining after removal of all carious tissue. **proximal c.,** a carious lesion beginning on a proximal (the mesial or distal) surface of a tooth. **pulp c.,** the pulp-filled central chamber in the crown of a tooth; called also *nerve c., cavum dentis* [NA], *cavum pulpae,* and *cavitas dentis.* **rectoischiadic c.,** fossa ischiorectalis. **Retzius's c.,** spatium retropubicum. **Rosenmüller's c.,** recessus pharyngeus. **segmentation c.,** the blastocoele. **c. of septum pellucidum,** cavum septi pellucidi. **serous c.,** a celomic cavity, like that enclosed by the pericardium, peritoneum, or pleura, not communicating with the outside of the body, and whose lining membrane secretes a serous fluid. **sigmoid c. of radius,** incisura ulnaris radii. **sigmoid c. of ulna, greater,** incisura trochlearis ulnae. **sigmoid c. of ulna, lesser,** incisura radialis ulnae. **simple c.,** a carious lesion that involves only one surface of a tooth in its preparation, designated according to the surface involved as buccal, distal, incisal, labial, lingual, mesial, or occlusal. **somatic c.,** the intraembryonic portion of the coelom. **somite c.,** myocoele. **splanchnic c.,** visceral c. **subarachnoid c.,** cavum subarachnoideale. **subdural c.,** cavum subdurale. **tension c's,** cavities of the lung in which the air pressure is greater than that of the atmosphere. Radiologically, they appear as large, spherical, thin-walled defects indicative of productive inflammatory reaction in the bronchus that drains the cavity or of partial stenosis due to peribronchial fibrosis. **thoracic c.,** the portion of the ventral body cavity situated between the neck and the respiratory diaphragm; called also *pectoral c., cavum thoracis* [NA], and *cavum pectoris.* **trigeminal c.,** cavum trigeminale. **tympanic c.,** middle ear. **uterine c.,** cavum uteri. **visceral c.,** one of the cavities of the body containing organs, such as the thoracic, abdominal, or pelvic cavity; called also *splanchnic c.* **yolk c.,** the space between the germ disk and the yolk of the developing ovum of some animals; called also *subgerminal c.*

cavography (ka-vog′rah-fe) venacavography.

cavosurface (ka′vo-sur″fis) the surface of a cavity, as of a tooth.

cavovalgus (ka″vo-val′gus) see *talipes cavovalgus.*

cavum (ka′vum) pl. *ca′va* [L.] A general term used to designate a cavity or space; see also *cavitas* and *cavity.* **c. abdom′inis** [NA], the cavity of the body, located between the diaphragm above and the pelvis below; called also *abdominal cavity.* See also *abdomen.* **c. articula′re** [NA], articular cavity: the minute space of a synovial joint, enclosed by the synovial membrane and articular cartilages. **c. con′chae** [NA], cavity of concha: the inferior part of the concha of the auricle, which leads into the external acoustic meatus; called also *innominate fossa of auricle.* **c. corona′le** [NA], the crown portion of the cavum dentis. **c. den′tis** [NA], the pulp-filled chamber in the crown of a tooth. Called also *c. pulpae, cavitas dentis,* and *nerve* or *pulp cavity.* **c. doug′lasi,** excavatio rectouterina. **c. epidura′le** [NA], epidural cavity: the space between the dura mater and the walls of the vertebral canal, containing venous plexuses and fibrous and alveolar tissue; called also *epidural space.* **c. infraglot′ticum** [NA], infraglottic cavity: the most inferior part of the laryngeal cavity, extending from the rima glottidis above to the cavity of the trachea below. **c. laryn′gis** [NA], laryngeal cavity: the space enclosed by the walls of the larynx. **c. meck′elii,** c. trigeminale. **c. mediastina′le ante′rius,** mediastinum anterius. **c. mediastina′le poste′rius,** mediastinum posterius. **c. medulla′re os′sium** [NA], the spacious cavity, containing marrow, in the diaphysis of a long bone; called also *medullary* or *marrow cavity,* and *medullary canal.* **c. na′si** [NA], nasal cavity: the proximal portion of the passages

of the respiratory system, extending from the nares to the pharynx. **c. na′si os′seum** [NA], bony nasal cavity: the space between the floor of the cranium and the roof of the mouth, extending between the pharynx posteriorly and the external nose anteriorly, and divided by a median septum; called also *bony cavity of nose.* **c. o′ris** [NA], oral cavity: the cavity of the mouth and the associated structures, including the cheek, palate, oral mucosa, the glands whose ducts open into the cavity, the teeth, and the tongue. **c. o′ris exter′num,** vestibulum oris. **c. o′ris pro′prium** [NA], oral cavity proper: the part of the oral cavity internal to the teeth. **c. pec′toris,** c. thoracis. **c. pel′vis** [NA], the pelvic cavity: the space within the walls of the pelvis. **c. pericar′dii** [NA], pericardial cavity: a potential space between the visceral portion (epicardium) and the parietal portion of the serous pericardium. **c. peritonae′i, c. peritone′i** [NA], peritoneal cavity: the potential space between the parietal and visceral layers of the peritoneum; called also *greater peritoneal cavity.* **c. pharyn′gis** [NA], pharyngeal cavity: the space enclosed by the walls of the pharynx; called also *faucial cavity,* and *cavity of pharynx.* **c. pleu′rae** [NA], pleural cavity: the potential space between the parietal and visceral pleurae. **c. pul′pae,** c. dentis. **c. rectoischiad′icum,** fossa ischiorectalis. **c. ret′zii,** spatium retropubicum. **c. sep′ti pellu′cidi** [NA], the median cleft between the two laminae of the septum pellucidum; variously called *cavity of septum pellucidum, camera septi pellucidi, Duncan's ventricle, fifth ventricle, first ventricle of cerebrum, pseudocele, rhomboid sinus, sinus rhomboideus cerebri, ventricle of Arantius, ventricle of Sylvius,* and *Vieussen's ventricle.* **c. subarachnoidea′le** [NA], subarachnoid cavity: the space between the arachnoidea and the pia mater, containing cerebrospinal fluid and bridged by delicate trabeculae; called also *subarachnoid space.* **c. subdura′le,** subdural cavity: a narrow, fluid-containing space, often only a potential space, between the dura mater and arachnoid; called also *subdural space.* **c. thora′cis** [NA], the thoracic cavity: the portion of the body cavity situated between the neck and the respiratory diaphragm; called also *c. pectoris* and *pectoral c.* **c. trigemina′le** [NA], trigeminal cavity: the small outpocketing of the dura mater surrounding the ganglion and divisions of the trigeminal nerve, and located at the end of the petrous portion of the temporal bone, which contains the trigeminal ganglion; called also *c. meckelii* and *Meckel's cavity.* **c. tym′pani,** NA alternative for *auris media.* **c. u′teri** [NA], cavity of uterus: the flattened space within the uterus, communicating on either side with the uterine tubes and below with the vagina. **c. ver′gae,** Verga's ventricle.

cavus (kav′us) [L. "hollow"] see *talipes cavus.*

cavy (ka′ve) a small rodent of the family Caviidae, the best known representative of which is the guinea pig (*Cavia cobaya*).

Caytine (ka′tēn) trademark for a preparation of protokylol hydrochloride.

Cazenave's disease, vitiligo (kahz-nahvz′) [Pierre Louis Alphée *Cazenave,* French dermatologist, 1795–1877] see *pemphigus foliaceus* and *alopecia areata.*

Cb chemical symbol for *columbium,* now called *niobium.*

C.B. abbreviation for L. *Chirurgiae Baccalaureus,* Bachelor of Surgery.

c.b.c. complete blood count.

CBF cerebral blood flow.

CBG corticosteroid-binding globulin; see *transcortin.*

CBS chronic brain syndrome.

C.C. chief complaint.

cc. cubic centimeter.

CCA chimpanzee coryza agent (respiratory syncytial virus).

C. C. 914 a thioarsenite, *p*-carbamido-phenyl-bis (carboxymethyl-mercapto) arsine, used in treatment of intestinal amebiasis.

C. C. 1037 a thioarsenite, *p*-carbamido-phenyl-bis (2-carboxyphenyl-mercapto) arsine, used in intestinal amebiasis.

CCC cathodal closure contraction.

CCCl cathodal closure clonus.

CCK cholecystokinin.

CCK-179 the methanesulfonate salts of equal parts of dihydroergocornine, dihydroergocristine, and dihydroergocryptine, used as an antihypertensive and as a vasodilator in the treatment of peripheral vascular diseases.

CCl₄ carbon tetrachloride.

CCl₃·CHO chloral.

CCl₃·CH(OH)₂ chloral hydrate.

c.cm. cubic centimeter.

CCNU code designation for lomustine.

CCTe cathodal closure tetanus.

C.D. abbreviation for L. *conjugata diagonalis,* the diagonal conjugate diameter of the pelvic inlet, and for *curative dose.*

C.D.₅₀ median curative dose; a dose that abolishes symptoms in 50 per cent of the test subjects.

Cd 1. chemical symbol for *cadmium.* 2. abbreviation for *caudal* or *coccygeal;* used in vertebral formulas.

cd candela.

CDC Center for Disease Control.

Ce chemical symbol for *cerium*.

ceasmic (se-as′mik) [Gr. *keasma* chip] characterized by the persistence after birth of embryonic fissures.

cebocephalus (se″bo-sef′ah-lus) a monster exhibiting cebocephaly.

cebocephaly (se″bo-sef′ah-le) [Gr. *kebos* monkey + *kephalē* head] a developmental anomaly characterized by a monkey-like head, the nose being defective and the eyes close together.

cecal (se′kal) [L. *caecalis*] 1. ending in a blind passage. 2. pertaining to the cecum. 3. pertaining to the blind spot in the field of vision.

cecectomy (se-sek′to-me) [*cecum* + Gr. *ektomē* excision] surgical removal of the cecum.

Cecil-Culp urethroplasty [Arthur Bond *Cecil*, Los Angeles surgeon, born 1885; Ormond Skinner *Culp*, American surgeon, born 1910] see under *urethroplasty*.

cecitis (se-si′tis) inflammation of the cecum.

cecocele (se′ko-sēl) a hernia containing part of the cecum.

cecocentral (se″ko-sen′tral) centrocecal.

cecocolic (se″ko-kol′ik) pertaining to the cecum and the colon.

cecocolon (se″ko-ko′lon) the cecum and colon considered as a unit.

cecocolopexy (se″ko-ko′lo-pek″se) an operation for fixing the cecum and ascending colon.

cecocolostomy (se″ko-ko-los′to-me) the surgical creation of an anastomosis between the cecum and the colon; also, the anastomosis so constructed. Called also *colocecostomy*.

cecofixation (se″ko-fik-sa′shun) cecopexy.

cecoileostomy (se″ko-il″e-os′to-me) [*cecum* + *ileum* + Gr. *stomoun* to provide with a mouth, or opening] ileocecostomy.

Cecon (se′kon) trademark for preparations of ascorbic acid.

cecopexy (se′ko-pek″se) [*cecum* + Gr. *pēxis* fixation] fixation or suspension of the cecum to correct excessive mobility of the organ; called also *cecofixation*.

cecoplication (se″ko-pli-ka′shun) [*cecum* + L. *plica* fold] plication of the cecal wall to correct ptosis or dilatation of the organ.

cecoptosis (se″kop-to′sis) [*cecum* + Gr. *ptōsis* falling] (*obs.*) ptosis or downward displacement of the cecum.

cecorrhaphy (se-kor′ah-fe) [*cecum* + Gr. *rhaphē* suture.] suture or repair of the cecum.

cecosigmoidostomy (se″ko-sig″moi-dos′to-me) formation of an artificial opening between the cecum and sigmoid, usually by surgical procedure; also, the opening so constructed.

cecostomy (se-kos′to-me) [*cecum* + Gr. *stomoun* to provide with a mouth, or opening] the surgical creation of an artificial opening or fistula into the cecum; also, the opening so constructed.

cecotomy (se-kot′o-me) [*cecum* + Gr. *tomē* a cutting] the operation of cutting into the cecum.

cecum (se′kum) [L. *caecum* blind, blind gut] 1. the first part of the large intestine, forming a dilated pouch into which open the ileum, the colon, and the appendix vermiformis; called also *blindgut, caput coli, head of blind colon, blind intestine,* and *intestinum caecum.* 2. any blind pouch or cul-de-sac. **cupular c. of cochlear duct, c. cupula′re duc′tus cochlea′ris** [NA], the closed blind apical end of the cochlear duct. **high c.,** a cecum situated higher up in the abdomen than normal. **mobile c., c. mo′bile,** abnormal mobility of the cecum and lower portion of the ascending colon, caused by incomplete rotation or faulty fixation of the cecum in embryonic development. **vestibular c. of cochlear duct, c. vestibula′re duc′tus cochlea′ris** [NA], a small blind outpouching at the vestibular end of the cochlear duct.

Cedilanid (se″dĭ-lan′id) trademark for a preparation of lanatoside C.

Cedilanid-D trademark for a preparation of deslanoside.

Cediopsylla (se″de-o-sil′ah) a genus of fleas, including some of the rabbit fleas.

cefaclor (sef′ah-klor) chemical name: $[6R-[6\alpha,7\beta(R^*)]]$-7-[(amino-phenylacetyl)amino]-3-chloro-8-oxo-5-thia-1-azabicyclo-[4.2.0]oct-2-ene-2-carboxylic acid; a semisynthetic cephalosporin antibiotic, $C_{15}H_{14}ClN_3O_4S$.

cefadroxil (sef″ah-droks′il) [USP] chemical name: $[6R-[6\alpha,7\beta(R^*)]]$-7-[[amino(4-hydroxyphenyl)acetyl]amino]-3-methyl-8-oxo-5-thia-1-azabicyclo[4.2.0]oct-2-ene-2-carboxylic acid; a semisynthetic cephalosporin antibiotic, $C_{16}H_{17}N_3O_5S$.

Cefadyl (sef′ah-dil) trademark for a preparation of cephapirin sodium.

cefamandole (sef″ah-man′dōl) chemical name: $[6R-[6\alpha,7\beta-(R^*)]]$-7-[(hydroxyphenylacetyl)amino]-3-[[(1-methyl-1H-tetrazol-5-yl)thio]methyl-8-oxo-5-thia-1-azabicyclo [4.2.0]oct-2-ene-2-carboxylic acid; a semisynthetic cephalosporin antibiotic, $C_{18}H_{18}N_6$-O_5S_2. **c. nafate,** the monosodium salt of cefamandole, $C_{19}H_{17}$-$N_6NaO_6S_2$.

cefaparole (sef″ah-pah-rōl″) chemical name: $[6R-[6\alpha,7\beta(R^*)]]$-7-[[amino(4-hydroxyphenyl)acetyl]amino]-3-[[5-methyl-1,3,4-thiadiaxol-2-yl)thio]methyl]-8-oxo-5-thio-1-azabicyclo[4.2.0]oct-2-ene-2-carboxylic acid; a semisynthetic cephalosporin antibiotic, $C_{19}H_{19}N_5O_5S_3$.

cefatrizine (sef″ah-tri′zēn) chemical name: $[6R-[6\alpha,7\beta(R^*)]]$-7-[[amino(4-hydroxyphenyl)acetyl]amino]-8-oxo-3-[(1H-1,2,3-triazol-4-ylthio)methyl]-5-thia-1-azabicyclo[4.2.0]oct-2-ene-2-carboxylic acid; a semisynthetic cephalosporin antibiotic, $C_{18}H_{18}N_6O_5S_2$.

cefazaflur sodium (sĕ-faz′ah-flor) chemical name: $(6R$-$trans)$-3[[(1-methyl-1H-tetrazol-5-yl)thio]methyl]-7-[(trifluoromethyl)thio]acetyl]anino]-5-thia-1-azabicyclo [4.2.0] oct-2-ene-2-carboxylic acid monosodium salt; a semisynthetic cephalosporin antibiotic, $C_{13}H_{12}F_3N_6NaO_4S_3$.

cefazolin (sĕ-faz′o-lin) chemical name: $(6R$-$trans)$-3-[[(5-methyl-1,3,4-thiadiazol-2-yl)thio]methyl]-8-oxo-7-[[(1H-tetrazol-1-yl)acetyl]-amino]-5-thia-azabicyclo [4.2.0]oct-2-ene-2-carboxylic acid. A semisynthetic analogue, $C_{14}H_{14}N_8O_4S_3$, of the natural antibiotic cephalosporin C, effective against a wide range of gram-negative and gram-positive bacteria. **c. sodium,** the monosodium salt of cepazolin, $C_{14}H_{13}N_8NaO_4S_3$, having the same actions as the base; used in the treatment of infections of the respiratory tract, genitourinary tract, skin, soft tissues, bones, joints, and blood due to sensitive pathogens, administered intramuscularly and intravenously. It is available for therapeutic use as *sterile cefazolin sodium* [USP].

ceforanide (sĕ-for′ah-ni″d) chemical name: $(6R$-$trans)$-7-[[[2-(aminomethyl)phenyl]acetyl]amino]-3-[[[1-(carboxymethyl-1H-tetrazol-5-yl]thio]methyl]-8-oxo-5-thio-1-azabicyclo[4.2.0]oct-2-2-carboxylic acid; an antibacterial, $C_{20}H_{21}N_7O_6S_2$.

cefoxitin (sĕ-foks′ĭ-tin) chemical name: $(6R$-$cis)$-3-[[(aminocarbonyl)oxy]methyl]-7-methoxy-8-oxo-7-[(2-thienylacetyl)amino]-5-thia-1-azabicyclo[4.2.0]oct-2-ene-2-carboxylic acid. A semisynthetic derivative of cephamycin C, an analogue of the cephalosporin antibiotic cephalothin, especially effective against gram-negative organisms, with strong resistance to degradation by β-lactamase.

Cel. Celsius (thermometric scale).

cel (sel) a unit of velocity, being the velocity of 1 cm. per second.

cel- see *celo-*.

celarium (sĕ-la′re-um) mesothelium.

Celbenin (sel′bĕ-nin) trademark for preparations of sodium methicillin.

-cele (sēl) 1. [Gr. *kēlē* hernia] a word termination denoting relationship to a tumor or swelling. 2. [Gr. *koilia* cavity] a word termination denoting relationship to a cavity; see also words spelled *-coele*.

celectome (se-lek′tōm) [Gr. *kēlē* tumor + *ektomē* excision] an instrument for removing a segment of tumor for examination.

celenteron (se-len′ter-on) 1. archenteron. 2. gastrovascular cavity.

Celestone (se-les′tōn) trademark for preparations of betamethasone.

celiac (se′le-ak) [Gr. *koilia* belly] pertaining to the abdomen.

celiaca (se-li′ah-kah) (*obs.*) disease of the abdominal organs, especially celiac disease in children.

celialgia (se″le-al′je-ah) [*celio-* + *-algia*] (*obs.*) pain in the abdomen.

celiectomy (se″le-ek′to-me) [*celio-* + Gr. *ektomē* excision] 1. surgical removal of an abdominal organ. 2. excision of the celiac branches of the vagus nerve for the relief of essential hypertension.

celio- (se′le-o) [Gr. *koilia* belly] a combining form denoting relationship to the abdomen. For words beginning thus, see also words beginning *celo-* and *coelo-*.

celiocentesis (se″le-o-sen-te′sis) [*celio-* + Gr. *kentēsis* puncture] puncture into the abdominal cavity, usually for the withdrawal of fluid.

celiocolpotomy (se″le-o-kol-pot′o-me) [*celio-* + Gr. *kolpos* vagina + *tome* a cutting] incision into the abdomen through the vagina.

celiodynia (se″le-o-din′e-ah) (*obs.*) celialgia.

celioelytrotomy (se″le-o-el″e-trot′o-me) [*celio-* + Gr. *elytron* sheath + *tomē* a cutting] (*obs.*) celiocolpotomy.

celioenterotomy (se″le-o-en″ter-ot′o-me) [*celio-* + *enterotomy*] incision through the abdominal wall into the intestine.

celiogastrotomy (se″le-o-gas-trot′o-me) [*celio-* + *gastrotomy*] incision through the abdominal wall into the stomach.

celiohysterectomy (se″le-o-his″ter-ek′to-me) [*celio-* + *hysterectomy*] 1. excision of the uterus through an abdominal incision. 2. cesarean hysterectomy.

celioma (se-le-o′mah) [*celio-* + *-oma*] a tumor of the abdomen, especially mesothelioma of the peritoneum.

celiomyalgia (se″le-o-mi-al′je-ah) (*obs.*) myocelialgia.

celiomyomectomy (se″le-o-mi″o-mek′to-me) [*celio-* + *myomectomy*] myomectomy by an abdominal incision.

celiomyomotomy (se″le-o-mi″o-mot′o-me) [*celio-* + *myomotomy*] incision into a muscular organ or tumor through the abdominal wall.

celiomyositis (se″le-o-mi″o-si′tis) [*celio-* + *myositis*] inflammation of the abdominal muscles.

celioncus (se″le-on′kus) (*obs.*). celioma.

celioparacentesis (se″le-o-par″ah-sen-te′sis) [*celio-* + *paracentesis*] paracentesis of the abdominal cavity, usually with a trocar or needle.

celiopathy (se″le-op′ah-the) [*celio-* + Gr. *pathos* disease] any abdominal disease.

celiophyma (se″le-o-fi′mah) (*obs.*) celioma.

celiopyosis (se″le-o-pi-o′sis) [*celio-* + *pyosis*] (*obs.*) suppuration in the abdominal cavity.

celiorrhaphy (se″le-or′ah-fe) [*celio-* + Gr. *rhaphē* suture] suture of the abdominal wall.

celiosalpingectomy (se″le-o-sal″pin-jek′to-me) [*celio-* + *salpingectomy*] excision of a uterine tube through an abdominal incision.

celiosalpingotomy (se″le-o-sal″pin-got′o-me) incision of a uterine tube through an incision in the abdominal wall.

celioscope (se′le-o-skōp″) [*celio-* + Gr. *skopein* to examine] an endoscope for examining the abdominal cavity.

celioscopy (se″le-os′ko-pe) examination of the abdominal cavity through a celioscope.

celiothelioma (se″le-o-the″le-o′mah) (*obs.*) mesothelioma of the peritoneum.

celiotomy (se″le-ot′o-me) [*celio-* + Gr. *tomē* a cutting] surgical incision into the abdominal cavity. **vaginal c.,** incision into the abdominal cavity through the vagina. **ventral c.,** incision into the abdominal cavity through the abdominal wall.

celitis (se-li′tis) any abdominal inflammation.

cell (sel) [L. *cella* compartment] **1.** any one of the minute protoplasmic masses that make up organized tissue, consisting of a nucleus which is surrounded by cytoplasm which contains the various organelles and is enclosed in the cell or plasma membrane. A cell is the fundamental, structural, and functional unit of living organisms. See Plates XI and XII. In some of the lower forms of life, e.g., bacteria, a morphological nucleus is absent, although nucleoproteins (and genes) are present. **2.** a small, more or less closed space. **A c.,** alpha c. **Abbé-Zeiss counting c.,** see *Thoma-Zeiss counting chamber,* under *chamber.* **absorptive c.,** intestinal, one of the cells of the intestinal epithelium, having a brush border made up of many closely packed parallel microvilli, and believed to be associated with absorption, particularly of macromolecules. **accessory c's,** cells that cooperate with T- and B-lymphocytes in initiation of the immune response; they have macrophage functions and process antigen for presentation to antibody-forming cells. **acid c.,** parietal c. **acidophilic c.,** a cell having an affinity for acid dyes; called also *acidocyte.* See also *acidophil.* **acinar c., acinous c.,** any of the cells lining an acinus, especially applied to the zymogen-secreting cells of the pancreatic acini. **acoustic hair c.,** any one of the cells provided with cilia that serve as sensory receptors in the organ of Corti; called also *auditory c.* **adelomorphous c.** (*obs.*), chief c. (def. 1). **adipose c.,** a fat cell. **adventitial c's,** macrophages that occur along the walls of blood vessels; called also *Marchand's c's* and *perithelial c's.* **agger nasi c's,** the cells of the anterior part of the ethmoid crest. **air c.,** one containing air, such as an alveolus of the lungs (alveolus pulmonis) or one of the air-containing cells of the auditory tube (cellulae pneumaticae tubae auditivae). **albuminous c.,** serous c. **algoid c's,** cells resembling algae, seen in cases of chronic diarrhea. **alkaline-manganese c.,** one similar to the Leclanché cell but containing a cell electrolyte of concentrated aqueous sodium hydroxide. **alpha c's,** 1. cells situated in the periphery of the islets of Langerhans, which secrete glucagon. 2. the acidophils of the adenohypophysis; see also *carminophil* and *orangeophil.* Called also *A c's.* **alveolar c.,** any cell of the walls of the pulmonary alveoli. Often restricted to the cells of the alveolar epithelium (type I and type II alveolar cells) and alveolar phagocytes. **alveolar c's, type I,** the flattened cells of the alveolar epithelium, distinguished by their greatly attenuated cytoplasm and paucity of organelles; called also *membranous pneumonocytes* and *squamous* or *small alveolar cells.* **alveolar c's, type II,** pleomorphic cells of the pulmonary alveolar epithelium that secrete surfactant and are distinguished by abundant cytoplasm containing numerous lipid-rich multilamellar bodies; called also *granular pneumonocytes* and *great* or *large alveolar cells.* **Alzheimer's c's,** 1. giant astrocytes with large prominent nuclei found in the brain in hepatolenticular degeneration and hepatic coma. 2. degenerated astrocytes. **amacrine c.,** see *amacrine,* def. 2. **ameboid c.,** any cell that is able to change its form and move about. See *migratory c.* and *wandering c.* **amine precursor uptake and decarboxylation (APUD) c's,** a group of apparently unrelated cells found in different organs which share a number of cytochemical and ultrastructural characteristics and which produce polypeptide hormones and neurotransmitters. Such cells contain amines,

concentrate the amino acid precursors of these amines, and decarboxylate them to their respective amines. The group includes basal granular cells of the intestine, parafollicular cells of the thyroid, pancreatic islet cells, and pituitary corticotrophs. **amphophilic c.,** one that stains readily with either acid or basic dyes; called also *amphocyte, amphophil, amphochromatophil,* and *amphochromaphil.* **Anichkov's (Anitschkow's) c.,** see *Anichkov's myocyte,* under *myocyte.* **antipodal c's,** a group of four cells in the early embryo. **apocrine c's,** see *apocrine.* **apolar c.,** a neuron with no processes or poles. **apotrophic c's,** hypothetical cells in the peripheral stump of a divided nerve, which attract young axons from the proximal stump to aid in regeneration. **APUD c's,** amine precursor uptake and decarboxylation c's. **argentaffin c's,** enterochromaffin cells (q.v.) whose granules stain readily with chromium and silver salts, located in the basilar portions of the glands of the gastrointestinal tract. Based upon their staining reactions with silver, these cells have been divided into two groups: those that reduce silver without pretreatment (*argentaffin c's*), and those that require prior exposure to a reducing substance (*argyrophilic c's*). See also *argentaffinoma.* **argyrophilic c's,** enterochromaffin cells that require exposure to a reducing substance before their granules will react with silver; they are located in the fundic and pyloric glands between the basement lamina and zymogenic cells. See also *argentaffin c's.* **Arias-Stella c's,** columnar cells in the endometrial epithelium which have hyperchromatic enlarged nuclei and which appear to be associated with chorionic tissue in an intrauterine or extrauterine site. **arkyochrome c.,** a neuron in which the Nissl bodies are arranged in a network. **Armanni-Ebstein c's,** epithelial cells in the terminal part of the first convoluted renal tubule containing deposits of glycogen: a lesion characteristic of diabetes. **Aschoff's c's,** a type of giant cell as seen in the rheumatic nodule in the myocardium. **auditory c's,** cells in the internal ear bearing the auditory hairs; called also *acoustic hair c.* **B c's,** 1. beta c's. 2. B-lymphocytes; see under *lymphocyte.* **balloon c's,** peculiar degenerated cells in the vesicles of herpes zoster and varicella. **band c.,** a late metamyelocyte in which the nucleus is in the form of a curved or coiled band, not having acquired the typical lobulate shape of the mature (segmented) neutrophil; called also *staff* or *stab cell,* and *band form.* **basal c.,** the name applied to the early keratinocyte, present in the basal layer of the epidermis; called also *foot c.* **basal granular c's,** a group of cells, including enterochromaffin cells (argentaffin and argyrophilic cells), and gastrin-secreting, L, and S cells, which have numerous cytoplasmic granules. They are found scattered throughout the gastrointestinal epithelium, the majority at the base of the epithelium, and because of the location of their granules in the basal cytoplasm, which suggests that they liberate their secretions into the extracellular space rather than into the lumen, they have been called *endocrine cells of the gut.* See also *amine precursor uptake and decarboxylation (APUD) c's.* **basket c.,** 1. a cell of the cerebellar cortex whose axon gives off brushes of fibrils, forming a basket-like nest in which the body of each Purkinje cell rests. 2. myoepithelial c's. Called also *basket.* **basophilic c.,** a cell staining readily with basic dyes; called also *basocyte* and *basophil.* **battery c.,** one of the chambers of a galvanic battery, containing its fluids and essential elements. **beaker c.,** goblet c. **Beale's ganglion c's,** bipolar cells with one process coiled around the other. **Bergmann's c's,** peculiar glial cells in the molecular layer of the cerebellar cortex having dendrites that extend outward through that layer. **berry c.,** a term applied to plasma cells and plasmacytoid reticulum cells whose cytoplasm contains numerous transparent bluish vesicles, most probably protein in nature; found in disorders associated with pronounced hypergammaglobulinemia. Called also *grape c.* and *morular c.* **beta c's,** 1. the cells composing the bulk of the islets of Langerhans and which secrete insulin. 2. the basophilic cells of the adenohypophysis; see also *gonadotrope* (def. 3) and *thyrotrope* (def. 2). Called also *B c's.* **Betz's c's,** large pyramidal ganglion cells forming one of the layers of the motor area of the gray matter of the brain; called also *giant pyramids* and *giant pyramidal c's.* **Bevan-Lewis c's,** certain pyramidal cells in the motor cortex of the brain. **bichromate c., dichromate c.,** Grenet c. **bipolar c.,** a nerve cell with two processes. **bipolar retinal c's,** neurons of the inner plexiform layer of the retina which transmit signals from cones and rods to the ganglion cells. Bipolar retinal cells include *rod bipolar cells,* connecting to rod cells; *midget bipolar cells,* each synapsing with a single cone pedicle; and *diffuse bipolar cells,* connecting with many cone pedicles. Cf. *ganglion c.* (def. 2). **bladder c's,** swollen cells in the epidermis of the tips of the fingers and toes of the embryo. Called also *Zander's c's.* **blast c.,** the least differentiated blood cell without commitment as to its particular series. **bloated c.,** a swollen fattened astrocyte. **blood c's,** see under *corpuscle.* **bone c.,** a nucleated cell occupying each a separate lacuna of bone; called also *osseous c.* and *bone corpuscle.* **border c's,** 1. a row of columnar supporting cells that delimit the inner boundary of the organ of Corti. 2. parietal c's. **Böttcher's c's,** small groups of polyhedral cells interposed between Claudius' cells and the basilar membrane of the cochlea. **breviradiate c's,** neuroglial cells that have short prolongations. **bristle c's,** the hair cells associated with the cochlear nerve. **bronchic c.,** an air cell of the lungs. **brood c.,** mother cell. **burr c.,** a form of spiculed mature red blood cell, the echinocyte, having multiple small projections evenly spaced over the cell circumference; observed in azotemia, gastric carcinoma, and bleeding peptic ulcer. **C c's,** cells in the islands of Langerhans, especially in the guinea pig, which contain no granules. **Cajal c.,** 1. an astrocyte. 2. one of the neuroglial cells arranged horizontally in the stratum zonale of the cerebral cortex. **caliciform c.,** goblet c. **cameloid c.,** an elliptocyte. **capsule c.,** amphicyte. **cartilage c's,** cells embedded in the lacunae of the cartilages; called also *chondrocyte.* **caryochrome c's,** karyochrome c's. **Caspersson type B c's,** cells rich in nucleolar ribonucleic acid and relatively poor in nuclear deoxyribonucleic acid. **castration c's,** vacuolated basophil cells observed in the anterior pituitary gland after castration. **caudate c's,** neuroglial cells of the gray matter having several streaming prolongations like the tail of a comet; called also *cometal c's.* **caveolated c's,** epithelial cells with thick, short, apical microvilli containing bundles of filaments extending down into the cytoplasm and with irregular tubules (caveolae) passing as invaginations from the apical surface between microvilli; found rarely in the small intestine and respiratory tract, it has been suggested that they function as chemoreceptors. **central c.,** chief c's (def. 1). **centroacinar c's,** the intra-acinar beginnings of the intralobular duct system of the pancreas. **chalice c.,** goblet c. **chief c's,** 1. epithelial cells, either columnar or cuboidal, that line the lower portions of the gastric glands and secrete pepsin; called also *adelomorphous c's, central c's, Heidenhain's c's, peptic c's,* and *zymogenic c's.* 2. pinealocytes. 3. the most abundant cells (see also *oxyphil c's*) of the parathyroid glands, being polygonal epithelial cells with a granular cytoplasm and vesicular nuclei, arranged in plates or cords, and sometimes divided into clear, or light, and dark forms, both of which are rich in glycogen: the clear cells are more numerous and have relatively large nuclei and clear cytoplasm with few granules, while the dark cells are smaller with smaller and darker nuclei and finely granular cytoplasm with many granules. Intermediate forms also exist. Called also *principal c's.* 4. the principal chromaffin cells of the paraganglia, each of which is surrounded by supporting cells. 5. chromophobe c's. **chromaffin c's,** cells that stain readily with chromium salts, especially the cells of the adrenal medulla and similar cells occurring in widespread small accumulations (paraganglia) throughout the body in various organs, whose cytoplasm characteristically shows fine brown granules when stained with potassium bichromate. Cf. *argentaffin c's.* **chromophobe c's, chromophobic c's,** small, faintly staining cells with scanty cytoplasm found often in clusters in the center of the cell cords in the adenohypophysis; the cytoplasm of these cells was formerly thought to be nongranular, but electron micrographs reveal that relatively few have no specific granules. **ciliated c.,** any cell with cilia. **Clara c's,** unciliated cells occurring at the boundary where alveolar ducts branch from the bronchioles. **Clarke's c's,** pigmented cells in the thoracic nucleus of the spinal cord. **Claudius' c's,** cuboidal cells, which along with Böttcher's cells, form the floor of the external spiral sulcus, external to the organ of Corti. **clear c's,** cells with empty-appearing cytoplasm. **cleavage c.,** any one of the cells derived from the fertilized ovum by mitosis; a blastomere. **clump c's,** round, thick, pigmented cells seen in the sphincter muscle of the iris. **collenchyma c's,** elongated living cells with walls thickened in the corners, which compose the collenchyma of plants. Cf. *schlerenchyma c's.* **columnar c.,** an elongate epithelial cell. **cometal c's,** caudate c's. **commissural c's,** heteromeral c's. **committed c.,** a lymphocyte which, after contact with antigen, is obligated to follow an individual course of development leading to antibody synthesis or immunological memory. **compound granule c.,** microglia. **cone c's,** retinal cone. **connective tissue c's,** a general name for the cellular elements of the fibrous and nonfibrous components of the various forms of connective tissue. **contractile fiber c's,** the spindle-shaped and nucleated cells which, collected into bundles, make up unstriated or smooth muscle. **corneal c.,** a modified connective tissue cell occupying each corneal space. **c's of Corti,** the cells of the organ of Corti. **counting c.,** see under *chamber.* **cover c.,** any cell that covers and protects other cells, especially any long epithelial cell of the outer layer of the taste buds; called also *encasing c.* **crescent c's,** crescents of Giannuzzi. **cribrate c.,** a cell whose walls are perforated with numerous sievelike pores. **Crooke's c's,** the basophils in Crooke's hyaline degeneration; see under *degeneration.* **cuboid c.,** an epithelial cell of which the transverse and vertical diameters are approximately equal. **Custer c's,** cells with long delicate protoplasmic processes replacing the lymphoid tissue of lymph nodes in reticuloendothelial disease. **cylindric c.,** columnar c. **D c's,** delta c's. **daughter c.,** any cell formed by the division of a mother cell. **Davidoff's c's,** Paneth's c's. **decidual c's,** connective-tissue cells of the uterine mucous membrane, enlarged and specialized during pregnancy. **Deiters' c's,** 1. the outer phalangeal cells of the organ of Corti; see under *supporting c's.* 2. neuroglial cells. **delomorphous c's** (*obs.*), parietal c's. **delta c's,** 1. cells in

the islets of Langerhans filled with small blue-staining secretory granules, which contain somatostatin. 2. gonadotropes. Called also *D c's.* **demilune c's,** crescents of Giannuzzi. **dendritic c's,** cells with long cytoplasmic processes in the lymph nodes and germinal centers of the spleen; such processes which extend along lymphoid cells retain antigen molecules for extended periods of time. **dentin c.,** odontoblast. **dome c's,** the large cells that compose the epitrichium of the fetus. **Dorothy Reed c's,** Reed-Sternberg c's. **Downey c's,** atypical lymphocytes of three types invariably present in infectious mononucleosis. Type I is a mature cell with a kidney-shaped or lobulated nucleus with vacuolated, basophilic foamy cytoplasm; type II cells contain plasmacytoid nuclei with less vacuolated and basophilic cytoplasm; type III has a finer chromatin pattern and one or two nucleoli. **dust c's,** alveolar macrophages. **effector c.,** any cell, such as an activated lymphocyte or plasma cell, which is instrumental in causing antigen disposal, accomplished by either a cell-mediated or a humoral immunological response. **electrochemical c., electromotive force c.,** a device consisting of an anode, a cathode, and one or more electrolyte phases that exhibits an electromotive force or potential drop between the two electrodes. **elementary c's, embryonic c's,** blastomere. **emigrated c.,** a leukocyte that has passed through the wall of a blood vessel into the neighboring tissue. **enamel c.,** ameloblast. **encasing c.,** cover c. **endocrine c's of gut,** basal granular c's. **endothelioid c's,** large protoplasmic cells frequently seen in disease of the blood-making organs and believed by some to be derived from the endothelial lining of the blood vessels and lymph vessels. **enterochromaffin c's,** a group of basal granular cells (q.v.) whose granules stain readily with silver and chromium salts, and which are sites of synthesis and storage of serotonin (5-hydroxytryptamine); included in the group are *argentaffin cells* and *agyrophilic cells.* **ependymal c's,** the cells of the ependyma; called also *ependymocytes.* **epidermic c's,** the cells of the epidermis. **epithelial c's,** cells that cover the surface of the body and line its cavities. **epithelioid c's,** 1. large polyhedral cells of connective tissue origin. 2. highly phagocytic, modified macrophages, resembling epithelial cells, having large, pale and vesicular nuclei with abundant, eosinophilic cytoplasm, which are characteristic of granulomatous inflammation; they may coalesce to form multinucleate giant cells. 3. pinealocytes. **erythroid c's,** blood cells of the erythrocytic series. **ethmoidal c's, bony,** cellulae ethmoidales osseae. **eukaryotic c.,** a cell with a true nucleus; see *eukaryote.* **fat c.,** a connective tissue cell specialized for the synthesis and storage of fat; such cells are bloated with globules of triglycerides, the nucleus being displaced to one side and the cytoplasm seen as a thin line around the fat droplet. Called also *adipose c., adipocyte,* and *lipocyte.* **fat-storing c's of liver,** lipid-accumulating, stellate cells located in the perisinusoidal space of the liver. **fatty granule c.,** microglia containing fat. **ferment c.,** a cell that secretes an enzyme causing fermentation. **Ferrata's c.,** hemohistioblast. **fiber c.,** any elongated and linear cell. **flagellate c.,** any cell having a flagellum, usually motile. **flame c's,** flagellate cells at the termination of collecting tubules of the excretory system of flatworms and nemerteans; so called because the beating of the flagella suggests a flickering flame. Called also *protonephridia* and *solanocytes.* **floor c's,** the cells of the floor of the arch of Corti. **foam c's,** 1. cells with a peculiar vacuolated appearance due to the presence of complex lipoids; such cells are seen notably in xanthoma and have, therefore, been termed *xanthoma c's.* Called also *lattice c.* 2. Mikulicz's c's. **follicle c's, follicular c's,** cells located in the epithelium of follicles, e.g., the cells of the thyroid follicles and ovarian follicles. Called also *follicular epithelial c's.* **follicular epithelial c's,** follicle c's. **foot c's,** 1. basal cells. 2. Sertoli's cells. **foreign body giant c's,** giant cells, resembling Langhans' giant cells, having clusters of nuclei scattered in an irregular pattern throughout the cytoplasm, characteristic of granulomatous inflammation due to invasion of the tissue by a foreign body. **formative c.,** a cell of the inner cell mass of the conceptus, a blastomere destined to form a part of the embryo, as distinct from a trophoblast cell. **Foulis' c's,** large nucleated epithelial cells seen in fluids from malignant ovarian cysts. **Fuller c.,** electromotive force cell resembling the Grenet cell, but employing amalgamated zinc and copper electrodes. **fusiform c.,** spindle c. **G c's,** granular enterochromaffin cells in the mucosa of the pyloric part of the stomach, which are the source of gastrin. **gametoid c's,** carcinoma cells resembling reproductive cells (gametes). **gamma c's of hypophysis,** chromophobic c's. **ganglion c.,** 1. a form of large nerve cell characteristic of ganglia; called also *gangliocyte.* 2. any of the nerve cells of the ganglion cell layer of the retina with their dendrites in the inner plexiform layer and their axons forming the optic nerve fiber. Ganglion cells include *diffuse ganglion cells,* synapsing with different types of bipolar retinal cells, and *midget ganglion cells,* synapsing with a single midget bipolar retinal cell. Cf. *bipolar retinal c's.* **Gaucher's c.,** a large and distinctive cell characteristic of Gaucher's disease, with one or more eccentrically placed nuclei and with fine wavy kerasin fibrils running parallel to the long axis of the cell, imparting a wrinkled, tissue-paper appearance to the gray or bluish opaque cytoplasm.

Plate XI

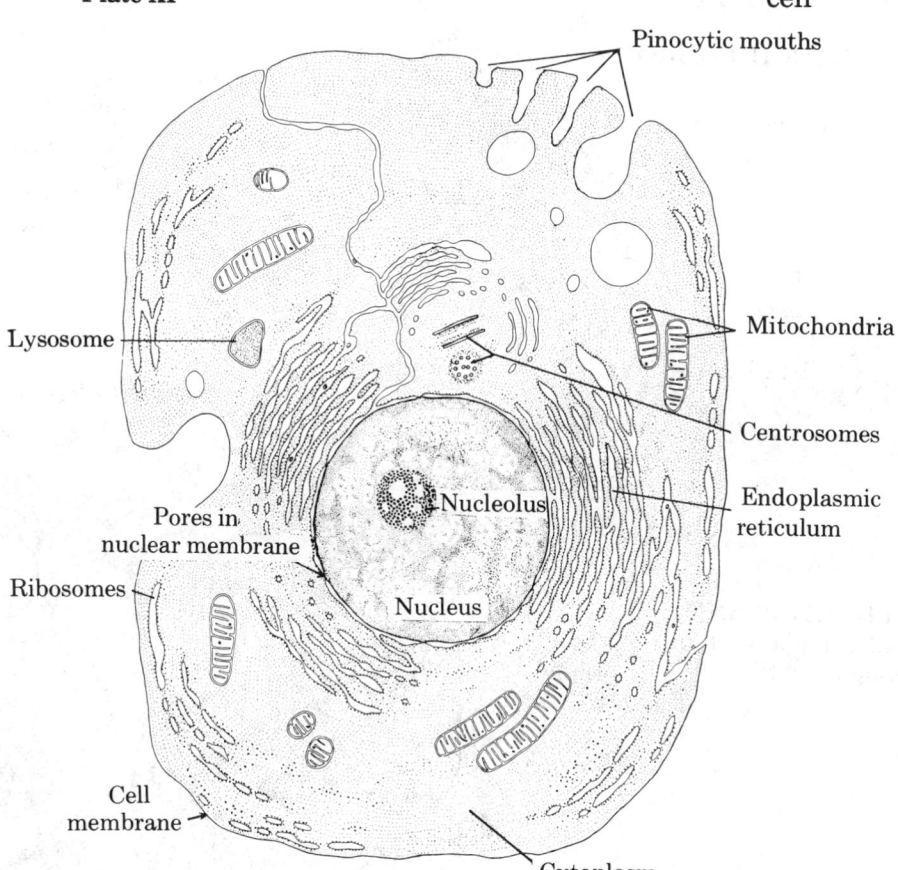

cell

Pinocytic mouths

Lysosome

Mitochondria

Centrosomes

Endoplasmic reticulum

Pores in nuclear membrane

Nucleolus

Ribosomes

Nucleus

Cell membrane

Cytoplasm

TYPICAL ANIMAL CELL

(Modified from Scientific American)

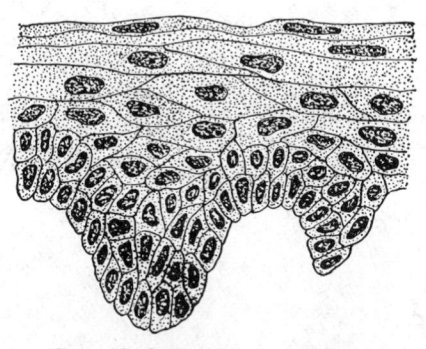

Stratified squamous, esophagus

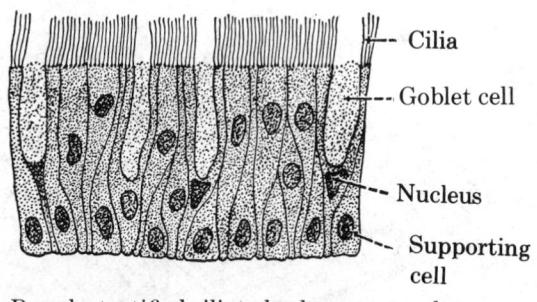

Cilia

Goblet cell

Nucleus

Supporting cell

Pseudostratified ciliated columnar, trachea

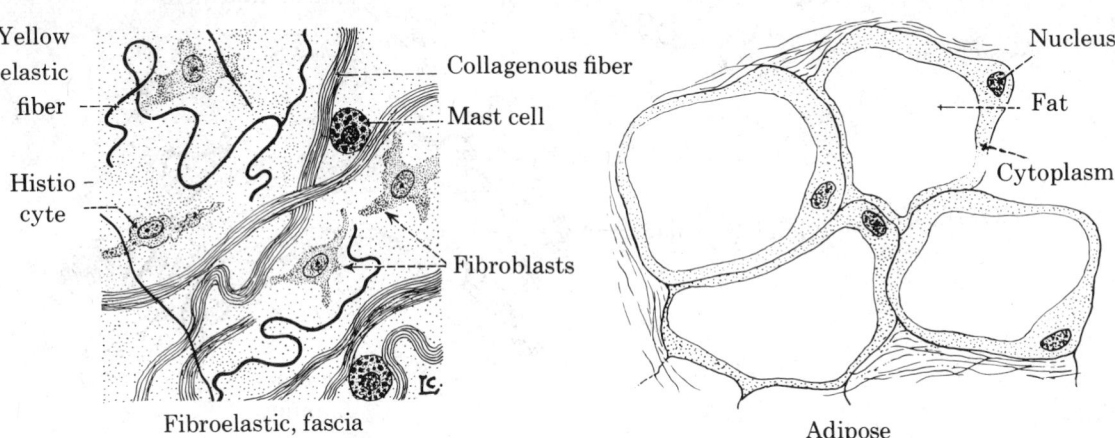

Yellow elastic fiber

Collagenous fiber

Mast cell

Histiocyte

Fibroblasts

Fibroelastic, fascia

Nucleus

Fat

Cytoplasm

Adipose

VARIOUS TYPES OF EPITHELIAL CELL

(King and Showers)

Plate XII

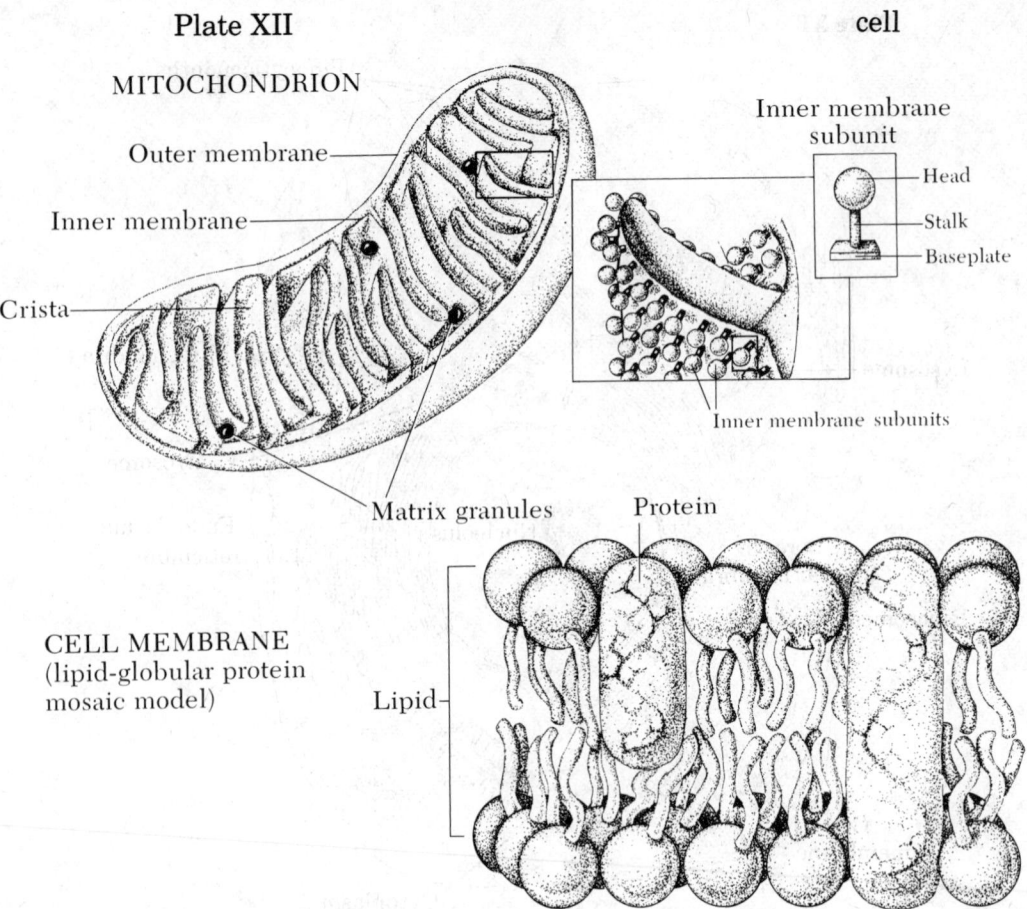

MITOCHONDRION

Outer membrane

Inner membrane

Crista

Matrix granules

Inner membrane subunit

Head

Stalk

Baseplate

Inner membrane subunits

Protein

CELL MEMBRANE
(lipid-globular protein
mosaic model)

Lipid

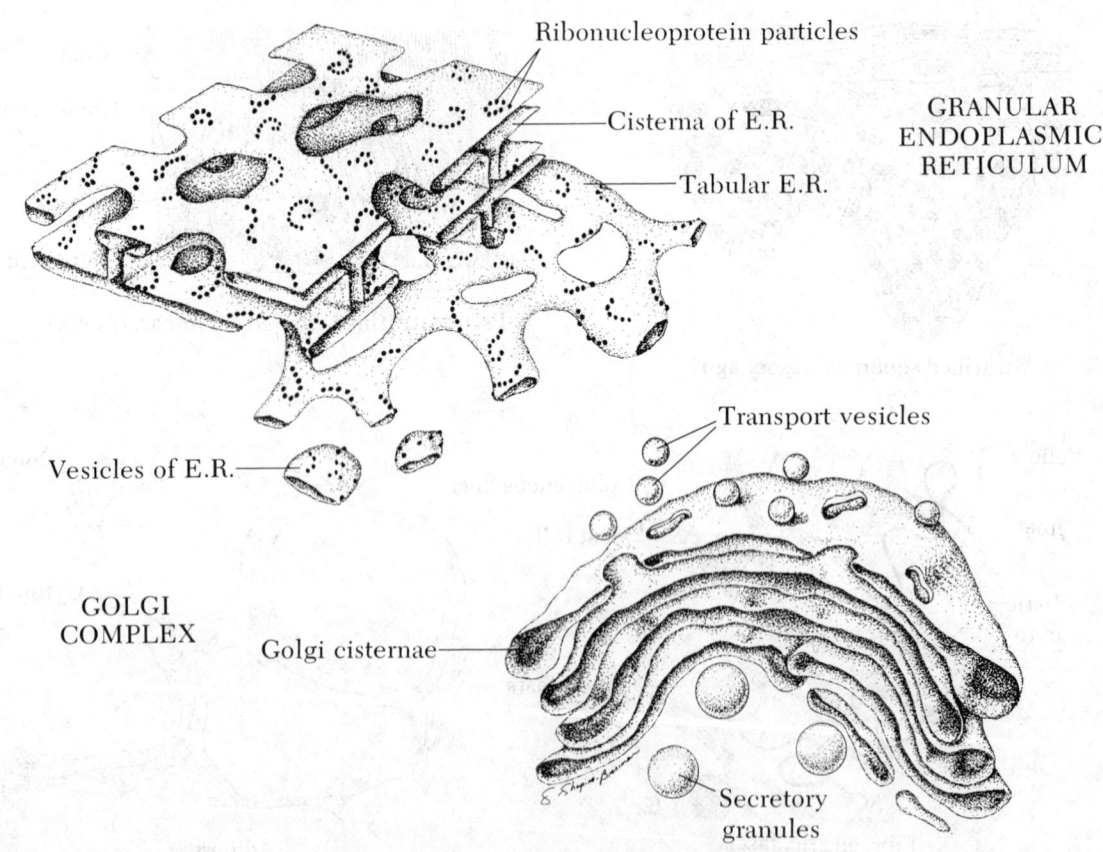

Ribonucleoprotein particles

Cisterna of E.R.

Tabular E.R.

GRANULAR
ENDOPLASMIC
RETICULUM

Vesicles of E.R.

Transport vesicles

GOLGI
COMPLEX

Golgi cisternae

Secretory
granules

CELL ORGANELLES AND CELL MEMBRANE

Gegenbaur's c., osteoblast. **germ c's,** the cells of an organism whose function it is to reproduce the kind, i.e., an ovum or spermatozoon, or an immature stage of either, called also *initial c's* and *sexual c's.* **germ c., primordial,** the earliest recognizable precursor in the embryo of an ovum or spermatozoon. **germinal c.,** a cell capable of dividing and differentiating. **ghost c.,** one that appears only as a shadowy outline; called also *shadow c.* **c's of Giannuzzi,** see under *crescent.* **giant c.,** 1. any very large cell, such as the megakaryocyte of bone marrow. 2. any of the very large, multinucleate, modified macrophages, which may be formed by coalescence of epithelioid cells or by nuclear division without cytoplasmic division of monocytes, e.g., those characteristic of granulomatous inflammation (*Langhans' giant c's*) and those that form around large foreign bodies (*foreign body giant c's*). **giant pyramidal c's,** Betz's c's. **Gierke's c's,** small, deeply staining nerve cells that constitute the chief cells of the substantia gelatinosa. **gitter c.,** microglia. **Gley's c's,** large glandular cells in the interstitial tissue of the testicle. **glia c.,** a cell of the neuroglia. **glitter c's,** polymorphonuclear leukocytes that stain a pale blue with gentian-violet-safranin and contain granules in the cytoplasm that exhibit brownian movement; their presence in urine may indicate pyelonephritis. **glomus c's,** the specific cells (type I) of the carotid body, which contain many dense-cored vesicles, and occur in clusters surrounded by other cells that have no cytoplasmic granules (type II). **goblet c.,** a unicellular mucous gland found in the epithelium of various mucous membranes, especially that of the respiratory passages and intestines. Droplets of mucigen collect in the upper part of the cell and distend it, while the basal end remains slender, and the cell assumes the shape of a goblet. Called also *beaker c.,caliciform c.,* and *chalice c.* See also *ptyocrinous.* **Golgi's c's,** see under *neuron.* **gonadotropic c.,** gonadotrope, def. 3. **Goormaghtigh c's,** juxtaglomerular c's. **granular c.,** the name applied to a keratinocyte in the stratum granulosum of the epidermis, when it has become flattened and rhomboidal in shape and contains a dense collection of variously sized darkly staining granules, before it dies and desquamates. **granule c's,** diminutive cells found in the granular layers of the cerebral and cerebellar cortices. **granulosa c's,** cells surrounding the vesicular ovarian follicle and forming the stratum granulosum and cumulus oophorus; after ovulation they are transformed to lutein cells. **granulosa-lutein c's,** lutien cells of the corpus luteum derived from granulosa cells. **grape c.,** berry c. **gravity c.,** an electromotive force cell like the Sieman and Halske, but the fluids are superimposed upon each other with no intervening diaphragm, being kept partly separate by the force of gravity; called also *Hill's c.* **Grenet c.,** an electromotive force cell with a carbon-collecting plate, the fluid and depolarizer being a solution of potassium dichromate; called also *bichromate c.* or *dichromate c.* **Grove c.,** a two-fluid galvanic cell charged with dilute sulfuric and nitric acids, employing zinc and platinum electrodes. **gustatory c's,** the taste cells. **gyrochrome c.,** see *gyrochrome.* **hair c's,** neuroepithelial cells with hairlike processes (kinocilia or stereocilia, or both) found in the organ of Corti, ampullar crest, and utricle and saccule of the inner ear; the hair cells receive afferent and efferent fibers of the cochlear nerve (organ of Corti) or the vestibular nerve. **hairy c.,** any of the abnormal large cells found in the blood in leukemic reticuloendotheliosis, having a round or oval nucleus, gray-blue cytoplasm, moderately clumped nuclear chromatin, small or not visible nucleoli, and numerous irregular cytoplasmic villi that give the cell a flagellated or hairy appearance. Called also *tricholeukocyte.* **Hammar's myoid c's,** myoid c's (def. 2). **Hargraves' c.,** LE c. **heart-disease c's, heart-failure c's, heart-lesion c's,** macrophages containing granules of iron, found in the pulmonary alveoli and sputum in congestive heart failure. **hecatomeral c's,** cells of gray matter of the spinal cord whose axis cylinder processes divide and send one branch into the white substance of the same side of the cord and another into the anterolateral columns of the other side. **heckle c.,** prickle c. **Heidenhain's c's,** the chief cells and *parietal cells* of the gastric glands. **HeLa c's,** cells of the first continuously cultured carcinoma strain, descended from a human cervical carcinoma; used in the study of life processes, including viruses, at the cell level. **helmet c.,** an abnormal red cell form resembling a helmet, seen in hemolytic anemia. **helper c.,** a subtype of T-lymphocytes which cooperate with B-lymphocytes for the synthesis of antibody to many antigens; these cells play an integral role in immunoregulation. **Henle's c's** (*obs.*), large granular nucleated cells in the seminiferous tubules. **Hensen's c's,** tall supporting cells arranged in rows adjacent to the last row of outer phalangeal cells, constituting the outer border of the organ of Corti. **hepatic c's,** the polyhedral epithelial cells that constitute the substance of an acinus of the liver; called also *liver c's.* **heteromeral c's,** nerve cells of the gray matter of the spinal cord whose axon processes pass to the white matter of the opposite side; called also *commissural c's.* **Hill's c.,** gravity c. **hilus c's,** groups of large epitheloid cells closely associated with vascular spaces and unmyelinated nerve fibers in the hilus of the ovary and the adjacent mesovarium; they seem to be histologically and functionally related to the Leydig cells of the testis. **Hodgkin's c's,** Reed-Sternberg c's. **Hofbauer c's,** large chromophilic cells in the chorionic villi that are probably macrophages. **horizontal c's,** neurons whose axons run horizontally for long distances in the outer plexiform layer of the retina; their dendrites synapse at various points with the rods and cones. There are two physiologic classes: *luminosity horizontal cells* respond to illumination of the photoreceptors by hyperpolarization; *chromaticity horizontal cells* may hyperpolarize or depolarize, depending on the wavelength of the light stimulus. **horn c's,** 1. epithelial cells that have lost their protoplasm, have sharp edges, and look horny. 2. any ganglion cell of the horns of the spinal cord. **Hortega c.,** microglia. **Hürthle c's,** large eosinophilic cells sometimes found in the thyroid gland; they seem to be parathyroid rests included by chance in thyroid tissue. See also *Hürthle cell tumor,* under *tumor.* **hyperchromatic c.,** one that stains more intensely than is typical of its cell type. **I-c.,** see mucolipidosis II. **immunologically competent c.,** immunocyte. **incasing c's,** a single layer of fusiform cells around the gustatory cells of the tongue. **indifferent c.,** a cell that has no characteristic structure, or that is not an essential part of the tissue in which it is found. **inflammatory c.,** a cell (neutrophil, macrophage, etc.) participating in the inflammatory response to a foreign substance. **initial c's,** germ c's. **integrator c.,** interneuron. **intercalary c's,** dark, rodlike structures between the other (secretory and nonsecretory) cells of the endosalpinx, which may be emptied secretory cells; called also *peg c's.* **intercapillary c's,** mesangial c's. **interdental c's,** cells found in the spiral limbus between the dentes acustici, which secrete the tectorial membrane of the cochlear duct. **interfollicular c's,** Hürthle c's. **interstitial c's,** 1. Leydig's c's. 2. masses of large epithelioid, lipid-containing cells in the ovarian stroma, believed to have a secretory function, derived from the theca interna of atretic ovarian follicles, and thus, in humans, more numerous during the first year of life when atresia is commonest. In women, they are either absent or poorly represented, but in some lower mammals, especially rodents, they are more prominent; see also *interstitial gland* (def. 2), under *gland.* 3. cells with elongated nuclei and long cytoplasmic processes, found in the perivascular areas and between the cords of pinealocytes in the pineal body, and regarded by some to be glial elements. 4. nerve cells with finely vacuolated protoplasm and short, branching processes that interlace with other processes to form an irregular feltwork in the enteric plexuses, submucosa, and interior of the villi of the intestinal tract. 5. fat-storing c's of liver. **islet c's,** cells composing the islets of Langerhans; see *islets of Langerhans.* **juvenile c.,** Schilling's name for a polymorphonuclear leukocyte in which the nuclear element is a single fragment no longer containing a definite nucleolus; called also *young form* and *metamyelocyte.* **juxtaglomerular c's,** specialized cells containing secretory granules, located in the tunica media of the afferent glomerular arterioles; they are receptors thought to stimulate secretion of the adrenal hormone aldosterone and to play a major role in renal autoregulation. Called also *apparatus of Goormaghtigh, Goormaghtigh c's, juxtaglomerular apparatus, sentinel c's, periarterial pad,* and *polkissen.* **K c's,** killer c's. **karyochrome c's,** cells of the chromatophil substance of neurons that contain much chromatin in the nucleus and a small amount of cytoplasm. **killer c's,** cells that are morphologically indistinguishable from small lymphocytes but which have cytotoxic activity against target cells coated with specific IgG antibody. They destroy foreign cells either by attacking them directly or by releasing nonspecific toxins. Killer cells have Fc receptors on their surfaces which combine with the Fc regions of IgG molecules bound through their Fab regions to cell surfaces. By this mechanism they bring about antibody-dependent cell-mediated cytotoxicity (ADCC), which can be measured *in vitro* by the release of ^{51}Cr from target cells. Called also *K c's* and *killer lymphocytes.* **Kulchitsky's c's,** argentaffin cells situated between the cells that line the glands of Lieberkühn of the intestine. **Kupffer's c's,** large star-shaped or pyramidal cells with a large oval nucleus and a small prominent nucleolus. These intensely phagocytic cells line the walls of the sinusoids of the liver and form a part of the reticuloendothelial system (q.v.). Called also *stellate c's of liver* and *von Kupffer's c's.* **L c's,** 1. cells from a strain (C3H) of mouse fibroblasts grown in tissue culture for many years; employed for their ability to support replication of many types of viruses. 2. argyrophilic basal granular cells with large cytoplasmic granules in the mucosa of the upper intestine; because of the resemblance of their ultrastructure to that of the alpha cells of the islets of Langerhans, they are believed by some to synthesize and secrete a glucagon-like hyperglycemic substance, enteroglucagon; called also *large granule c's.* **lacrimoethmoid c's,** the ethmoid cells situated under the lacrimal bone. **lactotropic c.,** mammotrope. **lacunar c.,** a variant of the Reed-Sternberg cell, typically having a single nucleus surrounded by an ample, pale-staining cytoplasm enclosed in a sharply defined cell membrane; it is primarily associated with nodular sclerosing Hodgkin's disease. **Langerhans' c's,** 1. dendritic clear cells of the granular layer of the epidermis that resemble melanocytes but lack tyrosinase. 2. irregular wandering cells in the intercellular spaces of the cornea. Called also *Langerhans' stellate corpuscles.* **Langhans' c's,** 1. polyhedral epithelial cells constituting cytotrophoblast (Langhans' layer). 2. Langhan's giant c's.

Langhans' giant c's, giant cells, resembling foreign body giant cells, having their nuclei arranged in a complete circle or in a horseshoe-shaped pattern at the periphery of the cells, characteristically seen in granulomatous inflammations, as occur in tuberculosis, syphilis, sarcoidosis, and deep fungal infections. **large granule c's,** L c's (def. 2). **LE c.,** a mature neutrophilic polymorphonuclear leukocyte, which has phagocytized a spherical, homogeneous-appearing inclusion, itself derived from another neutrophil; a characteristic of lupus erythematosus, but also found in analogous disorders of connective tissue. Called also *Hargraves' c.* **Leclanché c.,** an electromotive force cell employing a zinc cathode and an inert carbon anode and, as an electrolyte, a paste containing diamminedichlorozinc, ammonium chloride, manganese dioxide, and dimanganese trioxide monohydrate; the manganese dioxide acts as the depolarizer at the carbon anode. **Leishman's chrome c's,** basophil granular leukocytes occurring in black-water fever. **lepra c.,** a histiocyte in a leprous nodule that has been converted by the action of lepra bacilli into a sac containing degenerated protoplasm and bacilli; called also *Virchow's c.* **Leydig's c's,** 1. clusters of epithelioid cells constituting the endocrine tissue of the testis, which elaborate androgens, chiefly testosterone; called also *interstitial c's* or *interstitial c's of Leydig,* and *interstitial glands.* 2. mucous cells that do not pour their secretion out over the surface of the epithelium. **light c's,** parafollicular c's. **littoral c's,** flattened cells lining the walls of lymph or blood sinuses. **liver c's,** hepatic c's. **Loevit c.** (*obs.*), erythroblast. **longiradiate c's,** neuroglial cells having long prolongations. **luteal c's, lutein c's,** the plump, pale-staining, polyhedral cells of the corpus luteum; they include the granulosa lutein cells and the theca lutein cells. **lymph c.,** lymphocyte. **lymphadenoma c's,** Reed-Sternberg c's. **lymphoid c.,** cells of the immune system that react specifically with antigen and elaborate specific cell products; they comprise the lymphocytes and plasma cells. **malpighian c.,** keratinocyte. **Marchand's c.,** adventitial c. **marginal c's,** crescents of Giannuzzi. **Marié-Davy c.,** an electromotive force cell with a carbon collecting plate, the fluid, depolarizer, and amalgamator being a paste of mercuric or mercurous sulfate and water. **marrow c.,** any one of the immature blood cells that develop in the bone marrow; called also *myeloid c.* **Martinotti's c's,** fusiform cells with ascending axon processes in the polymorphic layer of the cerebral cortex. **mast c.,** a connective tissue cell whose specific physiologic function remains unknown; capable of elaborating basophilic, metachromatic cytoplasmic granules that contain histamine, heparin, and, in certain species, such as the rat and mouse, serotonin; called also *mastocyte* and *labrocyte.* **mastoid c's,** cellulae mastoideae. **matrix c's,** flat cells found in the lobules of sebaceous glands; they undergo a rather abrupt transformation into the pale, foamy-looking, fat-containing cells of the alveoli. **Mauthner's c.,** a large cell in the metencephalon of fishes and amphibians that gives rise to Mauthner's fiber. **megaspore mother c.,** any of the diploid cells developed in the megasporangium of plants which divide by meiosis to produce four haploid daughter cells (megaspores), usually only one of which survives to become a megagametophyte, or female gametophyte. **memory c's,** T-lymphocytes; see under *lymphocyte.* **Merkel's c's, Merkel-Ranvier c's,** 1. clear cells in the basal layer of the epidermis that contain catecholamine granules and resemble melanocytes. 2. menisci tactus. **Merkel tactile c.,** menisci tactus. **mesangial c's,** cells found in the mesangium, the connective tissue stalk in the glomerular capsule of the kidney. **mesenchymal c's,** the pluripotential cells constituting the mesenchymae. **mesothelial c's,** flattened epithelial cells of mesenchymal origin that line the serous cavities. **metallophil c's,** cells in which the cytoplasm has a great affinity for metal salts; these are cells of the reticuloendothelial system, and also a series of related cells that are not selectively stained by vital staining. **Meynert's c's,** solitary pyramidal cells in the cerebral cortex about the calcarine fissure. **microspore mother c.,** any of the diploid cells with large nuclei developed in the microsporangium of plants which divide by meiosis to produce four haploid microspores. **migratory c's,** ameboid cells found in blood and tissue spaces. See also *wandering c.* **Mikulicz's c's,** the cells in rhinoscleroma that contain the bacillus of the disease; called also *foam c's.* **mitral c's,** the pyramidal cells forming one of the layers of the olfactory bulb. **Mooser c.,** a large mononuclear (serosal) cell with numerous rickettsiae in the cytoplasm, observed in inflammatory exudate in murine typhus; called also *Neill-Mooser bodies.* **morular c.,** berry c. **mossy c's,** 1. protoplasmic astrocyte. 2. any of the cells of the oligodendroglia or of the microglia. **mother c.,** a cell that divides so as to form new or daughter cells; called also *brood c.* and *parent c.* **motor c.,** an efferent neuron, especially one of the cells of the spinal cord that has its axon continued into a motor nerve fiber. **Mott c.,** a plasma cell in which Russell bodies have formed in scleroma. **mouth c's,** squamous cells detached from the epithelium lining the oropharynx, found in the sputum. **mucoalbuminous c's, mucoserous c's,** trophochrome c's. **mucous c's,** cells that secrete mucus or mucin. **mucous neck c's,** cells found in the necks of gastric glands; they fill the spaces between the parietal cells and are filled with

pale transparent granules. **mulberry c.,** 1. a vacuolated plasma cell; see also *berry c.* 2. a rounded cell, with centrally placed nuclei and coarse cytoplasmic vacuoles near the outer border, developing at the periphery of a retrogressing corpus luteum. **c's of Müller,** see under *fiber.* **muscle c.,** any contractile cell peculiar to muscle. Smooth muscle cells are elongated spindle-shaped cells containing a single nucleus and longitudinally arranged myofibrils. For cardiac and skeletal muscle cells, see *muscle fiber,* under *fiber.* **myeloid c.,** marrow c. **myeloma c.,** a cell found in bone marrow and occasionally in peripheral blood of patients with multiple myeloma. In the more anaplastic forms, the cell is large, has abundant blue-staining cytoplasm with no perinuclear pallor, and has one or more moderately large and vesicular nuclei that may be centrally or eccentrically placed and may contain nucleoli. In better differentiated tumors, the cell is smaller and, except for the finer chromatic structure, greatly resembles a plasmacyte. **myoepithelial c's,** smooth muscle cells of epithelial origin occurring in certain glands such as the mammary gland, glands of the skin, glands of the eyelid, and salivary glands, which provide a contractile mechanism that may serve to narrow and empty the ducts; called also *basket c's.* **myoepithelioid c's,** juxtaglomerular c's; so called because they appear to be highly modified smooth muscle cells. **myoid c's,** 1. cells found in the seminiferous tubules of common laboratory rodents, which cytologically resemble smooth muscle and are presumed to be contractile and to be responsible for the rhythmic shallow contractions of the seminiferous tubules of these species; called also *peritubular contractile c's.* 2. striated muscles cells found in the thymus of nonmammalian vertebrates, especially reptiles and birds, and rarely in mammals; called also *Hammar's myoid c's.* **myointimal c.,** a smooth muscle cell occurring in the intima of an artery. **Nageotte's c's,** cells of the cerebrospinal fluid that become greatly increased in number in disease. **nerve c.,** a neuron, with its processes, collaterals, and terminations, regarded as a structural unit of the nervous system. See *neuron.* **Neumann's c's** (*obs.*), nucleated red cells in the bone marrow developing into erythrocytes. **neuroepithelial c's,** neuroglial c's. **neuroglia c's, neuroglial c's,** the cells of the supportive tissue of the central nervous system (neuroglia); these non-neural cells are of three kinds: astrocytes (macroglia), oligodendrocytes, and microglia. Called also *Deiters' c's* and *neuroepithelial c's.* See Plate accompanying *nerve.* **neuromuscular c.,** a form of cell chiefly or always seen in the lower animals, of which the outer part receives stimuli and the inner part is contractile. **neutrophilic c.,** a cell, particularly a leukocyte, stainable by neutral dyes; called also *neutrophil.* **nevus c.,** a small oval or cuboidal cell with a deeply staining nucleus and scanty pale cytoplasm, sometimes containing melanin granules, possibly derived from Schwann cells or from embryonal nevoblasts. Nevus cells are clustered in rounded masses (called *theques*) in the epidermis, and reach the dermis by a kind of centripetal extrusion (*abtropfung*). **niche c.,** septal c. **Niemann-Pick c's,** round, oval, or polyhedral cells present in the bone marrow and spleen in Niemann-Pick disease; they have foamy, lipid-containing cytoplasm, in the form of sphingomyelin, which gives a positive reaction with Sudan III and other fat stains. Called also *Pick's c's.* **NK c's,** natural killer cells; cells capable of mediating cytotoxic reactions without themselves being specifically sensitized against the target. **noble c's,** the differentiated cells of the organs and tissues of the body. **normal c.,** any cell found naturally in any part or organ free from disease. **nucleated c.,** any cell having a nucleus. **nucleated red c., nucleated red blood c.,** any of the immature forms of a red blood cell, as a normoblast. **null c's,** lymphocytes that lack the surface antigens characteristic of B- and T-lymphocytes. Such cells are seen in active systemic lupus erythematosus and other disease states. Called also *null lymphocytes.* **nurse c's, nursing c's,** Sertoli's c's. **oat c's, oat-shaped c's,** cells shaped like oat grains, seen in some kinds of carcinoma; also a characteristic of erythrocytes in sickle cell anemia. **olfactory c's,** a set of specialized and nucleated fusiform cells of the mucous membrane of the nose embedded among the epithelial cells; called also *Schultze's c's.* **osseous c.,** a bone cell. **osteoprogenitor c's,** relatively undifferentiated cells found on or near all of the free surfaces of bone, which, under certain circumstances, undergo division and transform into osteoblasts or coalesce to give rise to osteoclasts. **owl's eye c's,** desquamated renal epithelial cells. **oxyntic c's,** parietal c's. **oxyphil c's, oxyphilic c's,** acidophilic cells found, along with the more numerous chief cells, in the parathyroid glands; they increase in number with age, have small dark nuclei and abundant finely granular cytoplasm, and are larger and have many more mitochondria than the chief cells. **packed human blood c's** [USP], **packed red blood c's (human),** whole blood from which plasma has been removed; used therapeutically in blood transfusions. **Paget's c's,** degenerating cells, swollen, rounded, and pigmented, found in the epidermis in Paget's disease of the nipple and in extramammary Paget's disease. **palatine c's,** those parts of ethmoid cells that are extended into the palatine bone. **palisade c's** a compact layer of cylindrical chloroplast-bearing cells located in the mesophyll layer of a leaf, and so arranged that their long axes are at right angles to the epidermal surface of the leaf. **Paneth's c's,** narrow, pyramidal, or columnar epithelial cells with a round or oval nucleus close to the base of the cell, occurring in the fundus of the crypts of Lieberkühn; they contain large secretory granules that may contain peptidase. Called also *Davidoff's c's.* **para-follicular c's,** ovoid cells with an irregular nucleus and many brown or black cytoplasmic granules, which are located along with the principal cells of the thyroid follicles, in the follicular epithelium and interfollicular spaces, and which elaborate the polypeptide hormone calcitonin. They arise during embryonic life from the fifth pharyngeal pouches and are incorporated in the thyroid gland in mammals, but form discrete epithelial cell masses (*ultimobranchial bodies*) in submammalian vertebrates. Called also *C c's* and *light c's.* **paraluteal c's, paralutein c's,** theca-lutein c's. **parenchymal hepatic c's, parenchymal liver c's,** hepatic c's. **parent c.,** mother c. **parietal c's,** large spheroidal or pyramidal cells that are the source of gastric hydrochloric acid and are the site of intrinsic factor production; they are found scattered along the walls of the gastric glands, with their tapered ends pushed between the chief cells. Called also *acid c's, border c's, Heidenhain's c's, oxyntic c's,* and *delomorphous c's.* **pathologic c.,** any cell that results from a disease process or that belongs to or arises from a pathogenic microorganism. **pavement c's,** the flat cells composing pavement epithelium. **pediculated c's,** neuroglial cells that possess a pedicle implanted into a capillary wall. **peg c's,** intercalary c's. **peptic c's,** a name sometimes given to the chief cells of the stomach. **pericapillary c's,** perithelium. **pericellular c's,** neuroglial cells that surround a neuron. **perithelial c.,** adventitial c. **peritubular contractile c's,** myoid c's, def. 1. **perivascular c's,** cells accumulated around the outside of small blood vessels. **pessary c.,** a markedly hypochromic erythrocyte in which the hemoglobin is present merely as a narrow circumferential rim. **phalangeal c's,** elongated supporting cells of the organ of Corti with bases that rest on the basilar membrane adjacent to the pillar cells; the *inner* ones are arranged in a row on the inner surface of the inner pillar cells and surround the inner hair cells; the *outer* ones (*c's of Deiters*) support the outer hair cells. **pheochrome c's,** cells of the medulla of the adrenal gland that stain dark with chromium salts. **photoautotrophic c's,** green plant cells. **photoreceptor c's,** visual c's. **physaliferous c's,** spheroidal nucleated cells, containing glycogen or mucin, characteristic of chordoma. **Pick's c's,** Niemann-Pick c's. **pigment c.,** any cell containing pigment granules. **pillar c's,** elongated supporting cells in a double row (*inner* and *outer pillar c's*) in the organ of Corti, having their heads joined and their bases resting on the basilar membrane widely separated so as to form a tunnel (*inner tunnel* or *canal of Corti*) that extends the length of the cochlea. Called also *Corti's rods.* **pineal c.,** pinealocyte. **plasma c.,** a spherical or ellipsoidal cell, with a single, eccentrically placed nucleus containing clumped chromatin, an area of perinuclear clearing (hof), and generally abundant, sometimes vacuolated cytoplasm; plasma cells result from differentiation of sensitized small B-lymphocytes, and are the most active of any cell type in secreting antibody. See also *plasmacytic series,* under *series.* **pneumatic c's,** the cell-like structures of the petrous bone. **polar c's,** polar bodies, def. 1. **polychromatic c's, polychromatophil c's,** immature erythrocytes staining with both acid and basic stains so that their color is a diffuse mixture of blue-gray and pink. **polyhedral c's,** cells having a polyhedral shape. **polyplastic c.,** a cell made up of various structural elements; also one that passes through various modifications of form. **pre-B c's,** lymphoid cells that are immature and contain cytoplasmic IgM; they develop into B-lymphocytes. **prefollicle c's,** cells encapsulating the germ cells in the fetal ovary. **pregnancy c.,** altered chromophobe cell observed in the anterior pituitary in pregnant women. **prickle c.,** a cell with delicate radiating processes that connect with similar cells; the name applied to one of the dividing keratinocytes present in the stratum germinativum of the epidermis. Called also *heckel c.* **primary c.,** an irreversible (non-rechargeable) electromotive force cell, e.g., the Leclanché cell. **primitive granulosa c's,** prefollicle c's. **primitive wandering c.,** a small mononuclear cell of the embryo that arises from the mesoderm and subsequently by differentiation gives rise to wandering cells of the body (Saxer, Maximow). **primordial germ c's,** the earliest germ cells, originating extragonadally but migrating early in embryonic development. **principal c's,** 1. chief c's, def. 3. 2. the fundamental cells of an organ, which usually have a specific function. **prokaryotic c.,** a cell without a true nucleus; see *prokaryote.* **prolactin c.,** mammotrope. **prop c's,** Purkinje c's. **psychic c's,** the cells of the cerebral cortex. **pulmonary epithelial c's,** extremely thin nonphagocytic squamous cells with flattened nuclei, constituting the outer layer of the aveolar wall in the lungs. **pulpar c's,** the typical cells of the spleen substance. **Purkinje's c's,** large branching neurons in the middle layer of the cortex cerebelli; called also *prop c's* and *Purkinje's corpuscles.* **pyramidal c.,** one of the large multipolar pyramid-shaped ganglion cells of the cerebral cortex which, with their attached fibers, constitute the pyramidal neurons. **radial c's of Müller,** Müller's fibers. **red c., red blood**

c., one of the elements of the peripheral blood, an erythrocyte. Normally, in humans, the mature form is a non-nucleated, yellowish, biconcave disk, adapted, by virtue of its configuration and its hemoglobin content, to transport oxygen. **Reed c's, Reed-Sternberg c's,** giant histiocytic cells, typically multinucleate, most often binucleate with the two halves of the cell appearing as mirror-images of each other; the nuclei are enclosed in abundant amphophilic cytoplasm and contain prominent nucleoli. The presence of the cells is the common histiologic characteristic of Hodgkin's disease. A variant form is the lacunar cell (q.v.). Called also *Dorothy Reed's c's, Reed's c's, Sternberg-Reed c's, Hodgkin's c's, Sternberg's giant c's,* and *lymphadenoma c's.* **Renshaw c's,** interneurons in the ventromedial region of the ventral horn that make inhibitory connections with the motoneurons. **reserve c's,** cells of the basal or germinal layer of the bronchial epithelium. **residential c.,** a cell that does not wander, especially one of the cells of the substantia propria of the cornea. **resting c.,** a cell that is not undergoing karyokinesis. **resting wandering c.,** a fixed macrophage. **reticular c's,** the cells forming the reticular fibers of connective tissue; those forming the framework of lymph nodes, bone marrow, and spleen are part of the reticuloendothelial system and under appropriate stimulation may differentiate into macrophages. **reticuloendothelial c.,** see *reticuloendothelial system,* under *system.* **reticulum c.,** reticular c. **rhagiocrine c.,** macrophage. **Rieder's c.,** a myeloblast observed in acute leukemia, having a nucleus with several wide and deep indentations suggesting lobulation, which may represent asynchronism of nuclear and cytoplasmic maturation. **Rindfleisch's c's** (*obs.*), eosinophils. **rod c's,** 1. retinal rods. 2. microglia as observed in chronic diseases of the cerebral cortex and in dementia paralytica, in which the cells are markedly attenuated in form, their processes being confined mainly to the two extremities. 3. littoral c's. **Rohon-Beard c's,** giant ganglion cells in the spinal cord of some vertebrates. **Rolando's c's,** the ganglion cells of Rolando's gelatinous substance. **root c's,** cells of the nerve roots. **Rouget's c's,** contractile cells found upon the walls of capillaries; see *pericyte.* **round c.,** any cell having a spherical shape, especially a lymphocyte. **S c's,** 1. mucoid cells of the adenohypophysis that contain a cysteine-rich protein. 2. basal granular cells found predominantly in the duodenum, which have cytoplasmic granules and which may be the source of secretin production; called also *small granule c's.* **Sala's c's,** star-shaped cells of connective tissue in the fibers that form the sensory nerve endings situated in the pericardium. **sarcogenic c's,** the cells that are developed into muscle fiber. **satellite c's,** 1. neurilemmal elements encapsulating a ganglion cell. 2. free nuclei that accumulate around cells in certain diseases. 3. elongated cells that are closely associated with a muscle fiber; they are either flattened against the fiber or occupy shallow depressions in its surface. **scavenger c.,** a cell which absorbs and removes irritant products. **Schultze's c's,** olfactory c's. **Schwann's c.,** any of the large nucleated cells whose cell membrane spirally enwraps the axons of myelinated peripheral neurons and is the source of myelin; a single Schwann cell supplies the myelin sheath between two nodes of Ranvier. **sclerenchyma c's,** thick-walled, lignified, usually dead cells, which compose the sclerenchyma of plants. Cf. *collenchyma c's.* **segmented c.,** a mature granulocyte in which the nucleus is divided into definite lobes joined by a filamentous connection, as distinguished from a band cell. **seminal c's,** epithelial cells within the tubuli seminiferi. **seminoma c.,** a large, round to polygonal cell having a round, moderately large nucleus with clumped chromatin in the center of clear abundant cytoplasm and one or more nucleoli, occurring in fairly well-differentiated sheets or cords in classical seminoma of the testis. **sensory c.,** one of the neurons of the peripheral sense organs. **sentinel c's,** juxtaglomerular c's. **septal c.,** a name applied to alveolar cells occupying angular niches in the alveolar walls. **serous c.,** a cell concerned in the secretion of a watery fluid rich in protein, like the secretory cells of the parotid gland; called also *albuminous c.* **Sertoli's c's,** elongated cells in the tubules of the testes to which the spermatids become attached; they provide support, protection, and, apparently, nutrition until the spermatids become transformed into mature spermatozoa; called also *sustentacular c's, nurse* or *nursing c's, foot c's,* and *trophocytes.* **sexual c's,** germ c's. **Sézary c.,** a reticular lymphocyte characterized by a large convoluted or folded nucleus with a narrow rim of cytoplasm that may contain vacuoles; seen in many proliferative states of the reticuloendothelial system, and massively present in the skin and blood in the Sézary syndrome. **shadow c.,** ghost c. **sickle c.,** an erythrocyte shaped like a sickle or crescent, the abnormal shape caused by the presence of varying proportions of hemoglobin S; see *sickle cell anemia,* under *anemia.* **Siemens and Halske c.,** a battery cell with a copper anode and an anode electrolyte of aqueous copper sulfate that is separated from the anode compartment by a porous diaphragm with a papier-mâche packing. **signet-ring c.,** one in which the nucleus has been pressed to one side by an accumulation of intracytoplasmic mucin; see *Krukenberg's tumor* under *tumor.* **silver c's,** argentaffin c's. **skeletogenous c.,** an osteoblast. **small granule c's,** S c's, def. 2. **Smee c.,** an electromotive force cell consisting of a plate of zinc and one of platinized silver in a dilute solution of sulfuric acid. **smudge c's,** a name applied to disrupted leukocytes appearing during the course of preparation of peripheral blood smears. **Snell c.,** a one-fluid electromotive force cell having a collecting plate of platinized silver; its fluid is dilute sulfuric acid. **somatic c's,** the cells of the somatoplasm; undifferentiated body cells. **somatotropic c.,** somatotrope. **sperm c.,** a spermatozoon. **spermatogenic c's,** cells that produce sperm; called also *androgones.* **spermatogonial c.,** spermatogonium. **sphenoid c's,** the two large cavities or sinuses of the sphenoid bone; see *sinus sphenoidalis.* **spider c.,** 1. an astrocyte, especially a fibrous astrocyte. 2. a cell occurring in rhabdomyosarcoma; its nucleus, with a narrow rim of cytoplasm, is located in what appears to be a large vacuole, with thread-like processes radiating to the outer cell wall. **spindle c.,** a spindle-shaped cell; called also *fusiform c.* **spur c.,** a form of spiculed mature red blood cell, whose prototype is the acanthocyte of congenital abetalipoproteinemia, characterized by five to ten spiny projections of varying length distributed irregularly over the cell surface. **squamous c.,** a flat, scalelike epithelial cell. **stab c.,** band c. **staff c.,** band c. **star c's,** cells with large vacuoles in their cytoplasm and cytoplasmic bridges; seen in ameloblastoma. **stave c's,** littoral c's. **stellate c.,** any star-shaped cell, such as a Kupffer cell or astrocyte, having a large number of filaments extending from it in all directions. **stellate c's of liver,** Kupffer's c's. **stem c.,** a generalized mother cell whose descendants specialize, often in different directions, such as an undifferentiated mesenchymal cell which may be considered to be a progenitor of the blood and fixed-tissue cells of the bone marrow. **Sternberg's giant c's,** Reed-Sternberg c's. **Sternberg-Reed c's,** Reed-Sternberg c's. **stipple c.,** a red blood cell containing granules of varying size and shape, taking a basic or bluish stain with Wright's stain, as in punctate basophilia. **supporting c's,** cells that serve to provide support and protection and perhaps contribute to the nutrition of principal or other cells of certain organs; such cells are found in the labyrinth of the inner ear, organ of Corti, olfactory epithelium, taste buds, and seminiferous tubules (Sertoli's cells). Called also *sustentacular c's.* **suppressor c's,** lymphoid cells, especially T-lymphocytes, that inhibit humoral and cell-mediated immune responses to antigen. These cells play an integral role in immunoregulation and are believed to be operative in various autoimmune and other immunological disease states. **sustentacular c's,** supporting c's. **sympathicotrophic c's,** large epithelioid cells occurring in groups and connected with bundles of nonmyelinated nerve fibers in the hilus of the ovary. **sympathochromaffin c's,** small round cells in the fetal suprarenal gland, the forerunners of the sympathetic and medullary cells. **syncytial c.,** a cell whose cytoplasm is confluent with that of an adjacent cell. **synovial c's,** fibroblasts lying between the cartilaginous fibers in the synovial membrane of joints. **T c's,** T-lymphocytes; see under *lymphocyte.* **tactile c.,** corpuscula tactus. **tadpole c's,** cells with an elongated cytoplasmic tail. **target c.,** 1. an abnormally thin erythrocyte which, when stained, shows a dark center and a peripheral ring of hemoglobin, separated by a pale unstained ring containing less hemoglobin, as seen in certain congenital and acquired anemias, thalassemia, certain hemoglobinopathies, liver disease, especially obstructive jaundice, and other disorders, and the postsplenectomy state. Called also *target,* or *"Mexican hat," erythrocyte.* 2. any cell selectively affected by a particular agent, such as a hormone or drug. **tart c.,** a macrophage or monocytoid reticuloendothelial cell that contains a phagocytized nucleus with well preserved nuclear structure; the phagocytized nucleus, as distinguished from an LE cell inclusion, shows an intact chromatin pattern, chromatin that is more dense and tends to become vacuolated, and is frequently smaller than that in a true LE cell. **taste c's,** the interior cells of a taste bud hidden by the cover cells; called also *gustatory c's* and *taste corpuscles.* **tautomeral c's,** cells of the gray matter of the spinal cord whose axons pass into the white substance of the same side of the cord. **tegmental c's,** cells that cover any delicate structure. **tendon c's,** flattened tissue cells of connective tissue occurring in rows between the primary bundles of the tendons. **theca c's,** theca-lutein c's. **theca-lutein c's,** lutein cells derived from the theca interna; called also *paraluteal* or *paralutein c's.* **Thoma-Zeiss counting c.,** see under *chamber.* **thyroidectomy c's,** altered basophilic cells occurring in the anterior pituitary gland after thyroidectomy. **thyrotropic c.,** thyrotrope, def. 2. **totipotential c.,** an embryonic cell that is capable of developing into any variety of body cells. **touch c.,** corpuscula tactus. **Touton giant c's,** large multinucleated cells containing lipoid material found in the lesions of xanthoma and histiocytosis X. **trophochrome c's,** serous cells whose secretory granules give a staining reaction for mucus with mucicarmine; called also *mucoalbiminous c's* and *mucoserous c's.* **tubal air c's,** cellulae pneumaticae tubae auditivae. **Türk's c.,** a nongranular, mononuclear cell displaying morphologic characteristics of both an atypical lymphocyte and a plasma cell, observed in the peripheral blood during severe anemias, chronic infections, and leukemoid reactions; called also *Türk's irritation leukocyte.* **tympanic c's,** cellulae tympanicae. **type I c's,** alveolar c's, type I. **type II c's,** alveolar c's, type II.

Tzanck c., a degenerated epithelial cell caused by acantholysis, and found especially in pemphigus. **ultimobranchial c's,** parafollicular c's. **vacuolated c.,** a cell whose protoplasm contains vacuoles. **c's of van Gehuchten,** Golgi neurons of type II, i.e., neurons with short branching processes. **vasofactive c's, vasoformative c's,** cells that join with other cells to form blood vessels. **ventricular c.,** any of the columnar epithelial cells of the neural tube. **Vignal's c's,** embryonic connective tissue cells secreting myelin and associated with the formation of the axons of nerves in the fetus. **Virchow c's,** lepra c's. **visual c's,** the neuroepithelial elements of the retina, the outer specialized segments of which are the retinal rods and cones. **von Kupffer's c's,** Kupffer's c's. **wandering c's,** cells capable of ameboid movement, such as free macrophages, lymphocytes, mast cells, and plasma cells. **Warthin-Finkeldey c's,** the peculiar multinucleated giant cell present in tonsillar, nasopharyngeal, and appendiceal tissue in measles. **wasserhelle c's** [Ger.], water-clear c. **water-clear c.,** a large clear cell found in the parathyroid gland; these cells have a ballooned appearance and are especially numerous in adenoma of the gland. Called also *wasserhelle c.* **Wedl c's,** large swollen cells (bladder cells) formed by the capsular epithelium in cataract development. **white c., white blood c.,** leukocyte. **wing c's,** cells in the corneal epithelium with convex anterior surfaces and concave posterior surfaces. **xanthoma c.,** foam c. **Zander's c's,** bladder c's. **zymogenic c's,** chief c's, def. 1.

cella (sel′ah), pl. *cel′lae* [L.] [NA] an enclosure, or compartment. **c. latera′lis ventric′uli latera′lis** (*obs.*), the lateral part of the lateral ventricle of the brain. **c. me′dia ventric′uli latera′lis** (*obs.*), the central part of the lateral ventricle of the brain; called also *pars centralis.*

cellaburate (sel-ah-bur′āt) chemical name: cellulose acetate butanoate; a plastic filming agent.

cellae (sel′le) [L.] plural of *cella.*

cellase (sel′ās) an enzyme that acts upon cellose.

Cellase 1000 (sel′ās) trademark for a preparation of cellulase, used as a digestant adjunct.

Cellfalcicula (sel″fal-sik′u-lah) a genus of microorganisms of the family Spirillaceae, suborder Pseudomonadineae, order Pseudomonadales, made up of short, rod- or spindle-shaped cells with pointed ends, containing metachromatic granules. It includes three species, *C. fus′ca, C. muco′sa,* and *C. vi′ridis.*

Cellia (sel′e-ah) [Angelo *Celli,* Italian physician, 1857–1914] *Anopheles.*

cellicolous (sel-lik′ŏ-lus) [L. *cella* cell + *colere* to dwell] inhabiting cells.

celliferous (sel-lif′er-us) producing or bearing cells.

celliform (sel′ĭ-form) cell-like.

cellifugal (sel-lif′u-gal) cellulifugal.

cellipetal (sel-lip′e-tal) cellulipetal.

cellobiase (sel″lo-bi′ās) β-glucosidase.

cellobiose (sel″lo-bi′ōs) a disaccharide, $C_{12}H_{22}O_{11}$, formed from cellulose by the action of cellulase; called also *cellose.*

cellohexose (sel″o-hek′sōs) a crystalline hexasaccharide, $C_{36}H_{62}O_{31}$, obtained by the hydrolysis of cellulose.

celloidin (sĕ-loi′din) a concentrated preparation of pyroxylin, employed in microscopy for embedding specimens for section cutting.

cellon (sel′on) tetrachlorethane.

cellophane (sel′o-fān) a transparent tissue of regenerated cellulose used as a dialysis membrane and for bandages, compresses, etc.

cellose (sel′ōs) cellobiose.

cellotetrose (sel″o-tet′rōs) a crystalline tetrasaccharide, $C_{24}H_{42}O_{21}$, obtained by the hydrolysis of cellulose.

cellotriose (sel″o-tri′ōs) a crystalline trisaccharide, $C_{18}H_{32}O_{16}$, obtained by the hydrolysis of cellulose.

cellula (sel′lu-lah), pl. *cel′lulae* [L.] a small cell; [NA] a general term for a small, more or less enclosed space. **cel′lulae ethmoida′les** [NA], ethmoidal cells: air-containing spaces in the ethmoid bone, communicating with the infundibulum ethmoidale and the bulla ethmoidalis; classified, on the basis of their openings, as *cellulae anteriores, mediae,* and *posteriores,* and collectively forming the sinus ethmoidalis. **cel′lulae mastoi′deae** [NA], mastoid cells: the air spaces of the mastoid process of the temporal bone. **cel′lulae pneumat′icae tu′bae auditi′vae** [NA], air cells in the floor of the auditory tube close to the carotid canal, being similar to the air cells of the mastoid part of the temporal bone; called also *air cells of auditory tube; cellulae pneumaticae tubariae,* and *tubal air cells.* **cel′lulae pneumat′icae tuba′riae,** cellulae pneumaticae tubae auditivae. **cel′lulae tympan′icae** [NA], tympanic cells: spaces in the tympanic cavity between the bony projections from the floor, or jugular wall.

cellulae (sel′u-le) [L.] plural of *cellula.*

cellular (sel′u-lar) pertaining to, or made up of, cells.

cellularity (sel″u-lār′ĭ-te) the state of a tissue or other mass as regards the number of constituent cells.

cellulase (sel′u-lās) 1. an enzyme that hydrolyzes cellulose to cellobiose; it is secreted by certain bacteria and by fungi that destroy wood. 2. a concentrate of such enzymes derived from *Aspergillus niger* and used as a digestive aid.

cellule (sel′ūl) [L. *cellula*] a small cell; see also *cellula*. **c. claire,** clear cell.

cellulicidal (sel″u-lis′ĭ-dal) [L. *cellula* cellule + *caedere* to kill] destroying cells.

cellulifugal (sel″u-lif′u-gal) [L. *cellula* cellule + *fugere* to flee] directed away from a cell body.

cellulipetal (sel″u-lip′ĕ-tal) [L. *cellula* cellule + *petere* to seek] directed toward a cell body.

cellulitis (sel″u-li′tis) diffuse inflammation of the soft or connective tissue due to infection, in which a thin, watery exudate spreads through the cleavage planes of interstitial and tissue spaces; it may lead to ulceration and abscess. Called also *phlegmon*. **anaerobic c.,** inflammation of the subcutaneous tissue in which the infecting bacteria, most commonly *Clostridium perfringens*, proliferate and produce gas in the tissue (but not in muscle, as in gas gangrene). The onset is gradual, pain is absent, and systemic symptoms are not severe. **clostridial c.,** anaerobic c. **dissecting c.,** cellulitis with suppuration spreading between the layers of the involved tissue, as of the scalp. **dissecting c. of scalp,** perifolliculitis capitis abscedens et suffodiens. **finger c.,** felon. **gangrenous c.,** that leading to the death of the tissue associated with bacterial invasion and putrefaction. **gaseous c.,** inflammation due to a gas-producing organism; see *anaerobic c.* **indurated c.,** phlebitic induration. **orbital c.,** inflammation of the cellular tissue within the orbit. **pelvic c.,** parametritis. **periurethral c.,** see under *phlegmon*. **phlegmonous c.,** an infectious inflammatory process spreading by continuity through the skin and subcutaneous tissues, or more deeply, without sharp margination or localization. **streptococcus c.,** cellulitis due to streptococcus infection and frequently manifested as erysipelas. **ulcerative c.,** see under *lymphangitis*.

cellulofibrous (sel″u-lo-fi′brus) partly cellular and partly fibrous.

celluloid (sel″u-loid) a substance composed largely of pyroxylin and camphor; used in the arts and in surgery, and formerly in dentistry.

Cellulomonas (sel″lu-lo-mo′nas) [*cellulose* + Gr. *monas* a unit] a genus of microorganisms of the family Corynebacteriaceae, order Eubacteriales, made up of pleomorphic, gram-variable microorganisms found in soil.

celluloneuritis (sel″u-lo-nu-ri′tis) inflammation of neurons. **acute anterior c.,** Raymond's name for acute anterior poliomyelitis, polyneuritis, and Landry's paralysis, which he considered one disease.

cellulose (sel′u-lōs) a carbohydrate, $(C_6H_{10}O_5)_n$ the most abundant polysaccharide in nature, being a rigid, unbranched, long-chain polymer of glucose and forming the skeleton of most plant structures and of plant cells; it is a colorless, transparent solid, insoluble in water, alcohol, etc., but soluble in Schweitzer's reagent. **absorbable c.,** oxidized c. **c. acetate phthalate** [NF], a reduction product of phthalic anhydride and a partial acetate ester of cellulose; it is a free-flowing white powder used as a tablet-coating agent. **acid c.,** any combination of cellulose with carboxyl groups, such as pectinic acid; they are mostly gelatinous bodies. **microcrystalline c.** [NF], purified, partially depolymerized cellulose prepared by treating alpha cellulose, obtained as a pulp from fibrous plant material with mineral acids; used as a tablet and capsule diluent. **oxidized c.** [USP], cellulose partially oxidized and with a varying content of carboxylic acid groups, which confers some solubility in dilute alkali; it is insoluble in water. Dried in vacuum over phosphorus pentoxide, it is used as local hemostatic. Called also *absorbable c. and absorbable cotton*. **starch c.,** a nonlinear glucan polysaccharide obtained from waxy corn; not a true cellulose since it is not a β-glycoside; it is comparatively insoluble and said to be concentrated in the outer portion of starch grain. **tetranitrate c.,** $(C_{12}H_{16}N_4O_{18})_n$, the principle constituent of pyroxylin.

cellulosity (sel″u-los′ĭ-te) the condition of being composed of cells.

cellulotoxic (sel″u-lo-tok′sik) 1. toxic to cells. 2. produced by cell toxins.

cellulous (sel′u-lus) made up of cells.

Cellvibrio (sel-vib′re-o) a genus of microorganisms of the family Spirillaceae, suborder Pseudomonadineae, order Pseudomonadales, made up of straight or slightly curved rods sometimes joined in long chains or bundles. It includes four species, *C. flaves′cens, C. ful′vus, C. ochra′ceus,* and *C. vulga′ris*.

celo-, cel- 1. [Gr. *kēlē* hernia] a combining form denoting relationship to a tumor or swelling. 2. [Gr. *koilia* cavity] a combining form denoting relationship to a cavity. See also words beginning *celio-* and *coelo-*.

celom (se′lom) coelom.

celomic (se-lom′ik) coelomic.

Celontin (se-lon′tin) trademark for a preparation of methsuximide.

celophlebitis (se″lo-fle-bi′tis) [*celo-* (2) + *phlebitis*] inflammation of a vena cava.

celoschisis (se-los′kĭ-sis) [*celo-* (2) + *schisis* cleft] congenital fissure of the abdominal wall.

celoscope (sel′o-skōp) celioscope.

celoscopy (se-los′kŏ-pe) celioscopy.

celosomia (se-lo-so′me-ah) [*celo-* (1) + Gr. *sōma* body] a developmental anomaly characterized by eventration, fissure, or absence of the sternum, with hernial protrusion of the viscera.

celosomus (se″lo-so′mus) a fetus exhibiting celosomia; called also *kelosomus*.

celothel (se′lo-thel) mesothelium.

celothelioma (se″lo-the-le-o′mah) mesothelioma.

celothelium (se″lo-the′le-um) mesothelium.

celotomy (se-lot′o-me) herniotomy.

celovirus (sel′o-vi′rus) CELO virus.

celozoic (se″lo-zo′ik) [*celo-* (2) + *zōon* animal] inhabiting the intestinal cavities of the body; said of parasites.

Celsius scale, thermometer (sel′se-us) [Anders *Celsius*, Swedish astronomer, 1701–1744] see under *scale* and *thermometer*.

Celsus (sel′sus), Aurelius Cornelius (1st century A.D.) a celebrated Roman medical encyclopedist—"the Cicero of medicine." Of his many writings, only his *De re medicina* (in eight books) survives; the four classical signs (*Celsus' quadrilateral*) of inflammation—*calor* (heat), *dolor* (pain), *rubor* (redness), and *tumor* (swelling)—are mentioned in the third book of this work.

cement (se-ment′) [L. *cemen′tum*] 1. a substance that serves to produce solid union between two surfaces. 2. a filling material, such as zinc phosphate, used in dentistry to assist in retaining gold castings in prepared teeth and to insulate the tooth pulp from metallic and other fillings. 3. cementum. **acrylic resin dental c.,** a dental cement, dispensed as a powder or liquid, that is mixed as any other cement. The powder contains polymethyl methacrylate, a filler, a plasticizer, and a polymerization initiator. The liquid monomer is methyl methacrylate, with an inhibitor and an activator. **germicidal dental c.,** usually a zinc phosphate cement to which has been added copper or silver salts to render it bactericidal. **intercellular c.,** a mucilaginous substance that holds cells, and especially epithelial cells, together. **interprismatic c.,** the material that binds together the enamel prisms. **muscle c.,** the myoglia. **nerve c.,** the neuroglia. **silicate c.,** a dental cement used for semipermanent restorations on the basis of good early color and translucency. **silicophosphate c.,** a combination of zinc phosphate and silicate cement that is less translucent than silicate and stronger than zinc phosphate cement. **zinc-eugenol c.** [USP], a temporary, topical dental protective prepared by mixing 10 parts of the powder (composed of zinc acetate, zinc stearate, zinc oxide, and rosin) with 1 part of the liquid (composed of eugenol and cottonseed oil) to a thick paste immediately before use; applied to the cleaned carious lesion. **zinc phosphate c.,** the general purpose dental cement. The powder is zinc oxide with a small amount of modifier. The liquid consists essentially of phosphoric acid, with metallic salts as buffers, and approximately one-third water.

cementation (se″men-ta′shun) the attachment of anything by the means of cement, such as the use of cement in attaching restorative material to a natural tooth.

cementicle (se-men′tĭ-kel) a small, discrete globular mass of cementum in the region of a tooth root; called also *cementoexostosis*. **adherent c., attached c.,** one that is firmly connected with the cementum. **free c., interstitial c.,** one that is completely surrounded by connective tissue of the periodontal membrane.

cementification (se-men″tĭ-fĭ-ka′shun) cementogenesis.

cementin (se-men′tin) the material that sometimes unites the margins of squamous endothelial cells.

cementitis (se″men-ti′tis) inflammation of the cementum of a tooth.

cementoblast (se-men′to-blast) [*cementum* + Gr. *blastos* germ] a large cuboidal cell with spheroid or ovoid nucleus, found on the surface of cementum, between the fibers, which is active in the formation of cementum.

cementoblastoma (se-men″to-blas-to′mah) an odontogenic fibroma in which the cells are developing into cementoblasts, and there is only a small proportion of calcified tissue; called also *cementifying fibroma*.

cementoclasia (se-men″to-kla′se-ah) [*cementum* + Gr. *klasis* breaking] disintegration of the cementum of a tooth.

cementocyte (se-men′to-sīt) a cell found in lacunae of cellular cementum, frequently having long processes radiating from the cell body toward the periodontal surface of the cementum; called also *cement cell*.

cemento-exostosis (se-men″to-ek″sos-to′sis) cementicle.

cementogenesis (se-men″to-jen′ĕ-sis) [*cementum* + Gr. *genesis* formation] the development of the cementum on the root dentin of a tooth; called also *cementification*.

cementoma (se″men-to′mah) a mass of cementum lying free at the apex of a tooth, probably a reaction to injury rather than a neoplasm.

cementopathia (se-men′to-path′e-ah) periodontitis or periodontosis resulting from disease or defect of the cementum.

cementoperiostitis (se-men″to-per″e-os-ti′tis) periodontitis.

cementosis (se″men-to′sis) a condition characterized by proliferation of cementum; called also *dental exostosis*.

cementum (se-men′tum) [L.] [NA] the bonelike connective tissue covering the root of a tooth and assisting in tooth support; the intercellular substance is calcified and arranged in layers (lamellae). Called also *crusta petrosa dentis* and *substantia ossea dentis*.

cenadelphus (se″nah-del′fus) [Gr. *koinos* common + *adelphos* brother] a twin monster in which the two components are equally developed.

cenencephalocele (se″nen-sef′ah-lo-sēl) an encephalocele or protrusion of the brain without cystic condition.

cenesthesia (se″nes-the′ze-ah) [Gr. *koinos* common + *aisthēsis* perception] the general feeling or sense of conscious existence; the sense of normal functioning of the organs of the body.

cenesthesic (se″nes-the′sik) pertaining to cenesthesia.

cenesthesiopathy (se″nes-the″ze-op′ah-the) [*cenesthesia* + Gr. *pathos* disease + *-ia*] any disturbance of cenesthesia. Cf. *paracenesthesia*.

cenesthetic (se″nes-thet′ik) cenesthesic.

cenesthopathia (se″nes-tho-path′e-ah) cenesthesiopathy.

ceno- 1. [Gr. *kainos* new, fresh] a combining form denoting new; see also words beginning *caino-* and *kaino-*. 2. [Gr. *kenos* empty] a combining form denoting empty; see also words beginning *caeno-* and *keno-*. 3. [Gr. *koinos* shared in common] a combining form denoting relationship to a common feature or characteristic; see also words beginning *coeno-*, *coino-*, and *koino-*.

cenobium (se-no′be-um) [Gr. *koinobios* living in communion with others] a colony of independent cells or organisms held together by a common investment.

cenocyte (se′no-sīt) [*ceno-*(3) + Gr. *kytos* hollow vessel] 1. a multinucleate plant cell enclosed within a hollow wall, examples of which are found within the fungi and algae. 2. a multinucleate bit of cytoplasm in which the nuclei are not separated by walls. 3. a multinucleate plant protoplast.

cenogenesis (se″no-jen′ĕ-sis) [*ceno-* (1) + Gr. *genesis* production] the appearance of new features in development, in adaptive response to environmental conditions. Cf. *palingenesis*, def. 2.

Cenolate (sen′o-lāt) trademark for a preparation of ascorbic acid.

cenopsychic (se″no-si′kik) [*ceno-* (1) + Gr. *psychē* soul] of recent appearance in mental development.

cenosis (se-no′sis) [Gr. *kenōsis* an emptying, or emptiness] a morbid discharge.

cenosite (se′no-sīt) coinosite.

cenotic (se-not′ik) pertaining to or characterized by cenosis.

cenotoxin (se″no-tok′sin) kenotoxin.

cenotype (se′nŏ-tīp) [*ceno-* (3) + *type*] the original type from which all forms have arisen.

censor (sen′sor) 1. a member of a committee on ethics or for critical examination and supervision of a medical or other society. 2. in freudian terminology, the psychic influence that prevents unconscious thoughts and wishes from coming into consciousness unless they are disguised so as to be unrecognizable; called also *freudian c.* and *psychic c.*

censorship (sen′sor-ship) the operation of the censor.

center (sen′ter) [Gr. *kentron;* L. *centrum*] 1. the middle point of a body. 2. a collection of neurons concerned with performance of a particular function; see also *area*. **accelerating c.,** a center in the brain stem involved in acceleration of the heart; called also *cardioaccelerating c.* **acoustic c.,** auditory c. **anospinal c's,** the centers for contracting the sphincter ani, for relaxing it (defecation center), and for the anal reflex; all are in the lumbar enlargement. **apneustic c.,** a nerve center in the brain stem controlling normal respiration. **auditopsychic c.,** a center dealing with the interpretation of sounds, in the superior temporal gyrus. **auditory c.,** the center for hearing, in the more anterior of the transverse temporal gyri; called also *acoustic c.* **brain c.,** 1. an area of the cerebral cortex having a specialized structure or function. 2. a group of cells in the brain having a special function. See also *specific areas*, under *area*. **Broca's c.,** the speech center. **Budge's c.,** 1. ciliospinal center. 2. genital center. **cardioaccelerating c.,** accelerating c. **cardioinhibitory c.,** a center in the medulla oblongata that exerts an inhibitory influence on the heart by way of the vagus. **cardiomotor c.,** Tawara's name for the atrioventricular node, on the theory that the heart's impulse arises there. **cell c.,** centrosome. **cheirokinesthetic c.,** the center in the posterior part of the left second frontal gyrus, controlling movements concerned in writing. **c's of chondrification,**

dense aggregations of embryonic mesenchymal cells at sites of future cartilage formation; called also *protochondral tissue*. **ciliospinal c.,** a center in the lower cervical and upper dorsal portions of the spinal cord, connected with the dilatation of the pupil; called also *Budge's c.* **community health c.,** a health service delivery system providing a coordinated program of continuing mental health care to a specific population. **coordination c.,** a nerve center serving the function of coordination. **correlation c.,** a nerve center serving the function of correlation. **cortical c.,** any portion of the cerebral cortex that can be differentiated functionally from its neighbors; such a center is sometimes called area, field, or zone. **coughing c.,** a center in the medulla oblongata, situated above the respiratory center, which controls the act of coughing. **defecation c.,** see *anospinal c.* **deglutition c.,** a nerve center in the medulla oblongata that controls the function of swallowing. **dentary c.,** an ossification center of the mandible, giving origin to the lower border and outer plate. **C. for Disease Control (CDC),** an agency of the U.S. Department of Health and Human Services which serves as a center for the control, prevention, and investigation of diseases. **dominating c.,** the principal or controlling center of a group having a common function. **ejaculation c.,** the center that controls the erection of the penis and the normal discharge of semen; it is in the lumbar region of the spinal cord, and is itself regulated from the oblongata. Called also *erection c.* **epiotic c.,** the center of ossification that forms the mastoid process. **epiphyseal c.,** secondary c. of ossification. **erection c.,** ejaculation c. **eupraxic c.,** any cerebral center that controls the proper performance of any action or set of actions. **facial c.,** a center for face movements, located in the lower part of the ascending frontal convolution. **Flemming c.,** germinal c. **ganglionic c.,** any mass of gray matter between the lateral ventricles and the decussation of the anterior pyramids, including the thalami, striati, and other basal ganglia. **genital c., genitospinal c.,** the ejaculation center of the male or the parturition center of the female; said to be in the cord, near the second lumbar vertebra. Called also *Budge's c.* **germinal c.,** the area in the center of a lymph nodule containing aggregations of actively proliferating lymphocytes (classically, antibody-forming B-cells); it appears as a spherical mass surrounded by a capsule of elongated cells that is partially invested by a crescentic cap of small lymphocytes. Called also *Flemming c., noeud vital,* and *secondary nodule*. **glossokinesthetic c.,** the center in the posterior part of the left second frontal gyrus that controls movements concerned in articulate speech. **gustatory c.,** the cerebral center supposed to control taste, situated in the cortex of the uncinate convolution; called also *taste c.* **health c.,** 1. a community health organization for creating health work and coordinating the efforts of all health agencies. 2. an educational complex consisting of a medical school and various allied health professional schools. **heat-regulating c's,** thermoregulator c's. **inhibitory c.,** any nerve center that restrains any function or process or controls other centers. **kinetic c.,** the centrospheres of a fertilized ovum. **Kronecker's c.,** cardioinhibitory c. **Kupressoff's c.,** micturition c. **Lumsden's c.,** pneumotaxic c. **medullary c. of cerebellum,** corpus medullare cerebelli. **medullary respiratory c.,** a center in the medulla oblongata that coordinates respiratory movements. **micturition c.,** a center controlling the bladder and inhibiting the tension of the vesical sphincter, situated in the lumbar enlargement; called also *Kupressoff's c.* **motor c.,** any center that originates, controls, inhibits, or maintains a motor impulse. **nerve c.,** a collection of nerve cells in the central nervous system that are associated together in the performance of some particular function. **optic c.,** that point in a lens, or combination of lenses, where all rays that help to form a clear image cross the principal axis; in the eye, about 2 mm. back of the cornea (Fording). **ossification c.,** any point at which the process of ossification begins in a bone; in a long bone there is a *primary center* for the diaphysis and one *secondary center* for each epiphysis. **oval c., greater** (obs.), centrum semiovale. **panting c.,** polypneic c. **parenchymatous c.,** a nerve center situated in the substance of a viscus. **phrenic c.,** centrum tendineum. **pneumotaxic c.,** a center in the upper part of the pons that rhythmically inhibits inspiration independently of the vagi; called also *Lumsden's c.* **polypneic c.,** a center in the tuber cinereum that accelerates the rate of breathing. **pteriotic c.,** a center of ossification from which are developed the tegmen tympani and the covering of the lateral semicircular canal. **reaction c.,** germinal c. **rectovesical c.,** a cord reflex center for the rectum and bladder. **reflex c.,** any center in the brain or cord in which a sensory impression is changed into a motor impulse; the reflex centers already discovered are numerous. **respiratory c's,** a series of centers in the medulla and pons which coordinate respiratory movements; they include the pneumotaxic center, apneustic center, and the medullary respiratory center. **rotation c.,** the point or axis about which a body rotates. **semioval c.,** centrum semiovale. **sensory c.,** a center that receives or appreciates a sensory impulse. **Setchenow's (Sechenoff's) c's,** reflex inhibitory centers in the cord and oblongata. **sex-behavior c.,** the ventromedial nucleus of hypothalamus; see under *nucleus*. **soma-**

tic c., the pituitary gland; so called from the belief that it influences the growth of the whole body. **speech c.,** a center in the left (or right) inferior frontal gyrus; called also *Broca's c.* **sphenotic c.,** a center of ossification in the sphenoid bone for the lingula. **splenial c.,** one of the ossification centers of the mandible, forming a part of its inner plate. **sudorific c's, sweat c's,** centers in the spinal cord controlling diaphoresis, with a dominant center in the oblongata. **swallowing c.,** deglutition c. **taste c.,** the gustatory center. **tendinous c.,** centrum tendineum. **thermoregulatory c's,** hypothalamic centers regulating the conservation and dissipation of heat. **vasoconstrictor c.,** a center in the medulla oblongata that controls contraction of the blood vessels. **vasodilator c.,** a center in the medulla oblongata for dilating the blood vessels. **vasomotor c's,** centers in the tuber cinereum, oblongata, and cord, believed to regulate the caliber of the blood vessels and to cause their contraction and dilatation. **vesical c., vesicospinal c.,** the micturition center or rectovesical center. **vomiting c.,** a center in the lower central region of the medulla oblongata; its stimulation causes vomiting. **Wernicke's c.,** the central speech center; see under *area.* **word c., auditory,** a center in the left superior transverse temporal gyrus that controls the perception of words that are heard. **word c., visual,** one in the posterior part of the left parietal lobe; it appears to govern the perception of printed or written words.

centesimal (sen-tes'ĭ-mal) [L. *centesimus* hundredth] divided into hundredths or based upon divisions into hundredths.

centesis (sen-te'sis) [Gr. *kentēsis*] perforation or tapping, as with an aspirator, trocar, or needle. Used also as a word termination, affixed to a root indicating the part on which the operation is performed, as *abdominocentesis, thoracocentesis,* and the like.

centi- (sen'tĭ) [L. *centrum* a hundred] a combining form denoting (1) one hundredth of the unit designated by the root with which it is combined, as in centimeter, or (2) one hundred, as in centipede.

centibar (sen'tĭ-bar) a unit of atmospheric pressure, being one-hundredth part of a bar, or 10^{-2} bar.

centigrade (sen'tĭ-grād) [L. *centum* hundred + *gradus* a step] consisting of or having 100 gradations (steps or degrees); abbreviated C. See *Celsius (centigrade) scale,* under *scale.*

centigram (sen'tĭ-gram) one hundredth part of a gram (10^{-2} gram), or the equivalent of 0.1543 grain (Troy); abbreviated cg. or cgm.

centiliter (sen'tĭ-le''ter) one hundredth part of a liter (10^{-2} l.), or the equivalent of 0.33815 of a fluid ounce; abbreviated cl.

centimeter (sen'tĭ-me''ter) [Fr. *centimètre*] a unit of linear measure of the metric system, being one hundredth part of a meter (10^{-2} m.), or approximately 0.3937 inch; abbreviated cm. **cubic c.,** a unit of capacity, being that of a cube each side of which measures 1 cm.; abbreviated cc., cm.³, or cu. cm.

centinem (sen'tĭ-nem) (*obs.*) Pirquet's term for one one-hundredth of a nem.

centinormal (sen'tĭ-nor'mal) [L. *centum* hundred + *norma* rule] having a hundredth part of the standard strength.

centipede (sen'tĭ-pēd) an elongated arthropod of the class Chilopoda characterized by having one pair of legs to each body segment; they may have 15 to 173 pairs of legs. Centipedes paralyze and kill insects and small animals with their poison claws, which are modified legs of the first body segment. A few species are capable of penetrating the skin of man, causing painful bites. See *Scolopendra.*

centipoise (sen'tĭ-poiz) one one-hundredth of a poise.

centistoke (sen'tĭ-stōk) one one-hundreth of a stoke.

centiunit (sen''te-u'nit) one one-hundredth of the conventional unit.

centra (sen'trah) [L.] plural of *centrum.*

centrad (sen'trad) 1. toward the center or a center, especially toward the center of the body. 2. a measure of an angle of deviation, being 0.57 degree, or one one-hundredth part of a portion of the arc of a circle equal in length to the radius of the circle; called also *prism degree.*

centrage (sen'trāj) the condition in which the centers of the various refracting surfaces of the eye are in the same straight line.

central (sen'tral) situated at or pertaining to a center; not peripheral.

centralis (sen-tra'lis) [NA] a general term denoting a centrally located structure.

centraphose (sen'trah-fōz) any aphose, or sensation of darkness, originating in the optic or visual centers.

centration (sen-tra'shun) the inability to pay attention to more than one salient feature at a time; it is a normal stage in human intellectual development.

centraxonial (sen''trak-so'ne-al) having the axis in a central median line.

centre (sen'ter) center.

centrencephalic (sen''tren-sĕ-fal'ik) pertaining to the center of the encephalon; see under *system.*

centric (sen'trik) in orthodontics, pertaining to the bilaterally balanced position of the mandibular condyles and articular disks, with the two articular eminentia, the articular capsular structures and ligaments, and with the controlling musculature. This state may occur anywhere along the path of closure from open mouth to full tooth contact or habitual occlusion.

centriciput (sen-tris'ĭ-put) [*center* + L. *caput* head] the central part of the upper surface of the head, located between the occiput and sinciput.

centrifugal (sen-trif'u-gal) [*center* + L. *fugere* to flee] moving away from a center; moving away from the cerebral cortex; efferent or exodic.

centrifugalization (sen-trif''u-gal-ĭ-za'shun) centrifugation.

centrifugate (sen-trif'u-gāt) material subjected to centrifugation.

centrifugation (sen-trif''u-ga'shun) the process of separating the lighter portions of a solution, mixture, or suspension from the heavier portions by centrifugal force; called also *centrifugalization.* **density gradient c.,** ultracentrifugation in a liquid, such as cesium chloride solution, the density of which increases along the lines of centrifugal force, the substances under test seeking their level of density. **differential c.,** that based on the sedimentation coefficient of the substances under investigation; applied to homogenates to derive various subcellular fractions. **isopyknic c.,** that in which the solvent is of the same density as the substance to be isolated.

centrifuge (sen'trĭ-fūj) [*center* + L. *fugere* to flee] 1. a machine by which centrifugation is effected. 2. to subject to centrifugation. **microscope c.,** a high-speed centrifuge with a built-in microscope, permitting a specimen to be viewed under centrifugal force.

centrilobular (sen''trĭ-lob'u-lar) pertaining to the central portion of a lobule.

centriole (sen'trĭ-ōl) either of the two cylindrical organelles located in the centrosome and containing nine triplets of microtubules arrayed around their edges; centrioles migrate to opposite poles of the cell during cell division and serve to organize the spindles. They are capable of independent replication and of migrating to form basal bodies. **anterior c.,** proximal c. **distal c.,** that centriole of a spermatozoon which, after migrating to the cell surface and giving rise to a slender flagellum, returns to a position just caudal to the proximal centriole; called also *posterior c.* **posterior c.,** distal c. **proximal c.,** that centriole of a spermatozoon which migrates to a position in a depression in the wall of the posterior portion of the nucleus, with its axis at right angles to the main axis of the spermatozoon, and from which the axoneme extends; called also *anterior c.* **ring c.,** a dark annular structure at the posterior end of the middle piece of a spermatozoon; it is not a true centriole. Called also *annulus of spermatozoon.*

centripetal (sen-trip'e-tal) [*center* + L. *petere* to seek] moving toward a center; moving toward the cerebral cortex; afferent or esodic.

centro- (sen'tro) [Gr. *kentron;* L. *centrum*] a combining form denoting relationship to a center, or to a central location.

centrocecal (sen''tro-se'kal) pertaining to the central macular area and the blind spot; called also *cecocentral.*

Centrocestus (sen''tro-ses'tus) a genus of flukes. **C. cuspida'tus,** a fluke occurring in the Egyptian kite. *C. cuspidatus* var. *canina* is reported from dogs in Taiwan; it may be the same as *Stamnosoma formosanum.*

centrocinesia (sen''tro-si-ne'se-ah) centrokinesia.

centrocinetic (sen''tro-si-net'ik) centrokinetic.

centrodesmose (sen''tro-des'mōs) centrodesmus.

centrodesmus (sen''tro-des'mus) [*centro-* + Gr. *desmos* a band] the matter connecting the centrosomes of a cell and forming the beginning of the central spindle.

centrokinesia (sen''tro-ki-ne'se-ah) [*center* + Gr. *kinēsis* movement] movement originating from central stimulation.

centrokinetic (sen''tro-ki-net'ik) pertaining to, characterized by, or promoting centrokinesia.

centrolecithal (sen''tro-les'ĭ-thal) [*centro-* + Gr. *lekithos* yolk] having the yolk centrally located; see under *ovum.*

centrolobular (sen''tro-lob'u-lar) centrilobular.

centromere (sen''tro-mēr) the clear constricted portion of the chromosome at which the chromatids are joined and by which the chromosome is attached to the spindle during cell division. According to its location, a centromere is said to be metacentric (central), submetacentric (off center), or acrocentric (near one end). Called also *kinetochore* and *primary constriction.*

centromeric (sen''tro-mer'ik) pertaining to or resembling a centromere.

centron (sen'tron) a postulated preexistent spherical stromal structure in the lymph node cortex; cortical follicles result from the grouping of lymphoid cells in relation to the centron during antigen stimulation.

centronucleus (sen''tro-nu'kle-us) amphinucleus.

centro-osteosclerosis (sen″tro-os″te-o-skle-ro′sis) centrosclerosis.

centrophose (sen′tro-fōz) any phose, or sensation of light, originating in the visual centers.

centroplasm (sen′tro-plazm) the substance of the centrosome.

centrosclerosis (sen′tro-skle-ro′sis) [*center* + *osteosclerosis*] the filling of the marrow cavity of a bone with osseous material.

centrosome (sen′tro-sōm) [*centro-* + Gr. *sōma* body] the cell center; the centrosphere together with the two centrioles.

centrosphere (sen′tro-sfēr) [*centro-* + Gr. *sphaira* sphere] 1. a specialized area of condensed cytoplasm that contains the centrioles and plays an important part in mitosis; called also *cytocentrum, microcentrum, attractin sphere*, and *paranuclear body*. 2. centrosome.

centrostaltic (sen″tro-stal′tik) [*centro-* + Gr. *stellein* to send] pertaining to a center of motion.

centrotherapy (sen″tro-ther′ah-pe) externally applied treatment designed to act upon the nerve centers.

centrum (sen′trum), pl. *cen′tra* [L.; Gr. *kentron*] 1. [NA] a center. 2. the body of a vertebra. **c. media′num,** nucleus medialis centralis thalami. **c. ova′le ma′jus** (*obs.*), c. semiovale. **c. semiova′le,** semioval center: the white matter of the cerebral hemispheres which underlies the cerebral cortex and which, in horizontal sections superior to the corpus callosum, has a semioval shape; it contains projection, commissural, and association fibers; called also *greater oval center*. **c. tendin′eum** [NA], **c. tendin′eum [diaphrag′matis],** the trefoil-shaped aponeurosis, immediately below the pericardium, onto which the diaphragmatic fibers converge to insert; called also *central tendon of diaphragm, phrenic center,* and *tendinous center*. **c. tendin′eum perine′i** [NA], the fibromuscular mass in the median plane of the perineum where converge and attach the bulbospongiosus and sphincter ani externus muscles, the two levatores ani, and the two deep and the two superficial transverse perineal muscles; called also *perineal body* and *central tendon of perineum*. **c. ver′tebrae,** corpus vertebrae.

Centruroides (sen″troo-roi′dēz) a genus of subtropical and tropical American scorpions, some of which are poisonous.

Cenurus (sen-u′rus) *Coenurus*. **C. cerebra′lis,** *Coenurus cerebralis*.

cephacetrile sodium (sef′ah-sĕ-trīl) chemical name: 7-(2-cyanoacetamido-3-(hydroxymethyl)-8-oxo-5-thia-1-azabicyclo[4.2.0.]oct-2-ene-2-carboxylic acid acetate (ester) monosodium salt. An antibiotic, $C_{13}H_{12}N_3NaO_6S$, effective against a wide range of gram-positive and gram-negative bacteria.

Cephaelis (sef″a-e′lis) a genus of tropical shrubs and trees. *C. acuminata* and *C. ipecacuanha* are sources of *ipecac* (q.v.).

cephal- see *cephalo-*.

cephalad (sef′ah-lad) [Gr. *kephalē* head] toward the head; opposite to caudad.

cephalalgia (sef″ah-lal′je-ah) [Gr. *kephalalgia*] pain in the head; headache. Called also *cephalgia* and *cephalodynia*. **histamine c.,** former name for migrainous neuralgia. **pharyngotympanic c.,** Legal's disease. **quadrantal c.,** headache affecting one quadrant of the head.

cephaledema (sef″al-ĕ-de′mah) [*cephal-* + Gr. *oidēma* swelling] edema of the head.

cephalematocele (sef″al-ĕ-mat′o-sēl) cephalhematocele.

cephalematoma (sef″al-em″ah-to′mah) cephalhematoma.

cephalexin (sef″ah-lek′sin) [USP] chemical name: [6*R*-[6α,-8β(*R**)]]-7-[(aminophenylacetyl) amino]-3-methyl-8-oxo-5-thia-1-azabicyclo[4.2.0]oct-2-ene-2-carboxylic acid monohydrate. A semisynthetic analogue, $C_{16}H_{17}N_3O_4S \cdot H_2O$, of the natural antibiotic cephalosporin C, occurring as a white to off-white, crystalline powder, effective against a wide range of gram-negative and gram-positive bacteria; used in the treatment of infections of the urinary and respiratory tracts and of skin and soft tissues due to sensitive pathogens, administered orally.

cephalgia (sĕ-fal′je-ah) cephalalgia.

cephalhematocele (sef″al-he-mat′o-sēl) [*cephal-* + Gr. *haima* blood + *kēlē* tumor] a bloody tumor under the pericranium, communicating with one or more sinuses of the dura through the cranial bones. **Stromeyer's c.,** a subperiosteal cephalhematocele which communicates with veins and becomes filled with blood during strong expiratory efforts.

cephalhematoma (sef″al-he″mah-to′mah) [*cephal-* + *hematoma*] a subperiosteal hemorrhage limited to the surface of one cranial bone, a usually benign condition seen frequently in the newborn as a result of bone trauma. Called also *cephalohematoma*. **c. defor′mans,** a bulging of the anterior part of the skull due to hyperostosis, osteoporosis, and cavity formation in the bone.

cephalhydrocele (sef″al-hi′dro-sēl) [*cephal-* + *hydrocele*] a serous or watery accumulation under the pericranium. **c. traumat′ica,** Billroth's disease, def. 1.

cephalic (sĕ-fal′ik) [L. *cephalicus;* Gr. *kephalikos*] pertaining to the head, or to the head end of the body.

cephalin (sef′ah-lin) [Gr. *kephalē* head] any of a group of phosphoglycerides in which phosphatidic acid is linked to ethanolamine (phosphatidyl ethanolamine) or to serine (phosphatidyl serine); the cephalins are found particularly in brain and nervous tissue and have blood-coagulating properties.

cephalitis (sef″ah-li′tis) encephalitis.

cephalization (sef″al-i-za′shun) [Gr. *kephalē* head] the concentration or initiation of the growth tendency at the head end of the embryo.

cephalo-, cephal- [Gr. *kephalē* head] a combining form denoting relationship to the head.

cephalocathartic (sef″ah-lo-kah-thar′tik) [*cephalo-* + Gr. *kathartikos* purgative] cleansing or clearing the head.

cephalocaudad (sef″ah-lo-kaw′dad) 1. proceeding in a direction from the head toward the tail; caudad. 2. in both a cephalic and caudal direction.

cephalocaudal (sef″ah-lo-kaw′dal) [*cephalo-* + L. *cauda* tail] pertaining to the long axis of the body, in a direction from head to tail.

cephalocele (se-fal′o-sēl) [*cephalo-* + Gr. *kēlē* hernia] a protrusion of a part of the cranial contents. **orbital c.,** protrusion of the cranial contents through a defect in the orbital wall, named according to its contents as meningocele, encephalocele, etc.

cephalocentesis (sef″ah-lo-sen-te′sis) [*cephalo-* + Gr. *kentēsis* puncture] the surgical puncture of the head.

cephalocercal (sef″ah-lo-ser′kal) [*cephalo-* + Gr. *kerkos* tail] (*obs.*) cephalocaudal.

cephalochord (sef′ah-lo-kord″) [*cephalo-* + Gr. *chordē* cord] the intracranial portion of the embryonic notochord.

Cephalochordata (sef″ah-lo-kor-da′tah) a subphylum of primitive, small, fishlike chordates in which the notochord extends the entire length of the body; it includes the genus *Amphioxus*.

cephalochordate (sef″ah-lo-kor′dāt) any member of the Cephalochordata.

cephalocyst (sef′ah-lo-sist″) a larval cestode, such as a hydatid cyst.

cephalodactyly (sef″ah-lo-dak′tĭ-le) [*cephalo-* + Gr. *daktylos* a finger or toe] malformation of the head and digits. **Vogt's c.,** Apert-Crouzon disease.

cephalodiprosopus (sef″ah-lo-di-pros′o-pus) [*cephalo-* + Gr. *di* twice + *prosopus* face] a monster with a partially incomplete head attached to the head proper.

cephalodymia (sef″ah-lo-dim′e-ah) the condition of a cephalodymus.

cephalodymus (sef″ah-lod′ĭ-mus) [*cephalo-* + Gr. *didymos* twin] a twin monster with a single or united head.

cephalodynia (sef″ah-lo-din′e-ah) [*cephalo-* + Gr. *odynē* pain] cephalalgia.

cephalogenesis (sef″ah-lo-jen′ĕ-sis) [*cephalo-* + Gr. *gennan* to produce] the development of the head in the embryo.

cephaloglycin (sef″ah-lo-gli′sin) [USP] chemical name: [6*R*-[6α,7β(*R**)]]3-[(acetyloxy) methyl]-7-(aminophenylacetyl)amino]-8-oxo-5-thio-1-azabicyclo[4.2.0]oct-2-ene-2-carboxylic acid dihydrate. A semisynthetic analogue, $C_{18}H_{19}N_3O_6S \cdot 2H_2O$, of the natural antibiotic cephalosporin C, occurring as a white to off-white, crystalline powder, effective against a wide range of gram-negative and gram-positive bacteria; used in the treatment of acute and chronic urinary infections due to sensitive pathogens, administered orally.

cephalogram (sef′ah-lo-gram) an x-ray image of the anatomic structures of the head; cephalometric radiograph.

cephalogyric (sef″ah-lo-ji′rik) [*cephalo-* + Gr. *gyros* a turn] pertaining to turning motions of the head.

cephalohematocele (sef″ah-lo-he-mat′o-sēl) cephalhematocele.

cephalohematoma (sef″ah-lo-he″mah-to′mah) cephalhematoma.

cephaloma (sef-ah-lo′mah) (*obs.*) medullary carcinoma.

cephalomelus (sef″ah-lo-lom′ĕ-lus) [*cephalo-* + Gr. *melos* limb] a monster with an accessory limb growing from the head.

cephalomenia (sef″ah-lo-me′ne-ah) [*cephalo-* + Gr. *mēn* month] vicarious menstruation from the head, as in a nasal discharge at the menstrual period.

cephalomeningitis (sef″ah-lo-men″in-ji′tis) [*cephalo-* + *meningitis*] (*obs.*) inflammation of the membranes of the brain.

cephalometer (sef″ah-lom′ĕ-ter) [*cephalo-* + Gr. *metron* measure] an instrument for measuring the head; an orienting device for positioning the head for radiographic examination and measurement.

cephalometrics (sef″ah-lo-met′riks) cephalometry.

cephalometry (sef″ah-lom′ĕ-tre) scientific measurement of the dimensions of the head. In dentistry, certain combinations of linear and angular measurements developed from tracing the oriented lateral and frontal radiographic head film are used to assess craniofacial growth and development on a longitudinal basis and to determine the nature of orthodontic treatment response. **fetal c.,** measurement of the fetal skull *in utero* by means of x-ray films or by interpreting the echoes of ultrasonic radiation received from each side of the skull; useful in determining the proper time for elective termination of pregnancy.

cephalomotor (sef″ah-lo-mo′tor) [*cephalo-* + L. *motus* motion] moving the head; pertaining to motions of the head.

Cephalomyia (sef″ah-lo-mi′yah) *Oestrus.*

cephalonia (sef″ah-lo′ne-ah) a condition in which the head is abnormally large with sclerotic hyperplasia of the brain.

cephalont (sef′ah-lont) [*cephalo-* + Gr. *ōn* being] that stage of a developing gregarine protozoon in which it is attached to the epithelial host cell.

cephalopagus (sef″ah-lop′ah-gus) craniopagus.

cephalopathy (sef″ah-lop′ah-the) [*cephalo-* + Gr. *pathos* disease] any disease of the head.

cephalopelvic (sef″ah-lo-pel′vik) pertaining to the relationship of the fetal head to the maternal pelvis.

cephalopharyngeus (sef″ah-lo-fah-rin′je-us) musculus constrictor pharyngis superior; see *Table of Musculi.*

cephaloplegia (sef″ah-lo-ple′je-ah) [*cephalo-* + Gr. *plēgē* stroke] paralysis of the muscles about the head and face.

Cephalopoda (sef″ah-lop′ŏ-dah) [*cephalo-* + Gr. *pous* foot] the class of mollusks embracing the octopus, squid, cuttlefish, and nautilus.

cephalorhachidian (sef″ah-lo-rah-kid′e-an) (*obs.*) pertaining to the head and the spinal column.

cephaloridine (sef″ah-lor′ĭ-dēn) chemical name: (6*R-trans*)-1-[[2-carboxy-8-oxo-7-[(2-thienylacetyl)amino]-5-thia-1-azabicyclo-[4.2.0]oct-2-en-3-yl]methyl]pyridinium hydroxide inner salt. A semisynthetic analogue, $C_{19}H_{17}N_3O_4S_2$, of the natural antibiotic cephalosporin C, occurring as a white to off-white crystalline powder, effective against many gram-positive and some gram-negative bacteria; used in the treatment of infections of the bones, joints, skin, soft tissues, and major organ and tissue systems due to sensitive pathogens, administered intramuscularly or intravenously. Sterile cephaloridine, prepared in conformance with USP specifications, is suitable for parenteral use.

cephalosporin (sef″ah-lo-spōr′in) any of a group of broad-spectrum, relatively penicillinase-resistant antibiotics derived from the fungus *Cephalosporium*, which share the nucleus 7-aminocephalosporanic acid and are structurally related to the penicillins. The cephalosporins available for medicinal use are semisynthetic derivatives of the natural antibiotic *cephalosporin C.* **c. C,** chemical name: 7-(D-5-aminocarboxyvaleramido)-3-(hydroxymethyl)-3-oxo-5-thia-1-azabicyclo[4.2.0]oct-2-ene-2-carboxylic acid acetate. A cephalosporin isolated from *Cephalosporium acremonium,* $C_{16}H_{21}N_3O_8S$, which is the parent compound of a number of semisynthetic antibiotics, including cefazolin sodium, cephalexin, cephaloridine, cephaloglycin, cephalothin, cephapirin, and cephradine, used in the treatment of a wide range of infections due to sensitive gram-positive and gram-negative bacteria. **c. N,** adicillin. **c. P,** an antibacterial steroid, $C_{33}H_{50}O_8$; the crude form contains at least five components (P_1, P_2, P_3, P_4, P_5), P_1 being the major active substance.

cephalosporinase (sef″ah-lo-spōr′in-ās) an enzyme that hydrolyzes the CO—NH bond in the lactam ring of cephalosporin and converting it to an inactive product. Called also *β-lactamase II.*

cephalosporiosis (sef″ah-lo-spo″re-o′sis) infection with species of *Cephalosporium* (q.v.).

Cephalosporium (sef″ah-lo-spo′re-um) a genus of soil-inhabiting imperfect fungi of the family Moniliaceae, order Moniliales; some species are the source of a group of antibiotics, the cephalosporins. **C. falcifor′me,** *Acremonium kiliense.* **C. granulo′matis,** a species reported as causing gumma-like lesions in man.

cephalostat (sef″ah-lo-stat″) a head-positioning device which assures reproducibility of the relations between an x-ray beam, a patient's head, and an x-ray film in dental radiology.

cephalostyle (sef″ah-lo-stīl″) the cranial end of the notochord.

cephalotetanus (sef″ah-lo-tet′ah-nus) cerebral tetanus.

cephalothin (sef″ah-lo-thin″) chemical name: (6*R-trans*)-3-[(acetyloxy)methyl]-8-oxo-7-[(2-thienyl)amino]-5-thia-1-azabicyclo-[4.2.0]oct-2-ene-2-carboxylic acid. A semisynthetic analogue, $C_{16}H_{16}N_2O_6S_2$, of the natural antibiotic cephalosporin C, effective against a wide range of gram-positive and gram-negative bacteria. **c. sodium** [USP], the monosodium salt of cephalothin, $C_{16}H_{15}N_2$-NaO_6S_2, used in the treatment of those infections of the major organ and tissue systems of the body that are due to sensitive pathogens; it is administered parenterally.

cephalothoracic (sef″ah-lo-tho-ras′ik) pertaining to the head and thorax.

cephalothoracopagus (sef″ah-lo-tho′rah-kop′ah-gus) a twin monster united at the head, neck, and thorax. **c. disym′met-ros,** a cephalothoracopagus fused squarely in the frontal plane and presenting two broad anterior surfaces and two narrow posterior ones, with a common head bearing two faces, each being formed by the right and left halves of the different components. **c. monosym′metros,** a cephalothoracopagus with one com-

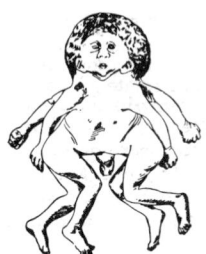

Cephalothoracopagus (Abt).

plete face formed by a right and a left half of the two components, the other face being only rudimentary.

cephalotome (sef′ah-lo-tōm) an instrument for cutting the fetal head.

cephalotomy (sef-ah-lot′o-me) [*cephalo-* + Gr. *temnein* to cut] 1. the cutting up of the fetal head to facilitate delivery. 2. dissection of the fetal head.

cephalotribe (sef′ah-lo-trīb″) [*cephalo-* + Gr. *tribein* to crush] (*obs.*) an instrument for use in cephalotripsy.

cephalotripsy (sef′ah-lo-trip″se) [*cephalo-* + Gr. *tripsis* a rubbing] (*obs.*) the crushing of the fetal head in order to facilitate delivery.

cephalotropic (sef″ah-lo-trop′ik) [*cephalo-* + Gr. *tropos* a turning] having an affinity for brain tissue.

cephalotrypesis (sef″ah-lo-tri-pe′sis) [*cephalo-* + Gr. *trypēsis* a boring] trephination of the cranium.

cephamycin (sef″ah-mi′sin) any of a family of naturally occurring antibacterial antibiotics derived from various species of *Streptomyces* or produced semisynthetically, which are resistant to degradation by *β*-lactamase. Cephamycins A, B, and C have been isolated.

cephapirin (sef-ah-pi′rin) chemical name: [6*R-trans*]-3-[(acetyloxy)methyl]-8-oxo-7-[[(4-pyridinylthio)acetyl]amino]-5-thia-1-aza-acid. A semisynthetic analogue, $C_{17}H_{16}N_3O_6S_2$, of the natural antibiotic cephalosporin, C effective against a wide range of gram-negative and gram-positive bacteria. **c. sodium,** the monosodium salt of cephapirin, $C_{17}H_{16}N_3NaO_6S_2$, used in the treatment of infections of the respiratory and genitourinary tracts, skin, soft tissues, bones, joints, and blood due to sensitive pathogens. It is administered intramuscularly and intravenously. Sterile cephapirin sodium [USP] conforms to FDA regulations concerning antibiotic drugs.

cephradine (sef′rah-dēn) [USP] chemical name: [6*R*-[6α,7β-(*R**)]]-7-[(amino-1,4-cyclohexadien-1-ylacetyl)amino]-3-methyl-8-oxo-5-thia-1-azabicyclo[4.2.0]oct-2-ene-carboxylic acid. A semisynthetic analogue, $C_{16}H_{19}N_3O_4S$, of the natural antibiotic cephalosporin C, effective against a wide range of gram-positive and gram-negative bacteria; used in the treatment of infections of the urinary tract, skin, and soft tissues due to sensitive pathogens, administered orally or by intramuscular or intravenous injection.

ceptor (sep′tor) 1. in Ehrlich's side-chain theory, receptors that have been thrown off into the blood stream. 2. any nervous apparatus that receives external stimuli or impressions and transfers them to the nerve centers. Cf. *beneceptor* and *nociceptor.* **chemical c.,** a ceptor that transforms proper stimuli into electrochemical reactions in the body. **contact c.,** a ceptor that receives stimuli of direct physical contact. **distance c.,** the nervous apparatus through which an individual perceives or is affected by his distant environment. **nerve c.,** ceptor, def. 2.

cera (se′rah) [L.] wax. **c. al′ba,** white wax. **c. fla′va,** yellow wax.

ceraceous (se-ra′shus) [L. *cera* wax] waxlike in appearance.

ceramics (sĕ-ram′iks) [Gr. *keramos* potters' clay] the modeling and processing of objects made of clay or similar material. **dental c.,** the employment of porcelain and similar materials in restorative dentistry; called also *ceramodontics.*

ceramidase (ser-am′ĭ-dās) an enzyme occurring in most mammalian tissue that catalyzes the reversible acylation-deacylation of ceramides.

ceramide (ser′ah-mīd) any of a group of naturally occurring sphingolipids in which the NH_2 group of sphingosine is acylated with a fatty acyl CoA derivative to form an *N*-acylsphingosine. **galactosyl c.,** cerebroside. **c. glucoside,** the major sphingolipid accumulated in Gaucher's disease; called also *glucocerebroside.* **c. trihexoside,** the major sphingolipid accumulated in Fabry's disease.

ceramidosis (ser-am″ĭ-do′sis)) accumulation of ceramides in tissues. **lactosyl c.,** ceramide lactosidosis.

ceramodontics (se-ram″o-don′tiks) dental ceramics.

cerasin (ser′ah-sin) a class of gums from cherry, plum, and other trees, containing carbohydrate; they are insoluble in cold water.

cerasine (ser′ah-sīn) a red azo dye, $C_{10}H_7 \cdot N{:}N \cdot C_{10}H_4(SO_2-ONa)_2 \cdot OH$, used as a cytoplasmic stain.

cerasus (ser'ah-sus) [L.] cherry, or cherry tree; see *Prunus*.

cerate (se'rāt) [L. *ceratum*, from *cera* wax] a medicinal preparation for external application, made with a basis of fat or wax, or both, intermediate in consistency between an ointment and a plaster. **simple c.,** a mixture of benzoinated lard and white wax, melted together. **Turner's c.,** calamine ointment.

ceratectomy (ser-ah-tek'to-me) keratectomy.

ceratin (ser'ah-tin) keratin.

ceratitis (ser"ah-ti'tis) keratitis.

cerato- for words beginning thus, see also those beginning *kerato-*.

ceratocricoid (ser"ah-to-kri'koid) pertaining to the posterior horn of the thyroid cartilage and the cricoid cartilage.

ceratocricoideus (ser"at-to-kri-koi'de-us) see *Table of Musculi*.

ceratohyal (ser"ah-to-hi'al) pertaining to a cornu minus of the hyoid bone.

ceratonosus (ser"ah-ton'o-sus) [Gr. *keras* cornea + *nosos* disease] any disease of the cornea.

ceratopharyn'geus (ser"at-o-fahr-in'je-us) see *Table of Musculi*.

Ceratophyllus (ser"ah-tof'ĭ-lus) [Gr. *keras* horn + *phyllon* leaf] a genus of fleas, now including only bird fleas, but formerly including those of birds and small mammals. **C. acu'tus,** *Diamanus montanus*. **C. fascia'tus,** *Nosopsyllus fasciatus*. **C. galli'nae,** a species that attacks chickens and man. **C. idahoen'sis,** *Oropsylla idahoensis*. **C. monta'nus,** *Diamanus montanus*. **C. punjaben'sis,** a rat flea of India. **C. silantiew'i,** *Oropsylla silantiewi*. **C. tesquo'rum,** a plague-transmitting flea of ground squirrels in the Russian steppes.

Ceratopogonidae (ser"ah-to-po-gon'ĭ-de) biting midges or sandflies.

ceratum (se-ra'tum) [L.] cerate.

cerberin, cerberine (ser'bĕ-rin) a poisonous alkaloid, $C_{32}H_{48}O_9$, from *Cerbera odallam*, a tree of Asia; a cardiotonic agent.

cercaria (ser-ka're-ah), pl. *cerca'riae* [Gr. *kerkos* tail] the final free-swimming larval stage of a trematode parasite, consisting of a body and tail. Cercariae encyst on aquatic vegetation and penetrate the skin of a fish or the tissues of an aquatic arthropod to form encysted metacercariae. (Cercariae of schistosomes penetrate directly into the skin of the definitive host without forming metacercariae.)

cercaricidal (ser-ka're-si'dal) destructive to cercariae.

cercarienhullenreaktion (ser-ka"re-en-hul"en-re-ak'shun) a test for *Schistosoma mansoni*, utilized in measuring the efficiency of chemotherapy against schistosomiasis. When cercariae of *S. mansoni* are placed *in vitro* in contact with sera of monkeys or men infected with *S. mansoni*, a transparent envelope is formed around each cercaria.

cerclage (sār-klahzh') [Fr. "an encircling"] encircling of a part with a ring or loop, such as encirclement of the incompetent cervix uteri, or the binding together of the ends of a fractured bone with a metal ring or wire loop (tiring).

cercocystis (ser"ko-sis'tis) cysticercoid.

cercoid (ser'koid) the last stage in the development of a tapeworm.

cercomonad (ser-kom'ŏ-nad) any protozoon of the genus *Cercomonas*.

Cercomonas (ser-kom'ŏ-nas) [Gr. *kerkos* tail + *monas* monad] a genus of biflagellate protozoa of the family Bodonidae, sometimes coprozoic. **C. hom'inis,** the name formerly given to the organisms now known as *Trichomonas hominis* and *Chilomastix mesnili*. **C. longicau'da,** a species coprozoic in humas feces.

cercopithecoid (ser"ko-pith'ĕ-koid) an Old World monkey, having a tail but not using it as a limb.

Cercopithecoidea (ser"ko-pith"ĕ-koid'e-ah) a superfamily of the order Primates (suborder Anthropoidea), characterized by nostrils that are close together and directed downward, including the Old World apes and monkeys, and man; formerly called *Catarrhina*.

Cercosphaera addisoni (ser"ko-sfēr'ah ad"ĭ-so'ni) *Microsporum audouini*.

Cercospora apii (ser"kos'por-ah a'pe-i) a fungus that is a common plant pathogen (celery blight) and that causes cercosporamycosis in man.

Cercosporalla vexans (ser"kos-pŏ-ral'ah vek'sanz) a species of molds of the Fungi Imperfecti, order Moniliales, family Moniliaceae, which has been reported to cause skin eruptions, probably a variant of *Trichophyton mentagrophytes*.

cercosporamycosis (ser"ko-spōr"ah-mi-ko'sis) a fungous disease of man in Indonesia characterized by subcutaneous, indurated verrucous lesions in which brown mycelium is seen.

cercus (ser'kus), pl. *cer'ci* [L.; Gr. *kerkos* tail] a bristle-like structure.

cerea flexibilitas (sēr'e-ah-flek"sĭ-bil'ĭ-tas) flexibilitas cerea.

cereal (se're-al) [L. *cerealis*] 1. Pertaining to edible grain. 2. any graminaceous plant bearing an edible seed; also the seed or grain of such a plant.

cerealin (se-re'ah-lin) an enzyme contained in grain extract and capable of converting starch into dextrose.

cerealose (se're-ah-lōs) a substance containing maltose and glucose, obtained by the action of enzymes on grains.

cerebellar (ser"ĕ-bel'ar) pertaining to the cerebellum.

cerebellifugal (ser"ĕ-bel-lif'ŭ-gal) [*cerebellum* + L. *fugere* to flee] tending or proceeding from the cerebellum.

cerebellipetal (ser"ĕ-bel-lip'ĕ-tal) [*cerebellum* + L. *petere* to seek] tending or moving toward the cerebellum.

cerebellitis (ser"ĕ-bel-li'tis) inflammation of the cerebellum.

cerebellofugal (ser"ĕ-bel-lof'ŭ-gal) cerebellifugal.

cerebello-olivary (ser"ĕ-bel"o-ol'ĭ-va-re) conducting or proceeding from the cerebellum to the olivary body.

cerebellopontile (ser"ĕ-bel"o-pon'tēl) conducting or proceeding from the cerebellum to the pons varolii.

cerebellopontine (ser"ĕ-bel"o-pon'tēn) cerebellopontile.

cerebellorubral (ser"ĕ-bel"o-ru'bral) conducting or proceeding from the cerebellum to the red nucleus.

cerebellorubrospinal (ser"ĕ-bel"o-roo"bro-spi'nal) conducting or proceeding from the cerebellum, to the red nucleus, and then to the spinal cord.

cerebellospinal (ser"ĕ-bel"o-spi'nal) conducting or proceeding from the cerebellum to the spinal cord.

cerebellum (ser"ĕ-bel'um) [L. dim. of *cerebrum* brain] [NA] the part of the metencephalon that occupies the posterior cranial fossa behind the brain stem, being a fissured mass consisting of a median lobe (vermis) and two lateral lobes (the hemispheres) connected with the brain stem by three pairs of peduncles. It is concerned in the coordination of movements.

cerebral (ser'ĕ-bral, sĕ-re'bral) pertaining to the cerebrum.

cerebration (ser"ĕ-bra'shun) [L. *cerebratio*] functional activity of the cerebrum. **unconscious c.,** mental action of which the subject has no consciousness.

cerebriform (sĕ-reb'rĭ-form) [L. *cerebrum* brain + *forma* form] resembling the brain or brain substance.

cerebrifugal (ser"ĕ-brif'u-gal) [*cerebrum* + L. *fugere* to flee] conducting or proceeding away from the brain, or cerebrum.

cerebripetal (ser"ĕ-brip'ĕ-tal) [*cerebrum* + L. *petere* to seek] conducting or proceeding toward the brain, or cerebrum.

cerebritis (ser"ĕ-bri'tis) inflammation of the cerebrum. **saturnine c.,** brain inflammation due to lead poisoning.

cerebrocardiac (ser"ĕ-bro-kar'de-ak) [*cerebrum* + L. *cardia* heart] pertaining to the brain and heart.

cerebrocentric (ser"ĕ-bro-sen'trik) [*cerebro-* + Gr. *kentrikos* of or from the center] relating to the concept, or designating, that control of the personality centers in the physical brain, as distinguished from the mind or the psychical system of the individual. Cf. *psychocentric*.

cerebrocerebellar (ser"ĕ-bro-ser"ĕ-bel'ar) pertaining to the cerebrum and the cerebellum.

cerebrocuprein (ser"ĕ-bro-ku'pre-in) a copper protein isolated from the human and bovine brain.

cerebrogalactose (ser"ĕ-bro-gah-lak'tos) galactose (of cerebrosides).

cerebrogalactoside (ser"ĕ-bro-gah-lak'to-sīd) cerebroside.

cerebrohyphoid (ser"ĕ-bro-hi'foid) [*cerebrum* + Gr. *hyphē* web + *eidos* form] resembling brain tissue.

cerebroid (ser'e-broid) resembling the brain substance.

cerebrology (ser"ĕ-brol'o-je) [*cerebrum* + *-logy*] the sum of knowledge regarding the brain.

cerebroma (ser"ĕ-bro'mah) any abnormal mass of brain substance.

cerebromacular (ser"ĕ-bro-mak'u-lar) pertaining to or affecting the brain and the macula retinae.

cerebromalacia (ser"ĕ-bro-mah-la'she-ah) [*cerebrum* + Gr. *malakos* soft] abnormal softening of the substance of the cerebrum.

cerebromedullary (ser"ĕ-bro-med'u-la-re) cerebrospinal.

cerebromeningeal (ser"ĕ-bro-mĕ-nin'je-al) pertaining to the brain and its membranes.

cerebromeningitis (ser"ĕ-bro-men"in-ji'tis) meningoencephalitis.

cerebron (ser'ĕ-bron) phrenosin.

cerebro-ocular (ser"e-bro-ok'u-lar) pertaining to the brain and the eye.

cerebropathia (ser"ĕ-bro-path'e-ah) [L.] cerebropathy. **c. psy'chica toxe'mica,** Korsakoff's psychosis.

cerebropathy (ser"ĕ-brop'ah-the) [*cerebrum* + Gr. *pathos* disease] any disorder of the brain.

cerebrophysiology (ser"ĕ-bro-fiz"e-ol'o-je) the physiology of the cerebrum.

cerebropontile (ser″ĕ-bro-pon′til) pertaining to the cerebrum and pons.

cerebropsychosis (ser″e-bro″si-ko′sis) [*cerebrum* + *psychosis*] (*obs.*) organic brain syndrome; see under *syndrome*.

cerebrorachidian (ser″ĕ-bro″rah-kid′e-an) cerebrospinal.

cerebrosclerosis (ser″ĕ-bro″skle-ro′sis) [*cerebrum* + *sclerosis*] morbid hardening of the substance of the cerebrum.

cerebrose (ser′e-brōs) galactose (of cerebrosides).

cerebroside (ser′ĕ-bro-sīd″) a general designation of an acid amide of a C_{24}, C_{18}, or C_{16} fatty acid with sphingosine or di-hydrosphingosine in glycosidic linkage with galactose or glucose. Kerasin and phrenosin are typical members of this class. It is abundant in membranes of nervous tissue, especially the myelin sheath, and is a major component of the cell coats of higher organisms. Called also *cerebrogalactoside, galactocerebroside,* and *glucocerebroside.*

cerebrosidosis (ser″ĕ-bro″si-do′sis) a lipoidosis in which the fatty accumulation in the body consists largely of kerasin, as in Gaucher's disease.

cerebrosis (ser″ĕ-bro′sis) any disease of the cerebrum.

cerebrospinal (ser″ĕ-bro-spi′nal) pertaining to the brain and spinal cord.

cerebrospinant (ser″ĕ-bro-spi′nant) any medicine or agent that affects the brain and spinal cord.

cerebrospinase (ser″e-bro-spi′nās) an oxidizing enzyme occurring in the cerebrospinal fluid.

cerebrostomy (ser″ĕ-bros′to-me) [*cerebrum* + Gr. *stoma* opening] the making of an artificial opening into the cerebrum.

cerebrotendinous (ser″ĕ-bro-ten′dĭ-nus) pertaining to the cerebrum and the tendons.

cerebrotomy (ser″ĕ-brot′o-me) [*cerebrum* + Gr. *temnein* to cut] the anatomy or dissection of the brain.

cerebrotonia (ser″ĕ-bro-to′ne-ah) [*cerebro-* + Gr. *tonos* tension + *-ia*] (*obs.*) a psychic type characterized by predominance of restraint, inhibition, and desire for concealment.

cerebrovascular (ser″ĕ-bro-vas′ku-lar) pertaining to the blood vessels of the cerebrum, or brain.

cerebrum (ser′ĕ-brum, sĕ-re′brum) [L.] 1. [NA] the main portion of the brain, occupying the upper part of the cranial cavity; its two hemispheres (see *cerebral hemisphere*, under *hemisphere*), united by the corpus callosum, form the largest part of the central nervous system in man. It is derived (developed) from the telencephalon of the embryo. 2. a term sometimes applied to the postembryonic prosencephalon and mesencephalon together or to the entire brain. **c. exsicca′tum,** the gray substance of the brain of calves, freed from fats, dried, and pulverized; used therapeutically in brain and nervous diseases.

cerecloth (sēr′kloth) cloth impregnated with wax and made antiseptic; used in dressings.

Cerenkov radiation (ka′ren-kov) [P. A. *Cerenkov,* Russian physicist] see under *radiation*.

cereoli (se-re′o-li) plural of *cereolus*.

cereolus (se-re′o-lus), pl. *cere′oli* [L., dim. of *cereus* wax taper] a medicated bougie.

cerevisia (ser″e-viz′e-ah), pl. and gen., *cerevis′iae* [L.] beer, ale, porter, or other brewed malt liquor. **cerevis′iae fermen′tum,** brewer's yeast. **cerevis′iae fermen′tum compres′sum,** compressed yeast.

cerevisiae (ser″e-viz′e-e) [L.] plural and genitive singular of *cerevisia.*

cerin (se′rin) cerotic acid.

Cerithidia (ser″ĭ-thid′e-ah) a genus of spiral-shelled snails found in brackish water in tropical and subtropical areas. **C. cing′ulata,** the chief intermediate host of *Heterophyes heterophyes;* it is found in Japan.

cerium (se′re-um) [L.] a metallic element: symbol, Ce; atomic number, 58; atomic weight, 140.12. **c. oxalate,** a white, insoluble powder, a mixture of the oxalates of cerium, neodymium, praseodymium, lanthanum, and other elements; sedative, tonic, and nervine; has been used as a sedative and antiemetic.

ceroid (se′roid) an insoluble, acid-fast, sudanophilic, lipid pigment found in the liver, the nervous system, and muscle.

cerolipoid (se″ro-li′poid) a waxy substance existing in plants.

cerolysin (se-rol′ĭ-sin) [L. *cera* wax + *-lysin*] a lysin that decomposes wax.

ceroma (se-ro′mah) [Gr. *kērōma* waxy mass] a tumor of tissue that has undergone a waxy degeneration.

ceroplasty (se′ro-plas″te) [L. *cera* wax + Gr. *plassein* to mold] the making of anatomical models in wax.

cerotin (ser′o-tin) ceryl alcohol.

certifiable (ser″tĭ-fi′ah-b'l) capable of being certified; said of infectious diseases, cases of which must by law be reported to the health officers.

cerulein (sĕ-roo′le-in) a decapeptide amide isolated from the skin of frogs; it is a peptide analogue of choleystokinin and gastrin; in mammals it is a powerful stimulant of gallbladder contraction.

ceruloplasmin (sĕ-roo″lo-plaz′min) an alpha₂-globulin of the plasma, being a glycoprotein in which approximately 96 per cent of the plasma copper is transported.

cerumen (sĕ-roo′men) [L. from *cera* wax] the waxlike secretion found within the external meatus of the ear; called also *earwax*. **impacted c.,** accumulated cerumen forming a solid mass that adheres to the wall of the external auditory canal. **inspissated c.,** dried earwax in the external canal of the ear.

ceruminal (sĕ-roo′mĭ-nal) of or pertaining to the cerumen.

ceruminolysis (sĕ-roo″mĭ-nol′ĭ-sis) the solution or disintegration of cerumen in the external auditory meatus.

ceruminolytic (sĕ-roo″mĭ-no-lit′ik) 1. pertaining to, characterized by, or promoting ceruminolysis. 2. an agent that dissolves cerumen in the external auditory canal.

ceruminoma (sĕ-roo″mĭ-no′mah) tumor of the ceruminous glands.

ceruminosis (sĕ-roo″mĭ-no′sis) excessive or disordered secretion of cerumen.

ceruminous (sĕ-roo′mĭ-nus) ceruminal.

ceruse (se′rōōs) [L. *cerussa*] the basic carbonate of lead; white lead.

cervical (ser′vĭ-kal) [L. *cervicalis,* from *cervix* neck] pertaining to the neck, or to the neck of any organ or structure.

cervicalis (ser″vĭ-ka′lis) [L.] cervical.

cervicectomy (ser″vĭ-sek′to-me) excision of the cervix uteri; called also *trachelectomy.*

cervicitis (ser″vĭ-si′tis) inflammation of the cervix uteri; called also *trachelitis*. **granulomatous c.,** granulomatous infections of the cervix, including tuberculosis, syphilis, and granuloma inguinale. **traumatic c.,** a nonspecific cervicitis resulting from such procedures as irradiation or cauterization.

cervicoaxillary (ser″vĭ-ko-ak′sĭ-lār-e) pertaining to the neck and axilla.

cervicobrachial (ser″vĭ-ko-bra′ke-al) pertaining to the neck and arm.

cervicobrachialgia (ser″vĭ-ko-brak′e-al′je-ah) pain in the neck radiating to the arm, due to compression of nerve roots of the cervical spinal cord.

cervicobuccal (ser″vĭ-ko-buk′al) buccocervical.

cervicocolpitis (ser″vĭ-ko-kol-pi′tis) inflammation of the cervix uteri and vagina. **c. emphysemato′sa,** colpitis emphysematosa with similar lesions occurring beneath the squamous mucosa of the cervix uteri.

cervicodorsal (ser″vĭ-ko-dor′sal) pertaining to the neck and the back.

cervicodynia (ser″vĭ-ko-din′e-ah) [*cervix* + Gr. *odynē* pain] pain in the neck.

cervicofacial (ser″vĭ-ko-fa′she-al) pertaining to the neck and face.

cervicolabial (ser″vĭ-ko-la′be-al) labiocervical.

cervicolingual (ser″vĭ-ko-ling′gwal) linguocervical.

cervico-occipital (ser″vĭ-ko-ok-sip′ĭ-tal) pertaining to the neck and occiput.

cervicoplasty (ser″vĭ-ko-plas′te) [*cervix* + Gr. *plassein* to form] plastic surgery on the neck.

cervicoscapular (ser″vĭ-ko-skap′u-lar) pertaining to the neck and scapula.

cervicothoracic (ser″vĭ-ko-tho-ras′ik) pertaining to the neck and thorax.

cervicovaginitis (ser″vĭ-ko-vaj′ĭ-ni′tis) inflammation involving both the cervix uteri and vagina.

cervicovesical (ser″vĭ-ko-ves′e-kal) pertaining to the cervix uteri and urinary bladder.

Cervilaxin (ser″vĭ-lak′sin) trademark for a preparation of relaxin.

cervimeter (ser-vim′ĕ-ter) [*cervix* + Gr. *metron* measure] an apparatus for measuring the cervix uteri.

cervix (ser′viks), pl. *cer′vices* [L.] neck; [NA] a term denoting the front portion of the collum, or neck (the part connecting the head and trunk), or a constricted part of an organ (e.g., cervix uteri). **c. of axon,** a constricted part of an axon, before the myelin sheath is added. **c. colum′nae posterio′ris, c. cor′nu,** the constricted part of the dorsal horn of gray matter in the spinal cord. **c. den′tis,** neck of the tooth (collum dentis [NA]). **c. glan′dis,** collum glandis penis. **incompetent c.,** one that is abnormally prone to dilate in the second trimester of pregnancy, resulting in premature expulsion of the fetus (middle trimester abortion). **c. mal′lei,** collum mallei. **tapiroid c.,** a uterine cervix with a peculiarly elongated anterior lip. **c. u′teri,** neck of uterus: the lower and narrow end of the uterus, between the isthmus and the ostium uteri. **c. vesi′cae** [NA], a constricted portion of the urinary bladder, formed by the meeting of its inferolateral surfaces proximal to the opening of the urethra.

ceryl (se′ril) a univalent aliphatic, straight-chain hydrocarbon radical having the formula $C_{26}H_{53}$.

c.e.s. central excitatory state; see under *state*.

cesarean (se-sa're-an) [L. *caesarea,* from *caedere* to cut] see under *section.*

Cesaris Demel bodies (cha'sar-is da'mel) [Antonio *Cesaris Demel,* Italian pathologist, born 1866] see under *body.*

cesium (se'ze-um) [L. *caesium,* from *caesius* blue] a rare univalent metallic element with an alkaline oxide; atomic number, 55; atomic weight, 132.905; symbol, Cs. Some of its salts and binary compounds are used like those of potassium.

Cestan-Chenais syndrome (ses-tan'shen-āz') [Raymond *Cestan,* French neurologist, 1872–1934] see under *syndrome.*

Cestan-Raymond syndrome (ses-tan'-ra-maw') [Etienne Jacques Marie Raymond *Cestan;* Fulgence *Raymond,* French neurologist, 1844–1910] Raymond-Cestan syndrome.

cesticidal (ses"tĭ-si'dal) destructive to cestodes.

Cestoda (ses-to'dah) a subclass of Cestoidea comprising the true tapeworms, which have a head or scolex, and segments or proglottides. Adult tapeworms are endoparasitic in the alimentary tract and associated ducts of various vertebrate hosts; their larval stages (cysticercus, coenurus, hydatid, sparganum) may be found in various organs or tissues. Of the eleven orders, two—Pseudophyllidea and Cyclophyllidea—contain species that parasitize man and other animals. Called also *Eucestoda.*

Cestodaria (ses-to-da're-ah) a subclass of tapeworms, the unsegmented tapeworms of the class Cestoidea, which are endoparasitic in the intestines and coelom of various primitive fishes and rarely in reptiles.

cestode (ses'tōd) 1. any tapeworm or platyhelminth of the class Cestoidea, especially those of the subclass Cestoda. 2. cestoid.

cestodiasis (ses"to-di'ah-sis) infection by cestodes.

cestodology (ses"to-dol'o-je) the scientific study of cestodes.

cestoid (ses'toid) [Gr. *kestos* girdle + *eidos* form] resembling a tapeworm.

Cestoidea (ses-toi'de-ah) a class of tapeworms (platyhelminths) characterized by the absence of a mouth and digestive tract and by the presence of a noncuticular layer covering their bodies. It comprises two subclasses: Cestodaria and Cestoda.

cetaben sodium (se'tah-ben) chemical name: 4-(hexadecylamino)benzoic acid sodium salt; an antihyperlipoproteinemic, $C_{23}H_{38}NNaO_2$.

cetaceum (sĕ-ta'se-um) spermaceti.

cetalkonium chloride (set-al-ko'ne-um) chemical name: *N*-hexadecyl-*N,N*-dimethylbenzene methanaminium chloride. A cationic quaternary ammonium surfactant, $C_{25}H_{46}ClN$, used as a topical anti-infective and disinfectant.

cetanol (se'tah-nol) a solid white alcohol, $C_{16}H_{33}OH$, from sperm oil.

cetiedil citrate (sĕ-ti'ĕ-dil) chemical name: 2-(hexahydro-1*H*-azepin-1-yl) ethyl ester α-cyclohexyl-α-hydroxy-1,2,3-propanetricarboxylate (1:1); a peripheral vasodilator, $C_{20}H_{31}NO_2S \cdot C_6H_8O_7$, which has been used in the treatment of arteritis, Raynaud's disease, and acrocyanosis.

cetocycline hydrochloride (se"to-si'klēn) chemical name: [4*R*-(4α,4aβ,12aβ)]-acetyl-4-amino-4a,12a-dihydro-3,10,11,12a-tetrahydroxy-6,9-dimethyl-1,12(4*H*,5*H*)-naphthacenedione; an antibacterial, $C_{22}H_{21}NO_7 \cdot HCl$.

cetohexazine (se-to-heks'ah-zēn) ketohexazine.

Cetraria (sĕ-tra're-ah) 1. a genus of lichens. 2. the official name of *C. islandica,* so-called Iceland moss; it is nutritious and useful in lung and bowel affections, and is a source of lichenin.

cetrimide (se'trĭ-mīd) cetrimonium bromide.

cetrimonium bromide (set"rĭ-mo'ne-um) a quaternary ammonium antiseptic and detergent composed of a mixture of tetradecyltrimethylammonium bromide with dodecyl- and hexadecyltrimethyl ammonium bromides, $C_{19}H_{42}BrN$, occurring as a white to creamy white powder; applied topically to the skin to cleanse wounds, as a preoperative disinfectant, and to treat seborrhea of the scalp; solutions are also used to cleanse utensils and to store surgical instruments. Abbreviated CTBA. Called also *cetrimide* and *cetyltrimethylammonium bromide.*

cetyl (se'til) a univalent alcohol radical, $CH_3(CH_2)_{14}CH_2.$

cetylpyridinium chloride (se"til-pi"rĭ-din'e-um) [USP] chemical name: 1-hexadecylpyridinium chloride. A cationic disinfectant, $C_{21}H_{38}ClN \cdot H_2O$, occurring as a white powder; used as a local anti-infective administered sublingually or applied topically to intact skin and mucous membranes, and as a preservative in pharmaceutical preparations.

cetyltrimethylammonium bromide (se"til-meth"il-ah-mo'ne-um) cetrimonium bromide.

Cevalin (se'vah-lin) trademark for preparations of ascorbic acid (vitamin C).

Cevex (se'veks) trademark for a liquid preparation of ascorbic acid (vitamin C).

Ce-Vi-Sol (se'vi-sol) trademark for a preparation of ascorbic acid for calibrated dropper dosage.

Ceylancyclostoma (se"lan-si-klos'to-mah) *Ancylostoma braziliense.*

ceyssatite (sēs'ah-tīt) [*Ceyssat,* a village of France] a white earth from France, useful as an adsorbent powder in eczema and hyperidrosis, and in preparing ointments and medicated pastes.

CF cardiac failure; Christmas factor (see under *factor.*)

C.F. carbolfuchsin; citrovorum factor.

Cf chemical symbol for *californium.*

cf. abbreviation for L. *confer* bring together, compare.

c.f.f. critical fusion frequency (flicker fusion threshold); see under *flicker.*

C.F.T. complement-fixation test; see under *fixation.*

CFU-C colony-forming unit–culture, a granulocytic precursor cell which grows in *in vitro* culture in the presence of appropriate stimulators.

CFU-E colony-forming unit–erythroid, a red cell precursor detectable in *in vitro* culture; it precedes the proerythroblast in development but follows the BFU-E.

CFU-S colony-forming unit–spleen, the pluripotential stem cell which gives rise to the erythroid, granulocytic, and megakaryocytic cell lines; so named because the cell gives rise to colonies of marrow cells in the spleen of irradiated mice.

CG trademark for a preparation of indocyanine green.

cg. centigram.

cgm. centigram.

C.G.S., c.g.s. abbreviation for *centimeter-gram-second* system, a system of measurements in which the units are based on the centimeter as the unit of length, the gram as the unit of mass, and the second as the unit of time.

C.H. crown-heel (length of fetus).

Ch¹ Christchurch chromosome; see under *chromosome.*

C.H.A. Catholic Hospital Association.

CH₄ methane.

C₂H₂ acetylene.

C₂H₄ ethylene.

C₆H₆ benzene.

Chabert's disease (shah-bārz') [Philebert *Chabert,* French veterinarian, 1737–1814] symptomatic anthrax.

Chabertia (shah-ber'te-ah) a genus of nematodes parasitic in animals. **C. ovi'na,** a species of worms, the large-mouth bowel worm, parasitic in the colon of sheep, goats, and cattle.

Chaddock's reflex (sign) (chad'oks) [Charles Gilbert *Chaddock,* St. Louis neurologist, 1861–1936] see under *reflex.*

chafe (chāf) to irritate the skin, as by the rubbing together of opposing folds.

Chagas' disease (chag'as) [Carlos *Chagas,* physician in Brazil, 1879–1934] see under *disease.*

Chagas-Cruz disease (chag'as-kruz) [Carlos *Chagas;* Oswald *Cruz,* Brazilian physician, 1871–1917] Chagas' disease.

Chagasia (chah-gas'e-ah) [Carlos *Chagas*] a subgenus of *Anopheles* mosquitoes of Central and South America.

chagasic (chah-gas'ik) pertaining to or due to Chagas' disease.

chagoma (chă-go'mah) a skin tumor occurrring in Chagas' disease.

Chagres fever (chag'res) [named from a river in Panama] see under *fever.*

Chailletia (ka-il-e'she-ah) a genus of trees and shrubs, nearly all tropical. **C. cymo'sa,** a species of South Africa that contains the poison fluoroacetic acid. **C. toxica'ria,** of West Africa, bears poisonous fruit and seeds.

Chain (chān), Ernst Boris. A German biochemist, born 1906; co-winner, with Sir Alexander Fleming and Sir Howard Walter Florey, of the Nobel prize for medicine in 1945 for his work on antibacterial substances produced by microorganisms.

chain (chān) a collection of objects linked together in linear fashion, or end to end, as the assemblage of atoms or radicals in a chemical compound, or an assemblage of individual bacterial cells. **branched c.,** an open chain of atoms, usually carbon, with one or more side chains attached to it. **closed c.,** several atoms linked together so as to form a ring, which may be

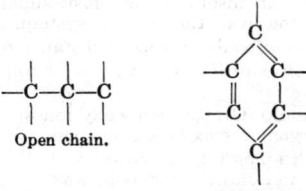

Open chain.   Closed chain.

saturated, as in cyclopentane, or aromatic, as in benzene. **food c.,** a sequence of organisms through which energy is transferred from its ultimate source in a plant; each organism eats the preceding and is eaten by the following member in the sequence. **heavy c.,** any of the large polypeptide chains of five classes that, paired with the light chains, make up the antibody molecule; see *immunoglobulin.* Heavy chains bear the antigenic determinants that differentiate the immunoglobulin classes. **J c.,** a polypeptide present in both IgM and certain IgA molecules that permits them to form polymers. **kappa c.,** a light polypeptide chain of immunoglobulin molecules; see *light c.* **lambda c.,** a light polypeptide chain found in immunoglobulin molecules; they are of two types, kappa and lambda, which are unrelated to immunoglobulin class differences. See *immunoglobulin.* Light chains have an N-terminal variable region related to the antibody combining site and a C-terminal constant region which is invariable with the exception of the Inv and Oz group allotypic markers. **nuclear c.,** a longitudinal array of nuclei occurring on an intrafusal fiber of muscle. **open c.,** several atoms united to form an open chain; compounds of this series are related to methane and are also called *fatty, aliphatic, acyclic,* or *paraffin* compounds. **side c.,** a chain of atoms attached to a larger chain or to a ring; called also *lateral c.* **sympathetic c.,** the sympathetic trunk (truncus sympathicus [NA]).

Chalara (kah-lar′ah) a genus of imperfect fungi of the order Moniliales, which causes many diseases of plants, such as oak wilt.

chalasia (kah-la′ze-ah) [Gr. *chalasis* relaxation] relaxation of a bodily opening, such as the cardiac sphincter, which is a cause of vomiting in infants.

chalastodermia (kah-las″to-der′me-ah) cutis laxa.

chalaza (kah-la′zah) [Gr. "lump"] a spiral band of albumin extending from either end of the yolk of a bird's egg to the shell.

chalazia (kah-la′ze-ah) [Gr.] plural of *chalazion.*

chalazion (kah-la′ze-on), pl. *chala′zia* or *chalazions* [Gr. "small lump"] an eyelid mass that results from chronic inflammation of a meibomian gland and shows a granulomatous reaction to liberated fat when subjected to histopathological examination; sometimes called *meibomian* or *tarsal cyst.*

chalazodermia (kah-laz″o-der′me-ah) cutis laxa.

chalcitis (kal-si′tis) chalkitis.

chalcone (kal′kōn) [Gr. *chalkos* copper or brass] any one of a group of yellow pigments that are substituted benzalacetophenone derivatives.

chalcosis (kal-ko′sis) [Gr. *chalkos* copper] the presence of copper deposits in the tissues. **c. cor′neae,** deposition of copper in the cornea resulting in a pigmented ring in the deeper layers; seen especially in metal workers. **c. len′tis,** sunflower cataract.

chalicosis (kal-ĭ-ko′sis) [Gr. *chalix* gravel] a disorder of the lungs or bronchioles (chiefly among stone-cutters), due to the inhalation of fine particles of stones; it is a form of pneumoconiosis. Called also *flint disease.*

chalinoplasty (kal′ĭ-no-plas″te) [Gr. *chalinos* a corner of the mouth + *plassein* to mold] plastic surgery of the angle of the mouth.

chalk (chawk) [L. *calx* or *creta*] 1. impure calcium carbonate. 2. prepared c. **French c.,** talc. **precipitated c.,** precipitated calcium carbonate. **prepared c.,** native calcium carbonate freed from most of its impurities by elutriation; used as an antacid, and has been used in the treatment of diarrhea and in the preparation of dentifrices.

chalkitis (kal-ki′tis) [Gr. *chalkos* brass] inflammation of the eyes caused by rubbing the eyes after the hands have been used on brass; called also *brassy eye.*

challenge (chal′enj) in immunology, (1) to administer antigen to evoke an immunologic response in a previously sensitized individual, or (2) an instance of so challenging.

chalone (kal′ōn) [Gr. *chalan* to relax] 1. a group of tissue-specific (but not species-specific) water-soluble substances that are produced within a tissue and that inhibit mitosis of cells of that tissue and whose action is reversible. 2. (*obs.*) a substance which neutralizes the action of a hormone; inhibitory hormone.

chalonic (kah-lon′ik) of or pertaining to a chalone.

chaluni (chal-oo′ne) pitted keratolysis.

chalybeate (kah-lib′e-āt) [L. *chalybs*; Gr. *chalyps* steel] containing or charged with iron: ferruginous or martial.

chamaecephalic (kam″e-se-fal′ik) pertaining to or characterized by chamaecephaly.

chamaecephaly (kam″e-sef′ah-le) [Gr. *chamai* low + *kephalē* head] the condition of having a low flat head, that is, a cephalic index of 70 or less.

chamaeprosopic (kam″ĕ-pro-sop′ik) pertaining to or characterized by chamaeprosopy.

chamaeprosopy (kam″ĕ-pros′o-pe) [Gr. *chamai* low + *prosōpon* face] the condition of having a low, broad face, i.e., a facial index of 90 or less.

chamber (chām′ber) [L. *camera*; Gr. *kamara*] an enclosed space or antrum. **Abbé-Zeiss counting c.,** Thoma-Zeiss counting c. **acoustic c.,** a soundproof room or enclosure used in measuring hearing. **air c.,** relief c. **air-equivalent ionization c.,** in radiology, a chamber in which the materials of the wall

and electrodes are such that ionizing radiations produce ionization essentially similar to that in a free air ionization chamber. **altitude c.,** a vacuum chamber used to simulate the effects of high altitude and low atmospheric pressure. **anterior c. of eye,** that portion of the aqueous-containing space between the cornea and the lens which is bounded in front by the cornea and part of the sclera, and behind by the iris, part of the ciliary body, and that part of the lens which presents through the pupil; called also *camera anterior bulbi* [NA]. **aqueous c.,** that part of the eyeball which is filled with aqueous humor; see *anterior c. of eye* and *posterior c. of eye.* **bubble c.,** an instrument designed to permit the use of superheated liquid to display the tracks of ionizing particles, the ions acting as nuclei for the production of small bubbles along the path of the particle. **cloud c.,** an instrument with a chamber containing air or other gas saturated with vapor, used in demonstrating the tracks produced by the passage of ionizing particles. **counting c.,** a space of definite thickness provided with a ruled base, into which blood samples of specific dilutions may be placed, for counting and quantitating the formed elements. **detonating c.,** a muffler surrounding the discharging balls of a static machine or resonator for deadening the sound of a spark discharge. **diffusion c.,** an apparatus for separating a substance by means of a semipermeable membrane. **c's of eye,** the various spaces in the eyeball; see *anterior c. of eye, posterior c. of eye,* and *vitreous c.* **Haldane c.,** an air-tight chamber in which animals may be confined for the performance of metabolic studies; called also *Haldane apparatus.* **c's of the heart,** the cavities of the atria and ventricles. **hyperbaric c.,** a compartment in which the air pressure may be raised to more than normal atmospheric pressure; used in treatment of gas gangrene and other anaerobic infections, or other conditions in which a high concentration of oxygen is desirable, and for studying the effects of pressure and decompression in animals and man. **ionization c.,** any chamber designed to permit measurement of the ionization of the gas contained in the chamber. **lethal c.,** a chamber that may be filled with gas, for killing small animals. **Petroff-Hauser counting c.,** a chamber containing a grid and so arranged as to hold a fixed volume of fluid; used to count microorganisms such as bacteria under high magnification. **posterior c. of eye,** that portion of the aqueous-containing space of the eye which is bounded in front by the iris, and behind by the lens and suspensory ligament; called also *camera posterior bulbi* [NA]. **pulp c.,** the natural cavity in the central portion of the tooth crown occupied by the dental pulp; called also *pulp cavity.* **relief c.,** the recess in the surface of a denture that rests on the oral structures, to reduce or eliminate pressure on the tissues at that particular site in the mouth. **standard ionization c.,** a chamber in which a delimited beam of radiation passes between the electrodes without striking them or other internal parts of the equipment. **Storm Van Leeuwen c.,** a room that can be kept free of airborne antigens for allergic patients. **thimble ionization c.,** a small thimble-shaped ionization chamber, usually with walls of organic material. **Thoma-Zeiss counting c.,** a device consisting of a receptacle in the bottom of a slide for a microscope, with ruled lines dividing the area into minute squares, to facilitate the counting of blood corpuscles or other cells; called also *Abbe-Zeiss counting c.* **tissue-equivalent ionization c.,** a chamber in which the walls, electrodes, and gas are so selected that ionizing radiations produce ionization essentially equivalent to the characteristics of the tissue under consideration. **vitreous c.,** the space in the eyeball enclosing the vitreous humor, bounded anteriorly by the lens and ciliary body, and posteriorly by the posterior wall of the eyeball. **Zappert's c.,** a form of counting chamber.

Chamberland filter (shahm-ber-lah′) [Charles Edouard *Chamberland,* French bacteriologist, 1851–1908] see under *filter.*

Chamberlen forceps [Peter (Pierre) *Chamberlen,* English obstetrician, 1560–1631] see under *forceps.*

chamecephalic (kam″ĕ-se-fal′ik) chamaecephalic.

chamecephaly (kam″ĕ-sef′ah-le) chamaecephaly.

chameprosopic (kam″e-pro-sop′ik) chamaeprosopic.

chameprosopy (kam″ĕ-pros′o-pe) chamaeprosopy.

Champetier de Ribes' bag (shahmp-te-a′ de rēbz′) [Camille Louis Antoine *Champetier de Ribes,* French obstetrician, 1848–1935] see under *bag.*

chancre (shang′ker) [Fr. for "canker," a destructive sore, from L. *cancer* crab] 1. the primary sore of syphilis, a painless, indurated, eroded papule occurring at the site of entry of the infection; called also *hard c., hunterian c.,* and *true c.* 2. the primary cutaneous lesion of such diseases as sporotrichosis and tuberculosis; see *sporotrichotic c.* and *tuberculous c.* **fungating c.,** chancroid characterized by fungoid granulations. **hard c., hunterian c.,** see *chancre.* **mixed c.,** a skin lesion due to simultaneous infection with *Treponema pallidum* (primary syphilis) and *Hemophilus ducreyi* (chancroid); called also *mixed sore.* **recurrent c., c. redux.** **c. re′dux,** chancre developing on the scar of a healed primary chancre, caused by organisms that remain in the scar; called also *monorecidive c., recurrent c.,* and *sclerosis redux.* **Rollet's c.,** mixed c. **soft c.,** chancroid. **sporotrichotic c.,** the primary lesion occurring at the site of inoculation in the cutaneous lymphatic form of sporotrichosis. **true c.,** see *chancre.* **tuberculous c.,** a brownish red papule which develops into an indurated nodule or plaque that may ulcerate, representing the initial cutaneous infection of the tubercle bacillus into the skin or, less often, into the mucosa of a previously unexposed individual, usually a child. Called also *primary inoculation complex* and *primary tuberculous complex.*

chancriform (shang′kre-form) resembling a chancre.

chancroid (shang′kroid) a nonsyphilitic venereal disease transmitted by direct contact, and caused by *Hemophilus ducreyi.* It begins as a painless macule on the genitalia, which enlarges and becomes pustular; an ulcer forms with a shaggy base and adjacent bubo formation. Called also *soft chancre.* See also *mixed chancre.* **phagedenic c.,** a variety attended by sloughing of the tissues. **serpiginous c.,** a variety which tends to spread in curved lines.

chancroidal (shang-kroi′dal) pertaining to chancroid.

chancrous (shang′krus) of the nature of chancre.

change (chānj) an alteration. **Armanni-Ebstein c.,** see under *lesion.* **Crooke's c's, Crooke-Russel c's,** see under *degeneration.* **harlequin color c.,** transient reddening of one half of the body longitudinally with simultaneous blanching of the other half; a temporary vasomotor disorder of the newborn.

Ch'ang Shan (chang′ shan) the Chinese name for the root of the shrub *Dichroa febrifuga* Lour. Basak, Aseru (Saxifragaceae), of China, Java, India, and the Philippines. The Chinese have used it for its antiparasitic, emetic, and antipyretic effect in malaria. It contains several isomeric active alkaloids, e.g., febrifugine, isofebrifugine, and α-, β-, and γ-dichroines.

channel (chan′el) [L. *canalis* a water pipe] that through which anything flows; a cut or groove. **blood c's,** narrow passages with no distinct walls, but containing blood; they are found in fresh granulation tissue. **central c.,** a long straight capillary that connects an arteriole to a venule. **lymph c's,** the smaller lymph sinuses; irregular in and about the lymphatic glands and around lymphatic vessels. **perineural c.,** a lymph channel that surrounds a nerve trunk. **thoroughfare c.,** a channel between terminal arterioles and venules, larger than a capillary.

Ch'an su (chan soo) the dried venom of various Chinese toads.

Chantemesse' reaction (shant-mes′) [André *Chantemesse,* French bacteriologist, 1851–1919] see under *reaction.*

Chaoborus (ka″o-bor′us) a genus of non–blood-sucking gnats of the family Culicidae; called also *Corethra.* **C. lacus′tris,** the Clear Lake gnat of California.

Chaos chaos (ka′os ka′os) *Pelomyxa carolinensis.*

Chaoul therapy, tube (showl) [Henri *Chaoul,* Lebanese radiologist in Berlin, 1887–1964] see under *therapy* and *tube.*

Chapman's mixture, pill (chap′manz) [Nathaniel *Chapman,* American physician, 1780–1853] see under *mixture* and *pill.*

chappa (chap′ah) a disease of West Africa somewhat resembling syphilis or yaws; it is characterized by the formation of marble-sized nodules beneath the skin which degenerate and give off scaly material.

chapped (chapt) roughened and cracked, or split open by the cold or frequent wetting, as chapped hands or lips.

Chaput's method (shap-ōōz′) [Henri *Chaput,* French surgeon, 1857–1919] see under *method.*

character (kar′ak-ter) a quality or attribute indicative of the nature of an object or an organism. In genetics, the expression of a gene or group of genes as seen in a phenotype. **acquired c.,** a noninheritable modification produced in an animal as a result of its own activities or of environmental influences. **compound c.,** a character that is dependent on two or more genes for its production. **dominant c.,** a mendelian character that develops when it is transmitted by a single gene. **imvic c's,** four important characters in the classification of the coliform organisms: they are indole, methyl-red, Voges-Proskauer reaction, and sodium citrate. **mendelian c's,** in genetics, the separate and distinct traits that are exhibited by an animal or plant, and are dependent on the genetic constitution of the organism; they may be recessive or dominant. See *Mendel's law,* under *law.* **primary sex c's,** those characters of the male and female that are concerned directly in reproduction. **recessive c.,** a mendelian character that develops only when it is transmitted by both genes determining the trait. **secondary sex c's,** those characters specific to the male or female organism but not directly concerned in reproduction. **sex-conditioned c.,** an autosomal trait whose full expression is conditioned by the sex of the individual, e.g., human baldness. **sex-influenced c.,** sex-conditioned c. **sex-limited c.,** a sex-linked or autosomal trait that is expressed in one sex only. **sex-linked c.,** one transmitted consistently to individuals of one sex only, being carried in the sex chromosome. **unit c.,** a trait transmitted from parent to offspring intact, i.e., without blending or mixing, though it may be either dominant or recessive.

characteristic (kar″ak-ter-is′tik) 1. character. 2. typical of an individual or other entity. **demand c's,** behavior exhibited by an experimental subject in his attempt to fulfill the expectations of the experimenter as he perceives them; it is believed that the experimenter unknowingly communicates these expectations

by subtle cues or by the design of the experiment itself. Called also *experimenter effects.*

characterization (kar″ak-ter-ĭ-za′shun) in prosthodontics, modification of the form and color of the denture base and teeth and of crown restorations to produce a more lifelike appearance. **denture c.,** see *characterization.*

characterology (kar″ak-ter-ol′o-je) the study of character and personality.

charas (chahr′as) ganja.

charbon (shar-baw′) [Fr. "coal"] anthrax. **c. symptomatique′,** blackleg.

charcoal (char′kōl) carbon prepared by charring wood or other organic material. **activated c.,** [USP], the residue from the destructive distillation of various organic materials, treated to increase its adsorptive powers; used as a general purpose antidote. Called also *carbo activatus.* **animal c.,** charcoal prepared from bone; called also *animal, ivory,* or *Paris black,* and *bone-black.* **purified animal c.,** charcoal prepared from bone and purified by removal of materials dissolved by hot hydrochloric acid and water; adsorbent and decolorizer.

Charcot's arthritis, etc. (shar-kōz′) [Jean Martin *Charcot,* French neurologist, 1825–1893] see under *arthritis, arthropathy, arthrosis, bath, cirrhosis, disease, fever, foot, gait, joint, syndrome,* and *triad.*

Charcot-Leyden crystals (shar-ko′ li′den) [J. M. *Charcot;* Ernst Victor von *Leyden,* German physician, 1832–1910] see under *crystal.*

Charcot-Marie atrophy (type) (shar-ko′ mah-re′) [J. M. *Charcot;* Pierre *Marie,* French physician, 1853–1940] progressive neuropathic (peroneal) muscular atrophy; see under *atrophy.*

Charcot-Marie-Tooth atrophy, disease, type (shar-ko′-mah-re′tooth) [J. M. *Charcot;* Pierre *Marie;* Howard Henry *Tooth,* English physician, 1856–1925] progressive neuropathic (peroneal) muscular atrophy.

Charcot-Neumann crystals (shar-ko′noy′mahn) see under *crystal.*

Charcot-Vigouroux sign (shar-ko′ve-goo-roo′) [J. M. *Charcot;* Romain *Vigouroux,* French physician of 19th century] Vigouroux's sign; see under *sign.*

charlatan (shar′lah-tan) [Fr.] a pretender to knowledge or skills that he does not possess, in medicine, a quack.

charlatanism (shar′lah-tan-izm) the pretension of knowledge and skills that one does not possess; in medicine, quackery.

charlatanry (shar′lah-tan-re) charlatanism.

Charles' law (sharlz) [Jacques Alexandre César *Charles,* French physicist, 1746–1823] see under *law.*

charley horse (char′le-hors) soreness and stiffness in a muscle caused by overstrain or contusion; the term is usually restricted to injuries of the quadriceps muscle.

Charlouis's disease (shar″loo-ēz′) [M. *Charlouis,* Dutch physician in Java] yaws.

Charrière scale (shar″e-ār′) [Joseph Frédéric Benoit *Charrière,* French instrument maker, 1803–1876] see under *scale.*

Charrin's disease (shar-raz′) [Albert *Charrin,* pathologist in Paris, 1857–1907] pyocyanic infection.

charring (char′ing) carbonization; in surgical diathermy, the reduction of tissue into a residue of carbon.

Chart. abbreviation for L. *char′ta,* paper.

chart (chart) 1. a simplified graphic representation of the fluctuation of some variable, as of pulse, temperature, and respiration, or a record of all the clinical data of a particular case. 2. to record graphically the fluctuation of some variable, or to record the clinical data of a particular case. **Amsler's c's,** a set of charts showing various geometric patterns in black and white, e.g., grids or parallel lines, used for detecting defects of the central visual field. **Guibor's c.,** a chart containing outline pictures for orthoptic training. **Hawley c.,** graded outlines of dental arch sizes based on the mesiodistal diameters of the six anterior teeth. **reading c.,** a chart bearing material printed in type of gradually increasing sizes; used in testing acuity of near vision. **Reuss' color c's,** charts with colored letters printed on colored backgrounds, used in testing color vision; called also *Reuss' tables.* **Snellen's c.,** a chart imprinted with block letters (Snellen's test type) in gradually decreasing sizes, identified according to distances at which they are ordinarily visible; used in testing visual acuity.

charta (kar′tah), pl. *char′tae* [L.; Gr. *chartēs*] 1. paper. 2. a piece of paper, medicated or otherwise. **c. explorato′ria caeru′lea,** blue litmus paper; see under *paper.* **c. explorato′ria lu′tea,** turmeric paper; paper stained with turmeric for use as a test paper. **c. explorato′ria ru′bra,** red litmus paper; see under *paper.*

chartaceous (kar-ta′shus) papyraceous.

chartula (kar′tu-lah), pl. *char′tulae* [L. dim. of *charta* paper] a small piece of paper, as for containing a dose of a medicinal powder.

chasma (kaz′mah) [L.; Gr. *chasma* a cleft]   a yawning; an opening.

chasmatoplasson (kaz-mat′o-plas″on)   plasson in an expanded condition. Cf. *pyknoplasson*.

chasmus (kas′mus) [L.; Gr. *chasma* a cleft]   chasma.

Chassaignac's tubercle (shas″ān-yahks′) [Charles Marie Édouard *Chassaignac*, French surgeon, 1804–1879]   *tuberculum caroticum vertebrae cervicalis IV.*

chaude-pisse (shōd-pēs) [Fr.]   a burning sensation experienced during micturition.

chauffage (sho-fahzh′) [Fr. *chauffer* to heat]   treatment with a cautery at low heat which is passed to and fro across the tissue about ¼ inch distant therefrom.

Chauffard's syndrome (sho-farz′) [Anatole Marie Emile *Chauffard*, French physician, 1855–1932]   see under *syndrome*.

Chauffard-Still syndrome (sho-far′stil) [Anatole Marie Emile *Chauffard*; Sir George Frederick *Still*, English physician, 1868–1941]   Chauffard's syndrome.

Chauliac (sho″le-ahk′), Guy de (1300–1368).   An eminent French surgeon who practiced in Avignon. His treatise on surgery (*Chirurgia magna*) was regarded as a standard work until Paré's time.

Chaussier's areola, line (sho″se-āz′) [François *Chaussier*, Parisian surgeon and anatomist, 1746–1828]   see under *areola* and *line*.

Chauveau's bacillus, bacterium (sho-vōz′) [Auguste *Chauveau*, Paris veterinarian, 1827–1917]   *Clostridium chauvoei.*

Ch.B.   abbreviation for L. *Chirur′giae Baccalau′reus*, Bachelor of Surgery.

C₂H₅Br C_2H_5Br ethyl bromide.

CHCl₃ $CHCl_3$ chloroform.

C₂H₄Cl₂ $C_2H_4Cl_2$ ethylene chloride.

C₂H₅Cl C_2H_5Cl ethyl chloride.

C₂H₅CO₂NH₂ $C_2H_5CO_2NH_2$ ethyl carbamate.

(CH₃·CO)₂O $(CH_3 \cdot CO)_2O$ acetic anhydride.

CH₃·COOH $CH_3 \cdot COOH$ acetic acid.

C₄H₉·COOH $C_4H_9 \cdot COOH$ valeric acid.

CHD   coronary heart disease.

Ch.D.   abbreviation for L. *Chirur′giae Doc′tor*, Doctor of Surgery.

ChE   cholinesterase.

Cheadle's disease (che′delz) [Walter Butler *Cheadle*, London pediatrician, 1835–1910]   infantile scurvy.

check-bite (chek′bīt)   a sheet of hard wax or modeling compound placed between the teeth in centric, eccentric, lateral, or protrusive occlusion, to be used as a check on the occlusion of the teeth in those positions in the articulator.

checkerboard (chek′er-bōrd)   a grid with margins which shows the gametes of each parent (in the margins) and their possible progeny (in the squares).

Chediak test (reaction) [Alejandro *Chediak*, Cuban physician]   see under *test*.

cheek (chēk)   a fleshy protuberance, especially the fleshy portion of the side of the face; called also *bucca* [NA]. Also applied to the fleshy mucous-membrane covered side of the oral cavity (bucca cavum oris [NA]).   **cleft c.,** facial cleft caused by developmental failure of union between the maxillary and primitive frontonasal processes.

cheesy (che′ze)   caseous, resembling cheese.

cheil-   see *cheilo-*.

cheilectomy (ki-lek′to-me) [*cheil-* + Gr. *ektomē* excision]   1. excision of a lip.   2. the operation of chiseling off the irregular bony edges of a joint cavity that interfere with motion.

cheilectropion (ki″lek-tro′pe-on) [*cheil-* + *ectropion*]   eversion of the lip.

cheilitis (ki-li′tis) [*cheil-* + *-itis*]   inflammation affecting the lips.   **actinic c., c. actin′ica,** pain and swelling of the lips and development of a scaly crust on the vermilion border after exposure to actinic rays; called also *acute solar c.*   **acute c.,** eczema of the lips.   **angular c.,** perlèche.   **apostematous c.,** see *c. glandularis.*   **commissural c.,** cheilitis affecting principally the angles (commissures) of the mouth.   **c. exfoliati′va,** seborrheic dermatitis affecting the vermilion border of the lips.   **c. glandula′ris,** a rare disease in which the lower lip becomes enlarged, firm, and finally everted, exposing the openings of the accessory salivary glands, which are inflamed and dilated, appearing as small red macules on the mucosa; the glands themselves are enlarged and sometimes nodular. It occurs in three basic types: The *simple type* is characterized by multiple painless, pin-head-sized lesions, with central depressions and dilated canals, and may develop into either of the other two types. The *superficial suppurative type* is characterized by painless swelling, induration, crusting, and superficial and deep ulcerations of the lip; called also *Baelz's disease.* The *deep suppurative type* is a basically deep-seated infection, with abscesses and fistulous tracts that eventually form scars; called also *apostematous c., c. glandularis apostematosa*, and *myxadenitis labialis.*   **c. glandula′ris**

apostemato′sa, see *c. glandularis.*   **c. granulomato′sa,** an inflammation of the lips marked by granular papules.   **impetiginous c.,** impetigo of the lips.   **migrating c.,** perlèche.   **solar c.,** involvement of the lips after exposure to actinic rays; such involvement may be acute (see *actinic c.*), or chronic, with alteration of the epithelium and sometimes fissuring or ulceration.   **c. venena′ta,** inflammation of the lips caused by a chemical irritant.

cheilo-, cheil- (ki′lo, kīl′) [Gr. *cheilos* lip; an edge, or brim]   a combining form denoting relationship to the lip, or to an edge or brim.

cheiloangioscopy (ki″lo-an″je-os′ko-pe) [*cheilo-* + Gr. *angeion* vessel + *skopein* to examine]   microscopical observation of the circulation in the blood vessels of the lip.

cheilocarcinoma (ki″lo-kar″sĭ-no′mah)   carcinoma of the lip.

cheilognathopalatoschisis (ki″lo-na″tho-pal″ah-tos′kĭ-sis)   cheilognathouranoschisis.

cheilognathoprosoposchisis (ki″lo-na″tho-pros″o-pos′kĭ-sis) [*cheilo-* + Gr. *gnathos* jaw + *prosōpon* face + *schisis* cleft]   a developmental anomaly characterized by presence of an oblique facial cleft continuing into the lip and upper jaw.

cheilognathoschisis (ki″lo-na-thos′kĭ-sis) [*cheilo-* + Gr. *gnathos* jaw + *schisis* cleft]   a developmental anomaly characterized by the presence of a cleft in the lip and jaw.

cheilognathouranoschisis (ki″lo-na″tho-u-rah-nos′kĭ-sis) [*cheilo-* + Gr. *gnathos* jaw + *ouranos* palate + *schisis* cleft]   a developmental anomaly characterized by the presence of a cleft in the lip, upper jaw, and palate.

cheiloncus (ki-long′kus)   (*obs.*) a tumor of the lip.

cheilophagia (ki″lo-fa′je-ah) [*cheilo-* + Gr. *phagein* to eat]   biting of the lips.

cheiloplasty (ki′lo-plas″te) [*cheilo-* + Gr. *plassein* to form]   surgical repair of a defect of the lip.

cheilorrhaphy (ki-lor′ah-fe) [*cheilo-* + Gr. *rhaphē* suture]   the operation of suturing the lip; surgical repair of a congenitally cleft lip.

cheiloschisis (ki-los′kĭ-sis) [*cheilo-* + Gr. *schisis* cleft]   harelip.

cheiloscopy (ki-los′ko-pe)   study of the surface configuration of the vermilion border of the lips to identify individual patterns (lip-print patterns).

cheilosis (ki-lo′sis) [*cheilo-* + *-osis*]   a condition marked by fissuring and dry scaling of the vermilion surface of the lips and angles of the mouth (perlèche); it is characteristic of riboflavin deficiency.   **angular c.,** perlèche.

cheilostomatoplasty (ki″lo-sto-mat′o-plas″te) [*cheilo-* + Gr. *stoma* mouth + *plassein* to form]   surgical restoration of the lips and mouth, as after trauma or the removal of a cancer.

cheilotomy (ki-lot′o-me) [*cheilo-* + Gr. *tomē* a cutting]   incision into the lip; also, cheilectomy.

cheir-   see *cheiro-*.

Cheiracanthium (ki″rah-can′the-um)   *Chiracanthium.*

Cheiracanthus (ki″rah-kan′thus)   *gnathostoma.*

cheiragra (ki-rag′rah) [*cheir-* + Gr. *agra* seizure]   gout of the hand, especially tophaceous gout with torsion of the fingers.

cheiralgia (ki-ral′je-ah)   pain in the hand.   **c. paresthet′ica,** isolated neuritis of the superficial ramus of the radial nerve.

cheirarthritis (ki″rar-thri′tis) [*cheir-* + *arthritis*]   inflammation of the joints of the hand and fingers.

cheiro-, cheir- [Gr. *cheir* hand]   a combining form denoting relationship to the hand. For words beginning with this root, see also those beginning *chir-* and *chiro-*.

cheirobrachialgia (ki″ro-bra″ke-al′je-ah)   a syndrome of paresthesia and pain in the arm, hand, and fingers; called also *cheirobrachialgia paresthetica.*

cheirocinesthesia (ki″ro-sin″es-the′ze-ah)   cheirokinesthesia.

cheirognomy (ki-rog′no-me) [*cheiro-* + Gr. *gnomōn* judge]   the study of the hand as a guide to characteristics of the individual.

cheirognostic (ki″rog-nos′tik) [*cheiro-* + Gr. *gnostikos* knowing]   pertaining to or characterized by the ability to distinguish stimuli as originating on the right or the left side of the body.

cheirokinesthesia (ki″ro-kin″es-the′ze-ah)   the subjective perception of the movements of the hand, especially in writing.

cheirokinesthetic (ki″ro-kin″es-thet′ik)   pertaining to or characterized by cheirokinesthesia.

cheirology (ki-rol′o-je)   dactylology.

cheiromegaly (ki-ro-meg′ah-le)   abnormal enlargement of the hands.

cheiroplasty (ki′ro-plas″te) [*cheiro-* + Gr. *plassein* to form]   plastic surgery on the hand.

cheiropodalgia (ki″ro-po-dal′je-ah) [*cheiro-* + Gr. *pous* foot + *algos* pain]   pain in the hands and feet.

cheiropompholyx (ki″ro-pom′fo-liks) [*cheiro-* + Gr. *pompholyx* a bubble]   pompholyx.

cheiroscope (ki′ro-skōp) [*cheiro-* + Gr. *skopein* to view]   an instrument used in the training of binocular vision, by which the image of a test object seen reflected in a mirror by the sound eye is projected by the other eye to a drawing board, where it is traced with a pencil guided by the hand of the subject.

cheirospasm (ki′ro-spazm) [*cheiro-* + Gr. *spasmos* spasm] spasm of the muscles of the hand.

chelate (ke′lāt) [Gr. *chēlē* claw] to combine with a metal in complexes in which the metal is part of a ring. By extension, a chemical compound in which a metallic ion is sequestered and firmly bound into a ring within the chelating molecule. Chelates are used in chemotherapeutic treatments for metal poisoning.

chelation (ke-la′shun) combination with a metal in complexes in which the metal is part of a ring.

chelen (ke′len) ethyl chloride.

chelicera (ke-lis′er-ah) a pair of pincer-like head appendages of spiders, scorpions, and other arachnids.

Chel-Iron (kēl′i-ron) trademark for preparations of ferrocholinate.

cheloid (ke′loid) keloid.

cheloma (ke-lo′mah) keloid.

chelonian (ke-lo′ne-an) [Gr. *chelōnē* tortoise] pertaining to turtles and tortoises, (order Chelonia).

chemabrasion (kēm-ah-bra′shun) superficial destruction and exfoliation of the epidermis and the upper layer of the dermis by application of a cauterant to the skin; done to remove scars, tattoos, pigmented nevi, etc. Called also *chemexfoliation.* See also *planing.*

chemanesia (kēm″ah-ne′ze-ah) the controlled and reversible amnesia induced by a drug, as in certain anesthesia procedures.

chemasthenia (kem″as-the′ne-ah) an asthenic condition of the chemical processes of the body.

chemexfoliation (kēm′eks-fo″le-a″shun) chemabrasion.

chemiatric (kem″e-at′rik) iatrochemical.

chemiatry (kem′e-ah-tre) [Gr. *chēmeia* chemistry + *iatreia* treatment] iatrochemistry.

chemical (kem′ĭ-kal) 1. of, or pertaining to, chemistry. 2. a substance composed of chemical elements, or obtained by chemical processes.

chemicobiological (kem″ĭ-ko-bi″o-loj′e-kal) biochemical.

chemicocautery (kem″ĭ-ko-kaw′ter-e) chemocautery.

chemicogenesis (kem″ĭ-ko-jen′ĕ-sis) [*chemistry* + Gr. *genesis* production] development of an ovum by chemical stimulation.

chemicophysical (kem″ĭ-ko-fiz′e-kal) pertaining to chemistry and physics; pertaining to physical chemistry.

chemicophysiologic (kem″ĭ-ko-fiz″e-o-loj′ik) pertaining to physiology and chemistry.

chemiluminescense (kem″ĭ-loo″mĭ-nes′ens) chemoluminescence.

cheminosis (kem″ĭ-no′sis) [*chemistry* + Gr. *nosos* disease] any disease due to chemical agents.

chemiosmosis (kem″e-os-mo′sis) chemosmosis.

chemiosmotic (kem″e-o-os-mot′ik) chemosmotic.

chemiotaxis (kem″e-o-tak′sis) chemotaxis.

chemiotherapy (kem″e-o-ther′ah-pe) chemotherapy.

chemism (kem′izm) chemical activity; chemical property or relationship.

chemisorption (kem″ĭ-sorp′shun) the chemical adsorption of one material by another, resulting in the production of a different chemical compound.

chemist (kem′ist) 1. an individual skilled in chemistry. 2. (British) a pharmacist.

chemistry (kem′is-tre) [Gr. *chēmeia*] the science that treats of the elements and atomic relations of matter, and of the various compounds of the elements. **analytical c.,** chemistry that deals with analysis of different elements in a compound. **applied c.,** the application of chemistry to industry and the arts; called also *industrial c.* **biological c.,** biochemistry. **colloid c.,** chemistry dealing with the nature and composition of colloids. **dental c.,** the chemistry of materials used in dental procedures and the processes to which they are subjected. **ecological c.,** the study of those chemical compounds synthesized by plants that serve no metabolic purpose but which, by reason of their toxic effect on insects and higher animals, influence a community of interacting plants and animals. **forensic c.,** use of chemical knowledge in the solution of legal problems. **industrial c.,** applied c. **inorganic c.,** that branch of the science of chemistry which deals with compounds that do not occur in the plant or animal worlds; called also *mineral c.* **medical c.,** chemistry as it relates to medicine. **metabolic c.,** biochemistry. **mineral c.,** inorganic c. **organic c.,** that branch of chemistry which deals with compounds that contain carbon. **pharmaceutical c.,** chemistry that deals with the composition and preparation of substances used in treatment of patients or diagnostic studies. **physical c.,** that branch of chemistry which deals with the relationship of chemical and physical properties. **physiological c.,** biochemistry. **structural c.,** chemical study of the structure of molecules.

surface c., in the field of catalysis, the study of chemical reactions between the outermost layer of atoms of a solid and molecules brought to the solid surface in the liquid or gaseous state. **synthetic c.,** that branch of chemistry which deals with the building up of chemical compounds from simpler substances or from the elements.

chemo- (ke′mo, kem′o) [Gr. *chēmeia* chemistry] a combining form denoting relationship to chemistry, or to a chemical.

chemoattractant (ke″mo-ah-trak′tant) a chemical (chemotactic) agent that induces an organism or a cell (e.g., a leukocyte) to migrate toward it.

chemoautotroph (ke″mo-aw′to-trōf) a chemoautotrophic microorganism.

chemoautotrophic (kem″o-aw″to-trof′ik) capable of synthesizing cell constituents from carbon dioxide by means of the energy derived from inorganic reactions.

chemobiotic (ke″mo-bi-ot′ik) the combination of a chemotherapeutic agent and an antibiotic, as of one or more of the sulfonamide compounds with penicillin.

chemocautery (ke″mo-kaw′ter-e) destruction of tissue by application of a caustic chemical substance.

chemocephalia (ke″mo-sĕ-fa′le-ah) chamaecephaly.

chemocephaly (ke″mo-sef′ah-le) chamaecephaly.

chemoceptor (ke′mo-sep-tor) chemoreceptor.

chemocoagulation (ke″mo-ko-ag″u-la′shun) coagulation or destruction of neoplasm by the application of chemicals.

chemodectoma (ke″mo-dek-to′mah) [*chemo-* + *dektos* to be received or accepted + *-oma*] any tumor of the chemoreceptor system, such as a tumor of the carotid body, aortic pulmonary bodies, or glomus jugulare; called also *nonchromaffin paraganglioma.*

chemodifferentiation (ke″mo-dif″er-en-she-a′shun) the invisible point of decision which foreruns and controls the actual differentiation of cells into the rudimentary organs of the embryo.

chemodynesis (ke″mo-di′nĕ-sis) the initiation of cytoplasmic streaming in plant cells by chemicals.

chemoheterotroph (ke″mo-het′er-o-trōf″) a microorganism, parasitic or saprophytic, deriving its energy and most of its carbon from the oxidation of preformed organic compounds.

chemoheterotrophic (ke″mo-het″er-o-trōf′ik) pertaining to a chemoheterotroph.

chemohormonal (ke″mo-hor-mo′nal) pertaining to drugs having hormone activity.

chemoimmunology (ke″mo-im-u-nol′o-je) the study of the chemical processes involved in immunity; immunochemistry.

chemokinesis (ke″mo-ki-ne′sis) [*chemo-* + Gr. *kinēsis* motion] increased activity of an organism due to the presence of a chemical substance.

chemokinetic (ke″mo-ki-net′ik) pertaining to or exhibiting chemokinesis.

chemolithotroph (ke″mo-lith′o-trōf) an organism that derives its energy from oxidation of inorganic compounds and its carbon from carbon dioxide.

chemolithotrophic (ke″mo-lith″o-trof′ik) deriving energy from the oxidation of inorganic compounds of iron, nitrogen, sulfur, or hydrogen; said of bacteria.

chemoluminescence (ke″mo-loo″mĭ-nes′ens) luminescence produced by the direct transformation of chemical energy into light energy.

chemolysis (ke-mol′ĭ-sis) [*chemo-* + Gr. *lysis* solution] chemical decomposition.

chemomorphosis (ke″mo-mor-fo′sis) [*chemo-* + Gr. *morphē* form] change of form due to chemical action.

chemonucleolysis (ke″mo-nu″kle-ol′ĭ-sis) [*chemo-* + *nucleo* nucleus + *lysis*] dissolution of the nucleus pulposus of an intervertebral disk by injection of a chemolytic agent, e.g., the enzyme chymopapain; used especially in the treatment of herniation of a disk.

chemoorganotroph (ke″mo-or′gah-no-trōf″) an organism that derives its energy and carbon from organic compounds.

chemoorganotrophic (ke″mo-or″gah-no-trof′ik) deriving energy from the oxidation of organic compounds; said of bacteria.

chemopallidectomy (ke″mo-pal″ĭ-dek′to-me) [*chemo-* + *pallidum* + *ektomē* excision] creation of a lesion of the globus pallidus by destruction of tissue by a chemical agent.

chemopallidothalamectomy (ke″mo-pal″ĭ-do-thal″ah-mek′-to-me) creation of a lesion of the globus pallidus and thalamus by a chemical agent.

chemopharmacodynamic (ke″mo-far″mah-ko-di-nam′ik) denoting the relationship between chemical constitution and biologic or pharmacologic activity.

chemophysiology (ke″mo-fiz-ĭ-ol′o-je) biochemistry.

chemoprophylaxis (ke″mo-pro″fi-lak′sis) [*chemo-* + Gr. *prophylax* an advanced guard] use of a chemotherapeutic agent as a means of preventing development of a specific disease. **primary c.,** prophylactic use of a chemotherapeutic agent before infection has occurred in an individual. **secondary c.,** prophylactic use of a chemotherapeutic agent in an individual after infection has occurred (with *Mycobacterium tuberculosis*, for example) but before disease has become manifest.

chemopsychiatry (ke″mo-si-ki′ah-tre) the use of drugs in the treatment of mental and emotional disorders; psychopharmacology.

chemoreception (ke″mo-re-sep′shun) [*chemo-* + L. *receptio*, from *recipere* to receive] the process of being sensitive to or perceiving chemical stimuli in the surrounding medium.

chemoreceptor (ke″mo-re-sep′tor) 1. a receptor adapted for excitation by chemical substances, e.g., olfactory and gustatory receptors, or a sense organ, as the carotid body or the aortic (supracardial) bodies, which is sensitive to chemical changes in the blood stream, especially reduced oxygen content, and reflexly increases both respiration and blood pressure. See *receptor*. 2. a supposed group of atoms in cell protoplasm having the power of fixing chemicals, in the same way as bacterial poisons are fixed. Called also *chemoceptor*.

chemoresistance (ke″mo-re-zis′tans) specific resistance acquired by cells to the action of chemicals.

chemosensitive (ke″mo-sen′sĭ-tiv) sensitive to changes in chemical composition.

chemosensory (ke″mo-sen′so-re) relating to the perception of chemical substances, as in odor detection.

chemoserotherapy (ke″mo-se′ro-ther′ah-pe) the treatment of disease with both drugs and serum.

chemosis (ke-mo′sis) [Gr. *chēmōsis*] excessive edema of the ocular conjunctiva.

chemosmosis (ke″mos-mo′sis) chemical action taking place through an intervening membrane.

chemosmotic (ke″mos-mot′ik) pertaining to chemosmosis.

chemosorption (kem″o-sorp′shun) chemisorption.

chemosphere (ke′mo-sfēr) the layer of the upper atmosphere where photochemical reactions become important (30–80 km.).

chemostat (ke′mo-stat) an apparatus in which the environment is so controlled that bacterial populations are maintained in a steady state of continuous cell division in a constant environment.

chemosterilant (ke″mo-ster′ĭ-lant) a chemical compound the ingestion of which causes sterility of an organism; such compounds have been used as a means of controlling various insects and other pests by inducing sterility in the male.

chemosurgery (ke″mo-sur′jer-e) the destruction of tissue by chemical agents; originally applied to chemical fixation of malignant, gangrenous, or infected tissue, with the use of frozen sections to facilitate systematic microscopic control of the extent of ablation.

chemosynthesis (ke″mo-sin′the-sis) [*chemo-* + Gr. *synthesis* putting together] the synthesis of carbohydrate from carbon dioxide and water as a result of the energy derived from chemical reactions, rather than from absorbed light. Such synthesis is carried out by certain bacteria and algae. Cf. *photosynthesis*.

chemosynthetic (ke″mo-sin-thet′ik) pertaining to or characterized by chemosynthesis.

chemotactic (ke″mo-tak′tik) of or pertaining to chemotaxis.

chemotaxin (ke″mo-tak′sin) a substance, e.g., a complement component, that induces chemotaxis.

chemotaxis (ke″mo-tak′sis) [*chemo-* + Gr. *taxis* arrangement] the movement of an organism or an individual cell, such as a leukocyte, in response to a chemical concentration gradient. **leukocyte c.,** the response of leukocytes to products formed in immunologic reactions, wherein leukocytes are attracted to and accumulate at the site of the reaction; it is a part of the inflammatory response. **negative c.,** movement of an organism from a region of high to a region of low concentration of a specific chemical compound or element; tactile irritability. **positive c.,** movement of an organism from a region of low to a region of high concentration of a specific chemical compound or element.

chemothalamectomy (ke″mo-thal-ah-mek′to-me) destruction of a portion of the thalamus by the introduction of chemical agents.

chemotherapeutic (ke″mo-ther-ah-pu′tik) pertaining to chemotherapy.

chemotherapeutics (ke″mo-ther-ah-pu′tiks) chemotherapy.

chemotherapy (ke″mo-ther′ah-pe) the treatment of disease by chemical agents; first applied to use of chemicals that affect the causative organism unfavorably but do not harm the patient.

chemotic (ke-mot′ik) 1. pertaining to or affected with chemosis. 2. an agent that increases the production of lymph in the ocular conjunctiva.

chemotrophic (ke″mo-trof′ik) deriving energy from the oxidation of organic (chemoorganotrophic) or inorganic (chemolithotrophic) compounds; said of bacteria.

chemotropic (ke″mo-trop′ik) of or pertaining to chemotropism.

chemotropism (ke-mot′ro-pizm) [*chemo-* + Gr. *tropos* a turning] an orienting response or a growth toward a chemical stimulus in plants and animals; chemotaxis.

chemurgy (kem′er-ge) [*chemo-* + Gr. *ergon* work] chemistry applied to the industrial use of raw organic products, especially agricultural products.

chenodeoxycholate (ke″no-de-ok-sĭ-ko′lāt) the salt or dissociated form of chenodeoxycholic acid; see under *acid*.

chenodiol (ke″no-di′ōl) chemical name: $3\alpha,7\alpha$-dihydroxy-5β-cholan-24-oic acid; an anticholelithogenic, $C_{24}H_{40}O_4$.

Chenopodium (ke″no-po′de-um) a genus of herbs of the temperate regions of the world; see also under *oil*.

chenotherapy (ke″no-ther′ah-pe) treatment with chenodeoxycholic acid, as for dissolution of gallstones.

cheoplastic (ke′o-plas″tik) pertaining to cheoplasty.

cheoplasty (ke′o-plas″te) [Gr. *chein* to pour + *plassein* to form] a method once used to mold artificial teeth with an alloy of tin, silver, and bismuth.

Cherchevski's (Cherchewski's) disease (sher- shev′skēz) [Mikhail *Cherchevski*, Russian physician] see under *disease*.

cheromania (ke″ro-ma′ne-ah) [Gr. *chairein* to rejoice + *mania* madness] (*obs.*) mania characterized by exaltation and cheerfulness.

Cheron's serum (sha-rawz′) [Jules *Cheron*, French gynecologist, 1837–1900] see under *serum*.

cherry (cher′e) [L. *cerasus*] the name of various rosaceous trees and species of the genus *Prunus*; see *Prunus virginiana*. **choke c.,** *Prunus virginiana*. **c. laurel,** an Old World evergreen cherry tree, *Prunus laurocerasus* L. (Rosaceae); the source of a preparation (cherry laurel water) formerly used as an antispasmodic, sedative, and anodyne, and for cough. **rum c.,** *Prunus serotina*. **wild c.,** 1. *Prunus serotina*. 2. [USP] the carefully dried stem bark of *P. serotina*, used in a syrup as a flavored vehicle for drugs; called also *wild black cherry bark*. See also under *syrup*.

cherubism (cher′ŭ-bizm) [*cherub* + *-ism*] hereditary and progressive bilateral swelling at the angle of the mandible, sometimes involving the entire jaw. The swelling imparts a cherubic look to the face, in some cases enhanced by upturning of the eyes. Called also *familial fibrous dysplasia of jaw* and *familial bilateral giant cell tumor*.

Chervin's treatment (method) (sher-vaz′) [Claudius *Chervin*, French teacher, 1824–1896] see under *treatment*.

chest (chest) the thorax. **alar c.,** flat chest. **barrel c.,** a rounded, bulging chest with abnormal increase in the anteroposterior diameter, showing little movement on respiration; seen in emphysema and in kyphosis. **blast c.,** pulmonary concussion and hemorrhage occurring as the result of injury by a blast. **cobbler's c.,** a chest showing a sinking in at the lower end of the sternum. **flail c.,** one whose wall moves paradoxically with respiration, owing to multiple fractures of the ribs. **flat c.,** deformity of the chest in which it is flattened from front to back; called also *alar c.* and *pterygoid c.* **foveated c.,** funnel chest. **funnel c.,** a chest in which there is funnel-shaped depression in the middle of the anterior thoracic wall, the deepest part being in the sternum; called also *foveated c., funnel breast, pectus excavatum* or *recurvatum, koilosternia, chonechondrosternon,* and *trichterbrust.* **keeled c.,** pigeon breast. **paralytic c.,** a long and narrow chest with emaciation so that the ribs stand out sharply under the skin. **phthinoid c.,** the same as *flat chest*; so called as indicating a tubercular diathesis. **pigeon c.,** pigeon breast. **pterygoid c.,** flat chest. **tetrahedron c.,** a chest that suggests a solid with four sides, each an equilateral triangle, the chest projecting in a peak between the nipples.

chestnut (chest′nut) 1. *Castanea*. 2. one of the masses of horn on the medial surface of the forearm and on the distal part of the medial surface of the tarsus of horses. **horse c.,** *Aesculus*.

Cheyletiella (sha″lĕ-te-el′lah) a genus of mites. **C. parasitov′orax,** a species infesting the cat or on other mites infesting cats, and which may cause a dermatosis in human beings.

Cheyne-Stokes asthma, etc. (chān′stōks) [John *Cheyne*, Scottish physician, 1777–1836; William *Stokes*, Irish physician, 1804–1878] see *cardiac asthma,* under *asthma,* and see under *nystagmus, psychosis,* and *respiration*.

CHF congestive heart failure.

CHI₃ iodoform.

C₂H₅I ethyl iodide.

Chiari's network (reticulum), syndrome (disease) (ke-ar′ēz) [Hans *Chiari*, Austrian pathologist, 1851–1916] see under *network*, and see *Budd-Chiari syndrome*, under *syndrome*.

Chiari-Arnold syndrome (ke-ar′e-ar′nold) [Hans von *Chiari*; Julius *Arnold*, Austrian pathologist, 1835–1915] Arnold-Chiari deformity.

Chiari-Frommel syndrome (disease) (ke-ar′e-from′el) [Johann Baptist *Chiari*, German obstetrician, 1817–1854; Richard *Frommel*, German gynecologist, 1854–1912] see under *syndrome*.

chiasm (ki′azm) [L., Gr. *chiasma*] a decussation or X-shaped crossing; see *chiasma*. **c. of digits of hand,** chiasma tendinum digitorum manus. **optic c.,** chiasma opticum. **tendinous c. of flexor digitorum sublimis muscle,** chiasma tendinum digitorum manus.

chiasma (ki-as′mah), pl. *chias′mata* [L.; Gr.] a decussation or X-shaped crossing. In genetics, the points at which members of a chromosome pair are in contact during the prophase of meiosis and because of which recombination, or crossing over, occurs on separation. In official anatomical nomenclature the crossing of two elements or structures, as the optic nerves. **c. op′ticum** [NA], the optic chiasm: the part of the hypothalamus formed by the decussation, or crossing, of the fibers of the optic nerve from the medial half of each retina; called also *optic decussation* and *decussation of optic nerve.* **c. ten′dinum digito′rum ma′nus** [NA], the crossing of the tendons of the flexor digitorum profundus through the tendons of the flexor digitorum sublimis; called also *c. of digits of hand* and *tendinous c. of flexor sublimis.*

chiasmal (ki-az′mal) chiasmatic.

chiasmata (ki-as′mah-tah) plural of *chiasma.*

chiasmatic (ki-az-mat′ik) resembling a chiasm; crosswise.

chiasmatypy (ki-az′mah-ti″pe) [Gr. *chiasma* a crossing + *type*] crossing over.

chiasmic (ki-az′mik) chiasmatic.

chiastometer (ki″as-tom′ĕ-ter) [Gr. *chiastos* crossed + *metron* measure] an apparatus for measuring any deviation of the optic axes from their normal parallelism.

chichism (che′chizm) a term in northern South America for pellagra.

chickenpox (chik′en-poks) a highly contagious disease caused by the herpes zoster virus and characterized by crops of vesicular eruptions confined mainly to the face and trunk, appearing over a period of a few days to a week, after an incubation period of 17–21 days. The lesions begin as macules, develop quickly into vesicles, and then become crusted. The disease is usually benign in children, but may be serious in infants, children with underlying malignancy, and adults; varicella pneumonia may occur, particularly in adults. Called also *varicella.*

chick-pea (chik′pe) the plant *Cicer arietinum* of Southern Europe whose seeds are used as food and may be toxic to certain individuals.

Chiene's operation (shēnz) [John *Chiene*, Scottish surgeon, 1843–1923] see under *operation.*

Chievitz's layer, organ (che′vits-ez) [Johan Henrik *Chievitz*, Danish anatomist, 1850–1901] see under *layer* and *organ.*

chigger (chig′er) the six-legged red larva of mites of the family Trombiculidae, which attach to the skin of their hosts, and whose bites produce a wheal, usually accompanied by intense itching and severe dermatitis. The habitat of these mites is tall grass and underbrush. *Eutrombicula alfreddugèsi* is the common chigger of the United States; *E. splendens* is a species found in southeastern localities; and *Trombicula autumnalis* is the chigger of Europe. Some species in the Asiatic-Pacific region are vectors of the rickettsiae of scrub typhus. Chiggers are to be distinguished from chigoes. Called also *bête rouge, harvest mite, mower's mite, red bug,* and *red mites.*

chigo (chig′o) chigoe.

chigoe (chig′o) the flea, *Tunga* (*Dermatophilus, Sarcopsylla, Pulex*) *penetrans,* of tropical and subtropical America and Africa. The pregnant female flea burrows into the skin of the feet (often beneath the nail), legs, or other part of the body, causing intense irritation and ulceration, and sometimes leading to spontaneous amputation of a digit. Chigoes are to be distinguished from chiggers. Called also *burrowing flea, chigo, jigger,* and *sand flea.*

chikungunya (chik″un-gun′yah) a febrile viral disease that occured in an outbreak of infection in the Newala district of Tanganyika in 1953; it resembles dengue, but without headache.

chilblain (chil′blān) [L. *pernio*] a recurrent localized itching, swelling and painful erythema on the fingers, toes, or ears, produced by mild frostbite; called also *pernio* and *erythema pernio.* **necrotized c.,** sarcoidosis.

child (chīld) the human young, from infancy to puberty. **preschool c.,** a child between two and six years of age. **school c.,** a child between six and ten to twelve years of age.

childbed (chīld′bed) the puerperal state or period.

childbirth (chīld′birth) the act or process of giving birth to a child; see *labor.*

childhood (chīld′hood) the period of life of the human young generally considered to extend from infancy to puberty.

chilitis (ki-li′tis) cheilitis.

chill (chil) a shivering or shaking; an attack of involuntary contractions of the voluntary muscles, accompanied by a sense of cold and pallor of the skin; called also *ague.* **brass c., brazier's c.,** see *brassfounder's fever.* **peritubular contractile c's, Bloom & Fawcett p. 807** myoid c's, (def. 1). **congestive c.,** pernicious malaria with gastrointestinal congestion and diarrhea, preceded by a chill. **creeping c.,** a chilly sensation, without any definite tremor or chattering of the teeth. **ner-**

vous c., a tremor due to some form of excitement and unaccompanied by alteration of temperature. **shaking c.,** a chill in which there is a definite tremor. **spelter c's,** see under *fever.* **urethral c.,** a chilly sensation, with or without tremor, sometimes following the passage of a catheter. **zinc c.,** spelter's fever.

chilo- for words beginning thus, see also words beginning *cheilo-.*

Chilodon (ki′lo-don) a genus of free-living ciliates, some species of which have been described as probable contaminants of human feces. *C. dentatus* has been found in the feces in a case of dysentery. *C. uncinatus* was found in the feces in a case of schistosomiasis.

Chilognatha (ki-log′nah-thah) an order of arthropods of the class Diplopoda, superclass Myriapoda, embracing the millipedes.

chilomastigiasis (ki″lo-mas″tĭ-gi′ah-sis) infection with *Chilomastix.*

Chilomastix (ki″lo-mas′tiks) a genus of minute piriform protozoa of the order Polymastigida, class Zoomastigophora, with three anterior flagella and a fourth undulating within the cleft formed by the cytosome; the organisms are found in the intestine of vertebrates. **C. mesnil′i,** a very common, widely distributed species found as a commensal in the colon and cecum of humans; both trophozoites and cystic stages are found in feces.

chilomastixiasis (ki″lo-mas″tik-si′ah-sis) chilomastigiasis.

Chilopoda (ki-lop′o-dah) [Gr. *cheilos* lip + *pous* foot] a class of the phylum Arthropoda, embracing the centipedes.

chimaera (ki-me′rah) chimera.

chimera (ki-me′rah) [Gr. *chimaira* a mythological fire-spouting monster with a lion's head, goat's body, and serpent's tail] an individual organism whose body contains cell populations derived from different zygotes, of the same or of different species, occurring spontaneously, as in twins (blood group chimeras), or produced artificially, as an organism which develops from combined portions of different embryos, or one in which tissues or cells of another organism have been introduced. Cf. *mosaic.* **heterologous c.,** a chimera in which the foreign cells or tissues are derived from an organism of a different species. **homologous c.,** a chimera in which the foreign cells or tissues are derived from an organism of the same species but of a different genotype. **isologous c.,** a chimera in which the foreign cells or tissues are derived from an identical organism of the same genotype, such as an identical twin. **radiation c.,** an organism that survives with immunologic characteristics of host and donor after a bone marrow graft from an antigenically different donor, the host having first been subjected to sublethal whole-body irradiation so that there is no immune response to foreign cells by the donor.

chimerism (ki-mēr′izm) the quality of being a chimera; in genetics, the presence in an individual of cells of different origin, as of blood cells derived from a dizygotic co-twin. Cf. *mosaicism.*

chimpanzee (chim-pan′ze, chim-pan-ze′) an anthropoid ape, *Pan troglodytes,* inhabiting the tropical rain forests of Africa, used for experimental purposes because of its susceptibility to some of the diseases of man and in behavioral studies because of its high level of intelligence.

chin (chin) the anterior prominence of the lower jaw; the mentum [NA]. **galoche c.** (gah-losh′) [Fr. "galosh"], a long pointed chin.

chinacrine (kin′ah-krin) quinacrine.

chincap (chin′kap) an extraoral orthodontic appliance for applying pressure to the chin, designed to exert an upward and backward force on the mandible in anterior cross-bite, skeletal Class III, and open bite malocclusions; also utilized for anchorage in some forms of malocclusion.

chiniofon (kin′e-o-fon) a canary yellow powder, containing 26.5–29.0 per cent iodine, formerly used as an antiprotozoan in amebic dysentery.

chionablepsia (ki″o-nah-blep′se-ah) [Gr. *chiōn* snow + *ablepsia* blindness] snow blindness.

chip (chip) a small piece, as of something broken off. **bone c's,** small pieces of bone, usually cancellous, generally used to fill in bony defects to facilitate recalcification.

chip-blower (chip-blo′er) chip syringe; see under *syringe.*

chir- see *chiro;* for words beginning thus, see also those beginning *cheir-* and *cheiro-.*

Chiracanthium (ki″rah-kan′the-um) a genus of venomous spiders, two species of which, *C. inclu′sum* and *C. diver′sium,* have produced local reactions in man in California and Hawaii, respectively.

chiro-, chir- (ki′ro, kīr′) [Gr. *cheir* hand] a combining form denoting relationship to the hand; for words beginning thus, see also those beginning *cheir-* and *cheiro-.*

chirobrachialgia (ki″ro-bra″ke-al′je-ah) cheirobrachialgia.

chirognostic (ki″rog-nos′tik) cheirognostic.

chiromegaly (ki″ro-meg′ah-le) cheiromegaly.

Chironomidae (ki″ro-nom′ĭ-de) a family of the suborder Nematocera, order Diptera, that comprises the true midges.

Chironomus (ki-ron′o-mus) a genus of gnatlike flies noted for their giant chromosomes.

chiroplasty (ki′ro-plas″te) cheiroplasty.

chiropodalgia (ki″ro-po-dal′je-ah) cheiropodalgia.

chiropodical (ki″re-pod′ĭ-kal) pertaining to chiropody (now called *podiatry*).

chiropodist (ki-rop′o-dist) podiatrist.

chiropody (ki-rop′o-de) podiatry.

chiropractic (ki″ro-prak′tik) [*chiro-* + Gr. *prattein* to do] a system of therapeutics based upon the claim that disease is caused by abnormal function of the nerve system. It attempts to restore normal function of the nerve system by manipulation and treatment of the structures of the human body, especially those of the spinal column. Called also *chiropraxis*.

chiropractor (ki″ro-prak′tor) a practitioner of chiropractic.

chiropraxis (ki″ro-prak′sis) chiropractic.

chiroscope (ki′ro-skōp) cheiroscope.

chirospasm (ki′ro-spazm) cheirospasm.

chirurgenic (ki″rur-jen′ik) [*chirurgery* + Gr. *gennan* to produce] arising as a result of a surgical procedure.

chirurgeon (ki-rur′jun) archaic term for a surgeon.

chirurgery (ki-rur′jer-e) [L. *chirurgia*, from Gr. *cheir* hand + *ergon* work] archaic term for surgery.

chirurgic (ki-rur′jik) archaic term for surgical.

chisel (chis′l) a cutting instrument with a beveled edge for planing or smoothing a surface, as during cavity preparations in teeth. **binangled c.,** one whose blade forms two angles before meeting with the shank.

chi-square (ki′skwār) see under *tests*.

chitin (ki′tin) [Gr. *chitōn* tunic] a white, insoluble, horny polysaccharide, $C_{30}H_{50}O_{19}N_4$, the principal constituent of the shells of arthropods and the shards of beetles and found in certain fungi. On hydrolysis it yields a linear homopolymer of β-(1→4)-2-acetamido-2-deoxy-D-glucose (an acetyl glucosamine). Next to cellulose, it is the most abundant natural polysaccharide.

chitinase (ki′tĭ-nās) an enzyme that catalyzes the hydrolysis of chitin to acetyl glucosamine.

chitinous (kit′ĭ-nus) composed of or of the nature of chitin.

chitobiose (ki″to-bi′ōs) a disaccharide composed of two glucosamine units, obtained by hydrolysis of de-acetylated chitin (chitosan).

chitosan (ki′to-san) a polysaccharide composed of repeating glucosamine units; obtained by de-acetylation of chitin and used in the preparation of chitobiose.

chitose (ki′tōs) a sugar, 2,5-anhydro-D-mannose, $C_6H_{12}O$, formed by the reduction of chitonic acid.

chitotriose (ki″to-tri′ōs) a trisaccharide composed of three glucosamine units; obtained from chitosan by hydrolysis.

chiufa (che-oo′fah) a gangrenous inflammation of the colon and rectum occurring in mountainous regions of South America and South Africa.

chlamydemia (klah-mĭ-de′me-ah) the presence of chlamydiae in the blood.

Chlamydia (klah-mid′e-ah) [Gr. *chlamys* cloak] a genus of the family Chlamydiaceae, order Chlamydiales, occurring as two species which cause a wide variety of diseases in man and animals. Called also *PLT group* and, formerly, *Miyagawanella, Bedsonia,* and *Chlamydozoon.* **C. psitta′ci,** a species, various strains of which cause psittacosis in man and psittacine birds and ornithosis in nonpsittacine birds; pneumonitis in cattle, sheep, swine, cats, goats, and horses; epizootic bovine abortion and enzootic abortion of ewes; enteritis of calves; sporadic encephalomyelitis of calves; epizootic chlamydiosis of hares and muskrats; and conjunctivitis of cattle, sheep, and guinea pigs. **C. tracho′matis,** a species various strains of which cause trachoma, inclusion conjunctivitis (or inclusion blennorrhea), "nonspecific" urethritis, proctitis, mouse pneumonitis, and lymphogranuloma venereum. It is differentiated from *C. psittaci* by its intracytoplasmic production of glycogen and susceptibility to sulfadiazine. Called also *TRIC group.*

chlamydia (klah-mid′e-ah), pl. *chlamyd′iae.* Any member of the genus *Chlamydia.*

Chlamydiaceae (klah-mid″e-a′se-e) a family of the order Chlamydiales consisting of small coccoid microorganisms that have a unique, obligately intracellular developmental cycle and are incapable of synthesizing ATP. They induce their own phagocytosis by host cells, in which they then form intracytoplasmic colonies. They are parasites of birds and mammals (including man), in which they cause a variety of diseases (see *Chlamydia*). They have also been isolated from sanguivorous arachnids and insects, but the role of arthropods in the transmission of chlamydial diseases is unclear. The family contains a single genus, *Chlamydia.*

chlamydiae (klah-mid′e-e) plural of *chlamydia.*

chlamydial (klah-mid′e-al) pertaining to or caused by *Chlamydia.*

Chlamydiales (klah-mid′e-al-ēz) an order of coccoid, gram-negative, parasitic microorganisms that multiply only within the cytoplasm of vertebrate host cells by a unique developmental cycle. It includes one family, Chlamydiaceae, which was formerly assigned to the order Rickettsiales.

chlamydiosis (klah-mid″e-o′sis) 1. a general term for any infection or disease caused by any species of *Chlamydia* (q.v.). 2. a term embracing psittacosis and ornithosis. **epizootic c.,** a fatal septicemia of muskrats and snowshoe hares caused by a strain of *Chlamydia psittaci.*

Chlamydobacteriaceae (klah-mi″do-bak-te″re-a′se-e) a family of Schizomycetes (order Chlamydobacteriales), made up of filamentous, alga-like cells, frequently showing false branching. It includes three genera: *Leptothrix, Sphaerotilus,* and *Toxothrix.*

Chlamydobacteriales (klah-mi″do-bak-te″re-a′lēz) an order of Schizomycetes, made up of nonpigmented alga-like bacteria occurring in filaments which may or may not be ensheathed, and which frequently show false branching as a result of lateral displacement of cells within a sheath. It includes three families: Chlamydobacteriaceae, Crenotrichaceae, and Peloplocaceae.

Chlamydophrys (klah-mid′o-fris) a genus of free-living or coprozoic protozoa. **C. anchel′ys, C. sterco′rea,** species of coprozoic protozoa found in the feces of man and various animals.

chlamydospore (klam′ĭ-do-spōr″) [Gr. *chlamys* cloak + *spore*] a thick-walled intercalary or terminal asexual spore formed by the rounding-up of a cell; it is not shed. See *spore*. Cf. *condium.*

Chlamydozoaceae (klam″ĭ-do″zo-a′se-e) a name formerly given the family Chlamydiaceae.

Chlamydozoon (klam″ĭ-do-zo′on) a name formerly given a genus of gram-negative microorganisms; see *Chlamydia.*

chloasma (klo-az′mah) [Gr. *chloazein* to be green] melasma. **c. gravida′rum,** melasma. **c. hepat′icum,** discoloration of the skin allegedly resulting from disorder of the liver; presumably indirectly due to accumulation of estrogen in the blood. **c. periora′le virgin′ium,** brownish or blackish pigmentation, associated with macular seborrhea, situated chiefly around the mouth but involving other parts of the face, and occurring in normal young girls at the time of the first menstrual period. **c. uteri′num,** melasma gravidarum.

chlophedianol hydrochloride (klo″fĕ-di′ah-nol) chemical name: 2-chloro-α-[(dimethylamino)ethyl]-α-phenylbenzenemethanol hydrochloride. An antitussive agent, $C_{17}H_{20}ClNO\cdot HCl$, occurring as a white, crystalline powder; administered orally.

chloracetization (klor-as″e-tĭ-za′shun) the production of local anesthesia by application of equal parts of chloroform and glacial acetic acid; no longer used.

chloracne (klor-ak′ne) an acneiform eruption caused by exposure to chlorine compounds.

chloral (klo′ral) [*chlor*ine + *-al*] 1. chemical name: trichloroacetaldehyde. A colorless, oily liquid, $Cl_3C\cdot CHO$, having a pungent, irritating odor, and prepared by the mutual action of alcohol and chlorine. It is used in the manufacture of chloral hydrate and DDT. 2. chloral hydrate. **c. betaine,** an adduct formed by the reaction of chloral hydrate with betaine, occurring as a white, crystalline powder, having actions and uses similar to those of chloral hydrate but having the advantage of eliminating undesirable gastrointestinal symptoms sometimes associated with chloral hydrate; administered orally. **butyl c.,** see *butylchloral hydrate.* **c. carmine,** a staining fluid made of carmine, 0.05 gm.; hydrochloric acid, 30 minims; alcohol, 20 cc.; and chloral hydrate, 25 gm. **c. hydrate** [USP], chemical name: 2,2,2-trichloro-1,1-ethanediol. A hypnotic and sedative, $C_2H_3Cl_3O_2$, occurring as colorless, transparent, or white crystals; administered orally.

chloralism (klo′ral-izm) a morbid condition caused by excessive use of chloral.

chloralization (klo″ral-ĭ-za′shun) 1. chloralism. 2. formerly, anesthesia by the use of chloral.

chloralose (klo′rah-lōs) chemical name: 1,2,O-(2,2,2-trichloroethylidene)-α-D-glucofuranose. A compound of chloral and glucose, $C_8H_{11}Cl_3O_6$, which has been used as a hypnotic, but is primarily used as a surgical anesthetic in laboratory animals, rodenticide for mice, and bird repellent on grain. Called also *α-chloralose.*

chlorambucil (klo-ram′bu-sil) [USP] chemical name: 4-[*p*-[bis(2-chloroethyl)amino]benzenebutanoic acid. A cytotoxic alkylating agent, $C_{14}H_{19}Cl_2NO_2$, occurring as an off-white, slightly granular powder; used as an antineoplastic in the palliative treatment of Hodgkin's disease, chronic lymphocytic leukemia, and lymphosarcoma, administered orally.

chloramine-T (klo′rah-mēn) chemical name: *N*-chloro-4-methylbenzenesulfonamide sodium salt. A chlorine derivative, $C_7H_7ClNNaO_2S$, which has been used in solution as a topical antiseptic to irrigate and dress wounds and as a mouthwash, and has been used to sterilize drinking water.

chloramphenicol (klo″ram-fen′ĭ-kol) [USP] chemical name: [R-(R*, R*)]-2, 2-dichloro-*N*-[2-hydroxy-1-(hydroxymethyl)-2-(4-nitrophenyl)ethyl]acetamide. A broad-spectrum antibiotic, $C_{11}H_{12}Cl_2N_2O_5$, originally derived for *Streptomyces venezuelae* and later shown to be elaborated by other spirochetes, and produced synthetically. It occurs as fine, white to grayish white or yellowish white, needle-like crystals or elongated plates, and is effective against rickettsiae, gram-positive and gram-negative bacteria, and certain spirochetes, being used especially in the treatment of typhus and other rickettsial infections and in typhoid, shigellosis, and related enteric diseases; used as an antibacterial, administered orally or applied topically to the conjunctiva, or as an antirickettsial, administered orally. **c. palmitate** [USP], the monopalmitic ester of chloramphenicol, $C_{27}H_{42}Cl_2N_2O_6$, occurring as a fine, white, unctuous, crystalline powder, having the same actions and uses as the base; administered orally. **c. sodium succinate,** the sodium succinate derivative of chloramphenicol, $C_{15}H_{15}Cl_2N_2NaO_8$, occurring as a light yellow powder, having the same actions and uses as the base; administered intravenously. Sterile chloramphenicol sodium [USP] conforms to FDA regulations concerning antibiotic drugs.

chlorate (klo'rāt) any salt of chloric acid.

chlorazanil hyrochloride (klo-rah'zah-nil) chemical name: *N*-(4-chlorophenyl)-1,3,5-triazine-2,4-diamine monohydrochloride; a diuretic, $C_9H_8ClN_5HCl$.

chlorbutol (klōr-bu'tol) chlorobutanol.

chlorcyclizine hydrochloride (klōr-si'klĭ-zēn) [USP] chemical name: 1-[(4-chlorophenyl)phenylmethyl]-4-methylpiperazine monohydrochloride. An antihistaminic, $C_{18}H_{21}ClN_2 \cdot HCl$, occurring as white, crystalline powder; administered orally.

chlordan (klōr'dān) chlordane.

chlordane (klōr'dān) a poisonous substance of the chlorinated hydrocarbon group, used as an insecticide; human poisoning may occur by percutaneous absorption, ingestion, or inhalation.

chlordantoin (klōr-dan'to-in) chemical name: 5-(1-ethylpentyl)-3-[(trichloromethyl)thio]-2,4-imidazolidinedione. An antifungal agent, $C_{11}H_{17}Cl_3N_2O_2S$, effective against various fungi, including *Candida albicans;* used topically in the treatment of fungal infections of the vulvovaginal region and of the skin.

chlordiazepoxide (klōr''di-az''ĕ-pok'sīd) [USP] chemical name: 7-chloro-*N*-methyl-5-phenyl-3*H*-1,4-benzodiazepin-2-amine-4-oxide.One of the benzodiazepine tranquilizers, $C_{16}H_{14}ClN_3O$, occurring as a yellow, crystalline powder; administered orally in the treatment of conditions in which anxiety, tension, and apprehension are prominent symptoms, in acute anxiety, and in chronic alcoholism or alcohol withdrawal. **c. hydrochloride** [USP], the monohydrochloride salt of chlordiazepoxide, $C_{18}H_{21}Cl-N_2 \cdot HCl$, occurring as a white, or almost white, crystalline powder; used for the same purposes as the base, administered orally, intravenously, or intramuscularly.

chlordimorine hydrochloride (klōr-dim'or-ēn) chemical name: 4-[3-[(3-chloro-4-biphenylyl)oxy]propyl]morpholine hydrochloride; an antifungal agent, $C_{19}H_{22}ClNO_2$.

chlorella (klo-rel'ah) a genus of fresh-water green algae which are the source of chlorellin and are used in studies of photosynthesis.

chlorellin (klo-rel'in) a bacteriostatic substance derived from fresh water algae of the genus *Chlorella.*

chloremia (klo-re'me-ah) [Gr. *chlōros* green + *haima* blood + *-ia*] 1. chlorosis. 2. hyperchloremia.

chlorenchyma (klo-ren'kĭ-mah) the chlorophyll-bearing tissue of plants.

chloretic (klo-ret'ik) an agent that accelerates the flow of bile.

Chloretone (klo're-tōn) trademark for a preparation of chlorobutanol.

chlorguanide (klōr-gwan'īd) proguanil.

chlorhexidine (klōr-heks'ĭ-dēn) chemical name: *N,N*''-bis(4-chlorophenyl)-3,12-diimino-2,4-11,13-tetraazatetradecanediimidamide. An antibacterial, $C_{22}H_{30}Cl_2N_{10}$, effective against a wide variety of gram-negative and gram-positive organisms. **c. acetate,** the diacetate salt of chlorhexidine, $C_{22}H_{30}Cl_2N_{10}O_4 \cdot 2C_2H_4$-$O_2$, occurring as a white, crystalline powder, having the same actions as the base; used mainly as a preservative for eye-drops. **c. gluconate,** the digluconate salt of chlorhexidine, $C_{22}H_{30}Cl_2$-$N_{10} \cdot 2C_6H_{12}O_7$, having the same actions as the base; used as a topical anti-infective for the skin and mucous membranes. **c. hydrochloride,** the dihydrochloride salt of chlorhexidine, C_{22}-$H_{30}Cl_2N_{10} \cdot 2HCl$, occurring as a white or almost white, crystalline powder, having the same actions as the base; used as a topical anti-infective for the skin and mucous membranes.

chlorhistechia (klōr''his-tek'e-ah) [*chloride* + Gr. *histos* tissue + *echein* to hold + *-ia*] the presence of an abnormally large amount of chloride in a tissue.

chlorhydria (klōr-hi'dre-ah) an excess of hydrochloric acid in the stomach.

chloric (klo'rik) [L. *chloricus*] derived from or containing pentavalent chlorine; a term used to distinguish those compounds which contain a smaller proportion of chlorine than the chlorous compounds, and forming salts known as chlorates.

chloride (klo'rīd) a salt of hydrochloric acid; any binary compound of chlorine in which the latter is the negative element. Formerly called *muriate.* **acid c.,** a substance formed by substituting chlorine for hydroxyl in an acid molecule. **ferric c.,** orange-yellow or brownish yellow pieces, $FeCl_3 \cdot 6H_2O$,

very soluble in water; used as a reagent and as a diagnostic aid in phenylketonuria; it was formerly used as a hematinic in the treatment of iron deficiency anemias, and has been used as a topical astringent and styptic. Called also *iron chloride.* **mercuric c.,** mercury bichloride. **mercurous c.,** calomel. **stannous c.,** chemical name: tin chloride ($SnCl_2$) dihydrate; a pharmaceutic aid, $SnCl_2 \cdot 2H_2O$.

chloridemia (klo''rĭ-de'me-ah) [*chloride* + Gr. *haima* blood + *-ia*] (*obs.*) hyperchloremia.

chloridimeter (klo''rĭ-dim'ĕ-ter) [*chloride* + Gr. *metron* measure] an instrument for measuring the chloride content of the urine or other fluid.

chloridimetry (klo''rĭ-dim'ĕ-tre) the determination of the chloride content of fluids.

chloridion (klo''rid-i'on) negatively ionic chlorine, the anion of hydrochloric acid and the chlorides.

chloridometer (klo''rĭ-dom'ĕ-ter) chloridimeter.

chloridorrhea (klor''īd-o-re'ah) diarrhea with an excess of chlorides in the stool.

chloriduria (klo''rĭ-du're-ah) [*chloride* + Gr. *ouron* urine + *-ia*] excess of chlorides in the urine.

chlorinated (klo'rĭ-nāt''ed) charged with chlorine.

chlorine (klor'ēn, klo'rēn, klo'rin) [L. *chlorum* or *chlorinum*, from Gr. *chlōros* green] a yellowish green, gaseous element, of suffocating odor; symbol, Cl; atomic number, 17; atomic weight, 35.453; specific gravity, 1.56. It is disinfectant, decolorant, and an irritant poison. It is used for disinfecting, fumigating, and bleaching, either in an aqueous solution or in the form of chlorinated lime. **c. dioxide,** an oxidizing and germicidal agent, ClO_2, used in the purification of water and for bleaching.

chlorinum (klo-ri'num) [L.] (*obs.*) chlorine.

chloriodized (klōr-i'o-dīzd) containing chlorine and iodine.

chlorisondamine chloride (klōr''i-son'dah-mēn) chemical name: 4,5,6,7-tetrachloro-1,3-dihydro-2-methyl-2-[2-(trimethylammonio)ethyl]-2*H*-isoindolium dichloride. An asymmetrical bisquaternary ammonium derivative with ganglionic blocking action, $C_{14}H_{20}Cl_6N_2$, used as an antihypertensive.

chlorite (klo'rīt) any salt of chlorous acid.

chlormadinone acetate (klōr-mah'dĭ-nōn) chemical name: 17-(acetyloxy)-6-chloro-pregna-4,6-diene-3,20-dione. A progestin, $C_{23}H_{29}ClO_4$, formerly used in oral contraceptive products.

chlormerodrin (klōr-mer'o-drin) chemical name: [3-[(aminocarbonyl)amino]-2-methoxypropyl]chloromercury. An orally effective mercurial diuretic, $C_5H_{11}ClHgN_2O_2$, occurring as a white powder. **c. Hg 197** [USP], chlormerodrin tagged with radioactive mercury (^{197}Hg); used as a diagnostic aid in renal function determination, administered intravenously. **c. Hg 203** [NF], chlormerodrin tagged with radioactive mercury (^{203}Hg); used as a diagnostic aid in renal function determination, administered intravenously.

chlormethazanone (klōr''meth-az'ah-nōn) chlormezanone.

chlormethyl (klōr-meth'il) methyl chloride.

chlormezanone (klōr-mez'ah-nōn) chemical name: 2-(4-chlorophenyl)tetrahydro-3-methyl-4*H*-1,3-thiazin-4-one. A muscle relaxant and tranquilizer, $C_{11}H_{12}ClNO_3S$, occurring as a white, crystalline powder; administered orally.

chloro- (klo'ro) [Gr. *chlōros* green] a combining form meaning green.

chloroazodin (klo''ro-a'zo-din) [USP] chemical name: *N,N*''-dichlorodiazenedicarboximidamide. An antibacterial, $C_2H_4Cl_2N_6$, which has been used as an antiseptic.

Chlorobacteriaceae (klo''ro-bak-te''re-a'se-e) a family of Schizomycetes (order Pseudomonadales, suborder Rhodobacteriineae), composed of microorganisms developing in environments containing considerable hydrogen sulfide and exposed to light, and containing green pigments resembling but not identical with chlorophylls. It includes six genera, *Chlorobacterium, Chlorobium, Chlorochromatium, Clathrochloris, Cylindrogloea,* and *Pelodictyon.*

Chlorobacterium (klo''ro-bak-te're-um) a genus of microorganisms of the family Chlorobacteriaceae, suborder Rhodobacteriineae, order Pseudomonadales, occurring as nonmotile, often slightly curved rod-shaped cells growing symbiotically on the outside of protozoa. The type species is *C. symbiot'icum.*

Chlorobium (klo-ro'be-um) a genus of microorganisms of the family Chlorobacteriaceae, suborder Rhodobacteriineae, order Pseudomonadales, occurring as spherical to rod-shaped cells, singly or in chains. It includes two species: *C. limi'cola* and *C. thiosulfato'philum.*

chlorobrightism (klo''ro-brīt'izm) chlorosis with albuminuria.

chlorobutanol (klo''ro-bu'tah-nol) [NF] chemical name: 1,1,1-trichloro-2-methyl-2-propanol. Colorless to white crystals, C_4H_7-Cl_3O, with a camphoraceous odor and taste; used as an antimicrobial preservative in various pharmaceutical solutions, especially injectables. It has been used as a local dental analgesic, hypnotic, antipruritic, sedative, somnifacient, and antiseptic.

Chlorochromatium (klo''ro-kro-ma'te-um) a genus of microorganisms of the family Chlorobacteriaceae, suborder Rhodobacteriineae, order Pseudomonadales, occurring as ovoid to rod-shaped cells with rounded ends, forming barrel-shaped aggregates about a large, colorless bacterium. The type species is *C. aggregat'um*.

chlorocruorin (klo″ro-kroo′o-rin) a green respiratory pigment occurring in certain marine worms.

chloroerythroblastoma (klo″ro-e-rith″ro-blas-to′mah) a new growth containing the elements of granulocytic sarcoma (chloroma) and erythrocytic sarcoma (erythroblastoma).

chloroethane (klo-ro-eth′ān) ethyl chloride.

chloroform (klo′ro-form) [L. *chloroformum;* from *chlorine* + *formyl*] [NF] a clear, colorless, volatile liquid, CHCl₃, with a strong ethereal smell and a sweetish, burning taste used as a solvent. It was once widely used as an inhalation anesthetic and analgesic, and as an antitussive, carminative, and counterirritant. Called also *trichlormethane*. **acetone c.,** chlorobutanol. **alcoholized c.,** a mixture of chloroform and alcohol. **Anschütz's c.,** a crystalline substance from which gentle heat liberates a vapor of pure chloroform; called also *salicylide chloroform*. **Pictet's c.,** chloroform purified by congelation at a very low temperature.

chloroformism (klo′ro-form″izm) 1. the habitual use of chloroform for its narcotic effect. 2. the anesthetic effect of the vapor of chloroform.

chloroformization (klo″ro-form″i-za′shun) the administration of chloroform.

chloroguanide hydrochloride (klor″o-gwan′īd) proguanil hydrochloride.

chlorolabe (klor′o-lāb) [*chloro-* + Gr. *lambanein* to take] name proposed for the pigment in retinal cones that is more sensitive to the green portion of the spectrum than are the other pigments (cyanolabe and erythrolabe).

chloroleukemia (klo″ro-lu-ke′me-ah) chloroma.

chlorolymphosarcoma (klo″ro-lim″fo-sar-ko′mah) chloroma; so called because mononuclear cells in the peripheral blood were thought to be lymphocytes rather than myeloblasts.

chloroma (klo-ro′mah) [*chloro-* + *-oma*] a malignant green-colored tumor arising from myeloid tissue, associated with myelogenous leukemia and occurring anywhere in the body. Besides containing green pigment, which has no clear metabolic role and is principally myeloperoxidase (verdoperoxidase), chloroma tissue demonstrates a bright red fluorescence under ultraviolet light. Called also *green cancer, chloroleukemia, chlorolymphosarcoma,* and *granulocytic sarcoma*.

***p*-chloromercuribenzoate** (klo″ro-mer″ku-re-ben′zo-āt) a univalent organic mercury compound that reacts with sulfhydryl groups on proteins, or other molecules, thereby often inhibiting their activities.

chloromethapyriline citrate (klo″ro-meth″ah-pi′rĭ-lēn) chlorothen citrate.

chlorometry (klo-rom′ĕ-tre) the quantitative determination of chlorine.

Chloromycetin (klo″ro-mi-se′tin) trademark for preparations of chloramphenicol.

chloromyeloma (klo″ro-mi-ĕ-lo′mah) chloroma attended with growths in the bone marrow.

chloronaphthalene (klo″ro-naf′thah-lēn) any of the products of the chlorination of naphthalene; exposure to such substances may cause halogen acne.

chloropenia (klo″ro-pe′ne-ah) [*chlorine* + Gr. *penia* poverty] (*obs.*) hypochloremia.

chloropenic (klo″ro-pe′nik) (*obs.*) hypochloremic.

chloropexia (klo″ro-pek′se-ah) the fixation of chlorine in the body tissues.

chlorophane (klo′ro-fān) [*chloro-* + Gr. *phainein* to show] a greenish yellow pigment obtainable from the retina.

***p*-chlorophenol** (klo″ro-fe′nol) parachlorophenol.

chlorophenothane (klo″ro-fe′no-thān) chemical name: 1,1′(2,2,2-trichloroethylidene)bis-4-chlorobenzene. An insecticide and larvicide, C₁₄H₉Cl₅, effective against a wide variety of insects, occurring as white crystals or as a white to slightly off-white powder; used as a topical pediculicide. Called also *DDT, dicophane, gesarol,* and *pentachlorin*.

chlorophyl (klo′ro-fil) chlorophyll.

chlorophylase (klo′ro-fil-ās) chlorophyll chlorophyllido-hydrolase: an esterase that occurs in green leaves and hydrolyzes chlorophyll.

chlorophyll (klo′ro-fil) [*chloro-* + Gr. *phyllon* leaf] the green coloring matter of plants by which photosynthesis is accomplished. There are many types: *chlorophyll a,* C₅₅H₇₂O₅N₄Mg, is bluish green in color and the major pigment in plants that release oxygen in photosynthesis; *chlorophyll b,* C₅₅H₇₀O₆N₄Mg, is yellowish green in color; *chlorophyll c* occurs in many marine algae; *chlorophyll d* occurs in red algae. The bacteriochlorophylls occur in phototrophic bacteria. Preparations of *water-soluble chlorophyll derivatives,* consisting mainly of the copper complex of the

sodium and/or potassium salts of chlorophyll, are applied topically to the skin for deodorization, for enhancement of normal tissue repair, and for relief of itching in various skin lesions. Preparations of the derivatives for oral administration were used to deodorize certain necrotic, ulcerative lesions, to control fecal and urinary odors in colostomy, ileostomy, or incontinence, and to deodorize urinary and fecal fistulas and breath and body odors not related to faulty hygiene.

chlorophyllin (klo′ro-fil-in) any of the water-soluble salts obtained by alkaline hydrolysis of chlorophyll with replacement of the methyl and phytyl ester groups by sodium or potassium.

chloropia (klo-ro′pe-ah) chloropsia.

Chloropidae (klo-rop′ĭ-de) a family of small to minute flies (order Diptera); two medically important genera are *Hippelates* and *Siphunculina*.

chloroplast (klo′ro-plast) [*chloro-* + Gr. *plastos* formed] any one of the chlorophyll-bearing bodies of plant cells; called also *chloroplastid*.

chloroplastid (klo″ro-plas′tid) chloroplast.

chloroprivic (klo″ro-pri′vik) [*chlorine* + L. *privare* to deprive] deprived of chlorides; due to loss of chlorides.

chloroprocaine hydrochloride (klo″ro-pro′kān) [USP] chemical name: 2-(diethylamino)ethyl ester benzoic acid monohydrochloride. A local anesthetic, C₁₇H₁₉ClN₂O₂·HCl, occurring as a white, crystalline powder; used in minor and general surgery for infiltration, field block, and regional nerve block, including caudal and epidural block.

chloroprocaine penicillin (klo″ro-pro′kān) see under *penicillin*.

chloropsia (klo-rop′se-ah) [*chloro-* + Gr. *opsis* vision + *-ia*] a visual defect in which all objects seen appear to have a greenish tinge.

Chloroptic (klōr-op′tik) trademark for preparations of chloramphenicol.

chloroquine (klo′ro-kwin) [USP] chemical name: N⁴-(7-chloro-4-quinolinyl)-N¹,N¹-diethyl 1,4-pentanediamine. A compound, C₁₈H₂₆ClN₃, occurring as a white or slightly yellow, crystalline powder; used as antimalarial in certain forms of malaria and as an antiamebic in extraintestinal amebiasis, administered intramuscularly. **c. phosphate** [USP], the phosphate salt of chloroquine, C₁₈H₂₆ClN₃·2H₃PO₄, occurring as a white, crystalline powder; used as an antimalarial for the suppression and treatment of certain forms of malaria, as an antiamebic in extraintestinal amebiasis, and as a lupus erythematosus suppressant, administered orally.

chlorosarcolymphadeny (klo″ro-sar″ko-lim-fad′ĕ-ne) (*obs.*) chloroma.

chlorosarcoma (klo″ro-sar-ko′mah) (*obs.*) chloroma.

chlorosarcomyeloma (klo″ro-sar″ko-mi″ĕ-lo′mah) (*obs.*) chloroma.

chlorosis (klo-ro′sis) a disorder, especially common during the nineteenth century and disappearing abruptly soon thereafter, generally affecting adolescent females, believed to be associated with iron deficiency anemia, and characterized by greenish yellow discoloration of the skin and by hypochromic erythrocytes.

Chlorostigma (klo″ro-stig′mah) a genus of plants, e.g., *C. stuckertianum* (Asclepiadaceae). Its alkaloid, chlorostigmine, has been used to stimulate the secretion of milk during lactation.

chlorostigmine (klōr″o-stig′mēn) a galactopoietic alkaloid from plants of the genus *Chlorostigma*.

chlorothen citrate (klo′ro-then) chemical name: N-[(5-chloro-2-thienyl)methyl]-N,N″-dimethyl-N-2-pyridinyl-1,2-ethanediamine dihydrogen citrate. An antihistaminic, C₁₄H₁₈ClN₃S·C₆H₈O₇, occurring as a white, crystalline powder; administered orally.

chlorothenium citrate (klo″ro-then′ĭ-um) chlorothen citrate.

chlorothiazide (klo″ro-thi′ah-zīd) [USP] chemical name: 6-chloro-2H-1,2,4-benzothiadiazine-7-sulfonamide-1,1-dioxide. An orally effective diuretic, C₇H₆ClN₃O₄S₂, occurring as a white or practically white, crystalline powder; used in the treatment of renal, hepatic, and drug-induced edema, edema and toxemia of pregnancy, and fluid retention associated with various conditions, and in hypertension. **c. sodium,** the monosodium salt of chlorothiazide, C₇H₅ClN₃NaO₄S₂, administered intravenously for the same purposes as the base.

chlorothymol (klo″ro-thi′mol) chemical name: 4-chloro-5-methyl-2-(1-methylethyl)phenol; a powerful germicide, C₁₀H₁₃ClO, which has been used as a topical antibacterial and fungicide.

chlorotic (klo-rot′ik) pertaining to, or affected with chlorosis.

chlorotrianisene (klo″ro-tri-an′ĭ-sēn) [USP] chemical name: 1,1′,1″-(1-chloro-1-ethenyl-2-ylidene)tris-4-methoxybenzene. A synthetic estrogen, C₂₃H₂₁ClO₃, occurring as small white crystals or as a crystalline powder; used to suppress lactation in postpartum women, for palliative treatment in inoperable prostatic carcinoma, and for replacement therapy of estrogen deficiency, administered orally.

chlorous (klo′rus) derived from or containing trivalent chlorine, as in chlorous acid, HClO₂; a term used to distinguish those compounds which contain a larger proportion of chlorine than the chloric compounds, and forming salts known as chlorites.

chlorovinyldichloroarsine (klo″ro-vin″il-di-klo″ro-ar′sin) lewisite.

chloroxine (klo-roks′ēn) chemical name: 5,7-dichloro-8-quinolinol. A synthetic antibacterial, $C_9H_5Cl_2NO$; used in the topical treatment of dandruff and seborrheic dermatitis of the scalp.

chloroxylenol (klo″ro-zi′lĕ-nōl) chemical name: 4-chloro-3,5-dimethylphenol. An antibacterial, C_8H_9ClO, which is most active against streptococci; used mainly as a disinfectant for the skin.

chlorphenesin (klōr-fen′ĕ-sin) chemical name: 3-(4-chlorophenoxy)-1,2-propanediol. An antibacterial, antifungal, and antitrichomonal agent, $C_9H_{11}ClO_3$, occurring as white or pale cream-colored crystals or crystalline masses; used in the treatment of tinea pedis and other fungal infections of the skin and in fungal and trichomonal infections of the vagina, applied topically or intravaginally. **c. carbamate,** a skeletal muscle relaxant, $C_{10}H_{12}ClNO_4$ occurring as a white, crystalline powder; used as an adjunct in the short-term treatment of skeletal muscle spasms, such as sprains, strains, and trauma to tendons and ligaments, administered orally.

chlorpheniramine (klōr″fen-ir′ah-mēn) chemical name: γ-(4-chlorophenyl)-N,N-dimethyl-2-pyridinepropanamine. An antihistaminic, $C_{16}H_{19}ClN_2$, derived from pheniramine. **c. maleate** [USP], the maleate salt of chlorpheniramine, $C_{16}H_{19}ClN_2 \cdot C_4H_4O_4$, occurring as a white, crystalline powder; administered orally or by subcutaneous injection for therapy and prophylaxis of conditions in which antihistamines may be effective. Called also *chlorprophenpyridamine maleate.*

chlorphenoxamine hydrochloride (klōr″fen-ok′sah-mēn) [USP] chemical name: 2-[1-(4-chlorophenyl)-1-phenylethoxy]-N,N-dimethylethanamine hydrochloride. An anticholinergic $C_{18}H_{23}Cl_2NO$, with weak antihistaminic action, occurring as needle-like crystals; used as a skeletal muscle relaxant in the treatment of Parkinson's disease, administered orally.

chlorphentermine hydrochloride (klōr-fen′ter-mēn) chemical name: 4-chloro-α,α-dimethylbenzeneethanamine hydrochloride. A sympathomimetic amine, $C_{10}H_{14}ClN \cdot HCl$, occurring as a white to off-white powder; used as an anorexic agent, administered orally.

chlorpromazine (klōr-pro′mah-zēn) [USP] chemical name: 2-chloro-N,N-dimethyl-10H-phenothiazine-10-propanamine. A phenothiazine derivative, $C_{17}H_{19}ClN_2S$, occurring as a white, crystalline solid; used as an antiemetic and tranquilizer, administered by rectal suppository. **c. hydrochloride** [USP], the hydrochloride of chlorpromazine, occurring as a white, crystalline powder, used orally, muscularly, or intravenously as a major tranquilizer.

chlorpropamide (klōr-pro′pah-mīd) [USP] chemical name: 4-chloro-N-[(propylamino)carbonyl]benzenesulfonamide. An orally effective hypoglycemic agent, $C_{10}H_{13}ClN_2O_3S$, occurring as a white, crystalline powder.

chlorprophenpyridamine (klōr″pro-fen-pi-rid′ah-mēn) chlorpheniramine.

chlorprothixene (klōr-pro-thiks′ēn) [USP] chemical name: (Z)-3-(2-chloro-9H-thioxanthen-9-ylidene)-N,N-dimethyl-1-propanamine. A drug, $C_{18}H_{18}ClNS$, occurring as a yellow crystalline powder, having sedative, antiemetic, antihistaminic, anticholinergic, and alpha-adrenergic blocking activity; used to control the symptoms of psychotic disorders, administered orally or by intramuscular injection.

chlorquinaldol (klōr-kwin′al-dol) chemical name: 5,7-dichloro-8-hydroxyquinaldine. A yellow, crystalline powder, $C_{10}H_7Cl_2NO$, insoluble in water; used as a topical keratoplastic, bactericide, and fungicide in dermatoses.

chlortetracycline (klōr″tet-rah-si′klēn) chemical name: 7-chloro-4-dimethylamino-1,4,4a,5,5a,6,11,12a-octahydro-3,6,10,12,12a-pentahydroxy-6-methyl-1,11-dioxo-2-naphthacenecarboxamide. A broad-spectrum antibiotic, $C_{22}H_{23}ClN_2O_8$, elaborated by *Streptomyces aureofaciens;* it was the first of the tetracycline group to be discovered. **c. hydrochloride** [USP], the monohydrochloride salt of chlortetracycline, $C_{22}H_{23}ClN_2O_8 \cdot HCl$, occurring as a yellow crystalline powder; a broad-spectrum antibiotic used as an antibacterial and antiprotozoal, administered orally, by intravenous injection, or applied topically to the conjunctiva.

chlorthalidone (klōr-thal′ĭ-dōn) [USP] chemical name: 2-chloro-5-(2,3-dihydro-1-hydroxy-3-oxo-1H-isoindol-1-yl)benzenesulfonamide. An orally effective diuretic, $C_{14}H_{11}ClN_2O_4S$, occurring as a white to yellowish white, crystalline powder; used in the treatment of edema associated with various conditions and in hypertension.

Chlor-Trimeton (klōr-tri′mĕ-ton) trademark for preparations of chlorpheniramine maleate.

chlorum (klo′rum) [L.] chlorine.

chloruremia (klo″roo-re′me-ah) [*chloride* + Gr. *ouron* urine + *haima* blood + *-ia*] (*obs.*) hyperchloremia.

chloruremic (klo″roo-re′mik) (*obs.*) hyperchloremic.

chloruresis (klor″u-re′sis) [*chloride* + Gr. *ourein* to urinate] the excretion of chlorides in the urine.

chloruretic (klor″u-ret′ik) 1. promoting the excretion of chlorides in the urine. 2. an agent that promotes the excretion of chlorides in the urine.

chloruria (klo-roo′re-ah) [*chloride* + Gr. *ouron* urine + *-ia*] presence of chlorides in the urine.

chlorzoxazone (klōr-zok′sah-zōn) chemical name: 5-chloro-2(3H)-benzoxazolone. A skeletal muscle relaxant, $C_7H_4ClNO_2$, occurring as a white or creamy white, glistening, crystalline powder; used to relieve discomfort of painful musculoskeletal disorders, administered orally.

Chlumsky's button (klum′skēz) [Vitezslav *Chlumsky,* Czech surgeon, 1867–1943] see under *button.*

Ch.M. abbreviation for L. *Chirurgiae Magister,* Master of Surgery.

$C_6H_5NH_2$ aniline.

$C_3H_5(NO_3)_3$ glyceryl trinitrate (nitroglycerin).

$C_5H_4N_4O_3$ uric acid.

$C_5H_{11}NO_2$ amyl nitrite.

C_8H_9NO acetanilid.

$C_9H_9NO_3$ hippuric acid.

$C_6H_2(NO_2)_3OH$ trinitrophenal (picric acid).

CH_2O formaldehyde.

CH_2O_2 formic acid.

CH_4O methyl alcohol.

$C_2H_2O_4$ oxalic acid.

$C_2H_4O_2$ acetic acid.

C_2H_6O ethyl alcohol.

C_3H_6O acetone.

$C_3H_6O_3$ lactic acid.

$C_3H_8O_3$ glycerin.

$C_4H_6O_2$ crotonic acid.

$C_4H_6O_5$ malic acid.

$C_4H_6O_6$ tartaric acid.

$C_4H_8O_2$ butyric acid; isobutyric acid.

$C_4H_{10}O$ ether (ethyl ether).

$C_5H_{10}O_2$ valeric acid.

$C_5H_{12}O$ amyl alcohol.

C_6H_6O phenol.

$C_6H_8O_7$ citric acid.

$(C_6H_{10}O_5)_n$ starch, glycogen, or other hexose polymers.

$C_6H_{12}O_6$ dextrose (d-glucose).

$C_7H_4O_7$ meconic acid.

$C_7H_6O_2$ benzoic acid.

$C_7H_6O_3$ salicylic acid.

$C_7H_6O_5$ gallic acid.

$C_{12}H_{22}O_{11}$ cane sugar.

$C_{15}H_{10}O_4$ chrysophanic acid.

$C_{18}H_{34}O_2$ oleic acid.

$C_{18}H_{36}O_2$ stearic acid.

choana (ko′a-nah), pl. *choa′nae* [L.; Gr. *choanē* funnel] 1. any funnel-shaped cavity or infundibulum. 2. [pl.] [NA] the paired openings between the nasal cavity and the nasopharynx; called also *choanae osseae* and *posterior nares.* **bony choanae, choa′nae os′seae,** see *choana,* def. 2. **primary c.,** the opening of the embryonic olfactory sac into the mouth. **secondary c.,** the definitive choana after the formation of the palate.

choanae (ko-a′ne) [L.] plural of *choana.*

choanal (ko′ah-nal) pertaining to a choana.

choanoid (ko′ah-noid) [Gr. *choanē* funnel + *eidos* form] funnel-shaped.

choanocyte (ko′ah-no″sīt) a unique type of cell having a flagellum surrounded by a thin cytoplasmic collar; characteristic of sponges and certain protozoa.

choanoflagellate (ko″ah-no-flaj′ĕ-lāt) any member of the order Choanoflagellida.

Choanoflagellida (ko″ah-no-flaj′ĕ-li″dah) an order of sedentary protozoa resembling sponges and having a single flagellum surrounded by a delicate cytoplasmic collar.

Choanotaenia (ko-a″no-te′ne-ah) a genus of tapeworms. **C. infundib′ulum,** an important tapeworm parasite of both chickens and turkeys.

choc (shok) [Fr.] shock.

chocolate (chok′o-lat) [L. *chocolata,* from Mexican *chocolatl*] a dried paste prepared from the kernels of the cacao, *Theobroma cacao,* with sugar and flavoring substances.

C_6H_5OH phenol.

choke (chōk) 1. to interrupt respiration by obstruction or compression, or the condition resulting from such interruption. 2. [pl.] a burning sensation beginning in the substernal region, with increasing uncontrollable urge to cough, and great apprehension and anxiety, leading to vasovagal attack, experienced during decompression. **ophthalmovascular c.,** interference with the blood supply of the retina due to pressure of the retinal vessels against one another. **thoracic c.,** in veterinary medicine, obstruction of the thoracic part of the esophagus with a foreign body. **water c.,** laryngeal spasm caused by fluid entering the larynx and especially by getting between the true and false vocal cords.

chol- see *chole-*.

cholagogic (ko″lah-goj′ik) stimulating the flow of bile to the duodenum.

cholagogue (ko′lah-gog) [*chol-* + Gr. *agōgos* leading] an agent that stimulates the flow of bile into the duodenum.

cholaligenic (ko-lal″ĭ-jen′ik) [*cholalic* acid + Gr. *gennan* to produce] (*obs.*) forming cholalic (cholic) acid from cholesterol—one of the functions of the liver.

Cholan-DH (ko′lan) trademark for preparations of dehydrocholic acid.

cholaneresis (ko″lah-ner′ĕ-sis) increase in the output or elimination of bile acids, their conjugates, or their salts.

cholangeitis (ko″lan-ji′tis) cholangitis.

cholangiectasis (ko-lan″je-ek′tah-sis) dilatation of a bile duct.

cholangioadenoma (ko-lan″je-o-ad″ĕ-no′mah) a benign adenoma of the liver made up of congeries of small alveoli with distinct lumina, lined by cubical or cylindrical cells resembling those of normal bile ducts.

cholangiocarcinoma (ko-lan″je-o-kar″sĭ-no′mah) cholangiocellular carcinoma.

cholangiocholecystocholedochectomy (ko-lan″ge-o-ko″le-sis″to-ko″le-do-kek′to-me) excision of hepatic duct, common bile duct, and gallbladder.

cholangioenterostomy (ko-lan″je-o-en″ter-os′to-me) [*chol-* + Gr. *angeion* vessel + *enteron* intestine + *stomoun* to provide with an opening, or mouth] surgical anastomosis of a bile duct to the intestine.

cholangiogastrostomy (ko-lan″je-o-gas-tros′to-me) [*chol-* + Gr. *angeion* vessel + *gastēr* stomach + *stomoun* to provide with an opening, or mouth] surgical anastomosis of a bile duct to the stomach.

cholangiogram (ko-lan′je-o-gram″) a roentgenogram of the gallbladder and bile ducts.

cholangiography (ko-lan″je-og′rah-fe) [*chol-* + Gr. *angeion* vessel + *graphein* to write] roentgenography of the biliary ducts after administration or injection of a contrast medium. **operative c.,** cholangiography performed during a surgical procedure on the gallbladder.

cholangiohepatitis (ko-lan″je-o-hep″ah-ti′tis) severe inflammation of the bile passages often associated with liver fluke infestation, which causes obstruction of the bile ducts.

cholangiohepatoma (ko-lan″je-o-hep″ah-to′mah) primary carcinoma of the liver of mixed liver cell and bile-duct cell origin; called also *hepatocholangiocarcinoma.*

cholangiojejunostomy (ko-lan″je-o-jĕ-ju-nos′to-me) surgical anastomosis of a bile duct to the jejunum. **intrahepatic c.,** surgical creation of an anastomosis between an intrahepatic bile duct and the jejunum; also, the anastomosis so constructed.

cholangiolar (ko″lan-je′o-lar) pertaining to a cholangiole.

cholangiole (ko-lan′je-ōl) [*chol-* + Gr. *angeion* vessel + *-ole* diminutive suffix] one of the fine terminal elements of the bile duct system, leaving the portal canal, and pursuing a course at the periphery of a lobule of the liver; called also *bile* or *biliary ductule* and, rarely, *bile capillary.*

cholangiolitis (ko-lan″je-o-li′tis) inflammation of the cholangioles.

cholangioma (ko-lan″je-o′mah) [*chol-* + Gr. *angeion* vessel + *-oma*] cholangiocellular carcinoma.

cholangiostomy (ko″lan-je-os′to-me) [*chol-* + Gr. *angeion* vessel + *stomoun* to provide with an opening, or mouth] fistulization of a bile duct.

cholangiotomy (ko″lan-je-ot′o-me) [*chol-* + Gr. *angeion* vessel + *tomē* a cutting] incision into a bile duct.

cholangitis (ko″lan-ji′tis) [*chol-* + Gr. *angeion* vessel + *-itis*] inflammation of a bile duct. **c. len′ta,** chronic infectious cholangitis without gallstones or biliary tract obstruction.

cholanopoiesis (ko″lah-no-poi-e′sis) the synthesis of bile acids or of their conjugates and salts by the liver.

cholanopoietic (ko″lah-no″poi-et′ik) 1. pertaining to or promoting cholanopoiesis. 2. an agent that promotes cholanopoiesis.

cholanthrene (ko-lan′thrēn) a pentacyclic hydrocarbon, $C_{20}H_{14}$, of great carcinogenicity.

cholate (ko′lāt) a salt or ester of cholic acid.

chole-, chol-, cholo- (ko′le, kōl, ko′lo) [Gr. *cholē* bile] a combining form denoting relationship to the bile.

cholebilirubin (ko″le-bil″e-ru′bin) a pigment, $C_{32}H_{50}O_{11}N_2$, differing from bilirubin, occurring in gallbladder bile; it gives a direct reaction to the Van den Bergh test.

Cholebrine (ko′le-brin) trademark for a preparation of iocetamic acid.

cholecalciferol (ko″le-kal-sif′er-ol) [USP] chemical name: activated 5,7-cholestadien-3β-ol. An antirachitic vitamin occurring as white, odorless crystals, $C_{27}H_{44}O$, soluble in alcohol, chloroform, and fatty oils; it undergoes metabolic conversion before exerting biological effects (see *dihydroxycholecalciferol*). Called also *activated 7-dehydrocholesterol* and *vitamin D₃.*

cholechromopoiesis (ko″le-kro″mo-poi-e′sis) the synthesis of bile pigments.

cholecyanin (ko″le-si′ah-nin) bilicyanin.

cholecyst (ko′le-sist) [*chole-* + Gr. *kystis* bladder] the gallbladder.

cholecystagogic (ko″le-sis″tah-goj′ik) cholecystokinetic.

cholecystagogue (ko″le-sis′tah-gog) a cholecystokinetic agent.

cholecystalgia (ko″le-sis-tal′je-ah) [*cholecyst* + *-algia*] 1. gallbladder colic due to impaction of a gallstone in the cystic duct. 2. pain due to inflammation of the gallbladder.

cholecystatony (ko″le-sis-tat′o-ne) atony of the gallbladder.

cholecystectasia (ko″le-sis″tek-ta′ze-ah) [*cholecyst* + Gr. *ektasis* distention] distention of the gallbladder.

cholecystectomy (ko″le-sis-tek′to-me) [*cholecyst* + Gr. *ektomē* excision] surgical removal of the gallbladder.

cholecystenteric (ko″le-sis″ten-ter′ik) pertaining to communication between the gallbladder and intestine; called also *cholecystointestinal.*

cholecystenteroanastomosis (ko″le-sis-ten″ter-o-ah-nas″to-mo′sis) cholecystenterostomy.

cholecystenterorrhaphy (ko″le-sis-ten″ter-or′ah-fe) suture of the gallbladder to the small intestine.

cholecystenterostomy (ko″le-sis″ten″ter-os′to-me) [*cholecyst* + Gr. *enteron* bowel + *stomoun* to provide with an opening, or mouth] surgical anastomosis of the gallbladder to the intestine.

cholecystgastrostomy (ko″le-sist-gas-tros′to-me) cholecystogastrostomy.

cholecystic (ko″le-sis′tik) pertaining to the gallbladder.

cholecystis (ko″le-sis′tis) [Gr. *chole* bile, gall + *kystis* bladder] the gallbladder.

cholecystitis (ko″le-sis-ti′tis) [*cholecyst* + *-itis*] inflammation of the gallbladder. **acute c.,** a form usually due to obstruction of the gallbladder outlet, with signs ranging from mild edema and congestion to severe infection with gangrene and perforation. **chronic c.,** inflammation of the gallbladder with relatively mild symptoms persisting over a long period. **c. emphysemato′sa,** emphysematous c. **emphysematous c.,** inflammation of the gallbladder caused by gas-producing organisms, characterized by gas in the gallbladder lumen and frequently infiltrating into the wall of the gallbladder and surrounding tissues; called also *gaseous c.* **follicular c.,** inflammation of the gallbladder in which there is conspicuous formation of lymphoid follicles, which commonly contain germinal centers. **gaseous c.,** emphysematous c. **c. glandula′ris prolif′erans,** a thickening of the wall of the chronically inflamed gallbladder, with formation of crypts which may develop into cysts.

cholecystnephrostomy (ko″le-sist″ne-fros′to-me) cholecystopyelostomy.

cholecystocholangiogram (ko″le-sis″to-ko-lan′je-o-gram) roentgenogram of the gallbladder and bile ducts.

cholecystocolonic (ko″le-sis″to-ko-lon′ik) pertaining to communication between the gallbladder and colon, as cholecystocolonic fistula.

cholecystocolostomy (ko″le-sis″to-ko-los′to-me) surgical anastomosis of the gallbladder to the colon; called also *colocholecystostomy.*

cholecystocolotomy (ko″le-sis″to-ko-lot′o-me) surgical incision of the gallbladder and colon.

cholecystoduodenostomy (ko″le-sis″to-du″o-dĕ-nos′to-me) surgical anastomosis of the gallbladder and the duodenum.

cholecystoenterostomy (ko″le-sis-to-en″ter-os′to-me) cholecystenterostomy.

cholecystogastric (ko″le-sis″to-gas′trik) pertaining to communication between the gallbladder and stomach, as a cholecystogastric fistula.

cholecystogastrostomy (ko″le-sis″to-gas-tros′to-me) surgical anastomosis between the gallbladder and the stomach.

cholecystogogic (ko″le-sis″to-goj′ik) cholecystokinetic.

cholecystogram (ko″le-sis′to-gram) a roentgenogram of the gallbladder.

cholecystography (ko″le-sis-tog′rah-fe) [*cholecyst* + Gr. *graphein* to write] roentgenography of the gallbladder.

cholecystoileostomy (ko″le-sis″to-il″e-os′to-me) surgical anastomosis of the gallbladder and the ileum.

cholecystointestinal (ko″le-sis″to-in-tes′tĭ-nal) cholecystenteric.

cholecystojejunostomy (ko″le-sis″to-jĕ-ju-nos′to-me) surgical anastomosis of the gallbladder and the jejunum.

cholecystokinase (ko″le-sis″to-ki′nās) an enzyme in the blood that catalyzes the decomposition of cholecystokinin.

cholecystokinetic (ko″le-sis″to-ki-net′ik) causing or promoting contraction of the gallbladder.

cholecystokinin (ko″le-sis″to-kin′in) [*cholecyst* + Gr. *kinein* to move] a polypeptide hormone secreted by the mucosa of the upper intestine which stimulates contraction of the gallbladder (with release of bile) and secretion of pancreatic enzymes. It is identical with pancreozymin. Abbreviated CCK.

cholecystolithiasis (ko″le-sis″to-lĭ-thi′ah-sis) [*cholecyst* + *lithiasis*] cholelithiasis.

cholecystolithotripsy (ko″le-sis″to-lith′o-trip″se) [*cholecyst* + *lithotripsy*] the crushing of gallstones within the gallbladder.

cholecystonephrostomy (ko″le-sis″to-ne-fros′to-me) cholecystopyelostomy.

cholecystopathy (ko″le-sis-top′ah-the) [*cholecyst* + Gr. *pathos* disease] any gallbladder disease.

cholecystopexy (ko″le-sis″to-pek″se) [*cholecyst* + Gr. *pēxis* fixation] suspension or fixation of the gallbladder by surgical means.

cholecystoptosis (ko″le-sis″to-to′sis) [*cholecyst* + Gr. *ptōsis* fall] downward or distal displacement of the gallbladder.

cholecystopyelostomy (ko″le-sis″to-pi″ĕ-los′to-me) surgical anastomosis of the gallbladder to the pelvis of the kidney; called also *cholecystonephrostomy*.

cholecystorrhaphy (ko″le-sis-tor′ah-fe) [*cholecyst* + Gr. *rhaphē* suture] suture or repair of the gallbladder.

cholecystosis (ko″le-sis-to′sis) any noninflammatory disease of the gallbladder. **hyperplastic c.,** abnormal increase in cellular structure of the gallbladder.

cholecystostomy (ko″le-sis-tos′to-me) [*cholecyst* + Gr. *stomoun* to provide with an opening, or mouth] the creation of an opening into the gallbladder for drainage.

cholecystotomy (ko″le-sis-tot′o-me) [*cholecyst* + Gr. *tomē* a cutting] surgical incision of the gallbladder; done for exploration, drainage (cholecystostomy), or removal of calculi.

cholecystotyphoid (ko″le-sis″to-ti′foid) typhoid fever complicated by acute cholecystitis.

choledochal (kol′ĕ-dok-al) pertaining to the common bile duct.

choledochectomy (kol″ĕ-do-kek′to-me) [*choledochus* + Gr. *ektomē* excision] excision of a portion of the common bile duct.

choledochendysis (kol″ĕ-do-ken′dĭ-sis) [*choledochus* + Gr. *endysis* entrance] choledochotomy.

choledochitis (kol″ĕ-do-ki′tis) inflammation of the common bile duct, or ductus choledochus.

choledochocele (ko-led′o-ko-sēl) a rare form of congenital cystic dilatation of the common bile duct in which the dilated portion is within the wall of the duct.

choledochocholedochostomy (ko-led″o-ko-kol″ĕ-do-kos′to-me) surgical formation of an anastomosis between two portions of the common bile duct.

choledochoduodenostomy (ko-led″o-ko-du″o-dĕ-nos′to-me) surgical anastomosis of the common bile duct to the duodenum.

choledochoenterostomy (ko-led″o-ko-en″ter-os′to-me) surgical anastomosis of the common bile duct to the intestine.

choledochogastrostomy (ko-led″o-ko-gas-tros′to-me) surgical anastomosis of the common bile duct and the stomach.

choledochogram (ko-led′ŏ-ko-gram″) a roentgenogram of the common bile duct.

choledochography (ko-led″o-kog′rah-fe) [*choledochus* + Gr. *graphein* to write] roentgenography of the common bile duct after the administration of opaque material.

choledochohepatostomy (ko-led″o-ko-hep″ah-tos′to-me) surgical anastomosis of the common bile duct to the hepatic duct.

choledochoileostomy (ko-led″o-ko-il-e-os′to-me) surgical anastomosis of the common bile duct and the ileum.

choledochojejunostomy (ko-led″o-ko-jĕ-ju-nos′to-me) surgical anastomosis of the common bile duct and the jejunum.

choledocholith (ko-led′ŏ-ko-lith″) a calculus in the common bile duct.

choledocholithiasis (ko-led″ŏ-ko-lĭ-thi′ah-sis) the occurrence of calculi in the common bile duct.

choledocholithotomy (ko-led″ŏ-ko-lĭ-thot′o-me) incision of the common bile duct for the removal of stone.

choledocholithotripsy (ko-led″o-ko-lith′o-trip″se) the crushing of a gallstone within the common bile duct.

choledochoplasty (ko-led″o-ko-plas′te) the performance of a plastic operation on the common bile duct; plastic repair of the duct following injury.

choledochorrhaphy (ko-led″o-kor′ah-fe) [*choledochus* + Gr. *rhaphē* suture] suture or repair of the common bile duct.

choledochoscope (ko-led″o-ko-skōp″) an instrument for direct inspection of the interior of the common bile duct by artificial light.

choledochostomy (ko-led″o-kos′to-me) [*choledochus* + Gr. *sto-*

moun to provide with an opening, or mouth] surgical formation of an opening into the common bile duct and drainage by catheter or T-tube.

choledochotomy (ko-led″o-kot′o-me) [*choledochus* + Gr. *tomē* a cutting] incision into the common bile duct for exploration or removal of a calculus; called also *choledochendysis*.

choledochus (ko-led′o-kus) [*chole-* + Gr. *dochos* receptacle] the ductus choledochus, or common bile duct.

Choledyl (ko-lēd′il) trademark for a preparation of oxtriphylline.

choleglobin (ko″le-glo′bin) a compound of globin and an open-ring iron porphyrin, being an intermediate in the formation of bile pigment from the catabolism of hemoglobin.

cholehematin (ko″le-hem′ah-tin) a red pigment (not a bile pigment) found in the bile of herbivorous animals; it is derived from chlorophyll and is the same as phylloerythrin and bilipurpurine.

cholehemia (ko″le-he′me-ah) (*obs.*) cholemia.

choleic (ko-le′ik) pertaining to or derived from the bile; see under *acid*.

cholelith (ko′le-lith) [*chole-* + Gr. *lithos* stone] a gallstone.

cholelithiasis (ko″le-lĭ-thi′ah-sis) [*chole-* + *lithiasis*] the presence or formation of gallstones.

cholelithic (ko″le-lith′ik) pertaining to or caused by gallstones.

cholelithotomy (ko″le-lĭ-thot′o-me) removal of gallstones through an incision in the gallbladder.

cholelithotripsy (ko″le-lith′o-trip-se) [*cholelith* + Gr. *tribein* to crush] the crushing of gallstones.

cholelithotrity (ko″le-lĭ-thot′rĭ-te) cholelithotripsy.

cholemesis (ko-lem′ĕ-sis) [*chole-* + Gr. *emein* to vomit] vomiting of bile.

cholemia (ko-le′me-ah) [*chole-* + Gr. *haima* blood + *-ia*] the presence of bile or bile pigments in the blood. **familial c., Gilbert's c.,** Gilbert's disease.

cholemic (ko-le′mik) pertaining to, marked by, or due to cholemia.

cholemimetry (ko″le-mim′ĕ-tre) determination of the amount of bile pigment in the blood.

choleophosphatase (ko″le-o-fos′fah-tās) an enzyme in the pancreas and in the intestinal juice which liberates choline from lecithin.

cholepathia (ko″le-path′e-ah) [*chole-* + Gr. *pathos* disease + *-ia*] a morbid condition of the biliary tract. **c. spas′tica** (*obs.*), a morbid condition of the biliary tract, characterized by spasm of the bile ducts.

choleperitoneum (ko″le-per″ĭ-to-ne′um) [*chole-* + *peritoneum*] the presence of bile in the peritoneum resulting from rupture of the bile passages; called also *biliary* or *bile peritonitis*, and *choleperitonitis*.

choleperitonitis (ko″le-per″ĭ-to-ni′tis) choleperitoneum.

cholepoiesis (ko″le-poi-e′sis) 1. the manufacture and secretion by the liver of bile constituents other than water. 2. the manufacture and secretion of bile salts by the liver.

cholepoietic (ko″le-poi-et′ik) [*chole-* + Gr. *poiein* to make] forming or secreting a constituent peculiar to bile; increasing the secretion of bile without a fall in its specific gravity.

choleprasin (ko″le-pra′sin) one of the pigments of bile isolated from gallstones.

cholera (kol′er-ah) [Gr., from *cholē* bile] an acute infectious disease caused by *Vibrio cholerae* and characterized by severe diarrhea with extreme fluid and electrolyte depletion, metabolic acidosis, and by vomiting, muscle cramps, and prostration. A specific toxin of the cholera vibrio blocks sodium absorption and promotes excretion of water and electrolytes. The resultant severe dehydration may lead to shock or renal failure. The disease, most commonly disseminated by contaminated drinking water, is endemic and epidemic in Asia. Called also *Asiatic c.* **Asiatic c.,** a term applied to epidemic outbreaks of cholera in Asia and associated with a high mortality rate; see *cholera*. **automatic c.,** that characterized by twitching movements of the fingers, toes, and occasionally the arms or legs preceding tonic muscle cramps after voluminous water and electrolyte loss. **bilious c.,** former term for mild cholera characterized by violent and painful vomiting and copious bilious stools. **chicken c.,** pasteurellosis in chickens; see *fowl c.* **dry c.,** c. sicca. **English c.** (*obs.*), c. morbus. **European c.,** bilious c. **fowl c.,** hemorrhagic septicemia caused by *Pasteurella multocida* and occurring in all species of domestic fowl, canaries, waterfowl, seagulls, game birds, and birds of prey, all over the world. **c. ful′minans,** c. sicca. **c. gallina′rium,** fowl c. **hog c.,** an infectious communicable disease of swine occurring in epizootics and caused by a virus; marked by fever, loss of appetite, emaciation, ulceration of the intestines, diarrhea, and ecchymoses in the kidney and on the skin of the ventral surface of the body; called also *swine fever.* **c. infan′tum,** a common, noncontagious diarrhea of young children prevailing in the summer months. **c. mor′bus,** a once popular name for an acute gastroenteritis, with diarrhea, cramps, and vomiting, occurring in summer or autumn; called also *summer c.* or *summer complaint.* **c. nos′tras,** bilious c. **c. nos′tras paratypho′sa,** former term for gastroenteritis paratyphosa B. **pancreatic c.,** a condition marked by profuse watery diarrhea, hypokalemia, and usually achlorhydria, due to an islet-cell tumor (other than beta cell) of the pancreas. **c. sic′ca, c. sid′erans,** cholera in which death takes place before diarrhea has occurred. **summer c.,** c. morbus. **typhoid c.,** a form of Asiatic cholera, marked by extreme depression. **winter c.** (*obs.*), a mild diarrheal disease of unknown cause, occurring in the winter months.

choleragen (kol′er-ah-jen) the exotoxin produced by the cholera vibrio, which is thought to stimulate electrolyte and water secretion into the small intestine in Asiatic cholera.

choleraic (kol″ĕ-ra′ik) of, pertaining to, or of the nature of cholera.

choleraphage (kol′er-ah-fāj) a bacteriophage that infects cholera bacilli.

choleresis (ko-ler′ĕ-sis) [*chole-* + Gr. *hairesis* a taking] the secretion of bile by the liver by either cholepoiesis or hydrocholeresis.

choleretic (ko″ler-et′ik) 1. stimulating the production of bile by the liver by either cholepoiesis or hydrocholeresis. 2. a choleretic agent.

choleria (ko-ler′e-ah) an irritable or hostile temperament.

choleric (kol′er-ik) hot-tempered; irascible.

choleriform (ko-ler′ĭ-form) choleroid.

cholerigenic (kol″er-ĭ-jen′ik) causing cholera.

cholerigenous (kol-er-ij′e-nus) causing cholera.

cholerine (kol′er-in) 1. the earliest stage of cholera. 2. a comparatively mild form of bilious cholera, sometimes closely simulating Asiatic cholera, but not often of a fatal issue.

cholerization (kol″er-i-za′shun) protective inoculation with cholera.

choleroid (kol′er-oid) [Gr. *cholera* + *eidos* form] resembling cholera.

choleromania (kol″er-o-ma′ne-ah) [*cholera* + Gr. *mania* madness] mania sometimes seen in cholera.

cholestane (ko′les-tān) a saturated steroid hydrocarbon, $C_{27}H_{48}$, with C-18 and C-19 methyl groups and an isooctyl side chain at C-17; obtained by reduction of cholesterol and other C_{27} steroids.

cholestanol (ko-les′tah-nol) a compound, $C_{27}H_{47}OH$, formed by the reduction of cholesterol. **beta-c.,** an isomer of coprosterol derived from cholesterol by bacterial action and found in the feces; called also *dihydrocholesterol.*

cholestasia (ko″le-sta′ze-ah) cholestasis.

cholestasis (ko″le-sta′sis) [*chole-* + Gr. *stasis* stoppage] stoppage or suppression of the flow of bile, having intrahepatic or extrahepatic causes.

cholestatic (ko″le-stat′ik) pertaining to or characterized by cholestasis.

cholesteatoma (ko″le-ste″ah-to′mah) [*chole-* + *steatoma*] a cystlike mass, with a lining of stratified squamous epithelium, usually of keratinizing type, filled with desquamating debris frequently including cholesterol. Cholesteatomas occur in the meninges, central nervous system, and bones of the skull, but are most common in the middle ear and mastoid region. **congenital c.,** epidermoidoma. **c. tym′pani,** cholesteatoma associated with chronic infection of the middle ear, formed of the outer desquamating layers of stratified squamous epithelium which has extended inward and upward to line the tympanum, epitympanum, and antrum.

cholesteatomatous (ko″le-ste″ah-to′mah-tus) relating to or of the nature of cholesteatoma.

cholesteatosis (ko″le-ste-ah-to′sis) fatty degeneration due to cholesterol esters.

cholestene (ko′les-tēn) an unsaturated hydrocarbon, $C_{27}H_{46}$, formed by the dehydrogenation of cholestane.

cholesteremia (ko-les″ter-e′me-ah) [*cholesterol* + Gr. *haima* blood + *-ia*] hypercholesterolemia.

cholesterin (ko-les′ter-in) cholesterol.

cholesterinemia (ko-les″ter-in-e′me-ah) hypercholesterolemia.

cholesterinosis (ko-les″ter-ĭ-no′sis) cholesterosis.

cholesterinuria (ko-les″ter-ĭ-nu′re-ah) cholesteroluria.

cholesterogenesis (ko-les″ter-o-jen′ĕ-sis) synthesis of cholesterol.

cholesterohistechia (ko-les″ter-o-his-tek′e-ah) [*cholesterol* + Gr. *histos* tissue + *echein* to hold + *-ia*] the presence of an abnormally large amount of cholesterol in a tissue.

cholesterohydrothorax (ko-les″ter-o-hi″dro-tho′raks) presence in the thoracic cavity of watery fluid that contains cholesterol crystals.

cholesterol (ko-les′ter-ol) [*chole-* + Gr. *stereos* solid] 1. a pearly, fatlike steroid alcohol, $C_{27}H_{45}OH$, crystallizing in the form of leaflets or plates from dilute alcohol, and found in animal fats

and oils, in bile, blood, brain tissue, milk, yolk of egg, myelin sheaths of nerve fibers, the liver, kidneys, and adrenal glands. It constitutes a large part of the most frequently occurring type of gallstones and occurs in atheroma of the arteries, in various cysts, and in carcinomatous tissue. Most of the body's cholesterol is synthesized in the liver, but some is absorbed from the diet. It is a precursor of bile acids and is important in the synthesis of steroid hormones. 2. [USP] a commercial preparation of cholesterol used as a pharmaceutic aid. Called also *cholesterin.*

cholesterolemia (ko-les″ter-ol-e′me-ah) [*cholesterol* + Gr. *haima* blood + *-ia*] hypercholesterolemia.

cholesteroleresis (ko-les″ter-ol-er′ĕ-sis) increased elimination of cholesterol in the bile.

cholesterolestersturz (ko-les″ter-ol-es′ter-stoorts) [Ger.] decrease in the proportion of esters in the blood cholesterol.

cholesterolopoiesis (ko-les″ter-ol″o-poi-e′sis) the synthesis of cholesterol by the liver.

cholesterolosis (ko-les″ter-ol-o′sis) cholesterosis.

cholesteroluria (ko-les″ter-ol-u′re-ah) [*cholesterol* + Gr. *ouron* urine + *-ia*] the presence of cholesterol in the urine; called also *cholesterinuria.*

cholesterosis (ko-les″ter-o′sis) a condition in which cholesterol is deposited in tissues in abnormal quantities. **extracellular c.,** a condition in which cholesterol is deposited in extracellular sites; it is marked by erythematous nodules of the acral areas, particularly the hands, and considered to be a variant of erythema elevatum diutinum.

choletelin (ko-let′ĕ-lin) [*chole-* + Gr. *telos* end] a yellow pigment, $C_{16}H_{18}N_2O_6$, the oxidation product of bilirubin; bilixanthine.

choletherapy (ko″le-ther′ah-pe) [*chole-* + *therapy*] treatment by the administration of bile salts.

choleuria (ko″le-u′re-ah) [*chole-* + Gr. *ouron* urine + *-ia*] choluria.

choleverdin (ko″le-ver′din) biliverdin.

choline (ko′lin) hydroxyethyl trimethyl ammonium hydroxide, $CH_2OH \cdot CH_2N^+(CH_3)_3$, derivable from many animal and some vegetable tissues and produced synthetically. Considered to be a vitamin of the B complex, it is the basic constituent of lecithin and prevents the deposition of fat in the liver; the acetic acid ester of choline (acetylcholine) is essential in synaptic transmission of nerve impulses. Choline is also oxidized to form betaine in methionine biosynthesis. Choline readily forms salts, several of which (*c. bitartrate, c. chloride,* and *c. dihydrogen citrate*) have been used in medicine as lipotropic agents in the treatment of fatty degeneration and hepatic cirrhosis. **c. acetylase,** choline acetyltransferase. **c. acetyltransferase,** acetyl CoA:choline O-acetyltransferase: an enzyme that brings about the synthesis of acetylcholine; called also *choline acetylase.* **c. magnesium trisalicylate,** a combination of choline salicylate and magnesium salicylate, used as an antiarthritic. **phosphatidyl c.,** lecithin. **c. salicylate,** the choline salt of salicylic acid, $C_{12}H_{19}NO_4$, having analgesic, antipyretic, and anti-inflammatory properties; used in conditions where salicylates, including aspirin, are indicated. It is administered orally. **c. theophyllinate,** oxtriphylline.

cholinergic (ko″lin-er′jik) 1. stimulated, activated or transmitted by choline (acetylcholine): a term applied to those nerve fibers which liberate acetylcholine at a synapse when a nerve impulse passes, i.e., the parasympathetic nerve endings. 2. an agent that produces such effects. Called also *parasympathomimetic.* Cf. *adrenergic.*

cholinesterase (ko″lin-es′ter-ās) an enzyme that catalyzes the hydrolysis of acetylcholine to choline and an anion; called also *pseudocholinesterase.* **serum c.,** cholinesterase. **true c.,** acetylcholinesterase.

cholinoceptive (ko″lin-o-sep′tiv) pertaining to the sites on effector organs that are acted upon by cholinergic transmitters.

cholinoceptor (ko″lin-o-sep′tor) cholinergic receptor; see under *receptor.*

cholinolytic (ko″lin-o-lit′ik) 1. blocking the action of acetylcholine, or of cholinergic agents. 2. an agent that blocks the action of acetylcholine in cholinergic areas, that is, organs supplied by parasympathetic nerves, and voluntary muscles.

cholinomimetic (ko″lĭ-no-mi-met′ik) having an action similar to that of acetylcholine; parasympathomimetic.

cholo- see *chole-.*

cholochrome (kol′o-krōm) [*cholo-* + Gr. *chrōma* color] any biliary pigment.

cholocyanin (kol″o-si′ah-nin) [*cholo-* + Gr. *kyanos* blue] bilicyanin.

chologenetic (kol″o-je-net′ik) [*cholo-* + Gr. *gennan* to produce] producing bile; cholepoietic.

Cholografin (ko″lo-gra′fin) trademark for preparations of iodipamide.

cholohematin (kol″o-hem′ah-tin) cholehematin, a brown bile pigment.

cholohemothorax (ko″lo-he″mo-tho′raks) [*cholo-* + Gr. *haima* blood + *thōrax* chest] presence of bile and blood in the thorax.

chololith (kol′o-lith) cholelith.

chololithiasis (kol″o-lĭ-thi′ah-sis) cholelithiasis.

chololithic (kol″o-lith′ik) cholelithic.

cholopoiesis (kol″o-poi-e′sis) cholepoiesis.

choloscopy (ko-los′ko-pe) [*cholo-* + Gr. *skopein* to examine] (*obs.*) examination of the biliary system or testing of the biliary function.

cholothorax (ko″lo-tho′raks) [*cholo-* + Gr. *thōrax* chest] cholohemothorax.

Choloxin (ko-lok′sin) trademark for a preparation of dextrothyroxine sodium.

choluria (ko-lu′re-ah) [*chol-* + Gr. *ouron* urine + *-ia*] the presence of bile in the urine; discoloration of the urine with bile pigments.

choluric (ko-lur′ik) pertaining to or marked by choluria.

chondodendrine (kon″do-den′drēn) bebeerine.

Chondodendron (kon″do-den′dron) a genus of climbing menispermaceous shrubs. **C. tomento′sum** Ruiz et Pavon, one of the sources of curare, or South American arrow poison. The major alkaloid is D-tubocurarine, which is used as a skeletal muscle relaxant in surgery, to control convulsion in strychnine toxicity and tetanus, and as a diagnostic aid in myasthenia gravis.

chondr- see *chondro-*.

chondral (kon′dral) pertaining to cartilage.

chondralgia (kon-dral′je-ah) chondrodynia.

chondralloplasia (kon″dral-lo-pla′ze-ah) [*chondr-* + Gr. *allos* other + *plassein* to form] dyschondroplasia.

chondrectomy (kon-drek′to-me) [*chondr-* + Gr. *ektomē* excision] surgical removal of a cartilage.

chondri- see *chondrio-*.

chondric (kon′drik) cartilaginous; of or relating to cartilage.

chondrichthyes (kon-drik′thĭ-ēz) [Gr. *chondros* cartilage + *ichthys* fish] a class of fishes with cartilaginous skeletons, includes sharks, skates, and their allies.

chondrification (kon″drĭ-fĭ-ka′shun) [*chondri-* + L. *facere* to make] the formation of cartilage; transformation into cartilage.

chondrigen (kon′drĭ-jen) chondrogen.

chondrin (kon′drin) a protein, resembling gelatin, from cartilage (Johannes Müller, 1837); it is considered to be a mixture of gelatin and mucin.

Chondrina (kon-dri′nah) a genus of snails that serves as a host of *Dicrocoelium dendriticum*.

chondrio- (kon′dre-o) [Gr. *chondrion*, diminutive of *chondros* (1) a granule (2) gristle or cartilage] a combining form denoting relationship (1) to a granule or (2) to cartilage; see also words beginning *chondro-*.

chondriome (kon′dre-ōm) a term sometimes used to denote the total mitochondrion content of a cell.

chondriosome (kon′dre-o-sōm″) [*chondrio-* + Gr. *sōma* body] mitochondrion.

chondritis (kon-dri′tis) [*chondr-* + *-itis*] inflammation of cartilage. **costal c.,** Tietze's syndrome. **c. intervertebra′lis calca′nea,** calcinosis intervertebralis.

chondro-, chondr- (kon′dro, kon′dr) [Gr. *chondros* cartilage] a combining form denoting relationship to cartilage; see also words beginning *chondri-* and *chondrio-*.

chondroadenoma (kon″dro-ad″ĕ-no′mah) adenochondroma.

chondroangioma (kon″dro-an″je-o′mah) a benign mesenchymoma containing chondromatous and angiomatous elements.

chondroblast (kon′dro-blast) [*chondro-* + Gr. *blastos* germ] a cell that arises from the mesenchyma and forms cartilage; called also *chondroplast*.

chondroblastoma (kon″dro-blas-to′mah) [*chondroblast* + *-oma*] a benign tumor composed of cells which arise from chondroblasts or their precursors and which tend to differentiate into cartilage cells; it occurs primarily in the epiphyses of adolescents. **benign c.,** chondroblastoma.

chondrocalcinosis (kon″dro-kal″sĭ-no′sis) [*chondro-* + L. *calx* lime + *-osis*] the presence of calcium salts, especially calcium pyrophosphate, in the cartilaginous structures of one or more joints; when accompanied by attacks of goutlike symptoms, it is known as *pseudogout*.

chondrocarcinoma (kon″dro-kar″sĭ-no′mah) carcinoma with chondromatous metaplasia.

chondroclast (kon″dro-klast) [*chondro-* + Gr. *klan* to break] a giant cell of the class that is believed associated with the absorption of cartilage.

Chondrococcus (kon″dro-kok′us) a genus of microorganisms of the family Myxococcaceae, found in dung of various animals.

chondrocostal (kon″dro-kos′tal) [*chondro-* + L. *costa* rib] of or pertaining to the ribs and costal cartilages.

chondrocranium (kon″dro-kra′ne-um) [*chondro-* + Gr. *kranion* head] the cartilaginous skull of the embryo.

chondrocyte (kon′dro-sīt) [*chondro-* + Gr. *kytos* hollow vessel] a mature cartilage cell embedded in a lacuna within the cartilage matrix. **isogenous c's,** cartilage cells that make up a single group.

chondrodermatitis (kon″dro-der″mah-ti′tis) an inflammatory process involving cartilage and skin; used almost exclusively to mean chondrodermatitis nodularis chronica helicis. **c. nodula′ris chron′ica hel′icis,** a condition marked by the presence of a painful nodule on the helix of the ear.

chondrodynia (kon″dro-din′e-ah) [*chondro-* + Gr. *odynē* pain] pain in a cartilage.

chondrodysplasia (kon″dro-dis-pla′ze-ah) [*chondro-* + *dysplasia*] enchondromatosis. **hereditary deforming c.,** enchondromatosis.

chondrodystrophia (kon″dro-dis-tro′fe-ah) [*chondro-* + *dys-* + Gr. *trophē* nutrition] chondrodystrophy. **c. calcif′icans congen′ita, c. congen′ita puncta′ta, c. feta′lis calcif′icans,** dysplasia epiphysealis punctata. **c. feta′lis,** achondroplasia.

chondrodystrophy (kon″dro-dis′tro-fe) a morbid condition characterized by abnormal development of cartilage. **familial c.,** hereditary deforming chondrodysplasia. **hereditary deforming c.,** dyschondroplasia. **hyperplastic c.,** chondrodystrophy with excessive growth of the epiphyses. **hypoplastic c.,** chondrodystrophy in which the bone is spongy and the epiphyses are irregularly developed. **hypoplastic fetal c.,** chondrodystrophia calcificans congenita. **c. mala′cia,** a form marked by softening of the epiphyseal cartilage.

chondroendothelioma (kon″dro-en″do-the″le-o′mah) a benign mesenchymoma containing chondromatous and endotheliomatous elements.

chondroepiphyseal (kon″dro-ep″ĭ-fiz′e-al) pertaining to the epiphyseal cartilages.

chondroepiphysitis (kon″dro-ep″ĭ-fiz-i′tis) inflammation involving the epiphyseal cartilages.

chondrofibroma (kon″dro-fi-bro′mah) [*chondroma* + *fibroma*] a fibroma with cartilaginous elements.

chondrogen (kon′dro-jen) [*chondro-* + Gr. *gennan* to produce] a substance regarded as the basis of cartilage and of the corneal tissue: boiling turns it into chondrin.

chondrogenesis (kon″dro-jen′ĕ-sis) [*chondro-* + Gr. *genesis* production] the formation of cartilage.

chondrogenic (kon″dro-jen′ik) giving rise to or forming cartilage.

chondroglossus (kon″dro-glos′us) see *Table of Musculi*.

chondroglucose (kon″dro-glu′kōs) a sugar formed by the action of hydrochloric acid on chondrin from cartilage.

chondrography (kon-drog′rah-fe) [*chondro-* + Gr. *graphein* to write] a description or account of the cartilages.

chondroid (kon′droid) resembling cartilage.

chondroitic (kon″dro-it′ik) pertaining to, derived from, or resembling cartilage; see also *acid*.

chondroitin (kon-dro′ĭ-tin) a mucopolysaccharide, $C_{18}H_{27}NO_{14}$, found in the cornea and differing from hyaluronic acid in that it contains acetylgalactosamine in place of acetylglucosamine. The sulfate ester occurs in 3 forms, *A* composed of glucuronic acid and sulfated galactosamine, *B* in which the uronic acid constituent is replaced by L-iduronic acid, and *C* which differs from chondroitin sulfate B in the position of the sulfate on the galactosamine residue. They are widespread in connective tissues, particularly cartilage. Chondroitin sulfate B is also called *dermatan sulfate*.

chondroitinuria (kon-dro″ĭ-tin-u′re-ah) the presence of chondroitic acid in the urine.

chondrolipoma (kon″dro-lĭ-po′mah) a benign mesenchymoma containing lipomatous and cartilaginous elements.

chondrology (kon-drol′o-je) [*chondro-* + *-logy*] the sum of knowledge in regard to the cartilages.

chondrolysis (kon-drol′ĭ-sis) [*chondro-* + Gr. *lysis* dissolution] the degeneration of cartilage cells that occurs in the process of intracartilaginous ossification.

chondroma (kon-dro′mah) [*chondro-* + *-oma*] a tumor or tumor-like growth of cartilage cells. It may remain within the substance of a cartilage or bone (*true chondroma*, or *enchondroma*) or may develop on the surface of a cartilage (*ecchondroma*, or *ecchondrosis*). **joint c.,** a mass of cartilage in the synovial membrane of a joint; see *synovial chondromatosis*. **c. sarcomato′sum,** chondrosarcoma. **synovial c.,** a cartilaginous body formed in a synovial membrane; see under *chondromatosis*. **true c.,** enchondroma.

chondromalacia (kon″dro-mah-la′she-ah) [*chondro-* + Gr. *malakia* softness] softening of the articular cartilage, most frequently in the patella. **c. feta′lis,** a condition in which the limbs of the stillborn fetus are soft and pliable due to softening of the epiphyseal cartilage. **c. patel′lae,** premature degeneration of the patellar cartilage, the patellar margins being tender so that pain is produced when the patella is pressed against the femur.

chondromatosis (kon″dro-mah-to′sis) multiple formation of chondromas. **synovial c.,** a rare condition in which cartilage is formed in the synovial membranes of joints, tendon sheaths, or bursa, by metaplasia of the connective tissue beneath the surface of the membrane. Some metaplastic foci on the surface of the membrane may become sessile, and then pedunculated, and finally become detached, producing a number of loose bodies. Called also *synovial chondrometaplasia.*

chondromatous (kon-drom′ah-tus) pertaining to or of the nature of cartilage.

chondromere (kon′dro-mēr) [*chondro-* + Gr. *meros* part] a cartilaginous vertebra of the fetal vertebral column.

chondrometaplasia (kon″dro-met″ah-pla′ze-ah) a condition characterized by metaplastic activity of the chondroblasts. **synovial c.,** synovial chondromatosis. **tenosynovial c.,** synovial chondromatosis affecting the sheath of a tendon.

chondromitome (kon″dro-mi′tōm) [*chondro-* + Gr. *mitos* thread] the paranucleus.

chondromucin (kon″dro-mu′sin) a dense homogeneous intercellular substance in cartilage, being a compound of a protein with chondroitic acid; called also *chondromucoid.*

chondromucoid (kon″dro-mu′koid) chondromucin.

chondromucoprotein (kon″dro-mu″ko-pro′te-in) the principal constituent of the ground substance of cartilage, a copolymer of a mucoprotein, chondroitin-4-sulfate (chondroitin sulfate A), and chondroitin-6-sulfate (chondroitin sulfate C).

Chondromyces (kon″dro-mi′sēz) [*chondro-* + Gr. *mykēs* fungus] a genus of bacteria of the family Polyangiaceae, found in animal manure and decaying fungi.

chondromyoma (kon″dro-mi-o′mah) a benign mesenchymoma containing myomatous and cartilaginous elements.

chondromyxoma (kon″dro-mik-so′mah) myxoma containing cartilaginous elements.

chondromyxosarcoma (kon″dro-mik″so-sar-ko′mah) a malignant mesenchymoma containing sarcomatous and cartilaginous elements.

chondronecrosis (kon″dro-nĕ-kro′sis) necrosis of cartilage.

chondro-osseous (kon″dro-os′e-us) composed of cartilage and bone.

chondro-osteodystrophy (kon″dro-os″te-o-dis′tro-fe) [*chondro-* + Gr. *osteon* bone + *dystrophy*] Morquio's syndrome.

chondropathia (kon″dro-path′e-ah) chondropathy. **c. tubero′sa,** Tietze's syndrome.

chondropathology (kon″dro-pah-thol′o-je) the pathology of disease of cartilage.

chondropathy (kon-drop′ah-the) [*chondro-* + Gr. *pathos* disease] disease of a cartilage.

chondrophyte (kon′dro-fīt) [*chondro-* + Gr. *phyton* a growth] a cartilaginous growth at the articular extremity of a bone.

chondroplasia (kon″dro-pla′ze-ah) the formation of cartilage by specialized cells (chondrocytes). **c. puncta′ta,** dysplasia epiphysealis punctata.

chondroplast (kon′dro-plast) [*chondro-* + Gr. *plassein* to form] chondroblast.

chondroplastic (kon″dro-plas′tik) pertaining to plastic operations on cartilage.

chondroplasty (kon′dro-plas″te) [*chondro-* + Gr. *plassein* to form] plastic surgery on cartilage; repair of lacerated or displaced cartilage.

chondroporosis (kon″dro-po-ro′sis) [*chondro-* + Gr. *poros* a passage] the formation of spaces or sinuses in the cartilages; it occurs normally during ossification.

chondroproteid (kon″dro-pro′te-id) chondroprotein.

chondroprotein (kon″dro-pro′te-in) any of a series of glycoproteins occurring in cartilage, comprising lardacein and chondromucoid; they yield chondroitic acid on decomposition.

chondrosamine (kon-dro′sam-in) a galactosamine, CH$_2$OH-(CHOH)$_3$CH(NH$_2$)CHO, which results from hydrolysis of chondrosin.

chondrosarcoma (kon″dro-sar-ko′mah) [*chondro-* + *sarcoma*] a malignant tumor derived from cartilage cells or their precursors; called also *chondroma sarcomatosum.* **central c.,** one developing in the interior of a bone; called also *enchondrosarcoma.* **mesenchymal c.,** a chondrosarcoma that is multicentric in origin.

chondrosarcomatosis (kon″dro-sar″ko-mah-to′sis) the formation of multiple chondrosarcomas.

chondrosarcomatous (kon″dro-sar-ko′mah-tus) pertaining to or of the nature of chondrosarcoma.

chondroseptum (kon″dro-sep′tum) [*chondro-* + *septum*] the cartilaginous part of the nasal septum.

chondrosin (kon′dro-sin) a disaccharide, 2-amino-2-deoxy-3-*O*-(β-D-glucopyranurosyl)-D-galactopyranose, (C$_{12}$H$_{21}$NO$_{11}$); the most common aldohexuronic acid in nature occurring as a structural unit. It is obtained by hydrolysis of chondroitins and chondroitin sulfates.

chondrosis (kon-dro′sis) [Gr. *chondros* cartilage] the formation of cartilaginous tissue.

chondroskeleton (kon″dro-skel′ĕ-ton) 1. a cartilaginous skeleton, as in certain fish. 2. that part of the skeleton composed of cartilage.

chondrosome (kon′dro-sōm) [*chondro-* + Gr. *sōma* body] chondriosome.

chondrosteoma (kon-dros″te-o′mah) osteochondroma.

chondrosternal (kon″dro-ster′nal) pertaining to the costal cartilages and the sternum.

chondrosternoplasty (kon″dro-ster′no-plas″te) surgical correction of funnel chest.

chondrotome (kon′dro-tōm) an instrument for cutting the cartilages.

chondrotomy (kon-drot′o-me) [*chondro-* + Gr. *temnein* to cut] the dissection or surgical division of cartilage.

chondrotrophic (kon″dro-trof′ik) [*chondro-* + Gr. *trophē* nutrition] having an influence on the formation or growth of cartilage.

chondroxiphoid (kon″dro-zi′foid) [*chondro-* + *xiphoid*] pertaining to the xiphoid process.

chondrus (kon′drus) the dried, sun-bleached plant of the seaweed *Chondrus crispus;* used as a protective agent for the skin; called also *carragen* or *carragheen, Irish moss, killeen, pearl moss,* and *salt rock moss.*

chonechondrosternon (ko″ne-kon′dro-ster′non) funnel chest.

Chopart's amputation (operation), articulation (joint) (sho-parz′) [François *Chopart,* French surgeon, 1743–1795] see under *amputation,* and see *articulatio tarsi transversa.*

chorangioma (ko-ran″je-o′mah) chorioangioma.

chord (kord) condyle c., condylar axis.

chorda (kor′dah), pl. *chor′dae* [L.; Gr. *chordē* + cord] [NA] any cord or sinew. **c. dorsa′lis,** notochord. **c. gubernac′-ulum,** gubernacular cord: a portion of the gubernaculum testis or of the round ligament of the uterus that develops in the inguinal crest and adjoining body wall. **c. mag′na,** tendo calcaneus. **c. obli′qua membra′nae interos′seae antebra′chii** [NA], a small ligamentous band extending from the lateral face of the tuberosity of the ulna to the radius a little distal to its tuberosity; called also *oblique cord of elbow joint,* and *Weitbrecht's cord* or *ligament.* **c. spermat′ica,** spermatic cord. **c. spina′lis,** spinal cord (medulla spinalis [NA]). **c. tendin′eae cor′dis** [NA], the tendinous cords that connect each cusp of the two atrioventricular valves to appropriate papillary muscles in the heart ventricles. **c. tym′pani** [NA], a nerve originating from the facial nerve (nervus intermedius) and distributed to the submandibular, sublingual, and lingual glands and the anterior two-thirds of the tongue; modality: parasympathetic and special sensory. **c. umbilica′lis,** umbilical cord. **c. voca′lis,** ligamentum vocale. **chor′dae willis′ii,** dural trabeculae, which are numerous fibrous bands that extend transversely across the inferior angle of the superior sagittal sinus.

chordae (kor′de) [L.] plural of *chorda.*

chordal (kor′dal) pertaining to any chorda (chiefly used of the notochord).

chorda-mesoderm (kor″dah-mez′o-derm) tissue of the dorsal lip of the blastopore, which gives rise to both notochord and mesoderm.

Chordata (kor-da′tah) [L. *chordatus* having a cord] a phylum of the animal kingdom comprising all animals that have a notochord during some stage of their development. It includes the subphyla Cephalochordata, Urochordata, and Vertebrata.

chordate (kor′dāt) 1. an animal belonging to the phylum Chordata. 2. having a notochord.

chordectomy (kor-dek′to-me) [*chordo-* + Gr. *ektomē* excision] excision of a vocal cord.

chordee (kor′de, kor′da) [Fr. *cordée* corded] downward bowing of the penis as a result of a congenital anomaly (hypospadias) or a urethral infection (gonorrhea); called also *gryposis penis.*

chorditis (kor-di′tis) inflammation of a vocal or spermatic cord. **c. canto′rum,** inflammation of the vocal cords in professional singers. **c. fibrino′sa,** acute laryngitis marked by the deposition of fibrin and the formation of erosions on the vocal cords. **c. nodo′sa,** c. tuberosa. **c. tubero′sa,** a condition marked by the formation of a small whitish nodule on one or both vocal cords, occurring in persons who use their voice excessively; called also *c. nodosa.* **c. voca′lis,** inflammation of the vocal cords. **c. voca′lis infe′rior,** chronic subglottic laryngitis.

chordo- (kor′do) [Gr. *chordē* cord] a combining form denoting relationship to a cord.

chordoblastoma (kor″do-blas-to′mah) [*chordo-* + Gr. *blastos* germ + *-oma*] a tumor, the cells of which tend to differentiate into cells like those of the notochord.

chordocarcinoma (kor″do-kar″sĭ-no′mah) chordoma.

chordoepithelioma (kor″do-ep″ĭ-the′le-o′mah) a chordoma.

chordoid (kor′doid) resembling the notochord.

chordoma (kor-do'mah) [*chordo-* + *-oma*] a malignant tumor arising from the embryonic remains of the notochord; called also *chordocarcinoma* and *chordoepithelioma.* Cf. *ecchordosis physaliphora.*

chordopexy (kor'do-pek"se) cordopexy.

chordosarcoma (kor"do-sar-ko'mah) chordoma.

chordoskeleton (kor"do-skel'ĕ-ton) [*chordo-* + *skeleton*] that portion of the bony skeleton which is formed around the notochord.

chordotomy (kor-dot'o-me) [*chordo-* + Gr. *tomē* a cutting] cordotomy, def. 2.

chorea (ko-re'ah) [L.; Gr. *choreia* dance] the ceaseless occurrence of a wide variety of rapid, highly complex, jerky movements that appear to be well coordinated but are performed involuntarily. **acute c.,** Sydenham's c. **automatic c.,** a disease characterized by the performance of actions which seem to be intentional, but which are really performed independently of the will in response to some impulse or external stimulus. **Bergeron's c.,** electric chorea of childhood, characterized by violent rhythmic spasms, but running a benign course; see also *c. major.* **button-makers' c.,** an occupation neurosis observed in button-makers. **chronic c., chronic progressive hereditary c.,** Huntington's c. **chronic progressive non-hereditary c.,** senile c. **c. cor'dis,** chorea with great irregularity of the heart's action. **dancing c.,** saltatory chorea. **degenerative c.,** Huntington's c. **diaphragmatic c.,** the utterance of a peculiar cry in cases of painless tic; called also *laryngeal c.* and *Schrötter's c.* **c. dimidia'ta,** hemichorea. **Dubini c.,** an acute, fatal form of electric chorea due to acute infection of the central nervous system; called also *Dubini's disease.* **electric c.,** a variety with violent and sudden movements. See *Bergeron's c., Dubini's c.,* and *Henoch's c.* **epidemic c.,** dancing mania. **c. fes'tinans,** old name for ataxia with festination; paralysis agitans. **fibrillary c.,** fibrillary contractions of various muscles; paramyoclonus. **c. gravida'rum,** Sydenham's chorea occurring in the early months of pregnancy, with or without a previous history of rheumatic disease; it may recur in subsequent pregnancies. **hemilateral c.,** hemichorea. **Henoch's c.,** chronic progressive electric chorea; see also *c. major.* **hereditary c.,** Huntington's c. **Huntington's c.,** a rare hereditary disease characterized by chronic progressive chorea and mental deterioration terminating in dementia; the age of onset is variable but usually occurs in the fourth decade of life. Death usually follows within 15 years. It is transmitted as an autosomal dominant trait. Called also *chronic* (*progressive hereditary*) *c., degenerative c.,* and *hereditary c.* **hyoscine c.,** chorea-like movements occurring in acute hyoscine (scopolamine) intoxication. **hysterical c.,** c. major. **imitative c.,** a pseudochorea, or neurotic affection; a kind of tic due to imitation. **c. insa'niens,** chorea with symptoms of insanity, chiefly seen in pregnant women; called also *maniacal c.* **juvenile c.,** Sydenham's c. **laryngeal c.,** diaphragmatic c. **limp c.,** chorea associated with extreme weakness; called also *c. mollis.* **local c.,** occupation neurosis. **c. ma'jor,** hysteria with continuous and somewhat regular oscillatory movements; called also *Bergeron's disease,* and *hysterical c.* **malleatory c.,** rhythmic chorea in which the patient performs persistent movements of hammering. **maniacal c.,** c. insaniens. **methodic c.,** a variety in which the movements take place at regular intervals. **mimetic c.,** that which is caused by imitation. **c. mi'nor,** Sydenham's c. **c. mol'lis,** limp c. **Morvan's c.** (*obs.*), fibrillary contractions of the muscles of the calves and posterior part of the thighs, sometimes extending to the trunk, but never affecting the neck and face. **c. noctur'na,** chorea in which the movements continue during sleep. **c. nu'tans,** nodding spasm, or chorea with nodding head movements. **one-sided c.,** hemichorea. **paralytic c.,** chorea in which immobility replaces movement; see *Huntington's c.* **posthemiplegic c.,** a form that affects the partially paralyzed muscles after hemiplegia; see *athetosis.* **prehemiplegic c.,** choreic movements that may precede an attack of hemiplegia. **rhythmic c.,** chorea major in which the patient performs persistent rhythmic movements. **rotary c.,** chorea major marked by rhythmic movements of the head or body. **saltatory c.,** rhythmic chorea with dancing movements; called also *dancing c.* **Schrötter's c.,** diaphragmatic c. **senile c.,** a benign, usually mild disorder of the elderly, marked by choreiform movements unassociated with mental disturbance. **simple c.,** Sydenham's c. **Sydenham's c.,** an acute, usually self-limited disorder of early life, usually between the ages of five and fifteen, or during pregnancy, and closely linked with rheumatic fever. It is characterized by involuntary movements that gradually become severe, affecting all motor activities including gait, arm movements, and speech. A mild psychic component is usually present. The disorder may be limited to one side of the body (hemichorea) or may take the form of muscular rigidity (paralytic chorea). Called also *St. Vitus' dance.*

choreal (ko're-al) choreic.

choreatic (ko"re-at'ik) choreic.

choreic (kŏ-re'ik) pertaining to, of the nature of, or characterized by chorea.

choreiform (kŏ-re'ĭ-form) [*chorea* + L. *forma* form] resembling chorea.

choreoathetoid (ko"re-o-ath'ĕ-toid) pertaining to or characterized by choreoathetosis.

choreoathetosis (ko"re-o-ath"ĕ-to'sis) a condition marked by choreic and athetoid movements.

choreoid (ko're-oid) choreiform.

choreomania (ko"re-o-ma'ne-ah) [Gr. *choreia* dance + *mania* madness] dancing mania.

choreophrasia (ko-re"o-fra'ze-ah) a condition in which the patient repeats phrases without regard to form or meaning.

chorial (ko're-al) of or relating to the chorion.

chorioadenoma (ko"re-o-ad"ĕ-no'mah) adenomatous tumor of the chorion. **c. destru'ens,** a form of hydatidiform mole in which molar chorionic villi penetrate into the myometrium and/or parametrium or, rarely, are transported to distant sites, most often the lungs; called also *invasive, metastasizing,* or *malignant mole.*

chorioallantoic (ko"re-o-al"an-to'ik) pertaining to the chorioallantois.

chorioallantois (ko"re-o-ah-lan'to-is) an extraembryonic structure derived from union of the chorion and allantois which by means of vessels in the associated mesoderm serves in gas exchange. In reptiles and birds, it is a membrane apposed to the egg shell; in many mammals, it forms the placenta.

chorioamnionitis (ko"re-o-am"ne-o-ni'tis) inflammation of fetal membranes.

chorioangiofibroma (ko"re-o-an"je-o-fi-bro'mah) angiofibroma of the chorion.

chorioangioma (ko"re-o-an"je-o'mah) an angiomatous tumor of the chorion.

chorioblastoma (ko"re-o-blas-to'mah) choriocarcinoma.

chorioblastosis (ko"re-o-blas-to'sis) overgrowth of the chorion.

choriocapillaris (ko"re-o-kap"ĭ-la'ris) [*chorioid* + L. *capillaris* capillary] lamina choriocapillaris.

choriocarcinoma (ko"re-o-kar"sĭ-no'mah) an epithelial malignancy of trophoblastic cells, formed by the abnormal proliferation of cuboidal and syncytial cells of the placental epithelium, without the production of chorionic villi. Almost all cases arise in the uterus, developing from hydatidiform mole (50 per cent), following abortion (25 per cent), or during normal pregnancy (22 per cent). The remainder occur in ectopic pregnancies and genital (ovarian and testicular) and extragenital teratomas. Called also *chorioblastoma, chorioepithelioma, chorionic carcinoma* or *epithelioma, deciduocellular sarcoma,* and *syncytioma malignum.*

choriocele (ko're-o-sēl) [*chorion* + Gr. *kēlē* hernia] protrusion of the eye through an aperture in the choroid.

chorioepithelioma (ko"re-o-ep"ĭ-the"le-o'mah) choriocarcinoma. **c. malig'num,** choriocarcinoma.

choriogenesis (ko"re-o-jen'ĕ-sis) [*chorio-* + Gr. *genesis* origin] the development of the chorion.

chorioid (ko're-oid) the choroid, def. 1.

chorioidea (ko"re-oi'de-ah) the choroid, def. 1.

chorioido- for words beginning thus, see those beginning *choroido-.*

chorioma (ko"re-o'mah) [*chorion* + *-oma*] any trophoblastic proliferation, benign or malignant.

choriomeningitis (ko"re-o-men"in-ji'tis) cerebral meningitis with lymphocytic infiltration of the choroid plexuses. **lymphocytic c.,** a form of viral meningitis usually occurring in adults 20 to 40 years of age during the fall and winter months.

chorion (ko're-on) [Gr.] 1. in human embryology, the cellular, outermost extraembryonic membrane, composed of trophoblast lined with mesoderm; it develops villi about 2 weeks after fertilization, is vascularized by allantoic vessels a week later, gives rise to the placenta, and persists until birth. 2. in mammalian embryology, the cellular, outer extraembryonic membrane, not necessarily developing villi. 3. endometrial stroma. 4. in biology, the noncellular membrane covering eggs of various animals, including fish and insects. See illustration under *amnion.* **c. frondo'sum,** the region of the chorion that bears villi; called also *shaggy c.* **c. lae've,** the smooth (nonvillous) and membranous part of the chorion. **primitive c.,** the chorion from its inception by addition of mesoderm to trophoblast through the stage in which it has many primitive villi. **shaggy c.,** c. frondosum.

chorionepithelioma (ko"re-on-ep"ĭ-the"le-o'-mah) choriocarcinoma.

chorionic (ko"re-on'ik) pertaining to the chorion.

chorioplacental (ko"re-o-plah-sen'tal) pertaining to the chorion and the placenta.

Chorioptes (ko"re-op'tēz) a genus of parasitic mites infesting the skin and hair of domestic animals and causing a sort of mange (*chorioptic acariasis* or *itch*).

chorioretinal (ko″re-o-ret′ĭ-nal) pertaining to the choroid and retina.

chorioretinitis (ko″re-o-ret′ĭ-ni′tis) inflammation of the choroid and retina.

chorioretinopathy (ko″re-o-ret″ĭ-nop′ah-the) a noninflammatory process involving both chorion and retina.

chorista (ko-ris′tah) [Gr. *chōristos* separated] defective development due to, or characterized by, displacement of the primordium.

choristoblastoma (ko-ris″to-blas-to′mah) [Gr. *chōristos* separated + *blastos* germ + *-oma*] choristoma.

choristoma (ko″ris-to′mah) [Gr. *chōristos* separated + *-oma*] a mass of tissue histologically normal for an organ or part of the body other than the site at which it is located; called also *aberrant rest* and *heterotopic tissue*.

choroid (ko′roid) [*chorion* + Gr. *eidos* form] 1. the thin, pigmented, vascular coat of the eye extending from the ora serrata to the optic nerve; it furnishes blood supply to the retina and conducts arteries and nerves to the anterior structures. Called also *choroidea* [NA] and *chorioidea*. 2. resembling the chorion or corium.

choroidal (ko-roi′dal) pertaining to the choroid.

choroidea (ko-roi′de-ah) [NA] the choroid, def. 1.

choroidectomy (ko″roi-dek′to-me) surgical removal or destruction of the choroid plexus of the lateral ventricles of the brain.

choroideremia (ko″roi-der-e′me-ah) [*choroid* + Gr. *erēmia* destitution] hereditary primary choroidal degeneration, transmitted as an X-linked trait and beginning in the first decade of life. In males, the earliest symptom is usually night blindness, followed by constricted visual field and eventual blindness as the degeneration of the pigment epithelium of the retina progresses to complete atrophy. In females, it is nonprogressive; usually there is normal vision and often an atypical pigmentary retinopathy.

choroiditis (ko″roid-i′tis) [*choroid* + *-itis*] inflammation of the choroid. **anterior c.,** that in which there are points of inflammation in the peripheral choroid. **areolar c.,** that which starts around or near the macula lutea and progresses toward the periphery. **areolar central c.,** Förster's c. **central c.,** a variety in which the inflammation is in the region of the macula lutea. **diffuse c., disseminated c.,** that which is characterized by spots scattered over the fundus. **Doyne's familial honeycombed c.,** a hereditary degenerative ocular abnormality marked by light-colored patches in the neighborhood of the optic disk and macula. **exudative c.,** that which is characterized by scattered patches of an exudate. **Förster's c.,** former term for a type of central choroiditis in which the spots are black at first, but later enlarge and become white; called also *areolar central c.* and *Forster's disease.* **c. gutta′ta seni′lis,** Tay's c. **metastatic c.,** a form due to metastasis in pyemia, meningitis, etc. **senile macular exudative c.,** disciform macular degeneration. **c. sero′sa,** glaucoma. **suppurative c.,** that which leads to the formation of pus. **Tay's c.,** degeneration of the choroid marked by irregular yellow spots around the macula lutea, and believed to be due to an atheromatous state of the arteries; seen in advanced life. Called also *c. guttata senilis* and *Tay's disease.*

choroidocyclitis (ko-roi″do-sik-li′tis) inflammation of the choroid and ciliary processes.

choroidoiritis (ko-roi″do-i-ri′tis) inflammation of the choroid coat and the iris.

choroidopathy (ko″roi-dop′ah-the) [*choroid* + Gr. *pathos* disease] any morbid process affecting the choroid.

choroidoretinitis (ko-roi″do-ret″ĭ-ni′tis) inflammation of the choroid and retina.

chorology (ko-rol′o-je) [Gr. *choros* place + *-logy*] the science of geographic distribution of organisms.

choromania (ko″ro-ma′ne-ah) [Gr. *choros* dance + *mania* madness] a morbid desire to dance.

chortosterol (kor-tos′ter-ol) [Gr. *chortis* grass] the sterol of grass; also a mixture of sterols found in the feces of the horse, hence *hippocoprosterol.*

Chr. Chromobacterium.

Christian's disease (syndrome) (kris′chanz) [Henry Asbury *Christian*, American physician, 1876–1951] Hand-Schüller-Christian disease.

Christian-Weber disease (kris′chan-web′er) [H. A. *Christian;* Frederick Parkes *Weber,* British physician, 1863–1962] nodular nonsuppurative panniculitis.

Christison's formula (kris′tĭ-sonz) [Sir Robert *Christison,* Scotch physician, 1797–1882] Trapp's formula; see under *formula.*

Christmas disease, factor [*Christmas,* for the name of the first patient with the disease who was studied in detail] see *coagulation Factor IX,* under *factor.*

chrom- see *chromo-.*

chromaffin (kro-maf′in) [*chromium-* + L. *affinis* having affinity for] taking up and staining strongly with chromium salts; said of certain cells occurring in the adrenal, coccygeal, and carotid glands, along the sympathetic nerves, and in various organs whose cytoplasmic granules give a brownish reaction with chromium salts. Called also *chromaphil.*

chromaffinity (kro″mah-fin′ĭ-te) the property of staining strongly with chrome salts.

chromaffinoblastoma (kro-maf″ĭ-no-blas-to′mah) (*obs.*) argentaffinoma.

chromaffinoma (kro″maf-ĭ-no′mah) any tumor containing chromaffin cells. **medullary c.,** pheochromocytoma.

chromaffinopathy (kro″maf-ĭ-nop′ah-the) [*chromaffin* + Gr. *pathos* disease] any disease of the chromaffin system.

chromaphil (kro′mah-fil) [*chrom-* + Gr. *philein* to love] chromaffin.

chromargentaffin (krōm″ar-jen′tah-fin) [*chromium* + L. *argentum* silver + L. *affinis* having affinity for] staining with chromium salts and impregnable with silver; said of certain cells of the mucous membrane of the intestinal tract. Cf. *enterochromaffin gland* and *argentaffinoma.*

chromate (kro′māt) 1. any salt of chromic acid. 2. to subject to the action of a salt of chromic acid.

chromatelopsia (kro″mat-el-op′se-ah) [*chrom-* + Gr. *atelēs* imperfect + *opsis* sight + *-ia*] imperfect perception of colors; called also *chromatodysopia.*

chromatic (kro-mat′ik) 1. pertaining to color; stainable with dyes. 2. pertaining to chromatin.

chromatid (kro′mah-tid) one of the two spiral filaments joined at the centromere which make up a chromosome, and which separate in cell division, each going to a different pole of the dividing cell and each becoming a chromosome of one of the two daughter cells. **nonsister c's,** the two chromatids of one homologous chromosome with respect to those of the other homologue. **sister c's,** the two chromatids of a chromosome held together by a centromere; dyads.

chromatin (kro′mah-tin) [Gr. *chrōma* color] the more readily stainable portion of the cell nucleus, forming a network of nuclear fibrils within the achromatin of a cell. It is a deoxyribonucleic acid attached to a protein (primarily histone) structure base and is the carrier of the genes in inheritance. It occurs in two interchangeable states, euchromatin and heterochromatin, and during cell division it coils and folds to form the chromosomes. Called also *chromoplasm.* **nucleolar-associated c., nucleolus-associated c.,** heterochromatin containing DNA, situated around, and sometimes extending into, the nucleolus of a cell. **sex c.,** the persistent mass of the material of the inactivated X chromosome in cells of normal females; called also *Barr body.* See *Lyon's hypothesis,* under *hypothesis.*

chromatinic (kro″mah-tin′ik) of or pertaining to the chromatin.

chromatin-negative (kro″mah-tin-neg′ah-tiv) lacking sex chromatin; characteristic of the nuclei of cells in a normal male.

chromatinolysis (kro″mah-tĭ-nol′ĭ-sis) [*chromatin* + Gr. *lysis* dissolution] chromatolysis.

chromatinorrhexis (kro″mat-ĭ-no-rek′sis) [*chromatin* + Gr. *rhēxis* rupture] splitting up of the chromatin.

chromatin-positive (kro″mah-tin-poz′ĭ-tiv) having sex chromatin (Barr body) in the nuclei of autosomal cells, a characteristic of the normal female.

chromatism (kro′mah-tizm) a hallucinatory perception of colored light.

Chromatium (kro-ma′te-um) a genus of microorganisms of the family Thiorhodaceae, suborder Rhodobacteriineae, order Pseudomonadales, made up of more or less ovoid, bean-shaped, or vibrio-shaped cells, or short rods, occurring singly. It includes 21 species.

chromatize (kro′mah-tīz) to charge with some chromium compound.

chromato- (kro′mah-to) [Gr. *chrōma, chrōmatos* color] 1. combining form denoting relationship to chromatin. 2. see *chromo-.*

chromatoblast (kro-mat′o-blast) [*chromato-* + Gr. *blastos* germ] a cell that can become a chromatophore, or bearer of pigment.

chromatocinesis (kro″mah-to-si-ne′sis) chromatokinesis.

chromatodysopia (kro″mah-to-dis-o′pe-ah) chromatelopsia.

chromatogenous (kro″mah-toj′ĕ-nus) [*chromato-* + Gr. *gennan* to produce] producing color or coloring matter.

chromatogram (kro-mat′o-gram) 1. the record produced by the bands of color in an adsorption column after a solution for analysis has been poured into an adsorbent-containing vertical glass tube, or the record produced in paper chromatography. 2. any graphical record of the results of a chromatographic separation.

chromatograph (kro-mat′o-graf) 1. the apparatus used in chromatography. 2. to analyze by chromatography.

chromatographic (kro″mah-to-graf′ik) pertaining to or produced by chromatography.

chromatography (kro″mah-tog′rah-fe) [*chromato-* + Gr. *graphein* to write] a method of separating and identifying the components of a complex mixture by differential movement through a two-phase system, in which the movement is effected by a flow of a liquid or a gas (mobile phase) which percolates through an adsorbent (stationary phase) or a second liquid phase, based on the physicochemical principles of adsorption, partition, ion exchange, or exclusion, or a combination of these principles. Chromatographic techniques may be classified according to the nature of the adsorbent employed, the physical characteristics of the mobile and stationary phases, or the type of technique employed. **adsorption c.,** that in which the adsorptive force is provided by molecules adhering to the surface of a solid packed in a column, spread as a thin film on a glass or plastic sheet, or as a coating inside a tube; the various components move through the stationary phase at different velocities, according to their degree of attraction to it, and are deposited at specific sites on the adsorbent. **column c.,** that in which the various solutes of a solution are allowed to travel down an adsorptive column, the individual components being adsorbed by the stationary phase; the most strongly adsorbed component will remain near the top of the column, and the other components will move to sites farther and farther down the column according to their affinity for the adsorbent. If the individual components are naturally colored, they will form bands or zones at different levels on the adsorption column. **electric c.,** electrochromatography. **exclusion c.,** that based on molecular size and, to some extent, molecular shape and hydration, in which the stationary phase consists of very small beads of special polymers, most often gel-forming hydrophilic beads, containing pores and channels, the size of which can be varied so that a molecule is either allowed to enter the gel beads or is excluded and flows along the spaces between the beads. Called also *gel-filtration c., gel-permeation c.,* and *molecular sieve c.* **filter paper c.,** paper c. **gas c.,** that in which an inert gas is used to move the vapors of the materials to be separated through a column of inert material. **gas-liquid c.,** that in which the substances to be separated are moved by an inert gas along a long tube filled with a finely divided inert solid coated with a nonvolatile oil; each component migrates at a rate determined by its solubility in oil and its vapor pressure. **gel-filtration c., gel-permeation c.,** exclusion c. **ion-exchange c.,** that utilizing resins to which are coupled either cations or anions that will exchange with other cations or anions in the material passed through their meshwork. **liquid-liquid c.,** partition c. **molecular sieve c.,** exclusion c. **paper c.,** a form of chromatography in which a sheet of blotting paper, usually filter paper, is substituted for the adsorption column. After separation of the components as a consequence of their differential migratory velocities, they are stained to make the chromatogram visible. Called also *filter paper c.* **partition c.,** a form of separation of solutes utilizing the partition of the solutes between two liquid phases, namely, the original solvent and the film of solvent on the adsorption column. **thin-layer c.,** chromatography through a thin layer of inert material, such as cellulose.

chromatoid (kro′mah-toid) having the tinctorial properties of chromatin; see also under *body.*

chromatokinesis (kro″mah-to-ki-ne′sis) [*chromatin* + Gr. *kinēsis* movement] movement of chromatin during the life and division of a cell.

chromatology (kro″mah-tol′o-je) [*chromato-* + *-logy*] the science of colors.

chromatolysis (kro″mah-tol′ĭ-sis) [*chromato-* + Gr. *lysis* dissolution] 1. the solution and disintegration of the chromatin of cell nuclei. 2. disintegration of the Nissl (chromophil) bodies of a nerve cell as the result of injury, or of fatigue or exhaustion; a part of the so-called axon reaction.

chromatolysm (kro-mat′o-lizm) chromatolysis.

chromatolytic (kro″mah-to-lit′ik) pertaining to chromatolysis.

chromatometer (kro″mah-tom′ĕ-ter) [*chromato-* + Gr. *metron* measure] an instrument for measuring color or color perception.

chromatopathy (kro″mah-top′ah-the) [*chromato-* + Gr. *pathos* disease] (*obs.*) any skin disease characterized by a disorder of pigmentation.

chromatopectic (kro″mah-to-pek′tik) chromopectic.

chromatopexis (kro″mah-to-pek′sis) chromopexy.

chromatophagus (kro″mah-tof′ah-gus) [*chromato-* + Gr. *phagein* to devour] destroying pigments.

chromatophil (kro′mah-to-fil″) a cell or element that stains easily.

chromatophile (kro′mah-to-fil″) 1. chromatophil. 2. chromatophilic.

chromatophilia (kro″mah-to-fil′e-ah) [*chromato-* + Gr. *philein* to love + *-ia*] the condition of staining easily.

chromatophilic (kro″mah-to-fil′ik) staining easily.

chromatophilous (kro″mah-tof′ĭ-lus) chromatophilic.

chromatophore (kro′mah-to-fōr″) [*chromato-* + Gr. *pherein* to bear] any pigmentary cell or color-producing plastid, such as those of the cutis or deep layers of the epidermis. Cf. *melanophore.*

chromatophoroma (kro″mah-to-fo-ro′mah) (*obs.*) malignant melanoma.

chromatophoromatosis (kro″mah-to-fo″ro-mah-to′sis) (*obs.*) malignant melanomatosis.

chromatophorotropic (kro″mah-to-fo″ro-trop′ik) having an influence or effect on chromatophores; applied to a principle of the pars intermedia of the pituitary.

chromatoplasm (kro′mah-to-plazm) the colored portions of the protoplasm of a pigmented cell.

chromatopseudopsis (kro″mah-to-su-dop′sis) [*chromato-* + Gr. *pseudēs* false + *opsis* vision] abnormal perception of color.

chromatopsia (kro″mah-top′se-ah) [*chromato-* + Gr. *opsis* vision + *-ia*] 1. a visual defect in which colorless objects appear to be tinged with color. 2. a visual defect in which various colors are imperfectly perceived; anomalous color vision.

chromatoptometer (kro″mah-top-tom′ĕ-ter) [*chromato-* + Gr. *op-* to see + *metron* measure] a device used in measuring color perception.

chromatoptometry (kro″mah-top-tom′ĕ-tre) the testing of the power of discriminating colors.

chromatosis (kro″mah-to′sis) (*obs.*) pigmentation, especially abnormal pigmentation of the skin.

chromatoskiameter (kro″mah-to-ski-am′ĕ-ter) an instrument for measuring the color sense.

chromatosome (kro-mat′o-sōm) [*chromato-* + Gr. *sōma* body] chromosome.

chromatotaxis (kro″mah-to-tak′sis) [*chromatin* + Gr. *taxis* arrangement] the attraction or influence of certain substances on the chromatin of a cell nucleus, causing destruction of the chromatin, while the cell body remains intact.

chromatotropism (kro″mah-tot′ro-pizm) [*chromato-* + Gr. *tropos* a turning] an orienting response to a color.

chromaturia (kro″mah-tu′re-ah) [*chromato-* + Gr. *ouron* urine + *-ia*] abnormal coloration of the urine.

1,2-chromene (kro′mēn) a plant pigment, a constituent of oxidized tocopherol; called also *1,2-benzopyran.*

chromesthesia (kro″mes-the′ze-ah) [*chrom-* + Gr. *aisthēsis* perception] the association of imaginary sensations of color with actual sensations of hearing, taste, or smell; see *photism.*

chromhidrosis (kro″mĭ-dro′sis) [*chrom-* + Gr. *hidrōs* sweat] the secretion of colored sweat.

chromicize (kro′mĭ-sīz) to treat with a chromium compound.

chromidia (kro-mid′e-ah) plural of *chromidium.*

chromidial (kro-mid′e-al) pertaining to or composed of chromidia.

chromidiation (kro″mid-e-a′shun) chromidiosis.

chromidien (kro-mid′e-en) [Ger.] that part of the extranuclear chromatin not concerned in the reproduction of the cell.

chromidiosis (kro-mid-e-o′sis) the outpouring of nuclear substance and chromatin from the nucleus into the cytoplasm of a cell.

chromidium (kro-mid′e-um), pl. *chromid′ia.* Any one of the granules of extranuclear chromatin seen in the cytoplasm of a cell, and staining deeply with basic stains.

chromidrosis (kro″mid-ro′sis) chromhidrosis.

chromiole (kro′me-ōl) one of the minute granules of chromatin composing the chromosomes (Eisen, 1899).

chromium (kro′me-um) [L.; Gr. *chrōma* color] a blue-whitish, brittle metal: atomic number, 24; atomic weight, 51.996; specific gravity, 7.1; symbol, Cr; several of its compounds are pigments, and the metal itself is used for weather-resistant plating. Chromium, which plays a role in glucose metabolism, is considered essential in trace amounts in nutrition. **c. oxide,** a substance used in dentistry as a polishing agent, especially for stainless steel; called also *chrome green.* **c. trioxide,** chromic acid, def. 2.

chromo-, chrom-, chromato- [Gr. *chrōma, chrōmatos* color] a combining form denoting relationship to color.

Chromobacterium (kro″mo-bak-te′re-um) a genus of microorganisms of the family Rhizobiaceae, order Eubacteriales, made up of small flagellated rods that characteristically produce a violet pigment which is soluble in alcohol but not in water or chloroform. It includes four species: *C. amythis′tinum, C. jan′thinum, C. marismor′tui,* and *C. viola′ceum.*

chromoblast (kro′mo-blast) [*chromo-* + Gr. *blastos* germ] an embryonic cell that develops into a pigment cell.

chromoblastomycosis (kro″mo-blas″to-mi-ko′sis) chromomycosis.

chromocenter (kro′mo-sen″ter) 1. karyosome. 2. a fused mass of heterochromatin with spokelike extensions of euchromatin, representing the chromosomes in the salivary glands of some insects.

chromocholoscopy (kro″mo-ko-los′ko-pe) [*chromo-* + Gr. *cholē* bile + Gr. *skopein* to examine] testing the biliary function by a pigment excretion test (methylthionine chloride).

chromoclastogenic (kro″mo-klas″to-jen′ik) giving rise to or inducing chromosomal disruption or damage.

chromocrinia (kro″mo-krin′e-ah) [*chromo-* + Gr. *krinein* to separate] the secretion or excretion of coloring matter.

chromocystoscopy (kro″mo-sis-tos′ko-pe) [*chromo-* + *cystoscopy*] examination of the interior of the bladder after administration of indigo carmine or other dye which is excreted in the urine, for identification and study of the activity of the ureteral orifices; called also *chromoureteroscopy* and *cystochromoscopy*.

chromocyte (kro′mo-sīt) [*chromo-* + Gr. *kytos* hollow vessel] any colored cell or pigmented corpuscle.

chromodacryorrhea (kro″mo-dak″re-o-re′ah) [*chromo-* + Gr. *dacryon* tear + *rhoia* flow] the shedding of bloody tears.

chromodiagnosis (kro″mo-di″ag-no′sis) [*chromo-* + *diagnosis*] 1. diagnosis by change of color. 2. diagnosis of functional derangements by observing the rate at which coloring matters, such as methylthionine chloride, are excreted. 3. diagnostic examination made through colored glass or sheets of colored gelatin.

chromoflavine (kro″mo-fla′vin) acriflavine.

chromogen (kro′mo-jen) any substance that may give origin to a coloring matter. **Porter-Silber c's,** 17-hydroxycorticosteroids, adrenocorticosteroids with a dihydroxyacetone side chain; so called because their concentration in urine can be determined by the Porter-Silber reaction employing sulfuric acid–phenylhydrazine reagent.

chromogene (kro′mo-jēn) [*chromo*some + *gene*] a gene that is located on a chromosome. Cf. *plasmagene*.

chromogenesis (kro″mo-jen′ě-sis) [*chromo-* + *genesis*] the formation of pigments or colors, as by bacterial action.

chromogenic (kro″mo-jen′ik) producing a pigment or coloring matter.

chromogranin (kro″mo-gran′in) a soluble protein constituent of the secretory granules of the chromaffin cells of the adrenal medulla.

chromoisomerism (kro″mo-i-som′er-izm)[*chromo-*+ *isomerism*] isomerism in which the isomers have different colors.

chromolipoid (kro″mo-lip′oid) lipochrome.

chromolysis (kro-mol′ĭ-sis) chromatolysis.

chromoma (kro-mo′mah) (*obs.*) an ulcerated malignant melanoma.

chromomere (kro′mo-mēr) [*chromo-* + Gr. *meros* part] 1. any one of the beadlike granules occurring in series along the chromonema of a chromosome; called also *idiomere*. 2. granulomere.

chromometer (kro-mom′ě-ter) [*chromo-* + Gr. *metron* measure] colorimeter.

chromomycosis (kro″mo-mi-ko′sis) a chronic fungal infection of the skin, producing wartlike nodules or papillomas that may or may not ulcerate; microscopically, they are characterized by round, brown bodies that reproduce by equatorial splitting and not by budding. The disease occurs sporadically in many areas of the world, and may be caused by *Phialophora verrucosa, Fonsecaea pedrosoi, F. compactum, Cladosporium carrioni,* and other fungi. Called also *chromoblastomycosis* and *dermatitis verrucosa*.

chromonar hydrochloride (kro′mo-nar) chemical name: [[3-[2-(diethylamino)-ethyl]4-methyl-2-oxo-2*H*-1-benzopyran-7-yl]oxy]acetic acid ethyl ester hydrochloride; a coronary vasodilator, $C_{20}H_{27}NO_5 \cdot HCl$. Called also *carbocromen hydrochloride*.

chromone (kro′mōn) [Gr. *chrōma* color] coumarin.

chromonema (kro′mo-ne′mah), pl. *chromone′mata* [*chromo-* + Gr. *nēma* thread] the coiled central thread of a chromatid, along which lie the chromomeres.

chromonemal (kro″mo-ne′mal) of or pertaining to a chromonema.

chromonemata (kro″mo-ne′mah-tah) plural of *chromonema*.

chromoneme (kro′mo-nēm) chromonema.

chromoparic (kro-mo-par′ik) [*chromo-* + L. *parere* to produce] producing or giving rise to color; chromogenic.

chromopathy (kro-mop′ah-the) chromatopathy.

chromopectic (kro″mo-pek′tik) pertaining to, characterized by, or promoting chromopexy.

chromopexic (kro″mo-pek′sik) chromopectic.

chromopexy (kro″mo-pek′se) [*chromo-* + Gr. *pēxis* fixation] the fixation of pigment, a term applied especially to the function of the liver in forming bilirubin.

chromophage (kro′mo-fāj) [*chromo-* + Gr. *phagein* to eat] pigmentophage.

chromophane (kro′mo-fān) [*chromo-* + Gr. *phainein* to show] a retinal pigment.

chromophil (kro′mo-fil) [*chromo-* + Gr. *philein* to love] any easily stainable cell, structure, or tissue.

chromophile (kro′mo-fīl) 1. chromophil. 2. chromophilic.

chromophilic (kro-mo-fil′ik) readily or easily stained; said especially of certain leukocytes and other histologic elements.

chromophilous (kro-mof′ĭ-lus) chromophilic.

chromophobe (kro′mo-fōb) [*chromo-* + Gr. *phobein* to be affrighted by + *ia*] any cell, structure, or tissue that does not stain readily; applied especially to the nonstaining cells of the anterior hypophysis (pituitary gland).

chromophobia (kro″mo-fo′be-ah) the quality of staining poorly with dyes.

chromophore (kro′mo-fōr) any chemical group whose presence gives a decided color to a compound and which unites with certain other groups (auxochromes) to form dyes; called also *color radical*.

chromophoric (kro″mo-fōr′ik) [*chromo-* + Gr. *pherein* to bear] 1. bearing color; said of chromogenic bacteria when the pigment is a component of the bacterial cell itself. 2. pertaining to a chromophore.

chromophorous (kro-mof′o-rus) chromophoric.

chromophose (kro′mo-fōs) [*chromo-* + *phose*] a subjective sensation of color.

chromophototherapy (kro″mo-fo″to-ther′ah-pe) [*chromo-* + Gr. *phōs* light + *therapeia* treatment] treatment with colored light.

chromoplasm (kro′mo-plazm) [*chromo-* + Gr. *plasma* something formed] chromatin.

chromoplast (kro′mo-plast) chromoplastid.

chromoplastid (kro″mo-plas′tid) [*chromo-* + *plastid*] any pigment-producing plastid other than a chloroplast.

chromoprotein (kro″mo-pro′te-in) [*chromo-* + *protein*] a colored conjugated protein. Examples are the red hemoglobin of the higher animals, the blue hemocyanin of many lower animals, and the red and blue pigments of seaweeds. Chromoproteins have respiratory functions and are closely related to the green chlorophyll of the higher plants.

chromopsia (kro-mop′se-ah) chromatopsia.

chromoptometer (kro″mop-tom′ě-ter) [*chromo-* + Gr. *op-* to see + *metron* measure] chromatoptometer.

chromoradiometer (kro″mo-ra″de-om′ě-ter) [*chromo-* + L. *radius* ray + Gr. *metron* measure] an apparatus once used for estimating radiation exposure by means of the color changes produced in slides placed next to the skin. **Holzknecht's c.,** an apparatus once used for estimating radiation exposure, consisting of a capsule which contains a substance color-sensitive to the roentgen ray. This capsule is placed in the pathway of the x-ray beam at the level of treatment. Following exposure the color is then compared with a color scale whose colors are numbered from 3 to 24. The quantities indicated by these numbers are known as *Holzknecht's units*.

chromoretinography (kro″mo-ret″ĭ-nog′rah-fe) [*chromo-* + *retina* + Gr. *graphein* to write] color photography of the retina.

chromorhinorrhea (kro″mo-ri″no-re′ah) [*chromo-* + Gr. *rhis* nose + Gr. *rhoia* a flow] the discharge of a pigmented secretion from the nose.

chromosantonin (kro″mo-san′to-nin) yellow santonin; an isomeric form produced when santonin is exposed to sunlight.

chromoscope (kro′mo-skōp) [*chromo-* + Gr. *skopein* to examine] an instrument for testing color perception.

chromoscopy (kro-mos′kŏ-pe) [*chromo-* + Gr. *skopein* to examine] 1. the testing of color vision. 2. diagnosis of renal function by the color of the urine following the administration of dyes. **gastric c.,** diagnosis of gastric function by the color of the gastric contents; a test for achylia gastrica.

chromosomal (kro″mo-so′mal) pertaining to chromosomes.

chromosome (kro″mo-sōm) [*chromo-* + Gr. *sōma* body] 1. in animal cells, a structure in the nucleus containing a linear thread of DNA, which transmits genetic information and is associated with RNA and histones; during cell division, the material (chromatin) composing the chromosome is compactly coiled, making it visible with appropriate staining and permitting its movement in the cell with minimal entanglement. Each organism of a species is normally characterized by the same number of chromosomes in its somatic cells, 46 being the number normally present in man, including the two (XX or XY) which determine the sex of the organism. See *illustration*. 2. in bacterial genetics, a closed circle of double-stranded DNA that contains the genetic material of the cell and is attached to the cell membrane; the bulk of the material forms a compact bacterial nucleus (called also *chromatinic body*). **accessory c's,** see *sex c's*. **bivalent c.,** see *bivalent, def. 2*. **Christchurch c.,** an autosome of Group G, with deletion of the short arms, first found in two siblings with chronic lymphocytic leukemia; now considered to be a variant found incidentally in patients with different defects. Symbol Ch¹. **daughter c's,** the name for chromatids when they reach the poles of the cell in the anaphase stage of mitosis. **gametic c.,** one in a haploid cell (gamete) consisting of a double strand of DNA. **giant c's,** 1. polytene c's. 2. lampbrush c's. **heterotypical c's,** see *sex c's*. **homologous c's,** the chromosomes of a matching pair in the diploid complement that contains the alleles of specific genes. **lampbrush c's,** giant chromosomes of the oocytes of many lower animals arranged like a cylindrical brush. **m-c.,** a small chromosome that conjugates only in the first spermatocyte division. **nucleolar c's,** those in relation to which the nucleoli reorganize during the telophase of mitosis. **odd c's,** see *sex c's*. **Ph¹ c., Philadelphia c.,** an abnormality of chromosome 22, characterized by shortening of its long arms (the

Human male chromosomes with Giemsa banding (Type G banding), arranged as a karyotype. (Courtesy of R. G. Worton in Thompson & Thompson)

missing portion usually translocated to chromosome 9) and present in marrow cells of most patients with chronic myelocytic leukemia. **polytene c's,** giant bundles of unseparated chromonemata occurring especially in the salivary glands of some insects; called also *giant c's.* **ring c.,** a chromosome in which both ends have been lost (deletion) and the two broken ends have reunited to form a ring-shaped figure. **sex c's,** chromosomes that are associated with the determination of sex, in mammals constituting an unequal pair, the X and the Y chromosome. **small c.,** m-c. **somatic c.,** an autosome: one in a diploid (tissue) cell of the body, consisting of a double strand of DNA. **supernumerary c.,** one or more extra chromosomes found inconstantly in wild populations of certain species of animals; they are not homologous to members of the regular set of chromosomes and apparently exert little influence on the phenotypic effect. **W c's, Z c's,** the sex chromosomes of certain insects, birds, and fishes, in which the female is heterogametic (i.e., has a W and a Z chromosome) and the males are homogametic (having only Z chromosomes). **X c.,** the female sex chromosome, being the differential sex chromosome carried by half the male gametes and all female gametes in man and other male-heterogametic species. **Y c.,** the male sex chromosome, being the differential sex chromosome carried by half the male gametes and none of the female gametes in man and in some other male-heterogametic species in which the homologue of the X chromosome has been retained.

chromospermism (kro″mo-sper′mizm) [*chromo-* + *sperm*] a colored condition of the sperm.

chromotherapy (kro″mo-ther′ah-pe) [*chromo-* + Gr. *therapeia* treatment] 1. treatment of disease by variously colored lights. 2. the therapeutic use of restricted areas of the spectrum; called also *beamtherapy.*

chromotoxic (kro″mo-tok′sik) [*chromo-* + Gr. *toxikon* poison] destructive to hemoglobin or due to the destruction of hemoglobin.

chromotrichia (kro″mo-trik′e-ah) [*chromo-* + Gr. *thrix* hair + *-ia*] coloration of the hair.

chromotrichial (kro″mo-trik′e-al) pertaining to the coloration of the hair.

chromotropic (kro″mo-trop′ik) [*chromo-* + Gr. *tropikos* turning] turning to or attracting color or pigment.

chromoureteroscopy (kro″mo-u-re″ter-os′ko-pe) chromocystoscopy.

chromourinography (kro″mo-u″rǐ-nog′rah-fe) diagnosis by

measuring the intensity of color and the time of appearance in the urine after injection of a dye.

chron- see *chrono-.*

chronaxia (kro-nak′se-ah) chronaxy.

chronaxie (kro′nak-se) chronaxy.

chronaximeter (kron″ak-sim′ĕ-ter) Lapicque's instrument for measuring chronaxy in nerve lesions.

chronaximetric (kron″ak-sǐ-met′rik) pertaining to chronaximetry.

chronaximetry (kron″ak-sim′ĕ-tre) the measurement of chronaxy.

chronaxy (kro′nak-se) [*chron-* + Gr. *axios* fit] the minimum time an electric current must flow at a voltage twice the rheobase to cause a muscle to contract.

chronic (kron′ik) [L. *chronicus,* from Gr. *chronos* time] persisting over a long period of time.

chronicity (kro-nis′ǐ-te) the quality of being chronic.

chroniosepsis (kron″e-o-sep′sis) a chronic form of sepsis.

chrono- [Gr. *chronos* time] a combining form denoting relationship to time.

chronobiologic, chronobiological (kron″o-bi″o-loj′ik; kron″o-bi″o-loj′ǐ-kal) pertaining to chronobiology; relating to the effects of time and biological rhythms on living systems.

chronobiologist (kron″o-bi-ol′o-jist) a specialist in chronobiology.

chronobiology (kron″o-bi-ol′ŏ-je) [*chrono-* + Gr. *bios* life + *-logy*] the scientific study of the effect of time on living systems; see *anachronobiology* and *catachronobiology.*

chronognosis (kron″og-no′sis) [*chrono-* + Gr. *gnōsis* knowledge] the subjective appreciation of the passage of time.

chronograph (kron′o-graf) [*chrono-* + Gr. *graphein* to write] an instrument for recording small intervals of time.

chronometry (kro-nom′ĕ-tre) [*chrono-* + Gr. *metrein* to measure] the measurement of time or intervals of time. **mental c.,** the measurement and study of the duration of mental processes.

chronomyometer (kron″o-mi-om′ĕ-ter) an apparatus for measuring chronaxy.

chronon (kro′non) a unit representing the persistence of genetic information throughout a lifetime; it is a function of gene redundancy and is reflected in the persistence of the resultant phenotypical trait. Cf. *ergon.*

chronophotograph (kron″o-fo′to-graf) [*chrono-* + *photograph*] one of a series of photographs of a moving object taken for the purpose of showing successive phases of the motion.

chronoscope (kron′o-skōp) [*chrono-* + Gr. *skopein* to examine] an instrument for measuring minute intervals of time.

chronosphygmograph (kron″o-sfig′mo-graf) Jaquet's instrument for observing the rhythm as well as the character of the pulse.

chronotaraxis (kro-no-tar-ak′sis) [*chrono-* + Gr. *taraxis* confusion] disorientation for time; observed as a transient symptom following thalamic or frontal lobe lesions.

chronotropic (kron″o-trop′ik) [*chrono-* + Gr. *tropikos* turning] affecting the time or rate, as the rate of contraction of the heart.

chronotropism (kro-not′ro-pizm) interference with the regularity of a periodic movement, such as the heart beat.

chrotoplast (kro′to-plast) [Gr. *chrōs* skin + *plassein* to form] a dermal or skin cell.

chrysalis (kris′ah-lis) [L.] the pupa of some insects, especially of a moth or butterfly.

chrysarobin (kris′ah-ro′bin) [L. *chrysarobinum,* from Gr. *chrysos* gold + *araroba*] a brownish to yellow-orange microcrystalline powder consisting of a mixture of the neutral principles extracted from Goa powder; a reduction product of chrysophanic acid, it is used topically in the treatment of psoriasis and other chronic skin disease.

chrysazin (kris′ah-zin) danthron.

chrysiasis (krĭ-si′ah-sis) [Gr. *chrysos* gold] the deposition of gold in the tissues; called also *auriosis.*

Chrysippus (kri-sip′us) **of Cnidos** (4th century B.C.) a Greek physician who was a teacher of Erasistratus.

chryso- (kris′o) [Gr. *chrysos* gold] a combining form denoting relationship to gold.

chrysoderma (kris′o-der′mah) [*chryso-* + Gr. *derma* skin] a permanent pigmentation of the skin due to gold deposit.

Chrysomonadina (kris″o-mon-ah-di′nah) an order of very small, free-swimming, chiefly ameboid protozoa of the class Phytomastigophora, subphylum Mastigophora, which usually have one or two flagella, and are found in fresh and marine waters. It includes the families Syncryptidae and Ochromonadidae.

Chrysomyia (kris″o-mi′yah) [*chryso-* + Gr. *myia* fly] a genus of flies of the family Calliphoridae, of Africa, Australia, and parts of Asia. **C. al′biceps,** a South African species whose larvae (wool maggots) live in the soiled wool of sheep. **C. bezzia′na,** a species widely distributed in Asia and Africa and frequently found in wounds of man and animals; it may cause severe and disfiguring myiasis in man. Called also *Cochliomyia bezziana.* **C. macella′ria,** *Cochliomyia hominivorax.*

chrysophoresis (kris″o-fo-re′sis) diffusion of gold particles to various organs of the body after therapeutic administration of preparations of gold, by macrophages and polymorphonuclear leukocytes.

Chrysops (kris′ops) [*chryso-* + Gr. *ōps* eye] a genus of blood-sucking tropical tabanid flies, the grove flies. **C. cecu′tiens,** a species that inflicts bites about the eyes of men and animals. **C. dimidia′ta,** a species of southwestern Africa that is an intermediate host of *Loa loa;* called also *mango* or *mangrove fly.* **C. disca′lis,** a common vector of tularemia in the western part of the United States; called also *deer fly.* **C. sila′cea,** an intermediate host of *Loa loa.*

chrysosis (kris-o′sis) chrysiasis.

Chrysosporium (kris-o-spor′rĭ-um) a genus of imperfect, keratinophilic, soil fungi, related to the dermatophytes; some species have been isolated from dermatophytosis. Formerly called *Aleurisma* and *Glenosporella.*

chrysotherapy (kris″o-ther′ah-pe) [*chryso-* + *therapy*] treatment with gold salts.

Chrysozona (kris″o-zo′nah) [*chryso-* + Gr. *zōne* girdle] a genus of tabanid flies. *C. ital′ica* and *C. pluvia′lis* are common in Europe; called also *Hematopota.*

chthonophagia (thon″o-fa′je-ah) [Gr. *chthōn* earth + *phagein* to eat] the morbid habit of eating clay or other earth; geophagia.

chthonophagy (thon-of′ah-je) chthonophagia.

chunk (chunk) in learning theory, a unit of information already stored in memory before beginning the learning of new material that includes the unit.

churus (chur′us) ganja.

Chvostek's anemia, sign (symptom) (vos′teks) [Franz *Chvostek,* Austrian surgeon, 1835–1884] see under *anemia* and *sign.*

Chvostek-Weiss sign (vos′tek-vīs′) [Franz *Chvostek;* Nathan *Weiss,* physician in Vienna, 1851–1883] Chvostek's sign.

chylangioma (ki″lan-je-o′mah) [*chyle* + *angioma*] a tumor made up of intestinal lymph vessels.

chylaqueous (ki-la′kwe-us) [*chyle* + L. *aqua* water] both chylous and watery.

chyle (kīl) [L. *chylus* juice] the milky fluid taken up by the lacteals from the food in the intestine during digestion. It consists of lymph and droplets of triglyceride fat (chylomicrons) in a stable emulsion. It passes into the veins by the thoracic duct, becoming mixed with the blood; called also *chylus* [NA].

chylectasia (ki″lek-ta′se-ah) [*chyle* + Gr. *ektasis* dilatation] dilatation of a chylous vessel; e.g., of a lacteal.

chylemia (ki-le′me-ah) [*chyle* + Gr. *haima* blood + *-ia*] the presence of chyle in the blood.

chylifacient (ki″lĭ-fa′shent) forming chyle.

chylifaction (ki″lĭ-fak′shun) [*chyle* + L. *facere* to make] the formation of chyle; called also *primary assimilation* and *chylopoiesis.*

chylifactive (ki″lĭ-fak′tiv) [*chyle* + L. *facere* to make] chylifacient.

chyliferous (ki-lif′er-us) [*chyle* + L. *ferre* to bear] 1. forming chyle. 2. conveying chyle.

chylification (ki″lĭ-fĭ-ka′shun) [*chyle* + L. *facere* to make] the formation of chyle.

chyliform (ki′lĭ-form) resembling chyle.

chylocele (ki′lo-sēl) [*chyle* + Gr. *kēlē* tumor] elephantiasis scroti. **parasitic c.,** elephantiasis scroti.

chylocyst (ki′lo-sist) [*chyle* + Gr. *kystis* bladder] the cisterna chyli.

chyloderma (ki″lo-der′mah) [*chyle* + Gr. *derma* skin] elephantiasis filarensis.

chyloid (ki′loid) resembling chyle.

chylology (ki-lol′o-je) the study of chyle.

chylomediastinum (ki″lo-me″de-as-ti′num) the presence of chyle in the mediastinum.

chylomicrograph (ki″lo-mi′kro-graf) a curve plotted from counts of chylomicrons.

chylomicron (ki″lo-mi′kron) a stable droplet containing 86 per cent triglyceride fat, 3 per cent cholesterol, 9 per cent phospholipids, and 2 per cent protein, found in the intestinal lymphatics (lacteals) and blood during and after meals; this is the form in which absorbed long-chain fats and cholesterol are transported from the intestine.

chylomicronemia (ki″lo-mi″kron-e′me-ah) [*chylomicron* + Gr. *haima* blood + *-ia*] an excess of chylomicrons in the blood.

chylopericarditis (ki″lo-per″ĭ-kar-di′tis) pericarditis with effusion of chyle into the pericardial sac.

chylopericardium (ki″lo-per″ĭ-kar′de-um) [*chyle* + *pericardium*] the presence of effused chyle in the pericardium.

chyloperitoneum (ki″lo-per″ĭ-to-ne′um) the presence of effused chyle in the peritoneal cavity.

chylophoric (ki″lo-for′ik) [*chyle* + Gr. *phoros* bearing] conveying chyle.

chylopleura (ki″lo-ploo′rah) chylothorax.

chylopneumothorax (ki″lo-nu″mo-tho′raks) the presence of chyle and air in the pleural cavity.

chylopoiesis (ki″lo-poi-e′sis) [*chyle* + Gr. *poiēsis* formation] chylifaction or chylification.

chylopoietic (ki″lo-poi-et′ik) concerned in the formation of chyle.

chylorrhea (ki″lo-re′ah) 1. discharge of chyle due to rupture of or injury to the thoracic duct. 2. chylous diarrhea, due to rupture of lymphatics in the small intestine.

chylosis (ki-lo′sis) the process of conversion of food into chyle and of absorption of the latter into the tissues.

chylothorax (ki″lo-tho′raks) [*chyle* + Gr. *thōrax* chest] the presence of effused chyle in the thoracic cavity; called also *chylopleura.*

chylous (ki′lus) pertaining to, mingled with, or of the nature of chyle.

chyluria (ki-lu′re-ah) [*chyle* + Gr. *ouron* urine + *-ia*] the presence of chyle in the urine, giving it a milky appearance, due to obstruction anywhere between the intestinal lymphatics and the thoracic duct, which causes rupture of renal lymphatics into the renal tubules. The chief cause of obstruction is filariasis due to infection with *Wuchereria bancrofti* (*tropical c.*). Called also *galacturia.* **c. trop′ica,** see *chyluria.*

chylus (ki′lus) [L. *juice*] [NA] the milky fluid taken up by the lacteals from the food in the intestine after digestion. See *chyle.*

Chymar (ki′mar) trademark for preparations of chymotrypsin.

chymase (ki′mās) an enzyme of the gastric juice, which accelerates the action of the pancreatic juice.

chyme (kīm) [Gr. *chymos* juice] the semifluid, homogeneous, creamy or gruel-like material produced by gastric digestion of food; called also *chymus.*

chymification (ki″mĭ-fĭ-ka′shun) [*chyme* + L. *facere* to make] the formation of chyme; gastric digestion.

chymodenin (ki″mo-de′nin) a polypeptide secreted by the duodenum that specifically stimulates pancreatic secretion of chymotrypsinogen.

chymopapain (ki″mo-pah-pa′in) a proteolytic enzyme (a sulfhydryl proteinase) from the latex of a chiefly tropical tree, *Carica papaya,* that curdles milk and breaks down the mucopolysaccharide-protein complexes in the nucleus pulposus; used in chemonucleolysis.

chymorrhea (ki″mo-re′ah) [*chyme* + Gr. *rhoia* flow] a discharge or flow of chyme.

chymosin (ki-mo′sin) rennin.

chymosinogen (ki″mo-sin′o-jen) renninogen.

chymotrypsin (ki″mo-trip′sin) 1. one of the proteolytic and milk-curdling enzymes of the pancreatic secretion, produced in the intestine by activation of chymotrypsinogen by trypsin. It is a protein endopeptidase that catalyzes the hydrolysis of native food proteins to peptones, polypeptides, and amino acids, by breaking the peptide linkages of the carboxyl groups of tyrosine and phenylalanine. There are two forms, A and B, having similar specificity. 2. [USP] a proteolytic enzyme preparation crystallized from an extract of the pancreas of the ox, *Bos taurus.* It is a white to yellowish white, crystalline powder; used for enzymatic zonulolysis in intracapsular lens extraction, applied by irrigation to the posterior chamber of the eye, under the iris. It has also been used to débride necrotic lesions and to reduce inflammation and edema, administered orally, buccally, and intramuscularly.

chymotrypsinogen (ki″mo-trip-sin′o-jen) a crystallizable pre-enzyme occurring in the pancreas and converted to chymotrypsin by trypsin.

chymous (ki′mus) pertaining to chyme.

chymus (ki′mus) chyme.

Chytridiales (ki-trid″ē-a′lēz) an order of usually aquatic fungi of the subclass Chytrididiomycetes, class Phycomycetes, most of which are parasites of algae, higher plants, microscopic animals, and fresh-water fungi, although some are saprophytic; they usually have a thallus that is not a true mycelium. It includes the genus *Chytridium.*

Chytridiomycetes (ki-trid′ē-o-mi-se′tēz) a subclass of phycomycetous fungi in which the reproductive cells most commonly have one flagellum and the cells walls are composed of chitin; it includes the order Chytridiales.

Chytridium (ki-trid′e-um) a genus of water molds of the order Chytridiales, subclass Chytridiomycetes, which are usually parasitic on plants.

C.I. color index; Colour Index.

Ci symbol for *curie* recommended by the International Commission on Radiological Units and Measurements.

Ciaccio's glands (chah′chō) [Giuseppe Vincenzo *Ciaccio,* Italian anatomist, 1824–1901] glandulae lacrimales accessoriae.

Ciaccio's method, stain (chah′chōz) [Carmelo *Ciaccio,* Palermo pathologist, born 1877] see *Table of Stains.*

Ciarrocchi's disease (char-ro′kēz) [Gaetano *Ciarrocchi,* Italian dermatologist, 1857–1924] see under *disease.*

Cib. abbreviation for L. *ci′bus,* food.

cibarian (sĭ-ba′re-an) [L. *cibus* food] pertaining to food.

cibisotome (sĭ-bis′o-tōm) [Gr. *kibisis* pouch + *tomē* cut] an instrument for opening the capsule of the lens in removing cataract.

cicatrectomy (sik″ah-trek′to-me) excision of a cicatrix.

cicatrices (sik-ah-tri′sēz) plural of *cicatrix.*

cicatricial (sik″ah-trish′al) pertaining to or of the nature of a cicatrix.

cicatricotomy (sik″ah-tri-kot′o-me) [*cicatrix* + Gr. *tomē* a cutting] incision of a cicatrix.

cicatrix (sik-a′triks; sik″ah-triks), pl. *cica′trices* [L.] a scar; the new tissue formed in the healing of a wound. **filtering c.,** a cicatrix following glaucoma operation through which the aqueous humor escapes. **hypertrophic c.,** a hard, rigid tumor formed by hypertrophy of the tissue of a cicatrix. **manometric c.,** a cicatrix of the drum membrane of the ear that moves in and out with variations of the intratympanic pressure. **vicious c.,** a cicatrix that causes deformity or impairs the function of an extremity.

cicatrizant (sik-at′rĭ-zant) an agent that promotes cicatrization.

cicatrization (sik″ah-trĭ-za′shun) the formation of a cicatrix or scar.

cicatrize (sik′ah-trīz) to heal by the formation of a scar or cicatrix.

ciclafrine hydrochloride (sik′lah-fēn) chemical name: 3-(1-oxa-4-azaspiro[4.6]undec-2-yl)phenol hydrochloride; an antihypotensive, $C_{15}H_{21}NO_2 \cdot HCl.$

ciclopirox olamine (si″klo-pēr′oks) chemical name: 6-cyclohexyl-1-hydroxy-4-methyl-2-(1*H*)-pyridinone compound with 2-aminoethanol (1:1); an antifungal, $C_{12}H_{17}NO_2 \cdot C_2H_7NO.$

cicloprofen (si″klo-pro′fen) chemical name: α-methyl-9*H*-fluorene-2-acetic acid; an anti-inflammatory, $C_{16}H_{14}O_2.$

Cicuta (sik′u-tah) a genus of umbelliferous plants, including the water hemlocks, long recognized for their poisonous qualities. **C. macula′ta** L., American water hemlock; its root is very poi-

sonous, containing cicutoxin. **C. viro′sa,** the highly poisonous European water hemlock, which contains cicutoxin.

cicutoxin (sik″u-toks′in) a very poisonous, highly unsaturated higher alcohol from *Cicuta.*

Cidex (si′deks) trademark for a preparation of glutaraldehyde.

CIF clone-inhibiting factor; see under *factor.*

ciguatera (se″gwah-ta′rah) [Sp. (orig. Taino) *cigua* a poisonous snail + *-era,* Sp. noun suffix] a form of ichthyosarcotoxism, marked by gastrointestinal and neurological symptoms due to ingestion of marine fish (e.g., grouper and snapper) that store the toxin in their tissues; it occurs in tropical and subtropical coastal areas. The term was formerly applied to all types of fish poisoning in the West Indies, where the name originated.

C.I.H. Certificate in Industrial Health.

cilia (sil′e-ah) [L.] plural of *cilium.*

ciliaris (sil″e-a′ris) [L., from *cilium*] see *Table of Musculi.*

ciliariscope (sil″e-ar′ĭ-skōp) [*ciliary* + Gr. *skopein* to examine] an instrument for examining the ciliary region of the eye.

ciliarotomy (sil″e-ar-ot′o-me) surgical division of the ciliary zone for glaucoma.

ciliary (sil′e-er″e) [L. *ciliaris,* from *cilium*] pertaining to or resembling the eyelashes or cilia; used particularly in reference to certain structures in the eye, as the ciliary (ciliaris) muscle, ciliary process, and ciliary ring.

Ciliata (sil″e-a′tah) a class of protozoa of the subphylum Ciliophora, characterized by the presence of cilia throughout the life cycle. It includes the subclasses Euciliatia and Protociliata.

ciliate (sil′e-āt) 1. having cilia. 2. any individual organism of the subphylum Ciliophora.

ciliated (sil′e-āt″ed) provided with cilia or with a fringe of hairs.

ciliectomy (sil″e-ek′to-me) [*cilia* + Gr. *ektomē* excision] 1. excision of a portion of the ciliary body. 2. excision of a portion of the ciliary margin of the eyelid with the roots of the lashes.

ciliogenesis (sil″e-o-jen′ĕ-sis) the formation or development of cilia.

Ciliophora (sil″e-of′o-rah) a subphylum of Protozoa characterized by the presence of cilia during some stage of development and usually possessing two kinds of nuclei (a micronucleus and a macronucleus). Most species are free-living, but several are parasitic. It includes the classes Ciliata and Suctoria. Called also *Infusoria.*

ciliophoran (sil″e-of′o-ran) 1. any individual of the subphylum Ciliophora. 2. of or pertaining to the subphylum Ciliophora.

ciliretinal (sil″e-o-ret′ĭ-nal) pertaining to the retina and the ciliary body.

cilioscleral (sil″e-o-skle′ral) pertaining to the ciliary apparatus and to the sclera.

ciliospinal (sil″e-o-spi′nal) pertaining to the ciliary body and the spinal cord; see under *center* and *reflex.*

ciliotomy (sil″e-ot′o-me) surgical division of the ciliary nerves.

cilium (sil′e-um), pl. *cil′ia* [L.] 1. an eyelid or its outer edge. 2. [pl.] [NA] the hairs growing on the edges of the eyelids; called also *eyelashes.* 3. a minute vibratile, hairlike process projecting from the free surface of a cell; composed of nine pairs of microtubules arrayed around a central pair, cilia are extensions of basal bodies. They beat rhythmically to move the cell about in its environment or to move fluid or mucous films over its surface. Ciliary movement consists of an *effective stroke,* in which the cilium stiffens and moves forward rapidly, and a *recovery stroke,* in which the cilium becomes flexible and bends. Cilia may all beat simultaneously (*isochronal rhythm*) or successive cilia in each row may start their beat sequentially producing a wavelike movement (*metachronal rhythm*). Cf. *flagellum.* **olfactory cilia,** see under *hair.*

cillo (sil′lo) cillosis.

Cillobacterium (sil″lo-bak-te′re-um) a genus of microorganisms of the tribe Lactobacilleae, family Lactobacillaceae, order Eubacteriales, made up of nonsporulating, anaerobic, gram-positive bacilli found in the intestinal tract and occasionally associated with purulent infections.

cillosis (sil-lo′sis) [L.] a spasmodic quivering of the eyelid; called also *cillo.*

cimbia (sim′be-ah) [L.] a white band running across the ventral surface of the crus cerebri.

cimetidine (si-met′ĭ-dēn) chemical name: *N*″-cyano-*N*-methyl-*N*′-[2-[[(5-methyl-1*H*-imidazol-4-yl)-methyl]thio]ethyl]guanidine. An antagonist to histamine H_2 receptors, $C_{10}H_{16}N_6S,$ which inhibits gastric acid secretion in response to all stimuli, and is effective especially in the treatment of peptic ulcer; administered orally, intravenously, and by intravenous infusion.

Cimex (si′meks) [L. "bug"] a genus of insects, the bedbugs, of the family Cimicidae. **C. boue′ti,** the tropical bedbug of West Africa and South America; called also *Leptocimex boueti.* **C. hemip′terus,** *C. rotundatus.* **C. lectula′rius,** the common bedbug that infests man in temperate areas; called also *Acanthia lectularia.* **C. pilosel′lus,** an American species found in bats.

C. pipistrel′la, a species that transmits a trypanosome disease of bats. **C. rotunda′tus,** a flattened, oval, reddish bedbug that infests man in the tropics; called also *C. hemipterus.*

cimex (si′meks), pl. *cim′ices* [L.] an individual of the genus *Cimex;* a bedbug.

cimices (sim′ĭ-sēz) plural of *cimex.*

cimicid (si′mĭ-sid) pertaining to insects of the family Cimicidae.

Cimicidae (si-mis′ĭ-de) a family of wingless, blood-sucking, hemipterous insects of the suborder Heteroptera, including the bedbugs and related forms. *Cimex, Haematosiphon, Leptocimes,* and *Oeciacus* are medically important genera.

Cimicifuga (sim″ĭ-sif′u-gah) [L. *cimex* bug + *fugare* to put to flight] a genus of ranunculaceous plants. The rootlets of *C. racemosa* (L.) Nutt. (black snakeroot or cohosh) are tonic and antispasmodic.

cimicosis (sim″ĭ-ko′sis) itching of the skin due to the bites of *Cimex lectularius* (bedbug).

cinanserin hydrochloride (sin-an′ser-in) chemical name: *N*-[2-[[3-(dimethyl-amino)propyl]thio]phenyl]-3-phenyl-2-propenamide monohydrochloride. A serotonin antagonist, $C_{20}H_{24}N_2OS\cdot HCl$, which has been used in the treatment of mania and schizophrenia.

cinching (sinch′ing) surgical shortening of an ocular muscle by plicating.

Cinchona (sin-ko′nah) [named from a countess of *Chinchon*] a genus of rubiaceous trees, all natives of South America, the source of the medicinally important quinoline alkaloids, quinine, quinidine, cinchonine, and cinchonidine. Mainly used for malaria and as cardiac depressants. The major species used are *C. succirubra* Pavon et Klotzsch and hybrids (red cinchona), *C. calisaya* Weddell, *C. Ledgeriana* (Howard) Moens et Trimen, and hybrids (yellow cinchona).

cinchona (sin-ko′nah) the dried bark of the stem or of the root of various species of *Cinchona.* It is the source of the medicinally important quinoline alkaloids *quinine, quinidine, cinchonine,* and *cinchonidine.* Cinchona was once widely used as an antimalarial but it has been largely replaced by its alkaloids. Called also *calisaya bark, cinchona bark, Jesuit's bark, Peruvian bark,* and *quinquina.*

cinchonidine (sin-ko′nĭ-dēn) chemical name: (8α,9*R*)-cinchonan-9-ol. An alkaloid of cinchona, $C_{19}H_{22}N_2O$, used as an antimalarial, chiefly in the form of the sulfate salt; administered orally.

cinchonine (sin′ko-nin) [L. *cinchonina*] chemical name: (9*S*)-cinchona-9-ol. An alkaloid of cinchona, $C_{19}H_{22}N_2O$, used as an antimalarial, chiefly in the form of the sulfate salt; administered orally.

cinchonism (sin′ko-nizm) the morbid or injurious effect of the injudicious use of cinchona bark or its alkaloids; it is attended by nausea, vomiting, headache, tinnitus aurium, deafness, symptoms of cerebral congestion, vertigo, and visual disturbances.

cinchophen (sin′ko-fen) chemical name: 2-phenyl-quinoline-4-carboxylic acid. An analgesic, antipyretic, and uricosuric agent, $C_{16}H_{11}NO_2$, formerly used in the treatment of gout and acute rheumatic fever. Called also *phenylcinchoninic acid* and *phenylquinoline carboxylic acid.*

cinclisis (sin′klĭ-sis) [Gr. *kinklisis* a wagging] a rapidly repeated movement, such as rapid breathing, or rapid winking.

cine- [Gr. *kinēsis* movement] a combining form denoting relationship to movement.

cineangiocardiography (sin″e-an″je-o-kar″de-og′rah-fe) the photographic recording of fluoroscopic images of the heart and great vessels by motion picture techniques.

cineangiograph (sin″ĕ-an′je-o-graf) a motion picture camera for photographing fluoroscopic images.

cineangiography (sin″e-an″je-og′rah-fe) the photographic recording of fluoroscopic images of the blood vessels by motion picture techniques. **radionuclide c.,** that in which a sample of human serum albumin labeled with a radioisotope (technetium 99) is injected into the peripheral blood and then a scintillation camera records emitted radiation over the chest area, the heart movements being shown on a video tube.

cinedensigraphy (sin″ĕ-den-sig′rah-fe) the recording of movements of internal body structures by means of x-rays and radiosensitive cells.

cinefluorography (sin″ĕ-floo″or-og′rah-fe) cineradiography.

cinemascopia (sin″ĕ-mah-sko′pe-ah) the use of motion picture records for the study of movements of the body.

cinemascopy (sin″ĕ-mas′ko-pe) cinemascopia.

cinematics (sin″ĕ-mat′iks) kinematics.

cinematization (sin″ĕ-mat-ĭ-za′shun) kineplasty.

cinematography (sin″ĕ-mah-tog′rah-fe) cineradiography.

cinematoradiography (sin″ĕ-mah-to-ra″de-og′rah-fe) cineradiography.

cinemicrography (sin″ĕ-mi-krog′rah-fe) the making of moving pictures of a small object through the lens system of a microscope. **time-lapse c.,** the taking of motion pictures of a minute object through a microscope at a slower than normal speed, so that with projection at normal speed the movements of the object appear to occur more rapidly.

cineol (sin′e-ol) eucalyptol.

cinepazet maleate (sin″ĕ-paz′et) chemical name: 4-[1-oxo-3-(3,4,5-trimethoxyphenyl)-2-propenyl]-1-piperazineacetic acid ethyl ester. A coronary vasodilator, $C_{20}H_{28}N_2O_6\cdot C_4H_4O_4$, which has been used in the treatment of angina of effort.

cinephlebography (sin″ĕ-flĕ-bog′rah-fe) cineradiography of the veins after administration of a contrast medium. In *ascending functional cinephlebography,* the contrast medium is introduced into a vein in the foot and its progress is observed as it courses through the tibial, popiteal, femoral, and iliac veins.

cineplastics (sin″ĕ-plas′tiks) kineplasty.

cineplasty (sin′ĕ-plas′te) kineplasty.

cineradiography (sin″ĕ-ra″de-og′rah-fe) the making of a motion picture record of the successive images appearing on a fluoroscopic screen; called also *cinefluorography, cinematography, cinematoradiography, cineroentgenofluorography,* and *cineroentgenography.*

cinerea (si-ne′re-ah) [L. *cinereus* ashen hued] the gray matter of the nervous system.

cinereal (sĭ-ne′re-al) pertaining to the gray matter of the brain or nervous system.

cineritious (sin″er-ish′us) [L. *cineritius*] ashen gray; of the color of ashes.

cineroentgenofluorography (sin″ĕ-rent″gen-o-floo″or-og′rah-fe) cineradiography.

cineroentgenography (sin″ĕ-rent″gen-og′rah-fe) cineradiography.

cinesalgia (sin″es-al′je-ah) [Gr. *kinēsis* motion + *-algia*] pain in a muscle when it is brought into action.

cinesi- for words beginning thus, see those beginning *kinesi-.*

cineto- for words beginning thus, see those beginning *kineto-.*

cineurography (sin″ĕ-u-rog′rah-fe) cineradiography of the urinary tract.

cingestol (sin-jes′tōl) chemical name: 19-nor-17α-pregn-5-en-20-yn-17-ol; a progestin, $C_{20}H_{28}O$.

cingula (sing′gu-lah) plural of *cingulum.*

cingule (sin′gūl) cingulum.

cingulectomy (sin″gu-lek′to-me) bilateral extirpation of the anterior half of the gyrus cinguli.

cingulotomy (sing″gu-lot′o-me) cingulumotomy.

cingulum (sin′gu-lum), pl. *cin′gula* [L. "girdle"] 1. [NA] an encircling structure or part; anything that encircles a body. Called also *cingule* and *girdle.* 2. [NA], a bundle of association fibers that partly encircles the corpus callosum not far from the median plane, the fibers of which interrelate the cingulate and hippocampal gyri. 3. the lingual lobe of an anterior tooth, making up the bulk of the cervical third of its lingual surface; called also *basal ridge.* **c. extremita′tis inferio′ris,** c. membri inferioris. **c. extremita′tis superio′ris,** c. membri superioris. **c. hemisphe′rii,** gyrus cinguli. **c. mem′bri inferio′ris** [NA], the encircling bony structure that supports the lower limbs, comprising the two ossa coxae, articulating with each other and with the sacrum, to complete the essentially rigid bony ring; called also *c. extremitatis inferioris, girdle of inferior extremity,* and *pelvic girdle.* **c. mem′bri superio′ris** [NA], the encircling bony structure supporting the upper limbs, comprising the clavicles and scapulae, articulating with each other and with the sternum and vertebral column, respectively; called also *c. extremitatis superioris, shoulder girdle, thoracic girdle,* and *girdle of superior extremity.*

cingulumotomy (sing″gu-lum-ot′o-me) the creation of precisely placed lesions in the cingulum of the frontal lobe, for relief of intractable pain; called also *cingulotomy.*

cinnamaldehyde (sin-ah-mal′dĕ-hīd) a yellowish oily liquid with a strong odor of cinnamon, C_9H_8O, used as a flavoring agent.

cinnamene (sin-am′en) styrol.

cinnamic (sĭ-nam′ik) of or relating to cinnamon; see under *acid.*

cinnamol (sin′ah-mol) styrol.

Cinnamomum (sin″ah-mo′mum) a genus of evergreen trees native to Asia. The wood of *C. camphora* is the source of camphor and the bark of *C. loureirii* of cinnamon.

cinnamon (sin′ah-mon) [L.; Gr. *kinnamon*] [NF] the dried bark of *Cinnamomum loureirii,* containing, in each 100 gm., not less than 2.5 ml. of volatile oil; used as a flavor in pharmaceutical preparations.

cinnarizine (sĭ-nar′ĭ-zēn) chemical name: 1-(diphenylmethyl)-4-(3-phenyl-2-propenyl)piperazine. An antihistamine, $C_{26}H_{28}N_2$, used chiefly in the treatment of nausea and vertigo associated with labyrinthine disorders and in the prevention and treatment of motion sickness.

cinnopentazone (sin-o-pen′tah-zōn) cintazone.

cinology (sĭ-nol′o-je) kinesiology.

cinometer (sĭ-nom′ĕ-ter) kinesimeter.

cinoplasm (sin′o-plazm)   kinoplasm.

cinoxacin (sin-oks′ah-sin)   chemical name: 1-ethyl-1,4-di-hydro-4-oxo-[1,3]dioxolo[4,5-*g*]cinnoline-3-carboxylic acid. An antibacterial, $C_{12}H_{10}N_2O_5$, which inhibits most gram-negative organisms.

cinoxate (sin-oks′āt)   chemical name: 3-(4-methoxyphenyl)-2-propenoic acid 2-ethoxyethyl ester; an ultraviolet screen, $C_{14}H_{18}$-O_4, applied topically to the skin.

cinromide (sin′ro-mīd)   chemical name: 3-(3-bromophenyl)-2-propenamide; an anticonvulsive, $C_{11}H_{12}BrNO$.

cintazone (sin′tah-zōn)   chemical name: 2-pentyl-6-phenyl-1*H*-pyrazolo[1,2-*a*]cinnoline-1,3(2*H*)-dione; an anti-inflammatory agent, $C_{22}H_{22}N_2O_2$. Called also *cinnopentazone*.

C.I.O.M.S.   Council for International Organizations of Medical Sciences.

cionectomy (si″o-nek′to-me) [Gr. *kiōn* uvula + *ektomē* excision] excision of the uvula or of a part of it; uvulectomy.

Cionella (si″o-nel′ah)   a genus of land snails that serve as hosts of *Dicrocoelium dentriticum*.

Cionellidae (si″o-nel′ĭ-de)   a family of garden snails (suborder Stylommatophora, subclass Euthyneura, class Gastropoda) that serve as hosts of *Dicrocoelium dendriticum*.

cionitis (si″o-ni′tis) [Gr. *kiōn* uvula + *-itis*]   inflammation of the uvula; uvulitis.

cionoptosis (si″on-op-to′sis) [Gr. *kiōn* uvula + Gr. *ptōsis* a falling] undue elongation of the uvula.

cionorrhaphy (si″ŏ-nor′ah-fe)   plastic repair of the uvula.

cionotome (si-on′o-tōm) [Gr. *kiōn* uvula + *tomē* cut]   a cutting instrument for amputating the uvula; uvulotome.

cionotomy (si″o-not′o-me) [Gr. *kiōn* uvula + *tomē* a cutting] surgical removal of part of the uvula; uvulotomy.

ciprocinonide (sip″ro-si′no-nīd)   chemical name: 21-[(cyclopropylcarbonyl)-oxy]-6α,9-difluoro-11β-hydroxy-16α,17-[(1-methylethylidene)bis(oxy)]pregna-1,4-diene-3,20-dione; an adrenocorticosteroid, $C_{28}H_{34}F_2O_7$.

ciprofibrate (si″pro-fi′brāt)   chemical name: 2-[4-(2,2-dichlorocyclopropyl)phenoxy]-2-2-methylpropanoic acid; an antihyperlipidemic, $C_{13}H_{14}Cl_2O_3$.

circadian (ser″kah-de′an) [L. *circa* about + *dies* a day]   pertaining to a period of about 24 hours; applied especially to the rhythmic repetition of certain phenomena in living organisms at about the same time each day (circadian rhythm).

circannual (ser-kan′u-al) [L. *circa* about + *annus* year]   occurring every year; applied especially to the rhythmic repetition of certain phenomena (e.g., the flowering of plants) in living organisms at about the same time each year.

circellus (ser-sel′us)   a small ring, or circle.

circinate (ser′sĭ-nāt)   resembling a ring, or circle.

circle (ser′k'l) [L. *circulus*]   a round figure, structure, or part. **arterial c. of iris, greater,** circulus arteriosus iridis major. **arterial c. of iris, lesser,** circulus arteriosus iridis minor. **arterial c. of Willis,** circulus arteriosus cerebri. **Berry's c's,** charts with circles on them for testing stereoscopic vision. **c. of Carus,** see under *curve*. **c. of confusion,** a disk representing the image of a theoretical point made by a lens. **defensive c.,** the coexistence of two conditions that tend to have an antagonistic or inhibitory effect on each other. **diffusion c.,** a confused image formed on the retina when the latter is not at the focus of the eye. **c. of dispersion, c. of dissipation,** the circular space on the retina within which the image of a luminous point is formed. **c. of Haller,** 1. circulus vasculosus nervi optici. 2. (*obs.*) valvula pylori. **c. of Hovius,** an intrascleral circular arrangement of anastomosing ciliary veins anterior to the vorticose veins, not far from the corneoscleral margin, occurring in mammals other than man; called also *circulus venosus hovii*. **Huguier's c.,** the circle formed about the junction of the cervix with the body of the uterus by the uterine arteries. **c. of iris, greater,** anulus iridis major. **c. of iris, lesser,** anulus iridis minor. **Latham's c.,** a circle 2 inches in diameter covering the area of pericardial dullness and situated midway between the left nipple and the lower end of the sternum. **Minsky's c's,** a device used for the graphic recording of eye lesions. **Pagenstecher's c.,** the circle formed on the abdominal wall by joining the points marking the positions occupied by a mobile abdominal tumor which has been manipulated throughout its entire range of motion. The center of such a circle indicates the point of attachment of the tumor. **Robinson's c.,** an arterial circle formed by anastomoses between the abdominal aorta, common iliac, hypogastric, uterine, and ovarian arteries. **sensory c.,** an area on the body within which it is impossible to distinguish separately the impressions arising from two sites of stimulation. **vascular c. of optic nerve,** circulus vasculosus nervi optici. **c's of Weber,** circles of points on the skin marking the points of tactile sense discrimination. **c. of Willis,** circulus arteriosus cerebri. **c. of Zinn,** circulus vasculosus nervi optici.

circlet (ser′klet)   a small circular structure.

circling (ser′kling)   movement in a circle, as manifested by animals with listeriosis.

circuit (ser′kit) [L. *circuitus*]   the round or course traversed by an electrical current. The circuit is said to be *closed* when it is continuous, so that the current may pass through it; it is *open*, *broken*, or *interrupted* when it is not continuous and the current cannot pass through it. **magnetic c.,** the closed path of magnetic lines. **open c.,** a circuit having some break in it so that current is not passing or cannot pass. **reflex c.,** a chain of neurons that function in a reflex act. **short c.,** 1. a current developed between two branches of another circuit at a point short of the terminals, so that the current does not reach the latter. 2. a communication between two portions of intestine, one above and the other below an obstruction.

circular (ser′ku-lar) [L. *circularis*]   shaped like a circle; occurring in a circle.

circulation (ser″ku-la′shun) [L. *circulatio*]   movement in a regular or circuitous course, as the movement of the blood through the heart and blood vessels. **allantoic c.,** fetal circulation through the umbilical vessels; called also *umbilical c.* **assisted c.,** pumping that aids the natural activity of the heart. **collateral c.,** that which is carried on through secondary channels after obstruction of the principal vessel supplying the part; called also *compensatory c.* **compensatory c.,** collateral c. **coronary c.,** that within the coronary vessels of the heart. **cross c.,** the circulation in a portion of the body of one animal of blood supplied from another animal. **derivative c.,** the passage of blood from arteries to the veins without going through capillaries. **enterohepatic c.,** the recurrent cycle in which bile salts and other substances excreted by the liver pass through the intestinal mucosa and become reabsorbed by the hepatic cells and re-excreted. **extracorporeal c.,** the circulation of blood outside the body, as through a heart-lung apparatus for carbon dioxide–oxygen exchange, or through an artificial kidney for removal of substances usually excreted in the urine. **fetal c.,** that propelled by the fetal heart through the fetus, umbilical cord, and placental villi. **first c.,** primitive c. **fourth c.,** the con-

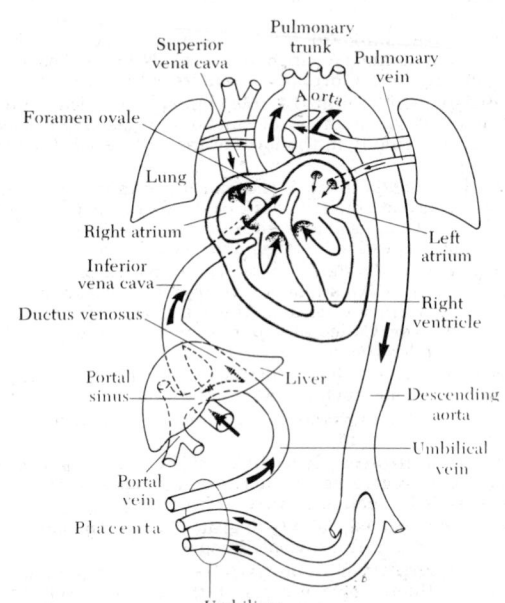

Schematic diagram of fetal circulation.

tinuous movement of lymphocytes from their sources in all the hematopoietic and connective tissues to the blood passing through all the tissues and organs, then to the lymph nodes, then into the lymph of the thoracic duct, and into the blood again. **greater c.,** systemic c. **hypophyseoportal c.,** that passing from the capillaries of the median eminence of the hypothalamus into the portal vessels to the sinusoids of the adenohypophysis. **intervillous c.,** the flow of maternal blood through the intervillous space. **lesser c.,** pulmonary c. **lymph c.,** the passage of the lymph through lymph vessels and glands. **omphalomesenteric c.,** vitelline c. **persistent fetal c.,** pulmonary hypertension in the postnatal period secondary to right-to-left shunting of the blood through the foramen ovale and ductus arteriosus. **placental c.,** the fetal circulation; also, the maternal circulation through the intervillous space of the placenta. **portal c.,** the circulation of blood from the capillaries of one organ through larger vessels to the capillaries of another organ, before returning through larger veins back to the heart, especially the passage of the blood from capillaries of the gastrointestinal tract and spleen through capillaries of the liver before entering the hepatic vein. See also *hypophyseoportal c.* **portoumbilical c.,** Cruveilhier-Baumgarten syndrome. **primitive c.,** the earliest circulation by which nutriment and oxygen are conveyed to the embryo; called also *first c.* **pulmonary c.,** that carrying the venous blood from the right ventricle to the lungs, and returning oxygenated blood to the left atrium of the heart; called also *lesser c.* **sinusoidal c.,** that occurring through the sinusoids of various organs. **systemic c.,** the general circulation, carrying oxygenated blood from the left ventricle to various tissues of the body, and returning the venous blood to the right atrium of the heart; called also *greater c.* **thebesian c.,** the circulation of blood through the thebesian veins. **umbilical c.,** allantoic c. **vitelline c.,** the circulation through the blood vessels of the yolk sac; called also *omphalomesenteric c.*

circulatory (ser′ku-lah-to″re) pertaining to the circulation.

circulus (ser′ku-lus), pl. *cir′culi* [L. "a ring"] a circle or circuit, used in anatomical nomenclature to designate such an arrangement, usually of arteries or veins. **c. arterio′sus cer′ebri** [NA], the important polygonal anastomosis formed by the internal carotid, the anterior and posterior cerebral arteries, the anterior communicating artery, and the posterior communicating arteries; called also *c. arteriosus [Willisi], circle of Willis,* and *c. Willisii.* **c. arterio′sus hal′leri,** c. vasculosus nervi optici. **c. arterio′sus i′ridis ma′jor** [NA], greater arterial circle of the iris: a circle of anastomosing arteries situated in the ciliary body along the ciliary margin of the iris. **c. arterio′sus i′ridis mi′nor** [NA], lesser arterial circle of the iris: a circle of anastomosing arteries in the iris near the pupillary margin. **c. arterio′sus [Willis′i],** c. arteriosus cerebri. **c. articula′ris vasculo′sus** [NA], an arrangement of anastomosing vessels encircling a joint. **c. umbilica′lis,** an arterial plexus in the subperitoneal tissue surrounding the navel. **c. vasculo′sus ner′vi op′tici** [NA], a circle of arteries in the sclera surrounding the site of entrance of the optic nerve; called also *c. vasculosus nervi optici [Halleri], c. arteriosus halleri, c. zinnii, circle of Haller,* and *circle of Zinn.* **c. veno′sus hal′leri,** plexus venosus areolaris. **c. veno′sus ho′vii,** circle of Hovius. **c. veno′sus rid′leyi,** sinus circularis. **c. willis′ii,** c. arteriosus cerebri. **c. zinn′ii,** c. vasculosus nervi optici.

circum- (ser′kum) [L.] a prefix signifying around.

circumanal (ser″kum-a′nal) surrounding the anus.

circumarticular (ser″kum-ar-tik′u-lar) around a joint.

circumaxillary (ser″kum-ak′sĭ-lār″e) around the axilla.

circumbulbar (ser″kum-bul′bar) surrounding the eyeball.

circumcallosal (ser″kum-kah-lo′sal) surrounding the corpus callosum.

circumcise (ser′kum-sīz) to perform circumcision.

circumcision (ser″kum-sizh′un) [L. *circumcisio* a cutting around] the removal of all or part of the prepuce, or foreskin. **female c.,** incision of the fold of the skin over the glans clitoridis; called also *clitoridotomy.* **pharaonic c.,** infibulation.

circumclusion (ser″kum-kloo′zhun) [L. *circumcludere* to shut in] compression of an artery by a wire and pin.

circumcorneal (ser″kum-kor′ne-al) around the cornea.

circumcrescent (ser″kum-kres′ent) [*circum-* + L. *crescere* to grow] growing around and over.

circumduction (ser″kum-duk′shun) [L. *circumducere* to draw around] the active or passive circular movement of a limb or of the eye.

circumference (ser-kum′fer-ens) [*circum-* + L. *ferre* to bear] the outer limit or margin of a rounded body. **articular c.,** circumferentia articularis; see specific names under *circumferentia.*

circumferentia (ser-kum″fer-en′she-ah) [L.] circumference. **c. articula′ris,** articular circumference: the rounded surface of a bone which is received into a depression of another bone with which it articulates. **c. articula′ris cap′itis ul′nae** [NA], articular circumference of head of ulna: the semilunar surface of the head of the ulna which articulates with the ulnar notch of the radius; called also *c. articularis capituli ulnae.* **c. articula′ris capit′uli ul′nae,** c. articularis capiti ulnae. **c. articula′ris ra′dii** [NA], the rounded surface of the head or capitulum of the radius which articulates with the radial notch of the ulna; called also *articular circumference of head of radius.*

circumferential (ser″kum-fer-en′shal) pertaining to or forming a circumference.

circumflex (ser′kum-fleks) [L. *circumflexus* bent about] curved like a bow.

circumflexus (ser″kum-flek′sus) [L.] bent about; circumflex.

circumgemmal (ser″kum-jem′al) [*circum-* + L. *gemma* bud] surrounding a bud; a term applied to that form of nerve ending in which an end-bud is surrounded by fibrils.

circuminsular (ser″kum-in′su-lar) [*circum-* + L. *insula* island] surrounding, situated, or occurring about the insula.

circumintestinal (ser″kum-in-tes′tĭ-nal) surrounding the intestine.

circumlental (ser″kum-len′tal) [*circum-* + L. *lens* lens] situated or occurring around the lens.

circumnuclear (ser″kum-nu′kle-ar) surrounding or occurring near the nucleus.

circumocular (ser″kum-ok′u-lar) [*circum-* + L. *oculus* eye] surrounding or occurring around the eye.

circumoral (ser″kum-o′ral) [*circum-* + L. *os, oris* mouth] around or near the mouth.

circumorbital (ser″kum-or′bĭ-tal) [*circum-* + L. *orbita* orbit] situated around or occurring near an orbit.

circumpolarization (ser″kum-po″lar-i-za′shun) [*circum-* + *polarization*] the rotation of a ray of polarized light to the right or left; cf. *optical rotation,* under *rotation.*

circumrenal (ser″kum-re′nal) [*circum-* + L. *ren* kidney] situated or occurring near a kidney.

circumscribed (ser″kum-skrībd) [*circum-* + L. *scribere* to write] bounded or limited; confined to a limited space.

circumscriptus (ser″kum-skrip′tus) [L.] circumscribed.

circumstantiality (ser″kum-stan″she-al′ĭ-te) a disturbance in the flow of thought in which the patient's conversation is characterized by unnecessary elaboration of many trivial details.

Circumstraint (sir′kum-strānt″) trademark for a device used to hold a baby for circumcision.

circumtractor (ser′kum-trak″tor) a self-retaining circular retractor (H. R. Arnold).

circumvallate (ser″kum-val′āt) [*circum-* + L. *vallare* to wall] surrounded by a trench or by a ridge; see *vallate papilla,* under *papilla.*

circumvascular (ser″kum-vas′ku-lar) [*circum-* + L. *vasculum* vessel] situated or occurring about the vessels.

circumvolute (ser″kum-vo′lūt) [*circum-* + L. *volutus* rolled] twisted about.

circumvolutio (ser″kum-vo-lu′she-o) a convolution, or the folding of one object about another. **c. crista′ta,** gyrus fornicatus.

cirrhogenous (sir-roj′ĕ-nus) producing cirrhosis or hardening.

cirrhonosus (sir-ron′o-sus) [Gr. *kirrhos* orange yellow + *nosos* disease] a fetal disease characterized by a golden-yellow staining of the pleura and peritoneum.

cirrhosis (sir-ro′sis) [Gr. *kirrhos* orange yellow] liver disease characterized pathologically by loss of the normal microscopic lobular architecture, with fibrosis and nodular regeneration; see *c. of the liver.* The term is sometimes used to refer to chronic interstitial inflammation of any organ. **acholangic biliary c.,** a liver ailment affecting children up to 12 years old, due to complete or partial agenesis of the intrahepatic, intralobular bile ducts, with manifestations similar to those in obstructive biliary cirrhosis. **alcoholic c.,** cirrhosis in the alcoholic, attributed by some to associated nutritional deficiency and by others to chronic excessive exposure to alcohol as a hepatotoxin. **atrophic c.,** cirrhosis in which the liver is decreased in size; it may be seen in the alcoholic, but is more common in posthepatitic or postnecrotic cirrhosis. **bacterial c.,** a variety said to be of microbic origin. **biliary c.,** cirrhosis of the liver due to obstruction or infection of the major extra- or intrahepatic bile ducts (except in *primary biliary c.*). It is marked by jaundice, abdominal pain, steatorrhea, and enlargement of the liver and spleen. See *primary* and *secondary biliary c.* **biliary c. of children,** secondary biliary cirrhosis due to congenital atresia of the bile ducts; called also *infantile liver.* See also *Indian childhood c.* **Budd's c.** (obs.), chronic hepatic enlargement once thought to be caused by intestinal intoxication. **calculus c.,** secondary biliary cirrhosis caused by the presence of gallstones. **cardiac c.,** fibrosis of the liver, probably following central hemorrhagic necrosis, in association with congestive heart disease. It is characterized by scarring about the central veins of the hepatic lobules. **cardiotuberculous c.** (obs.), Hutinel's disease. **Charcot's c.,** primary biliary c. **congestive c.,** cirrhosis of the liver with passive congestion. **Cruveilhier-Baumgarten c.,** see under *syndrome.* **fatty c.,** cirrhosis in which liver cells are infiltrated with fat (triglyceride), the infiltration usually being due to alcohol ingestion; Laennec's c. **Hanot's c.,** 1. primary biliary c. 2. secondary biliary c. **hypertrophic c.,** primary biliary c. **Indian childhood c.,** cirrhosis of the liver of unknown etiology occurring in children in India, characterized typically by insidious onset, stunting of growth, hepatomegaly, and a low inconstant fever. In the late stages, portal hypertension with ascites, evidence of collateral circulation, hematemesis, splenomegaly, and edema may be seen. Cf. *veno-occlusive disease of the liver,* under *disease.* **c. of kidney** (obs.), chronic interstitial nephritis. **Laennec's c.,** cirrhosis of the liver closely associated with chronic excessive alcohol ingestion. In the early stages, liver enlargment may reflect fatty infiltration of liver cells (fatty c.), with necrosis and inflammation due to acute alcohol injury; progressive fibrosis extending from portal areas separates uniform small regeneration nodules. See *c. of liver* for symptoms. **c. of liver,** a group of chronic diseases of the liver characterized by loss of normal hepatic lobular architecture with fibrosis, and by destruction of parenchymal cells and their regeneration to form nodules. The disease has a lengthy latent period, usually followed by the sudden appearance of abdominal swelling and pain, hematemesis, dependent edema, or jaundice. In advanced stages, ascites, jaundice, portal hypertension, and central nervous system disorders, which may end in hepatic coma, become prominent. Called also *chronic interstitial hepatitis.* **c. of lung,** see *diffuse interstitial pulmonary fibrosis,* under *fibrosis.* **malarial c.,** cirrhosis associated with malaria; the malaria is probably not an etiologic factor. **c. mam′mae,** chronic interstitial mastitis. **metabolic c.,** cirrhosis of the liver associated with metabolic diseases, such as hemochromatosis, Wilson's disease, glycogen storage disease, galactosemia, and disorders of amino acid metabolism. **multilobular c.,** postnecrotic c. **periportal c.,** postnecrotic c. **pigment c., pigmentary c.,** a condition marked by a slightly to moderately enlarged, chocolate-brown liver, the surface of which is diffusely nodular; it is the characteristic lesion of hemochromatosis. **pipe stem c.,** cirrhosis of the liver characterized by fibrotic scars around the large portal vessels; seen in hepatic schistosomiasis, in which fibrosis surrounds parasites or ova trapped in branches of the portal vein. **portal c.,** Laennec's c. **posthepatitic c.,** cirrhosis (usually macronodular) resulting as a sequel to acute hepatitis. **postnecrotic c.,** cirrhosis which follows submassive necrosis of the liver (subacute yellow atrophy) due to toxic or viral hepatitis. The reticulin framework of normal lobules collapses and may be replaced by broad bands of fibrous tissue separating regeneration nodules (multilobular liver) of varying size. Called also *multilobar c., periportal c., toxic c.,* and *healed yellow atrophy.* **primary biliary c.,** a rare form of biliary cirrhosis of unknown etiology, occurring without obstruction or infection of the major bile ducts, sometimes developing after the administration of such drugs as chlorpromazine and arsenicals. Affecting chiefly middle-aged women, it is characterized by chronic cholestasis with pruritus, jaundice, and hypercholesterolemia, with xanthomas, and malabsorption. Called also *Charcot's c., Hanot's c., disease,* or *syndrome, hypertrophic c., Todd's c.,* and *unilobular c.* **pulmonary c.,** see *diffuse interstitial pulmonary fibrosis,* under *fibrosis.* **secondary bilary c.,** cirrhosis of the liver resulting from chronic bile obstruction due to congenital atresia or stricture. **stasis c.,** a general term for cirrhosis due to obstruction of the outflow of the hepatic vein; see also *cardiac c., veno-occlusive disease,* and *Budd-Chiari syndrome.* **c. of stomach,** linitis plastica. **syphilitic c.,** cirrhosis of the liver due to congenital or tertiary syphilis. **Todd's c.,** primary biliary c. **toxic c.,** postnecrotic c. **unilobular c.,** primary biliary c. **vascular c.,** cirrhosis of the liver following upon obstruction of the hepatic vein, portal vein, or general hepatic circulation.

cirrhotic (sir-rot′ik) pertaining to or characterized by cirrhosis.

cirri (sir′ri) plural of *cirrus.*

cirrus (sir′rus), pl. *cir′ri* [L. "curl"] a slender, usually flexible, appendage, such as one of the stiff, spike-like organs of locomotion of ciliate protozoa, composed of fused cilia from several rows, or the muscular retractile copulatory organ of certain trematodes, or one of the short, tentacle-like projections around the mouth of cephalochordates that form a coarse sieve preventing entrance of large particles (e.g., sand) into the mouth.

cirsectomy (ser-sek′to-me) [Gr. *kirsos* varix + *ektomē* excision] excision of a portion of a varicose vein.

cirsenchysis (ser-sen′kĭ-sis) [Gr. *kirsos* varix + *enchysis* injection] treatment of varicose veins by injection of a sclerosing solution.

cirso- (ser′so) [Gr. *kirsos* varix] a combining form denoting relationship to a varix.

cirsocele (ser′so-sēl) [*cirso-* + Gr. *kēlē* tumor] varicocele.

cirsodesis (ser-sod′ĕ-sis) [*cirso-* + Gr. *desis* ligation] the ligation of varicose veins.

cirsoid (ser′soid) [*cirso-* + Gr. *eidos* form] resembling a varix.

cirsomphalos (ser-som′fah-los) [*cirso-* + *omphalos* navel] a varicose state of the navel; caput medusae.

cirsophthalmia (ser″sof-thal′me-ah) [*cirso-* + Gr. *ophthalmos* eye] a varicose state of the conjunctival vessels.

cirsotome (ser′so-tōm) [*cirso-* + Gr. *tomē* a cutting] a cutting instrument for use in operating on varicosities.

cirsotomy (ser-sot′o-me) [*cirso-* + Gr. *temnein* to cut] incision of varicose veins.

cis (sis) [L. "on the same side"] a prefix denoting on this side, on the same side, on the near side; in organic chemistry, having certain atoms or radicals on the same side; in genetics, having the two mutant genes of a pseudoallele on the same chromosome. Cf. *trans.*

cisclomiphene (sis-klo′mĭ-fēn) enclomiphene.

cismatan (sis′mah-tan) the seeds of *Cassia absus;* used in Egypt as a cure for ophthalmia.

cisplatin (sis′plah-tin) chemical name: (*SP-4-2*)diamminedichloroplatinum; an antineoplastic, $Cl_2H_6N_2Pt$, used in the treatment of metastatic testicular and ovarian cancer. Called also cis-*platinum* and *platinum diamminodichloride.*

***cis*-platinum** (sis-plat′ĭ-num) cisplatin.

11-*cis* retinal see *retinal.*

cissa (sis′ah) [Gr. *kissa* longing for strange food] pica.

Cissampelos (sis-am′pĕ-los) [Gr. *kissos* ivy + *ampelos* vine] a genus of menispermaceous climbing plants. *C. capensis* of Africa, is emetic and purgative. *C. pareira* L. is used by tropical American tribes for snakebites; also used as a diuretic, expectorant, emmenagogue, and febrifuge. It contains pelosine, an alkaloid.

cistern (sis′tern) a closed space serving as a reservoir for fluid; see also *cisterna.* **basal c.,** cisterna interpeduncularis. **cerebellomedullary c.,** cisterna cerebellomedullaris. **c. of chiasma, chiasmatic c.,** cisterna chiasmatis. **c. of fossa of Sylvius,** cisterna fossae lateralis cerebri. **great c.,** cisterna cerebellomedullaris. **interpeduncular c.,** cisterna interpeduncularis. **c. of lateral fossa of cerebrum,** cisterna fossae lateralis cerebri. **c. of Pecquet,** cisterna chyli. **posterior c.,** cisterna cerebellomedullaris. **subarachnoidal c's,** cisternae subarachnoideales. **c. of Sylvius,** cisterna fossae lateralis cerebri. **terminal c's,** pairs of transversely oriented channels that are confluent with the sarcotubules, which together with an intermediate T tubule constitute a triad of skeletal muscle. See also *T system,* under *system; T tubule,* under *tubule;* and *triad of skeletal muscle.*

cisterna (sis-ter′nah), pl. *cister′nae* [L.] [NA] a cistern: a closed space serving as a reservoir for lymph or other body fluid, especially one of the enlarged subarachnoid spaces containing cerebrospinal fluid. **c. am′biens,** one that connects the cisterna venae magnae cerebri with the cisterna interpeduncularis. **c. basa′lis,** c. interpeduncularis. **c. cerebellomedulla′ris** [NA], cerebellomedullary cistern: the enlarged subarachnoid space between the under surface of the cerebellum and the posterior surface of the medulla oblongata, and continuous below with the spinal subarachnoid space. It can be tapped by means of a needle inserted through the posterior atlanto-occipital membrane (cisternal puncture). Called also *c. magna,* and *great* or *posterior cistern.* **c. chiasmat′ica,** c. chiasmatis. **c. chias′matis** [NA], chiasmatic cistern: a subarachnoid space between the optic chiasma and the rostrum of the corpus callosum; called also *cistern of chiasma.* **c. chy′li** [NA], a dilated portion of the thoracic duct at its origin in the lumbar region; it receives several lymph-collecting vessels, including the intestinal, lumbar, and descending intercostal trunks. Called also *ampulla chyli, chylocyst, cistern of Pecquet, receptaculune chyli,* and *receptaculum Pecqueti.* **c. fos′sae latera′lis cer′ebri** [NA], cistern of lateral fossa of cerebrum: the space between the arachnoid and the lateral cerebral fossa; called also *c. fossae lateralis cerebri [Sylvii], cistern* or *fossa of Sylvius,* and *c. sulci lateralis.* **c. fos′sae Syl′vii,** fossae lateralis cerebri. **c. intercrura′lis profun′da,** c. interpeduncularis. **c. interpeduncula′ris** [NA], interpeduncular cistern: a dilatation of the subarachnoid space between the cerebral peduncles; called also *c. intercruralis profunda,* and *basal cistern.* **c. mag′na,** c. cerebellomedullaris. **perinuclear c.,** the space separating the inner from the outer nuclear membrane; called also *perinuclear space.* **cister′nae subarachnoida′les,** cisternae subarachnoideales. **cister′nae subarachnoidea′les** [NA], subarachnoidal cisterns: localized enlargements of the subarachnoid space, occurring in areas where the dura mater and arachnoid do not closely follow the contour of the brain with its covering pia mater, and serving as reservoirs of cerebrospinal fluid; called also *cisternae subarachnoidales.* **c. sul′ci latera′lis,** c. Sylvii, c. fossae lateralis cerebri. **c. ve′nae mag′nae cer′ebri,** the superior confluent of the subarachnoid space, lying in the angle between the splenium of the corpus callosum and the superior surfaces of the cerebellum and mesencephalon, and containing the great vein of the cerebrum. Called also *Bichat's* or *arachnoid canal.*

cisternae (sis-ter′ne) [L.] plural of *cisterna.*

cisternal (sis-ter′nal) pertaining to a cistern, especially the cisterna cerebellomedullaris.

cisternographic (sis″ter-no-graf′ik) pertaining to cisternography.

cisternography (sis″ter-nog′rah-fe) radiography of the basal cistern of the brain after subarachnoid injection of a contrast medium.

cistron (sis′tron) [L. *cis* on this side + *trans* on the other side + Gr. *on* neuter ending] the smallest unit of genetic material that must be intact to function as a transmitter of genetic information, i.e., to determine the sequence of amino acids of one polypeptide chain. The cistron is identified by the *cis-trans* test. The gene as traditionally conceived is identical to the cistron. Cf. *muton* and *recon.*

Citanest (si′tah-nest) trademark for preparations of prilocaine hydrochloride.

Citelli's syndrome (che-tel′ēz) [Salvatore *Citelli,* Italian laryngologist, 1875–1947] see under *syndrome.*

Citellus (si-tel′us) *Spermophilus.*

citrate (sit′rāt) any salt of citric acid. In biochemistry, the term is often used interchangeably with citric acid (see under *acid*) **cupric c.,** a bluish green, crystalline powder, $Cu_2C_6H_4O_7$; antiseptic and astringent. **ferric c.,** garnet-red scales or brown granules, $FeC_6H_5O_7 \cdot xH_2O$, used as a reagent; called also *iron citrate.*

citrated (sit′rāt-ed) containing a citrate, especially potassium citrate.

citreoviridin (si″tre-o-vir′ĭ-din) a toxic compound isolated from the fungus *Penicillium citreoviride,* said to have the empirical formula of $C_{23}H_{30}O_6$.

Citromyces (sit″ro-mi′sēz) [*citric acid* + Gr. *mykes* fungus] a name formerly used for some species of *Penicillium,* especially those which produce citric acid from sugars.

citron (sit′ron) [L. *citrus*] 1. the orange-like tree, *Citrus medica,* and its fruit. 2. in bacteriology, shaped like a lemon.

citronella (sit″ron-el′ah) a fragrant grass, *Cymbopogon (Andropogon) nardus* (L.) Rendle, the source of a volatile oil (citronella oil) used in perfumes and insect repellents.

citrophosphate (sit″ro-fos′fāt) a compound of a citrate and a phosphate.

citrulline (sit-rul′lin) alpha-amino delta-carbamido normal valeric acid, $NH_2 \cdot CO \cdot NH \cdot (CH_2)_3 \cdot CH(NH_2) \cdot COOH$; it is formed from ornithine and is itself converted into arginine in the urea cycle.

citrullinuria (sit-rul″lĭ-nu′re-ah) the presence of large amounts of citrulline in the urine, with increased levels of citrulline in both plasma and cerebrospinal fluid.

Citrullus (sĭ-trul′lus) a genus of curcurbitaceous plants, including *C. vulga′ris,* the watermelon, the seeds of which are the source of cucurbital and cucurbocitrin.

Citrus (sit′rus) [L.] a genus of rutaceous trees: *C. aurantifolia,* the lime; *C. aurantium,* the orange; *C. bergamia,* the bergamot; *C. limonum,* the lemon; *C. medica,* the citron; *C. sinensis,* the sweet orange.

citta (sit′ah) [Gr. *kitta* longing for strange food] pica.

cittosis (sit-to′sis) pica.

Civatte's poikiloderma (siv-ats′) [Achille *Civatte,* French dermatologist, 1877–1956] see under *poikiloderma.*

Civiale's operation (se″ve-alz′) [Jean *Civiale,* French physician, 1792–1867] see under *operation.*

Civinini's ligament, process (spine) (che″ve-ne′nēz) [Filippo *Civinini,* Italian anatomist, 1805–1844] see *ligamentum pterygospinale* and *processus pterygospinosus.*

Cl chemical symbol for *chlorine.*

cl. *centiliter.*

cladiosis (klad″e-o′sis) a fungal disease resembling sporotrichosis, marked by chains of subcutaneous nodules along the forearm, and from which an organism called *Scopulariopsis blochi* was isolated; the organism was later found to be a *Paecilomyces,* and was probably a contaminant. Called also *gummatous lymphangitis.*

Clado's anastomosis, etc. (klah′dōz) [Spiro *Clado,* French gynecologist, born 1856] see under *anastomosis, band, fossa,* and *point.*

Cladonia (klah-do′ne-ah) [Gr. *klados* branch] a genus of lichens. *C. rangiferina,* reindeer moss, was formerly used as a stomachic and pectoral.

Cladorchis watsoni (kla-dor′kis wat-so′ni) *Watsonius watsoni.*

cladosporiosis (klad″o-spo″re-o′sis) a general term for infection with *Cladosporium,* including black degeneration of the brain, chromomycosis, and tinea nigra.

Cladosporium (klad″o-spo′re-um) a genus of dematiacious Fungi Imperfecti of the order Moniliales. *C. herbarum* produces "black spot" on meat in cold storage. It will grow at a temperature of 18° F. (−8° C.). *C. carrioni* is an agent of chromomycosis. *C. wernecki* and *C. mansoni* are agents of tinea nigra. *C. trichoides* and other species cause black degeneration of the brain.

cladothricosis (klad″o-thrĭ-ko′sis) infection with *Cladothrix (Nocardia);* now called *nocardiosis.*

Cladothrix (klad′o-thriks) [Gr. *klados* branch + *thrix* hair] former name of a genus of bacteria, now discarded.

clairaudience (klār-aw′de-ens) [Fr. *clair* clear + *audience* a hearing] the subjective impression of sound; see *clairvoyance.*

clairsentience (klār-sen′she-ens) [Fr. *clair* clear + *sentience* perception] clairvoyance.

clairvoyance (klār-voi′ans) [Fr.] a form of extrasensory perception in which knowledge of objective events is acquired without the use of the senses; called also *clairsentience.* Cf. *telepathy.*

clamoxyquin hydrochloride (klah-moks′ĭ-kwin) chemical name: 5-chloro-7-[[[3-(diethylamino)propyl]amino]methyl]-8-quinolinol dihydrochloride; an antiamebic agent, $C_{21}H_{26}ClNO$, which has been used in intestinal amebiasis.

clamp (klamp) a surgical instrument for effecting compression. **Cope's c.,** a crushing clamp with several hinged segments for use in surgery of the colon and rectum. **cotton roll rubber dam c.,** a rubber dam clamp with a buccal and lingual wing or flange to hold cotton rolls in position in the mouth. **Crile's c.,** a rubber-shod clamp to secure temporary hemostasis in suture of blood vessels. **Doyen's c.,** a forceps with flexible blades for clamping tissues to control bleeding temporarily during operations on the gastrointestinal tract. **Gant's c.,** a right-angled

clamp used in operating for piles. **gingival c.,** a clamp for retracting gingival tissues. **Goldblatt's c.,** a clamp for the renal artery to produce experimental hypertension. **Herff's c.,** a variety of wound clamp. **Joseph's c.,** a clamp used after a nasal operation to improve the alignment of the mobilized fragments of the bony framework of the nose. **Martel's c.,** a crushing clamp used in resection of the colon. **Mikulicz's c.,** a clamp used for crushing the septum between the proximal and distal segments of the colon after exteriorization. **Payr c.,** a crushing clamp used in resections of the stomach, intestine, and colon. **pedicle c.,** clamp forceps, def. 1; see under *forceps.* **Pott's c's,** clamps used to grasp individual blood vessels. **Rankin c.,** a three-bladed clamp for crushing the colon during resection. **rubber dam c's,** metallic devices that are used to retain the rubber dam on a tooth. **Sehrt's c.,** a clamp for compressing the aorta or for compressing a limb to arrest hemorrhage; called also *Sehrt's compressor.* **voltage c.,** an electronic technique employing the feedback principle to impose a fixed potential difference across a cell membrane. **Willet's c.,** Willet's forceps. **Yellen c.,** a special clamp used for circumcision.

clang (klang) a harsh quality of a sound or of the voice.

clap (klap) gonorrhea.

clapotage (klap″o-tahzh′) clapotement.

clapotement (klah-pawt-maw′) [Fr.] a splashing sound heard on succussion; called also *clapotage.*

claquement (klak-maw′) [Fr.] a clapping or snapping. **c. d'ouverture,** opening snap.

clarificant (klar-if′ĭ-kant) an agent that clears liquids of turbidity.

clarification (klar″ĭ-fĭ-ka′shun) [L. *clarus* clear + *facere* to make] the clearing of a liquid from turbidity.

clarify (klar′ĭ-fi) [L. *clarificare* to render clear] to clear of turbidity or of suspended matter.

Clark II an irritant poison gas, diphenylcyanoarsine, $(C_6H_5)_2$-AsCN.

Clark's test (klarks) [Guy Wendell *Clark,* American biochemist, born 1887] see under *tests.*

Clark-Collip method (klark-kol′ip) [Earl Perry *Clark,* American biochemist, born 1892; James Bertram *Collip,* Canadian biochemist, born 1892] see under *method.*

Clarke's cells, nucleus (column) (klarks) [Jacob Augustus Lockhart *Clarke,* English anatomist and physician, 1817–1880] see under *cell,* and see *nucleus thoracicus.*

clasmatocyte (klaz-mat′o-sit) [Gr. *klasma* a piece broken off + *kytos* hollow vessel] Ranvier's name for certain branched cells in connective tissue that allegedly detach portions of their processes as a means of discharging their secretions. As now used the term is equivalent to the cell described under macrophage.

clasmatocytosis (klaz-mat″o-si-to′sis) an excess of clasmatocytes.

clasmatodendrosis (klaz-mat″o-den-dro′sis) [Gr. *klasma* a piece broken off + *dendron*] a breaking up of the protoplasmic expansions of astrocytes.

clasmatosis (klaz″mah-to′sis) [Gr. *klasma* a piece broken off] 1. the breaking off of parts of a cell. 2. the process of cytoplasmic fragmentation by which plasmacytes are said to release synthesized immunoglobulins.

clasmocytoma (klaz″mo-si-to′mah) reticulum cell sarcoma.

clasp (klasp) a device by which something is held, such as a part of a removable partial denture which retains and stabilizes the denture by contacting or partially surrounding an abutment tooth; called also *direct retainer.* **Adams c.,** a specially designed retention crib for assisting in retention of a removable appliance. **bar c.,** one with two or more separate arms located opposite to each other on the tooth, one acting as a retentive and the other as a reciprocal arm. **circumferential c.,** one that encircles without interruption more than half of the circumference of the abutment tooth. **Dujarier's c.,** a metal device for use in fractures of the calcaneus.

class (klas) 1. a taxonomic category subordinate to a phylum (or subphylum) and superior to an order. 2. in statistics, a group of variables all of which show a particular value or a value falling between certain limits. The *frequency of class* is the number of variables that it contains.

classic (klas′ik) of first class or rank; standard.

classification (klas″sĭ-fĭ-ka′shun) the systematic arrangement of similar entities on the basis of certain differing characteristics. **adansonian c.,** numerical taxonomy. **Angle's c.,** a classification of dental malocclusion based on the mesiodistal (anteroposterior) position of the mandibular dental arch and teeth relative to the maxillary dental arch and teeth; see under *malocclusion.* **Arneth's c.,** see under *formula.* **Broders' c.,** see under *index.* **Caldwell-Moloy c.,** classification of female pelves as gynecoid, android, anthropoid, and platypelloid; see under *pelvis.* **Denver c.,** the classification of human chromosomes on the basis of size and centromere position. Ideally, the 23 pairs of chromosomes are classified individually, but usually the best that can be done is to arrange them into seven groups, labeled A to G, in the order of decreasing length. **Jansky's c.,** a classification of ABO blood types designated by roman numerals I to IV, corresponding with types O, A, B, and AB, respectively. **Jensen's c.,** a classification of bacteria based upon the nutritive characteristics of the organisms. **Keith-Wagener-Barker c.,** a classification of hypertension and arteriolosclerosis based on retinal changes. Group 1, essential benign hypertension indicated by moderate arteriolar attenuation. Group 2, constant high blood pressure but no apparent effect on health, indicated by more definite arteriolar attenuation with localized constriction. Group 3, hypertension with retinal, renal, cerebral, and other symptoms, indicated by marked attenuation of the arterioles, cotton-wool exudates, and hemorrhages. Group 4, severe hypertension with severe nervous system, visual, and other organ disturbances, indicated by ophthalmoscopic signs of Group 3, with papilledema. **Kennedy c.,** a classification of partially edentulous conditions and partial dentures, based on the location of the edentulous spaces in relation to the remaining teeth. **Kraepelin's c.,** a classification of the manic-depressive and schizophrenic groups of mental disease. **Lancefield c.,** a serologic classification of the hemolytic streptococci based on the precipitin test, depending on the presence of group-specific cell-wall antigens (carbohydrates), and giving a strong indication of their predilections. They are grouped as follows: *group A,* primarily pathogenic for man; *group B,* almost exclusively found in bovine mastitis; *group C,* primarily pathogenic for lower animals; *group D,* isolated from cheese; *group E,* isolated from milk; *group F,* isolated from human throats; *group G,* isolated from man, dogs, and monkeys; *groups H, K, and O,* nonpathogenic from the respiratory tract of man. **McNeer c.,** a classification of gastric carcinoma as (1) polypoid, (2) ulcerocancerous, (3) ulcerating and infiltrating, and (4) infiltrating. **Migula's c.,** a classification of bacteria drawn up by Migula in 1900. **Moss' c.,** a classification of ABO blood types designated by roman numerals I to IV, corresponding with types AB, A, B, and O, respectively. **New York Heart Association (NYHA) c.,** a functional and therapeutic classification for prescription of physical activity for cardiac patients. Class I (or A): patients with no limitation of activities; they suffer no symptoms from ordinary activities. Class II (or B): patients with slight limitation of activity; they are comfortable at rest or with mild exertion. Class III (or C): patients with marked limitation of activity; they are comfortable only at rest. Class IV (or D): patients who should be at complete rest, confined to bed or chair; any physical activity brings on discomfort. **numerical c.,** see under *taxonomy.*

clastic (klas'tik) [Gr. *klastos* broken] 1. causing or undergoing a division into parts. 2. separable into parts, as an anatomical model.

clastogenic (klas″to-jen'ik) giving rise to or inducing disruption or breakages, as of chromosomes.

clastothrix (klas'to-thriks) [Gr. *klastos* broken + *thrix* hair] trichorrhexis nodosa.

clathrate (klăth'rāt) [L. *clathrare* to provide with a lattice] 1. having the shape or appearance of a lattice. 2. a clathrate compound; also, pertaining or relating to a clathrate compound. See under *compound.*

Clathrochloris (klath″ro-klo'ris) a genus of microorganisms of the family Chlorobacteriaceae, suborder Rhodobacteriineae, order Pseudomonadales, occurring usually as spherical cells arranged in chains and joined in trellis-like aggregates; the type species is *C. sulphu'rica.*

Clathrocystis (klath″ro-sis'tis) a genus name formerly given microorganisms, some of which are now classified in the genus *Lamprocystis.*

Clauberg's culture medium, test, unit (klaw'bergz) [Karl Wm. *Clauberg,* German bacteriologist, born 1893] see under *culture medium, test,* and *unit.*

Claude's hyperkinesis sign, syndrome (klawdz) [Henri *Claude,* French psychiatrist, 1869–1945] see under *sign* and *syndrome.*

claudicant (klaw'dĭ-kant) pertaining to or affected by claudication; by extension, sometimes used to denote a patient with intermittent claudication.

claudication (klaw″dĭ-ka'shun) [L. *claudicatio*] limping or lameness. **intermittent c.,** a complex of symptoms characterized by absence of pain or discomfort in a limb when at rest, the commencement of pain, tension, and weakness, after walking is begun, intensification of the condition until walking becomes impossible, and the disappearance of the symptoms after a period of rest. The condition is seen in occlusive arterial diseases of the limbs, such as thromboangiitis obliterans, and in compression of the cauda equina. Called also *Charcot's syndrome* and *angina cruris.* **venous c.,** intermittent claudication caused by venous stasis.

claudicatory (klaw'dĭ-kah-tor″e) pertaining to or marked by claudication.

Claudius' cell (klaw'de-us) [Friedrich Matthias *Claudius,* Austrian anatomist, 1822–1869] see under *cell.*

claustra (klaws'trah) [L.] plural of *claustrum.*

claustral (klaws'tral) pertaining to or of the nature of a claustrum.

claustrophilia (klaws″tro-fil'e-ah) a morbid desire to be shut in, to close all doors, windows, etc.

claustrophobia (klaws″tro-fo'be-ah) [L. *claudere* to shut + Gr. *phobein* to be affrighted by + *ia*] morbid dread of being shut up in a confined space.

claustrum (klaws'trum), pl. *claus'tra* [L. "a barrier"] [NA] the thin layer of gray matter lateral to the external capsule of the brain, dividing it from the white matter of the insula; it is mainly composed of spindle cells. Called also *claustrum of insula.* **c. gut'turis, c. o'ris,** palatum molle. **c. virgina'le,** hymen.

clausura (klaw-su'rah) [L. "closure"] atresia.

clava (kla'vah) [L. "stick"] tuberculum nuclei gracilis.

clavacin (kla'vah-sin) patulin.

claval (kla'val) pertaining to the clava (tuberculum nuclei gracilis [NA]).

clavate (kla'vāt) [L. *clavatus* club] pertaining to the clava (tuberculum nuclei gracilis [NA]); club-shaped.

clavelization (klav″ĕ-li-za'shun) [Fr. *clavelée* sheep-pox] inoculation with the virus of sheep-pox for the purpose of immunizing the host against the disease.

Claviceps (klav'ĭ-seps) [L. *clava* club + *caput* head] a genus of parasitic ascomycetous fungi of the family Clavicipitaceae, order Clavicipitales, which infest the seeds of various plants. *C. purpurea* is the source of the common ergot of rye. See *ergot,* def. 1.

Clavicipitaceae (klav″ĭ-sip″ĭ-ta'se-e) a family of fungi of the order Clavicipitales having long cylindrical asci and long filiform ascospores, including the genera *Claviceps* and *Cordyceps.*

Clavicipitales (klav″ĭ-sip″ĭ-ta'lēz) an order of ascomycetous fungi of the series Pyrenomycetes, in which the perithecia are formed in well-developed stroma and the asci have thick caps; it includes the family Clavicipitaceae.

clavicle (klav'ĭ-k'l) the bone articulating with the sternum and scapula; see *clavicula.*

clavicotomy (klav″ĭ-kot'o-me) [*clavicle* + Gr. *tomē* a cutting] the operation of cutting or dividing the clavicle.

clavicula (klah-vik'u-lah) [L. dim. of *clavis* key] [NA] the clavicle: a bone, curved like the letter *f,* that articulates with the sternum and scapula, forming the anterior portion of the shoulder girdle on either side; called also *collar bone.*

clavicular (klah-vik'u-lar) pertaining to the clavicle.

claviculus (klah-vik'u-lus), pl. *clavic'uli* [L. dim. of *clavus* nail] any one of Sharpey's fibers (a set of fibers that hold together the laminae of a bone).

claviformin (klav″ĭ-for'min) patulin.

clavipectoral (klav″ĭ-pek'to-ral) [L. *clavis* clavicle + *pectus* breast] pertaining to the clavicle and thorax.

clavus (kla'vus), pl. *cla'vi* [L. "nail"] a corn. **c. hyster'icus,** a sensation as if a nail were being driven into the head. **c. secali'nus,** ergot, def. 1.

clawfoot (klaw-fut) a high-arched foot with the toes hyperextended at the metatarsophalangeal joint and flexed at the distal joints; called also *gampsodactyly* and *griffe des orteils.*

clawhand (klaw-hand) flexion and atrophy of the hand and fingers; it occurs in lesions of the ulnar nerve, in leprosy, and in syringomyelia. Called also *main en griffe.*

Clawhand.

clay (kla) a native hydrated aluminum silicate, resulting from the decomposition of rocks caused by weathering; various forms of clays have been used in medicine, both externally and internally, since earliest times. **China c.,** kaolin.

clazolam (kla'zo-lam) chemical name: 2-chloro-5,9,10,14b-tetrahydro-5-methylisoquino[2,1-*d*][1,4]benzodiazepin-6(7*H*)-one; a minor tranquilizer, $C_{18}H_{17}ClN_2O.$

clazolimine (kla-zo'lĭ-mēn) chemical name: 1-(4-chlorophenyl)-2-imino-3-methyl-4-imidazolidinone; a diuretic, $C_{10}H_{10}ClN_3O.$

Cl₃C·CHO chloral.

clear (klēr) to remove cloudiness from microscopical specimens by the use of a clearing agent.

clearance (klēr'ans) 1. the act of clearing; specifically complete removal of a solute or substance from a specific volume of blood per unit of time, i.e., blood cleared of substance per minute, e.g., creatinine clearance of 120 ml. per minute. 2. the space existing between opposed structures. **blood-urea c.,** the volume of the blood cleared of urea per minute by renal elimination; called also *urea c.* **creatinine c.,** the volume of plasma cleared of creatinine after the parenteral administration of a specified amount of the substance (exogenous creatinine clearance); the volume of plasma cleared of creatinine occurring without parenteral administration, i.e., of creatinine synthesized within the body (endogenous creatinine clearance). **immune c.,** immune elimination. **interocclusal c.,** interocclusal distance. **inulin c.,** an expression of the renal efficiency in eliminating inulin from the blood; it approximates the glomerular filtration rate (G.F.R.). **iron plasma c.,** a term indicating the time (in minutes) required for 50 per cent of a measured quantity of radioactive iron, injected for test purposes, to be cleared from the plasma. **occlusal c.,** a condition in which the opposing occlusal surfaces may glide over one another without any interfering projection. **plasma c.,** an expression of the ability of the kidneys to completely remove various substances, e.g., urea, from the blood plasma on a single passage through the kidneys; it is determined by simultaneously measuring the concentration of the substance in question in the plasma and in the urine in conjunction with the rate of urine formation (ml. per minute). **urea c.,** blood-urea c.

clearer (klēr′er)   a clearing agent; an agent used in microscopy to remove the cloudiness from a specimen.

cleavage (klēv′ij)   the mitotic segmentation of the fertilized ovum, the size of the structure remaining unchanged, as the cleavage cells, or blastomeres, become smaller and smaller with each division. **accessory c.,** peripheral cleavage in telolecithal eggs due to polyspermy. **adequal c.,** a form in which the blastomeres are practically equal in size. **complete c.,** holoblastic c. **determinate c.,** cleavage following a precise pattern, each blastomere having a characteristic and unalterable fate, i.e., each blastomere becoming the precursor of a definite part of the embryo. **discoidal c.,** cleavage limited to the animal pole of highly telolecithal eggs. **equal c.,** a form in which the blastomeres are equal in size. **equatorial c.,** cleavage that occurs in a plane passing through the equator of the egg. **holoblastic c.,** a form in which the entire egg participates in cell division; called also *complete* or *total c.* **incomplete c.,** meroblastic c. **indeterminate c.,** that following a less rigid cleavage pattern, the blastomeres having more developmental possibilities than they usually show, each of which, when isolated, being capable of developing into a normal embryo. **latitudinal c.,** cleavage in planes passing at right angles to the egg axis. **meridional c.,** cleavage in planes passing through the egg axis. **meroblastic c.,** a form in which only the protoplasmic portions of the egg participate; called also *incomplete* or *partial c.* **partial c.,** meroblastic c. **superficial c.,** a form in which only the surface region of centrolecithal eggs participate. **total c.,** holoblastic c. **unequal c.,** a form in which the blastomeres about the vegetal pole remain larger in size than those nearer the animal pole.

cleft (kleft)   a fissure or elongated opening, especially one occurring in the embryo or derived from a failure of parts to fuse during embryonic development. **anal c.,** crena ani. **branchial c.,** any of the slit-like openings in the gills of fishes, formed between the branchial arches. Also, any of the homologous branchial grooves of the mammalian embryo. **cervical c′s,** clefts in the endocervical mucosa. **cholesterol c.,** a cleft in a section of tissue embedded in paraffin, due to the dissolving of cholesterol crystals. **clunial c.,** crena ani. **corneal c.,** see under *fissure.* **facial c.,** the clefts between the embryonic processes that normally unite to form the face. Failure of such union, depending on its site, causes such developmental defects as cleft cheek; cleft lip (harelip); cleft mandible; oblique facial cleft; and transverse facial cleft. **facial c., lateral,** a unilateral or bilateral cleft with complete fissure extending from the commissure of the mouth into the cheeks, usually to the anterior border of the masseter muscle. **facial c., oblique,** a fissure extending from the ala nasi to the lateral canthus of the eye, caused by failure of union of the maxillary and lateral nasal processes in the embryo. **facial c., transverse,** lateral facial c. **genital c.,** a depression of the external genital region of the fetus, which develops into the male urethra or the vestibule. **hyobranchial c.,** the cleft between the hyoid and the next succeeding arch in the developing embryo; called also *posthyoidean c.* **hyoid c.,** hyomandibular c. **hyomandibular c.,** the cleft between the mandibular and hyoid arches in the developing embryo; called also *hyoid c.* **interdental c.,** diastema. **intergluteal c.,** gluteal furrow. **Lanterman's c′s,** incisures of Lanterman. **Larrey's c.,** trigonum sternocostale. **Maurer's c′s,** Maurer's dots. **natal c.,** gluteal furrow. **posthyoidean c.,** hyobranchial c. **Schmidt-Lanterman c′s,** incisures of Lanterman. **synaptic c.,** a narrow extracellular cleft between the pre- and postsynaptic cell membranes at the synapse. **visceral c′s,** grooves between the branchial (visceral) arches of the embryo. **vulval c.,** rima pudendi.

clegs (klegz)   a common name for certain tabanid flies, the horseflies or gadflies.

cleid-   see *cleido-.*

cleidagra (kli-dag′rah) [*cleid-* + Gr. *agra* seizure]   gouty pain in the clavicle.

cleidal (kli′dal)   pertaining to or affecting the clavicle.

cleidarthritis (kli″dar-thri′tis) [*cleid-* + Gr. *arthron* joint]   gout in the clavicular region.

cleido-, cleid- (kli′do, klīd) [Gr. *kleis* bolt, hook; the collar bone (clavicle), so called from its hook shape]   combining form denoting relationship to the clavicle, or to something barred.

cleidocostal (kli″do-kos′tal)   pertaining to the clavicle and the ribs.

cleidocranial (kli″do-kra′ne-al) [*cleido-* + Gr. *kranion* head]   pertaining to the clavicle and the head.

cleidoic (kli-do′ik) [Gr. *kleidouchos* holding the keys]   isolated from the environment, self-contained, as the ova (eggs) of reptiles, birds, and primitive mammals, which are self-sufficient, having become a closed system, and, except for oxygen intake, developing at the expense of the substances stored inside the egg itself, directly into miniature adults without passing through a larval stage.

cleidomastoid (kli″do-mas′toid)   pertaining to the clavicle and the mastoid process.

cleidorrhexis (kli″do-rek′sis) [*cleido-* + Gr. *rhēxsis* rupture]   cleidotomy.

cleidotomy (kli-dot′o-me) [*cleido-* + Gr. *tomē* a cutting]   surgical division of the clavicle of the fetus in difficult labor, to facilitate passage of the shoulders through the birth canal; called also *cleidorrhexis.*

cleidotripsy (kli′do-trip″se) [*cleido-* + Gr. *tribein* to rub]   crushing of the fetal clavicle to facilitate delivery.

cleisagra (kli-sag′rah)   cleidagra.

cleisiophobia (kli″se-o-fo′be-ah) [Gr. *kleisis* closure + *phobia*] (*obs.*) claustrophobia.

cleistothecium (klis″to-the′se-um) [Gr. *kleisis* closure + *thēkē* case]   the fruiting body, or carp, produced by certain ascomycetes, in which there is no pore for the escape of ascospores, the spores being released after decay of the cleistothecium. Cf. *apothecium, gymnothecium,* and *perithecium.*

cleithrophobia (kli″thro-fo′be-ah)   (*obs.*) claustrophobia.

clemastine (klem′as-tēn)   chemical name: (+)-2-[2-[(*p*-chloro-α-methyl-α-phenylbenzyl)oxy]ethyl]-1-methylpyrrolidine; an antihistaminic, $C_{21}H_{26}ClNO$.   **c. fumarate,** a salt of clemastine, $C_{21}H_{26}ClNO \cdot C_4H_4O_4$; an antihistaminic used in the treatment of allergic rhinitis and allergic skin disorders.

Clematis (klem′ah-tis) [Gr. *klēmatis*]   a genus of ranunculaceous plants, many of them active poisons.

clemizole (klem′i-zōl)   chemical name: 1-[(4-chlorophenyl)methyl]-2-(1-pyrrolidinylmethyl)-1*H*-benzimidazole; an antihistaminic, $C_{19}H_{20}ClN_3$.   **c. hydrochloride,** the hydrochloride salt of clemizole, $C_{19}H_{20}ClN_3 \cdot HCl$, used as an antihistaminic in the treatment of skin allergies, food and cosmetic hypersensitivities, and serum sickness; administered orally.   **c. penicillin,** see under *penicillin.*

clenching (klench′ing)   a frequent oral neuromuscular response during sleep or occurring subconsciously when awake, the jaws being forcibly closed, and the teeth firmly in contact, with continuous pulsating contraction of the temporalis and pterygomassetric muscles. It is often associated with bruxism, and as with bruxism, nervous excitability and dental malocclusion are etiologic factors.

Cleocin (kle′o-sin)   trademark for preparations of clindamycin.

cleoid (kle′oid) [Anglo-Saxon *cle,* claw + Gr. *eidos* form]   a dental instrument, shaped like a claw, used for carving dental restorations.

cleptomania (klep″to-ma′ne-ah)   kleptomania.

cleptophobia (klep″to-fo′be-ah)   kleptophobia.

Clérambault-Kandinsky complex (syndrome) (kla″rah-bo′ kan-din′ske) [Gatian de *Clérambault,* French psychiatrist, 1872–1934; Viktor Kandinsky, 1849–1889]   see under *complex.*

Clethrionomys (kleth″re-on′o-mis)   a genus of voles. **C. glario′lus,** a species implicated as a reservoir of epidemic hemorrhagic fever.

click (klik)   a brief sharp sound; see also *clicking.* **ejection c′s,** see under *sound.* **Ortolani's c.,** a click felt when the thigh is abducted in flexion, in congenital dislocation of the hip. It results from the sliding of the femoral head over the acetabular rim. A click can also be felt when the head slips out of the acetabulum on the opposite maneuver. Called also *Ortolani's sign.* **systolic c′s,** short, dry clicking heart sounds during systole, indicative of various heart conditions.

clicking (klik′ing)   a series of clicks, such as the snapping, cracking, or crepitant noise evident on excursions of the mandibular condyle.

clid-, clido-   for words beginning thus, see those beginning *cleid-.*

clidinium bromide (kli-din′e-um) [USP]   chemical name: 3-[(hydroxydiphenylacetyl)oxy]-1-methyl-1-azoniabicyclo[2.2.2]octane bromide. A quaternary ammonium anticholinergic, $C_{22}H_{26}BrNO_3$, with pronounced antispasmotic and antisecretory effects on the gastrointestinal tract, occurring as a white or nearly white, crystalline powder; used as adjunctive therapy in the treatment of peptic ulcer and other gastrointestinal disorders, administered orally.

climacteric (kli-mak′ter-ik, kli″mak-ter′ik) [Gr. *klimaktēr* rung of ladder, critical point in human life] the syndrome of endocrine, somatic, and psychic changes occurring at the termination of the reproductive period in the female (menopause); it may also accompany the normal diminution of sexual activity in the male. Called also *climacterium*.

climacterium (kli″mak-te′re-um) climacteric. **c. prae′cox,** premature menopause.

climatology (kli″mah-tol′o-je) [Gr. *klima* the supposed slope of the earth from the equator to the pole + *logos* treatise] the science devoted to the study of the conditions of the natural environment (rainfall, daylight, temperature, humidity, air movement) prevailing in specific regions of the earth. **medical c.,** that concerned especially with the effect of climatic factors on man, on his functions and health, and on the treatment of his ills.

climatotherapeutics (kli″mah-to-ther″ah-pu′tiks) climatotherapy.

climatotherapy (kli″mah-to-ther′ah-pe) [*climate* + Gr. *therapeia* treatment] the treatment of disease by means of a favorable climate.

climax (kli′maks) [Gr. *klimax* a ladder, staircase] the acme, or period of greatest intensity, as in the course of a disease (crisis), or in sexual excitement (orgasm).

climograph (kli′mŏ-graf) [*climate* + Gr. *graphein* to write] a diagram representing the effect of climate on man.

clinarthrosis (klin″ar-thro′sis) [Gr. *klinein* to bend + *arthrōsis* a jointing] abnormal deviation in the alignment of the bones at a joint.

clindamycin (klin″dah-mi′sin) chemical name: 2S-*trans*-methyl-7-chloro-6, 7, 8-trideoxy-6-[[(1-methyl-4-propyl-2-pyrrolidinyl)carbonyl]amino]-1-thio-L-α-D-*galacto*-octopyranoside. A semisynthetic analogue of the natural antibiotic lincomycin from which it is produced by chlorination, $C_{18}H_{33}ClN_2O_5S$; it is effective primarily against gram-positive bacteria. **c. hydrochloride** [USP], the hydrated hydrochloride salt of clindamycin, $C_{18}H_{33}ClN_2O_5S \cdot HCl$, occurring as a white or practically white, crystalline powder; used primarily in the treatment of penicillin-resistant gram-positive infections and in patients allergic to penicillin; administered orally. **c. palmitate hydrochloride** [USP], a water-soluble hydrochloride salt of the ester of clindamycin and palmitic acid, $C_{34}H_{63}ClN_2O_6S \cdot HCl$, occurring as a white to off-white amorphous powder, having the same actions and uses as the hydrochloride salt; it is suitable for the preparation of solutions for oral administration. **c. phosphate** [USP], a water-soluble ester of clindamycin and phosphoric acid, $C_{18}H_{34}ClN_2O_8PS$, occurring as a white to off-white, hygroscopic, crystalline powder, having the same actions and uses as the hydrochloride salt; it is suitable for preparation of parenteral dosage forms, administered intramuscularly or intravenously.

cline (klīn) [Gr. *klinein* to slope] a continuous series of differences in structure or function exhibited by the members of a species along a line extending from one part of their range to another.

clinic (klin′ik) [Gr. *klinikos* pertaining to a bed] 1. a clinical lecture; examination of patients before a class of students; instruction at the bedside. 2. an establishment where patients are admitted for special study and treatment by a group of physicians practicing medicine together. **ambulant c.,** one for patients not confined to the bed. **dry c.,** a clinical lecture with the presentation of case histories but without the presence of the patients described.

clinical (klin′e-k'l) pertaining to a clinic or to the bedside; pertaining to or founded on actual observation and treatment of patients, as distinguished from theoretical or basic sciences.

clinician (klĭ-nish′an) an expert clinical physician and teacher. **nurse c.,** see under *nurse*.

clinicogenetic (klin″ĭ-ko-jĕ-net′ik) pertaining to the clinical manifestations of a chromosomal (genetic) abnormality.

clinicopathologic (klin″e-ko-path″o-loj′ik) pertaining both to the symptoms of disease and to its pathology.

Clinistix (klin′ĭ-stiks) trademark for an enzyme-impregnated strip of plastic used to test for sugar in the urine. The strip is dipped into the urine and results of positive or negative are indicated by the color of the strip.

Clinitest (klin′ĭ-test)) trademark for reagent tablets containing copper sulfate, used to test for the presence of sugar in the urine. Ten drops of water and 5 of urine are placed in a test tube. The tablet, which generates heat, is added and the solution is allowed to boil. After a few moments the color of the solution is compared to a color chart.

clinocephalism (kli-no-sef′ah-lizm) [Gr. *klinein* to bend + *kephalē* head] clinocephaly.

clinocephaly (kli″no-sef′ah-le) congenital flatness or concavity of the vertex of the head.

clinodactylism (kli″no-dak′tĭ-lizm) clinodactyly.

clinodactyly (kli″no-dak′tĭ-le) [Gr. *klinein* to bend + *daktylos* finger] permanent lateral or medial deviation or deflection of one or more fingers.

clinography (kli-nog′rah-fe) [Gr. *klinē* bed + *graphein* to write] a system of graphic representations of the temperature, symptoms, and pathologic manifestations exhibited by a patient.

clinoid (kli′noid) [Gr. *klinē* bed + *eidos* form] resembling a bed; bed-shaped, as the clinoid processes. See *processus clinoideus*.

clinology (kli-nol′ŏ-je) [Gr. *klinein* to recline + -*logy*] the science of the retrogression of an animal organism.

clinometer (kli-nom′ĕ-ter) [Gr. *klinein* to recline + *metron* measure] clinoscope.

clinoscope (kli′no-skōp) [Gr. *klinein* to recline + *skopein* to examine] an instrument for measuring an angle of deviation, as the torsion of the eyes when gazing at a fixed object; it is used for measuring paralysis of the ocular muscles. Called also *clinometer*.

clinostatic (kli″no-stat′ik) occurring when the patient lies down.

clinostatism (kli′no-stat″izm) [Gr. *klinē* bed + *stasis* position] a lying-down position of the body.

clinotherapy (kli″no-ther′ah-pe) treatment by keeping the patient in bed.

clioquinol (kli′o-kwin′ol) iodochlorhydroxyquin.

clioxanide (kli-oks′ah-nīd) chemical name: 2-(acetyloxy)-*N*-(4-chlorophenyl)-3,5-diiodobenzamide; an anthelmintic, $C_{15}H_{10}ClI_2$-NO_3.

clip (klip) a metallic device for approximating the edges of a wound or for the prevention of bleeding from small individual blood vessels.

ciprofen (kli′-pro′fen) chemical name: 3-chloro-α-methyl-4-(2-thienylcarbonyl)benzeneacetic acid; an anti-inflammatory, C_{14}-$H_{11}ClO_3S$.

cliseometer (klis″e-om′ĕ-ter) [Gr. *klisis* inclination + *metron* measure] an instrument for measuring the angle which the pelvic axis makes with the spinal column.

clisis (kli′sis) [Gr. *klisis* inclination] attraction or inclination.

Clistin (klis′tin) trademark for preparations of carbinoxamine maleate.

clithridium (klith-rid′e-um) [Gr. *kleithria* a keyhole] any bacterium having a shape like a keyhole or figure of 8.

clithrophobia (klith″ro-fo′be-ah) (*obs.*) claustrophobia.

clition (klit′e-on) [Gr. *kleitys* slope, clivus] the midpoint of the anterior border of the clivus.

Clitocybe (kli-tos′ĭ-be) a genus of club fungi of the family Agaricus, order Agaricales. *C. gigan′tea* is the source of clitocybine, *C. nebula′ris* the source of nebularine. The ingestion of *C. illu′dens*, the orange jack-o-lantern mushroom, causes mycetismus gastrointestinalis.

clitocybine (klit″o-si′bin) any one of a group of antibiotic substances obtained from a mushroom, *Clitocybe gigantea*, of the Agaricus family.

clitoral (klit′o-ral, kli′to-ral, klĭ-tor′al) pertaining to the clitoris.

clitorectomy (klit″o-rek′to-me) clitoridectomy.

clitoridauxe (kli′to-rid-awk′se) [*clitoris* + Gr. *auxe* increase] enlargement of the clitoris; clitorism.

clitoridean (kli″to-rid-e′an) clitoral.

clitoridectomy (kli″to-rĭ-dek′to-me) [*clitoris* + Gr. *ektomē* excision] excision of the clitoris; called also *clitorectomy*.

clitoriditis (kli″to-rĭ-di′tis) clitoritis.

clitoridotomy (kli″to-rĭ-dot′o-me) [*clitoris* + Gr. *tomē* cut] incision of the clitoris; female circumcision.

clitorimegaly (kli″to-rĭ-meg′ah-le) [*clitoris* + Gr. *megalē* great] an enlarged clitoris.

clitoris (klit′o-ris, kli′to-ris, klĭ-tor′is) [Gr. *kleitoris*] a small, elongated, erectile body, situated at the anterior angle of the rima pudendi; homologous with the penis in the male. Called also *coles femininus*.

clitorism (kli′to-rism) 1. hypertrophy of the clitoris. 2. persistent and usually painful erection of the clitoris.

clitoritis (kli″to-ri′tis) inflammation of the clitoris.

clitoromania (kli″to-ro-ma′ne-ah) (*obs.*) nymphomania.

clitoromegaly (kli″to-ro-meg′ah-le) clitorimegaly.

clitoroplasty (kli′to-ro-plas″te) plastic surgery of the clitoris.

clitorotomy (kli″to-rot′o-me) [*clitoris* + Gr. *tomē* a cut] surgical incision of the clitoris.

clival (kli′val) pertaining to the clivus.

clivography (kli-vog′rah-fe) radiographic visualization of the clivus, or posterior cranial fossa.

clivus (kli′vus) [L. "slope"] [NA] a bony surface in the posterior cranial fossa, sloping upward from the foramen magnum to the dorsum sellae, the lower part being formed by a portion of the basilar part of the occipital bone (c. ossis occipitalis) and the upper part by a surface of the body of the sphenoid bone (c. ossis sphenoidalis). Called also *c. blumenbachii*. **basilar c.,** c. **basila′ris,** c. ossis occipitalis. **c. blumenbach′ii,** clivus. **c. montic′uli,** declive. **c. os′sis occipita′lis,** the lower part of the clivus, formed by the basilar portion of the occipital bone; called also *basilar c.* or *c. basilaris,* and *basilar groove of occipital bone.* **c. os'sis sphenoida'lis,** the upper part of the clivus, formed by a surface of the body of the sphenoid bone; called also *basilar groove of sphenoid bone.*

clo (klo) a unit of measurement, being the insulation provided by man's normal everyday clothing and representing approximately the insulation provided by $\frac{1}{4}$ in. thickness of wool.

cloaca (klo-a'kah), pl. *cloa'cae* [L. "drain"] 1. in zoology, a common passage for fecal, urinary, and reproductive discharge in most lower vertebrates. 2. in mammalian embryology, the terminal end of the hindgut before division into rectum, bladder, and genital primordia. 3. in pathology, an opening in the involucrum of a necrosed bone. **congenital c.,** persistent c. **ectodermal c.,** that portion of the embryonic cloaca originally external to the cloacal membrane. **entodermal c.,** that portion of the embryonic cloaca originally internal to the cloacal membrane. **persistent c.,** the congenital persistence of a common cavity into which the intestinal, urinary, and reproductive ducts open; called also *congenital c.*

cloacal (klo-a'kal) pertaining to the cloaca.

cloacitis (klo″ah-si'tis) an infectious disease of fowls, marked by ulceration of the cloaca and a chronic discharge.

cloacogenic (klo″ah-ko-jen'ik) originating from the cloaca or from persisting cloacol remnants; said of a group of rare transitional-cell nonkeratinizing epidermoid anal cancers.

clobazam (klo'bah-zam) chemical name: 7-chloro-1-methyl-5-phenyl-1*H*-1,5-benzodiazepine-2,4(3*H*,5*H*)-dione; a minor tranquilizer, $C_{16}H_{13}ClN_2O_2$.

clock (klok) a device by which time may be measured. **biological c.,** the physiologic mechanism that governs the rhythmic occurrence of certain biochemical, physiological, and behavioral phenomena in plants and animals.

clocortolone (klo-kor'to-lōn) chemical name: 9-chloro-6α-fluoro-11β, 21-dihydroxy-16α-methylpregna-1,4-diene-3,20-dione. A glucocorticoid, $C_{22}H_{28}ClFO_4$, available as the 21-acetate, $C_{24}H_{30}$-ClFO$_5$, and as the 21-pivalate, $C_{27}H_{36}ClFO_5$, esters.

clodanolene (klo-dan'o-lēn) chemical name: 1-[[[5-(3,4-dichlorophenyl)-2-furanyl]methylene]amino]-2,4-imidazolidinedione; a skeletal muscle relaxant, $C_{14}H_9Cl_2N_3O_3$.

clodazon hydrochloride (klo'dah-zon) chemical name: 5-chloro-1-[3-(dimethylamino)propyl]-1,3-dihydro-3-phenyl-2*H*-benzimidazol-2-one monohydrochloride monohydrate; an antidepressant, $C_{18}H_{20}ClN_3O \cdot HCl \cdot H_2O$.

clofazimine (klo-fah'zĭ-mēn) chemical name: *N*,5-bis(4-chlorophenyl)-3,5-dihydro-3-[(1-methylethyl)imino]-2-phenazamine; an antibacterial, $C_{27}H_{22}Cl_2N_4$, having leprostatic and tuberculostatic actions.

clofedanol (klo-fed'ah-nōl) chlophedianol.

clofibrate (klo-fi'brāt) [USP] chemical name: 2-(4-chlorophenoxy)-2-methylpropanoic acid methyl ester. An antihyperlipidemic agent, $C_{12}H_{15}ClO_3$, occurring as a colorless to pale yellow liquid; used to reduce elevated serum lipids, administered orally.

clogestone acetate (klo-jes'tōn) chemical name: 3β-17-bis-(acetyloxy)-6-chloropregna-4,6-dien-20-one; a progestin, $C_{25}H_{33}Cl$-O$_5$.

clomacran phosphate (klo'mah-kran) chemical name: 2-chloro-9,10-dihydro-*N,N*-dimethyl-9-acridinepropanamine phosphate; a tranquilizer, $C_{18}H_{21}ClN_2 \cdot H_3PO_4$.

Clomid (klo'mid) trademark for a preparation of clomiphene citrate.

clomiphene citrate (klo'mĭ-fēn) [USP] chemical name: 2-[4-(2-chloro-1,2-diphenylethenyl)phenoxy]ethanamine. A synthetic gonad-stimulating principle structurally related to the proestrogen chlorotrianisene, occurring as a white to pale yellow powder and consisting of a mixture of the *cis-* and *trans*-isomers; used to induce ovulation in certain forms of anovulatory infertility, administered orally.

clomipramine hydrochloride (klo-mip'rah-mēn) chemical name: 3-[[[5-3-chloro-10,11-dihydro-*N*, *N*-dimethyl-5*H*-dibenz[*bf*]azepine-5-propanamine monohydrochloride; a tricyclic antidepressant, $C_{19}H_{23}ClN_2 \cdot HCl$.

clonal (klōn'al) of or pertaining to a clone; see also *clonal selection theory,* under *theory.*

clonality (klo-nal'ĭ-te) the ability to form clones.

clonazepam (klo-naz'ě-pam) chemical name: 5-(*o*-chlorophenyl)-1,3-dihydro-7-nitro-2*H*-1,4-benzodiazepin-2-one; an anticonvulsant, $C_{15}H_{10}ClN_3O_3$.

clone (klōn) [Gr. *klōn* young shoot or twig] 1. in microbiology, the asexual progeny of a single cell. 2. a group of plants which have been propagated vegetatively (i.e., by cutting or budding) from one single seedling or stock. The members of a clone are identical in character with one another, but they will not come true from seed. Called also *clonal variety.* 3. a strain of cells descended in culture or *in vivo* from a single cell; used also as a verb to denote the establishment or initiation of such a strain. **forbidden c.,** in the clonal selection theory, a clone of immunologically competent cells that may become reactive against self-antigens and cause autoimmune disease.

clonic (klon'ik) [Gr. *klonos* turmoil] pertaining to or of the nature of clonus.

clonicity (klo-nis'ĭ-te) the condition of being clonic.

clonicotonic (klon″e-ko-ton'ik) both clonic and tonic.

clonidine hydrochloride (klo'nĭ-dēn) chemical name: *N*-(2,6-dichlorophenyl)-4,5-dihydro-1*H*-imidazol-2-amine monohydrochloride. An adrenergic, $C_9H_9Cl_2N_3 \cdot HCl$, used as an antihypertensive; administered orally.

clonism (klon'izm) [Gr. *klonos* turmoil] a succession of clonic spasms.

clonismus (klo-niz'mus) clonism.

clonixeril (klo-niks'er-il) chemical name: 2-[(3-chloro-2-methylphenyl)amino]-2,3-dihydroxypropyl ester; an analgesic, $C_{16}H_{17}Cl$-N$_2O_4$.

clonixin (klo-niks'in) chemical name: 2-[(3-chloro-2-methylphenyl)amino]-3-pyridinecarboxylic acid; an analgesic, $C_{13}H_{11}Cl$-N$_2O_2$.

clonogenic (klo″no-jen'ik) [*clone* + Gr. *gennan* to produce] giving rise to a clone of cells.

clonograph (klon'o-graf) [*clonus* + Gr. *graphein* to write] an instrument for recording spasmodic movements of parts and tendon reflexes.

Clonopin (klon'o-pin) trademark for a preparation of clonazepam.

clonorchiasis (klo″nor-ki'ah-sis) infection of the biliary passages with the liver fluke *Clonorchis sinensis,* which may lead to inflammation of the biliary tree, proliferation of the biliary epithelium, and progressive portal fibrosis; extension into the liver parenchyma may lead to fatty changes and cirrhosis.

clonorchiosis (klo-nor″ke-o'sis) clonorchiasis.

Clonorchis sinensis (klo-nor″kis si-nen'sis) [Gr. *klōn* branch + *orchis* testicle] the common liver fluke of man in China, Japan, Korea, Taiwan, and Indochina. Adult worms inhabit the bile ducts. Larval development requires two intermediate hosts, the first a snail of the genus *Parafossarulus* or *Bithynia,* the second a fresh-water fish of the carp family. Human infection (see *clonorchiasis*) is acquired from the latter host. Called also *Opisthorchis sinensis* and *Distoma sinensis.*

clonospasm (klon'o-spazm) [Gr. *klonos* turmoil + *spasmos* spasm] clonic spasm.

Clonothrix (klo'no-thriks) [Gr. *klōn* branch + *thrix* hair] a genus of microorganisms of the family Crenotrichaceae, order Chlamydobacteriales, made up of colorless cylindrical cells occurring in attached trichomes which show false branching and are enclosed in sheaths encrusted with iron or manganese compounds. The type species is *C. putea'lis.*

clonus (klo'nus) [Gr. *klonos* turmoil] alternate muscular contraction and relaxation in rapid succession. **ankle c.,** a series of abnormal reflex movements of the foot, induced by sudden dorsiflexion of the foot, which causes alternate contraction and relaxation of the triceps surae muscle (gastrocnemius and soleus muscles); called also *foot c.* **anodal closure c. (ACCl),** clonic muscular contraction occurring at the anode when the electrical circuit is closed. **anodal opening c. (AOCl),** muscular contraction occurring at the anode when the electrical circuit is opened or broken. **cathodal closure c. (CCCl),** clonic muscular contraction occurring at the cathode when the electrical circuit is closed. **cathodal opening c. (COCl),** clonic muscular contraction occurring at the cathode when the electrical circuit is opened or broken. **foot c.,** ankle c. **patellar c.,** rhythmic jerking movement of the patella produced by grasping the patella between the thumb and forefinger and pushing it forcibly toward the foot one or more times; an abnormal reflex with alternate contraction and relaxation of the quadriceps muscle. **toe c.,** abnormal rhythmic movement of the great toe, induced by suddenly extending the first phalanx. **wrist c.,** spasmodic movement of the hand, which is induced by forcibly extending the hand at the wrist.

clopamide (klo-pah'mīd) chemical name: 3-(aminosulfonyl)-4-chloro-*N*-(2,6-dimethyl-1-piperidinyl)benzamide. A diuretic, C_{14}-H$_{20}ClN_3O_3S$, used in the treatment of edema associated with various disorders and in hypertension.

Clopane (klo'pān) trademark for preparations of cyclopentamine hydrochloride.

clopenthixol (klo″pen-thiks'ōl) chemical name: 4-[3-(2-chloro-9*H*-thioxanthen-9-ylidene)propyl]-1-piperazineethanol. A compound, $C_{22}H_{25}ClN_2OS$, having sedative, tranquilizing, antiemetic, antihistaminic, anticholinergic, and alpha-adrenergic blocking properties; it has been used as a tranquilizer in the treatment of schizophrenia.

clopidol (klo'pĭ-dōl) chemical name: 3,5-dichloro-2,6-dimethyl-4-pyridinol; a coccidiostat for poultry, $C_7H_7Cl_2NO$.

clopimozide (klo-pim'o-zīd) chemical name: 1-[1-[4,4-bis(4-fluorophenyl)butyl]-4-piperidinyl]-5-chloro-1,3-dihydro-2*H*-benzimidazol-2-one; a tranquilizer, $C_{28}H_{28}ClF_2N_3O$.

clopirac (klo'pĭ-rak) chemical name: 1-(4-chlorophenyl)-2,5-dimethyl-1*H*-pyrrole-3-acetic acid; an anti-inflammatory, $C_{14}H_{14}Cl$-NO$_2$.

cloprednol (klo-pred′nŏl)   chemical name: 6-chloro-11β,17,21-trihydroxypregna-1,4,6-triene-3,20-dione; a glucocorticoid, C_{21}-$H_{25}ClO_5$.

cloprostenol (klo-pros′tĕ-nŏl)   chemical name: (±)-(Z)-7-[(1R*,2R*,3R*,5S*)-2-[(E)-(3R*)-4-(m-chlorophenoxy)-3-hydroxy-1-butenyl]-3,5-dihydroxycyclopentyl]-5-heptenoic acid; a prostaglandin, $C_{22}H_{28}ClO_6$. Also available as the sodium salt.

Cloquet's canal, fascia, hernia, ligament, septum (klo-kāz′) [Jules Germain *Cloquet*, French surgeon, 1790–1883] see under *fascia*, and see *canalis hyaloidens, crural hernia; vestigium processus vaginalis*, and *septum femorale*.

Cloquet's ganglion (pseudoganglion) (klo-kāz′) [Hippolyte *Cloquet*, anatomist in Paris, 1787–1840]   see under *ganglion*.

clorazepate (klo-raz′ĕ-pāt)   chemical name: 7-chloro-2,3-dihydro-2,2-dihydroxy-5-phenyl-1H-1,4-benzodiazepine-3-carboxylic acid. One of the benzodiazepine tranquilizers, $C_{16}H_{13}ClN_2O_4$, derived from clorazepic acid. **c. dipotassium,** the dipotassium salt of clorazepic acid, $C_{16}H_{11}ClK_2N_2O_4$, used orally as a minor tranquilizer. **c. monopotassium,** the monopotassium salt of clorazepic acid, $C_{16}H_{10}ClKN_2O_3$; a minor tranquilizer.

clorexolone (klo-reks′o-lōn)   chemical name: 6-chloro-2-cyclohexyl-2,3-dihydro-3-oxo-1H-isoindole-5-sulfonamide. A diuretic, $C_{14}H_{11}ClO$, used in the treatment of edema associated with various disorders and in hypertension.

cloroperone hydrochloride (klo″ro-per′ōn)   chemical name: 4-[4-(4-chlorobenzoyl)-1-piperidinyl]-1-(4-fluorophenyl)-1-butanone hydrochloride; a tranquilizer, $C_{22}H_{23}ClFNO_2 \cdot HCl$.

clorophene (klo′ro-fēn)   chemical name: 4-chloro-2-(phenylmethyl)phenol. A disinfectant, $C_{14}H_{17}ClN_2O_3S$, effective against a wide variety of bacteria and fungi.

Clorpactin XCB (klōr-pak′tin)   trademark for a preparation of oxychlorosene.

clorprenaline hydrochloride (klōr-pren′ah-lēn)   chemical name: 2-chloro-α-[[1-methylethyl)amino]methyl]benzenemethanol monohydrochloride monohydrate. An adrenergic, $C_{11}H_{16}Cl$-$NO \cdot HCl \cdot H_2O$, used as a bronchodilator.

clortermine hydrochloride (klōr-ter′mēn)   chemical name: 2-chloro-α,α-dimethylbenzeneethanamine hydrochloride. An adrenergic, $C_{10}H_{14}ClN \cdot HCl$, used as an oral anorexic in the short-term treatment of exogenous obesity.

closantel (klo′san-tel)   chemical name: N-[5-chloro-4-[(4-chlorophenyl)-cyanomethyl]-2-methylphenyl]-2-hydroxy-3,5-diiodobenzamide; an anthelmintic, $C_{22}H_{14}Cl_2I_2N_2O_2$.

closiramine aceturate (klo-sēr′ah-mēn)   chemical name: 8-chloro-11-[2-(dimethylamino)ethyl]-6,11-dihydro-5H-benzo[5,6]cyclohepta[1,2-b]pyridine compound with N-acetylglycine (1:1); an antihistaminic, $C_{18}H_{21}ClN_2 \cdot C_4H_7NO_3$.

clostridia (klos-trid′e-ah)   plural of *clostridium*.

clostridial (klo-strid′e-al)   pertaining to or caused by clostridia.

clostridiopeptidase (klos-trid″e-o-pep′tĭ-dās)   an enzyme that hydrolyzes peptides, the A form (collagenase) hydrolyzing those containing proline, including collagen and gelatin, and the B form hydrolyzing peptides at bonds involving arginine residues.

Clostridium (klo-strid′e-um) [Gr. *klōstēr* spindle]   a genus of Schizomycetes, family Bacillaceae, order Eubacteriales, made up of obligate anaerobic or microaerophilic, gram-positive, spore-forming, rod-shaped bacteria, with spores of greater diameter than the vegetative cells. The spores may be central, terminal, or subterminal. Two hundred and five species have been differentiated on the basis of physiology, morphology, and toxin formation. **C. acetobutyl′icum,** a species found widely distributed in agricultural soils but not found to be pathogenic. **C. ag′ni,** a name once given type B of *C. perfringens,* which causes dysentery in lambs. **C. bifermen′tans,** a species found widely distributed in nature, occurring commonly in feces, sewage, and soil; variously reported as being associated with 4 to 54 per cent of cases of gas gangrene. See also *C. sordellii.* **C. botuli′num,** the agent causing botulism in man, wild ducks, and other waterfowl, limberneck of fowl, certain forms of forage poisoning in cattle and horses in Australia, and lamziekte of cattle in South Africa. It produces a powerful exotoxin that is resistant to proteolytic

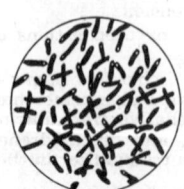

Clostridium botulinum.

digestion, and is divided into types A, B, C alpha and beta, D, and E on the basis of the immunological specificity of the toxin. Formerly called *Bacillus botulinus.* **C. butyr′icum,** a species isolated from the soil. **C. chauvoe′i,** the etiologic agent of blackleg, or symptomatic anthrax, in cattle and sheep; called also *C. feseri,* and *Chauveau's bacillus* or *bacterium.* **C. dif′ficile,** a species often occurring transiently in the gut of infants, but

whose toxin causes pseudomembranous enterocolitis in those receiving prolonged antibiotic therapy. **C. fe′seri,** *C. chauvoei.* **C. haemolyt′icum,** a species isolated from the blood and other tissues of cattle dying with bacillary hemoglobinuria, thought by some to be a type of *C. novyi.* **C. histolyt′icum,** a species found occasionally in feces and soil, originally isolated from necrotic war wounds; according to one report found in 6 per cent of cases of gas gangrene. **C. kluy′veri,** a species thought to be widely distributed in nature, which has been used in study of both microbial synthesis and microbial oxidation of fatty acids. **C. no′vyi,** a species that is an important cause of gas gangrene, being reported in 32 to 48 per cent of cases; three immunological types have been identified, designated A, B, and C. Formerly called *C. oedematiens* and *Bacillus oedematis maligni No. II.* **C. oedemat′iens,** *C. novyi.* **C. ovitox′icus,** a name once given type D of *C. perfringens,* which causes enterotoxemia of sheep. **C. palu′dis,** a name once given type C of *C. perfringens,* which causes struck in sheep. **C. parabotuli′num,** a species that is widely dispersed in soil and is pathogenic for animals, producing a powerful neurotoxin. **C. parabotuli′num e′qui,** *C. botulinum* type D. **C. pasteuria′num,** an anaerobic microorganism occurring in soil, which was the first nitrogen-fixing bacterium to be studied in pure culture. **C. pastoria′num,** *C. pasteurianum.* **C. perfrin′gens,** the most common etiologic agent of gas gangrene, variously reported as occurring in 39 to 83 per cent of cases; differentiable, on the basis of the distribution of nine different toxins and three other substances, which are enzymes, into several different types: type A (the cause of classic gas gangrene in man), B (lamb dysentery), C (struck in sheep), D (enterotoxemia in sheep), E (enterotoxemia

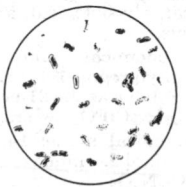 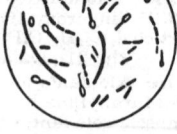

Clostridium perfringens.   *Clostridium tetani.*

in lambs and calves), F (enteritis necroticans in man). It has also been shown to cause a form of food poisoning; see *clostridial food poisoning,* under *poisoning.* Called also *C. welchii* and, formerly, *Bacillus capsulatum* or *welchii.* **C. sep′ticum,** a species commonly occurring in animal intestines and soil, strikingly pathogenic for various animals but reportedly associated with gaseous infections in man in only 4 to 24 per cent of cases. Six groups have been distinguished. Called also *Vibrio septicus, vibrion septique,* and *Ghon-Sacks bacillus.* **C. sordel′lii,** a name commonly given more toxic and virulent strains of *C. bifermentans.* **C. sporog′enes,** a species widely distributed in nature; a harmless saprophyte in pure culture, it is reportedly associated with pathogenic anaerobes in 37 to 72 per cent of gangrenous infections. **C. ter′tium,** a species found widely distributed in feces, sewage, and soil, and variously reported as present in 3 to 59 per cent of gangrenous infections. **C. tet′ani,** a common inhabitant of soil and human and horse intestines, and the cause of tetanus in man and domestic animals; its potent exotoxin is made up of two components, a neurotoxin, or tetanospasmin, and a hemolytic toxin, or tetanolysin. It is variously reported as associated with gangrene in 4 to 13 per cent of cases. Formerly called *Bacillus tetani.* **C. welch′ii,** British name for *C. perfringens.*

clostridium (klo-strid′e-um), pl. *clostrid′ia.*   a microorganism belonging to the genus *Clostridium.*

closure (klo′shur)   the act of shutting, or of bringing together two parts, one or both of which may be movable. **flask c.,** the bringing together of the two halves or parts of a flask in which a denture base is formed. **flask c., final,** the last closure of a flask before curing the denture-base material packed in the mold. **flask c., trial,** preliminary closure of the flask, to eliminate excess material and to ensure that the mold is completely filled. **velopharyngeal c.,** closure of nasal air escape by the elevation of the soft palate and contraction of the posterior pharyngeal wall.

closylate (klo′sĭ-lāt)   USAN contraction for p-chlorobenzesulfonate.

clot (klot)   a semisolidified mass, as of blood or lymph; called also *coagulum.* **agonal c., agony c.,** a blood clot formed in the heart during the death agony. **antemortem c.,** a blood clot formed in the heart or in a large vessel before death. **blood c.,** a coagulum formed of blood, either in or out of the body. **chicken fat c.,** a blood clot that appears yellow because of the settling out of the erythrocytes before clotting occurred. **currant jelly c.,** a clot of reddish color because of the presence of erythrocytes enmeshed in it. **distal c.,** a clot formed in a blood vessel distal to a ligature. **external c.,** a clot formed outside a blood vessel. **heart c.,** postmortem coagulation within the heart. **internal c.,** a blood clot formed within a blood vessel. **laminated c.,** a blood clot formed by successive

deposits, giving it a layered appearance; called also *stratified c.*
marantic c., a blood clot formed because of enfeebled circulation and general malnutrition. **muscle c.,** a clot formed by coagulation of muscle plasm. **passive c.,** a clot formed in the sac of an aneurysm through which the blood has stopped circulating. **plastic c.,** a clot formed from the intima of an artery at the point of ligation, permanently obstructing the artery. **postmortem c.,** a blood clot formed in the heart or in a large blood vessel after death. **proximal c.,** a clot formed in a blood vessel proximal to a ligature. **Schede's c.,** a blood clot formed in Schede's operation (def. 3); see under *operation.* **spider-web c.,** the fine fibrin clot that forms when a sample of fluid from a subject with tuberculous meningitis is allowed to stand, especially when it is warmed to 37° C. for a few hours. **stratified c.,** laminated c. **washed c., white c.,** a blood clot composed of fibrin and platelets.

clothiapine (klo-thi′ah-pēn) chemical name: 2-chloro-11-(4-methyl-1-piperazinyl)dibenzo[b,f][1,4]thiazepine; a tranquilizer, $C_{18}H_{18}ClN_3S$.

clotrimazole (klo-trim′ah-zōl) [USP] chemical name: 1-[(2-chlorophenyl)diphenylmethyl]-1H-imidazole. A broad-spectrum antifungal agent, $C_{22}H_{17}ClN_2$, applied topically to the skin in the treatment of candidiasis and various forms of tinea, and administered intravaginally in the treatment of vulvovaginal candidiasis.

clouding (klowd′ing) loss of clarity. **c. of consciousness,** loss of perception or comprehension of the environment, with loss of ability to respond properly to external stimuli.

Cloudman's melanoma S91 (klowd′manz) [Arthur M. *Cloudman,* American pathologist] see under *melanoma.*

Clouston's syndrome (klow′stonz) [H. R. Clouston] hidrotic ectodermal dysplasia.

clove (klōv) [L. *clavus* a nail or spike] an aromatic spice, the dried flower bud of *Eugenia caryophyllus;* formerly used as a carminative, for the relief of nausea and vomiting, and to stimulate digestion. See also *clove oil,* under *oil.*

clownism (klown′izm) the hysterical performance of grotesque actions.

cloxacillin sodium (kloks″ah-sil′in) [USP] chemical name: [[[3-(2α-chlorophenyl-5α-methyl-4-isoxazolyl]carbonyl]amino]-3,-3-dimethyl-7-oxo-4-thia-1-azabicyclo [3.2.0] heptane-2-carboxylic acid monosodium monohydrate. A semisynthetic penicillinase-resistant penicillin, $C_{19}H_{17}ClN_3NaO_5S \cdot H_2O$, occurring as a white, crystalline powder; used primarily in the treatment of infections due to penicillinase-producing staphylococci, administered orally.

cloxyquin (kloks′ĭ-kwin) chemical name: 5-chloro-8-quinolinol; an antibacterial, C_9H_6ClNO.

clozapine (klo′zah-pēn) chemical name: 8-chloro-11-(4-methyl-1-piperazinyl)-5H-dibenzo[b,e][1,4]diazepine; a sedative, $C_{18}H_{19}ClN_4$.

clubbing (klub′ing) a proliferative change in the soft tissues about the terminal phalanges of the fingers or toes, with no constant osseous changes.

clubfoot (klub′foot) a congenitally deformed foot; called also *reel foot.* See *talipes.*

clubhand (klub′hand) a hand deformity analogous to clubfoot; see *talipomanus.*

clump (klump) an aggregation as of bacteria caused by the action of agglutinins (agglutination).

clumping (klump′ing) the aggregation of particles, such as bacteria, into irregular masses. See *agglutination* (def. 3), and *Gruber's reaction,* under *reaction.*

cluneal (kloo′ne-al) pertaining to the buttocks.

clunis (kloo′nis), pl. *clu′nes* [L.] [NA] the buttock; see *nates.*

clupeine (kloo′pe-in) [L. *clupea* herring] a protamine obtainable from the spermatozoa of the herring.

cluttering (klut′er-ing) hurried nervous speech, marked by the dropping of syllables.

Clutton's joint (klut′unz) [Henry Hugh *Clutton,* London surgeon, 1850–1909] see under *joint.*

clysis (kli′sis) [Gr. *klysis*] 1. (*obs.*) the washing out of a body cavity. 2. the administration other than by the oral route of any one of several solutions to replace lost body fluid, supply nutriment, or raise blood pressure. 3. the solution so administered.

clysma (kliz′mah), pl. *clys′mata* [Gr. *klysma*] a clyster, or enema.

Clysodrast (kli′so-drast) trademark for a preparation of bisacodyl tannex.

clyster (klis′ter) [Gr. *klystēr* a syringe] an injection into the rectum; an enema.

clysterize (klis′ter-īz) [L. *clysterizare;* Gr. *klystēr*] to treat with enemas, or with injections into the rectum.

clytocybine (kli′to-si′bēn) clitocybine.

C.M. abbreviation for L. *Chirur′giae Ma′gister,* Master in Surgery.

Cm chemical symbol for *curium.*

cm. centimeter.

cm.² square centimeter.

cm.³ cubic centimeter.

CMA Certified Medical Assistant.

C.M.A. Canadian Medical Association.

CMI cell-mediated immunity.

c./min. cycles per minute.

c.mm. cubic millimeter.

C.M.R. cerebral metabolic rate.

c.m.s. abbreviation for L. *cras ma′ne sumen′dus,* to be taken tomorrow morning.

C.N. abbreviation for L. *cras noc′te,* tomorrow night.

C.N.A. Canadian Nurses' Association.

cnemial (ne′me-al) pertaining to the shin.

Cnemidocoptes (ne″mĭ-do-kop′tēz) *Knemidokoptes.*

cnemis (ne′mis) the lower leg, shin, or tibia.

cnemitis (ne-mi′tis) inflammation of the tibia.

cnemoscoliosis (ne″mo-sko″le-o′sis) [Gr. *knēmē* leg + *skoliōsis* crookedness] a lateral bending of the leg.

Cnidaria (ni-dah′re-ah) [Gr. *knide* a nettle] Coelenterata.

cnidarian (ni-dah′re-an) 1. of or pertaining to Cnidaria. 2. any member of Cnidaria.

Cnidian (ni′de-an) [*Cnidos,* site of one of the early Greek temples of medicine] 1. an early school of medicine in Greece that stressed the diagnosis and classification of disease. 2. a believer in or practitioner of the Cnidian theory of medicine.

cnidoblast (ni′dŏ-blast) the epidermal cells of coelenterates which contain the nematocysts, especially numerous on the tentacles.

cnidocil (ni′dŏ-sil) [Gr. *knide* nettle + L. *cilium hair*] a bristle-like process at one end of a cnidoblast, which, when stimulated, triggers the discharge of the nematocyst.

C.N.M. Certified Nurse-Midwife; see *nurse-midwife.*

CNOH cyanic acid.

CNS sulfocyanate.

C.N.S. central nervous system.

c.n.s. abbreviation for L. *cras noc′te sumen′dus,* to be taken tomorrow night.

CO carbon monoxide.

CO₂ carbon dioxide.

Co chemical symbol for *cobalt.*

co- a prefix signifying with, together.

C.O.A. Canadian Orthopaedic Association.

CoA coenzyme A.

coacervate (ko-as′er-vāt) [L. *coacervatus* heaped up] the viscous phase separating from a colloid-containing system in the phenomenon of coacervation.

coacervation (ko-as″er-va′shun) a phenomenon that involves both lyophilic and hydrophilic colloids, but particularly the latter, being the separation of microscopic liquid droplets when sols of two hydrophilic colloids of opposite electric charge are mixed. These droplets may later unite to form a viscous layer at the bottom of the container, constituting a new phase.

coadaptation (ko″ad-ap-ta′shun) [co- + L. *adapta′re* to adapt] the mutual, correlated, adaptive changes in two interdependent organs.

coadunation (ko″ad-u-na′shun) [L. co- together + ad to + u′nus one] union of dissimilar substances in one mass.

coadunition (ko″ad-u-nish′un) coadunation.

coagglutination (ko″ah-gloo″tĭ-na′shun) the aggregation of particulate antigens combined with agglutinins of more than one specificity.

coagglutinin (ko″ah-gloo′tĭ-nin) partial agglutinin.

coagula (ko-ag′u-lah) [L.] plural of *coagulum.*

coagulability (ko-ag″u-lah-bil′ĭ-te) the state of being capable of forming or of being formed into clots.

coagulable (ko-ag′u-lah-b'l) susceptible of being coagulated.

coagulant (ko-ag′u-lant) [L. *coagulans*] 1. promoting, accelerating, or making possible the coagulation of blood. 2. an agent that promotes or accelerates the coagulation of blood.

coagulase (ko-ag′u-lās) an antigenic substance of bacterial origin, produced chiefly by the staphylococci, that may be causally related to thrombus formation. See also under *tests.*

coagulate (ko-ag′u-lāt) [L. *coagulare*] 1. to cause to clot. 2. to become clotted.

coagulation (ko-ag″u-la′shun) [L. *coagulatio*] 1. the process of clot formation; see *blood c.* 2. in colloid chemistry, the solidification of a sol into a gelatinous mass; an alteration of a disperse phase or of a dissolved solid which causes the separation of the system into a liquid phase and an insoluble mass called the clot or curd. Coagulation is usually irreversible. 3. in surgery, the disruption of tissue by physical means to form an amorphous residuum, as in electrocoagulation and photocoagulation.

blood c., the sequential process by which the multiple coagulation factors of the blood interact, ultimately resulting in the formation of an insoluble fibrin clot; it may be divided into three stages: stage 1, the formation of intrinsic and extrinsic prothrombin converting principle; stage 2, the formation of thrombin; stage 3, the formation of stable fibrin polymers. **diffuse intravascular c., disseminated intravascular c. (DIC),** a disorder characterized by reduction in the elements involved in blood coagulation due to their utilization in widespread blood clotting within the vessels; the activation of the clotting mechanism may arise from any of a number of disorders. In the late stages, it is marked by profuse hemorrhaging. Called also *consumption coagulopathy* and *defibrination syndrome.* **electric c.,** electrocoagulation. **massive c.,** coagulation of the spinal fluid so as to form an almost solid clot; a condition seen in some cases of *Froin's syndrome* in meningomyelitis or tumor of the cord.

coagulative (ko-ag′u-la″tiv) associated with coagulation or promoting a process of coagulation; of the nature of coagulation.

coagulator (ko-ag″u-la′tor) a surgical device that utilizes electrical current or light to stop bleeding.

coagulogram (ko-ag′u-lo-gram″) a term used colloquially in clinical hematology to denote a series of laboratory tests measuring the various parameters of hemostasis.

coagulopathy (ko-ag″u-lop′ah-the) any disorder of blood coagulation. **consumption c.,** diffuse intravascular coagulation.

coagulum (ko-ag′u-lum), pl. *coag′ula* [L.] a clot or curd. **closing c.,** the clot that closes the gap made in the uterine lining by the implanting blastocyst; schlusskoagulum.

Coakley's operation (kōk′lēz) [Cornelius Godfrey *Coakley*, laryngologist in New York, 1862–1934] see under *operation.*

coalescence (ko-ah-les′ens) [L. *coalescere* to grow together] the fusion or blending of parts.

coapt (ko′apt) [L. *coaptare*] to approximate, as the edges of a wound or the ends of a fractured bone.

coarctate (ko-ark′tāt) [L. *coarctare* to straighten or tighten] 1. to press close together; contract. 2. pressed together; restrained.

coarctation (ko″ark-ta′shun) [L. *coarctatio,* from *cum* together + *arctare* to make tight] a condition of stricture or contraction. **c. of aorta,** a localized malformation characterized by deformity of the aortic media, causing narrowing, usually severe, of the lumen of the vessel. **c. of aorta, adult type,** a form characterized by a localized constriction at or below the insertion of the ductus arteriosus and distal to the aortic isthmus and left clavian artery, and by a closed ductus and absence of cyanosis. **c. of aorta, infantile type,** a form characterized by diffuse involvement of the aortic isthmus, by association with other anomalies, including a patent ductus, and by cyanosis. **reversed c.,** pulseless disease.

coarse (kōrs) not fine; not microscopical.

coarticulation (ko″ar-tik″u-la′shun)[L. *con* together + *articulare* to join] a synarthrosis.

coat (kōt) [L. *cot′ta* a tunic] a membrane or other structure covering or lining a part or organ; see also *tunic* and *tunica.* **adventitial c.,** tunica adventitia; see terms beginning thus under *tunica.* **adventitious c. of uterine tube,** tela subserosa. **albugineous c.,** tunica albuginea; see terms beginning thus under *tunica.* **buffy c.,** the thin yellowish layer of leukocytes overlying the packed red cells in centrifuged blood; called also *buffy crust* and *leukocytic cream.* **corneoscleral c.,** the corneosclera. **cremasteric c. of testis,** musculus cremaster. **dartos c.,** tunica dartos. **external c. of capsule of graafian follicle,** tunica externa thecae folliculi. **external c. of esophagus,** tunica adventitia esophagi. **external c. of ureter,** tunica adventitia ureteris. **external c. of vessels,** tunica externa vasorum. **external c. of viscera,** tunica adventitia. **extraneous c.,** a cement-like structure, constituting a visible cell wall, in some animal cells; it generally plays no role in permeability, but has other important functions. **fibrous c.,** tunica fibrosa; see terms beginning thus under *tunica.* **fibrous c. of corpus cavernosum of penis,** tunica albuginea corporum cavernosorum. **fibrous c. of eye,** tunica fibrosa bulbi. **fibrous c. of ovary,** theca folliculi. **fibrous c. of testis,** tunica albuginea testis. **internal c. of capsule of graafian follicle,** tunica interna thecae folliculi. **internal c. of pharynx of Luschka,** tela submucosa pharyngis. **mucous c.,** tunica mucosa; for various specific structures, see terms beginning thus under *tunica.* **muscular c.,** tunica muscularis; see terms beginning thus under *tunica.* **pharyngobasilar c.,** fascia pharyngobasilaris. **proper c.,** **proper c. of corium,** stratum reticulare corii. **proper c. of pharynx,** tela submucosa pharyngis. **proper c. of testis,** tunica albuginea testis. **sclerotic c.,** the sclera. **serous c.,** tunica serosa; see terms beginning thus under *tunica.* **submucous c.,** tela submucosa; see terms beginning thus under *tela.* **subserous c.,** tela subserosa; see terms beginning thus under *tela.* **vaginal c. of testis,** tunica vaginalis testis. **vascular c. of pharynx,** tela submucosa pharyngis. **vascular c. of stomach,** tela submucosa ventriculi. **vascular c. of viscera,** tela sub-

mucosa. **villous c. of small intestine,** tunica mucosa intestini tenuis. **white c.,** tunica albuginea.

Coats' disease, retinitis (kōts) [George *Coats,* London ophthalmologist, 1876–1915] exudative retinopathy.

cobalamin (ko-bal′ah-min) the cobalt-containing complex common to all members of the vitamin B_{12} group; frequently used generically to designate any substituted derivative, even cyanocobalamin. **c. concentrate** [USP], a dried, partially purified product resulting from the growth of selected *Streptomyces* cultures, containing in each gram not less than 500 μg. of cobalamin; used as a vitamin B_{12} supplement.

cobalt (ko′bawlt) [L. *cobaltum*] a metal, atomic number, 27; atomic weight 58.9332; symbol Co; the metal is used in magnetic alloys, and the compounds afford pigments. In animals, a deficiency of this element leads to anemia; an excess of normal dietary requirements leads to erythrocytosis. In the human, although cobalt has been used with limited transient effectiveness to treat the anemia of infection, and renal disease, its sole physiological function, most probably, is as a constituent of vitamin B_{12}. Radioisotopes of cobalt, particularly ^{60}Co, a gamma emitter, are used in experimental biology and medicine and in cancer therapy. **c. salipyrine,** a salicylate of cobalt and antipyrine, forming a pale red powder. **c. 60,** a radioactive isotope of cobalt, ^{60}Co, which has a half-life of 5.27 years, used as a source of radiation in the treatment of malignancies and in industrial radiography.

cobaltosis (ko″bal-to′sis) pneumoconiosis due to inhalation of and tissue reaction to cobalt dust.

cobaltous (ko-bawl′tus) pertaining to or containing cobalt in its bivalent state.

cobra (ko′brah) any of several extremely poisonous elapid snakes commonly found in Africa, Asia, and India, which are capable of expanding the neck region to form a hood, and have two comparatively short, erect, deep grooved fangs. A serum obtained from animals inoculated with cobra venom is used in counteracting the effects of bites by the cobra. See table accompanying *snake.* **black-necked c.,** *Naja nigricollis,* a species that usually does not bite but discharges venom by spitting when agitated; the venom is not poisonous but may cause severe irritation or even blindness if it enters the eyes. Called also *spitting c.* **Indian c.,** a yellowish to dark brown cobra, *Naja tripudians,* characterized by black and white markings that resemble a pair of spectacles on its hood; it sometimes attains a length of 6 feet. Called also *c. de capello* and *Naja naja.* **king c.,** a very large cobra, *Naja hannah,* sometimes reaching a length of 12 feet. **spitting c.,** black-necked c.

cobraism (ko′brah-izm) poisoning by cobra venom.

cobralysin (ko-bral′ĭ-sin) a hemolytic substance derived from the poison of the cobra.

COBS abbreviation for *cesarean-obtained barrier-sustained,* a term applied to animals delivered by cesarean section into a germ-free environment and maintained under the same conditions.

cobweb (kob′web) [A.S. abbreviation of *attercop,* poison head, and *web,* from *wefan*] the web of various kinds of spider; sometimes used as a styptic, in the moxa, and as a domestic remedy: a febrifuge and antispasmodic.

COC cathodal opening contraction.

coca (ko′kah) the leaves of *Erythroxylon coca,* a South American plant from which cocaine is obtained; once used as a central nervous system stimulant and still widely used in parts of South America as a euphoriant masticatory.

cocaine (ko′kān) [USP] chemical name: [1*R*-(*exo,exo*)]-3-(benzoyloxy)-8-methyl-8-azabicyclo[3.2.1]octane-2-carboxylic acid methyl ester. A crystalline alkaloid, $C_{17}H_{21}NO_4$, obtained from leaves of *Erythroxylon coca* (coca leaves) and other species of *Erythroxylon,* or by synthesis from ecgonine or its derivatives; used as a local narcotic anesthetic applied topically to mucous membranes. **c. hydrochloride** [USP], the hydrochloride salt of cocaine, $C_{17}H_{21}NO_4 \cdot HCl$, occurring as colorless crystals or a white crystalline powder; used as an anesthetic, applied topically to mucous membranes.

cocainism (ko′kān-izm) the morbid condition resulting from prolonged misuse of cocaine as a stimulant or a narcotic.

cocainist (ko′kān-ist) a person addicted to the habitual use of cocaine.

cocainization (ko″kān-ĭ-za′shun) the act of putting under the influence of cocaine.

cocainize (ko′kān-īz) to put under the influence of cocaine.

cocarboxylase (ko″kar-bok′sĭ-lās) phosphorylated thiamine.

cocarcinogen (ko-kar′sĭ-no-jen″) a factor that, in combination with other factors, produces cancer.

cocarcinogenesis (ko-kar″sĭ-no-jen′ĕ-sis) the development, according to one theory, of cancer only in preconditioned cells and as a result of conditions favorable to its growth.

cocardiform (ko-kar′dĭ-form) [Fr. *cocarde* a rosette worn as a decoration] shaped like a cockade.

coccal (kok′al) resembling or pertaining to cocci.

coccerin (kok′sĕ-rin) a wax from *Coccus*, the cochineal insect, being an ester of cocceryl alcohol and two acids, 13-keto-n-dotriacontanoic acid and n-triacontanoic acid; used as a biological stain.

cocci (kok′si) [L.] plural of *coccus*.

Coccidia (kok-sid′e-ah) an order of protozoa of the subphylum Sporozoa, commonly parasitic in the epithelial cells of the intestinal tract, but also found in the liver and other organs (see *coccidiosis*). It includes the genera *Eimeria, Haemogregarina, Isospora, Hepatozoon, Karyolysus*, and *Lankesterella*.

coccidia (kok-sid′e-ah) plural of *coccidium*.

coccidial (kok-sid′e-al) pertaining to coccidia.

coccidian (kok-sid′e-an) 1. pertaining to Coccidia. 2. any individual of the order Coccidia.

coccidioidal (kok-sid″e-oi′dal) caused by *Coccidioides*.

Coccidioides (kok-sid″e-oi′dēz) a genus of pathogenic imperfect fungi of the family Moniliaceae, order Moniliales. In soil it grows as a mycelium with arthrospores; in tissue as a spherule with endospores. *C. im′mitis* (*Blastomyces coccidioides, Blastomycoides immitis*) causes coccidioidomycosis.

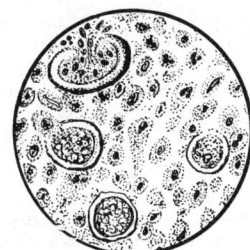

Coccidioides in tissue (de Rivas).

coccidioidin (kok″sid-e-oi′din) [USP] a sterile solution containing the by-products of growth products of *Coccidioides immitis*, injected intracutaneously as a test for coccidioidomycosis.

coccidioidoma (kok-sid″e-oi-do′mah) residual pulmonary granulomatous nodules seen roentgenographically as solid round foci in coccidioidomycosis.

coccidioidomycosis (kok-sid″e-oi″do-mi-ko′sis) a fungous disease caused by infection with *Coccidioides immitis*, occurring in a primary and a secondary form. Called also *coccidioidal granuloma, Posada′s mycosis, Posada-Wernicke disease, California disease*, and *desert fever*. The *primary* form is an acute, benign, self-limited respiratory infection due to inhalation of spores, and varying in severity from that of a common cold to symptoms resembling those accompanying influenza, with pneumonia, cavitation, high fever, and, rarely, erythema nodosum (bumps). Called also *desert rheumatism, San Joachim Valley fever*, and *valley fever*. The *secondary* form (or *progressive c.*) is a virulent and severe, chronic, progressive, granulomatous disease resulting in involvement of the cutaneous and subcutaneous tissues, viscera, central nervous system, and lungs, with anemia, phlebitis, and various allergic responses. This form may be caused by a new infection or by reactivation of arrested primary disease. **primary extrapulmonary c.,** coccidioidomycosis in which infection occurs by primary cutaneous inoculation, usually with secondary lymphadenopathy; called also *chancriform syndrome*.

coccidioidosis (kok-sid″e-oi-do′sis) coccidioidomycosis.

coccidiosis (kok″sid-e-o′sis) infection by coccidia. In man, the term is applied to the presence of *Isospora hominis* or *I. belli* in the stools; such infection is often asymptomatic, rarely causing a severe watery mucous diarrhea. In mammals, such as cattle, sheep, rabbits, swine, cats, and dogs, especially young animals, coccidiosis causes destruction of the intestinal mucosa, accompanied by diarrhea, intestinal hemorrhage, emaciation, and sometimes fatal dysentery. It is due principally to species of *Eimeria* and *Isosphora*. In domesticated mammals, four genera of coccidia are associated with disease: *Eimeria, Tyzzeria, Isospora*, and *Hepatozoon*. Among domesticated animals, coccidial infections cause greatest damage to poultry; *Eimeria* species are highly infective, producing high morbidity and mortality rates, especially in young birds.

coccidiostat (kok-sid′ĭ-o-stat″) any of a group of chemical agents, e.g., nitrofurazone, nitrophenide, nicarbazin, mixed in feed or drinking water to control coccidiosis in animals.

coccidiostatic (kok-sid″ĭ-o-stat′ik) 1. inhibiting the growth of coccidia. 2. an agent that inhibits the growth of coccidia; see *coccidiostat*.

Coccidium (kok-sid′e-um) [L.; dim. of Gr. *kokkos* berry] a former genus of sporozoons of the order Coccidia. **C. bigem′inum,** *Isospora bigemina*. **C. cunic′uli,** *Eimeria stiedae*. **C. hom′inis,** *Isospora hominis*. **C. ovifor′me,** *Eimeria stiedae*. **C. tenel′lum,** *Eimeria tenella*.

coccidium (kok-sid′e-um), pl. *coccid′ia*. Any organism of the order Coccidia.

coccigenic (kok′sĭ-jen′ik) caused by cocci.

coccillana (kok″sĭ-yah′nah) cocillana.

coccinella (kok″sĭ-nel′ah) cochineal.

coccinellin (kok″sĭ-nel′in) [L. *coccinellinum*] carmine; the coloring principle of cochineal.

coccobacillary (kok″o-bas′ĭ-ler″e) pertaining to or resembling a coccobacillus.

coccobacilli (kok″o-bah-sil′li) plural of *coccobacillus*.

Coccobacillus (kok″o-bah-sil′us) *Asterococcus*.

coccobacillus (kok″o-bah-sil′us), pl. *coccobacil′li*. An oval bacterial cell intermediate between the coccus and bacillus forms.

coccobacteria (kok″o-bak-te′re-ah) [Gr. *kokkos* berry + *baktērion* rod] a common name for the spheroid bacteria, or for the various bacterial cocci.

coccode (kok′ōd) a globular granule.

coccogenic (kok″o-jen′ik) coccigenic.

coccogenous (kok-oj′ĕ-nus) [*coccus* + Gr. *gennan* to produce] coccigenic.

coccoid (kok′oid) resembling a coccus; globose.

cocculin (kok′u-lin) picrotoxin.

cocculus (kok′u-lus) [L. dim. of *coccus*] a small berry. **c. in′dicus,** the dried berry or fruit of *Anamirta cocculus*, from which picrotoxin is derived.

Coccus (kok′us) [L.; Gr. *kokkos* berry] a genus of hemipterous insects, the source of cochineal, kermes, and lac.

coccus (kok′us), pl. *coc′ci* [L.] a spherical bacterial cell, usually slightly less than 1μ in diameter.

coccyalgia (kok″se-al′je-ah) coccygodynia.

coccycephalus (kok″se-sef′ah-lus) [Gr. *kokkyx* cuckoo + *kephalē* head] a monster whose head is beak shaped.

coccydynia (kok″sĕ-din′e-ah) coccygodynia.

coccygalgia (kok″se-gal′je-ah) coccygodynia.

coccygeal (kok-sij′e-al) pertaining to or located in the region of the coccyx.

coccygectomy (kok″se-jek′to-me) [*coccyx* + Gr. *ektomē* excision] excision of the coccyx.

coccygerector (kok″se-je-rek′tor) the ventral sacrococcygeal muscle.

coccygeus (kok-sij′e-us) [L.] pertaining to the coccyx.

coccygodynia (kok″se-go-din′e-ah) [*coccyx* + Gr. *odynē* pain] pain in the coccyx and neighboring region; called also *coccygalia*.

coccygotomy (kok″se-got′o-me) [*coccyx* + Gr. *tomē* a cutting] incision of the coccyx.

coccyodynia (kok″se-o-din′e-ah) coccygodynia.

coccyx (kok′siks) [Gr. *kokkyx* cuckoo, whose bill it is said to resemble] the small bone caudad to the sacrum in man, formed by union of four (sometimes five or three) rudimentary vertebrae, and forming the caudal extremity of the vertebral column. Called also *os coccygis* [NA], and *coccygeal, cuckoo*, or *pelvic bone*.

Cochicella (kok″ĭ-sel′ah) a genus of snails that serve as a host of *Dicrocoelium dentriticum*.

cochineal (koch″ĭ-nēl′) the dried female insects, *Coccus cacti*, enclosing the young larvae; formerly used as a coloring agent for pharmaceutical agents. It is the source of carmine and carminic acid.

cochl. abbreviation for L. *cochlea′re*, a spoonful. **cochl. amp.,** L. *cochlea′re am′plum*, a heaping spoonful. **cochl. mag.,** L. *cochlea′re mag′num*, a tablespoonful. **cochl. med.,** L. *cochlea′re me′dium*, a dessertspoonful. **cochl. parv.,** L. *cochlea′re par′vum*, a teaspoonful.

cochlea (kok′le-ah) [L. "snail shell"] 1. anything of a spiral form. 2. [NA] the essential organ of hearing; a spirally wound tube, resembling a snail shell, which forms part of the inner ear. Its base lies against the lateral end of the internal acoustic meatus and its apex is directed anterolaterally. Called also *acoustic labyrinth*. **membranous c.,** ductus cochlearis.

cochlear (kok′le-ar) of or pertaining to the cochlea.

cochleare (kok″le-a′re) [L.] spoon or spoonful. **c. am′plum** [L. "large spoon"], a heaping spoonful. **c. mag′num**, a tablespoon or tablespoonful. **c. me′dium**, a dessertspoon or dessertspoonful. **c. par′vum**, a teaspoon or teaspoonful.

Cochlearia (kok″le-a′re-ah) [L.] a genus of cruciferous plants. *C. armoracia* L. is the common horse radish, used as a condiment and appetite stimulant, and has also been used as a rubefacient and plaster, like mustard, because it contains sinigrin and myrosin, which yield on hydrolysis the counterirritant principle allyl isothiocyanate. **C. officina′lis,** a species once used as an antiscorbutic; called also *scurvy grass*.

cochleariform (kok″le-ar′ĭ-form) [L. *cochleare* spoon + *forma* form] shaped like a spoon.

cochleitis (kok″le-i′tis) inflammation of the cochlea.

cochleotopic (kok″le-o-top′ik) relating to the organization of the auditory pathways and auditory area of the brain.

cochleovestibular (kok″le-o-ves-tib′u-lar) pertaining to the cochlea and vestibule of the ear.

Cochliomyia (kok″le-o-mi′yah) [Gr. *kochlias* snail with a spiral shell + *myia* fly] a genus of flies of the family Calliphoridae. **C. america′na,** *C. hominivorax.* **C. bezzia′na,** *Chrysomyia bezziana.* **C. hominivo′rax,** the screw-worm fly, a bluish green fly that deposits its eggs during the warmest hours of the day on wounds of animals; the larvae, known as screw-worms, after hatching, burrow into the wound and feed on living tissue. Called also *C. americana* and *Chrysomyia macellaria.*

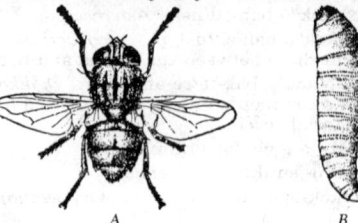

Cochliomyia hominivorax: A, adult; *B,* maggot. (x3).

cochlitis (kok-li′tis) cochleitis.

cocillana (ko″se-yah′nah) the bark of *Guarea rusbyi* (Britt.) Rusby (Meliaceae) used as an emetic, expectorant, and cathartic.

Cock's operation (koks) [Edward *Cock,* English surgeon, 1805–1892] see under *operation.*

cockade (kok-ād′) a rosette or knot of ribbons; by extension, a lesion with two or more concentric zones, as in erythema multiforme or relapsing tuberculoid leprosy.

Cockayne's syndrome (disease) (kok-ānz′) [E. A. *Cockayne,* British physician] see under *syndrome.*

cocktail (kok′tāl) a beverage concocted of various ingredients. **frostbite c.,** a solution of alcohol, procaine, and heparin, in 5 per cent glucose, once recommended in treatment of frostbite. **lytic c.,** a concoction of various drugs used to block the function of the autonomic nervous system at every level, thus inhibiting the homeostatic defense reactions of the organism and producing the state known as artificial hibernation. **McConckey c.,** an emulsion of cod liver oil and tomato juice. **Philadelphia c.,** Rivers′ c. **Rivers′ c.,** a solution of dextrose in isotonic saline solution, with thiamine chloride and insulin added, given by intravenous drip for detoxification in acute alcoholism.

COCl cathodal opening clonus.

cocoa (ko′ko) [NF] a powder prepared from the roasted, cured kernels of the ripe seed of *Theobroma cacao,* which contains caffeine and theobromine; used as a flavor in pharmaceutical preparations. See also *cocoa syrup,* under *syrup.*

coconscious (ko-ken′shus) not in the field of the conscious yet capable under favorable circumstances of being remembered.

coconsciousness (ko-kon′shus-nes) consciousness secondary to the main stream of consciousness, being made up of processes outside that stream.

cocontraction (ko″kon-trak′shun) the mutual coordination of antagonist muscles as of flexors and extensors in maintaining a straight limb.

coconut (ko′ko-nut) the fruit of *Cocos nucifera,* a palm tree whose sap affords palm wine or toddy, while the nut is an important article of food, and supplies great quantities of a valuable oil. See also under *oil.*

Coct. abbreviation for L. *coc′tio,* boiling.

coction (kok′shun) [L. *coctio,* a cooking] 1. the process of boiling. 2. digestion (def. 2).

cocto-immunogen (kok″to-ĭ-mu′no-jen) an immunogen that has been heated.

coctolabile (kok″to-la′bil) [L. *coctus* cooked + *labilis* perishable] destroyed or altered by heating to the boiling point of water.

coctoprecipitin (kok″to-pre-sip′ĭ-tin) [L. *coctus* cooked + *precipitin*] a precipitin produced by injection of a heated serum or other antigen (thermoprecipitinogen); it reacts not only with the heated antigen, but with the unheated one also.

coctoprotein (kok″to-pro′te-in) a heated protein.

coctostabile (kok″to-sta′bil) [L. *coctus* cooked + *stabilis* resisting] not altered by heating to the temperature of boiling water.

coctostable (kok″to-sta′b′l) coctostabile.

coculine (kok′u-lēn) sinomenine.

cocultivation (ko″kul-tĭ-va′shun) the culturing of cells (e.g., normal uninfected human cells) with infected or latently infected cells of the same kind.

code (kōd) [L. *codex* something written] 1. a set of rules governing one's conduct. 2. a system by which information can be communicated. **genetic c.,** the arrangement of nucleotides in the polynucleotide chain of a chromosome that governs the transmission of genetic information to proteins, i.e., determines the sequence of amino acids in the polypeptide chain making up each protein synthesized by the cell. Genetic information is coded in DNA by means of four bases (two purines: adenine and guanine; and two pyrimidines: thymine and cystosine). Each adjacent sequence of three bases (a codon) determines the insertion of a

specific amino acid. In RNA, uracil replaces thymine. **triplet c.,** the three-base sequence (nucleotide) in the DNA molecule which codes for one amino acid.

codehydrogenase I (ko″de-hi′dro-jen-ās″) nicotinamide adenine dinucleotide (NAD). **c. II,** nicotinamide-adenine dinucleotide phosphate (NADP).

codeine (ko′dēn) [L. *codeina*] [USP] chemical name: 7,8-didehydro-4,5α-epoxy-3-methoxy-17-methyl-morphinan-6α-ol monohydrate. A narcotic alkaloid obtained from opium or prepared by methylating morphine, $C_{18}H_{21}NO_3 \cdot H_2O$, occurring as colorless or white crystals or as a white, crystalline powder; used as an analgesic and antitussive, administered orally. Called also *methylmorphine.* **c. phosphate** [USP], the phosphate salt of codeine, $C_{18}H_{21}NO_3 \cdot H_3PO_4 \cdot \frac{1}{2}H_2O$, occurring as fine white, needle-shaped crystals or a white crystalline powder; used as a narcotic analgesic and antitussive; administered subcutaneously. **c. sulfate** [USP], white crystals or white crystalline powder, $(C_{18}H_{21}NO_3)_2 \cdot H_2SO_4 \cdot 3H_2O$; used as a narcotic analgesic, administered orally.

codex (ko′deks), pl. *cod′ices* [L.] an authorized medicinal formulary; especially the French Pharmacopoeia, *Codex medicamentarium.*

Codivilla's extension, operation (ko″di-vil′ahz) [Alessandro *Codivilla,* surgeon in Bologna, 1861–1912] see under *extension* and *operation.*

Codman's sign, triangle (kod′manz) [Ernest Amory *Codman,* Boston surgeon, 1869–1940] see under *sign* and *triangle.*

codominance (ko-dom′ĭ-nans) the full expression in a heterozygote of both alleles of a pair without either being influenced by the other, as in a person with blood group AB.

codominant (ko-dom′ĭ-nant) exhibiting codominance.

codon (ko′don) a series of three adjacent bases in one polynucleotide chain of a DNA or RNA molecule, which codes for a specific amino acid; called also *triplet.*

coe- for words beginning thus, see also words beginning *ce-.*

coefficient (ko″ĕ-fish′ent) 1. an expression of the change or effect produced by the variation in certain factors, or of the ratio between two different quantities. 2. in chemistry, a number or figure put before a chemical formula to indicate how many times the formula is to be multiplied. **absorption c.,** 1. the ratio of the linear rate of change of roentgen rays in a homogeneous material to the intensity at a given point (A. M. A.); see *linear absorption c.* and *mass absorption c.* 2. a number indicating the volume of a gas absorbed by a unit volume of a liquid at 0° C. and a pressure of 760 mm. Hg; called also *Bunsen c.* **activity c.,** the ratio of the activity (of an electrolyte) as measured by some property, such as the depression of the freezing point of a solution, to the true concentration (molality). It is usually less than 1 and increases as the solution becomes more dilute, approaching unity at infinite dilution, when the attractive forces between oppositely charged ions become negligible. **Amann's c.,** the normal proportion between the quantities of ethereal sulfates and the total nitrogen in the urine. It is expressed as follows: (eth. s. × 100)/urea in urine. **Ambard's c.,** see under *formula.* **Baumann's c.,** the ratio of the ethereal to the total sulfates in the urine. **biological c.,** the amount of potential energy consumed by the body when at rest. **Bouchard's c.,** 1. the ratio between the amount of urine and the total solids present in the urine. 2. urotoxic coefficient. **Bunsen c.,** absorption c., def. 2. **creatinine c.,** the figure obtained by dividing the total of milligrams of creatinine in the day's urine by the body weight expressed in kilograms. **cryoscopic c.,** the comparison of the freezing point depression of an electrolyte with that of an ideal nonelectrolyte of the same concentration (usually 1 molal of each). **c. of demineralization,** the proportion of mineral matter to the total dry residue of the urine; it averages 30 per cent. **distribution c.,** partition c. **c. of extinction,** that dilution of an antibody at which its specific activity is no longer manifest. **Falta's c.,** the percentage of ingested sugar eliminated from the system. **Haines' c.,** see under *formula.* **Häser's c.,** see under *formula.* **homogeneity c.,** in radiology, the ratio of the half-value layer and the additional thickness of the material needed to reduce a radiation beam to one fourth of its original exposure rate; it is unity for monoenergetic photons. **hygienic laboratory c.,** phenol c. **c. of inbreeding,** an expression of the probability that an individual has received both alleles of a pair from a single ancestor common to both parents, or of the proportion of loci at which he is homozygous. **isometric c. of lactic acid,** the ratio of the total isometric tension a muscle can produce before fatigue, to the milligrams of lactic acid it produced. **Lancet c.,** phenol c. **lethal c.** (*obs.*), that concentration of a disinfectant that will kill sporeless bacteria (*inferior lethal c.*) or bacterial spores (*superior lethal c.*) in water at a temperature of 20° to 25° C. **linear absorption c.,** in radiology, a factor expressing the fraction of a beam of x- or gamma-radiation absorbed in unit thickness of material. **Loebisch's c.,** see under *formula.* **Long's c.,** see under *formula.* **Maillard's c.,** a coefficient expressing the relationship between the urea and the total nitrogen of the urine. **mass absorption c.,** in radiology, the linear absorption coefficient per centimeter divided by the density of the absorber in grams per cubic centimeter. **osmotic c.,** a factor, φ, which corrects for the deviation in the behavior of a solute in question from ideal behavior defined by the ideal gas equation as applied to osmotic pressure. **c. of partage,** a number indicating the ratio between the amount of an acid absorbed by ether from an aqueous solution of the acid and the amount remaining in solution. Symbol C′. **partition c.,** the ratio in which a given substance distributes itself between two or more different phases; called also *distribution c.* **phenol c.,** a measure of the bactericidal activity of a chemical compound in relation to phenol. The test and test microorganisms are standardized (Rideal-Walker method, U. S. Department of Agriculture method), and the activity of the unknown is expressed as the ratio of dilution in which it kills in 10 minutes but not in 5 minutes, to the dilution of phenol (ca. 1:90) which kills in 10 minutes but not in 5 minutes under the specified conditions. It can be determined in the absence of organic matter, or in the presence of a standard amount of added organic matter. **c. of relationship,** an expression of the probability that two persons have inherited a certain gene from a common ancestor; or the proportion of all their genes that have been inherited from common ancestors. **Rideal-Walker c.,** see *phenol c.* **sedimentation c.,** the rate in centimeters per second per unit centrifugal field at which a particle (e.g., protein) in solution travels in the analytical ultracentrifuge. A rate of 1×10^{-13} cm./second/unit centrifugal field is defined as one Svedberg unit (S). **selection c.,** a measure of the disadvantage in survival value of a given genotype as compared with that of a standard genotype in a population. **temperature c.,** a number indicating the effect of temperature upon the velocity constant of a chemical reaction. Cf. *van't Hoff's rule,* under *rule.* **c. of thermal conductivity,** a number indicating the quantity of heat that passes in a unit of time through a unit thickness of a substance when the difference in temperature is 1° C. **c. of thermal expansion,** the change in volume per unit volume of a substance produced by a 1° C. temperature increase. **Trapp's c.,** see under *formula.* **urohemolytic c.,** the smallest degree of dilution necessary to render a specimen of urine hemolytic. **urotoxic c.,** a number expressing the toxicity of the urine; it is the quantity of urotoxic units produced per unit weight and eliminated in unit time. Called also *Bouchard's c.* **c. of variability,** the ratio of the standard deviation to the mean. **velocity c.,** a number expressing the rate of a reaction; the rate of transformation of a unit mass of a substance in a chemical reaction. **c. of viscosity,** the force necessary to slide tangentially a unit of area of smooth surface at unit velocity on another parallel surface separated from the first surface by a unit layer of viscous substance. **volume c.,** the volume of packed red cells per 100 ml. of blood. **Yvon's c.,** the ratio between the quantity of urea and the phosphates of the urine.

coel- (sēl) [Gr. *koilia* cavity] a combining form denoting relationship to a cavity or space; sometimes spelled *cel-.*

coelarium (se-la′re-um) [L., from Gr. *koilos* a hollow] the membrane that lines the body cavity of the embryo, or coelom; it consists of a parietal layer, the *exocoelarium,* and a visceral layer, the *endocoelarium.* Called also *mesothelium.*

-coele (sēl) [Gr. *koilia* cavity] a word termination denoting relationship to a cavity or space; sometimes spelled *-cele* and *-coel.*

Coelenterata (se-len″ter-a′tah) [Gr. *koilos* hollow + *enteron* intestine] a phylum of invertebrates that includes the hydras, jellyfish, sea anemones, and corals; called also *Cnidaria.*

coelenterate (se-len′ter-āt) 1. pertaining or belonging to the Coelenterata. 2. an individual of the phylum Coelenterata.

coelenteron (se-len′ter-on) archenteron.

coeliac (se′le-ak) celiac.

coeloblastula (se″lo-blas′tu-lah) [*coelo-* + Gr. *blastos* germ] the common type of blastula, consisting of a hollow sphere composed of blastomeres.

coelom (se′lom) [Gr. *koilōma*] the body cavity. In the mammalian embryo, it is situated between the somatopleure and the splanchnopleure; it is both extraembryonic and intraembryonic. From the intraembryonic portion arise the principal cavities of the trunk. Also spelled *celom.* Called also *coeloma* and *somatic cavity.* **extraembryonic c.,** the portion of the coelom external to the embryo, bordered by chorionic mesoderm and the mesoderm of the amnion and yolk sac; it communicates temporarily at the umbilicus with the intraembryonic coelom. Called also *exocoelom.*

coeloma (se-lo′mah) coelom.

coelomate (sēl′o-māt) 1. having a coelom. 2. an individual of the Eucoelomata; eucoelomate.

coelomic (se-lom′ik) pertaining to the coelom.

coelomyarian (se″lo-mi-a′re-an) designating a type of nematode musculature in which the muscle fibers are next to the hypodermis and perpendicular to it; myofibrils extend varying distances up the side of the muscle cell, partially enclosing the sarcoplasm.

coelosomy (se″lo-so′me) a developmental anomaly characterized by protrusion of the viscera from their presence outside the body cavity.

coelothel (se′lo-thel) [Gr. *koilos* hollow + *thēlē* nipple] mesothelium.

coeno- see *ceno-.*

coenurosis (se″nu-ro′sis) gid.

Coenurus (se-nu′rus) [Gr. *koinos* common + *oura* tail] a genus of certain tapeworm larvae. **C. cerebra′lis,** the larva of the *Multiceps multiceps,* found in the brain of sheep, goats, and other ruminants, and rarely in man.

coenurus (se-nu′rus) the larval stage of tapeworms of the genus *Multiceps,* a semitransparent, fluid-filled, bladder-like organism that contains multiple scoleces attached to the inner surface of its wall and that do not form brood capsules. It develops in various parts of the host body, especially in the central nervous system. Cf. *cystercicus* and *hydatid cyst.*

coenzyme (ko-en′zim) 1. an organic, dialyzable, thermostable molecule, usually containing phosphorus and some vitamin, and sometimes separable from the enzyme protein. A coenzyme and an apoenzyme must unite in order to function (as a holoenzyme). Formerly called *coferment* and *cohydrogenase.* 2. the prosthetic group (see under *group*) of an enzyme. **c. A,** a coenzyme consisting of adenine, ribose, three phosphate groups, pantothenic acid, and mercaptoethylamine, which plays a central role in metabolism by catalyzing the transfer of acyl groups (acetylation); abbreviated CoA. See also *acetylcoenzyme A.* **c. I,** nicotinamide-adenine dinucleotide (NAD). **c. II,** nicotinamide-adenine dinucleotide phosphate (NADP). **c. Q,** any of a group of related quinones with isoprenoid units in the side chains (the ubiquinones), occurring in the lipid fraction of mitochondria and serving, along with the cytochromes, as an intermediate in electron transport. They are similar in structure and function to vitamin K_1. **c. R,** biotin. **Warburg's c.,** nicotinamide-adenine dinucleotide phosphate (NADP).

coenzymometer (ko″en-zi-mom′ĕ-ter) an instrument that measures light absorption to determine enzyme activity.

COEPS cortically originating extrapyramidal system: pathways from the cortex to the spinal cord, the major ones being the corticostriatal and corticopallidal, corticothalamic, corticoreticular, and corticopontine pathways.

coetaneous (ko″ĕ-ta′ne-us) [L. *co* with + *aetas* age] having the same age.

coeur (ker) [Fr.] heart. **c. en sabot** (ker-on-să-bo′), a heart visible radiographically as having an increased transverse diameter, a convexity in the inferior line, and an elevation and rounded shape of the apex, so that its form suggests vaguely that of a wooden shoe; noted in tetralogy of Fallot.

coexcitation (ko-ek-si-ta′shun) simultaneous excitation.

cofactor (ko′fak-tor) an element or principle, as a coenzyme, with which another must unite in order to function. **platelet c. I,** Factor VIII; see *coagulation factors,* under *factor.* **platelet c. II,** Factor IX; see *coagulation factors,* under *factor.*

coferment (co-fer′ment) coenzyme.

coffee (kof′e) [L. *coffea, caffea*] the dried seeds of *Coffea arabica* L. and *C. liberica* (Rubiaceae), trees believed to have originated in Africa, but now growing in nearly all tropical regions: a drink made by decoction or infusion of the dried and roasted ripe seeds is invigorating, tonic, and conservant; useful in chronic asthma, headache, and opium poisoning. The active principles include caffeine in seed, coffee oil, sugars, protein, and numerous volatile flavor oils.

coffeurin (kof-e-u′rin) a substance said to be present in the urine after the free use of coffee.

Coffey-Humber treatment [Walter B. *Coffey,* American surgeon, 1868–1944; John D. *Humber,* American surgeon, born 1895] see under *treatment.*

cogener (ko′jĕ-ner) congener.

Cogentin (ko-jen′tin) trademark for preparations of benztropine mesylate.

cognition (kog-nish′un) [L. *cognitio,* from *cognoscere* to know] that operation of the mind by which we become aware of objects of thought or perception; it includes all aspects of perceiving, thinking, and remembering.

cognitive (kog′nĭ-tiv) of, pertaining to, or characterized by cognition.

cohesion (ko-he′zhun) [L. *cohaesio,* from *con* together + *haerere* to stick] the force that causes various particles to unite.

cohesive (ko-he′siv) uniting together, or characterized by cohesion.

Cohn's solution (kōnz) [Ferdinand Julius *Cohn,* German bacteriologist, 1828–1898] see under *solution.*

Cohn's test (kōnz) [Hermann Ludwig *Cohn,* German oculist, 1838–1906] see under *tests.*

$C_4O_6H_4NaK$ potassium sodium tartrate.

Cohnheim's areas, etc. (kōn′hīmz) [Julius Friedrich *Cohnheim,* German pathologist, 1839–1884] see under *area, field, frog,* and *theory.*

cohoba (ko-ho′bah) parica.

cohobation (ko″ho-ba′shun) the repeated distilling of a liquid from the same material; redistillation.

cohort (ko′hort) 1. a group of individuals sharing a statistical characteristic (e.g., date of birth) who are used in epidemiologic or other statistical studies of disease. 2. a taxonomic category approximately equivalent to a division, order, or suborder in various systems of classification.

cohosh (ko-hosh′) a North American (Algonkin) name for various medicinal plants, as *Actaea spicata,* or red cohosh; *Caulophyllum thalictroides,* or blue cohosh; and *Cimicifuga racemosa,* or black cohosh.

cohydrogenase (ko″hi-dro′jen-ās) coenzyme.

CoI coenzyme I (nicotinamide-adenine dinucleotide).

CoII coenzyme II (nicotinamide-adenine dinucleotide phosphate).

coil (koil) anything wound in a spiral. **paranemic c.,** a coil formed between two or more chromonemal threads which has freely separable subunits. **plectonemic c.,** a coil formed between two or more chromonemal threads which has intertwined subunits. **relational c.,** the stretched subunits of the plectonemic coil. **standard (somatic) c.,** a helical structure similar to the major coil of meiotic chromosomes but found in mitotic chromosomes.

coino- see *ceno-.*

coinosite (koi′no-sīt) [Gr. *koinos* common + *sitos* food] a free or unfixed commensal organism; called also *cenosite.*

coisogeneic (ko-i″so-jĕ-na′ik) of or relating to strains of inbred animals that are genetically identical except for a difference at a single genetic locus.

coital (ko′ĭ-tal) pertaining to coitus.

coition (ko-ish′un) coitus.

coitophobia (ko″ĭ-to-fo′be-ah) [*coitus* + Gr. *phobein* to be affrighted by + *ia*] morbid dread of coitus.

coitus (ko′ĭ-tus) [L. *coitio* a coming together, meeting] sexual connection per vaginam between male and female. **c. incomple′tus, c. interrup′tus,** coitus in which the penis is withdrawn from the vagina before ejaculation; a widely used but unreliable method of contraception. **c. reserva′tus,** coitus in which ejaculation is intentionally suppressed. **c. à la vache,** coitus from behind, with the woman in the knee-chest position.

Coix (ko′iks) [L.; Gr. *koix* a palm] a genus of grasses. *C. lacryma,* an Asiatic species, bears large seeds called *Job's tears,* which have been strung as beads for infants' use in teething; said to be anodyne and diuretic.

Col. abbreviation for L. *co′la,* strain.

col (kol) a small depression in the interdental tissues just below the interproximal contact area, connecting the buccal and lingual papillae.

Colace (ko′lās) trademark for a preparation of docusate sodium.

colamine (ko′lah-min) monoethanolamine.

colaspase (ko-las′pās) asparaginase.

Colat. abbreviation for L. *cola′tus,* strained.

colation (ko-la′shun) [L. *colatio*] 1. the process of straining or filtration. 2. the product of such a process.

colatorium (kol″ah-to′re-um), pl. *colato′ria* [L., from *colare* to strain] a strainer or colander; a sieve.

colature (ko′lah-tūr) [L. *colatura,* from *colare* to strain] a liquid obtained by straining.

colauxe (ko-lawk′se) [Gr. *kolon* colon + *auxē* increase] (*obs.*) dilatation of the colon.

colchicine (kol′chĭ-sin) [USP] chemical name: (*S*)-*N*-(5,6,7,9-tetrahydro-1,2,3,10-tetramethoxy-9-oxobenzo[*a*]heptalen-7-yl) acetamide. An alkaloid, $C_{22}H_{25}NO_6$, obtained from various species of *Colchicum,* occurring as pale yellow amorphous scales or powder; used as a gout suppressant, usually administered orally.

Colchicum (kol′chĭ-kum) a genus of Old World liliaceous trees, the meadow saffron, from whose corm or dried ripe seed colchicine is obtained.

cold (kōld) 1. privation, or relatively low degree, of heat. 2. common cold; a catarrhal disorder of the upper respiratory tract, which may be viral, a mixed infection, or an allergic reaction. It is marked by acute coryza, slight rise in temperature, chilly sensations, and general indisposition. **allergic c.,** hay fever. **common c.,** see *cold,* def. 2. **June c.,** hay fever. **rose c.,** a form of seasonal hay fever caused by the pollen of roses.

coldsore (kōld′sōr) see *herpes simplex.*

cole- see *coleo-.*

Cole's sign (kōlz) [Lewis Gregory *Cole,* American roentgenologist, 1874–1954] see under *sign.*

Cole's test (kōlz) [Sidney William *Cole,* English physiologist, born 1877] see under *tests.*

colectasia (ko″lek-ta′se-ah) (*obs.*) dilatation of the colon.

colectomy (ko-lek′to-me) [*colon* + Gr. *ektomē* excision] excision of a portion of the colon (*partial c.*) or of the whole colon (*complete* or *total c.*).

coleitis (kol″e-i′tis) [*cole-* + *-itis*] (*obs.*) vaginitis.

Coleman-Shaffer diet [Warren *Coleman,* New York physician, 1869–1948; Philip Anderson *Shaffer,* American biochemist, born 1881] see under *diet.*

coleo-, cole- (kol′e-o, kol′e) [Gr. *koleos* sheath] a combining form denoting relationship to the vagina, or to a sheath.

coleocele (kol′e-o-sēl″) [*coleo-* + Gr. *kēlē* hernia] (*obs.*) vaginal hernia.

coleocystitis (kol″e-o-sis-ti′tis) [*coleo-* + *cystitis*] (*obs.*) inflammation of the vagina and bladder.

Coleomitus (ko″le-o-mi′tus) a genus of Schizomycetes of the order Caryophanales, family Arthromitaceae.

Coleoptera (kol″e-op′ter-ah) [*coleo-* + Gr. *pteron* wing] an order of insects comprising the beetles.

coles (ko′lēz) [Gr. *kōlē*] the penis. **c. femini′nus,** the clitoris.

Colesiota (ko-le″se-o′tah) [J. D. W. A. *Coles*] a genus (incertae sedis) of microorganisms, occurring as a single species, *C. conjuncti′vae,* the agent causing infectious ophthalmia of sheep.

colestipol (ko-les′tĭ-pōl) chemical name: tetraethylenepentamine polymer with 1-chloro-2,3-epoxypropane; an antilipemic agent.

Colet. abbreviation for L. *cole′tur,* let it be strained.

Colettsia (ko-let′se-ah) [J. D. W. A. *Coles*] a genus (incertae sedis) of microorganisms occurring as a single species, *C. pe′coris,* a parasitic microorganism found in the conjunctiva of domestic animals.

Coley's toxin (fluid) (ko′lēz) [William Bradley *Coley,* surgeon in New York, 1862–1936] see under *toxin.*

colibacillemia (ko″lĭ-bas-ĭ-le′me-ah) the presence of *Escherichia coli* in the blood.

colibacillosis (ko″lĭ-bas-ĭ-lo′sis) infection with *Escherichia coli.* **c. gravida′rum,** severe infection with *Escherichia coli* during pregnancy.

colibacilluria (ko″lĭ-bas″ĭ-lu′re-ah) presence of *Escherichia coli* in the urine; called also *Albarrán's disease.*

colibacillus (ko″lĭ-bah-sil′us) *Escherichia coli.*

colic (kol′ik) [Gr. *kōlikos*] 1. pertaining to the colon. 2. acute abdominal pain; characteristically, intermittent visceral pain with fluctuations corresponding to smooth muscle peristalsis. **appendicular c.,** vermicular c. **biliary c.,** paroxysms of pain and other severe symptoms due to the passage of gallstones along the bile duct; called also *gallstone* or *hepatic c.,* and *cholecystalgia.* **bilious c.,** abdominal pain accompanied by the vomiting of bile. **copper c.,** a severe colic due to copper poisoning. **Devonshire c.,** lead colic. **endemic c.,** a dangerous form of colic peculiar to hot countries. **flatulent c.,** tympanites. **gallstone c.,** biliary c. **gastric c.,** pain in the stomach. **hepatic c.,** biliary c. **infantile c.,** benign paroxysmal abdominal pain during the first three months of life. **intestinal c.,** colic originating from the small bowel, characteristically periumbilical in location. **lead c.,** colic due to lead poisoning. **meconial c.** (*obs.*), colic of newborn infants. **menstrual c.,** severe abdominal pain at the menstrual period; dysmenorrhea. **nephric c.,** renal c. **ovarian c.,** ovarian pain. **painters' c.,** lead c. **pancreatic c.,** abdominal pain caused by obstruction of the excretory duct of the pancreas. **Poitou c.,** lead c. **renal c.,** pain produced by thrombosis or dissection of the renal artery, renal infarction, intrarenal mass lesions, the passage of a stone within the collecting system, or thrombosis of the renal vein; called also *nephric c.* **salivary c.,** pain in the region of the salivary gland occurring in cases of salivary calculus. **sand c.,** chronic indigestion in horses and cattle due to the presence in the stomach or intestine of sand taken in with food or drink. **saturnine c.,** lead c. **stercoral c.,** intestinal colic due to accumulation of feces. **tubal c.,** painful spasmodic contraction of the fallopian tube. **ureteral c.,** colicky pains due to obstruction of the ureter. **uterine c.,** severe abdominal pain arising in the uterus, usually at the menstrual period. **vermicular c.,** a condition of colic in the vermiform appendix occasioned by a catarrhal inflammation resulting from blocking of the outlet of the appendix; called also *appendicular c.* **verminous c.,** colic due to the presence of intestinal worms; called also *worm c.* **wind c.,** pain in the bowels due to their distention with air or gas. **worm c.,** verminous c. **zinc c.,** colic resulting from chronic zinc poisoning.

colica (kol′ĭ-kah) [L.] colic. **c. muco′sa,** mucous colitis. **c. pic′tonum,** lead colic. **c. scorto′rum** (*obs.*), severe colicky pain in the region of the fallopian tubes; seen in salpingitis.

colicin (kol′ĭ-sin) [*coli* (from *Escherichia coli*) + *-cin* (adapted from L. *caedere* to kill)] a protein secreted by colicinogenic strains of *Escherichia coli* and lethal to other strains of the same species. Specific colicins attach to specific receptors on the cell membrane with resulting impairment of macromolecule synthesis or energy production.

colicinogen (kol″ĭ-sin′o-jen) an episome in some strains of *Escherichia coli* that induces secretion of the corresponding colicin. Some colicinogens also serve as sex factors. Called also *colicinogenic factor* (*Cf*).

colicinogenic (kol″ĭ-sin″o-jen′ik) elaborating colicin; said of strains of *Escherichia coli.*

colicinogeny (kol″ĭ-sin-oj′ĕ-ne) the production of colicin; see *colicinogen.*

colicky (kol′ik-e) pertaining to or affected by colic.

colicoplegia (kol″ĭ-ko-ple′je-ah) [Gr. *kōlikos* colic + *plēgē* stroke] lead colic and lead paralysis together.

colicystitis (ko″lĭ-sis-ti′tis) cystitis dependent upon the presence of *Escherichia coli.*

colicystopyelitis (ko-lĭ-sis″to-pi″e-li′tis) [*colon* + Gr. *kystis* bladder + *pyelos* pelvis] inflammation of the bladder and kidney pelvis due to *Escherichia coli.*

coliform (ko′lĭ-form) [L. *colum* a sieve] 1. a collective term denoting enteric, fermentative gram-negative rods, and sometimes restricted to the lactose-fermenting, gram-negative enteric bacilli, i.e., *Escherichia, Klebsiella, Enterobacter,* and *Citrobacter.* 2. any organism of that group.

colinearity (ko″lin-e-ar′ĭ-te) the correspondence between the linear sequence of the nucleotide codons, the RNA, and the linear sequence of amino acids in the polypeptide coded for by that sequence; a concept implicit in the original Watson-Crick model of the DNA structure.

colinephritis (ko″lĭ-ne-fri′tis) nephritis due to the presence of *Escherichia coli.*

coliphage (kol′ĭ-fāj) any bacteriophage that infects *Escherichia coli.*

coliplication (ko″lĭ-pli-ka′shun) coloplication.

colipuncture (kol′ĭ-punk″tūr) colocentesis.

colisepsis (ko″lĭ-sep′sis) infection with *Escherichia coli.*

colistimethate sodium (ko-lis″tĭ-meth′āt) chemical name: colistinmethanesulfonic acid pentasodium. The pentasodium salt of the methanesulfonate derivative of colistin, $C_{58}H_{105}N_{16}Na_5O_{28}$-$S_5$, occurring as a white to slightly yellow, fine powder, having actions and uses similar to those of the base (colistin); administered intramuscularly or intravenously.

colistin (ko-lis′tin) a polypeptide antibiotic of the polymyxin (q.v.) group, produced by the growth of the soil bacterium *Bacillus polymyxa* var. *colistinus,* specifically effective against many gram-negative bacteria, especially *Pseudomonas aeruginosa,* but also useful against others, including *Escherichia coli* and species of *Aerobacter, Klebsiella, Shigella,* and *Brucella; Proteus* species are resistant. **c. sulfate** [USP], the sulfate salt of colistin, occurring as a white to cream-colored, hygroscopic powder; used in the treatment of various systemic, urinary tract, gastrointestinal, ophthalmic, and otic infections due to susceptible gram-negative bacteria, administered orally, parenterally, and topically.

colitides (ko-lit′ĭ-dēz) plural of *colitis.* Inflammatory disorders of the colon considered collectively.

colitis (ko-li′tis) inflammation of the colon. **amebic c.,** colitis due to *Entamoeba histolytica;* amebic dysentery. **antibiotic-associated c.,** see under *enterocolitis.* **balantidial c.,** colitis due to infestation with *Balantidium coli.* **c. cys′tica profun′da,** a condition marked by mucous retention cysts in the colic submucosa that are characteristic of the healing of chronic lesions of bacillary dysentery. **c. cys′tica superficia′lis,** a cystic condition of the colic mucous membrane sometimes seen in children with such chronic debilitating disease as leukemia, possibly the result of malnutrition and vitamin deficiency. **granulomatous c.,** transmural colitis with the formation of noncaseating granulomas. **c. gra′vis,** ulcerative c. **ischemic c.,** acute vascular insufficiency of the colon usually involving the portion supplied by the inferior mesenteric artery; symptoms include pain at the left iliac fossa, bloody diarrhea, low-grade fever, abdominal distention, and abdominal tenderness. The classic radiologic sign is thumbprinting due to localized elevation of the mucosa by submucosal hemorrhage or edema. Ulceration may follow. **mucous c.,** a chronic noninflammatory disease characterized by excessive secretion of mucus and disordered colonic motility with consequent colic, constipation, and/or diarrhea with the passage of mucus; it is a common disorder with a psychophysiologic basis. Called also *spastic* or *irritable colon,* and *irritable bowel* (or *colon*) *syndrome.* The term mucous colitis is sometimes restricted to cases in which diarrhea with considerable mucus is the major manifestation. **myxomembranous c.,** mucous c. **c. polypo′sa,** ulcerative colitis associated with the formation of pseudopolyps (edematous, inflamed islands of mucosa between areas of ulceration). **pseudomembranous c.,** see under *enterocolitis.* **regional c., segmental c.,** transmural or granulomatous inflammatory disease of the colon; regional enteritis involving the colon. It may be associated with ulceration, strictures, or fistulas. **transmural c.,** inflammation of the full thickness of the bowel, rather than mucosal and submucosal disease, usually with the formation of noncaseating granulomas. It may be confined to the colon, segmentally or diffusely, or may be associated with small bowel disease (regional enteritis). Clinically, it may resemble ulcerative colitis, but the ulceration is often longitudinal or deep, the disease is often segmental, stricture formation is common, and fistulas, particularly in the perineum, are a frequent complication. **c.**

ulcerati′va, ulcerative c., chronic, recurrent ulceration in the colon, chiefly of the mucosa and submucosa, of unknown cause; it is manifested clinically by cramping abdominal pain, rectal bleeding, and loose discharges of blood, pus, and mucus with scanty fecal particles. Complications include hemorrhoids, abscesses, fistulas, perforation of the colon, pseudopolyps and carcinoma.

colitose (kol′ĭ-tōs) an unusual sugar found to be a polysaccharide somatic antigen of *Salmonella* species.

colitoxemia (ko″lĭ-tok-se′me-ah) toxemia due to infection with *Escherichia coli.*

colitoxicosis (ko″lĭ-tok″sĭ-ko′sis) intoxication caused by *Escherichia coli.*

colitoxin (ko″lĭ-tok′sin) a substance contained in *Escherichia coli* that is the cause of colitoxicosis.

coliuria (ko″lĭ-u′re-ah) presence of *Escherichia coli* in the urine.

colla (kol′lah) [L.] plural of *collum.*

collacin (kol′ĭ-sin) degenerated collagenous tissue; collastin.

collagen (kol′ah-jen) [Gr. *kolla* glue + *gennan* to produce] the protein substance of the white fibers (collagenous fibers) of skin, tendon, bone, cartilage, and all other connective tissue; composed of molecules of tropocollagen (q.v.), it is converted into gelatin by boiling. See also under *disease.* **fibrous long-spacing (FLS) c.,** a form of collagen having a periodicity of about 240 nm. instead of the 64 nm. characteristic of the native fibers; found in the trabecular network of the eye and in aging collagen. **segment long-spacing (SLS) c.,** collagen occurring in segments about 240 nm. long instead of in fibers.

collagenase (kol-laj′ĕ-nās) an enzyme that catalyzes the degradation of collagen.

collagenation (kol-laj″ĕ-na′shun) the appearance of collagen in developing cartilage.

collagenic (kol″ah-jen′ik) 1. collagenous. 2. collagenogenic.

collagenitis (ko-laj′ĕ-ni′tis) inflammatory involvement of collagen fibers in the fiber component of connective tissue, characterized by pain, swelling, low-grade fever, and by increased erythrocyte sedimentation rate.

collagenoblast (kol-laj′ĕ-no-blast) a cell which arises from a fibroblast and which, as it matures, is associated with the production of collagen; it may also, at times, form cartilage and bone by metaplasia.

collagenocyte (kol-laj′ĕ-no-sīt″) a mature collagen-producing cell; see *collagenoblast.*

collagenogenic (kol″lah-jen-o-jen′ik) pertaining to or characterized by the production of collagen; forming collagen or collagen fibers.

collagenolysis (kol″ah-jen-ol′ĭ-sis) dissolution or digestion of collagen.

collagenolytic (kol-laj″ĕ-no-lit′ik) effecting the digestion of collagen.

collagenosis (kol-laj″ĕ-no′sis) collagen disease; see under *disease.*

collagenous (kol-laj′ĕ-nus) pertaining to collagen; forming or producing collagen.

collapse (kŏ-laps′) [L. *collapsus*] 1. a state of extreme prostration and depression, with failure of circulation. 2. abnormal falling in of the walls of any part or organ. **circulatory c.,** shock; circulatory insufficiency without congestive heart failure. **c. of the lung,** an airless or fetal state of all or a part of a lung, as seen in atelectasis from bronchial obstruction and in pneumothorax. **massive c.,** a condition in which an entire lung becomes airless, often due to obstruction of a main bronchus.

collar (kol′ler) an encircling band, generally around the neck. **Biett's c.,** a ring of epidermis around a papulolenticular syphilid. **Casal's c.,** see under *necklace.* **c. of pearls,** syphilitic leukoderma about the neck. **periosteal bone c.,** a band of spongy bone that forms around the middle of the diaphysis of early bones. **Spanish c.,** paraphimosis. **c. of Stokes,** an edematous thickening of the neck and soft parts of the thorax associated with dilatation of the veins from the neck to the diaphragm, seen in cases of obstruction of the superior vena cava. **venereal c., c. of Venus,** syphilitic leukoderma about the neck.

collarette (kol″er-et′) 1. a narrow rim of loosened keratin overhanging the periphery of a circumscribed skin lesion, attached to the normal surrounding skin, especially in miliaitasis and pityriasis rosea. 2. (*obs.*) collar-like dermatitis in pellagra. 3. ciliary zone. **c. of Biet,** the ring of scales that develops around the macular lesions of secondary syphilis.

collastin (kŏ-las′tin) degenerate collagenous tissue that stains like normal elastic tissue.

collateral (kŏ-lat′er-al) [L. *con* together + *la′tus* side] 1. secondary or accessory; not direct or immediate. 2. a small side branch, as of a blood vessel or nerve.

collenchyma (ko-leng′kĭ-mah) [Gr. *kolla* glue + *enchyma* infusion] supportive tissue occurring just beneath the epidermis of stems and leaf stalks of plants, composed of elongated living cells with walls thickened in the corner. Cf. *sclerenchyma*.

Colles' fascia, ligament, etc. (kol′ēz) [Abraham *Colles,* an Irish surgeon, 1773–1843] see *fascia diaphragmatis urogenitalis inferior* and *ligamentum inguinale reflexum,* and see under *fracture, law,* and *space.*

Colles-Baumès law (kol′ēz-bo-māz′) [Abraham *Colles;* Pierre Prosper François *Baumès,* French physician, 1791–1871] see *Colles' law,* under *law.*

Collet's syndrome (kol-lāz′) [Frédéric Justin *Collet,* Lyons laryngologist, born 1870] see under *syndrome.*

Collet-Sicard syndrome (kol-la′-se-kar′) [Frédéric Justin *Collet;* Jean Athanase *Sicard,* Paris neurologist, 1872–1929] Collet's syndrome.

colliculectomy (kŏ-lik″u-lek′to-me) [*colliculus* + Gr. *ektomē* excision] excision of the colliculus seminalis.

colliculi (kŏ-lik′u-li) plural of *colliculus.*

colliculitis (kŏ-lik″u-li′tis) inflammation about the colliculus seminalis.

colliculus (kŏ-lik′u-lus), pl. *collic′uli* [L.] a small elevation, or mound. **c. of arytenoid cartilage,** c. cartilaginis arytenoideae. **bulbar c.,** corpus spongiosum penis. **c. cartilag′-inis arytenoi′deae** [NA], colliculus of arytenoid cartilage: a small eminence on the anterior margin and anterolateral surface of the arytenoid cartilage; called also *c. cartilaginis arytaenoideae.* **c. cauda′lis** (*obs.*), c. inferior. **c. cauda′tus,** nucleus caudatus. **cervical c. of female urethra, of Barkow,** crista urethralis femininae. **c. crania′lis** (*obs.*), c. superior. **facial c., c. facia′lis** [NA], an elevation of the medial eminence above the medullary striae in the rhomboid fossa, caused by the internal genu of the facial nerve as it loops backward around the abducent nucleus. **inferior c., c. infe′rior lam′inae quadrigem′inae, c. infe′rior lam′inae tec′ti** [NA], the caudal of the two pairs of rounded eminences in the tectum of the mesencephalon; it is primarily concerned with auditory reflexes. Called also *inferior c.* and *c. inferior laminae quadrigeminae.* **seminal c., c. semina′lis** [NA], a prominent portion of the urethral crest on which are the opening of the prostatic utricle and, on either side of it, the orifices of the ejaculatory ducts; called also *caput gallinaginis, seminal crest,* and *seminal hillock.* **superior c., c. supe′rior lam′inae quadrigem′inae, c. supe′rior lam′inae tec′ti** [NA], the rostral of the two pairs of rounded eminences in the tectum of the mesencephalon; it is primarily concerned with visual reflexes.

collifixation (kol″ĭ-fik-sa′shun) collopexia.

colligation (kol″ĭ-ga′shun) 1. a form of mental composition in which the units maintain their own distinction. 2. the bringing together of isolated elements in a composite experience.

colligative (kol′ĭ-ga″tiv) in physical chemistry, depending on the number of molecules present in a given space, rather than on their size, molecular weight or chemical constitution.

collimation (kol″lĭ-ma′shun) a making parallel. In microscopy, the process of making light rays parallel; the process of aligning the optical axis of the optical system to the reference mechanical axes or surfaces of the instrument, or the adjustment of two or more optical axes with respect to each other. In radiology, the elimination of the peripheral (more divergent) portion of an x-ray beam by means of metal tubes, cones, or diaphragms interposed in the path of the beam.

collimator (kol′ĭ-ma″tor) a diaphragm or system of diaphragms made of an absorbing material, designed to define the dimensions and direction of a beam of radiation.

Collin's osteoclast (kol′inz) [Anatole *Collin,* Parisian instrument maker, 1831–1923] see under *osteoclast.*

Collinsonia (kol″in-so′ne-ah) [after Peter *Collinson,* 1694–1768] a genus of labiate herbs. C. *canadensis,* stoneroot or richweed, is tonic and diuretic.

Collip unit (kol′ip) [James Bertram *Collip,* Canadian biochemist, born 1892] see under *unit.*

colliquation (kol″lĭ-kwa′shun) [L. *con* together + *liquare* to melt] liquefactive degeneration of tissue. **ballooning c.,** liquefaction of cell protoplasm attended by edematous swelling. **reticulating c.,** liquefaction of cell protoplasm with the formation of reticulations.

colliquative (kŏ-lik′wah-tiv) [L. *con* together + *liquare* to melt] 1. characterized by an excessive fluid discharge. 2. marked by liquefaction of tissues.

collision (ko-lĭ′zhun) in obstetrics, the contact *in utero* of any parts of one twin with those of the co-twin, so that engagement of either is prevented.

collochemistry (kol″o-kem′is-tre) the chemistry of colloids.

collodiaphyseal (kol″o-di″ah-fiz′e-al) [L. *collum* neck + *diaphysis*] pertaining to the neck and shaft of a long bone, especially the femur.

collodion (ko-lo′de-on) [L. *collodium,* from Gr. *kollōdēs* glutinous] [USP] a clear or slightly opalescent, highly flammable, syrupy liquid compounded of pyroxylin, ether, and alcohol, which dries to a transparent, tenacious film; used as a topical protectant, applied

to the skin to close small wounds, abrasions, and cuts, to hold surgical dressings in place, and to keep medications in contact with the skin. **c. elastique,** flexible c. **flexible c.** [USP], a preparation of camphor, castor oil, and collodion, used for the same purposes as collodion but providing a flexible, contracting film. Called also *c. elastique.* **salicylic acid c.** [USP], a preparation containing between 9.5 and 11.5 per cent salicylic acid in flexible collodion; used as a topical keratolytic for warts and corns.

colloid (kol′oid) [Gr. *kollōdēs* glutinous] 1. glutinous or resembling glue. 2. a state of matter in which the matter is dispersed in or distributed throughout some medium called the dispersion medium. The matter thus dispersed is called the disperse phase of the colloid system. The particles of the disperse phase are larger than an ordinary crystalloid molecule, but are not large enough to settle out under the influence of gravity; and they resist diffusion; they range in size from 1 to 100 nm. or up to 500 or 1000 nm., the range being indefinite and arbitrary. There are two kinds of colloids: *suspension colloids* (suspensoids), in which the disperse phase consists of particles of any insoluble substance, as a metal, and the dispersion medium may be gaseous, liquid, or solid; and *emulsion colloids* (emulsoids), in which the dispersion medium is usually water and the disperse phase consists of highly complex organic substances, such as starch or glue, which absorb much water, swell, and become uniformly distributed throughout the dispersion medium in a manner not well understood. The former tend to be less stable than the latter. Cf. *crystalloid.* 3. the translucent, yellowish, gelatinous substance resulting from colloid degeneration. **amyl c., anodyne c.,** a local anodyne preparation containing ½ ounce each of amyl hydride and absolute alcohol, 1 grain aconitine, 6 grains veratrine, and 2 oz. of collodion. **antimony trisulfide c.,** antimony sulfide (Sb₂S₃), a pharmaceutic aid. **association c.,** a colloid in which the dispersed particles are each made up of many molecules. **bovine c.,** conglutinin. **dispersion c.,** see *colloid,* def. 2. **emulsion c.,** see *colloid,* def. 2. **hydrophilic c.,** emulsion c.; see *colloid,* def. 2. **hydrophobic c.,** suspension c.; see *colloid,* def. 2. **irreversible c.,** a colloid that cannot be dispersed. Cf. *reversible c.* **lyophilic c.,** emulsion c.; see *colloid,* def. 2. **lyophobic c.,** suspension c.; see *colloid,* def. 2. **lyotropic c.,** emulsion c.; see *colloid,* def. 2. **protective c.,** one that is able to prevent the precipitation of another colloid. **reversible c.,** a colloid that can be dispersed after having been precipitated or a gel that can be converted into a sol. **stable c.,** reversible c. **stannous sulfur c.,** a sulfur colloid containing stannous ions formed by reacting sodium thiosulfate with hydrochloric acid, then adding stannous ions; a diagnostic aid (bone, liver, and spleen imaging). **suspension c.,** see *colloid,* 2nd def. **thyroid c.,** the colloid found in the acini of the thyroid gland, consisting essentially of thyroglobulin.

colloidal (kŏ-loi′dal) of the nature of a colloid. **c-S,** an iron-oxide preparation used intravenously in severe infections.

colloidin (ko-loi′din) a jelly-like substance, C₉H₁₅NO₆, one of the products of colloid degeneration.

colloidoclasia (ko-loi″do-kla′se-ah) [*colloid* + Gr. *klasis* breaking up] a breaking up of the physical equilibrium of the colloids of the body, producing anaphylactic shock attributed to absorption into the blood of unchanged colloids; called also *colloidoclastic crisis.*

colloidoclasis (kŏ-loi″do-kla′sis) colloidoclasia.

colloidophagy (kol″oi-dof′ah-je) [*colloid* + Gr. *phagein* to eat] resorption of colloid by macrophages under the influence of the thyroid-stimulating hormone.

colloma (kŏ-lo′mah) [Gr. *kolla* glue + *-oma*] (*obs.*) mucinous carcinoma.

collonema (kol″o-ne′mah) [Gr. *kolla* glue] (*obs.*) see *mucinous carcinoma,* under *carcinoma.*

collopexia (kol″o-pek′se-ah) [L. *collum* neck + Gr. *pēxis* fixing.] (*obs.*) the surgical fixation of the uterine neck.

colloxylin (kŏ-lok′sĭ-lin) [Gr. *kolla* glue + *xylinos* woody] pyroxylin.

collum (kol′lum), pl. *col′la* [L.] [NA] 1. the neck: the portion of the body connecting the head and trunk; the lower front portion of the collum is called the cervix, and the back is called the nucha. 2. a general term applied to any necklike part of a body structure or organ. **c. anatom′icum hu′meri** [NA], anatomical neck of humerus: the somewhat constricted zone on the humerus just distal to the head, separating the articular surface from the tubercles. **c. chirur′gicum hu′meri** [NA], surgical neck of humerus: the region on the humerus just below the tubercles, where the bone becomes constricted. **c. cos′tae** [NA], neck of rib: the part of a rib extending from the head to the tubercle. **c. den′tis** [NA], the slightly constricted region of union of the crown and the root or roots of a tooth; called also *neck of tooth, cervix dentis,* and *dental neck.* **c. distor′tum,** torticollis. **c. fem′oris** [NA], neck of femur: the heavy column of bone connecting the head of the femur and the shaft. **c. follic′uli pi′li,** the narrow portion of a hair follicle between the hair bulb and the opening on the surface of the skin. **c. glan′dis pe′nis** [NA], neck of the glans penis: the constricted portion between the corona of the glans penis and the corpora cavernosa;

called also *cervix glandis*. **c. mal′lei** [NA], neck of malleus: the constricted portion of the malleus below the head; called also *cervix mallei*. **c. mandib′ulae** [NA], neck of mandible: the narrow portion supporting the condyle of the mandible; called also *c. processus condyloidei mandibulae*. **c. proces′sus condyloi′dei mandib′ulae,** c. mandibulae. **c. ra′dii** [NA], neck of radius: the somewhat constricted portion of the radius just distal to the head. **c. scap′ulae** [NA], neck of scapula: the somewhat constricted part of the scapula that surrounds the lateral angle. **c. ta′li** [NA], neck of talus: the constriction between the head and body of the talus. **c. val′gum,** coxa valga. **c. vesi′cae fel′leae** [NA], neck of gallbladder: the upper, constricted part of the gallbladder, between the body and the cystic duct.

collunaria (kol″u-na′re-ah) plural of *collunarium*.

collunarium (kol″u-na′re-um), pl. *colluna′ria* [L.] a nasal douche.

Collut. abbreviation for L. *collutorium* (mouth wash).

collutoria (kol″u-to′re-ah) [L.] plural of *collutorium*.

collutorium (kol″u-to′re-um), pl. *colluto′ria* [L.] collutory.

collutory (kol′u-to″re) [L. *colluto·ium*] a mouthwash or gargle. **Miller's c.,** a mouth wash containing benzoic acid, tincture of krameria, oil of peppermint.

Collyr abbreviation for L. *collyr′ium,* an eye wash.

collyria (ko-lir′e-ah) [L.] plural of *collyrium*.

Collyriculum (kol″le-rik′u-lum) a genus of trematode parasites. **c. fa′ba,** a trematode parasite forming subcutaneous cysts in chickens, turkeys, and sparrows.

collyrium (kŏ-lir′e-um), pl. *collyr′ia* [L.; Gr. *kollyrion* eye salve] a lotion for the eyes; an eye wash. **Beer's c.,** lead acetate, rose water, and spirit of rosemary.

coloboma (kol″o-bo′mah), pl. *colobomas* or *colobo′mata* [L.; Gr. *kolobōma*] an apparent absence or defect of some ocular tissue, usually resulting from a failure of a part of the fetal fissure to close. **atypical c's,** those involving areas of the eye which do

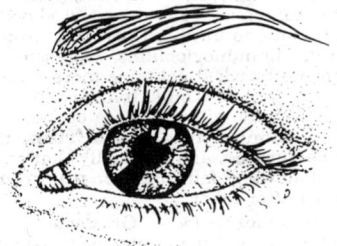

Coloboma of the iris.

not originate from the embryonic cleft. **bridge c.,** a variety of coloboma of the iris in which a strip of iris tissue bridges over the fissure. **c. of choroid,** fissure in the choroid coat due to persistence of a fetal fissure and causing a scotoma on the retina. **Fuchs's c.,** a small, crescent-shaped defect of the choroid, at the lower edge of the optic disk. **c. i′ridis, c. of iris,** a fissure of the iris, usually of the lower portion. **c. len′tis,** a defect in the lens of the eye in which the periphery is incomplete or indented. **c. lob′uli,** fissure of the ear lobe, which may occur as a congenital defect, or be acquired. **c. of optic nerve,** a defect attributed to the incomplete closure of the fetal fissure of the optic stalk. **c. palpebra′le,** a vertical fissure of an eyelid. **c. of retina, c. ret′inae,** a congenital fissure of the retina attributed to incomplete closure of the fetal fissure in the optic cup. **typical c's,** those that arise from faulty closure of the fetal fissure. **c. of vitreous,** a notch in the lower border of the vitreous.

colocecostomy (ko″lo-se-kos′to-me) [*colon* + *cecum* + Gr. *stomoun* to provide with an opening, or mouth] cecocolostomy.

colocentesis (ko″lo-sen-te′sis) [*colon* + Gr. *kentēsis* puncture] surgical puncture of the colon for the withdrawal of fluid or gas; called also *colopuncture*.

colocholecystostomy (ko″lo-ko″le-sis-tos′to-me) cholecystocolostomy.

coloclysis (ko″lo-kli′sis) [*colon* + Gr. *klysis* a drenching] irrigation of the colon.

coloclyster (ko″lo-klis′ter) an enema injected into the colon through the rectum.

colocolostomy (ko″lo-ko-los′to-me) [*colon* + *colostomy*] surgical formation of an anastomosis between two portions of the colon.

colocutaneous (ko″lo-ku-ta′ne-us) pertaining to the colon and skin, or communicating with the colon and the cutaneous surface of the body, as colocutaneous fistula.

colocynth (kol′o-sinth) [L. *colocynthis;* Gr. *kolokynthē*] the dried pulp of the unripe but full-grown fruit of *Citrullus colocynthus;* used as a drastic cathartic. Called also *bitter apple* and *bitter cucumber*.

colocynthidism (kol″o-sin′thĭ-dizm) poisoning by colocynth.

colocynthin (kol″o-sin′thin) a bitter, purgative glycoside, $C_{38}H_{54}O_{13}$, from colocynth.

colocynthis (kol″o-sin′this), gen. *colocyn′thidis* [L.] colocynth.

colodyspepsia (ko″lo-dis-pep′se-ah) dyspepsia due to reflex disturbance set up by the constipated colon.

coloenteritis (ko″lo-en″ter-i′tis) [*colon* + *enteritis*] enterocolitis.

colofixation (ko″lo-fik-sa′shun) the fixation or suspension of the colon in cases of ptosis.

Cologel (kol′o-jel) trademark for a preparation of methylcellulose.

colohepatopexy (ko″lo-hep′ah-to-pek″se) [*colon* + Gr. *hēpar* liver + *pēxis* fixation] fixation of the colon to the liver to prevent the formation of adhesions between the liver and the stomach, which occasionally occurs after removal of the gallbladder.

coloileal (ko″lo-il′e-al) ileocolic.

cololysis (ko-lol′ĭ-sis) [*colon* + Gr. *lysis* dissolution] the division of pericolic adhesions.

colometrometer (ko″lo-mĕ-trom′ĕ-ter) an apparatus for measuring the activity of the colon.

colon (ko′lon) [L.; Gr. *kolon*] [NA] that part of the large intestine which extends from the cecum to the rectum; sometimes used inaccurately as a synonym for the entire large intestine. **c. ascen′dens** [NA], **ascending c.,** the portion of the colon between the cecum and the right colic flexure. **c. descen′dens** [NA], **descending c.,** the portion of the colon between the left collic flexure and the sigmoid colon at the pelvic brim; the portion of the descending colon lying in the left iliac fossa is sometimes called the *iliac colon*. **giant c.,** megacolon. **iliac c.,** that part of the descending colon lying in the left iliac fossa and continuous with the sigmoid colon. **irritable c.,** see *mucous colitis,* under *colitis*. **lead-pipe c.,** a term applied to the radiological appearance of a diseased colon which has become shortened, contracted, and rigid owing to inflammatory fibrosis. In such a colon the normal haustral pattern is lost and function may be impaired. This is usually a consequence of chronic ulcerative or granulomatous colitis. **left c.,** the distal portion of the large intestine, developing embryonically from the hind gut and functioning in the storage and elimination from the body of nonabsorbed residue. **pelvic c.,** sigmoid c. **right c.,** the proximal portion of the large intestine, extending from the ileocecal valve usually to a point proximal to the left colic flexure, developing embryonically from the terminal portion of the midgut and functioning in absorption. **sigmoid c., c. sigmoi′deum** [NA], the S-shaped part of the colon which lies in the pelvis, extending from the pelvic brim to the third segment of the sacrum, and continuous above with the descending (or iliac) colon and below with the rectum; called also *pelvic c.* and *sigmoid flexure*. **spastic c.,** see *mucous colitis,* under *colitis*. **transverse c., c. transver′sum** [NA], the portion of the colon that runs transversely across the upper part of the abdomen, from the right to the left colic flexure.

colonalgia (ko″lon-al′je-ah) [*colon* + *-algia*] pain in the colon.

colonic (ko-lon′ik) pertaining to the colon.

colonitis (ko″lo-ni′tis) colitis.

colonization (ko″lŏ-nĭ-za′shun) innidiation.

Colonna's operation (kŏ-lōn′ah) [Paul *Colonna,* American orthopedic surgeon, 1892–1966] see under *operation*.

colonopathy (ko″lo-nop′ah-the) [*colon* + Gr. *pathos* disease.] any disease or disorder of the colon.

colonorrhagia (ko″lon-o-ra′je-ah) hemorrhage from the colon.

colonorrhea (ko″lon-o-re′ah) [*colon* + Gr. *rhoia* flow] mucous colitis.

colonoscope (ko-lon′o-skōp) [*colon* + Gr. *skopein* to examine] an elongated flexible endoscope which permits visual examination of the entire colon; called also *coloscope*.

colonoscopy (ko″lon-os′ko-pe) 1. endoscopic examination of the colon during laparotomy by insertion of a sigmoidoscope proximally and distally through a colotomy. 2. examination by means of the colonoscope. Called also *coloscopy*.

colony (kol′o-ne) [L. *colonia*] a collection or group of bacteria in a culture derived from the increase of an isolated single organism or group of organisms. **bitten c.,** a colony from the edge of which a portion has been removed as though bitten out, but has really been lysed out by the action of bacteriophage; called also *nibbled c.* **butyrous c.,** a colony of butter-like consistency. **D. c.,** dwarf c. **daughter c.,** a small bacterial colony formed as a papilla on the surface or in the margin of a normal colony. **disgonic c.,** a bacterial colony that grows feebly and slowly. **dwarf c.,** a bacterial colony smaller than normal and containing poorly developed forms; called also *D. colony*. **effuse c.,** one that is very thin and flat. **H c.** (Ger. *Hauch* film), a type of bacterial colony that spreads in a thin film over the culture medium. **M. c.,** mucoid c. **matte c.** (Ger. "mat"), a variant of the R. colony in β-hemolytic streptococci, indicating virulence. **mucoid c.,** a colony that is large, dome-shaped, and shiny, and may be drawn out in viscid strings by a needle; called also *M. colony.* **nibbled c.,** bitten c. **O c.** (Ger. *ohne Hauch* without film), a bacterial colony that is compact as contrasted with an H colony. **R. c., rough c.,** a bacterial colony showing a rough, wrinkled, granular, flattened surface; known as R-type. **S. c., smooth c.,** a bacterial colony showing the smooth, glistening, rounded, regular surface, normally shown by colonies of organisms; known as S-type. **satellite c.,** a bacterial colony that grows more vigorously in the immediate vicinity of a colony of some other organism, as *Hemophilus influenzae* near a colony of staphylococci; called also *bacterial satellite.*

colopathy (ko-lop'ah-the) colonopathy.

colopexia (ko''lo-pek'se-ah) colopexy.

colopexotomy (ko''lo-pek-sot'o-me) [*colon* + Gr. *pēxis* fixation + *tomē* a cutting] incision and fixation of the colon.

colopexy (ko'lo-pek''se) [*colon* + Gr. *pēxis* fixation] fixation or suspension of the colon by surgical means.

colophony (ko-lof'o-ne) [L. *colophonia;* Gr. *Kolophōn* (Colophon) a city of Asia Minor] former name of rosin.

coloplication (ko''lo-pli-ka'shun) [*colon* + L. *plica* fold] the operation of infolding or taking tucks in the wall of the colon in cases of dilatation to shorten or decrease its lumen.

coloproctectomy (ko''lo-prok-tek'to-me) surgical removal of the colon and rectum.

coloproctitis (ko''lo-prok-ti'tis) inflammation of the colon and rectum.

coloproctostomy (ko''lo-prok-tos'to-me) [*colon* + Gr. *prōktos* anus + *stomoun* to provide with an opening, or mouth] colorectostomy.

coloptosis (ko''lop-to'sis) [*colon* + Gr. *ptōsis* fall] downward displacement of the colon, a term based on the outmoded concept that variations in the position of abdominal organs are pathological.

colopuncture (ko'lo-punk''tūr) colocentesis.

Color. abbreviation for L. *colore'tur,* let it be colored.

color (kul'or) [L. *color, colos*] 1. a property of a surface or substance resulting from absorption of certain of the incident light rays and reflection of others falling within the range of wavelengths (roughly 370–760 mμ) adequate to excite the retinal receptors. 2. radiant energy within the range of adequate chromatic stimuli of the retina, that is, between the infrared and ultraviolet. 3. a sensory impression of one of the rainbow hues, excited by stimulation of the retinal receptors, notably the cones, by radiant energy of the appropriate wavelength. **complementary c's,** a pair of colors the sensory mechanisms for which are so linked that when they are mixed on the color wheel they cancel each other out, leaving neutral gray; complementary colors are also associated with each other in after-image and contrast. **confusion c's,** different colors that are likely to be mistakenly matched by individuals with defective color vision (e.g., violet and blue with defect of vision for red); for this reason they are combined in the design on charts used for detecting different types of color vision defects. **contrast c.,** an illusory tinge of complementary hue or brightness induced by a vivid hue or luminance on the area surrounding it in the visual field. **incidental c.,** that seen as an after-image. **metameric c's,** colors that appear identical to the normal eye, but which are the resultants of different combinations of chromatic stimuli or wavelengths. **Munsell's c's,** a set of standardized colors, representing 40 hues in varying degrees of brightness and saturation, identifiable by a simple letter-number formula. **primary c's,** a small number of fundamental colors, usually referred to the retinal receptor cones, mixture of varying proportions of the approximate stimuli of which will yield the 150 discriminable hues of normal human vision. According to (*a*) the Newton theory, the seven rainbow hues: violet, indigo, blue, green, yellow, orange, red; (*b*) the painter and printer: blue (cyan), yellow, red (or magenta); (*c*) the Helmholtzian theory (old school): red, green, blue (or violet); (*d*) the Hering theory: four paired complementary hues, red-green and blue-yellow, plus a black-white pair. (*e*) *Other theories list five to seven colors as primaries.* **pseudoisochromatic c's,** colors that appear the same to an individual with defective color vision; see *confusion c's.* **pure c.,** a color whose stimulus consists of homogeneous wavelengths, with little or no admixture of other hues. **saturation c.,** one that is high on the chroma or vividness scale, the farthest possible removed from gray.

coloration (kul''er-a'shun) the state of being colored; an arrangement of colors distinguishing a species. **protective c.,** coloration that blends with the background, making the organism less visible to predators. **warning c.,** brilliant, conspicuous coloration of poisonous or unpalatable animals, as a warning to potential predators.

colorectal (kol''o-rek'tal) pertaining to or affecting the colon and rectum.

colorectitis (ko''lo-rek-ti'tis) coloproctitis.

colorectostomy (ko''lo-rek-tos'to-me) [*colon* + *rectum* + Gr. *stomoun* to provide with an opening, or mouth] formation of an artificial opening between the colon and rectum; called also *coloproctostomy.*

colorectum (kol''o-rek'tum) the colon and rectum considered as a unit.

colorimeter (kul''or-im'ĕ-ter) [*color* + Gr. *metron* measure] an instrument for measuring color differences; especially one for measuring the color of the blood in order to determine the proportion of hemoglobin. Called also *chromometer.* **Duboscq's c.,** an apparatus for measuring concentration by comparing the tint of the substance in question against that of a standard. **titration c.,** a device using colorimetric technique to automatically stop titration at the end point.

colorrhaphy (ko-lor'ah-fe) [*colon* + Gr. *rhaphē* suture] suture or repair of the colon.

colorrhea (ko''lo-re'ah) a discharge of mucus from the colon.

coloscope (kol'o-skōp) colonoscope.

coloscopy (ko-los'ko-pe) colonoscopy.

colosigmoidostomy (ko''lo-sig''moi-dos'to-me) surgical creation of an artificial opening between the sigmoid and the proximal portion of the colon.

colostomy (ko-los'to-me) [*colon* + Gr. *stomoun* to provide with an opening, or mouth] the surgical creation of an opening between the colon and the surface of the body; also used to refer to the opening, or stoma, so created. **dry c.,** colostomy performed in the left half of the colon, the discharge from the stoma consisting of soft or formed fecal residue with no urine. **Hartmann's c.,** see under *procedure.* **ileotransverse c.,** surgical anastomosis between the ileum and the transverse colon. **wet c.,** colostomy in (*a*) the right half of the colon, the drainage from which is liquid in character, or (*b*) the left half of the colon following anastomosis of the ureters to the sigmoid or descending colon so that urine is also expelled through the same stoma.

colostric (ko-los'trik) pertaining to or occurring in colostrum.

colostrorrhea (ko-los''tro-re'ah) [L. *colostrum* + Gr. *rhoia* flow] spontaneous discharge of colostrum.

colostrous (ko-los'trus) [L. *colostrosus*] containing or filled with colostrum.

colostrum (kŏ-los'trum) [L.] the thin, yellow, milky fluid secreted by the mammary gland a few days before or after parturition. It contains up to 20 per cent protein, predominant among which are immunoglobulins, representing the antibodies found in maternal blood. It contains more minerals and less fat and carbohydrate than does milk. It also contains many colostrum corpuscles and usually will coagulate on boiling due to a large amount of lactalbumin. **c. gravida'rum,** the colostrum secreted before parturition, and especially that secreted during the first few days following delivery. **c. puerpera'rum,** the colostrum secreted after labor.

colotomy (ko-lot'o-me) [*colo-* + Gr. *tomē* a cutting] incision into the colon for removal of a foreign body, polyp, or other benign tumor. Cf. *colostomy.*

colotyphoid (ko''lo-ti'foid) typhoid fever in which there is follicular ulceration of the colon, with extensive lesions in the small intestine.

colovaginal (ko''lo-vaj'ĕ-nal) pertaining to or communicating with the colon and vagina, as a colovaginal fistula.

colovesical (ko''lo-ves'ĭ-kal) pertaining to or communicating with the colon and urinary bladder, as a colovesical fistula.

colp- see *colpo-.*

colpalgia (kol-pal'je-ah) [*colp-* + *-algia*] colpodynia; vaginodynia.

colpatresia (kol''pah-tre'ze-ah) [*colp-* + *atresia*] atresia or occlusion of the vagina.

colpectasia (kol-pek-ta'se-ah) [*colp-* + Gr. *ektasis* distention + *-ia*] distention or dilatation of the vagina.

colpectasis (kol-pek'tah-sis) colpectasia.

colpectomy (kol-pek'to-me) [*colp-* + Gr. *ektomē* excision] excision of the vagina.

colpeurynter (kol''pu-rin''ter) [*colp-* + Gr. *eurynein* to dilate] metreurynter.

colpeurysis (kol-pu'rĭ-sis) [*colp-* + Gr. *eurynein* to dilate] dilatation of the vagina.

colpismus (kol-piz'mus) [Gr. *kolpos* vagina] vaginismus.

colpitic (kol-pit'ik) pertaining to colpitis.

colpitis (kol-pi'tis) [*colpo-* + *-itis*] inflammation of the vagina; see also *vaginitis.* **c. emphysemato'sa, emphysematous c.,** inflammation of the vagina characterized by the presence of small gas-filled spaces in the lamina propria mucosae. **c. granulo'sa,** vaginitis verrucosa. **c. mycot'ica,** inflammation of the vagina due to the presence of fungi.

colpo-, colp- (kol'po, kolp) [Gr. *kolpos* a bosom or fold; vagina] a combining form denoting relationship to the vagina.

colpocele (kol'po-sēl) [*colpo-* + Gr. *kēlē* hernia] 1. hernia into the vagina. 2. colpoptosis.

colpoceliocentesis (kol''po-se''le-o-sen-te'sis) puncture of the abdominal cavity through the vagina, usually the posterior vault.

colpoceliotomy (kol''po-se''le-ot'o-me) [*colpo-* + Gr. *koilia* belly

+ *tomē* a cutting] incision into the abdomen through the vaginal wall.

colpocleisis (kol″po-kli′sis) [*colpo-* + Gr. *kleisis* closure] surgical closure of the vaginal canal.

colpocystitis (kol″po-sis-ti′tis) [*colpo-* + Gr. *kystis* bladder + *itis*] inflammation of the vagina and of the bladder.

colpocystocele (kol″po-sis′to-sēl) [*colpo-* + Gr. *kystis* bladder + *kēlē* hernia] hernia of the bladder into the vagina, of which the anterior wall becomes prolapsed.

colpocystoplasty (kol″po-sis′to-plas″te) [*colpo-* + Gr. *kystis* bladder + *plassein* to form] plastic operation for the repair of the vesicovaginal wall.

colpocystotomy (kol″po-sis-tot′o-me) [*colpo-* + Gr. *kystis* bladder + *tomē* cutting] incision into the bladder through the vaginal wall.

colpocystoureterocystotomy (kol″po-sis″to-u-re″ter-o-sis-tot′o-me) [*colpo-* + Gr. *kystis* bladder + *ourētēr* ureter + *cystotomy*] the operation of exposing the ureteral orifices by incising the walls of the bladder and vagina.

colpocytogram (kol″po-si′to-gram) a tabulation of the various types of cells observed in smears taken from the mucous membrane of the vagina.

colpocytology (kol″po-si-tol′o-je) the quantitative and differential study of cells exfoliated from the epithelium of the vagina.

colpodynia (kol″po-din′e-ah) [*colpo-* + Gr. *odynē* pain] pain in the vagina; called also *colpalgia* and *vaginodynia*.

colpoepisiorrhaphy (kol″po-ĕ-piz″e-or′ah-fe) [*colpo-* + Gr. *episeion* pubes + *rhaphē* stitch] (*obs.*) the operation of suturing the vagina and vulva.

colpohyperplasia (kol″po-hi-per-pla′ze-ah) [*colpo-* + *hyperplasia*] excessive growth of the mucous membrane and wall of the vagina. **c. cys′tica,** a variety characterized by the presence of cysts in the mucous membrane. **c. emphysemato′sa,** a variety characterized by the presence of small gas-filled spaces in the mucous membrane.

colpohysterectomy (kol″po-his″ter-ek′to-me) [*colpo-* + *hysterectomy*] (*obs.*) surgical removal of the uterus by a vaginal operation.

colpohysteropexy (kol″po-his′ter-o-pek″se) [*colpo-* + Gr. *hystera* uterus + *pēxis* fixation] (*obs.*) vaginal hysteropexy.

colpohysterorrhaphy (kol″po-his″ter-or′ah-fe) [*colpo-* + Gr. *hystera* uterus + *rhaphē* suture] (*obs.*) vaginal hysteropexy.

colpohysterotomy (kol″po-his-ter-ot′o-me) [*colpo-* + *hysterotomy*] (*obs.*) surgical incision of the vagina and uterus.

colpomicroscope (kol″po-mi′kro-skōp) an instrument especially designed for insertion in the vagina, for the microscopic examination of tissues of the cervix in situ; it has higher powers of magnification than the colposcope.

colpomicroscopic (kol″po-mi″kro-skop′ik) performed with the colpomicroscope, or pertaining to colpomicroscopy.

colpomicroscopy (kol″po-mi-kros′ko-pe) examination of tissues of the cervix in situ with the colpomicroscope.

colpomycosis (kol″po-mi-ko′sis) [*colpo-* + Gr. *mykēs* fungus] (*obs.*) colpitis mycotica.

colpomyomectomy (kol″po-mi″o-mek′to-me) [*colpo-* + *myomectomy*] myomectomy performed through a vaginal incision.

colpoperineoplasty (kol″po-per″ĭ-ne′o-plas″te) [*colpo-* + Gr. *perinaion* perineum + *plassein* to form] plastic surgery of the vagina and perineum.

colpoperineorrhaphy (kol″po-per″ĭ-ne-or′ah-fe) [*colpo-* + Gr. *perinaion* perineum + *rhaphē* suture] suture of the ruptured vagina and perineum; vaginoperineorrhaphy.

colpopexy (kol′po-pek″se) [*colpo-* + Gr. *pēxis* fixation] suture of a relaxed vagina to the abdominal wall; vaginofixation.

colpoplasty (kol′po-plas″te) [*colpo-* + Gr. *plassein* to shape] plastic surgery involving the vagina; called also *vaginoplasty*.

colpopoiesis (kol″po-poi-e′sis) [*colpo-* + Gr. *poiein* to make] the formation of a vagina by plastic operation.

colpopolypus (kol″po-pol′e-pus) [*colpo-* + *polypus*] (*obs.*) a vaginal polyp.

colpoptosis (kol″po-to′sis) [*colpo-* + Gr. *ptōsis* prolapse] prolapse or falling of the vagina; called also *colpocele*.

colporectopexy (kol″po-rek′to-pek″se) [*colpo-* + *rectum* + Gr. *pēxis* fixation] suspension of a prolapsed rectum by suture to the vaginal wall.

colporrhagia (kol″po-ra′je-ah) [*colpo-* + Gr. *rhēgnynai* to burst out] vaginal hemorrhage.

colporrhaphy (kol-por′ah-fe) [*colpo-* + Gr. *rhaphē* suture] 1. the operation of suturing the vagina. 2. the operation of denuding and suturing the vaginal wall for the purpose of narrowing the vagina.

colporrhexis (kol″po-rek′sis) [*colpo-* + Gr. *rhēxis* rupture] laceration of the vagina.

colposcope (kol′po-skōp) [*colpo-* + Gr. *skopein* to examine] originally a speculum for examining the vagina; now an instrument inserted into the vagina for examination of the tissues of the

vagina and cervix by means of a magnifying lens. Cf. *colpomicroscope.*

colposcopic (kol″po-skop′ik) relating to the colposcope or to colposcopy.

colposcopy (kol-pos′ko-pe) examination of the cervix and vagina by means of the colposcope.

colpospasm (kol′po-spazm) [*colpo-* + Gr. *spasmos* spasm] vaginal spasm.

colpostat (kol′po-stat) [*colpo-* + Gr. *statos* standing] an appliance for retaining something, such as radium, in the vagina.

colpostenosis (kol″po-stĕ-no′sis) [*colpo-* + Gr. *stenōsis* stricture] contraction or narrowing of the vagina.

colpostenotomy (kol″po-stĕ-not′o-me) [*colpo-* + Gr. *stenōsis* stricture + *tomē* a cutting] a cutting operation for stricture or atresia of the vagina.

colpotherm (kol′po-therm) [*colpo-* + Gr. *thermē* heat] an electrical apparatus for applying heat within the vagina.

colpotomy (kol-pot′o-me) [*colpo-* + Gr. *tomē* a cutting] incision of the vagina with entry into the cul-de-sac; called also *vaginotomy.* **posterior c.,** culdotomy.

colpoureterocystotomy (kol″po-u-re″ter-o-sis-tot′o-me) [*colpo-* + *ureter* + *cystotomy*] the exposure of the orifices of the ureters by cutting through the walls of the vagina and bladder.

colpoureterotomy (kol″po-u-re″ter-ot′o-me) incision of the ureter through the vagina, performed for the relief of ureteral stricture.

colpoxerosis (kol″po-ze-ro′sis) [*colpo-* + Gr. *xēros* dry] abnormal dryness of the vulva and vagina.

colterol mesylate (kōl′tĕ-rōl) chemical name: (+)-4-[2-[(1,1-dimethylethyl)amino]-1-hydroxyethyl] 1,2-benzenediol methanesulfonate (salt); a bronchodilator, $C_{12}H_{19}NO_3 \cdot CH_4O_3S$.

Coluber (kol′u-ber) a genus of nonvenomous snakes (family Colubridae) found in northeastern Asia and North America. *C. constrictor,* is the American blacksnake or black racer.

colubrid (kol′ŭ-brid) 1. any snake of the family Colubridae. 2. of or pertaining to the family Colubridae.

Colubridae (kol-u′brĭ-de) [L. *coluber* serpent] a family of snakes; most of the species are harmless, though the boomslang of South Africa is venomous. See table accompanying *snake.*

columbium (ko-lum′be-um) a former name of the element *niobium.*

columella (kol″u-mel′lah), pl. *columel′lae* [L.] 1. a little column. 2. in molds, the central axis of the spore case, around which the spores are arranged, especially in the series Gasteromycetes. Called also *columnella.* **c. coch′leae,** modiolus. **c. for′nicis** (*obs.*), columna fornicis. **c. na′si,** the fleshy distal margin of the nasal septum.

columellae (kol″u-mel′le) [L.] plural of *columella.*

column (kol′um) [L. *colum′na*] an anatomical part in the form of a pillar-like structure, sometimes used specifically for the gray column of the spinal cord; see also *columna.* **c's of abdominal ring,** thickened fibers of the aponeurosis of the external oblique muscle around the superficial abdominal ring. **anal c's,** columnae anales. **anterior c. of fauces,** arcus palatoglossus. **anterior c. of spinal cord,** columna anterior medullae spinalis. **anterolateral c.,** funiculus lateralis medullae spinalis. **c's of Bertin,** columnae renales. **c. of Burdach,** fasciculus cuneatus medullae spinalis. **Clarke's c. of spinal cord,** nucleus thoracicus. **dorsal c.,** columna vertebralis. **enamel c's,** prismata adamantina. **fat c's,** columns of fatty tissue extending from the cutaneous connective tissue to the hair follicles and sweat glands; called also *columnae adiposae* and *Warren's fat c's.* **fleshy c's of heart,** trabeculae carneae cordis. **c's of folds of tongue,** papillae foliatae. **fornix c., c. of fornix,** columna fornicis. **fractionating c.,** an apparatus for separating the volatile constituents of a solution by distillation. **fundamental c.,** fasciculi proprii. **c. of Goll,** fasciculus gracilis medullae spinalis. **c. of Gowers,** tractus spinocerebellaris anterior. **gray c's of spinal cord,** columnae griseae. **gray c. of spinal cord, anterior,** columna anterior medullae spinalis. **gray c. of spinal cord, lateral,** columna lateralis medullae spinalis. **gray c. of spinal cord, posterior,** columna posterior medullae spinalis. **c. of Kölliker,** sarcostyle, def. 2. **lateral c. of spinal cord,** columna lateralis medullae spinalis. **c. of Lissauer,** tractus dorsolateralis. **c's of Morgagni,** columnae anales. **muscle c.,** sarcostyle, def. 2. **c. of nose,** septum nasi. **positive c.,** a pinkish stream of light seen when a current of high potential is passed through a tube from which the air has been partly exhausted. **posterior c. of fauces,** arcus palatopharyngeus. **posterior c. of spinal cord,** columna posterior medullae spinalis. **posteroexternal c.,** the outer wider portion of the posterior column of the spinal cord. **posteromedian c. of medulla oblongata,** fasciculus gracilis medullae oblongatae. **posteromedian c. of spinal cord,** fasciculus gracilis medullae spinalis. **Rathke's c's,** two cartilages at the anterior end of the notochord. **rectal c's,** columnae anales. **renal c's of Bertin,** columnae renales. **c. of Rolando,** a name once given an elevation on the lateral side of the fasciculus cuneatus of the medulla oblongata. **c's of rugae of vagina,** columnae rugarum vaginae. **c. of Sertoli,** an elongated Sertoli cell in the parietal layer of the seminiferous tubules. **spinal c.,** columna vertebralis. **c. of Spitzka-Lissauer,** tractus dorsolateralis. **Stilling's c.,** nucleus thoracicus. **striomotor c.,** an efferent column of the anterior horn of the spinal cord supplying striated muscle. **Türck's c.,** tractus pyramidalis anterior. **c's of vagina,** columnae rugarum vaginae. **vertebral c.,** the columnar assemblage of the vertebrae from the cranium through the coccyx; called also *axon, columna vertebralis* [NA], *backbone, spine,* and *dorsal* or *spinal c.* **Warren's fat c's,** fat c's.

columna (ko-lum′nah), pl. *colum′nae* [L.] [NA]   column: a pillar-like structure; in anatomical nomenclature, used to designate a pillar-like structure or part. **colum′nae adipo′sae,** fat columns. **colum′nae ana′les** [NA], **colum′nae a′ni,** anal columns: vertical ridges or folds of mucous membrane at the upper half of the anal canal; called also *columnae rectales* [*Morgagnii*], *rectal columns, columns of Morgagni,* and *mucous folds of rectum.* **c. ante′rior medul′lae spina′lis** [NA], the ventral portion of the gray substance of the spinal cord; in transverse section it is seen as a horn. Called also *anterior column* or *horn of spinal cord.* **colum′nae berti′ni,** columnae renales. **colum′nae car′neae cor′dis,** trabeculae carneae cordis. **c. for′nicis** [NA], fornix column: either of the two columnar masses of fibers diverging from the anterior end of the body of the fornix to descend into the diencephalon; called also *anterior pillar of fornix, column of fornix,* and *columella fornicis.* **colum′nae gris′eae** [NA], the longitudinally oriented parts of the spinal cord in which the nerve cell bodies are found, comprising the gray substance of the spinal cord; called also *gray columns of spinal cord.* **c. latera′lis medul′lae spina′lis** [NA], the lateral portion of the gray matter of the spinal cord, in transverse section seen as a horn; it is present only in the thoracic and upper lumbar regions. Called also *lateral column* or *horn of spinal cord.* **c. na′si,** septum nasi. **c. poste′rior medul′lae spina′lis** [NA], the dorsal portion of the gray substance of the spinal cord, in transverse section seen as a horn; called also *posterior column* or *horn of spinal cord.* **colum′nae recta′les [Morgagn′ii],** columnae anales. **colum′nae rena′les** [NA], renal columns: inward extensions of the cortical structure of the kidney, between the renal pyramids; called also columnae renales [*Bertini*], *columnae bertini,* and *renal columns of Bertin.* **colum′nae rena′les [Berti′ni],** columnae renales. **c. ruga′rum ante′rior vagi′nae** [NA], a well-marked longitudinal ridge on the anterior wall of the vagina. **c. ruga′rum poste′rior vagi′nae** [NA], a well-marked longitudinal ridge on the posterior wall of the vagina. **colum′nae ruga′rum vagi′nae** [NA], columns of rugae of vagina: well-marked longitudinal ridges on either the anterior (c. rugarum anterior vaginae) or posterior (c. rugarum posterior vaginae) wall of the vagina; called also *columns of vagina.* **c. vertebra′lis** [NA], the columnar assemblage of the vertebrae from the cranium through the coccyx; called also *axon, vertebral, dorsal,* or *spinal column, backbone,* and *spine.*

columnae (ko-lum′ne) [L.]   plural of *columna.*

columnella (kol″um-nel′ah) [L.]   columella.

columning (kol″um-ing)   columnization.

columnization (kol″um-nǐ-za′shun)   the supporting of the prolapsed uterus with tampons.

Coly-Mycin M (kol′e-mi″sin)   trademark for preparations of colistimethate sodium.

Coly-Mycin S (kol′e-mi″sin)   trademark for a preparation of colistin sulfate.

colypeptic (ko″le-pep′tik)   kolypeptic.

coma (ko′mah) [L.; Gr. *kōma*]   1. a state of unconsciousness from which the patient cannot be aroused, even by powerful stimulation; called also *exanimation.* 2. the optical aberration produced when an image is received upon a screen which is not exactly at right angles to the line of propagation of the incident light. **agrypnodal c.,** c. vigil. **alcoholic c.,** stupor accompanying severe alcoholic intoxication. **alpha c.,** coma in which there are electroencephalographic findings of dominant alpha-wave activity. **apoplectic c.,** the stupor that accompanies stroke. **diabetic c.,** the coma of severe diabetic acidosis. **hepatic c., c. hepat′icum,** coma accompanying hepatic encephalopathy. **hyperosmolar nonketotic c.,** diabetic coma in which the level of ketone bodies is normal, due to hyperosmolarity of extracellular fluid resulting in dehydration of intracellular fluid; often a consequence of overtreatment with hyperosmolar solutions. **c. hypochlorae′micum,** coma occurring in disorders associated with sodium chloride loss. **irreversible c.,** brain death; see under *death.* **Kussmaul's c.,** the coma and air hunger of diabetic acidosis. **metabolic c.,** the coma accompanying metabolic encephalopathy. **c. somnolen′tium,** cataphora. **trance c.,** lethargy produced by hypnosis. **uremic c.,** lethargic state due to uremia. **c. vigil,** apparent wakefulness with absent or grossly diminished response to outside stimuli; called also *agrypnodal c.* and *akinetic autism.*

comatose (ko′mah-tōs)   pertaining to or affected with coma.

combing (kōm′ing)   hersage.

combustion (kom-bust′yun) [L. *combustio*]   rapid oxidation with emission of heat.

comedo (kom′ě-do), pl. *comedo′nes.*   A plug of keratin and sebum within the dilated orifice of a hair follicle, frequently containing the bacteria *Corynebacterium acnes, Staphylococcus albus,* and *Pityrosporon ovale;* called also *blackhead.* See also *acne vulgaris.*

comedocarcinoma (kŏ-me″do-kar-sǐ-no′mah)   an intraductal carcinoma of the breast, the central cells of which are degenerated and easily expressed from the cut surface of the tumor.

comedogenic (kom″ě-do-jen′ik)   producing comedones.

comedomastitis (kŏ-me″do-mas-ti′tis)   mammary duct ectasia.

comes (ko′mēz), pl. *com′ites* [L. *"companion"*]   an artery or vein that accompanies a nerve trunk, as arteria comitans nervi ischiadici.

comfimeter (kum-fim′ě-ter)   an apparatus devised by Leonard Hill to measure the cooling power of the atmosphere at body temperature; it is used as a guide to keeping comfortable conditions in rooms.

comfortization (kum″fort-i-za′shun)   the scientific application of physiological principles for the promotion of comfort in potentially stressful situations, as in aircraft design.

comites (kom′ǐ-tēz)   plural of *comes.*

commasculation (kom-mas″ku-la′shun)   homosexuality between men.

commensal (kŏ-men′sal) [L. *com-* together + *mensa* table]   1. living on or within another organism, and deriving benefit without injuring or benefiting the other individual.   2. an organism living on or within another, but not causing injury to the host. See *symbiosis.*

commensalism (kŏ-men′sal-izm″)   symbiosis (q.v.) in which one population (or individual) gains from the association and the other is neither harmed nor benefited.

comminuted (kom′ǐ-nūt″ed) [L. *comminutus,* from *com* together + *minuere* to diminish]   broken or crushed into small pieces, as a comminuted fracture.

comminution (kom″ǐ-nu′shun) [L. *comminutio*]   the act of breaking, or condition of being broken, into small fragments, as of a fractured bone.

Commiphora (kom-if′o-rah)   a genus of trees of the East Indies and Africa. *C. molmol* and other species yield myrrh. *C. opobalsamum* Engl. (Burseraceae) yields balsam of Gilead.

commissura (kom″mǐ-su′rah), pl. *commissurae* [L. *"a joining together"*] [NA]   commissure: a site of union of corresponding parts; a general term used to designate such a junction of corresponding anatomical structures, frequently, but not always, across the midplane of the body. **c. al′ba medul′lae spina′lis** [NA], the structure formed by fibers crossing from one side of the spinal cord to the other, anterior and posterior to the central canal; called also *white commissure of spinal cord.* **c. ante′rior al′ba medul′lae spina′lis,** the aggregate of fibers crossing from one side of the spinal cord to the other, anterior to the central canal; see *c. alba medullae spinalis* [NA]. **c. ante′rior cer′ebri** [NA], anterior commissure of cerebrum: the band of fibers passing transversely through the lamina terminalis and connecting the parts of the two cerebral hemispheres, and consisting of a pars anterior and a pars posterior. **c. ante′rior gris′ea medul′lae spina′lis,** a network of gray matter anterior to the central canal of the spinal cord. **c. bre′vis lobo′rum posteri-o′rum inferio′rum cerebel′li** (obs.), tuber vermis. **c. cerebel′li,** pons, def. 2. **c. for′nicis** [NA], commissure of fornix: a band of fibers connecting the hippocampi of the two sides through the body of the fornix; called also *c. hippocampi,* and *hippocampal commissure.* **c. habenula′rum** [NA], commissure of habenulae: a band of fibers of the stria medullaris that pass through the habenula of each side to decussate and terminate in the habenula of the other side. **c. hippocam′pi,** c. fornicis. **c. infe′rior [Gudde′ni],** see *commissurae supraopticae.* **c. labio′rum ante′rior** [NA], anterior commissure of labia: the junction of the two labia majora anteriorly, at the lower border of the pubic symphysis. **c. labio′rum o′ris** [NA], commissure of lips of mouth: the junction of the upper and lower lips at either side of the mouth. **c. labio′rum poste′rior** [NA], posterior commissure of labia: the apparent junction of the labia majora posteriorly, formed by the forward projection of the tendinous center of the perineum into the pudendal cleft. **c. labio′rum puden′di,** see *c. labiorum anterior* and *c. labiorum posterior.* **c. mag′na cer′ebri,** corpus callosum. **c. me′dia cer′ebri, c. mol′lis** (obs.), adhesio interthalamica. **c. oliva′rum,** see *fibrae arcuatae internae.* **c. palpebra′rum latera′lis** [NA], the lateral junction of the superior and inferior eyelids; called also *c. palpebrarum temporalis* and *lateral commissure of eyelids.* **c. palpebra′rum media′lis** [NA], the medial junction of the superior and inferior eyelids; called also *c. palpebrarum nasalis* and *medial commissure of eyelids.* **c. palpebra′rum nasa′lis,** c. palpebrarum medialis. **c. palpebra′rum tempora′lis,** c. palpebrarum lateralis. **c. poste′rior cer′ebri** [NA], posterior commissure of cerebrum: a large fiber bundle that crosses from one side of the brain to the other just dorsal to the point where the aqueduct opens into the third ventricle. **c. poste′rior medul′lae spina′lis,** a transverse bar of gray substance connecting the lateral crescents of gray matter and lying posterior to the central canal of the spinal cord. **c. supe′rior [Meyner′ti],** see *commissurae supraopticae.* **commissu′rae supraop′ticae** [NA], supraoptic commissures: commissural fibers that cross the midline of the human brain dorsal to the caudal border of the optic chiasma, connecting the medial geniculate body and inferior colliculus of one side with those of the opposite side; they represent the combined commissures of Gudden and Meynert.

commissurae (kom″mĭ-su′re) [L.] plural of *commissura.*

commissural (kom-mis′u-ral) pertaining to or acting as a commissure.

commissure (kom′ĭ-shur) a site of union of corresponding parts; see *commissura.* Used also with specific reference to the sites of junction between adjacent cusps of the valves of the heart. **anterior c. of cerebrum,** commissura anterior cerebri. **anterior c. of labia,** commissura labiorum anterior. **Forel′s c.,** a name once applied to a band that joins the subthalamic nucleus of each side. **c. of fornix,** commissura fornicis. **Gudden′s c.,** see *commissurae supraopticae.* **c. of habenulae,** commissura habenularum. **hippocampal c.,** commissura fornicis. **interthalamic c.,** adhesio interthalamica. **laryngeal c.,** the region of junction (anterior or posterior) of the two sides of the larynx. **lateral c. of eyelids,** commissura palpebrarum lateralis. **c. of lips of mouth,** commissura labiorum oris. **medial c. of eyelids,** commissura palpebrarum medialis. **Meynert′s c.,** see *commissurae supraopticae.* **middle c. of cerebrum,** adhesio interthalamica. **optic c.** (*obs.*), chiasma opticum. **posterior c.,** commissura posterior cerebri. **posterior c., chiasmatic,** see *commissurae supraopticae.* **posterior c. of labia,** commissura labiorum posterior. **superior c.,** see *commissurae supraopticae.* **supraoptic c's,** commissurae supraopticae. **white c. of spinal cord,** commissura alba medullae spinalis. **white c. of spinal cord, lateral,** funiculus lateralis medullae spinalis.

commissurorrhaphy (kom″ĭ-shur-or′ah-fe) [*commissure* + Gr. *rhaphē* a seam] suture of the component parts of a commissure, to decrease the size of the orifice.

commissurotomy (kom″ĭ-shur-ot′o-me) [*commissure* + Gr. *tomē* cutting] surgical incision or digital disruption of the component parts of a commissure to increase the size of the orifice; commonly utilized to separate the adherent, thickened leaflets of a stenotic mitral valve.

commitment (kŏ-mit′ment) the legal consignment of a mental patient to an institution for treatment.

commotio (kŏ-mo′she-o) [L. "disturbance"] a concussion; a violent shaking, or the shock which results from it. **c. cer′ebri,** concussion of the brain. **c. ret′inae,** edema around the macular region of the retina, caused by a severe blow to the eyeball, and producing a permanent central scotoma as a result of destruction of the delicate cones in the fovea. Called also *Berlin's disease* or *edema,* and *concussion of the retina.* **c. spina′lis,** concussion of the spine.

communicable (kŏ-mu′nĭ-kah-b'l) capable of being transmitted from one person or animal to another.

communicans (kŏ-mu′nĕ-kanz) [L.] communicating; used in anatomical nomenclature to denote a communicating structure, as a nerve.

communis (kŏ-mu′nis) [L.] common; [NA] a general term denoting a structure serving several branches.

community (kŏ-mu′nĭ-te) a body of individuals living in a defined area or having a common interest or organization. **biotic c.,** an assemblage of populations living in a defined area. **climax c.,** the final, stable, and mature community in a series that appears in succession, which is in equilibrium with the environmental conditions and is composed of a definite group of plant and animal species. The entire sequence of communities is called a *sere* and the individual transitional communities are *seral stages.* **seral c.,** see under *stage.* **therapeutic c.,** a specially structured mental hospital or ward employing group and milieu therapy and encouraging the patient to function within social norms.

Comolli′s sign (kom-ol′ēz) [Antonio *Comolli,* Italian pathologist, born 1879] see under *sign.*

Comp. abbreviation for L. *compos′itus,* compound.

compact (kom-pakt′) dense; having a dense structure.

compacta (kom-pak′tah) the more superficial and denser portion of the decidua basalis; stratum compactum.

compaction (kom-pak′shun) a complication of labor in twin births in which there is simultaneous full engagement of the leading fetal poles of both twins, so that the true pelvic cavity is filled and further descent is prevented. Cf. *interlocking.*

comparascope (kom-par′ah-skōp″) a device attached to a microscope for the purpose of comparing two slides.

comparator (kom′pah-ra″tor) a simple colorimeter consisting of a block of wood with holes in which to place the test tubes to be

compared, and transverse holes through which to view the colors; called also *comparator block.*

compartment (com-part′ment) a small enclosure within a larger space. **muscular c.,** lacuna musculorum. **vascular c.,** lacuna vasorum.

compartmentalization, compartmentation (kom″part-men″tah-li-za′shun; kom-part′men-ta′shun) the natural partitioning within cells due to the selectively permeable membranes which enclose each of the separate parts (mitochondria, lysosomes, Golgi complex, etc.), enabling each part to regulate its own contents.

compatibility (kom-pat″ĭ-bil′ĭ-te) [L. *compatibilis* accordant] the quality of being compatible.

compatible (kom-pat′ĭ-b'l) capable of harmonious coexistence; of medications, suitable for simultaneous administration without nullification or aggravation of the effects of either.

Compazine (kom′pah-zēn) trademark for preparations of prochlorperazine maleate.

compensation (kom″pen-sa′shun) [L. *compensatio,* from *cum* together + *pensare* to weigh] the counterbalancing of any defect of structure or function. In psychoanalysis, the mechanism by which an approved character trait is put forward to conceal from the ego the existence of an opposite trait. In cardiology, the maintenance of an adequate blood flow without distressing symptoms, accomplished by such cardiac and circulatory adjustments as tachycardia or cardiac hypertrophy, or increase of blood volume by sodium and water retention. **broken c.,** inability of the heart to maintain sufficient blood flow through the fissures, so that stagnation ensues and symptoms of stasis are produced. **dosage c.,** in genetics, the mechanism by which the effect of the two X chromosomes of the normal female is rendered identical to that of the one X chromosome of the normal male. See *Lyon hypothesis,* under *hypothesis.*

compensatory (kom-pen′sah-to″re) making good a defect or loss; restoring a just balance.

competence (kom′pĕ-tens) the ability of an organ or part to perform adequately any function required of it. In embryology, the ability of embryonic cells to differentiate into cell types determined by inductors. **embryonic c.,** the ability of embryonic tissue to respond normally to the influence of an inductor. **immunologic c.,** immunocompetence.

competition (kom″pĕ-tish′un) the phenomenon in which two structurally similar molecules "compete" for a single binding site on a third molecule. See *competitive inhibition,* under *inhibition.*

compimeter (kom-pim′ĕ-ter) an instrument for measuring the field of vision.

complaint (kom-plānt′) a symptom, disease, or disorder. **chief c.,** the symptom or group of symptoms about which the patient first consults the doctor; the presenting symptom. **summer c.,** cholera morbus.

complement (kom′plĕ-ment) a complex series of enzymatic proteins occurring in normal serum that interact to combine with antigen-antibody complex, producing lysis when the antigen is an intact cell. Complement comprises eleven discrete proteins, or nine functioning components symbolized as C1 through C9, with C1 being divided into subcomponents C1q, C1r, and C1s. Activated forms are indicated by a bar over the numeral (e.g., C$\overline{1}$), or over the numerals signifying a complex of components (e.g., C$\overline{567}$). Biologically active fragments of a component are designated by the lower-case *a* or *b* (e.g., C3a). The components combine in various sequences and interact to participate in biological activities such as cell lysis, anaphylotoxic activities, promotion of phagocytosis, etc. (see Plate XIII). The complement system is known to be activated by IgG and IgM and by the properdin system, cobra venom, and other factors. Called also *alexin.* See also under *fixation,* and see *alternative pathway,* under *pathway.* **dominant c.,** that one of several complements which exerts the specific action. **endocellular c.,** endocomplement.

complemental (kom″plĕ-men′tal) complementary.

complementary (kom″plĕ-men′tă-re) [L. *complere* to fill] supplying a defect, or helping to do so; making complete; accessory.

complementation (kom″ple-men-ta′shun) in genetics, the restoration of wild-type function as a result of two distinct mutations on the same chromosome. In virology, the interaction of two defective bacteriophages that results in the replication of both, as occurs in some mixed infections of bacterial cells. **interallelic c.,** intragenic c. **intercistronic c., intergenic c.,** the essentially full restoration of wild-type function in a *cis-trans* test when two mutations, in transportation, are located in two different cistrons (genes). **intracistronic c., intragenic c.,** the partial restoration of function sometimes seen in the *cis-trans* test when the two mutations are located at different sites within the same cistron.

complemented (kom′plĕ-ment″ed) joined with complement so as to be active.

complementoid (kom″plĕ-men′toid) in early immunological theory, a complement that has lost its activity, the zymotoxic group being destroyed, without affecting its binding property with amboceptors. A complementoid, produced by heating a complement, is capable of producing an anticomplement when injected.

complementophil (kom″plĕ-men′to-fil) [L. *complement* + Gr. *philein* to love] in early immunological theory, possessing an affinity for a complement, a term applied to that element of the amboceptor to which the complement becomes attached. See *Ehrlich's side-chain theory,* under *theory.*

complex (kom′pleks) [L. *complexus* woven together] 1. complicated; not simple. 2. the sum or combination of various things, like or unlike, as a *complex* of symptoms; see *syndrome.* 3. Jung's term for a group of associated, partially or wholly repressed ideas that can evoke emotional forces which influence an individual's behavior, usually outside his awareness. 4. that portion of an electrocardiographic tracing which represents the systole of an atrium or ventricle. **adrenochrome monosemicarbazone sodium salicylate c.,** carbazochrome salicylate. **anomalous c.,** a complex that varies from the normal type, as an electrocardiographic complex. **antigen-antibody c.,** molecules of antibody and antigen bound together in various molecular ratios, some of which are soluble and some of which are insoluble and precipitate out of solution. Complexes whose antibody Fc regions possess the capability may fix complement, reducing serum levels of complement components in patients with immune complex diseases. These complexes are the mediators of Type III hypersensitivity reactions such as Arthus reactions, and serum sickness and immune complex glomerulonephritis. **atrial c.,** the P wave of the electrocardiogram; see *electrocardiogram.* **avian leukosis c.,** see *avian leukosis,* under *leukosis.* **Cain c.,** the rivalry, competition, or destructive impulses between brothers. (*Genesis 4:* the first born of Adam and Eve, who murdered his brother Abel.) **calcarine c.,** calcar avis. **castration c.,** the fear (usually fantasied) of damage to sexual organs or of loss of sexual organs as punishment for forbidden sexual desires; called also *castration anxiety.* **Clérambault-Kandinsky c.,** a mental state in which the patient thinks his mind is controlled by some outside influence or by another person. **Diana c.** (*obs.*), masculine psychic tendencies in a female. (*Roman mythology:* goddess of the moon, chastity, and hunting, and protectress of women.) **EAHF c.,** the symptom complex of eczema, asthma, and hay fever. **Eisenmenger c.,** a defect of the interventricular septum with severe pulmonary hypertension, hypertrophy of the right ventricle, and latent or overt cyanosis. **Electra c.,** libidinous fixation of a daughter toward her father; some authors use Oedipus complex (q.v.) to refer equally to son-mother and daughter-father attachments while others reserve Oedipus complex for the former and Electra complex for the latter. (*Greek legend:* the daughter of Agamemnon and Clytemnestra, who incited her brother Orestes to kill their mother and their mother's former lover and new husband, Aegisthus, to avenge the murder of their father.) Called also *father c.* Cf. *Oedipus c.* **factor IX c.** [USP], a sterile, freeze-dried powder consisting of partially purified Factor IX fraction, as well as concentrated Factors II, VII, and X fractions, of venous plasma from healthy human donors. **father c.,** Electra c. **Ghon c.,** primary c. **Golgi c.,** a complex cuplike structure within cells, made up of several elements, each consisting of a number of flattened sacs (cisternae) with associated vacuoles and vesicles. Golgi complexes are membrane sites of the formation of the carbohydrate side chains of glycoproteins and mucopolysaccharides, and of other substances. The secretion vacuoles migrate through the cell membrane and release the glycoproteins and mucopolysaccharides, and thus play a role in internal and external secretion. Cytochemical studies have shown that they are also sites of formation of primary lysosomes and give rise to the acrosome of spermatozoa and the nematocyst of *Hydra.* Called also *Golgi apparatus* and *Golgi body.* **hapten-carrier c.,** the antigen formed by the coupling of a hapten and a carrier protein. **hemoglobin-haptoglobin c.,** the binding resulting from the extremely high affinity between haptoglobin and hemoglobin, so that no free hemoglobin is detectable in plasma unless extensive intravascular hemolysis has saturated all the available haptoglobin. **immune c.,** antibody combined with its specific antigen; if complement is fixed by the antigen-antibody complexes, deposition in tissues, such as renal glomeruli, may lead to inflammation and tissue injury. Use of the term *immune complex* usually denotes an association with disease, whereas the term *antigen-antibody complex* is usually used as the general term. **inclusion c's,** compounds in which molecules of one type are enclosed within cavities in the crystalline lattice of another substance. **inferiority c.,** a combination of emotionally charged feelings of inferiority that operate in the unconscious to produce timidity or, as a compensation, exaggerated aggressiveness and expression of superiority (superiority c.). **Jocasta c.,** libidinous fixation of a mother toward a son. (*Greek legend:* the queen of Thebes, who married her son, Oedipus.) Cf. *Lear c.* **jumped process c.,** dislocation of articular processes of spine. **junctional c.,** the intercellular arrangement between adjacent columnar epithelial cells, consisting of the zonula occludens, the zonula adherens, and the desmosome. **Lear c.,** libidinous fixation of a father toward his daughter. (Shakespeare's *King Lear.*) Cf. *Jocasta c.* **Lutembacher's c.,** see under *syndrome.* **major histocompatibility c.,** the chromosomal region containing the genes that control the histocompatibility antigens (see under *antigen*); in man, it is designated HLA. Abbreviated MHC. Immune response (IR) genes located in the I region of the MHC control the capacity to develop specific immune responses to thymus-dependent antigens. **Meyenburg's c's,** bile duct hamartomas. **mother c.,** Oedipus c. **Oedipus c.,** libidinous fixation of a son toward his mother. (*Greek legend:* the son of Jocasta and the Theban king, Laius, who, raised by a foster parent, killed his father and subsequently married his mother. Later, when he discovered the true relationship, he blinded himself [edipism].) Called also *mother c.* Cf. *Electra c.* **Parkinson-dementia c.,** a condition characterized by a gradually progressive parkinsonian state associated with progressive dementia. It occurs among the Chamorro population of Guam and is sometimes associated with the familial form of amyotrophic lateral sclerosis. **pore c.,** a nuclear pore and its annulus considered together. **primary c.,** 1. the combination of a parenchymal pulmonary lesion (*Ghon focus* or *tubercle*) and a corresponding lymph node focus, occurring in primary tuberculosis, usually in children; it may undergo cellular necrosis and eventually calcify. Similar lesions may also be associated with other mycobacterial infections and with fungal infections such as histoplasmosis and coccidiodomycosis. Called also *Ghon c.* and *Ranke c.* 2. the primary cutaneous lesion at the site of infection in the skin, e.g., chancre in syphilis and tuberculous chancre. **primary inoculation c., primary tuberculous c.,** tuberculous chancre. **Ranke c.,** primary c. **sex c.,** the correlation between the internal secretions and the sex functions. **superiority c.,** see *inferiority c.* **symptom c.,** a set of symptoms that occur together; the sum of signs of any morbid state; a syndrome. **synaptonemal c.,** a thick, threadlike structure formed during the zygotene (synaptic) stage of meiosis by the intertwining of two leptotene chromosomes so that they are indistinguishable separately. **ureterotrigonal c.,** ureterovesical junction. **urobilin c.,** a hypothetical substance consisting of a number of urobilinogen molecules linked together, which is the form in which urobilinogen exists in the blood and tissues. **ventricular c's,** the Q, R, S, and T waves of the electrocardiogram, representing ventricular electrical activity. **zymase c.,** the enzyme system of systems that function in alcoholic fermentation.

complexion (kom-plek′shun) [L. *complexio* combination] 1. the color and appearance of the skin of the face. 2. (*obs.*) physical constitution or bodily habit.

complexus (kom-plek′sus) [L. "encompassing"] musculus semispinalis capitis.

compliance (kom-pli′ans) a quality of yielding to pressure or force without disruption, or an expression of the measure of the ability to do so, as an expression of the distensibility of an air- or fluid-filled organ, e.g., the lung or urinary bladder, in terms of unit of volume change per unit of pressure change. Cf. *elastance.*

complicated (kom″plĭ-kāt′ed) [L. *complicare* to infold] involved; associated with other injuries, lesions, or diseases.

complication (kom″plĭ-ka′shun) [L. *complicatio* from *cum* together + *plicare* to fold] 1. a disease or diseases concurrent with another disease. 2. the concurrence of two or more diseases in the same patient.

complon (kom′plon) a cistron.

Compocillin-VK (com″po-sil′in) trademark for a preparation of penicillin V potassium.

component (kom-po′nent) a constituent element or part; specifically in neurology, a series of neurons forming a functional system for conducting the afferent and efferent impulses in the somatic and splanchnic mechanisms of the body. **anterior c.,** Angle's term for "a forward propelling force which is the result of meshing and pounding of the occlusal inclined planes of the teeth and the mesial inclination of the teeth." **group-specific c.,** a serum group of particular use in anthropological studies because of the great differences in gene frequency in different populations. **M c.,** a single species of homogeneous immunoglobulins of any class (IgA, IgG, etc.) appearing as a very narrow band on electrophoresis. It occurs in such diseases as multiple myeloma, macroglobulinemia of Waldenström, heavy chain disease, and lichen myxedematosus. **plasma thromboplastin c. (PTC),** Factor IX; see *coagulation factors,* under *factor.* **secretory c.,** see under *piece.* **somatic motor c.,** the system of neurons that conduct impulses to the somatic effectors (skeletal muscle) of the body. **somatic sensory c.,** the system of neurons conducting impulses from the somatic receptors. **splanchnic motor c.,** the system of neurons conducting impulses to the splanchnic (visceral) effectors (cardiac muscle, smooth muscle, and glands). **splanchnic sensory c.,** the system of neurons conducting impulses from the splanchnic receptors.

compos mentis (kom′pos men′tis) [L.] sound of mind; sane.

compound (kom-pownd) [L. *componere* to place together] 1. made of two or more parts or ingredients. 2. any substance made up of two or more kinds of materials. 3. in chemistry, a substance that consists of two or more chemical elements in union. **c. A,** 11-dehydrocorticosterone. **acyclic c.,** an open-chain compound; see under *chain.* **addition c.,** a compound formed by the union of two or more compounds or elements. **ali-**

Plate XIII   complement

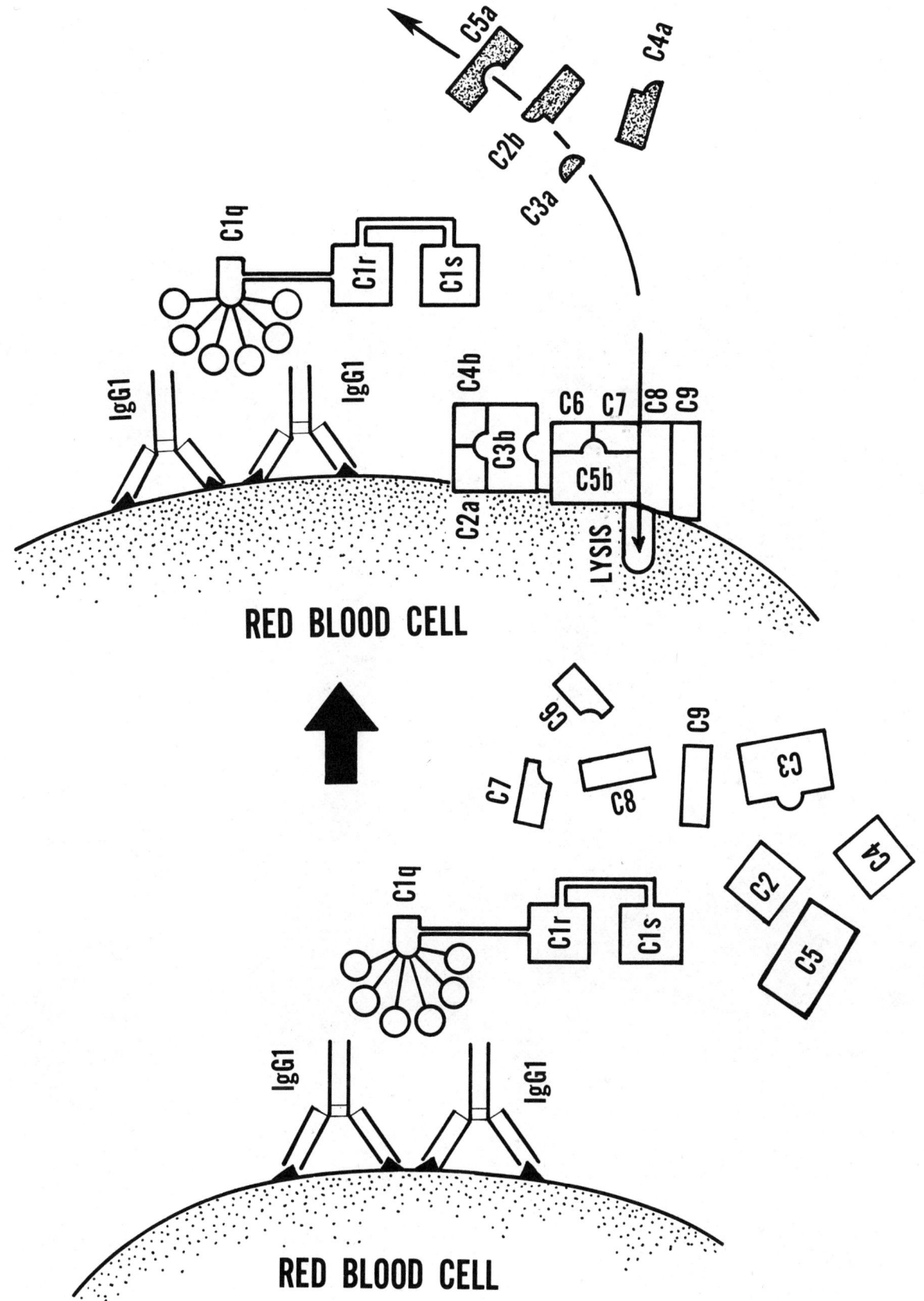

CLASSICAL COMPLEMENT ACTIVATION

Schematic representation of classical complement pathway: Two molecules of IgG, termed a "doublet," combine with homologous antigenic determinants on a red blood cell surface and activate the first complement component by interacting with C1q. This is followed by C1r and C1s activation. The reaction sequence of the classical complement pathway is C1,4,2,3,5,6,7,8,9. This biochemical pathway leads to the formation of a "hole" in the cell membrane, leading to cell swelling and lysis. Although C9 is not essential for lysis, it accelerates the lytic reaction. This in contrast to the alternative or properdin pathway which provides a mechanism to mediate the bactericidal and opsonic effects of complement without requiring specific antibody. From the C3 step forward both pathways follow a similar course.

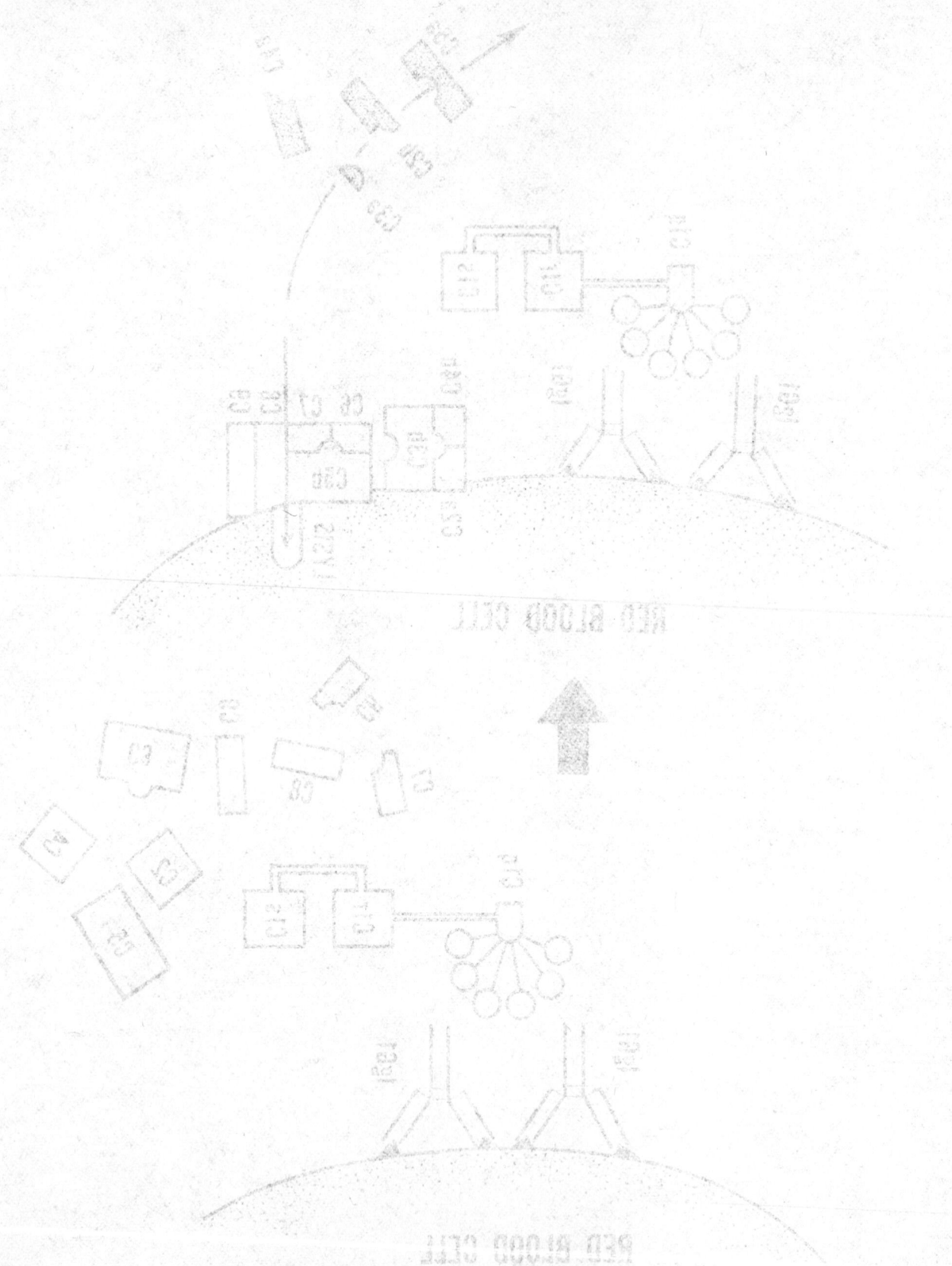

phatic c., an open-chain compound that does not contain multiple bonds; a saturated compound. See under *chain.* **APC c.,** a preparation of acetylsalicylic acid, phenacetin, and caffeine citrate. **aromatic c.,** a closed-chain compound that contains bonds similar to those in benzene; see under *chain.* **c. B,** corticosterone. **benzene c's,** aromatic compounds. **benzoin tincture c.,** see under *tincture.* **binary c.,** a compound whose molecule is composed of atoms of only two elements. **clathrate c's,** inclusion complexes in which molecules of one type are trapped within cavities of the crystalline lattice of another substance; called also *clathrates* or *occlusion c's.* **closed-chain c.,** see under *chain.* **coal-tar c.,** a closed-chain compound; see under *chain.* **condensation c.,** a compound that is formed by union of substances with the loss of one or more molecules, usually of low molecular weight, as water or ammonia. **cyclic c.,** a closed-chain compound; see under *chain.* **diazo c.,** a compound containing the group —N₂—. **c. E,** cortisone. **endothermic c.,** one whose formation is attended with absorption of heat. **energy-rich c's,** high-energy c's. **exothermic c.,** one whose formation is attended with loss of heat. **c. F,** cortisol. **fatty c.,** an open-chain compound; see under *chain.* **Grignard c.,** see under *reagent.* **heterocyclic c.,** a chemical substance that contains a ring-shaped nucleus composed of dissimilar elements. **high-energy c's,** a group of pyrophosphates that yield high levels of negative free energies on hydrolysis, and so are basic to the energy supply of living organisms. Among the most important are ATP, acetyl CoA, aminoacyl adenylates, phosphocreatinine, and phosphoenol pyruvate. Called also *energy-rich c's.* **Hurler-Scheie c.,** mucopolysaccharidosis I-H/S. **inorganic c.,** a compound that contains no carbon. **isocyclic c.,** a chemical substance that contains a ring-shaped nucleus composed of the same elements throughout. **isopropyl alcohol rubbing c.,** a solution containing 70 per cent isopropyl alcohol in water; used as a rubefacient. **Kendall's c. A.,** 11-dehydrocorticosterone. **Kendall's c. B.,** corticosterone. **Kendall's c. E,** cortisone. **Kendall's c. F,** cortisol. **low-energy c's,** compounds containing phosphate ester or other linkages that yield relatively low levels of negative free energies on hydrolysis, including AMP, glucose-1-phosphate, and glucose-6-phosphate. **nonpolar c's,** compounds in which electrons are shared equally by the two atoms forming a bond and which therefore do not ionize in solution, e.g., the paraffins, olefins, and cyclic compounds. **occlusion c's,** clathrate c's. **open-chain c.,** see under *chain.* **organic c.,** a compound of chemical elements containing carbon atoms. **organometallic c.,** one in which carbon is linked to a metal. **paraffin c.,** an open-chain compound; see under *chain.* **polar c's,** compounds in which the electrons are unequally shared by the two atoms forming the bond and which therefore may act as dipoles or, in some instances, completely ionize. They include the alcohols, water, ammonia, etc. **quaternary c.,** one composed of four elements. **quaternary ammonium c.,** see *tetraethylammonium.* **ring c.,** see *closed chain,* under *chain.* **saturated c.,** a compound in which the combining capacities of all the elements are satisfied. **substitution c.,** a compound formed by replacement of elements of a molecule by other elements. **ternary c., tertiary c.,** a compound composed of three elements. **unsaturated c.,** a compound in which the combining capacities of all the elements are not satisfied; see *unsaturated,* 2nd def. **Wintersteiner's c. F,** cortisone.

compress (kom′pres) [L. *compressus*] a pad or bolster of folded linen or other material, applied with pressure; it is sometimes medicated, and may be wet or dry, hot or cold. **cribriform c.,** one perforated with holes, like a sieve, to permit the escape of fluids from an underlying wound. **fenestrated c.,** one pierced with a hole for the discharge of purulent material or to permit inspection of the underlying wound. **graduated c.,** one composed of layers of gradually decreasing size. **Priessnitz c.,** a cold wet compress; called also *Priessnitz's bandage.*

compressibility (kom-pres″ĭ-bil′ĭ-te) the volume change per unit of a substance produced by a unit increase in pressure.

compression (kom-presh′un) [L. *compressio* from *comprimere* to squeeze together] 1. the act of pressing together; an action exerted upon a body by an external force which tends to diminish its volume and augment its density. 2. in embryology, the shortening or omission of certain stages during development. **c. of the brain,** a condition in which the brain is compressed by fractures, tumors, blood clots, abscesses, etc. **digital c.,** compression of a blood vessel by the fingers for the purpose of checking hemorrhage. **instrumental c.,** compression of a blood vessel by instruments. **pneumatic c.,** compression applied to a body part, e.g., the calf, by means of compressed air. **spinal c.,** a condition in which pressure is exerted on the spinal cord, as by a tumor, spinal fracture, etc.; its manifestations, which vary with location and degree of pressure, may include pain, paresthesias, and sensory and motor disturbances.

compressor (kom-pres′or) [L.] any agent by which compression may be achieved. **Deschamps' c.,** an instrument for the direct compression of an artery. **c. na′ris,** pars transversa musculi nasalis. **Sehrt's c.,** see under *clamp.* **shot c.,** a forceps for compressing split shot applied to sutures; see also *shotted suture,* under *suture.* **c. ure′thrae,** musculus sphincter ure-

thrae. **c. vagi′nae,** the bulbospongiosus muscle in the female.

compressorium (kom″pres-o′re-um), pl. *compresso′ria* [L.] a device for making graduated pressure upon objects under microscopic examination.

compromised (kom′pro-mīzd) lacking adequate resistance to infection, or lacking the ability to mount an adequate immune response, owing to a course of treatment (irradiation, etc.) or to an underlying disorder (leukemia, etc.).

Compton effect (komp′ton) [Arthur Holly *Compton,* American physicist, 1892–1962; winner of the Nobel prize in physics for 1927] see under *effect.*

compulsion (kom-pul′shun) an irresistible impulse to perform some act contrary to one's better judgment or will. **repetition c.,** in psychoanalytic theory, the impulse to reenact earlier emotional experiences.

compulsive (kom-pul′siv) pertaining to or characterized by compulsion.

con- [L.] a prefix signifying with or together.

conalbumin (kon″al-bu′min) a glucoprotein, formed by the acidification of egg white to pH 3.9, containing 2.1 per cent of mannose and 0.7 per cent of galactose; the noncrystalline part of egg albumin.

conamen (ko-na′men) [L. "an effort"] (*obs.*) attempted suicide.

conarial (ko-na′re-al) pertaining to the conarium.

conarium (ko-na′re-um) [L.; Gr. *kōnarion* a cone] the pineal body; so called from its conical shape.

conation (ko-na′shun) in psychology, the power that impels to effort of any kind; the conscious tendency to act.

conative (kon′ah-tiv) pertaining to the basic strivings of a person, as expressed in his behavior and actions.

conavanine (kon-ah-van′in) a basic amino acid from soy bean meal, α-amino-γ-guanidinoxybutyric acid.

concameration (kon-kam″er-a′shun) (*obs.*) an arrangement of connecting cavities or chambers.

concanavalin (kon″ka-nav′ah-lin) either of two phytohemagglutinins isolated along with canavalin from the meal of the Jack bean (*Canavalia ensiformis* D.C., and other species of *Canavalia*), which agglutinate the blood of mammals as a result of reaction with polyglucosans. *Concanavalin A* has been shown to inhibit the growth of ascites tumors.

concassation (kon″kah-sa′shun) the act of breaking up roots or woods into small pieces in order that their active principles may be more easily extracted by solvents.

concatenate (kon-kat′e-nāt) [L. *con* together + *catena* chain] to fasten or link together, as in a chain.

concatenation (kon-kat″e-na′shun) a series of events or objects occurring together or in sequence.

Concato's disease (kon-kah′tōz) [Luigi Maria *Concato,* Italian physician, 1825–1882] see under *disease.*

concave (kon′kāv) [L. *concavus*] having a rounded, somewhat depressed surface, resembling the hollowed inner surface of a segment of a sphere.

concavity (kon-kav′ĭ-te) [L. *concavitas,* from *con* together + *cavus* hollow] a hollowed-out area on the surface of an organ or other structure.

concavoconcave (kon-ka″vo-kon′kāv) concave on each of two opposite surfaces.

concavoconvex (kon-ka″vo-kon′veks) concave on one surface and convex on the opposite one.

conceive (kon-sēv′) 1. to become pregnant. 2. to take in, grasp, or form in the mind.

concentrate (kon′sen-trāt) [L. *con* together + *centrum* center] 1. to bring to a common center; to gather together at one point. 2. To increase the strength by diminishing the bulk of, as of a liquid; to condense. 3. A drug or other preparation that has been strengthened by the evaporation of its nonactive parts. **liver c.,** a dried, unfractionated product produced from a water extract derived from mammalian liver; used as a hematopoietic. **plant protease c.,** a concentrate of bromelains, proteolytic enzymes derived from pineapple plants; used to reduce inflammation and edema, and to accelerate tissue repair. **vitamin c.,** a concentrated medicinal preparation of a vitamin or vitamins.

concentration (kon″sen-tra′shun) [L. *concentratio*] 1. increase in strength by evaporation. 2. the ratio of the mass or volume of a solute to the mass or volume of the solution or solvent. Cf. *molarity, molality, normality,* and *mol fraction.* **hydrogen ion c.,** the degree of concentration of hydrogen ions in a solution; it is related approximately to the pH of the solution by the equation $(H^+) = 10^{-pH}$. **ionic c.,** the number of moles of an ion that are contained in the unit volume of a solution or in the unit mass of solvent. **limiting isorrheic c. (LIC),** the upper limit of urinary concentration at which a steady state consistent with effective physiologic regulation of solute and water balance can be maintained. **mass c.,** the mass of a constituent substance divided by the volume of the mixture, as milligrams per liter (mg/l), etc. **maximum urinary c. (MUC),** the highest attainable concentration of a solute or of the collective solutes of the urine. **MC c.,** the limiting living population density of microorganisms that is possible in any fluid culture medium. **minimal isorrheic c. (MIC),** the lower limit of urinary concentration at which a steady state consistent with effective physiologic regulation of solute and water balances can be maintained. **molar c.,** substance c. **substance c.,** the amount of a constituent substance in moles (millimoles or micromoles) divided by the volume of the mixture, as millimoles per liter (mmol./l.), etc. Called also *molar c.*

concentric (kon-sen′trik) [L. *concentricus,* from *con* together + *centrum* center] having a common center; extending out equally in all directions from a common center.

concept (kon′sept) the image of a thing as held in the mind. **second messenger c.,** the concept that a hormone (first messenger) activates adenyl cyclase in the surface membrane of its target tissue, increasing the intracellular level of cyclic AMP, which acts as a "second messenger" and carries out the work of the hormone within the target cell.

conception (kon-sep′shun) [L. *conceptio*] 1. the onset of pregnancy, marked by implantation of the blastocyst; the formation of a visable zygote. 2. concept.

conceptive (kon-sep′tiv) 1. able to become pregnant. 2. pertaining to conception.

conceptus (kon-sep′tus) [L.] the sum of derivatives of a fertilized ovum at any stage of development from fertilization until birth, including extraembryonic membranes as well as the embryo or fetus.

concha (kong′kah), pl. *con′chae* [L.; Gr. *konchē*] a shell; used in anatomical nomenclature to designate a structure or part that resembles a shell in shape. **c. of auricle, c. auric′ulae** [NA], the hollow of the auricle of the external ear, bounded anteriorly by the tragus and posteriorly by the anthelix. **c. bullo′sa,** a cystic distention of the middle nasal concha, sometimes seen in chronic rhinitis. **c. of cranium,** calvaria. **ethmoidal c., inferior,** c. nasalis media. **ethmoidal c., superior,** c. nasalis superior. **ethmoidal c., supreme,** c. nasalis suprema. **c. of eye,** orbita. **inferior nasal c.,** c. nasalis inferior. **inferior turbinate c.,** c. nasalis inferior. **middle nasal c.,** c. nasalis media. **c. nasa′lis infe′rior** [NA], inferior nasal concha: a thin bony plate with curved margins, articulating with the ethmoid, maxilla, and lacrimal and palatine bones, and forming the lower part of the lateral wall of the nasal cavity, and the mucous membrane covering the plate; called also *inferior spongy* or *turbinate bone* and *maxilloturbinal bone.* **c. nasa′lis me′dia** [NA], middle nasal concha: the

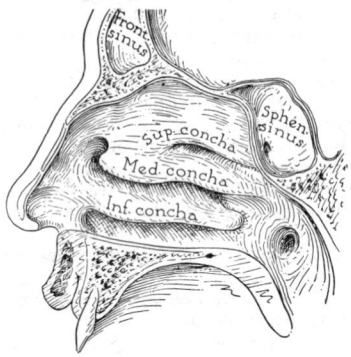

Nasal conchae (Anson).

lower of two bony plates projecting from the inner wall of the ethmoid labyrinth and separating the superior from the middle meatus of the nose, and the mucous membrane covering the plate; called also *inferior ethmoidal c., middle turbinate bone,* and *ethmoid cornu.* **c. nasa′lis supe′rior** [NA], superior nasal concha: the upper of two bony plates projecting from the inner wall of the ethmoid labyrinth and forming the upper boundary of the superior meatus of the nose, and the mucous membrane covering the plate; called also *superior ethmoidal c.* and *superior turbinate* or *spongy bone.* **c. nasa′lis supre′ma** [NA], supreme nasal concha: a thin bony plate occasionally found projecting from the inner wall of the ethmoid labyrinth above the bony superior nasal concha, and the mucous membrane covering the plate; called also *highest turbinate bone, supreme nasal* or *ethmoidal bone,* and *supreme ethmoidal c.* **nasoturbinal c.,** agger nasi. **sphenoidal c.,** 1. concha sphenoidalis. 2. ala minor ossis sphenoidalis. **c. sphenoida′lis** [NA], a thin curved plate of bone at the anterior and lower part of the body of the sphenoid bone, on either side, forming part of the roof of the nasal cavity; called also *sphenoturbinal bone* or *ossicles, Bertin's bone* or *ossicles,* and *sphenoidal c.* **superior nasal c.,** c. nasalis superior.

conchae (kong′ke) [L.] plural of *concha.*

conchiform (kong′kĭ-form) [L. *concha* shell + *forma* shape] shaped like one half of a bivalve shell.

conchiolin (kong-ki′o-lin) [Gr. *konchē* shell] a substance, isomeric with ossein, from the outer surface of shells of mollusks.

conchiolinosteomyelitis (kong-ki″o-lin-os″te-o-mi″ĕ-li′tis) a form of osteomyelitis occurring in pearl workers.

conchitis (kong-ki′tis) an inflammation of a concha.

conchoidal (kong-koi′dal) like a shell.

conchoscope (kong′ko-skōp) [Gr. *konchē* shell + Gr. *skopein* to examine] a speculum for examining the walls of the nasal cavity.

conchotome (kong′ko-tōm) [Gr. *konchē* shell + *tomē* a cutting] an instrument for the surgical removal of the nasal conchae.

conchotomy (kong-kot′o-me) incision of a nasal concha.

Concis. abbreviation for L. *conci′sus,* cut.

conclination (kon″klĭ-na′shun) [L. *con* together + *clinatus* leaning] inward rotation of the upper pole of the vertical meridian of each eye. Cf. *disclination.*

concoction (kon-kok′shun) [L. *concoctio*] 1. a mixture of medicinal substances usually prepared by the aid of heat. 2. the digestive process.

concomitant (kon-kom′ĭ-tant) [L. *concomitans,* from *cum* together + *comes* companion] accompanying; accessory; joined with another.

conconscious (kon-kon′shus) Prince's term to denote associated mental processes of which the subject is not aware.

concordance (kon-kor′dans) in genetics, the occurrence of a given trait in both members of a twin pair, as opposed to discordance.

concordant (kon-kor′dant) exhibiting concordance.

concrement (kon′kre-ment) [L. *concrementum*] a concretion, especially a calcified tubercle or similar mass.

concrescence (kon-kres′ens) [L. *con* together + *crescere* to grow] a growing together; a union of parts originally separate. In embryology, the flowing together and piling up of cells. In dentistry, the union of the roots of two approximating teeth by a deposit of cementum.

concrete (kon-krēt′) [L. *concretus*] 1. solid; tangible. 2. a mass of coalesced particles, solidified or hardened after having been more or less fluid.

concretio (kon-kre′she-o) [L.] concretion. **c. cor′dis, c. pericar′dii,** a form of adhesive pericarditis in which the pericardial cavity is obliterated.

concretion (kon-kre′shun) [L. *concretio,* from *cum* together + *crescere* to grow] 1. a calculus or inorganic mass in a natural cavity or in the tissues of an organism. 2. abnormal union of adjacent parts. 3. a process of becoming harder or more solid. **alvine c.,** a bezoar, or calculus, in the stomach or intestine. **calculous c.,** articular calculus. **preputial c.,** a concretion formed beneath a tight foreskin through deposit of urinary salts on the accumulated smegma. **prostatic c′s,** rounded and often lamellated masses of amyloid-like material present in many prostatic alveoli. **tophic c.,** tophus, def. 1.

concretism (kon-krēt′izm) thinking and behaving at simple and concrete (as contrasted with abstract) levels which are related to sensation.

concussion (kon-kush′un) [L. *concussio*] a violent jar or shock, or the condition which results from such an injury. **abdominal c., hydraulic,** abdominal injury produced in persons in the water by violent underwater explosions. **air c.,** see under *blast,* 3rd def. **c. of the brain,** loss of consciousness as the result of a blow to the head. In *mild* concussion there is transient loss of consciousness with possible impairment of the higher mental functions, such as retrograde amnesia and emotional lability. In *severe* concussion there is prolonged unconsciousness with impairment of the functions of the brain stem, such as transient loss of respiratory reflex, vasomotor activity, and dilatation of the pupils. Concussion is sometimes differentiated from contusion in that in the former the injury is functional, whereas in the latter it is organic. **c. of the labyrinth,** deafness with tinnitus, resulting from a blow on or explosion near the ear. **pulmonary c.,** mechanical damage to the lungs produced by an explosion. **c. of the retina,** commotio retinae. **c. of the spinal cord,** transient spinal cord dysfunction due to mechanical injury.

condensation (kon″den-sa′shun) [L. *condensatio,* from *con* together + *densare* to make thick] 1. the act of rendering, or process of becoming, more compact; in dentistry, the packing of filling materials into tooth cavities to eliminate voids within the cavity or filling. 2. a Freudian term for a fusion of events, thoughts or concepts to produce a new and simpler concept. 3. the process of passing from a gaseous to a liquid or solid phase.

condenser (kon-den′ser) [L. *condensare* to make thick, press close together] 1. a vessel or apparatus for condensing gases or vapors. 2. a device on a microscope used to supply illumination of the degree necessary for the specimen under study to be easily visible, and under the conditions necessary for the full resolving power of the instrument to be realized. 3. an apparatus by which charges of electricity can be accumulated, consisting of two conducting surfaces separated by a nonconductor. 4. in dentistry, an instrument used to pack a plastic filling material into the prepared cavity of a tooth. **Abbe's c.,** as originally designed, a two-lens condenser combination placed below the stage of a microscope. **cardioid c.,** a special type of condenser for illuminating a specimen in darkfield microscopy. **darkfield c.,** one with a central stop, permitting production of a hollow cone of light having its apex in the plane of the specimen. **paraboloid c.,** a special type of condenser for illuminating a specimen in darkfield microscopy.

condition (kon-dish′un) to train; to subject to conditioning.

conditioning (kon-dish′un-ing) learning in which a response is elicited by a neutral stimulus which previously has been repeatedly presented in conjunction with the stimulus that originally elicited the response. Called also *classical* or *respondent c.* **classical c.,** see *conditioning.* **instrumental c.,** learning in which a particular response is elicited by a stimulus because that response produces consequences which are rewarding to the organism; called also *operant c.* **operant c.,** instrumental c. **respondent c.,** see *conditioning.*

condom (kon′dum) [L. *condus* a receptacle; according to some authorities a corruption of *Condon,* the inventor] a sheath or cover for the penis, worn during coitus to prevent impregnation or infection.

conductance (kon-duk′tans) capacity for conducting or ability to convey; the unit of electrical conductance is the mho.

conduction (kon-duk′shun) [L. *conductio*] the transfer of sound waves, heat, nervous impulses, or electricity; see also under *system.* **aerial c.,** the passing of sound waves to the ear through the air. **aerotympanal c.,** the conduction of sound to the inner ear through the air and tympanum. **air c.,** the conduction of sound to the inner ear through the auditory canal and middle ear to the inner ear. **anomalous c.,** conduction of the sinus impulse which avoids the delay in passage through the normal atrioventricular node. **antidromic c.,** the conduction of a nerve impulse in a direction contrary to the normal direction, as from the axon toward the dendrites. **avalanche c.,** the conduction of nerve impulses which takes place when the terminals of one neuron come in contact with the bodies of several neurons, resulting in widespread discharge following relatively little input. **bone c.,** the conduction of sound to the inner ear through the bones of the skull; called also *cranial c., osteotympanic c.,* and *tissue c.* **concealed c.,** the conduction of a sinus impulse only part of the way through the conducting pathway of the heart so that a ventricular response is not elicited. **cranial c.,** bone conduction. **decremental c.,** the delay or failure of propagation of an impulse in the normal atrioventricular node resulting from progressive decrease in the rate of the rise and amplitude of the action potential as it spreads through the node. **delayed c.,** a nonspecific term indicating mild degree of atrioventricular heart block with an increase above the normal 0.2 second in the time interval between the atrial and ventricular contractions. **ephaptic c.,** the conduction of a nerve impulse across an ephapse, as opposed to synaptic conduction. **osteotympanic c.,** bone c. **saltatory c.,** the rapid passage of a potential from node (of Ranvier) to node of a myelinated nerve fiber, rather than along the full length of the membrane. **synaptic c.,** the conduction of a nerve impulse across a synapse. **tissue c.,** bone conduction.

conductivity (kon″duk-tiv′ĭ-te) the capacity of a body to conduct a current; when expressed in figures conductivity is the reciprocal of resistance. Gold, silver, and copper are good conductors.

conductor (kon-duk′tor) [L.] 1. a material that possesses conductivity; a substance that transmits electricity. 2. a grooved director for surgical use. 3. a healthy individual who may transmit some hereditary condition, as the daughter of a hemophiliac.

conduit (kon′doo-it) a channel for the passage of fluids. **ileal c.,** the surgical anastomsis of the ureters to one end of a detached segment of ileum, the other end being used to form a stoma on the abdominal wall.

conduplicato (kon-du″plĭ-ka′to) [L. *conduplicare* to double up] doubled up. **c. cor′poris,** a doubled-up attitude of a fetus in shoulder presentation.

condurangin (kon″du-rang′gin) either of two poisonous glycosides from condurango.

condurango (kon″du-rang′go) [Spanish American] the bark of condurango blanco, *Marsdenia (Gonolobus) condurango,* a South American asclepiadaceous plant; used as a bitter tonic and stomachic.

Condy's fluid (kon′dēz) [Henry Bollmann *Condy,* English physician of the 19th century] see under *fluid.*

condylar (kon′dĭ-lar) pertaining to a condyle.

condylarthrosis (kon″dil-ar-thro′sis) [*condyle* + Gr. *arthrōsis* joint] articulatio ellipsoidea.

condyle (kon′dīl) [L. *condylus;* Gr. *kondylos* knuckle] a rounded projection on a bone; see *condylus.* **extensor c. of humerus,** epicondylus lateralis humeri. **external c. of fe-**

mur, condylus lateralis femoris. **external c. of humerus,** epicondylus lateralis humeri. **external c. of tibia,** condylus lateralis tibiae. **fibular c. of femur,** condylus lateralis femoris. **flexor c. of humerus,** epicondylus medialis humeri. **c. of humerus,** condylus humeri. **internal c. of femur,** condylus medialis femoris. **internal c. of humerus,** epicondylus medialis humeri. **internal c. of tibia,** condylus medialis tibiae. **lateral c. of femur,** condylus lateralis femoris. **lateral c. of humerus,** epicondylus lateralis humeri. **lateral c. of tibia,** condylus lateralis tibiae. **c. of mandible,** processus condylaris mandibulae. **medial c. of femur,** condylus medialis femoris. **medial c. of humerus,** epicondylus medialis humeri. **medial c. of tibia,** condylus medialis tibiae. **c. of metacarpal bone,** caput ossis metacarpalis. **occipital c.,** condylus occipitalis. **radial c. of humerus,** epicondylus lateralis humeri. **c. of scapula,** angulus lateralis scapulae. **tibial c. of femur,** condylus medialis femoris. **ulnar c. of humerus,** epicondylus medialis humeri.

condylectomy (kon″dil-ek′to-me) [*condyle* + Gr. *ektomē* excision] excision of a condyle.

condyli (kon′dĭ-li) plural of *condylus.*

condylicus (kon-dil′ĭ-kus) pertaining to a condyle; condylar.

condylion (kon-dil′ĭ-on) [Gr. *kondylion* knob] the most lateral point on the surface of the caput mandibulae.

condyloid (kon′dĭ-loid) [*condyle* + Gr. *eidos* form] resembling a condyle or knuckle.

condyloma (kon″dĭ-lo′mah), pl. *condylo′mata* [Gr. *kondylōma,* knuckle or knob] 1. c. acuminatum. 2. rarely, c. latum. 3. in veterinary medicine, hyperplasia of the skin in cloven-hoofed animals, growing between the toes, caused by chronic inflammation. **c. acumina′tum,** a papilloma with a central core of connective tissue in a treelike structure covered with epithelium, usually occurring on the mucous membrane or skin of the external genitals or in the perianal region; although the lesions are usually few in number, they may aggregate to form large cauliflower-like masses. Caused by a virus, it is infectious, and autoinoculable. Called also *acuminate wart, verruca acuminata,* or *venereal wart.* **flat c.,** c. latum. **giant c. acumina′tum,** Buschke-Löwenstein tumor. **c. la′tum,** a broad and flat syphilitic condyloma located in warm, moist, intertriginous areas, especially about the anus and external genitals, it may become hypertrophic and erode to form a soft, red mass with a moist, weeping surface. Called also *flat c.* **pointed c.,** c. acuminatum.

condylomata (kon″dĭ-lo′mah-tah) plural of *condyloma.*

condylomatoid (kon″dĭ-lo′mah-toid) resembling a condyloma.

condylomatosis (kon″dĭ-lo′mah-to′sis) the presence of numerous condylomas.

condylomatous (kon″dĭ-lo′mah-tus) of the nature of a condyloma.

condylotomy (kon″dĭ-lot′o-me) [Gr. *kondylos* condyle + *temnein* to cut] surgical incision or division of a condyle or of condyles.

condylus (kon′dĭ-lus), pl. *con′dyli* [L.; Gr. *kondylos* knuckle] [NA] condyle: a rounded projection on a bone, usually for articulation with another. **c. hu′meri** [NA], condyle of humerus: the distal end of the humerus, including the various fossae as well as the trochlea and capitulum. **c. latera′lis fem′oris** [NA], lateral condyle of femur: the lateral of the two surfaces at the distal end of the femur that articulate with the superior surfaces of the head of the tibia; called also *external* or *fibular condyle of femur.* **c. latera′lis hu′meri,** epicondylus lateralis humeri. **c. latera′lis tib′iae** [NA], lateral condyle of tibia: the lateral articular eminence on the proximal end of the tibia; called also *external condyle of tibia.* **c. media′lis fem′oris** [NA], medial condyle of femur: the medial of the two surfaces at the distal end of the femur that articulate with the superior surfaces of the head of the tibia; called also *internal* or *tibial condyle of femur,* and *c. tibialis femoris.* **c. media′lis hu′meri,** epicondylus medialis humeri. **c. media′lis tib′iae** [NA], medial condyle of tibia: the medial articular eminence on the proximal end of the tibia; called also *internal condyle of tibia.* **c. occipita′lis** [NA], occipital condyle: one of two oval processes on the lateral portions of the occipital bone, on either side of the foramen magnum, for articulation with the atlas. **c. tibia′lis fem′oris,** c. medialis femoris.

cone (kōn) [Gr. *kōnos;* L. *conus*] 1. a solid figure or body with a circular base tapering to a point; specifically one of the conelike bodies of the retina; called also *conus.* See *retinal c's.* 2. in radiology, a conical or open-ended cylindrical structure attached over the portal of the x-ray tube housing, used as an aid in centering the radiation beam on the target field and as a guide to source-to-film distance; also, often designed to collimate primary and/or scattered radiation, and/or to retain disks for added filtration. 3. surgical cone. **acrosomal c.,** an axial body of the spermatozoon between the acrosomal granule and the nucleus. **adjusting c's,** a pair of hollow cones used in measuring the distance between the axes of the eyes when they are parallel. **antipodal c.,** the cone of rays opposite the spindle fibers of the amphiaster. **arterial c.,** conus arteriosus. **attraction c.,** fertilization c. **bifurcation c.,** the cone-shaped structure at the bifurcation of a dendrite. **cerebellar pressure c.,** a deformity of the brain caused by increased intracranial pressure, which forces the cerebellum downward into the spinal canal. **Dunham's c's,** see under *fan.* **ectoplacental c.,** the thickened trophoblast of the blastocyst in rodents which becomes the fetal portion of the placenta. **elastic c. of larynx,** conus elasticus laryngis. **ether c.,** originally an apparatus to be placed over the face for the administration of ether by inhalation, now used with various anesthetics. **fertilization c.,** a bulging of the cytoplasm in the ovum at the site of contact of a spermatozoon, which gradually engulfs the spermatozoon and then retracts, carrying the spermatozoon inward; called also *attraction c.* **growth c.,** a bulbous enlargement of the growing tip of a nerve axon. **Haller's c's,** lobuli epididymidis. **implantation c.,** the cone-shaped insertion of an axon in its neuron. **c. of light,** the triangular reflection of light seen on the membrana tympani; called also *Politzer's c. and light reflex.* **long c.,** in dental radiology, a tubular "cone" designed to establish an extended anode-to-skin distance, usually within a range of from 12 to 20 inches. **medullary c.,** conus medullaris. **ocular c.,** a cone of light in the eye, the base being on the cornea, the apex on the retina; called also *visual c.* **Politzer's c.,** c. of light. **pressure c.,** the area of compression exerted by a mass in the brain, as in uncal or transtentorial herniation. **primitive c.,** the conelike arrangement of the collecting tubules in the kidney. **retinal c's,** the highly specialized conical or flask-shaped outer segments of the visual cells; together with the retinal rods, they form the light-sensitive elements of the retina. Called also *cones, cone cells,* and *visual cones.* **sarcoplasmic c.,** the conical mass of sarcoplasm at each end of the nucleus of a smooth or cardiac muscle fiber. **short c.,** in dental radiology, a conical or a tubular "cone" having as one of its functions the establishment of an anode-to-skin distance of up to 9 inches. **surgical c.,** a cone of tissue removed surgically, as in partial excision of the cervix uteri. **terminal c. of spinal cord,** conus medullaris. **theca interna c.,** a wedge-shaped thickening of the theca interna projecting toward the ovarian surface, found only in growing follicles. **twin c's,** cone cells of the retina in which two cells are blended. **Tyndall c.,** the murky cone of scattered light seen when a colloid is viewed at right angles to the incident beam; it distinguishes colloids from crystalloids. **ureteral c.,** the upper conic part of the ureter; at ordinary rates of urine flow it is filled with urine during the resting phase of the renal pelvis and emptied during activity. **visual c.,** 1. ocular cone. 2. retinal cone.

cone-nose (kōn'nōs) see *Reduviidae.*

Conestron (kon-es'tron) trademark for a preparation of conjugated estrogens.

conexus (kŏ-nek'sus) [L. "connection, union"] a connecting structure. **c. intertendin'eus** [NA], tendinous junctions: narrow bands extending obliquely between the tendons of insertion of the extensor digitorum muscles on the back of the hand; called also *juncturae tendinum.* **c. interthalam'icus,** adhesio interthalamica.

confabulation (kon"fab-u-la'shun) the recitation of imaginary experiences to fill gaps in the memory, especially seen in organic psychoses, such as Korsakoff's psychosis; called also *fabrication.*

confectio (kon-fek'she-o) [L.] confection.

confection (kon-fek'shun) [L. *confectio*] a medicated conserve, sweetmeat, or electuary. **Damocrates' c.,** a confection of some thirty ingredients, the chief of which were agaric, frankincense, galbanum, cinnamon, garlic, gentian, ginger, opium, etc. **c. of senna,** a mild laxative containing powdered senna with other ingredients.

confertus (kon-fer'tus) [L.] close together; confluent.

configuration (kon-fig"u-ra'shun) 1. the general form of a body. 2. in gestalt psychology, an organized whole with interdependent parts so that the whole is more than the sum of its parts. **cis c.,** in genetics, the condition (coupling) in which the two mutant genes of a pseudoallele are on one chromosome and the two wild-type genes are on the homologous chromosome. Called also *cis position.* Cf. *trans c.* **trans c.,** in genetics, the condition (repulsion) in which each of two homologous chromosomes contains one mutant and one wild-type gene of a pseudoallele. Called also *trans position.* Cf. *cis c.*

confinement (kon-fin'ment) restraint within a specific area; used especially to designate the termination of pregnancy with delivery of the infant; see *labor.*

conflict (kon'flikt) a painful state of consciousness due to clash between opposing trends found to a certain extent in every person. **approach-approach c.,** conflict resulting from two available goals which are desirable but incompatible. **approach-avoidance c.,** conflict resulting from a single goal having both desirable and undesirable consequences. **avoidance-avoidance c.,** conflict resulting from the desire to avoid two equally distasteful alternatives. **extrapsychic c.,** that between the self and the external environment. **intrapsychic c.,** that between forces within the personality.

confluence (kon'floo-ens) [L. *confluens* running together] the meeting of streams; in embryology the flowing of cells, a compo-

nent process of gastrulation. **c. of sinuses,** confluens sinuum.

confluens (kon'floo-ens) [L.] a place of running together; the meeting of streams. **c. sin'uum** [NA], confluence of sinuses: the dilated point of confluence of the superior sagittal, straight, occipital, and two transverse sinuses of the dura mater, lodged in a depression at one side of the internal occipital protuberance; called also *torcular Herophili.*

confluent (kon'floo-ent) [L. *confluens* running together] becoming merged; not discrete.

confocal (kon-fo'kal) having the same focus.

conformation (kon"for-ma'shun) the particular shape of an entity, such as the shape a molecule assumes.

confrication (kon"fri-ka'shun) [L. *confricatio*] the rubbing of a drug to the condition of a powder.

confrontation (kon"frun-ta'shun) [L. *con* together + *frons* face] a technique in treating psychological disorders whereby the contradictory statements or actions of a patient are brought directly to his attention.

confusion (kon-fu'zhun) disturbed orientation in regard to time, place, or person, sometimes accompanied by disordered consciousness.

confusional (kon-fu'zhun-al) pertaining to, characterized by, or resulting in confusion.

cong. abbreviation for L. *con'gius,* gallon.

congelation (kon"jĕ-la'shun) [L. *congelatio*] frostbite or freezing.

congeneic (kon"jĕ-na'ik) of or relating to a strain of animals developed from an inbred (isogenic) strain by repeated matings with animals from another stock that have a foreign gene, the final congeneic strain then presumably differing from the original inbred strain by the presence of this gene.

congener (kon'jĕ-ner) [L. *con* together + *genus* race] something closely related to another thing, as a member of the same genus, a muscle having the same function as another, or a chemical compound closely related to another in composition and exerting similar or antagonistic effects, or something derived from the same source or stock. Also, a secondary product in alcohol fermentation that helps to determine the composition of the final product.

congeneric (kon"jĕ-ner'ik) pertaining to a congener.

congenerous (kon-jen'er-us) [L. *con* together + *genus* race] having a common action or function; derived from the same source. See *congener.*

congenital (kon-jen'ĭ-tal) [L. *congenitus* born together] existing at, and usually before, birth; referring to conditions that are present at birth, regardless of their causation. Cf. *hereditary.*

congested (kon-jest'ed) overloaded, as with blood; in a state of congestion.

congestin (kon-jes'tin) a toxic substance derived from the tentacles of sea anemones which, when injected into dogs, causes intense congestion of the splanchnic vessels, and hemorrhage; originally called *actinocongestin.* Cf. *medusocongestin.*

congestion (kon-jest'yun) [L. *congestio,* from *congerere* to heap together] excessive or abnormal accumulation of blood in a part. **active c.,** accumulation of blood in a part on account of the dilatation of the lumen of its blood vessels. **functional c.,** increased vascularization and flow of blood to an organ during the performance of its function. **hypostatic c.,** congestion of the lowest part of an organ by reason of the action of gravity when the circulation is much enfeebled. **neuroparalytic c.,** that which results from paralysis of the constrictor fibers of the vasomotor nerves. **neurotonic c.,** that which is due to irritation of the vasodilator nerves. **passive c.,** the congestion of a part due to the obstruction to the escape of blood from the part; called also *venous c.* **physiologic c.,** increased vascularization and blood flow that occurs during functional activity. **pulmonary c.,** engorgement of the pulmonary vessels, with transudation of fluid into the alveolar and interstitial spaces; it occurs in cardiac disease, infections, and certain injuries. **venous c.,** passive c.

congestive (kon-jes'tiv) pertaining to, characterized by, or resulting in congestion.

congius (kon'je-us) [L.] a gallon; abbreviated c. or cong.

conglobate (kon'glo-bāt) [L. *conglobatus*] forming a rounded mass or clump; said of certain glands.

conglobation (kon"glo-ba'shun) the act of forming, or the state of being formed, into a rounded mass.

conglomerate (kon-glom'er-āt) [L. *con* together + *glomerare* to heap] heaped together.

conglutin (kon-gloo'tin) a protein from almonds and from seeds of various leguminous plants.

conglutinant (kon-gloo'tĭ-nant) [L. *conglutinare* to glue together] promoting union, as of the lips of a wound.

conglutinatio (kon-gloo"tĭ-na'she-o) [L.] conglutination. **c. orific'ii exter'ni,** a condition in labor in which the circular fibers around the cervical os will not relax, and the cervix remains closed.

conglutination (kon-gloo″tĭ-na′shun) 1. agglutination of erythrocytes that is dependent upon both complement and antibodies; see *conglutinin.* 2. the adherence of tissues to each other.

conglutinin (kon-gloo′tĭ-nin) a factor present in fresh bovine and certain other sera that agglutinates erythrocytes in the presence of complement. It has been used as the indicator system in the conglutinating complement absorption test (CCAT) in the serodiagnosis of glanders, Q fever, and infection with microorganisms of the psittacosis-lymphogranuloma group (*Chlamydia*). Called also *bovine colloid.*

congressus (kon-gres′us) [L. "a coming together"] coitus.

CO(NH₂)₂ urea.

coni (ko′ni) [L.] plural of *conus.*

conic (kon′ik) conical.

conical (kon′e-kal) cone-shaped.

conidia (ko-nid′e-ah) plural of *conidium.*

conidial (ko-nid′e-al) pertaining to or of the nature of conidia; bearing conidia.

conidiophore (ko-nid′e-o-fōr) [L. *conidium* + Gr. *phoros* bearing] the branch of the mycelium of a fungus that bears conidia.

Conidiosporales (ko-nid″e-o-spo-ra′lēz) former name for Moniliales.

conidiospore (ko-nid′e-o-spōr) [Gr. *konidion* a particle of dust + *spore*] conidium.

conidium (ko-nid′e-um), pl. *conid′ia.* An asexual fungal spore shed at maturity (deciduous), and formed by splitting off from the summit of a conidiophore; called also *exospore.* See *spore.* Cf. *aleuriospore* and *chlamydospore* (def. 1).

coniine (co′ne-ēn) a poisonous, liquid alkaloid from *Conium maculatum* L. (poison hemlock), C₈H₁₇N.

coniofibrosis (ko″ne-o-fi-bro′sis) [Gr. *konis* dust + *fibrosis*] a form of pneumoconiosis marked by an exuberant growth of connective tissue caused by a specific irritant; it may occur in asbestosis, silicosis, and silicotuberculosis.

coniology (ko-ne-ol′ŏ-je) [Gr. *konis* dust + *-logy*] the scientific study of dust, its influence and its effects on plant and animal life.

coniolymphstasis (ko″ne-o-limf′stah-sis) a form of pneumoconiosis caused by dusts that act by blocking the lymphatics.

coniometer (ko″ne-om′ĕ-ter) konometer.

coniophage (ko′ne-o-fāj″) [Gr. *konis* dust + *phagein* to eat] a macrophage that ingests dust particles.

coniosis (ko″ne-o′sis) [Gr. *konis* dust] a disease state caused by the inhalation of dust, such as pneumoconiosis.

Coniosporium (ko″ne-o-spōr′e-um) a genus of saprophytic fungi. *C. cortica′le* (*Cryptostroma corticale*), which grows under the bark of certain trees, causes coniosporosis.

coniosporosis (ko″ne-o-spo-ro′sis) a condition characterized by asthmatic symptoms and acute pneumonitis, caused by inhalation of spores of *Coniosporium corticale*, a fungus which grows under the bark of certain trees; observed in workers engaged in peeling logs.

coniotomy (ko″ne-ot′o-me) incision through the conus elasticus laryngis.

coniotoxicosis (ko″ne-o-tok″sĭ-ko′sis) a form of pneumoconiosis in which the irritants affect the tissues directly.

Conium (ko-ni′um) [L.; Gr. *kōneion*] a genus of umbelliferous plants, the hemlocks. **C. macula′tum** L., poison hemlock; see *hemlock,* def. 2.

conization (kon″ĭ-za′shun) the removal of a cone of tissue, as in partial excision of the cervix uteri. **cold c.,** that done with a cold knife, as opposed to electrocautery, to better preserve the histologic elements.

conjugal (kon′ju-gal) [L. *con* together + *jugum* a yoke] pertaining to marriage; pertaining to husband and wife.

conjugata (kon″ju-ga′tah) [NA] the anteroposterior diameter of the superior aperture of the minor pelvis; see also *true conjugate diameter.* **c. anatom′ica,** true conjugate diameter. **c. diagona′lis,** diagonal conjugate diameter. **c. ve′ra,** true conjugate diameter. **c. ve′ra obstet′rica,** obstetric conjugate diameter.

conjugate (kon′ju-gāt) [L. *conjugatus* yoked together] 1. paired, or equally coupled; working in unison. 2. a conjugate diameter of the pelvic inlet; used alone usually to denote the true conjugate diameter. See under *diameter.* **anatomic c.,** true conjugate diameter; see under *diameter.* **diagonal c.,** see under *diameter.* **external c.,** see under *diameter.* **obstetric c.,** see under *diameter.*

conjugation (kon″ju-ga′shun) [L. *conjugatio* a blending] the act of joining together. In bacterial genetics, a form of sexual reproduction in which a donor bacterium (male) contributes some, or all, of its DNA (in the form of a replicated set) to a recipient (female), which then incorporates differing genetic information into its own chromosome by recombination, and passes the

recombined set on to its progeny by replication. In chemistry, the joining together of two compounds to produce another compound, such as the combination of a toxic product with some substance in the body to form a detoxified product, which is then eliminated.

conjugon (kon′ju-gon) an episome that promotes conjugation.

conjunctiva (kon″junk-ti′vah), pl. *conjuncti′vae* [L.] the delicate membrane that lines the eyelids (*palpebral conjunctiva*) and covers the exposed surface of the sclera (*bulbar* or *ocular conjunctiva*); called also *tunica conjunctiva* [NA].

conjunctival (kon″junk-ti′val) pertaining to the conjunctiva.

conjunctiviplasty (kon-junk′tĭ-vĭ-plas″te) conjunctivoplasty.

conjunctivitis (kon-junk″tĭ-vi′tis) inflammation of the conjunctiva, generally consisting of conjunctival hyperemia associated with a discharge. **actinic c.,** conjunctivitis produced by ultraviolet (actinic) rays, as that of Klieg lights, therapeutic lamps, or acetylene torches. **acute contagious c.,** a mucopurulent inflammation of the conjunctiva occurring in epidemic form and caused by *Hemophilus aegypticus;* called also *epidemic c., Sanders' disease,* and *pink eye.* **acute hemorrhagic c.,** a highly contagious disease, certain epidemics of which have been associated etiologically with enteroviruses, characterized by subconjunctival hemorrhage varying from minute petechiae to copious, and by sudden swelling of the eyelids and congestion, redness, and pain in the eye. **allergic c., anaphylactic c.,** hay fever. **angular c.,** conjunctivitis with characteristic reddening at the canthi, usually due to Morax-Axenfeld bacillus or *Staphylococcus aureus.* **arc-flash c.,** actinic conjunctivitis from electric welding. **atopic c.,** allergic conjunctivitis of the immediate type, due to such airborne allergens as pollens, dusts, spores, and animal hair. **atropine c.,** follicular conjunctivitis from continued use of atropine. **blennorrheal c.,** gonorrheal c. **calcareous c.,** c. petrificans. **catarrhal c.,** a mild form characterized by excessive mucous secretion. **chemical c.,** that due to exposure to chemical irritants. **croupous c.,** membranous c. **diphtheritic c.,** a purulent form due to *Corynebacterium diphtheriae;* diphtheria of the conjunctiva, a major cause of membranous conjunctivitis. **diplobacillary c.,** Morax-Axenfeld's c. **eczematous c.,** phlyctenular c. **Egyptian c.,** trachoma, def. 1. **epidemic c.,** acute contagious c. **follicular c.,** a form characterized by dense localized infiltrations of lymphoid tissue that occur as a response to irritation. **gonococcal c.,** gonorrheal c. **gonorrheal c.,** a severe form caused by infection with gonococci; called also *blennorrheal c.* and *gonoblennorrhea.* **granular c.,** trachoma. **inclusion c.,** conjunctivitis caused by an organism (*Chlamydia trachomatis*) of the psittacosis-lymphogranuloma venereum-trachoma group; it affects primarily newborn infants, beginning as an acute purulent conjunctivitis that leads to papillary hypertrophy of the palpebral conjunctiva. Called also *inclusion blennorrhea* and *swimming pool c.* **larval c.,** myiasis of the conjunctiva. **c. medicamento′sa,** conjunctivitis due to medication. **membranous c.,** a variety associated with the formation of a whitish-gray membrane; called also *croupous c.* **meningococcus c.,** conjunctivitis occurring as a complication of epidemic cerebrospinal meningitis. **molluscum c.,** conjunctivitis occurring as a complication of molluscum contagiosum. **Morax-Axenfeld's c.,** a form of conjunctivitis due to *Hemophilus duplex;* called also *diplobacillary c.* **c. necrot′icans infectio′sus,** an infectious conjunctivitis associated with unilateral swelling of the parotid and submaxillary glands; called also *Pascheff's c.* **c. nodo′sa, nodular c.,** ophthalmia nodosa. **Parinaud's c.,** Parinaud's oculoglandular syndrome. **Pascheff's c.,** c. necroticans infectiosus. **c. petrif′icans,** a variety of conjunctivitis marked by the formation of deposits of chalky concretions in the conjunctiva and attended with necrosis; called also *calcareous c.* **phlyctenular c.,** a variety marked by small vesicles or ulcers, each surrounded by a reddened zone; called also *eczematous c.* and *scrofular c.* See also *phlyctenulosis.* **prairie c.,** chronic conjunctivitis marked by white spots on the conjunctiva of the lids. **pseudomembranous c.,** inflammation of the conjunctiva in which a fibrous exudate forms a false membrane on the epithelial surface; it may result from diphtheria or hyperacute conjunctivitis of other etiology. **purulent c.,** a variety characterized by a discharge of pus. **scrofular c.,** phlyctenular c. **shipyard c.,** epidemic keratoconjunctivitis. **spring c.,** vernal c. **squirrel plague c.,** c. tularensis. **swimming pool c.,** inclusion c. **trachomatous c.,** trachoma, def. 1. **tularemic c., c. tularen′sis,** conjunctivitis associated with tularemia, caused by injection with *Francisella tularensis;* it begins with single or multiple necrotic papules, usually in the lower cul-de-sac, followed by generalized conjunctivitis with enlargement and tenderness of the associated lymph nodes, lasting about four weeks. Called also *squirrel plague c.* **uratic c.,** conjunctivitis marked by the deposit of crystals of uric acid or sodium urate in the conjunctiva. **vernal c.,** conjunctivitis characteristically occurring in the spring; called also *spring c., Fruehjahr,* and *spring catarrh.* **welder's c.,** conjunctivitis occurring in welders, caused by the glare from electric or acetylene torches. **Widmark's c.,** congestion of the inferior tarsal conjunctiva, with occasionally slight stippling of the cornea.

conjunctivodacryocystostomy (kon″junk-ti″vo-dak″re-o-sis-tos′to-me) surgical connection of the lacrimal sac directly to the conjunctival sac.

conjunctivoma (kon-junk″tĭ-vo′mah) a tumor of the eyelid made up of conjunctival tissue.

conjunctivoplasty (kon″junk-ti′vo-plas″te) [*conjunctiva* + Gr. *plassein* to form] repair of a defect of the conjunctiva by plastic operation.

conjunctivorhinostomy (kon″junk-ti″vo-ri-nos′to-me) surgical correction of total lacrimal canalicular obstruction: a dacryocystorhinostomy is done by suturing the posterior flaps, and the lacrimal caruncle is dissected out, preserving the conjunctiva.

Conn's syndrome (konz) [Jerome W. *Conn*, American internist, born 1907] primary hyperaldosteronism.

connatal (kon-na′tal) [L. *con* along with + *natus* birth] occurring at the time of birth; acquired at birth.

connate (kon′nāt) connatal.

connection (kŏ-nek′shun) 1. the act of connecting or state of being connected. 2. anything that connects; a connector. **clamp c.,** a short tubular branch connecting one cell of a hypha to another, formed by fusion during cell division in certain basidiomycetous fungi, and serving in the transfer of the two daughter nuclei of the parent cell to a newly formed cell.

connector (kŏ-nek′tor) anything serving as a link between two separate objects or units, such as the portion of a neural arc between the receptor and the effector. In dentistry, the portion of a fixed or removable partial denture that unites its components. **major c.,** a plate or bar, such as a labial, lingual, or palatal bar, that unites two or more bilateral parts of a removable partial denture. **minor c.,** a connecting link between the major connector or base of a partial denture and other units of the prosthesis, such as clasps, indirect retainers, and occlusal rests; called also *connector bar.*

Connell's suture (kŏn′elz) [Frank Gregory *Connell*, American surgeon, 1875–1968] see under *suture.*

connexus (kŏ-nek′sus) see *conexus.*

conoid (ko′noid) [Gr. *kōnoeidēs*] resembling or shaped like a cone. **Sturm's c.,** the changing shapes of the diffusion images of a point in various forms of astigmatism; the image may be an ellipse, a circle, or a sharp line.

Conolly's system (kon′ŏ-lēz) [John *Conolly*, English alienist, 1794–1866] see under *system.*

conomyoidin (ko″no-mi-oi′din) [Gr. *kōnos* cone + *mys* muscle + *eidos* form] a protoplasmic material within the cones of some retinas that expands and contracts under the influence of light, causing the cones to shift.

conophthalmus (kŏn″of-thal′mus) [Gr. *kōnos* cone + *ophthalmos* eye] staphyloma corneae, def 1.

Conorhinus (ko″no-ri′nus) [Gr. *kōnos* cone + *rhis* nose] a genus name formerly applied to insects of the family Reduviidae, now placed in the genera *Panstrongylus* and *Triatoma.*

conquinine (kon-kwin′in) quinidine.

Conradi's line (kon-rah′dez) [Andreas Christian *Conradi*, Norwegian physician, 1809–1869] see under *line.*

Conray (kon′ra) trademark for a preparation of iothalamate meglumine.

Cons. abbreviation for L. *conser′va,* keep.

consanguineous (kon″san-gwin′e-us) related by blood.

consanguinity (kon″san-gwin′ĭ-te) [L. *consanguinitas*] kinship; relationship by blood.

conscience (kon′shens) an individual's set of moral values. It corresponds to the conscious part of the superego (q.v.).

conscious (kon′shus) [L. *conscius* aware] capable of responding to sensory stimuli and having subjective experiences; awake; aware.

consciousness (kon′shus-nes) the state of being conscious; responsiveness of the mind to the impressions made by the senses. **collective c.,** the aggregation of the conscious processes of all the individuals in a group; shared ideas and experiences. **colon c.,** a condition in which the patient is aware of the colon and its activities, because of disturbance of the normal defecation reflex; embracing chronic constipation. **double c., dual c.,** see *multiple personality,* under *personality.* **noetic c.,** consciousness in which the experiences are largely cognitive.

conscious-sedation (kon′shus-se-da′shun) in dental anesthesia, a state of sedation in which the conscious patient is rendered free of fear, apprehension, and anxiety through the use of pharmacological agents.

consensual (kon-sen′shu-al) [L. *consensus* agreement] excited by reflex stimulation; used especially to designate the similar reaction of both pupils to a stimulus applied to only one.

conservative (kon-ser′vah-tiv) [L. *conservare* to preserve] designed to preserve health, restore function, and repair structures by nonradical methods, as conservative surgery. Cf. *radical.*

conserve (kon′serv) [L. *conserva*] a confection, electuary, or medicated sweetmeat.

consilia (kon-sil′e-ah) [L. pl. of *consilium* a deliberation, consultation] letters published by physicians of the 13th to 17th centu-

ries, outlining the symptomatology and treatment of diseases under their observation.

consolidant (kon-sol′ĭ-dant) [L. *consolidare* to make firm] 1. promoting the healing or union of parts. 2. an agent that promotes the healing or union of parts.

consolidation (kon-sol″ĭ-da′shun) [L. *consolidatio*] solidification; the process of becoming or the condition of being solid, as when the lung becomes firm as air spaces are filled with exudate in pneumonia.

consolute (kon′so-lūt) perfectly miscible.

consonance (kon′so-nans) [L. *consonantia*] agreement or harmony. **cognitive c.,** harmony of thoughts, beliefs, and behavior.

consonation (kon″so-na′shun) the presence of consonating rales; see under *rale.*

conspecific (kon″spĕ-sif′ik) 1. of or pertaining to the same species. 2. a member of the same species.

constancy (kon′stan-se) the state of being constant.

constant (kon′stant) [L. *constans* standing together] 1. not failing; remaining unaltered. 2. a datum, fact, or principle that is not subject to change. **Ambard's c.,** see *Ambard's formula,* under *formula.* **association c.,** a measure of the extent of a reversible association between two molecular species; called also *binding c.* **Avogadro's c.,** see under *number.* **binding c.,** association c. **decay c.,** the fraction of the number of atoms of a radionuclide which decay in unit time; symbol λ. Called also *disintegration c.* and *radioactive c.* **dielectric c.,** the dielectric value of any substance compared with air, which is taken as 1. **disintegration c.,** decay c. **dissociation c.,** the equilibrium constant for the dissociation of a weak acid into hydrogen ion and its conjugate base in solution. **equilibrium c.,** an expression of the relationship between the equilibrium activities of reactants and products of a reversible chemical reaction to one another. **Faraday's c.,** 1. the quantity of electricity contained in one mole of electrons; the value of the constant is 96,493.5 coulombs per mole of electrons. 2. the minimum amount of electricity necessary to electrodeposit one mole of a univalent metal. **gravitational c., c. of gravitation,** the constant of proportionality in the law of gravitation, equal to 6.67 × 10⁻¹¹ newton m.²/kg.²; symbol G. Called also *Newtonian constant of gravitation.* **Lapicque's c.,** the figure 0.37, used for converting noninductive resistance into direct current equivalents. **Michaelis c.,** a constant representing the substrate concentration at which the velocity of an enzyme reaction is half the maximal velocity; symbol K_m. **Newtonian c. of gravitation,** gravitational c. **Planck's c., quantum c.,** a constant, *h,* which represents the ratio of the energy of any quantum of radiation to its frequency; the value of *h* is 6.625 × 10⁻²⁷ erg seconds. **radioactive c.,** decay c. **sedimentation c.,** a measure, commonly expressed in Svedberg units, of the relative sedimentation rate of molecules under an induced gravitational field, as in a centrifuge; symbol S. **urea c.,** see *Ambard's formula,* under *formula.*

constipated (kon′stĭ-pāt″ed) affected with constipation.

constipation (kon″stĭ-pa′shun) [L. *constipatio* a crowding together] infrequent or difficult evacuation of the feces. **atonic c.,** constipation due to intestinal atony. **gastrojejunal c.,** constipation due to reflex inhibition from some disease of the gastrointestinal tract. **proctogenous c.,** constipation due to some abnormality of the defecation reflex resulting in failure of fecal masses in the rectum to excite impulses leading to their evacuation. **spastic c.,** constipation marked by spasmodic constriction of a portion of the intestine; seen in neurasthenia and lead poisoning.

constitution (kon″stĭ-tu′shun) [L. *constitutio*] 1. the make-up or functional habit of the body, determined by the genetic, biochemical, and physiologic endowment of the individual, and modified in great measure by environmental factors. Cf. *diathesis* and *type.* 2. in chemistry, the arrangement of atoms in a molecule. Cf. *atomic configuration.* **ideo-obsessional c.** (obs.), a peculiar psychic constitution marked by a tendency to worrying, fretting, exaggerated doubts, and excessive introspection. **lymphatic c.,** a condition of hyperplasia of the lymphatic system. **neuropathic c.,** that quality of mind and body once thought to predispose to nervous disease. **psychopathic c.** (obs.), a tendency toward mental imbalance. **vasoneurotic c.,** a constitution characterized by instability of the vasomotor mechanism.

constitutional (kon″stĭ-tu′shun-al) 1. affecting the whole constitution of the body; not local. 2. pertaining to the constitution.

constriction (kon-strik′shun) [L. *con* together + *stringere* to draw] 1. a constricted part or place; a stricture. 2. in psychiatry, a diminution in range of thinking or feeling, associated with diminished spontaneity. **apical c.,** that point of the apical portion of the root canal of a tooth having the narrowest diameter; it may be associated with the dentinocemental junction cementum alone or with dentin alone. **duodenopyloric c.,** the constriction marking the junction of the stomach and duodenum. **primary c.,** centromere. **Ranvier's c's,** nodes of Ranvier. **secondary c.,** in genetics, the narrowed heterochromatic area of the short arms of acrocentric autosomes by which a satellite is attached.

constrictive (kon-strik′tiv) causing constriction or having a tendency to constriction.

constrictor (kon-strik′tor) [L.] that which constricts, such as a muscle or an instrument by which a part may be constricted. See *Table of Musculi.* **c. isth′mi fau′cium,** musculus palatoglossus. **c. na′ris,** pars transversa musculi nasalis. **c. ure′thrae,** musculus sphincter urethrae. **c. vagi′nae,** the musculus bulbospongiosus in the female.

constructive (kon-struk′tiv) pertaining to any process of construction; in physiology, anabolic.

consult (kon-sult′) [L. *consultus*] to confer with another physician about a case.

consultant (kon-sul′tant) [L. *consultare* to counsel] a physician called in for advice and counsel.

consultation (kon″sul-ta′shun) [L. *consultatio*] a deliberation by two or more physicians with respect to the diagnosis or treatment in any particular case.

consumption (kon-sump′shun) [L. *consumptio* a wasting] 1. the act of consuming, or the process of being consumed. 2. a wasting away of the body; formerly applied especially to pulmonary tuberculosis. **galloping c.,** pulmonary tuberculosis that runs an exceptionally rapid course. **luxus c.,** the ingestion of excess protein which does not form part of the tissues but remains in the body as a reserve supply.

consumptive (kon-sump′tiv) 1. of the nature of or affected with consumption. 2. (*obs.*) a person affected with tuberculosis of the lungs.

Cont. abbreviation for L. *contu′sus,* bruised.

contact (kon′takt) [L. *contactus* a touching together] 1. a mutual touching of two bodies or persons. 2. an individual known to have been sufficiently near to an infected individual to have been exposed to the transfer of infectious material. 3. contactant. **balancing c.,** the contact between the upper and lower occlusal surfaces of the teeth (of the natural or artificial dentition) on the side opposite the working contact. **complete c.,** contact of the entire proximal surface of one tooth with the entire proximal surface of the adjacent tooth. **direct c., immediate c.,** the touching by a healthy person of a person having a communicable disease, the disease often being transmitted as a result. **indirect c.,** that achieved through some intervening medium, as the propagation of a communicable disease through the air or by means of fomites. **initial c.,** the first meeting of the upper and lower teeth when the jaws are brought together. **mediate c.,** indirect c. **occlusal c.,** the contact between the upper and lower teeth when the jaws are closed in habitual occlusion. **occlusal c., deflective,** a condition in which the mandible is diverted from a normal path of closure to centric jaw relation by abnormal contact between upper and lower teeth. **occlusal c., interceptive,** a condition in which the normal movement of the mandible is stopped or deviated by an initial or premature contact of the teeth. **occlusal c., premature,** occlusal c., interceptive. **proximal c., proximate c.,** touching of the proximal surfaces of two adjoining teeth. **weak c.,** contact in which the proximal surface of one tooth barely touches that of the adjacent tooth, enhancing the packing of food between the teeth. **working c.,** the contact between the upper and lower teeth (of the natural or artificial dentition) on the side toward which the mandible has been moved in mastication.

contactant (kon-tak′tant) an allergen capable of inducing delayed contact-type hypersensitivity of the animal or human epidermis after one or more episodes of contact.

contactologist (kon″tak-tol′o-jist) an individual skilled in contactology.

contactology (kon″tak-tol′o-je) the specialized field of knowledge related to the use and prescription of contact lenses.

contagion (kon-ta′jun) [L. *contagio* contact, infection] 1. the communication of disease from one person to another. 2. a contagious disease. 3. a contagium. **direct c., immediate c.,** communication of disease by direct contact with a sick person. **mediate c.,** communication of a disease from a sick to a well person through an intervening object or person. **psychic c.,** communication of psychological symptoms through mental influence.

contagiosity (kon″ta″je-os′i-te) the quality of being contagious.

contagious (kon-ta′jus) [L. *contagiosus*] capable of being transmitted from one person to another.

contagium (kon-ta′je-um), pl. *conta′gia* [L.] (*obs.*) any virus or other infectious agent that may transmit a disease.

contaminant (kon-tam′ĭ-nant) something that causes contamination.

contamination (kon-tam″ĭ-na′shun) [L. *contaminatio,* from *con* together + *tangere* to touch] 1. the soiling or making inferior by contact or mixture as by the introduction of organisms in a wound, or sewage in a stream. 2. the deposition of radioactive material in any place where it is not desired, and particularly where its presence may be harmful or constitute a radiation hazard.

content (kon′tent) that which is contained within a thing. **latent c.,** the hidden part of a dream or thought, which can be discovered only by free association or by some other appropriate technique. **manifest c.,** the outward form of a dream as remembered by the dreamer.

contiguity (kon″tĭ-gu′ĭ-te) [L. *contiguus* in contact] contact or close proximity; the quality of being contiguous.

contiguous (kon-tig′u-us) [L. *contiguus*] in contact or nearly so.

Contin. abbreviation for L. *continue′tur,* let it be continued.

continence (kon′tĭ-nens) [L. *continentia*] the ability to refrain from yielding to desire, as self-restraint with respect to sexual indulgence. **fecal c.,** the ability to retain the contents of the colon until conditions are proper for defecation. **urinary c.,** the ability to retain the contents of the bladder until conditions are proper for urination.

continent (kon′tĭ-nent) able to refrain from yielding to normal impulses, as sexual desire, or from the urge to defecate or urinate.

continued (kon-tin′ūd) having no remission, intermission, or interruption.

continuity (kon″tĭ-nu′ĭ-te) [L. *continuitas,* uninterrupted succession] the quality of being without interruption or separation.

continuous (kon-tin′u-us) [L. *continuus*] not interrupted; having no interruption.

contologist (kon-tol′o-jist) contactologist.

contology (kon-tol′o-je) contactology.

contour (kon′toor) [Fr.] 1. the normal outline or configuration of the body or of a part. 2. to shape a solid along certain desired lines. **height of c.,** in dentistry, the line encircling a tooth at its greatest bulge with reference to a predetermined path of insertion for a removable partial denture.

contoured (kon′toord) 1. having an irregularly undulating outline or surface; said of bacterial colonies. 2. shaped along certain desired lines, as a dental or other prosthesis or plastic restoration.

contra- (kon′trah) [L. *contra* against] a prefix signifying against, opposed.

contra-angle (kon″trah-ang′g'l) an angulation by which the working point of a surgical instrument is brought close to the long axis of its shaft; it may involve two, three, or four bends, or angles, in its shank.

contra-aperture (kon″trah-ap′er-chūr) [*contra-* + L. *apertura* opening] a second opening made in an abscess to facilitate the discharge of its contents.

contraception (kon″trah-sep′shun) the prevention of conception or impregnation. **intrauterine c.,** prevention of conception by use of a device inserted in the uterus; see under *device*.

contraceptive (kon″trah-sep′tiv) 1. diminishing the likelihood of, or preventing, conception. 2. an agent that diminishes the likelihood of or prevents conception. **intrauterine c.,** see under *device*. **oral c.,** a hormonal compound taken orally in order to block ovulation and prevent the occurrence of pregnancy.

contract (kon-tract′) [L. *contractus,* from *contrahere* to draw together] 1. to shorten, or reduce in size, as a muscle. 2. to acquire or incur.

contractile (kon-trak′tĭl) [L. *con* together + *trahere* to draw] having the power or tendency to contract in response to a suitable stimulus.

contractility (kon″trak-til′ĭ-te) capacity for becoming short in response to a suitable stimulus. **cardiac c.,** the property of the cardiac muscle cells or tissues to shorten in response to an appropriate stimulus. **galvanic c.,** galvanocontractility. **idiomuscular c.,** a contractility peculiar to wasted or degenerated muscles. **neuromuscular c.,** normal, as distinguished from idiomuscular, contractility.

contraction (kon-trak′shun) [L. *contractus* drawn together] 1. a shortening or reduction in size; in connection with muscles contraction implies shortening and/or development of tension. 2. a morbid or pathologic shortening or shrinkage. 3. in orthodontics, unusual narrowness of the dental arch. **anodal closure c.** (ACC), contraction of the muscles at the anode when the electrical circuit is closed. **anodal opening c.** (AOC), contraction of the muscles at the anode when the electrical circuit is broken. **automatic ventricular c.,** a ventricular contraction caused by an impulse arising in the atrioventricular node; called also *escaped ventricular c.* **Braxton Hicks c's,** Hicks' sign; see under *sign*. **carpopedal c.,** the condition resulting from chronic shortening of the muscles of the fingers, toes, arms, and legs in tetany. **cathodal closure c.** (CCC), contraction of muscles at the cathode when the electrical circuit is closed. **cathodal opening c.** (COC), contraction of the muscles at the cathode when the electrical circuit is opened. **cicatricial c.,** the shrinkage and spontaneous closing of open skin wounds. **clonic c.,** contraction of a muscle alternating with periods of relaxation. **closing c.,** contraction occurring at the point of application of the stimulus when the electrical circuit is closed. **Dupuytren's c.,** Dupuytren's contracture. **Dupuytren's c., false,** a contracted state of the palm and fingers due to injury of the palmar fascia. **escaped ventricular c.,** automatic ventricular c. **fibrillary c's,** abnormal spontaneous contractions occurring successively in different bundles of the fibers of a diseased muscle. **galvanotonic c.,** a sustained muscular contraction produced by a continuous electrical current. **Gowers' c.,** front tap c. **Hicks' c's,** see under *sign.* **hourglass c.,** contraction of an organ (as the stomach or uterus) at or near the middle. **idiomuscular c.,** a contraction produced by direct electrical stimulation of a wasted muscle. **isometric c.,** muscle contraction without appreciable shortening or change in distance between its origin and insertion. **isotonic c.,** muscle contraction without appreciable change in the force of contraction; the distance between the muscle's origin and insertion becomes less. **myotatic c.,** contraction or irritability of a muscle brought into play by sudden passive stretching or by tapping on its tendon. **opening c.,** contraction occurring at the point of application of the stimulus when the electrical circuit is opened. **palmar c.,** Dupuytren's contracture. **paradoxical c.,** the contraction of a muscle caused by the passive approximation of its extremities. **postural c.,** that state of muscular tension and contraction which just suffices to maintain the posture of the body. **premature c.,** extrasystole. **rheumatic c.,** tetany, def. 1. **segmentation c.,** see under *movement.* **tetanic c.,** sustained contraction of a muscle without intervals of relaxation; called also *tonic c.* Symbol ADTe. **tone c.,** a muscular contraction developing slowly and showing a prolonged phase of relaxation. **tonic c.,** tetanic c. **twitch c.,** the all-or-none response of muscle cells to a single stimulus. **uterine c.,** contraction of the uterus during labor.

contracture (kon-trak′tūr) [L. *contractura*] a condition of fixed high resistance to passive stretch of a muscle, resulting from fibrosis of the tissues supporting the muscles or the joints, or from disorders of the muscle fibers. **Dupuytren's c.,** shortening, thickening, and fibrosis of the palmar fascia, producing a flexion deformity of a finger; sometimes associated with long-standing epilepsy. Applied also to flexion deformity of a toe caused by involvement of the plantar fascia. **ischemic c.,** contracture and degeneration of a muscle due to interference with the circulation from pressure, as by a tight bandage, or from injury or cold. **organic c.,** one that is permanent and continuous. **postpoliomyelitic c.,** any distortion of a joint following an attack of poliomyelitis, due to partial or complete paralysis of one muscle or group of muscles, allowing overuse of an opposing muscle or group of muscles, such as flexion contracture of the knee and paralysis of the quadriceps muscle group. **veratrin c.,** peculiar type of muscular contraction produced by injecting a muscle with veratrin. **Volkmann's c.,** a contraction of the fingers and sometimes of the wrist, with loss of power, developing rapidly after a severe injury in the region of the elbow joint or improper use of a tourniquet. A similar phenomenon may develop in the distal extremity and involve the foot when similar vascular damage is sustained to the muscles of the leg; called also *ischemic muscular atrophy* and *Volkmann's syndrome.*

contraextension (kon″trah-eks-ten′shun) counterextension.

contrafissura (kon-trah-fis-su′rah) contrafissure.

contrafissure (kon″trah-fish′ur) a fracture in a part opposite the site of a blow.

contraincision (kon″trah-in-sizh′un) counterincision to promote drainage.

contraindicant (kon″trah-in′dĭ-kant) rendering any particular line of treatment undesirable or improper.

contraindication (kon″trah-in″dĭ-ka′shun) any condition, especially any condition of disease, which renders some particular line of treatment improper or undesirable.

contrainsular (kon″trah-in′su-lar) having an inhibiting influence on insular secretion.

contralateral (kon″trah-lat′er-al) [*contra-* + L. *latus* side] situated on, pertaining to, or affecting the opposite side, as opposed to ipsilateral.

contraparetic (kon″trah-pah-ret′ik) 1. counteracting paresis. 2. a preparation useful in the treatment of paresis.

contrasexual (kon″trah-seks′u-al) pertaining to or characteristic of the opposite sex.

contrast (kon′trast) comparison in order to distinguish differences. In radiology, the visual differentiability of variations in photographic or film density produced on a radiograph by the structural composition of the object or objects radiographed. **high c.,** short-scale c. **long-scale c., low c.,** that degree of contrast which limits visual differentiation to those image densities produced by relatively disparate structural features. **short-scale c.,** that degree of contrast which favors visual differentiation of image densities produced by objects or object components with relatively comparable structural features.

contrastimulant (kon″trah-stim′u-lant) [*contra-* + *stimulant*] 1. counteracting or opposing stimulation. 2. a depressant medicine.

contrastimulism (kon″trah-stim′u-lizm) the systematic use of contrastimulant medicines or appliances.

contrastimulus (kon″trah-stim′u-lus) [*contra-* + *stimulus*] a remedy, force, or agent that opposes stimulation.

contravolitional (kon″trah-vo-lish′un-al) done in opposition to the will; involuntary.

contrecoup (kon-tr-koo′) [Fr. "counterblow"] injury resulting from a blow on another site, such as a fracture of the skull caused by a blow on the opposite side.

contrectation (kon″trek-ta′shun) [L. *contrectare* to handle] the fondling of a person of the opposite sex.

Cont. rem. abbreviation for L. *continue′tur reme′dium,* let the medicine be continued.

control (kon-trōl′) [Fr. *contrôle* a register] 1. the governing or limitation of certain objects or events. 2. a standard against which experimental observations may be evaluated, as a procedure identical in all respects to the experimental procedure except for absence of the one factor that is being studied. **associative automatic c.,** nerve impulses that arise in the corpus striatum and act upon the final common pathway, and thus upon the muscles. **aversive c.,** in behavior therapy, the use of unpleasant stimuli to change undesirable behavior. **birth c.,** deliberate limitation of childbearing by measures designed to control fertility and to prevent conception; see also *contraception.* **feedback c.,** a physiological control mechanism operating to regulate the metabolic processes of a cell and thus maintain a constant internal environment, in which the accumulation of the product of a reaction leads to a decrease in its rate of production or a deficiency of the product leads to an increase in its rate of production. **idiodynamic c.,** nerve impulses from the cells of the ventral gray column and the motor nuclei of the brain that maintain the muscles in their normal trophic condition. **reflex c.,** control of muscular activity by nerve impulses transmitted to the muscles by one of the reflex arcs by which reflex action is maintained. **sex c.,** regulation of the sex of future offspring by artificial means. **stimulus c.,** any influence exerted by the environment on behavior. **synergic c.,** nerve impulses transmitted to the common pathway from the cerebellum for the regulation of the muscular activity of the synergic units of the body. **tonic c.,** nerve impulses transmitted to the final common pathway through the reflex arc for the maintenance of the muscle tone. **vestibuloequilibratory c.,** nerve impulses from the semicircular canals, saccule, and utricle for the maintenance of body equilibrium. **volitional c., voluntary c.,** impulses from the motor area of the cerebral cortex that direct muscular action under the influence of the will.

Controlled Substances Act a federal law enacted in 1970 that regulates the prescribing and dispensing of psychoactive drugs, including narcotics, according to five schedules based on their abuse potential, medical acceptance, and ability to produce dependence; it also establishes a regulatory system for the manufacture, storage, and transport of the drugs in each schedule. Drugs covered by this Act include opium and its derivatives, opiates, hallucinogens, depressants, and stimulants.

contund (kon-tund′) [L. *contundere*] to bruise.

contuse (kon-tūz′) to bruise.

contusion (kon-tu′zhun) [L. *contusio,* from *contundere* to bruise] a bruise; an injury of a part without a break in the skin. **brain c.,** contusion with loss of consciousness as a result of direct trauma to the head, usually associated with fracture of the skull. See also *concussion of the brain.* **contrecoup c.,** a contusion resulting from a blow on one side of the head with damage to the cerebral hemisphere on the opposite side by transmitted force. **c. of spinal cord,** organic injury to the cord due to a blow to the vertebral column, with resultant transient or prolonged dysfunction below the level of the lesion. See also *concussion of spinal cord.*

contusive (kon-tu′siv) producing a bruise.

conular (kon′u-lar) cone-shaped.

Conus (ko′nus) a genus of mollusks, some species of which are able to inflict a poisoned wound.

conus (ko′nus), pl. *co′ni* [L.; Gr. *kōnos*] 1. a cone; [NA] a general term denoting a structure resembling a cone in shape. 2. posterior staphyloma of the myopic eye. **c. arterio′sus** [NA], the anterosuperior portion of the right ventricle of the heart, which is delimited from the rest of the ventricle by the supraventricular crest and which joins the pulmonary trunk, thus forming the outflow tract for blood in the right ventricle. Called also *arterial cone* and *infundibulum* (*of heart*). **distraction c.,** a crescentic white area at the temporal edge of the papilla of the optic nerve sometimes seen with the ophthalmoscope in myopic eyes. **c. elas′ticus laryn′gis** [NA], elastic cone of larynx: the lower part of the fibroelastic membrane of the larynx. **co′ni epididym′idis,** NA alternative for *lobuli epididymidis.* **c. medulla′ris** [NA], medullary cone: the cone-shaped lower end of the spinal cord, at the level of the upper lumbar vertebrae; called also *c. terminalis* and *terminal cone of spinal cord.* **myopic c.,** posterior staphyloma of the myopic eye. **supertraction c.,** a gray or yellowish ring on the nasal side of the optic papilla sometimes seen with the ophthalmoscope, especially in myopic eyes. **c. termina′lis,** c. medullaris. **co′ni vasculo′si,** lobuli epididymidis.

convalescence (kon″vah-les′ens) [L. *convalescere* to become strong] the stage of recovery following an attack of disease, a surgical operation, or an injury.

convalescent (kon″vah-les′ent) 1. pertaining to or characterized by convalescence. 2. a patient who is recovering from a disease, surgical operation, or injury.

convection (kon-vek′shun) [L. *convectio,* from *convehere* to convey] transmission of heat in liquids or gases by a circulation carried on by the heated particles.

convergence (kon-ver′jens) 1. inclination toward a common point. In embryology, the movement of cells from the periphery toward the midline during gastrulation. In physiology, the coordinated movement of the two eyes toward fixation of the same near point. In evolution, development of similar structures or organisms in unrelated taxa. 2. the point of meeting of convergent lines. **accommodative c.,** that portion of convergence initiated by the stimulus to accommodation. **far point of c.,** the point of intersection of the lines of sight at minimum convergence. **fusional c.,** convergence resulting from the attempt to keep the visual stimulus on the fovea of both eyes. **near point of c.,** the point of intersection of the lines of sight at maximum convergence. **negative c.,** outward deviation of the visual axes. **positive c.,** inward deviation of the visual axes. **proximal c.,** convergence induced by the sense of nearness of an object. **tonic c.,** the continuous convergence maintained by the tone of the medial rectus muscle in the primary position.

convergent (kon-ver′jent) [L. *con* together + *vergere* to incline] meeting at or tending toward a common point.

convergiometer (kon-ver″je-om′ĕ-ter) an instrument for measuring latent strabismus.

conversion (kon-ver′zhun) [L. *con* with + *versio* turning] 1. a freudian term for the process by which emotions become transformed into physical (motor or sensory) manifestations. 2. manipulative correction of any malposition of a fetal part during the course of labor, especially correction of face or brow presentation to occiput presentation. **Mantoux c.,** a term denoting the change from a tuberculin-negative to a tuberculin-positive state, as determined by the intracutaneous injection of a solution of tuberculin; the opposite of Mantoux reversion.

convertase (kon-ver′tās) an enzyme that converts a substance to its active state. **C3 c.,** the activated form of complement components C4 and C2 (written C4̄2̄), a peptidase that splits C3 to C3a and C3b.

convertin (kon-ver′tin) Factor VII; see *coagulation factors,* under *factor.*

convex (kon′veks) [L. *convexus*] having a rounded, somewhat elevated surface, resembling a segment of the external surface of a sphere. **low c.,** having a rounded, slightly elevated surface, resembling a segment of the external surface of a sphere of long radius.

convexity (kon-vek′sĭ-te) [L. *convexitas*] 1. the condition of being convex. 2. a rounded, somewhat elevated area on the surface of an organ or other structure.

convexobasia (kon-vek″so-ba′se-ah) [*convex* + *base* of the skull] a deformity of the occipital bone, which is bent forward by the spine; seen in osteitis deformans.

convexoconcave (kon-vek″so-kon′kāv) convex on one surface and concave on the other.

convexoconvex (kon-vek″so-kon′veks) convex on each of two opposite surfaces.

convoluted (kon′vo-lūt-ed) [L. *convolutus*] rolled together or coiled.

convolution (kon-vo-lu′shun) [L. *convolutus* rolled together] a tortuous irregularity or elevation caused by a structure being infolded upon itself, as the convolutions of the brain; see also *gyrus.* **Broca's c.,** the inferior frontal gyrus of the left hemisphere of the cerebrum; called also *Broca's gyrus* or *region.* **c's of cerebrum,** gyri cerebri. **Heschl's c.,** the anterior transverse temporal gyrus; see *gyri temporales transversi,* under *gyrus.* **occipitotemporal c.,** gyrus occipitotemporalis lateralis. **Zuckerkandl's c.,** gyrus paraterminalis.

convolutional (kon″vo-lu′shun-al) of or pertaining to a convolution or convolutions.

convolutionary (kon″vo-lu′shun-a-re) convolutional.

convulsant (kon-vul′sant) 1. producing or causing convulsions. 2. an agent that causes convulsions.

convulsibility (kon-vul″sĭ-bil′ĭ-te) capability of being convulsed.

convulsion (con-vul′shun) [L. *convulsio,* from *convellere* to pull together] a violent involuntary contraction or series of contractions of the voluntary muscles. **central c.,** a convulsion not excited by any external cause, but due to a lesion of the central nervous system; called also *essential c.* and *spontaneous c.* **clonic c.,** a convulsion marked by alternating contracting and relaxing the muscles. **coordinate c.,** a convulsion marked by clonic movements similar to natural, purposeful movements. **crowing c.,** laryngismus stridulus. **epileptiform c.,** any convulsion attended with loss of consciousness. **essential c.,** central c. **febrile c's,** those associated with high fever, occurring in infants and children. **hysterical c.,** any spasmodic movement attendant upon a hysterical disorder. **hysteroid c.,** hysteroepilepsy. **local c.,** any minor spasm affecting but

one muscle or only one part or member. **mimetic c., mimic c.,** facial spasm or tic. **puerperal c.,** involuntary spasms in women just before, during, or just after, childbirth. **salaam c.,** nodding spasm. **spontaneous c.,** central c. **tetanic c.,** a tonic spasm without loss of consciousness; see *tetanus* (def. 2) and *tetany* (def. 1). **tonic c.,** prolonged contraction of the muscles, as a result of an epileptic discharge. **uremic c.,** one due to uremia, or retention in the blood of material that should have been expelled by the kidneys.

convulsivant (kon-vul′sĭ-vant) convulsant.

convulsive (kon-vul′siv) pertaining to, characterized by, or of the nature of convulsion.

Cooke's formula (count, criterior, index) [William Edmond *Cooke,* 1881–1939] see under *formula.*

Cooley's anemia, disease [Thomas Benton *Cooley,* American pediatrician, 1871–1945] see *thalassemia.*

Coolidge tube (koo′lij) [William David *Coolidge,* American physicist, born 1873] see under *tube.*

cooling (kōōl′ing) the process of reducing the temperature, especially the body temperature of patients and experimental animals. See also *hypothermia.* **peritoneal c.,** reduction of body temperature achieved experimentally by circulation of a cooled irrigation fluid through the peritoneal cavity. **pleural c.,** reduction of body temperature accomplished experimentally by circulation of a cooled irrigation fluid through the pleural cavity.

Coombs' test (kōōmz) [R. R. A. *Coombs,* British immunologist] see under *tests.*

Cooper's disease, etc. (koo′perz) [Sir Astley Paston *Cooper,* English surgeon, 1768–1841] see under *breast, disease, fascia, hernia, ligament, operation,* and *testis.*

Cooperia (koo-pe′re-ah) a genus of parasitic nematodes. **C. oncoph′ora, C. pectina′ta, C. puncta′ta,** species of parasitic nematodes sometimes occurring in the small intestine of cattle.

cooperid (koo′per-id) a parasitic namatode of the genus *Cooperia.*

Coopernail's sign (koo′per-nālz) [George Peter *Coopernail,* American physician, born 1876] see under *sign.*

coordination (ko-or″dĭ-na′shun) the harmonious functioning of interrelated organs and parts; applied especially to the process of the motor apparatus of the brain which provides for the co-working of particular groups of muscles for the performance of definite adaptive useful responses.

coossification (ko-os″ĭ-fĭ-ka′shun) the action or state of being joined together by ossification.

coossify (ko-os″ĭ-fi) to grow together by ossification.

copaiba (ko-pi′bah) the resinous juice (balsam) of various leguminous trees of tropical America, especially *Copaifera officinalis* and *C. langsdorffii* Leguminosae; it was formerly used for gonorrhea and chronic inflammation of mucous membranes and as a diaphoretic and expectorant. Called also *balsam of copaiba.*

copal (ko-pal′) [Mex.] the commercial name of many resinous substances of extremely varied origin and character; the original copals came from trees of tropical America, chiefly of the leguminous species *Hymenea courbaril* L. and various species of *Trachylobium.* It is used in various varnishes and cements and in dentistry for modeling compounds and varnishes for cavities.

coparaffinate (ko-par′ah-fin-āt) a mixture of water-insoluble isoparaffinic acids partially neutralized with isoctyl hydroxybenzyldialkyl amines; used as an anti-infective for the skin.

COPD chronic obstructive pulmonary disease.

cope (kōp) the upper half of a flask used in the casting art; applied in prosthetic dentistry to the upper or cavity side of a denture flask.

copepod (ko′pĕ-pod) [Gr. *kōpē* oar + *pous* foot] an individual member of Copepoda.

Copepoda (ko-pep′ŏ-dah) [Gr. *kōpē* oar + *pous* foot] a subclass of minute aquatic arthropods (class Crustacea) that are intermediate hosts of *Diphyllobothrium* and *Dracunculus;* ingestion of copepods infected with the early larval stages of *Spirometra mansonoides* may cause human sparganosis.

Copernicia (ko″per-nish′e-ah) a genus of palms, including *C. cerifera* Mart., a South American species, which is the source of carnauba wax.

coping (kōp′ing) a thin metal covering or cap, such as the plate of metal applied over the prepared crown or root of a tooth preparatory to attaching an artificial crown; called also *cope* and *thimble.* **long c.,** one placed on a tooth that has been reduced only as much as necessary to receive the crown or overdenture. **short c.,** one placed on a tooth that has been reduced in vertical height to within 0.5 to 1.0 mm. above the gingival margin, after root canal therapy. **transfer c.,** a covering or cap of metal, acrylic resin, or other material, used to position a die in an impression.

copiopia (kop-e-o′pe-ah) [Gr. *kopos* fatigue + *opsis* sight] eyestrain from overwork or improper use of the eyes.

copodyskinesia (kop″o-dis″ki-ne′ze-ah) [Gr. *kopos* fatigue + *dys-* + *kinēsis* motion] (*obs.*) any difficulty of movement due to fatigue from the habitual performance of some particular action; occupation neurosis.

copolymer (ko-pol′ĭ-mer) a polymer containing monomers of more than one kind.

copper (kop′er) [L. *cuprum;* Gr. *Kypros*] a reddish, malleable metal; atomic number, 29; atomic weight, 63.54; symbol Cu, with poisonous salts. Copper is essential in nutrition, being a component of various proteins, including ceruloplasmin, erythrocuprein, cytochrome *c* oxidase, tyrosinase, etc. Deficiency, which is rare, may result in hypochromic microcytic anemia, neutropenia, and bone changes. **c. abietinate,** a copper salt in green scales, soluble in oil; used as an anthelmintic and vermifuge in veterinary practice. **c. citrate,** see *cupric citrate,* under *citrate.* **c. iodide,** cuprous iodide, CuI. **c. oxyphosphate,** a salt of copper, zinc phosphate, and glacial acetic acid, occasionally used as a temporary filling material for tooth cavities; called also *green precipitate.* **c. phenolsulfonate,** green prismatic crystals, $(OH \cdot C_6H_4 \cdot SO_2O)_2Cu \cdot 6H_2O.$ **c. sulfate,** cupric sulfate; see under *sulfate.*

copperas (kop′er-as) commercial ferrous sulfate, $FeSO_4 \cdot 7H_2O$; disinfectant and deodorizer. See also *ferrous sulfate,* under *sulfate.*

copperhead (kop′er-hed) 1. a venomous snake (a pit viper), *Agkistrodon contortrix,* of the United States, having a brown to copper-colored body with dark bands. 2. a very venomous elapid snake, *Denisonia superba,* of Australia, Tasmania, and the Solomon Islands. See table accompanying *snake.*

copracrasia (kop″rah-kra′se-ah) [Gr. *kopros* dung + *akrasia* want of self control] fecal incontinence.

copragogue (kop′rah-gog) [Gr. *kopros* dung + *agōgos* leading] cathartic.

coprecipitin (ko″pre-sip′ĭ-tin) a precipitin in the same serum with one or more other precipitins.

copremesis (kop-rem′ĕ-sis) [Gr. *kopros* dung + *emesis* vomiting] the vomiting of fecal material.

copro- (kop′ro) [Gr. *kopros* dung] a combining form denoting relationship to feces.

coproantibody (kop″ro-an′tĭ-bod′e) an antibody (chiefly IgA) present in the intestinal tract, associated with immunity to enteric infection.

coprodaeum (kop″ro-de′um) [*copro-* + Gr. *hodiaos* on the way] the large dorsal passage in the proximal part of the cloaca in monotremes, into which the intestine opens.

coprodeum (kop″ro-de′um) coprodaeum.

coprolagnia (kop″ro-lag′ne-ah) [*copro-* + Gr. *lagneia* lust] a form of paraphilia in which sexual excitement is associated with feces or defecation.

coprolalia (kop″ro-la′le-ah) [*copro-* + Gr. *lalia* babble] the use of foul language, particularly of words relating to the feces; called also *coprophrasia, eschrolalia,* and *coprolalomania.*

coprolalomania (kop″ro-lal″o-ma′ne-ah) coprolalia.

coprolith (kop′ro-lith) [*copro-* + Gr. *lithos* a stone] a hard fecal concretion.

coprology (kop-rol′o-je) [*copro-* + *-logy*] the study of the feces.

coproma (kop-ro′mah) [*copro-* + *-oma*] stercoroma.

Copromastix (kop″ro-mas′tiks) a genus of coprozoic protozoa of the order Polymastigida, class Zoomastigophora, having four equally long anterior flagella and a trailing flagellum. **C. prowazek′i,** a species found in rat and human feces in Brazil.

Copromonas (kop-rom′o-nas) a genus of elongate, ovoid, uniflagellate protozoa of the order Euglenoidina, class Phytomastigophora, which are coprozoic in the feces of toads, frogs, and man. **C. subti′lis,** a piriform coprozoic flagellate found in the feces of frogs and sometimes in the human stool.

coprophagia (kop″ro-fa′je-ah) coprophagy.

coprophagous (kop-rof′ah-gus) feeding on dung, or feces.

coprophagy (kop-rof′ah-je) [*copro-* + Gr. *phagein* to eat] the ingestion of dung, or feces.

coprophil (kop′ro-fil) a coprophilic microorganism.

coprophile (kop′ro-fil) 1. coprophil. 2. coprophilic.

coprophilia (kop″ro-fil′e-ah) [*copro-* + Gr. *philia* affection] a psychopathologic interest in filth, especially in feces and in defecation.

coprophiliac (kop″ro-fil′e-ak) an individual exhibiting coprophilia.

coprophilic (kop″ro-fil′ik) 1. pertaining to or characterized by coprophilia. 2. inhabiting dung or feces; said of bacteria.

coprophilous (kop-rof′ĭ-lus) coprophilic.

coprophobia (kop″ro-fo′be-ah) [*copro-* + Gr. *phobein* to be affrighted by + *ia*] abnormal repugnance to defecation and to feces.

coprophrasia (kop″ro-fra′ze-ah) (*obs.*) coprolalia.

coproporphyria (kop″ro-por-fir′e-ah) hereditary porphyria characterized by excessive excretion of coproporphyrin, chiefly in the feces; usually a symptomless condition, but attacks resembling those of acute intermittent porphyria may be precipitated by drugs.

coproporphyrin (kop″ro-por′fir-in) [*copro-* + *porphyrin*] a porphyrin, $C_{36}H_{38}O_8N_4$, formed in the intestine from bilirubin and found in the feces and in the urine in coproporphyrinuria; each of its four pyrrole groups has a methyl and a propionate side chain. Called also *stercoporphyrin.*

coproporphyrinogen (kop″ro-por′fĭ-rin′o-jin) the fully reduced, colorless compound, readily giving rise to coproporphyrin by oxidation.

coproporphyrinuria (kop″ro-por″fir-in-u′re-ah) the presence of coproporphyrin in the urine.

coprostanol (kop″ro-sta′nol) a saturated sterol, $C_{27}H_{48}O$, found in feces, probably reduced from cholesterol; called also *coprosterin* and *coprosterol.*

coprostasis (kop-ros′tah-sis) [*copro-* + Gr. *stasis* stoppage] impaction of the feces in the intestine.

coprostasophobia (kop″ro-sta″so-fo′be-ah) [*coprostasis* + *phobia*] (*obs.*) morbid dread of fecal stasis.

coprosterin (kop″ro-ste′rin) [*copro-* + *sterin*] coprostanol.

coprosterol (kop″ro-ste′rol) coprostanol.

coprozoa (kop″ro-zo′ah) [*copro-* + Gr. *zōon* animal] protozoa which are found in fecal matter outside the body, but which do not inhabit the intestine.

coprozoic (kop″ro-zo′ik) living in fecal material; found in fecal material.

Coptis (kop′tis) [L.] a genus of ranunculaceous plants. *C. tee′ta,* an Asiatic species, is tonic. *C. trifo′lia* (goldthread), of North America, was formerly used as a bitter tonic.

coptosystole (kop″to-sis′to-le) [Gr. *koptein* to cut + *systole*] (*obs.*) the cutting off of a ventricular systole.

copula (kop′u-lah) [L.] 1. any connecting part or structure. 2. copula linguae. **c. lin′guae,** a median ventral elevation on the embryonic tongue formed by union of the second branchial arches; it represents the future root of the tongue.

copulation (kop″u-la′shun) [L. *copulatio*] sexual union between male and female; usually used in reference to animals lower than man.

Coq. abbreviation for L. *co′que,* boil.

Coq. in s. a. abbreviation for L. *co′que in sufficien′te a′qua,* boil in sufficient water.

Coq. s. a. abbreviation for L. *co′que secun′dum ar′tem,* boil properly.

coquille (ko-kēl′) [Fr.] a glass or lens shaped like a watch crystal.

cor (kor), gen. *cor′dis* [L.] [NA] the muscular organ that maintains the circulation of the blood; see *heart.* **c. adipo′sum,** a heart that has undergone fatty degeneration or that has an accumulation of fat around it; called also *fat,* or *fatty, heart.* **c. arterio′sum,** the left side of the heart, so called because it contains oxygenated (arterial) blood. **c. bilocula′re,** a congenital anomaly characterized by failure of formation of the atrial and ventricular septums, the heart having only two chambers, a single atrium and a single ventricle, and a common atrioventricular valve. **c. bovi′num** [L. "ox heart"], a greatly enlarged heart due to a hypertrophied left ventricle; called also *c. taurinum* and *bucardia.* **c. dex′trum** [L. "right heart"], the right atrium and ventricle. **c. hirsu′tum,** c. villosum. **c. mo′bile** (*obs.*), an abnormally movable heart. **c. pen′dulum,** a heart so movable that it seems to be hanging by the great blood vessels. **c. pseudotrilocula′re biatria′tum,** a congenital cardiac anomaly in which the heart functions as a three-chambered heart because of tricuspid atresia, the right ventricle being extremely small or rudimentary and the right atrium greatly dilated. Blood passes from the right to the left atrium and thence to the left ventricle and aorta. **c. pulmona′le,** heart disease due to pulmonary hypertension secondary to disease of the lung, or its blood vessels, with hypertrophy of the right ventricle. **c. sinis′trum** [L. "left heart"], the left atrium and ventricle. **c. tauri′num,** c. bovinum. **c. triatria′tum,** a congenital anomaly caused by failure of incorporation of the embryonic common pulmonary vein into the left atrium, the pulmonary veins emptying into an accessory chamber superior to the true left atrium and communicating with it by a small opening, which obstructs pulmonary venous flow, thus simulating mitral stenosis, Called also *triatrial heart.* **c. trilocula′re,** three-chambered heart. **c. trilocular′e biatria′tum,** a congenital anomaly caused by failure of formation of the ventricular septum, the heart having two atria, communicating, by the tricuspid and mitral valves, with a single ventricle. **c. trilocula′re biventricula′re,** a three-chambered heart with one atrium and two ventricles. **c. veno′sum,** the right side of the heart, so called because it contains blood that has given up most of its oxygen (venous blood). **c. villo′sum** [L. "hairy heart"], a roughened state of the pericardium caused by exudate on its surface, occurring in pericarditis; called also *c. hirsutum.*

coracidia (kor″ah-sid′e-ah) plural of *coracidium.*

coracidium (kor″ah-sid′e-um), pl. *coracidia.* The individual free-swimming or free-crawling, spherical, ciliated embryo of tapeworms of the order Pseudophyllidea.

coracoacromial (kor″ah-ko-ah-kro′me-al)   pertaining to the coracoid and acromion processes.

coracoclavicular (kor″ah-ko-klah-vik′u-lar)   pertaining to the coracoid process and the clavicle.

coracohumeral (kor″ah-ko-hu′mer-al)   pertaining to the coracoid process and the humerus.

coracoid (kor′ah-koid) [Gr. *korakoeidēs* crowlike]   1. like a raven's beak. 2. the coracoid process (processus coracoideus scapulae [NA]).

coracoiditis (kor″ah-koi-di′tis)   a painful condition in the region of the scapula and of the coracoid process, with deltoid atrophy; attributed to injury of the coracoid process.

coracoradialis (kor″ah-ko-ra″de-a′lis)   caput breve musculi bicipitis brachii.

coracoulnaris (kor″ah-ko-ul-na′ris)   the fibers of the biceps muscle attached to the fascia of the forearm.

coralliform (ko-ral′ĭ-form) [L. *corallum* coral + *forma* shape]   having the form of a coral; branching like a coral.

corallin (kor′ah-lin)   aurin.   **yellow c.,** the sodium salt of aurin, occurring as yellow masses with a greenish metallic luster, which turns red in solution; called also *corallin yellow.*

coralloid (kor′ah-loid)   coralliform.

Coramine (ko′rah-min)   trademark for preparations of nikethamide.

corasthma (kor-az′mah)   hay fever.

Corbus' disease (kor′bus) [Budd Clarke *Corbus,* American urologist, 1876–1954]   balanitis gangrenosa.

cord (kord) [L. *chorda;* Gr. *chordē* string]   any long, rounded, flexible structure; see also *chorda.*   **Bergmann's c's,** striae medullares ventriculi quarti; see under *stria.*   **Billroth's c's,** red pulp c's.   **dental c.,** a cordlike mass of cells from which the enamel organ develops.   **enamel c.,** a vertical extension of the enamel knot in a developing tooth, connecting the enamel knot with the outer dental epithelium, a temporary structure which disappears before enamel formation begins.   **Ferrein's c's,** the inferior, or true, vocal cords (plica vocalis [NA]).   **ganglionated c.,** truncus sympathicus.   **genital c.,** in the embryo, the midline fused caudal part of the two urogenital ridges, each containing a mesonephric and paramesonephric duct.   **gubernacular c.,** chorda gubernaculum.   **hepatic c's,** anastomosing plates of hepatic cells radiating outward from the central vein and composing the parenchyma of a hepatic lobule; called also *hepatic cell c's.*   **lateral c.,** see *fasciculus lateralis plexus brachialis,* under *fasciculus.*   **lumbosacral c.,** truncus lumbosacralis.   **lymph c's,** medullary c's (def. 1).   **medial c.,** see *fasciculus medialis plexus brachialis,* under *fasciculus.*   **medullary c's,** 1. strands of dense lymphoid tissue surrounded by the sinuses of the medulla of a lymph node; called also *lymph c's.* 2. rete c's.   **nephrogenic c.,** a longitudinal cord, formed by fusion of the nephrotome plates, that gives rise to the mesonephric tubule and part of the metanephric tubules.   **nerve c.,** any nerve trunk or bundle of nerve fibers.   **oblique c. of elbow joint,** chorda obliqua membranae interosseae antebrachii.   **ovigerous c's,** rete cords of the primitive ovary that resolve into eggs and their follicles.   **Pflüger's c's,** 1. the ovarian tubes. 2. the salivary tubes.   **posterior c.,** see *fasciculus posterior plexus brachialis,* under *fasciculus.*   **psalterial c.,** stria vascularis ductus cochlearis.   **red pulp c's,** the masses of red pulp of the spleen; called also *Billroth's c's* and *splenic c's.*   **rete c's,** strands of primordial cells in the medulla of the embryonic gonads that connect with some of the mesonephric tubules, and from which the rete ovarii or the rete testis develop; called also *medullary c's* and *sex c's.*   **scirrhous c.,** chronic infection of the stump of the spermatic cord of a castrated horse caused by bacterial infection, with discharge of pus and sometimes formation of a tumor-like mass with numerous weeping sinuses.   **sex c's,** rete c's.   **sexual c's,** the seminiferous tubules of the early fetus.   **spermatic c.,** the structure that extends from the abdominal inguinal ring to the testis, comprising the ductus deferens, testicular artery, pampiniform plexus, and nerves, as well as various other vessels, enclosed by its various coverings (tunicae funiculi spermatici et testis); called also *funiculus spermaticus* [NA], and *chorda spermatica.*   **spinal c.,** that part of the central nervous system which is lodged in the vertebral canal; it extends from the foramen magnum, where it is continuous with the medulla oblongata, to the upper part of the lumbar region. It ends between the twelfth thoracic and third lumbar vertebrae, often at or adjacent to the disc between the first and second lumbar vertebrae. It is composed of an inner core of gray substance in which nerve cells predominate, and an outer layer of white substance in which myelinated nerve fibers predominate, and is enclosed in three protective membranes, or meninges: the dura mater, the arachnoid, and the pia mater. Thirty-one spinal nerves originate from the spinal cord: 8 cervical, 12 thoracic, 5 lumbar, 5 sacral, and 1 coccygeal. The spinal cord conducts impulses to and from the brain, and controls many automatic muscular activities (reflexes). Called also *chorda spinalis* and *medulla spinalis* [NA]. See Plate X, under *brain.*   **splenic c's,** red pulp c's.   **testis**

c's, the rete cords of the embryonic testis.   **umbilical c.,** the flexible structure connecting the umbilicus of the embryo and fetus with the placenta and giving passage to the umbilical arteries and vein. In the newborn it measures about 50 cm. in length. First formed during the fifth embryonic week from the allantoic stalk, it contains the omphalomesentric duct and the allantois. Called also *funiculus umbilicalis* [NA] and *chorda umbicalis.*   **vocal c., false,** a fold of mucous membrane covering muscle in the larynx and separating the ventricle from the vestibule; called also *plica vestibularis* [NA], *plica ventricularis, false vocal fold,* and *vestibular fold.*   **vocal c., true,** a fold of mucous membrane covering the vocalis muscle in the larynx forming the inferior boundary of the ventricle. Called also *plica vocalis* [NA], *vocal fold,* and *Ferrein's c.*   **Weitbrecht's c.,** chorda obliqua membranae interosseae antebrachii.   **Wilde's c's,** a name once applied to the transverse striae of the corpus callosum (striae transversae corporis callosi [NA]).   **Willis' c's,** numerous fibrous bands (dural trabeculae) that extend transversely across the inferior angle of the superior sagittal sinus; called also *chordae Willisii.*

cordal (kor′dal)   pertaining to a cord; used specifically in referring to the vocal cord, or the plica vocalis.

cordate (kor′dāt) [L. *cor* heart]   heart-shaped.

cordectomy (kor-dek′to-me) [cord + Gr. *ektomē* excision]   excision of a cord, as a vocal cord.

cordial (kord′yal) [L. *cordialis*]   1. stimulating the heart; invigorating. 2. an aromatized alcoholic liqueur.

cordiale (kor-de-a′le) [L.]   cordial.

cordiform (kor′dĭ-form) [L. *cor* heart + *forma* form]   heart-shaped.

corditis (kor-di′tis)   inflammation of the spermatic cord.

cordopexy (kor′do-pek″se) [cord + Gr. *pēxis* fixation]   the operation of displacing outward the vocal cord for bilateral vocal cord paralysis.

cordotomy (kor-dot′o-me)   1. section of a vocal cord. 2. interruption of the lateral spinothalamic tract of the spinal cord, usually in the anterolateral quadrant, for relief of intractable pain; it may be done by open surgery or percutaneously by sterotaxic surgery. Also spelled *chordotomy.*

Cordran (kor′dran)   trademark for a preparation of flurandrenolide.

Cordyceps (kor′dĭ-seps)   a genus of ascomycetous fungi of the family Clavicipitaceae, order Clavicipitales; certain species produce fatal disease of caterpillars.   **C. sinen′sis,** a parasite of insect larvae; in Chinese medicine ("hea-tsao-taog-chung") it is reputed to be a drug coagulant; called also *Sphaeria sinensis.*

Cordylobia (kor″dĭ-lo′be-ah)   a genus of flies of the family Calliphorida.   **C. anthropoph′aga,** a species of flies of Africa the larvae (cayor worms) of which burrow under the skin of man and animals, causing a myiasis; called also *tumbu fly.*

core (kōr)   1. the central part of anything, such as the central mass of necrotic matter in a boil. 2. a bar of iron around which a wire is wound to form an induction coil or electromagnet. 3. a metal casting, usually with a post in the canal of a root, designed to retain an artificial crown. 4. a sectional record, usually of plaster of Paris or one of its derivatives, of the relationships of parts, such as teeth, metallic restorations, or copings.

core-, coro- (kōr′e, kōr′o) [Gr. *korē* pupil]   a combining form denoting relationship to the pupil of the eye; see also words beginning *irid-* and *irido-.*

coreclisis (kōr″e-kli′sis) [core- + Gr. *kleisis* closure]   iridencleisis.

corectasis (kōr-ek′tah-sis) [core- + Gr. *ektasis* a dilatation]   dilatation of the pupil.

corectome (kōr-ek′tōm) [core- + Gr. *tomē* a cutting]   a cutting instrument used in performing iridectomy (corectomy).

corectomedialysis (ko-rek″to-me″de-al′ĭ-sis) [core- + Gr. *ektemnein* to excise + *dialysis* separating]   the operation of forming an artificial pupil by detaching the iris from the ciliary ligament.

corectomy (ko-rek′to-me) [core- + Gr. *ektomē* excision]   iridectomy.

corectopia (kōr-ek-to′pe-ah) [core- + Gr. *ek* out + *topos* place]   abnormal situation of the pupil.

coredialysis (ko″re-di-al′ĭ-sis) [core- + Gr. *dialysis* separating]   the surgical separation of the external margin of the iris from the ciliary body; called also *iridodialysis.*

corediastasis (ko″re-di-as′tah-sis) [core- + Gr. *diastasis* distention]   the dilatation or a dilated state of the pupil.

coregonin (ko-reg′o-nin)   a protamine obtained from the sperm of the white fish.

corelysis (ko-rel′ĭ-sis) [core- + Gr. *lysis* dissolution]   operative destruction of the pupil; especially the surgical detachment of adhesions of the pupillary margin of the iris from the lens.

coremorphosis (kōr″e-mor-fo′sis) [core- + Gr. *morphōsis* formation]   the surgical formation of an artificial pupil.

corenclisis (kōr″en-kli′sis) [core- + Gr. *enkleiein* to inclose]   iridencleisis.

coreometer (ko″re-om′ĕ-ter) [core- + Gr. *metron* measure] pupillometer.

coreometry (ko″re-om′ĕ-tre) pupillometry.

coreoplasty (ko′re-o-plas″te) [core- + Gr. *plassein* to form] any plastic operation on the iris.

corepressor (ko″re-pres′sor) a small molecule which combines with an aporepressor to form the substance that controls the synthesis of an enzyme.

corestenoma (ko″re-ste-no′mah) [core- + Gr. *stenōma* contraction] an abnormally contracted state of the pupil. **c. congen′itum,** a congenital condition in which the pupil is partially occluded by excrescences which meet, leaving scattered small openings.

Corethra (ko-re′thrah) *Chaoborus.*

coretomedialysis (ko″re-to-me-dĭ-al′ĭ-sis) [core- + Gr. *temnein* to cut + *dialysis* separation] the formation of an artificial pupil by a combined cutting and tearing operation upon the iris.

coretomy (ko-ret′o-me) [core- + Gr. *temnein* to cut] iridotomy.

Cori cycle, ester (ko′re) [Carl Ferdinand *Cori,* born 1896, and Gerty Theresa *Cori,* 1896–1955: American biochemists; co-winners, with Bernardo Alberto Houssay, of the Nobel prize for medicine and physiology in 1947] see *glucose-lactate cycle,* under *cycle,* and see under *ester.*

coriaceous (ko-re-a′shus) [L. *corium* leather] resembling leather; leathery, tough; said of bacterial cultures.

coriander (ko″re-an′der) [L. *coriandrum*] the dried ripe fruit of the umbelliferous plant *Coriandrum sativum;* formerly used as a weak carminative and aromatic, but now used as a flavor.

Coriaria (ko-re-a′re-ah) a genus of Old World poisonous coriariaceous plants (shrubs and small trees), containing coriamyrtin; they are also noted for their content of dyes and tannins.

coriin (ko′re-in) a substance formed by treating fibrous connective tissue with alkalis.

corium (ko′re-um) [L. "hide"] [NA] the dermis: the layer of the skin deep to the epidermis, consisting of a dense bed of vascular connective tissue; called also *cutis vera* and *true skin.*

corm (korm) [L. *cormus*] a solid bulblike expansion of a plant stem below the surface of the ground.

cormethasone acetate (kor-meth′ah-sōn) chemical name: 21-(acetyloxy)-6,6,9-trifluoro-11β, 17-dihydroxy-16α-methylpregna-1,4-diene-3,20-dione; a topical anti-inflammatory, $C_{24}H_{29}F_3O_6$.

corn (korn) [L. *cornu* horn] 1. a horny induration and thickening of the stratum corneum of the skin of the toes, caused by friction and pressure from poorly fitting shoes or hose; it forms a conical mass pointing down into the corium, producing pain and inflammation. There are two kinds: the *hard corn,* usually located on the outside of the little toe or on the upper surfaces of the other toes, and the *soft corn,* found between the toes, most often the fourth and fifth toes, kept softened by moisture. Called also *clavus.* 2. the seeds of a variety of certain cereal grains, especially *Zea mays* L., Gramineae, used as both animal and human food. Corns yield corn oil, used as a solvent for injections, and corn starch, used as an absorbent and dusting powder. 3. a bruise on the bottom of a horse's foot between the wall of the heel and the bar. **hard c.,** see *corn,* def. 1 **soft c.,** See *corn,* def. 1.

cornea (kor′ne-ah) [L. *corneus* horny] [NA] the transparent structure forming the anterior part of the fibrous tunic of the eye. It consists of five layers: (1) the anterior corneal epithelium, continuous with that of the conjunctiva, (2) the anterior limiting layer, (Bowman's membrane), (3) the substantia propria, (4) the posterior limiting layer, (Descemet's membrane), and (5) the endothelium of the anterior chamber, called also *keratoderma.* **conical c.,** keratoconus. **c. farina′ta,** degeneration of the cornea marked by fine dustlike stippling. **flat c.,** the configuration of the cornea when a shallow ocular chamber is present or when the eyeball is atrophic. **c. globo′sa,** buphthalmos. **c. gutta′ta,** a degenerative condition of the cornea due to dystrophy of the endothelial cells; called also *dystrophia endothelialis corneae.* **c. opa′ca,** the sclerotic coat of the eye. **c. pla′na,** cogenital flatness of the cornea. **sugar-loaf c.** (*obs.*), keratoconus. **c. verticilla′ta,** Fleischer's vortex.

corneal (kor′ne-al) [L. *cornealis*] pertaining to the cornea.

corneitis (kor″ne-i′tis) keratitis.

corneoblepharon (kor″ne-o-blef′ah-ron) [cornea + Gr. *blepharon* eyelid] adhesion between the eyelid and cornea.

corneoiritis (kor″ne-o-i-ri′tis) inflammation of the cornea and iris.

corneosclera (kor″ne-o-skle′rah) the cornea and sclera regarded as forming one organ.

corneoscleral (kor″ne-o-skle′ral) affecting or pertaining to both the cornea and the sclera.

corneous (kor′ne-us) [L. *corneus*] hornlike, or horny; consisting of keratin.

corner (kor′ner) the third incisor on either side of each jaw in the horse.

Corner's tampon [Edred Moss *Corner,* British surgeon, 1873–1950] see under *tampon.*

Corner-Allen test, unit [George Washington *Corner,* American anatomist, born 1889; Willard Myron *Allen,* American gynecologist, born 1904] see under *tests* and *unit.*

Cornet's forceps (kor′nets) [Georg *Cornet,* German bacteriologist, 1858–1915] a cover glass forceps.

corneum (kor′ne-um) [L. "horny"] the horny layer of the skin (stratum corneum epidermidis [NA]).

corniculate (kor-nik′u-lāt) shaped like a small horn.

corniculum (kor-nik′u-lum) [L. dim. of *cornu*] cartilago corniculata.

cornification (kor″nĭ-fĭ-ka′shun) [L. *cornu* horn + *facere* to make] 1. conversion into keratin, or horn. 2. conversion of epithelium to the stratified squamous type.

cornified (kor′nĭ-fĭd) converted into horny tissue (keratin); keratinized.

Corning's anesthesia (method), puncture (kor′nings) [James Leonard *Corning,* New York neurologist, 1855–1923] see *spinal anesthesia* (def. 1), under *anesthesia,* and *lumbar puncture,* under *puncture.*

cornoid (kor′noid) [L. *cornu* horn + *eidos* form] resembling horn; see under *lamella.*

cornu (kor′nu), pl. *cor′nua* [L. "horn"] a hornlike excrescence or projection; used in anatomical nomenclature to designate a structure resembling a horn in shape, especially in section. Called also *horn.* **c. Ammo′nis** [L. "horn of Ammon"], hippocampus. **c. ante′rius medul′lae spina′lis** [NA], the horn-shaped structure seen in transverse section of the spinal cord, formed by the anterior column of the cord (columna anterior medullae spinalis); called also *anterior horn of spinal cord.* **c. ante′rius ventric′uli latera′lis** [NA], anterior horn of lateral ventricle: the part of the lateral ventricle that extends forward from the pars centralis into the frontal lobe; called also *antecornu.* **cor′nua cartilag′inis thyroi′deae,** the horns of the thyroid cartilage; see *c. inferius cartilaginis thyroideae* and *c. superius cartilaginis thyroideae.* **c. cer′vi,** the horn of a stag or deer; hart's horn. **coccygeal c., c. coccy′geum** [NA], **c. of coccyx,** coccygeal horn: either of the cranial pair of rudimentary articular processes of the coccyx that articulate with the cornua of the sacrum. **c. cuta′neum,** cutaneous horn. **ethmoid c.,** concha nasalis media. **c. infe′rius cartilag′inis thyroi′deae** [NA], inferior horn of thyroid cartilage: the inferior extension of the posterior border of the thyroid cartilage. **c. infe′rius mar′ginis falcifor′mis** [NA], inferior horn of falciform margin: the distal edge of the falciform margin of the saphenous hiatus, deep to the great saphenous vein. **c. infe′rius ventric′uli latera′lis** [NA], inferior horn of lateral ventricle: the part of the lateral ventricle that extends forward from the pars centralis and the posterior horn into the temporal lobe; called also *inferior horn of cerebrum.* **c. latera′le medul′lae spina′lis** [NA], the horn-shaped structure seen in transverse section of the spinal cord, formed by the lateral column of the cord (columna lateralis medullae spinalis); called also *lateral horn of spinal cord.* **c. ma′jus os′sis hyoi′dei** [NA], greater horn of hyoid bone: a bony projection passing backward and upward from either side of the body of the hyoid bone; called also *lateral horn of hyoid bone.* **c. mi′nus os′sis hyoi′dei** [NA], lesser horn of hyoid bone: a small conical eminence projecting upward on either side of the hyoid bone at the angle of junction between the body and the greater horns; called also *superior horn of hyoid bone.* **c. occipita′le,** c. posterius ventriculi lateralis. **cor′nua os′sis hyoi′dei,** the horns of the hyoid bone; see *c. majus ossis hyoidei* and *c. minus ossis hyoidei.* **c. poste′rius medul′lae spina′lis** [NA], the horn-shaped structure seen in transverse section of the spinal cord, formed by the posterior column of the cord (columna posterior medullae spinalis); called also *posterior horn of spinal cord.* **c. poste′rius ventric′uli latera′lis** [NA], posterior horn of lateral ventricle: the part of the lateral ventricle that extends posteriorly from the pars centralis into the occipital lobe; called also *c. occipitale.* **sacral c., c. sacra′le** [NA], sacral horn: either of the two hook-shaped processes extending downward from the arch of the last sacral vertebra; called also *coccygeal eminence.* **cor′nua of spinal cord,** the horn-shaped structures seen in transverse section of the spinal cord; see *columna anterior medullae spinalis, columna lateralis medullae spinalis,* and *columna posterior medullae spinalis.* **c. supe′rius cartilag′inis thyroi′deae** [NA], superior horn of thyroid cartilage: the superior extension of the posterior border of the thyroid cartilage. **c. supe′rius mar′ginis falcifor′mis** [NA], superior horn of falciform margin: the proximal end of the falciform margin of the saphenous hiatus; called also *Scarpa's ligament.* **c. us′tum** [L. "burnt horn"], the burnt or charred horn of the deer or stag, formerly used in medicine as an antacid.

cornua (kor′nu-ah) [L.] plural of *cornu.*

cornual (kor′nu-al) pertaining to a cornu or to cornua.

cornuate (kor′nu-āt) cornual.

cornucommissural (kor″nu-kŏ-mis′u-ral) pertaining to a cornu and to a commissure.

cornucopia (kor″nu-ko′pe-ah) [L. *cornu copiae* "horn of plenty"] an extension of the choroid plexus into each of the lateral recesses of the fourth ventricle.

Cornus (kor′nus) [L.] a genus of cornaceous trees and shrubs of both hemispheres; the cornels or dogwoods. The dried root bark of many, especially that of *C. florida*, the common dogwood of North America, was once used as an astringent bitter and tonic.

coro (ko′ro) koro.

coro- see *core-*.

corodiastasis (ko″ro-di-as′tah-sis) corediastasis.

corolla (ko-rol′ah) [L. "little crown"] the inner set of leaves of a floral envelope, the individual portions of which are called *petals*.

corometer (ko-rom′ĕ-ter) pupillometer.

corona (ko-ro′nah), pl. *coronas*, or *coro′nae* [L.; Gr. *korōnē*] a crown; used in anatomical nomenclature to designate a crownlike eminence or encircling structure. **c. cilia′ris** [NA], the region on the anterior inner surface of the ciliary body of the eye from which radiate the ciliary processes. **c. clin′ica** [NA], clinical crown: the portion of a tooth which is exposed above the gingiva. **dental c., c. den′tis** [NA], the portion of a tooth that is covered by enamel and is separated from the root or roots at the cementoenamel junction; called also *anatomical crown*. **c. glan′dis pe′nis** [NA], **c. of glans penis,** the rounded proximal border of the glans penis, separated from the corpora cavernosa penis by the neck of the glans. **c. radia′ta,** 1. [NA] the radiating crown of projection fibers which pass from the internal capsule to every part of the cerebral cortex. 2. an investing layer of radially elongated follicular cells surrounding the zona pellucida of an ovum. **c. seborrhe′ica** (*obs.*), a red line or band along the upper border of the forehead and temples sometimes seen in severe cases of dermatitis seborrheica or pityriasis capitis, and often portending the development of frank psoriasis. **c. ven′eris,** a ring of syphilitic sores around the forehead, sometimes deeply affecting the bones of the head. **Zinn's c.,** circulus vasculosus nervi optici.

coronad (kor′ŏ-nad) toward the crown of the head or any corona.

coronae (ko-ro′ne) [L.] plural of *corona*.

coronal (ko-rŏ′nal) [L. *coronalis*] 1. pertaining to the crown of the head or to any corona. 2. situated in the direction of the coronal suture; said of a longitudinal plane or section passing through the body at right angles to the median plane. See under *plane*. Called also *coronalis* [NA].

coronale (kor-o-na′le) 1. the point of the coronal suture at the end of the maximum frontal diameter. 2. the frontal bone (os frontale [NA]).

coronalis (kor″o-na′lis) [L.] coronal; [NA] a term used to denote a structure situated in the direction of the coronal suture.

coronaritis (kor″o-nah-ri′tis) coronary arteritis.

coronary (kor′ŏ-na-re) [L. *corona;* Gr. *korōnē*] encircling in the manner of a crown; a term applied to vessels, nerves, ligaments, etc. The term usually denotes the arteries that supply the heart muscle and, by extension, a pathologic involvement of them.

coronavirus (kor″o-nah-vi′rus) any of a group of morphologically similar, ether-sensitive viruses, probably RNA, causing infectious bronchitis of birds, hepatitis in mice, gastroenteritis in swine, and respiratory infections in humans; called coronaviruses because of their resemblance, under the electron microscope, to a corona or crown.

corone (kŏ-ro′ne) [L.; Gr. *korōnē* anything hooked or curved] the coronoid process of the mandible (processus coronoideus mandibulae [NA]).

coroner (kor′o-ner) an officer who holds inquests in regard to violent, sudden, or unexplained deaths.

coronet (kor′o-net) the lower part of the pastern of a horse, where the horn joins the skin.

coronion (ko-ro′ne-on) the tip of the coronoid process of the mandible.

coronitis (kor-o-ni′tis) inflammation of the coronary band or cushion of the horse hoof or the claw of cloven-hoofed animals.

coronoid (kor′o-noid) [Gr. *korōnē* anything hooked or curved, a kind of crown + *oid*] 1. shaped like a crow's beak. 2. crown-shaped.

coronoidectomy (kor″o-noi-dek′to-me) surgical removal of the coronoid process of the mandible.

coroparelcysis (ko″ro-par-el′sĭ-sis) [*coro-* + Gr. *parelkein* to draw aside] the drawing aside of the pupil in partial corneal opacity in order to bring it under a transparent portion.

coroplasty (ko′ro-plas″te) coreoplasty.

coroscopy (ko-ros′ko-pe) [*coro-* + Gr. *skopein* to examine] retinoscopy.

corotomy (ko-rot′o-me) [*coro-* + Gr. *temnein* to cut] iridotomy.

corpora (kor′po-rah) [L.] plural of *corpus*.

corporal (kor′po-ral) corporeal.

corporeal (kor-po′re-al) pertaining to the body.

corporic (kor-po′rik) [L. *corpus* body] affecting the body, or corpus, of an organ.

corps (kōr) [Fr., from L. *corpus*] 1. an organized body, or group of individuals. 2. corpus. **medical c.,** the surgeon officers of the army or navy, comprising a surgeon general, medical directors, medical inspectors, surgeons, passed assistant surgeons, and assistant surgeons. **c. ronds,** Darier's name for round, double contoured bodies seen in keratosis follicularis.

corpse (korps) [L. *corpus* body] a dead body; used to refer specifically to a human body in the early period after death. Cf. *cadaver*.

corpulency (kor′pu-len″se) [L. *corpulentia*] undue fatness or obesity.

corpus (kor′pus), pl. *cor′pora*, gen. *cor′poris* [L. "body"] a discrete mass of material, as of specialized tissue; used in anatomical nomenclature to designate the entire organism, and applied also to the main portion of an anatomical part, structure, or organ. **c. adipo′sum buc′cae** [NA], adipose body of cheek: a thick layer of fat external to the buccinator muscle, containing the buccal glands; the main portion of fatty tissue in the cheek. Called also *fatty ball of Bichat, sucking cushion,* and *sucking* or *suctorial pad*. **c. adipo′sum fos′sae ischiorecta′lis** [NA], adipose body of the ischiorectal fossa: a pad of fat found in the ischiorectal fossa. **c. adipo′sum infrapatella′re** [NA], infrapatellar fatty body: a mass of fibrous fatty tissue inferior to the patella, in the angle between the deep surface of the patellar ligament and the tibia. **c. adipo′sum or′bitae** [NA], adipose body of orbit: a mass of fatty tissue in the posterior part of the orbit, around the optic nerve, extraocular muscles, and vessels. **c. al′bicans** (pl. *cor′pora albican′tia*) [NA], white fibrous tissue that replaces the regressing corpus luteum in the human ovary in the latter half of pregnancy, or soon after ovulation when pregnancy does not supervene; called also *c. fibrosum*. **c. alie′num,** a foreign body. **c. amygdaloi′deum** [NA], the amygdaloid body: a small, ovoid complex of nuclei partly covered by the pyriform cortex, within the tip of the temporal lobe, anterior to the inferior horn of the lateral ventricle of the brain; it is part of the limbic system and is sometimes classified as one of the basal ganglia. The amygdala has olfactory connections, is reciprocally connected to the limbic cortex, and projects fibers to the hippocampus, the septum, the thalamus, and especially to the hypothalamus. Called also *amygdala* and *nucleus amygdalae*. **cor′pora amyla′cea** [L. "starchy bodies"], small hyaline masses of degenerate cells found in the prostate, neuroglia, etc. Called also *amylaceous bodies* or *corpuscles, amyloid bodies* or *corpuscles, colloid corpuscles,* and *corpora versicolorata*. **cor′pora aran′tii** [L. "bodies of Arantius"], nodules of aortic valve; see *noduli valvularum semilunarium*. **cor′pora atret′ica,** ovarian follicles that never mature, but undergo degeneration; called also *pseudolutein body*. **cor′pora bigem′ina** (sing. *cor′pus bigem′inum*), corpora quadrigemina. **c. calca′nei,** the body of the calcaneus. **c. callo′sum** [NA], an arched mass of white matter, found in the depths of the longitudinal fissure, composed of transverse fibers connecting the cerebral hemispheres and consisting, from the anterior to the posterior, of rostrum, genu, trunk, and splenium; called also *commissura magna cerebri*. **c. caverno′sum clitor′idis** [NA], cavernous body of clitoris: a column of erectile tissue on either side [dextrum et sinistrum], the two fusing to form the body of the clitoris (c. clitoridis). **c. caverno′sum pe′nis** [NA], cavernous body of penis: one of the columns of erectile tissue forming the dorsum and sides of the penis; called also *spongy body of penis*. **c. caverno′sum ure′thrae viril′is,** c. spongiosum penis. **c. cilia′re** [NA], **c. cilia′ris,** the ciliary body: the thickened part of the vascular tunic of the eye anterior to the ora serrata, connecting the choroid with the iris; it is composed of the ciliary crown, ciliary processes and folds, ciliary orbiculus, the ciliary muscle, and a basal lamina. **c. clitor′idis** [NA], the main part of the clitoris, formed by the two fused corpora cavernosa, which are embedded anteriorly in the floor of the vestibule of the vagina. **c. coccyg′eum** [NA], an arteriovenous anastomotic structure along the course of the median sacral artery. **c. cos′tae** [NA], the part of a rib extending between its dorsally placed tubercle and its ventral extremity; called also *shaft of rib*. **c. denta′tum cerebel′li,** nucleus dentatus. **c. denta′tum oli′vae,** nucleus olivaris. **c. epididym′idis** [NA], the middle part of the epididymis, which is formed by the convolutions of the single ductus epididymidis. **c. fem′oris** [NA], the main part or shaft of the femur. **c. fibro′sum,** c. albicans. **c. fib′ulae** [NA], the principal part or shaft of the fibula. **c. fimbria′tum** [L. "fringed body"], a narrow band of white substance bordering the lateral edge of the lower cornu of the lateral ventricle of the cerebrum. **c. fimbria′tum hippocam′pi,** fimbria hippocampi. **cor′pora fla′va** [L. "yellow bodies"], waxy bodies found in the central nervous system and elsewhere, thought to be formed by the transformation of nerve cells. **c. for′nicis** [NA], body of fornix: the middle part of the fornix of the cerebrum, formed by fusion of the two lateral halves under the corpus callosum. **c. genicula′tum latera′le** [NA], the lateral geniculate body: an eminence of the metathalamus produced by the underlying lateral geniculate nucleus, just lateral to the medial geniculate body. It relays visual impulses from the optic tract to the calcarine cortex. Called also *optic thalamus*. **c. genicula′tum media′le** [NA], the medial geniculate body: an eminence of the metathalamus produced by the underlying medial geniculate nucleus, just lateral to the superior colliculus. It relays auditory impulses from the lateral lemniscus to the auditory cortex. **c. glan′dulae bulboure-**

thra′lis, the body of the bulbourethral gland. **c. glan′dulae sudorif′erae** [NA], the coiled secretory part of a sweat gland, found in the deep part of the corium; called also *coil* or *acinus of the sweat gland.* **c. glandula′re prosta′tae,** substantia glandularis prostatae. **c. glandulo′sum,** a spongy eminence surrounding the orifice of the female urethra. **c. hemor-rhag′icum,** 1. an ovarian follicle containing blood. 2. a corpus luteum containing a blood clot. **c. Highmo′ri, c. high-moria′num** [L. "body of Highmore"], mediastinum testis. **c. hu′meri** [NA], the main part or shaft of the humerus. **c. hypothalam′icum,** nucleus subthalamicus. **c. incu′dis** [NA], the central part of the incus, which contains an excavation in which the head of the malleus articulates. **c. interpedun-cula′re,** nucleus interpeduncularis. **c. lin′guae** [NA], the larger anterior part of the tongue, in the floor of the mouth. **c. lu′teum** (pl. *cor′pora lu′tea*) [L. "yellow body"] [NA], a yellow glandular mass in the ovary formed by an ovarian follicle that has matured and discharged its ovum; if the ovum has been impregnated, the corpus luteum increases in size and persists for several months (*true c. luteum, c. luteum of pregnancy, c. luteum graviditatis*); if impregnation has not taken place, the corpus luteum degenerates and shrinks (*false c. luteum, c. luteum of menstruation, c. luteum menstruationis*). The corpus luteum secretes progesterone. Called also *yellow body of ovary.* Cf. *corpus albicans,* def. 1. **cor′pora lu′tea atret′ica,** corpora lutea in which regressive changes have occurred. **c. Luy′sii,** nucleus subthalamicus. **c. malpig′hii,** the stratum malpighii. **c. mamilla′re** [NA], the mamillary body: either of the pair of small spherical masses situated close together in the interpeduncular space rostral to the posterior perforated substance and forming part of the hypothalamus; called also *bulla fornicis* or *bulla of fornix,* and *mamillary eminence.* **c. mam′mae** [NA], the essential mass of the mammary gland, exclusive of the glandular elements, which is thickest beneath the nipple and thinner toward the periphery; see illustration accompanying *mammary gland,* under *gland.* **c. mandib′ulae** [NA], body of mandible: the horizontal horseshoe-shaped portion of the mandible. **c. max-il′lae** [NA], body of maxilla: the large central portion of the maxilla, roughly pyramidal in shape, to which four major processes are connected; it contains the maxillary sinus. **c. medulla′re cerebel′li** [NA], medullary body of cerebellum: the white substance of the cerebellum; called also *center of cerebellum.* **c. medulla′re ver′mis,** arbor vitae cerebelli. **c. muco′-sum,** stratum mucosum. **c. nu′clei cauda′ti** [NA], the part of the caudate nucleus lying in the floor of the pars centralis of the lateral ventricle of the brain, extending posteriorly from the head and continuous with the tail. **c. of Oken,** mesonephros. **cor′pora oryzoi′dea** (sing. *cor′pus oryzoi′deum*), rice bodies. **c. os′sis hyoi′dei** [NA], body of hyoid bone: the central portion of the hyoid bone to which the large and small horns are attached; called also *basihyal* and *basihyoid.* **c. os′sis il′ii** [NA], **c. os′-sis il′ium,** the inferior portion of the ilium, which forms roughly the superior two-fifths of the acetabulum; called also *body of ilium.* **c. os′sis isch′ii** [NA], the thick, irregular, prismatic part of the ischium. Its superior end participates in the acetabulum, and from its inferior end the ramus of the ischium projects. It incorporates what was formerly called the superior ramus; called also *body of ischium.* **c. os′sis metacarpa′lis** [NA], the main part or shaft of a metacarpal bone. **c. os′sis metatarsa′lis** [NA], the main part or shaft of a metatarsal bone. **c. os′sis pu′bis** [NA], body of pubic bone: the irregular mass of the pubic bone that lies alongside the median plane, articulating with the similar portion of the opposite pubic bone. From it extend the superior and inferior rami of the pubic bone. **c. os′sis sphenoida′lis** [NA], body of sphenoid bone: the central, cuboidal part of the sphenoid bone to which the great wings, small wings, and pterygoid processes are attached; it contains the sphenoidal sinuses. Called also *c. sphenoidale.* **c. pampinifor′me,** epoophoron. **c. pancrea′tis** [NA], body of pancreas: the triangularly prismatic portion of the pancreas, extending from the neck on the right to the tail on the left. **cor′pora paraaor′tica** [NA], para-aortic bodies: exclaves of glandular cells of sympathetic origin (chromaffin cells) found near the sympathetic ganglia along the aorta in the abdominal cavity; they serve as chemoreceptors responsive to oxygen, carbon dioxide, and hydrogen ion concentration, that help to control respiration. See also *paraganglion.* **c. pe′nis** [NA], the free part of the penis between the root and the glans, consisting chiefly of the paired corpora cavernosa and the unpaired corpus spongiosum penis; called also *shaft of penis.* **c. phalan′gis digito′rum ma′nus** [NA], the main part or shaft of each phalanx of the fingers. **c. phalan′gis digito′-rum pe′dis** [NA], the main part or shaft of each phalanx of the toes. **c. pinea′le** [NA], the pineal body: a small, somewhat flattened, cone-shaped body in the epithalamus, lying above the superior colliculi below the splenium of the corpus callosum. Arising embryologically from the ependyma of the third ventricle and consisting of glial cells and pinealocytes, it appears to be the major or unique site of melatonin biosynthesis in most mammals, including man. The effect of melatonin on the body and the exact function of the corpus pineale remain obscure. Called also *pineal gland.* **c. pontobulba′re,** a ridge running obliquely across the restiform body just caudal to the ridge formed by the cochlear

nuclei. **c. pyramida′le medul′lae,** pyramis medullae oblongatae. **cor′pora quadrigem′ina** (sing. *cor′pus quad-rigem′inum*), four rounded eminences on the posterior surface of the mesencephalon; called also *bigeminal* or *quadrigeminal bodies,* and *corpora bigemina.* See also *colliculus.* **c. ra′dii** [NA], the main part or shaft of the radius. **cor′pora restifor′mia** (sing. *cor′pus restifor′mis*), see *pedunculus cerebellaris inferior.* **c. rhomboida′le,** nucleus dentatus. **cor′pora san-toria′na,** cartilago corniculata. **c. spongio′sum pe′nis** [NA], the column of erectile tissue that forms the urethral surface of the penis, and in which the urethra is found; its distal expansion forms the glans penis. Called also *c. cavernosum urethrae virilis* and *spongy body of male urethra.* **c. spongio′sum ure′-thrae mulie′bris,** the submucous layer of the female urethra. **c. ster′ni** [NA], body of sternum: the second or principal portion of the sternum, located between the manubrium above and the xiphoid process below; called also *gladiolus.* **c. stria′tum** (pl. *cor′pora stria′ta*) [NA], the striate body: one of the components of the basal ganglia; specifically, a subcortical mass of gray and white substance in front of and lateral to the thalamus in each cerebral hemisphere. The gray substance of this structure is arranged in two principal masses, the caudate nucleus and the lentiform nucleus; the striate appearance on section of the area being produced by connecting bands of gray substance passing from one of these nuclei to the other through the white substance of the internal capsule. **c. subthalam′icum,** nucleus subthalamicus. **c. ta′li** [NA], body of talus: the roughly quadrilateral portion of the talus, which presents several surfaces for articulation with the calcaneus, tibia, and fibula. **c. tib′iae** [NA], the main part or shaft of the tibia. **c. trapezoi′deum** [NA], the trapezoid body: a mass of transverse fibers extending through the central part of the pons and forming a part of the path of the cochlear nerve. **c. tritic′eum,** cartilago triticea. **c. ul′nae** [NA], the main part or shaft of the ulna. **c. un′guis** [NA], nail plate: the large distal, exposed portion of the nail of a digit. **c. u′teri** [NA], that part of the uterus above the isthmus and below the orifices of the uterine tubes. **c. ventric′-uli** [NA], body of stomach: that part of the stomach between the fundus and the pyloric portion. **cor′pora versicolora′ta,** corpora amylacea. **c. ver′tebrae** [NA], the body of a vertebra; called also *centrum vertebrae* and *intravertebral body.* **c. vesi′cae fel′leae** [NA], body of gallbladder: that part of the gallbladder between the fundus and the neck. **c. vesi′cae urina′riae** [NA], that part of the urinary bladder between the apex and the fundus. **c. vesic′ulae semina′lis,** body of small vesicle: the main portion of the seminal vesicle. **c. vit′-reum** [NA], the vitreous body: the transparent substance that fills the part of the eyeball between the lens and the retina; called also *hyaloid body, crystalline* or *vitreous humor,* and *humor cristallinus.* **c. Wolf′fi,** mesonephros.

corpuscle (kor′pus′l) any small mass or body; see also *corpuscu-lum.* **Alzheimer's c's,** compound granular corpuscles in the oligodendroglia of the brain. **amylaceous c's, amyloid c's,** corpora amylacea. **articular c's,** corpuscula articularia. **axile c., axis c.,** the central part of a tactile corpuscle. **Ba-bès-Ernst c's,** metachromatic granules. **basal c.,** see under *body.* **Bennet's large c's,** Nunn's gorged c's. **Bennet's small c's,** Drysdale's c's. **blood c's,** formed elements of the blood; i.e., erythrocytes and leukocytes. **blood c., red,** erythrocyte. **blood c., white,** leukocyte. **bone c.,** bone cell. **bridge c.,** desmosome. **bulboid c's,** corpuscula bulboidea. **Burckhardt's c's,** peculiar yellowish bodies found in trachoma secretion. **cancroid c's** (*obs.*), a nodular epithelioma. **cartilage c.,** cartilage cell. **cement c.,** cementocyte. **chorea c's,** a name given peculiar round hyaline bodies, concentrically laminated and strongly refractile, found in the perivascular sheaths of the vessels of the corpora striata and internal capsule in chorea. **chromophil c.,** Nissl's body. **chyle c.,** a lymphocyte found in chyle. **colloid c's,** corpora amylacea. **colostrum c's,** large rounded bodies in colostrum, containing droplets of fat and sometimes a nucleus; they apparently are phagocytic cells of the mammary gland, present for the first two weeks after parturition. Called also *Donné's bodies* or *corpuscles.* **concentric c's,** Hassall's c's. **corneal c's,** star-shaped connective tissue cells within the corneal spaces; called also *Toynbee's* and *Virchow's c's.* **Dogiel's c.,** a sensory end-organ found in the mucous membrane of the eyes, nose, mouth, and genitals. **Donné's c's,** colostrum c's. **Drysdale's c's,** transparent microscopical cells seen in the fluid of ovarian cysts; called also *Bennet's c's.* **dust c's,** hemoconia. **Eichhorst's c's,** a name once given a peculiar variety of microcytes seen in pernicious anemia. **genital c's,** corpuscula genitalia. **ghost c.,** phantom c. **Gierke's c's,** roundish bodies found in the nervous system, probably identical with Hassall's corpuscles. **Gluge's c's,** granular corpuscles occurring in diseased nerve tissue. **Golgi's c's,** encapsulated end-organs found in a tendon at its junction with the muscular fibers, which mediate tension differences to the innervating nerve fibers. **Golgi-Mazzoni c's,** tactile corpuscles found in the subcutaneous tissue of the fingertips, resembling pacinian corpuscles, but possessing fewer lamellae and a relatively larger cone, and having the contained nerve fibers more extensively branched. **Grandry's c's, Gran-**

dry-Merkel c's, Merkel's c's. **Guarnieri's c's,** see under *body*. **Hassall's c's,** spherical or ovoid bodies found in the medulla of the thymus, composed of concentric arrays of epithelial cells which contain keratohyalin and bundles of cytoplasmic filaments. Called also *Hassall's bodies, concentric c's, Leber's c's* and *thymus c's.* **Herbst's c's,** peculiar sensory end-organs in the skin of the bill and in the mucous membrane of the tongue of the duck. **Jaworski's c's,** spiral mucous bodies seen in the secretion of the stomach in hyperchlorhydria. **Krause's c's,** corpuscula bulboidea. **lamellar c's, lamellated c's,** corpuscula lamellosa. **Langerhans's stellate c's,** see under *cell*. **Laveran's c's,** former name for the malarial parasite, *Plasmodium*. **Leber's c's,** Hassall's c's. **lingual c.,** an encapsulated terminal sensory nerve ending in a lingual papilla. **Lostorfer's c's,** granular bodies observed in the blood in syphilis; called also *Lostorfer's bodies.* **lymph c's,** lymphocytes observed in lymph. **lymphoid c's,** lymphocytes observed in tissues. **malpighian c's of kidney,** corpuscula renis. **malpighian c's of spleen,** see *folliculi lymphatici lienales.* **Mazzoni's c's,** sensory nerve endings resembling Krause's corpuscles. **meconium c's,** epithelial cells containing many coarse yellow granules, observed in the lower part of the small intestine in a fetus. **Meissner's c's,** corpuscula tactus. **Merkel's c's,** tactile corpuscles in the submucosa of the tongue and mouth, each consisting of a sheath which is continuous with the sheath of Henle of the nerve. Enclosed within the sheath are two flattened epithelial cells between the opposed surfaces of which is a biconvex disk continuous with the end of the neurofibrils. Called also *Grandry-Merkel c's* and *Merkel's disks.* **Miescher's c's,** Rainey's c's. **milk c's,** delicate particles of fat suspended in the serum of the milk. **molluscous c's,** molluscum bodies. **mucous c's,** bodies resembling leukocytes occurring in mucus. **nerve c's,** the sheath cells lying between the neurilemma and the medullary sheath. **Norris' c's,** colorless, transparent disks in the blood serum. **Nunn's gorged c's,** epithelial cells found in ovarian cysts that have undergone a high degree of fatty degeneration; called also *Bennet's large c's.* **Pacini's c's, pacinian c's,** lamellated nerve endings (corpus-

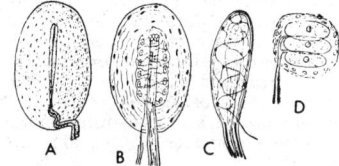

Sense corpuscles. *A*, Herbst's corpuscle from the tongue of a duck. *B*, Pacinian corpuscle from the mesentery of a cat. *C*, Krause's corpuscle. *D*, Merkel's corpuscle.

cula lameosa) that are concerned in the perception of pressure. **Paschen's c's,** see under *body*. **Paterson's c's,** molluscum bodies. **pessary c.,** see under *cell*. **phantom c.,** an artifactual red cell from which the hemoglobin has been dissolved. **Purkinje's c's,** see under *cell*. **pus c.,** one of the cells of pus, chiefly neutrophilic leukocytes. **Rainey's c's,** sarcosporidian cysts. **red c.,** erythrocyte. **renal c's,** corpuscula renis. **reticulated c's,** erythrocytes which on proper staining show filamentous reticulations filling a greater part of the cell. **Röhl's marginal c's,** small bodies seen in the margins of erythrocytes of animals after the administration of chemotherapeutic substances. **Ruffini's c's,** lamellated nerve endings (corpuscula lamellosa) that are concerned in the perception of pressure and of warmth. **salivary c's,** white blood cells found in the saliva. **Schwalbe's c.,** caliculus gustatorius. **sensitized c.,** a given kind of blood corpuscle laden with an antibody specific for that variety of corpuscle; if erythrocytes sensitized with specific antibody (hemolysin) are brought into contact with complement, hemolysis takes place. **shadow c.,** phantom c. **splenic c's,** folliculi lymphatici lienales. **tactile c's,** corpuscula tactus. **taste c's,** taste cells. **tendon c's,** flattened cells of connective tissue occurring in rows between the primary bundles of the tendons. **terminal nerve c's,** corpuscula nervosa terminalia. **thymus c's,** Hassall's c's. **Timofeew's c's,** a specialized form of pacinian corpuscle found in the submucosa of the membranous and prostatic portions of the urethra. **touch c's,** corpuscula tactus. **Toynbee's c's,** corneal c's. **Traube's c.,** phantom c. **Tröltsch's c's,** connective tissue spaces lined with flattened endothelial cells, and appearing like corpuscular bodies among the radial fibers of the membrana tympani. **typhic c's,** cells of Peyer's patches that have undergone degeneration in typhoid fever. **Valentin's c's,** small amyloid bodies found in nerve tissue. **Vater's c's, Vater-Pacini c's,** corpuscula lamellosa. **Virchow's c's,** corneal c's. **Wagner's c's,** corpuscula tactus. **Weber's c.,** utriculus prostaticus. **white c.,** leukocyte. **Zimmermann's c.** (*obs.*), achromocyte.

corpuscula (kor-pus′ku-lah) [L.] plural of *corpusculum*.

corpuscular (kor-pus′ku-lar) pertaining to or of the nature of corpuscles.

corpusculum (kor-pus′ku-lum), pl. *corpus′cula* [L. dim. of *corpus*] a small mass or body; used as a general term in anatomical

nomenclature to designate certain small discrete masses of specialized tissue, especially of nerve tissue. **corpus′cula articula′ria** [NA], articular corpuscles: encapsulated nerve endings found within joints; called also *corpuscula nervorum articularia*. **corpus′cula bulbifor′mia,** corpuscula bulboidea. **corpus′cula bulboi′dea** [NA], bulboid corpuscles: small encapsulated nerve endings found in the skin, mucous membranes, conjunctiva, and heart, at varying levels; called also *bulbs of Krause, corpuscula bulbiformis,* and *Krause's corpuscles.* **corpus′cula genita′lia** [NA], genital corpuscles: small encapsulated nerve endings occurring in the mucous membrane in the genital region; called also *corpuscula nervorum genitalia.* **corpus′cula lamello′sa** [NA], lamellar or lamellated corpuscles: large encapsulated nerve endings, which are the most complicated of the nerve endings and are found throughout the body. Concerned with the perception of different sensations, various such endings are named for the men who originally described them, e.g., *Pacini's corpuscles* and *Ruffini's corpuscles.* Called also *Vater's* and *Vater-Pacini corpuscles.* **corpus′cula nervo′rum articula′ria,** corpuscula articularia. **corpus′cula nervo′rum genita′lia,** corpuscula genitalia. **corpus′cula nervo′rum termina′lia,** corpuscula nervosa terminalia. **corpus′cula nervo′sa termina′lia** [NA], terminal nerve corpuscles: nerve endings characterized by a fibrous capsule of varying thickness that is continuous with the endoneurium; for different named varieties, see under *corpuscle.* Called also *corpuscula nervorum terminalia* and *encapsulated nerve endings.* **corpus′cula re′nis** [NA], renal corpuscles: bodies forming the beginnings of the nephrons, each consisting of a tuft of capillaries (the glomerulus), surrounded by an expanded portion of the renal tubule (the glomerular capsule); called also *glomerular corpuscles, acinus renalis* [*malpighii*]*, acinus renis* [*malpighii*]*, malpighian bodies of kidneys,* and *malpighian* or *renal tufts.* **corpus′cula tac′tus** [NA], tactile corpuscles: medium-sized encapsulated nerve endings found in the skin, most commonly in the palms and soles; called also *tactile* or *touch cells,* and *Meissner's oval, tactile,* or *touch corpuscles.* **c. tritic′eum,** cartilago triticea.

correction (kŏ-rek′shun) [L. *correctio* straightening out; amendment] a setting right, as the provision of specific lenses for the improvement of vision, or an arbitrary adjustment made in values or devices in performance of experimental procedures.

corrector (kor-rek′tor) something that corrects or sets right. **function c.,** a removable orthodontic appliance utilizing oral and facial muscle forces to move teeth and possibly change the relationship of dental arches; called also *Fränkel appliance.*

correlation (kor″ĕ-la′shun) in neurology, those combinations of the afferent impulses within the sensory centers which provide for the integration of the impulses into appropriate responses (Herrick). In statistics, the degree of association of variable phenomena, as intelligence and birth order.

correspondence (kor″e-spon′dens) the condition of being in agreement, or conformity. **anomalous retinal c.,** a condition in which disparate points on the retinas of the two eyes come to be associated sensorially; abbreviated A.R.C. **harmonious retinal c.,** the condition in which corresponding points on the retinas of the two eyes are associated sensorially. **retinal c.,** the state regarding the impingement of images on the retinas of the two eyes.

Corrigan's cautery, etc. (kor′e-ganz) [Sir Dominic John *Corrigan*, physician in Dublin, 1802–1880] see under *cautery, disease, line, pulse, respiration,* and *sign.*

corrigent (kor′ĕ-jent) [L. *corrigens* correcting] 1. amending or rendering milder. 2. any agent that favorably modifies the action of a drug which is too powerful or harsh, or that improves its taste.

corrin (kor′in) a tetrapyrrole ring system resembling the porphyrin ring system of hemoglobin, but in which a pair of the rings is joined directly rather than through a methene bridge, with cobalt being bound to the inner four nitrogen atoms. The cobalamins contain a corrin ring system.

corroid (kor′oid) a compound, such as the cobalamins, containing a corrin ring system.

corrosion (kŏ-ro′zhun) [L. *corrosio*] the slow destruction of the texture or substance of a tissue, as by the action of a corrosive substance.

corrosive (kŏ-ro′siv) [L. *con* with + *rodere* to gnaw] 1. destructive to the texture or substance of the tissues. 2. a substance that destroys the texture or substance of the tissues. Called also *caustic* and *escharotic.*

corrugator (cor′u-ga″tor) [L. *con* together + *ruga* wrinkle] that which wrinkles; a muscle that wrinkles.

corset (kor′set) an orthopedic device that encircles and supports a part, as worn in certain spinal injuries or deformities.

Cort. abbreviation for L. *cor′tex*, bark.

Cortate (kor′tāt) trademark for preparations of desoxycorticosterone acetate.

Cort-Dome (kort′dōm) trademark for preparations of hydrocortisone.

Cortef (kor′tef) trademark for preparations of hydrocortisone.

Cortenema (kor-ten′ĕ-mah) trademark for a preparation of hydrocortisone.

cortex (kor′teks), gen. *cor′ticis*, pl. *cor′tices* [L. "bark, rind, shell"] 1. an external layer, as the bark of a tree, or the rind of a fruit. 2. [NA] the outer layer of an organ or other body structure, as distinguished from the internal substance. **adrenal c.,** the outer, firm, yellowish layer that comprises the larger part of the adrenal (suprarenal) gland, the zona glomerulosa, the zona fasciculata, and the zona reticularis; it secretes, in response to release of corticotropin by the pituitary gland, many steroid hormones, including mineralocorticoids, glucocorticoids, androgens, 17-ketosteroids, and progestins (see *adrenal gland,* under *gland*). Called also *cortex glandulae suprarenalis* [NA], *substantia corticalis glandulae suprarenalis,* and *cortical substance of suprarenal gland.* **cerebellar c., c. cerebel′li** [NA], **c. of cerebellum,** the superficial gray matter of the cerebellum; called also *substantia corticalis cerebelli* and *cortical substance of cerebellum.* **cerebral c., c. cer′ebri** [NA], **c. of cerebrum,** the thin layer of gray matter on the surface of the cerebral hemisphere, folded into gyri with about two-thirds of its area buried in the depths of the fissures. It reaches its highest development in man, where it is responsible for the higher mental functions, for general movement, for visceral functions, perception, and behavioral reactions, and for the association and integration of these functions. Many classifications have been suggested: it has been divided into neopallium, archipallium, paleopallium according to supposed phylogenetic and ontogenetic differences; into areas according to the presence of six cell layers (see *neopallium*) or according to differences in the structure and arrangement of cell and fiber layers; and into functional areas such as motor, sensory, and association areas. Called also *pallium.* **c. glan′dulae suprarena′lis** [NA], the outer, firm yellowish layer that comprises the larger part of the suprarenal gland; called also *adrenal cortex* (q.v.), *cortical substance of suprarenal gland,* and *substantia corticalis glandulae suprarenalis.* **heterotypical c.,** the portion of the cerebral cortex containing fewer than the six cell layers of the homotypical cortex; see *archipallium.* **homotypical c.,** the portion of the cerebral cortex containing all six cell layers; see *neopallium.* **c. of kidney,** renal c. **c. len′tis** [NA], the softer, external part of the lens of the eye; called also *substantia corticalis lentis* and *cortical substance of lens.* **motor c.,** the area of the frontal lobe of the cerebral cortex concerned with primary motor control of the body; Brodmann's area 4. **c. no′di lymphat′ici** [NA], the outer portion of a lymph node, consisting mainly of dense lymphatic tissue and follicles; called also *substantia corticalis lymphoglandulae* and *cortical substance of lymph nodes.* **nonolfactory c.,** neopallium. **olfactory c.,** archipallium. **piriform c.,** the cortex of the piriform lobe or area. **provisional c.,** the cortex of the fetal adrenal gland that undergoes involution in early fetal life. **renal c., c. re′nis** [NA], cortex of kidney; the outer part of the substance of the kidney, composed mainly of glomeruli and convoluted tubules; called also *substantia corticalis renis* and *cortical substance of kidney.* **somesthetic c.,** postcentral area; see under *area.* **striate c.,** the primary visual cortex: the part of the occipital lobe of the cerebral cortex containing the line of Gennari and receiving the fibers of the optic radiation from the lateral geniculate body; it is the primary receptive area for vision. Called also *striate area* and *area striata.* **c. of thymus,** the outer part of each lobule of the thymus; it consists chiefly of closely packed lymphocytes (thymocytes) and surrounds the medulla. **visual c.,** the area of the occipital lobe of the cerebral cortex concerned with vision; it consists of the primary visual cortex (Brodmann's area 17; see *striate c.*) and two other areas (Brodmann's areas 18 and 19) whose role is not as well defined, although area 18 is linked to the opposite hemisphere by the corpus callosum.

cortexone (kor-tek′sōn) desoxycorticosterone.

Corti's arch, membrane, organ, etc. [Alfonso *Corti,* Italian anatomist, 1822–1888] see under *arch, canal, cell, fiber, ganglion, rod,* and *tunnel,* and see *membrana tectoria ductus cochlearis* and *organum spirale.*

cortiadrenal (kor′te-ad-re′nal) corticoadrenal.

cortical (kor′tĭ-kal) [L. *corticalis*] pertaining to or of the nature of a cortex or bark.

corticalosteotomy (kor″tĭ-kal-os″te-ot′o-me) osteotomy through the bone cortex at the base of the dentoalveolar segment, which serves to weaken the resistance of the bone to the application of orthodontic forces.

corticate (kor′tĭ-kāt) possessing a cortex or bark.

corticectomy (kor″tĭ-sek′to-me) excision of an area of cerebral cortex (scar or microgyrus) in the treatment of focal epilepsy.

cortices (kor′tĭ-sēz) [L.] plural of *cortex.*

corticifugal (kor″tĭ-sif′u-gal) [*cortex* + L. *fugere* to flee] proceeding, conducting, or moving away from the cortex.

corticipetal (kor″tĭ-sip′e-tal) [*cortex* + L. *petere* to seek] proceeding, conducting, or moving toward the cortex.

corticoadrenal (kor″tĭ-ko-ad-re′nal) pertaining to the adrenal cortex.

corticoafferent (kor″tĭ-ko-af′fer-ent) conveying impressions from the lower levels inward and upward to the cerebral cortex; said of certain nerve fibers.

corticoautonomic (kor″tĭ-ko-aw″to-nom′ik) denoting the relationship of autonomic function to definite areas in the cerebral cortex.

corticobulbar (kor″tĭ-ko-bul′bar) pertaining to or connecting the cerebral cortex and the medulla oblongata and/or brain stem.

corticocerebral (kor″tĭ-ko-ser′e-bral) pertaining to the cerebral cortex.

corticodiencephalic (kor″tĭ-ko-di″en-se-fal′ik) pertaining to or connecting the cerebral cortex and the diencephalon.

corticoefferent (kor″tĭ-ko-ef′er-ent) carrying impressions outward and downward from the cerebral cortex; said of certain nerve fibers.

corticofugal (kor″tĭ-kof′u-gal) corticifugal.

corticoid (kor′tĭ-koid) any of the steroids of the adrenal cortex; a corticosteroid (q.v.).

corticomesencephalic (kor″tĭ-ko-mes″en-se-fal′ik) pertaining to or connecting the cerebral cortex and the mesencephalon.

corticopeduncular (kor″tĭ-ko-pe-dung′ku-lar) pertaining to the cortex and the peduncles of the brain.

corticopetal (kor″tĭ-kop′e-tal) corticipetal.

corticopleuritis (kor″tĭ-ko-ploo-ri′tis) inflammation of the visceral pulmonary pleura.

corticopontine (kor″tĭ-ko-pon′tin) pertaining to or connecting the cerebral cortex and the pons.

corticospinal (kor″tĭ-ko-spi′nal) pertaining to or connecting the cortex of the brain and the spinal cord.

corticosteroid (kor″tĭ-ko-ste′roid) any of the steroids elaborated by the adrenal cortex (excluding the sex hormones of adrenal origin) in response to the release of corticotropin (adrenocorticotropic hormone) by the pituitary gland, or any of the synthetic equivalents of these steroids. They are divided, according to their predominant biological activity, into two major groups: *glucocorticoids,* chiefly affecting carbohydrate, fat, and protein metabolism, and *mineralocorticoids,* affecting the regulation of electrolyte and water balance. Some corticosteroids exhibit both types of activity in varying degrees, and others exert only one type of effect. The corticosteroids are used clinically for hormonal replacement therapy, for suppression of ACTH secretion by the anterior pituitary, as antineoplastic and anti-inflammatory agents, and to suppress the immune response. Called also *adrenocortical hormone* and *corticoid.*

corticosterone (kor″tĭ-kos′ter-ōn) chemical name: $11\beta,21$-dihydroxypregn-4-ene-3,20-dione. A natural mineralocorticoid with some glucocorticoid activity, $C_{21}H_{30}O_4$, possessing life-maintaining properties in adrenalectomized animals and several other activities peculiar to the adrenal cortex. It is similar to 11-deoxycorticosterone, but its life-maintaining and sodium-retaining potencies are less. Called also *(Kendall's) compound B.*

corticosuprarenaloma (kor″tĭ-ko-su″prah - re″nal - o′ mah) (*obs.*) adenoma or carcinoma of the adrenal cortex.

corticosuprarenoma (kor″tĭ-ko-su″prah-re-no′mah) (*obs.*) adenoma or carcinoma of the adrenal cortex.

corticotensin (kor″tĭ-ko-ten′sin) a low-molecular-weight polypeptide purified from kidney extract that exhibits a vasopressor effect when given intravenously.

corticothalamic (kor″tĭ-ko-thah-lam′ik) pertaining to or connecting the cerebral cortex and the thalamus.

corticotrope (kor′ti-ko-trop) any of a group of ACTH-secreting, irregularly stellate chromophobe cells of the anterior pituitary gland, having cell processes extending between and partially surrounding neighboring cells and a few extremely small cytoplasmic granules. Called also *corticotroph.*

corticotrophic (kor″tĭ-ko-trof′ik) corticotropic.

corticotrophin (kor′tĭ-ko-tro′fin) corticotropin.

corticotropic (kor″tĭ-ko-trop′ik) exerting a specific effect upon the cortex of the adrenal gland; called also *adrenocorticotropic.*

corticotropin (kor″tĭ-ko-tro′pin) a peptide hormone secreted by the anterior pituitary gland that acts primarily on the adrenal cortex, stimulating its growth and its secretion of corticosteroids. The production of corticotropin is increased during times of stress. A sterile preparation [USP] of the same principle(s) derived from the anterior pituitary of those mammals used for food by man is administered parenterally for diagnostic testing of adrenocortical function and to stimulate the adrenal cortex to release its hormones, especially cortisol (hydrocortisone), in the treatment of several diseases, e.g., allergies, rheumatic disorders, and collagen, dermatologic, ophthalmic, hematologic, and neoplastic diseases, etc. It is used in veterinary medicine in the treatment of ketosis. Called also *adrenocorticotropic hormone (ACTH)* and *adrenocorticotropin.*

cortilymph (kor′tĕ-limf″) [organ of *Corti* + *lymph*] the fluid filling the intercellular spaces of the organ of Corti.

cortin (kor′tin) an extract from the adrenal cortex containing a mixture of hormones having glucocorticoid and mineralocorticoid activity.

cortisol (kor′tĭ-sol) chemical name: 11β,17α,21-trihydroxy-pregn-4-ene-3,20-dione. The major natural glucocorticoid (q.v.) elaborated by the human adrenal cortex, or hydrocortisone [USP], as it is usually referred to pharmaceutically. See *hydrocortisone* for therapeutic uses. Called also (*Kendall's*) *compound F.*

cortisone (kor′tĭ-sōn) chemical name: 17α,21-dihydroxy-4-pregnene-3,11,20-trione. A natural glucocorticoid (q.v.), with significant mineralocorticoid properties, $C_{21}H_{28}O_5$; believed to be both a precursor and a metabolite of cortisol (hydrocortisone). The human adrenal cortex secretes only minute amounts of cortisone; the synthetic hormone exerts its pharmaceutical effects through its metabolic conversion to cortisol. **c. acetate** [USP], an ester of cortisone (q.v.), $C_{23}H_{30}O_6$, occurring as a white or practically white, crystalline powder; used as an anti-inflammatory in various conditions, including allergies and the collagen diseases. It is also used as replacement therapy in adrenocortical deficiencies, including Addison's disease and hypopituitarism, administered intramuscularly or orally, and is applied topically to treat steroid-responsive inflammatory conditions of the eye and skin.

cortivazol (kor-ti′vah-zōl) chemical name: 11β-17,21-trihydroxy-6,16α-dimethyl-2′-phenyl-2′H-pregna-2, 4, 6-trieno [3,2-c]-20-one 21-acetate; a glucocorticoid, $C_{32}H_{38}N_2O_5$.

Cortone (kor′tōn) trademark for preparations of cortisone acetate.

Cortril (kor′tril) trademark for preparations of hydrocortisone.

Cortrophin (kor-tro′fin) trademark for preparations of corticotropin.

Cortrosyn (kor′tro-sin) trademark for a preparation of cosyntropin.

corundum (kŏ-run′dum) native aluminum oxide.

coruscation (kor″us-ka′shun) a glittering sensation, as of flashes of light before the eyes.

Corvisart's disease (kor″ve-sarz′) [Baron Jean Nicolas *Corvisart* des Marest, French physician, 1755–1821] see under *disease.*

corybantiasm (kor″ĕ-ban′te-azm) corybantism.

corybantism (kor″ĕ-ban′tizm) [Gr. *Korybas* a reveller] wild, frenzied, and sleepless delirium.

corydaline (kŏ-rid′ah-lēn) an alkaloid, $C_{22}H_{27}NO_4$, from *Corydalis tuberosa*; a diuretic and tonic.

corydalis (kŏ-rid′ah-lis) [L. from Gr. *korys* helmet] the dried tuber of *Dicentra cucullaria* (L.) Bernh., or of *D. canadensis* (DC.) Walp., Fumariaceae, perennial herbs distributed throughout Ontario to Kentucky and Missouri. Also known as squirrel corn and turkey corn. It contains several isoquinoline type alkaloids, e.g., corydaline, bulbocapnine, corytuberine, etc. Bulbocapnine has been used for various muscle tremors and for vestibular nystagmus. The plant extract was once used as a tonic, antiperiodic, diuretic, and alterative.

corymbiform (ko-rim′bĭ-form) [Gr. *korymbos* the cluster of ivy flower + *form*] clustered; said of lesions grouped around a single, usually larger, lesion, as in tinea versicolor or late secondary syphilis.

corymbose (kor′im-bōs) corymbiform.

Corynebacteriaceae (ko-ri″ne-bak-te″re-a′se-e) a family of Schizomycetes (order Eubacteriales), made up of usually nonmotile rods, sometimes showing marked variation in form, and sometimes beaded or banded with metachromatic granules. It includes six genera, *Arthrobacter, Cellulomonas, Corynebacterium, Erysipelothrix, Listeria,* and *Microbacterium.*

Corynebacterium (ko-ri″ne-bak-te″re-um) [Gr. *korynē* club + *baktērion* little rod] a genus of microorganisms of the family Corynebacteriaceae, order Eubacteriales, made up of straight to slightly curved rods, which are generally aerobic but may be microaerophilic or even anaerobic; 144 species have been described. **C. ac′nes,** a diptheroid bacillus, differing from the diphtheria bacillus in being nontoxigenic and microaerophilic, and in producing a pink pigment in culture. It is found on the skin, and is usually present in acne lesions in association with other bacteria, especially *Staphylococcus albus* and *Pityrosporon ovale.* **C. belfan′tii,** a species considered to be a possible cause of ozena; it may be a nontoxogenic form of the mitis type of *C. diphtheriae.* **C. diphthe′riae,** the specific etiologic agent of diphtheria, producing a potent exotoxin, and separable into three types—mitis, gravis, and intermedius, which are now thought to be without

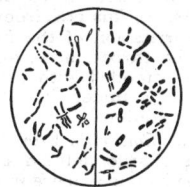

Corynebacterium diphtheriae.

pathological significance. Called also *Klebs-Löffler bacillus.* **C. enzy′micum,** a diphtheria-like bacillus found largely in, and of

uncertain pathogenicity for, man, but the etiologic agent of an epidemic ophthalmia of sheep. **C. e′qui,** an etiologic agent of pneumonia in foals, occurring as coccoid and bacillary forms, the former being acid-fast. **C. hofman′nii,** a species of diptheroid bacilli occurring in the human throat. **C. infantisep′ticum,** *Listeria monocytogenes.* **C. minutis′simum,** a species that causes erythrasma. **C. murisep′ticum,** a diphtheria-like bacillus producing septicemic disease in mice, but apparently nonpathogenic for other animals. **C. necroph′orum,** *Fusobacterium necrophorum.* **C. o′vis,** *C. pseudotuberculosis.* **C. par′vulum,** *Listeria monocytogenes.* **C. par′vum,** a species first isolated in the blood of a woman with postpartal fever; used by injection in treating malignant ascitic and pleural infusions. **C. pseudodiphtherit′icum,** a microorganism present in the upper respiratory tract, morphologically indistinguishable from the diphtheria bacillus but nonpathogenic and nontoxigenic; called also *Hofmann's bacillus.* **C. pseudotuberculo′sis-o′vis,** a weakly toxigenic diphtheria-like bacillus whose toxin is unrelated to diphtheria toxin; nonpathogenic for man, but pathogenic for domestic animals, in which it produces a caseous lymphadenitis and ulcerative lymphangitis, referred to as pseudotuberculosis. Called also *Preisz-Nocard bacillus* and *C. ovis.* **C. pyog′enes,** a diphtheria-like bacillus producing an exotoxin less potent than diphtheria toxin and differing from it immunologically; a common cause of purulent infections in lower animals, but nonpathogenic for man. **C. rena′le,** a diphtheria-like bacillus closely related to *C. pseudotuberculosis,* and pathogenic for lower animals, in which it produces purulent infections of the urinary tract. **C. ten′uis,** the etiologic agent of trichomycosis axillaris. **C. xero′se, C. xero′sis,** a species of diphtheroid bacilli which occurs in the normal eye and has been isolated from a form of conjunctivitis known as xerosis.

coryneform (ko-ri″nĕ-form) denoting or resembling organisms of the family Corynebacteriaceae.

corytuberine (ko″re-tu′ber-ēn) a crystalline alkaloid, $C_{19}H_{21}$-$NO_4 \cdot 5H_2O$, from commercial corydaline.

coryza (kŏ-ri′zah) [L.; Gr. *koryza*] an acute catarrhal condition of the nasal mucous membrane, with a profuse discharge from the nostrils. **allergic c.,** hay fever. **c. foe′tida,** ozena. **infectious avian c.,** an acute respiratory disease of chickens characterized by nasal discharge, sneezing, and edema of the face, and caused by *Hemophilus gallinarum.* Infection of the lower respiratory tract sometimes occurs. **c. oedemato′sa,** a serous inflammation of the inferior and middle turbinate bones.

coryzavirus (kŏ-ri″zah-vi′rus) one of a group of viral agents isolated from patients with the common cold and believed to be an etiologic agent of the common cold; now called *rhinovirus.*

C.O.S. Canadian Ophthalmological Society; Clinical Orthopaedic Society.

Coschwitz' duct (kosh′vits) [Georgius Daniel *Coschwitz,* German physician, 1679–1729] see under *duct.*

cosensitize (ko-sen′sĭ-tīz) to sensitize to two or more sensitizing agents.

Cosmegen (kos-mĕ-jen) trademark for a preparation of dactinomycin.

cosmesis (koz-me′sis) [Gr. *kosmēsis*] (*obs.*) the art of increasing and preserving beauty.

cosmetic (koz-met′ik) [Gr. *kosmētikos*] 1. beautifying; tending to preserve, restore, or confer comeliness. 2. a beautifying substance or preparation.

cosmetology (koz″mĕ-tol′o-je) the study of the proper care of the body from the point of view of cleanliness and comeliness.

cosmic (koz′mik) [Gr. *kosmikos* pertaining to the world] pertaining to the universe; expansive and vast.

costa (kos′tah), pl. *cos′tae* [L. "rib"], [NA] 1. one of the paired bones, twelve on each side, that extend from the thoracic vertebrae toward the median line on the ventral aspect of the trunk; a rib. 2. a thin, firm, rodlike structure running along the base of the undulating membrane of flagellates, such as *Trichomonas,* which is probably a supporting structure. **c. fluc′tuans,** floating rib: one of the lowest two ribs on either side, whose ventral tips ordinarily have no attachment. **c. fluc′tuans dec′ima,** Stiller's sign. **cos′tae spu′riae** [NA], the lower five ribs on either side: the ventral tips of the upper three of the five pairs connect with the costal cartilages of the superiorly adjacent ribs; the ventral tips of the lower two pairs ordinarily have no attachment. Called also *false ribs.* **cos′tae ve′rae** [NA], true ribs: the upper seven ribs on either side, which are connected to the sides of the sternum by their costal cartilages.

costae (kos′te) [L.] plural of *costa.*

costal (kos′tal) [L. *costalis*] pertaining to a rib or ribs.

costalgia (kos-tal′je-ah) [*costa* + *-algia*] pain in the ribs.

costalis (kos-ta′lis) [L.] costal; used in anatomical nomenclature to denote relationship to a rib.

costatectomy (kos″tah-tek′to-me) costectomy.

costectomy (kos-tek′to-me) [*costa* + Gr. *ektomē* excision] the operation of excising or resecting a rib.

Costen's syndrome (kos'tenz) [James Bray *Costen*, St. Louis oto-laryngologist, 1895–1962] temporomandibular joint syndrome.

costicartilage (kos"tĭ-kar'tĭ-lij) [*costa* + *cartilage*] the carti-lage of a rib.

costicervical (kos"tĭ-ser've-kal) pertaining to or connecting the ribs and the neck.

costiferous (kos-tif'er-us) [*costa* + L. *ferre* to carry] bearing a rib, as the thoracic vertebrae of man.

costiform (kos'tĭ-form) shaped like a rib.

costispinal (kos-tĭ-spi'nal) pertaining to or connecting the ribs and spine.

costive (kos'tiv) 1. pertaining to, characterized by, or producing constipation. 2. an agent that depresses intestinal motility.

costiveness (kos'tiv-nes) constipation.

costo- (kos'to) [L. *costa* rib] a combining form denoting relation-ship to the ribs.

costocentral (kos"to-sen'tral) pertaining to a rib and the cen-trum (body) of a vertebra.

costocervicalis (kos"to-ser"vĭ-ka'lis) [*costo-* + *cervicalis*] mus-culus iliocostalis cervicis; see *Table of Musculi*.

costochondral (kos"to-kon'dral) pertaining to a rib and its cartilage.

costoclavicular (kos"to-klah-vik'u-lar) pertaining to the ribs and clavicle.

costocoracoid (kos"to-kor'ah-koid) pertaining to the ribs and coracoid process.

costogenic (kos"to-jen'ik) [*costo-* + Gr. *gennan* to produce] arising from a rib, especially from defect of the marrow of the ribs.

costoinferior (kos"to-in-fe're-or) pertaining to the lower ribs.

costophrenic (kos"to-fren'ik) pertaining to the ribs and dia-phragm.

costopleural (kos"to-plu'ral) pertaining to the ribs and the pleura.

costopneumopexy (kos"to-nu'mo-pek"se) [*costo-* + Gr. *pneumōn* lung + *pēxis* fixing] the operation of anchoring the lung to a rib.

costoscapular (kos"to-skap'u-lar) pertaining to the ribs and the scapula.

costoscapularis (kos"to-skap"u-la'ris) musculus serratus an-terior; see *Table of Musculi*.

costosternal (kos"to-ster'nal) pertaining to a rib and to the sternum.

costosternoplasty (kos"to-ster'no-plas"te) surgical repair of funnel chest, a segment of rib being used to support the sternum.

costosuperior (kos"to-su-pe're-or) pertaining to the upper ribs.

costotome (kos'to-tōm) [*costo-* + Gr. *temnein* to cut] a knife for dividing ribs or costal cartilages.

costotomy (kos-tot'o-me) [*costo-* + Gr. *tomē* a cut] incision or division of a rib or costal cartilage.

costotransverse (kos"to-trans-vers') lying between the ribs and transverse processes of the vertebrae.

costotransversectomy (kos"to-trans"ver-sek'to-me) excision of a part of a rib with the transverse process of a vertebra.

costovertebral (kos"to-ver'tĕ-bral) pertaining to a rib and a vertebra.

costoxiphoid (kos"to-zi'foid) connecting the ribs and the xiph-oid cartilage.

cosyntropin (ko-sin-tro'pin) α^{1-24}-corticotropin: a synthetic corticotropin used in the screening of adrenal insufficiency on the basis of plasma cortisol response after intramuscular or intrave-nous injection.

Cotard's syndrome (ko-tarz') [Jules *Cotard*, French neurologist, 1840–1889] see under *syndrome*.

cotarnine chloride (ko-tar'nēn) chemical name: 7,8-dihydro-4-methoxy-6-methyl-1,3-dioxolo[4,5-*g*]isoquinolinium chloride. A substance, $C_{12}H_{14}ClNO_3$, prepared by oxidation of noscapine with dilute nitric acid; formerly used as a hemostatic agent.

Cotazym (kot'ah-zīm) trademark for a preparation of pancreli-pase.

COTe. cathodal opening tetanus.

cothromboplastin (ko-throm"bo-plas'tin) Factor VII; see *co-agulation factors*, under *factor*.

cotinine (ko'tĭ-nēn) the major urinary metabolite of nicotine.
c. fumarate, an antidepressant, $(C_{10}H_{12}N_2O)_2 \cdot C_4H_4O_4$.

co-trimoxazole (ko"tri-moks'ah-zōl) a mixture of trimetho-prim and sulfamethoxazole.

Cotte's operation (kots) [Gaston *Cotte*, Lyons surgeon, 1879–1951] see under *operation*.

Cotting's operation (kot'ingz) [Benjamin Eddy *Cotting*, Ameri-can surgeon, 1812–1898] see under *operation*.

cotton (kot'n) [L. *gossypium*] a textile material derived from the seeds of one or more of the cultivated varieties of *Gossypium*.
absorbent c., purified c. **collodion c.,** pyroxylin. **gun**

c., pyroxylin. **gun c., soluble,** pyroxylin. **purified c.** [USP], the hair of the seed of cultivated varieties of *Gossypium hirsutum* Linné, or other species of *Gossypium*, freed from impurities, deprived of fatty matter, bleached, and sterilized; used as a surgical dressing. Called also *absorbent cotton*, and *gossypium asepticum*, *depuratum*, or *purificatum*. **salicylated c.,** puri-fied cotton charged with salicylic acid, an antiseptic dressing. **styptic c.,** cotton impregnated with a styptic solution and dried.

cottonpox (kot'n-poks) variola minor.

cotton-wool (kot'n-wool) raw nonabsorbent cotton, or espe-cially the absorbent form prepared by removing the cottonseed oil.

Cotugno's disease (ko-toon'yoz) [Domenico *Cotugno*, Italian anatomist, 1736–1822] sciatica. See also *Cotunnius*.

Cotunnius' aqueduct, etc. (ko-tun'e-us) [Domenico *Cotugno*, Italian anatomist, 1736–1822] see under *aqueduct, canal, nerve,* and *space.*

coturnism (ko-tur'nizm) food poisoning caused by ingestion of meat of the European migratory quail, genus *Coturnix*, and marked by such symptoms as difficult breathing, impaired speech, nausea, weakness and loss of feeling in the legs, and partial paralysis, and sometimes resulting in death; the causative toxin, which occurs in only some of the quail, is unidentified.

co-twin (ko-twin) a twin; usually applied in twin studies to identify pairs of twins.

cotyledon (kot"ĭ-le'don) [Gr. *kotylēdōn*] 1. the seed leaf of the embryo of a plant. 2. any one of the subdivisions of the uterine surface of a discoidal placenta. 3. one of the tufted areas of a ruminant's placenta.

cotyledontoxin (kot"ĭ-le"don-tok'sin) a toxic, neutral nonal-kaloidal, nonglucosidal, non-nitrogenous, amorphous substance obtained from the herbaceous plants *Cotyledon ventricosa* and *C. wallchii.*

Cotylogonimus (kot"ĭ-lo-gon'ĭ-mus) [Gr. *kotylē* cup + *gonimos* productive] *Heterophyes.*

cotyloid (kot"ĭ-loid) [Gr. *kotyloeides* cup shaped] 1. cup-shaped. 2. pertaining to the cotyloid cavity (acetabulum).

cotylopubic (kot"ĭ-lo-pu'bik) relating to the cotyloid cavity (ac-etabulum) and the os pubis.

cotylosacral (kot"ĭ-lo-sa'kral) relating to the cotyloid cavity (acetabulum) and the sacrum.

cotype (ko-tīp) any strain of microorganisms (of the same taxon), other than a holotype, from the collection of the bacteriolo-gist who originally described the taxon.

couch grass (kowch' gras) the perennial grass *Agropyrum* (*Triticum*) *repens* (L.) Beauv. (Gramineae); its long roots are diuretic and have been used in cystitis, and possess demulcent and antitussive properties.

couching (kowch'ing) surgical displacement of the lens in cata-ract; called also *abaissement, cataractopiesis,* and *depression of cataract.*

cough (kawf) [L. *tussis*] 1. a sudden noisy expulsion of air from the lungs, usually produced to keep the airways of the lungs free of foreign matter; see also under *reflex*. 2. to produce such an expulsion of air. **aneurysmal c.,** a variety of cough associ-ated with aortic aneurysm, and sometimes with paralysis of one vocal cord. **Balme's c.,** cough on lying down, seen in obstruc-tion of the nasopharynx. **barking c.,** the barklike cough of early youth, as in croup. **compression c.,** a deep resonant cough caused by compression of a bronchus; it resembles in character the cough of a dog and is sometimes called *dog c.* **dog c.,** see *compression c.* **dry c.,** one that is not accompa-nied with expectoration. **ear c.,** a reflex cough caused by dis-ease of the ear, when Arnold's nerve is stimulated. **extrapul-monary c.,** a cough due to causes outside the lungs. **hack-ing c.,** a short, frequent, shallow, and feeble cough. **mechan-ical c.,** expulsion of air from the lungs produced by use of an exsufflator, with effects similar to those of a natural cough. **minute gun c.,** whooping cough with the paroxysms occurring close together. **Morton's c.,** a persistent cough in pulmonary tuberculosis which brings on vomiting and thus causes loss of nourishment. **privet c.,** an allergic cough noted in China and attributed to the pollen of privet. **productive c.,** a cough that is effective in removing material from the respiratory tract. **reflex c.,** a cough due to the irritation of some remote organ. **stomach c.,** a cough caused by reflex irritation from stomach disorder. **Sydenham's c.,** hysterical spasm of the respiratory muscles. **tea taster's c.,** cough in tasters of tea, attributed to inhaling fungi, such as *Candida, Aspergillus,* etc., from tea leaves. **trigeminal c.,** a cough due to irritation of the fibers of the trigeminal nerve distributed to the throat, nose, and external meatus of the ear. **wet c.,** one attended with expectoration. **whooping c.,** see *whooping cough,* under *W.* **winter c.,** chronic bronchitis recurring in the winter.

coulomb (koo'lom) [after C. A. de *Coulomb*, French physicist, 1736–1806] the unit of electrical charge, defined as the quan-tity of electrical charge transferred by one ampere in one second; called also *absolute c.* See also *faraday*. **international c.,** the former standard of electrical charge, equal to 0.999835 absolute coulomb.

Coumadin (koo-mah-din) trademark for preparations of sodium warfarin.

coumamycin (koo-mah-mi′sin) coumermycin.

coumarin (koo′mah-rin) 1. chemical name: 2H-1-benzopyran-2-one. A principle, $C_9H_6O_2$, with a bitter taste and an odor resembling that of vanilla beans, derived from tonka bean, sweet clover, and other plants, and also prepared synthetically. Coumarin contains a factor, dicumarol (3,3′-methylenebis[4-hydroxy-2H-1-benzopyran-2-one], which inhibits the hepatic synthesis of the vitamin K–dependent coagulation factors (prothrombin, Factors VII, IX, and X), and a number of its derivatives are used widely as anticoagulants in the treatment of disorders in which there is excessive or undesirable clotting, such as thrombophlebitis, pulmonary embolism, and certain cardiac conditions. 2. any derivative of coumarin or any synthetic compound with coumarin-like actions.

coumermycin (koo-mer-mi′sin) chemical name: 5-methylpyrrole-2-carboxylic acid, diester with 3,3′-[(3-methylpyrrole-2,4-diyl) bis (carbonylimino] bis [4-hydroxy-8-methyl-7-[(tetrahydro-3,4-dihydroxy-5-methoxy-6,6-dimethylpyran-2-yl)oxy] coumarin]; an antibacterial agent, $C_{55}H_{59}N_5O_{20}$, isolated from *Streptomyces hazeliensis* var. *hazeliensis* and from *S. rishiriensis*.

Councilman's bodies (lesions) (kown′sil-man) [William Thomas *Councilman*, American pathologist, 1854–1933] see under *body*.

Councilmania (kown″sil-ma′ne-ah) [William Thomas *Councilman*] *Entamoeba*. **C. dissim′ilis**, *Entamoeba coli*. **C. lafleu′ri**, *Entamoeba coli*.

count (kownt) [L. *computare* to reckon] a numerical computation or indication. **Addis c.**, the determination of the number of red blood cells, white blood cells, epithelial cells, casts, and the protein content in an aliquot of a twelve-hour urine specimen, used in the diagnosis and management of kidney disease. **Arneth c.**, see under *formula*. **blood c.**, determination of the number of formed elements in a measured volume of blood, usually a cubic millimeter (as red blood cell, white blood cell, or platelet count.) **complete blood c.**, a series of tests of the peripheral blood, including the hematocrit (per cent), the amount of hemoglobin (grams per cent), the white cell count (per cubic millimeter), and the proportions of the different white cells as they appear on a blood smear. **differential c.**, a count made by observation, on the stained blood smear, of the proportion of the different types of leukocytes (or other cells), expressed in percentages. **direct platelet c.**, determination of the total number of platelets per cubic millimeter of blood, in a counting chamber, with the use of conventional light or phase microscopy. **filament-nonfilament c.**, determination of the number of juvenile and mature leukocytes, as in the differential blood count. **indirect platelet c.**, calculation of the total number of platelets per cubic millimeter of blood by determining, in a peripheral blood smear, the ratio of platelets to erythrocytes, and computing the number of platelets from the total red cell count. **parasite c.**, determination of the number of parasites per unit volume of fluid, as, in malaria, the number of plasmodia per cubic millimeter of blood. **Schilling blood c.** (*obs.*), a differential blood count in which the neutrophils are divided into four groups: myelocytes, juvenile cells (or young forms), staff cells, and segmented forms. **staff c.** (*obs.*), Schilling blood c.

counter (kown′ter) an instrument or apparatus by which numerical value is computed; in radiology, a device for enumerating ionizing events. **Coulter c.**, an automatic photoelectric instrument used in the enumeration of formed peripheral blood elements, based on the principle that cells are poor electrical conductors compared with saline solution. **Geiger c., Geiger-Müller c.**, a highly sensitive amplifying device that indicates the presence of ionizing particles. **proportional c.**, a gas-filled radiation detection tube in which the pulse produced is proportional to the number of ions formed in the gas by the primary ionizing particle. **Quebec bacteria colony c.**, a bacteria colony counter in which an oblique light illuminates the colonies so that they appear as brilliant spots or points on subdued background. **scintillation c.**, an instrument for indicating the emission of ionizing particles, making possible the determination of the concentration of radioactive isotopes in the body or other substance; the radiation is absorbed by a phosphor crystal, which emits minute flashes of light that are detected and amplified by a photomultiplier tube.

counterbalance (kown″ter-bal′ans) counterpoise; offset. **renal c.**, compensatory hypertrophy of a normal kidney or part of a kidney accompanied by the tendency of its diseased mate or part to remain in a relatively atrophic state.

countercurrent (kown′ter-ker′ent) flowing in an opposite direction; see also under *mechanism*.

counterdie (kown′ter-di) the reverse image of a die, usually made of a softer and lower fusing metal than the die.

counterelectrophoresis (kown″ter-e-lek″tro-fo-re′sis) counterimmunoelectrophoresis.

counterextension (kown″ter-eks-ten′shun) traction in a proximal direction coincident with traction in the opposite direction.

counterimmunoelectrophoresis (kown″ter-im″u-no-e-lek″-tro-fo-re′sis) a technique in which antigen and antibody are placed in opposing wells in a buffered diffusion system and subjected to an electric field; the antigen (e.g., HB_sAg) and antibody (e.g., anti-HB_s) will migrate (toward the anode and cathode, respectively) rapidly toward each other and form a visible precipitin line. Called also *counterelectrophoresis*.

counterincision (kown″ter-in-sizh′un) a second incision usually made to promote drainage, but occasionally to relieve tension on the edges of a clean wound during closure.

counterinvestment (kown″ter-in-vest′ment) anticathexis.

counterirritant (kown″ter-ir′ĭ-tant) 1. producing a counterirritation. 2. any agent which causes counterirritation.

counterirritation (kown″ter-ir″ĭ-ta′shun) a superficial irritation; an irritation that is intended to relieve some other irritation.

counteropening (kown″ter-o′pen-ing) a second incision made across an earlier one to promote drainage.

counterphobia (kown″ter-fo′be-ah) the seeking out of situations or objects which one fears or has feared.

counterphobic (kown″ter-fo′bik) pertaining to or characterized by counterphobia.

counterpoison (kown′ter-poi′zn) a poison given to counteract another poison.

counterpulsation (kown″ter-pul-sa′shun) a technique for assisting the circulation and decreasing the work of the heart, by synchronizing the force of an external pumping device with cardiac systole and diastole. **intra-aortic balloon c.**, circulatory support provided by a balloon inserted into the thoracic aorta, which is inflated during diastole (enhancing coronary perfusion pressure) and deflated during systole (enhancing peripheral perfusion because of maximal dilation of systemic arterial vessels during diastole).

counterpuncture (kown′ter-punk″chur) a second opening made opposite another.

counterstain (kown′ter-stān) a stain applied to render the effects of another stain more discernible.

countersuggestion (kown″ter-sug-jes′chun) in psychiatry, a technique, often employed with negativistic patients, of suggesting the opposite of what the therapist intends.

countertraction (kown″ter-trak″shun) traction opposed to another traction; employed in the reduction of fractures.

countertransference (kown″ter-trans-fer′ens) in psychoanalysis, the emotional reaction aroused in the physician by the patient; cf. *transference*.

coup (koo) [Fr.] stroke. **c. de fouet** (koo-duh-fwa′) [Fr. "stroke of the whip"], rupture of the plantaris muscle accompanied by a sharp disabling pain. **en c. de sabre** (ahn-koo-duh-sahb′) [Fr. "saber stroke"], resembling the scar of a saber wound; used to designate such a lesion of linear scleroderma on the forehead and scalp. **c. de sang** (koo-duh-sang′), congestion of the brain. **c. de soleil** (koo-duh-sŏ-la′), sunstroke. **c. sur coup** (koo-ser-koo′) ["blow on blow"], the administration of a drug in small doses at short intervals, to secure rapid, complete, or continuous action; abbreviated C.S.C.

couple (kup′l) 1. two equal forces operating on an object in parallel but opposite directions. 2. an area of contact between two dissimilar metals, producing a difference in electrical potential.

coupling (kup′ling) a pairing or joining. In genetics, the occurrence on the same chromosome in a double heterozygote of the two mutant alleles of interest. Cf. *repulsion*. In cardiology, the serial occurrence of a normal heart beat followed closely by a premature beat. **excitation-contraction c.**, the coupling of the action potential to muscle constriction by means of calcium ions which diffuse rapidly into the myofibrils and catalyze the chemical reactions that promote the contractile sliding of actin and myosin filaments. **fixed c.**, coupling in which the premature heart beats follow the preceding normal beats at identical intervals.

courap (koo-rap′) a disease of the skin occurring in India, with eruption and itching of the armpits, groin, breast, and face.

courbature (koor′bah-tūr) [Fr.] 1. aching of the muscles. 2. decompression sickness.

Cournand (kōōr′nand), André Frédéric. American physiologist, born in France in 1895; co-winner, with Werner T. O. Forssmann and Dickinson W. Richards, of the Nobel prize in medicine and physiology for 1956, for the development of new techniques to measure more precisely lung and heart function.

courses (kor′sez) (*obs.*) menses.

Courvoisier's law (sign) (koor-vwah″ze-āz′) [Ludwig Georg *Courvoisier*, Swiss surgeon, 1843–1918] see under *law*.

Courvoisier-Terrier syndrome (koor-vwah″ze-a′-ter-ya′) [L. G. *Courvoisier*; Louis Félix *Terrier*, Paris surgeon, 1837–1908] see under *syndrome*.

Coutard's method (koo-tarz′) [Henri *Coutard*, French radiologist in United States, 1876–1950] see under *method*.

couvade (koo-vad′) a custom of primitive peoples, in which the husband feigns illness during his wife's parturient and puerperal periods.

Couvelaire uterus (koo″vel-ār′) [Alexandre *Couvelaire*, Paris obstetrician, 1873–1948] see *uteroplacental apoplexy*, under *apoplexy*.

couvercle (koo′ver-kl) [Fr.]   a blood clot formed outside a vessel.

couveuse (koo-vuz′) [Fr.]   (*obs.*) incubator.

covalence (ko-vāl′ens)   the number of electron pairs an atom can share with other atoms.

covalent (ko-vāl′ent)   see under *bond*.

covariance (ko-va′re-ans)   the expected value of the product of the deviations of corresponding values of two random variables from their respective means.

cover (kov′er)   1. to provide protection against, as by prophylaxis.   2. the prophylaxis so provided.

coverglass (kov′er-glas)   a thin glass plate that covers a mounted microscopical object or a culture.

coverslip (kov′er-slip)   coverglass.

cowage (kow′aj)   1. a perennial herb, *Mucuna pruriens* DC. (Leguminosae), of the East Indies.   2. the hairs of the cowage pods, which cause severe itching, are used medicinally as a vermifuge, anthelmintic, and counterirritant in admixture with such vehicles as honey. Also used as "itching powders" of joke-shop fame.

Cowdria (kow′dre-ah) [Edmund Vincent *Cowdry*, American anatomist and zoologist, born 1888]   a genus of the tribe Ehrlichieae, family Rickettsiaceae, order Rickettsiales.   **C. ruminan′tium,** the etiologic agent of heartwater (q.v.) of sheep, goats, and cattle; it is nonpathogenic for man.

cowl (kowl)   caul.

Cowper's gland, ligament (kow′perz) [William *Cowper*, English surgeon, 1666–1709]   see *glandula bulbourethralis* and *fascia pectinea*.

cowperian (kow-pe′re-an)   described by or named in honor of William Cowper.

cowperitis (kow″per-i′tis)   inflammation of Cowper's glands (glandula bulbourethralis).

cowpox (kow′poks)   a mild eruptive skin disease of milk cows, usually confined to the udder and teats, caused by vaccinia virus. The disease is transmissible to man by inoculation and contact. See *vaccinia*.

coxa (kok′sah) [L.] [NA]   the part of the body lateral to and including the hip joint. Also loosely used to denote the hip joint.   **c. adduc′ta, c. flex′a,** c. vara.   **c. mag′na,** a condition marked by broadening of the head and neck of the femur.   **c. pla′na,** osteochondrosis of the capitular epiphysis of the femur; see under *osteochondrosis*.   **c. val′ga,** deformity of the hip in which the angle formed by the axis of the head and the neck of the femur and the axis of its shaft is materially increased.   **c. va′ra,** deformity of the hip in which the angle formed by the axis of the head and neck of the femur and the axis of its shaft is materially decreased; called also *c. adducta* and *c. flexa*.   **c. va′ra lux′ans,** fissure of the neck of the femur with dislocation of the head developing from coxa vara.

coxalgia (kok-sal′je-ah) [L. *coxa* hip + *-algia*]   1. hip-joint disease.   2. pain in the hip.

coxarthria (koks-ar′thre-ah)   coxitis.

coxarthritis (koks″ar-thri′tis)   coxitis.

coxarthrocace (koks″ar-throk′ah-se)   fungus disease of the hip joint.

coxarthropathy (koks″ar-throp′ah-the) [L. *coxa* hip + Gr. *arthron* joint + *pathos* disease]   hip-joint disease.

coxarthrosis (koks-ar-thro′sis)   degenerative joint disease or osteoarthritis of the hip joint.

Coxiella (kok″se-el′lah) [Herald Rae *Cox*, American bacteriologist, born 1907]   a genus of microorganisms of the tribe Rickettsieae, family Rickettsiaceae, order Rickettsiales, occurring as a single species.   **C. burnet′ii,** the etiologic agent of Q fever, transmitted by *Haemaphysalis, Ixodes, Dermacentor,* and *Amblyomma* ticks, and also acquired by inhalation of infectious dust and other materials from animal reservoirs of infection.

coxitis (kok-si′tis)   inflammation of the hip joint; called also *coxarthritis*.   **c. fu′gax,** a transient benign coxitis.   **senile c.,** degenerative arthritis of the hip joint.

coxodynia (kok″so-din′e-ah)   coxalgia, def. 2.

coxofemoral (kok″so-fem′o-ral) [L. *coxa* hip + *femur* thigh]   pertaining to the hip and thigh.

coxotomy (kok-sot′o-me)   the operation of opening the hip joint.

coxotuberculosis (kok″so-tu-ber″ku-lo′sis) [L. *coxa* hip + *tuberculosis*]   tuberculous disease of the hip joint.

coxsackievirus (kok-sak′e-vi″rus) [Coxsackie, N.Y., where it was first identified]   one of a heterogeneous group of enteroviruses producing, in man, a disease resembling poliomyelitis, but without paralysis; separable into two groups: A, producing degenerative lesions of striated muscle and B, producing leptomeningitis in infant mice. A number of different serotypes have also been identified. Also written *Coxsackie virus*.

cozymase (ko-zi′mās)   nicotinamide-adenine dinucleotide (NAD); see under *dinucleotide*.

C.P.   chemically pure; candle power.

cp   centipoise.

CPC   clinicopathological conference.

C.P.H.   Certificate in Public Health.

CPK   creatine phosphokinase.

C. Ped.   Certified Pedorthist.

c.p.m.   counts per minute, an expression of the particles emitted after administration of a radioactive material such as ^{131}I.

CPR   cardiopulmonary resuscitation.

c.p.s.   cycles per second.

CR   conditioned reflex (response).

C.R.   crown-rump; in embryology, the usual axis of measurement of an embryo or fetus.

Cr   chemical symbol for *chromium*.

crab (krab)   a vernacular term for *Phthirus pubis*.

crack (krak)   an incomplete split, break, or fissure.   **sand c.,** a crack originating at the ground level in a horse's hoof, sometimes causing lameness. When situated on the inside of the hoof it is termed *quarter c.;* when in the fore part of the hoof it is *toe c.*

crackle (krak′l)   a small sharp sound.   **pleural c's,** superficial crepitation heard in the early stages of acute fibrinous pleurisy.

cradle (kra′dl)   a frame placed over the body of a bed patient for application of heat or cold or for protecting injured parts from contact with the bed clothes.   **electric c., heat c.,** a tunnel- or hood-shaped cradle equipped with electric light bulbs, for application of heat to the body of a patient.   **ice c.,** a device for lowering a patient's body temperature.

Crafts' test (krafts) [Leo Melville *Crafts*, American neurologist, 1863–1938]   see under *tests*.

Craigia (kra′ge-ah) [Charles Franklin *Craig*, U. S. Army surgeon, 1872–1950]   a genus of flagellate protozoa, originally named *Paramoeba* by Craig. The organisms have been the subject of much controversy, but its flagellate stages are thought by Wenyon to be *Chilomastix mesnili*, and its ameboid stages *Entamoeba coli*.

Cramer's splint (krah′merz) [Friedrich *Cramer*, German surgeon, 1847–1903]   see under *splint*.

cramp (kramp)   a painful spasmodic muscular contraction, especially a tonic spasm.   **accessory c.,** spastic torticollis due to a lesion of the accessory nerve.   **heat c.,** a form of heat exhaustion in which muscular spasm is attended by pains, dilated pupils, and weak pulse; seen in those who labor in intense heat (stokers, miners, cane-cutters) and lose much water and salt. Called also *Edsall's disease*.   **intermittent c.,** intermittent abnormal contractions of a muscle, as in tetanus or tetany.   **recumbency c's,** cramping of muscles in legs and feet occurring while resting or during light sleep.   **stoker's c.,** heat c.   **writers' c.,** an occupation neurosis which is characterized by spasmodic contraction of the muscles of the fingers, hand, and forearm, together with neuralgic pain therein; it comes on whenever an attempt is made to write. Called also *graphospasm*.

Crampton's muscle (kramp′tonz) [Sir Philip *Crampton*, Irish surgeon, 1777–1858]   see under *muscle*.

Crampton's test (kramp′tonz) [Charles Ward *Crampton*, American physician, born 1877]   see under *tests*.

craniad (kra′ne-ad) [L. *cranium* head + *ad* toward]   in a cranial direction; toward the anterior (in animals) or superior (in humans) end of the body.

cranial (kra′ne-al) [L. *cranialis*]   pertaining to the cranium, or to the anterior (in animals) or superior (in humans) end of the body.

cranialis (kra″ne-a′lis) [L.]   pertaining to the cranium, or to the superior end of the body; [NA] a term used to denote relationship to the superior end of the body.

craniamphitomy (kra″ne-am-fit′o-me) [*cranium* + Gr. *amphi* around + *tome* a cutting]   division of the entire circumference of the skull for securing decompression.

Craniata (kra-ne-a′tah)   the subphylum of the Chordata containing the species with a true skull and spinal column; the vertebrates.

craniectomy (kra″ne-ek′to-me) [*cranium* + Gr. *ektome* excision]   excision of a part of the skull.   **linear c.,** excision of a strip of the skull, done for the relief of microcephalus.

cranio- (kra′ne-o) [L. *cranium*; Gr. *kranion* skull]   a combining form denoting relationship to the cranium or skull.

cranioacromial (kra″ne-o-ah-kro′me-al)   pertaining to the cranium and acromion.

cranioaural (kra″ne-o-aw′ral)   pertaining to the cranium and the ear.

craniobuccal (kra′ne-o-buk′al)   pertaining to the head and mouth.

craniocele (kra′ne-o-sēl″) [*cranio-* + Gr. *kele* hernia]   a protrusion of any part of the cranial contents through a defect in the skull.

craniocerebral (kra″ne-o-ser′e-bral) pertaining to the cranium and the cerebrum.

cranioclasis (kra″ne-ok′lah-sis) [*cranio-* + Gr. *klasis* fracture] craniotomy, def. 2.

cranioclast (kra′ne-o-klast″) [*cranio-* + Gr. *klan* to break] an instrument for performing craniotomy (def. 2).

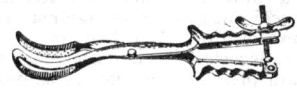

A cranioclast.

cranioclasty (kra′ne-o-klas″te) craniotomy, def. 2.

craniocleidodysostosis (kra″ne-o-kli″do-dis″os-to′sis) [*cranio-* + Gr. *kleis* clavicle + *dys-* bad + *osteon* bone] cleidocranial dysostosis.

craniodidymus (kra″ne-o-did′ĭ-mus) [*cranio-* + Gr. *didymos* twin] a monster with two heads.

craniofacial (kra″ne-o-fa′shal) pertaining to the cranium and the face.

craniofenestria (kra″ne-o-fĕ-nes′tre-ah) [*cranio-* + L. *fenestra* an opening] defective development of the bones of the vault of the fetal skull, marked by areas in which no bone is formed.

craniognomy (kra-ne-og′no-me) [*cranio-* + Gr. *gnōmōn* an interpreter or judge] the study of the shape of the head.

craniograph (kra′ne-o-graf″) [*cranio-* + Gr. *graphein* to write] an instrument for outlining the skull.

craniography (kra″ne-og′rah-fe) the study of the skull by means of photographs, charts, etc.

craniolacunia (kra″ne-o-lah-ku′ne-ah) [*cranio-* + L. *lacuna* a hollow + *-ia*] defective development of the bones of the vault of the fetal skull marked by depressed areas on the inner surfaces of the bones.

craniology (kra″ne-ol′o-je) [*cranio-* + *-logy*] the scientific study of skulls.

craniomalacia (kra″ne-o-mah-la′she-ah) [*cranio-* + Gr. *malakia* softness] abnormal softness of the skull.

craniomeningocele (kra″ne-o-mĕ-nin′go-sēl) [*cranio-* + Gr. *mēninx* membrane + *kēlē* hernia] protrusion of cerebral membranes through a defect in the skull.

craniometer (kra″ne-om′ĕ-ter) [*cranio-* + Gr. *metron* measure] an instrument for use in craniometry.

craniometric (kra″ne-o-met′rik) pertaining to craniometry.

craniometry (kra″ne-om′ĕ-tre) [*cranio-* + Gr. *metrein* to measure] the scientific measurement of the dimensions of the bones of the skull and face.

craniopagus (kra″ne-op′ah-gus) [*cranio-* + Gr. *pagos* a thing fixed] a double monster united by the heads; called also *cephalopagus*. **c. occipita′lis,** craniopagus in which fusion is in the occipital region. **c. parasit′icus,** craniopagus in which a parasitic head is attached to the head of the autosite. **c. parieta′lis,** craniopagus in which fusion is in the parietal region.

craniopathy (kra″ne-op′ah-the) [*cranio-* + Gr. *pathos* disease] any disease of the skull. **metabolic c.,** a condition characterized by lesions of the calvarium with multiple metabolic changes and marked by headache, obesity, and visual disturbances.

craniopharyngeal (kra″ne-o-fah-rin′jĕ-al) pertaining to the cranium and the pharynx.

craniopharyngioma (kra″ne-o-fah-rin″je-o′mah) a tumor arising from cell rests derived from the hypophyseal stalk or Rathke's pouch, frequently associated with increased intracranial pressure, and showing calcium deposits in the capsule or in the tumor proper. Called also *craniopharyngeal duct tumor, Rathke's (pouch) tumor, suprasella cyst,* and *pituitary adamantinoma* or *ameloblastoma.*

craniophore (kra′ne-o-fōr) [*cranio-* + Gr. *phoros* bearing] a device for holding a skull during measurement of its diameters and angles.

cranioplasty (kra′ne-o-plas″te) [*cranio-* + Gr. *plassein* to mold] any plastic operation on the skull; surgical correction of defects of the skull.

craniopuncture (kra′ne-o-punk″tūr) puncture of the skull for exploratory purposes in cranial disease.

craniorachischisis (kra″ne-o-rah-kis′kĭ-sis) [*cranio-* + Gr. *rhachis* spine + *schisis* fissure] congenital fissure of the skull and vertebral column.

craniosacral (kra″ne-o-sa′kral) 1. pertaining to the skull and the sacrum. 2. pertaining to the parasympathetic nerves.

cranioschisis (kra″ne-os′kĭ-sis) [*cranio-* + Gr. *schisis* fissure] congenital fissure of the skull.

craniosclerosis (kra″ne-o-skle-ro′sis) [*cranio-* + Gr. *sklēros* hard] thickening of the bones of the skull.

cranioscopy (kra″ne-os′ko-pe) [*cranio-* + Gr. *skopein* to examine] diagnostic examination of the head.

craniospinal (kra″ne-o-spi′nal) pertaining to the cranium and spine.

craniostenosis (kra″ne-o-ste-no′sis) [*cranio-* + Gr. *stenōsis* narrowing] deformity of the skull caused by premature fusion of the cranial sutures, with consequent cessation of growth, the nature of the deformity depending on the sutures involved in the process.

craniostosis (kra″ne-os-to′sis) [*cranio-* + Gr. *osteon* bone] congenital ossification of the cranial sutures.

craniosynostosis (kra″ne-o-sin″os-to′sis) premature closure of the sutures of the skull.

craniotabes (kra″ne-o-ta′bēz) [*cranio-* + L. *tabes* a wasting] reduction in the mineralization of the skull, with abnormal softness of the bone, usually located in the occipital and parietal bones along the lambdoidal sutures.

craniotome (kra′ne-o-tōm″) [*cranio-* + Gr. *tomē* a cutting] an instrument for use in performing craniotomy.

craniotomy (kra″ne-ot′o-me) [*cranio-* + Gr. *tomē* a cut] 1. any operation on the cranium. 2. an operation to decrease the size of the head of a dead fetus and facilitate delivery by puncturing the skull and removing its contents; encephalotomy.

craniotonoscopy (kra″ne-o-to-nos′ko-pe) [*cranio-* + Gr. *tonos* tone + Gr. *skopein* to examine] auscultatory percussion of the head.

craniotopography (kra″ne-o-to-pog′rah-fe) [*cranio-* + *topography*] the study of the relations of the surface of the skull to the various parts of the brain beneath.

craniotrypesis (kra″ne-o-trĭ-pe′sis) [*cranio-* + Gr. *trypēsis* a piercing] trephination of the skull.

craniotympanic (kra″ne-o-tim-pan′ik) pertaining to the skull and the tympanum.

cranitis (kra-ni′tis) inflammation of the cranial bones.

cranium (kra′ne-um), pl. *cra′nia* [L.; Gr. *kranion* the upper part of the head] the skeleton of the head, variously construed as including all of the bones of the head, all of them except the mandible, or the eight bones which form the vault that lodges the brain. See also *cranial bones,* under *bone.* **c. bif′idum,** congenital cleft of the cranium. **c. bif′idum occul′tum,** congenital cleft of the cranium without associated abnormality of the brain or meninges, detectable only roentgenographically. **cerebral c., c. cerebra′le,** those portions of the bones of the head that contribute to the brain case. **visceral c., c. viscera′le,** those portions of the bones of the head that form the skeleton of the face; this includes the mandible and hyoid bone.

crapulent, crapulous (krap′u-lent, krap′u-lus) [L. *crapulentus, crapulosis* drunken] due to excess in eating or drinking.

craquelé (krak-la′) [Fr.] profusely cracked; see *eczema craquelé.*

crasis (kra′sis) [L.; Gr. *krasis* mixture] the individual temperament or constitution.

crassamentum (kras″ah-men′tum) [L.] a clot, as of blood.

Crast. abbreviation for L. *cras′tinus,* for tomorrow.

crater (kra′ter) a circular area of depression surrounded by an elevated margin.

crateriform (kra-ter′ĭ-form) [L. *crater* bowl + *forma* shape] depressed or hollowed, like a bowl.

craterization (kra″ter-i-za′shun) the operation of excising a craterlike piece from a bone.

craunology (kraw-nol′o-je) crenology.

craunotherapy (kraw″no-ther′ah-pe) crenotherapy.

cravat (krah-vat′) [Fr. *cravate*] a bandage made by folding a triangular piece of cloth from its apex toward the base.

craw-craw (kraw′kraw) an obstinate form of skin disease occurring in West Africa, and affecting chiefly the thighs and genitals, though it may spread over the whole body; it is caused by *Onchocerca volvulus* and is related to dermatitis nodosa.

crazing (kra′zing) minute cracks on the surface of plastic or porcelain dental restorations.

cream (krēm) the oily or fatty part of milk from which butter is prepared, or a fluid mixture of similar consistency; in pharmaceutical preparations, a semisolid emulsion of the oil-in-water or water-in-oil type, ordinarily used topically. **acrisorcin c.** [USP], acrisorcin in a suitable water-miscible base, containing not less than 90 per cent and not more than 110 per cent of acrisorcin; used as a topical antifungal agent. **benzocaine c.** [USP], a mixture containing 90 to 100 per cent of the labeled amount of benzocaine; used as a local anesthetic, applied topically to the skin and mucous membranes. **betamethasone c.** [USP], a mixture containing 90 to 115 per cent of the labeled amount of betamethasone in a suitable water-miscible base; used topically as an anti-inflammatory glucocorticoid. **betamethasone dipropionate c.** [USP], a mixture containing betamethasone dipropionate equivalent to 90 to 110 of the labeled amount of betamethasone in a suitable cream base; used topically as an anti-inflammatory. **betamethasone valerate c.** [USP], a mixture containing betamethasone valerate equivalent to 95 to 115 per cent of the labeled amount of betamethasone in a suitable cream base; used topically as an anti-inflammatory glucocorticoid. **clotrimazole c.** [USP], a cream containing not less than 90 per cent and not more than 110 per cent of the labeled amount of clotrimazole; used as a topical antifungal agent. **cold c.** [USP], a preparation of spermaceti, white wax, mineral oil, sodium borate, and purified water; used as a topical emollient for minor skin irritations and as a water-in-oil emulsion ointment base. **cortisol acetate c.** [USP], a mixture containing between 90 and 110 per cent of the labeled amount of total steroids in a suitable cream base; used as a topical anti-inflammatory steroid. **crotamiton s.** [USP], a preparation containing 93 to 107 per cent of the labeled amount of crotamiton; used as a scabicide, applied topically to the skin. **cyclomethycaine sulfate c.** [USP], a preparation containing 90 to 110 per cent of the labeled amount of cyclomethycaine sulfate in a suitable cream base; used as a local anesthetic, applied topically. **desoximetasone c.** [USP], a preparation containing between 90 and 110 per cent of the labeled amount of desoximetasone in an emollient cream base; used topically as a corticosteroid anti-inflammatory. **dexamethasone sodium phosphate c.,** a cream containing dexamethasone sodium phosphate equivalent to 90 to 115 per cent of the labeled amount of dexamethasone phosphate; used topically as an anti-inflammatory glucocorticoid. **dibucaine c.** [USP], a mixture containing between 90 and 110 per cent of the labeled amount of dibucaine in a suitable cream base; used topically as a local anesthetic. **dienestrol c.** [USP], a mixture containing between 90 to 110 per cent of the labeled amount of dienestrol in a suitable water-miscible base; used topically for its estrogenic effect in the treatment of postmenopausal and senile vulvovaginitis, atrophic vaginitis, pruritus vulvae due to atrophic changes in the vulval epithelium, dyspareunia associated with atrophic vaginal epithelium, and prior to plastic pelvic surgery in menopausal cases. **dioxybenzone and oxybenzone c.** [USP], a preparation usually containing 3 per cent dioxybenzone and 3 per cent oxybenzone; used as a sunscreening agent, applied topically to the skin. **flumethasone pivalate c.** [USP], a preparation containing not less than 90 per cent and not more than 110 per cent of flumethasone pivalate in a suitable cream base; used topically as an anti-inflammatory glucocorticoid. **fluocinolone acetonide c.** [USP], a cream containing 90 to 110 per cent of the labeled amount of fluocinolone acetonide; used as an anti-inflammatory in steroid-responsive dermatoses, applied topically. **fluocinonide c.** [USP], a preparation containing 90 to 110 per cent of the labeled amount of fluocinonide; used as an anti-inflammatory in steroid-responsive dermatoses, applied topically. **fluorometholone c.** [USP], a cream containing 90 to 110 per cent of the labeled amount of fluorometholone; used topically as an anti-inflammatory in the treatment of steroid-responsive dermatoses. **fluorouracil c.** [USP], a preparation containing 90 to 110 per cent of the labeled amount of fluorouracil; used as an antineoplastic in the treatment of actinic keratoses, applied topically. **flurandrenolide c.** [USP], a cream containing 85 to 115 per cent of the labeled amount of flurandrenolide; used as a topical anti-inflammatory in the treatment of steroid-responsive dermatoses. **gamma benzene hexachloride c.,** lindane c. **gentamicin sulfate c.** [USP], a mixture containing 90 to 135 per cent of the labeled amount of gentamicin sulfate, expressed in terms of gentamicin, in a suitable semisolid vehicle; used as a topical antibacterial. **gentian violet c.** [USP], a preparation containing, in each 100 gm., 1.20 to 1.60 gm. of gentian violet, calculated as hexamethylpararosaniline chloride; applied intravaginally in the treatment of vulvovaginal candidiasis. **hydrocortisone c.** [USP], a mixture containing 90 to 110 per cent of the labeled amount of hydrocortisone in a suitable cream base; used topically as an anti-inflammatory in the treatment of steroid-responsive dermatosis. **hydroquinone c.** [USP], a cream containing 94 to 106 per cent of the labeled amount of the hydroquinone; used as a depigmenting agent. **iodochlorhydroxyquin c.** [USP], a mixture containing 90 to 100 per cent of the labeled amount of iodochlorhydroxyquin in a suitable cream base; used as a topical anti-infective in the treatment of a wide range of dermatoses, including all types of eczema. **iodochlorhydroxyquin and hydrocortisone c.** [NF], a preparation containing 90 to 110 per cent of the labeled amounts of iodochlorhydroxyquin and hydrocortisone; used topically for its local anti-infective effect and for the anti-inflammatory and antipruritic activity of glucocorticoids in a wide range of dermatoses. **leukocytic c.,** buffy coat. **lindane c.** [USP], a mixture containing 90 to 100 per cent of the labeled amount of lindane in a suitable cream base; used topically as a pediculicide and scabicide. Called also *gamma benzene hexachloride c.* **mafenide acetate c.** [USP], a preparation containing 90 to 110 per cent of mafenide acetate in terms of the labeled amount of mafenide; used as a topical anti-infective for adjunctive therapy in patients with second and third-degree burns. **methylprednisolone acetate c.** [USP], a mixture containing 90 to 110 per cent of the labeled amount of methylprednisolone acetate in a cream base; used as a topical glucocorticoid. **Moynihan's c.,** a mixture consisting of as much bismuth carbonate in 1:1000 aqueous solution of HgI_2 as will make a thick paste; used as a wound dressing. **nystantin c.** [USP], a cream containing 90 to 130 per cent of the labeled amount of nystatin, the labeled amount being 100,000 nystatin units per gram of cream. **neomycin sulfate and dexamethasone sodium phosphate c.,** a preparation containing neomycin sulfate equivalent to 90 to 135 per cent of the labeled amount of neomycin base, and

dexamethasone sodium phosphate equivalent to 90 to 115 per cent of the labeled amount of dexamethasone sodium phosphate; used topically for its broad-spectrum antibacterial effects, and for the anti-inflammatory and antipruritic activity of glucocorticoids in a wide range of dermatoses. **nitrofurazone c.** [USP], a mixture containing 95 to 105 per cent of the labeled amount of nitrofurazone in a suitable, emulsified, water-miscible base, used topically as a local anti-infective against a wide variety of gram-negative and gram-positive bacteria in the treatment of many skin lesions, especially second and third degree burns, and to aid healing and prevent infection of skin grafts. **piperazine estrone sulfate vaginal c.** [USP], a mixture containing 90 to 120 percent of the labeled amount of piperazine estrone sulfate in a suitable cream base; used as an estrogen. **pramoxine hydrochloride c.** [USP], a mixture containing 90 to 110 per cent of the labeled amount of pramoxine hydrochloride in a suitable water-miscible base; used topically as a local anesthetic. **prednisolone c.** [USP], a mixture containing 90 to 110 per cent of the labeled amount of prednisolone in a suitable cream base; used as a topical glucocorticoid. **c. of tartar,** potassium bitartrate. **tetracaine hydrochloride c.** [USP], a mixture containing the equivalent of 1 per cent of tetracaine in a suitable water-miscible base; used as a local anesthetic, applied to the skin. **tolnaftate c.** [USP], a cream containing 90 to 110 per cent of the labeled amount of tolnaftate; used topically as an antifungal in the treatment of various forms of tinea of the skin. **tretinoin c.** [USP], a mixture containing 90 to 130 per cent of the labeled amount of tretinoin; used as a topical keratolytic agent. **triacetin c.,** a cream containing 90 to 110 per cent of the labeled amount of triacetin; used topically as a local antifungal. **triamcinolone acetonide c.** [USP], a mixture containing 90 to 115 per cent of the labeled amount of triamcinolone acetonide in a suitable cream base; used as a topical anti-inflammatory in steroid-responsive dermatoses. **triclobisonium chloride c.,** a cream containing 90 to 110 per cent of the labeled amount of triclobisonium chloride; used intravaginally as a local anti-infective, primarily in the treatment of gynecological infections due to susceptible organisms.

Creamalin (krem'ah-lin) trademark for preparations of aluminum hydroxide gel.

creamometer (kre-mom'ĕ-ter) ⌊cream + Gr. *metron* measure] an instrument for the determination of the percentage of cream in milk.

crease (krēs) a line or slight linear depression (in anatomical terminology). **palmar c., flexion c.,** any of the normal grooves across the palm which accommodate flexion of the hand by separating folds of tissue. In certain congenital anomalies, there is only a single transverse (simian) crease. **simian c.,** a single transverse palmar crease formed by fusion of the proximal and distal palmar creases; seen in congenital disorders such as Down's syndrome; called also *simian line.* **Sydney c.,** a proximal transverse palmar crease that extends to the ulnar border of the hands; called also *Sydney line.*

creasote (kre'ah-sōt) creosote.

creatinase (kre-at'ĭ-nās) an enzyme that catalyzes the transformation of creatine into urea and ammonia.

creatine (kre'ah-tin) [Gr. *kreas* flesh] N-methyl-guanidinoacetic acid. A crystallizable nitrogenous compound synthesized in the body, phosphorylated creatine (see *phosphocreatine*) being an important storage form of high-energy phosphate. **c. kinase,** ATP:creatine phosphotransferase. An enzyme of skeletal muscle and the myocardium and of brain tissue that catalyzes the transfer of a phosphate group from phosphocreatine to ADP, producing creatine and ATP. It occurs as three isoenzymes each having two components labeled M and B: the form in brain tissue is BB, in skeletal muscle MM, and in myocardial tissue both MM and MB. The form normally found in serum is virtually all MM isoenzyme. **c. phosphate,** phosphocreatine.

creatinemia (kre″ah-tĭ-ne'me-ah) [*creatin* + Gr. *haima* blood + *-ia*] excess of creatine in the blood.

creatininase (kre″ah-tin'ĭ-nās) creatinine amidinohydrolase; an enzyme that decomposes creatinine into urea and methyl glycocoll.

creatinine (kre-at'ĭ-nin) an anhydride of creatine, $NH \cdot C(:NH) \cdot N(CH_3) \cdot CH_2$, being the end product of creative metabolism, found in muscle and blood and excreted in the urine.

creatinuria (kre-at″ĭ-nu're-ah) increased concentration of creatine in the urine.

creatorrhea (kre″ah-to-re'ah) [Gr. *kreas* flesh + *rhoia* flow] the presence of undigested muscle fibers in the feces.

creatotoxism (kre″ah-to-tok'sism) meat poisoning.

creatoxicon (kre″ah-tok'se-kon) kreotoxicon.

creatoxin (kre″ah-tok'sin) kreotoxin.

crèche (kresh) [Fr.] a day nursery for infants.

Credé's ointment (kra-dāz') [Benno C. *Credé,* German surgeon, 1847–1929] see under *ointment.*

Credé's method (maneuver) (kra-dāz′) [Karl Sigmund Franz *Credé*, German gynecologist, 1819–1892] see under *method*.

cremaster (kre-mas′ter) [L.; Gr. *kremasthai* to suspend] musculus cremaster; see *Table of Musculi*. **internal c. of Henle,** fibers of the gubernaculum testis, inserted in elements of the fetal spermatic cord.

cremasteric (kre″mas-ter′ik) pertaining to the cremaster.

cremation (kre-ma′shun) [L. *crematio* a burning] the burning or incineration of dead bodies.

crematorium (kre″mah-to′re-um) an establishment for the burning of dead bodies.

cremnocele (krem′no-sēl) vaginolabial hernia.

cremor (kre′mor) [L.] cream. **c. tar′tari** ["cream of tartar"], potassium bitartrate.

crena (kre′nah), pl. *cre′nae* [L.] [NA] a notch or cleft. **c. a′ni** [NA], the anal cleft: the cleft between the buttocks on which the anus opens; variously called *c. clunium, clunial cleft,* and *rima ani* or *clunium*. **c. clu′nium,** c. ani. **c. cor′dis,** sulcus interventricularis anterior.

crenae (kre′ne) [L.] plural of *crena*.

crenate, crenated (kre′nāt, kre′nāt-ed) [L. *crenatus*] scalloped or notched.

crenation (kre-na′shun) the formation of abnormal notching in the edge of an erythrocyte; the notched appearance of an erythrocyte caused by its shrinkage after suspension in a hypertonic solution. Cf. *echinosis.*

Crenated erythrocytes (Hill).

crenilabrin (kren-il-a′brin) a protamine obtained from the sperm of the cunner (fish).

crenocyte (kre′no-sīt) a crenated erythrocyte.

crenocytosis (kre″no-si-to′sis) the presence of crenated erythrocytes in the blood.

crenology (kre-nol′o-je) [Gr. *krēnē* spring + *-logy*] the science of therapeutic springs.

crenotherapy (kren″o-ther′ah-pe) [Gr. *krēnē* spring + *therapeia* treatment] treatment by water from mineral springs.

Crenothrix (kre′no-thriks) [Gr. *krēnē* spring + *thrix* hair] a genus of microorganisms of the family Crenotrichaceae, order Chlamydobacteriales, made up of disc-shaped to cylindrical cells occurring in attached trichomes which are unbranched or show false branching, and are enclosed in plainly visible sheaths, encrusted at the base with iron or manganese oxides. The type species is *C. poly′spora.*

Crenotrichaceae (kre″no-tri-ka′se-e) a family of Schizomycetes, order Chlamydobacteriales, made up of firmly attached trichomes, showing differentiation of base and tip, enclosed in sheaths that may be encrusted with oxides of iron or manganese. It includes three genera: *Clonothrix, Crenothrix,* and *Phragmidiothrix.*

crenulation (kren″u-la′shun) crenation.

creophagism, creophagy (kre-of′ah-jism; kre-of′ah-je) [Gr. *kreas* flesh + *phagein* to eat] the use of flesh as food.

creosol (kre′o-sol) [*creosote* + L. *oleum* oil] chemical name: 2-methoxy-4-methylphenol. A colorless oily liquid, the methyl ether of methyl catechol, $CH_3 \cdot O \cdot C_6H_3(OH)CH_3$, one of the active constituents of creosote.

creosote (kre′o-sōt) a mixture of phenols obtained by distilling wood tar, mainly beech *Fagus sylvatica* L. (Fagaceae). The liquid is colorless to yellowish, very refractive and oily, and has an empyreumatic odor. It is used externally as an antiseptic and internally in chronic bronchitis as an expectorant. **c. carbonate,** a clear, viscid liquid, a mixture of carbonates of various constituents of creosote, used as an expectorant and antiseptic.

creotoxin (kre″o-tok′sin) kreotoxin.

creotoxism (kre″o-tok′sizm) kreotoxism.

crepitant (krep′ĭ-tant) [L. *crepitare* to rattle] rattling or crackling.

crepitation (krep″ĭ-ta′shun) [L. *crepitare* to crackle] 1. a sound like that made by rubbing the hair between the fingers, or like that made by throwing fine salt into a fire. 2. the noise made by rubbing together the ends of a fractured bone.

crepitus (krep′ĭ-tus) [L.] 1. the discharge of flatus from the bowels. 2. crepitation. 3. a crepitant rale. **articular c.,** joint c. **bony c.,** the crackling sound produced by the rubbing together of fragments of fractured bone. **false c.,** joint c. **c. in′dux,** a crepitant rale, or crackling sound, heard in pneumonia at the beginning of the process of solidification of the lung. **joint c.,** the grating sensation caused by the rubbing together of the dry synovial surfaces of joints; called also *articular c.* **c. re′dux,** crepitus heard in the resolving stage of pneumonia.

silken c., a sensation as of two pieces of silk rubbed between the fingers, felt on moving a joint affected with hydrarthrosis.

crepuscular (kre-pus′ku-lar) [L. *crepusculum* twilight] referring to twilight, as a twilight state; also imperfectly luminous or glimmering.

crescent (kres′ent) [L. *crescens*] 1. shaped like a new moon. 2. a crescent-shaped structure. **articular c.,** a crescent-shaped articular fibrocartilage. **epithelial c.,** a more or less crescentic mass of epithelial cells between the glomerular tuft and the inside of Bowman's capsule in glomerulonephritis. **c's of Giannuzzi,** darkly staining crescents surrounding the mucous tubules, appearing in sections of mixed (mucous and albuminous) glands, and formed by the outnumbered albuminous cells pushed to the blind ends of the terminal portions or into saccular outpocketings. Called also *demilunes of Heidenhain; Giannuzzi's bodies, cells,* or *demilunes; crescent, demilune,* or *marginal cells;* and *semilunar bodies.* **gray c.,** an area on some amphibian eggs from which pigment retreats; it is dorsal and opposite to the point of sperm entry, giving the first visible sign of the dorsoventral axis. **malarial c's,** the gametocytes of *Plasmodium falciparum;* they may be male (microgametocytes) or female (macrogametocytes). Called also *flagellated bodies.* **myopic c.,** a crescentic posterior staphyloma in the fundus of the eye in myopia. **c's of spinal cord** (*obs.*), either of the two lateral bands of gray substance in the spinal cord, each made up of the anterior and posterior horn of the respective side. **sublingual c.,** the crescent-shaped area on the floor of the mouth, formed by the lingual wall of the mandible and the adjacent part of the floor of the mouth.

crescentic (krě-sen′tik) resembling a crescent.

cresol (kre′sol) a mixture of isomeric cresols, $CH_3C_6H_4OH$, obtained from coal tar and containing not more than 5 per cent of phenol; it is a poisonous, colorless, or yellowish to brownish yellow, or pinkish liquid, and is more powerful disinfectant and antiseptic than phenol; used chiefly to sterilize instruments, dishes, utensils, and other inanimate objects. Called also *cresylic acid* and *tricresol.*

cresolphthalein (kre″sol-thal′e-in) an acid-base indicator that is colorless at pH 7.2 and red at 8.8.

cresomania (kre″so-ma′ne-ah) [*Croesus,* king of Lydia in 6th century B.C., renowned for his great wealth] (*obs.*) hallucinations consisting in the imagination of the possession of great wealth.

cresorcin (kre-sor′sin) chemical name: 2,4-dihydroxytoluene. A crystalline derivative from cresol, $C_7H_8O_2$.

cresorcinol (kre-sor′sin-ol) cresorcin.

cresoxydiol (kres-ok″se-di′ol) mephenesin.

cresoxypropanediol (kres-ok″se-pro-pān′de-ol) mephenesin.

crest (krest) [L. *crista*] a projection or projecting structure, or ridge, especially one surmounting a bone at its border; see also *crista* and *ridge*. **acoustic c.,** crista ampullaris. **acusticofacial c.,** the embryonic cell mass from which develop the ganglia of the seventh and eighth cranial nerves. **ampullar c., ampullary c.,** crista ampullaris. **anterior c. of fibula,** margo anterior fibulae. **anterior c. of tibia,** margo anterior tibiae. **arcuate c. of arytenoid cartilage,** crista arcuata cartilaginis arytenoideae. **basilar c.,** crista basilaris ductus cochlearis. **basilar c. of occipital bone,** tuberculum pharyngeum. **buccinator c.,** crista buccinatoria. **cerebral c's of cranial bone,** juga cerebralia ossium cranii; see under *jugum.* **c. of cochlear window,** crista fenestrae cochleae. **conchal c. of maxilla,** crista conchalis maxillae. **conchal c. of palatine bone,** crista conchalis ossis palatini. **cross c.,** a ridge of enamel extending across the face of a tooth. **deltoid c.,** tuberositas deltoidea humeri. **dental c.,** the maxillary ridge passing along the alveolar processes of the fetal maxillary bones. **ethmoid c. of maxilla,** crista ethmoidalis maxillae. **ethmoid c. of palatine bone,** crista ethmoidalis ossis palatini. **femoral c.,** linea aspera femoris. **fimbriated c.,** plica fimbriata. **frontal c.,** crista frontalis. **frontal c., external,** linea temporalis ossis frontalis. **frontal c., internal,** crista frontalis. **glandular c. of larynx,** ligamentum vestibulare. **gluteal c.,** tuberositas glutea femoris. **c. of greater tubercle of humerus,** crista tuberculi majoris. **c. of hypotrochanteric fossa,** tuberositas glutea femoris. **iliac c.,** crista iliaca. **iliopectineal c. of iliac bone,** linea arcuata ossis ilii. **iliopectineal c. of pelvis,** linea terminalis pelvis. **iliopectineal c. of pubis,** eminentia iliopubica. **c. of ilium,** crista iliaca. **infratemporal c.,** crista infratemporalis. **infundibuloventricular c.,** crista supraventricularis. **inguinal c.,** a prominence on the inguinal body wall in the embryo, participating in the formation of the gubernaculum testis. **interosseous c. of fibula,** margo interosseus fibulae. **interosseous c. of radius,** margo interosseus radii. **interosseous c. of tibia,** margo interosseus tibiae. **interosseous c. of ulna,** margo interosseus ulnae. **intertrochanteric c.,** crista intertrochanterica. **intertrochanteric c., anterior,** linea intertrochanterica. **jugular c. of great wing of sphenoid bone,** margo zygomaticus alae majoris. **lacrimal c., anterior,** crista lacrimalis anterior. **lacrimal c., posterior,** crista lacrimalis posterior. **c. of larger tubercle,** crista tuberculi majoris. **lateral c. of**

fibula, margo posterior fibulae. **c. of lesser tubercle,** crista tuberculi minoris. **c. of little head of rib,** crista capitis costae. **malar c. of great wing of sphenoid bone,** margo zygomaticus alae majoris. **c. of matrix of nail,** cristae matricis unguis. **medial c. of fibula,** crista medialis fibulae. **mental c., external,** protuberantia mentalis. **mitochondrial c's,** complex infoldings in the mitochondrial cavity which originate in a membrane outside the cavity. **nasal c. of maxilla,** crista nasalis maxillae. **nasal c. of palatine bone,** crista nasalis ossis palatini. **c. of neck of rib,** crista colli costae. **neural c.,** a cellular band dorsolateral to the neural tube that gives origin to the cranial and spinal ganglia and many other structures. **obturator c. (anterior),** crista obturatoria. **occipital c., external,** crista occipitalis externa. **occipital c., internal,** eminentia cruciformis. **orbital c.,** margo supraorbitalis ossis frontalis. **palatine c. (of palatine bone),** crista palatina. **pectineal c. of femur,** linea pectinea femoris. **pharyngeal c. of occipital bone,** tuberculum pharyngeum. **pubic c., c. of pubis,** crista pubica. **radial c.,** margo interosseus radii. **c. of ridge,** the highest continuous surface of the ridge, but not necessarily the center of the ridge; the top of a residual or alveolar ridge. **rough c. of femur,** linea aspera femoris. **sacral c.,** crista sacralis mediana. **sacral c., articular,** crista sacralis intermedia. **sacral c., external,** crista sacralis lateralis. **sacral c., intermediate,** crista sacralis intermedia. **sacral c., lateral,** crista sacralis lateralis. **sacral c., medial,** crista sacralis mediana. **seminal c.,** colliculus seminalis. **c. of smaller tubercle,** crista tuberculi minoris. **sphenoidal c.,** crista sphenoidalis. **spinal c. of Rauber,** processus spinosus vertebrarum. **c. of spinous processes of sacrum,** crista sacralis mediana. **supinator c., c. of supinator muscle,** crista musculi supinatoris. **supramastoid c.,** the superior border of the posterior root of the zygomatic process of the temporal bone. **supraventricular c.,** crista supraventricularis. **temporal c. of frontal bone,** linea temporalis ossis frontalis. **terminal c. of right atrium,** crista terminalis atrii dextri. **tibial c.,** margo anterior tibiae. **transverse c. of internal auditory meatus,** crista transversa. **trigeminal c.,** the embryonic cell mass from which the trigeminal ganglion develops. **turbinal c. of maxilla, inferior,** crista conchalis maxillae. **turbinal c. of maxilla, superior,** crista ethmoidalis maxillae. **turbinal c. of palatine bone, inferior,** crista conchalis ossis palatini. **turbinal c. of palatine bone, superior,** crista ethmoidalis ossis palatini. **ulnar c.,** margo interosseus ulnae. **urethral c., female,** crista urethralis femininae. **urethral c., male,** crista urethralis masculini. **c. of vestibule,** crista vestibuli. **zygomatic c. of great wing of sphenoid bone,** margo zygomaticus alae majoris.

crestomycin sulfate (kres-to-mi′sin) paromomycin sulfate.

cretin (kre′tin; kret′in) [Fr.] a person affected with cretinism.

cretinism (kre′tin-izm) a chronic condition due to congenital lack of thyroid secretion, marked by arrested physical and mental development, dystrophy of the bones and soft parts, and lowered basal metabolism. It is the congenital form of this deficiency, while myxedema is the acquired form. Called also *cretinoid idiocy* and *myxedematous infantilism.* **athyreotic c.,** cretinism due to thyroid aplasia or destruction of the thyroid of the fetus *in utero;* called also *sporadic nongoitrous c.* **goitrous c.,** cretinism co-existing with severe hypothyroidism, and characterized by goiter. **spontaneous c., sporadic c.,** cretinism in a person not descended from cretins, and who has not lived in a region where cretinism prevails; called also *athyreotic c.* **sporadic goitrous c.,** a genetically determined condition in which enlargement of the thyroid gland is associated with deficiency in the supply of circulating thyroid hormone. **sporadic nongoitrous c.,** athyreotic c.

cretinistic (kre″tin-is′tik) pertaining to cretinism.

cretinoid (kre′tin-oid) resembling a cretin; resembling cretinism.

cretinous (kre′tin-us) affected with cretinism.

Creutzfeldt-Jakob disease (syndrome) (kroits′felt-yak′ob) [Hans Gerhard *Creutzfeldt,* German psychiatrist, 1885–1964; Alfons Maria *Jakob,* German psychiatrist, 1884–1931] see under *disease.*

crevice (krev′is) [Fr. *crever* to split] a longitudinal fissure. **gingival c.,** the space between the surface of the cervical enamel of a tooth and the overlying unattached gingiva; called also *subgingival space.*

crevicular (kre-vik′u-lar) pertaining to a crevice, especially the gingival crevice.

CRF corticotropin releasing factor.

crib (krib) 1. a removable anchorage for orthodontic appliances. 2. a fixed orthodontic appliance used to control oral problem habits involving lips, tongue, or fingers. **clinical c.,** a crib in which an infant is placed for observation. **tongue c.,** an appliance used to eliminate visceral (infantile) swallowing and thrusting and to stimulate the mature or somatic tongue posture and function.

cribbing (krib′ing) a bad habit of some horses in which the an-

imal grasps the manger or other object with the incisor teeth, arches the neck, makes peculiar movements with the head, and swallows quantities of air; called also *windsucking.*

cribra (krib′rah) [L.] plural of *cribrum.*

cribral (krib′ral) pertaining to the cribrum, or sieve-like structure.

cribrate (krib′rāt) [L. *cribratus*] perforated, as a sieve.

cribration (krib-ra′shun) 1. the quality of being cribrate. 2. the process or act of sifting or passing through a sieve, as a drug.

cribriform (krib′rĭ-form) [*cribrum* + L. *forma* form] perforated with small apertures like a sieve.

cribrum (kri′brum), pl. *cri′bra* [L. "sieve"] lamina cribrosa ossis ethmoidalis. **cri′bra orbita′lia of Welcker,** small apertures in the lamina cribrosa ossis ethmoidalis, which give the bone a porous appearance and are thought to transmit veins from the diplöe to the orbit.

Cricetus (kri-se′tus) a genus of rodents; see *hamster.*

Crichton-Browne's sign (kri′ton-brownz) [Sir James *Crichton-Browne,* English physician, 1840–1938] see under *sign.*

Crick (krik) Francis Harry Compton. English biologist, born 1916; co-winner, with Maurice Wilkins and James Dewey Watson, of the Nobel prize in medicine and physiology for 1962, for the discovery of the molecular structure of deoxyribonucleic acid.

cricoarytenoid (kri″ko-ar″ĭ-te′noid) pertaining to or extending between the cricoid and arytenoid cartilages.

cricoid (kri′koid) [Gr. *krikos* ring + *eidos* form] 1. resembling a ring; ring shaped. 2. the cricoid cartilage (cartilago cricoidea [NA]).

cricoidectomy (kri″koi-dek′to-me) excision of the cricoid cartilage.

cricoidynia (kri″koi-din′e-ah) [Gr. *krikos* ring + *odynē* pain] pain in the cricoid cartilage.

cricopharyngeal (kri″ko-fah-rin′je-al) pertaining to the cricoid cartilage and the pharynx.

cricothyreotomy (kri″ko-thi″re-ot′o-me) [Gr. *krikos* ring + *thyreos* shield + *tomē* a cutting] incision through the cricoid and thyroid cartilages.

cricothyroid (kri-ko-thi′roid) pertaining to or connecting the cricoid and thyroid cartilages.

cricothyroidotomy (kri″ko-thi″roi-dot′o-me) cricothyreotomy.

cricothyrotomy (kri″ko-thi-rot′o-me) incision through the skin and cricothyroid membrane to secure a patent airway for emergency relief of upper airway obstruction.

cricotomy (kri-kot′o-me) [Gr. *krikos* ring + *tomē* a cutting] incision of the cricoid cartilage.

cricotracheotomy (kri″ko-tra″ke-ot′o-me) incision of the cricoid cartilage and trachea.

cri du chat (kre-du-shah) [Fr. "cat's cry"] see under *syndrome.*

Crile-Matas operation (krīl-mat′as) [George Washington *Crile,* Cleveland surgeon, 1864–1943; Rudolph *Matas,* New Orleans surgeon, 1860–1957] see under *operation.*

criminology (krim″ĭ-nol′o-je) [L. *crimen* crime + -*logy*] the scientific study of crime and criminals.

crines (kri′nēz) [L.] plural of *crinis.*

crinin (krin′in) [Gr. *krinein* to separate] a substance that stimulates glandular secretion.

crinis (kri′nis), pl. *cri′nes* [L.] hair; see also *capilli.* **c. cap′itis,** the hair of the head. **c. pu′bis,** the pubic hair.

crinogenic (kri″no-jen′ik, krin″o-jen′ik) [Gr. *krinein* to separate + *gennan* to produce] stimulating secretion.

crinology (kri-nol′o-je) the scientific study of secretion and secretions.

crinophagy (krin-of′ah-je) [Gr. *krinein* to separate + *phagein* to eat] the intracytoplasmic digestion of the contents (peptides, proteins) of secretory vacuoles, after the vacuoles fuse with lysosomes.

Crinum (kri′num) a genus of amaryllidaceous plants; the root of *C. asiaticum,* of India, has properties like those of squill.

crisis (kri′sis), pl. *cri′ses* [L.; Gr. *krisis*] 1. the turning point of a disease for good or evil; especially, a sudden change, usually for the better, in the course of an acute disease. A disease terminates by crisis when recovery is indicated by a sudden and definite decrease in the intensity of the symptoms. Cf. *lysis* (def. 4). 2. a sudden paroxysmal intensification of symptoms in the course of a disease. **addisonian c., adrenal c.,** the symptoms accompanying an acute onset or worsening of Addison's disease, viz., fatigue, nausea and vomiting, loss of weight, hypotension, fever, and collapse. **anaphylactoid c.,** symptoms resembling those of anaphylaxis due to colloidoclasia. **aplastic c.,** a transient condition, marked by sudden disappearance of erythroblasts from the bone marrow, developing under various circumstances, including certain hemolytic states and infections. **asthmatic c.,** status asthmaticus. **blast c.,** a sudden, severe change in the course of chronic myelocytic leukemia in which the clinical picture resembles that in acute myelocytic leukemia, with an increase in the proportion of myeloblasts. Recent evidence suggests that in some cases the blast cells may be lymphoblasts. **bronchial c.,** a paroxysm of dyspnea in the course of a case of tabes dorsalis. **cardiac c.,** a severe paroxysm of palpitation of the heart occurring in tabes dorsalis. **celiac c.,** an attack of severe watery diarrhea and vomiting producing dehydration and acidosis which sometimes occurs in the infantile form of nontropical sprue. **clitoris c.,** an attack of sexual excitement occurring in women with tabes dorsalis. **colloidoclastic c.,** colloidoclasia. **deglobulinization c.,** a condition observed in congenital spherocytic anemia, characterized clinically by the acute onset of fever, abdominal pain, and vomiting, associated with reticulocytopenia, leukopenia, thrombocytopenia, erythroblastopenia. **Dietl's c.,** sudden severe attack of nephralgia or gastric pain, chills, fever, nausea and vomiting, and general collapse; said to be due to partial turning of the kidney upon its pedicle. **false c.,** pseudocrisis. **febrile c.,** an attack of chilliness, fever, and sweating. **gastric c.,** a paroxysm of intense abdominal pain in tabes dorsalis. **genital c. of newborn,** a condition characterized by estrinization of the vaginal mucosa and hyperplasia of the breasts, under the influence of transplacentally acquired estrogens. **glaucomatocyclitic c.,** a relatively uncommon, recurrent, unilateral form of secondary open angle glaucoma, lasting one to two weeks, and rarely producing permanent damage to the optic disk or to the outflow facility. It is characterized by high intraocular pressure and marked depression of outflow facility, with minimal inflammatory signs and symptoms. **hepatic c.,** an attack of intense pain in the region of the liver. **identity c.,** a period in the psychosocial development of an individual, usually occurring during adolescence, manifested by a loss of the sense of the sameness and historical continuity of one's self, and inability to accept the role the individual perceives as being expected of him by society. **intestinal c.,** gastric c. **laryngeal c.,** paroxysmal spasm of the larynx in the earlier course of tabes dorsalis. **Lundvall's blood c.** (*obs.*), a term used by Lundvall to designate a shift from leukopenia to leukocytosis in patients with dementia praecox. **nefast c.,** the peculiar onset of severe and unaccountable symptoms in experimental icterogenous spirochetosis. **nephralgic c.,** a paroxysm of pain in the ureter in a case of tabes dorsalis. **nitritoid c.,** a group of symptoms sometimes following the injection of arsphenamine, consisting of redness of the face, dyspnea, a feeling of distress, cough, and precordial pain. The condition is named from its resemblance to the symptoms of amyl nitrite poisoning. **ocular c.,** a sudden attack of intense pain in the eyes, with lacrimation, photophobia, etc. **oculogyric c.,** a crisis occurring in epidemic encephalitis or postencephalitic parkinsonism in which the eyeballs become fixed in one position for minutes or hours. **parkinsonian c.,** a condition sometimes observed in parkinsonism, superficially resembling akinetic mutism or coma vigil, the patient lying stiff and motionless, and making no spontaneous communication. **Pel's c's,** ocular crises in tabes dorsalis. **pharyngeal c.,** a sudden attack occurring in tabes dorsalis, marked by peculiar sensations in the pharynx and involuntary swallowing movements. **rectal c.,** a severe seizure of rectal pain in tabes dorsalis. **renal c.,** an attack of pain resembling renal colic, occurring in tabes. **salt-depletion c.,** salt-losing syndrome. **salt-losing c.,** see under *syndrome.* **tabetic c.,** a painful paroxysm with functional disturbance occurring in the course of tabes dorsalis. **thoracic c.,** an attack of pain resembling angina pectoris, but with spasmodic contracture of the muscles of the chest and arms in tabes dorsalis. **thyroid c., thyrotoxic c.,** a sudden and dangerous increase of the symptoms of thyrotoxicosis. **vesical c.,** a severe seizure of pain in the bladder in cases of tabes dorsalis. **visceral c.,** a paroxysm of shooting pain in any viscus occurring in a case of tabes dorsalis.

Crismer's test (kris′merz) [Leon *Crismer,* Belgian chemist, born 1858] see under *tests.*

crispation (kris-pa′shun) [L. *crispare* to curl] slight convulsive or spasmodic muscular contractions producing a creeping sensation.

crista (kris′tă), pl. *cris′tae* [L.] [NA] a projection or projecting structure, or ridge, especially one surmounting a bone or its border; called also *crest* and *ridge.* **c. acus′tica,** c. ampullaris. **c. ampulla′ris** [NA], ampullar crest: the most prominent part of a localized thickening of the membrane that lines the ampullae of the semicircular ducts, covered with neuroepithelium containing endings of the vestibular nerve; called also *c. acoustica* or *acoustic crest.* **c. ante′rior fib′ulae,** margo anterior fibulae. **c. ante′rior tib′iae,** margo anterior tibiae. **c. arcua′ta cartilag′inis arytenoi′deae** [NA], arcuate crest of arytenoid cartilage: a ridge on the external surface of the arytenoid cartilage between the triangular pit and the oblong pit. **c. basila′ris duc′tus cochlea′ris** [NA], basilar crest: the triangular eminence on the spiral ligament to which the basilar membrane is attached. **c. buccinato′ria,** buccinator crest: a ridge running from the base of the coronoid process of the mandible to a point near the last molar tooth, giving attachment to the buccinator muscle. **c. cap′itis cos′tae** [NA], **c. capit′uli cos′tae,** crest of head of rib: a horizontal crest dividing the articular surface of the head of the rib into two facets, for articulation with the depression on the bodies of two adjacent vertebrae; called

also *crest of little head of rib, cuneiform eminence of head of rib,* and *interarticular ridge of head of rib.* **c. col′li cos′tae** [NA], crest of neck of rib: a crest on the superior border of the neck of a rib, giving attachment to the anterior costotransverse ligament; called also *ridge of neck of rib.* **c. concha′lis maxil′lae** [NA], conchal crest of maxilla: an oblique ridge on the nasal surface of the body of the maxilla, just anterior to the lacrimal sulcus, which articulates with the inferior nasal concha; called also *inferior turbinal crest of maxilla.* **c. concha′lis os′sis palati′ni** [NA], conchal crest of palatine bone: a sharp transverse ridge, near the posterior edge of the palatine bone, which articulates with the inferior concha; called also *inferior turbinal crest of palatine bone.* **cris′tae cu′tis** [NA], ridges of the skin produced by the projecting papillae of the corium on the palm or sole, producing a finger- or foot-print that is characteristic of the individual; called also *dermal ridges.* **c. div′idens,** limbus foraminis ovalis. **c. ethmoida′lis maxil′lae** [NA], ethmoidal crest of maxilla: a low, oblique ridge on the medial surface of the frontal process of the maxilla, which articulates with the middle nasal concha; called also *superior turbinal crest of maxilla.* **c. ethmoida′lis os′sis palati′ni** [NA], ethmoidal crest of palatine bone: a ridge near the upper end of the medial surface of the palatine bone, which articulates with the middle concha; called also *superior turbinal crest of palatine bone.* **c. falcifor′mis,** c. transversa. **c. fenes′trae coch′leae** [NA], crest of cochlear window: the ledge of bone that overhangs the cochlear window of the middle ear. **c. fronta′lis** [NA], the frontal crest: a median ridge on the internal surface of the frontal bone, extending upward from the foramen cecum to unite with the sulcus for the superior sagittal sinus; called also *internal frontal crest.* **c. gal′li** [NA], a thick triangular process projecting upward from the cribriform plate of the ethmoid bone; the falx cerebri attaches to it. **c. hel′icis,** crus helicis. **c. ili′aca** [NA], **c. il′ii,** the iliac crest: the thickened, expanded upper border of the ilium; called also *crest of ilium.* **c. infratempora′lis** [NA], infratemporal crest: a crest separating the temporal surface of the great wing of the sphenoid bone into a temporal portion above and an infratemporal portion below. **c. interos′sea fib′ulae,** margo interosseus fibulae. **c. interos′sea ra′dii,** margo interosseus radii. **c. interos′sea tib′iae,** margo interosseus tibiae. **c. interos′sea ul′nae,** margo interosseus ulnae. **c. intertrochanter′ica** [NA], intertrochanteric crest: a prominent ridge running obliquely downward and medialward from the summit of the greater trochanter on the posterior surface of the neck of the femur to the lesser trochanter; called also *intertrochanteric ridge, linea intertrochanterica posterior,* and *posterior intertrochanteric line.* **c. lacrima′lis ante′rior** [NA], anterior lacrimal crest: the lateral margin of the groove on the posterior border of the frontal process of the maxilla. **c. lacrima′lis poste′rior** [NA], posterior lacrimal crest: a vertical ridge dividing the lateral or orbital surface of the lacrimal bone into two parts, and forming one margin of the fossa for the lacrimal sac. **c. latera′lis fib′ulae,** margo posterior fibulae. **c. margina′lis** [NA], marginal ridge; see under *ridge.* **cris′tae ma′tricis un′guis** [NA], crests of matrix of nail: vascular longitudinal ridges in the nail matrix. **c. media′lis fib′ulae** [NA], medial crest of fibula: the long crest on the posterior surface of the body of the fibula, which separates the origin of the tibialis posterior muscle from that of the flexor hallucis longus muscle; called also *oblique line of fibula* and *posterointernal border of fibula.* **mitochondrial cristae, cris′tae mitochondria′les,** numerous narrow, transverse infoldings of the inner membrane of a mitochondrion. **c. mus′culi supinato′ris** [NA], crest of supinator muscle: a strong ridge forming the posterior margin of the supinator fossa below the radial notch of the ulna, and with it giving attachment to the supinator muscle; called also *supinator crest* or *ridge.* **c. nasa′lis maxil′lae** [NA], nasal crest of maxilla: a ridge, raised along the medial border of the palatine process of the maxilla, with which the vomer articulates. **c. nasa′lis os′sis palati′ni** [NA], nasal crest of palatine bone: a thick ridge projecting upward from the medial part of the horizontal plate of the palatine bone and articulating with the posterior part of the vomer. **c. obturato′ria** [NA], obturator crest: the inferior border of the superior ramus of the os pubis, a strong ridge of bone beginning near the pubic tubercle and extending to the anterior part of the gap in the rim of the acetabulum, forming part of the circumference of the obturator foramen, and giving attachment to the obturator membrane. **c. occipita′lis exter′na** [NA], external occipital crest: a variable crest of bone that sometimes extends from the external occipital protuberance toward the foramen magnum; called also *median* or *middle nuchal line.* **c. occipita′lis inter′na** [NA], internal occipital crest: a median ridge on the internal surface of the occipital bone extending from the midpoint of the cruciform eminence toward the foramen magnum. **c. palati′na** [NA], palatine crest: a transverse crest often seen on the inferior surface of the horizontal plate of the palatine bone a short distance anterior to the posterior border. **c. pu′bica** [NA], pubic crest: the thick, rough, anterior border of the body of the pubic bone. **cris′tae sacra′les articula′res,** see *crista sacralis intermedia.* **c. sacra′lis interme′dia** [NA], intermediate sacral crest: either of two indefinite crests just medial to the dorsal sacral foramina, formed by fusion of the articular processes of the sacral vertebrae; called also *articular sacral crest*. **c. sacra′lis latera′lis** [NA], lateral sacral crest: either of two series of tubercles lateral to the dorsal sacral foramina, representing the transverse processes of the sacral vertebrae; called also *external sacral crest*. **c. sacra′lis me′dia, c. sacra′lis media′na** [NA], medial sacral crest: a median ridge on the dorsal surface of the sacrum, formed by the remnants of the spinous processes of the upper four sacral vertebrae; called also *sacral crest, crest of spinous processes of sacrum*, and *tubercular ridge of sacrum*. **c. sphenoida′lis** [NA], sphenoidal crest: a median ridge on the anterior surface of the body of the sphenoid bone, articulating with the perpendicular plate of the ethmoid. **c. spira′lis,** labium limbi vestibulare laminae spirales. **c. supraventricula′ris** [NA], supraventricular crest: a ridge on the inner surface of the right ventricle of the heart, marking off the conus arteriosus; called also *infundibuloventricular crest*. **c. tempora′lis,** linea temporalis ossis frontalis. **c. termina′lis a′trii dex′tri** [NA], terminal crest of right atrium: a ridge on the internal surface of the right atrium of the heart, located to the right of the orifices of the superior and inferior venae cavae. The pectinate muscles of the right atrium are attached at this crest. It corresponds to a groove on the external surface, the sulcus terminalis. **c. transver′sa** [NA], transverse crest: a ridge of bone that divides the fundus of the internal acoustic meatus into a superior and an inferior fossa; called also *c. falciformis* and *transverse crest of internal acoustic meatus*. **c. transversa′lis** [NA], transverse ridge; see under *ridge*. **c. triangula′ris** [NA], triangular ridge; see under *ridge*. **c. tuber′culi majo′-ris** [NA], crest of greater tubercle (of the humerus): a projection on the greater tubercle of the humerus, forming one lip of the intertubercular groove; called also *crest of larger tubercle, pectoral ridge*, and *external, outer*, or *posterior bicipital ridge*. **c. tuber′culi mino′ris** [NA], crest of lesser tubercle: a projection on the lesser tubercle of the humerus, forming one lip of the intertubercular groove; called also *crest of smaller tubercle*, and *anterior* or *internal bicipital ridge*. **c. tympan′ica,** a ridge on the tympanic ring. **c. ul′nae,** margo interosseus ulnae. **c. urethra′lis femini′nae** [NA], female urethral crest: a prominent longitudinal fold of the mucosa along the posterior wall of the female urethra; called also *c. urethralis muliebris* and *cervical crest of female urethra (of Barkow)*. **c. urethra′lis·mas-culi′nae** [NA], male urethral crest: a median elevation along the posterior wall of the urethra in the male, lying between the prostatic sinuses; called also *c. urethralis virilis*. **c. urethra′lis mulie′bris,** crista urethralis femininae. **c. urethra′lis vir′ilis,** c. urethralis masculinae. **c. vestib′uli** [NA], crest of vestibule: a ridge between the spherical and elliptical recesses of the vestibule, dividing posteriorly to bound the cochlear recess.

cristae (kris′te) [L.] plural of *crista*.

cristal (kris′tal) pertaining to a crest or ridge.

Cristispira (kris″tĭ-spi′rah) [L. *crista* crest + Gr. *speira* coil] a genus of microorganisms of the family Spirochaetaceae, order Spirochaetales, made up of coarse, flexuous, spiral cells with cross striations and a thin membrane on one side, extending the whole length of the body; found in the intestinal tracts of mollusks. It contains three species: *C. anodon′tae, C. balbia′nii*, and *C. pin′nae*.

Critchett's operation (krich′ets) [George *Critchett*, ophthalmic surgeon, in London, 1817–1882] see under *operation*.

criterion (kri-te′re-on) [Gr. *kritērion* a means for judging] a standard by which something may be judged.

crith (krith) [Gr. *krithē* barleycorn, the smallest weight] the unit of weight for gases, being the weight of a liter of hydrogen gas at 0° C. and pressure equivalent to that of a column of mercury 760 mm. high.

Crithidia (krĭ-thid′e-ah) a genus of parasitic protozoa of the family Trypanosomatidae, order Protomastigida, found in the digestive tract of arthropods and other invertebrates. The adult form is similar to the leptomonads, but the flagellum arises from the kinetoplast just in front of the nucleus, and is attached to the body by an undulating membrane. The organisms go through a leishmanial stage, which is enclosed in a spherical cyst that is discharged by the host in the feces. After ingestion by another host, the cysts develop into a leptomonad form and finally attain the adult form.

crithidia (krĭ-thid′e-ah) 1. any organism of the genus *Crithidia*. 2. any individual of the family Trypanosomatidae when exhibiting the typical crithidial (epimastigote) form during its life cycle.

crithidial (krĭ-thid′e-al) 1. pertaining to the genus *Crithidia*. 2. denoting a morphologic stage in the development of certain protozoa of the family Trypanosomatidae; see *epimastigote*.

critical (krit′ĭ-kl) pertaining to or of the nature of a crisis; in danger of death; in sufficient quantity as to constitute a turning point, as a critical mass or critical concentration.

CRM cross-reacting material; see under *material*.

C.R.N.A. Certified Registered Nurse Anesthetist.

crocein (kro′se-in) any one of a series of bright red stains.

crocidismus (kro″se-diz′mus) [Gr. *krokē* a tuft of wool] carphology.

Crocq's disease (kroks) [Jean B. *Crocq*, Belgian physician, 1868–1925] acrocyanosis.

crofilicon A (kro-fil′kon) chemical name: 2-methyl-2-propenoic acid 2,3-dihydroxypropyl ester polymer with methyl-2-2-propenoate; a contact lens material (hydrophobic), $(C_7H_{12}O_4)_x(C_5H_8O_2)_y$.

Crohn's disease (krōnz) [Burrill Bernard *Crohn*, New York physician, born 1884] see under *disease*.

cromoglycate (kro″mo-gli′kāt) a salt of cromoglycic acid; the disodium salt, cromolyn sodium, is used in the treatment of bronchial asthma.

cromolyn (kro′mŏ-lin) cromoglycic acid. **c. sodium** [USP], chemical name: 5,5′-[(2-hydroxy-1,3-propanediyl)bisoxy)]bis[4-oxo-4*H*-1-benzopyran-2-carboxylic acid]disodium salt. The disodium salt of cromoglycic acid, $C_{23}H_{14}Na_2O_{11}$, which interferes with allergic histamine release; administered by inhalation in the prophylactic treatment of bronchial asthmas and rhinitis associated with allergy.

Cronin Lowe test (reaction) [E. *Cronin Lowe*, British physician] see under *tests*.

Crooke's changes [Arthur Carleton *Crooke*, British pathologist] hyalinization of the cytoplasm of the basophilic cells of the anterior lobe of the pituitary gland, disappearance of their basophilic granules, ballooning of their nuclei, enlargement and multinucleation of the cells.

Crookes's space, tube [Sir William *Crookes*, English physicist, 1832–1919] see under *space* and *tube*.

crop (krop) a dilatation of the gullet of birds at the base of the neck, where food is stored, softened with fluids, and passed to the stomach in small amounts.

cropropamide (kro-pro′pah-mīd) chemical name: *N*-[1-(dimethylcarbamoyl)propyl]-*N*-propylcrotonamide; an analgesic, $C_{13}H_{24}N_2O_2$. See also *prethcamide*.

cross (kros) 1. any figure or structure in the shape of a cross. 2. any organism produced by crossbreeding; a method of crossbreeding. **clavicular c.,** a wooden or metallic cross applied to the back by a figure-of-8 bandage or web straps over the shoulders to extend the latter and thus reduce overriding fragments of a fractured clavicle; a belt or bandage is worn around the waist to hold the lower projection of the cross tightly against the spine. **dihybrid c.,** one in which the parents have different genes determining two particular traits. **monohybrid c.,** one in which the parents have different genes involving only one particular trait. **phage c.,** a phage (bacteriophage) having genes from two or more parental phages as a result of infection by the parent phages of a single bacterial cell; it is a result of recombination. Also, the process of an instance of the formation of a phage cross. **polyhybrid c.,** one in which the parents have different genes determining more than three particular traits. **Ranvier's c's,** dark, cross-shaped markings at the nodes of Ranvier, seen on longitudinal section after staining with silver nitrate. **silver c.,** a crosslike marking seen at the nodes of certain bundles of medullated nerve fibers. **trihybrid c.,** one in which the parents have different genes determining three particular traits. **two-factor c.,** recombination involving two genetic markers. **yellow c.,** 2,2′-dichlorodiethyl sulfide.

crossbite (kros′bīt) malocclusion in which the mandibular teeth are in buccal version (or in complete lingual version in posterior segments) to the maxillary teeth, bilaterally, unilaterally, or involving only a pair of opposing teeth, so that opposing occlusal surfaces are not in contact in habitual occlusion. Also written *cross bite*. **anterior c.,** that in which one or more primary or permanent maxillary incisors is lingual to the mandibular incisors. **buccal c.,** that in which the maxillary molar is buccal to its mandibular antagonist. **lingual c.,** crossbite in which the maxillary or mandibular molar is lingual to its antagonist. **posterior c.,** that in which one or more primary or permanent posterior teeth are locked in an abnormal relation with the opposing teeth of the opposite arch; it may be buccal or lingual crossbite and may be accompanied by a shift of the mandible. **scissors-bite c.,** that in which the mandibular arch is entirely lingual to the maxillary arch. **telescoping c.,** scissors-bite c.

crossbreeding (kros′brēd-ing) hybridization; the mating of animals or plants of different strains or species.

cross-bridges (kros-brij′ez) in A bands of myofibrils, the intertwining of the thick and the thin filaments to form the dark striations.

crossed (krost) shaped or arranged like a cross; decussating.

cross-eye (kros′i) esotropia.

crossfoot (kros′foot) talipes varus.

crossing over (kros′ing o′ver) the exchanging of genetic material between nonsister chromatids of the paired homologous chromosomes during the pachytene stage of the first meiotic division, resulting in new combinations of genes; called also *chiasmatypy*.

crossmatching (kros-mach′ing) see under *matching*.

cross-over (kros-o′ver) the result of the reciprocal exchange of genetic material between chromosomes; see *crossing over*.

cross-reactivation (kros″re-ak-tĭ-va′shun) the activation of an inactive virus particle by another active or inactive virus particle in the same cell.

cross-reactivity (kros″re-ak-tiv′ĭ-te) the degree to which an antibody participates in cross-reactions (see under *reaction*).

cross-sensitization (kros-sen″sĭ-ti-za′shun) sensitization to a substance induced by exposure to another substance having cross-reacting antigens.

crossway (kros′wā) the path by which something crosses; *decussation.*

crotalid (krot′ah-lid) 1. any snake of the family Crotalidae; a pit viper. 2. of or pertaining to the family Crotalidae.

Crotalidae (kro-tal′ĭ-de) a family of venomous snakes, the pit vipers, characterized by front, movable, hollow fangs, and a depression or pit between the nostril and the eye. It includes the genera *Agkistrodon* (copperhead and water moccasin), *Bothrops* (fer-de-lance), *Crotalus* (rattlesnake), *Lachesis* (bushmaster), and *Trimeresurus* (habu). See table accompanying *snake.*

crotalin (kro′tah-lin) a protein found in the venom of rattlesnakes and certain other serpents; formerly used hypodermically in the treatment of epilepsy.

crotaline (krot′ah-lin) crotalid.

crotalism (kro′tal-izm) a disease of animals caused by eating leguminous plants of the genus *Crotalaria,* which are in low bottom land. The disease is characterized by congestion and hemorrhage of the liver and spleen, emaciation, weakness, and stupor. Called also *bottom disease.*

crotalotoxin (kro″tah-lo-tok′sin) a poisonous substance from rattlesnake venom.

Crotalus (krot′ah-lus) [L. from Gr. *krotalon* rattle] a genus of rattlesnakes of the family Crotalidae. *C. horridus* is the common rattlesnake of the eastern United States; *C. adamanteus* is the diamondback rattlesnake of Georgia, Alabama, and Florida; *C. atrox* is the western diamondback rattlesnake of the Southwest and adjacent areas of Mexico; and *C. viridis* is the prairie rattlesnake. See table accompanying *snake.*

crotamine (kro′tah-mēn) a toxic protein occurring in the venom of some *Crotalus* species.

crotamiton (kro″tah-mi′ton) [USP] chemical name: *N*-ethyl-*N*-(2-methylphenyl)-2-butenamide. A scabicide, $C_{13}H_{17}NO$, occurring as a light yellow, oily liquid; applied topically to the skin.

crotaphion (kro-taf′e-on) [Gr. *krotaphos* the temple] a craniometric point at the tip of the great wing of the sphenoid.

crotchet (kroch′et) [Fr. *crochet*] *(obs.)* a hook used in delivering the fetus after craniotomy.

crotethamide (kro-teth′ah-mīd) chemical name: *N*-[1-[(dimethylamino)carbonyl]propyl]-*N*-ethyl-2-butenamide; an analgesic, $C_{12}H_{22}N_2O_2$. See also *prethcamide.*

crotin (kro′tin) a poisonous substance (phytotoxin) derived from the seeds of *Croton tiglium;* see *crotinism.*

Croton (kro′ton) [L.; Gr. *krotōn* tick] a genus of euphorbiaceous shrubs, some of which are popular as ornamentals. Certain species are used medically in parts of Mexico and South America, and others, e.g., *C. texensis* (Texas C.) and *C. capitatus,* are poisonous to livestock. *C. eluteria* Benn. is a source of cascarilla bark (tonic and bitter), while *C. tiglium* yields croton oil (see under *oil*), a drastic purgative and counterirritant that can cause pustular eruptions on the skin.

crotonism (kro′ton-izm) poisoning by croton oil, characterized by burning of the mouth and sometimes emesis, followed by severe watery diarrhea and colic; sometimes accompanied by headache, somnolence, vertigo, prostration, and collapse. Death from circulatory or respiratory failure may occur.

crotoxin (kro-tok′sin) a crystalline neurotoxic principle from the venom of the rattlesnake, *Crotalus terrificus.*

crounotherapy (kroo″no-ther′ah-pe) [Gr. *krounos* spring + *therapeia* treatment] crenotherapy.

croup (kroōp) a condition resulting from acute obstruction of the larynx caused by allergy, foreign body, infection, or new growth, occurring chiefly in infants and children, and characterized by resonant barking cough, hoarseness, and persistent stridor. Called also *angina trachealis, exudative angina,* and *laryngostasis.* **catarrhal c.,** croup accompanied by a catarrhal discharge. **diphtheritic c.,** croup associated with infection by *Corynebacterium diphtheriae.* **false c.,** laryngismus stridulus. **membranous c., pseudomembranous c.,** croup associated with a fibrinous exudate forming a membrane-like deposit, usually caused by *Corynebacterium diphtheriae;* called also *laryngeal diphtheria.* **spasmodic c.,** laryngismus stridulus.

croupous (kroo′pus) of the nature of croup, or attended with an exudation like that of croup.

croupy (kroōp′e) affected with or resembling croup.

Crouzon's disease (kroo-zonz′) [Octave Crouzon, French neurologist, 1874–1938] craniofacial dysostosis.

crowding (krowd′ing) the condition in which the teeth are crowded and assume such altered positions as overlapping, displacement in various directions, torsiversion, etc.

crown (krown) [L. *corona*] 1. the topmost part of an organ or other structure, such as the top of the head, or the upper part of a tooth (corona dentis [NA]); see *anatomical c.* 2. an artificial crown replacing the natural crown of a tooth. **anatomical c.,** the portion of a tooth that is covered by enamel; see *corona dentis* [NA]. **artificial c.,** a restoration of metal, porcelain, or plastic which reproduces the surface anatomy of the clinical crown of a tooth and which is affixed to the remains of the natural tooth structure. **bell c.,** a tooth crown whose circumference at the occlusal surface is larger than usual in relation to the size of the circumference at the crown cervix. **cap c.,** an artificial crown that is applied like a cap over the remaining natural crown of a tooth; called also *shell c.* **Carmichael c.,** partial veneer c. **ciliary c.,** corona ciliaris. **clinical c.,** that portion of a tooth which is exposed beyond the gingiva. **collar c.,** an artificial crown attached by a metal ferrule to a natural tooth root. **Davis c.,** an artificial porcelain crown attached by a pin inserted into both the crown and the natural root of the tooth; called also *post c.* **extra-alveolar c.,** that portion of a tooth which is mesial or distal to the attachment of the tooth in the alveolus. **full c., full veneer c.,** a dental restoration that completely reproduces the clinical crown of a natural tooth. **half-cap c.,** an artificial crown attached by a metal band which covers only the lingual surface of the tooth that supports it; called also *open-face c.* **jacket c.,** a resin or porcelain restoration that is applied over the clinical crown of a tooth and usually terminates at or under the gingiva. **open-face c.,** half-cap c. **partial veneer c.,** a restoration applied to the proximal and lingual surfaces and the occlusal surface or incisal edge of a tooth, used as a retainer for a bridge or as a single-unit restoration on a carious or fractured tooth; called also *Carmichael c.* and *three-quarter c.* **physiological c.,** the portion of a tooth that is exposed distal to the gingival crevice or to the margin of the gum; it may or may not coincide with the anatomical crown, which is the portion covered by enamel. **post c.,** Davis c. **Richmond c.,** a factory-made porcelain dental restoration with a gold retentive post in the root canal and a soldered back, introduced in the late 1870's. **shell c.,** cap c. **three-quarter c.,** partial veneer c. **veneered c.,** an artificial crown that bears a thin layer of resin or porcelain on the buccal or labial surface, attached to or bonded to the metal casting; called also *window c.* **window c.,** veneered c.

crowning (krown′ing) that phase in the second stage of labor when a large segment of the fetal scalp is visible at the vaginal orifice, the perineum being distended and the anus opened.

CRP C-reactive protein; see under *protein.*

CRS Chinese restaurant syndrome.

cruces (kroo′sēz) [L.] plural of *crux.*

crucial (kroo′shal) [L. *crucialis*] 1. *(obs.)* cruciate. 2. severe, searching, and decisive.

cruciate (kroo′she-āt) shaped like a cross.

crucible (kroo′sĭ-bl) [L. *crucibulum*] a vessel for melting refractory substances.

cruciform (kroo′sĭ-form) [*crux* + L. *forma* form] shaped like a cross.

crude (kroōd) [L. *crudus* raw] raw or unrefined.

cruentation (kroo″en-ta′shun) [L. *cruor* blood] in medieval jurisprudence, the supposed bleeding of the corpse in the presence of the murderer.

crufomate (kroo′fo-māt) chemical name: methylphosphoramidic acid 2-chloro-4-(1,1-dimethylethyl)phenyl methyl ester; a veterinary anthelmintic, $C_{12}H_{19}ClNO_3P$.

cruor (kroo′or), pl. *cruo′res* [L.] a blood clot.

crura (kroo′rah) [L.] plural of *crus.*

crural (kroor′al) pertaining to the leg or to a leglike structure (crus).

crureus (kroo-re′us) musculus vastus intermedius; see *Table of Musculi.*

crus (krus), pl. *cru′ra* [L.] [NA] 1. the leg, from knee to foot. 2. a general term used to designate a leglike part. **ampullary crura of semicircular duct,** crura membranacea ampullaria ductus semicircularis. **ampullary osseous crura,** crura ossea ampullaria. **anterior c. of anterior inguinal ring,** c. mediale anuli inguinalis superficialis. **anterior c. of internal capsule,** c. anterius capsulae internae. **anterior c. of stapes,** c. anterius stapedis. **c. ante′rius cap′sulae inter′nae** [NA], anterior crus of internal capsule: the part of the internal capsule of the brain that separates the caudate and the lentiform nuclei. Called also *anterior limb of internal capsule* and *pars frontalis capsulae internae.* **c. ante′rius stape′dis** [NA], anterior crus of stapes: the anterior of the two bony limbs in the middle ear that connect the base and head of the stapes; called also *anterior limb of stapes.* **cru′ra anthel′icis** [NA], **crura of anthelix,** the two ridges on the external ear marking the superior termination of the anthelix and bounding the triangular fossa; called also *limbs of anthelix.* **c. bre′ve incu′dis** [NA], short crus of incus: the backward-projecting process on the incus that is connected to the posterior wall of the tympanic cavity; called also *short limb of incus.* **c. cerebel′li ad pon′-**

tem, pedunculus cerebellaris medius. **c. cer′ebri** [NA], the ventral part of the cerebral peduncle, composed of descending fiber tracts that pass from the cerebral cortex to form the longitudinal fascicles of the pons, including the corticospinal, corticopontine, and corticobulbar tracts; called also *basis pedunculi cerebri.* **c. clitor′idis** [NA], **c. of clitoris,** the continuation of each corpus cavernosum clitoridis, diverging posteriorly to be attached to the pubic arch. **common membranous c. of semicircular duct,** c. membranaceum commune ductus semicircularis. **common osseous c.,** c. osseum commune. **c. commu′ne cana′lis semicircula′ris,** c. osseum commune. **c. dex′trum diaphrag′matis** [NA], right crus of diaphragm; a fibromuscular band arising from the upper three or four lumbar vertebrae, and ascending along with the left crus, to insert into the central tendon of the diaphragm. **crura of diaphragm, cru′ra diaphrag′matis,** see *c. dextrum diaphragmatis* and *c. sinistrum diaphragmatis.* **c. of diaphragm, left,** c. sinistrum diaphragmatis. **c. of diaphragm, right,** c. dextrum diaphragmatis. **external c. of anterior inguinal ring,** c. laterale anuli inguinalis superficialis. **c. fascic′uli atrioventricula′ris** [dex′trum et sinis′trum] [NA], either branch (right or left) of the atrioventricular bundle, arising from the main trunk of the bundle at the superior end of the muscular part of the interventricular septum and descending on either side to be distributed to the respective ventricle of the heart. **c. for′nicis** [NA], **c. of fornix,** either of the two flattened bands of white substance of the brain that are in close contact with the splenium and that unite under the posterior part of the body of the corpus callosum to form the body of the fornix. **c. glan′dis clitor′idis,** frenulum clitoridis. **c. hel′icis** [NA], **c. of helix,** the anterior termination of the helix of the external ear located above the entrance to the external acoustic meatus; called also *crista helicis.* **c. infe′rius an′nuli inguina′lis subcuta′nei,** c. laterale anuli inguinalis superficialis. **internal c. of anterior inguinal ring,** c. mediale anuli inguinalis superficialis. **internal c. of greater alar cartilage of nose,** c. mediale cartilaginis alaris majoris. **lateral c. of greater alar cartilage,** c. laterale cartilaginis alaris majoris. **lateral c. of superficial inguinal ring,** c. laterale anuli inguinalis superficialis. **c. latera′le an′uli inguina′lis superficia′lis** [NA], lateral crus of superficial inguinal ring: the part of the superficial inguinal ring that blends with the inguinal ligament as it goes to the pubic tubercle; called also *c. inferius annuli inguinalis subcutanei,* and *external* or *posterior c. of anterior inguinal ring.* **c. latera′le cartilag′inis ala′ris majo′ris** [NA], lateral crus of greater alar cartilage: the part of the greater alar cartilage that curves laterally around the naris and helps maintain its contour. **long c. of incus,** c. longum incudis. **c. lon′gum in′cudis** [NA], long crus of incus: a process on the incus directed downward and inward, parallel with the manubrium of the malleus; called also *long limb of incus.* **medial c. of external inguinal ring,** ligamentum inguinale reflexum. **medial c. of greater alar cartilage,** c. mediale cartilaginis alaris majoris. **medial c. of superficial inguinal ring,** c. mediale anuli inguinalis superficialis. **c. media′le an′uli inguina′lis superficia′lis** [NA], medial crus of superficial inguinal ring: the part of the superficial inguinal ring that is attached to the symphysis and that blends with the fundiform ligament of the penis; called also *superior c. of subcutaneous inguinal ring, c. superius annuli inguinalis subcutanei,* anterior or *interior c. of anterior inguinal ring,* and *anterior* or *internal inguinal ligament.* **c. media′le cartilag′inis ala′ris majo′ris** [NA], medial crus of greater alar cartilage: the part of the greater alar cartilage, loosely attached to its fellow of the opposite side, and helping to form the mobile septum of the nose; called also *internal c. of greater alar cartilage.* **cru′ra membrana′cea** [NA], the membranous crura: the two ends of each semicircular duct of the ear, both opening into the utricle. See *crura membranacea ampullaria ductus semi-circularis, c. membranaceum commune ductus semicircularis,* and *c. membranaceum simplex ductus semicircularis.* **cru′ra membrana′cea ampulla′ria duc′tus semicircula′ris** [NA], ampullary membranous crura of semicircular duct: the end of each semicircular duct of the ear, in which the membranous ampulla is situated. **c. membrana′ceum commu′ne duc′tus semicircula′ris** [NA], common membranous crus of semicircular duct: the joined nonampullary ends of the anterior and posterior semicircular duct of the ear. **c. membrana′ceum sim′plex duc′tus semicircula′ris** [NA], simple membranous crus of semicircular duct: the nonampullary end of the lateral semicircular duct of the ear, opening into the utricle. **membranous crura,** crura membranacea. **cru′ra os′sea** [NA], osseous crura: those parts of the bony semicircular canals of the ear that lodge the correspondingly named parts of the membranous crura of the semicircular ducts; see *crura ossea ampullaria, c. osseum commune,* and *c. osseum simplex.* **cru′ra os′sea ampulla′ria** [NA], ampullary osseous crura: the parts of the bony semicircular canals of the ear that lodge the crura membranacea ampullaria ductus semicircularis. **osseous crura,** crura ossea. **c. os′seum commu′ne** [NA], common osseous crus: the part of the bony semicircular canals of the ear that lodges the crus membranaceum commune ductus semicircularis; called also *c. commune canalis*

semicircularis. **c. os′seum sim′plex** [NA], simple osseous crus: that part of the bony semicircular canals of the ear that lodges the crus membranaceum simplex ductus semicircularis; called also *c. simplex canalis semicircularis.* **c. pe′nis** [NA], **c. of penis,** the continuation of each corpus cavernosum penis, diverging posteriorly to be attached to the pubic arch. **posterior c. of anterior inguinal ring,** c. laterale anuli inguinalis superficialis. **posterior c. of internal capsule,** c. posterius capsulae internae. **posterior c. of stapes,** c. posterius stapedis. **c. poste′rius cap′sulae inter′nae** [NA], posterior crus of internal capsule: the part of the internal capsule of the brain that separates the thalamus from the lentiform nucleus; it includes a pars sublentiformis and a pars retrolentiformis. Called also *posterior limb of internal capsule* and *pars occipitalis capsulae internae.* **c. poste′rius stape′dis** [NA], posterior crus of stapes: the posterior of the two bony limbs that connect the base and head of the stapes in the middle ear; called also *posterior limb of stapes.* **short c. of incus,** c. breve incudis. **simple membranous c. of semicircular duct,** c. membranaceum simplex ductus semicircularis. **simple osseous c.,** c. osseum simplex. **c. sim′plex cana′lis semicircula′ris,** c. osseum simplex. **c. sinis′trum diaphrag′matis** [NA], left crus of diaphragm: a fibromuscular band arising from the upper two or three lumbar vertebrae, and ascending along with the right crus, to insert into the central tendon of the diaphragm. **superior c. of cerebellum,** pedunculus cerebellaris superior. **superior c. of subcutaneous inguinal ring,** c. mediale anuli inguinalis superficialis. **c. supe′rius an′nuli inguina′lis subcuta′nei,** c. mediale anuli inguinalis superficialis.

crust (krust) [L. *crusta*] a formed outer layer, especially an outer layer of solid matter formed by the drying of a bodily exudate or secretion; called also *scab.* **milk c.,** crusta lactea.

crusta (krus′tah), pl. *crus′tae* [L.] 1. a crust. 2. crus cerebri. **c. lac′tea,** seborrhea of the scalp of nursing infants; called also *cradle cap* and *milk crust.* **c. petro′sa den′tis,** the cementum.

Crustacea (krus-ta′she-ah) [L. from *crusta* shell] a large class of arthropods including the lobsters, crabs, shrimps, wood lice, water fleas, and barnacles.

crustaceorubin (krus-ta″se-o-roo′bin) a brown-black pigment (chromoprotein) found in lobster shells and eggs and in certain crabs; called also *zoonerythrin, tetra-erythrin,* and *vitellorubin.*

crustae (krus′te) [L.] plural of *crusta.*

crustal (krus′tal) pertaining to the crusta.

crustosus (krus-to′sus) [L.] crusted; said of certain lesions of the skin.

crutch (kruch) a device of wood or metal, ordinarily long enough to reach from the armpit to the ground, with a concave surface fitting under the arm and a cross bar for the hand, used for supporting the weight of the body. **Canadian c.,** a crutch consisting of two uprights extending halfway between the elbow and shoulder, with a cross piece for the hand and a curved upper arm part against which the subject leans his upper arm.

Cruveilhier's atrophy (paralysis), disease, joint (kroo-vāl-yāz′) [Jean *Cruveilhier,* French pathologist, 1791–1874; he held the first chair of pathology in the Paris faculty] see *spinal muscular atrophy,* under *atrophy,* see under *disease,* and see *articulatio atlantooccipitalis.*

Cruveilhier-Baumgarten syndrome (cirrhosis) (kroo-vāl-yā′-baum′gar-ten)[Jean *Cruveilhier;* Paul Clemens von *Baumgarten,* German pathologist, 1848–1928] see under *syndrome.*

crux (kruks), pl. *cru′ces* [L.] cross. **c. of heart,** the intersection of the walls separating the right and left sides and the atrial and ventricular chambers of the heart. **cru′ces pilo′rum** [NA], crosslike figures formed by the pattern of hair growth, the hairs lying in opposite directions.

Cruz's trypanosomiasis (kruz) [Oswaldo *Cruz,* Brazilian physician, 1871–1917] Chagas' disease.

Cruz-Chagas disease (kruz-chag′as) [Oswald *Cruz;* Carlos *Chagas,* physician in Brazil, 1879–1934] Chagas' disease.

cry (kri) 1. a sudden loud, involuntary vocal sound. 2. to utter such a sound. 3. to weep. **arthritic c., articular c.,** night c. **cephalic c.,** a shrill, high-pitched penetrating cry of the newborn suggesting intracranial damage of some severity. **epileptic c.,** a loud scream that often occurs at the onset of an epileptic attack. **hydrocephalic c.,** the loud cry of a patient with acute tuberculous meningitis. **joint c.,** night c. **night c.,** a shrill cry uttered by a child in sleep, often heard in beginning joint disease; called also *arthritic, articular,* or *joint c.*

cryalgesia (kri″al-je′ze-ah) [*cryo-* + Gr. *algēsis* pain] pain due to the application of cold.

cryanesthesia (kri″an-es-the′ze-ah) [*cryo-* + *anesthesia*] loss of the power of perceiving cold.

Cryer's elevator (kri′erz) [Matthew Henry *Cryer,* American surgeon, 1840–1921] see under *elevator.*

cryesthesia (kri″es-the′ze-ah) [*cryo-* + Gr. *aisthēsis* perception] abnormal sensitiveness to cold.

crymo- (kri′mo) [Gr. *krymos* frost] a combining form denoting relationship to cold.

crymoanesthesia (kri″mo-an-es-the′ze-ah) [crymo- + anesthesia] refrigeration anesthesia.

crymodynia (kri″mo-din′e-ah) [crymo- + Gr. odyne pain] rheumatic pain coming on in cold or damp weather.

crymophilic (kri″mo-fil′ik) psychrophilic.

crymophylactic (kri″mo-fi-lak′tik) cryophylactic.

crymotherapeutics (kri″mo-ther″ah-pu′tiks) cryotherapy.

crymotherapy (kri″mo-ther′ah-pe) cryotherapy.

cryo- (kri′o) [Gr. kryos cold] a combining form denoting relationship to cold.

cryoanalgesia (kri″o-an″al-je′ze-ah) the relief of pain by application of cold by cryoprobe to peripheral nerves.

cryobank (kri′o-bank″) a facility for freezing and preserving semen at low temperatures, usually by immersion in liquid nitrogen at −196.5° C.

cryobiology (kri″o-bi-ol′ŏ-je) [cryo- + Gr. bios life + -logy] the science dealing with the effect of low temperatures on biological systems.

cryocardioplegia (kri″o-kar″de-o-ple′je-ah) cessation of contraction of the myocardium produced by application of cold during cardiac surgery.

cryocautery (kri″o-kaw′ter-e) [cryo- + cautery] cold cautery.

cryocrit (kri′o-krit) [cryo- + Gr. krinein to separate] the percentage of the total volume of blood serum or plasma occupied by cryoprecipitable protein after deposition by centrifugation.

cryoextraction (kri″o-eks-trak′shun) the application of low temperature in the removal of a cataractous lens; it is accomplished with an instrument (cryoprobe) whose extremely cold tip forms an adhesion (iceball) with the lens, thus permitting removal of the lens.

cryoextractor (kri″o-eks-trak′tor) a cryoprobe used in cryoextraction.

cryofibrinogen (kri″o-fi-brin′o-jen) [cryo- + fibrinogen] fibrinogen with the abnormal physical property of precipitating in the cold (4° C.) and subsequently redissolving at 37° C.

cryofibrinogenemia (kri″o-fi-brin″o-jen-e′me-ah) the presence of cryofibrinogen in the blood; see cryofibrinogen.

cryogammaglobulin (kri″o-gam″ah-glob′u-lin) cryoglobulin.

cryogen (kri′o-jen) [cryo- + Gr. gennan to produce] a substance used for lowering temperatures.

cryogenic (kri″o-jen′ik) pertaining to or causing the production of low temperatures.

cryoglobulin (kri″o-glob′u-lin) an abnormal globulin that precipitates at low temperatures (i.e., 4° C.) and redissolves upon warming to body temperature; called also cryogammaglobulin.

cryoglobulinemia (kri″o-glob″u-lin-e′me-ah) the presence of cryoglobulin in the blood, which is precipitated in the microvasculature upon exposure to cold temperature; the clinical condition is marked by restricted blood flow through the skin of areas exposed to the cold, e.g., the digits, nose, and ears, where painful ischemia and even infarction may occur.

cryohydrate (kri″o-hi′drāt) [cryo- + hydrate] a eutectic mixture, especially one having water as one of its constituents.

cryohypophysectomy (kri″o-hi″po-fiz-ek′to-me) destruction of the hypophysis by the application of cold.

cryometer (kri-om′ĕ-ter) [cryo- + Gr. metron measure] a thermometer for measuring very low temperatures.

cryopathy (kri-op′ah-the) [cryo- + Gr. pathos disease] any morbid condition caused by cold.

cryophilic (kri″o-fil′ik) [cryo- + Gr. philein to love] psychrophilic.

cryophylactic (kri″o-fi-lak′tik) [cryo- + Gr. phylaxis a guarding] resistant to very low temperatures; said of bacteria.

cryoprecipitability (kri″o-pre-sip″ĭ-tah-bil′ĭ-te) the quality of being readily precipitated by reduced temperature (cold).

cryoprecipitate (kri″o-pre-sip′ĭ-tāt) [cryo- + precipitate] any precipitate that results from cooling, as cryoglobulin or antihemophilic factor.

cryoprecipitation (kri″o-pre-sip″ĭ-ta′shun) the precipitation of a substance in solution (e.g., antihemophilic factor in blood plasma) on exposure to lowered temperature.

cryopreservation (kri″o-pres″er-va′shun) [cryo- + preservation] the maintaining of the viability of excised tissue or organs by storing at very low temperatures.

cryoprobe (kri′o-prōb) an instrument for applying extreme cold to tissue.

cryoprotective (kri″o-pro-tek′tiv) capable of protecting against injury due to freezing, as glycerol protects frozen red blood cells.

cryoprotein (kri″o-pro′te-in) [cryo- + protein] any blood protein that precipitates on cooling, as cryoglobulin or cryofibrinogen.

cryoscope (kri′o-skōp) an apparatus for performing cryoscopy.

cryoscopical (kri″o-skop′e-kl) pertaining to cryoscopy.

cryoscopy (kri-os′ko-pe) [cryo- + Gr. skopein to examine] examination of liquids, based on the principle that the freezing point

of solutions varies according to the amount and the nature of the substance contained in them in solution.

cryospray (kri′o-spra) the use of a liquid nitrogen spray in cryosurgery.

cryostat (kri′o-stat) [cryo- + Gr. histanai to halt] 1. a device by which temperature can be maintained at a very low level. 2. in pathology and histology, a chamber containing a microtome for sectioning frozen tissue.

cryosurgery (kri′o-sur′jer-e) destruction of tissue by the application of extreme cold; utilized in some forms of intracranial and cutaneous surgery.

cryothalamectomy (kri″o-thal″ah-mek′to-me) destruction of a portion of the thalamus by application of extreme cold; see cryosurgery.

cryotherapy (kri″o-ther′ah-pe) [cryo- + Gr. therapeia treatment] the therapeutic use of cold.

cryotolerant (kri″o-tol′er-ant) able to withstand unusually low temperatures.

crypt (kript) [L. crypta, from Gr. kryptos hidden] a blind pit or tube on a free surface; see also crypta [NA]. **alveolar c.,** the bony compartment surrounding a developing tooth. **anal c's,** sinus anales. **dental c.,** the space occupied by a developing tooth. **enamel c.,** a space bounded by the dental ledges on either side and usually by the enamel organ; it is filled with mesenchyma. **c's of Fuchs,** c's of iris. **c's of Haller,** glandulae preputiales. **c's of iris,** pitlike depressions found in the iris, in the region of the circulus arteriosus minor; called also c's of Fuchs. **c's of Lieberkühn,** glandulae intestinales. **c's of Littre,** glandulae preputiales. **Luschka's c's,** deep indentations of the gallbladder mucosa which penetrate into the muscular layer of the organ. **c. of Morgagni,** 1. fossa navicularis urethrae. 2. see sinus anales. **mucous c's of duodenum,** glandulae duodenales. **odoriferous c's of prepuce,** glandulae preputiales. **c's of palatine tonsil,** fossulae tonsillares tonsillae palatinae. **c's of pharyngeal tonsil,** fossulae tonsillares tonsillae pharyngeae. **synovial c.,** a pouch in the synovial membrane of a joint. **c's of tongue,** deep, irregular invaginations from the surface of the lingual tonsil. **tonsillar c's,** cryptae tonsillares tonsillae pharyngeae. **tonsillar c's of palatine tonsil,** cryptae tonsillares tonsillae palatinae. **tonsillar c's of pharyngeal tonsil,** cryptae tonsillares tonsillae pharyngeae. **c's of Tyson,** glandulae preputiales.

crypt- (kript) see crypto-.

crypta (krip′tah), pl. cryp′tae [L.] [NA] a crypt: a blind pit or tube on a free surface. **cryp′tae muco′sae,** see glandula mucosa. **cryp′tae muco′sae duode′ni,** glandulae duodenales. **cryp′tae odorif′erae, cryp′tae praeputia′les,** glandulae preputiales. **cryp′tae tonsilla′res tonsil′lae palati′nae** [NA], tonsillar crypt of palatine tonsils: the blind ends of the tonsillar fossulae on the palatine tonsils; called also tonsillar crypts. **cryp′tae tonsilla′res tonsil′lae pharyn′geae** [NA], tonsillar crypts of pharyngeal tonsils: the blind ends of the tonsillar fossulae of the pharyngeal tonsils. **cryp′tae ure′thrae mulie′bris,** glandulae urethrales urethrae femininae.

cryptae (krip′te) [L.] plural of crypta.

cryptanamnesia (kript″an-am-ne′ze-ah) cryptomnesia.

cryptectomy (krip-tek′to-me) [crypt- + Gr. ektome excision] excision or obliteration of a crypt.

cryptenamine (krip-ten′ah-mīn) a mixture of ester alkaloids derived from a nonaqueous extract of Veratrum viride Ait. (Liliaceae); it forms a white amorphous powder that possesses antihypertensive properties, and contains several alkaloids, including protoveratrines A and B, neogermitrine, germitrine, germerine, etc. **c. acetates,** a mixture of the acetate salts of cryptenamine, administered intravenously or intramuscularly in the management of eclampsia and hypertensive encephalopathy. **c. tannates,** a mixture of the tannate salts of cryptenamine, administered orally to control moderate to severe hypertension.

cryptesthesia (krip″tes-the′ze-ah) [crypt- + Gr. aisthesis perception] subconscious appreciation or perception of occurrences not ordinarily perceptible to the senses.

cryptic (krip′tik) [Gr. kryptikos hidden] concealed, hidden, larval.

cryptitis (krip-ti′tis) inflammation of a crypt. **anal c.,** inflammation of the anal crypts, with pain and tenderness (especially during bowel movements), pruritus, and spasm of the anal sphincter; it may progress to abscess of the crypt.

crypto- (krip′to) [Gr. kryptos hidden] a combining form meaning hidden or concealed, or denoting relationship to a crypt.

Cryptobia (krip-tōb′e-ah) [Gr. kryptos hidden + bios life] a genus of protozoa of the family Cryptobiidae, order Protomonadina, found as parasites in the reproductive organs of invertebrates, especially mollusks, but also in the blood and digestive tract of fish; called also Trypanoplasma. It includes the species: C. abramidis, found in the bream (Abramis brama); C. borreli and C. cyprini, found in the blood of various fish; C. helicis, found in the reproductive organs of various pulmonate snails; T. intestinalis, found in a salt-water fish (*Bax boops*)—the first trypanosome-like organism to be found outside the blood; *T. truttae*, found in the trout (*Salmo fario*); and *T. ventriculi*, found in the lump-sucker (*Cyclopterus umpus*).

Cryptobiidae (krip″to-bi′ĭ-de) a family of parasitic, trypanosome-like protozoa of the order Protomonadina, class Zoomastigophora, characterized by the presence of two flagella: one is anterior and free and the other is attached to the body, forming the outer edge of an undulating membrane. It includes the genus *Cryptobia*.

cryptocephalus (krip″to-sef′ah-lus) [*crypto-* + Gr. *kephalē* head] a monster with an inconspicuous head.

Cryptococcaceae (krip″to-kok-ka′se-e) a family of the Fungi Imperfecti, order Moniliales, the members of which are yeastlike throughout most or all of their life cycle; it includes a number of pathogenic genera, such as *Crytococcus, Candida, Geotrichum, Trichosporon,* and *Pityrosporon.*

cryptococcosis (krip″to-kok-o′sis) an infection by *Cryptococcus neoformans* which may involve the skin, lungs, or other parts, but has a predilection for the brain and meninges. The cutaneous form is marked by acneiform lesions; called also *European blastomycosis*. The generalized form invades the central nervous system; less often the lungs, liver, spleen and joints. It is fatal if left untreated. Called also *torulosis,* and *Busse-Buschke disease.*

Cryptococcus (krip″to-kok′us) [*crypto-* + Gr. *kokkos* berry] a genus of asexual yeastlike organisms of the family Cryptococcaceae, which usually have a capsule and do not form pseudomycellium as do the *Candida*. Formerly called *Atelosaccharomyces* and *Torula*. **C. capsula′tus,** former name for *Histoplasma capsulatum*. **C. gilchris′ti,** former name for *Blastomyces dermatitidis*. **C. histolyt′icus,** *C. neoformans*. **C. hom′inis,** *C. neoformans*. **C. meningit′idis,** *C. neoformans*. **C. neofor′mans,** a species causing an infection in humans; see *cryptococcosis*. Formerly called *C. histolytians, hominis,* and *meningitidis,* and *Debaryomyces neoformans hominis* and *Torula histolytica*.

cryptocrystalline (krip″to-kris′tah-lĭn) [*crypto-* + *crystalline*] composed of crystals of microscopic size.

Cryptocys′tis trichodec′tis a name erroneously applied to the cysticercoid larval form of the tapeworm *Dipylidium caninum* when it was first discovered in the body cavity of the dog louse, *Trichodectes*.

cryptodeterminant (krip″to-de-ter′min-ant) hidden determinant.

cryptodidymus (krip″to-did′ĭ-mus) [*crypto-* + Gr. *didymos* twin] a teratism in which one twin is concealed within the body of the other.

cryptoempyema (krip″to-em″pi-e′mah) [*crypto-* + *empyema*] empyema that is difficult to aspirate, being loculated or interlobar.

cryptogam (krip′to-gam) [*crypto-* + Gr. *gamos* marriage] any one of the lower plants that have no true flowers, but propagate by spores.

cryptogenetic (krip″to-jĕ-net′ik) cryptogenic.

cryptogenic (krip″to-jen′ik) [*crypto-* + Gr. *gennan* to produce] of obscure, doubtful, or unascertainable origin. Cf. *phanerogenic*.

cryptoglioma (krip″to-gli-o′mah) [*crypto-* + *glioma*] one of the stages in the development of glioma of the retina, marked by shrinking of the eyeball due to cyclitis, which masks the presence of the growth.

cryptoleukemia (krip″to-lu-ke′me-ah) [*crypto-* + *leukemia*] an archaic term previously applied to a hyperplastic blood process in which there were no abnormal cells in the blood stream.

cryptolith (krip′to-lith) [*crypto-* + Gr. *lithos* stone] a calculus or concretion in a crypt.

cryptomenorrhea (krip″to-men″o-re′ah) [*crypto-* + *menorrhea*] a condition in which the symptoms of menstruation are experienced but no external bleeding occurs, as in cases of imperforate hymen.

cryptomere (krip′to-mēr) [*crypto-* + Gr. *meros* part] a cystic or saclike condition.

cryptomerorachischisis (krip″to-me″ro-rah-kis′kĭ-sis) [*crypto-* + Gr. *meros* part + *rhachis* spine + *schisis* cleavage] spina bifida occulta.

cryptomnesia (krip″tom-ne′ze-ah) [*crypto-* + Gr. *mnasthai* to be mindful] the recall of events not recognized as part of one's conscious experience.

cryptomnesic (krip″tom-ne′sik) hidden in the memory; pertaining to or characterized by cryptomnesia.

cryptomonad (krip″to-mon′ad) any of the algae of the order Cryptophyceae.

cryptoneurous (krip″to-nu′rus) [*crypto-* + Gr. *neuron* nerve] having no definite or distinct nervous system.

cryptophthalmia (krip″tof-thal′me-ah) cryptophthalmos.

cryptophthalmos (krip″tof-thal′mos) [*crypto-* + Gr. *ophthalmos* eye] a developmental anomaly in which the skin is continuous over the eyeballs without any indication of the formation of eyelids; called also *ankyloblepharon totale.*

cryptophthalmus (krip″tof-thal′mus) cryptophthalmos.

Cryptophyceae (krip″to-fi′se-e) [*crypto-* + Gr. *phykos* seaweed] an order of light brown, biflagellate, protozoon-like algae of uncertain taxonomic classification.

cryptopine (krip′to-pin) [*crypto-* + Gr. *opion* opium] a minor alkaloidal constituent, $C_{21}H_{23}NO_5$, of opium, of *Corydalis sempervirens* (L.) Pers., and of *Dicentra* spp. (Fumariaceae).

cryptoplasmic (krip″to-plaz′mik) occurring in a concealed form; said of an infection in which the infecting organism has concealed itself; occult.

cryptopodia (krip″to-po′de-ah) [*crypto-* + Gr. *pous* foot] a condition characterized by swelling of the lower part of the leg and dorsum of the foot so as to cover all but the soles of the feet.

cryptopsychic (krip″to-si′kik) of concealed or vague psychic significance.

cryptopsychism (krip″to-si′kizm) parapsychology.

cryptopyic (krip″to-pi′ik) [*crypto-* + Gr. *pyon* pus] attended by concealed suppuration.

cryptoradiometer (krip″to-ra″de-om′ĕ-ter) [*crypto-* + L. *radius* ray + Gr. *metron* measure] an apparatus for measuring the penetrative power of roentgen rays.

cryptorchid (krip-tor′kid) [*crypto-* + Gr. *orchis* testis] pertaining to or characterized by cryptorchidism; by extension, sometimes used to designate an individual exhibiting cryptorchidism.

cryptorchidectomy (krip″tor-kĭ-dek′to-me) [*cryptorchid* + Gr. *ektomē* excision] excision of an undescended testis.

cryptorchidism (krip-tor′kĭ-dizm) a developmental defect characterized by failure of the testes to descend into the scrotum.

cryptorchidopexy (krip-tor″kĭ-do-pek′se) orchiopexy.

cryptorchidy (krip-tor″kĭ-de) cryptorchidism.

cryptorchism (krip-tor′kizm) cryptorchidism.

cryptorrhea (krip″to-re′ah) [*crypto-* + Gr. *rhoia* flow] abnormal activity of an endocrine organ.

cryptorrheic (krip″to-re′ik) cryptorrhetic.

cryptorrhetic (krip″to-ret′ik) 1. pertaining to the internal secretions. 2. pertaining to cryptorrhea.

cryptoscope (krip′to-skōp) [*crypto-* + Gr. *skopein* to examine] a fluoroscope. **Satvioni's c.,** one of the early forms of fluoroscope.

cryptoscopy (krip-tos′ko-pe) fluoroscopy.

cryptosterol (krip-tos′ter-ol) a triterpenic sterol, $C_{30}H_{50}O$, from yeast; it also occurs in wool fat (see *lanosterol*).

Cryptostroma (krip″to-stro′mah) a genus of fungi. **C. cortica′le,** *Coniosporium corticale.*

cryptotia (krip-to′she-ah) a rare anomaly in which the superior portion of the auricle is buried in the scalp.

cryptotoxic (krip″to-tok′sik) [*crypto-* + *toxic*] having hidden toxic properties; said of a solution normally nontoxic, but which may become toxic when the colloidal balance is disturbed.

cryptoxanthin (krip″to-zan′thin) a yellow carotenoid widely distributed in nature (egg yolk, green grass, yellow corn, etc.), which can be converted into vitamin A in the body.

cryptozoite (krip″to-zo′īt) [*crypto-* + Gr. *zōon* animal] a malarial sporozoite in the exo-erythrocytic stage as it lives in the tissues before entering the blood to attack a blood corpuscle.

cryptozygous (krip-toz′ĭ-gus) [*crypto-* + Gr. *zygon* yoke] having the face no wider than the cranium, so that the zygomatic arches are concealed by the bulging of the cranium when the skull is viewed from above. Cf. *phenozygous*.

Crys. crystal.

crystal (kris′tal) [Gr. *krystallos* ice] a naturally produced angular solid of definite form in which the ultimate units from which it is built up are systematically arranged; they are usually evenly spaced on a regular space lattice. **asthma c's,** Charcot-Leyden c's. **blood c's,** hematoidin crystals in the blood. **Böttcher's c's,** microscopic crystals seen on adding a drop of solution of ammonium phosphate to a drop of prostatic fluid. **Charcot-Leyden c's,** crystalline structures, protein in nature, found wherever eosinophilic leukocytes are undergoing fragmentation, e.g., in the bronchial secretions in bronchial asthma and in stools in some cases of intestinal parasitism. Called also *asthma, leukocytic,* and *Leyden's c's.* **Charcot-Neumann c's,** minute cyrstals of spermine phosphate found in semen and various animal tissues. **coffin lid c's,** peculiar indented crystals of ammoniomagnesium phosphate from alkaline urine; called also *knife rest c's.* **Dubos crude c's** (obs.), tyrothricin. **dumbbell c's,** crystals of calcium oxalate occurring in the urine. **ear c.,** statolith, def. 1; see *statoconia*. **Florence c's,** crystals formed by the action of iodine on any liquid containing lecithin, as in semen. **hedgehog c's,** a spiny form of uric acid concretions. **knife rest c's,** coffin lid c's. **leukocytic c's, Leyden's c's,** Charcot-Leyden c's. **liquid c's,** certain liquids which manifest some of the optical properties of crystals and the hydrodynamic properties of fluids, e.g., phosphatidyl choline. **Lubarsch's c's,** crystals in the testis resembling sperm crystals. **Platner's c's,** crystals of the salts of the bile acids. **c's of Reinke,** conspicuous crystals contained in interstitial cells of the human testis. They are 2–3 μ thick and up to 20 μ in length with variable shapes, are isotropic in polarized light, and have the solubility and staining properties of protein. They seem to be composed of closely compacted microtubules. **rock c.,** quartz; a transparent form of silicon dioxide (silica), SiO_2; used for lenses. **sperm c's, spermin c's** crystals of spermine phosphate in the semen. **Teichmann's c's,** crystals of hemin. **thorn-apple c's,** yellow or reddish brown spheres of ammonium urate which are covered with sharp spicules or prisms, as found in the urine. **Virchow's c's,** yellow or orange crystals of hematoidin sometimes seen in extravasated blood. **whetstone c's,** crystals of xanthine sometimes seen in urine.

crystalbumin (kris″tal-bu′min) 1. an albuminous substance found in an aqueous extract of the crystalline lens. 2. a general term for crystallizable albumins of the type of egg albumin and serum albumin.

crystalli (kris-tal′e) chickenpox.

crystallin (kris-tal′lin) a globulin existing in the crystalline lens of the eye. *Alpha c.* is precipitated by dilute acetic acid; *beta c.* is not.

crystalline (kris′tah-lin) resembling a crystal in nature or clearness.

crystallitis (kris-tah-li′tis) phakitis.

crystallization (kris″tah-li-za′shun) the formation of crystals; conversion to a crystalline form. **fern-leaf c.,** crystallization of cervical mucus in a fernlike pattern, observable during the first half of the menstrual cycle and said to be most conspicuous at the time of ovulation.

crystallography (kris″tah-log′rah-fe) [*crystal* + Gr. *graphein* to write] the science dealing with the study of crystals. **x-ray c.,** the determination of the three-dimensional structure of molecules by means of diffraction patterns produced by x-rays.

crystalloid (kris′tah-loid) [*crystal* + Gr. *eidos* form] 1. resembling a crystal. 2. a noncolloid substance; a substance which, in solution, passes readily through animal membranes, lowers the freezing point of the solvent containing it, and is generally capable of being crystallized. Cf. *colloid,* def. 1. **Charcot-Böttcher c's,** slender spindle-shaped crystals 10 to 25 μ long, commonly found in Sertoli cells of the human testis but not in other species.

crystalloiditis (kris-tah-loi-di′tis) phakitis.

crystalluria (kris-tah-lu′re-ah) the excretion of crystals in the urine, producing renal irritation.

Crysticillin (kris″ti-sil′in) trademark for preparations of penicillin G procaine.

Crystodigin (kris″to-dig′in) trademark for preparations of digitoxin.

CS cesarean section; conditioned stimulus.

CS₂ carbon disulfide.

Cs chemical symbol for *cesium.*

C.S.A.A. Child Study Association of America.

C.S.C. coup sur coup.

C.S.F. cerebrospinal fluid.

C.S.G.B.I. Cardiac Society of Great Britain and Ireland.

C.S.M. cerebrospinal meningitis.

CST convulsive shock therapy; see *shock therapy,* under *therapy.*

CT computerized tomography.

C.T.A. Canadian Tuberculosis Association.

CTBA cetrimonium bromide.

cteinophyte (ti′no-fīt) [Gr. *kteinein* to kill + *phyton* plant] a fungus that has a destructive influence upon its host; limited to chemical rather than parasitic activity.

Ctenocephalides (te″no-se-fal′ĭ-dēz) a genus of fleas. **C. ca′nis,** a species frequently found on dogs, which may transmit the dog tapeworm to man; formerly called *Pulex serraticeps.* **C. fe′lis,** a species commonly found parasitic on cats.

Ctenophthalmus (te″nof-thal′mus) a genus of fleas. **C. agry′tes,** the European mouse flea.

Ctenopsyllus (te″no-sil′us) (*obs.*) *Leptopsylla.* **C. seg′nis,** *Leptopsylla segnis.*

Ctenus (te′nus) a genus of spiders. *C. ferus* is the South American wandering spider whose bite causes great pain. In severe cases, weakness and irregularity of the heart beat, breathing difficulty, and temporary blindness may occur; some deaths have occurred in young children.

C-terminal (ter′min-al) the end of the peptide chain carrying the free alpha carboxyl group of the last amino acid, conventionally written to the right.

Ctesias (te′se-as) (5th century B.C.) a Greek physician who was a contemporary of Hippocrates, and who was said by Galen to have written the Cnidian aphorisms.

ctetology (te-tol′ŏ-je) [Gr. *ktētos* acquired + *-logy*] that branch of biology which treats of acquired characters.

ctetosome (tet′o-sōm) [Gr. *ktētos* acquired + Gr. *sōma* body] a supernumerary chromosome; a sex chromosome.

CTP cytidine triphosphate.

Cu chemical symbol for *copper* (L. *cuprum*).

cuajani (kwah-hah′ne) an expectorant preparation from *Prunus occidentalis.*

cubeb (ku′beb) [L. *cubeba;* Arabic *kabāba*] the dried, unripe, almost fully grown fruit of *Piper cubeba* L.f. (Piperaceae), the tailed pepper or Java pepper, found throughout Southern Asia, which contains 10–18 per cent volatile oil, cubebin, resins, fat, and wax. Formerly used to stimulate healing of mucous membranes, and as a diuretic and urinary antiseptic.

cubebin (ku-be′bin) an inactive crystalline principle, $C_{10}H_{10}O_3$, from cubeb; formerly used as a urinary antiseptic.

cubebism (ku′beb-izm) poisoning by cubeb (*Piper cubeba*), characterized by nausea, vomiting, diarrhea, fever with or without skin eruptions, prostration, arthralgia, irritation of the kidneys, soft pulse, loss of consciousness, miosis, delirium, and coma. In severe poisonings, death from respiratory failure may occur.

cubicle (ku′bǐ-k'l) a compartment in a larger area, such as a dormitory or a ward, separated from similar adjoining compartments and from the rest of the room by low partitions.

cubilose (ku′bǐ-lōs) [L. *cubile* nest] a mucilaginous and nutritious principle from the edible nest of the swiftlet, *Collocalia esculenta,* of southern Asia; it is an excretion from the stomach of the bird.

cubit (ku′bit) [L. *cubitus*] a unit of measure, being the distance from the joint between the arm and forearm (elbow) to the tip of the middle finger; ranging, according to various systems of measurement, between 46 and 53 cm.

cubital (ku′bǐ-tal) 1. pertaining to the elbow. 2. pertaining to the ulna or to the forearm.

cubitalis (ku-bǐ-ta′lis) [L.] cubital.

cubitocarpal (ku″bǐ-to-kar′pal) pertaining to the ulna and the carpus.

cubitoradial (ku″bǐ-to-ra′de-al) pertaining to the ulna and the radius.

cubitus (ku′bǐ-tus) [L.] 1. [NA] the bend of the arm; the joint between the arm and forearm; the elbow. 2. the upper limb distal to the humerus: the elbow, forearm, and hand. 3. ulna. **c. val′gus,** deformity of the elbow (judged with the palm facing forward), in which it deviates away from the midline of the body when extended. **c. va′rus,** deformity of the elbow, due to lateral angulation of the joint and accompanied by deviation of the forearm toward the midline of the body when the forearm is extended; called also *gun stock deformity.*

cuboid (ku′boid) [Gr. *kyboeidēs*] 1. resembling a cube. 2. the cuboid bone (os cuboideum [NA]).

cuboidal (ku-boi′dal) resembling a cube.

cu. cm. cubic centimeter.

cucoline (ku′ko-lēn) sinomenine.

cucullaris (ku-ku-la′ris) [L. *cucullus* hood] musculus trapezius; see *Table of Musculi.*

cucumber (ku′kum-ber) [L. *cucumis*] the edible fruit of various species of *Cucumis,* chiefly *C. sativus* L., the seeds of which are diuretic and whose juice is used as an astringent in various cosmetic formulations. **bitter c.,** colocynth.

Cucumis (ku′kum-is) a genus of curcurbitaceous plants which includes several edible species, as well as some which have medicinal properties, e.g., *C. sativus* L., the cucumber (q.v.).

Cucurbita (ku-ker′bǐ-tah) a genus of curcurbitaceous plants, including *C. pepo* L., the pumpkin (q.v.).

cucurbitol (ku-ker′bǐ-tol) a sterol, $C_{24}H_{40}O_4$, obtained from watermelon seeds.

cucurbitula (ku″ker-bit′u-lah) [L. dim. of *cucurbita,* a gourd] a cupping glass. **c. cruen′ta** [L. "bloody cup"], a cupping glass applied to draw blood. **c. sic′ca** [L. "dry cup"], a cupping glass that does not draw blood.

cucurbocitrin (ku″ker-bo-sit′rin) an extract from watermelon seeds; it has been tried in the treatment of hypertension.

cudbear (kud′bār) a red-brown powder, obtained from lichens, such as *Lecanora tartarea;* and used as a coloring matter in pharmacy.

cudding (kud′ing) quidding.

cuff (kuf) a small bandlike structure encircling a part. **musculotendinous c.,** one formed by intermingled muscle and tendon fibers; see *rotator c.* **rotator c.,** a musculotendinous structure about the capsule of the shoulder joint, formed by the inserting fibers of the supraspinatus, infraspinatus, teres minor, and subscapularis muscles, blending with the capsule, and providing mobility and strength to the shoulder joint.

cuffing (kuf′ing) the formation of a cufflike surrounding border, such as collections of leukocytes surrounding blood vessels, noted in certain viral diseases.

Cuignet's method (ke-ēn-yāz′) [Ferdinand Louis Joseph *Cuignet,* French opthalmologist, born 1823] skiametry.

cuirass (kwe-ras′) [Fr. *cuirasse* breastplate] a covering for the chest. **tabetic c.,** an area of diminished sense of touch encircling the chest of a patient with tabes dorsalis.

Cuj., cuj. abbreviation for L. *cu'jus,* of which.

cul-de-sac (kul'dĕ-sahk') [Fr.] a blind pouch or cecum. **conjunctival c.,** the fold formed by the junction of the palpebral and the ocular conjunctiva. **Douglas' c.,** excavatio rectouterina. **dural c.,** the terminal portion of the dural sac.

culdocentesis (kul''do-sen-te'sis) [*cul-de-sac* + *centesis*] aspiration of fluid from the rectouterine excavation by puncture of the vaginal wall.

culdoscope (kul'do-skōp) an endoscope for performing culdoscopy.

culdoscopy (kul-dos'ko-pe) visual examination of the female pelvic viscera by means of an endoscope introduced into the pelvic cavity through the posterior vaginal fornix.

culdotomy (kul-dot'o-me) [*cul-de-sac* + Gr. *tomē* a cutting] incision into the cul-de-sac (pouch of Douglas); called also *posterior colpotomy.*

Culex (ku'leks) [L. "gnat"] a genus of culicine mosquitoes characterized by short palpi and by holding the body parallel to the surface on which it rests while the head and beak are bent at an angle to the body. Many species occurring throughout the world are vectors of various disease-producing agents. Species include *C. annuliros'tris, C. fat'igans, C. moles'tus, C. pi'piens, C. quinquefascia'tus, C. tarsa'lis,* and *C. tritaeniorhyn'cus,* among many others.

culicicide (ku-lis'ĭ-sīd) culicide.

Culicidae (ku-lis'ĭ-de) a family of insects of the suborder Nematocera, order Diptera, including the mosquitoes. There are ten tribes, of which three are of particular medical interest: Anophelini, Culicini, and Megarhinini.

culicidal (ku-lĭ-si'dal) destructive to gnats and mosquitoes.

culicide (ku'lĭ-sīd) [L. *culex* gnat + *caedere* to kill] an agent destructive to gnats and mosquitoes.

culicifuge (ku-lis'ĭ-fūj) [L. *culex* gnat + *fugare* to put to flight] a preparation that repels gnats and mosquitoes.

Culicinae (ku-lĭ-si'ne) a subfamily of the Culicidae, the true mosquitoes, containing the tribes Anophelini, Culicini, and Megarhinini.

culicine (ku'lĭ-sin, ku'lĭ-sīn) 1. a member of the genus *Culex* or related genera. 2. pertaining to, involving, or affecting mosquitoes of the genus *Culex* or related genera.

Culicini (ku-lĭ-si'ni) a tribe of the subfamily Culicinae containing many genera, the most important of which are *Aedes, Culex, Mansonia, Psorophora, Theobaldia,* and *Wyeomyia.*

Culicoides (ku-lĭ-koi'dēz) a genus of biting flies of the family Heleidae. *C. aus'teni* and *C. gra'hami* are intermediate hosts of the parasitic roundworm *Dipetalonema perstans. C. fu'cens* and possibly other species are intermediate hosts of *Mansonella ozzardi.*

Culiseta (ku''lĭ-se'tah) a genus of culicine mosquitoes; formerly called *Theobaldia.* **C. inora'ta,** a vector of the Cache Valley virus in Utah. **C. melanu'ra,** a vector of the viruses causing eastern and western equine encephalitides.

Cullen's sign (kul'enz) [Thomas Stephen *Cullen,* Baltimore surgeon, 1868–1953] see under *sign.*

culling (kul'ing) the process of selective removal. The term is applied to the removal from the circulation, by the spleen, of abnormal erythrocytes, such as those occurring in congenital spherocytosis, or to the selective separation of other elements or organisms.

culmen (kul'men), pl. *cul'mina* [L. "ridge"] [NA] the part of the vermis of the cerebellum between the lobulus centralis and the primary fissure; called also *culmen monticuli.*

culmina (kul'mĭ-nah) [L.] plural of *culmen.*

Culp ureteropelvioplasty [Ormond Skinner *Culp,* American surgeon, born 1910] see under *urethroplasty.*

cult (kult) a system of treating disease based on some special and unscientific theory of disease causation.

cultivation (kul''tĭ-va'shun) [L. *cultivatio*] the propagation of living organisms, applied especially to the propagation of cells in artificial media.

culturable (kul'chur-ah-b'l) capable of being cultured.

cultural (kul'tu-ral) pertaining to a culture.

culture (kul'tūr) [L. *cultura*] 1. the propagation of microorganisms or of living tissue cells in special media conducive to their growth. 2. a growth of microorganisms or other living cells. 3. to induce the propagation of microorganisms or living tissue cells in media conducive to their growth. See also *culture medium.* **attenuated c.,** a culture of microorganisms that have altered virulence. **cell c.,** a growth of cells *in vitro;* although the cells proliferate they do not organize into tissue. **chorioallantoic c.,** the cultivation of microorganisms, cells, or tissues on the chorioallantois of the developing chick. **continuous flow c.,** the cultivation of bacteria in a continuous flow of fresh medium to maintain bacterial growth in logarithmic phase. **direct c.,** one made by direct transfer from a natural source to an artificial medium. **flask c.,** one grown on a medium contained in a flask. **fractional c.,** a technique for obtaining a single species of microorganisms from a culture containing more than one. **hanging-block c.,** one grown on a block of agar medium fastened to a coverglass, which is then inverted over a hollow slide.

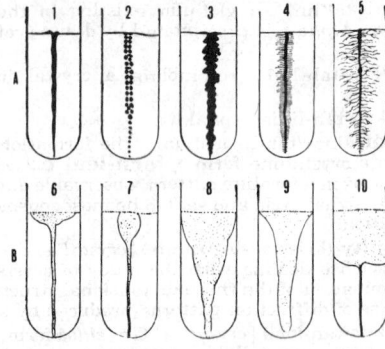

Types of growth in stab cultures. A, Nonliquefying: 1, filiform (*B. coli*); 2, beaded (*Str. pyogenes*); 3, echinate (*Bact. acidi-lactici*); 4, villous (*Bact. murisepticum*); 5, arborescent (*B. mycoides*). B, Liquefying: 6, crateriform (*B. vulgare,* 24 hours); 7, napiform (*B. subtilis,* 48 hours); 8, infundibuliform (*B. prodigiosus*); 9, saccate (*Msp. finkleri*); 10, stratiform (*Ps. fluorescens*). (Frost.)

hanging-drop c., a culture in which the material to be cultivated is inoculated into a drop of fluid attached to a coverglass, which is inverted over a hollow slide. **mixed leukocyte c., mixed lymphocyte c.,** see under *reaction.* **needle c.,** stab c. **plate c.,** one grown on a medium, usually agar or gelatin, on a Petri dish. **primary c.,** a cell or tissue culture started from material taken directly from an organism, as opposed to that from an explant in an organism. **pure c.,** a culture of a single species of cell, without presence of any contaminants. **sensitized c.,** a bacterial culture to which has been added its specific antiserum. **shake c.,** a culture made by inoculating warm liquid agar culture medium in a tube to allow the development of separated colonies in the solidified medium on incubation; especially applicable to obligate anaerobes. **slant c.,** one made on a slanting surface of a solidified medium in a tube, the tube being tilted to provide a greater surface area for growth. **slope c.,** slant c. **smear c.** (*obs.*), one made by smearing the inoculating material on the surface of the medium. **stab c.,** one in which the medium is inoculated by a needle thrust deeply into its substance; called also *needle c.* and *thrust c.* **stock c.,** a permanent culture from which transfers may be made. **streak c.,** one in which the medium is inoculated by drawing an infected wire across it. **suspension c.,** a culture in which cells multiply while suspended in a suitable medium. **thrust c.,** stab c. **tissue c.,** the maintaining or growing of tissue, organ primordia, or the whole or part of an organ *in vitro* so as to preserve its architecture and/or function. **tube c.,** one made in a test tube. **type c.,** a culture of any species of microorganism usually maintained in a central collection of type or standard cultures.

culture medium (kul'tūr me'de-um) any substance or preparation used for the cultivation of living cells; see *Table of Culture Media.*

TABLE OF CULTURE MEDIA

Abbreviations used in this table are: a. = agar, b. = broth, c. = culture medium, m. = medium.

acetate differential a., a sodium acetate-inorganic salt medium containing bromthymol blue, for the differentiation of *Shigella* from *Salmonella* and coliform bacteria; *Shigella* does not grow on this medium.

agar c., one in which agar is used as the solidifying agent.

albumin b. (Dubos), a liquid medium containing peptone, asparagine, inorganic salts, and Tween 80, enriched with serum albumin, for the culture of tubercle bacilli and other mycobacteria as a submerged diffuse growth.

Anderson's m., chocolate agar–tellurite medium; an enriched medium for cultivation of the diphtheria bacillus.

antibiotic c. 1, seed a.

antibiotic c. 5, streptomycin assay agar with yeast extract.

antibiotic c. 9 and 10, see *polymyxin test a.*

antibiotic c. 11, neomycin assay a.

antibiotic c. 12, nystatin assay a.

Aronson's c., an alkaline medium for the isolation of the cholera spirillum, consisting of agar, meat extract, peptone, sodium chloride, sodium carbonate, cane sugar, dextrin, basic fuchsin, sodium sulfite, and water.

asparagin c., 1. a synthetic medium containing asparagin, disodium acid phosphate, ammonium lactate, and sodium chloride; called also *Fränkel* and *Voges' asparagin c.* 2. a synthetic medium containing asparagin, ammonium lactate, sodium chloride, magnesium sulfate, calcium chloride, monopotassium acid phosphate, and glycerin; called also *Uschinsky's c.*

Avery's c., a glucose meat infusion broth containing 5 per cent of sterile defibrinated rabbit blood.

azide violet blood a., a beef heart infusion culture medium containing tryptose, sodium azide, and crystal violet (which inhibits the growth of streptococci, staphylococci, and micrococci), used as a selective medium for the isolation of *Erysipelothrix rhusiopathiae.*

bacteriostasis a., a medium containing peptone, beef extract, sodium chloride, and agar, used to maintain stock cultures of test organisms and to test antibacterial activity.

Balamuth's c., a monophasic culture medium used for the growth of *Entamoeba histolytica;* it consists of buffered aqueous egg yolk infusion with or without liver extract.

Barile-Yaguchi-Eveland (BYE) a., a simplified culture medium containing brain-heart infusion and yeast extract, used for the cultivation of *Mycoplasma.*

basal c., any medium usually composed of meat extract broth and agar as follows: meat extract 3 gm., peptone 5 gm., sodium chloride 5 gm. (included if for serological work or if enriched with blood), and agar 15 gm. (omitted if liquid medium is desired), per liter of distilled water.

beef infusion c., see *infusion m.*

beer wort c., crushed malt macerated in water, then filtered and sterilized.

bile c., bile salt c., nutrient broth containing dextrose and sodium taurocholate and sufficient litmus solution to color it a deep purple.

bismuth sulfite a., Wilson-Blair c.

blood c. (Kracke), a liquid medium containing brain suspension in meat infusion broth with dextrose, peptone, and citrate, and buffered with phosphate at pH 7.4, for the enrichment culture of pathogenic bacteria present in the blood in bacteremias.

Boeck and Drbohlav's c., a culture medium for amoeba containing sodium chloride, calcium chloride, potassium chloride, sodium bicarbonate, and glucose; called also *Les c.*

Bordet-Gengou a., an agar base containing infusion from potato, peptone, sodium chloride, and agar, enriched with blood and glycerol, for isolation of *Hemophilus pertussis* and *Mycobacterium tuberculosis.* Also used without peptone to enhance selectivity of *H. pertussis.*

boric acid b., a liquid culture medium containing peptone, lactose, and boric acid, buffered with phosphate, used in the presumptive test for *Escherichia coli* in water and food.

brain-heart infusion m., a medium containing calf brain and beef heart infusion, peptone, dextrose, and phosphate buffer, used in the liquid state (broth) for blood culture, and solidified with agar for the culture of pathogenic bacteria, especially streptococci and pneumococci; with the addition of the antibiotics penicillin and streptomycin, or chloramphenicol and cycloheximide, it is used as a selective medium for the isolation of fungi.

Braun's c., Endo agar.

brilliant green a., a selective medium containing yeast extract, peptone, sodium chloride, lactose, saccharose, agar, and brilliant green, for the detection of *Salmonella* in foods.

brilliant green–bile a., a selective differential culture medium containing peptone, lactose, bile salts, decolorized fuchsin, and brilliant green, for the culture of coliform bacteria from water and food samples.

bromcresol purple desoxycholate (BCP-D) a., a selective differential microbial culture medium containing lactose and sucrose, bromcresol purple as an indicator, and desoxycholate as an inhibitor; used for the isolation of *Shigella* and *Salmonella.*

Brucella a., a culture medium containing pancreatic digest of casein, peptic digest of animal tissue, yeast autolysate, and dextrose, for the isolation of *Brucella* from blood, dairy products, and foods according to the APHA standard methods.

buffered desoxycholate glucose (BDG) b., a liquid culture medium inhibitory to gram-positive bacteria, used as a presumptive medium for the detection of gram-negative enteric bacilli in water and food specimens.

carbohydrate b., a plain broth or a peptone solution that contains only one carbohydrate.

Cary-Blair transport m., an agar medium containing thioglycollate, phosphate, and sodium chloride, for the collection of clinical specimens containing *Shigella, Salmonella,* or *Pasteurella.*

Casman a., a liquid culture medium containing beef extract, peptones, nicotinamide, dextrose, *p*-aminobenzoic acid, and corn starch enriched with 5 per cent sterile defibrinated rabbit blood, used for the isolation of *Hemophilus* species, especially *H. vaginalis.*

Chapman-Stone a., a culture medium containing peptone, yeast extract, gelatin, and mannitol, made selective for staphylococci by high content of sodium chloride (5.5 per cent); used for the isolation of food-poisoning staphylococci.

charcoal a., a beef heart infusion–peptone culture medium con-

taining soluble starch, yeast extract, and Norit (charcoal), for stock culture maintenance and vaccine production of *Bordetella pertussis.*

chlamydospore a., an inorganic salt medium containing polysaccharide, biotin, and trypan blue, for the identification of *Candida albicans* by favoring the formation of chlamydospores which are stained blue by the dye.

chocolate c., nutrient bouillon or agar to which fresh blood has been added and which is then heated, the red blood changing to a chocolate brown color; used for growing the influenza organism.

Clark and Lubs c., MR-VP broth.

Clauberg's a., a culture medium consisting of ox or sheep serum (coagulated) with glycerol and potassium tellurite.

clostrisel c., a culture medium containing peptones, dextrose, cystine, thioglycollate, formaldehyde sulfoxylate, neomycin, and azide, used as a highly selective medium for the isolation of pathogenic clostridia.

coagulase-mannitol a., a brain-heart infusion/tryptic soy agar containing mannitol and bromcresol purple, enriched with 10 per cent sterile human plasma for the culture of pathogenic staphylococci; coagulase-positive, mannitol-fermenting strains show an opaque yellow zone around the colonies, and coagulase-negative, mannitol-positive strains show a clear yellow zone.

corn meal a., an inorganic salt culture medium containing corn meal, used for the identification of *Candida albicans* by favoring the production of chlamydospores. With dextrose added, it is used for cultivation of fungi, but not for chlamydospore production.

Corper's c., a culture medium for tubercle bacilli consisting of glycerolated pieces of potato that have been soaked in crystal violet solution.

Craig's c. (for intestinal protozoa), a mixture of sterile human or rabbit serum and Locke's solution.

cystine-heart a., beef heart infusion containing peptone, dextrose, L-cystine, and agar, used in diagnostic bacteriology, especially for the cultivation of *Pasteurella tularensis.*

Czapek-Dox a., an inorganic salt-sucrose-nitrate medium, used either as broth or solidified with agar for the cultivation of fungi; called also *Czapek-Dox c.*

decarboxylase c., a liquid culture medium containing beef extract, peptone, and acid-base indicator (cresol red and/or bromcresol purple) to which is added an amino acid (commonly lysine, arginine, or ornithine), for the determination of the amino acid decarboxylase activity as a differential character of bacteria, especially Enterobacteriaceae.

deoxycholate-citrate m., one of the most widely used mediums for isolation of *Salmonella* and dysentery bacilli, containing meat infusion 1000 ml., peptone 10 gm., agar 20 gm., lactose 10 gm., sodium citrate 20.6 gm., sodium deoxycholate 5 gm., lead chloride (0.35% aqueous) 1 ml., ferric ammonium citrate 2 gm., and neutral red (1% aqueous) 2 ml.

deoxycholate citrate lactose saccharose (DCLS) a., a selective differential medium containing sodium thiosulfate and neutral red as the indicator, used for the isolation of gram-negative enteric bacilli. Gram-positive bacteria and coliforms are inhibited, *Shigella* and *Salmonella* appearing as colorless or slightly pink translucent colonies.

dextrose a., a culture medium containing beef extract, peptone, dextrose, sodium chloride, and agar.

dextrose starch a., a culture medium containing peptone, dextrose, soluble starch, and gelatin, for the cultivation of gonococci, meningococci, and other bacteria which do not ferment starch.

Dieudonné's c., an alkaline blood agar used for the isolation of the cholera vibrio.

differential c., a medium, usually solid, whose composition is designed to show physiological characteristics by typical colonial morphology.

Dorset's egg c., a culture medium consisting of whole eggs in isotonic salt solution and glycerol, solidified by coagulated egg, for the nonselective culture of tubercle bacilli; called also *egg c.*

Dubos' c., albumin b.

Durham's c., inosite-free b.

egg c., 1. Dorsett egg c. 2. (Lubenau) Dorset's egg medium with added glycerin. 3. (Petroff) a meat juice prepared by extracting chopped beef with glycerin solution and filtering, to which is added whole eggs, well mixed, and gentian violet.

egg albumin c., 1. (inspissated) a mixture of egg white, distilled water, sodium hydroxide, and glucose; filtered and coagulated in an inclined position. 2. (Tarchanoff and Kolesnikoff) unbroken eggs are placed in dekanormal sodium hydroxide for ten days, the shell removed and the contents cut into slices, washed in running water two hours, placed in Petri dishes, and sterilized.

egg-meat c. (Rettger), a medium prepared from ground lean meat and egg whites, heated separately, but mixed before tubing, with calcium carbonate added to stabilize the reaction; anaerobes may be grown in this mixture without anaerobic precautions.

Eijkman lactose b., a culture medium containing peptone and lactose, for the identification of coliform bacteria in water when incubated at 45.5° C. according to the APHA standard method.

Eisenberg's milk-rice c., see *milk-rice c.*

EMB a., eosin–methylene blue a.

Emerson a., a culture medium containing beef extract, yeast extract, peptone, and dextrose (cycloheximide may be added), for the culture of fungi, especially actinomyces and streptomyces, producing antibiotic substances. A fluid form (broth) is prepared by substituting meat peptone for beef extract.

Endo a., an agar culture medium containing lactose and decolorized fuchsin as an indicator of aldehyde production during the fermentation of lactose; used as a differential medium for the culture of enteric bacilli. Lactose-fermenting coliform bacterial colonies appear red, and nonlactose-ferments uncolored or pink. With the addition of chlortetracycline-HCl, 100 μg. per milliliter, the medium is selective for the isolation of *Candida albicans.* Called also *fuchsin agar, fuchsin-sulfite agar,* and *Braun's c.*

enriched c., one to which the nutrients, such as blood, serum, dextrose, or peptone, have been added.

eosin–methylene blue (EMB) a., a differential culture medium containing peptone, lactose, sucrose, eosin Y, and methylene blue, used especially for the isolation of *Shigella.*

eosin–methylthionine chloride c., eosin–methylene blue agar.

esculin c., a medium containing esculin and iron citrate on which the colon bacillus produces a black colony.

ethyl violet azide b., a culture medium containing peptone, dextrose, sodium azide, and ethyl violet, used as a highly selective medium for the culture of enterococci, especially in water examination.

extract a., FDA m.

FDA m., a culture medium containing beef extract and peptic digest of animal tissue, used in the solid (agar) form for the maintenance of standard cultures and in the liquid (broth) form for nonfastidious bacteria used in phenol coefficient and similar tests; called also *extract agar.*

Fildes c., see under *enrichment.*

fish b., a nutritive broth in which fish water is used in place of meat extract.

Fletcher m., a liquid culture medium containing peptone, and beef extract enriched with 20 per cent fresh pooled rabbit serum, for the isolation, cultivation, and maintenance of *Leptospira;* medium 92 of the APHA Diagnostic Procedures and Reagents.

Forget-Fredette a., a selective culture medium containing Trypticase soy broth and sodium azide, used for the isolation of spore-forming and nonspore-forming obligate anaerobic bacteria.

formate ricinoleate m., a culture medium containing sodium formate, sodium ricinoleate, lactose, and peptone, for the detection of coliform bacteria in milk, water, etc., according to APHA standard methods.

Fränkel and Voges' asparagin c., see *asparagin c.,* def. 1.

fuchsin a., fuchsin sulfite a., Endo agar.

gelatin a., nutrient bouillon solidified with gelatin and agar.

gelatin c., one in which gelatin is used as the solidifying agent.

glucose-formate b., nutrient broth containing glucose and sodium formate; called also *Kitasato's b.*

glycerin b., nutrient broth containing glycerin.

glycerinated potato c., potato culture medium in which the wedges of potato have been soaked, and in which the cotton pads at the bottom are moistened with a 25 per cent solution of glycerin.

glycerin-potato b., a cold water extract of grated potatoes containing glycerin.

haricot b., an extract of kidney beans with salt and cane sugar.

Hershell's c., malt extract solution.

hormone c., a bacteriological culture medium made without filtration; it is thought that the filter material removes by adsorption or by some other process constituents which enhance the nutritive value of the medium.

Hoyle's m., a chocolate agar–tellurite medium used for cultivation of diphtheria bacillus.

indicator c., 1. a differential culture medium designed to reflect or accentuate physiological characteristics of a bacterium by characteristic colonial morphology. 2. a culture medium containing carbohydrate and an acid-base indicator.

infusion m., a bacterial culture medium containing infusion of fresh meat (commonly veal or beef), peptone, and sodium chloride, used as a liquid medium (broth) or solidified with agar, for the culture of more fastidious bacteria, and as a base for media enriched with blood, serum, ascitic fluid, etc.

inosite-free b., nutrient bouillon in which *Escherichia coli* or some other sugar-fermenting organism has grown and thus removed all sugars; it is then clarified and sterilized. Called also *Durham's c.*

iron b., nutrient broth containing ferric tartrate or ferric lactate.

Jordan tartrate c., phenol red medium with sodium potassium tartrate added.

Kendall's c., a culture medium prepared from animal or human small intestine, previously extracted with alcohol and benzol, and therefore relatively protein-rich and peptone-free.

KF streptococcal m., a bacterial culture medium containing peptone, yeast extract, sodium glycerophosphate, maltose, lactose, and sodium azide, which may be used in liquid form or solidified with agar for the culture of fecal streptococci.

Kitasato's b., glucose-formate b.

Kligler iron a., a selective differential bacterial culture medium containing peptone, lactose, dextrose, ferric ammonium citrate, sodium thiosulfate, and phenol red as an indicator, for the differentiation of enteric bacilli.

Koser citrate b., an inorganic salt medium containing sodium citrate, for testing for the utilization of citrate by enteric bacilli.

Krumwiede triple sugar a., a differential bacterial culture medium containing dextrose, lactose, and sucrose with phenol red as an indicator, used in the differentiation and identification of enteric bacilli on the basis of their ability to ferment the contained sugars.

Kulp c., tomato juice a.

lactose-litmus b., nutrient broth containing lactose and sufficient litmus to color it a deep purple.

lauryl sulfate b., a selective enrichment culture medium containing peptone, sodium lauryl sulfate, and lactose, for the detection of coliform bacteria according to the APHA standard methods.

lead b., nutrient broth containing lead acetate.

Les c., Boeck and Drbohlav's c.

Levine's EMB a., Levine's eosin–methylene blue a., a differential culture medium containing peptone, lactose, eosin Y, and methylene blue, for the isolation of enteric bacilli according to APHA and USP standard methods.

Li-Rivers c., Tyrode's solution containing minced chick embryo for the cultivation of filtrable viruses and toxoplasmata.

litmus-milk c., milk culture medium containing sufficient litmus solution to give it a deep lavender color.

litmus-whey c., see under *gelatin.*

Littman a., a culture medium containing peptone, oxgall, dextrose, crystal violet, and streptomycin, for the isolation of fungi; streptomycin is omitted for the culture of *Nocardia.*

Loeffler m., a culture medium consisting of infusion broth enriched by the addition of beef serum and whole egg and solidified by coagulation of serum and egg, used for the isolation of diphtheria bacilli.

Löwenstein's c., a culture medium containing monopotassium phosphate, sodium citrate, magnesium sulfate, asparagin, glycerin, starch, egg yolk, and Congo red or malachite green, for culturing tubercle bacilli in blood.

Löwenstein-Jensen c., a modified Löwenstein culture medium containing asparagine, glycerol, malachite green as an inhibitor, and whole egg, for the culture of tubercle bacilli; the medium is solidified by the heat coagulation of the egg.

L.S.U. m., a lactose-saccharose-urea agar buffered medium, containing a triple indicator system, designed for the isolation of *Salmonella* and *Shigella* by incubation from feces directly and from enrichment broths.

MacConkey a., a selective differential culture medium containing peptone, lactose, bile salts, neutral red, and crystal violet, for the isolation of coliform bacteria; called also *MacConkey's bile salt a.*

MacConkey b., a culture medium containing peptone, oxgall, lactose, and bromcresol purple, used in the presumptive test for the presence of coliform bacteria in water.

malachite green b., nutrient broth with malachite green.

malt a., a solution of malt extract solidified with agar, for the culture of yeasts and molds.

malt extract a., a culture medium containing maltose, dextrin, glycerol, and peptone, for the cultivation of yeasts and molds.

malt extract b., a nutritive medium made by dissolving powdered malt extract in water; adjusting the reaction to plus 1.5 to phenolphthalein and heating in the autoclave for fifteen minutes, filtering through paper and sterilizing.

mannitol salt a., a selective medium containing peptone, mannitol, and 7.5 per cent sodium chloride, with phenol red as an indicator, for the isolation of pathogenic staphylococci.

Martin's b., a preparation of peptone from digested pig stomach and cattle or rabbit serum.

meat extract m., one prepared with commercial meat extract.

meat infusion m., infusion m.

membrane filter m., any of a variety of liquid culture media used for the isolation of bacteria by the membrane filter method.

milk c., milk, usually in test tubes, free from cream, and sterilized for use as a culture medium.

milk-rice c., a mixture of nutrient broth and milk solidified with rice powder, used for growing chromogenic bacteria. Called also *Eisenberg's milk-rice c.* or *Soyka's.*

mineral salts a., a medium containing ammonium nitrate, monopotassium phosphate, dipotassium phosphate, magnesium sulfate, ferrous sulfate, and dried agar, for the culture of *Chaetomium globosum* and *Aspergillus niger.*

Monsur's a., a selective differential tellurite-containing agar medium used for the isolation of *V. cholerae.*

motility test m., a culture medium containing beef extract and peptone, partially solidified by the inclusion of 0.4 per cent agar, used for the detection of motility of enteric bacilli in stab culture.

MR-VP b., a broth culture medium containing peptone, dextrose, and phosphate, for the culture and differentiation of coliform bacteria for the methyl red and Voges-Proskauer tests according to the APHA standard methods; called also *Clark and Lub c.*

Mueller-Hinton a., a solid beef-infusion culture medium containing starch and agar, used for the primary isolation of *Neisseria.* A broth medium is prepared by omitting the agar.

Mycoplasma a., a beef heart infusion medium enriched with horse serum and yeast extract which may be made selective by the inclusion of penicillin and thallium acetate, for the isolation of *Mycoplasma.*

Naegeli's c., see under *solution.*

Neill's m., a chocolate agar–tellurite medium used in Great Britain.

neomycin assay a., a culture medium containing beef extract, yeast extract, peptone, pancreatic digest of casein, and dextrose, for the assay of the neomycin content of pharmaceutical preparations according to FDA and USP requirements; called also *antibiotic c. 11.*

neutral red c., glucose agar containing neutral red.

NIH agar m., a culture medium containing pancreatic digest of casein, yeast extract, dextrose, and cystine, specified in the requirements for sterility testing by the National Institutes of Health; called also *sterility test c.*

nitrate b., nutrient broth containing sodium nitrate, for testing for the bacterial reduction of nitrate to nitrite.

N.N.N. c., a medium containing agar, salt, and rabbit blood, for growing *Leishmania donovani.*

Noguchi's c., an enriched culture medium containing sterile fresh rabbit kidney tissue, for the culture of spirochetes.

nutrient c., a bacterial culture medium containing beef extract, peptone, and sodium chloride, used as a liquid medium (nutrient broth) or solidified with agar (nutrient agar, plain agar) for the culture of nonfastidious organisms.

nystatin assay a., a culture medium containing beef extract, yeast extract, peptone, and dextrose, for the assay of the mycostatic activity of pharmaceutical preparations according to FDA and USP requirements; called also *antibiotic c. 12.*

oleic a. (Dubos), an agar medium containing peptone, asparagine, and inorganic salts to which is added oleic acid complex containing 0.05 per cent oleic acid in 5 per cent serum albumin fraction V. The albumin may be replaced with normal beef serum. Used for the culture of tubercle bacilli and other mycobacteria.

Omeliansky's nutritive c., a synthetic medium containing potassium phosphate, magnesium sulfate, ammonium sulfate, sodium chloride, and precipitated chalk; for growing cellulose-fermenting organisms.

Pai's c., a medium for the cultivation of diphtheria bacilli.

Parietti's b., nutrient broth containing small amounts of a mixture of hydrochloric acid and phenol solution.

Park and Williams' chocolate c., chocolate c.

Pasteur's c., see under *solution.*

peptone water c., peptone water.

Petragnani c., a culture medium containing milk, potato flour, potato, whole egg and egg yolk, and malachite green, for the culture of tubercle bacilli; the medium is solidified by heat coagulation of the egg.

Petroff's synthetic c., a synthetic medium for growing the tubercle bacillus.

Petruschky's c., litmus whey.

phenol red m., a culture medium containing peptone and phenol red, which may be used in liquid (broth) or solid (agar) form, containing a test sugar, commonly dextrose, lactose, maltose, mannitol, sucrose, etc., used for testing fermentation reactions; with added sodium potassium tartrate (tartrate c.), it may be used for the tartrate reaction of *Salmonella.*

phenylalanine a., a culture medium containing yeast extract and DL-phenylalanine, for the differentiation of enteric bacilli on the basis of the production of phenylpyruvic acid, which is tested for with ferric chloride.

Pike streptococcal b., a liquid selective enrichment medium containing peptones, yeast extract, dextrose, and sodium azide and crystal violet as inhibitory agents, for the isolation of β-hemolytic streptococci.

polymyxin test a's, culture medium containing peptones and dextrose in the base agar, and polysorbate 80 in the seed agar, used in the cylinder plate assay method of polymyxin B according to FDA and USP methods. The base agar is antibiotic culture medium 9, and the seed agar antibiotic culture medium 10.

potato blood a., Bordet-Gengou a.

potato dextrose a., a culture medium containing potato infusion and dextrose, for the culture of yeasts and molds.

proof a., Sabouraud a.

Proskauer-Beck m., a nonselective liquid medium containing asparagine and citrate, for the culture of tubercle bacilli for metabolic and related studies.

protein-free c., a synthetic medium containing calcium chloride, magnesium sulfate, monopotassium acid phosphate, potassium aspartate, sodium chloride, ammonium lactate, and glycerin; called also *Uschinsky's c.*

rice extract a., an extract of white rice solidified with agar, for the identification of *Candida albicans* by favoring the production of chlamydospores.

Robertson's c., a beef heart infusion medium.

Rogosa SL m., a selective culture medium containing tryptose, yeast extract, dextrose, arabinose, sucrose, acetate, citrate, and sorbitan mono-oleate, which may be used in either liquid form or solidified with agar for the culture of lactobacilli.

Rosenow's veal-brain b., a mixture of nutrient bouillon, glucose, and Andrade's indicator, with a few small pieces of crushed calf brain and a few small pieces of crushed marble, autoclaved at 10 pounds.

rosolic acid-peptone c., Dunham's solution containing alcoholic solution of rosolic acid.

Russell's double sugar a., a culture medium containing beef extract, dextrose, lactose, sodium chloride, phenol red, and agar; used to differentiate gram-negative enteric bacilli.

Sabouraud a., a culture medium containing agar, peptone, and dextrose or maltose, pH 5.6, used for the cultivation of fungi; called also *proof a.*

saccharose-mannitol a., nutrient agar containing saccharose, D-mannitol, peptone, beef extract, and phenol red, pH 7.5; used to differentiate enteric bacteria.

Salmonella-Shigella (SS) a., a selective differential culture medium containing beef extract, peptone, lactose, bile salts, sodium and ferric citrates, thiosulfate neutral red, and brilliant green, used for the primary isolation of enteric bacilli, especially *Salmonella* and *Shigella.*

seed a., a culture medium containing peptone, pancreatic digest of casein, yeast extract, beef extract, and dextrose, used for the cylinder plate method of antibiotic assay according to the FDA and USP methods; called also *antibiotic c. 1.* Adjusted to a high pH, it is known as *neomycin assay agar* (q.v.).

selective c., a liquid or solid culture medium that contains inhibitory substances (dyes, tellurite, bile salts, etc.), which allow the growth of the desired microorganism while inhibiting the growth of contaminants.

selenite b., a differential and selective culture medium.

selenite-cystine b., a liquid enrichment medium containing tryptone, lactose, cystine, and sodium acid selenite, for the detection of *Salmonella* in foods, according to FDA and APHA methods.

semisolid c., 1. a culture medium containing 0.5 per cent agar to give it a semisolid consistency; see *motility test medium.* 2. a culture medium containing agar or gelatin that is liquid in the warm state and solid when cooled.

serum b., a mixture of horse serum and nutrient broth.

silicate jelly c., a synthetic medium containing ammonium sulfate, ammonium phosphate, calcium chloride, potassium phosphate, and sodium carbonate, solidified with silicic acid; for the growth of nitrogen-fixing bacteria.

Simmons' citrate a., an inorganic salt medium containing sodium citrate and bromthymol blue, for the differentiation of enteric bacilli on the basis of citrate utilization.

Snyder a., a culture medium containing peptone, dextrose, and bromcresol green, pH 4.8, used for lactobacillus counts as an indicator of dental caries activity.

Soyka's milk-rice c., see *milk-rice c.*

spirit blue a., a culture medium containing tryptone, yeast extract, and spirit blue, to which is added an emulsion of an appropriate lipid for the culture and study of lipolytic microorganisms; colonies of lipolytic bacteria develop a deep blue color beneath and surrounding the colony.

Spirolate b., a culture medium containing peptone, yeast extract, dextrose, thioglycollate, and cysteine, enriched with 10 per cent rabbit or bovine serum, for the mass culture of the Reiter treponeme.

standard methods a., a culture medium containing pancreatic digest of casein, yeast extract, and dextrose, for bacterial counts of milk, etc., according to APHA standard methods.

sterility test b., a culture medium containing pancreatic digest of casein, yeast extract, dextrose, and thioglycollate and cystine, used as an alternative to thioglycollate medium for sterility testing according to NIH and USP methods.

sterility test c., NIH a.

streptomycin assay a. with yeast extract, a culture medium containing beef extract, yeast extract, and peptone, for the assay of streptomycin in accordance with the requirements of FDA and USP; called also *antibiotic c. 5.*

Stuart b., a culture medium containing inorganic salts, asparagine, and thiamine, enriched with rabbit serum containing hemoglobin, and used for the isolation and culture of *Leptospira.*

sugar b., a nutrient or infusion broth containing a sugar and bromthymol blue or bromcresol purple, for the determination of the fermentation characteristics of bacteria.

sulfite a., a culture medium containing peptone and sodium sulfite, for the detection of sulfide-producing thermophilic bacteria in foods according to APHA standard methods.

sulfite polymyxin sulfadiazine (SPS) a., a culture medium containing peptone, yeast extract, iron citrate, sodium sulfite, polymyxin, and sulfadiazine, used as a moderately selective medium for the isolation of *Clostridium welchii* (*perfringens*) from foods.

tartrate c., see *phenol red c.*

TB charcoal a., an agar medium containing yeast extract, peptone, asparagine, citrate, dextrose, oleic acid, charcoal, and ethyl violet, for the culture of tubercle bacilli.

TCBS a., thiosulfate citrate bile salts sucrose a.

tellurite a., a culture medium containing peptones, dextrose, and sodium tellurite, for the primary culture of diphtheria bacilli.

tellurite glycine a., a culture medium containing peptone, yeast extract, mannitol, lithium chloride, and glycine, for the isolation of coagulase-positive staphylococci.

tetrathionate b., a selective enrichment medium containing yeast extract, tryptose, dextrose, mannitol, desoxycholate and brilliant green as inhibitory agents, and sodium thiosulfate, which is converted to tetrathionate by the addition of iodine immediately prior to use; for the isolation of *Salmonella* and related bacteria.

tetrathionate enrichment b., a nutritive enrichment broth.

thiosulfate citrate bile salts sucrose (TCBS) a., a selective medium containing peptone, yeast extract, citrate, thiosulfate, oxgall, sodium cholate, and sucrose, for the primary isolation of *Vibrio cholerae.*

Tindale's m., a base composed of proteose-peptone, sodium chloride, and agar to which is added as enrichment of bovine serum, sodium hydroxide, L-cystine, sodium thiosulfate, and potassium tellurite; used to detect *Corynebacterium diphtheriae,* which form grayish-black colonies surrounded by a black halo.

Todd-Hewitt b., a culture medium containing beef heart infusion, peptone, and dextrose, for the production of streptococcal hemolysin.

tomato juice a., a culture medium containing tomato juice, peptone, and peptonized milk, for the cultivation of lactobacilli; called also *Kulp's c.*

triple sugar iron a., a culture medium containing peptone, lactose, sucrose, dextrose, ferrous ammonium sulfate, sodium thiosulfate, and phenol red, for the differentiation of enteric bacilli.

Trudeau m., an egg yolk–potato medium.

urea a., a culture medium containing peptone, dextrose, urea, and phenol red, for the differentiation of enteric bacilli on the basis of urease activity.

urease test b., a phosphate-buffered culture medium containing yeast extract, urea, and phenol red, used to determine urease activity in the differentiation of *Proteus* from other enteric bacilli.

Uschinsky's c., see *asparagin c.,* def. 2, and *protein-free c.*

veal infusion c., see *infusion m.*

Venkatraman-Ramikrishnan m., a sea-salt–containing medium used as a transport medium for *Vibrio cholerae.*

wheat b., a nutritive medium made from wheat flour, magnesium sulfate, potassium nitrate, and glucose, in water.

Wilson-Blair c., an agar culture medium containing beef extract, peptone, dextrose, brilliant green, and bismuth sulfite, for the primary isolation of the typhoid bacillus; called also *bismuth sulfite agar.*

Winogradsky's c., 1. *for growing nitrifying organisms:* potassium phosphate, magnesium sulfate, calcium chloride, sodium chloride, and ammonium sulfate, in water. 2. *for growing nitrosifying organisms:* ammonium sulfate, potassium sulfate, and basic magnesium carbonate.

wort a., a solid medium containing malt extract, peptone, maltose, dextrin, and glycerol, used in the cultivation of yeasts.

wort b., the fluid form of wort agar, prepared by omitting the agar.

yeast autolysate c., a solution prepared by incubating yeast in water, kept sterile with chloroform, filtered, and solidified with agar.

zein a., an inorganic salt medium containing the extractives of zein, used for the identification of *Candida albicans* by favoring the production of chlamydospores.

---

cumidine (ku'mĭ-din) chemical name: 4-amino-1-isopropylbenzene. A liquid base, $C_3H_7 \cdot C_6H_4 \cdot NH_2$, derived from cumic acid.

cu. mm. cubic millimeter.

cumulative (ku'mu-la''tiv) [L. *cumulus* heap] increasing by successive additions, the total being greater than the expected sum of its parts.

cumuli (ku'mu-li) [L.] plural of *cumulus.*

cumulus (ku'mu-lus), pl. *cu'muli* [L.] a little mound. **c. ooph'orus** [NA], **ovarian c., c. ova'ricus,** a solid mass of follicular cells surrounding the ovum in the side of a developing vesicular ovarian follicle: called also *discus oophorus, ovigerus,* or *proligerus;* and *germ* or *germ-bearing hillock.*

cuneate (ku'ne-āt) [L. *cuneus* wedge] wedge-shaped.

cunei (ku'ne-i) [L.] plural of *cuneus.*

cuneiform (ku-ne'ĭ-form) [L. *cuneus* wedge + *forma* form] shaped like a wedge.

cuneihysterectomy (ku''ne-i-his''ter-ek'to-me) [L. *cuneus* wedge + *hysterectomy*] *(obs.)* the excision of a wedge-shaped piece from the uterine tissue for the correction of anteflexion.

cuneocuboid (ku''ne-o-ku'boid) pertaining to the cuneiform and cuboid bones.

cuneonavicular (ku''ne-o-nah-vik'u-lar) pertaining to the cuneiform and navicular bones.

cuneoscaphoid (ku''ne-o-skaf'oid) cuneonavicular.

cuneus (ku'ne-us), pl. *cu'nei* [L. "wedge"] a wedge-shaped lobule of the occipital lobe of the cerebrum on its medial aspect, between the parietooccipital and calcarine sulci.

cuniculi (ku-nik'u-li) [L.] plural of *cuniculus.*

cuniculus (ku-nik'u-lus), pl. *cunic'uli* [L. "rabbit," "rabbit-burrow"] the burrow of an itch mite, *Sarcoptes scabiei,* in the skin.

Cunila (ku-ni'lah) a genus of labiate plants. *C. origanoides* (L.) Butt., of North America (dittany), is the source of a diuretic and diaphoretic tea used by American Indians and early settlers.

cunnilinctus (kun''ĭ-link'tus) cunnilingus.

cunnilinguism (kun''ĭ-ling'gwizm) the practice of cunnilingus.

cunnilingus (kun''ĭ-ling'gus) [L. *cunnus* vulva + *lingere* to lick] oral stimulation of the female genitalia.

cunnus (kun'us) [L.] pudendum femininum.

CuO cupric oxide.

Cu₂O cuprous oxide.

cuorin (ku'o-rin) a mono-aminodiphosphatide lipoid compound isolated from the heart muscle.

cup (kup) 1. a cupping glass. 2. a cup-shaped part or structure. **Diogenes c.,** poculum Diogenis. **dry c.,** a cupping glass applied to the intact skin in order to induce a flow of blood to the area. **glaucomatous c.,** a form of ocular disk depression peculiar to glaucoma. **Montgomery's c's** *(obs.),* the dilated canals of the tubular glands of the uterus. **ocular c.,** caliculus ophthalmicus. **ophthalmic c.,** caliculus ophthalmicus. **optic c.,** 1. physiologic cup. 2. caliculus ophthalmicus. **physiologic c.,** a depression in the center of the optic disk; called also *excavatio papillae nervi optici* [NA] and *optic c.* **wet c.,** a cupping glass applied to the incised skin in order to abstract blood.

cupola (ku'po-lah) cupula.

cupped (kupt) hollowed out like a cup.

cupping (kup'ing) 1. the application of a cupping glass. 2. the formation of a cup-shaped depression. **pathologic c.,** depression of the optic disk due to disease.

cuprammonia (ku''prah-mo'ne-ah) Schweitzer's reagent.

cupremia (ku-pre'me-ah) [L. *cuprum* copper + Gr. *haima* blood + *-ia*] the presence of copper in the blood.

cupric (ku'prik) containing copper in its divalent form ($>$Cu), and yielding divalent ions (Cu^{++}) in aqueous solution. For cupric compounds, see under the salt, e.g., sulfate.

Cuprimine (kup'rĭ-mēn) trademark for a preparation of penicillamine.

cuprimyxin (kup''rĭ-mik'sin) chemical name: bis(6-methoxy-1-phenazinol-5,10-dioxidato-O^1,O^{10})copper; a veterinary antibacterial and antifungal, $C_{26}H_{18}CuN_4O_8$.

cupriuria (ku''pre-u're-ah) the presence of copper in the urine.

cuprous (ku'prus) containing copper in its monovalent form (Cu^+).

cupruresis (ku''proo-re'sis) [L. *cuprum* copper + Gr. *ourēsis* a making water] the urinary excretion of copper.

cupruretic (ku''proo-ret'ik) [L. *cuprum* copper + Gr. *ourētikos* promoting urine] pertaining to or promoting the urinary excretion of copper.

cupula (ku'pu-lah), pl. *cu'pulae* [L.] a small inverted cup or dome-shaped cap over some structure. **c. of ampullary crest,** c. cristae ampullaris. **c. of cochlea, c. coch'leae** [NA], the rounded or dome-shaped apex of the spiral cochlear duct. **c. cris'tae ampulla'ris** [NA], a cap of viscid, gelatinous fluid over the crista of the ampulla of the ear; in fixed material this cap stains slightly and is thus differentiated from the rest of the ampullar fluid. Called also *c. of ampullary crest.* **c. of pleura, c. pleu'rae** [NA], the domelike roof of the pleural cavity on either side, extending up through the superior aperture of the thorax.

cupulae (ku'pu-le) [L.] plural of *cupula.*

cupulogram (ku'pu-lo-gram'') the record, in the form of a tracing, made during cupulometry.

cupulolithiasis (ku''pu-lo-lĭ-thi'ah-sis) the presence of calculi in the cupula of the posterior semicircular duct, a cause of benign paroxysmal positional vertigo.

cupulometry (ku''pu-lom'e-tre) a method of testing vestibular function in which subjects are accelerated and decelerated in a rotational chair and the duration of postrotational vertigo and nystagmus are plotted against angular deceleration.

curage (ku-rahzh') [Fr.] curettage, especially when a finger, rather a curet, is used.

curare (koo-rah're) [South American] a term applied to a wide variety of highly toxic extracts from numerous botanical sources, including various species of *Strychnos;* used originally as arrow poisons in South America. A form extracted from *Chondodendron tomentosum* has been used for the reduction of spasms in tetanus and in shock treatments, in plastic muscular rigidity, spastic paralysis, and similar conditions, and also as an adjunct to general anesthesia. Cf. *tubocurarine.*

curaremimetic (koo-rah''re-mi-met'ik) having an action similar to that of curare, or producing similar effects.

curari (koo-rah're) curare.

curariform (ku-ra'rĭ-form) resembling curare.

curarization (ku''rar-i-za'shun) administration of curare until the physiologic effect of the drug is produced.

curative (kūr'ah-tiv) [L. *curare* to take care of] tending to overcome disease and promote recovery.

curb (kurb) a thickening of the metatarsocalcaneal ligament of the horse, causing a swelling at the back of the hock joint and resulting in lameness.

curcumin (kur'ku-min) an orange-yellow, crystalline substance, $C_{21}H_{20}O_6$, which is the coloring principle of turmeric.

curd (kurd) the coagulum of milk, consisting mainly of casein. **alum c.,** a coagulum formed by agitating milk containing a piece of alum. **alum c. of Riverius,** a coagulum prepared with white of an egg and drachm of alum.

cure (kūr) [L. *curatio,* from *cura* care] 1. the course of treatment of any disease, or of a special case. 2. the successful treatment of a disease or wound. 3. a system of treating diseases. 4. a medicine effective in treating a disease. **Banting c.,** see under *treatment.* **diet c.,** treatment by the systematic regulation of the diet. **economic c.,** cure of a disease which, while not complete, is sufficient to restore the patient to his wage-earning capacity. **faith c.,** an ancient form of psychotherapy: cure by belief or faith as produced by faith-healers, and shamans. **gold c.** (*obs.*), Keeley c. **grape c.,** the use of an exclusive diet of grapes; called also *ampelotherapy* and *botryotherapy.* **hunger c.,** the treatment of disease by severe fasting; limotherapy. **Karell's c.,** see under *treatment.* **Keeley c.** (*obs.*), a proprietary method of treatment for the alcohol and opium habits; called also *gold c.* **liman c.,** a method of treatment that was practiced at Odessa, consisting of bathing in the water of "limans," or sheets of water that have been isolated from the sea and converted into salt lakes: used in cases of scrofula, rickets, chronic rheumatism, and chronic skin diseases. **milk c.,** an exclusive diet of milk as a means of treatment. **mind c.,** psychotherapy. **potato c.,** treatment of foreign bodies in the alimentary canal by ingesting mashed potatoes. **radical c.,** 1. a complete and permanent cure. 2. a treatment involving extensive surgery. **rest c.,** Weir Mitchell treatment. **starvation c.,** the treatment of a disease by a diet markedly restricted in calories. **thirst c.,** treatment by restricting the intake of fluids. **water c.,** hydrotherapy. **whey c.,** treatment by drinking whey. **work c.,** the treatment of neurasthenia by systematically arranged work.

curet (ku-ret′) [Fr. *curette* scraper] 1. an instrument for removing material from the uterine cavity. 2. to remove growths or other material from the wall of a cavity or other surface with a spoon-shaped instrument. **Hartmann's c.,** an instrument for removing adenoids.

curettage (ku″rĕ-tahzh′) [Fr.] the removal of growths or other material from the wall of a cavity or other surface, as with a curet; called also *curettement.* **medical c.,** the induction of bleeding from the endometrium by administration and withdrawal of any progestational agent. **periapical c.,** removal with a curet of diseased periapical tissue without excision of the root tip. **suction c.,** vacuum c. **vacuum c.,** removal of the uterine contents, after dilatation, by means of a hollow curet introduced into the uterus, through which suction is applied. Called also *suction c., vacuum aspiration,* and *vacuum extraction.*

curette (ku-ret′) [Fr.] curet.

curettement (ku-ret′ment) curettage. **physiologic c.,** enzymatic débridement.

curie (ku′re) [Marie Sklodowska *Curie,* Polish chemist in Paris, 1867–1934, the discoverer of radium, and Pierre *Curie,* 1859–1906, co-winners, with A. H. Becquerel, of the Nobel prize in physics for 1903, for studies on spontaneous radioactivity; Mme. Curie also received the Nobel prize in chemistry in 1911 for discovery and isolation of radium] a unit of radioactivity, defined as the quantity of any radioactive nuclide in which the number of disintegrations per second is 3.700×10^{10}. Abbreviated c and Ci.

Curie's law, therapy (ku′rez) [Pierre *Curie,* French scientist, 1859–1906] see under *law* and *therapy.*

curiegram (ku′re-gram) a print made by radium emanation on a sensitized plate.

curie-hour (ku′re-owr″) a unit of dose equivalent to that obtained by exposure for one hour to radioactive material disintegrating at the rate of 3.7×10^{10} atoms per second. Abbreviated c-hr.

curietherapy (ku″re-ther′ah-pe) originally, radium or radon therapy; but now applied to therapy given by emanations from any radioactive source.

curing (kūr′ing) a method or process of preparing for use, as by aging, heating, etc. **denture c.,** the process by which the denture-base materials are hardened to the form of a denture in a denture mold.

curioscopy (ku″re-os′ko-pe) the detection and mapping of objects by means of the nuclear radiations coming from them.

curium (ku′re-um) [Pierre and Marie *Curie*] the chemical element of atomic number 96, atomic weight 247, symbol Cm, obtained by cyclotron bombardment of uranium and plutonium.

curling (kur′ling) shaped like a curl or coil, as the appearance of the esophagus in diffuse esophageal spasm.

Curling's ulcer (kur′lingz) [Thomas Blizard *Curling,* English physician, 1811–1888] see under *ulcer.*

current (kur′ent) [L. *currens* running] 1. anything that flows. 2. the stream of electricity that moves along a conductor. An electric current is due to a difference of potential between two points, this difference being measured in volts. The volume of flow depends on the difference of potential and the resistance to be overcome and is measured in amperes. The quantity of current is

measured in coulombs. **abnerval c.,** an electric current passing from a nerve to and through a muscle. **action c.,** the current generated in a cell membrane of a nerve or muscle by the action potential; it serves to depolarize adjacent membrane areas beyond the threshold, thus initiating a repetition of the action potential process along the nerve fiber. Called also *nerve-action c.* **alternating c.,** a current that periodically flows in opposite directions. Abbreviated A.C. **ascending c.,** centripetal c. **axial c.,** the central colored part of the blood current. **centrifugal c.,** an electric current in the body with the positive pole near the nerve center and the negative at the periphery; called also *descending c.* **centripetal c.,** an electric current passing through the body with the positive electrode on the nerve or at the periphery and the negative near the nerve center: called also *ascending c.* **coagulating c.,** an electric current applied by a needle, ball, or other type of electrode to coagulate tissue. **compensating c.,** an electric current for neutralizing the intensity of a muscle current. **d'Arsonval c.,** a high-frequency, low-voltage current of comparatively high amperage. See also *high-frequency c.* **demarcation c.,** c. of injury. **descending c.,** centrifugal c. **De Watteville c.,** a combined galvanic and faradic current. **direct c.,** a current that flows in one direction only. When used medically it is called the galvanic current; this current has distinct and important polarity and marked secondary chemical effects. **electric c.,** the flow of electricity through a conductor. **electrotonic c.,** a current induced in the sheath of a nerve by a current passing through the conducting part of that nerve, or by an action potential in an adjacent nerve. **fulguration c.,** high-frequency current used in destruction of superficial skin lesions. **galvanic c.,** a steady direct current. **high-frequency c.,** an alternating current having a frequency of interruption or change of direction sufficiently high so that tetanic contractions are not set up when it is passed through living contractile tissues; see *d'Arsonval c.* **induced c.,** electricity in a circuit generated by proximity to another current, i.e., by induction. **c. of injury,** the current flowing between pathologically depolarized areas of excitable tissue (as of the heart) and the normally polarized areas, the injury tissue being negative with respect to the normal tissue. Called also *demarcation c.* **Leduc c.,** an interrupted direct current, each pulse of which is approximately of the same current strength and same duration; formerly used as a general anesthetic agent. **Morton's c.** (*obs.*), a type of alternating high-frequency current produced by a static machine; called also *static induced c.* **nerve-action c.,** action c. **Oudin c.,** a high-frequency current of higher voltage than the high-frequency currents used for ordinary diathermy treatment. **saturation c.,** the maximum current across an x-ray tube which utilizes for the production of x-rays all the electrons available at the cathode. **static induced c.,** Morton's c. **surgical c.,** an electric current used to achieve surgical dissection or fulguration. **Tesla's c.** (*obs.*), a high-frequency current of higher voltage than that of the high-frequency currents used for ordinary diathermy treatment, but not so high as that of the Oudin current.

curricula (kur-rik′u-lah) [L.] plural of *curriculum.*

curriculum (kur-rik′u-lum), pl. *curric′ula* [L.] a regular and established course of study.

Curschmann's disease, mask, spiral (koorsh′manz) [Heinrich *Curschmann,* physician in Leipzig, 1846–1910] see *perihepatitis chronica hyperplastica,* and see under *mask* and *spiral.*

curse (kers) an infliction thought to be invoked by a malevolent spirit. **Ondine's c.,** impairment of automatic control of respiration, sometimes due to encephalitis, with voluntary control remaining intact.

Curtius' syndrome (kur′tĭ-us) [Friedrich *Curtius,* German internist, born 1896] see under *syndrome.*

curtometer (kur-tom′ĕ-ter) (*obs.*) cyrtometer.

curvatura (kur″vah-tu′rah), pl. *curvatu′rae* [L.] [NA] a nonangular deviation from a straight course in a line or surface. **c. ventric′uli ma′jor** [NA], greater curvature of stomach: the left or lateral and inferior border of the stomach, marking the inferior junction of the anterior and posterior surfaces. **c. ventric′uli mi′nor** [NA], lesser curvature of stomach: the right or medial border of the stomach, marking the superior junction of the anterior and posterior surfaces.

curvature (kur′vah-tūr) [L. *curvatura*] deviation from a rectilinear direction. **gingival c.,** the curved line following the crest of the gingiva where it is attached to the tooth. **greater c. of stomach,** curvatura ventriculi major. **lesser c. of stomach,** curvatura ventriculi minor. **occlusal c.,** curve of occlusion; see under *curve.* **Pott's c.,** abnormal posterior curvature of the vertebral column caused by tuberculous caries. **spinal c.,** deviation of the spine from its normal direction or position; see *kyphosis, lordosis, scoliosis.*

curve (kurv) [L. *curvum*] a nonangular deviation from a straight course in a line or surface. **alignment c.,** the dental curve determined by a line passing through the center of the teeth and paralleling the dental arch. **anti-Monson c.,** reverse c. **audibility c.,** a plotting of the relationship between frequency and the intensity of sound waves necessary to elicit a sensation. **Barnes's c.,** the segment of a circle whose center is the promontory of the sacrum, the concavity being directed dorsally. **buccal c.**, the portion of the curve of occlusion from the mesial surface of the first premolar to the distal surface of the third molar. **c. of Carus**, the normal axis of the pelvic outlet; called also *circle of Carus*. **compensating c.**, the anteroposterior and lateral curvature in the alignment of the occlusal surfaces and incisal edges of artifical teeth, which is used to develop balanced occlusion. **Damoiseau's c.**, Ellis' line. **dental c.**, c. of occlusion. **dissociation c., oxygen**, oxygen-hemoglobin dissociation c. **dose-effect c., dose-response c.**, a curve indicating the relationship between dose of radiation and the degree of a particular biological effect produced. **dromedary c.**, a temperature or other curve showing two phases of elevation separated by a phase of depression. **dye-dilution c.**, a graph representing the concentration of a fixed dose of a dye (as in the systemic circulation) at specific time intervals; used in studies of cardiac output. **c. of Ellis and Garland**, Ellis' line. **frequency c.**, a curve representing graphically the probabilities of different numbers of recurrences of an event; called also *probability c*. **Garland's c.**, Ellis' line. **gaussian c.**, normal curve of distribution. **growth c.**, the curve obtained by plotting increase in size or numbers against the elapsed time, as a measure of the growth of a child, or the multiplication of microorganisms. **Harrison's c.**, see under *groove*. **inverted-U c. of arousal**, a curve which plots the effects of arousal on a given individual; studies of such curves show that the capacity of sensory stimulation to guide behavior is poor when arousal is very low or very high. **isodose c's**, diagrams delimiting body areas receiving equal quantities of radiation in radiotherapy. **labial c.**, that portion of the curve of occlusion between the distal surfaces of the two canine teeth in the dental arch. **logistic c.**, in biometry, an S-shaped curve to describe the growth of a population in an area of fixed limits. **Monson c.**, a curve of occlusion conforming to a segment of the surface of a sphere 8 inches in diameter, with its center in the region of the glabella. **muscle c.**, myogram. **normal c. of distribution**, the symmetrical bell-shaped curve that is usually produced by plotting a single variable. **c. of occlusion**, a curved line determined by the occlusal surfaces and incisal edges of the existing teeth, when viewed from the lateral aspect; called also *dental curve, occlusal curvature*, and *Spee's curve*. **oxygen dissociation c., oxygen-hemoglobin dissociation c., oxyhemoglobin dissociation c.**, a graphic curve representing the normal variation in the amount of oxygen which combines with hemoglobin as a function of the partial pressures of oxygen and carbon dioxide. The dissociation curve is said to shift to the right when less than a normal amount of oxygen is taken up by the blood at a given P_{O_2}, and to shift to the left when more than a normal amount is taken up. Factors influencing the shape of the curve include changes in the blood pH, P_{CO_2}, and temperature, the presence of carbon monoxide, alterations in the constituents of the erythrocytes, and certain disease states. **Price-Jones c.**, a graphic curve representing the variation in the size of the red blood corpuscles. **probability c.**, frequency c. **pulse c.**, sphygmogram. **reverse c.**, a curve of occlusion which is convex upward. **Spee's c.**, c. of occlusion. **temperature c.**, a graphic tracing showing variations in body temperature. **tension c's**, lines observed in the arrangement of the cancellous tissue of bones, depending on the directions of tension exerted on the bones. **visibility c.**, a plotting of the relationship between wavelength and the intensity of light necessary to elicit a sensation. **Wunderlich's c.**, the typical variation shown by the temperature in a patient with typhoid fever.

cuscamidine (kus-kam′ĭ-din) a cinchona alkaloid.

cuscamine (kus-kam′in) a cinchona alkaloid.

cuscohygrine (kus-ko-hi′grin) an alkaloid, $C_{13}H_{24}ON_2$, from cusco leaves; called also *bellaradine*.

Cushing's disease, law, syndrome, etc. (koosh′ingz) [Harvey Williams *Cushing*, Boston surgeon, 1869–1939] see under *disease, law, operation, phenomenon*, and *syndrome*.

Cushing's suture (koosh′ingz) [Hayward W. *Cushing*, Boston surgeon, 1854–1934] see under *suture*.

cushingoid (koosh′ing-oid) resembling Cushing's syndrome; said of signs and symptoms.

cushion (koosh′un) a fleshy, padlike anatomical structure. **coronary c.**, see under *band*. **digital c.**, a wedge-shaped mass of white and elastic fibers, containing fat and cartilage, overlying the frog of a horse's foot. **endocardial c's**, elevations on the atrioventricular canal of the embryonic heart, which later fuse with the free edge of the septum primum to separate the right and left atria. **c. of epiglottis**, 1. petiolus epiglottidis. 2. tuberculum epiglotticum. **eustachian c., c. of eustachian orifice**, torus tubarius. **intimal c's**, longitudinal thickenings of the intima of certain arteries, e.g., the penile arteries, formed by prominent local concentrations of smooth muscle fibers; they serve functionally as valves, controlling blood flow by occluding the lumen of the artery. **Passavant's c.**, see under *bar*. **plantar c.**, a wedge-shaped mass of elastic tissue overlying the frog of a horse's foot. **sucking c.**, corpus adiposum buccae.

cuskohygrine (kus″ko-hi′grin) cuscohygrine.

cusp (kusp) [L. *cuspis* point] a tapering projection; especially (*a*) one of the triangular segments of a cardiac valve (see under *cuspis*), or (*b*) a notably pointed or rounded eminence making up a divisional part of the masticating surface of a tooth, usually designated according to its position in relation to the axial surfaces of the tooth. Called also *cuspis dentis* [NA] and *tuberculum* (pl. *tubercula*) *coronae dentis*. Those of the maxillary first molar are: mesiobuccal, mesiolingual, distobuccal, and distolingual. **aortic c.**, cuspis anterior valvae atrioventricularis sinistrae. **Carabelli c.**, a fifth, or supplemental, cusp, sometimes found lingual to the mesiolingual cusp of the maxillary first molar tooth; called also *Carabelli's tubercle*. **semilunar c.**, any of the semilunar segments of the aortic valve (having posterior, right, and left cusps) or the pulmonary valve (having anterior, right, and left cusps); called also *valvula semilunaris*.

cuspid (kus′pid) 1. having one cusp or point. 2. a canine tooth.

cuspidate (kus′pĭ-dāt) [L. *cuspidatus*] having a cusp or cusps.

cuspides (kus′pĭ-dēz) [L.] plural of *cuspis*.

cuspis (kus′pis), pl. *cus′pides* [L.] 1. a tapering projection or structure, applied especially to one of the triangular segments of a cardiac valve. 2. a cusp of a tooth. **c. ante′rior val′vae atrioventricula′ris dex′trae** [NA], the anterior of the cusps of the right atrioventricular valve; called also *c. anterior valvulae tricuspidalis*. **c. ante′rior val′vae atrioventricula′ris sinis′trae** [NA], the anterior of the cusps of the left atrioventricular valve; called also *c. anterior valvulae bicuspidalis* and *aortic cusp*. **c. ante′rior val′vulae bicuspida′lis**, c. anterior valvae atrioventricularis sinistrae. **c. ante′rior val′vulae tricuspida′lis**, c. anterior valvae atrioventricularis dextrae. **c. den′tis** [NA], a notably pointed or rounded eminence of the masticating surface of a tooth; see *cusp*. **c. media′lis val′vulae tricuspida′lis**, c. septalis valvae atrioventricularis dextrae. **c. poste′rior val′vae atrioventricula′ris dex′trae** [NA], the posterior of the cusps of the right atrioventricular valve; called also *c. posterior valvulae tricuspidalis*. **c. poste′rior val′vae atrioventricula′ris sinis′trae** [NA], the posterior of the cusps of the left atrioventricular valve; called also *c. posterior valvulae bicuspidalis*. **c. poste′rior val′vulae bicuspida′lis**, c. posterior valvae atrioventricularis sinistrae. **c. poste′rior val′vulae tricuspida′lis**, c. posterior valvae atrioventricularis dextrae. **c. septa′lis val′vae atrioventricula′ris dex′trae** [NA], the cusp of the right atrioventricular valve which is attached to the membranous interventricular septum; called also *c. medialis valvulae tricuspidalis*.

cutaneous (ku-ta′ne-us) [L. *cutis* skin] pertaining to the skin.

cutdown (kut′down) creation of a small, incised opening, especially over a vein (venous cutdown), to facilitate venipuncture and permit the passage of a needle or cannula for the withdrawal of blood or administration of fluids.

Cuterebra (ku-ter-e′brah) a genus of botflies of the family Oestridae (often included in the family Cuterebridae), whose larvae commonly infest rodents.

Cuterebridae (ku″te-reb′rĭ-de) a family of New World batflies (order Diptera), the larvae of which parasitize various mammals, including man.

cuticle (ku′te-kl) [L. *cuticula*, from *cutis* skin] 1. a layer of more or less solid substance which covers the free surface of an epithelial cell. 2. eponychium (def. 1). **dental c.**, cuticula dentis. **enamel c.**, cuticula dentis. **keratose c.**, the outer surface layer of the pigment cells of the eye. **c. of root sheath**, a layer of cells lining the hair follicles.

cuticula (ku-tik′u-lah), pl. *cutic′ulae* [L. "little skin"] 1. a horny secreted layer. 2. (*obs.*) epidermis. **c. den′tis** [NA], the dental cuticle: the calcified epithelial remnants on the enamel of a tooth following the complete formation of the enamel; called also *enamel cuticle* and *Nasmyth's membrane*.

cuticulae (ku-tik′u-le) [L.] plural of *cuticula*.

cuticularization (ku-tik″u-lar-i-za′shun) the growth of new skin over a wound; epithelialization.

cuticulin (ku-tik′u-lin) a lipoprotein containing a large amount of fatty material, which is a constituent of the epicuticle and procuticle of certain arthropods and crustaceans.

cuticulum (ku-tik′u-lum) cuticula. **Flechsig's c.**, a layer of flat cells on the external surface of the neuroglia.

cutidure (ku′tĭ-dūr) coronary band.

cutiduris (ku″tĭ-du′ris) coronary band.

cutin (ku′tin) [L. *cutis* skin] 1. a waxy substance which, combined with cellulose, forms the cuticle of plants. 2. a preparation of the gut of the ox used as a substitute for catgut and silk and as a dressing for wounds.

cutinization (ku″tin-i-za′shun) the operation of lining a cavity, such as a fistulous cavity in bone, with skin.

cutireaction (ku″tĕ-re-ak′shun) [L. *cutis* skin + *reaction*] an inflammatory or irritative reaction on the skin, occurring in certain infectious diseases, on the application to or injection into the skin of a preparation of the organism causing the disease. Such reactions occur in glanders, leprosy, syphilis, tinea, tuberculosis, typhoid fever, etc. Called also *cutaneous reaction*, and *dermoreaction*. See the following reactions or tests: *Deehan's typhoid* *reaction, Dick test, Lautier's test, Lignière's test, Moro's reaction, Noguchi's luetin reaction, pallidin reaction, Pirquet's reaction, Schick test, typhoidin test.* **differential c.,** cutaneous inoculation at one and the same time of old tuberculin, a filtrate of human tubercle bacilli, and a filtrate of bovine tubercle bacilli in order to determine whether the patient is tuberculous or not, and if he is, whether the infection is human or bovine. **von Pirquet's c.,** Pirquet reaction.

cutis (ku′tis) [L.] [NA]   the skin: the outer protective covering of the body, consisting of the epidermis and the corium, or dermis, and resting upon the subcutaneous tissues. **c. anseri′na** [L. "goose skin"], a transitory localized change in the skin surface caused by elevation of the hair follicles as a result of contraction of the arrectores pilorum muscles, a reflection of sympathetic nerve discharge. Called also *gooseflesh.* **c. elas′tica,** Ehlers-Danlos syndrome. **c. hyperelas′tica,** Ehlers-Danlos syndrome. **c. lax′a,** a congenital hereditary disorder in which the skin and subcutaneous tissues hypertrophy, the skin hanging in folds as a result; it is usually transmitted as an autosomal recessive trait, but a dominant mode of inheritance has been reported. Called also *chalazodermia, c. pendula,* and *dermatolysis.* **c. marmora′ta,** a transitory mottling of the skin sometimes occurring on exposure of the skin to cold. Cf. *livedo reticularis.* **c. pen′dula** [L. "hanging skin"], c. laxa. **c. pen′silis,** c. laxa. **c. rhomboida′lis nu′chae,** a thickened and furrowed condition of skin exposed for many years to the sun, especially on the back of the neck. **c. ver′ticis gyra′ta,** enlargement and thickening of the skin of the scalp, which lies in folds resembling gyri and sulci of the brain.

cuvette (ku-vet′) [Fr. dim. of *cuve* vat or tub]   a glass container, generally possessing well-defined characteristics with regard to dimensions (particularly thickness) and optical properties, and generally used to examine colored and colorless solutions free of turbidity, but also used to examine the light scattering of turbid suspensions, such as bacterial suspensions. Its area of usefulness is determined to a large extent by the chemical composition of the glass: a *silica cuvette* is used for examination of materials in the ultraviolet region of the spectrum; a *Pyrex cuvette* is used for examination of materials in the visible range.

Cuvier's canal, duct (sinus) (koo′ve-āz) [Georges Léopold Chrétien Frédéric Dagobert, Baron de la *Cuvier,* French naturalist, 1769–1832]   see *ductus venosus,* and see under *duct.*

CV   cardiovascular.

C.V.   abbreviation for L. *cras ves′pere,* tomorrow evening, and L. *conjuga′ta ve′ra,* true conjugate diameter of the pelvic inlet.

CVA   costovertebral angle; cerebrovascular accident; cardiovascular accident.

C.V.D.   color-vision-deviant (showing anomalies of color vision), or color vision deviate (an individual showing anomalies of color vision).

C.V.O.   abbreviation for L. *conjuga′ta ve′ra obstet′rica,* obstetric conjugate diameter of the pelvic inlet.

CVP   central venous pressure.

CVS   cardiovascular system.

Cwt.   hundredweight.

Cx.   cervix; convex.

Cy   symbol for *cyanogen.*

cyan-   see *cyano-.*

cyanamide (si-an′ah-mīd)   1. carbamic acid nitril, CN·NH₂ or NH·C·NH, the anhydride of urea. 2. calcium cyanamide.

cyanate (si′ah-nāt)   a salt of cyanic acid which contains the radical CNO.

cyanhematin (si″an-hem′ah-tin)   a compound of cyanogen and hematin.

cyanhemoglobin (si″an-he″mo-glo′bin)   a compound formed in the blood by the action of hydrocyanic acid on hemoglobin; it gives the blood a bright red color.

cyanide (si′ah-nīd)   any binary compound of cyanogen; the term is often used alone to mean hydrogen cyanide (see under *hydrogen*). **mercuric c.,** a colorless, very poisonous salt, Hg(CN)₂.

cyanin (si′ah-nin)   a coumarin glycoside, $C_{27}H_{30}O_{16}$; its aglycon is cyanidin, and it is used as an indicator with a pH of 7 to 8.

cyanmethemoglobin (si″an-met″he-mo-glo′bin)   a crystalline substance formed by the action of hydrocyanic acid on methemoglobin in the cold or on oxyhemoglobin at the body temperature: the pigment most widely employed in clinical hemoglobinometry.

cyanmetmyoglobin (si″an-met-mi″o-glo′bin)   a compound formed from metmyoglobin by addition of the cyanide ion to yield reduction to the ferrous state.

cyano-, cyan- (si′ah-no; si′an) [Gr. *kyanos* blue]   a combining form denoting blue.

cyanoalcohol (si″ah-no-al′ko-hol)   cyanohydrin.

Cyanobacteria (si″ah-no-bak-tēr′e-ah)   Cyanophyceae.

cyanocobalamin (si″ah-no-ko-bal′ah-min)   a water-soluble hematopoietic vitamin (vitamin B₁₂), $C_{63}H_{88}CoN_{14}O_{14}P$, found in the liver, fish meal, eggs, and other natural products, or produced from cultures of *Streptomyces griseus,* which combines with

intrinsic factor for intestinal absorption and which is needed for maturation of erythrocytes. Absence of intrinsic factor leads to malabsorption of cyanocobalamin and results in pernicious anemia. The official preparation, prepared in accordance with USP specifications, is used in the prophylaxis and treatment of pernicious anemia and other macrocytic anemias, usually administered intramuscularly or subcutaneously. Called also *antipernicious anemia factor, extrinsic factor,* and *LLD factor.* See also *Castle's factor,* under *factor.* **radioactive c.,** cyanocobalamin in which a portion of the molecules contain cobalt of mass number 57 (⁵⁷Co), 58 (⁵⁸Co), or 60 (⁶⁰Co), used as a diagnostic aid in pernicious anemia.

cyanocrystallin (si″ah-no-kris′tal-lin)   a blue coloring matter from the integument of decapods.

cyanoform (si-an′o-form)   a crystalline substance, CH(CN)₃, formed by the action of potassium cyanide on chloroform.

cyanogen (si-an′o-jen) [*cyano-* + Gr. *gennan* to produce]   the radical CN—; also NCCN (dicyanogen dicyan, ethanedinitrile), the latter an exceedingly poisonous gas. Symbol Cy. **c. bromide,** a highly toxic lacrimatory war gas, BrCN. **c. chloride,** a gas, ClCN, used for fumigating houses, ships, etc. It is as lethal for rats and other vermin as hydrocyanic acid, but less dangerous to man, as it causes lacrimation.

cyanogenesis (si″ah-no-jen′e-sis) [*cyano-* + Gr. *genesis* production]   the formation or production of cyanogen or hydrocyanic acid.

cyanogenetic (si″ah-no-jĕ-net′ik)   producing cyanogen or hydrocyanic acid.

cyanohydrin (si″ah-no-hi′drin)   a compound formed by the addition of hydrocyanic acid to the aldehyde or ketone group; called also *cyanoalcohol.*

cyanolabe (si′ah-no-lāb″) [*cyano-* + Gr. *lambanein* to take]   name proposed for the pigment in retinal cones that is more sensitive to the blue range of the spectrum than are the other retinal pigments. Cf. *chlorolabe* and *erythrolabe.*

cyanophil (si-an′o-fil)   1. cyanophilous. 2. a cell or other histologic element readily stainable with blue.

cyanophilous (si″ah-nof′ĭ-lus) [*cyano-* + Gr. *philein* to love]   stainable with blue dyes.

cyanophoric (si″ah-no-fōr′ik)   yielding hydrocyanic acid; e.g., the glycoside amygdalin yields HCN on hydrolysis.

cyanophose (si′ah-no-fōz) [*cyano-* + Gr. *phōs* light]   a blue phose.

Cyanophyceae (si″ah-no-fi′se-e) [*cyano-* + Gr. *phykos* seaweed]   in some systems of classification, a division of the kingdom Procaryotae that includes the blue-green algae (blue-green bacteria), which are unicellular or filamentous microorganisms that are immobile or move by gliding, and usually reproduce by fission. They are photosynthetic and fix nitrogen in both soil and aquatic environments, and are often used as indicators of eutrophication of lakes and streams. Called also *Cyanobacteria* and *Schizophyceae.*

cyanopia (si″ah-no′pe-ah)   cyanopsia.

cyanopsia (si″ah-nop′se-ah) [*cyano-* + Gr. *opsis* vision + *-ia*]   a visual defect in which all objects appear to have a blue tinge.

cyanopsin (si″ah-nop′sin) [*cyano-* + Gr. *opsis* vision]   a visual pigment of bluish tint found in the retinal cones of some animals and important for vision.

cyanose (si′ah-nōs″) [Fr.]   cyanosis. **c. tardive′,** tardive cyanosis.

cyanosed (si″ah-nōsd)   cyanotic.

cyanosis (si″ah-no′sis) [Gr. *kyanos* blue]   a bluish discoloration, applied especially to such discoloration of skin and mucous membranes due to excessive concentration of reduced hemoglobin in the blood. **autotoxic c.,** enterogenous c. **c. bul′bi,** 1. congenital violet flecks in the sclera (Liebisch). 2. bluish discoloration of the white of the eye in cyanosis (Hirschfeld). **central c.,** cyanosis produced as a result of arterial unsaturation, the aortic blood carrying reduced hemoglobin. **enterogenous c.,** a syndrome due to absorption of nitrites and sulfides from the intestine, principally marked by methemoglobinemia and/or sulfhemoglobinemia associated with cyanosis. It is accompanied by severe enteritis, abdominal pain, constipation or diarrhea, headache, dyspnea, dizziness, syncope, anemia, and, occasionally, digital clubbing and indicanuria. Called also *Stokvis' disease, Stokvis-Talma syndrome, van den Bergh's disease,* and *autotoxic cyanosis.* **false c.,** cyanosis due to the presence of pigment and not to deficient oxygenation of the blood. **hereditary methemoglobinemic c.,** cyanosis caused by a structural variant in the hemoglobin molecule, i.e., one of the M hemoglobins, or by a deficiency of NADH-methemoglobin diaphorase, inherited as an autosomal recessive trait. **c. lie′nis,** passive congestion of the spleen. **peripheral c.,** cyanosis produced as a result of an excessive amount of reduced hemoglobin in the venous blood, caused by extensive oxygen extraction at the capillary level. **pulmonary c.,** central cyanosis caused by poor oxygenation of the blood in the lungs. **c. ret′inae,** distinct cyanosis of the retina, observable in some cases of cyanotic congenital heart disease, patent ductus arteriosus, and other congenital cardiac anomalies.

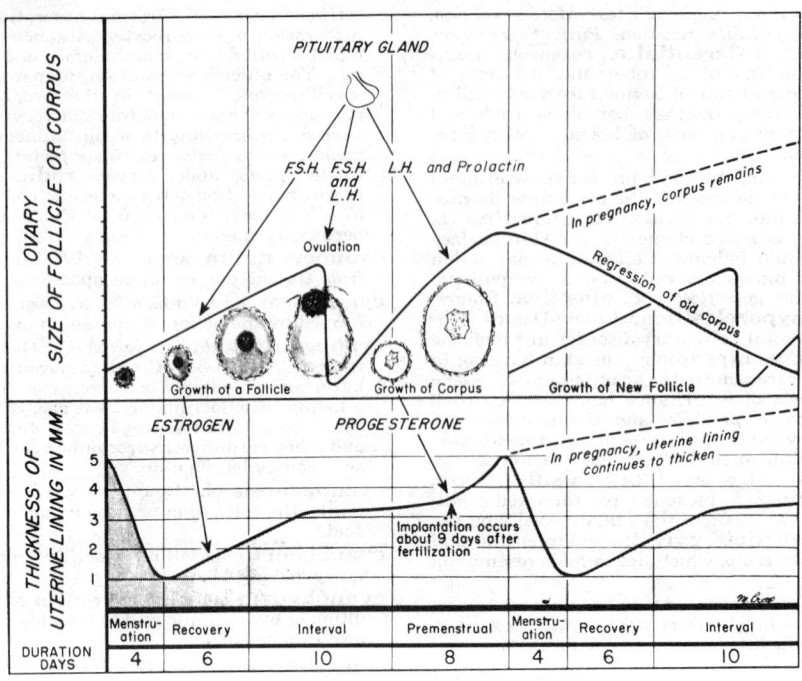

CHANGES IN MENSTRUAL CYCLE IN HUMAN FEMALE

Solid lines indicate course of events when ovum is not fertilized; dotted lines indicate course of events when fertilization occurs. Actions of hormones of pituitary and ovary in regulating the cycle are indicated by arrows. (Villee.)

shunt c., central cyanosis caused by mixing of unoxygenated blood with the arterial blood in the heart or great vessels. **tardive c.,** cyanosis in congenital heart disease which appears only after cardiac failure has developed; called also *cyanose tardive.*

cyanotic (si-ah-not′ik) pertaining to or characterized by cyanosis.

Cyantin (si-an′tin) trademark for a preparation of nitrofurantoin.

cyanuria (si″ah-nu′re-ah) the passage of blue urine.

cyanurin (si″ah-nu′rin) [*cyan-* + Gr. *ouron* urine] indigo blue found in the urine on the addition of a mineral acid to it.

Cyath. abbreviation for L. *cy′athus,* a glassful.

cybernetics (si″ber-net′iks) [Gr. *kybernētēs* helmsman] the science of the processes of communication and control in the animal and in the machine.

cycasin (si′kah-sin) a toxic principle, methylazoxymethanol β-glucoside, $C_8H_{16}N_2O_7$, from the seeds of *Cycas revoluta* Thumb. and *C. circinalis* L., (Cycadaceae), native to Guam; it is neoplastic to the liver, kidneys, intestine, and lungs.

cyclacillin (si-klah-sil′in) chemical name: 6-(1-aminocyclohexanecarboxamido) - 3, 3 - dimethyl - 7 - oxo - 4 - thia - 1- azabicyclo-[3.2.0]heptane-2-carboxylic acid; an antibacterial agent, $C_{15}H_{23}N_3$-O_4S, effective against a wide range of gram-negative and gram-positive organisms.

Cyclaine (si′klān) trademark for preparations of hexylcaine hydrochloride.

cyclamate (si′klah-māt) any salt of cyclamic acid. Cyclamate calcium and cyclamate sodium were once used widely as non-nutritive sweeteners, but because of an association with bladder tumors in animals they were banned as food additives in the United States in 1969.

Cyclamen (sik′lah-men) [L.] a genus of primulaceous plants. *C. europaeum* L., has an acrid, cathartic root, and is listed as a poisonous plant by European references, although it is a fairly common house plant in the United States.

cyclamin (sik′lah-min) a glycoside, $C_{20}H_{34}O_{10}$, from *Cyclamen europaeum;* it is strongly purgative and emetic.

Cyclamycin (si′klah-mi″sin) trademark for a preparation of troleandomycin.

cyclandelate (si-klan′dĕ-lāt) chemical name: α-hydroxybenzeneacetic acid 3,3,5-trimethylcyclohexyl ester. An antispasmodic, $C_{17}H_{24}O_3$, with a direct effect on vascular smooth muscle, occurring as a white to pale yellow, crystalline powder; used as a vasodilator mainly in peripheral vascular diseases, administered orally.

cyclarthrodial (sik″lar-thro′de-al) pertaining to a cyclarthrosis.

cyclarthrosis (sik″lar-thro′sis) [Gr. *kyklos* circle + *arthrosis*] a joint that permits rotation.

cyclase (si′klās) an enzyme that catalyzes the formation of a cyclic phosphodiester. **adenyl c., adenylate c.,** see under *adenyl.*

cyclazocine (si″klah-zo′sĕn) chemical name: 3-(cyclopropylmethyl)-1,2,3,4,5,6-hexahydro-6,11-dimethyl-2,6-methano-benzazocin-8-ol. A narcotic antagonist, $C_{18}H_{25}NO$, which has been used as an analgesic and in the treatment of narcotic dependence.

cycle (si′kl) [Gr. *kyklos* circle] a round or succession of observable phenomena, recurring usually at regular intervals and in the same sequence. **aberrant c.,** one that shows variation in the interval or the sequence of events. **anovulatory c.,** a sexual cycle in which no ovum is discharged. **asexual c.,** generation by budding or division of the parent organism. **biliary c.,** Schiff's biliary c. **Calvin c.,** a dark reaction occurring in photosynthesis in plants in which carbon dioxide is affixed to a five-carbon sugar molecule and subsequently reduced to form other sugars. **carbon c.,** the steps by which carbon (in the form of carbon dioxide) is extracted from the atmosphere by living organisms and ultimately returned to the atmosphere. It comprises a series of interconversions of carbon compounds beginning with the production of carbohydrates by plants during photosynthesis, proceeding through animal consumption, and ending and beginning again in the decomposition of the animal or plant or in the exhalation of carbon dioxide by animals. **cardiac c.,** a complete cardiac movement or heart beat. The period from the beginning of one heart beat to the beginning of the next; the systolic and diastolic movement, with the interval between them. **cell c.,** the cycle of biochemical and morphological events occurring in a reproducing cell population; it consists of: the *S phase,* occurring toward the end of interphase, in which DNA is synthesized; the *G_2 phase,* a relatively quiescent period; the *M phase,* consisting of the four phases of mitosis; and the *G_1 phase* of interphase, which lasts until the *S phase* of the next cycle. **chewing c.,** masticating c. **citric acid c.,** tricarboxylic acid c. **Cori c.,** the cycle in carbohydrate metabolism in which muscle glycogen is converted to lactate (glycolysis) during muscle activity and is carried by the blood to the liver, where it is converted to glucose (gluconeogenesis); the glucose is then carried by the blood to muscle, where it is converted to muscle glycogen. Called also *glucose-lactate c.* **cytoplasmic c.,** that stage in the life of a parasite during which it lives in cytoplasm of the cells of the host. **Embden-Meyerhof c.,** see under *pathway.* **endogenous c.,** that portion of the life of a parasite which is spent within the body of its host. **estrous c.,** the recurring periods of heat, or estrus, in the adult female of most mammals and the correlated changes in the reproductive tract from one period to the next. See also *metestrus, diestrus,* and *proestrus.* **exogenous c.,** that part of the life of a parasite which is spent outside the body of its definitive host. **forced c.,** a cardiac cycle that is interrupted by a forced beat. **gastric c.,** rhythmical alterations in the shape of the stomach due to peristaltic waves.

Plate XIV

cycle

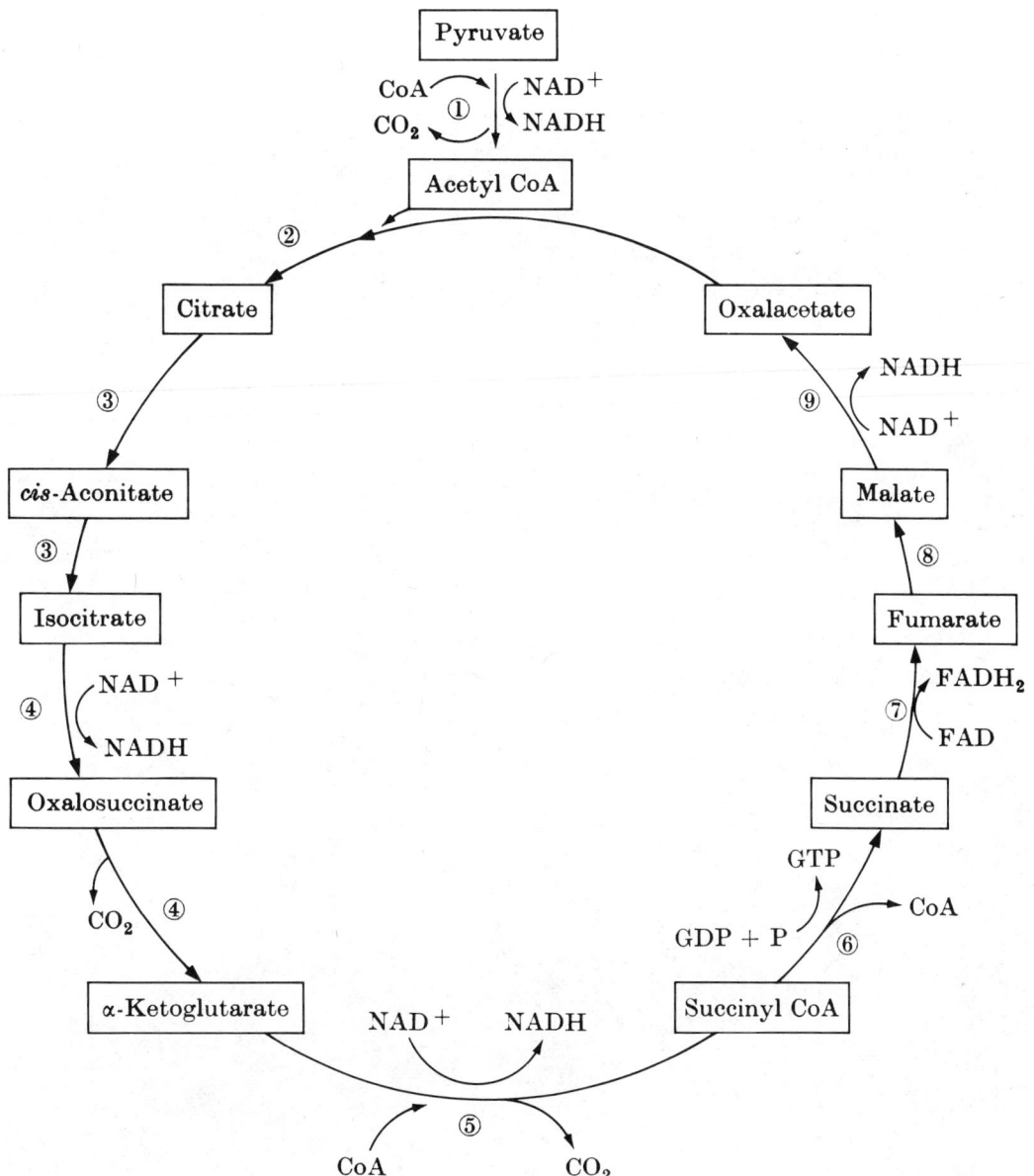

TRICARBOXYLIC ACID (KREBS) CYCLE

Diagrammatic representation of reactions by which carbon chains of sugars, fatty acids, and amino acids are metabolized to yield carbon dioxide, water, and high-energy phosphate bonds. Key to enzymes (circled numbers): 1 = pyruvate dehydrogenase. 2 = citrate synthase. 3 = aconitrate dehydrogenase. 4 = isocitric dehydrogenase. 5 = α-ketoglutarate dehydrogenase. 6 = succinyl-CoA synthetase. 7 = succinate dehydrogenase. 8 = fumarate hydratase (furmarase). 9 = malate dehydrogenase. (Mazur and Harrow.)

genesial c., the reproductive period of a woman's life. **glucose-lactate c.,** Cori c. **glyoxylate c.,** a metabolic pathway by which certain microorganisms and plants convert fat to carbohydrate, the enzymes of which are contained in microbodies known as *glyoxosomes;* it is a modification of the tricarboxylic acid cycle but differs in that two auxiliary enzymes (isocitratase and malate synthetase) are used and two molecules of acetyl coenzyme A instead of one are required. **Golgi's c.,** that cycle in the life of a plasmodium which is passed in human blood. Cf. *Ross's c.* **gonotrophic c.,** the interval in the life of an insect between the time of feeding to deposition of the ova. **hair c.,** the successive phases in the production of hair, from initiation of its growth to its loss from the follicle, consisting of anagen, catagen, and telogen. **Hodgkin c.,** a regenerative, circular sequence of events between depolarization and permeability to sodium occurring in excitable cells: depolarization increases permeability to sodium, thus increasing the entry of sodium (Na^+) into the cell, and the increased concentration of Na^+ further depolarizes the membrane. **intranuclear c.,** that stage in the life of a microorganism during which it lives in the nuclei of the cells of the host. **isohydric c.,** the series of chemical reactions in the erythrocyte, in which the uptake of CO_2 and the release of O_2 is accomplished without the production of an excess of hydrogen ions (H^+). **Krebs' c.,** tricarboxylic acid c. **Krebs-Henseleit c.,** urea c. **life c.,** the successive events in the life history of an organism; for example, the entire life of a protozoan blood parasite, including the endogenous and exogenous cycles. **mammary c.,** the rhythmic growth of mammary glands after menarche occurring in coordination with the ovarian cycle. **masticating c.,** a complete course of movement of the mandible performed in mastication of food, from midline position back to the midline. Called also *chewing c.* **menstrual c.,** the period of the regularly recurring physiologic changes in the endometrium, occurring during the reproductive period of human females and a few primates, culminating in partial shedding of the endometrium and some bleeding per vagina (menstruation); see illustration. **mosquito c.,** that period of the life of a malarial parasite that is spent in the body of the mosquito host. **nitrogen c.,** the steps by which nitrogen is extracted from the nitrates of soil and water, incorporated as amino acids and proteins in living organisms, and ultimately reconverted to nitrates: (1) conversion of nitrogen to nitrates by bacteria; (2) the extraction of the nitrates by plants and the building of amino acids and proteins by adding an amino group to the carbon compounds produced in photosynthesis; (3) the ingestion of plants by animals, and (4) the return of nitrogen to the soil in animal excretions or on the death and decomposition of plants and animals. **oogenetic c.,** ovarian c. **ornithine c.,** urea c. **ovarian c.,** the sequence of physiologic changes in the ovary, including development and rupture of the follicle, discharge of the ovum, and corpus luteum formation and regression; called also *oogenetic c.* **pregnancy c.,** cycle of physiologic changes in reproductive organs during pregnancy. **reproductive c.,** the cycle of physiologic changes occurring in the reproductive organs, from the time of fertilization of the ovum through gestation and parturition. **restored c.,** a cardiac cycle following a returning cycle and taking up the normal rhythm. **returning c.,** a cardiac cycle that begins with an extrasystole. **Ross's c.,** that cycle in the development of a plasmodium which is passed in the mosquito. Cf. *Golgi's c.* **Schiff's biliary c.,** the cycle in which bile salts in the bile are absorbed by the intestinal villi and are then conveyed back to the liver, where they are used over again; see also *enterohepatic circulation,* under *circulation.* **schizogenic c., schizogenous c.,** the asexual cycle in protozoa during which growth and segmentation occur. **sex c., sexual c.,** 1. the physiologic changes recurring regularly in the genital organs of female mammals when pregnancy does not supervene. 2. the period of sexual reproduction in an organism that also reproduces asexually. **sporogenic c., sporogenous c.,** the sexual cycle in protozoa that is usually passed in another host, often an insect. **tricarboxylic acid c.,** the cyclic metabolic mechanism by which the complete oxidation of the acetyl moiety of acetyl-coenzyme A is effected; see *diagram.* Called also *Krebs' c.* and *citric acid c.* **urea c.,** a cyclic series of reactions that produce urea, a major route for removal of the ammonia produced in the metabolism of amino acids in the liver and kidney: arginine is hydrolyzed (catalyzed by arginase) to ornithine and urea in the soluble cytoplasm, the ornithine then being converted to citrulline in the mitochondria by the addition of the carbamyl group from carbamyl phosphate, and subsequently to arginine by the transfer of nitrogen from aspartate. The arginine is again hydrolyzed to ornithine and urea, and so on. Called also *ornithine c.* and *Krebs-Henseleit c.* **uterine c.,** the phenomena occurring in the endometrium during the estrous or menstrual cycle, preparing it for implantation of the blastocyst. **vaginal c.,** the rhythmic alteration occurring in the epithelial lining of the vagina in conjunction with the ovarian cycle.

cyclectomy (sik-lek'to-me) [Gr. *kyklos* circle, ciliary body + *ektomē* excision] 1. excision of a piece of the ciliary body. 2. excision of a portion of the ciliary border of the eyelid.

cyclencephalus (sik″len-sef'ah-lus) [Gr. *kyklos* circle + *enke-*

phalos brain] a monster with the cerebral hemispheres blended into one.

cyclic (si'klik, sik'lik) [Gr. *kyklikos*] pertaining to or occurring in a cycle or cycles; the term is applied to chemical compounds that contain a ring of atoms in the nucleus. See *closed chain,* under *chain.*

cyclicotomy (sik″le-kot'o-me) cyclotomy.

cyclindole (si-klin'dōl) chemical name: 2,3,4,9-tetrahydro-*N,N*-dimethyl-1*H*-carbazol-3-amine; an antidepressant, $C_{14}H_{18}N_2$.

cyclitis (sik-li'tis) [Gr. *kyklos* ciliary body + *-itis*] inflammation of the ciliary body. **heterochromic c.,** chronic cyclitis producing difference in the color of the two irides, the inflamed eye having the lighter iris. **plastic c.,** cyclitis with exudation of fibrinous matter into the anterior chamber. **pure c.,** inflammation of the ciliary body without involvement of the iris. **purulent c.,** suppuration in the ciliary body. **serous c.,** simple inflammation of the ciliary body.

cyclizine (si'klĭ-zēn) [USP] chemical name: 1-(diphenylmethyl)-4-methylpiperazine. An antihistaminic, $C_{18}H_{22}N_2$, occurring as a white, or creamy white, crystalline powder; used in the form of the lactate salt as an antiemetic and antinauseant, especially for the prevention and relief of motion sickness, administered intramuscularly. **c. hydrochloride** [USP], the monohydrochloride salt of cyclizine, $C_{18}H_{22}N_2 \cdot HCl$, occurring as a white, crystalline powder or small, colorless crystals, having the same actions and uses as the base; administered orally. **c. lactate,** see *cyclizine.*

cyclo- (si'klo) [Gr. *kyklos* circle] a combining form denoting round or recurring; see *cyclic.* Often used with particular reference to the eye, or to the ciliary body of the eye.

cycloanemization (si″klo-an″ĕ-mi-za'shun) Kettesy's name for his procedure of obstructing the long ciliary arteries in the surgical treatment of glaucoma.

cyclobarbital (si″klo-bar'bĭ-tal) chemical name: 5-(1-cyclohexen-1-yl)-5-ethylbarbituric acid. A short-acting barbiturate, $C_{12}H_{16}N_2O_3$, mainly used as a hypnotic; administered orally. **c. calcium,** the calcium salt of cyclobarbital, $C_{24}H_{30}CaN_4O_6$, having actions and uses similar to those of the base; administered orally.

cyclobendazole (si″klo-ben'dah-zōl) chemical name: [5-(cyclopropylcarbonyl)-1*H*-benzimidazol-2-yl]carbamic acid methyl ester; an anthelmintic, $C_{13}H_{13}N_3O_3$.

cyclobenzaprine hydrochloride (si″klo-ben'zah-prēn) [USP] chemical name: 3-(5*H*-dibenzo[*a,d*]cyclohepten-5-ylidene)-*N,N*-dimethyl-1-propanamine hydrochloride; a muscle relaxant, $C_{20}H_{21}N \cdot HCl$.

cyclocephalus (si″klo-sef'ah-lus) [*cyclo-* + Gr. *kephalē* head] a cyclops.

cycloceratitis (si″klo-ser'ah-ti'tis) cyclokeratitis.

cyclochoroiditis (si″klo-ko″roid-i'tis) [*cyclo-* + *choroid*] inflammation of the choroid and ciliary body.

cyclocryotherapy (si″klo-kri″o-ther'ah-pe) freezing of the ciliary body; done in the treatment of glaucoma.

cyclocumarol (si″klo-koo'mah-rōl) chemical name: 3,4-dihydro-2-methoxy-2-methyl-4-phenyl-2*H*,5*H*-pyrano[3,2-*c*][1]benzopyran-5-one; an anticoagulant, $C_{20}H_{18}O_4$.

cyclodamia (si″klo-da'me-ah) [*cyclo-* + Gr. *damnao* I subdue] subdued or suppressed accommodation of the eyes.

cyclodialysis (si″klo-di-al'ĭ-sis) [*cyclo-* + Gr. *dialysis* dissolution] the operative formation of a communication between the anterior chamber of the eye and the suprachoroidal space; done in the treatment of glaucoma.

cyclodiathermy (si″klo-di'ah-ther″me) destruction of a portion of the ciliary body by diathermy; employed as therapy in cases of glaucoma.

cycloduction (si″klo-duk'shun) [*cyclo-* + *duction*] the duction of the eyeball produced by the oblique muscle.

cycloelectrolysis (si″klo-e″lek-trol'ĭ-sis) destruction of the ciliary body by passage of an electric current.

cyclogeny (si-kloj'ĕ-ne) [*cyclo-* + Gr. *gennan* to produce] the developmental cycle of a microorganism.

cyclogram (si'klo-gram) a graph or chart of the visual field made with the cycloscope (1st def.).

cycloguanide embonate (si-klo-gwan'īd) cycloguanil pamoate.

cycloguanil pamoate (si-klo-gwan'il) chemical name: 1-(4-chlorophenyl)-1,6-dihydro-6,6-dimethyl-1,3,5-triazine-2,4-diamine. A metabolite of the antimalarial drug proguanil, $C_{45}H_{44}Cl_2N_{10}O_6$, and itself having potent antimalarial effects. Called also *c. embonate* and *cycloguanide embonate.*

Cyclogyl (si'klo-jil) trademark for a preparation of cyclopentolate hydrochloride.

cyclohexanehexol (si″klo-heks″ān-heks'ōl) inositol.

cyclohexanol (si″klo-hek'sah-nol) the monohydroxy derivative of the saturated six-carbon-ring hydrocarbon cyclohexane.

cycloheximide (si″klo-heks'ĭ-mīd) chemical name: 3-[2-(3,5-dimethyl-2-oxocyclohexyl)-2-hydroxyethyl]glutarimide. An antibiotic substance, $C_{15}H_{23}NO_4$, isolated from *Streptomyces griseus*, and used as an agricultural fungicide and in selective media for fungi. It inhibits most saprophytic fungi, while allowing dermatophytes and most systemic fungi to grow, and inhibits nuclear division of karyotic organisms but has no effect on prokaryotic cells (bacteria).

cycloid (si'kloid) 1. containing a ring of atoms; said of organic chemical compounds. 2. cyclothymic. 3. cyclothyme.

cycloisomerase (si″klo-i-som'er-ās) an enzyme that catalyzes intramolecular lyase reactions.

cyclokeratitis (si″klo-ker-ah-ti'tis) [*cyclo-* + *keratitis*] inflammation of the cornea and ciliary body; called also *Dalrymple's disease.*

cyclo-ligase (si″klo-li'gās) an enzyme that catalyzes the formation of carbon-nitrogen, C—N bonds, and the breakdown of a pyrophosphate bond, as of ATP.

cyclomastopathy (si″klo-mas-top'ah-the) [*cyclo-* + Gr. *mastos* breast + *pathos* disease] an affection of the mammae, presenting excessive connective tissue overgrowth or epithelial proliferation or both in response to growth stimuli or as a manifestation of abnormal involution following normal response. Cf. *eccyclomastoma.*

cyclomethycaine sulfate (si″klo-meth'ĭ-kān) [USP] chemical name: 4-(cyclohexyloxy)benzoic acid 3-(2-methyl-1-piperidinyl)-propyl ester sulfate (1:1). A local anesthetic, $C_{22}H_{33}NO_3 \cdot H_2SO_4$, occurring as a white, crystalline powder; applied topically to relieve burning, itching, and pain originating in the rectal, vaginal, urethral, or nasal mucous membranes or associated with skin lesions, and also used to facilitate various diagnostic procedures, such as bronchoscopy, sigmoidoscopy, tracheal intubation, etc.

cyclopentamine hydrochloride (si″klo-pen'tah-mēn) [USP] chemical name: *N,α*-dimethylcyclopentaneethanamine hydrochloride. An adrenergic, $C_9H_{19}N \cdot HCl$, occurring as a white, crystalline powder; used as a vasoconstrictor to reduce nasal congestion, applied topically to the nasal mucous membranes.

cyclopentane (si″klo-pen'tān) a hydrocarbon, C_5H_{10}, in which all five carbon atoms are in a single ring.

cyclopentenophenanthrene (si″klo-pen-tēn″o-fĕ-nan'thrēn) a polycyclic nucleus present in sterols, bile acids, sex hormones, cardiac poisons, and saponins.

cyclopenthiazide (si″klo-pen-thi'ah-zīd) chemical name: 6-chloro-3-(cyclopentylmethyl)-3,4-dihydro-2*H*-1,2,4-benzothiadiazine-7-sulfonamide 1,1-dioxide. An orally effective diuretic, $C_{13}H_{18}ClN_3O_4S_2$, used in the treatment of edema associated with various disorders and in hypertension.

cyclopentolate hydrochloride (si″klo-pen'to-lāt) [USP] chemical name: 2-dimethylaminoethyl-1-hydroxy-α-phenylcyclopentaneacetate hydrochloride. An anticholinergic, $C_{17}H_{25}NO_3 \cdot HCl$, occurring as a white, crystalline powder; used to produce cycloplegia and mydriasis by instillation into the eye.

cyclophenazine hydrochloride (si″klo-fen'ah-zēn) chemical name: 10-[3-(4-cyclopropyl-1-piperazinyl)propyl]-2-(trifluoromethyl)phenothiazine dihydrochloride; a tranquilizer, $C_{23}H_{26}F_3N_3S \cdot 2HCl$.

cyclophoria (si″klo-fo're-ah) heterophoria in which there is deviation of the eye from the anteroposterior axis in the absence of visual fusional stimuli. See *excyclophoria* and *incyclophoria*. Cf. *cyclotropia.* **accommodative c.,** cyclophoria due to oblique astigmatism. **minus c., negative c.,** incyclophoria. **plus c., positive c.,** excyclophoria.

cyclophorometer (si″klo-fo-rom'ĕ-ter) an instrument for measuring cyclophoria.

cyclophosphamide (si″klo-fos'fah-mīd) [USP] chemical name: *N,N*-bis (2-chloroethyl) tetrahydro-2*H*-1, 3, 2-oxazaphosphorin-2-amine 2 oxide monohydrate. A cytotoxic alkylating agent derived from mechlorethanamine hydrochloride (nitrogen mustard), $C_7H_{15}Cl_2N_2O_2P \cdot H_2O$, occurring as a white, crystalline powder, used as an antineoplastic in the treatment of many types of malignancies, including Hodgkin's disease, leukemias, multiple myeloma, ovarian sarcoma, and lymphosarcoma; usually administered orally or intravenously. Also used as an immunosuppressant.

cyclophrenia (si″klo-fre'ne-ah) (*obs.*) cyclothymia.

Cyclophyllidea (si″klo-fil-lid'e-ah) an order of tapeworms of the subclass Cestoda, class Cestoidea, comprising seven families that are habitually or accidentally parasitic in man: Taeniidae, Hymenolepididae, Dilepididae, Davaineidae, Anoplocephalidae, Linstowiidae, and Mesocestoididae.

cyclopia (si-klo'pe-ah) [Gr. *kyklos* circle + *ōpo* eye + *-ia*] a developmental anomaly characterized by a single orbit, with the globe absent or rudimentary, apparently normal, or duplicated, and the nose absent or present as a tubular appendage located above the orbit.

cyclopin (si'klo-pin) a proteinaceous constituent of *Penicillium cyclopium* that has been shown to inhibit the multiplication of representative members of group A and B arboviruses.

cycloplegia (si″klo-ple'je-ah) [*cyclo-* + Gr. *plēgē* stroke] paralysis of the ciliary muscle; paralysis of accommodation.

cycloplegic (si″klo-ple'jik) 1. pertaining to, characterized by, or causing cycloplegia. 2. an agent that causes cycloplegia.

cyclopropane (si″klo-pro'pān) a colorless, inflammable and explosive gas, C_3H_6, with characteristic odor and pungent taste; used by inhalation as a general anesthetic.

Cyclops (si'klops) a genus of minute crustacean species of which are hosts to *Dracunculus* and *Diphyllobothrium*.

cyclops (si'klops) [Gr. *kyklōps* one of a race of one-eyed giants] a monster exhibiting cyclopia; called also *cyclocephalus.* **c. hypogna'thus,** a modified cyclops, lacking the typical proboscis, with ears abnormally low, rudimentary mandible, and tiny orifice of the buccal cavity.

cyclopterin (si-klop'ter-in) a protamine derived from the spermatozoa of the lump-sucker, *Cyclopterus lumpus.*

cycloscope (si'klo-skōp) [*cyclo-* + Gr. *skopein* to examine] a form of perimeter for mapping the visual fields.

cyclose (si'klōs) any of a class of carbohydrates which are polyhydroxy cyclohexanes; they include inositol and phytol.

cycloserine (si″klo-ser'ēn) [USP] chemical name: (*R*)-4-amino-3-isoxazolidinone. A broad-spectrum antibiotic, $C_3H_6N_2O_2$, with tuberculostatic activity, produced by growth of *Streptomyces orchidaceus* or obtained by synthesis, occurring as a white to pale yellow, crystalline powder; effective against many gram-negative and gram-positive bacteria, it is used in the treatment of tuberculosis, pulmonary and extrapulmonary, and sometimes in urinary tract infections due to susceptible pathogens, administered orally.

cyclosis (si-klo'sis) [Gr. *kyklōsis* a surrounding, enclosing] movement of the cytoplasm within a cell, without deformation of the cell wall; called also *cytoplasmic* or *protoplasmic streaming.*

cyclospasm (si'klo-spazm) spasm of accommodation of the eyes.

Cyclospasmol (si″klo-spaz'mol) trademark for preparations of cyclandelate.

cyclostat (si'klŏ-stat) a cylinder of glass in which an experimental animal is rotated about its vertical axis.

cyclotate (si'klo-tāt) USAN contraction for 4-methylbicyclo-[2.2.2]oct-2-ene-1-carboxylate.

cyclotherapy (si″klo-ther'ah-pe) [*cyclo-* + Gr. *therapeia* treatment] use of the bicycle in treatment.

cyclothiazide (si″klo-thi'ah-zīd) [USP] chemical name: 3-bicyclo[2.2.1]hept-5-en-2-yl-6-chloro-3,4-dihydro-2*H*-1,2,4-benzo-thiadiazone-7-sulfonamide 1,1-dioxide. An orally effective diuretic, $C_{14}H_{16}ClN_3O_4S_2$, occurring as a white to nearly white powder; used in the treatment of edema associated with various conditions and in hypertension.

cyclothyme (si'klo-thīm) an individual with a cyclothymic personality or exhibiting cyclothymia; called also *cycloid, cyclothymiac,* and *cyclothymic.*

cyclothymia (si″klo-thīm'e-ah) [*cyclo-* + Gr. *thymos* spirit] 1. cyclothymic personality. 2. a condition characterized by a predisposition to alternating moods of elation and mild depression.

cyclothymiac (si″klo-thim'e-ak) cyclothyme.

cyclothymic (si″klo-thi'mik) 1. of or pertaining to a cyclothymic personality. 2. of, pertaining to, or characterized by cyclothymia. 3. cyclothyme. Called also *cycloid.*

cyclothymosis (si″klo-thi-mo'sis) (*obs.*) any mental disease of the cyclothymic and manic-depressive group (Southard).

cyclotol (si'klo-tol) a polyhydroxy cyclohexane, such as inositol.

cyclotome (si'klo-tōm) a cutting instrument for use in cyclotomy or other operations upon the eye.

cyclotomy (si-klot'o-me) [*cyclo-* + Gr. *temnein* to cut] division of or incision of the ciliary muscle.

cyclotron (si'klo-tron) an apparatus for accelerating protons or deuterons to high energies by a combination of a constant magnet and an oscillating electric field.

cyclotropia (si″klo-tro'pe-ah) [*cyclo-* + Gr. *tropos* a turning] a form of strabismus (q.v.) in which there is permanent deviation of an eye around the anteroposterior axis even in the presence of visual fusional stimuli, resulting in diplopia. Cf. *cyclophoria.* **minus c., negative c.,** incyclotropia. **plus c., positive c.,** excyclotropia.

cycrimine hydrochloride (si'krĭ-mīn) [USP] chemical name: α-cyclopentyl-α-phenyl-1-piperidinepropanol hydrochloride. An anticholinergic, $C_{19}H_{29}NO \cdot HCl$, occurring as a white solid; used in the treatment off parkinsonism, administered orally.

cyema (si-e'mah) [Gr. *kyēma* embryo] the product of conception during all its stages.

cyemology (si″e-mol'o-je) embryology.

cyesedema (si″e-sĕ-de'mah) [Gr. *kyēsis* conception + *edema*] (*obs.*) a peculiar bloating of the body, especially of the face, sometimes seen in pregnant women.

cyesiognosis (si-e″se-og-no'sis) [Gr. *kyēsis* conception + *gnōsis* knowledge] (*obs.*) diagnosis of pregnancy.

cyesiology (si-e″se-ol′o-je) [Gr. *kyēsis* conception + *-logy*] (*obs.*) the sum of knowledge regarding pregnancy.

cyesis (si-e′sis) [Gr. *kyēsis*] pregnancy.

cyestein (si-es′te-in) a skinlike formation sometimes seen on the surface of urine of a pregnant woman.

cyesthein (si-es′the-in) cyestein.

cyl. cylinder; cylindrical lens.

cylicotomy (sil″e-kot′o-me) [Gr. *kylix* cup + *tomē* a cutting] surgical division of the ciliary muscle.

cylinder (sil′in-der) [Gr. *kylindros* a roller] a solid body shaped like a column, especially a cylindrical cast or cylindrical lens. **Bence Jones c's,** cylindrical gelatinous bodies forming the contents of the seminal vesicles; called also *Jones c's,* and *Lallemand's, Lallemand-Trousseau,* or *Trousseau-Lallemand bodies.* **crossed c's,** two cylindrical lenses at right angles to each other. **Külz's c.,** coma cast. **Leydig's c's,** bundles of muscular fibers separated by partitions of protoplasm. **Ruffini's c's,** Ruffini's corpuscles. **terminal c's,** brushes of Ruffini. **urinary c.,** a urinary cast.

cylindrarthrosis (sil″in-drar-thro′sis) [*cylinder* + Gr. *arthrōsis* joint] a joint in which the articular surfaces are cylindrical, as in the proximal radioulnar joint or the odontoid process and atlas.

cylindraxile (sil″in-drak′sil) an axon, def. 2.

cylindrical (sǐ-lin′drǐ-k'l) pertaining to or shaped like a cylinder.

cylindriform (sǐ-lin′drǐ-form) cylindrical.

cylindrocellular (sil″in-dro-sel′u-lar) composed of or containing cylindrical cells.

cylindrodendrite (sil″in-dro-den′drīt) a collateral branch of an axon.

Cylindrogloea (sǐ-lin″dro-gle′ah) a genus of microorganisms of the family Chlorobacteriaceae, suborder Rhodobacteriineae, order Pseudomonadales, occurring as small ovoid to rod-shaped cells, forming cylindrical aggregates about a filamentous, colorless bacterium. The type species is *C. bacterif′era.*

cylindroid (sil′in-droid) [Gr. *kylindroeidēs* cylindrical] 1. resembling, or shaped like a cylinder. 2. a cast in the urine, of various origins and of various forms, generally resembling hyaline casts, but differing from the latter in that they taper to a slender tail which is often twisted or curled upon itself; called also *mucous* or *spurious* (*tube*) *cast.*

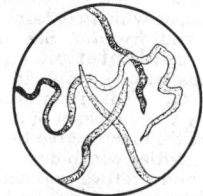

Cylindroids.

cylindroma (sil″in-dro′mah) 1. adenoid cystic carcinoma. 2. cutaneous or dermal cylindroma, a benign tumor of the skin consisting of cylindrical masses of epithelial cells surrounded by a thick band of hyaline material, believed to be related to, or derived from the hair follicle or the sweat glands; the microscopic appearance resembles that of adenoid cystic carcinoma. It occurs in a nonhereditary form, manifested by a solitary lesion, usually on the scalp and face, and in a dominantly inherited form, manifested by numerous lesions of various sizes on the scalp, sometimes covering the scalp completely (*turban tumors*).

cylindromatous (sil″in-drom′ah-tus) pertaining to or of the nature of cylindroma.

cylindrosarcoma (sǐ-lin″dro-sar-ko′mah) (*obs.*) a tumor containing both cylindromatous and sarcomatous elements.

Cylindrothorax (sǐ-lin″dro-tho′raks) a genus of beetles. **C. melanoceph′ala,** a blister beetle of Africa that secretes cantharidin, which if rubbed into the skin causes a severe dermatitis.

cylindruria (sil″in-droo′re-ah) [Gr. *kylindros* cylinder + *ouron* urine + *-ia*] the presence of tube casts in the urine.

cylite (si′līt) benzyl bromide.

cyllosis (sil-lo′sis) [Gr. *kyllōsis*] clubfoot or similar deformity of the foot or leg.

cyllosoma (sil″lo-so′mah) [Gr. *kyllos* lame + *sōma* body] a monster with lower lateral abdominal eventration and absence or imperfect development of the lower limb on the side having the eventration.

cyllosomus (sil″lo-so′mus) cyllosoma.

cymarose (si′mah-rōs) a rare sugar, 2,6-deoxy-3-methoxyaldohexose, $CH_3(CHOH)_3CH(OCH_3)CH_2CHO$, from hydrolysis of various strophanthin glycosides.

cymba (sim′bah), pl. *cym′bae* [L.; Gr. *kymbē*] a boat-shaped structure. **c. con′chae auric′ulae** [NA], the upper part of the concha of the auricle.

cymbiform (sim′bǐ-form) [L. *cymba* boat + L. *forma* form] boat-shaped; scaphoid.

cymbo- (sim′bo) [L. *cymba,* Gr. *kymbē,* boat] a combining form denoting boat-shaped.

cymbocephalia (sim″bo-se-fa′le-ah) scaphocephaly.

cymbocephalic (sim″bo-se-fal′ik) [*cymbo-* + *kephalē* head] scaphocephalic.

cymbocephalous (sim″bo-sef′ah-lus) scaphocephalic.

cymbocephaly (sim″bo-sef′ah-le) scaphocephaly.

cyme (sīm) a form of inflorescence composed of a flat-topped cluster of blossoms.

cymograph (si′mo-graf) kymograph.

cyn- see *cyno-.*

cynanche (sǐ-nan′ke) [*cyn-* + Gr. *anchein* to choke] severe sore throat with threatened suffocation. **c. malig′na,** a gangrenous or putrid sore throat, often diphtheritic or scarlatinal. **c. tonsilla′ris,** peritonsillar abscess.

cynanthropy (sǐ-nan′thro-pe) [*cyn-* + Gr. *anthrōpos* man] delusion in which the patient considers himself a dog or behaves like a dog.

cynarase (si′nar-ās) an enzyme derived from the plant *Cynara.*

cynic (sin′ik) [Gr. *kynikos*] see *risus sardonicus.*

cyno-, cyn- [Gr. *kyōn* dog] a combining form denoting relationship to a dog, or doglike.

cynocephalic (si″no-se-fal′ik) [*cyno-* + Gr. *kephalē* head] having a head shaped like that of a dog.

cynodont (si′no-dont) [*cyno-* + Gr. *odous* tooth] a canine tooth.

cynomolgus (sin-o-mol′gus) a monkey of the genus *Macaca,* especially *M. irus,* used in laboratory research.

Cynomyia (si″no-mi′yah) a genus of blue-bottle flies that deposit their ova in decaying meat and in wounds.

Cynomys (si′no-mis) a genus of prairie dogs species of which harbor plague-transmitting fleas.

cynophobia (si″no-fo′be-ah) [*cyno-* + Gr. *phobein* to be affrighted by + *ia*] morbid fear of dogs.

cynorexia (si″no-rek′se-ah) [*cyno-* + Gr. *orexis* appetite] morbidly excessive hunger; bulimia.

cyogenic (si″o-jen′ik) [Gr. *kyos* fetus + *gennan* to produce] producing pregnancy.

Cyon's experiment, nerve (se′onz) [Elie de Cyon (Il′ia Faddeevich Tsion), a Russian physiologist, 1842–1912] see under *experiment* and *nerve.*

cyonin (si′o-nin) [Gr. *kyos* fetus] a general term for gonad-stimulating hormones of placental origin.

cyophoria (si″o-fo′re-ah) [Gr. *kyos* fetus + *phoros* bearing] pregnancy.

cyophoric (si″o-for′ik) pertaining to pregnancy.

cyophorin (si-of′o-rin) (*obs.*) kyestein.

cyopin (si′o-pin) [Gr. *kyanos* blue + *pyon* pus] the substance responsible for the color of blue pus.

cyotrophy (si-ot′ro-fe) [Gr. *kyos* fetus + *trophē* nutrition] nutrition of the fetus.

Cyperus (si-pe′rus) [L.; Gr. *kypeiros* rush] a genus of grasslike sedges or rushes. See *adrue.*

cypho- (si′fo) for words beginning thus, see those beginning *kypho-.*

cypionate (sip′e-o-nāt) USAN contraction for cyclopentanepropionate.

cypothrin (si′po-thrin) chemical name: 3,3-dimethylcyano-(3-phenoxyphenyl) methyl ester spiro[cyclopropane-1,1′-[1*H*-indene]-2-carboxylic acid; a veterinary anthelmintic, $C_{28}H_{23}NO_3$.

cyprazepam (si-prah′zĕ-pam) chemical name: 7-chloro-2-[(cyclopropylmethyl) amino] -5-phenyl-3*H* -1,4-benzodiazepine 4-oxide; a tranquilizer, $C_{19}H_{18}ClN_3O$.

cypridology (sip″re-dol′o-je) [Gr. *kypris* love, passion + *-logy*] venereology.

cypridopathy (sip″re-dop′ah-the) [Gr. *kypris* love, passion + *pathos* disease] a venereal disease.

cyprinin (sip′rǐ-nin) a toxic substance derived from the milt of the carp, *Cyprinus carpio.*

cyproheptadine hydrochloride (si″pro-hep′tah-dēn) [USP] chemical name: 4-(5*H*-dibenzo[*a,d*]cyclohepten-5-ylidene)-1-methylpiperidine hydrochloride sesquihydrate. A serotonin and histamine antagonist with anticholinergic and sedative properties, $C_{21}H_{21}N·HCl·1\frac{1}{2}H_2O$, occurring as a white to slightly yellow, crystalline powder; used as an antihistaminic for relief of symptoms of allergy and as an antipruritic for relief of itching associated with various skin disorders, administered orally.

cyproquinate (si-pro-kwin′āt) chemical name: 6,7-bis(cyclopropylmethoxy)-4-hydroxy-3-quinolinecarboxylic acid ethyl ester; a coccidiostat for poultry, $C_{20}H_{23}NO_5$.

cyproterone acetate (si-pro′ter-ōn) chemical name: 6-chloro-1β,2β -dihydro-17- hydroxy-3′*H* -cyclopropa[1,2]pregna-1,4,6-triene-3,20-dione acetate. A synthetic antiandrogenic steroid, C_{24}-

$H_{29}ClO_4$, which has been used in the treatment of male sexual disorders.

cyrtograph (sir'to-graf) [Gr. *kyrtos* bent + *graphein* to write] a cyrtometer that registers the movements of the chest wall.

cyrtometer (sir-tom'ĕ-ter) [Gr. *kyrtos* bent + *metron* measure] a device for use in measuring the curves and curved surfaces of the body.

cyrtosis (sir-to'sis) [Gr. *kyrtōsis*] 1. kyphosis. 2. distortion of the bones.

Cys cysteine.

Cys-Cys cystine.

cyst (sist) [Gr. *kystis* sac, bladder] 1. any closed cavity or sac, normal or abnormal, lined by epithelium, and especially one that contains a liquid or semisolid material. 2. a stage in the life cycle of certain parasites, during which they are enclosed within a protective wall; see, for example, *hydatid c.* and *multilocular c.* **adventitious c.,** a cyst formed about a foreign body or an exudate; called also *false c.* **allantoic c.,** urachal c. **alveolar c's,** dilatations of pulmonary alveoli, which may fuse by breakdown of their septa to form large air cysts (pneumatoceles). **alveolar hydatid c.,** a hydatid cyst formed by the larvae of the tapeworm *Echinococcus multilocularis;* see *hydatid disease, alveolar,* under *disease.* **amnionic c.,** cystlike processes containing amniotic fluid resulting from adhesion of amnionic folds. **aneurysmal bone c.,** a solitary lesion of bone that typically causes a bulging of the overlying cortex bearing some resemblance to the saccular protrusion of the aortic wall in aortic aneurysm. **angioblastic c.,** an ingrowth of the mesenchymal tissue having blood-forming power in an embryo. **apical c.,** an epithelium-lined cyst in the bone at the apex of a tooth with an infected or devitalized pulp. **apoplectic c.,** a cyst formed in a part by extravasation of blood. **arachnoid c.,** a fluid-filled cyst between the layers of the leptomeninges, lined with arachnoid membrane, most commonly occurring in the sylvian fissure; called also *leptomeningeal c.* **atheromatous c.,** keratin cyst, called also *sebaceous cyst.* **Baker's c.,** a swelling behind the knee, caused by escape of synovial fluid which has become enclosed in a sac of membrane; popliteal bursitis; synovial cyst of the popliteal space. **Blessig's c's,** cystic spaces that frequently appear at the periphery of the retina close to the ora serrata without significant effect on vision; called also *Blessig's lacunae, Blessig's spaces, cystoid degeneration,* and *Iwanoff's c's.* **blood c.,** a cyst containing extravasated blood. **blue dome c.,** a benign retention cyst of the breast containing straw-colored fluid that shows a blue color when unopened; see *cystic disease of breast,* under *disease.* **Boyer's c.,** a painless and gradual enlargement of the subhyoid bursa. **branchial c., branchial cleft c., branchiogenetic c., branchiogenous c.,** a cyst arising in the lateral aspect of the neck, from epithelial remnants of a branchial cleft, usually located between the second and third branchial arches. **bronchial c's,** bronchogenic c. **bronchogenic c.,** a spherical cyst of bronchial origin lined with bronchial epithelium which may contain secretory elements, generally found in the mediastinum or the lung. It may contain air, and if communication with the trachea or a bronchus exists, may periodically evacuate fluid contents into the air passages, resulting in attacks of voluminous expectoration. Infection will lead to mediastinal or pulmonary abscess. Called also *bronchial c.* **bronchopulmonary c.,** bronchogenic cyst of the lung. **bursal c.,** a cyst derived from a serous bursa. **butter c.,** 1. a necrotic mass in a lipoma. 2. a retention cyst of the mammary gland filled with the products of the alteration of milk, such as butyric acid. **cervical c.,** a branchial or thyroglossal cyst. **chocolate c.,** one having dark, syrupy contents, resulting from collection of hemosiderin following local hemorrhage, such as sometimes occurs after mastectomy or in the ovary in ovarian endometriosis; called also *endometrial c.* and *Sampson's c.* **choledochal c.,** a congenital cystic dilatation of the common bile duct which may cause pain in the right upper quadrant, jaundice, fever, or vomiting, or be asymptomatic. **choledochus c.,** a dilatation of the lower end of the common bile duct, usually recognized during childhood. **chyle c.,** an abnormal sac of the mesentery containing chyle. **ciliated epithelial c.,** a cyst lined with ciliated epithelium; they occur in the gastrointestinal tract (enterocystoma), in the hair, thorax, lung, and genital organs. **colloid c.,** a cyst that contains jelly-like material, particularly in the third ventricle. **compound c.,** multilocular c. **corpus luteum c.,** a cyst of the ovary formed by a serous accumulation developed from a corpus luteum. **craniobuccal c.,** a cyst of Rathke's pouch. **craniopharyngeal duct c.,** cysts originating in the vestiges of the craniopharyngeal duct; they are closely related to craniopharyngiomas. **cutaneous c., cuticular c.,** a cyst of the skin. **daughter c.,** a small parasitic cyst developed from the wall of a larger one, as from the hydatid cyst of the tapeworm *Echinococcus granulosus;* called also *secondary c.* **dental c.,** one derived from some portion of the odontogenic apparatus. **dentigerous c.,** an odontogenic cyst surrounding the coronal portion of a tooth and originating after the crown is completely formed. **dermoid c.,** a teratoma, usually benign, representing a disorder of embryologic development, characterized by the presence of mature

ectodermal elements, consisting of a fibrous wall lined with stratified epithelium, and containing a keratinous material and hair and sometimes other elements, such as bone, tooth, and nerve tissue; they are most often found in the ovary, but also commonly occur in the skin of the head and neck. Called also *benign cystic teratoma, cystic teratoma, mature teratoma,* and *dermoid.* See also *malignant teratoma.* **dilatation c.,** a cyst formed by dilation of a previously existing cavity. **distention c.,** a collection of watery fluid in a normal, but distended cavity. **echinococcus c.,** hydatid c. **endometrial c.,** a chocolate cyst, particularly in the ovary, lined with endometrium. **endothelial c.,** a cyst whose sac has an endothelial lining. **enteric c., enterogenous c.,** a cyst of the intestine arising or developing from some fold or pouch along the intestinal tract. **ependymal c.,** a circumscribed dilatation of some part of the ependyma. **epidermal c., epidermal inclusion c., epidermoid c.,** an epithelial cyst of the skin due to proliferation of surface epidermal cells within the corium, arising from occluded pilosebaceous follicles and containing a laminated, cheesy, odoriferous keratinous material. Called also *sebaceous c.* and *wen.* See also *pilar c.* **epithelial c.,** 1. any cyst lined by keratinizing stratified squamous epithelium, found most often in the skin, and including epidermal, pilar, and dermoid cysts, milia, and steatomas. 2. epidermal c. **eruption c.,** a dentigerous cyst that causes a clinically evident bulging of the overlying alveolar ridge. **extravasation c.,** a cyst formed by hemorrhage into the tissues. **exudation c.,** a cyst formed by an exudate collected in a closed cavity. **false c.,** an adventitious cyst. **fissural c.,** one arising along a line of fusion of the various embryonic processes; according to location, those of the oral region are classified as median palatal, median anterior maxillary, globulomaxillary, and nasoalveolar. **follicular c.,** one due to the occlusion of the duct of a follicle or small gland; especially a cyst formed by the enlargement of a graafian follicle as a result of accumulated transudate. **ganglionic c.,** subchondral c. **Gartner's c., gartnerian c.,** a cystic tumor developed from Gartner's duct (ductus epoophori longitudinalis [NA]). **gas c.,** a small cyst filled with gas, of bacterial origin. **globulomaxillary c.,** a cyst occurring within the maxilla at the junction of the globular portion of the medial nasal process and the maxillary process, usually between the lateral incisor and the canine tooth. **granddaughter c.,** a cyst sometimes seen within a daughter cyst (q.v.). **hemorrhagic c.,** an encapsulated mass of extravasated blood. **hydatid c.,** the larval cyst stage of the tapeworms *Echinococcus granulosus,* and *E. multilocularis,* which contains daughter cysts, each of which contains many scoleces; called also *echinococcus c.* and *hydatid.* See *hydatid disease, unilocular,* under *disease.* **implantation c.,** a cyst formed from a piece of skin that has become implanted into the deep tissues. **incisive canal c.,** median anterior maxillary c. **inclusion c.,** one formed by the inclusion of a small portion of epithelium or mesothelium within connective tissue. **intraepithelial c's,** round or oval cavities which develop in the epithelium of the ureter, bladder, and urethra and contain a peculiar colloid substance. **intraluminal c's,** duplications of the bowel, or retention cysts, which are an infrequent cause of intrinsic obstruction in the newborn. **intrapituitary c's,** Rathke's c's. **involution c.,** mammary duct ectasia. **iodine c.,** see *Iodamoeba buetschlii.* **Iwanoff's c's,** Blessig's c's. **keratinizing c., keratinous c.,** any cyst containing keratinous material; see *epithelial c.* **lacteal c.,** a cyst of the breast due to obstruction of a lactiferous duct; called also *milk c.* **lateral c.,** a periodontal cyst along the lateral surface of the root of a tooth. **leptomeningeal c.,** arachnoid c. **lutein c.,** a cyst of the ovary developed from a corpus luteum. **median anterior maxillary c.,** a cyst in or near the incisive canal, arising from proliferation of epithelial remnants of the nasopalatine duct; called also *incisive canal c.* and *nasopalatine duct c.* **median mandibular c.,** a very rare cyst occurring in the midline of mandible, of disputed origin. **median palatal c.,** one located in the midline of the hard palate, between the lateral palatal processes. **meibomian c.,** a cyst of the meibomian gland, sometimes applied to a chalazion. **mesenteric c.,** a congenital thin-walled cyst of the abdomen between the leaves of the mesentery, which may be of wolffian or lymphatic duct origin; as it enlarges, it may cause colicky pain and intestinal obstruction. **milk c.,** lacteal c. **morgagnian c.,** hydatid of Morgagni. **mother c.,** a cyst enclosing other cysts, as in the cyst stage of *Echinococcus granulosus.* **mucous c.,** a retention cyst that contains mucus. **multilocular c.,** a cyst containing several loculi or spaces; a hydatid cyst composed of many small irregular cavities, which may contain scoleces but generally little fluid, and which tend to enlarge by budding since they have a poorly developed hyaline cuticle, as in *Echinococcus multilocularis;* called also *alveolar c.* **myxoid c.,** a nodular lesion usually overlying a distal interphalangeal finger joint in the dorsolateral or dorsomesial position, consisting of focal mucinous degeneration of the collagen of the dermis; not a true cyst, lacking an epithelial wall, it does not communicate with the underlying synovial space. Called also *synovial c.* and *synovial ganglion.* **Naboth's c's, nabothian c's,** Naboth's follicles. **nasoalveolar c.,** a fissural cyst arising outside the bones at the junction of the globular portion of the medial nasal process, the lateral nasal process, and the maxillary process, sometimes secondarily involving the maxilla; called also *nasolabial c.* **nasolabial c.,** nasoalveolar c. **nasopalatine duct c.,** median anterior maxillary c. **necrotic c.,** a cyst containing necrotic matter. **neural c.,** a cyst or cystlike structure occurring in the central nervous system, as a soapsuds cyst or a porencephalic cyst. **neurenteric c.,** a cyst of the posterior mediastinum containing tissues from the nervous system and other organs, and connecting with the spinal dura mater. **nevoid c.,** an abnormal cyst with vascular walls. **odontogenic c.,** any cyst derived from odontogenic epithelium and therefore found exclusively in the jaws; primordial, dentigerous, and periodontal cysts fall into this classification. **oil c.,** a cyst containing oily matter, due to fatty degeneration of the epithelial lining. **omental c's,** cysts similar in all respects to mesenteric ones except that they are confined to the omentum. **oophoritic c.,** a cyst of the ovary proper. **osseous hydatid c's,** hydatid cysts formed by the larvae of *Echinococcus granulosus* and occurring in bone, which may become weakened and eroded by the exuberant growth. **pancreatic c.,** a retention cyst of the pancreatic duct; called also *pancreatic ranula.* Cf. *pancreatic pseudocyst.* **paranephric c.,** a cyst of the fatty tissue surrounding the kidney. **parapyelitic c's,** apparently congenital cysts of uncertain etiology occurring in the kidney sinus, usually in a small cluster, and causing pelvic compression and local deformity, with pain, hematuria, infection, and pyuria. **parasitic c.,** a cyst formed by the larva of a parasite, such as a hydatid cyst. **parent c.,** a mother cyst. **parovarian c.,** a cyst of the epoophoron. **pearl c.,** a cyst or a solid mass of epithelial cells in the iris caused by implantation of an eyelash, cotton, or other foreign particle. **pericardial c.,** a benign tumor containing clear fluid, almost always located immediately adjacent to the pericardium; such cysts must be differentiated from the more serious mediastinal tumors. **periodontal c.,** a cyst occurring adjacent to a tooth root, either apical or lateral. **periodontal c., apical,** radicular c. **pilar c.,** an epithelial cyst clinically indistinguishable from an epidermal cyst, almost always found on the scalp, and arising from the outer root sheath of the hair follicle. Called also *sebaceous c., tricholemmal c.,* and *wen.* **piliferous c., pilonidal c.,** a hair-containing sacrococcygeal dermoid cyst or sinus which often opens at a postanal dimple. Cf. *coccygeal sinus,* under *sinus.* **placental c.,** a grayish white, disklike cyst of the placenta, resulting from degeneration of trophoblastic cells. **porencephalic c.,** a cyst occurring in the brain substance in porencephaly. **preauricular c., congenital,** a cyst resulting from imperfect fusion of the first and second branchial arches in formation of the auricle, communicating with a pitlike depression just in front of the helix and above the tragus (ear pit). **primordial c.,** a rare type of odontogenic cyst developing before calcified enamel or dentin is formed, and found in place of a tooth. **proliferous c.** (*obs.*), multilocular c. **proligerous c.** (*obs.*), cystadenocarcinoma. **pseudomucinous c.,** see under *cystadenoma.* **psorospermal c's,** sarcosporidian cysts. **pyelogenic renal c.,** calyceal diverticulum. **radicular c.,** an epithelium-lined sac, which may contain cholesterol, at the apex of a tooth; called also *apical periodontal c., radiculodental c.,* and *root c.* **radiculodental c.,** radicular c. **Rathke's c's,** groups of epithelial cells forming small colloid-filled cysts in the pars intermedia of the pituitary gland. **residual c.,** a cyst in the maxilla or mandible which remains or forms after the tooth with which it was once associated has been removed. **retention c.,** one caused by retention of glandular secretion. **root c.,** radicular c. **Sampson's c.,** chocolate c. **sanguineous c.,** a cyst containing blood. **sarcosporidian c's,** cylindrical cysts containing banana-shaped spores of the parasites, found in the muscles of those infected with the protozoan *Sarcocystis,* and which may become large enough to be grossly visible. Called also *sarcocysts, Miescher's tubules,* and *Rainey's corpuscles.* **sebaceous c.,** 1. epidermal c. 2. pilar c. **secondary c.,** a daughter cyst. **secretory c.,** a cyst produced by retention of the normal secretion of a gland. **seminal c.,** a cyst containing semen. **serous c.,** a cyst containing a thin liquid or serum. **soap c.,** a collection of yellow fatty matter encysted in the breast. **soapsuds c's,** cysts that stud the cerebral cortex in cryptococcosis. **solitary bone c.,** a pathologic bone space in the metaphyses of long bones of growing children; of disputed origin, it may be either empty or filled with fluid and have a delicate connective tissue lining. **springwater c.,** pericardial c. **sterile c.,** a true hydatid cyst that fails to produce brood capsules; called also *acephalocyst.* **subchondral c.,** a bone cyst within the fused epiphysis beneath the articular plate; it is lined with a membrane (probably modified synovia) which contains a mucinous material. Called also *ganglionic c.* **sublingual c.,** ranula. **subsynovial c.,** one caused by the distention of a synovial follicle. **suprasellar c.,** craniopharyngioma. **synovial c.,** myxoid c. **tarry c.,** 1. a corpus luteum cyst resulting from hemorrhage into a corpus luteum. 2. a bloody cyst resulting from endometriosis. **tarsal c.,** a cyst in the tarsus of the lid, sometimes applied to a chalazion. **thecal c.,** distention of a sheath of a tendon. **theca-lutein c.,** a cyst of the ovary in which the lutein cells lining the cystic cavity are theca interna cells. **thymic c's,** rare unilocular or multilocular cysts of the upper anterior mediastinum containing tissue resembling that of the thymus; they are congenital in origin. **thyroglossal c., thyrolingual c.,** a cyst in the neck caused by persistence of portions of, or by lack of closure of, the primitive thyroglossal duct. **Tornwaldt's c.,** bursa pharyngea. **trichilemmal c.,** pilar c. **true c.,** any cyst that is not a normal structure and not formed by the dilatation of a passage or cavity. **tubular c.,** tubulocyst. **umbilical c.,** vitellointestinal c. **unicameral c.,** unilocular c. **unicameral bone c.,** solitary bone c. **unilocular c.,** a cyst containing but one cavity. Cf. *multilocular c.* **urachal c.,** a form of cystic dilatation of the urachus; called also *allontoic c.* **urinary c.,** a cyst containing urine. **vitelline c.,** a congenital cyst lined with ciliated epithelium occurring along the gastrointestinal canal; the remains of the omphalomesenteric duct. Called also *enterocystoma.* **vitellointestinal c.,** a cystlike tumor at the umbilicus, caused by persistence of a portion of the umbilical duct; called also *umbilical c.* **wolffian c.,** a cyst of the broad ligaments of the uterus, regarded as developed from vestiges of the wolffian body (mesonephros).

cyst- see *cysto-.*

cystadenocarcinoma (sis-tad″e-no-kar″si-no′mah) carcinoma and cystadenoma.

cystadenoma (sis″tad-e-no′mah) [*cyst-* + *adenoma*] adenoma associated with cystoma. **c. adamanti′num,** ameloblastoma. **mucinous c.,** a multilocular tumor produced by the epithelial cells of the ovary and having mucin-filled cavities; the great majority of these tumors are benign. **papillary c.,** any tumor producing patterns which are both papillary and cystic. **papillary c. lymphomato′sum,** papillary adenocystoma lymphomatosum. **c. par′tim sim′plex par′tim papillif′erum** (*obs.*), papillary cystadenoma. **pseudomucinous c.,** mucinous c.; so called because the cavity contents were thought to be pseudomucin. **serous c.,** a cystic tumor of the ovary, containing thin, clear, yellow serous fluid and varying amounts of solid tissue, with a malignant potential several times greater than that of mucinous cystadenoma.

cystadenosarcoma (sis-tad″e-no-sar-ko′mah) (*obs.*) cystadenoma blended with sarcoma.

cystalgia (sis-tal′je-ah) [*cyst-* + *-algia*] pain in the bladder.

cystathionase (sis″tah-thi′o-nās) cystathionine γ-lyase. **β-c.,** cystathionine β-lyase. **γ-c.,** cystathionine γ-lyase.

cystathionine (sis″tah-thi′o-nīn) an unsymmetrical thio-ether of homocysteine and serine, $COOH \cdot CH(NH_2) \cdot CH_2 \cdot CH_2 \cdot S \cdot CH_2 \cdot CH(NH_2) \cdot COOH$, which serves as an intermediate in the transfer of a sulfur atom from methionine to cysteine. **c. β-lyase,** a pyridoxal-phosphate enzyme that catalyzes the hydrolysis of cystathionine to pyruvate, ammonia, and homocysteine. Called also *β-cystathionase.* **c. γ-lyase,** a pyridoxal-phosphate enzyme that catalyzes the hydrolysis of cystathionine to cysteine, ammonia, and 2-oxobutyrate. It also catalyzes the conversion of (*a*) homoserine to 2-oxobutyrate, H_2O, and ammonia, (*b*) cystine to thiocysteine, pyruvate, and ammonia, and (*c*) cysteine to pyruvate ammonia, and hydrogen sulfide. Called also *cystathionase* and *γ-cystathionase.*

cystathioninuria (sis″tah-thi″o-nīn-u′re-ah) a hereditary disorder of cystathionine metabolism marked by increased concentrations of cystathionine in the urine, due to deficiency of γ-cystathionase; mental retardation is associated in some instances.

cystatrophia (sis″tah-tro′fe-ah) [*cyst-* + Gr. *atrophia* atrophy] atrophy of the bladder.

cystauchenitis (sis″taw-kĕ-ni′tis) [*cyst* + Gr. *auchēn* neck + *-itis*] inflammation of the neck of the bladder.

cystauchenotomy (sis″taw-kĕ-not′o-me) [*cyst-* + Gr. *auchēn* neck + *tomē* cut] surgical incision of the neck of the bladder.

cystauxe (sis′tauk-se) enlargement of the bladder.

cystectasia, cystectasy (sis-tek-ta′ze-ah; sis-tek′tah-se) [*cyst-* + Gr. *ektasis* dilatation] slitting of the membranous portion of the urethra and dilatation of the neck of the bladder for the extraction of stone.

cystectomy (sis-tek′to-me) [*cyst-* + Gr. *ektomē* excision] 1. excision of a cyst. 2. excision of the bladder (*complete* or *total c.*) or resection of the bladder (*partial c.*).

cysteine (sis-te′in) chemical name: 2-amino-3-mercaptopropionic acid. A sulfur-containing amino acid produced by the enzymatic or acid hydrolysis of proteins. It is easily oxidized to cystine, is sometimes found in the urine, and has limited detoxification properties. Called also *thioaminopropionic acid.* **c. hydrochloride,** a compound suggested for the treatment of cutaneous ulcers.

cystelcosis (sis″tel-ko′sis) [*cyst-* + Gr. *helkōsis* ulceration] ulceration of the bladder.

cystencephalus (sis″ten-sef′ah-lus) [*cyst-* + Gr. *enkephalos* brain] a monster with a membranous sac in place of a brain.

cystendesis (sis″ten-de′sis) [*cyst-* + Gr. *endesis* suturation] suture of a wound of the gallbladder or of the urinary bladder.

cysterethism (sis-ter′e-thizm) [*cyst-* + Gr. *erethismos* irritation] irritability of the bladder.

cysthypersarcosis (sist-hi″per-sar-ko′sis) [*cyst-* + Gr. *hyper* over + *sarkōsis* growth of flesh]   a thickening of the muscular coat of the bladder.

cysti-   see *cysto-*.

cystic (sis′tik) [Gr. *kystis* bladder]   1. pertaining to a cyst.   2. pertaining to the urinary bladder or to the gallbladder.

cysticerci (sis″tĭ-ser′si)   plural of *cysticercus*.

cysticercoid (sis″tĭ-ser′koid)   a form of larval tapeworm resembling *Cysticercus*, but having the cyst small, almost devoid of fluid, and provided with a caudal appendage, as in *Hymenolepis*.

cysticercosis (sis″tĭ-ser-ko′sis)   infection with cystercerci. In man, it is an infection with the larval forms (*Cysticercus cellulosae*) of *Taenia solium*, which penetrate the intestinal wall and invade such tissues as the subcutaneous tissue, brain, eye, muscle, heart, liver, lung, and peritoneum. Brain involvement may result in epilepsy, increased intracranial pressure, etc.

Cysticercus (sis″tĭ-ser′kus) [Gr. *kystis* bladder + *kerkos* tail]   a former genus of larval forms of tapeworms, with such species names as *C. acantho′trias, C. bo′vis* (beef tapeworm), *C. cellulo′sae* (pork tapeworm), *C. fasciola′ris, C. o′vis,* and *C. tenuicollis.* **C. bo′vis,** the larva of *Taenia saginata.* **C. cellulo′sae,** the larva of *Taenia solium;* see also *cysticercosis.* **C. o′vis,** the larva of *Taenia ovis.* **C. tenuicol′lis,** the larva of *Taenia hydatigena.*

cysticercus (sis″tĭ-ser′kus)   pl *cysticer′ci.*   a larval form of tapeworm, consisting of a single scolex enclosed in a bladder-like cyst; cf. *hydatid cyst,* under *cyst.*

cysticolithectomy (sis″tĭ-ko″lĭ-thek′to-me) [Gr. *kystis* bladder + *lithos* stone + *ektomē* excision]   removal of a stone from the cystic duct.

cysticolithotripsy (sis″tĭ-ko-lith′o-trip-se)   crushing of a calculus within the cystic duct.

cysticorrhaphy (sis″tĭ-kor′ah-fe) [*cystic duct* + *rhaphē* suture]   suture or repair of the cystic duct.

cysticotomy (sis″tĭ-kot′o-me) [*cystic duct* + Gr. *tomē* a cutting]   incision into the cystic duct.

cystides (sis′tĭ-dēz)   plural of *cystis.*

cystido-   see *cysto-*.

cystidoceliotomy (sis″tĭ-do-se″le-ot′o-me)   cystidolaparotomy.

cystidolaparotomy (sis″tĭ-do-lap″ah-rot′o-me) [*cystido-* + *laparotomy*]   incision of the bladder through the abdominal wall; called also *cystidoceliotomy.*

cystidotrachelotomy (sis″tĭ-do-tra-kel-ot′o-me) [*cystido-* + Gr. *trachēlos* neck + *tomē* a cutting]   incision of the neck of the bladder.

cystifellotomy (sis″tĭ-fel-lot′o-me) [*cysti-* + L. *fel* bile + Gr. *tomē* a cutting]   cholecystotomy.

cystiferous (sis-tif′er-us)   cystigerous.

cystiform (sis′tĭ-form) [*cysti-* + L. *forma* form]   having the form or appearance of a cyst.

cystigerous (sis-tij′er-us) [*cysti-* + L. *gerere* to bear]   containing cysts.

cystine (sis′tēn, sis′tin)   chemical name: 3,3′-dithiobis (2-aminopropanoic acid). An amino acid, $[S \cdot CH_2 \cdot CH(NH_2) \cdot COOH]_2$, produced by the digestion or acid hydrolysis of proteins. It is sometimes found in the urine and in the kidneys in the form of minute hexagonal crystals, frequently forming a cystine calculus in the bladder. Cystine is the chief sulfur-containing compound of the protein molecule, and is readily reduced to two molecules of cysteine (hence, also called *dicysteine*).

cystinemia (sis′tĭ-ne′me-ah) [*cystine* + Gr. *haima* blood + *-ia*]   presence of cystine in the blood.

cystinosis (sis″tĭ-no′sis) [*cystine* + *-osis*]   a hereditary disorder of childhood, usually appearing after 6 months of age, marked by osteomalacia, aminoaciduria, phosphaturia, and deposition of cystine throughout the tissues of the body, including the liver, bone marrow, spleen, and cornea. As the most common cause of Fanconi's syndrome (def. 2), cystinosis is associated with proximal renal tubular dysfunction and with stunting of growth, vitamin D–resistant rickets, acidosis, and corneal opacities. Called also *cystine storage disease* and *Lignac-Fanconi s.*

cystinuria (sis″tĭ-nu′re-ah) [*cystine* + *urine*]   a hereditary condition of persistent excessive urinary excretion of cystine and three other dibasic amino acids: lysine, ornithine, and arginine; it is due to impairment of renal transport in tubular reabsorption of these amino acids. The predominant clinical manifestation is the formation of urinary cystine calculi.

cystinuric (sis″tĭ-nu′rik)   pertaining to or affected with cystinuria.

cystirrhagia (sis″tĭ-ra′je-ah)   cystorrhagia.

cystirrhea (sis″tĭ-re′ah)   cystorrhea.

cystis (sis′tis), pl. *cys′tides* [Gr. *kystis*]   a pouch or sac; a cyst. **c. fel′lea,** gallbladder.

cystistaxis (sis″tĭ-stak′sis) [*cysti-* + Gr. *staxis* dripping]   oozing of blood from the mucous membrane into the bladder.

cystitis (sis-ti′tis)   inflammation of the urinary bladder. **aller-** gic c., cystitis resulting from some unusual hypersensitivity, characterized by a large number of mononuclear leukocytes and eosinophils in the bladder mucosa and musculature, and in the urinary sediment. **bacterial c.,** bacterial infection of the bladder. **catarrhal c., acute,** cystitis resulting from injury, irritation by foreign bodies, gonorrhea, etc., and marked by burning in the bladder, pain in the urethra, and painful micturition. **c. col′li,** inflammation involving the neck of the bladder. **croupous c.,** diphtheritic c. **cystic c., c. cys′tica,** cystitis with the formation of multiple submucosal cysts in the bladder wall. **diphtheritic c.,** cystitis due to infection by *Corynebacterium diphtheriae,* and characterized by the formation of a false membrane; called also *croupous c.* **c. emphysemato′sa,** an unusual inflammation of the bladder, characterized by the presence of gas-filled vesicles and cysts in the bladder mucosa and musculature. **eosinophilic c.,** cystitis characterized by the presence of large numbers of eosinophils in the urinary sediment. **exfoliative c.,** cystitis with sloughing of the bladder mucosa. **c. follicula′ris,** cystitis in which the mucosa of the bladder is studded with nodules containing lymph follicles. **c. glandula′ris,** cystitis in which the mucosa contains mucin-secreting glands, observed more frequently in cases of exstrophy of the bladder, and sometimes leading to malignant degeneration. **incrusted c.,** an intense cystitis characterized by deposition of phosphatic or other inorganic salts on the chronically inflamed bladder wall, generally at the site of ulcerations, granulations, or tumors. **interstitial c., chronic,** a condition of the bladder occurring predominantly in women, with an inflammatory lesion, usually in the vertex, and involving the entire thickness of the wall, appearing as a small patch of brownish red mucosa, surrounded by a network of radiating vessels. The lesions, known as Fenwick-Hunner or Hunner ulcers, may heal superficially, and are notoriously difficult to detect. Typically, there is urinary frequency and pain on bladder filling and at the end of micturition. Called also *panmural c., submucous c.,* and *panmural fibrosis of the bladder.* **mechanical c.,** cystitis resulting from irritation by a vesical calculus, manipulation, or a foreign body in the bladder. **panmural c.,** interstitial c., chronic. **c. papillomato′sa,** cystitis characterized by the presence of papillomatous growths on the inflamed mucous membrane. **c. seni′lis femina′rum,** a chronic cystitis occurring in elderly women, marked by abnormal frequency of micturition, with tenesmus and burning. **submucous c.,** interstitial c., chronic.

cystitome (sis′tĭ-tōm) [*cysti-* + Gr. *temnein* to cut]   an instrument for opening the capsule of the lens of the eye; called also *kibisitome.*

cystitomy (sis-tit′o-me) [*cysti-* + Gr. *tomē* a cut]   the surgical division of the capsule of the lens; capsulotomy.

cysto-, cyst-, cysti-, cystido- [Gr. *kystis, kystides* a sac or bladder]   combining form denoting a relationship to a sac, cyst, or bladder, most frequently used in reference to the urinary bladder.

cystoadenoma (sis″to-ad″e-no′mah)   cystadenoma.

cystoblast (sis′to-blast) [*cysto-* + Gr. *blastos* germ]   the layer of cells that lines the amniotic cavity of the early embryo on the side of the enveloping layer.

cystocarcinoma (sis″to-kar″sĭ-no′mah)   carcinoma associated with cysts.

cystocele (sis′to-sēl) [*cysto-* + Gr. *kēlē* hernia]   hernial protrusion of the urinary bladder through the vaginal wall; called also *cystic hernia.*

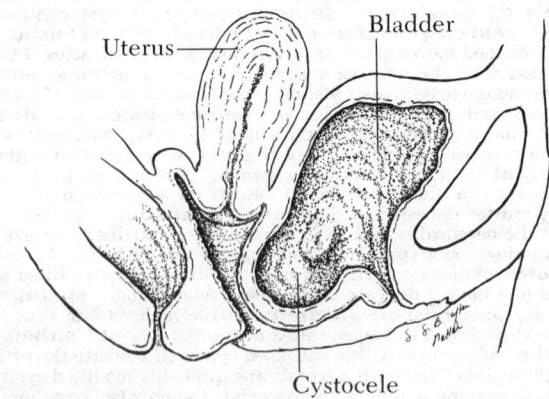

Uterus — Bladder
Cystocele

cystochrome (sis′to-krōm) [*cysto-* + Gr. *chrōma* color]   a mixture of indigo carmine and methenamine; used by intramuscular or intravenous injection for the indigo carmine test of renal function.

cystochromoscopy (sis″to-kro-mos′ko-pe)   chromocystoscopy.

cystocolostomy (sis″to-ko-los′to-me) [*cysto-* + *colostomy*]   the surgical creation of a permanent passage from the bladder to the colon.

Cysto-Conray (sis″to-kon′ra) trademark for preparations of iothalamate meglumine.

cystodiaphanoscopy (sis″to-di″ah-fah-nos′ko-pe) [*cysto-* + *diaphanoscopy*] examination within, or transillumination of, the urinary bladder by means of a diaphanoscope.

cystoduodenostomy (sist″o-du-od″ĕ-nos′to-me) internal drainage of an adjacent cyst into the duodenum.

cystodynia (sis″to-din′e-ah) [*cysto-* + Gr. *odynē* pain] pain in the urinary bladder.

cystoelytroplasty (sis″to-e-lit′ro-plas″te) [*cysto-* + Gr. *elytron* sheath + *plassein* to form] surgical repair of vesicovaginal injuries.

cystoenterocele (sis″to-en′ter-o-sēl) hernia of a portion of the bladder and of the intestine.

cystoepiplocele (sis″to-e-pip′lo-sēl) hernia of a portion of the bladder and of the omentum.

cystoepithelioma (sis″to-ep″ĭ-the″le-o′mah) a tumor containing cystic and epitheliomatous elements.

cystofibroma (sis″to-fi-bro′mah) [L.] fibroma containing cysts.

cystogastrostomy (sis″to-gas-tros′to-me) surgical anastomosis of an adjacent cyst to the stomach.

Cystografin (sis″to-graf′in) trademark for a preparation of diatrizoate meglumine.

cystogram (sis′to-gram) a roentgenogram of the bladder.

cystography (sis-tog′rah-fe) [*cysto-* + Gr. *graphein* to write] roentgenography of the bladder after injection of the organ with opaque solution. **delayed c.**, cystography in which film exposures are made at varying intervals up to 30 minutes or longer; useful in the study of urinary reflux. **voiding c.**, radiography of the bladder while the patient is urinating.

cystoid (sis′toid) [*cysto-* + Gr. *eidos* form] 1. resembling a cyst. 2. a cystlike, circumscribed collection of softened material, differing from a true cyst in having no enclosing capsule.

cystojejunostomy (sis″to-je-ju-nos′to-me) surgical anastomosis of an adjacent cyst to the jejunum.

cystolith (sis′to-lith) [*cysto-* + Gr. *lithos* stone] a vesical calculus.

cystolithectomy (sis″to-lĭ-thek′to-me) [*cysto-* + Gr. *lithos* stone + *ektomē* excision] the removal of a calculus by cutting into the urinary bladder. The term has been used erroneously for excision of a gallstone from the gallbladder.

cystolithiasis (sis″to-lĭ-thi′ah-sis) [*cysto-* + Gr. *lithos* stone] the development of calculi in the urinary bladder.

cystolithic (sis″to-lith′ik) pertaining to vesical calculi.

cystolithotomy (sis″to-lĭ-thot′o-me) cystolithectomy.

cystolutein (sis″to-lu″te-in) [*cysto-* + L. *luteus* yellow] a yellow pigment from certain ovarian cysts.

cystoma (sis-to′mah) [*cysto-* + *-oma*] a tumor containing cysts of neoplastic origin; a cystic tumor. **myxoid c.** (*obs.*), mucinous cystadenoma. **c. sero′sum sim′plex**, simple cyst of the ovary.

cystomatitis (sis″to-mah-ti′tis) inflammation of one or more of the cysts of a cystoma.

cystomatous (sis-to′mah-tus) relating to or containing cystoma.

cystometer (sis-tom′ĕ-ter) [*cysto-* + Gr. *metron* measure] an instrument for studying the neuromuscular mechanism of the bladder by means of measurements of pressure and capacity.

cystometrogram (sis″to-met′ro-gram) the tracing recorded by cystometrography.

cystometrography (sis″to-mĕ-trog′rah-fe) the graphic recording of the pressure exerted at varying degrees of filling of the urinary bladder.

cystometry (sis-tom′ĕ-tre) the study of bladder efficiency by means of the cystometer.

Cystomonas (sis-tom′o-nas) *Bodo.*

cystomorphous (sis″to-mor′fus) [*cysto-* + Gr. *morphē* form] shaped like a cyst or bladder.

cystomyoma (sis″to-mi-o′mah) (*obs.*) myoma with cystic degeneration.

cystomyxoadenoma (sis″to-mik″so-ad″e-no′mah) (*obs.*) adenomyoma with cystic degeneration.

cystomyxoma (sis″to-mik-so′mah) (*obs.*) mucinous cystadenoma.

cystonephrosis (sis″to-nĕ-fro′sis) [*cysto-* + Gr. *nephros* kidney] cystiform dilatation or enlargement of the kidney.

cystoneuralgia (sis″to-nu-ral′je-ah) [*cysto-* + *neuralgia*] neuralgia of the bladder.

cystoparalysis (sis″to-pah-ral-ĭ-sis) cystoplegia.

cystopexy (sis″to-pek′se) [*cysto-* + Gr. *pēxis* fixation] fixation of the bladder to the abdominal wall in the treatment of cystocele; vesicofixation.

cystophorous (sis-tof′o-rus) [*cysto-* + Gr. *phoros* bearing] containing cysts.

cystophotography (sis″to-fo-tog′rah-fe) the photographing of the inside of the bladder.

cystophthisis (sis-tof′thĭ-sis) [*cysto-* + Gr. *phthisis* consumption] tuberculosis of the bladder.

cystoplasty (sis′to-plas″te) [*cysto-* + Gr. *plassein* to mold] any plastic or reconstructive operation on the bladder. **augmentation c.**, enlargement of the bladder by grafting to it a detached segment of intestine (ileum, cecum, or sigmoid).

cystoplegia (sis″to-ple′je-ah) [*cysto-* + Gr. *plēgē* stroke] paralysis of the bladder; called also *cystoparalysis.*

cystoproctostomy (sis″to-prok-tos′to-me) [*cysto-* + Gr. *proktos* rectum + *stomoun* to provide with an opening, or mouth] the surgical creation of a communication between the urinary bladder and rectum; called also *cystorectostomy.*

cystoptosis (sis″top-to′sis) [*cysto-* + Gr. *ptōsis* a falling] prolapse of a part of the inner coat of the bladder into the urethra.

cystopyelitis (sis″to-pi-e-li′tis) inflammation involving both the urinary bladder and the pelvis of the kidney.

cystopyelography (sis″to-pi″ĕ-log′rah-fe) roentgenography of the urinary bladder and the pelvis of the kidney.

cystopyelonephritis (sis″to-pi″e-lo-ne-fri′tis) [*cysto-* + Gr. *pyelos* pelvis + *nephros* kidney + *-itis*] combined cystitis and pyelonephritis.

cystoradiography (sis″to-ra″de-og′rah-fe) [*cysto-* + *radiography*] radiography of the bladder.

cystorectostomy (sis″to-rek-tos′to-me) cystoproctostomy.

cystorrhagia (sis″to-ra′je-ah) [*cysto-* + Gr. *rhēg-nynai* to burst forth] hemorrhage from the bladder.

cystorrhaphy (sis-tor′ah-fe) [*cysto-* + Gr. *rhaphē* suture] the operation of suturing the bladder.

cystorrhea (sis″to-re′ah) [*cysto-* + Gr. *rhoia* flow] catarrh of the bladder.

cystosarcoma (sis″to-sar-ko′mah) a variant of mammary fibroadenoma, usually of large size, with an unusually cellular, sarcoma-like stroma; it is locally aggressive, and sometimes metastasizes. Called also *c. phylloides* and *c. phyllodes.*

cystoschisis (sis-tos′kĭ-sis) [*cysto-* + Gr. *schisis* fissure] fissure of the bladder.

cystoscirrhus (sis″to-skir′us) [*cysto-* + Gr. *skirrhos* scirrhus] (*obs.*) infiltrating scirrhous carcinoma of the urinary bladder.

cystosclerosis (sis″to-skle-ro′sis) a cyst that has undergone sclerosis or fibrosis.

cystoscope (sis′to-skōp″) [*cysto-* + Gr. *skopein* to examine] an endoscope for visual examination of the bladder.

cystoscopic (sis″to-skop′ik) pertaining to cystoscopy, or performed with the cystoscope.

cystoscopy (sis-tos′ko-pe) direct visual examination of the urinary tract with a cystoscope. **air c.**, cystoscopy in which the bladder is distended with air. **water c.**, cystoscopy in which the bladder is distended with water.

cystose (sis′tōs) resembling or containing a cyst or cysts.

cystospasm (sis′to-spazm) [*cysto-* + Gr. *spasmos* spasm] spasm of the bladder.

Cystospaz (sis′to-spaz) trademark for preparations of hyoscyamine.

cystospermitis (sis″to-sper-mi′tis) [*cysto-* + Gr. *sperma* semen] inflammation of a seminal vesicle.

cystostaxis (sis″to-stak′sis) cystistaxis.

cystostomy (sis-tos′to-me) [*cysto-* + Gr. *stoma* opening] the formation of an opening into the bladder. **tubeless c.**, suprapubic cystostomy in which a fistula of combined skin and bladder flap is created to enable the collection of urine in a reservoir without using a cystostomy tube.

cystotome (sis′to-tōm) [*cysto-* + Gr. *tomē* a cutting] 1. an instrument for incising the bladder. 2. cystitome.

cystotomy (sis-tot′o-me) surgical incision of the urinary bladder; vesicotomy. **suprapubic c.**, the operation of cutting into the bladder by an incision just above the pubic symphysis.

cystotrachelotomy (sis″to-tra″kel-ot′o-me) [*cysto-* + Gr. *trachēlos* neck + *tomē* a cut] surgical incision of the neck of the bladder.

cystoureteritis (sis″to-u-re″ter-i′tis) inflammation involving the urinary bladder and ureters.

cystoureterogram (sis″to-u-re′ter-o-gram) a roentgenogram of the urinary bladder and ureters.

cystoureteropyelitis (sis″to-u-re″ter-o-pi″e-li′tis) inflammation involving the urinary bladder, ureter, and pelvis of the kidney.

cystoureteropyelonephritis (sis″to-u-re″ter-o-pi″e-lo-ne-fri′tis) combined inflammation of the bladder, ureter, and pelvis and pyramids of the kidney.

cystourethritis (sis″to-u″re-thri′tis) inflammation of the bladder and urethra.

cystourethrocele (sis″to-u-re′thro-sēl) prolapse of the female urethra and bladder.

cystourethrogram (sis″to-u-re′thro-gram) a roentgenogram of the urinary bladder and urethra.

cystourethrography (sis″to-u-re-throg′rah-fe) roentgenography of the urinary bladder and urethra. **chain c.,** that in which a sterile beaded metal chain is introduced via a modified catheter into the bladder and urethra; used in evaluating anatomical relationships of the bladder and urethra. **voiding c.,** cystourethrography in which radiographs are made before, during, and after voiding.

cystourethroscope (sis″to-u-re′thro-skōp″) an instrument for examining the bladder and posterior urethra.

cystous (sis′tus) cystose.

cyt- see *cyto-*.

cytapheresis (sīt″ah-fĕ-re′sis) [*cyt-* + Gr. *aphairesis* removal] a procedure in which cells of one or more kinds (leukocytes, platelets, etc.) are separated from whole blood and retained, the plasma and other formed elements being retransfused into the donor; it includes leukapheresis and thrombocytapheresis.

cytarabine (si-tār′ah-bēn) [USP] chemical name: 4-amino-1-β-D-arabinofuranosyl-2(1*H*)-pyrimidinone. A synthetic nucleoside of cytosine and arabinose isomeric with cytidine, $C_9H_{13}N_3O_5$, which inhibits DNA synthesis and hence has cytotoxic and antiviral properties and which occurs as a white to off-white, crystalline powder; used as an antineoplastic, primarily for induction of remission in acute granulocytic leukemia and secondarily for the acute leukemias of adults and children, administered intravenously and subcutaneously. It has also been used in the treatment of herpesvirus infections. Called also *arabinosylcytosine, ara-C,* and *cytosine arabinoside.* **c. hydrochloride,** the hydrochloride of cytarabine, an antiviral agent.

cytarme (sit-ar′me) [Gr. *kytos* cell + *armē* union] the flattening of rounded blastomeres at the conclusion of cleavage.

cytase (si′tās) [Gr. *kytos* hollow vessel + *-ase*] 1. Metchnikoff's term for the complement regarded as an enzyme; see also *alexin.* 2. an enzyme occurring in the seeds of various plants, having the power of making soluble the material of the cell wall.

cytaster (si′tas-ter) [Gr. *kytos* hollow vessel + *astēr* star] aster.

-cyte (sīt) [Gr. *kytos* hollow vessel, anything that contains or covers] a word termination denoting a cell, the type of which is designated by the root to which it is affixed, as *elliptocyte, erythrocyte, leukocyte,* etc.

Cytellin (si-tel′in) trademark for a preparation of sitosterols.

cythemolysis (si″thĕ-mol′ĭ-sis) hemolysis.

cytheromania (sith″er-o-ma′ne-ah) [Gr. *Kythereia* Venus + *mania* madness] nymphomania.

cytidine (si′tĭ-dēn) a nucleoside from nucleic acid; on hydrolysis it yields cytosine and ribose. **c. triphosphate (CTP),** an energy-rich nucleotide that provides energy in the biosynthesis of certain cellular constituents.

cytisine (sit′ĭ-sin) [Gr. *kytisos* laburnum] a highly toxic alkaloid, $C_{11}H_{14}N_2O$, from *Cytisus laburnum,* the laburnum tree of Europe, and others of the same genus; formerly used as an antiemetic and antitussive. Called also *baptitoxine, laburnine, sophorine,* and *ulexine.* See also *cytisism.*

cytisism (sit′ĭ-sizm) poisoning by *Cytisus laburnum,* the laburnum tree of Europe, characterized by burning in the mouth and pharynx, thirst, nausea, vomiting, diarrhea, prostration, and irregular pulse; sometimes accompanied by aphasia, visual disturbances, delirium, and unconsciousness. Death from respiratory paralysis may occur.

Cytisus (sit′ĭ-sus) a genus of leguminous trees of Europe, northern Africa, and southern Asia. *C. scopa′rius* (L.) Link., or scotch broom, is the source of scoparin and scoparius. Called also *Sarothamnus.*

cyto-, cyt- [Gr. *kytos* hollow vessel; anything that contains or covers] a combining form denoting relationship to a cell.

cytoanalyzer (si″to-an″ah-li′zer) an electronic optical apparatus for the detection of malignant cells in smears.

cytoarchitectonic (si″to-ar″kĭ-tek-ton′ik) pertaining to cellular structure or the arrangement of cells in a tissue.

cytoarchitectural (si″to-ar″kĭ-tek′tu-ral) cytoarchitectonic.

cytoarchitecture (si″to-ar″kĭ-tek″tūr) the organization of cells in the structure of an organ or tissue, especially that in the cerebral cortex.

cytobiology (si″to-bi-ol′o-je) [*cyto-* + *biology*] the biology of cells.

cytobiotaxis (si″to-bi-o-tak′sis) [*cyto-* + Gr. *bios* life + *taxis* arrangement] cytoclesis.

cytoblast (si′to-blast) [*cyto-* + Gr. *blastos* germ] Schleiden's name for the cell nucleus.

cytoblastema (si″to-blas-te′mah) [*cyto-* + *blastema*] Schleiden's name for the mother liquid from which cells were said to form.

cytocentrum (si″to-sen′trum) [*cyto-* + Gr. *kentron* center] centrosome.

cytocerastic (si″to-se-ras′tik) cytokerastic.

cytochalasin (si″to-kal′ah-sin) any of a group of fungal metabolites that affect the motility of polymorphonuclear leukocytes. **c. B,** a cytochalasin that causes the disappearance of cytoplasmic microfilaments and inhibits certain cellular processes, e.g., cytokinesis.

cytochemism (si″to-kem′izm) [*cyto-* + *chemism*] chemical activity of cells.

cytochemistry (si″to-kem″is-tre) [*cyto-* + *chemistry*] the identification and localization of the different chemical compounds and their activities within the cell.

cytochrome (si′to-krōm) [*cyto-* + Gr. *chrōma* color] 1. any of a class of hemoproteins whose principal biologic function is electron transport by virtue of a reversible valency change of its heme iron; cytochromes, which are widely distributed in animal and plant tissues, are distinguished according to their prosthetic group as *a, b, c,* and *d.* 2. a neuron having an ill-developed cell body, in which the stained nucleus appears to be completely surrounded, and does not exceed in size the nucleus of a leukocyte. **c. aa_3,** c. *c* oxidase. **c. b_5 reductase,** a flavoprotein that transfers electrons from NADPH (or NADH) to cytochrome b_5, as in the liver microsomal desaturation of fatty acids. **c. *c* oxidase,** a copper-containing cytochrome of the *a* type which receives electrons from cytochrome *c* and transfers them to oxygen, enabling the oxygen to combine with hydrogen ions to form water. Called also *c. aa_3.*

cytochylema (si″to-ki-le′mah) [*cyto-* + Gr. *chylos* juice] hyaloplasm, def. 1.

cytocidal (si″to-si′dal) destructive to cells.

cytocide (si″to-sīd) [*cyto-* + L. *caedere* to kill] an agent that destroys cells.

cytocinesis (si″to-si-ne′sis) cytokinesis.

cytoclasis (si-tok′lah-sis) [*cyto-* + Gr. *klasis* a breaking] the destruction of cells.

cytoclastic (si″to-klas′tik) pertaining to, characterized by, or causing cytoclasis.

cytoclesis (si″to-kle′sis) [*cyto-* + Gr. *klēsis* a call] a form of energy, totally unrelated to electricity, light, heat, or sound, which is generated by living tissues; the vital principle in all living tissues (M. Kelly). The term was first introduced in 1923 by Frederic Wood Jones, who defined it as the influence of body cells on other body cells; the "call of cell to cell." Called also *cytobiotaxis.*

cytocletic (si″to-klet′ik) pertaining to cytoclesis.

cytoctony (si-tok′to-ne) [*cyto-* + Gr. *ktonos* murder] the killing of cells; specifically the killing by viruses of cells in culture.

cytocyst (si′to-sist) [*cyto-* + Gr. *kystis* sac] (*obs.*) a cystlike structure enclosing a mass of merozoites, being the remains of the host cell in which the merozoites were formed; seen in malaria.

cytode (si′tōd) [*cyto-* + Gr. *eidos* form] a non-nucleated cell or cell element.

cytodendrite (si″to-den′drīt) [*cyto-* + *dendrite*] dendrite.

cytodesma (si″to-dez′mah) [*cyto-* + Gr. *desma* band] the lamellar or bridgelike tissues binding animal cells together (Studnicka).

cytodiagnosis (si″to-di″ag-no′sis) [*cyto-* + *diagnosis*] diagnosis of disease based on the examination of cells. **exfoliative c.,** the examination of cells that have desquamated from the external or internal surfaces of the body as a means of detecting cancer.

cytodiagnostic (si″to-di″ag-nos′tik) pertaining to or subserving cytodiagnosis.

cytodieresis (si″to-di-er′ĕ-sis) [*cyto-* + Gr. *diairesis* division] cell division, i.e., meiosis or mitosis.

cytodifferentiation (si″to-dif″er-en″she-a′shun) the development of specialized structures and functions in embryonic cells.

cytodistal (si″to-dis′tal) [*cyto-* + *distal*] denoting that part of an axon remote from the cell of origin.

cytoflav (si′to-flav) a phosphoric acid ester of riboflavin, found in the liver and in the heart.

cytoflavin (si″to-fla′vin) a flavin that was first isolated from heart muscle; it is the phosphoric acid ester of riboflavin.

cytogene (si′to-jēn) [*cyto-* + *gene*] a self-perpetuating cytoplasmic particle that traces its origin to the genes of the nucleus.

cytogenesis (si″to-jen′ĕ-sis) [*cyto-* + Gr. *genesis* origin] the origin and development of cells.

cytogenetical (si″to-jĕ-net′ĕ-kal) pertaining to cytogenetics.

cytogeneticist (si″to-je-net′ĭ-sist) a specialist in cytogenetics.

cytogenetics (si″to-jĕ-net′iks) the branch of genetics devoted to study of the cellular constituents concerned in heredity, that is, the chromosomes. **clinical c.,** the scientific study of the relationship between chromosomal aberrations and pathological conditions.

cytogenic (si-to-jen′ik) 1. pertaining to cytogenesis. 2. forming or producing cells.

cytogenous (si-toj′ĕ-nus) [*cyto-* + Gr. *gennan* to produce] producing cells.

cytogeny (si-toj′ĕ-ne) 1. cytogenesis. 2. cell lineage.

cytoglomerator (si″to-glom″er-a′tor) an apparatus for processing blood before freezing it for storage, and after thawing it.

cytoglucopenia (si″to-gloo″ko-pe′ne-ah) cytoglycopenia.

cytoglycopenia (si″to-gli″ko-pe′ne-ah) [*cyto-* + *glucose* + Gr. *penia* poverty] deficient glucose content of body or blood cells.

cytogony (si-tog′ŏ-ne) [*cyto-* + Gr. *gonos* seed] cytogenic reproduction.

cytohistogenesis (si″to-his″to-jen′ĕ-sis) [*cyto-* + Gr. *histos* web + *genesis* formation] the development of the structure of cells.

cytohistologic (si″to-his″to-loj′ik) involving both cytologic and histologic methods.

cytohistology (si″to-his-tol′o-je) the combination of cytologic and histologic methods.

cytohormone (si″to-hor′mōn) [*cyto-* + *hormone*] a cell hormone.

cytohyaloplasm (si″to-hi′ah-lo-plazm″) [*cyto-* + Gr. *hyalos* crystal + *plasma* plasm] the clear substance of cytoplasm.

cytohydrolist (si″to-hi′dro-list) [*cyto-* + *hydrolist*] an enzyme that breaks up the cell wall by hydrolysis.

cytoid (si′toid) [*cyto-* + Gr. *eidos* form] resembling a cell.

cyto-inhibition (si″to-in″hĭ-bish′un) [*cyto-* + L. *inhibere* to restrain] the action of phagocytic cells in protecting bacteria or viruses which they have ingested from lysis or chemical destruction by chemotherapeutic agents.

cytokalipenia (si″to-kal″ĭ-pe′ne-ah) [*cyto-* + L. *kalium* potassium + Gr. *penia* poverty] deficient potassium content of body or blood cells.

cytokerastic (si″to-kĕ-ras′tik) [*cyto-* + Gr. *kerastos* mixed] pertaining to the development of cells from a lower to a higher order.

cytokinesis (si″to-ki-ne′sis) [*cyto-* + Gr. *kinēsis* motion] the changes that take place in the cytoplasm during cell division; division of the cytoplasm, a process synchronized in eukaryotic cells with nuclear division (mitosis).

cytokinin (si″to-ki′nin) any of a class of phytohormones (N⁶-substituted adenines) whose principal functions are the induction of cell division (cytokinesis) and the regulation of differentiation of tissue (organogenesis).

cytolist (si′to-list) cytolysin.

cytologic (si″to-loj′ik) pertaining to cytology.

cytologist (si-tol′o-jist) a specialist in cytology.

cytology (si-tol′o-je) [*cyto-* + *-logy*] the study of cells, their origin, structure, function, and pathology. **aspiration biopsy c. (ABC),** the microscopic study of cells obtained from superficial or internal lesions by suction through a fine needle. **exfoliative c.,** microscopic examination of cells desquamated from a body surface or lesion as a means of detecting malignancy and microbiologic changes, to measure hormonal levels, etc. Such cells may be obtained by such procedures as aspiration, washing, smear, and scraping, and the technique may be applied to vaginal secretions, sputum, urine, abdominal fluid, prostatic secretion, etc.

cytolymph (si′to-limf) [*cyto-* + *lymph*] hyaloplasm, def. 1.

cytolysate (si-tol′ĭ-sāt) a preparation of lyzed cells. **blood c.,** hemolysate.

cytolysin (si-tol′ĭ-sin) a substance or antibody that produces dissolution of cells. Cytolysins that have a specific action for certain cells are named accordingly, as *hemolysins,* etc.

cytolysis (si-tol′ĭ-sis) [*cyto-* + Gr. *lysis* dissolution] the dissolution or destruction of cells. **immune c.,** cell lysis produced by antibody with the participation of complement.

cytolysosome (si″to-li′so-sōm) autophagosome.

cytolytic (si″to-lit′ik) pertaining to, characterized by, or causing cytolysis.

cytoma (si-to′mah) [*cyto-* + *-oma*] a cell tumor, as a sarcoma.

cytomachia (si″to-mak′e-ah) [*cyto-* + Gr. *machē* fight] the struggle between bacteria and the protective cells of the body.

cytomegaloviruria (si″to-meg″ah-lo-vi-roo′re-ah) presence in the urine of cytomegaloviruses.

cytomegalovirus (si″to-meg″ah-lo-vi′rus) one of a group of highly host-specific herpesviruses that infect man, monkeys, or rodents, with the production of unique large cells bearing intranuclear inclusions. Also termed *salivary gland virus.* The virus specific for man causes cytomegalic inclusion disease, and it has been associated with a syndrome resembling infectious mononucleosis.

Cytomel (si′to-mel) trademark for a preparation of liothyronine sodium.

cytomere (si′to-mēr) [*cyto-* + Gr. *meros* part] 1. one of the bodies formed in coccidian reproduction by division of the trophozoite, each cytomere becoming the center of merozoite formation. 2. that part of the sperm which is composed of cytoplasm; called also *chondriomere* and *plastomere.*

cytometaplasia (si″to-met″ah-pla′ze-ah) [*cyto-* + Gr. *metaplasis* change] alteration in the form or function of a cell.

cytometer (si-tom′ĕ-ter) [*cyto-* + Gr. *metron* measure] a device for counting blood cells, as a hemocytometer.

cytometry (si-tom′ĕ-tre) the counting of blood cells; blood counting.

cytomitome (si″to-mi′tōm) [*cyto-* + Gr. *mitos* thread] a fibril or fibrillary structure in the cytoplasm.

cytomorphology (si″to-mor-fol′o-je) the morphology of cells.

cytomorphosis (si″to-mor-fo′sis) [*cyto-* + Gr. *morphōsis* a shaping] the series of changes through which cells go in the process of formation, development, senescence, etc.

cytomycosis (si″to-mi-ko′sis) [*cyto-* + Gr. *mykēs* fungus] former term for disseminated histoplasmosis with hepatosplenomegaly, anemia, leukopenia, and fatal outcome.

cyton (si′ton) the cell body of a neuron.

cytonecrosis (si″to-nĕ-kro′sis) death of individual cells.

cytopathic (si″to-path′ik) pertaining to or characterized by pathological changes in cells.

cytopathogenesis (si″to-path″o-jen′ĕ-sis) the production of pathological changes in cells.

cytopathogenetic (si″to-path″o-jĕ-net′ik) pertaining to or characterized by cytopathogenesis.

cytopathogenic (si″to-path″o-jen′ik) capable of producing pathological changes in cells.

cytopathogenicity (si″to-path″o-jĕ-nis′ĭ-te) the quality of being capable of producing pathological changes in cells.

cytopathologic, cytopathological (si″to-path″o-loj′ik; si″-to-path″o-loj′ĭ-kal) relating to cytopathology; denoting the changes in cells in disease.

cytopathologist (si″to-pah-thol′o-jist) an expert in the study of cells in disease; a cellular pathologist.

cytopathology (si″to-pah-thol′o-je) [*cyto-* + Gr. *pathos* disease + *-logy*] the study of cells in disease; cellular pathology.

cytopenia (si″to-pe′ne-ah) [*cyto-* + Gr. *penia* poverty] deficiency in the cellular elements of the blood.

Cytophaga (si-tof′ah-gah) [*cyto-* + Gr. *phagein* to eat] a genus of schizomycetes (family Cytophagaceae), species of which dissolve vegetable fiber and hydrolyze cellulose.

Cytophagaceae (si″to-fah-ga′se-e) a family of Schizomycetes, order Myxobacterales, made up of saprophytic soil microorganisms, many of which decompose cellulose; it includes a single genus, *Cytophaga.*

cytophagocytosis (si″to-fag″o-si-to′sis) cytophagy.

cytophagous (si-tof′ah-gus) [*cyto-* + Gr. *phagein* to eat] devouring or consuming cells; said of phagocytes.

cytophagy (si-tof′ah-je) the ingestion of cells by phagocytes.

cytopharynx (si″to-far′inks) the depression in the body of certain flagellates and ciliates through which food matter is received.

cytopherometric (si″to-fer″o-met′rik) see under *tests.*

cytophil (si′to-fil) an element or substance that has an affinity for cells.

cytophilic (si-to-fil′ik) [*cyto-* + Gr. *philein* to love] having an affinity for cells, as cytophilic antibodies.

cytophotometer (si″to-fo-tom′ĕ-ter) a photometer for measuring localization of organic compounds within cells by measuring the light intensity through selected stained areas of cytoplasm.

cytophotometric (si″to-fo″to-met′rik) pertaining to or accomplished by cytophotometry.

cytophotometry (si″to-fo-tom′ĕ-tre) the study of organic compounds within cells by means of the cytophotometer. Called also *microfluorometry.*

cytophylactic (si″to-fi-lak′tik) pertaining to cytophylaxis.

cytophylaxis (si″to-fi-lak′sis) [*cyto-* + Gr. *phylaxis* a guarding] 1. the protection of cells. 2. increase of cellular activity.

cytophyletic (si″to-fi-let′ik) [*cyto-* + Gr. *phylē* a tribe] pertaining to the genealogy of cells.

cytophysics (si″to-fiz′iks) the physics of cell activity.

cytophysiology (si″to-fiz-e-ol′o-je) [*cyto-* + *physiology*] the physiology of the cell.

cytopigment (si′to-pig″ment) any pigment found in cells.

cytopipette (si″to-pi-pet′) a pipette for taking cytological smears.

cytoplasm (si′to-plazm″) [*cyto-* + Gr. *plasma* plasm] the protoplasm of a cell exclusive of that of the nucleus; it consists of a continuous aqueous solution (cytosol) and the organelles and inclusions suspended in it (phaneroplasm), and is the site of most of the chemical activities of the cell. Cf. *nucleoplasm.*

cytoplasmic (si″to-plaz′mik) pertaining to or contained in the cytoplasm.

cytoplast (si′to-plast) a cell from which the nucleus has been removed and which remains viable for a time.

cytoproximal (si″to-prok′sĭ-mal) [*cyto-* + *proximal*] denoting that part of an axon nearer to the cell of origin.

cytoreticulum (si″to-rĕ-tik′u-lum) [*cyto-* + L. *reticulum* network] spongioplasm.

cytorrhyctes (si″to-rik′tēz) [*cyto-* + Gr. *oryssein* to dig] cell inclusions, found in various diseases, which may be specific protozoan pathogens, or they may be manifestations of cell reactions to the parasite of the disease, or they may be degenerations caused by the disease. See *Siegel's organism,* under *organism.*

Cytosar (si'to-sar) trademark for preparations of cytarabine.

cytoscopy (si-tos'ko-pe) [cyto- + Gr. skopein to examine] examination of cells.

cytosiderin (si″to-sid'er-in) intracellular pigment due probably to derangement of iron metabolism.

cytosine (si'to-sēn) a base, oxyaminopyrimidine, $C_4H_5N_3O$, a component of nucleic acid. **c. arabinoside,** cytarabine. **5-hydroxymethyl c.,** a pyrimidine that replaces cytosine in the DNA of certain coliphages.

cytoskeletal (si″to-skel'ĕ-tal) of or pertaining to the cytoskeleton.

cytoskeleton (si″to-skel'ĕ-ton) a conspicuous internal reinforcement in the cytoplasm of a cell, consisting of tonofibrils, terminal web, or other microfilaments.

cytosol (si'to-sol) the liquid medium of the cytoplasm, i.e., cytoplasm minus organelles and nonmembranous insoluble components.

cytosolic (si″to-sol'ik) pertaining to or contained in the cytosol.

cytosome (si'to-sōm) [cyto- + Gr. sōma body] 1. the body of a cell apart from its nucleus. 2. multilamellar body.

cytospongium (si″to-spon'je-um) [cyto- + Gr. spongos sponge] spongioplasm.

cytost (si'tost) [Gr. kytos hollow vessel] a specific toxin given off from a cell as a result of injury to it; a specific agent given off from broken-down tissue.

cytostasis (si-tos'tah-sis) [cyto- + Gr. stasis halt] the closure of capillaries by white blood corpuscles in the early stages of inflammation.

cytostatic (si″to-stat'ik) [cyto- + Gr. statikos bringing to a stand-still] 1. suppressing the growth and multiplication of cells. 2. an agent that suppresses cell growth and multiplication.

cytostome (si'to-stōm) [cyto- + Gr. stoma mouth] the cell mouth; the aperture through which food enters certain protozoa.

cytostromatic (si″to-stro-mat'ik) [cyto- + stroma] pertaining to the stroma of a cell.

cytotactic (si″to-tak'tik) pertaining to cytotaxis.

cytotaxigen (si″to-taks'ĭ-jen) a substance that mediates chemotaxis of cells indirectly by inducing cytotaxin formation; thus antigen-antibody complexes are cytotaxigenic because when added to serum they fix complement, resulting in the liberation of chemotactic factors derived from complement.

cytotaxin (si″to-taks'in) a substance that directly mediates the chemotaxis of cells.

cytotaxis (si-to-tak'sis) [cyto- + Gr. taxis arrangement] the movement and arrangement of cells with respect to a specific source of stimulation.

cytotherapy (si″to-ther'ah-pe) [cyto- + Gr. therapeia treatment] 1. treatment by the administration of animal cells. 2. the therapeutic use of a cytolytic or cytotoxic serum.

cytothesis (si-toth'ĕ-sis) [cyto- + Gr. thesis placing] the restitution of injured cells to their normal condition.

cytotoxic (si″to-tok'sik) pertaining to, resulting from, or having the action of a cytotoxin.

cytotoxicity (si″to-tok-sis'ĭ-te) the quality of being capable of producing a specific toxic action upon cells of special organs.

cytotoxicosis (si″to-tok″se-ko'sis) a condition produced by a cytotoxin or by poisoning cells.

cytotoxin (si″to-tok'sin) [cyto- + toxin] a toxin or antibody that has a specific toxic action upon cells of special organs; cytotoxins are named according to the special variety of cell for which they are specific, as nephrotoxin.

cytotrochin (si″to-tro'kin) [cyto- + Gr. trochia track] that element of a tropic substance that carries the active element to the cell.

cytotrophoblast (si″to-trof'o-blast) [cyto- + Gr. trophē nutrition + blastos germ] the cellular (inner) layer of the trophoblast; called also Langhans' layer.

cytotropic (si″to-trop'ik) [cyto- + Gr. tropos a turning] attracting cells; possessing an affinity for cells; said especially of the antibodies responsible for immediate-type allergic reactions. See also under antibody.

cytotropism (si-tot'ro-pizm) 1. cell movement in response to external stimulation. 2. the tendency of viruses, bacteria, drugs, etc. to exert their effect upon certain cells of the body.

Cytoxan (si-tok'san) trademark for preparations of cyclophosphamide.

cytozoic (si″to-zo'ik) living within or attached to cells; said of parasites.

cyttarrhagia (sit″ah-ra'je-ah) [Gr. kyttaros cell of a honey-comb + rhēgnynai to burst forth] alveolar hemorrhage.

cytula (sit'u-lah) the impregnated ovum.

cytuloplasm (sit'u-lo-plazm″) the combined ovoplasm and spermoplasm in a cytula.

cyturia (sĭ-tu're-ah) [Gr. kytos hollow vessel + ouron urine + -ia] the presence of cells of any sort in the urine.

Czermak's spaces (lines) (chār'mahks) [Johann Nepomuk Czermak, Bohemian physician, 1828–1873] spatia interglobularia.

Czerny's anemia (chār'nēz) [Adalbert Czerny, German pediatrician, 1863–1941] see under anemia.

Czerny's suture (chār'nēz) [Vincenz Czerny, surgeon in Heidelberg, 1842–1916] see under suture.

Czerny-Lembert suture (char'ne-lah-bar') [Vincenz Czerny; Antoine Lembert, French surgeon, 1802–1851] see under suture.

D

D symbol for deuterium.

D. 1. abbreviation for L., dosis, dose; da, give; detur, let it be given; dexter, right; also for deciduous, density, died, didymium, diopter, distal, dorsal (in vertebral formulas), and duration. 2. a symbol for the unit of vitamin D potency.

D_{37} the dose necessary to reduce the surviving fraction, as of cells, to e^{-1} or 0.37, where the biological activity declines exponentially as a function of dose.

D- (de) chemical prefix (small capital) which specifies that the substance corresponds in configuration to the standard substance D-glyceraldehyde, that is, belongs to the same configurational family. In carbohydrate nomenclature, the symbol refers to the configurational family of the highest numbered asymmetric carbon atom, as in D-glucose. In amino acid nomenclature, under rules adopted in 1947, the symbol refers to the configurational family to which the lowest numbered asymmetric carbon atom, i.e., the 2-carbon atom or α-carbon atom, belongs, as in D-threonine. Opposed to L-.

D_g- (de-sub-je) see D-; this chemical prefix (with the subscript g) is occasionally used to emphasize that the rules of carbohydrate nomenclature are being employed, as in D_g-glucosaminic acid. The subscript refers to the standard substance glyceraldehyde. Opposed to L_g-.

D_s- (de-sub-es) see D-; this chemical prefix (with the subscript s) is used where needed in amino acid nomenclature to avoid possible confusion with carbohydrate nomenclature, as in D_s-threonine. The subscript refers to the standard substance serine. Opposed to L_s-.

d- (de-) 1. chemical abbreviation for dextro- (i.e., right or clockwise), with reference to the direction in which the plane of polarized light is rotated when passed through a solution of the substance or through the substance itself if a liquid: opposed to l- (levo-). 2. a prefix used with one of the additional symbols (+) or (−), especially in amino acid nomenclature in the literature from 1923 until 1947 or a little later, with reference to the configurational family to which the 2-carbon or α-carbon atom of the amino acid belongs, the actual direction of the rotation in a specified solvent being indicated by the plus or minus sign, as in d(−)-alanine; opposed to l(+)- or l(−)-, as in l(+)-alanine or l(−)-cystine. Now replaced by D-.

δ,Δ the fourth letter of the Greek alphabet; see delta.

D.A. developmental age.

d'Abano, Pietro see Peter of Abano.

Dabney's grip (dab'nēz) [William Cecil Dabney, American physician, 1849–1894] epidemic pleurodynia.

Daboia (dah-boi'ah) a genus of snakes. **D. russel'li,** Russell's viper (Vipera russelli).

D and C dilation and curettage (dilation of the cervix and curettage of the uterus).

d'Acosta see Acosta.

DaCosta's disease, syndrome [Jacob Mendes DaCosta, American physician, 1833–1900] see misplaced gout and neurocirculatory asthenia.

dacry- see dacryo-.

dacryadenalgia (dak″re-ad-ĕ-nal'je-ah) dacryoadenalgia.

dacryadenitis (dak″re-ad-ĕ-ni'tis) dacryoadenitis.

dacryadenoscirrhus (dak″re-ad″ĕ-no-skir'us) [dacry- + Gr. adēn gland + skirrhos scirrhus] (obs.) scirrhous carcinoma of a lacrimal gland.

dacryagogatresia (dak″re-ah-gog″ah-tre'ze-ah) [dacry- + Gr.

agōgos leading + *atresia*] atresia, imperforation, or closure of a lacrimal duct.

dacryagogic (dak″re-ah-goj′ik) 1. inducing a flow of tears; dacryogenic. 2. serving as a duct for the secretion of the lacrimal glands.

dacryagogue (dak′re-ah-gog″) [*dacry-* + Gr. *agōgos* leading] 1. an agent that induces a flow of tears. 2. a lacrimal duct.

dacrycystalgia (dak″re-sis-tal′je-ah) dacryocystalgia.

dacrycystitis (dak″re-sis-ti′tis) dacryocystitis.

dacryelcosis (dak″re-el-ko′sis) dacryohelcosis.

dacryo-, dacry- [Gr. *dakryon* tear] a combining form denoting relationship to tears.

dacryoadenalgia (dak″re-o-ad″ĕ-nal′je-ah) [*dacryo-* + Gr. *adēn* gland + *algos* pain + *-ia*] pain in a lacrimal gland.

dacryoadenectomy (dak″re-o-ad″ĕ-nek′to-me) excision of a lacrimal gland.

dacryoadenitis (dak″re-o-ad″ĕ-ni′tis) inflammation of a lacrimal gland.

dacryoblennorrhea (dak″re-o-blen″o-re′ah) [*dacryo-* + Gr. *blennos* mucus + *rhein* to flow] mucous discharge from the lacrimal ducts, as in chronic dacryocystitis.

dacryocanaliculitis (dak″re-o-kan″ah-lik″u-li′tis) inflammation of the lacrimal ducts.

dacryocele (dak′re-o-sēl″) dacryocystocele.

dacryocyst (dak′re-o-sist″) [*dacryo-* + Gr. *kystis* sac] the lacrimal sac.

dacryocystalgia (dak″re-o-sis-tal′je-ah) pain in a lacrimal sac.

dacryocystectasia (dak″re-o-sis″tek-ta′ze-ah) [*dacryocyst* + Gr. *ektasis* dilatation + *-ia*] dilatation of the lacrimal sac.

dacryocystectomy (dak″re-o-sis-tek′to-me) [*dacryocyst* + Gr. *ektomē* excision] excision of the wall of the lacrimal sac.

dacryocystis (dak″re-o-sis′tis) the lacrimal sac.

dacryocystitis (dak″re-o-sis-ti′tis) inflammation of the lacrimal sac.

dacryocystitome (dak″re-o-sis′tĭ-tōm) [*dacryocyst* + Gr. *temnein* to cut] an instrument for incising strictures of the lacrimal duct.

dacryocystoblennorrhea (dak″re-o-sis″to-blen″o-re′ah) a chronic catarrhal inflammation of the lacrimal sac, with constriction of the lacrimal duct.

dacryocystocele (dak″re-o-sis′to-sēl) [*dacryocyst* + Gr. *kēlē* hernia] hernial protrusion of the lacrimal sac; called also *dacryocele.*

dacryocystoptosis (dak″re-o-sis″top-to′sis) [*dacryocyst* + Gr. *ptōsis* fall] prolapse or downward displacement of the lacrimal sac.

dacryocystorhinostenosis (dak″re-o-sis″to-ri″no-stĕ-no′sis) narrowing of the duct leading from the lacrimal sac to the nasal cavity.

dacryocystorhinostomy (dak″re-o-sis″to-ri-nos′to-me) [*dacryocyst* + Gr. *rhis* nose + *stomoun* to provide with an opening, or mouth] surgical creation of a communication between the lacrimal sac and the nasal cavity; called also *dacryorhinocystotomy* and *Toti's operation.*

dacryocystorhinotomy (dak″re-o-sis″to-ri-not′o-me) passage of a probe through the lacrimal sac into the nasal cavity.

dacryocystostenosis (dak″re-o-sis″to-stĕ-no′sis) narrowing of the lacrimal sac.

dacryocystostomy (dak″re-o-sis-tos′to-me) [*dacryocyst* + Gr. *stomoun* to provide with an opening, or mouth] surgical creation of a new opening into the lacrimal sac.

dacryocystosyringotomy (dak″re-o-sis″to-sir″in-got′o-me) [*dacryocyst* + Gr. *syrinx* tube + *tomē* a cutting] incision of the lacrimal sac and duct.

dacryocystotome (dak″re-o-sis′to-tōm) an instrument for incising the lacrimal sac.

dacryocystotomy (dak″re-o-sis-tot′o-me) incision of the lacrimal sac; called also *Ammon's operation.*

dacryogenic (dak″re-o-jen′ik) promoting the secretion of tears.

dacryohelcosis (dak″re-o-hel-ko′sis) [*dacryo-* + Gr. *helkōsis* ulceration] ulceration of the lacrimal sac or lacrimal duct.

dacryohemorrhea (dak″re-o-hem″o-re′ah) [*dacryo-* + Gr. *haima* blood + *rhein* to flow] the discharge of tears mixed with blood.

dacryolith (dak′re-o-lith″) [*dacryo-* + Gr. *lithos* stone] a concretion in the lacrimal sac or duct.

dacryolithiasis (dak″re-o-lĭ-thi′ah-sis) [*dacryo-* + *lithiasis*] the presence of calculi in the lacrimal sac or duct.

dacryoma (dak″re-o′mah) a tumor-like swelling caused by obstruction of the lacrimal duct.

dacryon (dak′re-on) [Gr. *dakryon* tear] a cranial point at the juncture of the lacrimal and frontal bones, and the maxilla.

dacryops (dak′re-ops) [*dacry-* + Gr. *ōps* eye] 1. a watery state of the eye. 2. distention of a lacrimal duct by contained fluid.

dacryopyorrhea (dak″re-o-pi″o-re′ah) [*dacryo-* + Gr. *pyon* pus + *rhein* to flow] the discharge of tears mixed with pus.

dacryopyosis (dak″re-o-pi-o′sis) [*dacryo-* + Gr. *pyōsis* suppuration] suppuration of the lacrimal sac and duct.

dacryorhinocystotomy (dak″re-o-ri″no-sis-tot′o-me) dacryocystorhinotomy.

dacryorrhea (dak″re-o-re′ah) [*dacryo-* + Gr. *rhein* to flow] an overabundant flow of tears.

dacryoscintigraphy (dak″re-o-sin-tig′rah-fe) scintigraphy of the lacrimal ducts.

dacryosinusitis (dak″re-o-si″nus-i′tis) inflammation of the lacrimal duct and ethmoid sinus.

dacryosolenitis (dak″re-o-so-lĕ-ni′tis) [*dacryo-* + Gr. *sōlēn* duct + *-itis*] inflammation of a lacrimal duct.

dacryostenosis (dak″re-o-stĕ-no′sis) [*dacryo-* + Gr. *stenōsis* a narrowing] stricture or narrowing of a lacrimal duct.

dacryosyrinx (dak″re-o-sir′inks) [*dacryo-* + Gr. *syrinx* tube] 1. a lacrimal duct (canaliculus lacrimalis [NA]). 2. a lacrimal fistula. 3. a syringe for irrigating the lacrimal ducts.

Dactil (dak′til) trademark for preparations of piperiodolate hydrochloride.

dactinomycin (dak″tĭ-no-mi′sin) [USP] a highly toxic antibiotic, $C_{62}H_{86}N_{16}O_{16}$, of the actinomycin group, actinomycin D, occurring as a bright red, crystalline powder; used as an antineoplastic in the palliative treatment of Wilms' tumor, rhadomyosarcoma, and testicular and uterine carcinoma, administered intravenously.

dactyl (dak′til) [Gr. *daktylos* a finger] a digit; a finger or toe.

dactyl- see *dactylo-.*

dactylate (dak′tĭ-lāt) possessing finger-like processes.

dactyledema (dak″til-ĕ-de′mah) edema or swelling of the fingers or toes.

dactylion (dak-til′e-on) (*obs.*) webbing together or union of fingers.

dactylitis (dak″tĭ-li′tis) [*dactyl-* + *-itis*] inflammation of a finger or toe. **d. strumo′sa,** d. tuberculosa. **d. syphilit′ica,** syphilitic periostitis of a finger or toe. **d. tuberculo′sa,** tuberculous inflammation of a finger or toe; called also *d. strumosa.*

dactylium (dak-til′e-um) (*obs.*) dactylion.

dactylo-, dactyl- [Gr. *daktylos* a finger] a combining form denoting relationship to a digit, usually referring to a finger but sometimes to the toes.

dactylocampsodynia (dak″tĭ-lo-kamp″so-din′e-ah) [*dactylo-* + Gr. *kampsis* bend + *odynē* pain] painful flexure of the fingers.

dactylogram (dak-til′o-gram) [*dactylo-* + Gr. *gramma* mark] a fingerprint taken for purposes of identification.

dactylography (dak″tĭ-log′rah-fe) [*dactylo-* + Gr. *graphein* to write] the study of fingerprints.

dactylogryposis (dak″tĭ-lo-grĭ-po′sis) [*dactylo-* + Gr. *grypōsis* a hooking] a permanent curving of the fingers.

dactylology (dak″til-ol′o-je) [*dactylo-* + Gr. *logos* discourse] use of movements of the hands and fingers as a means of communication between individuals; called also *cheirology* and *dactylophasia.*

dactylolysis (dak″tĭ-lol′ĭ-sis) [*dactylo-* + Gr. *lysis* a loosening] 1. surgical correction of syndactyly. 2. loss or amputation of a digit. **d. spontan′ea,** the spontaneous loss of fingers and toes, as in ainhum or in leprosy.

dactylomegaly (dak″tĭ-lo-meg′ah-le) [*dactylo-* + Gr. *megaleia* largeness] abnormally large fingers or toes.

dactylophasia (dak″tĭ-lo-fa′ze-ah) [*dactylo-* + Gr. *phasis* speech] dactylology.

dactyloscopy (dak″tĭ-los′ko-pe) [*dactylo-* + Gr. *skopein* to examine] examination of fingerprints for purposes of identification.

dactylospasm (dak′tĭ-lo-spazm) [*dactylo-* + Gr. *spasmos* spasm] spasm or cramp of a finger or toe.

dactylosymphysis (dak″tĭ-lo-sim′fĭ-sis) [*dactylo-* + *symphysis*] (*obs.*) a growing together of fingers or toes; syndactyly.

dactylus (dak′tĭ-lus) [Gr. *daktylos* finger] a digit; a finger or toe.

DADDS diacetyl diaminodiphenylsulfone; see *acedapsone.*

Dagenan (dag′ĕ-nan) trademark for sulfapyridine.

D.A.H. disordered action of the heart. See *neurocirculatory asthenia,* under *asthenia.*

dahlia (dahl′yah) the term for certain unspecified mixtures of methylated and ethylated pararosanilins and rosanilins; C.I.42530. Sometimes used as a basic dye for violet staining. Called also *Hofmann's* or *iodine violet.* **d. B.,** see *gentian violet,* under *violet.*

dahlin (dah′lin) inulin.

dahllite (dahl′īt) a complex salt, $CaCO_3 \cdot 2Ca_3(PO_4)_2$, formerly believed to be the principal inorganic constituent of bone and teeth.

Dakin's fluid (antiseptic solution) (da′kinz) [Henry Drysdale *Dakin,* New York chemist, 1880–1952] diluted sodium hypochlorite solution.

Dakin-Carrel method (da′kin-kar-el′) [Henry Drysdale *Dakin;*

Alexis *Carrel*, French surgeon, 1873–1944] see *Carrel treatment*, under *treatment*.

dakinization (da″kin-i-za′shun) (*obs.*) treatment with Dakin's fluid.

dakryon (dak′re-on) dacryon.

Dale's reaction (phenomenon) (dāl) [Sir Henry Hallett *Dale*, British physiologist and pharmacologist, 1875–1968; co-winner in 1936, with Otto Loewi, of the Nobel prize for medicine and physiology, for their work on the chemical transmission of nerve impulses] see under *reaction*.

daledalin tosylate (dah-lĕ′dah-lin) chemical name: 3-methyl-3-[3-(methylamino)propyl]-1-phenylindoline mono-*p*-toluenesulfonate; an antidepressant, $C_{19}H_{24}N_2 \cdot C_7H_8O_3S$.

Dalmane (dal′mān) trademark for a preparation of flurazepam hydrochloride.

Dalrymple's disease, sign (dal′rim-pelz) [John *Dalrymple*, an English oculist, 1804–1852] see *cyclokeratitis*, and see under *sign*.

dalton (dawl′ton) [John *Dalton*, English chemist and physicist, 1766–1844: the founder of the atomic theory] an arbitrary unit of mass, being $\frac{1}{12}$ the mass of the nuclide of carbon-12, equivalent to 1.657×10^{-24} gm. Called also *atomic mass unit*.

Dalton's law (dawl′tonz) [John *Dalton*] see under *law*.

Dalton-Henry law (dawl′ton hen′re) [John *Dalton*; Joseph *Henry*, American physicist, 1797–1878] see under *law*.

daltonism (dawl′ton-izm) [John *Dalton*] a name applied to defective perception of red and green.

Dam (dam), Carl Peter Henrik. A Danish biochemist, born 1895; co-winner in 1943, with Edward Adelbert Doisy, of the Nobel prize for medicine and physiology, for the discovery of vitamin K.

dam (dam) a thin sheet of latex rubber used to isolate teeth from the fluids of the mouth during dental therapy; also used occasionally in surgical procedures to separate certain tissues or structures. Often called *rubber dam*. **rubber d.,** see *dam*.

Damalinia (dam″ah-lin′e-ah) a genus of parasitic insects of the order Mallophaga, the biting lice; several species were formerly classified in the genus *Trichodectes*. *D. bo′vis* infests cattle, *D. cap′re* the goat, *D. e′qui* and *D. pilo′sus* the horse, and *D. herm′si* and *D. o′vis* infest sheep.

damiana (dah″me-ah′nah) the leaves of *Turnera aphrodisiaca* (*T. diffusa*) and *Haplopappus discoideus*, Mexican plants; said to be tonic, analeptic, diuretic, and aphrodisiac. Called also *turnera*.

dammar (dam′ar) a transparent resin of *Dammara orientalis*, *D. alba*, *Hopea micrantha*, *H. splendida*, *Shorea* spp., and other trees; used in varnishes, as a mounting medium in microscopy, and for the preservation of animal and vegetable specimens.

dämmerschlaf (dem′er-shlaf) [Ger.] twilight sleep.

Damoiseau's curve, sign (dam-wah-zōz′) [Louis Hyacinthe Céleste *Damoiseau*, French physician, 1815–1890] see *Ellis's line*, under *line*.

damp (damp) foul air or noxious gas(es) in a mine. **after-d.,** a gaseous mixture formed in a mine by the explosion of fire damp or dust; it contains nitrogen, carbon dioxide, and usually carbon monoxide. **black d., choke d.,** a nonrespirable atmosphere sometimes formed in a mine by the gradual absorption of the oxygen and the giving off of carbon dioxide by the coal. **cold d.,** foggy vapor charged with carbon dioxide. **fire d.,** light explosive hydrocarbon gases, chiefly methane, CH_4, found in coal mines. **white d.,** carbon monoxide.

damping (damp′ing) the steady diminution of the amplitude of vibration of a specific form of energy, as of electricity or sound waves.

Dana's operation (da′nahz) [Charles Loomis *Dana*, neurologist in New York, 1852–1935] see under *operation*.

danazol (dah′nah-zōl) [USP] chemical name: 17α-pregna-2,4-dien-20-yno[2,3-*d*]isoxazol-17-ol. An anterior pituitary suppressant, $C_{22}H_{27}NO_2$, which has been used in the treatment of endometriosis, gynecomastia, fibrocystic mastitis, precocious puberty, and pubertal breast hypertrophy.

dance (dans) movement of a rhythmic, or of an unusual or exaggerated type. **brachial d.,** writhing of tortuous brachial arteries under the skin, sometimes observed in elderly arteriosclerotic patients. **hilar d.,** striking abnormal pulsation of hilar vessels. **hilus d.,** marked pulsations of the hilus shadows of both lungs on roentgen examination; seen in pulmonic regurgitation. **St. Anthony's d., St. Guy's d., St. John's d., St. Vitus' d.,** Sydenham's chorea. **St. Vitus' d. of the voice,** stuttering.

Dancel's treatment (dah-selz′) [Jean François *Dancel*, French physician, born 1804] see under *treatment*.

D and C dilation and curettage (dilation of the cervix and currettage of the uterus).

dander (dan′der) small scales from the hair or feathers of animals, which may be the cause of allergy in sensitive persons.

dandruff (dan′druf) 1. dry scaly material desquamated from the scalp; the term is applied to that normally desquamated from the epidermis of the scalp as well as to the excessive scaly material

associated with disease, as in seborrheic dermatitis. 2. seborrheic dermatitis of the scalp; called also *pityriasis sicca*.

Dandy-Walker syndrome (deformity) (dan′de-wok′er) [Walter Edward *Dandy*, American surgeon, 1886–1946; Arthur Earl *Walker*, American surgeon, born 1907] see under *syndrome*.

daniell (dan′yel) [John Frederick *Daniell*, English scientist, 1790–1845] a unit of electromotive force equal to 1.124 volts.

Danilone (dan′ĭ-lōn) trademark for a preparation of phenindione.

Danlos' syndrome (disease) (dan′los) [Henri Alexandre *Danlos*, French dermatologist, 1844–1912] Ehlers-Danlos syndrome.

DANS 1-dimethylaminonaphthalene-5-sulphonyl chloride. A fluorochrome that gives an apple green fluorescence in ultraviolet light resembling fluorescein isothiocyanate. It is employed in immunofluorescence studies of tissues and cells.

danthron (dan′thron) [USP] chemical name: 1,8-dihydroxy-9,10-anthracenedione. A cathartic, $C_{14}H_8O_4$, occurring as an orange, crystalline powder; administered orally.

dantrolene sodium (dan′tro-lēn) chemical name: 1-[[[5-(4-nitrophenyl)-2-furanyl]methylene]amino]-2,4-imidazolidinedione sodium salt tetrahydrate. A skeletal muscle relaxant, $C_{14}H_9N_4$-NaO, used as an antispasmodic in conditions such as stroke, multiple sclerosis, and cerebral palsy.

Danysz's phenomenon (effect) (dan′ēz) [Jan *Danysz*, Polish pathologist in Paris, 1860–1928] see under *phenomenon*.

Daphne (daf′ne) [Gr. *daphnē* bay tree] a genus of trees and shrubs. *D. gnidium* and *D. mezereum* L. (Thymelaeaceae), the principal medicinal species, are vesicatory and purgative. Toxic glycosides have caused the plant *D. mezereum* to be listed as poisonous; its attractive berries have poisoned children and livestock. See *mezereum*.

daphnetin (daf-ne′tin) the aglycon of daphnin, $C_9H_6O_4$, 7,8-dihydroxycoumarin.

Daphnia (daf′ne-ah) a genus of fresh-water crustaceans, called water fleas, often used in biological research.

daphnin (daf′nin) glycoside, $C_{15}H_{16}O_9 + 2H_2O$, from *Daphne mezereum*; 7,8-dihydroxycoumarin-7-β-D-glucoside.

daphnism (daf′nizm) poisoning by species of *Daphne*.

dapsone (dap′sōn) [USP] chemical name: 4,4′-sulfonylbisbenzenamine. An antibacterial, $C_{12}H_{12}N_2O_2S$, occurring as a white or creamy white, crystalline powder. It is the parent compound of a group of sulfonamide-like sulfones, including acedapsone, acetosulfone sodium, glucosulfone sodium, sulfoxone sodium, and solapsone. Dapsone and its derivatives are bacteriostatic for a broad spectrum of gram-negative and gram-positive organisms, including *Mycobacterium tuberculosis* and *M. leprae*, and have suppressive action on *Plasmodium falciparum*. Dapsone is used as a leprostatic, especially in tuberculoid and lepromatous leprosy, as a dermatitis herpetiformis suppressant, and in the prophylaxis of falciparum malaria; administered orally. Called also *diaminodiphenylsulfone* or *DDS*.

Daranide (dar′ah-nīd) trademark for a preparation of dichlorphenamide.

Daraprim (dar′ah-prim) trademark for a preparation of pyrimethamine.

Darbid (dar′bid) trademark for a preparation of isopropamide iodide.

Dar es Salaam bacterium (dahr es sah-lahm′) [*Dar es Salaam*, East Africa, where it was isolated in 1922] see under *bacterium*.

Dare's method (dārz) [Arthur *Dare*, Philadelphia physician, born 1868] see under *method*.

Daricon (dar′ĭ-kon) trademark for a preparation of oxyphencyclimine hydrochloride.

Darier's disease (dar′e-āz) [Ferdinand Jean *Darier*, French dermatologist, 1856–1938] keratosis follicularis.

Darkshevich's fibers, nucleus (ganglion) (dark-sha′vich-ez) [Liverij Osipovich *Darkshevich*, Russian neurologist, 1858–1925] see under *fiber* and *nucleus*.

Darling's disease (dar′lingz) [Samuel Taylor *Darling*, American physician, 1872–1925] histoplasmosis.

darmous (dahr′moos) North African name for fluorine poisoning.

darnel (dar′nel) a rye grass, *Lolium temulentum* L. (Gram.), the seeds of which contain a narcotic poison. Ingestion of flour contaminated with darnel may produce vertigo, staggering, vomiting, visual disturbances, burning pain in the mouth, and prostration.

d'arsonvalism, d'arsonvalization (dar′sonval″izm, dar″son-val″i-za′shun) [A. *d'Arsonval*, French physicist, 1851–1940] (*obs.*) a high-frequency treatment: the therapeutic use of high-frequency damped electromagnetic oscillations of relatively high voltage and low current.

Dartal (dar′tal) trademark for a preparation of thiopropazate dihydrochloride.

dartoic (dar-to′ik) of the nature of a dartos; having a slow, involuntary contractility like that of the dartos.

dartoid (dar′toid) resembling the dartos.

dartos (dar′tos) [Gr. "flayed"] tunica dartos.

dartre (dartr) [Fr.] a term formerly applied to various skin disorders, especially the herpetic (vesicular) or eczematous, having a common cause.

dartrous (dar′trus) 1. of, pertaining to, or resembling the dartos. 2. pertaining to dartre.

Darvon (dar′von) trademark for a preparation of propoxyphene hydrochloride.

darwinism (dar′wĭ-nizm) [Charles Robert *Darwin*, English naturalist, 1809–1882] the theory of evolution according to which higher organisms have been developed from lower ones through the influence of natural selection.

dasymeter (das-im′ĕ-ter) an instrument for measuring the density of a gas.

Dasypus (das′e-pus) [Gr. *dasypous* a rough foot] a genus of tropical armadillos, species of which are reservoirs of *Trypanosoma cruzi*, including *D. novemcincta*, the nine-banded armadillo.

data (da′tah) [L., plural of *datum*] the material or collection of facts on which a discussion or an inference is based.

Datura (da-tu′rah) a genus of solanaceous plants, the most famous of which is *D. stramonium* L. Its chief constituents are hyoscyamine and scopolamine, which give the herb anticholinergic properties. The powdered leaf is also incorporated into "asthma powders," which are burned as is or in cigarettes for asthma relief; the smoke carries the alkaloids to the bronchi, causing their relaxation. In large doses, asthma powders may induce intoxication with visual disturbances. **D. me′tel,** a source of scopolamine.

daturine (da-tu′rin) hyoscyamine.

daturism (da-tu′rizm) poisoning caused by plants of the genus *Datura*, which contain several solanaceous alkaloids of the tropane configuration; principal among these are atropine, hyoscyamine, and hyoscine (scopolamine).

Daubenton's angle, line, plane (do-bon-tonz′) [Louis Jean Marie *Daubenton*, French physician and naturalist, 1716–1800] see under *angle, line,* and *plane*.

dauernarkose (dow′er-nar-kōs) [Ger.] prolonged sleep.

dauerschlaf (dow′er-shlaf) [Ger.] prolonged sleep.

daughter (daw′ter) 1. decay product; see under *product*. 2. arising from cell division, as a daughter cell.

daunomycin (daw-no-mi′sin) daunorubicin.

daunorubicin (daw″no-ru′bĭ-sin) chemical name: (8*S*-*cis*)-8-acetyl-10-[(3-amino-2,3,6-trideoxy-α-L-lyxo-hexopyranosyl)oxy]-7,8,-9,10-tetrahydro-6,8,11-trihydroxy-1-methoxy-5,12-naphthacenedione. An antibiotic with antineoplastic, immunosuppressive, and antibacterial properties, $C_{27}H_{29}NO_{10}$, isolated from *Streptomyces peucetius*. Called also *daunomycin* and *rubidomycin*. **d. hydrochloride,** the hydrochloride salt of daunorubicin, $C_{27}H_{29}$-$NO_{10} \cdot HCl$, having the same actions as the base; it has been used investigationally in the treatment of acute myelogenous and acute lymphocytic leukemia.

Davainea (da-va′ne-ah) [Casimir Joseph *Davaine*, French physician, 1812–1882] a genus of tapeworms of the family Davaineidae. **D. proglotti′na,** a species found in fowls.

Davaineidae (da-va-ne′ĭ-de) a family of relatively small tapeworms of the order Cyclophyllidea, subclass Cestoda, which parasitize mammals and birds. *Davainea* and *Raillietina* are medically important genera.

David's disease (dah-vidz′) 1. [Jean Pierre *David*, French surgeon, 1737–1784] tuberculosis of the spine. 2. [W. *David*, German physician, born 1890] see under *disease*, def. 2.

Davidoff's (Davidov's) cells (da′vid-ofs) [M. von *Davidoff*, histologist in Munich, d. 1904] Paneth's cells.

Davidsohn's sign (da′vid-sōnz) [Hermann *Davidsohn*, Prussian physician, 1842–1911] see under *sign*.

Daviel's operation, spoon (dav-e-elz′) [Jacques *Daviel*, French oculist, 1696–1762, the originator of the modern treatment of cataract by extraction of the lens] see under *operation* and *spoon*.

Davis graft (da′vis) [John Staige *Davis*, American surgeon, 1872–1946] a pinch graft.

Davy's test (da′vez) [Edmund William *Davy*, Irish physician, 1826–1899] see under *tests*.

Dawbarn's sign [Robert Hugh Mackay *Dawbarn*, New York surgeon, 1860–1915] see under *sign*.

Day's test (dāz) [Richard Hance *Day*, American physician, 1813–1892] see under *tests*.

dazadrol maleate (da′zah-drōl) chemical name: α-(4-chlorophenyl)-α-(4,5-dihydro-1*H*-imidazol-2-yl)-2-pyridine methanol(*Z*)-2-butenedioate (1:1) (salt); an antidepressant, $C_{15}H_{14}ClN_3O \cdot C_4H_4$-$O_4$.

dB, db decibel.

DBA dibenzanthracene.

DBE (*obs.*) a synthetic estrogen, $(C_2H_5 \cdot O \cdot C_6H_4)_2 C{:}C(Br) \cdot C_6H_5$.

DBI trademark for preparations of phenformin hydrochloride.

D.C. direct current; Doctor of Chiropractic.

D & C dilatation and curettage (dilatation of the cervix and curettage of the uterus).

DCA desoxycorticosterone acetate.

D.Cc. double concave.

D.C.F. *direct centrifugal flotation;* see *Lane method,* under *method*.

D.C.H. Diploma in Child Health.

DCI dichloroisoproterenol.

D.C.O.G. Diploma of the College of Obstetricians and Gynaecologists (British).

D.Cx. double convex.

d.d. abbreviation for L. *de′tur ad,* "let it be given to."

DDS diaminodiphenylsulfone; see *dapsone*.

D.D.S. Doctor of Dental Surgery.

D.D.Sc. Doctor of Dental Science.

DDT chlorophenothane.

de- Latin prefix often signifying down or from; it is sometimes negative or privative, and frequently intensive.

deacetyllanatoside C (de-as″ĕ-til-lah-nat′o-sīd) deslanoside.

deacidification (de″ah-sid″ĭ-fĭ-ka′shun) the act or art of correcting or destroying acidity or of neutralizing an acid.

deactivation (de″ak-tĭ-va′shun) the process of making or becoming inactive, as the removal or loss of radioactivity from a previously radioactive material.

deacylase (de-as′il-ās) a hydrolase that catalyzes the removal of an acyl group. **acetyl-CoA d.,** acetyl-CoA hydrolase. **acyl-lysine d.,** a hydrolase that catalyzes the hydrolysis of ε-*N*-acyl-L-lysine to a fatty acid ion and L-lysine.

dead (ded) 1. destitute of life; see also *death*. 2. numb.

deaf (def) lacking the sense of hearing or having profound hearing loss.

deafferentate (de-af′er-en-tāt″) to eliminate or interrupt afferent nerve impulses, as by destruction of the afferent pathway.

deafferentation (de-af″er-en-ta′shun) the elimination or interruption of afferent nerve impulses, as by destruction of the afferent pathway.

deaf-mute (def-mūt′) an individual who is unable to hear or speak; it has been demonstrated that deaf individuals thought to be mute can learn to speak.

deaf-mutism (def-mūt′izm) the absence both of the sense of hearing and of the faculty of speech.

deafness (def′nes) lack of the sense of hearing, or profound hearing loss. Moderate loss of hearing is often called *hearing loss*. See also *hearing loss*, under *H*. **Alexander's d.,** see under *hearing loss*. **apoplectiform d.,** Meniere's disease in which the hearing impairment is sudden in onset and fluctuates, and ultimately severe and permanent deafness may occur. **bass d.,** deafness to certain low tones. **boilermakers' d.,** that caused by working in places where the noise level is extremely high. **central d.,** deafness due to causes in the auditory pathways or in the auditory center. **conduction d.,** see under *hearing loss*. **cortical d.,** deafness due to a lesion of cortical brain substance. **functional d.,** apparent deafness without organic lesion. **hysterical d.,** that which may appear or disappear in a hysterical patient without discoverable cause. **labyrinthine d.,** that which is due to disease of the labyrinth. **malarial d.,** that which occurs as a result of malarial poisoning. **Michel's d.,** congenital deafness due to total lack of development of the inner ear. **midbrain d.,** deafness dependent on injury of the fillet tract of the tegmentum. **Mondini's d.,** congenital deafness due to dysgenesis of the organ of Corti, with partial aplasia of the bony and membranous labyrinth and a resultant flattened cochlea. **music d.,** inability to recognize musical notes; amusia. **nerve d., neural d.,** that which is due to a lesion of the auditory nerve or the central neural pathways. **organic d.,** deafness due to defect in the ear or auditory apparatus. **pagetoid d.,** that occurring in osteitis deformans (Paget's disease) of the bones of the skull. **paradoxic d.,** see under *hearing loss*. **perceptive d.,** sensorineural d. **postlingual d.,** deafness acquired after the development of speech. **prelingual d.,** deafness acquired before the development of speech. **Scheibe's d.,** congenital deafness due to aplasia of the saccule and cochlear duct. **sensorineural d.,** deafness due to a lesion in the sensory mechanism (cochlea) of the ear or to a lesion in the acoustic nerve or the central neural pathways or to a combination of such lesions. See also *Rinne test*, under *tests*. **tone d.,** sensory amusia. **toxic d.,** deafness caused by the effect of poisons. **vascular d.,** that due to disease of blood vessels of the inner ear. **word d.,** a form of receptive aphasia in which sounds are heard, but convey no meaning to the mind, due to disease of the auditory center of the brain; called also *acoustic* or *auditory aphasia, aphememesthesia, auditory amnesia,* and *logokophosis*.

dealbation (de″al-ba′shun) bleaching.

dealcoholization (de-al″ko-hol-ĭ-za′shun) the removal of alcohol from an object or substance.

deallergization (de-al″er-ji-za′shun) the desensitization of an allergic individual to any particular allergen.

deamidase (de-am′ĭ-dās) an enzyme that splits amides to form carboxylic acid plus ammonia.

deamidation (de-am″ĭ-da′shun) deamidization.

deamidization (de-am″ĭ-di-za′shun) liberation of the ammonia from an amide.

deaminase (de-am′ĭ-nās) an enzyme that causes deamination, or the removal of the amino group from organic compounds. **adenosine d.,** an enzyme that catalyzes the change of adenosine to inosine and ammonia. **adenylic acid d.,** an enzyme that catalyzes the change of adenylic acid into inosine 5-phosphoric acid and ammonia. **cytidine d.,** an enzyme that catalyzes the change of cytidine into uridine and ammonia. **guanine d.,** guanine aminohydrolase: an enzyme that catalyzes the hydrolysis of guanine into xanthine and ammonia; called also *guanase.* **guanosine d.,** an enzyme that catalyzes the change of guanosine into xanthosine and ammonia. **guanylic acid d.,** an enzyme that catalyzes the change of guanylic acid into xanthylic acid and ammonia.

deamination (de-am″ĭ-na′shun) removal of the amino group, —NH_2, from a compound.

deaminization (de-am″ĭ-ni-za′shun) deamination.

Deaner (de′ner) trademark for a preparation of deanol acetamidobenzoate.

deanol acetamidobenzoate (de′ah-nol as″et-am′ĭ-do-ben′zo-āt) chemical name: 4-(acetylamino)benzoic acid compounded with 2-(dimethylamino)ethanol (1:1). A cerebral stimulant with parasympathomimetic activity, $C_{13}H_{20}N_2O_4$, occurring as a white or nearly white, crystalline powder; used as an antidepressant in the treatment of certain behavior and/or learning disorders in children.

deaquation (de″ah-kwa′shun) [L. *de* from + *aqua* water] removal of water from anything; dehydration.

Dearg. pil. (*obs.*) abbreviation for L. *deargen′tur pil′ulae,* let the pills be silvered.

dearterialization (de″ar-te″re-al-ĭ-za′shun) (*obs.*) 1. the conversion of arterial into venous blood. 2. interruption of the supply of oxygenated blood to a part or organ.

dearticulation (de″ar-tik″u-la′shun) dislocation of a joint.

death (deth) the cessation of life; permanent cessation of all vital bodily functions. For legal and medical purposes, the following definition of death has been proposed—the irreversible cessation of all of the following: (1) total cerebral function, (2) spontaneous function of the respiratory system, and (3) spontaneous function of the circulatory system. **apparent d.,** a state of complete interruption of bodily processes from which the patient can be resuscitated. **black d.,** former name for bubonic plague. **brain d.,** irreversible brain damage as manifested by absolute unresponsiveness to all stimuli, absence of all spontaneous muscle activity, including respiration, shivering, etc., and an isoelectric electroencephogram for 30 minutes, all in the absence of hypothermia or intoxication by central nervous system depressants. Called also *irreversible coma.* **cell d.,** complete degeneration or necrosis of cells. **cot d., crib d.,** sudden infant death syndrome; see under *syndrome.* **fetal d.,** stillbirth; death in utero; failure of the product of conception to show evidence of respiration, heart beat, or definite movement of a voluntary muscle after expulsion from the uterus, with no possibility of resuscitation. **fetal d., early,** fetal death occurring during the first 20 weeks of gestation. **fetal d., intermediate,** fetal death occurring during the twenty-first to twenty-eighth weeks of gestation. **fetal d., late,** fetal death occurring after 28 weeks of gestation. **functional d.,** total, permanent destruction of the central nervous system, with vital functions being sustained by artificial means. **genetic d.,** 1. failure of a given gene or genotype to be transmitted to progeny because of the death or sterility of the bearer of the gene or genotype. 2. failure of any organism to survive owing to its genetic makeup. **liver d.,** death due to failure of hepatic function. **local d.,** death of a part of the body. **molecular d.,** caries, catastasis, or the last stage of a catabolic process. **somatic d.,** cessation of all vital cellular activity. **voodoo d.,** a phenomenon seen among many primitive peoples in which the affected individual dies after transgressing a taboo or becoming convinced that he is bewitched.

Deaur. pil. (*obs.*) abbreviation for L. *deauren′tur pil′ulae,* let the pills be gilded.

Deaver's incision (de′verz) [John Blair *Deaver,* American surgeon, 1855–1931] see under *incision.*

debanding (de-band′ing) the removal of fixed orthodontic appliances.

Debaryomyces (de″bar-e-o-mi′sēz) a genus of ascomycetous fungi of the family Saccharomycetaceae. **D. hansen′ii,** a species which changes sugars into oxalic acid; called also *Saccharomyces hansenii.* **D. hom′inis, D. neofor′mans,** former name for *Cryptococcus neoformans.*

debility (de-bil′ĭ-te) lack or loss of strength.

débouchement (da-bōōsh-maw′) [Fr.] an opening out.

Debrisan (dĕ-bri′san) trademark for dextranomer.

Débove's disease, membrane, treatment (dĕ-bōvz′) [Georges Maurice *Débove,* French physician, 1845–1920] see *splenomegaly,* and see under *membrane* and *treatment.*

débride (da-brēd′) to remove foreign material and contaminated or devitalized tissue, usually by sharp dissection.

débridement (da-brēd′maw) [Fr.] the removal of foreign material and devitalized or contaminated tissue from or adjacent to a traumatic or infected lesion until surrounding healthy tissue is exposed. Cf. *épluchage.* **enzymatic d.,** removal of fibrinous or purulent exudate by application of a nontoxic and nonirritating enzyme which is capable of lysing fibrin, denatured collagen, and elastin, but does not destroy normal tissue. **surgical d.,** débridement by mechanical methods, usually sharp dissection.

debris (dĕ-bre′) [Fr.] accumulated fragments; rubbish. In dentistry, soft foreign matter loosely attached to the surface of a tooth. **word d.,** sounds made by an aphasic patient in attempting to talk.

Debrisan (dĕ-bri′san) trademark for dextranomer.

debrisoquin sulfate (deb-ris′o-kwin) chemical name: 3,4 - dihydro - 2 (1 *H*) - isoquinolinecarboxamidine sulfate; an antihypertensive agent, $C_{10}H_{13}N_3 \cdot \frac{1}{2}H_2SO_4$.

Deb. spis. abbreviation for L. *deb′ita spissitu′dine,* of the proper consistency.

debt (det) something owed. **oxygen d.,** the extra oxygen that must be used in the oxidative energy processes after a period of strenuous exercise to reconvert lactic acid to glucose, and decomposed ATP and creatine phosphate to their original states.

Dec. abbreviation for L. *decan′ta,* pour off.

deca- [Gr. *deka* ten] a combining form designating ten; used in naming units of measurement to indicate a quantity 10 times the unit designated by the root with which it is combined.

decacurie (dek″ah-ku′re) a unit of radioactivity, being ten curies.

Decaderm (dek′ah-derm) trademark for a preparation of dexamethasone.

Decadron (dek′ah-dron) trademark for preparations of dexamethasone.

Deca-Durabolin (de″ka-dur-ab′o-lin) trademark for a preparation of nandrolone decanoate.

decagram (dek′ah-gram) [*deca-* + *gram*] ten grams, or 154.32 grains troy.

decalcification (de″kal-sĭ-fi-ka′shun) 1. the loss of calcium salts from a bone or tooth. 2. the process of removing calcareous matter.

decalcify (de-kal′sĭ-fi) [L. *de* priv. + *calx* lime] to deprive of calcium salts.

decaliter (dek′ah-le″ter) [*deca-* + *liter*] ten liters, or 610.28 cubic inches.

decameter (dek′ah-me″ter) [*deca-* + *meter*] ten meters.

decamethonium (dek″ah-mĕ-tho′ne-um) chemical name: *N,N,N,N′,N′,N′*-hexamethyl-1,10-decanediaminium. A bisquaternary ammonium compound, $C_{16}H_{38}N_2$, structurally analogous to tubocurarine. **d. bromide** [USP], the bromide salt of decamethonium, $C_{16}H_{38}Br_2N_2$, occurring as a white crystalline powder; used as a skeletal muscle relaxant during surgical anesthesia, to aid endotracheal intubation, in obstetrics, and in electroconvulsive therapy, administered intravenously. **d. iodide,** the iodide salt of decamethonium, $C_{16}H_{38}I_2N_2$, which has been used for the same purposes as the bromide salt.

decane (dek′ān) a hydrocarbon, $C_{10}H_{22}$, from paraffin.

decannulation (de-kan″u-la′shun) removal of a cannula, especially of a tracheostomy cannula.

decanormal (dek″ah-nor′mal) [*deca-* + *normal*] having ten times the strength of normal; said of solutions.

decantation (de″kan-ta′shun) [*de-* + L. *canthus* tire of a wheel] the pouring of a clear supernatant liquid from a sediment.

decapeptide (dek″ah-pep′tīd) a peptide containing ten amino acids.

decapitation (de-kap″ĭ-ta′shun) [*de-* + L. *caput* head] the removal of the head, as of an animal, a fetus, or a bone; beheading.

decapitator (de-kap′ĭ-ta″tor) an instrument for removing the head of a fetus in embryotomy.

Decapoda (de-kah-po′dah) [Gr. *deka* ten + *pous* foot] an order of *Crustacea,* including the crabs, lobsters, shrimps, etc., which have five pairs of legs upon the thorax.

Decapryn (dek′kal-prin) trademark for preparations of doxylamine succinate.

decapsulation (de-kap″su-la′shun) removal of the capsule, especially of the renal capsule.

decarbazine (dah-kar′bah-zēn) chemical name: 5-(3,3-dimethyl-1-triazenyl)-1*H*-imidazole-4-carboxamide. A synthetic antineoplastic, $C_6H_{10}N_6O_3$, used in the treatment of metastatic malignant melanoma, Hodgkin's disease, soft-tissue sarcoma, and neuroblastoma, administered intravenously. Abbreviated DTIC.

decarbonization (de-kar″bon-i-za′shun) (*obs.*) the removal of carbon from the blood in the lungs by the substitution of oxygen for carbon dioxide.

decarboxylase (de″kar-bok′sĭ-lās) any of the lyase class of enzymes that catalyze the removal of carbon dioxide from the carboxyl group of alpha keto acids. **acetoacetate d.,** acetoacetate carboxy-lyase: an enzyme that catalyzes the removal of carbon dioxide from acetoacetate to form acetone. **acetolactate d.,** an enzyme that catalyzes the removal of carbon dioxide from acetolactate to form acetoin.

decarboxylation (de″kar-bok″sĭ-la′shun) removal of the carboxyl group.

decavitamin (dek″ah-vi′tah-min) [USP] a combination of vitamins in capsular or tablet form, each of which contains vitamins A and D, ascorbic acid, calcium pantothenate, cyanocobalamin, folic acid, niacinamide, pyridoxine hydrochloride, riboflavin, thiamine hydrochloride, and a suitable form of alpha tocopherol.

decay (de-ka′) [*de-* + L. *cadere* to fall] 1. the gradual decomposition of dead organic matter. 2. the process or stage of decline, as in aging. **beta d.,** disintegration of the nucleus of an unstable radionuclide in which the mass number is unchanged, but the atomic number is increased or decreased by 1, as result of emission of a negatively or positively charged (beta) particle and a neutrino. **radioactive d.,** disintegration of the nucleus of an unstable nuclide by the spontaneous emission of charged particles and/or photons; called also *radioactive disintegration*.

deceit (de-sēt) misrepresentation; deception. **facial d.,** in psychology, misrepresentation, in terms of facial expressiveness, of one's true emotional state; see also *falsifying, modulating,* and *qualifying*.

deceleration (de-sel″er-a′shun) decrease in speed or rate.

decentered (de-sen′terd) denoting a lens in which the visual axis does not pass through the optical center of the lens.

decentration (de″sen-tra′shun) [*de-* + L. *centrum* center] the act or process of removing from a center.

deceration (de″se-ra′shun) [*de-* + L. *cera* wax] the removal of paraffin from a tissue section prepared for the microscope.

decerebellation (de-ser″ĕ-bel-la′shun) removal of the cerebellum.

decerebrate (de-ser′ĕ-brāt) 1. to eliminate cerebral function by transecting the brain stem between the superior colliculi and the vestibular nuclei or by ligating the common carotid arteries and the basilar artery at the center of the pons. 2. an animal so prepared. 3. a person with brain damage resulting in neurologic signs similar to those of a decerebrated animal. See also *decerebrate rigidity,* under *rigidity*.

decerebration (de″ser-ĕ-bra′shun) [*de-* + *cerebrum*] the act of decerebrating.

decerebrize (de-ser′ĕ-brīz) to decerebrate (def. 1).

dechloridation (de-klo″rĭ-da′shun) the removal of chloride, or salt.

dechlorination (de-klo″rĭ-na′shun) dechloridation.

dechlorurant (de-klo′roo-rant) an agent that causes dechloruration.

dechloruration (de-klo″roo-ra′shun) diminution of excretion of chlorates in the urine.

decholesterinization (de″ko-les″ter-in-i-za′shun) decholesterolization.

decholesterolization (de″ko-les″ter-ol-i-za′shun) extraction of cholesterol from the blood.

Decholin (de′ko-lin) trademark for preparations of dehydrocholic acid.

deci- [L. *decem* ten] a combining form designating one-tenth; used in naming units of measurement to indicate one-tenth of the unit designated by the root with which it is combined (10⁻¹).

decibel (des′ĭ-bel) a unit used to express the ratio of two powers, usually electric or acoustic powers, equal to one-tenth the common logarithm of the ratio of the powers. One decibel is equal approximately to the smallest difference in acoustic power that the human ear can detect. Abbreviated dB and db. See also *bel*.

decidua (de-sid′u-ah) [L., from *deciduus* falling off] the endometrium of the pregnant uterus, all of which, except the deepest layer, is shed at parturition. Called also *membranae deciduae* [NA], *caduca, decidual* or *deciduous membrane,* and *tunica decidua*. **basal d., d. basa′lis** [NA], the portion of the decidua directly underlying the chorionic vesicle and attached to the myometrium; called also *d. serotina* and *membrana serotina*. **capsular d., d. capsula′ris** [NA], the portion of the decidua directly overlying the chorionic vesicle and facing the uterine cavity; called also *reflex d.* and *d. reflexa*. **menstrual d., d. menstrua′lis,** the hyperemic mucosa of the uterus that is shed during the menstrual period. **parietal d., d. parieta′lis** [NA], the portion of the decidua lining the uterus elsewhere than at the site of attachment of the chorionic vesicle; called also *d. vera*. **reflex d., d. reflex′a,** d. capsularis. **d. seroti′na,** d. basalis. **d. subchoria′lis,** the maternal component of the tissue

comprising the closing ring of Winkler-Waldeyer. **true d.,** d. parietalis. **d. tubero′sa papulo′sa,** a cast of the uterine cavity expelled at abortion. **d. ve′ra,** d. parietalis.

decidual (de-sid′u-al) pertaining to the decidua.

deciduate (de-sid′u-āt) characterized by shedding.

deciduation (de-sid″u-a′shun) the shedding of the decidua.

deciduitis (de-sid″u-i′tis) a bacterial disease leading to alterations in the decidua.

deciduoma (de-sid″u-o′mah) [*decidua* + *-oma*] an intrauterine mass containing decidual cells. **Loeb's d.,** a tumor-like structure resembling the maternal placenta, produced in the uteri of guinea pigs by the action of progesterone. **d. malig′num,** choriocarcinoma.

deciduomatosis (de-sid″u-o-mah-to′sis) formation of decidual tissue in the nonpregnant state.

deciduosarcoma (de-sid″u-o-sar-ko′mah) (*obs.*) choriocarcinoma.

deciduosis (de-sid″u-o′sis) the presence of decidual tissue or of tissue resembling the endometrium of pregnancy in an ectopic site.

deciduous (de-sid′u-us) [L. *deciduus,* from *decidere* to fall off] falling off or shed at maturity; the term is used to designate the teeth of the first dentition in animals and man.

decigram (des′ĭ-gram) the tenth part of a gram; 1.544 grains.

deciliter (des′ĭ-le″ter) one tenth of a liter, equal to 6.1028 cubic inches.

decimeter (des′ĭ-me″ter) one tenth of a meter, equal to 3.937 linear inches.

decinem (des′ĭ-nem) (*obs.*) Pirquet's term for one tenth of a nem or the nutritive value of 1 decigram of milk; abbreviated dn.

decinormal (des″ĭ-nor′mal) [L. *decimus* tenth + *norma* rule] having one tenth of the normal strength.

decipara (des″ĭ-par′ah) [L. *decem* ten + *parere* to produce] a woman who has had ten pregnancies which resulted in viable offspring; also written Para X.

decision (de-siz′un) a judgment, conclusion, or verdict. **Durham d.,** see under *rule*.

deckplatte (dek′plaht-tĕ) [Ger.] roof plate; see under *plate*.

declination (dek″lĭ-na′shun) [L. *declinare* to decline] deviation from a normally vertical position, as rotation of the eye about its anteroposterior axis so that its vertical meridian lies to the temporal (*positive d.*) or to the nasal side (*negative d.*) of its proper position.

declinator (dek′lĭ-na″tor) an instrument by which parts (as the meninges of the brain) are held aside during an operation.

decline (de-klīn) 1. the period or stage of the abatement of a disease or paroxysm. 2. a gradual deterioration or wasting away of the physical and mental faculties.

declive (de-klīv′) [Fr. *déclive;* L. *declivis*] [NA] the part of the vermis of the cerebellum just caudal to the primary fissure; called also *d. monticuli cerebelli*.

declivis (de-kli′vis) [L.] declive.

Declomycin (dek′lo-mi″sin) trademark for preparations of demeclocycline.

decoagulant (de″ko-ag′u-lant) 1. reducing the amount of existing coagulants or procoagulants in the blood. 2. a substance which inhibits coagulation of blood by reducing the amount of existing coagulants or procoagulants.

Decoct. abbreviation for L. *decoc′tum,* a decoction.

decoction (de-kok′shun) [L. *decoctum,* from *de* down + *coquere* to boil] 1. the act or process of boiling. 2. a medicine or other substance prepared by boiling. Called also *apozem*. **d. of the woods,** Zittmann's decoction. **Zimmermann's d.,** a cathartic decoction of rhubarb, potassium bitartrate, barley, water, and syrup. **Zittmann's d.,** a decoction of sarsaparilla, calomel, cinnabar, alum, senna, licorice, anise seed, and fennel.

decoctum (de-kok′tum) [L.] a decoction.

decollation (de″kol-la′shun) [*de-* + L. *collum* neck] decapitation, or beheading; removal of the head, chiefly of the fetus in difficult labor.

decoloration (de-kul″or-a′shun) 1. removal of color; bleaching. 2. lack or loss of color.

decolorize (de-kul′or-īz) to free from color; to bleach.

decompensation (de″kom-pen-sa′shun) 1. failure of compensation; cardiac decompensation is marked by dyspnea, venous engorgement, and edema. 2. in psychiatry, failure of defense mechanisms resulting in progressive personality disintegration.

decomplementize (de-kom′ple-men″tīz) to remove complement from.

decomposition (de″kom-po-zish′un) [*de-* + L. *componere* to put together] the separation of compound bodies into their constituent principles by whatever process. **anaerobic d.,** the breakdown of organic compounds in the absence of oxygen. In animals, the process is known as *glycolysis;* in plants and microorganisms, *fermentation*. **d. of movement,** lack of coordination characterized by irregularity in the successive flexion and extension of joints in performing a movement with the limb.

decompression (de″kom-presh′un) the removal of pressure, particularly the slow lessening of pressure on deep-sea divers and caisson workers to prevent the onset of bends, and the reduction of pressure on persons as they ascend to great heights. See also under *sickness*. **abdominal d.**, the removal of pressure from the abdomen during the first stage of labor. **cardiac d.**, d. of heart. **cerebral d.**, removal of a flap of the skull and incision of the dura mater for the purpose of relieving intracranial pressure. **explosive d.**, decompression more rapid than that corresponding to a rate of ascent greater than 5000 feet per minute. **d. of heart,** pericardiotomy with evacuation of a hematoma; called also *d. of pericardium*. **Heyns′ d.,** a method of abdominal decompression using a partial vacuum. **nerve d.,** relief of pressure on a nerve by surgical removal of the constricting fibrous or bony tissue. **d. of pericardium,** d. of heart. **d. of rectum,** proctostomy for imperforate anus. **d. of spinal cord,** relief of pressure on the spinal cord by means of surgery; the pressure may be due to hematoma, bone fragments, etc. **subtemporal d.,** cerebral decompression after removal of a portion of the temporal bone.

deconditioning (de″kon-dish′un-ing) a change in cardiovascular function after prolonged periods of weightlessness, probably related to a shift of a quantity of blood from the lower limbs to the thorax, resulting in reflex diuresis and a reduction of blood volume.

decongestant (de″kon-jes′tant) 1. tending to reduce congestion or swelling. 2. an agent that reduces congestion or swelling.

decongestive (de″kon-jes′tiv) reducing congestion.

decontamination (de″kon-tam-ĭ-na′shun) the freeing of a person or an object of some contaminating substance such as war gas, radioactive material, etc.

decoquinate (de-ko-kwin′āt) chemical name: 6-(decyloxy)-7-ethoxy-4-hydroxy-3-quinolinecarboxylic acid ethyl ester, a coccidiostat effective against the sporozoan *Eimeria*, $C_{24}H_{35}NO_5$; used in poultry.

decortication (de″kor-tĭ-ka′shun) [*de-* + L. *cortex* bark] 1. the removal of bark, hull, husk, or shell from a plant, seed, or root, as in pharmacy. 2. removal of portions of the cortical substance of a structure or organ, as of the brain, kidney, lung, etc. **arterial d.,** periarterial sympathectomy. **chemical d., enzymatic d.,** removal of cortical substance by chemical agents or enzymes. **d. of lung,** removal of the visceral pleura to permit the lung to expand. **renal d.,** removal of the capsule of the kidney; decapsulation of the kidney.

decrement (dek′re-ment) [L. *decrementum*] 1. subtraction, or decrease; the amount by which a quantity or value is decreased. 2. the stage of decline of a disease; see *stadium decrementi.*

decrepitate (de-krep′ĭ-tāt) 1. to roast or calcine certain substances (salt, crystals, etc.) until crackling occurs, or until crackling ends. 2. to explode with a crackling noise upon heating, owing to the release of entrapped water as steam.

decrepitation (de-krep″ĭ-ta′shun) the explosion or crackling of certain substances (salt, crystals, etc.) upon heating.

decrudescence (de″kroo-des′ens) diminution or abatement of the intensity of symptoms.

decrustation (de″krus-ta′shun) the detachment of a crust.

dectaflur (dek′tah-floor) chemical name: 9-octadecenylamine hydrofluoride; a dental caries prophylactic, $C_{18}H_{37}N \cdot HF$.

Decub. abbreviation for L. *decu′bitus,* lying down.

decubation (de″ku-ba′shun) [*de-* + L. *cubare* to lie down] the period in the course of an infectious disease from the disappearance of the symptoms to complete recovery and the end of the infectious period. Cf. *incubation.*

decubital (de-ku′bĭ-tal) pertaining to decubitus (decubitus ulcer).

decubitus (de-ku′bĭ-tus), pl. *decu′bitus* [L. "a lying down"] 1. an act of lying down; also the position assumed in lying down. 2. decubitus ulcer; see under *ulcer*. **d. acu′tus,** a severe decubitus ulcer on a paralyzed side in hemiplegia. **Andral′s d.,** decubitus on the sound side; a position assumed in the early stages of pleurisy. **dorsal d.,** lying in the supine position. **lateral d.,** lying on the side, as for radiologic examinations; designated right lateral decubitus when the subject lies on his right side and left lateral decubitus when on his left side. **ventral d.,** lying on the stomach.

decumbin (de-kum′bin) a toxic substance obtained from *Penicillium decumbens,* which causes respiratory distress and hemorrhage; the oral LD_{50} for rats is about 275 mg./kg.

decurrent (de-kur′ent) [L. *decurrere* to run down] extending or moving from above downward.

decussate (de-kus′āt) [L. *decussare* to cross in the form of an X] 1. to cross or intersect in the form of the letter X. 2. crossing in the form of the letter X.

decussatio (de″kus-sa′she-o), pl. *decussatio′nes* [L.] [NA] decussation; [NA] a general term for the intercrossing of fellow parts or structures in the form of an X. See also *chiasma* and *commissura.* **d. bra′chii conjuncti′vi,** d. pedunculorum cerebellarium su-

periorum. **d. lemnis′ci, d. lemnisco′rum** [NA], decussation of lemniscus; the region at the caudal end of the medulla oblongata in which the fibers from the nucleus cuneatus and the nucleus gracilis on each side intersect as they cross the midline before ascending as the medial lemniscus. Called also *d. sensoria* [NA alternative] and *decussation of fillet.* **d. moto′ria,** NA alternative for *d. pyramidum.* **d. nervo′rum trochlea′rium** [NA], decussation of trochlear nerves: the crossing of the fibers of the trochlear nerves in the superior medullary velum. **d. pedunculo′rum cerebella′rium superio′rum** [NA], decussation of superior cerebellar peduncles: the crossing of the fibers of the superior cerebellar peduncles within the tegmentum of the mesencephalon. Called also *d. brachii conjunctivi.* **d. pyram′idum** [NA], pyramidal decussation: the anterior part of the lower medulla oblongata in which most of the fibers of each pyramid intersect as they cross the midline and descend as the lateral corticospinal tracts. Called also *d. motoria* [NA alternative], *decussation of pyramids,* and *motor decussation.* **d. senso′ria,** NA alternative for *d. lemniscorum.* **decussatio′nes tegmen′ti** [NA], **decussatio′nes tegmento′rum,** decussations of tegmentum: crossing fibers in the midbrain, including the ventral tegmental decussation of the rubrospinal and rubroreticular tracts, and the dorsal tegmental decussation of the tectospinal tract. Called also *tegmental decussations.*

decussation (de″kus-sa′shun) a crossing over; see *decussatio.* **d. of fillet,** decussatio lemniscorum. **Forel′s d.,** the ventral tegmental decussation of the rubrospinal and rubroreticular tracts in the mesencephalon. **fountain d. of Meynert,** the dorsal tegmental decussation of the tectospinal tract in the mesencephalon. **d. of lemniscus,** decussatio lemniscorum. **motor d.,** decussatio pyramidum. **optic d., d. of optic nerves** (*obs.*), chiasma opticum. **pyramidal d., d. of pyramids,** decussatio pyramidum. **d. of superior cerebellar peduncles,** decussatio pedunculorum cerebellarium superiorum. **tegmental d′s, d′s of tegmentum,** decussationes tegmenti. **d. of trochlear nerves,** decussatio nervorum trochlearium.

decussationes (de″kus-sa″she-o′nēz) [L.] plural of *decussatio.*

decussorium (de″kus-so′re-um) an instrument for depressing the dura mater in trephining.

dedentition (de″den-tish′un) [*de-* + L. *dens* tooth] the shedding or loss of teeth.

dedifferentiation (de-dif″er-en″she-a′shun) anaplasia.

de d. in d. abbreviation for L. *de di′e in di′em,* from day to day.

dedolation (ded″o-la′shun) 1. a sensation as if the limbs had been bruised. 2. the removal of a thin piece of skin by an oblique cut.

de Duve (dĕ doōv′), Christian Rene. Belgian biochemist in U.S., born 1917; co-winner, with Albert Claude and George E. Palade, of Nobel prize in medicine or physiology for 1974, for his work in development of cell fractionation and discovery of lysosomes.

deemanate (de-em′ah-nāt) to deprive of the property of giving off radioactive emanations.

Deen′s test (dēnz) [Izaac Abrahamszoon van *Deen,* Dutch physiologist, 1804–1869] see under *tests.*

deep (dēp) situated far beneath the surface; not superficial.

de-epicardialization (de″ep-ĭ-kar″dĭ-al-ĭ-za′shun) a surgical procedure for the relief of intractable angina pectoris, in which epicardial tissue is destroyed by phenolization or the application of other caustic agents to promote the development of collateral circulation.

Deetjen′s bodies (dāt′yenz) [Hermann *Deetjen,* German physician, 1867–1915] blood platelets.

DEF an expression of dental caries experience in deciduous teeth, *D* representing the number of teeth indicated for filling; *E* the number indicated for extraction; *F* the number of filled teeth.

defatigation (de-fat″ĭ-ga′shun) overstrain or fatigue of muscular or nervous tissue.

defatted (de-fat′ed) deprived of fat, as a food.

defaunate (de-fawn′āt) [*de-* + L. *fauna* animal life] to remove or destroy an animal population; sometimes applied to removal of hookworms from the intestinal tract, delousing, etc.

defecation (def″e-ka′shun) [L. *defaecare* to deprive of dregs] 1. the removal of impurities, as chemical defecation. 2. the evacuation of fecal material from the rectum. **fragmentary d.,** the evacuation of small pieces of feces.

defect (de′fekt) an imperfection, failure, or absence. **acquired d.,** an imperfection arising secondarily, after birth. **aortic septal d.,** a congenital anomaly in which there is abnormal communication between the ascending aorta and pulmonary artery just above the semilunar valves; called also *aorticopulmonary fenestration, aorticopulmonary septal d.,* and *aorticopulmonary window.* **aorticopulmonary septal d.,** aortic septal d. **atrial septal d′s, atrioseptal d′s,** congenital cardiac anomalies in which there is persistent patency of the atrial septum due to failure of fusion between either the septum secundum or the septum primum and the endocardial cushions. In *ostium secundum defect* there is a rim of septum all around the defect. In *ostium* *primum defect,* which is an incomplete form of atrioventricularis communis, there is no septum at the base of the defect, between the mitral and tricuspid valves; it is usually associated with a cleft mitral cusp and occasionally with a cleft tricuspid valve. **birth d.,** congenital d. **congenital d.,** birth defect; a structural or chemical imperfection present at birth. **cortical d.,** a benign, symptomless, circumscribed rarefaction of cortical bone, detected radiographically; called also *subperiosteal cortical d.* **ectodermal d., congenital,** a rare hereditary condition affecting chiefly males and marked by a smooth glossy skin, total absence of sweat glands, abnormality of the teeth, and defective hair formation. Saddle nose, prominent frontal bones, large chin, and thick lips are characteristic. It is transmitted as an X-linked trait, and possibly as an autosomal recessive in rare instances. Called also *anhidrotic ectodermal dysplasia* and *Christ-Siemens* or *Christ-Siemens-Touraine syndrome.* Cf. *hidrotic ectodermal dysplasia.* **endocardial cushion d's,** a spectrum of septal defects resulting from imperfect fusion of the endocardial cushions, and ranging from persistent ostium primum to persistent common atrioventricular canal; see *atrial septal d's* and *atrioventricularis communis.* **filling d.,** any localized defect in the contour of the stomach, duodenum, or intestine, as seen in the roentgenogram after a barium enema, due to a lesion of the wall projecting into the lumen or to an object in the lumen. **neural-tube d.,** a developmental anomaly resulting in anencephaly or spina bifida. **ostium primum d.,** see *atrial septal d.* **ostium secundum d.,** see *atrial septal d.* **retention d.,** a defect in the power of recalling or remembering names, numbers, or events. **salt-losing d.,** see under *syndrome.* **septal d.,** a defect in one of the cardiac septa, resulting in an abnormal communication between the opposite chambers of the heart. **subperiosteal cortical d.,** cortical d. **ventricular septal d.,** a congenital cardiac anomaly in which there is persistent patency of the ventricular septum in either the muscular or fibrous portions, most often due to failure of the bulbar septum to completely close the interventricular foramen.

defective (de-fek′tiv) 1. imperfect. 2. a person lacking in some physical, mental, or moral quality.

defeminization (de-fem″ĭ-ni-za′shun) loss of female sexual characteristics.

defense (de-fens′) behavior directed to the protection of the individual from injury. **character d.,** any character trait, e.g., a mannerism, attitude, or affectation, which serves as a defense mechanism. **insanity d.,** a legal concept that a person cannot be convicted of a crime if he lacked criminal responsibility by reason of insanity at the time of commission. See *M'Naghten rule* and *Durham rule,* under *rule,* and *American Law Institute Formulation,* under *formulation.* **muscular d.,** the muscular tension and rigidity which accompanies a localized inflammation (as in appendicitis) or passage of a kidney stone. **ur d.,** see *ur-defense.*

deferens (def′er-enz) [L.] deferent; see *ductus deferens.*

deferent (def′er-ent) [L. *deferens* carrying away] conveying anything away, as from a center.

deferentectomy (def″er-en-tek′to-me) surgical removal of a ductus deferens.

deferential (def″er-en′shal) pertaining to the ductus deferens.

deferentitis (def″er-en-ti′tis) inflammation of the ductus deferens.

deferoxamine (dĕ-fer-oks′ah-mēn) chemical name: *N′*-[5-[[4-[[5-(acetylhydroxyamino) pentyl] amino] -1,4-dioxobutyl] hydroxyamino]pentyl]-*N*-(5-aminopentyl)-*N*-hydroxybutanediamide. A chelating agent, isolated from *Streptomyces pilosus,* $C_{25}H_{48}N_6O_8$, which binds with iron to form a soluble complex. Called also *desferrioxamine.* **d. hydrochloride,** the hydrochloride salt of deferoxamine, $C_{25}H_{48}N_6O_8 \cdot HCl.$ **d. mesylate,** [USP], the water-soluble mesylate salt of deferoxamine, $C_{25}H_{48}N_6O_8 \cdot CH_3SO_3H$, occurring as a white to off-white powder, having the same actions as the base; used as an antidote to iron poisoning, usually administered by intramuscular injection or by intravenous infusion. *Sterile deferoxamine mesylate,* prepared in conformance with USP specifications, is suitable for parenteral use.

defervescence (def″er-ves′ens) [L. *defervescere* to cease boiling] the period of abatement of fever.

defervescent (def″er-ves′ent) 1. causing reduction of fever. 2. an agent that acts to reduce fever.

defibrillation (de-fib″rĭ-la′shun) termination of atrial or ventricular fibrillation, usually by electroshock. 2. separation of the fibers of a tissue by blunt dissection.

defibrillator (de-fib″rĭ-la′tor) [*de-* + *fibrillation*] an electronic apparatus used to counteract atrial or ventricular fibrillation by the application of brief electroshock to the heart, directly or through electrodes placed on the chest wall.

defibrinated (de-fi′brĭ-nāt″ed) deprived of fibrin.

defibrination (de-fi″brĭ-na′shun) removal of fibrin from the blood; see also under *syndrome.*

deficiency (de-fish′en-se) a lack or defect. **17-hydroxylase d.,** see under *syndrome.* **kappa-chain d.,** deficiency in immunoglobulin molecules with kappa light chains. **mental d.,**

see under *retardation.* **oxygen d.,** anoxemia; hypoxia. **thymus-dependent d.,** a defect in cell-mediated immunity with relatively intact humoral immunity, due to aplasia or dysplasia of the thymus and the resultant lack of T(thymus-dependent)-lymphocytes, as in Nezelof's syndrome and DiGeorge's syndrome. **thymus-independent d.,** a defect in the proliferation of B(thymus-independent)-lymphocytes, including agammaglobulinemia and dysgammaglobulinemia. **vitamin d.,** see specific vitamins.

deficit (def′ĭ-sit) a lack or deficiency. **oxygen d.,** see *anoxia, anoxemia,* and *hypoxia.* **pulse d.,** the difference between the heart rate and the pulse rate in atrial fibrillation, resulting from failure of some of the ventricular contractions to produce peripheral pulse waves.

Definate (def′ĭ-nāt) trademark for a preparation of docusate sodium.

definition (def″ĭ-nish′un) the clear determination of the limits of anything, as of a disease process or a microscopical image. See also *resolution,* def. 2.

definitive (de-fin′ĭ-tiv) established with certainty. In embryology, denoting acquisition of final differentiation or character. In parasitology, denoting the host in which a parasite reaches the sexual stage.

deflection (de-flek′shun) a turning aside; in psychoanalysis, an unconscious diversion of ideas from conscious attention.

defloration (def″lo-ra′shun) [L. *deflora′tio*] the rupturing of the hymen in sexual intercourse, in vaginal examination, or by sexual manipulation.

deflorescence (def″lo-res′ens) the disappearance of the eruption in any exanthematous disease.

defluvium (de-floo′ve-um) [L.] defluxio. **postpartum d.,** loss of hair by the mother after delivery. **d. un′guium,** onychomadesis.

defluxio (de-fluk′se-o) [L.] 1. a flowing down. 2. a disappearance.

defluxion (de-fluk′shun) [L. *defluxio*] 1. a sudden disappearance. 2. a copious discharge, as of catarrhal fluid. 3. a falling out, as of the hair.

deformability (de-form″ah-bil′ĭ-te) the ability of cells, such as erythrocytes, to change shape as they pass through narrow spaces, such as the microvasculature.

deformation (de″for-ma′shun) 1. deformity, especially an alteration in shape and/or structure of a previously normally formed part. 2. the process of adapting in shape or form, as the change in shape of erythrocytes as they pass through capillaries.

deforming (de-form′ing) causing or producing deformity.

deformity (de-for′mĭ-te) distortion of any part or general disfigurement of the body; malformation. **Åkerlund d.,** a deformity of the duodenal cap in the radiograph in duodenal ulcer, consisting of an indentation (incisura) in addition to the niche. **Arnold-Chiari d.,** a congenital anomaly in which the cerebellum and medulla oblongata, which is elongated and flattened, protrude down into the spinal canal through the foramen magnum; it may be associated with many other defects, including spina bifida occulta and meningomyelocele. Called also *Arnold-Chiari malformation* or *syndrome.* **boutonnière d.,** a deformity of the finger characterized by flexion of the proximal interphalangeal joint and hyperextension of the distal joint; called also *buttonhole d.* **buttonhole d.,** 1. boutonnière d. 2. see *buttonhole mitral stenosis,* under *stenosis.* **crossbar d.,** the stiffening of a segment of the lesser curvature of the stomach, usually due to the healing of a deep penetrating ulcer. **Dandy-Walker d.,** see under *syndrome.* **funnel d.,** a funnel-shaped mitral orifice occurring as a result of fusion and shortening of the chordae tendineae. **gun stock d.,** cubitus varus. **Ilfeld-Holder d.,** prominent scapula with difficulty in raising the arm. **lobster-claw d.,** a developmental anomaly characterized by an abnormal cleft between the central metacarpal bones, the soft tissues of the digits being fused into two masses, one on either side of the cleft. **Madelung's d.,** radial deviation of the hand secondary to overgrowth of the distal ulna or shortening of the radius; called also *carpus curvus.* **recurvatum d.,** a deformity of the proximal interphalangeal joint in which the joint extends when pressure is exerted between the thumb and middle finger. **reduction d.,** congenital absence of a portion or all of a body part, especially the limbs. **rocker-bottom d.,** see under *foot* (def. 1). **rolled edge d.,** a highly characteristic deformity of the aortic valve cusps caused by syphilis. **seal-fin d.,** ulnar deviation of the fingers in rheumatoid arthritis. **silver fork d.,** the peculiar deformity seen in Colles' fracture; see illustration under *fracture.* Called also *Velpeau's deformity.* **Sprengel's d.,** congenital elevation of the scapula, due to failure of descent of the scapula to its normal thoracic position during fetal life. **swan-neck d.,** a finger deformity in which the proximal interphalangeal joint is hyperextended and the distal interphalangeal joint is flexed. **ulnar drift d.,** a deformity occurring when the proximal phalanx dislocates toward the volar aspect of the metacarpal head and at the same time deviates to the ulnar side of the hand. **Velpeau's d.,** silver fork deformity. **Volkmann's d.,** see under *disease.*

defundation (de″fun-da′shun) [*de-* + L. *fundus*] excision of the fundus of the uterus along with the uterine tubes; called also *defundectomy.*

defundectomy (de″fun-dek′to-me) defundation.

Deg. degeneration; degree.

degassing (de-gas′ing) 1. removal of a gas from a person or an object. 2. treatment of a person or an object subjected to the fumes of gas. 3. in dentistry, the heating of gold in a flame to drive off any contaminating gases and increase its cohesive properties.

degeneracy (de-jen′er-ah-se) a state characterized by deterioration of the powers of body and mind; called also *Nordan's disease* or *nordanism.*

degenerate 1. (de-jen′er-āt) to change from a higher to a lower type or form. 2. (de-jen′er-it) characterized by degeneration. 3. (de-jen′er-it) a person whose moral or physical state is below the normal.

degeneratio (de-jen″er-a′she-o) [L.] degeneration. **d. mi′-cans,** glistening degeneration.

degeneration (de-jen″er-a′shun) [L. *degeneratio*] deterioration; change from a higher to a lower form; especially change of tissue to a lower or less functionally active form. When there is chemical change of the tissue itself, it is *true* degeneration; when the change consists in the deposit of abnormal matter in the tissues, it is *infiltration.* Called also *retrogression.* **Abercrombie's d.,** amyloid d. **adipose d.,** fatty d. **adiposogenital d.,** adiposogenital dystrophy. **albuminoid d., albuminous d.,** cloudy swelling; see under *swelling.* **amyloid d.,** degeneration with the deposit of lardacein in the tissues; it indicates impairment of nutritive function, and is seen in wasting diseases. Also known as *Abercrombie's d.* or *syndrome, Virchow's d., bacony d., cellulose d., hyaloid d., lardaceous d.,* and *waxy d.* **angiolithic d.,** one characterized by mineral deposits and hyaline changes in the coats of the vessels. **Armanni-Ehrlich's d.,** hyaline degeneration of the epithelial cells of Henle's loops; seen in diabetes. **ascending d.,** wallerian degeneration affecting centripetal nerve fibers and progressing toward the brain or spinal cord. **atheromatous d.,** atheroma (def. 2). **axonal d.,** the reaction of a nerve cell to injury to its axon; it consists of central chromatolysis and eccentricity of the nucleus. **bacony d.,** amyloid d. **basic d., basophilic d.,** basophilia, def. 1. **black d. of brain,** a fungous disease caused by species of *Cladosporium,* especially *C. tricoides,* which is named for the most apparent pathological sign. On tissue section of the brain, multiseptate, brown distorted hyphae are seen. **blastophthoric d.,** blastophthoria. **calcareous d.,** degeneration with infiltration of calcareous materials into the tissues; called also *earthy d.* **caseous d.,** caseation, def. 2. **cellulose d.,** amyloid d. **cerebromacular d., cerebroretinal d.,** degeneration of brain cells and of the macula retinae, as in Tay-Sachs disease. **cheesy d.,** caseation, def. 2. **chitinous d.,** amyloid d. **colloid d.,** the assumption by the tissues of a gumlike or gelatinous character; called also *gelatiniform d.* **colloid d. of choroid,** Tay's choroiditis. **comma d.,** progressive degeneration of the nervous matter of the comma tract (interfascicular fasciculus). **congenital macular d.,** a hereditary form of macular degeneration transmitted as an autosomal dominant trait, and characterized by the presence of a cystlike lesion that in the early stages resembles egg yolk; called also *vitelliform d. of Best.* **corticostriatal-spinal d.,** Creutzfeldt-Jakob syndrome. **crenation d.,** a condition in which the cells of the corium become irregular and toothed; it is seen in granuloma fungoides. **Crooke's hyaline d.,** degeneration of basophils of the pituitary gland, in which they lose their specific granulations and the cytoplasm becomes progressively hyalinized; a constant finding in Cushing's syndrome, but also occurring in Addison's disease. **cystic d.,** degeneration with the formation of cysts. **cystoid d.,** Blessig's cysts. **descending d.,** wallerian degeneration extending peripherally along nerve fibers. **disciform macular d.,** a form of macular degeneration occurring in persons over 40 years of age, in which sclerosis involving the macula and retina is produced by hemorrhages between Bruch's membrane and the pigment epithelium; called also *senile macular exudative choroiditis, senile disciform d.,* and *Kuhnt-Junius disease.* **Doyne's familial colloid d., Doyne's honeycomb d.,** see under *choroiditis.* **dystrophic d.,** degeneration arising from defective or faulty nutrition. **earthy d.,** calcareous d. **elastoid d.,** amyloid degeneration of the elastic tissue of arteries. **familial colloid d.,** Doyne's familial honeycombed choroiditis. **fascicular d.,** degeneration of paralyzed muscles due to lesion in the motor ganglion cells of the central tube of gray matter of the cord. **fatty d.,** deposit of fat globules in a tissue; called also *adipose d.* **fibrinous d.,** necrosis with deposit of fibrin within the cells of the tissue. **fibroid d.,** degeneration into fibrous tissue. **fibrous d.,** fibrosis. **gelatiniform d.,** colloid d. **glassy d.,** a peculiar change occurring in the heart muscle and other muscles in fevers. **glistening d.,** degeneration of glia tissue characterized by the formation of glistening masses; called also *degeneratio micans* and *Rosenthal's d.* **glycogenic d.,** a form of degeneration in which abnormal amounts of glycogen accumulate in the cells, as in glycogenosis. **Gombault's d.,**

progressive hypertrophic interstitial neuropathy. **granulovascular d.,** a condition in which the ganglion cells become filled with vacuoles containing condensed granules of protoplasm. **gray d.,** degeneration of the white substance of the spinal cord, in which it loses myelin and assumes a gray color. **hematohyaloid d.,** a form of hyaline degeneration of thrombi due to conglutination of the red cells or blood platelets. **hemoglobinemic d.,** an archaic term applied to accumulation of hemoglobin in the center of the erythrocyte. **hepatolenticular d.,** a rare progressive disease, inherited as an autosomal recessive trait, and due to a defect in the metabolism of copper; a pigmented ring (Kayser-Fleischer ring) at the outer margin of the cornea is pathognomonic. The disease is characterized by degenerative changes in the brain, especially the basal ganglia, and by cirrhosis of the liver, splenomegaly, involuntary movements, tremor, muscular rigidity, spastic contractures, psychic disturbances, dysphagia, and increasing weakness and emaciation. Called also *familial hepatitis, hepatolenticular disease, lenticular d., progressive lenticular d., Strümpell-Westphal pseudosclerosis, Westphal-Strümpell disease* or *pseudosclerosis,* and especially *Wilson's degeneration, disease,* or *syndrome.* **Holmes's d.,** primary progressive cerebellar d. **Horn's d.,** degeneration with nuclear proliferation in striated muscles. **hyaline d.,** a regressive cellular change in which the cytoplasm take on a homogeneous glassy eosinophilic appearance. Also used loosely to describe the histologic appearance of tissues. Called also *vitreous d.* and *hyalinosis.* **hyaloid d.,** amyloid d. **hydropic d.,** a variety in which the epithelial cells absorb much water. **lardaceous d.,** amyloid d. **lattice d. of retina,** a frequently bilateral, usually benign asymptomatic condition, characterized by patches of fine gray or white lines that intersect at irregular intervals in the peripheral retina, usually associated with numerous, round, punched-out areas of retinal thinning or retinal holes. **lenticular d.,** hepatolenticular d. **lipoidal d.,** a condition somewhat resembling fatty degeneration or infiltration but in which the extraneous material is lipoid. **macular d.,** degenerative changes in the macula retinae. **Mönckeberg's d.,** see under *arteriosclerosis.* **mucinoid d.,** a term used to include both mucoid and colloid degeneration; called also *mucinous d.* and *myelinic d.* **mucinous d.,** mucous d. **mucoid d.,** degeneration accompanied by deposit of myelin and lecithin in the cells. **mucous d.,** a form in which mucus accumulates in epithelial tissues. **myelinic d.,** mucoid d. **myxomatous d.,** degeneration in which mucus accumulates in connective tissues. **Nissl d.,** degeneration of a nerve cell after division of the nerve fiber supplying it. **olivopontocerebellar d.,** familial cerebellar degeneration occurring in the young or middle aged, characterized by extensive atrophy of the middle cerebellar peduncles and of the ventral surface of the pons, with loss of myelin in the white matter of the cerebellum and of cells in the olivary nuclei, the nuclei pontis, and the Purkinje and granular cell layers of the cerebellum. **pallidal d.,** degeneration of the globus pallidus. **parenchymatous d.,** cloudy swelling. **Paschutin's d.,** the degeneration peculiar to diabetes. **pigmental d., pigmentary d.,** that in which cells of affected tissue become abnormally pigmented. **polypoid d.,** the development, on a mucous membrane, of polypoid growths. **primary progressive cerebellar d.,** a familial disease marked by motor disorders and due to cerebellar degeneration, occurring in adults between the ages of thirty and forty and progessing slowly to a fatal termination; called also *Holmes' d.* **progressive lenticular d.,** hepatolenticular d. **Quain's d.,** fibrous degeneration of the muscles of the heart. **red d.,** degeneration of a uterine leiomyoma during pregnancy, marked by the formation of soft red areas due to necrosis and edema. **retrograde d.,** axon reaction. **rim d.,** degeneration of the spinal cord affecting the periphery only. **Rosenthal's d.,** glistening d. **sclerotic d.,** a variety of hyaline degeneration affecting connective tissue, especially the intima of arteries. **secondary d.,** wallerian d. **senile d.,** the widespread degenerative changes, principally fibroid and atheromatous, that occur in old age. **senile disciform d.,** disciform macular d. **spongy d. of central nervous system, spongy d. of white matter,** a rare hereditary form of leukodystrophy, transmitted as an autosomal recessive trait, characterized by early onset, widespread demyelination and vacuolation of the cerebral white matter that gives rise to a spongy appearance, severe mental retardation, megalocephaly, atony of the neck muscles, spasticity of the arms and legs, and blindness, with death usually occurring at about 18 months of age. Called also *Canavan's disease.* **subacute combined d. of spinal cord,** degeneration of both the posterior and lateral columns of the spinal cord caused by vitamin B₁₂ deficiency; a progressive disease, most often affecting persons over forty years of age, it is usually associated with pernicious anemia. The symptoms include paresthesias, ataxia, unsteadiness of gait, and sometimes emotional disorders. Called also *Lichtheim's disease* or *syndrome, Putnam-Dana syndrome,* and *posterolateral sclerosis.* **trabecular d.,** a change in the walls of the bronchi, which become thin and wasted in respect to the muscular and mucous elements, while the stroma is increased in volume. **transneuronal d.,** atrophy of certain neurons after interruption of afferent axons or death of other neurons to which they send their efferent output. **traumatic**

d., degeneration of a divided nerve up to the nearest node of Ranvier. **Türck's d.,** secondary parenchymatous degeneration of nerve tracts of the cord. **uratic d.,** degeneration marked by the deposit of urates or uric acid. **vacuolar d.,** the formation of vacuoles in the cells of a tissue. **Virchow's d.,** amyloid d. **vitelliform d. of Best, vitelliform macular d.,** congenital macular degeneration in which the lesions have a "fried-egg" appearance. **vitreous d.,** hyaline d. **wallerian d.,** fatty degeneration of a nerve fiber which has been severed from its nutritive centers; called also *secondary d.* **waxy d.,** amyloid d. **Wilson's d.,** hepatolenticular d. **Zenker's d.,** necrosis and hyaline degeneration of striated muscle; called also *Zenker's necrosis.*

degenerative (de-jen′er-a-tiv) of or pertaining to degeneration.

degenitalize (de-gen′ĭ-tal-īz) in psychoanalysis, to remove the genital aspects of an affect.

degerm (de-germ′) disinfect.

degloving (de-gluv′ing) intra-oral surgical exposure of the bony mandibular chin; it can be performed in the posterior region if necessary.

Deglut. abbreviation for L. *deglutia′tur,* let it be swallowed.

deglutible (de-gloo′tĭ-bl) capable of being swallowed.

deglutition (deg″loo-tish′un) [L. *deglutitio*] the act of swallowing.

deglutitive (de-gloo′tĭ-tiv) deglutitory.

deglutitory (de-gloo′tĭ-to″re) pertaining to or promoting deglutition.

degradation (deg-rah-da′shun) the reduction of a chemical compound to one less complex, as by splitting off one or more groups.

degranulation (de-gran″u-la′shun) the process of losing granules; said of certain granular cells.

degree (de-gre′) 1. a grade or rank awarded scholars by a college or university. 2. a unit of measure of temperature. 3. a unit of measure of arcs and angles. **prism d.,** centrad, def. 2.

degrowth (de′groth) decrease in the mass of living matter because of use of the proteins of the protoplasm to produce energy by the organism.

degustation (de″gus-ta′shun) [L. *degustatio*] the act or function of tasting.

dehab (de′hahb) surra.

dehematize (de-hem′ah-tīz) [*de-* + Gr. *haima* blood] to deprive of blood.

dehemoglobinize (de″hem-o-glo′bĭ-nīz) to remove hemoglobin from the red blood corpuscles.

dehepatized (de-hep′ah-tīzd) having the liver removed.

Dehio's test (da′he-ōz) [Karl Konstantinovich *Dehio,* Russian physician, 1851–1927] see under tests.

dehiscence (de-his′ens) [L. *dehiscere* to gape] a splitting open. **root d.,** the absence of all or a portion of the bony covering of the buccal or lingual aspect of the root of a tooth. **d. of uterus,** occult rupture of the uterus following cesarean section. **wound d.,** separation of the layers of a surgical wound; it may be partial and superficial only, or complete with total disruption. **Zuckerkandl's d's,** small gaps occasionally seen in the papyraceous layer of the ethmoid bone.

dehumanization (de-hu″man-i-za′shun) [*de-* + L. *humanus* human] loss of the qualities of humanity, as in some severe psychotic conditions.

dehumidifier (de″hu-mid′ĭ-fi″er) an apparatus by which the content of moisture in the air is reduced.

dehydrant (de-hi′drant) 1. reducing hydration. 2. an agent that removes or reduces body water.

dehydrase (de-hi′drās) a term formerly applied to both the dehydrogenases and the dehydratases.

dehydratase (de-hi′drah-tās) any lyase (hydro-lyase) that catalyzes the removal of H_2O, leaving double bonds (or adding groups to double bonds).

dehydrate (de-hi′drāt) to remove water from (a compound, the body, etc.).

dehydration (de″hi-dra′shun) [L. *de* away + Gr. *hydōr* water] 1. removal of water from a substance. 2. the condition that results from excessive loss of body water. Called also *anhydration, deaquation,* and *hypohydration.* **absolute d.,** water content below the normal or below a standard amount. **hypernatremic d.,** a condition in which electrolyte losses are disproportionately smaller than water losses. **relative d.,** dehydration resulting from increased osmotic pressure of the body fluids. **voluntary d.,** that resulting when thirst does not stimulate sufficient replacement of water loss.

dehydroandrosterone (de-hi″dro-an-dros′ter-ōn) former name for dehydroepiandrosterone.

dehydrobilirubin (de-hi″dro-bil-ĭ-ru′bin) biliverdin.

dehydrocholaneresis (de-hi″dro-ko″lan-er′ĕ-sis) increase in the output of dehydrocholic acid in the bile.

dehydrocholate (de-hi″dro-ko′lāt) a salt of dehydrocholic acid.

dehydrocholesterol (de-hi″dro-ko-les′ter-ol) a sterol found in the skin which, when properly irradiated, forms vitamin D. **7-d., activated,** cholecalciferol.

11-dehydrocorticosterone (de-hi″dro-kor-tĭ-kos′ter-ōn) chemical name: 21-hydroxypregn-4-ene-3,11,20-trione. A steroid, $C_{21}H_{28}O_4$, from the adrenal cortex, which has a slight effect on protein and carbohydrate metabolism. Also produced synthetically, it is used like cortisone as a glucocorticoid and as an antiallergic agent. Called also *Kendall's compound A.*

dehydrocorydaline (de-hi″dro-kŏ-rid′ah-lin) a yellowish crystalline alkaloid, $C_{22}H_{23}O_4N$, from the roots of species of *Corydalis.*

dehydroepiandrosterone (de-hi″dro-ep″ĭ-an-dros′ter-ōn) an androgen, $C_{19}H_{28}O_2$, occurring in normal human urine and synthesized from cholesterol; abbreviated DHA. Called also *dehydroisoandrosterone* and, formerly, *dehydroandrosterone.*

dehydrogenase (de-hi′dro-jen-ās) an enzyme which mobilizes the hydrogen of a substrate so that it can pass to a hydrogen acceptor. Cf. *coenzyme.* Dehydrogenases are variously designated according to their specific activity, or the substrate acted upon. **acetaldehyde d.,** a flavoprotein that catalyzes the conversion of acetaldehyde to acetic acid and H_2O_2. **acetoin d.,** acetoin: NAD oxidoreductase. An enzyme that catalyzes the conversion of acetoin and nicotinamide-adenine dinucleotide (NAD) to diacetyl and reduced nicotinamide-adenine dinucleotide. **aerobic d.,** one that transfers hydrogen directly to oxygen. **alcohol d.,** one that catalyzes the dehydrogenation of ethyl alcohol to acetaldehyde. **anaerobic d.,** one that is linked with a carrier. **beta-hydroxybutyric d.,** one that catalyzes the dehydrogenation of beta-hydroxybutyric acid to acetoacetic acid. **fatty acid d.,** one that catalyzes the removal of hydrogen from higher fatty acids. **formic d.,** an enzyme that catalyzes the change of formic acid into carbon dioxide and hydrogen. **glucose d.,** an enzyme that catalyzes the oxidation of glucose to gluconic acid. **glucose-6-phosphate d. (G6PD),** an enzyme of the pentose phosphate pathway which, with $NADP^+$ as coenzyme, catalyzes the dehydrogenation of glucose-6-phosphate to 6-phosphogluconolactone. Called also *Robison ester d.* and *Zwischenferment.* **glutamate d.,** glutamic acid d. **glutamic acid d.,** an enzyme that catalyzes the change of glutamic acid into ketoglutaric acid and ammonia. **glycerolphosphate d.,** an enzyme that catalyzes the oxidation of glycerolphosphate into phosphoglyceric acid. **hexose d.,** an enzyme that catalyzes the oxidation of hexose to hexonic acid. **lactate d., (LDH),** an enzyme that catalyzes the interconversion of lactate and pyruvate. It is widespread in tissues and is particularly abundant in kidney, skeletal muscle, liver, and myocardium. It appears in elevated concentrations when these tissues are injured. **malate d.,** one that catalyzes the dehydrogenation of malic acid to oxalacetic acid. **pyruvic d.,** an enzyme complex that catalyzes the oxidation of pyruvic acid. **Robison ester d.,** glucose-6-phosphate d. **succinic d.,** one that catalyzes the change of succinic acid into fumaric acid. **xanthine d.,** an enzyme that catalyzes the oxidation of xanthine to uric acid.

dehydrogenate (de-hi″dro-jen-āt) to remove hydrogen from.

dehydrogenation (de-hi″dro-jen-a′shun) indirect oxidation due to removal of hydrogen by the reaction of a hydrogen acceptor.

dehydroisoandrosterone (de-hi″dro-i″so-an-dro′ster-ōn) dehydroepiandrosterone.

dehydromorphine (de-hi″dro-mor′fin) pseudomorphine.

dehydropeptidase (de-hi″dro-pep′tĭ-dās) aminoacylase.

dehydroretinal (de-hi″dro-ret′ĭ-nal) the aldehyde of dehydroretinol, derived from the visual pigment porphyropsin, found in fresh-water fishes and certain vertebrates and amphibians. Its metabolic role is analogous to that of rhodopsin in other animals. Called also *retinal₂.*

dehydroretinol (de-hi″dro-ret′ĭ-nol) vitamin A₂, the form, $C_{20}H_{28}O$, of vitamin A found in the retina and liver of fresh-water fishes and certain invertebrates and amphibians; it differs from retinol (vitamin A₁) in having one more conjugated double bond and has approximately one-third the biological activity of retinol. Called also *retinol₂.*

dehypnotize (de-hip′no-tīz) to arouse from the hypnotic state.

deiodination (de-i″o-din-a′shun) the loss or removal of iodine from a compound.

deionization (de-i″on-i-za′shun) the production of a mineral-free state by the removal of ions, especially by use of ion-exchange resins.

deiteral (di′ter-al) pertaining to Deiters' nucleus.

Deiters' cells, etc. (di′terz) [Otto Friedrich Carl *Deiters,* German anatomist, 1834–1863] see under *cell, frame, nucleus, phalanx, process,* and *tract.*

déjà entendu (da-zhah′ on″ton-doo′) [Fr. "already heard"] the feeling that one has heard or perceived something previously although it is in fact new to one's experience.

déjà éprouvé (da-zhah′ a″proo-va′) [Fr. "already tested"] a feeling that something a person has never engaged in has been done.

déjà fait (da-zhah′ fa) [Fr. "already done"] a feeling that what is happening has happened before.

déjà pensé (da-zhah′ pon-sa′) [Fr. "already thought"] a feeling that one has thought the same thoughts before.

déjà raconté (da-zhah′ rak″on-ta′) [Fr. "already told"] a feeling that one's forgotten experience has been told to him by someone else.

déjà vécu (da-zhah′ va-koo′) [Fr. "already lived"] an illusory feeling that a new experience has been previously encountered.

déjà voulu (da-zhah′ voo-loo′) [Fr. "already desired"] a feeling that one has entertained the same desires before.

déjà vu (da-zhah′ voo′) [Fr. "already seen"] an illusion in which a new situation is incorrectly viewed as a repetition of a previous situation.

dejecta (de-jek′tah) excrement.

dejection (de-jek′shun) [L. *dejectio*] 1. a mental state marked by depression and melancholy. 2. discharge of feces; defecation. 3. excrement; feces.

Dejerine's disease, etc. (deh″zher-ēnz′) [Joseph Jules *Dejerine*, French neurologist, 1849–1917] see under *disease, sign, syndrome*, and *type*.

Dejerine-Klumpke paralysis, syndrome (deh″zher-ēn′ klump′ke) [Augusta *Dejerine-Klumpke*, French neurologist, 1859–1927] Klumpke's paralysis.

Dejerine-Landouzy dystrophy (type) (deh″zher-ēn′ lan-doo′ze) [J. J. *Dejerine*; Louis Théophile Joseph *Landouzy*, French physician, 1845–1917] see *Landouzy-Dejerine dystrophy*, under *dystrophy*.

Dejerine-Lichtheim phenomenon (deh″zher-en′ lict′hīm) [J. J. *Dejerine*; Ludwig *Lichtheim*, German physician, 1845–1928] Lichtheim sign.

Dejerine-Roussy syndrome (deh″zher-ēn′ roo-se′) [J. J. *Dejerine*; Gustav *Roussy*, French pathologist, 1874–1948] thalamic syndrome.

Dejerine-Sottas atrophy, disease, syndrome (deh″zher-ēn′ sot′tahz) [J. J. *Dejerine*; Jules *Sottas*, French neurologist, born 1866] progressive hypertrophic interstitial neuropathy.

deka- (dek′ah) [Gr. *deka* ten] a combining form meaning ten; for words beginning thus, see also those beginning *deca-*.

dekanem (dek′ah-nem) [(*obs.*) ten nems; abbreviated Dn.

delacrimation (de-lak″rĭ-ma′shun) [L. *de* from + *lacrima* tear] excessive and abnormal flow of tears.

delactation (de″lak-ta′shun) 1. weaning. 2. the cessation of lactation.

Delafield's fluid, hematoxylin (del′ah-fēldz) [Francis *Delafield*, pathologist in New York, 1841–1915] see under *fluid*, and see *Table of Stains*.

Delalutin (del″ah-lu′tin) trademark for a preparation of hydroxyprogesterone caproate.

delamination (de″lam-ĭ-na′shun) [L. *de* apart + *lamina* plate] separation into layers, as the separation of blastoderm into epiblast and hypoblast during chick embryo development.

Delatestryl (del″ah-tes′tril) trademark for a preparation of testosterone enanthate.

Delbet's sign (del-bāz′) [Pierre *Delbet*, French surgeon, 1861–1925] see under *sign*.

de-lead (de-led′) to remove lead from a tissue, as from the bones in lead poisoning by the administration of edetate disodium calcium.

Delestrogen (del-es′tro-jen) trademark for a preparation of estradiol valerate.

deleterious (del″ĕ-te′re-us) [Gr. *dēlētērios*] hurtful; injurious.

deletion (de-le′shun) removal; in genetics, a loss of genetic material from a chromosome. **antigenic d.,** loss or masking of antigenic determinants in daughter cells of cells whose parent tissue normally carries them; it may result from neoplastic or other mutational change in the parent tissue or may be due to loss or repression of genetic material from the cell.

delimitation (de-lim″ĭ-ta′shun) [*de-* + L. *limitare* to limit] 1. the process of limiting or of becoming limited. 2. ascertainment of the limits and extent of some diseased tissue or process, or the spread of a disease in a host or a community.

delinquency (de-lin′kwen-se) antisocial, illegal or criminal conduct.

delinquent (de-lin′kwent) 1. characterized by antisocial, illegal, or criminal conduct. 2. an individual whose conduct is antisocial, illegal, or criminal, especially a minor exhibiting such behavior (**juvenile d.).**

deliquescense (del″ĕ-kwes′ens) [L. *deliquescere* to grow moist] the condition of becoming moist or liquefied as a result of the absorption of water from the air.

deliquescent (del″ĕ-kwes′ent) having a tendency to form an aqueous solution or become liquid by the absorption of moisture from the air.

délire (da-lēr′) [Fr.] delirium; frenzy. **d. de toucher** (da-lēr′

duh too-sha′), an unreasonable and irresistable impulse to handle or to feel various objects.

deliria (de-lir′ĭ-ah) plural of *delirium*.

deliriant (de-lir′ĭ-ant) 1. capable of producing delirium. 2. a drug which may produce delirium. 3. a delirious person.

delirifacient (de-lir″ĭ-fa′she-ent) [L. *delirium* + *facere* to make] 1. capable of causing delirium. 2. a drug which may produce delirium.

delirious (de-lir′ĭ-us) suffering from delirium.

delirium (de-lir′ĭ-um) pl. *delir′ia* [*de-* + L. *lira* furrow or track; i.e., "off the track"] a mental disturbance marked by illusions, hallucinations, short unsystematized delusions, cerebral excitement, physical restlessness and incoherence, and having a comparatively short course. Delirium usually reflects a toxic state. **active d.,** delirium accompanied by maniacal movements. **acute d.,** a suddenly appearing and severe delirium lasting only a short time. **afebrile d.,** delirium not attended by, nor occurring in the course of, fever. **d. alcohol′icum,** d. tremens. **Bell's d.,** (*obs.*), acute d. **chronic alcoholic d.,** Korsakoff's psychosis. **d. cor′dis,** atrial fibrillation. **exhaustion d.,** delirium due to strain or exhaustion from metabolic or nutritional disturbance; called also *infection exhaustion psychosis*. **febrile d.,** the delirium of fever. **low d.,** delirium marked by confusion of ideas and slowness of mental action rather than by excitement. **macromaniacal d.** (*obs.*), macroptic d. **macroptic d.** (*obs.*), a psychosensory disturbance in which the patient believes that his body or limbs, or both, have assumed enormous proportions. **micromaniacal d.** (*obs.*), microptic d. **microptic d.** (*obs.*), a psychosensory disturbance in which the patient believes that his body or limbs, or both, have assumed minute proportions. **oneiric d.,** oneirism. **d. schizophrenoi′des,** delirium accompanied by reactions typical of schizophrenia. **senile d.,** a syndrome occurring in old age, usually of acute onset, and characterized by disorientation, insomnia, hallucinations, and aimless wandering, sometimes associated with senile psychosis. **d. si′ne delir′io** [L. "delirium without delirium"], delirium tremens without hallucinations and mental distress, but with all the physical symptoms present. **specific febrile d.,** febrile d. **toxic d.,** delirium caused by poisons. **traumatic d.,** that which follows severe head injury; superficially the patient is alert, but there is marked disorientation, memory defect, and confabulation. **d. tre′mens,** an acute mental disturbance marked by delirium with trembling and great excitement, and attended by anxiety, mental distress, sweating, gastrointestinal symptoms, and precordial pain. It is one of the forms of alcoholic psychosis and is ordinarily seen following withdrawal from heavy alcohol intake, but may occur despite continued drinking. It is also seen in opium addiction. Called also *d. alcoholicum*.

delitescence (del″ĭ-tes′ens) [L. *delitescere* to lie hidden] 1. sudden disappearance of symptoms or of objective signs of a disease or of a lesion. 2. the period of latency or incubation of a poison or morbific agent.

deliver (de-liv′er) 1. to aid in the process of childbirth. 2. to remove, as the fetus or placenta, or the lens of the eye.

delivery (de-liv′er-e) 1. expulsion or extraction of the child and the after-birth; see also *labor*. 2. removal of a part, as the lens of the eye. **abdominal d.,** delivery of an infant through an incision made into the intact uterus through the abdominal wall. **breech d.,** delivery of an infant in breech presentation; see *breech extraction*, under *extraction*. **forceps d.,** extraction of the child from the maternal passages by application of forceps to the child's head, without injury to the child or to the mother. **forceps d., high,** forceps delivery in which the forceps is applied to the head before engagement has taken place. **forceps d., low,** forceps delivery in which the forceps is applied when the scalp is or has been visible at the introitus without separating the labia, the skull has reached the pelvic floor, and the sagittal suture is in the anteroposterior diameter of the pelvis; called also *outlet forceps d.* **forceps d., outlet,** forceps d., low. **midforceps d.,** the application of forceps when the fetal head is engaged, but the conditions for outlet (low) forceps delivery have not been met; any forceps delivery requiring artificial rotation. **postmature d.,** delivery of a postmature infant. **postmortem d.,** birth of a child after the death of the mother. **premature d.,** birth of a premature infant. **spontaneous d.,** birth of an infant without any aid from an attendant. **vaginal d.,** delivery of an infant through the normal openings of the uterus and vagina.

dell (del′) a slight depression or dimple.

delle (del′eh) the clear area in the center of a stained erythrocyte.

dellen (del′en) saucer-shaped excavations at the periphery of the cornea, usually on the temporal side, probably caused by insufficiency of the limbal circulation; called also *Fuchs' dimples*.

delling (del′ing) the formation of a slight depression; dimpling.

delmadinone acetate (del-mad′ĭ-nōn) chemical name: 17-(acetyloxy)-6-chloro-pregna-1,4,6-triene-3,20-dione. A progestin, antiandrogen, and antiestrogen, $C_{23}H_{27}ClO_4$, used in veterinary medicine.

delomorphic (del″o-mor′fik) delomorphous.

delomorphous (del″o-mor′fus) [Gr. *dēlos* evident + *morphē* form] having definitely formed and well-defined limits, as a cell or tissue.

Delore's method (da-lorz′) [Xavier *Delore*, French physician, 1828–1916] see under *method*.

Delorme's operation (dĕ-lormz′) [Edmond *Délorme*, Paris surgeon, 1847–1929] see under *operation*.

delousing (de-lows′ing) the freeing from lice; destruction of lice.

Delpech's abscess (del-pesh′ez) [Jacques Mathieu *Delpech*, French surgeon, 1777–1832] see under *abscess*.

Delphian node (*Delphi*, a town of ancient Greece, the location of the sanctuary and (Delphian) oracle of Apollo) see under *node*.

delphine (del′fin) delphinine.

delphinine (del′fĭ-nin) a poisonous alkaloid, $C_{33}H_{45}NO_9$, from the seeds of *Delphinium staphisagria;* formerly used for the most part externally to relieve pain in neuralgia, rheumatism, and paralysis. Called also *delphine.*

Delphinium (del-fin′e-um) [L.] a genus of ranunculaceous plants, including *D. consolida,* or larkspur, the seeds of which are diuretic, emmenagogue, and poisonous. The seeds of *D. staphisagria,* or stavesacre, were used for destroying lice. See *staphisagria.*

delphinoidine (del″fĭ-noid′in) an alkaloid from the seeds of *Delphinium staphisagria.*

delphisine (del′fĭ-sin) an alkaloid, isomeric with delphinine, from seeds of *Delphinium staphisagria.*

delta (del′tah) [Gr. letter *delta* δ, Δ] 1. a triangular space. 2. the fourth letter of the Greek alphabet; see *alpha.* **Galton's d.,** a triangular arrangement of the lines of a fingerprint near the base. **d. mesoscap′ulae,** the triangular area at the root of the spine of the scapula.

Delta-Cortef (del′tah kor″tef) trademark for a preparation of prednisolone.

deltacortisone (del″tah-kor′tĭ-sōn) prednisone.

Deltalin (del′tah-lin) trademark for a preparation of synthetic vitamin D_2.

Deltasone (del′tah-sōn) trademark for a preparation of prednisone.

deltoid (del′toid) [L. *deltoides* triangular] triangular in outline, as the deltoid muscle.

Deltra (del′trah) trademark for prednisone.

de lunatico inquirendo (de lu-nat′ĭ-ko in-kwĭ-ren′do) [L.] a commission, board, inquisition, or jury appointed by a court for the investigation of the mental condition of a person whose sanity has been disputed.

delusion (de-lu′zhun) [L. *delusio,* from *de* from + *ludus* a game] a false personal belief based on incorrect inference about external reality and firmly maintained in spite of incontrovertible and obvious proof or evidence to the contrary; it is not a belief that is accepted by other members of the person's culture or subculture (i.e., it is not an article of religious faith). Cf. *illusion.* **depressive d.,** delusion in which the patient experiences feelings of uneasiness, unworthiness, and futility. **expansive d.,** a pathologically unreasonable belief in one's own greatness, goodness, or power, encountered in the manic form of manic-depressive psychosis. **d. of grandeur,** delusional conviction of one's own importance, power, wealth, etc., as in megalomania, dementia paralytica, and paranoid schizophrenia. **d. of negation,** the delusion that some part of the body is missing or that the world has ceased to exist. **nihilistic d.,** a delusion which denies the existence of something or everything. **d. of persecution,** a morbid belief on the part of a patient that he is being mistreated, slandered, and injured by secret enemies, as in paranoia and paranoid schizophrenia. **d. of reference,** idea of reference. **somatic d.,** a delusion that there is some alteration in a bodily organ or its function. **systematized d.,** a delusion formulated in a logical manner; a delusion which has a logical structure, especially characteristic of true paranoia. **unsystematized d.,** a delusion made up of disconnected parts.

delusional (de-lu′zhun-al) pertaining to or characterized by delusions.

Delvinal (del′vĭ-nal) trademark for preparations of vinbarbital.

Demansia (de-man′sĭ-ah) a genus of venomous elapid snakes, including the brown snake of Australia and New Guinea. See table accompanying *snake.*

demarcation (de″mar-ka′shun) [L. *demarcare* to limit] the marking off or ascertainment of boundaries. **surface d.,** any dividing line apparent on the surface of a solid body, such as the boundary between living and necrotic tissue.

Demarquay's sign (dem-ar-kāz′) [Jean Nicholas *Demarquay,* a French surgeon, 1811–1875] see under *sign.*

demasculinization (de-mas″ku-lin-i-za′shun) the loss of normal male characters, with testicular atrophy and involution of the prostate.

Dematiaceae (de-mat″ĭ-a′se-e) a family of imperfect fungi of the order Moniliales, producing simple conidiophores, and having dark brown or black conidia, spores, or hyphae. It includes the

genera *Acremoniella, Arthrographis, Auerobasidium, Alternaria, Chalara, Cladosporium, Dematium, Fonsecaea, Madurella,* and *Phialophora.*

dematiacious (de-mat″ĭ-a′shus) of or pertaining to a fungus of the family Dematiaceae.

Dematium (de-ma′she-um) a genus of soil and wood-rotting dematiaceous fungi, species of which have been reported to be isolated from human lesions, but are of questionable significance.

deme (dēm) [Gk. *dēmos* common people] a population of very similar organisms interbreeding in nature and occupying a circumscribed area; called also *genetic population.*

demecarium bromide (dem″e-ka′re-um) [USP] chemical name: 3,3′-[1,10-decanediylbis[(methylimino)carbonyloxy]]bis[*N,-N,N*-trimethylbenzenaminium]dibromide. A potent, long-acting cholinesterase inhibitor, $C_{32}H_{52}Br_2N_4O_4$, occurring as a white or slightly yellow, crystalline powder; applied topically to the conjunctiva in the treatment of glaucoma and convergent strabismus.

demeclocycline (dem″e-klo-si′klēn) [USP] chemical name: 7-chloro-4*S*-(dimethylamino)-1,4α,4aα,5,5aα,6β,11,12α-octahydro-3,6,10,12,12a-pentahydroxy-1,11-dioxo-2-naphthacenecarboxamide. A broad-spectrum oral antibiotic of the tetracycline group, $C_{21}H_{21}ClN_2O_8$, produced by a mutant strain of *Streptomyces aureofaciens* or semisynthetically, occurring as a yellow, crystalline powder. It also inhibits the effect of antidiuretic hormone on the renal tubules. Called also *demethylchlortetracycline.* **d. hydrochloride** [USP], the monohydrochloride salt of demeclocycline, $C_{21}H_{21}ClN_2O_8 \cdot HCl$, occurring as a yellow, crystalline powder; administered orally. It is also used as a diuretic.

dement (de-ment′) a person affected with dementia, i.e., one who has lost mental faculties once possessed (used often in contrast with *ament*).

demented (de-ment′ed) deprived of reason, mentally deteriorated.

dementia (de-men′she-ah) [de- + L. *mens* mind] organic loss of intellectual function; called also *aphrenia, amnesia,* and *athymia.* **Alzheimer's d.,** presenile d. **Binswanger d.,** a form of presenile dementia caused by demyelination of the subcortical white matter of the brain accompanying sclerotic changes in the blood vessels supplying it; called also *encephalitis subcorticalis chronica.* **dialysis d.,** a progressive encephalopathy marked by dysarthria with nominal aphasia, dementia, myoclonic jerking, grand mal seizures, and psychosis, occurring in persons undergoing chronic hemodialysis, and probably due to high levels of aluminum in the water used in the dialysis fluid. **epileptic d.,** see under *psychosis.* **d. myoclon′ica,** mental deterioration occurring in paramyoclonus multiplex. **paralytic d., d. paralyt′ica,** a chronic syphilitic meningoencephalitis, characterized by degeneration of the cortical neurons, progressive dementia, and a generalized paralysis which, if untreated, is ultimately fatal. Called also *general paresis, general paralysis of the insane, paretic dementia, cerebral tabes,* and *syphilitic meningoencephalitis.* **d. paranoi′des,** paranoid schizophrenia. **paretic d.,** dementia paralytica. **d. prae′cox,** in the U.S., an obsolete term for schizophrenia; commonly used in Europe to denote process schizophrenia as opposed to reactive schizophrenia. **d. praeseni′lis, presenile d.,** dementia of unknown etiology beginning at middle age and characterized by cortical atrophy and secondary ventricular dilatation; called also *Alzheimer's disease, dementia,* or *sclerosis.* **primary d.,** dementia occurring independently of any other form of psychosis. **d. pugilis′tica,** cerebral concussion caused by repeated blows to the head, as in a boxer. **secondary d.,** dementia following and due to some other form of psychosis. **semantic d.,** inability to experience values and meaning in life. **senile d.,** senile psychosis. **tabetic d.,** that which sometimes follows tabes dorsalis. **terminal d.,** dementia coming on as a final result of nervous or mental disease. **toxic d.,** that which is due to excessive use of some poison.

Demerol (dem′er-ol) trademark for preparations of meperidine (pethidine) hydrochloride.

demethylation (de″meth-ĭ-la′shun) the removal of a methyl group, —CH_3, from a compound.

demethylchlortetracycline (de-meth″il-klōr″tet-rah-si′klēn) demeclocycline.

demi- [Fr. *demi;* L. *demidius* half] a prefix signifying half.

demibain (dem′e-bān) [Fr.] sitz bath.

demifacet (dem″e-fas′et) a small plane surface on either of two bones which both articulate with a third bone. **inferior d. for head of rib,** fovea costalis inferior. **superior d. for head of rib,** fovea costalis superior.

demigauntlet (dem-e-gawnt′let) a form of bandage for the hand and fingers.

demilune (dem′e-lūn) 1. a half moon, or crescent. 2. crescentic; crescent shaped. **d's of Adamkiewicz,** crescent-shaped cells beneath the neurilemma of medullated nerve fibers. **d's of Giannuzzi, d's of Heidenhain,** crescents of Giannuzzi.

demimonstrosity (dem″e-mon-stros′ĭ-te) malformation of a part which does not prevent the exercise of its function.

demineralization (de-min″er-al-i-za′shun) excessive elimination of mineral or inorganic salts, as in pulmonary tuberculosis, cancer, and osteomalacia.

demipenniform (dem″e-pen′ĭ-form) feather-shaped as to one of the two margins; said of certain muscles.

Democritus (de-mok′rĭ-tus) **of Abdera** (5th century B.C.) a Greek philosopher who was the first to state that everything in nature, including the body and the soul, is made up of atoms of different sizes and shapes, the movements of which are the cause of life and mental activity.

demodectic (dem-o-dek′tik) pertaining to, or caused by, *Demodex.* See also *mange.*

Demodex (dem′o-deks) [Gr. *dēmos* fat + *dēx* worm] a genus of mites or acarids which cause follicular mange. **D. ca′nis,** the

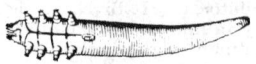

Demodex folliculorum (x 100) (Brumpt).

cause of follicular mange in dogs. **D. e′qui,** a species causing mange in horses. **D. folliculo′rum,** the hair follicle mite: a species found in hair follicles of man, and in sebaceous secretions, especially of the face and nose; called also *Acarus folliculorum, face mite,* and *follicle mite.*

Demodicidae (dem″o-dik′ĭ-de) a family of minute follicular mites (order Acarina) that parasitize the skin of various mammals, including man.

demodicidosis (dem″o-dis″ĭ-do′sis) infestation with *Demodex.*

demodicosis (dem″o-dĭ-ko′sis) 1. demodectic mange. 2. demodicidosis.

demogram (de′mo-gram) a graphic representation, in grid form, of the population of a given area according to the time period and the age and sex of the individuals comprising it.

demography (de-mog′rah-fe) [Gr. *dēmos* people + *graphein* to write] the study of mankind collectively; especially of their geographical distribution and physical environment. **dynamic d.,** collective physiology of communities, with statistics of births, marriages, deaths, etc. **static d.,** collective anatomy of communities and study of their environment.

demoniac (de-mo′ne-ak) 1. frenzied. 2. a lunatic.

demonology (de″mon-ol′o-je) [*demon* + *-logy*] the earlier approach to problems of mental disorder, by which evil spirits were believed to possess the patient and exorcisms constituted the treatment.

demonomania (de″mon-o-ma′ne-ah) [Gr. *daimōn* demon + *mania* madness] monomania in which the patient considers himself possessed of devils; called also *demonopathy.*

demonopathy (de″mon-op′ah-the) demonomania.

demonophobia (de″mon-o-fo′be-ah) [Gr. *daimōn* demon + *phobein* to be affrighted by + *ia*] morbid fear of demons.

demonstrator (dem′on-stra″tor) [L.] an instructor who teaches individuals or small groups by using dissections or other aids.

De Morgan's spots (de-mor′ganz) [Campbell *De Morgan,* English physician, 1811–1876] cherry angiomas.

demorphinization (de-mor″fin-i-za′shun) the gradual depriving of one addicted to morphine of the drug until the addiction is cured.

Demours' membrane (da-moorz′) [Pierre *Demours,* French ophthalmologist, 1702–1795] lamina limitans posterior corneae.

demoxepam (dem-oks′ĕ-pam) chemical name: 7-chloro-1,3-dihydro-5-phenyl-2*H*-1,4-benzodiazepin-2-one 4-oxide. A minor tranquilizer, $C_{15}H_{11}ClN_2O_2$, which is an active metabolite of chlordiazepoxide.

demucosation (de″mu-ko-sa′shun) removal of the mucous membrane from a part.

demulcent (de-mul′sent) 1. soothing; bland; allaying the irritation of inflamed or abraded surfaces. 2. a soothing, mucilaginous, or oily medicine or application. Called also *lenitive.*

de Musset see *Musset.*

de Mussy's point (sign) (dŭ-mis-sēz′) [Noel François Odon Guéneau *de Mussy,* French physician, 1813–1885] see under *point.*

demustardization (de-mus″tard-i-za′shun) 1. removal of mustard gas from a person. 2. treatment of a person subjected to the fumes of mustard gas.

demutization (de″mu-ti-za′shun) [*de-* + L. *mutus* mute] the teaching of the deaf to communicate by lip reading or by dactylology.

demyelinate (de-mi′ĕ-lin-āt) to destroy or remove the myelin sheath of a nerve or nerves.

demyelination (de-mi″ĕ-li-na′shun) destruction, removal, or loss of the myelin sheath of a nerve or nerves.

demyelinization (de-mi″ĕ-lin-i-za′shun) demyelination.

denarcotize (de-nar′ko-tīz) to deprive of a narcotic drug in the process of treating addiction.

denasality (de″na-zal′ĭ-te) hyponasality.

denatality (de″na-tal′ĭ-te) decrease in the number of births in proportion to the population.

denatonium benzoate (de-nah-to′nĭ-um) [NF] chemical name: *N*-[2-[(2,6-dimethylphenyl)amino]-2-oxoethyl]-*N,N*-diethyl-benzenemethanaminium benzoate. An alcohol denaturant, $C_{28}H_{34}N_2O_3$, occurring as a white, crystalline powder; used as a pharmaceutic aid.

denaturant (de-na′chur-ant) a denaturing agent.

denaturation (de-na″chur-a′shun) the destruction of the usual nature of a substance, as the addition of methanol or acetone to alcohol to render it unfit for drinking, or the change in the physical properties of proteins caused by heat or certain chemicals. **protein d.,** disruption of the configuration (tertiary structure) of a protein, as by heat, change in pH, or other physical or chemical means, resulting in alteration of the physical properties and loss of biological activity of the protein.

denatured (de-na′tūrd) having undergone denaturation.

dendr-, dendro- [Gr. *dendron* tree] a combining form denoting a relationship to a tree or treelike structure.

dendraxon (den-drak′son) [Gr. *dendron* tree + *axon*] a nerve cell whose axon breaks up into terminal filaments almost immediately after leaving the cell. Cf. *inaxon.*

dendric (den′drik) dendritic.

dendriceptor (den′drĭ-sep″tor) one of the sensitive points at the ends of the branching processes of a dendrite, capable of being stimulated by the axon endings of other neurons.

Dendrid (den′drid) trademark for a preparation of idoxuridine.

dendriform (den′drĭ-form) branched, or tree-shaped.

dendrite (den′drīt) [Gr. *dendron* tree] one of the threadlike extensions of the cytoplasm of a neuron (q.v.); in unipolar and bipolar neurons, they resemble axons structurally, but typically, as in multipolar neurons, they branch into treelike processes. Dendrites comprise most of the receptive surface of a neuron. Called also *cytodendrite, dendron, neurodendrite,* and *neurodendron.* Cf. *axon* (def. 2), *collateral* (def. 2), and *telodendron.*

dendritic (den-drit′ik) 1. branched like a tree. 2. pertaining to or possessing dendrites.

dendro- see *dendr-.*

dendroarcheology (den″dro-ar″ke-ol′o-ge) dendrochronology.

Dendroaspis (den-dro-as′pis) a genus of extremely venomous elapid snakes of Africa, including the deadly mamba, which are related to cobras but do not have a dilatable hood. See table accompanying *snake.*

Dendrochium (den-dro-ke′um) a genus of imperfect fungi (family Stilbaceae, order Moniliales), including *D. tox′icum,* the etiologic agent of dendrodochiotoxicosis in the U.S.S.R.

dendrochronology (den″dro-kron-ol′o-ge) determination of the age of a tree by observation of the annual growth rings in the trunk.

dendrodendritic (den″dro-den-drit′ik) referring to a synapse between dendrites of two neurons.

dendrodochiotoxicosis (den-dro″do-ke-o-tok″sĭ-ko′sis) an intoxication reported within the U.S.S.R. caused by the fungus *Dendrodochium toxicum.* Mycotoxications of this type are especially common in horses, but may affect humans as well.

dendroid (den′droid) [Gr. *dendron* tree + *eidos* form] branching like a tree or shrub.

dendron (den′dron) [Gr.] a dendrite.

dendrophagocytosis (den″dro-fag″o-si-to′sis) the absorption by microglia cells of broken portions of degenerating astrocytes.

denervate (de-ner′vāt) to deprive of a nerve supply.

denervation (de″ner-va′shun) resection of or removal of the nerves to an organ or part.

dengue (deng′e; Spanish, dān-ga) [Sp.] an infectious, eruptive, febrile disease, marked by severe pains in the head, eyes, muscles, and joints, sore throat, catarrhal symptoms, and sometimes a cutaneous eruption and painful swellings of the parts. The disease comes on suddenly after an incubation period of from three to six days. The symptoms increase in severity for two or three days, then decrease somewhat, only to increase again on the fourth or fifth day, at which time the eruption appears. Dengue occurs epidemically and sporadically in India, Japan, the South Pacific, the Caribbean, and northern South America. It is caused by a virus, and is transmitted by the bite of the mosquitoes urban *Aedes aegypti,* sylvan *A. albopictus,* and urbosylvan *A. polynesiensis.* **hemorrhagic d.,** dengue with hemorrhagic manifestations; the attack rate is highest in young children. Called also *Philippine hemorrhagic fever, Southeast Asian hemorrhagic fever,* and *Thai hemorrhagic fever.*

denial (dĕ-ni′al) a defense mechanism in which the existence of intolerable actions, ideas, wishes, impulses and affects are unconciously denied.

denicotinized (de-nik′o-tin-īzd) deprived of nicotine.

denidation (den″ĭ-da′shun) [*de-* + L. *nidus* nest] degeneration and expulsion of the uterine mucous membrane (endometrium) in the menstrual cycle.

Denigès's test (den-ĭ-zhāz′) [Georges *Denigès*, French chemist, 1859–1951] see under *tests*.

Denis' method (den′is) [Wiley Glover *Denis*, American biochemist, born 1879] see under *method*.

Denisonia (den-ĭ-so′nĭ-ah) a genus of very venomous elapid snakes, including *D. super′ba*, the copperhead of Australia, Tasmania, and the Solomons. See table accompanying *snake*.

denitrification (de-ni″trĭ-fi-ka′shun) the setting free of gaseous nitrogen from nitrites and nitrates, as by certain soil bacteria, which results in deprivation of nitrogen for plant growth.

denitrifier (de-ni′trĭ-fi″er) a bacterium that causes denitrification.

denitrify (de-ni′trĭ-fi) to remove nitrogen from any substance; see *denitrification*.

denitrogenation (de-ni″tro-jĕ-na′shun) removal of the dissolved nitrogen from the body, as a preventive of caisson disease, aeroembolism, etc.

Denman's spontaneous evolution (version, method) (den′manz) [Thomas *Denman*, English obstetrician, 1733–1815] see under *evolution*.

denofungin (de″no-fun′jin) an antibiotic substance produced by a variant of *Streptomyces hygroscopicus*, which has antifungal and antibacterial properties.

Denonvilliers' aponeurosis, fascia, operation (den-aw-vēl-yāz′) [Charles Pierre *Denonvilliers*, surgeon in Paris, 1808–1872] see *septum rectovesicale*, and see under *fascia* and *operation*.

dens (dens), pl. *den′tes* [L.] a tooth or toothlike structure; [NA] a general term for a tooth or the teeth (dentes), the small bonelike structures of the jaws, serving in mastication of food and production of certain sounds in speech. See also *tooth*. **den′tes acus′tici** [NA], elevations along the free surface and margin of the labium limbi vestibulare; called also *auditory teeth of Huschke* and *hair teeth*. **den′tes acu′ti**, the incisor teeth (dentes incisivi [NA]). **d. ax′is** [NA], tooth of axis: the toothlike process that projects from the superior surface of the body of the axis, ascending to articulate with the atlas; called also *d. epistrophei*, *odontoid bone*, *odontoid apophysis*, *odontoid process of axis*, and *tooth of epistropheus*. **den′tes cani′ni** [NA], the canine teeth: the four teeth, one on either side in each jaw, immmediately lateral to the lateral incisors; called also *cuspids* or *cuspid teeth*, and *cynodonts*. **dentes de Chiaie**, teeth having mottled enamel; dental fluorosis. **den′tes decid′ui** [NA], the deciduous teeth: the teeth of the first dentition; called also *milk teeth*, *primary teeth*, and *temporary teeth*. **d. epistro′phei**, d. axis. **den′tes incisi′vi** [NA], incisor teeth: the four front teeth of each jaw, called also *dentes acuti* and *primary teeth*. **d. in den′te**, a malformed tooth resulting from invagination of the crown before it is calcified; so named because severe invagination of enamel and dentin gives the appearance of a "tooth within a tooth." Called also *d. invaginatus*. **d. invagina′tus**, dens in dente. **den′tes mola′res** [NA], molar teeth: the grinders, or double teeth, situated in the back part of either jaw, having the largest and most efficient chewing surfaces. **den′tes permanen′tes** [NA], permanent teeth: the teeth of the second dentition. **den′tes premola′res** [NA], premolar teeth: the two permanent teeth on either side of each jaw, between the canine teeth and the molars, called also *bicuspids*, or *bicuspid teeth*. **d. sapien′tiae**, d. serotinus. **d. seroti′nus** [NA], the aftermost tooth on each side of each jaw, being the last of the molar teeth to appear; called also *d. sapientiae*, *third molar*, and *wisdom tooth*.

densimeter (den-sim′ĕ-ter) [L. *densus* dense + *metron*] densitometer.

densitometer (den″sĭ-tom′ĕ-ter) 1. an apparatus for determining the density of a liquid. 2. an instrument for determining the degree of darkening of developed photographic or x-ray film by means of a photocell which measures light transmission through a given area of the film. Called also *densimeter*. **gas d.**, an apparatus for measuring specific gravity of a gas. **ultrasonic d.**, an apparatus for determining the thickness or density of a substance or structure as measured by the time required for an ultrasonic signal directed at it to reach a receiver.

densitometry (den″sĭ-tom′ĕ-tre) determination of variations in density by comparison with that of another material, or with a certain standard.

density (den′sĭ-te) [L. *densitas*] 1. the quality of being compact or dense. 2. the quantity of matter in a given space based on the ratio of mass to volume. 3. the quantity of electricity in a given area or in a given volume or in a given time. 4. the degree of darkening of exposed and processed photographic or x-ray film, expressed as the logarithm of the opacity of a given area of the film. **arciform d.**, a trough-shaped body separating the synaptic ribbon and the membrane of the cone pedicle or of the rod spherule in the retina. **background d.**, in radiography, the density of a processed film due to factors other than the radiation exposure received through the recorded objects or structures, e.g., inherent (film) density, scatter radiation, or fogging. **inherent d.**, the density of a processed film due to inherent factors such as the density of the film base, emulsion gelatin, etc. **ionization d.**, the number of ion pairs per unit volume.

densography (den-sog′rah-fe) the exact determination of the contrast densities in a roentgen negative by a photoelectric cell.

dent-, denta- see *dento-*.

dentagra (den-tag′rah, den′tah-grah) [dent- + Gr. *agra* seizure] 1. a forceps or key for extracting teeth. 2. odontalgia.

dental (den′tal) [L. *dentalis*] 1. pertaining to a tooth or teeth. 2. a letter or sound made by or in part by the front teeth.

dentalgia (den-tal′je-ah) odontalgia.

dentaphone (den′tah-fōn) [denta- + Gr. *phōne* sound] an instrument by means of which persons with hearing loss are enabled to hear sounds propagated through the medium of the teeth.

dentata (den-ta′tah) the second cervical vertebra or axis, so called from its toothlike process.

dentate (den′tāt) [L. *dentatus*] having teeth or projections like saw teeth on the edges.

dentatothalamic (den-ta″to-thah-lam′ik) pertaining to or connecting the dentate nucleus and the thalamus.

dentatum (den-ta′tum) [L. "toothed"] the nucleus dentatus.

dentes (den′tēz) [L.] plural of *dens*.

denti- see *dento-*.

dentia (den′she-ah) [L.] a condition relating to development or eruption of the teeth. Used also as a combining form, denoting relationship to the teeth. **d. prae′cox**, premature eruption of the teeth; the presence of teeth in the mouth at birth. **d. tar′da**, delayed eruption of the teeth, beyond the usual time for their appearance.

dentibuccal (den-tĭ-buk′al) pertaining to the teeth and cheek.

denticle (den′tĭ-kl) [L. *denticulus* a little tooth] 1. a small toothlike process. 2. a relatively large body of calcified substance in the pulp chamber of a tooth. **adherent d., attached d.,** a calcified formation in a pulp chamber partially fused with the dentin. **embedded d.,** interstitial d. **false d.,** a calcified formation in the pulp chamber of a tooth that does not show the structure of true dentin. **free d.,** a calcified formation in a tooth completely surrounded by the dental pulp. **interstitial d.,** a calcified formation within a tooth, completely surrounded by dentin. **true d.,** a calcified formation in the pulp chamber of a tooth that consists of dentin and shows traces of dentinal tubules and odontoblasts.

denticulated (den-tik′u-lāt″ed) [L. *denticulatus*] having minute teeth.

dentification (den″tĭ-fi-ka′shun) the formation of tooth substance.

dentiform (den′tĭ-form) shaped like a tooth.

dentifrice (den′tĭ-fris) [L. *dentifricium*] a preparation composed of an inorganic abrasive, detergent, humectant, binder, and flavoring agent, intended to clean and polish the teeth; it may contain a therapeutic agent, such as fluoride, to inhibit dental caries.

dentigerous (den-tij′er-us) [denti- + L. *gerere* to carry] bearing teeth.

dentilabial (den″tĭ-la′be-al) [denti- + L. *labium* lip] pertaining to the teeth and lips.

dentilingual (den″tĭ-ling′gwal) [denti- + L. *lingua* tongue] pertaining to the teeth and tongue.

dentimeter (den-tim′ĕ-ter) [denti- + Gr. *metron* measure] an instrument for measuring teeth.

dentin (den′tin) [L. *dens* tooth] the chief substance or tissue of the teeth, which surrounds the tooth pulp and is covered by enamel on the crown and by cementum on the roots of the teeth. Called also *dentinum* [NA] and *substantia eburnea dentis*. Similar to bone, but harder and denser, it consists of a solid organic substratum, infiltrated with lime salts. Dentin is permeated by numerous branching spiral canaliculi or tubules which contain processes of the connective tissue cells (odontoblasts) that line the pulp cavity. Sometimes spelled *dentine*. Called also *substantia dentalis propria*, *proper substance of tooth*, *ivory*, *ebur dentis*, *membrana eboris of Kölliker*, and *ivory membrane*. **adventitious d.,** secondary d. **circumpulpar d.,** the inner portion of the dentin, adjacent to the pulp chamber, consisting of thinner fibrils. **cover d.,** the peripheral portion of the dentin, adjacent to the enamel or cementum, consisting of coarser fibers than the circumpulpar dentin; called also *mantle d.* **hereditary opalescent d.,** the brown opalescent-appearing dentin observed in dentinogenesis imperfecta. **interglobular d.,** imperfectly calcified dentinal matrix situated between the calcified globules near the periphery of the dentin. **intermediate d.,** the soft matrix of the predentin. **irregular d.,** secondary d. **mantle d.,** cover d. **opalescent d.,** dentin giving an unusual translucent or opalescent appearance to the teeth, as in dentinogenesis imperfecta. **primary d.,** the dentin formed before the eruption of a tooth. **reparative d.,** dentin produced in response to strong pulp irritation such as may be associated with caries invasion or injurious operative procedures; it has no tubular pattern and often demonstrates cellular inclusions. **sclerotic d.,** transparent d. **secondary d.,** new dentin formed in response to stimuli associated with the normal aging process or with pathological conditions such as caries or injury, or cavity preparation; such dentin is highly irregular in nature. Called also *adventitious d.* and *irregular d.* **sensitive d.,** dentin that is highly sensitive owing to distal irritation of the dentinal tubules. **tertiary d.,** reparative d. **transparent d.,** dentin in which some dentinal tubules have become sclerotic or calcified (dental sclerosis), producing the appearance of translucency; called also *sclerotic d.*

dentinal (den′tĭ-nal) pertaining to dentin.

dentinalgia (den″tĭ-nal′je-ah) (*obs.*) pain in the dentin.

dentine (den′tēn) dentin.

dentinification (den-tin″ĭ-fi-ka′shun) (*obs.*) dentinogenesis.

dentinoblast (den′tĭ-no-blast) [*dentin* + Gr. *blastos* germ] a cell that forms dentin.

dentinoblastoma (den″tĭ-no-blas-to′mah) dentinoma.

dentinogenesis (den″tĭ-no-jen′ĕ-sis) [*dentin* + Gr. *genesis* formation] the formation of dentin. **d. imperfec′ta,** a hereditary condition characterized by defective formation and calcification of the dentin, giving the teeth a brown or blue opalescent appearance; it is transmitted as an autosomal dominant trait. Called also *odontogenesis imperfecta.*

dentinogenic (den″tĭ-no-jen′k) forming or producing dentin.

dentinoid (den′tĭ-noid) 1. resembling dentin. 2. (*obs.*) dentinoma. 3. predentin.

dentinoma (den″tĭ-no′mah) a tumor of odontogenic origin, consisting mainly of dentin.

dentinosteoid (den″tin-os′te-oid) a tumor composed of or containing dentin and bone.

dentinum (den-ti′num) [NA] dentin: the chief substance or tissue of the teeth. See *dentin.*

dentiparous (den-tip′ah-rus) bearing teeth.

dentist (den′tist) a person who has recieved a degree in dentistry and is authorized to practice dentistry.

dentistry (den′tis-tre) 1. that department of the healing arts which is concerned with the teeth, oral cavity, and associated structures, including the diagnosis and treatment of their diseases and the restoration of defective and missing tissue. 2. the work done by dentists, such as the creation of restorations, crowns, and bridges, and surgical procedures performed in and about the oral cavity. 3. the practice of the dental profession collectively. Called also *odontology.* **cosmetic d., esthetic d.,** that aspect of dental practice concerned with the repair and restoration of carious, broken, or defective teeth in such a manner as to improve their appearance. **forensic d.,** dental jurisprudence. **geriatric d.,** gerodontics. **operative d.,** that phase of dentistry concerned with restoration of parts of the teeth that are defective through disease, trauma, or abnormal development to a state of normal function, health, and esthetics. **pediatric d.,** pedodontics. **preventive d.,** that phase of dentistry concerned with maintenance of a normal masticating mechanism by fortifying the oral cavity against damage and disease. **prosthetic d.,** prosthodontics. **psychosomatic d.,** that phase of dentistry which considers the mind-body relationship.

dentition (den-tish′un) [L. *dentitio*] the teeth in the dental arch; ordinarily used to designate the natural teeth in position in their alveoli. **artificial d.,** an artificial substitute for the natural dentition; see *denture.* **deciduous d.,** the teeth which erupt first and are later replaced by the permanent teeth or dentition; called also *primary d.* **delayed d.,** retarded dentition. **mixed d.,** the complement of teeth in the jaws after eruption of some of the permanent teeth, before all of the deciduous teeth are shed; called also *transitional d.* **natural d.,** the natural teeth in the dental arch, considered collectively; it may comprise deciduous or permanent teeth, or a mixture of the two, present at one time. **permanent d.,** the teeth which erupt and take their places after the deciduous teeth are lost; called also *secondary d.* **precocious d.,** abnormally accelerated appearance of the deciduous or permanent teeth. **prediciduous d.,** cornified epithelial structures found in the mouth before the eruption of the true deciduous teeth. **primary d.,** deciduous d. **retarded d.,** abnormally delayed appearance of the deciduous or permanent teeth; called also *delayed d.* **secondary d.,** permanent d. **transitional d.,** mixed d.

dento-, dent-, denta-, denti- [L. *dens* tooth] a combining form denoting relationship to a tooth or to the teeth. Cf. *odonto-.*

dentoalveolar (den″to-al-ve′o-lar) pertaining to a tooth and its alveolus.

dentoalveolitis (den″to-al″ve-o-li′tis) periodontal disease.

dentofacial (den″to-fa′shal) of or pertaining to the teeth and alveolar process and the face.

dentography (den-tog′rah-fe) odontography.

dentoid (den′toid) odontoid.

dentoidin (den-toi′din) the organic or albuminous ground substance of a tooth.

dentolegal (den″to-le′gal) pertaining to dental jurisprudence.

dentoliva (den″to-li′vah) [*dento-* + L. *oliva* olive] (*obs.*) the olivary nucleus.

dentoma (den-to′mah) dentinoma.

dentomechanical (den″to-mĕ-kan′i-k′l) pertaining to the mechanics or to the biomechanics of dentistry.

dentonomy (den-ton′o-me) odontonomy.

dentosurgical (den″to-sur′jĭ-k′l) pertaining to or used in dentistry and surgery.

dentotropic (den″to-trop′ik) turning toward or having an affinity for tissues composing the teeth.

dentulous (den′tu-lus) possessing natural teeth.

denture (den′chur) [Fr.; L. *dens* tooth] an entire set of natural or artificial teeth; ordinarily used to designate an artificial replacement for missing natural teeth and adjacent tissues. **acrylic resin d.,** a denture made of acrylic resin. **basal surface d.,** impression surface. **clasp d.,** a removable partial denture which is retained and stabilized by means of clasps. **complete d.,** an appliance replacing all the teeth of one jaw, as well as associated structures of the jaw; called also *full d.* **continuous gum d.** (*obs.*), a dental substitute in which the teeth are implanted in tinted base material fused to a platinum base. **duplicate d.,** a second denture intended to be a copy of the first denture. **full d.,** complete d. **immediate d., immediate-insertion d.,** an artificial denture made before all the teeth are extracted, and placed immediately after the final extraction. **implant d.,** a denture constructed with a metal framework (substructure) which is embedded within the underlying soft tissues, in contact with the bone, giving stability to and retaining the teeth and overlying material (superstructure) of the appliance. **interim d.,** a denture to be used for a short interval of time for reasons of esthetics, mastication, occlusal support, convenience, or to condition the patient to the acceptance of an artificial substitute for missing natural teeth until more definite prosthetic dental treatment can be provided. **overlay d.,** a complete denture supported both by soft tissue (mucosa) and by a few remaining natural teeth that have been altered, as by insertion of a long or short coping, to permit the denture to fit over them; called also *overdenture.* **partial d.,** a prosthetic appliance replacing one or more missing teeth in one jaw, and receiving its support and retention from the underlying tissues and/or some or all of the remaining teeth. **partial d., distal extension,** a removable partial denture that is retained by natural teeth at one end of the base segments only, a portion of the functional load being carried by the residual ridge. **partial d., fixed,** an appliance for replacement of one or more natural teeth, supported by natural teeth or roots to which it is permanently attached, so that it is not readily removed by patient or dentist; called also *fixed bridge.* **partial d., removable,** an appliance for the replacement of one or more natural teeth, so constructed that it may readily be removed and replaced in the mouth; called also *removable bridge.* **partial d., unilateral,** an appliance for the replacement of one or more natural teeth all on the same side of the jaw. **permanent d.,** a term applied to a denture that is constructed and inserted after the oral tissues have healed and the condition of the alveolar ridges has become fairly stabilized. **provisional d.,** an interim denture used for the purpose of conditioning the patient to the acceptance of an artificial substitute for missing natural teeth. **temporary d.,** interim d. **transitional d.,** a partial denture which is to serve as a temporary prosthesis and to which teeth will be added as more teeth are lost and which will be replaced after postextraction tissue changes have occurred; it may become an interim denture when all of the teeth have been removed from the dental arch. **trial d.,** a denture fabricated for placement in the patient's mouth for verification of its esthetic qualities, the making of records, or other procedures before the final denture is completed.

Denucé's ligament (den-u-sāz′) [Jean Henri Maurice *Denucé,* French surgeon, 1859–1924] see under *ligament.*

denucleated (de-nu′kle-āt″ed) deprived of the nucleus; called also *anucleated.*

denudation (den″u-da′shun) [L. *denudare* to make bare] the act of laying bare; removal of the epithelial covering from any surface, by surgery, trauma, or pathologic change.

denutrition (de″nu-trish′un) a withdrawal or failure of the nutritive processes, with consequent atrophy and degeneration.

Denys' tuberculin (den-ēs′) [Joseph *Denys,* Belgian bacteriologist (Louvain), died 1932] tuberculin bouillon filtrate.

deodorant (de-o′der-ant) [L. *de* from + *odorare* to perfume] 1. removing undesirable or offensive odors. 2. a substance that masks offensive odors. Called also *antibromic.*

deodorize (de-o′der-īz) [L. *de* from + *odor* odor] to neutralize or absorb odor.

deodorizer (de-o′der-īz-er) a deodorizing agent.

deolepsy (de′o-lep″se) [L. *deus* god + Gr. *lēpsis* seizure] belief that one is possessed by a god.

deontology (de″on-tol′o-je) [Gr. *deonta* things that ought to be done + *-logy*] the science of professional duties and etiquette.

deoppilant (de-op′ĭ-lant) removing obstructions.

deoppilation (de-op″ĭ-la′shun) [L. *de* away + *oppilatio* obstruction] the removal of obstructions.

deorsumduction (de-or″sum-duk′shun) [L. *deorsum* downward + *ducere* to lead] the turning down of a part, as of the eyes.

deorsumvergence (de-or″sum-ver′jens) a downward movement, especially of the eyes.

deorsumversion (de-or″sum-ver′zhun) [L. *deorsum* downward + *vertere* to turn] an act of turning or directing downward, especially the simultaneous and equal downward turning of both eyes.

deossification (de-os″ĭ-fi-ka′shun) [L. *de* from + *os* bone + *facere* to make] loss of or removal of the mineral elements of bone.

deoxidation (de-ok″sĭ-da′shun) [L. *de* from + *oxygen*] the removal of oxygen from a chemical compound.

deoxidize (de-ok′sĭ-dīz) to deprive of chemically combined oxygen.

deoxy- (de-ok′se) a prefix used in naming chemical compounds, to designate a compound containing one less atom of oxygen than the reference substance. For words beginning thus see also those beginning *desoxy-*.

deoxycholaneresis (de-ok″se-ko″lan-er′ĕ-sis) increase in the output of deoxycholic acid in the bile.

deoxycorticosterone (de-ok″se-kor″te-kos′ter-ōn) desoxycorticosterone.

deoxygenation (de-ok″sĭ-jen-a′shun) the act of depriving of oxygen.

2-deoxy-D-glucose (de-ok″se-gloo′kōs) an antimetabolite of glucose that has antiviral properties by virtue of its inhibition of the glycosylation of glycoproteins and glycolipids; radioactive 2-deoxyglucose is also used to determine the rate of energy metabolism in cells, since cells (e.g., neurons) adjust their rate of glucose (or 2-deoxyglucose) uptake to fill their metabolic needs.

deoxyhemoglobin (de-ok″se-he″mo-glo′bin) hemoglobin not combined with oxygen, formed when oxyhemoglobin releases its oxygen; called also *deoxygenated* or *reduced hemoglobin*.

deoxyribonuclease (de-ok″se-ri″bo-nu′kle-ās) [*deoxyribonucleic* acid + *-ase*] an enzyme which catalyzes the hydrolysis (depolymerization) of deoxyribonucleic acid (DNA). See also *dornase*.

deoxyribonucleoprotein (de-ok″se-ri″bo-nu″kle-o-pro′te-in) a nucleoprotein in which the nucleic acid sugar is D-2-deoxyribose.

deoxyribonucleoside (de-ok″se-ri″bo-nu′kle-o-sīd) a nucleoside having a purine or pyrimidine base bonded to deoxyribose.

deoxyribonucleotide (de-ok″se-ri″bo-nu′kle-o-tīd) a nucleotide consisting of a purine or a pyrimidine base bonded to deoxyribose, which in turn is bound to a phosphate group.

deoxyribose (de-ok″se-ri′bōs) an aldopentose, $CH_2 \cdot OH \cdot \cdot (CHOH)_2 \cdot CH_2 \cdot CHO$, found in deoxyribonucleic acids (DNA), deoxyribonucleotides, and deoxyribonucleosides.

Dep. abbreviation for L. *depura′tus*, purified.

depancreatize (de-pan′kre-ah-tīz) to remove the pancreas.

dependence (de-pend′ens) the psychophysical state of an addict in which the usual or increasing doses of the drug are required to prevent the onset of withdrawal symptoms.

dependency (de-pen′den-se) the quality of being dependent.

depepsinized (de-pep′sin-īzd) deprived of pepsin; peptically inactivated: said of gastric juice.

depersonalization (de-per″sun-al-i-za′shun) alteration in the perception of the self so that the usual sense of one's own reality is temporarily lost or changed. It may be a manifestation of depersonalization neurosis or another mental illness. It can occur also in normal persons but is then mild and without significant impairment.

dephosphorylation (de-fos″for-i-la′shun) [*de-* + *phosphorylation*] removal of the trivalent PO_3 group from organic molecules.

depigmentation (de″pig-men-ta′shun) the removal of pigment, generally of melanin; frequently used to mean hypopigmentation.

depilate (dep′ĭ-lāt) [L. *de* away + *pilus* hair] to remove the hair from.

depilation (dep″ĭ-la′shun) epilation.

depilatory (de-pil′ah-to-re) [L. *de* from + *pilus* hair] 1. having the power to remove the hair. 2. an agent for removing or destroying the hair. **Martin's d.,** a soft mass containing calcium hydrosulfide, prepared from 2 parts slaked lime and 3 parts water, by passing into the mixture hydrogen sulfide as long as it is absorbed.

deplasmolysis (de″plaz-mol′ĭ-sis) return to the initial volume, after plasmolysis, of the protoplasm of a cell in hypertonic solution.

deplasmolyze (de-plaz′mo-līz) to undergo deplasmolysis.

deplete (de-plēt′) [L. *deplere* to empty] to empty; to unload; to cause depletion.

depletion (de-ple′shun) [L. *deplere* to empty] 1. the act or process of emptying; removal of a fluid, as the blood. 2. exhausted state which results from excessive loss of blood. **plasma d.,** plasmapheresis.

depolarization (de-po″lar-i-za′shun) the process or act of neutralizing polarity. In neurophysiology, the reversal of the resting potential in excitable cell membranes when stimulated, i.e., the

tendency of the cell membrane potential to become positive with respect to the potential outside the cell.

depolarize (de-po′lar-īz) [L. *de* from + *polus* pole] to reduce toward a nonpolarized condition; to deprive of polarity. See *depolarization*.

depolarizer (de-po′lar-īz″er) 1. a chemical agent placed in a galvanic cell for preventing the accumulation of gas upon either of the plates. 2. a substance that reduces the voltage across a biological membrane. 3. a muscle relaxant that produces striated muscle paralysis by altering the electrical state of the muscle receptor, thus blocking muscle response to nerve impulse.

depolymerization (de-pol″ĕ-mer-i-za′shun) the conversion of a compound into one of smaller molecular weight and different physical properties without changing the percentage relationships of the elements composing it.

depolymerize (de-pol′ĕ-mer-īz) to cause to undergo depolymerization.

Depo-Provera (dep″o-pro-ver′ah) trademark for a preparation of medroxyprogesterone acetate for intramuscular injection.

deposit (de-poz′it) [L. *de* down + *ponere* to place] 1. sediment or dregs. 2. extraneous inorganic matter collected in the tissues or in a viscus or cavity. 3. in dentistry, hard or soft material adherent to the surface of a tooth.

depot (de′po, dep′o) [Fr. *dépôt* from L. *depositum*] a body area in which a substance, e.g., a drug, can be accumulated, deposited, or stored and from which it can be distributed. **fat d.,** a site in the body in which large quantities of fat are stored, as in adipose tissue.

Depo-Testosterone (de″po-tes-tos′ter-ōn) trademark for a sustained-action preparation of testosterone.

depravation (dep″rah-va′shun) [L. *depravare* to vitiate; *de* down + *pravus* bad] deterioration; a change for the worse.

depraved (de-prāvd′) vitiated or perverted.

deprementia (dep″re-men′she-ah) (*obs.*) a psychosis marked by depression, impairment of memory, etc.

depressant (de-pres′ant) 1. diminishing functional activity. 2. an agent that reduces functional activity and the vital energies in general by producing muscular relaxation and diaphoresis. **cardiac d.,** an agent that depresses the rate or force of contraction of the heart.

depressed (de-prest′) carried below the normal level; associated with depression.

depression (de-presh′un) [L. *depressio; de* down + *premere* to press] 1. a hollow or depressed area; downward or inward displacement. 2. a lowering or decrease of functional activity. 3. a psychiatric syndrome consisting of dejected mood, psychomotor retardation, insomnia, and weight loss, sometimes associated with guilt feelings and somatic preoccupations, often of delusional proportions. **agitated d.,** psychotic depression accompanied by more or less constant activity. Called also *melancholia agitata*. **anaclitic d.,** impairment of an infant's physical, social, and intellectual development which sometimes follows a sudden separation from the mothering person for long periods of time; called also *hospitalism*. **atrial d.** (*obs.*), great lowering in the sphygmographic tracing of the venous pulse, representing the diastole of the right atrium. **aversion d.** (*obs.*), depression characterized by aversion to the facts of the illness and to the medical attention which it involves. **d. of cataract,** couching. **congenital chondrosternal d.,** a congenital, deep, funnel-shaped depression in the anterior chest wall. **groove d.,** a depression of the parietal or frontal bones of a newborn due to compression against the maternal symphysis pubis or sacral promontory during delivery; normal contour is usually regained spontaneously. **involutional d.,** see under *melancholia*. **otic d.,** auditory pit. **pacchionian d's,** granular foveolae. **postdormital d.,** mental depression following awakening from sleep. **precordial d.,** epigastric fossa, def. 1. **pterygoid d.,** pterygoid fovea. **radial d.,** radial fossa of humerus. **reactive d.,** depression caused by some external situation, and relieved when that situation is removed. **retarded d.,** the depressive phase of manic-depressive psychosis. **situational d.,** reactive d. **supratrochlear d.,** a slight depression on the anterior surface of the femur, above the trochlea. **systolic d.** (*obs.*), a falling of the precordial region of the chest observed during the systole. **ventricular d.,** that part of the venous pulse tracing which lies between the ventricular and atrial waves.

depressive (de-pres′iv) causing depression.

depressomotor (de-pres″o-mo′tor) [L. *deprimere* to press down + *motor* mover] 1. retarding or abating motion. 2. an agent which lessens or depresses motor activity.

depressor (de-pres′or) [L.] that which depresses, as a muscle, agent, instrument, or apparatus which depresses, or an afferent nerve whose stimulation causes a fall of blood pressure. **d. an′guli o′ris,** see *Table of Musculi*. **d. epiglot′tidis,** a portion of the thyroepiglottic muscle which depresses the epiglottis. **d. la′bii inferio′ris,** see *Table of Musculi*. **tongue d.,** an instrument for pressing the tongue against the floor of the mouth.

deprimens oculi (dep′re-menz ok′u-le) [L.] musculus rectus inferior bulbi.

deprivation (dep-rĭ-va′shun) [L. *de* from + *privare* to remove] loss or absence of parts, organs, powers, or things that are needed. **emotional d.,** deprivation of adequate and appropriate interpersonal and/or environmental experience, usually in the early development years. **sensory d.,** deprivation of usual external stimuli and the opportunity for perception.

deprostil (dĕ-pros′til) chemical name: 15-hydroxy-15-methyl-9-oxoprostan-1-oic acid; a prostaglandin that inhibits gastric secretion, $C_{21}H_{38}O_4$.

deproteinization (de-pro″te-in-i-za′shun) removal of protein.

depside (dep′sīd) one of a class of compounds which are products of the condensation of two or more molecules of the hydroxyacids of benzene, e.g., tannic acid.

depth (depth) an expression of the distance separating the upper and lower surfaces of an object. **focal d.,** the measure of the power of a lens to yield clear images of objects at different distances from it.

depula (dep′u-lah) [L., from Gr. *depas* goblet] in zoology, the developing egg in the stage succeeding the blastula and preceding the gastrula.

depurant (dep′u-rant) 1. cleansing or purifying. 2. an agent that cleanses or purifies.

depurate (dep′u-rāt) [L. *depurare* to purify] to cleanse, refine, or purify.

depurative (dep′u-ra″tiv) tending to purify or cleanse; called also *pellant*.

depurator (dep′u-ra″tor) 1. an agent that cleanses or purifies. 2. (*obs.*) a vacuum-producing apparatus for stimulating the excretory function of the skin.

der- (der) [Gr. *derē* neck] combining form denoting relationship to the neck.

deradelphus (der″ah-del′fus) [*der-* + Gr. *adelphos* brother] a monster made up of twins fused at or near the navel, and having only one head.

deranencephalia (der-an″en-sĕ-fa′le-ah) [*der-* + *an* neg. + Gr. *enkephalos* brain] monstrosity marked by defect of the brain and upper part of the spinal cord.

derangement (de-rānj′ment) 1. mental disorder. 2. disarrangement of a part or organ. **Hey's internal d.,** partial dislocation of the knee, marked by great pain and spasm of the muscles.

Dercum's disease (der′kumz) [Francis Xavier *Dercum*, American physician, 1856–1931] adiposis dolorosa.

derealization (de-re″al-ĭ-za′shun) a mental state characterized by a peculiar change in awareness of the external world, creating a feeling of unreality.

dereism (de′re-izm) [L. *de* away + *res* thing] mental activity in which fantasy runs on unhampered by logic and experience.

dereistic (de″re-is′tik) pertaining to or characterized by dereism.

derencephalocele (der″en-sĕ-fal′o-sēl) [*der-* + Gr. *enkephalos* brain + *kēlē* hernia] protrusion of the brain substance through a slit in one or more of the cervical vertebrae.

derencephalus (der″en-sef′ah-lus) [*der-* + Gr. *enkephalos* brain] a monster with rudimentary skull bones and bifid cervical vertebrae, the brain resting in the bifurcation.

derepression (de″re-presh′un) 1. elevation of the level of an enzyme above the normal, either by lowering of the corepressor concentration or by a mutation that decreases the formation of aporepressor or the response to the complete repressor. 2. in genetic theory, the inhibition of the repressor substance produced by the regulator genes with the result that the operator gene is free to initiate the process of polypeptide formation; called also *gene d.* Cf. repression, def. 3. **gene d.,** derepression, def. 2.

dericin (der′ĭ-sin) a light-colored oil derived from castor oil and used as a vehicle for menthol; called also *florizine*.

derism (de′rizm) dereism.

derivant (der′ĭ-vant) derivative.

derivation (der″ĭ-va′shun) [L. *derivatio*, from *derivare* to draw off] 1. the origin or source of a substance. 2. a lead in electrocardiography. 3. (*obs.*) the process or act of drawing off, as the withdrawal of blood, or the removal of a disease process from one part of the body to another part.

derivative (de-riv′ah-tiv) 1. producing or causing a derivation. 2. a chemical substance derived from another substance either directly or by modification or partial substitution. 3. an agent which withdraws blood from the seat of a disease.

derma (der′mah) [Gr.] the skin, usually with special reference to the dermis or corium.

derma- see *dermato-*.

dermabrader (der-mah-brād′er) any device used for dermabrasion.

dermabrasion (der-mah-bra′shun) planing of the skin done by mechanical means, e.g., sandpaper, wire brushes, etc. See *planing*.

Dermacentor (der″mah-sen′tor) [*derma-* + Gr. *kentein* to prick, stab] a genus of ticks which are important as transmitters of

disease. **D. albipic′tus,** a species of brown ticks widely distributed in the United States, parasitic on cattle, horses, deer, elk, and moose. Called also *winter tick*. **D. anderso′ni,** a reddish

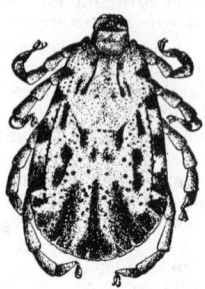

Dermacentor andersoni (Chandler).

brown tick which is responsible for transmitting Rocky Mountain spotted fever, Colorado tick fever, and tularemia to man and for causing tick paralysis. Its hosts include deer, elk, antelope, grizzly bear, porcupine, prairie dog, and various species of rabbits. Called also *D. venustus, Rocky Mountain wood tick,* and *mountain wood tick*. **D. hal′li,** a yellow-brown tick found on peccaries in Texas. **D. hun′teri,** a brown tick found on Rocky Mountain sheep in southwestern United States, particularly in southwestern Arizona. **D. margina′tus,** a species that is the vector of a type of tick-borne hemorrhagic fever in Siberia. **D. ni′tens,** *Anocentor nitans*. **D. nuttal′lii,** a tick which transmits Siberian tick typhus. **D. occidenta′lis,** a brown tick found widely distributed along the west coast of the United States, from southwestern Oregon to southern California, the principal hosts being the cow, horse, deer, dog, and man; called also *Pacific coast dog tick*. **D. parumaper′tus,** a reddish brown tick which is found widely distributed in the southwestern United States, found on deer and coyotes, and abundant on various species of rabbits. **D. reticula′tus,** a tick which attacks sheep and oxen, occurring in Europe, Asia, and America; a vector of canine babesiosis in southern Europe. **D. sylva′rum,** a tick which transmits Siberian tick typhus. **D. varia′bilis,** a dark brown tick found along the California coast and widely distributed east of the Rocky Mountains, the dog being the principal host of the adults, which are found also on cattle, horses, rabbits, and man; it is the principal vector of Rocky Mountain spotted fever in the central and eastern United States. Called also *American dog tick* and *dog tick*. **D. venus′tus,** *D. andersoni*.

Dermacentroxenus (der″mah-sen″trok-se′nus) [*Dermacentor* + Gr. *xenos* a guest-friend] a genus name formerly given microorganisms parasitic in ticks, now included in the genus Rickettsia; later used as the name of a subgenus including the species *R. a′kari, R. austra′lis, R. cono′rii, R. rickett′sii,* and *R. siberica.* **D. a′kari,** *Rickettsia akari.* **D. austra′lis,** *Rickettsia australis.* **D. cono′ri,** *Rickettsia conorii.* **D. orienta′lis,** *Rickettsia tsutsugamushi.* **D. pijpe′ri,** *Rickettsia conorii.* **D. rickett′si,** *Rickettsia rickettsii.* **D. siber′icus,** a name proposed for the tick-borne agent causing tick typhus in Siberia, thought to be identical with *Rickettsia conorii.* **D. ty′phi,** *Rickettsia typhi.*

dermad (der′mad) toward the integument.

dermal (der′mal) of or pertaining to the skin.

dermamyiasis (der″mah-mi-i′ah-sis) [*derma-* + Gr. *myia* fly] dermatomyiasis.

Dermanyssidae (der″mah-nis′ĭ-de) a family of mites (order Acarina) parasitizing mammals, reptiles, and birds, whose bite may cause a painful dermatitis in man; *Dermanyssus* is the type genus.

Dermanyssus (der″mah-nis′sus) [*derma-* + Gr. *nyssein* to prick] a genus of mites of the family Dermanyssidae. **D. galli′nae,** the bird mite, poultry (chicken or fowl) mite, or chicken louse, which sometimes infests man.

dermaskeleton (der″mah-skel′ĕ-ton) exoskeleton.

dermat- see *dermato-*.

dermatergosis (der″mat-er-go′sis) [*dermat-* + Gr. *ergon* work] any occupational disease or lesion of the skin.

dermatic (der-mat′ik) dermal.

dermatitides (der″mah-tit′ĭ-dēz) plural of *dermatitis*.

dermatitis (der″mah-ti′tis), pl. *dermatit′ides* [*dermato-* + *-itis*] inflammation of the skin. **actinic d.,** dermatitis resulting from exposure to actinic radiation, such as that from the sun, ultraviolet waves, or x or gamma radiation. **allergic d.,** 1. any inflammation of the skin believed to be due to allergy. 2. atopic d. **ammonia d.,** a form of diaper dermatitis that has been attributed to irritation of the skin due to the ammonia decomposition products of urine. **ancylostome d.** (*obs.*), ground itch. **d. artefac′ta,** a condition of the skin characterized by lesions that are self-inflicted by the patient, as by heat, chemicals, or other physical or mechanical means. **ashy d.,** erythema dyschromicum perstans. **atopic d.,** a chronic pruritic eruption occurring in adolescents and adults, of unknown etiology although allergic, hereditary, and psychogenic factors appear to be involved. The lesions occur chiefly on the flexural surfaces of the knees and elbows, but may involve other areas, and are marked by lichenification, excoriations, and crusting. In infants and young children the condition is sometimes called *infantile eczema* or (in Britain) *Besnier's prurigo.* Called also *allergic d., flexural eczema,* and *disseminated neurodermatitis.* **berlock d., berloque d.,** phototoxic dermatitis, typically on the neck, face, and breast, occurring as drop-shaped or quadrilateral patches or streaks, induced by sequential exposure to perfume and other toilet articles and then to sunlight. Called also *perfume d.* **bhiwanol d.,** dhobie itch. **brown-tail moth d.,** a cutaneous irritation produced by the hairs of the brown-tail moth, *Euproctis chrysorrhoea;* called also *brown-tail rash.* **brucella d.,** dermatitis occurring in veterinarians and stockmen who come in contact with cows affected with infectious abortion (brucellosis). **d. calor'ica,** inflammation of the skin due to heat or cold; cf. *erythema abigne.* **caterpillar d.,** a transient but sometimes painful dermatitis caused by contact with caterpillars, with resultant penetration of the skin by their hairs (setae). **contact d.,** 1. an acute allergic inflammation of the skin caused by contact with various substances of a chemical, animal, or vegetable nature to which delayed hypersensitivity has been acquired; when severe, it is called *d. venenata.* 2. primary-irritant (nonallergic) d. **contagious pustular d.,** see *contagious acne,* under *acne* and see *orf.* **cosmetic d.,** allergic contact dermatitis caused by some ingredient in a cosmetic preparation. **dhobie mark d.,** dhobie itch. **diaper d.,** dermatitis localized to the area in contact with the diaper in infants, the folds of skin being spared. The manifestations vary from diffuse erythema to nodular lesions. Called also *Jacquet's d.* or *erythema, napkin erythema, napkin-area d.,* and *gluteal erythema.* **d. dysmenorrhoe'ica,** a rosacea-like eruption on the cheeks of women, recurring during or just before painful menstrual periods. **d. escharot'ica,** see *primary irritant d.* **d. exfoliati'va,** exfoliative d. **d. exfoliati'va neonato'rum,** exfoliative dermatitis supervening in bullous impetigo of the newborn; it may be identical to toxic epidermal necrolysis. Both conditions may be caused by staphylococci of phage group two, although a toxic drug reaction is also suspected in the etiology of toxic epidermal necrolysis. Called also *Ritter's disease.* **exfoliative d.,** a skin disorder evolving from any of several preceding skin disorders, such as drug eruption or psoriasis, and characterized by virtually universal erythema with desquamation, scaling, itching, and loss of hair. **exudative discoid and lichenoid d.,** a disease seen in older men, characterized by itching oval or disk-shaped plaques, which later becomes a widespread dermatitis, followed by oozing and lichenification. **d. gangreno'sa infan'tum,** a condition of unknown etiology occurring in infants and marked by bullous or pustular eruption followed by disseminated gangrene of the skin; not infrequently confused with *ecthyma gangrenosum.* **d. gestatio'nis,** herpes gestationis. **grass d.,** meadow d. **halowax d.,** chloracne. **d. hemostat'ica,** stasis dermatitis. **d. herpetifor'mis,** chronic dermatitis marked by grouped, symmetrical, erythematous, papular, vesicular, eczematous, or bullous lesions occurring in successive crops in varied combinations, accompanied by burning and itching; a granular deposition of IgA around the lesion occurs in almost every case. Called also *Duhring's disease.* Cf. *herpes gestationis.* **d. hiema'lis,** dermatitis coming on with cold weather; cf. *pruritus hiemalis.* **d. hypostat'ica,** stasis dermatitis. **industrial d.,** contact dermatitis, sometimes of the primary-irritant type, but usually of the delayed hypersensitivity type, caused by material handled by the patient in the course of his employment; called also *occupational d.* **d. infectio'sa eczematoi'des, infectious eczematoid d.,** a pustular eczematoid eruption frequently following or occurring coincidentally with some pyogenic process. **insect d.,** dermatitis caused by the irritant hairs of certain insects, especially moths and caterpillars. **io-moth d.,** dermatitis caused by the irritant hairs of the larva of *Automeris io.* **Jacquet's d.,** diaper d. **d. lichenoi'des chron'ica atroph'icans** (*obs.*), lichen sclerosus et atrophicus. **livedoid d.,** a condition due to temporary or prolonged local ischemia resulting from accidental arterial obliteration from intragluteal administration of medications, marked by severe local pain, swelling, livedoid changes, and local increase in temperature; fever, tachycardia, dyspnea, and albuminuria also occur, and gangrene may supervene. **marine d.,** swimmer's itch occurring in persons wading or swimming in salt water; called also *seabather's eruption.* **meadow d., meadow-grass d.,** phototoxic dermatitis marked by an eruption of vesicles and bullae arranged in streaks and bizarre configurations, caused by exposure to sunlight after contact with meadow grass, usually *Agrimonia eupatoria.* Called also *grass d.* and *d. striata pratensis bullosa.* **d. medicamento'sa,** drug eruption. **d. micropapulo'sa erythemato'sa hyperidrot'ica na'si** (*obs.*), granulosis rubra nasi. **mollus'cum d.,** a dermatitis ranging from very mild to moderately severe, of unknown cause, occasionally seen in association with molluscum contagiosum. **napkin area d.,** diaper d. **occupational d.,** dermatitis caused by material employed in the patient's occupation; called also *industrial d.* **onion mite d.,** dermatitis af-

fecting handlers of decaying onions, caused by the onion mite, *Acarus rhyzoglypticus hyacinthi.* **d. papilla'ris capilli'tii,** keloidal folliculitis. **d. pediculoi'des ventrico'sus,** grain itch. **perfume d.,** berlock d. **perioral d.,** a papular, sometimes pustular, dermatitis of unknown etiology, confined to the nasolabial fold areas, upper lip, and chin, and occurring almost exclusively in women between the ages of 20 and 35. **photocontact d.,** allergic contact dermatitis caused by the action of sunlight on skin sensitized by contact with a substance capable of causing this reaction, such as a halogenated salicylanilide, sandalwood oil, or hexachlorophene. **phototoxic d.,** erythema followed by hyperpigmentation of sun-exposed areas of the skin, resulting from sequential exposure to agents containing photosensitizing substances, such as coal tar and certain perfumes, drugs, or plants containing psoralens, and then to sunlight. **pigmented purpuric lichenoid d.,** dermatitis of the extremities, especially the legs, characterized by papules which become purpuric or pigmented. **poison ivy d., poison oak d., poison sumac d.,** see *rhus d.* **precancerous d.,** Bowen's disease. **primary irritant d.,** skin inflammation induced by a substance acting as an irritant rather than as a sensitizer or allergen, so that all persons are affected similarly on initial contact. When severe, it is called also *d. escharotica,* or *chemical burn.* **purpuric pigmented lichenoid d.,** pigmented pururic lichenoid d. **radiation d.,** radiodermatitis. **rat-mite d.,** dermatitis resulting from the bite of *Ornithonyssus bacoti.* **d. re'pens,** acrodermatitis continua. **rhus d.,** allergic contact dermatitis due to exposure to plants of the genus *Rhus* (*Toxicodendron*) (poison ivy, poison oak, poison sumac), which contain urushiol, a potent skin-sensitizing agent. **roentgen-ray d.,** radiodermatitis. **sabra d.,** a dermatitis somewhat resembling scabies, affecting those who handle the fruit of cacti (sabra or prickly pear) and Indian figs in Israel; thought to be due to the penetration of minute thorns or hairs into the skin. **schistosome d.,** swimmer's itch. **seborrheic d., d. seborrheica,** a chronic inflammatory disease of the skin of unknown etiology, characterized by moderate erythema, dry, moist, or greasy scaling, and yellow crusted patches on various areas, including the mid-parts of the face, ears, supraorbital regions, umbilicus, genitalia, and especially the scalp, where it is manifested by small patches of scales that progress to involve the entire scalp, with exfoliation of an excessive amount of dry scales (dandruff). The condition is usually accompanied by itching. Called also *eczema seborrheicum, seborrheic eczema,* and *seborrhea.* **d. skiagraph'ica,** radiodermatitis. **stasis d.,** an often chronic, usually eczematous dermatitis, which initially involves the inner aspect of the lower leg just above the internal malleolus and which later may involve the entire lower leg or portions thereof, characterized by edema, pigmentation, and commonly ulceration; it is due to venous insufficiency. Called also *d. hemostatica, d. hypostatica,* and *stasis eczema.* **straw-mat d.** (*obs.*), grain itch. **d. stria'ta praten'sis bullo'sa,** meadow d. **swimmer's d.,** swimmer's itch. **uncinarial d.,** ground itch. **vanilla d.,** dermatitis from handling vanilla beans. **d. vegetans,** a chronic, benign, vegetative pyoderma having histologic features of pemphigus vulgaris, and marked by the growth of fungating masses on eczematous areas, which may be bordered by pustules and vesicles; it is probably due to a superimposed staphylococcal infection. Called also *benign pemphigus vegetans, Hallopeau type of pemphigus vegetans, pyoderma vegetans, pyoderma verrucosum,* and *pyodermatitis vegetans.* Cf. *pemphigus vegetans.* **d. venena'ta,** see *contact d.* **verminous d.,** stephanofilariasis. **d. verruco'sa** (*obs.*), chromomycosis. **vesicular d.,** a sometimes fatal disease, believed to be eczematous in nature, affecting young poultry that range over unbroken prairie sod, marked by the formation of blisters and scabs on the feet and legs; called also *sod disease.* **weeping d.,** eczema. **x-ray d.,** radiodermatitis.

dermato-, derma-, dermat-, dermo- [Gr. *derma, dermatos* skin] combining forms denoting relationship to the skin.

dermatoarthritis (der″mah-to-ar-thri′tis) skin disease associated with arthritis. **lipid d., lipoid d.,** multicentric reticulohistiocytosis.

dermatoautoplasty (der″mah-to-aw′to-plas″-te) [*dermato-* + Gr. *autos* self + *plassein* to mold] the grafting on denuded areas of skin taken from some other portion of the patient's own body.

Dermatobia (der″mah-to′be-ah) [*dermato-* + Gr. *bios* life] a genus of botflies of the family Oestridae. **D. hom'inis,** the hu-

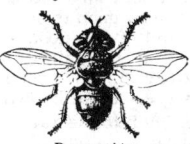

Dermatobia.

man botfly of South America whose larvae (called ver macaque or ver moyocuil) are parasitic in the skin of man, mammals and birds; the eggs are deposited by the female on the bodies of mosquitoes, flies or ticks and by them transported to the host.

dermatobiasis (der″mah-to-bi′ah-sis) the presence of *Dermatobia* in the body.

dermatocandidiasis (der″mah-to-kan″dĭ-di′ah-sis) cutaneous candidiasis.

dermatocele (der′mah-to-sēl″) [*dermato-* + Gr. *kēlē* hernia] cutis laxa.

dermatochalasis, dermatochalazia (der″mah-to-kal′ah-sis; der″mah-to-kal-ah′zi-ah) [*dermato-* + Gr. *chalasthai* to become slack] cutis laxa.

dermatoconjunctivitis (der″mah-to-kon-junk″tĭ-vi′tis) inflammation of the conjunctiva and of the skin around the eyes.

dermatodysplasia (der″mah-to-dis-pla′ze-ah) a condition characterized by abnormal development of the skin.

dermatofibroma (der″mah-to-fi-bro′mah) a fibrous tumor-like nodule of the dermis. **d. protu′berans,** a large-sized molluscum growth that tends to recur after incision; called also *dermatofibrosarcoma protuberans.*

dermatofibrosarcoma (der″mah-to-fi″bro-sar-ko′mah) a fibrosarcoma of the skin. **d. protu′berans,** dermatofibroma protuberans.

dermatofibrosis (der″mah-to-fi-bro′sis) a condition characterized by fibrotic changes in the skin. **d. lenticula′ris dissemina′ta,** a hereditary condition of the skin associated with osteopoikilosis and marked by the presence of papular fibromas over the back, arms, and thighs. Called also *Buschke-Ollendorff syndrome.*

dermatogen (der-mat′o-jen) a skin antigen that may be associated with any skin disease.

dermatoglyphics (der″mah-to-glif′iks) [*dermato-* + Gr. *glyphein* to carve] the study of the patterns of ridges of the skin of the fingers, palms, toes, and soles; of interest in anthropology and law enforcement as a means of establishing identity and in medicine, both clinically and as a genetic indicator, particularly of chromosomal abnormalities.

dermatograph (der-mat′o-graf) [*dermato-* + Gr. *graphein* to write] (*obs.*) 1. an instrument for marking or writing on the skin, as in marking the boundaries of the body. 2. dermograph.

dermatographia (der″mah-to-graf′e-ah) dermatographism.

dermatographic (der″mah-to-grof′ik) pertaining to or characterized by dermatographism.

dermatographism (der″mah-tog′rah-fizm) urticaria due to physical allergy, in which moderately firm stroking or scratching of the skin with a dull instrument produces a pale, raised welt or wheal, with a red flare on each side; see also *white d.* and *black d.* **black d.,** black or greenish streaking of the skin caused by deposit of fine metallic particles abraded from jewelry by various dusting powders. **white d.,** linear blanching of (usually erythematous) skin of persons with atopic dermatitis in response to firm stroking with a blunt instrument.

dermatoheteroplasty (der″mah-to-het′er-o-plas″te) [*dermato-* + Gr. *heteros* other + *plassein* to form] the grafting of skin derived from an individual of another species.

dermatoid (der′mah-toid) [*dermato-* + Gr. *eidos* form] (*obs.*) dermoid, def. 1.

dermatologic, dermatological (der″mah-to-loj′ik, der″mah-to-loj′ĭ-kal) pertaining to dermatology; of or affecting the skin.

dermatologist (der″mah-tol′o-jist) a physician who limits his practice to the diagnosis and treatment of skin disorders.

dermatology (der″mah-tol′o-je) the medical specialty concerned with the diagnosis and treatment of diseases of the skin.

dermatolysis (der″mah-tol′ĭ-sis) [*dermato-* + Gr. *lysis* loosening] cutis laxa. **d. palpebra′rum,** blepharochalasis.

dermatome (der′mah-tōm) [*derma-* + Gr. *temnein* to cut] 1. an instrument for cutting thin skin slices for skin grafts. 2. the area of skin supplied with afferent nerve fibers by a single posterior spinal root; called also *dermatomic area.* 3. the lateral portion of a mesodermal somite; the cutis plate. **Brown d.,** an electric dermatome, the first to be developed, for cutting thick-split skin grafts; it enables the surgeon to rapidly remove long strips of skin. **Castroviejo d.,** an electric dermatome used for cutting mucous membrane grafts for the treatment of eyelid and socket deformities and as an adjunct in the removal of tattoos after the initial excision has been done using either the Brown or Padgett dermatomes. It has a tiny cutting head with special blades and skims to control the thickness of the cut. **Padgett d.,** an instrument for cutting thin- or thick-split skin grafts which enables the surgeon to cut a sheet of skin of any size up to 4 × 7½ inches and of any desired thickness. **Reese d.,** an instrument for cutting split-skin grafts of 0.008 to 0.034 inch in thickness. **Stryker d.,** an electric dermatome similar to and having the same uses as the Brown dermatome.

dermatomegaly (der″mah-to-meg′ah-le) cutis laxa.

dermatomere (der′mah-to-mēr″) [*dermato-* + Gr. *meros* part] any segment or metamere of the embryonic integument.

dermatomic (der″mah-tom′ik) pertaining to a dermatome.

dermatomyces (der″mah-to-mi′sēz) dermatophyte.

dermatomycin (der″mah-to-mi′sin) any of several antigens

derived from fungi and used in the diagnosis, prophylaxis, and treatment of dermatomycosis.

dermatomycosis (der″mah-to-mi-ko′sis) [*dermato-* + Gr. *mykes* fungus] a superficial infection of the skin or its appendages by fungi. The term includes dermatophytosis and the various clinical forms of tinea, as well as deep fungous infections.

dermatomyiasis (der″mah-to-mi-i′ah-sis) infestation of the skin by flies or fly maggots.

dermatomyoma (der″mah-to-mi-o′mah) [*dermato-* + *myoma*] a dermal leiomyoma.

dermatomyositis (der″mah-to-mi″o-si′tis) [*dermato-* + Gr. *mys* muscle + *-itis*] a nonsuppurative inflammation of the skin, subcutaneous tissue, and muscles, with necrosis of muscle fibers; one of the so-called collagen or connective tissue diseases. There is underlying cancer in as many as 50 per cent of adult cases. When the skin lesions are absent, it is known as *polymyositis.*

dermatoneurology (der″mah-to-nu-rol′o-je) [*dermato-* + Gr. *neuron* nerve + *-logy*] the study of the nerves of the skin in health and disease.

dermato-ophthalmitis (der″mah-to-of″thal-mi′tis) inflammation of the skin and of the eye, including the conjunctiva, cornea, etc.

dermatopathic (der″mah-to-path′ik) pertaining or attributable to disease of the skin, as dermatopathic lymphadenopathy.

dermatopathology (der″mah-to-pah-thol′o-je) microscopic anatomic pathology of the skin.

dermatopathy (der″mah-top′ah-the) [*dermato-* + Gr. *pathos* disease] dermopathy.

Dermatophagoides (der″mah-tof″ah-goi′dēs) a genus of sarcoptiform mites, usually found on the skin of chickens. **D. pteronyssi′mus,** the house dust mite, which acts as an antigen and produces an allergic asthmatic reaction in atopic persons. **D. scheremetew′skyi,** a species that attacks man and causes a mange-like inflammation.

dermatopharmacology (der″mah-to-fahr″mah-kol′o-je) pharmacology as applied to dermatologic disorders.

dermatophiliasis (der″mah-to-fĭ-li′ah-sis) 1. tungiasis. 2. dermatophilosis.

dermatophilosis (der″mah-to-fi-lo′sis) an actinomycotic disease caused by *Dermatophilus congolense,* affecting cattle, sheep, horses, goats, deer, and sometimes man. In man, it is characterized by nonpainful pustules on the hands and arms; the lesions break down and form shallow red ulcers which regress spontaneously, leaving some scarring. In sheep, it is characterized by exudative red scaling lesions that form pyramidal masses and is known as *lumpy wool, strawberry rot foot,* and formerly *streptotricosis.*

Dermatophilus (der″mah-tof′ĭ-lus) 1. *Tunga.* 2. a genus of pathogenic actinomycetes. **D. congolen′sis,** the etiologic agent of dermatophilosis. **D. pen′etrans** *Tunga penetrans,* or chigoe.

dermatophylaxis (der″mah-to-fi-lak′sis) [*dermato-* + Gr. *phylaxis* a guarding] (*obs.*) protection against skin infection; protection of the skin against infection.

dermatophyte (der′mah-to-fīt″) [*dermato-* + Gr. *phyton* plant] a fungus parasitic upon the skin; the term embraces the imperfect fungi of the genera *Microsporum, Epidermophyton,* and *Trichophyton.* Called also *cutaneous fungus* and *dermatomyces.*

dermatophytid (der″mah-tof′ĭ-tid) a secondary skin eruption which is an expression of hypersensitivity to a dermatophyte, especially *Epidermophyton,* infection, occurring on an area far from the site of infection; called also *epidermophytid* and *mycid.*

dermatophytosis (der″mah-to-fi-to′sis) a fungous infection of the skin, or infection caused by a dermatophyte; often used specifically to designate such an infection of the skin of the feet (tinea pedis). Called also *dermomycosis* and *epidermomycosis.*

dermatoplastic (der″mah-to-plas′tik) pertaining to dermatoplasty.

dermatoplasty (der′mah-to-plas″te) [*dermato-* + Gr. *plassein* to form] a plastic operation on the skin; operative replacement of destroyed or lost skin.

dermatopolyneuritis (der″mah-to-pol″e-nu-ri′tis) acrodynia.

dermatorrhagia (der″mah-to-ra′je-ah) discharge of blood into or from the skin. **d. parasit′ica,** a disease of the skin of horses, asses, and mules in Europe and Asia, marked by hard elevations formed by accumulations of blood between the layers of the skin, and caused by the presence of a parasitic filarial worm, *Parafilaria multipapillosa.* Called also *summer bleeding.*

dermatorrhexis (der″mah-to-rek′sis) [*dermato-* + Gr. *rhēxis* a breaking] rupture of the skin capillaries, as in Ehlers-Danlos syndrome.

dermatosclerosis (der″mah-to-skle-ro′sis) [*dermato-* + Gr. *sklērōsis* hardening.] scleroderma.

dermatoses (der″mah-to′sēz) plural of *dermatosis.*

dermatosis (der″mah-to′sis), pl. *dermato′ses* [*dermat-* + *-osis*] any skin disease, especially one not characterized by inflammation. **acute febrile neutrophilic d.,** a rare condition usually affecting women, characterized by a nonpruritic eruption of painful, raised, partly confluent, red nodules or plaques, 0.5 to 4 cm. broad, primarily on the arms; associated with acute high fever and moderate neutrophil leukocytosis, it may persist for several months. Called also *Sweet's syndrome.* **angioneurotic d.** (*obs.*), angioneurotic edema. **ashy d. of Ramirez,** erythema dyschromicum perstans. **Bowen's precancerous d.,** Bowen's disease. **chick nutritional d.,** a disease of chicks due to a deficiency of pantothenic acid, marked by eruptions on the head and feet. **d. cinecien'ta,** erythema dyschromicum perstans. **d. cine'rea per'stans,** erythema dyschromicum perstans. **industrial d.,** occupational dermatitis. **lichenoid d.,** a skin disease characterized by the appearance of small, firm, discrete papules. **d. papulo'sa ni'gra,** a variety of seborrheic keratosis observed principally in Negroes, with multiple miliary pigmented papules usually on the upper lateral aspect of the cheek, but sometimes occurring more widely on the face and neck. **precancerous d.,** any skin condition in which the lesions, such as warts, moles, or other excrescences, are likely to undergo malignant degeneration. **progressive pigmentary d.,** a slowly progressive purpuric and pigmentary disease of the skin affecting chiefly the shins, ankles, and dorsum of the feet; called also *Schamberg's d.* or *disecse.* **Schamberg's d.,** progressive pigmentary d. **stasis d.,** see under *dermatitis.* **subcorneal pustular d.,** a chronic, superficial, pustular disorder with a chronic relapsing course, resembling dermatitis herpetiformis, and chiefly affecting women in middle life, with sterile pustular blebs beneath the horny layer of the epidermis on the trunk and in the major skin folds. Called also *Sneddon-Wilkinson disease.* **Unna's d.** (*obs.*), seborrheic dermatitis. **d. veg'etans,** a hereditary disease of young pigs characterized by raised skin lesions, abnormalities of the hooves, and pneumonia.

dermatosome (der'mah-to-sōm") [*dermato-* + Gr. *sōma* body] a thickening on each spindle fiber in the equatorial region during mitosis.

dermatosparaxis (der"mah-to-spah-rak'sis) [*dermato-* + Gr. *sparaxis, sparagmos* a tearing] a disease of cattle and sheep in which the skin is fragile and very easily torn; it is related to the Ehlers-Danlos syndrome of humans, and evidence indicates that the defect may reside in an abnormally low activity of the enzyme procollagen peptidase.

dermatotherapy (der"mah-to-ther'ah-pe) [*dermato-* + Gr. *therapeia* treatment] treatment of the skin and its diseases.

dermatothlasia (der"mah-to-thla'ze-ah) [*dermato-* + Gr. *thlasis* bruising] (*obs.*) a morbid tendency to injure the skin by pinching and bruising.

dermatotome (der'mah-to-tōm) [*dermato-* + Gr. *temnein* to cut] dermatome, defs. 1 and 3.

dermatotropic (der"mah-to-trop'ik) [*dermato* + Gr. *tropos,* turning toward or affecting] preferentially infecting, infesting, or affecting the skin; said of certain microorganisms.

dermatozoiasis (der"mah-to-zo-i'ah-sis) dermatozoonosis.

dermatozoon (der"mah-to-zo'on) [*dermato-* + Gr. *zōon* animal] any animal parasite of the skin; an ectoparasite.

dermatozoonosis (der"mah-to-zo"o-no'sis) [*dermato-* + Gr. *zōon* animal + *nosos* disease] a skin disease caused by a dermatozoon; called also *dermatozoiasis.*

dermenchysis (der-men'ki-sis) [*derma-* + Gr. *enchysis* pouring in] the hypodermic administration of medicines.

dermic (der'mik) dermal.

dermis (der'mis) NA alternative for the corium.

dermitis (der-mi'tis) [*derma-* + *-itis*] (*obs.*) dermatitis.

dermo- see *dermato-.*

dermoanergy (der"mo-an'er-je) lack of hypersensitivity response by skin to (administered) antigen; absence of immunologic (allergic) reactivity in skin.

dermoblast (der'mo-blast) [*dermo-* + Gr. *blastos* germ] that part of the mesoblast which develops into the true skin or corium.

dermochrome (der'mo-krōm) [*dermo-* + Gr. *chrōma* color] (*obs.*) a colored illustration of the skin or of a skin disease.

dermocyma (der"mo-si'mah) [*dermo-* + Gr. *kyma* fetus] a monstrosity in which one fetus is inclosed within another.

dermocymus (der"mo-si'mus) dermocyma.

dermoglyphics (der"mo-glif'iks) dermatoglyphics.

dermograph (der'mo-graf) (*obs.*) the elevated mark or wheal which appears on the skin in dermographism.

dermographia (der"mo-graf'e-ah) [*dermo-* + Gr. *graphein* to write] dermatographism.

dermographic (der"mo-graf'ik) dermatographic.

dermographism (der-mog'rah-fizm) dermatographism.

dermohygrometer (der"mo-hi-grom'ĕ-ter) an instrument for measuring skin resistance without inducing a constant current into the skin.

dermoid (der'moid) [*derma-* + Gr. *eidos* form] 1. resembling the skin. 2. a dermoid cyst. **corneal d.,** a tumorous growth upon the cornea of animals; its surface contains hairs. **implantation d.,** a dermoid cyst resulting from an injury by which a portion of the epiblastic structure is driven into the body.

inclusion d., a dermoid cyst due to the inclusion of foreign tissue in the closure of a developmental cleft. **thyroid d.,** a dermoid cyst considered to arise from a retention cyst of the persistent thyroid duct or of the thyrolingual duct. **tubal d.,** a dermoid cyst of the oviduct.

dermoidectomy (der"moid-ek'to-me) [*dermoid* + Gr. *ektomē* excision] excision of a dermoid cyst.

dermolipoma (der"mo-lĭ-po'mah) a congenital yellow fatty growth beneath the bulbar conjunctiva.

dermolysin (der-mol'ĭ-sin) a substance, circulating in the blood, capable of dissolving the skin.

dermometer (der-mom'ĕ-ter) the instrument used in dermometry.

dermometry (der-mom'ĕ-tre) [*dermo-* + Gr. *metron* measure] the measurement of areas of skin resistance to a passage of direct electric current; these areas will correspond to the areas of sensory loss.

dermomycosis (der"mo-mi-ko'sis) [*dermo-* + Gr. *mykēs* fungus] dermatophytosis.

dermomyotome (der"mo-mi'o-tōm) [*dermo-* + *myo-* + *-tome*] all but the sclerotome of a mesodermal somite; the primordium of skeletal muscle and, perhaps, of corium.

dermoneurotropic (der"mo-nu"ro-trop'ik) having an affinity for the skin and nervous tissue.

dermopathic (der"mo-path'ik) dermatopathic.

dermopathy (der-mop'ah-the) [*dermo-* + Gr. *pathos* disease] any skin disorder. **diabetic d.,** any of several cutaneous manifestations of diabetes marked by papular, erosive, ulcerated, pigmented, macular, or cicatricial lesions of the shins, apparently occurring as a result of a specific angiitis of small blood vessels; the term is sometimes broadened to include bullae in diabetics, especially bullae of the toes, feet, and ankles, and necrobiosis lipoidica diabeticorum. Called also *diabetid.*

dermophylaxis (der"mo-fi-lak'sis) dermatophylaxis.

dermophyte (der'mo-fīt) dermatophyte.

dermoplasty (der'mo-plas"te) dermatoplasty.

dermoreaction (der"mo-re-ak'shun) cutireaction.

dermoskeleton (der"mo-skel'ĕ-ton) exoskeleton.

dermostosis (der"mos-to'sis) [*dermo-* + Gr. *osteon* bone] (*obs.*) osteomas of the skin.

dermosynovitis (der"mo-sin-o-vi'tis) [*dermo-* + *synovitis*] inflammation of skin overlying an inflamed bursa or tendon sheath.

dermotoxin (der"mo-tok'sin) a toxin of staphylococci which produces a necrotic area in the skin when injected.

dermotropic (der"mo-trop'ik) dermatotropic.

dermovaccine (der"mo-vak'sin) [*dermo-* + *vaccine*] vaccine virus maintained by dermal inoculations and prepared from scrapings of skin lesions; called also *dermovirus.*

dermovascular (der"mo-vas"ku-lar) [*dermo-* + *vas* vessel] pertaining to the blood vessels of the skin.

dermovirus (der"mo-vi"rus) dermovaccine.

derodidymus (der"o-did'ĭ-mus) dicephalus.

Deronil (der'o-nil) trademark for a preparation of dexamethasone.

derrengadera (der"en-gah-da'rah) [Sp. "*crooked*"] murrina.

Derrien's test (dār"e-anz') [Eugène *Derrien,* French chemist, 1879–1931] see under *tests.*

derriengue (der"e-eng'geh) [Sp.] a paralytic form of rabies in cattle of South America (from Mexico to north of Argentina) causing severe economic losses; it is transmitted by vampire bats (*Desmodus rotundus*).

derris (der'is) a plant of the South Sea Islands; extracts of the leaves and dried root are used as insecticides. Cf. *rotenone.*

desalination (de"sal-ĭ-na'shun) [L. *de* from + *sal* salt] the removal of salt from a substance.

desalivation (de"sal-ĭ-va'shun) the depriving of saliva.

desanimania (des"an-ĭ-ma'ne-ah) [L. *dis-* neg. + *animus* mind + *mania* madness] (*obs.*) amentia, or mindless insanity.

desaturase (de-sach'u-rās) any enzyme that catalyzes desaturation of a fatty acid.

desaturation (de-sach"er-a'shun) the process of introducing a double bond between carbon atoms of a fatty acid.

Desault's bandage (apparatus), sign (dĕ-sōz') [Pierre Joseph *Desault,* French surgeon, 1744–1795] see under *bandage* and *sign.*

Descemet's membrane (des-ĕ-māz') [Jean *Descemet,* French anatomist, 1732–1810] lamina limitans posterior corneae.

descemetitis (des"ĕ-mĕ-ti'tis) inflammation of Descemet's membrane.

descemetocele (des"ĕ-met'o-sēl) [*Descemet's membrane* + Gr. *dēlē* hernia] herniation of Descemet's membrane.

descendens (de-sen'denz) [L.] [NA] a general term denoting a descending structure or part. **d. cervica'lis, d. cer'vicis,** the inferior root of the ansa cervicalis.

descending (de-send'ing) [L. *descendere* to go down] extending downward.

descensus (de-sen'sus), pl. *descen'sus* [L.] the process of descending or falling. **d. tes'tis** [NA], the descent of the testis from its fetal position in the abdominal cavity to the scrotum; it normally occurs during the last three months of fetal life and is essential to spermatogenesis. **d. u'teri,** prolapse of the uterus. **d. ventric'uli,** gastroptosis.

Deschamps' compressor, needle (da-shawz') [Joseph François Louis *Deschamps*, French surgeon, 1740–1824] see under *compressor* and *needle*.

descinolone acetonide (des-in'o-lōn) chemical name: 9-fluoro-11β,16α,17-trihydroxypregna-1,4-diene-3,20-dione cyclic 16,17-acetal with acetone; a glucocorticoid, $C_{24}H_{31}FO_5$.

desensitization (de-sen''sĭ-ti-za'shun) 1. the prevention or reduction of immediate hypersensitivity reactions by administration of graded doses of allergen. 2. in behavior therapy, the treatment of phobias and related disorders by intentionally exposing the patient, in imagination or in real life, to emotionally distressing stimuli. Common forms of desensitization include flooding (q.v.), implosion (q.v.), and systematic desensitization (q.v.). **systematic d.,** a form of desensitization therapy in which the patient is taught to relax and is then exposed, in imagination, to the mildest or least anxiety-provoking stimuli first; as treatment progresses he is exposed progressively to stronger anxiety-provoking stimuli until he can tolerate the most extreme stimuli.

desensitize (de-sen'sĭ-tīz) 1. to deprive of sensation; paralysis of a sensory nerve by section or blocking. 2. to remove antibody from sensitized cells for the purpose of preventing allergy or anaphylaxis.

desequestration (de''se-kwes-tra'shun) (*obs.*) the release of sequestered material, such as release into the general circulation of blood formerly withheld from it, by either physiological or mechanical means.

deserpidine (de-ser'pĭ-dēn) chemical name: 17α-methoxy-18β-[(3,4,5-trimethoxybenzoyl)oxy]-3β-20α-yohimban-16β-carboxylic acid methyl ester. An alkaloid of *Rauwolfia canescens*, $C_{32}H_{38}N_2$-O_8, occurring as a white to light yellow, crystalline powder; used as an antihypertensive and tranquilizer, administered orally.

desexualize (de-seks'u-al-iz'') to deprive of sexual characters; to castrate.

Desferal (des'fer-al) trademark for a preparation of deferoxamine mesylate.

desferrioxamine (des-fer'e-oks'ah-mēn) deferoxamine.

deshydremia (des''hi-dre'me-ah) [L. *de* from + Gr. *hydōr* water + *haima* blood + *-ia*] deficiency of the watery element of the blood.

desiccant (des'ĭ-kant) 1. promoting dryness; causing to dry up. 2. an agent that promotes dryness. Called also *exsiccant*.

desiccate (des'ĭ-kāt) [L. *desiccare* to dry up] to render thoroughly dry.

desiccation (des''ĭ-ka'shun) the act of drying up. **electric d.,** the treatment of a tumor or other disease by drying up the part by the application of a monopolar electric current (short spark) of high frequency and high tension.

desiccative (des'ĭ-ka''tiv) causing to dry up.

desiccator (des'ĭ-ka''tor) a closed vessel for containing apparatus or chemicals that are to be kept free from moisture.

desipramine hydrochloride (des-ip'rah-mēn) [USP] chemical name: 10,11-dihydro-*N*-methyl-5*H*-dibenz[*b,f*]azepine-5-propanamine monohydrochloride. A metabolite of imipramine, C_{18}-$H_{22}N_2 \cdot HCl$, occurring as a white to off-white, crystalline powder; used as an antidepressant, administered orally.

-desis [Gr. "binding"] a word termination indicating a binding or fusion, as in pleurodesis.

Desjardins' point (da''zhar-danz') [Abel *Desjardins*, French surgeon] see under *point*.

deslanoside (des-lan'o-sīd) [USP] a digitalis glycoside, $C_{47}H_{74}$-O_{19}, occurring as white crystals or as a white crystalline powder; used as a cardiotonic where digitalis is recommended, administered intramuscularly or intravenously. Called also *deacetyl-lanatoside C*.

desm- see *desmo-*.

desmalgia (des-mal'je-ah) [*desmo-* + *-algia*] pain in a ligament; called also *desmodynia*.

desmectasis (des-mek'tah-sis) [*desmo-* + Gr. *ektasis* stretching] the stretching of a ligament.

desmepithelium (des''mep-ĭ-the'le-um) [*desmo-* + *epithelium*] the endothelial lining of blood vessels, lymphatics, and synovial membranes.

desmid (des'mid) unicellular, free-floating, aquatic algae characterized by symmetrical, curved, spiny or lacey bodies with a median constriction dividing the cell into two equal halves.

desmiognathus (des''me-o-nath'us) [Gr. *desmios* binding + *gnathos* jaw] a monster with a parasitic head attached to the jaw or neck; called also *dicephalus parasiticus*.

desmitis (des-mi'tis) [*desmo-* + *-itis*] inflammation of a ligament.

desmo-, desm- [Gr. *desmos* band, ligament] a combining form denoting relationship to a band, bond, or ligament.

Desmobacteriaceae (des''mo-bak-te''re-a'se-e) a family of Schizomycetes in the Lehmann and Newmann outline classification of bacteria.

desmocranium (des''mo-kra'ne-um) [*desmo-* + *cranium*] the mass of mesoderm at the cranial end of the notochord in the early embryo, forming the earliest stage of the skull.

desmocyte (des'mo-sīt) [*desmo-* + Gr. *kytos* hollow vessel] fibroblast.

desmocytoma (des''mo-si-to'mah) fibroma.

desmodynia (des''mo-din'e-ah) [*desmo-* + Gr. *odynē* pain] desmalgia.

desmogenous (des-moj'ĕ-nus) [*desmo-* + Gr. *gennan* to produce] of ligamentous origin.

desmography (des-mog'rah-fe) [*desmo-* + Gr. *graphein* to write] a description of the ligaments.

desmohemoblast (des''mo-hem'o-blast) [*desmo-* + Gr. *haima* blood + *blastos* germ] mesenchyme.

desmoid (des'moid) [*desmo-* + Gr. *eidos* form] 1. a fibromatous tumor arising in the muscle sheath, usually of the abdominal wall, and closely resembling fibrosarcoma; desmoids are not encapsulated, are locally invasive, and rarely metastasize. Called also *desmoid tumor*. 2. fibrous or fibroid.

desmolase (des'mo-lās) an enzyme that catalyzes the addition or removal of some chemical group to or from a substrate without hydrolysis, oxidation, or reduction, the group being taken up from or liberated in the free state.

desmology (des-mol'o-je) [*desmo-* + *-logy*] 1. the study of ligaments, their structure and function. 2. the art of bandaging.

desmoma (des-mo'mah) [*desmo-* + *-oma*] desmoid tumor.

desmon (des'mon) [Gr. *desmos* band] see *amboceptor*.

desmoneoplasm (des''mo-ne'o-plazm) [*desmo-* + *neoplasm*] a connective tissue tumor (q.v.).

desmopathy (des-mop'ah-the) [*desmo-* + Gr. *pathos* disease] any disease of the ligaments.

desmopexia (des''mo-pek'se-ah) [*desmo-* + Gr. *pēxis* fixation] (*obs.*) the operation of suturing the round ligaments to the abdominal wall or to the vaginal wall for the correction of uterine displacement.

desmoplasia (des''mo-pla'ze-ah) the formation and development of fibrous tissue.

desmoplastic (des''mo-plas'tik) [*desmo-* + Gr. *plassein* to form] characterized by or causing the growth of fibrous tissue; producing or forming adhesions.

desmopressin (des''mo-pres'in) chemical name: 1-(3-mercaptopropionic acid)-8-*D*-argininevasopressin; a potent synthetic analogue of vasopressin used as an antidiuretic in diabetes insipidus.

desmopyknosis (des''mo-pik-no'sis) [*desmo-* + Gr. *pyknōsis* condensation] Dudley's operation of shortening the round ligaments by fastening them to an oval denuded area on the anterior vaginal wall.

desmorrhexis (des''mo-rek'sis) [*desmo-* + Gr. *rhēxis* rupture] rupture of a ligament.

desmosine (des'mo-sin) one of two unusual amino acids found in elastin, the other being isodesmosine.

desmosis (des-mo'sis) [*desmo-* + *-osis*] a disease of the connective tissue.

desmosome (des'mo-sōm) [*desmo-* + Gr. *sōma* body] a small, discrete, circular, dense body that forms the site of attachment between certain epithelial cells, especially those of stratified epithelium of the epidermis. It consists of local differentiations of the apposing cell membranes, with a dense cytoplasmic plaque underlying each membrane, toward which numerous tonofilaments converge; a dense lamina may occur within the intercellular gap. Called also *macula adherens*. See also *intercellular bridge*, under *bridge*. **half d.,** hemidesmosome.

desmosterol (des-mos'ter-ol) the immediate precursor of cholesterol in the biosynthetic pathway, 24-dehydrocholesterol; normally not present in the blood in amounts that can be detected by ordinary means.

desmotomy (des-mot'o-me) [*desmo-* + Gr. *tomē* a cutting] the cutting or division of ligaments.

desmotropism (des-mot'ro-pizm) tautomerism.

desoleolecithin (des-o''le-o-les'ĭ-thin) one of the components, the other being oleic acid, into which lecithin is split by the action of cobra venom.

desomorphine (des''o-mor'fin) chemical name: 4,5a-epoxy-17-methylmorphinan-3-ol; a narcotic analgesic, $C_{17}H_{21}NO_2$.

desonide (des'o-nīd) chemical name: 11β,21-dihydroxy-16α,17-[(1-methylethylidene)bis(oxy)]pregna-1,4-diene-3,20-dione. A synthetic corticosteroid, $C_{24}H_{36}O_6$, used as an anti-inflammatory in the treatment of steroid-responsive dermatoses, applied topically.

desorb (de-sorb) to remove a substance from the state of absorption or adsorption.

desorption (de-sorp'shun) the process or state of being desorbed.

desoximetasone (des-ok''se-met'a-sōn) [USP] chemical name: 9-fluoro-11β-21-dihydroxy-16α-methylpregna-1,4-diene-3,20-dione. A corticosteroid, $C_{22}H_{29}FO_4$, having anti-inflammatory, antipruritic, and vasoconstrictive actions; applied topically for the relief of inflammatory manifestations of corticosteroid-responsive dermatoses.

desoxy- a prefix used in names of chemical compounds. See also words beginning *deoxy-*.

desoxycorticosterone (des-ok''se-kor''te-kos'ter-ōn) chemical name: 21-hydroxypregn-4-ene-3,20-dione. A mineralocorticoid, $C_{21}H_{30}O_3$, which has no glucocorticoid activity. It is secreted in small amounts by the human adrenal cortex. Called also *deoxycorticosterone* and *desoxycortone*. **d. acetate** [USP], an ester of desoxycorticosterone, $C_{23}H_{32}O_4$, occurring as a white or creamy white, crystalline powder; used for replacement therapy in adrenocortical insufficiency in Addison's disease and in the treatment of salt-losing adrenogenital syndrome, administered by intramuscular injection or by implantation of pellets subcutaneously. Called also *cortexone* and *desoxycortone acetate*. **d. pivalate** [USP], an ester of desoxycorticosterone, $C_{26}H_{38}O_4$, occurring as a white to creamy white, crystalline powder; used the same as the acetate ester, administered in a repository type of intramuscular injection. **d. trimethylacetate,** d. pivalate.

desoxycortone (des''ok-se-kōr'tōn) desoxycorticosterone. **d. acetate,** desoxycorticosterone acetate.

desoxyephedrine (des''ok-se-ef'ĕ-drin) methamphetamine.

desoxymorphine (des''ok-se-mor'fin) a product of the reduction of morphine.

Desoxyn (des-ok'sin) trademark for preparations of methamphetamine hydrochloride.

desoxyphenobarbital (des-ok''se-fe''no-bar'bĭ-tal) primidone.

desoxyribonuclease (des-ok''se-ri''bo-nu'kle-ās) deoxyribonuclease.

desoxyribose (des''ok-se-ri'bōs) deoxyribose.

desoxy-sugar (des-ok''se-shoog'ar) a sugar having one oxygen atom less than the parent monosaccharide.

despeciate (de-spe'se-āt) to undergo despeciation; to subject to (as by chemical treatment), or to undergo, loss of species antigenic characteristics.

despeciation (de-spe''se-a'shun) deviation from or loss of species characteristics.

despecification (de-spes''ĭ-fĭ-ka'shun) the process of reducing the antigenicity of heterologous antisera used therapeutically, by treating them with enzymes such as pepsin to remove the antigenic Fc regions of the immunoglobulin molecules. This leaves $F(ab')_2$ fragments which contain both antigen binding regions of each immunoglobulin molecule.

d'Espine's sign (des-pēnz') [Jean Henri Adolphe *d'Espine*, French physician, 1846–1930] see under *sign*.

despumation (des''pu-ma'shun) [L. *de* away + *spuma* froth] the removal of froth or scum from the surface of a liquid.

desquamation (des''kwah-ma'shun) [L. *de* from + *squama* scale] the shedding of epithelial elements, chiefly of the skin, in scales or small sheets; exfoliation. **furfuraceous d.,** desquamation in branlike scales. **lamellar d. of the newborn,** see under *exfoliation.*

desquamative (des-kwam'ah-tiv) pertaining to or characterized by desquamation.

desquamatory (des-kwam'ah-to-re) desquamative.

dest. abbreviation for L. *destil'la* distil, and *destilla'tus* distilled.

desthiobiotin (des''thi-o-bi'o-tin) biotin in which the sulfur has been replaced by two atoms of hydrogen. It is an analogue, $CH_2 \cdot CH \cdot NH \cdot CO \cdot NH \cdot CH \cdot CH_2 \cdot (CH_2)_4 \cdot COOH$, of ascorbic acid which competitively inhibits the activity of the latter.

destil. abbreviation for L. *destil'la,* distil.

destructive (de-struk'tiv) characterized by or causing destruction.

desulfhydrase (de''sulf-hi'drās) an enzyme that splits cysteine into hydrogen sulfide, ammonia, and pyruvic acid; called also *desulfurase.*

Desulfovibrio (de-sul''fo-vib're-o) a genus of microorganisms of the family Spirillaceae, suborder Pseudomonadineae, order Pseudomonadales, made up of actively motile, slightly curved rods of variable length, usually occurring singly but sometimes in short chains. It includes three species, *D. aestua'rii, D. desulfur'icans,* and *D. rubentschi'kii.*

desulfurase (de-sul'fu-rās) desulfhydrase.

Det. abbreviation for L. *de'tur,* let it be given.

detachment (de-tach'ment) [Fr. *détacher* to unfasten; to separate] the condition of being unfastened, disconnected, or separated. **d. of retina, retinal d.,** a condition in which the inner layers of the retina (neural retina) are separated from the pigment epithelium.

detector (de-tek'tor) a device by which the presence of something, or the existence of a certain condition, is discovered. **lie d.,** polygraph. **radiation d.,** any device for converting radiant energy to a form more readily observable.

deterenol hydrochloride (dě-ter'ĕ-nōl) chemical name: (+)-4-hydroxy-α-[[(1-methylethyl)amino]methyl]benzenemethanol hydrochloride; an adrenergic, $C_{11}H_{17}NO_2 \cdot HCl$, used in ophthalmology.

detergent (de-ter'jent) [L. *detergere* to cleanse] 1. purifying, cleansing. 2. an agent which purifies or cleanses.

determinant (de-ter'mĭ-nant) [L. *determinare* to bound, limit, or fix] a factor that establishes the nature of an entity or event. See also *biophore.* **antigenic d.,** the structural component of an antigen molecule that is responsible for specific interaction with antibody (immunoglobulin) molecules elicited by the same or a related antigen. Antigenic determinants consist of chemically active surface groupings of amino acids in globular proteins and sugar side chains in polysaccharides. Called also *antigenic determinant group,* or *epitope.* A small portion of the determinant group critical in establishing specificity is called the *immunodominant point.* Antibodies produced in response to immunization with a carrier protein to which specific chemical groups (haptens) have been introduced artificially by conjugation show reactive specificity for antigenic determinant groups that are frequently identical or nearly identical in structure to the hapten. **germ-cell d.,** oosome. **hidden d.,** an antigenic determinant located in an unexposed region of a molecule so that it is prevented from interacting with receptors on lymphocytes, or with antibody molecules, and is unable to induce an immune response. Such hidden determinants may appear following stereochemical alterations of molecular structure.

determination (de-ter''mĭ-na'shun) establishment of the exact nature of an entity or event. **embryonic d.,** the loss of pluripotency in any part of an embryo and its start on the way toward an unalterable fate. **sex d.,** the process by which the sex of an organism is fixed, associated, in man, with the presence or absence of the Y chromosome.

determiner (de-ter'min-er) determinant.

determinism (de-ter'min-izm) the theory that all phenomena are the result of antecedent conditions and that nothing occurs by chance. **psychic d.,** the theory that mental processes are always determined by motives.

dethyroidism (de-thi'roid-izm) a condition produced by abolition of the function of the thyroid gland.

dethyroidize (de-thi'roid-īz) to deprive of the function of the thyroid gland by chemical or surgical means.

Det. in dup., Det. in 2 plo. abbreviations for L. *de'tur in du'plo,* let twice as much be given.

detonation (de''to-na'shun) [L. *de* intensive + *tonare* to thunder] loudly explosive combustion.

detorsion (de-tor'shun) 1. the correction of a curvature or deformity; as the reduction of torsion of the testis. 2. a deficiency in a normal twisting as may occur in the early development of the heart.

detoxicate (de-tok'sĭ-kāt) detoxify.

detoxication (de-tok''sĭ-ka'shun) detoxification.

detoxification (de-tok''sĭ-fi-ka'shun) 1. reduction of the toxic properties of poisons. 2. treatment designed to free an addict from his drug habit. **metabolic d.,** reduction of the toxic properties of a substance by chemical changes induced in the body, producing a compound which is less poisonous or is more readily eliminated.

detoxify (de-tok'sĭ-fi) to remove the toxic quality of a substance.

Detre's reaction (det'erz) [László *Detre,* Hungarian physician, 1875–1939] differential cutireaction.

detrition (de-trish'un) [L. *de* away + *terere* to wear] a wearing away, as of the teeth, by friction.

detritivorous (de''trĭ-tiv'o-rus) subsisting on particulate matter (detritus), a mode of existence important in certain, such as aquatic, ecosystems.

detritus (de-tri'tus) [L., from *deterere* to rub away] particulate matter produced by or remaining after the wearing away or disintegration of a substance or tissue; designated as organic or nonorganic, depending on the nature of the original material. See also *biodetritus.*

detruncation (de''trun-ka'shun) [L. *de* off + *truncus* trunk] decapitation, or decollation; beheadal, chiefly of the fetus.

detrusor (de-tru'sor) [L. *detrudere* to push down] [NA] a general term for any body part that pushes down. **d. uri'nae,** collective term for the bundles of smooth muscle forming the muscular wall of the urinary bladder; they are arranged in a longitudinal and a circular layer and, on contraction, serve to expel the urine. Called also *detrusor muscle.*

D. et s. abbreviation for L. *de'tur et signe'tur,* let it be given and labeled.

detubation (de''tu-ba'shun) removal or withdrawal of a tube.

detumescence (de″tu-mes′ens) [L. *de* down + *tumescere* to swell] the subsidence of swelling, or turgor.

deutan (doo′tan) an individual exhibiting deuteranomalopia or deuteranopia, marked by derangement or loss of the red-green sensory mechanism but without noticeable shift or shortening of the spectrum or luminancy loss in the long-wave (red) end; includes those with the commoner and less severe types of color vision defect. Cf. *protan*.

deutencephalon (doo″ten-sef′ah-lon) [Gr. *deuteros* second + *enkephalos* brain] (*obs.*) diencephalon.

deuteranomalopia (doo″ter-ah-nom″ah-lo′pe-ah) [Gr. *deuteros* second + *anōmalos* irregular + *ōpē* sight + *-ia*] a problematic variant of normal color vision, in which none of the constituents for complete chromatic perception are lacking, but a greater than usual proportion of thallium green light to lithium red is required to match a fixed sodium yellow. The defect may be congenital or acquired, and occurs in different degrees of severity. Sometimes called "green weakness," and viewed as a transitional stage to "green blindness." Cf. the correlative terms *protanomalopia* and *tritanomalopia*.

deuteranomalopsia (doo″ter-ah-nom″ah-lop′se-ah) deuteranomalopia.

deuteranomalous (doo″ter-ah-nom′ah-lus) pertaining to or characterized by deuteranomaly (deuteranomalopia).

deuteranomaly (doo″ter-ah-nom′ah-le) deuteranomalopia.

deuteranope (doo″ter-ah-nōp″) an individual exhibiting deuteranopia; a color deviant.

deuteranopia (doo″ter-ah-no′pe-ah) [Gr. *deuteros* second + *an*- neg. + *ōpē* sight + *-ia*] defective color vision of the dichromatic type, characterized by retention of the sensory mechanism for two hues only (blue and yellow) of the normal 4-primary quota, and lacking that for red and green and their derivatives, without loss of luminance or shift or shortening of the spectrum. Coined by von Kries (1897) to replace "green blindness." Cf. the correlative terms *protanopia*, *tritanopia*, and *tetartanopia*, in which the color vision deficiency is in the first, third, and fourth primary, respectively. Called also *aglaucopsia* or *aglaukopsia*.

deuteranopic (doo″ter-ah-nop′ik) pertaining to or characterized by deuteranopia.

deuteranopsia (doo″ter-ah-nop′se-ah) deuteranopia.

deuterate (du′ter-āt) to treat (combine) with deuterium.

deuterion (doo-te′re-on) deuteron.

deuterium (du-te′re-um) [Gr. *deuteros* second] the mass two isotope of hydrogen, symbol ²H, or D. It is available as a gas or as heavy water and is used as a tracer or indicator in studying fat and amino acid metabolism; called also *heavy hydrogen* (see *hydrogen*). Cf. *protium* and *tritium*. **d. oxide,** heavy water; see under *water*.

deutero-, deuto- [Gr. *deuteros* second] combining form meaning second.

deuteroconidium (doo″ter-o-ko-nid′e-um) [*deutero-* + *conidium*] a reproductive element derived from a hemispore.

deuterofat (doo′ter-o-fat) a fat containing deuterium.

deuterohemin (du″ter-o-hem′in) a derivative of hemin, $C_{30}H_{28}O_4N_4FeCl$.

deuterohemophilia (doo″ter-o-he″mo-fil′e-ah) a group of hemorrhagic disorders resembling classical hemophilia, due to coagulation factor deficiency or to the action of certain anticoagulants. See individual coagulation factors, under *factor*.

Deuteromyces (doo″ter-o-mi′zēz) Deuteromycetes.

Deuteromycetae (doo″ter-o-mi-se′te) Deuteromycetes.

deuteromycete (doo″ter-o-mi′sēt) any individual fungus of the Deuteromycetes; an imperfect fungus.

Deuteromycetes (doo″ter-o-mi-se′tēz) [*deutero-* + Gr. *mykēs* fungus] a class of the Eumycetes in which the perfect (sexual) stage is unknown; the Fungi Imperfecti. Called also *Deuteromyces* and *Deuteromycetae*.

deuteron (doo′ter-on) the nucleus of deuterium, or heavy hydrogen; deuterons are used as bombing particles for nuclear disintegration.

deuteropathic (doo″ter-o-path′ik) occurring secondarily to some other disease.

deuteropathy (doo″ter-op′ah-the) [*deutero-* + Gr. *pathos* disease] a disease that is secondary to another disease.

deuteropine (doo″ter-o′pin) an alkaloid, $C_{20}H_{21}O_3N$, from opium.

deuteroplasm (doo″ter-o-plazm″) [*deutero-* + Gr. *plasma* something formed] the passive or inactive materials in protoplasm, especially reserve foodstuffs, such as yolk. Cf. *energid*.

deuteroporphyrin (doo″ter-o-por′fi-rin) a hemin-porphyrin derivative, $C_{30}H_{30}O_4N_4$.

deuterosome (doo″ter-o-sōm″) [*deutero-* + Gr. *sōma* body] a cytoplasmic organelle of ciliating epithelial cells that plays a role in the formation of ciliary basal bodies, being the precursor of the procentriole.

deuterostome (doo′ter-o-stōm″) an animal belonging to the Deuterostomia.

Deuterostomia (doo″ter-o-sto′mĭ-ah) [*deutero-* + Gr. *stoma* mouth + *-ia*] a series of the Eucoelomata, including the echinoderms, hemichordates, and chordates, in all of which the site of the blastopore is posterior—far from the mouth, which forms a new structure unrelated to the blastopore.

deuterotocia (doo″ter-o-to′se-ah) [*deutero-* + Gr. *tokos* birth] asexual reproduction in which the female produces offspring of both sexes.

deuterotoky (doo″ter-ot′o-ke) deuterotocia.

deuterotoxin (doo″ter-o-tok′sin) (*obs.*) the second of the three groups into which toxins may be divided on the basis of their affinity for antitoxin. It has less affinity for antitoxin than has prototoxin and more than has tritotoxin.

deuthyalosome (doo″thi-al′o-sōm) [Gr. *deuteros* second + *hyalos* glass + *sōma* body] the matured nucleus of an ovum.

deuto- see *deutero-*.

deutomerite (doo″to-me′rit) [*deuto-* + Gr. *meros* portion] the posterior portion of certain gregarine protozoa. Cf. *protomerite*.

deuton (doo′ton) deuteron.

deutonephron (doo″to-nef′ron) [*deuto-* + Gr. *nephros* kidney] mesonephros.

deutoplasm (doo′to-plazm) deuteroplasm.

deutoplasmolysis (doo″to-plaz-mol′ĭ-sis) destruction or disintegration of deutoplasm.

Deutschländer's disease (doich′len-derz) [Karl Ernst Wilhelm *Deutschländer*, surgeon in Hamburg, 1872–1942] 1. see under *disease*. 2. march foot.

devasation (de″vas-a′shun) [L. *de* away + *vas* vessel] (*obs.*) devascularization. **senile cortical d.,** interruption of the circulation to the cerebral cortex as a result of arteriosclerosis of the blood vessels.

devascularization (de-vas″ku-lar-i-za′shun) interruption of the circulation of blood to a part caused by obstruction or destruction of the blood vessels supplying it.

Devegan (dev′e-gan) trademark for a preparation of acetarsone.

development (de-vel′op-ment) the process of growth and differentiation. **arrested d.,** cessation of the development process at some stage prior to its normal completion. **cognitive d.,** the development of intelligence, conscious thought, and problem solving ability that begins in infancy. **mosaic d.,** the development of an embryo in a fixed, unalterable way, local regions being independent portions of a mosaic whole. **postnatal d.,** that which occurs after birth. **prenatal d.,** that which occurs before birth. **psychosexual d.,** 1. a general term for the developing sexuality of the individual as affected by biological, cultural, and emotional influences from prenatal life onward through the life cycle. 2. in psychoanalysis, libidinal maturation from infancy through adulthood (including the oral, anal, and genital stages). **psychosocial d.,** the development of the personality, including the acquisition of social attitudes and skills, from infancy through maturity. **regulative d.,** the development of an embryo, the determination of the various organs and parts being gradually attained through the action of inductors.

developmental (de-vel″op-men′tal) pertaining to development.

Deventer's diameter (de-ven′terz) [Hendrik van *Deventer*, Dutch obstetrician, 1651–1724] see *diameter obliqua pelvis*.

Devergie's attitude, disease (dev-er-zhēz′) [Marie Guillaume Alphonse *Devergie*, French physician, 1798–1879] see under *attitude*, and see *pityriasis rubra pilaris*.

deviant (de′ve-ant) [L. *deviare* to turn aside] 1. varying from a determinable standard. 2. an individual with characteristics varying from what is considered normal, or standard. **color d.,** an individual whose color perception varies from the norm, usually lacking discrimination of a pair of primaries (red-green or blue-yellow); see *deuteranope, protanope,* and *tritanope*. **sex d.,** an individual exhibiting paraphilia; i.e., one whose sexual behavior varies from that normally considered socially or biologically acceptable. Called also *paraphiliac*.

deviation (de″ve-a′shun) [L. *deviare* to turn aside] a turning away from the regular standard or course. In ophthalmology, a tendency for the visual axes of the eyes to fall out of alignment due to muscular imbalance. **animal d.,** the attracting of zoophilous mosquitos from human beings by the proximity of animals preferred by the insects. **axis d.,** the direction of the mean QRS complex in the electrocardiogram; changes may be due to alteration in the anatomical position of the heart or to intraventricular conduction (ventricular preponderance). **complement d.,** inhibition of complement-mediated immune hemolysis in the presence of excess antibody. Called also *Neisser-Wechsberg phenomenon*. **conjugate d.,** deflection of two similar parts, as the eyes, in the same direction at the same time. **Hering-Hellebrand d.,** any deviation of the horopter from the circle. **immune d.,** modification of the immune response to an antigen by previous inoculation of the same antigen. **latent d.,** heterophoria. **manifest d.,** strabismus. **mini-**

mum d., the smallest deflection of a ray of light that can be produced by a given prism. **primary d.,** deviation of the visual axis of the squinting eye in strabismus when the sound eye fixates. **secondary d.,** deviation of the visual axis of the sound eye in strabismus when the squinting eye fixates. **sexual d.,** paraphilia. **skew d.,** downward and inward rotation of the eye on the side of the cerebellar lesion and upward and outward deviation on the opposite side. **squint d.,** squint angle; see under *angle*. **standard d.,** in standardized tests, a measure of deviations from a central value, determined as the square root of the average of the squares of all deviations from the mean; symbol σ. **strabismic d.,** deviation of the visual axis of an eye in strabismus. **d. to the left,** shift to the left. **d. to the right,** shift to the right.

device (dĕ-vīs′) something contrived for a specific purpose. **central-bearing d.,** a device that provides a central point of bearing, or support, between upper and lower occlusion rims, consisting of a contacting point attached to one occlusion rim and a plate that provides the surface on which the bearing point rests or moves. **central-bearing tracing d.,** a central-bearing device for making a tracing and/or for support between occlusion rims. **contraceptive d.,** one used to prevent conception, as a diaphragm or condom to prevent entrance of spermatozoa into the uterine cervix, or one inserted into the uterus (intrauterine contraceptive device) to prevent implantation of a fertilized ovum. **intrauterine d. (IUD),** a coil, loop, T, or triangle of plastic or metallic substance inserted into the uterus to prevent conception. **left ventricular assist d.,** a circulatory support device consisting of a pump with afferent and efferent conduits attached to the left ventricular apex and the ascending aorta, repectively, each conduit containing a porcine valve to ensure unidirectional blood flow; the pump rests on the external chest wall and is connected to an external pneumatic power source and control circuit.

deviometer (de″ve-om′ĕ-ter) [*deviation* + Gr. *metron* measure] an instrument for measuring the amount of deviation in strabismus.

devisceration (de-vis″er-a′shun) [L. *de* away + *viscus* viscus] the removal of viscera. Cf. *evisceration*.

devitalization (de-vi″tal-i-za′shun) the deprivation of vitality or life, as of a tissue. **pulp d.,** the destruction of vitality of the pulp of a tooth.

devitalize (de-vi′tal-īz) [L. *de* from + *vita* life] to deprive of vitality or of life.

devolution (dev″o-lu′shun) [L. *de* down + *volvere* to roll] 1. the reverse of evolution. 2. catabolic change.

devolutive (dev′o-lu″tiv) characterized by devolution; specifically applied to a type of mental defect due to intercurrent destructive factors, based on the Jacksonian concept that the most recently (from the standpoint of evolution) acquired cerebral functions are the first to be impaired by states of ill health. Cf. *evolutive*.

devorative (dev′o-ra″tiv) [L. *devorare* to devour] (*obs.*) intended to be swallowed without chewing.

De Vries' theory (de-vrēz′) [Hugo *de Vries*, botanist in Amsterdam, 1848–1935] see *theory of mutations*.

dewatered (de-wah′terd) having the water removed; a term applied to sludge from which the water has been removed by drying or pressing.

dewclaw (doo′klaw) a vestigial digit or claw in an animal.

dewlap (du′lap) a heavy fold of skin on the ventral aspect of the neck in animals.

deworming (de-werm′ing) the destruction and removal of worms from an infected individual.

dexamethasone (dek″sah-meth′ah-sōn) [USP] chemical name: 9-fluoro-11β,17, 21-trihydroxy-16α-methylpregna-1,4-diene-3, 20-dione. A synthetic glucocorticoid, $C_{22}H_{29}FO_5$, occurring as a white to practically white, crystalline powder; used primarily as an anti-inflammatory in various conditions, including the collagen diseases and allergic states, administered orally or topically. It is also used in certain neoplastic diseases, soft tissue disorders, and hemolytic anemias, and is the basis of a screening test in the diagnosis of Cushing's syndrome. **d. acetate** [USP], an ester of dexamethasone, $C_{24}H_{31}FO_6 \cdot H_2O$, occurring as a clear, white to off-white, odorless powder, having actions and uses similar to those of the base. **d. sodium phosphate** [USP], an ester of dexamethasone, $C_{22}H_{28}FNa_2O_8P$, occurring as a white or slightly yellow, crystalline powder, having actions and uses similar to those of the base; administered by intra-articular, soft tissue, intravenous or intramuscular injection, by inhalation, or applied topically to the skin and conjunctiva.

dexamisole (deks-am′ĭ-sōl) chemical name: (*R*)-2,3,5,6,-tetrahydro-6-phenyl-imidazo[2,1-*b*]thiazole; an antidepressant, $C_{11}H_{12}N_2S$.

dexbrompheniramine (deks″brōm-fen-ir′ah-mēn) chemical name: γ-(4-bromophenyl)-*N,N*-dimethyl-2-pyridinepropanamine. The bromine analogue of dexchlorpheniramine, $C_{16}H_{19}BrN_2$, an antihistaminic drug. **d. maleate** [USP], the maleate salt of dexbrompheniramine, $C_{16}H_{19}BrN_2 \cdot C_4H_4O_4$, occurring as a white,

crystalline powder; administered orally for therapy and prophylaxis of conditions in which antihistamines may be effective.

dexchlorpheniramine (deks″klōr-fen-ir′ah-mēn) chemical name: γ-(4-chlorophenyl)-*N,N*-dimethyl-2-pyridinepropanamine. The dextrorotatory isomer of chlorpheniramine, $C_{16}H_{19}ClN_2$, an antihistaminic drug. **d. maleate** [USP], the maleate salt of dexchlorpheniramine, $C_{16}H_{19}ClN_2 \cdot C_4H_4O_4$, occurring as a white, crystalline powder; administered orally for therapy and prophylaxis of conditions in which antihistamines may be effective.

dexclamol hydrochloride (deks′klah-mōl) chemical name: (±)-2,3α,4,4aα,8,9,13bβ,14-octahydro-3-(1-methyl ethyl)-1*H*-benzo[6,7]cyclohepta[1,2,3-*de*]pyrido[2,1-*a*]isoquinoline-3-ol hydrochloride; a sedative, $C_{24}H_{29}NO \cdot HCl$.

Dexedrine (dek′sĕ-drēn) trademark for preparations of dextroamphetamine sulfate.

dexetimide (dek-set′ĭ-mīd) chemical name: (*S*)-3-phenyl-1′-(phenylmethyl)-[3,4′-biperidine]-2,6-dione. An anticholinergic, $C_{23}H_{26}N_2O_2$, which has been tried as an antiparkinsonian agent.

deximafen (dek-sim′ah-fen) chemical name: (+)-2,3,5,6-tetrahydro-5-phenyl-1*H*-imidazo[1,2-*a*]imidazol; an antidepressant, $C_{11}H_{13}N_3$.

dexiocardia (dek″se-o-kar′de-ah) dextrocardia.

dexiotropic (dek″se-o-trop′ik) [Gr. *dexios* on the right + *tropos* a turning] wound in a spiral from left to right, as a shell.

dexivacaine (dek-siv′ah-kān) chemical name: (+)-1-methyl-2′,6′-pipecoloxylidide; an anesthetic, $C_{15}H_{22}N_2O$.

Dexon (dek′son) trademark for a synthetic suture material, polyglycolic acid, a polymer that is completely absorbable and nonirritating.

Dexoval (dek′so-val) trademark for a preparation of methamphetamine hydrochloride.

dexpanthenol (deks-pan′thě-nōl) chemical name: (*R*)-2,4-dihydroxy-*N*-(3-hydroxypropyl)-3,3-dimethylbutamide. The D(+) form of *panthenol* (pantothenyl alcohol), $C_9H_{19}NO_4$, the alcoholic analogue of pantothenic acid. It is claimed to be a precursor of coenzyme A, and is administered intravenously or intramuscularly to increase peristalsis in atony and paralysis of the lower intestine and orally to help relieve gas retention and abdominal distention in certain conditions. It is also applied topically to the skin to stimulate healing of the lesions of various dermatologic lesions such as burns, infected wounds, eczema, diaper rash, etc.

dexpropranolol hydrochloride (deks″-pro-pran′o-lōl) chemical name: 1-[(1-methylethyl)amino]-3-(1-naphthalenyloxy)-2-propanol hydrochloride. The dextrorotatory isomer of propranolol, $C_{16}H_{21}NO_2 \cdot HCl$, having cardiac depressant properties similar to those of the parent compound; used as an antiarrhythmic.

dexter (dek′ster) [L.] right; [NA] a term denoting the right-hand one of two similar structures, or the one situated on the right side of the body.

dextrad (deks′trad) toward the right side.

dextral (deks′tral) 1. right as opposed to left; right-handed. 2. a right-handed person.

dextrality (deks-tral′ĭ-te) [L. *dexter* right] the preferential use, in voluntary motor acts, of the right member of the major paired organs of the body, as the right eye, hand, or foot.

dextran (dek′stran) a water-soluble polysaccharide of glucose (dextrose) produced by the action of *Leuconostoc mesenteroides* on sucrose; used as a plasma volume extender. Specific preparations are designated according to their average molecular weight divided by 1000, as *dextran 40, dextran 45,* and so on.

dextranomer (deks-tran′o-mer) a preparation of highly hydrophilic dextran polymers occurring as small beads, used in débridement of secreting wounds, such as venous stasis ulcers; the sterilized beads are poured over secreting wounds to absorb wound exudates and prevent crust formation.

dextransucrase (deks″tran-soo′krās) an enzyme that synthesizes dextran from sucrose.

dextrates (deks′trāts) a tablet binder and diluent, composed of a mixture of sugars (approximately 92 per cent dextrose monohydrate and 8 per cent high saccharides; dextrose equivalent is 95 to 97 per cent) resulting from the controlled enzymatic hydrolysis of starch.

dextraural (deks-traw′ral) [L. *dexter* right + *auris* ear] hearing better with the right ear than with the left.

dextriferron (deks″trĭ-fer′on) [NF] a complex of ferric hydroxide and partially hydrolyzed dextrin used in the treatment of iron-deficiency anemia.

dextrin (deks′trin) [L. *dexter* right] any one, or the mixture, of the intermediate products $(C_6H_{10}O_5)_n$, formed during the hydrolysis of starch, which are dextrorotatory, soluble in water, and precipitable by alcohol. Commercial dextrin or starch sugar is a white or yellowish powder, in aqueous solution forming mucilage. See *erythrodextrin*.

dextrin-1,6-glucosidase (deks″trin-glu-ko′sĭ-dās) dextrin 6-glucanohydrolase: an enzyme which catalyzes the hydrolysis of α-1-6-glucan links in dextrins containing short 1,6-linked side chains; called also *amylo-1,6-glucosidase* and *debranching enzyme*.

dextrinase (deks'trin-ās) an enzyme that catalyzes the conversion of starch into isomaltose.

dextrinate, dextrinize (deks'trin-āt; deks'trin-īz) to convert into dextrin.

dextrinose (deks'trin-ōs) isomaltose.

dextrinosis (deks″trĭ-no'sis) accumulation in the tissues of an abnormal polysaccharide. **limit d.,** glycogen storage disease, type III; see under *disease.*

dextrinuria (deks″trin-u're-ah) [*dextrin* + Gr. *ouron* urine + *-ia*] the presence of dextrin in the urine.

dextro- [L. *dexter* right] 1. a combining form denoting relationship to the right. 2. chemical prefix, for which the symbol (+)- is frequently substituted, used to emphasize that the substance is the dextrorotatory enantiomorph, whether the configurational family is known or not. This practice avoids possible confusion with the occasional erroneous use of *d-* standing alone to designate the configurational family to which the substance belongs. Opposed to *levo-.*

dextroamphetamine (dek″stro-am-fet'ah-mēn) chemical name: (*S*)-α-methylbenzeneethanamine. The dextrorotatory isomer of amphetamine, which has substantially more central nervous system stimulating effect than the levorotatory form (levamphetamine) or racemic forms of amphetamine. Abuse of this drug may lead to dependence; see *amphetamine,* def. 1. **d. phosphate** [USP], a white, crystalline powder, $C_9H_{13}N \cdot H_3PO_4$, having the same actions as the base, used chiefly for its central stimulant effects in the treatment of mental depression, psychopathic states, narcolepsy, hyperkinetic behavior disorders in children, and exogenous obesity; administered orally. **d. sulfate** [USP], a white, crystalline powder, $(C_9H_{13}N)_2 \cdot H_2SO_4$, having the same actions and uses as the phosphate salt; administered orally.

dextrocardia (deks″tro-kar'de-ah) location of the heart in the right hemithorax, with the apex pointing to the right, occurring with transposition (situs inversus) of the abdominal viscera, or without such transposition (*isolated d.*). **mirror-image d.,** location of the heart in the right side of the chest, the atria being transposed and the right ventricle lying anteriorly and to the left of the left ventricle, usually associated with complete situs inversus. **secondary d.,** displacement of the heart to the right as a result of disease of the pleura, diaphragm, or lungs.

dextrocardiogram (deks″tro-kar'de-o-gram) [L. *dexter* right + *cardiogram*] that part of the normal cardiogram which represents the action of the right side of the heart.

dextrocerebral (deks″tro-ser'e-bral) [L. *dexter* right + *cerebrum*] having the right hemisphere of the brain more active than the left.

dextroclination (deks″tro-klĭ-na'shun) [L. *dexter* right + L. *clinatus* leaning] rotation of the upper poles of the vertical meridians of the two eyes to the right; called also *dextrocycloduction* and *dextrotorsion.* Cf. *levoclination.*

dextrocompound (deks″tro-kom'pound) a dextrorotatory compound.

dextrocular (deks-trok'u-lar) right eyed; affected with dextrocularity.

dextrocularity (deks″trok-u-lar'ĭ-te) [L. *dexter* right + *oculus* eye] the condition of having greater visual power in the right eye and, therefore, using it more than the left.

dextrocycloduction (deks″tro-si″klo-duk'shun) dextroclination.

dextroduction (deks″tro-duk'shun) [L. *dexter* right + *ducere* to draw] movement of either eye to the right.

dextrogastria (deks″tro-gas'tre-ah) [L. *dexter* right + Gr. *gastēr* stomach] displacement of the stomach to the right, being simple displacement or situs inversus.

dextroglucose (deks″tro-glu'kōs) dextrose.

dextrogram (deks'tro-gram) [*dextro-* + Gr. *graphein* to record] an electrocardiographic tracing showing right axis deviation, indicative of right ventricular hypertrophy.

dextrogyral (deks″tro-ji'ral) [L. *dexter* right + *gyrare* to turn] dextrorotatory.

dextrogyration (deks″tro-ji-ra'shun) a turning to the right or motion to the right; said of movements of the eye and of the plane of polarization.

dextromanual (deks″tro-man'u-al) [L. *dexter* right + *manus* hand] right handed.

dextromenthol (deks″tro-men'thol) an oxidation product of menthol.

dextromethorphan hydrobromide (dek″stro-meth'or-fan) [USP] chemical name: 3-methoxy-17-methyl-9α,13α,14α-morphinan hydrobromide monohydrate. An antitussive, $C_{18}H_{25}NO \cdot HBr \cdot H_2O$, occurring as practically white crystals or as a crystalline powder; administered orally.

dextropedal (deks-trop'ĕ-dal) [L. *dexter* right + *pes* foot] using the right leg in preference to the left.

dextroposition (deks″tro-po-zish'un) displacement to the right.

dextropropoxyphene (dek″stro-pro-pok'se-fēn) propoxyphene.

dextrorotary (deks″tro-ro'tah-re) dextrorotatory.

dextrorotatory (deks″tro-ro'tah-to-re) [L. *dexter* right + *rotare* to turn] turning the plane of polarization, or rays of light, to the right; called aslo *dextrogyral.*

dextrose (deks'trōs) chemical name: *D*-glucose monohydrate. A monosaccharide, $C_6H_{12}O_6H_2O$, known as *glucose* (q.v.) in biochemistry and physiology. The official preparation [USP] is usually obtained by the hydrolysis of starch, and occurs as colorless crystals or as a white, crystalline or granular powder; it is used chiefly as a fluid and nutrient replenisher, usually administered by intravenous infusion. It is also used as a diuretic and alone or in combination with other agents for various other clinical purposes.

dextrosinistral (deks″tro-sin'is-tral) [L. *dexter* right + *sinister* left] extending from right to left. The term is also applied to a person naturally left-handed but trained to use the right hand in certain performances.

dextrosozone (deks″tro-so'zōn) glucosazone.

Dextrostix (dek'stro-stiks) trademark for a reagent strip designed for determination of blood-glucose levels with the use of fingertip venous blood.

dextrosuria (deks″tro-su're-ah) [*dextrose* + Gr. *ouron* urine + *-ia*] the presence of dextrose (d-glucose) in the urine; called also *glucosuria.*

dextrothyroxine sodium (deks″tro-thi-rok'sin) [USP] chemical name: *O*-(4-hydroxy-3,5-diiodophenyl)-3,5-diiodo-*D*-tyrosine monosodium salt hydrate. The sodium salt of the dextrorotatory isomer of thyroxine, $C_{15}H_{10}I_4NNaO_4 \cdot xH_2O$, occurring as a light yellow to buff-colored powder; used as an oral anticholesteremic, mainly to treat hypercholesteremia in euthyroid patients.

dextrotorsion (deks″tro-tor'shun) dextroclination.

dextrotropic (deks″tro-trop'ik) [L. *dexter* right + Gr. *tropos* a turning] turning to the right; see also *dexiotropic.*

dextroversion (deks″tro-ver'shun) [L. *dexter* right + *vertere* to turn] 1. version to the right side; especially movement of the eyes to the right. 2. location of the heart in the right hemithorax, the left ventricle remaining on the left as in the normal position, but lying anterior to the right ventricle.

dextroverted (deks″tro-vert'ed) turned to the right.

dezocine (dez'o-sēn) chemical name: (−)-13*S**-amino-5,6,7,8,-9,10,11α,12-octahydro-5α-methyl-5,11-methanobenzocyclodecen-3-ol; an analgesic, $C_{16}H_{23}NO.$

DFDT a powerful insecticide, difluoro-diphenyl-trichloroethane; called also *GIX.*

DFP diiopropyl fluorophosphate, see *isoflurophate.*

dg decigram.

DHA dehydroepiandrosterone.

D.H.E.45 trademark for dihydroergotamine.

d'Herelle phenomenon (dĕ-rel') [Felix Hubert *d'Herelle* of the Pasteur Institute, Paris, 1873–1949] see *Twort-d'Herelle phenomenon,* under *phenomenon.*

D.Hg., D.Hy. Doctor of Hygiene.

dhobie itch (do'be) [Hindu "laundryman"] see under *itch.*

dhurrin (du'rin) a cyanogenetic glycoside, $C_{14}H_{17}NO_7$, from sorghum which hydrolyzes into parahydroxy benzaldehyde, glucose, and hydrocyanic acid.

di- [Gr. *dis* twice, double] 1. a prefix meaning twice. 2. a variant spelling of *de-, dia-,* and *dis-.*

dia- [Gr. *dia* through] a prefix meaning through, between, apart, across, or completely.

diabetes (di″ah-be'tēz) [Gr. *diabētēs* a syphon, from *dia* through + *bainein* to go] a general term referring to disorders characterized by excessive urine excretion (polyuria), as in diabetes mellitus and diabetes insipidus. When used alone, the term refers to diabetes mellitus. **adult-onset d.,** maturity-onset d. **d. albuminurin'icus,** diabetes with nephrotic syndrome. **alloxan d.,** a condition resembling diabetes, produced by the injection of 100–200 mg. of alloxan per kilogram of body weight. **artificial d.,** puncture or other type of experimental d. **brittle d.,** diabetes that is difficult to control, characterized by unexplained oscillation between hypoglycemia and acidosis. **bronze d., bronzed d.,** hemochromatosis. **chemical d.,** a mild abnormality of carbohydrate tolerance manifested by hyperinsulinemia or hyperglycemia only when the patient is subjected to stress loads of glucose; called also *latent d.* **experimental d.,** diabetes induced experimentally; artificial d. **gestational d.,** that in which onset or recognition of impaired glucose tolerance occurs during pregnancy. **gouty d.,** diabetes associated with the gouty diathesis. **growth-onset d.,** juvenile d. **d. in'nocens,** a condition marked by the presence of glycosuria which is not associated with pancreatic disease. **d. inosi'tus,** diabetes in which the sugar of the urine is inositol; inosituria. **d. insip'idus,** a metabolic disorder due to injury of the neurohypophyseal system, which results in a deficient quantity of antidiuretic hormone being released or produced, and thus in failure of tubular reabsorption of water in the kidney. As a consequence, there is the passage of a large amount of urine of low specific gravity, and great thirst; it is often attended by voracious appetite, loss of strength, and emaciation. It may be inherited, acquired, or idiopathic. Another form occurs (nephrogenic diabetes insipidus) in which the renal tubules are refractory to the antidiuretic effect of vasopressin. **d. insip′idus, nephrogenic,** a rare congenital and familial form of diabetes insipidus, resulting from failure of the renal tubules to reabsorb water; there is excessive production of antidiuretic hormone but the tubules fail to respond to it. **insulin-deficient d.,** juvenile d. **juvenile d., juvenile-onset d.,** severe diabetes mellitus, usually having an abrupt onset before the age of 25 and tending to be difficult to control and unstable ("brittle"); plasma insulin is often deficient and ketoacidosis occurs frequently, and oral hypoglycemics and diet are almost never effective, daily injections of insulin being required in almost all patients. Called also *growth-onset d.* and *ketosis-prone d.* **ketosis-prone d.,** juvenile d. **ketosis-resistant d.,** maturity-onset d. **Lancereaux's d.,** diabetes mellitus with marked emaciation. **latent d.,** chemical d. **lipoatrophic d.,** diabetes characterized by deficiency or absence of fat storage in the body. **lipoplethoric d.,** maturity-onset d. **lipuric d.,** diabetes marked by the presence of fat in the urine. **masked d.,** obesity without glycosuria; at a later stage it passes into diabetes mellitus. **maturity-onset d.,** a mild, often asymptomatic, form of diabetes mellitus with onset usually after 40 years of age, most often in overweight persons; although pancreatic insulin reserve is diminished, it is almost always sufficient, except under stressful conditions, to prevent ketoacidosis, and dietary control and/or oral hypoglycemics are usually effective. Called also *adult-onset d.* and *ketosis-resistant d.* **d. melli′tus,** a metabolic disorder in which the ability to oxidize carbohydrates is more or less completely lost, usually due to faulty pancreatic activity, especially of the islets of Langerhans, and consequent disturbance of normal insulin mechanism. This produces hyperglycemia with resulting glycosuria and polyuria giving symptoms of thirst, hunger, emaciation, and weakness and also imperfect combustion of fats with resulting acidosis, sometimes leading to dyspnea, lipemia, ketonuria, and finally coma. It is frequently associated with progressive disease of the small vessels (microangiopathy), particularly by affecting the eye (diabetic retinopathy) and kidney, and atherosclerosis, and there may also be pruritus and lowered resistance to pyogenic infections. Called also *Willis' disease.* See also *juvenile d.* and *maturity-onset d.* **Mosler's d.,** inosituria with polyuria. **neurogenous d.,** a form due to certain lesions of the brain. **overflow d.,** the loss of sugar into the urine when it is steadily administered intravenously in amounts greater than can be utilized by the body; dogs can thus utilize about 7 gm. per kilogram of body weight per hour. All above this passes into the urine. **overt d.,** diabetes manifested by symptoms, as opposed to chemical diabetes. **pancreatic d.,** d. mellitus. **phlorhizin d.,** a form produced by administering phlorhizin. **phosphate d.,** a genetically determined failure of renal tubular reabsorption of phosphates, resulting in osteomalacia; it is believed to be due to impairment of the ability to utilize vitamin D. **piqûre d.,** puncture d. **puncture d.,** a form produced by puncturing the floor of the fourth ventricle in the medulla oblongata; called also *piqûre d.* **renal d.,** diabetes thought to be dependent on defective renal function; renal glycosuria. **skin d.,** Urbach's term for the "syndrome of therapy-resistant, recurrent or chronic dermatosis, a high fasting skin sugar level together with a normal blood sugar curve, and pronounced improvement of the skin disease, as well as a drop in the high skin sugar level, on a low carbohydrate diet, sometimes combined with insulin." **steroid d., steroidogenic d.,** diabetes induced by sustained administration of glucocorticoids. **subclinical d.,** a state characterized by an abnormal glucose-tolerance test but without any clinical signs of diabetes. **temporary d.,** a temporary state characterized by an abnormality shown on the glucose-tolerance test, which later becomes normal. **toxic d.,** diabetes due to poisoning.

diabetic (di″ah-bet′ik) 1. pertaining to or affected with diabetes. 2. a person affected with diabetes. See under *diabetes* for specific forms.

diabetid (di″ah-be′tid) diabetic dermopathy.

diabetogenic (di″ah-bet″o-jen′ik) [*diabetes* + Gr. *gennan* to produce] producing diabetes.

diabetogenous (di″ah-be-toj′ĕ-nus) produced by diabetes.

diabetograph (di″ah-be′to-graf) [*diabetes* + Gr. *graphein* to write] an instrument used in urinalysis, with a graduated scale to show the proportion of glucose present.

diabetometer (di″ah-be-tom′ĕ-ter) [*diabetes* + Gr. *metron* measure] a polariscope for use in estimating the percentage of sugar in the urine.

Diabinese (di-ab′ĭ-nēs) trademark for chlorpropamide.

diabolepsy (di-ab′o-lep″se) [L. *diab′olus* devil + Gr. *lēpsis* a taking hold, a seizure] (*obs.*) a state in which the subject believes he is possessed by a devil, or that he is endowed with supernatural powers.

diabrosis (di″ah-bro′sis) [*dia-* + Gr. *brōsis* eating] perforation resulting from a corrosive process; perforating ulceration.

diabrotic (di″ah-brot′ik) [Gr. *diabrōtikos*] 1. ulcerative; caustic. 2. a corrosive or escharotic agent.

diacele (di′ah-sēl) (*obs.*) the third ventricle of the cerebrum (ventriculus tertius cerebri [NA]).

diacetate (di-as′ĕ-tāt) any salt of acetoacetic acid.

diacetemia (di″as-ĕ-te′me-ah) [*diacetic acid* + Gr. *haima* blood + *-ia*] the presence of acetoacetic acid (diacetic acid) in the blood.

diaceticaciduria (di″ah-set″ik-as″ĭ-du′re-ah) diaceturia.

diacetonuria (di-as″ĕ-to-nu′re-ah) diaceturia.

diaceturia (di″as-ĕ-tu′re-ah) [*diacetic acid* + Gr. *ouron* urine + *-ia*] the excretion of acetoacetic acid (diacetic acid) in the urine; called also *acetoacetic aciduria.*

diacetyl (di-as′ĕ-til) a yellow liquid, 2,3-butane-dione, CH_3-$COCOCH_3$, having the odor of butter. **d. peroxide,** a compound, $CH_3CO \cdot O \cdot O \cdot CO \cdot CH_3$, used in solution as an antiseptic.

diacetylmorphine (di″ah-se″til-mor′fēn) heroin; a white, bitterish, crystalline powder, $C_{17}H_{17}(O \cdot OC \cdot CH_3)_2 \cdot NO$, the diacetic acid ester of morphine, formerly used as an analgesic and narcotic. Because it is highly addictive, the importation of heroin and its salts into the United States, as well as its use in medicine, is illegal. Called also *acetomorphine* and *dimorphine.* **d. hydrochloride,** a white, crystalline powder, $C_{17}H_{17}(O \cdot CO \cdot CH_3)_2ON \cdot HCl \cdot H_2O$. See *diacetylmorphine.*

Diachlorus (di-ah-klo′rus) a genus of tabanid flies of South America.

diachorema (di″ah-ko-re′mah) [Gr. *diachōrēma*] excrement; feces.

diachoresis (di-ah-ko-re′sis) defecation.

diachylon (di-ak′ĭ-lon) [*dia-* + Gr. *chylos* juice] a plaster consisting essentially of lead oleate mixed with small amounts of glycerin and oleic acid; used as an adhesive for excoriated surfaces and wounds.

diacid (di-as′id) [Gr. *dis* twice + *acid*] having two replaceable hydrogen atoms; a dibasic acid, having the acid activity of two molecules of a monobasic acid.

diaclasis (di-ak′lah-sis) [*dia-* + Gr. *klasis* fracture] osteoclasis.

diaclast (di′ah-klast) an instrument for perforating the fetal skull in craniotomy.

diacrinous (di-ak′rĭ-nus) [Gr. *diakrinein* to separate] giving off secretion directly, as from a filter; said of gland cells, as those of the kidney. Opposed to *ptyocrinous.*

diacrisis (di-ak′rĭ-sis) [Gr. *diakrisis* separation] 1. diagnosis. 2. a disease marked by a morbid state of the secretions. 3. a critical discharge or excretion.

diacritic (di-ah-krit′ik) [*dia-* + Gr. *krinein* to judge] distinguishing; diagnostic.

diactinic (di″ak-tin′ik) transmitting chemically active rays.

diactinism (di-ak′tin-izm) [*dia-* + Gr. *aktis* ray] the property of transmitting chemically active rays.

diad (di′ad) 1. (*obs.*) having a valency or combining power of two. 2. dyad.

diaderm (di′ah-derm) [*dia-* + Gr. *derma* skin] the blastoderm during that stage in which it consists of an ectoderm and an entoderm.

diadermic (di-ah-der′mik) 1. pertaining to the diaderm. 2. through the skin.

diadochocinesia (di-ad″ŏ-ko-si-ne′se-ah) diadochokinesia.

diadochocinetic (di-ad″ŏ-ko-si-net′ik) diadochokinetic.

diadochokinesia (di-ad″ŏ-ko-ki-ne′se-ah) [Gr. *diadochos* succeeding + *kinēsis* motion] the function of arresting one motor impulse and substituting for it one that is diametrically opposite.

diadochokinesis (di-ad″ŏ-ko-ki-ne′sis) diadochokinesia.

diadochokinetic (di-ad″ŏ-ko-ki-net′ik) pertaining to diadochokinesia.

Diadol (di′ah-dol) trademark for a preparation of allobarbital.

Diafen (di′ah-fen) trademark for a preparation of diphenylpyraline hydrochloride.

diagnose (di′ag-nōs) to make a diagnosis of; to recognize the nature of an attack of disease.

diagnosis (di″ag-no′sis) [*dia-* + Gr. *gnōsis* knowledge] 1. the art of distinguishing one disease from another. 2. the determination of the nature of a case of disease. **biological d.,** diagnosis by tests performed on animals, as by the Aschheim-Zondek test. **clinical d.,** diagnosis based on signs, symptoms, and laboratory findings during life. **cytohistologic d.,** cytologic diagnosis. **cytologic d.,** the diagnosis of disease, both benign and malignant, by study of exfoliated cells; called also *cytohistologic d.* **differential d.,** the determination of which one of two or more diseases or conditions a patient is suffering from, by systematically comparing and contrasting their clinical findings. **direct d.,** pathologic diagnosis by observing structural lesions or pathognomonic symptoms. **d. ex juvan′tibus,** diagnosis based on the results of treatment. **d. by exclusion,** recognition of a disease by excluding all other known diseases. **laboratory d.,** diagnosis based on the findings of various laboratory examinations or measurements. **niveau d.** [Fr. "level diagnosis"], localization of the exact level of a lesion; as, for instance, of an intervertebral tumor. **pathologic d.,** diagnosis by observing the structural lesions present. **physical d.,** determination of disease by inspection, palpation, percussion, and auscultation. **provocative d.,** the induction of a condition for the purpose of diagnosis, as the induction of a fit in a doubtful case of epilepsy. **roentgen d.,** diagnosis made by means of roentgen rays. **serum d.,** diagnosis by means of the analysis of serums; immunodiagnosis.

diagnostic (di″ag-nos′tik) pertaining to or subserving diagnosis; distinctive of or serving as a criterion of a disease, as signs and symptoms.

diagnosticate (di″ag-nos′te-kāt) diagnose.

diagnostician (di″ag-nos-tish′an) an expert in diagnosis.

diagnostics (di″ag-nos′tiks) the science and practice of diagnosis of disease.

diagnosticum (di″ag-nos′te-kum) a preparation used in tests and experiments. **Ficker's d.,** an emulsion of killed typhoid bacilli for use in the Gruber reaction.

diagram (di′ah-gram) a graphic representation, in simplest form, of an object or concept, made up of lines and lacking entirely any pictorial elements. **vector d.,** a diagram representing the direction and magnitude of electromotive forces of the heart for one entire cycle, based on analysis of the scalar electrocardiogram.

diagrammatic (di″ah-grah-mat′ik) pertaining to or of the nature of a diagram.

diagraph (di′ah-graf) [*dia-* + Gr. *graphein* to write] an instrument for recording outlines; used in craniometry, etc.

diakinesis (di″ah-ki-ne′sis) [*dia-* + Gr. *kinēsis* motion] the stage of first meiotic prophase in which the nucleolus and nuclear envelope disappear and the spindle fibers form.

Dial (di′al) trademark for a preparation of allobarbital.

dial (di′al) [L. *dialis* daily, from *dies* day] a circular area with graduations around the circumference and a centrally fixed pointer for indicating values of time, pressure, etc. **astigmatic d.,** a diagram arranged like the face of a watch used to determine the presence and axis of astigmatism.

Dialister (di″ah-lis′ter) a genus of minute gram-negative rod-shaped bacteria found in the respiratory tract. They pass some bacteria-proof filters, and at one time *D. pneumosintes* was thought to be etiologically related to epidemic influenza.

diallyl (di-al′il) 1. any compound containing two allyl molecules. 2. a liquid unsaturated hydrocarbon, $CH_2:CH\cdot CH_2\cdot\cdot CH_2\cdot CH:CH_2$, having the odor of radishes. **d. sulfide,** allyl sulfide.

diallylbisnortoxiferin dichloride (di-al″il-bis-nor-tok′sifer-in) alcuronium chloride.

Dialog (di′ah-log) trademark for a preparation of allobarbital and acetaminophen.

Dialume (di′ah-loom) trademark for a preparation of dried aluminum hydroxide gel.

dialurate (di-al′u-rāt) a salt of dialuric acid.

dialysance (di″ah-li′sans) [*dialysis* + *-ance* suffix denoting action or process] the minute rate of net exchange of a substance between blood and bath fluid, per unit blood-bath concentration gradient; a parameter in artifical kidney kinetics (nonfiltration) functionally equivalent to the clearance of the natural kidney.

dialysate (di-al′ĭ-sāt) the material that passes through the membrane in dialysis.

dialysis (di-al′ĭ-sis) [*dia-* + Gr. *lysis* dissolution] the process of separating crystalloids and colloids in solution by the difference in their rates of diffusion through a semipermeable membrane: crystalloids pass through readily, colloids very slowly or not at all. See also *hemodialysis*. **Abderhalden's d.,** Abderhalden's reaction. **cross d.,** dialytic parabiosis. **equilibrium d.,** a technique employed to measure primary interaction of hapten and antibody. A container is employed in which two cells are separated by cellophane. Antibody is placed in one cell and hapten in the opposite one. The hapten will pass through the cellophane until, at equilibrium, an equivalent number of free hapten molecules is present in either cell on opposite sides of the membrane. In the cell containing antibody, additional hapten is present, combined with the antibody molecules. The use of radiolabeled hapten molecules permits calculation of the ratio of bound to free hapten, thus permitting determination of the association constant of hapten antibody reactions. **lymph d.,** removal of urea and other elements from lymph collected from the thoracic duct, treated outside the body, and later reinfused. **peritoneal d.,** dialysis through the peritoneum, the dialyzing solution being introduced into and removed from the peritoneal cavity as either a continuous or an intermittent procedure. **d. ret′inae,** a tear in the retina at the ora serrata.

dialyzable (di-ah-līz′ah-b'l) capable of dialysis or of passing through a membrane.

dialyzed (di′ah-līzd) separated or prepared by dialysis.

dialyzer (di′ah-līz″er) an apparatus for effecting dialysis; see *hemodialyzer.*

Diamanus (di″ah-ma′nus) a genus of fleas. **D. monta′nus,** a flea of rodents in the western United States which has been implicated in the transmission of sylvatic plague; formerly called *Ceratophyllus acustus, C. montanus,* and *Oropsylla montana.*

diameter (di-am′e-ter) the length of a straight line passing through the center of a circle and connecting opposite points on its circumference; hence the distance between two specified opposite points on the periphery of a structure such as the cranium or pelvis. **anteroposterior d.,** the distance between two points located on the anterior and posterior aspects, respectively, of the structure being measured; such as the true conjugate diameter of the pelvis, or the occipitofrontal diameter of the skull. **anterotransverse d.** (of the cranium), temporal d. **Baudelocque's d.,** external conjugate diameter. **biischial d.,** transverse diameter of pelvic outlet. **biparietal d.,** the distance between the two parietal eminences. **bisacromial d.,** the distance between the outermost points of the shoulder. **bisiliac d.,** the distance between the two most remote points of the iliac crests. **bispinous d.,** the distance between the opposite spines of the ischia. **bitemporal d.,** the distance between the two extremities of the coronal suture. **buccolingual d.,** the distance from the buccal to the lingual surface of a tooth crown at its widest point or greatest curvature. **cervicobregmatic d.,** the distance between the center of the anterior fontanel and the junction of the neck with the floor of the mouth. **coccygeopubic d.,** the distance from the tip of the coccyx to the under margin of the symphysis pubis. **conjugate d.,** the distance between two specified opposite points on the periphery of the pelvic inlet, usually used in reference to the true conjugate diameter. **conjugate d., anatomic,** the true conjugate diameter. **conjugate d., diagonal,** a diameter of the pelvic inlet: the distance from the posterior surface of the pubis to the tip of the sacral promontory; called also *conjugata diagonalis* and *diagonal conjugate.* **conjugate d., external,** the distance from the depression under the last lumbar spine to the upper margin of the pubis; called also *external conjugate* and *Baudelocque's d.* or *line.* **conjugate d., internal,** true conjugate d. **conjugate d., obstetric,** the shortest anteroposterior diameter of the pelvic inlet; the distance from a point 1 cm. below the top of the pubis to the tip of the sacral promontory, measuring 11 to 13 cm. in the normal pelvis. So called because it is intimately concerned in the process of labor. Called also *obstetric conjugate* and *conjugata vera obstetrica.* **conjugate d., true,** the anteroposterior diameter of the superior aperture of the minor pelvis (pelvic inlet), measured from the superior margin of the symphysis pubis to the sacrovertebral angle; called also *conjugata* [NA], *conjugata anatomica, conjugata vera, anatomic, internal,* or *true conjugate,* and *anatomic conjugate d.* **cranial d's,** distances measured between certain landmarks of the skull, such as the *biparietal d., bitemporal d., cervicobregmatic d., frontomental d., occipitofrontal d., occipitomental d.,* and *suboccipitobregmatic d.* **craniometric d.,** any line connecting two craniometric points of the same name. **extracanthic d.,** the distance between the lateral points of junction of the upper and lower eyelids of the two eyes. **frontomental d.,** the distance from the forehead to the chin. **fronto-occipital d.,** occipitofrontal d. **intercanthic d.,** the distance between the medial points of junction of the upper and lower eyelids of the two eyes. **intercristal d.,** the distance between the middle points of the iliac crests. **intertuberal d.,** the distance between the sciatic notches. **longitudinal d., inferior,** the distance from the foramen cecum to the internal occipital protuberance. **mento-occipital d.,** occipitomental d. **mentoparietal d.,** the distance from the chin to the vertex of the skull. **d. obli′qua pel′vis** [NA], **oblique diameter of pelvis,** the oblique diameter of the superior aperture of the minor pelvis, measured from one sacroiliac articulation to the iliopubic eminence of the other side. Designated right or left depending on the sacroiliac joint used for reference; the left is uniformly 0.5 cm. shorter than the right. **occipitofrontal d.,** the distance from the external occipital protuberance to the most prominent midpoint of the frontal bone; called also *fronto-occipital d.* **occipitomental d.,** the distance from the external occipital protuberance to the most prominent midpoint of the chin; called also *mento-occipital d.* **parietal d.,** the distance between tuberosities of parietal bones; called also *posterotransverse d.* **pelvic d.,** any diameter of the pelvis. **posterotransverse d.,** parietal d. **pubosacral d.,** true conjugate d. **pubotuberous d.,** the distance from the tuberosity of the ischium to a point on the superior ramus of the pubis which is located directly perpendicular to the tuberosity. **sacropubic d.,** the distance from the tip of the sacrum or coccyx to the lower margin of the symphysis pubis. **sagittal d.,** the distance from the glabella to the external occipital protuberance. **suboccipitobregmatic d.,** the distance from the lowest posterior point of the occiput to the center of the anterior fontanel. **temporal d.,** the distance between the tips of the alae magnae; called also *anterotransverse d.* **d. transver′sa pel′vis** [NA], transverse diameter of pelvis: the greatest distance from side to side of the superior aperture of the minor pelvis. **transverse d.,** the distance between two points located on the opposite sides of the body part being measured, such as the biparietal diameter of the head. **transverse d. of pelvis,** d. transversa pelvis. **transverse**

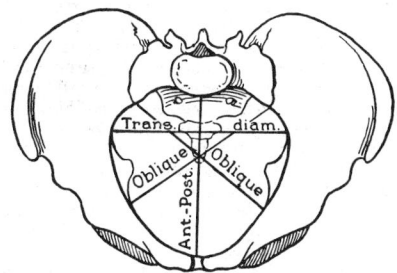

Diameters of pelvic inlet (see also pelvic planes) (Moloy).

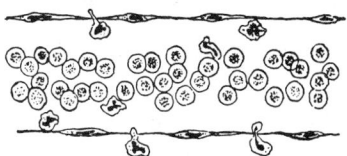

Diapedesis of leukocytes (Williams).

d. of pelvic outlet, the distance between the medial surfaces of the ischial tuberosities (average length 11 cm.); called also *biischial d.* **vertebromammary d.,** the anteroposterior diameter of the chest. **vertical d.,** the distance between two points situated on the upper and lower aspects of the structure being measured, such as the distance between the occipital foramen and the vertex of the skull.

diamide (di-am′id) [L. *di* two + *amide*] 1. a compound which contains two amido groups. 2. hydrazine.

diamidine (di-am′ĭ-dēn) a compound that contains two amidine groups.

diamido- a prefix indicating the possession of two amido groups.

diamine (di′ah-mēn″; di″ah-min′) [L. *di* two + *amine*] 1. a compound which contains two amino groups. 2. hydrazine sulfate, $N_2H_8HSO_4$, used as a germicide. **diethylene d.,** piperazine.

diaminoacridine (di-am″ĭ-no-ak′rĭ-din) proflavine.

diaminodiphenylsulfone (di-am″ĭ-no-di-fen″il-sul′fōn) dapsone. **diacetyl d.,** acedapsone.

diaminodiphosphatide (di-am″ĭ-no-di-fos′fah-tīd″) a phosphatide containing two atoms of nitrogen and two of phosphorus to the molecule.

diaminomonophosphatide (di-am″ĭ-no-mon″o-fos′fah-tīd″) a phosphatide containing two atoms of nitrogen and one of phosphorus to the molecule.

diaminuria (di-am″ĭ-nu′re-ah) the presence of diamines in the urine.

diamniotic (di″am-ne-ot′ik) having or developing within separate amniotic cavities, as diamniotic twins.

diamocaine cyclamate (di-ah′mo-kān) chemical name: 1-(2-anilinoethyl)-4-[2-(diethylamino)ethoxy]-4-phenylpiperidine; a local anesthetic, $C_{37}H_{63}N_5O_7S_2$.

diamonds (di′ah-munz) an urticarial form of swine erysipelas characterized by well-defined quadrangular or rhombic patches on the skin.

diamorphine (di″ah-mor′fēn) diacetylmorphine.

diamorphosis (di″ah-mor-fo′sis) (*obs.*) growth into normal shape.

Diamox (di′ah-moks) trademark for preparations of acetazolamide.

diamthazole dihydrochloride (di-am′thah-zōl) chemical name: 6-(2-diethylaminoethoxy)-2-dimethylaminobenzothiazole dihydrochloride. An antifungal agent, $C_{15}H_{25}Cl_2N_3OS$, effective against species of *Trichophyton* and *Microsporum* and *Candida albicans;* it has been used in the treatment of various forms of tinea, applied topically.

diamylene (di-am′ĭ-lēn) dipentene.

Diana complex (di-an′ah) [in Roman mythology, the goddess of the moon, hunting, and chastity] see under *complex.*

Dianabol (di-an′ah-bol) trademark for methandrostenolone.

diandry (di-an′dre) [*di*-(1) + Gr. *anēr, andros* man] triploidy in which the extra haploid set is of paternal origin.

dianhydroantiarigenin (di″an-hi′dro-an″te-ar′ĭ-jen″in) an aglycone, $C_{23}H_{28}O_5$, from antiarin.

dianoetic (di″ah-no-et′ik) [*dia*- + Gr. *nous* mind] pertaining to the intellectual functions, especially to reasoning.

diantebrachia (di″an-te-bra′ke-ah) a developmental anomaly characterized by duplication of a forearm.

diapamide (di-ap′ah-mīd) chemical name: 4-chloro-*N*-methyl-3-(methylsulfamoyl)benzamide; a diuretic and antihypertensive, $C_9H_{11}ClN_2O_3S$.

Diaparene (di-ap′ah-rēn) trademark for preparations of methylbenzethonium chloride.

diapause (di′a-pawz) [*dia*- + Gr. *pausis* pause] a state of inactivity and arrested development accompanied by greatly decreased metabolism, as in many eggs, insect pupae, and plant seeds; it is a mechanism for surviving adverse winter conditions.

diapedesis (di″ah-pĕ-de′sis) [*dia*- + Gr. *pēdan* to leap] the outward passage through intact vessel walls of corpuscular elements of the blood; called also *diapiresis* and *emigration.*

diapedetic (di″ah-pĕ-det′ik) pertaining to or characterized by diapedesis.

diaphane (di′ah-fān) [Gr. *diaphanēs* transparent] a minute electric lamp for use in transillumination.

diaphaneity (di″ah-fah-ne′ĭ-te) transparency.

diaphanometer (di-af″ah-nom′ĕ-ter) [Gr. *diaphanēs* transparent + Gr. *metron* measure] an instrument for testing milk, urine, and other fluids by means of transmitted light.

diaphanometry (di-af″ah-nom′ĕ-tre) the measurement of the transparency of a fluid.

diaphanoscope (di-af′ah-no-skōp″) [Gr. *diaphanēs* transparent + *skopein* to examine] an instrument for transilluminating a body cavity; called also *electrodiaphane* and *electrodiaphanoscope.*

diaphanoscopy (di-af″ah-nos′ko-pe) examination with the diaphanoscope; transillumination; called also *electrodiaphanoscopy.*

diaphemetric (di″ah-fĕ-met′rik) [*dia*- + Gr. *haphē* touch + *metron* measure] pertaining to the measurement of tactile sensibility.

diaphorase (di-af′o-rās) a flavoprotein that catalyzes the oxidation of nicotinamide-adenine dinucleotide (NAD) or nicotinamide-adenine dinucleotide phosphate (NADP).

diaphoresis (di″ah-fo-re′sis) [Gr. *diaphorēsis*] perspiration, especially profuse perspiration.

diaphoretic (di″ah-fo-ret′ik) [Gr. *diaphorētikos*] 1. pertaining to, characterized by, or promoting diaphoresis. 2. an agent that promotes diaphoresis.

diaphragm (di′ah-fram) 1. the musculomembranous partition separating the abdominal and thoracic cavities, and serving as a major inspiratory muscle; called also *diaphragma* [NA], *midriff,* and *diaphragmatic muscle.* 2. any separating membrane or structure. 3. a disk with one or more openings in it, or with an adjustable opening, mounted in relation to a lens or source of radiation by which part of the light or radiation may be excluded from the area. 4. a contraceptive device of molded rubber or other soft plastic material with a metal spring rim that is coated with a spermicidal agent; it is fitted over the cervix uteri prior to intercourse to prevent the entrance of spermatozoa by both mechanical and chemical means. Called also *contraceptive d.* and *vaginal d.* **accessory d.,** diaphragma urogenitale. **Akerlund d.,** a spiral type of diaphragm used in roentgenography. **Bucky d., Bucky-Potter d.,** a diaphragm used in roentgenography to prevent the secondary rays from reaching the film, thereby securing better contrast and definition. **contraceptive d.,** see diaphragm, def. 4. **d. of mouth** musculus mylohyoideus. **optic d.,** the iris of the eye; so called because it regulates the amount of light entering the eye. **oral d.,** musculus mylohyoideus. **pelvic d., d. of pelvis,** diaphragma pelvis. **polyarcuate d.,** one showing abnormal scalloping of margins on radiographic visualization. **Potter-Bucky d.,** Bucky d. **secondary d.,** diaphragma urogenitale. **d. of sella turcica,** diaphragma sellae. **urogenital d.,** diaphragma urogenitale. **vaginal d.,** see *diaphragm* (def. 4).

diaphragma (di″ah-frag′mah), pl. *diaphragmata* [Gr. "a partition-wall, barrier"] [NA] the diaphragm: the musculomembranous partition separating the abdominal and thoracic cavities, and serving as a major thoracic muscle. Called also *midriff* and *diaphragmatic muscle.* Also used in anatomical nomenclature in the names of other separating structures. **d. o′ris,** musculus mylohyoideus. **d. pel′vis** [NA], pelvic diaphragm: the portion of the floor of the pelvis formed by the coccygei and levatores ani muscles and their fasciae. **d. sel′lae** [NA], diaphragm of sella turcica: a ring-shaped fold of dura mater covering the sella turcica, and containing an aperture for passage of the infundibulum of the hypophysis. **d. urogenita′le** [NA], urogenital diaphragm: the musculomembranous layer superficial to the pelvic diaphragm, extending between the ischiopubic rami and surrounding the urogenital ducts. Called also *accessory* or *secondary diaphragm, Camper's ligament, deep fascia of perineum* or *deep perineal fascia,* and *fascia of urogenital trigone.*

diaphragmalgia (di″ah-frag-mal′je-ah) [*diaphragm* + Gr. *algos* pain + *-ia*] pain in the diaphragm.

diaphragmata (di″ah-frag′mah-tah) [Gr.] plural of *diaphragma.*

diaphragmatic (di″ah-frag-mat′ik) pertaining to or of the nature of a diaphragm.

diaphragmatitis (di″ah-frag″mah-ti′tis) diaphragmitis.

diaphragmatocele (di″ah-frag-mat′o-sēl) [*diaphragm* + Gr. *kēlē* hernia] diaphragmatic hernia.

diaphragmitis (di″ah-frag-mi′tis) inflammation of the diaphragm.

diaphragmodynia (di″ah-frag″mo-din′e-ah) [*diaphragm* + Gr. *odynē* pain] diaphragmalgia.

diaphysary (di-af′ĭ-zār-e) diaphyseal.

diaphyseal (di″ah-fiz′e-al) pertaining to or affecting the shaft of a long bone (diaphysis).

diaphysectomy (di″ah-fiz-ek′to-me) [*diaphysis* + Gr. *ektomē* excision] excision of a portion of the shaft of a long bone.

diaphyses (di-af′ĭ-sēz) [Gr.] plural of *diaphysis*.

diaphysial (di″ah-fiz′e-al) diaphyseal.

diaphysis (di-af′ĭ-sis), pl. *diaph′yses* [Gr. "the point of separation between stalk and branch"] 1. [NA] the elongated cylindrical portion (the shaft) of a long bone, between the ends or extremities (the epiphyses), which are usually articular and wider than the shaft; it consists of a tube of compact bone, enclosing the medullary (marrow) cavity. Called also *shaft*. 2. the portion of a long bone formed from a primary center of ossification.

diaphysitis (di″ah-fiz-i′tis) inflammation of a diaphysis. **tuberculous d.,** inflammation involving intermediate segments of the shafts of long bones, caused by the tubercle bacillus.

Diapid (di′ah-pid) trademark for a preparation of lypressin.

diapiresis (di″ah-pi-re′sis) [Gr. *diapeirein* to drive through] diapedesis.

diaplacental (di″ah-plah-sen′tal) through the placenta.

diaplasis (di-ap′lah-sis) [Gr.] the setting of a fracture or the reduction of a dislocation.

diaplastic (di″ah-plas′tik) pertaining to the setting of a fracture or the reduction of a dislocation.

diapophysis (di-ah-pof′ĭ-sis) [*dia-* + Gr. *apophysis* outgrowth] the superior or articular part of a transverse process of a vertebra.

Diaptomus (di-ap′to-mus) a genus of copepod crustaceans, species of which act as hosts of the larvae of *Diphyllobothrium latum*.

diapyesis (di″ah-pi-e′sis) suppuration.

diapyetic (di″ah-pi-et′ik) promoting suppuration.

diarrhea (di″ah-re′ah) [*dia-* + Gr. *rhein* to flow] abnormal frequency and liquidity of fecal discharges. **d. ablactato′rum** (*obs.*), a diarrhea of infants at the time they are weaned. **d. al′ba** (*obs.*), a disease of hot countries, affecting children especially; thought to be of filarial origin. **cachectic d.,** diarrhea associated with cachexia; it may be due to malabsorption, or both the diarrhea and the cachexia may be manifestations of an underlying disease, e.g., neoplasm. **choleraic d.,** acute diarrhea with serous stools, accompanied by circulatory collapse, thus resembling cholera. **chronic bacillary d.,** Johne's disease. **d. chylo′sa,** diarrhea in which the discharge consists of a yellowish white, mucopurulent substance that resembles chyle in gross appearance. **Cochin-China d.,** 1. sprue (def. 1). 2. strongyloidiasis. **colliquative d.,** profuse diarrhea, producing a state of dehydration, sometimes seen in the late stages of pulmonary tuberculosis. **congenital chloride d.,** familial chloride d. **crapulous d.,** that due to excess in eating or drinking. **critical d.,** diarrhea occurring at the crisis of a disease or producing a crisis. **dientameba d.,** a mild though chronic diarrhea caused by infection with *Dientamoeba fragilis*. **dysenteric d.,** diarrhea with mucous and bloody stools. **enteral d.,** diarrhea due to infection within the gastrointestinal tract. **epidemic d. of newborn,** a contagious diarrhea occurring in epidemics among newborn infants in hospitals; called also *neonatal d.* **familial chloride d.,** severe watery diarrhea with an excess of chloride in the stool, beginning in early infancy and marked by distended abdomen, lethargy, and retarded growth and mental development. It is accompanied by alkalosis and hypokalemia, and maternal hydramnios is often associated. The disorder is due to impairment of chloride-bicarbonate exchange in the lower bowel. Called also *congenital chloride d.* and *familial chloridorrhea.* **fermental d., fermentative d.,** diarrhea caused by fermentation due to microorganisms. **flagellate d.,** diarrhea marked by the presence of flagellate organisms (*Giardia*) in the stools. **gastrogenic d.,** diarrhea due to gastric disorder. **hill d.,** a chronic diarrhea peculiar to hot climates and occurring only at elevations of several thousand feet: named from the hill districts of India; it is considered by some to be identical with sprue. **infantile d.,** summer diarrhea. **inflammatory d.,** diarrhea in which there is an inflammation of the intestine due to bacterial action. **irritative d.,** diarrhea due to irritation of the intestine by improper food, poisons, purgatives, etc. **lienteric d.,** diarrhea with fluid stools containing undigested food. **mechanical d.,** diarrhea due to mechanical obstruction to the portal circulation, producing gastrointestinal hyperemia. **morning d.,** a condition marked by diarrhea in the morning only. **mucous d.,** a kind characterized by the presence of mucus in stools. **neonatal d.,** epidemic diarrhea of the newborn. **osmotic d.,** diarrhea resulting from the presence of osmotically active nonabsorbable solutes, e.g., magnesium sulfate, in the intestine. **d. pancreat′ica,** the diarrhea that accompanies parenchymatous degeneration or cystic disease of the pancreas. **pancreatogenous fatty d.,** a diarrhea in which the stools contain an excessive amount of fat due to dysfunction of the

pancreas. **paradoxical d.,** stercoral d. **parenteral d.,** diarrhea due to infections outside the gastrointestinal tract, such as tuberculosis, syphilis, etc. **putrefactive d.,** diarrhea due to putrefaction of the intestinal contents. **serous d.,** discharge of feces softened by copious serous fluid; called also *watery d.* **stercoral d.,** diarrhea accompanied by colic and following two or three days of constipation; called also *paradoxical d.* **summer d.,** acute diarrhea in children during great heat of summer; called also *infantile d.* **traveler's d.,** diarrhea occurring among travelers, particularly in those visiting tropical or subtropical areas where sanitation is suboptimal; it is currently considered to be due to infection with enteropathogenic *Escherichia coli.* In Mexico, it is also called *turista.* **trench d.,** a form of diarrhea and dysentery that occurred in troops in the trenches. **tropical d.,** see *sprue;* def. 1. **tubercular d.,** a variety of diarrhea peculiar to cases of tuberculosis. **tubular d.,** mucous colitis. **virus d.,** a specific infectious condition manifested by diarrhea in infants and by stomatitis and diarrhea in older children. **watery d.,** serous d. **white d.,** 1. a form in which the stools contain a thin, white mucus. 2. an infectious disease of young chickens marked by loss of appetite, dullness, and diarrhea, the discharges of which leave white lumps around the cloaca; it is caused by *Salmonella pullorum.* Called also *pullorum disease.*

diarrheal (di″ah-re′al) pertaining to or marked by diarrhea.

diarrheic (di″ah-re′ik) diarrheal.

diarrheogenic (di″ah-re″o-jen′ik) [*diarrhea* + Gr. *gennan* to produce] giving rise to diarrhea.

diarthric (di-ar′thrik) [*di-* + Gr. *arthron* a joint] pertaining to or affecting two different joints.

diarthrodial (di″ar-thro′dĭ-al) of the nature of a diarthrosis.

diarthroses (di″ar-thro′sēz) plural of *diarthrosis*.

diarthrosis (di″ar-thro′sis), pl. *diarthroses* [Gr. *diarthrōsis* a movable articulation] junctura synovialis. **d. rotato′ria,** a joint characterized by mobility in a rotary direction.

diarticular (di″ar-tik′u-lar) diarthric.

diaschisis (di-as′kĭ-sis) [*dia-* + Gr. *schizein* to split] the loss of function and electrical activity caused by cerebral lesions in areas which are remote from the lesion but which are neuronally connected to it; called also *Monakow's theory.*

diascope (di′ah-skōp) [*dia-* + Gr. *skopein* to examine] a glass or clear plastic plate, usually a flat blade or microscope slide, pressed against the skin to permit observation of changes produced in the underlying skin after the blood vessels are emptied and the skin is blanched.

diascopy (di-as′ko-pe) 1. examination with the diascope. 2. transillumination.

Diasone (di′ah-sōn) trademark for a preparation of sulfoxone sodium.

diasostic (di″ah-sos′tik) hygienic.

diaspironecrobiosis (di-as″pi-ro-nek″ro-bi-o′sis) [*dia-* + Gr. *speirein* to sow + *necrobiosis*] disseminated necrobiosis.

diaspironecrosis (di-as″pi-ro-ne-kro′sis) disseminated necrosis.

diastalsis (di″ah-stal′sis) [*dia-* + Gr. *stalsis* contraction] (*obs.*) a downward moving wave of contraction with a preceding wave of inhibition occurring in the digestive tube.

diastaltic (di″ah-stal′tik) (*obs.*) 1. pertaining to diastalsis. 2. performed reflexly; reflex.

diastase (di′ah-stās) [Gr. *diastasis* separation] a white, amorphous, soluble enzyme produced during the germination of seeds, and contained in malt; it converts starch into maltose and then into dextrose. **pancreatic d.,** see *amylase.* **taka d.,** see *Taka-Diastase.* **d. ve′ra,** pancreatin.

diastatic (di″as-ta′sik) diastatic.

diastasimetry (di″as-tah-sim′ĕ-tre) the estimation of the diastatic power (carbohydrase activity) of a substance.

diastasis (di-as′tah-sis) [Gr.] 1. a form of dislocation in which there is separation of two bones normally attached to each other without the existence of a true joint; as in separation of the pubic symphysis. Also, separation beyond the normal between associated bones, as between the ribs, or the ulna and radius. 2. diastasis cordis. Called also *divarication.* **d. cor′dis,** the rest period of the cardiac cycle, which occurs just before systole. **iris d.,** iridodiastasis. **d. rec′ti abdom′inis,** separation of the rectus muscles of the abdominal wall, sometimes occurring during pregnancy.

diastasuria (di″ah-stās-u′re-ah) the presence of diastase in the urine.

diastatic (di″ah-stat′ik) 1. pertaining to diastase. 2. pertaining to diastasis.

diastem (di′ah-stem) diastema.

diastema (di″ah-ste′mah), pl. *diastem′ata* [Gr. *diastēma* an interval] [NA] a general term for a space or cleft. In dentistry, a space between two adjacent teeth in the same dental arch. In cytology, a narrow zone in the equatorial plane through which the cytosome divides in mitosis. **anterior d.,** a space between the incisor teeth, generally one between the maxillary central incisors.

diastemata (di″ah-stem′ah-tah) pl. of *diastema*.

diastematocrania (di″ah-stem″ah-to-kra′ne-ah) [Gr. *diastēma* an interval + *kranion* cranium] congenital longitudinal fissure of the cranium.

diastematomyelia (di″ah-stem″ah-to-mi-e′le-ah) [Gr. *diastēma* an interval + *myelos* marrow] a congenital defect, often associated with spina bifida, in which the spinal cord is split into halves by a bony spicule or fibrous band, each half being surrounded by a dural sac.

diastematopyelia (di″ah-stem″ah-to-pi-e′le-ah) [Gr. *diastēma* an interval + *pyelos* pelvis] congenital median fissure of the pelvis.

diaster (di′as-ter) [*di-* two + Gr. *astēr* star] amphiaster.

diastereoisomer (di″ah-ster″e-o-i′so-mer) a compound exhibiting, or capable of exhibiting, diastereoisomerism.

diastereoisomeric (di″ah-ster″e-o-i″so-mer′ik) exhibiting diastereoisomerism.

diastereoisomerism (di″ah-ster″e-o″i′i-som′er-izm) a special type of optical isomerism in which the respective molecules of the compounds do not, at any time, exhibit a mirror-image (or enantiomorphic) relationship to one another. For example, the relationship between either *dextro-* or *levo*-tartaric acid and *meso*-tartaric acid is called diastereoisomeric. Diastereoisomers, in contrast to enantiomorphs, differ in both physical and chemical properties.

Diastix (di′ah-stiks) trademark for a reagent strip designed for the quantitative determination of glucose in urine.

diastole (di-as′to-le) [Gr. *diastolē* a drawing asunder; expansion] the dilatation, or period of dilatation, of the heart, especially of the ventricles; it coincides with the interval between the second and the first heart sound.

diastolic (di″ah-stol′ik) of or pertaining to the diastole.

diastomyelia (di-as″to-mi-e′le-ah) diastematomyelia.

diastrophic (di″-ah-strahf′ik) [Gr. *diastrephein* distortion] bent or curved; said of structures, such as bones, deformed in such manner.

diataxia (di″ah-tak′se-ah) [*di-* two + *ataxia*] ataxia affecting both sides of the body. **cerebral d., d. cerebra′lis infanti′lis**, infantile cerebral ataxic paralysis.

diathermal (di″ah-ther′mal) pertaining to diathermy; heated by high-frequency electromagnetic radiation.

diathermic (di″ah-ther′mik) pertaining to diathermy; permeable to high-frequency electromagnetic radiation.

diathermy (di′ah-ther″me) [*dia-* + Gr. *thermē* heat] heating of the body tissues due to their resistance to the passage of high-frequency electromagnetic radiation, electric currents, or ultrasonic waves. In *medical d.* (thermopenetration) the tissues are warmed but not damaged; in *surgical d.* (electrocoagulation) tissue is destroyed. **short wave d.**, the therapeutic heating of the body tissues by means of an oscillating electromagnetic field of high frequency; the frequency varies from 10 million to 100 million cycles per second and the wavelength from 30 to 3 meters. **ultrashort wave d.**, diathermy in which the wavelength used is less than 10 meters.

diathesis (di-ath′ĕ-sis) [Gr. "arrangement, disposition"] a constitution or condition of the body which makes the tissues react in special ways to certain extrinsic stimuli and thus tends to make the person more than usually susceptible to certain diseases. Cf. *constitution* (def. 1) and *type*. **aneurysmal d.**, propensity for the formation of multiple aneurysms. **asthenic d.**, a low state of general vitality. **bilious d.**, nonspecific gastrointestinal symptoms once attributed to disordered bile secretion or biliary tract disease. **contractural d.**, tendency to contractures having a hysterical basis. **cystic d.**, a tendency to the development of multiple cysts in an organ. **fibroplastic d.**, a tendency of the body to develop connective tissue in excess in response to trauma. **gouty d.**, predisposition to gout; status arthriticus. **hemorrhagic d.**, a predisposition to abnormal hemostasis. **hemorrhagic d. of newborn**, hemorrhagic disease of newborn. **inopectic d.**, a bodily predisposition to embolism and thrombosis. **lupus d.**, a predisposition, probably genetic, to systemic lupus erythematosus. **neuropathic d.**, a congenital predisposition to nervous instability, a concept originated in 19th century French and German psychiatry; called also *psychopathic d.* **ossifying d.**, a tendency to the formation of bony deposits in the muscles. **oxalic d.**, one characterized by unusual amounts of oxalic acid in the urine; called also *Bird's disease.* **psychopathic d.**, neuropathic d. **spasmodic d., spasmophilic d.**, spasmophilia; a condition of abnormal excitability of the peripheral motor nerves, tending to tetany and general convulsions. **uric acid d.**, a tendency to the collection of uric acid and urates in the tissues, resulting in gout, diabetes, etc.

diathetic (di″ah-thet′ik) of or pertaining to a diathesis.

diatom (di′ah-tom) any unicellular microscopical form of alga having a wall of silica and belonging to the family Diatomaceae.

Several species are toxic, causing the "red blooms" or "red tides." The skeletal siliceous remains of many others are mined from deposits and used as filtering and abrasive agents; see *infusorial earth*, under *earth*.

diatomaceous (di″ah-to-ma′shus) composed of diatoms; said of earth composed of the siliceous skeletons of diatoms. See *infusorial earth*, under *earth*.

diatomic (di″ah-tom′ik) [*di-* + *atom*] 1. made up of two atoms. 2. dibasic. 3. diatomaceous.

diatrizoate (di″ah-tri-zo′āt) any salt of diatrizoic acid. **d. meglumine** [USP], a radiopaque medium, $(C_7H_{11}NO_5 \cdot C_{11}H_9I_3 - N_2O_4)$, available in solution, consisting of diatrizoate meglumine in water for injection or of diatrizoic acid in water for injection, prepared with the aid of meglumine; used intra-arterially in angiocardiography, aortography, cerebral angiography, and peripheral arteriography, intravenously in angiocardiography, excretory urography, and venography, and unilaterally in retrograde pyelography. **d. sodium** [USP], a radiopaque medium, $C_{11}H_8I_3N_2NaO_4$, available in solution, consisting of diatrizoate sodium in water for injection or of diatrizoic acid in water for injection, prepared with the aid of sodium hydroxide; used in cholangiography, intravenously in excretory urography, hysterosalpingography, and unilaterally in retrograde pyelography.

diauchenos (di-awk′ĕ-nos) a dicephalic monster with two necks.

diauxic (di-awk′sik) pertaining to or characterized by diauxie; implying two periods of growth separated by a lag period.

diauxie (di-awk′se) [*di-* + Gr. *auxein* to increase in size] a phenomenon of bacterial growth in which an organism given a mixture of organic compounds first grows exclusively on one until that compound is exhausted, and then, after a lag during which it forms induced enzymes for utilizing the second compound, resumes growth on the latter.

diaveridine (di″ah-ver′ĭ-dēn) chemical name: 5-[(3,4-dimethoxyphenyl)methyl]-2,4-pyrimidinediamine. An antiprotozoal and antibacterial, $C_{13}H_{16}ClN_2O$; used as a coccidiostat in poultry.

diaxon (di-ak′son) [*di-* + *axon*] a nerve cell having two axons or axis-cylinder processes.

diaxone (di-ak′sōn) diaxon.

diazepam (di-az′ĕ-pam) [USP] chemical name: 7-chloro-1,3-dihydro-1-methyl-5-phenyl-2*H*-1,4-benzodiazepin-2-one. One of the benzodiazepine tranquilizers, $C_{16}H_{13}ClN_2O$, occurring as an off-white to yellow, crystalline powder. It is administered orally, intravenously, or intramuscularly as a sedative, and is also used as a skeletal muscle relaxant, to produce anesthesia, as an anticonvulsant, and in the management of alcohol withdrawal symptoms and delirium tremens.

diazine (di-az′in) any compound containing a ring of four carbon and two nitrogen atoms.

diazo- (di-az′o) a prefix indicating possession of the group —N=N—.

diazobenzene (di-az″o-ben′zēn) a univalent organic radical, $C_6H_5N_2$.

diazoma (di″ah-zo′mah) [Gr. *diazōma* that which is put round] the diaphragm.

diazomethane (di-az″o-meth′ān) an extremely poisonous yellow gas, N_2CH_2, used in organic synthesis.

diazonal (di″ah-zo′nal) 1. situated across or bridging two zones. 2. pertaining to a diazone.

diazone (di′ah-zōn) one of the dark bands, alternating with white bands (*parazones*), formed by the layers of enamel prisms and seen in cross section of a tooth.

diazosulfobenzol (di-az″o-sul′fo-ben′zol) a substance which acts upon certain principles in the urine to form aniline colors.

diazotization (di-az″o-ti-za′shun) conversion into a diazo compound.

diazotize (di-az′o-tīz) to introduce the diazo group into a compound.

diazoxide (di-az-ok′sīd) [USP] chemical name: 7-chloro-3-methyl-2*H*-1,2,4-benzothiadiazine. An antihypertensive, $C_8H_7ClN_2O_2S$, structurally related to chlorothiazide but having no diuretic properties, occurring as white or cream-colored crystals or crystalline powder; administered intravenously. Because it inhibits release of insulin, it is also administered orally in the treatment of hypoglycemia due to hyperinsulinism.

dibasic (di-bā′sik) [*di-* + Gr. *basis* base] containing two hydrogen atoms replaceable by bases, and thus yielding two series of salts, as H_2SO_4.

Dibenamine (di-ben′ah-mēn) trademark for a preparation of dibenzylchlorethamine.

dibenzanthracene (di-benz-an′thrah-sēn) an aromatic polycyclic hydrocarbon, $C_{22}H_{14}$, capable, when injected into the body, of producing epithelial tumors. Abbreviated DBA.

dibenz-dibutyl anthraquinol (di-benz″di-bu′til an″thrah-kwin′ol) a carcinogenic and estrogenic substance, 1,2,5,6-dibenz-9,10,di-n-butyl anthraquinol.

dibenzepin hydrochloride (di-benz′ĕ-pin) chemical name:

10-[2-(dimethylamino)ethyl]-5,10-dihydro-5-methyl-11*H*-dibenzo-[*b*,*e*][1,4]diazepin-11-one monohydrochloride; a tricyclic antidepressant, $C_{18}H_{21}N_3O \cdot HCl$.

dibenzothiazine (di-ben″zo-thi′ah-zēn) phenothiazine.

dibenzylchlorethamine (di″ben-zil-klōr-eth′ah-mēn) chemical name: N-(2-chloroethyl)dibenzylamine. An alpha-adrenergic blocking agent, $C_{16}H_{18}ClN$, which has been used in the treatment of peripheral vascular disorders and in the diagnosis of pheochromocytoma.

Dibenzyline (di-ben′zĭ-lēn) trademark for a preparation of phenoxybenzamine hydrochloride.

diblastula (di-blas′tu-lah) [*di-* + *blastula*] a blastula in which the ectoderm and entoderm are both present.

dibothriocephaliasis (di-both″re-o-sef″ah-li′ah-sis) diphyllobothriasis.

Dibothriocephalus (di-both″re-o-sef′ah-lus) [*di-* + Gr. *bothrion* pit + *kephalē* head] Diphyllobothrium.

dibrachia (di-bra′ke-ah) [*di-* + Gr. *brachion* arm] a developmental anomaly characterized by duplication of an arm.

dibrachius (di-bra′ke-us) a twin monster having only two arms.

dibromide (di-bro′mīd) any bromide which combines two atoms of bromine with one of another element or radical.

dibromoketone (di-bro″mo-ke′tōn) methyl dibromoethyl ketone, $CH_3COCHBrCH_2Br$, a war gas.

dibromsalan (di-brom′sah-lan) chemical name: 5-bromo-N-(4-bromophenyl)-2-hydroxybenzamide. A disinfectant with antibacterial and antifungal activities, $C_{13}H_9Br_2NO_2$, used mainly in medicated soaps.

dibucaine (di′bu-kān) [USP] chemical name: 2-butoxy-N-[2-(diethylamino)ethyl]-4-quinolinecarboxamide. A potent local anesthetic, $C_{20}H_{29}N_3O_2$, occurring as a white to off-white powder; applied topically to the skin and mucous membranes. **d. hydrochloride** [USP], the monohydrochloride salt of dibucaine, $C_{20}H_{29}N_2O_2 \cdot HCl$, occurring as colorless or white to off-white crystals or as a white to off-white, crystalline powder, having the same actions as the base; administered in the form of an aerosol spray to produce anesthesia of the skin and mucous membranes or injected into the subarachnoid space to produce spinal anesthesia.

Dibuline (di′bu-lēn) trademark for a preparation of dibutoline sulfate.

dibutoline sulfate (di-bu′to-lēn) chemical name: bis[ethyl(2-hydroxyethyl)dimethylammonium]sulfate bis(dibutylcarbamate). A quaternary ammonium anticholinergic, $C_{30}H_{66}N_4O_8S$, used as a cycloplegic and gastrointestinal antispasmodic, administered intramuscularly or subcutaneously.

dibutyl (di-būt′il) a hydrocarbon, C_8H_{18}, occurring in mineral oil.

DIC disseminated intravascular coagulation.

dicacodyl (di-kak′o-dĭl) cacodyl.

dicalcic (di-kal′sik) having in each molecule two atoms of calcium.

dicalcium phosphate (di-kal′se-um fos′fāt) dibasic calcium phosphate; see under *calcium*.

dicamphendion (di″kam-fen′de-on) a substance, $(C_{10}H_{14}O)_2$, obtained by the action of metallic sodium upon bromocamphor, dicamphor being produced at the same time.

dicamphor (di-kam′for) a principle in colorless needles, $(C_{10}H_{15}O)_2$, produced at the same time and from the same materials as dicamphendion.

dicarbonate (di-kar′bon-āt) bicarbonate.

dicelous (di-se′lus) [*di-* + Gr. *koilos* hollow] 1. hollowed on both sides. 2. having two cavities. 3. amphicelous.

dicentric (di-sen′trik) pertaining to, developing from, or having two centers. In genetics, having two centromeres.

dicephalous (di-sef′ah-lus) having two heads.

dicephalus (di-sef′ah-lus) [*di-* + Gr. *kephalē* head] a monster with two heads. **d. di′pus dibra′chius,** a monster with two heads but only two feet and two arms. **d. di′pus tetrabra′chius,** a monster with only two legs, but with varying degrees of fusion of the upper trunk, each component having a head and pair of arms. **d. di′pus tribra′chius,** a monster with two heads, two feet, but with a median third arm or arm rudiment. **d. dipy′gus,** anakatadidymus. **d. parasit′icus,** desmiognathus. **d. tri′pus tribra′chius,** a monster with a common trunk, but with two heads, three arms, and three legs, the third limbs being either rudimentary or complete.

dicephaly (di-sef′ah-le) a developmental anomaly characterized by the presence of two heads.

dicheilia (di-ki′le-ah) the appearance of a double lip, owing to folding of the oral mucosa.

dicheiria (di-ki′re-ah) [*di-* + Gr. *cheir* hand] a developmental anomaly characterized by duplication of a hand.

dicheirus (di-ki′rus) an individual exhibiting dicheiria.

dichlordioxydiamidoarsenobenzol (di-klor″di-ok″se-di-am″ĭ-do-ar″sĕ-no-ben′zol) arsphenamine.

dichlorhydrin (di″klor-hi′drin) a colorless fluid, $CH_2Cl \cdot CHOH \cdot CH_2Cl$, used as a solvent for resins and prepared by heating anhydrous glycerin with sulfur monochloride.

dichloride (di-klo′rīd) a combination of a base or a metal with two atoms of chlorine.

dichlorisone (di-klōr′ĭ-sōn) chemical name: 9,11β-dichloro-17,21-dihydroxy pregna-1,4-diene-3,20-dione. A glucocorticoid, $C_{21}H_{26}Cl_2O_4$, used in the treatment of steroid-responsive pruritic or allergic inflammations, applied topically.

dichlorodiethyl sulfide (di-klo″ro-di-eth′il) chemical name: bis(2-chloroethyl)sulfide. Mustard gas, $(CH_2ClCH_2)_2S$, a vesicant gas once employed in war. It produces blistering and subsequent sloughing of the skin with involvement of the eyes and respiratory tract. Death results from bronchopneumonia. Called also *yellow cross* and *yperite*.

dichlorodifluoromethane (di-klo″ro-di-floor″o-meth′ān) [NF] a clear, colorless gas with a faint, ethereal odor, CCl_2F_2, used as an aerosol propellant, and also as a refrigerant.

dichloroformoxime (di-klo″ro-for-mok′sim) a suffocating war gas, CCl_2:N·OH; called also *phosgene oxime*.

dichloroisoproterenol (di-klo″ro-i″so-pro-ter′ĕ-nol) chemical name: 3,4-dichloro-α-(isopropylaminomethyl)benzyl alcohol. A beta-adrenergic blocking agent, $C_{11}H_{15}Cl_2NO$, used in the treatment of various cardiac disorders.

dichlorotetrafluoroethane (di-klo″ro-tet″rah-floor″o-eth′ān) [NF] chemical name: 1,2-dichlorotetrafluoroethane. A clear, colorless gas with a faint ethereal odor, $CClF_2$-$CClF_2$, used as an aerosol propellant.

dichlorphenamide (di″klor-fen′ah-mīd) [USP] chemical name: 4,5-dichloro-1,3-benzenedisulfonamide. A carbonic anhydrase inhibitor, $C_6H_6Cl_2N_2O_4S_2$, occurring as a white or practically white, crystalline powder; used mainly to reduce intraocular pressure in glaucoma, administered orally.

dichlorvos (di-klor′vos) chemical name: phosphoric acid 2,2-dichloroethenyl dimethyl ester; an organophorous insecticide and anthelmintic, $C_4H_7Cl_2O_4P$.

dichogeny (di-koj′ĕ-ne) [Gr. *dicha* in two + *gennan* to produce] development of tissues in different ways in accordance with changes in conditions affecting them.

dichorial (di-ko′re-al) dichorionic.

dichorionic (di″ko-re-on′ik) having two distinct chorions; said of dizygotic twins.

dichotomization (di-kot″ŏ-mi-za′shun) dichotomy.

dichotomy (di-kot′o-me) [Gr. *dicha* in two + *tomē* a cutting] the process or result of division into two parts.

dichroic (di-kro′ik) exhibiting dichroism.

dichroine (di-kro′ēn) an alkaloid from Ch'ang Shan, the root of the shrub *Dichroa febrifuga* Lour. (Saxifragaceae), having three isomeric forms α-, β-, and γ-dichroine.

dichroism (di′kro-izm) [*di-* + Gr. *chroa* color] the quality or condition of presenting one color in reflected and another in transmitted light.

dichromasy (di-kro′mah-se) dichromatism, def. 1.

dichromat (di′kro-mat) an individual exhibiting dichromatopsia.

dichromate (di-kro′māt) any salt containing the bivalent Cr_2O_7 radical.

dichromatic (di″kro-mat′ik) pertaining to or characterized by dichromatism.

dichromatism (di-kro′mah-tism) 1. the quality of existing in or exhibiting two different colors. 2. dichromatopsia.

dichromatopsia (di″kro-mah-top′se-ah) [*di-* + Gr. *chrōma* color + *opsis* vision + *-ia*] a condition characterized by ability to perceive only two of the 160 colors discriminable by the normal eye; usually a complementary blue and yellow or, rarely, a red and green.

dichromic (di-kro′mik) pertaining to two colors.

dichromophil (di-kro′mo-fil) amphophilic; also, an amphophilic element.

dichromophilism (di″kro-mof′ĭ-lizm) capacity for double staining, that is, with both acid and basic dyes.

dichuchwa a type of nonvenereal syphilis found among the Bantus.

dick (dik) a vesicant war gas, ethyldichlorarsine, $C_2H_5 \cdot AsCl_2$, causing sneezing and pulmonary edema.

Dick serum, test (reaction), toxin (dik) [George Frederick Dick, 1881–1967, and Gladys Rowena Henry Dick, 1881–1963, American physicians] see under *serum* and *tests*, and see *erythrogenic toxin*, under *toxin*.

dicliditis (dik″lĭ-di′tis) [Gr. *diklis* double door + *-itis*] (obs.) inflammation of a valve, especially one of the heart valves.

diclidostosis (dik″lid-os-to′sis) [Gr. *diklis* double door + *osteon* bone + *-osis*] ossification of the valves of the veins.

diclofenac sodium (di-klo′fen-ak) chemical name: 2-[(2,6-dichlorophenyl)amino]benzeneacetic acid monosodium salt. An analgesic, antipyretic, and anti-inflammatory, $C_{14}H_{10}Cl_2NNaO_2$, used in the treatment of rheumatic and other inflammatory disorders.

dicloralurea (di″klor-al″u-re′ah)· chemical name: *N,N′*-bis-2,2,2-trichloro-1-hydroxyethyl)urea; a food additive for animal feed, $C_5H_6Cl_6N_2O_3$.

dicloxacillin sodium (di-kloks″ah-sil′in) [USP] chemical name: [2*S*-(2α,5α,6β)]-6[[3-(2,6-dichlorophenyl)-5-methyl-4-isoxazolyl]carbonyl] amino]-3,3-dimethyl-7-oxo-4-thia-1-azabicyclo[3.-2.0]heptane-2-carboxylic acid monosodium salt monohydrate. A semisynthetic penicillinase-resistant penicillin, $C_{19}H_{16}Cl_2N_3Na$-$O_5S\cdot H_2O$, occurring as a white to off-white, crystalline powder; used primarily in the treatment of infections due to penicillinase-resistant staphylococci, administered orally. It is also available as *sterile dicloxacillin sodium* [USP].

Dicodid (di-ko′did) trademark for preparations of hydrocodone bitartrate.

dicoelous (di-se′lus) [*di-* + Gr. *koilos* hollow] 1. hollowed on each of two sides. 2. having two cavities.

dicophane (di′ko-fān) chlorophenothane.

dicoria (di-ko′re-ah) [*di-* + Gr. *korē* pupil] doubleness of the pupil.

dicotyledon (di-kot″ĭ-le′don) [Gr. *dis* twice + *kotylēdon* a cup-shaped hollow] a flowering plant with embryos having two seed leaves, or cotyledons.

dicoumarin (di-koo′mah-rin) dicumarol.

dicroceliasis (dik″ro-se-li′ah-sis) infection with *Dicrocoelium*.

Dicrocoelium (dik″ro-se′le-um) [Gr. *dikroos* forked + *koilia* bowel] a genus of trematodes. **D. dendrit′icum,** a lancet-shaped fluke infesting the liver of cattle and sheep in Europe, North and South America, and northern Africa; it has been found in the human bilary passages. **D. hos′pes,** a species found in the gallbladder of cattle in the Soudan. **D. lanceola′tum,** *D. dendriticum.* **D. macrosto′mum,** a species found in the gallbladder of guinea fowl in Egypt.

dicrotic (di-krot′ik) [Gr. *dikrotos* double beating] pertaining to or characterized by dicrotism, as the dicrotic notch.

dicrotism (di′krŏ-tizm) the quality of having two sphygmographic waves or elevations to one beat of the pulse.

Dictyocaulus (dik″te-o-kaw′lus) a genus of nematode parasites of the bronchial tree of horses, sheep, goats, deer, and cattle. **D. fila′ria,** a species that infects the bronchial tree of sheep, goats, and cattle, and causes hoose; called also *Strongylus filaria.* **D. vivipa′rus,** a species that infects the bronchial tree of cattle and deer, and causes hoose; called also *Strongylus micrurus.*

dictyokinesis (dik″te-o-ki-ne′sis) [Gr. *diktyon* net + *kinēsis* movement] the migration and distribution of the dictyosomes to the daughter cells in mitosis.

dictyoma (dik″te-o′mah) [Gr. *diktyon* net (retina) + *-oma*] diktyoma.

dictyosome (dik′te-o-sōm) [Gr. *diktyon* net + *soma* body] a stack of membranous lamellae or cisternae with attached tubules and vesicles in the cytoplasm of various cells; see also *Golgi complex,* under *complex.*

dictyotene (dik′te-o-tēn) [Gr. *diktyon* net + *-tene*] the protracted stage resembling suspended prophase in which the primary oocyte persists from late fetal life until discharged from the ovary at or after puberty.

dicumarol (di-koo′mah-rol) [USP] chemical name: 3,3′-methylenebis[4-hydroxy-2*H*-1-benzopyran-2-one]. One of the coumarin anticoagulants, $C_{19}H_{12}O_6$, occurring as a white or creamy white, crystalline powder, originally isolated from spoiled sweet clover but now produced synthetically; it acts by inhibiting the hepatic synthesis of vitamin K–dependent coagulation factors (prothrombin, Factors II, VII, IX, and X); administered orally. It is the etiologic agent of the hemorrhagic disease in animals known as *sweet clover disease.* Called also *bishydroxycoumarin* and *dicoumarin.*

Dicurin (di-kur′in) trademark for a preparation of merethoxylline.

dicyclic (di-si′klik) pertaining to or having two cycles; in chemistry, having a molecular structure containing two rings.

dicyclomine hydrochloride (di-si′klo-mēn) [USP] chemical name: [bicyclohexyl]-1-carboxylic acid 2-(diethylamino)ethyl ester. An anticholinergic, $C_{19}H_{35}NO_2\cdot HCl$, occurring as a fine, white, crystalline powder; used as an antispasmodic in the treatment of functional gastrointestinal disorders, administered orally or intramuscularly.

dicysteine (di′sis-te′in) cystine.

didactic (di-dak′tik) [Gr. *didaktikos*] conveying instruction by lectures and books rather than by practice.

didactylism (di-dak′til-izm) [*di-* + Gr. *daktylos* finger] the condition of having only two digits on a hand or foot.

didactylous (di-dak′tĭ-lus) having only two digits on a hand or foot.

didelphia (di-del′fe-ah) [*di-* + Gr. *delphys* uterus] the condition characterized by presence of a double uterus.

didelphic (di-del′fik) pertaining to or possessing a double uterus.

Didelphis (di-del′fis) [*di-* + Gr. *delphys* uterus] a genus of marsupials, the opossums, species of which are reservoirs of *Trypanosoma cruzi* in South America.

didermoma (di″der-mo′mah) bidermoma.

Didrex (di′dreks) trademark for a preparation of benzphetamine hydrochloride.

didymalgia (did″ĭ-mal′je-ah) orchialgia.

didymitis (did″ĭ-mi′tis) orchitis.

didymodynia (did″ĭ-mo-din′e-ah) orchialgia.

didymous (did′ĭ-mus) occurring in pairs.

didymus (did′ĭ-mus) [Gr. *didymos* double, twofold, twain] a testis. Sometimes used as a word termination to designate a fetus with a duplication of parts or one consisting of conjoined symmetrical twins. See also *-pagus.*

die (di) a form to be used in the construction of something, as a positive reproduction of the form of a prepared tooth in a suitable hard substance, such as metal or a specially prepared artificial stone. See *counterdie.* **amalgam d.,** a model of a tooth in silver or copper amalgam, used for making an inlay or crown. **plated d.,** one formed by electroplating the surface of an impression with copper or silver. **stone d.,** a positive reproduction of a tooth or other structure, created in artificial stone, for use in making a dental prosthesis.

Dieb. alt. abbreviation for L. *die′bus alter′nis,* on alternate days.

Dieb. tert. abbreviation for L. *die′bus ter′tiis,* every third day.

diechoscope (di-ek′o-skōp) [*di-* + Gr. *ēchō* echo + *skopein* to examine] an instrument for the simultaneous perception of two different sounds in auscultation.

diecious (di-e′shus) [*di-* + Gr. *oikos* house] sexually distinct; denoting species in which male and female genitals do not occur in the same individual. In botany, having staminate and pistillate flowers on separate plants.

Dieffenbach's amputation, operation (de′fen-bahks) [Johann Friedrich *Dieffenbach,* Prussian surgeon, 1792–1847] see under *operation.*

dieldrin (di-el′drin) chemical name: 3,4,5,6,9,9-hexachloro-1a,2,2a,3,6,6a,7,7a-octahydro-2,7:3,6-dimethanonaphth[2,3-*b*]oxirene. A chlorinated insecticide, $C_{12}H_8Cl_6O$, of particular value against the sheep tick *Melophagus ovinus,* and also used to control vectors of insect-borne diseases, especially mosquitoes. Inhalation, ingestion, or skin contact with dieldrin may cause poisoning.

dielectric (di″ĕ-lek′trik) transmitting electric effects by induction, but not by conduction. The term is applied to an insulating substance through or across which electric force is acting or may act, by induction without conduction.

dielectrolysis (di″e-lek-trol′ĭ-sis) [Gr. *dia* through + *electrolysis*] electrolysis of a drug, the current being passed through a diseased portion of the body, so that the drug passes through the part.

diembryony (di-em′bre-on″e) [*di-* + *embryon* embryo] the production of two embryos from a single egg.

diencephalic (di″en-se-fal′ik) pertaining to the diencephalon.

diencephalohypophysial (di″en-sef″ah-lo-hi″po-fiz′e-al) pertaining to the diencephalon and the pituitary gland.

diencephalon (di″en-sef′ah-lon) [*dia-* + Gr. *enkephalos* brain] 1. [NA] the posterior part of the prosencephalon, consisting of the hypothalamus and thalamus (including the epithalamus); the subthalamus is often recognized as a distinct division. Called also *betweenbrain* and *'tween brain.* See Plate accompanying *brain.* See also *brain stem,* under *B.* 2. the posterior of the two brain vesicles formed by specialization of the prosencephalon in the developing embryo.

-diene a suffix used in chemistry to denote an unsaturated hydrocarbon containing two double bonds.

diener (de′ner) [Ger. "man-servant"] a man-of-all-work in a laboratory.

dienestrol (di″ēn-es′trol) [USP] chemical name: 4,4′-(1,2-diethylidene-1,2-ethanediyl)bisphenol. A synthetic estrogen, C_{18}-$H_{18}O_2$, occurring as colorless, white, or practically white, needle-like crystals or as a white or practically white, crystalline powder; administered orally in the management of menopausal symptoms, in the treatment of functional uterine bleeding, as a postpartum antigalactagogue, for palliative therapy in certain female breast cancers, and in the management of prostatic carcinoma, and applied locally in the treatment of postmenopausal and senile vulvovaginitis, atrophic vaginitis, pruritus vulvae due to atrophic changes in the vulval epithelium, dyspareunia associated with atrophic vaginal epithelium, and prior to plastic pelvic surgery in menopausal patients.

Dientamoeba (di″ent-ah-me′bah) a genus of small protozoa of the class Sarcodina, order Amoebida, commonly found in the colon and appendix of man; it possesses one or two vesicular nuclei with endosomes made up of several chromatin granules. **D. frag′i-**

lis, a possibly pathogenic species which has been associated with diarrhea; it is not known to cause ulceration of the bowel.

dieresis (di-er'ĕsis) [Gr. *diairesis* a taking] 1. the division or separation of parts normally united. 2. in surgery, the operative separation of parts by incision, electrosurgery, or cautery.

diesophagus (di-e-sof'ah-gus) doubling of the esophagus.

diestrum (di-es'trum) diestrus.

diestrus (di-es'trus) a short period of sexual quiescence occurring between metestrus and proestrus in female mammals. **gestational d.,** the period of sexual inactivity occurring during gestation in female mammals. **lactational d.,** the period of sexual inactivity occurring during lactation in female mammals.

diet (di'et) [Gr. *diaita* way of living] the customary allowance of food and drink taken by any person from day to day, particularly one especially planned to meet specific requirements of the individual, and including or excluding certain items of food. **absolute d.,** fasting. **acid-ash d.,** a diet to produce acidification of the urine, consisting of meat, fish, eggs and cereals, with little fruit and vegetables and no cheese or milk; used in prophylaxis of some types of urolithiasis. **adequate d.,** one that enables an animal to grow, mature, and reproduce in a normal manner. Cf. *optimal d.* **alkali-ash d.,** a diet of fruit, vegetables, and milk with as little as possible of meat, fish, eggs, and cereals. **balanced d.,** one containing all the nutritive factors in proper proportion for adequate nutrition. **Banting d.,** see under *treatment.* **basal d.,** one which is just sufficient to meet the caloric requirements of basal metabolism. **basic d.,** a diet which contains a preponderant proportion of alkaline ash; used for some types of urinary calculus. **bland d.,** one that is free from any irritating or stimulating foods. **Coleman-Shaffer d.,** a diet once used in typhoid fever, composed of eggs, cream, cocoa, milk sugar, and bread and butter; it has a high carbohydrate ratio and is rich in protein. The food is administered in small quantities, but frequently. **diabetic d.,** a diet prescribed in the treatment of diabetes mellitus, usually limited in the amount of sugar or readily available carbohydrate. **elemental d.,** one consisting of a well-balanced, residue-free mixture of all essential and nonessential amino acids combined with simple sugars, electrolytes, trace elements, and vitamins. **elimination d.,** a procedure to identify food allergy in which foods are sequentially omitted in order to detect the one or ones responsible for symptoms. **Feingold d.,** a diet proposed for hyperactive children which excludes artificial colors, artificial flavors, preservatives, and salicylates. **Giordano-Giovannetti d.,** a low protein diet given to alleviate gastrointestinal symptoms of chronic renal failure. **gluten-free d.,** a diet deficient in the cereal protein gluten; used as a specific treatment for celiac disease (gluten enteropathy). **gouty d.,** one for mitigation of gout, restricting nitrogenous, especially high-purine foods, and substituting dairy products, with prohibition of wines and liquors. **high calorie d.,** one that furnishes more calories than needed for the maintenance of weight, often more than 3500–4000 calories per day. **high fat d.,** ketogenic d. **high fiber d.,** one relatively high in dietary fibers, which decreases bowel transit time and relieves constipation. **high protein d.,** one containing large amounts of protein, consisting largely of meats, fish, milk, legumes, and nuts. **Karell d.,** a diet for nephritis and cardiac conditions, consists of 800 ml. of milk per day; the milk diet, running from six days to a week, is amplified gradually by the use of eggs, dry toast, meat, rice, and vegetables. **Keith's low ionic d.,** a diet for chronic nephritis based on decrease in the water content, reduction of the amount of sodium, and the minimum water content kept constant from day to day. **Kempner's d.,** a diet consisting of only rice, fruit juices, and sugar, supplemented with vitamins and iron; for hypertension and chronic renal disease. **ketogenic d.,** one containing a large amount of fat with minimal amounts of protein and carbohydrate, the object of such a diet being to produce ketosis; called also *high fat d.* **light d.,** a simple mixed diet suitable for convalescents. **low calorie d.,** one containing fewer calories than needed for the maintenance of weight, e.g., less than 1200 calories per day for an adult. **low fat d.,** one containing limited amounts of fat. **low oxalate d.,** one with no potatoes, beans, or fiber vegetables, and no sweet fruit, tea, chocolate, or sweets; used for the prevention of oxalate stones in the urinary tract. **low purine d.,** one for mitigation of gout, omitting meat, fowl, and fish and substituting milk, eggs, cheese, and vegetable protein. **low residue d.,** a diet which gives the least possible fecal residue: such as gelatin, sucrose, dextrose, broth, hard-boiled egg, meat, liver, rice, and cottage cheese. **low salt d.,** a diet which contains very little sodium chloride; prescribed by some for hypertension and for edematous states. **Meulengracht d.,** a full-feeding diet for peptic ulcer. **Minot-Murphy d.,** see under *treatment.* **Moro-Heisler d.,** a diet of grated raw apple for diarrheal conditions in infants. **optimal d.,** a diet that produces the most desirable growth, the most successful reproduction, and the maintenance of the best possible health; Cf. *adequate d.* **Petrén's d.,** a diet once used to diabetics, consisting of extremely small amounts of protein and carbohydrate and very large amounts of fat, chiefly butter. **protein-sparing d.,** one consisting only of liquid proteins or liquid mixtures of proteins,

vitamins, and minerals, and containing no more than 600 calories; it is designed to maintain a favorable nitrogen balance. **provocative d.,** a diet designed to include the most common allergenic foods, from which they are eliminated one by one, as a means of determining the offending substances in cases of food allergy. **purine-free d.,** see *low-purine d.* **rachitic d.,** an inadequate diet which will bring about rickets in an experimental animal. The animal is kept in a room from which all daylight is excluded and the diet consists of whole wheat flour, 33 per cent; yellow maize, 33 per cent; wheat gluten, 15 per cent; gelatin powder, 15 per cent; calcium carbonate, 3 per cent; sodium chloride, 1 per cent; and tap water, ad libitum. **rice d.,** Kempner's d. **salt-free d.,** see *low-salt d.* **Schemm d.,** a low-sodium, neutral and acid-ash diet for patients with congestive heart failure. **Schmidt d.,** a daily diet consisting of 1.5 liters of milk, 100 gm. of zwieback, 2 eggs, 50 gm. of butter, 125 gm. of beef, 190 gm. of boiled potato, and gruel made from 80 gm. of oatmeal. It contains 102 gm. of protein, 111 gm. of fat, and 191 gm. of carbohydrate, supplying 2234 calories. It is used to facilitate examination of the stools in diarrhea of various causation. **Schmidt-Strassburger d.,** Schmidt d. **Sippy d.,** a diet for peptic ulcer and for conditions in which the patient is unable to take bulky foods. It consists of nothing but milk and cream for the first few days, with the addition of crackers, cereals, and eggs on the third day; the amounts increasing gradually until during the later days of the diet puréed vegetables are included. On the twenty-eighth day the patient is placed on the regular ward diet. **smooth d.,** one which avoids the use of foods containing roughage. **subsistence d.,** a diet on which one can just live. **Taylor's d.,** a preparation of white of egg, olive oil, and sugar, given when the urine is to be tested for chlorides. **Wilder's d.,** a low-potassium diet formerly used in Addison's disease.

dietary (di'ĕ-ta"re) a regular or systematic scheme of diet.

dietetic (di"ĕ-tet'ik) [Gr. *diaitetikos*] pertaining to diet or proper food.

dietetics (di"ĕ-tet'iks) the science or study and regulation of the diet.

diethazine hydrochloride (di-eth'ah-zēn) chemical name: *N,N*-diethyl-10*H*-phenothiazine-10-ethanamine hydrochloride. An anticholinergic, $C_{18}H_{23}ClN_2S$, which has been used as an antiparkinsonian agent.

diethylamine (di"eth-il-am'in) a nonpoisonous liquid ptomaine, $NH(C_2H_5)_2$, from decaying fish and putrid sausages.

diethylcarbamazine citrate (di-eth"il-kar-bam'ah-zēn) [USP] chemical name: *N,N*-diethyl-4-methyl-1-piperazinecarboxamide. An antifilarial agent, $C_{10}H_{21}N_3O \cdot C_6H_8O_7$, occurring as a white crystalline powder, highly effective against microfilariae of certain nematodes, such as *Wuchereria bancrofti, Loa loa,* and *Onchocerca volvulus;* administered orally.

diethylene diamine (di-eth"il-ēn di-am'in) piperazine.

diethylmalonylurea (di-eth"il-mal"o-nil-u-re'ah) (obs.) barbital.

diethylpropion hydrochloride (di-eth'il-pro'pe-on) [USP] chemical name: 2-(diethylamino)-1-phenyl-1-propanone hydrochloride. An adrenergic, $C_{13}H_{19}NO \cdot HCl$, structurally related to amphetamine, methamphetamine, and ephedrine, occurring as a white to off-white, fine crystalline powder; used as an anorexic, administered orally.

diethylstilbestrol (di-eth"il-stil-bes'trol) [USP] chemical name: (*E*)-4,4'-(1,2-diethyl-1,2-ethenediyl)bis-phenol. A synthetic nonsteroidal estrogen, $C_{18}H_{20}O_2$, occurring as a white, crystalline powder, having estrogenic activity similar to but greater than that of estrone. It is used for many purposes, e.g., to relieve menopausal symptoms, to suppress lactation, in amenorrhea, dysmenorrhea, senile vaginitis, and pruritus vulvae, in the palliative treatment of female breast carcinoma, and to relieve the symptoms of prostatic carcinoma; administered orally, intravaginally, or intramuscularly. Formerly used to prevent threatened or habitual abortion and premature labor. Women who have been exposed *in utero* to diethylstilbestrol show characteristic changes in the cervix and vagina and are subject to an increased risk of vaginal or cervical carcinoma. Called also *estrostilben* and *stilbestrol.* **d. diphosphate** [USP], an ester of diethylstilbestrol, $C_{18}H_{22}O_8P_2$, occurring as an off-white, crystalline powder, having the same actions as the base; used in the treatment of prostatic carcinoma, administered intravenously. **d. dipropionate,** an ester of diethylstilbestrol, $C_{24}H_{28}O_4$, occurring as a white, crystalline powder, having actions and uses similar to those of the base; administered orally, intravaginally, or intramuscularly.

diethyltoluamide (di-eth"il-tol-u'ah-mīd) [USP] chemical name: *N,N*-diethyl-3-methylbenzamide. An arthropod repellent, $C_{12}H_{17}NO$, occurring as a colorless liquid; applied topically to the skin and to the clothing.

diethyltryptamine (di-eth"il-trip'tah-min) chemical name: N_2N-diethyltryptamine. A hallucinogenic substance closely related to dimethyltryptamine, but prepared synthetically. Abbreviated DET.

dietitian (di-ĕ-tish'an) a person trained in the scientific use of diet in health and disease.

Dietl's crisis (de′tlz) [Józef *Dietl*, physician in Cracow, 1804–1878] see under *crisis.*

dietotherapy (di″ĕ-to-ther′ah-pe) dietetic treatment.

dietotoxic (di″ĕ-to-tok′sik) having the quality of dietotoxicity.

dietotoxicity (di″ĕ-to-tok-sis′ĭ-te) a quality in certain food substances which renders them toxic when used in an unbalanced diet.

Dieudonné's medium (agar, culture) (dyuh-don-āz′) [Adolf *Dieudonné*, serologist in Munich, 1864–1945] see under *culture medium.*

Dieulafoy's aspirator, theory, triad (dyuh-lah-fwahz′) [Georges *Dieulafoy*, physician in Paris, 1839–1911] see under *aspirator, theory,* and *triad.*

difenoxamide hydrochloride (di″fen-oks′ah-mīd) chemical name: 4-[[(2,5-dioxo-1-pyrrolidinyl)oxy]carbonyl]-α,α,4-triphenyl-1-piperidinebutanenitrile monohydrochloride; an antiperistaltic, $C_{32}H_{31}N_3O_4 \cdot HCl$.

difenoxin (di″fen-oks′in) chemical name: 1-(3-cyano-3,3-diphenylpropyl)-4-phenylisonipecotic acid; an antiperistaltic, $C_{28}H_{28}N_2O_2$.

differential (dif″er-en′shal) [L. *differre* to carry apart] pertaining to a difference or differences.

differentiate (dif″er-en′she-āt) 1. to distinguish, on the bases of differences. 2. to develop specialized form, character, or function differing from that of surrounding cytoplasm, cells, or tissue or from the original type.

differentiation (dif″er-en″she-a′shun) 1. the distinguishing of one thing or disease from another. 2. the act or process of acquiring completely individual characters, as occurs in the progressive diversification of cells and tissues of the embryo. 3. increase in morphological or chemical heterogeneity. **correlative d.,** differentiation caused by factors outside the tissue itself, as by an inductor; called also *dependent d.* **dependent d.,** correlative d. **functional d.,** differentiation which results from the functioning of the tissue of a part. **invisible d.,** the development toward a fixed fate, through chemodifferentiation, by cells that show no visible signs of this determination. **regional d.,** the appearance of regional differences within a field of development. **self d.,** differentiation produced by factors solely within the tissue or part.

diffluence (dif′loo-ens) the act of becoming fluid or of flowing readily.

diffluent (dif′loo-ent) [L. *diffluere* to flow off] easily flowing away or dissolving; deliquescent; temporary.

diffraction (dĭ-frak′shun) [L. *dis-* apart + *frangere* to break] the bending or breaking up into its component parts of a ray of light. **d. grating,** a strip of glass ruled closely with fine lines for use in the spectroscope. **x-ray d.,** a technique for studying the cell based on the diffraction of radiations when they encounter small obstacles; used especially in the study of inorganic and organic crystals, in which it is possible to determine the precise spatial relationships between the constituent atoms.

diffusate (dĭ-fu′zāt) material that has passed through a membrane.

diffuse (dĭ-fūs′) [L. *dis-* apart + *fundere* to pour] 1. not definitely limited or localized; widely distributed. 2. (dĭ-fūz′) to pass through or to spread widely through a tissue or structure.

diffusible (dĭ-fūz′ĭ-b'l) susceptible of becoming widely spread.

diffusiometer (dĭ-fu″ze-om′ĕ-ter) an apparatus for measuring the speed of diffusion.

diffusion (dĭ-fu′zhun) 1. the process of becoming diffused, or widely spread; the spontaneous movement of molecules or other particles in solution, owing to their random thermal motion, to reach a uniform concentration throughout the solvent, a process requiring no addition of energy to the system. 2. dialysis. **double d.,** an immunodiffusion test in which both antigen and antibody diffuse into a common area so that, if the antigen and antibody are interacting, they combine to form bands of precipitate. **exchange d.,** the process in which diffusion of a molecule across a membrane in one direction brings about diffusion of another molecule in the opposite direction. **facilitated d.,** diffusion across a cell membrane or other biological membrane in which the molecules to be transported form complexes with specific carriers in the membrane, are shuttled across the membrane by the complex, and then released on the other side. **free d.,** diffusion in which there is no obstacle such as a membrane. **gel d.,** a test in which antigen and antibody diffuse toward one another through a gel medium to form a precipitate. **impeded d.,** diffusion in which the rate is slowed down by the difficulty of passing through a membrane.

diflorasone diacetate (di-flor′ah-sōn) chemical name: 17,21-bis(acetyloxy)-6α,9-difluoro-11β-hydroxy-16β-methylpregna-1,4-diene-3,20-dione; a topical corticosteroid, $C_{26}H_{32}F_2O_7$, used as a cream or ointment in treatment of certain dermatoses.

difluanine hydrochloride (di-floo′ah-nēn) chemical name: 1-(2-anilinoethyl)-4-[4,4-bis(*p*-fluorophenyl)butyl] piperazine; a central nervous system stimulant, $C_{28}H_{33}F_2N_3 \cdot 3HCl$.

diflucortolone (di″floo-kor′to-lōn) chemical name: 6α,9-di-fluoro-11β,21-dihydroxy-16α-methylpregna-1,4-diene-3, 20-dione; a glucocorticoid, $C_{22}H_{28}F_2O_4$. **d. pivalate,** the pivalate salt of diflucortolone, a glucocorticoid.

diflumidone sodium (di-floo′mĭ-dōn) chemical name: 3′-benzoyl-1,1-difluoromethanesulfonanilide sodium salt; an anti-inflammatory agent, $C_{14}H_{10}F_2NNaO_3S$.

diflunisal (di-floo′nĭ-sil) chemical name: 2′,4′-difluoro-4-hydroxy-[1,1′-biphenyl]-3-carboxylic acid; an anti-inflammatory, $C_{13}H_8F_2O_3$.

difluprednate (di-floo-pred′nāt) chemical name: 6α,9-difluoro-11β,17,21-trihydroxypregna-1,4-diene-3,20-dione 21-acetate 17-butyrate; an anti-inflammatory agent, $C_{27}H_{34}F_2O_7$.

diftalone (dif′tah-lōn) chemical name: phthalazino[2,3-*b*]phthalazine-5,12-(7*H*,14*H*)-dione; an anti-inflammatory, $C_{16}H_{12}N_2O_2$.

Dig. abbreviation for L. *digera′tur*, let it be digested.

digametic (di″gah-met′ik) 1. pertaining to or producing gametes or sex cells of two different types, female (ova) and male (spermatozoa). 2. heterogametic.

digastric (di-gas′trik) [*di-* + Gr. *gastēr* belly] 1. having two bellies. 2. musculus digastricus.

digenesis (di-jen′ĕ-sis) alternation of generation.

digenetic (di″jĕ-net′ik) [*di-* + Gr. *genesis* generation] having two stages of multiplication, one sexual in the mature forms, the other asexual in the larval stages; said of flukes and many other parasites.

digestant (di-jes′tant) 1. assisting or stimulating digestion. 2. an agent that assists or stimulates digestion.

digestion (di-jest′yun) [L. *digestio*, from *dis-* apart + *gerere* to carry] 1. the process or act of converting food into chemical substances that can be absorbed and assimilated. 2. the subjection of a body to prolonged heat and moisture, so as to disintegrate and soften it. **artificial d.,** that which is performed outside the body. **biliary d.,** the digestive effect of the bile upon food. **gastric d.,** that which is carried on in the stomach by aid of the gastric juice; called also *peptic d.* and *chymification.* **gastrointestinal d.,** the gastric and intestinal digestions together; called also *primary d.* **intercellular d.,** digestion carried on within an organ by secretions from the cells of the organ. **intestinal d.,** that which is carried on in the intestine. **intracellular d.,** digestion carried on within a single cell. **lipolytic d.,** the splitting of fat into fatty acid and glycerol. **pancreatic d.,** that which is performed by the pancreatic secretion. **parenteral d.,** digestion taking place somewhere else in the body than in the alimentary canal, as in the blood or under the skin. **peptic d.,** gastric d. **primary d.,** gastrointestinal d. **salivary d.,** the change of starch into maltose by the saliva. **sludge d.,** the biochemical process by which organic matter in sludge is gasified, liquefied, mineralized, or converted into more stable organic matter.

digestive (di-jes′tiv) 1. pertaining to digestion. 2. digestant.

digit (dij′it) [L. *digitus*] a finger or toe.

digital (dij′ĭ-tal) 1. of, pertaining to, or performed with, a finger. 2. resembling the imprint of a finger. 3. pertaining to numerical methods or discrete variables.

digitalin (dij″ĭ-tal′in) 1. true digitalin; a cardiac glycoside, $C_{36}H_{56}O_{14}$, from the seeds of *Digitalis purpurea.* 2. any of several mixtures of digitalis glycosides extracted from the leaves or seeds.

Digitaline Nativelle (dij″ĭ-tal′ēn na″tĭ-vel′) trademark for a preparation of digitoxin.

Digitalis (dij″ĭ-ta′lis) [L. from *digitus* finger, because of the finger-like leaves of the corolla of its flowers] a genus of herbs. *D. purpu′rea* is the purple foxglove whose leaves furnish digitalis. *D. lana′ta* is a Balkan species which yields digoxin and lanatoside.

digitalis (dij″ĭ-tal′is) 1. [USP] the dried leaf of *Digitalis purpurea*, the purple foxglove, the main systemic effects of which are manifested by an increase in the strength of the heart beat while decreasing its rate. When digitalis is prescribed *powdered digitalis* (see below) is to be dispensed. Called also *d. leaf.* 2. [NA] a general term for any finger-like structure. **d. leaf,** digitalis (def. 1). **powdered d.** [USP], **prepared d.,** the standardized preparation to be dispensed when digitalis is prescribed; principally used in the treatment of congestive heart failure but also used in other cardiac disorders, administered orally.

digitalization (dij″ĭ-tal-i-za′shun) the administration of digitalis in a dosage schedule designed to produce and then maintain optimal therapeutic concentrations of its cardiotonic glycosides.

digitaloid (dij″ĭ-tal-oid) resembling or related to digitalis.

digitalose (dij″ĭ-tal-ōs) a hexose sugar, 6-desoxy-*d*-allose, $CH_3(CHOH_3)CH(O \cdot CH_3) \cdot CHO$, from digitalin.

digitate (dij′ĭ-tāt) having several finger-like processes.

digitatio (dij″ĭ-ta′she-o), pl. *digitatio′nes* [L.] a finger-like process. **digitatio′nes hippocam′pi,** see *pes hippocampi.*

digitation (dij″ĭ-ta′shun) 1. a finger-like process, as of a muscle. 2. surgical creation of a functioning digit by making a cleft between two adjacent metacarpal bones, after amputation of some or all of the fingers.

digitationes (dij″ĭ-ta″she-o′nez) [L.] plural of *digitatio*.

digiti (dij′ĭ-ti) [L.] plural of *digitus*.

digitiform (dij′ĭ-tĭ-form) resembling a finger; finger-like.

digitigrade (dij′ĭ-tĭ-grād″) [L. *digitus* finger or toe + *gradi* to walk] characterized by walking on the toes; applied to animals whose digits only touch the ground, the posterior part of the foot being more or less raised, such as horses and cattle. Cf. *plantigrade*.

digitogenin (dij″ĭ-toj′ĕ-nin) a sapogenin, $C_{27}H_{44}O_5$, from digitonin.

digitonin (dij″ĭ-to′nin) [USP] a saponin, $C_{55}H_{90}O_{29}$, from *Digitalis purpurea*, which possesses no cardiotonic action; used as a reagent to precipitate free cholesterol.

digitoplantar (dij″ĭ-to-plan′tar) [L. *digitus* finger or toe + *planta* sole] pertaining to the toes and the sole of the foot.

digitoxin (dij″ĭ-tok′sin) [USP] chemical name: 3β-[(O-2,6-dideoxy-β-D-*ribo*-hexopyranosyl-(1 → 4)-O-2,6-dideoxy-β-D-*ribo*-hexopyranosyl-(1→4)-2,6-dideoxy-β-D-*ribo*-hexopyranosyl)oxy]-14-hydroxy-card-5β-20(22)-enolide. A cardiac glycoside, $C_{41}H_{64}$- O_{13}, obtained for *Digitalis purpurea, D. lanata,* and other *Digitalis* species, occurring as a white or pale buff, microcrystalline powder. It has actions and uses similar to thɔse of digitalis, administered orally, intramuscularly, or intravenously.

digitoxose (dij″ĭ-tok′sōs) a hexose sugar, $CH_3(CHOH)_3CH_2$- CHO, derived from several of the digitalis glycosides.

digitus (dij′ĭ-tus), pl. *dig′iti* [L.] digit: a finger or a toe. **d. anula′ris** [NA], the fourth digit, or ring finger, of the hand. **d. hippocrat′icus,** clubbed finger. **d. I,** the first digit; NA alternative for *hallux* (great toe) and *pollex* (thumb). **d. II,** 1. [NA] the second digit of the hand. 2. NA alternative for *index* (finger). **d. III,** 1. [NA] the third digit of the foot. 2. NA alternative for *d. medius.* **d. IV,** 1. [NA] the fourth digit of the foot. 2. NA alternative for *d. anularis.* **d. mal′leus,** mallet finger. **dig′iti ma′nus** [NA], the digits of the hand; the fingers. **d. me′dius** [NA], the middle, or third, finger of the hand. **d. min′imus** [NA], the fifth digit of the hand or foot; the little finger (*d. minimus manus*) or toe (*d. minimus pedis*). **d. mor′tuus** [L. "dead finger"], a numb, mottled finger, as seen in acrocyanosis; called also *waxy* or *white finger.* **dig′iti pe′dis** [NA], the digits of the foot; the toes. **d. postmin′imus,** an appendage ranging from a small round mass of fat and connective tissue to a longer mass containing bones and with a nail at its distal end, attached by a small pedicle to the soft tissue covering the lateral surface of the little finger or toe. **d. recel′lens** (*obs.*), trigger finger. **d. V,** the fifth digit of the hand or foot; NA alternative for *d. minimus.* **d. val′gus,** deviation of a digit in the radial direction, or toward the digit of next higher number. **d. va′rus,** deviation of a digit in the ulnar direction, or toward the digit of next lower number.

diglossia (di-glos′e-ah) [*di-* + Gr. *glōssa* tongue] bifid tongue.

diglutathione (di-glu″tah-thi′ōn) an oxidized form of glutathione.

diglyceride (di-glis′er-id) a glyceride containing two fatty acid molecules in ester linkage.

dignathus (dig-na′thus) [*di-* + Gr. *gnathos* jaw] a monster with two lower jaws.

digoxin (di-goks′in) [USP] chemical name: 3β-[(O-2,6-dideoxy-β-D-*ribo*-hexopyranosyl-(1→4)-O-2,6-dideoxy-β-D-*ribo*-hexopyranosyl-(1 → 4)-2,6-dideoxy-β-*ribo*-hexopyranosyl)oxy]-12β,14-dihydroxy-card-5β-20(22)-enolide. A cardiotonic glycoside, $C_{41}H_{64}O_{14}$, obtained from the leaves of *Digitalis lanata,* occurring as clear to white crystals or white crystalline powder. It may be used for the same purposes as digitalis, administered orally, intramuscularly, or intravenously.

Digramma brauni (di-gram′ah braw′ni) a larval tapeworm belonging to the family Diphyllobothriidae, reported from man in Roumania; formerly called *Diplogonoporus brauni.*

digyny (di′jĕ-ne) [*di-*(1) + Gr. *gynē* woman] triploidy in which the extra haploid set is of maternal origin.

diheterozygote (di-het″er-o-zi′gōt) an individual heterozygous for two pairs of genes.

dihexyverine hydrochloride (di″heks-ĭ-ver′ēn) chemical name: 2-piperidinoethyl ester of bicyclohexyl-1-carboxylic acid hydrochloride; an anticholinergic, $C_{20}H_{35}NO_2 \cdot HCl$, which has been used as an antispasmodic in uterine hypermotility and intestinal muscle spasm.

dihomocinchonine (di-ho″mo-sin′ko-nin) an alkaloid, $C_{38}H_{44}$- O_2N_4, from cinchona.

dihybrid (di-hi′brid) the offspring of parents who differ in two characters.

dihydrate (di-hi′drāt) [*di-* + Gr. *hydōr* water] 1. any compound containing two hydroxyl groups. 2. any compound containing two molecules of water.

dihydrated (di-hi′drāt-ed) compounded with two molecules of water.

dihydric (di-hi′drik) having two hydrogen atoms in each molecule.

dihydrocholesterol (di-hi″dro-ko-les′ter-ol) cholestanol.

dihydrocodeine (di-hi″dro-ko′dēn) chemical name: 4,5α-epoxy-3-methoxy-17-methylmorphinan-6α-ol: a narcotic analgesic and antitussive, $C_{18}H_{23}NO_3$; called also *drocode.*

dihydrocodeinone bitartrate (di-hi″dro-ko′de-ĭ-nōn) hydrocodone bitartrate.

dihydrocoenzyme I reduced nicotinamide adenine dinucleotide (NAD); see under *dinucleotide.*

dihydrocollidine (di-hi″dro-kol′ĭ-din) an oily base, $C_8H_{11}NH_2$, from decaying flesh and fish; regarded as a ptomaine.

dihydrodiethylstilbestrol (di-hi″dro-di-eth″il-stil-bes′trol) hexestrol.

dihydroergocornine (di-hi″dro-er″go-kor′nin) an ergot derivative that has sympatholytic and adrenolytic properties.

dihydroergocristine (di-hi″dro-er″go-kris′tin) an ergot derivative that has sympatholytic and adrenolytic properties.

dihydroergocryptine (di-hi″dro-er″go-krip′tin) an ergot derivative that has sympatholytic and adrenolytic properties.

dihydroergotamine mesylate (di-hi″dro-er-got′ah-mēn) [USP] chemical name: 9-10-dihydro-12′-hydroxy-2′-methyl-5′α-(phenylmethyl)-ergotaman-3′,6′,18-trione monomethanesulfonate. An antiadrenergic, $C_{34}H_{41}N_5O_8S$, produced by the catalytic hydrogenation of ergotamine; used as a vasoconstrictor in the treatment of migraine.

dihydrofolliculin (di-hi″dro-fol-lik′u-lin) estradiol.

dihydrol (di-hi″drol) the associated water molecule, $(H_2O)_2$.

dihydrolutidine (di-hi″dro-lu′tĭ-din) an oily, poisonous, caustic base, $C_7H_{11}N$, from rancid cod liver oil.

dihydromorphinone (di-hi″dro-mor′fĭ-nōn) hydromorphone hydrochloride.

dihydroporphyrin (di-hi″dro-por′fĭ-rin) the form of porphyrin that, together with iron, acts as the prosthetic heme group of cytochrome *c.*

dihydrostreptomycin (di-hi″dro-strep″to-mi′sin) an antibiotic substance, $C_{21}H_{41}N_7O_{12}$, produced by the hydrogenation of streptomycin; no longer used in medicine because of its toxicity.

dihydrotachysterol (di-hi″dro-tak-is′tĕ-rol) [USP] chemical name: 9,10-secoergosta-5,7,22-trien-3β-ol. A synthetic reduction product of tachysterol, $C_{28}H_{46}O$, occurring as colorless or white crystals, or white, crystalline powder; used as an antihypocalcemic agent in the treatment of hypocalcemic tetany, administered orally. Called also *A.T. 10.*

dihydrotestosterone (di-hi″dro-tes-tos′ter-ōn) 7β-hydroxy-5α-androstan-3-one (DHT), a powerful androgenic hormone, C_{19}- $H_{30}O_2$, formed in peripheral tissue by the action of the enzyme 5α-reductase on testosterone; it is thought to be the essential androgen responsible for external virilization during embryogenesis, for development of most male secondary characteristics at puberty, and for adult male sexual function. A semisynthetic preparation is called *stanolone* (q.v.).

dihydrotheelin (di-hi″dro-the′ĕ-lin) estradiol.

dihydroxyacetone (di″hi-drok″se-as′ĕ-tōn) one of the trioses, the ketotriose, $CH_2OH \cdot CO \cdot CH_2OH$; formed by the oxidation of glycerin with nitric acid; used as a humectant. **d. phosphate,** a triosephosphate, $CH_2OH \cdot CO \cdot CH_2O \cdot PO(OH)_2$, which is produced in the splitting of fructose-1,6-diphosphate in glycolysis.

dihydroxyaluminum (di″hi-drok″se-ah-lu′mĭ-num) an aluminum compound having two hydroxyl groups in the molecule. **d. aminoacetate** [USP], chemical name: (glycinato-*N,O*)dihydroxyaluminum. A basic aluminum salt of aminoacetic acid, $C_2H_6AlNO_4 \cdot xH_2O$, occurring as a white powder; used as a gastric antacid. Available in tablets and as a magma. Called also *aluminum aminoacetate.* **d. sodium carbonate** [USP], chemical name: [carbonato(2-)-*O,O′*]dihydroxy-aluminate(1–)sodium hydrate. An aluminum salt of sodium carbonate, CH_2AlNa- $O_5 \cdot xH_2O$, occurring as a fine, white powder; used as a gastric antacid in tablet form.

dihydroxycholecalciferol (di″hi-drok″se-ko″le-kal-sif′ĕ-rol) a group of active metabolites of cholecalciferol (vitamin D_3) numbered according to the carbon atom(s) on which a hydroxyl group is substituted. 1,25-Dihydroxycholecalciferol, synthesized in the kidney from 25-hydroxycholecalciferol, is the most active derivative; it increases intestinal absorption of calcium and phosphate, enhances bone resorption, and prevents rickets and, because of these activities at sites distant from the site of its synthesis, is considered to be a hormone. Called also *1,25-dihydroxyvitamin D_3.* Another form, *24,25-dihydroxycholeciferol,* is almost inert.

dihydroxyestrin (di-hi″drok′se-es-trin) estradiol.

dihydroxyfluorane (di″hi-drok″se-floo′o-rān) fluorescein.

3,4-dihydroxyphenylalanine (di-hi-drok″se-fen″il-al′ah-nēn) dopa.

dihydroxyvitamin D_3 (di″hi-drok″se-vi′tah-min) see *dihydroxycholecalciferol.*

dihysteria (di″his-te′re-ah) [*di-* + Gr. *hystera* uterus + *-ia*] the condition of having a double uterus.

diiodide (di-i′o-dīd) a combination of a base or a metal with two atoms of iodine.

diiodohydroxyquin (di″i-o″do-hi-drok′se-kwin) iodoquinol.

3,5-diiodothyronine (di″i-o″do-thi′ro-nēn) chemical name: 3-[4-(p-hydroxyphenoxy)-3,5-diiodophenyl] alanine. An organic iodine-containing compound, $C_{15}H_{13}I_2NO_4$, used in the manufacture of thyroxine.

diiodotyrosine (di″i-o″do-ti′ro-sēn) chemical name: 2-amino-3-(3,5-diiodo-4-hydroxyphenol)-proprionic acid. A precursor of the thyroid hormone thyroxine; an organic iodine-containing compound liberated from thyroglobulin by hydrolysis, and thought to be formed by the iodination of monoiodotyrosine. Called also *iodogorgoric acid.*

dikaryon (di-ka′re-on) [*di-* + Gr. *karyon* kernel] a growth stage in the mycelium of fungi, especially Basidiomycetes, in which each cell has two haploid nuclei.

dikaryote (di-kar′e-ōt) a cell having two haploid nuclei.

dikaryotic (di″kar-e-ot′ik) pertaining to the dikaryon or to a dikaryote.

diketone (di-ke′tōn) a ketone containing two carbonyl groups.

diketopiperazine (di-ke″to-pi-per′ah-zin) a closed-ring compound produced by the condensation of two amino acids, the carboxyl group of each combining with the amino group of the other.

diktyoma (dik″te-o′mah) [Gr. *diktyon* net + *-oma*] a benign or malignant tumor of the ciliary epithelium with characteristics resembling those of embryonic retinal tissue.

dikwakwadi (dik″wak-wad′e) witkop.

dil. abbreviation for L. *dil′ue,* dilute or dissolve.

dilaceration (di-las″er-a′shun) [L. *dilaceratio*] a tearing apart, as of a cataract; see *discission.* In dentistry, a condition due to injury to a tooth during its developmental period and characterized by a crease or band at the junction of the crown and root, or by tortuous roots with abnormal curvatures.

Dilantin (di-lan′tin) trademark for preparations of phenytoin.

dilatancy (di-la′tan-se) an unusual behavior observed in cytoplasm (and in some physical systems) during which its viscosity and applied force both increase.

dilatant (di-la′tant) exhibiting dilatancy.

dilatation (dil-ah-ta′shun) 1. the condition, as of an orifice or tubular structure, of being dilated or stretched beyond the normal dimensions. 2. the act of dilating or stretching. **digital d.,** digital dilation. **gastric d.,** d. of the stomach. **d. of the heart,** enlargement of the cavities of the heart, with thinning of its walls. **idiopathic d.,** dilatation of a vessel or other channel, especially of the pulmonary artery, not associated with any other abnormality. **post-stenotic d.,** dilatation of a vessel distal to a stenosed segment or valve, often seen in the pulmonary artery distal to valvular pulmonary stenosis. **prognathic d., prognathion d.,** dilatation of the pyloric end of the stomach greater than that of the fundus, giving a protruding appearance in the roentgen-ray picture. **d. of the stomach,** distention of the stomach with retained secretions, food, and/or gas due to obstruction, ileus, or denervation; called also *gastric d.*

dilatator (dil″ah-ta′tor) [L.] that which dilates, as a muscle.

dilation (di-la′shun) 1. the action of dilating or stretching. 2. dilatation. **digital d.,** the expansion or stretching of a cavity or orifice by means of a finger.

dilator (di-la′tor) 1. [NA] a general term for a structure (muscle) that dilates. 2. an instrument used in enlarging an orifice or canal by stretching. **anal d.,** an instrument for dilating or stretching the anal sphincter. **Arnott's d.,** a distensible cylinder of oiled silk for urethral strictures. **Bailey d.,** an instrument designed especially for use in dilating the aortic valve in cardiac surgery. **Barnes's d.,** see under *bag.* **Einhorn's d.,** a metal dilator used to stretch the cardioesophageal region in cardiospasm. **Hegar's d's,** a series of bougies of varying sizes for dilating the ostium uteri. **Kollmann's d.,** a metallic, expandable urethral dilator. **laryngeal d.,** a bougie-like instrument which is used for distending a stenosed larynx. **Starck d.,** an expandable rubber-covered metal frame used to dilate the cardioesophageal region.

Dilaudid (di-law′did) trademark for preparations of hydromorphone hydrochloride.

dilecanus (di″lĕ-ka′nus) [*di-* + Gr. *lekanē* a dish] dipygus.

Dilepididae (dil″ĕ-pid′ĭ-de) a family of medium-sized or small tapeworms of the order Cyclophyllidea, subclass Cestoda, which parasitize mammals, birds, and snakes. The genus *Dipylidium* is of medical importance.

diltiazem hydrochloride (dil-ti′ah-zem) chemical name: (+)-*cis*-3-(acetyloxy)-5-[2-(dimethylamino)ethyl]-2,3-dihydro-2-4-methoxyphenyl)-1,5-benzothiazepin-4(5H)one monohydrochloride. A coronary vasodilator, $C_{22}N_2O_4S \cdot HCl$, used in the symptomatic treatment of angina of effort.

Diluc. abbreviation for L. *dilu′culo,* at daybreak.

diluent (dil′u-ent) [L. *diluere* to wash] 1. diluting. 2. an agent that dilutes or renders less potent or irritant.

dilut. abbreviation for L. *dilu′tus,* diluted.

dilution (di-lu′shun) 1. the art or process of diluting or the state of being diluted. 2. a diluted or attenuated medicine. 3. in homeopathy, the diffusion of a given quantity of a medicinal agent in ten or one hundred times the same quantity of water. **doubling d.,** a serial dilution in which the dilution in each tube is double that of the preceding tube. **nitrogen d.,** the addition of nitrogen to inspired air to lower its oxygen tension, producing an alveolar oxygen tension equal to a desired oxygen pressure. **serial d.,** 1. the progressive dilution of a substance in a series of tubes in predetermined ratios. 2. a method of obtaining a pure bacterial culture by rapid transfer of an exceedingly small amount of material from one nutrient medium to a succeeding one of the same volume.

dim. abbreviation for L. *dimid′ius,* one half.

dimargarin (di-mar′gar-in) a glyceride having two molecules of margaric acid combined with a molecule of glycerin.

Dimastigamoeba (di-mas″tig-ah-me′bah) *Naegleria.*

dimefadane (di-mef′ah-dān) chemical name: *N,N*-dimethyl-3-phenyl-1-indanamine; an analgesic, $C_{17}H_{19}N$.

dimefilcon A (di″mĕ-fil′kon) chemical name: 2-hydroxyethyl methacrylate polymer with methyl methacrylate and ethylenebis-(oxyethylene)dimethacrylate; a contact lens material (hydrophilic), $(C_6H_{10}O_3)_x \cdot (C_5H_8O_2)_y \cdot (C_{14}H_{22}O_6)_z$.

dimefline hydrochloride (di-mef′lēn) chemical name: 8-[(dimethylamino)methyl]-7-methoxy-3-methylflavone hydrochloride; a respiratory stimulant, $C_{20}H_{21}NO_3 \cdot HCl$.

dimelia (di-me′le-ah) [*di-* + Gr. *melos* limb] a developmental anomaly characterized by duplication of a limb.

dimelus (di-me′lus) a fetus exhibiting dimelia.

dimenhydrinate (di″men-hi′drĭ-nāt) [USP] chemical name: 8-chloro-3,7-dihydro-1,3-dimethyl-1H-purine-2,6-dione compound with 2-(diphenylmethoxy)-*N,N*-dimethylethanamine. An antiemetic, $C_{17}H_{21}NO \cdot C_7H_7ClN_4O_2$, occurring as a white, crystalline powder; used in the treatment of motion sickness and in other conditions in which nausea may be a feature, administered orally.

dimension (dĭ-men′shun) a numerical expression, in appropriate units, of a linear measurement of an object, such as an organ or body part. **vertical d.,** the distance between two points, measured perpendicular to the horizontal. In prosthodontics, the distance between two arbitrarily selected points on the face, one above and one below the mouth, usually in the midline, measured with the jaws in centric occlusion (*occlusal vertical d.*) or in rest position (*rest vertical d.*).

dimer (di′mer) 1. a compound formed by combination of two identical simpler molecules. 2. a capsomer having two structural subunits. **thymine d.,** two adjacent thymine residues linked together by a covalent bond along a single polynucleotide of DNA, which may lead to inactivation of the DNA molecule. It results from exposure to ultraviolet radiation and may be reversed by photoreactivation.

dimercaprol (di″mer-kap′rol) [USP] chemical name: 2,3-dimercaptopropanol. A metal complexing agent, $C_3H_8OS_2$, occurring as a colorless or almost colorless liquid; used as an antidote to poisoning by arsenic, gold, and mercury, and sometimes other metals, administered intramuscularly. It has also been used in the treatment of hepatolenticular degeneration.

dimeric (di′mer-ik) exhibiting the characteristics of a dimer.

dimerous (dim′er-us) [*di-* + Gr. *meros* part] made up of two parts.

dimetallic (di″mĕ-tal′ik) containing two atoms or equivalents of a metallic element in the molecule.

Dimetane (di′mĕ-tān) trademark for preparations of brompheniramine maleate.

dimethicone (di-meth′ĭ-kōn) 1. a silicone oil consisting of dimethylsiloxane polymers with viscosities from 0.65 to 3,000,000 centistokes at 25° C. The term is used with a numeric suffix which indicates the approximate viscosity of the various grades in centistokes, e.g., the viscosity of dimethicone 200 in centistokes is 190 to 210. Dimethicones are used as ingredients of ointments and other preparations for topical application to protect the skin against water-soluble irritants. 2. simethicone. **activated d.,** simethicone. **d. 350,** a grade of dimethicone having a viscosity of approximately 350 in centistokes at 25° C; a prosthetic aid for soft tissues.

dimethindene maleate (di″meth-in′dēn) [USP] chemical name: *N,N*-dimethyl-3-[1-(2-pyridinyl)-1H-indene-2-ethanamine (Z)-2-butenedioate. An antihistaminic, $C_{20}H_{24}N_2 \cdot C_4H_4O_4$, occurring as a white to off-white, crystalline powder; administered orally.

dimethisoquin hydrochloride (di″mĕ-thi′so-kwin) [USP] chemical name: 2-[(3-butyl-1-isoquinolinyl)oxy]-*N,N*-dimethylethanamine monohydrochloride. A local anesthetic, $C_{17}H_{24}N_2O \cdot HCl$, occurring as a white to off-white, crystalline powder; applied topically to relieve pain, itching, and burning of the skin.

dimethisterone (di″meth-is′ter-ōn) chemical name: 17-hydroxy-6-methyl-17-(1-propynyl)androst-4-en-3-one monohydrate. An orally effective progestin, $C_{23}H_{32}O_2 \cdot H_2O$, occurring as a white, crystalline powder, having actions and uses similar to those of progesterone; used alone or as the progestin component in combination with ethinyl estradiol as an oral contraceptive.

dimethoxanate hydrochloride (di″mě-thok′sĭ-nāt) chemical name: 10H-phenothiazine-10-carboxylic acid 2-[2-(dimethylamino)ethoxy]ethyl ester hydrochloride; an antitussive, $C_{19}H_{22}N_2O_3S \cdot HCl$.

2,5-dimethoxy-4-methylamphetamine (di″mě-thok″se-meth″il-am-fet′ah-mēn) a hallucinogenic compound derived from amphetamine; abbreviated DOM and popularly called STP.

3,4-dimethoxyphenylethylamine (di-mě-thok″se-fen″il-eth″-il-am′in) a substance characteristically found in the urine of schizophrenics; abbreviated DMPE.

dimethylacetal (di″meth-il-as′ě-tal) a colorless, volatile liquid, ethylidene dimethyl ether, $CH_3 \cdot CH(OCH_3)_2$, formerly used as an inhalation anesthetic.

dimethylamine (di-meth″il-am′in) a gaseous and liquid ptomaine, $(CH_3)_2NH$, from decaying gelatin, decomposing yeast, rotten fish, etc.

p-dimethylaminoazobenzene (di-meth″il-am″ĭ-no-az″o-ben′zēn) a carcinogenic dye, $C_6H_5N_2C_6H_4 \cdot N(CH_3)_2$; used as an indicator in Töpfer's test for free hydrochloric acid in gastric juice. It has a pH range of 2.9 to 4, being red at 2.9 and yellow at 4. Called also *butter yellow.*

Dimethylane (di-meth′ĭ-lān) trademark for a preparation of promoxolane.

dimethylarsine (di-meth″il-ar′sin) cacodyl hydride.

dimethylbenzene (di-meth″il-ben′zēn) xylene.

dimethyl carbate (di-meth′il kar′bāt) chemical name: *cis*-5-norbornene-2,3-dicarboxylic acid dimethyl ester; an insect repellent, $C_{11}H_{14}O_4$.

dimethylcarbinol (di-meth″il-kar′bĭ-nol) isopropyl alcohol.

dimethylethylpyrrole (di-meth″il-eth″il-pir′ol) a substituted pyrrole obtained from bilirubin.

dimethylguanidine (di-meth″il-guan′ĭ-din) a ptomaine, $CH_3 \cdot NH \cdot C(:NH) \cdot NH \cdot CH_3$, found in small amounts in the urine.

dimethylketone (di-meth″il-ke′ton) acetone.

dimethylphenanthrene (di-meth″il-fe-nan′thrēn) a carcinogenic and weakly estrogenic hydrocarbon.

dimethylphosphine (di-meth″il-fos′fēn) a phosphine extremely destructive to infusorial life, $(CH_3)_2PH$.

dimethyl phthalate (di-meth″il-thal′āt) chemical name: 1,2-benzenedicarboxylic acid dimethyl ester. A clear, colorless, oily liquid, $C_6H_4(COO \cdot CH_3)_2$, the normal methyl ester of phthalic acid; used as an insect repellent.

dimethyl sulfate (di-meth′il sul′fāt) an industrial poison and war gas, $(CH_3)_2SO_4$, causing nystagmus, convulsions, and death from pulmonary complications.

dimethyl sulfoxide (di-meth′il sul-fok′sīd) chemical name: sulfinylbis[methane]: an alkyl sulfoxide, C_2H_6OS, practically odorless in its purified form. As a highly polar organic liquid, it is a powerful solvent, dissolving most aromatic and unsaturated hydrocarbons, organic compounds, and many other substances. Its biologic activities include the ability to penetrate plant and animal tissues and to preserve living cells during freezing. It has been used investigationally as a topical analgesic and anti-inflammatory agent and as an agent to increase the penetrability of other substances. It is available as a 50 per cent solution for direct instillation into the bladder for treatment of interstitial cystitis. Abbreviated DMSO.

dimethyltryptamine (di-meth″il-trip′tah-mēn) chemical name: $N,N,$dimethyltryptamine. A hallucinogenic substance, $C_{12}H_{16}N_2$, derived from the apocynaceous plant *Prestonia amazonica* (Benth.) Macbride (*Haemadictyon amazonicum* Spruce and Benth.) which is native to parts of South America and the West Indies. Abbreviated DMT.

dimetria (di-me′tre-ah) [*di-* + Gr. *mētra* womb] uterus duplex.

diminution (dim″ĭ-nu′shun) reduction or decrease in size or substance.

Dimmer's keratitis (dim″erz) [Friedrich *Dimmer*, Austrian ophthalmologist, 1855–1926] keratitis nummularis.

Dimocillin (di-mo-sil′in) trademark for preparations of sodium methicillin.

dimorphic (di-mor′fik) dimorphous.

dimorphism (di-mor′fizm) [*di-* + Gr. *morphē* form] the property of having or existing in two forms, as fungi that can grow as molds or yeasts. See also *dysmorphism,* def. 2. **physical d.,** the property of certain solids of existing in two crystalline or allotropic forms. **sexual d.,** 1. physical or behavioral differences associated with sex. 2. the condition of having some of the properties of both sexes, as in the early embryo and in some hermaphrodites.

dimorphobiotic (di-mor″fo-bi-ot′ik) [*di-* + Gr. *morphē* form + *biōsis* life] showing alternation of generations and having a parasitic and a nonparasitic stage in the complete life history.

dimorphous (di-mor′fus) [*di-* + Gr. *morphē* form] occurring in two distinct forms; having the property of dimorphism.

dimoxamine hydrochloride (di-mok′sah-mēn) chemical name: (R)-α-ethyl-2,5-dimethoxy-4-methylbenzene ethanamine hydrochloride; a memory adjuvant, $C_{13}H_{21}NO_2 \cdot HCl$.

dimoxyline phosphate (di-mok′-sĭ-lēn) dioxyline phosphate.

dimple (dim′pl) a slight depression, as in the flesh of the cheek or chin. **Fuchs' d's,** dellen. **postanal d.,** coccygeal foveola. **sacrococcygeal d.,** sacral bald spot.

dimpling (dim′pling) the formation of slight depressions or dimples.

dineric (di-ner′ik) [*di-* + Gr. *nēros* liquid] denoting a solution made up of two immiscible solvents with a single solute soluble in each.

dineuric (di-nu′rik) having two neurons or axons; said of nerve cells.

dinical (din′ĭ-kl) [Gr. *dinos* whirl, giddiness] pertaining to dizziness; relieving dizziness.

dinitrate (di-ni′trāt) a compound of a base or a metal with two nitrate groups, as in lead dinitrate, $Pb(NO_3)_2$.

dinitrated (di-ni′trāt-ed) compounded with or containing two nitrate (NO_3) or nitro (NO_2) groups.

dinitroaminophenol (di-ni″tro-am″ĭ-no-fe′nol) a phenol, $C_6H_2(NO_2)_2 \cdot OH$, found in the blood after poisoning with trinitrophenol, forming red granules, free or in the leukocytes. Called also *aminodinitrophenol* and *picramic acid.*

dinitrobenzene (di-ni″tro-ben′zēn) a poisonous substance, $C_6H_4(NO_2)_2$, whose fumes may cause breathlessness and final asphyxia.

dinitrocellulose (di-ni″tro-sel′u-lōs) pyroxylin.

dinitrochlorobenzene (di-ni″tro-klōr″o-ben′zēn) chemical name: 1-chloro-2,4-dinitrobenzene. A compound, $C_6H_3(NO_2)_2Cl$, derived by chlorination of nitrobenzene, used to apply sensitizing dosages to test the ability of an organism to develop delayed-contact allergic reactions (type IV or delayed hypersensitivity).

dinitrocresol (di-ni″tro-kre′sol) a poisonous cresol compound, $CH_3C_6H_2(NO_2)_2OH$, used as an insecticide. Dinitro-*o*-cresol has an effect similar to that of α-dinitrophenol.

dinitrofluorobenzene (di-ni″tro-floo″o-ro-ben′zēn) a substance that induces contact hypersensitivity following application to the skin. Employed to prepare hapten-carrier conjugates, it introduces 2,4-dinitrophenyl groups into substances whose molecules have free-NH_2 groups. Abbreviated DNFB.

dinitrogen (di-ni′tro-gen) containing two nitrogen atoms. **d. monoxide,** nitrous oxide.

dinitrophenol (di-ni″tro-fe′nol) any one of six isomeric compounds, $C_6H_3(OH)(NO_2)_2$, used in making dyes. 2,4-Dinitrophenol was formerly suggested for administration in the treatment of myxedema and obesity, but it has been reported as a cause of agranulocytosis and cataracts, and is now used only as a reagent and indicator and frequently as a hapten.

dinitroresorcinol (di-ni″tro-re-sor′sin-ol) a green coal tar derivative, $C_6H_2(NO_2)_2(OH)_2$, used in preparing degenerated nerve tissue for study.

Dinobdella (di″nob-del′ah) a genus of leeches of the family Gnathobdellidae, species of which attack the larynx of cattle in India when swallowed in drinking water.

Dinoflagellata (di″no-flaj″ě-la′tah) [Gr. *dinos* whirl + *flagellum* whip] an order of minute, chiefly marine, plantlike protozoa of the class Phytomastigophora, subphylum Mastigophora, with two or more flagella in grooves, transverse and longitudinal, which cause the organism to rotate as it advances. They generally have a cellulose covering and numerous green, yellow, or brown chromatophores. Dinoflagellates may be present in seawater in vast numbers, causing a discoloration known as "red tide" or "red water," which may cause the death of many fish and various invertebrates. It includes the genera *Gonyaulax* and *Gymnodinium.*

dinoflagellate (di-no-flaj′ě-lāt) 1. of or pertaining to the order Dinoflagellata. 2. any individual of the order Dinoflagellata.

dinogunellin (di″no-gun′el-lin) the toxic lipoprotein found in the roe of the Japanese blenny *Stichaeus* (*Dinogunellus*) *grigorjewi.*

dinoprost (di′no-prōst) chemical name: (5Z,9α,11α,13E,15S)-9,11,15-trihydroxyprosta-5,13-dien-1-oic acid. A prostaglandin of the F type, $C_{20}H_{34}O_5$, the main action of which is to stimulate the myometrium to contract. Called also *prostaglandin $F_{2α}$*. **d. trometamol,** d. tromethamine. **d. tromethamine,** the tromethamine salt of dinoprost, $C_{20}H_{34}O_5 \cdot C_4H_{11}NO_3$, having the same actions as the base; used as an oxytocic for induction of labor, termination of pregnancy, missed abortion, fetal death, and hydatidiform mole. It is administered intravenously, extra-amniotically, or intra-amniotically. Called also *d. trometanol* and *prostaglandin $F_{2α}$*.

dinoprostone (di″no-prōst′ōn) chemical name: (5Z,11α,13E,15S)-11,15-dihydroxy-9-oxo-prosta-5,13-diene-1-oic. A prostaglandin of the E type, $C_{20}H_{32}O_5$, with oxytoxic activity and uses similar to those of dinoprost; administered orally, intravenously, or extra-amniotically. Called also *prostaglandin E_2*.

D. in p. aeq. abbreviation for L. *div'ide in par'tes aequa'les,* divide into equal parts.

dinsed (din'sed) chemical name: *N-N'*-ethylenebis[3-nitrobenzenesulfonamide]. A coccidiostat for use in poultry, $C_{14}H_{14}N_4O_8S_2$.

dinucleotide (di-nu'kle-o-tīd) one of the cleavage products into which a polynucleotide may be split; a dinucleotide itself may be split into two mononucleotides.

Diocles (di'ŏ-klēz) **of Carystus** (4th century B.C.) an eminent Greek physician and able anatomist who belonged to the Dogmatist school.

diocoele (di'o-sēl) [*di-* + Gr. *koilos* hollow] (*obs.*) the cavity of the diencephalon; the third ventricle of the cerebrum.

Dioctophyma (di-ok"to-fi'mah) a genus of nematodes of the superfamily Dioctophymoidea. **D. rena'le,** the kidney worm, the largest nematode known, found commonly in dogs, cattle, horses, and other animals, but rarely in man; red in color and 35 cm. (males) to 103 cm. (females) in length, they are found usually in the pelvis of the kidney or free in the peritoneal cavity. The parasite is highly destructive to kidney tissue and may cause death. Called also *Eustrongylus gigas.*

Dioctophymoidea (di-ok"to-fi"moi'de-ah) a superfamily of aphasmids, including the genus *Dioctophyma.*

dioctyl calcium sulfosuccinate (di'ok'til) docusate calcium.

dioctyl sodium sulfosuccinate (di'ok'til) docusate sodium.

Diodon (di'o-don) a genus of tetraodontiform fishes of the family Diodontidae; some species are poisonous when ingested.

Diodoquin (di"o-do'kwin) trademark for a preparation of iodoquinol.

Diodrast (di'o-drast) trademark for a preparation of iodopyracet for injection.

dioecious (di-e'shus) diecious.

diogenism (di-oj'ĕ-nizm) [from *Diogenes,* a Greek philosopher of the 5th century B.C. noted for his contempt of the common aims and conditions of life] an effort or tendency to get rid of the refinements of civilization and to lead a life closer to nature.

diolamine (di-ol'ah-mēn) USAN contraction for diethanolamine.

Dioloxol (di"o-lok'sol) trademark for a preparation of mephenesin.

Dionosil (di-on'o-sil) trademark for preparations of propyliodone.

diopsimeter (di"op-sim'ĕ-ter) [Gr. *diopsis* vision + *metron* measure] a device for measuring the field of vision.

diopter (di-op'ter) [Gr. *dioptra* optical instrument for measuring angles] the refractive power of a lens with a focal distance of one meter; assumed as a unit of measurement for refractive power (Monoyer, Donders). **prism d.,** a unit of prismatic deviation; deflection of one centimeter at a distance of one meter.

dioptometer (di"op-tom'ĕ-ter) [*dioptric* + Gr. *metron* measure] an instrument for use in testing ocular refraction.

dioptometry (di"op-tom'ĕ-tre) the measurement of refraction and accommodation of the eye.

dioptoscopy (di"op-tos'ko-pe) [*dioptric* + Gr. *skopein* to examine] measurement of ocular refraction by means of the ophthalmoscope.

dioptre (di-op'ter) diopter.

dioptric (di-op'trik) [Gr. *dioptrikos* belonging to the use of the *dioptra*] pertaining to refraction or to transmitted and refracted light; refracting.

dioptrics (di-op'triks) the science of refracted light.

dioptrometer (di"op-trom'ĕ-ter) dioptometer.

dioptrometry (di"op-trom'ĕ-tre) dioptometry.

dioptroscopy (di"op-tros'ko-pe) dioptoscopy.

dioptry (di'op-tre) diopter.

Dioscorea (di"os-ko're-ah) a genus of plants, the Mexican yams, family Dioscoreaceae. The dried rhizome of *D. villosa* L., which contains saponin and acrid resins, was once used for its diaphoretic, expectorant, and diuretic properties. Several species of *Dioscorea,* e.g., *D. villosa, D. floribunda,* and *D. tokoro,* are used as sources of diosgenin, an important saponin precursor in the synthesis of several medically important steroids, e.g., pregnenolone and progesterone. **D. mexica'na,** the source of botogenin.

Dioscorides (di"ŏ-skōr'ĭ-dēz) **of Anazarbos** (1st century A.D.) a noted botanist and pharmacologist whose encyclopedia of materia medica was widely used for centuries after his death. See also under *granule.*

diose (di'ōs) the simplest sugar, a monosaccharide containing two carbon atoms in the molecule: $CH_2OH—CHO$. Called also *glycolic aldehyde.*

diosgenin (di-os'jen-in) an aglycone of the saponin dioscin, Δ^5-20β_F,22α-$_F$,25α_F-spirosten-3-β-ol; $C_{27}H_{42}O_3$. Obtained from several species of *Dioscorea,* it is a precursor in the synthesis of pregnenolone, progesterone, and other medically useful steroids.

diospyrobezoar (di"os-pi"ro-be'zōr) a bezoar made up of persimmon fibers.

diovulatory (di-ov'u-lah-to"re) ordinarily discharging two ova in one ovarian cycle.

dioxane (di-ok'sān) diethylene dioxide, a clear fluid, used for dehydrating and clearing tissues preparatory to paraffin embedding; it is an industrial poison.

dioxide (di-ok'sīd) 1. a binary compound containing two oxide ions, such as silicon dioxide, SiO_2. 2. an oxide of a non-metal with a valence of four, such as sulfur dioxide, SO_2.

dioxin (di-ok'sin) any of the heterocyclic hydrocarbons present as a trace contaminant in herbicides, especially the chlorinated dioxin 2,3,7,8-tetrachlorodibenzo-para-dioxin, thought to have oncogenic and teratogenic properties.

dioxybenzone (di-oks"ĭ-ben'zōn) [USP] chemical name: (2-hydroxy-4-methoxyphenyl)(2-hydroxyphenyl)methanone. A sunscreening agent, $C_{14}H_{12}O_4$, occurring as an off-white to yellow powder; applied topically to the skin.

dioxygenase (di-ok"sĕ-jen'āse) an oxidative enzyme which catalyzes the incorporation of two atoms of oxygen into one molecule of substrate.

dioxyline phosphate (di-ok'sĭ-lēn) chemical name: 1-(4-ethoxy-3-methoxybenzyl)-6,7-dimethoxy-3-methylisoquinoline. A synthetic analogue of papaverine, $C_{22}H_{25}NO_4$, occurring as a white, crystalline powder; used as a vasodilator, mainly in the treatment of vascular spasm associated with acute myocardial infarction, angina of effort, peripheral vascular disease in which there is a vasospastic element, and peripheral and pulmonary embolism, administered orally. Called also *dimoxyline phosphate.*

Dipaxin (di-pak'sin) trademark for a preparation of diphenadione.

dipentene (di-pen'tēn) any terpene found in volatile oils; called also *diamylene.*

dipeptidase (di-pep'tĭ-dās) a peptidase which catalyzes the hydrolysis of the peptide linkage in a dipeptide.

dipeptide (di-pep'tīd) a peptide which, on hydrolysis, yields two amino acids.

diperodon (di-per'o-don) [USP] chemical name: 3-(1-piperidinyl)-1,2-propanediolbis(phenylcarbamate)(ester) monohydrate. A local anesthetic, $C_{22}H_{27}N_3O_4 \cdot H_2O$, occurring as a white to cream-colored powder; applied topically to the skin for abrasions, irritations, and pruritus and intrarectally for relief of discomfort associated with hemorrhoids. **d. hydrochloride,** the monohydrochloride salt of diperodon, $C_{22}H_{27}N_3O_4 \cdot HCl$, having the same actions and uses as the base.

Dipetalonema (di-pet"ah-lo-ne'mah) a genus of nematodes of the superfamily Filarioidea. **D. per'stans,** a filarial nematode up to 80 mm. long, found in the tropical regions of South America and Africa and in Panama, transmitted by the bites of small flies of the genus *Culicoides.* The adults inhabit the pleural and peritoneal tissues, while the larval forms (microfilariae) are found in the peripheral blood. Although considered to be nonpathogenic, they have been implicated as the cause of such symptoms as eosinophilia, abdominal and pectoral pain, enlargement of the spleen and liver, and fever followed by urticaria and edema of the lower limbs and scrotum. Called also *Acanthocheilonema perstans* and *Filaria perstans.* **D. recondi'tum,** a species found in the perirenal fat pad of dogs; called also *Filaria recondita.* **D. streptocer'ca,** a filarial worm found in man and chimpanzees in equatorial Africa, transmitted by the bite of small flies of the genus *Culicoides.* The microfilariae, which may be found in scarification smears, are sometimes confused with those of *Onchocerca volvulus.* It produces a pruritic rash resembling that of onchocerciasis. Called also *Acanthocheilonema streptoceria.*

dipetalonemiasis (di-pet"ah-lo-ne-mi'ah-sis) infection with the nematode *Dipetalonema perstans* or *D. streptocerca.*

diphallia (di-fal'e-ah) [*di-* + Gr. *phallos* penis] duplication of the penis.

diphallus (di'fal-lus) a double penis.

diphasic (di-fa'zik) [*di-* + Gr. *phasis* phase] occurring in two phases or stages. Cf. *monophasic* and *triphasic.*

diphebuzol (di-feb'u-zol) phenylbutazone.

diphemanil methylsulfate (di-fe'mah-nil) [USP] chemical name: 4-(diphenylmethylene)-1,1-dimethylpiperidinium methyl sulfate. A quaternary ammonium anticholinergic, $C_{21}H_{27}NO_4S$, occurring as a white or nearly white, crystalline powder; used in the treatment of peptic ulcer, gastric hyperacidity, and hypermotility in gastritis and pylorospasm, and in the treatment of hyperhidrosis, administered orally.

diphenadione (di-fen"ah-di'ōn) [USP] chemical name: 2-(diphenylacetyl)-1*H*-indene-1,3-(2*H*)-dione. One of the indanedione anticoagulants, $C_{23}H_{16}O_3$, occurring as yellow crystals or as a yellow, crystalline powder; administered orally.

diphenhydramine hydrochloride (di"fen-hi"drah-mēn) [USP] chemical name: 2-(diphenylmethoxy)-*N,N*-dimethylethanamine hydrochloride. An antihistaminic, $C_{17}H_{21}NO \cdot HCl$, occurring as a white, crystalline powder; used in the symptomatic management of allergic symptoms and also for its sedative, antiemetic, antitussive, local anesthetic, and anticholinergic (antispasmodic) effects, administered orally, intramuscularly, and intravenously.

diphenidol (di-fen′ĭ-dōl) chemical name: α,α-diphenyl-1-piperidinebutanol. An antiemetic, $C_{21}H_{27}NO$, used for the treatment of vertigo and to control nausea and vomiting; administered rectally. **d. hydrochloride,** the hydrochloride salt of diphenidol, $C_{21}H_{27}NO \cdot HCl$, having the same actions and uses as the base; administered orally or intramuscularly. **d. pamoate,** the pamoate salt of diphenidol, $(C_{21}H_{27}NO)_2 C_{23}H_{16}O_6$, having the same actions as the base.

diphenoxylate hydrochloride (di″fen-ok′sĭ-lāt) [USP] chemical name: 1-(3-cyano-3,3-diphenylpropyl)-4-phenyl-4-piperidinecarboxylic acid ethyl ester monohydrochloride. An antiperistaltic derived from meperidine, $C_{30}H_{32}N_2O_2 \cdot HCl$; used as an antidiarrheal, administered orally.

diphenyl (di-fe′nil) a colorless compound, $C_6H_5C_6H_5$, found in coal tar and used as fungistat in containers for shipping oranges. Called also *biphenyl.*

diphenylamine (di-fen″il-am′in) chemical name: *N*-phenylbenzeneamine. A compound, $(C_6H_5)_2NH$, used as a test for oxidizing agents, such as nitric acid and chlorine, and, in veterinary medicine, in the prevention and treatment of screw-worm infestation.

diphenylaminearsine chloride (di-fen″il-am″in-ar′sin klo′rīd) a toxic smoke for war use, $NH(C_6H_4)_2AsCl$; called also *adamsite.*

diphenylamino-azo-benzene (di-fen″il-am″ĭ-no-az″o-ben′zēn) an indicator with a pH range of 1.2 to 2.1.

diphenylchlorarsine (di-fen″il-klor-ar′sin) sneezing gas, $(C_6H_5)_2AsCl$, a toxic smoke once used in war, causing sneezing, coughing, headache, salivation, and vomiting; called also *Clark I* and *DA.*

diphenylcyanarsine (di-fen″il-si″an-ar′sin) a lethal war gas, $(C_6H_5)_2AsCN$; called also *Clark II.*

diphenylhydantoin (di-fen″il-hi-dan′to-in) phenytoin.

diphenylpyraline hydrochloride (di-fen″il-pi′rah-lēn) [USP] chemical name: 4-(diphenylmethoxy)-1-methylpiperidine hydrochloride. An antihistaminic, $C_{19}H_{23}NO \cdot HCl$, occurring as a white powder; used to relieve the symptoms of allergic reactions, administered orally.

diphonia (di-fo′ne-ah) [*di-* + Gr. *phōnē* voice] a condition in which two different tones are produced in speaking; double voice.

diphosgene (di-fos′jēn) a gas, $ClCOOCCl_3$, which is intensely irritating to the lungs, producing pulmonary edema.

2,3-diphosphoglycerate (di-fos′fo-glis′er-āt) 2,3-bisphosphoglycerate.

diphosphopyridine nucleotide (di-fos′fo-pir′ĭ-dēn) DPN; former name of nicotinamide-adenine dinucleotide (NAD).

diphosphothiamin (di-fos″fo-thi′ah-min) the coenzyme that is involved in the decarboxylation of α-keto acids.

diphtheria (dif-the′re-ah) [Gr. *diphthera* membrane + *-ia*] an acute infectious disease caused by the toxigenic gram-positive bacillus *Corynebacterium diphtheriae,* affecting primarily the membranes of the nose, throat, or larynx, and characterized by the formation of a gray white pseudomembrane. It is attended by fever and pain of varying degree and, in the laryngeal form, by aphonia and respiratory obstruction. Myocarditis and cranial or peripheral neuritis are complications resulting from the effects of toxin released from the local site. A cutaneous form also occurs (see below). **avian d.,** fowlpox. **Bretonneau's d.,** diphtheria. **calf d.,** a contagious disease of young calves in which grayish patches form in the mouth and throat, caused by *Fusobacterium necrophorum.* Called also *necrotic laryngitis.* **cutaneous d.,** ulcerated skin lesions with raised margins, often involving underlying connective tissue and muscle as well; it is usually not accompanied by nasal or pharyngeal lesions. **false d.,** pseudodiphtheria. **faucial d.,** membranous pharyngitis with lesions limited to the tonsils, or involving the tonsils, tonsillar pillars, and soft palate. **fowl d.,** fowlpox. **gangrenous d.,** diphtheria attended with gangrene of the skin or mucous membrane, or both. **d. gra′vis,** malignant d. **laryngeal d.,** membranous croup. **laryngotracheal d.,** diphtheria in which the infection invades the larynx and trachea, with edema, congestion, and development of a pseudomembrane. **malignant d.,** an often fatal form beginning with rigors and marked by massive swelling in the neck (bull neck), tonsillar enlargement, and sometimes purpura. Called also *d. gravis.* **nasal d.,** diphtheria in which the infection is mainly in the nasal passages. **pharyngeal d.,** that which is especially manifested on the mucous membrane of the pharynx. **septic d.,** diphtheria rendered especially severe by secondary infection with pyogenic cocci. **surgical d.,** wound d. **umbilical d.,** diphtherial infection of the umbilical cord in the newborn. **wound d.,** formation of a false membrane on the surface of a wound.

diphtherial (dif-the′re-al) pertaining to or derived from diphtheria.

diphtheric (dif-the′rik) diphtheritic.

diphtherin (dif′the-rin) 1. (*obs.*) diphtheria toxin. 2. a polyvalent diphtheritic antigen for use in anaphylactic skin test.

diphtheritic (dif″the-rit′ik) pertaining to or affected with diphtheria.

diphtheritis (dif″the-ri′tis) diphtheria.

diphtheroid (dif′ther-oid) 1. resembling diphtheria or the diphtheria bacillus. 2. any member of *Corynebacterium* other than *C. diphtheriae.* 3. pseudodiphtheria. 4. former name for organisms now in the genus *Propionibacterium.*

diphtherotoxin (dif″thĕ-ro-tok′sin) see *diphtheria toxin,* under *toxin.*

diphthongia (dif-thon′je-ah) [*di-* + Gr. *phthongos* sound] the production of double vocal sounds; called also *diplophonia.*

Diphylets (di′fĭ-let) trademark for a preparation dextroamphetamine sulfate.

diphyllobothriasis (di-fil″o-both-ri′ah-sis) the state of being infected with tapeworms of the genus *Diphyllobothrium;* formerly called *dibothriocephaliosis.*

Diphyllobothriidae (di-fil″o-both-re′ĭ-de) a family of tapeworms of the order Pseudophyllidea, subclass Cestoda, which are parasitic in man and other fish-eating vertebrates. The genera *Diphyllobothrium, Diplogonoporus,* and *Spirometra* are of medical importance.

Diphyllobothrium (di-fil″o-both′re-um) [*di-* + Gr. *phyllon* leaf + *bothrion* pit] a genus of large tapeworms of the family *Diphyllobothriidae,* order Pseudophyllidea; formerly called *Bothriocephalus* and *Dibothriocephalus.* **D. corda′tum,** the heartheaded tapeworm; a small species found in dogs and in seals in Greenland and very rarely in man. **D. erina′cei,** a species found in the adult form in the dog and other carnivores; formerly called *D. mansoni.* **D. la′tum,** the broad tapeworm or fish tapeworm; a very large tapeworm found in the intestines of man and (somewhat smaller) in cats, dogs, mink, bears, and other fish-eating mammals. It may be ¾ inch wide and 30 feet long. The head is marked with two grooves or suckers (bothria). It has two intermediate hosts: the first a crustacean, the second a fish.

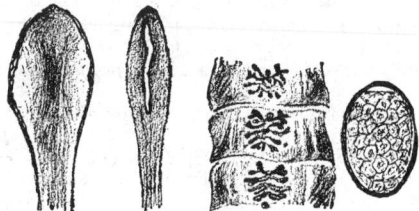

Diphyllobothrium latum: head, segments, and egg (de Rivas).

Infection in man, acquired by eating inadequately cooked fish, may result in a clinical and blood picture resembling that of pernicious anemia. Formerly called *D. taenioides.* Called also *Dibothriocephalus latus.* **D. manso′ni,** *D. erinacei.* **D. mansonoi′des,** a species whose migrating larvae (spargana) are one of the causes of sparganosis. **D. par′vum,** a species found in man in Tasmania, Japan, Rumania, Iran, and Minnesota; possibly identical with *D. latum.* **D. taenioi′des,** *D. latum.*

diphyodont (dif′ĭ-o-dont″) [*di-* + Gr. *phyein* to produce + *odous* tooth] having two dentitions, a deciduous and a permanent.

dipipanone hydrochloride (di-pip′ah-nōn) chemical name: *dl*-4,4-diphenyl-6-piperidinoheptan-3-one hydrochloride. An analogue of methadone, $C_{24}H_{31}NO \cdot HCl$, occurring as a white, crystalline powder; used as an analgesic, administered subcutaneously, intramuscularly, and intravenously.

dipivefrin (dĭ-piv′ĕ-frin) chemical name: (+)-4-[1-hydroxy-2-(methylamino)ethyl]-1,2-phenylene ester 2,2-dimethylpropanoic acid; an ophthalmic adrenergic, $C_{19}H_{29}NO_5.$

diplacusia (dip″lah-ku′ze-ah) diplacusis.

diplacusis (dip″lah-ku′sis) [Gr. *diplous* double + *akousis* hearing] the perception of a single auditory stimulus as two sounds, as a result of a pathologic condition involving the cochlea; called also *double disharmonic hearing.* **binaural d.,** different perception of a single auditory stimulus by the two ears; the difference may be in tone (disharmonic d.) or in timing (echo d.). **d. binaura′lis dysharmon′ica,** disharmonic d. **d. binaura′lis echo′ica,** echo d. **disharmonic d.,** a form of diplacusis in which a given pure tone is heard differently in the two ears. **echo d.,** a form in which a sound of brief duration is heard in the one ear a fraction of a second later than in the other ear. **monaural d., d. monaura′lis,** a form in which a pure tone is heard in the same ear as a split tone of two frequencies.

diplasmatic (di″plaz-mat′ik) [*di-* + Gr. *plasma* something formed] containing substances besides protoplasm; said of cells.

diplegia (di-ple′je-ah) [*di-* + Gr. *plēgē* stroke] paralysis affecting like parts on both sides of the body; bilateral paralysis. **atonic-astatic d.,** diplegia characterized by hypotonia instead of spasticity. **facial d.,** paralysis affecting both sides of the face. **facial p., congenital,** Möbius syndrome. **infantile**

d., birth palsy. **masticatory d.,** paralysis of all the muscles which take part in mastication. **spastic d.,** Little's disease.

diplegic (di-ple′jik) pertaining to or marked by diplegia.

diplo- (dip′lo) [Gr. *diploos* double] a combining form meaning double, twin, twofold, or twice.

diploalbuminuria (dip″lo-al-bu″mĭ-nu′re-ah) [*diplo-* + *albuminuria*] the presence of both physiologic and pathologic albuminuria.

diplobacilli (dip″lo-bah-sil′i) plural of *diplobacillus.*

diplobacillus (dip″lo-bah-sil′us), pl. *diplobacil′li* [*diplo-* + *bacillus*] a short, rod-shaped organism occurring in pairs; diplobacterium. **Morax's d.,** *Hemophilus duplex.*

diplobacteria (dip″lo-bak-te′re-ah) plural of *diplobacterium.*

diplobacterium (dip″lo-bak-te′re-um), pl. *diplobacteria* [*diplo-* + *bacterium*] diplobacillus.

diploblastic (dip″lo-blas′tik) [*diplo-* + Gr. *blastos* germ] made up of two germ layers.

diplocardia (dip″lo-kar′de-ah) [*diplo-* + Gr. *kardia* heart] a condition in which the right and left heart are somewhat separated by a fissure.

diplocephalus (dip″lo-sef′ah-lus) dicephalus.

diplocephaly (dip″lo-sef′ah-le) dicephaly.

diplococcal (dip″lo-kok′al) pertaining to or caused by diplococci.

diplococci (dip″lo-kok′si) plural of *diplococcus.*

diplococcoid (dip″lo-kok′oid) 1. resembling diplococci. 2. an organism that resembles a diplococcus.

Diplococcus (dip″lo-kok′us) [*diplo-* + *coccus*] former name for a genus of the tribe Streptococceae, order Eubacteriales, the species of which have been assigned to other genera. **D. con-stella′tus,** a microaerophilic or obligate anaerobe normally found in the mouth and intestinal tract. **D. mag′nus,** a microaerophilic or obligate anaerobe normally found in the mouth and intestinal tract. **D. morbillo′rum,** a microaerophilic or obligate anaerobe normally found in the mouth and intestinal tract. **D. muco′sus,** a type of diplococcus considered by some to be a separate species, characterized by production of a heavily mucoid growth, and differentiable with difficulty from *Streptococcus mucosus.* **D. paleopneumo′niae,** a species closely resembling *D. pneumoniae* except that is an obligate anaerobe, occurring normally in the buccopharyngeal cavity and said to be highly pathogenic. **D. plagarumbel′li,** an obligate anaerobe found in septic wounds. **D. pneumo′niae,** *Streptococcus pneumoniae.*

diplococcus (dip″lo-kok′us), pl. *diplococ′ci.* 1. a spherical bacterium occurring predominantly in pairs as a consequence of incomplete separation following cell division in a single plane; the organism may also be lanceolate (pneumococcus) or coffee-bean-shaped (gonococcus). 2. an organism of the genus *Diplococcus.* **d. of Morax-Axenfeld,** *Hemophilus duplex.* **d. of Neisser,** *Neisseria gonorrhoeae.* **Weichselbaum's d.,** *Neisseria meningitidis.*

diplocoria (dip″lo-ko′re-ah) [*diplo-* + Gr. *korē* pupil] double pupil.

Diplodia (dĭ-plo′de-ah) a genus of imperfect fungi producing the dry-rot or corn-stalk disease of corn.

diplodiatoxicosis (dip″lo-dĭ″ah-tok″sĭ-ko′sis) a form of mycotoxicosis caused by fungi of the genus *Diplodia.*

Diplodinium (dip″lo-din′e-um) a genus of ciliate protozoa of the subclass Euciliata, species of which are parasitic in the stomachs of cattle.

diploë (dip′lo-e) [Gr. *diploē* fold] [NA] the loose osseous tissue between the two tables of the cranial bones.

diploetic (dip″lo-et′ik) of or pertaining to the diploë.

Diplogaster (dip′lo-gas″ter) [*diplo-* + Gr. *gastēr* stomach] a genus of free-living coprozoic nematodes which may, in fecal examination, be confused with hookworms or *Strongyloides.*

diplogenesis (dip″lo-jen′ĕ-sis) [*diplo-* + Gr. *genesis* production] the production of a double monster.

Diplogonoporus (dip″lo-go-nop′o-rus) [*diplo-* + Gr. *gonos* seed + *poros* passage] a genus of tapeworms of the family Diphyllobothriidae, characterized by the possession of two sets of reproductive organs in each segment. **D. brau′ni,** former name for *Digramma brauni.* **D. gran′dis,** a common parasite of whales that has been found in man in Japan; it may be up to 10 meters long, and may cause diarrhea or constipation, and secondary anemia.

diplogram (dip′lo-gram) [*diplo-* + Gr. *gramma* a writing] a roentgenogram containing two exposures.

diploic (dip-lo′ik) 1. double. 2. diploetic.

diploid (dip′loid) [Gr. *diploos* twofold] 1. having two sets of chromosomes, as normally found in the somatic cells of higher organisms. Cf. *haploid* (def. 1). 2. an individual or cell having two full sets of homologous chromosomes. Symbol, 2N.

diploidy (dip′loi-de) the state of having two full sets of homologous chromosomes.

diplokaryon (dip″lo-kar′e-on) [*diplo-* + Gr. *karyon* nucleus] a nucleus which has twice the diploid number of chromosomes.

diplomate (dip′lo-māt) a person who has received a diploma or certificate. In medicine the term refers particularly to a holder of a certificate of the National Board of Medical Examiners or of one of the American Boards in the Specialties.

Diplomonadina (dip″lo-mon″ah-di′nah) a suborder of flagellate protozoa of the order Polymastigida, having two nuclei and bilateral symmetry; it includes the genus *Giardia.* Formerly called *Diplozoa.*

diplomyelia (dip″lo-mi-e′le-ah) [*diplo-* + Gr. *myelos* marrow + *-ia*] lengthwise fissure and seeming doubleness of spinal cord.

diplon (dip′lon) [Gr. *diploos* double] deuteron.

diplonema (dip″lo-ne′mah) [*diplo-* + Gr. *nema* thread] the double chromosomes in the diplotene stage.

diploneural (dip″lo-nu′ral) [*diplo-* + Gr. *neuron* nerve] (obs.) having a double nerve supply.

diplont (dip′lont) [Gr. *diploō* to double + *ōn* being] a diploid individual.

diplopagus (dip-lop′ah-gus) [Gr. *diploos* double + *pagos* a thing fixed] a double monster in which the component parts are equal to and the symmetrical equivalents of one another; called also *duplicitas symmetros.*

diplophase (dip′lo-fāz) that phase in the life history of certain organisms in which the nuclei are diploid.

diplophonia (dip″lo-fo′ne-ah) [*diplo-* + Gr. *phōnē* voice] diphthongia.

diplopia (dĭ-plo′pe-ah) [*diplo-* + Gr. *ōpē* sight + *-ia*] the perception of two images of a single object; called also *ambiopia, double vision,* and *binocular polyopia.* **binocular d.,** the perception of a separate image of a single object by each of the two eyes. **crossed d.,** double vision in which the image belonging to the right eye is displaced to the left of the image belonging to the left eye, as occurs in exotropia (divergent squint). **direct d.,** double vision in which the image belonging to the right eye appears to the right of the image belonging to the left eye, as occurs in esotropia (convergent squint). **heteronymous d.,** crossed d. **homonymous d.,** direct d. **horizontal d.,** diplopia in which the images lie in the same horizontal plane, being either crossed or direct. **monocular d.,** the perception by the same eye of two images of a single object, due to double pupil, early cataract, irregular astigmatism, or displacement of the lens. **paradoxical d.,** crossed d. **torsional d.,** double vision in which the upper pole of the vertical axis of one image is inclined toward or away from that of the other. **vertical d.,** double vision in which one image appears to be above the other.

diplopiometer (dĭ-plo″pe-om′ĕ-ter) [*diplopia* + Gr. *metron* measure] an instrument for measuring diplopia.

Diplopoda (di-plop′o-dah) [*diplo-* + Gr. *pous* foot] a class of arthropods of the superclass Myriapoda, which comprises the millipedes.

Diplopylidium (dip″lo-pi-lid′e-um) a genus of small tapeworms of the family *Dilepididae,* species of which are parasites of birds and mammals.

diploscope (dip′lo-skōp) [*diplo-* + Gr. *skopein* to examine] an apparatus for the study of binocular vision.

diplosomatia (dip″lo-so-ma′she-ah) [*diplo-* + Gr. *sōma* body] a condition in which complete twins are joined at some part of their bodies.

diplosome (dip′lo-sōm) [*diplo-* + Gr. *sōma* body] the two centrioles of mammalian cells; called also *paired allosomes.*

diplotene (dip′lo-tēn) the stage of the first meiotic prophase, following the pachytene, in which the two chromosomes in each bivalent begin to repel one another and a split occurs between the chromosomes, which are then held together by regions where exchanges have taken place (chiasmata) during crossing over. See also *leptotene, pachytene* and *zygotene.*

diploteratology (dip″lo-ter″ah-tol′o-je) [*diplo-* + *teratology*] the sum of what is known regarding joined twin monstrosities.

Diplozoa (dip″lo-zo′ah) [*diplo-* + Gr. *zōon* animal] former name for *Diplomonadina.*

Dipluridae (dip-lu′rĭ-de) a family of spiders (suborder Orthognatha); two genera, *Atrax* and *Trechona,* have been shown to be harmful to man.

dipodia (di-po′de-ah) [*di-* + Gr. *pous* foot] a developmental anomaly characterized by duplication of a foot.

dipole (di′pōl) 1. a molecule having charges of equal and opposite signs but in which the center of the positive charge does not coincide with that of the negative charge, a property which enables the molecule to be bound electrostatically by both positively and negatively charged groups. See *polar compounds,* under *compound.* 2. a pair of electric charges or magnetic poles separated by a short distance.

dipotassium phosphate (di″po-tas′e-um fos′fāt) potassium phosphate.

dipping (dip′ing) palpation of the liver by a quick depressing movement of the fingers with the hand flat across the abdomen.

dippoldism (dip′ol-dizm) [Dippold, a German school teacher] flagellation, def. 2.

Diprosone (di-pro′sōn) trademark for preparations of betamethasone dipropionate.

diprosopus (di-pros′o-pus) [*di-* + Gr. *prosōpon* face] a monster with a single trunk and normal limbs, but with varying degrees of duplication of the face. **d. tetrophthal′mus,** a monster hav-

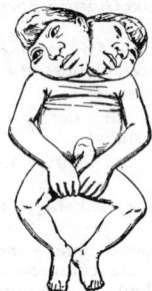

Diprosopus (Gould and Pyle).

ing two fused faces, the median eye of each being fused into a common orbit.

diprotrizoate (di″pro-tri′zo-āt) chemical name: 3,5-dipropionamido-2,4,6-triiodobenzoate; used as a contrast medium in roentgenography of the urinary tract.

dipsesis (dip-se′sis) [Gr. *dipsēsis* a thirst, longing] thirst.

dipsetic (dip-set′ik) [Gr. *dipsētikos* thirsty; provoking thirst] pertaining to, characterized by, or producing dipsesis.

dipsia (dip′se-ah) [Gr. *dipsa* thirst + *-ia*] thirst; often used as a word termination, denoting a condition relative to thirst, or the physiological state of the body leading to the ingestion of fluids.

dipsogen (dip′so-jen) [Gr. *dipsa* thirst + *gennan* to produce] an agent or measure that induces thirst and promotes the ingestion of fluids.

dipsogenic (dip-so-jen′ik) engendering thirst.

dipsomania (dip″so-ma′ne-ah) [Gr. *dipsa* thirst + *mania* madness] alcoholism.

dipsophobia (dip″so-fo′be-ah) [Gr. *dipsa* thirst + *phobein* to be affrighted by] morbid fear of alcoholic liquor.

dipsosis (dip-so′sis) [Gr. *dipsa* thirst + *-osis*] morbid thirst.

dipsotherapy (dip″so-ther′ah-pe) [Gr. *dipsa* thirst + *therapeia* treatment] treatment by strict limitation of the amount of water to be ingested.

dipstick (dip′stik) a strip of cellulose chemically impregnated to render it sensitive to protein, glucose, or other substances in the urine.

Diptera (dip′ter-ah) [Gr. *dipteros* two winged] an order of insects including the flies, gnats, and mosquitoes.

Dipterocarpus (dip″ter-o-kar′pus) [Gr. *dipteros* two winged + *karpos* fruit] a genus of trees from southern Asia, affording gurjun balsam.

dipterous (dip′ter-us) 1. having two wings. 2. pertaining to insects of the order Diptera.

dipus (di′pus) [*di-* + Gr. *pous* foot] a conjoined twin monster with only two feet.

dipygus (di-pi′gus) [*di-* + Gr. *pygē* rump] a monster with double pelvis. **d. parasit′icus,** gastrothoracopagus dipygus.

dipylidiasis (dip″ĭ-lĭ-di′ah-sis) infection with *Dipylidium caninum.*

Dipylidium (dip″ĭ-lid′e-um) [Gr. *dipylos* having two entrances] a genus of tapeworms of the family Dilepididae, found in cats and other small carnivores. **D. cani′num,** a common tapeworm of dogs and cats, the larval stage living in fleas (*Ctenocephalides canis*) and lice (*Trichodectes canis*) of dogs, as well as in *Pulex irritans,* which thus act as vectors; it has been found in man. Called also *Taenia elliptica.*

dipyridamole (di″pi-rid′ah-mōl) chemical name: 2,2′2″,2‴-(4,8-dipiperidinopyrimido[5,4-*d*]pyrimidine-2,6-diyldinitrilo)tetraethanol. A coronary vasodilator, $C_{24}H_{40}N_8O_4$, occurring as a yellow, crystalline powder; administered orally.

dipyrithione (di″pēr-ĭ-thi-ōn) chemical name: 2,2′-dithiobispyridine 1,1′-dioxide; an antibacterial and antifungal, $C_{10}H_8N_2O_2$-S_2.

dipyrone (di′pi-rōn) chemical name: [(2,3-dihydro-1,5-dimethyl-3-oxo-2-phenyl-1*H*-pyrazol-4-yl)methylamino] methanesulfonic acid sodium salt monohydrate. A pyrazole derivative, $C_{13}H_{18}N_3NaO_5S$, which is an effective analgesic and antipyretic, but is seldom used because of an association with cases of fatal agranulocytosis. Called also *methylmelubrine* and *noramidopyrine.*

direct (di-rekt′) [L. *directus*] 1. straight; in a straight line. 2. performed immediately and without the intervention of subsidiary means.

director (di-rek′tor) [L. *dirigere* to direct] any person, thing, or device that guides or directs. **grooved d.,** a grooved instrument used to guide the direction and depth of a surgical incision.

dirhinic (di-ri′nik) pertaining to both nasal cavities.

dirigomotor (dir″ĭ-go-mo′tor)[L. *dirigere* to direct + *motor* mover] controlling muscular activity.

Dirofilaria (di″ro-fĭ-la′re-ah) a genus of filarial nematodes with very long filiform bodies and a striated cuticle. **D. im-mit′is,** the heartworm, a species found in the right heart and veins of the dog, wolf, and fox; it is of worldwide distribution in tropical and subtropical areas. Called also *Filaria immitis.* **D. magalhae′si,** a species found in the heart of a child in Brazil; it is probably identical with *D. immitis.* **D. re′pens,** a species found in the subcutaneous connective tissues of dogs and occasionally of man.

dirofilariasis (di″ro-fil″ah-ri′ah-sis) infection with a parasite of the genus *Dirofilaria.*

Dir. prop. abbreviation for L. *directio′ne pro′pria,* with a proper direction.

dis- a prefix denoting (1) reversal or separation [L. *dis-* apart], or (2) duplication [Gr. *dis* twice, doubly].

disability (dis″ah-bil′ĭ-te) 1. a lack of the ability to function normally, physically or mentally; incapacity. 2. anything that causes disability. 3. as defined by the federal government: "inability to engage in any substantial gainful activity by reason of any medically determinable physical or mental impairment which can be expected to last or has lasted for a continuous period of not less than 12 months." **developmental d.,** a substantial handicap having its onset before the age of 18 years and of indefinite duration, and attributable to mental retardation, autism (when found to be closely related to and requiring treatments similar to that of mental retardation), cerebral palsy, epilepsy, or other neuropathy.

disaccharidase (di-sak′ah-rĭ-dās″) an enzyme that hydrolyzes disaccharides.

disaccharide (di-sak′ah-rīd) any of a class of sugars that yield two monosaccharides on hydrolysis and have the general formula $C_n(H_2O)_{n-1}$ or $C_{12}H_{22}O_{11}$. They include sucrose, lactose, and maltose. Formerly called *biose, disaccharose,* and *hexabiose.* **reducing d's,** disaccharides that can reduce Fehling's solution or other reagents, owing to the presence of a functional aldehyde group.

disacchariduria (di-sak″ah-ri-du′re-ah) presence of a disaccharide (lactose or sucrose) in the urine.

disaccharose (di-sak′ah-rōs) disaccharide.

disacidify (dis″ah-sid′ĭ-fi) to remove an acid from, or to neutralize an acid in, a mixture.

disaggregation (dis″ag-re-ga′shun) failure of the hysterical mind to connect new sensations with each other.

disarticulation (dis″ar-tik″u-la′shun) [L. *dis-* apart + *articulus* joint] amputation or separation at a joint.

disassimilate (dis″ah-sim′ĭ-lāt) dissimilate.

disassimilation (dis″ah-sim″ĭ-la′shun) [*dis-* + *assimilation*] dissimilation.

disazo (dis-az′o) diazo-.

disc (disk) [L. *discus*] disk.

disc- see disco-.

discharge (dis-charj′) 1. a setting free, or liberation. 2. matter or force set free. 3. an excretion or substance evacuated. **brush d.,** in electrotherapeutics, the spark discharge from a static machine or an induction coil; because of its slight ability to penetrate solid matter it was confused with x-rays by early investigators. Called also *spark x-rays.* **disruptive d.,** the passing of a current through an insulating medium due to the breakdown of the medium under the electrostatic stress. **epileptic d.,** the pathophysiological events underlying epilepsy. **nervous d., neural d.,** the propagated excitation produced by stimulation of a center in the nervous system. **systolic d.,** see *stroke volume,* under *volume.*

dischronation (dis″kro-na′shun) [L. *dis-* apart + Gr. *chronos* time] a dislocation in the consciousness of time.

disci (dis′i) [L.] plural of *discus.*

disciform (dis′ĭ-form) [L. *discus* disk + *forma* shape] in the form of a disk.

discission (dis-sizh′un) [L. *discissio; dis-* apart + *scindere* to cut] incision, or cutting into, as of a soft cataract. **d. of cataract,** the surgical rupturing of the capsule so that the aqueous humor may gain access to the lens of the eye. **d. of cervix uteri,** incisions on each side of the cervix uteri, formerly done for the relief of stenosis of the cervix. **posterior d.,** incision of the capsule of a cataract from behind.

discitis (dis-ki′tis) diskitis.

disclination (dis″klĭ-na′shun) [L. *dis-* apart + *clinatus* leaning] outward rotation of the upper pole of the vertical meridian of each eye; called also *abtorsion.* Cf. *conclination.*

disco-, disc- [L. *discus;* Gr. *diskos*] a combining form denoting relationship to a disk, or disk-shaped. See also words beginning *disko-*.

discoblastic (dis″ko-blas′tik) [*disco-* + Gr. *blastos* germ] pertaining to a discoblastula or to discoidal cleavage.

discoblastula (dis″ko-blas′tu-lah) the specialized blastula formed by cleavage of a fertilized telolecithal ovum, consisting of a cellular cap—the germinal disk, or blastoderm—separated by the blastocoele from a floor of uncleaved yolk.

discogastrula (dis″ko-gas′troo-lah) a modified, flattened gastrula formed by discoidal cleavage of a highly telolecithal ovum.

discogenetic (dis″ko-jĕ-net′ik) discogenic.

discogenic (dis″ko-jen′ik) [*disco-* + Gr. *gennan* to produce] caused by derangement of an intervertebral disk.

discogram (dis′ko-gram) diskogram.

discography (dis-kog′rah-fe) diskography.

discoid (dis′koid) [Gr. *diskos* disk + *eidos* form] 1. shaped like a disk. 2. a disklike medicated tablet. 3. a dental instrument with a disklike or circular blade, used for carving dental restorations.

discoidectomy (dis″koid-ek′to-me) diskectomy.

Discomyces (dis″ko-mi′sēz) [*disco-* + Gr. *mykēs* fungus] a name formerly given to certain organisms now included under *Streptomyces*.

Discomycetes (dis″ko-mi-se′tēz) [*disco-* + Gr. *mykēs* fungus] a series of ascomycetous fungi of the subclass Euascomycetidae, including the order Pezizales; their fruiting body is an apothecium.

discopathy (dis-kop′ah-the) [*disco-* + Gr. *pathos* disease] disease of an intervertebral cartilage (disk). **traumatic d.,** rupture of an intervertebral disk due to physical trauma.

discophorous (dis-kof′o-rus) [*disco-* + Gr. *phoros* bearing] possessing a disklike organ or part.

discoplacenta (dis″ko-plah-sen′tah) a discoid placenta.

discord (dis′kord) [L. *discordia*] a simultaneous assemblage of two or more inharmonious sounds.

discordance (dis-kor′dans) in genetics, the occurrence of a given trait in only one member of a twin pair, as opposed to *concordance*.

discordant (dis-kor′dant) exhibiting discordance.

discoria (dis-ko′re-ah) dyscoria.

discrepancy (dis-krep′an-se) disagreement or inconsistency. **tooth size d.,** lack of harmony of size of individual or groups of teeth when related to those within the same arch or the opposing arch.

discrete (dis-krēt′) [L. *discretus; discernere* to separate] made up of separated parts or characterized by lesions which do not become blended.

discus (dis′kus), pl. *dis′ci* [L.; Gr. *diskos*] a circular or rounded flat plate; used as a general term in anatomical nomenclature to designate such a structure. Called also *disc* or *disk*. **d. articula′ris** [NA], the articular disk: a pad composed of fibrocartilage or dense fibrous tissue found in some synovial joints; it extends into the joint from a marginal attachment at the articular capsule and in some cases completely divides the joint cavity into two separate compartments. Called also *interarticular disk*. **d. articula′ris articulatio′nis acromioclavicula′ris** [NA], articular disk of acromioclavicular articulation: a pad of fibrocartilage, sometimes present, commonly imperfect, within the articular cavity of the acromioclavicular joint. Called also *Weitbrecht's cartilage* and *meniscus of acromioclavicular joint.* **d. articula′ris articulatio′nis mandibula′ris,** discus articularis articulationis temporomandibularis. **d. articula′ris articulatio′nis radioulna′ris dista′lis** [NA], articular disk of distal radioulnar articulation: a triangular pad of fibrocartilage, attached at its base to the radius and at its apex to the base of the styloid process of the ulna; it usually separates the articular cavity of the distal radioulnar joint from that of the radiocarpal joint. Called also *cartilago triqueta, meniscus of inferior radioulnar joint,* and *triquetal* or *triquetrous cartilage.* **d. articula′ris articulatio′nis sternoclavicula′ris** [NA], articular disk of sternoclavicular articulation: a pad of fibrocartilage, the circumference of which is connected to the articular capsule of the sternoclavicular joint; it is attached superiorly to the clavicle and inferiorly to the first costal cartilage near its union with the sternum, and divides the joint cavity into two parts. Called also *meniscus of sternoclavicular joint.* **d. articula′ris articulatio′nis temporomandibula′ris** [NA], articular disk of temporomandibular joint: a plate of fibrocartilage or fibrous tissue that divides the temporomandibular joint into two separate cavities; its circumference is connected to the articular capsule. Called also *d. articularis articulationis mandibularis* and *meniscus of temporomandibular joint.* **d. interpu′bicus** [NA], interpubic disk: a midline plate of fibrocartilage interposed between the symphysial surfaces of the pubic bones, these surfaces being covered by a thin layer of hyaline cartilage; called also *lamina fibrocartilaginea interpubica.* **dis′ci intervertebra′les** [NA], intervertebral disks: the 23 plates of fibrocartilage found, from the axis to the sacrum, between the bodies of adjacent vertebrae, each consisting of a fibrous ring (anulus fibrosus)

enclosing a pulpy center (nucleus pulposus); called also *fibrocartilagines intervertebrales,* and *intervertebral cartilages, fibrocartilage,* or *ligaments.* **d. lentifor′mis** (*obs.*), subthalamic nucleus. **d. ner′vi op′tici** [NA], the optic disk: the intraocular portion of the optic nerve formed by fibers converging from the retina and appearing as a pink to white disk. Called also *d. opticus, nerve head, optic papilla,* and *papilla nervi optici.* **d. ooph′orus,** cumulus oophorus. **d. op′ticus,** d. nervi optici. **d. ovig′erus, d. prolig′erus,** cumulus oophorus.

discussive (dis-kus′iv) discutient.

discutient (dis-ku′she-ent) [L. *discutere* to dissipate] 1. scattering; causing a disappearance. 2. a remedy which so acts. Called also *discussive.*

disdiaclast (dis-di′ah-klast) [Gr. *dis* twice + *diaklan* to break through] any of the doubly refracting elements of the contractile substance of muscle.

disdiadochokinesia (dis-di-ad″ŏ-ko-ki-ne′se-ah) dysdiadochokinesia.

disease (dĭ-zēz′) [Fr. *dès* from + *aise* ease] any deviation from or interruption of the normal structure or function of any part, organ, or system (or combination thereof) of the body that is manifested by a characteristic set of symptoms and signs and whose etiology, pathology, and prognosis may be known or unknown. **accumulation d.,** thesaurismosis. **Acosta's d.,** acute mountain sickness. **acute d.,** a disease characterized by a swift onset and short course. **acute demyelinating d.,** postinfection encephalitis. **Adams' d., Adams-Stokes d.,** a condition caused by heart block and characterized by sudden attacks of unconsciousness, with or without convulsions; called also *Adams-Stokes syndrome* or *syncope, Stokes-Adams d., syndrome,* or *syncope, Morgagni-Adams-Stokes syndrome,* and *Stokes' syndrome.* See also *heart block.* **adaptation d.,** any metabolic disorder occurring as the result of adaptation or resistance to severe physical or psychologic stress. **Addison's d.,** a disease characterized by a bronzelike pigmentation of the skin, severe prostration, progressive anemia, low blood pressure, diarrhea, and digestive disturbance; it is due to disease (hypofunction) of the adrenal glands and, in the absence of replacement therapy (cortisol), is usually fatal. Called also *melasma suprarenale* and *bronzed disease* or *skin.* **adult celiac d.,** the adult form of celiac disease, or nontropical sprue. **airsac d.,** infectious sinusitis of turkeys. **akamushi d.,** scrub typhus. **Akureyri d.,** benign myalgic encephalomyelitis; named for a town in northern Iceland where more than 1000 cases occurred in 1948. **Albarrán's d.,** colibacilluria. **Albers-Schönberg d.,** osteopetrosis. **Aleutian mink d.,** a chronic, progressive disease of mink, probably of viral origin, marked by inappetance, weight loss, lethargy, polydipsia, and hemorrhages. **Alexander's d.,** an infantile form of leukodystrophy, characterized histologically by the presence of eosinophilic material at the surface of the brain and around its blood vessels, resulting in brain enlargement. **alkali d.,** 1. botulism in ducks. 2. a disease of livestock; see *selenium poisoning,* under *poisoning.* **allogeneic d.,** graft-versus-host reaction occurring in immunosuppressed animals receiving injections of allogeneic lymphocytes. **Almeida's d.,** South American blastomycosis. **Alper's d.,** poliodystrophia cerebri. **alpha-chain d.,** heavy chain disease characterized by a serum paraprotein composed of incomplete heavy chains without light chains of IgA. Free incomplete alpha chains appear in the serum and patients exhibit severe malabsorption syndrome with chronic diarrhea, steatorrhea, weight loss, hypocalcemia and lymphadenopathy; this is by far the most prevalent of the relatively rare heavy chain diseases. **altitude d.,** high-altitude sickness. **Alzheimer's d.,** presenile dementia. **Anders' d.,** adiposis tuberosa simplex. **Andersen's d.,** glycogen storage d. (type IV). **Andes d.,** chronic mountain sickness. **Andrews' d.** (*obs.*), pustular bacterid. **angiospasmodic d.** (*obs.*), a disease marked by spasms of various vessels of the body. **Apert's d.,** acrocephalosyndactylia. **Apert-Crouzon d.,** a hereditary disorder, transmitted as an autosomal dominant trait, consisting of the hand and foot malformations associated with Apert's syndrome (see *acrocephalosyndactyly*) together with the facial characteristics of Crouzon's disease (see *craniofacial dysostosis,* under *dysostosis*). Called also *acrocephalosyndactyly type II* and *Vogt's cephalodactyly.* **Aran-Duchenne d.,** spinal muscular atrophy. **arc-welders' d.,** siderosis (def. 1). **Armstrong's d.,** lymphocytic choriomeningitis. **atopic d.,** atopy. **Aufrecht's d.** (*obs.*), parenchymatous alterations in the liver and kidney in infectious jaundice. **Aujeszky's d.,** pseudorabies. **Australian X d.,** an acute epidemic encephalitis of viral origin observed in Australia during the summer months between 1917 and 1926, which resembled Japanese B encephalitis both symptomatically and pathologically; the virus appeared to be a variant of Japanese B encephalitis virus, but the culture was lost before it could be identified. See also *Murray Valley encephalitis,* under *encephalitis.* **autoimmune d.,** any of a group of disorders in which tissue injury is associated with humoral or cell-mediated responses to the body's own constituents; they may be systemic (e.g., systemic lupus erythematosus) or organ specific (e.g., autoimmune thyroiditis). **aviators' d.,** high-altitude sickness. **Ayerza's d.,** a form of polycythemia vera marked by chronic cyanosis, chronic dyspnea, chronic bronchitis, bronchiectasis, enlargement of liver and spleen, hyperplasia of bone marrow, and associated with sclerosis of the pulmonary artery. **Baastrup's d.**, kissing spine. **Baelz's d.**, see *cheilitis glandularis.* **Ballingall's d.** (*obs.*), maduromycosis. **Baló's d.**, an atypical form of Schilder's disease in which the demyelination is arranged in concentric rings around a central circle; called also *encephalitis periaxialis concentrica* and *leukoencephalitis periaxialis concentrica.* **Bamberger's d.**, 1. saltatory spasm or tic of the lower extremities. 2. Concato's d. **Bamberger-Marie d.**, hypertrophic pulmonary osteoarthropathy. **Bamle d.**, epidemic pleurodynia. **Bang's d.**, infectious abortion in cattle caused by *Brucella abortus.* **Bannister's d.** (*obs.*), angioneurotic edema. **Banti's d.**, originally described as a primary disease of the spleen associated with splenomegaly and pancytopenia, but later considered secondary to portal hypertension; called also *congestive splenomegaly, Klemperer's d.,* and *splenic anemia.* **barbed-wire d.**, the condition seen in prisoners of war who fall victims of confinement in prison camps. **Barcoo d.**, desert sore. **Barlow's d.**, infantile scurvy. **barometer-maker's d.**, chronic mercurial poisoning in makers of barometers, due to the inhalation of the fumes of mercury. **Barraquer's d.**, lipodystrophia progressiva. **Barthélemy's d.** (*obs.*), papulonecrotic tuberculid. **Basedow's d.**, Graves' d. **Basel d.** (*obs.*), an epidemic form of keratosis follicularis occurring in Switzerland. **Bateman's d.** (*obs.*), molluscum contagiosum. **Batten's d., Batten-Mayou d.**, the juvenile form of cerebral sphingolipidosis with pigmentation of the macula and pallor of the optic disk. **bauxite workers' d.**, bauxite pneumoconiosis. **Bayle's d.**, paralytic dementia. **Bazin's d.**, erythema induratum. **Beard's d.**, neurasthenia. **Beau's d.**, cardiac insufficiency. **Beauvais' d.**, rheumatoid arthritis. **Beck's d.**, a disease affecting young people in Siberia and marked by fatigue and swelling of the phalanges; later all the joints of the body become enlarged and normal growth is retarded. **Bekhterev's d.**, rheumatoid spondylitis. **Begbie's d.**, Graves' d. **Béguez César d.**, Chédiak-Higashi syndrome. **Behçet's d.**, see under *syndrome.* **Behr's d.**, degeneration of the macula retinae in adult life. **Beigel's d.** (*obs.*), piedra. **Bell's d.** (*obs.*), acute delirium. **Benson's d.**, asteroid hyalosis. **Berger's d.**, IgA glomerulonephritis. **Bergeron's d.**, see under *chorea.* **Berlin's d.**, commotio retinae. **Bernhardt's d., Bernhardt-Roth d.**, meralgia paraesthetica. **Besnier-Boeck d.**, sarcoidosis. **Best's d.**, congenital macular degeneration. **Bettlach May d.**, a fatal disease affecting adult honeybees, principally in Switzerland, marked by paralysis with inability to fly, caused by ingestion of the pollen of certain buttercups, which contains a poisonous substance. **Biedl's d.**, see *Laurence-Moon-Biedl syndrome,* under *syndrome.* **Bielschowsky-Jansky d.**, the late infantile form of cerebral sphingolipidosis. **Biermer's d.**, pernicious anemia. **Biett's d.** (*obs.*), discoid lupus erythematosus. **Bilderbeck's d.**, acrodynia. **Billroth's d.**, 1. meningocele due to skull fracture and tearing of the arachnoid; called also *cephalhydrocele traumatica* and *spurious meningocele.* 2. lymphoma. **Binswanger's d.**, see under *dementia.* **Bird's d.**, oxalic diathesis. **black d.**, infectious necrotic hepatitis of sheep; a fatal disease of sheep, and occasionally of man, in the United States (in Montana) and in Australia (in New South Wales, Victoria, Tasmania), marked by necrotic areas in the liver; it is caused by *Clostridium novyi.* **blinding filarial d.**, onchocerciasis caused by *Onchocerca volvulus* (q.v.). **Blocq's d.**, astasia-abasia. **Bloodgood's d.**, cystic d. of breast. **Blount's d.**, osteochondrosis deformans tibiae. **blue d.**, 1. an old term for congenital heart disease; see *morbus caeruleus.* 2. Rocky Mountain spotted fever. **blue nose d.**, a disease of horses, apparently due to photosensitization following the ingestion of certain meadow plants, in which there is usually a blue discoloration of muzzle, sloughing of nonpigmented skin, and frequently intense excitement. **Boeck's d.**, sarcoidosis. **border d. of sheep**, a disease of unknown etiology and very high mortality that affects sheep on the English-Welsh border; it is manifested by an increase in the amount of hair in the fleece, slow growth, diminished stature, slight abnormality of head shape, and a slightly swaying gait. **Borna d.**, a fatal enzootic encephalitis of horses, cattle, and sheep, caused by a virus; called also *enzootic encephalitis of horses, equine encephalitis,* and *crazy d.* **Bornholm d.**, epidemic pleurodynia. **Bostock's d.**, hay fever. **bottom d.**, crotalism. **Bouchard's d.**, dilatation of the stomach from inefficiency of the gastric muscles. **Bouchet-Gsell d.**, swineherd's d. **Bouillaud's d.**, rheumatic endocarditis. **Bourneville's d.**, tuberous sclerosis. **Bouveret's d.**, paroxysmal tachycardia. **Bowen's d.**, intraepidermal squamous cell carcinoma, often occurring in multiple primary sites; called also *Bowen's precancerous dermatosis* and *precancerous dermatitis.* **Bradley's d.**, epidemic nausea and vomiting. **brancher glycogen storage d.**, glycogen storage d. (type IV). **Breda's d.**, yaws. **Breisky's d.**, kraurosis vulvae. **Bretonneau's d.**, diphtheria. **Bright's d.**, a broad descriptive term once used for kidney disease with proteinuria, usually glomerulonephritis. **Brill's d.**, a recrudescence of typhus occurring as long as 70 years after the initial acute episode of epidemic typhus. In the United States, it is seen

primarily in middle-aged or elderly immigrants from Russia, Poland, and neighboring countries. It is milder than the primary infection, owing to the persistence of specific antibody of the IgG class. Called also *Brill-Zinsser d., benign typhus,* and *recrudescent typhus.* **Brill-Symmers d.**, giant follicular lymphoma. **Brill-Zinsser d.**, Brill's d. **Brinton's d.**, linitis plastica. **Brion-Kayser d.**, paratyphoid, def. 2. **brisket d.**, a disease resembling mountain sickness in man, affecting young cattle living at altitudes above 7600 feet; it is sometimes seen in sheep and has been produced experimentally in pigs. **broad-beta d.**, familial hyperlipoproteinemia (type III); so called because on electrophoresis the lipoproteins show a broad band of beta lipoproteins. **Brodie's d.**, 1. chronic synovitis, especially of the knee, with a pulpy degeneration of the parts affected. 2. hysterical pseudofracture of the spine. **bronzed d.**, Addison's d. **Brown-Séquard d.**, see under *syndrome.* **Brown-Symmers d.**, fatal acute serous encephalitis in children. **Bruck's d.**, a condition marked by deformity of bones, multiple fractures, ankylosis of joints, and atrophy of muscles. **Brushfield-Wyatt d.**, see under *syndrome.* **Budd's d.** (*obs.*), Budd's cirrhosis. **Budd-Chiari d.**, see under *syndrome.* **Buerger's d.**, thromboangiitis obliterans. **Buerger-Grütz d.**, idiopathic hyperlipemia. **buffalo d.**, 1. barbone. 2. buffalo encephalitis. **Buhl's d.**, an acute sepsis affecting newborn infants, marked by hemorrhages into the skin, mucous membranes, and navel attended with cyanosis and jaundice; there are also hemorrhages in the intestinal organs. **Bury's d.** (*obs.*), erythema elevatum diutinum. **Buschke's d.**, cryptococcosis. **bush d.**, a disease of sheep and cattle in certain parts of New Zealand, marked by progressive anemia; it is due to an iron or an iron and copper deficiency. **Busquet's d.**, exostoses on the dorsum of the foot due to osteoperiostitis of the metatarsal bones. **Buss d.**, a viral encephalomyelitis with pleuritis affecting cattle in the United States and Japan, marked by dullness, labored breathing, cough, diarrhea, staggering gait, and, sometimes, drooling of saliva and a discharge from the nose; called also *sporadic bovine encephalomyelitis.* **Busse-Buschke d.**, cryptococcosis. **Cacchi-Ricci d.**, sponge kidney. **Caffey's d.**, infantile cortical hyperostosis. **caisson d.**, decompression sickness. **California d.**, coccidioidomycosis. **caloric d.**, any disease due to exposure to high temperature. **Calvé-Perthes d.**, osteochondrosis of the capitular epiphysis of the femur. **Camurati-Engelmann d.**, diaphyseal dysplasia. **Canavan's d.**, spongy degeneration of the central nervous system; see under *degeneration.* **canine parvovirus d.**, an acute, often fatal gastroenteritis of dogs caused by a parvovirus related to the virus of feline panleukopenia or of mink enteritis. **Carrión's d.**, an infectious disease occurring in the valleys of the Andes Mountains in Peru, Chile, Bolivia, and Colombia. It appears in an acute febrile anemic stage (*Oroya fever*) followed in several weeks by a nodular skin eruption (*verruga peruana*). It is caused by *Bartonella bacilliformis,* which is transmitted by the sandfly, *Phlebotomus verrucarum,* but may also be transmitted by *P. noguchi.* Called also *bartonellosis* and *bartonelliosis.* **Castellani's d.**, bronchospirochetosis. **cat-scratch d.**, see under *fever.* **Cavare's d.**, familial periodic paralysis. **Cazenave's d.**, pemphigus foliaceus. **celiac d.**, a malabsorption syndrome affecting both children and adults, precipitated by the ingestion of gluten-containing foods; its etiology is unknown but a hereditary factor has been implicated. Pathologically, the proximal intestinal mucosa loses its villous structure, surface epithelial cells exhibit degenerative changes, and the absorptive function of these cells is severely impaired. It is characterized by diarrhea in which the stools are bulky, frothy, fatty (steatorrhea), and fetid (occasionally, malabsorption may be associated with the passage of a single bulky stool without diarrhea); abdominal distention; flatulence; weight loss; asthenia; deficiency of vitamins B, D, and K; and electrolyte depletion. Called also *gluten enteropathy* and *nontropical sprue.* In the *infantile form* the onset is insidious, and is marked by irritability, loss of appetite, weakness, extreme wasting, growth retardation, and celiac crisis. The *adult form* is marked by extreme lassitude, fatigue, difficulty in breathing, clubbing of the fingers, bone pain, cramping of the muscles, tetany, abdominal distention during the day, megacolon, tympanitis, and skin pigmentation. Until recently it was thought that the infantile form and the adult form were different entities, but it is now believed that they are the same. **central core d. of muscle**, a rare hereditary disease, transmitted as an autosomal dominant trait, in which severe hypotonia arrests motor development in infancy, but the course is benign and by school age affected children can walk; histologically, the diagnostic feature is a central core in each muscle fiber. **Chabert's d.**, blackleg. **Chagas' d.**, a form of trypanosomiasis that runs an acute course in children and a chronic course in adults. Widely distributed in Central and South America, it is caused by *Trypanosoma cruzi,* which is transmitted by *Panstrongylus megistus, P. infestans,* and other reduviid bugs. The acute disease is marked initially by an erythematous nodule (chagoma) at the site of inoculation and by regional lymphadenopathy; in later stages, after the organisms invade tissues via the circulation, it may be marked by myxedema and cardiac and neurologic symptoms. In the chronic phase, which occurs after a latent period of years, the most important manifestation is heart disease (chagasic myocarditis) but neurological and gastrointestinal disorders (e.g., megacolon) also occur. Various animals, including armadillos, cats, bats, foxes, and guinea pigs, serve as reservoir hosts. Called also *South American trypanosomiasis*. **Chagas-Cruz d.**, Chagas' d. **Charcot's d.**, neuropathic arthropathy. **Charcot-Marie-Tooth d.**, progressive neuropathic (peroneal) muscular atrophy. **Charlouis' d.**, yaws. **Charrin's d.**, infection with *Pseudomonas aeruginosa*. **Chédiak-Higashi d.**, see under *syndrome*. **Cherchevski's (Cherchewski's) d.**, ileus of nervous origin. **Chester's d.**, xanthomatosis of the long bones with spontaneous fractures. **Chiari's d.**, Budd-Chiari syndrome. **Chiari-Frommel d.**, see under *syndrome*. **Chicago d.**, North American blastomycosis. **chignon d.** (*obs.*), piedra. **Christian's d.**, Hand-Schüller-Christian d. **Christian-Weber d.**, nodular nonsuppurative panniculitis. **Christmas d.**, hemophilia B. **chronic d.**, one which is slow in its progress and of long continuance. **chronic granulomatous d.**, chronic suppurative lymphadenitis, eczematoid dermatitis, hepatosplenomegaly, and chronic pulmonary disease associated with a genetically determined defect in the intracellular bactericidal function of leukocytes. **chronic obstructive pulmonary d. (COPD)**, any disorder, e.g., asthma, chronic bronchitis, and pulmonary emphysema, marked by persistent obstruction of bronchial air flow. **chronic respiratory d. of poultry**, a common respiratory disease of chickens caused by mycoplasma, and marked by distressed breathing, swelling of the face, and discharge from the nostrils; abbreviated C.R.D. **chylopoietic d.** (*obs.*), one which affects the digestive organs. **Ciarrocchi's d.** (*obs.*), erosio interdigitalis blastomycetica. **circling d.**, listeriosis. **climatic d.**, any disease thought to be produced by a change of climate. **coast d.**, a disease of domestic animals similar to enzootic marasmus (q.v.), occurring in Tasmania. **Coats' d.**, chronic progressive exudative retinopathy usually occurring in male children and young adults. **Cogan's d.**, see under *syndrome*. **collagen d.**, any of a group of diseases that, although clinically distinct and not necessarily related etiologically, have in common widespread pathologic changes in the connective tissue; they include lupus erythematosus, dermatomyositis, scleroderma, polyarteritis nodosa, thrombotic purpura, rheumatic fever, and rheumatoid arthritis. **comb d.**, favus of fowl. **combined immunodeficiency d.**, deficiency of lymphoid cells that mediate both humoral (B-lymphocytes) and cellular (T-lymphocytes) immunity. **combined system d.**, subacute combined degeneration of the spinal cord; see under *degeneration*. **communicable d.**, a disease the causative agent of which may pass or be carried from one person to another directly or indirectly. **complicating d.**, one which occurs in the course of some other disease as a complication. **compressed-air d.**, decompression sickness. **Concato's d.**, progressive malignant polyserositis with large effusions into the pericardium, pleura, and peritoneum. **Conor and Bruch's d.**, boutonneuse fever. **Conradi's d.**, dysplasia epiphysealis punctata. **constitutional d.**, one that involves a system of organs or one characterized by widespread symptoms. **contagious d.**, a disease that is communicable by contact with an individual suffering from it or with some secretion of such an individual, or with an object touched by him. Cf. *infectious d.* **Cooley's d.**, see β-thalassemia. **Cooper's d.** (*obs.*), chronic cystic disease of the breast. **Corbus' d.**, gangrenous balanitis. **Cori's d.**, glycogen storage d. (type III). **cornstalk d.**, toxic encephalomalacia of dietary origin affecting horses. **corridor d.**, a disease resembling East Coast fever, affecting African buffalo and cattle, caused by the protozoan parasite *Theileria lawrencei*, which is transmitted by ticks. **Corrigan's d.**, aortic insufficiency; see also *insufficiency of the valves*. **Corvisart's d.**, 1. chronic hypertrophic myocarditis. 2. tetralogy of Fallot associated with right aortic arch. **Cotugno's d.**, sciatica. **covering d.**, dourine. **Cowden's d.**, a hereditary disease characterized by multiple ectodermal, mesodermal, and endodermal nevoid and neoplastic anomalies. Papules of the face and oral mucosa are the most characteristic lesion; other changes occur in the skin, in the thyroid (goiter, adenoma, carcinoma), the breast (fibrocystic disease), the gastrointestinal system, and the nervous system. Called also *multiple hamartoma syndrome*. **coxsackievirus A d.**, herpangina. **crazy d.**, Borna disease. **crazy chick d.**, 1. avian encephalomalacia. 2. avian encephalomyelitis. **creeping d.**, a condition marked by cutaneous lesions similar to those seen in larva migrans, but produced by nematodes of the genus *Gnathostoma*. **Creutzfeldt-Jakob d.**, a rare, usually fatal, transmissible spongiform viral encephalopathy, occurring in middle life, in which there is partial degeneration of the pyramidal and extrapyramidal systems accompanied by progressive dementia and sometimes wasting of the muscles, tremor, athetosis, and spastic dysarthria. Called also *Creutzfeldt-Jakob syndrome*, *Jakob's disease*, *Jakob-Creutzfelt disease*, and *spastic pseudoparalysis*. **Crigler-Najjar d.**, see under *syndrome*. **Crocq's d.** (*obs.*), acrocyanosis. **Crohn's d.**, a chronic granulomatous inflammatory disease of unknown etiology, involving any part of the gastrointestinal tract from mouth to anus, but commonly involving the terminal ileum with scarring and thickening of the bowel wall; it frequently leads to intestinal

obstruction and fistula and abscess formation and has a high rate of recurrence after treatment. Called also *regional enteritis* or *ileitis*. **Crouzon's d.**, craniofacial dysostosis. **Cruveilhier's d.**, 1. spinal muscular atrophy. 2. Cruveilhier's ulcer. **Cruz-Chagas d.**, Chagas' d. **Csillag's d.** (*obs.*), lichen sclerosus et atrophicus. **Curschmann's d.** (*obs.*), perihepatitis chronica plastica. **Cushing's d.**, Cushing's syndrome in which the hyperadrenocorticism is secondary to excessive pituitary secretion of adrenocorticotropic hormone. **cystic d. of breast**, a form of mammary dysplasia with formation of cysts of various size containing a semitransparent, turbid fluid that imparts a brown to blue color (blue dome cyst) to the unopened cysts; considered to be due to abnormal hyperplasia of the ductal epithelium and dilatation of the ducts of the mammary gland, occurring as a result of an exaggeration and distortion of the cyclic breast changes that normally occur in the menstrual cycle. Called also *chronic cystic mastitis, fibrocystic disease, fibrocystic disease of breast*, and *Schimmelbusch's disease*. **cystic d. of lung**, a condition in which there are abnormally large air spaces in the lung parenchyma; the term is sometimes applied to cystic emphysema. Called also *pseudocysts of lung* and *pulmonary pseudocysts*. **cysticercus d.**, infection with larval forms (*Cysticercus cellulosae*) of *Taenia solium* (the pork tapeworm). **cystine d., cystine storage d.**, cystinosis. **cytomegalic inclusion d.**, an infection due to cytomegalovirus and marked by nuclear inclusion bodies in enlarged infected cells. In the congenital form, there is hepatosplenomegaly with cirrhosis, and microcephaly with mental or motor retardation. Acquired disease may cause a clinical state similar to infectious mononucleosis. When acquired by blood transfusion, postperfusion syndrome (q.v.) results. Called also *salivary gland disease*. **Czerny's d.**, periodic hydrarthrosis of the knee. **Daae's d., Daae-Finsen d.**, epidemic pleurodynia. **DaCosta's d.**, 1. misplaced gout. 2. neurocirculatory asthenia. **Dalrymple's d.**, cyclokeratitis. **dancing d.**, tarantism. **Danlos' d.**, *Ehlers-Danlos syndrome*. **Darier's d.**, keratosis follicularis. **Darling's d.**, histoplasmosis. **David's d.**, 1. [J. P. David.] tuberculosis of the spine. 2. [W. David.] an unexplained form of hemorrhagic disease in women, marked by severe bleeding from the gums and mucous membranes, attributed, without definite basis, to deficiency of ovarian hormone. **debrancher glycogen storage d.**, glycogen storage d. (type II). **deer fly d.**, tularemia. **deficiency d.**, a condition produced by dietary or metabolic deficiency; the term includes all diseases—e.g., kwashiorkor, beriberi, scurvy, pellagra, calcium deficiency, etc.—caused by an insufficient supply of the essential nutrients, i.e., protein (or amino acids), vitamins, and minerals. **degenerative joint d.**, osteoarthritis. **Degos' d.**, malignant papulosis. **Dejerine's d.**, Dejerine-Sottas d., progressive hypertrophic interstitial neuropathy. **demyelinating d.**, any condition characterized by destruction of myelin. **deprivation d.**, deficiency d. **de Quervain's d.**, painful tenosynovitis due to relative narrowness of the common tendon sheath of the abductor pollicis longus and the extensor pollicis brevis. **Dercum's d.**, adiposis dolorosa. **Deutschländer's d.**, 1. tumor of the metatarsal bones. 2. march foot (fracture). **Devergie's d.** (*obs.*), pityriasis rubra pilaris. **Devic's d.**, neuromyelitis optica. **diamond-skin d.**, the urticarial and mildest form of swine erysipelas. **Di Guglielmo d.**, erythremic myelosis. **Dimitri's d.**, Sturge-Weber syndrome. **diverticular d.**, a general term embracing the prediverticular state, diverticulosis, and diverticulitis. **Döhle's d.**, syphilitic aortitis. **Down's d.**, see under *syndrome*. **drug d.**, 1. a morbid condition due to long-continued use of a drug. 2. in homeopathy, the group of symptoms seen after the administration of a drug for the purpose of proving. **Dubin-Sprinz d.**, Dubin-Johnson syndrome. **Dubini's d.**, see under *chorea*. **Dubois' d.**, the development of multiple abscesses in the thymus gland in congenital syphilis. **Duchenne's d.**, 1. spinal muscular atrophy. 2. bulbar paralysis. 3. tabes dorsalis. **Duchenne-Aran d.**, spinal muscular atrophy. **Duchenne-Griesinger d.**, pseudohypertrophic muscular dystrophy. **Duhring's d.**, dermatitis herpetiformis. **Dukes' d.**, a febrile disease of childhood characterized by an exanthematous eruption, probably a mild form of scarlet fever; called also *fourth d.* **Duplay's d.** (*obs.*), subacromial or subdeltoid bursitis; see *calcific tendinitis*, under *tendinitis*. **Dupré's d.**, meningism, def. 1. **Durand's d.**, a viral disease, characterized by headache and by upper respiratory, meningeal, and gastrointestinal symptoms. **Durand-Nicolas-Favre d.**, lymphogranuloma venereum. **Durante's d.**, osteogenesis imperfecta. **Duroziez's d.**, congenital mitral stenosis. **Dutton's d.** (*obs.*), trypanosomiasis. **Eales's d.**, a condition marked by recurrent hemorrhages into the retina and vitreous, affecting mainly males in the second and third decades of life. **Ebstein's d.**, 1. hyaline degeneration and necrosis of the epithelial cells of the renal tubules; seen in diabetes. 2. see under *anomaly*. **echinococcus d.**, hydatid d. **Economo's d.**, lethargic encephalitis. **Eddowes' d.**, see under *syndrome*. **Edsall's d.**, heat cramp. **Ehlers-Danlos d.**, see under *syndrome*. **Eichstedt's d.** (*obs.*), tinea versicolor. **elevator d.**, respiratory distress affecting persons who work in grain elevators. **endemic d.**, a disease which is at all times present in a small number of persons in a particular region. **Engelmann's d.,** diaphyseal dysplasia. **Engel-Recklinghausen d.,** osteitis fibrosa cystica. **English d.,** rickets. **Engman's d.** (*obs.*), infectious eczematoid dermatitis. **enzootic d.,** a disease which is at all times present in a small number of animals in a particular region. **eosinophilic endomyocardial d.,** Löffler's endocarditis. **epidemic d.,** a disease which affects a large number of people in some particular region within a short period of time. **epizootic d.,** a disease which affects a large number of animals in some particular region within a short period of time. **Epstein's d.,** pseudodiphtheria. **Erb's d.,** progressive muscular dystrophy. **Erb-Charcot d.,** Erb's spastic paraplegia. **Erb-Goldflam d.,** myasthenia gravis. **Erb-Landouzy d.,** muscular dystrophy. **Eulenburg's d.,** myotonia congenita. **extrapyramidal d.,** any of a group of clinical disorders marked by abnormal involuntary movements, alterations in muscle tone, and postural disturbances and involving lesions of the extrapyramidal tract; it includes parkinsonism, chorea, athetosis, etc. **extensor process d.,** buttress foot. **Fabry's d.,** a rare hereditary sphingolipidosis in which glycolipids (chiefly ceramide trihexoside) are deposited in various tissues, especially the kidneys; it is marked by vasomotor disturbances, edema, enlargement of the heart, especially the left ventricle, and moderate hypertension; by urinary abnormalities (albuminuria, and some erythrocytes, leukocytes, and casts); and by cutaneous lesions (diffuse, purpuric, and nodular, or generalized angiomatous). Muscles may also be affected, and there may be ocular involvement. The metabolic defect is deficiency of an α-galactosidase, transmitted as an X-linked recessive trait. Called also *angiokeratoma corporis diffusum* and *Fabry's syndrome.* **Fahr-Volhard d.,** malignant nephrosclerosis. **Fallot's d.,** tetralogy of Fallot. **Fanconi's d.,** see under *syndrome.* **Farber's d.,** one of the sphingolipidoses, a rare hereditary disorder of ceramide metabolism due to deficiency of the enzyme ceramidase and marked by hoarseness, aphonia, and a brownish desquamating dermatitis beginning at about three months of age, followed by foam cell infiltration of bones and joints, resulting in deformations; granulomatous reaction in lymph nodes, heart, lung, and kidneys; and psychomotor retardation. It is transmitted as an autosomal recessive trait. **fat-deficiency d.,** a condition characterized by cessation of growth and skin lesions that result when essential fatty acids (arachidonic and linoleic acid) are absent from the diet. **fatigue d.,** occupation neurosis. **Fauchard's d.,** periodontitis. **Favre-Durand-Nicholas d.,** lymphogranuloma venereum. **Fede's d.,** Riga-Fede d. **Feer's d.,** acrodynia. **Fenwick's d.,** idiopathic atrophic gastritis, first described by Fenwick in a patient with pernicious anemia. **fibrocystic d., fibrocystic d. of breast,** cystic d. of breast. **fibrocystic d. of the pancreas,** cystic fibrosis of the pancreas (q.v. under *fibrosis*). **Fiedler's d.,** leptospiral jaundice. **fifth d.,** erythema infectiosum. **fifth venereal d.,** lymphogranuloma venereum. **Filatov's d.,** infectious mononucleosis. **Filatov-Dukes d.,** Dukes' d. **file-cutters' d.,** lead poisoning from inhaling particles of lead which arise from the bed of lead used in file cutting. **finger and toe d.,** a disease of cabbage and other cruciferous plants caused by *Plasmodiophora brassicae*; called also *root hernia.* **fish-handler's d.** (*obs.*), erysipeloid. **fish-skin d.** (*obs.*), ichthyosis. **fishslime d.,** septicemia following a puncture wound made by the spine of a fish. **Flajani's d.,** exophthalmic goiter. **Flatau-Schilder d.,** Schilder's d. **flax-dresser's d.,** a pulmonary disorder seen in flax-dressers, and caused by inhaling particles of flax. **flecked retina d.,** a group of retinal disorders, including fundus flavimaculatus, fundus albipunctatus, drusen, and congenital macular degeneration, all suspected of being primary abnormalities of the retinal pigment epithelium. **Fleischner's d.,** osteochondritis affecting the middle phalanges of the hand. **flint d.,** chalicosis. **fluke d.,** infection with flukes; see *Trematoda.* **focal d.,** one which is localized at one or more foci. **Fölling's d.,** phenylketonuria. **foot-and-mouth d.,** an acute, naturally occurring, extremely contagious viral disease of wild and domestic animals, chiefly cattle, pigs, sheep, goats, and other ruminants, and very rarely of man. It is marked by an eruption of vesicles on the lips, buccal cavity, pharynx, legs, and feet; sometimes the skin of the udder or teats is involved. Called also *hoof-and-mouth d.; aftosa; contagious, epizootic,* or *malignant aphthae; aphthous fever;* and *aphthobullous, epidemic,* or *epizootic stomatitis.* **Fordyce's d.,** glycogen storage d. (type III). **Fordyce's d.,** 1. a developmental anomaly characterized by enlarged and ectopic sebaceous glands that appear as minute yellowish papules (Fordyce's spots or granules) on the oral mucosa. 2. Fox-Fordyce d. **Förster's d.,** see under *choroiditis.* **Fothergill's d.,** 1. scarlatina anginosa. 2. trigeminal neuralgia. **Fournier's d.,** fulminating gangrene of the scrotum. **fourth d.,** Dukes' d. **fourth venereal d.,** 1. specific gangrenous and ulcerative balanoposthitis; see under *balanoposthitis.* 2. granuloma inguinale. **Fox-Fordyce d.,** a persistent and recalcitrant itchy papular eruption, limited chiefly to the axillae and the pubes, due to inflammation of the apocrine sweat glands. **Francis' d.,** tularemia. **Frankl-Hochwart's d.,** polyneuritis cerebralis menieriformis. **Frei's d.,** lymphogranuloma venereum. **Freiberg's d.,** osteochondrosis

of the head of the second metatarsal. **Friedländer's d.,** endarteritis obliterans. **Friedreich's d.,** 1. paramyoclonus multiplex. 2. Friedreich's ataxia. **fright d.,** canine hysteria; psychic disturbance in dogs marked by symptoms of fright and by hysterical barking and running. **Frommel's d.,** Chiari-Frommel syndrome. **functional d.,** a disease involving functions without tissue damage. **functional cardiovascular d.,** neurocirculatory asthenia. **Fürstner's d.,** pseudospastic paralysis with tremor. **Gaisböck's d.,** stress polycythemia. **Gamna's d.,** a form of splenomegaly, with thickening of the splenic capsule and the presence of small brownish areas (Gamna nodules) which are usually surrounded by a hematogenous zone; ferruginous pigment is deposited in the splenic pulp. **Gamstorp's d.,** adynamia episodica hereditaria. **Gandy-Nanta d.,** siderotic splenomegaly. **gannister d.,** pneumoconiosis due to the inhalation of dust by workers in the manufacture of refractory brick or fire clay. **garapata d.,** relapsing fever. **Garré's d.,** sclerosing nonsuppurative osteomyelitis. **Gaucher's d.,** a group of hereditary disorders of glucocerebroside metabolism characterized by the presence of Gaucher's cells in the marrow and by splenomegaly, hepatomegaly, and erosion of the cortices of the long bones and pelvis. The adult form is associated with moderate anemia and thrombocytopenia, and yellowish pigmentation of the skin. In the infantile form, there is, in addition, marked impairment of the central nervous system. The juvenile form is characterized by rapidly progressing systemic manifestations but moderate involvement of the central nervous system. The disorder is transmitted as an autosomal recessive and, possibly in some instances, as an autosomal dominant trait. Called also *Gaucher's splenomegaly, kerasin thesaurismosis,* and *cerebroside lipoidosis.* **Gee's d., Gee-Herter d., Gee-Herter-Heubner d.,** childhood celiac disease; nontropical sprue. **Gee-Thaysen d.,** adult celiac disease; the adult form of nontropical sprue. **genetotrophic d.,** inborn error of metabolism; see under *metabolism.* **Gensoul's d.,** Ludwig's angina. **Gerhardt's d.,** erythromelalgia. **Gerlier's d.,** a disease of the nerves and nerve centers attacking farm laborers and stablemen, and characterized by pain, paresis, vertigo, ptosis, and muscular contractions; called also *endemic paralytic vertigo, paralyzing vertigo,* and *Gerlier's syndrome.* **Gibert's d.** (*obs.*), pityriasis rosea. **Gibney's d.,** see under *perispondylitis.* **Gierke's d.,** see *glycogen storage d.* (*type I*). **Gilbert's d.,** a familial, benign elevation of unconjugated bilirubin levels without evidence of liver damage or hematologic abnormalities. Called also *constitutional hepatic dysfunction, familial cholemia, familial nonhemolytic jaundice,* and *Gilbert's cholemia* or *syndrome.* **Gilchrist's d.,** North American blastomycosis. **Gilles de la Tourette's d.,** see under *syndrome.* **Glanzmann's d.,** see *thrombasthenia.* **Glasser's d.,** a disease mainly affecting pigs 5 to 14 weeks old, in which swelling of the hocks or knee joints, or both, is accompanied by fever, lameness, and a disinclination to move: if untreated, death usually results. It is caused by a strain of *Hemophilus influenzae.* **Glénard's d.** (*obs.*), splanchnoptosis. **Glisson's d.,** rickets. **glycogen d.,** glycogen storage d. **glycogen storage d.,** a group of chronic, genetically determined metabolic disorders of childhood. Called also *glycogen d., glycogenosis, glycogenic thesaurismosis,* and *glycogenic hepatomegaly.* Many types have been recognized, including the following: In *type I,* a deficiency in glucose-6-phosphatase results in liver and kidney involvement, with hepatomegaly, hypoglycemia, hyperuricemia, and gout. Called also *Gierke's* (*von Gierke's*) d. and *hepatorenal glycogenosis.* In *type II,* a defect in α-1,4-glucosidase (acid maltase) results in generalized glycogen accumulation, with cardiomegaly, cardiorespiratory failure, and death. Affected children appear imbecilic and are hypotonic. Called also *cardiomegalia glycogenica diffusa, generalized glycogenosis,* and *Pompe's d.* In *type III,* a rare defect in the debranching enzyme amylo-1,6-glucosidase affects the heart and liver, with hepatomegaly, hypoglycemia, acidosis, stunted growth, and doll facies. Called also *Forbes' d.* and *limit dextrinosis.* In *type IV,* a rare defect in the branching enzyme amylo-1:4, 1:6-transglucosidase results in hepatomegaly and splenomegaly, with progressive hepatic failure and death. Called also *amylopectinosis* and *Andersen's d.* In *type V,* deficiency of muscle phosphorylase affects the skeletal muscles, with muscle cramps and a depressed blood lactate level during exercise. Called also *McArdle's d.* and *myophosphorylase deficiency glycogenosis.* In *type VI,* a deficiency of liver phosphorylase is manifested in the liver and leukocytes, with hepatomegaly, moderate hypoglycemia, mild acidosis, and growth retardation. Called also *Hers' d.* In *type VII,* a deficiency in phosphofructokinase affects muscle and erythrocytes, with temporary weakness and cramping of skeletal muscle after exercise. In *type VIII,* the enzyme deficiency is unknown but the liver and brain are affected, with hepatomegaly, truncal ataxia, and nystagmus; the neurologic deterioration progressing to hypertonia, spasticity, and death. In *type IX,* a deficiency in liver phosphorylase kinase results in marked hepatomegaly, which may disappear in early adulthood. In *type X,* a lack of activity of cyclic AMP–dependent kinase affects the liver and muscle, with mild clinical symptoms. **Goldflam's d., Goldflam-Erb d.,** myasthenia gravis. **Goldstein's d.,** hereditary hemorrhagic telangiectasia. **Graefe's d.,** ophthalmoplegia progressiva. **graft-versus-host d.,** graft-versus-host reaction. **grass d.,** a usually fatal disease of horses occurring after they have been put to graze on grass, usually between May and July; first seen in Scotland, it has spread to Wales, England, and Sweden. It is marked by dysphagia, severe diarrhea, dehydration, interrupted peristalsis, and priapism. Called also *grass sickness.* **Graves' d.,** a disorder of the thyroid of unknown etiology, occurring most often in women, and characterized by exophthalmos, enlarged pulsating thyroid gland, marked acceleration of the pulse rate, a tendency to profuse sweats, nervous symptoms (including fine muscular tremors, restlessness, and irritability), psychic disturbances, emaciation, and increased metabolic rate. Called also *Basedow's d., Begbie's d., cachexia exophthalmica, exophthalmic goiter, hyperthyroidism, Parry's d., Stokes' d., thyroid cachexia, thyrotoxicosis, tachycardia strumosa exophthalmica,* and *toxic goiter.* **greasy pig d.,** seborrhea of piglets, which is thought to be associated with a vitamin B deficiency. **Greenfield's d.,** see *metachromatic leukodystrophy,* under *leukodystrophy.* **Greenhow's d.** (*obs.*), vagabonds' d. **Griesinger's d.** (*obs.*), hookworm d. **grinder's d.,** pneumoconiosis of grinders. **Gross's d.,** encysted rectum; saccular dilatation of anal wall with retained inspissated feces. **di Guglielmo's d.,** acute erythremic myelosis. **guinea worm d.,** dracunculiasis. **Guinon's d.,** Gilles de la Tourette's syndrome. **Gull's d.,** atrophy of the thyroid with myxedema. **Günther's d.,** congenital erythropoietic porphyria. **H d.,** Hartnup d. **Habermann's d.,** pityriasis lichenoides et varioliformis acuta. **Haff d.,** a condition affecting fishermen of the Koenigsberg (Frisches) Haff, a lagoon joining the Baltic Sea. The men are suddenly seized with severe pain in the limbs, great weariness, and myoglobinuria. The disease is said to be the result of poisoning by arsine introduced into the Haff through the waste water of cellulose factories. Several epidemics occurred prior to World War II. **Haglund's d.,** bursitis in the region of the Achilles tendon. **Hagner's d.,** an obscure bone disease somewhat resembling acromegaly (Pierre Marie described this obscure bone disease in the two Hagner brothers). **Hailey-Hailey d.,** benign familial pemphigus. **Hall's d.** (*obs.*), spurious hydrocephalus in children. **Hallervorden-Spatz d.,** see under *syndrome.* **Hamman's d.,** interstitial emphysema of the lungs due to spontaneous rupture of the alveoli. Called also *Hamman's syndrome.* **Hammond's d.,** athetosis. **Hand's d.,** Hand-Schüller-Christian d. **hand-foot-and-mouth d.,** a mild, highly infectious viral disease of children, characterized by vesicular lesions in the mouth and on the hands and feet. **Hand-Schüller-Christian d.,** a chronic idiopathic form of histiocytosis, sometimes with accumulation of cholesterol, characterized classically by the triad of: defects in the membranous bones, exophthalmos, and diabetes insipidus. In most cases this triad is not seen, but there is multiple-system, soft tissue, and bone involvement. Called also *chronic idiopathic xanthomatosis* and *cholesterol thesaurismosis.* **Hanot's d.,** 1. primary biliary cirrhosis. 2. secondary biliary cirrhosis. **Hansen's d.,** leprosy. **Hansen's d., benign,** the tuberculoid type of leprosy. **Hansen's d., malignant,** the lepromatous type of leprosy. **d. of the Hapsburgs,** hemophilia. **Harada's d.,** see under *syndrome.* **hard pad d.,** hyperkeratosis of the footpads of young dogs, occurring in canine distemper. **Hartnup d.,** a condition characterized by hereditary pellagra-like skin rash, with transient cerebellar ataxia, constant renal aminoaciduria, and other bizarre biochemical abnormalities; the defect involves the intestinal and renal transport of neutral alpha-amino acids and is transmitted as an autosomal recessive trait. **Hashimoto's d.,** struma lymphomatosa. **heart d.,** any organic, mechanical, or functional abnormality of the heart; it may be valvular, myocardial, or neurogenic. **heartwater d.,** see *heartwater.* **heavy-chain d.,** a condition marked by the presence of heavy-chain subunits of immunoglobulins in the serum. In the IgG (γ-chain) form, symptoms include weakness, weight loss, lymphadenopathy, and recurrent bacterial infections. The IgA (α-chain) form occurs mostly in the Middle East and is marked by abdominal lymphoma and malabsorption syndrome. In the IgM (μ-chain) form, the spleen, liver, and abdominal lymph nodes are primarily involved and there are vacuolated plasma cells in the bone marrow and Bence Jones proteinuria. **Heberden's d.,** 1. rheumatism of the smaller joints, accompanied by nodules in or about the distal interphalangeal joints. 2. angina pectoris. **Heerfordt's d.,** uveoparotid fever. **Heine-Medin d.,** the major form of poliomyelitis, with involvement of the central nervous system and perhaps paralysis; see *poliomyelitis.* **Heller-Döhle d.,** syphilitic aortitis. **helminthic d.,** a disease caused by worms. **hemoglobin d.,** any of a group of heredity molecular diseases, characterized by the presence of various abnormal hemoglobins, e.g., hemoglobin C, D, E, H, or S, in the red blood cells, in which the homozygous form is manifested by hemolytic anemia. See also *sickle cell anemia,* under *anemia,* and see individual hemoglobins, under *hemoglobin.* **hemoglobin C–thalassemia d.,** a hereditary disorder involving simultaneous heterozygosity for hemoglobin C and thalassemia, manifested by mild hemolytic anemia and persistent splenomegaly; called also *hemoglobin C–thalassemia.* **hemoglobin E–thalassemia d.,** a hereditary condition involving simultaneous heterozygosity for hemoglobin E and thalassemia, manifested by mild hemolytic anemia and persistent

splenomegaly; called also *hemoglobin E–thalassemia.* **hemolytic d. of newborn,** erythroblastosis fetalis. **hemorrhagic d., epidemic,** epidemic hemorrhagic fever; see under *fever.* **hemorrhagic d. of the newborn,** a self-limited hemorrhagic disorder of the first days of life, caused by a deficiency of the vitamin K–dependent blood coagulation factors II, VII, IX, and X. **Henderson-Jones d.,** osteochondromatosis characterized by the presence of numerous cartilaginous foreign bodies in the joint cavity or in the bursa of a tendon sheath. **hepatolenticular d.,** see under *degeneration.* **hepatorenal glycogen storage d.,** glycogen storage d. (type I). **hereditary d.,** one that is transmitted genetically from parents to children. **heredoconstitutional d.,** an inherited pathologic condition which does not progress. **heredodegenerative d.,** a disease of the central nervous system characterized by specific loss of neural tissue due to hereditary influence. **Hers' d.,** glycogen storage d. (type VI). **Herter's d., Herter-Heubner d.,** the infantile form of nontropical sprue. **Heubner's d.,** syphilitic endarteritis of the cerebral vessels; called also *Heubner's specific endarteritis.* **Hildenbrand's d.,** typhus. **hip-joint d.,** tuberculosis of the hip joint. **Hippel's d.,** see *von Hippel's d.* **Hippel-Lindau d.,** see *von Hippel-Lindau d.* **Hirschfeld's d.,** acute diabetes mellitus. **Hirschsprung's d.,** congenital megacolon. **His's d., His-Werner d.,** trench fever. **hock d.,** perosis. **Hodara's d.** (*obs.*), a kind of trichorrhexis nodosa seen in women in Istanbul. **Hodgkin's d.,** a malignant condition characterized by painless, progressive enlargement of the lymph nodes, spleen, and general lymphoid tissue; other symptoms may include anorexia, lassitude, weight loss, fever, pruritus, night sweats, and anemia. The characteristic histologic feature is presence of Reed-Sternberg cells. Hodgkin's disease is usually classified as: (1) diffuse, according to the number of lymphocyte and histiocytes (lymphocytes predominant; mixed cellularity; lymphocytes depleted) and (2) nodular sclerosing (marked by birefringent bands of collagen and the presence of the lacunar cells). The condition, which affects twice as many males as females and usually occurs between the ages of 15 and 34 or after 50, is considered by many to be neoplastic in origin, but neither an infectious origin nor an immune response to the development of Reed-Sternberg cells has been excluded. **Hodgson's d.,** an aneurysmal dilatation of the proximal part of the aorta, often accompanied by dilatation or hypertrophy of the heart. **Hoffa's d.,** traumatic proliferation of fatty tissue (solitary lipoma) in the knee joint (Albert Hoffa, 1904). **hoof-and-mouth d.,** foot-and-mouth d. **hookworm d.,** a condition due to infection with *Ancylostoma duodenale* or *Necator americanus,* nematode worms that closely resemble each other. (In dogs, the disease is caused by *Uncinaria stenocephala.*) The disease occurs in practically all tropical and subtropical countries, including the southern United States and the West Indies. In temperate regions, it may occur in mines and tunnels, where conditions of temperature and moisture resemble the tropics. The larvae of the parasite live in soil and gain entrance to the digestive tract indirectly by way of the skin of the feet or legs or directly with contaminated food or water. The percutaneous infection is followed by a transitory eruption known as "ground itch." From here the parasites are carried by the blood to the lungs, ascend the trachea, are swallowed, and settle in the small intestine, where they attach to the intestinal mucosa and ingest blood. Symptoms, which vary with diet and with severity of infection, may include abdominal pain, diarrhea, and colic or nausea. Anemia is seen only in moderate to severe infections or when other adverse nutritional factors operate in conjuction with the parasite-induced blood loss. **Horton's d.,** migrainous neuralgia. **Huchard's d.,** continued arterial hypertension, thought to be a cause of arteriosclerosis. **Hünermann's d.,** dysplasia epiphysealis punctata. **hunger d., hungry d.,** excessive hunger accompanied by weakness and nervousness caused by hyperinsulism. **Hunt's d.,** 1. dyssynergia cerebellaris myoclonica. 2. Ramsay Hunt syndrome, def. 1. **Huntington's d.,** see under *chorea.* **Hurler's d.,** see under *syndrome.* **Hutchinson's d.,** 1. prurigo estivalis. 2. angioma serpiginosum. 3. pompholyx. 4. Tay's choroiditis. **Hutchinson-Boeck d.,** sarcoidosis. **Hutchinson-Gilford d.,** progeria. **Hutinel's d.,** tuberculous pericarditis with cirrhosis of the liver in children. **hyaline membrane d.,** a disorder affecting newborn infants (usually premature) characterized pathologically by the development of a hyalin-like membrane lining the terminal respiratory passages. Extensive atelectasis is attributed to lack of surfactant. See *respiratory distress syndrome of newborn,* under *syndrome.* **hydatid d.,** an infection, usually of the liver, caused by larval forms (hydatid cysts) of tapeworms of the genus *Echinococcus,* and characterized by the development of expanding cysts. See *hydatid d., alveolar,* and *hydatid d., unilocular.* Called also *hydatidosis, echinococcus d.,* and *echinococcosis.* **hydatid d., alveolar,** infection with larval forms (hydatid cysts) of *Echinococcus multilocularis,* characterized by invasion and destruction of the host's tissues as the cysts undergo endogenous budding to form an aggregate of innumerable small cysts which honeycomb the affected organ (the liver in over 90 per cent of cases) and may metastasize. **hydatid d., unilocular,** infection with the larval forms (hydatid cysts) of *Echinococcus granulosis,* characterized by the formation of single or multiple expanding cysts which are unilocular in nature; as the cysts expand they may give rise to symptoms of related space-occupying lesions in the tissues or organs affected. **hydrocephaloid d.,** a condition similar to hydrocephalus, but marked by depression of the fontanels, due to diarrhea or some other wasting disease with dehydration. **Iceland d., Icelandic d.,** benign myalgic encephalomyelitis. **I-cell d.,** mucolipidosis II. **idiopathic d.,** one not consequent upon any other disease, and of which the cause is unknown. **immune-complex d.,** 1. disease induced by the deposition of or association with antigen-antibody-complement complexes in the microvasculature of tissues, such as peripheral capillary glomerular basement membranes and mesangial areas of renal glomeruli. Fixation of complement component C3 by the complexes initiates inflammation. Called also *immune deposit disease.* 2. serum sickness. **inborn lysosomal d's,** lysosomal storage d. **inclusion d.,** any disease in which cell inclusions are found. **infantile celiac d.,** the infantile form of celiac disease, or nontropical sprue. **infectious d.,** a disease due to organisms ranging in size from viruses to parasitic worms; it may be contagious in origin, result from nosocomial organisms, or be due to endogenous microflora from the nose and throat, skin, or bowel. **inflammatory bowel d.,** a general term for those inflammatory diseases of the bowel of unknown etiology, including Crohn's disease and ulcerative colitis. **inherited d.,** one transmitted genetically, from parents to offspring. **insect-borne d's,** diseases caused by microorganisms which are transmitted by insects, the principal ones being dengue, encephalitis, filariasis, kala-azar, leishmaniasis, malaria, nagana, phlebotomas fever, plague, relapsing fever, Rocky Mountain spotted fever, surra, Texas fever, trypanosomiasis, tularemia, typhus, and yellow fever. **intercurrent d.,** a disease occurring during the course of another disease with which it has no connection. **interstitial d.,** one in which the stroma of an organ is mainly affected. **iron storage d.,** hemochromatosis. **Isambert's d.,** acute miliary tuberculosis of the larynx and pharynx. **island d.,** scrub typhus. **Isle of Wight d.,** paralysis of the muscles of flight in honey bees caused by the presence of the mite *Acarapis woodi* in the tracheae of the bees. **itch d.,** a dermatomycosis of horses probably caused by the mold *Microsporum canis.* **Jaffe-Lichtenstein d.,** cystic osteofibromatosis; a form of polyostotic fibrous dysplasia characterized by an enlarged medullary cavity with a thin cortex, which is filled with fibrous tissue (fibroma). **Jakob's d., Jakob-Creutzfeldt d.,** Creutzfeldt-Jakob syndrome. **Jaksch's d.,** anemia pseudoleukemica infantum. **Janet's d.,** psychasthenia. **Jansen's d.,** metaphyseal dysostosis. **Jensen's d.,** retinochoroiditis juxtapapillaris. **Johne's d.,** a usually fatal form of chronic enteritis due to *Mycobacterium paratuberculosis,* chiefly affecting cattle but also sheep, goats, and deer. It remotely resembles a tuberculous infection, and is marked by intermittent or persistent diarrhea, progressive emaciation, anemia, and extreme weakness. Called also *chronic dysentery of cattle, bovine leprosy,* and *paratuberculosis.* **Johnson-Stevens d.,** see *Stevens-Johnson syndrome.* **Jourdain's d.,** suppurative inflammation of the gums and alveolar processes. **jumping d.,** Gilles de la Tourette's syndrome. **Jüngling's d.,** sarcoidosis. **juvenile Paget's d.,** hyperphosphatasia. **Kahlbaum's d.,** catatonic schizophrenia. **Kahler's d.,** multiple myeloma. **Kaiserstuhl d.,** a form of chronic arsenic poisoning that occurred in the Kaiserstuhl wine district of Germany. **Kalischer's d.,** Sturge-Weber syndrome. **Kaschin-Beck d.,** Kashin-Beck d. **Kashin-Beck d.,** a slowly progressive, chronic, disabling, degenerative disease of the peripheral joints and spine, which principally occurs in children and is endemic in eastern Siberia, northern China, and Korea. It is believed to be caused by the ingestion of cereal grains infected with *Fusarium sporotrichiella.* Called also *osteoarthritis deformans endemica.* **Katayama d.,** schistosomiasis japonica. **Kawasaki d.,** mucocutaneous lymph node syndrome. **Kayser's d.,** hepatolenticular degeneration. **Kedani d.,** scrub typhus. **Kempf's d.,** acute homosexual panic. **Kienböck's d.,** 1. slowly progressive osteochondrosis of the semilunar (carpal lunate) bone; it may affect other bones of the wrist. Called also *lunatomalacia.* 2. traumatic cavity formation in the spinal cord; called also *traumatic syringomyelia.* **Kimberley horse d.,** a disease of horses in the Kimberley district of northeastern Western Australia occurring during the wet season (January to April), due to grazing on *Crotolaria* spp. It is marked by cirrhosis of the liver, dullness, wasting, irritability, biting of other horses, gnawing fence posts, constant yawning, and muscular spasms leading to uncontrollable galloping, which gradually merges into aimless walking with a slow staggering gait and low stiff carriage of the head. Called also *walk-about d.* **Kimura's d.,** angiolymphoid hyperplasia. **kinky hair d.,** Menkes' syndrome. **Kinnier Wilson d.,** hepatolenticular degeneration. **Kirkland's d.,** an acute infection of the throat with regional lymphadenitis. **kissing d.,** popular term for infectious mononucleosis. **Klebs' d.,** glomerulonephritis. **Klemperer's d.,** Banti's d. **Klippel's d.,** arthritic general pseudoparalysis; see under *pseudoparalysis.* **knight's d.,** infection of the perianal region following a minute abrasion of the skin, so called historically because of the frequency of its occurrence in horsemen. **Koenig-**

Wichman d. (*obs.*), chronic bullous disease (pemphigus). **Köhler's bone d.,** 1. osteochondrosis of the tarsal navicular bone in children; called also *tarsal scaphoiditis, epiphysitis juvenilis, osteoarthrosis juvenilis,* and *os naviculare pedis retardatum.* 2. a disease of the second metatarsal bone, with thickening of its shaft and changes about its articular head, characterized by pain in the second metatarsophalangeal joint on walking or standing. Called also *Köhler's second d.,* and *juvenile deforming metatarsophalangeal osteochondritis.* See also *osteochondrosis.* **Köhler's second d.,** Köhler's bone d., def. 2. **Köhler-Pellegrini-Stieda d.,** Pellegrini's d. **Kokka d.,** epidemic hemorrhagic fever. **Korsakoff's d.,** see under *psychosis.* **Koshevnikoff's (Koschewnikow's, Kozhevnikov's) d.,** epilepsia partialis continua. **Krabbe's d.,** a familial form of leukoencepalopathy in which a sphingolipid (ceramide galactoside) accumulates in the tissues owing to deficiency of β-galactosidase. It begins in infancy with irritability, fretfulness, and rigidity, followed by tonic seizures, convulsions, quadriplegia, blindness, deafness, dysphagia, and progressive mental deterioration. Pathologically, there is rapidly progressive cerebral demyelination and large globoid bodies (swollen with accumulated cerebroside) in the white substance. Called also *globoid, globoid cell,* and *Krabbe's leukodystrophy.* **Krishaber's d.,** a neurosis characterized by tachycardia, insomnia, lightheadedness or vertigo, and hyperesthesia; called also *cerebrocardiac syndrome.* **Kufs' d.,** the late juvenile form of cerebral sphengolipidosis. **Kugelberg-Welander d.,** a hereditary juvenile form of muscular atrophy, usually transmitted as an autosomal recessive trait, due to lesions of the anterior horns of the spinal cord. It is marked by onset in the first or second decade, principally between two and seventeen years, atrophy and weakness of the proximal muscles of the lower extremities and pelvic girdle, followed by involvement of the distal muscles and muscular twitchings. Cf. *Werdnig-Hoffman paralysis.* **Kuhnt-Junius d.,** disciform macular degeneration. **Kümmell's d.,** compression fracture of vertebra; a complex of symptoms coming on in a few weeks after spinal injury, and consisting of pain in the spine, intercostal neuralgia, motor disturbances of the legs, and a gibbus of the spine which is painful on pressure and easily reduced by extension; post-traumatic spondylitis. Called also *Kümmell-Verneuil d.* **Kümmell-Verneuil d.,** Kümmell's d. **Kussmaul's d., Kussmaul-Maier d.,** periarteritis nodosa. **Kyasanur Forest d.,** a highly fatal arboviral disease of monkeys in the Kyasanur Forest in India, communicable to man, in whom it produces hemorrhagic symptoms. **Kyrle's d.,** hyperkeratosis follicularis in cutem penetrans. **Laennec's d.,** 1. see under *cirrhosis.* 2. dissecting aneurysm. **Lafora's d.,** myoclonus epilepsy. **Lancereaux-Mathieu d.,** leptospiral jaundice. **Landouzy's d.,** leptospiral jaundice. **Landry's d.,** acute febrile polyneuritis. **Lane's d.,** chronic intestinal stasis; small bowel obstruction in chronic constipation. **Langdon-Down's d.,** Down's syndrome. **Larrey-Weil d.,** leptospiral jaundice. **Larsen's d., Larsen-Johansson d.,** a disease of the patella in which the x-ray shows an accessory center of ossification in the lower pole of the patella. **Lasègue's d.,** persecution mania. **Lauber's d.,** fundus albipunctatus. **laughing d.,** kuru. **leaf-curl d.,** a viral disease of plants characterized by curling or crinkling of the leaves. **Leber's d.,** 1. Leber's optic atrophy; see under *atrophy.* 2. Leber's congenital amaurosis; see under *amaurosis.* **Legal's d.,** a disease affecting the pharyngotympanic region, and marked by headache and local inflammatory changes; called also *pharyngotympanic cephalalgia.* **Legg's d., Legg-Calvé d., Legg-Calvé-Perthes d., Legg-Calvé-Waldenström d.,** osteochondrosis of the capitular epiphysis of the femur; see *osteochondrosis.* **legionnaires' d.,** a highly fatal disease caused by a gram-negative bacillus (*Legionella pneumophila*), which is not spread by person-to-person contact and is characterized by high fever, gastrointestinal pain, headache, and pneumonia; there may also be involvement of the kidneys, liver, and nervous system. The etiologic agent was identified after an outbreak occurred in the summer of 1976 at an American Legion convention in Philadelphia, Pennsylvania. **Leiner's d.,** erythroderma desquamativum. **Leloir's d.** (*obs.*), discoid lupus erythematosus. **Lenegre's d.,** acquired complete heart block due to primary degeneration of the conduction system. **Leriche's d.,** post-traumatic osteoporosis. **Letterer-Siwe d.,** a nonlipid reticuloendotheliosis of early childhood, probably an autosomal recessive trait, characterized by a hemorrhagic tendency, eczematoid skin eruption, hepatosplenomegaly with lymph node enlargement, and progressive anemia. **Lev's d.,** acquired complete heart block due to sclerosis of the cardiac skeleton. **Lewandowsky-Lutz d.,** epidermodysplasia verruciformis. **Leyden's d.,** a form of periodic vomiting. **Libman-Sacks d.,** atypical verrucous endocarditis. **Lichtheim's d.,** subacute combined degeneration of the spinal cord; see under *degeneration.* **Lignac's d., Lignac-Fanconi d.,** Fanconi syndrome, def. 2. **Lindau's d., Lindau-von Hippel d.,** von Hippel-Lindau d. **Lipschütz's d.,** ulcus vulvae acutum. **Little's d.,** congenital spastic stiffness of the limbs, a form of cerebral spastic paralysis dating from birth and due to lack of development of the pyramidal tracts; it may be associated with various disorders, including birth trauma, fetal anoxia, or illness of the mother during pregnancy. Clinically, it is characterized by muscular weakness, walking difficulties, and, usually, by convulsions, bilateral athetosis, and mental deficiency. Called also *spastic diplegia.* **Lobo's d.,** keloidal blastomycosis. **Lobstein's d.,** see *osteogenesis imperfecta.* **local d.,** a condition which originates in and remains confined to one part. **loco d.,** locoism. **Lorain's d.,** hypophyseal infantilism. **Lowe's d.,** oculocerebrorenal syndrome. **Luft's d.,** a hypermetabolic disorder of striated muscle caused by an abnormal quantity and type of mitochondria producing excessive cellular respiration; it is characterized by profuse perspiration, asthenia, progressive weakness, and an abnormally increased basal metabolic rate. **lumpy skin d.,** a highly infectious viral disease of cattle in Africa, which may result in permanent sterility or death, marked by the formation of nodules in the skin and sometimes in the mucous membranes. **lung fluke d.,** parasitic hemoptysis. **lunger d.,** pulmonary adenomatosis, def. 2. **Lutembacher's d.,** see under *syndrome.* **Lutz-Splendore-Almeida d.,** South American blastomycosis. **Lyell's d.,** toxic epidermal necrolysis. **lymphocystic d. of fish,** a disease of fish marked by the formation on the skin of spherical nodules caused by a virus. **lysosomal storage d.,** any of a group of storage diseases due to congenital absence of one of the lysosomal enzymes, leading to engorgement of lysosomes by material that the enzyme would normally degrade; the term includes the glycogenoses, sphingolipidoses, mucopolysaccharidoses, etc. Called also *inborn lysosomal d.* and *lysosomal enzymopathy.* **McArdle's d.,** glycogen storage d. (type V). **Mackenzie's d.,** x disease, def. 1. **MacLean-Maxwell d.,** a chronic condition of the calcaneus marked by enlargement of its posterior third and attended by pain on pressure. **Madelung's d.,** 1. see under *deformity.* 2. see under *neck.* **Magitot's d.,** osteoperiostitis of the alveoli of the teeth. **Maher's d.,** paracolpitis. **Majocchi's d.,** purpura anularis telangiectodes. **Malassez's d.,** cyst of the testis. **Malibu d.,** surfers' nodules. **Manson's d.,** see under *schistosomiasis.* **maple bark d.,** a granulomatous interstitial pneumonitis caused by inhalation of spores from *Cryptostroma corticale,* a mold found beneath the bark of maple logs. **maple syrup urine d.,** a genetotrophic disease involving an enzyme defect in the metabolism of the branched chain amino acids, the plasma and urinary levels of the keto acids valine, leucine, and isoleucine being greatly increased. Clinical features include mental and physical retardation, feeding difficulties, and a characteristic odor of the urine, from which the disorder derives its name. It is transmitted as an autosomal recessive trait. Called also *branched-chain ketoaciduria* or *ketoaminoacidemia.* **Marburg d., Marburg virus d.,** a severe, often fatal, viral disease first reported in Marburg, Germany, among laboratory workers exposed to African green monkeys. It is characterized by skin lesions, conjunctivitis, enteritis, hepatitis, encephalitis, and renal failure. **March's d.,** Graves' d. **Marchiafava-Bignami d.,** progressive degeneration of the corpus callosum characterized by progressive intellectual deterioration, emotional disturbances, confusion, hallucinations, tremor, rigidity, and convulsions. It is a very rare disorder affecting chiefly middle-aged male alcoholics, especially those who consume excessive amounts of crude red wine. **Marchiafava-Micheli d.,** paroxysmal nocturnal hemoglobinuria; see under *hemoglobinuria.* **Marek's d.,** a lymphoproliferative disease of chickens caused by a herpesvirus. Lymphoid cell infiltrations are most common in the peripheral nerves and gonads, but widespread infiltrations may also be found in any of the visceral organs, skin, muscle, and the iris of the eye. Perivascular cuffing of blood vessels in the brain and spinal cord frequently occurs. The location of the lesions dictates the clinical signs, such as paralysis, general depression, and blindness. It was once included in the avian leukosis complex. Called also, according to the symptoms manifested, *acute leukosis, fowl paralysis, ocular lymphomatosis, neural lymphomatosis, neurolymphomatosis gallinarum, range paralysis,* and *skin leukosis.* **margarine d.,** erythema multiforme due to an emulsifier in oleomargarine; it occurred as an explosive epidemic outbreak in Germany and Holland, thought at the time to be infectious in origin. **Marie's d.,** 1. acromegaly. 2. hypertrophic pulmonary osteoarthropathy. **Marie-Bamberger d.,** hypertrophic pulmonary osteoarthropathy. **Marie-Strümpell d.,** rheumatoid spondylitis. **Marie-Tooth d.,** progressive neuropathic (peroneal) muscular atrophy. **Marion's d.,** congenital obstruction of the posterior urethra due to muscular hypertrophy of the bladder neck or absence of the plexiform dilator fibers in the urinary tract. **Marsh's d.,** Graves' d. **Martin's d.,** periosteoarthritis of the foot from excessive walking. **mast cell d.,** urticaria pigmentosa. **Mathieu's d.,** leptospiral jaundice. **Maunier-Kuhn d.,** a form of cutis laxa in which slackness of the eyelids and ears occurs in childhood, followed by tracheomegaly and bronchomegaly. **Maxcy's d.,** a rickettsial infection endemic in the southeastern part of the United States. **M component d.,** any disease in which the M component appears; see under *component.* **Medin's d.,** see *poliomyelitis.* **Mediterranean d.,** see *β-thalassemia.* **medullary cystic d.** familial juvenile nephronophthisis. **Meige's d.,** Milroy's d. **Meleda d.,** mal de Meleda. **Menetrier's d.,** giant hypertrophic gastritis. **Meniere's d.,**

hearing loss, tinnitus, and vertigo resulting from nonsuppurative disease of the labyrinth with the histopathologic feature of endolymphatic hydrops (distention of the membranous labyrinth). **Menkes' d.,** see under *syndrome.* **mental d.,** see under *disorder.* **Merzbacher-Pelizaeus d.,** familial centrolobar sclerosis. **metabolic d.,** one caused by some defect in the chemical reactions of the cells of the body. **metazoan d.,** a disease caused by metazoan parasites, such as nematodes, cestodes, trematodes, and arthropods. **Meyer's d.,** adenoid vegetations of the pharynx. **Meyer-Betz d.,** a rare familial disease of unknown etiology, marked by attacks of myoglobinuria, which may be precipitated by strenuous exertion or possibly by an infection, and which results in tenderness, swelling, and weakness of muscles of varying intensity. It may occur with or without diffuse chronic myopathy or dystrophy. Called also *idiopathic, spontaneous,* or *familial myoglobinuria.* **miasmatic d.,** one due to malarial infection. **microdrepanocytic d.,** sickle cell–thalassemia d. **Miescher's d.,** elastosis perforans serpiginosa. **Mikulicz's d.,** a benign, self-limited lymphocytic infiltration and enlargement of the lacrimal and salivary glands of uncertain etiology (possibly an autoimmune response), usually affecting middle-aged or older women. It is considered by some to be identical with Sjögren's syndrome; others suggest that it is a different form of the same malady, with a common etiology. When associated with sarcoidosis, malignant lymphoma, or collagen disease, the similar clinical picture is called *Mikulicz's syndrome.* **milk-borne d's,** diseases caused by organisms transmitted in milk; the principal ones are cholera, diphtheria, dysentery, food infections, foot-and-mouth disease, summer diarrhea, brucellosis, scarlet fever, septic sore throat, tuberculosis, and typhoid fever. **milky d., milky-white d.,** a fatal infection of beetle larvae due to *Bacillus papilliae* or *B. lentimorbus,* in which the "blood" of the larvae appears milky white as a result of the profuse multiplication and sporulation of the bacilli. The infection may be produced deliberately in Japanese beetles to control their population. **Miller's d.,** osteomalacia. **Mills' d.,** ascending hemiplegia that eventually develops into quadriplegia; its etiology is unknown. **Milroy's d.,** congenital hereditary lymphedema of the legs caused by chronic lymphatic obstruction; other areas, including the arms, trunk, and face may be involved. Called also *Meige's d., Milroy's edema, Nonne-Milroy-Meige syndrome,* and *congenital lymphedema.* **Minamata d.,** a severe neurologic disorder caused by alkyl mercury poisoning, usually characterized by peripheral and circumoral paresthesia, ataxia, dysarthria, and loss of peripheral vision, and leading to severe permanent neurologic and mental disabilities or death. It was prevalent between 1953 and 1958 among those who ate sea food from Minamata Bay, Japan, which contained an excess of alkyl mercury compounds. **Minor's d.,** hematomyelia involving the central parts of the spiral cord. **mish d.,** a dysentery in Syria caused by eating apricots. **Mitchell's d.,** erythromelalgia. **mixed connective tissue d.,** a disorder combining features of scleroderma, myositis, systemic lupus erythematosus, and rheumatoid arthritis, and marked serologically by the presence of antibody against extractable nuclear antigen. **Möbius' d.,** periodic migraine with paralysis of the oculomotor muscles. **Moeller-Barlow d.,** subperiosteal hematoma in rickets. **molecular d.,** any disease in which the pathogenesis can be traced to a single molecule, usually a protein, which is either abnormal in structure or present in reduced amounts; the classical example is abnormal hemoglobin in sickle cell anemia. **Molten's d.,** Pictou d. **Mondor's d.,** phlebitis affecting the large subcutaneous veins normally crossing the lateral chest region and breast from the epigastric or hypochondriac region to the axilla, occurring in both males and females. **Monge's d.,** chronic mountain sickness. **Morel-Kraepelin d.,** schizophrenia. **Morgagni's d.,** hyperostosis frontalis interna. **Morquio's d.,** see under *syndrome.* **Morquio-Ullrich d.,** Morquio's syndrome. **Morton's d.,** see under *toe.* **Morvan's d.,** a form of syringomyelia marked by painless ulceration of the tips of the fingers (paronychia) and analgesic paralysis and atrophy of the forearms and hands. **mosaic d's,** infectious diseases of plants caused by viruses and characterized by mottling of the foliage. **Moschcowitz's d.,** thrombotic thrombocytopenic purpura. **motor neuron d.,** any disease of a motor neuron, including spinal muscular atrophy, progressive bulbar paralysis, amyotrophic lateral sclerosis, and lateral sclerosis. **mountain d.,** see under *sickness.* **Mozer's d.,** myelosclerosis in adults. **Mucha's d., Mucha-Habermann d.,** pityriasis lichenoides et varioliformis acuta. **mucosal d.,** a disease of cattle, due to the virus of bovine virus diarrhea; ulcerations in the mouth may be the only sign, but often there is fever, diarrhea, loss of appetite, and a drop in milk yield. **mule spinner's d.,** warts or ulcers of the skin, especially of the scrotum, which tend to become malignant; so called because they were found chiefly among the operators of spinning mules in cotton mills. **Münchmeyer's d.,** a diffuse progressive ossifying polymyositis. **Murray Valley d.,** see under *encephalitis.* **mushroom picker's d., mushroom worker's d.,** an allergic respiratory disease closely resembling farmer's lung, developing in persons working with moldy compost prepared for growing mushrooms in closed areas, especially in those handling the dried material after harvesting.

mushy chick d., omphalitis of birds; see under *omphalitis.*
Myà's d. (*obs.*), congenital dilatation of the colon. **Nadia d.,** a disease of unknown etiology that affected residents of the Nadia District of West Bengal in 1964. It was marked by burning sensations of the hands and feet, anorexia, diarrhea, and lethargy, followed by hyperkeratosis of the soles with black pigmentation and fissures, and by facial erythema. **Nairobi d.,** an infectious disease of sheep and goats in Africa, especially in the region around Nairobi, marked by acute hemorrhagic gastroenteritis, green, watery diarrhea, mucopurulent nasal discharge, and breathing difficulty; it is caused by a virus transmitted by the ticks *Rhipicephalus appendiculatus* and *Amblyomma variegatum.* **nanukayami d.,** nanukayami. **naronian d.,** an endemic intermittent fever once prevalent at Narenta (Bosnia, Yugoslavia). **navicular d.,** necrotic inflammation of the navicular bone in horses, causing intermittent lameness; called also *grog.* **New-castle d.,** an influenza-like viral disease of birds, including domestic fowl, characterized by respiratory and gastrointestinal or pneumonic and encephalitic symptoms. First seen near Newcastle, England, the infection is also transmissible to man by contact with infected birds. Called also *avian influenza.* **Nicolas-Favre d.,** lymphogranuloma venereum. **Nidoko d.,** epidemic hemorrhagic fever. **Niemann's d.,** Niemann-Pick d. **Niemann-Pick d.,** a hereditary disease characterized by massive hepatosplenomegaly, brownish yellow discoloration of the skin, nervous system involvement, and presence in the liver, spleen, lungs, lymph nodes, and bone marrow of foamy reticular cells or histiocytes which store phospholipids, chiefly lecithin and sphingomyelin. Called also *lipid histiocytosis, Niemann's d., Pick's d., phosphatide thesaurismosis* or *lipoidosis, sphingomyelinosis, sphingomyelin lipidosis.* **nodule d., nodular worm d.,** a disease of sheep and cattle, caused by a minute worm,*OEsophagostomum columbianum,* which infests the intestines, becoming embedded in the mucous membrane, where it causes the formation of nodules of varying size. **Nordau's d.,** degeneracy. **Norrie's d.,** a hereditary disorder consisting of bilateral blindness from retinal malformation, mental retardation, and deafness, transmitted as an X-linked trait; called also *atrophia bulborum hereditaria.* **nosema d.,** a disease of bees caused by *Nosema apis,* characterized by dysentery and paralysis. Cf. *pébrine.* **Novy's rat d.,** a viral disease discovered by Novy in his stock of experimental rats. **oasthouse urine d.,** Smith-Strang d. **occupational d.,** one due to factors involved in one's employment, e.g., various forms of pneumoconiosis or dermatitis. **Oguchi's d.,** a form of congenital night blindness occurring in Japan. **Ohara's d.,** a disease observed in Japan, probably identical with tularemia. **oid-oid d.,** [from disc*oid* and lichen-*oid*] Sulzberger-Garbe syndrome. **Ollier's d.,** enchondromatosis. **Olmer's d.,** boutonneuse fever. **Ondiri's d.,** bovine infectious petechial fever. **Opitz's d.,** thrombophlebitic splenomegaly: enlargement of the spleen due to thrombosis of the splenic vein. **Oppenheim's d.,** amyotonia congenita. **organic d.,** one associated with demonstrable change in a bodily organ or tissue. **Oriental lung fluke d.,** parasitic hemoptysis. **Ormond's d.,** retroperitoneal fibrosis. **Osgood-Schlatter d.,** osteochondrosis of the tuberosity of the tibia; called also *apophysitis tibialis adolescentium, Schlatter's d.,* and *Schlatter-Osgood d.* See also *osteochondrosis.* **Osler's d.,** 1. polycythemia vera. 2. hereditary hemorrhagic telangiectasia. **Osler-Vaquez d.,** polycythemia vera. **Osler-Weber-Rendu d.,** hereditary hemorrhagic telangiectasia. **Otto's d.,** osteoarthritic protrusion of the acetabulum; arthrokatadysis. **overeating d.,** pulpy kidney d. **Owren's d.,** Factor V deficiency; see *coagulation factors,* under *factor.* **ox-warble d.,** see *larva migrans.* **Paas' d.,** a familial disorder marked by skeletal deformities such as coxa valga, shortening of phalanges, scoliosis, spondylitis, etc. **Paget's d.,** 1. osteitis deformans. 2. an inflammatory cancerous affection of the areola and nipple, usually associated with carcinoma of the lactiferous ducts and deeper structures of the breast, and occurring usually in middle-aged women. 3. see *Paget's d., extramammary.* **Paget's d., extramammary,** a counterpart of Paget's disease of the breast, which usually involves the vulva, and sometimes other sites, such as the perianal and axillary regions. **Panner's d.,** osteochondrosis of the capitellum of the humerus. **parenchymatous d.,** one which attacks the parenchyma of an organ. **Parkinson's d.,** paralysis agitans. **parrot d.,** psittacosis. **Parrot's d.,** see under *pseudoparalysis.* **Parry's d.,** Graves' d. **Parsons' d.,** Graves' d. **Patella's d.,** pyloric stenosis in tuberculous patients following fibrous stenosis. **Pavy's d.,** cyclic proteinuria. **Payr's d.,** constipation with left upper quadrant pain attributed to kinking of an adhesion between the transverse and descending colon with obstruction; probably a manifestation of the irritable colon syndrome rather than an organic lesion. Called also *splenic flexure syndrome.* **pearl d.,** tuberculosis of the peritoneum and mesentery of cattle. **pearl-worker's d.,** recurrent inflammation of bone with hypertrophy, seen in persons who work in pearl dust. **Pel-Ebstein d.,** Hodgkin's d. **Pelizaeus-Merzbacher d.,** familial centrolobar sclerosis. **Pellegrini's d., Pellegrini-Stieda d.,** a condition characterized by a semilunar bony formation in the upper portion of the medial lateral ligament of the knee, due to traumatism; called also *Köhler-Pelle-*

grini-Stieda d. and *Stieda's d.* **periodic d.,** a condition characterized by regularly recurring and intermittent episodes of fever, edema, arthralgia, or gastric pain and vomiting, continuing for years without further development in otherwise healthy individuals. **periodontal d.,** any disease or disorder of the periodontium; see *periodontitis* and *periodontosis.* **Perrin-Ferraton d.,** snapping hip. **Perthes' d.,** osteochondrosis of the capital femoral epiphysis; see *osteochondrosis.* **Peyronie's d.,** induration of the corpora cavernosa of the penis, producing a fibrous chordee; called also *fibrous cavernitis, penis plastica,* and *penile induration.* **Pfeiffer's d.,** infectious mononucleosis. **Phocas' d.,** chronic glandular mastitis with the formation of numerous small nodules. **Pick's d.** 1. (Arnold Pick) lobar atrophy of the brain. 2. (Friedel Pick) ascites and fibrotic liver disease associated with constrictive pericarditis; called also *pericardial pseudocirrhosis of the liver.* 3. (Ludwig Pick) Niemann-Pick d. **Pictou d.,** cirrhosis of the liver in horses and cattle in Nova Scotia due to ingestion of *Senecio jacobeus,* the ragwort; called also *Molten's d.* and *Winton d.* **pink d.,** acrodynia. **Pinkus' d.,** lichen nitidus. **plaster-of-Paris d.,** atrophy of a limb which has been enclosed in a plaster-of-Paris splint. **Plummer's d.,** the development of toxicity (hyperthyroidism) in simple adenoma of the thyroid. **pneumatic hammer d.,** vasospastic disease in the hands resulting from use of a pneumatic hammer. **policeman's d.,** tarsalgia. **polycystic d. of kidneys,** a heritable disorder marked by cysts scattered throughout both kidneys. It occurs in two unrelated forms: The *infantile* form, transmitted as an autosomal recessive trait, may be congenital or appear at any time during childhood. There is a high perinatal mortality rate, and almost all cases lead to hypertension. In older children cystic and fibrotic disease of the liver may be associated. The *adult* form, transmitted as an autosomal dominant trait, is marked by progressive deterioration of renal function. Called also *polycystic kidneys* and *polycystic renal d.* **polycystic ovary d.,** Stein-Leventhal syndrome. **polycystic renal d.,** polycystic kidney d. **polyhedral d's,** infectious diseases of insects, especially caterpillars, caused by viruses. **Pompe's d.,** glycogen storage d. (type II). **Poncet's d.,** tuberculous rheumatism. **Posada-Wernicke d.,** coccidioidomycosis. **Pott's d.,** tuberculosis of the spine. **pregnancy d.,** pregnancy toxemia in ewes. **Preiser's d.,** osteoporosis and atrophy of the carpal scaphoid due to trauma or to fracture which has not been kept immobilized. **Pringle's d.,** adenoma sebaceum. **Profichet's d.,** see under *syndrome.* **pullet d.,** pyelonephritis of young hens of unknown etiology, characterized by loss of appetite, diarrhea with watery or whitish evacuations, and sometimes darkening of the comb; affected birds appear drowsy. **pullorum d.,** see *white diarrhea* (def. 2), under *diarrhea.* **pulpy kidney d.,** a fatal enterotoxemia usually seen in young animals, chiefly lambs, but which may affect sheep, goats, and cattle of any age; it is caused by *Clostridium perfringens* type D. Pathologically, the kidneys are mottled and soft in consistency and the cortex is jelly-like or almost semifluid; the liver is severely congested with small hemorrhages diffusely scattered over its surface. **pulseless d.,** progressive obliteration of the brachiocephalic trunk and the left subclavian and left common carotid arteries above their origin in the aortic arch, leading to loss of pulse in both arms and carotids and to symptoms associated with ischemia of the brain (syncope, transient hemiplegia, etc.), eyes (transient blindness, retinal atrophy, etc.), face (muscular atrophy, etc.), and arms (claudication, etc.). Called also *arteritis brachiocephalica* or *brachiocephalic arteritis, Martorell's syndrome, reversed coarctation,* and *Takayasu's disease* or *syndrome.* **Purtscher's d.,** traumatic angiopathy of the retina with edema, hemorrhage, and exudation, usually following crush injuries of the chest; called also *Purtscher's angiopathic retinopathy.* **Pyle's d.,** metaphyseal dysplasia. **pyramidal d.,** buttress foot. **Quervain's d.** see *de Quervain's d.* **Quincke's d.,** angioneurotic edema. **rag-sorter's d.,** anthrax. **railroad d.,** transit tetany. **Ramsay Hunt d.,** see under *syndrome,* def. 1. **rat-bite d.,** see under *fever.* **Raynaud's d.,** 1. a primary or idiopathic vascular disorder characterized by bilateral attacks of Raynaud's phenomenon. The disease affects females more frequently than males. Called also *Raynaud's gangrene.* See *Raynaud's phenomenon,* under *phenomenon.* 2. paralysis of the throat muscles following parotiditis; called also *local asphyxia.* **Recklinghausen's d.,** neurofibromatosis. **Recklinghausen's d. of bone,** osteitis fibrosa cystica. **Recklinghausen-Applebaum d.,** hemochromatosis. **Reclus' d.,** 1. a painless cystic enlargement of the mammae, marked by multiple dilatations of the acini and ducts. 2. cellulitis with induration. **redwater d.,** bacillary hemoglobinuria. **Reed-Hodgkin d.,** Hodgkin's d. **Refsum's d.,** a hereditary disease associated with a defect in the metabolism of phytanic acid, manifested chiefly by chronic polyneuritis, retinitis pigmentosa, and cerebellar signs (including mild ataxia), with persistent elevation of protein in the cerebrospinal fluid. There may be ichthyosis, nerve deafness, and electrocardiographic abnormalities. It is transmitted as an autosomal recessive trait. Called also *heredopathia atactica polyneuritiformis* and *Refsum's syndrome.* **Reichmann's d.** (*obs.*), gastrosuccorrhea. **Reiter's d.,** nongonococcal urethritis followed by conjunctivitis and arthritis, of unknown etiology, and occurring predominantly in males; it is frequently associated with keratoderma blenorrhagica, stomatitis, ulceration of the glans penis, and balanitis. Called also *Reiter's syndrome.* **Rendu-Osler-Weber d.,** hereditary hemorrhagic telangiectasia. **Renikhet d.** (*obs.*), Newcastle d. in chickens. **rheumatic heart d.,** the most important manifestation of and sequel to rheumatic fever (q.v.), consisting chiefly of valvular deformities. **rheumatoid d.,** a systemic condition best known by its articular involvement (rheumatoid arthritis) but emphasizing nonarticular changes, e.g., pulmonary interstitial fibrosis, pleural effusion, and lung nodules. **Ribas-Torres d.,** variola minor. **rice d.,** beriberi. **Riedel's d.,** see under *struma.* **Riga-Fede d.,** granuloma of the frenum linguae in children, occurring after abrasion by the lower central incisors; called also *Fede's d., Riga's d.,* and *cachectic aphthae.* **Riggs' d.,** compound periodontitis. **Ritter's d.,** dermatitis exfoliativa neonatorum. **Robles' d.,** onchocerciasis, caused by *Onchocerca volvulus* (q.v.). **Roger's d.,** a ventricular septal defect; the term is usually restricted to small, asymptomatic defects. **Rokitansky's d.,** acute yellow atrophy of the liver; see under *atrophy.* **rolling d.,** a disease of laboratory mice characterized by lateral rolling movements, by neurolysis and by a polymorphonuclear leukocytic reaction in the brain; it is caused by a potent neurolytic exotoxin produced by *Mycoplasma neurolyticum.* **Romberg's d.,** facial hemiatrophy. **Rose d.,** the urticarial form of swine erysipelas. **Rossbach's d.,** hyperchlorhydria. **Rot's d., Rot-Bernhardt d.,** meralgia paresthetica. **Roth's d.,** meralgia paraesthetica. **Roth-Bernhardt d.,** meralgia paraesthetica. **Rougnon-Heberden d.,** angina pectoris. **round heart d.,** a disease of unknown etiology which causes sudden death in apparently healthy poultry; a greatly enlarged heart is seen post mortem. **Roussy-Lévy's d.,** a type of familial ataxia marked by disorders of gait, clubfoot, and lack of tendon reflexes. **Rubarth's d.,** hepatitis contagiosa canis. **Rummo's d.** (*obs.*), downward displacement of the heart; cardioptosis. **runt d.,** a syndrome produced experimentally by injecting immunologically competent cells into genetically foreign hosts that are unable to reject these elements, resulting in gross retardation of host development and fatal consequences; called also *graft vs. host reaction.* **Rust's d.,** tuberculous spondylitis of the cervical vertebrae. **Ruysch's d.,** Hirschsprung's d. **saccharine d.,** a term proposed for any disease resulting from the overconsumption of refined carbohydrate foods in combination with the removal of dietary fiber and protein, including diabetes, cardiovascular disease, constipation, obesity, peptic ulcer, etc. **Sachs' d.,** Tay-Sachs d. **sacroiliac d.,** chronic tuberculous inflammation of the sacroiliac joint. **St. Agatha's d.,** mastitis. **St. Aignon's d.** (*obs.*), favus. **St. Anthony's d.,** 1. chorea. 2. vernacular name for ergotism. **St. Appolonia's d.,** toothache. **St. Avertin's d.,** epilepsy. **St. Avidus' d.,** deafness. **St. Blasius' d.,** peritonsillar abscess. **St. Dymphna's d.,** insanity. **St. Erasmus' d.,** colic, def. 2. **St. Fiacre's d.,** hemorrhoids. **St. Gervasius' d.,** rheumatism. **St. Gotthard's tunnel d.** (*obs.*), hookworm d. **St. Hubert's d.,** rabies. **St. Job's d.,** syphilis. **St. Mathurin's d.,** idiocy. **St. Modestus' d.,** chorea. **St. Roch's d.,** plague. **St. Sement's d.,** syphilis. **St. Valentine's d.,** epilepsy. **St. Zachary's d.,** mutism. **salivary gland d.,** cytomegalic inclusion d. **Sander's d.,** a form of paranoia. **Sanders' d.,** epidemic keratoconjunctivitis. **Sandhoff's d.,** a variant of Tay-Sachs disease marked by a progressively more rapid course, due to a defect in the enzymes hexosaminidase A and B. Unlike Tay-Sachs disease, it is not confined to Ashkenazic Jews. **sandworm d.,** larva migrans. **San Joaquin Valley d.,** coccidioidomycosis. **sartian d.,** a facial skin disease endemic in Turkestan, resembling cutaneous leishmaniasis; called also *Turkestan ulcer.* **Saunders' d.,** a dangerous condition seen in infants having digestive disturbances to whom is given a large percentage of carbohydrates; it is marked by vomiting, cerebral symptoms, and depression of circulation. **Schamberg's d.,** progressive pigmentary dermatosis. **Schanz's d.,** traumatic inflammation of the tendo achillis. **Schaumann's d.,** sarcoidosis. **Scheuermann's d.,** osteochondrosis of vertebral epiphyses in juveniles; see *osteochondrosis.* **Schilder's d.,** a subacute or chronic form of leukoencephalopathy of children and adolescents. Clinical symptoms include blindness, deafness, bilateral spasticity, and progressive mental deterioration. There is massive destruction of the white substance of the cerebral hemispheres, cavity formation, and glial scarring. The disease usually occurs sporadically, but a familial form has been reported. Called also *encephalitis periaxialis diffusa, progressive subcortical encephalopathy, Flatau-Schilder disease,* and *Schilder's encephalitis.* **Schimmelbusch's d.,** cystic d. of breast. **Schlatter's d., Schlatter-Osgood d.,** Osgood-Schlatter d. **Schmorl's d.,** 1. herniation of the nucleus pulposus into an adjacent ventral body. 2. necrobacillosis of wild and domestic rabbits, rats, and other wild animals, due to infection with *Fusobacterium necrophorum* (Schmorl's bacillus); it is characterized by abscesses on various parts of the body, or by areas of necrosis around the mouth, nose, eyelids, throat, and chest. **Scholz's d.,** a familial form of leukoencephalopathy transmitted as an X-linked recessive trait. Beginning at about

eight years of age, it is characterized by demyelination of the white substance of the brain, sensory aphasia, cortical blindness, deafness, weakness and spasticity of the limbs, complete paralysis, and dementia. **Schönlein's d.,** see under *purpura.* **Schönlein-Henoch d.,** see under *purpura.* **Schottmüller's d.,** paratyphoid, def. 2. **Schridde's d.** (*obs.*), congenital generalized dropsy. **Schroeder's d.,** a condition characterized by hypertrophic endometrium and excessive uterine bleeding, probably due to deficiency of the gonadotropic hormone. **Schüller's d.,** 1. Hand-Schüller-Christian disease. 2. osteoporosis circumscripta cranii. **Schüller-Christian d.,** Hand-Schüller-Christian d. **Schultz's d.,** agranulocytosis. **Schwediauer's d.,** see *Swediaur's d.* **secondary d.,** 1. a morbid condition occurring subsequent to or as a consequence of another disease. 2. one due to introduction of incompatible immunologically competent cells into a host rendered incapable of rejecting them by heavy exposure to ionizing radiation. **Seitelberger's d.,** infantile neuroaxonal dystrophy. **self-limited d.,** one which by its very nature runs a limited and definite course. **Selter's d.,** acrodynia. **senecio d.,** cirrhosis of the liver occurring as the result of poisoning by the plant *Senecio.* **septic d.,** one which arises from the development of pyogenic or putrefactive organisms. **serum d.,** see under *sickness.* **Sever's d.,** epiphysitis of the calcaneus. **severe combined immunodeficiency d. (SCID),** a group of rare congenital disorders in which the functional capacities of both the humoral (B-lymphocyte) and cell-mediated (T-lymphocyte) components of the immune system are absent or severely depressed. The disorder occurs in several genetic forms, including one involving deficiency of adenosine deaminase. Affected persons are susceptible to severe candidiasis and to pneumonias caused by viruses, low-grade pathogenic bacteria, and *Pneumocystis carinii.* **Shaver's d.,** bauxite pneumoconiosis. **shimamushi d.,** scrub typhus. **shipyard d.,** epidemic keratoconjunctivitis. **Shichito d.,** scrub typhus. **shuttlemaker's d.,** a condition in shuttlemakers, marked by faintness, shortness of breath, headache, nausea, etc., attributed to inhaling the dust of poisonous wood from which the shuttles (devices used in weaving) are made. **sickle-cell d.,** any of the diseases associated with the presence of hemoglobin S, including sickle cell anemia, sickle cell–hemoglobin C or D disease, and sickle cell–thalassemia disease. **sickle cell–hemoglobin C d.,** a genetically determined anemia in which the red cells contain both hemoglobin S and hemoglobin C. **sickle cell–hemoglobin D d.,** a genetically determined anemia characterized by the presence of both hemoglobin S and hemoglobin D in red blood cells. **sickle cell–thalassemia d.,** a hereditary anemia involving simultaneous heterozygosity for hemoglobin S and thalassemia. Called also *microdrepanocytosis, microdrepanocytic d., hemoglobin S–thalassemia, sickle cell–thalassemia,* and *thalassemia–sickle cell disease.* **silo-filler's d.,** pulmonary inflammation, often with acute pulmonary edema, caused by inhalation of the irritant gases (especially oxides of nitrogen) which collect in recently filled silos. **Simmonds' d.,** panhypopituitarism. **Simons' d.,** lipodystrophia progressiva. **sixth d.,** exanthema subitum. **sixth venereal d.,** lymphogranuloma venereum. **Sjögren's d.,** see under *syndrome.* **Skevas-Zerfus d.,** sponge-diver's d. **sleeping d.,** narcolepsy. **sleepy foal d.,** a form of equulosis affecting foals within the first three days of life, due to infection with *Actinobacillus equuli,* characterized by sudden onset, extreme prostration, and death usually within 12 hours. **Smith's d.,** mucous colitis. **Smith-Strang d.,** a defect in methionine absorption transmitted as an autosomal recessive trait, in which the urine has a characteristic odor resembling that of the interior of an oasthouse due to alpha-hydroxybutyric acid formed by bacterial action on the unabsorbed methionine; it is characterized by white hair, mental retardation, convulsions, and attacks of hyperpnea. Called also *methionine malabsorption syndrome* and *oasthouse urine d.* **Sneddon-Wilkinson d.,** subcorneal pustular dermatosis. **sod d.,** vesicular dermatitis. **specific d.,** any disease, such as syphilis, due to a characteristic morbific agency. **Spencer's d.,** a form (probably viral) of epidemic gastroenteritis. **Spielmeyer-Vogt d.,** the juvenile form of cerebral sphingolipidosis. **sponge-diver's d.,** a condition encountered by divers in the Mediterranean who come in contact with the stinging tentacles of sea anemones of the genera *Sagartia* and *Actinia,* which are frequently attached to the base of sponges; it is marked by burning, itching, erythema, necrosis, and ulceration. Called also *Skevas-Zerfus d.* **Stanton's d.,** melioidosis. **Stargardt's d.,** hereditary degeneration of the macula lutea occurring between the ages of six and twenty, marked by rapid loss of visual acuity and by abnormal appearance and pigmentation of the macular area. **Steinert's d.,** myotonic dystrophy. **Sterbe d.,** a disease of horses in South Africa; a serum prepared from horses affected with this disease is said to be curative of malarial poisoning. **sterility d.,** a deficiency disease observed in experimental animals and due to a lack of vitamin E in the diet. **Sternberg's d.,** Hodgkin's d. **Sticker's d.,** erythema infectiosum. **Stieda's d.,** Pellegrini's d. **stiff lamb d.,** a disease of lambs due to vitamin E deficiency; also, a polyarthritis in lambs due to infection with *Erysipelothrix insidiosa,* marked by stiffness and lameness; called also *white muscle d.* **Still's d.,** a variety of chronic polyarthritis affecting children and marked by enlargement of lymph nodes, generally of the spleen, and irregular fever; called also *juvenile rheumatoid arthritis.* **Stokes' d.,** Graves' d. **Stokes-Adams d.,** Adams-Stokes d. **Stokvis' d.,** enterogenous cyanosis; see under *cyanosis.* **storage d.,** a metabolic disorder in which some substance accumulates or is stored in certain cells in unusually large amounts; the stored substances may be lipids, proteins, carbohydrates, or other substances. See, for example, *glycogen storage d., mucopolysaccharidosis,* and *proteinosis.* Formerly called *thesaurismosis.* **storage pool d,** a blood coagulation disorder due to failure of the platelets to release ADP in response to aggregating agents (collagen, epinephrine, exogenous ADP, thrombin, etc.). It is characterized by mild bleeding episodes, prolonged bleeding time, and reduced aggregation response to collagen or thrombin. **structural d.,** any disease in which there are microscopic changes. **Strümpell's d.,** 1. a hereditary form of lateral sclerosis (q.v. under *sclerosis*) in which the spasticity is principally limited to the legs; called also *Strümpell type.* 2. polioencephalomyelitis. **Strümpell-Leichtenstern d.,** hemorrhagic encephalitis. **Strümpell-Marie d.,** rheumatoid spondylitis. **Stühmer's d.,** balanitis xerotica obliterans. **Sturge's d., Sturge-Weber-Dimitri d.,** Sturge-Weber syndrome. **Stuttgart d.,** a nonjaundiced type of canine leptospirosis caused by *Leptospira canicola;* called also *canine typhus.* **Sudeck's d.,** post-traumatic osteoporosis. **Sutton's d.,** 1. [R. L. Sutton, Sr.] (a) halo nevus; (b) periadenitis mucosa necrotica recurrens. 2. [R. L. Sutton, Jr.] granuloma fissuratum. **Sutton and Gull's d.** (*obs.*), arteriocapillary fibrosis. **Swediaur's (Schwediauer's) d.,** inflammation of the calcaneal bursa. **sweet clover d.,** a hemorrhagic disease of animals, especially cattle, caused by ingestion of spoiled sweet clover, which contains the anticoagulant dicumarol. **Swift's d.,** acrodynia. **Swift-Feer d.,** acrodynia. **swineherd's d.,** a benign meningitis caused by *Leptospira pomona* and *L. hyos,* seen in those who work with swine or pork. **Sylvest's d.,** epidemic pleurodynia. **Symmers' d.,** giant follicular lymphoma. **systemic d.,** one affecting a number of organs and tissues. **systemic mast cell d.,** systemic mastocytosis. **Takahara's d.,** acatalasia. **Takayasu's d.,** pulseless d. **Talfan d.,** infectious porcine encephalomyelitis. **Talma's d.,** myotonia acquisita. **Tangier d.,** a familial disorder first observed in inhabitants of Tangier Island on the Chesapeake Bay, characterized by a deficiency of high-density lipoproteins in the blood serum, with storage of cholesterol esters in the tonsils and other tissues. **tarabagan d.,** plague in humans resulting from the bite of an ectoparasite of the Mongolian marmot (tarabagan). **tartaric d.,** gout and calculus (Paracelsus). **Tay's d.,** see under *choroiditis.* **Tay-Sachs d.,** the infantile form of cerebral sphingolipidosis in which symptoms become noticeable at about 4 to 6 months of age. A progressive disorder, it is characterized by degeneration of brain cells and the macula (with formation of a cherry-red spot on both retinas) and eventually by dementia, blindness, paralysis, and death. Affecting chiefly Ashkenazic Jewish children, it is inherited as an autosomal recessive trait and is due to an error of lipid metabolism in which a defect in hexosaminidase A results in accumulation of ganglioside GM_2 in the brain. Called also *Sachs' d.* and GM_2 *gangliosidosis.* A variant of Tay-Sachs disease is known as *Sandhoff's disease* (q.v.). **teart d. in cattle,** a diarrhea that affects cattle that graze on certain pastures in England, due to the presence of molybdenum in the herbage. **Teschen d.,** infectious porcine encephalomyelitis. **thalassemia–sickle cell d.,** sickle cell–thalassemia d. **Thaysen's d.,** nontropical sprue, or celiac disease. **Theiler's d.,** spontaneous encephalomyelitis of mice, caused by invasion of the nervous system by a common viral infection of the intestinal tract; called also *Theiler's mouse encephalomyelitis* and *murine encephalomyelitis.* **Thiemann's d.,** familial avascular necrosis of the phalangeal epiphysis, beginning in childhood or adolescence and resulting in deformity of the interphalangeal joints; called also *familial osteoarthropathy of the fingers.* Similar lesions may occur in the great toes and first tarsometatarsal joints, in which case it is known as *osteochondritis ossis metacarpi et metatarsi.* **Thomsen's d.,** myotonia congenita. **Thomson's d.,** a hereditary condition characterized by developmental hyperkeratotic lesions and xerodermatous changes; see also *Rothmund-Thomson syndrome,* under *syndrome.* **thyrocardiac d.,** thyrotoxic heart d. **thyrotoxic heart d.,** heart disease associated with hyperthyroidism, marked by atrial fibrillation, cardiac enlargement, and congestive heart failure; called also *thyrocardiac d.* **Tietze's d.,** see under *syndrome.* **Tillaux's d.,** mastitis with the formation of multiple tumors in the breast. **Tommaselli's d.,** pyrexia and hematuria due to excessive use of quinine. **Tooth d.,** progressive neuropathic (peroneal) muscular atrophy. **Tornwaldt's (Thornwaldt's) d.,** see under *bursitis.* **Tourette's d.,** Gilles de la Tourette's syndrome. **Traum's d.,** infectious abortion (brucellosis) in swine. **Trevor's d.,** dysplasia epiphysealis hemimelica. **trophoblastic d.,** a group of disorders that have their origin in the placenta, including hydatidiform mole, chorioadenoma destruens, and gestational choriocarcinoma. **tsetse-fly d.,** nagana. **tsutsugamushi d.,** scrub typhus. **tunnel d.,** 1. (*obs.*) hookworm d. 2. decompression sickness. **twin-lamb d.,** pregnancy tox-

emia in ewes. **Tyzzer's d.,** a disease caused by *Bacillus piliformis* and characterized by necrotic lesions of the liver and intestine; originally described in Japanese waltzing mice, it also affects rats, rabbits, gerbils, dogs, and man. **Underwood's d.,** sclerema. **Unna's d.** (*obs.*), seborrheic dermatitis. **Unverricht's d.,** progressive familial myoclonic epilepsy. **Urbach-Oppenheim d.** (*obs.*), necrobiosis lipoidica diabeticorum. **Urbach-Wiethe d.,** lipoid proteinosis. **vagabonds' d., vagrants' d.,** discoloration of the skin in persons subjected to louse (*Pediculus humanus corporis*) bites over long periods; called also *parasitic melanoderma.* **van Buren's d.,** Peyronie's disease. **Vaquez' d., Vaquez-Osler d.,** polycythemia vera. **veld d., veldt d.,** heartwater. **venereal d.,** a contagious disease, most commonly acquired in sexual intercourse or other genital contact; the venereal diseases include syphilis, gonorrhea, chancroid, granuloma inguinale, lymphogranuloma venereum, genital herpesvirus infection, and balanitis gangraenosa. **veno-occlusive d. of the liver,** an acute or chronic condition encountered predominantly in children, characterized by partial or complete occlusion of the branches of the hepatic veins by endophlebitis and thrombosis, leading to centrilobular necrosis, fibrosis, and portal hypertension with ascites; it was first observed in children in Jamaica and probably resulted from the toxic action of alkaloids ingested in bush tea. Called also *serous hepatosis.* **vent d.,** rabbit syphilis. **Verneuil's d.,** syphilitic disease of the bursae. **Verse's d.,** calcinosis intervertebralis. **vibration d.,** blanching and diminished flexion of the fingers with loss of perception of cold, heat, and pain and osteoarthritic changes in joints of the arm, due to continuous use of vibrating tools. **Vidal's d.,** lichen simplex chronicus. **Vincent's d.,** necrotizing ulcerative gingivostomatitis. **Vogt's d.,** see under *syndrome.* **Vogt-Spielmeyer d.,** the juvenile form of cerebral sphingolipidosis. **Volkmann's d.,** a congenital deformity of the foot due to a tibiotarsal dislocation; called also *Volkmann's deformity.* **Voltolini's d.,** an acute purulent inflammation of the internal ear with violent pain, followed by involvement of the meninges with subsequent fever, delirium, and unconsciousness. **von Economo's d.,** lethargic encephalitis. **von Gierke's d.,** glycogen storage d. (type I). **von Hippel's d.,** angiomatosis confined principally to the retina; when associated with hemangioblastoma of the cerebellum, it is known as *von Hippel-Lindau d.* **von Hippel-Lindau d.,** hereditary phakomatosis characterized by congenital angiomatosis of the retina and cerebellum; there may also be similar lesions of the spinal cord and cysts of the pancreas, kidneys, and other viscera. Neurologic symptoms, including seizures and mental retardation, may be present. Called also *cerebroretinal* or *retinocerebral angiomatosis,* and *Lindau-von Hippel d.* **von Jaksch's d.,** anemia pseudoleukemica infantum. **von Recklinghausen's d.,** see *Recklinghausen's d.* **von Willebrand's d.,** a congenital hemorrhagic diathesis, inherited as an autosomal dominant trait, characterized by a prolonged bleeding time, a deficiency of coagulation Factor VIII, and often impairment of adhesion of platelets on glass beads, associated with epistaxis and increased bleeding after trauma or surgery, menorrhagia, and postpartum bleeding. Called also *angiohemophilia, Minot-von Willebrand syndrome, pseudohemophilia, vascular hemophilia,* and *Willebrand's syndrome.* **Vrolik's d.,** osteogenesis imperfecta congenita. **Wagner's d.,** colloid milium; see under *milium.* **Waldenström's d.,** osteochondrosis of the capital femoral epiphysis; see *osteochondrosis.* **walk-about d.,** Kimberley horse d. **Wartenberg's d.,** 1. cheiralgia paresthetica. 2. brachialgia statica paresthetica. 3. partial thenar atrophy. **Wassilieff's d.,** leptospiral jaundice. **wasting d.,** any disease marked especially by progressive emaciation and weakness. **Weber's d.,** Sturge-Weber syndrome. **Weber-Christian d.,** nodular nonsuppurative panniculitis. **Weber-Dimitri d.,** Sturge-Weber syndrome. **Wegner's d.,** osteochondritic separation of the epiphyses in hereditary syphilis. **Weil's d.,** leptospiral jaundice. **Weir Mitchell's d.,** erythromelalgia. **Wenckebach's d.** (*obs.*), cardioptosis. **Werdnig-Hoffmann d.,** see under *paralysis.* **Werlhof's d.,** idiopathic thrombocytopenic purpura. **Werner-His d.,** trench fever. **Werner-Schultz d.,** agranulocytosis. **Wernicke's d.,** see under *encephalopathy.* **Wesselsbron d.,** a mosquito-borne viral disease causing death of lambs and abortion and death in ewes in Africa; it is communicable to man, in whom it causes a mild febrile illness. **Westphal-Strümpell d.,** see under *pseudosclerosis.* **Whipple's d.,** a malabsorption syndrome characterized by diarrhea, steatorrhea, skin pigmentation, arthralgia and arthritis, lymphadenopathy, and central nervous system lesions. The intestinal mucosa is infiltrated with macrophages containing PAS-positive material (the remnants of bacillary microorganisms which invade the lamina propria). **white heifer d.,** a condition reputed to most commonly occur in white heifers, usually of the Shorthorn breed, in which there is a rubber-like sheet of fibrous tissue and membrane stretching across the posterior part of the vagina; the converage may be partial or complete. Called also *persistent hymen.* **white muscle d.,** 1. muscular dystrophy in calves, caused by vitamin E deficiency. 2. stiff lamb d. **white-spot d.,** lichen sclerosus et atrophicus; sometimes used erroneously for guttate morphea or guttate scleroderma. **Whitmore's d.,** melioidosis. **Whytt's**

d., tuberculous meningitis causing acute hydrocephalus. **Willis' d.,** diabetes mellitus. **Wilson's d.,** [S.A.K. Wilson] hepatolenticular degeneration. **Winckel's d.,** a fatal disease of newborn infants characterized by jaundice, hemoglobinuria, hemorrhage, bloody urine, cyanosis, polyuria, collapse, and convulsions. **Winkler's d.** (obs.), chondrodermatitis nodularis chronica helicis. **winter vomiting d.,** outbreaks of vomiting which have been observed in various countries. **Winton d.,** Pictou d. **Witkop's d., Witkop-Von Sallmann d.,** hereditary benign intraepithelial dyskeratosis. **Wolman's d.,** primary familial xanthomatosis in infants, associated with involvement and calcification of the adrenal glands, failure to thrive, vomiting, diarrhea, hepatomegaly, splenomegaly, foam cells in the bone marrow and other tissues, and early death; it is transmitted as an autosomal recessive trait. **woolsorters' d.,** pulmonary anthrax. **x d.,** 1. Mackenzie's name for a series of morbid symptoms of unknown origin, consisting of a feeling of general ill health with sensitiveness to cold, dyspepsia, intestinal disorder, and disturbance of respiration and of the action of the heart. 2. hyperkeratosis (3rd def.). 3. aflatoxicosis. **Zahorsky's d.,** exanthema subitum. **Ziehen-Oppenheim d.,** dystonia musculorum deformans. **zymotic d.,** a disease due to the action of an enzyme, as of a morbific germ or a ptomaine.

disengagement (dis″en-gāj′ment) liberation of the fetus, or parts thereof, from the vaginal canal.

disequilibrium (dis-e″kwĭ-lib′re-um) a disturbed state of equilibrium, either physical or mental. **linkage d.,** a genetic phenomenon in which certain phenotypic combinations are much more common than would be expected on the basis of gene frequencies of individual genes.

disesthesia (dis″es-the′ze-ah) dysesthesia.

disgerminoma (dis-jer″mĭ-no′mah) dysgerminoma.

dish (dish) a shallow vessel of glass or other material for laboratory work. **culture d.,** a shallow glass vessel for making bacterial cultures. **dappen d.,** a small heavy ten-sided piece of glass, each end of which is ground into a small cup for mixing dental medicaments or fillings. **evaporating d.,** a laboratory vessel, usually wide and shallow, in which material is evaporated by exposure to heat. **Petri d.,** a shallow glass receptacle for growing bacterial cultures. **Stender d.,** a vessel of various forms and sizes, used in preparing and staining histologic specimens.

disharmony (dis-har′mo-ne) lacking harmony; discordant. **occlusal d.,** a condition in which (a) contacts of opposing occlusal surfaces of teeth are not in harmony with other tooth contacts and with the anatomic and physiologic control of the mandible, or (b) occlusions do not coincide with their respective jaw relations.

disimmune (dis″ĭ-mūn′) deprived of immunity.

disimmunity (dis″ĭ-mu′nĭ-te) the state that results from the loss of immunity.

disimmunize (dis-im′u-niz) to deprive of immunity.

disimpaction (dis″im-pak′shun) (obs.) the relief or removal of an impaction.

disinfect (dis″in-fekt′) [dis- + L. inficere to corrupt] to free from pathogenic organisms, or to render them inert.

disinfectant (dis″in-fek′tant) 1. freeing from infection. 2. an agent that disinfects; applied particularly to agents used on inanimate objects. Cf. antiseptic. **coal-tar d.,** creosote.

disinfection (dis″in-fek′shun) the act of disinfecting. **concomitant d., concurrent d.,** immediate disinfection and disposal of discharges and infective matter all through the course of a disease. **terminal d.,** disinfection and destruction of infectious material after the recovery of a patient from an infectious disease or after his death.

disinfestation (dis″in-fes-ta′shun) the extermination or destruction of insects, rodents, or other animal forms which might transmit infection and which are present on the person or clothing of an individual or in his surroundings; defaunation.

disinhibition (dis″in-hĭ-bish′un) the abolition of inhibition; in an experimental animal, the revival of an extinguished conditioned reflex or response by a stimulus to which the animal is unaccustomed.

disinomenine (di″sĭ-nom′ĕ-nin) an alkaloid, $C_{19}H_{25}O_4N$, formed by the oxidation of sinomenine.

disinsected (dis″in-sekt′ed) freed from insects or vermin.

disinsection (dis″in-sek′shun) disinsectization.

disinsectization (dis″in-sek″ti-za′shun) removal of insects from; extermination of insects or vermin.

disinsector (dis″in-sek′tor) an apparatus for the removal of insects or vermin from patients or their clothing.

disinsertion (dis″in-ser′shun) 1. rupture of a tendon from its insertion into a bone. 2. detachment of the retina at its periphery; retinodialysis.

disintegrant (dis-in′tĕ-grant) disintegrator; an agent used in the pharmaceutical preparation of tablets, which causes them to disintegrate and release their medicinal substances on contact with moisture.

disintegration (dis″in-tĕ-gra′shun) [dis- + L. integer entire]

the process of breaking up or decomposing. **radioactive d.,** see under decay.

Disipal (dis′ĭ-pal) trademark for a preparation of orphenadrine hydrochloride.

disjoint (dis-joint′) to disarticulate.

disjunction (dis-junk′shun) the act or state of being disjoined. In genetics, the moving apart of bivalent chromosomes at first anaphase of meiosis. **craniofacial d.,** Le Fort III fracture; see under fracture.

disk (disk) [L. discus; Gr. diskos] a circular or rounded flat plate; also disc. **A d.,** A band; see under band. **abrasive d.,** a dental disk with abrasive particles attached to one or both of its surfaces or its edge. **Amici's d.,** Z band; see under band. **anangioid d.,** a retinal disk without blood vessels. **anisotropic d., anisotropous d.,** A band; see under band. **articular d.,** 1. a pad of fibrocartilage or dense fibrous tissue found in some synovial joints; see discus articularis, and for names of articular disks of particular joints, see entries beginning discus articularis, under discus. 2. meniscus articularis. **Bardeen's primitive d.,** the embryonic structure which develops into the intervertebral ligament. **Blake's d's,** disks of paper for pasting over drumhead perforations. **blastodermic d.,** the early germinal disk during the period of cleavage. **blood d.,** see platelet. **Bowman's d's,** flat, disklike plates which make up striated muscle fibers. **carborundum d.,** a dental disk charged with carborundum. **choked d.,** papilledema. **ciliary d.,** orbiculus ciliaris. **cloth d.,** a dental disk made of one or more round pieces of cloth. **cupped d.,** a pathologically depressed optic disk. **cutting d.,** a dental disk charged with an abrasive material and used for grinding or reducing teeth. **cuttlefish d.,** a dental disk charged with powdered cuttlefish bone. **dental d.,** a thin, circular piece of paper or other material, usually operated by a dental engine, and used in procedures on the teeth or dental restorations. It may be used for carrying polishing powders, such as chalk, pumice, rouge, or whiting, or be specially treated with such substances as cuttlefish bone, emery, garnet, or sand, for fine cutting or polishing. **diamond d.,** a dental disk charged with small diamond particles. **ectodermal d.,** an elongated plate of epithelial cells developed from the inner cell mass in the human conceptus about a week after fertilization. **embryonic d.,** a flattish area in a cleaved ovum in which the first traces of the embryo are seen; called also germinal d. and gastrodisk. **emery d.,** a dental disk charged with emery powder. **Engelmann's d.,** H band; see under band. **gelatin d.,** a disk or lamella of gelatin, variously medicated; used chiefly in eye diseases. **germinal d.,** embryonic d. **Hensen's d.,** H band; see under band. **I d.,** the light disk or band of a striated muscle fiber; called also isotropic disk or J disk. **interarticular d.,** articular d., def. 1. **intercalated d.,** dense bands that extend in a serrated fashion transversely across cardiac muscle fibers, separating one fiber from another but containing contact specializations, including desmosomes and gap junctions. **intermediate d.,** Z band; see under band. **interpubic d.,** discus interpubicus. **intervertebral d's,** layers of fibrocartilage between the bodies of adjacent vertebrae, consisting of a fibrous ring enclosing a pulpy center; called also disci intervertebrales [NA], intervertebral cartilages, fibrocartilagines intervertebrales, and intervertebral fibrocartilages. **intra-**

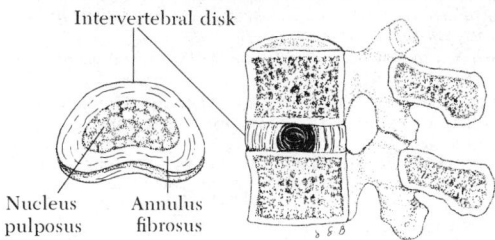

Intervertebral disk

Nucleus pulposus   Annulus fibrosus

articular d., fibrous structures within the capsules of diarthrodial joints. **isotropic d., J d.,** I band; see under band. **M d.,** M band; see under band. **Merkel's d's,** Merkel's corpuscles. **micrometer d.,** a glass disk, engraved with a scale, used in an ocular in making microscopical measurements. **Newton's d.,** a disk which is divided into seven sectors that are colored the seven primary colors of the spectrum and which, when rotated rapidly, appears to be white. **optic d.,** discus nervi optici. **Placido's d.,** a disk having concentric circles marked on it; used in examining the cornea. **polishing d.,** a dental disk charged with a polishing agent rather than an abrasive material; used for polishing teeth or fillings. **proligerous d.,** cumulus oophorus. **Q d.,** A band; see under band. **Ranvier's tactile d's,** terminations of nerve fibers in cup-shaped bodies in the transparent substance between Grandry's corpuscles. **Rekoss d.,** the rotating device for quickly changing the lenses in the ophthalmoscope. **sandpaper d.,** a dental disk charged with pulverized silica. **Schiefferdecker's d's,** a substance in neurons staining black with silver nitrate, assumed to occupy the space in Ranvier's nodes between Schwann's sheath and the axon. **slipped d.,** popular name for herniation of an intervertebral disk. **stenopeic d.,** an opaque disk having a narrow slit; used for testing for astigmatism. **stroboscopic d.,** a disk used in eye examinations to produce distortion of objects seen. **tactile d.,** a disklike nerve termination in a tactile cell, as in an end-organ of a nerve of special sense. **thin d.,** Z band; see under *band.* **transverse d.,** A band; see under *band.* **Z d.,** Z band; see under *band.*

disk- see *disko-.*

diskectomy (dis-kek′to-me) excision of an intervertebral disk.

diskiform (dis′ki-form) in the shape of a disk.

diskitis (dis-ki′tis) inflammation of a disk, particularly of an interarticular disk.

disko-, disk- [L. *discus;* Gr. *diskos*] a combining form denoting relationship to a disk, or disk-shaped, see also words beginning *disco-.*

diskogram (dis′ko-gram) a roentgenogram of an intervertebral disk.

diskography (dis-kog′rah-fe) roentgenography of the spine for visualization of an intervertebral disk, after injection into the disk itself of an absorbable contrast medium.

dislocatio (dis″lo-ka′she-o) [L.] dislocation. **d. erec′ta,** subglenoid dislocation of the shoulder with the arm in a vertical position and the hand on top of the head.

dislocation (dis″lo-ka′shun) [*dis-* + L. *locare* to place] the displacement of any part, more especially of a bone; see Plate. Called also *luxation.* **Bell-Dally d.,** nontraumatic dislocation of the atlas. **closed d.,** simple d. **complete d.,** one which completely separates the surfaces of a joint. **complicated d.,** one which is associated with other important injuries. **compound d.,** one in which the joint communicates with the external air. **congenital d.,** one which exists from or before birth. **consecutive d.,** one in which the luxated bone has changed its position since its first displacement. **divergent d.,** one in which the ulna and radius are dislocated separately. **fracture d.,** dislocation complicated by fracture of, or adjacent to, a joint. **habitual d.,** one which often recurs after replacement. **incomplete d.,** a subluxation; a slight displacement. Called also *partial d.* **intrauterine d.,** one which occurs to the fetus in utero. **Kienböck's d.,** isolated dislocation of the semilunar bone. **d. of the lens,** displacement of the crystalline lens of the eye. **Lisfranc's d.,** dislocation of the forefoot at the tarsometatarsal joints. **Monteggia's d.,** dislocation of the hip joint in which the head of the femur is near the anterosuperior spine of the ilium. **Nélaton's d.,** dislocation of the ankle in which the talus is forced up between the end of the tibia and the fibula. **old d.,** a dislocation in which inflammatory or fibrotic changes have occurred. **open d.,** compound d. **partial d.,** incomplete d. **pathologic d.,** one which results from paralysis, synovitis, infection, or other disease. **primitive d.,** one in which the bones remain as originally displaced. **recent d.,** one in which there is no complicating inflammation. **simple d.,** one in which the joint is not penetrated by a wound. **Smith's d.,** upward and backward dislocation of the metatarsals and the medial cuneiform bone. **subastragalar d.,** separation of the calcaneus and the navicular bone from the talus. **subspinous d.,** dislocation of the head of the humerus into the space below the spine of the scapula. **traumatic d.,** one due to an injury or to violence.

dismemberment (dis-mem′ber-ment) amputation of a limb or a portion of it.

dismutase (dis-mu′tās) any of a group of enzymes that have the ability to catalyze the reaction of two molecules of the same compound to yield two molecules in different oxidation states. **superoxide d.,** an enzyme present in aerobic and facultative bacteria but not in anaerobes, which catalytically converts superoxides by the reaction $2O_2^- + 2H^+ \rightarrow H_2O_2 + O_2$.

dismutation (dis″mu-ta′shun) a complex enzymic process that results simultaneously in oxidation and reduction or also in decarboxylation.

disocclude (dis″o-klood′) to grind a tooth so that it does not touch its antagonist in the other jaw in any of the movements of mastication.

disodium (di-so′de-um) having two atoms of sodium in each molecule.

disome (di′sōm) [*di-* + Gr. *sōma* body] a chromosome set having paired members.

Disomer (di′so-mer) trademark for preparations of dexbrompheniramine maleate.

disomus (di-so′mus) [*di-* + Gr. *sōma* body] a double-bodied monster.

disopyramide (di-so-pēr′ah-mīd) [USP] chemical name: α-[2-[bis(1-methylethyl)amino]ethyl]-α-phenyl-2-pyridineacetamide. A cardiac depressant with anticholinergic properties, $C_{21}H_{29}N_3O$, used as an antiarrhythmic. **d. phosphate,** the phosphate salt of disopyramide, $C_{21}H_{29}N_3O \cdot H_3PO_4$, having the same actions and uses as the base, administered orally.

disorder (dis-or′der) a derangement or abnormality of function; a morbid physical or mental state. **affective d's,** 1. any of a group of mental disorders in which a disturbance of affect is predominant, including depressive neurosis, the major affective disorders, and psychotic depressive reaction. 2. major affective d. **behavior d.,** a type of behavior deviation marked by impulsive, antisocial acts; the term has been used to refer to any abnormal behavior. Called also *conduct d.* **behavior d's of childhood and adolescence,** a group of personality disorders occurring during childhood and adolescence, characterized by overactivity, inattentiveness, shyness, feelings of rejection, over-aggressiveness, timidity, or delinquency; they are less severe than psychoses but more resistant to treatment than transient situational disturbances because they are more stabilized and internalized. **brain d.,** see *organic brain syndrome,* under *syndrome.* **character d.,** a personality disorder characterized by maladaptive behavior, emotional responses that are socially unacceptable, and minimal feelings of anxiety or other symptoms that usually accompany neuroses. **conduct d.,** behavior d. **functional d.,** a disorder not associated with clearly defined physical cause or structural change, i.e., having no detectable organic basis. Called also *functional illness.* **major affective d.,** any of a group of psychoses, including involutional melancholia and the various forms of manic-depressive psychosis, characterized by a severe disorder of mood, either extreme depression or elation or both, which do not seem to be attributable entirely to precipitating life experiences. Called also *affective psychosis.* **mental d.,** any psychiatric illness or disease, whether functional or of organic origin; called also *mental disease* or *illness* and *emotional illness.* **personality d.,** a mental disorder which stems from the personality of the individual and in which there is minimal feeling of subjective anxiety and little or no feeling of distress. **personality d., epileptoid,** see *explosive personality,* under *personality.* **personality d., histrionic,** see *hysterical personality,* under *personality.* **psychophysiologic d., psychosomatic d.,** a group of disorders characterized by physical symptoms and demonstrable structural and/or physiological changes in which emotional factors are believed to play a major etiologic or pathogenic role. Typically a single organ system is involved, usually under autonomic control.

disorganization (dis-or″gan-i-za′shun) the process of destruction of any organic tissue; any profound change in the tissues of an organ or structure which causes the loss of most or all of its proper characters.

disorientation (dis-o″re-en-ta′shun) the loss of proper bearings, or a state of mental confusion as to time, place, or identity. **spatial d.,** a condition in which a pilot or other air crew member is unable to determine accurately his spatial attitude in relation to the surface of the earth; it occurs only in conditions of poor visibility or when vision is otherwise restricted and results from vestibular illusions. Called also *pilot's vertigo.*

disoxidation (dis″ok-se-da′shun) deoxidation.

dispar (dis′par) [L.] unequal.

disparasitized (dis-par′ah-si-tīzd) freed from parasites.

disparate (dis′pah-rat) [L. *disparatus, dispar* unequal] not situated alike; not exactly paired; dissimilar in kind.

dispensary (dis-pen′sah-re) [L. *dispensarium,* from *dispensare* to dispense] 1. a place where medical or dental skill, treatment, and remedies are provided for the indigent ambulant sick at little or no cost to them. 2. any place where drugs and medicines are actually dispensed.

dispensatory (dis-pen′sah-to-re) [L. *dispensatorium*] a treatise on the qualities and composition of medicines. **D. of the United States of America,** a collection of monographs on unofficial drugs and drugs recognized by the United States Pharmacopoeia, the British Pharmacopoeia, and the National Formulary, and on general tests, processes, reagents, and solutions of the U.S.P. and N.F., as well as drugs used in veterinary medicine.

dispense (dis-pens′) [L. *dispensare, dis-* out + *pensare* to weigh] to prepare and distribute medicines to those who are to use them.

dispermine (di-sper′min) piperazine.

dispermy (di′sper-me) the penetration of two spermatozoa into one ovum.

dispersate (dis′pur-sāt) a suspension of finely divided particles of a substance.

disperse (dis-pers′) [L. *dis-* apart + *spargere* to scatter] to scatter the component parts, as of a tumor or the fine particles in a colloid system; also the particles so dispersed.

dispersible (dis-per′si-b'l) capable of being dispersed.

dispersion (dis-per′shun) [L. *dispersio*] 1. the act of scattering or separating; the condition of being scattered. 2. the incorporation of the particles of one substance into the body of another, comprising solutions, suspensions, and colloid solutions. 3. a colloid solution. **colloid d.,** a colloid solution. **molecular d.,** solution, def. 1.

dispersity (dis-per′si-te) the degree of dispersion of a colloid, i.e., the degree to which the dimensions of the disperse particles have been reduced.

Plate XV   dislocation

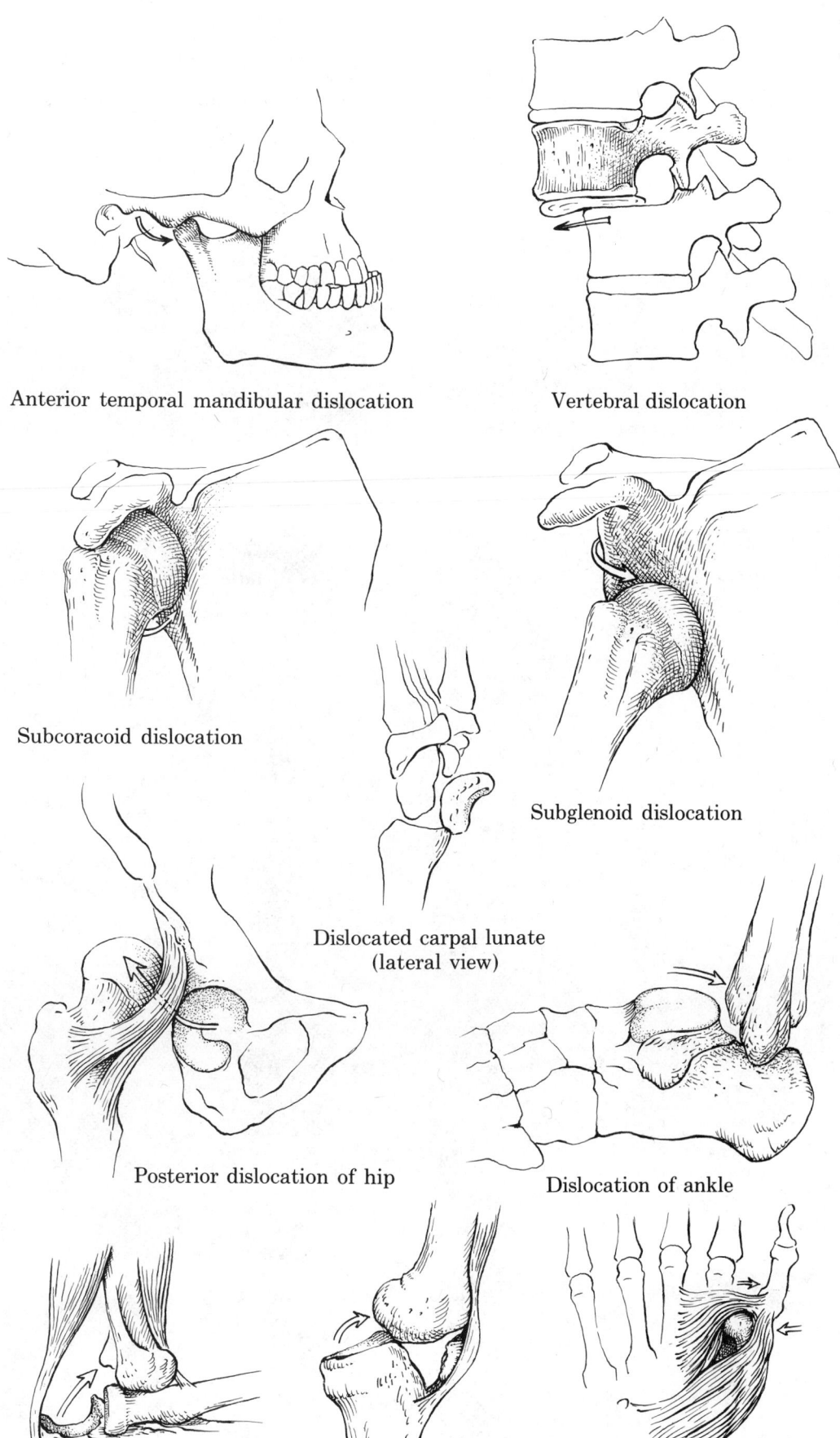

Anterior temporal mandibular dislocation   Vertebral dislocation

Subcoracoid dislocation

Subglenoid dislocation

Dislocated carpal lunate
(lateral view)

Posterior dislocation of hip   Dislocation of ankle

H. Goodwin

Posterior dislocation of elbow   Posterior dislocation of knee   Dislocation of thumb

VARIOUS TYPES OF DISLOCATION

dispersoid (dis-per′soid) a colloid in which the dispersity is relatively great.

dispersonalization (dis-per″son-al-i-za′shun) depersonalization.

dispert (dis′pert) a medicinal preparation obtained from a vegetable drug or endocrine gland by extracting its therapeutical constituents in the cold and then reducing the product to a dry concentrated form.

Dispholidus (dis-fol′ĭ-dus) a genus of venomous colubrid snakes. *D. ty′pus* is the boomslang of South Africa. See table accompanying *snake*.

dispira (di-spi′rah) [*di-* + Gr. *speira* coil] dispireme.

dispireme (di-spi′rem, di-spi′rēm) [*di-* + Gr. *speirēma* coil] the stage of cell division which follows the diaster; so called because the cytoplasm is divided into two parts, in each of which the chromatin appears to assume the form of a coil. See *mitosis*.

displaceability (dis-plās″ah-bil′ĭ-te) the quality of being susceptible to movement from an initial position, or the degree to which such movement is possible.

displacement (dis-plās′ment) 1. removal from the normal position or place; ectopia. 2. percolation. 3. a mental mechanism in which the emotional charge attached to one set of ideas is displaced (transferred) onto other, initially unrelated, ideas. 4. in dentistry, the malposition of the crown and root of one or more teeth from the normal line of occlusion; also the deflection of the mandible from its normal path of closure, i.e., posterior displacement. **condylar d.,** an abnormal position of the head of the mandibular condyle in the fossa due to a deviation or shift of the mandible, which is often the result of malocclusion. **fetal d.,** a group of cells which, during fetal development, has become displaced from its normal relations. **fish-hook d.,** a form of displacement of the stomach in which the orifice of the pylorus faces directly upward, and the duodenum runs upward and to the right to join the pylorus at an angle, producing a constricting hook; there is no evidence that such displacement causes symptoms. **gallbladder d.,** wandering gallbladder. **tissue d.,** change in the position of tissues as the result of pressure or other force.

dispore (di′spōr) one of two spores, as the basidia of higher fungi; opposed to tetraspore (four-spored basidium).

disporous (di′spo-rus) having two spores, as the basidia of the higher fungi.

disposition (dis″po-zish′un) a tendency either physical or mental toward certain diseases.

disproportion (dis″pro-por′shun) a lack of the proper relationship between two elements or factors. **cephalopelvic d.,** a condition in which the head of the fetus is too large for the pelvis of the mother.

disruption (dis-rup′shun) the act of separating forcibly, or the state of being abnormally separated.

disruptive (dis-rup′tiv) bursting apart; rending.

Disse's spaces (dis′ez) [Joseph *Disse,* German anatomist, 1852–1912] see under *space.*

dissect (dĭ-sekt′, di-sekt′) [L. *dissecare* to cut up] to cut apart, or separate; applied especially to the exposure of structures of a cadaver, for anatomical study.

dissection (dĭ-sek′shun) [L. *dissectio*] 1. the act of dissecting. 2. a part or whole of an organism prepared by dissecting. **aortic d.,** dissecting aneurysm. **blunt d.,** dissection accomplished by separating tissues along natural cleavage lines, without cutting. **sharp d.,** dissection accomplished by incising tissues with a sharp edge.

dissector (dĭ-sek′tor) 1. one who dissects. 2. a handbook used as a guide for the act of dissecting.

disseminated (dis-sem′ĭ-nāt″ed) [L. *dis-* apart + *seminare* to sow] scattered; distributed over a considerable area.

dissepiment (dis-sep′ĭ-ment) partition; separation.

dissimilate (dis-sim′ĭ-lāt) [L. *dis-* neg. + *similare* to make alike] to decompose a substance into simpler compounds, for the production of energy or of materials that can be eliminated.

dissimilation (dis″sim-ĭ-la′shun) the act or process of dissimilating (see *dissimilate*); the reverse of assimilation.

dissociable (dis-so′shĕ-b'l) easily separable into component parts; separable from associations.

dissociant (dis-so′she-ant) a strain of microorganisms derived by bacterial dissociation.

dissociated (dis-so′she-āt″ed) split off from consciousness. Cf. *dissociation* (def. 3).

dissociation (dis-so″she-a′shun) [L. *dis-* neg. + *sociatio* union] 1. the act of separating or state of being separated. 2. resolution by heat of a molecule into two or more simpler molecules. 3. a defect of mental integration in which one or more groups of mental processes become separated off from normal consciousness and, thus separated, function as a unitary whole. Cf. *unconscious.* **albuminocytologic d.,** increase of protein with normal cell count in the spinal fluid. **atrial d.,** independent beating of the left and right atria, each with normal rhythm or with various combinations of normal rhythm, atrial flutter, or atrial fibrilla-

tion. **atrioventricular d.,** control of the atria by one pacemaker and of the ventricles by another, independent pacemaker; when the ventricular rate is more rapid than the atrial rate, ventriculoatrial (retrograde) block is present but atrioventricular conduction (anterograde) usually is not impaired. **auriculoventricular d.,** atrioventricular d. **bacterial d.,** the change, due to mutation and selection, in colonial morphology (usually from mucoid or smooth to rough) of bacteria in culture on laboratory media; called also *microbic d.* **interference d., d. by interference,** control of the atria by the sinoatrial node or other atrial pacemaker and of the ventricles by a lower pacemaker (atrioventricular dissociation) with a phasic rhythm related to capture of the ventricle (anterograde) or atrium (retrograde) by conduction from the pacemaker in the other chamber; called also *atrioventricular interference d.* **microbic d.,** bacterial d. **peripheral d.,** sensory disturbance in which touch, superficial pain, and temperature sensibility are diminished in the hands and feet; seen in polyneuritis. **syringomyelic d.,** loss of pain and temperature sense due to a lesion in the region of the central canal of the spinal cord implicating the spinothalamic fibers with preservation of other sensory modalities. **tabetic d.,** disturbance of the vibratory and muscle-tendon sensibility due to lesion of the dorsal columns.

dissogeny (dĭ-soj′ĕ-ne) [Gr. *dissos* twofold + *gennan* to produce] the state of having sexual maturity in both a larval and an adult stage.

dissolution (dis″so-lu′shun) [L. *dissolutio, dissolvere* to dissolve] 1. the process in which one substance is dissolved in another. 2. separation of a compound into its components by chemical action. 3. liquefaction. 4. the process of loosening, or of relaxing. 5. death.

dissolve (diz-zolv′) 1. to cause a substance to pass into solution. 2. to pass into solution.

dissolvent (diz-zol′vent) 1. a solvent medium. 2. a medicine capable of dissolving concretions within the body. 3. solvent; capable of dissolving substances.

dissonance (dis′so-nans) discord or disagreement. **cognitive d.,** discord or disharmony of thoughts, beliefs, and behavior.

Dist. abbreviation for L. *distil′la,* distil.

distad (dis′tad) in a distal direction.

distal (dis′tal) [L. *distans* distant] remote; farther from any point of reference; opposed to proximal. In dentistry, used to designate a position on the dental arch farther from the median line of the jaw.

distalis (dis-ta′lis) distal; [NA] a term denoting remoteness from the point of origin or attachment of an organ or part.

distally (dis′tal-le) in a distal direction.

distance (dis′tans) the measure of space intervening between two objects or two points of reference. **angular d.,** the aperture of the angle made at the eye by lines drawn from the eye to two objects. **cone-surface d.,** in radiology, the distance measured along the central beam from the distal end of the cone to the surface of the irradiated object. **focal d.,** the distance from the focal point to the optical center of a lens or the surface of a concave mirror. **infinite d.,** in ophthalmology, a distance of 20 feet or more: so called because rays entering the eye from an object at that distance are practically as parallel as if they came from a point at an infinite distance. **interarch d.,** 1. the vertical distance between the maxillary and mandibular arches (alveolar or residual) under certain conditions of vertical dimension that must be specified. 2. the vertical distance between the maxillary and mandibular ridges; called also *interridge d.* **interocclusal d.,** the distance between the occluding surfaces of the maxillary and mandibular teeth when the mandible is in physiologic rest position; called also *interocclusal rest space, gap,* or *clearance,* and *free way space.* **interocular d.,** the distance between the two eyes, usually used in reference to the interpupillary distance. **interpediculate d.,** the distance between the vertebral pedicles as measured on the roentgenogram. **interpupillary d.,** the distance between the centers of the pupils of the two eyes when the visual axes are parallel; in practice usually measured from the lateral margin of one pupil to the medial margin of the other. **interridge d.,** interarch d. **map d.,** see *map unit,* under *unit.* **object-film d.,** in radiology, the distance from the site or plane being radiographed, to the surface of the film. Unless otherwise specified, this distance should be construed as being measured along the central ray. **source-cone d.,** in radiology, the distance measured along the central ray from the front surface of the source of radiation to the distal end of the cone. **target-skin d.,** the distance intervening between the anode from which roentgen rays are deflected and the skin of the body surface interposed in their path. **working d.,** the distance between the front lens of a microscope and the object when the instrument is correctly focused.

distemper (dis-tem′per) a name for several infectious diseases of animals, especially canine distemper. **canine d.,** a specific infectious respiratory and sometimes gastrointestinal disease of dogs characterized by fever, dullness, loss of appetite, and a discharge from the eyes and nose. It is caused by a virus and it is also infectious for foxes and ferrets. **cat d.,** panleukopenia. **colt d.,** strangles, def. 1.

distemperoid (dis-tem′per-oid) an attenuated canine distemper virus that has been subjected to several passages in ferrets; called also *Green's distemperoid.*

distensibility (dis-ten″sĭ-bil′ĭ-te) capability of being distended.

distention (dis-ten′shun) the state of being distended or enlarged; the act of distending.

distichia (dis-tik′e-ah) distichiasis.

distichiasis (dis″tĭ-ki′ah-sis) [Gr. *distichia* a double line] the presence of a double row of eyelashes on an eyelid, one or both of which are turned in against the eyeball.

distichous (dis′tĭ-kus) arranged in two vertical rows; said of the arrangement of leaves where the leaf at one node is opposite to those just above and below it.

distil, distill (dis-til′) [L. *destillare; de* from + *stillare* to drop] to volatilize by heat and then cool and condense the evaporated matter, as to purify a substance or to separate a volatile substance from other less volatile substances.

distillate (dis′til-lāt) material that has been obtained by distillation.

distillation (dis-til-la′shun) vaporization; the process of vaporizing and condensing a substance to purify the substance or to separate a volatile substance from less volatile substances. **destructive d., dry d.,** decomposition of a solid by heating in the absence of air, which results in volatile liquid products. **fractional d.,** that which is attended by the successive separation of volatilizable substances in the order of their respective volatility. **molecular d.,** a process of purification applied to drugs and pharmaceuticals during which the crude material is evaporated under high vacuum of about one millionth of an atmosphere, and the condensate is caught on a cooled surface held close in front of the evaporating layer. The process is applied currently to vitamins A, D, and E, to animal and vegetable sterols and hormones, and to drugs and intermediates. **vacuum d.,** distillation under reduced pressure to avoid the decomposition which might occur at atmospheric pressure.

distobuccal (dis″to-buk′al) pertaining to or formed by the distal and buccal surfaces of a tooth, or by the distal and buccal walls of a tooth cavity.

distobucco-occlusal (dis″to-buk″o-ŏ-kloo′zal) pertaining to or formed by the distal, buccal, and occlusal surfaces of a tooth.

distobuccopulpal (dis″to-buk″o-pul′pal) pertaining to or formed by the distal, buccal, and pulpal walls of a tooth cavity.

distocervical (dis″to-ser′vĭ-kal) 1. pertaining to the distal surface of the neck of a tooth. 2. distogingival.

distoclination (dis″to-kli-na′shun) deviation of a tooth from the vertical, in the direction of the tooth next distal (posterior) to it in the dental arch.

distoclusal (dis″to-kloo′zal) disto-occlusal.

distoclusion (dis″to-kloo′zhun) a malrelation of the dental arches in which the mandibular arch is in a posterior (distal) position in relation to the maxillary arch; called also *posteroclusion.*

distogingival (dis″to-jin′jĭ-val) pertaining to or formed by the distal and gingival walls of a tooth cavity; called also *distocervical.*

distolabial (dis″to-la′be-al) pertaining to or formed by the distal and labial surfaces of a tooth, or the distal and labial walls of a tooth cavity.

distolabioincisal (dis″to-la″be-o-in-si′zal) pertaining to or formed by the distal, labial, and incisal surfaces of a tooth.

distolingual (dis″to-ling′gwal) pertaining to or formed by the distal and lingual surfaces of a tooth, or the distal and lingual walls of a tooth cavity.

distolinguoincisal (dis″to-ling″gwo-in-si′zal) pertaining to or formed by the distal, lingual, and incisal surfaces of a tooth.

distolinguo-occlusal (dis″to-ling″gwo-ŏ-kloo′zal) pertaining to or formed by the distal, lingual, and occlusal surfaces of a tooth.

distolinguopulpal (dis″to-ling″gwo-pul′pal) pertaining to or formed by the distal, lingual, and pulpal walls of a tooth cavity.

Distoma (dis′to-mah) [*di-* + Gr. *stoma* mouth] former name of a genus of trematode worms; as now used, a general term including various genera of trematodes or flukes, such as *Paragonimus, Fasciola,* etc. **D. bus′ki,** *Fasciolopsis buski.* **D. conjunc′tum,** *Amphimerus noverca.* **D. feli′neum,** *Opisthorchis felineus.* **D. haemato′bium,** *Schistosoma haematobium.* **D. hepat′icum,** *Fasciola hepatica.* **D. heteroph′yes,** *Heterophyes heterophyes.* **D. rin′geri,** *Paragonimus westermani.* **D. sinen′sis,** *Clonorchis sinensis.* **D. westerman′i,** *Paragonimus westermani.*

distomatosis (dis″to-mah-to′sis) distomiasis.

distomia (dis-to′me-ah) the presence of two mouths.

distomiasis (dis″to-mi′ah-sis) infection by trematodes or flukes. **hemic d.,** schistosomiasis. **hepatic d.,** infection by *Opisthorchis, Dicrocoelium, Fasciola hepatica,* or *Fasciola gigantica.* **intestinal d.,** infection by *Fasciolopsis* or other intestinal flukes. **pulmonary d.,** parasitic hemoptysis.

distomolar (dis″to-mo′lar) a supernumerary molar; any tooth found distal to a third molar.

Distomum (dis′to-mum) distoma.

distomus (di-sto′mus) [*di-* + Gr. *stoma* mouth] a fetus having a double mouth.

disto-occlusal (dis″to-ŏ-kloo′zal) pertaining to or formed by the distal and occlusal surfaces of a tooth, or the distal and occlusal walls of a tooth cavity.

disto-occlusion (dis″to-ŏ-kloo′zhun) distoclusion.

distoplacement (dis-to-plās′ment) displacement of a tooth distally.

distopulpal (dis″to-pul′pal) pertaining to or formed by the distal and pulpal walls of a tooth cavity.

distopulpolabial (dis″to-pul″po-la′be-al) pertaining to or formed by the distal, pulpal, and labial walls of a tooth cavity.

distopulpolingual (dis″to-pul″po-ling′gwal) pertaining to or formed by the distal, pulpal, and lingual walls of a tooth cavity.

distortion (dis-tor′shun) [L. *dis-* apart + *torsio* a twisting] the state of being twisted out of a natural or normal shape or position. In psychiatry, a mechanism through which material offensive to the superego is replaced by disguised transformations of the original material. In radiology, deviation of a radiographic image from the true outline or shape of an object or structure. **parataxic d.,** distortions in judgment and perception, particularly in interpersonal relations, based upon the need to perceive objects and relationships in accord with a pattern from earlier experience.

distortor (dis-tor′tor) [L.] that which distorts. **d. o′ris,** musculus zygomaticus minor; see *Table of Musculi.*

distoversion (dis″to-ver′zhun) the position of a tooth which is farther than normal from the median line of the face along the dental arch.

distractibility (dis″trak-tĭ-bil′ĭ-te) a morbid or abnormal variation of attention; inability to fix attention on any subject.

distraction (dĭ-strak′shun) [L. *dis-* apart + *tractio* a drawing] 1. a state in which the attention is diverted from the main portion of an experience or is divided among various portions of it. 2. a form of dislocation in which the joint surfaces have been separated without rupture of their binding ligaments and without displacement. 3. excessive space between fracture fragments due to interposed tissue or too forceful traction. 4. surgical separation of the two parts of a bone after the bone is transected. 5. in orthodontics, unusual width of the dontal arch.

distress (dĭ-stres′) [L. *distringere* to draw apart] physical or mental anguish or suffering. **idiopathic respiratory d. of newborn,** see *respiratory distress syndrome of newborn,* under *syndrome.*

distribution (dis″trĭ-bu′shun) [L. *distributio*] 1. the specific location or arrangement of continuing or successive objects or events in space or time. 2. the branching, as of an artery, to supply various tissues. 3. the geographical range of an organism or disease. 4. in statistics, a set of numbers representing instances of a variable arranged according to their value. **Bernouilli d.,** a mathematical formula for calculating the theoretical distribution of male and female children to be born to any given set of parents. **dose d.,** in radiology, a representation of the variation of dose with position in any region of an irradiated object.

districhiasis (dis″trĭ-ki′ah-sis) [Gr. *dis* double + Gr. *thrix* hair + *-iasis*] a condition in which two hairs grow from a single follicle.

distrix (dis′triks) [Gr. *dis* double + Gr. *thrix* hair] the splitting of hairs at their distal ends.

disturbance (dis-tur′bans) a departure or divergence from that which is considered normal. **emotional d.,** mental disorder. **sexual orientation d.,** a condition in which the affected individual's sexual interests are primarily directed towards persons of the same sex and the individual is either disturbed by, in conflict with, or wishes to change his or her sexual orientation; it is to be distinguished from homosexuality and lesbianism. **transient situational d.,** a transient mental disorder, occurring as a reaction to overwhelming environmental stress. If symptoms persist after the stress is relieved, the diagnosis of another mental disorder is indicated.

disubstituted (di-sub′stĭ-tūt-ed) having two atoms in each molecule replaced by other atoms or radicals.

disulfate (di-sul′fāt) a compound containing two sulfate ions or radicals, as in titanium disulfate, $Ti(SO_4)_2$ (not to be confused with bisulfate).

disulfide (di-sul′fīd) a compound of a base with two atoms of sulfur; see also under *bond.*

disulfiram (di-sul′fi-ram) [USP] chemical name: tetraethylthioperoxydicarbonic diamide $[(H_2N)C(S)]_2S_2$. An antioxidant, $C_{10}H_{20}N_2S_4$, occurring as a white to off-white, crystalline powder, which inhibits the oxidation of the acetaldehyde metabolized from alcohol, resulting in high concentrations of acetaldehyde in the body. Extremely uncomfortable symptoms occur when alcohol is ingested subsequent to the oral administration of disulfiram (see *mal rouge*); used to produce an aversion to alcohol in the treatment of chronic alcoholism. Called also *tetraethylthiuram disulfide.*

dithiazanine iodide (di″thi-az′ah-nēn) chemical name: 3-ethyl-2-[5-(3-ethyl-2-(3H)-benzothiazolinylidene)-1,3-pentadienyl]-benzothiazolium iodide. A dark green crystalline powder, $C_{23}H_{23}$-IN_2S_2, used as an anthelminthic against strongylids and whipworms.

dithio (di-thi′o) the chemical group —S_2—.

dithiol (di-thi′ol) a chemical compound containing two sulfhydryl (thiol) radicals.

dithranol (dith′rah-nōl) anthralin.

dithymol diiodide (di-thi″mol di-i′o-dīd) thymol iodide.

Ditropan (di′tro-pan) trademark for a preparation of oxybutynin hydrochloride.

Ditropenotus aureoviridis (di″tro-pĕ-no′tus aw″re-o-vir′ĭ-dis) former name for *Pyemotes ventricosus.*

Dittel's operation (dit′elz) [Leopold Ritter von *Dittel*, Vienna urologist, 1815–1898] see under *operation.*

Dittrich's plugs (dit′riks) [Franz *Dittrich*, German pathologist, 1815–1859] see under *plug.*

Ditylenchus (dit-ĕ-len′kus) a genus of small nematodes. **D. dip′saci,** the stem and bulb eelworm, a parasite of various grains, grasses, and bulbs, such as lilies, hyacinths, gladioli, narcissi, and onions; when ingested with the latter, it may be found as a pseudoparasite in the feces. Called also *Anguillulina putrifaciens.*

diurea (di-u-re′ah) a crystalline substance, $C_2H_4N_4O_2$, 1,2,4,5-tetrazine-3,6-dione, derivable from two molecules of urea, slightly soluble in ethanol or water. Called also *p-urazine* or *urazin.*

diureide (di-u′re-id) see *ureide.*

diurese (di″u-rēs′) the act of effecting diuresis.

diureses (di″u-re′sēz) plural of *diuresis.*

diuresis (di″u-re′sis) pl. *diure′ses* [Gr. *diourein* to urinate, to pass in urine] increased excretion of urine. **tubular d.,** diuresis resulting from the presence of nonabsorbable or poorly absorbable, osmotically active substances (mannitol, urea, glucose, etc.) in the renal tubules.

diuretic (di″u-ret′ik) [Gr. *diourētikos* promoting urine] 1. increasing the excretion of urine. 2. an agent that promotes the excretion of urine. **cardiac d.,** a drug that causes diuresis by increasing the force of the heart beat. **hemopiesic d.,** one that acts by raising the blood pressure. **hydragogue d.,** one that promotes a copious discharge of water from the kidneys. **loop d.,** any diuretic (e.g., furosemide and ethacrynic acid) that appears to exert its action on the sodium reabsorption mechanism of the ascending limb of the loop of Henle, resulting in excretion of urine isotonic with plasma. **mechanical d.,** any agent that acts favorably by washing out the urinary tubules. **osmotic d.,** a low-molecular-weight substance, e.g., mannitol, capable of remaining in high concentrations in the renal tubules and thereby contributing to the osmolality of the glomerular filtrate. **thiazide d.,** any of a group of synthetic compounds that effect diuresis by enhancing the excretion of sodium and chloride.

diuria (di-u′re-ah) [L. *dies* day + *urine*] frequency of urination during the day.

Diuril (di′u-ril) trademark for preparations of chlorothiazide.

diurnal (di-er′nal) [L. *dies* day] occurring during the day.

diurnule (di-ern′ūl) [L. *diurnus* daily] a pill or other preparation containing the complete allowance of a medicine for one day.

Div. abbreviation for L. *div′ide,* divide.

divagation (di″vah-ga′shun) incoherent speech.

divalent (di-va-lent) [Gr. *dis* twice + *valent*] 1. bivalent. 2. carrying an electronic charge of two units.

divarication (di-var″ĭ-ka′shun) separation; divergence; diastasis.

divergence (di-ver′jens) a spreading or tending apart; in ophthalmology, the simultaneous abduction of both eyes. **negative vertical d.** (–V.D.), the condition in which the visual line of the left eye deviates upward or the visual line of the right eye deviates downward. **positive vertical d.** (+V.D.), the condition in which the visual line of the right eye deviates upward, or the visual line of the left eye deviates downward.

divergent (di-ver′jent) [L. *divergens; dis-* apart + *vergere* to tend] tending apart; deviating or radiating away from a common point.

diversine (di-ver′sin) an amorphous sinomenine alkaloid, C_{20}-$H_{27}O_5N$.

diversion (di-ver′zhun) a turning aside. **antigenic d.,** the change in the antigenic structure of tumor cells or tissue to that normally found in different cells or tissue.

diverticula (di″ver-tik′u-lah) [L.] plural of *diverticulum.*

diverticular (di″ver-tik′u-lar) pertaining to or resembling a diverticulum.

diverticularization (di″ver-tik″u-lar-i-za′shun) the act of forming diverticula, pockets, etc.

diverticulectomy (di″ver-tik″u-lek′to-me) [*diverticulum* + Gr. *ektomē* excision] excision of a diverticulum.

diverticuleve (di″ver-tik′u-lēv) an instrument for lifting up a bladder diverticulum so that the subjacent bladder wall may be separated.

diverticulitis (di″ver-tik-u-li′tis) inflammation of a diverticulum, especially inflammation related to colonic diverticula which may undergo perforation with abscess formation. Sometimes called *left-sided* or *L-sided appendicitis.*

diverticulogram (di″ver-tik′u-lo-gram) [*diverticulum* + Gr. *gramma* mark] a roentgenogram of a diverticulum.

diverticulopexy (di″ver-tik″u-lo-pek′se) surgical fixation of a diverticulum in a new position following its separation from the initial adjacent or adherent structures.

diverticulosis (di″ver-tik″u-lo′sis) the presence of diverticula, particularly of colonic diverticula, in the absence of inflamation. Cf. *diverticulitis.*

diverticulum (di″ver-tik′u-lum), pl. *divertic′ula* [L. *divertere* to turn aside] a circumscribed pouch or sac of variable size occurring normally or created by herniation of the lining mucous membrane through a defect in the muscular coat of a tubular organ. **acquired d.,** any diverticulum produced secondarily, mechanically or by disease. **allantoic d.,** the entodermal sacculation that becomes the allantois; called also *allantoic vesicle.* **divertic′ula ampul′lae duc′tus deferen′tis** [NA], sacculations in the wall of the ampulla of the ductus deferens. **caliceal d., calyceal d.,** an epithelial-lined cavity in the kidney, situated peripherally to a calix and connected to it by a narrow isthmus, the lining of the cavity being continuous with that of the calix. **cervical d.,** one derived from an embryonic branchial groove or pouch. **diverticula of colon, colonic diverticula,** acquired herniations of the mucosa of the colon through the muscular layers of the bowel wall, which may become inflamed (see *diverticulitis*). **false d.,** an intestinal diverticulum due to the protrusion of the mucous membrane through a tear in the muscular coat. **functional d.,** a benign, radiological entity, in which a diverticulum-like shadow is demonstrated by contrast medium, although subsequent laparotomy shows no sign of any corresponding anomaly. **ganglion d.,** a hernial protrusion of the synovial membrane through a tendon sheath. **Ganser's d.,** multiple pulsion diverticula of the sigmoid flexure. **Graser's d.,** false diverticulum of the sigmoid flexure. **Heister's d.,** bulbus venae jugularis superior. **hepatic d.,** one arising from the embryonic duodenum and forming the liver, gallbladder, and bile ducts. **d. il′ei ve′rum,** Meckel's d. **intestinal d.,** a pouch or sac formed by hernial protrusion of the mucous membrane through a defect in the muscular coat of the intestine. **Kirchner's d.,** a diverticulum of the eustachian tube. **laryngeal d.,** a diverticulum of the laryngeal mucous membrane. **Meckel's d.,** an occasional sacculation or appendage of the ileum, derived from an unobliterated yolk stalk; called also *d. ilei verum.* **Nuck's d.,** processus vaginalis peritonei. **pancreatic diverticula,** two outpocketings from the embryonic duodenum, later forming the pancreas and its ducts. **Pertik's d.,** an unusually deep recessus pharyngeus. **pharyngoesophageal d.,** a diverticulum at the junction of the pharynx and esophagus; called also *Zenker's d.* **pituitary d.,** Rathke's pouch. **pressure d., pulsion d.,** a sac or pouch formed by hernial protrusion of the mucous membrane through the muscular coat (as of the colon or esophagus) as a result of pressure from within. **Rokitansky's d.,** a traction diverticulum of the esophagus. **supradiaphragmatic d.,** a diverticulum of the esophagus situated just above the diaphragm. **synovial d.,** a hernial protrusion of the synovial membrane of a joint or a tendon sheath. **thyroid d.,** an outpouching of the ventral floor of the embryonic pharynx that becomes the thyroid gland. **diverticula of trachea, tracheal diverticula,** pouches projecting from the trachea. **traction d.,** a localized distortion, angulation, or funnel-shaped bulging of the full thickness of the wall of the esophagus, caused by adhesions resulting from some external lesion. **vesical d.,** diverticulum of the bladder. **Zenker's d.,** pharyngoesophageal d.

divi-divi (div″e-div′e) the leguminous pods of *Caesalpinia coriaria* (Jacq.) Willd., plants of South America; the seeds contain tannin and gallic acid and have been used as an astringent and in tanning.

divinyl (di-vi′nil) a gaseous hydrocarbon, vinyl ethylene, $CH_2{:}CH{\cdot}CH{:}CH_2$. **d. oxide,** vinyl ether.

division (dĭ-vizh′un) [L. *divisio*] the act of separating into two or more parts. **cell d.,** the fission of a cell. **cell d., direct,** see *amitosis.* **cell d., indirect,** see *meiosis* and *mitosis.* **craniosacral d.,** see *pars parasympathica systematis nervosi autonomici.* **equational d.,** the second meiotic division, essentially mitotic in type, characterized by the separation of sister chromatids. The latter are genetically identical since they are longitudinally-split reduplications of individual chromosomes. **maturation d.,** meiosis. **reduction d.,** the first meiotic division, so called because at this stage the chromosome number per cell is reduced from diploid to haploid. **thoracicolumbar d., thoracolumbar d.,** see *pars sympathica systematis nervosi autonomici.*

divulse (dĭ-vuls′) to pull apart forcibly.

divulsion (dĭ-vul′shun) [L. *dis-* apart + *vellere* to pluck]   the act of separating or pulling apart.

divulsor (dĭ-vul′sor)   an instrument for dilating the urethra.

Dixon Mann   see *Mann.*

dizygotic (di″zi-got′ik)   pertaining to or derived from two separate zygotes, as dizygotic (fraternal) twins.

dizygous (di-zi′gus)   dizygotic.

dizziness (diz′ĭ-nes)   a disturbed sense of relationship to space; a sensation of unsteadiness with a feeling of movement within the head; giddiness; lightheadedness; dysequilibrium. Cf. *vertigo.*

DL- (de-el)   chemical prefix (small capitals) denoting that the substance is an equimolecular mixture of two enantiomorphs, one of which corresponds in configuration to D-glyceraldehyde, the other to L-glyceraldehyde.

dl- (de-el)   chemical prefix formerly used to denote that the substance is an equimolecular mixture of the dextrorotatory and levorotatory enantiomorphs, such as is produced by chemical synthesis without resolution or by the process of racemization. The sign $\pm$ is currently used.

DLE   discoid lupus erythematosus.

DM   diastolic murmur.

D.M.   see *diphenylamine-arsine chloride.*

D.M.D.   Doctor of Dental Medicine.

dmelcos (dmel′kos)   a culture of Ducrey's bacillus (*Hemophilus ducreyi*) grown on gelose and sterilized; formerly used as a test for chancroid, and injected into patients with paresis to induce high temperature.

DMF   an expression of the accumulated dental caries experience in permanent teeth, *D* representing the number of carious teeth; *M* the number of missing teeth; and *F* the number of filled teeth.

DMPE   3,4-dimethoxyphenylethylamine.

D.M.R.D.   Diploma in Medical Radio-Diagnosis (British).

D.M.R.T.   Diploma in Medical Radio-Therapy (British).

DMSO   dimethyl sulfoxide.

DMT   dimethyltryptamine.

DN   dibucaine number.

Dn.   dekanem.

dn.   decinem.

DNA   deoxyribonucleic acid (see under *acid*).   **recombinant DNA,** DNA that has been artificially introduced into a cell so that it alters the genotype and phenotype of the cell and is replicated along with the natural DNA.

DNase   deoxyribonuclease.

D.N.B.   dinitrobenzene; Diplomate of the National Board (of Medical Examiners).

DNCB   dinitrochlorobenzene.

D.O.   Doctor of Osteopathy; diamine oxidase.

D₂O   the symbol for heavy water.

D.O.A.   dead on arrival.

Dobell's solution (do-belz′) [Horace Benge *Dobell,* English physician, 1828–1917]   sodium borate solution; see under *solution.*

Dobie's globule, layer (line) (do′bēz) [William Murray *Dobie,* English physician, 1828–1915]   see under *globule,* and see *Z band,* under *band.*

dobutamine (do-bu′tah-mēn)   chemical name: (+)-[2-[[3-(4-hydroxyphenyl)-1-methylpropyl]amino]ethyl]-1,2-benzenediol. A synthetic catecholamine, $C_{18}H_{23}NO_3$, used as an adrenergic with cardiotonic actions.   **d. hydrochloride,** the hydrochloride salt of dobutamine, $C_{18}H_{23}NO_3 \cdot HCl$, having the same actions as the base.

Doca (do′kah)   trademark for desoxycorticosterone acetate.

Dochmius duodenalis (dok′me-us du″o-dĕ-na′lis)   former name for *Ancylostoma duodenale.*

Docibin (do′si-bin)   trademark for a crystalline preparation of vitamin B_{12}; see *cyanocobalamin.*

docimasia (do″se-ma′ze-ah) [Gr. *dokimazein* to examine]   an assay or examination; an official test.   **auricular d.,** Wreden's sign.   **hepatic d.,** the search for glycogen or glucose in the liver.   **pulmonary d.,** determination as to whether air has entered the lungs of a dead infant, as an indication whether it was born dead or alive.

docimastic (do″se-mas′tik)   pertaining to docimasia; of the nature of an assay or test.

dock (dok)   to remove part or all of the tail of an animal.

doconazole (do-ko′nah-zōl)   chemical name: *cis*-1-[[4-[(1,1′-biphenyl]-4-yloxy)methyl]-2-(2,4-dichlorophenyl)-1,3-dioxolan-2-yl]methyl]1*H*-imidazole; an antifungal, $C_{26}H_{22}Cl_2N_2O_3$.

doctor (dok′tor) [L. "teacher"]   1. a practitioner of the healing arts, one who has received a degree from a college of medicine, osteopathy, dentistry, or veterinary medicine, licensed to practice by a state.   2. a holder of a diploma of the highest degree from a university, qualified as a specialist in a particular field of learning.

doctrine (dok′trin)   a theory supported by authorities and hav-

ing general acceptance.   **Arrhenius' d.,** see under *theory.* **Flourens' d.,** see under *theory.*   **Monro-Kellie d.,** the quantity of blood within the cranium must be approximately constant at all times, in health or disease; the doctrine refers to quantity of blood not to blood flow.   **neuron d.,** the doctrine that the nervous system is entirely cellular, that its cells are distinctive as to morphological type and functional characteristics, and that its cells are not in protoplasmic continuity but are juxtaposed without a significant amount of intervening extracellular substance.

docusate calcium (dok′u-sāt) [USP]   chemical name: sulfobutanedioic acid 1,4-bis(2-ethylhexyl) ester calcium salt. An ionic surfactant, $C_{40}H_{74}CaO_{14}S_2$, occurring as a white, amorphous powder; used as a fecal softener, administered orally. Called also *dioctyl calcium sulfosuccinate.*

docusate sodium (dok′u-sāt) [USP]   chemical name: sulfobutanedioic acid 1,4-bis(2-ethylhexyl)ester sodium salt. An anionic surfactant, $C_{20}H_{37}NaO_7S$, with wetting, detergent, emulsifying, and dispersing properties, occurring as a white, waxlike plastic solid; used as a fecal softener, administered orally or rectally, and for its solubilizing action as a tablet disintegrant. It has also been used for its dispersing and emulsifying properties in dermatological preparations. Called also *dioctyl sodium sulfosuccinate.*

dodecadactylitis (do″dek-ah-dak″tĭ-li′tis) [*dōdecadactylon* + *-itis*]   duodenitis.

dodecadactylon (do″dek-ah-dak′tĭ-lon) [Gr. *dōdeka* twelve + *daktylos* finger, from its length]   the duodenum.

Döderlein's bacillus (ded′er-līnz) [Albert Siegmund Gustav *Döderlein,* German obstetrician and gynecologist, 1860–1941]   see under *bacillus.*

Dogiel's corpuscles (do-zhe-elz′) [Jean von *Dogiel,* Russian physiologist, 1830–1916]   see under *corpuscle.*

dögling (deg′ling) [Danish and German]   the northern bottlenosed whale (*Hyperoodon ampullatus*).

Dogmatist (dog′mah-tist)   1. the first of the post-hippocratic schools of medicine, in which the open-minded spirit of Hippocrates' teaching became merged with a strict formalism which cared more for rigid doctrine than for investigation. The most important members of this school—Diocles of Carystus and Praxagoras of Cos—were, however, far more enlightened than the label "Dogmatist" would seem to imply.   2. a believer in or practitioner of the Dogmatist theory of medicine.

Döhle's disease, inclusion bodies (de′lēz) [Paul *Döhle,* German pathologist, 1855–1928]   see *syphilitic aortitis,* under *aortitis,* and see under *body.*

Döhle-Heller aortitis (de′lĕ-hel′er) [K.G.P. *Döhle;* Arnold Ludwig Gotthilf *Heller,* Kiel pathologist, 1840–1913]   syphilitic aortitis.

doigt (dwa) [Fr.]   finger or toe.   **d. mort** [Fr.], dead finger.

Doisy (doi′se), Edward Adelbert.   An American biochemist, born 1893; co-winner, with Carl Peter Henrik Dam, of the Nobel prize for medicine and physiology in 1945, for the isolation and synthesis of vitamin K.

dol (dōl) [L. *do′lor* pain]   a unit of pain intensity.

dolabrate (do-lab′rāt) [L. *dolabra* ax]   ax-shaped.

dolabriform (do-lab′rĭ-form)   dolabrate.

Dold's test (reaction) (dolts) [Hermann *Dold,* German bacteriologist, born 1882]   see under *test.*

Doléris' operation (dol-a-rēz′) [Jacques Amédée *Doléris,* French gynecologist, 1852–1938]   see under *operation.*

dolicho- (dol′ĭ-ko) [Gr. *dolichos* long]   a combining form meaning long.

dolichocephalia (dol″ĭ-ko-sĕ-fa′le-ah)   dolichocephaly.

dolichocephalic, dolichocephalous (dol″ĭ-ko-se-fal′ik; dol″ĭ-ko-sef′ah-lus) [*dolicho-* + Gr. *kephalē* head]   long headed; having a cephalic index of 75.9 or less. Called also *mecocephalic.*

dolichocephalism (dol″ĭ-ko-sef′ah-lizm)   dolichocephaly.

dolichocephaly (dol″ĭ-ko-sef′ah-le)   the quality of being dolichocephalic.

dolichocolon (dol″ĭ-ko-ko′lon) [*dolicho-* + *colon*]   an abnormally long colon.

dolichocranial (dol″ĭ-ko-kra′ne-al)   having a cranial index of 74.9 or less.

dolichoderus (dol″ĭ-ko-dēr′us) [*dolicho-* + Gr. *dere* neck]   an individual with a long neck.

dolichofacial (dol″ĭ-ko-fa′shal)   having a long face.

dolichogastry (dol″ĭ-ko-gas′tre) [*dolicho-* + Gr. *gastēr* stomach] (*obs.*)   a term once proposed to replace gastroptosis, because the condition is one of stretching of the center of the stomach.

dolichohieric (dol″ĭ-ko-hi-er′ik)   having a sacral index below 100.

dolichokerkic (dol″ĭ-ko-ker′kik)   having a radiohumeral index above 80.

dolichoknemic (dol″ĭ-ko-ne′mik)   having a tibiofemoral index of 83 or above.

dolichomorphic (dol″ĭ-ko-mor′fik) [*dolicho-* + Gr. *morphē* form] built along lines that tend toward the slender or longer type.

dolichopellic, dolichopelvic (dol″ĭ-ko-pel′ik; dol″ĭ-ko-pel′vik) [*dolicho-* + Gr. *pella* bowl] having a pelvic index of 95 or above.

dolichoprosopic (dol″ĭ-ko-pro-sop′ik) dolichofacial.

dolichosigmoid (dol″ĭ-ko-sig′moid) [*dolicho-* + *sigmoid*] (*obs.*) an abnormally long sigmoid flexure.

dolichostenomelia (dol″ĭ-ko-ste″no-me′le-ah) [*dolicho-* + Gr. *stenos* narrow + *melos* limb] arachnodactyly.

dolichuranic (dol″ĭk-u-ran′ik) [*dolicho-* + Gr. *ouranos* palate] having a maxilloalveolar index of 109.9 or less.

Döllinger's ring (del′ing-erz) [Johann Ignaz Josef *Döllinger*, German physiologist, 1770–1841] Schwalbe's ring.

Dolophine (do′lo-fēn) trademark for preparations of methadone hydrochloride.

dolor (do′lor), pl. *dolo′res* [L.] pain; one of the cardinal signs of inflammation. **d. cap′itis,** headache. **d. cox′ae,** coxalgia, def. 2. **dolo′res praesagien′tes,** false pains late in pregnancy, similar to those experienced during menstruation, indicating that labor is imminent. **d. va′gus,** wandering pain.

dolores (do-lo′rēz) plural of *dolor.*

dolorific (do″lor-if′ik) producing or causing pain.

dolorimeter (do″lor-im′ĕ-ter) an instrument for measuring pain in dols.

dolorimetry (do″lor-im′ĕ-tre) [L. *dolor* pain + Gr. *metrein* to measure] the measurement of pain.

dolorogenic (do-lor″o-jen′ik) dolorific.

DOM 2,5-dimethoxy-4-methylamphetamine.

Domagk (do′mak), Gerhard. A German physician and biochemist, 1895–1964; winner of the Nobel prize for medicine in 1939, for his work on the chemotherapy of infectious diseases.

domain (do′mān) in immunology, any of the homology regions of heavy or light polypeptide chains of immunoglobulins.

domaria (do-mar′ĭ-ah) yaws.

domazoline fumarate (do″mah-zo′lēn) chemical name: 2-[3,6-dimethoxy-2,4-dimethylphenyl)methyl]-4,5-dihydro-1*H*-imidazole (*E*)-2-butenedioate (1:1); an anticholinergic, $C_{14}H_{20}N_2O_2 \cdot C_4H_4O_4$.

Domeboro (dōm′bor-o) trademark for preparations of aluminum subacetate.

domiciliary (dom″ĭ-sil′e-ār″e) [L. *domus* house] pertaining to or carried on in the house or place of permanent residence, as domiciliary treatment.

dominance (dom′ĭ-nans) 1. the supremacy, or superior manifestation, in a specific situation of one of two or more competitive or mutually antagonistic factors. 2. the appearance, in a heterozygote, of one of two alternative parental characters; see *Mendel's law*, under *law*. **cerebral d.,** the dominance of one cerebral hemisphere over the other, in cerebral functions, demonstrated by laterality in voluntary motor acts. **incomplete d.,** failure of one gene to be competely dominant, the heterozygotes showing a phenotype intermediate between the two parents; called also *partial d.* and *semidominance.* **lateral d.,** the preferential use, in voluntary motor acts, of ipsilateral members of the major paired organs of the body (arm, ear, eye, and leg). **ocular d.,** the preferential use of one eye over the other, in vision. **one-sided d.,** lateral d. **partial d.,** incomplete d.

dominant (dom′ĭ-nant) 1. exerting a ruling or controlling influence; in genetics, capable of expression when carried by only one of a pair of homologous chromosomes. 2. a dominant allele or trait.

domiphen bromide (do′mĭ-fen) chemical name: *N,N*-dimethyl-*N*-(2-phenoxyethyl)-1-dodecanaminium bromide. A quaternary ammonium compound, $C_{22}H_{40}BrNO$, occurring as colorless to faintly yellow, crystalline flakes, effective against a wide range of gram-negative and gram-positive bacteria and against certain fungi; used as a topical anti-infective and to disinfect instruments and utensils.

domperidone (dom-per′ĭ-dōn) chemical name: 5-chloro-1-[1-[3-(2,3-dihydro-2-oxo-1*H*-benzimidazol-1-yl)propyl]-4-piperidinyl]-1,3-dihydro-2*H*-benzimidazol-2-one; an antiemetic, $C_{22}H_{24}ClN_5O_2$.

Donath's phenomenon (test) (do′naths) [Julius *Donath*, German immunologist, 1870–1950] see under *phenomenon.*

Donath-Landsteiner test (do′nath-land′sti-ner) [Julius *Donath*; Karl *Landsteiner*, Austrian physician in New York, 1868–1943] see under *test.*

donaxine (do-nak′sēn) gramine.

Donders' glaucoma, law (don′derz) [Franciscus Cornelius *Donders*, Dutch physician and ophthalmologist, 1818–1889] see *glaucoma simplex*, and see under *law.*

Donec alv. sol. fuerit abbreviation for L. *do′nec al′vus solu′ta fu′erit*, until the bowels are opened (i.e., until a bowel movement occurs).

donee (do-ne′) recipient; host (def. 2).

Don Juan (don-joo′an, or don-hwan) a man who is sexually promiscuous.

Don Juanism (don-hwan′izm) sexual promiscuousness in the male.

Donnan's equilibrium (don′anz) [Frederick George *Donnan*, English chemist, 1870–1956] see under *equilibrium.*

Donné's corpuscles (bodies), test (don-āz′) [Alfred *Donné*, French physician, 1801–1878] see *colostrum corpuscle*, under *corpuscle*, and see under *tests.*

donor (do′nor) 1. an individual organism that supplies living tissue to be used in another body, as a person who furnishes blood for transfusion, or an organ for transplantation in a histocompatible recipient. 2. in chemistry, a substance or compound which contributes part of itself, as an atom or radical, to another substance (acceptor). **general d.,** universal d. **hydrogen d.,** a substance or compound that gives up hydrogen to another substance (the hydrogen acceptor). **universal d.,** a person with group O blood (International Classification); such blood (blood cells preferred, rather than whole blood) is sometimes used in emergency transfusion.

Donovan bodies (don′o-van) [Charles *Donovan*, Irish physician, formerly in Sanitary Service in India, 1863–1951] 1. *Calymmatobacterium granulomatis.* 2. Leishman-Donovan bodies.

Donovania (don-o-va′ne-ah) [Charles *Donovan*] a genus of schizomycetes, included in the order Eubacteriales, suborder Eubacteriineae, family Parvobacteriaceae, tribe Pasteurelleae. **D. granulo′matis,** a gram-negative, pleomorphic, rod-shaped microorganism that is not cultivable on non-viable media but grows in the yolk, yolk sac, and amniotic fluid of the chick embryo. It is serologically related to *Klebsiella pneumoniae* and coliform bacilli, and is grouped with *Pasteurella, Malleomyces,* and *Actinobacillus* by some workers. It is the causative agent of granuloma inguinale in man. Called also *Calymmatobacterium granulomatis* and *Donovan body.*

donovanosis (don″o-vah-no′sis) granuloma inguinale.

dopa (do′pah) an amino acid, 3,4-dihydroxyphenylalanine, produced by oxidation of tyrosine by tyrosinase; it is the precursor of dopamine and an intermediate product in the biosynthesis of norepinephrine, epinephrine, and melanin. L-dopa (*levodopa* [USP]), the naturally occurring form, is used in the treatment of parkinsonism.

dopamantine (do″pah-man′tēn) chemical name: *N*-[2-(3,4-dihydroxyphenyl) ethyl] tricyclo [3,3,1,1³,⁷] decane-1-carboxamide; an antiparkinsonian agent, $C_{19}H_{25}NO_3$.

dopamine (do′pah-mēn) chemical name: 4-(2-aminoethyl)-1,2-benzenediol. A monoamine, $C_8H_{11}NO_2$, formed in the body by the decarboxylation of dopa; it is an intermediate product in the synthesis of norepinephrine, and acts as a neurotransmitter in the central nervous system. **d. hydrochloride,** the hydrochloride salt of dopamine, $C_8H_{11}NO_2 \cdot HCl$, used to correct hemodynamic balance in the treatment of shock syndrome; administered intravenously.

dopaminergic (do″pah-mēn-er′jik) activated or transmitted by dopamine; pertaining to tissues or organs affected by dopamine.

dopa-oxidase (do″pah-ok′sĭ-dās) an enzyme that oxidizes dihydroxyphenylalanine (dopa) to melanin in the skin, producing pigmentation; called also *dopase.*

Dopar (do′par) trademark for a preparation of levodopa.

dopase (do′pās) dopa-oxidase.

Doppler effect (phenomenon, principle) (dop′lerz) [Christian Johann *Doppler*, Austrian physicist and mathematician, 1803–1853] see under *effect.*

Doppler's operation (dop′lerz) [Karl *Doppler*, Vienna surgeon] see under *operation.*

Dopram (do′pram) trademark for a preparation of doxapram hydrochloride.

Dopter's serum (dop-terz′) [Charles Henri Alfred *Dopter*, French bacteriologist, 1875–1950] see under *serum.*

dorastine hydrochloride (dor′as-tēn) chemical name: 8-chloro-2,3,4,5-tetrahydro-2-methyl-5-[2-(6-methyl-3-pyridyl)-ethyl]-1*H*-pyrido[4,3-*b*]indole dihydrochloride; an antihistaminic, $C_{20}H_{22}ClN_3 \cdot 2HCl$.

Dorbane (dor′bān) trademark for a preparation of danthron.

Dorendorf's sign (dor′en-dorfs) [Hans *Dorendorf*, German physician, born 1866] see under *sign.*

Doriden (dor′ĭ-den) trademark for preparations of glutethimide.

dormancy (dor′man-se) the state of being dormant; in bacteriology, the property exhibited by some bacteria of lying dormant for a time before starting growth.

dormant (dor′mant) [L. *dormire* to sleep] sleeping, inactive, quiescent.

dormifacient (dor″mĭ-fa′shent) [L. *dormire* to sleep + *facere* to make] producing sleep; counteracting the conditions which tend to prevent sleep.

dornase (dor′nās) a shortened term for *deoxyribonuclease;* used also as a word termination, as in *streptodornase.* **pan-**

creatic d., a stabilized preparation of deoxyribonuclease, prepared from beef pancreas: used as an aerosol to reduce tenacity of pulmonary secretions.

Dornavac (dor′nah-vak)   trademark for a preparation of pancreatic dornase.

Dorno's rays (dor′no) [Carl Wilhelm *Dorno,* Swiss climatologist, 1865–1942]   see under *ray.*

Dorn-Sugarman test [John H. *Dorn,* American obstetrician; Edward J. *Sugarman,* American chemist]   see under *tests.*

dorsa (dor′sah) [L.]   plural of *dorsum.*

Dorsacaine (dor′sah-kān)   trademark for a preparation of benoxinate hydrochloride.

dorsad (dor′sad)   toward the back or dorsal aspect.

dorsal (dor′sal) [L. *dorsalis;* from *dorsum* back]   1. pertaining to the back or to any dorsum.   2. denoting a position more toward the back surface than some other object of reference; same as posterior in human anatomy.

dorsalgia (dor-sal′je-ah) [*dorsum* + *-algia*]   pain in the back.

dorsalis (dor-sa′lis) [L.]   dorsal; [NA] a term denoting a position closer to the back surface. Cf. *posterior.*

dorsi- (dor′si)   see *dorso-.*

dorsiduct (dor′si-dukt) [*dorsi* + L. *ducere* to draw]   to draw toward the back or dorsum.

dorsiflexion (dor″si-flek′shun) [*dorsi-* + *flexion*]   backward flexion or bending, as of the hand or foot.

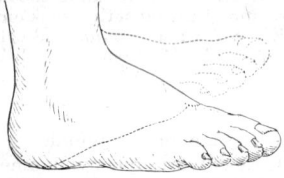

Dorsiflexion of foot (Hauser).

dorsimesal (dor″si-mes′al)   dorsomesial.

dorsispinal (dor″si-spi′nal)   pertaining to the back and vertebral column.

dorso-, dorsi- [L. *dorsum* back]   combining form denoting relationship to a dorsum or to the back (posterior) aspect of the body.

dorsoanterior (dor″so-an-te′re-or)   having the back of the fetus toward the front of the mother.

dorsocephalad (dor″so-sef′ah-lad) [*dorso-* + Gr. *kephalē* head]   directed toward the back of the head.

dorsodynia (dor″so-din′e-ah)   dorsalgia.

dorsointercostal (dor″so-in″ter-kos′tal)   situated in the back and between the ribs.

dorsolateral (dor″so-lat′er-al)   pertaining to the back and to the side.

dorsolumbar (dor″so-lum′bar)   pertaining to the back and the loins.

dorsomedian (dor″so-me′de-an)   the median line of the back.

dorsomesial (dor″so-me′se-al)   pertaining to the median line of the back.

dorsonasal (dor″so-na′sal)   pertaining to the bridge of the nose.

dorsonuchal (dor″so-nu′kal)   pertaining to the back of the neck.

dorsoposterior (dor″so-pos-te′re-or)   having the back of the fetus directed toward the mother's back.

dorsoradial (dor″so-ra′de-al)   pertaining to the radial or outer side of the back of the forearm or hand.

dorsoscapular (dor″so-skap′u-lar)   pertaining to the posterior surface of the scapula.

dorsoventrad (dor″so-ven′trad) [*dorso-* + *venter* belly]   directed from the dorsal toward the ventral aspect.

dorsoventral (dor″so-ven′tral)   1. pertaining to the back and belly surfaces of the body.   2. passing from the back to the belly surface.

dorsum (dor′sum), pl. *dor′sa* [L.] [NA]   1. the back.   2. the aspect of an anatomical part or structure corresponding in position to the back; posterior, in the human.   **d. of foot,** d. pedis.   **d. of hand,** d. manus.   **d. lin′guae** [NA], the superior surface of the tongue.   **d. ma′nus** [NA], the back of the hand; the surface opposite the palm.   **d. na′si** [NA], **d. of nose,** that part of the external surface of the nose formed by junction of the lateral surfaces.   **d. pe′dis** [NA], the upper surface of the foot; the surface opposite the sole.   **d. pe′nis** [NA], **d. of penis,** the anterior, more extensive surface of the dependent penis, opposite the urethral surface.   **d. of scapula,** facies dorsalis scapulae.   **d. sel′lae** [NA], the quadrilateral plate on the sphenoid bone that forms the posterior boundary of the sella turcica; the posterior clinoid processes project from its superior extremity, and it is continuous inferiorly with the clivus.   **d. of testis,** margo posterior testis.   **d. of tongue,** d. linguae.

dosage (do′sij)   the determination and regulation of the size, frequency, and number of doses.

dose (dōs) [Gr. *dosis* a giving]   a quantity to be administered at one time, such as a specified amount of medication, or a given quantity of roentgen ray or other radiation.   **absorbed d.,** the amount of energy from ionizing radiations absorbed per unit mass of matter, expressed in rads.   **air d.,** the intensity of a roentgen-ray (x-ray) or gamma-ray beam in air, expressed in roentgens. Sometimes called *exposure d.*   **average d.,** the quantity of an agent which will usually produce the therapeutic effect for which it is administered.   **booster d.,** an amount of immunogen (vaccine, toxoid, or other antigen preparation), usually smaller than the amount given originally, injected at an appropriate time interval after primary immunization to sustain the immune response to that immunogen (e.g., to maintain protection of the individual against infectious disease agents). See also *anamnestic reaction,* under *reaction.*   **cumulative d., cumulative radiation d.,** the total dose resulting from repeated exposures to radiation.   **curative d.,** a dose that is sufficient to restore normal health.   **curative d., median,** a dose that abolishes symptoms in 50 per cent of the test subjects. Abbreviated C.D.$_{50}$.   **daily d.,** the total amount of a drug administered in a 24-hour period.   **depth d.,** the intensity of radiation at a given depth in an irradiated body, expressed as a percentage of that at the surface of the body nearest the portal of entry.   **divided d.,** a fraction of the total quantity of the drug prescribed, to be given at intervals, usually during a twenty-four hour period.   **doubling d.,** in radiation biology, the dose of ionizing radiation which will result in a doubling of the current rate of spontaneous biological changes, such as mutations or cancers of various kinds, in a population.   **effective d.,** that quantity of a drug which will produce the effects for which it is administered; abbreviated E.D.   **effective d., median,** a dose that produces the desired effect in 50 per cent of a population. Abbreviation ED$_{50}$.   **emergency d.,** an immunizing injection given immediately after an injury.   **epilating d.,** the amount of radiation necessary to cause temporary or permanent loss of hair.   **erythema d.,** the amount of radiation which, when applied to the skin, causes temporary reddening of the skin.   **exit d.,** the intensity of radiation emerging from the body at the surface opposite the portal of entry.   **exposure d.,** air d.   **fatal d.,** lethal d.   **fractional d's,** amounts of an agent less than that usually administered, given at shorter intervals than usual.   **infective d.,** that amount of pathogenic microorganisms that will cause infection in suseptible subjects. Abbreviated I.D.   **infective d., median,** the amount of pathogenic microorganisms that will produce infection in 50 per cent of the test subjects. Abbreviated I.D.$_{50}$.   **integral d., integral absorbed d.,** in radiation biology, the total energy absorbed by an individual or other biological object during exposure to radiation, expressed in gram-rads (100 ergs).   **intoxicating d.,** the dose of sensitinogen required to bring on an allergic reaction.   **L + d.,** the smallest amount of diphtheria toxin which will kill a 250-gm. guinea pig within four days when mixed with one unit of diphtheria antitoxin before being injected subcutaneously.   **lethal d.,** the amount of an agent, such as radiation, which will or may be sufficient to cause death. Called also *fatal d.*   **lethal d., median,** the amount of pathogenic bacteria, bacterial toxin, or other poisonous substance, required to kill 50 per cent of uniformly susceptible animals inoculated with it. In radiology, the amount of ionizing radiation that will kill, within a specified period, 50 per cent of individuals in a large group or population. Abbreviated L.D.$_{50}$.   **lethal d., minimum,**   1. the amount of toxin which will just kill the experimental animal; abbreviated M.L.D.   2. the smallest quantity of diphtheria toxin which will kill a guinea pig of 250-gm. weight in four to five days when injected subcutaneously.   **Lf d.,** the amount of diphtheria toxin which in the shortest time produces precipitation when mixed with one standard unit of antitoxin.   **limes nul d., L$_0$ d.,** the amount of diphtheria toxin which is exactly neutralized by one standard unit of antitoxin.   **Lr d.,** the amount of diphtheria toxin which, when mixed with one standard unit of antitoxin, will produce a minimal skin reaction in a guinea pig.   **maintenance d.,** a dose (often a daily dose or dosage regimen) sufficient to maintain at the desired level the influence of a drug achieved by earlier administration of larger amounts.   **maximum d.,** the largest quantity of an agent that may be safely administered to the average patient.   **maximum permissible d.,** the largest amount of ionizing radiation that a person may receive according to recommended limits in current radiation protection guides; abbreviated M.P.D.   **median tissue culture infective d.,** that quantity of a cytopathogenic agent (virus) that will produce a cytopathic effect in 50 per cent of the cultures inoculated. Abbreviated TCID$_{50}$.   **minimal d., minimum d.,** the smallest quantity of an agent that is likely to produce an appreciable effect.   **optimal d., optimum d.,** the quantity of an agent which will produce the effect desired without unfavorable effects.   **organ tolerance d.,** in radiology, that amount of radiation which can be administered without appreciable damage to a normal organ; abbreviated OTD.   **permissible d.,** that amount of ionizing radiation that, in the light of current knowledge, is not expected to lead to appreciable bodily injury and is allowable according to current radiation protection guides; see also *maximum permissible d.* **priming d.,** a quantity several times larger than the maintenance dose, used at the initiation of therapy to rapidly establish the desired blood and tissue levels of the drug. **radiation absorbed d.,** see *absorbed d.* and *rad²*. **reacting d.,** the second dose of sensitizing antigen administered to an animal; it is followed by an immediate hypersensitive (e.g., anaphylactic or allergic) response. Cf. *sensitizing d.* **sensitizing d.,** the first dose of sensitizing antigen (e.g., protein) administered to an animal in the induction of a hypersensitivity (e.g., anaphylactic or allergic) response; cf. *reacting d.* **skin d.,** 1. the air dose of radiation at the skin surface, comprising primary radiation plus backscatter. 2. the absorbed dose in the skin. **therapeutic d.,** a quantity several times larger than the maintenance dose, used in vitamin therapy when a marked deficiency exists. **threshold d.,** the minimum dose of ionizing radiation that will produce a detectable degree of any given effect. **threshold erythema d.,** the single skin dose that will produce in 80 per cent of those tested, a faint but definite erythema within 30 days, and in the other 20 per cent, no visible reaction. Abbreviated T.E.D. **tissue d.,** the absorbed dose of radiation in a tissue or organ, expressed in rads. **tolerance d.,** the largest quantity of an agent, such as x-ray energy, that may be administered without harm. **toxic d.,** the amount of an agent which will cause toxic symptoms. **volume d.,** integral d.

dosimeter (do-sim′ĕ-ter) in radiology, an instrument used to detect and measure exposure to radiation, commonly a pencil-sized ionization chamber with a built-in electrometer used in monitoring exposure of personnel. Called also *dosage meter.*

dosimetric (do″se-met′rik) of or pertaining to dosimetry.

dosimetrist (do-sim-ĕ′trist) one who plans an optimum radiation treatment technical dosage pattern, or establishes a summation isodose pattern for the radiation treatment by means of isodose curves or other data supplied by a radiation physicist.

dosimetry (do-sim′ĕ-tre) [Gr. *dosis* dose + *metron* measure] the determination by scientific methods of the amount, rate, and distribution of radiation emitted from a source of ionizing radiation.

dosis (do′sis) [L., Gr. "a giving"] dose. **d. curati′va,** the minimum amount of a therapeutic agent that will effect a cure. **d. ef′ficax,** d. curativa. **d. refrac′ta,** fractional dose. **d. tolera′ta,** the largest amount of a therapeutic agent that can be given with safety.

dossier (dos′e-a) [Fr.] the accumulated records of a patient's case history.

dot (dot) a small spot or speck. **Gunn's d's,** white dots seen about the macula lutea on oblique illumination. **Maurer's d's,** irregular dots, staining red with Leishman's stain, seen in erythrocytes infected with *Plasmodium falciparum;* called also *Maurer's clefts.* **Mittendorf's d.,** a congenital anomaly manifested as a small gray or white opacity just inferior and nasal to the posterior pole of the lens, representing the remains of the lenticular attachment of the hyaloid artery; it does not affect vision. **Schüffner's d's,** minute granules observed in erythrocytes infected with *Plasmodium vivax* when stained by certain methods, such as Romanowsky's or Wright's stain; called also *Schüffner's granules* or *punctuation.* **Trantas' d's,** small, white calcareous looking dots in the limbus of the conjunctiva in vernal conjunctivitis.

dotage (do′tij) feebleness of mind in old age; senility; senile psychosis.

dotard (do′tard) a person who is weak minded from old age.

dothiepin hydrochloride (do-thi′ĕ-pin) chemical name: 3-dibenzo[*b,e*]thiepin-11(6*H*)-ylidene-*N*,*N*-dimethyl-1-propanamine; a tricyclic antidepressant, C₁₉H₂₁NS·HCl.

double bind (dub′l bīnd) in psychiatry, a type of communication in which one individual directs contradictory verbal remarks to another who is unable to perceive the lack of congruence and cannot respond effectively or escape from the situation. Also, the situation produced by such interaction.

double-blind (dŭ′b′l-blīnd′) denoting a study of the effects of a specific agent in which neither the administrator nor the recipient, at the time of administration, knows whether the active or an inert substance is given.

doublet (dub′let) a combination of two similar or complementary entities, as a combination of two components into a single lens, or of two microtubules in a cilium. **Wollaston's d.,** a microscopical lens consisting of a combination of two planoconvex lenses for correcting chromatic aberration.

douche (doōsh) [Fr.] a stream of water directed against a part of the body or into a cavity. **air d.,** a current of air blown into a cavity, particularly into the tympanum, for opening the eustachian tube. **alternating d.,** transition douche. **fan d.,** water applied to the body in a fan-shaped spray. **jet d.,** water applied to the body in a single stream. **Scotch d.,** a jet douche of alternating hot and cold water. **Tivoli d.,** a reclining bath in which a hot douche is employed over the patient's abdomen. **transition d.,** a douche of alternating hot and cold water; called also *alternating d.* **Weber's d.,** a nasal douche.

Douglas's cry, etc. (dug′las) [James *Douglas*, Scottish anatomist in London, 1675–1742] see under *cry, cul-de-sac, fold, ligament, line, pouch, space,* and *septum.*

douglascele (dug′lah-sēl) posterior vaginal hernia.

douglasitis (dug-lah-si′tis) inflammation of Douglas' pouch (excavatio rectouterina).

dourine (doo-rēn′) a contagious disease of donkeys and horses, characterized by swelling of lymph glands, genital inflammation, and paralysis of hind limbs. It is caused by *Trypanosoma equiperdum* and spread by sexual contact. Called also *covering disease.*

Dover's powder (do′verz) [Thomas *Dover*, English physician, 1660–1742] ipecac and opium powder.

dowel (dow′l) a peg or pin, generally of metal, for fastening an artificial crown or core to the root of a natural tooth, or for fastening a die into a working model for the construction of a crown, inlay, or partial denture; called also *post.*

down (down) lanugo.

Down's syndrome (disease) (downz) [John Langdon Haydon *Down*, English physician, 1828–1896] see under *syndrome.*

downgrowth (down′grōth) a growing downward; something that grows downward. **epithelial d.,** see under *ingrowth.*

doxapram hydrochloride (dok′sah-pram) [USP] chemical name: 1-ethyl-4-[2-(4-morpholinyl)ethyl]-3,3-diphenyl-2-pyrrolidinone monohydrochloride monohydrate. A respiratory stimulant, C₂₄H₃₀N₂O₂·HCl·H₂O, occurring as a white to off-white, crystalline powder; used in the treatment of postanesthetic respiratory depression, administered intravenously.

doxaprost (doks′ah-prost) chemical name: (13*E*)-15-hydroxy-15-methyl-9-oxoprost-13-en-1-oic acid; a bronchodilator, C₂₁H₃₆O₄.

doxepin hydrochloride (dok′sĕ-pin) [USP] chemical name: 3-dibenz[*b,e*]oxepin-11(6*H*)ylidene-*N*,*N*-dimethyl-1-propanamine hydrochloride. A tricyclic compound, C₁₉H₂₁NO·HCl, occurring as a white crystalline powder, having marked antianxiety and significant antidepressant activity; administered orally. It is also used as an antipruritic in veterinary medicine.

Doxinate (dok′si-nāt) trademark for a preparation of dioctyl sulfosuccinate sodium.

doxogenic (dok″so-jen′ik) [Gr. *doxe* opinion + *gennan* to produce] caused by one's own mental conceptions, as doxogenic disease.

doxorubicin (dok″so-ru′bi-sin) chemical name: (8*S*-cis)-10-[(3-amino-2,3,6-trideoxy-α-L-lyxo-hexopyranosyl)oxy]-7,8,9,10-tetrahydro-6,8,11-trihydroxy-8-(hydroxyacetyl)-1-methoxy-5, 12-naphthacenedione. An antineoplastic antibiotic, C₂₇H₂₉NO₁₁, isolated from *Streptomyces peucetius* var. *caesius;* used in the treatment of various neoplastic conditions, including leukemia, sarcomas, lymphomas, neuroblastomas, and Wilms' tumor, administered venously. **d. hydrochloride** [USP], the hydrochloride salt of doxorubicin, C₂₇H₃₀ClNO₄, having the same actions, uses, and route of administration as the base.

doxycycline (dok″se-si′klēn) [USP] chemical name: 4α*S*-(dimethylamino)-1,4,4aα,5,5aα,6,11,12a-octahydro-3,5α,10,12aα-pentahydroxy-6α-methyl-1,11-dioxo-2-naphthacenecarboxamide monohydrate. A semisynthetic broad-spectrum antibacterial of the tetracycline (q.v.) group, C₂₂H₂₄N₂O₈·H₂O, derived from methacycline, it occurs as a yellow crystalline powder; administered orally. **d. calcium,** a complex prepared from doxycycline hyclate and calcium chloride, having the same actions and uses as the hyclate salt; administered orally. **d. hyclate [USP], d. hydrochloride,** a salt, (C₂₂H₂₄N₂O₈·HCl)₂·C₂H₆O·H₂O, occurring as a yellow crystalline powder, having the antibacterial effects of other tetracyclines; administered orally.

Doxy-II (dok′se) trademark for a preparation of doxycycline.

doxylamine succinate (dok-sil′ah-mēn) [USP] chemical name: *N*,*N*-dimethyl-2-[1-phenyl-1-(2-pyridinyl)ethoxy]ethanamine butanedioate (1:1). An antihistaminic, C₁₇H₂₂N₂O·C₄H₆O₄, occurring as a white or creamy white powder; administered orally.

Doyen's clamp, operation (dwah-yahz′) [Eugene Louis *Doyen*, surgeon in Paris, 1859–1916] see under *clamp* and *operation.*

Doyère's eminence (hillock) (dwa-yārz′) [Louis Michel François *Doyère*, French physiologist, 1811–1863] see under *eminence.*

Doyne's familial honeycombed choroiditis (doinz) [Robert Walter *Doyne*, Oxford ophthalmologist, 1857–1916] see under *choroiditis.*

D.P. abbreviation for L. *directio′ne prop′ria* ["with proper direction"]; Doctor of Pharmacy; Doctor of Podiatry.

D.P.H. Diploma in Public Health.

D.P.M. Diploma in Psychological Medicine; Doctor of Podiatric Medicine.

DPN diphosphopyridine nucleotide; now called *nicotinamide adenine dinucleotide* (NAD).

DPT diphtheria-pertussis-tetanus (vaccine).

DR reaction of degeneration; see under *reaction.*

dr. dram.

drachm (dram) [Gr. *drachmē*] dram.

dracontiasis (drak″on-ti′ah-sis) [Gr. *drakontion* (little dragon) tapeworm] dracunculiasis.

dracuncular (drah-kung′ku-lar) pertaining to or caused by nematodes of the genus *Dracunculus*.

dracunculiasis (drah-kung″ku-li′ah-sis) the state of being infected with nematodes of the genus *Dracunculus;* called also *guinea worm disease.*

Dracunculoidea (drah″kung-ku-loi′de-ah) a superfamily of phasmid nematodes including the genus *Dracunculus*.

dracunculosis (drah-kung″ku-lo′sis) dracunculiasis.

Dracunculus (drah-kung′ku-lus) [L. "little dragon"] a genus of nematode parasites of the superfamily Dracunculoidea. **D. medinen′sis,** the guinea worm or Medina worm, a threadlike worm, 30 to 120 cm. long, which inhabits the subcutaneous and intermuscular tissues of man and several domestic animals in India, Africa, and Arabia. Its embryos are discharged through an opening in the skin upon contact with water, in which they enter the bodies of a small crustacean, *Cyclops*, where they undergo larval development. Called also *dragon* or *serpent worm;* formerly called *Filaria medinensis*.

draft (draft) a potion; dose. **black d.,** the compound infusion of senna. **effervescing d.,** one which contains an acid and sodium or potassium bicarbonate. **mustard d.,** a mild rubefacient paste of mustard and flour. **Riverius' d.,** Rivière's potion.

drag (drag) the lower or cast side of a denture flask to which the cope is fitted.

dragée (drah-zha′) [Fr. "sugar-plum"] a sugar-coated pill, or medicated confection.

Dragendorff's test (drag′en-dorfs) [Georg Johann Noël *Dragendorff*, German physician, 1836–1898] see under *tests*.

drain (drān) any device by which a channel or open area may be established for the exit of fluids or purulent material from any cavity, wound, or infected area. **cigarette d.,** a drain made by drawing a strip of gauze or surgical sponge into a tube of gutta-percha. **controlled d.,** a drain made by pressing a square of gauze into the wound and then packing with gauze strips, the ends of which, together with the corners of the square, are left projecting from the wound. **Mikulicz's d.,** a drain formed by pushing a single layer of gauze into a wound or cavity, then packing with several thick wicks of gauze as the original layer is forced farther and farther into the defect. **Mosher d.,** a truncated cone of copper mesh, used in the drainage of brain wounds. **Penrose d.,** cigarette d. **quarantine d.,** one left in place after laparotomy to drain the peritoneal cavity. **stab wound d.,** drainage accomplished by bringing out the drain through a small separate wound adjacent to the major operative incision. **Wylie d.,** a stem pessary of hard rubber having a groove along the stem.

drainage (drān′ij) the systematic withdrawal of fluids and discharges from a wound, sore, or cavity. **basal d.,** withdrawal of the cerebrospinal fluid from the basal subarachnoid space for the relief of intracranial pressure. **button d.,** drainage of a peritoneal transudate by means of a special button affixed to all layers of the abdominal wall. **capillary d.,** drainage effected by strands of hair, catgut, spun glass, or other material of tiny diameter which induces capillary attraction. **closed d.,** drainage of an empyema cavity carried out with protection against the entrance of outside air into the pleural cavity. **closed pleural d.,** continuous aspiration of the pleural cavity by means of an intercostal drainage tube passing into an airtight receiving vessel to which suction is applied. **continuous suction d.,** see *Wangensteen d.* **Monaldi's d.,** a method of suction drainage of tuberculous cavities of the lungs. **open d.,** drainage of an empyema cavity through an opening in the chest wall into which one or more rubber drainage tubes are inserted, the opening not being sealed against the entrance of outside air. **postural d.,** therapeutic drainage in bronchiectasis and lung abscess by placing the patient with the head downward so that the trachea will be inclined downward and below the affected area. **suction d.,** closed drainage of a cavity, with a suction apparatus attached to the drainage tube. **through d.,** drainage achieved by passing a perforated tube or other type of drain through a cavity, so that irrigation may be effected by injecting fluid into one aperture and letting it escape through another. **tidal d.,** drainage of the urinary bladder by an apparatus which alternately fills the bladder to a predetermined extent and then empties it by a combination of siphonage and gravity flow. **Wangensteen d.,** continuous drainage by suction through an indwelling gastric or duodenal tube; for treatment of intestinal obstruction, paralytic ileus, etc.

dram (dram) a unit of weight which, in the apothecaries' system, equals 60 grains, or ⅛ ounce; in the avoirdupois system it equals 27.34 grains, or 1/16 ounce. Symbol ℨ; abbreviated dr. Called also *drachm*. **fluid d.,** a unit of capacity (liquid measure) of the apothecaries' system, being 60 minims, or the equivalent of 3.697 ml. Abbreviated fl.dr.

Dramamine (dram′ah-mēn) trademark for preparations of dimenhydrinate.

dramatism (dram′ah-tizm) pompous and dramatic speech and behavior in mental disorder.

dramatization (dram″ah-ti-za′shun) that part of the dream-work in which the manifest content of the dream is an action or situation.

drastic (dras′tik) [Gr. *drastikos* effective] 1. acting powerfully or thoroughly. 2. a violent purgative.

draught (draft) draft.

dream (drēm) a conscious series of images, emotions, or thoughts that occur during sleep, usually during the rapid eye movement (R.E.M.) stage of sleep. **clairvoyant d.,** one that seems to reveal a real event to the sleeper. **day d.,** wishful, purposeless reveries, without regard to reality. **wet d.,** a slang term for nocturnal emission.

Drechsel's test (drek′selz) [Edmund *Drechsel*, Swiss chemist, 1843–1897] see under *tests*.

drench (drench) a draft of medicine given to an animal by pouring it into its mouth.

Drepanidotaenia (drep″ah-nid-o-te′ne-ah) a genus of tapeworms parasitic in birds. *D. lanceola′ta* (*Hymenolepis lanceolata*) is a tapeworm of ducks and geese once reported from man.

drepanocyte (drep′ah-no-sīt″) [Gr. *drepanē* sickle + *kytos* cell] a sickle cell.

drepanocytemia (drep″ah-no-si-te′me-ah) sickle cell anemia.

drepanocytic (drep″ah-no-si′tik) pertaining to drepanocytes (sickle cells); having sickle-shaped cells.

drepanocytosis (drep″ah-no-si-to′sis) an occurrence of drepanocytes in the blood.

Drepanospira (drep″ah-no-spi′rah) [Gr. *drepanē* sickle + *speira* coil] a genus of Spirillaceae parasitic on protozoa.

Dresbach's anemia (syndrome) (dres′bahks) [Melvin *Dresbach*, American physician, 1874–1946] elliptocytosis.

dresser (dres′er) a surgical assistant who dresses wounds, etc.

dressing (dres′ing) any of various materials utilized for covering and protecting a wound. See also *bandage*. **adhesive absorbent d.,** a sterile individual dressing consisting of a plain absorbent compress affixed to a film or fabric coated with a pressure-sensitive adhesive substance. **antiseptic d.,** a dressing of gauze impregnated with an antiseptic material. **bolus d.,** tie-over d. **cocoon d.,** a dressing of gauze affixed to the surrounding skin by collodion or other liquid adhesive in such fashion that its elevated appearance resembles a cocoon. **cross d.,** transvestism. **dry d.,** dry gauze or absorbent cotton applied to a wound. **fixed d.,** a dressing impregnated with plaster of Paris, starch, or silicate of soda, utilized to secure fixation of the part when the material dries. **Lister's d.,** gauze impregnated with phenol, once used for covering or packing a wound. **occlusive d.,** one which seals a wound from contact with air or bacteria. **paraffin d.,** a dressing of gauze impregnated with paraffin. **pressure d.,** one by which pressure is exerted on the area covered to prevent the collection of fluids in the underlying tissues; most commonly used after skin grafting and in the treatment of burns. **protective d.,** a light dressing to prevent exposure to injury or infection. **stent d.,** a dressing in which is incorporated a mold or stent, to maintain position of a graft. **tie-over d.,** a dressing placed over a skin graft or other sutured wound, and tied on by the sutures which have been made of sufficient length for that purpose; called also *bolus d.*

Dressler's disease (dres′lerz) [*Dressler*, physician in Wurzburg] intermittent hemoglobinuria.

drift (drift) a chance variation, as in gene frequency from one generation to another; the smaller the population, the greater are the random variations. Called also *genetic d.* or *random genetic d.* **antigenic d.,** change in the antigenic structure of a virus strain, probably resulting from natural selection of virus variants circulating among an immune or partially immune population. **genetic d.,** see *drift*. **random genetic d.,** see *drift*.

drill (dril) a rotating cutting instrument for making holes in hard substances, such as bones or teeth. **bur d.,** see *bur*. **cannulated d.,** a drill with a hole through the center of its long axis, to be used over a guide wire. **dental d.,** see *bur*.

Drinalfa (drin-al′fah) trademark for preparations of methamphetamine hydrochloride.

drinidene (dri′nĭ-dēn) chemical name: 2-(aminomethylene)-2,3-dihydro-1*H*-inden-1-one; an analgesic, $C_{10}H_9NO$.

drink (drink) a quantity of liquid taken in one or a series of successive swallows; to take a drink. **sham d.,** a drink, as by an esophagostomized dog, in which swallowed water fails to be ingested or retained in the stomach.

Drinker respirator (drink′er) [Philip *Drinker*, American public health engineer, born 1894] see under *respirator*.

drip (drip) the slow, drop by drop, infusion of a liquid. **alkalinized milk d. of Winkelstein,** a method of treating certain cases of ulcers, in which a mixture of 5 gm. of sodium bicarbonate in 1 quart of whole milk is allowed to drip into the stomach through a small nasal or oral tube at the rate of 30 drops per minute, producing constant achlorhydria. **intravenous d.,**

continuous intravenous instillation, drop by drop, of saline or other solution. **Murphy d.,** see *Murphy method,* 2d def., under *method.* **nasal d.,** a method of giving fluid slowly to dehydrated infants through a catheter inserted into the nose and pushed down into the esophagus. **postnasal d.,** the dripping of discharges from the postnasal region into the pharynx due to hypersecretion of mucus in the nasal or nasopharyngeal mucosa or to chronic sinusitis.

Drisdol (driz'dol) trademark for preparations of ergocalciferol.

drive (drīv) the force which activates human impulses.

drobuline (dro'bu-lēn) chemical name: $(\pm)$-α-[[(1-methylethyl)-amino]methyl-γ-phenylbenzenepropanol; a cardiac depressant with antiarrhythmic action, $C_{19}H_{25}NO$.

drocarbil (dro-kar'bil) chemical name: arecoline N-acetyl-4-hydroxy-m-arsanilate. An odorless powder, $C_{16}H_{23}AsN_2O_7$, freely soluble in water; used as an anthelmintic in veterinary medicine.

drocinonide (dro-sin'o-nīd) chemical name: 9-fluoro-11β,21-dihydroxy-16α-17-[(1-methylethylidene)bis(oxy)]-5α-pregnane-3,-20-dione; an anti-inflammatory, $C_{24}H_{35}FO_6$.

drocode (dro'kod) dihydrocodeine.

Drolban (drol'ban) trademark for a preparation of dromostanolone propionate.

dromo- (drom'o) [Gr. *dromos* a course] a combining form denoting relation to conduction, or to running.

dromograph (drom'o-graf) [*dromo-* + Gr. *graphein* to record] an instrument for recording conduction or flow.

dromostanolone propionate (dro"mo-stan'o-lōn) [USP] chemical name: 2α-methyl-17β-(1-oxopropoxy)-5α-androstan-3-one. An adrogenic, anabolic steriod, $C_{23}H_{36}O_3$, occurring as a white to creamy white, crystalline powder; used as an antineoplastic agent in the palliative treatment of advanced metastatic, inoperable breast cancer in certain postmenopausal women, administered intramuscularly.

dromotropic (drom"o-trop'ik) affecting the conductivity of a nerve fiber.

dromotropism (dro-mot'ro-pizm) [Gr. *dromos* a course + *tropē* a turn, turning] the quality or property of affecting the conductivity of a nerve fiber. **negative d.,** the property of diminishing the conductivity of a nerve. **positive d.,** the property of increasing the conductivity of a nerve.

drop (drop) [L. *gutta*] a minute sphere of liquid as it hangs or falls. **ear d's,** medicated oil or water to be dropped into the external auditory meatus. **enamel d.,** enameloma. **eye d's,** a medicated solution to be dropped into the conjunctival sac. **foot d.,** footdrop. **Hoffmann's d's,** ether spirit. **nose d's,** a medicated solution to be dropped into the nose. **d. phalangette,** a condition in which the terminal phalanx of a finger or toe is permanently flexed, as in baseball finger or mallet finger. **wrist d.,** wristdrop.

dropacism (drop'ah-sizm) [Gr. *drōpax* plaster] the removal of hairs by means of a plaster.

droperidol (dro-per'ĭ-dol) [USP] chemical name: 1-[1-[4-(4-fluorophenyl)-4-oxobutyl]-1,2,3,6-tetrahydro-4-pyridinyl]-1,3-dihydro-2H-benzimidazol-2-one. A drug of the butyrophenone series, $C_{22}H_{22}FN_3O_2$, occurring as a white to light tan, amorphous or microcrystalline powder; used for its antianxiety, sedative, and antiemetic effects as a premedication prior to surgery and during induction and maintenance of anesthesia, administered intravenously or intramuscularly. A combination of droperidol and fentanyl citrate (known as *Innovar*) is administered intramuscularly to produce neuroleptanalgesia.

droplet (drop'let) a diminutive drop, such as the particles of moisture expelled from the mouth in coughing, sneezing, or speaking, which may carry infection to others through the air.

dropper (drop'er) a pipet or tube for dispensing liquid in drops.

dropping (drop'ing) the limping gait of a horse, which is due to a neurologic disorder affecting the extensors of the limb.

dropsical (drop'sĭ-kal) affected with or pertaining to dropsy.

dropsy (drop'se) [L. *hydrops,* from Gr. *hydōr* water] the abnormal accumulation of serous fluid in the cellular tissue or in a body cavity; see also *hydrops.* **abdominal d.,** ascites. **acute anemic d.,** epidemic d. **d. of amnion,** hydramnios. **articular d.,** hydrarthrosis. **d. of belly,** ascites. **d. of brain,** hydrocephalus. **cardiac d.,** gross edema related to heart failure. **d. of chest,** hydrothorax. **cutaneous d.,** edema. **epidemic d.,** a disease epidemic in India, Mauritius, and Fiji among the natives only, characterized by fever, anemia, and diarrhea, and followed by sudden edema; called also *argemone oil poisoning.* **famine d.,** nutritional edema. **d. of head,** hydrocephalus. **hepatic d.,** that which is due to disease of the liver. **nutritional d.,** nutritional edema. **d. of pericardium** (*obs.*), hydropericardium. **peritoneal d.,** ascites. **renal d.,** anasarca due to kidney disease. **salpingian d.,** hydrosalpinx. **war d.,** nutritional edema. **wet d.,** beriberi.

Drosophila (dro-sof'ĭ-lah) [Gr. *drosos* dew + *philein* to love] a genus of flies; the fruit flies. **D. melanogas'ter,** a small fly often seen about decaying fruit; used extensively in experimental genetics.

drosopterin (dro-sop'ter-in) any of a group of bright red pteridine pigments of the eye of *Drosophila* which are readily decomposed by light.

drowning (drown'ing) suffocation and death resulting from filling of the lungs with water or other substance or fluid, so that gas exchange becomes impossible. **secondary d.,** delayed death from drowning, due to such complications as pulmonary alveolar inflammation.

droxacin sodium (droks'ah-sin) chemical name: 5-ethyl-2,3,5,8-tetrahydro-8-oxo-furo[2,3-*g*]quinoline-7-carboxylic acid sodium salt; an antibacterial, $C_{14}H_{12}NNaO_4$.

droxifilcon A (droks"ĭ-fil'kon) chemical name: 2-hydroxyethyl methacrylate polymer with ethylenebis(oxyethylene)dimethacrylate and 1-vinyl-2-pyrrolidinone; a hydrophilic contact lens material, $(C_6H_{10}O_3)_x(C_{14}H_{22}O_6)_yI(C_6H_9NO)_z$.

Dr.P.H. Doctor of Public Health.

drug (drug) 1. any chemical compound that may be used on or administered to humans or animals as an aid in the diagnosis, treatment, or prevention of disease or other abnormal condition, for the relief of pain or suffering, or to control or improve any physiologic or pathologic condition. 2. a narcotic. **antagonistic d.,** one that tends to counteract or neutralize the effect of another. **crude d.,** the whole drug with all its ingredients. **habit-forming d.,** any drug, such as alcohol, tobacco, morphine, cocaine, opium, that produces dependence, whether physical or psychic.

drug-fast (drug'fast) drug-resistant.

druggist (drug'ist) pharmacist.

drug-resistant (drug're-zis"tant) resistant to the action of drugs; said of microorganisms. Called also *drug-fast.*

drum (drum) 1. the middle ear (auris media [NA]). 2. membrane tympani.

drumhead (drum'hed) the tympanic membrane (membrana tympani [NA]).

Drummond's sign (drum'unds) [Sir David *Drummond,* English physician, 1852–1932] see under *sign.*

drumstick (drum'stik) a nuclear lobule attached by a slender strand to the nucleus of a small proportion of polymorphonuclear leukocytes of normal females but not of normal males.

drupe (droop) [L. *drupa* an overripe olive] stone fruits in which the outer part of the ovary wall forms a skin, the middle part becomes fleshy and juicy, and the inner part forms a hard pit or stone around the seed; e.g., peaches, plums, apricots.

drusen (droo'sen) [Ger., pl. of *Druse* stony nodule, geode] 1. hyaline excrescences in Bruch's membrane (lamina basalis choroideae); they usually result from aging, but sometimes occur with other pathologic conditions. 2. rosettes of granules occurring in the lesions of actinomycosis.

Drysdale's corpuscles (driz'dālz) [Thomas Murray *Drysdale,* American gynecologist, 1831–1904] see under *corpuscle.*

Dryvax (dri'vaks) trademark for a preparation of smallpox vaccine.

D.S.C. Doctor of Surgical Chiropody.

DT duration tetany.

D.T.D abbreviation for L. *da'tur ta'lis do'sis,* give of such a dose.

DTIC dacarbazine.

DTIC-Dome (dōm) trademark for a preparation of dacarbazine.

D.T.P. distal tingling on percussion; see *Tinel's sign,* under *sign.*

dualism (du'al-izm) [L. *duo* two] 1. the theory that there are two distinct stem cells for blood cell formation: one for the lymphatic cells and the other for the myeloid cells. 2. the theory that human beings are made up of two independent systems, mind and body, and that psychic and physical phenomena are fundamentally independent and different in nature.

dualist (du'al-ist) an adherent of the dualistic theory.

dualistic (du"al-is'tik) 1. twofold. 2. pertaining to dualism.

Duane's syndrome, test (du-ānz') [Alexander *Duane,* ophthalmologist in New York, 1858–1926] see under *syndrome* and *test.*

duazomycin (du-az"o-mi'sin) an antibiotic substance with antineoplastic properties, produced by *Streptomyces ambofaciens;* formerly called *duazomycin A.* **d. A,** former name for duazomycin. **d. B,** former name for azotomycin. **d. C,** former name for ambomycin.

dubi (doo'be) the native name on the Gold Coast for yaws.

Dubini's chorea (disease) (du-be'nēz) [Angelo *Dubini,* Italian physician, 1813–1902] see under *chorea.*

Dubois's abscess, disease (du-bwahz') [Paul *Dubois,* French obstetrician, 1795–1871] see under *abscess* and *disease.*

Dubois's method (treatment) (du-bwahz') [Paul Charles *Dubois,* Swiss psychiatrist, 1848–1918] see under *method.*

DuBois-Reymond's law (dŭ-bwah"ri-maw') [Emil Heinrich *Du-Bois-Reymond,* German physiologist, 1818–1896] see under *law.*

Duboisia (du-boi′se-ah) a genus of solanaceous plants; *D. myoporoi′des* yields hyoscyamine and scopolamine.

Dubos enzyme (crude crystals, lysin), medium (doo-bos′) [René Jules *Dubos*, French biochemist in America, born 1901] see *tyrothricin*, and see under *culture medium*.

Duboscq colorimeter (du-bosk′) [Louis Jules *Duboscq*, French optician, 1817–1886] see under *colorimeter*.

Duchenne's disease, etc. (du-shenz′) [Guillaume Benjamin Amand *Duchenne*, French neurologist, 1806– 1875] see under *disease, dystrophy, paralysis, trocar*, and *type*.

Duchenne-Aran muscular atrophy (disease, type) (du-shen′ar-an′) [G. B. A. *Duchenne*; F. A. *Aran*] spinal muscular atrophy; see under *atrophy*.

Duchenne-Erb paralysis, syndrome (du-shen′airb) [G. B. A. *Duchenne*; Wilhelm Heinrich *Erb*, German internist, 1840–1921] Erb-Duchenne paralysis.

Duchenne-Landouzy dystrophy (type) [G. B. A. *Duchenne*; L. T. J. *Landouzy*] facioscapulohumeral muscular dystrophy; see under *dystrophy*.

Duckworth's phenomenon (sign) (duk′worths) [Sir Dyce *Duckworth*, British physician, 1840–1928] see under *phenomenon*.

Ducobee (doo′ko-be) trademark for preparations of vitamin B₁₂; see *cyanocobalamin*.

Ducrey's bacillus (doo-krāz′) [Augosto *Ducrey*, Italian dermatologist, 1860–1940] *Hemophilus ducreyi*.

duct (dukt) [L. *ductus*, from *ducere* to draw or lead] a passage with well-defined walls, especially a tube for the passage of excretions or secretions; called also *ductus* [NA]. **aberrant d.**, any duct that is not usually present or that takes an unusual course or direction, such as the ductulus aberrans superior. **acoustic d.**, meatus acusticus externus. **adipose d.**, an elongated sac in the cellular tissue filled with fat. **alimentary d.**, thoracic d. **allantoic d.**, allantoic stalk. **alveolar d's**, ductuli alveolares. **d. of Arantius**, ductus venosus. **archinephric d.**, pronephric d. **arterial d.**, ductus arteriosus. **Bartholin's d.**, ductus sublingualis major. **Bellini's d's**, tubuli renales recti. **Bernard's d.**, ductus pancreaticus accessorius. **bile d., common**, ductus choledochus. **bile d's, interlobular**, ductuli interlobulares. **biliary d's, biliferous d's**, the passages for the conveyance of bile in and from the liver. **Blasius' d.**, ductus parotideus. **Bochdalek's d.**, ductus thyroglossus. **d. of Botallo**, ductus arteriosus. **branchial d's**, drawn-out branchial grooves 2, 3, and 4, which open into the temporary cervical sinus of the embryo. **canalicular d's**, ductus lactiferi. **cervical d.**, the opening from the exterior into the temporary cervical sinus of the embryo. **choledochus d.**, ductus choledochus. **chyliferous d.**, thoracic d. **cloacal d.**, Reichel's cloacal d. **cochlear d.**, 1. a spirally arranged membranous tube in the bony canal of the cochlea; see *canalis cochlearis* [NA]. 2. canalis spiralis cochleae. **common bile d.**, the duct formed by union of the cystic duct and the hepatic duct; called also *ductus choledochus* [NA]. **Coschwitz' d.**, a supposed salivary duct forming an arch over the dorsum of the tongue, proved by von Haller to be a vein. **cowperian d.**, ductus glandulae bulbourethralis. **craniopharyngeal d.**, hypophyseal d. **d's of Cuvier**, common cardinal veins: two short venous trunks in the fetus opening into the atrium of the heart; the right one becomes the superior vena cava; called also *Cuvier's sinuses* and *ductus cuvieri*. **cystic d.**, ductus cysticus. **deferent d.**, ductus deferens. **efferent d.**, a duct that gives outlet to a glandular secretion. **ejaculatory d.**, ductus ejaculatorius. **endolymphatic d.**, ductus endolymphaticus. **d. of epididymis**, ductus epididymidis. **d. of epoophoron**, ductus epoophori longitudinalis. **excretory d.**, one that is merely conductive and not secretory. **excretory d. of bulbourethral gland**, ductus glandulae bulbourethralis. **excretory d. of seminal vesicle**, ductus excretorius vesiculae seminalis. **excretory d. of testis**, ductus deferens. **frontonasal d.**, nasofrontal d. **galactophorous d's**, ductus lactiferi. **gall d's**, biliary d's. **d. of gallbladder**, ductus cysticus. **Gartner's d.**, ductus epoophori longitudinalis. **gasserian d.**, ductus paramesonephricus. **genital d.**, genital canal. **gutteral d.**, auditory tube. **Haller's aberrant d.**, a small coiled tube extending from the lower part of the canal of the epididymis; called also *ductus aberrans halleri*. **Hensen's d.**, ductus reuniens. **hepatic d., common**, ductus hepaticus communis. **hepatic d., left**, ductus hepaticus sinister. **hepatic d., right**, ductus hepaticus dexter. **hepaticopancreatic d.**, ductus pancreaticus. **hepatocystic d.**, ductus choledochus. **d. of His**, ductus thyroglossus. **hypophyseal d.**, an embryonic structure composed of the elongated Rathke's pouch joining the infundibulum of the embryonic hypophysis; called also *craniopharyngeal duct*. **incisive d., incisor d.**, ductus incisivus. **intercalated d.**, a slender initial portion of the duct system interposed between an acinus of a gland and a secretory duct. **interlobular d's**, channels located between different lobules of a gland; see *ductuli interlobulares*. **lacrimal d.**, canaliculus lacrimalis. **lacrimonasal d.**, ductus nasolacrimalis. **lactiferous d's**, ductus lactif-

eri. **Leydig's d.**, d. mesonephricus. **lingual d.**, a depression on the dorsum of the tongue at the apex of the terminal sulcus. **longitudinal d. of epoophoron**, ductus epoophori longitudinalis. **Luschka's d's**, tubular structures in the wall of the gallbladder, some connected with bile ducts but none connected with the lumen of the gallbladder; they may be aberrant bile ducts. **lymphatic d's**, channels for conducting lymph. **lymphatic d., left**, thoracic d. **lymphatic d., right**, ductus lymphaticus dexter. **mammary d's, mammillary d's**, ductus lactiferi. **mesonephric d.**, ductus mesonephricus. **metanephric d.**, ureter. **milk d's**, ductus lactiferi. **d. of Müller, müllerian d.**, ductus paramesonephricus. **nasal d.**, ductus nasolacrimalis. **nasofrontal d.**, a duct in the lateral wall of the nasal cavity extending from the infundibulum of the ethmoid bone to the frontal sinus; called also *frontonasal d.* **nasolacrimal d.**, ductus nasolacrimalis. **nasopharyngeal d.**, the lumen of the nasopharynx. **nephric d.**, ureter. **omphalomesenteric d.**, the narrow tube connecting the umbilical vesicle (yolk sac) with the midgut of the embryo; called also *omphalomesenteric canal, umbilical duct, vitelline duct, vitellointestinal duct*, and *yolk stalk*. **ovarian d.**, tuba uterina. **pancreatic d.**, ductus pancreaticus. **pancreatic d., accessory, pancreatic d., minor**, ductus pancreaticus accessorius. **papillary d's**, tubuli renales recti. **paramesonephric d.**, ductus paramesonephricus. **paraurethral d's**, ductus paraurethrales. **parotid d.**, ductus parotideus. **d. of Pecquet**, thoracic d. **perilymphatic d's**, ductus perilymphatici. **primordial d.**, ductus paramesonephricus. **pronephric d.**, the duct of the pronephros, which later serves as the mesonephric duct (ductus mesonephricus); called also *archinephric d.* or *canal*. **d's of prostate gland, prostatic d's**, ductuli prostatici. **Rathke's d.**, that part of the ductus paramesonephricus lying between its main part and the sinus pocularis. **Reichel's cloacal d.**, the cleft between Douglas' septum and the cloaca in the embryo. **renal d.**, ureter. **d's of Rivinus**, ductus sublinguales minores. **Rokitansky-Aschoff d's**, see under *sinus*. **sacculoutricular d.**, ductus utriculosaccularis. **salivary d's**, the ducts that convey the saliva: they are the ductus parotideus, ductus submandibularis, ductus sublingualis major, and ductus sublinguales minores. **d. of Santorini**, ductus pancreaticus accessorius. **Schüller's d's**, ductus paraurethrales. **secretory d.**, a smaller duct that is tributary to an excretory duct of a gland and that also has a secretory function. **semicircular d's**, the long ducts of the membranous labyrinth of the ear; called also *ductus semicirculares* [NA]. **semicircular d., anterior**, ductus semicircularis anterior. **semicircular d., lateral**, ductus semicircularis lateralis. **semicircular d., posterior**, ductus semicircularis posterior. **semicircular d., superior**, ductus semicircularis anterior. **seminal d's**, passages for the conveyance of spermatozoa and semen, including the ductus deferens, ductus excretorius vesiculae seminalis, and ductus ejaculatorius. **d. of seminal vesicle**, ductus excretorius vesiculae seminalis. **Skene's d's**, ductus paraurethrales. **spermatic d.**, ductus deferens. **d. of Steno, Stensen's d.**, ductus parotideus. **sublingual d's**, the ducts of the sublingual salivary glands, including the ductus sublingualis major and ductus sublinguales minores. **sublingual d., major**, ductus sublingualis major. **sublingual d's, minor**, ductus sublinguales minores. **submandibular d., submaxillary d. of Wharton**, ductus submandibularis. **suderiferous d., sweat d.**, ductus sudoriferus. **tear d's**, the ducts conveying the secretion of the lacrimal glands. **testicular d.**, ductus deferens. **thoracic d.**, the canal that ascends from the cisterna chyli to the junction of the left subclavian and left internal jugular vein; called also *ductus thoracicus* [NA], *alimentary d., chyliferous d., d. of Pecquet, left lymphatic d.*, and *Van Hoorne's canal*. **thoracic d., right**, ductus thoracicus dexter. **thyroglossal d., thyrolingual d.**, ductus thyroglossus. **umbilical d.**, yolk stalk. **urogenital d's**, the ductus paramesonephricus and ductus mesonephricus. **utriculosaccular d.**, ductus utriculosaccularis. **d. of Vater**, ductus thyroglossus. **vitelline d., vitellointestinal d.**, yolk stalk. **Walther's d's**, ductus sublinguales minores. **Wharton's d.**, ductus submandibularis. **d. of Wirsung**, ductus pancreaticus. **d. of Wolff, wolffian d.**, ductus mesonephricus.

ductal (duk′tal) pertaining to a duct.

ductile (duk′til) [L. *ductilis*, from *ducere* to draw, to lead] susceptible of being drawn out, as into a wire.

ductless (dukt′les) having no excretory duct.

ductule (dukt′ul) a minute duct, especially that part or branch of a duct which is nearest the alveolus of a gland; called also *ductulus* [NA]. **aberrant d's**, ductules that are not usually present, or that follow an unusual course or direction; see *ductuli aberrantes* [NA]. **aberrant d., superior**, ductulus aberrans superior. **alveolar d's**, ductuli alveolares. **bile d's, biliary d's**, 1. ductuli biliferi [NA]. 2. cholangioles. **efferent d's of testis**, ductuli efferentes testis. **excretory d's of lacrimal gland**, ductuli excretorii glandulae lacrimalis. **interlobular d's**, ductuli interlobulares. **d's of prostate**, ductuli prostatici. **transverse d's of epoophoron**, ductuli transversi epoophori.

ductuli (duk′tu-li) [L.] plural of *ductulus*.

ductulus (duk′tu-lus), pl. *duc′tuli* [L.] [NA] ductule: a general term for a minute duct; applied especially to branches of ducts nearest to the alveoli of a gland, or the smallest beginnings of the duct system of an organ. **duc′tuli aberran′tes** [NA], aberrant ductules: blind vestiges of mesonephric tubules standing in relation to the epididymis. **d. aber′rans supe′rior** [NA], superior aberrant ductule: a narrow tube of variable length that lies in the epididymis and is connected with the rete testis; called also *ductus aberrans*. **duc′tuli alveola′res** [NA], alveolar ductules: small passages connecting the respiratory bronchioles and the alveolar sacs; see Plate XLVI accompanying *system*. Called also *alveolar ducts*. **duc′tuli bili′feri** [NA], biliary ductules: the small channels that connect the interlobular ducts with the right and left hepatic ducts; called also *bile ductule* and *ductus biliferi*. **duc′tuli efferen′tes tes′tis** [NA], efferent ductules of testis: ductules entering the head of the epididymis from the rete testis. **duc′tuli excreto′rii glan′dulae lacrima′lis** [NA], excretory ductules of lacrimal gland: numerous ductules that traverse the palpebral part of the lacrimal gland and open into the superior fornix of the conjunctiva. **duc′tuli interlobula′res** [NA], interlobular ductules: small channels between the hepatic lobules, draining into the bile ductules; called also *ductus interlobulares*, and *interlobular biliary canals* or *bile ducts*. **duc′tuli prostat′ici** [NA], ductules of prostate gland: minute ducts from the prostate gland that open on either side into or near the prostatic sinuses on the posterior wall of the urethra; called also *ductus prostatici, ducts of prostate gland*, and *prostatic ducts*. **duc′tuli transver′si epooph′ori** [NA], transverse ductules of epoophoron: the remains of the mesonephric ducts, opening into the longitudinal duct of the epoophoron.

ductus (duk′tus), pl. *duc′tus* [L.] [NA] a duct: a general term for a passage with well defined walls, especially such a channel for the passage of excretions or secretions. **d. aber′rans**, ductulus aberrans superior. **d. aber′rans hal′leri**, Haller's aberrant duct. **d. Aran′tii**, d. venosus. **d. arterio′sus** [NA], arterial duct: a fetal blood vessel connecting the pulmonary artery directly to the descending aorta; called also *arterial canal, Botallo's duct*, and *pulmoaortic canal*. **d. arteriosus, patent**, abnormal persistence of an open lumen in the ductus arteriosus after birth, the direction of flow being from the aorta to the pulmonary artery, resulting in recirculation of arterial blood through the lungs. **d. arteriosus, reversed**, abnormal persistence of an open lumen in the ductus arteriosus after birth with obstruction of the small vessels of the lungs, the direction of flow being from the pulmonary artery to the aorta, resulting in the return of venous blood to the systemic circulation (the reverse of the normal post-fetal circulation); characterized clinically by cyanosis, especially of the feet. **d. bilif′eri**, ductuli biliferi. **d. choled′ochus** [NA], choledochous duct: the duct formed by union of the common hepatic and the cystic duct which empties into the duodenum at the major duodenal papilla, along with the pancreatic duct; called also *common bile duct, hepatic funiculus*, and *hepatocystic duct*. **d. cochlea′ris** [NA], cochlear duct: a spirally arranged membranous tube in the bony canal of the cochlea along its outer wall, lying between the scala tympani below and the scala vestibuli above; called also *cochlear canal, membranous cochlea, scala media*, and *scala of Löwenberg*. **d. cow′peri**, d. glandulae bulbourethralis. **d. cuvi′eri**, ducts of Cuvier. **d. cys′ticus** [NA], cystic duct: the passage connecting the neck of the gallbladder and the common bile duct; called also *duct of gallbladder*. **d. def′erens** [NA], deferent duct: the excretory duct of the testis, which unites with the excretory duct of the seminal vesicle to form the ejaculatory duct; called also *vas deferens, excretory duct of testis, spermatis duct*, and *testicular duct*. **d. ejaculato′rius** [NA], ejaculatory duct: the canal formed by union of the ductus deferens and the excretory duct of the seminal vesicle. It enters the prostatic part of the urethra on the colliculus seminalis. **d. endolymphat′icus** [NA], endolymphatic duct: a canal connecting the utriculosaccular duct with the endolymphatic sac; called also *aqueductus vestibuli* [NA alternative], and *aqueductus endolymphaticus*. **d. epididym′idis** [NA], duct of epididymus: the single tube into which the coiled ends of the efferent ductules of the testis open, the convolutions of which make up the greater part of the epididymis; called also *canal of epididymus*. **d. epooph′ori longitudina′lis** [NA], longitudinal duct of epoophoron: a closed rudimentary duct lying parallel to the uterine tube, into which 10 to 15 transverse ducts of the epoophoron open; it is a remnant of the part of the mesonephros which participates in formation of the reproductive organs. Called also *duct of epoophoron* and *Gartner's canal* or *duct*. **d. excreto′rius glan′dulae bulboure-thra′les**, ductus glandulae bulbourethralis. **d. excreto′rius vesic′ulae semina′lis** [NA], excretory duct of seminal vesicle: the duct that drains the seminal vesicle and unites with the ductus deferens to form the ejaculatory duct. **d. glan′dulae bulbourethra′lis** [NA], duct of bulbourethral gland: a duct passing from the bulbourethral gland through the urogenital diaphragm into the bulb of the penis and entering the spongy part of the urethra; called also *d. cowperi, cowperian duct*, and *d. excretorius glandulae bulbourethralis*. **d. hepat′icus commu′nis** [NA], common hepatic duct: the duct which is formed by union of the

right and left hepatic ducts, and in turn joins the cystic duct to form the common bile duct. **d. hepat′icus dex′ter** [NA], right hepatic duct: the duct that drains the right lobe and part of the caudate lobe of the liver. **d. hepat′icus sin′ister** [NA], left hepatic duct: the duct that drains the left and the quadrate lobe and part of the caudate lobe of the liver. **d. inci′sivus** [NA], incisive duct: a passage sometimes found in the incisive canal that interconnects the nasal and oral cavities during embryonic development; it occasionally fails to close. Called also *incisor canaliculis* and *incisor duct*. **d. interlobula′res**, ductuli interlobulares. **d. lacrima′les**, canaliculus lacrimalis. **d. lactif′eri** [NA], lactiferous ducts: channels conveying the milk secreted by the lobes of the breast to and through the nipples; called also *mammary ducts*. **d. lingua′lis**, a depression on the dorsum of the tongue, at the apex of the terminal sulcus. **d. lo′bi cauda′ti dex′ter** [NA], the right duct of the caudate lobe of the liver. **d. lo′bi cauda′ti sinis′ter** [NA], the left duct of the caudate lobe of the liver. **d. lymphat′icus dex′ter** [NA], right lymphatic duct: a vessel draining the lymph from the upper right side of the body, receiving lymph from the right subclavian, jugular, and mediastinal trunks when those vessels do not open independently into the right brachiocephalic vein. **d. mesoneph′ricus** [NA], mesonephric duct: an embryonic duct which initiated in association with rudiments of the pronephric kidney, is taken over as excretory duct by the mesonephros, and develops into the epididymis, the ductus deferens and its ampulla, the seminal vesicles, and the ejaculatory duct in the male and into vestigial structures in the female. Called also *d. Wolffi, wolffian duct, duct of Wolff, Leydig's duct*, and *canal of Oken*. **d. Muel′leri**, ductus paramesonephricus. **d. nasolacrima′lis** [NA], nasolacrimal duct: the passage that conveys the tears from the lacrimal sac into the interior nasal meatus; called also *lacrimonasal* or *nasal duct*. **d. pancrea′ticus** [NA], pancreatic duct: the main excretory duct of the pancreas, which usually unites with the common bile duct before entering the duodenum at the major duodenal papilla; called also *duct* or *canal of Wirsung*, and *hepatopancreatic duct*. **d. pancrea′ticus accesso′rius** [NA], accessory pancreatic duct: a small inconstant duct draining a part of the head of the pancreas into the minor duodenal papilla; called also *minor pancreatic duct*, and *duct of Santorini* or *Bernard*. **d. paramesoneph′ricus** [NA], paramesonephric duct: either of the paired embryonic ducts arising as a peritoneal pocket, extending caudally to join the urogenital sinus, and developing into uterine tubes, uterus, and vagina in the female and into a vestigial structure (appendix testis) in the male. Called also *d. Muelleri, duct of Müller* or *müllerian duct*, and *gasserian* or *primordial duct*. **d. paraurethra′les** [NA], paraurethral ducts: inconstantly present ducts in the female, which drain a group of the urethral glands into the vestibule; called also *Guérin's glands, Schüller's ducts, Skene's ducts* or *glands*, and *paraurethral glands*. **d. paroti′deus** [NA], parotid duct: the duct that drains the parotid gland and empties into the oral cavity opposite the second superior molar; called also *Blasius' duct, Stensen's canal* or *duct*, and *duct* or *canal of Steno*. **patent d. arteriosus**, see *d. arteriosus, patent*. **d. perilymphat′ici** [NA], perilymphatic duct: a small canal that connects the scala tympani with the subarachnoid space. Called also *aqueductus cochleae* [NA alternative]. **d. prostat′ici**, ductuli prostatici. **d. reu′niens** [NA], a small canal leading from the saccule to the cochlear duct; called also *canalis reuniens, Hensen's canal* or *duct*, and *Reichert's canal*. **reversed d. arteriosus**, see *d. arteriosus, reversed*. **d. semicircula′res** [NA], semicircular ducts: the long ducts of the membranous labyrinth of the ear, corresponding to the semicircular canals of the bony labyrinth and designated anterior, posterior, and lateral, according to the canal they occupy. Their diameter is only one-fourth that of the bony canals containing them, and each is affixed by one wall to the endosteal lining of the canal. They give information about angular acceleration and deceleration. Called also *membranous semicircular canal*. **d. semicircula′ris ante′rior** [NA], anterior semicircular duct: the semicircular duct occupying the anterior semicircular canal; called also *d. semicircularis superior*, or *superior semicircular duct*. See *ductus semicirculares*. **d. semicircula′ris latera′lis** [NA], lateral semicircular duct: the semicircular duct occupying the lateral semicircular canal; see *ductus semicirculares*. **d. semicircula′ris poste′rior** [NA], posterior semicircular duct: the semicircular duct occupying the posterior semicircular canal; see *ductus semicirculares*. **d. semicircula′ris supe′rior**, d. semicircularis anterior. **d. spermat′icus**, d. deferens. **d. sublingua′lis ma′jor** [NA], major sublingual duct: the duct that drains the sublingual gland and opens alongside the submandibular duct on the sublingual caruncle; called also *Bartholin's duct*. **d. sublingua′les mino′res** [NA], minor sublingual ducts: the ducts that drain the sublingual gland and open along the crest of the sublingual fold; called also *canals* or *ducts of Rivinus*, and *Walther's ducts*. **d. submandibula′ris** [NA], **d. submaxilla′ris [Wharto′ni]**, submandibular duct: the duct that drains the submandibular gland and opens at the sublingual caruncle; called also *submaxillary duct of Wharton*, and *Wharton's duct*. **d. sudorif′erus** [NA], sudoriferous duct: the duct that leads from the body of a sweat gland to the surface of the skin; called also *sweat duct*. **d. thora′cicus** [NA], thoracic duct: the vessel that ascends from the cisterna chyli to the junction of the left subclavian and left internal jugular veins; it acts as a channel for the collection of the lymph from the portions of the body below the diaphragm and from the left side of the body above the diaphragm. Called also *alimentary* or *chyliferous duct, left lymphatic duct, duct of Pecquet*, and *Van Hoorne's canal*. **d. thora′cicus dex′ter** [NA], right thoracic duct: a lymphatic channel formed by union of the right jugular, subclavian, and bronchomediastinal trunks and opening into the right brachiocephalic vein. **d. thyroglos′sus** [NA], thyroglossal duct: a duct in the embryo extending between the thyroid primordium and the posterior part of the tongue; called also *duct of His* or *Vater, Bochdalek's duct, His' canal*, and *thyrolingual duct*. **d. utriculosaccula′ris** [NA], utriculosaccular duct: a narrow duct uniting the utricle and saccule of the membranous labyrinth; called also *sacculoutricular duct* or *canal* and *utriculosaccular canal*. **d. veno′sus** [NA], a major blood channel that develops through the embryonic liver from the left umbilical vein to the inferior vena cava; called also *canal* or *duct of Arantius, canal of Cuvier*, and *ductus Arantii*. **d. Wolf′fi**, ductus mesonephricus.

Duddell's membrane (dud′elz) [Benedict *Duddell*, English physician of the 18th century] lamina limitans posterior corneae.

Dugas' test (sign) (doo′gahz) [Louis Alexander *Dugas*, American physician, 1806–1884] see under *tests*.

Duhot's line (dŭ-hōz′) [Robert *Duhot*, urologist and dermatologist in Brussels, born 1867] see under *line*.

Duhring's disease (du′rings) [Louis Adolphus *Duhring*, dermatologist in Philadelphia, 1845–1913] dermatitis herpetiformis.

Dührssen's incisions, operation (dēr′senz) [Alfred *Dührssen*, German gynecologist, 1862–1933] see under *incision* and *operation*.

Dujarier's clasp (du-zah-re-az′) see under *clasp*.

Duke's method, test (dūks) [William Waddell *Duke*, pathologist in Kansas City, Missouri, 1883–1945] see *bleeding time*, under *time*, and see under *tests*.

Dukes' disease (dūks) [Clement *Dukes*, English physician, 1845–1925] exanthema subitum.

Dulbecco (dūl-bāk′o) Renato. Italian-born American (biologist) born 1914; co-winner, with David Baltimore and Howard Temin, of the Nobel prize in medicine and physiology for 1975, for discoveries concerning the interaction between tumor viruses and the genetic material of host cells and the role of reverse transcriptase.

dulcite, dulcitol (dul′sīt dul′sĭ-tol) [L. *dulcis* sweet] a polyhydric alcohol, $CH_2OH(CHOH)_4CH_2OH$, occurring in various plants.

dulcose (dul′kōs) dulcite.

dull (dul) not resonant on percussion.

dullness, dulness (dul′nes) diminished resonance on percussion; also a peculiar percussion sound which lacks the normal resonance. **Gerhardt's d.**, see under *triangle*. **Grocco's triangular d.**, Grocco's sign, def. 1. **postcardial d.** (*obs.*), dullness on percussion on the back over the site of the heart. **shifting d.**, dullness on abdominal percussion, the level of which shifts as the patient is rolled from side to side; indicative of free fluid in the abdominal cavity. **tympanitic d.**, resonance of a dull and diminished quality.

dulse (duls) a coarse red seaweed used as a food in Scotland and other northern countries.

dumas (du′mas) a native name for tubba in Ceylon.

dumb (dum) unable to speak; mute.

dumbbell (dum′bel) a dumbbell-shaped body; a mass consisting of two spherical portions connected by a narrow isthmus. **d's of Schäfer**, microscopic bodies found in striated muscular tissue.

dumbness (dum′nes) [L. *surditas*] mutism, or aphasia.

dummy (dum′e) 1. (Brit.) placebo. 2. pontic.

Dumontpallier's test (du″maw-pal-yāz′) [Victor Alphonse Amédée *Dumontpallier*, French physician, 1826–1899] see under *tests*.

dumping (dump′ing) see under *syndrome*.

Dunbar's serum (dun′barz) [William Phillips *Dunbar*, American physician, 1863–1922] see under *serum*.

Duncan's folds, position, ventricle (dun′kanz) [James Matthews *Duncan*, British gynecologist, 1826–1890] see under *fold* and *position*, and see *cavum septi pellucidi*.

Duncan's method (dun′kanz) [Charles H. *Duncan*, American physician, born 1880] autotherapy.

Dunfermline scale (dun-ferm′lin) [*Dunfermline*, a city in Scotland where the scheme was devised] see under *scale*.

Dunham's fans (cones, triangles) (dun′amz) [Henry Kennon *Dunham*, American physician, 1872–1944] see under *fan*.

duodenal (du″o-de′nal) of, pertaining to, or situated in, the duodenum.

duodenectomy (du″o-dĕ-nek′to-me) [*duodenum* + Gr. *ektomē* excision] excision of the duodenum, total or partial.

duodenitis (du″od-ĕ-ni′tis) inflammation of the duodenal mucosa.

duodeno- (du″o-de′no) [L. *duodeni* twelve] a combining form denoting relationship to the duodenum.

duodenocholangeitis (du″o-de″no-ko-lan″je-i′tis) inflammation of the duodenum and common bile duct.

duodenocholecystostomy (du″o-de″no-ko″le-sis-tos′to-me) surgical creation of a communication between the gallbladder and the duodenum.

duodenocholedochotomy (du″o-de″no-ko″led-o-kot′o-me) surgical incision of the duodenum and common bile duct.

duodenocolic (du″o-de″no-kol′ik) pertaining to the duodenum and colon.

duodenocystostomy (du″o-de″no-sis-tos′to-me) [*duodeno-* + Gr. *kystis* bladder + *stomoun* to provide with an opening or mouth] surgical formation of a communication between the duodenum and the gallbladder.

duodenoduodenostomy (du″o-de″no-du″o-de-nos′to-me) anastomosis of the two portions of a divided duodenum.

duodenoenterostomy (du″o-de″no-en″ter-os′to-me) surgical formation of a communication from the duodenum to another part of the small intestine.

duodenogram (du-od′ĕ-no-gram″) a roentgenogram of the duodenum.

duodenohepatic (du-od″ĕ-no″hĕ-pat′ik) pertaining to the duodenum and the liver.

duodenoileostomy (du″o-de″no-il″e-os′to-me) surgical formation of a communication between the duodenum and the ileum.

duodenojejunostomy (du″o-de″no-jĕ-joo-nos′to-me) surgical formation of a communication between the duodenum and the jejunum.

duodenolysis (du″o-dĕ-nol′ĭ-sis) the operation of loosening the duodenum from adhesions.

duodenopancreatectomy (du″o-de″no-pan″kre-ah-tek′to-me) pancreatoduodenectomy.

duodenorrhaphy (du″o-dĕ-nor′ah-fe) [*duodeno-* + Gr. *rhaphē* suture] the operation of suturing the duodenum.

duodenoscope (du″o-de′no-skōp) an endoscope for examining the duodenum.

duodenoscopy (du″od-ĕ-nos′ko-pe) [*duodeno-* + Gr. *skopein* to examine] endoscopic examination of the duodenum.

duodenostomy (du″od-ĕ-nos′to-me) [*duodeno-* + Gr. *stomoun* to provide with an opening or mouth] surgical formation of a permanent orifice into the duodenum.

duodenotomy (du″od-ĕ-not′o-me) [*duodeno-* + Gr. *tomē* a cutting] incision of the duodenum.

duodenum (du″o-de′num, du-od′ĕ-num) [L. *duode′ni* twelve at a time] [NA] the first or proximal portion of the small intestine, extending from the pylorus to the jejunum; so called because it is about 12 fingerbreadths in length.

duoparental (du″o-pah-ren′tal) [L. *duo* two + *parens* parent] pertaining to or derived from two parents or sexual elements.

Duphalac (du′fah-lak) trademark for a preparation of lactulose.

Duphaston (du-fas′ton) trademark for a preparation of dydrogesterone.

Duplay's bursitis (disease, syndrome) operation (doo-plāz′) [Simon Emanuel *Duplay*, French surgeon, 1836–1924] see under *bursitis* and *operation*.

duplication (du″plĭ-ka′shun) a doubling; in genetics, the presence of an extra segment of chromosome existing as a separate fragment or attached to a member of the normal chromosome complement. **incomplete d. of spinal cord**, diastematomyelia.

duplicitas (du-plis′ĭ-tas) [L.] a doubling, or duplication. **d. ante′rior**, katadidymus. **d. asym′metros**, heteropagus. **d. comple′ta**, a double monster in which each component is completely or almost completely developed. **d. crucia′ta**, conjoined twins with fused heads, each face being a joint product whose midplane forms a right angle with that of the body. **d. incomple′ta**, a double monster in which the two components are not completely developed. **d. infe′rior**, anadidymus. **d. me′dia**, a double monster in which the duplication is restricted to the middle region of the body. **d. paralle′la**, a double monster consisting of two components united in the sagittal plane. **d. poste′rior**, anadidymus. **d. supe′rior**, katadidymus. **d. sym′metros**, diplopagus.

duplitized (du′plĭ-tīzd) double coated; a term applied to x-ray films.

dupp (dup) a syllable used to represent the second sound of the heart in auscultation; it is shorter and higher pitched than the first sound. See *lubb* and *lubb-dupp*.

Dupré's disease, syndrome (du-prāz′) [Ernest Pierre *Dupré*, French physician, 1862–1921] meningism, def. 1.

Dupuy-Dutemps' operation (du-pue′-du-tahm′) [Louis *Dupuy-Dutemps*, Paris ophthalmologist, born 1871] see under *operation*.

Dupuytren's contracture, etc. (du-pwe-trahnz′) [Baron Guillaume *Dupuytren*, a celebrated French surgeon, 1777–1835] see under *amputation, contracture, enterotome, fracture, hydrocele, sign*, and *splint*.

dura (du′rah) [L. "hard"] dura mater.

Durabolin (du-rab′o-lin) trademark for a preparation of nandrolone phenpropionate.

Duracillin (du″rah-sil′in) trademark for preparations of penicillin G procaine.

dural (du′ral) pertaining to the dura mater.

dura mater (du′rah ma′ter) [L. "hard mother"] the outermost, toughest, and most fibrous of the three membranes (meninges) covering the brain and spinal cord; called also *pachymeninx*. **d. m. of brain, d. m. enceph′ali** [NA], the dura mater covering the brain, composed of two mostly fused layers: an endosteal outer layer (endocranium) adherent to the inner aspect of the cranial bones, and an inner, meningeal layer. Venous sinuses and the trigeminal ganglion are located between the layers. **d. m. of spinal cord, d. m. spina′lis** [NA], the dura mater covering the spinal cord; it is separated from the periosteum of the enclosing vertebrae by an epidural space containing blood vessels and fibrous and areolar tissue.

duramatral (du-rah-ma′tral) (*obs.*) dural.

Duran-Reynals' permeability factor [Francisco *Duran-Reynals*, American bacteriologist, 1899–1958] hyaluronidase.

Durand's disease (du-ranz′) [Paul *Durand*, French physician, born 1895] see under *disease*.

Durand-Nicolas-Favre disease [J. *Durand*, Joseph *Nicolas*, M. *Favre*, French physicians] lymphogranuloma venereum.

Duranest (du′rah-nest) trademark for a preparation of etidocaine hydrochloride.

durapatite (dur-ap′ah-tīt) chemical name: hydroxylapatite; a prosthetic aid, $Ca_5HO_{13}P_3$.

duraplasty (du′rah-plas-te) [*dura mater* + Gr. *plassein* to form] a plastic operation on the dura mater; graft of the dura.

Dürck's nodes (derks) [Hermann *Dürck*, Munich pathologist, born 1869] see under *node*.

Dur. dolor. abbreviation for L. *duran′te dolo′re*, while the pain lasts.

Duret's lesion (du-rāz′) [Henri *Duret*, French neurological surgeon, 1849–1921] see under *lesion*.

Durham decision (dur′ham) see under *decision*.

Durham's tube (dur′hamz) [1. Arthur Edward *Durham*, English surgeon, 1834–1895. 2. Herbert Edward *Durham*, English bacteriologist, 1866–1945] see under *tube*.

duroarachnitis (du″ro-ar″ak-ni′tis) inflammation of the dura mater and arachnoid.

Duroziez' disease, murmur (sign) (du-ro″ze-ez′) [Paul Louis *Duroziez*, French physician, 1826–1897] see under *disease* and *murmur*.

dust (dust) fine, dry particles of earth or any other substance small enough to be blown by the wind. **blood d. (of Müller)**, hemokonia. **chromatin d.**, small red granules, smaller than Howell's bodies, sometimes seen at the periphery of stained erythrocytes. **ear d.**, statoconia.

Dutton's disease, relapsing fever, spirochete (dut′unz) [Joseph Everett *Dutton*, English physician, 1877–1905] see *trypanosomiasis* and *Borrelia duttonii*, and see under *fever*.

Duttonella (dut-o-nel′ah) [J. Everett *Dutton*] *Trypanosoma*.

Duval's nucleus (du-valz′) [Mathias Marie *Duval*, French anatomist, 1844–1907] see under *nucleus*.

Duverney's foramen, gland (du-ver-nāz′) [Joseph Guichard *Duverney*, French anatomist, 1648–1730] see *foramen epiploicum* and *glandula bulbourethralis*.

d.v. double vibrations (a unit for the measurement of the frequency of sound waves).

D.V.M Doctor of Veterinary Medicine. Also abbreviated V.M.D.

dwale (dwāl) belladonna leaf.

dwarf (dwarf) an abnormally undersized person. **achondroplastic d.**, a type of dwarf, having a relatively large head with saddle nose and brachycephaly, short extremities, and usually lordosis; see also *achondroplasia*. **Amsterdam d.**, a dwarf affected with de Lange's syndrome. **asexual d.**, an adult dwarf with deficient sexual development. **ateliotic d.**, a dwarf whose skeleton is infantile with persistent nonunion between epiphyses and diaphyses. **bird-headed d., bird-headed d. of Seckel**, a dwarf with a proportionately small head, a narrow birdlike face with a beaklike protrusion of the nose, large eyes, antimongoloid slant of the palpebral fissures, and receding lower jaw; called also *nanocephalic d.* **Brissaud's d.**, one with infantile myxedema. **cretin d.**, a thyroid-deficient dwarf; see *cretinism*. Called also *hypothyroid d.* **diastrophic d.**, a dwarf with progressive structural deformities of the bones and joints, including scoliosis, bilateral clubfoot, deformity of the thumb, micromelia, joint contractures and subluxations, malformation of the pinna with calcification of the cartilage, premature calcification of the costal cartilages, and cleft palate. **geleophysic d.**, a dwarf with a peculiar but pleasant facial appearance and bone

dysplasia, especially of the hands and feet. **hypophyseal d.**, pituitary d. **hypothyroid d.**, cretin d. **infantile d.**, a person with marked retardation of mental and physical development. **Levi-Lorain d.**, pituitary d. **micromelic d.**, a dwarf with very small limbs. **nanocephalic d.**, bird-headed d. **normal d.**, a person who is abnormally undersized, but is perfectly formed. **Paltauf's d.**, pituitary d. **phocomelic d.**, a dwarf in whom the diaphyses of the long bones are abnormally short. **physiologic d.**, normal d. **pituitary d.**, a dwarf whose retarded development is due to hypofunction of the anterior pituitary; called also *hypophyseal d., Levi-Lorain d.*, and *Paltauf's d.* **primordial d., pure d.**, normal d. **rachitic d.**, a person dwarfed by rickets, having a high forehead with prominent bosses, bent long bones, and Harrison's sulcus or groove. **renal d.**, a dwarf whose failure to achieve normal bone maturation is due to renal failure. **Russell d.**, see under *syndrome*. **sexual d.**, a dwarf with normal sexual development. **Silver d.**, see under *syndrome*. **thanatophoric d.**, a micromelic dwarf having very short ribs and bones of the extremities, and vertebral bodies that are greatly reduced in height with wide intervertebral spaces; death usually occurs in the first few hours of life. **true d.**, normal d.

dwarfism (dwarf′izm) the state of being a dwarf; underdevelopment of body. See various forms under *dwarf*. **deprivation d.**, lack of growth due to psychosocial upset, with resumption of growth when the source of stress is removed; it is believed to be due to cessation of secretion of the growth-hormone releasing factor. Called also *maternal deprivation syndrome*. **Robinow d.**, see under *syndrome*.

Dy chemical symbol for *dysprosium*.

dyad (di′ad) a double chromosome resulting from the halving of a tetrad.

dyaster (di′as-ter) amphiaster.

Dyclone (di′klōn) trademark for preparations of dyclonine hydrochloride.

dyclonine hydrochloride (di′klo-nēn) [USP] chemical name: 1-(4-butoxyphenyl)-3-(1-piperidinyl)-1-propanone. A local anesthetic having significant bactericidal and fungicidal activity, $C_{18}H_{27}NO_2 \cdot HCl$, occurring as a white, crystalline powder or as white crystals; applied topically to the skin and mucous membranes.

dydrogesterone (di″dro-jes′ter-ōn) [USP] chemical name: (9β,10α)-pregna-4,6-diene-3,20-dione. An orally effective, synthetic progestin, $C_{21}H_{28}O_2$, occurring as a white to pale yellow, crystalline powder; used mainly in the diagnosis and treatment of primary amenorrhea and severe dysmenorrhea, and in combination with estrogen in dysfunctional menorrhagia.

dye (di) any of various colored substances that contain auxochromes and thus are capable of coloring substances to which they are applied; used for staining and coloring, as test reagents, and as therapeutic agents in medicine. **acid d., acidic d.**, one which is acidic in reaction and usually unites with positively charged ions of the material acted upon; called also *anionic d.* **amphoteric d.**, one containing both reactive basic and reactive acidic groups, and staining both acidic and basic elements. **anionic d.**, acid d. **basic d.**, one which is basic in reaction and unites with negatively charged ions of material acted upon; called also *cationic d.* **cationic d.**, basic d. **metachromatic d.**, a dye that stains tissues two or more colors. **orthochromatic d.**, a dye that stains tissues a single color. **vital d.**, one that penetrates living cells and colors certain structures, without serious injury to the cells.

Dymelor (di′mě-lor) trademark for a preparation of acetohexamide.

dynamic (di-nam′ik) [Gr. *dynamis* power] pertaining to or manifesting force.

dynamics (di-nam′iks) that phase of mechanics which deals with the motions of material bodies taking place under different specific conditions.

dynamization (di″nam-i-za′shun) (*obs.*) the hypothetical increase of medicinal effectiveness by dilution and trituration.

dynamo- (di′nah-mo) [Gr. *dynamis* power] a combining form denoting relationship to power or strength.

dynamogenesis (di″nah-mo-jen′ĕ-sis) [*dynamo-* + Gr. *genesis* production] the development of energy or force, as in muscle or nerves.

dynamogenic (di″nah-mo-jen′ik) [*dynamo-* + Gr. *gennan* to produce] producing or favoring the development of power; pertaining to the development of power, as in muscle or nerves.

dynamogeny (di-nah-moj′ĕ-ne) dynamogenesis.

dynamograph (di-nam′o-graf) [*dynamo-* + Gr. *graphein* to write] a self-registering dynamometer.

dynamometer (di″nah-mom′ĕ-ter) [*dynamo-* + Gr. *metron* measure] an instrument for measuring the force of muscular contraction. **squeeze d.**, one by which the grip of the hand is measured.

dynamoneure (di-nam′o-nūr) [*dynamo-* + Gr. *neuron* nerve] a spinal neuron connected with the muscles; a spinal motoneuron.

dynamopathic (di-nam″o-path′ik) [*dynamo-* + Gr. *pathos* disease] affecting function; functional.

dynamophore (di-nam′o-fōr) [*dynamo-* + Gr. *phoros* carrying] food or any substance that supplies energy to the body.

dynamoscope (di-nam′o-skop) [*dynamo-* + Gr. *skopein* to examine] a device for performing dynamoscopy.

dynamoscopy (di″nah-mos′ko-pe) the observation of the performance of function by an organ or structure, as of muscle action or of kidney function by ureteral catheterization.

Dynapen (di′nah-pen) trademark for a preparation of dicloxacillin sodium.

dyne (dīn) the C.G.S. unit of force, being that amount of force which, when acting continuously upon a mass of 1 gram, will impart to it an acceleration of 1 cm. per second per second.

dynein (di′ne-in) a protein from the microtubules of cilia and flagella; which functions as an ATP-splitting enzyme, and is essential to the motility of cilia and flagella.

dyphylline (di-fil′in) chemical name: 7-(2,3-dihydroxypropyl)-3,7-dihydro-1,3-dimethyl-1*H*-purine-2,6-dione. A theophylline derivative, $C_{10}H_{14}N_4O_4$, occurring as a white, amorphous powder, having the peripheral vasodilator, bronchodilator, diuretic, and myocardial stimulant effects of the parent compound; used chiefly in the treatment of acute bronchial asthma and reversible bronchospasm associated with chronic bronchitis and emphysema; administered orally or intramuscularly. Called also *glyphylline* and *hyphylline*.

Dyrenium (di-ren′ĭ-um) trademark for a preparation of triamterene.

dys- [Gr. *dys-*] a combining form signifying difficult, painful, bad, disordered, abnormal; the opposite of *eu-*.

dysacousia (dis″ah-koo′ze-ah) [*dys-* + Gr. *akousis* hearing + *-ia*] dysacusis.

dysacousis (dis″ah-koo′sis) dysacusis.

dysacousma (dis″ah-kōōs′mah) dysacusis.

dysacusis (dis″ah-koo′sis) [*dys-* + Gr. *akousis* hearing] 1. a hearing impairment in which there is distortion of frequency or intensity. 2. a condition in which certain sounds produce discomfort; called also *auditory dysesthesia*.

dysadaptation (dis″ad-ap-ta′shun) dysaptation.

dysadrenalism (dis″ad-re′nal-izm) any disorder of adrenal function, whether of decreased function (hypoadrenalism, hypoadrenocorticism) or heightened function (hyperadrenalism, hyperadrenocorticism).

dysadrenia (dis″ad-re′ne-ah) dysadrenalism.

dysallilognathia (dis-al″il-lo-na′the-ah) a condition characterized by disproportion of the maxilla and mandible.

dysanagnosia (dis″an-ag-no′se-ah) a form of dyslexia in which certain words cannot be recognized.

dysantigraphia (dis″an-te-gra′fe-ah) loss of power to copy writing; it is due to a lesion of the association path between the word-seeing center and the word-writing center.

dysaphia (dis-a′fe-ah) [*dys-* + Gr. *haphē* touch] impairment of the sense of touch.

dysaptation (dis″ap-ta′shun) defective power of accommodation of the iris and retina to light variations.

dysarteriotony (dis-ar-te″re-ot′o-ne) [*dys-* + Gr. *artēria* artery + *tonos* tension] abnormality of blood pressure.

dysarthria (dis-ar′thre-ah) [*dys-* + Gr. *arthroun* to utter distinctly + *-ia*] imperfect articulation of speech due to disturbances of muscular control which result from damage to the central or peripheral nervous system. Cf. *anarthria*. **d. litera′lis,** stuttering. **d. syllaba′ris spasmod′ica,** stuttering.

dysarthric (dis-ar′thrik) characterized by or pertaining to dysarthria.

dysarthrosis (dis″ar-thro′sis) [*dys-* + Gr. *arthrōsis* joint] 1. deformity or malformation of a joint. 2. dysarthria.

dysautonomia (dis″aw-to-no′me-ah) [*dys-* + Gr. *autonomia* freedom to use its own laws] a hereditary condition characterized by defective lacrimation, skin blotching, emotional instability, motor incoordination, total absence of pain sensation, and hyporeflexia; seen almost exclusively in Jews, it is transmitted as an autosomal recessive trait. Called also *familial autonomic dysfunction* and *Riley-Day syndrome*.

dysbarism (dis′bar-izm) a general term applied to any clinical syndrome caused by difference between the surrounding atmospheric pressure and the total gas pressure in the various tissues, fluids, and cavities of the body, including such conditions as barotitis media, barosinusitis, or expansion of gases in the hollow viscera.

dysbasia (dis-ba′ze-ah) [*dys-* + Gr. *basis* step] difficulty in walking, especially that due to nervous lesion. **d. angiosclerot′ica, d. angiospas′tica, d. intermit′tens angiosclerot′ica** (*obs.*), intermittent claudication. **d. lordot′ica progressi′va,** dystonia musculorium deformans. **d. neurasthen′ica intermit′tens,** distorted walking of psychologic origin.

dysbetalipoproteinemia (dis-ba″tah-lip″o-pro″te-in-e′me-ah) the accumulation of abnormal β-lipoproteins in the blood. **familial d.,** familial hyperlipoproteinemia, type III.

dysbolism (dis′bo-lizm) [*dys-* + *metabolism*] a condition arising from an error in metabolism not necessarily of a disease nature, as in incomplete oxidation of tyrosine, giving a reddish color to the urine.

dysboulia (dis-bu′le-ah) dysbulia.

dysboulic (dis-bu′lik) dysbulic.

dysbulia (dis-bu′le-ah) [*dys-* + Gr. *boulē* will + *-ia*] abnormal weakness or disturbance of the will (volition).

dysbulic (dis-bu′lik) pertaining to or characterized by dysbulia.

dyscalculia (dis″kal-ku′le-ah) impairment of the ability to do mathematical problems because of brain injury or disease.

dyscephaly (dis-sef′ah-le) malformation of the cranium and bones of the face. **mandibulo-oculofacial d.,** oculomandibulofacial syndrome.

dyschesia (dis-ke′se-ah) dyschezia.

dyschezia (dis-ke′ze-ah) [*dys-* + Gr. *chezein* to go to stool + *-ia*] difficult or painful evacuation of feces from the rectum.

dyschiasia (dis-ki-a′se-ah) any disorder of sense localization.

dyschiria (dis-ki′re-ah) [*dys-* + Gr. *cheir* hand + *-ia*] derangement of the power to tell which side of the body has been touched; see *achiria*, *allochiria*, and *synchiria*.

dyscholia (dis-ko′le-ah) [*dys-* + Gr. *cholē* bile + *-ia*] a disordered condition of the bile.

dyschondroplasia (dis″kon-dro-pla′ze-ah) [*dys-* + Gr. *chondros* cartilage + *plassein* to form + *-ia*] enchondromatosis.

dyschondrosteosis (dis″kon-dros″te-o′sis) a form of dyschondroplasia that may produce micromelia.

dyschromasia (dis″kro-ma′ze-ah) dyschromatopsia.

dyschromatopsia (dis″kro-mah-top′se-ah) [*dys-* + Gr. *chrōma* color + *opsis* vision + *-ia*] disorder of color vision.

dyschromia (dis-kro′me-ah) [*dys-* + Gr. *chrōma* color] any disorder of pigmentation of the skin or hair.

dyschronism (dis-kro′nizm) separate in time; disturbance of any time relation.

dyschylia (dis-ki′le-ah) disorder of the chyle.

dyscinesia (dis-si-ne′se-ah) dyskinesia.

dyscoimesis (dis″koi-me′sis) dyskoimesis.

dyscoria (dis-ko′re-ah) [*dys-* + Gr. *korē* pupil] abnormality of the form or shape of the pupil or in the reaction of the two pupils.

dyscorticism (dis-kor′tĭ-sizm) disordered functioning of the adrenal cortex.

dyscrasia (dis-kra′ze-ah) [Gr. *dyskrasia* bad temperament] a term formerly used to indicate a depraved state of the humors, now used generally to indicate a morbid condition, especially one which involves an imbalance of component elements. **blood d.,** any abnormal or pathological condition of the blood. **lymphatic d.,** 1. lymphatism (2nd def.). 2. Hodgkin's disease.

dyscrasic (dis-kra′sik) dyscratic.

dyscratic (dis-krat′ik) [Gr. *dyskratos*] pertaining to or characterized by dyscrasia.

dyscrinism (dis-kri′nizm) [*dys-* + Gr. *krinein* to separate] (*obs.*) endocrine disorder; perversion of the secretion of any endocrine gland or the state resulting from such perversion.

dysdiadochocinesia (dis″di-ad″ŏ-ko″si-ne′se-ah) dysdiadochokinesia.

dysdiadochocinetic (dis″di-ad″ŏ-ko-si-net′ik) dysdiadochokinetic.

dysdiadochokinesia (dis″di-ad″ŏ-ko-ki-ne′se-ah) derangement of the function of diadochokinesia.

dysdiadochokinetic (dis″di-ad″ŏ-ko-ki-net′ik) pertaining to or characterized by dysdiadochokinesia.

dysdipsia (dis-dip′se-ah) [*dys-* + Gr. *dipsa* thirst] difficulty in drinking.

dysecoia (dis″ĕ-koi′ah) dysacusis.

dysembryoma (dis-em″bre-o′mah) teratoma.

dysembryoplasia (dis-em″bre-o-pla′se-ah) [*dys-* + Gr. *embryon* embryo + *plasis* formation + *-ia*] malformation occurring during embryonic life.

dysemia (dis-e′me-ah) [*dys-* + Gr. *haima* blood + *-ia*] (*obs.*) disorder of the blood.

dysencephalia splanchnocystica (dis-en″sĕ-fa′le-ah splank″no-sis′tĭ-kah) Meckel's syndrome.

dysendocrinia (dis-en″do-krin′e-ah) (*obs.*) dysendocrisiasis.

dysendocriniasis (dis-en″do-krĭ-ni′ah-sis) (*obs.*) dysendocrisiasis.

dysendocrinism (dis″en-dok′rĭ-nizm) (*obs.*) dysendocrisiasis.

dysendocrisiasis (dis-en″do-kris-i′ah-sis) [*dys-* + Gr. *endon* within + *krinein* to separate] (*obs.*) disorder of hormonal secretions.

dysenteric (dis″en-ter′ik) pertaining to or of the nature of dysentery.

dysenteriform (dis″en-ter′ĭ-form) resembling dysentery.

dysentery (dis′en-ter″e) [L. *dysenteria*, from Gr. *dys-* + *enteron* intestine] a term given to a number of disorders marked by inflammation of the intestines, especially of the colon, and attended by pain in the abdomen, tenesmus, and frequent stools containing blood and mucus. The causative agent may be chemical irritants, bacteria, protozoa, or parasitic worms. There are two specific varieties, the *amebic* and the *bacillary*. **amebic d.,** dysentery due to ulceration of the bowel caused by invasion of the mucosa by *Entamoeba histolytica;* called also *intestinal amebiasis* and *amebic colitis.* **asylum d.,** dysentery occurring in a closed community. **bacillary d.,** an infectious disease caused by bacteria of the genus *Shigella*, and marked by intestinal pain, tenesmus, diarrhea with mucus and blood in the stools, and more or less toxemia; it is especially prevalent in tropical countries, but it frequently occurs elsewhere. Called also *Flexner's d.* and *Japanese d.* **balantidial d.,** dysentery caused by *Balantidium coli.* **bilharzial d.,** dysentery caused by the parasitic worm *Schistosoma haematobium* (*Bilharzia haematobia*). **catarrhal d.,** sprue, def. 1. **chronic d. of cattle,** Johne's disease. **ciliary d., ciliate d.,** dysentery due to ciliate organisms, such as *Balantidium coli.* **epidemic d.,** a variety that becomes epidemic and is often fatal. **flagellate d.,** dysentery due to a flagellate organism, such as *Giardia lamblia* or *Trichomonas.* **Flexner's d.,** bacillary d. **fulminant d.,** bacillary dysentery marked by collapse and toxemia and followed by death. **giardiasis d.,** giardiasis. **institutional d.,** bacillary dysentery affecting patients in an institution, especially in mental hospitals. **Japanese d.,** bacillary d. **lamb d.,** a highly fatal form of enterotoxemia affecting young lambs, caused by *Clostridium perfringens* type B, and marked by ulcerative inflammation of the intestine and fetid diarrhea, sometimes tinged with blood; it is also frequently seen in young foals and calves. **malarial d.,** that which is complicated with intermittent febrile attacks. **malignant d.,** a form in which the symptoms are all very intense and progress rapidly to a fatal ending. **protozoal d.,** amebic and balantidial dysentery. **schistosomal d.,** dysentery accompanying intestinal schistosomiasis. **scorbutic d.,** that which is an accompaniment of scurvy. **Sonne d.,** bacillary dysentery occurring in temperate regions, caused by group D dysentery bacillus, *Shigella sonnei.* **spirillar d.,** dysentery caused by spirilla in the intestines. **sporadic d.,** dysentery occurring in scattered cases that have apparently no connection. **swine d.,** a contagious form of enteritis due to *Vibrio coli*, marked by grayish feces. **viral d.,** a virus-caused dysentery occurring in epidemics and marked by acute watery diarrhea. **winter d.,** see under *scours.*

dysequilibrium (dis″e-kwĭ-lib′re-um) any derangement of proper balance.

dyserethesia (dis″er-e-the′ze-ah) [*dys-* + Gr. *erethizein* to irritate] impairment of sensibility to stimuli.

dyserethism (dis-er′e-thizm) dyserethesia.

dysergasia (dis″er-ga′ze-ah) [*dys-* + Gr. *ergon* work] Meyer's term for a behavior disorder due to defective brain support and including disorientative and hallucinatory states and delirious reactions.

dysergastic (dis″er-gas′tik) Meyer's term for psychic disorders due to inadequate support or metabolism of the brain (disorientation, hallucination, fears, dreamy states, etc.).

dysergia (dis-er′je-ah) [*dys-* + Gr. *ergon* work] motor incoordination due to defect of efferent nerve impulse.

dysesthesia (dis″es-the′ze-ah) [*dys-* + Gr. *aisthēsis* perception] 1. impairment of any sense, especially of that of touch. 2. an unpleasant abnormal sensation produced by normal stimuli. **auditory d.,** dysacusis (def. 2).

dysesthetic (dis″es-thet′ik) pertaining to or characterized by dysesthesia.

dysfunction (dis-funk′shun) disturbance, impairment, or abnormality of the functioning of an organ. **constitutional hepatic d.,** Gilbert's disease. **constitutional d. of liver,** Gilbert's disease. **minimal brain d.,** a diagnostic term for children and adolescents who have some central nervous system deficits which affect their behavior and ability to learn; they exhibit hyperkinesis, distractability, emotional lability, poor coordination, but have normal or above normal intelligence and no signs of major neurologic or psychiatric disturbance. **d. of uterus,** inertia uteri.

dysgalactia (dis″gah-lak′te-ah) [*dys-* + Gr. *gala* milk] disordered milk secretion.

dysgammaglobulinemia (dis-gam″mah-glob″u-lĭ-ne′me-ah) an immunological deficiency state characterized by selective deficiencies of one or more, but not all, classes of immunoglobulins, resulting in heightened susceptibility to infectious diseases vulnerable to immunoglobulin-associated defense mechanisms. It may result from failure of synthesis or functional abnormality of immunoglobulins. The dysgammaglobulinemias have been classified into seven types. Cf. *agammaglobulinemia.*

dysgenesia (dis″jĕ-ne′ze-ah) [*dys-* + Gr. *gennan* to generate + *-ia*] impairment of the powers of procreation.

dysgenesis (dis-jen′ĕ-sis) defective development. **epiphyseal d.,** a condition in which epiphyseal centers may be irregularly formed or appear to be fragmented or stippled. **gonadal d.,** a general term for a variety of gonadal developmental anomalies, including gonadal aplasia, Turner's syndrome, hermaphroditism, and pseudohermaphroditism. **mixed gonadal d.,** a condition in which there is a testis on one side and a streak gonad on the other; those affected typically show some degree of virilization and ambiguous genitalia, and a uterus, vagina, and at least one fallopian tube are usually present. The most common karyotype is a mosaic, 45,XO/46,XY. **seminiferous tubule d.,** Klinefelter's syndrome.

dysgenic (dis-jen′ik) detrimental to the race or tending to counteract race improvement.

dysgenics (dis-jen′iks) [*dys-* + Gr. *gennan* to produce] the study of racial deterioration. Cf. *eugenics.*

dysgenitalism (dis-jen′ĭ-tal-izm) an abnormality of genital development, as eunuchism.

dysgenopathy (dis″jen-op′ah-the) [*dys-* + Gr. *gennan* to produce + *pathos* disease] a disorder of bodily development.

dysgerminoma (dis″jer-mĭ-no′mah) [*dys-* + *germ* + *-oma*] a malignant ovarian neoplasm, thought to be derived from primordial germ cells of the sexually undifferentiated embryonic gonad; it is the counterpart of the classical seminoma (q.v.) of the testis, to which it is both grossly and histologically identical. Called also *ovarian seminoma.*

dysgeusia (dis-gu′ze-ah) [*dys-* + Gr. *geusis* taste] perversion of the sense of taste.

dysglandular (dis-glan′du-lar) due to or marked by disordered functioning of glands, particularly the endocrine glands.

dysglobulinemia (dis-glob″u-lin-e′me-ah) [*dys-* + *globulin* + Gr. *haima* blood + *-ia*] any disorder of the blood globulins.

dysglycemia (dis″gli-se′me-ah) [*dys-* + Gr. *glykys* sweet + *haima* blood + *-ia*] any derangement of the sugar content of the blood.

dysgnathia (dis-na′the-ah) any oral abnormality extending beyond the teeth to involve the maxilla or mandible, or both, as opposed to eugnathia.

dysgnathic (dis-nath′ik) [*dys-* + Gr. *gnathos* jaw] pertaining to or characterized by abnormality of the maxilla and mandible.

dysgnosia (dis-no′se-ah) [Gr. *dysgnōsia* difficulty of knowing] any disorder of intellectual function.

dysgonesis (dis″go-ne′sis) [*dys-* + Gr. *gonē* seed] a functional disorder of the genital organs.

dysgonic (dis-gon′ik) seeding badly; said of bacterial cultures that grow poorly on culture media.

dysgrammatism (dis-gram′ah-tizm) partial impairment of the ability to speak grammatically because of brain injury or disease.

dysgraphia (dis-gra′fe-ah) [*dys-* + Gr. *graphein* to write] inability to write properly; it may be part of a language disorder caused by a disturbance of the parietal lobe or of the motor system. Called also *status dysgraphicus.*

dyshematopoiesis (dis-hem″ah-to″poi-e′sis) defective blood formation.

dyshematopoietic (dis-hem″ah-to-poi-et′ik) pertaining to or characterized by dyshematopoiesis.

dyshemopoiesis (dis-he″mo-poi-e′sis) dyshematopoiesis.

dyshemopoietic (dis-he″mo-poi-et′ik) dyshematopoietic.

dyshepatia (dis-hĕ-pa′she-ah) [*dys-* + Gr. *hēpar* liver] disordered liver function. **lipogenic d.,** a liver disorder of children due to excessive fats in the diet.

dyshesion (dis-he′shun) [*dys-* + L. *haesio*, from *haerere* to stick] 1. disordered cell adherence. 2. loss of intercellular cohesion, a characteristic of malignancy, as determined by aspiration biopsy cytology.

dyshidrosis (dis-hid-ro′sis) [*dys-* + Gr. *hidrōsis* a sweating] 1. pompholyx. 2. any disorder of the eccrine sweat glands.

dyshormonal (dis-hōr′mo-nal) due to hormone or endocrine disturbance.

dyshormonic (dis-hōr-mon′ik) dyshormonal.

dyshormonism (dis-hōr′mōn-izm) disturbance of the hormone secretions.

dyshydrosis (dis-hid-ro′sis) dyshidrosis.

dyshypophysia (dis″hi-po-fiz′e-ah) (*obs.*) dyspituitarism.

dyshypophysism (dis″hi-pof′ĭ-sizm) (*obs.*) dyspituitarism.

dysidrosis (dis-id-ro′sis) dyshidrosis.

dysimmunity (dis-ĭ-mu′nĭ-te) disordered or misdirected immunity.

dysinsulinism (dis-in′su-lin-izm) (*obs.*) a condition caused by disordered secretion of insulin.

dysinsulinosis (dis-in″su-lĭ-no′sis) (*obs.*) dysinsulinism.

dysjunction (dis-junk′shun) see *disjunction.*

dyskaryosis (dis-kar′e-o′sis) abnormal changes in cell nuclei, such as those observed in epithelial cells of the cervix during pregnancy.

dyskaryotic (dis″kar-e-ot′ik) [*dys-* + Gr. *karyon* nucleus] pertaining to, characterized by, or promoting dyskaryosis.

dyskeratoma (dis″ker-ah-to′mah) a dyskeratotic tumor. **warty d.,** a solitary brownish red nodule with a soft, yellowish, central keratotic plug, most commonly occurring on the face, neck, scalp, or axilla, or in the mouth; histologically it resembles an individual lesion of keratosis follicularis.

dyskeratosis (dis″ker-ah-to′sis) abnormal, premature, or imperfect keratinization of the keratinocytes. **d. congen′ita,** a rare congenital syndrome, probably transmitted as a sex-linked recessive trait, consisting of atrophy and pigmentation of the skin, nail dystrophy, and leukoplakia; carcinoma may supervene and blood dyscrasias are common. **hereditary benign intra-epithelial d.,** a congenital hereditary disease, transmitted as an autosomal dominant trait, characterized by foamy gelatinous plaques on the conjunctiva and white thickenings resembling leukoplakia on the oral mucosa; photophobia is common in children, and blindness may occur. Called also *Witkop's* or *Witkop-Von Sallmann disease.*

dyskeratotic (dis″ker-ah-tot′ik) of, relating to, or affected by dyskeratosis.

dyskinesia (dis″ki-ne′ze-ah) [Gr. *dyskinēsia* difficulty of moving] impairment of the power of voluntary movement, resulting in fragmentary or incomplete movements. **d. al′gera,** a condition in which movement is painful; seen in hysteria. **biliary d.,** derangement of the filling and emptying mechanism of the gallbladder. **d. intermit′tens,** disability of the limbs, coming on intermittently, and due to impairment of the circulation. **occupational d.,** occupation neurosis. **orofacial d.,** tardive dyskinesia affecting primarily the mouth and face. **d. tar′da, tardive d.,** a form marked typically by involuntary repetitive movements of the facial, buccal, oral, and cervical musculature, affecting chiefly the elderly; it is induced by long-term administration of neuroleptic (antipsychotic) agents and may persist after withdrawal of the agent.

dyskinetic (dis″ki-net′ik) pertaining to or characterized by dyskinesia.

dyskoimesis (dis″koi-me′sis) [*dys-* + Gr. *koimēsis* sleeping] difficulty in getting to sleep.

dyslalia (dis-la′le-ah) [*dys-* + Gr. *lalein* to talk + *-ia*] impairment of utterance with abnormality of the external speech organs.

dyslexia (dis-lek′se-ah) [*dys-* + Gr. *lexis* diction] an inability to read understandingly, due to a central lesion.

dyslipidoses (dis″lip-ĭ-do′sēz) plural of *dyslipidosis.*

dyslipidosis (dis″lip-ĭ-do′sis), pl. *dyslipido′ses.* A general designation applied to a localized or systemic disturbance of fat metabolism.

dyslipoidosis (dis-lip″oi-do′sis), pl. *dyslipoido′ses.* Dyslipidosis.

dyslipoproteinemia (dis-lip″o-pro″te-in-e′me-ah) the presence of abnormal lipoproteins in the blood.

dyslochia (dis-lo′ke-ah) [*dys-* + Gr. *lochia* lochia] disordered lochial discharge.

dyslogia (dis-lo′je-ah) [*dys-* + Gr. *logos* understanding] impairment of the reasoning power; also impairment of the speech, due to mental disorders.

dysmaturity (dis-mah-tūr′ĭ-te) placental dysfunction. **pulmonary d.,** Wilson-Mikity syndrome.

dysmegalopsia (dis″meg-ah-lop′se-ah) [*dys-* + Gr. *megas* big + *opsis* vision] a disturbance of the visual appreciation of the size of objects, in which they appear larger than they are.

dysmelia (dis-me′le-ah) [*dys-* + Gr. *melos* limb + *-ia*] malformation of a limb or limbs as a result of a disturbance in embryonic development; the term includes defects of excessive development as well as reduction deformities. See also *amelia* and *phocomelia.*

dysmenorrhea (dis″men-o-re′ah) [*dys-* + Gr. *mēn* month + *rhein* to flow] painful menstruation. **acquired d.,** secondary d. **congestive d.,** that which is accompanied by great congestion of the uterus. **essential d.,** painful menstruation for which there is no demonstrable cause; called also *primary d.* **inflammatory d.,** that which comes from or is due to inflammation. **d. intermenstrua′lis,** intermenstrual pain. **mechanical d.,** that which is believed to be due to mechanical interference with the flow, as from clots or flexion of the uterus. **membranous d.,** that which is characterized by membranous exfoliations derived from the uterus. **obstructive d.,** that which is due to mechanical obstruction to the discharge of the menstrual fluid. **ovarian d.,** neuralgic pain which is due to ovarian disease. **primary d.,** essential d. **psychogenic d.,** dysmenorrhea due to disturbance of psychic control. **secondary d.,** dysmenorrhea due to a definite pelvic lesion. **spasmodic d.,** that which is due to spasmodic uterine contractions. **tubal d.,** that which is due to disease of the oviduct, such as chronic salpingitis. **uterine d.,** that which arises from a uterine lesion.

dysmetabolism (dis″mĕ-tab′o-lizm) defective metabolism.

dysmetria (dis-me′tre-ah) [*dys-* + Gr. *metron* measure] a condition in which there is improper measuring of distance in muscular acts; disturbance of the power to control the range of movement in muscular action. In *hypermetria,* voluntary muscular movement overreaches the intended goal, and in *hypometria,* voluntary muscular movement falls short of reaching the intended goal.

dysmetropsia (dis″mĕ-trop′se-ah) [*dys-* + Gr. *metron* measure + *opsis* vision] defect in the visual appreciation of the measure or size of objects.

dysmimia (dis-mim′e-ah) [*dys-* + Gr. *mimia* imitation] impairment of the power of expressing thought by gestures.

dysmnesia (dis-ne′se-ah) [*dys-* + Gr. *mnēmē* memory] impaired memory.

dysmnesic (dis-ne′zik) characterized by impairment or disorder of memory.

dysmorphic (dis-mor′fik) characterized by dysmorphism.

dysmorphism (dis-mor′fizm) [*dys-* + Gr. *morphē* form] 1. allomorphism. 2. the condition of appearing under different morphologic forms; for example, some fungi grow differently under parasitic and under saprophytic conditions. 3. an abnormality in morphological development, as a congenital malformation.

dysmorphophobia (dis-mor″fo-fo′be-ah) [Gr. *dysmorphos* deformed + *phobia*] morbid fear of deformity or of becoming deformed.

dysmorphopsia (dis″mor-fop′se-ah) [Gr. *dysmorphos* deformed + *opsis* vision + *-ia*] defective vision, with distortion of the shape of objects perceived.

dysmorphosis (dis″mor-fo′sis) [Gr. *dysmorphos* deformed] malformation.

dysmyotonia (dis″mi-o-to′ne-ah) [*dys-* + Gr. *mys* muscle + *tonos* tension] muscular dystonia; abnormal tonicity of muscle.

dysnomia (dis-no′me-ah) [*dys-* + Gr. *onoma* name] partial nominal aphasia; cf. *anomia.*

dysodontiasis (dis″o-don-ti′ah-sis) [*dys-* + Gr. *odous* tooth + *-iasis*] defective, delayed, or difficult eruption of the teeth.

dysoemia (dis-e′me-ah) [*dys-* + Gr. *oimos* road, path] a medicolegal term for death from obscure causes, traceable to chronic mineral poisoning.

dysontogenesis (dis″on-to-jen′ĕ-sis) [*dys-* + *ontogenesis*] defective embryonic development.

dysontogenetic (dis″on-to-jĕ-net′ik) pertaining to or characterized by dysontogenesis.

dysopia (dis-o′pe-ah) [*dys-* + Gr. *ōpē* sight + *-ia*] defective vision. **d. al′gera,** disturbances of vision due to pains in the eyes and head on looking at objects.

dysopsia (dis-op′se-ah) dysopia.

dysorexia (dis″o-rek′se-ah) [*dys-* + Gr. *orexis* appetite] impaired or deranged appetite.

dysorganoplasia (dis-or″gan-o-pla′se-ah) [*dys-* + Gr. *organon* organ + *plasis* formation] disordered development of an organ.

dysoria (dis-or′e-ah) [*dys-* + Gr. *oros* serum] any abnormality of vascular permeability.

dysoric (dis-or′ik) pertaining to or affected with dysoria.

dysosmia (dis-oz′me-ah) [*dys-* + Gr. *osmē* smell] defect or impairment of the sense of smell.

dysosteogenesis (dis-os″te-o-jen′ĕ-sis) defective bone formation; dysostosis.

dysostosis (dis″os-to′sis) [*dys-* + Gr. *osteon* bone] defective ossification; defect in the normal ossification of fetal cartilages. **cleidocranial d.,** a rare hereditary condition in which there is defective ossification of the cranial bones, with large fontanels and delayed closing of the sutures; complete or partial absence of the clavicles, so that the shoulders may be brought together, or nearly together, in front; and dental and vertebral anomalies. It is transmitted as an autosomal dominant trait. Called also *cleidocranial dysplasia.* **d. cleidocrania′lis congen′ita,** cleidocranial d. **craniofacial d.,** a hereditary disorder characterized by acrocephaly, exophthalmos, hypertelorism, strabismus, parrot-beaked nose, and hypoplastic maxilla with relative mandibular prognathism. It is transmitted as an autosomal dominant trait. Called also *Crouzon's disease.* **d. enchondra′lis epiphysa′ria,** dysplasia epiphysealis multiplex. **mandibulofacial d.,** a hereditary disorder occurring in two forms: the complete form (Franceschetti's syndrome) is characterized by antimongoloid slant of the palpebral fissures, coloboma of the lower lid, micrognathia and hypoplasia of the zygomatic arches, and microtia. It is transmitted as an autosomal dominant trait. The incomplete form (Treacher Collins syndrome) is characterized by the same anomalies in less pronounced degree. It occurs sporadically, but an autosomal dominant mode of transmission is suspected. **mandibulofacial d. with epibulbar dermoids,** oculoauriculovertebral dysplasia. **metaphyseal d.,** a skeletal abnormality in which the epiphyses are normal, or nearly so, and the metaphyseal tissues are replaced by masses of cartilage, producing interference with endochondral bone formation, and expansion and thinning of the metaphyseal cortices. Called also *Jansen's disease* and *metaphyseal chondrodysplasia.* **d. mul′tiplex,** Hurler's syndrome. **Nager's acrofacial d.,** a congenital condition in which mandibulofacial dysostosis is associated with limb deformities consisting of absence of the radius, radioulnar synostosis, and hypoplasia or absence of the thumbs. **orodigitofacial d.,** orofaciodigital syndrome.

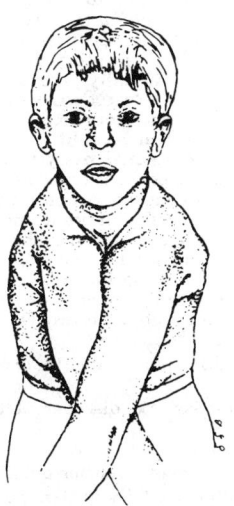

Cleidocranial dysostosis.

dysoxidative (dis-ok′sĭ-da″tiv) due to deficient oxidation.

dysoxidizable (dis-ok′sĭ-diz″ah-b'l) [*dys-* + *oxidizable*] not easily oxidizable.

dyspancreatism (dis-pan′kre-ah-tizm″) disorder of the function of the pancreas.

dysparathyroidism (dis″par-ah-thi′roid-izm) (*obs.*) disorder of parathyroid function.

dyspareunia (dis″pah-roo′ne-ah) [Gr. *dyspareunos* badly mated] difficult or painful coitus.

dyspepsia (dis-pep′se-ah) [*dys-* + Gr. *peptein* to digest] impairment of the power or function of digestion; usually applied to epigastric discomfort following meals. **acid d.,** a variety associated with excessive acidity of the stomach. **appendicular d., appendix d.,** dyspeptic symptoms occurring in chronic appendicitis. **atonic d.** (*obs.*), a form ascribed to a lack of tone in the digestive organs; a nonspecific symptom of gastrointestinal dysfunction. **catarrhal d.,** a variety accompanied by gastric inflammation. **chichiko d.,** a condition of farinaceous malnutrition found in badly nourished infants who are fed mostly on solutions of polished rice powder. **cholelithic d.,** the sudden dyspeptic attacks characteristic of gallbladder disturbance. **colon d.,** functional disturbance of the large intestine, giving rise to the symptoms of dyspepsia. **fermentative d.,** that characterized by the fermentation of ingested food. **flatulent d.,** that which is associated with the formation of gas in the stomach, especially upper abdominal discomfort accompanied by frequent belching. **functional d.,** that which is either atonic or of reflex or nervous origin. **gastric d.,** that which originates within the stomach. **intestinal d.,** that which arises in the intestines. **nervous d.,** dyspepsia which is functional in origin. **ovarian d.,** a form of reflex indigestion due to ovarian disease. **reflex d.,** that which is due to reflex influence from some disease of an organ not directly concerned in digestion. **salivary d.** (*obs.*), dyspepsia due to defective or deficient saliva.

dyspeptic (dis-pep′tik) pertaining to or affected with dyspepsia.

dysperistalsis (dis″per-ĭ-stal′sis) [*dys-* + *peristalsis*] painful or abnormal peristalsis.

dysphagia (dis-fa′je-ah) [*dys-* + Gr. *phagein* to eat] difficulty in swallowing. **contractile ring d.,** dysphagia due to an overactive interior esophageal sphincteric mechanism which gives rise to painful sticking sensations under the lower sternum. **d. inflammato′ria,** dysphagia due to inflammation of the pharynx or esophagus. **d. luso′ria,** dysphagia resulting from compression of the esophagus caused by an anomalous right subclavian artery that arises from the descending aorta and passes behind the esophagus. **d. nervo′sa,** esophagospasm. **d. paralyt′ica,** dysphagia due to paralysis of the pharyngeal or esophageal muscles. **sideropenic d.,** Plummer-Vinson syndrome. **d. spas′tica,** esophagospasm. **tropical d.,** entalação. **vallecular d.,** dysphagia caused by the lodgment of food in the valleculae. **d. valsalvia′na,** dysphagia due to subluxation of the major cornu of the hyoid bone.

dysphagy (dis′fah-je) dysphagia.

dysphasia (dis-fa′ze-ah) [*dys-* + Gr. *phasis* speech] impairment of speech, consisting in lack of coordination and failure to arrange words in their proper order; due to a central lesion.

dysphemia (dis-fe′me-ah) stuttering or other speech disorder due to psychoneurosis.

dysphonia (dis-fo′ne-ah) [*dys-* + Gr. *phōnē* voice] any impairment of voice; a difficulty in speaking. **d. clerico′rum,** any impairment of voice; a difficulty in speaking, such as that which

may be experienced by those who speak at length, e.g., clergymen. **dysplatic d.,** chronic hoarseness due to malformation of the larynx. **d. pli′cae ventricula′ris,** a condition in which phonation is performed with the false vocal cords (ventricular bands). **d. pu′berum,** the harsh, irregular utterance of puberty, and of the change of voice in youth. **spastic d., d. spas′tica,** difficulty in speaking due to excessively vigorous adduction of the vocal cords against each other, so that the voice is hoarse, soft, and strained.

dysphonic (dis-fon′ik) pertaining to or characterized by dysphonia.

dysphoretic (dis″fo-ret′ik) 1. dysphoric. 2. dysphoriant.

dysphoria (dis-fo′re-ah) [Gr. "excessive pain, anguish, agitation"] disquiet; restlessness; malaise.

dysphoriant (dis-fo′re-ant) 1. producing a condition of dysphoria. 2. an agent that produces dysphoria.

dysphoric (dis-for′ik) pertaining to or characterized by dysphoria.

dysphrasia (dis-fra′ze-ah) [*dys-* + Gr. *phrasis* speech + *-ia*] imperfection of utterance due to a central or cerebral defect.

dysphrenia (dis-fre′ne-ah) [*dys-* + Gr. *phrēn* mind + *-ia*] any secondary (functional) psychosis as distinguished from an idiopathic (organic) brain disease (Kahlbaum).

dysphylaxia (dis″fi-lak′se-ah) [*dys-* + Gr. *phylaxis* watching] a condition marked by too early waking.

dyspigmentation (dis″pig-men-ta′shun) a disorder of pigmentation of the skin or hair.

dyspinealism (dis-pin′e-al-izm) (*obs.*) disordered function of the pineal gland.

dyspituitarism (dis″pĭ-tu′ĭ-tar-izm″) a condition due to disordered activity of the pituitary body. See *hyperpituitarism* and *hypopituitarism.*

dysplasia (dis-pla′se-ah) [*dys-* + Gr. *plassein* to form] abnormality of development; in pathology, alteration in size, shape, and organization of adult cells. **anhidrotic ectodermal d.,** congenital ectodermal defect. **anteroposterior facial d.,** defective development resulting in abnormal anteroposterior relationship of the maxilla and mandible to each other or to the cranial base. **basal d.,** malocclusion involving abnormal relationships of components of the maxilla and mandible, with the teeth reflecting that relationship. **bronchopulmonary d.,** a chronic lung disease of infants, possibly related to oxygen toxicity or barotrauma, characterized by bronchiolar metaplasia and interstitial fibrosis. **d. of cervix,** cellular deviations from the normal in the epithelium of the uterine cervix, which may begin as basal cell hyperplasia and progress to anaplasia; its relationship to cervical carcinoma has not been established. **chondroectodermal d.,** achondroplasia occurring in association with defective development of skin, hair, and teeth, polydactyly, and defect of the cardiac septum. **cleidocranial d.,** see under *dysostosis.* **congenital alveolar d.,** respiratory distress syndrome of newborn; see under *syndrome.* **craniocarpotarsal d.,** see under *dystrophy.* **craniodiaphyseal d.,** a hereditary condition transmitted as an autosomal recessive trait, in which progressive cranial and facial hyperostosis results in striking distortion. **craniometaphyseal d.,** metaphyseal dysplasia associated with overgrowth of the head bones, leontiasis ossea, and hypertelorism. **cretinoid d.,** abnormality of development characteristic of cretinism, consisting of retarded ossification and smallness of the internal and sex organs. **dental d.,** abnormality of development producing abnormal relationship of a varying number of teeth with their opposing members. **dentin d., dentinal d.,** a condition affecting both primary and secondary dentition, in which the teeth have short distorted roots, many with periapical rarefactions, no pulp chambers or small demilune-shaped chambers, and normal dentin in the upper crown with atypical osteodentin and tubular dentin in the lower crown; the affected teeth are normal in color or slightly brown to blue-brown and are commonly malaligned in the arch. Called also *rootless teeth.* **diaphyseal d.,** a condition characterized by thickening of the cortex of the mid-shaft area of the long bones, progressing toward the epiphyses, the thickening sometimes occurring also in the flat bones; excessive growth in length of bones of the extremities usually results in abnormal stature. Called also *diaphyseal sclerosis* and *Engelmann's disease.* **ectodermal d.,** congenital ectodermal defect. **encephalo-ophthalmic d.,** a developmental structural defect of the eye related to faulty development of the brain. **epiphyseal d.,** faulty growth and ossification of the epiphyses, with roentgenographically apparent stippling and decreased stature, not associated with thyroid disease. Called also *stippled epiphyses.* See *d. epiphysealis hemimelica, d. epiphysealis multiplex,* and *d. epiphysealis punctata.* **d. epiphysea′lis hemimel′ica,** a rare condition characterized by swellings in the extremities, usually on the inner and outer aspects of the ankles and knees, made up of bone covered with epiphyseal cartilage, and leading to limitation of motion of the joints. Called also *tarsoepiphyseal aclasis* and *Trevor's disease.* **d. epiphysea′lis mul′tiplex,** a developmental abnormality of various epiphyses, which appear late and are mottled, flattened, fragmented, and usually hypoplastic; the digits are short and thick, with blunt ends, and stature may be diminished owing to flattening deformities at the hips, knees, and ankles. Called also *dysostosis enchondralis epiphysaria.* **d. epiphysea'lis puncta'ta,** a rare hereditary condition marked by radiographic appearance of multiple punctate opacities (stippling) in the epiphyses, usually present at birth, and by dwarfism, flexion contractures, cataract, dulled intellect, short blunt fingers, and general weakness. Frequently infants are stillborn or die of associated anomalies in the first year. Called also *Conradi's disease, chondrodystrophia calcificans congenita, chondrodystrophia congenita punctata, chondrodystrophia fetalis calcificans,* and *stippled epiphyses.* **faciogenital d.,** Aarskog's syndrome. **fibrous d. (of bone),** a disease of bone marked by thinning of the cortex and replacement of bone marrow by gritty fibrous tissue containing bony spicules, producing pain, disability, and gradually increasing deformity. Only one bone may be involved (*monostotic fibrous d.*), with the process later affecting several or many bones (*polyostotic fibrous d.*). When associated with melanotic pigmentation of the skin and endocrine disorders, it is known as *Albright's syndrome.* **fibrous d. of jaw,** cherubism. **hereditary bone d.,** a condition characterized by kyphoscoliosis, generalized osteopenia without fractures, slender long bones, arachnodactyly, congenital contractures, underdeveloped musculature, and abnormally formed ears; it appears to be inherited as an autosomal dominant. **hidrotic ectodermal d.,** a hereditary condition, transmitted as an autosomal dominant trait, marked by generalized hypotrichosis, dystrophy of the nails, and hyperpigmentation; hyperkeratosis of the palms and soles and mental deficiency may also occur. Called also *Clouston's syndrome.* Cf. *congenital ectodermal defect.* **d. linguofacia'lis,** orodigitofacial dysostosis. **metaphyseal d.,** a disturbance in enchondral bone growth, failure of modeling causing the ends of the shafts to remain larger than normal in circumference; called also *Pyle's disease.* See also *craniometaphyseal d.* **multiple epiphyseal d.,** d. epiphysealismultiplex. **oculoauricular d.,** oculoauriculovertebral d. **oculoauriculovertebral (OAV) d.,** a congenital condition in which colobomas of the upper eyelid, epibulbar dermoids, bilateral accessory auricular appendages anterior to the ears, and vertebral anomalies are frequently associated with characteristic facies, consisting of asymmetry of the skull, prominent frontal bossing, low hairline, mandibular hypoplasia, low set ears, and, sometimes, hemifacial microstomia. Called also *Goldenhar's syndrome, oculoauricular d., mandibulofacial dysostosis with epibulbar dermoids,* and *OAV syndrome.* **oculodentodigital (ODD) d.,** a rare hereditary condition transmitted as an autosomal dominant trait, characterized by bilateral microphthalmos, abnormally small nose with anteverted nostrils, hypotrichosis, dental anomalies, camptodactyly, syndactyly, and missing phalanges of the toes. Called also *dysplasia oculodentodigitalis syndrome, Meyer-Schwickerath and Weyers syndrome, oculodento-osseous syndrome,* and *ODD syndrome.* **oculovertebral d.,** a congenital syndrome consisting of microphthalmia, anophthalmia, cryptophthalmia, or coloboma with small orbit; unilateral maxillary dysplasia and dysplastic soft tissue causing facial scoliosis and dental malocclusion, macrostomia, and alveolar malformations; and vertebral malformations and costal anomalies. Called also *Weyers-Thier syndrome.* **ophthalmomandibulomelic d.,** a hereditary syndrome transmitted as an autosomal dominant trait, consisting of blindness caused by corneal opacities, temporomandibular fusion, absent coronoid process, obtuse mandibular angle, radiohumeral and radioulnar dislocations, and aplasia of the lateral condyle of the humerus, radial head, and distal ulna. **progressive diaphyseal d.,** diaphyseal d. **skeletodental d.,** abnormality of development producing not only abnormal relationship of varying numbers of apposing teeth, but also abnormal relationship of the maxilla and mandible to each other or to the base of the skull. **spondyloepiphyseal d.,** a hereditary dysplasia of the vertebrae and extremities resulting in dwarfism of the short-trunk type, often with shortened limbs due to epiphyseal abnormalities. In the delayed onset form, the principal feature is precocious osteoarthritis. There are several forms, including autosomal dominant, autosomal recessive, and X-linked forms, the dominant form often being associated with such ocular anomalies as myopia and detached retina. **thymic d.,** any of a group of hereditary disorders, some transmitted as an autosomal recessive trait and others as an X-linked recessive trait, characterized by faulty development of the thymus, which may be associated with (*a*) normal serum immunoglobulin levels and impaired cell-mediated immunity (Nezelof's syndrome), (*b*) Swiss type agammaglobulinemia and impairment of both cell-mediated and humoral immunity, or (*c*) variable deficiencies of immunoglobulins, the severity being dependent on the degree of the deficiency. **ureteral neuromuscular d.,** megaloureter.

dysplastic (dis-plas'tik) 1. marked by dysplasia. 2. having a body form which does not belong to one of the three main classes, athletic, asthenic, or pyknic.

dyspnea (disp'ne-ah) [Gr. *dyspnoia* difficulty of breathing] difficult or labored breathing. **cardiac d.,** distressful breathing caused by heart disease. **exertional d.,** dyspnea provoked by physical effort or exertion. **expiratory d.,** difficulty in breathing caused by hindrance to the free egress of air from the lungs. **functional d.,** respiratory distress not caused by or-

ganic disease and unrelated to exertion but associated with anxiety states; see also *sighing d.* **inspiratory d.,** difficulty in breathing caused by hindrance to the free ingress of air into the lungs. **nocturnal d.,** respiratory distress that is minimal in the morning, and may gradually progress until it becomes quite disturbing at night. **nonexpansional d.,** difficulty in breathing caused by inadequate expansion of the chest. **orthostatic d.,** difficulty in breathing experienced when in the erect position. **paroxysmal nocturnal d.,** a form of respiratory distress related to posture (especially reclining at night) and usually attributed to congestive heart failure with pulmonary edema. **renal d.,** difficulty in breathing attributable to kidney disease. **sighing d.,** a syndrome characterized by intermittent deep sighing respirations, the depth of inspiration being greatly increased, without significant alteration in the respiratory rate and without wheezing; it is associated with functional or emotional rather than organic disorders, and is characteristic of functional dyspnea.

dyspneic (disp-ne'ik) pertaining to or characterized by dyspnea.

dyspoiesis (dis"poi-e'sis) a disorder of formation, as of blood cells.

dysponderal (dis-pon'der-al) [*dys-* + L. *pondus* weight] pertaining to disorder of weight, either obesity or underweight.

dysponesis (dis"po-ne'sis) [*dys-* + Gr. *ponēsis* toil, exertion] a reversible physiopathologic state consisting of unnoticed, misdirected neurophysiologic reactions to various agents (environmental events, bodily sensations, emotions, and thoughts) and the repercussions of these reactions throughout the organism. These errors in energy expenditure, which are capable of producing functional disorders, consist mainly of covert errors in action-potential output from the motor and premotor areas of the cortex and the consequences of that output.

dyspragia (dis-pra'je-ah) [Gr. *dyspragia* ill success] painful performance of any function. **d. intermit'tens angiosclerot'ica intestina'lis,** intestinal (abdominal) angina.

dyspraxia (dis-prak'se-ah) [Gr. *dyspraxia* ill success] partial loss of ability to perform coordinated acts.

dysprosium (dis-pro'se-um) one of the rare earth elements, atomic number 66, atomic weight 162.50, symbol Dy.

dysprosody (dis-pros'o-de) disturbance of stress, pitch, and rhythm of speech.

dysproteinemia (dis-pro"te-in-e'me-ah) [*dys-* + *protein* + Gr. *haima* blood + *-ia*] derangement of the protein content of the blood.

dysraphia, dysraphism (dis-ra'fe-ah; dis'rah-fizm) [*dys-* + Gr. *raphē* seam] incomplete closure of a raphe; defective fusion, e.g., of the neural tube.

dysrhaphia, dysrhaphism (dis-ra'fe-ah; dis'rah-fizm) dysraphia.

dysrhythmia (dis-rith'me-ah) [*dys-* + Gr. *rhythmos* any regularly recurring motion + *-ia*] disturbance of rhythm, as abnormality of rhythm in speech: *d. pneumophra'sia* is defective breath grouping; *d. proso'dia* is defective placement of stress; *d. to'nia* is defective inflection. **cerebral d.,** disturbance or irregularity in the rhythm of the brain waves as recorded by electroencephalography; called also *electroencephalographic d.* **electroencephalographic d.,** cerebral d. **esophageal d.,** diffuse esophageal spasm.

dyssebacea (dis"se-ba'she-ah) [*dys-* + *sebum*] disorder of sebaceous follicles; specifically a condition seen (but not exclusively) in riboflavin deficiency, marked by greasy, branny seborrhea on the midface, with erythema in the nasal folds, canthi, or other folds of the skin, or in all three.

dyssocial (dis-so'shal) denoting a personality disorder that is not antisocial, but is characterized by disregard for social codes, by predation, and by more or less criminality. See *dyssocial personality,* under *personality.*

dyssomnia (dis-som'ne-ah) [*dys-* + L. *somnus* sleep] any disorder of sleep.

dysspermia (dis-sper'me-ah) [*dys-* + Gr. *sperma* seed + *-ia*] impairment of the spermatozoa, or of the semen.

dysstasia (dis-sta'se-ah) [*dys-* + Gr. *stasis* standing] difficulty in standing.

dysstatic (dis-stat'ik) pertaining to or characterized by dysstasia.

dyssymbolia (dis"sim-bo'le-ah) failure of conceptual thinking so that thoughts can not be intelligently formulated in language.

dyssymboly (dis-sim'bo-le) dyssymbolia.

dyssymmetry (dis-sim'ĕ-tre) a condition characterized by absence of symmetry.

dyssynergia (dis"sin-er'je-ah) [*dys-* + Gr. *synergia* cooperation] disturbance of muscular coordination. **biliary d.,** failure of coordinated action of the different parts of the biliary system. **d. cerebella'ris myoclon'ica,** dyssynergia cerebellaris progressiva associated with myoclonus epilepsy; called also *Hunt's disease.* **d. cerebella'ris progressi'va,** a condition marked by generalized intention tremors associated with disturbance of muscle tone and of muscular coordination; due to disorder of cerebellar function. Called also *Ramsay Hunt syndrome.*

dyssystole (dis-sis′to-le) [*dys-* + *systole*] (*obs.*) abnormal cardiac systole, especially asystole.

dystaxia (dis-tak′se-ah) [*dys-* + Gr. *taxis* arrangement] difficulty in controlling voluntary movements; partial ataxia.

dystectia (dis-tek′she-ah) [*dys-* + L. *tectum* roof] defective closure of the neural tube, resulting in such malformations as anencephaly, porencephaly, meningocele, spina bifida, etc.

dysteleology (dis″te-le-ol′o-je) 1. the study of apparently useless organs or parts. 2. lack of purposefulness, or of contribution to the final result.

dysthymia (dis-thim′e-ah) 1. [*dys-* + Gr. *thymos* mind] mental depression; also, any intellectual anomaly. 2. [*dys-* + Gr. *thymos* thymus] the condition allegedly produced by disordered thymus secretion in childhood.

dysthymiac (dis-thi′me-ak) an individual exhibiting dysthymia.

dysthyreosis (dis″thi-re-o′sis) dysthyroidism.

dysthyroid, dysthyroidal (dis-thi′roid; dis″thi-roid′al) denoting defective functioning of the thyroid gland.

dysthyroidea (dis″thi-roi′de-ah) dysthyroidism.

dysthyroidism (dis-thi′roid-izm) imperfect development and function of the thyroid gland.

dystimbria (dis-tim′bre-ah) defect in quality or resonance of the voice.

dystithia (dis-tith′e-ah) [*dys-* + Gr. *tithēnē* a nurse + *-ia*] difficulty in breast feeding.

dystocia (dis-to′se-ah) [*dys-* + Gr. *tokos* birth] abnormal labor or childbirth. **cervical d.,** dystocia caused by mechanical obstruction at the ostium uteri. **constriction ring d., contraction ring d.,** difficult labor caused by contraction of an area of circular muscle fibers, which may occur at various levels of the parturient uterus. **fetal d.,** that which is due to the shape, size, or position of the fetus. **maternal d.,** that which is due to some condition inherent in the mother. **placental d.,** difficulty in delivering the placenta.

dystonia (dis-to′ne-ah) [*dys-* + Gr. *tonos*] disordered tonicity of muscle. **d. defor′mans progressi′va,** d. musculorum deformans. **d. lenticula′ris,** dystonia due to a lesion of the lenticular nucleus. **d. musculo′rum defor′mans,** a rare, chronic, hereditary disease marked by involuntary, irregular, clonic contortions of the muscles of the trunk and extremities. The symptoms appear chiefly on walking, at which time the contortions twist the body forward and sideways in a grotesque fashion (tortipelvis). An autosomal recessive form occurs before puberty, principally among Jews; the autosomal dominant form has a later onset and is not as consistent in severity. Called also *Ziehen-Oppenheim disease, dystonia deformans progressiva, dysbasia lordotica progressiva,* and *torsion dystonia* or *neurosis.* **torsion d.,** d. musculorum deformans.

dystonic (dis-ton′ik) pertaining to or characterized by dystonia.

dystopia (dis-to′pe-ah) [*dys-* + Gr. *topos* place] malposition; faulty placement of an organ.

dystopic (dis-top′ik) misplaced; out of its normal place.

dystopy (dis′to-pe) dystopia.

dystrophia (dis-tro′fe-ah) [L.] dystrophy. **d. adipo′sa cor′-neae,** primary fatty degeneration of the cornea. **d. adiposogenita′lis,** adiposogenital dystrophy. **d. brevicol′-lis,** a condition of dwarfism characterized especially by shortness of the neck. **d. diffu′sa,** diffuse atrophy, as of the alveolar bone, in advanced periodontal disease. **d. endothelia′lis cor′neae,** cornea guttata. **d. epithelia′lis cor′neae,** dystrophy of the epithelium of the cornea marked by erosions; called also *Fuchs′ dystrophy.* **d. hypophysopri′va chron′ica,** the condition produced by partial removal of the hypophysis (pituitary gland) and marked by obesity, increased carbohydrate tolerance, hypothermia, hypoplasia of the sex glands, retardation of skeletal growth, and mental dullness. **d. mesoderma′lis congen′ita hyperplas′tica,** Weill-Marchesani syndrome. **d. myoton′ica,** myotonic dystrophy; see under *dystrophy.* **d. periosta′lis hyperplas′tica familia′ris,** a familial condition marked by acrocephaly, with thickening of the bones. **d. un′guium,** dystrophy of the nails; changes in the texture, structure, and/or color of the nails due to no demonstrable cause, but presumed to be attributable to some disturbance of nutrition. **d. un′guis media′na canalifor′mis,** a fissure or deep groove close to the middle of a nail, usually the thumb nail, starting at the cuticle and extending (with growth of the nail) to the free edge. Spontaneous recovery after months or years is not unusual, nor is relapse. Called also *solenonychia.*

dystrophic (dis-trof′ik) pertaining to or characterized by dystrophy.

dystrophodextrin (dis″trof-o-deks′trin) [*dys-* + Gr. *trophē* nutrition + *dextrin*] a starchlike material said to exist in normal blood.

dystrophoneurosis (dis-trof″o-nu-ro′sis) [*dys-* + Gr. *trophē* nutrition + *neurosis*] 1. any nervous disorder due to poor nutri-

tion. 2. impairment of nutrition which is caused by nervous disorder.

dystrophy (dis′tro-fe) [L. *dystrophia,* from *dys-* + Gr. *trephein* to nourish] any disorder arising from defective or faulty nutrition, especially the muscular dystrophies. **adiposogenital d.,** a condition characterized by adiposity of the feminine type, genital hypoplasia, changes in secondary sex characters, and metabolic disturbances; seen with lesions of the hypothalamus. Called also *Fröhlich′s syndrome.* **Albright′s d.,** pseudopseudohypoparathyroidism. **asphyxiating thoracic d.,** a congenital hereditary syndrome transmitted as an autosomal recessive trait, in which chondrodystrophy of the rib cage, usually causing asphyxia early in the newborn period, occurs in association with defects of the phalanges and pelvis; called also *Jeune′s syndrome* and *thoracic-pelvic-phalangeal dystrophy.* **Becker′s d., Becker′s muscular d.,** a form closely resembling pseudohypertrophic muscular dystrophy but having a late onset and slowly progressive course; it is transmitted as an X-linked recessive trait. **Biber-Haab-Dimmer d.,** lattice d. **corneal d.,** see *granular corneal d., lattice d., macular corneal d., Salzmann′s nodular corneal d., cornea guttata, dystrophia epithelialis corneae,* and *dystrophia adiposa cornea.* **craniocarpotarsal d.,** a congenital anomaly transmitted as an autosomal dominant trait, consisting of characteristic flattened, masklike facies; microstomia, the lips protruding as in whistling; deep-set eyes with hypertelorism; camptodactyly with ulnar deviation of the fingers; and talipes equinovarus. Called also *Freeman-Sheldon syndrome, whistling face syndrome,* and *whistling face–windmill vane hand syndrome.* **Dejerine-Landouzy d.,** Landouzy-Dejerine d. **distal muscular d.,** late distal hereditary myopathy. **Duchenne type muscular d.,** pseudohypertrophic muscular d. **Duchenne-Landouzy d.,** Landouzy-Dejerine d. **Erb′s d.,** pseudohypertrophic muscular d. **facioscapulohumeral muscular d.,** Landouzy-Dejerine d. **familial osseous d.,** Morquio′s syndrome. **Fuchs′ d.,** dystrophia epithelialis corneae. **Gowers type muscular d.,** late distal hereditary myopathy. **granular corneal d. (Groenouw′s type I),** a dominately transmitted form of corneal dystrophy occurring during the first decade and characterized by the presence of small opacities in the superficial layers of the cornea, which form a granular disk. **hypophyseal d.,** hypopituitarism. **infantile neuroaxonal d.,** progressive hereditary degenerative encephalopathy transmitted as an autosomal recessive trait, beginning in infancy with muscular hypotonia and arrest of development in late infancy, followed by dementia, blindness, spasticity, and ataxia. Pathologically it is characterized by widespread focal swellings and degeneration of the axons with scattered spheroids in the brain. Called also *Seitelberger′s disease* and *spastic amaurotic axonal idiocy.* **Landouzy′s d.,** Landouzy-Dejerine d. **Landouzy-Dejerine d.,** a relatively benign form of muscular dystrophy in which there is marked atrophy of the muscles of the face, shoulder girdle, and arm, producing a facial expression called myopathic face. Most patients enjoy a normal life-span. The disorder is transmitted as an autosomal dominant. Called also *facioscapulohumeral muscular d.* or *atrophy.* **lattice d. (of cornea),** hereditary dystrophy of the cornea marked clinically by linear lesions having a filamentous interwoven appearance and histologically by fusiform areas of hyaline degeneration and dense deposits of hyalin between the epithelium and Bowman′s membrane; called also *Biber-Haab-Dimmer d.* **Leyden-Moebius d.,** limb-girdle muscular d. **limb-girdle muscular d.,** a slowly progressive form of muscular dystrophy affecting either sex and usually beginning in childhood, sometimes in maturity or later; it is characterized by weakness and wasting in the shoulder or pelvic girdle. Called also *Leyden-Moebius d.* or *type.* **macular corneal d. (Groenouw′s type II),** a recessively transmitted form of corneal dystrophy occurring during the first or second decade and characterized by the presence of macular opacities with indistinct irregular borders, between which the stroma is cloudy. **median canaliform d. of the nail,** dystrophia unguis mediana canaliformis. **muscular d.,** a group of genetically determined, painless, degenerative myopathies characterized by weakness and atrophy of muscle without involvement of the nervous system. There are three main types: pseudohypertrophic muscular dystrophy, Landouzy-Dejerine dystrophy, and limb-girdle muscular dystrophy. Rarer forms are distal muscular dystrophy, ocular myopathy, and myotonic dystrophy. Called also *Erb′s* or *Erb-Landouzy disease, idiopathic muscular atrophy,* and *myodystrophia.* **myotonic d.,** a rare, slowly progressive, hereditary disease transmitted as an autosomal dominant trait, characterized by myotonia followed by atrophy of the muscles (especially those of the face and neck), cataracts, hypogonadism, frontal balding, and cardiac abnormalities; called also *dystrophia myotonica, myotonia atrophica,* and *Steinert′s disease.* **oculocerebrorenal d.,** see under *syndrome.* **papillary and pigmentary d.** (Darier) (*obs.*), acanthosis nigricans. **progressive muscular d.,** muscular d. **progressive tapetochoroidal d.,** choroideremia. **pseudohypertrophic muscular d.,** a chronic progressive disease affecting the shoulder and pelvic girdles, commencing in early childhood. It is characterized by increasing weakness, pseudohypertrophy of the muscles followed by atrophy, lordosis, and a peculiar swaying gait with the legs kept wide apart. The disorder is transmitted as a sex-linked recessive trait, and affected individuals, predominantly males, rarely survive to maturity; death is usually due to respiratory weakness or heart failure. Called also *Duchenne's muscular d.* or *type, Erb's d.* or *paralysis, pseudohypertrophic muscular atrophy* or *paralysis,* and *Zimmerlin's d.* or *type.* **reflex sympathetic d.,** a disturbance of the sympathetic nervous system marked by pallor or rubor, pain, sweating, edema, or skin atrophy following sprain, fracture or injury to nerves or blood vessels. **Salzmann's nodular corneal d.,** a progressive hypertrophic degeneration of the epithelial layer of the cornea, Bowman's membrane, and the outer portion of the corneal stroma. **Simmerlin's d.,** limb-girdle muscular d. **tapetochoroidal d.,** choroideremia. **thoracic-pelvic-phalangeal d.,** asphyxiating thoracic d. **thyroneural d.,** a condition marked by chorea, athetosis, rigidity, ataxia, and other indications of disturbed function of the autonomic nervous system with mental and thyroid defects. **wound d.,** a syndrome of defective protein metabolism (hypoproteinemia) that sometimes develops after severe injury.

dystropic (dis-tro′pik) [*dys-* + Gr. *tropos* a turning] characterized by abnormal behavior.

dystropy (dis′tro-pe) abnormal behavior.

dystrypsia (dis-trip′se-ah) [*dys-* + *trypsin* + *-ia*] derangement of intestinal or pancreatic digestion due to lack of trypsin.

dysuresia (dis-u-re′se-ah) dysuria.

dysuria (dis-u′re-ah) [*dys-* + Gr. *ouron* urine + *-ia*] painful or difficult urination. **psychic d.,** difficulty in passing the urine in the presence of other persons. **spastic d.,** difficult urination due to spasm of the bladder.

dysuriac (dis-u′re-ak) an individual exhibiting dysuria.

dysuric (dis-u′rik) pertaining to dysuria.

dysvitaminosis (dis″vi-tah-min-o′sis) a disorder due to an excess or deficiency of a vitamin.

dyszoospermia (dis-zo-o-sper′me-ah) [*dys-* + *zoospermia*] a disorder of spermatozoon formation.

E

E. emmetropia; eye; electromotive force; experimenter.

Ea a god of the Babylonians and Assyrians, said to be the earliest deity associated with the art of healing.

EAC an abbreviation used in studies of complement in which E represents erythrocyte, A antibody, and C complement.

EACA epsilon-aminocaproic acid; see *ε-aminocaproic acid,* under *acid.*

ead. abbreviation for L. *ea′dem,* the same.

Eagle test (e′gl) [Harry *Eagle,* American physician, born 1905] see under *test.*

EAHF eczema, asthma, hay fever; see *EAHF complex,* under *complex.*

Eales' disease (ēlz) [Henry *Eales,* British physician, 1852–1913] see under *disease.*

EAP epiallopregnanolone.

Ea. R. abbreviation for Ger. *Entartungs-Reaktion,* reaction of degeneration.

ear (ēr) [L. *auris;* Gr. *ous*] the organ of hearing and of equilibrium, consisting of the external ear, the middle ear, and the internal ear; called also *auris* [NA]. See Plate XVI. **acute e.,** acute middle ear catarrh, otitis media catarrhalis acuta. **aviator's e.,** barotitis media. **Aztec e.,** an ear in which the lobule is wanting, the whole ear looking as if it were pushed forward and downward. **bat e.,** lop e. **beach e.,** maceration and inflammation of the auditory canal as a result of ocean bathing. **Blainville e's,** asymmetry of the two ears. **Cagot e.,** an ear in which the lobule is wanting. **cat's e.,** an ear that is folded over on itself. **cauliflower e.,** a partially deformed auricle caused by injury and subsequent perichondritis. **cup e.,** a protruding ear which in its milder form presents a poorly developed or unformed antihelical crus with deficient or faulty development of the superior helix, and exaggerated overdevelopment of its deep "cup-shaped," concave concha. In the severe forms, the ear is smaller than normal and the helical rim is shortened to such an extent that the helix margin, or fold, cups forward and over the scapha as a hood. **Darwin's e.,** an ear having an eminence on the edge of the helix. **diabetic e.,** mastoiditis complicating diabetes. **external e.,** the pinna and external meatus together (auris externa [NA]). **glue e.,** a chronic condition marked by a collection of fluid of high viscosity in the middle ear, due to obstruction of the eustachian tube. **hairy e's,** hypertrichosis pinnae auris. **Hong Kong e.,** otomycosis. **hot weather e.,** an otitis externa, especially of the meatus, which is rather common in the hot and humid tropics and is often caused by *Pseudomonas aeruginosa.* **inner e., internal e.,** the labyrinth, comprising the vestibule, cochlea, and semicircular canals (auris interna [NA]). **insane e.** (*obs.*), hematoma of the ear. **lop e.,** deformity of the external ear in which the conchal portion grows at a right angle to the head; called also *bat e.* **middle e.,** the space medial to the tympanic membrane (mesotympanum), the epitympanum, and the hypotympanum; auris media [NA]. It contains the auditory ossicles and connects with the mastoid cells and auditory tubes. Called also *drum, eardrum, tympanic cavity, cavum tympani,* and *tympanum.* **Morel e.,** a deformed ear marked by abnormal development of the helix, anthelix, and scaphoid fossa, so that the folds of the ear seem obliterated, and the ear is smooth, large, and often prominent, with a thin edge. **Mozart e.,** congenital fusion of the crura of the anthelix and the helix. **outer e.,** external e. **prizefighter e.,** cauliflower e. **satyr e.,** one with a pointed pinna. **scroll e.,** one in which the pinna is rolled up. **Singapore e.,** otomycosis. **Stahl e., No. 1,** a deformed ear in which the helix is broad and coalesces with the anthelix; the fossa ovalis and fossa scaphoidea are scarcely to be seen, and the lower portion of the helix is obliterated. **Stahl e., No. 2,** a deformed ear in which there are three instead of two crura anthelicis. **swimmer's e.,** otitis externa. **tank e.,** a condition like beach ear from bathing in swimming pools. **tropical e.,** a local infection of the external auditory meatus prevalent in tropical and semitropical countries. **Wildermuth's e.,** a deformed ear with prominent anthelix and poorly developed helix.

earache (ēr′āk) pain in the ear; otalgia.

eardrum (ēr′drum) 1. the middle ear (auris media [NA]). 2. membrana tympani.

ear-minded (ēr-mind′ed) remembering chiefly the impressions perceived by hearing. Cf. *audile.*

earth (erth) 1. the soil and other pulverulent substances forming the ground. 2. any amorphous, easily pulverizable mineral. **alkaline e.,** any oxide of the alkaline earth metals. **diatomaceous e.,** infusorial earth. **fuller's e.,** an impure aluminum silicate having decolorizing and purifying properties. **infusorial e.,** a silicious earth composed mostly of the frustules and fragments of diatoms. By boiling with dilute hydrochloric acid, washing, and calcining, it can be so purified as to be a very pure form of silica, SiO_2 (terra silicea purificata). It is often mixed with clay and used in various industries. Called also *diatomaceous e.* **silicious e., purified** [NF], a form of silica (*infusorial e.*), SiO_2, purified by boiling with acid, washing, and calcining; used as a pharmaceutical filtering agent.

earwax (ēr′waks) cerumen.

E.B. elementary body.

Ebbinghaus test (eb′ing-hows) [Hermann *Ebbinghaus,* psychologist in Halle, 1850–1909] see under *tests.*

Eberth's lines (ā′berts) [Karl Joseph *Eberth,* pathologist in Halle, 1835–1926] see under *line.*

Eberthella (e″ber-thel′ah) [K. J. *Eberth*] a former genus name applied to bacteria now included in the genus *Salmonella;* see *Salmonella typhosa.*

Ebner's fibrils, glands, reticulum (eb′nerz) [Victor *Ebner* von Rofenstein, histologist in Vienna, 1842–1925] see under the nouns.

ebonation (e″bo-na′shun) [L. *e* out + *bone*] the removal of fragments of bone after injury.

ébranlement (a-brahnl-maw′) [Fr.] removal of a polyp by twisting the pedicle of the tumor.

ebrietas (e-bri′ĕ-tas) [L.] drunkenness; inebriety.

ebriety (e-bri′ĕ-te) drunkenness; inebriety.

Ebstein's angle, anomaly, disease (eb′stīnz) [Wilhelm *Ebstein,* physician in Göttingen, 1836–1912] see *cardiohepatic angle,* under *angle,* and see under *anomaly* and *disease.*

ebullition (eb-u-lish′un) [L. *ebullire* to boil] 1. the process or condition of boiling. 2. the motion of a boiling liquid.

ebur (e′bur) [L.] ivory. **e. den′tis,** dentin.

eburnation (e″bur-na′shun) [L. *ebur* ivory] the conversion of a bone into an ivory-like mass. In osteoarthritis, the thinning of the articular cartilage due to disorganization and fragmentation of the superficial tissue and extension of degenerative changes to the deeper part of the cartilage, resulting in exposure of the subchondral bone, which becomes denser and the surface of which becomes worn and polished. In dentistry, a condition of exposed dentin which is hard, and yellow, brown or black in color, with a polished look.

eburneous (e-bur′ne-us) resembling ivory.

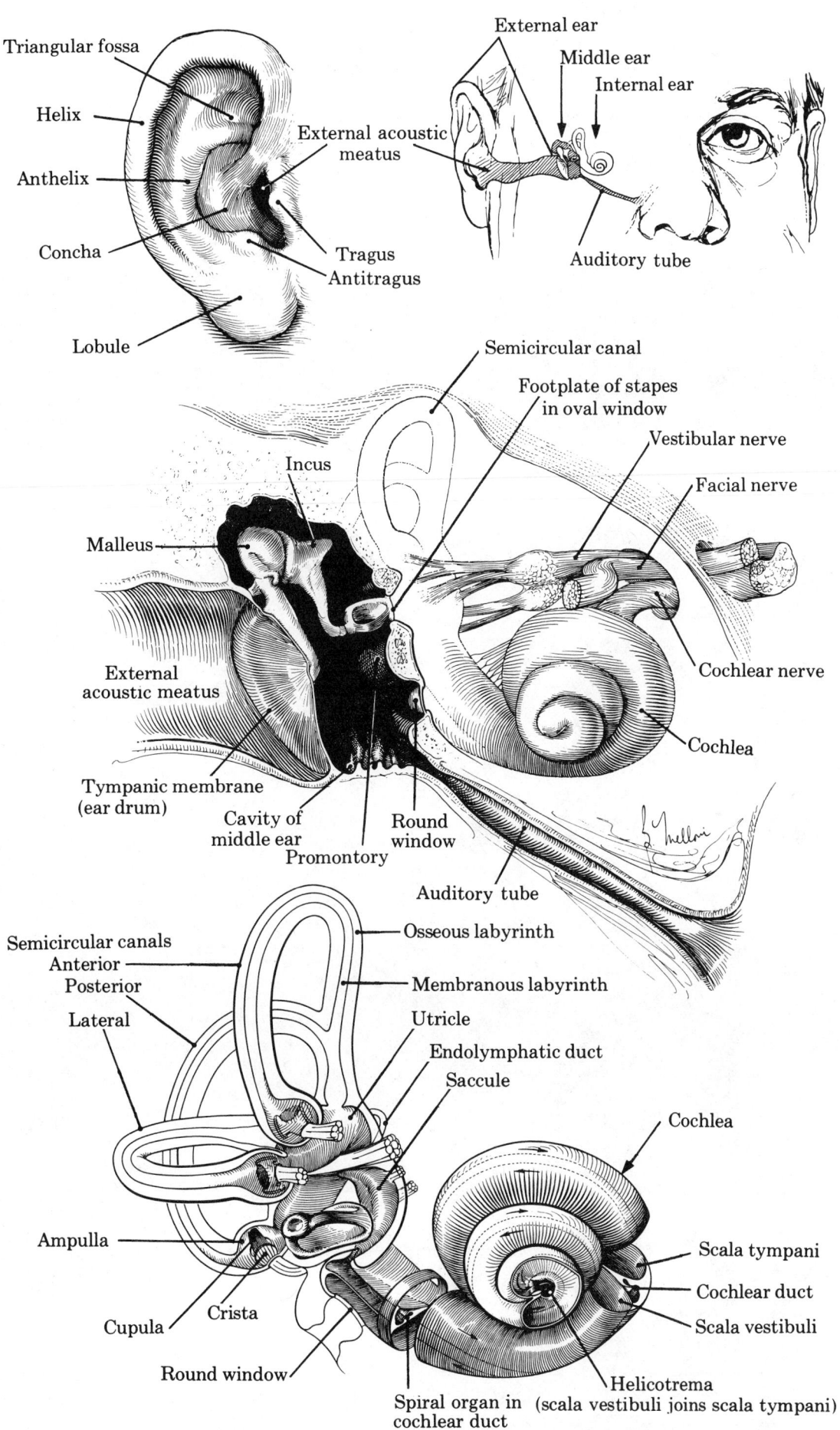

EXTERNAL AND INTERNAL STRUCTURES OF EAR

eburnitis (e″bur-ni′tis) [L. *eburnus* of ivory + *-itis*] increased hardness and density of dentin.

EBV Epstein-Barr virus.

écarteur (ā-kar-ter′) [Fr.] a retractor.

ecaudate (e-kaw′dāt) [L. *e* without + *cauda* tail] without a tail.

ecbolic (ek-bol′ik) [Gr. *ekbolikos* throwing out] oxytocic.

ecbovirus (ek″bo-vi′rus) [from *enteric cytopathic bovine orphan* + *virus*] an enteric orphan virus isolated from cattle; also written *ECBO virus.*

eccentric (ek-sen′trik) 1. situated or occurring away from a center. 2. proceeding from a center.

eccentrochondroplasia (ek-sen″tro-kon″dro-pla′se-ah) Morquio's syndrome.

eccentro-osteochondrodysplasia (ek-sen″tro-os″te-o-kon″-dro-dis-pla′se-ah) [Gr. *ekkentros* from the center + *osteon* bone + *chondros* cartilage + *dys-* + *plassein* to form] Morquio's syndrome.

eccephalosis (ek″sef-ah-lo′sis) [Gr. *ek* out + *kephalē* head] craniotomy.

ecchondroma (ek″kon-dro′mah) [Gr. *ek* out + *chondros* cartilage + *-oma*] a hyperplastic growth of cartilage tissue developing on the surface of a cartilage or projecting under the periosteum of a bone; called also *ecchondrosis.*

ecchondrosis (ek″kon-dro′sis) ecchondroma.

ecchondrotome (ek-kon′dro-tōm) [Gr. *ek* out + *chondros* cartilage + *tomē* a cutting] a knife for excising cartilaginous tissue.

ecchordosis physaliphora (ek″kor-do′sis fis″ah-lif′o-rah) gelatinous nodules of heterotopic notochordal tissue projecting from the clivus or dorsum sellae. True tumors (chordomas) may arise from these or from intraosseous remnants of the notochord.

ecchymoma (ek-ĭ-mo′mah) a swelling due to a bruise and formed by subcutaneous extravasation of blood.

ecchymosed (ek′ĭ-mōsd) characterized by ecchymosis.

ecchymoses (ek″ĭ-mo′sēz) [Gr.] plural of *ecchymosis.*

ecchymosis (ek″ĭ-mo′sis), pl. *ecchymo′ses* [Gr. *ekchymōsis*] a small hemorrhagic spot, larger than a petechia, in the skin or mucous membrane forming a nonelevated, rounded or irregular, blue or purplish patch. **cadaveric e's,** stains seen on the more dependent portions of the body after death, giving the appearance of bruises.

ecchymotic (ek-ĭ-mot′ik) pertaining to or of the nature of an ecchymosis.

Eccles (ek′k'lz), John Carew. Australian physiologist, born 1903; co-winner, with Alan Lloyd Hodgkin and Andrew Fielding Huxley, of the Nobel prize in medicine and physiology for 1963, for discoveries concerning the ionic mechanisms involved in excitation and inhibition in the peripheral and central portions of the nerve cell membrane.

eccoprotic (ek″o-prot′ik) [Gr. *ek* out + *kopros* dung] cathartic.

eccrine (ek′rin) exocrine, with special reference to ordinary sweat glands.

eccrinology (ek-rĭ-nol′o-je) [Gr. *ekkrinein* to secrete + *-logy*] the study or science of secretions and excretions.

eccrisiology (ek-kris″e-ol′o-je) eccrinology.

eccrisis (ek′rĭ-sis) [Gr. *ek* out + *krisis* separation] the excretion or expulsion of waste products.

eccritic (ek-krit′ik) [Gr. *ekkritikos*] 1. promoting excretion. 2. an agent that promotes excretion.

eccyesis (ek″si-e′sis) [Gr. *ek* out + *kyēsis* pregnancy] ectopic pregnancy.

ecdemic (ek-dem′ik) [Gr. *ekdēmos* gone on a journey] not endemic; applied to a disease caused by a factor originating far from the place in which the disease is observed.

ecdovirus (ek″do-vi′rus) [from *enteric cytopathic dog orphan* + *virus*] an enteric orphan virus isolated from dogs; also written *ECDO virus.*

ecdysiasm (ek-di′sĭ-azm) [Gr. *ekdyein* to strip off one's clothes] an abnormal tendency to take off one's clothes.

ecdysis (ek′dĭ-sis) [Gr. *ekdysis* a getting out] desquamation or sloughing; especially the shedding of an outer covering and the development of a new one such as occurs in certain arthropods, crustaceans, lizards, and snakes. Called also *molting.*

ecdysone (ek-di′son) [Gr. *edkysis* a getting out] the hormone produced in the prothoracic glands of arthropods that induces molting (ecdysis) and metamorphosis.

ECF extracellular fluid.

ECF-A abbreviation for eosinophil chemotactic factor of anaphylaxis, a primary mediator of Type I anaphylactic hypersensitivity. It is an acidic peptide (molecular weight 500) released by mast cells, which attracts eosinophils to areas where it is present.

ECG electrocardiogram.

ecgonine (ek′go-nin) chemical name: 3β-hydroxy-2β-tropane-carboxylic acid. The final basic product, $C_9H_{15}NO_3$, obtained by hydrolysis of cocaine and several related alkaloids.

echeosis (ek″e-o′sis) [Gr. *ēchē* loud sound] a neurosis produced by continuous loud or harassing noises.

echidnase (e-kid′nās) [Gr. *echidna* viper + *-ase*] an enzyme found in the venom of vipers.

echidnin (e-kid′nin) [Gr. *echidna* viper] serpent venom, or a nitrogenous poisonous principle from it.

Echidnophaga (ek″id-nof′ah-gah) a genus of fleas. **E. gallina′cea,** the sticktight flea, which collects in dense masses on the heads of chickens, in the ears of other animals, and which may also parasitize man.

echidnotoxin (e-kid′no-tok′sin) a poisonous principle in the venom of vipers.

echidnovaccine (e-kid′no-vak′sēn) [Gr. *echidna* viper + *vaccine*] viper venom that has been deprived of its poisonous power by heating; it is used as a vaccine against venom.

Echinacea (ek″ĭ-na′se-ah) [Gr. *echinos* hedgehog] a genus of composite plants, the cone flowers. The dried rhizome and roots of *E. angustifo′lia* and *E. purpu′rea* have tonic properties.

echinate (ek′ĭ-nāt) echinulate.

echinenone (e-kin′ĕ-nōn) a carotenoid provitamin prepared from the sex glands of sea urchins and which in the body becomes vitamin A.

echino- (e-ki′no) [Gr. *echinos* a prickly husk; hedgehog] a combining form denoting relationship to spines, or spiny.

Echinochasmus (e-ki″no-kaz′mus) [*echino-* + Gr. *chasma* open mouth] a genus of parasitic intestinal flukes. **E. perfolia′tus,** the causative agent of echinostomiasis in Japan.

echinochrome (e-ki′no-krōm) a brown respiratory pigment found in sea urchins.

echinococciasis (e-ki″no-kok-ki′ah-sis) hydatid disease.

echinococcosis (e-ki″no-kok-o′sis) hydatid disease.

echinococcotomy (e-ki″no-kok-kot′o-me) [*echinococcus* + Gr. *tomē* a cutting] evacuation of an echinococcus (hydatid) cyst.

Echinococcus (e-ki″no-kok′us) [*echino-* + Gr. *kokkos* berry] a genus of small tapeworms of the family Taeniidae. **E. alveola′ris,** *E. multilocularis.* **E. granulo′sus,** a small tapeworm parasitic in dogs and wolves and occasionally in cats. Its larva, known as the hydatid, may develop in nearly all mammals, forming hydatid tumors or cysts in the liver, lungs, kidneys, and other organs. See *hydatid disease, unilocular,* under *disease.* **E. multilocula′ris,** a species whose adults usually parasitize the fox and wild rodents, although man is sporadically infected. It resembles *E. granulosis,* but the larvae form alveolar or multilocular cysts rather than unilocular cysts. See *hydatid disease, alveolar,* under *disease.*

echinocyte (e-ki′no-sīt) [*echino-* + Gr. *kytos* hollow vessel] a burr cell.

echinoderm (e-kin′o-derm) one of the Echinodermata.

Echinodermata (e-ki″no-der′mah-tah) [*echino-* + Gr. *derma* skin] a phylum of the animal kingdom, including starfishes, sea urchins, etc.

Echinolaelaps (e-ki″no-le′laps) a genus of mites found on rats and in stable litter; its bite causes intense itching. Called also *Laelaps* or *Lelaps.* **E. echidni′nus,** a mite that acts as an intermediate host of *Hepatozoon muris* and *H. perniciosum.*

echinophthalmia (e-kin″of-thal′me-ah) [*echino-* + *ophthalmia*] inflammation of the eyelids marked by projection of the lashes.

Echinorhynchus (e-ki″no-ring′kus) [*echino-* + Gr. *rhynchos* beak] a former genus of parasitic worms. **E. gi′gas, E. hom′inis,** *Macracanthorhynchus hirudinaceus.* **E. monilifor′mis,** *Moniliformis moniliformis.*

echinosis (ek″ĭ-no′sis) [Gr. *echinos* hedgehog + *-osis*] irregularity in the form of an erythrocyte, giving it a spiny appearance. Cf. *crenation.*

Echinostoma (ek″ĭ-nos′to-mah) [*echino-* + Gr. *stoma* mouth] a genus of parasitic flukes. *E. revolu′tum* is found in the intestines of ducks and geese and has been reported in man in Taiwan and Indonesia. *E. iloca′num* has been found in the feces of natives of Java and the Philippine Islands. *E. lindoen′sis* occurs in Celebes; *E. perfolia′tum* in Japan.

echinostomiasis (e-kin″o-sto-mi′ah-sis) infection by flukes of the genus *Echinostoma* or of related genera of the family Echinostomatidae.

echinulate (e-kin′u-lāt) [L. *echinus* hedgehog] having small prickles or spines; applied in bacteriology to cultures showing toothed or pointed outgrowths.

Echis (e′kis) a genus of small venomous vipers ranging from India to North Africa.

echo (ek′o) [Gr. *ēchō* a returned sound] repetition of a sound as a result of reverberation of sound waves; also the reflection of ultrasonic, radio, and radar waves. Sometimes used to refer to repetition of movement. **amphoric e.,** a resonant repetition of a sound heard on auscultation of the chest, occurring at an appreciable interval after the vocal sound. **metallic e.,** a peculiar ringing repetition of the heart sounds sometimes heard in patients with pneumopericardium and pneumothorax.

echoacousia (ek″o-ah-koo′ze-ah) [*echo* + Gr. *akousis* hearing +

-ia] the subjective experience of hearing echoes after normally heard sounds.

echocardiogram (ek″o-kar′de-o-gram″) the record produced by echocardiography.

echocardiography (ek″o-kar″de-og′rah-fe) a method of graphically recording the position and motion of the heart walls or the internal structures of the heart and neighboring tissue by the echo obtained from beams of ultrasonic waves directed through the chest wall. Called also *ultrasonic cardiography.*

echoencephalogram (ek″o-en-sef′ah-lo-gram″) the record produced by echoencephalography.

echoencephalograph (ek″o-en-sef′ah-lo-graf) the instrument used in echoencephalography.

echoencephalography (ek″o-en-sef″ah-log′rah-fe) a diagnostic technique in which pulses of ultrasonic waves are beamed through the head from both sides, and echoes from the midline structures of the brain are recorded as graphic tracings; shifts from the midline may indicate a centrally placed mass.

echogenic (ek″o-jen′ik) in ultrasonography, giving rise to reflections (echoes) of ultrasound waves.

echogram (ek′o-gram) the record made by echography.

echographia (ek-o-gra′fe-ah) [*echo* + Gr. *graphein* to write + *-ia*] an aphasic condition in which the patient can copy writing, but cannot write to express ideas.

echography (ĕ-kog′rah-fe) ultrasonography; the use of ultrasound as a diagnostic aid. Ultrasound waves are directed at the tissues, and a record is made, as on an oscilloscope, of the waves reflected back through the tissues, which indicate interfaces of different acoustic densities and thus differentiate between solid and cystic structures.

echokinesis (ek″o-ki-ne′sis) [*echo* + Gr. *kinesis* motion] echopraxia.

echolalia (ek″o-la′le-ah) [*echo* + Gr. *lalia* speech, babble] the repetition by a patient of words addressed to him; called also *echophrasia.* **delayed e.,** echolalia, the onset of which does not follow immediately after the stimulus; it may occur days or weeks later.

echolalus (ek″o-la′lus), pl. *echola′li* [L.] a person who in a hypnotized state repeats meaninglessly the words he hears.

echolucent (ek″o-loo′sent) permitting the passage of ultrasonic waves without giving rise to echoes, the representative areas appearing black on the sonogram.

echomimia (ek″o-mim′e-ah) [*echo* + Gr. *mimia* imitation] echopraxia.

echomotism (ek″o-mo′tizm) [*echo* + L. *motio* movement] echopraxia.

echopathy (ek-op′ah-the) [*echo* + Gr. *pathos* disease] a neurosis marked by the senseless repetition of words or actions of others.

echophonocardiography (ek″o-fo″no-kar″de-og′rah-fe) the combined use of echocardiography and phonocardiography.

echophony (ek-of′o-ne) [*echo* + Gr. *phōne* voice] an echo-like sound heard immediately after a vocal sound on auscultation of the chest.

echophotony (ek″o-fot′o-ne) [*echo* + Gr. *phōs* light + *tonos* tone] the association of certain colors with certain sounds.

echophrasia (ek″o-fra′se-ah) echolalia.

echopraxia (ek″o-prak′se-ah) the spasmodic and involuntary imitation of the movements of another.

echopraxis (ek″o-prak′sis) [*echo* + Gr. *prassein* to perform] echopraxia.

echo-ranging (ek″o-ranj′ing) in ultrasonography, the determining of the position or depth of a body structure on the basis of the time interval between the moment an ultrasonic pulse is transmitted and the moment its echo is received.

echothiophate iodide (ek″o-thi′o-fāt) [USP] chemical name: 2-[(diethoxyphosphinyl)thio]-*N,N,N*-trimethylethaminium iodide. A cholinergic, $C_9H_{23}INO_3PS$, occurring as a white, crystalline solid; used as a miotic in certain forms of glaucoma, applied topically to the conjunctiva.

echovirus (ek″o-vi′rus) [*enteric cytopathic human orphan* + *virus*] an enteric orphan RNA virus isolated from man, separable into many serotypes, certain of which are associated with human disease, especially aseptic meningitis; also written *ECHO virus.* **e. 28,** a serotype isolated from patients with mild respiratory disease, pathogenic for man but not for conventional laboratory animals, including the suckling mouse and monkey, by the intracerebral route; also written *ECHO 28 virus.*

Eck's fistula (eks) [Nicolai Vladimirovich *Eck,* Russian physiologist, 1847–1908] see under *fistula.*

Ecker's fissure (ek′erz) [Alexander *Ecker,* German anatomist, 1816–1887] see under *convolution* and *fissure.*

Ecker's fluid (ek′erz) [Enrique E. *Ecker,* American bacteriologist, born 1859] Rees and Ecker diluting fluid; see under *fluid.*

eclabium (ek-la′be-um) [Gr. *ek* out + L. *labium* lip] eversion of the lips or of a lip.

Eclabron (ek′lah-bron) trademark for preparations of guaithylline.

eclampsia (ĕ-klamp′se-ah) [Gr. *eklampein* to shine forth] convulsions and coma occurring in a pregnant or puerperal woman, associated with preeclampsia, i.e., with hypertension, edema, and/or proteinuria. **puerperal e.,** that occurring after childbirth. **uremic e.,** eclampsia due to uremia.

eclampsism (ĕ-klamp′sizm) preeclampsia.

eclamptic (ĕ-klamp′tik) pertaining to or of the nature of eclampsia.

eclamptism (ĕ-klamp′tizm) the condition due to the autointoxication incident to pregnancy, and marked by headache, visual impairment, and sometimes by convulsions.

eclamptogenic (ĕ-klamp″to-jen′ik) causing convulsions.

eclectic (ĕ-klek′tik) [Gr. *eklektikos* selecting] designating a sect or school which professes to select what is best from all other systems of medicine. See *eclecticism.*

eclecticism (ĕ-klek′tĭ-sizm) [Gr. *eklegein* to pick out] a once popular system of medicine which treats diseases by the application of single remedies to known pathologic conditions, without reference to nosology, special attention being given to developing indigenous plant remedies.

eclipse (e-klips′) in virology, that period of the infective cycle during which infected bacterial cells contain no detectable infective bacteriophage.

eclysis (ek′lĭ-sis) mild syncope.

ecmnesia (ek-ne′ze-ah) [Gr. *ek* out of + *mnēmē* memory] forgetfulness of recent events with normal memory for more remote ones.

ecmovirus (ek″mo-vi′rus) [from *enteric cytopathic monkey orphan* + *virus*] an enteric orphan virus isolated from monkeys; also written *ECMO virus.*

ecochleation (e-kok″le-a′shun) 1. excision of the cochlea. 2. enucleation.

ecogenetics (ek″o-jĕ-net′iks) the study of the relationship between genetic factors and the nature of response to an environmental agent.

ecoid (e′koid) (*obs.*) the colorless framework of a red blood corpuscle.

ecologist (e-kol′o-jist) an individual skilled in ecology.

ecology (e-kol′o-je) [Gr. *oikos* house + *-logy*] the science of organisms as affected by the factors of their environments; study of the environment and life history of organisms. **human e.,** application of the ecologic approach to the study of human societies.

ecomania (e″ko-ma′ne-ah) [Gr. *oikos* house + *mania* madness] an attitude of mind that is dominating toward members of the family but humble toward those in authority.

econazole nitrate (ĕ-kon′ah-zōl) chemical name: 1-[2-[(4-chlorophenyl)methoxy]-2-(2,4-dichlorophenyl)ethyl]-1*H*-imidazole. A broad-spectrum antifungal with some antibacterial activity, $C_{18}H_{15}Cl_3N_2O \cdot HNO_3$; used topically in the treatment of infections due to susceptible organisms, including dermatophytes, and in vaginal candidiasis.

Economo's disease (encephalitis) (a-kon′o-mōz) [Constantin von *Economo,* Austrian neurologist, 1876–1931] encephalitis lethargica.

economy (e-kon′o-me) [Gr. *oikos* house + *nomos* law] the management of domestic affairs. **animal e.,** the system of operation of the bodily processes in organic bodies; also the body as an organized whole. **token e.,** a program of treatment in behavior therapy, usually conducted in a hospital setting, in which the patient may earn tokens by engaging in appropriate personal and social behavior, or lose tokens by inappropriate or antisocial behavior; tokens may be exchanged for tangible rewards (food snacks, clothing, etc.) or for special privileges (watching television, passes to leave the hospital, etc.).

ecoparasite (e″ko-par′ah-sīt) ecosite.

écorché (a″kor-sha′) [Fr.] a painting or sculpture of a man or other animal exhibited as deprived of its skin, so that the muscles are exposed for study.

ecostate (e-kos′tāt) [L. *e* without + *costa* rib] ribless; without ribs.

ecosystem (ek″o-sis′tem) the fundamental unit in ecology, comprising the living organisms and the nonliving elements interacting in a certain defined area.

ecotaxis (ek′o-tak″sis) [Gr. *oikos* house + *taxis* arrangement] the movement or "homing" of a circulating cell, e.g., a lymphocyte, to a specific anatomical compartment.

ecotone (ek′o-tōn) a transition region where adjacent biomes blend, containing some organisms from each of the adjacent biomes plus some that are characteristic of, and perhaps restricted to, the ecotone; this region tends to have more species and to be more densely populated than either adjacent biome.

Ecotrin (ek′o-trin) trademark for a preparation of aspirin.

écouvillon (a-koo″ve-yaw′) [Fr.] a stiff brush or swab used for swabbing cavities and inflammatory lesions.

écouvillonage (a-koo″ve-yŏ-nahzh′) [Fr.] the scrubbing of a cavity or an infected area.

ecphoria (ek-fo′re-ah) [Gr. *ekphoros* to be made known + *-ia*] the revival of an engram, or memory trace.

ecphorize (ek′fo-rīz) to revive an engram, or memory trace, and bring it into the consciousness.

ecphory (ek′fo-re) ecphoria.

ecphyadectomy (ek″fi-ah-dek′to-me) [Gr. *ekphyas* appendix + *ektomē* excision] (*obs.*) appendectomy.

ecphyaditis (ek″fi-ah-di′tis) [Gr. *ekphyas* appendix + *-itis*] appendicitis.

ecphylactic (ek″fi-lak′tik) pertaining to or marked by ecphylaxis.

ecphylaxis (ek″fi-lak′sis) [Gr. *ek* out of + *phylaxis* a guarding] a condition of impotency of the antibodies in the blood.

écrasement (a-krahz-maw′) [Fr.] removal by means of the écraseur.

écraseur (e-krah-zer′) [Fr. "crusher"] an instrument containing a chain or cord to be looped about a part and then tightened in order to transect the portion enclosed within the loop.

ECS electroconvulsive shock; see *shock therapy*, under *therapy*.

ecsomatics (ek″so-mat′iks) [Gr. *ek* out + *sōma* body] the study by laboratory methods of the materials removed from the body.

ecsovirus (ek″so-vi′rus) [from *enteric cytopathic swine orphan + virus*] an enteric orphan virus isolated from swine; also written *ECSO virus*.

ecstasy (ek′stah-se) [Gr. *ekstasis*] a kind of trance or state of fixed contemplation with mental exaltation, partial abeyance of most of the functions, and rapt expression of countenance.

ecstatic (ek-stat′ik) pertaining to or characterized by ecstasy.

ecstrophy (ek′stro-fe) [Gr. *ekstrephein* to turn inside out] exstrophy.

E.C.T. electroconvulsive therapy.

ectacolia (ek″tah-ko′le-ah) ectasia of a portion of the colon.

ectad (ek′tad) [Gr. *ektos* without] outward; the reverse of inward.

ectal (ek′tal) [Gr. *ektos* without] superficial or external.

ectasia (ek-ta′ze-ah) [Gr. *ektasis* + *-ia*] dilatation, expansion, or distention. **alveolar e.,** overdistention of the pulmonary alveoli. **annuloaortic e.,** dilatation of the proximal aorta and the fibrous ring of the heart at the aortic orifice, marked by aortic regurgitation and, when severe, by dissecting aneurysm; it is often associated with Marfan's syndrome. **corneal e.,** keratectasia. **diffuse arterial e.,** racemose aneurysm. **hypostatic e.,** dilatation of a blood vessel from the effect of gravity on the blood. **mammary duct e.,** a condition characterized chiefly by dilatation of the collecting ducts of the mammary gland, inspissation of breast secretion, intraductal inflammation, and marked periductal and interstitial chronic inflammatory reaction in which plasma cells are prominent; a benign process associated with atrophy of the duct epithelium, it generally occurs during or after the menopause. **papillary e.,** a circumscribed dilatation of the capillaries, forming a red spot on the skin. **scleral e.,** see under *staphyloma*. **tubular e.,** a congenital, usually bilateral and diffuse condition of the renal medulla characterized by dilated collecting tubules and medullary cysts.

ectasis (ek′tah-sis) ectasia.

ectasy (ek′tah-se) ectasia.

ectatic (ek-tat′ik) distended or stretched; distensible.

ectental (ek-ten′tal) [Gr. *ektos* without + *entos* within] pertaining to the ectoderm and entoderm, and to their line of junction.

ecterograph (ek′ter-o-graf) [Gr. *ektos* outside + *graphein* to write] an apparatus for recording graphically the movements of the intestines.

ectethmoid (ek-teth′moid) [Gr. *ektos* without + *ethmoid*] one of the paired lateral masses of the ethmoid bone.

ecthyma (ek-thi′mah) [Gr. *ekthyma*] a shallowly ulcerative form of impetigo, usually on the shins or forearms; it is usually secondary to minor trauma and often results in scarring. **e. contagio′sum,** contagious pustular dermatitis of sheep caused by a virus, which sometimes infects human beings; orf. **e. gangreno′sum,** a *Pseudomonas* infection in the newborn resembling dermatitis gangrenosa infantum (q.v.). **e. infecti-o′sum,** orf. **e. syphilit′icum,** an ecthymiform eruption in tertiary syphilis.

ecthymiform (ek-thi′mĭ-form) resembling ecthyma.

ecthyreosis (ek-thi″re-o′sis) [Gr. *ek* out + *thyroid*] absence of the thyroid gland or loss of the function of the gland.

ecto- [Gr. *ektos* outside] a prefix denoting situated on, without, or on the outside.

ectoantigen (ek″to-an′te-jen) an antigen which seems to be loosely attached to the outside of bacteria so that it can be readily removed by shaking them in physiologic sodium chloride solution; also an antigen formed in the ectoplasm of a bacterium.

ectobiology (ek″to-bi-ol′o-je) the study of the properties and biochemical constitution of the cell surface and the specific enzymes at the surface.

ectoblast (ek′to-blast) [*ecto-* + Gr. *blastos* germ] 1. the ectoderm. 2. an external membrane; a cell wall.

ectocardia (ek-to-kar′de-ah) [*ecto-* + Gr. *kardia* heart] congenital displacement of the heart, either inside or outside the thorax.

ectocervical (ek″to-ser′vĭ-kal) of or pertaining to the ectocervix.

ectocervix (ek″to-ser′viks) the portio vaginalis cervicis, the part of the uterine cervix lined with stratified squamous epithelium; called also *exocervix*.

ectocinerea (ek″to-sĭ-ne′re-ah) [*ecto-* + *cinerea*] (*obs.*) the cortical gray matter of the brain.

ectocinereal (ek″to-sĭ-ne′re-al) (*obs.*) relating to the ectocinerea.

ectocolon (ek″to-ko′lon) [Gr. *ektasis* dilatation + *kolon* colon] dilatation of the colon.

ectocolostomy (ek″to-ko-los′to-me) [*ecto-* + *colostomy*] (*obs.*) the surgical formation of an opening into the colon through the abdominal wall.

ectocommensal (ek″to-kom-men′sal) a commensal organism that lives outside the body of its symbiotic companion, but cannot be separated from it.

ectocondyle (ek″to-kon′dīl) the external condyle of a bone.

ectocuneiform (ek″to-ku-ne′ĭ-form) the lateral cuneiform bone.

ectocytic (ek″to-si′tik) [*ecto-* + Gr. *kytos* hollow vessel] outside the cell.

ectoderm (ek′to-derm) [*ecto-* + Gr. *derma* skin] the outermost of the three primary germ layers of the embryo. From it are developed the epidermis and the epidermal tissues, such as the nails, hair, and glands of the skin, the nervous system, the external sense organs, as the ear, eye, etc., and the mucous membrane of the mouth and anus. Cf. *entoderm* and *mesoderm*. **amniotic e.,** the inner layer of the amnion (and covering of the umbilical cord) that is continuous with body ectoderm. **basal e.,** trophoblast covering the eroded uterine tissue that faces the placental sinuses. **blastodermic e.,** the external layer of a blastula or blastodisk; called also *primitive e.* **chorionic e.,** the trophoblast. **extraembryonic e.,** a derivative of epiblast or ectoderm located outside the body of the embryo. **neural e.,** the region of the ectoderm destined to become the neural tube; neuroderm. **primitive e.,** blastodermic e.

ectodermal (ek″to-der′mal) [*ecto-* + Gr. *derma* skin] pertaining to or derived from the ectoderm.

ectodermatosis (ek″to-der″mah-to′sis) ectodermosis.

ectodermic (ek″to-der′mik) ectodermal.

ectodermoidal (ek″to-der-moid′al) of the nature of or resembling the ectoderm.

ectodermosis (ek″to-der-mo′sis) a disorder based on congenital maldevelopment of the organs of ectodermal derivation, i.e., nervous system, retina, eyeball, and skin. **e. erosi′va pluri-orificia′lis,** Stevens-Johnson syndrome.

ectoentad (ek″to-en′tad) from without inward.

ectoenzyme (ek″to-en′zīm) an enzyme secreted from a cell into the surrounding medium; an extracellular enzyme. Cf. *endoenzyme*.

ectogenic (ek″to-jen′ik) ectogenous.

ectogenous (ek-toj′ĕ-nus) [*ecto-* + Gr. *gennan* to produce] introduced from without; arising from causes outside the organism, as an infectious disease.

ectoglia (ek-tog′le-ah) [*ecto-* + Gr. *glia* glue] the thin, external marginal layer of the early medullary tube of the embryo.

ectoglobular (ek″to-glob′u-lar) [*ecto-* + *globule*] (*obs.*) formed outside the blood cells.

ectogony (ek-tog′o-ne) the influence exerted on the mother by the developing embryo. Improperly called *metaxenia*.

ectohormone (ek″to-hor′mōn) a hormone secreted to the outside of the body, as a pheromone.

ectolecithal (ek″to-les′ĭ-thal) [*ecto-* + Gr. *lekithos* yolk] having the yolk situated peripherally; see under *ovum*.

ectolysis (ek-tol′ĭ-sis) [*ectoplasm* + *lysis*] lysis of the ectoplasm.

ectomere (ek′to-mēr) [*ecto-* + Gr. *meros* part] any of the blastomeres which share in the formation of the ectoderm.

ectomesoblast (ek″to-mes′o-blast) the layer of cells which has not yet become differentiated into ectoblast and mesoblast.

-ectomize (ek′to-mīz) [Gr. *ektomē* excision + *-izein* to render] a word termination meaning to deprive by excision, as in *thyroidectomize*, *adrenalectomize*, etc. By extension, used in terms to designate destruction or deprivation by other methods as well.

ectomorph (ek′to-morf) an individual having a type of body build in which tissues derived from the ectoderm predominate: there is a preponderance of linearity and fragility, with large surface area, thin muscles and subcutaneous tissue, and slightly developed digestive viscera, as contrasted with endomorph and mesomorph.

ectomorphic (ek″to-mor′fik) pertaining to or characteristic of an ectomorph.

ectomorphy (ek′to-mor″fe) [ectoblast + Gr. *morphē* form] the condition of being an ectomorph.

ectomy (ek′to-me) [Gr. *ektomē*] excision of an organ or part. Used as a word termination to indicate excision of the structure or organ designated by the root to which it is affixed, as *appendectomy, tonsillectomy*, etc. By extension, used in terms to designate destruction or deprivation by other methods as well.

ectonuclear (ek″to-nu′kle-ar) outside the nucleus of a cell.

ectopagus (ek-top′ah-gus) [ecto- + Gr. *pagos* something fixed] a double monster connected along the side of the body, so that the components are definitely right and left, the inner arms and/or legs being represented by a bilateral median limb.

ectoparasite (ek″to-par′ah-sīt) [ecto- + *parasite*] a parasite that lives on the outside of the body of the host.

ectopectoralis (ek″to-pek″to-ra′lis) musculus pectoralis major.

ectoperitoneal (ek″to-per″ĭ-to-ne′al) relating to the external or abdominal surface of the peritoneum.

ectoperitonitis (ek″to-per″ĭ-to-ni′tis) [ecto- + *peritonitis*] inflammation of the external or abdominal side of the peritoneum.

ectophyte (ek′to-fīt) [ecto- + Gr. *phyton* plant] a vegetable parasite or species living on the outside of the body of its host.

ectopia (ek-to′pe-ah) [Gr. *ektopos* displaced + *-ia*] displacement or malposition, especially if congenital. **e. cloa′cae,** exstrophy of cloaca. **e. cor′dis,** congenital displacement of the heart outside the thoracic cavity. **e. cor′dis, pectoral,** location of the heart outside the chest wall, through a fissure in the lower sternum. **e. cor′dis abdomina′lis,** location of the heart in the abdominal cavity. **crossed renal e.,** a condition in which the two kidneys are on the same side of the body, one ureter crossing the midline. **e. i′ridis,** displacement of the iris, with resultant abnormal smallness of the pupil. **e. len′tis,** displacement of the crystalline lens of the eye. **e. pupil′lae congen′ita,** congenital displacement of the pupil. **renal e., e. re′nis,** displacement of the kidney. **e. tes′tis,** dislocation of the testicle. **e. vesi′cae,** exstrophy of the bladder.

ectopic (ek-top′ik) 1. pertaining to or characterized by ectopia. 2. located away from normal position, as in ectopic pregnancy. 3. arising from an abnormal site or tissue.

ectopism (ek′to-pizm) anatopism.

ectoplacenta (ek-to-plah-sen′tah) [ecto- + Gr. *placenta* cake] the actively growing trophoblast that becomes the placenta in rodents.

ectoplasm (ek′to-plazm) [ecto- + Gr. *plasma* a thing formed] plasma membrane.

ectoplasmatic (ek″to-plaz-mat′ik) pertaining to ectoplasm.

ectoplast (ek′to-plast) cell membrane.

ectoplastic (ek″to-plas′tik) [ecto- + Gr. *plassein* to shape] having a formative power on the surface, as *ectoplastic* cells.

ectopotomy (ek″to-pot′o-me) [Gr. *ektopos* displaced + Gr. tomē a cutting] operation for extrauterine pregnancy.

ectopterygoid (ek″to-ter′ĭ-goid) musculus pterygoideus lateralis.

ectopy (ek′to-pe) ectopia.

ectosarc (ek′to-sark) [ecto- + Gr. *sarx* flesh] plasma membrane.

ectoscopy (ek-tos′ko-pe) [ecto- + Gr. *skopein* to examine] a diagnostic method based on observation of chest and abdominal movements, and said to be capable of determining the outlines of the lungs and of localized internal conditions.

ectosite (ek′to-sīt) (*obs.*) ectoparasite.

ectoskeleton (ek″to-skel′ĕ-ton) exoskeleton.

ectosphere (ek′to-sfēr) the outer zone of the centrosome.

ectosteal (ek-tos′te-al) pertaining to or situated on the outside of a bone.

ectostosis (ek″to-sto′sis) [ecto- + Gr. *osteon* bone] ossification beneath the perichondrium of a cartilage or the periosteum of a bone.

ectosuggestion (ek″to-sug-jes′chun) a suggestion originating from outside. Cf. *autosuggestion*.

ectosymbiont (ek″to-sim′be-ont) a symbiont that lives outside the body of the organism with which it is biologically related.

ectothrix (ek′to-thriks) [ecto- + Gr. *thrix* hair] a fungus which grows inside the hair shaft but also produces a sheath of arthrospores on the outside of the hair. Such fungi include *Trichophyton verrucosum* (*large-spored e.*) and *T. mentagrophytes, Microsporum audouinii, M. canis,* and *M. gypseum* (*small-spored e's*).

ectotoxemia (ek″to-tok-se′me-ah) [ecto- + *toxemia*] (*obs.*) toxemia produced by a substance introduced from outside the body.

ectotoxin (ek″to-tok′sin) (*obs.*) exotoxin.

Ectotrichophyton (ek″to-tri-kof′ĭ-ton) [ecto- + Gr. *thrix* hair + *phyton* plant] former name for a genus of fungi, now included in the genus *Trichophyton*.

ectozoa (ek″to-zo′ah) [Gr.] plural of *ectozoon*.

ectozoal (ek″to-zo′al) pertaining to or caused by ectozoa.

ectozoon (ek″to-zo′on), pl. *ectozo′a* [ecto- + Gr. *zōon* animal] ectoparasite.

ectro- [Gr. *ektrōsis* miscarriage] a combining form signifying congenital absence of a part.

ectrodactylia (ek″tro-dak-til′e-ah) ectrodactyly.

ectrodactylism (ek″tro-dak′tĭ-lism) ectrodactyly.

ectrodactyly (ek″tro-dak′tĭ-le) [Gr. *ektrōsis* abortion + *daktylos* finger] congenital absence of all or of only part of a digit (*partial e.*).

ectrogenic (ek″tro-jen′ik) pertaining to or characterized by ectrogeny.

ectrogeny (ek-troj′ĕ-ne) [Gr. *ektrōsis* abortion + *gennan* to produce] congenital absence or defect of a part.

ectromelia (ek″tro-me′le-ah) [ectro- + Gr. *melos* limb + *-ia*] gross hypoplasia or aplasia of one or more long bones of one or more limbs; the term includes amelia, hemimelia, and phocomelia. **infectious e.,** a disease of mice caused by a poxvirus and characterized by gangrene and often loss of one or more of the feet and sometimes of other external parts, and by necrotic areas in the liver, spleen, and other organs; called also *mousepox*.

ectromelic (ek″tro-mel′ik) pertaining to or characterized by ectromelia.

ectromelus (ek-trom′ĕ-lus) [Gr. *ektrōsis* abortion + *melos* limb] an individual exhibiting ectromelia.

ectrometacarpia (ek″tro-met″ah-kar′pe-ah) [Gr. *ektrōsis* abortion + *metacarpus* + *-ia*] congenital absence of a metacarpal bone.

ectrometatarsia (ek″tro-met″ah-tar′se-ah) [Gr. *ektrōsis* abortion + *metatarsus* + *-ia*] congenital absence of a metatarsal bone.

ectrophalangia (ek″tro-fah-lan′je-ah) congenital absence of one or more phalanges of a digit.

ectropion (ek-tro′pe-on) [Gr. "an everted eyelid"; *ektropē* a turning aside] the turning outward (eversion) of an edge or margin, as of the eyelid, resulting in exposure of the palpebral conjunctiva. **cervical e.,** eversion of uterine cervix. **e. cicatri′ceum, cicatricial e.,** eversion of the margin of an eyelid caused by contraction of scar tissue in the lid or by contraction of the skin. **flaccid e.,** ectropion of the lower lid resulting from reduced tone of the orbicularis oculi muscle. **e. luxu′rians,** e. sarcomatosum. **paralytic e., e. paralyt′icum,** eversion of the margin of the lower eyelid as a result of paralysis of the facial nerve, and loss of contractile power of the orbicularis oculi muscle. **e. of pigment layer,** proliferation of the cells in the posteriorly situated pigment layer of the iris, leading to their migration around the pupillary margin to encroach upon the anterior surface of the iris. **e. sarcomato′sum,** eversion of an eyelid resulting from chronic thickening of the palpebral conjunctiva; called also *e. luxurians*. **senile e., e. seni′lis,** eversion of the lower eyelid associated with relaxation of the fibers of the palpebral portion of the orbicularis oculi muscle as a concomitant of age, or occurring as a result of atrophic changes in the skin. **spastic e., e. spas′ticum,** ectropion caused by tonic spasm of the orbicularis oculi muscle. **e. u′veae,** eversion of the margin of the pupil, often congenital (*e. u′veae congen′itum*), and frequently due to the presence of a newly formed membrane on the anterior layer of the iris, or to the formation of connective tissue in the stroma, particularly in diabetes. Called also *iridectropium*.

ectropionize (ek-tro′pe-ŏ-nīz″) to put into a state of eversion.

ectropium (ek-tro′pe-um) ectropion.

ectrosis (ek-tro′sis) [Gr. *ektrōsis*] 1. abortion. 2. treatment that arrests the development of disease.

ectrosyndactylia (ek″tro-sin″dak-til′e-ah) ectrosyndactyly.

ectrosyndactyly (ek″tro-sin-dak′tĭ-le) [Gr. *ektrōsis* abortion + *syn* together + *daktylos* finger] a condition in which some of the digits are missing and those that remain are webbed, so that they are more or less attached.

ectrotic (ek-trot′ik) 1. pertaining to or producing abortion. 2. arresting the development of a disease.

ectylurea (ek″til-u-re′ah) chemical name: cis-(2-ethylcrotonyl)-urea. A white crystalline powder, $C_7H_{12}N_2O_2$, used as a sedative.

ectyonin (ek″tĭ-on′in) an antimicrobial substance obtained from the sponge *Microciona prolifera*.

ectype (ek′tīp) an unusual type of physical or mental constitution.

ectypia (ek-ti′pe-ah) deviation from type; the possession of an unusual type of constitution.

eczema (ek′zĕ-mah) [Gr. *ekzein* to boil out] 1. a superficial inflammatory process involving primarily the epidermis, characterized early by redness, itching, minute papules and vesicles, weeping, oozing, and crusting, and later by scaling, lichenification, and often pigmentation. It is not a disease entity or an acceptable diagnosis. 2. atopic dermatitis. **allergic e.** (*obs.*), allergic dermatitis. **atopic e.** (*obs.*), 1. see under *dermatitis*. 2. atopic dermatitis. **e. cap′itis** (*obs.*), seborrheic dermatitis or allergic contact dermatitis of the scalp. **contact e.,** contact dermatitis (def. 1). **e. ep′ilans** (*obs.*), eczema with loss of hair. **facial**

e. of ruminants, a photosensitive disease of ruminants, particularly in New Zealand, due to ingestion of the spores of the mold *Pithomyces chartarum* (class Deuteromycetes), which contain sporidesmin. **flexural e.,** atopic dermatitis. **e. herpet'icum,** disseminated herpes simplex; see also *Kaposi's varicelliform eruption.* **impetiginous e.,** infectious eczematoid dermatitis. **infantile e.,** atopic dermatitis in infants. Called also *Besnier's prurigo* (in Britain). **e. intertri'go,** intertrigo. **e. margina'tum,** tinea cruris. **nummular e., e. nummula're,** eczema in which the patches are coin shaped; it may be a form of neurodermatitis. **orbicular e.,** nummular e. **seborrheic e., e. seborrhoe'icum** (*obs.*), seborrheic dermatitis. **solar e., e. sola're** (*obs.*), polymorphous light eruption. **stasis e.,** stasis dermatitis. **e. vaccina'tum,** a serious and generalized vesiculopustular eruption caused by the vaccinia virus, superimposed upon a preexisting chronic dermatitis, usually atopic dermatitis. See also *Kaposi's varicelliform eruption.*

eczematid, eczematide (ek-zem'ah-tid) loosely, an eczematous lesion not caused by external contact-type allergy, or by infection in the involved area; the term has different uses in different countries and little currency in the United States.

eczematization (ek-zem″ah-ti-za'shun) persistent eczema-like lesions of the skin, usually due to the continued trauma of scratching.

eczematogenic (ek-zem″ah-to-jen'ik) causing eczema.

eczematoid (ek-zem'ah-toid) resembling eczema.

eczematous (ek-zem'ah-tus) affected with or of the nature of eczema.

E.D. erythema dose; effective dose.

ED$_{50}$ median effective dose; a dose that produces the desired effect in 50 per cent of a population.

edathamil (ĕ-dath'ah-mil) edetate. **calcium disodium e.,** edetate calcium disodium. **e. disodium,** edetate disodium.

Eddowes' syndrome (disease) (ed'ōz) [Alfred *Eddowes*, British physician, 1850–1946] see under *syndrome.*

Edebohls' operation, position (ed'e-bōlz) [George Michael *Edebohls*, New York surgeon, 1853–1908] see under *operation* and *position.*

Edecrin (ĕ-dek'krin) trademark for preparations of ethacrynic acid.

Edelman, Gerald Maurice. American biochemist, born 1929, co-winner, with Rodney Porter, of the Nobel prize in physiology and medicine for 1972, for his work on the chemical structure of antibodies.

Edelmann's anemia, cell (a'del-manz) [Adolf *Edelmann*, physician in Vienna, 1885–1939] see under *anemia,* and see *kinetocyte.*

edema (ĕ-de'mah) [Gr. *oidēma* swelling] the presence of abnormally large amounts of fluid in the intercellular tissue spaces of the body; usually applied to demonstrable accumulation of excessive fluid in the subcutaneous tissues. Edema may be localized, due to venous or lymphatic obstruction or to increased vascular permeability, or it may be systemic due to heart failure or renal disease. Collections of edema fluid are designated according to the site, e.g., ascites (peritoneal cavity), hydrothorax (pleural cavity), and hydropericardium (pericardial sac). Massive generalized edema is called *anasarca.* **acute circumscribed e., acute essential e.,** angioneurotic e. **alimentary e.,** nutritional edema. **ambulant e.** (*obs.*), Calabar swelling; see under *swelling.* **angioneurotic e.,** recurring attacks of transient edema suddenly appearing in areas of the skin or mucous membranes and occasionally of the viscera, often associated with dermatographism, urticaria, erythema, and purpura. In the hereditary form, transmitted as an autosomal dominant trait, it tends to involve more visceral lesions than the sporadic form, especially of the respiratory and gastrointestinal tracts; two types of the familial form have been identified: one involves failure of synthesis of the inhibitor of complement component C1, the other involves the synthesis of an abnormal protein. Called also *acute circumscribed e., Milton's e., Quincke's e., wandering e., angioedema,* and *giant urticaria.* **e. artefac'tum,** edema that is artificially produced. **Berlin's e.,** commotio retinae. **blue e.,** a puffed, bluish appearance of a limb in hysterical paralysis. **brain e.,** an excessive accumulation of fluid in the brain substance (*wet brain*); it may be due to various causes, including trauma, tumor, and increased permeability of the capillaries occurring as a result of anoxia or exposure to toxic substances. **brown e.,** hardening and infiltration of the lung with a brownish fluid. **e. bullo'sum vesi'cae,** a condition of the mucous lining of the bladder marked by the formation of clear vesicles with small white particles floating between them. **Calabar e.,** Calabar swellings. **e. cal'idum,** inflammatory e. **cardiac e.,** a manifestation of congestive heart failure, caused by increased venous and capillary pressures and often associated with the retention of sodium by the kidneys. **circumscribed e.,** angioneurotic e. **dependent e.,** edema affecting most seriously the lowermost or dependent parts of the body. **famine e.,** nutritional e. **fingerprint e.,** edema in which the whorls of the fingerprint are clearly visible after circumferential manipulation of a pressure point on the forehead or sternum, considered indicative of

intracellular fluid excess. **e. frig'idum,** noninflammatory e. **e. fu'gax,** transient accumulation of fluid in a specific region. **gaseous e.,** edema accompanied with gas formation, as in gas bacillus infection and subcutaneous emphysema. **giant e.,** angioneurotic e. **hepatic e.,** edema due to faulty functioning of the liver. **high-altitude pulmonary e.,** pulmonary edema caused by hypoxia that develops as a result of prolonged exertion after ascending quickly to high altitudes without the benefit of acclimatization; seen especially in mountain climbers. **Huguenin's e.,** acute congestive edema of the brain. **hunger e.,** nutritional e. **hydremic e.,** edema in conditions marked by hydremia. **hysterical e.,** blue e. **idiopathic e.,** edema of unknown cause affecting women, occurring intermittently over a period of years and usually worse during the premenstrual phase; it is associated with increased aldosterone secretion. **inflammatory e.,** a form due to inflammation, and attended with redness and pain. **insulin e.,** edema which sometimes follows the injection of insulin. **invisible e.,** the accumulation of a considerable amount of fluid in the subcutaneous tissues before it becomes demonstrable. **local intracutaneous e.,** urticaria. **e. of lung,** pulmonary e. **lymphatic e.,** edema associated with obstruction of the lymph vessels. **malignant e.,** edema marked by rapid extension, with destruction of tissue and formation of a gas. **migratory e.,** angioneurotic e. **Milroy's e.,** see under *disease.* **Milton's e.,** angioneurotic e. **mucous e.,** myxedema. **e. neonato'rum,** a disease of premature and feeble infants that resembles sclerema and is marked by spreading edema with cold, livid skin. **nephrotic e.,** edema occurring in nephrosis and in the intermediate stage of diffuse nephritis. **neuropathic e.,** pseudolipoma. **noninflammatory e.,** edema without redness and pain, occurring from passive congestion or from lowered serum osmolarity. **nonpitting e.,** edema in which the tissues cannot be pitted by pressure. **nutritional e.,** a disorder of nutrition due to long-continued diet deficiency of protein and/or calories, and marked by anasarca and edema; called also *alimentary e., famine e., war e., hunger e.,* and *nutritional, famine,* or *war dropsy.* **paroxysmal pulmonary e.,** pulmonary edema marked by nocturnal attacks of difficult respiration, audible rales, wheezes, and cough, caused by acute left ventricular failure, usually associated with hypertensive heart disease. **passive e.,** edema occurring because of obstruction to vascular or lymphatic drainage from the area. **periodic e.,** angioneurotic e. **periretinal e.,** central serous retinopathy. **Pirogoff's e.,** malignant e. **pitting e.,** edema in which the tissues show prolonged existence of the pits produced by pressure. **placental e.,** the presence of fluid in the villi of the placenta, the villi being club-shaped and irregularly swollen. **prehepatic e.,** edema occurring in prehepatic hypoproteinemia. **pulmonary e.,** abnormal, diffuse, extravascular accumulation of fluid in the pulmonary tissues and air spaces due to changes in hydrostatic forces in the capillaries or to increased capillary permeability; it is characterized clinically by intense dyspnea and, in the intra-alveolar form, by voluminous expectoration of frothy pink serous fluid and, if severe, by cyanosis. **purulent e.,** a swelling due to the effusion of a purulent fluid. **Quincke's e.,** angioneurotic e. **renal e.,** edema due to nephritis and the consequent hypoproteinemia. **rheumatismal e.,** painful red edematous swellings on the limbs in rheumatism, due to subcutaneous exudation. **salt e.,** edema produced by an increase of sodium chloride in the diet. **solid e.,** myxedema. **solid e. of lungs,** a rubbery consistency and gelatinous appearance of the lungs sometimes associated with hypertensive left ventricular failure and uremia. **terminal e.,** pulmonary edema which frequently develops as an agonal event from circulatory failure. **toxic e.,** edema caused by a poison. **vasogenic e.,** edema characterized by increased permeability of capillary endothelial cells; the most common form of brain edema. **venous e.,** edema in which the effused liquid comes from the blood. **vernal e. of lung,** edema of the lung occurring in spring and considered to be allergic. **wandering e.,** angioneurotic e. **war e.,** nutritional e.

edemagen (ĕ-de'mah-jen) an irritant that elicits edema by causing capillary damage but not the cellular response of true inflammation. Cf. *inflammagen.*

edematigenous (ĕ-dem″ah-tij'ĕ-nus) edematogenic.

edematization (ĕ-dem″ah-ti-za'shun) the process of becoming or of making edematous.

edematogenic (ĕ-dem″ah-to-jen'ik) producing or causing edema.

edematous (ĕ-dem'ah-tus) pertaining to or affected by edema.

Edentata (e″den-ta'tah) an order of mammals including armadillos, tree sloths, and anteaters.

edentate (e-den'tāt) edentulous.

edentia (e-den'she-ah) [L. *e* without + *dens* tooth] absence of the teeth.

edentulate (e-den'tu-lāt) edentulous.

edentulous (e-den'tu-lus) [L. *e* without + *dens* tooth] without teeth; having lost the natural teeth.

edetate (ed'ĕ-tāt) any salt or ester of edetic acid (ethylenediaminetetraacetic acid, EDTA). Formerly called *edathamil.* **e.**

calcium disodium [USP], **calcium disodium e.,** chemical name: disodium [[N,N'-1,2-ethanediylbis[N-(carboxymethyl)-glycinato]](4–)-N,N',$O,O',O^N,O^{N'}$calciate (2–). A metal complexing agent, $C_{10}H_{12}CaN_2NaO_8 \cdot xH_2O$, consisting of a mixture of the dihydrate and tetrahydrate calcium disodium salt of edetic acid, used intramuscularly or intravenously in the diagnosis and treatment of lead poisoning. Called also *calcium disodium edathamil, calcium EDTA, sodium calciumedetate,* and *sodium calcium edetate.* **e. disodium** [USP], **disodium e.,** chemical name: N,N'-1,2-ethanediylbis[N-(carboxymethyl)glycine disodium salt. A metal complexing agent, $C_{10}H_{14}N_2Na_2O_8 \cdot 2H_2O$, used as a chelating pharmaceutic aid. It is also used in poisoning with lead and other heavy metals and, because of its affinity for calcium, in the treatment of hypercalcemia. Called also *edathamil disodium.* **e. sodium,** the tetrasodium salt of edetic acid, $C_{10}H_{12}N_2NaO_8$, used as a chelating agent. **e. trisodium,** the trisodium salt of edetic acid, $C_{10}H_{13}N_2NaO_8$, sometimes used similarly to edetate disodium.

edge (ej) a thin side or border. **cutting e.,** the angle formed by the merging of two flat surfaces, by which something may be cut, such as the blade of a knife, or the incisal surface of an anterior tooth. **denture e.,** see under *border.* **incisal e.,** the junction of the labial surface of an anterior tooth with a flattened linguoincisal surface created by occlusal wear.

edge-strength (ej' strength) the resistance offered by an edge to a fracturing force, applied especially in dentistry to such resistance offered by the edge of an amalgam restoration.

Edinger's law, nucleus (ed'ing-gerz) [Ludwig *Edinger,* German neurologist, 1855–1918] see under *law* and *nucleus.*

Edinger-Westphal nucleus (ed'ing-ger-vest'fahl) [L. *Edinger;* Carl Friedrich Otto *Westphal,* German neurologist, 1833–1890] nucleus accessorius.

edipism (ed'ĭ-pizm) [from *Oedipus,* King of Thebes. See *Oedipus complex*] intentional injury of one's own eyes.

edisylate (ĕ-dis'ĭ-lāt) USAN contraction for 1,2-ethanedisulfonate.

Edlefsen's reagent test (ed'lef-senz) [Gustav J. J. F. *Edlefsen,* German physician, 1842–1910] see under *reagent.*

EDR effective direct radiation; electrodermal response.

edrophonium chloride (ed''ro-fo'ne-um) [USP] chemical name: N-ethyl-3-hydroxy-N,N-dimethylbenzenaminium chloride. A cholinergic, $C_{10}H_{16}ClNO$, occurring as a white, crystalline powder; used as an antidote for curare principles, as a diagnostic aid in myasthenia gravis, and in the treatment of myasthenic crises, administered intramuscularly and intravenously.

Edsall's disease (ed'salz) [David Linn *Edsall,* American physician, 1869–1945] heat cramp.

EDTA see *edetate.*

educable (edj'u-kah-b'l) capable of being educated; the term is used with special reference to persons with mild mental retardation (I.Q. approximately 52–67) who are capable of achieving an academic level of the fourth to fifth grade and may be able to be self-supporting. Cf. *trainable.*

eduction (e-duk'shun) [L. *e* (*ex*) from + *ducere* to lead] the process of leading out from or the dissipation of a former state, as the restoration to normal physiological state of an anesthetized patient.

edulcorant (e-dul'ko-rant) sweetening.

edulcorate (e-dul'ko-rāt) to sweeten.

EEE eastern equine encephalomyelitis.

EEG electroencephalogram.

eelworm (ēl'wurm) (*obs.*) any roundworm, such as ascaris.

E.E.N.T. eye-ear-nose-throat.

EFA essential fatty acids.

effacement (ĕ-fās'ment) the obliteration of the cervix in labor when it is so changed that only the thin external os remains.

effect (ĕ-fekt') the result produced by an action. **additive e.,** the combined effect produced by the action of two or more agents, being equal to the sum of their separate actions. **anachoretic e.,** see *anachoresis.* **Anrep e.,** augmented resistance to outflow in the heart. **Blinks e's,** brief enhancement in photosynthesis which follows shifts from a long wavelength to a shorter wavelength. **Bohr e.,** displacement of the oxyhemoglobin dissociation curve by a change in partial pressure of carbon dioxide or in pH. **Braid e.,** in hypnosis, alternating pupillary size (constriction then dilation), wavy pupil motion, eyelid closure, general tonic rigidity, specific catalepsies associated with rises in pulse rate, hypersuggestibility, and stupor. **Bruce e.,** the blocking of pregnancy in a newly impregnated female mouse by a pheromone (the odor of a strange male). **clasp-knife e.,** a sudden complete flexion of the limb in the lengthening reaction. **Compton e.,** the change in the wavelength of x- or gamma-radiation due to the interaction of an incident photon with an orbital electron of an atom, which produces a recoil electron and a scattered photon of reduced energy. **contrary e.,** Hata's phenomenon. **Crabtree e.,** the inhibition of oxygen consumption on the addition of glucose to tissues or microorganisms having a high rate of aerobic glycolysis; the converse of the Pasteur effect.

Danysz e., see under *phenomenon.* **Deelman e.,** scarification of the skin in artificial carcinogenesis tends to localize the subsequent carcinomata at the scarified area. **Doppler e.,** the relationship of the apparent frequency of waves, as of sound, light, and radio waves, to the relative motion of the source of the waves and the observer, the frequency increasing as the two approach each other and decreasing as they move apart. **Emerson e.,** the photosynthetic efficiency of a long wavelength of light is enhanced by simultaneous exposure of plant cells to shorter wavelengths of light. **experimenter e's,** demand characteristics, see under *characteristic.* **Fahraeus-Lindqvist e.,** the marked fall in blood viscosity when the diameter of the tube used in measuring is less than 1 mm. **Hallberg e.,** the crests and troughs of ultrashort standing-wave field have opposite electrical signs. **Hallwachs e.,** photoelectrical e. **heel e.,** a variation in roentgen ray intensity output along the longitudinal tube axes in relation to the film. **interpolar e.,** the effect of an electric current throughout the whole region of the body between the two electrodes or poles, as contrasted with polar effects. **isomorphic e.,** Koebner phenomenon. **Mierzejewski e.,** the disharmonious development of gray and white matter of the brain, the gray being in excess. **Nagler e.,** gas-filled tubes, placed in high frequency fields, will act as rectifiers, causing a unidirectional current. **Orbeli e.,** see under *phenomenon.* **Pasteur e.,** the decrease in the rate of glucose utilization glycolysis and the suppression of lactate accumulation by tissues or microorganisms in the presence of oxygen. Cf. *Crabtree e.* **photechic e.,** Russell e. **photoelectrical e.,** the ejection of electrons from matter when light of short wavelengths falls upon it; called also *Hallwachs e.* **placebo e.,** the nonspecific psychologic or psychophysiologic effect produced by a placebo. **polar e.,** the effect of the electric current which is manifested at one of the poles. **position e.,** in genetics, the changed effect produced by alteration of the relative positions of various genes on the chromosomes. **pressure e.,** the sum of the changes that are due to obstruction of tissue drainage by pressure. **Raman e.,** when a substance is irradiated with monochromatic light, the spectrum which the substance scatters contains, in addition to a line of the same wavelength as the incident radiation, lines which are satellites of the primary line moving with it when the wavelength of the primary radiation is altered. **Russell e.,** the rendering of a photographic plate developable by agents other than light; called also *photechic effect.* **side e.,** see under *S.* **Somogyi e.,** a rebound phenomenon occurring in diabetes: overtreatment with insulin induces hypoglycemia, which initiates the release of epinephrine, ACTH, glucagon, and growth hormone, which stimulate lipolysis, gluconeogenesis, and glycogenolysis, which, in turn, result in a rebound hyperglycemia and ketosis. **Soret e.,** when a solution is maintained for some time in a temperature gradient, a difference in concentration develops along the temperature gradient. **specific dynamic e.,** see under *action.* **Staub-Traugott e.,** a second dose of dextrose by mouth to a normal person one hour after a first dose does not elevate the blood sugar level. **Tyndall e.,** see under *phenomenon.* **Whitten e.,** initiation and synchronization of the estrous cycles and reduction of the frequency of reproductive abnormalities in female mice by the odor (pheromone) of a male mouse placed among them; when more than four female mice are placed together in a cage their estrous cycles become very erratic. **Wolff-Chaikoff e.,** the inhibition of the synthesis of thyroid hormone after administration of large doses of iodide, first demonstrated in the rat. **Zeeman e.,** separation of a single line in the spectrum by suitable magnetic fields.

effectiveness (ĕ-fek'tiv-nes) the ability to produce a specific result or to exert a specific measurable influence. **relative biological e.,** an expression of the effectiveness of other types of radiation in comparison with that of gamma or roentgen rays. Abbreviated RBE.

effector (ef-fek'tor) a muscle or gland which contracts or secretes, respectively, in direct response to nerve impulses. **allosteric e.,** an enzyme inhibitor or activator that has its effect at a site other than the catalytic site of the enzyme; see also under *site,* and see *allosteric.*

effemination (ĕ-fem''ĭ-na'shun) feminization.

efferent (ef'er-ent) [L. *ex* out + *ferre* to bear] centrifugal; conveying away from a center, as an efferent nerve.

efferential (ef''er-en'shal) efferent.

effervescent (ef-er-ves'ent) [L. *effervescens*] bubbling; sparkling; giving off gas bubbles.

efficiency (e-fish'en-se) ability to accomplish a desired effect or to perform a certain action. **visual e.,** the ratio of the resolving power of the eye that is being tested to that of a normal eye.

effleurage (ef-loo-rahzh') [Fr.] stroking movement in massage; frottage.

efflorescence (ef''lo-res'ens) [L. *efflorescentia*] a rash or eruption; any skin lesions, especially numerous and conspicuous lesions.

efflorescent (ef''lo-res'ent) [L. *efflorescere* to bloom] becoming powdery in consequence of losing water of crystallization.

effluve (ef-lōōv′) a conductive discharge of a high voltage current through a dielectric.

effluvia (ef-floo′ve-ah) plural of *effluvium*.

effluvium (ef-floo′ve-um), pl. *efflu′via* [L. "a flowing out"] 1. an outflowing, or shedding, especially of the hair. 2. an exhalation or emanation, applied especially to one of noxious character. **anagen e.,** abnormal loss of hair in the anagen phase, sometimes resulting from administration of cytotoxic drugs, as in chemotherapy of cancer, or from administration of colchicine or methotrexate. **telluric e.,** an emanation arising from the earth; see *miasma* and *tellurium*. **telogen e.,** falling out of the hair resulting from the mass precipitation of telogen, caused by a variety of stresses such as parturition, surgical shock, febrile illness, or severe emotional stress.

effraction (ef-frak′shun) a breaking open; a weakening.

effumability (ef″u-mah-bil′ĭ-te) [L. *ex* out + *fumus* smoke] the property of being easily volatilized.

effuse [L. *effusus*, from *ex* out + *fundere* to pour] 1. (ĕ-fūs′) spread out, profuse; said of bacterial growth that is thin, veily, and unusually widely spread. 2. (ĕ-fūz′) to pour out and spread widely.

effusion (ĕ-fu′zhun) [L. *effusio* a pouring out] 1. the escape of fluid into a part or tissue, as an exudation or a transudation. 2. an effused material, which may be classified according to protein content as an exudate or transudate. **hemorrhagic e.,** an effusion of bloody liquid. **pleural e.,** the presence of liquid in the pleural space.

Efudex (ef′u-deks) trademark for a preparation of fluorouracil.

egagropilus (e″gah-grop′ĭ-lus) [Gr. *aigagros* wild goat + *pilos* felt] trichobezoar.

egersimeter (e″ger-sim′ĕ-ter) an instrument for testing the electric excitability of nerves and muscles and for measuring chronaxia.

egersis (e-ger′sis) [Gr.] abnormal wakefulness; insomnia.

egesta (e-jes′tah) [L. *e* out + *gerere* to bear] undigested material thrown out from the body.

egestion (e-jes′chun) the casting out of material which is indigestible.

egg (eg) [L. *ovum*] 1. an ovum; a female gamete. 2. an oocyte. 3. a female reproductive cell at any stage before fertilization and its derivatives after fertilization and even after some development.

Eggleston's method (eg′el-stunz) [Cary *Eggleston*, New York physician, 1884–1966] see under *method*.

egilops (e′jĭ-lops) [Gr. *aix* goat + *ōps* eye] perforating abscess at the inner canthus of the eye.

eglandulous (e-gland′u-lus) [L. *e* without + *glandula* glandule] having no glands.

ego (e′go) [L. *ego* I] that portion of the psyche which possesses consciousness, maintains its identity, and recognizes and tests reality; the conscious sense of the self.

ego-alien (e″go-āl′yen) ego-dystonic.

egobronchophony (e″go-bron-kof′o-ne) [Gr. *aix* goat + *bronchophony*] increased vocal resonance with high-pitched bleating quality of the transmitted voice, detected by auscultation of the lungs, especially over lung tissue compressed by pleural effusion.

egocentric (e″go-sen′trik) [L. *ego* I + *centric*] having all one's ideas centered on one's self. Cf. *allocentric*.

ego-dystonic (e″go-dis-ton′ik) denoting any impulse, idea, or the like, that is repugnant to and inconsistent with an individual's conception of himself. Called also *ego-alien*. Cf. *ego-syntonic*.

egoism (e′go-izm) a self-seeking for advantage at the expense of others; overevaluation of the self.

egomania (e″go-ma′ne-ah) [Gr. *egō* I + *mania* madness] morbid self-esteem.

egophony (e-gof′o-ne) [Gr. *aix* goat + *phōnē* voice] egobronchophony.

ego-syntonic (e″go-sin-ton′ik) denoting any impulse, idea, or the like, that is in harmony with an individual's conception of himself. Cf. *ego-dystonic*.

egotism (e′go-tizm) overevaluation of one's self.

egotropic (e″go-trop′ik) [Gr. *egō* I + *tropos* a turning] egocentric.

EHBF estimated hepatic blood flow.

Ehlers-Danlos syndrome (disease) (a′lerz-dan′los) [Edvard *Ehlers*, Danish dermatologist, 1863–1937; Henri Alexandre *Danlos*] see under *syndrome*.

Ehrenritter's ganglion (er′en-rit″erz) [Johann *Ehrenritter*, Austrian anatomist, died 1790] ganglion superius nervi glossopharyngei.

Ehrlich's reaction, etc. (ār′lik) [Paul *Ehrlich*, German bacteriologist, 1854–1915; co-winner, with Elie Metchnikoff, of the Nobel prize for medicine and physiology in 1908, in recognition of his work in immunity] see under *body*, *granule*, *reaction*, *stain*, *test*, and *theory*, and see arsphenamine.

Ehrlich-Hata preparation, remedy, treatment [Paul *Ehr-*

lich; Sahachiro *Hata*, Japanese physician, 1872–1938] arsphenamine.

Ehrlich-Heinz granules (ār′lik hīnts) [Paul *Ehrlich;* Robert *Heinz*, German pathologist, 1865–1924] Ehrlich's granules.

Ehrlichia (ār-lik′e-ah) [Paul *Ehrlich*] a genus of the tribe Ehrlichieae, family Rickettsiaceae, order Rickettsiales. Three species, *E. ca′nis*, *E. bo′vis*, and *E. ovi′na*, produce disease in dogs, cattle, and sheep, respectively, but are nonpathogenic for man.

Ehrlichieae (ār″lĭ-ki′e-e) a tribe of the family Rickettsiaceae, order Rickettsiales, class Microtatobiotes, made up of rickettsia-like organisms adapted to existence in invertebrates, chiefly arthropods, and pathogenic for certain vertebrates, but not for man. It includes three genera, *Cowdria*, *Ehrlichia*, and *Neorickettsia*.

Eichhorst's atrophy (type), corpuscles (ik′horsts) [Hermann Ludwig *Eichhorst*, Swiss physician, 1849–1921] see under *atrophy* and *corpuscle*.

Eichstedt's disease (ik′stets) [Karl Ferdinand *Eichstedt*, physician in Greifswald, 1816–1892] tinea versicolor.

Eicken's method (i′kenz) [Carl von *Eicken*, German laryngologist and otologist, 1873–1960] see under *method*.

eiconometer (i″ko-nom′ĕ-ter) eikonometer.

eicosanoate (i-ko″sah-no′āt) systematic name for arachidate, denoting that it has twenty (*eicosa* twenty) carbon atoms in a straight chain.

eidetic (i-det′ik) [Gr. *eidos* that which is seen; form or shape] pertaining to or characterized by exact visualization of events or of objects previously seen. By extension, sometimes used to designate an individual possessing such an ability.

eidogen (i′do-jen) [Gr. *eidos* form + *genesthai* produced] a substance elaborated by a second grade inductor, which is capable of modifying the form of an embryonic organ already in the process of formation.

eidoptometry (i″dop-tom′ĕ-tre) [Gr. *eidos* form + *optos* seen + *metron* measure] measurement of the acuteness of vision for the perception of form.

Eijkman's test (ik′manz) [Christiaan *Eijkman*, Dutch physiologist, 1858–1930; discoverer of the causative agent in beriberi, proponent of the vitamin theory, and co-winner, with F. G. Hopkins, of the Nobel prize for medicine in 1929 for his discovery of the antineuritic vitamin] see under *tests*.

Eikenella (i″ken-el′ah) a genus of facultative gram-negative, rod-shaped bacteria which inhabit the oral cavity and upper respiratory tract; *E. corrodens* can cause abscess formation.

eikonometer (i″ko-nom′ĕ-ter) [Gr. *eikōn* image + *metron* measure] an instrument used in making an examination for aniseikonia.

eiloid (i′loid) [Gr. *eilein* to roll up + *eidos* form] having a coiled appearance.

Eimeria (i-me′re-ah) [Gustav Heinrich Theodor *Eimer*, German zoologist, 1843–1898] a genus of sporozoan parasites of the order Coccidia in which an oocyst contains four spores and each spore two sporozoites; various species are parasitic in the epithelial cells of man and animals, the oocysts being found in the feces. **E. a′vium,** *E. tenella*. **E. caviae,** a species found in guinea pigs. **E. clupea′rum,** a species found almost constantly in the livers of herrings (*Clupea harengus*) and to a lesser extent in the livers of sprat (young herring) and mackerel (*Scomber scomber*). **E. falcifor′mis,** a species found in mice. **E. max′ima,** a species that infects the small intestine of fowl. **E. meleagri′dis,** a species found in the intestines of turkeys. **E. mieschul′zi,** a species found in feces of laboratory rats. **E. nec′atrix,** a species that causes a chronic coccidiosis of fowl. **E. per′forans,** a species causing intestinal coccidiosis in rabbits. **E. sardi′nae,** a species found in large numbers in the testes of sprats (young herrings), to some extent in the "soft roes" of adult herrings (*Clupea harengus*), and in tinned sardines. **E. sti′edae,** a species found in the liver of rabbits. **E. tenel′la,** a species causing bloody diarrhea in fowls; see *white diarrhea*, under *diarrhea*. **E. zur′ni,** a species causing intestinal coccidiosis in cattle and severe diarrhea in calves.

Einhorn's saccharimeter (in′hornz) [Max *Einhorn*, physician in New York, 1862–1953] see under *saccharimeter*.

einsteinium (in-sti′ne-um) [Albert *Einstein*, theoretical physicist, born in Germany, became a naturalized citizen of Switzerland, then of the United States, 1879–1955; winner of Nobel prize for physics in 1921] the chemical element of atomic number 99, atomic weight 254, symbol Es, originally discovered in debris from a thermonuclear explosion in 1952.

Einthoven's formula, galvanometer, triangle (in′to-venz) [Willem *Einthoven*, Dutch physiologist, 1860–1927; winner of the Nobel prize for medicine in 1924 for his discovery of the mechanism of the electrocardiogram] see under *formula*, *galvanometer*, and *triangle*.

eisanthema (īs-an′the-mah) [Gr. *eis* into + *anthein* to bloom] an eruption on a mucous membrane.

Eisenia (i-se′ne-ah) a genus of chaelopod worms. *E. foe′tida*, a species reportedly found in the urine of man.

Eisenmenger's complex (i'sen-meng''erz) [Victor *Eisenmenger*, German physician, 1864–1932] see under *complex*.

eisodic (i-sod'ik) [Gr. *eis* into + *hodos* way] afferent or centripetal.

Eitelberg's test (i'tel-bergz) [Abraham *Eitelberg*, Austrian physician, born 1847] see under *tests*.

eiweissmilch (i'vīs-milkh) [Ger.] albumin milk; see under *milk*.

ejaculate (e-jak'u-lāt) 1. to expel suddenly, especially semen. 2. the semen expelled in a single ejaculation; ejaculum.

ejaculatio (e-jak''u-la'she-o) [L.] ejaculation. **e. defi'ciens,** defective ejaculation. **e. prae'cox,** ejaculation of the semen immediately after the beginning of the sexual act. **e. retarda'ta,** unduly delayed ejaculation.

ejaculation (e-jak''u-la'shun) [L. *ejaculatio*] a sudden act of expulsion, as of the semen. **premature e.,** ejaculatio praecox.

ejaculator (e-jak'u-la''tor) [L.] that which or one who ejaculates. **e. sem'inis,** musculus bulbospongiosus.

ejaculatory (e-jak'u-lah-to''re) [L. *ejaculatorius*] pertaining to ejaculation.

ejaculum (e-jak'u-lum) the semen discharged in a single ejaculation in the male, consisting of the secretions of Cowper's gland, epididymis, ductus deferens, seminal vesicles, and prostate, and containing the spermatozoa. Called also *ejaculate*.

ejecta (e-jek'tah) [L. pl.; from *e* out + *jacere* to cast] materials which have been cast out from the body. Excrementitious material; refuse.

ejection (e-jek'shun) 1. the act of ejecting or the state of being ejected. 2. something ejected. **milk e.,** let-down reflex.

ejector (e-jek'tor) an apparatus for effecting the forcible expulsion or removal of a material or body. **saliva e.,** an apparatus for removal of saliva and water from the mouth of the patient during operations on the teeth.

Ejusd. abbreviation for L. *ejus'dem,* of the same.

eka- (e'kah) [Sanscrit, "one" or "first"] a prefix added to the name of a known chemical element as a provisional designation of the unknown element which should occur next in the same group in the periodic system.

eka-iodine (e'kah i'o-dīn) the name formerly used to designate element 85, now officially known as astatine.

EKG electrocardiogram.

ekiri (e-ki'ri) an acute cerebral and cardiovascular disorder occurring in children with shigellosis in Japan.

ekphorize (ek'fo-rīz) ecphorize.

EKY electrokymogram.

elaborate (e-lab'o-rāt) [L. *elabora're* to work out] to produce complex substances out of simpler materials.

elaboration (e-lab''o-ra'shun) 1. the process of producing complex substances out of simpler materials. 2. in psychiatry, an unconscious mental process of expansion and embellishment of detail, especially of a symbol or representation in a dream; called also *secondary e.*

elacin (el'ah-sin) degenerated elastic tissue.

elaeo- for words beginning thus, see those beginning *eleo-*.

elaioma (e-le-o'mah) eleoma.

elaiometer (e''la-om'ĕ-ter) eleometer.

elaiopathia (e''la-o-path'e-ah) elaiopathy.

elaiopathy (e''la-op'ah-the) [Gr. *elaion* oil + *pathos* disease] a diffuse fatty edema, usually attacking the joints of the lower extremities, the effect of contusions or distortions incurred in war, and attributed to the formation of an irritating oily substance and its action upon the subcutaneous cellular tissue (C. Blondi, 1917). **pathomimic e.,** the simulation of disease produced by the injection of liquid petrolatum subcutaneously.

elaioplast (e-la'o-plast) [Gr. *elaion* oil + *plassein* to form] a fat-producing plastid.

elantrine (el'an-trēn) chemical name: 3-(5,6-dihydro-5-methyl)-11*H*-dibenz[*b,e*]azepin-11-ylidine-*N,N*-dimethyl-1-propanamine. An anticholinergic, $C_{20}H_{24}N_2$, which has been used in the treatment of drug-induced extrapyramidal syndrome.

elapid (el'ah-pid) 1. any snake of the family Elapidae. 2. of or pertaining to the family Elapidae.

Elapidae (e-lap'ĭ-de) a family of usually terrestrial, venomous snakes, which have cylindrical tails and front fangs that are short, stout, immovable, and grooved. It includes cobras, kraits, coral snakes, Australian copperheads, Australian blacksnakes, brown snakes, tiger snakes, death adders, and mambas.

Elaps (e'laps) *Micruris.*

elasmobranch (e-las'mo-brank) [Gr. *elasmos* plate + L. *branchia* gill] 1. any cartilaginous fish having platelike gills, each gill slit opening independently on the body surface, such as sharks, skates, rays, and sawfish. 2. of or pertaining to elasmobranchs.

elassosis (el''ah-so'sis) [Gr. *elassōn* smaller, less] a diminutive type of mitosis characteristic of the small cells of the thymus.

elastance (e-las'tans) the quality of recoiling on removal of

pressure without disruption, or an expression of the measure of the ability to do so, as an expression of the recoil of an air- or fluid-filled organ, e.g., the lung or urinary bladder, in terms of unit of pressure change per unit of volume change. It is the reciprocal of compliance.

elastase (e-las'tās) an enzyme of the protease class formed from the zymogen proelastase, which is secreted by the pancreas; it catalyzes the hydrolysis of peptide bonds; it is so named because it was once thought to attack elastin preferentially.

elastic (e-las'tik) [L. *elasticus*] 1. susceptible of being stretched, compressed, or distorted, and then tending to assume its original shape; resilient. 2. an elastic band, as that placed around a tooth in dental procedures. **intermaxillary e.,** elastic material used to produce traction between the upper and lower teeth as one element of the corrective process. **intramaxillary e.,** elastic material applied within the same dental arch to achieve space closure. **vertical e.,** elastic material applied in a direction perpendicular to the occlusal plane, connecting one arch wire to the other, usually for approximating teeth to improve intercuspation.

elastica (e-las'tĭ-kah) [L.] 1. gum elastic or caoutchouc. 2. a general term for elastic tissue of the body, such as that found in the tunica media of blood vessels. 3. tunica media.

elasticin (e-las'tĭ-sin) elastin.

elasticity (e''las-tis'ĭ-te) the quality or condition of being elastic. **physical e. of muscle,** the physical quality of muscle of being elastic, of yielding to passive physical stretch. **physiologic e. of muscle,** the biologic quality, unique to muscle, of being able to change and resume size under neuromuscular control. **total e. of muscle,** the combined effect of physical and physiologic elasticity of muscle.

elastin (e-las'tin) a yellow scleroprotein, the essential constituent of yellow elastic connective tissue: it is brittle when dry, but when moist is flexible and elastic.

elastinase (e-las'tin-ās) elastase.

elastofibroma (e-las''to-fi-bro'mah) a tumor consisting of both elastin and fibrous elements. **e. dor'si,** a tumor-like nodule of subscapular soft tissue, occurring in old age, consisting of an elastin-filled central core and a surrounding elastase-resistant matrix impregnated with elastin.

elastogel (e-las'to-jel) a gel which possesses great elasticity.

elastoid (e-las'toid) a substance formed by the hyaline degeneration of the internal elastic lamina of blood vessels; seen in the vessels of the uterus after delivery.

elastoidosis, nodular (e-las''toi-do'sis) a condition characterized by comedones and yellowish, circumscribed, thickened plaques around the orbits or nose, or the nape. Called also *Favre-Racouchot syndrome*.

elastolysis (e''las-tol'ĭ-sis) the digestion of elastic substance or tissue. **perifollicular e.,** a form of anetoderma occurring around hair follicles and caused by elastase produced by staphylococci within the follicles.

elastolytic (e-las''to-lit'ik) capable of catalyzing the digestion of elastic tissue.

elastoma (e''las-to'mah) a tumor or focal excess of elastic tissue fibers or abnormal collagen fibers of the skin. **juvenile e.,** a form of connective tissue nevi (q.v.) characterized by hyperplasia of the elastic tissue of the skin. **Miescher's e.,** elastosis perforans serpiginosa.

elastomer (e-las'to-mer) a soft rubber-like material; synthetic rubber. A rubber base impression material, e.g., silicone and mercaptan.

elastometer (e''las-tom'ĕ-ter) an instrument for determining the elasticity of tissues, and thus measuring the degree of edema.

elastometry (e''las-tom'ĕ-tre) the measurement of elasticity.

elastomucin (e-las''to-mu'sin) a polysaccharide component of elastic tissue.

elastopathy (e''las-top'ah-the) deficiency of elastic tissue.

Elastoplast (e-las'to-plast) trademark for an elastic bandage.

elastorrhexis (e-las''to-rek'sis) rupture of fibers composing elastic tissue.

elastose (e-las'tōs) an albumose formed by treating elastin with ferments, acids, or alkalis.

elastosis (e''las-to'sis) 1. degeneration of elastic tissue. 2. degenerative changes in the dermal connective tissue with increased amounts of elastotic material having the staining properties of elastin. 3. any disturbance of the dermal connective tissue. **actinic e.,** degeneration of the elastic tissue of the dermis due to constant exposure to sunlight; called also *solar e.* **e. intrapapilla're,** e. perforans serpiginosa. **e. perfo'rans serpigino'sa, perforating e.,** an elastic tissue defect, occurring alone or in association with various other disorders, including Down's syndrome, pseudoxanthoma elasticum, Ehlers-Danlos syndrome, Marfan's syndrome, and acrogeria, in which elastomas are extruded through small keratotic papules in the epidermis; the lesions are usually arranged in arcuate serpiginous clusters on the sides of the nape, face, or arms. Called also *e. intrapapillare, Miescher's disease* or *elastoma*, and *reactive perforating e.* **re-**

active perforating e., e. perforans serpiginosa. **senile e., e. seni′lis,** a dermatosis marked by degeneration in the elastic and collagen fibers of the skin in old age. **solar e.,** actinic e.

elastotic (e″las-tot′ik) 1. pertaining to or characterized by elastosis. 2. resembling elastic tissue; having the staining properties of elastin.

elater (el′ah-ter) a specialized structure of certain plants, such as liverworts and slime molds, which aids in the distribution of spores.

elation (e-la′shun) emotional excitement marked by speeding up of mental and bodily activity.

Elavil (el′ah-vil) trademark for preparation of amitriptyline hydrochloride.

elbow (el′bo) [L. *cubitus*] 1. the bend of the arm; the joint that connects the arm and forearm; called also *cubitus* [NA]. 2. any angular bend. **baseball pitchers′ e.,** a disorder of the elbow in baseball pitchers due to a piece of cartilage or bone torn from the head of the radius. **capped e.,** hygroma of the elbow; a swelling of the bursa or a hard, fibrous mass on the point of the elbow in horses or cattle. Called also *shoe boil*. **dropped e.,** radial paralysis (def. 2). **golfer′s e.,** pain due to medical epicondylitis, the lesion being in the origin of the flexor muscles. **little leaguer′s e.,** medial epicondylitis of the elbow due to repeated stress on the flexor muscles of the forearm, a frequent problem of adolescent ballplayers. **miners′ e.,** enlargement of the bursa over the point of the elbow (olecranon bursitis) caused by resting the weight of the body on the elbow as in mining. **nursemaids′ e.,** pulled e. **pulled e.,** subluxation of the head of the radius distally under the annular ligament; called also *nursemaid′s e.* and *Goyrand′s injury*. **tennis e.,** a painful condition localized to the outer aspect of the elbow, due to inflammation or irritation of the extensor tendon attachment to the lateral humeral condyle; called also *external humeral epicondylitis*, and *radiohumeral bursitis* or *epicondylitis*.

elcosis (el-ko′sis) helcosis.

Eldadryl (el′dah-dril) trademark for a preparation of diphenhydramine hydrochloride.

El debab the native name in Algeria for surra.

Eldecort (el′dĕ-kort) trademark for preparations of hydrocortisone.

elder (el′der) the plants, *Sambucus nigra* L., of Europe, S. *canadensis*, L. (Caprifoliaceae), of America, and other congeneric species; the flowers, which contain a volatile oil, have been used in dressing wounds, burns, ulcers, etc., and as a diaphoretic, laxative and diuretic.

Eldodram (el′do-dram) trademark for a preparation of dimenhydrinate.

Eldopaque (el′do-pāk) trademark for preparations of hydroquinone.

Eldoquin (el′do-kwin) trademark for a preparation of hydroquinone.

eldrin (el′drin) rutin.

elective (e-lek′tiv) 1. tending to combine with or act on one substance rather than another. 2. subject to the choice or decision of the patient or physician; applied to procedures that are advantageous to the patient but not urgent.

Electra complex (e-lek-trah) see under *complex*.

electro- [Gr. *ēlektron* amber] a combining form denoting relationship to electricity.

electroacupuncture (e-lek″tro-ak″u-pung′-cher) acupuncture in which the needles are stimulated electrically.

electroaffinity (e-lek″tro-ah-fin′ĭ-te) electronegativity.

electroanalgesia (e-lek″tro-an″al-je′ze-ah) the reduction of pain by electrical stimulation of a peripheral nerve or the dorsal column of the spinal cord.

electroanalysis (e-lek″tro-ah-nal′ĭ-sis) chemical analysis performed by the aid of the electric current.

electroanesthesia (e-lek″tro-an″es-the′ze-ah) anesthesia, either local or general, induced by electricity.

electroappendectomy (e-lek″tro-ap″en-dek′to-me) excision of the appendix by transection of its base by electrosurgical means.

electroaugmentation (e-lek″tro-awg″men-ta′shun) electrical pacing of the heart.

electrobasograph (e-lek″tro-ba′so-graf) [*electro-* + Gr. *basis* step + *graphein* to record] an apparatus for recording the duration of weight bearing on the respective part while walking, i.e., a record of the gait.

electrobiology (e-lek″tro-bi-ol′o-je) [*electro-* + *biology*] the study of electric phenomena in living tissue.

electrobioscopy (e-lek″tro-bi-os′ko-pe) [*electro-* + Gr. *bios* life + *skopein* to examine] the determination of the presence or absence of life by means of an electric current.

electrocardiogram (e-lek″tro-kar′de-o-gram″) [*electro-* + Gr. *kardia* heart + *gramma* mark] a graphic tracing of the variations in electrical potential caused by the excitation of the heart muscle and detected at the body surface. The normal electrocardiogram shows deflections resulting from atrial and ventricular

activity. The first deflection, P, is due to excitation of the atria. The QRS deflections are due to excitation (depolarization) of the ventricles. The T wave is due to recovery of the ventricles (repolarization). The U wave is a potential undulation of unknown origin immediately following the T wave, seen in normal electrocardiograms and accentuated in hypokalemia. Abbreviated ECG or EKG. See also *lead* ². **scalar e.,** a conventional tracing

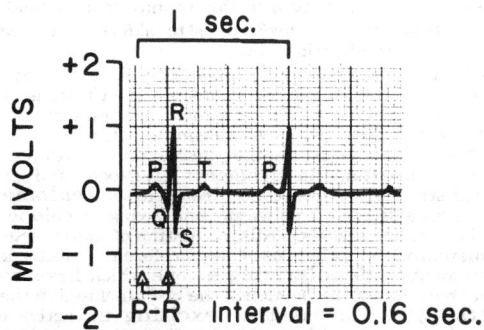

Normal electrocardiogram (Guyton).

showing only changes in magnitude of voltage and polarity (positive and negative) with time.

electrocardiograph (e-lek″tro-kar′de-o-graf″) an instrument for performing electrocardiography, i.e., for making electrocardiograms.

electrocardiography (e-lek″tro-kar″de-og′rah-fe) the making of graphic records of the variations in electrical potential caused by electrical activity of the heart muscle and detected at the body surface, as a method for studying the action of the heart muscle; see *electrocardiogram*. **intracardiac e.,** that performed by introducing an electrode through a cardiac catheter. **precordial e.,** an electrocardiographic technique in which potentials over the chest wall near the surface of the heart are recorded; see *precordial leads*, under *lead* ².

electrocardiophonogram (e-lek″tro-kar″de-o-fo′no-gram) (*obs.*) a record of the heart sounds made by an electrocardiophonograph.

electrocardiophonograph (e-lek″tro-kar″de-o-fo′no-graf) (*obs.*) an apparatus for recording electrically the heart sounds.

electrocardioscopy (e-lek″tro-kar-de-os′ko-pe) [*electro-* + Gr. *kardia* heart + *skopein* to examine] (*obs.*) electrocardiography by means of a cathode-ray oscillograph which throws a record on a luminous screen.

electrocatalysis (e-lek″tro-kah-tal′ĭ-sis) the catalytic effect produced by electricity on the bodily processes.

electrocautery (e-lek″tro-kaw′ter-e) an apparatus for cauterizing tissue, consisting of a platinum wire in a holder which is heated to a red or white heat when the instrument is activated by an electric current.

electrochemistry (e-lek″tro-kem′is-tre) study of chemical changes produced by electric action.

electrocholecystectomy (e-lek″tro-ko″-le-sis-tek′to-me) excision of the gallbladder by electrosurgical means.

electrocholecystocausis (e-lek″tro-ko″le-sis″to-kaw′sis) electrosurgical cauterization of the gallbladder.

electrochromatography (e-lek″tro-kro″mah-tog′rah-fe) electrophoresis.

electrocision (e-lek″tro-sizh′un) excision of malignant growths after the application to them of oscillatory electricity.

electrocoagulation (e-lek″tro-ko-ag″u-la′shun) coagulation of tissue usually accomplished by means of a biterminal high frequency electric current.

electrocochleogram (e-lek″tro-kok′le-o-gram) the record obtained by electrocochleography.

electrocochleograph (e-lek″tro-kok′le-o-graf″) the instrument used in electrocochleography.

electrocochleographic (e-lek″tro-kok′le-o-graf′ik) pertaining to or accomplished by electrocochleography.

electrocochleography (e-lek″tro-kok″le-og′rah-fe) measurement of electrical potentials (cochlear microphonics and action potentials of the eighth cranial nerve) in response to acoustic stimuli applied by an electrode to the external acoustic canal or to the promontory or the round window through the tympanic membrane.

electrocontractility (e-lek″tro-kon-trak-til′ĭ-te) contractility in response to electric stimulation.

electroconvulsive (e-lek″tro-con-vul′siv) inducing convulsions by means of electric shock; see under *therapy*.

electrocorticogram (e-lek″tro-kor′tĭ-ko-gram″) the record obtained by electrocorticography.

electrocorticography (e-lek″tro-kor′tĭ-kog′rah-fe) electroencephalography with the electrodes applied directly to the cortex of the brain.

electrocryptectomy (e-lek″tro-krip-tek′to-me) diathermic destruction of tonsillar crypts.

electrocution (e-lek″tro-ku′shun) the taking of life by passage of electric current through the body.

electrocystography (e-lek″tro-sis-tog′rah-fe) the recording of changes of electric potential in the human urinary bladder.

electrocystoscope (e-lek″tro-sis′to-skōp) a cystoscope equipped with an electric light.

electrode (e-lek′trōd) [Gr. *ēlektron* amber + *hodos* way] a medium used between an electric conductor and the object to which the current is to be applied. In electrotherapy, an instrument with a point or surface from which to transmit an electric current to the body of a patient or to another instrument. **active e.**, one smaller in size than an indifferent electrode, and producing electrical stimulation in a concentrated area. **calomel e.**, an electrode capable of both collecting and giving up chloride ions in neutral or acidic aqueous media, consisting of mercury in contact with mercurous chloride; used as a reference electrode in pH measurements. **depolarizing e.**, one which has a resistance greater than that of the portion of the body inclosed in the circuit. **dispersing e.**, indifferent e. **exciting e.**, active e. **impregnated e.**, one with an absorbent tip impregnated with prescribed medicament. **indifferent e.**, one larger in size than an active electrode, and dispersing electrical stimulation over a larger area. **localizing e.**, active e. **multiple point e.**, an electrode possessing multiple contact points. **point e.**, an electrode with a metallic point for use in applying an electric current to a small area. **silent e.**, indifferent e. **therapeutic e.**, active e.

electrodeposition (e-lek″tro-de″po-zish′un) the deposition of metal by electric action (electroplating), sometimes employed in dentistry for the copper coating of inlay impressions, etc.

electrodermal (e-lek″tro-der′mal) pertaining to the electrical properties of the skin, especially to changes in its resistance.

electrodermatome (e-lek″tro-der′mah-tōm) an electrical dermatome for cutting off even layers of large areas of skin in a short time; used in skin grafting, shaving scars, etc.

electrodesiccation (e-lek″tro-des″ĭ-ka′shun) dehydration of tissue by the use of a high frequency electric current; see *fulguration.*

electrodiagnosis (e-lek″tro-di″ag-no′sis) the use of electrical devices in the diagnosis of pathologic conditions.

electrodiagnostics (e-lek″tro-di″ag-nos′tiks) the science and practice of electrodiagnosis.

electrodialysis (e-lek″tro-di-al′ĭ-sis) dialysis under the influence of an electric field.

electrodialyzer (e-lek″tro-di″ah-li′zer) a blood dialyzer utilizing an applied electric field and semipermeable membranes for separating the colloids from the solution.

electrodiaphake (e-lek″tro-di-af′ah-ke) an instrument for removing the lens by diathermy.

electrodiaphane (e-lek″tro-di′ah-fān) diaphanoscope.

electrodiaphanoscope (e-lek″tro-di-af′ah-no-skōp″) diaphanoscope.

electrodiaphany (e-lek″tro-di-af′ah-ne) [*electro-* + Gr. *diaphainein* to show through] diaphanoscopy.

electroencephalogram (e-lek″tro-en-sef′ah-lo-gram″) a re-

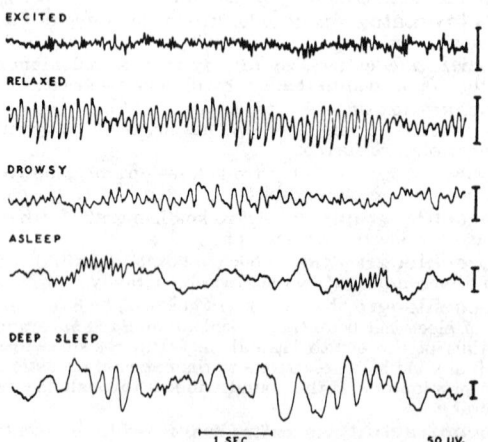

EXCITED

RELAXED

DROWSY

ASLEEP

DEEP SLEEP

1 SEC.   50 μV.

Electroencephalogram

Recordings made while the subject was excited, relaxed, and in various stages of sleep. During excitement the brain waves are rapid and of small amplitude, whereas in sleep they are much slower and of greater amplitude. The regular waves characteristic of the relaxed state are called alpha waves. (From Jasper, in Epilepsy and Cerebral Localization, by Penfield and Erickson.)

cording of the potentials on the skull generated by currents emanating spontaneously from nerve cells in the brain. The dominant frequency of these potentials is about 8 to 10 cycles per second and the amplitude about 10 to 100 microvolts. Variations in wave characteristics correlate well with neurological conditions and so have been useful as diagnostic criteria. Abbreviated EEG. **flat e., isoelectric e.,** one in which no brain waves are recorded, indicating a complete lack of brain activity.

electroencephalograph (e-lek″tro-en-sef′ah-lo-graf″) an instrument for performing electroencephalography.

electroencephalography (e-lek″tro-en-sef′ah-log′rah-fe) the recording of the electric currents developed in the brain, by means of electrodes applied to the scalp, to the surface of the brain (*intracranial e.*), or placed within the substance of the brain (*depth e.*). See *electroencephalogram.*

electroencephaloscope (e-lek″tro-en-sef′ah-lo-skōp) an instrument for detecting brain potentials at many different sections of the brain and displaying them on a cathode-ray tube.

electroendosmosis (e-lek″tro-en″dos-mo′sis) endosmosis under the influence of an electric field.

electroenterostomy (e-lek″tro-en″ter-os′to-me) enterostomy performed by electrosurgical technique.

electroexcision (e-lek″tro-ek-siz′zhun) excision performed by electrosurgical means.

electrofluoroscopy (e-lek″tro-floo″o-ros′ko-pe) (*obs.*) fluoroscopic electrocardiography.

electrofocusing (e-lek″tro-fo′kus-ing) isoelectric focusing.

electrogastroenterostomy (e-lek″tro-gas″tro-en-ter-os′to-me) gastroenterostomy performed by electrosurgical means.

electrogastrogram (e-lek″tro-gas′tro-gram) the graphic record obtained by electrogastrography.

electrogastrograph (e-lek″tro-gas′tro-graf) an instrument for recording the electrical activity of the stomach by means of swallowed gastric electrodes.

electrogastrography (e-lek″tro-gas-trog′rah-fe) the recording of the electrical activity of the stomach as measured between its lumen and the surface of the body.

electrogoniometer (e-lek″tro-go″ne-om′ĕ-ter) an instrument for measuring angular positions, as of a finger, arm, limb.

electrogram (e-lek′tro-gram) any record produced by changes in electric potential. **His bundle e.,** an intracardiac electrocardiogram of potentials in the bundle of His, done through a cardiac catheter.

electrograph (e-lek′tro-graf) electrogram.

electrography (e″lek-trog′rah-fe) [*electro-* + Gr. *graphein* to record] the graphic recording of changes in electric potential, as in electrocardiography, electroencephalography, etc.

electrogustometry (e-lek″tro-gus-tom′ĕ-tre) the testing of the sense of taste by application of galvanic stimuli to the tongue.

electrohemostasis (e-lek″tro-he-mos′tah-sis) [*electro-* + *hemostasis*] the arrest of hemorrhage by the application of a high frequency current to coagulate the bleeding point or surface.

electrohysterogram (e-lek″tro-his′ter-o-gram) the graphic record obtained by electrohysterography.

electrohysterography (e-lek″tro-his″ter-og′rah-fe) the recording of the changes in electric potential associated with contractions of the uterine muscle.

electroimmunodiffusion (e-lek″tro-im″u-no-dif-u′zhun) immunodiffusion accelerated by application of an electric current; serum proteins in an alkaline medium, having a negative charge, move toward the positive pole, whereas gamma globulins, having a lesser negative charge, move toward the negative pole through the action of osmosis. Called also *immunoelectro-osmophoresis* and *counterimmunoelectro-osmophoresis.*

electrokinetic (e-lek″tro-ki-net′ik) pertaining to motion produced by an electric current.

electrokymogram (e-lek″tro-ki′mo-gram) the graphic record produced by electrokymography; abbreviated EKY.

electrokymograph (e-lek″tro-ki′mo-graf) an instrument for graphically recording motion of or changes in density of organs by recording variations in intensity of a small beam of roentgen rays; it consists of three essential parts—a fluoroscope, a pick-up unit, and a recording instrument; used especially for showing motion of the cardiac silhouette.

electrokymography (e-lek″tro-ki-mog′rah-fe) the photography on x-ray film of the motion of the heart or of other moving structures which can be visualized radiologically. See *electrokymograph.*

electrolepsy (e-lek′tro-lep″se) electric chorea.

electrolithotrity (e-lek″tro-lĭ-thot′rĭ-te) the disintegration of calculi by the application of electric current.

electrolysis (e″lek-trol′ĭ-sis) [*electro-* + Gr. *lysis* dissolution] destruction by passage of a galvanic electric current, as in disintegration of a chemical compound in solution or removal of excessive hair from the body.

electrolyte (e-lek′tro-līt) [*electro-* + Gr. *lytos* that may be dissolved] a substance that dissociates into ions when fused or in solution, and thus becomes capable of conducting electricity; an ionic solute. **amphoteric e.,** a compound which dissociates into both hydrogen (H$^+$) and hydroxyl (OH$^-$) ions; called also *ampholyte.* **colloidal e.,** an electrolyte in which one or more of the ionic components is of macromolecular dimensions.

electrolytic (e-lek″tro-lit″ik) pertaining to or characterized by electrolysis.

electrolyzable (e-lek′tro-līz″ah-bl) susceptible of being decomposed by electric current.

electromagnet (e-lek″tro-mag′net) a temporary magnet made by passing an electric current through a coil of wire, surrounding a core of soft iron.

electromagnetism (e-lek″tro-mag′net-izm) magnetism produced by an electric current.

electromanometer (e-lek″tro-man-om′ĕ-ter) an instrument for measuring the pressure of gases or liquids by electronic methods.

electrometer (e″lek-trom′ĕ-ter) [*electro-* + Gr. *metron* measure] an electrostatic instrument for measuring the difference in potential between two points. In radiology, it is used to measure changes in the potential of charged electrodes due to ionization occasioned by radiation.

electrometrogram (e-lek″tro-met′ro-gram) [*electro-* + Gr. *mētra* uterus + *gramma* mark] an apparatus for recording changes in electric potential associated with contraction of the uterine muscle.

electromigratory (e-lek″tro-mi′grah-to″re) moving under the influence of electric current.

electromotive (e-lek″tro-mo′tiv) causing electric activity to be propagated along a conductor.

electromyogram (e-lek″tro-mi′o-gram) the record obtained by electromyography.

electromyograph (e-lek″tro-mi′o-graf) the instrument used in electromyography.

electromyography (e-lek″tro-mi-og′rah-fe) [*electro-* + *myography*] the recording and study of the intrinsic electrical properties of skeletal muscle (1) by means of surface or needle electrodes to determine merely whether the muscle is contracting or not (useful in kinesiology) or (2) by insertion of a needle electrode into the muscle and observing by cathode-ray oscilloscope and loud-speaker the action potentials spontaneously present in a muscle (abnormal) or induced by voluntary contractions, as a means of detecting the nature and location of motor unit lesions; or (3) recording the electrical activity evoked in a muscle by electrical stimulation of its nerve (called also *electroneuromyography*), a procedure useful for study of several aspects of neuromuscular function, neuromuscular conduction, extent of nerve lesion, reflex responses, etc. Abbreviated EMG. **ureteral e.,** recording of the action potentials produced by peristalsis of the ureter.

electron (e-lek′tron) the unit or "atom" of negative electricity. It is equivalent to 4.77×10^{-10} absolute electrostatic units or 1.59×10^{-20} absolute electromagnetic units, and its mass when moving at moderate speed is $\frac{1}{1845}$ that of a hydrogen atom or 9×10^{-28} grams. Electrons flowing in a conductor constitute an electric current; when ejected from a radioactive substance, the beta rays; and when revolving about the nucleus of an atom they determine all of its physical and chemical properties except mass and radioactivity. Cf. *atom.* **emission e.,** one of the electrons which give radioactivity to the atom. **free e.,** an electron which is not bound to the nucleus of an atom but may move from one atom nucleus to another. **valency e.,** one of the electrons involved in the binding of an atom to other atoms.

electronarcosis (e-lek″tro-nar-ko′sis) anesthesia produced by passing an electric current through the brain by electrodes placed on the temples; used in treating a wide variety of psychiatric disorders in the U.S.S.R. It differs from electroconvulsive therapy in not producing convulsions.

electron-dense (e-lek′tron-dens″) in electron microscopy, having a density that prevents electrons from penetrating.

electronegative (e-lek″tro-neg′ah-tiv) bearing a negative electric charge.

electronegativity (e-lek″tro-neg″ah-tiv′ĭ-te) the relative power of an atom to attract electrons.

electroneurography (e-lek″tro-nu-rog′rah-fe) the measurement of the conduction velocity and latency of peripheral nerves.

electroneurolysis (e-lek″tro-nu-rol′ĭ-sis) neurolysis by means of the electric needle.

electroneuromyography (e-lek″tro-nu″ro-mi-og′rah-fe) electromyography in which the nerve of the muscle under study is stimulated by application of an electric current.

electronic (e″lek-tron′ik) pertaining to or carrying electrons.

electronics (e″lek-tron′iks) the science which treats of the conduction of electricity through gases, solids, or a vacuum.

electron-microscopic (e-lek′tron-mi-kro-skop′ik) visible under the electron microscope.

electron-microscopical (e-lek′tron-mi″kro-skop′ĭ-kal) observable with the aid of an electron microscope; of such size as to be so observed.

electronograph (e″lek-tron′o-graf) electron micrograph.

electronystagmogram (e-lek″tro-nis-tag′mo-gram) the record obtained by electronystagmography.

electronystagmograph (e-lek″tro-nis-tag′mo-graf) an instrument for recording eye movements induced by electrical stimulation; abbreviated ENG.

electronystagmography (e-lek″tro-nis″tag-mog′rah-fe) the recording of changes in the corneoretinal potential due to eye movements that provide objective documentation of induced and spontaneous nystagmus.

electro-oculogram (e-lek″tro-ok′u-lo-gram″) the electroencephalographic tracings made by moving the eyes a constant distance between two fixation points, inducing a deflection of fairly constant amplitude; abbreviated EOG.

electro-oculography (e-lek″tro-ok″u-log′rah-fe) the production and interpretation of electro-oculograms.

electro-olfactogram (e-lek″tro-ol-fak′to-gram) a recording of electrical potential changes detected by an electrode placed on the surface of the olfactory mucosa as the mucosa is subjected to an odorous stimulus. Abbreviated EOG.

electro-osmosis (e-lek″tro-oz-mo′sis) the movement of a solution past a stationary colloid material when an electric potential is applied; see also *iontophoresis.*

electroparacentesis (e-lek″tro-par″ah-sen-te′sis) puncture of the eyeball with a needle, using galvanic current and holding the needle in position until bubbles of hydrogen appear in the aqueous humor.

electropathology (e-lek″tro-pah-thol′o-je) [*electro-* + Gr. *pathos* disease + *-logy*] the study of pathologic conditions of the body as revealed by electricity.

electropherogram (e-lek″tro-fer′o-gram) electrophoretogram.

electrophile (e-lek′tro-fil) an electron acceptor that is covalently bonded to a nucleophile.

electrophilic (e-lek″tro-fil′ik) having an affinity for electrons; serving as an electrophile.

electrophoregram (e-lek″tro-fo′rĕ-gram) electrophoretogram.

electrophoresis (e-lek″tro-fo-re′sis) the movement of charged particles suspended in a liquid under the influence of an applied electric field. Also, the technique of separating materials that utilizes this phenomenon. **counter e.,** counterimmunoelectrophoresis. **disc e.,** gel electrophoresis in which a discontinuity of pH or gel pore size is introduced near the point of origin, producing a very thin starting zone and sharp separations. **gel e.,** that in which a gel, such as agar gel, is the diffusion medium. **moving boundary e.,** electrophoresis in which the number of distinct moving boundaries in a suspension and their rates of spread are monitored by an optical system. **paper e.,** that in which ions migrate along a strip of porous filter paper saturated with an electrolyte when a potential gradient is applied across the length of the strip. **thin-layer e.,** that in which the particles migrate through a thin layer of inert material (cellulose acetate, agar gel, etc.) under the influence of an electric field. **zone e.,** electrophoresis in which a supporting medium such as paper or starch granules immobilizes the solvent. This allows complete separation of components of different electrophoretic mobility, which is ordinarily not possible in moving boundary electrophoresis because of convective mixing.

electrophoretic (e-lek″tro-fo-ret′ik) pertaining to electrophoresis.

electrophoretogram (e-lek″tro-fo-ret′o-gram) the record produced on or in a supporting medium by bands of material which have been separated by the process of electrophoresis. Called also *electropherogram* and *electrophoregram.*

electrophorus (e-lek-trof′o-rus) [*electro-* + Gr. *phoros* bearing] an instrument for obtaining static electricity by means of induction.

electrophotometer (e-lek″tro-fo-tom′ĕ-ter) an instrument equipped with a photoelectric sensor for colorimetric determinations.

electrophysiologic (e-lek″tro-fis″ĭ-o-loj′ik) pertaining to electrophysiology.

electrophysiology (e-lek″tro-fiz″e-ol′o-je) the science of physiology in its relations to electricity; the study of the mechanisms of the production of electrical phenomena, and their consequences, in the living organism; the electrical phenomena involved in physiological processes.

electroplax (e-lek′tro-plaks) the electric units of the specialized organs in the muscle fibers of electric fish.

electroplexy (e-lek′tro-plek″se) [*electro-* + Gr. *plēgē* stroke] electric shock.

electropositive (e-lek″tro-poz′ĭ-tiv) [*electro-* + *positive*] bearing a positive electric charge.

electroradiometer (e-lek″tro-ra-de-om′ĕ-ter) an electroscope for measuring radiant energy.

electroresection (e-lek″tro-re-sek′shun) excision by electrosurgical means.

electroretinogram (e-lek″tro-ret′ĭ-no-gram) the record obtained by electroretinography; abbreviated ERG.

electroretinograph (e-lek″tro-ret′in-o-graf) an instrument for measuring the electrical response of the retina to light stimulation; abbreviated ERG.

electroretinography (e-lek″tro-ret′ĭ-nog′rah-fe) the recording of the changes in electric potential in the retina after stimulation by light.

electrosalivogram (e-lek″tro-sah-li′vo-gram) a graphic record or curve showing the action potential of the salivary glands.

electroscission (e-lek″tro-sizh′un) cutting tissue by use of the electric cautery.

electroscope (e-lek′tro-skōp) [electro- + Gr. skopein to examine] an instrument for measuring the intensity of radiation by detecting the motion imparted to charged strips suspended from a conductor.

electrosection (e-lek″tro-sek′shun) an incision made by electrosurgical means.

electroselenium (e-lek″tro-sĕ-le′ne-um) a form of colloidal selenium.

electroshock (e-lek″tro-shok) shock produced by application of electric current to the brain; see electroconvulsive therapy, under therapy.

electrosleep (e-lek′tro-slēp) see cerebral electrotherapy under electrotherapy.

electrosol (e-lek′tro-sol) a colloidal solution of a metal obtained by passing electric sparks through distilled water between poles formed of the metal.

electrosome (e-lek′tro-sōm) (obs.) a chrondriosome considered as a center of chemical activity.

electrospectrogram (e-lek″tro-spek′tro-gram) a record produced in electrospectrography.

electrospectrography (e-lek″tro-spek-trog′rah-fe) the isolation and recording of the constituent wave systems that are merged in an electroencephalogram.

electrospinogram (e-lek″tro-spi′no-gram) a tracing of the action potential of the spinal cord.

electrostatic (e-lek″tro-stat′ik) pertaining to static electricity.

electrostenolysis (e-lek″tro-stĕ-nol′ĭ-sis) the oxidation and reduction which occur on opposite surfaces of a high resistance membrane in a solution when there is a steep electric potential gradient across the membrane, reduction occurring on the surface facing the anode.

electrostethograph (e-lek″tro-steth′o-graf) (obs.) an apparatus for recording the amplified heart sounds over the chest.

electrostimulation (e-lek″tro-stim″u-la′shun) electrical stimulation of tissues, as for therapeutic or experimental purposes.

electrostriatogram (e-lek″tro-stri-āt′o-gram) a record of waves derived by the bipolar technique from the several structures of the corpus striatum.

electrosurgery (e-lek″tro-sur′jer-e) surgery performed by electrical methods; the active electrode may be a needle, bulb, or disk.

electrosyneresis (e-lek″tro-sin-ĕ-re′sis) immunofiltration.

electrosynthesis (e-lek″tro-sin″thĕ-sis) chemical reactions effected by means of electricity.

electrotaxis (e-lek″tro-tak′sis) [electro- + Gr. taxis arrangement] the movement of organisms or cells under the influence of electric currents.

electrothanasia (e-lek″tro-thah-na′ze-ah) [electro- + Gr. thanatos death] death by electricity; electrocution.

electrotherapeutics (e-lek″tro-ther-ah-pu′tiks) treatment of disease by means of electricity.

electrotherapeutist (e-lek″tro-ther-ah-pu′tist) a physician who specializes in the therapeutic use of electricity.

electrotherapist (e-lek″tro-ther′ah-pist) a person trained in using electricity for therapeutic purposes.

electrotherapy (e-lek″tro-ther′ah-pe) electrotherapeutics. **cerebral e.,** the use of low intensity electricity, usually employing positive pulses or direct current, in the treatment of insomnia, anxiety, and neurotic depression. It has been called electrosleep, a misleading term because the treatment does not induce sleep.

electrotherm (e-lek′tro-therm) [electro- + Gr. thermē heat] an electrosurgical appliance used for cutting.

electrotome (e-lek′tro-tōm) [electro- + Gr. tomē a cut] an electric surgical cutting instrument.

electrotomy (e-lek-trot′o-me) electroexcision with low current, high voltage, and high frequency; a procedure in which the tissues are not coagulated.

electrotonic (e-lek″tro-ton′ik) 1. pertaining to electrotonus. 2. denoting the direct spread of current in tissues by electrical conduction, without the generation of new current by action potentials.

electrotonus (e-lek-trot′o-nus) the altered electrical state of a nerve or muscle cell when a constant electric current is passed through it.

electrotrephine (e-lek″tro-tre′fin) a form of trephine operated by electricity.

electrotropism (e″lek-trot′ro-pizm) [electro- + Gr. tropos a turning, change] the tendency of a cell or organism to react in a definite manner in response to an electric stimulus. **negative e.,** the tendency of a cell to be repelled by an electric stimulus. **positive e.,** the tendency of a cell to be attracted by an electric stimulus.

electroultrafiltration (e-lek″tro-ul″trah-fil-tra′shun) ultrafiltration in an electric field.

electroureterogram (e-lek″tro-u-re′ter-o-gram) the record obtained by electroureterography.

electroureterography (e-lek″tro-u-re″ter-og′rah-fe) electromyography in which the action potentials produced by peristalsis of the ureter are recorded.

electrovagogram (e-lek″tro-va′go-gram) vagogram.

electrovalence (e-lek″tro-va′lens) 1. the number of charges an atom acquires by the gain or loss of electrons in forming an ionic bond. 2. the bonding resulting from such a transfer of electrons.

electrovalent (e-lek″tro-va′lent) pertaining to electrovalence or to an electrovalent (ionic) bond.

electroversion (e-lek″tro-ver′zhun) the act of electrically terminating a cardiac dysrhythmia.

electrovert (e-lek′tro-vert) to apply electricity to the heart or precordium to depolarize the heart and terminate a cardiac dysrhythmia.

electuary (e-lek′tu-a-re) [L. electuarium, from e out + legere to select] a medicinal preparation consisting of a powdered drug made into a paste with honey or syrup; a confection. Called also lincture and linctus. **e. of senna,** a mixture of senna, syrup, and tamarind pulp.

eledoisin (el-ĕ-doi′sin) chemical name: L-pyroglutamyl-L-prolyl-L-seryl-L-lysyl-L-aspartyl-alanyl-phenylalanyl-L-isoleucyl-glycyl-L-leucyl-L-methioninamide. An endecapeptide, $C_{54}H_{85}N_{13}$-$O_{15}S$, from the posterior salivary gland of a species of small octopus (Eledone), which is a precursor of a large group of biologically active peptides. It has vasodilator, hypotensive, and extravascular smooth muscle stimulant properties.

eleidin (el-e′ĭ-din) a substance of peculiar nature, allied to keratin and protoplasm, found in the cells of the stratum lucidum of the skin.

element (el′ĕ-ment) [L. elementum] 1. any of the primary parts or constituents of a thing. 2. in chemistry, a simple substance which cannot be decomposed by chemical means and which is made up of atoms which are alike in their peripheral electronic configurations and so in their chemical properties, and also in the number of protons in their nuclei, but which may differ in the number of neutrons in their nuclei and so in their atomic weight and in their radioactive properties. [See accompanying Table of Elements.] **anatomic e.,** morphological e. **appendicular e's,** a set of cartilaginous rods attached to the chondral skull of the embryo; from them are developed the ear bones, the hyoid, and the styloid process. **electronegative e.,** any chemical element that adds electrons (or tends to add electrons) during chemical combination. **electropositive e.,** a chemical element that loses electrons (or tends to lose electrons) during chemical combination. **F e.,** see under factor. **formed e's (of the blood),** erythrocytes, leukocytes, and platelets. **labile e.,** tissue cells which continue to multiply during the life of the individual. **morphological e.,** any cell, fiber, or other of the ultimate structures which go to make up tissues and organs. **radioactive e.,** a chemical element which spontaneously transmutes into another element with emission of corpuscular or electromagnetic radiations. The natural radioactive elements are all those with atomic number above 83, and some other elements, such as potassium (at. no. 19) and rubidium (at. no. 37), which are very weakly radioactive. **rare earth e's,** elements of the lanthanum series, comprising elements with atomic numbers 57 to 71. **sarcous e.,** any of the elementary granules into which the primitive fibril of an elementary muscle fiber is divisible. **stable e.,** 1. a chemical element which does not spontaneously transmute into another element with emission of corpuscular or electromagnetic radiations; the stable elements are those with atomic number below 84, except for a few, such as potassium and rubidium, which are weakly radioactive. 2. a tissue cell of mature tissues which does not alter by mitosis. **tissue e.,** morphological e. **trace e's,** chemical elements that are distributed throughout the tissues in very small amounts and are either essential in nutrition, such as cobalt, copper, magnesium, manganese, and zinc, or may be harmful, such as selenium. **tracer e's,** see radioactive tracer, under tracer. **transcalifornium e's,** the elements with atomic numbers higher than that of californium, and discovered subsequent to its discovery in 1950. They are einsteinium 99, fermium 100, mendelevium 101, nobelium 102, and lawrencium 103. **transuranic e's, transuranium e's,** the elements with atomic numbers higher than that of uranium. Applied originally to neptunium 93, plutonium 94, americium 95,

TABLE OF ELEMENTS

NAME	SYMBOL	AT. NO.	AT. WT.*	NAME	SYMBOL	AT. NO.	AT. WT.*
Actinum	Ac	89	(227)	Mercury	Hg	80	200.59
Aluminum	Al	13	26.982	Molybdenum	Mo	42	95.94
Americium	Am	95	(243)	Neodymium	Nd	60	144.24
Antimony	Sb	51	121.75	Neon	Ne	10	20.183
Argon	Ar	18	39.948	Neptunium	Np	93	(237)
Arsenic	As	33	74.922	Nickel	Ni	28	58.71
Astatine	At	85	(210)	Niobium	Nb	41	92.906
Barium	Ba	56	137.34	Nitrogen	N	7	14.007
Berkelium	Bk	97	(247)	Nobelium	No	102	(253)
Beryllium	Be	4	9.012	Osmium	Os	76	190.2
Bismuth	Bi	83	208.980	Oxygen	O	8	15.999
Boron	B	5	10.811	Palladium	Pd	46	106.4
Bromine	Br	35	79.909	Phosphorus	P	15	30.974
Cadmium	Cd	48	112.40	Platinum	Pt	78	195.09
Calcium	Ca	20	40.08	Plutonium	Pu	94	(242)
Californium	Cf	98	(249)	Polonium	Po	84	(210)
Carbon	C	6	12.011	Potassium	K	19	39.102
Cerium	Ce	58	140.12	Praseodymium	Pr	59	140.907
Cesium	Cs	55	132.905	Promethium	Pm	61	(147)
Chlorine	Cl	17	35.453	Protactinium	Pa	91	(231)
Chromium	Cr	24	51.996	Radium	Ra	88	(226)
Cobalt	Co	27	58.933	Radon	Rn	86	(222)
Copper	Cu	29	63.54	Rhenium	Re	75	186.2
Curium	Cm	96	(247)	Rhodium	Rh	45	102.905
Dysprosium	Dy	66	162.50	Rubidium	Rb	37	85.47
Einsteinium	Es	99	(254)	Ruthenium	Ru	44	101.07
Erbium	Er	68	167.26	Rutherfordium	Rf	104	(261)
Europium	Eu	63	151.96	Samarium	Sm	62	150.35
Fermium	Fm	100	(253)	Scandium	Sc	21	44.956
Fluorine	F	9	18.998	Selenium	Se	34	78.96
Francium	Fr	87	(223)	Silicon	Si	14	28.086
Gadolinium	Gd	64	157.25	Silver	Ag	47	107.870
Gallium	Ga	31	69.72	Sodium	Na	11	22.990
Germanium	Ge	32	72.59	Strontium	Sr	38	87.62
Gold	Au	79	196.967	Sulfur	S	16	32.064
Hafnium	Hf	72	178.49	Tantalum	Ta	73	180.948
Hahnium	Ha	105	(260)	Technetium	Tc	43	(99)
Helium	He	2	4.003	Tellurium	Te	52	127.60
Holmium	Ho	67	164.930	Terbium	Tb	65	158.924
Hydrogen	H	1	1.008	Thallium	Tl	81	204.37
Indium	In	49	114.82	Thorium	Th	90	232.038
Iodine	I	53	126.904	Thulium	Tm	69	168.934
Iridium	Ir	77	192.2	Tin	Sn	50	118.69
Iron	Fe	26	55.847	Titanium	Ti	22	47.90
Krypton	Kr	36	83.80	Tungsten	W	74	183.85
Lanthanum	La	57	138.91	Uranium	U	92	238.03
Lawrencium	Lw	103	(257)	Vanadium	V	23	50.942
Lead	Pb	82	207.19	Xenon	Xe	54	131.30
Lithium	Li	3	6.939	Ytterbium	Yb	70	173.04
Lutetium	Lu	71	174.97	Yttrium	Y	39	88.905
Magnesium	Mg	12	24.312	Zinc	Zn	30	65.37
Manganese	Mn	25	54.938	Zirconium	Zr	40	91.22
Mendelevium	Md	101	(256)				

* Atomic weights are corrected to conform with the 1961 values of the Commission on Atomic Weights, expressed to the fourth decimal point, rounded off to the nearest thousandth. The numbers in parentheses are the mass numbers of the most stable or most common isotope.

curium 96, berkelium 97, and californium 98, the term now, by definition, includes the transcalifornium elements as well.

elementary (el″ĕ-men′tah-re) not resolvable or divisible into simpler parts or components; see also under *particle*.

elemi (el″ĕ-me) [Turkish *eleme* hand picked] a resinous substance, of extremely various origin, the best coming from *Canarium commune*, of the Philippine Islands. It furnishes a volatile oil, and was formerly used externally, generally in an ointment, for ulcers and sores.

eleo- (el′e-o) [Gr. *elaion* oil] combining form denoting relationship to oil.

eleoma (el″e-o′mah) [*eleo-* + *-oma*] a tumor or swelling caused by the injection of oil into the tissues.

eleometer (el″e-om′ĕ-ter) [*eleo-* + Gr. *metron* measure] an instrument for determining percentage of oil in a mixture, also specific gravity of oils.

eleopathy (el″e-op′ah-the) elaiopathy.

eleoplast (el-e′o-plast) [*eleo-* + Gr. *plastos* formed] a globular body made up of granular protoplasm and containing drops of oil.

eleopten (el″e-op′ten) [*eleo-* + Gr. *ptēnos* volatile] the more volatile constituent of a volatile oil, as distinguished from its stearopten.

eleosaccharum (el″e-o-sak′ah-rum), pl. *eleosacch′ara* [Gr. *elaion* oil + *sakcharon* sugar] a mixture of sugar with a volatile oil; an oil sugar. Called also *oleosaccharum*.

eleotherapy (el″e-o-ther′ah-pe) [*eleo-* + *therapy*] oleotherapy.

elephantiasic (el″ĕ-fan″te-as′ik) pertaining to elephantiasis.

elephantiasis (el″ĕ-fan-ti′ah-sis) ["elephant disease"] a chronic filarial disease due to infection of the lymphatic channels with the nematode *Wuchereria bancrofti* or *Brugia malayi*, and characterized by inflammation and obstruction of the lymphatics and hypertrophy of the skin and subcutaneous tissues. The legs and external genitals are principally affected, the disease beginning in attacks of dermatitis, with enlargement of the part, attended by chills and fever (elephantoid fever) and followed by the formation of ulcers and tubercles, with thickening, discoloration, and fissuring of the skin. The disease is most common in tropical regions. The term elephantiasis is often applied to hypertrophy and thickening of the tissues from any cause. **e. arab′icum,** elephantiasis. **e. chirur′gica,** Halsted's name for massive edema of the arm after mastectomy. **congenital e.,** Milroy's disease. **e. filarien′sis,** true elephantiasis due to filariasis. **e. gingi′vae,** fibromatosis gingivae. **e. graeco′rum** (*obs.*), leprosy. **e. leishmania′na,** the edema and hypertrophy of tissues caused by leishmaniasis. **lymphangiectatic e.,** elephantiasis of a part due to lymphangiectasis. **e. neuromato′sa,** neurofibroma. **nevoid e.,** a variety marked by great dilatation of the lymph vessels. **e. nos′tras,** that due to either chronic recurrent streptococcal erysipelas or chronic recurrent cellulitis. **e. oc′uli,** thickening and protrusion of the eyelids. **e. scro′ti,** that in which the scrotum is the principal seat of the disease; called also *parasitic chylocele*, and *lymph scrotum*.

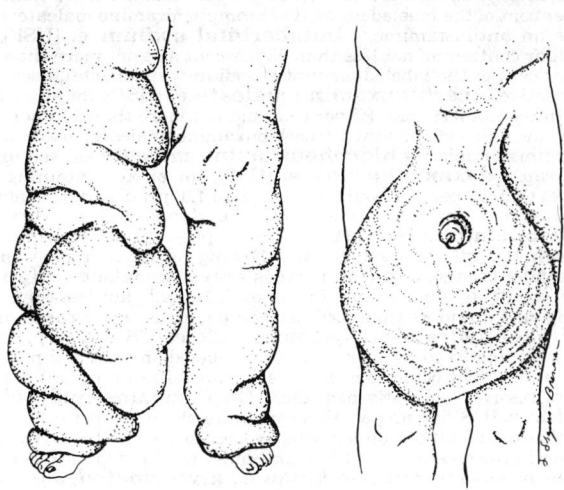

Elephantiasis of the legs and of the scrotum.

elephantoid (el″ĕ-fan′toid) relating to or resembling elephantiasis.

Elettaria cardamomum (L.) Maton (Zingiberaceae) (el″ĕ-ta′re-ah kar″dah-mo′mum) a species of plants of tropical areas of the Old World, which afford cardamom and grains of paradise.

eleutheromania (e-lu″ther-o-ma′ne-ah) [Gr. *eletheria* freedom] abnormal enthusiasm for freedom.

elevation (el″ĕ-va′shun) a raised area, or point of greater height. **dicrotic e.** (*obs.*), the secondary rise of a dicrotic pulse wave in the sphygmogram. **tactile e's,** toruli tactiles.

elevator (el′ĕ-va″tor) [L. *elevare* to lift] an instrument for elevating tissues, for removing osseous fragments, or roots of teeth. **Cryer's e.,** a dental instrument for removing the roots of molar teeth; furnished in pairs, one for mesial and one for distal roots, which are reversed for use on opposite sides of the jaw. **malar e.,** an instrument used to elevate or reposition the zygomatic bone and/or arch. **periosteum e.,** a flat steel bar for separating the attachments of the periosteum to bone. **screw e.,** a dental instrument designed to be screwed into a root canal for subsequent removal of the root, usually of the apical third.

elfazepam (el-faz′ĕ-pam) chemical name: 7-chloro-1-[2-(ethylsulfonyl)ethyl]-5-(2-fluorophenyl)-1,3-dihydro-2H-1,4-benzodiazepin-2-one; a veterinary appetite stimulant, $C_{19}H_{18}ClFN_2O_3S$.

eliminant (e-lim′ĭ-nant) 1. causing an evacuation. 2. an agent that promotes evacuation.

elimination (e-lim″ĭ-na′shun) [L. *eliminatio,* from *e* out + *limen* threshold] 1. the act of expulsion or of extrusion, especially of expulsion from the body. 2. omission or exclusion, as in an elimination diet. Cf. *excretion.* **immune e.,** the period of accelerated degradation of antigen (e.g., foreign gamma globulin) as a result of its removal and destruction by antibodies. Also, a technique for determining antibody response by measuring the rate of removal of labeled antigen from the circulation of an immunized animal. Called also *immune clearance.*

elinguation (e″lin-gwa′shun) [L. *e* out + *lingua* tongue] the removal of the tongue.

elinin (el′ĭ-nin) a lipoprotein fraction of red cells containing the Rh and A and B factors.

Elipten (e-lip′ten) trademark for a preparation of aminoglutethimide.

elixir (e-lik′ser) [L., from Arabic] a clear, sweetened, usually hydroalcoholic liquid containing flavoring substances and sometimes active medicinal agents, used orally as a vehicle or for the effect of the medicinal agent contained. **acetaminophen e.** [USP], an elixir containing not less than 95 per cent and not more than 105 per cent of the labeled amount of acetaminophen, $C_8H_9NO_2$; used as an analgesic and antipyretic. **amobarbital e.** [USP], an elixir containing not less than 95.0 per cent and not more than 105.0 per cent of the labeled amount of amobarbital; used as a sedative and hypnotic. **aprobarbital e.,** an elixir containing not less than 92.5 per cent and not more than 107.5 per cent of aprobarbital; used as a sedative. **aromatic e.** [NF], a preparation containing orange, lemon, coriander, and anise oils, syrup, talc, and alcohol in purified water; used as a flavored vehicle for pharmaceutical preparations. **aromatic e., red,** aromatic elixir colored by addition of amaranth solution. **benzaldehyde e., compound,** a preparation of benzaldehyde, vanillin, orange flower water, alcohol, simple syrup, and water; used as a vehicle for pharmaceutical preparations. **bromodiphenhydramine hydrochloride e.** [USP], an elixir containing not less than 93 per cent and not more than 107 per cent of the labeled amount of bromodiphenhydramine hydrochloride; used as an antihistaminic. **brompheniramine maleate e.** [USP], an elixir containing not less than 95 per cent and not more than 105 per cent of the labeled amount of brompheniramine maleate; used as an antihistaminic. **butabarbital sodium e.** [USP], an elixir containing not less than 95 per cent and not more than 105 per cent of the labeled amount of sodium butabarbital; used as a sedative. **carbinoxamine maleate e.** [USP], an elixir containing not less than 95 per cent and not more than 105 per cent of the labeled amount of carbinoxamine maleate; used as an antihistaminic. **chlorpheniramine maleate e.,** see under *syrup.* **dexamethasone e.** [USP], an elixir containing not less than 90 per cent and not more than 110 per cent of the labeled amount of dexamethasone; used as a glucocorticoid. **dextroamphetamine sulfate e.** [USP], a preparation containing, in each 100 ml., between 90 and 110 mg. of dextroamphetamine sulfate; used as a central nervous system stimulant. **digoxin e.** [USP], an elixir containing, in each 100 ml., not less than 4.60 mg. and not more than 5.40 mg. of digoxin; used as a cardiotonic. **diphenhydramine hydrochloride e.** [USP], a preparation containing 94 to 106 per cent of the labeled amount of diphenhydramine hydrochloride; used as an antihistaminic, antiemetic, antitussive, and antispasmodic. **fluphenazine hydrochloride e.** [USP], a preparation containing 95 to 105 per cent of the labeled amount of fluphenazine hydrochloride; used as a tranquilizer in the treatment of the manifestations of psychotic disorders, and as an antiemetic. **gentian e., glycerinated,** a preparation of gentian and taraxacum fluidextracts, compound cardamon tincture, raspberry syrup, sweet orange peel tincture, phosphoric

acid, ethyl acetate, glycerin, sucrose, and alcohol, in purified water; used as a flavored vehicle for drugs. **high-alcoholic e.,** see *iso-alcoholic e.* **homatropine methylbromide e.,** a preparation containing 90 to 110 per cent of the labeled amount of homatropine methylbromide; used as an anticholinergic to reduce spasms and inhibit secretions, especially in gastrointestinal disorders. **e. I. Q. & S., iron, quinine, and strychnine e.,** a preparation of iron, quinine, and strychnine, with compound orange spirit, alcohol, glycerin, and purified water; used as a bitter tonic. **iso-alcoholic e.** [NF], a mixture of low-alcoholic elixir and high-alcoholic elixir to produce a solution whose strength is suitable for the medicament for which it serves as a vehicle. *Low-alcoholic e.:* compound orange spirit 10 ml., alcohol 100 ml., glycerin 200 ml., sucrose 320 gm., and sufficient purified water to make a total of 1000 ml. *High-alcoholic e.:* compound orange spirit 4 ml., saccharin 3 gm., glycerin 200 ml., and sufficient alcohol to make a total of 1000 ml. **low-alcoholic e.,** see *iso-alcoholic e.* **methenamine e.** [USP] an elixir containing 90 to 110 per cent of the labeled amount of methenamine; used as a urinary antibacterial. **oxtriphylline e.** [USP], an elixir containing between 90 and 110 per cent of the labeled amount of oxtriphylline; used as a bronchodilator. **pentobarbital e.** [USP], an elixir containing between 92.5 and 107.5 per cent of the labeled amount of pentobarbital; used as a sedative and hypnotic. **pentobarbital sodium e.** [USP], pentobarbital sodium 4.0 gm., glycerin 450.0 ml., alcohol 150.0 ml., orange oil 0.75 ml., caramel 2 gm., syrup 150.0 ml., diluted hydrochloric acid 6.0 ml., and sufficient purified water to make a total of 1000 ml.; used as a sedative and hypnotic. **pepsin e., lactated,** a water preparation containing a proteolytic enzyme from the glandular layer of the fresh stomach of the hog, with lactic acid, glycerin, alcohol, orange oil, and amaranth solution. **phenobarbital e.** [USP], an elixir containing between 92.5 and 107.5 per cent of the labeled amount of phenobarbital; used as a sedative, hypnotic, and anticonvulsant. **potassium chloride e.** [USP], an elixir containing between 90 and 110 per cent of the labeled amount of potassium chloride, KCl; used as an electrolyte replenisher. **potassium gluconate e.** [USP], an elixir containing 97 to 103 per cent of the labeled amount of potassium gluconate; used as an electrolyte replenisher in the prophylaxis and treatment of hypokalemia. **reserpine e.,** [USP], an elixir containing between 90 and 110 per cent of the labeled amount of reserpine; used as an antihypertensive agent. **secobarbital e.** [USP], an elixir containing, in each 100 ml., not less than 417 mg. and not more than 461 mg. of secobarbital in a suitable, flavored solution; used as a hypnotic. **terpin hydrate e.** [USP], terpin hydrate 17 gm., sweet orange peel tincture 20 ml., benzaldhyde 50 μl., glycerin 400 ml., alcohol 430 ml., syrup 100 ml., and sufficient purified water to make 1000 ml.; used as an expectorant. **terpin hydrate and codeine e.** [USP], 2 gm. of codeine dissolved in a sufficient quantity of terpin hydrate elixir to make 1000 ml.; used as an expectorant and antitussive. **terpin hydrate and dextromethorphan hydrobromide e.** [USP], 2 gm. of dextromethorphan hydrobromide dissolved in a sufficient quantity of terpin hydrate elixir to make 1000 ml.; used as an expectorant and antitussive. **theophylline sodium glycinate e.** [USP], an elixir containing an amount of theophylline between 47 and 54 per cent of the labeled amount of theophylline sodium glycinate; used as a bronchodilator and smooth muscle relaxant. **three bromides e.,** a mixture of ammonium, potassium, and sodium bromides, amaranth solution and compound benzaldehyde elixir; occasionally used as a sedative in grand mal seizures. See also *bromide.* **trihexyphenidyl hydrochloride e.** [USP], an elixir containing, in each 100 ml., not less than 37.2 mg. and not more than 42.8 mg. of trihexyphenidyl hydrochloride; used as an antiparkinsonian agent. **tripelennamine citrate e.** [USP], an elixir containing, in each 100 ml., not less than 705 mg. and not more than 795 mg. of tripelennamine citrate; used as an antihistaminic in the symptomatic treatment of allergic disorders.

Elixophyllin (e-lik″so-fil′in) trademark for preparations of theophylline.

Elkosin (el′ko-sin) trademark for preparations of sulfisomidine.

elkosis (el′ko-sis) helcosis.

Ellermann-Erlandsen test (method) (el′er-mahn-ār′land-sen) [Vilhelm *Ellermann,* Copenhagen pathologist, 1871–1924; Alfred Wilhelm Erland *Erlandsen,* Copenhagen hygienist, 1878–1918] tuberculin titer test; see under *test.*

Elliot's operation (el′e-ots) [Col. Robert Henry *Elliot,* of the Indian Medical Service, 1864–1936] see under *operation.*

Elliot's position [John Wheelock *Elliot,* American surgeon, 1852–1925] see under *position.*

Elliot's sign [George T. *Elliot,* American dermatologist, 1851–1935] see under *sign.*

ellipsin (e-lip′sin) the insoluble constituents of cells which remain after the removal of the soluble proteins.

ellipsis (e-lip′sis) [Gr. "a leaving out"] in psychiatry, the omission of words or of ideas by a patient in the course of psychoanalysis.

ellipsoid (e-lip′soid) any structure having a spindle shape, especially (*a*) any of the spindle-shaped masses of cells surrounding the second portion of the arterioles of the spleen (see *sheathed artery,* under *artery*) or (*b*) the outer refractile portion of the inner section of the retinal rods and cones.

elliptocytary (e-lip″to-si′tah-re)   pertaining to elliptocytes.

elliptocyte (e-lip′to-sīt)   an elliptical erythrocyte.

elliptocytosis (e-lip″to-si-to′sis)   a hereditary disorder in which the greater proportion of erythrocytes are elliptical in shape, and which is characterized by varying degrees of increased red cell destruction and anemia.

elliptocytotic (e-lip″to-si-tot′ik)   pertaining to or characterized by elliptocytosis.

Ellis's line (curve), sign (el′ĭ-sez) [Calvin *Ellis,* Boston physician, 1826–1883]   see under *line* and *sign.*

Ellis-Garland line (el′is-gar′land) [Calvin *Ellis;* George Minot *Garland,* American physician, 1849–1926]   Ellis' line.

Eloesser flap (el-es′er) [Leo *Eloesser,* San Francisco surgeon, born 1881]   see under *flap.*

elongation (e″long-ga′shun)   the process or condition of increasing in length.

Elorine (el′o-rēn)   trademark for a preparation of tricyclamol chloride.

Elsberg's test (els′bergz) [Charles Albert *Elsberg,* New York surgeon, 1871–1948]   see under *solution* and *test.*

Elschnig's bodies (pearls) (elsh′nig) [Anton *Elschnig,* German ophthalmologist, 1863–1939]   see under *body.*

Elsner's asthma (els′nerz) [Christoph Friedrich *Elsner,* German physician, 1749–1820]   angina pectoris.

eluate (el′u-āt)   the substance separated out by, or the product of, elution or elutriation.

elucaine (ĕ-lu′kān)   chemical name: α-(diethylamino)methyl]-benzenemethanol benzoate (ester); an anticholinergic (gastric), $C_{19}H_{23}NO_2$.

eluent (el′u-ent)   a solution used in elution.

elurophobia (e-lu″ro-fo′be-ah)   (*obs.*) ailurophobia.

elution (e-lu′shun) [L. *e* out + *luere* to wash]   in chemistry, the separation of material by washing, as in the freeing of an enzyme from its absorbent.   **membrane e.,** a method of selecting cells in which a culture of cells is collected on a membrane filter, over which a fresh warm culture fluid is then slowly passed, washing off excess cells and leaving only adsorbed cells at a particular developmental stage.

elutriation (e-lu″tre-a′shun) [L. *elutriare* to wash out]   the operation of pulverizing substances and mixing them with water in order to separate the heavier constituents, which settle out in solution, from the lighter constituents.

Ely's operation (e′lēz) [Edward Talbot *Ely,* American otologist, 1850–1885]   see under *operation.*

Ely's test (sign) (e′lēz) [Leonard Wheeler *Ely,* American orthopedic surgeon, 1868–1944]   see under *test.*

elytro- (el′ĭ-tro) [Gr. *elytron* a covering, sheath]   a combining form denoting relationship to the vagina or to a sheath; for words beginning thus, see those beginning colpo-.

Elzholz's bodies, mixture (elts′holts-ez) [Adolf *Elzholz,* alienist in Vienna, 1863–1925]   see under *body* and *mixture.*

Em. *emmetropia.*

emaciation (e-ma″se-a′shun) [L. *emaciare* to make lean]   excessive leanness; a wasted condition of the body.

emailloblast (e-māl′o-blast) [Fr. *émail* enamel + Gr. *blastos* germ]   ameloblast.

eman (em′an)   a unit for expressing the concentration of radium emanation in solution: it is the concentration present when one tenth of a millimicrocurie of radium emanation is dissolved in 1 liter of air or water, or 10^{-10} curie.

emanation (em-ah-na′shun) [L. *e* out + *manare* to flow]   that which is given off, such as a gaseous disintegration product given off from radioactive substances or an effluvium.   **actinium e.,** one member of the radioactive series derived from actinium. It is produced from actinium X, has an atomic weight of 218, its atomic number is 86, and by the loss of alpha particles it becomes actinium A. Called also *actinon.*   **radium e.,** radon.   **thorium e.,** one member of the radio-active series derived from thorium. It is produced from thorium X, has an atomic weight of 220, its atomic number is 86, and by the loss of alpha particles it changes into thorium A. Called also *thoron.*

emanator (em′ah-na″tor)   an instrument for giving off and applying to the body radioactive emanations.

emanatorium (em″ah-na-to′re-um)   an institute for treating diseases by radioactive emanations.

emancipation (e-man″sĭ-pa′shun) [L. *emancipare* to release, give up]   the establishment of local autonomy within restricted fields of a developing embryo.

emasculation (e-mas″ku-la′shun) [L. *emasculare* to castrate]   1. excision of the penis. 2. castration.

Embadomonas (em″bah-dom′o-nas)   *Retortamonas.*

embalming (em-bahm′ing)   the treatment of the dead body with antiseptics and preservatives, to prevent putrefaction.

embarrass (em-bar′as)   to impede the function of; to obstruct.

embedding (em-bed′ing)   the fixation of a tissue specimen in a firm medium, in order to keep it intact during the cutting of thin sections.

Embelia (em-be′le-ah)   a genus of myrtaceous East Indian climbing plants.   **E. ri′bes, E. robus′ta,** species whose fruit has been used for its anthelminthic and cathartic principles.

embelin (em′bĕ-lin)   chemical name: 2,5-dihydroxy-3-undecyl-*p*-benzoquinone. An active principle, $CH_3(CH_2)_{10}\cdot C_6HO_2(OH)_2$, from *Embelia ribes,* formerly used as a teniacide.

emboitement (aw-bwat′maw) [Fr. "encasement"]   the supposed encasement of miniature individuals within the germ cells of predecessors, advanced as one theory of preformation.

embolalia (em″bo-la′le-ah)   embololalia.

embole (em′bo-le) [Gr. *embolē* a throwing in]   1. the reducing of a dislocated limb. 2. emboly.

embolectomy (em″bo-lek′to-me) [*embolus* + Gr. *ektomē* excision]   surgical removal of an embolus from a blood vessel.

embolemia (em″bo-le′me-ah) [*embolus* + Gr. *haima* blood + *-ia*]   (*obs.*) the presence of emboli in the blood.

emboli (em′bo-li) [L.]   plural of *embolus.*

embolia (em-bo′le-ah)   embole.

embolic (em-bol′ik)   pertaining to an embolus or to embolism.

emboliform (em-bol′ĭ-form)   1. shaped like a wedge. 2. resembling an embolus.

embolism (em′bo-lizm) [L. *embolismus,* from Gr. *en* in + *ballein* to throw]   the sudden blocking of an artery by a clot or foreign material which has been brought to its site of lodgment by the blood current.   **air e.,** that due to air bubbles entering the veins after trauma or surgical procedures.   **amniotic fluid e.,** embolism due to amniotic fluid forced into the maternal circulation near the end of normal pregnancy by strong uterine contractions.   **bacillary e.,** obstruction of a vessel by an aggregation of bacilli.   **bland e.,** that in which the thrombotic plug is composed of nonseptic material.   **bone marrow e.,** embolism caused by material from a fractured long bone.   **capillary e.,** blocking of the capillaries with bacteria.   **cerebral e.,** embolism of a cerebral artery.   **coronary e.,** embolism of one of the coronary arteries.   **crossed e.,** paradoxical e.   **direct e.,** embolism occurring in the direction of the blood stream.   **fat e.,** embolism of fat that has entered the circulation, especially after fractures of large bones.   **infective e.,** embolism in which the embolus is infective.   **lymph e., lymphogenous e.,** embolism of a lymph vessel.   **miliary e.,** that which affects at the same time many small blood vessels.   **multiple e.,** embolism by a number of small emboli.   **oil e.,** fat e.   **pantaloon e.,** saddle e.   **paradoxical e.,** blockage of a systemic artery by a thrombus originating in a systemic vein, which has passed through a defect that permits direct communication between the right and the left side of the heart, notably an open foramen ovale; called also *crossed e.*   **plasmodium e.,** the occlusion of a coronary artery by *Plasmodium falciparum.*   **pulmonary e.,** the closure of the pulmonary artery or one of its branches by an embolus, sometimes associated with infarction of the lung.   **pyemic e.** (*obs.*), infective e.   **retinal e.,** embolism of the central artery of the retina.   **saddle e.,** an embolism lodging at the bifurcation of the aorta, causing sudden severe pain of the legs, abdomen, and back, with numbing and coldness. Called also *pantaloon e.*   **spinal e.,** embolism of an artery in the spinal cord.   **trichinous e.,** embolism due to trichinae.   **tumor e.,** embolism due to tumor fragments, especially from cancer of the stomach.   **venous e.,** embolism in which the clot or plug originates in the veins.

embolization (em″bo-li-za′shun)   1. the process or condition of becoming an embolus.   2. therapeutic introduction of a substance into a vessel in order to occlude it.   **poppet e.,** the embolization of the ball of a poppet valve used as a heart valve prosthesis.

embololalia (em″bŏ-lo-la′le-ah) [Gr. *emballein* to insert + *lalia* babble]   the interpolation of meaningless words or phrases into the speech; called also *embolophrasia.*

embolomycotic (em″bŏ-lo-mi-kot′ik)   pertaining to or marked by an infectious embolus.

embolophrasia (em″bŏ-lo-fra′ze-ah) [Gr. *emballein* to insert + *phrasis* utterance]   embololalia.

embolus (em′bo-lus), pl. *em′boli* [Gr. *embolos* plug]   1. a clot or other plug brought by the blood from another vessel and forced into a smaller one, thus obstructing the circulation.   2. the emboliform nucleus of the cerebellum. See illustration on following page.   **air e.,** a bubble of air obstructing a blood vessel.   **cancer e.,** a small mass of cells detached from a cancer and carried by the blood stream to lodge in a distant location.   **cellular e.,** one consisting of tissue cells of various kinds.   **fat e.,** one composed of oil or fat.   **foam e.,** one formed by a mixture of a gas and blood.   **obturating e.,** one completely blocking a vessel.   **riding e., saddle e., straddling e.,** one at the bifurcation of an artery, blocking both branches.

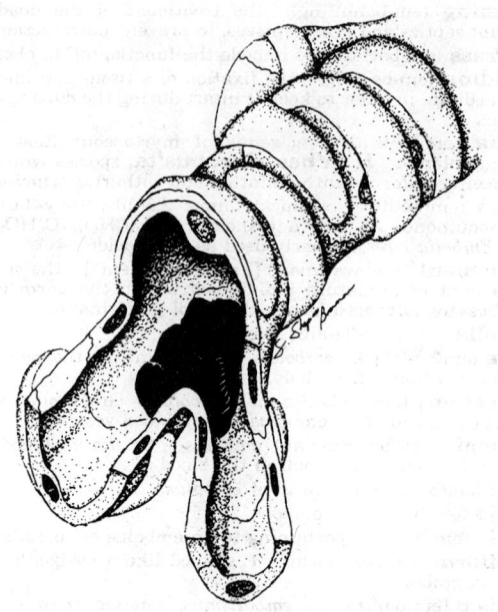

Embolus impacted at site of branching of an artery.

emboly (em′bo-le) [Gr. *embolē* a throwing in] the invagination of the blastula by which the gastrula is formed.

embouchment (aw-boosh-maw′) [Fr.] the opening of one vessel into another.

embrasure (em-bra′zhur) the interproximal space occlusal to the area of contact of adjacent teeth in the same dental arch. Cf. *interproximal space.* **buccal e.,** the embrasure opening out toward the cheek between molar and premolar teeth. **labial**

e., the embrasure opening toward the lips between canine and incisor teeth. **lingual e.,** one of the embrasure openings on the lingual sides of the teeth. **occlusal e.,** the space between the marginal ridges of approximating teeth, mesially and distally, and the point of contact and the occlusal plane.

embrocation (em-bro-ka′shun) [L. *embrocatio*] 1. the application of a liquid medicament to the surface of the body. 2. a liquid medicine for external use.

embryectomy (em″bre-ek′to-me) [*embryo* + Gr. *ektomē* excision] excision of the embryo in extrauterine pregnancy.

embryo (em′bre-o) [Gr. *embryon*] 1. in plants, the element of the seed that develops into a new individual. 2. in animals, those derivatives of the fertilized ovum that eventually become the offspring, during their period of most rapid development, i.e., after the long axis appears until all major structures are represented. In man, the developing organism is an embryo from about two weeks after fertilization to the end of seventh or eighth week. **hexacanth e.,** the six-hooked embryo, or onchosphere, characteristic of most tapeworms of man and domestic animals. **Janošík's e.,** a human embryo having three aortic arches and two gill pouches. **presomite e.,** the embryo at any stage prior to the appearance of the first somite. **previllous e.,** the conceptus before the chorionic villi develop. **somite e.,** the embryo at any stage between the appearances of the first and the last somites. **Spee's e.,** a 1.5 mm. human embryo, horizon IX, about 20 days old as described by Spee.

embryoblast (em′bre-o-blast″) [*embryo* + Gr. *blastos* germ] inner cell mass.

embryocardia (em″bre-o-kar′de-ah) [*embryo* + Gr. *kardia* heart] a symptom in which the sounds of the heart resemble those of fetal life, there being very little difference in the quality of the first and second sounds.

embryoctony (em″bre-ok′tŏ-ne) [*embryo* + Gr. *kteinein* to kill] the artificial destruction of the living embryo, or fetus.

embryogenesis (em″bre-o-jen′ĕ-sis) [*embryo* + *genesis*] the development of a new individual by means of sexual reproduction, that is, from a fertilized ovum; the process of embryo formation.

embryogenetic (em″bre-o-jĕ-net′ik) embryogenic.

embryogenic (em″bre-o-jen′ik) 1. pertaining to the development of the embryo. 2. producing an embryo.

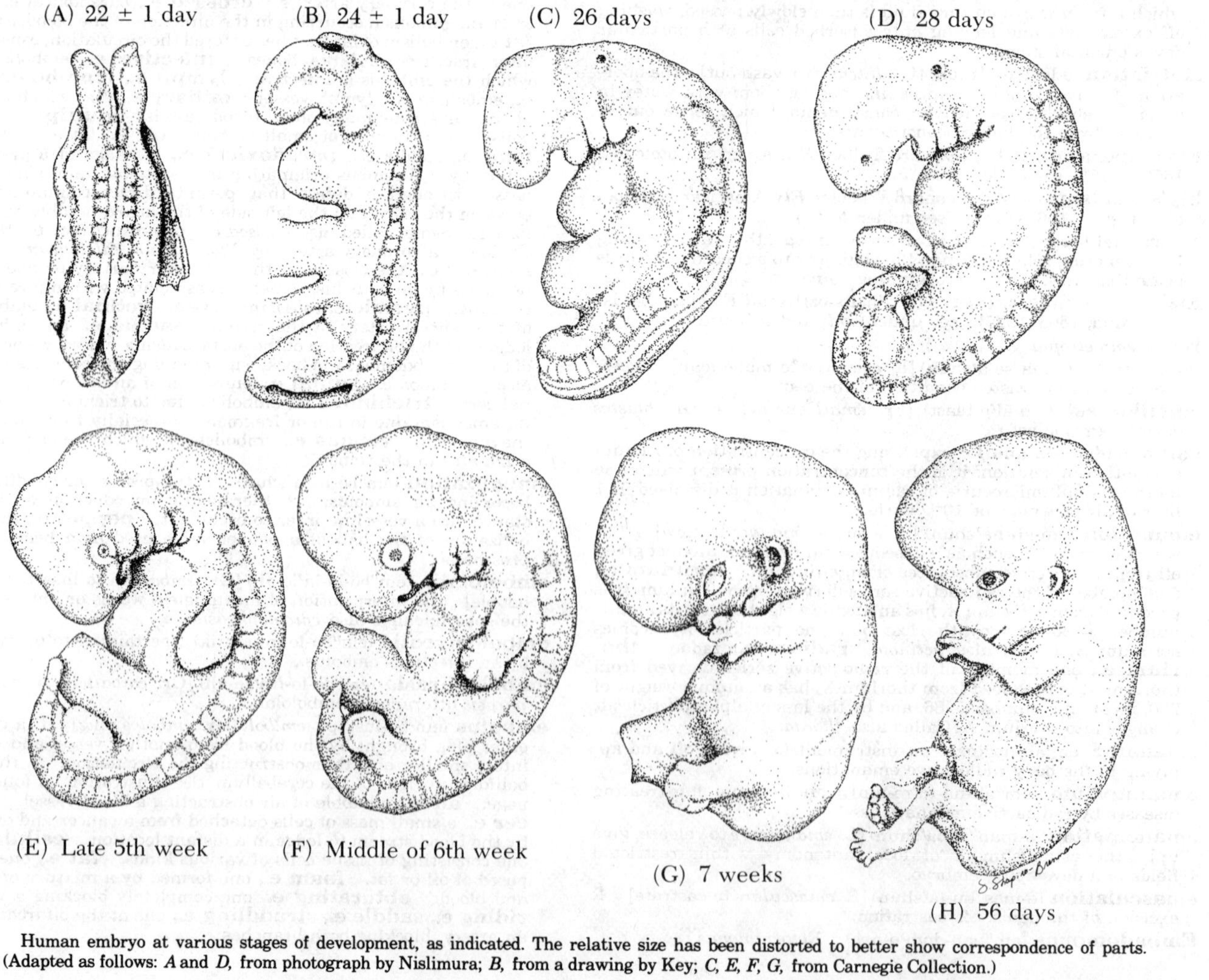

(A) 22 ± 1 day   (B) 24 ± 1 day   (C) 26 days   (D) 28 days

(E) Late 5th week   (F) Middle of 6th week

(G) 7 weeks

(H) 56 days

Human embryo at various stages of development, as indicated. The relative size has been distorted to better show correspondence of parts. (Adapted as follows: *A* and *D,* from photograph by Nislimura; *B,* from a drawing by Key; *C, E, F, G,* from Carnegie Collection.)

embryogeny (em″bre-oj′ĕ-ne) [*embryo* + Gr. *gennan* to produce] the production or origin of the embryo.

embryograph (em′bre-o-graf) [*embryo* + Gr. *graphein* to write] a combination of a microscope and a camera lucida; used in drawing figures of the embryo.

embryography (em″bre-og′rah-fe) [*embryo* + Gr. *graphein* to write] 1. a treatise or description of the embryo. 2. the drawing of an embryo by means of the embryograph.

embryoid (em′bre-oid) [*embryo* + Gr. *eidos* form] resembling an embryo.

embryoism (em′bre-o-izm) the condition of being an embryo.

embryologist (em″bre-ol′o-jist) an expert in embryology.

embryology (em″bre-ol′o-je) [*embryo* + *-logy*] the science of the development of the individual during the embryonic stage and, by extension, in several or even all preceding and subsequent stages of the life cycle. **causal e.**, experimental e. **comparative e.**, embryology applied with a comparative view to various species studied with reference to their taxonomy and the principle that ontogeny recapitulates phylogeny. **descriptive e.**, the study of embryos and fetuses and their components with reference to anatomical and chronological sequence so as to define stages and report the course of development. **experimental e.**, analysis of the factors and relations in development, obtained by subjecting embryos to experimental procedures; called also *causal embryology.*

embryoma (em″bre-o′mah) 1. a general term applied to neoplasms thought to be derived from embryonic cells or tissues, including dermoid cysts, teratomas, embryonal carcinomas and sarcomas, nephroblastomas, hepatoblastomas, etc. 2. a former term for neoplasms once thought to be derived from cells of a blighted ovum. **e. of kidney,** Wilms' tumor.

embryomorphous (em″bre-o-mor′fus) [*embryo* + Gr. *morphē* form] having a form suggestive of an embryo; said of certain abnormal tissue elements supposed to be relics of a conceptus.

embryonal (em′bre-o-nal) pertaining to the embryo.

embryonate (em′bre-o-nāt) 1. pertaining to or resembling an embryo. 2. containing an embryo. 3. impregnated; fecundated.

embryonic (em″bre-on′ik) of or pertaining to the embryo.

embryoniform (em″bre-on′ĭ-form) resembling an embryo.

embryonism (em′bre-o-nizm) embryoism.

embryonization (em″bre-o-ni-za′shun) reversion to the embryonic form on the part of a tissue or cell.

embryonoid (em′bre-o-noid″) resembling an embryo.

embryony (em′bre-o-ne) the production of an embryo.

embryopathia (em″bre-o-path′e-ah) embryopathy. **e. rubeola′ris,** developmental anomalies observed in infants of mothers who had rubeola during pregnancy.

embryopathology (em″bre-o-pah-thol′o-je) the study of abnormal embryos or of defective development.

embryopathy (em″bre-op′ah-the) [*embryo-* + Gr. *pathos* disease] a morbid condition of the embryo or a disorder resulting from abnormal embryonic development. **rubella e.,** congenital deformities in an infant due to rubella in the mother during early pregnancy.

embryophore (em′bre-o-fōr) the inner egg shell surrounding the embryo, as seen in the eggs of *Taenia* found in the feces.

embryoplastic (em″bre-o-plas′tik) [*embryo* + Gr. *plassein* to shape.] pertaining to or concerned in the formation of an embryo.

embryoscope (em″bre-o-skōp) [*embryo* + Gr. *skopein* to examine] an instrument for observing the embryo.

embryotocia (em″bre-o-to′se-ah) [*embryo* + Gr. *tokos* birth.] abortion.

embryotome (em′bre-o-tōm) a cutting instrument used in embryotomy.

embryotomy (em″bre-ot′o-me) [*embryo* + Gr. *tomē* a cutting] 1. the dismemberment of a fetus in the uterus or vagina to facilitate delivery. 2. the dissection of embryos and fetuses.

embryotoxon (em″bre-o-tok′son) [*embryo* + Gr. *toxon* a bow, or anything arched] a ringlike opacity of the margin of the cornea. **anterior e.,** embryotoxon. **posterior e.,** a developmental anomaly in which there is a ringlike opacity at Schwalbe's ring, with thickening and anterior displacement of the latter; it is seen in Axenfeld's syndrome and Rieger's syndrome.

embryotroph (em′bre-o-trōf″) [*embryo* + Gr. *trophē* nourishment] the total nutriment (histotroph and hemotroph) made available to the embryo.

embryotrophy (em″bre-ot′ro-fe) [*embryo* + Gr. *trophē* nourishment] the nutrition of the embryo.

embryulcia (em″bre-ul′se-ah) [Gr. *embryoulkia*] the instrumental removal of the fetus from the uterus.

embryulcus (em″bre-ul′kus) [Gr. *embryoulkos*] a blunt hook for use in embryulcia.

EMC encephalomyocarditis (virus).

emedullate (e-med′u-lāt) [L. *e* out + *medulla* marrow] to remove bone marrow.

emeiocytosis (e″me-o-si-to′sis) emiocytosis.

emergency (e-mer′jen-se) [L. *emergere* to raise up] an unlooked for or sudden occasion; an accident; an urgent or pressing need.

emergent (e-mer′jent) 1. pertaining to an emergency. 2. coming into being through consecutive stages of development, as in emergent evolution.

emery (em′er-e) an abrasive substance consisting of corundum and various impurities, such as iron oxide.

emesia (ĕ-me′ze-ah) emesis.

emesis (em′ĕ-sis) [Gr. *emein* to vomit] vomiting; an act of vomiting. Also used as a word termination, as in *hematemesis.* **e. gravida′rum,** the vomiting of pregnancy.

ematatrophia (em″ĕ-tah-tro′fe-ah) [Gr. *emetos* vomiting + *atrophia* atrophy] atrophy or wasting due to persistent vomiting.

emetic (ĕ-met′ik) [Gr. *emetikos*; L. *emeticus*] 1. bringing on or causing the act of vomiting. 2. an agent that causes vomiting. **central e.,** one carried by the blood stream to the vomiting center, upon which it acts; called also *indirect e.* and *systemic e.* **direct e.,** one that acts directly on the stomach; called also *mechanical e.* **indirect e.,** central e. **mechanical e.,** direct e. **systemic e.,** central e. **tartar e.,** antimony potassium tartrate.

emeticology (ĕ-met″ĭ-kol′o-je) the sum of knowledge regarding emetics.

emetine (em′ĕ-tin) chemical name: 6′,7′,10-11-tetramethoxy-emetan; an alkaloid, $C_{29}H_{40}N_2O_4$, obtained from ipecac or prepared by methylation of cephaeline. **e. and bismuth iodide,** a complex iodide of emetine and bismuth, occurring as a reddish-orange powder; used as an antiamebic in amebic dysentery, administered orally. **e. hydrochloride** [USP], the dihydrochloride salt of emetine, $C_{29}H_{40}N_2O_4 \cdot HCl$, occurring as a white or very slightly yellowish, crystalline powder; used as an antiamebic, administered subcutaneously or intramuscularly.

emetocathartic (em″ĕ-to-kah-thar′tik) 1. both emetic and cathartic. 2. an agent that is both emetic and cathartic.

emetology (em″ĕ-tol′o-je) emeticology.

E.M.F. electromotive force; erythrocyte maturation factor.

EMG *electromyogram.*

emigration (em″ĭ-gra′shun) [L. *e* out + *migrare* to wander] the escape of leukocytes through the walls of small blood vessels; diapedesis.

emilium tosylate (ĕ-mil′e-um) chemical name: N-ethyl-3-methoxy-N,N-dimethylbenzenemethanaminium salt with 4-methylbenzenesulfonic acid (1:1); a cardiac depressant with antiarrhythmic action, $C_{19}H_{27}NO_4S$.

eminence (em′ĭ-nens) a prominence or projection, especially one upon the surface of a bone; called also *eminentia* [NA]. **antithenar e.,** hypothenar. **arcuate e.,** eminentia arcuata. **articular e. of temporal bone,** tuberculum articulare ossis temporalis. **bicipital e.,** tuberositas radii. **canine e.,** a prominent bony ridge overlying the root of either canine tooth on the labial surface of both the maxilla and the mandible. **capitate e.,** capitulum humeri. **e. of cartilage of Santorini,** tuberculum corniculatum. **caudate e. of liver,** processus caudatus hepatis. **coccygeal e.,** cornu sacrale. **cochlear e. of sacral bone,** promontorium ossis sacri. **collateral e. of lateral ventricle,** eminentia collateralis ventriculi lateralis. **e. of concha,** eminentia conchae. **cruciate e., cruciform e. of occipital bone,** eminentia cruciformis. **cuneiform e. of head of rib,** crista capitis costae. **deltoid e.,** tuberositas deltoidea humeri. **Doyère's e.,** the papilla marking the entrance of a nerve filament into a muscle fiber; called also *Doyère's hillock.* **facial e. of eminentia teres,** colliculus facialis. **frontal e.,** tuber frontale. **genital e.,** genital tubercle. **gluteal e. of femur,** tuberositas glutea femoris. **hypobranchial e.,** copula linguae. **hypothenar e.,** hypothenar. **e. of humerus,** capitulum humeri. **iliopectineal e., iliopubic e.,** eminentia iliopubica. **intercondylar e., intercondyloid e., intermediate e.,** eminentia intercondylaris. **jugular e.,** tuberculum jugulare ossis occipitalis. **mamillary e.,** corpus mamillare. **medial e. of rhomboid fossa,** eminentia medialis fossae rhomboideae. **median e. (of hypothalamus),** a raised area on the infundibulum at the floor of third ventricle of the brain. Continuous below with the infundibular stem or stalk, it contains the primary capillary network of the hypophyseal portal system. **nasal e.,** the prominence above the root of the nose. **oblique e. of cuboid bone,** tuberositas ossis cuboidei. **occipital e.,** a ridge a lateral ventricle of the embryonic brain, corresponding to the occipital fissure in the adult. **olivary e. of sphenoid bone,** tuberculum sellae turcicae. **parietal e.,** tuber parietale. **postchiasmatic e.,** an inconstant protuberance on the floor of the third ventricle posterior to the optic chiasm; called also *postfundibular e.* **postfundibular e.,** postchiasmatic e. **pyramidal e.,** eminentia pyramidalis. **radial e. of wrist,** eminentia carpi radialis. **e. of scapha,** eminentia scaphae. **e. of superior semicircular canal,** eminentia arcuata. **terete e.,** eminentia medialis fossae rhomboideae. **thenar e.,** thenar. **thyroid e.,** prominentia laryngea. **triangular**

e., e. of triangular fossa of auricle, eminentia fossa triangularis auriculae. **e. of triquetral fossa,** eminentia fossae triangularis auriculae. **trochlear e.,** trochlea humeri. **ulnar e. of wrist,** eminentia carpi ulnaris. **vagal e.,** trigonum nervi vagi.

eminentia (em″ĭ-nen′she-ah), pl. *eminen′tiae* [L.] [NA] an eminence: a general term for a prominence or projection, especially one on the surface of a bone. **e. abducen′tis** (*obs.*), colliculus facialis. **e. arcua′ta** [NA], arcuate eminence: an arched prominence on the internal surface of the petrous part of the temporal bone in the floor of the middle cranial fossa, marking the position of the superior semicircular canal. It is particularly prominent in young skulls. Called also *eminence of superior semicircular canal.* **e. articula′ris os′sis tempora′lis,** tuberculum articulare ossis temporalis. **e. capita′ta,** capitulum humeri. **e. car′pi radia′lis,** an eminence on the palmar surface of the radial side of the wrist, formed by the tubercles on the scaphoid and trapezium bones; called also *radial eminence of wrist.* **e. car′pi ulna′ris,** an eminence on the palmar surface of the ulnar side of the wrist, formed by the pisiform bone and the hook of the hamate bone; called also *ulnar eminence of wrist.* **e. ciner′ea cuneifor′mis,** trigonum nervi vagi. **e. collatera′lis ventric′uli latera′lis** [NA], collateral eminence of lateral ventricle: an elevation in the floor of the inferior horn of the lateral ventricle, produced by the collateral sulcus. **e. con′chae** [NA], eminence of concha: the projection on the medial surface of the auricle that corresponds to the concha on the lateral surface. **e. crucia′ta,** e. cruciformis. **e. crucifor′mis** [NA], cruciform eminence of occipital bone: the cross-shaped bony prominence on the internal surface of the squama of the occipital bone, at the intersection of the ridges associated with the sulci of the superior sagittal sinus and the transverse sinuses. Called also *e. cruciata, internal occipital crest,* and *cruciate line.* **e. facia′lis,** colliculus facialis. **e. fallo′pii,** a ridge on the inner wall of the tympanum, showing the position of the facial nerve. **e. fos′sae triangula′ris auric′ulae** [NA], eminence of triangular fossa of auricle: the protuberance on the medial surface of the auricle of the ear that corresponds to the triangular fossa on the lateral surface. Called also *agger perpendicularis, e. triangularis, eminence of triquetral fossa,* and *triangular eminence.* **e. grac′ilis,** fasciculus gracilis medullae oblongatae. **e. hypoglos′si,** trigonum nervi hypoglossi. **e. iliopectin′ea,** e. iliopubica. **e. iliopu′bica** [NA], iliopubic eminence: a diffuse enlargement just anterior to the acetabulum, marking the junction of the ilium with the superior ramus of the pubis; called also *e. iliopectinea, iliopectinal eminence, iliopubic tuber* or *tubercle,* and *iliopectinal tubercle* or *crest of pubis.* **e. intercondyla′ris** [NA], **e. intercondyloi′dea, e. interme′dia,** intercondylar eminence: an eminence on the proximal extremity of the tibia, surmounted on either side by a prominent tubercle, on to the sides of which the articular facets are prolonged; called also *intermediate eminence* and *tuberculum intercondyloideum.* **e. jugula′ris,** tuberculum jugulare ossis occipitalis. **e. latera′lis cartilag′inis cricoi′deae,** facies articularis thyroidea. **e. media′lis fos′sae rhomboi′deae** [NA], medial eminence of rhomboid fossa: an eminence in the medial part of the floor of the fourth ventricle, bounded laterally by the sulcus limitans and produced by the facial colliculus and the trigone of the hypoglossal nerve. Called also *e. teres* and *terete eminence.* **e. papilla′ris,** e. pyramidalis. **e. pyramida′lis** [NA], pyramidal eminence: the hollow elevation in the posterior wall of the middle ear, which contains the stapedius muscle; called also *e. papillaris.* **e. sca′phae** [NA], eminence of scapha: the prominence on the medial side of the auricle of the external ear that corresponds to the scapha on the lateral side. **e. styloi′dea,** prominentia styloidea. **e. sym′physis,** the prominent lower border of the middle of the chin. **e. te′res,** e. medialis fossae rhomboideae. **e. triangula′ris,** e. fossae triangularis auriculae. **e. trigem′ina, e. trigem′ini,** tuberculum eminentia. **e. va′gi,** trigonum nervi vagi.

emiocytosis (e″me-o-si-to′sis) the ejection of material from a cell, as the process in which beta granules of the pancreas, which store insulin, are ejected into the extracellular fluid when appropriate stimuli for insulin secretion are applied.

emissaria (em″ĭ-sa′re-ah) [L.] plural of *emissarium.*

emissarium (em″ĭ-sa′re-um), pl. *emissa′ria* [L.] an emissary vein; see *venae emissariae.* **e. condyloi′deum,** vena emissaria condyloidea. **e. mastoi′deum,** vena emissaria mastoidea. **e. occipita′le,** vena emissaria occipitalis. **e. parieta′le,** vena emissaria parietalis.

emissary (em′ĭ-sa″re) [L. *emissarium* drain] affording an outlet, referring especially to the venous outlets from the dural sinuses through the skull.

emission (e-mish′un) [L. *emissio,* a sending out] a discharge; specifically an involuntary discharge of semen. **nocturnal e.,** reflex emission of the semen during sleep. **thermionic e.,** the emission of electrons and ions by incandescent bodies.

emissivity (e″mis-siv′ĭ-te) the ratio of emissive power (of radiant energy) of a surface to that of a black surface having the same temperature.

emmenagogic (ĕ-men″ah-goj′ik) inducing menstruation.

emmenagogue (ĕ-men′ah-gog) [Gr. *emmēna* menses + *agōgos* leading] an agent or measure that induces menstruation. **direct e.,** an agent that induces menstruation by acting directly upon the reproductive organs. **indirect e.,** an agent or measure that acts to induce menstruation by relieving another condition of which amenorrhea is a secondary result.

emmenia (ĕ-me′ne-ah) [Gr. *emmēna*] the menses.

emmenic (ĕ-men′ik) pertaining to the menses; menstrual.

emmeniopathy (ĕ-me″ne-op′ah-the) [Gr. *emmēnios* menses + *pathos* disease] any disorder of menstruation.

emmenology (em″ĕ-nol′o-je) [Gr. *emmēna* menses + *-logy*] the sum of knowledge regarding menstruation and its disorders.

Emmert-Gellhorn pessary (em′ert-gel′horn) [Frederick Victor *Emmert,* St. Louis surgeon, born 1897; George *Gellhorn,* St. Louis gynecologist, 1870–1936] see under *pessary.*

Emmet's operation (em′ets) [Thomas Addis *Emmet,* gynecologist in New York, 1818–1919] see under *operation.*

emmetrope (em′ĕ-trōp) an individual who has no refractive error of vision (emmetropid).

emmetropia (em-ĕ-tro′pe-ah) [Gr. *emmetros* in proper measure + *ōpē* sight + *-ia*] a state of proper correlation between the refractive system of the eye and the axial length of the eyeball, rays of light entering the eye parallel to the optic axis being brought to a focus exactly on the retina.

emmetropic (em″ĕ-trop′ik) pertaining to or characterized by emmetropia.

Emmonsia (ĕ-mon′se-ah) a genus of imperfect, saprophytic, soil fungi of the order Moniliales, family Moniliaceae. Two species, *E. cres′cens* and *E. par′va,* cause adiospiromycosis in rodents and man. Called also *Haplosporangium.*

emodin (em′o-din) [from *Rheum emodi,* a Himalayan rhubarb] a purgative compound, trihydroxymethyl anthraquinone, from rhubarb, aloes, senna, and cascara sagrada.

emollient (e-mol′e-ent) [L. *emolliens* softening, from *e* out + *mollis* soft] 1. softening or soothing; called also *malactic.* 2. an agent which softens or soothes the skin, or soothes an irritated internal surface; called also *malagma.*

emotiometabolic (e-mo″she-o-met″ah-bol′ik) inducing metabolic activity as a result of emotion.

emotiomotor (e-mo″she-o-mo′tor) inducing some activity as a result of emotion.

emotiomuscular (e-mo″she-o-mus′ku-lar) pertaining to muscular activity due to emotion.

emotion (e-mo′tion) [L. *emovere* to disturb] a state of mental excitement characterized by alteration of feeling tone and by physiological behavioral changes.

emotional (e-mo′shun-al) pertaining to the emotions.

emotiovascular (e-mo″she-o-vas′ku-lar) producing a vascular change as a result of emotion.

emotive (e-mo′tiv) marked by emotion; exciting emotion.

emotivity (e″mo-tiv′ĭ-te) the capacity for emotion; the capacity for reacting to a stimulus.

Emp. abbreviation for L. *emplas′trum,* a plaster.

empacho (em-pah′cho) a Mexican term for chronic indigestion in children with diarrhea.

empasma (em-paz′mah) [Gr. *en* in + *passein* to sprinkle] a powder for external use.

empathic (em-path′ik) pertaining to or characterized by empathy.

empathize (em′pah-thīz) to experience or feel empathy; to enter into another person's feelings.

empathy (em′pah-the) [Gr. *en* into + *pathos* feeling] the recognition of and entering into the feelings of another person.

emperipolesis (em-per″ĭ-po-le′sis) [Gr. *en-* + *peripolēsis* a going about] lymphocytic penetration of and movement within another cell. Cf. *peripolesis.*

emphlysis (em′flĭ-sis) [Gr. *en* in + *phlysis* eruption] (*obs.*) an exanthematous disease in which the lesions become scabby.

emphraxis (em-frak′sis) [Gr.] a stoppage or obstruction.

emphysatherapy (em″fiz-ah-ther′ah-pe) [Gr. *emphysan* to inflate + *therapeia* treatment] the injection of gas into an organ or bodily cavity for therapeutic purposes.

emphysema (em″fĭ-se′mah, em″fĭ-ze′mah) [Gr. "an inflation"] a pathological accumulation of air in tissues or organs; applied especially to such a condition of the lungs (see *pulmonary e.*). **alveolar e.,** overdistention of the alveolar spaces in the lungs. **alveolar duct e.,** distention of the alveolar ducts as seen in elderly individuals, often producing little or no functional disturbance. **atrophic e.,** overdistention and stretching of lung tissues due to atrophic changes, especially loss of elastic tissue. **bullous e.,** single or multiple large cystic alveolar dilatations of lung tissue; see also *paraseptal e.* **centriacinar e., centrilobular e.,** focal dilatations of air spaces distributed throughout the lung in the midst of grossly normal lung tissue; the dilatations affect respiratory bronchioles rather than alveoli. **chronic hypertrophic e.,** panacinar e. **compensating e.,** compensatory e., overdistention of lung tissue which fills a void produced by contraction, atelectasis, surgical resection, fibrosis, or otherwise reduced volume of another part of the lung. **cutaneous e.,** subcutaneous e. **cystic e.,** dilatations of lung tissue characterized by multiple alveolar cysts. **diffuse e.,** panacinar e. **ectatic e.,** vesicular e. **false e.,** deformity of the thoracic cage which simulates the form associated with pulmonary emphysema (increased anterior-posterior diameter, elevated rib angle, etc.); the lungs may or may not be normal. Called also *skeletal e.* **focal-dust e.,** a form of pulmonary emphysema associated with inhalation of environmental dusts, producing dilatation of the terminal and respiratory bronchioles. **gangrenous e.,** a malignant emphysema of microbic origin. **generalized e.,** pulmonary emphysema affecting all portions of both lungs in a similar manner. **glass blower's e.,** emphysema of the lungs attributed to overstrain in glass blowers. **hypertrophic e.,** a discarded term for chronic obstructive pulmonary edema (atrophy rather than hypertrophy is involved). **hypoplastic e.,** pulmonary emphysema due to a developmental abnormality resulting in reduced number of alveoli, which are abnormally large; it may affect a pulmonary segment, lobe, or an entire lung. **idiopathic unilobar e.,** a syndrome characterized by emphysematous expansion of one lobe of the lung, with the production of dyspnea and cyanosis. **interlobular e.,** accumulation of air in interlobar spaces, between the lobes of lungs. **interstitial e.,** presence of air in the peribronchial and interstitial tissues of the lungs; called also *Hamman's disease.* **intestinal e.,** a condition marked by accumulation of gas under the serous tunic of the intestine. **lobar e.,** emphysema involving fewer than all the lobes of the affected lung. **lobar e., infantile,** a condition characterized by overinflation, commonly affecting one of the upper lobes and causing respiratory distress in early life; called also *congenital lobar e.* **e. of lungs,** pulmonary e. **mediastinal e.,** pneumomediastinum. **obstructive e.,** overinflation of the lungs associated with partial bronchial obstruction which interferes with exhalation. **obstructive e., localized,** overinflation of a lobe or segment of lung, often due to partial bronchial obstruction; called also *obstructive pulmonary overinflation.* **panacinar e., panlobular e.,** generalized obstructive emphysema affecting all lung segments, with atrophy and dilatation of the alveoli and destruction of the vascular bed. **paracicatricial e.,** alveolar distention occurring in the vicinity of pulmonary scars. **paraseptal e.,** alveolar distention localized to the lung periphery, including the interlobar septa; a form of bullous emphysema. **pulmonary e.,** a condition of the lung characterized by increase beyond normal in the size of air spaces distal to the terminal bronchioles, either from dilatation of the alveoli (*panacinar e.*), or from destruction (*interstitial e.*) of their walls. **pulmonary e. of cattle, acute,** fog fever. **senile e.,** pulmonary emphysema due to dilatation of the alveoli occurring with age. **skeletal e.,** false e. **small-lunged e.,** atrophic e. **subcutaneous e.,** the presence of air or gas in the subcutaneous tissues of the body. **surgical e.,** subcutaneous emphysema following surgical operation. **traumatic e.,** subcutaneous, interstitial, or mediastinal emphysema due to trauma. **unilateral e.,** emphysema affecting only one lung, frequently due to congenital defects in circulation; called also *hyperlucent lung.* **vesicular e.,** panlobular e.

emphysematous (em″fi-sem′ah-tus) of the nature of or affected with emphysema.

Empiric (em-pir′ik) [Gr. *empeirikos* experienced] 1. the second of the post-hippocratic schools of medicine, which arose in the second century, B.C., under the leadership of Philinos of Cos and Serapion of Alexandria. As opposed to the Dogmatists, the Empirics declared that the search for the ultimate causes of phenomena was vain, but they were active in endeavoring to discover the immediate causes. They paid particular attention to the totality of symptoms. In their search for a line of treatment to benefit a particular set of symptoms they employed the "tripod of the Empirics": (1) their own chance observations—their own experience; (2) learning obtained from contemporaries and predecessors—the experience of others; and (3), in cases of new diseases, the formation of conclusions from other diseases which they resembled—analogy. The Empirics paid great attention to clinical observation, and were guided in their methods of treatment almost entirely by experience. 2. a believer in or practitioner of the Empiric school of medicine.

empiric (em-pir′ik) 1. empirical. 2. a practitioner whose skill is based on experience.

empirical (em-pir′e-kal) based on experience.

empiricism (em-pir′ĭ-sizm) [Gr. *empeirikos,* experienced] 1. the method of the Empiric school of medicine; opposed to rational medicine. 2. reliance on mere experience; empirical practice. 3. quackery.

Empirin (em′pĭ-rin) trademark for tablets containing acetylsalicylic acid, phenacetin, and caffeine.

emplastic (em-plas′tik) [Gr. *emplastikos* stopping up] 1. adhesive or glutinous. 2. a constipating medicine.

emplastrum (em-plas′trum) [L.; Gr. *emplastron*] resin plaster; adhesive plaster. See *plaster.*

emporiatrics (em-po″re-at′riks) [Gr. *emporos* one who goes on shipboard as a passenger + *iatrikē* medicine] that branch of medicine which treats of the health problems of travelers about the world.

emprosthotonos (em″pros-thot′o-nos) [Gr. *emprosthen* forward + *tonos* tension] a form of tetanic spasm in which the head and feet are brought forward and the body is rendered tense; called also *episthotonos.*

emprosthotonus (em″pros-thot′o-nus) emprosthotonos.

emptysis (emp′tĭ-sis) [Gr.] expectoration, especially of blood.

Empusa (em-pu′sah) former name for *Entomophora.*

empyema (em″pi-e′mah) [Gr. *empyema*] accumulation of pus in a cavity of the body; when used without a descriptive qualifier, it refers to thoracic empyema (q.v.). **e. artic′uli,** acute suppurative synovitis. **e. benig′num,** thoracic empyema in which fever is absent and there is a fair condition of general health. **e. of the chest,** thoracic e. **e. of gallbladder,** cholecystitis in which the contents of the acutely inflamed gallbladder are turbid, or appear to be frankly purulent. **interlobar e.,** empyema situated between two lobes of the lung. **latent e.,** empyema unaccompanied by any symptoms. **loculated e.,** pus in a group of loculi. **mastoid e.,** suppurative inflammation of the mucous lining of the cavities of the mastoid process. **metapneumonic e.,** empyema developing some time after the subsidence of the pneumonia; cf. *synpneumonic e.* **e. necessita′tis,** empyema in which the pus can make a spontaneous escape. **e. of pericardium,** purulent pericarditis. **pneumococcal e.,** that which is due to the pneumococcus, *Streptococcus pneumoniae.* **pulsating e.,** thoracic empyema in which the movements of the heart produce a visible vibration of the chest wall. **putrid e.,** empyema in which the pus has become more or less decomposed. **streptococcal e.,** a form due to *Streptococcus pyogenes.* **synpneumonic e.,** empyema which arises during the course of pulmonary inflammation. Cf. *metapneumonic e.* **thoracic e.,** suppurative inflammation of the pleural space; called also *pyothorax.* **tuberculous e.,** a form of empyema due to *Mycobacterium tuberculosis.*

empyemic (em″pi-e′mik) pertaining to or of the nature of empyema.

empyesis (em″pi-e′sis) [Gr. *empyēsis* suppuration] 1. an accumulation of pus, as one behind the iris, or in the anterior chamber of the eye. 2. any disease characterized by phlegmonous vesicles becoming filled with purulent fluid.

empyocele (em′pi-o-sēl) [Gr. *empyein* to suppurate + *kēlē* tumor] a collection of pus at the umbilicus.

empyreuma (em″pi-roo′mah) [Gr. *empyreuma* a live coal] the peculiar odor of animal or vegetable matter when charred in a closed vessel.

empyreumatic (em″pi-roo-mat′ik) pertaining to empyreuma; pertaining to or produced by destructive distillation of organic matter.

E.M.S. Emergency Medical Service (British).

emul. abbreviation for L. *emul′sum* emulsion.

emulgent (e-mul′jent) [L. *emulgere* to milk or drain out] 1. effecting a straining or purifying process. 2. a renal artery or vein. 3. a medicine that stimulates the flow of bile or urine.

emulsifier (e-mul″si-fi′er) an agent used to produce an emulsion.

emulsify (e-mul′sĭ-fi) to convert or to be converted into an emulsion.

emulsin (e-mul′sin) a hydrolyzing enzyme which splits amygdalin and other beta glycosides; called also *beta glucosidase.*

emulsion (e-mul′shun) [L. *emulsio, emulsum*] a preparation of one liquid distributed in small globules throughout the body of a second liquid. The dispersed liquid is the discontinuous phase, and the dispersion medium is the continuous phase. When oil is the dispersed liquid and an aqueous solution is the continuous phase, it is known as an oil-in-water emulsion, whereas when water or aqueous solution is the dispersed phase and oil or oleaginous substance is the continuous phase, it is known as a water-in-oil emulsion. Pharamaceutical emulsions for which official standards have been promulgated include cod liver oil emulsion, cod liver oil emulsion with malt, liquid petrolatum emulsion, and phenolphthalein in liquid petrolatum emulsion. **bacillary e.,** New tuberculin in which the pulverized tubercle bacilli are permitted to settle as much as they will, but are not removed by centrifugation; the supernatant is then mixed with equal parts of glycerin. **Butschli e.,** a preparation of potassium carbonate and rancid olive oil, used in microscopical work. **chylomicron e.,** the finely dispersed emulsion of fat which is found in the blood. **hexachlorophene cleansing e.** [USP], an emulsion containing between 90 and 110 per cent of the labeled amount of hexachlorophene in a suitable aqueous vehicle; used as a topical anti-infective and detergent. **kerosene e.,** an emulsion of kerosene in soap solution, used as an insecticide. **liquid petrolatum e.,** mineral oil e. **mineral oil e.** [USP], an emulsion of mineral oil, acacia, syrup, vanillin, and alcohol in purified water, used as a cathartic; called also *liquid petrolatum e.* **photographic e.,** a light- and radiation-sensitive gelatinous coating incorporating silver halide which is applied to film. **Pusey's e.,** a preparation of powdered tragacanth, glycerin, phenol, oil of bergamot, and olive oil in water, used in infantile eczema.

emulsive (e-mul′siv) 1. capable of emulsifying a substance. 2. susceptible of being emulsified. 3. affording an oil on pressure.

emulsoid (e-mul′soid) an emulsion colloid.

emulsum (e-mul′sum), pl. *emul′sa* [L.] an emulsion.

emunctory (e-munk′to-re) [L. *emungere* to cleanse] 1. excretory or depurant. 2. any excretory organ or duct.

E-Mycin (e-mi′sin) trademark for a preparation of erythromycin.

emylcamate (e-mil′kah-māt) chemical name: 3-methyl-3-pentanol carbamate. A white crystalline powder, $C_7H_{15}NO_2$, freely soluble in alcohol, used as a tranquilizer.

enamel (en-am′el) the white, compact, and very hard substance that covers and protects the dentin of the crown of a tooth; called also *enamelum* [NA] and *substantia adamantina dentis*. **brown e., hereditary,** amelogenesis imperfecta. **curled e.,** enamel in which the columns are bent. **dwarfed e.,** enamel that is less thick than normal; called also *nanoid e.* **gnarled e.,** enamel in which the rods run in bundles, each bundle having a different direction and intertwining with its neighbors. Cf. *straight e.* **hypoplastic e.,** incomplete or defective development of the enamel of the teeth. **mottled e.,** dental fluorosis. **nanoid e.,** dwarfed e. **straight e.,** enamel in which the rods pursue an almost straight course. Cf. *gnarled e.*

enameloblast (en-am′el-o-blast) ameloblast.

enameloblastoma (en-am″el-o-blas-to′mah) ameloblastoma.

enameloma (en-am″el-o′mah) [*enamel* + *-oma*] a tiny globule of enamel, firmly adherent to a tooth, most frequently found near or in the bifurcation or trifurcation of the roots, or on the root surface near the cemento-enamel junction.

enamelum (e-nam′el-um) [NA] enamel: the white, compact, and very hard substance that covers and protects the dentin of the crown of a tooth; called also *substantia adamantina dentis* and *adamantine layer.*

enanthate (en-an-thāt) USAN contraction for heptanoate.

-enanthem (en-an′them) enanthema.

enanthema (en″an-the′ma), pl. *enanthe′mas, enanthem′ata* [Gr. *en* in + *anthema* a blossoming] an eruption upon a mucous surface.

enanthematous (en″an-them′ah-tus) pertaining to or of the nature of an enanthema.

enanthrope (en-an′thrōp) [Gr. *en* in + *anthrōpos* man] any source of disease situated within the human body.

enantiobiosis (en-an″te-o-bi-o′sis) [Gr. *enantios* opposite + *bios* life] the condition in which organisms living together antagonize one another's development. Cf. *symbiosis,* def. 1.

enantiomer (en-an′te-o-mer) one of a pair of compounds showing mirror-image isomerism, an enantiomorph.

enantiomorph (en-an′te-o-morf″) [Gr. *enantios* opposite + *morphē* form] a compound exhibiting, or capable of exhibiting, enantiomorphism; an enantiomorphic isomer.

enantiomorphic (en-an″te-o-mor′fik) pertaining to or exhibiting enantiomorphism.

enantiomorphism (en-an″te-o-mor′fizm) [Gr. *enantios* opposite + *morphē* form] a special type of optical isomerism in which a nonsuperimposable, mirror-image relationship exists at all times between the respective molecules of the compounds. Enantiomorphic isomers always rotate the plane of polarized light to the same degree but in opposite directions; otherwise most of their chemical and physical properties are identical, the principal exceptions being biological reactions catalyzed by enzymes. The molecules are always asymmetric, very often as the result of possession of one or more asymmetric carbon atoms. Thus lactic acid, CH_3-CHOHCOOH, possessing one such carbon atom, exists in a *dextro* and a *levo* form. The molecules of some enantiomorphic compounds (e.g., certain biphenyl or spirane compounds) are asymmetric as a whole, but do not possess any asymmetric carbon atoms. Cf. *diastereoisomerism.*

enantiopathia (en-an″te-o-path′e-ah) [Gr. *enantios* opposite + *pathos* suffering] 1. any disease or morbid process antagonistic to or curative of another. 2. the curing of one disease by inducing another of an opposite kind.

enantiopathic (en-an″te-o-path′ik) inducing opposite feelings.

enantiopathy (en-an″te-op′ah-the) enantiopathia.

Enantiothamnus (en-an″te-o-tham′nus) a former genus of yeastlike imperfect fungi. *E. braulti* was once isolated in Algeria from pyogenic nodules with a central opening.

enarkyochrome (en-ar′ke-o-krōm) [Gr. *en* in + *arkys* network + *chrōma* color] an arkyochrome nerve cell containing a single network of chromatin substance.

enarthritis (en″ar-thri′tis) inflammation of an enarthrosis.

enarthrodial (en″ar-thro′de-al) of or pertaining to an enarthrosis.

enarthrosis (en″ar-thro′sis) [Gr. *en* in + *arthrosis* joint] a joint in which the globular head of one bone is received into a socket in another, as in the hip joint.

en bloc (aw blok′) [Fr.] in a lump; as a whole.

encanthis (en-kan′this) [Gr. *en* in + *kanthos* the angle of the eye] a small red excrescence on the semilunar fold of the conjunctiva and inner lacrimal caruncle.

encapsulated (en-kap′su-lāt-ed) [Gr. *en* in + L. *capsula* a little box] enclosed within a capsule.

encapsulation (en-kap′su-la′shun) 1. any act of inclosing in a capsule. 2. a physiologic process of inclosure in a sheath made up of a substance not normal to the part.

encapsuled (en-kap′sūld) encapsulated.

encarditis (en″kar-di′tis) endocarditis.

encatarrhaphy (en″kat-ar′ah-fe) enkatarrhaphy.

enceinte (aw-sawt′) [Fr.] pregnant; with child.

encelialgia (en″se-le-al′je-ah) [Gr. *en* in + *koilia* belly + *-algia* pain] pain in an abdominal viscus.

enceliitis (en-se″le-i′tis) [Gr. *en* in + *koilia* belly + *-itis*] inflammation of an intra-abdominal organ.

encelitis (en″se-li′tis) enceliitis.

encephalalgia (en-sef″ah-lal′je-ah) [*encephalo-* + *-algia*] pain within the head.

encephalasthenia (en-sef″al-as-the′ne-ah) [*encephalo-* + Gr. *astheneia* weakness] (*obs.*) mental fatigue; psychasthenia.

encephalatrophy (en-sef″ah-lat′ro-fe) [*encephalo-* + *atrophy*] atrophy of the brain.

encephalauxe (en″sef-ah-lawk′se) [*encephalo-* + Gr. *auxē* increase] hypertrophy of the brain.

encephalemia (en-sef″ah-le′me-ah) [*encephalo-* + Gr. *haima* blood + *-ia*] congestion of the brain.

encephalic (en″se-fal′ik) 1. pertaining to the encephalon. 2. within the skull.

encephalitic (en″sef-ah-lit′ik) pertaining to or affected with encephalitis.

encephalitides (en″sef-ah-lit′ĭ-dēz) [Gr.] plural of *encephalitis.*

encephalitis (en″sef-ah-li′tis), pl. *encephalit′ides* [*encephalo-* + *-itis*] inflammation of the brain. **e. A,** lethargic e. **acute disseminated e.,** postinfection e. **acute necrotizing e.,** morphological term for encephalitis characterized by a particularly destructive reaction in the brain. **Australian X e.,** see under *disease.* **e. B,** Japanese B e. **benign myalgic e.,** see under *encephalomyelitis.* **Binswanger's e.,** see under *dementia.* **bovine e.,** encephalitis of cows caused by microorganisms of the psittacosis-lymphogranuloma venereum group (*Chlamydia*). **buffalo e.,** a viral encephalitis of the Asiatic water buffalo. **e. C,** St. Louis e. **California e.,** an acute viral encephalitis caused by an arbovirus, primarily a disease of children. **Central European e.,** Russian spring-summer e. **chronic subcortical e.,** Binswanger's dementia. **cortical e., e. cortica′lis,** encephalitis affecting the cortex of the brain only. **Dawson's e.,** subacute sclerosing panencephalitis. **eastern equine e.,** see under *encephalomyelitis.* **Economo's e.,** lethargic e. **enzootic e. of horses,** Borna disease. **epidemic e., e. epidem′ica,** a viral encephalitis occurring epidemically in several types (see *influenzal e., Japanese B e., lethargic e., Russian spring-summer e.,* and *St. Louis e.*). **equine e.,** see *equine encephalomyelitis,* under *encephalomyelitis,* and *Borna disease,* under *disease.* **forest-spring e.,** Russian spring-summer e. **fox e.,** a viral disease of foxes, raccoons, and coyotes. **Hayem's e.,** e. hyperplastica. **hemorrhagic e.,** herpes encephalitis in which there is inflammation of the brain with hemorrhagic foci and perivascular exudate; called also *Strümpell-Leichtenstern type of encephalitis.* **hemorrhagic arsphenamine e.,** a rapidly progressive form which sometimes follows the administration of arsphenamine. **e. hemorrha′gica supe′rior,** Wernicke's encephalopathy. **herpes e., herpes simplex e., herpetic e.,** a disease caused by herpesvirus, resembling equine encephalomyelitis. See *hemorrhagic e.* **e. hyperplas′tica,** an acute nonsuppurating form of encephalitis; called also *Hayem's encephalitis.* **Ilhe′us e.,** a viral encephalitis transmitted by mosquitoes in Brazil. See also under *virus.* **infantile e.,** inflammation of the brain in children from infectious disease. **influenzal e.,** encephalitis occurring as a complication of influenza. **Japanese B e.,** a form of epidemic encephalitis occurring in Japan and other Pacific islands, China, Manchuria, U.S.S.R., and probably much of the Far East; it may occur as a symptomless, subclinical infection, or an acute meningoencephalomyelitis with cortical damage and cord lesions resembling those of poliomyelitis. Called also *e. B.* and *Russian autumnal e.* See also under *virus.* **lead e.,** encephalitis with marked cerebral edema, caused by lead poisoning. **Leichtenstern's e.,** hemorrhagic e. **lethargic e., e. lethar′gica,** a form of epidemic encephalitis, the original type described by von Economo, characterized by increasing languor, apathy, and drowsiness, passing into lethargy; observed in various parts of the world between 1915 and 1926. Called also *e. A, Economo's e.* or *disease,* and *Vienna e.* **Murray Valley e.,** a viral encephalitis that occurred epidemically in 1950 and 1951 in the Murray Valley, Victoria, Australia, believed to be a recrudescence of Australian X disease; a few cases occurred in 1956 and it has been reported in New Guinea. **e. neonato′rum,** encephalitis in the newborn. **e. periaxia′lis concen′trica,** Baló's disease. **e. periaxia′lis diffu′sa,** Schilder's disease. **postinfection e.,** an acute disease of the central nervous system seen in persons who are convalescing from infectious diseases, usually one of viral origin; called also *acute disseminated e., acute disseminated encephalomyelitis, acute demyelinating disease,* and *acute perivascular myelinoclasis.* **postvaccinal e.,** acute encephalitis sometimes occurring after vaccination; called also *vaccinal e.* **Powassan e.,** a form reported from Canada, caused by a tickborne virus and closely resembling Russian spring-summer encephalitis. **purulent e., pyogenic e.,** suppurative e. **Russian autumnal e.,** Japanese B e. **Russian endemic e., Russian forest-spring e.,** Russian spring-summer e. **Russian spring-summer e.,** a form of epidemic encephalitis which is acquired in forests from infected ticks (*Ixodes persulcatus*), but is also transmitted in other ways, as by ingestion of the flesh of infected mammals and birds, or milk of infected goats. It ranges in severity from mild to fatal cases, with degenerative changes in organs other than those of the nervous system. See also under *virus.* **Russian tick-borne e., Russian vernal e.,** Russian spring-summer e. **St. Louis e.,** a viral disease first observed in Illinois in 1932, closely similar to western equine encephalomyelitis clinically, occurring in late summer and early fall and transmitted usually by mosquitoes of the genus *Culex;* it ranges from an abortive type of infection to severe disease. Called also *e. C.* see also under *virus.* **Schilder's e.,** see under *disease.* **Semliki Forest e.,** a form due to a virus transmitted by mosquitoes in the Semliki Forest of western *Uganda.* See also under *virus.* **e. sid′erans,** a form of epidemic encephalitis terminating fatally in a few hours. **subacute inclusion body e.,** subacute sclerosing panencephalitis. **e. subcortica′lis chron′ica,** Binswanger's dementia. **summer e.,** Japanese B e. **suppurative e.,** encephalitis accompanied by suppuration and abscess formation; called also *purulent e.* and *pyogenic e.* **toxoplasmic e.,** encephalitis due to infection with *Toxoplasma.* **vaccinal e.,** postvaccinal e. **van Bogaert e.,** subacute sclerosing panencephalitis. **Venezuelan equine e.,** see under *encephalomyelitis.* **vernal e.,** Russian spring-summer e. **vernoestival e.,** Russian spring-summer e. **Vienna e.,** lethargic e. **von Economo's e.,** lethargic e. **western equine e.,** see under *encephalomyelitis.* **West Nile e.,** a mild, febrile, sporadic disease of viral origin, probably transmitted by the mosquito *Culex univittatus,* occurring chiefly in the summer; frequently, infection does not lead to encephalitis. It may be of sudden onset, and symptoms may include drowsiness, severe frontal headache, maculopapular rash, abdominal pain, loss of appetite, nausea, and generalized lymphadenopathy. It was first reported in Uganda, but is widespread in Africa and has been reported in Israel. See also under *virus.* **woodcutter's e.,** Russian spring-summer e.

encephalitogen (en-sef″ah-lit′o-jen) any agent that causes encephalitis.

encephalitogenic (en-sef″ah-lit-o-jen′ik) [*encephalitis* + Gr. *gennan* to produce] causing encephalitis.

Encephalitozoon (en″sĕ-fal″ĭ-to-zo′on) [*encephalitis* + Gr. *zōon* animal] *Nosema.* **E. cunic′uli,** *Nosema cuniculi.* **E. rabi′ei,** Negri bodies.

encephalization (en-sef″ah-li-za′shun) the developmental process by which the cerebral cortex has taken over the functions of the lower (spinal) centers.

encephalo- (en-sef′ah-lo) [Gr. *enkephalos* brain] a combining form denoting relationship to the brain.

encephalo-arteriography (en-sef″ah-lo-ar-te″re-og′rah-fe) a combination of encephalography and arteriography for examining the blood supply of the brain.

encephalocele (en-sef′ah-lo-sēl″) [*encephalo-* + Gr. *kēlē* hernia] hernia of the brain, manifested by protrusion of brain substance through a congenital or traumatic opening of the skull.

encephaloclastic (en-sef″ah-lo-klas′tik) [*encephalo-* + Gr. *klastōs* broken] exhibiting the residues of a destructive lesion in the brain; see under *porencephaly,* def. 2.

encephalocoele (en-sef″ah-lo-se′le) [*encephalo-* + Gr. *koilos* hollow] 1. the entire cavity of the cranium. 2. the ventricles and other spaces of the brain.

encephalocystocele (en-sef″ah-lo-sis′to-sēl) [*encephalo-* + Gr. *kystis* sac, bladder + *kēlē* hernia] hernia of the brain, the protrusion being distended by a collection of fluid communicating with the ventricle; called also *hydrencephalocele.*

Encephalocytozoon (en-sef″ah-lo-si″to-zo′on) [*encephalo-* + Gr. *kytos* hollow vessel + *zōon* animal] *Nosema.*

encephalodialysis (en-sef″ah-lo-di-al′ĭ-sis) [*encephalo-* + Gr. *dialysis* loosening] softening of the brain.

encephalodysplasia (en-sef″ah-lo-dis-pla′se-ah) any congenital anomaly of the brain.

encephalogram (en-sef′ah-lo-gram″) the film made by encephalography.

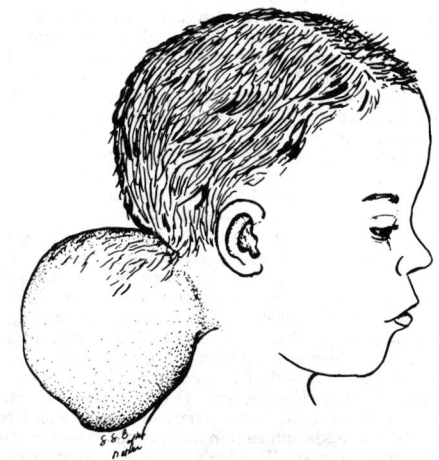

Encephalocele (after Netter).

encephalography (en-sef″ah-log′rah-fe) [*encephalo-* + Gr. *graphein* to write] roentgenography demonstrating the intracranial fluid-containing spaces after the withdrawal of cerebrospinal fluid and introduction of air or other gas; it includes pneumoencephalography and ventriculography.

encephaloid (en-sef′ah-loid) [*encephalo-* + Gr. *eidos* form] 1. resembling the brain or brain substance. 2. medullary carcinoma.

encephalolith (en-sef′ah-lo-lith″) [*encephalo-* + Gr. *lithos* stone] a brain calculus.

encephalology (en″sef-ah-lol′o-je) [*encephalo-* + *-logy*] the sum of knowledge regarding the brain, its functions, and its diseases.

encephaloma (en″sef-ah-lo′mah) 1. any swelling or tumor of the brain. 2. medullary carcinoma.

encephalomalacia (en-sef″ah-lo-mah-la′she-ah) [*encephalo-* + Gr. *malakia* softness] softening of the brain. **avian e.,** a disease of young chickens due to vitamin E deficiency, in which there is ataxia, incoordination, paralysis, and severe encephalomalacia in several areas of the brain, especially the cerebellum. It must be differentiated from avian encephalomyelitis. Called also *crazy chick disease.*

encephalomeningitis (en-sef″ah-lo-men″in-ji′tis) [*encephalo-* + *meningitis*] meningoencephalitis.

encephalomeningocele (en-sef″ah-lo-me-ning′go-sēl) [*encephalo-* + Gr. *mēninx* membrane + *kēlē* hernia] meningoencephalocele.

encephalomeningopathy (en-sef″ah-lo-men″in-gop′ah-the) meningoencephalopathy.

encephalomere (en-sef′ah-lo-mēr″) [*encephalo-* + Gr. *meros* part] any one of the succession of segments which make up the embryonic brain.

encephalometer (en-sef″ah-lom′e-ter) [*encephalo-* + Gr. *metron* measure] an instrument used in locating certain of the regions of the brain.

encephalomyelitis (en-sef″ah-lo-mi″ĕ-li′tis) inflammation involving both the brain and the spinal cord. **acute disseminated e.,** postinfection encephalitis. **avian e.,** a viral disease of chickens under six weeks old, marked by weakness of the legs followed by partial or complete paralysis of the legs, trembling of the head and neck, and degeneration of the neurons in the pons, medulla, and anterior horns of the spinal cord. Clinically, it resembles avian encephalomalacia and must be differentiated from that condition. Called also *crazy chick disease* and *epidemic tremor.* **benign myalgic e.,** a disease, usually occurring in epidemics, characterized by headache, unusual muscular pain, lymphadenopathy, low-grade fever, and fatigability; paresthesias are common, sensory loss less so. Called also *epidemic neuromyasthenia* and *Iceland* (or *Icelandic*) *disease.* **equine e.,** a viral disease of horses and mules, communicable to man, occurring as summer epizootics in the Western Hemisphere. Three forms are recognized: *eastern equine e., western equine e.,* and *Venezuelan equine e.* Called also *equine encephalitis.* See also under *virus.* **equine e., eastern,** a viral disease similar to western equine encephalomyelitis, but occurring in the United States in a region extending from New Hampshire to Texas and as far west as Wisconsin, and in Canada, Mexico, the Carribean, and parts of Central and South America. Abbreviated EEE. **equine e., Venezuelan,** a viral disease of horses and mules first observed in Colombia in 1935, the causative agent being isolated in Venezuela in 1938. It has since been reported in other South American countries and in Mexico, Texas, and Florida. The infection in man resembles influenza, with little or no indication of central nervous system involvement. Abbreviated VEE.

equine e., western, a viral disease of horses and mules, communicable to man, occurring chiefly as a meningoencephalitis, with little involvement of the medulla or spinal cord; observed west of the Mississippi River in the United States, but present also along the Gulf and Atlantic coasts. Abbreviated WEE. **experimental allergic e.,** acute encephalomyelitis marked by perivascular accumulation of lymphocytes and macrophages accompanied by demyelination and occurring about 10 days after repeated injections of brain or spinal cord tissue incorporated into Freund's complete adjuvant. It resembles postvaccination encephalomyelitis in man. T-cells rather than B-cell products appear to be responsible for this autoimmune disease process. **granulomatous e.,** a disease marked by granulomas and necrosis of the walls of the cerebral and spinal ventricles. **infectious porcine e.,** a highly fatal encephalomyelitis of swine, caused by a picornavirus, and characterized by a flaccid ascending paralysis, similar in character to the paralysis of human poliomyelitis. First reported in the Teschen district of Czechoslovakia, it occurs throughout Europe. Called also *porcine encephalomyelitis, porcine poliomyelitis, Talfan disease,* and *Teschen disease.* **Mengo e.,** a form of encephalomyelitis the virus of which was first isolated from animals in the Mengo region of Uganda. See also under *virus.* **mouse e., murine e.,** Theiler's disease. **porcine e.,** infectious porcine e. **postinfectious e., postvaccinal e.,** inflammation of the brain and spinal cord following vaccination or infection, as with vaccinia virus. **sporadic bovine e.,** Buss disease. **Theiler's mouse e.,** Theiler's disease. **toxoplasmic e.,** encephalomyelitis due to infection with *Toxoplasma.* **viral e., virus e.,** encephalomyelitis caused by a virus. See *equine e.*

encephalomyelocele (en-sef″ah-lo-mi-el′o-sēl) [*encephalo-* + Gr. *myelon* spinal cord + *kēlē* hernia] abnormality of the foramen magnum and absence of the laminae and spinal processes of the cervical vertebrae, with herniation of meninges, brain substance, and spinal cord.

encephalomyeloneuropathy (en-sef″ah-lo-mi″ĕ-lo-nu-rop′-ah-the) disease involving the brain, spinal cord, and peripheral nerves.

encephalomyelopathy (en-sef″ah-lo-mi″ĕ-lop′ah-the) [*encephalo-* + Gr. *myelos* marrow + *pathos* disease] any disease or diseased condition of the brain and spinal cord. **postinfection e.,** demyelination secondary to common viral diseases such as measles, varicella, rubella, mumps, and influenza. **postvaccinial e.,** demyelination complicating the reaction to vaccination against smallpox.

encephalomyeloradiculitis (en-sef″ah-lo-mi″ĕ-lo-rah-dik″u-li′tis) inflammation of the brain, spinal cord, and spinal nerve roots.

encephalomyeloradiculoneuritis (en-sef″ah-lo-mi″ĕ-lo-rah-dik″u-lo-nu-ri′tis) acute febrile polyneuritis.

encephalomyeloradiculopathy (en-sef″ah-lo-mi″ĕ-lo-rah-dik″u-lop′ah-the) disease involving the brain, spinal cord, and spinal nerve roots.

encephalomyocarditis (en-sef″ah-lo-mi″o-kar-di′tis) a viral disease characterized by degenerative and inflammatory changes in skeletal and cardiac muscle, and lesions of the central nervous system resembling those of poliomyelitis.

encephalon (en-sef′ah-lon) [Gr. *enkephalos*] [NA] the brain: that part of the central nervous system contained within the cranium, comprising the prosencephalon, mesencephalon, and rhombencephalon; it is derived (developed) from the anterior part of the embryonic neural tube. See illustration accompanying *brain.* See also *cerebrum.*

encephalonarcosis (en-sef″ah-lo-nar-ko′sis) [*encephalo-* + Gr. *narkē* stupor] stupor due to brain disease.

encephalopathia (en-sef″ah-lo-path′e-ah) encephalopathy. **e. alcohol′ica,** polioencephalitis haemorrhagica superior.

encephalopathic (en-sef″ah-lo-path′ik) pertaining to encephalopathy.

encephalopathy (en-sef″ah-lop′ah-the) [*encephalo-* + Gr. *pathos* illness] any degenerative disease of the brain. **biliary e.,** kernicterus. **bilirubin e.,** kernicterus. **boxer's e.,** traumatic e. **demyelinating e.,** a degenerative disease of the brain characterized by demyelination; see *Schilder's disease,* under *disease.* **dialysis e.,** a degenerative disease of the brain associated with long-term use of hemodialysis, marked by speech disorders and constant myoclonic jerks, progressing to global dementia, with associated psychological changes; it is probably due to high levels of aluminum in the water used in the dialysis fluid. Called also *progressive dialysis e.* **hepatic e.,** a condition usually occurring secondarily to advanced disease of the liver but also seen in the course of any severe disease or in patients with portacaval shunts. It is marked by disturbances of consciousness which may progress to deep coma (hepatic coma), psychiatric changes of varying degree, flapping tremor, and fetor hepaticus. Called also *portal-systemic encephalopathy.* **hypernatremic e.,** a severe hemorrhagic encephalopathy induced by the hyperosmolarity accompanying hypernatremia and dehydration. **hypertensive e.,** a complex of cerebral phenomena (headache, convulsions, coma, etc.) occurring in the course of malignant

hypertension. **hypoglycemic e.,** metabolic encephalopathy induced by severe hypoglycemia, as in glycogen storage disease, oversecretion or overdose of insulin, etc. **lead e.,** brain disorder caused by lead poisoning; called also *saturnine e.* **metabolic e.,** neuropsychiatric disturbances due to metabolic brain disease. It may occur primarily as a result of hypoxia, ischemia, or hypoglycemia, or secondarily to disease of other organs, such as the kidney, lung, or liver. **mink e.,** a progressive viral disease of the central nervous system of mink, characterized by locomotor incoordination, progressing to semicoma and death within three to eight weeks. **myoclonic e. of childhood,** a neurologic disorder of unknown etiology with onset between ages one and three, characterized by myoclonus of trunk and limbs and by opsoclonus, with ataxia of gait, and intention tremor; some cases have been associated with occult neuroblastoma. Called also *Kinsbourne syndrome.* **portal-systemic e., portasystemic e.,** hepatic e. **progressive dialysis e.,** dialysis e. **progressive subcortical e.,** Schilder's disease; see under *disease.* **saturnine e.,** lead e. **spongiform e.,** encephalopathy involving extensive vacuolization of the cerebral cortex; the term embraces Creutzfeldt-Jakob syndrome, kuru, scrapie of sheep, and mink encephalopathy. Called also *status spongiosus.* **subacute spongiform e.,** transmissible spongiform e. **transmissible spongiform e., transmissible spongiform virus e.,** any of a group of transmissible infections of the nervous system caused by a slow virus, including Creutzfeldt-Jakob syndrome, kuru, scrapie, and mink encephalopathy, characterized pathologically by neuronal loss, astrogliosis, and extensive vacuolization of the cerebral cortex. Called also *subacute spongiform e.* **traumatic e.,** a syndrome due to cumulative punishment absorbed in the boxing ring, characterized by the general slowing of mental functions, occasional bouts of confusion, and scattered memory loss. **Wernicke's e.,** an inflammatory hemorrhagic form of encephalopathy with lesions of the hypothalamus, mamillary bodies, and periventricular and periaqueductal regions, caused by a thiamine deficiency with chronic alcoholism as a contributing factor, but also occurring as a complication of disease of the gastrointestinal tract and sometimes of hyperemesis gravidarum. It is characterized by paralysis of the eye muscles (chiefly the external recti), diplopia, nystagmus, ataxia, and mental changes ranging from deterioration and forgetfulness to delirium tremens and Korsakoff's psychosis. Called also *polioencephalitis hemorrhagica superior.*

encephalophyma (en-sef″ah-lo-fi′mah) [*encephalo-* + Gr. *phyma* growth] (*obs.*) any tumor of the brain.

encephalopsy (en-sef′ah-lop′se) [*encephalo-* + Gr. *opsis* vision] a condition in which the patient associates certain colors with certain words, numbers, flavors, etc.

encephalopuncture (en-sef″ah-lo-punk′tūr) surgical puncture of the brain.

encephalopyosis (en-sef″ah-lo-pi-o′sis) [*encephalo-* + Gr. *pyōsis* suppuration] suppuration or abscess of the brain.

encephalorachidian (en-sef″ah-lo-rah-kid′e-an) [*encephalo-* + Gr. *rhachis* spine] cerebrospinal.

encephaloradiculitis (en-sef″ah-lo-rah-dik′u-li″tis) inflammation of the roots of spinal nerves and of the brain.

encephalorrhagia (en-sef″ah-lo-ra′je-ah) [*encephalo-* + Gr. *rhēgnynai* to burst out] hemorrhage within the brain or from the brain, especially cerebral pericapillary hemorrhage.

encephalosclerosis (en-sef″ah-lo-skle-ro′sis) [*encephalo-* + Gr. *sklērōsis* hardness] hardening of the brain.

encephaloscope (en-sef′ah-lo-skōp) a speculum for examining cavities (such as abscess cavities) in the brain.

encephaloscopy (en-sef″ah-los′ko-pe) [*encephalo-* + Gr. *skopein* to examine] inspection or examination of the brain.

encephalosepsis (en-sef″ah-lo-sep′sis) [*encephalo-* + Gr. *sēpsis* decay] gangrene of brain tissue.

encephalosis (en-sef″ah-lo′sis) [*encephalo-* + *-osis*] any organic brain disease; as used by Winkelman, the term indicates a degenerative process as distinguished from true encephalitis.

encephalospinal (en-sef″ah-lo-spi′nal) pertaining to the brain and spinal column.

encephalothlipsis (en-sef″ah-lo-thlip′sis) [*encephalo-* + Gr. *thlipsis* pressure] compression of the brain.

encephalotome (en-sef′ah-lo-tōm) an instrument for performing encephalotomy.

encephalotomy (en-sef″ah-lot′o-me) [*encephalo-* + Gr. *tomē* a cutting] 1. the destruction of the head of a fetus in order to facilitate delivery. 2. the dissection or anatomy of the brain.

encheiresis (en″ki-re′sis) [Gr. *en* in + *cheir* hand] any manipulation, especially the introduction of a bougie, sound, or catheter.

enchondral (en-kon′dral) endochondral.

enchondroma (en″kon-dro′mah) [Gr. *en* in + *chondros* cartilage + *-oma*] a benign growth of cartilage arising in the metaphysis of a bone; called also *true chondroma* and *enchondrosis.* When multiple bones are involved, the condition is called *enchondromatosis.* **multiple congenital e.,** enchondromatosis.

enchondromatosis (en-kon″dro-mah-to′sis) a condition characterized by hamartomatous proliferation of cartilage cells within the metaphysis of several bones, causing thinning of the overlying cortex and distortion of the growth in length; called also *multiple* or *skeletal e., dyschondroplasia,* and *Ollier's disease.* In combination with multiple cutaneous or visceral hemangiomas, the disorder is known as *Maffucci's syndrome.* **multiple e., skeletal e.,** enchondromatosis.

enchondromatous (en″kon-dro′mah-tus) of the nature of or pertaining to enchondroma.

enchondrosarcoma (en-kon″dro-sar-ko′mah) central chondrosarcoma.

enchondrosis (en″kon-dro′sis) 1. an outgrowth from cartilage. 2. an enchondroma.

enchylema (en″ki-le′mah) [Gr. *en* in + *chylos* juice] hyaloplasm, def. 1.

enchyma (en′kĭ-mah) [Gr. *en* in + *chymos* juice] the substance elaborated from absorbed nutritive materials; the formative juice of the tissues.

enclave (en′klāv, aw-klahv′) [Fr.] a tissue detached from its normal connection and enclosed within another organ or tissue.

enclitic (en-klit′ik) [Gr. *enklinein* to incline] having the planes of the fetal head inclined to those of the maternal pelvis; not synclitic.

enclomiphene (en-klo′mĭ-fēn) chemical name: (*E*)-2-[4-(2-chloro-1,2-diphenylethenyl)phenoxy]-*N,N*-diethylethanamine; the *cis*-isomer of the gonad-stimulating principle clomiphene citrate (q.v.), $C_{26}H_{28}ClNO$. Called also *cisclomiphene.* Cf. *zuclomiphene.*

encolpism (en-kol′pizm) [Gr. *en* in + *kolpos* vagina] medication administered via the vagina.

encopresis (en-ko-pre′sis) incontinence of feces not due to organic defect or illness.

encranial (en-kra′ne-al) (*obs.*) situated within the cranium.

encranius (en-kra′ne-us) [Gr. *en* in + *kranion* skull] a teratoid parasitic twin located within the cranium of the autosite.

encyesis (en″si-e′sis) [Gr. *en* in + *kyēsis* pregnancy] normal uterine pregnancy.

encyopyelitis (en-si″o-pi″ĕ-li′tis) [*encyesis* + *pyelitis*] dilatation of the ureters and/or renal pelvis during normal pregnancy with associated edema, but seldom with all the classical signs of inflammation.

encysted (en-sist′ed) [Gr. *en* in + *kystis* sac, bladder] enclosed in a sac, bladder, or cyst.

encystment (en-sist′ment) the process or condition of being or becoming encysted.

end- see *endo-.*

endadelphos (en″ah-del′fos) [*end-* + Gr. *adelphos* brother] a monster in which a parasitic twin is inclosed within the body of the autosite, or within a tumor upon the larger twin.

Endamoeba (en″dah-me′bah) a genus of amebae of the order Amoebida, class Rhizopoda, parasitic in the intestines of invertebrates, having a large central area of the nucleus devoid of chromatic material, surrounded by a wide zone of chromatin granules and a thick nuclear membrane. Cf. *Entamoeba.* **E. blat′tae,** a species found in the intestine of the cockroach.

endangiitis (en″dan-je-i′tis) inflammation of the endangium; intimitis.

endangium (en″dan′je-um) [*end-* + Gr. *angeion* vessel] the innermost coat of a blood vessel (tunica intima vasorum [NA]).

endaortic (en″da-or′tik) pertaining to the interior of the aorta.

endaortitis (end″a-or-ti′tis) inflammation of the lining membrane of the aorta. **bacterial e.,** the formation of bacterial vegetations on the endothelial surface of the aorta.

endarterectomize (end″ar-ter-ek′to-mīz) to subject to endarterectomy.

endarterectomy (end″ar-ter-ek′to-me) excision of the thickened, atheromatous tunica intima of an artery. **gas e.,** endarterectomy performed by utilizing high-pressure carbon dioxide to remove plaque deposits from the coronary blood vessels in the treatment of atherosclerosis.

endarterial (end″ar-te′re-al) within an artery.

endarteritis (end″ar-ter-i′tis) [*end-* + Gr. *artēria* artery + *-itis*] inflammation of the tunica intima of an artery; intimitis. Cf. *arteritis* and *periarteritis.* **e. defor′mans,** (*obs.*), chronic endarteritis characterized by fatty degeneration of the arterial tissues, with the formation of deposits of lime salts. **Heubner's specific e.,** see under *disease.* **e. oblit′erans,** endarteritis in which the lumina of the smaller vessels become narrowed or obliterated as a result of proliferation of the tissue of the intimal layer; called also *arteritis obliterans* and *Friedländer's disease.* **e. prolif′erans,** overgrowth of fibrous tissue in the internal layers of the aorta.

endarterium (end″ar-te′re-um) [*end-* + Gr. *artēria* artery] the tunica intima of an artery.

endarteropathy (end″ar-ter-op′ah-the) disorder of the innermost coat (tunica intima) of an artery. **digital e.,** disorder of the tunica intima of the arteries of the digits, associated with

Raynaud's phenomenon and nutritional lesions of the pulp of the fingers.

end-artery (end′ar-ter-e) an artery that does not anastomose with other arteries.

endaural (end-aw′ral) within the ear.

end-body (end′bod-e) end-piece.

endbrain (end′brān) telencephalon.

end-brush (end′brush) the brushlike or tufted arrangement sometimes forming the termination of the process of a nerve cell.

end-bud (end′bud) 1. an ovoid or spheroid body located at the termination of a nerve fiber, and dispersed in the skin, mucous membranes, muscles, joints, and connective tissue of the internal organs. End-buds show a wide diversity, from simple end knobs to complex sensory end organs with connective tissue sheaths. Called also *end-bulb.* For names of specific types see under *corpuscle.* 2. tail bud (def. 1); see under *bud.*

end-bulb (end′bulb) end-bud, def. 1.

endchondral (end-kon′dral) endochondral.

endeictic (en-dīk′tik) [Gr. *endeixis* a pointing out] symptomatic.

endemia (en-de′me-ah) any endemic disease.

endemial (en-de′me-al) endemic.

endemic (en-dem′ik) [Gr. *endēmos* dwelling in a place] 1. present in a community at all times. 2. a disease of low morbidity that is constantly present in a human community, but clinically recognizable in only a few.

endemiology (en-de″me-ol′o-je) [*endemic* + *-logy*] the field of science dealing with all the factors relating to the occurrence of endemic disease.

endemoepidemic (en″dĕ-mo-ep″ĭ-dem′ik) endemic, but occasionally becoming epidemic.

endemy (en′dĕ-me) any endemic disease.

endepidermis (end″ep-ĭ-der′mis) the epithelium or internal epidermis.

endergic (end-er′jik) [*end-* + Gr. *ergon* work] taking in work: a term applied to chemical reactions in which the products have a higher free energy than the reactants.

endergonic (end″er-gon′ik) [*end(o)-* + Gr. *ergon* work] characterized by or accompanied by the absorption of energy; said of chemical reactions that require energy in order to proceed, so that the products have a higher free energy than the reactants. Opposed to *exergonic.*

enderon (en′der-on) [Gr. *en* in + *deros* skin] the deeper part of the skin or mucous membrane, as distinguished from the epithelium or epidermis.

enderonic (en″der-on′ik) pertaining to the enderon or derived from it.

Enders (en′derz), John Franklin. United States microbiologist, born 1897; co-winner, with Thomas H. Weller and Frederick C. Robbins, of the Nobel prize in medicine and physiology for 1954, for the discovery that poliomyelitis viruses multiply in human tissue.

end-feet button-like or knoblike terminal enlargements of naked nerve fibers which end in relation to the dendrite of another cell; called also *terminal buttons, boutons terminaux,* and *synaptic knobs.* **e. of Held,** end-feet.

end-flake (end′flāk) end-plate.

ending (end′ing) a termination or finish, especially the peripheral termination of a nerve or nerve fiber. **annulospiral e's,** wide, ribbon-like sensory nerve endings which are wrapped around the fibers of a muscle spindle. **club e. of Bartelmez,** a type of nerve fiber ending in the vertebrate central nervous system, terminating abruptly on the dendrite of another neuron. **encapsulated nerve e's,** corpuscula nervosa terminalia. **epilemmal e's,** sensory nerve endings in striated muscle in which the nerve endings are in close contact with the muscle fibers but do not penetrate the sarcolemma. **flower-spray e's,** branched, slender sensory nerve endings on the sarcolemma of muscle spindles. **free nerve e's,** terminationes nervorum liberae. **grape e's,** sensory nerve endings in muscle which have the form of terminal swellings. **nerve e's,** the fine branchlike terminations of axons.

end-nuclei (end-nu′kle-i) terminal nuclei; see under *nucleus.*

endo-, end- [Gr. *endon* within] prefix denoting an inward situation, within.

endoabdominal (en″do-ab-dom′ĭ-nal) pertaining to the interior of the abdomen.

endoaneurysmorrhaphy (en″do-an″u-riz-mor′ah-fe) [*endo-* + Gr. *aneurysma* aneurysm + *rhaphē* suture] Matas' operation for aneurysm by opening the aneurysmal sac and closing the internal orifices by suture.

endoangiitis (en″do-an-je-i′tis) endangiitis.

endoantitoxin (en″do-an-te-tok′sin) (*obs.*) an antitoxin contained within the elaborating cell.

endoaortitis (en″do-a″or-ti′tis) endaortitis.

endoappendicitis (en″do-ah-pen″dĭ-si′tis) inflammation of the mucous membrane lining the vermiform appendix.

endoarteritis (en″do-ar″ter-i′tis) endarteritis.

endoauscultation (en″do-aws″kul-ta′shun) auscultation of the stomach and thoracic organs by means of a tube passed into the stomach.

endobacillary (en″do-bas′ĭ-lār-e) contained within a bacillus.

endobiotic (en″do-bi-ot′ik) [endo- + Gr. biōsis living] living parasitically within the tissues of the host.

endoblast (en′do-blast) [endo- + Gr. blastos germ] entoderm.

endoblastic (en″do-blas′tik) entodermic.

endobronchitis (en″do-brong-ki′tis) inflammation of the epithelial lining of the bronchi.

endocardial (en″do-kar′de-al) [endo- + Gr. kardia heart] 1. situated or occurring within the heart. 2. pertaining to the endocardium.

endocardiopathy (en″do-kar″de-op′ah-the) any noninflammatory disease of the endocardium.

endocarditic (en″do-kar-dit′ik) pertaining to endocarditis.

endocarditis (en″do-kar-di′tis) exudative and proliferative inflammatory alterations of the endocardium, characterized by the presence of vegetations on the surface of the endocardium or in the endocardium itself, and most commonly involving a heart valve, but sometimes affecting the inner lining of the cardiac chambers or the endocardium elsewhere. It may occur as a primary disorder, or as a complication of or in association with another disease. **atypical verrucous e.,** nonbacterial endocarditis found in association with systemic lupus erythematosus, in which the vegetations consist of necrotic debris, fibrinoid material, and trapped, disintegrating, fibroblastic and inflammatory cells. Called also *Libman-Sacks e.* or *disease, e. benigna,* and *nonbacterial verrucous e.* **bacterial e.,** infectious endocarditis (q.v.), acute or subacute, caused by various bacteria, including streptococci, staphylococci, enterococci, gonococci, gram-negative bacilli, etc. **e. benig′na,** atypical verrucous e. **e. chorda′lis,** endocarditis affecting particularly the chordae tendineae. **chronic e.,** chronic deforming disease of the heart valves. **constrictive e.,** Löffler's e. **fungal e.,** mycotic e. **infectious e., infective e.,** endocarditis caused by infection with microorganisms, especially bacteria and fungi, and sometimes other organisms, such as spirochetes, rickettsiae, and the etiologic agent of psittacosis. It has been classified according to course as acute and subacute: the *acute* form, which may be due to staphylococci, pneumococci, gonococci, streptococci, and other bacteria and microorganisms, usually involves a normal heart valve, has a high mortality rate with or without treatment, and causes rapid destruction and metastases; the *subacute* form, which may be caused by viridans streptococci, fungi, or other organisms, usually affects a previously damaged heart valve, produces additional damage slowly, and responds well to therapy. **e. len′ta,** the subacute form of infectious endocarditis. **Libman-Sacks e.,** atypical *verrucous e.* **Löffler's e., Löffler's parietal fibroplastic e.,** endocarditis associated with eosinophilia, marked by fibroplastic thickening of the endocardium, and resulting in congestive heart failure, persistent tachycardia, hepatomegaly, splenomegaly, serous effusions into the pleural cavity, edema of the legs, and edema and ascites of the arms; called also *constrictive e.* and *eosinophilic endomyocardial disease.* **malignant e.,** a term sometimes applied to a rapidly fatal form of acute infectious endocarditis marked by ulcerated valvular lesions (*ulcerative e.*); called also *septic e.* **marantic e.,** nonbacterial thrombotic e. **mural e.,** a form affecting the lining of the walls of the heart chambers, as distinguished from *valvular e.;* called also *parietal e.* **mycotic e.,** infectious endocarditis (q.v.), usually subacute, due to various fungi, most commonly *Candida* (especially *C. albicans*), *Aspergillus* and *Histoplasma.* Called also *fungal e.* **nonbacterial thrombotic e.,** endocarditis in which the vegetations, single or multiple, consist of fibrin and other blood elements. **nonbacterial verrucous e.,** atypical verrucous e. **parietal e.,** mural e. **prosthetic valve e.,** infective endocarditis as a complication of implantation of a prosthetic valve in the heart; the vegetations usually occur along the line of suture. **pulmonic e.,** endocarditis involving the pulmonic valve. **rheumatic e.,** endocarditis associated with rheumatic fever; called also *Bouillaud's disease.* **rickettsial e.,** endocarditis caused by invasion of the heart valves with *Coxiella burnetii;* it is a sequela of Q fever, usually occurring in persons who have had rheumatic fever. **right-side e.,** primary acute endocarditis of the right side of the heart. **septic e.,** malignant e. **syphilitic e.,** endocarditis resulting from extension of syphilitic infection from the aorta. **tuberculous e.,** a rare form of endocarditis in which the endocardium is involved by extension of a tuberculous perimyocarditis or of miliary tuberculosis. **ulcerative e.,** see *malignant e.* **valvular e.,** endocarditis affecting the membrane over the valves of the heart only, as distinguished from *mural e.* **vegatative e., verrucous e.,** endocarditis, infectious or noninfectious, the characteristic lesions of which are vegetations or verrucae on the endocardium. **viridans e.,** the subacute form of infectious endocarditis due to infection with viridans streptococci.

endocardium (en″do-kar′de-um) [endo- + Gr. kardia heart] [NA] the endothelial lining membrane of the cavities of the heart and the connective tissue bed on which it lies.

endoceliac (en″do-se′le-ak) [endo- + Gr. koilia cavity] inside one of the body cavities.

endocellular (en″do-sel′u-lar) within a cell.

endocervical (en″do-ser′vĭ-kal) pertaining to the interior of the cervix uteri.

endocervicitis (en″do-ser″vĭ-si′tis) [endo- + L. cervix neck] inflammation of the mucous membrane of the cervix uteri; called also *endotrachelitis.*

endocervix (en″do-ser′viks) 1. the mucous membrane lining the canal of the cervix uteri. 2. the region of the opening of the uterine cervix into the uterine cavity.

endochondral (en″do-kon′dral) situated, formed, or occurring within cartilage.

endochorion (en″do-ko′re-on) [endo- + Gr. chorion chorion] the inner chorionic layer.

endochrome (en′do-krōm) [endo- + Gr. chrōma color] the coloring matter within a cell.

endocolitis (en″do-ko-li′tis) inflammation of the mucous membrane of the colon.

endocommensal (en″do-kom-men′sal) a commensal organism which lives inside the body of its symbiotic companion.

endoconidiotoxicosis (en″do-ko-nĭd″e-o-tok″sĭ-ko′sis) a form of mycotoxicosis caused by a fungus of the genus *Endoconidium.*

endocorpuscular (en″do-kor-pus′ku-lar) situated within a corpuscle.

endocranial (en″do-kra′ne-al) situated within the cranium.

endocraniosis (en″do-kra″ne-o′sis) intracranial hyperostosis described by Morgagni.

endocranitis (en″do-kra-ni′tis) inflammation of the endocranium.

endocranium (en″do-kra′ne-um) [endo- + Gr. kranion skull] the endosteal outer layer of the dura mater of the brain.

endocrinasthenia (en″do-krin″as-the′ne-ah) a hormonal imbalance resulting in a psychosis or psychoneurosis.

endocrinasthenic (en″do-krin″as-then′ik) pertaining to or marked by endocrinasthenia.

endocrine (en′do-krīn, en′do-krin) [endo- + Gr. krinein to separate] 1. secreting internally; applied to organs and structures whose function is to secrete into the blood or lymph a substance (hormone) that has a specific effect on another organ or part. See also under *system.* 2. pertaining to internal secretions; hormonal. Cf. *exocrine.*

endocrinic (en″do-krin′ik) endocrinous.

endocrinism (en-dok′rĭ-nism) endocrinopathy.

endocrinium (en″do-krin′e-um) the endocrine system.

endocrinologist (en″do-krĭ-nol′o-jist) an individual skilled in endocrinology, and in the diagnosis and treatment of disorders of the glands of internal secretion, i.e., the endocrine glands.

endocrinology (en″do-krĭ-nol′o-je) [endocrine + -logy] the study of the endocrine system and its role in the physiology of the body.

endocrinopath (en″do-krin′o-path) a person with a disorder of the endocrine system.

endocrinopathic (en″do-krin″o-path′ik) pertaining to or characterized by endocrinopathy.

endocrinopathy (en″do-krĭ-nop′ah-the) [endocrine + Gr. pathos disease] any disease due to disorder of the endocrine system; hormonal imbalance.

endocrinosis (en″do-krĭ-no′sis) a disordered condition due to dysfunction of the endocrine system.

endocrinosity (en″do-krĭ-nos′ĭ-te) the quality or state of secreting internally, or of being endocrine.

endocrinotherapy (en″do-kri″no-ther′ah-pe) treatment of disease by the administration of endocrine preparations; hormonotherapy.

endocrinotropic (en″do-kri″no-trop′ik) having an endocrine tendency.

endocrinous (en-dok′rĭ-nus) of or pertaining to an internal secretion or to a gland producing such a secretion, i.e., to an endocrine gland.

endocritic (en″do-krit′ik) endocrine.

endocuticle (en″do-ku′tĭ-kl) [endo- + L. cuticula] the inner layer of the procuticle in certain crustaceans and arthropods, which is almost entirely composed of protein and chitin.

endocyclic (en″do-sik′lik) a term applied to cyclic compounds in which the bond occurs in the ring.

endocyst (en′do-sist) the inner, germinative, or embryonic membrane of the hydatid cyst.

endocystitis (en″do-sis-ti′tis) inflammation of the lining membrane of the bladder.

endocyte (en′do-sīt) [endo- + Gr. kytos hollow vessel] any cell inclusion.

endocytosis (en″do-si-to′sis) [endo- + Gr. *kytos* a hollow vessel] the uptake by a cell of material from the environment by invagination of its plasma membrane; it includes both phagocytosis and pinocytosis.

endoderm (en′do-derm) [endo- + Gr. *derma* skin] entoderm.

endodermal (en″do-der′mal) entodermal.

Endodermophyton (en″do-der-mof′ĭ-ton) [endo- + Gr. *derma* skin + *phyton* a growth] the former name of a genus of fungi, now called *Trichophyton*.

endodermoreaction (en″do-der″mo-re-ak′shun) Trambusti's reaction.

endodiascope (en″do-di′ah-skōp) a roentgen-ray tube which may be placed inside a body cavity for roentgenography and radiotherapy.

endodiascopy (en″do-di-as′ko-pe) [endo- + Gr. *dia* through + *skopein* to examine] roentgenoscopic examination of a body cavity by means of an endodiascope.

endodontia (en″do-don′she-ah) endodontics.

endodontics (en″do-don′tiks) [end- + Gr. *odous* tooth + -*ics*] that branch of dentistry which is concerned with the etiology, prevention, diagnosis, and treatment of diseases and injuries that affect the tooth pulp, root, and periapical tissue. Called also *endodontology*.

endodontist (en″do-don′tist) a dentist who specializes in endodontics; called also *endodontologist*.

endodontitis (en″do-don-ti′tis) [endo- + Gr. *odous* tooth] pulpitis.

endodontium (en″do-don′she-um) the dental pulp.

endodontologist (en″do-don-tol′o-jist) endodontist.

endodontology (en″do-don-tol′o-je) endodontics.

endodyogeny (en″do-di-oj′ĕ-ne) reproduction by the formation of two daughter cells within the wall of the mother cell (internal budding), the progeny being released by rupture of the mother cell, as in the protozoan *Toxoplasma*.

endoectothrix (en″do-ek′to-thriks) a ringworm fungus which produces spores both on the interior and exterior of the hairs.

endoenteritis (en″do-en″ter-i′tis) inflammation of the mucous membrane of the intestine.

endoenzyme (en″do-en′zīm) an intracellular enzyme; an enzyme that is retained in a cell and does not normally diffuse out of the cell into the surrounding medium. Cf. *ectoenzyme*.

endoepidermal (en″do-ep″ĭ-der′mal) within the epidermis.

endoepithelial (en″do-ep″ĭ-the′le-al) within the epithelium.

endoergic (en″do-er′jik) characterized by or accompanied by the absorption of free energy; requiring energy for its completion, as a chemical reaction to which energy must be supplied if it is to proceed. Cf. *exoergic* and *exothermic*.

endoesophagitis (en″do-e-sof″ah-ji′tis) inflammation of the lining membrane of the esophagus.

endoexoteric (en″do-ek″so-ter′ik) [endo- + Gr. *exōterikos* pertaining to the outside] resulting from certain causes internal to the body, and from others of external origin.

endofaradism (en″do-far′ah-dizm) the application of alternating current to an internal organ, as to the stomach.

endogalvanism (en″do-gal′vah-nizm) the application of direct current to an internal organ, as to the stomach.

endogamous (en-dog′ah-mus) characterized by endogamy.

endogamy (en-dog′ah-me) [endo- + Gr. *gamos* marriage] 1. fertilization by the union of separate cells having the same chromatin ancestry; called also *pedogamy*. Cf. *autogamy* (def. 1) and *exogamy* (def. 1). 2. restricting marriage to persons within the community; inbreeding.

endogastric (en″do-gas′trik) pertaining to the interior of the stomach.

endogastritis (en″do-gas-tri′tis) inflammation of the mucous membrane of the stomach.

endogenetic (en″do-jĕ-net′ik) endogenous.

endogenic (en″do-jen′ik) endogenous.

endogenote (en″do-je′nōt) in bacterial genetics, the recipient cell's own complement of genetic information, as opposed to the exogenote introduced by transduction.

endogenous (en-doj′ĕ-nus) [endo- + Gr. *gennan* to produce] 1. growing from within. 2. developing or originating within the organism, or arising from causes within the organism.

endoglobar (en″do-glo′bar) endoglobular.

endoglobular (en″do-glob′u-lar) situated or occurring within the blood corpuscles.

endognathion (en″do-na′the-on) [endo- + Gr. *gnathos* jaw] the inner segment of the incisive bone.

endogonidium (en″do-go-nid′e-um) a gonidium developed within a cell, especially in the algal component of a lichen.

endoherniorrhaphy (en″do-her″ne-or′ah-fe) an operation for the repair of hernia similar in technic to endoaneurysmorrhaphy.

endointoxication (en″do-in-tok″sĭ-ka′shun) poisoning caused by an endogenous toxin.

endolabyrinthitis (en″do-lab″ĭ-rin-thi′tis) inflammation of the membranous labyrinth.

endolaryngeal (en″do-lah-rin′je-al) [endo- + Gr. *larynx*] situated or occurring within the larynx.

endolarynx (en′do-lar″inks) the interior or cavity of the larynx.

Endolimax (en″do-li′maks) [endo- + Gr. *leimax* a snail] a genus of small amebae of the order Amoebida, class Rhizopoda, distinguished by a vesicular nucleus containing a comparatively large irregular endosome, and by the absence of chromatin granules lining the nuclear membrane; found in the colon of man and other mammals, birds, amphibians, and cockroaches. Cf. *Endamoeba* and *Entamoeba*. **E. na′na,** a commensal common in the intestine of man and in lower animals.

endolymph (en′do-limf) [endo- + *lymph*] the fluid contained in the membranous labyrinth of the ear; it is entirely separate from the perilymph. Called also *endolympha*[NA], *liquor scarpae, liquor of Scarpa,* and *Scarpa's fluid*.

endolympha (en″do-lim′fah) [NA] the endolymph.

endolymphatic (en″do-lim-fat′ik) pertaining to the endolymph.

endolysin (en-dol′ĭ-sin) [endo- + *lysin*] a bactericidal substance existing in cells, acting directly on bacteria. **leukocytic e.,** leukin, def. 1.

endolysis (en-dol′ĭ-sis) [endo- + Gr. *lysis* dissolution] dissolution or breaking up of the cytoplasm of a cell.

endomastoiditis (en″do-mas″toi-di′tis) inflammation within the mastoid cavity and cells.

endomesoderm (en″do-mes′o-derm) [endo- + Gr. *mesos* middle + *derma* skin] mesoderm originating from the entoderm of the two-layered blastodisk.

endometrectomy (en″do-mĕ-trek′to-me) [endo- + Gr. *mētra* womb + *ektomē* excision] extirpation of the uterine mucosa.

endometria (en″do-me′tre-ah) [Gr.] plural of *endometrium*.

endometrial (en″do-me′tre-al) pertaining to the endometrium.

endometrioid (en″do-me′tre-oid) resembling endometrium.

endometrioma (en″do-me″tre-o′mah) a solitary, non-neoplastic mass containing endometrial tissue.

endometriosis (en″do-me″tre-o′sis) [endometrium + -*osis*] a condition in which tissue more or less perfectly resembling the uterine mucous membrane (the endometrium) and containing typical endometrial granular and stromal elements occurs aberrantly in various locations in the pelvic cavity; called also *adenomyosis externa* and *endometriosis externa*. **e. exter′na,** endometriosis. **e. inter′na,** adenomyosis. **ovarian e., e. ova′rii,** occurrence in the ovary of tissue resembling the uterine mucous membrane, either in the form of small superficial islands or in the form of endometrial ("chocolate") cysts of various sizes; called also *adenoma endometrioides ovarii*. **stromal e.,** adenomyosis in which all or nearly all of the tissue infiltrating the myometrium consists of stroma. **e. uteri′na,** adenomyosis. **e. ves′icae,** endometriosis involving the bladder.

endometriotic (en″do-me″tre-ot′ik) pertaining to or characterized by endometriosis.

endometritis (en″do-mĕ-tri′tis) [endometrium + -*itis*] inflammation of the endometrium. **bacteriotoxic e.,** endometritis caused by the toxins of bacteria, as distinguished from that caused by the presence of the organisms themselves. **decidual e.,** inflammation of the decidua of pregnancy. **exfoliative e.,** endometritis with the casting off of portions of the membrane. **glandular e.,** endometritis of the uterine glands. **membranous e.,** endometritis with an exudate which forms a false membrane. **puerperal e.,** endometritis following childbirth. **syncytial e.,** a benign tumor-like lesion with infiltration of the uterine wall by large syncytial trophoblastic cells; called also *syncytioma*. **tuberculous e.,** inflammation of the endometrium due to infection by *Mycobacterium tuberculosis*, with the presence of tubercles; usually the uterine tubes are also involved. **e. tubero′sa papulo′sa,** a cast of the uterine cavity expelled at abortion.

endometrium (en-do-me′tre-um), pl. *endome′tria* [endo- + Gr. *metra* uterus] the inner mucous membrane of the uterus, the thickness and structure of which vary with the phase of the menstrual cycle. It is functionally divisible into three layers: the stratum basale, stratum spongiosum, and stratum compactum; the latter two layers together form the *stratum functionale*. Accepted by NA as an alternative term for *tunica mucosa uteri*. **Swiss-cheese e.,** hyperplasia of the endometrium, under the influence of progesterone, in which the glands vary in size and shape, producing an appearance like that of Swiss cheese, with its large and small holes.

endometry (en-dom′ĕ-tre) [endo- + Gr. *metron* measure] the measurement of the capacity of a cavity.

endomitosis (en″do-mi-to′sis) reproduction of nuclear elements not followed by chromosome movements and cytoplasmic division; called also *endopolyploidy*.

endomitotic (en″do-mi-tot′ik) pertaining to or characterized by endomitosis.

endomixis (en″do-miks′is) [endo- + Gr. *mixis* mixture] the disintegration of the macronucleus and its subsequent reorganization following the division of the micronucleus, occasionally observed in a protozoan organism. It may to some extent take the place of conjugation.

endomorph (en′do-morf) an individual having the type of body build in which tissues derived from the endoderm predominate. There is relative preponderance of soft roundness throughout the body, with large digestive viscera and accumulations of fat, and with large trunk and thighs and tapering extremities, as contrasted with ectomorph and mesomorph (def. 1).

endomorphic (en″do-mor″fik) pertaining to or characterized by endomorphy.

endomorphy (en′do-mor″fe) [*endo* derm + Gr. *morphē* form] the condition of being an endomorph.

Endomyces (en″do-mi′sēz) [*endo-* + Gr. *mykēs* fungus] a genus of ascomycetous fungi of the order Endomycetales, which includes a number of yeasts from soil, nectar, and decaying fruit. **E. al′bicans,** former name for *Candida albicans.* **E. capsula′tus, E. epidermat′idis, E. epider′midis,** former name for *Blastomyces dermatitidis.*

Endomycetales (en″do-mi″sĕ-ta′lēz) an order of mostly saprophytic ascomycetous fungi of the subclass Hemiascomycetidae in which the zygote results from fusion of two cells and immediately forms an ascus; it includes the family Saccharomycetaceae.

endomyocarditis (en″do-mi″o-kar-di′tis) [*endo-* + Gr. *mys* muscle + *kardia* heart] inflammation of the endocardium and myocardium.

endomysium (en″do-mis′e-um) [*endo-* + Gr. *mys* muscle] the sheath of delicate reticular fibrils which surrounds each muscle fiber.

endonasal (en″do-na′zal) within the nose.

endoneural (en″do-nu′ral) pertaining to or situated within a nerve.

endoneurial (en″do-nu′re-al) pertaining to the endoneurium.

endoneuritis (en″do-nu-ri′tis) inflammation of the endoneurium.

endoneurium (en″do-nu′re-um) [*endo-* + Gr. *neuron* nerve] the interstitial connective tissue in a peripheral nerve, separating the individual nerve fibers; called also *epilemma.*

endoneurolysis (en″do-nu-rol′ĭ-sis) [*endo-* + Gr. *neuron* nerve + *lysis* dissolution] hersage.

endonuclear (en″do-nu′kle-ar) within a cell nucleus.

endonuclease (en″do-nu′kle-ās) a nuclease that cleaves internal bonds of polynucleotides (nucleic acids). **restriction e's,** enzymes that cleave large DNA molecules into discrete fragments at particular sites in specific sequences of four to six nucleotides.

endonucleolus (en″do-nu-kle′o-lus) a nonstaining spot near the center of the nucleolus of a cell.

endo-oxidase (en″do-ok′sĭ-dās) oxidase occurring within a cell, such as a bacterium.

endoparasite (en″do-par′ah-sīt) [*endo-* + *parasite*] a parasite that lives within the body of its host.

endopelvic (en″do-pel′vik) within the pelvis.

endopeptidase (en″do-pep′tĭ-dās) a proteolytic enzyme that is capable of hydrolyzing peptide linkages initially in the interior of the peptide chain, as well as terminal linkages.

endoperiarteritis (en″do-per″ĭ-ar″ter-i′tis) (*obs.*) inflammation involving both the internal and the external coat of an artery.

endopericardial (en″do-per″ĭ-kar′de-al) pertaining to the endocardium and pericardium.

endopericarditis (en″do-per″ĭ-kar-di′tis) inflammation involving both the endocardium and pericardium.

endoperimyocarditis (en″do-per″ĭ-mi″o-kar-di′tis) inflammation of the endocardium, pericardium, and myocardium.

endoperineuritis (en″do-per″ĭ-nu-ri′tis) inflammation of the endoneurium and perineurium.

endoperitoneal (en″do-per″ĭ-to-ne′al) within the peritoneum.

endoperitonitis (en″do-per″ĭ-to-ni′tis) inflammation of the serous lining of the peritoneal cavity.

endophasia (en″do-fa′ze-ah) the silent reproduction of a word or words; see also *aphasia.*

endophlebitis (en″do-fle-bi′tis) [*endo-* + Gr. *phleps* vein + *-itis*] inflammation of the intima of a vein. **e. hepat′ica oblit′erans,** Budd-Chiari syndrome. **proliferative e.,** phlebosclerosis.

endophthalmitis (en″dof-thal-mi′tis) [*endo-* + *ophthalmitis*] inflammation involving the ocular cavities and their adjacent structures. **e. phaco-aller′gica, e. phaco-anaphylac′tica, e. phacogenet′ica,** endophthalmitis occurring as a reaction to lens material which has escaped through the lens capsule.

endophylaxination (en″do-fi-lak″si-na′shun) resistance to infection developed entirely within the body of the animal possessing it.

endophyte (en′do-fīt) [*endo-* + Gr. *phyton* plant] a parasitic plant organism living within the body of its host.

endophytic (en″do-fit′ik) [*endo-* + Gr. *phyein* to grow] 1. pertaining to an endophyte. 2. growing inward; proliferating on the interior or inside of an organ or other structure, as a tumor.

endoplasm (en′do-plazm) [*endo-* + Gr. *plasma* something formed] the central portion of the cytoplasm of a cell. Cf. *ectoplasm.*

endoplasmic (en″do-plas′mik) composed of or pertaining to endoplasm; see under *reticulum.*

endoplast (en′do-plast) [*endo-* + Gr. *plassein* to form] the nucleus of a cell; see *nucleus,* def. 1.

endoplastic (en″do-plas′tik) entoplastic.

endopolyploid (en″do-pol′e-ploid) having reduplicated chromatin within an intact nucleus, with or without an increase in the number of chromosomes (applied only to cells and tissues); see also *endomitosis.*

endopolyploidy (en″do-pol′e-ploi″de) [*endo-* + *polyploidy*] 1. endomitosis. 2. polysomaty. 3. autopolyploidy resulting from a previous endomitotic cycle. See also *polysomaty.*

endopredator (en″do-pred′ah-tor) an individual or species that lives within the body of an organism of another species which it feeds upon and destroys.

endoradiography (en″do-ra″de-og′rah-fe) the radiographic demonstration of the condition of internal organs and cavities by means of radiopaque materials.

endoradiosonde (en″do-ra″de-o-sond′) a small radio transmitter inserted within a body cavity or tube, as within the intestinal lumen to measure the pressure.

endoreduplication (en″do-re-du″plĭ-ka′shun) replication of the chromosomes without subsequent cell division.

end-organ (end′or-gan) one of the larger, encapsulated endings of the sensory nerves; for names of specific types, see under *corpuscle.*

endorhinitis (en″do-ri-ni′tis) [*endo-* + Gr. *rhis* nose] inflammation of the lining membrane of the nasal passages.

endorphin (en-dor′fin, en′dor-fin) [*endo*genous + *mo*rphine] a group of endogenous brain substances (polypeptides) that bind to opiate receptors in various areas of the brain and thereby raise the pain threshold; they occur in various forms, including α-, β-, and γ-endorphin (β-endorphin being the most potent) and the enkephalins.

endosalpingitis (en″do-sal″pin-ji′tis) [*endosalpinx* + *-itis*] inflammation of the endosalpinx.

endosalpingoma (en″do-sal″pin-go′mah) adenomyoma of the uterine tube.

endosalpingosis (en″do-sal″pin-go′sis) 1. endometriosis of the uterine tube. 2. ovarian endometriosis in which the abnormal mucosa resembles tubal mucosa rather than endometrial mucosa.

endosalpinx (en″do-sal′pinks) [*endo-* + Gr. *salpinx* tube] the mucous membrane lining the uterine tube, arranged in longitudinal rugae, or folds, and continuous with the mucous lining of the uterus (tunica mucosa tubae uterinae [NA]).

endosarc (en′do-sark) endoplasm.

endoscope (en′do-skōp) [*endo-* + Gr. *skopein* to examine] an instrument for the examination of the interior of a hollow viscus, such as the bladder.

endoscopic (en″do-skop′ik) performed by means of an endoscope; pertaining to endoscopy.

endoscopy (en-dos′ko-pe) visual inspection of any cavity of the body by means of an endoscope. **peroral e.,** examination of organs accessible to observation through an endoscope passed through the mouth. **transcolonic e.,** examination of the lumen of the colon by means of an endoscope inserted through an incision in its wall.

endosecretory (en-do-se′kre-to-re) [*endo-* + *secretory*] pertaining to the internal secretions; secreting internally; endocrine.

endosepsis (en″do-sep′sis) septicemia originating within the organism.

endosite (en′do-sīt) (*obs.*) an endoparasite.

endoskeleton (en″do-skel′ĕ-ton) [*endo-* + Gr. *skeleton*] the bony and cartilaginous skeleton of the body, exclusive of that part of the skeleton which is of dermal origin; called also *neuroskeleton.*

endosmometer (en″dos-mom′ĕ-ter) [*endosmosis* + Gr. *metron* measure] an instrument for determining the rate and extent of endosmosis.

endosmosis (en″dos-mo′sis) [*endo-* + Gr. *ōsmos* impulsion] a movement in liquids separated by a membranous or porous septum, by which one fluid passes through the septum into the cavity which contains another fluid of a different density. Cf. *exosmosis.*

endosmotic (en″dos-mot′ik) of the nature of endosmosis.

endosome (en′do-sōm) a body thought to consist of deoxyribonucleic acid, observed in the vesicular nucleus of certain protozoan cells.

endosperm (en′do-sperm) a substance containing reserve food materials, formed within the embryo sac of plants.

endospore (en'do-spōr) [endo- + Gr. *sporos* seed] 1. a spore produced in the hyphae or cell, as in a spherule of *Coccidioides immitis*. 2. the inner wall of a spore. 3. a thick-walled body formed within certain bacteria which is able to withstand for prolonged periods various adverse environmental conditions; under favorable conditions, it will quickly germinate to form a vegetative bacterium. See also *spore*.

endosporium (en''do-spōr'e-um) the inner layer of the envelope of a spore.

endosteal (en-dos'te-al) pertaining to the endosteum; occurring or located within a bone.

endosteitis (en-dos''te-i'tis) inflammation of the endosteum.

endosteoma (en-dos''te-o'mah) [endo- + Gr. *osteon* bone + *-oma*] a tumor in the medullary cavity of a bone.

endostethoscope (en''do-steth'o-skōp) a stethoscope passed into the esophagus for auscultating the heart.

endosteum (en-dos'te-um) [endo- + Gr. *osteon* bone] the tissue lining the medullary cavity of a bone.

endostitis (en''dos-ti'tis) endosteitis.

endostoma (en''dos-to'mah) endosteoma.

endosymbiont (en''do-sim'be-ont) [endo- + symbiont] a symbiont which lives within the cells of its partner.

endosymbiosis (en''do-sim''bi-o'sis) the state achieved between a virus and its host cell in which cellular division is inhibited but the cell is not immediately destroyed.

endotendineum (en''do-ten-din'e-um) [endo- + L. *tendo, tendines*, after Gr. *tenon*] the delicate connective tissue separating the secondary bundles (fascicles) of a tendon.

endotenon (en''do-ten'on) [endo- + Gr. *tenōn* tendon] endotendineum.

endothelia (en''do-the'le-ah) [Gr.] plural of *endothelium*.

endothelial (en''do-the'le-al) pertaining to or made up of endothelium.

endothelialization (en''do-the''le-al-ĭ-za'shun) the healing of the inner surfaces of vessels or grafts by endothelial cells.

endotheliitis (en''do-the-le-i'tis) inflammation of the endothelium.

endothelioblastoma (en''do-the''le-o-blas-to'mah) [endothelium + Gr. *blastos* germ + *-oma*] a tumor derived from primitive vasoformative tissue with formation of usually small and slit-like vascular spaces lined by prominent endothelial cells; the term, which now includes hemangioendothelioma, angiosarcoma, lymphangioendothelioma, and lymphangiosarcoma, was applied formerly to such tumors arising from mesothelial tissue as well.

endotheliochorial (en''do-the''le-o-ko're-al) [endothelium + chorion] denoting a type of placenta in which syncytial trophoblast embeds maternal vessels bared to their endothelial lining.

endotheliocyte (en''do-the''le-o-sīt'') [endothelia + Gr. *kytos* hollow vessel] a term for the large mononuclear phagocytic wandering cells of the circulating blood and tissues which are supposed by some to be derived from proliferating vascular endothelium. Called also *endothelial phagocyte*.

endotheliocytosis (en-do-the''le-o-si-to'sis) an abnormal increase in the number of endotheliocytes.

endothelioid (en''do-the'le-oid) resembling endothelium.

endotheliolysin (en''do-the''le-ol'ĭ-sin) an antibody capable of causing disintegration of endothelial tissue.

endotheliolytic (en''do-the''le-o-lit'ik) capable of destroying endothelial tissue.

endothelioma (en''do-the''le-o'mah) [endothelium + *-oma*] a tumor which originates from the endothelial linings of blood vessels (*hemangioendothelioma*), lymphatics (*lymphangioendothelioma*), or serous cavities (*mesothelioma*). **e. cap'itis,** a large multiple hemangioma on the scalp. **e. cu'tis,** endothelioma of the skin, manifested as violaceous papules. **dural e.,** meningioma.

endotheliomatosis (en''do-the''le-o-mah-to'sis) the formation of multiple and diffuse endotheliomas in a tissue.

endotheliomyoma (en''do-the''le-o-mi-o'mah) (*obs.*) a vascular leiomyoma.

endotheliosarcoma (en''do-the''le-o-sar-ko'mah) Kaposi's sarcoma.

endotheliosis (en''do-the''le-o'sis) proliferation of endothelium.

endotheliotoxin (en''do-the''le-o-tok'sin) a specific toxin which acts on the endothelium of capillaries and small veins, producing hemorrhage. Cf. *hemorrhagin*.

endothelium (en''do-the'le-um), pl. *endothe'lia* [endo- + Gr. *thēlē* nipple] [NA] the layer of epithelial cells that lines the cavities of the heart and of the blood and lymph vessels, and the serous cavities of the body, originating from the mesoderm. **e. cam'erae anterio'ris bul'bi** [NA], **e. cam'erae anterio'ris oc'uli,** the mesothelial layer covering the posterior surface of the posterior limiting lamina of the cornea; it was once believed to extend to the anterior surface of the stroma of the iris. **corneal e.,** the portion of the endothelium of the anterior chamber of the eye that covers the posterior surface of the cornea. **ex-**

traembryonic e., endothelium which arises outside of the body of the embryo, such as that lining the vitelline vessels.

endothermal (en''do-ther'mal) endothermic.

endothermic (en''do-ther'mik) characterized by or accompanied by the absorption of heat, as a chemical reaction accompanied by absorption of heat and to which heat must be supplied if it is to proceed: storing up heat or energy in a potential form. Cf. *endoergic* and *exothermic*.

endothermy (en'do-ther''me) [endo- + Gr. *thermē* heat] diathermy.

endothoracic (en''do-tho-ras'ik) within the thorax; situated internal to the ribs.

endothrix (en'do-thriks) [endo- + Gr. *thrix* hair] a dermatophyte whose growth and spore production are confined chiefly within the shaft of the hair, without formation of conspicuous external spores; such fungi include *Trichophyton tonsurans* and *T. violaceum*.

endothyroidopexy (en''do-thi-roi'do-pek''se) endothyropexy.

endothyropexy (en-do-thi'ro-pek-se) the operation of freeing the thyroid from the trachea, dislocating it forward, and fixing it to one side in a pocket between the sternocleidomastoid muscle and the skin.

endotoxemia (en''do-toks-e'me-ah) the presence of endotoxins in the blood, which may result in shock.

endotoxic (en''do-tok'sik) pertaining to or possessing endotoxin.

endotoxicosis (en''do-tok''sĭ-ko'sis) (*obs.*) poisoning caused by an endotoxin.

endotoxin (en''do-tok'sin) a heat-stable toxin present in the bacterial cell but not in cell-free filtrates of cultures of intact bacteria. They are found primarily in gram-negative organisms, in which they are identical with the somatic antigen. They occur in the cell wall as a lipopolysaccharide complex extractable in trichloracetic acid and glycols. The endotoxins are pyrogenic and increase capillary permeability, the activity being substantially the same regardless of the species of bacteria from which they are derived. Called also *bacterial pyrogen*.

endotoxoid (en''do-tok'soid) a toxoid prepared from endotoxin.

endotracheal (en''do-tra'ke-al) [endo- + *trachea*] 1. within or through the trachea. 2. performed by passage through the lumen of the trachea.

endotracheitis (en''do-tra-ke-i'tis) inflammation of the mucosa of the trachea.

endotrachelitis (en''do-tra-kel-i'tis) [endo- + Gr. *trachēlos* neck] endocervicitis.

endotrypsin (en''do-trip'sin) [endo- + *trypsin*] a digestive ferment derived from yeast and resembling trypsin in its action.

endourethral (en''do-u-re'thral) within the urethra.

endouterine (en''do-u'ter-in) within the uterus.

endovaccination (en''do-vak''sĭ-na'shun) [endo- + *vaccination*] the administration of vaccines by the mouth.

endovasculitis (en''do-vas''ku-li'tis) [endo- + L. *vasculum* vessel] endangiitis.

endovenitis (en''do-ve-ni'tis) endophlebitis.

endovenous (en''do-ve'nus) intravenous.

Endoxan (en-dok'san) trademark for a preparation of cyclophosphamide.

end-piece (end'pēs) in early immunological theory, the pseudoglobulin fraction of guinea pig serum, which corresponds to the C2 component of complement.

end-plate (end'plāt) a flattened discoid expansion at the neuromuscular junction, where a myelinated motor nerve fiber joins a skeletal muscle fiber. It contains two kinds of receptors, one that combines with acetylcholine and another that combines with acetylcholinesterase, which inactivates acetylcholine.

end-pleasure (end'plezh-er) the pleasure produced by the sexual orgasm, as contrasted with the fore-pleasure which precedes it.

end point (end' point) in titration, the highest dilution of a substance that produces a reaction with a given volume of another substance.

end product (end prod'ukt) the chemical compound resulting from the completion of a sequence of metabolic reactions.

Endrate (en'drāt) trademark for preparations of edetate disodium.

endrin (en'drin) chemical name: 1,2,3,4,4,10,10-hexachloro-6,7-epoxy-1,4,4a,5,6,7,8,8a-octahydro-1,4,5,8-endo-endo-dimethanonaphthalene; a highly toxic insecticide of the chlorinated hydrocarbon group.

endrysone (en'drĭ-sōn) chemical name: 11β-hydroxy-6α-methylpregna-1,4-diene-3,20-dione; a topical anti-inflammatory for use in ophthalmology, $C_{22}H_{30}O_3$.

Enduron (en'du-ron) trademark for a preparation of methyclothiazide.

endyma (en'dĭ-mah) ependyma.

-ene a suffix used in chemistry to indicate an unsaturated hydrocarbon containing one double bond.

enema (en′e-mah), pl. *enemas* or *enem′ata* [Gr.] a clyster or injection; a liquid injected or to be injected into the rectum. **analeptic e.,** an enema consisting of a pint of tepid water containing ½ teaspoonful of salt; called also *thirst e.* **barium e.,** a suspension of barium administered as a clyster and retained in the intestines during roentgenologic examination, the presence of deformities of the intestine, produced by neoplasm or other abnormality, being demonstrated by filling defects revealed by the column of radiopaque barium. Called also *contrast e.* **blind e.,** the insertion of a soft-rubber tube into the rectum to aid in the expulsion of flatus. **contrast e.,** barium e. **double contrast e.,** injection and evacuation of a suspension of barium, followed by inflation of the intestines with air under light pressure; used in mucosal relief roentgenography. **flatus e.,** an enema made of ½ oz. of magnesium sulfate, 1 oz. of glycerin, and 4 oz. of warm water. **Fleet e.,** trademark for an enema containing, in each 100 ml., 16 gm. sodium biphosphate and 6 gm. sodium phosphate, packaged in a plastic squeeze bottle fitted with a 2-inch, prelubricated rectal tube. **hydrocortisone e.** [USP], a suspension containing 100 mg. of hydroxycortisone per 60 ml.; used in the treatment of various conditions responsive to the anti-inflammatory action of glucocorticoids. **nutrient e., nutritive e.,** an enema of predigested nutrient matter. **pancreatic e.,** an enema containing pancreatin. **soapsuds e.,** an enema made by dissolving 2 oz. of soap in a pint of warm water. **sodium phosphate and biphosphate e., sodium phosphate e.** [USP], a solution of sodium phosphate and sodium biphosphate, or sodium phosphate and phosphoric acid in purified water, containing in each 100 ml., 5.7 to 6.3 gm. of sodium phosphate and 15.2 to 16.8 gm. of sodium biphosphate; used as a cathartic. **theophylline olamine e.** [USP], an enema containing an amount of anhydrous theophylline equivalent to 72 to 78 per cent of the labeled amount of theophylline olamine and an amount of monethanolamine equivalent to 22 to 28 per cent of the labeled amount of theophylline olamine. **thirst e.,** analeptic enema. **turpentine e.,** an enema of 1 pint of soapsuds containing 2 oz. olive oil and 1 oz. turpentine.

enemator (en′ĕ-ma″tor) an apparatus for giving enemas.

energetics (en″er-jet′iks) the study of energy; the science of energy.

energid (en′er-jid) living, active protoplasm, as distinguished from deuteroplasm.

energizer (en′er-jīz″er) that which gives energy to, activates, or charges. **psychic e.,** a popular term for an antidepressant agent.

energometer (en″er-gom′ĕ-ter) an apparatus for studying the pulse.

energy (en′er-je) [Gr. *energeia*] the capacity to operate or work; power to produce motion, to overcome resistance, and to effect physical changes. **atomic e.,** energy that can be liberated by changes in the nucleus of an atom (as by fission of a heavy nucleus or fusion of light nuclei into heavier ones with accompanying loss of mass). **binding e.,** energy equal to the difference between the weight of the nucleus of an atom and the sum of the weights of its constituent particles. **biologic e., biotic e.,** the form of energy peculiar to living matter; i.e., energy produced by biologic processes. **chemical e.,** energy which shows itself in chemical transformations. **free e.,** the energy equal to the maximum amount of work that can be obtained from a process occurring under conditions of fixed temperature and pressure. **kinetic e.,** energy in action or engaged in producing work or motion. **nuclear e.,** atomic e. **e. of position, potential e.,** energy at rest or not manifested in actual work. **radiant e.,** the energy of electromagnetic waves, such as radio waves, visible light, x-rays, and gamma rays.

enervation (en″er-va′shun) [L. *enervatio*] 1. lack of nervous energy; languor. 2. removal of a nerve or a section of a nerve.

enflagellation (en″flaj-el-la′shun) the formation of flagella.

enflurane (en′floo-rān) [USP] chemical name: 2-chloro-1-(difluoromethoxy)-1,1,2-trifluoroethane; a stable nonflammable liquid, $C_3H_2ClF_5O$, used as an inhalation anesthetic.

ENG electronystagmography.

engagement (en-gāj′ment) in obstetrics, the entrance of the fetal head, or presenting part, into the superior pelvic strait and beginning descent through the pelvic canal.

engastrius (en-gas′tre-us) [Gr. *en* in + *gastēr* belly] a monster in which a parasitic twin is contained within the abdomen of the autosite.

Engel's alkalimetry (eng′elz) [Rodolphe Charles *Engel*, Alsatian chemist, 1850–1916] see under *alkalimetry.*

Engelmann's disease (eng′el-mahnz) [Guido *Engelmann*, German surgeon, born 1876] diaphyseal dysplasia.

Engelmann's disk (eng′el-mahnz) [Theodor Wilhelm *Engelmann*, a German physiologist, 1843–1909] H band; see under *band.*

engine (en′jin) a machine by which energy is converted into mechanical motion. **dental e.,** a machine operated by elec-

tricity, water, or compressed air, for activating burs (drills), burnishers, or other instruments held in the handpiece and used by dentists in procedures on the teeth. **high-speed e.,** originally, a dental engine capable of turning the bur in the handpiece at a rate of more than 10,000 revolutions per minute; now often used to denote an engine (sometimes called *ultraspeed e.*) that turns the bur more than 100,000 revolutions per minute. **surgical e.,** a machine similar to the dental engine, used in surgery. **ultraspeed e.,** a dental engine that turns burs at a rate of more than 100,000 revolutions per minute; see also *high-speed e.*

englobe (en-glōb′) phagocytize; to absorb within the substance of a globe.

Engman's disease (eng′manz) [Martin Feeney *Engman*, dermatologist in St. Louis, 1869–1953] dermatitis infectiosa eczematoides.

engorged (en-gorjd′) distended or swollen with fluids.

engorgement (en-gorj′ment) hyperemia; local congestion; excessive fullness of any organ, vessel, or tissue due to accumulation of fluids, especially that due to accumulation of blood.

engram (en′gram) [Gr. *en* in + *gramma* mark] a lasting mark or trace. The term is applied to the definite and permanent trace left by a stimulus in nerve tissue. See *engraphia.* In psychology it is the lasting trace left in the psyche by anything that has been experienced psychically; a latent memory picture.

engraphia (en-graf′e-ah) the process hypothesized in the theory that stimuli leave definite traces (engrams) on the protoplasm which, when regularly repeated, induce a habit that persists after the stimuli cease.

enhancement (en-hans′ment) in immunology, (1) the successful establishment and prolonged survival (or delayed rejection) of a tumor allograft in the host as a consequence of contact with specific antibody, or (2) various specific and nonspecific means to increase the level of an immune response (immunoenhancement).

enhematospore (en-hem′ah-to-spōr″) [Gr. *en* in + *haima* blood + *sporos* spore] (*obs.*) merozoite.

enhemospore (en-hem′o-spōr) merozoite.

enhexymal (en-hek′sĭ-mal) hexobarbital.

Enhydrina (en″hi-dri′nah) a genus of sea snakes. **E. schisto′sa,** a venomous sea snake commonly found in Indo-Pacific waters.

eniotypy (en″ĭ-o-ti′pe) [Gr. *enioi* some + *typos* type] polymorphism in which a macromolecular gene-product is present in some individuals of a species and not in others; it is detectable since the isologous antibody has wide cross-reactivity, whereas the heterologous antibody has no reactivity, with the serum of deficient animals.

enkatarrhaphy (en″kah-tar′ah-fe) [Gr. *enkatarrhaptein* to sew in] the operation of burying a structure by suturing together the sides of the tissues adjacent to it.

enkephalin (en-kef′ah-lin) either of two naturally occurring pentapeptides (methionine enkephalin and leucine enkephalin) isolated from the brain, that have potent opiate-like effects and probably serve as neurotransmitters; classified as endorphins, they occur in nerve endings of brain tissue, spinal cord, and the gastrointestinal tract and bind to the same receptor sites as do opiates.

enlargement (en-larj′ment) an increase in the size of an organ or part; see *hypertrophy* and *hyperplasia.* **cardiac e.,** dilatation or hypertrophy of the heart, due to compensatory mechanisms or secondary to disease. **gingival e.,** an increase in size of the gingiva due to hypertrophy or hyperplasia. **e. of heart,** cardiac e.

enol (e′nol) one of two tautomeric forms of a substance, the other being the keto form. The enol is formed from the keto by migration of hydrogen from the adjacent carbon atom to the carbonyl group:

$$\begin{array}{ll} \text{R.CH} & \text{R.CH}_2 \\ \parallel & \mid \\ \text{R.C.OH} & \text{R.C:O} \\ \text{enol form} & \text{keto form} \end{array}$$

enolase (e′no-lās) an enzyme in glycolytic systems that changes phosphoglyceric acid into phosphopyruvic acid.

enology (e-nol′o-je) [Gr. *oinos* wine + *-logy*] the scientific study of the production and composition of wine.

enophthalmos (en-of-thal′mos) [Gr. *en* in + *ophthalmos* eye] a backward displacement of the eyeball into the orbit.

enophthalmus (en″of-thal′mus) enophthalmos.

enorganic (en-or-gan′ik) existing as a permanent quality of the organism.

enostosis (en″os-to′sis) [Gr. *en* in + *osteon* bone] a morbid bony growth developed within the cavity of a bone or on the internal surface of the bone cortex.

Enovid (en-o′vid) trademark for preparations of mestranol and norethynodrel.

enoxidase (e-nok′sĭ-dās) [Gr. *oinos* wine + *oxidase*] an oxidizing ferment found in spoiled wines.

en plaque (ahn-plak′) [Fr.] in the form of a plaque or plate.

enpromate (en′pro-māt) chemical name: 1,1-diphenyl-2-propynyl cyclohexanecarbamate; an antineoplastic agent, $C_{22}H_{23}NO_2$.

enrichment (en-rich′ment) the addition of nutrients, as to culture media; the medium resulting from such addition. **Fildes e.,** a sterile enzymatic digest of sheep blood added to liquid or solid culture media for the cultivation of *Hemophilus* species; called also *Fildes culture medium.*

ens (enz) [L.] a thing. **e. mor′bi,** the nature or essential principle of a disease considered apart from its causation; the pathology of a disease as distinguished from its etiology.

ensiform (en′sĭ-form) [L. *ensis* sword + *forma* form] shaped like a sword; xiphoid.

ensisternum (en″sis-ter′num) [L. *ensis* sword + *sternum*] xiphoid process (processus xiphoideus [NA]).

ensomphalus (en-som′fah-lus) [Gr. *en* in + *sōma* a body + *omphalos* navel] a double monster with blended bodies, two separate navels, and two umbilical cords.

enstrophe (en′stro-fe) [Gr. *enstrephein* to turn in] inversion, especially of the margin of the eyelids.

E.N.T. ear, nose, and throat.

ent- see *ento-.*

entad (en′tad) toward the center; inwardly.

ental (en′tal) [Gr. *entos* within] inner; central.

entalação (en″tah-lah-sah′yo) a complication of Chagas′ disease in which megaesophagus with severe dysphagia occurs as a result of involvement of the intramural nervous plexus of the esophagus; it may be due to direct action of *Trypanosoma cruzi* on the ganglion cells or to a toxic substance elaborated by the parasite. The intramural nervous plexuses of the colon, duodenum, and other tubular organs may also be affected and result in pathologic dilatation. Called also *tropical cardiospasm* and *tropical dysphagia.*

entamebiasis (en″tah-me-bi′ah-sis) infection with *Entamoeba.*

Entamoeba (en″tah-me′bah) a genus of amebae of the order Amoebida, class Rhizopoda, parasitic in the intestine of vertebrates. They are distinguished by a more or less spherical nucleus with a relatively small chromosome near its center, and numerous chromatic granules lining the nuclear membrane. Several species, including *E. co′li, E. gingiva′lis, E. hartman′ni,* and *E. histolyt′ica,* are commonly parasitic in man. Cf. *Endamoeba.* **E. bucca′lis,** *E. gingivalis.* **E. buetsch′lii,** *Iodamoeba buetschlii.* **E. co′li,** a nonpathogenic form found in the intestinal tract of

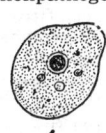 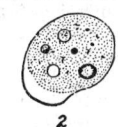

1, *Entamoeba coli.* 2, *E. histolytica.* (de Rivas.)

man; called also *Amoeba coli.* **E. gingiva′lis,** a species found in the mouth, about the gums, and in the tartar of the teeth; called also *E. buccalis,* and *Amoeba buccalis* or *dentalis.* **E. hartman′ni,** a nonpathogenic form found in the intestinal tract of man; it is similar in appearance to *E. histolytica,* but smaller. **E. histolyt′ica,** the only species with pathogenic potential for man, causing amebic dysentery and amebic abscess of the liver; it invades the bowel mucosa, causing ulceration and may be carried to other organs by the blood stream. **E. inva′dens,** a tissue-invading pathogenic parasite of snakes. **E. na′na,** *Endolimax nana.* **E. polec′ki,** an intestinal parasite of hogs, sheep, monkeys, and cattle; it has rarely been found in man. **E. tetrage′na** (*obs.*), *E. histolytica.* **E. tropica′lis** (*obs.*), *E. histolytica.*

entasia (en-ta′ze-ah) [Gr. *entasis*] a constrictive spasm; spasmodic muscular action.

entasis (en′tah-sis) entasia.

entelechy (en-tel′ĕ-ke) [Gr. *entelecheia* actuality] 1. completion; full development or realization; the complete expression of some function. 2. a supposed vital principle operating in living creatures as a directive spirit.

entepicondyle (en-tep″ĭ-kon′dīl) the internal epicondyle of the humerus.

enteque (en-ta′ka) chronic hemorrhagic septicemia of unknown etiology affecting chiefly cattle and sometimes horses and sheep in the Argentine. It occurs in two forms: the *intestinal* form, marked by wasting, diarrhea, and death within three to four months, and a *wasting* form, (*e. seca*), marked by progressive emaciation, anemia, inflammation of the joints, and calcification of the lungs.

enter- see *entero-.*

enteraden (en-ter′ad-en) [*enter-* + Gr. *adēn* gland] any intestinal gland.

enteradenitis (en″ter-ad″ĕ-ni′tis) [*enteraden* + *-itis*] inflammation of the intestinal glands.

enteral (en′ter-al) [Gr. *enteron* intestine] within, by way of, or pertaining to the small intestine.

enteralgia (en″ter-al′je-ah) [*enter-* + *-algia*] pain or neuralgia of the intestine.

enteramine (en″ter-am′in) serotonin.

enterangiemphraxis (en″ter-an″je-em-frak′sis) [*enter-* + Gr. *angeion* vessel + *emphraxis* stoppage] (*obs.*) obstruction of the intestinal blood vessels.

enterauxe (en″ter-awk′se) [*enter-* + Gr. *auxē* increase] (*obs.*) hypertrophy of the intestinal wall.

enterectasis (en″ter-ek′tah-sis) [*enter-* + Gr. *ektasis* extension] distention of the intestines.

enterectomy (en″ter-ek′to-me) [*enter-* + Gr. *ektomē* excision] excision of a part of the intestine; resection of the intestine.

enterelcosis (en″ter-el-ko′sis) [*enter-* + Gr. *helkōsis* ulceration] (*obs.*) ulceration of the intestine.

enterepiplocele (en″ter-e-pip′lo-sēl) enteroepiplocele.

enteric (en-ter′ik) [Gr. *enterikos* intestinal] pertaining to the small intestine.

enteric-coated (en-ter″ik-kōt′ed) a term designating a special coating applied to tablets or capsules which prevents release and absorption of their contents until they reach the intestines.

entericoid (en-ter′ĭ-koid) resembling enteric or typhoid fever.

enteritis (en″ter-i′tis) [*enter-* + *-itis*] inflammation of the intestine, applied chiefly to inflammation of the small intestine; see also *enterocolitis.* **e. anaphylac′tica,** hemorrhagic inflammation of both the large and the small intestine following a second dose of anaphylactogen in sensitized dogs. **cat e.,** panleukopenia. **choleriform e.,** an acute, cholera-like diarrheal disease with a high case fatality rate, prevalent in epidemic and endemic form in the Western Pacific area since 1938, caused by the El Tor or Celebes vibrio, immunologically identical with the cholera vibrio. **chronic cicatrizing e.,** Crohn′s disease. **e. cys′tica chron′ica,** a form marked by cystic dilatation of the intestinal glands, due to closure of the openings of their ducts. **diphtheritic e.,** enteritis characterized by the presence of a false membrane and severe ulceration of the mucosa beneath the membrane. **feline e.,** panleukopenia. **e. gra′vis,** an often fatal disease characterized by acute onset of severe abdominal pain, nausea, vomiting, and bloody diarrhea, with mucosal necrosis and hemorrhage and edema of the submucosa, most prominent in the jejunum and proximal ileum. **infectious feline e.,** panleukopenia. **e. membrana′cea, membranous e., mucomembranous e., mucous e., myxomembranous e.,** mucous colitis. **e. necrot′icans,** an inflammation of the intestines in man, caused by *Clostridium perfringens* type F, and characterized by necrosis. **e. nodula′ris,** enteritis with enlargement of the lymph nodes. **pellicular e.,** mucous colitis. **phlegmonous e.,** a condition with symptoms resembling those of peritonitis; it may be secondary to other intestinal diseases, as chronic obstruction, strangulated hernia, carcinoma, etc. **e. polypo′sa,** enteritis marked by polypoid growths in the intestine, due to proliferation of the connective tissue. **protozoan e.,** enteritis in which the intestine is infested with protozoan organisms of various species. **pseudomembranous e.,** pseudomembranous enterocolitis. **regional e., segmental e.,** Crohn′s disease. **specific feline e.,** panleukopenia. **streptococcus e.,** primary phlegmonous enteritis, due to *Streptococcus pyogenes.* **terminal e.,** Crohn′s disease. **tuberculous e.,** enteritis secondary to advance pulmonary tuberculosis, believed to be caused by the swallowing of large amounts of positive sputum; now rare due to antibiotic tuberculosis therapy.

entero-, enter- [Gr. *enteron* intestine] a combining form denoting relationship to the intestines.

enteroanastomosis (en″ter-o-ah-nas″to-mo′sis) the surgical formation of an anastomosis between two portions of the intestine.

enteroantigen (en″ter-o-an′tĭ-jen) an antigen derived from the intestine.

enteroapokleisis (en″ter-o-ap″o-kli′sis) [*entero-* + Gr. *apokleisis* a shutting out] the surgical exclusion of a segment of the intestine.

Enterobacteriaceae (en″ter-o-bak-te″re-a′se-e) a family of Schizomycetes, order Eubacteriales, made up of gram-negative rod-shaped organisms, occurring as plant or animal parasites, or as saprophytes. It includes five tribes, Erwinieae, Escherichieae, Proteeae, Salmonelleae, and Serratieae.

enterobacteriotherapy (en″ter-o-bak-te″re-o-ther′ah-pe) treatment by vaccine made from intestinal bacteria.

enterobiasis (en″ter-o-bi′ah-sis) infection with nematode worms of the genus *Enterobius,* especially *E. vermicularis.*

enterobiliary (en″ter-o-bil′e-er-e) pertaining to the small intestine and the bile passages.

Enterobius (en″ter-o′be-us) [*entero-* + Gr. *bios* life] a genus of intestinal nematode worms of the superfamily Oxyuroidea. **E. vermicula′ris,** the seatworm, threadworm, or pinworm, a small white worm parasitic in the upper part of the large intestine, and occasionally in the female genitals and bladder. Infection is frequent in children, sometimes causing itching. Formerly called *Ascaris vermicularis* or *Oxyuris vermicularis*.

enterocele (en'ter-o-sēl") [*entero-* + Gr. *kēlē* hernia] 1. any hernia of the intestine through intact vaginal mucosa. 2. posterior vaginal hernia.

enterocentesis (en"ter-o-sen-te'sis) [*entero-* + Gr. *kentēsis* puncture] surgical puncture of the intestine.

enterochirurgia (en"ter-o-ki-rur'je-ah) [*entero-* + Gr. *cheirourgia* surgery] surgery of the intestine.

enterocholecystostomy (en"ter-o-ko"le-sis-tos'to-me) [*entero-* + Gr. *cholē* bile + *kystis* bladder + *stoma* mouth] formation of an opening from the gallbladder into the small intestine; it may be created surgically or occur spontaneously by rupture due to an impacted stone.

enterocholecystotomy (en"ter-o-ko"lo-sis-tot'o-me) [*entero-* + *cholecystotomy*] incision into the gallbladder and the intestine.

enterocinesia (en"ter-o-si-ne'ze-ah) [*entero-* + Gr. *kinēsis* motion] peristalsis.

enterocinetic (en"ter-o-si-net'ik) pertaining to or stimulating peristalsis.

enterocleisis (en"ter-o-kli'sis) [*entero-* + Gr. *kleisis* closure] 1. closure of a wound in the intestine. 2. occlusion of the lumen of the intestine. **omental e.,** closure of an intestinal perforation by suturing the omentum over the defect.

enteroclysis (en"ter-ok'lĭ-sis) [*entero-* + Gr. *klysis* a drenching] the injection of a nutrient or medicinal liquid into the bowel.

enteroclysm (en"ter-o-klizm) [*entero-* + Gr. *klysmos* a clyster] enteroclysis.

enterococcemia (en"ter-o-kok-se'me-ah) [*enterococcus* + Gr. *haima* blood + *-ia*] the presence of enterococci in the blood.

enterococci (en"ter-o-kok'si) [Gr.] plural of enterococcus.

enterococcus (en"ter-o-kok'us), pl. *enterococ'ci* [*entero-* + *coccus*] any streptococcus of the human intestine; the enterococcus group includes *Streptococcus faecalis, S. durans, S. liquefaciens,* and *S. zymogenes.*

enterocoel (en'ter-o-sīl) enterocoele.

enterocoele (en"ter-o-se'le) [*entero-* + Gr. *koilia* belly] the body cavity formed by the outpouchings from the archenteron, typically found in echinoderms and chordates. Cf. *schizocoele.*

enterocoelom (en"ter-o-se'lom) enterocoele.

enterocoelomate (en"ter-o-sēl'o-māt) 1. having an enterocoele. 2. any of a group of animals, such as echinoderms and chordates, having a body cavity (enterocoele) derived from the archenteron.

enterocolectomy (en"ter-o-ko-lek'to-me) resection of the intestines, including the ileum, cecum, and ascending colon.

enterocolitis (en"ter-o-ko-li'tis) [*entero-* + *colitis*] inflammation involving both the small intestine and the colon; see also *enteritis.* **antibiotic-associated e.,** that in which treatment with antibiotics alters the bowel flora and results in diarrhea or pseudomembranous enterocolitis. Called also *antibiotic-associated colitis.* **hemorrhagic e.,** an inflammation of the small intestine and colon, characterized by hemorrhagic breakdown of the intestinal mucosa with inflammatory-cell infiltration. **necrotizing e.,** pseudomembranous e. **pseudomembranous e.,** an acute inflammation of the bowel mucosa with the formation of pseudomembranous plaques overlying an area of superficial ulceration, and the passage of the pseudomembranous material in the feces; it may result from shock and ischemia or be associated with antibiotic therapy. Called also *necrotizing e.* and *pseudomembranous colitis* or *enteritis.* **regional e.,** Crohn's disease.

enterocolostomy (en"ter-o-ko-los'to-me) [*entero-* + Gr. *kolon* colon + *stomoun* to provide with an opening, or mouth] the surgical formation of a communication between the small intestine and the colon; also, the opening so constructed.

enterocrinin (en"ter-ok'rĭ-nin) an extract of the mucosa of the small intestine, said to be a physiological hormone, which stimulates the intestine to secretory activity.

enterocutaneous (en"ter-o-ku-ta'ne-us) pertaining to or communicating with the intestine and the cutaneous surface of the body, as an enterocutaneous fistula.

enterocyst (en'ter-o-sist") [*entero-* + Gr. *kystis* sac, bladder] a benign cyst proceeding from the subperitoneal tissue.

enterocystocele (en"ter-o-sis'to-sēl) [*entero-* + Gr. *kystis* bladder + *kēlē* hernia] hernia of the bladder and intestine.

enterocystoma (en"ter-o-sis-to'mah) [*entero-* + Gr. *kystis* cyst + *-oma*] vitelline cyst.

enterocyte (en'ter-o-sīt") an intestinal epithelial cell.

enterodynia (en"ter-o-din'e-ah) [*entero-* + Gr. *odynē* pain] pain in the intestine.

enteroenterostomy (en"ter-o-en"ter-os'to-me) surgical anastomosis between two segments of the intestine.

enteroepiplocele (en"ter-o-e-pip'lo-sēl) [*entero-* + Gr. *epiploon* omentum + *kēlē* hernia] hernia of the small intestine and omentum.

enterogastric (en"ter-o-gas'trik) of or pertaining to the intestine and stomach.

enterogastritis (en"ter-o-gas-tri'tis) [*entero-* + Gr. *gastēr* stomach + *-itis*] gastroenteritis.

enterogastrone (en"ter-o-gas'trōn) [*entero-* + *gastro-* + *chalone*] a hormone of the duodenum which mediates the humoral inhibition of gastric secretion and motility produced by the ingestion of fat; called also *anthelone E.*

enterogenous (en"ter-oj'ĕ-nus) [*entero-* + Gr. *gennan* to produce] 1. arising from the primitive foregut. 2. originating within the small intestine.

enteroglucagon (en"ter-o-gloo'kah-gon) [*entero-* + *glucagon*] a glucagon-like hyperglycemic agent released by the mucosa of the upper intestine in response to the ingestion of glucose, and believed by some to be synthesized and secreted by the L cells. It is immunologically distinct from pancreatic glucagon but has similar activities. Called also *intestinal glucagon.*

enterogram (en'ter-o-gram") a tracing made by an instrument of the movements of the intestine.

enterograph (en'ter-o-graf) [*entero-* + Gr. *graphein* to write] an instrument for recording the intestinal movements.

enterography (en"ter-og'rah-fe) 1. recording of the intestinal movements by means of an enterograph. 2. a description of the intestines.

enterohepatitis (en"ter-o-hep-ah-ti'tis) [*entero-* + Gr. *hēpar* liver + *-itis*] 1. inflammation of the bowel and liver. 2. histomoniasis of turkeys.

enterohepatocele (en"ter-o-hep'ah-to-sēl") an infantile umbilical hernia which contains intestines and liver.

enterohepatopexy (en"ter-o-hep"ah-to-pek'se) fixation to the liver of a seromuscular flap of a defunctionalized loop of the proximal small intestine, a step in autotransplantation of the liver.

enterohydrocele (en"ter-o-hi'dro-sēl) [*entero-* + *hydrocele*] hernia with hydrocele.

enteroidea (en"ter-oi'de-ah) the intestinal fevers; the fevers caused by intestinal bacteria, including typhoid fever, paratyphoid fever, etc.

enterointestinal (en"ter-o-in-tes'tĭ-nal) [*entero-* + *intestine*] intestino-intestinal.

enterokinase (en"ter-o-ki'nās) enteropeptidase.

enterokinesia (en"ter-o-ki'ne'se-ah) peristalsis.

enterokinetic (en"ter-o-ki-net'ik) pertaining to or stimulating peristalsis.

enterokinin (en"ter-o-ki'nin) an extract of the mucosa of the small intestine, said to be a physiological hormone, which stimulates intestinal motility.

enterolith (en'ter-o-lith") [*entero-* + Gr. *lithos* stone] an intestinal calculus; any concretion found in the intestine.

enterolithiasis (en"ter-o-lĭ-thi'ah-sis) [*entero-* + *lithiasis*] a condition characterized by the presence of intestinal calculi.

enterology (en"ter-ol'o-je) [*entero-* + *-logy*] the sum of what is known regarding the intestines.

enterolysis (en"ter-ol'ĭ-sis) [*entero-* + Gr. *lysis* dissolution] the operative division of adhesions between loops of intestine or between the intestine and abdominal wall.

enteromegalia (en"ter-o-mĕ-ga'le-ah) enteromegaly.

enteromegaly (en"ter-o-meg'ah-le) [*entero-* + Gr. *megaleia* bigness] enlargement of the intestine.

enteromere (en'ter-o-mēr") [*entero-* + Gr. *meros* part] any segment of the embryonic alimentary tract.

enteromerocele (en"ter-o-me'ro-sēl) [*entero-* + Gr. *mēros* thigh + *kēlē* hernia] femoral hernia.

Enteromonas (en"ter-o-mo'nas) a genus of extremely small, spherical or piriform protozoa of the order Polymastigida, class Zoomastigophora, having three anterior flagella and a fourth trailing from the posterior end of the body. *Tricercomonas* is believed to be identical with this organism. **E. hom'inis,** a species found as a commensal in the human intestine.

enteromycodermitis (en"ter-o-mi"ko-der-mi'tis) [*entero-* + Gr. *myxa* mucus + *derma* skin] endoenteritis.

enteromycosis (en"ter-o-mi-ko'sis) [*entero-* + Gr. *mykēs* fungus + *-osis*] disease of the intestine due to bacteria or fungi. **e. bacteria'cea,** a general name for certain infections of the intestine due to nonspecific bacteria.

enteromyiasis (en"ter-o-mi-i'ah-sis) [*entero-* + Gr. *myia* fly] presence of larvae of flies in the intestine.

enteron (en'ter-on) [Gr.] the gut or alimentary canal; usually used in medicine with specific reference to the small intestine.

enteroneuritis (en"ter-o-nu-ri'tis) inflammation of the nerves of the intestine.

enteronitis (en"ter-o-ni'tis) enteritis. **polytropous e.** (*obs.*), acute infectious gastroenteritis.

enteroparesis (en"ter-o-par'e-sis) [*entero-* + Gr. *paresis* relaxation] relaxation of the intestine resulting in dilatation.

enteropathogen (en″ter-o-path′o-jen) a microorganism which causes a disease of the intestines.

enteropathogenesis (en″ter-o-path″o-jen′ĕ-sis) the production of disease or disorder of the intestines.

enteropathogenic (en″ter-o-path″o-jen′ik) pertaining to or effective in production of disease of the intestines.

enteropathy (en″ter-op′ah-the) [*entero-* + Gr. *pathos* illness] any disease of the intestine. **gluten e.,** nontropical sprue. **protein-losing e.,** a nonspecific term referring to conditions associated with excessive enteric loss of plasma protein. It occurs in extensive ulceration (e.g., inflammatory bowel disease), diffuse mucosal disease (e.g., adult celiac disease) in which there is more rapid desquamation of mucosal epithelial cells, and in intestinal lymphatic obstruction (intestinal lymphangiectasia).

enteropeptidase (en″ter-o-pep′tĭ-dās) an enzyme of the intestinal juice which activates the proteolytic enzyme of the pancreatic juice by converting trypsinogen into trypsin. Called also *enterokinase.*

enteropexy (en′ter-o-pek″se) [*entero-* + Gr. *pēxis* fixation] surgical fixation of the intestine to the anterior or posterior abdominal wall, or occasionally of one segment to another.

enteroplasty (en′ter-o-plas″te) [*entero-* + Gr. *plassein* to mold] plastic surgery of the intestine, especially to enlarge the caliber of a constricted segment or area of bowel.

enteroplegia (en″ter-o-ple′je-ah) [*entero-* + Gr. *plēgē* stroke] adynamic ileus.

enteroproctia (en″ter-o-prok′she-ah) [*entero-* + Gr. *prōktos* anus] the condition of having an artificial anus.

enteroptosia (en″ter-op-to′se-ah) enteroptosis.

enteroptosis (en″ter-op-to′sis) [*entero-* + Gr. *ptōsis* fall] descent or downward displacement of the intestine in the abdominal cavity; a term based on the outmoded concept that variation of position of abdominal organs are pathological.

enteroptotic (en″ter-op-tot′ik) pertaining to or characterized by enteroptosis.

enteroptychia, enteroptychy (en″ter-o-ti′ke-ah; en″ter-o-ti′ke) [*entero-* + Gr. *ptychē* a fold] plication of the intestine, an operation for the prevention of intestinal adhesions.

enterorenal (en″ter-o-re′nal) pertaining to the intestine and the kidney.

enterorrhagia (en″ter-o-ra′je-ah) [*entero-* + Gr. *rhēgnynai* to burst forth] hemorrhage from the intestine.

enterorrhaphy (en″ter-or′ah-fe) [*entero-* + Gr. *rhaphē* suture] repair or suture of the intestine. **circular e.,** the suturing of two completely divided portions of intestine after invaginating one segment over the other so that they are joined end to end.

enterorrhea (en″ter-o-re′ah) diarrhea.

enterorrhexis (en″ter-o-rek′sis) [*entero-* + Gr. *rhēxis* rupture] rupture of the intestine.

enteroscope (en′ter-o-skōp″) [*entero-* + Gr. *skopein* to examine] an endoscope for examining the lumen of the intestine.

enterosepsis (en″ter-o-sep′sis) [*entero-* + Gr. *sēpsis* putrefaction] intestinal sepsis due to putrefaction of the contents of the intestines.

enterosite (en′ter-o-sīt″) (*obs.*) an intestinal parasite.

enterosorption (en″ter-o-sorp′shun) accumulation of a substance in the bowel by virtue of its passage from the circulating blood; occurring when its exsorption exceeds its insorption.

enterospasm (en′ter-o-spazm″) [*entero-* + Gr. *spasmos* spasm] a spasm of the intestine.

enterostasis (en″ter-o-sta′sis) [*entero-* + Gr. *stasis* stoppage] intestinal stasis.

enterostaxis (en″ter-o-stak′sis) [*entero-* + Gr. *staxis* dripping] slow hemorrhage through the intestinal mucous membrane.

enterostenosis (en″ter-o-stĕ-no′sis) [*entero-* + Gr. *stenōsis* contraction] narrowing or stricture of the intestine.

enterostomal (en″ter-o-sto′mal) relating to or having undergone enterostomy.

enterostomy (en″ter-os′to-me) [*entero-* + Gr. *stomoun* to provide with an opening, or mouth] the formation of a permanent opening into the intestine through the abdominal wall, usually by surgical means; also, the opening so created. **gun-barrel e.,** enterostomy in which the two segments of the divided intestine are parallel to one another as they emerge through the abdominal wall, like the tubes of a double-barreled shotgun.

enterotome (en′ter-o-tōm″) [*entero-* + Gr. *tomē* a cutting] an instrument for cutting the intestine. **Dupuytren's e.,** a cutting forceps used in making an artificial anus.

enterotomy (en″ter-ot′o-me) [*entero-* + Gr. *tomē* a cutting] incision into the intestine.

enterotoxemia (en″ter-o-tok-se′me-ah) a condition characterized by presence in the blood of toxins produced in the intestines. **hemorrhagic e.,** struck. **infectious e. of sheep,** pulpy kidney disease (q.v., under *disease*) of sheep.

enterotoxication (en″ter-o-tok″sĭ-ka′shun) enterotoxism.

enterotoxigenic (en″ter-o-tok″sĭ-jen′ik) producing or containing a toxin specific for the cells of the intestinal mucosa.

enterotoxin (en″ter-o-tok′sin) 1. a toxin specific for the cells of the intestinal mucosa. 2. a toxin arising in the intestine. 3. an exotoxin that is protein in nature and relatively heat stable, produced by staphylococci, primarily by coagulase-positive *Staphylococcus pyogenes* var. *aureus.* Enterotoxin, which on ingestion produces violent vomiting and diarrhea, is the primary factor in staphylococcal food poisoning.

enterotoxism (en″ter-o-tok′sizm) autointoxication of enteric origin.

enterotropic (en″ter-o-trop′ik) [*entero-* + Gr. *tropos* a turning] having a special affinity for or exerting its principal effect upon the intestines.

enterotyphus (en″ter-o-ti′fus) typhoid fever.

enterovaginal (en″ter-o-vaj′ĭ-nal) pertaining to or communicating with the intestine and the vagina, as an enterovaginal fistula.

enterovenous (en″ter-o-ve′nus) communicating between the intestinal lumen and the lumen of a vein.

enterovesical (en″ter-o-ves′ĭ-kal) pertaining to or communicating with the intestine and urinary bladder, as an enterovesical fistula.

Entero-Vioform (en″ter-o-vi′o-form) trademark for a preparation of iodochlorhydroxyquin.

enteroviral (en″ter-o-vi′ral) pertaining to or caused by enteroviruses.

enterovirus (en″ter-o-vi′rus) one of a subgroup of the picornaviruses infecting the gastrointestinal tract and discharged in the excreta, including poliovirus, the coxsackieviruses, and the echoviruses.

enterozoic (en″ter-o-zo′ik) relating to or caused by an enterozoon.

enterozoon (en″ter-o-zo′on), pl. *enterozo′a* [*entero-* + Gr. *zōon* animal] an animal parasite or species inhabiting or infecting the intestinal canal.

enteruria (en″ter-u′re-ah) [*entero-* + Gr. *ouron* urine + *-ia*] the presence of fecal constituents in the urine.

enthalpy (en′thal-pe) [Gr. *en* within + *thalpein* to warm] the heat content or chemical energy of a physical system; it is a thermodynamic function equal to the internal energy plus the product of the pressure and volume.

enthesis (en′the-sis) [Gr. "a putting in; insertion"] 1. the use of artificial material in the repair of a defect or deformity of the body. 2. the site of attachment of a muscle or ligament to bone.

enthesitis (en-thĕ-si′tis) inflammation of the muscular or tendinous attachment to bone.

enthetic (en-thet′ik) [Gr. *enthetikos* fit for implanting] 1. pertaining to enthesis. 2. introduced from without.

enthetobiosis (en-thet″o-bi-o′sis) [Gr. *enthesis* a putting in + *biōsis* way of life] dependency on a mechanical implant, as on an artificial cardiac pacemaker.

enthlasis (en′thlah-sis) [Gr. "a dent caused by pressure"] comminuted fracture of the skull, with depression of the bony fragments.

entiris (en-ti′ris) [Gr. *entos* within + *iris* iris] the posterior pigment layer of the iris.

entity (en′tĭ-te) [L. *ens* being] an independently existing thing; a reality.

ento-, ent- [Gr. *entos* inside] a prefix signifying within, or inner.

entoblast (en′to-blast) [*ento-* + Gr. *blastos* germ] 1. entoderm. 2. a cell nucleolus.

entocele (en′to-sēl) [*ento-* + Gr. *kēlē* hernia] an internal hernia.

entochondrostosis (en″to-kon″dros-to′sis) [*ento-* + Gr. *chondros* cartilage + *osteon* bone] the development of bone taking place within cartilage.

entochoroidea (en″to-ko-roid′e-ah) [*ento-* + Gr. *chorioeidēs* choroid] the inner layer of the choroid coat of the eye.

entocnemial (en″tok-ne′me-al) on the inner side of the tibia.

entocone (en′to-kōn) [*ento-* + Gr. *kōnos* cone] the medial posterior cusp of a maxillary molar.

entoconid (en″to-ko′nid) [*ento-* + Gr. *kōnos* cone] the medial posterior cusp of a mandibular molar.

entocornea (en″to-kor′ne-ah) [*ento-* + *cornea*] lamina limitans posterior cornea.

entocranial (en″to-kra′ne-al) endocranial.

entocuneiform (en″to-ku′ne-ĭ-form) os cuneiform mediale.

entocyte (en′to-sīt) [*ento-* + Gr. *kytos* hollow vessel] the cell contents.

entoderm (en′to-derm) [*ento-* + Gr. *derma* skin] the innermost of the three primary germ layers of the embryo; from it are derived the epithelium of the pharynx, respiratory tract (except the nose), the digestive tract, bladder and urethra. Called also *endoderm, endoblast, entoblast,* and *hypoblast.* Cf. *ectoderm* and *mesoderm.*

primitive e., the primary internal layer of the gastrula that becomes both gut and yolk sac. **yolk-sac e.,** the epithelial lining of the yolk sac.

entodermal (en″to-der′mal)   pertaining to or derived from the entoderm.

entodermic (en″to-der′mik)   entodermal.

entoectad (en″to-ek′tad) [ento- + Gr. *ektos* without]   directed or proceeding from within outward.

entome (en′tōm) [Gr. *entemnein* to cut in]   an instrument for cutting urethral strictures.

entomere (en′to-mēr) [ento- + Gr. *meros* part]   a blastomere destined to become entoderm.

entomesoderm (en″to-mes′o-derm)   endomesoderm.

entomion (en-to′me-on) [Gr. *entomē* notch]   the point at the tip of the mastoid angle of the parietal bone in the parietal notch of the temporal bone.

entomo- (en′to-mo) [Gr. *entomon* insect]   a combining form denoting relationship to an insect, or to insects.

Entomobrya (en″to-mo-bri′ah)   a genus of insects, the spring tails, of the order Collembola, Australian species of which cause irritation by their bite.

entomogenous (en″to-moj′ĕ-nus) [entomo- + Gr. *gennan* to produce]   1. derived from insects, their bites, emanations, etc. 2. growing in the body of an insect.

entomologist (en″to-mol′o-jist)   an expert in entomology.

entomology (en″to-mol′o-je) [entomo- + *-logy*]   that branch of zoology which deals with the study of insects. **medical e.,** that concerned with insects that cause disease or serve as vectors of microorganisms that cause disease in man.

entomophilous (en″to-mof′ĭ-lus) [entomo- + Gr. *philein* to love]   fertilized by insect-borne pollen; said of certain flowers.

Entomophthora (en″to-mof′thor-ah) [entomo- + Gr. *phthora* destruction, death]   a genus of phycomycetous fungi of the order Entomophthorales, which comprises pathogens of insects and spiders. Formerly called *Empusa*. **E. corona′ta,** a parasite of spiders, termites, and other insects, which causes a subcutaneous infection of the nose (rhinoentomophthoromycosis) in man, and has been isolated from nasal polyps in horses. **E. mus′cae,** a species developing in the bodies of flies, thus destroying them.

Entomophthoraceae (en″to-mof″tho-ra′se-e)   a family of fungi of the order Entomophthorales, subclass Zygomycetes, found as parasites on man, horses, and insects; it includes the genera *Basidiobolus* and *Entomophthora*.

Entomophthorales (en″to-mof″tho-ra′lēz)   an order of phycomycetous fungi of the subclass Zygomycetes, which are typically parasites of insects, but may cause entomophthoromycosis in man; it includes the family Entomophthoraceae.

entomophthoromycosis (en″to-mof″tho-ro-mi-ko′sis)   any disease caused by phycomycetous fungi of the order Entomophthorales, such as rhinoentomophthoromycosis and subcutaneous phycomycosis.

Entomospira (en″to-mo-spi′rah) [entomo- + Gr. *speira* coil]   a genus name formerly given certain spirochetal microorganisms, now included in the genus *Borrelia*.

entophthalmia (en″tof-thal′me-ah)   inflammation of the inner parts of the eyeball.

entophyte (en′to-fīt) [ento- + Gr. *phyton* plant]   endophyte.

entopic (en-top′ik) [Gr. *en* in + *topos* place]   occurring in the proper place, as opposed to ectopic.

entoplasm (en′to-plazm) [ento- + Gr. *plasma* something formed]   1. endoplasm. 2. (*obs.*) the blue-staining, or nonchromatinic, portion of certain bacteria.

entoplastic (en″to-plas′ik) [ento- + Gr. *plastikos* formative]   having a formative power lodged within.

entoptic (en-top′tik) [ento- + Gr. *optikos* seeing]   denoting visual phenomena which have their seat within the eye.

entoptoscope (en-top′to-skōp)   an instrument for examining the media of the eyes, to ascertain their transparency.

entoptoscopy (en″top-tos′ko-pe) [ento- + Gr. *ōps* eye + *skopein* to examine]   the observation of the interior of the eye and its light and shadows.

entoretina (en″to-ret′ĭ-nah) [ento- + *retina*]   the internal or nervous portion of the retina, disposed in five layers, which are named respectively outer molecular, inner nuclear, inner molecular, ganglion, and nerve fiber layers.

entorganism (ent-or′gan-izm) [ento- + *organism*]   endoparasite.

entosarc (en′to-sark) [ento- + Gr. *sarx* flesh]   endoplasm.

entosthoblast (en-tos′tho-blast) [Gr. *entosthen* from within + *blastos* germ]   the hypothetical nucleus of the nucleolus.

entostosis (ent″os-to′sis) [ento- + Gr. *osteon* bone]   enostosis.

entotympanic (en″to-tim-pan′ik)   within the tympanum of the ear.

entozoa (en″to-zo′ah) [Gr.]   plural of *entozoon*.

entozoal (en″to-zo′al)   pertaining to or caused by entozoa.

entozoon (en″to-zo′on), pl. *entozo′a* [ento- + Gr. *zōon* animal]   a parasitic animal organism living within the body of its host.

entripsis (en-trip′sis) [Gr. *en* in + *tripsis* rubbing]   inunction.

entropion (en-tro′pe-on) [Gr. *en* in + *tropein* to turn]   the turning inward (inversion) of an edge or margin, as of the margin of the eyelid, with the tarsal cartilage turned inward toward the eyeball; called also *blepharelosis*. **e. cicatric′eum, cicatricial e.,** inversion of the margin of an eyelid caused by contraction of scar tissue in the palpebral conjunctiva or underlying tarsus. **spastic e., e. spas′ticum,** inversion of the eyelid caused by tonic spasm of the orbicularis oculi muscle. **e. u′veae,** inversion of the margin of the pupil, usually the result of an iritis attended with exudate, and occurring rarely as a congenital condition.

entropionize (en-tro′pe-o-nīz″)   to put into a state of entropion or inversion; to turn inward.

entropium (en-tro′pe-um)   entropion.

entropy (en′tro-pe) [Gr. *entropē* a turning inward]   1. diminished capacity for spontaneous change, as occurs in aging. 2. the measure of that part of the heat or energy of a system which is not available to perform work; entropy increases in all natural (spontaneous and irreversible) processes.

entsulfon sodium (ent′sul-fon)   chemical name: 2-[2-[2-[4-(1,1,3,3-tetramethylbutyl)phenoxy]ethoxy]ethonesulfonic acid sodium salt; a detergent, $C_{20}H_{33}NaO_6S$.

entwicklungsmechanik (ent″wik-lungs″mĕ-kan′ik)   [Ger. "developmental mechanics"]   mechanisms of embryological development, as revealed by experimental study.

entypy (en′ti-pe) [Gr. *entypē* pattern]   a method of gastrulation in which the entoderm lies external to the amniotic ectoderm.

enucleate (e-nu′kle-āt) [L. *enucleare*]   to remove whole and clean, as a tumor from its envelope or the eyeball; see *enucleation*.

enucleated (e-nu′kle-āt″ed)   removed; said of an organ, tumor, or cell nucleus.

enucleation (e-nu″kle-a′shun) [L. *e* out + *nucleus* kernel]   the removal of an organ, of a tumor, or of another body in such a way that it comes out clean and whole, like a nut from its shell. Used in connection with the eye, it denotes removal of the eyeball after the eye muscles and optic nerve have been severed.

enuresis (en″u-re′sis) [Gr. *enourein* to void urine]   involuntary discharge of the urine; often used alone with specific reference to involuntary discharge of urine occurring during sleep at night (*bed-wetting; nocturnal enuresis*).

enuretic (en″u-ret′ik)   1. pertaining to enuresis. 2. an agent which causes enuresis. 3. a person who exhibits enuresis.

envelope (en′vĕ-lōp)   an encompassing structure or membrane. In virology, a coat surrounding the capsid and usually furnished at least partially by the host cell. In bacteriology, the cell wall and the plasma membrane considered together. **cell e.,** the plasma membrane and the cell wall considered together. **egg e.,** egg membrane; see under *membrane*. **nuclear e.,** the condensed double layer of lipids and proteins enclosing the cell nucleus and separating it from the cytoplasm; its two concentric membranes, inner and outer, are separated by a perinuclear space. Called also *nuclear membrane*.

envenomation (en-ven″o-ma′shun)   the poisonous effects caused by the bites, stings, or effluvia of insects and other arthropods, or the bites of snakes.

environment (en-vi′ron-ment) [Fr. *environner* to surround, to encircle]   the sum total of all the conditions and elements which make up the surroundings and influence the development of an individual.

envy (en′ve)   a desire to have another's possessions or qualities for oneself. **penis e.,** in psychoanalytic theory, the desire of the female to possess a penis; more generally, the female wish for male attributes.

Enzactin (en-zak′tin)   trademark for preparations of triacetin.

enzootic (en″zo-ot′ik) [Gr. *en* in + *zōon* animal]   1. present in an animal community at all times, but occurring in only small numbers of cases. 2. a disease of low morbidity which is constantly present in an animal community.

Enzopride (en′zo-prīd)   trademark for a preparation of nadide.

enzygotic (en″zi-got′ik)   developed from the same fertilized ovum.

enzymatic (en″zi-mat′ik)   relating to, caused by, or of the nature of an enzyme.

enzyme (en′zīm) [Gr. *en* in + *zymē* leaven]   a protein produced in a cell and capable of greatly accelerating by its catalytic action the chemical reaction of a substance (the substrate) for which it is often specific. Enzymes perform this function without being destroyed or altered. They are divided into six main groups: oxidoreductases, transferases, hydrolases, lyases, isomerases, and ligases. **activating e.,** an enzyme that activates a given amino acid by attaching it to the corresponding transfer ribonucleic acid (t-RNA). **adaptive e.,** induced e. **adding e.,** enzymes that catalyze the addition of a fragment to a molecule, e.g., the addition of CO_2 to a molecule, with the formation of a new carboxyl group. **allosteric e.,** one containing an allosteric site; see under *site*. **amylolytic e.,** one that catalyzes the conversion of starch into sugar. **autolytic e.,** one that produces autolysis or digestion of the cell in which it exists. **bacterial e.,** an enzyme existing in or secreted by a bacterium. **brancher e., branching e.,** α-glucan-branching glycosyltransferase; see under *glycosyltransferase*. **catheptic e.,** cathepsin. **clotting e., coagulating e.,** an enzyme, such as rennin and fibrin ferment, that catalyzes the conversion of soluble into insoluble proteins; called also *curdling e.* **constitutive e.,** one produced by a microorganism regardless of the presence or absence of the specific substrate. Cf. *induced e.* **converting e.,** an enzyme that catalyzes the conversion of angiotensin I to angiotensin II; it occurs in the blood plasma and in high concentrations in the lungs. **curdling e.,** clotting e. **debrancher e., debranching e.,** dextrin-1-6-glucosidase. **digestive e.,** a substance that catalyzes the process of digestion. **extracellular e.,** one that exists outside of the cell secreting it. **fat-splitting e.,** lipolytic e. **glycolytic e.,** one that catalyzes the conversion of sugar to pyruvic acid. **hydrolytic e.,** one that catalyzes hydrolysis; a hydrolase. **induced e.,** one whose production requires or is markedly stimulated by a specific small molecule, the *inducer*, which is the substrate of the enzyme or a compound structurally related to it. The inducers studied first were substrates whose utilization thus became possible; hence these enzymes were known earlier as *adaptive enzymes*. Cf. *constitutive e.* **inducible e.,** induced e. **inhibitory e.,** one whose action blocks another reaction or a reaction sequence. **intracellular e.,** one that is contained within the cell secreting it. **inverting e.,** one that catalyzes the hydrolysis of sucrose. **lipolytic e.,** one that catalyzes the hydrolysis of fat; called also *fat-splitting e.* and *steatolytic e.* **malic e.,** an enzyme that catalyzes the decarboxylation of malate to pyruvate with the accompanying conversion of NADP to NADP and H⁺. **microsomal e's,** enzymes associated with the thin tubular network of endoplasmic reticulum (or microsomes) of cells, especially such enzymes of the liver. **milk-curdling e.,** rennin. **mucolytic e.,** one that catalyzes the hydrolytic depolymerization of mucopolysaccharides. **old yellow e.,** a flavoprotein found in yeast, reduced NADP dehydrogenase, that catalyzes the oxidation of NADP by cytochrome C. **oxidation e.,** oxidase. **proteolytic e.,** one that catalyzes the hydrolysis of proteins and various split products of protein, the final product being small peptides and amino acids. **Q e.,** α-glucan-branching glycosyltransferase; see under *glycosyltransferase*. **receptor-destroying e.,** one that renders red cells insusceptible to viral hemolysis by destroying its receptors. **redox e.,** one that catalyzes oxidation-reduction reactions. **reducing e.,** reductase. **repressible e.,** one whose rate of production is decreased as the concentration of certain metabolites is increased. **respiratory e.,** an enzyme system that catalyzes the oxidation of a substrate by oxygen of the air. **restriction e.,** any of the enzymes that catalyze the splitting of a gene from the DNA molecule; specific enzymes split off specific genes. **Schardinger's e.,** xanthine oxidase. **splitting e.,** one that catalyzes the splitting of a fragment from a molecule, e.g., the splitting out of CO₂ from a carboxyl group (decarboxylation). **steatolytic e.,** lipolytic e. **transferring e.,** one which catalyzes the transfer of various radicals between molecules; a transferase. **urea e.,** urease. **uricolytic e.,** one that catalyzes the conversion of uric acid into urea. **yellow e's,** a number of flavoproteins which have been isolated from various sources and which take part in oxidations and reductions.

enzymic (en-zim′ik) enzymatic.

enzymoimmunoelectrophoresis (en″zi-mo-im″mu-no-e-lek″-tro-fo-re′sis) immunoelectrophoresis for the detection and identification of proteins with enzymatic activity, utilizing selective stains for enzymes, rather than a protein stain such as amido black.

enzymology (en″zi-mol′o-je) the study of enzymes and enzymatic action.

enzymolysis (en″zi-mol′ĭ-sis) [*enzyme* + Gr. *lysis* dissolution] the disintegrative action or reaction produced by an enzyme.

enzymopathy (en″zi-mop′ah-the) an inborn error of metabolism consisting of defective or absent enzymes, as in the glycogen storage diseases or the mucopolysaccharidoses. **lysosomal e.,** lysosomal storage disease.

enzymosis (en″zi-mo′sis) [*enzyme* + *-osis*] (*obs.*) fermentation induced by an enzyme.

enzymuria (en″zi-mu′re-ah) [*enzyme* + *urine*] the presence of enzymes in the urine.

EOG electro-olfactogram.

EOM extraocular movement.

eonism (e′o-nizm) [Chevalier *d'Eon*, French political adventurer, 1728–1810; having adopted woman's dress when sent on a secret mission to Russia in 1755, he was later forced by decree of Louis XVI to wear such apparel to the end of his life] transvestism in the male.

eopsia (e-op′se-ah) [Gr. *ēōs* dawn + *opsis* vision] orthropsia.

eosin (e′o-sin) [Gr. *ēōs* dawn] a rose-colored stain or dye: typically the sodium salt of tetrabromfluorescein, $C_{20}H_6Br_4Na_2O_5$, C.I.

45380. Commercially, several other red coal tar dyes are called eosin. All the eosins are bromine derivatives of fluorescin. Eosin is an important plasma stain, used especially with hematoxylin, methylene blue, and methyl green. **e. B, e. I bluish,** dibromodinitrofluorescein, a dye having staining properties similar to eosin, but of a distinctly bluer shade. **ethyl e.,** the ethyl ester of eosin. **water-soluble e., e. W or W S, yellowish e., e. Y,** eosin.

eosinocyte (e″o-sin′o-sīt) eosinophil.

eosinopenia (e″o-sin-o-pe′ne-ah) [*eosinophil* + Gr. *penia* poverty] abnormal deficiency of eosinophilic leukocytes in the blood.

eosinophil (e″o-sin′o-fil) [*eosin* + Gr. *philein* to love] a structure, cell, or histologic element readily stained by eosin, especially a granular leukocyte with a nucleus that usually has two lobes connected by a slender thread of chromatin, and cytoplasm containing coarse, round granules that are uniform in size; called also *acidocyte, eosinocyte, eosinophilic leukocyte,* and *Rindfleisch's cell.*

eosinophile (e″o-sin′o-fīl) 1. eosinophil. 2. eosinophilic.

eosinophilia (e″o-sin″o-fil′e-ah) [*eosin* + Gr. *philein* to love] 1. the formation and accumulation of an abnormally large number of eosinophils in the blood. 2. the condition of being readily stained with eosin. **Löffler's e.,** see under *syndrome*. **pulmonary infiltration e.,** infiltration of the pulmonary parenchyma by eosinophils, as in Löffler's syndrome. **tropical e., tropical pulmonary e.,** a disease occurring in certain parts of India, characterized clinically by anorexia, malaise, cough, leukocytosis, and an absolute increase in eosinophils; called also *Weingarten's disease* or *syndrome, eosinophilic lung,* and *Frimodt-Möller and Barton disease.*

eosinophilic (e″o-sin″o-fil′ik) readily stainable with eosin.

eosinophilopoietin (e″o-sin″o-fil″o-poi′ĕ-tin) a peptide of low molecular weight that induces production of eosinophils.

eosinophilosis (e″o-sin″o-fĭ-lo′sis) eosinophilia, def. 1. **pulmonary e., tropical e.,** tropical eosinophilia.

eosinophilotactic (e″o-sin″o-fil″o-tak′tik) having the power of attracting eosinophils; chemotactic for eosinophils.

eosinophilous (e″o-sin-of′ĭ-lus) eosinophilic.

eosinotactic (e″o-sin″o-tak′tik) [*eosinophil* + Gr. *taktikos* regulating] exhibiting an influence on eosinophilic cells, either repelling them (*negatively e.*) or attracting them (*positively e.*).

eosolate (e-o′so-lāt) acetyl guaiacol trisulfonate; the silver salt is used as an antiseptic.

ep- see *epi-*.

epacmastic (ep″ak-mas′tik) pertaining to the epacme.

epacme (ep-ak′me) [Gr. *epakmazein* to come to its height] in evolution, the stage or period of development.

epactal (e-pak′tal) [Gr. *epaktos* brought in] 1. supernumerary 2. a wormian bone; see *ossa suturarum*.

epallobiosis (ep-al″lo-bi-o′sis) [*epi-* + Gr. *allo-* other + *biōsis* way of life] dependency on an external life-support system, as on a heart-lung machine or hemodialyzer.

eparsalgia (ep″ar-sal′je-ah) [Gr. *epairein* to lift + *-algia*] any painful disorder due to overstrain of a part, including dilatation of the heart, hernia, enteroptosis, coughing, etc.

eparterial (ep″ar-te′re-al) [Gr. *epi* upon + *artēria* artery] over an artery; applied especially to the first branch of the right primary bronchus which is so situated.

epaxial (ep-ak′se-al) [Gr. *epi* upon + *axis*] situated upon or above an axis.

epencephal (ep″en-sef′al) epencephalon.

epencephalic (ep″en-se-fal′ik) pertaining to the epencephalon.

epencephalon (ep″en-sef′ah-lon) [Gr. *epi* upon + *enkephalos* brain] 1. cerebellum. 2. metencephalon.

ependopathy (ep″en-dop′ah-the) ependymopathy.

ependyma (ĕ-pen′dĭ-mah) [Gr. *ependyma* upper garment] [NA] the lining membrane of the ventricles of the brain and of the central canal of the spinal cord.

ependymal (ĕ-pen′dĭ-mal) pertaining to or composed of ependyma.

ependymitis (ĕ-pen″dĭ-mi′tis) inflammation of the ependyma.

ependymoblast (ĕ-pen′dĭ-mo-blast) an embryonic ependymal cell; an ependymal spongioblast.

ependymoblastoma (ĕ-pen″dĭ-mo-blas-to′mah) a malignant tumor composed of primitive ependymal cells; some neuropathologists classify such tumors as malignant ependymoma.

ependymocyte (ĕ-pen′dĭ-mo-sīt″) [*ependyma* + Gr. *kytos* hollow vessel] an ependymal cell.

ependymocytoma (ĕ-pen″dĭ-mo-si-to′mah) ependymoma.

ependymoma (ĕ-pen″dĭ-mo′mah) a neoplasm composed of differentiated ependymal cells; most ependymomas are slow growing and benign, but malignant varieties occur.

ependymopathy (ĕ-pen″dĭ-mop′ah-the) disease of the ependyma.

eperythrozoon (ep″ĕ-rith″ro-zo′on) [Gr. *epi* upon + *erythros* red + *zōon* animal] a genus of microorganisms of the family

Bartonellaceae, order Rickettsiales, occurring as seven species, of limited pathogenicity, which infect rodents, cattle, sheep, and swine.

eperythrozoonosis (ep″ĕ-rith″ro-zo″o-no′sis)   infection with organisms of the genus *Eperythrozoon.*

ephapse (e-faps′) [Gr. *ephapsis* a touching]   a point of lateral contact (other than a synapse) between nerve fibers across which impulses are conducted directly through the nerve membranes from one fiber to the other. Cf. *synapse.*

ephaptic (e-fap′tik)   denoting the conduction of a nerve impulse across an ephapse, as opposed to synaptic conduction.

epharmony (ep-har′mo-ne)   development in complete harmony with environment; harmonic relation between structure and environment.

ephebiatrics (ĕ-fe″be-at′riks) [Gr. *ephēbos* one arrived at puberty + *iatrikē* surgery, medicine]   that department of medicine which deals especially with the diagnosis and treatment of the diseases of youth (18–25 years).

ephebic (ĕ-feb′ik) [Gr. *ephēbikos* pertaining to puberty]   pertaining to youth or the period of puberty and adolescence.

ephebogenesis (ef″ĕ-bo-jen′ĕ-sis) [Gr. *ephēbos* one arrived at puberty + *genesis*]   the bodily changes occurring at puberty.

ephebogenic (ef″e-bo-jen′ik)   pertaining to or caused by ephebogenesis.

ephebology (ef″ĕ-bol′o-je) [Gr. *ephēbos* one arrived at puberty + *-logy*]   the study of puberty.

Ephedra (e-fed′rah) [Gr. *epi* upon + *hedra* seat]   a genus of low, branching, gnetaceous shrubs indigenous to China and India. *E. equisetina, E. sinica, E. vulgaris,* and other species, known as *ma huang* in China, furnish ephedrine.

ephedrine (ĕ-fed′rin, ef′ĕ-drin) [USP]   chemical name: [*R*-(*R**, *S**)]-α-[1-(methylamino)ethyl]benzenemethanol. An adrenergic, $C_{10}H_{15}NO$, obtained from *Ephedra* species or prepared synthetically, occurring as an unctuous, almost colorless solid or white crystals or granules. Its principal uses, in the form of the hydrochloride or sulfate salt, are: to decongest the nasal mucosa in allergic states and to relax bronchiolar muscles in bronchial asthma; to stimulate the central nervous system in narcolepsy and in poisoning by central nervous system depressants; to prevent hypotension during spinal and infiltration anesthesia; and as a mydriatic.   **e. hydrochloride** [USP], the hydrochloride salt of ephedrine, $C_{10}H_{15}NO \cdot HCl$, occurring as fine, white crystals or as a powder, having the same actions, uses, and routes of administration as the sulfate salt.   **e. sulfate** [USP], the sulfate salt of ephedrine, $(C_{10}H_{15}NO)_2H_2SO_4$, occurring as fine, white crystals or powder, having the same actions as the base; administered orally, parenterally, or intranasally.

ephelides (ĕ-fel′ĭ-dēz) [Gr.]   plural of *ephelis.*

ephelis (ĕ-fe′lis), pl. *ephel′ides* [Gr. *ephēlis*]   a freckle.

ephemera (ĕ-fem′er-ah) [Gr. *ephēmeros* short-lived]   a transitory condition or thing.

ephemeral (ĕ-fem′er-al)   short-lived; transient.

Ephemerida (e″fĕ-mer′ĭ-dah)   a family of flies (class Insecta), the exuviae of which may cause sensitization and severe asthmatic paroxysms when inhaled.

ephippium (ep-hip′e-um) [Gr. *epi* upon + *hippos* horse]   (*obs.*) sella turcica.

Ephynal (ef′ĭ-nal)   trademark for a preparation of vitamin E; see *tocopherol.*

epi-, ep- [Gr. *epi* on]   a prefix denoting on, upon, or over.

epiallopregnanolone (ep″ĭ-al″o-preg-nan′o-lōn)   a male sex hormone extracted from pregnancy urine, which aids in the development of male sex characteristics; abbreviated EAP.

epiandrosterone (ep″ĭ-an-dros′ter-ōn)   chemical name: 3β-hydroxy-17-androstanone. An androgenic steroid, one of the urinary 17-ketosteroids, less active than androsterone and excreted in small amounts in normal human urine. Called also *isoandrosterone.*

epiblast (ep′ĭ-blast) [*epi-* + Gr. *blastos* germ]   1. ectoderm.   2. ectoderm, except for the neural plate.

epiblastic (ep″ĭ-blas′tik)   pertaining to or arising from the epiblast; ectodermal.

epiblepharon (ep″ĭ-blef′ah-ron) [*epi-* + Gr. *blepharon* eyelid]   a developmental anomaly in which a horizontal fold of skin stretches across the border of the eyelid, pressing the eyelashes inward against the eyelid.

epibole (e-pib′o-le)   epiboly.

epiboly (e-pib′o-le) [Gr. *epibolē* cover]   a method of gastrulation by which the smaller blastomeres at the animal pole of the fertilized ovum grow over and enclose the cells of the vegetal hemisphere.

epibulbar (ep″ĭ-bul′bar)   upon the eyeball.

epicanthal, epicanthic (ep″ĭ-kan′thal; ep″ĭ-kan′thik)   1. pertaining to the epicanthus.   2. overlying the canthus.

epicanthine (ep″ĭ-kan′thin)   epicanthal.

epicanthus (ep″ĭ-kan′thus) [*epi-* + Gr. *kanthos* canthus]   a ver-

tical fold of skin on either side of the nose, sometimes covering the inner canthus. It is present as a normal characteristic in persons of certain races and sometimes occurs as a congenital anomaly in others. Called also *epicanthic fold, palpebronasal fold,* and *plica palpebronasalis* [NA].

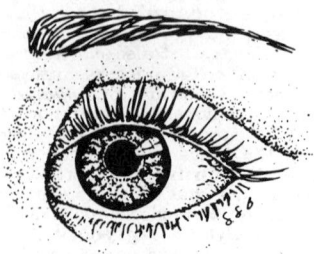

Epicanthus.

epicarcinogen (ep″ĭ-kar-sin′o-jen)   an agent that increases the effect of a carcinogen.

epicardia (ep″ĭ-kar′de-ah)   the lower portion of the esophagus, extending from the hiatus esophagi to the cardia.

epicardial (ep″ĭ-kar′de-al)   pertaining to the epicardium or to the epicardia.

epicardiectomy (ep″ĭ-kar″de-ek′to-me)   surgical removal of the epicardium, usually performed in constrictive pericarditis to permit greater diastolic filling of the heart.

epicardiolysis (ep″ĭ-kar-de-ol′ĭ-sis) [*epicardium* + Gr. *lysis* dissolution]   the operation of separating the visceral layer of the pericardium (epicardium) from the myocardium.

epicardium (ep″ĭ-kar′de-um) [*epi-* + Gr. *kardia* heart]   NA alternative for *lamina visceralis pericardii,* the layer of serous pericardium on the surface of the heart.

epicauma (ep″ĭ-kaw′mah) [Gr. *epikauma*]   a spot on the cornea of the eye.

Epicauta (ep″ĭ-kaw′tah)   a genus of blister beetles that secrete cantharidin, which if rubbed into the skin, causes severe vesicular dermatitis. *E. pennsylva′nica* and *E. vitta′ta* are found in eastern United States, *E. cine′rea* in southwestern United States, and *E. tormento′sa* and *E. sapphiri′na* in Africa.

epicele (ep′ĭ-sēl)   (*obs.*) epicoele.

epicentral (ep″ĭ-sen′tral)   attached to the centrum of a vertebra.

epichitosamine (ep″ĭ-ke-to′sah-min)   D-2-aminomannose: a hexosamine homologous with glucosamine, but containing mannose instead of D-glucose.

epichordal (ep″ĭ-kor′dal)   situated dorsad of the notochord.

epichorion (ep″ĭ-ko′re-on) [*epi-* + *chorion*]   that part of the uterine mucosa which incloses the implanted conceptus.

epicillin (ep-ĭ-sil′in)   chemical name: [2S-[2α,5α,6β(*S**)]]-6-[(amino-1,4-cyclohexadien-1-ylacetyl)amino]-3,3-dimethyl-7-oxo-4-thia-1-azabicyclo[3.2.0]heptane-2-carboxylic acid. An antibacterial, $C_{16}H_{21}N_3O_4S$, effective against various gram-negative and gram-positive organisms.

epicoele (ep′ĭ-sēl) [*epi-* + Gr. *koilia* hollow]   (*obs.*) the cavity of the myelencephalon.

epicoeloma (ep″ĭ-se-lo′mah)   the portion of the coeloma nearest the notochord.

epicomus (e-pik′o-mus) [*epi-* + Gr. *komē* hair]   a monster with a parasitic twin joined at the summit of the head.

epicondylalgia (ep″ĭ-kon-dĭ-lal′je-ah) [*epicondyle* + *-algia*]   pain in the muscles or tendons attached to the epicondyle of the humerus; see also *tennis elbow,* under *elbow.*

epicondyle (ep″ĭ-kon′dĭl) [*epi-* + Gr. *kondylos* condyle]   an eminence upon a bone, above its condyle; called also *epicondylus* [NA].   **external e. of femur,** epicondylus lateralis femoris.   **external e. of humerus,** epicondylus lateralis humeri.   **internal e. of femur,** epicondylus medialis femoris.   **internal e. of humerus,** epicondylus medialis humeri.   **lateral e. of femur,** epicondylus lateralis femoris.   **lateral e. of humerus,** epicondylus lateralis humeri.   **medial e. of femur,** epicondylus medialis femoris.   **medial e. of humerus,** epicondylus medialis humeri.

epicondyli (ep″ĭ-kon′dĭ-li) [L.]   plural of *epicondylus.*

epicondylian, epicondylic (ep″ĭ-kon-di′le-an; ep″ĭ-kon-dil′ik)   pertaining to an epicondyle.

epicondylitis (ep″ĭ-kon″dĭ-li′tis)   inflammation of the epicondyle or of the tissues adjoining the epicondyle of the humerus.   **external humeral e., radiohumeral e.,** tennis elbow.

epicondylus (ep″ĭ-kon′dĭ-lus), pl. *epicon′dyli* [L.] [NA]   epicondyle: a general term for an eminence upon a bone, above its condyle.   **e. latera′lis fem′oris** [NA], lateral epicondyle of femur: a projection from the distal end of the femur, above the lateral condyle, for the attachment of collateral ligaments of the knee. Called also *external epicondyle of femur.*   **e. latera′lis**

hu′meri [NA], lateral epicondyle of humerus: a projection from the distal end of the humerus, giving attachment to a common tendon of origin of the extensor carpi radialis brevis, extensor digitorum communis, extensor digiti quinti proprius, extensor carpi ulnaris, and supinator muscles. Called also *external epicondyle of humerus, external, extensor, lateral,* or *radial condyle of humerus,* and *condylus lateralis humeri.*   **e. media′lis fem′oris** [NA], medial epicondyle of femur: a projection from the distal end of the femur, above the medial condyle, for the attachment of collateral ligaments of the knee; called also *internal epicondyle of femur.*   **e. media′lis hu′meri** [NA], medial epicondyle of humerus: a projection from the distal end of the humerus, giving attachment to the pronator teres above; a common tendon of origin of the flexor carpi radialis, palmaris longus, flexor digitorum sublimis, and flexor carpi ulnaris muscles in the middle, and the ulnar collateral ligament below. Called also *condylus medialis humeri, internal epicondyle of humerus,* and *flexor, internal, medial,* or *ulnar condyle of humerus.*

epicoracoid (ep″ĭ-kor′ah-koid)   situated above the coracoid process.

epicorneascleritis (ep″ĭ-kor″ne-ah-skle-ri′tis)   a chronic inflammatory condition affecting the cornea and sclera.

epicostal (ep″ĭ-kos′tal) [*epi-* + L. *costa* rib]   situated upon a rib.

epicotyl (ep″ĭ-kot′il)   the part of the stem of a plant embryo or seedling above the cotyledons and below the leaves.

epicranium (ep″ĭ-kra′ne-um) [*epi-* + Gr. *kranion* skull]   the integument, aponeurosis, and muscular expansions of the scalp.

epicrisis (ep″ĭ-kri′sis) [*epi-* + *crisis*]   1. a second or supplementary crisis.   2. a critical analysis or discussion of a case of disease after its termination.

epicritic (ep″ĭ-krit′ik) [Gr. *epikrisis* determination]   relating to or serving the purpose of accurate determination; applied to cutaneous nerve fibers that serve the purpose of perceiving fine variations of touch or temperature. See under *sensibility.*

epicuticle (ep″ĭ-ku′tĭ-kl) [*epi-* + L. *cuticula*]   the thin, flexible, colorless, outermost layer of the exoskeleton of certain crustaceans and arthropods, composed of wax and cuticulin.

epicystitis (ep″ĭ-sis-ti′tis) [*epi-* + Gr. *kystis* bladder]   inflammation of the structures above the bladder.

epicystotomy (ep″ĭ-sis-tot′o-me) [*epi-* + Gr. *kystis* bladder + *tomē* a cutting]   suprapubic operation for stone in the bladder.

epicyte (ep′ĭ-sīt) [*epi-* + Gr. *kytos* hollow vessel]   1. see *cell membrane,* under *membrane.*   2. alveolar cell.

epidemic (ep″ĭ-dem′ik) [Gr. *epidēmios* prevalent]   1. attacking many people in any region at the same time; widely diffused and rapidly spreading.   2. a disease of high morbidity which is only occasionally present in a human community.   3. a season of the extensive prevalence of any particular disease.

epidemicity (ep″ĭ-dĕ-mis′ĭ-te)   the quality of being widely diffused and rapidly spreading throughout a community.

epidemiogenesis (ep″ĭ-de″me-o-jen′ĕ-sis)   the spread of a communicable disease to epidemic proportions.

epidemiography (ep″ĭ-de″me-og′rah-fe) [*epidemic* + Gr. *graphein* to write.]   a treatise upon or an account of epidemics.

epidemiology (ep″ĭ-de″me-ol′o-je) [*epidemic* + *-logy*]   1. the study of the relationships of the various factors determining the frequency and distribution of diseases in a human community.   2. the field of medicine concerned with the determination of the specific causes of localized outbreaks of infection, such as hepatitis, of toxic disorders, such as lead poisoning, or any other disease of recognized etiology.

epiderm (ep′ĭ-derm)   epidermis.

epidermal (ep′ĭ-der′mal)   pertaining to the epidermis.

epidermatitis (ep″ĭ-der-mah-ti′tis)   a term sometimes used to denote an inflammation restricted to the epidermis; in actuality the inflammation also invariably affects the dermis.

epidermatoplasty (ep″ĭ-der-mat′o-plas″te) [*epidermis* + Gr. *plassein* to form]   skin grafting done with pieces of epidermis with the underlying outer layer of the corium.

epidermicula (ep″ĭ-der-mik′u-lah)   a very thin membrane or cuticula, such as that covering a hair.

epidermidalization (ep″ĭ-der″mid-ah-li-za′shun)   development of epidermic cells (stratified epithelium) from mucous cells (columnar epithelium).

epidermides (ep″ĭ-der″mĭ-dēz) [Gr.]   plural of *epidermis.*

epidermidolysis (ep″ĭ-der″mi-dol′ĭ-sis)   (*obs.*) epidermolysis.

epidermis (ep″ĭ-der′mis), pl. *epider′mides* [*epi-* + Gr. *derma* skin] [NA]   the outermost and nonvascular layer of the skin, derived from the embryonic ectoderm, varying in thickness from 0.07 to 0.12 mm., except on the palms and soles where it may be 0.8 and 1.4 mm., respectively. On the palmar and plantar sufaces, it exhibits maximal cellular differentiation and layering, and comprises, from within outward, five layers: (1) a *basal layer* (stratum basale epidermidis), composed of columnar cells arranged perpendicularly;   (2) a *prickle-cell* or *spinous layer* (stratum spinosum epidermidis), composed of flattened polyhedral cells with short processes or spines;   (3) a *granular layer* (stratum granulosum

epidermidis), composed of flattened granular cells;   (4) a *clear layer* (stratum lucidum epidermidis), composed of several layers of clear, transparent cells in which the nuclei are indistinct or absent; and   (5) a *horny layer* (stratum corneum epidermidis), composed of flattened, cornified, non-nucleated cells. In the thinner epidermis of the general body surface, the basal, prickle-cell, and horny layers are constantly present and the granular layer is usually identifiable, but the clear layer is usually absent. Called also *cuticle.*

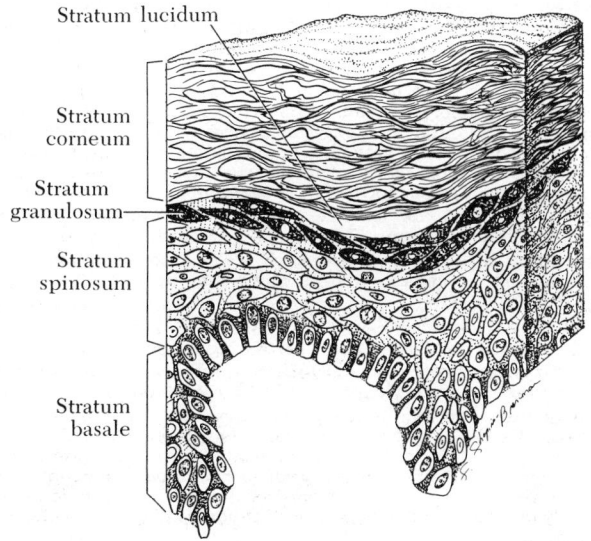

Section of epidermis.

epidermitis (ep″ĭ-der-mi′tis)   epidermatitis.

epidermization (ep″ĭ-der″mi-za′shun)   1. the process of covering or of becoming covered with epidermis.   2. skin grafting.

epidermodysplasia (ep″ĭ-der″mo-dis-pla′se-ah)   faulty development of the epidermis.   **e. verrucifor′mis,** a condition once believed to be a precancerous genodermatosis, but now known to be caused by a virus identical with or closely related to the virus of common warts; the lesions resemble those of verruca plana in appearance and morphology, but are red or red-violet and widespread, and have a tendency to become malignant. Called also *Lewandowsky-Lutz disease.*

epidermoid (ep″ĭ-der′moid)   1. resembling the epidermis.   2. any tumor occurring in a noncutaneous site (such as the skull, brain, or meninges) and formed by inclusion of epidermal elements, e.g., an intracranial cholesteatoma.

epidermoidoma (ep″ĭ-der″moi-do′mah)   a cerebral or meningeal tumor formed by inclusion of ectodermal elements at the time of closure of the neural groove.

epidermolysis (ep″ĭ-der-mol′ĭ-sis) [*epidermis* + Gr. *lysis* dissolution]   a loosened state of the epidermis, with formation of blebs and bullae either spontaneously or after trauma.   **e. acquisi′ta,** e. acquisita bullosa.   **e. bullo′sa,** a group of genetically transmitted diseases of the skin, marked by the development of bullae and vesicles, often at the site of trauma; the group includes *e. bullosa dystrophica, e. bullosa simplex,* and probably other variants. Called also *e. bullosa hereditaria.*   **e. bullo′sa acquisi′ta,** a nonhereditary condition marked by blisters at sites of trauma and by milia, involvement of mucous membranes, and usually nail dystrophy.   **e. bullo′sa dystroph′ica,** epidermolysis bullosa marked by severe scarring after healing of the lesions, occurring in three forms. In the *dominantly inherited form,* the lesions develop over the joints and may involve the mucous membranes of the mouth, tongue, esophagus, and pharynx; the scarring may be associated with loss of the nails, adhesions between the digits, contractures, clawlike hands, dwarfism, and baldness. In the *recessively inherited form,* the clinical manifestations are similar to those in the dominantly inherited form, but more severe, and the lesions may develop spontaneously or following mild irritation. In the *recessively inherited lethal form,* numerous large lesions are present at birth, which soon rupture, leaving extensive denuded areas; death usually occurs no later than three months of age.   **e. bullo′sa heredita′ria,** e. bullosa.   **e. bullo′sa leta′lis,** polydysplastic e. bullosa.   **e. bullo′sa sim′plex,** a relatively mild form of epidermolysis bullosa, transmitted as an autosomal dominant trait, in which the lesions are superficial, develop on any part of the skin subject to repeated trauma, and usually heal without scarring.   **dysplastic e. bullosa,** polydysplastic e. bullosa.   **hyperplastic e. bullo′sa,** a syndrome transmitted as an autosomal dominant trait, with onset of both traumatic and spontaneous bullae at any age through puberty, which heal with scarring, often severe.   **polydysplastic e. bullo′sa,** a recessively inherited disorder in which bullae are present at birth or soon after, scarring is severe, mucous membranes are often involved, and death from inanition or infection by the age of 30 is the usual result. Called also *Hallopeau-Siemens syndrome*, *dysplastic e. bullosa dystrophica*, and *e. bullosa letalis*. **toxic bullous e.,** bullous epidermolysis in which the epidermis peels off in large sheets; it has been attributed to an allergic response to drugs.

epidermolytic (ep″ĭ-der-mo-lit′ik) pertaining to or characterized by epidermolysis.

epidermomycosis (ep″ĭ-der″mo-mi-ko′sis) dermatophytosis.

epidermophytid (ep″ĭ-der-mof′ĭ-tid) dermatophytid.

epidermophytin (ep″ĭ-der-mof′ĭ-tin) a filtrate of *Epidermophyton* cultures that induces a hypersensitivity reaction of the tuberculin type; employed in the treatment of epidermophytosis.

Epidermophyton (ep″ĭ-der-mof′ĭ-ton) [*epidermis* + Gr. *phyton* plant] a monotypic genus of imperfect fungi (dermatophytes) of the order Moniliales, family Moniliaceae. **E. flocco′sum,** a species that attacks both skin and nails but not hair, and one of the causative organisms of tinea cruris, tinea pedis (athlete's foot), and onychomycosis; formerly called *Acrothesium floccosum*.

epidermophytosis (ep″ĭ-der″mo-fi-to′sis) infection by fungi, especially of the genus *Epidermophyton;* dermatophytosis.

epidermopoiesis (ep″ĭ-der″mo-poi-e′sis) the formation of epidermis, as in the embryo or during wound healing.

epidermotropic (ep″ĭ-der-mo-trop′ik) having a special affinity for or exerting a particular effect upon the epidermis.

epididymal (ep″ĭ-did′ĭ-mal) pertaining to the epididymis.

epididymectomy (ep″ĭ-did′ĭ-mek′to-me) [*epididymis* + Gr. *ektomē* excision] surgical removal of the epididymis.

epididymis (ep″ĭ-did′ĭ-mis), pl. *epididym′ides* [*epi-* + Gr. *didymos* testis] [NA] the elongated cordlike structure along the posterior border of the testis, whose elongated coiled duct provides for storage, transit, and maturation of spermatozoa and is continuous with the ductus deferens. It consists of a head (caput epididymis), body (corpus epididymis), and tail (cauda epididymis). Called also *parorchis*.

epididymitis (ep″ĭ-did′ĭ-mi′tis) inflammation of the epididymis. **spermatogenic e.,** an inflammatory reaction to spermatozoa that have escaped from the lumen of the epididymal tubules into the tissues of the epididymis.

epididymodeferentectomy (ep″ĭ-did′ĭ-mo-def″er-en-tek′to-me) excision of the epididymis and ductus deferens.

epididymodeferential (ep″ĭ-did′ĭ-mo-def″er-en′shal) pertaining to the epididymis and ductus deferens.

epididymo-orchitis (ep″ĭ-did′ĭ-mo-or-ki′tis) inflammation of the epididymis and testis.

epididymotomy (ep″ĭ-did′ĭ-mot′o-me) [*epididymis* + Gr. *tomē* a cut] incision of the epididymis.

epididymovasectomy (ep″ĭ-did′ĭ-mo-vaz-ek′to-me) excision of the epididymis and a large portion of the ductus deferens.

epididymovasostomy (ep-e-did″ĭ-mo-vaz-os′to-me) [*epididymo-* + *vas* vessel + Gr. *stomoun* to provide with an opening, or mouth] surgical creation of a new communication between the epididymis and a formerly distal portion of the vas (ductus) deferens.

epidural (ep″ĭ-du′ral) situated upon or outside the dura mater.

epidurography (ep″ĭ-du-rog′rah-fe) radiography of the spine after a radiopaque medium has been injected into the epidural space.

epiestriol (ep″i-es′tre-ol) an estrogenic steroid found in pregnant women.

epifascial (ep″ĭ-fash′e-al) upon a fascia.

epigamous (ĕ-pig′ah-mus) [*epi-* + Gr. *gamos* marriage] occurring after fertilization; a term descriptive of the erroneous theory that the sex of an embryo is determined by external factors acting on the embryo during its development.

epigaster (ep″ĭ-gas′ter) [*epi-* + Gr. *gastēr* belly] the hindgut: the embryonic structure from which the large intestine is formed.

epigastralgia (ep″ĭ-gas-tral′je-ah) [*epigastrium* + *-algia*] pain in the epigastrium.

epigastric (ep″ĭ-gas′trik) [*epi-* + Gr. *gastēr* belly] pertaining to the epigastrium.

epigastrium (ep″ĭ-gas′tre-um) [Gr. *epigastrion*] the upper middle region of the abdomen, located within the sternal angle; called also *regio epigastrica* [NA].

epigastrius (ep″ĭ-gas′tre-us) [*epi-* + Gr. *gastēr* belly] a double monster in which the parasite is small and forms a tumor upon the epigastrium of the autosite.

epigastrocele (ep″ĭ-gas′tro-sēl) [*epigastrium* + Gr. *kēlē* hernia] hernia in the epigastric region.

epigenesis (ep″ĭ-jen′ĕ-sis) [*epi-* + *genesis*] the development of an organism from an undifferentiated cell, consisting in the successive formation and development of organs and parts that do not preexist in the fertilized egg; opposed to the erroneous theory of preformation.

epigenetic (ep″ĭ-jĕ-net′ik) pertaining to epigenesis.

epigenetics (ep″ĭ-jĕ-net′iks) the science concerned with the analysis of development.

epiglottectomy (ep″ĭ-glot-tek′to-me) epiglottidectomy.

epiglottic (ep″ĭ-glot′ik) pertaining to the epiglottis.

epiglottidean (ep″ĭ-glo-tid′e-an) pertaining to the epiglottis.

epiglottidectomy (ep″ĭ-glot″ĭ-dek′to-me) [*epiglottis* + Gr. *ektomē* excision] excision of the epiglottis.

epiglottiditis (ep″ĭ-glot″ĭ-di′tis) inflammation of the epiglottis.

epiglottis (ep″ĭ-glot′is) [*epi-* + Gr. *glōttis* glottis] [NA] the lidlike cartilaginous structure overhanging the entrance to the larynx and serving to prevent food from entering the larynx and trachea while swallowing.

epiglottitis (ep″ĭ-glot-ti′tis) epiglottiditis.

epignathous (ĕ-pig′nah-thus) of the nature of an epignathus.

epignathus (ĕ-pig′nah-thus) [*epi-* + Gr. *gnathos* jaw] a fetal tumor arising from the soft or hard palate in the region of Rathke's pouch, filling the buccal cavity and protruding from the mouth. Because the tumor sometimes shows a certain degree of organization, it has been considered a parasitic fetus.

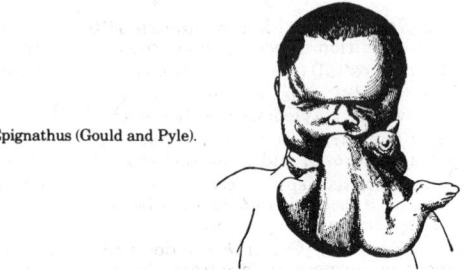

Epignathus (Gould and Pyle).

epigonal (ĕ-pig′o-nal) [*epi-* + Gr. *gonē* seed] situated on an embryonic gonad.

epiguanine (ep″ĭ-gwan′in) one of the purine bodies found in the urine after the ingestion of theobromine (cocoa). It is 7-methyl-2-amino-6-oxypurine, $C_6H_7N_5O$.

epihydrinaldehyde (ep″ĭ-hi″drin-al′dĕ-hīd) a chemical compound, one of the substances that give rancid fats their disagreeable odor.

epihyoid (ep″ĭ-hi′oid) situated upon the hyoid bone.

epilamellar (ep″ĭ-lah-mel′ar) situated upon the basement membrane.

epilate (ep′ĭ-lāt) to remove hair by the roots.

epilation (ep″ĭ-la′shun) [L. *e* out + *pilus* hair] the removal of hair by the roots.

epilemma (ep″ĭ-lem′ah) [*epi-* + Gr. *lemma* scale] the endoneurium.

epilemmal (ep″ĭ-lem′al) pertaining to the epilemma (endoneurium).

epilepsia (ep″ĭ-lep′se-ah) [L.; Gr. *epilēpsia*] epilepsy. **e. cursi′va,** cursive epilepsy. **e. gra′vior, e. major,** grand mal epilepsy. **e. minor, e. mi′tior,** minor epilepsy. **e. nu′tans,** head nodding attacks in children, a minor form of astatic seizure. **e. partia′lis contin′ua,** continuous clonic movements of a limited part of the body, due to an abnormal neuronal discharge. **e. procursi′va,** cursive epilepsy. **e. rotato′ria,** an epileptic seizure in which the body rotates. **e. tar′da,** epilepsy beginning in middle age or later.

epilepsy (ep′ĭ-lep″se) [Gr. *epilēpsia* seizure] paroxysmal transient disturbances of brain function that may be manifested as episodic impairment or loss of consciousness, abnormal motor phenomena, psychic or sensory disturbances, or perturbation of the autonomic nervous system. Symptoms are due to paroxysmal disturbance of the electrical activity of the brain. On the basis of origin, epilepsy is idiopathic (cryptogenic, essential, genetic) or symptomatic (acquired, organic). On the basis of clinical and electroencephalographic phenomenon, four subdivisions are recognized: (1) *grand mal e.* (major e., haut mal e.)—subgroups: generalized, focal (localized), jacksonian (rolandic), (2) *petit mal e.,* (3) *psychomotor e.* (temporal lobe e., psychic, psychic equivalent, or variant)—subgroups: psychomotor proper (tonic with adversive or torsion movements or masticatory phenomena), automatic (with amnesia), and sensory (hallucinations, or dream states or déjà vu), (4) *autonomic e.* (diencephalic), with flushing, pallor, tachycardia, hypertension, perspiration, or other visceral symptoms. Called also *epilepsia*. **abdominal e.,** paroxysmal abdominal pain, the expression of an abnormal neuronal discharge from the brain. **acquired e.,** epilepsy due to cerebral disease acquired after birth; see *symptomatic e.* **activated e.,** epileptic seizures induced by electrical or drug stimulation for the purpose of observing the pattern of clinical and electroencephalographic response. **automatic e.,** automatisms, often ambulatory with quasipurposive acts, but with amnesia for the events. **Bravais-jacksonian e.,** jacksonian e. **cortical e.,** seizure phenomena originating in the cerebral cortex. **cryptogenic e.,** idiopathic e. **cursive e.,** psychomotor epilepsy manifested by running. **diurnal e.,** epileptic attacks occurring in the daytime or when the patient is awake. **essential e.**, idiopathic e. **focal e.**, minor epileptic seizures in which the seizures are predominantly one-sided or local, or present localized features. **focal e.**, **chronic**, epilepsia partialis continua. **focal e.**, **minor**, an epileptic attack consisting of the aura without convulsions; called also *paraepilepsy.* **gelastic e.**, epilepsy in which there are episodes of uncontrollable mirthless laughter. **generalized e.**, epilepsy in which the seizures are generalized; they may have a focal onset or be generalized from the beginning. **generalized flexion e.**, hypsarrhythmia. **grand mal e.**, epilepsy, frequently preceded by an aura, in which a sudden loss of consciousness is immediately followed by generalized convulsions; called also *grand mal, major e.,* and *haut mal e.* Cf. *petit mal e.* **haut mal e.**, grand mal e. **hysterical e.**, seizures associated with hysteria, which may mimic epilepsy. **idiopathic e.**, epilepsy of unknown origin, possibly associated with some inherited predisposition for seizures; called also *cryptogenic e., essential e.,* and *genetic e.* **jacksonian e.**, epilepsy characterized by unilateral clonic movements that start in one group of muscles and spread systematically to adjacent groups, reflecting the march of the epileptic activity through the motor cortex. The seizures are due to a discharging focus in the contralateral motor cortex; called also *Bravais-jacksonian e.* and *rolandic e.* **Koshevnikoff's (Koschewnikow's, Kozhevnikov's) e.**, epilepsia partialis continua. **larval e.**, unerupted epileptic seizures, represented only by characteristic waves in the electroencephalogram; called also *latent e.* **laryngeal e.**, tussive syncope. **latent e.**, larval e. **localized e.**, focal e. **major e.**, grand mal e. **matutinal e.**, epileptic seizures occurring in the morning on awakening. **menstrual e.**, epileptic seizures associated with menstruation. **minor e.**, slight epileptic attacks consisting of brief impairment or loss of consciousness, or localized motor or sensory symptoms, as in petit mal epilepsy and psychomotor epilepsy. Called also *epilepsia minor* or *epilepsia mitior.* **musicogenic e.**, reflex epilepsy occurring in response to a musical stimulus. **myoclonus e.**, slowly progressive hereditary epilepsy beginning in childhood and characterized by attacks of intermittent or continuous clonus of muscle groups, resulting in difficulties in voluntary movement; there is mental deterioration, sometimes progressing to complete dementia, and the presence of Lafora bodies in various cells, including those of the nervous system, retina, heart, muscle, and liver. It is transmitted as an autosomal recessive trait. Called also *Lafora's disease, progressive familial myoclonic e., Unverricht's disease or syndrome,* and *myoclonia epileptica.* **nocturnal e.**, epileptic attacks occurring at night or while the patient is asleep. **organic e.**, symptomatic e. **petit mal e.**, epilepsy in which there is sudden momentary loss of consciousness with only minor myoclonic jerks, seen especially in children, and accompanied by 3-c.p.s. spike and wave discharges on the electroencephalogram; called also *petit mal* and *absence seizure.* Cf. *grand mal e.* **photogenic e.**, epilepsy in which seizures are induced by a flickering light. **physiologic e.**, biologic or electrobiologic seizures based on physiologic and not on organic or structural abnormalities of the brain. **post-traumatic e.**, recurring convulsions due to head injury. **procursive e.**, cursive e. **progressive familial myoclonic e.**, myoclonus e. **psychic e.**, a seizure manifested by a predominance of psychic or psychotic features; called also *psychic equivalent.* **psychomotor e.**, epileptic seizures associated with disease of the temporal lobe and characterized by variable degrees of impairment of consciousness, the patient performing a series of coordinated acts which are out of place, bizarre, and serve no useful purpose and for which he is amnesic. **reflex e.**, an epileptic seizure occurring in response to a sensory (tactile, visual, auditory, or musical) stimulus. **rolandic e.**, see *jacksonian e.* **sensory e.**, seizures manifested by hallucinations of sight, smell, or taste. **serial e.**, seizures occurring in series, with return of consciousness between the individual attacks. **sleep e.**, narcolepsy. **spinal e.**, a succession of clonic and tonic spasms in spastic paraplegia. **symptomatic e.**, acquired epileptic seizures caused by disease of the central nervous system itself, a generalized systemic disorder, such as hypoglycemia or uremia, or poisoning, as with lead or pentylenetetrazol; called also *organic e.* **tardy e.**, epilepsia tarda. **temporal lobe e.**, psychomotor e. **thalamic e.**, epilepsy ascribed to disease of the thalamus. **tonic e.**, a seizure characterized by generalized rigidity. **traumatic e.**, epileptic seizures occurring as the result of trauma (gunshot wound or other injury) to the brain. **uncinate e.**, epileptic seizures originating in the uncinate region of the temporal lobe, associated with hallucinations of smell and taste.

epileptic (ep″ĭ-lep′tik) [Gr. *epilēptikos*] 1. pertaining to or affected with epilepsy. 2. a person affected with epilepsy.

epileptiform (ep″ĭ-lep′tĭ-form) [Gr. *epilēptikos* + [L.] *forma* shape] 1. resembling epilepsy or its manifestations. 2. occurring in severe or sudden paroxysms.

epileptogenic (ep″ĭ-lep-to-jen′ik) [*epilepsy* + Gr. *gennan* to produce] producing epileptic attacks.

epileptogenous (ep″ĭ-lep-toj′ĕ-nus) epileptogenic.

epileptoid (ep″ĭ-lep′toid) epileptiform.

epileptologist (ep″ĭ-lep-tol′o-jist) a practitioner who makes a special study of epilepsy.

epileptology (ep″ĭ-lep-tol′o-je) the study of epilepsy.

epilesional (ep″ĭ-le′zhun-al) occurring on or introduced on the surface of a lesion, as epilesional scarification.

epiloia (ep″ĭ-loi′ah) tuberous sclerosis.

epimandibular (ep″ĭ-man-dib′u-lar) [*epi-* + [L.] *mandibulum* jaw] situated upon the lower jaw.

epimastigote (ep″ĭ-mas′tĭ-gōt) [*epi-* + Gr. *mastix* whip] the morphologic stage in the development of certain protozoa of the family Trypanosomatidae, characterized by a flagellum arising from a blepharoplast situated just in front of the nucleus and resembling the typical adult form of *Crithidia;* called also *crithidial stage* or *form.* Cf. *amastigote, promastigote,* and *trypomastigote.*

epimenorrhagia (ep″ĭ-men″o-ra′je-ah) too frequent and too excessive menstruation.

epimenorrhea (ep″ĭ-men″o-re′ah) abnormally frequent menstruation; menstrual irregularity in which the patient has a menstrual cycle less than the normal twenty-eight days.

epimer (ep′ĭ-mer) either of two diastereomers that differ in the configuration around one asymmetric carbon atom.

epimerase (ĕ-pim′er-āse″) an isomerase that catalyzes the inversion of asymmetric groups in substrates (epimers) having more than one center of asymmetry. **aldose 1-e.**, an enzyme that catalyzes the conversion of α-D- to β-D-glucose; called also *mutarotase* and *aldose mutarotase.* **diaminopimelate e.**, an enzyme that catalyzes the conversion of 2-6-LL-diaminopimelate to *meso*-diaminopimelate. **3-hydroxybutyryl-CoA e.**, an enzyme that catalyzes the conversion of L-3- to D-3-hydroxybutyryl-CoA. **hydroxyproline e.**, an enzyme that catalyzes the conversion of L-hydroxyproline to D-allohydroxyproline. **ribulosephosphate 3-e.**, an enzyme of the liver that catalyzes the conversion of D-ribulose-5-phosphate to D-xylulose-5-phosphate. **UDP-arabinose e.**, an enzyme that catalyzes the conversion of UDP-L-arabinose to UDP-D-xylose. **UDP-glucose e.**, an enzyme that catalyzes the conversion of UDP-glucose to UDP-galactose by inverting the H and OH groups. **UDP-glucuronate e.**, an enzyme that catalyzes the isomerization of UDP-D-glucuronate to UDP-D-galacturonate.

epimere (ep′ĭ-mēr) [*epi-* + Gr. *meros* a part] the dorsal portion of a somite, from which is formed muscles innervated by the dorsal ramus of a spinal nerve.

epimerite (ep″ĭ-mer′ĭt) [*epi-* + Gr. *meros* part] an organelle of certain gregarine protozoa by which they attach to epithelial cells.

epimerization (ĕ-pim″er-i-za′shun) the changing of one epimeric form of a compound into another, as by enzymatic action.

epimestrol (ep″ĭ-mes′trōl) chemical name: 3-methoxyestra-1,3,5(10)-triene-16α,17α-diol; an anterior pituitary activator, $C_{19}H_{26}O_3$.

epimicroscope (ep″ĭ-mi′kro-skōp) *(obs.)* a microscope in which the specimen is illuminated by light passing though a condenser built around the objective.

epimorphic (ep″ĭ-mor′fik) pertaining to or characterized by epimorphosis.

epimorphosis (ep″ĭ-mor-fo′sis) [*epi-* + Gr. *morphē* form] the regeneration of a part of an organism by proliferation at the cut surface.

Epimys (ep′ĭ-mis) [*epi-* + Gr. *mys* mouse] *Rattus.*

epimysium (ep″ĭ-mis′e-um) [*epi-* + Gr. *mys* muscle] the fibrous sheath about an entire muscle; called also *perimysium externum* or *external perimysium.*

Epinal (ep′ĭ-nal) trademark for a preparation of epinephryl borate.

epinephrectomy (ep″ĭ-nĕ-frek′to-me) adrenalectomy.

epinephrine (ep″ĭ-nef′rin) chemical name: 4-[1-hydroxy-2-(methylamino)ethyl]-1,2-benzenediol. A hormone, $C_9H_{13}NO_3$, secreted by the adrenal medulla in response to splanchnic stimulation, and stored in the chromaffin granules; it is released also in response to hypoglycemia. It is a potent stimulator of the sympathetic nervous system (adrenergic receptors), and a powerful vasopressor, increasing blood pressure, stimulating the heart muscle, accelerating the heart rate, and increasing cardiac output. It also increases such metabolic activities as glycogenolysis and glucose release. The official preparation [USP], produced synthetically as the levorotatory form (*l*-form), occurs as white to nearly white, microcrystalline powder or granules, and is used chiefly as a topical vasoconstrictor, cardiac stimulant, and bronchodilator; administered intranasally, orally, and parenterally, or by inhalation. Called also *adrenaline* (Great Britain). **e. bitartrate** [USP], the bitartrate salt of epinephrine, $C_9H_{13}NO_3 \cdot C_4H_6O_6$, occurring as a white, or grayish white or light brownish gray, crystalline powder, having the same actions as the base; applied topically to the conjunctiva to reduce intraocular pressure in the management of chronic simple (open-angle) glaucoma and administered by inhalation as a bronchodilator.

epinephrinemia (ep″ĭ-nef″rĭ-ne′me-ah) the presence of epinephrine in the blood.

epinephritis (ep″ĭ-nĕ-fri′tis) [*epi-* + Gr. *nephros* kidney] inflammation of an adrenal gland.

epinephroma (ep″ĭ-nĕ-fro′mah) (*obs.*) renal cell carcinoma.

epinephros (ep″ĭ-nef′ros) [*epi-* + Gr. *nephros* kidney] an adrenal gland (glandula suprarenalis [NA]).

epinephryl borate (ep-ĭ-nef′ril) chemical name: (*S*)-2-hydroxy-α-[(methylamino)methyl]-1,3,2-benzodioxaborole-5-methanol. A compound containing epinephrine as a borate complex, $C_9H_{12}BNO_4$; used as an adrenergic in ophthalmology.

epineural (ep″ĭ-nu′ral) situated upon a neural arch.

epineurial (ep″ĭ-nu′re-al) pertaining to the epineurium.

epineurium (ep″ĭ-nu′re-um) [*epi-* + Gr. *neuron* nerve] the connective tissue covering of a peripheral nerve.

epinosic (ep″ĭ-no′sik) [*epi-* + Gr. *nosos* disease] pertaining to some secondary advantage because of illness.

epinosis (ep″ĭ-no′sis) a psychic or imaginary state of illness secondary to an original illness. Cf. *paranosis.*

epionychium (ep″e-o-nik′e-um) eponychium.

epiorchium (ep″e-or′ke-um) lamina visceralis tunicae vaginalis testis.

epiotic (ep″e-ot′ik) [*epi-* + Gr. *ous* ear] situated on or above the ear.

epipastic (ep″ĭ-pas′tik) [*epi-* + Gr. *passein* to sprinkle] 1. suitable for use as a dusting powder. 2. a powder to be sprinkled upon the surface of the body.

epipharyngeal (ep″ĭ-fah-rin′je-al) nasopharyngeal.

epipharyngitis (ep″ĭ-far″in-ji′tis) nasopharyngitis.

epipharynx (ep″ĭ-far′inks) nasopharynx.

epiphenomenon (ep″ĭ-fĕ-nom′ĕ-non) [*epi-* + Gr. *phainomenon* phenomenon] an accessory, exceptional, or accidental occurrence in the course of an attack of any disease.

epiphora (ĕ-pif′o-rah) [Gr. *epiphora* sudden burst] an abnormal overflow of tears down the cheek, mainly due to stricture of the lacrimal passages; called also *illacrimation.*

epiphyseal (ep″ĭ-fiz′e-al) pertaining to or of the nature of an epiphysis.

epiphyses (ĕ-pif′ĭ-sēz) [Gr.] plural of *epiphysis.*

epiphysial (ep″ĭ-fiz′e-al) epiphyseal.

epiphysiodesis (ep″ĭ-fiz″e-od′ĕ-sis) [*epiphysis* + Gr. *desis* a binding] the operation of fixing a separated epiphysis to its diaphysis to produce healing and fusion of the epiphyseal plate.

epiphysioid (ep″ĭ-fiz′e-oid) resembling epiphyses; a term applied to carpal and tarsal bones which develop like epiphyses from centers of ossification.

epiphysiolysis (ep″ĭ-fiz″e-ol′ĭ-sis) [*epiphysis* + Gr. *lysis* loosening] separation of an epiphysis from its bone; especially slipping of the upper femoral epiphysis.

epiphysiometer (ep″ĭ-fis″e-om′ĕ-ter) an instrument for measuring the epiphyses, used in the diagnosis of rickets.

epiphysiopathy (ep″ĭ-fiz″e-op′ah-the) [*epiphysis* + Gr. *pathos* disease] 1. any disease of the pineal body. 2. any disease of an epiphysis of a bone.

epiphysis (ĕ-pif′ĭ-sis), pl. *epiph′yses* [Gr. "an ongrowth; excrescence"] [NA] 1. the end of a long bone, usually wider than the shaft, and either entirely cartilaginous or separated from the shaft by a cartilaginous disk. 2. part of a bone formed from a secondary center of ossification, commonly found at the ends of long bones, on the margins of flat bones, and at tubercles and processes; during the period of growth, epiphyses are separated from the main portion of the bone by cartilage. Called also *apophysis ossium.* **capital e.,** the epiphysis at the head of a long bone. **e. cer′ebri,** pineal body. **slipped e.,** dislocation of the epiphysis of a bone, as of the epiphysis of the head of the femur. **stippled epiphyses,** 1. dysplasia epiphysealis punctata. 2. epiphyseal dysplasia.

epiphysitis (ĕ-pif″ĭ-si′tis) inflammation of an epiphysis or of the cartilage that separates it from the main bone. **vertebral e.,** osteochondrosis (q.v.) of the vertebra.

epiphyte (ep′ĭ-fīt) [*epi-* + Gr. *phyton* plant] 1. a plant organism growing upon another plant. 2. a plant organism parasitic upon the exterior of the human or an animal body.

epiphytic (ep″ĭ-fit′ik) 1. pertaining to or caused by epiphytes. 2. a widely diffused outbreak of an infectious disease in plants.

epipial (ep″ĭ-pi′al) situated on the pia mater.

epipleural (ep″ĭ-ploo′ral) situated on a pleural element, or pleurapophysis.

epiplo- [Gr. *epiploon*] a combining form denoting relationship to the epiploon (omentum).

epiplocele (ĕ-pip′lo-sēl) [*epiplo-* + Gr. *kēlē* hernia] a hernia that contains omentum.

epiploectomy (ĕ-pip″ĭ-plo-ek′to-me) [*epiplo-* + Gr. *ektomē* excision] omentectomy; excision of the omentum.

epiploenterocele (ĕ-pip″lo-en′ter-o-sēl) [*epiplo-* + Gr. *enteron* intestine + *kēlē* hernia] hernia containing intestine and omentum.

epiploic (ep″ĭ-plo′ik) omental.

epiploitis (ĕ-pip″lo-i′tis) omentitis.

epiplomerocele (ĕ-pip″lo-me′ro-sēl) [*epiplo-* + Gr. *mēros* thigh + *kēlē* hernia] femoral hernia containing omentum.

epiplomphalocele (ep″ĭ-plom-fal′o-sēl″) [*epiplo-* + Gr. *omphalos* navel + *kēlē* hernia] umbilical hernia containing omentum.

epiploon (ĕ-pip′lo-on) [Gr.] the omentum. **great e.,** omentum majus. **lesser e.,** omentum minus.

epiplopexy (ĕ-pip′lo-pek″se) [*epiplo-* + Gr. *pēxis* fixation] omentopexy.

epiploplasty (ĕ-pip′lo-plas″te) [*epiplo-* + Gr. *plassein* to form] utilization of the epiploon (omentum) to cover raw surfaces in abdominal surgery; omentoplasty.

epiplorrhaphy (e″pip-lor′ah-fe) [*epiplo-* + Gr. *rhaphē* suture] omentorrhaphy; suture of the omentum.

epiplosarcomphalocele (ĕ-pip″lo-sar″kom-fal′o-sēl) [*epiplo-* + Gr. *sarx* flesh + *omphalos* navel + *kēlē* hernia] an umbilical hernia complicated with a local fleshy excrescence.

epiploscheocele (e″pip-los′ke-o-sēl″) [*epiplo-* + Gr. *oscheon* scrotum + *kēlē* hernia] scrotal hernia containing omentum.

epipygus (ep″ĭ-pi′gus) pygomelus.

epipyramis (ep″ĭ-pir′ah-mis) a small supernumerary carpal bone sometimes found between the triquetrum, lunate, hamate, and capitate bones; called also *epitriquetrum.*

epirizole (ĕ-pēr′ĭ-zōl) chemical name: 4-methoxy-2-(5-methoxy-3-methyl-1*H*-pyrazol-1-yl)-6-methylpyrimidine; an analgesic and anti-inflammatory, $C_{11}H_{14}N_4O_2$.

epirotulian (ep″ĭ-ro-tu′le-an) [*epi-* + L. *rotula* patella] upon the patella.

episarkin (ep″ĭ-sar′kin) one of the alloxur bases, $C_4H_6N_3O$, occurring in the normal urine and in excess in the urine of leukemia.

episclera (ep″ĭ-skle′rah) the loose connective tissue forming the external surface of the sclera.

episcleral (ep″ĭ-skle′ral) 1. overlying the sclera. 2. of or pertaining to the episclera.

episcleritis (ep″ĭ-skle-ri′tis) inflammation of tissues overlying the sclera; also inflammation of the outermost layers of the sclera. **e. partia′lis fu′gax,** sudden hyperemia of the sclera and overlying conjunctiva, lasting a short time.

episclerotitis (ep″ĭ-skle″ro-ti′tis) episcleritis.

episio- (ĕ-piz′e-o) [Gr. *epision* the region of the pubes] a combining form denoting relationship to the vulva.

episioclisia (ĕ-piz″e-o-kli′se-ah) [*episio-* + Gr. *kleisis* closure] (*obs.*) surgical closure of the vulva.

episioelytrorrhaphy (ĕ-piz″e-o-el″ĕ-tror′ah-fe) [*episio-* + *elytrorrhaphy*] (*obs.*) the operation of narrowing the vulva and vagina to support a prolapsed uterus.

episioperineoplasty (ĕ-piz″e-o-per″ĭ-ne′o-plas″te) [*episio-* + *perineum* + Gr. *plassein* to form] plastic repair of the vulva and perineum.

episioperineorrhaphy (ĕ-piz″e-o-per″ĭ-ne-or′ah-fe) the suturing of the vulva and perineum for the support of a prolapsed uterus.

episioplasty (ĕ-piz′e-o-plas″te) [*episio-* + Gr. *plassein* to shape] plastic repair of the vulva.

episiorrhaphy (ĕ-piz″e-or′ah-fe) [*episio-* + Gr. *rhaphē* suture] 1. the suturing of the labia majora. 2. the sewing up of a lacerated perineum.

episiostenosis (ĕ-piz″e-o-stĕ-no′sis) [*episio-* + Gr. *stenōsis* contraction] the narrowing of the vulvar orifice.

episiotomy (ĕ-piz″e-ot′o-me) [*episio-* + Gr. *tomē* a cutting] surgical incision into the perineum and vagina for obstetrical purposes.

episode (ep′ĭ-sōd) a noteworthy happening or series of happenings occurring in the course of continuous events, as an episode of illness; a separate but not unrelated incident. **acute schizophrenic e.,** the acute onset of schizophrenic symptoms, often associated with confusion, perplexity, ideas of reference, emotional turmoil, excitement, fear, depression, or dreamlike dissociation. **psycholeptic e.,** a sudden and vivid psychic experience to which a patient attributes the beginning of his illness, and which so possesses his mind that he is unable to shake it off.

episome (ep′ĭ-sōm) in bacterial genetics, any accessory extrachromosomal replicating genetic element that can exist either autonomously or integrated with the chromosome, e.g., the F factor, colicinogens, conjugons, and (drug) resistance transfer factor.

epispadia (ep″ĭ-spa′de-ah) epispadias.

epispadiac (ep″ĭ-spa′de-ak) pertaining to or exhibiting epispadias; by extension, sometimes used to designate an individual exhibiting epispadias.

epispadial (ep″ĭ-spa′de-al) pertaining to epispadias.

epispadias (ep″ĭ-spa′de-as) [*epi-* + Gr. *spadōn* a rent] congenital absence of the upper wall of the urethra, occurring in various degrees of severity in both sexes, but affecting males more commonly, the urethral opening being anywhere on the dorsum of the penis, and manifested as a groove or cleft without a covering. **balanic e., balanitic e.,** incomplete epispadias in which the

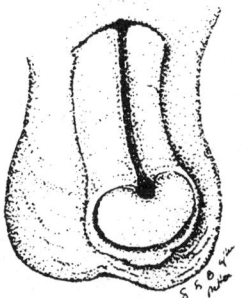

Epispadias (after Netter).

urethral opening is above and behind the glans, the dorsum of the penis usually being indented to its tip, but the opening may end at the corona or proximal to it. Called also *glandular e.* **clitoric e.,** incomplete epispadias in which the urethra opens cephalad to the clitoris or into it. **complete e.,** epispadias in which the urethra is entirely open to the bladder neck in males, and there may be complete failure of fusion of the anterior urethral wall in the female; it is frequently associated with exstrophy of the bladder. **glandular e.,** balanic e. **incomplete e.,** epispadias in which the bladder does not entirely open to the outside; designated according to the location of urethral opening in the male as *balanic* and *penile,* and in the female as *clitoric* and *subsymphyseal.* **penile e.,** incomplete epispadias in which the urethral orifice is somewhere between the postglandular sulcus and the suspensory ligament, but is usually at the base of the penis. **penopubic e.,** complete epispadias in which the urethral opening is at the junction of the penis and pubis; unless associated with exstrophy of the bladder, the urethral passage emerges between the corpora cavernosa under the pubic symphysis. **subsymphyseal e.,** incomplete epispadias in which the urethral opening is beneath the symphysis.

epispastic (ep″ĭ-spas′tik) [*epi-* + Gr. *span* to draw] (*obs.*) vesicant.

epispinal (ep″ĭ-spi′nal) situated upon the spinal cord or the spinal column.

episplenitis (ep″ĭ-splĕ-ni′tis) [*epi-* + Gr. *splēn* spleen + *-itis*] inflammation of the capsule of the spleen.

epistasis (ĕ-pis′tah-sis) [*epi-* + Gr. *stasis* a standing] 1. suppression of a secretion or excretion, as of blood, menses, or lochia. 2. a scum or pellicle on the surface of urine. 3. the interaction between genes at different loci, as a result of which one hereditary character is unexpressed, or is masked by the superimposition of another upon it. Cf. *dominance.*

epistasy (e-pis′tah-se) [*epi-* + Gr. *stasis* a standing] epistasis.

epistatic (ep″ĭ-stat′ik) 1. pertaining to or characterized by epistasis. 2. superimposed.

epistaxis (ep″ĭ-stak′sis) [Gr.] nosebleed; hemorrhage from the nose. **Gull's renal e.,** essential hematuria.

epistemology (ep″ĭ-stĕ-mol′o-je) [Gr. *epistēmē* knowledge + *-logy*] the science of the methods and validity of knowledge.

episternal (ep″ĭ-ster′nal) 1. situated on or over the sternum. 2. pertaining to the episternum.

episternum (ep″ĭ-ster′num) [*epi-* + Gr. *sternon* sternum] a bone present in reptiles and monotremes that may be represented as part of the manubrium, or first piece of the sternum.

episthotonos (e″pis-thot′o-nos) emprosthotonos.

epistropheus (ep″ĭ-stro′fe-us) [Gr. "the pivot"] the second cervical vertebra (axis [NA]).

epitarsus (ep″ĭ-tar′sus) [*epi-* + *tarsus*] a congenital anomaly of the eye consisting of a fold of conjunctiva passing from the fornix to near the lid border; called also congenital *pterygium.*

epitaxy (ep″ĭ-tak′se) the oriented growth and binding of a crystalline substance on a substrate of another crystalline compound, as in the embryonic formation of bone.

epitela (ep″ĭ-te′lah) [*epi-* + L. *tela* web] the delicate tissue of Vieussen's valve (velum medullare superius).

epitendineum (ep″ĭ-ten-din′e-um) the fibrous sheath covering a tendon.

epitenon (ep″ĭ-te′non) [*epi-* + Gr. *tenōn* tendon] the connective tissue covering a tendon within its sheath.

epithalamic (ep″ĭ-thah-lam′ik) 1. overlying the thalamus. 2. pertaining to the epithalamus.

epithalamus (ep″ĭ-thal′ah-mus) [NA] the part of the diencephalon just superior and posterior to the thalamus, comprising the pineal body, the habenula, and habenular trigone; the stria medullaris thalami is sometimes considered to belong to it.

epithalaxia (ep″ĭ-thah-lak′se-ah) [*epithelium* + Gr. *allaxis* ex-

change] desquamation of the epithelium, especially of the intestinal mucosa.

epithelia (ep″ĭ-the′le-ah) plural of *epithelium.*

epithelial (ep″ĭ-the′le-al) pertaining to or composed of epithelium.

epithelialization (ep″ĭ-the″le-al-i-za′shun) healing by the growth of epithelium over a denuded surface.

epithelialize (ep″ĭ-the′le-al-iz″) to cover with epithelium.

epitheliitis (ep″ĭ-the′le-i′tis) inflammation of epithelium.

epithelio- (ep″ĭ-the′le-o) a combining form denoting relationship to the epithelium.

epithelioblastoma (ep″ĭ-the″le-o-blas-to′mah) [*epithelio-* + Gr. *blastos* cell + *-oma*] (*obs.*) an undifferentiated carcinoma.

epithelioceptor (ep″ĭ-the″le-o-sep′tor) the region in a gland cell which receives a nerve stimulus from the end-organ of the nerve fibril.

epitheliochorial (ep″ĭ-the″le-o-ko′re-al) [*epithelium* + *chorion*] denoting a type of placenta in which the chorion is apposed to the uterine epithelium but does not erode it.

epitheliofibril (ep″ĭ-the″le-o-fi″bril) one of the fibrils which run through the cytoplasm of epithelial cells.

epitheliogenetic (ep″ĭ-the″le-o-jĕ-net′ik) [*epithelio-* + Gr. *gennan* to produce] due to epithelial proliferation.

epitheliogenic (ep″ĭ-the″le-o-jen′ik) tending to produce epithelium.

epithelioglandular (ep″ĭ-the′le-o-glan′du-lar) pertaining to the epithelial cells of a gland.

epithelioid (ep″ĭ-the′le-oid) resembling epithelium.

epitheliolysin (ep″ĭ-the-le-ol′ĭ-sin) a cytolysin formed in the serum of an animal when epithelial cells from an animal of a different species are injected. The epitheliolysin has the power of destroying epithelial cells of an animal of the same species as that from which the epithelial cells were originally taken.

epitheliolysis (ep″ĭ-the′le-ol′ĭ-sis) [*epithelio-* + Gr. *lysis* dissolution] destruction of epithelial cells.

epitheliolytic (ep″ĭ-the′le-o-lit′ik) pertaining to, characterized by, or causing epitheliolysis.

epithelioma (ep″ĭ-the″le-o′mah) any tumor derived from epithelium; formerly a synonym of carcinoma. **e. adamanti′num,** ameloblastoma. **e. adenoi′des cys′ticum,** trichoepithelioma. **basal cell e.,** basal cell carcinoma. **benign calcifying e.,** pilomatricoma. **calcified e., calcifying e., calcifying e. of Malherbe,** pilomatricoma. **chorionic e.,** choriocarcinona. **columnar e., cylindrical e.,** one composed of columnar cells arranged in glandlike tubules; when benign, it is *adenoma,* and when malignant, *adenocarcinoma.* **e. contagio′sum,** fowlpox. **diffuse e.,** infiltrating carcinoma. **glandular e.,** a variety consisting of gland cells and affecting mucous surfaces; when benign, it is *adenoma,* and when malignant, *adenocarcinoma.* **Malherbe's e., Malherbe's calcifying e.,** pilomatricoma. **malignant e.,** carcinoma. **multiple benign cystic e.,** trichoepithelioma. **multiple self-healing squamous e.,** multiple keratoacanthoma. **suprarenal e.** (*obs.*), renal cell carcinoma.

epitheliomatosis (ep″ĭ-the″le-o-mah-to′sis) the state of being subject to or afflicted with epitheliomas.

epitheliomatous (ep″ĭ-the″le-o′mah-tus) pertaining to or of the nature of epithelioma.

epitheliomuscular (ep″ĭ-the″le-o-mus′ku-lar) composed of epithelium and muscle.

epitheliosis (ep″ĭ-the″le-o′sis) 1. proliferation of the epithelium of the conjunctiva. 2. Borrel's name for a disease in which the causative agent is a virus which exhibits a special affinity for the epithelial structures of the body, including variola, vaccinia, sheeppox, molluscum contagiosum, and contagious epithelioma of birds. **e. desquamati′va conjuncti′vae,** a condition resembling trachoma occurring in the Samoan Islands.

epitheliotoxin (ep″ĭ-the″le-o-tok′sin) a cytotoxin which destroys epithelial cells.

epitheliotropic (ep″ĭ-the″le-o-trop′ik) having a special affinity for epithelial cells.

epithelite (ep″ĭ-the′līt) a lesion produced as a reaction to irradiation, in which the epithelium is replaced by a fibrous exudate.

epithelium (ep″ĭ-the′le-um), pl. *epithe′lia* [*epi-* + Gr. *thēlē* nipple] [NA] the covering of internal and external surfaces of the body, including the lining of vessels and other small cavities. It consists of cells joined by small amounts of cementing substances. Epithelium is classified into types on the basis of the number of layers deep and the shape of the superficial cells. **e. ante′rius cor′neae** [NA], **anterior e. of cornea,** the outer epithelial layer of the cornea, consisting of stratified squamous epithelium continuous with that of the conjunctiva; called also *e. corneae* or *corneal e.* **Barrett's e.,** the columnar epithelium of the esophagus seen in Barrett's syndrome. **capsular e.,** the outer, or parietal, layer of the renal glomerular capsule, composed of simple squamous epithelium, and separated from the inner, or visceral, layer by the capsular (Bowman's) space. Cf. *glomerular e.*

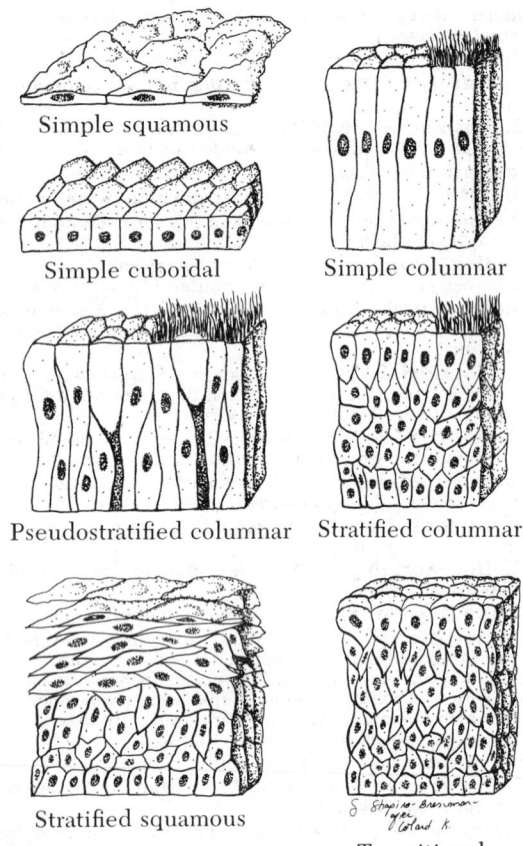

Simple squamous

Simple cuboidal

Simple columnar

Pseudostratified columnar

Stratified columnar

Stratified squamous

Transitional

Epithelium of different types (after Colard Keene, in Bloom and Fawcett).

ciliated e., any type bearing vibratile cilia on the free surface. **columnar e.,** a type composed of tall prismatic cells. **e. cor′neae, corneal e.,** e. anterius corneae. **cubical e., cuboidal e.,** a type composed of cells which have a cubical shape. **e. duc′tus semicircula′ris** [NA], the inner, simple, low epithelium lining the semicircular ducts. **enamel e.,** in the developing tooth, the inner or internal layer of cells (ameloblasts) of the enamel organ that deposit the organic matrix of enamel, plus the outer or external layer of cuboidal cells. The reduced enamel epithelium is the remains of both layers after enamel formation is complete. **false e.,** the lining of joint cavities. **germinal e.,** thickened peritoneal epithelium covering the gonad from earliest development; formerly thought to give rise to the germ cells, hence the name. **gingival e.,** the stratified squamous epithelial covering of the gingival tissues, varying in architecture according to location, functional demands, and adaptation. **glandular e.,** epithelium made up of glandular or secreting cells. **glomerular e.,** the inner, or visceral, layer of the renal glomerular capsule, overlying the capillaries, composed of podocytes, and separated from the outer, or parietal, layer by the capsular (Bowman's) space. Cf. *capsular e.* **laminated e.,** stratified e. **e. of lens, e. len′tis** [NA], the cuboidal epithelium on the front of the lens; called also *subscapular e.* **mesenchymal e.,** the epithelium which lines the subdural and subarachnoid spaces, the perilymphatic spaces in the inner ear, and the chamber of the eye. **olfactory e.,** pseudostratified epithelium lining the olfactory region of the nasal cavity, and containing the receptors for the sense of smell. **pavement e.,** epithelium composed of a single layer of flat cells. **pigmentary e., pigmented e.,** epithelium containing granules of pigment. **protective e.,** epithelium that forms a protective covering, as the epidermis. **pseudostratified e.,** a type of epithelium which occurs in the large excretory ducts of the parotid and several other glands and in the male urethra. The nuclei are spaced at different levels and the cells are quite variable in shape, giving the appearance of a stratified epithelium. **pyramidal e.,** columnar epithelium whose cells have been modified by pressure into truncated pyramids. **respiratory e.,** the pseudostratified epithelium that lines all but the finer divisions of the respiratory tract. **rod e.,** epithelium the cells of which are rod-shaped. **seminiferous e.,** stratified epithelium lining the seminiferous tubules of the testis. **sense e., sensory e.,** epithelium having relation with a special sense organ; neuroepithelium. **simple e.,** a type composed of a single layer of cells. **squamous e.,** epithelium composed of flattened platelike cells. **stratified e.,** epithelium in which the cells are arranged in several layers; called also *laminated e.* **subcapsular e.,** 1. the epithelioid lining of the capsule of ganglia. 2. epithelium lentis.

sulcular e., the stratified squamous epithelium forming the covering of the soft tissue wall of the gingival sulcus or crevice. **tessellated e.,** simple squamous epithelium. **transitional e.,** epithelium that was originally thought to represent a transitional form between stratified squamous and columnar epithelium, found characteristically in the mucous membrane of the excretory passages of the urinary system; in the contracted condition it consists of many cell layers, whereas in the stretched condition usually only two layers can be distinguished.

epithelization (ep″ĭ-the″li-za′shun)   epithelialization.

epithelize (ep″ĭ-the′līz)   epithelialize.

epithesis (ĕ-pith′ĕ-sis) [Gr. "a laying on"]   1. the surgical correction of deformity or of crooked limbs.   2. a splint or other appliance to be worn.

epithiazide (ep″ĭ-thi′ah-zīd)   chemical name: 6-chloro-3,4-dihydro-3-[[(2,2,2-trifluoroethyl)thio]-methyl]-2H,1,2,4-benzothiadiazine-7-sulfonamide 1,1-dioxide; an antihypertensive and diuretic, $C_{10}H_{11}ClF_3N_3O_4S_3$.

epitonic (ep″ĭ-ton′ik) [Gr. *epitonos* strained]   abnormally tense or tonic; exhibiting an abnormal degree of tension or of tone.

epitope (ep′ĭ-tōp)   an antigenic determinant (see under *determinant*) of known structure. Cf. *paratope.*

epitoxoid (ep″ĭ-tok′soid)   (obs.) any toxoid that has less affinity for an antitoxin than does the corresponding toxin.

epitoxonoid (ep″ĭ-tok′so-noid)   (obs.) a toxonoid which has the least affinity for its corresponding antitoxin.

Epitrate (ep′ĭ-trāt)   trademark for a preparation of epinephrine bitartrate.

epitrichium (ep″ĭ-trik′e-um) [*epi-* + Gr. *trichion* hair]   periderm, def. 1.

epitriquetrum (ep″ĭ-tri-kwe′trum)   epipyramis.

epitrochlea (ep″ĭ-trok′le-ah) [*epi-* + Gr. *trochilia*, L. *trochlea* pulley]   the inner condyle of the humerus.

epituberculosis (ep″ĭ-tu-ber″ku-lo′sis)   a form of primary tuberculosis in children, producing mild symptoms despite large, usually lobar, consolidations as seen roentgenographically; probably due to bronchial compression by enlarged hilar lymph nodes, with atelectasis.

epiturbinate (ep″ĭ-ter′bĭ-nāt)   the soft tissue covering a nasal concha (turbinate bone).

epitympanic (ep″ĭ-tim-pan′ik)   1. situated upon or over the tympanum.   2. pertaining to the epitympanum (recessus epitympanicus [NA]).

epitympanum (ep″ĭ-tim′pah-num)   recessus epitympanicus.

epitype (ep′ĭ-tīp)   a group of related epitopes.

epityphlitis (ep″ĭ-tif-li′tis) [*epi-* + Gr. *typhlon* cecum + *-itis*]   1. appendicitis.   2. paratyphlitis.

epityphlon (ep″ĭ-ti′flon) [*epi-* + Gr. *typhlon* cecum]   the vermiform appendix.

epivaginitis (ep″ĭ-vaj″ĭ-ni′tis)   a venereal disease of cattle, probably of viral origin, in Kenya, southern Africa, and the United States, marked in cows by vaginal inflammation and discharge and by sterility. In bulls it is marked by epididymitis.

epizoa (ep″ĭ-zo′ah) [Gr.]   plural of *epizoon.*

epizoic (ep″ĭ-zo′ik)   pertaining to or caused by epizoa.

epizoicide (ep″ĭ-zo′ĭ-sīd) [*epizoon* + L. *caedere* to kill]   an agent that destroys epizoa.

epizoon (ep″ĭ-zo′on), pl. *epizo′a* [*epi-* + Gr. *zōon* animal]   an animal parasite living upon the exterior of the body of the host.

epizootic (ep″ĭ-zo-ot′ik)   1. attacking many animals in any region at the same time; widely diffused and rapidly spreading.   2. a disease of high morbidity which is only occasionally present in an animal community.

epizootiology (ep″ĭ-zo-ot″e-ol′o-je)   the study of epizootics; the field of science dealing with the relationships of the various factors which determine the frequencies and distributions of infectious diseases among animals.

épluchage (a″ploo-shahzh′) [Fr. "cleaning," "picking"]   removal of the contused and contaminated tissues of a wound. Cf. *débridement.*

epontic (ĕ-pon′tik)   growing on any surface, plant, animal, or mineral.

eponychia (ep″o-nik′e-ah) [*eponychium* + *-ia*]   (obs.) a purulent blister, involving the epidermis at the groove of the nail. Cf. *felon* and *paronychia.*

eponychium (ep″o-nik′e-um) [*epi-* + Gr. *onyx* nail]   1. [NA] the narrow band of epidermis that extends from the nail wall onto the nail surface; commonly called *cuticle.*   2. the horny fetal epidermis at the site of the future nail.

eponym (ep′o-nim) [Gr. *epōnymos* named after]   a name or phrase formed from or including the name of a person, as Hodgkin's disease.

eponymic, eponymous (ep″o-nim′ik; ĕ-pon′ĭ-mus)   named for some person; pertaining to an eponym.

epoophorectomy (ep″o-of″o-rek′to-me) [*epi-* + Gr. *ōophoron* ovary + *ektomē* excision]   surgical removal of the epoophoron.

epoophoron (ep″o-of′o-ron) [epi- + Gr. ōophoron ovary] [NA] a vestigial structure associated with the ovary, consisting of a more cranial group of mesonephric tubules and a corresponding portion of the mesonephric duct; called also corpus pampiniforme, pampiniform body, parovarium, and Rosenmüller's body or organ.

epornithology (ep-or″nĭ-thol′o-je) the scientific study of diseases of high morbidity which are only occasionally present in a bird community.

epornitic (ep″or-nit′ik) [epi- + Gr. ornis bird] 1. attacking many birds in any region at the same time. 2. a disease of high morbidity which is only occasionally present in a bird population.

epoxy (ĕ-pok′se) 1. containing one atom of oxygen bound to two different carbon atoms. 2. a resin composed of epoxy polymers and characterized by adhesiveness, flexibility, and resistance to chemical actions.

epoxytropine tropate (e-pok″se-tro′pēn tro′pāt) methscopolamine.

Eppy (ep′e) trademark for a preparation of epinephryl borate.

EPR electrophrenic respiration.

Eprolin (ep′ro-lin) trademark for a preparation of vitamin E, consisting of a concentrate of distilled natural tocopherols.

EPS exophthalmos-producing substance.

EPSP excitatory postsynaptic potential.

Epstein's disease, pearls (ep′stīnz) [Alois Epstein, a pediatrician in Prague, 1849–1918] see pseudodiphtheria, and see under pearl.

Epstein's nephrosis, syndrome (ep′stīnz) [Albert Arthur Epstein, New York physician, 1880–1965] see under nephrosis, and see nephrotic syndrome, under syndrome.

Epstein-Barr virus (ep′stīn-bar′)[Michael Anthony Epstein, English physician, born 1921; Y. Barr] see under virus.

eptatretin (ep″tah-tre′tin) a potent cardiostimulant obtained from the branchial heart of the Pacific hagfish Eptatretus stouti and reported to be a highly unstable aromatic amine. Its chemical structure has not been fully defined, but it is not a catecholamine or other commonly occurring biochemical.

epulides (ep-u′lĭ-dēz) [Gr.] plural of epulis.

epulis (ep-u′lis), pl. epu′lides [Gr. epoulis a gumboil] a generic term applied to any tumor of the gingiva. **congenital e. of newborn,** a pedunculated lesion of the gingiva, present at birth, arising on the crest of the alveolar ridge or process, and usually occurring in the incisor region. **e. fibromato′sa,** a fibroma arising from the alveolar periosteum and the periodontal ligament. **e. fissura′ta,** granuloma fissuratum. **giant cell e., e. gigantocellula′ris,** peripheral giant cell reparative granuloma of gingiva. **e. granulomato′sa,** a small growth on the gingiva resulting from mechanical irritation or infection.

epuloerectile (ep″u-lo″e-rek′tīl) both epuloid and erectile.

epulofibroma (ep″u-lo″fi-bro′mah) a fibroma of the gingiva.

epuloid (ep′u-loid) resembling an epulis.

epulosis (ep″u-lo′sis) [Gr. epoulōsis] cicatrization.

epulotic (ep″u-lot′ik) [Gr. epoulōtikos] pertaining to, characterized by, or promoting cicatrization.

Equanil (ek′wah-nil) trademark for preparations of meprobamate.

equate (e′kwāt) to make equal or equivalent. In color vision, the physiologic faculty of combining two colors to match a third, as to combine red and green to make a homogeneous yellow.

equation (e-kwa′zhun) [L. aequatio, from aequare to make equal] an expression made up of two members connected by the sign of equality, =. **Ambard's e.,** see under formula. **Arrhenius' e.,** an equation describing the temperature dependence of a reaction rate constant, $k = Ae^{-E_a/RT}$, where k is the rate constant, E_a the activation energy, R the gas constant, T the absolute temperature, A the preexponential factor. **Ayala's e.,** see under quotient. **chemical e.,** an equation that expresses a chemical reaction, the symbols on the left of the equation denoting the substances before, and those on the right those after, the reaction. **Harden and Young e.,** an equation showing the chemical reaction in the fermentation of glucose to carbon dioxide, alcohol, and hexose diphosphate. **Henderson-Hasselbalch e.,** a formula for calculating the pH of a buffer solution such as blood plasma, $pH = pK' + \log\frac{(BA)}{(HA)}$. (HA) is the concentration of a weak acid; (BA) the concentration of a weak salt of this acid; pK′ the buffer system. **Nernst e.,** an equation for determining the value of a transmembrane potential at ionic equilibrium. **personal e.,** the more or less constant difference in the results of observation depending upon the personal qualities of observers. **Poiseuille e., (Hagenbach extension)** an equation for the volume flow (V) of a fluid through a capillary tube in terms of the pressure drop P, the radius R, and the length L of the system, and the viscosity η, of the fluid:

$$V = \frac{P\pi R^4}{8\eta L}$$

Ussing e., a method for determining active transport across a biologic membrane, by considering the unidirectional fluxes.

equator (e-kwa′tor) [L. aequator equalizer] an imaginary line encircling a globe, equidistant from the poles. Used in anatomical nomenclature to designate such a line on a spherical organ, dividing the surface into two approximately equal parts. Called also aequator. **e. bul′bi oc′uli** [NA], an imaginary line encircling the eyeball equidistant from the anterior and the posterior poles, dividing the eye into anterior and posterior halves. Called also e. of eyeball. **e. of cell,** the boundary of the plane of separation of a dividing cell. **e. of crystalline lens,** e. lentis. **e. of eyeball,** e. bulbi oculi. **e. of lens, e. len′tis** [NA], the rounded peripheral margin of the lens at which the anterior and posterior surfaces meet.

equatorial (e″kwah-to′re-al) pertaining to an equator; occurring at the same distance from each extremity of an axis.

equiaxial (e″kwe-ak′se-al) having axes of the same length.

equicaloric (e″kwi-kah-lōr′ik) isocaloric.

Equidae (ek′wĭ-de) [L. equus horse] a family of perissodactyl mammals containing a single living genus, Equus, which includes horses, asses, zebras, and onagers.

equilateral (e″kwĭ-lat′er-al) having sides that are equal or identical; called also isolateral.

equilibration (e″kwĭ-lĭ-bra′shun) the achievement of a balance between opposing elements or forces. **mandibular e.,** 1. the act or acts performed to place the mandible in equilibrium. 2. a condition in which all of the forces acting upon the mandible are neutralized. 3. a term applied to adjustive grinding of an interfering tooth structure during the functional stroke. **occlusal e.,** a modification of the occlusal forms of teeth to equalize occlusal stress, to produce simultaneous occlusal contacts, or to achieve harmonious occlusion.

equilibrator (e″kwĭ-lĭ-bra′tor) an apparatus used to produce or maintain a state of balance between opposing forces.

equilibrium (e″kwĭ-lib′re-um) [L. aequus equal + libra balance] a state of balance or equipoise; a condition in which opposing forces exactly counteract each other. **acid-base e.,** see under balance. **body e.,** the condition in which the materials taken into the body are balanced by corresponding excretions. **carbon e.,** the condition in which the total carbon of the excreta is balanced by the carbon of the food. **colloid e.,** a stable condition of the colloids of the body fluids; disturbance of such equilibrium produces colloidoclastic shock or anaphylactoid crisis. **Donnan's e.,** the conditions which exist at equilibrium when two solutions are separated by a membrane which is permeable to some of the ions of the solutions, but not to all of them. There is a complex distribution of the ions between the two solutions, an electrical potential develops between the two sides of the membrane and the two solutions vary in osmotic pressure. Called also Gibbs-Donnan e. **dynamic e.,** the condition of balance between varying, shifting, and opposing forces which is characteristic of living processes. **fluid e.,** see under balance. **genetic e.,** the condition that exists when the gene pool in a population is constant in successive generations (unless altered by selection or mutation); i.e., the frequency of each allele in the population remains unchanged in successive generations. **Gibbs-Donnan e.,** Donnan e. **Hardy-Weinberg e.,** the stabilizing point at which all the factors of the sex ratio are present in a theoretically ideal genotype frequency. **nitrogen e., nitrogenous e.,** the condition in which the body is metabolizing and excreting as much nitrogen as it is receiving in the food; called also protein e. **nutritive e.,** physiologic e. **physiologic e.,** the condition in which the amount of material taken into the body exactly equals the amount discharged. **protein e.,** nitrogen e. **radioactive e.,** the fixed ratio between a radioactive element and one of its disintegration products that results after the lapse of a suitable time, owing to their half value periods. That of uranium and radium is as 2,380,000 to 1. **water e.,** fluid balance.

equilin (ek′wil-in) chemical name: 3-hydroxyestra-1,3,5(10),7-tetraen-17-one. A conjugated estrogen, $C_{18}H_{20}O_2$, isolated from urine of pregnant horses.

equimolar (e″kwi-mo′lar) containing the same number of moles, or having the same molarity.

equimolecular (e″kwĭ-mo-lek′u-lar) containing the same number of molecules; said of solutions.

equination (e″kwĭ-na′shun) [L. equinus equine] inoculation with the virus of horsepox.

equine (e′kwīn) [L. equus a horse] pertaining to, characteristic of, or derived from the horse.

equinophobia (e-kwi″no-fo′be-ah) [L. equinus relating to horses + Gr. phobos fear + -ia] (obs.) morbid fear of horses.

equinovarus (e-kwi″no-va′rus) talipes equinovarus.

equinus (e-kwi′nus) talipes equinus.

equipotential (e″kwĭ-po-ten′shal) [L. *aequus* equal + *potentia* ability, power] possessed of similar and equal power; capable of developing in the same way and to the same extent.

equipotentiality (e″kwe-po-ten″she-al′ĭ-te) the quality or state of having similar and equal power; the capacity for developing in the same way and to the same extent.

equisetosis (ek″wĭ-sĕ-to′sis) poisoning of horses from eating equisetum.

equisetum (ek″wĭ-se′tum) a common weed, *E. arvense*, horsetail or jointed rush, that causes a form of poisoning in horses that eat it with hay. It is used as a diuretic drug in eclectic practice.

equivalence (e-kwiv′ah-lens) 1. the condition of being equivalent. In immunology, the ratio of antigen to antibody concentration at which maximal antigen-antibody combination takes place, yielding a precipitate or aggregate. 2. see *equivalent weight*, under *weight*.

equivalent (e-kwiv′ah-lent) [L. *aequivalens*, from *aequus* equal + *valere* to be worth] 1. having the same value; neutralizing or counterbalancing each other. 2. chemical equivalent. 3. in medicine, a symptom that replaces one that is usual in a given disease. **aluminum e.,** the thickness of pure aluminum affording the same radiation attenuation, under specified conditions, as the material or materials being considered. **bursa-e.,** see under *bursa*. **bursal e. tissue,** see under *tissue*. **chemical e.,** that weight in grams of a substance which will produce or react with one mole of hydrogen ion or one mole of electrons; called also *gram e.* **combustion e.,** the heat value of a gram of fat or carbohydrate burned outside the body. It measures the amount of potential energy of the substance available, in the form of food, for the production of heat or the supply of energy. **concrete e.,** the thickness of concrete having a density of 2.35 gm./cm.^{3} which would afford the same radiation attenuation, under specified conditions, as the material or materials being considered. **dose e.,** in radiation biology, the product of absorbed dose in rads and the modifying factors, namely the quality factor (QF), distribution factor (DF), and any other necessary factors. The unit of dose equivalent is the rem. **endosmotic e.,** the number which represents the quantity of water that will pass through a diaphragm by endosmosis in the same time that a unit of any other given substance will pass in the other direction by exosmosis. **epileptic e.,** a disturbance, mental or bodily, that may take the place of an epileptic attack. **gold e.,** the amount of protective colloid, expressed in milligrams, which is just enough to prevent the precipitation of 10 ml. of a 0.0055 per cent gold solution by 1 ml. of a 10 per cent sodium chloride solution. **gram e.,** chemical e. **isodynamic e.,** the ratio, from a food-energy standpoint, between carbohydrate and fat. It is 9.3 to 4.1, or 2.3 to 1; that is, one part of fat is equivalent to 2.3 parts of sugar or starch. **Joule's e.,** the mechanical equivalent of heat or the amount of work expended in raising a pound of water through 1° F.; 772 foot-pounds. Symbol J. **lead e.,** the thickness of pure lead which would afford the same radiation attenuation, under specified conditions, as the material or materials under consideration. **lethal e.,** a gene carried in the heterozygous state which, if homozygous, would be lethal, or any combination of genes which would be lethal to 100 percent of homozygotes; for example, a combination of two genes in the heterozygous state either of which in the homozygous state would be lethal to 50 per cent of the carriers. **neutralization e.,** the equivalent weight of an acid as determined by neutralization with a base regarded as a primary standard. **protein e.,** the protein content of a food plus the nonprotein content that can be converted into protein in the animal body. **psychic e.,** psychic epilepsy. **starch e.,** a number (nearly 2.4) expressing the amount of oxygen which a given weight of fat will require for its complete combustion as compared with the amount required by the same weight of starch. **toxic e.,** the amount of poison per kilogram of body weight necessary to kill an animal. **ventilation e.,** 1. the ratio of the total volume of ventilation to the volume of expired carbon dioxide per unit of time. 2. the ratio of the total volume of ventilation to the volume of oxygen absorbed by the lungs per unit of time. **water e.,** the product of the weight of an animal by its specific heat, it being also the number which represents the specific thermal capacity of an equal weight of water.

equulosis (ek″kwoo-lo′sis) [L. *equulus* a foal + *-osis*] a purulent arthritis, synovitis, and enteritis, often with formation of kidney abscesses, affecting primarily young foals but occasionally mature horses and caused by *Actinobacillus equuli*. When manifested as extreme prostration, it is known as *sleepy foal disease* (q.v.).

Equus (ek′wus) the single living genus of the family Equidae, including horses, asses, and zebras.

Er chemical symbol for *erbium*.

E.R.A. Electroshock Research Assocation.

erabutoxin (ĕ-rab″u-tok′sin) the active toxic principle of the venom of the sea snake *Laticauda semifasciata*.

erasion (e-ra′zhun) [L. *erasio*] removal by scraping, or curettage. **e. of a joint,** arthrectomy.

Erasistratus (er″ah-sis′trah-tus) **of Chios** (c. 300 B.C.) a celebrated Greek anatomist and physician who practiced chiefly in Alexandria. He dissected the human body, and observed the association between ascites and hepatic cirrhosis. He also made many physiological observations, and has been called "The Father of Physiology."

Eratyrus (er″ah-ti′rus) a genus of reduviid bugs that transmit Chagas' disease.

Erb (erb), Wilhelm Heinrich. A celebrated German internist (1840–1921). See *progressive muscular dystrophy* and *pseudohypertrophic muscular dystrophy*, under *dystrophy*, *Erb's spastic paraplegia*, under *paraplegia*, *Erb-Duchenne paralysis*, under *paralysis*, and see under *point, sclerosis, sign*, and *syndrome*.

Erb-Charcot disease (erb′shar-ko′) [W. H. *Erb*; Jean Martin *Charcot*, French neurologist, 1825–1893] Erb's spastic paraplegia.

Erb-Duchenne paralysis (erb′du-shen′) [Willhelm Heinrick *Erb*; Guillaume Benjamen Amand *Duchenne*, French neurologist, 1806–1875] see under *paralysis*.

Erb-Goldflam disease (erb′golt′flahm) [W. H. *Erb*; Samuel V. *Goldflam*, Polish neurologist, 1825–1932] myasthenia gravis.

Erben's phenomenon, reflex (sign) (er′benz) [Siegmund *Erben*, neurologist in Vienna, born 1863] see under *phenomenon* and *reflex*.

ERBF effective renal blood flow; see under *flow*.

erbium (er′be-um) a rare metallic element: symbol, Er; atomic number, 68; atomic weight, 167.26.

Erdmann's reagent (erd′manz) [Hugo *Erdmann*, German chemist, 1862–1910] see under *reagent*.

erectile (ĕ-rek′tīl) capable of erection; see under *tissue*.

erection (ĕ-rek′shun) [L. *erectio*] the condition of being made rigid and elevated; as erectile tissue when filled with blood.

erector (ĕ-rek′tor) [L.] [NA] a general term for a structure that erects, as a muscle which raises or holds up a part.

eremacausis (er″ĕ-mah-kaw′sis) [Gr. *ērema* gently + *kausis* burning] the slow oxidation, combustion, or decay of organic matter.

eremophobia (er″ĕ-mo-fo′be-ah) [Gr. *erēmos* solitary + *phobein* to be affrighted by + *ia*] (*obs.*) morbid fear of being alone.

erepsin (e-rep′sin) [Gr. *ereptesthai* to feed on] former term for a group of enzymes (peptidases) in the small intestines which catalyze the hydrolysis of partially digested proteins to produce amino acids.

erethism (er′ĕ-thizm) [Gr. *erethisma* stimulation] excessive irritability or sensibility to stimulation, particularly with reference to the sexual organs but including any body parts. Also a psychic disturbance marked by irritability, emotional instability, depression, shyness, and fatigue, as in chronic mercury poisoning.

erethismic (er″ĕ-thiz′mik) erethistic.

erethisophrenia (er″ĕ-thiz″o-fre′ne-ah) [Gr. *erethizein* to irritate + *phrēn* mind] exaggerated mental excitability.

erethistic (er″ĕ-this′tik) [Gr. *erethistikos*] pertaining to, characterized by, or producing erethism.

erethitic (er″ĕ-thit′ik) Hunt's term for the excitatory temperament, marked by great activity of mind and body, i.e., responsive, impulsive, emotional, quick tempered, and restless. Cf. *kolytic*.

Erethmapodites (ĕ-reth″mah-pod′ĭ-tēz) a genus of mosquitoes, species of which transmit Rift Valley fever.

ereuth- for words beginning thus, see those beginning *eryth-*.

ERG electroretinogram.

erg (erg) [Gr. *ergon* work] a unit of work or energy, being the work performed when a force of 1 dyne moves its point of operation through a distance of 1 centimeter; equivalent to 2.4×10^{-8} gram calories, or to 0.624×10^{12} electron volts.

ergasia (er-ga′se-ah) [Gr. "work"] 1. a hypothetical substance which stimulates the activity of body cells. 2. Meyer's term for any mentally integrated function, activity, reaction, or attitude of the individual; psychobiological functioning.

ergasiatrics, ergasiatry (er-ga″ze-at′riks; er″gah-si′ah-tre) Meyer's term for psychiatry.

ergasiology (er-ga″se-ol′o-je) [*ergasia* + *-logy*] objective psychobiology.

ergasiomania (er-ga″se-o-ma′ne-ah) [*ergasia* + Gr. *mania* madness] (*obs.*) 1. an insane desire to be continually at work. 2. undue eagerness to perform surgical operations.

ergasiophobia (er-ga″se-o-fo′be-ah) [*ergasia* + Gr. *phobein* to be affrighted by + *ia*] 1. (*obs.*) morbid aversion to work. 2. undue fear of performing surgical operations.

ergasthenia (er″gas-the′ne-ah) [Gr. *ergon* work + *astheneia* weakness] (*obs.*) a condition of debility from overwork.

ergastic (er-gas′tik) [Gr. *ergastikos*] 1. having potential energy; a term applied to passive material formed or stored by a cell, such as starch, fat, and cellulose. 2. pertaining to ergasia.

ergastoplasm (er-gas′to-plazm) [*ergasia* + *plasm*] 1. granular endoplasmic reticulum. 2. (*obs.*) Garnier's concept of cytoplasm, the fibrillar or flocculent masses found in many gland cells and elsewhere.

ergo- (er′go) [Gr. *ergon* work] a combining form denoting relationship to work.

ergobasine (er″go-ba′sin) ergonovine.

ergocalciferol (er-go-kal-sif′er-ol) [USP] chemical name: 9,10-secoergosta-5,7,10(19),22-tetraen-3β-ol. An activation product, $C_{28}H_{44}O$, of ergosterol, produced by ultraviolet irradiation or electronic bombardment, occurring in white odorless crystals, insoluble in water but soluble in alcohol, chloroform, ether, and fatty oils; used chiefly as an oral antirachitic vitamin. Called also *calciferol, activated ergosterol, viosterol,* and *vitamin D₂*.

ergocardiogram (er″go-kar′de-o-gram) the graphic record obtained by ergocardiography.

ergocardiography (er″go-kar″de-og′rah-fe) the recording of moment-to-moment electromotive forces of the heart while the subject is engaging in muscular activity.

ergocornine (er″go-kor′nēn) an alkaloid, $C_{31}H_{39}N_5O_5$, from ergot, once used in peripheral vascular disorders.

ergocristine (er″go-kris′tēn) an alkaloid, $C_{35}H_{39}N_5O_5$, from ergot, once used in peripheral vascular disorders.

ergocryptine (er″go-krip′tēn) an alkaloid, $C_{32}H_{41}N_5O_5$, from ergot, once used in peripheral vascular disorders.

ergodynamograph (er″go-di-nam′o-graf) [*ergo-* + Gr. *dynamis* force + *graphein* to record] an apparatus for recording the force exhibited and the work done in muscular contraction.

ergoesthesiograph (er″go-es-the′se-o-graf) [*ergo-* + Gr. *aisthēsis* sensation + *graphein* to record] an apparatus for recording graphically muscular reactions to various stimuli.

ergogenic (er″go-jen′ik) [*ergo-* + Gr. *gennan* to produce] tending to increase work output.

ergogram (er′go-gram) [*ergo-* + Gr. *gramma* a mark] a tracing made by an ergograph.

ergograph (er′go-graf) [*ergo-* + Gr. *graphein* to record] an instrument for recording work done in muscular exertion. **Mosso's e.** (1890), an apparatus for recording the force and frequency of flexion of the fingers.

ergographic (er″go-graf′ik) pertaining to the ergograph.

ergomaniac (er″go-ma′ne-ak) [*ergo-* + Gr. *mania* madness] a person morbidly desirous of being continually at work.

Ergomar (er′go-mar) trademark for a preparation of ergotamine tartrate.

ergometer (er-gom′ĕ-ter) [*ergo-* + Gr. *metron* measure] a dynamometer. **bicycle e.,** an apparatus for measuring the muscular, metabolic, and respiratory effects of exercise.

ergometrine (er″go-met′rin) ergonovine.

ergon (er′gon) a unit representing the stability of a particular gene throughout a lifetime; it is a function of the ratio of the adenine-thymine to guanine-cytosine content of the gene and is reflected in the persistence of the resultant phenotypical trait. Cf. *chronon.*

ergonomics (er″go-nom′iks) [*ergo-* + Gr. *nomos* law] the science relating to man and his work, embodying the anatomic, physiologic, psychologic, and mechanical principles affecting the efficient use of human energy.

ergonovine (er″go-no′vin) chemical name: D-lysergic acid 1-hydroxy-methylethylamide. A water-soluble alkaloid, $C_{19}H_{23}N_3O_2$, from ergot or produced synthetically; used as an oxytocic and to relieve migraine headache. Called also *ergobasine, ergometrine, ergostetrine,* and *ergotocine*. **e. maleate** [USP], the bimaleate salt of ergonovine, $C_{19}H_{23}N_3O_2 \cdot C_4H_4O_4$, occurring as a grayish white to faintly yellow odorless powder; used as an oxytocic, administered orally, intramuscularly, or intravenously. It is also used in the treatment of migraine.

ergophore (er″go-fōr) [*ergo-* + Gr. *phoros* bearing] in Ehrlich's side-chain theory, the group of atoms in a molecule that brings about the specific activity of the substance, as of a toxin, agglutinin, or the like, after the molecule has been properly anchored by the haptophore.

ergoplasm (er′go-plazm) ergastoplasm.

ergosome (er′go-sōm) polyribosome.

ergostat (er′go-stat) a machine to be worked for muscular exercise.

ergosterol (er-gos′tĕ-rol) a sterol, $C_{28}H_{43} \cdot OH$, occurring in animal and plant tissues which, on irradiation with ultraviolet rays, becomes a potent antirachitic substance, ergocalciferol (vitamin D₂). The substance was originally isolated by Tanret from ergot and named accordingly. **activated e., irradiated e.,** ergocalciferol.

ergostetrine (er″go-stet′rin) ergonovine.

ergot (er′got) [Fr.; L. *ergota*] 1. the dried sclerotium of *Claviceps purpurea,* which is developed on rye plants (*Secale cereale*); ergot alkaloids are used as oxytocics and in the treatment of migraine. 2. (*obs.*) calcar avis. 3. a small mass of horn in the tuft of hair at the flexion surface of the fetlock in horses.

ergotamine (er-got′ah-min) an alkaloid derived from ergot, consisting of lysergic acid, ammonia, proline, phenylalanine, and pyruvic acid combined in amide linkages; used in the treatment of migraine. **e. tartrate** [USP], the tartrate salt of ergotamine, $(C_{33}H_{35}H_5O_5)_2 \cdot C_4H_6O_6$, occurring as colorless crystals or as a yellowish crystalline powder; used as an analgesic in the treatment of migraine.

ergotaminine (er″go-tam′ĭ-nēn) an isomer, $C_{33}H_{35}N_5O_5$, of ergotamine.

ergotherapy (er″go-ther′ah-pe) [*ergo-* + Gr. *therapeia* treatment] treatment of disease by physical effort.

ergothioneine (er″go-thi′′o-ne′in) the trimethylbetaine of thiolhistidine, $C_3HN_2(SH) \cdot CH_2 \cdot CH \cdot CO \cdot ON(CH_3)_3 \cdot 2H_2O$, found in ergot and in the blood and in abnormal amounts in the urine of cancer patients; called also *thionene* and *erythrothioneine*.

ergotism (er′got-izm) chronic poisoning from excessive or misdirected use of ergot as a medicine, or from eating ergotized grain; it is marked by cerebrospinal symptoms, spasms, and cramps, or by a kind of dry gangrene.

ergotized (er′got-īzd) diseased or otherwise affected by ergot.

ergotocine (er″go-to′sēn) ergonovine.

ergotoxicosis (er″go-tok″si-ko′sis) a form of mycotoxicosis caused by one of the ergot (*Claviceps*) species.

ergotoxine (er″go-tok′sēn) a toxic crystalline alkaloid originally isolated from ergot (*Claviceps purpurea*), consisting of a mixture of ergocornine, ergocristine, and ergocryptine, which exert both oxytocic and adrenergic blocking effects. Because of the variability of these effects, neither ergotoxine nor its constituents are currently used in medicine.

Ergotrate (er′go-trāt) trademark for preparations of ergonovine maleate.

ergusia (er-ju′se-ah) a hypothetical lipoid substance which, liberated from a cell, reduces surface tension and enables the cell to migrate.

Erichsen's ligature, sign (test) (er′ik-senz) [Sir John Eric *Erichsen,* English surgeon, 1818–1896] see under *ligature* and *spine.*

Eriodictyon (er″e-o-dik′te-on) [Gr. *erion* wool + *diktyon* net] a genus of hydrophyllaceous plants. *E. califor′nicum* H. & A. Greene (*E. glutino′sum*), also known as yerba santa or mountain balm, was once used in bronchitis. See *eriodictyon.*

eriodictyon (er″e-o-dik′te-on) [NF] the dried leaf of *Eriodictyon californicum;* its fluidextract is used as a flavor and its aromatic syrup as a vehicle for dispensing drugs.

erisiphake (er-is′ĭ-fāk) erysiphake.

Eristalis (er-is′tah-lis) a genus of flies, the hover flies, of the family Syrphidae. **E. tenax,** the "drone fly," the "rat-tail" maggots (larvae), which occasionally cause intestinal and nasal myiasis.

Erlanger's sphygmomanometer (er′lang-erz) [Joseph *Erlanger,* American physiologist, 1874–1965, noted for his work on the nervous system; co-winner, with Herbert Spencer Gasser, of the Nobel prize for medicine in 1944] see under *sphymomanometer.*

Erlenmeyer flask (ār′len-mi″er) [Emil Richard August Carl *Erlenmeyer,* German chemist, 1825–1909] see under *flask.*

Erni's sign (er′nēz) [H. *Erni,* Swiss physician, 1859–1937] see under *sign.*

erntefieber (ern′te-fe″ber) [Ger. "harvest-fever"] schlammfieber.

erode (e-rōd′) to wear away.

erogenous (ĕ-roj′ĕ-nus) erotogenic; arousing erotic feelings; see also under *zone.*

erose (e-rōs′) [L. *erodere* to gnaw off] having an irregularly toothed edge.

erosio (e-ro′se-o) [L.] erosion. **e. interdigita′lis blastomycet′ica** or **saccharomycet′ica,** an eroded lesion occurring in the interdigital webs of the fingers, almost always between the third and fourth fingers, especially in cannery workers, housewives, or waitresses, caused by *Candida* (*Monilia*) *albicans.*

erosion (e-ro′zhun) [L. *erosio,* from *erodere* to eat out] an eating or gnawing away; a kind of ulceration. In dentistry, the wasting away or loss of substance of a tooth by a chemical process that does not involve known bacterial action. In dermatology, a gradual breakdown or very shallow ulceration of the skin which involves only the epidermis and heals without scarring. **cervical e.,** a condition caused by irritation and characterized by destruction of the squamous epithelium of the vaginal portion of the cervix; the eroded area is covered by columnar epithelium. **dental e.,** the disintegration of tooth substance on surfaces free from attrition by mastication.

erosive (e-ro′siv) 1. causing, characterized by, or producing erosion. 2. an agent that produces erosion.

erotic (ĕ-rot′ik) [Gr. *erōtikos*] pertaining to sexual love or to lust.

eroticism (e-rot′ĭ-sizm) erotism.

eroticize (ĕ-rot′ĭ-sīz) erotize.

eroticomania (ĕ-rot″ĭ-ko-ma′ne-ah) erotomania.

erotism (er′o-tizm) a sexual instinct or desire; the expression of one's instinctual energy or drive, especially the sex drive. **anal e.,** fixation of libido at (or regression to) the anal phase of infantile development, said in psychoanalytic theory to produce egotistic, dogmatic, stubborn, miserly character. **muscle e.,** erotism stimulated by muscular exercise. **oral e.,** 1. fixation of libido at (or regression to) the oral phase of infantile development, said in psychoanalytic theory to produce passive, insecure, sensitive character. 2. the pleasure derived from the use of the mouth for other than nutritional satisfactions.

erotize (er′o-tīz) to endow with erotic or libidinous instinct or energy.

eroto- (e-ro′to) [Gr. *erōs* love] a combining form denoting relationship to love or sexual desire.

erotogenesis (ĕ-ro″to-jen′ĕ-sis) the formation or production of erotic feeling.

erotogenic (ĕ-ro″to-jen′ik) [*eroto-* + Gr. *gennan* to produce] producing erotic feelings; erogenous. See also under *zone.*

erotology (er″o-tol′o-je) [*eroto-* + *-logy*] the study of love.

erotomania (ĕ-rot″to-ma′ne-ah) [*eroto-* + Gr. *mania* madness] morbid exaggeration of sexual behavior or reaction; preoccupation with sexuality.

erotomaniac (ĕ-ro″to-ma′ne-ak) a person exhibiting erotomania.

erotopath (ĕ-ro′to-path) a person exhibiting erotopathy.

erotopathy (er″o-top′ah-the) [*eroto-* + Gr. *pathos* disease] disorder of the sexual impulse.

erotophobia (ĕ-ro″to-fo′be-ah) [*eroto-* + Gr. *phobein* to be affrighted by + *ia*] morbid dislike of sexual love.

erotosexual (ĕ-ro″to-seks′u-al) pertaining to sexual love.

ERPF effective renal plasma flow; see under *flow.*

erratic (ĕ-rat′ik) [L. *errare* to wander] 1. roving or wandering. 2. eccentric; deviating from an accepted course of thought or conduct.

errhine (er′in) [Gr. *en* in + *rhis* nose] 1. promoting a nasal discharge. 2. a medicine that promotes nasal discharge or secretion.

error (er′or) a defect in structure or function; a deviation. **inborn e. of metabolism,** see under *metabolism.*

Ertron (er′tron) trademark for preparations of ergocalciferol (vitamin D₂).

eructatio (e″ruk-ta′she-o) [L., from *eructare* to belch] eructation. **e. nervo′sa,** nervous eructation.

eructation (ĕ-ruk-ta′shun) [L. *eructatio*] the act of belching, or of casting up wind from the stomach through the mouth. **nervous e.,** a gastric neurosis marked by air swallowing followed by belching.

eruption (e-rup′shun) [L. *eruptio* a breaking out] 1. the act of breaking out, appearing, or becoming visible, as eruption of the teeth. 2. visible efflorescence lesions of the skin due to disease, and marked by redness, prominence, or both; a rash. See also *exanthem.* **bullous e.,** an eruption of large blebs or blisters. **continuous e.,** eruption of a tooth beyond the normal so that the length of the clinical crown may be increased or the periodontium may be extruded with the tooth. **creeping e.,** a dermatitis caused by the burrowing of nematodes or larvae in the deeper layers of the skin; see *larva migrans.* **drug e.,** an eruption or a solitary skin lesion caused by a drug taken internally; called also *drug rash* and *dermatitis medicamentosa.* **fixed e.,** a circumscribed inflammatory skin lesion(s) that recurs at the same site(s) over a period of months or years; each attack lasts only a few days but leaves residual pigmentation which is cumulative. **fixed drug e.,** a drug eruption that recurs at the same site; see *fixed e.* **Kaposi's varicelliform e.,** a generalized and serious vesiculopustular eruption of viral origin, superimposed upon a preexisting atopic dermatitis; it may be caused by the virus of herpes simplex (eczema herpeticum) or vaccinia (eczema vaccinatum). Called also *pustulosis vacciniformis* (or *varioliformis*) *acuta.* **macular e.,** an eruption in the form of spots, due to hemorrhage, congestion, or increased or diminished pigmentation. **maculopapular e.,** an eruption consisting of both macules and papules; sometimes used loosely when only one or the other is present. **passive e.,** the apparent continued eruption of the teeth that is actually due to gingival recession. **petechial e.,** an eruption in the form of very minute spots, due to hemorrhage; a purpura. **polymorphous e.,** an eruption characterized by lesions in many different stages of evolution, from incipient through mature to healing. **polymorphous light e.,** a rather uniform skin eruption, though highly variable in different patients, confined to sun-exposed surfaces of the skin, not attributable to photosensitizing applications or medications, or to systemic disease, and typically initiated and aggravated by exposure to sunlight. **sandworm e.,** larva migrans. **seabather's e.,** marine dermatitis. **serum e.,** an eruption or exanthem accompanying serum sickness. **surgical e.,** the uncovering of a partially erupted tooth to permit its further eruption into the oral cavity by surgically removing overlying tissue, teeth, and/or bone.

eruptive (e-rup′tiv) pertaining to or characterized by eruption.

ERV expiratory reserve volume; see under *volume.*

Erwinia (er-win′e-ah) [*Erwin F. Smith*, American bacteriologist, 1854–1927] a genus of microorganisms of the tribe Erwinieae, family Enterobacteriaceae, order Eubacteriales. The 16 described species are pathogenic for plants, causing dry necroses, galls, or wilts, or soft rots.

Erwinieae (er″wĭ-ni′e-e) a tribe of the family Enterobacteriaceae, order Eubacteriales, made up of motile rods normally not requiring organic nitrogen compounds for growth and producing acid, with or without visible gas, from a variety of sugars. It includes a single genus, *Erwinia.*

erysipelas (er″ĭ-sip′ĕ-las) [Gr. *erythros* red + *pella* skin] a contagious disease of skin and subcutaneous tissue due to infection with *Streptococcus pyogenes* and marked by redness and swelling of affected areas, with constitutional symptoms; sometimes accompanied by vesicular and bullous lesions. **coast e.** (erisipela de la costa), onchocerciasis. **gangrenous e.,** a variety characterized by sloughing; it is fatal if not treated early with penicillin or other antibiotics. **e. gra′ve inter′num,** erysipelas in the vagina, uterus, and peritoneum; a form of puerperal fever. **malignant e.,** one of the forms of puerperal fever. **surgical e.,** erysipelas that occurs following a surgical operation. **swine e.,** a contagious disease affecting young swine in Europe, caused by *Erysipelothrix insidiosa.* Of great economic importance, it occurs in four clinical forms: An *acute septicemic form,* marked by high fever, lesions of the internal organs and viscera, and a high mortality rate. An *urticarial form,* marked by sudden onset, high fever, general debility, formation of reddish to purplish quadrangular or rhomboid blotches on the neck and body and sometimes by involvement of the viscera; this is the mildest form and is rarely fatal. Called also *diamonds, diamond skin disease, rose disease,* and *rouget du porc.* A *chronic form,* marked by difficulty in breathing, vegetative endocarditis, and ultimately death. An *arthritic form,* marked by stunting of growth; this form may occur alone or may complicate other forms of the disease, and is not usually fatal. **traumatic e.,** erysipelas that starts in a wound. **zoonotic e.** (*obs.*), erysipeloid.

erysipelatous (er″ĭ-sĭ-pel′ah-tus) pertaining to or of the nature of erysipelas.

erysipeloid (er″ĭ-sip′ĕ-loid) [*erysipelas* + Gr. *eidos* form] 1. an infective dermatitis or cellulitis due to infection with *Erysipelothrix rhusiopathiae;* it usually begins in a wound (often the result of a prick by a fish bone) and remains localized, rarely becoming generalized and septicemic. Called also *fish-handler's disease.* 2. loosely used to mean erysipelas-like.

Erysipelothrix (er″ĭ-sip′ĕ-lo-thriks″) [*erysipelas* + Gr. *thrix* hair] a genus of microorganisms of the family Corynebacteriaceae, order Eubacteriales, containing a single species, *E. insidiosa* (*E. rhusiopathiae*). This species, occurring as gram-positive rods and filaments, is the causative agent of swine erysipelas, and also infects sheep, turkeys, and rats. An erythematous-edematous lesion, commonly on the hand, resulting from contact with infected meat, hides, or bones, represents the usual type of infection in man (see *erypipeloid*). Called also *swine rotlauf bacillus.*

erysipelotoxin (er″ĭ-sip″ĕ-lo-tok′sin) the toxin of erysipelas.

Erysiphaceae (er-is″ĭ-fa′se-e) a family of fungi of the order Erysiphales, series Pyrenomycetes, which are plant pathogens and include the genus *Erysiphe.*

erysiphake (er-is″ĭ-fāk) [Gr. *erysis* a drawing + *phakos* lentil] an instrument for removing the lens in cataract by suction. Cf. *phacoerysis.*

Erysiphales (er-is″ĭ-fa′lēz) the powdery mildews, an order of ascomycetous fungi of the series Pyrenomycetes, subclass Euascomycetidae, which are parasitic on higher plants and usually have closed ascocarps and large spherical stalked asci; it includes the family Erysiphaceae.

Erysiphe (er-is″ĭ-fe) a genus of ascomycetous fungi of the family Erysiphaceae, order Erysiphales, including *E. polygoni,* the powdery mildews; its imperfect (sexual) stage is *Oidium.*

erythema (er″ĭ-the′mah) [Gr. *erythēma* flush upon the skin] a name applied to redness of the skin produced by congestion of the capillaries, which may result from a variety of causes, the etiology or a specific type of lesion often being indicated by a modifying term. **e. ab ig′ne,** redness of the skin caused by exposure to radiant heat; called also *e. calore* and *e. caloricum.* **e. a ca′lore,** e. ab igne. **acrodynic e.,** a condition characterized by reddened painful areas on the palms and soles. **e. annula′re,** a type of erythema multiforme in which the areas of redness are ring shaped; see also *e. annulare centifugum.* **e. annula′re centrif′ugum,** a chronic variant of erythema multiforme, with single or multiple edematous and erythematous papules, occurring usually on the thighs and lower legs, the lesions enlarging peripherally and clearing in the center, to produce annular lesions, which may coalesce; the condition may persist for years, with incomplete remissions and exacerbations. Called also *e. gyratum (perstans* or *repens*) and *e. figuratum (perstans).* **e. annula′re rheumat′icum,** an exanthem associated with rheumatic endocarditis, characterized by red or bluish red semicircles or rings over the abdomen, the sides of the thorax, and the back; called also *e. marginatum rheumaticum.* **e. arthrit′icum epidem′icum,** Haverhill fever. **e. calor′icum,** e. ab igne. **e. chron′icum mi′grans,** an annular erythema caused by the bite of a tick (*Ixodes*); it begins as an erythematous plaque several weeks after the bite and spreads peripherally with central clearing. **diaper e.,** see under *dermatitis.* **e. dyschro′micum per′stans,** a chronic, progressive, pigmenting dermatosis which has a predilection for the folds and creases, reported chiefly from South America and Texas and consisting of transient erythema followed by ashen or brownish gray pigmentation, with small islands of hypopigmentation in pigmented areas. Called also *dermatosis cinecienta, ashy dermatosis of Ramirez,* and *dermatosis cinera perstans.* **e. eleva′tum di-u′tinum,** firm, red, persistent, nodular elevations that are symmetrically distributed on the skin. Affected areas may include the backs of the hands, wrists, elbows, and rarely the ankles and buttocks. **epidemic e.,** acrodynia. **epidemic arthritic e.,** Haverhill fever. **e. figura′tum (perstans),** e. annulare centrifugum. **e. fu′gax,** redness of the skin that comes and goes quickly. **gluteal e.,** diaper dermatitis. **e. gyra′tum (perstans** or **repens),** e. annulare centrifugum. **e. indura′tum,** a chronic necrotizing vasculitis, usually occurring on the calves of young women, which was thought to be a form of tuberculosis of the skin complicated by vasculitis, but now the role of tuberculosis is in dispute; called also *Bazin's disease, tuberculosis cutis indurativa,* and *tuberculosis indurativa.* **e. infecti-o′sum,** a mildly contagious disease, sometimes occurring in epidemics, and marked by a rose-colored, coarsely lace-like macular rash; it occurs chiefly in children between the ages of four and twelve. Called also *fifth disease.* **e. i′ris,** a type of erythema multiforme in which the lesions form concentric rings, producing a target-like appearance. **Jacquet's e.,** diaper dermatitis. **e. margina′tum,** a type of erythema multiforme in which the reddened areas are disk shaped, with elevated edges. **e. margina′tum rheumat′icum,** e. annulare rheumaticum. **e. mi′grans,** geographic tongue. **Milian's e.,** a scarlatiniform eruption with malaise and fever, occurring seven to nine days after injection of arsphenamine, or as a toxic reaction to other drugs; called also *ninth-day e.* **e. multifor′me,** a symptom complex characterized by vivid erythematous, urticarial, bullous, more or less purpuric lesions which appear suddenly in a symmetrical distribution, usually on the face, neck, forearms, legs, and dorsal surfaces of the hands and feet. The lesions may appear as separate rings (*e. annulare*), as vesicles or bullae (*e. bullosum*), as concentric rings (*e. iris*), in round patches with elevated edges (*e. margina-tum*), or in variously figured arrangements (*e. figuratum*). The disease has also been classified according to severity as a mild form (*Hebra's disease*) and the severe form (*Stevens-Johnson syndrome*), with constitutional symptoms, involvement of the oronasal and anogenital mucosa and the eyes, and visceral involvement. Invidividual attacks are usually self-limited, but recurrences are the rule. The severe form may be fatal. **e. multiforme exudati′vum** (*obs.*), e. multiforme. **napkin e.,** diaper dermatitis. **e. neonato′rum,** a usually temporary diffuse redness of the skin of a newborn infant. **e. neonato′rum tox′icum,** erythema of a toxic origin in a newborn infant. **nine-day e.,** Milian's e. **e. nodo′sum,** an acute inflammatory skin disease marked by tender red nodules, usually on the shins, more rarely on the arms and face, due to exudation of blood and serum; the lesions may appear in successive patches during a period of several weeks. The disorder is thought to be an allergic reaction, sometimes to tuberculotoxin, streptococcal infection, drugs, psittacosis, or coccidioidomycosis. **e. nodo′sum lepro′sum,** a form of lepra reaction occurring in lepromatous and sometimes borderline leprosy, marked by the occurrence of tender, inflamed subcutaneous nodules, usually in crops. The reactions resemble multifocal Arthus reactions. When severe, such reactions may lead to ulcerations of the skin, acute neuritis, acute iridocyclitis, and orchitis. **e. nodo′sum syphilit′icum,** erythema nodosum occurring in congenital and in secondary syphilis. **palmar e.,** redness of the palms, occurring in certain disease states, including cirrhosis of the liver, tuberculosis, and nutritional deficiencies; during pregnancy; and rarely as a hereditary condition. **e. papulo′sum,** reddish or violaceous macules or papules. **e. paratrim′ma** (*obs.*), a skin inflammation, the first stage of an incipient decubitus ulcer. **e. per′nio,** chilblain. **e. streptog′enes,** pityriasis alba. **symptomatic e.,** erythema occurring secondarily to some systemic condition. **toxic e., e. tox′icum,** a generalized, diffuse erythematous eruption or a widespread erythematomacular eruption occurring as a result of administration of a drug, or caused by bacterial toxins or other toxic substances; called also *e. venenatum.* **e. tox′icum neonato′rum,** a self-limited urticarial condition affecting infants in the first few days of life. **e. traumat′icum,** redness of the skin caused by friction, pressure, or a blow. **e. venena′tum,** toxic e.

erythematopultaceous (er-ĭ-the″mah-to-pul-ta′shus) characterized by redness of the skin or mucous membrane, a condition caused by capillary congestion.

erythematous (er″ĭ-them′ah-tus) characterized by erythema.

erythemogenic (er″ĭ-the″mo-jen′ik) causing erythema.

erythermalgia (er″ĭ-ther-mal′je-ah) erythromelalgia.

Erythraea (er″ĭ-thre′ah) [Gr. *erythraios* red] a genus of red-flowered gentianaceous plants. *E. centau′rium,* the lesser centaury, and various other species are tonic and stomachic.

erythralgia (er″ĭ-thral′je-ah) [*erythro-* + *-algia*] erythromelalgia.

erythrasma (er″ĭ-thraz′mah) a chronic bacterial infection of major folds of the skin, marked by red or brownish patches on the skin. Affected areas may include the inner thighs, the scrotum, the axilla, and the area between the toes. The condition is caused by *Corynebacterium minutissimum.*

erythredema polyneuropathy (ĕ-rith″rĕ-de′mah pol″e-nu-ro-p′ah-the) [*erythro-* + Gr. *oidēma* swelling] acrodynia.

erythremia (er″ĭ-thre′me-ah) [*erythro-* + Gr. *haima* blood] polycythemia vera.

erythremomelalgia (er-ith″rĕ-mo-mel-al′je-ah) [Gr. *erythrēma* redness + *melos* limb + *-algia*] erythromelalgia.

erythrin (er′ith-rin) a depside chromogen $C_{20}H_{22}O_{11}$, from *Roccella tinctoria* and other lichens.

Erythrina (er″ĭ-thri′nah) a genus of tropical shrubs and trees of the legume family, long used in native medicines. Several species yield the alkaloids α-erythroidine and β-erythroidine.

erythrism (ĕ-rith′rizm) redness of the hair and beard with a ruddy complexion.

erythristic (er″ĭ-thris′tik) characterized by erythrism.

erythritol (ĕ-rith′rĭ-tol) chemical name: tetrahydroxybutane. A polyhydric alcohol, $CH_2OH(CHOH)_2CH_2OH$, occurring in algae, lichens, grasses, and several fungi; it is about twice as sweet as sucrose. Called also *erythrol.* See also *erythrityl.*

erythrityl (ĕ-rith′rĭ-til) the univalent radical C_4H_9 from erythritol. **e. tetranitrate,** chemical name: erythritol tetranitrate. A synthetic compound, $C_4H_6(NO_3)_4$, with actions similar to those of nitroglycerin. Percussion or excessive heat can cause undiluted erythrityl tetranitrate to explode. The official pharmaceutical preparations, prepared in accordance with USP standards, are used as a coronary vasodilator in the prophylaxis of angina pectoris and in long-term treatment of coronary insufficiency, administered orally or sublingually.

erythro- (ĕ-rith′ro) [Gr. *erythros* red] a combining form meaning red, or denoting a relationship to red.

Erythrobacillus (ĕ-rith″ro-bah-sil′us) a genus of small aerobic nonpathogenic bacterial organisms which produce red or pink pigments; it has been replaced by the genus *Serratia.*

erythroblast (ĕ-rith′ro-blast) [*erythro-* + Gr. *blastos* germ] a term used by Ehrlich to indicate any type of nucleated erythrocyte, but now more generally, and somewhat inaccurately, used to designate an immature cell from which a red corpuscle develops. The precise position assigned to it in the red cell lineage varies with the specific theory of blood maturation being propounded. **acidophilic e.,** orthochromatic normoblast. **basophilic e.,** basophilic normoblast. **early e.,** basophilic normoblast. **definitive e's,** basophil cells in the primordium of the liver that give rise to the mature non-nucleated erythrocytes; cf. *primitive e's.* **eosinophilic e.,** orthochromatic normoblast. **intermediate e.,** polychromatic normoblast. **late e.,** orthochromatic normoblast. **orthochromatic e.,** orthochromatic normoblast. **oxyphilic e.,** orthochromatic normoblast. **polychromatic e.,** polychromatic normoblast. **primitive e's,** cells arising from the blood islands of the yolk sac which are the precursors of the nucleated erythrocytes characteristic of the early embryo; cf. *definitive e's.*

erythroblastemia (ĕ-rith″ro-blas-te′me-ah) the presence in the peripheral blood of abnormally large numbers of nucleated red cells; erythroblastosis.

erythroblastic (ĕ-rith″ro-blas′tik) of, or relating to, erythroblasts.

erythroblastoma (ĕ-rith″ro-blas-to′mah) a tumor-like mass composed of nucleated red blood corpuscles.

erythroblastomatosis (ĕ-rith″ro-blas″to-mah-to′sis) a condition marked by the formation of erythroblastomas.

erythroblastopenia (ĕ-rith″ro-blas″to-pe′ne-ah) abnormal deficiency of the erythroblasts; see *aplastic crisis,* under *crisis.*

erythroblastosis (ĕ-rith″ro-blas-to′sis) 1. the presence of erythroblasts in the circulating blood; erythroblastemia. 2. a disease of fowl classified in the avian leukosis complex, marked by an increase in the number of immature red blood cells in the circulating blood; called also *erythroleukosis.* **e. feta′lis, e. neonato′rum,** hemolytic anemia of the fetus or newborn infant, caused by the transplacental transmission of maternally formed antibody, usually secondary to an incompatibility between the blood group of the mother and that of her offspring, characterized by accelerated destruction of erythrocytes and consequent jaundice and by increased red cell regeneration (nucleated red cells in the blood) and hepatosplenomegaly. In infants with severe jaundice, kernicterus may result. The most severe form is *hydrops fetalis.* Called also *hemolytic disease of newborn.*

erythroblastotic (ĕ-rith″ro-blas-tot′ik) pertaining to or characterized by erythroblastosis.

erythrocatalysis (ĕ-rith″ro-kah-tal′ĭ-sis) erythrokatalysis.

erythrochloropia (ĕ-rith″ro-klo-ro′pe-ah) [*erythro-* + Gr. *chlōros* green + *ōps* eye] ability to distinguish red and green, but not blue or yellow.

erythrochloropsia (ĕ-rith″ro-klo-rop′se-ah) erythrochloropia.

erythrochromia (ĕ-rith″ro-kro′me-ah) [*erythro-* + Gr. *chrōma,* color] hemorrhagic pigmentation of the spinal fluid, giving it a red color.

Erythrocin (ĕ-rith′ro-sin) trademark for a preparation of erythromycin.

erythroclasis (er″ĕ-throk′lah-sis) [*erythro-* + Gr. *klasis* a breaking] fragmentation or splitting up of red blood cells.

erythroclastic (ĕ-rith″ro-klas′tik) pertaining to, characterized by, or producing erythroclasis.

erythrocruorin (ĕ-rith″ro-kroo′o-rin) a respiratory protein from the blood of the marine worm, *Spirographis spallanzanii,* and certain other worms.

erythrocuprein (ĕ-rith″ro-koo′prin) a copper-protein compound, contained in the erythrocytes, the function of which is unknown.

erythrocyanogenia (ĕ-rith″ro-si″ah-no-je′ne-ah) (*obs.*) erythrocyanosis.

erythrocyanosis (ĕ-rith″ro-si″ah-no′sis) [*erythro-* + Gr. *kyanōsis* dark blue color] coarsely mottled bluish red discoloration on the legs and thighs of adolescent girls, or sometimes older women or fat, prepubertal boys; the condition is worse in winter, when chilblains may appear. Treatment is ineffective. Called also *e. crurum puellaris, e. crurum puellarum,* and *e. supramalleolaris.*

erythrocytapheresis (ĕ-rith″ro-si″tah-fer′ĕ-sis) [*erythrocyte* + Gr. *aphairesis* removal] the withdrawal of blood, separation and retention of red blood cells, and retransfusion of the remainder into the donor.

erythrocyte (ĕ-rith′ro-sīt) [*erythro-* + Gr. *kytos* hollow vessel] one of the elements found in peripheral blood; called also *red blood cell* or *corpuscle.* Normally, in the human, the mature form is a non-nucleated, yellowish, biconcave disk, adapted, by virtue of its configuration and its hemoglobin content, to transport oxygen. For immature forms in the erythrocytic series, see *normoblast.* **achromic e.,** a colorless erythrocyte; see *achromocyte.* **basophilic e.,** one that takes the basic stain; see *basophilia* (def. 1). **burr e.,** burr cell. **crenated e.,** an erythrocyte that shows a scalloped border. **hypochromic e.,** one that contains less than the normal concentration of hemoglobin and as a result appears paler than normal; it is usually also microcytic. Cf. *normochromic e.* **immature e.,** any erythrocyte prior to achievement of its complete development; see *normoblast* and *rubicyte.* **"Mexican hat" e.,** target cell. **normochromic e.,** one of normal color with a normal concentration of hemoglobin; cf. *hypochromic e.* **nucleated e.,** any of the immature forms of an erythrocyte, e.g., a normoblast. **orthochromatic e.,** one that takes only the acid stain. **polychromatic e., polychromatophilic e.,** an erythrocyte that, on staining, shows various shades of blue, combined with tinges of pink. **target e.,** see under *cell.*

erythrocythemia (ĕ-rith″ro-si-the′me-ah) an increase in the number of erythrocytes in the blood, as in erythrocytosis and polycythemia vera.

erythrocytic (ĕ-rith″ro-sit′ik) 1. pertaining to, characterized by, or of the nature of erythrocytes. 2. pertaining to the erythrocytic series; see under *series.*

erythrocytoblast (ĕ-rith″ro-si′to-blast) erythroblast.

erythrocytolysin (ĕ-rith″ro-si-tol′ĭ-sin) a substance that causes dissolution and escape of hemoglobin.

erythrocytolysis (ĕ-rith″ro-si-tol′ĭ-sis) [*erythrocyte* + Gr. *lysis* dissolution] dissolution of erythrocytes and escape of the hemoglobin.

erythrocytometer (ĕ-rith″ro-si-tom′ĕ-ter) [*erythrocyte* + Gr. *metron* measure] a device for measuring or counting erythrocytes.

erythrocytometry (ĕ-rith″ro-si-tom′ĕ-tre) the measurement or counting of erythrocytes.

erythrocyto-opsonin (ĕ-rith″ro-si″to-op-so′nin) [*erythrocyte* + *opsonin*] hemopsonin.

erythrocytopenia (ĕ-rith″ro-si″to-pe′ne-ah) erythropenia.

erythrocytophagous (ĕ-rith″ro-si-tof′ah-gus) pertaining to or characterized by erythrocytophagy.

erythrocytophagy (ĕ-rith″ro-si-tof′ah-je) [*erythrocyte* + Gr. *phagein* to devour] the engulfment or consumption of erythrocytes by other cells, such as the histiocytes of the reticuloendothelial system.

erythrocytopoiesis (ĕ-rith″ro-si″to-poi-e′sis) erythropoiesis.

erythrocytorrhexis (ĕ-rith″ro-si″to-rek′sis) [*erythrocyte* + Gr. *rhēxis* rending] a morphological change in erythrocytes, consisting in the escape from the cells of round, shiny granules and the splitting off of particles.

erythrocytoschisis (ĕ-rith″ro-si-tos′kĭ-sis) [*erythrocyte* + Gr. *schisis* division] a morphological change in erythrocytes, con-

sisting in the degeneration of the cells into disklike bodies similar to the blood platelets.

erythrocytosis (ĕ-rith″ro-si-to′sis) increase in the total red cell mass secondary to any of a number of nonhematopoietic systemic disorders in response to a known stimulus (*secondary polycythemia* [q.v.]), in contrast to erythremic or primary polycythemia (polycythemia vera). **leukemic e., e. megalosplen′ica,** polycythemia vera. **stress e.,** see under *polycythemia.*

erythrocyturia (ĕ-rith″ro-si-tu′re-ah) hematuria.

erythrodegenerative (ĕ-rith″ro-de-jen′er-a″tiv) characterized by degeneration of erythrocytes.

erythroderma (ĕ-rith″ro-der′mah) [*erythro-* + Gr. *derma* skin] abnormal redness of the skin, usually applied to a condition of abnormal redness over widespread areas of the body, a phase of exfoliative dermatitis. **congenital ichthyosiform e.,** a condition now recognized as two distinct diseases, one bullous (with dominant inheritance) and the other nonbullous (with recessive inheritance); see *epidermolytic hyperkeratosis* (the bullous form) and *lamellar ichthyosis* (the nonbullous form). Called also *e. ichthyosiforme congenitum.* **e. desquamati′vum,** a condition affecting chiefly newborn breast-fed infants, resembling and probably identical with severe seborrheic dermatitis, and characterized by generalized exfoliative dermatitis and marked erythroderma; called also *Leiner's disease.* **e. ichthyosifor′me congen′itum,** congenital ichthyosiform e. **lymphomatous e.,** widespread redness of the skin occurring as a manifestation of lymphoma. **maculopapular e.,** a reddish eruption composed of macules and papules. **e. psoriat′icum,** a generalized psoriasis vulgaris, showing the clinical characteristics of exfoliative dermatitis. **Sézary e.,** see under *syndrome.*

erythrodermia (ĕ-rith″ro-der′me-ah) erythroderma.

erythrodextrin (ĕ-rith″ro-dek′strin) a dextrin, *e*-dextrin, which is turned red by iodine and changed by various digestive enzymes into maltose.

erythrodontia (ĕ-rith″ro-don′she-ah) [*erythro-* + Gr. *odous* tooth] reddish brown pigmentation of the teeth.

erythrogen (ĕ-rith′ro-jen) a fatty, crystalline compound from diseased bile.

erythrogenesis (ĕ-rith″ro-jen′ĕ-sis) the production of erythrocytes. **e. imperfec′ta,** congenital hypoplastic anemia, def. 1.

erythrogenic (ĕ-rith″ro-jen′ik) [*erythro-* + Gr. *gennan* to produce] 1. producing erythrocytes. 2. producing a sensation of red. 3. producing or causing erythema.

erythrogone (ĕ-rith′ro-gōn) promegaloblast.

erythrogonium (ĕ-rith″ro-go′ne-um) [*erythrocyte* + Gr. *gonē* seed] promegaloblast.

erythrogranulose (ĕ-rith″ro-gran′u-lōs) an amylodextrin colored red by iodine.

erythroid (er″ĭ-throid) 1. of a red color; reddish. 2. pertaining to the developmental series of cells ending in erythrocytes.

β-erythroidine (ĕ-rith″roi-din) an alkaloid, $C_{16}H_{19}NO_3$ from *Erythrina americana:* it has a curare-like action.

erythrokatalysis (ĕ-rith″ro-kah-tal′ĭ-sis) [*erythro-* + Gr. *katalysis* dissolution] the dissolution of erythrocytes; erythrocytolysis.

erythrokeratodermia (ĕ-rith″ro-ker″ah-to-der′me-ah) a reddening and hyperkeratosis of the skin. **e. figura′ta varia′bilis, e. varia′bilis,** a rare hereditary disorder transmitted as an autosomal dominant trait and characterized by circumscribed erythematous and hyperkeratotic plaques on the skin which vary in size and shape within hours or days. They appear shortly after birth and persist into adolescence or adulthood.

erythrokinetics (ĕ-rith″ro-ki-net′iks) [*erythrocyte* + Gr. *kinētikos* of or for putting in motion] the quantitative, dynamic study of *in vivo* production and destruction of erythrocytes.

erythrol (er′ith-rol) erythritol. **e. tetranitrate,** erythrityl tetranitrate.

erythrolabe (ĕ-rith′ro-lāb) [*erythro-* + Gr. *lambanein* to take] name proposed for the pigment in retinal cones that is more sensitive to the red range of the spectrum than are the other pigments (chlorolabe and cyanolabe).

erythrolein (er″ĭ-thro′le-in) the ether-soluble fraction of the acid-precipitable part of the water-soluble pigments of litmus, occurring as a red oily substance.

erythroleukemia (ĕ-rith″ro-lu-ke′me-ah) a malignant blood dyscrasia, one of the myeloproliferative disorders, characterized by neoplastic proliferation of erythroblastic and myeloblastic elements, with atypical erythroblasts and myeloblasts in the peripheral blood, and showing a variable (acute or chronic) clinical course. Called also *di Guglielmo's disease* or *syndrome.* Cf. *erythremic myelosis.*

erythroleukoblastosis (ĕ-rith″ro-lu″ko-blas-to′sis) icterus gravis neonatorum.

erythroleukosis (ĕ-rith″ro-lu-ko′sis) 1. a condition seen in malaria in which the erythrocytes are changed into brassy bodies. 2. erythroblastosis, def. 2.

erythroleukothrombocythemia (ĕ-rith″ro-lu″ko-throm″bo-si-the′me-ah) di Guglielmo's term for hyperplasia of the erythroblastic, leukoblastic, and megakaryocytic tissue, with the appearance of immature cells in the blood.

erythrolitmin (e-rith″ro-lit′min) the alcohol-soluble fraction of the acid-precipitable part of the water-soluble pigments of litmus, occurring as a bright red powder.

erythrolysin (er″ĭ-throl′ĭ-sin) erythrocytolysin.

erythrolysis (er″ĭ-throl′ĭ-sis) erythrocytolysis.

erythromania (ĕ-rith″ro-ma′ne-ah) [erythro- + Gr. mania madness] excessive and uncontrollable blushing.

erythromelalgia (ĕ-rith″ro-mel-al′je-ah) [erythro- + Gr. melos limb + -algia] a disease affecting chiefly the extremities of the body, the feet more often than the hands, and marked by paroxysmal, bilateral vasodilatation, particularly of the extremities, with burning pain, and increased skin temperature and redness; called also erythermalgia, acromelalgia, and Gerhardt's, Mitchell's, or Weir Mitchell's disease. **e. of the head,** a severe recurring headache caused by vascular dilatation, both induced by and cured by doses of histamine.

erythrometer (er″ĭ-throm′ĕ-ter) [erythro- + Gr. metron measure] 1. an instrument or color scale for measuring degrees of redness. 2. erythrocytometer.

erythrometry (er″ĭ-throm′ĕ-tre) 1. the measurement of the degree of redness. 2. erythrocytometry.

erythromycin (ĕ-rith″ro-mi′sin) [USP] an intermediate spectrum macrolide antibiotic, $C_{37}H_{67}NO_{13}$, produced by Streptomyces erythreus, occurring as a slightly yellow, crystalline powder, effective against most gram-positive and certain gram-negative bacteria, such as Neisseria and Hemophilus influenzae, and against spirochetes, some rickettsias, and Entamoeba, and highly effective against Mycoplasma pneumoniae; used in the treatment of infections due to susceptible organisms, especially in patients allergic to penicillin, in penicillin-resistant infections, and in legionnaire's disease, administered orally or topically. **e. B,** berythromycin. **e. estolate** [USP], the lauryl sulfate ester of propionyl erythromycin, $C_{40}H_{71}NO_{14} \cdot C_{12}H_{26}O_4S$, occurring as a white, crystalline powder, having the same actions and uses as the base; administered orally. **e. ethylcarbonate,** a salt of erythromycin, $C_{40}H_{71}NO_{15}$, used for oral administration. **e. ethylsuccinate** [USP], a salt of erythromycin, $C_{43}H_{75}NO_{16}$, occurring as a white or slightly yellow crystalline powder, having the same actions and uses as the base; administered orally or intramuscularly. **e. gluceptate** [USP], a salt of erythromycin, $C_{37}H_{67}NO_{13} \cdot C_7H_{14}O_8$, occurring as a white powder, having the same actions and uses as the base; administered by intravenous infusion. **e. lactobionate** [USP], a salt of erythromycin, $C_{37}H_{67}NO_{13} \cdot C_{12}H_{22}O_{12}$, occurring as white or slightly yellow crystals or powder, having the same actions and uses as the base; administered by intravenous infusion. **e. propionate,** a salt of erythromycin, $C_{40}H_{71}NO_{14}$, suitable for oral use. **e. propionate lauryl sulfate,** former name for e. estolate. **e. stearate** [USP], a salt of erythromycin, $C_{37}H_{67}NO_{13} \cdot C_{18}H_{36}O_2$, suitable for oral use.

erythromyeloblastosis (ĕ-rith″ro-mi″ĕ-lo-blas-to′sis) a neoplastic disease of chickens caused by a fowl tumor virus.

erythron (er′ĭ-thron) [Gr. erythros red] the circulating erythrocytes in the blood, their precursors, and all the elements of the body concerned in their production; it is the counterpart of the leukon and thrombon.

erythroneocytosis (ĕ-rith″ro-ne″o-si-to′sis) [erythro- + Gr. neos new + kytos hollow vessel] the presence of immature erythrocytes in the blood.

erythronoclastic (ĕ-rith″ro-no-klas′tik) causing lysis or destruction of erythron.

erythroparasite (ĕ-rith″ro-par′ah-sīt) a parasite of erythrocytes.

erythropathy (er″ĭ-throp′ah-the) [erythro- + Gr. pathos disease] an archaic term for any disorder of the erythrocytes.

erythropenia (ĕ-rith″ro-pe′ne-ah) [erythro- + Gr. penia poverty] deficiency in the number of erythrocytes; called also erythrocytopenia.

erythrophage (ĕ-rith′ro-fāj) [erythro- + Gr. phagein to eat] a phagocyte that takes up erythrocytes and blood pigments.

erythrophagia (ĕ-rith″ro-fa′je-ah) erythrocytophagy.

erythrophagocytosis (ĕ-rith″ro-fag″o-si-to′sis) erythrocytophagy.

erythrophagous (er″ĭ-throf′ah-gus) erythrocytophagous.

erythropheresis (ĕ-rith″ro-fĕ-re′sis) [erythro- + Gr. aphairesis removal] erythrocytapheresis.

erythrophil (ĕ-rith′ro-fil) [erythro- + Gr. philein to love] 1. a cell or other element that is easily stained red. 2. erythrophilous.

erythrophilous (er″ĭ-throf′ĭ-lus) easily stained with red.

Erythrophloeum (ĕ-rith″ro-fle′um) [erythro- + Gr. phloios bark] a genus of leguminous trees. E. guineen′se affords casca or Mancona bark, an African ordeal poison.

erythrophobia (ĕ-rith″ro-fo′be-ah) [erythro- + phobia] 1. a neurotic manifestation marked by blushing on the slightest provocation. 2. morbid fear of blushing. 3. morbid aversion to red.

erythrophobic (ĕ-rith″ro-fo′bik) having no affinity for red dye (acid fuchsin).

erythrophore (ĕ-rith′ro-fōr) [erythro- + Gr. phoros bearing] a chromatophore containing granules of a red or brown alcohol-resistant pigment; called also allophore.

erythrophose (ĕ-rith′ro-fōz) [erythro- + Gr. phōs light] any red phose.

erythrophyll (ĕ-rith′ro-fil) [erythro- + Gr. phyllon leaf] a red coloring matter occurring in plants.

erythropia (er″ĕ-thro′pe-ah) erythropsia.

erythroplasia (ĕ-rith″ro-pla′ze-ah) a condition of the mucous membrane characterized by erythematous papular lesions. **e. of Queyrat,** squamous cell carcinoma in situ that manifests as a circumscribed, velvety, erythematous papular lesion on the glans penis, coronal sulcus, or prepuce, leading to scaling and superficial ulceration. **Zoon's e.,** a benign condition similar to erythroplasia of Queyrat, occurring on the mucosal and cutaneous surfaces of the glans penis (plasma cell balanitis) or vulva (plasma cell vulvitis); it is characterized by epidermal atrophy, spongiosis, and plasma cell infiltration of the dermis.

erythroplastid (ĕ-rith″ro-plas′tid) a red blood cell of mammalian animals, characterized by having no nucleus.

erythropoiesis (ĕ-rith″ro-poi-e′sis) [erythro- + Gr. poiēsis making] the production of erythrocytes.

erythropoietic (ĕ-rith″ro-poi-et′ik) pertaining to, characterized by, or promoting erythropoiesis.

erythropoietin (ĕ-rith″ro-poi′ĕ-tin) a glycoprotein hormone secreted chiefly by the kidney in the adult and by the liver in the fetus, which acts on stem cells of the bone marrow to stimulate red blood cell production (erythropoiesis).

erythroprosopalgia (ĕ-rith″ro-pros″o-pal′je-ah) [erythro- + Gr. prosōpon face + -algia] a nervous disorder, analogous to erythromelalgia, marked by redness and pain in the face.

erythropsia (er″ĭ-throp′se-ah) [erythro- + Gr. opsis vision + -ia] a visual defect in which all objects appear to have a red tinge.

erythropsin (er″ĕ-throp′sin) [erythro- + Gr. opsis vision] rhodopsin.

erythropyknosis (ĕ-rith″ro-pik-no′sis) [erythro- + pyknosis] pyknosis.

erythrorrhexis (ĕ-rith″ro-rek′sis) [erythro- + Gr. rhēxis rupture] erythrocytorrhexis.

erythrose (er′ĭ-thrōs) one of the aldotetroses. **e. péribuccale pigmentaire′,** Brocq's name for a condition marked by erythema and brownish pigmentation around the mouth and on the chin and cheeks, developing in apparently normal girls at puberty, and waxing and waning with each menstrual period. A photodynamic substance in cosmetics is suspected to be the causative agent. Called also erythrosis pigmentata faciei.

erythrosedimentation (ĕ-rith″ro-sed″ĭ-men-ta′shun) the sedimentation of erythrocytes.

erythrosin (ĕ-rith′ro-sin) a red compound, $C_{13}H_{18}O_6N_2$, used as a histologic stain.

erythrosine sodium (ĕ-rith′ro-sin) [USP] chemical name: 3′,6′-dihydroxy-2′,4′,5′,7′-tetraiodospiro [isobenzofuran-1(3H),9′-[9H]xanthen]-3-one disodium salt monohydrate. A coloring agent, $C_{20}H_6I_4Na_2O_5 \cdot H_2O$, occurring as a red or brownish red powder; used to disclose plaque on teeth; applied topically in solution, or tablets containing erythrosine sodium are chewed, after which the mouth is rinsed with water.

erythrosis (er″ĭ-thro′sis) 1. a reddish or purplish discoloration of the skin and mucous membranes seen in polycythemia vera. 2. hyperplasia of the hematopoietic tissue. **e. pigmenta′ta fa′ciei,** erythrose peribuccale pigmentaire.

erythrostasis (ĕ-rith″ro-sta′sis) the stoppage of erythrocytes in the capillaries, as in sickle cell anemia.

erythrothioneine (ĕ-rith″ro-thi″o-ne′in) ergothioneine.

erythrulose (ĕ-rith′roo-lōs) a ketose sugar, $C_4H_8O_4$, formed by the oxidation of erythrol.

erythruria (er″ĭ-throo′re-ah) [erythro- + Gr. ouron urine + -ia] the passing of red urine.

Es chemical symbol for einsteinium.

es (es) [L. esse to be] Nietzsche's term for the metaphysical incomprehensible something at the very bottom of human nature, being lower than the conscious ego and even lower than the freudian subconscious.

Esbach's method, reagent (test) (es′bahks) [Georges Hubert Esbach, a physician in Paris, 1843–1890] see under method and reagent.

escape (es-kāp′) the act of becoming free. **nodal e.,** extrasystole in which the atrioventricular node is the pacemaker. **vagal e.,** the exhaustion of or adaptation to neural chemical mediators in the regulation of systemic arterial pressure. **ventricular e.,** extrasystole in which a ventricular pacemaker becomes effective before the sinoatrial pacemaker; it usually occurs with slow sinus rates and often, but not necessarily, with increased vagal tone.

escarronodulaire (es″kar-ro′nod″u-lār′) [Fr.] boutonneuse fever.

eschar (es′kar) [Gr. *eschara* scab] 1. a slough produced by a thermal burn, by a corrosive application, or by gangrene. 2. the lesion seen in certain rickettsioses; see *tache noire.* **neuropathic e.** (*obs.*), a decubitus ulcer in disease of the spinal cord.

escharotic (es-kah-rot′ik) [Gr. *escharōtikos*] 1. corrosive; capable of producing an eschar. 2. a corrosive or caustic agent.

Escherich's bacillus, sign (reflex), test (esh′er-iks) [Theodor *Escherich,* German physician, 1857–1911] see *Escherichia coli,* and under *sign* and *tests.*

Escherichia (esh″er-i′ke-a) a genus of microorganisms of the tribe Escherichieae, family Enterobacteriaceae, order Eubacteriales, made up of gram-negative, motile or nonmotile short rods, widely distributed in nature, and occasionally pathogenic for man. **E. aures′cens,** a species of organisms isolated from human feces, from an infected eye, and from contaminated water supplies, characterized by the ability to produce yellow-orange carotenoid pigments. **E. co′li,** a species of organisms constituting the greater part of the intestinal flora of man and other animals. Characteristically positive to indol and methyl red tests, and negative to the Voges-Proskauer and citrate tests. Divided into physiological types on the basis of sucrose and salicin fermentation by some workers. Separable into serotypes on the basis of distribution of heat-stable O antigens, envelope antigens of varying heat stability, and flagellar antigens that are heat labile. Usually nonpathogenic, but pathogenic strains, often hemolytic, and predominantly certain serotypes are common. Pathogenic strains are the cause of scours in calves and the hemorrhagic septicemia Winckel's disease in newborn children, are one of the most frequently encountered causes of urinary tract infection and of epidemic diarrheal disease, especially in children, and are found infrequently in localized suppurative processes. They often become the predominant bacteria in the flora of the mouth and throat during antibiotic therapy. See Plate VII, accompanying *bacterium.* Called also *colibacillus* or *colon bacillus,* and *Escherich's bacillus.* **E. freun′dii,** a species normally found in soil and water, as well as in the intestinal tract of man and other animals; certain strains have been confused with salmonellas. **E. interme′dia,** a species widely distributed in nature, being found, like others of the genus, in soil, water, and the intestinal tract of man and other animals.

Escherichieae (esh″ĕ-rik′e-e) a tribe of the family Enterobacteriaceae, order Eubacteriales, made up of motile or nonmotile rods that ferment glucose and lactose with the production of acid and visible gas. It comprises the coliform bacteria and includes five genera, *Aerobacter, Alginobacter, Escherichia, Klebsiella,* and *Paracolobactrum.*

eschrolalia (es-kro-la′le-ah) [Gr. *aischros* shameful + *lalia* babble] coprolalia.

Eschscholtzia (esh-skŏlt′ze-ah) a genus of papaveraceous plants. *E. califor′nica* Cham. (California poppy) is a hypnotic and anodyne.

escin (es′kin) a strongly hemolytic saponin derived from horse-chestnut.

escorcin (es-kor′sin) a brown powder, $C_9H_6O_4$, prepared from a substance extracted from the horse chestnut; used in detecting corneal and conjunctival lesions.

Escudero's test (es-koo-da′rŏz) [Pedro *Escudero,* Buenos Aires physician, born 1877] see under *test.*

esculapian (es″ku-la′pe-an) aesculapian.

esculent (es′ku-lent) edible; fit for eating.

esculin (es′ku-lin) [L. *aesculus* horse-chestnut] a coumarin glycoside, $C_6H_{11}O_5O \cdot C_9H_4O(O:) \cdot OH$, from *Aesculus hippocastanum* L. (Hippocastanaceae) (horse-chestnut) bark, having febrifuge properties.

escutcheon (es-kuch′an) [L. *scutum* a shield] the pattern of distribution of the pubic hair.

eseptate (e-sep′tāt) having no septa.

eserine (es′er-in) [*esere,* an African name of the Calabar bean] physostigmine.

E.S.F. erythropoietic stimulating factor.

Esidrix (es′ĭ-driks) trademark for a preparation of hydrochlorothiazide.

-esis (e′sis) a word termination denoting state or condition; see *-sis.*

Eskabarb (es′kah-barb) trademark for a preparation of phenobarbital.

Eskadiazine (es″kah-di′ah-zēn) trademark for a preparation of sulfadiazine.

Eskalith (es′kah-lith) trademark for a preparation of lithium carbonate.

esmarch (es′mark) an Esmarch bandage.

Esmarch's bandage, tourniquet, tube (es′marks) [Johann

Friedrich August von *Esmarch,* German surgeon, 1823–1908] see under *bandage, tourniquet,* and *tube.*

eso- [Gr. *esō* inward] a combining form meaning within.

esocataphoria (es″o-kat-ah-fo′re-ah) [*eso-* + *cataphoria*] the condition in which the visual axis turns downward and inward.

esocine (es′o-sin) a protamine from the sperm of the pike, *Esox lucius.*

esodeviation (e″so-de″ve-a′shun) a turning inward.

esodic (ĕ-sod′ik) [Gr. *es* toward + *hodos* way] (*obs.*) afferent, as esodic nerves.

esoethmoiditis (es″o-eth″moi-di′tis) [*eso-* + *ethmoiditis*] inflammation within the sinuses of the ethmoid bone.

esogastritis (es″o-gas-tri′tis) [*eso-* + *gastritis*] inflammation of the mucous membrane of the stomach.

esophagalgia (ĕ-sof″ah-gal′je-ah) [*esophagus* + *-algia*] pain in the esophagus.

esophageal (ĕ-sof″ah-je′al, ĕ-so-fa′je-al) pertaining to or belonging to the esophagus.

esophagectasia (ĕ-sof″ah-jek-ta′se-ah) [*esophagus* + Gr. *ektasis* distention + *-ia*] dilatation of the esophagus.

esophagectasis (ĕ-sof″ah-jek′tah-sis) esophagectasia.

esophagectomy (ĕ-sof″ah-jek′to-me) [*esophagus* + Gr. *ektomē* excision] excision of a portion of the esophagus.

esophagism (ĕ-sof′ah-jism) esophagospasm. **hiatal e.,** cardiospasm.

esophagismus (ĕ-sof″ah-jiz′mus) esophagospasm.

esophagitis (ĕ-sof″ah-ji′tis) [*esophagus* + *-itis*] inflammation of the esophagus. **e. dis′secans superficia′lis,** infection of the esophagus, with sloughing of the squamous epithelial lining in the form of a tubular cast. **peptic e.,** inflammation of the esophagus caused by a reflux of acid and pepsin from the stomach; usually associated with hiatus hernia, duodenal ulcer, indwelling tubes, or prolonged vomiting. **reflux e.,** peptic e. **thrush e.,** esophagitis due to extension of oral thrush.

esophagobronchial (ĕ-sof″ah-go-brong′ke-al) pertaining to or communicating with the esophagus and a bronchus.

esophagocardiomyotomy (ĕ-sof″ah-go-kar″de-o-mi-ot′o-me) incision through the muscular coats of the esophagus and cardiac part of the stomach, the incision extending equal distances above and below the esophagogastric junction; done in achalasia of the esophagus. Called also *cardiomyotomy.*

esophagocele (ĕ-sof″ah-go-sēl″) [*esophagus* + Gr. *kēlē* hernia] abnormal distention of the esophagus; hernia of the esophagus: protrusion of the mucous and submucous coats of the esophagus through a rupture in the muscular coat, producing a pouch or diverticulum.

esophagocologastrostomy (ĕ-sof″ah-go-ko″lo-gas-tros′to-me) surgical creation of a new communication between the esophagus and stomach, with interposition of a segment of colon.

esophagocoloplasty (ĕ-sof″ah-go-ko′lo-plas″te) excision of a portion of the esophagus and its replacement by a segment of the colon.

esophagoduodenostomy (ĕ-sof″ah-go-du″o-de-nos′to-me) surgical anastomosis between the esophagus and the duodenum.

esophagodynia (ĕ-sof″ah-go-din′e-ah) [*esophagus* + Gr. *odynē* pain] pain in the esophagus.

esophagoenterostomy (ĕ-sof″ah-go-en″ter-os′to-me) [*esophagus* + Gr. *enteron* intestine + *stomoun* to provide with an opening, or mouth] formation of an anastomosis between the esophagus and small intestine, usually by surgical means following total gastrectomy.

esophagoesophagostomy (ĕ-sof″ah-go-ĕ-sof″ah-gos′to-me) anastomosis between two formerly remote parts of the esophagus.

esophagofundopexy (ĕ-sof″ah-go-fun″do-pek′se) surgical fixation of the fundus of the stomach to the esophagus.

esophagogastrectomy (ĕ-sof″ah-go-gas-trek′to-me) excision of the esophagus and stomach, usually the distal portion of the esophagus and the entire stomach.

esophagogastric (ĕ-sof″ah-go-gas′trik) pertaining to the esophagus and the stomach.

esophagogastroanastomosis (ĕ-sof″ah-go-gas″tro-ah-nas″to-mo′sis) surgical formation of an anastomosis between the esophagus and the stomach.

esophagogastromyotomy (ĕ-sof″ah-go-gas″tro-mi-ot′o-me) incision through the muscular coats of the esophagus and stomach.

esophagogastroplasty (ĕ-sof″ah-go-gas′tro-plas″te) plastic repair of the esophagus and stomach; cardioplasty.

esophagogastroscopy (ĕ-sof″ah-go-gas-tros′ko-pe) [*esophagus* + Gr. *gastēr* stomach + *skopein* to examine] endoscopic examination of the esophagus and the stomach.

esophagogastrostomy (ĕ-sof″ah-go-gas-tros′to-me) [*esophagus* + Gr. *gastēr* stomach + *stomoun* to provide with an opening, or mouth] surgical creation of an artificial communication between the stomach and esophagus.

esophagogram (ĕ-sof′ah-go-gram) a roentgenogram of the esophagus.

esophagography (ĕ-sof″ah-gog′rah-fe) roentgenography of the esophagus.

esophagojejunogastrostomosis (ĕ-sof″ah-go-je″ju-no-gas″-tros-to-mo′sus) the operation of mobilizing a loop of jejunum and implanting its proximal end in the esophagus and its distal end in the stomach: done in cases of esophageal stricture.

esophagojejunogastrostomy (ĕ-sof″ah-go-je-ju″no-gas-tros′-to-me) esophagojejunogastrostomosis.

esophagojejunoplasty (ĕ-sof″ah-go-jĕ-joo′no-plas″te) restoration of the esophagus with a segment of jejunum.

esophagojejunostomy (ĕ-sof″ah-go-je-ju-nos′to-me) surgical anastomosis between the esophagus and the jejunum.

esophagolaryngectomy (ĕ-sof″ah-go-lar″in-jek′to-me) en bloc excision of the upper cervical esophagus and larynx.

esophagology (ĕ-sof″ah-gol′o-je) the study and treatment of diseases of the esophagus.

esophagomalacia (ĕ-sof″ah-go-mah-la′she-ah) [esophagus + Gr. malakia softness] softening of the walls of the esophagus.

esophagometer (ĕ-sof″ah-gom′ĕ-ter) [esophagus + Gr. metron measure] an instrument for measuring the length of the esophagus.

esophagomycosis (ĕ-sof″ah-go-mi-ko′sis) [esophagus + Gr. mykēs fungus] any disease of the esophagus caused by fungi.

esophagomyotomy (ĕ-sof″ah-go-mi-ot′o-me) incision through the muscular coat of the esophagus, the term usually referring clinically to incision through the muscular coat of the distal part of the esophagus.

esophagopharynx (ĕ-sof″ah-go-făr′inks) the distal portion of the pharynx where the fibers of the inferior constrictor are arranged in circular form.

esophagoplasty (ĕ-sof′ah-go-plas″te) [esophagus + Gr. plassein to form] a plastic operation on the esophagus.

esophagoplication (ĕ-sof″ah-go-pli-ka′shun) the operation of narrowing the esophagus by folding in its wall.

esophagoptosis (ĕ-sof″ah-gop-to′sis) [esophagus + Gr. ptōsis falling] prolapse of the esophagus.

esophagorespiratory (ĕ-sof″ah-go-rĕ-spir′ah-to″re) pertaining to or communicating with the esophagus and respiratory tract (the trachea or a bronchus).

esophagoscope (ĕ-sof′ah-go-skōp) [esophagus + Gr. skopein to examine] an instrument for inspecting the lumen of the esophagus and carrying out diagnostic and therapeutic maneuvers such as taking biopsy specimens and removing foreign bodies.

esophagoscopy (ĕ-sof″ah-gos′ko-pe) endoscopic examination of the esophagus.

esophagospasm (ĕ-sof′ah-go-spazm″) [esophagus + spasm] spasm of the esophagus.

esophagostenosis (ĕ-sof″ah-go-stĕ-no′sis) [esophagus + Gr. stenōsis constriction] stricture or constriction of the esophagus.

esophagostoma (e″sof-ah-gos′to-mah) [esophagus + Gr. stoma mouth] the external opening of an artificial passage leading into the esophagus.

esophagostomiasis (ĕ-sof″ah-go-sto-mi′ah-sis) infestation with nematodes of the genus Oesophagostomum.

esophagostomy (ĕ-sof″ah-gos′to-me) [esophagus + Gr. stomoun to provide with an opening, or mouth] the creation of an opening into the esophagus.

esophagotome (e″so-fag′o-tōm) a cutting instrument for use in esophagotomy.

esophagotomy (ĕ-sof″ah-got′o-me) [esophagus + Gr. tomē a cutting] incision of the esophagus.

esophagotracheal (ĕ-sof″ah-go-tra′ke-al) pertaining to or communicating with esophagus and trachea.

esophagram (ĕ-sof′ah-gram) esophagogram.

esophagus (ĕ-sof′ah-gus) [Gr. oisophagos, from oisein to carry + phagēma food] [NA] the musculomembranous passage extending from the pharynx to the stomach. Called also gullet. **Barrett's e.**, see under syndrome.

esophoria (es″o-fo′re-ah) [eso- + Gr. phorein to bear] a form of heterophoria in which there is a deviation of the visual axis of an eye toward that of the other eye after the visual fusional stimuli have been eliminated; called also esodeviation.

esophoric (es″o-for′ik) pertaining to or characterized by esophoria.

esosphenoiditis (es″o-sfe″noi-di′tis) [eso- + sphenoid + -itis] osteomyelitis of the sphenoid bone.

esotoxin (es″o-tok′sin) (obs.) endotoxin.

esotropia (es″o-tro′pe-ah) [eso- + Gr. trepein to turn] strabismus in which there is manifest deviation of the visual axis of an eye toward that of the other eye, resulting in diplopia. Called also cross-eye and convergent or internal strabismus.

esotropic (es″o-trop′ik) pertaining to or characterized by esotropia.

ESP extrasensory perception.

espnoic (esp-no′ik) [Gr. es into + pnoē vapor, blast] pertaining to the injection of vapors or gases.

esponja (es-pong′ah) cutaneous habronemiasis.

esproquin hydrochloride (es′pro-kwin) chemical name: 2-[3-(ethylsulfinyl)propyl]-1,2,3,4-tetrahydroisoquinoline hydrochloride; an adrenergic, $C_{14}H_{21}NOS\cdot HCl$.

espundia (es-poon′de-ah) mucocutaneous leishmaniasis.

esquillectomy (es″kwil-lek′to-me) [Fr. esquille fragment + Gr. ektomē excision] excision of fragments of bone following fractures caused by projectiles.

E.S.R. erythrocyte sedimentation rate.

essence (es′ens) [L. essentia quality or being] 1. that which is or necessarily exists as the cause of the properties of a body. 2. a solution of a volatile oil in alcohol. **e. of peppermint,** peppermint spirit; see under spirit.

essentia (ĕ-sen′she-ah) [L.] essence.

essential (ĕ-sen′shal) [L. essentialis] 1. constituting the necessary or inherent part of a thing; giving a substance its peculiar and necessary qualities. 2. idiopathic; self-existing; having no obvious external exciting cause; said of a disease. 3. indispensable; required in the diet, as essential fatty acids.

Esser's graft, operation (es′erz) [Johannes Fredericus Samuel Esser, Holland surgeon, 1878–1946] see under graft, and see epithelial inlay, under inlay.

E.S.T. electroshock therapy; see electroconvulsive therapy, under therapy.

ester (es′ter) any compound formed from an alcohol and an acid by the removal of water; the esters are named as if they were salts of the acid. Called also compound ether. **acetoacetic e.,** the ethyl ester of acetoacetic acid, $CH_3\cdot CO\cdot CH_2\cdot CO\cdot O\cdot C_2H_5$, a colorless liquid used for synthesis of a great variety of compounds. **Cori e.,** glucose 1-phosphate; a glucopyranose 1-monophosphate, $CH_2\cdot OH\cdot CH(CHOH)_3\cdot CHO\cdot PO(OH)_2$. See hexosephosphoric esters. **Embden e.,** glucopyranose-6-phosphoric acid; see hexosephosphate. **Harden-Young e.,** fructofuranose diphosphate, $(OH)_2PO\cdot CH_2O\cdot CHO(CHOH)_2CH\cdot CH_2O\cdot PO(OH)_2$; called also hexose diphosphate. See hexosephosphoric esters. **hexosephosphoric e's,** esters concerned in the chemical processes of muscle contraction and the fermentation of glucose by yeast; they are the Cori ester, the Harden-Young ester, the Neuberg ester, and the Robison ester. **Neuberg e.,** fructose 6-phosphate; a fructofuranose monophosphate, $CH_2OH\cdot CHO\cdot(CHOH)_2\cdot CH\text{--}CH_2O\cdot PO(OH)_2$. See hexosephosphoric e's. **Robison e.,** glucose 6-phosphate; a glucopyranose 6-monophosphate, $CHOH(CHOH)_3\cdot CH\cdot CH_2O\cdot PO(OH)_2$. See hexosephosphoric e's.

esterapenia (es″ter-ah-pe′ne-ah) [esterase + Gr. penia poverty] deficiency in the cholinesterase content of the blood.

esterase (es′ter-ās) an enzyme that catalyzes the hydrolysis of an ester into its alcohol and acid. **C1 e.,** the activated form of complement component C1, which acts on components C4 and C2 to form C3 convertase.

esterification (es-ter″ĭ-fi-ka′shun) the process of converting an acid into an ester.

esterify (es-ter′ĭ-fi) to combine with an alcohol with elimination of a molecule of water, forming an ester.

esterize (es′ter-īz) to convert, or be converted, into an ester.

esterolysis (es″ter-ol′ĭ-sis) [ester + Gr. lysis dissolution] the hydrolysis of an ester into its alcohol and acid.

esterolytic (es″ter-o-lit′ik) effecting or pertaining to esterolysis.

Estes' operation (es′tēz) [William Lawrence Estes, Jr., American surgeon, 1885–1940] see under operation.

esthematology (es″them-ah-tol′o-je) [Gr. aisthēma sensation + -logy] the science of the senses and sense organs.

esthesia (es-the′ze-ah) [Gr. aisthēsis perception] perception, feeling, or sensation.

esthesic (es-the′sik) [Gr. aisthēsis perception] pertaining to the mental perception of sensations.

esthesio- (es-the′ze-o) [Gr. aisthēsis perception, sensation] a combining form denoting relationship to feeling or to the perceptive faculties. Also spelled aesthesio-.

esthesioblast (es-the′ze-o-blast″) [esthesio- + Gr. blastos germ] a ganglioblast; an embryonic cell of the spinal ganglia.

esthesiodic (es-the″ze-od′ik) esthesodic.

esthesiogen (es-the′ze-o-jen) [esthesio- + Gr. gennan to produce] a substance which is supposed to produce symptoms of excitation when brought near or into a sensory zone.

esthesiogenic (es-the″ze-o-jen′ik) producing sensation.

esthesiology (es-the″ze-ol′o-je) [esthesio- + -logy] the science of sensation and the senses.

esthesiomene (es-the″ze-om′ĕ-ne) esthiomene.

esthesiometer (es-the″ze-om′ĕ-ter) [esthesio- + Gr. metron measure] an instrument for measuring tactile sensibility; tactometer.

esthesioneure (es-the′ze-o-nūr) [*esthesio-* + Gr. *neuron* nerve] a sensory neuron.

esthesioneuroblastoma (es-the″ze-o-nu″ro-blas-to′mah) a radiosensitive glioma occurring in the nasal cavity.

esthesioneurosis (es-the″ze-o-nu-ro′sis) [*esthesio-* + *neurosis*] any disorder of the sensory nerves.

esthesionosus (es-the″ze-on′o-sus) [*esthesio-* + Gr. *nosos* disease] esthesioneurosis.

esthesiophysiology (es-the″ze-o-fiz″e-ol′o-je) the physiology of sensation and the sense organs.

esthesodic (es″thĕ-zod′ik) [*esthesio-* + Gr. *hodos* path] conducting or pertaining to the conduction of sensory impulses.

esthetic (es-thet′ik) [Gr. *aisthēsis* sensation] 1. pertaining to sensation. 2. pertaining to beauty, or the improvement of appearance. Also spelled *aesthetic.*

esthetics (es-thet′iks) the branch of philosophy dealing with beauty. In dentistry, a philosophy concerned especially with the appearance of a dental restoration, as achieved through its color and/or form. Also spelled *aesthetics.*

esthiomene (es″the-om′ĕ-ne) [Gr. *esthiomenos* eroded] a chronic ulceration and elephantiasis of the labia and clitoris due to lymphogranuloma venereum.

Estinyl (es′tĭ-nil) trademark for a preparationn of ethinyl estradiol.

estival (es′tĭ-val, ĕ-sti′val) [L. *aestivus,* from *aestas* summer] pertaining to or occurring in summer.

estivation (es″tĭ-va′shun) [L. *aestivus,* from *aestas* summer] the dormant state of decreased metabolism in which certain animal species, as some tropical amphibians, survive a hot, dry summer; summer dormancy. Cf. *hibernation.*

estivoautumnal (es″tĭ-vo-aw-tum′nal) pertaining to the summer and autumn; formerly applied, in the United States, to a form of malaria; see *falciparum malaria,* under *malaria.*

Estlander's operation (est′land-erz) [Jakob August *Estlander,* Finnish surgeon, 1831–1881] see under *operation.*

estolate (es′to-lāt) USAN contraction for propionate lauryl sulfate.

eston (es′ton) aluminum acetate.

Estrace (es′trās) trademark for a preparation of estradiol.

estradiol (es″trah-di′ol, es-tra′de-ol) chemical name: estra-1,3,5(10)-triene-3,17β-diol. The most potent naturally occurring ovarian and placental estrogen in human subjects, $C_{18}H_{24}O_2$, the chief functions of which are to prepare the uterus for implantation of the fertilized ovum and to induce and maintain the female secondary sex characteristics; it has also been isolated from hog ovaries and the urine of pregnant mares and has been produced semisynthetically. Estradiol exists in two isomeric forms: the most active isomer is *estradiol-17β* (formerly called β-estradiol), much less active *estradiol-17α* (formerly called α-estradiol). The official preparation [NF], occurring as white or creamy white, small crystals or crystalline powder, is administered by intramuscular injection or implanted subcutaneously in pellets. For functions and uses, see *estrogen.* Called also (rarely) *dihydroxyestrin, dihydrofolliculin,* and *dihydrotheelin.* **e. benzoate** [NF], an ester of estradiol, $C_{25}H_{28}O_3$, occurring as a white to creamy white, crystalline powder; injected intramuscularly in oil solution. **e. cypionate** [NF], chemical name: estradiol 17-cyclopentanepropionate. A white to practically white, crystalline powder, $C_{26}H_{36}O_3$, used intramuscularly as an estrogen. **e. dipropionate,** the dipropionyl ester of estradiol, which is said to be absorbed slowly. **e. enanthate,** an ester of estradiol, $C_{25}H_{36}O_3$, administered intramuscularly. **ethinyl e.** [USP], chemical name: 19-norpregna-1,3,5(10)-trien-20-yne-3,17α-diol. An orally effective semisynthetic derivative of estradiol, $C_{20}H_{24}O_2$, occurring as a white to creamy white, crystalline powder, which is one of the most potent estrogens. It is also used as the estrogen component in combination with progestins in many oral contraceptives. **e. undecylate,** an ester of estradiol, $C_{29}H_{44}O_3$, injected intramuscularly in oil solution. **e. valerate** [USP], an ester of estradiol, $C_{23}H_{32}O_3$, occurring as a white, crystalline powder; injected intramuscularly in oil solution.

estramustine (es″trah-mus′tēn) chemical name: 3-[bis(2-chlorothyl)carbamate]estra-1,3,5(10)-triene-3,17β-diol; an antineoplastic, $C_{23}H_{31}Cl_2NO_3$.

estrane (es′trān) the parent hydrocarbon, $C_{18}H_{30}$, of the estrogenic steroids.

estrapentaene (es″trah-pen′tah-ēn) a steroid nucleus with five double bonds and one methyl group, $C_{18}H_{20}$.

estratetraene (es″trah-tet′rah-ēn) a steroid nucleus with four double bonds and one methyl group, $C_{18}H_{22}$.

estratriene (es″trah-tri′ēn) a steroid nucleus with three double bonds and one methyl group, $C_{18}H_{24}$.

Estraval (es-trah-val) trademark for preparations of estradiol valerate.

estrazinol hydrobromide (es-trah′zĭ-nōl) chemical name:

(±)-3-methoxy-8-aza-19-nor-17α-1,3,5(10)-trien-20-yn-17-ol hydrobromide; an estrogen, $C_{20}H_{25}NO_2 \cdot HBr$.

estrenol (es′trĕ-nol) a crystalline estrogenic steroid, $C_{18}H_{24}O$, 3-hydroxy Δ1,3,5-estratriene.

estriasis (es-tri′ah-sis) oestriasis.

Estridae (es′trĭ-de) Oestridae.

estrin (es′trin) estrogen.

estrinization (es″trin-ĭ-za′shun) production of the cellular changes in the vaginal epithelium characteristic of estrus.

estriol (es′tre-ol) chemical name: estra-1,3,5(10)-triene-3,16α,-17β-triol. A reduction product of estradiol and estrone, $C_{18}H_{24}O_3$, having relatively weak estrogenic activity and detectable in high concentrations in the urine, especially human pregnancy urine. The official preparation [USP], rarely used clinically, occurring as a white, microcrystalline powder, is administered orally. For uses, see *estrogen.* Called also *trihydroxyestrin.*

estrofurate (es-tro-fūr′āt) chemical name: 21,23-epoxy-19, 24-dinorchola-1,3,5(10),7,20,22-hexaene-3,17α-diol 3-acetate; an estrogen, $C_{24}H_{26}O_4$.

estrogen (es′tro-jen) a generic term for estrus-producing steroid compounds; the female sex hormones. In humans, estrogen is formed in the ovary, the adrenal cortex, the testis, and the fetoplacental unit, and it has various functions in both sexes. It is responsible for the development of the female secondary sex characteristics, and during the menstrual cycle it acts on the female genitalia to produce an environment suitable for the fertilization, implantation, and nutrition of the early embryo. Estrogen is used in oral contraceptives and as a palliative in cancer of the breast after menopause, and of the prostate; other uses include the relief of the discomforts of menopause, inhibition of lactation, and treatment of osteoporosis, threatened abortion, ovarian disease, and severe menorrhagia. See also *estradiol, estrone,* and *estriol.* **conjugated e's** [USP], a mixture of the sodium salts of the sulfate esters of estrogenic substances, principally estrone and equilin, that are of the type excreted by pregnant mares, occurring as a buff-colored, amorphous powder; the actions and uses are those of estrogens (q.v.), administered orally. **esterified e's** [USP], a mixture of the sodium salts of esters of estrogenic substances, principally estrone, that are of the type excreted by pregnant mares, occurring as a white or buff-colored, amorphous powder; the actions and uses are those of estrogens (q.v.), administered orally.

estrogenic (es-tro-jen′ik) producing estrus; having the properties of, or similar to, an estrogen.

estrogenicity (es″tro-jĕ-nis′ĭ-te) the quality of exerting or the ability to exert an estrus-producing or an estrogenic effect.

estrogenous (es-troj′ĕ-nus) estrogenic.

estrone (es′trōn) chemical name: 3-hydroxyestra-1,3,5(10)-triene-17-one. An oxidation product of estradiol, $C_{18}H_{22}O_2$, the first of the estrogens isolated in pure form, found in human pregnancy urine, male human urine, human plasma, mare pregnancy urine, stallion urine, human ovarian follicular fluid and placenta, and palm kernel oil; also produced synthetically. Less potent than estradiol but more so than estriol, it is secreted by the ovary but circulating estrone is for the most part derived from peripheral metabolism of estradiol and especially androstenedione. The official preparation [NF], occurring as small, white crystals or as a white to creamy white, crystalline powder, is administered by intramuscular injection. For uses, see *estrogen.* Called also *folliculin, ketohydroxyestrone, ketohydroxyestrin,* and *thelykinin.* **piperazine e. sulfate** [USP], chemical name: 3-(sulfooxy)estra-1,3,5(10)-trien-17-one compound with piperazine (1:1). A preparation of pure crystalline estrone, solubilized as the sulfate and stabilized with piperazine, occurring as a white to yellowish white, fine crystalline powder; for uses see *estrogen.*

estrophilin (es″tro-fil′in) a cell protein that acts as a receptor for estrogen, found in estrogenic target tissue and in estrogen-dependent tumors and metastases.

estrostilben (es″tro-stil′ben) diethylstilbestrol.

estrous (es′trus) pertaining to estrus.

estrual (es′troo-al) pertaining to estrus.

estruation (es″troo-a′shun) estrus.

Estrugenone (es″troo-jen′on) trademark for a preparation of estrone.

estrum (es′trum) estrus.

estrus (es′trus) [L. *oestrus* gadfly; Gr. *oistros* anything that drives mad, any vehement desire] the recurrent, restricted period of sexual receptivity in female mammals other than human females, marked by intense sexual urge. See also *estrous cycle,* under *cycle.*

estuarium (es″tu-a′re-um) [L.] a vapor bath.

e.s.u. electrostatic unit.

esylate (es′ĭ-lāt) USAN contraction for ethanesulfonate.

Et ethyl group.

etafedrine hydrochloride (et-ah-fed′rin) chemical name: α-[1-(ethylmethylamino)ethyl]benzylmethanol hydrochloride; an adrenergic, $C_{12}H_{19}NO \cdot HCl$, administered orally in the treatment of bronchial asthma.

etafilcon A (et″ah-fil′kon) chemical name: 2-hydroxyethyl methacrylate polymer with sodium methacrylate and 2-ethyl-2-(hydroxymethyl)-1,3-propanediol trimethacrylate; a hydrophilic contact lens material, $(C_6H_{10}O_3)_x \cdot (C_4H_5NaO_2)_y \cdot (C_{18}H_{28}O_6)_z$.

Etamon (et′ah-mon) trademark for a preparation of tetraethyl-ammonium chloride.

état (a-tah′) [Fr.] state, condition. **é. criblé** (a-tah′ krēb-la′), 1. a condition in which the necrotic Peyer's patches in typhoid fever are riddled with small, irregular perforations. 2. status cribralis. **é. lacunaire** (a-tah′ lah-ku-nār′), status lacunaris. **é. mammelonné** (a-tah′ mah-mel-un-a′), hyperplasia of the mucous membrane of the stomach in chronic gastritis, resulting in the formation of small elevations. **é. marbré** (a-tah′ mar-bra′), status marmoratus. **é. vermoulu** (a-tah′ vār-moo-lu′) ["worm-eaten state"], an irregularly ulcerated condition of the surface of the brain, sometimes seen in advanced arteriosclerosis.

etazolate hydrochloride (ĕ-taz′o-lāt) chemical name: 1-eth-yl-4-[(1-methylethylidene) hydrazino] -1 H-pyrazolo [3,4- b] pyridine-5-carboxylic acid ethyl ester monohydrochloride; a tranquilizer, $C_{14}H_{19}N_5O_2 \cdot HCl$.

Eternod's sinus (a-ter-nōz′) [Auguste François Charles *Eternod,* Swiss histologist, 1854–1932] see under *sinus.*

eterobarb (ĕ-tēr′o-barb) chemical name: 5-ethyl-1,3-bis(methoxymethyl)-5-phenyl-2,4,6(1 H, 3 H, 5 H)-pyrimedinetrione; a barbiturate with anticonvulsant properties, $C_{16}H_{20}N_2O_5$.

ethacrynate sodium (eth-ah-kri′nāt) [USP], chemical name: [2,3-dichloro-4-(2-methylene-1-oxobutyl)phenoxy] acetic acid sodium salt. The sodium salt of ethycrynic acid, $C_{13}H_{11}Cl_2NaO_4$, used intravenously as a diuretic.

ethal (eth′al) cetyl alcohol.

ethambutol hydrochloride (ĕ-tham′bu-tōl) [USP] chemical name: $[R-(R^*,R^*)]$-2,2′-(1,2-ethanediyldiimino) bis - 1 - butanol dihydrochloride. An antibacterial, $C_{10}H_{24}N_2O_2 \cdot 2HCl$, occurring as a white crystalline powder, specifically effective against *Mycobacterium,* including *M. tuberculosis;* used in conjunction with one or more other antituberculous drugs in the treatment of pulmonary tuberculosis, administered orally.

Ethamide (eth′ah-mīd) trademark for a preparation of ethoxzolamide.

ethamivan (eth-am′ĭ-van″) [USP] chemical name: *N,N*-diethyl-4-hydroxy-3-methoxybenzamide. A central nervous system stimulant and analeptic, $C_{12}H_{17}NO_3$, occurring as a white or practically white, crystalline powder; used as a respiratory stimulant, administered intravenously.

ethamsylate (ĕ-tham′sĭ-lāt) chemical name: 2,5-dihydroxybenzenesulfonic acid compound with *N*-ethylethanamine; a hemostatic agent, $C_6H_6O_5S \cdot C_4H_{11}N$.

ethanal (eth′ah-nal) acetaldehyde.

ethane (eth′ān) a hydrocarbon of the methane series, C_2H_6, forming a constituent of natural gas, which occurs as a colorless, odorless, flammable gas.

ethanedial (eth-ān-di′al) glyoxal.

ethanol (eth′ah-nol) alcohol.

ethanolamine (eth″ah-nol′ah-mēn) monoethanolamine.

ethanolism (eth′ah-nol″izm) ethanol-induced hypoglycemia.

ethaverine hydrochloride (eth″ah-ver′ēn) chemical name: 1-[(3,4-diethoxyphenyl)methyl]-6,7-diethoxyisoquinoline. The tetrahydroxy analogue of papaverine, $C_{24}H_{29}NO_4 \cdot HCl$, used as an antispasmodic in peripheral and vascular insufficiency associated with arterial spasm and as a smooth muscle relaxant in spasticity of the gastrointestinal and genitourinary tracts; administered orally.

ethchlorvynol (eth-klōr′vĭ-nol) [USP] chemical name: 1-chloro-3-ethyl-1-penten-4-yn-3-ol. A nonbarbiturate sedative and hypnotic, C_7H_9ClO, occurring as a colorless to yellow, slightly viscous liquid; administered orally.

ethene (eth-ēn′) ethylene.

ethenoid (eth′ĕ-noid) containing an ethylene linkage.

etheogenesis (e″thĕ-o-jen′ĕ-sis) [Gr. *etheos* bachelor + *genesis* production] nonsexual reproduction in male gametes of protozoa.

ether (e′ther) [L. *aether,* Gr. *aithēr* "the upper and purer air"] 1. [USP] chemical name: diethyl ether. A colorless, transparent, mobile, very volatile liquid, $C_2H_5 \cdot O \cdot C_2H_5$, with a characteristic odor, and highly inflammable: used by inhalation as a general anesthetic. Called also *ethyl ether* and *ethyl oxide.* 2. any of a class of organic compounds characterized by the linkage of hydrocarbon groups by an oxygen atom bonded to two carbon atoms. 3. a hypothetical fluid of the utmost tenuity which was once thought to fill all space and to serve as a medium for the transmission of waves of heat and light. **acetic e.,** ethyl acetate. **anesthetic e.,** an organic oxide, usually aliphatic or alicyclic, or mixed, that vaporizes freely and whose vapors induce unconsciousness and surgical anesthesia when inhaled. 2. the British term for ethyl ether. **chloric e.** (*obs.*), a mixture of chloroform and alcohol. **complex e.,** a chemical compound derived from two different alcohol radicals by the elimination of water. **compound e.,** ester. **dibromomethyl e.,** a war

gas, $BrCH_2OCH_2Br$, that irritates the lungs and affects the functioning of the semicircular canals. **dichloromethyl e.,** a form of mustard gas, $(CH_2Cl)_2O$. **diethyl e.,** ether (def. 2). **dimethyl e.,** a liquid, $CH_3 \cdot O \cdot CH_3$, used as a solvent and refrigerant. **enanthic e.,** pelargonic e. **ethyl e.,** ether (def. 2). **ethyl-vinyl e.,** an aliphatic organic oxide, $CH_3 \cdot CH_2 \cdot O \cdot CH:CH_2$, whose vapors produce surgical anesthesia when inhaled. **formic e.,** ethyl formate. **hydriodic e.,** ethyl iodide. **hydrobromic e.,** ethyl bromide. **hydrochloric e.,** ethyl chloride. **luminiferous e.,** ether (def. 1). **mixed e.,** complex e. **nitrofurfuryl methyl e.,** 2-(methoxymethyl)-5-nitrofuran; used as a topical fungicide and sporicide in skin infections. **nitrous e.,** ethyl nitrite. **oenanthic e.,** pelargonic e. **pelargonic e.,** an ether of pelargonic acid; it is an oily liquid with the odor of quinces. **petroleum e.,** petroleum benzin. **pyroacetic e.,** acetone. **simple e.,** a chemical compound derived from two identical alcohol radicals by the elimination of water. **sulfuric e.,** see *ether* (def. 2). **thio e.,** an ether in which sulfur replaces oxygen. **thioallylic e.,** allyl sulfide. **vinyl e.** [USP], a clear colorless liquid, $CH_2:CH \cdot O \cdot CH:CH_2$, with a characteristic odor, administered by inhalation to produce general anesthesia. Called also *divinyl oxide.*

ethereal (e-the′re-al) 1. pertaining to, prepared with, containing, or resembling ether. 2. evanescent; delicate.

etherification (e″ther-ĭ-fi-ka′shun) the formation of an ether from alcohol.

etherion (e-the′re-on) (*obs.*) 1. a gas said to have been discovered in 1898 in the atmosphere; said to be about $\frac{1}{1000}$ part as dense as hydrogen, and to exist in less than $\frac{1}{1000000}$ part of its proportion in the air. 2. Mathews' name for one of the minute spheres once believed to make up the ether.

etherism (e′ther-izm) etheromania.

etherization (e″ther-i-za′shun) the administration of ether by inhalation, and the consequent production of anesthesia.

etherize (e′ther-iz) to put under the anesthetic influence of ether.

etheromania (e″ther-o-ma′ne-ah) uncontrollable addiction to the use of ether as a stimulant.

etherometer (e″ther-om′ĕ-ter) [*ether* + Gr. *metron* measure] a device for administering ether by which the number of drops per minute can be accurately controlled.

etherrausch (a′ter-rowsh) [Ger.] (*obs.*) see *rausch.*

ethical (eth′ĭ-kal) in accordance with the principles which govern right conduct.

ethics (eth′iks) [Gr. *ēthos* the manner and habits of man or of animals] the rules or principles which govern right conduct. **medical e.,** the values and guidelines that should govern decisions in medicine.

ethidene (eth′ĭ-dēn) ethylidene. **e. chloride,** ethylene dichloride. **e. diamine,** a harmful ptomaine, $C_2H_8N_2$, from fish.

ethidium (ĕ-thid′e-um) homidium.

ethinamate (ĕ-thin′ah-māt) [USP] chemical name: 1-ethynyl-cyclohexanol carbamate. A short-acting nonbarbiturate sedative, $C_9H_{13}NO_2$, occurring as a white powder; used as a hypnotic, administered orally.

ethinyl (eth′ĭ-nil) ethynyl. **e. estradiol,** see under *estradiol.* **e. trichloride,** trichloroethylene.

Ethiodol (ĕ-thi′o-dol) trademark for a preparation of ethiodized oil, used as a contrast medium.

ethionamide (ĕ-thi″on-am′ĭd) [USP] chemical name: 2-ethyl-4-pyridine-carbothioamide. An antibacterial, $C_8H_{10}N_2S$, occurring as a bright yellow powder, effective against *Myobacterium tuberculosis;* used in conjunction with one or more other antituberculous drugs in the treatment of pulmonary tuberculosis, administered orally.

ethionine (ĕ-thi′o-nin) the ethyl homologue of methionine.

ethisterone (ĕ-this′ter-ōn) chemical name: 17α-hydroxypregn-4-en-20-yn-3-one; a semisynthetic progestin, $C_{21}H_{28}O_2$, which may be considered a derivative of both progesterone and of testosterone. Called also *anhydrohydroxyprogesterone, pregneninolone,* and *ethinyl testosterone.*

ethmocarditis (eth″mo-kar-di′tis) [Gr. *ēthmos* sieve + *kardia* heart + *-itis*] inflammation of the connective tissue of the heart.

ethmocephalus (eth″mo-sef′ah-lus) [Gr. *ēthmos* sieve + *kephalē* head] a monster with an imperfect head, more or less union of the eyes, and a rudimentary nose, which may often be displaced upward.

ethmofrontal (eth″mo-fron′tal) pertaining to the ethmoid and frontal bones.

ethmoid (eth′moid) [Gr. *ēthmos* sieve + *eidos* form] cribriform; sievelike.

ethmoidal (eth-moi′dal) of or pertaining to the ethmoid bone.

ethmoidectomy (eth″moi-dek′to-me) [*ethmoid* + Gr. *ektomē* excision] excision of the ethmoid cells or of a portion of the ethmoid bone.

ethmoiditis (eth″moi-di′tis) inflammation of the ethmoid bone.

ethmoidotomy (eth″moi-dot′o-me)   surgical incision into the ethmoid sinus.

ethmolacrimal (eth″mo-lak′rĭ-mal)   pertaining to the ethmoid and the lacrimal bones.

ethmomaxillary (eth″mo-mak′sĭ-lār-e)   pertaining to the ethmoid and maxillary bones.

ethmonasal (eth″mo-na′zal)   pertaining to the ethmoid and nasal bones.

ethmopalatal (eth″mo-pal′ah-tal)   pertaining to the ethmoid and palatine bones.

ethmosphenoid (eth″mo-sfe′noid)   pertaining to the ethmoid and sphenoid bones.

ethmoturbinal (eth″mo-tur′bĭ-nal)   pertaining to the superior and middle nasal conchae.

ethmovomerine (eth″mo-vo′mer-in)   pertaining to the ethmoid bone and the vomer.

ethmyphitis (eth″mĕ-fi′tis) [Gr. ēthmos sieve + hyphē tissue] inflammation of the cellular tissue; cellulitis.

ethnic (eth′nik) [Gr. ethnikos of a nation; national]   pertaining to a social group who share cultural bonds (religious, national, etc.) or physical (racial) characteristics.

ethnics (eth′niks) [Gr. ethnikos of a nation; national]   ethnology.

ethnobiology (eth″no-bi-ol′o-je)   the scientific study of physical characteristics of different races of mankind.

ethnography (eth-nog′rah-fe) [Gr. ethnos race + graphein to write]   a description of the races of men. Cf. anthropography.

ethnology (eth-nol′o-je) [Gr. ethnos race + -logy]   the science which deals with the races of men, their descent, relationship, etc.

ethobrom (eth′o-brōm)   tribromoethanol.

ethocaine (eth′o-kān)   procaine hydrochloride.

ethoglucid (eth″o-glu′sid)   chemical name: triethylene glycol diglycidyl ether. A clear colorless viscous liquid, $C_{12}H_{22}O_6$, with antineoplastic properties.

ethoheptazine citrate (eth″o-hep′tah-zēn)   chemical name: ethylhexahydro-1-methyl-4-phenyl-1H-azepine-4-carboxylate dihydrogen citrate. An analgesic, $C_{16}H_{23}NO_2 \cdot C_6H_8O_7$, used to control mild or moderate pain; administered orally.

ethohexadiol (eth″o-heks-a′de-ol)   chemical name: 2-ethyl-1,3-hexamediol. An arthropod repellant, $C_8H_{18}O_2$, applied topically to the skin and clothing.

ethological (eth″o-loj′ĭ-kal)   pertaining to ethology.

ethologist (e-thol′o-jist)   an individual skilled in ethology.

ethology (e-thol′o-je) [Gr. ethos the manners and habits of man, or of animals + -logy]   The scientific study of animal behavior, particularly in the natural state, the evolution of behavior, and its biologic significance.

ethomoxane hydrochloride (eth″o-moks′ān)   chemical name: N-butyl-8-ethoxy-2,3-dihydro-1,4-benzodioxin-2-methanamine hydrochloride; a tranquilizer, $C_{15}H_{23}NO_3 \cdot HCl$.

ethonam nitrate (eth′o-nam)   chemical name: 1-(1,2,3,4-tetrahydro-1-naphthalenyl)-1H-imidazole-5-carboxylic acid ethyl ester mononitrate; an antifungal agent, $C_{16}H_{18}N_2O_2 \cdot HNO_3$.

ethopropazine hydrochloride (eth″o-pro′pah-zēn) [USP]   chemical name: N,N-diethyl-α-methyl-10H-phenothiazine-10-ethanamine monohydrochloride. A phenothiazine derivative, $C_{19}H_{24}N_2S \cdot HCl$, occurring as a white to slightly off-white, crystalline powder, having anticholinergic, antihistaminic, adrenergic-blocking, ganglion-blocking, local anesthetic, and central nervous system depressant effects; used as an antiparkinsonian agent, administered orally. Called also isothiazine hydrochloride and phenopropazine hydrochloride.

ethosuximide (eth″o-suk′sĭ-mĭd) [USP]   chemical name: 3-ethyl-3-methyl-2,5-pyrrolidinedione. An anticonvulsant, $C_7H_{11}NO_2$, occurring as a white to off-white crystalline powder or waxy solid; used in the treatment of petit mal epilepsy, administered orally.

ethotoin (ĕ-tho′to-in)   chemical name: 3-ethyl-5-phenyl-2,4-imidazolidinedione. An anticonvulsant, $C_{11}H_{12}N_2O_2$, occurring as a white, crystalline powder; used in the treatment of grand mal epilepsy and psychomotor seizures, administered orally. Called also ethylphenylhydantoin.

ethoxazene hydrochloride (ĕ-thok′sah-zēn)   chemical name: 4-[(4-ethoxyphenyl)azo]-1,3-benzenediamine hydrochloride. A local analgesic, $C_{14}H_{16}N_4O \cdot HCl$, occurring as a reddish powder; used to relieve pain associated with urinary tract infections, administered orally.

ethoxzolamide (eth″oks-zol′ah-mīd) [USP]   chemical name: 6-ethoxy-2-benzothiazolesulfonamide. A carbonic anhydrase inhibitor, $C_9H_{10}N_2O_3S_2$, occurring as a white to slightly yellow, crystalline powder; used as a diuretic in mild to moderate congestive heart failure and as an adjunct in the treatment of glaucoma and epilepsy, administered orally.

Ethrane (eth′rān)   trademark for a preparation of enflurane.

Ethril (eth′ril)   trademark for preparations of erythromycin stearate.

ethybenztropine (eth″ĭ-benz-tro′pēn)   chemical name: endo-3-(diphenylmethoxy)-8-ethyl-8-azabicyclo[3.2.1]octane. An anti-

cholinergic with high antihistaminic action, $C_{22}H_{27}NO$, which has been used as an antiparkinsonian agent and in the treatment of drug-induced extrapyramidal syndrome.

ethyl (eth′il) [ether + Gr. hylē matter]   the univalent alcohol radical, $CH_3 \cdot CH_2$. Symbol Et.   **e. acetate** [NF], a transparent, colorless liquid, $CH_3COOC_2H_5$, used as a flavoring agent in pharmaceutical preparations. Called also acetic ether, naphtha aceti, and vinegar naphtha.   **e. aminobenzoate**, benzocaine. **e. biscoumacetate**, chemical name: 4-hydroxy-α-(4-hydroxy-2-oxo-2H-1-benzopyran-3-yl)-2-oxo-2H-1-benzopyran-3-acetic acid ethyl ester. One of the synthetic, orally effective coumarin anticoagulants, $C_{22}H_{16}O_8$.   **e. bromide**, a colorless volatile liquid, C_2H_5Br, of sweetish taste and ethereal odor, used as an inhalation anesthetic; called also hydrobromic ether.   **e. butyrate**, the butyric acid ester of ethyl alcohol, $C_3H_7 \cdot CO \cdot O \cdot C_2H_5$, with the odor of pineapple.   **e. carbamate**, urethan.   **e. carbinol**, propyl alcohol.   **e. chaulmoograte**, a mixture of the ethyl esters of the unsaturated fatty acids—chaulmoogric and hydnocarpic—of chaulmoogra oil, used in the treatment of leprosy and sarcoidosis.   **e. chloride** [USP], chemical name: chloroethane. A colorless, mobile, extremely volatile liquid, C_2H_5Cl; used as a local anesthetic, applied topically as a spray on intact skin. Called also chelen and hydrochloric ether.   **e. cyanide**, a colorless liquid, C_2H_5CN; called also propionitril.   **e. diacetate**, a substance which has been used in urinary tests.   **e. dibunate**, chemical name: 3,6-bis(1,1-dimethylethyl)naphthalenesulfonic acid ethyl ester; an antitussive $C_{20}H_{28}O_3S$.   **e. ether**, see ether (def. 2).   **e. formate**, a volatile liquid, $HCOOC_2H_5$, used as a solvent and flavoring agent, and formerly as an anesthetic. Called also formic ether.   **e. iodide**, a colorless liquid, CH_3CH_2I, used as a reagent; called also hydriodic ether.   **e. linoleate**, ethyl, (9,12)-cis, cis-octadecadienoate: a lipid occurring on the skin of warm-blooded animals and responsible for its passive water-holding capacity; also prepared synthetically.   **e. mercaptan**, a thioalcohol, C_2H_5SH, which has a revolting odor and contributes to the odor of feces.   **e. nitrate**, a compound, $CH_3 \cdot CH_2 \cdot NO_3$, formerly used as a vasodilator.   **e. nitrite**, $C_2H_5NO_2$, a liquid which is mixed with alcohol to form ethyl nitrite spirit. Called also nitrous ether.   **e. oleate** [NF], chemical name: (Z)-9-octadecenoic acid ethyl ester. A mobile, practically colorless liquid, $C_{20}H_{38}O_2$, consisting of esters of ethyl alcohol and high-molecular-weight fatty acids; used as a vehicle for pharmaceutical preparations.   **e. orange**, a dye, the sodium salt of diethylaniline-azo-benzene-sulfonic acid, $C_6H_4 \cdot N(C_2H_5)_2 \cdot N_2 \cdot C_6H_4 \cdot SO_2 \cdot ONa$; used as an indicator, being turned red by acids and yellow by alkalis.   **e. oxide**, ether, def. 1.   **e. pelargonate**, the pelargonic acid ester of ethyl alcohol, $C_8H_{17} \cdot CO \cdot O \cdot C_2H_5$.   **e. phenylcinchoninate**, a yellowish powder once used in gout. **e. phenylephrine**, see ethylphenylephrine.   **e. salicylate**, the salicylic acid ester of ethyl alcohol, $CH_3 \cdot CH_2 \cdot O \cdot CO \cdot C_6H_4OH$, formerly used internally for rheumatism and as a counterirritant. **e. urethan**, a compound which inhibits cellular respiration and interferes with a large number of enzymes in the cell.

ethylaldehyde (eth″il-al′dĕ-hīd)   acetaldehyde.

ethylamine (eth″il-am′in)   a liquid ptomaine, $CH_3CH_2NH_2$, from decaying plant tissue, possessing many of the properties of ammonia.   **e. sulfonic acid**, taurine.   **e. urate**, a remedy formerly employed in the treatment of gout and gravel.

ethylate (eth′il-āt)   any compound of ethyl alcohol in which the hydrogen of the hydroxyl is replaced by a base.

ethylation (eth″il-a′shun)   the act of combining or causing to combine with the ethyl radical.

ethylcellulose (eth″il-sel′u-lōs) [NF]   chemical name: cellulose ethyl ester. A free-flowing, white to light tan powder, used as a tablet binder in pharmaceutical preparations.

ethylene (eth′ĭ-lēn)   a colorless gas, $CH_2{=}CH_2$, somewhat lighter than air, and having a slightly sweet taste and odor; used for inducing general anesthesia. Called also aethylenum, ethene, and olefiant gas.   **e. dichloride**, a colorless heavy liquid, $C_2H_4Cl_2$, with a pungent odor, used as a solvent; called also ethidine chloride.   **e. oxide**, a bactericidal agent, occurring as a colorless gas with a pleasant ethereal odor; used as a disinfectant, especially for disposable equipment.

ethylenediamine (eth″ĭ-lēn-di′ah-mēn) [USP]   chemical name: 1,2-ethanediamine. A clear, colorless or slightly yellow liquid, $C_2H_8N_2$, having an ammonia-like odor and a strong alkaline reaction; used as a component of aminophylline injection.

ethylenediaminetetraacetate (eth″ĭ-lēn-di″ah-mēn-tet-ras′ĕ-tāt)   edetate.

ethylestrenol (eth″il-es′trĕ-nōl)   chemical name: 19-nor-17α-pregn-4-en-17β-ol; an anabolic-androgenic steroid, $C_{20}H_{32}O$.

ethylic (e-thil′ik)   pertaining to or derived from ethyl.

ethylidene (eth′il-ĭ-dēn)   the bivalent radical, $CH_3 \cdot CH$; called also ethidene.

ethylmorphine hydrochloride (eth″il-mor′-fen)   chemical name: 7,8-didehydro-4,5α-epoxy-3-ethoxy-17-methylmorphinan-6α-ol hydrochloride. The chloride salt of the ethyl ester of morphine, $C_{10}H_{15}NO_3 \cdot HCl$, having some of the actions of morphine and codeine; used as a chemotic in the treatment of glaucoma, iritis, and corneal ulcers, applied topically to the conjunctiva. It has also been used as an antitussive.

ethylnoradrenaline (eth″il-nor-ah-dren′ah-lin) ethylnorepinephrine.

ethylnorepinephrine hydrochloride (eth″ĭl-nor-ep″ĭ-nef′-rin) [USP] chemical name: 4-(2-amino-1-hydroxybutyl)-1,2-benzendiol hydrochloride. A synthetic adrenergic, $C_{10}H_{15}NO_3 \cdot HCl$, used for the relief of bronchospasm in bronchial asthma; administered intramuscularly or subcutaneously.

ethylnorsuprarenin (eth″il-nor-su″prah-ren′in) ethylnorepinephrine.

ethylparaben (eth″il-par′ah-ben) [NF] chemical name: 4-hydroxybenzoic acid ethyl ester. An antifungal agent, $C_9H_{10}O_3$, occurring as small, colorless crystals or white powder; used as a preservative in pharmaceutical preparations.

ethylphenylhydantoin (eth″il-fen″il-hi-dan′to-in) ethotoin.

ethylstibamine (eth″il-sti″bah-mēn) neostibosan.

ethynodiol diacetate (ĕ-thi″no-di′ōl) [USP] chemical name: 19-norpregn-4-en-20-yne-3β,17α-diol diacetate. A progestin, $C_{24}H_{32}O_4$, occurring as a white, crystalline powder; used in combination with an estrogen as an oral contraceptive.

ethynyl (eth″ĭ-nil) the radical —C≡CH, when it occurs in organic compounds; called also *ethinyl*.

etidocaine hydrochloride (ĕ-te′do-kān) chemical name: (±)N-(2,6-dimethylphenyl)-2-(ethylpropylamino)butanamide hydrochloride. A local anesthetic of the amide type, $C_{17}H_{28}N_2O \cdot HCl$, used for percutaneous infiltration anesthesia, peripheral nerve blocks, and caudal and epidural blocks.

etidronate disodium (ĕ-tĭ-dro′nāt) chemical name: (1-hydroxyethylidene) bisphosphoric acid disodium dihydrogen salt; a bone calcium regulator, $C_2H_6Na_2O_7P_2$, used orally in the symptomatic treatment of osteitis deformans and as a pharmaceutic aid.

etiocholanolone (e″te-o-ko-lan′o-lōn) a reduced form of testosterone excreted in the urine.

etiogenic (e″te-o-jen′ik) [Gr. *aitia* cause + *gennan* to produce] causative.

etiolation (e″te-o-la′shun) [Fr. *étioler* to blanch] 1. a blanching or paleness of color in a plant due to lack of chlorophyll when grown in the dark. 2. the process by which the skin becomes pale when deprived of sunlight.

etiologic, etiological (e″te-o-loj′ik; e″te-o-loj′e-kal) pertaining to etiology, or to the causes of disease.

etiology (e″te-ol′o-je) [Gr. *aitia* cause + *-logy*] the study or theory of the factors that cause disease and the method of their introduction to the host; the cause(s) or origin of a disease. Cf. *pathogenesis*.

etiopathology (e″te-o-pah-thol′o-je) pathogenesis.

etioporphyrin (e″te-o-por′fir-in) a porphyrin, $C_{32}H_{38}N_4$, obtained from hematoporphyrin; a tetramethyl-tetraethylporphine.

etiotropic (e″te-o-trop′ik) [Gr. *aitia* cause + *tropos* turning] directed against the cause of a disease.

etoformin hydrochloride (et″o-for′min) chemical name: N-butyl-N‴-ethylimidodicarbonimidic diamide monohydrochloride; an antidiabetic, $C_8H_{19}N_5 \cdot HCl$.

etomidate (ĕ-tom′ĭ-dāt) chemical name: (+)-1-(1-phenylethyl)-1H-imidazole-5-carboxylic acid ethyl ester; a hypnotic, $C_{14}H_{16}N_2O_2$.

etoprine (et′o-prēn) chemical name: 5-(3,4-dichlorophenyl)-6-ethyl-2,4-pyrimidinediamine; an antineoplastic, $C_{12}H_{12}Cl_2N_4$.

etoxadrol hydrochloride (ĕ-toks′ah-drōl) chemical name: (+)-2-(2-ethyl-2-phenyl-1,3-dioxolan-4-yl) piperidine hydrochloride; an anesthetic, $C_{16}H_{23}NO_2 \cdot HCl$.

etozolin (et″o-zo′lin) chemical name: [3-methyl-4-oxo-5-(1-piperidinyl)-2-thiazolidinylidene]acetic acid ethyl ester; a diuretic, $C_{13}H_{20}N_2O_3S$.

etrohysterectomy (e″tro-his-ter-ek′to-me) [Gr. *ētron* hypogastrium + *hysterectomy*] (*obs.*) hypogastric excision of uterus.

etrotomy (e-trot′o-me) [Gr. *ētron* hypogastrium + *temnein* to cut] suprapubic incision.

etryptamine acetate (e-trip′tah-min) chemical name: 3-(2-aminobutyl) indole acetate. A compound, $C_{12}H_{16}N_2 \cdot C_2H_4O_2$, formerly used as a central stimulant, now removed from the market because of serious toxic reactions.

Eu chemical symbol for *europium*.

eu- (u) [Gr. *eu* well] a combining form meaning well, easily, or good; the opposite of *dys-*.

euallele (u-ah-lēl′) a mutation occurring in the same codon of a particular cistron in two homologous chromosomes.

euallelic (u-ah-le′lik) pertaining to a euallele.

euangiotic (u″an-je-ot′ik) [*eu-* + Gr. *angeion* vessel] well supplied with blood vessels.

Euascomycetidae (u-as″ko-mi-se″tĭ-de) a subclass of ascomycetous fungi in which the asci most commonly develop from hyphae, and functional sex organs are usually present; it includes the series Plectomycetes, Pyrenomycetes, and Discomycetes.

Eubacteriales (u″bak-te″re-a′lēz) an order of Schizomycetes, comprising the true bacteria, which are simple, undifferentiated, rigid, spherical or rod-shaped cells. It includes 13 families, *Achromobacteraceae*, *Azotobacteraceae*, *Bacillaceae*, *Bacteroidaceae*, *Brevibacteriaceae*, *Brucellaceae*, *Corynebacteriaceae*, *Enterobacteriaceae*, *Lactobacillaceae*, *Micrococcaceae*, *Neisseriaceae*, *Propionibacteriaceae*, and *Rhizobiaceae*.

Eubacterium (u″bak-te′re-um) a genus of microorganisms of the tribe Lactobacilleae, family Lactobacillaceae, order Eubacteriales, nonsporulating, gram-positive anaerobic bacilli found in the intestinal tract as parasites and as saprophytes in soil and water. Occasionally found in purulent lesions but of questionable primary pathogenicity.

eubiotics (u″bi-ot′iks) [*eu-* + Gr. *bios* life] the science of healthy living.

eucaine (u′kān) chemical name: 2,2,6-trimethyl-4-piperidinol benzoate ester. A substance, $C_{15}H_{21}NO_2$, closely resembling cocaine in action and composition, but less depressant to the heart; formerly used as a local anesthetic. In veterinary medicine, the hydrochloride is used as a substitute for cocaine. Called also *benzamine*.

eucalyptol (u″kah-lip′tol) a colorless liquid with a characteristic aromatic, camphoraceous odor, and a cooling, pungent, spicy taste, obtained from eucalyptus oil and other sources, used as a flavoring agent, expectorant, and local antiseptic, and formerly as a vermifuge. Used in veterinary medicine as an inhalant in bronchitis and as an expectorant.

Eucalyptus (u″kah-lip′tus) [*eu-* + Gr. *kalyptos* covered] a genus of myrtaceous trees and shrubs, chiefly Australian, of many species; on distillation, the leaves yield eucalyptus oil, the major constituent of which is eucalyptol. Called also *blue gum*.

eucapnia (u-kap′ne-ah) [*eu-* + Gr. *kapnos* smoke] the condition in which the carbon dioxide tension of the blood is normal.

eucaryon (u-kar′e-on) eukaryon.

eucaryosis (u″kar-e-o′sis) eukaryosis.

Eucaryotae (u-kar″e-o′te) [*eu-* + Gr. *karyon* nucleus] in some systems of classification, a kingdom of organisms that includes higher plants and animals, fungi, protozoa, and most algae (except blue-green algae), which are made up of eukaryotic cells, i.e., which have a true nucleus. Also written *Eukaryotae*. Cf. *Prokaryotae*.

eucaryote (u-kar′e-ōt) eukaryote.

eucaryotic (u″kar-e-ot′ik) eukaryotic.

eucatropine hydrochloride (u-kat′ro-pēn) [USP] chemical name: α-hydroxybenzeneacetic acid 1,2,2,6-tetramethyl-4-piperidinyl ester hydrochloride. An anticholinergic, $C_{17}H_{25}NO_3 \cdot HCl$, occurring as a white, granular powder; used as a mydriatic, applied topically to the eye.

Eucestoda (u-ses-to′dah) Cestoda.

euchlorhydria (u″klōr-hi′dre-ah) [*eu-* + *chlorhydric acid*] the presence of the normal proportion of free hydrochloric acid in the gastric juice.

eucholia (u-ko′le-ah) [*eu-* + Gr. *cholē* bile] normal condition of the bile.

euchromatic (u-kro-mat′ic) of or relating to euchromatin.

euchromatin (u-kro′mah-tin) that state of chromatin (q.v.) in which it stains lightly, is genetically active, and is considered to be partially or fully uncoiled; cf. *heterochromatin*.

euchromatopsy (u-kro′mah-top″se) [*eu-* + Gr. *chrōma* color + *opsis* vision] normal color vision.

euchromosome (u-kro′mo-sōm) [*eu-* + *chromosome*] autosome.

euchylia (u-kil′e-ah) [*eu-* + Gr. *chylos* chyle] a normal condition of the chyle.

Euciliatia (u-sil″e-a′she-ah) a subclass of protozoa of the class Ciliata, subphylum Ciliophora; they are usually free-living, but some are commensalistic, endosymbiotic, or epizoic, and a few are parasitic, including the intestinal ciliates of warm-blooded animals. It includes the genera *Balantidium*, *Nyctotherus*, *Ichthyophthirius*, *Tetrahymena*, and *Paramecium*.

eucoelom (u-se′lom) [*eu-* + *coelom*] coelom.

Eucoelomata (u″se-lo-ma′tah) the major division of the higher invertebrates, the coelomates, including mollusks, annelids, arthropods, echinoderms, and chordates, which all have a separate mouth and anus, a true coelom, and a well-developed circulatory system. It is divided into two series, the Deuterostomia and the Protostomia.

eucoelomate (u-sēl′o-māt″) any member of the Eucoelomata; a coelomate.

eucolloid (u-kol′oid) a colloid in which each dispersed particle consists of a single large molecule.

eucrasia (u-kra′se-ah) [*eu-* + Gr. *krasis* mixture] 1. a state of health; proper balance of different factors constituting a healthy state. 2. a state in which there is a decreased bodily reaction to ingested or injected drugs, proteins, etc.

eudiaphoresis (u-di″ah-fo-re′sis) [*eu-* + *diaphoresis*] (*obs.*) an easy, natural, or comforting escape of perspiration.

eudiemorrhysis (u″di-ĕ-mor′ĭ-sis) [*eu-* + Gr. *dia* through +

haima blood + *rhysis* flow] the normal flow of blood through the capillaries.

eudiometer (u″de-om′ĕ-ter) [Gr. *eudia* fine weather + *metron* measure] an instrument used in testing the purity of the air.

eudipsia (u-dip′se-ah) [*eu-* + Gr. *dipsa* thirst + *-ia*] ordinary, mild thirst.

euergasis (u″er-ga′ze-ah) [*eu-* + *ergasia*] normal psychobiological functioning.

euesthesia (u″es-the′ze-ah) [*eu-* + Gr. *aisthēsis* perception] a normal state of the senses.

Euflagellata (u-flaj″ĕ-la′tah) Mastigophora.

euflavine (u-fla′vin) acriflavine.

eugamy (u′gah-me) [Gr. *eu* well + *gamos* marriage] the union of gametes, each of which contains the proper (haploid) complement of chromosomes.

eugenetics (u″jĕ-net′iks) eugenics.

Eugenia (u-je′ne-ah) an extensive genus of myrtaceous trees and shrubs. *E. caryophyllata* Thunb. furnishes clove, clove oil.

eugenicist (u-jen′ĭ-sist) a person who is versed in eugenics.

eugenics (u-jen′iks) [*eu-* + Gr. *gennan* to generate] the study and control of procreation as a means of improving the hereditary characteristics of a race; called also *orthogenics.* Cf. *dysgenics.* **negative e.,** that concerned with prevention of reproduction (procreation) by individuals possessing inferior or undesirable traits. **positive e.,** that concerned with promotion of optimal mating of individuals possessing superior or desirable traits.

eugenism (u′jen-izm) that condition of heredity and environment which tends to produce healthy and happy existence.

eugenist (u-jen′ist) eugenicist.

eugenol (u′jen-ol) [USP] chemical name: 2-methoxy-4-(2-propenyl)phenol. A dental analgesic, $C_{10}H_{12}O_2$, occurring as a colorless or pale yellow liquid, obtained from clove oil or other natural sources; applied topically to dental cavities and also used as a component of dental protectives. Called also *allylguaiacol, caryophyllic acid,* and *eugenic acid.*

eugenothenics (u-je″no-then′iks) the study of race improvement by the regulation of both heredity and environment.

Euglena (u-gle′nah) [*eu-* + Gr. *glēnē* pupil of the eye] a genus of green flagellate protozoa of the order Euglenoidina, class Phytomastigophora, commonly found in great abundance in stagnant water. They have a pellicle usually marked by spiral or longitudinal striations; those with a thin pellicle are very plastic. *E. viridis* and *E. gracilis* are common species.

euglenoid (u-gle′noid) 1. pertaining to the order Euglenoidina. 2. any individual of the order Euglenoidina.

Euglenoidina (u-gle″noi-di′nah) an order of plantlike flagellate protozoa of the subclass Phytomastigophora, class Mastigophora, which typically have green chromatophores, one flagellum protruding from an anterior gullet, and a small stigma located anteriorly; they are usually found in fresh water, although some inhabit salt or brackish water, and a few are parasitic. It includes the genera *Euglena* and *Copromonas.* In botany, these difficult to classify organisms, are assigned to the algae.

euglobulin (u-glob′u-lin) one of a class of globulins characterized by being insoluble in water but soluble in saline solutions; see also under *globulin.*

euglycemia (u″gli-se′me-ah) a normal level of glucose in the blood.

euglycemic (u″gli-se′mik) pertaining to, characterized by, or conducive to euglycemia.

eugnathia (u-na′the-ah) any oral abnormality limited to the teeth and their immediate alveolar supports.

eugnathic (u-nath′ik) [*eu-* + Gr. *gnathos* jaw] pertaining to or characterized by a normal state of the maxilla and mandible.

eugnosia (u-no′se-ah) [*eu-* + Gr. *gnōsis* perception] ability to recognize and synthesize sensory stimuli into a normal perception.

eugnostic (u-nos′tik) pertaining to eugnosia.

eugonic (u-gon′ik) [*eu-* + Gr. *gonē* seed] growing luxuriantly; said of bacterial cultures.

euhydration (u-hi-dra′shun) a normal state of body water content; absence of absolute or relative hydration or of dehydration.

eukaryon (u-kar′e-on) [*eu-* + Gr. *karyon* nucleus] 1. a highly organized nucleus bounded by a nuclear membrane, a characteristic of cells of higher organisms. Cf. *prokaryon.* 2. eukaryote.

eukaryosis (u″kar-e-o′sis) [*eu-* + Gr. *karyon* nucleus + *-osis*] the state of having a true nucleus, the nuclear material being surrounded by a membrane and the cytoplasm containing organelles; generally a characteristic of all cell types except bacteria and blue-green algae. Cf. *prokaryosis.*

Eukaryotae (u-kar″e-o′te) Eucaryotae.

eukaryote (u-kar′e-ōt) an organism whose cells have a true nucleus, i.e., one bounded by a nuclear membrane, within which lie the chromosomes combined with proteins, and that exhibit mitosis; eukaryotic cells also contain many membrane-bound compartments (organelles) in which cellular functions are per-

formed. The cells of higher plants and animals, fungi, protozoa, and most algae are eukaryotic. Cf. *prokaryote.*

eukaryotic (u″kar-e-ot′ik) pertaining to a eukaryon or a eukaryote or to eukaryosis.

eukeratin (u-ker′ah-tin) a true keratin found in hair, nails, feathers, and horns.

eukinesia (u″ki-ne′se-ah) [Gr. *eu* well + *kinēsis* movement + *-ia*] the state of possessing normal or proper motor function or activity; normal or proper mobility.

eukinesis (u″ki-ne′sis) eukinesia.

eukinetic (u″ki-net′ik) pertaining to or characterized by eukinesia.

eulachon (u′lah-kon) the candle-fish, *Thaleichthys pacificus;* its oil is used like cod liver oil.

eulaminate (u-lam′ĭ-nāt) having the normal number of lamina, as certain areas of the cerebral cortex.

Eulenburg's disease (oil′en-burgz) [Albert *Eulenburg,* German neurologist, 1840–1917] myotonia congenita.

eumenorrhea (u″men-o-re′ah) [*eu-* + Gr. *mēn* menses + *rhoia* flow] normal menstruation.

Eumetazoa (u-met″ah-zo′ah) in some classifications, a subdivision of the Metazoa comprising all multicellular animals with organ systems, a mouth, and a digestive cavity. Cf. *Parazoa.*

eumetria (u-me′tre-ah) [Gr. "good measure," "good proportion"] a normal condition of nerve impulse, so that a voluntary movement just reaches the intended goal; the proper range of movement.

eumorphics (u-mor′fiks) a branch of orthopedics which deals with the reestablishment of normal or proper form.

eumorphism (u-mor′fizm) [*eu-* + Gr. *morphē* form] retention of the normal form of a cell.

Eumycetes (u″mi-se′tēz) a taxonomic division comprising the true or proper fungi. It includes three classes of perfect fungi (Ascomycetes, Phycomycetes, and Basidiomycetes) and all the imperfect fungi (Deuteromycetes, or Fungi Imperfecti). Called also *Eumycophyta.*

eumycin (u-mi′sin) an antibiotic isolated from *Bacillus subtilis* which has *in vitro* activity against diphtheria and tubercle bacilli and some fungi.

Eumycophyta (u-mi″ko-fi′tah) Eumycetes.

eunoia (u-noi′ah) [*eu-* + Gr. *nous* mind] alertness of mind and will.

eunuch (u′nuk) [Gr. *eunouchos* a castrated person, employed in Asia, and later in Greece, to take charge of the women and act as a chamberlain] a man or boy deprived of the testes or the external genital organs, especially one castrated before puberty (so that male secondary sex characteristics fail to develop).

eunuchism (u′nuk-izm) [Gr. *eunouchismos* castration] the condition of being a eunuch or of undeveloped sexual organs in which testicular hormones are not produced. **pituitary e.,** loss of sexual power due to derangement of the pituitary secretion.

eunuchoid (u′nŭ-koid) [Gr. *eunouchoeidēs*] 1. resembling a eunuch; having the characteristics of a eunuch. 2. a cryptorchid person with defective masculinity of appearance, causing him to resemble a eunuch.

eunuchoidism (u′nŭ-koi″dizm) a deficiency of the testes or of the testicular secretion, with impaired sexual power and eunuch-like symptoms. **female e.,** hypogonadism in which the ovaries fail to function at puberty, resulting in infertility, absence of development of secondary sex characteristics, infantile sexual organs, and excessive growth of the long bones. **hypergonadotropic e.,** that associated with high levels of gonadotropins, as in Klinefelter's syndrome. **hypogonadotropic e.,** that due to lack of gonadotropin secretion.

euosmia (u-os′me-ah) [*eu-* + Gr. *osmē* smell] 1. normal state of the sense of smell. 2. a pleasant odor.

eupancreatism (u-pan′kre-ah-tizm″) a normal condition of the pancreatic function.

eupatorin (u″pah-to′rin) 3′,5-dihydroxy-4′,6,7-trimethoxyflavone; an active (emetic) principle from *Eupatorium perfoliatum.*

Eupatorium (u″pah-to′re-um) a genus of composite-flowered plants. The leaves and tops of *E. perfoliatum,* boneset or thoroughwort, are tonic, diuretic, diaphoretic, and stomachic. The ingestion of *E. rugosum* (*E. urticaefolium*), the white snakeroot, which contains the toxic principle tremetol, causes a disease known as trembles in cattle and sheep.

eupepsia (u-pep′se-ah) [*eu-* + Gr. *pepsis* digestion + *-ia*] good digestion; particularly the presence of a normal amount of pepsin in the gastric juice. Cf. *dyspepsia.*

eupepsy (u′pep-se) eupepsia.

eupeptic (u-pep′tik) pertaining to, characterized by, or promoting eupepsia. Cf. *dyspeptic.*

euperistalsis (u-per″ĭ-stal′sis) normal or painless peristalsis.

euphenic (u-fen′ik) improving the phenotype; pertaining to euphenics.

euphenics (u-fen′iks) [*eu-* + Gr. *phainein* to appear] the improvement of phenotype by chemical or surgical means or by manipulation of the environment (e.g., nutrition); analogous to eugenics.

Euphorbia (u-for′be-ah) an extensive genus of euphorbiaceous trees, shrubs, and herbs, the spurges, which are actively poisonous, emetic, and cathartic. including *E. antisyphilitica* Zucca., the source of candelilla wax.

euphoretic (u″fo-ret′ik) 1. pertaining to, characterized by, or producing a condition of euphoria. 2. an agent that produces euphoria.

euphoria (u-fo′re-ah) [Gr. "the power of bearing easily"] bodily comfort; well-being; absence of pain or distress. In psychiatry, an abnormal or exaggerated sense of well-being, particularly common in the manic state.

euphoriant (u-fo′re-ant) euphoretic.

euphoric (u-fo′rik) characterized by euphoria.

euphorigenic (u-fōr′ĭ-jen′ik) tending to produce euphoria.

euphoristic (u″fo-ris′tik) causing euphoria.

euphoropsia (u″fōr-op′se-ah) [*euphoria* + Gr. *opsis* vision] comfortable vision.

euplastic (u-plas′tik) [*eu-* + Gr. *plastikos* plastic] readily becoming organized; adapted to the formation of tissue, as in embryonic development or wound healing.

euploid (u′ploid) [*eu-* + *-ploid*] 1. having a balanced set or sets of chromosomes, in any number. 2. an individual or cell having a balanced set or sets of chromosomes, in any number.

euploidy (u-ploi′de) the state of having a balanced set or sets of chromosomes, in any number.

eupnea (ūp-ne′ah) [*eu-* + Gr. *pnein* to breathe] easy or normal respiration.

eupneic (ūp-ne′ik) pertaining to or characterized by eupnea.

eupractic (u-prak′tic) [*eu-* + Gr. *praktikos* active, able, effective] pertaining to, characterized by, or promoting eupraxia.

eupraxia (u-prak′se-ah) [Gr. "good conduct"] intactness of reproduction of coordinated movements.

eupraxic (u-prak′sik) 1. concerned in the proper performance of a function. 2. eupractic.

euprocin hydrochloride (u′pro-sin) chemical name: (8α,-9R)-10,11-dihydro-6′-(3-methylbutoxy) cinchonan-9-ol dihydrochloride; a topical anesthetic, $C_{24}H_{34}N_2O_2 \cdot 2HCl$.

Euproctis (u-prok′tis) a genus of moths. **E. chrysorrhoe′a (phaeorrhoe′a),** the brown-tail moth, which is the cause of brown-tail rash.

eupyrene (u-pi′rēn) having a normal nucleus or chromatic material; said of certain spermatozoa.

eupyrexia (u″pi-rek′se-ah) a slight fever in the early stage of an infection, regarded as an attempt on the part of the individual to combat the infection.

eupyrous (u′pi-rus) eupyrene.

Eurax (u′raks) trademark for preparations of crotamiton.

Euresol (u′rĕ-sol) trademark for a preparation of resorcinol monoacetate.

eurhythmia (u-rith′me-ah) [Gr. "harmony"] 1. harmonious relationships in body or organ development. 2. regularity of the pulse.

europium (u-ro′pe-um) a rare element, atomic number 63, atomic weight 151.96, symbol Eu.

Eurotiaceae (u-ro″she-a′se-e) a family of ascomycetous fungi of the order Eurotiales, series Plectomycetes, containing the perfect, or sexual, stages of certain species of *Aspergillus* and *Penicillium*, and also the genus *Allescheria*.

Eurotiales (u-ro″she-a′lēz) an order of ascomycetous fungi (series Plectomycetes, subclass Euascomycetidae), in which the asci are irregularly arranged within the primitive cleistothecium.

Eurotium (u-ro′she-um) [Gr. *eurōs* mold] a genus of ascomycetous fungi or molds of the family Eurotiaceae, order Eurotiales. The imperfect (sexual) stage of these fungi includes some of the aspergilli. **E. malig′num,** former name for *Aspergillus fumigatus*. **E. re′pens,** a species sometimes seen on bread and on preserved fruits, and rarely found in human pulmonary infections. Its imperfect stage is *Aspergillus repens*.

Eurotransplant (u″ro-trans′plant) an international organization for the preservation and transport of organs for use in transplantation in European nations.

eury- (u′re) [Gr. *eurys* wide] a combining form meaning wide or broad.

eurycephalic (u″re-sĕ-fal′ik) [*eury-* + Gr. *kephalē* head] having a wide head.

eurycephalous (u″re-sef′ah-lus) eurycephalic.

eurycranial (u″re-kra′ne-al) eurycephalic.

eurygnathic (u″rig-nath′ik) pertaining to or characterized by eurygnathism.

eurygnathism (u-rig′nah-thizm) [*eury-* + Gr. *gnathos* jaw] the state of having a wide jaw.

euryon (u′re-on) [Gr. *eurys* wide] the point at either end of the greatest transverse diameter of the skull.

euryopia (u″re-o′pe-ah) [*eury-* + Gr. *ōps* eye] abnormally wide opening of the eyes.

Eurypelma (u″re-pel′mah) a genus of tarantulas. **E. hent′zii,** an American tarantula.

euryphotic (u″re-fo′tik) [*eury-* + Gr. *phōs* light] able to see in a wide range of light intensity.

eurysomatic (u″re-so-mat′ik) [*eury-* + Gr. *sōma* body] having a squat, thick-set body.

eurythermic (u″re-ther′mik) [*eury-* + Gr. *thermē* heat] able to grow through a wide range of temperature; said of bacteria.

Euscorpius (u-skor′pe-us) a genus of scorpions. **E. ital′icus,** the black scorpion of Europe and North Africa.

Eusimulium (u″sĭ-mu′le-um) a genus of flies of the family Simuliidae, various species of which are common hosts of *Onchocerca volvulus,* a filarial worm parasitic in man.

eusitia (u-sit′e-ah) [*eu-* + Gr. *sitos* food] normal appetite.

eusplanchnia (u-splank′ne-ah) [Gr. *eu* well + *splanchna* viscera + *-ia*] a normal condition of the internal organs.

eusplenia (u-sple′ne-ah) normal splenic function.

Eustace Smith's murmur [*Eustace Smith*, London physician, 1835–1914] see under *murmer*.

eustachian (u-sta′ke-an) [named after Bartolommeo *Eustachio* (L. *Eustachius*), an Italian anatomist, 1524–1574] see under *canal, cartilage, tube,* and *valve*.

eustachitis (u″sta-ki′tis) inflammation of the eustachian tube.

eustachium (u-sta′ke-um) the eustachian tube (tuba auditiva [NA]).

eusthenia (u-sthen′e-ah) [*eu-* + Gr. *sthenos* strength] a condition of normal strength and activity.

eusthenuria (u″sthen-u′re-ah) [*eu* + G. *sthenos* strength + *ouron* urine + *-ia*] a normal state of the urine as regards osmolality.

Eustrongylus (u-stron′jĭ-lus) genus of nematode parasites of aquatic birds. **E. gi′gas,** Dioctophyma renale.

eusystole (u-sis′to-le) [*eu-* + *systole*] a normal state of the systole of the heart.

eusystolic (u″sis-tol′ik) pertaining to or characterized by eusystole.

Eutamias (u-tam′e-as) the western chipmunk, which harbors the plague-infected fleas, *Monopsyllus eumolpi,* and has been found infected with plague.

eutectic (u-tek′tik) [Gr. *eutēktos* easily melted or dissolved] melting readily; said of a mixture that melts at a lower temperature than any of its ingredients.

eutelegenesis (u-tel″ĕ-jen′ĕ-sis) [*eu-* + Gr. *tēle* far off + *genesis* reproduction] artificial insemination by semen of a donor selected because of special characteristics for the production of superior offspring.

eutelolecithal (u-tel″o-les′ĭ-thal) [*eu-* + *telolecithal*] having deutoplasm greatly in excess of the cell protoplasm; said of the ova of birds and many reptiles. Cf. *oligolecithal* and *telolecithal*.

euthanasia (u″thah-na′zhe-ah) [*eu-* + Gr. *thanatos* death] 1. an easy or painless death. 2. mercy killing; the deliberate ending of life of a person suffering from an incurable and painful disease.

euthenic (u-then′ik) conducive to race improvement through environment.

euthenics (u-then′iks) [Gr. *euthēnia* well-being] the science of race improvement through the regulation of environment. Cf. *eugenics*.

eutherapeutic (u-ther″ah-pu′tik) [*eu-* + *therapeutic*] having good therapeutic properties.

Eutheria (u-the′rĭ-ah) [*eu-* + Gr. *thērion* beast, animal] in some systems of classification, a subclass of the Mammalia and in others an infraclass of the subclass Theria, including all the true placental mammals, and excluding the monotremes and marsupials.

eutherian (u-the′rĭ-an) any member of the Eutheria.

euthermic (u-ther′mik) [Gr. *euthermos* very warm] characterized by the proper temperature; promoting warmth.

Euthroid (u′throid) trademark for a preparation of liothrix.

euthymism (u-thi′mizm) a normal condition of thymus activity.

Euthyneura (u″thĕ-nu′rah) a subclass of hermaphroditic mollusks (class Gastropoda) found chiefly in fresh-water or terrestrial habitats; many species are primary or intermediate hosts of various pathogens.

euthyphoria (u″the-fo′re-ah) [Gr. *euthys* straight + *pherein* to bear] normal relationship of the visual axis, without deviation when fusion is prevented.

euthyroid (u-thi′roid) having a normally functioning thyroid gland.

euthyroidism (u-thi′roid-ism) a condition of normal thyroid function.

eutocia (u-to′se-ah) [Gr. *eutokia*] normal labor, or childbirth.

Eutonyl (u′to-nil) trademark for a preparation of pargyline hydrochloride.

eutopic (u-top′ik) [*eu*- + Gr. *topos* place] situated normally; arising from the normal site or tissue. Cf. *ectopic*.

Eutriatoma (u′′tri-at′o-mah) a genus of reduviid bugs, species of which transmit Chagas' disease.

Eutrichomastix cuniculi (u′′trik-o-mas′tiks ku-nik′u-li) a parasitic flagellate protozoon of the order Polymastigida, which resembles a trichomonad; found in rabbits.

Eutrombicula (u′′trom-bik′u-lah) a subgenus of *Trombicula;* see *chigger*. **E. alfreddugé′si,** the common chigger of the United States; called also *Trombicula irritans.* **E. splen′-dens,** a troublesome species found in southeastern localities.

eutrophia (u-tro′fe-ah) [*eu*- + Gr. *trophē* nourishment + *-ia*] a state of normal (good) nutrition.

eutrophic (u-trof′ik) pertaining to, characterized by, or conducive to good nutrition.

eutrophication (u′′tro-fi-ka′shun) the accidental or deliberate promotion of excessive growth (multiplication) of an organism to the disadvantage of other organisms in the same ecosystem by oversupplying it with nutrients.

euvolia (u-vo′le-ah) normal water content or volume of a given body compartment, e.g., extracellular euvolia.

euxanthon (u-zan′thon) chemical name: 1,7-dihydroxyxanthon. A ketone, dioxydiphenylene ketone oxide, $CO(C_6H_3OH)_2O$, obtained from Indian yellow.

eV, ev electron volt.

evacuant (e-vak′u-ant) [L. *evacuans* making empty] 1. emptying; serving to clear the bowels. 2. a remedy which empties any organ; a cathartic, emetic, or diuretic.

evacuation (e-vak′′u-a′shun) [L. *evacuatio,* from *e* out + *vacuus* empty] 1. an emptying, as of the bowels. 2. a dejection or stool; material discharged from the bowels.

evacuator (e-vak′u-a-tor) an instrument for removing fluid or small particles from a body cavity or container; formerly applied to one for compelling evacuation of the bowels or bladder.

evagination (e-vaj′′ĭ-na′shun) an outpouching of a layer or part. **optic e.,** optic vesicle (vesicula ophthalmica [NA]).

evanescent (ev′′ah-nes′ent) [L. *evanescere* to vanish away] vanishing; passing away quickly; unstable; unfixed.

evaporation (e-vap′′o-ra′shun) [L. *e* out + *vaporare* to steam] conversion of a liquid or solid into vapor.

Eve's method (ēvz) [Frank Cecil *Eve,* English physician, 1871–1952] a method of artificial respiration; see under *respiration, artificial.*

eventration (e′′ven-tra′shun) [L. *eventratio* disembowelment, from *e* out + *venter* belly] 1. protrusion of the bowels from the abdomen. 2. removal of the abdominal viscera. **diaphragmatic e.,** elevation of the dome of the diaphragm, usually the result of paralysis of a phrenic nerve. **umbilical e.,** omphalocele.

Eversbusch's operation (a′värz-boosh′′ez) [Oskar *Eversbusch,* German ophthalmologist, 1853–1912] see under *operation.*

eversion (e-ver′zhun) [L. *eversio*] a turning inside out; a turning outward, as of the foot.

evert (e-vert′) [L. *e* out + *vertere* to turn] to turn inside out; to turn outward.

evertor (e-ver′tor) a muscle that turns a part outward.

Evex (e′veks) trademark for a preparation of esterified estrogens.

évidement (a-vēd-maw′) [Fr.] the operation of scooping out a cavity or diseased portion of an organ.

évideur (a-ve-dur′) [Fr.] an instrument for performing évidement.

evil (e′vil) an illness or disease. **poll e.,** an abscess behind the ears of a horse, caused by a dual infection of the supra-atlantal bursa by *Brucella* and *Actinomyces.* **quarter e.,** blackleg. **St. John's e.,** epilepsy. **St. Main's e.,** scabies. **St. Martin's e.,** alcoholism.

Evipal (ev′ĭ-pal) trademark for a preparation of hexobarbital.

eviration (e′′vi-ra′shun) [L. *e* out + *vir* man] 1. castration. 2. a form of paranoia in which the patient believes he is a woman, and assumes feminine qualities (Krafft-Ebing).

evisceration (e-vis′′er-a′shun) [L. *evisceratio; e* out + *viscus* the inside of the body] extrusion of the viscera, or internal organs; disembowelment. When used in connection with the eye, it denotes removal of the contents of the eyeball, with the sclera being left intact.

evocation (ev′′o-ka′shun) [L. *e* out + *vocare* to call] the calling forth of morphogenetic potentialities through contact with organizer material.

evocator (ev′o-ka′′ter) a chemical substance emitted by an organizer region of an embryo that evokes a specific morphogenetic response from competent embryonic tissue in contact with it.

evolution (ev′′o-lu′shun) [L. *evolutio,* from *e* out + *volvere* to roll]

1. an unrolling. 2. a process of development in which an organ or organism becomes more and more complex by the differentiation of its parts; a continuous and progressive change according to certain laws and by means of resident forces. 3. preformation. Cf. *devolution.* **bathmic e.,** evolution due to something in the organism itself independent of environment; called also *orthogenic e.* **convergent e.,** the appearance of similar forms and/or functions in two or more lines not sufficiently related phylogenetically to account for the similarity. **Denman's spontaneous e.,** a mechanism of spontaneous version in shoulder presentations in which the head rotates behind, and as the breech descends the shoulder ascends in the pelvis, the breech finally coming down and emerging. Called also *Denman's spontaneous version.* **determinate e.,** orthogenesis, def. 2. **emergent e.,** the assumption that each step in evolution produces something new and something that could not be predicted from its antecedents. **organic e.,** the origin and development of species; the theory that existing organisms are the result of descent with modification from those of past times. **orthogenic e.,** bathmic e. **saltatory e.,** evolution showing sudden changes; mutation or saltation. **spontaneous e.,** the unaided expulsion of a transversely placed fetus without the process of version or turning.

evolutive (ev′′o-lu′tiv) relating to evolution; specifically applied to a type of mental defect characterized by retardation of the evolutionary process.

evulsio (e-vul′se-o) [L., from *e* out + *vellere* to pluck] evulsion. **e. ner′vi op′tici,** the tearing out of the optic nerve from the eyeball.

evulsion (e-vul′shun) [L. *evulsio*] extraction by force; see *avulsion.*

Ewart's sign (u′arts) [William *Ewart,* English physician, 1848–1929] see under *sign.*

Ewing's tumor (sarcoma) (u′ingz) [James *Ewing,* New York pathologist, 1866–1943] see under *tumor.*

ex- (eks) [L. *ex;* Gr. *ex* out, away from] a prefix meaning away from, without, or outside; it is sometimes used to denote completely, as in *exacerbation.*

exacerbation (eg-zas′′er-ba′shun) [*ex*- + L. *acerbus* harsh] increase in the severity of a disease or any of its symptoms.

exairesis (eks-er′ĕ-sis) [Gr. "a taking out"] exeresis; surgical removal.

exaltation (eg′′zawl-ta′shun) an abnormal mental state, marked by a feeling of great importance and ecstatic spiritual elevation.

examination (eg-zam′′ĭ-na′tion) [L. *examinare*] inspection or investigation, especially as a means of diagnosing disease, qualified according to the methods employed, as physical examination, roentgen examination, cystoscopic examination, etc. **double-contrast e.,** radiologic examination of the stomach using first a high concentration of contrast medium and then (after the stomach empties) a lower concentration of contrast material. The lower concentration is sometimes used first.

exangia (eks-an′je-ah) [*ex*- + Gr. *angeion* vessel] (*obs.*) dilatation of a blood vessel.

exania (ek-sa′ne-ah) [*ex*- + L. *anus*] prolapse of the rectum.

exanimation (eg-zan′′ĭ-ma′shun) unconsciousness; coma.

exanthem (eg-zan′them) [Gr. *exanthēma*] 1. any eruptive disease or eruptive fever. 2. the eruption which characterizes an eruptive fever; see *eruption.* Called also *rash.* **Boston e.,** a rash associated with echovirus 16, without lymphadenopathy. **e. subi′tum,** exanthema subitum. **syphilitic e.,** see under *roseola.* **vesicular e.,** a viral disease of swine marked by the formation of vesicles on the snout, lips, tongue, feet, and teats. A local eruption may be produced experimentally in horses by injection into the tongue.

exanthema (eg′′zan-the′mah), pl. *exanthe′mas, exanthem′ata* [Gr. *exanthēma*] exanthem. **e. subitum,** an acute, mild viral disease of infants and young children, marked by high, continuous or remittent fever that lasts for three to four days and then falls by crisis; just before or shortly after the fever subsides, a macular or maculopapular rash starts on the trunk and spreads to other areas of the body. Called also *roseola infantum* or *infantilis,* and *sixth disease.*

exanthemata (eg′′zan-them′ah-tah) plural of *exanthema.*

exanthematous (eg′′zan-them′ah-tus) pertaining to, characterized by, or of the nature of an exanthem.

exanthrope (ek′zan-thrōp) [*ex*- + Gr. *anthrōpos* man] any source of disease not situated within the human body.

exanthropic (ek′′zan-throp′ik) of the nature of an exanthrope; not situated within the human body.

exarteritis (eks′′ar-tĕ-ri′tis) [*ex*- + *arteritis*] (*obs.*) inflammation of the outer arterial coat.

exarticulation (eks′′ar-tik-u-la′shun) [*ex*- + L. *articulus* joint] amputation at a joint; removal of a portion of a joint.

excalation (eks′′kah-la′shun) absence or exclusion of one member of a normal series, such as a vertebra.

excarnation (eks′′kar-na′shun) [*ex*- + L. *caro, carnis* flesh] removal of superfluous fleshy tissue from a preparation.

excavatio (eks″kah-va′she-o), pl. *excavatio′nes* [L., from *ex* out + *cavus* hollow] excavation: [NA] a general term for a hollowed-out space, or pouchlike cavity. **e. dis′ci** [NA], a depression in the center of the optic disk; called also *optic* or *physiological cup* and *e. papillae nervi optici.* **e. papil′lae ner′vi op′tici,** e. disci. **e. rectouteri′na** [NA], rectouterine excavation: a sac or recess formed by a fold of the peritoneum dipping down between the rectum and the uterus; called also *cavum douglasi, cul-de-sac of Douglas, pouch of Douglas, Douglas' space,* and *rectouterine, rectovaginal, uterovesical,* or *vesicouterine pouch.* **e. rectovesica′lis** [NA], rectovesical excavation: the space between the rectum and the bladder in the peritoneal cavity of the male; called also *rectovesical pouch.* **e. vesicouteri′na** [NA], vesicouterine excavation: the space between the bladder and the uterus in the peritoneal cavity; called also *uterovesical* or *vesicouterine pouch.*

excavation (eks″kah-va′shun) [L. *excavatio*] 1. the act of hollowing out. 2. a hollowed-out space, or pouchlike cavity. **atrophic e.,** the cupping of the optic disk, caused by atrophy of the optic nerve fibers. **dental e.,** removal of carious material from a tooth in preparation for filling. **glaucomatous e.,** marked cupping of the optic disk, due to abnormally high intraocular pressure. **ischiorectal e.,** fossa ischiorectalis. **e. of optic disk, physiologic e.,** excavatio papillae nervi optici. **rectoischiadic e.,** fossa ischiorectalis. **rectouterine e.,** excavatio rectouterina. **rectovesical e.,** excavatio rectovesicalis. **vesicouterine e.,** excavatio vesicouterina.

excavationes (eks″kah-va″she-o′nēz) [L.] plural of *excavatio.*

excavator (eks′kah-va″tor) a form of scoop or gouge for surgical use. **dental e.,** an instrument for removing carious material from a tooth. **spoon e.,** a dental excavator with a spoon-shaped blade at its end, for removing dental caries.

excelsin (ek-sel′sin) a crystalline globulin from the Brazil nut.

excementosis (ek-se″men-to′sis) hyperplasia of the cementum of the root of a tooth.

excerebration (ek″ser-ĕ-bra′shun) [*ex-* + L. *cerebrum* brain] the removal of the brain, chiefly that of the fetus in embryotomy.

excernent (ek-ser′nent) [L. *excernere* to sift, to separate] causing an evacuation or discharge.

excess (ek-ses′, ek′ses) the state of exceeding that which is normal, sufficient, or needed; superfluous. **antigen e.,** the presence of more than enough antigen molecules to bind all available antibody combining sites in a mixture of antigen and homologous antibody molecules. Antigen-antibody complexes formed in conditions of antigen excess have the capacity to induce immunological injury to tissues and cells and constitute part of the pathogenesis of certain immune complex diseases.

exchange (eks-chānj) 1. the substitution of one thing for another. 2. to substitute one thing for another. **plasma e.,** the removal of plasma from withdrawn blood, usually to a greater extent than in plasmapheresis, with retransfusion of the formed elements into the donor; done for removal of circulating antibodies or abnormal plasma constituents. The plasma removed is replaced by type-specific frozen plasma or albumin.

exchanger (eks-chānj′er) an apparatus by which something may be exchanged. **heat e.,** a device which is placed in the circuit of extracorporeal circulation, to induce rapid cooling and rewarming of blood.

excipient (ek-sip′e-ent) [L. *excipiens,* from *ex* out + *capere* to take] any more or less inert substance added to a prescription in order to confer a suitable consistency or form to the drug; a vehicle.

excise (ek-sīz′) to cut out or off.

excision (ek-sizh′un) [L. *excisio,* from *ex* out + *caedere* to cut] removal, as of an organ, by cutting.

excitability (ek-sīt″ah-bil′ĭ-te) readiness to respond to a stimulus; irritability.

excitable (ek-sīt′ah-b'l) [L. *excitabilis*] susceptible of stimulation; responding to a stimulus.

excitant (ek-sīt′ant) any agent that produces excitation of the vital functions, or of those of the brain.

excitation (ek″si-ta′shun) [L. *excitatio,* from *ex* out + *citare* to call] an act of irritation or stimulation or of responding to a stimulus; a condition of being excited; the addition of energy, as the excitation of a molecule by absorption of photons. **anomalous atrioventricular e.,** Wolff-Parkinson-White syndrome. **direct e.,** electrostimulation of a muscle by placing the electrode on the muscle itself. **indirect e.,** electrostimulation of a muscle by placing the electrode on its nerve.

excitatory (ek-si′tah-to″re) 1. tending to excitation or stimulation. 2. tending to disassimilation.

excitoanabolic (ek-si″to-an″ah-bol′ik) stimulating anabolism.

excitocatabolic (ek-si″to-kat″ah-bol′ik) stimulating catabolism.

excitoglandular (ek-si″to-glan′du-lar) causing glands to secrete.

excitometabolic (ek-si″to-met″ah-bol′ik) producing metabolic changes.

excitomotor (ek-si″to-mo′tor) 1. tending to produce motion or motor function. 2. an agent that induces motion or functional activity.

excitomotory (ek-si″to-mo′to-re) excitomotor.

excitomuscular (ek-si″to-mus′ku-lar) stimulating muscular activity.

excitonutrient (ek-si″to-nu′tre-ent) exciting or stimulating nutrition.

excitor (ek-si′tor) a nerve, the stimulation of which excites greater action in the part which it supplies.

excitosecretory (ek-si″to-se-kre′to-re) producing increased secretion.

excitovascular (ek-si″to-vas′ku-lar) causing vascular changes.

exclave (eks′klāv) [*ex-* + L. *clavis* key, by analogy with *enclave*] a detached part of an organ, as of the pancreas or of some other gland.

exclusion (eks-kloo′zhun) [L. *exclusio,* from *ex* out + *claudere* to shut] elimination, rejection, or extrusion. Specifically, an operation in which a portion of an organ is separated from the remainder but is not removed from the body.

excochleation (eks-kok″le-a′shun) [*ex-* + L. *cochlea* spoon] the operation of curetting or scooping out a cavity.

exconjugant (eks-kon′ju-gahnt) [L. *ex* + *conjugare* to unite] a protozoon that has just undergone conjugation.

excoriation (eks-ko″re-a′shun) [L. *excoriare* to flay, from *ex* out + *corium* skin] any superficial loss of substance, such as that produced on the skin by scratching. **neurotic e.,** a self-induced skin lesion, inflicted by the fingernails or other physical means.

excrement (eks′krĕ-ment) [L. *excrementum,* from *ex* out + *cernere* to sift, to separate] fecal matter; matter cast out as waste from the body; called also *ordure.*

excrementitious (eks″krĕ-men-tish′us) pertaining to or of the nature of excrement; fecal.

excrescence (eks-kres′ens) [*ex-* + L. *crescere* to grow] any abnormal outgrowth; a projection of morbid origin. **cauliflower e.** (*obs.*), condyloma acuminatum. **fungating e., fungous e.,** a fungous growth in the umbilicus after separation of the umbilical cord; granuloma of the umbilicus. **Lambl's e's,** small papillary projections on the cardiac valves seen post mortem on many adult hearts.

excrescent (eks-kres′ent) resembling or of the nature of an excrescence.

excreta (eks-kre′tah) [L., pl.] excretion products; waste materials excreted by the body.

excrete (eks-krēt′) [L. *excernere*] to throw off or eliminate, as waste matter, by a normal discharge.

excretin (eks′kre-tin) a crystalline compound, $C_{20}H_{36}O$, derivable from human feces.

excretion (eks-kre′shun) [L. *excretio*] 1. the act, process, or function of excreting. 2. material which is excreted. Cf. *elimination.* **pseudouridine e.,** increased excretion of pseudouridine in the urine of gouty patients, the significance of which remains to be established; a greater turnover of some forms of RNA has been suggested, possibly adding to the hyperuricemia of gout.

excretory (eks′kre-to-re) of, pertaining to, or subserving excretion.

excurrent (eks-kur′ent) excretory; efferent.

excursion (eks-kur′zhun) [L. *excursio,* from *ex* out + *currere* to run] movements occurring from a normal, or rest, position of a movable part in performance of a function, as those of the mandible to attain functional contact between the cusps of the mandibular and maxillary teeth in mastication, or of the chest wall in respiration. **lateral e.,** sideward movement of the mandible between the position of closure and that in which the tips of the cusps of opposing teeth are in vertical proximity. **protrusive e.,** movement of the mandible between the position of closure and that in which the incisal edges of the anterior teeth are in vertical approximation. **retrusive e.,** the slight backward and return movement of the mandible between the position of closure and one slightly posterior, more often present with mandibular overclosure.

excursive (eks-kur′sive) pertaining to or characterized by excursion.

excyclophoria (ek″si-klo-fo′re-ah) cyclophoria in which the upper pole of the vertical axis of the eye deviates away from the midline of the face and toward the temple; called also *positive* (or *plus*) *cyclophoria.* Cf. *incyclophoria.*

excyclotropia (ek″si-klo-tro′pe-ah) cyclotropia in which the upper pole of the vertical axis of the eye deviates away from the midline of the face, and toward the temple; called also *positive* (or *plus*) *cyclotropia.*

excystation (ek″sis-ta′shun) escape from a cyst or envelope; especially a stage in the life cycle of parasites occurring after the cystic form has been swallowed by the host.

exelcin (ek-sel′sin) a substance extracted from Brazil nut.

exelcymosis (ek″sel-si-mo′sis) [*ex-* + Gr. *helkyein* to draw] extraction, as of a tooth.

exemia (ek-se′me-ah) [*ex-* + Gr. *haima* blood + *-ia*] loss of fluid from the blood vessels, the red cells being left behind. Cf. *hemoconcentration.*

exencephalia (eks″en-sĕ-fa′le-ah) exencephaly.

exencephalon (eks″en-sef′ah-lon) exencephalus.

exencephalous (eks″en-sef′ah-lus) characterized by exencephaly.

exencephalus (eks″en-sef′ah-lus) [*ex-* + Gr. *enkephalos* brain] a monster exhibiting exencephaly.

exencephaly (eks″en-sef′ah-le) [*ex-* + Gr. *enkephalos* brain] a developmental anomaly characterized by an imperfect cranium, the brain lying outside of the skull.

exenteration (eks-en″ter-a′shun) [*ex-* + Gr. *enteron* bowel] surgical removal of the inner organs; commonly used to indicate radical excision of the contents of a body cavity, as of the pelvis. Used in connection with the eye, it denotes removal of the entire contents of the orbit. **pelvic e.,** excision of the organs and adjacent structures of the pelvis. **pelvic e., anterior,** excision en masse of the bladder, lower ureters, vagina, adnexa, pelvic lymph nodes, and pelvic peritoneum, with implantation of the ureters into the intact pelvic colon. **pelvic e., posterior,** excision en masse of the pelvic colon, uterus, vagina, and adnexa, with or without pelvic lymph node excision, the lower urinary tract being undisturbed. **pelvic e., total,** excision en masse of the bladder, lower ureters, vagina, uterus, adnexa, and the pelvic and lower sigmoid colon, with excision of the pelvic lymph nodes and removal of all the pelvic peritoneum.

exenterative (eks-en′ter-ah-tiv) pertaining to or requiring exenteration, as exenterative surgery.

exenteritis (eks-en″ter-i′tis) inflammation of the peritoneal covering of the intestine; visceral peritonitis.

exercise (ek′ser-sīz) the performance of physical exertion for improvement of health or the correction of physical deformity. **active e.,** motion imparted to a part by voluntary contraction and relaxation of the muscles controlling the part. **active assisted e.,** motion imparted to a part of the body by voluntary contraction of muscles controlling the part, assisted by a therapist or by some other means. **active resistive e.,** that performed voluntarily by the patient against resistance. **corrective e.,** the scientific use of bodily movement to maintain or restore normal function in diseased or injured tissues. **free e.,** active exercise in which no aid is derived from external forces. **isometric e.,** active exercise performed against stable resistance, without change in the length of the muscle. **isotonic e.,** active exercise without appreciable change in the force of muscular contraction, with shortening of the muscle. **muscle-setting e.,** voluntary contraction and relaxation of skeletal muscles without movement of the associated part of the body; called also *static e.* **passive e.,** motion imparted to a segment of the body by another individual, machine, or other outside force, or produced by voluntary effort of another segment of the patient's own body. **static e.,** muscle-setting e. **therapeutic e.,** corrective e. **underwater e.,** exercise performed in a pool or a large tub. Cf. *Hubbard tank.*

exeresis (eks-er′ĕ-sis) [Gr. *exairesis* a taking out] surgical removal or excision.

exergic (ek-ser′jik) [*ex-* + Gr. *ergon* work] giving out work; a term applied to chemical reactions which occur with a decrease in free energy. Cf. *endergic.*

exergonic (ek″ser-gon′ik) [*ex(o)-* + Gr. *ergon* work] characterized or accompanied by the release of energy; said of chemical reactions that release free energy, so that the products have a lower free energy than the reactants. Opposed to *endergonic.*

exesion (eg-ze′zhun) [L. *exedere* to eat out] the gradual destruction of superficial parts of a tissue.

exfetation (eks″fe-ta′shun) [*ex-* + L. *fetus*] ectopic or extrauterine pregnancy.

exflagellation (eks″flaj-ĕ-la′shun) [*ex-* + L. *flagellum*] the protrusion or formation of flagelliform gametes (male gametes) from a microgametocyte in malaria and in some related sporozoons.

exfoliatio (eks″fo-le-a′she-o) [L., from *ex-* + *folium* leaf] exfoliation. **e. area′ta lin′guae,** geographic tongue.

exfoliation (eks″fo-le-a′shun) [L. *exfoliatio*] a falling off in scales or layers. **lamellar e. of the newborn,** a rare congenital disorder transmitted as an autosomal recessive trait, in which the infant (collodion baby) is born completely covered with a collodion or parchment-like membrane that peels off within twenty-four hours, after which there may be complete healing, or the scales may re-form and the process repeated. In the more severe form, the infant (harlequin fetus) is completely covered with thick, horny, armor-like scales, and is usually stillborn or dies shortly after birth. Some consider the disorder to be a form of lamellar ichthyosis (q.v.). Called also *ichthyosis congenita, ichthyosis fetalis, lamellar desquamation of the newborn,* and *lamellar ichthyosis of the newborn.*

exfoliative (eks-fo′le-a″tiv) characterized by exfoliation.

exhalation (eks″hah-la′shun) [L. *exhalatio,* from *ex* out + *halare* to breathe] 1. the giving off of watery or other vapor, or of an

effluvium. 2. a vapor or other substance exhaled or given off. 3. the act of breathing out.

exhale (eks-hāl′) [*ex-* + L. *halare* to breathe] 1. to expel from the lungs by breathing. 2. to give off a watery or other vapor.

exhaustion (eg-zawst′yun) [*ex-* + L. *haurire* to drain] 1. privation of energy with consequent inability to respond to stimuli; lassitude. 2. withdrawal. 3. condition of emptiness caused by withdrawal. 4. emptying by a process of withdrawal. **heat e.,** an effect of excessive exposure to heat occurring commonly among workers in furnace rooms, foundries, etc., although it may occur from exposure to the sun's heat. It is marked by subnormal temperature, with dizziness, headache, nausea, and sometimes delirium and/or collapse. Distinguished from heat stroke, in which the body temperature may be dangerously elevated. Called also *heat prostration.* Cf. *sunstroke.* **heat e., anhidrotic, heat e., type II,** tropical anhidrotic asthenia. **nervous e.,** depression of vital functions due to excessive demands upon the nervous energy; neurasthenia.

Exhib. abbreviation for L. *exhibea′tur,* let it be given.

exhibition (ek″sĭ-bish′un) administration of a drug.

exhibitionism (ek″sĭ-bish′ŭ-nizm″) an abnormal tendency to display one's body or parts for the purpose, conscious or unconscious, of attracting sexual interest; it is most commonly seen in males and when severe leads to exposure of the genitals, sometimes accompanied by sexual gratification.

exhibitionist (ek″sĭ-bish′ŭ-nist) an individual who is addicted to exhibitionism.

exhilarant (eg-zil′ar-ant) [L. *exhilarare* to gladden] (*obs.*) 1. causing elevation or gladness. 2. an enlivening or elating agent.

exhumation (eks″hu-ma′shun) [*ex-* + L. *humus* earth] disinterment; removal of the dead body from the earth after burial.

exitus (ek′sĭ-tus) pl. *exitus* [L. "a going out"] 1. death. 2. an exit or outlet. **e. pel′vis,** apertura pelvis inferior.

Exna (eks′nah) trademark for a preparation of benzthiazide.

Exner's plexus (eks′nerz) [Siegmund *Exner,* Austrian physiologist, 1846–1926] see under *plexus.*

exo- (ek′so) [Gr. *exō* outside] a prefix meaning outside, or outward.

exoantigen (ek″so-an′te-jen) ectoantigen.

exobiology (ek″so-bi-ol′o-je) the science concerned with the study of life on planets other than the earth.

exocardia (ek″so-kar′de-ah) ectocardia.

exocardial (ek″so-kar′de-al) situated, occurring, or developed outside the heart.

exocarp (ek′so-karp) the outer layer of the pericarp of a flower.

exocataphoria (ek″so-kat″ah-fo′re-ah) [*exo-* + *cataphoria*] the condition in which the visual axis turns downward and outward.

exocele (ek′so-sēl) extraembryonic coelom.

exocervix (ek″so-ser′viks) ectocervix.

exochorion (ek″so-ko′re-on) that part of the chorion which is derived from the ectoderm, as in those species in which extraembryonic membranes form by folding.

exocoelom (ek″so-se′lom) [*exo-* + *coelom*] extraembryonic coelom.

exocoeloma (ek″so-se-lo′mah) extraembryonic coelom.

exocolitis (ek″so-ko-li′tis) [*exo-* + *colitis*] inflammation of the outer coat of the colon.

exocrine (ek′so-krin) [*exo-* + Gr. *krinein* to separate] 1. secreting outwardly via a duct; the opposite of endocrine. 2. denoting such a gland or its secretion. See also under *gland.*

exocrinology (ek″so-krĭ-nol′o-je) the study of substances secreted externally by individual organisms which effect integration of a group of organisms.

exocrinosity (ek″so-krĭ-nos′ĭ-te) the quality or state of secreting externally.

exocuticle (ek″so-ku′tĭ-kl) [*exo-* + L. *cuticula*] the outer layer of the procuticle of certain crustaceans and arthropods, which contains cuticulin, chitin, and phenolic substances that are oxidized to produce the dark pigment of the cuticle.

exocyclic (ek-so-si′klik) a term applied to cyclic chemical compounds having their double bond in the side chain.

exocytosis (eks″o-si-to′sis) 1. the discharge from a cell of particles that are too large to diffuse through the wall; the opposite of endocytosis. 2. the aggregation of migrating leukocytes in the epidermis as part of the inflammatory response.

exodeviation (ek″so-de″ve-a′shun) a turning outward; in ophthalmology, exotropia.

exodic (ek-sod′ik) [*ex-* + Gr. *hodos* way] centrifugal or efferent.

exodontia (ek″so-don′she-ah) exodontics.

exodontics (ek″so-don′tiks) that branch of dentistry dealing with extraction of the teeth.

exodontist (ek″so-don′tist) a dentist who practices exodontics.

exoenzyme (ek″so-en′zīm) an extracellular enzyme; an enzyme that acts outside of the cells in which it originates.

exoergic (ek″so-er′jik) characterized by or accompanied by loss of free energy; releasing energy, as in a chemical reaction during and by which energy is released; energy releasing. Cf. *endoergic* and *endothermic.*

exoerythrocytic (ek″so-ĕ-rith″ro-si′tik) outside the erythrocyte, a term applied to stages in the development of malarial parasites which takes place in tissue cells instead of in erythrocytes.

exogamy (ek-sog′ah-me) [*exo-* + Gr. *gamos* marriage] 1. protozoan fertilization by the union of elements that are not derived from the same cell. Cf. *autogamy* (def. 1) and *endogamy* (def. 1). 2. marriage outside a particular group.

exogastric (ek″so-gas′trik) pertaining to the external surface of the stomach.

exogastritis (ek″so-gas-tri′tis) inflammation of the external coat of the stomach.

exogastrula (ek″so-gas′troo-lah) [*exo-* + *gastrula*] a gastrula in which invagination is hindered and the mesentoderm bulges outward.

exogastrulation (eks″o-gas″troo-la′shun) the evagination to the exterior (or turning inside out) of the gut due to an interference with the normal processes of gastrulation, which can occur if the morula is cut transversely below the equator. It is usually followed by a migration of mesenchyme cells into the interior.

exogenetic (ek″so-jĕ-net′ik) [*exo-* + Gr. *gennan* to produce] exogenous.

exogenic (ek″so-jen′ik) exogenous.

exogenote (eks″o-je′nōt) in bacterial genetics, the extra piece of genetic information introduced by transduction into the recipient cell. Cf. *endogenote.*

exogenous (eks-oj′ĕ-nus) [*exo-* + Gr. *gennan* to produce] growing by additions to the outside; developed or originating outside the organism, as exogenous disease.

exognathia (ek″sog-na′the-ah) prognathism.

exognathion (ek″sog-na′the-on) [*exo-* + Gr. *gnathos* jaw] the maxilla exclusive of the premaxilla.

exohemophylaxis (ek″so-he″mo-fi-lak′sis) [*exo-* + Gr. *haima* blood + *phylaxis* a guarding] a procedure consisting of mixing arsphenamine with some of the patient's blood and then injecting the mixture, the object being to reduce the sensitiveness of the blood.

exohysteropexy (ek″so-his′ter-o-pek″se) [*exo-* + Gr. *hystera* uterus + *pēxis* fixation] (*obs.*) uterine fixation by implanting the fundus in the abdominal wall.

exolever (ek″so-le′ver) a lever-like instrument for extracting tooth roots.

exometer (eks-om′ĕ-ter) an apparatus for measuring the fluorescent quality of the roentgen ray in comparison with units of candle power.

exomphalos (eks-om′fah-los) [*ex-* + Gr. *omphalos* navel] 1. hernia of the abdominal viscera into the umbilical cord. 2. congenital umbilical hernia.

exomysium (eks″o-mis′e-um) perimysium.

exonuclease (ek″so-nu′kle-ās) a nuclease that cleaves single mononucleotides from the end of a polynucleotide chain.

exopathic (ek″so-path′ik) of the nature of an exopathy; originating outside the body.

exopathy (eks-op′ah-the) [*exo-* + Gr. *pathos* disease] a disease originating in some cause lying outside the organism; exogenous disease.

exopeptidase (ek″so-pep′tĭ-dās) a proteolytic enzyme the action of which is limited to terminal peptide linkages.

exophoria (ek-so-fo′re-ah) [*exo-* + Gr. *phorein* to bear] a form of heterophoria in which there is deviation of the visual axis of one eye away from that of the other eye in the absence of visual fusional stimuli. Called also *exodeviation.*

exophoric (ek″so-for′ik) pertaining to or characterized by exophoria.

exophthalmic (ek″sof-thal′mik) of or pertaining to or characterized by exophthalmos.

exophthalmogenic (ek″sof-thal″mo-jen′ik) causing or producing exophthalmos.

exophthalmometer (ek″sof-thal-mom′ĕ-ter) an instrument for measuring the amount of exophthalmos.

exophthalmometric (ek″sof-thal″mo-met′rik) pertaining to exophthalmometry.

exophthalmometry (ek″sof-thal-mom′ĕ-tre) measurement of the extent of protrusion of the eyeball in exophthalmos.

exophthalmos (ek″sof-thal′mos) [*ex-* + Gr. *ophthalmos* eye] abnormal protrusion of the eyeball. **endocrine e.,** exophthalmos associated with disorder of an endocrine gland, commonly thyrotoxicosis. **malignant e.,** severe exophthalmos in which there is marked edema and infiltration of the orbital tissues and extraocular muscles, proptosis, and stare. It was formerly attributed to overactivity of thyrotropin, and so is also called *thyrotropic e.* **pulsating e.,** exophthalmos with pulsation and bruit, often due to aneurysm pushing the eye forward. **thyrotoxic**

e., a mild form due to thyrotoxicosis. **thyrotropic e.,** malignant e.

exophthalmus (ek″sof-thal′mus) exophthalmos.

exophytic (ek″so-fit′ik) [*exo-* + Gr. *phyein* to grow] growing outward; in oncology, proliferating on the exterior or surface epithelium of an organ or other structure, in which the growth originated.

exoplasm (ek′so-plazm) [*exo-* + Gr. *plasma* something formed] plasma membrane.

exopneumopexy (ek″so-nu′mo-pek″se) [*exo-* + Gr. *pneumōn* lung + *pēxis* fixation] (*obs.*) the operation of exteriorization and fixation of the lung.

exorbitism (ek-sor′bĭ-tizm) exophthalmos.

exormia (ek-sor′me-ah) [*ex-* + Gr. *hormē* rush] (*obs.*) any papular disease of the skin.

exosepsis (ek″so-sep′sis) [*ex-* + Gr. *sēpsis* decay] septic poisoning which does not originate within the organism.

exoserosis (ek″so-se-ro′sis) an oozing of serum or exudate, as in moist skin diseases and edema.

exoskeleton (ek″so-skel′ĕ-ton) [*exo-* + *skeleton*] a hard structure developed on the outside of the body, as the shell of a crustacean. In vertebrates the term is applied to structures produced by the epidermis, as hair, nails, hoofs, teeth, etc.

exosmose (ek′sos-mōs) to diffuse from within outward.

exosmosis (ek″sos-mo′sis) [*ex-* + Gr. *ōsmos* impulsion] diffusion or osmosis from within outward; movement outward through a diaphragm or through vessel walls. Cf. *endosmosis.*

exosplenopexy (ek″so-sple′no-pek″se) [*exo-* + Gr. *splēn* spleen + *pēxis* fixation] suture of the spleen to the outside of the body or within the layers of the wound.

exospore (ek′so-spōr) conidium.

exosporium (ek″so-spo′re-um) the external layer of the envelope of a spore.

exostosectomy (ek-sos″to-sek′to-me) excision of an exostosis.

exostosis (ek″sos-to′sis) [*ex-* + Gr. *osteon* bone] a benign bony growth projecting outward from the surface of a bone, characteristically capped by cartilage. **e. bursa′ta,** an exostosis from the epiphyseal portion of a bone, consisting of bone and cartilaginous tissue covered by a connective-tissue capsule. **e. cartilagin′ea,** a variety of osteoma consisting of a layer of cartilage developing beneath the periosteum of a bone. **dental e.,** cementosis. **hereditary multiple exostoses,** multiple e. **ivory e.,** a bony growth of great density. **multiple exostoses,** a hereditary disorder characterized by exostoses near the extremities of diaphyses of long bones, which may be cartilaginous or osteocartilaginous growths. Transmitted as an autosomal dominant, it is generally benign, although sarcomatous changes have occurred. Called also *multiple cartilaginous exostoses.* **multiple cartilaginous exostoses,** multiple exostoses. **osteocartilaginous e.,** osteochondroma.

exostotic (ek″sos-tot′ik) pertaining to or of the nature of exostosis.

exoteric (ek″so-ter′ik) [Gr. *exōterikos* outer] generated or developed outside the organism; exogenous.

exothelioma (ek″so-the″le-o′mah) meningioma.

exothermal (ek″so-ther′mal) exothermic.

exothermic (ek″so-ther′mik) [*exo-* + Gr. *thermē* heat] characterized or accompanied by the evolution of heat, as in a chemical reaction during and by which heat is released; liberating heat or energy from its potential forms. Cf. *endothermic* and *exoergic.*

exothymopexy (ek″so-thi′mo-pek″se) [*exo-* + *thymus* + Gr. *pēxis* fixation] enucleation of the thymus gland from its fossa and suture to the sternum.

exothyroidopexy (ek″so-thi-roi′do-pek″se) exothyropexy.

exothyropexia (ek″so-thi″ro-pek′se-ah) exothyropexy.

exothyropexy (ek″so-thi′ro-pek-se) [*exo-* + *thyroid* + Gr. *pēxis* fixation] (*obs.*) the operation of drawing out the enlarged thyroid gland through an incision and letting it shrivel on the outside.

exotic (eg-zot′ik) of foreign origin; not native.

exotoxic (ek″so-tok′sik) [*exo-* + *toxic*] pertaining to or produced by an exotoxin.

exotoxin (ek″so-tok′sin) [*exo-* + *toxin*] a toxic substance formed by bacteria that is found outside the bacterial cell, or free in the culture medium. Exotoxins are heat-labile, and protein in nature. They are detoxified with retention of antigenicity by treatment with formaldehyde (formol toxoid), and are the most poisonous substances known to man; the LD_{50} of crystalline botulinum type A toxin for the mouse is 4.5×10^{-9} mg.

exotropia (ek″so-tro′pe-ah) [*exo-* + Gr. *tropos* a turning + *-ia*] strabismus in which there is permanent deviation of the visual axis of one eye away from that of the other, resulting in diplopia; called also *divergent* or *external strabismus,* and *walleye.* **intermittent e.,** a condition alternating between phoria and tropia, with a tendency to shift to exotropia.

exotropic (ek″so-tro′pik) 1. turning outward. 2. pertaining to or characterized by exotropia.

expander (ek-span'der) [L. *expandere* to spread out] extender. **plasma volume e.,** artificial plasma extender.

expansion (ek-span'shun) [L. *expandere* to spread out] 1. the process or state of being increased in extent, surface, or bulk. 2. a region or area of increased bulk or surface. **e. of the arch,** widening of the dental arch in orthodontics. **clonal e.,** an immunological response in which lymphocytes stimulated by antigen proliferate and amplify the population of relevant cells. **cubical e.,** increase in volume by an increase in all dimensions. **hygroscopic e.,** an increase in dimensions of a body or substance as a result of absorption of moisture. **setting e.,** the increase in dimensions of a material, such as plaster of Paris, which occurs concurrently with its hardening. **thermal e.,** an increase in dimensions of a body or substance as a result of an increase in its temperature. **wax e.,** increase in the dimensions of a wax pattern for a dental restoration to compensate for shrinkage of the gold during the casting process.

expansiveness (ek-span'siv-nes) behavior marked by euphoria, loquacity, and grandiosity.

expectancy (ek-spek'tan-se) the probability of occurrence of a specific event. **life e.,** the number of years, based on statistical averages, that a given person of a specific age or class may reasonably expect to continue living.

expectation (ek"spek-ta'shun) [L. *expectare,* from *ex* out + *spectare* to look at] that which may be anticipated, or looked forward to.

expectorant (ek-spek'to-rant) [*ex-* + L. *pectus* breast] 1. promoting the ejection, by spitting, of mucus or other fluids from the lungs and trachea. 2. an agent that promotes the ejection of mucus or exudate from the lungs, bronchi, and trachea; sometimes extended to all remedies that quiet cough (antitussives). **liquefying e.,** an expectorant that promotes the ejection of mucus from the respiratory tract by decreasing its viscosity. **stimulant e.,** an expectorant that stimulates secretion of mucus by the respiratory tract mucosa. **Stokes's e.,** a preparation of ammonium carbonate, fluidextracts of senna and of squill, and camphorated tincture of opium in syrup of tolu.

expectoration (ek-spek"to-ra'shun) 1. the act of coughing up and spitting out materials from the lungs, bronchi, and trachea. 2. sputum.

experiment (ek-sper'ĭ-ment) [L. *experimentum* "proof from experience"] a procedure done in order to discover or to demonstrate some fact or general truth. **bulbocapnine e.,** the experimental injection of the alkaloid bulbocapnine into animals, which produces in them the motor phenomena typical of catatonia. **check e.,** crucial e. **control e.,** an experiment that is made under standard conditions, to test the correctness of other observations; see also *control.* **crucial e.,** an experiment so designed and so prepared for by previous work that it will definitely settle some point. **Cyon's e.,** the application of a stimulus to an intact anterior spinal nerve root, which induces a stronger contraction of muscle than the same stimulus to the peripheral end of a divided nerve root. **defect e.,** observation of an embryo, after destruction of a region or part, to ascertain the effect on development. **Goltz's e.,** the striking of a frog on the abdomen, which produces stoppage of the heart's action. **Küss's e.,** injection of a solution of opium or belladonna into the bladder, which produces no symptoms of poisoning and thus proves the impermeability of the bladder epithelium to these substances. **Mariotte's e.,** (to demonstrate the blind spot of the eye), the eye is fixed on the center of a cross marked on a card on which is also marked a large spot; the card is moved to or from the face, and at a certain distance the image of the spot will disappear. **Müller's e.,** the converse of Valsalva's maneuver, i.e., making a forced inspiratory effort with the glottis closed. **Nussbaum's e.,** ligation of the renal arteries of an animal in order to isolate the glomeruli of the kidneys from the circulation. **O'Beirne's e.,** injecting air or water into a loop of intestine passed through a hole in a sheet of paper to demonstrate the causation of strangulated hernia. **Scheiner's e.,** the experiment of looking at an object through two pin holes close together in a card: if the object is in focus, only one image is observed; if it is not, two or more images are seen. **Stensen's e.,** the experiment of cutting off the blood supply from the lumbar region of the spinal cord of an animal by compressing the abdominal aorta; it produces paralysis of the posterior parts of the body. **Toynbee's e.,** the experiment of partially exhausting the air in the tympanic cavity by swallowing while the nose and mouth are closed. **Valsalva's e.,** see under *maneuver.*

expirate (eks'pĭ-rāt) expired gas (or air); the gas expired in one expiration is called *single expirate.*

expiration (eks"pĭ-ra'shun) [*ex-* + L. *spirare* to breathe] 1. the act of breathing out, or expelling air from the lungs. 2. termination, or death.

expiratory (eks-pi'rah-to"re) subserving or pertaining to expiration.

expire (ek-spīr') 1. to breathe out. 2. to die, or terminate.

expirium (eks-pi're-um) (*obs.*) an expiration.

expiscation (eks"pis-ka'shun) (*obs.*) the long-continued study of symptoms for diagnostic purposes.

explant 1. (eks-plant') to take from the body and place in an artificial medium for growth. 2. (eks'plant) tissue taken from its original site and transferred to an artificial medium for growth.

explode (eks-plōd') [L. *explodere,* from *ex* out + *plaudere* to clap the hands] 1. to undergo sudden and violent decomposition or combustion. 2. to burst; to spread rapidly, as an epidemic.

exploration (eks"plo-ra'shun) [L. *exploratio,* from *ex* out + *plorare* to cry out] investigation or examination for diagnostic purposes.

exploratory (eks-plo'rah-to"re) [L. *exploratorius*] pertaining to exploration or investigation.

explorer (eks-plor'er) an instrument for use in exploration, particularly for foreign bodies.

explosion (eks-plo'zhun) [L. *explosio*] 1. the act of exploding. 2. a sudden and violent outbreak, as of emotion. 3. the discharge of a neural cell.

explosive (eks-plo'siv) characterized by explosions, or by sudden and violent outbreaks.

exponent (eks'po-nent) a symbol placed above and at the right of another symbol to indicate the power to which the latter is to be raised, as, x^2.

exposure (eks-po'zhur) 1. the act of laying open, as surgical exposure. 2. the condition of being subjected to something, as to infectious agents, extremes of weather or radiation, which may have a harmful effect. 3. in radiology, a measure of the amount of ionizing radiation at the surface of the irradiated object, e.g., the body.

expressate (eks-pres'āt) the material forced out by expression.

expression (eks-presh'un) [L. *expressio*] 1. the aspect or appearance of the face as determined by the physical or emotional state. 2. the act of squeezing or evacuating by pressure; a term used in pharmacy, surgery, and obstetrics. **early e.,** in obstetrics, manipulation of the uterus so as to exert pressure on the placenta lying in the vagina. **Kristeller e.,** see under *method.*

expressivity (eks"pres-siv'ĭ-te) [L. *expressus*] the extent to which a heritable trait is manifested by an individual carrying the principal gene or genes that determine it.

expulsive (ek-spul'siv) [*ex-* + L. *pellere* to drive] driving or forcing out; tending to expel.

exsanguinate (eks-sang'gwĭ-nāt) [*ex-* + L. *sanguis* blood] 1. to deprive of blood. 2. bloodless; anemic.

exsanguination (eks-sang"wĭ-na'shun) extensive loss of blood due to internal or external hemorrhage.

exsanguine (eks-sang'win) bloodless.

exsanguinotransfusion (eks-sang"gwĭ-no-trans-fu'zhun) exchange transfusion.

exsect (ek-sekt') to excise; to cut out.

exsection (ek-sek'shun) excision.

exsector (ek-sek'tor) a cutting instrument for use in performing exsections (excisions).

exsiccant (ek-sik'ant) desiccant.

exsiccate (ek'sĭ-kāt) [L. *exsiccare,* from *ex* out + *siccus* dry] desiccate.

exsiccation (ek"sĭ-ka'shun) the act of drying; in chemistry, the deprival of a crystalline substance of its water of crystallization.

exsomatize (ek-so'mah-tīz) [*ex-* + Gr. *sōma* body] to remove from the body.

exsorption (ek-sorp'shun) the movement of substances out of cells, especially the movement of substances out of the blood, through the intestinal epithelial cells, and into the intestinal lumen.

exstrophy (ek'stro-fe) [*ex-* + Gr. *strephein* to turn oneself] the congenital eversion or turning inside out of an organ, as the bladder. **e. of the bladder,** a developmental anomaly marked by absence of a portion of the lower abdominal wall and the anterior vesical (urinary bladder) wall, with eversion of the posterior vesical wall through the deficit and with an open pubic arch and widely separated ischia connected by a fibrous band. Called also *ectopia vesicae.* **e. of cloaca, cloacal e.,** a developmental anomaly in which two segments of bladder (hemibladders) are separated by an area of intestine with a mucosal surface, which appears as a large red tumor in the midline of the lower abdomen. Called also *ectopia cloacae.*

exsufflation (ek"suf-fla'shun) [*ex-* + L. *sufflatio* a blowing up] the act of exhausting the air content of a cavity by artificial or mechanical means, especially such action upon the lungs by means of an exsufflator.

exsufflator (ek"suf-fla'tor) an apparatus which, by the sudden production of negative pressure, can reproduce in the bronchial tree the effects of a natural, vigorous cough.

ext. extract.

extender (ek-sten'der) [*ex-* + L. *tendere* to stretch] something which enlarges or prolongs. **artificial plasma e.,** a substance which can be transfused, to maintain fluid volume of the blood in event of great necessity, supplemental to the use of whole blood and plasma.

extension (ek-sten′shun) [L. *extensio*] 1. the movement by which the two ends of any jointed part are drawn away from each other. 2. a movement which brings the members of a limb into or toward a straight condition. **Bardenheuer's e.,** extension for fractured limbs with longitudinal, transverse, and rotary pulls, designed to produce extension in all the directions in which the muscles which cause the displacement act. **Buck's e.,** the extension of a fractured leg by weights, the foot of the bed being raised so that the body makes counterextension. **Codivilla's e.,** extension of a fractured limb in which the attachment to the bone is by means of calipers or a nail passed through the lower end of the bone. **nail e.,** extension exerted on the distal fragment of a fractured bone by means of a nail or pin (Steinmann pin) driven into the fragment. **e. per contigui′tatem,** the spreading of a morbid process through one tissue or part into one adjacent to it. **e. per continui′tatem,** the spreading of a morbid process throughout a single tissue or part. **e. per sal′tam,** the spreading of a morbid condition from one part to a part or tissue distant from it, with normal tissues intervening; metastasis. **ridge e.,** an intraoral surgical operation for deepening the labial, buccal, and/or lingual sulci so as to increase the relative intraoral height of the alveolar ridge to facilitate denture retention. **Steinmann's e.,** see *nail e.*

extensometer (eks″ten-som′ĕ-ter) [L. *extensus* extension + Gr. *metron* measure] an instrument for measuring distortion of specimens under test.

extensor (eks-ten′sor) [L.] [NA] a general term for any muscle that extends a joint.

exterior (eks-te′re-or) [L.] situated on or near the outside; outer.

exteriorize (eks-te′re-or-īz) 1. to form a correct mental reference of the image of an object seen. 2. in psychiatry, to turn one's interest outward. 3. to transpose an internal organ to the exterior of the body.

extern (eks′tern) a medical student or graduate in medicine who assists in the care of patients in a hospital but does not reside in the hospital.

external (eks-ter′nal) [L. *externus* outside] situated or occurring on the outside; many anatomical structures formerly called external are now more correctly termed lateral.

externalia (eks″ter-na′le-ah) the external genitals.

externalize (eks-ter′nah-līz) to direct outwardly an internal conflict.

externe (eks′tern) extern.

externus (eks-ter′nus) external; [NA] a term denoting a structure farther from the center of a part or cavity.

exteroceptive (eks″ter-o-sep′tiv) Sherrington's term for the external surface field of distribution of receptor organs; see *interoceptive, proprioceptive,* and *receptor* (def. 3).

exteroceptor (eks″ter-o-sep′tor) a sensory nerve terminal which is stimulated by the immediate external environment, such as those in the skin and mucous membranes; cf. *interoceptor, proprioceptor,* and *receptor* (def. 3).

exterofection (eks″ter-o-fek′shun) the response of the body made to changes in external environment, effected by the cerebrospinal system.

exterofective (eks″ter-o-fek′tiv) responding to external stimuli; a term applied by Cannon to the cerebrospinal nervous system.

exterogestate (eks″ter-o-jes′tāt) 1. developing outside the uterus, but still requiring complete care to meet all physical needs. 2. an infant during the period of exterior gestation.

extima (eks′tĭ-mah) [L.] outermost.

extinction (eks-ting′shun) in psychology, the disappearance of a conditioned response as a result of nonreinforcement; also, the process by which this is accomplished.

extinguish (eks-ting′gwish) [L. *extinguere*] to render extinct.

extirpation (ek″ster-pa′shun) [L. *extirpare* to root out, from *ex* out + *stirps* root] complete removal or eradication of an organ or tissue. **e. of pulp, pulp e.,** complete removal of the dental pulp from the pulp chamber and root canal of a tooth.

Exton's reagent, test (eks′tonz) [William Gustav *Exton,* American physician, 1876–1943] see under *reagent* and *tests*.

Exton-Rose glucose tolerance test (eks′ton-rōz′) [William Gustav *Exton;* Anton Richard *Rose,* American biochemist, born 1877] see under *tests*.

extorsion (eks-tor′shun) [L. *ex* from + *torsio* twisting] tilting of the upper part of the vertical meridian of the eye away from the midline of the face.

extra- (eks′trah) [L.] a prefix meaning outside of, beyond, or in addition.

extra-adrenal (eks″trah-ah-dre′nal) situated or occurring outside the adrenal gland.

extra-anthropic (eks″trah-an-throp′ik) exanthropic.

extra-articular (eks″trah-ar-tik′u-lar) [*extra-* + L. *articulus* joint] situated or occurring outside a joint.

extrabronchial (eks″trah-brong′ke-al) outside or independent of the bronchial tubes; usually used in contrast to intrabronchial.

extrabuccal (eks″trah-buk′al) outside the mouth.

extrabulbar (eks″trah-bul′bar) outside or away from a bulb, as the medulla oblongata or the urethral bulb.

extracapsular (eks″trah-kap′su-lar) situated or occurring outside a capsule.

extracardial (eks″trah-kar′de-al) outside the heart.

extracarpal (eks″trah-kar′pal) just outside the region of the wrist.

extracellular (eks″trah-sel′u-lar) outside a cell or cells.

extracerebral (eks″trah-ser′ĕ-bral) situated or having its origin outside the cerebrum.

extracorporal (eks″trah-kor′po-ral) extracorporeal.

extracorporeal (eks″trah-kor-po′re-al) [*extra-* + L. *corpus* body] situated or occurring outside the body.

extracorpuscular (eks″trah-kor-pus′ku-lar) outside the corpuscles.

extracorticospinal (eks″trah-kor′tĭ-ko-spi′nal) outside the corticospinal tract; see under *tract*.

extracranial (eks″trah-kra′ne-al) outside the cranium.

extract (eks′trakt) [L. *extractum*] a concentrated preparation of a vegetable or animal drug obtained by removing the active constituents therefrom with a suitable menstruum, evaporating all or nearly all the solvent, and adjusting the residual mass or powder to a prescribed standard. Extracts are prepared in three forms: semiliquid or of syrupy consistency, pilular or solid, and as dry powder. **allergenic e.,** an extract of the protein of any substance to which a person may be sensitive; used for diagnosis or desensitization therapy in conditions due to hypersensitivity. They are prepared from a great variety of substances, from food to fungi, and from house dust to horse serum. **animal e.,** one prepared from material of animal origin. **beef e.,** a concentrate from beef broth, used in compounding certain prescriptions; called also *extractum carnis.* **belladonna e.** [USP], a preparation, available in pilular and powdered form, containing in each 100 grams, 1.15–1.35 gm. of the alkaloids of belladonna leaf; used as an anticholinergic for the same purposes as atropine and hyoscyamine. **cascara sagrada e.** [USP], a powdered preparation of cascara sagrada, each gram of which represents 3 gm. of cascara sagrada; a cathartic. Called also *Rhamnus purshiana e.* **cell-free e.,** the solution obtained by rupturing cells and removing all particulate matter. **chondodendron tomentosum e.,** an alcoholic extract of a desiccated substance (curare) obtained from the bark and stem of *Chondodendron tomentosum;* used in producing relaxation of skeletal muscle. **chondrus e.,** a tan powder prepared from chondrus, used as a protective; called also *Irish moss e.* **colocynth e.,** a powdered preparation each gram of which represents 4 gm. of colocynth; formerly used as a cathartic. **colocynth e., compound,** a preparation of colocynth extract with finely powdered ipomea, aloe, and cardamon seed; formerly used as a cathartic. **compound e.,** one prepared from more than one drug. **dry e.,** powdered e. **glycyrrhiza e.,** a brown powder prepared from the rhizome and roots of species of *Glycyrrhiza,* used as a flavoring agent; called also *licorice root e.* **glycyrrhiza e., pure,** [USP], a preparation of the dried rhizome and roots of varieties of *Glycyrrhiza glabra,* used in the compounding of aromatic cascara sagrada fluidextract; called also *pure licorice root e.* **Goulard's e.,** lead subacetate solution. **henbane e.,** hyoscyamus e. **hyoscyamus e.,** a preparation of hyoscyamus, formerly used as an anticholinergic for the same purposes as atropine. **Irish moss e.,** chondrus e. **licorice root e.,** glycyrrhiza e. **licorice root e., pure,** glycyrrhiza e., pure. **liver e.,** a brownish, somewhat hygroscopic powder prepared from mammalian livers; used as a hematopoietic. **liver e., liquid,** liver solution. **e. of male fern,** aspidium oleoresin; see under *oleoresin.* **malt e.,** a product containing dextrin, maltose, a small amount of glucose, and amylolytic enzymes, obtained by extracting the partially and artificially germinated grain of one or more varieties of *Hordeum vulgare* (barley); used as a nutritive and emulsifying agent. **nux vomica e.,** a powder prepared from nux vomica, each 100 gm. of which contains 7–7.75 gm. of strychnine. **ox bile e.,** a brownish to greenish yellow powder or granules, with a characteristic odor and bitter taste, prepared from the fresh bile of the ox and containing not less than 45 per cent of cholic acid; used as a choleretic. **oxgall e., powdered,** ox bile e. **parathyroid e.,** parathyroid injection. **pilular e.,** an extract prepared as a plastic mass, with liquid glucose, malt extract, or glycerin being used as a diluent. **poison ivy e.,** an extract of the fresh leaves of poison ivy, *Rhus (Toxicodendron) radicans* L., used in desensitization for prevention of rhus dermatitis due to poison ivy. **poison ivy e., alum precipitated,** a repository form of a pyridine extract of poison ivy, *Rhus (Toxicodendron) radicans* L., used to counteract rhus dermatitis due to poison ivy. **poison oak e.,** an extract of the fresh leaves of poison oak, *Rhus (Toxicodendron) diversiloba* L., used for desensitization in prevention of rhus dermatitis due to poison oak. **pollen e.,** a preparation of the pollen of certain plants, such as ragweed, used in the diagnosis and treatment of inhalant allergy. **powdered e.,** an extract prepared in a dry powdered form, with starch, sucrose, lactose, powdered glycyrrhiza, magnesium carbonate, magnesium oxide, or calcium phosphate being used as a diluent. Called also *dry e.* **Rhamnus purshiana e.,** cascara sagrada e. **rice polishings e.,** a preparation of rice polishings, used as a source of vitamin B_1, or thiamine. **semiliquid e.,** one evaporated to a syrupy consistency. **solid e.,** pilular e. **tikitiki e.,** rice polishings e. **trichinella e.,** an aqueous extract of specially treated larvae of *Trichinella spiralis,* usually obtained from inoculated rodents; used as a skin test for trichinella infection. **yeast e.,** a powder prepared from a water-soluble, peptone-like derivative of yeast cells (*Saccharomyces*).

extraction (eks-trak′shun) [L. *ex* out + *trahere* to draw] 1. the process or act of pulling or drawing out. 2. the preparation of an extract. **breech e.,** extraction of the infant from the uterus in breech presentation, i.e., when the buttocks of the fetus is presented in labor. **breech e., partial,** extraction of the remainder of the infant's body after it has been extruded from the uterus by natural forces as far as the umbilicus. **breech e., total,** extraction of the entire body of the infant from the uterus in cases of breech presentation. **e. of a cataract,** the surgical removal of a cataractous lens. **flap e.,** extraction of cataract by an incision which makes a flap of cornea. **serial e.,** the selective extraction of deciduous teeth during an extended period of time to allow autonomous adjustment; this procedure often involves eventual extraction of the first premolar teeth. **tooth e.,** the removal of a tooth. **vacuum e.,** see under *aspiration.*

extractive (eks-trak′tiv) any substance present in an organized tissue, or in a mixture in a small quantity, and requiring to be extracted by a special method.

extractor (eks-trak′tor) an instrument used for removing a calculus or foreign body.

extractum (eks-trak′tum), gen. *extrac′ti,* pl. *extrac′ta* [L., from *ex* out + *trahere* to draw] an extract. **e. car′nis,** beef extract. **e. fel′lis bo′vis,** ox bile extract. **e. hep′atis,** liver extract. **e. nu′cis vom′icae,** nux vomica extract. **e. perpoliti-o′num ory′zae,** rice polishings extract.

extracystic (eks″trah-sis′tik) outside a cyst or the bladder.

extradural (eks″trah-du′ral) situated or occurring outside the dura mater.

extraembryonic (eks″trah-em″bre-on′ik) external to the embryo proper, as the extraembryonic coelom or extraembryonic membranes.

extraepiphyseal (eks″trah-ep″ĭ-fiz′e-al) away from, or unconnected with, an epiphysis.

extragenic (eks″trah-jen′ik) occurring outside a gene, or in a gene other than the one in question.

extragenital (eks″trah-jen′ĭ-tal) unrelated to, not originating in, or remote from the genital organs.

extrahepatic (eks″trah-hĕ-pat′ik) situated or occurring outside the liver.

extraligamentous (eks″trah-lig″ah-men′tus) occurring outside a ligament.

extramalleolus (eks″trah-mal-le′o-lus) the outer malleolus of the ankle joint.

extramarginal (eks″trah-mar′jĭ-nal) below the limit of consciousness.

extramastoiditis (eks″trah-mas″toi-di′tis) inflammation of the outer surface of the mastoid process and of the superincumbent tissues.

extramedullary (eks″trah-med′u-la″re) situated or occurring outside any medulla, especially the medulla oblongata.

extrameningeal (eks″trah-mĕ-nin′je-al) occurring outside the meninges.

extramural (eks″trah-mu′ral) [L. *extra* + *murus* wall] situated or occurring outside the wall of an organ or structure.

extraneous (eks-tra′ne-us) [L. *extraneus* external] existing or belonging outside the organism.

extranuclear (eks″trah-nu′kle-ar) situated or occurring outside a cell nucleus.

extraocular (eks″trah-ok′u-lar) situated outside the eye.

extraoculogram (eks″trah-ok′u-lo-gram) a graphic representation of the changes in the corneofundal electric potential of the eye, recorded by means of electrodes applied to the skin on either side of the orbit; useful in determining disturbances in the metabolic activity of the eye.

extraosseous (eks″trah-os′e-us) occurring outside a bone or bones.

extraparenchymal (eks″trah-par-en″kĭ-mal) occurring or formed outside the parenchyma.

extrapelvic (eks″trah-pel′vik) unconnected with the pelvis.

extrapericardial (eks″trah-per″ĭ-kar′de-al) outside the pericardium.

extraperineal (eks″trah-per″ĭ-ne′al) away from the perineum.

extraperiosteal (eks″trah-per″e-os′te-al) outside or independent of the periosteum.

extraperitoneal (eks″trah-per″ĭ-to-ne′al) situated or occurring outside the peritoneal cavity.

extraplacental (eks″trah-plah-sen′tal) outside of or independent of the placenta.

extraplantar (eks″trah-plan′tar) on the outside of the sole of the foot.

extrapleural (eks″trah-ploo′ral) outside the pleural cavity.

extrapolation (eks″trap-o-la′shun) inference of a value(s) on the basis of that which is known or has been observed.

extraprostatic (eks″trah-pros-tat′ik) not connected with the prostate gland.

extraprostatitis (eks″trah-pros″tah-ti′tis) paraprostatitis.

extrapsychic (eks″tra-si′kik) occurring outside the mind; taking place between the mind and the external environment.

extrapulmonary (eks″trah-pul′mo-na″re) not connected with the lungs.

extrapyramidal (eks″trah-pi-ram′ĭ-dal) outside of the pyramidal tracts; see under *system.*

extrarectus (eks″trah-rek′tus) musculus rectus lateralis bulbi.

extraserous (eks″trah-se′rus) outside a serous cavity.

extrasomatic (eks″trah-so-mat′ik) unconnected with the body.

extrasuprarenal (eks″trah-su″prah-re′nal) extra-adrenal.

extrasystole (eks″trah-sis′to-le) a premature contraction of the heart that is independent of the normal rhythm and arises in response to an impulse in some part of the heart other than the sinoatrial node; called also *premature beat.* **atrial e.,** an ex-

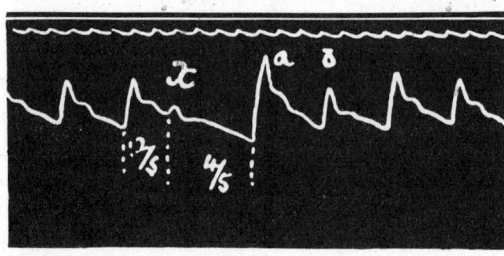

Tracing of the radial pulse in a patient suffering from occasional extrasystoles. The extrasystole occurs at *x.* Note the compensatory pause of four fifths of a second and the large pulse wave terminating this pause (Hay).

trasystole in which the stimulus is thought to arise in the atrium elsewhere than at the sinus. **auriclar e.,** former name for *atrial e.* **atrioventricular e.,** one in which the stimulus is supposed to arise in the atrioventricular node; called also *nodal e.* **auriculoventricular e.,** former name for *atrioventricular e.* **infranodal e.,** ventricular e. **interpolated e.,** a contraction taking place between two normal heart beats. **nodal e.,** atrioventricular e. **retrograde e.,** a premature ventricular contraction followed by a premature atrial contraction, due to transmission of the stimulus backward, usually over the bundle of His. **ventricular e.,** one in which either a pacemaker or re-entry site is in the ventricular structure.

extrathoracic (eks″trah-tho-ras′ik) outside the thorax.

extratracheal (eks″trah-tra′ke-al) situated or occurring outside the trachea.

extratubal (eks″trah-tu′bal) outside a tube.

extratympanic (eks″trah-tim-pan′ik) outside the tympanum of the ear.

extrauterine (eks″trah-u′ter-ĭn) situated or occurring outside the uterus.

extravaginal (eks″trah-vaj′ĭ-nal) outside the vagina.

extravasation (eks-trav″ah-sa′shun) [*extra-* + L. *vas* vessel] 1. a discharge or escape, as of blood, from a vessel into the tissues. 2. the process of being extravasated. 3. blood or other substance which has been extravasated. **punctiform e.,** extravasation which causes a tissue to be covered with minute bloody points.

extravascular (eks″trah-vas′ku-lar) situated or occurring outside a vessel or the vessels.

extraventricular (eks″trah-ven-trik′u-lar) situated or occurring outside a ventricle.

extraversion (eks″trah-ver′zhun) 1. the turning outward or objectifying of personal interests, emotions, or psychic trends. 2. (*obs.*) in orthodontics, an unusually wide dental arch.

extravert (eks′trah-vert) extrovert.

extremital (eks-trem′ĭ-tal) pertaining to or situated at an extremity.

extremitas (eks-trem′ĭ-tas), pl. *extremita′tes* [L.] 1. [NA] a general term denoting the distal or terminal portion of elongated or pointed structures. 2. the arm or leg (membrum [NA]. Called also *extremity.* **e. acromia′lis clavic′ulae** [NA], acromial extremity of clavicle: the lateral end of the clavicle, which articulates with the acromion of the scapula; called also *external*

Plate XVII   eye

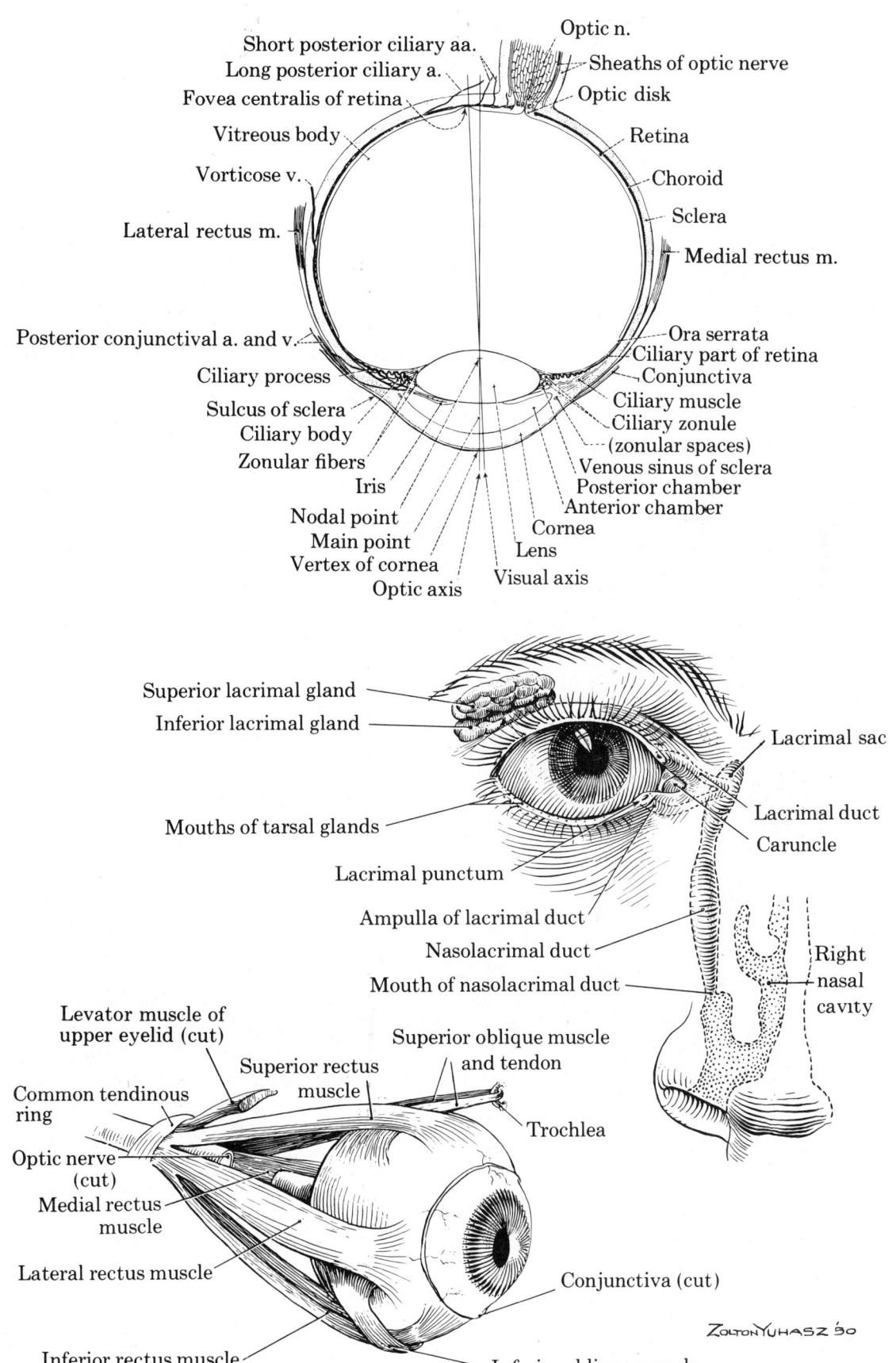

Short posterior ciliary aa.
Long posterior ciliary a.
Fovea centralis of retina
Vitreous body
Vorticose v.
Lateral rectus m.
Posterior conjunctival a. and v.
Ciliary process
Sulcus of sclera
Ciliary body
Zonular fibers
Iris
Nodal point
Main point
Vertex of cornea
Optic axis

Optic n.
Sheaths of optic nerve
Optic disk
Retina
Choroid
Sclera
Medial rectus m.
Ora serrata
Ciliary part of retina
Conjunctiva
Ciliary muscle
Ciliary zonule
(zonular spaces)
Venous sinus of sclera
Posterior chamber
Anterior chamber
Cornea
Lens
Visual axis

Superior lacrimal gland
Inferior lacrimal gland
Mouths of tarsal glands
Lacrimal punctum
Ampulla of lacrimal duct
Nasolacrimal duct
Mouth of nasolacrimal duct

Lacrimal sac
Lacrimal duct
Caruncle
Right nasal cavity

Levator muscle of
upper eyelid (cut)
Common tendinous ring
Optic nerve (cut)
Medial rectus muscle
Lateral rectus muscle
Inferior rectus muscle

Superior rectus muscle
Superior oblique muscle and tendon
Trochlea
Conjunctiva (cut)
Inferior oblique muscle

ZOLTON YUHASZ '90

THE EYE AND RELATED STRUCTURES

or *scapular extremity of clavicle.* **e. ante′rior lie′nis** [NA], anterior extremity of spleen: the lower pole of the spleen, which is situated anterior to the upper pole; called also *e. inferior lienis* and *cauda lienis.* **e. infe′rior,** membrum inferius. **e. infe′rior lie′nis,** e. anterior lienis. **e. infe′rior re′nis** [NA], inferior extremity of kidney: the lower, smaller pole of the kidney; called also *caput lienis* and *head of spleen.* **e. infe′rior tes′tis** [NA], inferior extremity of testis: the lower end of the testis, which is attached to the tail of the epididymis. **e. poste′rior lie′nis** [NA], posterior extremity of spleen: the uppermost pole of the spleen, situated somewhat posterior to the lower pole; called also *e. superior lienis.* **e. sterna′lis clavic′ulae** [NA], sternal extremity of clavicle: the medial end of the clavicle, which articulates with the sternum; called also *internal extremity of clavicle.* **e. supe′rior,** membrum superius. **e. supe′rior lie′nis,** e. posterior lienis. **e. supe′rior re′nis** [NA], superior extremity of kidney: the upper, larger pole of the kidney. **e. supe′rior tes′tis** [NA], superior extremity of testis: the upper end of the testis, which is attached to the head of the epididymis. **e. tuba′ria ova′rii** [NA], tubal extremity of ovary: the upper end of the ovary, related to the free end of the uterine tube. **e. uteri′na ova′rii** [NA], uterine extremity of ovary: the lower end of the ovary, directed toward the uterus; called also *pelvic extremity.*

extremitates (eks-trem″ĭ-ta′tēz) [L.] plural of *extremitas.*

extremity (eks-trem′ĭ-te) 1. a distal or terminal portion; for names of specific anatomical structures, see official terms under *extremitas.* 2. an arm or leg (membrum [NA]); sometimes applied specifically to a hand or foot. **cartilaginous e. of rib,** cartilago costalis. **external e. of clavicle,** extremitas acromialis claviculae. **fimbriated e. of fallopian tube,** fimbria ovarica. **internal e. of clavicle,** extremitas sternalis claviculae. **lower e.,** membrum inferius. **pelvic e. of ovary,** extremitas uterina ovarii. **proximal e. of phalanx of finger,** basis phalangis digitorum manus. **proximal e. of phalanx of toe,** basis phalangis digitorum pedis. **scapular e. of clavicle,** extremitas acromialis claviculae. **upper e.,** membrum superius. **uterine e. of ovary,** extremitas uterina ovarii.

extrinsic (eks-trin′sik) [L. *extrinsecus* situated on the outside] coming from or originating outside; having relation to parts outside the organ or limb in which found.

extro- [L. *extra* outside of, beyond] a prefix meaning outward, outside.

extrogastrulation (eks″tro-gas″troo-la′shun) the formation of an embryonic monster by gastrular evagination instead of invagination.

extrophia (eks-tro′fe-ah) exstrophy.

extrospection (eks″tro-spek′shun) [*extra-* + L. *spectare* to look] the continued habit of inspecting one's own skin, associated with mysophobia.

extroversion (eks″tro-ver′zhun) [L. *extroversio,* from *extra* outside + *vertere* to turn] 1. a turning inside out; exstrophy. 2. extraversion.

extrovert (eks′tro-vert) a person whose interest is turned outward toward external values.

extrude (eks-trood′) 1. to force out, or to occupy a position distal to that normally occupied. 2. in dentistry, to occupy a position occlusal to that normally occupied (said of an over-erupted tooth).

extrudoclusion (eks-troo″do-kloo′zhun) extrusion, def. 2.

extrusion (eks-troo′zhun) 1. a pushing out; a forcing out or expulsion. 2. in dentistry, the condition of a tooth when it extends too far in an occlusal direction.

extubate (eks-tu′bāt) [*ex-* + L. *tuba* tube] to remove a tube from.

extubation (eks″tu-ba′shun) the removal of a previously inserted tube.

exuberant (eg-zu′ber-ant) [L. *exuberare* to be very fruitful] copious or excessive in production; showing excessive proliferation.

exudate (eks′u-dāt) [L. *exsudare* to sweat out] material, such as fluid, cells, or cellular debris, which has escaped from blood vessels and has been deposited in tissues or on tissue surfaces, usually as a result of inflammation. An exudate, in contrast to a transudate, is characterized by a high content of protein, cells, or solid materials derived from cells. **cotton-wool e's,** see under *spot.*

exudation (eks″u-da′shun) 1. the escape of fluid, cells, and cellular debris from blood vessels and their deposition in or on the tissues, usually as the result of inflammation. 2. an exudate.

exudative (eks-oo′dah-tiv) of or pertaining to a process of exudation.

exulcerans (eks-ul′ser-anz) [L.] ulcerating.

exulceratio (eks-ul′ser-a′she-o) [L.] ulceration. **e. sim′plex,** superficial ulceration.

exumbilication (eks″um-bil″ĭ-ka′shun) [*ex-* + *umbilicus*] 1. marked protrusion of the navel. 2. umbilical hernia.

exutory (eks-u′tor-e) [L. *exutum,* from *exuere* to lay aside; remove] (*obs.*) 1. drawing off. 2. an agent that draws off.

exuviae (eks-u′ve-e) [L., pl.] (*obs.*) 1. cast-off epidermis. 2. a slough (def. 1).

exuviation (eks-u″ve-a′shun) [L. *exuere* to divest oneself of] the shedding of any epithelial structure, as of the deciduous teeth.

ex vivo (eks″ve′vo) outside the living body; denoting removal of an organ (e.g., the kidney) for reparative surgery, after which it is returned to the original site.

eye (i) [L. *oculus;* Gr. *ophthalmos*] the organ of vision. Called also *oculus* [NA]. In shape the eyeball (bulbus oculi [NA]) is of a large sphere, with the segment of a smaller sphere, the *cornea,* in front. It is composed of three coats—the *sclera* and *cornea,* the *choroid,* and the *retina*—each coat being divided into several layers. Within the three coats are the refracting media—namely, the *aqueous humor,* the *crystalline lens,* and the *vitreous humor.* The scleric, or external coat, is white and fibrous. Posteriorly the fibers of the optic nerve enter through small perforations in the *lamina cribrosa.* The inner surface is attached to the choroid by delicate connective tissue, the *lamina fusca.* The *cornea* is composed of five layers, the internal layer being a serous membrane, sometimes called *Descemet's membrane.* The uvea, or middle coat, is chiefly composed of blood vessels and pigment. Anteriorly, it terminates near the periphery of the lens in folds called the *ciliary processes.* The *retina,* or internal coat, is chiefly composed of nerve tissue, and is made up of three principal layers. The external layer, or Jacob's membrane, is composed of terminal nerve cells, which, from their shape, are called the *rods* and *cones.* The *iris* is a curtain with a central perforation, the *pupil,* and is composed of smooth muscular fibers arranged both in a circular and in a radiating manner. It varies in color, and is suspended in the aqueous humor in front of the lens. The *ciliary ligament* is a ring of connective tissue fibers surrounding the iris. The *ciliary muscle* surrounds the periphery of the iris and controls the convexity of the lens during accommodation. The *aqueous humor* fills the cavity between the cornea in front and the lens behind. The *vitreous humor* fills the space back of the lens, and is a clear, jelly-like substance containing mucin. It is surrounded by the *hyaloid membrane.* The *lens,* or *crystalline humor,* is a double convex transparent body between the vitreous and aqueous humors, and is held in place by an elastic *capsule* and *suspensory* ligament. The arteries of the eye are the short ciliary, the long ciliary, the anterior ciliary, and the central artery of the retina. The nerves are the optic and the long and short ciliary nerves. See Plate XVII. **blear e.,** blepharitis ciliaris. **Bright's e.,** the eye as affected in chronic disease of the kidney. **cinema e.,** Klieg e. **compound e.,** the multifaceted eye of insects. **crab's e's,** concretions from the digestive tract of a crawfish. **crossed e's,** esotropia. **cystic e.,** a malformed eye consisting of a cystic structure. **dark-adapted e.,** an eye that has undergone the changes produced by adequate exposure to darkness; it is more sensitive to very weak light. **epiphyseal e.,** a modification of the parapineal organ of certain lower vertebrates to form an eyelike structure lying subepidermally on the median dorsal aspect of the head; it is a photoreceptor rather than an image forming eye, enabling the organism to respond to darkness or to light. Called also *parietal e., parietal body,* and *pineal e.* **exciting e.,** the eye that is primarily injured and from which the influences start which involve the other eye in sympathetic ophthalmia; called also *primary e.* **fixating e.,** in strabismus, the eye directed toward the object of vision. **hare's e.** (*obs.*), lagophthalmos. **hop e.,** conjunctivitis in hop pickers caused by irritation from the spinelike hairs of the hop plant. **Klieg e.,** a condition marked by conjunctivitis, edema of the eyelids, lacrimation, and photophobia due to exposure to intense lights (Klieg lights); called also *cinema e.* **light-adapted e.,** an eye that has undergone the changes produced by adequate exposure to rather strong light; it is less sensitive to weak light. **median e.,** an organ on the top of the head of many reptiles; it plays an important role in the response to light. **monochromatic e.,** an eye that can perceive only one color. **Nairobi e.,** a form of conjunctivitis in East Africa produced by the juice of crushed blister beetles. **parietal e.,** a modification of the parietal body in some lower vertebrates, to form a second dorsal median eye. Cf. *epiphyseal e.* **pineal e.,** epiphyseal e. **pink e.,** acute contagious conjunctivitis. **primary e.,** exciting e. **reduced e., schematic e.,** 1. an apparatus with two refracting elements, one representing the cornea and the other the lens. 2. a diagrammatic illustration of the structure of the eye. **secondary e.,** sympathizing e. **shipyard e.,** epidemic keratoconjunctivitis. **Snellen's reform e.,** an artificial eye composed of two concavoconvex plates with an empty space between. **squinting e.,** in strabismus, the eye the visual axis of which deviates from the object of vision while the sound eye fixates. **sympathizing e.,** the uninjured eye which becomes secondarily involved in sympathetic ophthalmia; called also *secondary e.* **wall e.,** 1. leukoma of the cornea. 2. exotropia.

eyeball (i′bawl) the globe or ball of the eye; called also *bulbus oculi* [NA] and *orb.* See *eye.*

eyebrow (i′brow) 1. the transverse elevation at the junction of the forehead and the upper eyelid, consisting of five layers: skin, subcutaneous tissue, a layer of interwoven fibers of the orbicularis oculi and occipitofrontalis muscles, a submuscular areolar layer, and pericranium; called also *supercilium* [NA]. 2. the hairs growing on the transverse elevation at the junction of the forehead and the upper eyelid; called also *supercilia* [NA].

eyecup (i'kup) 1. a small vessel for the application of cleansing or medicated solution to the exposed area of the eyeball. 2. physiologic cup. 3. caliculus ophthalmicus.

eyeglass (i'glas) a lens for aiding the sight.

eyeground (i'ground) the fundus of the eye as revealed by ophthalmoscopical examination.

eyelash (i'lash) one of the hairs growing at the edge of an eyelid; collectively called *cilia* [NA].

eyelet (i'let) an orthodontic attachment welded or soldered for better rotational control.

eyelid (i'lid) either of the two movable folds (upper and lower) that protect the anterior surface of the eyeball; called also *palpebra* [NA]. **third e.,** the nictitating membrane; see under *membrane.*

eye-minded (i-mīnd'ed) remembering chiefly the impressions made on the eye.

eyepiece (i'pēs) the lens or system of lenses in a microscope (or telescope) that is nearest to the eye of the user and that serves to further magnify the image produced by the objective. **com-** parison e., an eyepiece which presents, as though in juxtaposition, the images of separate objects being transmitted through two different objectives. **compensating e.,** an eyepiece especially designed to correct chromatic and spherical aberrations of the light rays produced by the objective. **demonstration e.,** a device consisting of two eyepieces which may be affixed to the eyepiece tube of a microscope, permitting two observers to see the same field simultaneously. **huygenian e.,** a negative eyepiece consisting of two planoconvex lenses, the convexities being directed toward the objective. **negative e.,** a combination of two lenses, one of which is below the plane in which the real image from the objective is formed. **positive e.,** a single lens combination, consisting of two planoconvex lenses or of an achromatic doublet or triplet, the combination being above the plane in which the real image from the objective is formed. **Ramsden's e.,** a positive eyepiece consisting of two planoconvex lenses with the convexities turned toward each other. **widefield e.,** a positive eyepiece consisting of a doublet and a single element, giving a wider field of view than that afforded by other eyepieces.

eyepoint (i'point) a point above the eyepiece in which all the beams of light emerging from the microscope intersect.

eyespot (i'spot) the light-sensitive pigmented spot of certain invertebrates.

eyestrain (i'strān) fatigue of the eye from overuse or from uncorrected defect in focus of the eye.

F

F chemical symbol for *fluorine;* symbol for *gilbert.*

F. Fahrenheit; fiat; field of vision; French (catheter size); formula.

F₁ 1. the "first filial generation," produced by crossing two individuals. 2. a fluorescent substance found in small amounts in normal urine, and in larger quantities in the urine of pellagrins; said to be present in larger amounts after the ingestion of thiamine.

F₂ 1. the "second filial generation," produced by mating two members of the F₁ generation. 2. a substance in urine which develops fluorescence after alkali is added; it may appear in small amounts in normal urine or in large amounts in the urine of normal persons after the ingestion of nicotinic acid.

FA fatty acid.

F and R force and rhythm (of pulse).

Fab [*fragment, antigen- binding*] either of two segments of the IgG molecule, obtained by treatment of the antibody molecule with papain, which retain the ability to combine with antigen. See also *Fc.*

Fabc fragment antigen and complement binding; that part of an IgG molecule which remains following removal of pFc′ fragment from the Fc fragment region by the enzyme plasmin.

fabella (fah-bel'lah), pl. *fabel'lae* [L. "little bean"] a sesamoid fibrocartilage occasionally found on the gastrocnemius muscle; it is visible roentgenographically as a small bony shadow behind the knee joint.

fabellae (fah-bel'le) [L.] plural of *fabella.*

Faber's anemia, syndrome (fah'berz) [Knud Helge *Faber,* Danish physician, 1862–1956] see *achylanemia,* and see *hypochromic anemia,* under *anemia.*

fabism (fa'bizm) [L. *faba* bean] favism.

fabrication (fab"rĭ-ka'shun) the telling of imaginary events or tales as if they were true; confabulation.

Fabricius (fah-bris'e-us) **(of Aquapendente),** Hieronymus [It. Girolamo *Fabrizio*] (1537–1619) an Italian anatomist and surgeon who was the pupil and successor (at Padua) of Gabriele Falloppio. He was the teacher of William Harvey, and the first demonstrator of the valves of the veins.

Fabry's disease (syndrome) (fah'brez) [Johannes *Fabry,* German dermatologist, 1860–1930] see under *disease.*

F.A.C.D. Fellow of the American College of Dentists.

face (fās) [L. *facies*] 1. the anterior, or ventral, aspect of the head from the forehead to the chin, inclusive. 2. any presenting aspect, or surface. See also *facies.* **adenoid f.,** adenoid facies. **bovine f.,** facies bovina. **cleft f.,** macrostomia. **cow f.,** facies bovina. **dish f., dished f.,** a facial deformity characterized by a prominence of the forehead, a recession of the midface and lower half of the nose, a lengthening of the upper lip, and a prognathic chin; called also *facies scaphoidea.* **frog f.,** flatness of the face due to intranasal disease. **hippocratic f.,** facies hippocratica. **moon f., moon-shaped f.,** the peculiar rounded face observed in various conditions, such as Cushing's syndrome, or following administration of adrenal corticoids.

face-bow (fās'bo) a device used in dentistry to record the positional relationship of the maxillary arch to the temporomandibular joints (or opening axis of the jaw) and to orient dental casts in this same relationship to the opening axis of the articulator. **adjustable axis f.-b.,** one that can be adjusted to permit location of the axis of rotation of the mandible. **kinematic f.-b.,** adjustable axis f.-b.

faceometer (fās-om'ě-ter) an instrument for measuring the dimensions of the face.

facet (fas'et) [Fr. *facette*] a small plane surface on a hard body, as on a bone; see also *fovea.* **articular f.,** a small plane surface on a bone at the site where it articulates with another structure; see terms beginning *facies articularis,* under *facies.* **articular f. of atlas, circular,** fovea dentis atlantis. **articular f. of atlas, inferior,** fovea articularis inferior atlantis. **articular f. of atlas, superior,** fovea articularis superior atlantis. **articular f. of axis, anterior,** facies articularis anterior axis. **articular f's for rib cartilages,** incisurae costales sterni. **f. of calcaneus, posterior, medial,** facies articularis talaris media calcanei. **clavicular f.,** incisura clavicularis sterni. **costal f., anterior, costal f., inferior,** facies articularis tuberculi costae. **costal f., posterior, costal f., superior,** facies articularis capitis costae. **costal f's of sternum,** incisurae costales sterni. **costal f. of vertebra, superior,** fovea costalis superior. **lateral f's of sternum,** incisurae costales sterni. **locked f's of spine,** dislocation of articular processes of the spine. **malleolar f. of tibia, internal,** facies articularis malleolaris tibiae. **squatting f.,** a smooth area observed on the anterior surface of the lower end of the tibia in races whose members habitually sit in the squatting position. **f. for tubercle of rib,** fovea costalis transversalis.

facetectomy (fas"ě-tek'to-me) [*facet* + Gr. *ektomē* excision] excision of the articular facet of a vertebra.

facette (fah-set') [Fr.] facet.

facial (fa'shal) [L. *facialis*] of or pertaining to the face.

facies (fa'she-ēz), pl. *fa'cies* [L.] 1. a term used in anatomical nomenclature to designate (*a*) the anterior, or ventral, aspect of the head, from forehead to chin, inclusive, and (*b*) a specific surface of a body structure, part, or organ. 2. the expression or appearance of the face. **f. abdomina'lis,** the expression of the face characteristic of abdominal disease: it is pinched, anxious, and furrowed, with the nose and upper lip drawn up. **adenoid f.,** the dull expression, with open mouth, sometimes seen in children with adenoid growths. **f. ante'rior antebra'chii** [NA], the ventral, or front, surface of the forearm; called also *f. volaris antibrachii.* **f. ante'rior bra'chii** [NA], the ventral, or front, surface of the upper arm. **f. ante'rior cor'neae** [NA], the anterior surface of the cornea. **f. ante'rior cru'ris** [NA], the ventral, or front, surface of the leg. **f. ante'rior den'tium premola'rium et mola'rium,** the contact surface of the premolar and molar teeth that is directed toward the midline of the dental arch. **f. ante'rior fem'oris** [NA], the ventral, or front, surface of the thigh. **f. ante'rior glan'dulae suprarena'lis** [NA], the anterior, or front, surface of the adrenal gland. **f. ante'rior i'ridis** [NA], the anterior surface of the iris, directed toward the anterior chamber of the eye. **f. ante'rior latera'lis hu'meri** [NA], the anterolateral surface of the humerus, which provides attachment for the deltoid muscle and lateral part of the brachialis muscle. **f. ante'rior len'tis** [NA], the surface of the lens directed toward the anterior surface of the eye. **f. ante′rior maxil′lae** [NA], the surface of the body of the maxilla that is directed forward and somewhat laterally; it is bounded roughly by the infraorbital margin, root of the frontal process, nasal notch, alveolar process, and zygomatic process. **f. ante′rior media′lis hu′meri** [NA], the surface of the humerus that begins above at the intertubercular groove and spreads out inferiorly to form the wide smooth area for origin of the brachialis muscle; called also *anteromedial surface of humerus.* **f. ante′rior palpebra′rum** [NA], the anterior, or external, surface of the eyelids. **f. ante′rior pancre′atis** [NA], the front, or anterior, surface of the pancreas, directed toward the ventral surface of the body. **f. ante′rior par′tis petro′sae os′sis tempora′lis** [NA], the surface of the petrous part of the temporal bone that forms the posterior portion of the floor of the middle cranial fossa; called also *f. anterior pyramidis ossis temporalis.* **f. ante′rior patel′lae** [NA], the slightly convex, longitudinally striated anterior, or front, surface of the patella, which is perforated by small openings for the nutrient vessels. **f. ante′rior prosta′tae** [NA], the anterior, or ventral, surface of the prostate, separated from the pubic symphysis by the pudendal venous plexus. **f. ante′rior pyram′idis os′sis tempora′lis,** f. anterior partis petrosae ossis temporalis. **f. ante′rior ra′dii** [NA], the anterior, or volar, surface of the radius, which gives attachment to the flexor pollicis longus and pronator quadratus muscles; called also *f. volaris radii.* **f. ante′rior re′nis** [NA], the anterior, peritoneum-covered surface of the kidney which is directed toward the viscera. **f. ante′rior ul′nae** [NA], the front, or anterior, surface of the ulna; called also *f. volaris ulnae.* **f. anterolatera′lis cartilag′inis arytenoi′deae** [NA], the external surface of the arytenoid cartilage, which bears the triangular pit, the oblong pit, and the arcuate crest. **f. articula′ris acromia′lis clavic′ulae** [NA], the smooth area on the lateral end of the clavicle for articulation with the acromion of the scapula. **f. articula′ris acro′mii** [NA], a small variable area on the acromion of the scapula, for articulation with the acromial end of the clavicle. **f. articula′ris ante′rior ax′is** [NA], anterior articular facet of axis: an oval facet on the ventral surface of the odontoid process of the axis, articulating with the fovea dentis of the atlas; called also *f. volaris ulnae.* **f. anterolatera′lis cartilag′inis arytenoi′deae** [NA], the external surface of the arytenoid cartiarticula′ris ante′rior epistroph′ei, f. articularis anterior axis. **f. articula′ris arytenoi′dea cartilag′inis cricoi′deae** [NA], the surface of the cricoid cartilage that articulates with the arytenoid cartilage. **f. articula′ris calca′nea ante′rior ta′li** [NA], the small surface on the head of the talus that rests upon the anterior articular surface of the calcaneus. **f. articula′ris calca′nea me′dia ta′li** [NA], the convex part of the head of the talus that articulates with the sustentaculum tali of the calcaneus. **f. articula′ris calca′nea poste′rior ta′li** [NA], a transverse concavity on the inferior surface of the talus, articulating with the calcaneus. **f. articula′ris cap′itis cos′tae** [NA], the surface on the head of a rib where it articulates with the body of a vertebra. Typically it is divided into two facets by a transverse crest, the lower facet articulating with the corresponding vertebra, and the upper facet with the suprajacent vertebra. The articular surfaces of the heads of the first, tenth, eleventh, and twelfth ribs generally consist of only one facet. Called also *f. articularis capituli costae,* and *posterior* or *superior costal facet.* **f. articula′ris cap′itis fib′ulae** [NA], the medial surface of the head of the fibula, which articulates with the lateral condyle of the tibia; called also *f. articularis capituli fibulae.* **f. articula′ris capit′uli cos′tae,** f. articularis capitis costae. **f. articula′ris capit′uli fib′ulae,** f. articularis capitis fibulae. **f. articula′ris car′pea ra′dii** [NA], the concave part of the distal end of the radius, which articulates with the lunate and scaphoid carpal bones; called also *carpal articular surface of radius.* **f. articula′ris cartilag′inis arytenoi′dea** [NA], the surface of the arytenoid cartilage that articulates with the cricoid cartilage. **f. articula′ris cuboi′dea calca′nei** [NA], the saddle-shaped area on the anterior surface of the calcaneus where it articulates with the cuboid bone; called also *cuboid articular surface of calcaneus.* **f. articula′ris fibula′ris tib′iae** [NA], the articular surface on the posteroinferior aspect of the lateral condyle of the tibia, which articulates with the head of the fibula. **f. articula′ris fos′sae mandibula′ris,** f. articularis ossis temporalis. **f. articula′res inferio′res atlan′tis,** see *fovea articularis inferior atlantis.* **f. articula′ris infe′rior tib′iae** [NA], the surface on the distal end of the tibia where it articulates with the talus. **f. articula′res inferio′res vertebra′rum,** the surfaces on the inferior articular processes of the vertebrae. **f. articula′ris malleola′ris tib′iae** [NA], the lateral aspect of the medial malleolus, which articulates with the talus; called also *fovea of lateral malleolus* and *internal malleolar facet of tibia.* **f. articula′ris malle′oli fib′ulae** [NA], the anterosuperior surface of the lateral malleolus, which articulates with the lateral side of the talus; called also *lateral malleolar fovea of fibula.* **f. articula′ris me′dia calca′nei,** f. articularis talaris media calcanei. **f. articula′ris navicula′ris ta′li** [NA], the surface of the head of the talus that articulates with the navicular bone. **f. articula′ris os′sis tempora′lis** [NA], the articular surface found in the deep part of the mandibular fossa of the temporal bone; called also *f. articularis fossae mandibularis.* **f. articula′ris os′sium** [NA], the surface by which a bone articulates with another; called also *articular surface.* **f. articula′ris patel′lae** [NA], the posterior, or back, surface of the patella, which is largely covered by a thick cartilaginous layer. **f. articula′ris poste′rior ax′is** [NA], a smooth groove on the dorsal surface of the odontoid process of the axis, which lodges the transverse ligament of the atlas; called also *f. articularis posterior epistrophei.* **f. articula′ris poste′rior calca′nei,** f. articularis talaris posterior calcanei. **f. articula′ris poste′rior epistroph′ei,** f. articularis posterior axis. **f. articula′ris sterna′lis clavic′ulae** [NA], a triangular surface on the medial end of the clavicle for articulation with the sternum. **f. articula′ris supe′rior tib′iae** [NA], the surface on the proximal end of the tibia that articulates with the condyles of the femur; called also *condyloid surface of tibia.* **f. articula′res superio′res vertebra′rum,** the articular facets on the superior articular processes of the vertebrae. **f. articula′ris tala′ris ante′rior calca′nei** [NA], the small area on the superior surface of the calcaneus just anterior to the middle articular surface, which articulates with the talus; called also *f. articularis anterior calcanei.* **f. articula′ris tala′ris me′dia calca′nei** [NA], the area on the superior surface of the calcaneus just in front of the calcaneal sulcus, which articulates with the talus; called also *f. articularis media calcanei* and *medial posterior facet of calcaneus.* **f. articula′ris tala′ris poste′rior calca′nei** [NA], the area on the superior surface of the calcaneus just posterolateral to the calcaneal sulcus, which articulates with the talus; called also *f. articularis posterior calcanei.* **f. articula′ris thyroi′dea cartilag′inis cricoi′deae** [NA], the surface of the cricoid cartilage that articulates with the thyroid cartilage; called also *eminentia lateralis cartilaginis cricoideae.* **f. articula′ris tuber′culi cos′tae** [NA], the convex facet on the costal tubercle that articulates with the transverse process of a vertebra; called also *anterior* or *inferior costal facet.* **f. auricula′ris os′sis il′ii** [NA], **f. auricula′ris os′sis il′ium,** a somewhat ear-shaped area on the sacropelvic surface of the ilium, which articulates with the auricular surface of the sacrum to form the sacroiliac joint. **f. auricula′ris os′sis sa′cri** [NA], the broad irregular surface on the superior half of the lateral aspect of the sacrum, which articulates with the ilium; called also *auricular surface of sacrum.* **f. bovi′na** [L. "cow face"], a term sometimes applied to the appearance of the face in craniofacial dysostosis; called also *bovine* or *cow face.* **f. bucca′lis den′tis,** buccal surface: the surface of a posterior tooth that is directed outward toward the cheek. **f. cerebra′lis a′lae mag′nae, f. cerebra′lis a′lae majo′ris** [NA], the smooth, concave part of the great wing of the sphenoid bone that forms the anterior part of the floor of the middle cranial fossa, lying in front of the petrous and squamous parts of the temporal bone. **f. cerebra′lis os′sis fronta′lis,** f. interna ossis frontalis. **f. cerebra′lis os′sis parieta′lis,** f. interna ossis parietalis. **f. cerebra′lis squa′mae tempora′lis, f. cerebra′lis par′tis squamo′sae os′sis tempora′lis** [NA], the inner surface of the squamous part of the temporal bone, forming the lateral wall of the middle cranial fossa. **f. co′lica lie′nis** [NA], the surface of the spleen that is in contact with the colon. **f. contac′tus den′tis** [NA], contact surface: the surface of a tooth that is in contact with an adjacent tooth in the same dental arch. **f. convex′a cer′ebri,** f. superolateralis cerebri. **f. costa′lis pulmo′nis** [NA], the surface area of each lung adjacent to the rib cage. **f. costa′lis scap′ulae** [NA], the anteromedially facing, concave surface of the scapula; called also *anterior* or *costal surface of scapula.* **f. diaphragmat′ica cor′dis** [NA], the surface of the heart (within the pericardium) that rests on the diaphragm and is directed inferiorly and somewhat posteriorly; it is formed by the two ventricles, the left ventricle contributing a little more than the right. **f. diaphragmat′ica hep′atis** [NA], the surface of the liver that lies in contact with the diaphragm, being composed of the superior, anterior, right, and posterior aspects. **f. diaphragmat′ica lie′nis** [NA], the convex posterolateral surface of the spleen which is directed toward the diaphragm. **f. diaphragmat′ica pulmo′nis** [NA], the surface area of each lung that is adjacent to the diaphragm. **f. dista′lis den′tis** [NA], distal surface: the proximal or contact surface of a tooth that is farthest from the midline of the dental arch. **f. doloro′sa,** the facial expression of a patient experiencing pain or severe sickness. **f. dorsa′lis antibra′chii,** f. posterior antebrachii. **f. dorsa′les digito′rum ma′nus** [NA], the posterior, or back (dorsal), surfaces of the fingers. **f. dorsa′les digito′rum pe′dis** [NA], the superior, or upper (dorsal), surfaces of the toes. **f. dorsa′lis os′sis sac′ri** [NA], the markedly convex and rough posterior, or dorsal, surface of the sacrum, which gives origin to the sacrospinalis and multifidus muscles; called also *posterior surface of sacrum.* **f. dorsa′lis ra′dii,** f. posterior radii. **f. dorsa′lis scap′ulae** [NA], the convex posterior surface of the scapula, which is divided into two unequal parts (superior and inferior) by the spine of the scapula; called also *dorsum* or *posterior surface of scapula.* **f. dorsa′lis ul′nae,** f. posterior ulnae. **f. exter′na os′sis fronta′lis** [NA], the external surface of the squama of the frontal bone; called also *f. frontalis ossis frontalis.*

f. ex'terna os'sis parieta'lis [NA], the externally directed surface of the parietal bone; called also *f. parietalis ossis parietalis*. **f. facia'lis den'tis,** NA alternative for *f. vestibularis dentis*. **f. fibula'ris cru'ris,** NA alternative for *f. lateralis cruris*. **f. fronta'lis os'sis fronta'lis,** f. externa ossis frontalis. **f. gas'trica lie'nis** [NA], the surface of the spleen that is in contact with the stomach. **f. glu'tea os'sis il'ii** [NA], the large external, or dorsal, surface of the ala of the ilium, on which are located the three gluteal lines; called also *gluteal surface of ilium*. **f. hepat'ica,** a thin face with sunken eyeballs, sallow complexion, and yellow conjunctivae, characteristic of certain chronic disorders of the liver. **f. hippocrat'ica,** a drawn, pinched, and pale appearance of the face, indicative of approaching death. **Hutchinson's f.,** a peculiar appearance in ophthalmoplegia externa, the eyeballs being fixed, the eyebrows raised, and the lids drooping. **f. infe'rior cer'ebri** [NA], the lower, or inferior, surface of the cerebrum; called also *basis cerebri* and *basis encephali*. **f. infe'rior hemisphe'rii cerebel'li** [NA], the inferior surface of the cerebellar hemisphere, formed by the inferior semilunar lobule, the biventral lobule, the tonsilla, and the flocculus. **f. infe'rior hemisphe'rii cer'ebri** [NA], the part of the cerebral hemisphere that rests on the tentorium and in the anterior and middle cranial fossae. **f. infe'rior hep'atis,** f. visceralis hepatis. **f. infe'rior lin'-guae** [NA], the under surface of the body of the tongue. **f. infe'rior pancre'atis** [NA], the inferior surface of the pancreas. **f. infe'rior par'tis petro'sae os'sis tempora'lis** [NA], f. infe'rior pyram'idis os'sis tempora'lis, that surface of the petrous part of the temporal bone which appears on the external surface of the base of the cranium. **f. inferolatera'lis prosta'tae** [NA], the convex inferolateral surface of the prostate, separated from the superior fascia of the pelvic diaphragm by a venous plexus. **f. infratempora'lis maxil'lae** [NA], the posterior convex surface of the body of the maxilla, bounded roughly by the inferior orbital fissure, the zygomatic process and associated ridge, maxillary tuberosity, and posterior margin of the nasal surface. **f. interloba'res pulmo'nis** [NA], the surface area of each lung lying within the oblique and horizontal fissures. **f. inter'na os'sis fronta'lis** [NA], the vertically situated, concave cerebral surface of the frontal bone; in its midline the sagittal sulcus is seen superiorly and the frontal crest inferiorly. Called also *f. cerebralis ossis frontalis*. **f. inter'na os'sis parieta'lis** [NA], the internal, or cerebral, surface of the parietal bone; called also *f. cerebralis ossis parietalis*. **f. intestina'lis u'teri** [NA], the convex posterior surface of the uterus, adjacent to the intestine. **f. labia'lis den'tis,** labial surface: the surface of an anterior tooth that is directed outward toward the lip. **f. latera'lis bra'chii** [NA], the outer, or lateral, surface of the upper arm. **f. latera'lis cru'ris** [NA], the outer, or lateral, surface of the leg; called also *f. fibularis cruris* [NA alternative]. **f. latera'lis den'tium incisivo'rum et canino'rum,** the contact surface of the incisor and canine teeth that is directed away from the midline of the dental arch. **f. latera'les digito'rum ma'nus** [NA], the lateral surfaces of the fingers; called also *facies radiales digitorum manus* [NA alternative], *margines radiales digitorum manus,* and *radial margins of fingers*. **f. latera'les digito'rum pe'dis** [NA], the lateral surfaces of the toes; called also *margines laterales digitorum pedis*. **f. latera'lis fem'oris** [NA], the outer, or lateral, surface of the thigh. **f. latera'lis tib'ulae** [NA], the area between the anterior and posterior borders of the body of the fibula. **f. latera'lis os'sis zygomat'ici** [NA], the anterior convex surface of the zygomatic bone; called also *f. malaris ossis zygomatici*. **f. latera'lis ova'rii** [NA], the surface of the ovary in contact with the lateral pelvic wall. **f. latera'lis ra'dii** [NA], the surface of the radius that gives attachment to the supinator and pronator teres muscles proximally, and underlies the tendons of the extensor carpi radialis longus and brevis muscles distally. **f. latera'lis tes'tis** [NA], the surface of the testis that is directed away from its fellow of the opposite side. **f. latera'lis tib'iae** [NA], the surface of the body of the tibia between the interosseous and anterior borders; called also *external border of tibia*. **leonine f., f. leonti'na** [L. "lion's face"], a peculiar, deeply furrowed, lion-like appearance of the face, seen in certain cases of advanced lepromatous leprosy; see *leontiasis*. **f. lingua'lis den'tis** [NA], lingual surface: the surface of a tooth that faces inward toward the tongue. **f. luna'ta acetab'uli** [NA], the articular portion of the acetabulum. **f. mala'ris os'sis zygomat'ici,** f. lateralis ossis zygomatici. **f. malleola'ris latera'lis ta'li** [NA], the large triangular facet on the talus that articulates with the lateral malleolus. **f. malleola'ris media'lis ta'li** [NA], the narrow facet on the talus continuous with the superior surface; it articulates with the medial malleolus. **Marshall Hall's f.,** the facies of hydrocephalus: a triangular face with a broad forehead and prominent frontal bones. **f. masticato'ria den'tis,** masticatory surface: 1. f. occlusalis dentis. 2. the occlusal surface of a tooth upon which mastication can occur; called also *working occlusal surface*. **f. maxilla'ris a'lae majo'ris** [NA], a small surface on the inferior part of the great wing of the sphenoid bone above the pterygoid processes; it is perforated by the foramen rotundum. Called also *f. sphenomaxillaris alae magnae*. **f.**

maxilla'ris lam'inae perpendicula'ris os'sis palati'ni [NA], **f. maxilla'ris par'tis perpendicula'ris os'sis palati'ni,** the lateral surface of the perpendicular plate of the palatine bone, which is in relation to the maxilla. Posteriorly and inferiorly it contains the greater palatine sulcus, which forms the greater palatine canal with a corresponding groove on the maxilla. **f. media'lis bra'chii** [NA], the inner, or medial, surface of the upper arm. **f. media'lis cartilag'inis arytenoi'deae** [NA], the surface of the arytenoid cartilage that faces medially, toward the opposite arytenoid cartilage. **f. media'lis cer'ebri** [NA], the surface of the cerebrum parallel to and facing the median plane. **f. media'lis cru'ris** [NA], the inner, or medial, surface of the leg; called also *f. tibialis cruris* [NA alternative]. **f. media'lis den'tium incisivo'rum et canino'rum,** the contact surface of the incisor and canine teeth that is directed toward the midline of the dental arch. **f. media'les digito'rum ma'nus** [NA], the medial surfaces of the fingers; called also *facies ulnares digitorum manus* [NA alternative], *margines ulnares digitorum manus,* and *ulnar margins of fingers*. **f. media'les digito'rum pe'dis** [NA], the medial surfaces of the toes; called also *margines mediales digitorum pedis*. **f. media'lis fem'oris** [NA], the inner, or medial, surface of the thigh. **f. media'lis fib'ulae** [NA], the narrow area on the body of the fibula between the interosseous and anterior borders. **f. media'lis hemisphe'rii cer'ebri** [NA], the surface of the cerebral hemisphere parallel to and facing both the median plane and the corresponding surface of the opposite hemisphere. **f. media'lis ova'rii** [NA], the side of the ovary in contact with the fimbriated end of the uterine tube and the intestine. **f. media'lis pulmo'nis** [NA], the surface area of each lung lying medially next to the vertebral column and mediastinum; called also *f. mediastinalis pulmonis*. **f. media'lis tes'tis** [NA], the surface of the testis that is directed toward its fellow of the opposite side. **f. media'lis tib'iae** [NA], the slightly convex surface of the body of the tibia between the anterior and medial borders. **f. media'lis ul'nae** [NA], the smooth, rounded, internal surface of the ulna. **f. mediastina'lis pulmo'nis,** f. medialis pulmonis. **f. mesia'lis den'tis** [NA], mesial surface: the contact or proximal surface of the incisor or canine tooth that is closest to the midline of the dental arch. **mitral f., mitrotricuspid f.,** the appearance of the face of some patients with mitral disease of long duration, marked by rosy, flushed cheeks and dilated capillaries. **moon f.,** see under *face*. **myasthenic f.,** the characteristic facial expression in myasthenia gravis, caused by ptosis and weakness of the facial muscles. **myopathic f.,** the peculiar facial expression produced by relaxation of the facial muscles, as in Landouzy-Dejerine dystrophy. **f. nasa'lis lam'inae horizonta'lis os'sis palati'ni** [NA], the superior surface of the horizontal part of the palatine bone; it forms the posterior part of the floor of the nasal cavity. Called also *f. nasalis partis horizontalis ossis palatini*. **f. nasa'lis lam'inae perpendicula'ris os'sis palati'ni** [NA], the medial surface of the perpendicular plate of the palatine bone; it articulates with the middle and inferior nasal conchae. Called also *f. nasalis partis perpendicularis ossis palatini*. **f. nasa'lis maxil'lae** [NA], the surface of the body of the maxilla that helps form the lateral wall of the nasal cavity; it is bounded roughly by the following: medial margin of the orbital surface, medial margin of the infratemporal surface, the palatine process, and the nasal notch. **f. nasa'lis par'tis horizonta'lis os'sis palati'ni,** f. nasalis laminae horizontalis ossis palatini. **f. nasa'lis par'tis perpendicula'ris os'sis palati'ni,** f. nasalis laminae perpendicularis ossis palatini. **f. occlusa'lis den'tis** [NA], occlusal surface: the surface of a posterior tooth which comes in contact with structures of the opposite jaw when the jaws are closed. **f. orbita'lis a'lae mag'nae, f. orbita'lis a'lae majo'ris** [NA], the quadrilateral surface on the great wing of the sphenoid bone that forms the major part of the lateral wall of the orbit; called also *orbital border* or *surface of sphenoid bone*. **f. orbita'lis maxil'lae** [NA], a triangular surface on the body of the maxilla that forms the greater part of the floor of the orbit. **f. orbita'lis os'sis fronta'lis** [NA], the triangularly shaped plates of the frontal bone that form most of the roof of each orbit and the floor of the anterior cranial fossa; they are separated by the ethmoidal notch. **f. orbita'lis os'sis zygomat'ici** [NA], the part of the zygomatic bone that helps form the lateral wall of the orbit. **f. [os'sea] cra'nii,** the bony skeleton of the face. **f. palati'na lam'inae horizonta'lis os'sis palati'ni** [NA], **f. palati'na par'tis horizonta'lis os'sis palati'ni,** the inferior surface of the horizontal part of the palatine bone; it forms the posterior part of the hard palate. **f. palma'res digito'rum ma'nus** [NA], the ventral, or front (palmar), surfaces of the fingers; called also *f. volares digitorum manus*. **f. parieta'lis os'sis parieta'lis,** f. externa ossis parietalis. **Parkinson's f., parkinsonian f.,** a stolid masklike expression of the face, with infrequent blinking, pathognomonic of parkinsonism; see also *parkinsonian syndrome*, under *syndrome*, and see *paralysis agitans*. **f. patella'ris fem'oris,** the smooth anterior continuation of the condyles that forms the surface of the femur articulating with the patella; called also *anterior intercondylar fossa of femur*, and *patellar fossa of femur*. **f. pelvi'na os'sis sac'ri** [NA], the smooth, concave, ventrocaudally directed surface of the sacrum that helps form the posterior wall of the pelvis; called also *anterior surface of sacrum.* **f. planta′res digito′rum pe′dis** [NA], the inferior, or lower (plantar), surfaces of the toes. **f. poplit′ea fem′oris** [NA], the triangular area forming the superior part of the floor of the popliteal fossa; called also *planum popliteum femoris.* **f. poste′rior antebra′chii** [NA], the dorsal, or back, surface of the forearm; called also *f. dorsalis antibrachii.* **f. poste′rior bra′chii** [NA], the dorsal, or back, surface of the upper arm. **f. poste′rior cartilag′inis arytenoi′deae** [NA], the concave dorsal surface of the arytenoid cartilage, to which various laryngeal muscles are attached. **f. poste′rior cor′neae** [NA], the posterior surface of the cornea, which forms the anterior boundary of the anterior chamber. **f. poste′rior cru′ris** [NA], the dorsal, or back, surface of the leg. **f. poste′rior den′tium premola′rium et mola′rium,** posterior surface of premolar and molar teeth: the contact surface of the premolar and the molar teeth that is directed away from the midline of the dental arch. **f. poste′rior fem′oris** [NA], the dorsal, or back, surface of the thigh. **f. poste′rior fib′ulae** [NA], the large area between the posterior and interosseous borders of the body of the fibula, presenting the medial crest. **f. poste′rior glan′dulae suprarena′lis** [NA], the portion of the adrenal gland that is directed toward the posterior body wall. **f. poste′rior hep′atis,** pars posterior facies diaphragmaticae hepatis. **f. poste′rior hu′meri** [NA], the surface of the humerus that is subdivided obliquely by the radial groove to give attachment to the lateral and medial heads of the triceps muscle. **f. poste′rior i′ridis** [NA], the posterior surface of the iris, directed toward the posterior chamber of the eye. **f. poste′rior len′tis** [NA], the posterior surface of the lens, directed toward the vitreous body of the eye. **f. poste′rior palpebra′rum** [NA], the internal surface of the eyelids in contact with the eyeball and covered by the conjunctiva. **f. poste′rior pancre′atis** [NA], the posterior surface of the pancreas. **f. poste′rior par′tis petro′sae os′sis tempora′lis** [NA], the surface of the petrous part of the temporal bone that forms part of the anterior portion of the floor of the posterior cranial fossa; called also *f. posterior pyramidis ossis temporalis.* **f. poste′rior prosta′tae** [NA], the dorsal surface of the prostate, separated by fascia from the anterior wall of the rectum. **f. poste′rior pyram′idis os′sis tempora′lis,** f. posterior partis petrosae ossis temporalis. **f. poste′rior ra′dii** [NA], the posterior surface of the radius, which gives attachment to the supinator, abductor pollicis longus, and extensor pollicis brevis muscles; called also *f. dorsalis radii.* **f. poste′rior re′nis** [NA], the dorsal surface of the kidney, directed toward the posterior body wall, and not covered by peritoneum. **f. poste′rior tib′iae** [NA], the surface of the body of the tibia between the medial and interosseous borders; in the proximal third presenting the soleal line. **f. poste′rior ul′nae** [NA], the posterolaterally directed surface of the ulna; called also *f. dorsalis ulnae.* **Potter f.,** the facial appearance characteristic of bilateral renal agenesis: flattened nose, receding chin, wide interpupillary space, and large, low-set ears. **f. pulmona′lis cor′dis** [NA], the surface of the heart that faces the lung. **f. radia′les digito′rum ma′nus,** NA alternative for *f. laterales digitorum manus.* **f. rena′lis glan′dulae suprarena′lis** [NA], the surface of the adrenal gland that is directed toward the kidney, being separated from it by a layer of fat; called also *basis glandulae suprarenalis* and *inferior margin of suprarenal gland.* **f. rena′lis lie′nis** [NA], the surface of the spleen that is in contact with the left kidney. **f. sacropelvi′na os′sis il′ii** [NA], an irregular area on the inner surface of the ala of the ilium, posterior to the iliac fossa; it contains the iliac tuberosity and the auricular surface. Called also *sacropelvic surface of the ilium.* **f. scaphoi′dea,** dish face. **f. sphenomaxilla′ris a′lae mag′nae,** f. maxillaris alae majoris. **f. sternocosta′lis cor′dis** [NA], the convex surface of the heart, which in general is directed anteriorly and somewhat superiorly, being formed mainly by the right ventricle, and to a lesser degree by the left ventricle and the atria. **f. supe′rior hemisphe′rii cerebel′li** [NA], the superior surface of the cerebellar hemisphere, consisting of the ala of the lobulus centralis, the lobulus quadrangularis, the lobulus simplex, and the superior semilunar lobule. **f. supe′rior hep′atis,** pars superior faciei diaphragmaticae hepatis. **f. supe′rior troch′leae ta′li** [NA], the broad, smooth surface of the talus that articulates with the tibia. **f. superolatera′lis cer′ebri** [NA], the convex outer surface of the cerebrum, which faces the calvaria; called also *f. convexa cerebri.* **f. symphys′eos os′sis pu′bis, f. symphysia′lis** [NA], the rough, ovoid, medial surface of the body of the pubic bone, by which it articulates at the pubic symphysis with its fellow of the opposite side. **f. tempora′lis a′lae mag′nae, f. tempora′lis a′lae majo′ris** [NA], the lateral and inferior surface of the great wing of the sphenoid bone, divided by the infratemporal crest into a superior part that forms a portion of the wall of the temporal fossa, and an inferior part that forms part of the wall of the infratemporal fossa. **f. tempora′lis os′sis fronta′lis** [NA], the slightly concave surface of the frontal bone that forms the upper part of the wall of the temporal fossa and gives attachment to the anterosuperior part of the temporalis muscle. **f. tempora′lis os′sis zygomat′ici** [NA], the internal, concave surface of the zygomatic bone, facing the temporal and infratemporal fossae. **f. tempora′lis par′tis squamo′sae** [NA], **f. tempora′lis squa′mae tempora′lis,** the external surface of the squamous part of the temporal bone, the anterior part of which forms a portion of the temporal fossa. **f. tibia′lis cru′ris,** NA alternative for *f. medialis cruris.* **typhoid f., f. typho′sa,** the vacant and bewildered, often wild and defiant expression, with face flushed and a dusky, leaden hue, seen in early stages of typhoid fever. **f. ulna′res digito′rum ma′nus,** NA alternative for *f. mediales digitorum manus.* **f. urethra′lis pe′nis** [NA], the surface of the penis overlying the urethra, and opposite the dorsum penis. **f. vesica′lis u′teri** [NA], the flat anterior surface of the uterus, adjacent to the urinary bladder. **f. vestibula′ris den′tis** [NA], vestibular surface: the surface of a tooth that is directed outward toward the vestibule of the mouth, including the buccal and labial surfaces; called also *f. facialis dentis* [NA alternative] or *facial surface.* **f. viscera′lis hep′atis** [NA], the posteroinferior surface of the liver, which is in contact with various abdominal viscera; called also *f. inferior hepatis.* **f. viscera′lis lie′nis** [NA], the surface of the spleen which comes in contact with various other viscera, including the colon (facies colica), kidney (facies renalis), and stomach (facies gastrica). **f. vola′ris antibra′chii,** f. anterior antebrachii. **f. vola′res digito′rum ma′nus,** f. palmares digitorum manus. **f. vola′ris ra′dii,** f. anterior radii. **f. vola′ris ul′nae,** f. anterior ulnae.

facilitation (fah-sil″ĭ-ta′shun) [L. *facilis* easy] the promotion or hastening of any natural process; the reverse of inhibition; specifically, the effect of a nerve impulse acting across a synapse, and resulting in an increase in the efficacy of subsequent impulses in that nerve fiber, or impulses in other convergent nerve fibers, in exciting the postsynaptic element. See *law of facilitation.* **Wedensky f.,** facilitation across a block; when there is a complete block to nerve conduction the threshold of the nerve below the block to electric stimulation is lowered.

facilitative (fah-sil′ĭ-ta″tiv) in pharmacology, denoting a reaction arising as an indirect result of drug action, as development of an infection after the normal microflora has been altered by an antibiotic.

facilitory (fah-sil′ĭ-tōr-e) making easier; promoting or hastening a natural process; acting so as to render a neural element more easily excitable.

facing (fās′ing) a piece of porcelain or resin fashioned to represent the facial surface of a tooth and reinforced by metal so as to restore the full form of the natural tooth.

facio- (fa′she-o) [L. *facies* face] a combining form denoting relationship to the face.

faciobrachial (fa″she-o-bra′ke-al) [*facio-* + Gr. *brachiōn* arm] pertaining to the face and arm.

faciocephalalgia (fa″she-o-sef″ah-lal′je-ah) [*facio-* + Gr. *kephalē* head + *-algia*] neuralgic pain in the face and neck attributed to disorders of the autonomic (vegetative) nervous system.

faciocervical (fa″she-o-ser′vĕ-kal) [*facio-* + L. *cervix* neck] pertaining to or affecting the face and neck.

faciolingual (fa″she-o-ling′gwal) [*facio-* + L. *lingua* tongue] pertaining to the face and tongue.

facioplasty (fa″she-o-plas′te) [*facio-* + Gr. *plassein* to form] plastic surgery of the face.

facioplegia (fa″she-o-ple′je-ah) [*facio-* + Gr. *plēgē* stroke] facial paralysis.

facioscapulohumeral (fa″she-o-skap″u-lo-hu′mer-al) pertaining to the face, scapula, and arm.

faciostenosis (fa″she-o-stĕ-no′sis) failure of the midface to grow.

F.A.C.O.G. Fellow of the American College of Obstetricians and Gynecologists.

F.A.C.P. Fellow of the American College of Physicians.

F.A.C.S. Fellow of the American College of Surgeons.

F.A.C.S.M. Fellow of the American College of Sports Medicine.

F-actin see *actin.*

factitial (fak-tish′al) produced by artificial means; unintentionally produced.

factitious (fak-tish′us) [L. *factitiosus*] artificial; not natural.

factor (fak′tor) [L. "maker"] an agent or element that contributes to the production of a result, such as a chemical compound that is essential to a reaction (e.g., a coagulation factor); a quantity or symbol employed in a specific formula or, in the study of heredity, a particular gene; a property of immunoglobulins by which they can be identified by a given set of reagents. **accelerator f.,** see *Factor V,* under *coagulation f′s.* **accessory f., accessory food f.,** a vitamin. **activation f.,** see *Factor XII,* under *coagulation f′s.* **adrenocorticotropic releasing f. (ACTH-RF),** corticotropin releasing f. **aldosterone stimulating f.,** a hypothetical hormone of the diencephalon that stimulates the elaboration of aldosterone by the zona glomerulosa of the adrenal cortex. **alpha f.,** a name formerly given the hormone(s) that governs the estrous phase of the ovarian cycle; see *estrogenic hormones,* under *hormone.* **anabolism-promot-**

ing f., a principle which enhances protein utilization, permitting growth or tissue restitution with a lower level of protein intake than possible without it, an activity noted in various antibiotics and ataractics. Abbreviated APF. **animal protein f.,** an element in animal proteins found to be essential to maximal growth of animals; vitamin B_{12}. Abbreviated APF. **antiachromotrichia f.,** pantothenic acid. **antiacrodynia f.,** pyridoxine. **antialopecia f.,** inositol. **antianemia f.,** cyanocobalamin. **antianemia f. for chicks,** a vitamin, folic acid, in spinach and other green leaves, which prevents anemia in chicks. **anti-black tongue f.,** niacin. **anticanities f., antidermatitis f. of chicks,** pantothenic acid. **antidermatitis f. of rats,** pyridoxine. **anti-egg white f.,** biotin. **anti-gray hair f.,** pantothenic acid. **antihemophilic f.,** 1. see *Factor VIII,* under *coagulation f's.* Abbreviated AHF. 2. [USP] a sterile freeze-dried powder containing the Factor VIII fraction obtained from suitable whole-blood donors. **antihemophilic f., cryo-precipitated** [USP], a sterile, frozen concentrate of human antihemophilic factor prepared from the Factor VIII–rich cryoprotein fraction of human venous plasma obtained from suitable whole-blood donors from a single unit of plasma derived from whole blood or by plasmapheresis, collected and processed in a closed system. Called also *human antihemophilic f.* **antihemophilic f., human,** antihemophilic f., def. 2. **antihemophilic f. A,** see *Factor VIII,* under *coagulation f's.* **antihemophilic f. B,** see *Factor IX,* under *coagulation f's.* **antihemophilic f. C,** see *Factor XI,* under *coagulation f's.* **antihemorrhagic f.,** vitamin K. **antineuritic f.,** thiamine. **antinuclear f. (ANF),** an autoantibody against constituents of cell nuclei that may be demonstrated by immunofluorescence and is present in the sera of patients with systemic lupus erythematosus and occasionally in rheumatoid arthritis and other collagen diseases. **antipellagra f.,** niacin. **anti-pernicious anemia f.,** cyanocobalamin. **antirachitic f.,** vitamin D. **antiscorbutic f.,** ascorbic acid. **antisterility f.,** vitamin E. **antistiffness f.,** a factor present in raw cream, crude molasses, and unheated cane juice, lack of which in animals causes stiffness of the wrist, and later emaciation, weakness, and death. **antixerophthalmia f., antixerotic f.,** vitamin A. **f. B,** a complement component C3 proactivator which participates in the alternative pathway of complement activation. The factor B-C3b complex is split by factor D, which leads to formation of C3 convertase, which in turn acts in the alternative pathway. **beta f.,** former name for progesterone. **Bittner milk f.,** mouse mammary tumor virus. **blastogenic f. (BF),** lymphocyte transforming f. **bone f.,** a fundamental factor in periodontoclasia, being the systemic regulatory influence upon the response of alveolar bone to local irritants. **Bx f.,** aminobenzoic acid. **C f.,** a factor found in the soluble part of cytoplasm which promotes the contraction of mitochondria. **C3 nephritic f.,** a gamma globulin (not an immunoglobulin) in the plasma of certain individuals with membranoproliferative glomerulonephritis with hypocomplementemia. C3 nephritic factor initiates the alternative pathway of complement activation and stabilizes alternative pathway C3 convertase. **Castle's f.,** intrinsic factor, the mucoprotein in gastric juice necessary for the absorption of cyanocobalamin. **chemotactic f.,** the substance that brings about chemotaxis. **chick antidermatitis f.,** pantothenic acid. **chick antipellagra f.,** pantothenic acid. **chick growth f. S,** strepogenin. **Christmas f.,** see *Factor IX,* under *coagulation f's.* **chromotrichial f.,** aminobenzoic acid. **citrovorum f.,** folinic acid. **clone-inhibiting f. (CIF),** a lymphokine that exhibits a direct cytostatic effect against actively growing tissue-culture tumor cell lines. **coagulation f's,** substances in the blood that are essential to the clotting process and hence, to the maintenance of normal hemostasis. They are designated by Roman numerals, to which the notation "a" is added to indicate the activated state. Platelet factors, designated by Arabic numerals, also play a role in coagulation. *Factor I,* fibrinogen: a high-molecular-weight plasma protein which is converted to fibrin through the action of thrombin. Deficiency of this factor results in afibrinogenemia or hypofibrinogenemia. Several molecular forms of this factor have been recognized. *Factor II,* prothrombin: a protein present in the plasma that, in theoretical hematology, is converted to thrombin by extrinsic prothrombin converting principle. More than one molecular form has been detected. Deficiency of this factor leads to hypoprothrombinemia. *Factor III,* tissue thromboplastin: a material derived from several sources in the body (brain, lung, etc.) and important in the formation of extrinsic prothrombin converting principle in the extrinsic pathway of blood coagulation. Called also *tissue factor. Factor IV,* calcium: a factor required in many phases of blood coagulation. *Factor V,* proaccelerin: a heat- and storage-labile material, present in plasma but not in serum, functioning in both the intrinsic and extrinsic pathways of blood coagulation. Deficiency of this factor, an autosomal recessive trait, leads to a rare hemorrhagic tendency, known as Owen's disease or parahemophilia, which varies greatly in severity. Called also *accelerator globulin (AcG)* and *labile factor. Factor VI,* a factor (accelerin) previously thought to be an activated form of Factor V. It no longer is considered in the scheme of hemostasis, and hence it is assigned neither a name

nor a function at this time. *Factor VII,* proconvertin: a heat- and storage-stable factor participating only in the extrinsic pathway of blood coagulation. Deficiency of this factor which may be hereditary (autosomal recessive) or acquired (associated with vitamin K deficiency) results in a hemorrhagic tendency. Called also *prothrombokinase, autoprothrombin I, serum prothrombin conversion accelerator (SPCA),* and *stable factor. Factor VIII,* antihemophilic factor (AHF): a relatively storage-labile factor participating only in the intrinsic pathway of blood coagulation. Deficiency of this factor, when transmitted as a sex-linked recessive trait, causes classical hemophilia (hemophilia A). More than one molecular form of this factor has been discovered. Called also *antihemophilic globulin (AHG)* and *antihemophilic factor A. Factor IX,* plasma thromboplastin component (PTC): a relatively storage-stable substance involved only in the intrinsic pathway of blood coagulation. Deficiency of this factor results in a hemorrhagic syndrome called hemophilia B or Christmas disease, which is similar to classical hemophilia (hemophilia A). More than one molecular form has been discovered. Called also *autoprothrombin II, Christmas factor,* and *antihemophilic factor B. Factor X,* Stuart factor: a storage-stable factor that participates in both the intrinsic and extrinsic pathways of blood coagulation. Deficiency of this factor may cause a systemic coagulation disorder (Factor X deficiency). Called also *autoprothrombin C, Prower factor, Stuart-Prower factor,* and *thrombokinase. Factor XI,* plasma thromboplastin antecedent (PTA): a stable factor involved in the intrinsic pathway of blood coagulation. Deficiency of this factor results in a systemic blood-clotting defect called hemophilia C or Rosenthal's syndrome, that may resemble classical hemophilia. Called also *antihemophilic factor C. Factor XII,* Hageman factor: a stable factor activated by contact with glass or other foreign surfaces, which initiates the intrinsic process of blood coagulation *in vitro.* Deficiency of this factor results in prolonged *in vitro* blood clotting but overt clinical bleeding is rare. Called also *glass, contact,* or *activation factor. Factor XIII,* fibrin stabilizing factor (FSF): a factor that polymerizes fibrin monomers so that they become stable and insoluble in urea, thus enabling fibrin to form a firm blood clot. Deficiency of this factor produces a clinical hemorrhagic diathesis. Called also *fibrinase* and *Laki-Lorand factor (LLF).* The inactive form is also known as *protransglutaminase,* and the active form as *transglutaminase. platelet factor 1,* adsorbed Factor V from the plasma. *platelet factor 2,* an accelerator of the thrombin-fibrinogen reaction, attached to platelets. *platelet factor 3,* a substance, probably a lipoprotein, extracted from platelets, which contributes to the interaction of plasma coagulation proteins in the generation of intrinsic prothrombin converting principle. *platelet factor 4,* an intracellular protein component of blood platelets, capable of neutralizing the antithrombic activity of heparin in the fibrinogen-fibrin reaction and the inhibitory effect of heparin in the thromboplastin generation test. **coenzyme f.,** diaphorase. **contact f.,** see *Factor XII,* under *coagulation f's.* **corticotropin releasing f. (CRF),** a factor elaborated by the hypothalamus at the median eminence, which stimulates the release of corticotropin by the anterior pituitary gland. **Curling f.,** griseofulvin. **f. D,** a factor which, when activated (D̄) serves as a serine esterase that participates in the alternative pathway of complement activation by splitting factor B from C3b. **Day's f.,** folic acid. **diabetogenic f.,** a substance of unknown constitution associated with extracts of growth hormone from the anterior pituitary which, when injected into normal dogs, causes them to become diabetic. **diffusion f.,** hyaluronidase. **Duran-Reynals f.,** hyaluronidase. **eluate f.,** pyridoxine. **erythrocyte maturation f. (E.M.F.),** a former name for vitamin B_{12} (cyanocobalamin). **erythropoietic stimulating f. (E.S.F.),** a name given a factor in the body which stimulates the production of erythrocytes; probably identical with erythropoietin. **extrinsic f.,** vitamin B_{12} (cyanocobalamin). **F f.,** the episome which determines the mating type of conjugating bacteria, being present in the donor (male) bacterium and absent in the recipient (female); called also *F element, sex f.,* and *fertility f.* **fermentation L. casei f.,** folic acid. **fertility f.,** F f. **fibrin stabilizing f.,** see *Factor XIII,* under *coagulation f's.* **filtrate f., filtrate f. II,** pantothenic acid. **follicle stimulating hormone releasing f. (FRF, FSHRF),** gonadotropin releasing hormone. **galactopoietic f.,** prolactin. **gastric anti-pernicious anemia f., gastric intrinsic f.,** intrinsic f. **glass f.,** see *Factor XII,* under *coagulation f's.* **glucose tolerance f.,** a biologically active complex of chromium and nicotinic acid that facilitates the reaction of insulin with receptor sites on tissues. **gonadotropin releasing f. (GnRF),** see under hormone. **growth hormone releasing f. (GRF),** a postulated hormone elaborated by the median eminence of the hypothalamus, which stimulates the release of growth hormone from the anterior pituitary gland. Called also *growth hormone releasing hormone (GH-RH)* and *somatotropin releasing hormone (SRF).* **f. H,** biotin. **Hageman f. (HF),** see *Factor XII,* under *coagulation f's.* **histamine releasing f.,** a lymphokine that is produced by sensitized lymphocytes on stimulation by antigen and that leads to histamine release by basophils. **HL-A f's,** a single genetic system of closely related human histocompatibility antigens that are present on leukocytes. The expression of these antigens is determined by two closely linked loci termed LA and

Four. **hyperglycemic-glycogenolytic f.,** see *glucagon.* **f. I,** 1. see under *coagulation f's.* 2. pyridoxine. **f. II,** 1. see under *coagulation f's.* 2. pantothenic acid. **f. III,** see under *coagulation f's.* **inhibiting f's,** factors elaborated by one structure (as by the hypothalamus) that inhibit the release of hormones by another structure (as by the anterior pituitary gland), including melanocyte-stimulating hormone inhibiting factor and prolactin inhibiting factor. The term is applied to substances of unknown chemical structure, while substances of established chemical identity are called *inhibiting hormones* (see under *hormone*). **intermediate lobe inhibiting f.,** melanocyte-stimulating hormone inhibiting f. **intrinsic f.,** a glycoprotein secreted by the parietal cells of the gastric glands, necessary for the absorption of vitamin B_{12} (cyanocobalamin, extrinsic factor). Lack of intrinsic factor, with consequent deficiency of vitamin B_{12}, results in pernicious anemia. **f. IV,** see under *coagulation f's.* **f. IX,** see under *coagulation f's.* **labile f.,** see *Factor V,* under *coagulation f's.* **Lactobacillus casei f.,** folic acid. **Lactobacillus lactis Dorner f.,** cyanocobalamin. **lactogenic f.,** prolactin. **Laki-Lorand f.,** see *Factor XIII,* under *coagulation f's.* **LE f.,** an immunoglobulin (a 7S antibody) that reacts with leukocyte nuclei, found in the serum of patients with systemic lupus erythematosus. **lethal f's,** disorders of genetic material which lead to the death of the zygote, or of the individual developing from it before attaining the age of reproduction. This can be a matter of lethal genes or deficiencies due to missing sections. **leukocyte inhibitory f. (LIF),** a lymphokine that prevents polymorphonuclear leukocytes from migrating. **leukocyte mitogenic f. (LMF),** a lymphokine substance causing blast transformation and synthesis of DNA in normal lymphocytes. **leukocytosis promoting f.,** Menkin's name for a substance or factor liberated by injured cells, which is responsible for the leukocytosis accompanying inflammatory processes; abbreviated LPF. **leukopenic f.,** Menkin's name for a factor in inflammatory exudates which may be the cause of the initial leukopenia accompanying inflammatory processes. **liver filtrate f.,** pantothenic acid. **liver Lactobacillus casei f.,** folic acid. **LLD f.,** cyanocobalamin. **luteinizing hormone releasing f. (LRF),** a factor elaborated by the hypothalamus at the median eminence, which stimulates the release of luteinizing hormone by the anterior pituitary gland; called also *LH releasing f.* **lymph node permeability f. (LNPF),** a substance from normal lymph nodes which produces vascular permeability. **lymphocyte transforming f. (LTF),** a lymphokine that causes transformation and clonal expansion of nonsensitized lymphocytes; called also *blastogenic f., mitogenic f.,* and *recruitment f.* **lysogenic f.,** bacteriophage. **macrophage-activating f.,** a factor released by sensitized lymphocytes that induces in macrophages an increased content of lysosomal enzymes, more aggressive phagocytosis, and increased mitotic activity. **Marsh f., Marsh-Bendall f.,** a soluble muscle protein, derived from the sarcoplasmic reticulum, which produces muscle relaxation by interfering with the enzymatic (ATPase) breakdown of ATP and consequently with contraction of the muscle; called also *relaxing f.* **maturation f.,** a substance that causes cells to mature (differentiate). **mauve f.,** a substance in the urine that yields a mauve color on paper chromatography; see *malvaria.* **melanocyte stimulating hormone inhibiting f. (MIF),** a factor elaborated by the hypothalamus at the median eminence, which inhibits the release of melanocyte-stimulating hormone by the anterior pituitary gland; called also *intermediate lobe inhibiting f.* and *MSH inhibiting f.* **melanocyte stimulating hormone releasing f. (MRF, MSHRF),** a factor elaborated by the hypothalamus at the median eminence, which stimulates release of melanocyte-stimulating hormone by the anterior pituitary gland. **migration inhibiting f. (MIF),** a lymphokine released from sensitized lymphocytes which inhibits the migration of macrophages. **milk f.,** mouse mammary tumor virus. **mitogenic f.,** lymphocyte transforming f. **modifying f's,** polygenes, or multiple factors, which affect the degree of expressivity of another gene; called also *modifiers* or *modifying genes.* **mouse antialopecia f.,** inositol. **mouse mammary tumor f.,** see under *virus.* **MSH inhibiting f.,** melanocyte-stimulating hormone inhibiting f. **müllerian regression f., müllerian duct inhibitory f.,** a factor postulated to be present in the male embryo which inhibits development of the wolffian ducts. **multiple f's,** in heredity, two or more genes which cooperate or blend or cumulate to produce a certain character. **myocardial depressant f. (MDF),** a peptide formed in response to a fall in systemic blood pressure, that has a negatively inotropic effect on myocardial muscle fibers. **N f.,** a factor occurring in yeast, meat, liver, and wheat germ, the absence of which from an otherwise complete diet causes rats to voluntarily consume more alcohol than they do when factor N is present in the diet. **Nebenthau f.,** a chemical group, N:C(OH)·CH₂, derived from urea; an essential constituent of the barbituric acid hypnotics. **necrotizing f.,** necrotoxin. **nerve growth f.,** a protein consisting of two identical polypeptide chains associated with two gamma subunits (enzymes) and two alpha subunits; first isolated from mouse sarcoma and later from snake venom and mouse salivary glands, it stimulates the growth of sensory and sympathetic nerve cells and of the

adrenal medulla and has been found to be secreted by a variety of normal and neoplastic cells, including those of man. Abbreviated NGF. **Norit eluate f.,** folic acid. **osteoclast activating f.,** a lymphokine substance produced by lymphocytes which facilitates bone resorption. **pellagra-preventive f.,** niacin. **platelet f's,** factors important in hemostasis which are contained in or attached to the platelets. See *platelet factors 1, 2, 3,* and *4,* under *coagulation f's.* See also *platelet cofactors,* under *cofactor.* **platelet activating f. (PAF),** an immunologically produced substance which leads to clumping and degranulation of blood platelets. **P.-P. f.,** niacin. **prolactin inhibiting f. (PIF),** a factor elaborated by the hypothalamus at the median eminence, which inhibits the secretion of prolactin by the anterior pituitary gland. **prolactin releasing f. (PRF),** a factor(s) elaborated by the hypothalamus at the median eminence, which stimulates the release of prolactin by the anterior pituitary gland. In human subjects, thyrotropin releasing hormon (protirelin) can act as a prolactin releasing factor. **proliferation inhibiting f. (PIF),** a lymphokine that inhibits mitosis in tissue-culture cells. **Prower f.,** see *Factor X,* under *coagulation f's.* **f. R,** folic acid. **R f.,** the bacterial plasmid (R plasmid) responsible for resistance to antibiotics; it is transmitted to other bacterial cells by conjugation, as well as to the progeny of any cell containing it. The portions required for replication and transmission are called resistance transfer factors (RTF), to which are attached various R genes mediating specific resistances. **rat acrodynia f.,** pyridoxine. **recruitment f.,** lymphocyte transforming f. **reducing f.,** ascorbic acid. **relaxing f.,** Marsh f. **releasing f's,** factors elaborated in one structure (as in the hypothalamus) that effect the release of hormones from another structure (as from the anterior pituitary gland), including corticotropin releasing factor, melanocyte stimulating hormone releasing factor, and prolactin releasing factor. The term is applied to substances of unknown chemical structure, while substances of established chemical identity are called *releasing hormones* (see under *hormone*). **resistance-inducing f.,** see *Rubin's test* (def. 2), under *tests.* **resistance transfer f.,** see *R f.* **restropic f.,** an unidentified substance in extracts of the anterior pituitary claimed to stimulate the reticuloendothelial system. **Rh f., Rhesus f.,** antigens (agglutinogens) present on the membrane of red blood cells; see *blood group.* **rheumatoid f.,** a protein (IgM) of high molecular weight, detectable by serological tests, which is found in the serum of most patients with rheumatoid arthritis and in other related and unrelated diseases and sometimes in apparently normal persons. Abbreviated RF. **f. S,** biotin. **separation f.,** the ratio of the relative concentration of two isotopes after processing, to their relative concentration before processing. **sex f.,** F f. **Simon's septic f.,** decrease of eosinophils and increase of neutrophils in the blood in pyogenic infections. **SLR f.,** folic acid. **somatotropin releasing f. (SRF),** growth hormone releasing f. **spreading f.,** hyaluronidase. **stable f.,** see *Factor VII,* under *coagulation f's.* **Streptococcus lactis R f.,** folic acid. **Stuart f., Stuart-Prower f.,** see *Factor X,* under *coagulation f's.* **sulfation f.,** somatomedin. **thyrotropin releasing f. (TRF),** see under *hormone.* **transfer f. (TF),** a factor occurring in sensitized lymphocytes that has the capacity to transfer delayed hypersensitivity to a normal (nonreactive) individual. **Trapp's f.,** the last two figures expressive of the specific gravity of urine; when multiplied by 2 they give the number of parts of solids per 1000. **tumor-angiogenesis f.,** a factor produced by cancer cells of solid tumors that stimulates the growth of blood vessels into the tumor. **tumor necrosis f.,** a glycopeptide appearing in the blood in the presence of endotoxins; it is capable of producing *in vitro* necrosis of tumor cells but not of normal cells. **f. U,** folic acid. **f. V,** 1. see under *coagulation f's.* 2. nicotinamide-adenine dinucleotide phosphate (NADP); see under *dinucleotide.* **f. VI,** see under *coagulation f's.* **f. VII,** see under *coagulation f's.* **f. VIII,** see under *coagulation f's.* **f. W,** biotin. **Wills f.,** folic acid. **f. X,** 1. see under *coagulation f's.* 2. biotin. **f. XI,** see under *coagulation f's.* **f. XII,** see under *coagulation f's.* **yeast eluate f.,** pyridoxine. **yeast filtrate f.,** pantothenic acid. **yeast L. casei f.,** folic acid.

facultative (fak′ul-ta″tiv) not obligatory; pertaining to or characterized by the ability to adjust to particular circumstances or to assume a particular role.

faculty (fak′ul-te) [L. *facultas*] 1. any normal power or function, especially a mental one. 2. the corps of professors and instructors of a college or university. **fusion f.,** the power of blending into one the two images viewed by the two eyes.

FAD flavin adenine dinucleotide.

fading (fād′ing) an illness of puppies marked by progressive weakness which makes suckling impossible, a falling body temperature, and paddling movements; it usually results in death within a few days of birth.

fae- for words beginning thus, see those beginning *fe-*.

Faget's law (sign) (fazh-āz′) [Jean Charles *Faget,* French physician, 1818–1884] see under *law.*

fagopyrism (fag-op′ĭ-rizm) [L. *fagopyrum* buckwheat] poisoning by buckwheat.

Fahraeus phenomenon, reaction, test (fah-re′us) [Robin

Fahraeus, Swedish pathologist, born 1888] see *erythrocyte sedimentation rate*, under *rate*.

Fahrenheit scale, thermometer (far'en-hīt) [Gabriel Daniel *Fahrenheit*, German physicist, 1686–1736] see under *scale* and *thermometer*.

failure (fāl'yer) inability to perform. **heart f.,** see under *H*. **kidney f.,** renal f. **renal f.,** the inability of a kidney to excrete metabolites at normal plasma levels under conditions of normal loading, or the inability to retain electrolytes under conditions of normal intake. In the acute form, it is marked by uremia and usually by oliguria or anuria, with hyperkalemia and pulmonary edema. **respiratory f.,** a persistent condition of abnormally low arterial oxygen tension (PaO_2) or abnormally high carbon dioxide tension ($PaCO_2$).

faint (fānt) syncope.

falcadina (fal″kah-de′nah) a disease of Istria, a peninsula in the Adriatic, characterized by the formation of papillomas.

falcate (fal′kāt) falciform.

falces (fal′sēz) [L.] plural of *falx*.

falcial (fal′shal) pertaining to a falx.

falciform (fal′sĭ-form) [L. *falx* sickle + *forma* form] shaped like a sickle.

falcular (fal′ku-lar) [L. *falx* sickle] sickle-shaped.

fallopian aqueduct (arch), artery, ligament, tube (fal-lo′pe-an) [Gabriele *Falloppio* (L. *Fallopius*), 1523–1562; an important Italian anatomist, pupil of Vesalius, and later professor at Padua] see *canalis facialis, arteria uterina, ligamentum inguinale,* and *tuba uterina*.

Fallot's tetralogy (disease, syndrome, tetrad), trilogy (fal-ōz′) [Étienne-Louis Arthur *Fallot*, French physician, 1850–1911] see *tetralogy of Fallot* and *trilogy of Fallot*.

fallout (fawl′out) the settling to the earth's surface of radioactive fission products that have been projected into the atmosphere by the explosion of a nuclear device.

false (fawls) [L. *falsus*] not true; not genuine; apparent, but not real.

false-negative (fawls′neg′ah-tiv) 1. denoting a test result that wrongly excludes an individual from a diagnostic or other category. 2. an individual so excluded. 3. an instance of a false-negative result.

false-positive (fawls′pos′ĭ-tiv) 1. denoting a test result that wrongly assigns an individual to a diagnostic or other category. 2. an individual so categorized. 3. an instance of a false-positive result.

falsification (fawl″sĭ-fĭ-ka′shun) a deliberate misstatement or misrepresentation. **retrospective f.,** unconscious distortion of past experiences to conform to present emotional needs.

falsifying (fawl″sĭ-fi′ing) in psychology, signifying a form of facial deceit in which an individual pretends to experience a feeling not present, shows no feeling when aroused, or substitutes signs of one emotional reaction for those of another.

Falta's coefficient, triad (fahl′taz) [Wilhelm *Falta*, Vienna physician, born 1875] see under *coefficient* and *triad*.

falx (falks), pl. *fal′ces* [L. "sickle"] a sickle-shaped organ or structure; used as a general term in anatomical nomenclature to designate such a structure. **aponeurotic f., f. aponeurot′ica,** f. inguinalis. **f. cerebel′li** [NA], **f. of cerebellum,** the small fold of dura mater in the midline of the posterior cranial fossa, projecting forward toward the vermis of the cerebellum. **f. cer′ebri** [NA], **f. of cerebrum,** the sickle-shaped fold of dura mater that extends downward in the longitudinal cerebral fissure and separates the two cerebral hemispheres. **inguinal f., f. inguina′lis** [NA], the united tendons of the transverse and internal oblique muscles going to the linea alba and pectineal line of the pubic bone; called also *Henle's ligament* and *tendo conjunctivus*. **ligamentous f., f. ligamento′sa,** processus falciformis ligamenti sacrotuberosi. **f. sep′ti,** NA alternative for *valvula foraminis ovalis*.

F.A.M.A. Fellow of the American Medical Association.

fames (fa′mēz) [L.] hunger.

familial (fah-mil′e-al) [L. *familia* family] occurring in or affecting more members of a family than would be expected by chance.

family (fam′ĭ-le) 1. a group of individuals descended from a common ancestor. 2. a taxonomic subdivision subordinate to an order (or suborder) and superior to a tribe (or subfamily). **Jukes f.,** the fictitious name of a family located mostly in New York State, which exhibited a high degree of crime, immorality, disease, and poverty; their history covers five generations. **Kallikak f.,** the fictitious name of a New Jersey family whose sociological history dates from the American Revolution; there are two branches: one consisting mostly of intelligent and respectable individuals, the other exhibiting a high incidence of mental deficiency and immorality. **systematic f.,** see *family* (def. 2). **Zero f.,** a Swiss family of three branches, two of which are respected and one very unfit; a very complete history from the 17th century.

famotine hydrochloride (fam′o-tēn) chemical name: 1-[(4-chlorophenoxy)methyl]-3,4-dihydroisoquinoline hydrochloride; an antiviral agent, $C_{16}H_{14}ClNO \cdot HCl$.

fan (fan) an area, figure, or structure resembling an open fan. **Dunham's f's,** formations seen in the roentgenogram of the lung in silicosis, made up of nodules connected by fine lines in a pyramidal arrangement; called also *Dunham's cones* or *triangles*.

F and R force and rhythm (of pulse).

fang (fang) 1. the root of a tooth. 2. a carnassial tooth of a carnivore or the envenomed tooth of a serpent.

fango (fan′go) volcanic mud.

fangotherapy (fan″go-ther′ah-pe) the therapeutic use of fango in packs or baths.

Fannia (fan′e-ah) a genus of flies (family Muscidae), the larvae of which have caused both intestinal and urinary myiasis in man. In some systems of classification, it is included in the family Anthomyiidae. **F. canicula′ris,** the lesser house fly: a species of small grayish flies, visibly different from the housefly; they lay their eggs on decaying vegetable matter or animal manure, from which the eggs or larvae may gain access to human hosts. **F. scala′ris,** a species of flies, the latrine flies, similar to but larger than *F. canicularis,* and commonly depositing its eggs on excrement, rather than on vegetable matter.

fantascope (fan′tah-skōp) [*fantasy* + Gr. *skopein* to examine] an apparatus for enabling a person to converge the eyes, and so observe certain phenomena of binocular vision.

fantast (fan′tast) a psychopathic person in whom fantasy and day-dreaming usurp the place of real experience and activity.

fantasy (fan′tah-se) [Gr. *phantasia* imagination; the power by which an object is made apparent to the mind] a psychic mechanism by which a harsh reality is converted into an imaginary experience that satisfies unconscious wishes or expresses unconscious conflicts.

fantridone hydrochloride (fan′trĭ-dōn) chemical name: 5-[3-(dimethylamino)propyl]-6(5*H*)-phenanthridinone monohydrochloride monohydrate; an antidepressant, $C_{18}H_{20}N_2O \cdot HCl \cdot H_2O$.

Fantus' antidote (fan′tus) [Bernard *Fantus*, Chicago pharmacologist, 1874–1940] see under *antidote*.

F.A.P.H.A. Fellow of the American Public Health Association.

Farabeuf's amputation, triangle (far″ah-bufs′) [Louis Hubert *Farabeuf,* French surgeon, 1841–1910] see under *amputation* and *triangle*.

farad (far′ad) [Michael *Faraday*] the unit of electrical capacity. The capacity of a condenser which, charged with 1 coulomb, gives a difference of potential of 1 volt. This unit is so large that one-millionth part of it has been adopted as a practical unit called a microfarad.

faraday (far′ah-da) the quantity of electrical charge associated with one gram equivalent of an electrochemical reaction, equal to about 96,510 coulombs.

Faraday's constant, law, dark space (far′ah-dāz) [Michael *Faraday,* English physicist, 1791–1867] see under *constant, law,* and *space*.

faradic (fah-rad′ik) pertaining to faradism.

faradimeter (far″ah-dim′ĕ-ter) [*farad* + Gr. *metron* measure] an instrument for measuring faradic electricity.

faradism (far′ah-dizm) 1. induced current. 2. induced current in a rapidly alternating current. 3. faradization. **surging f.,** a faradic current of gradually increasing and decreasing amplitude.

faradization (far″ah-di-za′shun) the therapeutic use of an interrupted current for the stimulation of muscles and nerves. Such a current is derived from an induction coil.

faradocontractility (far″ah-do-kon″trak-tik′ĭ-te) contractility in response to faradic stimulus.

faradopalpation (far″ah-do-pal-pa′shun) galvanopalpation.

farcy (far′se) cutaneous glanders, the more chronic and constitutional lymphatic form of glanders, marked by thickening of the superficial lymph vessels; see *glanders*. **button f.,** farcy characterized by the formation of small tubercular nodules in the skin of the limbs, thorax, and abdomen. **cattle f.,** a disease of cattle caused by infection with *Nocardia farcinica,* and characterized by the formation of cheesy nodules in the subcutaneous tissue and the organs. **cryptococcus f.,** lymphangitis epizootica. **Japanese f., Neapolitan f.,** lymphangitis epizootica. **f. pipes,** acute farcy along the lymphatic vessels. **water f.,** inflammation of the lymphatics of a horse's leg.

fardel-bound (far′del-bownd) having an inflamed abomasum and distended omasum, so that chewing of the cud is impossible; a condition affecting cattle and sheep.

farina (fah-re′nah) [L.] 1. meal or flour. 2. a starchy food prepared from cereal grains, usually from wheat. **f. ave′na,** oatmeal. **f. trit′ici,** wheaten flour.

farinaceous (far″ĭ-na′shus) [L. *farinaceus*] 1. of the nature of flour or meal. 2. starchy; containing starch.

farinometer (far″ĭ-nom′ĕ-ter) an instrument for determining the percentage of gluten in flour.

farnoquinone (far-no-kwin′ōn) menaquinone.

Farr's law (farz) [William *Farr*, English medical statistician, 1807–1883] see under *law*.

Farr's tubercles (farz) [John Richard *Farre*, an English physician, 1775–1862] see under *tubercle*.

Farre's white line (farz) [Arthur *Farre*, British obstetrician, 1811–1887] see under *line*.

farsighted (far-sīt′ed) hyperopic.

farsightedness (far-sīt′ed-nes) hyperopia.

fasc. abbreviation for L. *fascic′ulus*, bundle.

fascia (fash′e-ah), pl. *fas′ciae* [L. "band"] 1. [NA] a sheet or band of fibrous tissue such as lies deep to the skin or forms an investment for muscles and various organs of the body. 2. (*obs.*) a bandage. **abdominal f., internal,** f. transversalis. **Abernethy's f.,** f. iliaca. **f. adher′ens,** that portion of the junctional complex of the cells of an intercalated disk which is the counterpart of the zonula adherens of epithelial cells, but instead of being beltlike it has multiple, moderately extensive but discontinuous areas with irregular and variable outlines. **anal f.,** f. diaphragmatis pelvis inferior. **anoscrotal f.,** f. perinei superficialis. **antebrachial f., f. antebra′chii** [NA], the investing fascia of the forearm; called also (*deep*) *f. of forearm.* **aponeurotic f.,** deep f. **f. of arm,** f. brachii. **f. axilla′ris** [NA], **axillary f.,** the investing fascia of the armpit which passes between the lateral borders of the pectoralis major and latissimus dorsi muscles. **bicipital f.,** aponeurosis musculi bicipitis brachii. **brachial f., f. bra′chii** [NA], the investing fascia of the arm. **buccinator f., f. buccopharyn′gea** [NA], **buccopharyngeal f.,** a fibrous membrane forming the external covering of the constrictor muscles of the pharynx, and passing forward superiorly to the surface of the buccinator muscle. **Buck's f.,** the deep fascia of the penis, being continuous with Colles' fascia of the perineum and with Scarpa's fascia of the abdominal wall. **bulbar f., f. bul′bi [Teno′ni],** vagina bulbi. **f. of Camper,** the superficial layer of the superficial fascia of the abdomen. **cervical f.,** f. cervicalis. **cervical f., deep,** f. nuchae. **f. cervica′lis** [NA], the fascia of the neck, comprising a superficial layer deep to the skin, a pretracheal layer anterior to the trachea, and a prevertebral layer anterior to the vertebrae; it also forms a sheath enclosing the carotid vessels and vagus nerve. Called also *f. colli, cervical f.,* and *f. of neck.* **f. cine′rea** (*obs.*), gyrus fasciolaris. **clavipectoral f., f. clavipectora′lis** [NA], a fascial sheet investing the subclavius muscle, attached to the clavicle above and continuing to the pectoralis minor muscle below; called also *f. coracoclavicularis* and *coracoclavicular f.* **f. clitor′idis** [NA], **f. of clitoris,** the dense fibrous tissue that encloses the two corpora cavernosa of the clitoris. **Cloquet's f.,** the condensation of extraperitoneal tissue closing the femoral ring (septum femorale). **Colles' f.,** f. diaphragmatis urogenitalis inferior. **f. col′li,** f. cervicalis. **fasciae of colon,** teniae coli. **Cooper's f.,** 1. fascia cremasterica. 2. see *fibrae intercrurales.* **coracoclavicular f., f. coracoclavicula′ris, coracocostal f.,** f. clavipectoralis. **cremasteric f., f. cremaster′ica** [NA], the thin covering of the spermatic cord formed by the investing fascia of the cremasteric muscle; it is adjacent to the external surface of the internal spermatic fascia. Called also *Cooper's f.* and *intercolumnar f.* **cribriform f.,** 1. fascia cribrosa. 2. septum femorale. **cribro′sa** [NA], cribriform fascia: the part of the superficial fascia of the thigh that covers the saphenous opening. **crural f., f. cru′ris** [NA], the investing fascia of the leg; called also *crural aponeurosis.* **Cruveilhier's f.,** f. perinei superficialis. **dartos f. of scrotum,** tunica dartos. **deep f.,** a dense, firm, fibrous membrane investing the trunk and limbs, and giving off sheaths to the various muscles; called also *aponeurotic f.* **deep f. of arm,** f. brachii. **deep f. of back,** f. thoracolumbalis. **deep f. of forearm,** f. antebrachii. **deep f. of perineum,** diaphragma urogenitale. **deep f. of thigh,** f. lata femoris. **Denonvilliers' f.,** septum rectovesicale. **f. denta′ta hippocam′pi, dentate f.,** gyrus dentatus. **f. diaphrag′matis pel′vis infe′rior** [NA], the fascia that covers the lower surface of the coccygeus and levator ani muscles, forming the medial wall of the ischiorectal fossa; called also *ischiorectal f.* and *ischiorectal aponeurosis.* **f. diaphrag′matis pel′vis supe′rior** [NA], the fascia on the upper surface of the levator ani and coccygeus muscles. **f. diaphrag′matis urogenita′lis infe′rior** [NA], the investing fascia on the superficial surface of the urogenital diaphragm, which is continuous with the fascia covering the external oblique muscle and the sheath of the rectus abdominis; called also *ischioprostatic aponeurosis or fascia,* and *membrana perinei.* **f. diaphrag′matis urogenita′lis supe′rior** [NA], the investing fascia on the deep surface of the urogenital diaphragm, continuous with the membranous layer of the subcutaneous tissue covering the front and sides of the lower part of the abdomen; called also *rectal f.* and *rectovesical f.* **dorsal f., deep,** f. thoracolumbalis. **dorsal f. of foot,** f. dorsalis pedis. **dorsal f. of hand, f. dorsa′lis ma′nus** [NA], the investing fascia of the back of the hand. **f. dorsa′lis pe′dis** [NA], the investing fascia on the dorsum of the foot. **endoabdominal f.,** f. transversalis. **endopelvic f., f. endopelvi′na,** a name given to fascia forming part of the general

layer lining the pelvic walls and serving as a packing for the pelvic organs, as well as ensheathing the blood vessels, various specific parts of which have been known by various names. **endothoracic f., f. endothora′cica** [NA], the fascial sheet beneath the serous lining of the thoracic cavity. **extrapleural f.,** a prolongation of the endothoracic fascia sometimes found at the root of the neck, which is important as possibly modifying the auscultatory sounds at the apex of the lung. **femoral f.,** f. lata femoris. **fibroareolar f.,** f. superficialis. **f. of forearm,** f. antebrachii. **f. of Gerota, Gerota's f.,** a fibrous capsule enclosing the kidney and extending for a variable distance down the ureter. **hypogastric f.,** f. pelvis. **iliac f.,** 1. fascia iliaca. 2. arcus iliopectineus. **f. ili′aca** [NA], a strong fascia covering the inner surface of the iliac and psoas muscles. **f. iliopectin′ea, iliopectineal f.,** arcus iliopectineus. **infundibuliform f.,** f. spermatica interna. **intercolumnar f.,** 1. fascia cremasterica. 2. see *fibrae intercrurales.* **ischioprostatic f.,** f. diaphragmatis urogenitalis inferior. **ischiorectal f.,** f. diaphragmatis pelvis inferior. **f. la′ta fem′oris** [NA], the external investing fascia of the thigh. **f. of leg,** f. cruris. **longitudinal f., anterior,** ligamentum longitudinale anterius. **longitudinal f., posterior,** ligamentum longitudinale posterius. **lumbodorsal f., f. lumbodorsa′lis,** f. thoracolumbalis. **masseteric f., f. masseter′ica** [NA], a layer of fascia covering the masseter muscle. **muscular fasciae of eye, fas′ciae muscula′res bul′bi** [NA], **fas′ciae muscula′res oc′uli,** the sheets of fascia investing the extraocular muscles, continuous with the vagina bulbi. **f. of nape,** f. nuchae. **f. of neck,** f. cervicalis. **f. nu′chae** [NA], **nuchal f.,** the fascia on the muscles in the dorsal region of the neck. **obturator f., f. obturato′ria** [NA], the part of the parietal fascia of the pelvis covering the internal obturator muscle. **orbital fasciae, fas′ciae orbita′les** [NA], fibrous tissue surrounding the posterior part of the eyeball, supporting and binding together the structures within the orbit. **palmar f.,** aponeurosis palmaris. **palpebral f., f. palpebra′lis,** septum orbitale. **parietal f. of pelvis,** f. pelvis parietalis. **parotid f., f. parotide′a** [NA], a layer of cervical fascia enclosing the parotid gland. **f. parotideomasseter′ica,** the fascia enclosing the parotid gland and masseter muscle; separately called *f. parotidea* and *f. masseterica* [NA]. **f. pectin′ea, pectineal f.,** the pubic portion of the fascia lata; called also *Cowper's ligament.* **pectoral f., f. pectora′lis** [NA], the sheet of fascia investing the pectoralis major muscle. **pelvic f.,** f. pelvis. **pelvic f., parietal,** f. pelvis parietalis. **pelvic f., visceral,** f. pelvis visceralis. **pelviprostatic f.,** f. prostatae. **f. pel′vis** [NA], pelvic fascia: an inclusive term for the fascia that forms part of the general layer lining the walls of the pelvis and invests the pelvic organs; called also *hypogastric f.* **f. pel′vis parieta′lis** [NA], the fascia on the wall of the pelvis that covers the muscles which pass from the interior of the pelvis to the thigh. **f. pel′vis viscera′lis** [NA], visceral fascia of pelvis: the fascia that covers the organs and vessels of the pelvis. **f. pe′nis profun′da** [NA], the firm inner fascial layer that surrounds the corpora cavernosa and the corpus spongiosum collectively. **f. pe′nis superficia′lis** [NA], the loose external layer of fascial tissue of the penis, continuous with the tunica dartos and with the superficial perineal fascia. **perineal f., deep,** diaphragma urogenitale. **perineal f., middle,** f. diaphragmatis urogenitale superior. **perineal f., superficial,** f. perinei superficialis. **f. perine′i superficia′lis** [NA], superficial fascia of perineum: the subcutaneous tissue of the urogenital region, comprising a superficial fatty and a deep membranous layer; called also *Cruveilhier's f.* **pharyngobasilar f., f. pharyngobasila′ris** [NA], a strong fibrous membrane in the wall of the pharynx, lined internally with mucous membrane and incompletely covered on its outer surface by the overlapping constrictor muscles of the pharynx. It blends with the periosteum at the base of the skull. Called also *pharyngeal* or *pharyngobasilar aponeurosis,* and *aponeurosis pharyngis* or *pharyngobasilaris.* **phrenicopleural f., f. phrenicopleura′lis** [NA], the fascial layer on the upper surface of the diaphragm, beneath the pleura. **plantar f.,** aponeurosis plantaris. **prevertebral f., f. prevertebra′lis,** lamina prevertebralis. **proper f. of neck, f. pro′pria col′li,** f. cervicalis. **f. pro′pria coo′peri,** fascia spermatica interna. **f. prosta′tae** [NA], **f. of prostate,** the reflection of the superior fascia of the pelvic diaphragm onto the prostate. **rectal f.,** f. diaphragmatis pelvis superior. **rectoabdominal f.,** vagina musculi recti abdominis. **rectovesical f.,** f. diaphragmatis pelvis superior. **Richet's f.,** a fold of extraperitoneal fascia enveloping the obliterated umbilical vein. **scalene f.,** membrana suprapleuralis. **Scarpa's f.,** 1. the deep, membranous layer of subcutaneous abdominal fascia. 2. see *fibrae intercrurales.* **semilunar f.,** aponeurosis musculi bicipitis brachii. **Sibson's f.,** membrana suprapleuralis. **spermatic f., external,** f. spermatica externa. **spermatic f., internal,** f. spermatica interna. **f. spermat′ica exter′na** [NA], external spermatic fascia: the thin outer covering of the spermatic cord, which is continuous with the investing fascia of the external oblique muscle. **f. spermat′ica inter′na** [NA], internal spermatic fascia: the thin innermost covering of the spermatic cord, derived from the transversalis fascia of the abdominal wall;

called also *tunica vaginalis communis* [*testis et funiculi spermatici*]. **subperitoneal f.,** 1. fascia subperitonealis. 2. tela subserosa peritonei. **f. subperitonea'lis** [NA], the thin layer of connective tissue separating the peritoneum from the transversalis fascia. **superficial f.,** 1. fascia superficialis. 2. subcutaneous tissue (tela subcutanea [NA]). **superficial f. of perineum,** f. perinei superficialis. **f. superficia'lis,** a fascial sheet lying directly beneath the skin. **f. superficia'lis perine'i,** f. perinei superficialis. **f. of Tarin,** f. tari'ni, gyrus dentatus, def. 1. **temporal f., f. tempora'lis** [lam'ina profun'da et lam'ina superficia'lis] [NA], a strong fibrous sheet covering the temporal muscle; it has a deep and a superficial part which attach inferiorly to the zygomatic arch. Called also *temporal aponeurosis.* **f. of Tenon,** vagina bulbi. **f. of thigh,** f. lata femoris. **f. thoracolumba'lis** [NA], **thoracolumbar f.,** the fascia of the back that attaches medially to the vertebral column for its entire length and blends laterally with the aponeurosis of the transversus abdominis muscle; inferiorly it attaches to the iliac crest and the sacrum. Called also *f. lumbodorsalis* and *lumbodorsal f.* **thyrolaryngeal f.,** fascia investing the thyroid body and attaching to the cricoid cartilage. **f. transversa'lis** [NA], **transverse f.,** part of the inner investing layer of the abdominal wall, continuous with the fascia of the other side behind the rectus abdominis and the rectus sheath, and continuous also with the diaphragmatic fascia, iliac fascia, and the parietal pelvic fascia. **triangular f. of abdomen,** ligamentum inguinale reflexum. **triangular f. of Macalister,** musculus pyramidalis. **triangular f. of Quain,** ligamentum inguinale reflexum. **Tyrrell's f.,** septum rectovesicale. **f. of urogenital trigone,** diaphragma urogenitale. **visceral f. of pelvis,** f. pelvis visceralis. **volar f.,** aponeurosis palmaris.

fasciae (fash'e-e) [L.] plural of *fascia.*

fasciagram (fash'e-ah-gram) a roentgenogram obtained by fasciagraphy.

fasciagraphy (fash″e-ag'rah-fe) roentgenography of fasciae after the injection of air into them.

fascial (fash'e-al) pertaining to or of the nature of a fascia.

fasciaplasty (fash'e-ah-plas″te) [*fascia* + Gr. *plassein* to form] a plastic operation on a fascia.

fascicle (fas'ĭ-k'l) a small bundle or cluster, especially of nerve or muscle fibers; see also *fasciculus.* **longitudinal f's of cruciform ligament,** fasciculi longitudinales ligamenti cruciformis atlantis.

fascicular (fah-sik'u-lar) 1. pertaining to a fascicle. 2. fasciculated.

fasciculated (fah-sik'u-lāt-ed) clustered together or occurring in bundles.

fasciculation (fah-sik″u-la'shun) 1. the formation of fasciculi. 2. a small local contraction of muscles, visible through the skin, representing a spontaneous discharge of a number of fibers innervated by a single motor nerve filament.

fasciculi (fah-sik'u-li) [L.] plural of *fasciculus.*

fasciculus (fah-sik'u-lus), pl. *fascic'uli* [L. dim. of *fascis* bundle] a fascicle: a small bundle or cluster; [NA] a general term for a small bundle of nerve, muscle, or tendon fibers. **f. aberrans of Monakow,** tractus rubrospinalis. **f. acus'ticus** (*obs.*), striae medullares ventriculi quarti. **f. ante'rior pro'prius [Flech'sigi],** a name given the fasciculi proprii of the anterior funiculus of the spinal cord; called also *Flechsig's f.* **f. anterolatera'lis superficia'lis [Gower'si],** tractus spinocerebellaris anterior. **f. arcua'tus,** f. longitudinalis superior cerebri. **f. atrioventricula'ris** [NA], a small band of atypical cardiac muscle fibers originating in the atrioventricular node; see *bundle of His.* **f. of Burdach,** f. longitudinalis posterior cerebri. 2. pars temporalis radiationis corporis callosi. **cerebellospinal f., f. cerebellospina'lis,** tractus spinocerebellaris posterior. **f. cerebrospina'lis ante'rior,** tractus pyramidalis anterior. **cerebrospinal f., lateral, f. cerebrospina'lis latera'lis,** tractus pyramidalis lateralis. **cuneate f. of Burdach,** f. cuneatus medullae spinalis. **cuneate f. of medulla oblongata,** f. cuneatus medullae oblongatae. **cuneate f. of spinal cord,** f. cuneatus medullae spinalis. **f. cunea'tus [Burda'chi],** f. cuneatus medullae spinalis. **f. cunea'tus medul'lae oblonga'tae** [NA], cuneate fasiculus of medulla oblongata: the continuation into the medulla oblongata of the fasciculus cuneatus of the spinal cord; called also *funiculus cuneatus medullae oblongatae.* **f. cunea'tus medul'lae spina'lis** [NA], the lateral portion of the posterior funiculus of the spinal cord, composed of ascending fibers that terminate in the nucleus cuneatus of the medulla oblongata; called also *cuneate f. of spinal cord* or *of Burdach,* and *f. cuneatus* [*Burdachi*]. **dorsolateral f., f. dorsolatera'lis,** tractus dorsolateralis. **f. exi'lis,** a cluster of muscle fibers connecting the flexor pollicis longus with the medial condyle of the humerus, or with the coronoid process of the ulna. **extrapyramidal motor f.,** rubrospinal tract. **fibrous f. of biceps muscle,** aponeurosis musculi bicipitis brachii. **Flechsig's f.,** 1. fasciculus anterior proprius. 2. fasciculus lateralis proprius. **f. of Foville,** a term that has been applied to the tractus spinocerebellaris posterior, but which more properly relates to the stria

terminalis. **f. of Goll,** f. gracilis medullae spinalis. **f. of Gowers,** tractus spinocerebellaris anterior. **f. gra'cilis [Gol'li],** f. gracilis medullae spinalis. **f. gra'cilis medul'lae oblonga'tae** [NA], the continuation into the medulla oblongata of the fasciculus gracilis of the spinal cord; called also *posteromedian column of medulla oblongata.* **f. gra'cilis medul'lae spina'lis** [NA], the median portion of the posterior funiculus of the spinal cord, composed of ascending fibers that terminate in the nucleus gracilis of the medulla oblongata; called also *f. gracilis* [*Golli*] and *column of Goll.* **interfascicular f., f. interfascicula'ris,** a collection of fibers situated between the fasciculus gracilis and the fasciculus cuneatus, containing some of the descending branches of the fibers of the medial division of the dorsal roots of the spinal nerves; called also *Schultze's bundle* and *comma tract of Schultze.* **f. latera'lis plex'us brachia'lis** [NA], the lateral cord of the brachial plexus, formed by the union of the anterior divisions of the superior and middle trunks, C5 through C7, and from which arise the lateral pectoral and musculocutaneous nerves and the lateral root of the median and the ulnar nerves. **f. latera'lis pro'prius [Flech'sigi],** a name given the white fibers (part of the fasciculi proprii) lateral to the gray matter of the spinal cord; called also *Flechsig's f.* **f. lenticula'ris,** the dorsal part of the ansa lenticularis lying between the subthalamic nucleus and the zona incerta, and consisting chiefly of nerve fibers that arise in the globus pallidus, reach the thalamus by traversing the H field (Forel's field), and enter the fasciculus thalamicus; called also *field H₂.* **longitudinal f., dorsal,** f. longitudinalis dorsalis. **longitudinal f., medial,** f. longitudinalis medialis. **longitudinal f. of cerebrum, inferior,** f. longitudinalis inferior cerebri. **longitudinal f. of cerebrum, superior,** f. longitudinalis superior cerebri. **longitudinal fasciculi of colon,** see *teniae coli.* **longitudinal fasciculi of cruciform ligament,** fasciculi longitudinales ligamenti cruciformis atlantis. **longitudinal f. of medulla oblongata, posterior,** f. longitudinalis medialis. **f. longitudina'lis dorsa'lis** [NA], dorsal longitudinal fasiculus: a lightly myelinated fiber bundle that runs in the periventricular gray substance throughout the extent of the mesencephalon, near the medial longitudinal fasciculus; called also *Schutz's bundle.* **f. longitudina'lis infe'rior cer'ebri** [NA], inferior longitudinal f. of cerebrum: a bundle of association fibers interconnecting the cortex of the occipital and temporal lobes, extending through the occipital and temporal lobes of the cerebrum, and consisting chiefly of geniculocalcarine projection fibers. **fascic'uli longitudina'les ligamen'ti crucifor'mis atlan'tis** [NA], longitudinal fasciculi of cruciform ligament: vertical midline longitudinal fibers that, together with the transverse ligament of the atlas, form the cruciform ligament of the atlas. The fibers arise in two groups from the root of the dens—one group extending cranially to the anterior margin of the foramen magnum, the other caudally to the body of the axis. **f. longitudina'lis media'lis** [NA], medial longitudinal fasiculus: a fiber tract extending between the mesencephalon and the upper part of the spinal cord; it lies close to the median plane, just ventral to the central gray matter, and interconnects the vestibular nuclei with motor nuclei, chiefly those of the third, fourth, sixth, and eleventh cranial nerves. **f. longitudina'lis media'lis medul'lae oblonga'tae,** the portion of the fasciculus longitudinalis medialis within the medulla oblongata. **f. longitudina'lis media'lis pon'tis,** the portion of the fasciculus longitudinalis medialis within the pons. **fascic'uli longitudina'les pon'tis** [NA], **fascic'uli longitudina'les [pyramida'les] pon'tis,** a former term for the corticopontine fibers (corticopontine tract), together with the corticonuclear and corticopontine fibers of the pyramidal tract in the pars ventralis pontis. **f. longitudina'lis supe'rior cer'ebri** [NA], superior longitudinal fasciculus of cerebrum: a bundle of association fibers in the cerebrum, extending from the frontal lobe to the posterior end of the lateral sulcus, and interrelating the cortex of the frontal, temporal, parietal, and occipital lobes; called also *f. arcuatus.* **maculary f.,** a system of nerve fibers originating in the macula lutea; some are uncrossed (on the temporal side) and others are crossed fibers (on the nasal side of the retina). **mamillothalamic f., f. mamillothalam'icus** [NA], a stout bundle of fibers from the mamillary body to the anterior nucleus of the thalamus; called also *f. thalamomamillaris* [*Vicq d'Azyri*], *thalamomamillary bundle,* and *bundle of Vicq d'Azyr.* **f. margina'lis ventra'lis** (*obs.*), a fasciculus made up of the tectospinal tract and the vestibulospinal tract. **f. media'lis plex'us brachia'lis** [NA], the medial cord of the brachial plexus, formed by the anterior division of the inferior trunk, C8 through T1, and from which arise the medial pectoral, medial brachial cutaneous, and medial antebrachial cutaneous nerves, and the medial root of the ulnar and the median nerves. **Meynert's f.,** f. retroflexus. **Monakow's f.,** tractus rubrospinalis. **f. occipitofronta'lis infe'rior,** a collection of association fibers in the inferior part of the extreme capsule near the uncinate fasciculus, connecting various inferior gyri of the temporal and frontal lobes. **f. occipitofronta'lis supe'rior,** f. subcallosus. **olivary f.** (*obs.*), the fibers that enclose the olivary body. **oval f.,** an area of descending fibers in the posterior funiculus of the spinal cord near the posterior septum; called also *median root zone.* **f.**

poste′rior plex′us brachia′lis [NA], the posterior cord of the brachial plexus, formed by the union of the posterior divisions of the superior, middle, and inferior trunks, C5 through C8 and sometimes T1, and from which arise the subscapular, thoracodorsal, radial, and axillary nerves. **fascic′uli pro′prii** [NA], that part of the white matter of the spinal cord bordering the gray matter, and containing fibers that travel for a distance of only a few segments of the cord. **pyramidal f., anterior,** former name for *tractus pyramidalis anterior.* **pyramidal f., direct,** former name for *tractus pyramidalis anterior.* **pyramidal f., lateral,** former name for *tractus pyramidalis lateralis.* **f. pyramida′lis ante′rior,** former name for *tractus pyramidalis anterior.* **f. pyramida′lis latera′lis,** former name for *tractus pyramidalis lateralis.* **fascic′uli pyramida′les medul′lae oblonga′tae,** fibrae pyramidales medullae oblongatae. **f. retroflex′us** [NA], one that begins in the habenular nuclei, and extends downward and forward to the interpeduncular nucleus; called also *Meynert's bundle, fasciculus,* or *tract,* and *habenulopeduncular tract.* **f. of Rolando,** an elevation on the lateral side of the fasciculus cuneatus of the medulla oblongata, produced by the underlying gray matter; called also *funiculus of Rolando.* **f. rotun′dus** (*obs.*), tractus solitarius medullae oblongatae. **septomarginal f.,** a collection of fibers situated near the posterior median septum of the spinal cord, containing some of the descending branches of the fibers of the medial division of the dorsal roots of the spinal nerves. **solitary f.,** tractus solitarius medullae oblongatae. **subcallosal f.,** f. subcallosus. **f. subcallo′sus** [NA], subcallosal fasciculus: a collection of association fibers lying just internal to the intersection of the internal capsule and corpus callosum, interconnecting the cortex of the occipital and temporal lobes with that of the insula and frontal lobe, and probably comprising a significant part of the tapetum. Called also *f. occipitofrontalis superior.* **sulcomarginal f., f. sulcomargina′lis,** a layer of descending branches from the midbrain tectum situated in the anterior funiculus of the spinal cord, along the border of the anterior fissure. **f. te′res** (*obs.*), f. longitudinalis medialis pontis. **f. thalam′icus,** a bundle of nerve fibers lying dorsal to the zona incerta, and comprising dentatothalamic, rubrothalamic, and pallidothalamic fibers; the latter fibers reach it by way of the fasciculus lenticularis (field H₂) and the H field (Forel's field). It is separated from the fasciculus lenticularis by the zona incerta. Called also *field H₁.* **f. thalamomamilla′ris** [Vicq d'Azyri], f. mamillothalamicus. **fascic′uli transver′si aponeuro′sis palma′ris** [NA], transverse fasciculi of palmar aponeurosis: the transverse fascial bands that support the webs between the fingers. **fascic′uli transver′si aponeuro′sis planta′ris** [NA], transverse fasciculi of plantar aponeurosis: transverse bundles in the plantar aponeurosis near the toes. **f. of Türck,** tractus pyramidalis anterior. **unciform f., uncinate f., f. uncina′tus** [NA], a collection of association fibers which interconnect the cortex of the orbital surface of the frontal lobe with the parahippocampal gyrus and perhaps with the amygdala; other temporofrontal connections probably also exist. **f. of Vicq d'Azyr,** f. mamillothalamicus.

fasciectomy (fas″e-ek′to-me) [*fascia* + Gr. *ektomē* excision] excision of fascia.

fasciitis (fas″e-i′tis) inflammation of fascia. **exudative calcifying f.,** calcinosis. **necrotizing f.,** a gas-forming, fulminating, necrotic infection of the superficial and deep fascia, resulting in thrombosis of the subcutaneous vessels and gangrene of the underlying tissues; a dark patch appears on the overlying skin, which breaks down and discharges large amounts of necrotic material. It is usually caused by multiple pathogens and is frequently associated with diabetes mellitus. **nodular f.,** proliferative f. **perirenal f.,** retroperitoneal fibrosis. **proliferative f.,** a benign reactive proliferation of fibroblasts with a distinct microscopic pattern superficially resembling that of sarcoma; the lesions are located in the subcutaneous tissues and commonly associated with the deep fascia. **pseudosarcomatous f.,** a benign soft-tissue tumor occurring subcutaneously and sometimes arising from deep muscle and fascia, and histologically resembling a malignant sarcoma.

fasciodesis (fas″e-od′ĕ-sis) [L. *fascia* + Gr. *desis* binding] the operation of suturing a fascia to skeletal attachment.

Fasciola (fah-si′o-lah) [L. *fasciola* a band] a genus of flukes. **F. cer′vi,** former name for *Paramphistomum cervi.* **F. gigan′tica,** the giant liver fluke of Africa, Asia, and Hawaii, which occasionally infects man. **F. hepat′ica,** the common liver fluke of sheep, oxen, goats, horses, and other herbivorous animals. It is occasionally found in the human liver, where it may cause dangerous symptoms by obstructing the biliary passages and by invasion of the liver parenchyma. Several snails of the genus *Lymnaea* act as invertebrate hosts. Called also *Distoma hepaticum.* **F. heteroph′yes,** *Heterophyes heterophyes.* **F. mag′na,** *Fascioloides magna.*

fasciola (fah-se′o-lah, fah-si′o-lah), pl. *fasci′olae* [L., dim. of *fascia*] 1. a small band or striplike structure. 2. a small bandage. **f. cine′rea, f. cine′rea cin′guli,** gyrus fasciolaris. **f. denta′ta** (*obs.*), gyrus dentatus.

fasciolae (fah-se′o-le, fah-si′o-le) [L.] plural of *fasciola.*

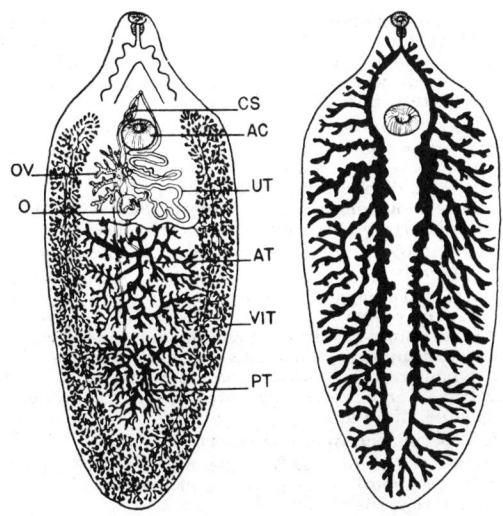

Fasciola hepatica (adult form). *Left,* Reproductive systems: *AC,* acetabulum; *AT,* anterior testis; *CS,* cirrus sac; *O,* ootype; *OV,* ovary; *PT,* posterior testis; *UT,* uterus; *VIT,* vitellaria. *Right,* Multibranched intestinal caeca. (Cheng.)

fasciolar (fah-se′o-lar, fah-si′o-lar) pertaining to a fasciola.

Fascioletta (fas″e-o-let′tah) a genus of parasitic flukes. **F. ilioca′na,** *Echinostoma iliocanum.*

fascioliasis (fas″e-o-li′ah-sis) infection with *Fasciola hepatica* or *F. gigantea.*

Fascioloides (fas″e-o-loi′dēz) a genus of flukes. **F. mag′na,** the large American liver fluke found in the liver and lungs of herbivorous animals in North America; formerly called *Fasciola magna.*

fasciolopsiasis (fas″e-o-lop-si′ah-sis) the state of being infected with flukes of the genus *Fasciolopsis.*

Fasciolopsis (fas″e-o-lop′sis) [*fasciola* + Gr. *opsis* appearance] a genus of trematode worms. **F. bus′ki,** a trematode worm found in the small intestine of residents in many parts of Asia. It is the largest of the intestinal flukes, and may cause nausea, diarrhea, and a malabsorption syndrome if present in large numbers. The intermediate hosts are the snails *Planorbis coenosus* and various species of *Segmentina.* Other names given this species are *F. fuelleborni* from Calcutta and Egypt, *F. goddardi* and *F. spinifera* from China, and *F. rathouisi* from Asia. Formerly called *Distoma buski.*

fascioplasty (fash′e-o-plas″te) plastic operation on fascia.

fasciorrhaphy (fash″e-or′ah-fe) [*fascia* + Gr. *rhaphē* suture] the repair of lacerated fascia.

fasciotomy (fash″e-ot′o-me) [*fascia* + Gr. *temnein* to cut] surgical incision or transection of fascia.

fascitis (fah-si′tis) fasciitis.

fast (fast) 1. immovable, or unchangeable; resistant to the action of a specific drug, stain, or destaining agent. 2. abstention from food.

fastidium (fas-tid′e-um) [L. "loathing, disgust"] repugnance to food.

fastigatum (fas″tĭ-ga′tum) [L.] pointed; sharpened to a point.

fastigial (fas-tij′e-al) of or pertaining to the fastigium.

fastigium (fas-tij′e-um) [L. "gable end"] 1. the highest point in the roof of the fourth ventricle of the brain, at the junction between the superior medullary velum and the nodulus. 2. the acme, or highest point, as of a fever.

fastness (fast′nes) the quality, in bacteria, of being resistant to the action of specific stains or inhibitors.

fat (fat) 1. adipose tissue; a white or yellowish tissue which forms soft pads between various organs of the body, serves to smooth and round out bodily contours, and furnishes a reserve supply of energy. 2. an ester of glycerol with fatty acids, usually oleic acid, palmitic acid, or stearic acid; tri-acyl glycerol; neutral fat. **bound f.,** masked f. **brown f.,** brown adipose tissue. **chyle f.,** fat in the form of an extremely fine emulsion taken into the chyle by the lymphatics of the intestine. **corpse f.,** adipocere. **fetal f.,** a term sometimes used in pathology to refer to brown adipose tissue. **grave f.,** adipocere. **masked f.,** fat that can be detected in a cell or tissue by chemical methods but is not revealed by staining methods; called also *bound f.* **milk f.,** the suspension in milk which tends to separate out as cream. **molecular f.,** fat occurring in fine specks within the cells. **moruloid f., mulberry f.,** brown adipose tissue. **neutral f.,** see *fat* (def. 2). **polyunsaturated f.,** a fat containing fatty acid that has more than one double bond in its carbon chain.

saturated f., one containing fatty acid that has only single bonds in its carbon chain. **unsaturated f.,** a fat containing fatty acid that has one or more double bonds in its carbon chain. **wool f.,** anhydrous lanolin. **wool f., hydrous,** lanolin. **wool f., refined,** anhydrous lanolin.

fatal (fa′tal) causing death; deadly; mortal; lethal.

fate (fāt) [L. *fatum* what is ordained by the gods] the ultimate disposition or decreed outcome. In pharmacology, the intermediate and ultimate disposition of a drug in the body. **prospective f.,** the development normally achieved by any region of the egg or early embryo when there is no interference.

fatigability (fat″ĭ-gah-bil′ĭ-te) easy susceptibility to fatigue.

fatigue (fah-tēg′) [Fr.; L. *fatigatio*] a state of increased discomfort and decreased efficiency resulting from prolonged or excessive exertion; loss of power or capacity to respond to stimulation. **combat f.,** disabling physical and emotional fatigue occurring in association with military combat; also formerly used (World War II) as a synonym for *combat neurosis.* Called also *battle f.* **stimulation f.,** an increase in the threshold of a neural element due to repeated stimulation.

fatty (fat′e) pertaining to or characterized by fat.

fauces (faw′sēz) [L., pl. of *faux* "a gorge, narrow pass"] [NA] the passage from the mouth to the pharnyx, including both the lumen and its boundaries; the throat.

Fauchard's disease (fo-sharz′)[Pierre *Fauchard,* French dentist, 1678–1761] periodontitis.

faucial (faw′shal) pertaining to the fauces.

faucitis (faw-si′tis) inflammation of the fauces.

Faught's sphygmomanometer (fawtz) [Francis Ashley *Faught,* American chemist, born 1881] see under *sphygmomanometer.*

fauna (faw′nah) [L. *Faunus* mythical deity of herdsmen] the animal life present in or characteristic of a given region or locality. It may be discernible with the unaided eye (macrofauna), or only with the aid of a microscope (microfauna).

Fauvel's granules (fo-velz′) [Sulpice Antoine *Fauvel,* French physician, 1813–1884] see under *granule.*

fava (fa′vah) *Vicia faba* L. (Leguminosae).

faveolar (fa-ve′o-lar) pertaining to the faveolus (foveola).

faveolate (fa-ve′o-lāt) [L. *faveolus,* from *fa′vus* honeycomb] honeycombed; alveolate.

faveoli (fa-ve′o-li) [L.] plural of *faveolus.*

faveolus (fa-ve′o-lus), pl. *fave′oli* [L.] foveola.

favid (fa′vid) a secondary skin eruption due to allergy in favus.

favism (fa′vism) [Italian *fava* bean] an acute hemolytic anemia caused by ingestion of fava beans or inhalation of the pollen of the plant *Vicia faba* (*fava*), occurring in certain individuals, usually as a result of a hereditary biochemical lesion of the erythrocytes and a consequent enzyme deficiency. See *glucose-6-phosphate dehydrogenase anemia,* under *anemia.*

favus (fa′vus) [L. "honeycomb"] a distinctive type of tinea capitis, caused by *Trichophyton schoenleini,* and characterized by the formation of yellow, cup-shaped crusts composed of dense mats of mycelia and epithelial debris, which enlarge to form prominent honeycomb-like masses. **f. circina′tus,** favus occurring in a circinate patch. **f. of fowl,** a chronic dermatomycosis affecting the comb of fowl, caused by *Trichophyton gallinae;* called also *comb disease,* usually in male birds. **f. herpet′icus,** a very rare form favus in which the lesion is papulovesicular and studded with small yellow points. **f. herpetifor′mis,** mouse favus. **mouse f.,** a disease of mice, caused by the fungus *Trichophyton mentagrophytes* var. *quinkeanum;* it may be transmitted to man. **f. mu′rium,** mouse f.

Fc [*fragment, crystallizable*] one of the two segments of the IgG molecule obtained by treatment of the antibody molecule with papain; it is crystallizable and contains most of the antigenic determinants. See also *Fab.*

Fc′ a fragment produced in minute quantities following papain digestion of immunoglobulin molecules, in addition to the usual Fc fragments. It is a dimer that is not bonded covalently. It contains the principal part of the C terminal portion of two Fc fragments, lacking the terminal 13 amino acids.

F.D. focal distance; fatal dose (now called lethal dose [LD]).

Fd the heavy chain portion of a Fab fragment following papain digestion of an IgG molecule. The variable segment of an Fd fragment is part of the antigen-binding site of the Fab region of an antibody molecule.

FDA Food and Drug Administration, a division of the Department of Health and Human Services.

F.D.A. fronto-dextra anterior (right frontoanterior, a position of the fetus); Food and Drug Administration.

F.D.I. abbreviation for *Fédération Dentaire Internationale* [Fr. International Dental Association].

F.D.P. fronto-dextra posterior (right frontoposterior, a position of the fetus).

F.D.T. fronto-dextra transversa (right frontotransverse, a position of the fetus).

Fe chemical symbol for *iron* (L. *ferrum*).

FE$_{Na}$ excreted fraction of filtered sodium; see under *test.*

fear (fēr) a normal emotional response, in contrast to anxiety and phobia, to consciously recognized and external sources of danger, which is manifested by alarm, apprehension, or disquiet.

febantel (feb′an-tel) chemical name: [[2-[(methoxyacetyl)-amino]-4-(phenylthio)phenyl]carbonimidoyl]biscarbamic acid dimethyl ester; a veterinary antihelmintic, $C_{20}H_{22}N_4O_6S$.

Feb. dur. abbreviation for L. *feb′re duran′te,* while the fever lasts.

febricant (feb′ri-kant) causing fever.

febricide (feb′ri-sīd) [*febris* + L. *caedere* to kill] 1. lowering bodily temperature in fever. 2. an agent that reduces fever.

febricity (fe-bris′ĭ-te) feverishness; the quality of being febrile.

febricula (fe-brik′u-lah) [L.] a slight or temporary attack of fever of indefinite origin or pathology.

febrifacient (feb″ri-fa′shent) [*febris* + L. *facere* to make] producing fever.

febrific (fĕ-brif′ik) producing fever.

febrifugal (fĕ-brif′ŭ-gal) [*febris* + L. *fugare* to put to flight] dispelling or relieving fever.

febrifuge (feb′ri-fūj) an agent that reduces body temperature in fever; antipyretic.

febrifugine (feb-rif′u-jin) an antimalarial alkaloid, $C_{16}H_{19}O_3$-N_3, from Ch'ang Shan.

febrile (feb′ril) [L. *febrilis*] pertaining to or characterized by fever.

febris (fe′bris) [L.] fever. **f. endem′ica rose′ola,** dengue. **f. entericoi′des,** entericoid fever. **f. meliten′sis,** brucellosis. **f. quinta′na,** trench fever. **f. recur′rens,** relapsing fever. **f. ru′bra,** scarlet fever. **f. sudora′lis,** brucellosis. **f. un′dulans,** brucellosis. **f. uveoparotide′a,** uveoparotid fever. **f. wolhyn′ica,** trench fever.

fecal (fe′kal) pertaining to or of the nature of feces.

fecalith (fe′kah-lth) [*feces* + Gr. *lithos* stone] an intestinal concretion formed around a center of fecal matter.

fecaloid (fe′kal-oid) resembling fecal matter.

fecaloma (fe″kah-lo′mah) [*feces* + *-oma*] stercoroma.

fecaluria (fe″kah-lu′re-ah) [*feces* + Gr. *ouron* urine + *-ia*] the presence of fecal matter in the urine.

feces (fe′sēz) [L. *faeces,* pl. of *faex* refuse] the excrement discharged from the intestines, consisting of bacteria, cells exfoliated from the intestines, secretions, chiefly of the liver, and a small amount of food residue.

Fechner's law (fek′nerz) [Gustav Theodor *Fechner,* Prussian natural philosopher, 1801–1887] see under *law.*

FeCO$_3$ ferrous carbonate.

fecula (fek′u-lah) [L. *faecula* lees, dregs] 1. lees or sediment. 2. starch; also the starchy part of a seed.

feculent (fek′u-lent) [L. *faeculentus*] 1. having dregs or a sediment. 2. excrementitious.

fecundate (fe′kun-dāt) [L. *fecundere* to make fruitful] to impregnate or fertilize.

fecundatio (fe″kun-da′she-o) [L.] fecundation. **f. ab ex′tra,** impregnation occurring without entrance of the penis into the vagina.

fecundation (fe″kun-da′shun) [L. *fecundatio*] impregnation or fertilization. **artificial f.,** artificial insemination.

fecundity (fĕ-kun′dĭ-te) [L. *fecunditas*] ability to produce offspring rapidly and in large numbers. In demography, the physiological ability to reproduce, as opposed to fertility.

Fede's disease (fa′daz) [Francesco *Fede,* an Italian physician, 1832–1913] Riga-Fede disease.

Federici's sign (fe-de-re′chēz) [Cesare *Federici,* an Italian physician, 1838–1892] see under *sign.*

feeblemindedness (fe″b′l-mīnd′ed-nes) former name for mental retardation. The feebleminded were divided into three grades: idiots, with a mental age below two years; imbeciles, with a mental age between two and seven years; and morons, with a mental age between seven and twelve years.

feedback (fēd′bak) the return of some of the output of a system as input so as to exert some control in the process; see also *endproduct inhibition,* under *inhibition.* **alpha f.,** see under *biofeedback.* **negative f.,** the condition of maintaining a constant output of a system by exertion of an inhibitory control on a key step in the system by a product of that system. **positive f.,** a condition causing the output of a system to increase continually by exertion of a stimulatory effect on a key step in the system by a product of that system.

feed-forward (fēd-for′ward) the anticipatory effect that one intermediate in a metabolic or endocrine control system exerts on another intermediate further along in the pathway; such effect may be stimulatory (positive f.) or inhibitory (negative f.).

feeding (fēd′ing) the taking or giving of food. **artificial f.,** feeding of a baby with food other than mother's milk. **breast**

f., breast-feeding. **extrabuccal f.,** the administration of nutriment other than by mouth. **Finkelstein's f.,** feeding of infants based upon decrease in the milk sugar of the food. **forced f., forcible f.,** the administration of food by force to those who cannot or will not receive it. **sham f.,** feeding in which the food is chewed and swallowed but does not enter the stomach, because of diversion to the exterior by an esophageal fistula or other device.

Feer's disease (fairz) [Emil *Feer,* Swiss pediatrician, 1864–1955] acrodynia.

fee-splitting (fe-split′ing)   the division of moneys received by a specialist, such as a surgeon, between himself and the physician who referred the patient to him.

feet (fēt)   see *foot.*

Fehleisen's streptococcus (fa′lis-enz) [Friedrich *Fehleisen,* German (later American) physician, 1854–1924]   *Streptococcus pyogenes.*

Fehling's solution, test (fa′lingz) [Hermann Christian von *Fehling,* German chemist, 1812–1885]   see under *solution* and *tests.*

fel (fel), gen. *fel′lis* [L. "bile," "gall"]   the bile.   **f. bo′vis,** ox bile. **f. bo′vis purifica′tum, f. tau′ri purifica′tum,** ox bile extract.

Felderstruktur (fel″der-shtrook′tur) [Ger.]   the term used to describe the pattern of organization of the myofilaments in cardiac and red skeletal muscles, in which the myofilaments are not associated in discrete myofibrils, but instead form a continuous field interrupted by mitochondria. Cf. *Fibrillenstruktur.*

Feleky's instrument (fa-la′kēz) [Hugó von *Feleky,* Budapest urologist, 1860–1932]   see under *instrument.*

Felicola (fel-ĭ-ko′lah)   a genus of parasitic insects of the order Mallophaga, the biting lice. It includes *F. subrostratus,* a parasite of cats.

feline (fe′lin) [L. *feles* cat]   pertaining to, characteristic of, or derived from a cat.

Felix Vi serum (fa′liks) [Arthur *Felix,* Prague bacteriologist, 1887–1956]   see under *serum.*

Felix-Weil reaction (fa′liks-vīl) [Arthur *Felix,* Prague bacteriologist, 1887–1956; Edmund *Weil,* German physician in Prague, 1880–1922]   Weil-Felix reaction.

fellatio (fĕ-la′she-o) [L. *fellare* to suck]   oral stimulation or manipulation of the penis.

felo-de-se (fa″lo-da-sa′) [Sp. "felon of one's self"]   a person who commits suicide.

felon (fel′on)   a purulent infection or abscess involving the pulp of the distal phalanx of the finger. Cf. *paronychia* and *eponychia.* **bone f.,** a subperiosteal felon causing necrosis of the bone. **deep f.,** a term which includes subcutaneous, thecal, and subperiosteal felons.   **frog f.,** an abscess in the web space of the hand. **subcutaneous f.,** a deep felon situated beneath the skin. **subcuticular f., subepithelial f.,** a pustule located between the cuticle and the true skin.   **subperiosteal f.,** a felon involving the periosteum of the terminal phalanx.   **superficial f.,** subcuticular felon.   **thecal f.,** a felon that involves the synovial sheath, producing a suppurative tenosynovitis.

Felsules (fel′sulz)   trademark for a preparation of chloral hydrate.

Felton's serum, unit (fel′tunz) [Lloyd D. *Felton,* Boston physician, 1885–1953]   see under *serum* and *unit.*

feltwork (felt′werk)   a complex of closely interwoven fibers, as of nerve fibrils.   **Kaes' f.,** a dense network of nerve fibers in the cerebral cortex.

Felty's syndrome (fel′tēz) [Augustus Roi *Felty,* American physician, born 1895]   see under *syndrome.*

female (fe′māl) [L. *femella* young woman]   1. an individual organism of the sex that bears young or that produces ova or eggs. 2. feminine.

feminine (fem′ĭ-nin)   pertaining to the female sex, or possessing qualities normally characteristic of the female.

femininity (fem″ĭ-nin′ĭ-te)   womanhood; the possession of normal female qualities by a woman.

feminism (fem′ĭ-nizm)   the appearance or existence of female secondary sex characters in the male.   **mammary f.,** gynecomastia.

Feminone (fem′ĭ-nōn)   trademark for a preparation of ethinyl estradiol.

feminization (fem″ĭ-ni-za′shun)   1. the normal induction or development of female sex characters. 2. the induction or development of female secondary sex characters in the male.   **testicular f.,** a condition in which the subject is phenotypically female but lacks nuclear sex chromatin and is of XY chromosomal sex; the uterus and tubes are absent or rudimentary, and the gonads are typically testes and may be abdominal or inguinal in position. The *incomplete* form is marked by partial fusion of the labioscrotal folds and clitoromegaly, and at puberty, variable feminization and partial virilization may both take place.

feminonucleus (fem″ĭ-no-nu-kle′us)   the female pronucleus.

Fem. intern.   abbreviation for L. *femor′ibus inter′nus,* at the inner side of the thighs.

femme (fahm) [Fr.]   woman.   **sage f.** (sahzh-fahm′) [Fr. "wise woman"], a midwife.

Femogen (fem′o-gen)   trademark for preparations of esterified estrogens.

femora (fem′o-rah) [L.]   plural of *femur.*

femoral (fem′or-al) [L. *femoralis*]   pertaining to the femur, or to the thigh.

femorocele (fem′o-ro-sēl″) [L. *femur* thigh + Gr. *kēlē* hernia]   femoral hernia.

femoroiliac (fem″o-ro-il′e-ak)   pertaining to the femur and the ilium.

femorotibial (fem″o-ro-tib′e-al)   pertaining to the femur and the tibia.

femto- [Danish *femten* fifteen]   a combining form used in naming units of measurement to indicate one-quadrillionth (10^{-15}) of the unit designated by the root with which it is combined.

femur (fe′mur), pl. *fem′ora* [L.]   1. [NA] the bone that extends from the pelvis to the knee, being the longest and largest bone in the body; its head articulates with the acetabulum of the hip bone, and distally the femur, along with the patella and tibia, forms the knee joint. See Plate accompanying *skeleton.* Called also *thigh bone* and *femoral bone.* 2. the proximal portion of the lower member of the body, situated between the pelvis and the knee; the thigh.

fenalamide (fen-al′ah-mīd)   chemical name: ethyl *N*-[2-(diethylamino)ethyl]-2-ethyl-2-phenylmalonamate; a smooth muscle relaxant, $C_{19}H_{30}N_2O_3$.

fenbendazole (fen-ben′dah-zōl)   chemical name: [5-(phenylthio)-1*H*-benzimidazol-2-yl] carbamic acid methyl ester; an anthelmintic, $C_{15}H_{13}N_3O_2S$.

fenbufen (fen-bu′fen)   chemical name: γ-oxo-[1,1′-biphenyl]-4-butanoic acid; an anti-inflammatory, $C_{16}H_{14}O_3$.

fenclofenac (fen-klo′fen-ak)   chemical name: 2-(2,4-dichlorophenoxy)benzeneacetic acid; an anti-inflammatory, $C_{14}H_{10}Cl_2O_3$.

fenclonine (fen′klo-nēn)   chemical name: DL-3-(4-chlorophenyl)alanine; a serotonin inhibitor, $C_9H_{10}ClNO_2$.

fenclorac (fen-klor′ak)   chemical name: α,3-dichloro-4-cyclohexylbenzeneacetic acid; an anti-inflammatory, $C_{14}H_{16}Cl_2O_2$.

fendosal (fen′do-sal)   chemical name: 5-(4,5-dihydro-2-phenyl-3*H*-benz[*e*]indol-3-yl)-2-hydroxy-5-benzoic acid; an anti-inflammatory, $C_{25}H_{19}NO_3$.

fenestra (fĕ-nes′trah), pl. *fenes′trae* [L. "window"]   a window-like opening; [NA] a general term for an opening or open area. Also, an opening in a bandage or cast, or in the blade of a forceps. **f. choled′ocha,** the perforation in the medial descending portion of the duodenum through which enter the common bile duct and the pancreatic duct.   **f. of cochlea, f. coch′leae** [NA], a round opening in the inner wall of the middle ear inferior to and a little posterior to the fenestra vestibuli; it is covered by the secondary tympanic membrane. Called also *round window.* **f. nov-ova′lis,** a surgically created oval window in the lateral semicircular canal in Lempert's fenestration operation.   **f. ova′lis,** f. vestibuli.   **f. rotun′da,** f. cochleae.   **f. vestib′uli** [NA], an oval opening in the inner ear, which is closed by the base of the stapes; called also *f. ovalis* and *oval window.*

fenestrae (fĕ-nes′tre) [L.]   plural of *fenestra.*

fenestrate (fen′es-trāt)   to pierce with one or more openings.

fenestrated (fen′es-trāt″ed) [L. *fenestratus*]   pierced with one or more openings.

fenestration (fen″es-tra′shun) [L. *fenestratus* furnished with windows]   1. the act of perforating, or the condition of being perforated. 2. the surgical creation of a new opening in the labyrinth of the ear for the restoration of hearing in cases of otosclerosis. **alveolar plate f.,** a condition in which a round or oval, window-like defect exists in the cortical plate of bone overlying a portion of the root of a tooth. Such defects are most common over the buccal aspect of the roots of teeth, particularly in those instances in which the alveolar bone over the root is unusually thin. **aortopulmonary f.,** aortic septal defect.

fenestrel (fen-es′trel)   chemical name: 5-ethyl-6-methyl-4-phenyl-3-cyclohexene-1-carboxylic acid; an estrogen, $C_{16}H_{20}O_2$.

fenethylline hydrochloride (fen-eth′ĭ-lin)   chemical name: 7-[2-[(α-methylphenethyl)amino]ethyl]theophylline monohydrochloride; a central nervous system stimulant, $C_{18}H_{23}N_5O_2\cdot$-HCl.

fenfluramine hydrochloride (fen-floor′ah-mēn)   chemical name: *N*-ethyl-α-methyl-3-(trifluoromethyl)benzeneethanamine hydrochloride. An adrenergic, $C_{12}H_{16}F_3N\cdot HCl$, used as an anorexic in the short-term treatment of exogenous obesity; administered orally.

fenisorex (fen-i′so-reks)   chemical name: *cis*-7-fluoro-3,4-dihydro-1-phenyl-1*H*-2-benzopyran-3-methanamine; an anorexic, $C_{16}H_{16}FNO$.

fenmetozole hydrochloride (fen-met′o-zōl)   chemical name: 2-[(3,4-dichlorophenoxy)methyl]-4,5-dihydro-1*H*-imidazole monohydrochloride; an antidepressant and narcotic antagonist, $C_{10}H_{10}$-$Cl_2N_2O \cdot HCl$.

fenobam (fen'o-bam)   chemical name: N-(3-chlorophenyl)-N'-(4,5-dihydro-1-methyl-4-oxo-1H-imidazol-2-yl)urea; a tranquilizer, $C_{11}H_{11}ClN_4O_2$.

fenoprofen (fen-o-pro'fen)   chemical name: $(\pm)$-α-methyl-3-phenoxybenzeneacetic acid; an anti-inflammatory, analgesic, and antipyretic, $C_{15}H_{14}O_3$.   **f. calcium** [USP], the calcium salt of fenoprofen, $C_{30}H_{26}CaO_6 \cdot 2H_2O$, having the same actions as the base; used for relief of the signs and symptoms of rheumatoid arthritis and osteoarthritis, administered orally.

fenoterol (fen''o-ter'ōl)   chemical name: 3,5-dihydroxy-α-[[(p-hydroxy-α-methylphenethyl)amino]methyl]benzyl alcohol; a bronchodilator, $C_{17}H_{21}NO_4$.

fenpipalone (fen-pip'ah-lōn)   chemical name: 5-[2-(3,6-dihydro-4-phenyl-1(2H)-pyridinyl)ethyl]-3-methyl-2-oxazolidinone; an anti-inflammatory, $C_{17}H_{22}N_2O_2$.

fenspiride hydrochloride (fen-spēr'īd)   8-(2-phenethyl)-1-oxa-3,8-diazaspiro[4.5]decan-2-one monohydrochloride. An antiadrenergic compound, $C_{15}H_{20}N_2O_2 \cdot HCl$, used as a bronchodilator.

fentanyl citrate (fen'tah-nil) [USP]   chemical name: N-phenyl-N-[1-(2-phenylethyl)-4-piperidineyl] propanamide 2-hydroxy-1,2,3-propanetricarboxylate (1:1). A narcotic analgesic, $C_{22}H_{28}N_2$-$O \cdot C_6H_8O_7$, derivative of piperidine, occurring as a white, crystalline powder or white, glistening crystals; used mainly preoperatively, postoperatively, and during surgery, administered intravenously or intramuscularly. A combination of fentanyl citrate and droperidol (known as *Innovar*) is administered intramuscularly to produce neuroleptanalgesia.

fenticlor (fen'tĭ-klor)   chemical name: 2,2'-thiobis[4-chlorophenol]. A topical anti-infective, $C_{12}H_8Cl_2O_2S$, which has been used in candidial and dermatophytic infections of the skin and mucous membranes.

fenugreek (fen'u-grēk) [L. *faenum graecum* Greek hay]   the leguminous annual herb, *Trigonella foenumgraecum* L., grown in Southern Europe, India, and Northern Africa for its oily seeds, which are used in making curry. The seeds are used in veterinary medicine in poultices, ointments, and plasters, and to flavor medicinal powders that are mixed with the food of livestock. See also *trigonelline*.

Fenwick's disease (fen'wiks) [Samuel *Fenwick*, English physician, 1821–1902]   see under *disease*.

Fe_2O_3 ferric oxide.

$Fe(OH)_3$ ferric hydroxide.

feosol (fe'o-sol)   trademark for preparations of ferrous sulfate.

feral (fe'ral) [L. *feralis*]   savage; wild; deadly; living in the wild state, especially after having been domesticated.

fer-de-lance (fār-dĕ-lahs') [Fr. "lance head"]   a large venomous snake, *Bothrops atrox*, of South and Central America, Mexico and the West Indies; see table accompanying *snake*.

Féréol's nodes (fa''ra-ōlz') [Louis Henri Felix *Féréol*, French physician, 1825–1891]   see under *node*.

Fergon (fer'gon)   trademark for preparations of ferrous gluconate.

Fergusson's incision (operation), speculum (fer'gus-unz) [Sir William *Fergusson*, British surgeon, 1808–1877]   see under *incision* and *speculum*.

Fer-In-Sol (fer'in-sōl)   trademark for a preparation of ferrous sulfate.

ferment [L. *fermentum* leaven]   1. (fer-ment') to undergo fermentation; the term is applied to decomposition of carbohydrates. 2. (fer'ment) any substance that causes fermentation in other substances with which it comes in contact; see *enzyme*.   **chemical f.,** a ferment that is not a living organism; an enzyme.   **curdling f.,** rennin.   **defensive f's,** see *Abderhalden's reaction*, under *reaction*.   **diastatic f.,** an enzyme that changes starch into sugar.   **digestive f.,** a ferment which participates in the digestion of food.   **fibrin f.,** thrombin.   **lactic f.,** a ferment or enzyme that decomposes lactose into lactic acid and carbon dioxide.   **milk-curdling f.,** rennin.   **organized f.** (*obs.*), a living plant or animal organism, such as a microbe, which acts as a ferment.   **protective f.,** a ferment formed in the body as a result of the presence in the blood of foreign substances, and capable of splitting up the foreign substance and thus protecting the organism. Called also *abwehrfermente* and *protective enzyme*. Cf. *Abderhalden's reaction*, under *reaction*.   **soluble f., unorganized f.,** an enzyme that can be extracted, isolated, and purified.   **urea f.,** see *urease*.   **Warburg's f.,** see under *enzyme*.

fermental (fer-men'tal)   pertaining to or arising from a ferment or enzyme.

fermentation (fer''men-ta'shun) [L. *fermentatio*]   the anaerobic enzymatic conversion of organic compounds, especially carbohydrates, to simpler compounds, especially to ethyl alcohol, resulting in energy in the form of adenosine triphosphate (ATP); the process is used in the production of alcohol, bread, vinegar, and other food or industrial products. It differs from respiration in that organic substances rather than molecular oxygen are used as electron acceptors.   **acetic f.,** the conversion of a weak alcoholic solution into acetic acid or vinegar.   **alcoholic f.,** the production of ethyl alcohol from carbohydrates.   **ammoniacal f.,** the formation of ammonia and carbon dioxide from urea by urease.   **amylic f.,** the fermentation which produces amyl alcohol from sugar.   **butyric f.,** the change of carbohydrates, milk, etc., into butyric acid.   **caseous f.,** the coagulation of soluble casein under the influence of rennin.   **dextran f.,** the fermentation by which dextrose is converted into dextran.   **diastatic f.,** the change of starch into glucose, under the influence of ptyalin, the glycolytic enzyme, etc.   **frog spawn f.,** dextran f.   **lactic f., lactic acid f.,** the conversion of sugars to lactic acid by various bacteria; the souring of milk.   **propionic f.,** the production of propionic acid from sugars or lactic acid by certain bacteria.   **stormy f.,** the rapid fermentation of milk produced by *Clostridium perfringens*, marked by rupture of the clotted milk by the pressure of the gas which develops.   **viscous f.,** the production of gummy substances, as in the urine, in milk, and in wine, under the influence of various bacilli.

fermentemia (fer''men-te'me-ah) [*ferment* + Gr. *haima* blood + *-ia*]   the presence of a ferment in the blood.

fermentogen (fer-men'to-jen) [*ferment* + Gr. *gennan* to produce]   a substance which may be converted into an enzyme; a zymogen.

fermentoid (fer-men'toid) [*ferment* + Gr. *eidos* form]   an enzyme that has been altered so as to lose its active properties; a denatured enzyme.

fermentum (fer-men'tum) [L. "ferment"]   yeast.

fermium (fer'me-um) [Enrico *Fermi*, Italian physicist, 1901–1954; winner of the Nobel prize for physics in 1938]   the chemical element number 100, atomic weight 253, symbol Fm, originally discovered in debris from thermonuclear explosion in 1952.

ferning (fern'ing)   the appearance of a fernlike pattern in a dried specimen of cervical mucus, an indication of the presence of estrogen; called also *fern phenomenon*.

-ferous [L. *ferre* to bear]   a word termination meaning bearing or producing.

Ferrata's cell (fer-at'az) [Adolfo *Ferrata*, Italian physician, 1880–1946]   hemohistioblast.

ferrated (fer-āt'ed)   charged with iron.

ferredoxin (fer''ĕ-dok'sin)   a nonheme iron-containing protein, also having a high sulfide content and a very low redox potential; the ferredoxins participate in electron transport in photosynthesis, nitrogen fixation, and various other biological processes.

Ferrein's canal, cord, etc. (fer'inz) [Antoine *Ferrein*, French physician, 1693–1769]   see under *canal, cord, foramen, ligament, pyramid, tube,* and *tubule*.

ferri (fer'e) [L. gen. of *ferrum*]   see *iron*.

ferri-albuminic (fer''e-al-bu-min'ik)   containing iron and albumin.

Ferribacterium (fer''re-bak-te're-um)   a genus of microorganisms of the family Siderocapsaceae, suborder Pseudomonadineae, order Pseudomonadales, occurring as rods with rounded or square ends, singly, or in pairs or short chains. It includes two species, *F. du'plex* and *F. rectangula're*.

ferric (fer'ik) [L. *ferrum*]   containing iron in its plus-three oxidation state, Fe(III) (sometimes designated Fe^{3+}). For ferric compounds see under the salt, e.g., arsenate and citrate.   **f. oxide, red** [NF], a red pigment used as a pharmaceutic aid in preparations for application to the skin.   **f. oxide, yellow** [NF], a yellow pigment used as a pharmaceutic aid in preparations for application to the skin.

Ferrier's treatment (method) (fer'e-erz) [P. *Ferrier*, French physician]   see under *treatment*.

ferrihemochrome (fer''e-he'mo-krōm)   the ferric compound of hemochrome.

ferritin (fer'ĭ-tin)   the iron-apoferritin complex, which is one of the chief forms in which iron is stored in the body; it occurs at least in the gastrointestinal mucosa, liver, spleen, bone marrow, and reticuloendothelial cells generally.

Ferrobacillus (fer''o-bah-sil'us)   a genus of microorganisms of the family Siderocapsaceae, suborder Pseudomonadineae, order Pseudomonadales, occurring as short rod-shaped cells, singly or in pairs, which oxidize ferrous iron to the ferric state. The type species is *F. ferroox'idans*.

ferrocholinate (fer''o-ko'lin-āt)   a chelate prepared by reacting equimolar quantities of freshly precipitated ferric chloride with choline dihydrogen citrate, the metallic ion being sequestered and firmly bound into a ring within the molecule; used in the treatment of iron-deficiency anemias. Called also *iron choline citrate*.

ferroflocculation (fer''o-flok''u-la'shun)   a flocculation test for malaria, performed with a fine-grained iron antigen; see *Henry's test*, under *tests*.

ferrohemochrome (fer''o-he'mo-krōm)   the ferrous compound of hemochrome.

ferrokinetics (fer''ro-ki-net'iks)   the turnover, or rate of change, of iron in the body.

Ferrolip (fer'o-lip) trademark for preparations of ferrocholinate.

ferroprotein (fer″o-pro′te-in) a protein combined with an iron-containing radical; the ferroproteins are respiratory carriers. Cf. *Warburg's enzyme*, under *enzyme*, and *cytochrome* (def. 1.).

ferrosilicon (fer″o-sil′ĭ-kon) an alloy of iron and silicon made by electrothermal reduction, and used for the deoxidation of steel.

ferrosoferric (fer-o″so-fer′ik) combining a ferrous with a ferric compound; containing iron in two different oxidation states, as in the oxide Fe_3O_4.

ferrotherapy (fer″o-ther′ah-pe) [*ferrum* + *therapy*] therapeutic use of iron and iron compounds.

ferrous (fer′us) containing iron in its plus-two oxidation state, Fe(II) (sometimes designated Fe^{2+}). For ferrous compounds see under the salt, e.g., arsenate and sulfate.

ferruginous (fer-u′jĭ-nus) [L. *ferruginosus; ferrugo* iron rust] 1. containing iron or iron rust; chalybeate. 2. of the color of iron rust.

ferrule (fer′ool) a ring or band of metal applied to the root or crown of a tooth in order to strengthen it, or to protect the margin of the prepared area during placement of a restoration.

ferrum (fer′um) [L.] iron.

Ferry-Porter law (fer′re-por′ter) [Edwin Sidney *Ferry*, American scientist, born 1868; T.C. *Porter*, English scientist] see under *law*.

fertile (fer′til) [L. *fertilis*] fruitful; susceptible of being developed into a new individual (of ova); not sterile or barren.

fertility (fer-til′ĭ-te) 1. the capacity to conceive or induce conception. 2. the ratio of the number of births per year to the number of women of child-bearing age; see *birth rate*, under *rate*.

fertilization (fer′tĭ-lĭ-za′shun) the act of rendering gametes fertile or capable of further development; fecundation. Fertilization begins with contact between spermatozoon and ovum, leading to their fusion, which stimulates the completion of ovum maturation with release of the second polar body. Male and female pronuclei then form and perhaps merge; synapsis follows, which restores the diploid number of chromosomes and results in biparental inheritance and the determination of sex. The process of fertilization leads to the formation of a zygote and ends with the initiation of its cleavage. **cross f.,** the fertilization of one flower by the pollen of another; allogamy. **external f.,** union of the gametes outside the bodies of the originating organisms, as in most fish. **internal f.,** union of the gametes inside the body of the female, the sperm having been transferred from the body of the male by an accessory sex organ or other means.

fertilizin (fer″tĭ-li′zin) a substance of the plasma membrane and gelatinous coat of the ovum of some species. It is considered to possess the specific receptor groups that bind the spermatozoon to the ovum. In sea-urchins, it has been characterized chemically as a glycoprotein of about 300,000 molecular weight.

Ferv. abbreviation for L. *fer′vens*, boiling.

fervescence (fer-ves′ens) [L. *fervescere* to become hot] development of an increased body temperature, or fever.

fescue (fes′ku) 1. any of the grasses belonging to the genus *Festuca*. 2. a condition resembling ergotism, affecting cattle and sometimes sheep, in New Zealand, Australia, and the United States, grazing on tall fescue (*Festuca arunincea*) contaminated by a fungus which contains a toxic principle similar to ergot; it is characterized by lameness of the hind feet, which may progress to necrosis of the affected extremities, sometimes involving the ears or tail. Called also *fescue foot*.

Fesotyme (fe′so-tīm) trademark for a preparation of ferrous sulfate.

fester (fes′ter) to suppurate superficially.

festinant (fes′tĭ-nant) accelerating.

festination (fes″tĭ-na′shun) [L. *festinatio*] an involuntary tendency to take short accelerating steps in walking (festinating gait), as in paralysis agitans and other neurologic diseases.

festoon (fes-toon′) a carving in the base material of a denture that simulates the contours of the natural tissues being replaced by the denture.

festschrift (fest′shrift) [Ger.] a memorial volume; a book made up of articles contributed by pupils or associates and friends of a scientist or leader, published usually to honor some special occasion, such as a birthday or other anniversary.

fetal (fe′tal) of or pertaining to a fetus; pertaining to *in utero* development after the embryonic period.

fetalism (fe′tal-izm) fetalization.

fetalization (fe″tal-i-za′shun) the retention, into adult life, of bodily characters which at some earlier stage of evolutionary history were actually only infantile and were rapidly lost as the organism attained maturity.

fetation (fe-ta′shun) 1. the development of a fetus within the uterus. 2. pregnancy.

feticide (fe′tĭ-sid) [*fetus* + L. *caedere* to kill] the destruction of the fetus.

fetid (fe′tid) [L. *foetidus*] having a rank or disagreeable smell.

fetish (fet′ish, fe′tish) an object believed to be endowed with supernatural powers or regarded with unreasoning devotion; an object (a shoe, stocking, etc.) or a part of the body (a lock of hair, etc.) charged with special erotic interest.

fetishism (fet′ish-izm, fe′tish-izm) the worship or adoration of an inanimate object as a symbol of a loved person; the displacement of erotic interest to a fetish.

fetishist (fet′ish-ist, fe′tish-ist) a person who secures erotic gratification from a fetish.

fetlock (fet′lok) the metacarpophalangeal and metatarsophalangeal regions in the horse.

fetoglobulin (fe″to-glob′u-lin) fetoprotein.

fetography (fe-tog′rah-fe) [*fetus* + Gr. *graphein* to write] roentgenography of the fetus in utero.

fetology (fe-tol′o-je) that branch of medicine dealing with the fetus *in utero*.

fetometry (fe-tom′ĕ-tre) [*fetus* + Gr. *metron* measure] the measurement of the fetus, especially of the diameters of its head. **roentgen f.,** measurement of the fetal head in the uterus by means of the roentgen ray.

fetoplacental (fe″to-plah-sen′tal) pertaining to the fetus and placenta.

fetoprotein (fe″to-pro′tēn) a fetal antigen that also occurs in adults in certain diseases; α_1-fetoprotein appears in the serum of patients with hepatoma and embryonal adenocarcinoma; γ-fetoprotein in that of patients with a variety of neoplasms, including sarcomas and leukemias; and β-fetoprotein (found to be identical with normal liver ferritin) in fetal liver and in adults with a variety of liver diseases. Called also *fetoglobulin*.

fetor (fe′tor) [L.] stench, or offensive odor. **f. ex o′re,** halitosis. **f. hepat′icus,** the peculiar odor of the breath characteristic of hepatic disease; liver breath. **f. o′ris,** halitosis.

fetoscope (fe′to-skōp) 1. a specially designed stethoscope for listening to the fetal heart beat. 2. an endoscope for viewing the fetus *in utero*.

fetoscopic (fe″to-skop′ik) pertaining to or accomplished by fetoscopy.

fetoscopy (fe-tos′ko-pe) viewing of the fetus *in utero* by means of the fetoscope.

fetoxylate hydrochloride (fĕ-toks′ĭ-lāt) chemical name: 2-phenoxyethyl 1-(3-cyano-3,3-diphenylpropyl)-4-phenylisonipecotate monohydrochloride; a smooth muscle relaxant, $C_{36}H_{36}H_2O_3$·-HCl.

fetuin (fe′tu-in) a low-molecular-weight globulin which constitutes nearly the total globulin in the blood of the fetus and newborn of ungulates.

fetus (fe′tus) [L.] the unborn offspring of any viviparous animal; specifically, the unborn offspring in the postembryonic period, after major structures have been outlined, in man from seven or eight weeks after fertilization until birth. **f. acardi′acus,** acardius. **f. amor′phus,** holoacardius amorphus. **calcified f.,** lithopedion. **f. compres′sus,** f. papyraceus. **harlequin f.,** a fetus entirely covered with thick, horny, armor-like plates, the severest form of lamellar exfoliation of the newborn (see under

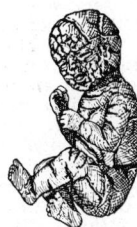

Harlequin fetus (Arey).

exfoliation); it is usually stillborn or dies shortly after birth. **ichthyosis f.,** harlequin f. **f. in fe′tu,** a small, imperfect fetus, incapable of independent life, contained within the body of another fetus, the autosite. **mummified f.,** a shriveled and dried-up fetus. **paper-doll f., papyraceous f.,** f. papyraceus. **f. papyra′ceus,** a dead fetus pressed flat by the growth of a living twin. **parasitic f.,** an incomplete minor fetus attached to a larger, more completely developed fetus, or autosite. **f. sanguinolen′tis,** a dead fetus which has undergone maceration. **sireniform f.,** a sirenomelus, or sympus apus.

Feulgen test (reaction) (foil′gen) [Robert *Feulgen*, German physiologic chemist, 1884–1955] see under *test*.

fever (fe′ver) [L. *febris*] 1. elevation of body temperature above the normal; pyrexia. It may be due to such physiological stress as ovulation, excess thyroid hormone secretions, vigorous exercise, central nervous system lesions, or to infection by microorganisms, or to a host of noninfectious processes, as that accompanying inflammation or resulting from release of pyrogenic materials, as in leukemia. 2. any disease characterized by fever. **abortus f.,** brucellosis. **absorption f.,** a fever often seen during the first twelve hours after parturition. **Aden f.,** dengue. **ady-**

namic f., asthenic f. **African coast f.,** East Coast f. **African tick f.,** relapsing fever caused by *Borrelia duttonii.* **algid pernicious f.,** pernicious malaria with symptoms of collapse. **American mountain f.,** Colorado tick f. **Andaman A f.,** a leptospiral fever occurring in the Netherlands East Indies. **aphthous f.,** foot-and-mouth disease. **Argentinian hemorrhagic f.,** an acute, sometimes fatal disease caused by the Junin virus, characterized by chills, fever, severe myalgia, leukopenia, hemorrhagic manifestations, shock, renal involvement, and neurologic abnormalities. Called also *mal de rostrojos* and *Junin f.* **artificial f.,** elevation of bodily temperature produced by artificial means, as by external heat or the injection of typhoid vaccine or malarial parasites. **aseptic f.,** fever associated with aseptic wounds, presumably due to the disintegration of leukocytes or to the absorption of avascular or traumatized but uninfected tissue. **Assam f.,** kala-azar. **asthenic f.,** a fever with nervous depression, feeble pulse, and a cool, moist skin. **Australian Q f.,** see *Q fever.* **autumn f.,** nanukayami. **Bangkok hemorrhagic f.,** dengue. **biduotertian f.,** tertian malaria with two broods of parasites segmenting on alternate days, so that the febrile paroxysms are nearly continuous. **biliary f. of dogs,** canine piroplasmosis. **biliary f. of horses,** a disease of horses due to infection with *Nuttalia equi* or *Babesia caballi,* marked by high fever, jaundice, hemoglobinuria, gastrointestinal disturbances, and rapid emaciation; called also *equine biliary f.* and *equine piroplasmosis.* **bilious f.** (*obs.*), fever accompanied by the vomiting of bile. **bilious f. of cattle,** gallsickness. **black f.,** 1. Rocky Mountain spotted f. 2. kala-azar. **blackwater f.,** a dangerous complication of falciparum malaria, characterized by the passage of dark red to black urine, severe toxicity, and high mortality, especially for Europeans; called also *West African f.* amd *hemolytic malaria.* **blue f.,** Rocky Mountain spotted f. **Bolivian hemorrhagic f.,** a hemorrhagic fever occurring in Bolivia, which is clinically identical with Argentinian hemorrhagic fever (q.v.), but is caused by the Machupo virus. **bouquet f.,** dengue. **boutonneuse f.,** a disease endemic in the Mediterranean area, the Crimea, Africa, and India, due to infection with *Rickettsia conorii,* which is transmitted by the tick *Rhipicephalus sanguineus;* it is marked by chills, fever, primary skin lesions (tache noir or eschar), and a rash appearing on the second to fourth day; called also *Conor and Bruch's disease* and *escharonodulaire.* Known also by various names according to geographical area, e.g., *Indian tick typhus, Kenya fever,* and *Marseilles fever.* **bovine epizootic f.,** ephemeral f. of cattle. **bovine infectious petechial f.,** a disease of cattle in Kenya, characterized by hemorrhages of the visible mucous membranes, fever, and diarrhea; there may be severe conjunctivitis and protrusion of the eyeball, and death within one to three days is not uncommon. The cause is believed to be a rickettsial-like organism, *Cytoectes ondiri,* spread by a biting insect. Called also *Ondiri disease.* **brain f.,** inflammation of the brain or meninges, or both together. **brassfounder's f.,** metal fume fever (q.v.) caused by fumes of any of several metals, most commonly zinc, copper, or magnesium; called also *brass* or *brazier's chill.* **Brazilian f., Brazilian spotted f.,** Rocky Mountain spotted f. **breakbone f.,** dengue. **buck f.,** the condition of suddenly being given one's great opportunity and being unable to act appropriately. **Bullis f.,** a febrile disease observed in soldiers who had been at Camp Bullis, Texas, in 1942, marked by very low white blood cell count with neutropenia, postorbital and occipital headache, and constant lymphadenitis. It is probably caused by an unclassified species of *Rickettsia,* and transmitted by the bites of the Lone Star tick, *Amblyomma americanum.* Called also *Lone Star f.* and *Texas tick f.* **Bushy creek f.,** pretibial f. **Bwamba f.,** a mild febrile viral disease of sudden onset, occurring in Uganda; it is marked by headache, backache, mild conjunctivitis, and rash. **cachectic f., cachexial f.,** kala-azar. **Cameroon f.,** malaria. **camp f.,** typhus. **canicola f.,** Stuttgart disease. **carbuncular f.,** a variety of anthrax affecting cattle and horses, marked by the formation of circumscribed swellings in the skin, which at first are hard, hot, and painful, but later become gangrenous. **catarrhal f.,** herpetic f. **cat-bite f.,** an infectious disease of man transmitted by the bite of a cat, caused by *Pasteurella multocida,* and marked by the formation of an abscess at the site of inoculation. NOTE: Not to be confused with cat-scratch fever, which has also been called cat-bite fever. **cat-scratch f.,** a benign, subacute, regional lymphadenitis resulting from the scratch or bite of a cat or a scratch from a surface contaminated by a cat; it is marked by a primary papular eruption at the site of inoculation which may develop into a small ulcer. Occasionally, a menignoencephalitis results. A virus is suspected as the cause. Cf. *cat-bite f.* **central f.,** sustained fever resulting from damage to the thermoregulatory centers of the hypothalamus. **Central Asian hemorrhagic f.,** a tickborne hemorrhagic fever occurring in Kazakhstan and Uzbekistan, U.S.S.R; it is thought to be transmitted by the tick *Hyalomma anatolicum.* **cerebrospinal f.,** epidemic cerebrospinal meningitis. **cesspool f.,** typhoid f. **Chagres f.,** originally, a severe type of malaria occurring along the Chagres River in Panama; it is also applied to fever caused by the Chagres virus, which occurs in Panama. Called also *Panama f.* **Charcot's f.,** intermittent hepatic f. **child-**

bed f., puerperal f. **Choix f.,** a disease observed in northern Mexico, identical with Rocky Mountain spotted fever. **Colombian tick f.,** a variety of spotted fever occurring in Colombia, identical with Rocky Mountain spotted fever. **Colorado tick f.,** a nonexanthematous febrile disease occurring in the Rocky Mountain regions of the United States where the tick vector (*Dermacentor andersoni*) of the causative virus is prevalent. **Congolian red f.,** murine typhus. **continued f.,** one which does not vary more than 1.0° to 1.5° F. in twenty-four hours. **continuous f.,** persistently elevated body temperature, showing no or little variation and never falling to normal during any 24-hour period. **Corsican f.,** a sort of malaria occurring in Corsica. **cotton-mill f.,** byssinosis. **Crimean hemorrhagic f.,** a hemorrhagic fever transmitted by the tick *Hyalomma marginatum,* occurring in the Crimea and the Lower Don and Volga River Valleys of the U.S.S.R. **Cyprus f.,** brucellosis. **dandy f.,** dengue. **deer fly f.,** tularemia. **dehydration f.,** 1. inanition f. 2. fever due to loss of body water or inadequate fluid intake, sometimes occurring as a postoperative complication. **dengue f.,** dengue. **desert f.,** the primary stage of coccidioidomycosis. **digestive f.,** a slight rise of temperature during the process of digestion. **double continued f.,** a fever resembling typhoid fever occurring in China. **double quartan f.,** a form of malaria in which the paroxysms occur on two successive days with a one day interval. **drug f.,** a febrile reaction marked by prolonged temperature elevation during the course of administration of a drug, such as an antibiotic, antineoplastic, vaccine, etc.; it may be associated with vasculitis affecting small vessels, and usually disappears rapidly on discontinuance of the drug. **Dumdum f.,** kala-azar. **dust f.,** brucellosis. **Dutton's relapsing f.,** the central African form of relapsing fever caused by *Borrelia duttonii.* **East Coast f.,** a form of piroplasmosis of cattle in Africa, caused by *Theileria (Piroplasma) parva,* and marked by high fever and swelling of the lymph nodes. The organism is transmitted by the bite of several ticks of the genus *Rhipicephalus.* Called also *African Coast f., Rhodesian f., Rhodesian red-water f., Rhodesian tick f.,* and *lymphadenosis aleucaemica parasitaria.* **elephantoid f.,** a recurrent acute febrile condition occurring with filariasis; it may be associated with elephantiasis or lymphangitis. **enteric f.,** 1. typhoid f. 2. paratyphoid (def. 2). **entericoid f.,** any fever which resembles typhoid fever in its clinical manifestations. **ephemeral f.,** a slight fever persisting or lasting only a day or two. **ephemeral f. of cattle,** stiff sickness; three-day sickness: an acute infectious disease symptomatically resembling a benign form of African horse sickness, which affects cattle in South Africa. It is characterized by high fever, stiffness, and lameness, and is thought to be of viral origin. **epidemic catarrhal f.,** influenza. **epidemic hemorrhagic f.,** an acute infectious disease characterized by fever, purpura, peripheral vascular collapse, and acute renal failure, caused by a filtrable agent thought to be transmitted to man by mites or chiggers; called also *hemorrhagic nephrosonephritis, hemorrhagic f. with renal syndrome,* and *nephropathia epidemica.* **equine biliary f.,** biliary f. of horses. **eruptive f.,** any fever accompanied by an eruption on the skin. **eruptive Mediterranean f.,** boutonneuse f. **essential f.,** fever for which no cause has been found. **estivoautumnal f.,** a type of falciparum malaria that was formerly endemic in the United States. **etiocholanolone f.,** a rare disorder in which periodic fever is accompanied by high plasma levels of unconjugated etiocholanolone; it may be associated or confused with other disorders, such as adrenogenital syndrome and familial Mediterranean fever. **exanthematic f. of Marseille,** boutonneuse f. **exanthematous f.,** eruptive f. **familial Mediterranean f.,** a hereditary disease transmitted in an autosomal recessive manner, usually occurring in Armenians and Sephardic Jews, and characterized by short recurrent attacks of fever with pain in the abdomen, chest, or joints and erythema resembling that seen in erysipelas; it is sometimes complicated by amyloidosis. Called also *benign paroxysmal peritonitis, periodic peritonitis, familial recurrent polyserositis,* and *periodic* or *recurrent polyserositis.* **famine f.,** 1. relapsing fever. 2. typhus. **Far East hemorrhagic f.,** epidemic hemorrhagic f. **fatigue f.,** a febrile attack due to overexercise and the absorption of waste products. **ferment f.,** a fever produced by the subcutaneous injection of an enzyme. **field f.,** harvest f. **five-day f.,** trench f. **flood f.,** a highly fatal, acute adenomatoid reaction in the lungs of cattle, believed to be a response to chemicals generated in the rumen by cattle grazing on "fog" (second growth pasture grasses). **food f.,** sudden fever with digestive disturbance lasting from a few days to some weeks; once attributed to intestinal autointoxication, these symptoms may be due to viral gastroenteritis. **Fort Bragg f.,** pretibial f. **foundryman's f.,** metal fume f. **Gibraltar f.,** brucellosis. **glandular f.,** infectious mononucleosis. **goat f., goat's milk f.,** brucellosis. **Hankow f.,** schistosomiasis japonica. **harvest f.,** a form of spirochetosis affecting harvest workers; it is marked by fever, conjunctivitis, stupor, diarrhea, vomiting, and abdominal pains, and is caused by *Leptospira grippotyphosa;* called also *field f.* **Hasami f.,** a mild fever of Japan caused by *Leptospira autumnalis.* **Haverhill f.,** the bacillary form of rat-bite fever (q.v.), caused by *Streptobacillus moniliformis*, and transmitted through contaminated raw milk and its products. It was first reported in an epidemic in Haverhill, Massachusetts in 1925. **hay f.**, a seasonal variety of allergic rhinitis, marked by acute conjunctivitis with lacrimation and itching, swelling of the nasal mucosa, nasal catarrh, sudden attacks of sneezing, and often with asthmatic symptoms. It is regarded as an anaphylactic or allergic condition excited by a specific allergen (e.g., a pollen) to which the individual is sensitized. Known by various names, including *allergic conjuctivitis* and *pollenosis*. Cf. *nonseasonal allergic rhinitis*. **hay f., nonseasonal, hay f., perennial**, nonseasonal allergic rhinitis. **hectic f.**, a daily recurring fever with profound sweating, chills, and flushed countenance. **hemoglobinuric f.**, malaria attended with hemoglobinuria; see *blackwater f.* **hemorrhagic f's**, a group of viral diseases of diverse etiology but having many similar clinical characteristics; increased capillary permeability, leukopenia, and thrombocytopenia are common to all. Hemorrhagic fevers are characterized by sudden onset, fever, headache, generalized myalgia, backache, conjunctivitis, and severe prostration, followed by various hemorrhagic symptoms, which result in focal inflammatory reaction and necrosis resulting in mild leukocytosis. **hemorrhagic f. with renal syndrome**, epidemic hemorrhagic f. **herpetic f.**, primary infection with herpes simplex virus, with diffuse involvement of mucous membranes of the mouth and lips and the surrounding skin; fever and sometimes chills occur. **Herxheimer's f.**, a fever that sometimes accompanies a Jarisch-Herxheimer reaction. **hospital f.**, epidemic typhus. **hyperpyrexial f.**, a fever with very high temperature (104 to 107° F.). **hysterical f.**, an irregular elevation of temperature without general symptoms, sometimes seen in hysteria. **icterohemorrhagic f.**, leptospiral jaundice. **Ikwa f.**, trench f. **inanition f.**, a transitory fever that frequently occurs in infants during the first few days of life; it is believed to be due to dehydration and is also called *dehydration f.* **induced f.**, fever brought on artificially, as by the injection of malarial organisms or typhoid vaccine. **intermenstrual f.**, fever sometimes seen in women between menstrual periods. **intermittent f.**, an attack of malaria or other fever characterized by recurring paroxysms of elevated temperature separated by intervals during which the temperature is normal. **intermittent hepatic f.**, a fever occurring intermittently as the result of intermittent impaction of stone in the common duct and inflammation of the bile ducts; called also *Charcot fever* and *Charcot syndrome*. **inundation f.**, scrub typhus. **irritation f.**, a febrile condition due to the presence of irritant materials in the body. **island f.**, scrub typhus. **Jaccoud's dissociated f.**, fever with slow and irregular pulse in tuberculosis meningitis of adults. **jail f.**, epidemic typhus. **Japanese flood f., Japanese river f.**, scrub typhus. **jungle f.**, falciparum malaria occurring in the East Indies. **jungle yellow f.**, a form of yellow fever endemic in parts of Africa and South America; it occurs in or near uncut forest or jungle. **Junin f.**, Argentinian hemorrhagic f. **Kagami f.**, infectious mononucleosis. **Katayama f.**, fever associated with severe schistosomal infections accompanied by hepatosplenomegaly and by eosinophilia. **Kedani f.**, scrub typhus. **Kenya f.**, Kenya typhus. **Kew Gardens spotted f.**, rickettsialpox. **Kinkiang f.**, schistosomiasis japonica. **Korean hemorrhagic f.**, epidemic hemorrhagic fever. **Korin f.**, epidemic hemorrhagic f. **kriim f.**, an endemic fever of Iceland, Faroe, and Greenland. **Kumaon f.**, form of typhus in India. **Kyoto f.**, a seven-day fever occurring in Kyoto, Japan. **land f.**, a set of symptoms resembling seasickness sometimes experienced when, after an ocean voyage, the ship enters a relatively landlocked body of water. **Lassa f.**, a highly fatal, acute, febrile disease caused by an extremely virulent arenavirus, occurring in West Africa, and characterized by progressively increasing prostration, sore throat, ulcerations of the mouth or throat, rash, and general aches and pains. **lechuguilla f.**, a disease of sheep and goats in western Texas, marked by toxic encephalitis, nephritis, photosensitization, listlessness, icterus, and a yellow discharge from the eyes and nostrils; it is caused by eating the plant *Agave lechuguilla*. Commonly called *swellhead*. **lent f.**, typhoid f. **leprotic f.**, the irregular febrile disturbances seen in the early stages of lepromatous leprosy; a form or a part of the lepra reaction. **Levant f.**, a fever endemic in the Levant; by some believed to be of malarial origin. **Lone Star f.**, Bullis f. **lung f.**, lobar or other pneumonia. **macular f.**, 1. a fever characterized by the presence of macules. 2. former term for typhus. **malarial f.**, malaria. **Malta f., Maltese f.**, brucellosis. **Manchurian f.**, a disease similar to typhoid fever or typhus, occurring in Manchuria. **Marseilles f.**, boutonneuse f. **marsh f.**, 1. leptospiral jaundice. 2. malaria. **Mediterranean f.**, 1. brucellosis. 2. boutonneuse f. **Mediterranean exanthematous f.**, boutonneuse f. **Mediterranean yellow f.**, leptospiral jaundice. **metal fume f.**, an occupational disorder occurring in those engaged in welding and other metallic operations and due to inhalation of volatilized metals; it is characterized by sudden onset of thirst and a metallic taste in the mouth, followed by high fever, muscular aches and pains, shaking chills, headache, weakness, diaphoresis, and leukocytosis. The symptoms usually subside

within 24 to 48 hours, but repeated attacks are common. The disorder includes *brassfounder's f.* (*brass chill, brazier's chill, brassfounders's ague*) and *spelter's f.* (*spelter's chill, zinc chill, zinc fume f.*). Cf. *polymer fume f.* **Meuse f.**, trench f. **mianeh f.**, a form of relapsing fever in Iran. **milk f.**, 1. a fever said to attend the establishment of lactation after delivery. 2. an endemic fever said to be caused by the use of unwholesome cow's milk. 3. a form of paralysis affecting cows near delivery; usually accompanied by hypocalcemia, it is due to a metabolic disorder. Called also *parturient apoplexy, parturient fever*, and *parturient paralysis*. **Mossman f.**, a febrile disease endemic in Queensland, Australia, caused by *Leptospira australis*. **mountain f.**, 1. Colorado tick fever. 2. Rocky Mountain spotted fever. 3. brucellosis. **mountain tick f.**, Colorado tick fever. **mud f.**, leptospiral jaundice. **muma f.**, a term applied to elephantoid fever in Samoa. **Murchison-Pel-Ebstein f.**, a type of fever typical of Hodgkins's disease, characterized by irregular episodes of pyrexia of several days' duration, with intervening periods in which the temperature is normal. **nanukayami f.**, nanukayami. **Neapolitan f.**, brucellosis. **night-soil f.**, typhoid f. **nine-mile f.**, a name formerly given to Q fever in mice and laboratory workers; see *Q fever*. **Omsk hemorrhagic f.**, an acute febrile viral disease occurring in Russia, closely resembling Kyasanur forest disease, and characterized by fever, headache, hemorrhagic manifestations, and a high incidence of bronchopneumonia; ticks of the genus *Dermacentor* serve as the vector. **O'nyong-nyong f.**, an epidemic, febrile, viral disease resembling dengue, which occurs in Kenya and Uganda. **Oroya f.**, the acute febrile anemic stage of Carrión's disease. **Pahvant Valley f.**, tularemia. **paludal f.**, malaria. **Panama f.**, Chagres f. **pappataci f.**, phlebotomus f. **paratyphoid f.**, paratyphoid. **parenteric f.**, a disease clinically resembling typhoid fever and paratyphoid fever, but not caused by *Salmonella*. **parrot f.**, psittacosis. **parturient f.**, milk f., def. 3 **Pel-Ebstein f.**, a cyclic fever occasionally seen in Hodgkin's disease and also associated with other diseases, characterized by irregular episodes of pyrexia of several days duration, with intervening afebrile periods lasting for days or weeks. Called also *Murchison-Pel-Ebstein f., Pel-Ebstein pyrexia*, and *Pel-Ebstein symptom*. **periodic f.**, a hereditary condition characterized by repetitive febrile episodes and autonomic disturbances, occurring in precise or irregular cycles of days, weeks, or months. Transmitted as an autosomal dominant trait, it may begin at any time of life and may last for decades with temporary remissions, or may cease. See also *etiocholanolone f.* and *familial Mediterranean f.* **petechial f.**, cerebrospinal meningitis. **Pfeifer's glandular f.**, infectious mononucleosis. **pharyngoconjunctival f.**, a febrile disease caused by an adenovirus, occurring in epidemic form, largely in school children, and characterized by fever, pharyngitis, rhinitis, conjunctivitis, and enlarged cervical lymph nodes; called also *Beal's disease*. **Philippine hemorrhagic f.**, hemorrhagic dengue. **phlebotomus f.**, a febrile disease of short duration, resembling dengue in many of its symptoms, occurring in Mediterranean and Middle East countries, and caused by Naples and Sicilian sandfly fever viruses, which are transmitted by the sandfly, *Phlebotomus papatasii*. Called also *pappataci f.* and *sandfly f.* **pinta f.**, a disease observed in northern Mexico, identical with Rocky Mountain spotted fever. **pneumonic f.**, pneumonia. **polyleptic f.**, relapsing f. **polymer fume f.**, an occupational disorder due to exposure to the products of combustion of polymers, chiefly polytef (also known as Teflon or paratetrafluoroethylene), the manifestations of which are quite similar to those of metal fume fever (q.v.). Called also *Teflon shakes*. **Pomona f.**, a leptospiral infection occurring in Australia, caused by *Leptospira pomona*. **Pontiac f.**, a self-limited disease first noted in an outbreak in 1968 in a single building in Pontiac, Michigan, marked by fever, cough, muscle aches, chills, headache, chest pain, confusion, and pleuritis; it is now known to be caused by a strain of *Legionella pneumophila*. **pretibial f.**, a leptospiral infection marked by a rash on the pretibial region accompanied by lumbar and postorbital pain, malaise, coryza, and fever; it is caused by *Leptospira autumnalis*. Called also *Bushy creek f.* and *Fort Bragg f.* **prison f.**, typhus. **protein f.**, heightened temperature produced by the injection of protein material into the body. **puerperal f.**, septicemia accompanied by fever, in which the focus of infection is a lesion of the mucous membrane of the parturient canal due to trauma during childbirth; the etiologic agent is usually a streptococcus. Called also *childbed f.*, and *puerperal sepsis* or *septicemia*. **pulmonary f.**, pneumonia. **pythogenic f.**, typhoid f. **Q f.** [Q for *query*] a generally self-limited rickettsial infection caused by *Coxiella burnetti* (*Rickettsia diaporica*), characterized by fever, headache, constitutional symptoms, and pneumonitis. Unlike other rickettsial infections, Q fever is usually acquired by inhalation of the agent and it is not marked by a rash. First described in Australia, but worldwide in distribution, it includes Balkan grippe in the Mediterranean area. Called also *Australian Q f., hiberno-vernal bronchopneumonia* and *nine-mile f.* **quartan f.**, see under *malaria*. **quintan f., quintana f.**, trench f. **quotidian f.**, a fever that recurs every day; see under *malaria*. **rabbit f.**, tularemia. **rat-bite f.**, either of two clinically similar but etiologically distinct, acute infectious diseases, usually transmitted through the bite of a rat, and occurring in a bacillary form caused by *Streptobacillus moniliformis,* and in a spirillary form caused by *Spirillum minor.* In the bacillary form, usually after a latent period of less than ten days, the initial wound heals promptly without inflammation, but after a week or ten days the bite site becomes inflamed, painful, and indurated, followed by adenitis, chills, vomiting, headache, high fever, morbilliform eruption, especially on the hands and feet, and polyarthritis that is often severe. This form also may be associated with ingestion of contaminated raw milk or its products (*Haverhill fever*), in which case there is no initial wound, the first symptoms being systemic. In the spirillary form (*sodoku*), the latent period is most commonly greater than ten days, inflammation recurs at the primary wound site, the rash is less evident than in the bacillary form, arthritis is rare, and the fever is commonly of the relapsing type. **recurrent f.,** relapsing f. **red f.,** dengue. **red f. of Congo,** murine typhus. **red-water f.,** Texas f. **relapsing f.,** any one of a group of acute infectious diseases caused by various species of *Borrelia,* transmitted by lice (*Pediculus humanus*) and ticks (*Ornithodoros*), and marked by alternating periods of fever and apyrexia, each lasting from five to seven days. The disease begins abruptly with chill, headache, neuromuscular pains, fever, and sometimes vomiting. During the febrile periods there is enlargement of the liver and spleen. The organism causing the disease varies in different countries. **remittent f.,** a fever in which the diurnal variation is 2° F. or more, but in which the temperature never falls to a normal level; see *malaria.* **rheumatic f.,** a febrile disease occurring as a delayed sequela of infections with group A hemolytic streptococci and characterized by multiple focal inflammatory lesions of the connective tissue structures, especially of the heart, blood vessels, and joints (polyarthritis), and by the presence of Aschoff bodies in the myocardium and skin. Typically, the onset is signalled by the sudden occurrence of fever and joint pain, followed by manifestations of heart and pericardial disease, abdominal pain, skin changes, and chorea. Atypical manifestations, particularly in adults, are not uncommon. Called also *acute articular rheumatism, acute rheumatic fever* or *arthritis,* and *polyarthritis rheumatica acuta.* **Rhodesian f.,** East Coast f. **rice-field f.,** a fever affecting workers in the rice harvest in Italy and in Sumatra; it is caused by a species of *Leptospira.* **Rift Valley f.,** a febrile disease caused by an arbovirus, transmitted by mosquitoes of the genera *Aedes, Culex,* and *Erethmapodites* and also by contact with tissues and secretions of diseased animals; the symptoms resemble those of dengue. First observed in the Rift Valley of Kenya, it is now seen in Uganda, Natal, and South Africa. It is rarely fatal to man. In animals, it is also known as enzootic hepatitis. **Rio Grande f.,** brucellosis. **river f. of Japan,** scrub typhus. **Robles' f.,** a condition characterized by irregular fever and mild general symptoms, and continuing from two weeks to three months. It occurs in British Honduras. Not to be confused with Robles' disease (onchocerciasis). **rock f.,** brucellosis. **Rocky Mountain spotted f.,** infection with *Rickettsia rickettsii,* transmitted by various ticks, including *Dermacentor andersoni, D. variabilis, Amblyomma americanum,* and the rabbit tick *Haemaphysalis leporispalustris.* First reported in Rocky Mountain states, the disease has since reported in the eastern U.S. and most other states, as well as in Canada, Mexico, Colombia, and Brazil. The infection follows tick bite by a few days and begins with fever, muscle pain, and weakness, with headache followed in two to four days by a macular petechial eruption that begins on the hands and feet and spreads centripetally to the trunk and face. The sensorium is clouded. The localization of rickettsiae in the intima of arterioles is responsible for microangiopathic thrombohemolytic anemia, nephritis, and meningoencephalitis. Called also *Choix f., pinta f.,* and *tickborne typhus.* It is also known by various names according to geographic area. **Roman f.,** a virulent type of malaria which prevailed in the Campagna of Rome, a low plain surrounding the city. **Russian headache f.,** a dengue-like disease. **sakushu f.,** seven-day fever occurring in autumn epidemics in the Okayama Prefecture of Japan. **Salinem f.,** see under *infection.* **Salonica f.,** trench f. **salt f.,** fever associated with excess of salt in the body, due to the retention by the salt of the water normally eliminated in perspiration. **sandfly f.,** phlebotomus f. **San Joaquin f.,** the primary stage of coccidioidomycosis. **scarlet f.,** infection due to Group A β-hemolytic streptococci, and rarely to other serological types of β-hemolytic streptococci that elaborate erythrogenic toxin. It affects mainly the pharynx, but may affect the skin (wound and burn scarlet fever) or birth canal (puerperal scarlet fever). The signs are those of streptococcal infection (pharyngotonsillitis, cellulitis) or those of endometritis, followed by those of toxic origin, including headache, abdominal pain, nausea, and rarely lymphocytic meningitis and hepatitis, and a cutaneous eruption. The skin lesions are a combination of a generalized flush on the trunk and proximal parts of the extremities and cheeks, and of a pinpoint papular eruption on all parts except the face. The skin folds, such as the antecubital fossae and inguinal folds, are hemorrhagic and nonblanching. The rash may last only a few hours, but typically lasts two to three days before fading. Superficial flaking appears over much of the involved area; confluent peeling over fingers and toes is characteristic. The disease is much milder now than in the past, and septic complications such as otitis media, mastoiditis, and suppurative lymphadenitis are rare. Immune-complex nephritis and rheumatic fever are complications derived from Group A streptococcal infection. Called also *febris rubra* and *scarlatina.* See also *erythrogenic toxin,* under *toxin.* **septic f.,** fever due to septicemia. **seven-day f.,** 1. a fever affecting Europeans in India, and marked by symptoms similar to those of dengue. 2. benign leptospirosis. 3. nanukayami. 4. sakushu f. **sheep f.,** heartwater. **shin bone f.,** trench f. **ship f.,** epidemic typhus. **shipping f.,** a disease of cattle caused by *Pasteurella haemolytica* in association with a virus; infection occurs when the resistance of the animal is lowered by stress. **shoddy f.,** a febrile disease, with cough, dyspnea, and headache, caused by dust in shoddy factories. **shouten f.,** a disease which is probably a form of dengue. **slime f.,** leptospiral jaundice. **slow f.,** brucellosis. **solar f.,** dengue. **Songo f.,** epidemic hemorrhagic f. **South African tick-bite f.,** an infection in South Africa caused by *Rickettsia conorii,* the etiologic agent of boutonneuse fever, transmitted by the ixodid ticks, *Haemaphysalis leachi, Rhipicephalus evertsi, R. appendiculatus, Amblyomma hebraeum,* and *Hyalomma aegypticum.* **South American hemorrhagic f.,** see *Argentinian hemorrhagic f.* and *Bolivian hemorrhagic f.* **spelter's f.,** metal fume fever caused by fumes in zinc smelters; called also *spelter's chill, zinc chill,* and *zinc fume f.* **spirillum f.,** sodoku or rat-bite fever due to *Spirillum minus.* **spotted f.,** a febrile disease typically characterized by a skin eruption, such as Rocky Mountain spotted fever, boutonneuse fever, and other infections caused by tick-borne rickettsiae, and typhus and epidemic cerebrospinal meningitis. **sthenic f.,** fever characterized by a full, strong pulse, hot and dry skin, high temperature, thirst, and active delirium. **stiff-neck f.,** epidemic cerebrospinal meningitis. **stockyards f.,** a complex of bacterial and viral diseases of the respiratory system of cattle. **Sumatran mite f.,** a form of scrub typhus transmitted by larvae of *Trombicula deliensis.* **sun f.,** dengue. **swamp f.,** 1. leptospiral jaundice. 2. equine infectious anemia. 3. malaria. **swine f.,** hog cholera. **swine f., African,** a viral disease similar to but more severe than hog cholera, and caused by an immunologically distinct agent; recognized first in Africa and found also in western Europe, Cuba, Brazil, the Dominican Republic, and Haiti. **tertian f.,** see under *malaria.* **tetanoid f.,** cerebrospinal meningitis. **Texas f.,** an infectious disease of cattle caused by the presence in the blood of *Babesia bigemina,* which is introduced by the bite of the ticks *Boophilus annulatus* and *B. microplus.* Called also *bovine piroplasmosis* and *red-water f.* **Texas tick f.,** Bullis f. **Thai hemorrhagic f.,** hemorrhagic dengue. **therapeutic f.,** pyretotherapy, def. 1. **thermic f.,** sunstroke. **three-day f.,** phlebotomus f. **threshing f.,** irritation of the respiratory tract, headache, and fever, occurring in workers at threshing grain. **tibialgic f.,** trench f. **tick f.,** any infectious disease transmitted by the bite of a tick; the causative parasite may be a rickettsia, as in Rocky Mountain spotted fever; a *Babesia,* as in Texas fever; a *Borrelia,* as in relapsing fever; or a virus, as in Colorado tick fever. **Tobia f.,** a disease observed in Colombia, identical with Rocky Mountain spotted fever. **Tokushima f.,** infectious mononucleosis. **traumatic f.,** one which follows a wound or injury. **trench f.,** a self-limited louseborne rickettsial disease due to *Rochalimaea quintana,* transmitted by the body louse, *Pediculus humanus,* and characterized by intermittent fever, generalized aches and pains, particularly severe in the shins, chills, sweating, vertigo, malaise, typhus-like rash, and multiple relapses. Conditions for spread were met principally during World War I. Called also *quintan f., five-day f., Meuse f., shin bone f., Wolhynia f.,* and *His-Werner disease.* **trypanosome f.,** trypanosomiasis. **tsutsugamushi f.,** scrub typhus. **twelve-day f. of Nigeria,** a dengue-like or typhus-like fever, characterized by abundant rash for several weeks, slight albuminuria, and fever terminating by lysis. **typhoid f.,** infection by *Salmonella typhosa* involving primarily the lymphoid follicles of the ileum. The disease may begin abruptly with chills and fever; there is bacteremia, abdominal distention, splenomegaly, and later bacilluria. Rose-colored macules appear transiently on the skin in the early stage of the disease. Perforation of the bowel occurs in about 5 per cent of untreated cases. **typhoid f., abenteric,** formerly, typhoid fever in which the intestinal tract was thought not to be involved. **typhoid f., ambulatory,** a form in which the symptoms are not severe enough to confine the patient to bed. **typhoid f., apyretic,** a form in which the fever does not rise above 100° F., often remaining normal. **typhomalarial f.,** a fever showing typhoid symptoms, but believed to be malarial in origin; called also *febris undulans.* **typhus f.,** see *typhus.* **undulant f.,** brucellosis. **urethral f., urinary f.,** fever following the use of the urethral bougie, catheter, or sound. **uveoparotid f.,** a manifestation of sarcoidosis, marked by chronic inflammation of the parotid gland and the uvea; it is attended also by chronic iridocyclitis, unilateral facial paralysis, lassitude, and a subfebrile temperature. Called also *febris uveoparotidea* and *Heerfordt's disease.* **Uzbekistan hemorrhagic f.,** a disease related to, and possibly identical with, Crimean hemorrhagic fever; it may be transmitted by the tick *Hyalomma anatolicum.* **vaccinal f.,** the slight fever that sometimes follows vaccination. **valley f.,** the primary stage of coccidioidomycosis. **van der Scheer's f.**, trench f. **Walcheren f.**, severe malaria endemic in Holland. **war f.**, epidemic typhus. **West African f.**, blackwater f. **West Nile f.**, see under *encephalitis*. **Whitmore's f.**, melioidosis. **Wolhynia f.**, trench f. **wound f.**, traumatic f. **Yangtze Valley f.**, schistosomiasis japonica. **yellow f.**, an acute infectious disease due to a virus, transmitted to man by mosquitoes which acquire the infection either from man (urban type) or from animals (jungle type). It occurs endemically primarily in the tropical regions of South America and Africa, and occasionally in Central America and other areas. It is marked by fever, jaundice, and albuminuria, the jaundice resulting from necrosis of the liver. *Urban yellow fever* affects chiefly persons living in close contact with one another, and is transmitted by *Aedes aegypti*, which usually breeds near human habitations. *Jungle* (or *sylvan*) *yellow fever* most often affects those working in or living near forests; it has a variety of mosquito vectors, including several species of *Haemagogus* in South America, and *Aedes africanus* and *A. simpsoni* in Central Africa. Called also *fievre jaune, gelb fieber,* and *virus amaril.* **zinc fume f.**, spelter's f.

F.F.A. free fatty acids.
F.F.T. flicker fusion threshold.
F.h. abbreviation for L. *fi′at haus′tus,* let a draught be made.
fiat (fi′at), pl. *fi′ant* [L.] let there be made.
fiber (fi′ber) 1. an elongated, threadlike structure; see also *fibra* [NA]. 2. in nutrition, the sum of the constituents of the diet that are not digested by gastrointestinal enzymes; see *dietary f.* **A f's,** myelinated fibers of the somatic nervous system having a diameter of 1μ to 22μ and a conduction velocity of 5 to 120 meters per second; they include the alpha, beta, delta, and gamma fibers. **accelerating f's, accelerator f's,** adrenergic fibers that transmit the impulses that accelerate the heart beat; called also *augmentor f's* and *cardiac accelerator f's.* **accessory f's,** those fibers of the zonule of Zinn running perpendicularly to the chief fibers and not reaching the lens of the eye; supporting the fibers running from the ciliary body to the chief fibers and bracing them, including the interciliary fibers and the orbiculociliary fibers. Called also *auxiliary fibers.* **adrenergic f's,** nerve fibers that liberate epinephrine-like substances at the time of passage of nerve impulses across a synapse. **alpha f's,** motor and proprioceptive fibers of the A type having conduction velocities of 70 to 120 meters per second and ranging from 13μ to 22μ in diameter. **alveolar f's,** fibers of the periodontal ligament extending from the cementum of the tooth root to the walls of the alveolus, distinguished as alveolar crest, horizontal, oblique, and apical fibers. Called also *cementoalveolar f's.* **alveolar crest f's,** fibers of the periodontal ligament extending from the cementum of the tooth root to the alveolar crest. **anastomosing f's, anastomotic f's,** fibers extending from one muscle bundle or nerve trunk to another. **apical f's,** fibers of the periodontal ligament extending from the cementum of the apical portion of the tooth root to the deepest portion of the alveolus. **archiform f's,** fibrae intercrurales. **arcuate f's, external,** fibrae arcuatae externae. **arcuate f's, internal,** fibrae arcuatae internae. **arcuate f's of cerebrum,** fibrae arcuatae cerebri. **argentaffin f's, argentophil f's, argentophilic f's,** reticular f's. **asbestos f's,** fibers formed in degenerating hyaline cartilage by ossification of the collagen fibers. **association f's,** nerve fibers that interconnect portions of the cerebral cortex within a hemisphere. Short association fibers interconnect neighboring gyri; long fibers interconnect more widely separated gyri and are arranged into bundles or fasciculi. **astral f.,** see under *ray.* **augmentor f's,** accelerating f's. **auxiliary f's,** accessory f's. **axial f.,** the axon of a nerve fiber. **B f's,** myelinated preganglionic autonomic axons having a fiber diameter ≤3μ and a conduction velocity of 3 to 15 meters per second. **basilar f's,** fibers that form the middle layer of the zona arcuata and the zona pectinata of the basilar membrane in the inner ear; called also *auditory strings.* **Bergmann's f's,** processes which radiate from the molecular layer of the cerebellum and enter the pia. **Berneheimer's f's,** a tract of nerve fibers connecting the optic tract to Luys' body. **beta f's,** touch and temperature fibers of the A type having conduction velocities of 30 to 70 meters per second and ranging from 8μ to 13μ in diameter. **bone f's,** Sharpey's f's. **Brücke's f's,** fibrae meridionales musculi ciliaris. **bulbospiral f's,** spiral muscular fibers forming a portion of the musculature of the atria and ventricles of the heart. **Burdach's f's,** nerve fibers connected with Burdach's nucleus (nucleus cuneatus). **C f's,** unmyelinated postganglionic fibers of the autonomic nervous system, also the unmyelinated fibers found at the dorsal roots, and at free nerve endings, which have a conduction velocity of 0.6 to 2.3 meters per second and a diameter of 0.3μ to 1.3μ. **capsular f's,** the nerve fibers within the internal capsule of the brain. **cardiac accelerator f's,** accelerating f's. **cardiac depressor f's,** vagal fibers to the heart which when activated cause a decrease in cardiac output. **cardiac pressor f's,** sympathetic nerve fibers to the heart which when activated cause an increase in cardiac output. **cemental f's,** the fibers of the periodontal membrane extending from the cementum to the zone of the

intermediate plexus, where their terminations are interspersed with the terminations of the alveolar group of periodontal fibers. **cementoalveolar f's,** alveolar f's. **cerebrospinal f's,** the fibers in the internal capsule of the brain which run from the motor region of the cortex to the pyramids of the medulla oblongata. **chief f's,** those fibers of the zonule of Zinn which run from the ciliary body to the lens, including the orbiculoposterocapsular, the orbiculoanterocapsular, the cilioposterocapsular, and cilioequatorial fibers; called also *principal* or *main f's,* and *white f's.* **cholinergic f's,** nerve fibers that liberate acetylcholine at the synapse. **chromatic f.,** the long fiber of chromatin into which the nucleus is resolved during the early stages of karyokinesis and which afterward separates into the chromosomes. **chromosomal f.,** traction f. **cilioequatorial f's,** those chief fibers which pass from the summits of the ciliary processes to the equator of the lens. **cilioposterocapsular f's,** the most numerous of the chief zonular fibers, arising from the tips and sides of the ciliary processes, passing posteriorly and crossing the anteriorly directed fibers, to insert into the posterior capsule anterior to the insertion of the orbiculoposterocapsular fibers. **circular f's of ciliary muscle,** fibrae circulares musculi ciliaris. **circular f's of eardrum,** see *stratum circulare membranae tympani.* **climbing f's, clinging f's,** afferent fibers arising in part from the middle cerebellar peduncle and passing through the granular layer of the cerebellar cortex to terminate on Purkinje cell dendrites. Called also *tendril f's.* Cf. *mossy f's.* **collagen f's, collagenic f's,** collagenous f's. **collagenous f's,** the soft, flexible, white fibers which are the most characteristic constituent of all types of connective tissue, consisting of the protein collagen, and composed of bundles of fibrils that are in turn made up of smaller units (microfibrils) which show a characteristic crossbanding with a major periodicity of 65 nm. See also *fibrous long-spacing collagen* and *segment long-spacing collagen,* under *collagen,* and see also *tropocollagen.* **collateral f's of Winslow,** fibrae intercrurales. **commissural f's,** the nerve fibers which pass between the cortex of opposite hemispheres of the brain, or between two sides of the brain stem or spinal cord. **cone f's,** the fiber-like extensions of the retinal cells on either side of their nuclei. *Outer cone fibers* connect the cone nucleus to the inner segment in the region of the fovea; *inner cone fibers* run from the cone nucleus through the outer part of the anterior plexiform layer and terminate in a cone pedicle. **continuous f's,** the spindle fibers in mitosis which extend from pole to pole. **Corti's f's,** rods of Corti. **corticobulbar f's, corticonuclear f's,** fibrae corticonucleares. **corticopontine f's,** tractus corticopontinus. **corticospinal f's,** fibrae corticospinales. **dark f's,** muscle fibers rich in sarcoplasm and having a dark appearance. **Darkshevich's f's,** nervous fibers of the cerebrum running from the optic tract to the habenular ganglion. **decussating f's,** any set of interconnecting fibers. **dendritic f's,** fibers which pass in a tree-like form from the cortex to the white substance of the brain. **dentinal f's,** Tomes' f's. **dentinogenic f's,** Korff's f's. **depressor f's,** 1. nerve fibers which, when stimulated reflexly, cause a diminished vasomotor tone and thereby a decrease in arterial pressure. 2. cardiac depressor f's. **dietary f.,** that part of whole grains, vegetables, fruits, and nuts that resists digestion in the gastrointestinal tract; it consists of carbohydrate (cellulose, etc.) and lignin. **Edinger's f's,** fibers in the cerebrum of amphibia, forming part of the visual paths. **elastic f's,** yellowish fibers of elastic quality traversing the intercellular substance of connective tissue; called also *yellow f's.* **endogenous f's,** nerve fibers of the spinal cord which arise from cells the bodies of which are situated inside the cord. **exogenous f's,** fibers of the spinal cord which arise from cells the bodies of which are situated outside the cord. **extraciliary f's,** see *fleece.* **extrafusal f's,** ordinary muscle fibers, as opposed to the intrafusal fibers of the muscle spindle. **forklike f's,** branching fibers in the tunica media of arteries. **gamma f's,** A fibers that conduct touch and pressure impulses and innervate the intrafusal fibers of the muscle spindle; they conduct at velocities of 15 to 40 meters per second and range from 3μ to 7μ in diameter. **Gerdy's f's,** the fibers of the superficial ligament connecting the clefts of the palmar surfaces of the fingers. **gingival f's,** the collagen fibers which make up the gingival corium and support the gingivae. They are attached and adapted to the tooth surface and act as a barrier to the apical migration of the epithelial attachment. **Goll's f's,** fibers extending from Goll's nucleus (nucleus gracilis) to the vermis of the cerebellum. **Gottstein's f's,** the external hair cells, and nerve fibers associated with them, forming a part of the expansion of the auditory nerve in the cochlea. **Gratiolet's radiating f's,** radiatio optica. **gray f's,** unmyelinated nerve fibers, found largely, but not exclusively, in the sympathetic nerves; called also *f's of Remak.* **hair f.,** any one of the horny fibers, each containing relics of a nucleus, which make up the main substance of a hair. **half-spindle f's,** spindle fibers in mitosis which extend from one pole to the chromosomes. **Henle's f's,** the fibers of the fenestrated membrane which exists in certain arteries between the external and middle coats; some are elastic, others nucleated. **Herxheimer's f's,** minute spiral fibers in the stratum mucosum of the skin; called also *Herxheimer's spirals.* **heterodesmotic f's,** white fibers connecting dissimilar gray structures of the nervous system. **homodesmotic f's,** white fibers connecting similar gray structures of the central nervous system. **horizontal f's,** fibers of the periodontal ligament extending horizontally from the cementum of the tooth root to the walls of the alveolus. **impulse-conducting f's,** Purkinje's f's. **interciliary f's,** those accessory fibers running between the ciliary processes. **intercolumnar f's,** fibrae intercrurales. **intercrural f's,** fibrae intercrurales. **internuncial f's,** fibers connecting nerve cells. **interzonal f's,** the delicate fibers of achromatin forming the central spindle during karyokinesis. **intrafusal f's,** modified muscle fibers which, surrounded by fluid and enclosed in a connective tissue envelope, compose the muscle spindle. **James f.,** junctional tissue or a tract which bypasses the atrioventricular node, thus permitting ventricular pre-excitation. **Korff's f's,** thickened radial argentophilic collagen fibers at the periphery of the pulp of a tooth, entering the dentin and condensing to form the matrix; called also *dentinogenic f's.* **lattice f's,** reticular f's. **f's of lens,** fibrae lentis. **light f's,** muscle fibers poor in sarcoplasm and therefore more transparent than dark fibers. **longitudinal f's of pons,** fasciculi longitudinales pontis. **Luschka's f's,** fibers of the levator ani muscle that meet between the anus and the vagina in the perineal body. **Mahaim f's,** fibers arising from the proximal main atrioventricular bundle, which allow early excitation of the base of the ventricular septum. **main f's,** chief f's. **mantle f.,** any one of the cytoplasmic filaments which assist in drawing the daughter chromosomes toward the poles of the central spindles. **Mauthner's f.,** an axon that extends from the metencephalon to the caudal end of the spinal cord of fishes and amphibians, and provides the final common path for impulses to the tail. **medullated f's,** *myelinated f's.* **meridional f's of ciliary muscle,** fibrae meridionales musculi ciliaris. **moss f's, mossy f's,** thick afferent nerve fibers arising from the inferior cerebellar peduncle and passing into the cerebellar cortex to terminate in numerous branches or mosslike appendages around the cells of the granular layer. Cf. *climbing f's.* **motor f.,** a fiber in a mixed nerve which transmits impulses to a muscle fiber. **Müller's f's,** elongated neuroglial cells traversing all the layers of the retina and forming its most important supporting element; called also *sustentacular f's, cells of Müller,* and *radial cells of Müller.* **muscle f.,** any of the cells of skeletal or cardiac muscle tissue. Skeletal muscle fibers are cylindrical multinucleate cells containing contracting myofibrils, across which run transverse striations, enclosed in a sarcolemma. Cardiac muscle fibers contain one or sometimes two nuclei and myofibrils and are separated from one another by an intercalated disk; although striated, cardiac muscle fibers branch to form an interlacing network. See also *muscle cell,* under *cell.* **muscle f's, intermediate,** muscle fibers having characteristics intermediate between red and white muscle fibers. **muscle f's, red,** the small dark fibers that predominate in red muscle (q.v.). **muscle f's, white,** the large pale fibers that predominate in white muscle (q.v.). **myelinated f's, myelinated nerve f's,** grayish white nerve fibers whose axons are encased in a myelin sheath, which may in turn be enclosed by a neurilemma; called also *medullated f's* and *medullated nerve f's.* Cf. *unmyelinated f's.* **Nélaton's f's,** Nélaton's sphincter. **nerve f.,** a slender process of a neuron, especially the prolonged axon which conducts nerve impulses away from the cell. Nerve fibers are classified on the basis of the presence or absence of a myelin sheath as myelinated or unmyelinated. **neuroglial f.,** one of the fibrillar structures embedded in the cytoplasm and expansions of neuroglial cells. **nonmedullated f's,** unmyelinated f's. **oblique f's,** fibers of the periodontal ligament which extend obliquely from the cementum of the tooth root to the alveolar bone. **oblique f's of stomach,** fibrae obliquae ventriculi. **odontogenic f's,** the fibers forming the layer of connective tissue of the matrix of a tooth surrounding the pulp. **olivocerebellar f's,** see *tractus olivocerebellaris.* **orbiculoanterocapsular f's,** those chief fibers which have the most posterior and internal position, lying in close relation to the anterior boundary of the vitreous. **orbiculociliary f's,** those accessory fibers which pass from the pars orbicularis to the ciliary processes. **orbiculoposterocapsular f's,** those chief fibers which spring from the prolongation of the hyaloid membrane investing the ciliary ring. **osteocollagenous f's,** fibers gathered together into bundles and united by a special binding substance in the interstitial substance of bone. **osteogenetic f's,** osteogenic f's. **osteogenic f's,** precollagenous fibers formed by osteoclasts and becoming the fibrous component of bone matrix. **oxytalan f.,** a connective tissue fiber, resistant to acid hydrolysis, found in structures subjected to mechanical stress, such as tendons, ligaments, adventitia, and connective tissue sheaths that surround the skin appendages. **perforating f's,** Sharpey's f's. **periventricular f's,** fibrae periventriculares. **pilomotor f's,** unmyelinated nerve fibers going to the small muscles of the hair follicles. **postcommissural f's,** the fibers of the posterior commissure lying just behind the pineal body. **postganglionic f's,** fibers constituting a postganglionic neuron. **precollagenous f's,** a name given reticular fibers on the supposition that they are immature collagenous fibers.

precommissural f's (*obs.*), fibers of the anterior commissure in the lamina terminalis. **preganglionic f's,** fibers constituting a preganglionic neuron. **pressor f's,** 1. nerve fibers which, when stimulated reflexly, cause or increase vasomotor tone. 2. cardiac pressor f's. **principal f's,** 1. chief f's. 2. fibers of the periodontal ligament, which are collagen fibers arranged in bundles along the length of the root of a tooth, and suspend and anchor the tooth to the alveolus. They include the transseptal, alveolar crest, horizontal, oblique, and apical fibers. **projection f's,** a term applied to all the bundles of axons which connect the cerebral cortex with the subcortical centers, the brain stem, and the spinal cord; called also *projection tract.* **Prussak's f's,** two short fibers from the end of the short process of the malleus to the notch of Rivinus. **Purkinje's f's,** modified cardiac muscle fibers in the subendothelial tissue that rapidly transmit impulses in the heart and serve to coordinate contraction of the heart; dense networks of these fibers form the sinoatrial and atrioventricular nodes. **pyramidal f's of medulla oblongata,** fibrae pyramidales medullae oblongatae. **radiating f's of anterior chondrosternal ligaments,** ligamenta sternocostalia radiata. **radiating f's of eardrum,** see *stratum radiatum membranae tympani.* **radicular f's,** fibers in the roots of the spinal nerves. **Rasmussen's nerve f's,** efferent fibers in both the vestibular and cochlear divisions of the eighth cranial nerve, which originate bilaterally from the vicinity of the superior olive. **Reissner's f.,** a highly refractive longitudinal fiber in the central canal of the spinal cord. **f's of Remak,** gray f's. **reticular f's,** immature connective tissue fibers, staining with silver, forming the reticular framework of lymphoid and myeloid tissue and occurring also in the interstitial tissue of glandular organs, the papillary layer of the skin, and elsewhere; called also *argentaffin f's, argentophilic f's, lattice f's,* and *Gitterfasern.* **Retzius' f's,** the stiff filaments of Deiters' cells in the organ of Corti. **Ritter's f.,** a fiber in the axis of a retinal rod, probably a nerve fiber. **rod f's,** the fiber portion of the rod cells of the retina. **Rolando's f's** (*obs.*), fibrae arcuatae externae. **Sappey's f's,** smooth muscle fibers in the check ligaments of the eye near their orbital attachments. **Sharpey's f's,** 1. collagenous fibers that pass from the periosteum and are embedded in the outer circumferential and interstitial lamellae of bone; called also *bone f's.* 2. terminal portions of principal fibers that insert into the cementum of a tooth. Called also *perforating f's.* **short association f's,** fibers in the cerebrum that connect adjacent gyri. **sinospiral f's,** spiral muscular fibers forming a portion of the musculature of the atria and ventricles of the heart. **spindle f's,** the microtubules radiating from the centrioles during mitosis and forming a spindle-shaped configuration. See *spindle.* **Stilling's f's,** a term applied, probably incorrectly, to association fibers of the cerebellum; more correctly refers to the reticular formation of the medulla oblongata. **sudomotor f's** unmyelinated nerve fibers going to the sweat glands. **sustentacular f's,** Müller's f's. **T f.,** a nerve fiber that branches at right angles from the axon of a nerve cell. **tendril f's,** climbing f's. **Tomes' f's,** branching processes of the odontoblasts in the dentinal canals; called also *dentinal f's.* **traction f's,** the fibers of the spindle in mitosis along which the daughter chromosomes move apart; called also *chromosomal f's.* **transilient f's,** short association fibers, especially those that pass from one gyrus to another not next to it. **transseptal f's,** fibers of the periodontal ligament extending interproximally over the interdental septum, their ends being embedded in the cementum of adjacent teeth. **transverse f's of pons,** fibrae pontis transversae. **ultraterminal f.,** a thin unmyelinated twig given off from the ramifications of the axon in the motor plate. **unmyelinated f's, unmyelinated nerve f's,** nerve fibers (axons) that lack the myelin sheath but may be enclosed by a neurilemma. Called also *nonmedullated f's* and *nonmedullated nerve f's.* Cf. *myelinated f's.* **varicose f's,** certain myelinated fibers which have no neurilemma; after death a fluid accumulates between the myelin and the axon, giving the fibers a varicose appearance. **vasomotor f's,** unmyelinated nerve fibers going chiefly to arteriolar muscles. **von Monakow's f's,** ansa lenticularis. **Weissmann's f's,** fibers within the muscle spindle. **white f's,** collagenous f's. **yellow f's,** elastic f's. **zonular f's,** fibrae zonulares.

fibercolonoscope (fi″ber-ko-lōn′-o-skōp) a fiberscope for viewing the colon.

fibergastroscope (fi″ber-gas′tro-skōp) a fiberscope for viewing the stomach.

fiber-illuminated (fi′ber-il-loo″min-a′ted) transmitting light by means of bundles of glass or plastic fibers, utilizing a lens system to transmit the image; said of endoscopes of such design.

fiberoptic (fi″ber-op′tik) pertaining to fiberoptics; coated with glass or plastic fibers having special optical properties.

fiberoptics (fi″ber-op′tiks) the transmission of an image along flexible bundles of coated parallel glass or plastic fibers that propagate light by internal reflections.

fiberscope (fi′ber-skōp) a flexible endoscope whose lumen is coated with glass or plastic fibers having special optical properties; see *fiberoptics.*

Fibiger (fi′bĭ-ger) Johannes Andreas Grib, Danish pathologist,

1867–1928; winner of the Nobel prize in physiology and medicine for 1926.

fibra (fi′brah), pl. *fi′brae* [L.] [NA] a fiber: a general term designating an elongated, threadlike structure. **fi′brae annula′res,** see *pars anularis vaginae fibrosae digitorum manus* and *pars anularis vaginae fibrosae digitorum pedis.* **fi′brae arcua′tae cer′ebri** [NA], arcuate fibers of cerebrum: short association fibers within the cerebral cortex, connecting adjacent gyri; called also *fibrae propriae.* **fi′brae arcua′tae exter′nae** [NA], external arcuate fibers: fibers that arise from the arcuate nuclei and run laterally over the surface of the medulla oblongata to reach the cerebellum by way of the inferior cerebellar peduncle. **fi′brae arcua′tae inter′nae** [NA], internal arcuate fibers: fibers that arise from the nucleus cuneatus and nucleus gracilis and pass ventromedially around the central gray substance of the medulla oblongata to form the decussation of the medial lemnisci. **fi′brae cerebello-oliva′res,** see *tractus olivocerebellaris.* **fi′brae circula′res mus′culi cilia′ris** [NA], circular fibers: fibers forming a fairly discrete portion of the ciliary muscle and extending around the apex of the ciliary body close to the root of the iris. Called also *Müller's muscle.* **fi′brae corticonuclea′res** [NA], corticonuclear fibers: longitudinal fibers of the pyramidal tract that arise in the cerebral cortex, descend in the internal capsule, and synapse in the various motor nuclei of the mesencephalon, pons, and medulla oblongata. Called also *corticobulbar fibers.* **fi′brae corticoponti′nae** [NA], corticopontine fibers: former NA term for *tractus corticopontinus.* **fi′brae corticoreticula′res** [NA], nerve fibers that arise chiefly in the sensorimotor areas of the cerebral cortex, descend with corticospinal fibers, and synapse with cells of the reticular formation, especially in the pons and medulla oblongata. **fi′brae corticospina′les** [NA], corticospinal fibers: longitudinal fibers that arise in the cerebral cortex, descend in the internal capsule, mesencephalon, pons, and pyramids of the medulla oblongata and which form, upon reaching the spinal cord, the pyramidal (corticospinal) tracts. **fi′brae intercrura′les** [NA], intercrural fibers: fibers joining the medial and lateral crura of the superficial inguinal ring; called also *Cooper's* or *Scarpa's fascia, Todd's process,* and *collateral fibers of Winslow.* **fi′brae len′tis** [NA], fibers of lens: long bands, derived from the epithelium, that make up the substance of the lens. **fi′brae meridiona′les [Brue′ckei],** fibrae meridionales musculi ciliaris. **fi′brae meridiona′les mus′culi cilia′ris** [NA], meridional fibers of ciliary muscle: fibers of the ciliary muscle that run from the pectinate ligament toward the ciliary processes; called also *fibrae meridionales [Brueckei]* and *Brücke's fibers.* **fi′brae obli′quae ventric′uli** [NA], oblique fibers of stomach: the inner, obliquely coursing fibers of the muscular tunic of the stomach. **fi′brae periventricula′res** [NA], periventricular fibers: fibers that arise from the hypothalamus, then descend in the central gray matter through the tegmentum of the mesencephalon and the reticular formation of the pons and medulla oblongata; some are found in the dorsal longitudinal fasciculus. **fi′brae pon′tis profun′dae,** the more deeply situated of the fibrae pontis transversae. **fi′brae pon′tis superficia′les,** the more superficial of the fibrae pontis transversae. **fi′brae pon′tis transver′sae** [NA], transverse fibers of pons: fibers within the ventral part of the pons which arise from the pontine nuclei and run laterally to form the middle cerebellar peduncles. Most of these fibers cross the midline. **fi′brae pro′priae,** fibrae arcuatae cerebri. **fi′brae pyramida′les medul′lae oblonga′tae,** former NA term for the portion of the pyramidal tract in the ventromedial part of the medulla oblongata; called also *fasciculi pyramidales medulla oblongatae* or *pyramidal fibers of medulla oblongata.* **fi′brae zonula′res** [NA], zonular fibers: the fibers that anchor the lens capsule to the ciliary body and the retina; called also *aponeurosis of Zinn.*

fibrae (fi′bre) [L.] plural of *fibra.*

fibre (fi′ber) fiber.

fibrescope (fi′ber-skōp) fiberscope.

fibril (fi′bril) [L. *fibrilla*] a minute fiber or filament; often a component of a compound fiber. **border f's,** myoglia. **collagen f's,** delicate fibrils of collagen in connective tissue, usually cemented together in wavy bundles. Cf. *fibroblast.* **dentinal f's,** component fibrils of the dentinal matrix. **Dirck's f's,** fibrils of elastic tissue binding together the layers of elastic fibers of the tunica media of an artery. **Ebner's f's,** threadlike fibrils in the dentin and in the cementum of a tooth. **fibroglia f's,** see *fibroglia.* **muscle f., muscular f.,** myofibril. **nerve f.,** an axon. **side f. of Golgi,** a delicate twig given off at right angles from a neuraxon near its junction with the ganglion cells. **Tomes' f's,** see under *fiber.*

fibrilla (fi-bril′ah), pl. *fibril′lae* [L.] a fibril.

fibrillae (fi-bril′e) [L.] plural of *fibrilla.*

fibrillar, fibrillary (fi′brĭ-lar, fi′brĭ-lār-e) pertaining to a fibril or to fibrils.

fibrillated (fi′brĭ-lāt-ed) made up of fibrils.

fibrillation (fi-brĭ-la′shun) 1. the quality of being fibrillar. 2. a small, local involuntary contraction of muscle, invisible under the skin, resulting from spontaneous activation of single muscle cells or muscle fibers. 3. the initial degenerative changes in osteoarthritis, characterized by softening of the articular cartilage and development of vertical clefts between groups of cartilage cells. **atrial f.,** atrial arrhythmia characterized by rapid randomized contractions of the atrial myocardium, causing a totally irregular, often rapid ventricular rate. **auricular f.,** atrial f. **ventricular f.,** arrhythmia characterized by fibrillary contractions of the ventricular muscle due to rapid repetitive excitation of myocardial fibers without coordinated contraction of the ventricle, an expression of randomized circus movement or of an ectopic focus with a very rapid cycle.

Fibrillenstruktur (fib″ril-len-shtrook′tur) [Ger.] the term used to describe the pattern of separate myofibrils that is typical of white skeletal muscles. Cf. *Felderstruktur.*

fibrilloblast (fi-bril′o-blast) [*fibril* + Gr. *blastos* germ] odontoblast.

fibrillogenesis (fi-bril″o-jen′ĕ-sis) the formation of fibrillae.

fibrillolysis (fi″brĭ-lol′ĭ-sis) the destruction or dissolution of fibrils or fibrillae.

fibrillolytic (fi″bril-o-lit′ik) destroying or dissolving fibrillae.

fibrin (fi′brin) the insoluble protein formed from fibrinogen by the proteolytic action of thrombin during normal clotting of blood. Fibrin forms the essential portion of the blood clot. **gluten f.,** a form of fibrin from the seeds of various plants. **Henle's f.,** fibrin formed by precipitating semen with water. **myosin f.,** an insoluble variety of myosin, probably actomyosin. **stroma f.,** fibrin obtained from the stroma of blood corpuscles. **vegetable f.,** gluten f.

fibrinase (fi′brin-ās) Factor XIII; see *coagulation factors,* under *factor.*

fibrinocellular (fi″brĭ-no-sel′u-lar) made up of fibrin and cells.

fibrinogen (fi-brin′o-jen) [*fibrin* + Gr. *gennan* to produce] 1. Factor I; see *coagulation factors,* under *factor.* 2. human fibrinogen: a sterile fraction of normal human plasma, dried from the frozen state, which in solution has the property of being converted into soluble fibrin when thrombin is added; administered by intravenous infusion to increase the coagulability of the blood.

fibrinogenase (fi″brin-oj′ĕ-nās) [*fibrinogen* + *-ase*] thrombin.

fibrinogenemia (fi-brin″o-jĕ-ne′me-ah) hyperfibrinogenemia.

fibrinogenesis (fi″brĭ-no-jen′ĕ-sis) the production or formation of fibrin.

fibrinogenic (fi″brĭ-no-jen′ik) producing or causing the formation of fibrin.

fibrinogenolysis (fi″brĭ-no-jĕ-nol′ĭ-sis) [*fibrinogen* + Gr. *lysis* dissolution] the dissolution or inactivation of fibrinogen in the blood.

fibrinogenolytic (fi″brĭ-no-jen″o-lit′ik) pertaining to or inducing fibrinogenolysis.

fibrinogenopenia (fi-brin″o-jen″o-pe′ne-ah) deficiency of fibrinogen in the blood.

fibrinogenopenic (fi″brin-o-jen″o-pe′nik) pertaining to or caused by fibrinogenopenia.

fibrinogenous (fi″brĭ-noj′ĕ-nus) caused by fibrin, or resulting from the formation of fibrin.

fibrinoid (fi′brĭ-noid) [*fibrin* + Gr. *eidos* form] 1. resembling fibrin. 2. a homogeneous, eosinophilic, refractile, relatively acellular material with some of the tinctorial properties of fibrin.

fibrinokinase (fi″brĭ-no-ki′nās) a non-water-soluble plasminogen activator derived from animal tissues; called also *tissue activator.*

fibrinolysin (fi″brĭ-nol′ĭ-sin) 1. plasmin. 2. a commercial preparation of proteolytic enzyme formed from profibrinolysin by the action of physical agents or by specific bacterial kinases; used to promote dissolutions of thrombi. **seminal f.,** an enzyme in human semen that liquefies the clotted semen.

fibrinolysis (fi″brĭ-nol′ĭ-sis) [*fibrin* + Gr. *lysis* dissolution] the dissolution of fibrin by enzymatic action.

fibrinolytic (fi″brĭ-no-lit′ik) pertaining to, characterized by, or causing fibrinolysis.

fibrinopenia (fi″brĭ-no-pe′ne-ah) [*fibrin* + Gr. *penia* poverty] deficiency of fibrinogen in the blood.

fibrinopeptide (fi″brĭ-no-pep′tid) a substance split off from fibrinogen, during coagulation, by the action of thrombin.

fibrinoplastic (fi″brĭ-no-plas′tik) of the nature of fibrinoplastin.

fibrinoplastin (fi″brĭ-no-plas′tin) paraglobulin. **Schmidt's f.,** paraglobulin.

fibrinoplatelet (fi″brin-o-plāt′let) composed of fibrin and platelets, as a blood clot.

fibrinopurulent (fi″brĭ-no-pu′roo-lent) characterized by the presence of both fibrin and pus.

fibrinorrhea (fi″brĭ-no-re′ah) a profuse discharge containing fibrin.

fibrinoscopy (fi-brĭ-nos′ko-pe) [*fibrin* + Gr. *skopein* to examine] inoscopy.

fibrinose (fi′brĭ-nōs) an albumose derived from fibrin.

fibrinous (fi′brĭ-nus) pertaining to or of the nature of fibrin.

fibrinuria (fi″brin-u′re-ah) the presence of fibrin in the urine.

fibro- (fi′bro) [L. *fibra* fiber] a combining form denoting relationship to fibers.

fibroadenia (fi″bro-ah-de′ne-ah) [*fibro-* + Gr. *adēn* gland] fibroid degeneration of gland tissue, especially the reduction in lymphocytes and increase in stroma in the malpighian bodies in Banti's disease.

fibroadenoma (fi″bro-ad″ĕ-no′mah) adenoma containing fibrous tissue. **giant f. of the breast,** a fibroadenoma of large size that may involve much of the mammary gland.

fibroadenosis (fi″bro-ad″ĕ-no′sis) a nodular condition of the breast not due to neoplasm.

fibroadipose (fi″bro-ad′ĭ-pōs) both fibrous and fatty.

fibroangioma (fi″bro-an″je-o′mah) an angioma containing much fibrous tissue. **nasopharyngeal f.,** see under *angiofibroma.*

fibroareolar (fi″bro-ah-re′o-lar) [*fibro-* + L. *areola*] both fibrous and areolar.

fibroatrophy (fi″bro-at′ro-fe) a combination of fibrosis and atrophy.

fibroblast (fi′bro-blast) [*fibro-* + Gr. *blastos* germ] 1. a connective tissue cell; a flat elongated cell with cytoplasmic processes at each end, having a flat, oval, vesicular nucleus. Fibroblasts, which differentiate into chondroblasts, collagenoblasts, and osteoblasts, form the fibrous tissues in the body, tendons, aponeuroses, supporting and binding tissues of all sorts. Called also *fibrocyte* and *desmocyte.* 2. collagenoblast; the collagen-producing cell. Such cells also proliferate at the site of chronic inflammation. **pericryptal f's,** flattened fibroblasts forming a sheath around the intestinal glands of the colon.

fibroblastic (fi″bro-blas′tik) 1. pertaining to fibroblasts. 2. fibroplastic.

fibroblastoma (fi″bro-blas-to′mah) a tumor arising from a fibroblast; such tumors are now differentiated as fibromas or fibrosarcomas. **perineural f.,** a tumor arising from the connective tissue sheath of a neuron, as an acoustic neuroma.

fibrobronchitis (fi″bro-brong-ki′tis) croupous bronchitis.

fibrocalcific (fi″bro-kal-sif′ik) pertaining to or characterized by partially calcified fibrous tissue.

fibrocarcinoma (fi″bro-kar″sĭ-no′mah) scirrhous carcinoma.

fibrocartilage (fi″bro-kar′tĭ-lij) a type of cartilage made up of typical cartilage cells (chondrocytes), with parallel thick, compact collagenous bundles forming the interstitial substances, separated by narrow clefts enclosing the encapsulated cells; called also *stratified cartilage.* For names of specific structures composed of such tissue, see under *fibrocartilago.* **basal f.,** fibrocartilago basalis. **basilar f.,** synchondrosis sphenooccipitalis. **circumferential f.,** fibrocartilage that forms a rim about a joint cavity. **connecting f.,** a disk of fibrocartilage that attaches opposing bones to each other by synchondrosis; called also *spongy f.* **cotyloid f.,** labrum acetabulare. **elastic f.,** fibrocartilage containing elastic fibers. **interarticular f.,** an articular disk (def. 1); see terms beginning *discus articularis,* under *discus.* **intervertebral f's,** disci intervertebrales. **semilunar f's,** crescent-shaped structures resting on the articulating surfaces of the upper end of the tibia, increasing the concavity of the tibial condyles and acting as cushions or shock absorbers; the lateral and medial menisci. **spongy f.,** connecting f. **stratiform f.,** cartilage such as that lining the bony grooves lodging certain tendons. **white f.,** fibrocartilage in which strong bundles of white fibrous tissue predominate. **yellow f.,** fibrocartilage containing bundles of yellow elastic fibers but with little or no white fibrous tissue.

fibrocartilagines (fi″bro-kar″tĭ-laj′ĭ-nēz) [L.] plural of *fibrocartilago.*

fibrocartilaginous (fi″bro-kar″tĭ-laj′ĭ-nus) pertaining to or composed of fibrocartilage.

fibrocartilago (fi″bro-kar″tĭ-lah′go), pl. *fibrocartilag′ines* [L.] [NA] fibrocartilage: a general term for an anatomical structure composed of cartilage the matrix of which contains a considerable amount of fibrous tissue; called also *stratified cartilage.* **f. basa′lis,** basal fibrocartilage: the cartilage that fills the foramen lacerum of the skull. **f. basila′ris,** synchondrosis sphenoocipitalis. **fibrocartilag′ines interverteb′les,** disci intervertebrales. **f. navicula′ris,** a fibrocartilaginous facet on the dorsal surface of the plantar calcaneonavicular ligament that helps form the articular cavity for the head of the talus.

fibrocaseous (fi″bro-ka′se-us) both fibrous and caseous.

fibrocellular (fi″bro-sel′u-lar) partly fibrous and partly cellular.

fibrochondritis (fi″bro-kon-dri′tis) [*fibro-* + *chondritis*] inflammation of a fibrocartilage.

fibrochondroma (fi″bro-kon-dro′mah) [*fibro-* + *chondroma*] chondroma that contains areas of fibrosis.

fibrocollagenous (fi″bro-kol-laj′ĕ-nus) both fibrous and collagenous; pertaining to or composed of fibrous tissue mainly composed of collagen.

fibrocyst (fi′bro-sist) [*fibro-* + Gr. *kystis* sac, bladder] cystic fibroma.

fibrocystic (fi″bro-sis′tik) characterized by the development of cystic spaces, especially in relation to some duct or gland, accompanied by an overgrowth of fibrous tissue.

fibrocystoma (fi″bro-sis-to′mah) cystic fibroma.

fibrocyte (fi′bro-sīt) [*fibro-* + Gr. *kytos* hollow vessel] fibroblast.

fibrocytogenesis (fi″bro-si″to-jen′ĕ-sis) [*fibrocyte* + Gr. *genesis* production] the development of connective tissue fibrils.

fibrodysplasia (fi″bro-dis-pla′se-ah) fibrous dysplasia.

fibroelastic (fi″bro-e-las′tik) composed of fibrous and elastic tissue.

fibroelastosis (fi″bro-e″las-to′sis) overgrowth of fibroelastic elements. **endocardial f.,** a condition characterized by hypertrophy of the wall of the left ventricle and conversion of the endocardium into a thick fibroelastic coat, with the capacity of the ventricle sometimes reduced, but often increased.

fibroenchondroma (fi″bro-en″kon-dro′mah) enchondroma containing fibrous elements.

fibroepithelioma (fi″bro-ep″ĭ-the″le-o′mah) a tumor composed of fibrous and epithelial elements. **premalignant f.,** a fibroepithelioma manifested as an elevated skin-colored sessile lesion, usually occurring on the lower trunk or lumbosacral region in persons of middle age or older, and composed of interlacing ribbons of cells that extend downward from the surface to form an epithelial meshwork upon a hyperplastic mesodermal stroma. It may occur in association with superficial basal cell carcinoma, and may eventually transform into a true basal cell carcinoma. Called also *premalignant fibroepithelial tumor.*

fibrofascitis (fi″bro-fah-si′tis) fibrositis.

fibrofatty (fi″bro-fat′e) both fibrous and fatty.

fibrofibrous (fi″bro-fi′brus) joining or connecting fibers.

fibrogenesis (fi″bro-jen′ĕ-sis) [*fibro-* + *genesis*] the development of fibers. **f. imperfec′ta os′sium,** a rare collagen disorder causing osteomalacia, with progressive skeletal pain and tenderness.

fibrogenic (fi″bro-jen′ik) conducive to the development of fibers.

fibroglia (fi-brog′le-ah) [*fibro-* + Gr. *glia* glue] border fibrils in close relation to the surface of fibroblasts, and thought by some to be transformations of the ectoplasm.

fibroglioma (fi″bro-gli-o′mah) a glioma containing an excessive amount of fibrous tissue.

fibrohemorrhagic (fi″bro-hem″o-raj′ik) attended with hemorrhage and fibrin formation.

fibrohistiocytic (fi″bro-his″te-o-sit′ik) having fibrous and histiocytic elements.

fibroid (fi′broid) [*fibro-* + Gr. *eidos* form] 1. having a fibrous structure; resembling a fibroma. 2. a fibroma. 3. leiomyoma; *fibroids* is a colloquial clinical term for leiomyoma uteri.

fibroidectomy (fi″broid-ek′to-me) [*fibroid* + Gr. *ektomē* excision] excision of a fibroid tumor (myoma) of the uterus.

fibroin (fi-bro′in) a white albuminoid, $C_{15}H_{23}N_3O_6$, from spiders' webs and the cocoons of insects.

fibrolipoma (fi″bro-lĭ-po′mah) [*fibro-* + Gr. *lipos* fat + *-oma*] lipoma containing an excess of fibrous tissue.

fibrolipomatous (fi″bro-lĭ-po′mah-tus) pertaining to fibrolipoma.

fibroma (fi-bro′mah) a tumor composed mainly of fibrous or fully developed connective tissue; called also *fibroid.* **ameloblastic f.,** an odontogenic tumor characterized by the simultaneous proliferation of both epithelial and mesenchymal tissue, without the formation of enamel or dentin. **f. caverno′sum,** a cavernous hemangioma containing an excess of fibrous tissue. **cementifying f.,** cementoblastoma; a tumor usually occurring in the mandible of older persons and consisting of fibroblastic tissue containing masses of cementum-like tissue. **chondromyxoid f.,** a rare, benign, slowly growing tumor of bone of chondroblastic origin, usually affecting the large long bones of the lower extremity; it has distinct histological characteristics and is sometimes mistaken for chondrosarcoma. **concentric f.,** a uterine fibroma surrounding the uterine cavity. **f. cu′tis,** fibroma of the skin. **cystic f.,** a fibroma that has undergone cystic degeneration. **f. du′rum,** hard f. **hard f.,** one composed of fibrous tissue with few cells; called also *f. durum.* **intracanalicular f.,** fibroadenoma of the breast. **juvenile nasopharyngeal f.,** nasopharyngeal angiofibroma. **f. mol′le,** soft fibroma. **f. mucino′sum,** a fibroma affected with mucoid degeneration. **f. myxomato′des,** a myxofibroma. **nonosteogenic f.,** a common degenerative and proliferative lesion of the medullary and cortical tissues of bone, occurring most commonly near the ends of the diaphyses of the large long bones, particularly of the lower extremities, often causing no symptoms and discovered only incidentally in roentgenograms of the skeleton made for other reasons. **odontogenic f.,** a benign tumor of the jaw, arising from the embryonic portion of the tooth germ, the dental papilla, or dental follicle, or originating later from the periodontal membrane. **ossifying f., ossifying f. of bone,** a benign, relatively slow-growing, central bone tumor, usually of the jaws, especially the mandible, which is composed of fibrous connective tissue within which bone is formed. **osteogenic f.,** osteoblastoma. **parasitic f.,** a pedunculated, subperitoneal fibroid of the uterus which obtains part or all of its blood supply from the omentum. **f. pen′dulum,** a pendulous fibroma of the skin. **rabbit f.,** a naturally occurring benign viral disease of the wild cottontail rabbit, which is transmissible to laboratory rabbits, and marked by the development of fibromas that regress; called also *Shope f.* **recurrent digital f. of childhood,** digital fibromatosis. **f. sarcomato′sum,** fibrosarcoma. **Shope f.,** rabbit f. **soft f.,** one containing copious cells; called also *f. molle.* **telangiectatic f.,** angiofibroma. **f. thecocellula′re xanthomato′des,** theca cell tumor. **f. xantho′ma,** fibroxanthoma.

fibromatogenic (fi-bro″mah-to-jen′ik) producing or causing the formation of fibroma.

fibromatoid (fi-bro′mah-toid) [*fibroma* + Gr. *eidos* form] resembling fibroma; fibroma-like.

fibromatosis (fi″bro-mah-to′sis) the formation of a fibrous, tumor-like nodule arising from the deep fascia with a tendency to local recurrence, as in desmoid tumor. **f. col′li,** a firm, fusiform, fibrous mass in the midportion of the sternocleidomastoid muscle, usually occurring between two weeks and two months of age, and commonly disappearing in four to eight months; in some instances, torticollis may develop. It is believed by some to be a small hematoma due to injury to the muscle at birth. **congenital generalized f.,** a condition in which multiple small, firm, spherical or ovoid fibromas of the subcutaneous and muscle tissues, the viscera, and osseous systems are characteristically present at birth. Visceral involvement may be responsible for various symptoms, such as intestinal obstruction, diarrhea due to diffuse involvement of the intestines, and respiratory disturbances. Death frequently occurs during the neonatal period or early infancy. **digital f.,** a rare, often recurrent, condition of infancy and early childhood, in which one or more fibromas occur on the lateral or dorsal aspects of the fingers and toes; histologically, the lesions are composed of fibrous connective tissue and abundant collagen, and contain characteristic virus-like, black intracellular inclusions. Called also *recurrent digital fibroma of childhood.* **f. gingi′vae, gingival f.,** noninflammatory fibrous hyperplasia of the gingiva manifested as a dense, diffuse, smooth or nodular overgrowth of the gingival tissues, sometimes to the point that the crowns of the teeth are hidden. It usually appears at the time of tooth eruption. Most cases are hereditary (autosomal dominant) and are associated with hypertrichosis. Called also *elephantiasis gingivae* and *macrogingivae.* **infantile digital f.,** digital f. **palmar f.,** fibromatosis involving the palmar fascia, and resulting in Dupuytren's contracture. **plantar f.,** fibromatosis involving the plantar fascia manifested as single or multiple nodular swellings, sometimes accompanied by pain but usually unassociated with contractures. **subcutaneous pseudosarcomatous f.,** proliferative fasciitis. **f. ventric′uli,** linitis plastica.

fibromatous (fi-bro′mah-tus) pertaining to or of the nature of fibroma.

fibromectomy (fi″bro-mek′to-me) [*fibroma* + Gr. *ektomē* excision] excision of a fibroma.

fibromembranous (fi″bro-mem′brah-nus) composed of membrane containing much fibrous tissue.

fibromuscular (fi″bro-mus′ku-lar) composed of fibrous and muscular tissue.

fibromyitis (fi″bro-mi-i′tis) [*fibro-* + Gr. *mys* muscle + *-itis*] inflammation and fibrous degeneration of a muscle.

fibromyoma (fi″bro-mi-o′mah) [*fibro* + Gr. *mys* muscle + *-oma*] leiomyoma. **f. u′teri,** leiomyoma uteri.

fibromyomectomy (fi″bro-mi″o-mek′to-me) excision of a fibromyoma (leiomyoma).

fibromyositis (fi″bro-mi″o-si′tis) [*fibro-* + Gr. *mys* muscle + *-itis*] inflammation of fibromuscular tissue. **nodular f.,** a disease marked by inflammation and the formation of nodules in the muscles.

fibromyotomy (fi″bro-mi-ot′o-me) incision into a fibromyoma (leiomyoma).

fibromyxoma (fi″bro-mik-so′mah) myxofibroma.

fibromyxosarcoma (fi″bro-mik″so-sar-ko′mah) myxosarcoma or myxoid liposarcoma that is undergoing fibrosis.

fibronectin (fi″bro-nek′tin) [*fibro-* + L. *nexus* a connecting] an adhesive glycoprotein: one form circulates in plasma, acting as an opsonin; another is a cell-surface protein which mediates cellular adhesive interactions. Fibronectins are important in connective tissue, where they cross-link to collagen, and they are also involved in aggregation of platelets.

fibroneuroma (fi″bro-nu-ro′mah) neurofibroma.

fibronuclear (fi″bro-nu′kle-ar) made up of nucleated fibers.

fibro-osteoma (fi″bro-os″te-o′mah) an ossifying fibroma.

fibropapilloma (fi″bro-pap″ĭ-lo′mah) a papilloma containing much fibrous tissue; called also *fibroepithelial papilloma.*

fibropituicyte (fi″bro-pĭ-tu″ĭ-sīt) see *pituicyte.*

fibroplasia (fi″bro-pla′se-ah) the formation of fibrous tissue, as occurs normally in the healing of wounds and abnormally in some tissues. **retrolental f.,** a bilateral retinopathy occurring in premature infants treated with excessively high concentrations of oxygen, characterized by vascular dilatation, proliferation, and tortuosity, edema, and retinal detachment, with ultimate conversion of the retina into a fibrous mass that can be seen as a dense retrolental membrane; usually, growth of the eye is arrested and may result in microophthalmia, and blindness may occur. Called also *retinopathy of prematurity, RLF,* and *Terry's syndrome.*

fibroplastic (fi″bro-plas′tik) [*fibro-* + Gr. *plassein* to form] giving origin to fibrous tissue.

fibroplastin (fi″bro-plas′tin) paraglobulin.

fibroplate (fi′bro-plāt) an interarticular fibrocartilage.

fibropolypus (fi″bro-pol′ĭ-pus) a polyp containing fibrous elements.

fibropurulent (fi-bro-pu′roo-lent) characterized by the presence of both fibers and pus.

fibroreticulate (fi″bro-re-tik′u-lāt) composed of a network of fibers.

fibrosarcoma (fi″bro-sar-ko′mah) a sarcoma derived from fibroblasts that produce collagen. **odontogenic f.,** a malignant tumor of the jaws, originating from one of the mesenchymal components of the tooth or tooth germ, and histologically identical with other fibrosarcomas; the malignant counterpart of odontogenic fibroma.

fibrosclerosis (fi″bro-skle-ro′sis) fibrosis associated with sclerosis. **multifocal f.,** any of a group of disorders of unknown etiology characterized by fibrosis, including mediastinal, hilar, and retroperitoneal fibrosis, Reidel's struma, and sclerosing cholangitis.

fibrose (fi′brōs) 1. to form fibrous tissue. 2. fibrous.

fibroserous (fi″bro-se′rus) composed of both fibrous and serous elements.

fibrosis (fi-bro′sis) the formation of fibrous tissue; fibroid or fibrous degeneration. **African endomyocardial f.,** endomyocardial f. **congenital hepatic f.,** a developmental disorder of the liver marked by formation of irregular broad bands of fibrous tissue containing multiple cysts formed by disordered terminal bile ducts, chiefly in the portal areas, resulting in vascular constriction, which leads to portal hypertension. It may be associated with polycystic renal disease. **cystic f.,** cystic f. of the pancreas. **cystic f. of the pancreas,** a generalized, hereditary disorder of infants, children, and young adults, in which there is widespread dysfunction of the exocrine glands; characterized by signs of chronic pulmonary disease (due to excess mucus production in the respiratory tract), pancreatic deficiency, abnormally high levels of electrolytes in the sweat, and occasionally by biliary cirrhosis. Pathologically, the pancreas shows obstruction of the pancreatic ducts by amorphous eosinophilic concretions, with consequent deficiency of pancreatic enzymes, resulting in steatorrhea and azotorrhea. The degree of involvement of organs and glandular systems may vary greatly, with consequent variations in the clinical picture. It is transmitted as an autosomal recessive trait. Called also *fibrocystic disease of the pancreas* and *mucoviscidosis.* **diatomite f.,** a form of silicosis caused by inhalation of diatomaceous earth (silicon dioxide). **diffuse interstitial pulmonary f.,** idiopathic pulmonary f. **endomyocardial f.,** idiopathic myocardiopathy occurring endemically in various regions of Africa and rarely in other areas, characterized by cardiomegaly, marked thickening of the endocardium with dense, white fibrous tissue that frequently extends to involve the inner third or half of the myocardium, and congestive heart failure. Called also *African endomyocardial f.* **graphite f.,** a form of silicosis caused by the inhalation of graphite, which may contain as much as 10 per cent silicon dioxide. **idiopathic pulmonary f.,** chronic inflammation and progressive fibrosis of the pulmonary alveolar walls, with steadily progressive dyspnea, resulting finally in death from oxygen lack or right heart failure. Called also *diffuse interstitial pulmonary f.* The acute, rapidly fatal form is often called *Hamman-Rick syndrome.* **idiopathic retroperitoneal f.,** retroperitoneal f. **mediastinal f.,** development of whitish, hard fibrous tissue in the upper mediastinum, causing compression, distortion, or obliteration of the superior vena cava, and sometimes constriction of the bronchi and large pulmonary vessels. **neoplastic f.,** proliferative f. **nodular subepidermal f.,** the formation, beneath the epidermis, of multiple fibrous nodules as the result of productive inflammation. **panmural f. of the bladder,** chronic interstitial cystitis. **periureteric f.,** progressive development of fibrous tissue, spreading laterally from the great midline vessels, gradually engulfing, distorting, and finally causing strangulation of one or both ureters. **postfibrinous f.,** fibrosis occurring in tissues in which fibrin has been deposited. **proliferative f.,** fibrosis in which the fibrous elements continue to proliferate after the original causative factor has ceased to operate; called also *neoplastic f.* **pulmonary f.,** see *idiopathic pulmonary f.* **replacement f.,** the development of fibrous tissues to replace tissue that has been damaged. **retroperitoneal f.,** deposition of fibrous tissue in the retroperitoneal space, producing vague abdominal discomfort, and often causing blockage of the ureters, with resultant hydronephrosis and impaired renal function, which may result in renal failure. **root sleeve f.,** fibrosis and thickening of the dura mater resulting from prolonged nerve root pressure. **f. u'teri,** a morbid condition characterized by overgrowth of the smooth muscle and increase in the collagenous fibrous tissue, producing a thickened, coarse, tough myometrium.

fibrositis (fi″bro-si′tis) [*fibrous* tissue + *-itis*] inflammatory hyperplasia of the white fibrous tissue of the body, especially of the muscle sheaths and facial layers of the locomotor system; it is marked by pain and stiffness. Called also *fibrofascitis* and *muscular rheumatism.*

fibrothorax (fi″bro-tho′raks) a condition characterized by adhesion of the two layers of pleura, the lung being covered by a thick layer of nonexpansible fibrous tissue; often a consequence of traumatic hemothorax or of effusion.

fibrotic (fi-brot′ik) pertaining to or characterized by fibrosis.

fibrotuberculosis (fi″bro-tu-ber″ku-lo′sis) fibroid phthisis.

fibrous (fi′brus) composed of or containing fibers.

fibrovascular (fi″bro-vas′ku-lar) both fibrous and vascular.

fibroxanthoma (fi″bro-zan-tho′mah) a type of xanthoma containing fibromatous elements.

fibula (fib′u-lah) [L. "buckle"] [NA] the outer and smaller of the two bones of the leg, which articulates proximally with the tibia and distally is joined to the tibia in a syndesmosis. See Plate accompanying *skeleton.*

fibular (fib′u-lar) pertaining to the fibula; peroneal.

fibularis (fib″u-la′ris) fibular; [NA] a term designating relationship to the fibula.

fibulocalcaneal (fib″u-lo-kal-ka′ne-al) pertaining to the fibula and calcaneus.

F.I.C.D. Fellow of the International College of Dentists.

ficin (fi′sin) [L. *ficus* fig] a highly active, crystallizable proteinase from the sap of fig trees which catalyzes the hydrolysis of many proteins at acid (4.1) pH, the clotting of milk, and "digestion" of some living worms, e.g., whipworms. Ficin is used as a protein digestant and to enhance the agglutination of red blood cells with IgG antibodies (e.g., Rh antibodies). It also shows esterase activity. It has been used in dogs as a trichuricide.

Fick's bacillus (fiks) [Rudolph Armin *Fick,* German physician, 1866–1939] *Proteus vulgaris.*

Fick principle (formula, method) (fik) [Adolph Eugen *Fick,* German physiologist, 1829–1901] see under *principle.*

Ficker's diagnosticum (fik′erz) [Philipp Martin *Ficker,* German bacteriologist, 1868–1950] see under *diagnosticum.*

F.I.C.S. Fellow of the International College of Surgeons.

fidicinales (fi-dis″ĭ-na′lez) [pl., from L. *fidicen, fidicinis,* a player on the harp] musculi lumbricales manus.

fieber (fe′ber) [Ger.] fever. **gelb f.,** yellow fever. **rück′fall f.,** relapsing fever.

Fiedler's disease, myocarditis (fēd′lerz) [Carl Ludwig Alfred *Fiedler,* German physician, 1835–1921] see *leptospiral jaundice,* under *jaundice,* and see *acute isolated myocarditis,* under *myocarditis.*

field (fēld) 1. an area or open space, as an operative field or visual field. 2. a range of specialization in knowledge, study, or occupation. 3. in embryology, the developing region within a range of modifying factors. **absolute f.,** that area of the cerebral cortex injury which always causes paralysis or spasm. **auditory f.,** the space or range within which stimuli may be perceived as sound. **Cohnheim's f's,** see under *area.* **f. of consciousness,** the total sum of experiences at a given instant. **dark-f.,** see under *microscope,* and see *ultramicroscope.* **f. of fixation,** the region bounded by the utmost limits of central or clear vision, the eye being allowed to move, but the head being fixed. **Flechsig's f.,** the myelinogenetic field. **Forel's f.,** the complex field of nerve fibers (the H field) that lies medial to the subthalamic nucleus and zona incerta, immediately rostral to the red nucleus. It contains pallidofugal, dentatothalamic, and rubrothalamic fibers, principally in the form of two fiber bundles: the fasciculus lenticularis (field H_2), which enters the H field, and the fasciculus thalamicus (field H_1), which leaves it. **gamma f.,** any area subjected to radiation from an unshielded or slightly shielded gamma radiation source. **H f.,** see *Forel's f.* **f. H_1,** fasciculus thalamicus. **f. H_2,** fasciculus lenticularis. **high-power f.,** the area of a slide visible under the high magnification system of a microscope. **individuation f.,** a region in which an organizer influences adjacent tissue to become a part of a total embryo. **Krönig's f.** (*obs.*), the area of resonance on the chest due to the apices of the lungs. **low-power f.,** the area of a slide visible under the low magnification system of a microscope. **magnetic f.,** that portion of space about a magnet in which its action is perceptible. **f. of a microscope,** the area that can be seen through a microscope at one time. The *high-power field* is that area which is visible under the high-power objective; the *low-power field* is that which is visible under low power. **morphogenetic f.,** an embryonic region, larger than its main deriv-

atives, out of which definite structures normally develop. **myelinogenetic f.,** a collection of fibers in the neuraxis which at a definite stage of development receive myelin sheaths; called also *Flechsig's field.* **penumbra f.,** the region of free space which is irradiated by primary photons coming from only part of the radiation source. **primary nail f.,** a flat area on the terminal phalanx in the embryo where the nail is to develop. **relative f.,** an area of the cerebral cortex in which a lesion may or may not cause paralysis. **surplus f.,** the portion of the field of vision in partial hemianopia which passes beyond the point of fixation. **f. of vision,** that portion of space which the fixed eye can see. **f. of vision, cribriform,** a field of vision over which a number of isolated scotomas lie dispersed. **f. of vision, overshot,** a condition in which the line of separation between the halves of the field of vision does not pass through the point of fixation. **visual f.,** the area within which stimuli will produce the sensation of sight with the eye in a straight-ahead position. **Wernicke's f.,** see under *area.*

Fielding's membrane (fēld′ingz) [George Hunsley *Fielding,* English anatomist, 1801–1871] the tapetum, def. 2.

fièvre (fe-evr′) [Fr.] fever. **f. boutonneuse** (fe-evr′ booton-uz′), boutonneuse fever. **f. caprine** (fe-evr′ kah-prēn), brucellosis. **f. exanthematique de Marseille** (fe-evr′ eks-an″thĕ-mah-tēk′) boutonneuse fever. **f. jaune** (fe-evr′ zhōn), yellow fever. **f. récurrente** (fe-evr′ ra″kuh-rant′), relapsing fever.

FIGLU formiminoglutamic acid.

figuratum (fig″u-ra′tum) [L.] figured; a term used to describe skin lesions that have a geometric, usually circular or annular, pattern.

figure (fig′ūr) [L. *figura,* from *fingere* to shape or form] 1. an object of a particular form. 2. a number, or numeral. **fortification f's,** a form of migraine aura characterized by scintillating, colored lights or zigzag luminous bands suggestive of the walls of a turret. **Minkowski's f.,** a numerical expression of the relation between dextrose and nitrogen in the urine on a pure meat diet, and when fasting. It is 2.8:1. **mitotic f's,** stages of chromosome aggregation exhibiting a pattern characteristic of mitosis. **Purkinje's f's,** see under *image.* **Stifel's f.,** a black disk having a white spot in the center, used for locating and measuring the blind spot in the eye. **Zöllner's f's,** see under *line.*

fila (fi′lah) [L.] plural of *filum.*

filaceous (fi-la′shus) made up of filaments.

filament (fil′ah-ment) [L. *filamentum*] a delicate fiber or thread. **acrosomal f.,** a long, thin, rigid filament projecting from the head of a spermatozoon; it is formed by elongation of the central part of the acrosome in preparation for the fertilization process, and is used to make contact with and to penetrate the cell membrane of the ovum. **axial f.,** axoneme. **linin f.,** a network of linin spread throughout the cell nucleus. **lymphatic anchoring f's,** filaments that attach the endothelial cells of lymphatic capillaries to the connective tissue between surrounding tissue cells. **root f's of spinal nerves,** fila radicularia nervorum spinalium. **spermatic f.,** end piece, def. 2. **terminal f.,** 1. filum terminale. 2. end piece (def. 2). **terminal f. of spinal dura mater,** filum durae matris spinalis.

filamenta (fil″ah-men′tah) [L.] plural of *filamentum.*

filamentous (fil-ah-men′tus) composed of long, threadlike structures; said of bacterial colonies.

filamentum (fil″ah-men′tum), pl. *filamen′ta* [L.] a filament.

filar (fi′lar) [L. *filum* thread] threadlike; filamentous.

Filaria (fi-la′re-ah) [L. *filum* thread] a former loosely applied generic name for members of the superfamily Filarioidea. **F. bancrof′ti,** *Wuchereria bancrofti.* **F. conjuncti′vae,** a species, possibly identical with *Dirofilaris conjunctivae,* found in the eye of horses and asses, and sometimes in man; called also *F. palpebralis.* **F. demarquay′i,** *Mansonella ozzardi.* **F. diur′na,** *Loa loa.* The name was actually applied to the microfilaria (*microfilaria diurna*). **F. equi′na,** *Setaria equina.* **F. immit′is,** *Dirofilaria immitis.* **F. jun′cea,** *Mansonella ozzardi.* **F. lo′a,** *Loa loa.* **F. medinen′sis,** *Dracunculus medinensis.* **F. noctur′na,** *Wuchereria bancrofti.* **F. ozzar′di,** *Mansonella ozzardi.* **F. palpebra′lis,** *F. conjunctivae.* **F. per′stans,** *Dipetalonema perstans.* **F. recon′dita,** *Dipetalonema reconditum.* **F. san′guinis-hom′inis,** *Wuchereria bancrofti.* **F. vol′vulus,** *Onchocerca volvulus.*

filaria (fi-la′re-ah), pl. *fila′riae* [L. *filum* thread] a nematode worm of the superfamily Filarioidea. **Bancroft's f.,** *Wuchereria bancrofti.* **Brug's f.,** *Brugia malayi.*

filariae (fi-la′re-e) [L.] plural of *filaria.*

filarial (fi-la′re-al) pertaining to, caused by, or denoting filariae.

filariasis (fil″ah-ri′ah-sis) a diseased state due to the presence of filariae within the body. **Bancroft's f., f. bancrof′ti, bancroftian f.,** infection with the filarial worm *Wuchereria bancrofti,* the adults of which reside in the lymphatic system, producing recurrent lymphangitis with fibrosis and obstruction. In extensive obstruction, chronic edema may result, progressing to elephantiasis. The disease is transmitted by mosquitoes, which harbor the larval forms (microfilariae). **Brug's f., Malayan f., ma′layi,** infection with the filarial worm *Brugia malayi,* the adult forms of which reside in the lymphatics, lymph nodes, and connective tissue; symptoms range from asymptomatic adenitis, to periodic attacks of fever and lymphangitis, to elephantiasis, especially of the legs and feet. The disease is transmitted by mosquitoes. **Ozzard's f.,** infection with *Mansonella ozzardi.*

filaricidal (fĭ-lăr″ĭ-sīd′al) [*filaria* + L. *caedere* to kill] destructive to filariae.

filaricide (fĭ-lăr′ĭ-sīd) an agent that is destructive to filariae.

filariform (fĭ-lăr′ĭ-form) threadlike; resembling filariae; denoting that developmental stage in the life cycle of certain nematodes which is characterized by the possession of an esophagus of uniform diameter and which is often, as in hookworms, the infective stage.

Filarioidea (fĭ-lăr″e-oi′de-ah) a superfamily or order of nematode parasites, the adults being threadlike worms which invade the tissues and body cavities where the female deposits embryonated eggs (prelarvae) known as microfilariae. These microfilariae are ingested by blood-sucking insects in whom they pass their developmental stage and are returned to man by the bites of such insects. The filariae of man belong to the genera *Wuchereria, Onchocerca, Loa, Dipetalonema, Mansonella, Dirofilaria,* and *Brugia.*

Filatov's (Filatow's) disease (fĭ-lat′ofs) [Nils Fédorovich *Filatov,* pediatrician in Moscow, 1847–1902] infectious mononucleosis.

Filatov-Dukes disease (fi-lat′of-dūks) [Nils Fédorovich *Filatov;* Clement *Dukes,* English physician, 1845–1925] Dukes' disease.

Fildes' law (fil′dez) [Paul Gordon *Fildes,* English bacteriologist, born 1882] see under *law.*

file (fīl) a surgical or a dental instrument with a finely serrated surface, for reducing surplus hard substance such as bone or materials used in dental restorations, or for smoothing roughened surfaces.

filicin (fil′ĭ-cin) a compound found in aspidium.

filiform (fil′ĭ-form, fi′lĭ-form) [L. *filum* thread + *forma* form] 1. thread shaped. 2. an extremely slender bougie.

filioparental (fil″e-o-pah-ren′tal) pertaining to the relationships between children and their parents.

filipin (fi′lĭ-pin) chemical name: 4,6,8,10,12,14,16,27-octahydroxy-3-(1-hydroxyethyl)-17,28-dimethyloxacyclooctacosa-17,19,-21,23,25-pentaen-2-one; an antifungal antibiotic, $C_{35}H_{58}O_{11}$. Called also *filipin III.*

Filipovitch's (Filipowicz's) sign (fĭ-le′po-vich″ez) [Casimir *Filipovitch,* Polish physician] see under *sign.*

filipuncture (fil′ĭ-punk-tūr) [L. *filum* thread + *punctura* puncture] (*obs.*) the insertion of a wire or thread into an aneurysm.

filix (fi′liks), pl. *fil′ices* [L.] a fern. **f. mas,** male fern; see *aspidium.*

fillet (fil′et) 1. a loop, as of cord or tape, for making traction. 2. in the nervous system, a long band of nerve fibers, such as the medial lemniscus.

filling (fil′ing) 1. the material inserted into a prepared tooth cavity, usually gold, amalgam, cement, or a synthetic resin. 2. the restoration of the crown with appropriate material after removal of the carious tissue from a tooth. **complex f.,** a filling for a complex cavity. **composite f.,** a filling that consists of a composite resin. **compound f.,** a filling for a cavity that involves two surfaces of a tooth. **direct f.,** one that is formed and completed directly in the tooth cavity. **direct resin f.,** a direct filling made from a synthetic resin. **indirect f.,** one that is constructed on a die that has been made from an accurate impression of the tooth and that is then inserted into the tooth cavity. **permanent f.,** a filling intended to provide complete function while the tooth remains in the oral cavity. **retrograde f.,** an amalgam or other restoration placed in the apical portion of a tooth to seal the root canal following surgical removal of a periapical lesion. **root canal f.,** a filling placed in the root canal of a tooth to obliterate the space once occupied by the dental pulp. **temporary f.,** a filling placed in a tooth cavity with the intention of removing it within a short period of time.

film (film) 1. a thin layer or coating. 2. a thin sheet specially processed for use in photography or roentgenography; used also to designate such a sheet after exposure to light rays or other radiant energy to which it is sensitive. **bite-wing f.,** an x-ray film for radiography of oral structures, with a protruding tab to be held between the upper and lower teeth. **fixed blood f.,** a thin film of blood spread on a slide, dried quickly, and fixed. **gelatin f., absorbable** [USP], a sterile, nonantigenic, absorbable, water-insoluble gelatin film, used as a local hemostatic. **lateral jaw f.,** a radiograph showing either the ramus or the body of the mandible. **occlusal f.,** a radiograph showing topographic and cross-sectional views of the maxillary or mandibular dental structure and adjacent tissue. **periapical f.,** a radiograph showing a particular tooth and the tissues adjacent to the apex of its root. **spot f.,** a radiograph of a small anatomic area obtained (*a*) by rapid exposure during fluoroscopy to provide a permanent record of a transiently observed abnormality, or (*b*)

by limitation of radiation passing through the area to improve definition and detail of the image produced. **sulfa f.,** a film made from an emulsion of sulfadiazine, sulfanilamide, and methyl cellulose; used as a dressing for burns, cuts, and skin grafts. **x-ray f.,** a sheet specially prepared for use in roentgenography after exposure to roentgen rays and appropriate processing; a roentgenogram.

film badge (film baj) a pack of radiographic film or films, used for the detection and approximate measurement of radiation exposure of personnel.

filopod (fil′o-pod) filopodium.

filopodia (fi″lo-po′de-ah) plural of *filopodium.*

filopodium (fi″lo-po′de-um), pl. *filopo′dia* [L. *filum* thread + Gr. *pous* foot] a slender, pointed pseudopodium composed of ectoplasm. Cf. *axopodium, lobopodium,* and *rhizopodium.*

filopressure (fi′lo-presh″ūr) [L. *filum* thread + *pressura* pressure] the compression of a blood vessel by a thread.

filovaricosis (fi′lo-var″ĭ-ko′sis) the development of varicosities on the axon of a nerve fiber.

filter (fil′ter) [L. *filtrum*] 1. a device for the straining of water or other liquid. 2. in radiology, a solid screen usually of varying thickness of metal (aluminum, copper, tin, lead, etc.) which when placed in the pathway of the radiation beam prevents transmission of beta particles and photons of longer wavelengths. **Berkefeld f.,** a bacterial filter made of infusorial earth, available in three porosities: V (*viel,* or coarse), N (normal), and W (*wenig,* or fine). Most bacteria are removed by the V filter; all are usually removed by the N; and the W is used for exceedingly small organisms. **Chamberland f.,** a bacterial filter made of unglazed porcelain, available in several graded porosities, L1, L2, L3, etc., the L3 being roughly equivalent to the Berkefeld N. **Coors f.,** a bacterial filter cylinder of unglazed porcelain. **Gooch f.,** a platinum or porcelain crucible the bottom of which is perforated with holes and covered with a layer of asbestos fibers. **intermittent sand f.,** a sand filter to which sewage is applied for only a short time and then is allowed to drain away so that aeration and oxidation may take place. **mechanical f.,** a filter of sand or other porous material through which water is forced rapidly to remove gross particles; these particles may be the precipitate caused by the addition of some coagulant. **Millipore f.,** trademark for a device used to filter nutrient solutions as they are administered intravenously. **Pasteur-Chamberland f.,** a hollow column of unglazed porcelain through which liquids are forced by pressure or by vacuum exhaustion. **percolating f.,** trickling f. **roughing f., scrubbing f.,** a coarse-grained filter through which turbid water is passed to remove the larger particles and thus protect the sand filter from clogging. **Seitz f.,** one in which the filtering element is an asbestos pad, which is the equivalent of the Berkefeld N filter. **sintered glass f.,** a filter of sintered glass, available in various porosities, sometimes designed C (coarse), M (medium), F (fine), and UF (ultrafine); only the ultrafine is bacteria-proof. **slow sand f.,** a filter made of sand and gravel through which water passes slowly and is purified largely by the action of the microorganisms growing on the surface of the grains of sand near the top of the filter. **sprinkling f.,** a trickling filter in which the sewage is applied by spray. **trickling f.,** beds of porous material on which sewage is distributed and allowed to percolate through to drains laid on a tight floor; the purpose is to so oxidize the organic material as to make it nonputrescible. Called also *percolating f.* **umbrella f.,** a filter used in transvenous caval interruption for the prevention of pulmonary embolism. **Wood's f.,** see under *light.*

filterable (fil′ter-ah-b'l) capable of passing through the pores of a filter; said of elements that can pass through a filter which will not permit the passage of the usual microorganisms.

filtrable (fil′trah-b'l) filterable.

filtrate (fil′trāt) a liquid that has passed through a filter. **glomerular f.,** the ultrafiltrate of plasma that passes across the membranes of the malpighian corpuscles of the kidney to the lumen of Bowman's capsule.

filtration (fil-tra′shun) 1. the passage of a liquid through a filter, accomplished by gravity, pressure, or vacuum (suction). 2. in radiology, the use of a solid screen usually made of metal (aluminum, copper, tin, lead, etc.) to absorb beta particles and photons of longer wavelengths. **gel f.,** column chromatography in which high molecular weight substances are separated according to molecular size.

fil′trum ventric′uli [L.] a depression between the two projections formed in the lateral wall of the vestibule of the larynx by the arytenoid and cuneiform cartilages; called also *Merkel's filtrum.*

filum (fi′lum), pl. *fi′la* [L.] [NA] a threadlike structure or part. **fi′la anastomot′ica ner′vi acus′tici,** an anastomotic filament between the vestibulocochlear and facial nerves in the internal acoustic meatus. **f. du′rae ma′tris spina′lis** [NA], filum of spinal dura mater: the downward prolongation of dura mater from the apex of the dural sac; joined by the filum terminale, it blends with the periosteum on the back of the coccyx. Called also *central ligament, coccygeal ligament,* or *terminal* *filament of spinal dura mater.* **fi′la olfacto′ria,** nervi olfactorii. **fi′la radicula′ria nervo′rum spina′lium** [NA], the threadlike filaments by which the dorsal and ventral roots of each spinal nerve are attached to the spinal cord; called also *root filaments of spinal nerves.* **f. of spinal dura mater,** f. durae matris spinalis. **f. termina′le** [NA], terminal filament: a slender, threadlike prolongation of the spinal cord from the conus medullaris to the apex of the dural sac, where it fuses with the filum of the dura mater, and extends to the back of the coccyx as the coccygeal ligament, where it blends with the periosteum.

fimbria (fim′bre-ah) [L. *fimbriae* (pl.) a fringe] 1. a fringe, border, or edge; [NA] a general term for such a structure. 2. in microbiology, one of the minute filamentous appendages of certain bacteria; they are considerably smaller and less rigid than flagella and are associated with antigenic properties of the cell surface; called also *pilus.* **f. hippocam′pi** [NA], the band of white matter along the medial edge of the ventricular surface of the hippocampus; called also *corpus fimbriatum hippocampi.* **ovarian f., f. ova′rica** [NA], the longest of the processes that make up the fimbriae tubae uterinae, extending along the free border of the mesosalpinx; called also *fimbriated extremity.* **fim′briae of tongue,** plica fimbriata. **fim′briae tu′bae uteri′nae** [NA], **fimbriae of uterine tube,** the numerous divergent fringelike processes on the distal part of the infundibulum of the uterine tube.

Fimbriaria (fim″bre-a′re-ah) a genus of tapeworms of the family Hymenolepididae, which are parasites of anseriform birds. **F. fasciola′ris,** a tapeworm infecting wild and domestic fowl.

fimbriated (fim′bre-āt-ed) [L. *fimbriatus*] fringed.

fimbriation (fim″bre-a′shun) the formation of or the possession of fimbriae.

fimbriatum (fim″bre-a′tum) [L.] fringed.

fimbriocele (fim′bre-o-sēl″) [*fimbria* + Gr. *kēlē* hernia] hernia containing fimbriae of the uterine tube.

Finckh test (fink) [Johann *Finckh,* German psychiatrist, born 1873] see under *tests.*

finder (fīnd′er) a device on a microscope to facilitate the finding of some object in the field.

finding (fīnd′ing) an observation; a condition discovered.

finger (fing′ger) any of the five digits of the hand. **baseball f.,** partial permanent flexion of the terminal phalanx of a finger caused by a ball or other object striking the end or back of the finger, resulting in rupture of the attachment of the extensor tendon; called also *mallet f.* **blubber f.,** seal f. **bolster f′s,** the swollen fingers that result from a *Candida* infection in workers who handle sugar. **Brodie's f.** (*obs.*), herpes zoster infection of the finger. **clubbed f.,** a deformity produced by proliferation of the soft tissues about the terminal phalanx, with no constant osseous changes; seen in various cases of chronic disease of the thoracic organs. **dead f.,** a numb, mottled finger, as one seen in acrocyanosis. **drop f.,** mallet f. **drumstick f.,** clubbed f. **first f.,** the thumb. **giant f.,** macrodactyly. **hammer f.,** mallet f. **hippocratic f′s,** enlargement of the terminal phalanges, with coarse nails curving over the ends of the fingers (hippocratic nails); see *hypertrophic pulmonary osteoarthropathy,* under *osteoarthropathy.* **index f.,** the second digit of the hand, the thumb being considered the first; the forefinger. **insane f.,** chronic felon in certain cases of confirmed insanity. **lock f.,** one that is fixed in a flexed position, owing to the presence of a small fibrous growth in the sheath of the flexor tendon. **Madonna f′s,** the thin, delicate fingers seen in pituitary acromicria. **mallet f.,** permanent flexion of the distal phalanx; called also *drop* or *hammer f.* See also *baseball f.* **ring f.,** the fourth digit of the hand. **seal f.,** a disease of unknown etiology clinically resembling erysipeloid, occurring in handlers of seals and seal skins; called also *blubber f.* **snapping f.,** trigger f. **spider f.,** arachnodactyly. **spring f.,** a condition in which flexion and extension of the finger beyond certain points are difficult. **trigger f.,** a finger liable to be affected with a momentary spasmodic arrest of flexion or extension, followed by a snapping into place; it is due to stenosing tendovaginitis, or a nodule in the flexor tendon (see *lock f.*). **tulip f′s,** a very rare condition in which the fingers are affected by dermatitis after handling tulip bulbs. **washerwoman's f′s,** the dry shrunken fingers of patients with fatal cases of cholera. **waxy f.,** dead f. **webbed f′s,** fingers united to a greater or less extent by a fold of skin; syndactyly. **white f.,** dead f.

fingeragnosia (fing″ger-ag-no′se-ah) [*finger* + *agnosia*] inability to recognize, indicate on command, name, or choose the individual fingers of one's own hand or of the hands of others.

finger and toe (fing′er and tōw) 1. finger and toe disease. 2. a condition affecting various animals, in which finger-like tumors develop in various organs of the body.

fingernail (fing′er-nāl) the nail of a finger; see *unguis* [NA].

fingerprint (fing′ger-print) 1. an impression of the cutaneous ridges of the fleshy distal portion of a finger, made by applying ink and pressing the finger on paper; such records (as well as prints of hand or foot) are used as means of establishing identification. 2. in biochemistry, a photomicrograph obtained by fingerprinting;

also, the characteristic positioning of the peptide fragments of a protein subjected to fingerprinting.

fingerprinting (fing″ger-print′ing) a technique for determining the structure of a protein in which the protein is split into peptides by digestion with protease and the fragments are separated in one direction by electrophoresis and at right angles by chromatography. After staining, the peptide fragments are seen to be in characteristic locations.

finger-sucking (fing′ger-suk′ing) see *thumb-sucking.*

Finikoff's treatment (method) (fin′ĭ-kofs) [Aleksandr Paulovick *Finikoff,* Leningrad surgeon, born 1886] see under *treatment.*

Finkelstein's albumin milk, feeding [Heinrich *Finkelstein,* German pediatrician, 1865–1942] see *albumin milk,* under *milk,* and see under *feeding.*

Finkler-Prior spirillium (fink′ler-pri′or) [Dittmar *Finkler,* German bacteriologist, 1852–1912; J. *Prior,* German bacteriologist, 19th century] *Vibrio proteus.*

Finney's pyloroplasty (operation) (fin′ēz) [John M. T. *Finney,* Baltimore surgeon, 1863–1942] see under *pyloroplasty.*

Finochietto's stirrup (fe-no″ke-at′ōz) [Enrique *Finochietto,* surgeon in Buenos Aires, 1880–1948] see under *stirrup.*

Finsen bath, lamp (apparatus), light (rays), treatment (fin′sen) [Niels Ryberg *Finsen,* Danish physician, 1860–1904; the first to discover the curative effects of ultraviolet rays, and winner of the Nobel prize for medicine and physiology in 1903] see under *bath, lamp, light,* and *treatment.*

fire (fīr) fever; inflammation. **St. Anthony's f.** (*obs.*), 1. ergotism. 2. erysipelas. **St. Francis' f.** (*obs.*), erysipelas.

firpene (fir′pēn) pinene.

first aid (ferst ād) emergency care and treatment of an injured person before definitive medical and surgical management can be secured.

Fischer's sign (fish′erz) [Louis *Fischer,* pediatrician in New York, 1864–1945] see under *sign.*

Fischer's test [Emil *Fischer,* German chemist, 1852–1919] see under *tests.*

Fishberg concentration test (fish′berg) [Arthur Maurice *Fishberg,* American physician, born 1898] see under *tests.*

fishpox (fish′poks) a hyperplastic epidermal disease of viral origin occurring in fresh-water and marine fish.

fissile (fis′il) capable of being split; fissionable.

fission (fish′un) [L. *fissio*] 1. the act of splitting. 2. a form of asexual reproduction in which the cell divides into two or more daughter parts, each of which becomes a new, independent organism; it is seen chiefly among the protists. See also *binary f.* and *multiple f.* 3. the splitting of the nucleus of an atom, releasing a great quantity of kinetic energy. **binary f.,** fission of a cell in which the cell divides into two approximately equal daughter parts. **cellular f.,** see *fission,* 2nd def. **multiple f.,** fission of a cell in which the cell divides into a number of daughter cells. **nuclear f.,** see *fission,* 3rd def.

fissionable (fish′un-ah-b′l) capable of undergoing fission.

fissiparous (fi-sip′ah-rus) [L. *fissus* cleft + *parere* to produce] propagated by fission.

fissula (fis′u-lah) [L., dim. of *fissum*] a little cleft. **f. an′te fenes′tram,** an irregular ribbon of connective tissue that extends through the bony otic capsule from the vestibule just anterior to the oval window, to the tympanic cavity near the processus cochleariformis.

fissura (fis-su′rah), pl. *fissu′rae* [L.] [NA] fissure: a general term for a cleft or groove, especially a deep fold in the cerebral cortex that involves its entire thickness. **f. in a′no,** anal fissure. **f. antitragohelici′na** [NA], antitragohelicine fissure: a fissure in the auricular cartilage between the cauda helicis and the antitragus; called also *posterior fissure of auricle.* **f. au′ris congen′ita,** preauricular fistula; see under *fistula.* **f. calcari′na,** sulcus calcarinus. **fissu′rae cerebel′li** [NA], the numerous shallow grooves in the cortex of the cerebellum, on the surface and within the deep fissures, which divide the cortex into folia; called also *sulci cerebelli* and *sulci of cerebellum.* **f. cer′ebri latera′lis [Syl′vii],** sulcus lateralis cerebri. **f. choroi′dea** [NA], choroid fissure: the line in the lateral ventricle along which the choroid plexus invaginates. **f. collatera′lis,** sulcus collateralis. **f. hippocam′pi,** sulcus hippocampi. **f. horizonta′lis cerebel′li** [NA], horizontal fissure of cerebellum: the fissure that separates the superior from the inferior semilunar lobule of the cerebellum. Called also *sulcus horizontalis cerebelli* and *great horizontal fissure.* **f. horizonta′lis pulmo′nis dex′tri** [NA], horizontal fissure of right lung: the cleft that extends forward from the oblique fissure in the right lung, separating the upper and middle lobes. **f. ligamen′ti te′retis** [NA], fissure for ligamentum teres: the fossa on the visceral surface of the liver lodging the ligamentum teres in the adult, and helping separate the right and left lobes of the liver; called also *fossa venae umbilicalis, fissure of round ligament,* and *umbilical fissure.* **f. ligamen′ti veno′si** [NA], fissure for ligamentum venosum: a fossa on the posterior part of the diaphragmatic surface of the liver lodging the ligamentum venosum in the adult. **f. longitudina′lis cer′ebri** [NA], longitudinal fissure of cerebrum: the deep fissure between the cerebral hemispheres extending inferiorly to the corpus callosum. **f. media′na [ante′rior] medul′lae oblonga′tae** [NA], anterior median fissure of medulla oblongata: the longitudinal fissure in the median plane of the anterior aspect of the medulla oblongata, continuous with the anterior median fissure of the spinal cord; it separates the pyramids and is partially obliterated below by their decussation. **f. media′na [ante′rior] medul′lae spina′lis** [NA], anterior median fissure of spinal cord; the deep longitudinal fissure in the median plane of the anterior aspect of the spinal cord; it contains the anterior spinal artery ensheathed in the linea splendens. Called also *anteromedian groove of spinal cord* and *Haller's line*. **f. media′na poste′rior medul′lae oblonga′tae,** sulcus mediana posterior medullae oblongatae. **f. obli′qua pulmo′nis** [NA], oblique fissure of lung: 1. the cleft that separates the lower from the middle lobe in the right lung. 2. the cleft that separates the upper from the lower lobe in the left lung. **f. orbita′lis infe′rior** [NA], inferior orbital fissure: a cleft in the inferolateral wall of the orbit bounded by the great wing of the sphenoid and the orbital process of the maxilla; it transmits the infraorbital and zygomatic nerves and the infraorbital vessels. Called also *inferior sphenoidal fissure* and *sphenomaxillary fissure*. **f. orbita′lis supe′rior** [NA], superior orbital fissure: an elongated cleft between the small and great wings of the sphenoid bone, which transmits various nerves and vessels; called also (*superior*) *sphenoidal fissure*. **f. parietooccipita′lis,** sulcus parietooccipitalis. **f. petrooccipita′lis** [NA], petrooccipital fissure: a fissure extending backward from the foramen lacerum to the jugular foramen, between the basioccipital and the posterior and inner border of the petrous portion of the temporal bone; called also *petrobasilar fissure*. **f. petrosquamo′sa** [NA], petrosquamous fissure: a slight fissure of varying distinctness in the floor of the middle cranial fossa, marking the line of fusion between the squamous and petrous portions of the temporal bone. **f. petrotympan′ica** [NA], petrotympanic fissure: a narrow transversely running slit just posterior to the articular surface of the mandibular fossa of the temporal bone; an arteriole and the chorda tympani nerve pass through it, and it lodges a portion of the malleus. Called also *glaserian, tympanic,* or *tympanosquamous fissure*. **f. posterolatera′lis cerebel′li** [NA], posterolateral fissure: the fissure which separates the nodulus from the uvula and the flocculus from the tonsilla of the cerebellum. **f. pri′ma cerebel′li** [NA], primary fissure: the fissure that separates the anterior from the posterior lobe in the cerebellum; it lies between the culmen and declive of the vermis, and between the part of the hemisphere that is continuous with the culmen and the lobulus simplex in the hemisphere. **f. pterygoi′dea,** pterygoid fissure: a fissure on the inferior portion of each pterygoid process where the pyramidal process of the palatine bone is inserted between the diverging medial and lateral pterygoid plates; called also *palatine* or *pterygoid notch,* and *palatine* or *pterygoid incisure*. **f. pterygomaxilla′ris** [NA], pterygomaxillary fissure: a cleft just behind the inferior orbital fissure between the lateral pterygoid plate and the maxilla; called also *pterygopalatine fissure*. **f. secun′da cerebel′li** [NA], secondary fissure: a fissure that lies between the uvula of the cerebellum and the pyramid. **f. sphenooccipita′lis,** sphenooccipital fissure: the fissure between the basilar part of the occipital bone and the body of the sphenoid bone; called also *basilar* or *occipitosphenoidal fissure*. **f. sphenopetro′sa** [NA], sphenopetrosal fissure: a fissure in the floor of the middle cranial fossa between the posterior edge of the great wing of the sphenoid bone and the petrous part of the temporal bone; called also *angular* or *petrosphenoidal fissure*. **f. transver′sa cer′ebri** [NA], transverse fissure of cerebrum: the fissure between the dorsal surface of the diencephalon and the ventral surface of the cerebral hemispheres, produced by the folding back of the hemispheres during their development; called also *great* (*transverse*) *fissure of cerebrum* and *fissure of Bichat*. **f. tympanomastoi′dea** [NA], tympanomastoid fissure: an external fissure on the inferior and lateral aspect of the skull between the tympanic portion and the mastoid process of the temporal bone; the auricular branch of the vagus nerve often passes through it. Called also *petromastoid fissure*. **f. tympanosquamo′sa** [NA], tympanosquamous fissure: a line seen on the posterior wall of the external acoustic meatus at the junction between the tympanic and squamous parts of the temporal bone.

fissurae (fis-su′re) [L.] plural of *fissura*.

fissural (fish′u-ral) pertaining to a fissure.

fissure (fish′ūr) [L. *fissura*] 1. any cleft or groove, normal or otherwise; especially a deep fold in the cerebral cortex which involves the entire thickness of the brain wall. See *fissura*. Cf. *sulcus*. 2. in dentistry, a fault in the surface of a tooth caused by the imperfect joining of the enamel of the different lobes; to be distinguished from a groove or sulcus (A.D.A.). Called also *enamel f.* **abdominal f.,** a congenital cleft in the abdominal wall. **adoccital f.,** an inconstant sulcus which crosses the caudal part of the precuneus and joins the occipital fissure. **Ammon's f.,** a pear-shaped aperture in the sclera at an early fetal period. **amygdaline f.,** a slight groove inconstantly present

near the extremity of the temporal lobe. **anal f., f. in a′no,** a painful linear ulcer at the margin of the anus. **angular f.,** fissura sphenopetrosa. **antitragohelicine f.,** fissura antitragohelicina. **ape f.** (*obs.*), any fissure in the human brain that is found also in apes, especially the sulcus lunatus. **f. of aqueduct of vestibule,** apertura externa aqueductus vestibuli. **f. of auricle, posterior,** fissura antitragohelicina. **auricular f. of temporal bone,** fissura tympanomastoidea. **basilar f.,** fissura sphenooccipitalis. **basisylvian f.,** the part of the lateral sulcus between the temporal lobe and the orbital surface of the frontal bone. **f. of Bichat,** fissura transversa cerebri. **branchial f's,** see under *cleft*. **Broca's f.,** a term loosely applied to the anterior and ascending rami of the cerebral lateral sulcus which invade the left inferior frontal gyrus. **Burdach's f.,** the groove between the lateral surface of the insula and the inner surface of the operculum. **calcarine f.,** sulcus calcarinus. **callosal f.,** sulcus corporis callosi. **callosomarginal f.,** sulcus cinguli. **central f.,** sulcus centralis cerebri. **cerebral f's, f's of cerebrum,** sulci cerebri. **cerebral f., lateral,** sulcus lateralis cerebri. **choroid f.,** 1. a ventral fissure formed by invagination of the optic vesicle and its stalk in the embryo, permitting the ingrowth of the mesoblast for the formation of the vitreous humor, etc. 2. fissura choroidea. **collateral f.,** sulcus collateralis. **corneal f.,** the cleft or groove in the scleral margin into which the limbus corneae fits; called also *rima cornealis* and *corneal cleft*. **craniofacial f.,** a vertical fissure separating the mesethmoid into two parts. **dentate f.,** sulcus hippocampi. **f. of ductus venosus,** fossa ductus venosi. **Ecker's f.,** sulcus occipitalis transversus. **enamel f.,** a fault in the enamel surface of a tooth; see *fissure* (def. 2). **entorbital f.,** a sulcus occasionally seen between the orbital and olfactory sulci. **ethmoid f.,** meatus nasi superior. **glaserian f.,** fissura petrotympanica. **f. of glottis,** rima glottidis. **great f. of cerebrum,** fissura transversa cerebri. **great horizontal f.,** fissura horizontalis cerebelli. **Henle's f's,** spaces filled with connective tissue between the muscular fibers of the heart. **hippocampal f., f. of hippocampus,** sulcus hippocampi. **horizontal f. of cerebellum,** fissura horizontalis cerebelli. **horizontal f. of right lung,** fissura horizontalis pulmonis dextri. **inferofrontal f.,** sulcus frontalis inferior. **intercerebral f.,** one separating the two hemispheres of the brain. **interparietal f.,** sulcus intraparietalis. **intratonsillar f.,** fossa supratonsillaris. **lacrimal f.,** sulcus lacrimalis ossis lacrimalis. **lateral f. of cerebrum,** sulcus lateralis cerebri. **f. for ligamentum teres,** fissura ligamenti teretis. **f. for ligamentum venosum,** fissura ligamenti venosi. **longitudinal f.,** 1. fissura longitudinalis cerebri. 2. tenia omentalis. **longitudinal f. of cerebellum,** vallecula cerebelli. **longitudinal f. of cerebrum,** fissura longitudinalis cerebri. **mandibular f's,** the two lowest facial fissures of the embryo. **maxillary f.,** a groove on the maxilla for the maxillary process of the palatal bone. **median f. of medulla oblongata, anterior,** fissura mediana anterior medullae oblongatae. **median f. of medulla oblongata, posterior,** sulcus medianus posterior medullae oblongatae. **median f. of spinal cord, anterior,** fissura mediana anterior medullae spinalis. **median f. of spinal cord, posterior,** sulcus medianus posterior medullae spinalis. **f. of Monro,** sulcus hypothalamicus. **oblique f. of lung,** fissura obliqua pulmonis. **occipital f.,** sulcus parietooccipitalis. **occipitosphenoidal f.,** fissura sphenooccipitalis. **oral f.,** rima oris. **orbital f., inferior,** fissura orbitalis inferior. **orbital f., superior,** fissura orbitalis superior. **f. of palpebrae,** rima palpebrarum. **Pansch's f.,** sulcus interparietalis. **paracentral f., anterior** (*obs.*), sulcus precentralis. **parietooccipital f.,** sulcus parietooccipitalis. **parietosphenoid f.,** incisura parietalis ossis temporalis. **parietotal f.** (*obs.*), the posterior portion of the sulcus intraparietalis. **petrobasilar f.,** fissura petrooccipitalis. **petromastoid f.,** fissura tympanomastoidea. **petrooccipital f.,** fissura petrooccipitalis. **petrosal f., superficial,** hiatus canalis nervi petrosi majoris. **petrosphenoidal f.,** fissura sphenopetrosa. **petrosquamosal f., petrosquamous f.,** fissura petrosquamosa. **petrotympanic f.,** fissura petrotympanica. **portal f.,** porta hepatis. **postcentral f.,** sulcus postcentralis. **posterolateral f.,** fissura posterolateralis cerebelli. **precentral f.,** sulcus precentralis. **precuneal f.,** a sulcus in the precuneus. **prepyramidal f.,** a fissure between the pyramis vermis and the uvula vermis. **presylvian f.,** the anterior branch of the lateral cerebral sulcus. **primary f.,** fissura prima cerebelli. **pterygoid f.,** fissura pterygoidea. **pterygomaxillary f.,** fissura pterygomaxillaris. **pterygopalatine f.,** fissura pterygomaxillaris. **pterygopalatine f. of palatine bone,** sulcus palatinus major ossis palatini. **pterygotympanic f.,** fissura petrotympanica. **pudendal f., f. of pudendum,** rima pudendi. **retrocuticular f.,** a fissure in the oral epithelium made by a tooth at the time of eruption. **f. of Rolando,** sulcus centralis cerebri. **f. of round ligament,** fissura ligamenti teretis. **sagittal f. of liver,** fossa sagittalis sinistra hepatis. **Santorini's f's,** incisurae cartilaginis meatus acustici. **Schwalbe's f.,** fissura choroidea. **secondary f.,** fissura secunda cerebelli. **sphe-**

noidal f., fissura orbitalis superior. **sphenoidal f., inferior,** fissura orbitalis inferior. **sphenoidal f., superior,** fissura orbitalis superior. **sphenomaxillary f.,** 1. fissura orbitalis inferior. 2. fossa pterygopalatina. **sphenooccipital f.,** fissura sphenoccipitalis. **sphenopetrosal f.,** fissura sphenopetrosa. **squamotympanic f.,** fissura petrotympanica. **subfrontal f.,** sulcus frontalis inferior. **subsylvian f.** (*obs.*), 1. an occasional fissure on the ventral surface of the frontal lobe of the brain. 2. ramus posterior sulci lateralis cerebri. **subtemporal f.,** an occasional fissure in the inferior and middle temporal convolutions. **superfrontal f.,** sulcus frontalis superior. **supertemporal f.,** sulcus temporalis superior. **sylvian f., f. of Sylvius,** sulcus lateralis cerebri. **tentorial f.** (*obs.*), sulcus collateralis. **transtemporal f.,** an occasional short fissure on the lateral surface of the temporal lobe. **transverse f.,** porta hepatis. **transverse f. of cerebrum,** fissura transversa cerebri. **transverse f. of cerebrum, great,** fissura transversa cerebri. **transverse occipital f.,** sulcus occipitalis transversus. **tympanic f.,** fissura petrotympanica. **tympanomastoid f.,** fissura tympanomastoidea. **tympanosquamous f.,** 1. fissura tympanosquamosa. 2. fissura petrotympanica. **umbilical f.,** fissura ligamenti teretis. **f. of the venous ligament,** fossa ductus venosi. **f. of the vestibule,** rima vestibuli. **zygal f.,** a fissure that consists of two portions united by a third portion. **zygomaticosphenoid f.,** a fissure between the orbital surface of the great wing of the sphenoid bone and the zygomatic bone.

fistula (fis′tu-lah), pl. *fistulas* or *fis′tulae* [L. "pipe"] an abnormal passage or communication, usually between two internal organs, or leading from an internal organ to the surface of the body; frequently designated according to the organs or parts with which it communicates, as anovaginal, bronchocutaneous, hepatopleural, pulmonoperitoneal, rectovaginal, urethrovaginal, and the like (see illustrations). Such passages are frequently created experimentally for the purpose of obtaining body secretions for physiologic study. **abdominal f.,** an abnormal passage lead-

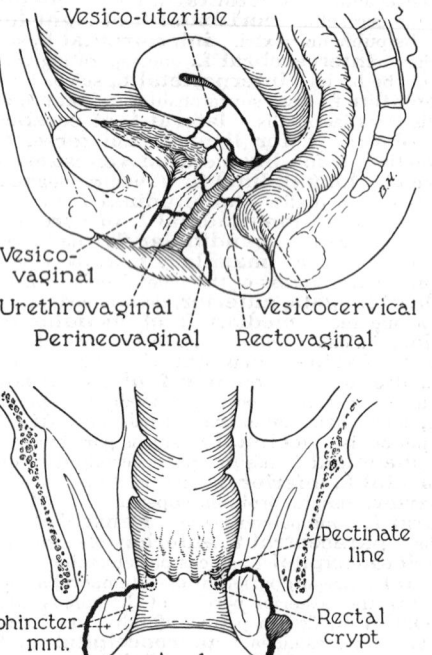

Various types of fistulae, designated according to site or to the organs with which they communicate.

ing from one of the hollow abdominal viscera to the surface of the abdomen. **alveolar f.,** dental f. **amphibolic f.,** an opening made into the gallbladder of an animal in order to obtain bile for study, with the common bile duct left intact so that the bile may flow through it when the fistula is closed. **anal f., f. in a′no,** one opening on the cutaneous surface near the anus, which may or may not communicate with the rectum. **arteriovenous f.,** an abnormal communication between an artery and a vein; it may result from injury (*traumatic arteriovenous f.*), or occur as a congenital abnormality (*congenital arteriovenous fistula*). **f. au′ris congen′ita,** preauricular f., congenital. **biliary f.,** an abnormal passage communicating with the biliary tract. **f. bimuco′sa,** a complete fistula of the anus, both ends of which open on the mucous surface of the anal canal. **blind f.,** a fistula that is open at one end only; it may open only upon the cutaneous surface of the body (*external blind f.*), or on an internal

mucous surface (*internal blind f.*). Called also *incomplete f.* **branchial f.,** an abnormal passage resulting from failure of closure of a branchial cleft; called also *cervical f.* **cervical f.,** 1. branchial f. 2. an abnormal passage communicating with the canal of the cervix uteri. **f. cervicovagina′lis laqueat′ica,** a fistula in the vaginal portion of the cervix uteri, communicating with the cervical canal and the vagina. **f. ciba′lis,** the esophagus. **f. col′li congen′ita,** a congenital fistula in the neck, opening into the pharynx. **colonic f.,** an abnormal passage communicating with the colon and the cutaneous surface of the body (*external colonic f.*), or with the colon and another hollow organ (*internal colonic f.*). **complete f.,** an abnormal passage in the body, each end of which opens on a mucous surface or on the cutaneous surface of the body. **f. cor′neae,** an orifice remaining after failure of a corneal ulcer to heal. **coronary arteriovenous f.,** a congenital condition in which there is an abnormal communication between a coronary artery and vein. **coronary artery f.,** a congenital condition in which there is an abnormal communication between a coronary artery and the right heart, or with the pulmonary or bronchial arteries. **craniosinus f.,** a fistula between the intracranial space and one of the paranasal sinuses, permitting the escape of cerebrospinal fluid into the nose. **dental f.,** an abnormal passage communicating with the apical periodontal area of a tooth, which permits egress on the mucous membrane or the skin of an inflammatory or suppurative discharge; called also *alveolar f.* **Eck's f.,** an artificial communication made between the portal vein and the vena cava (Eck, 1877). **Eck's f. in reverse,** an artificial communication created to route all the blood from the posterior (lower) part of the body through the portal vein and liver. **external f.,** an abnormal communication between a hollow organ and the external surface of the body. **fecal f.,** a colonic fistula opening on the external surface of the body and discharging feces. **gastric f.,** an abnormal passage communicating with the stomach; often applied to an artificially created opening through the abdominal wall into the stomach (gastrostoma). **gingival f.,** a dental fistula opening on the gingiva. **hepatic f.,** an abnormal communication between the liver and another body part or organ. **horseshoe f.,** a semicircular fistulous tract near the anus, both openings being on the cutaneous surface. **incomplete f.,** blind f. **internal f.,** an abnormal communication between two internal organs. **intestinal f.,** an abnormal passage communicating with the intestine, often designating an artificially created opening through the abdominal wall into the intestine. **lacrimal f.,** an abnormal passage communicating with the lacrimal sac or duct. **lacteal f.,** an abnormal passage communicating with a lacteal duct. **lymphatic f., f. lymphat′ica,** an abnormal passage communicating with a lymphatic vessel. **Mann-Bollman f.,** an artificial opening into an isolated segment of intestine, the proximal end of which is sutured to the abdominal wall and the distal end attached by end-to-side anastomosis to the duodenum or other part of the small intestine. **parietal f.,** an abnormal passage in the body wall, ending blindly or communicating with an internal organ or body cavity. **pharyngeal f.,** an abnormal passage communicating with the pharynx. **pilonidal f.,** pilonidal sinus. **preauricular f., congenital,** an epidermal-lined tract communicating with a pitlike depression just in front of the helix and above the tragus (ear pit), resulting from imperfect fusion of the first and second branchial arches in formation of the auricle; called also *f. auris congenita.* **pulmonary f.,** an abnormal passage communicating with the lung. **pulmonary arteriovenous f., congenital,** a congenital anomaly characterized by existence of a direct communication between the pulmonary arterial and venous systems, allowing unoxygenated blood to enter the systemic circulation. **rectovaginal f.,** one between the rectum and vagina. **rectovesical f.,** one between the rectum and urinary bladder. **salivary f.,** an abnormal passage communicating with a salivary duct. **spermatic f.,** an abnormal passage communicating with the seminal ducts. **stercoral f.,** fecal f. **submental f.,** a salivary fistula opening below the chin. **Thiry's f.,** an artificial opening into an isolated segment of intestine, the proximal end of which is sutured to the abdominal wall and the distal end is closed. **Thiry-Vella f.,** an artificial opening into an internal closed loop of intestine, which communicates with the abdominal wall through an intestinal segment interposed between the surface and the loop. **thoracic f.,** an abnormal passage communicating with the thoracic cavity. **tracheal f.,** an abnormal passage communicating with the trachea. **umbilical f.,** an abnormal passage communicating with the gut or with the urachus at the umbilicus. **urachal f.,** an abnormal passage communicating with the urachus. **urinary f.,** an abnormal passage communicating with the urinary tract. **Vella's f.,** an artificial opening into an isolated segment of intestine, both open ends of which are sutured to the abdominal wall. **vesical f.,** an abnormal passage communicating with the urinary bladder. **vesicovaginal f.,** one from the bladder to the vagina.

fistulae (fis′tu-le) plural of *fistula.*

fistulatome (fis′tu-lah-tōm″) [*fistula* + Gr. *temnein* to cut] an instrument for incising a fistula; syringotome.

fistulectomy (fis″tu-lek′to-me) [*fistula* + Gr. *ektomē* excision] excision of a fistulous tract.

fistulization (fis″tu-li-za′shun) 1. the process of becoming fistulous. 2. the surgical creation of an opening into a hollow organ, cavity, or abscess; the creation of a communication between two structures which were not previously connected.

fistuloenterostomy (fis″tu-lo-en″ter-os′to-me) the operation of making a biliary fistula empty permanently into the intestine.

fistulotomy (fis″tu-lot′o-me) incision of a fistula.

fistulous (fis′tu-lus) [L. *fistulosus*] pertaining to or of the nature of a fistula.

fit (fit) 1. an episode characterized by inappropriate and involuntary motor or psychic activity. See also *epilepsy*. 2. the adaptation of one structure into another, as the adaptation of any dental restoration to its site in the mouth. **running f.,** 1. fright disease. 2. cursive epilepsy.

Fitz's law, syndrome (fitz′ez) [Reginald Heber *Fitz*, physician in Boston, 1843–1913] see under *law* and *syndrome*.

Fitz Gerald method, treatment [William Henry Hope *Fitz Gerald*, American physician, 1872–1939] zone therapy.

fix (fiks) to fasten or hold firm; see *fixation*.

fixateur (fēks-ah-ter′) [Fr.] Metchnikoff's term for antibody or amboceptor.

fixation (fik-sa′shun) [L. *fixatio*] 1. the act or operation of holding, suturing, or fastening in a fixed position. 2. the condition of being held in a fixed position. 3. in psychiatry, the cessation of the development of personality at a stage short of complete maturity. 4. in microscopy, the treatment of material so that its structure may be examined in greatest detail with minimal alteration of the normal state, and also to provide information concerning the chemical properties (as of cell constituents) by interpretation of fixation reactions. 5. in chemistry, the process whereby a substance is removed from the gaseous or solution phase and localized. 6. in ophthalmology, direction of the gaze so that the visual image of the object falls on the fovea centralis. 7. in film processing, the chemical removal of all undeveloped salts of the film emulsion, as on x-ray films. **alexin f.,** complement f. **autotrophic f.,** the cyclic mechanism whereby carbon dioxide is fixed into organic linkage by autotrophic organisms, e.g., plants and autotrophic bacteria. **binocular f.,** training both eyes on the same object as in ordinary vision. **Bovin f.,** an acetic fixation which destroys the mitochrondria of the cell. **complement f., f. of the complement,** when antigen unites with its specific antibody, complement, if present is taken into the combine and becomes inactive or fixed. Its presence or absence as free, active complement can be shown by adding sensitized blood cells to the mixture. If free complement is present, hemolysis occurs; if not, no hemolysis is observed. This reaction is the basis of many serologic tests for infection, including the Wassermann test for syphilis, and reactions for gonococcus infection, glanders, typhoid fever, tuberculosis, amebiasis, etc. Called also *Bordet-Gengou phenomenon* and *Neisser-Wechsberg phenomenon.* **elastic band f.,** the stabilization of fractured segments of the jaws by means of intermaxillary elastic bands applied to splints or appliances. **external pin f.,** a method for stabilizing fractures by means of pins drilled into the bony parts through the overlying skin and connected by metal bars. **external pin f., biphase,** external pin fixation in which the rigid metal bar connector is replaced with an acrylic bar adapted at the time of the reduction. **father f.,** inordinate attachment of a person to the male parent. **freudian f.,** arrest of an emotional progression at some intermediate level of psychosexual development. **internal f.,** the fastening together of the ends of a fractured bone by means of wires, plates, screws, or nails applied directly to the fractured bone. **intraosseous f.,** the open reduction and stabilization of fractured bony parts by direct fixation to one another with surgical wires, screws, pins, and/or plates. **maxillomandibular f.,** the fixation of fractures of the maxilla or mandible in a functional relationship with the opposing dental arch, through the use of elastics, wire ligatures, arch bars, or other splints. **mother f.,** inordinate attachment of a person to the female parent. **nasomandibular f.,** mandibular immobilization, especially for edentulous jaws, using maxillomandibular splints; a circummandibular wire is connected with an intraoral interosseous wire passed through a hole drilled into the anterior nasal spine of the maxilla. **nitrogen f.,** the union of the free atmospheric nitrogen with other elements to form chemical compounds, such as ammonia and nitrates or amino groups. It is done mostly by certain organisms in the soil and in the roots of legumes, by electric power in special machines, and by catalysis. **parent f.,** inordinate attachment of an individual for a parent, persisting into adult life and preventing normal development of interest in a person of the opposite sex. **skeletal f.,** immobilization of the ends of a fractured bone by metal wires or plates applied directly to the bone (*internal skeletal fixation*) or on the body surface (*external skeletal fixation*).

fixative (fik′sah-tiv) 1. an agent employed in the preparation of a histologic or pathologic specimen, for the purpose of maintaining the existing form and structure of all its constituent elements. Great numbers of such agents are used, the most important being composed of formalin, potassium bichromate, bichloride of mercury, osmic acid, glutaraldehyde, or picric acid (trinitrophenol), alone or in various combinations. See also *fluid* and *solution.* 2. see *amboceptor.* **glutaraldehyde f.,** a fixative used in specimen preparation for electron microscopy that does not simultaneously stain the tissue. **Kaiserling's f.,** see under *solution.* **Maximow's f.,** a solution composed of Zenker's fixative, formol, and osmic acid, used in preserving vertebrate cells for study with the visible light microscope. **Zenker's f.,** a fixative solution containing corrosive mercuric chloride, potassium bichromate, sodium sulfate, glacial acetic acid, and water; the sodium sulfate is frequently omitted. The most widely used variations of this fixative are the modifications by Maximow, by Helly, and by Custer, in which formalin replaces the acetic acid. **Zenker-formol f.,** a solution composed of Zenker's fixative with added formalin; see *Helly's fluid*, under *fluid*.

fixator (fiks-a′tor) antibody.

Fl. fluid.

F.L.A. fronto-laeva anterior (left frontoanterior—a position of the fetus).

F.l.a. abbreviation for L. *fi′at le′ge ar′tis*, let it be done according to rule.

flabellum (flah-bel′um) [L. a "little fan"] (*obs.*) a set of radiating fibers in the corpus striatum.

flaccid (flak′sid) [L. *flaccidus*] weak, lax, and soft.

flacherie (flash-er-e′) [Fr.] a fatal disease of silkworms occurring in two forms: an infectious form due to a small nonoccluded virus and a noninfectious form due to environmental changes, such as a sudden increase in temperature and humidity. It is marked by diarrhea, weakness, flaccidity, and death, after which the body quickly turns dark and the tissues liquefy. See also *gattine.*

Flack's node, test (flaks) [Martin William Flack, physiologist in London, 1882–1931] see *Keith-Flack's node,* under *node,* and see under *tests.*

flagella (flah-jel′ah) [L.] plural of *flagellum.*

flagellar (flah-jel′ar) of or relating to a flagellum.

Flagellata (flaj″ĕ-la′tah) Mastigophora.

flagellate (flaj′ĕ-lāt) 1. any microorganism having flagella as organs of locomotion. 2. any protozoan of the subphylum Mastigophora. 3. having flagella. 4. to practice flagellation.

flagellation (flaj″ĕ-la′shun) 1. a form of massage by tapping a part with the fingers. 2. whipping or being whipped to achieve erotic pleasure. 3. the protrusion of flagella; exflagellation.

flagelliform (flah-jel′ĭ-form) [L. *flagellum* whip + *forma* shape] shaped like a flagellum, or lash.

flagellin (flah′jel-in) a protein occurring in the flagella of bacteria; it is similar to keratin, myosin, and fibrinogen.

flagellosis (flaj″ĕ-lo′sis) infection with a flagellate protozoon.

flagellospore (flah-jel′o-spōr) zoospore.

flagellula (flah-jel′u-lah) zoospore.

flagellum (flah-jel′um) pl. *flagel′la* [L. "whip"] a long, mobile, whiplike projection from the free surface of a cell, serving as a locomotor organelle; it is composed of nine pairs of microtubules arrayed around a central pair. Arising from basal bodies, flagella are common to all mastigophoran protozoa and occur in such specialized cells as spermatozoa. Bacterial flagella are thinner and simpler, being composed of tightly wound chains of strands that contain flagellin. Bacteria having a single flagellum are *monotrichous,* those with two or more at one end are *lophotrichous,* those with one flagellum at each end are *amphitrichous,* and those with flagella around the entire surface are *peritrichous.* Cf. *cilium,* def. 3.

Flagyl (flag′l) trademark for a preparation of metronidazole.

flail (flāl) exhibiting abnormal or paradoxical mobility, as flail joint, flail chest, or flail valve.

Flajani's disease (flah-jan′ēz) [Giuseppe *Flajani*, Italian surgeon, 1741–1808] Graves' disease.

flame (flām) 1. the luminous, irregular appearance usually accompanying combustion caused by the light emitted from energetically excited chemical species, or an appearance resembling it. 2. to render an object sterile by exposure to a flame. **capillary f's,** telangiectatic spots sometimes seen on the face of a newborn infant; called also *stork bites.* **manometric f.,** a gas flame in an enclosed box arranged so that it pulsates with the vibration of air caused by sound; such pulsations may be seen on a mirror or recorded photographically (flame picture).

flange (flanj) a projecting border or edge; in dentistry, that part of the denture base which extends from around the embedded teeth to the border of the denture. **buccal f.,** the portion of the flange of a denture that occupies the buccal vestibule of the mouth and extends distally from the buccal notch. **denture f.,** see *flange.* **labial f.,** the portion of the flange of a denture that occupies the labial vestibule of the mouth. **lingual f.,** the portion of the flange of a mandibular denture which occupies the space adjacent to the residual ridge and next to the tongue.

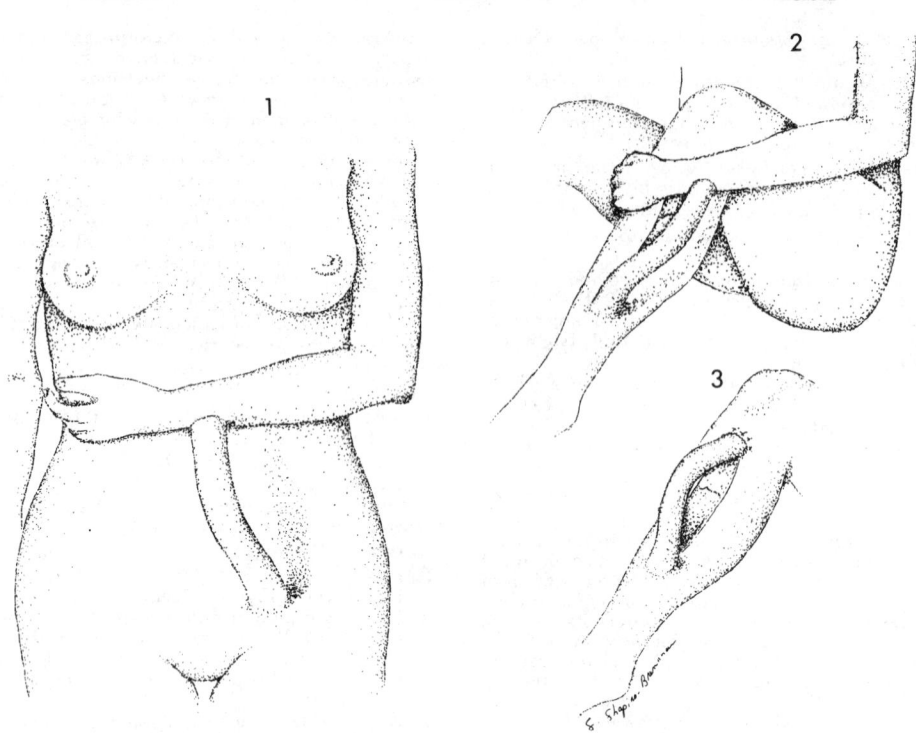

Tubed pedicle flap raised from the abdomen and (1) sutured to the arm to preserve blood supply, (2) transferred from abdomen to leg, and (3) from arm to leg.

flank (flank) the part of the body below the ribs and above the ilium.

flap (flap) 1. a mass of tissue for grafting, usually including skin, only partially removed from one part of the body so that it retains its own blood supply during its transfer to a new location; used to repair defects in an adjacent or distant part of the body. 2. an uncontrolled movement. **Abbé f.,** a triangular surgical flap taken from the median portion of the lower lip, and used to correct defects of the upper lip. **advancement f.,** sliding f. **bilobed f.,** Zimany's bilobed flap. **bipedicle f.,** a pedicle flap with two vascular attachments. **circular f.,** a surgical flap of somewhat circular outline. **cross-arm f.,** a surgical flap cut from one arm and attached to the other to repair a defect. **cross-leg f.,** a surgical flap cut from one leg and attached to the other to repair a defect. **delayed transfer f.,** a surgical flap that is partially raised from its bed and then later replaced; done to force the flap to develop further collateral circulation through the pedicle. **direct transfer f.,** immediate transfer f. **distant f.,** a pedicle flap brought from a distant area and transplanted by bringing the donor area and the recipient site into close approximation; called also *Italian f.* **double-end f.,** a pedicle flap or rope flap. **double pedicle f.,** bipedicle f. **envelope f.,** a mucoperiosteal flap retracted from a horizontal linear incision (as along the free gingival margin) with no vertical component of that incision. **Estlander f.,** a surgical flap cut from the corner of the upper lip, and used for repair of lateral defects of the lower lip. **free f.,** an island flap detached from the body and reattached at the distant recipient site by microvascular anastomosis. **French f.,** sliding f. **gauntlet f.,** pedicle f. **Gillies' f.,** rope f. **immediate transfer f.,** a surgical flap that is applied to the recipient site immediately after it is elevated from its bed; called also *direct transfer f.* **Indian f.,** interpolated f. **interpolated f.,** a pedicle flap that is twisted or rotated on its base and placed into a contiguous area; called also *Indian f.* **island f.,** a skin flap consisting of the skin and subcutaneous tissue with a pedicle made up of only the nutrient vessels. **Italian f.,** distant f. **jump f.,** a flap cut from the abdomen and attached to a flap of the same size on the forearm; the forearm flap is transferred later to some other part of the body to fill a defect there. **Langenbeck's pedicle mucoperiosteal f.,** von Langenbeck's bipedicle mucoperiosteal f. **lingual tongue f.,** a combination flap used to repair fistulae of the hard palate: a palatal flap forms the floor of the nose, and a flap taken from the back or edge of the tongue forms the palatal surface. **local f.,** a surgical flap cut from the tissue neighboring the defect. **mucoperiosteal f.,** a flap of mucosal tissue, including the periosteum, reflected from bone. **liver f.,** asterixis. **musculocutaneous f.,** a surgical flap cut from skin and muscle. **myocutaneous f.,** a compound flap of skin and muscle with adequate vascularity to permit sufficient tissue to be transferred to the recipient site. **pedicle f.,** a flap consisting of the full thickness of the skin and the subcutaneous tissue, attached by a pedicle. **rope f.,** a bipedicle flap made by elevating a long strip of tissue from its bed except at the two extremities, the cut edges then being sutured together to form a tube; called also *tube* or *tunnel f.,* and *Gillies' f.* **rotation f.,** a pedicle flap whose width is increased by transforming the edge of the flap distal to the defect into a curved line; the flap is then rotated and a counterincision is made at the base of the curved line, which increases the mobility of the flap. **skin f.,** a full-thickness mass or flap of tissue containing epidermis, dermis, and subcutaneous tissue. **sliding f.,** a flap carried to its new position by a sliding technique of surgical advancement. **surgical f.,** a mass of tissue partially detached from one part of the body but carrying with it its own nutrient blood vessels or at least a portion of them, and attached, directly or as a jump flap, to a remote part, for repair of a defect. **tube f., tubed pedicle f.,** rope f. **tunnel f.,** rope f. **von Langenbeck's bipedicle mucoperiosteal f.,** a bipedicle flap of the conjoined mucoperiosteal tissues, used for closure of a cleft palate. **V-Y f.,** a flap in which the incision is made in the shape of a V and is sutured in the shape of a Y so as to lengthen an area of tissue; or conversely the incision is Y-shaped and the closure V-shaped to shorten an area of tissue. **Z-f.,** a flap in which the incision is made in the shape of a Z so as to distribute contraction into more than one direction; often used to correct scars. **Zimany's bilobed f.,** a surgical flap consisting of a large lobe that is transposed into the primary defect and a smaller second lobe that is transposed to fill the secondary defect produced by mobilization of the large lobe.

flaps (flaps) severe swelling of the lips in horses.

flare (flār) 1. the red outermost zone of the "triple response" (Sir Thomas Lewis) urticarial wheal reaction, a manifestation of immediate, as opposed to delayed, allergy or hypersensitivity. 2. a spreading flush or area of redness on the skin, spreading out around an infective lesion or extending beyond the main point of reaction to an irritant. 3. sudden exacerbation of a disease.

flash (flash) excess material extruded from a mold, as in the packing of a denture by the compression technique.

flask (flask) 1. a container, such as a narrow-necked vessel of glass for containing liquid. 2. a metal case in which the materials used in the creation of artificial dentures are placed for processing. 3. to place a denture in a flask for processing. **casting f.,** refractory f. **crown f.,** a small, sectional, boxlike metal case in which a sectional mold of plaster of Paris or of artificial stone is made for compressing and curing plastics on small dental restorations. **culture f.,** a flask for growing cultures of bacteria or of other cells. **denture f.,** a boxlike case of metal which can be tightly closed, and in which dentures or other resinous restorations can be compressed and cured. **Erlenmeyer f.,** a glass flask with a conical body, broad base, and narrow neck. **refractory f.,** a metal tube in which a refractory mold is made for casting metal dental restorations or appliances; called also *casting f.* **volumetric f.,** a narrow-necked vessel of glass calibrated to contain or deliver an exact volume at a given temperature.

flasking (flask′ing) the act of investing a pattern for a dental prosthesis.

flat (flat) 1. lying in one plane; having an even surface. 2. having little or no resonance. 3. slightly below the normal pitch of a musical tone. **optical f.,** a glass plate so perfectly flat that only an interferometer can measure its unevenness.

Flatau's law (flat-owz′) [Edward *Flatau*, Polish neurologist, 1869–1932] see under *law*.

flatfoot (flat′foot) a condition in which one or more of the arches of the foot have flattened out; called also *pes planovalgus, pes planus,* and *pes valgus.* **rocker-bottom f.,** see under *foot.*

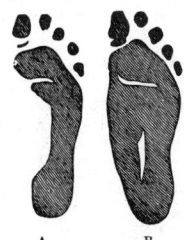

Print of soles (*A*) of normal foot and (*B*) of one with flatfoot (Albert).

spastic f., a painful form of flatfoot due to spasm of the peroneal muscles.

flatness (flat′nes) a peculiar sound lacking resonance, heard on percussing a part that is abnormally solid.

flatulence (flat′u-lens) [L. *flatulentia*] the presence of excessive amounts of air or gases in the stomach or intestine, leading to distention of the organs.

flatulent (flat′u-lent) [L. *flatulentus*] pertaining to or characterized by flatulence; distended with gas.

flatus (fla′tus) [L. "a blowing"] 1. gas or air in the gastrointestinal tract. 2. gas or air expelled through the anus. **f. vagina′lis,** noisy expulsion of gas from the vagina.

flatworm (flat′werm) any worm belonging to the phylum Platyhelminthes.

flav-, flavo- [L. *flavus* yellow] a combining form meaning yellow.

flavanoid (fla′vah-noid) flavonoid.

flavanone (fla′vah-nōn) colorless, flavonoid compounds formed by reduction of the 2:3 double bond of a flavone; they occur in free

form or as glycosides. A subgroup, the *flavanonols,* have a 3-hydroxy group and seldom occur as glycosides.

flavanonol (fla′vah-non-ol) a subgroup of flavanone (q.v.).

flavescent (flah-ves′ent) [L. *flavescere* to become gold colored] yellowish.

flavin (fla′vin) [L. *flavus* yellow] any one of a group of water-soluble pigments widely distributed in animals and plants, including riboflavin and yellow enzymes, and characterized by a yellow color, an intense green fluorescence, and the isoalloxazine nucleus. **f.-adenine dinucleotide (FAD),** a coenzyme that is a condensation product of riboflavin phosphate and adenylic acid; it forms the prosthetic group of certain enzymes (flavoproteins), including D-amino acid oxidase and xanthine oxidase, and is important in electron transport in mitochondria. **f. mononucleotide (FMN),** a derivative of riboflavin consisting of a three-ring system (isoalloxazine) attached to the alcohol (ribitol); it acts as a coenzyme for a number of oxidative enzymes (flavoproteins), including L-amino acid oxidase and cytochrome *c* reductase; called also *riboflavin phosphate.*

flavine (fla′vīn) acriflavine hydrochloride.

flavivirus (fla″ve-vi′rus) a subcategory of togaviruses; the type species is the yellow fever virus.

Flavobacterium (fla″vo-bak-te′re-um) a genus of microorganisms of the family Achromobacteraceae, order Eubacteriales, made up of gram-negative rod-shaped bacteria characteristically producing yellow, orange, red, or yellow-brown pigmentation, and found in soil and water. It includes 26 species, some of which are said to be pathogenic.

flavoenzyme (fla″vo-en′zīm) any enzyme containing a flavin nucleotide (FMN or FAD) as a prosthetic group; called also *flavoprotein.*

flavone (fla′vōn) a colorless crystalline substance, the 4-keto series of flavonoids, able to reverse increased capillary fragility. Numerous yellow dyestuffs having similar properties are derived from it.

flavonoid (fla′vo-noid) a generic term for a group of aromatic oxygen heterocyclic compounds derived from 2-phenylbenzopyran or its 2,3-dehydro derivative. They are widely distributed in higher plants, one subgroup, the anthocyanins, accounting for the majority of yellow, red, and blue pigmentation. Another subgroup, varying somewhat in structure, has physiologic properties formerly referred to as "vitamin P" activity, now called *bioflavonoids,* e.g., citrin, rutin, etc. The flavonoids are grouped in order of increasing oxidation state: catechins; leucoanthocyanidins and flavanones, flavanols, flavones, and anthocyanidins; and flavonols.

flavonol (fla′vo-nol) a yellow crystalline flavonoid, formed by introduction of an OH group at C-3 of a flavone; it is grouped with the flavones and isoflavones.

flavoprotein (fla″vo-pro′te-in) any enzyme containing a flavin nucleotide (FAD or FMN) as a prosthetic group; called also *flavoenzyme.*

flavor (fla′vor) 1. that quality of any substance which affects the taste. 2. a pharmaceutical or other preparation for improving the taste of a food or medicine.

flavoxanthin (fla″vo-zan′thin) a minor, yellow, carotenoid pigment, $C_{40}H_{56}O_3$, from the petals of ranunculaceous plants, structurally related to vitamin A but having no vitamin A activity.

flavoxate hydrochloride (fla-voks′āt) chemical name: 3-methyl-4-oxo-2-phenyl-4*H*-1-benzopyran-8-carboxylic acid 2-(1-piperidinyl)ethyl ester hydrochloride. A smooth muscle relaxant, $C_{24}H_{25}NO_4 \cdot HCl$, occurring as an off-white, crystalline powder; used as an antispasmodic for the urinary system, administered orally.

Flaxedil (flaks′ĕ-dil) trademark for a preparation of gallamine triethiodide.

flaxseed (flaks′sēd) linseed.

flazalone (fla′zah-lōn) chemical name: *p*-fluorophenyl-4-(*p*-fluorophenyl)-4-hydroxy-1-methyl-3-piperidyl ketone; an anti-inflammatory agent, $C_{19}H_{19}F_2NO_2.$

fld. fluid.

fl.dr. fluid dram.

flea (fle) any insect of the order *Siphonaptera;* many are parasitic and may act as carriers of disease. The genera of medical importance are: *Cediopsylla, Ceratophyllus, Ctenocephalides, Ctenophthalmus, Leptopsylla, Diamanus, Echidnophaga, Hoplopsyllus, Monopsyllus, Neopsylla, Nosopsyllus, Oropsylla, Pulex, Rhopalopsyllus, Tunga, Xenopsylla.* **Asiatic rat f.,** *Xenopsylla cheopis.* **burrowing f.,** *Tunga penetrans.* **cat f.,** *Ctenocephalides felis.* **cavy f.,** *Rhopalopsyllus cavicola.* **chigoe f.,** *Tunga penetrans.* **common f.,** *Pulex irritans.* **common rat f.,** *Nosopsyllus fasciatus.* **dog f.,** *Ctenocephalides canis.* **European mouse f.,** *Ctenophthalmus agrytes.* **European rat f.,** *Nosopsyllus fasciatus.* **human f.,** *Pulex irritans.* **Indian rat f.,** *Xenopsylla astia.* **jigger f.,** *Tunga penetrans.* **mouse f.,** *Leptopsylla segnis.* **sand f.,** *Tunga penetrans.* **squirrel f.,** *Hoplopsyllus anomalus.* **sticktight f.,** *Echidnophaga gallinacea.* **suslik f.,** any of several species of fleas which infest Russian ground squirrels. **tropical rat f.,** *Xenopsylla cheopis.*

flecainide acetate (flĕ-ka′nīd) chemical name: *N*-(2-piperidinylmethyl)-2,5-bis(2,2,2-trifluoroethoxy)benzamide monoacetate; a cardiac depressant with antiarrhythmic action, $C_{17}H_{20}F_6N_2O_3 \cdot C_2H_4O_2.$

Flechsig's area, etc. (flek′sigz) [Paul Emil *Flechsig,* neurologist in Leipzig, 1847–1929] see under *area, column, cuticulum, fasciculus, field,* and *law.*

fleck (flek) a flake, particle, speckle, or spot. **tobacco f's,** Gamna-Gandy nodules.

fleckfieber (flek-fe′ber) [Ger.] epidemic typhus; see under *typhus.*

fleckmilz (flek′milts) [Ger.] a condition of the spleen in malignant nephrosclerosis in which necrotic follicles appear as translucent areas.

flection (flek′shun) flexion.

fleece (flēs) a network of interlacing fibers. **f. of Stilling,** the lacework of white fibers surrounding the dentate nucleus.

Fleischl's test (fli'shelz) [Ernst von *Fleischl* von Marxow, Austrian pathologist, 1846–1891] see under *tests*.

Fleischmann's hygroma (flīsh'manz) [Godfried *Fleischmann*, German anatomist, 1777–1853] see under *hygroma*.

Fleitmann's test (flīt'manz) [Theodore *Fleitmann*, German chemist] see under *tests*.

Fleming (flem'ing), Sir Alexander. A Scottish bacteriologist, 1881–1955; co-winner, with Ernst Boris Chain and Sir Howard Walter Florey, of the Nobel prize in medicine and physiology for 1945 for the discovery of penicillin and its curative effect in infectious disease.

flemingen (flĕ-min'jin) any of several chalcone dyes from waras; a natural dyestuff (C.I. natural yellow 22) from shrubs of the genus *Flemingia*.

Flemming's center, solution (fixing fluid) [Walther *Flemming*, German anatomist, 1843–1905] see *germinal center*, under *center*, and see under *solution*.

flesh (flesh) the soft, muscular tissue of the animal body. **goose f.**, cutis anserina. **proud f.**, exuberant amounts of soft, edematous, granulation tissue that may develop during the healing of large surface wounds.

fletazepam (flĕ-taz'ĕ-pam) chemical name: 7-chloro-5-(2-fluorophenyl)-2,3-dihydro-1-(2,2,2-trifluoroethyl)-1*H*-1,4-benzodiazepine; a skeletal muscle relaxant, $C_{17}H_{13}ClF_4N_2$.

fletcherism (flech'er-izm) [Horace *Fletcher*, American dietitian, 1849–1919] the thorough mastication of solid food and the taking of liquids by sips.

flex (fleks) [L. *flexus* bent] to bend or put in a state of flexion.

flexibilitas (flek-sĭ-bil'ĭ-tas) [L.] flexibility. **f. ce'rea**, a cataleptic state in which the limbs retain any position in which they may be placed.

flexibility (flek″sĭ-bil'ĭ-te) [L. *flexibilitas*] the quality of being flexible. **waxy f.**, flexibilitas cerea.

flexible (flek'sĭ-bl) [L. *flexibilis, flexilis*] readily bent without tendency to break.

flexile (fleks'il) flexible.

fleximeter (fleks-im'ĕ-ter) an instrument for measuring the amount of flexion of a joint.

flexion (flek'shun) [L. *flexio*] the act of bending or condition of being bent.

Flexner's bacillus, dysentery, serum (fleks'nerz) [Simon *Flexner*, American pathologist, 1863–1946] see *Shigella flexneri*, see *bacillary dysentery*, under *dysentery*, and see *antimeningococcus serum*, under *serum*.

flexor (flek'sor) [L.] any muscle that flexes a joint; see Table of *Musculi*. **f. retinac'ulum**, see *retinaculum flexorum manus* and *retinaculum musculorum flexorum pedis*.

flexuose (fleks'u-ōs) winding or wavy.

flexura (flek-shoo'rah), pl. *flexu'rae* [L.] flexure: a bending; [NA] a general term for a bent portion of a structure or organ. **f. co'li dex'tra** [NA], right flexure of colon: the bend in the large intestine at which the ascending colon becomes the transverse colon; called also *f. hepatica coli* and *hepatic flexure of colon*. **f. co'li sinis'tra** [NA], left flexure of colon: the bend in the large intestine at which the transverse colon becomes the descending colon; called also *f. lienalis coli* and *splenic flexure of colon*. **f. duode'ni infe'rior** [NA], inferior flexure of duodenum: the bend in the duodenum at which the descending duodenum becomes horizontal or transverse. Called also *inferior angle of duodenum*. **f. duode'ni supe'rior** [NA], superior flexure of duodenum: the bend in the first or superior part of the duodenum; called also *superior angle of duodenum*. **f. duodenojejuna'lis** [NA], duodenal flexure: the bend in the small intestine at the junction between the duodenum and jejunum; the suspensory muscle of the duodenum attaches to this point. **f. hepat'ica co'li**, f. coli dextra. **f. liena'lis co'li**, f. coli sinistra. **f. perinea'lis rec'ti** [NA], perineal flexure of rectum: the dorsal and caudal bend at the caudal end of the rectum. **f. sacra'lis rec'ti** [NA], sacral flexure of rectum: the dorsal first bend in the rectum.

flexurae (flek-shoo're) [L.] plural of *flexura*.

flexural (flek'shur-al) pertaining to or affecting a flexure.

flexure (flek'sher) a bending; a bent portion of a structure or organ; see *flexura*. **basicranial f.**, pontine f. **caudal f.**, the bend at the aboral end of the embryo; called also *sacral f.* **cephalic f.**, the curve in the midbrain of the embryo; called also *cranial f.* **cerebral f.**, one of the bends in the embryonic brain; called also *nuchal f.* **cervical f.**, a bend in the neural tube of the embryo at the junction of the brain and spinal cord. **cranial f.**, cephalic f. **dorsal f.**, one of the flexures of the embryo in the mid-dorsal region. **duodenojejunal f.**, flexura duodenojejunalis. **hepatic f. of colon**, flexura coli dextra. **inferior f. of duodenum**, flexura duodeni inferior. **left f. of colon**, flexura coli sinistra. **lumbar f.**, the ventral curvature of the back in the lumbar region. **mesencephalic f.**, a flexure in the neural tube of the vertebrate embryo at the level of the mesencephalon. **nuchal f.**, cervical f. **perineal f. of rectum**, flexura perinealis recti. **pontine f.**, a flexure

in the hindbrain of the embryo; called also *basicranial f.* **right f. of colon**, flexura coli dextra. **sacral f.**, caudal f. **sacral f. of rectum**, flexura sacralis recti. **sigmoid f.**, sigmoid colon. **splenic f. of colon**, flexura coli sinistra. **superior f. of duodenum**, flexura duodeni superior.

flicker (flik'er) the visual sensation produced by intermittent flashes of light occurring at a certain rate. The flashes may appear to flicker or to be steady according to the rate of interruption (*flicker phenomenon*). The number of flashes per second at which the light just appears to be continuous is known as the *flicker fusion threshold* (*fusion frequency; critical fusion frequency*). The *flicker test*, determination of the flicker fusion threshold, is sometimes used in the diagnosis of existent or incipient high blood pressure and certain forms of heart disease, or to determine the effect of a drug on blood vessel spasm. A low threshold indicates disease.

Fliess treatment (therapy) (flēs) [Wilhelm *Fliess*, Berlin physician, 1858–1928] see under *treatment*.

flight of ideas a condition in which the patient talks almost continuously and jumps repeatedly from one subject to another before the first topic is concluded; sometimes seen in acute manic states and acute schizophrenia.

Flint's arcade, law (flints) [Austin *Flint*, American physiologist, 1836–1915] see under *arcade* and *law*.

Flint's murmur (flints) [Austin *Flint*, American physician, 1812–1886] see under *murmur*.

floaters (flo'ters) "spots before the eyes"; deposits in the vitreous of the eye, usually moving about and probably representing fine aggregates of vitreous protein occurring as a benign degenerative change. Called also *vitreous f's* and *muscae volitantes*.

floccilegium (flok″sĭ-le'je-um) floccillation.

floccillation (flok″sĭ-la'shun) [L. *floccilatio*] the picking at bedclothes by a delirious patient.

floccose (flok'ōs) [L. *floccosus* full of flocks of wool] woolly; said of a bacterial growth which is composed of short, curved chains variously oriented.

floccular (flok'u-lar) pertaining to the flocculus.

flocculation (flok″u-la'shun) a colloid phenomenon in which the disperse phase separates in discrete, usually visible, particles rather than in a continuous mass, as in coagulation. **Ramon f.**, a method of standardizing antitoxic sera by the *in vitro* precipitation of toxin and antitoxin when mixed.

floccule (flok'ūl) flocculus. **toxoid-antitoxin f.**, a suspension of the precipitate formed when toxoid and antitoxin are mixed.

flocculent (flok'u-lent) containing downy or flaky masses.

flocculi (flok'u-li) plural of *flocculus*.

flocculoreaction (flok″u-lo-re-ak'shun) a serum reaction characterized by flocculation.

flocculus (flok'u-lus), pl. *floc'culi* [L. "tuft"] 1. a small tuft, as of wool or similar material, or a small mass of other fibrous material such as one of the flakes of a flocculent solution. 2. [NA] a small lobe on the lower side of either cerebellar hemisphere, continuous with the nodule of the vermis. Called also *floccule*. 3. the floccular portion of the flocculonodular lobe. **accessory f., f. seconda'rii, secondary f.**, a small lobe sometimes seen near the flocculus in the inferior process of the cerebellum.

floctafenine (flok″tah-fen'ēn) chemical name: 2-[[8-(trifluoromethyl)-4-quinolinyl]amino]benzoic acid; an analgesic, $C_{20}H_{17}F_3N_2O_4$.

Flood's ligament (fludz) [Valentine *Flood*, Irish surgeon, 1800–1847] see under *ligament*.

flooding (flud'ing) in behavior therapy, a form of desensitization (q.v.) for the treatment of phobias and related disorders in which the patient is repeatedly exposed, in imagination or real life, to emotionally distressing stimuli of high intensity. Cf. *implosion* and *systematic densensitization*.

Flor. abbreviation for L. *flo'res*, flowers.

flora (flo'rah) [L. *Flora*, the goddess of flowers] the plant life present in or characteristic of a special location; it may be discernible with the unaided eye (macroflora), or only with the aid of a microscope (microflora). **intestinal f.**, the bacteria normally residing within the lumen of the intestine.

florantyrone (flo-ran'tĭ-rōn) chemical name: γ-oxo-8-fluoranthenebutyric acid. A hydrocholeretic agent, $C_{20}H_{14}O_3$, occurring as yellow, crystalline platelets; administered orally in the treatment of chronic cholecystitis, cholangitis, and biliary dyskinesia, and in the prevention of cholelithiasis.

Floraquin (flor'ah-kwin) trademark for a preparation of iodoquinal.

Florence's crystals, test (reaction) (flor-ahns') [Albert *Florence*, French physician, 1851–1927] see under *crystal* and *tests*.

florentium (flo-ren'she-um) former name for promethium.

flores (flo'rēz) [L., pl. of *flos* flower] 1. the blossoms or flowers of a plant. 2. a drug after sublimation. **f. benzoi'ni**, benzoic acid. **f. sul'furis**, sublimed sulfur.

Florey unit (flor'ē) [Sir Howard W. *Florey*, English pathologist, born 1898; co-winner, with Ernst Boris Chain and Sir Alexander Fleming, of the Nobel prize for medicine in 1945 for the discovery of penicillin] see *Oxford unit*, under *unit*.

florid (flor′id) [L. *floridus* blossoming] 1. in full bloom; occurring in fully developed form. 2. having a bright red color.

Floridin (flor′ĭ-din) trademark for a preparation of fuller's earth.

florigen (flor′ĭ-jen) a hypothetical flower-producing hormone of unknown chemical composition, believed to be produced in the leaves and transported in the phloem to the buds.

Florinef (flor′ĭ-nef) trademark for preparations of fludrocortisone acetate.

florizine (flor′ĭ-zēn) dericin.

Floropryl (flor′o-pril) trademark for preparations of isoflurophate.

Florschütz formula (flor′shitz) [Georg *Florschütz*, German physician, born 1859] see under *formula*.

Flourens' theory (doctrine) (floo-ranz′) [Marie Jean Pierre *Flourens*, French physiologist, 1794–1867] see under *theory*.

flow (flo) the amount of a fluid that flows through an organ or part in a specified time. **effective renal blood f.,** that portion of the total renal blood flow that perfuses functional renal tissue, e.g., the glomeruli; abbreviated ERBF. **effective renal plasma f.,** the amount of blood plasma perfusing functional renal tissue each minute, as measured by clearance methods (normally about 600 ml./min.); abbreviated ERPF. **gene f.,** transfer of genes from one population to another by migration and miscegenation. **total renal blood f.,** the volume of blood that passes each minute into the renal arteries (normally 1200 ml./min.); abbreviated TRBF.

Flower's index (flow′erz) [Sir William Henry *Flower*, British physician, 1831–1899] dental index; see under *index*.

flowers (flow′erz) 1. the blossoms of a plant. 2. a sublimed drug, as sulfur or benzoin. **f. of arsenic,** arsenic trioxide. **f. of benzoin,** benzoic acid. **f. of camphor,** powdered camphor prepared by sublimation. **pyrethrum f's,** the dried powdered flowers of the perennial herbs *Chrysanthemum (Pyrethrum) cinerariaefolium* (Trév.) Vis., indigenous to Dalmatia and Montenegro, and *C. coccineum* and *C. marschalli*, indigenous to western Asia; they are used in the preparation of insecticides, and have been used as a scabicide. Called also *Dalmatian*, or *Persian, insect powder*. **f. of sulfur,** sublimed sulfur.

flowmeter (flo′me-ter) an apparatus for measuring the rate of flow of liquids or gases. **blood f.,** an instrument for determining the rate of blood flow in the arteries or veins.

flow tract (flo′trakt) the path of the blood within the chambers of the heart. In the *left flow tract*, blood enters the left atrium through the pulmonary veins, flows through the mitral valve into the left ventricle, and passes through the aortic valve and on into the aorta and systemic circulation. In the *right flow tract*, blood enters the right atrium through the venae cavae, flows through the tricuspid valve into the right ventricle, and passes through the pulmonary valve and on into the pulmonary artery and the pulmonary circulation.

floxacillin (floks″ah-sil′in) chemical name: 6-[3-(2-chloro-6-fluorophenyl)-5-methyl-4-isoxazolecarboxamido]-3, 3-dimethyl-7-oxo-4-thia-1-azabicyclo[3.2.0]heptane-2-carboxylic acid. A penicillinase resistant, semisynthetic penicillin, $C_{19}H_{17}ClFN_3O_5S$, which has been used primarily in the treatment of infections due to benzylpenicillin-resistant staphylococci. Called also *flucloxacillin*.

floxuridine (floks-ur′ĭ-dēn) [USP] chemical name: 2′-deoxy-5-fluorouridine. An antineoplastic that acts as an antimetabolite similarly to fluorouracil, $C_9H_{11}FN_2O_5$, occurring as a white to off-white solid; used in the palliative management of carcinoma in certain patients, administered by intra-arterial infusion. Abbreviated FUDR. *Sterile floxuridine* [USP] is lyophilized floxuridine suitable for intra-arterial infusion.

fl.oz. fluidounce; see under *ounce*.

F.L.P. fronto-laeva posterior (left fronto posterior—a position of the fetus).

F.L.T. fronto-laeva transversa (left frontotransverse—a position of the fetus).

flu (floo) popular name for *influenza*.

Fluax (floo′aks) trademark for a preparation of influenza virus vaccine.

fluazacort (floo-az′ah-kort) chemical name: 21-(acetyloxy)-9-fluoro-11β,21-hydroxy-5′βH-pregna-4,6-dieno[17,16-d]-oxazole-3,20-dione; an anti-inflammatory, $C_{25}H_{30}FNO_6$.

flubendazole (floo-ben′dah-zōl) chemical name: [5-(4-fluoro-benzoyl)-1H-benzimidazol-2-yl]carbamic acid methyl ester; an antiprotozoal, $C_{16}H_{12}FN_3O_3$.

flucindole (floo-sin′dōl) chemical name: 6,8-difluoro-2,3,4,9-tetrahydro-N,N-dimethyl-1H-carbazol-3-amine; a tranquilizer, $C_{14}H_{16}F_2N_2$.

flucloronide (floo-klor′o-nīd) chemical name: 9,11β-dichloro-6α-fluoro-21-hydroxy-16α,17-[(1-methylethylidene)bis(oxy)]-pregna-1,4-diene-3,20-dione. A synthetic glucocorticoid, $C_{24}H_{29}Cl_2FO_5$, used in the treatment of steroid-responsive dermatoses.

flucloxacillin (floo″kloks-ah-sil′in) floxacillin.

Flucort (floo′kort) trademark for a preparation of flumethasone.

flucrylate (floo′krĭ-lāt) chemical name: 2,2,2-trifluoro-1-methylethyl 2-cyanoacrylate; a tissue adhesive, $C_7H_6F_3NO_2$.

fluctuant (fluk′tu-ant) 1. showing varying levels. 2. conveying the sensation of or exhibiting wavelike motion on palpation, owing to a liquid content.

fluctuation (fluk″tu-a′shun) [L. *fluctuatio*] 1. a variation, as about a fixed value or mass. 2. a wavelike motion, as of a fluid in a cavity of the body after succussion.

flucytosine (flu-si′to-sēn″) [USP] chemical name: 5-fluorocytosine. An antifungal, $C_4H_4FN_3O$, occurring as a white to off-white, crystalline powder; used in the treatment of serious infections, such as septicemia, endocarditis, and urinary tract infections, due to *Candida* and/or *Cryptococcus* species, administered orally.

fludalanine (floo-dal′ah-nēn) chemical name: 3-fluoro-d-alanine-2-d; an antibacterial, $C_3H_5DFNO_2$.

fludazonium chloride (floo″dah-zo′ne-um) chemical name: 1-[2-(2,4-dichlorophenyl)-2-[(2,4-dichlorophenyl)methoxy]ethyl]-3-[2-(4-fluorophenyl)-2-oxoethyl]-1H-imidazolium chloride; a topical anti-infective, $C_{26}H_{20}Cl_5FN_2O_2$.

fludorex (floo′do-reks) chemical name: β-methoxy-N-methyl-m-(trifluoromethyl)phenethylamine; an anorexic and antiemetic, $C_{11}H_{14}F_3NO$.

fludrocortisone acetate (floo″dro-kor′tĭ-sōn) [USP] chemical name: 21-(acetyloxy)-9α-fluoro-11β17α-dihydroxy-pregn-4-ene-3,20-dione. A synthetic corticosteroid with significant mineralocorticoid and glucocorticoid activity, $C_{23}H_{31}FO_6$, occurring as white to pale yellow crystals or crystalline powder; used mainly in replacement therapy of the mineralocorticoid in Addison's deficiency disease and in salt-losing adrenogenital syndrome; administered orally. Called also *fluohydrisone* and *fluohydrocortisone*.

flufenisal (floo-fen′ĭ-sal) chemical name: 4′-fluoro-4-hydroxy-3-biphenylcarboxylic acid acetate; an analgesic, $C_{15}H_{11}FO_4$.

flügelplatte (fle″gel-plah′teh) [Ger.] lamina alaris.

Fluhmann's test (floo′manz) [C. Frederic *Fluhmann*, American gynecologist, born 1898] see under *tests*.

fluid (floo′id) [L. *fluidus*] 1. a liquid or a gas. 2. composed of elements or particles which freely change their relative positions without their separating. See also *liquid, liquor*, and *solution*. **allantoic f.,** the fluid contained in the allantois. **Altmann's f.,** a histologic fixing fluid composed of equal parts of 2 per cent osmic acid solution and a 5 per cent potassium dichromate solution. **amniotic f.,** fluid within the amniotic cavity produced by the amnion at the very earliest period of fetation and later by lungs and kidneys; at first crystal clear, it later becomes cloudy. The amount at term normally varies from 500 to 2000 ml. Called also *aqua* or *liquor amnii*, and, popularly, *waters*. **ascitic f.,** the serous fluid which accumulates in the peritoneal cavity in ascites. **Bamberger's f.,** an albuminous mercuric solution for use in the treatment of syphilis. **bleaching f.,** a fluid prepared by passing chlorine gas into an emulsion of calcium hydrate. **Bouin's f.,** a histologic fixing fluid consisting of formaldhyde solution, glacial acetic acid, and saturated solution of trinitrophenol (picric acid). **Burnett's disinfecting f.,** a strong aqueous solution of zinc chloride. **Callison's f.,** a solution of distilled water, Löffler's aniline methylene blue, solution of formaldehyde, glycerin, ammonium oxalate, and sodium chloride; used as a diluent in counting red blood corpuscles. **Carrel-Dakin f.,** diluted sodium hypochlorite solution. **cerebrospinal f. (C.S.F.),** the fluid contained within the four ventricles of the brain, the subarachnoid space, and the central canal of the spinal cord; it is formed by the choroid plexus and brain parenchyma, is circulated through the ventricles into the subarachnoid space, and is absorbed into the venous system. Called also *liquor cerebrospinalis* [NA]. **chlorpalladium f.,** a decalcifying fluid for anatomical and other specimens, containing palladium chloride and hydrochloric acid; called also *Waldeyer's f.* **Coley's f.,** see under *toxin*. **Condy's f.,** a disinfecting solution of sodium and potassium permanganates. **Dakin's f.,** a buffered aqueous solution of sodium hypochlorite used as a bactericide; see *sodium hypochlorite solution*, under *solution*, and *Carrel-Dakin treatment*, under *treatment*. **decalcifying f.,** a solution of formic acid and formalin. **Delafield's f.,** a fixing fluid for delicate histologic tissues, containing osmic acid, chromic acid, acetic acid, and alcohol. **Ecker's f.,** Rees and Ecker diluting f. **extracellular f.,** a general term for all the body fluids outside the cells, including the interstitial fluid, plasma, lymph, cerebrospinal fluid, etc. Extracellular fluid consists of ultrafiltrates of the blood plasma and transcellular fluid, i.e., fluid produced by active cellular secretion. It provides a constant external environment for the cells. **Flemming's fixing f.,** Flemming's solution. **follicular f.,** liquor folliculi. **formol-Müller f.,** Müller's fluid to which formaldehyde has been added. **Gauvain's f.,** a mixture of guaiacol, iodoform, ether, and sterile olive oil; formerly for lavage in empyema. **Helly's f.,** a histologic fixative consisting of Zenker's fluid in which the glacial acetic acid is replaced by formalin; the most widely used formula consists of 9 parts Zenker stock solution and 1 part neutral formalin (Zenker-Helly-Maximow) and is usually called *Zenker-formol fixative.* **interstitial f.,** the extracellular fluid that bathes the cells of most tissues but which is not within the confines of the blood or lymph vessels and is not a transcellular fluid; it is formed by filtration through the blood capillaries and is drained away as lymph. It is the extracellular fluid volume minus the lymph volume, the plasma volume, and the transcellular fluid volume. **intracellular f.,** the portion of the total body water with its dissolved solutes which are within the cell membranes. **Kaiserling's f.,** see under *solution.* **labyrinthine f.,** perilymph. **Lang's f.,** a hardening fluid containing corrosive mercuric chloride, sodium chloride, and acetic acid, in water. **Locke's f.,** see under *solution.* **Mitchell's f.,** a mixture of sodium chloride, bromine, hydrochloric acid, and water acted on by an electric current; formerly advocated for treatment of pulmonary tuberculosis. **Morton's f.,** a mixture of iodine, potassium iodide, and glycerin; formerly used by injection in spinal meningocele. **Müller's f.,** a hardening solution consisting of potassium dichromate, sodium sulfate, and water. **Parker's f.,** a hardening fluid composed of formaldehyde and alcohol. **Pasteur's f.,** see under *solution.* **pericardial f.,** liquor pericardii. **Piazza's f.,** a blood-coagulating fluid composed of sodium chloride and ferric chloride in water. **Pitfield's f.,** a diluting fluid for counting leukocytes, made by dissolving acacia gum in distilled water and adding glacial acetic acid and gentian violet. **Rees and Ecker diluting f.,** a solution of sodium citrate, formaldehyde solution, brilliant cresyl blue, and distilled water, used as a diluting fluid for blood platelets. **Scarpa's f.,** endolymph (of the ear). **Schaudinn's f.,** a hardening fluid consisting of mercury bichloride, alcohol, and distilled water. **seminal f.,** semen, def. 2. **serous f.,** normal lymph of a serous cavity. **synovial f.,** synovia. **Tellyesniczky's f.,** a fixing solution consisting of potassium dichromate, water, and glacial acetic acid. **Thoma's f.,** a decalcifying fluid for histologic work, consisting of alcohol and pure nitric acid. **tissue f.,** interstitial f. **Toison's f.,** see under *solution.* **transcellular f.,** that portion of the extracellular fluid produced by active cellular secretion. **ventricular f.,** that portion of the cerebrospinal fluid contained in the cerebral ventricles. **von Behring's f.,** tulase. **Waldeyer's f.,** chlorpalladium f. **Wickersheimer's f.,** a fluid composed of arsenic trioxide, sodium chloride, and the sulfate, carbonate, and nitrate of potassium in a mixture of water, alcohol, and glycerin; used for preserving anatomical specimens. **Zenker's f.,** see under *fixative.*

fluidextract (floo″id-ek′strakt) a liquid preparation of a vegetable drug containing alcohol as a solvent or as a preservative, or both, of such strength that each milliliter contains the extraction of 1 gm. of the standard drug which it represents. The official preparations are *aromatic cascara f.* [USP], *cascara sagrada f.* [USP], *glycyrrhiza f.* [NF], and *senna f.* [USP], all of which are used as cathartics, and *eriodictyon f.* [NF], used as a flavoring agent for pharmaceutical preparations.

fluidextractum (floo″id-eks-trak′tum), gen. *fluidextrac′ti,* pl. *fluidextrac′ta* [L.] fluidextract.

fluidism (floo′id-izm) humoralism.

fluidounce (floo-id-ouns′) fluid ounce; see under *ounce.*

fluidrachm (floo″id-ram′) fluid dram; see under *dram.*

fluidram (floo″id-ram′) fluid dram; see under *dram.*

Flu-Imune (floo″ĭ-mūn′) trademark for a preparation of influenza virus vaccine.

fluke (flook) any trematode worm; see *Trematoda.* **blood f.,** *Schistosoma.* **intestinal f's,** see *Echinostoma, Fasciolopsis, Gastrodiscoides, Heterophyes, Metagonimus,* and *Watsonius.* **liver f's,** see *Clonorchis, Dicrocoelium, Fasciola,* and *Opisthorchis.* **lung f.,** see *Paragonimus.*

flumen (floo′men), pl. *flu′mina* [L.] a stream. **flu′mina pilo′rum** [NA], hair streams: continuous lines formed by the pattern of hair growth on various parts of the body, the hairs lying in the same direction.

flumequine (floo′mĕ-kwin) chemical name: 9-fluoro-6,7-dihydro-5-methyl-1-oxo-1*H*,5*H*-benzo[*ij*]quinolizine-2-carboxylic acid; an antibacterial, $C_{14}H_{12}FNO_3$.

flumethasone pivalate (floo-meth′ah-sōn) [USP] chemical name: 21-(2,2-dimethyl-1-oxopropoxy)-6α,9-difluoro-6,9-difluoro-11β,17-dihydroxy-16α-methylpregna-1,4-diene-3,20-dione. A synthetic glucocorticoid, $C_{27}H_{36}F_2O_6$, occurring as a white to off-white, crystalline powder; used as a topical anti-inflammatory in steroid-responsive dermatoses.

flumethiazide (floo″mĕ-thi′ah-zīd) chemical name: 6-trifluoromethyl-2*H*-1,2,4-benzothiadiazine-7-sulfonamide-1,1-dioxide; a thiazide diuretic, $C_8H_6F_3N_3O_4S_2$.

flumina (floo′mĭ-nah) [L.] plural of *flumen.*

flumizole (floo′mĭ-zōl) chemical name: 4,5-bis(4-methoxyphenyl)-2-(trifluoromethyl)-1*H*-imidazole; an anti-inflammatory, $C_{18}H_{15}F_3N_2O_2$.

flumoxonide (floo-mok′so-nīd) chemical name: 6α,9-difluoro-11β-hydroxy-21,21-dimethoxy-16α,17-[(1-methylethylidene)bis-

(oxy)]pregna-1,4-diene-3,20-dione; an adrenocortical steroid, $C_{26}H_{34}F_2O_7$.

flunarizine hydrochloride (floo-nar′ĭ-zēn) chemical name: (*E*)-1-[bis-(*p*-fluorophenyl)methyl]-4-cinnamylpiperazine dihydrochloride; a vasodilator, $C_{26}H_{26}F_2N_2 \cdot 2HCl$.

flunidazole (floo-ni′dah-zōl) chemical name: 2-(*p*-fluorophenyl)-5-nitroimidazole; an antiprotozoal agent, $C_{11}H_{10}FN_3O_3$.

flunisolide (floo-nis′o-līd) chemical name: 6α-fluoro-11β,21-dihydroxy-16α,17-[(1-methylethylidene)bis(oxy)]pregna-1,4-diene-3,20-dione; a glucocorticoid, $C_{24}H_{31}FO_6$. **f. acetate,** the 21-acetate ester of flunisolide, $C_{26}H_{33}FO_7$; an anti-inflammatory.

flunitrazepam (floo″ni-trāz′ĕ-pam) chemical name: 5-(2-fluorophenyl)-1,3-dihydro-1-methyl-7-nitro-2*H*-1,4-benzodiazepin-2-one; a hypnotic and induction agent in anesthesia, $C_{16}H_{12}FN_3O_3$.

flunixin (floo-nik′sin) chemical name: 2-[[2-methyl-3-(trifluoromethyl)phenyl]amino]-3-pyridinecarboxylic acid; an anti-inflammatory and analgesic, $C_{14}H_{11}F_3N_2O_2$. **f. meglumine,** the meglumine salt of flunixin, $C_{14}H_{11}F_3N_2O_2 \cdot C_7H_{17}NO_5$; an anti-inflammatory and analgesic.

fluocinolone acetonide (floo″o-sin′o-lon) [USP] chemical name: 6α,9-difluoro-11β,21-dihydroxy-16α,17-[(1-methylethylidene)bis(oxy)]pregna-1,4-diene,3,20-dione. A synthetic glucocorticoid, $C_{24}H_{30}F_2O_6$, occurring as a white or practically white, crystalline powder; used as a topical anti-inflammatory in steroid-responsive dermatoses.

fluocinonide (floo″o-sin′o-nīd) [USP] The 21-acetate ester of fluocinolone acetonide, occurring as a white to cream-colored, crystalline powder, which has anti-inflammatory, antipruritic, and vasoconstrictive properties; used topically in the treatment of certain dermatoses.

fluocortin butyl (floo″o-kor′tin) chemical name: 6α-fluoro-11β-hydroxy-16α-methyl-3,20-dioxopregna-1,4-dien-21-oic acid butyl ester; an anti-inflammatory, $C_{26}H_{35}FO_5$.

Fluogen (floo′o-jen) trademark for a preparation of influenza virus vaccine.

fluohydrisone (floo″o-hi′drĭ-sōn) fludrocortisone.

fluohydrocortisone (floo″o-hi″dro-kor′ti-sōn) fludrocortisone.

Fluonid (floo′o-nid) trademark for preparations of fluocinolone acetonide.

fluor (floo′or) [L. a "flux"] a discharge. **f. al′bus,** leukorrhea.

fluorane (floo′or-ān) the parent compound of fluorescein and related dyes; 9-hydroxy-9-xanthene-*o*-benzoic acid lactone.

fluorescein (floo″o-res′e-in) chemical name: resorcinolphthalein. The simplest of the fluorane dyes and the parent compound of eosin; used intravenously in tests to assess by its fluorescence the adequacy of the circulation, and combined with radioactive iodine in localization of brain tumors, etc. Called also *dihydroxyfluorane.* **f. isocyanate,** a form capable of being conjugated to protein and hence used as a label in fluorescent antibody staining procedures. **sodium f.** [USP], **soluble f.,** chemical name: resorcinolphthalein sodium. An odorless, water-soluble, orange-red powder, $C_{20}H_{10}Na_2O_5$, used in dilute solution to reveal corneal lesions and as a test of circulation in the extremities and retina. Called also *uranin.*

fluoresceinuria (floo″o-res″e-in-u′re-ah) the presence of fluorescein in the urine.

fluorescence (floo″o-res′ens) [first observed in *fluor spar*] the property of emitting light while exposed to light, the wavelength of the emitted light being only slightly longer than that of the light absorbed. Cf. *phosphorescence.* **secondary f.** fluorescence in tissues which is induced by staining with fluorescent dyes (*fluorochromes*). Cf. *autofluorescence.*

fluorescent (floo″o-res′ent) exhibiting fluorescence.

fluorescin (floo″o-res′in) a reduced form of fluorescein used to detect oxidative activity. As the sodium salt, it may be used for the same purposes as sodium fluorescein.

fluoridation (floo″or-ĭ-da′shun) treatment with fluorides; specifically, the addition of fluoride to the public water supply as part of the public health program to prevent or reduce the incidence of dental caries.

fluoride (floo′o-rīd) a binary compound of fluorine (q.v.). **stannous f.** [NF], a compound, SnF_2, containing not less than 71.2 per cent stannous tin and between 22.3 and 25.5 per cent fluoride; applied topically to the teeth as a dental caries prophylactic.

fluoridization (floo″or-ĭ-di-za′shun) 1. application of fluoride solution to the teeth. 2. fluoridation.

fluoridize (floo-or′ĭ-dīz) 1. to apply a solution of fluoride to the teeth as a means of controlling or preventing caries. 2. to add fluorides to a substance.

fluorimeter (floo″o-rim′ĕ-ter) fluorometer.

fluorimetry (floo″o-rim′ĕ-tre) fluorometry.

fluorine (floo′ŏ-rēn) [from *fluor spar,* from which it is derived] a nonmetallic, gaseous element, belonging to the halogen group; symbol, F; atomic number, 9; atomic weight, 18.998. Fluorine, in the form of fluoride, is incorporated into the structure of bone and teeth and provides protection against dental caries; an excess of fluorine may result in fluorosis.

fluoroacetate (floo″or-o-ah′sě-tāt) a salt of fluoroacetic acid (see under *acid*).

fluorochrome (floo′or-o-krōm) a fluorescent compound, as a dye, used to mark protein with a fluorescent label.

fluorocyte (floo′or-o-sīt) a reticulocyte showing red fluorescence.

fluorography (floo″or-og′rah-fe) photofluorography.

Fluoromar (floor′o-mar) trademark for a preparation of fluroxene.

fluorometer (floo″or-om′ě-ter) 1. an apparatus for measuring the quantity of rays given out by a roentgen-ray tube. 2. an attachment to the fluoroscope, enabling the operator to secure a correct and undistorted shadow of the object and to locate exactly the position of the object. 3. the instrument used in fluorometry, consisting of an energy source (e.g., a mercury arc lamp or xenon lamp) to induce fluorescence, monochromators for selection of the wavelength, and a detector; called also *fluorimeter*.

fluorometholone (floor″o-meth′o-lōn) [USP] chemical name: 9-fluoro-11β,17-dihydroxy-6α-(methylpregna-1,4-diene-3,20-dione. A synthetic glucocorticoid, $C_{22}H_{29}FO_4$, occurring as a white to yellowish white, crystalline powder; used as a topical anti-inflammatory in steroid-responsive dermatoses.

fluorometry (floo″o-rom′ě-tre) an analytical technique for identifying minute amounts of a substance by detection and measurement of the characteristic wavelength of the light it emits during fluorescence. Called also *fluorimetry*.

fluoronephelometer (floo″o-ro-nef″ě-lom′ě-ter) an instrument for analysis of a solution by measuring the light scattered or emitted by it. Called also *nefluorophotometer*.

***p*-fluorophenylalanine** (floo″o-ro-fen″il-al′ĭ-nīn) a modified molecule of phenylalanine that binds to enzymes but is incapable of performing the functions of the natural molecule and thus acts as an antagonist.

fluorophosphate (floo″or-o-fos′fāt) an organic compound containing fluorine and phosphorus. **diisopropyl f.,** isofluorophate.

fluorophotometry (floo″o-ro-fo-tom′ě-tre) the measurement of light given off by fluorescent substances. **vitreous f.,** the measurement of light given off by intravenously injected fluorescein that has leaked through the retinal vessels into the vitreous; done to detect the breakdown of the blood-retinal barrier, an early ocular change in diabetes mellitus.

Fluoroplex (floo′oro-pleks) trademark for a preparation of fluorouracil.

fluororoentgenography (floo″o-ro-rent″gen-og′rah-fe) photofluorography.

fluoroscope (floo′ŏ-ro-skōp) [*fluorescence* + Gr. *skopein* to examine] a device used for examining deep structures by means of roentgen rays; it consists of a screen (*fluorescent screen*) covered with crystals of calcium tungstate on which are projected the shadows of x-rays passing through the body placed between the screen and the source of irradiation. **biplane f.,** a fluoroscope by which examinations can be made in two planes, horizontal and vertical.

fluoroscopical (floo″o-ro-skop′ĭ-kal) pertaining to fluoroscopy.

fluoroscopy (floo″or-os′ko-pe) examination by means of the fluoroscope.

fluorosilicate (floo″o-ro-sil′ĭ-kāt) a compound of silicon and some other base with fluorine, such as sodium silicofluoride; fluorosilicates are sometimes used as insecticides, and are very toxic when ingested. Called also *silicofluoride*.

fluorosis (floo″o-ro′sis) a condition due to exposure to excessive amounts of fluorine or its compounds. Fluoride intoxication may occur as a result of such factors as accidental ingestion of fluoride-containing insecticides and rodenticides, chronic inhalation of industrial dusts or gases containing fluorides, or prolonged ingestion of water containing large amounts of fluorides; it is characterized by skeletal changes, consisting of combined osteosclerosis and osteomalacia (osteofluorosis) and by mottled enamel of the teeth when exposure occurs during enamel formation (see *dental f.*). A similar condition is seen in cattle, sheep, and other livestock, and is due to the same factors that cause intoxication in humans and also to ingestion of animal feed containing toxic levels of fluorides and grazing on pastures contaminated with fluorides in industrial dusts or gases. Called also *chronic endemic f.* and *chronic fluoride*, or *fluorine, poisoning*. **dental f.,** a form of enamel hypoplasia, largely of the permanent teeth, resulting from ingestion of excessive amounts of fluoride in the natural water supply used for drinking and for food preparation during the period of enamel calcification; it is manifested by a mottled discoloration of the tooth enamel, the affected teeth having a dull, chalky white appearance on eruption and later, in areas with higher fluoride concentration, may show a brown stain. Called also *mottled enamel.* **endemic f., chronic,** fluorosis.

fluorouracil (floo″o-ur′ah-sil) [USP] chemical name: 5-fluoro-2,4(1*H*,3*H*)-pyrimidinedione. A pyrimidine analogue that acts as

an antimetabolite to uracil, $C_4H_3FN_2O_2$, occurring as a white to practically white, crystalline powder; used as an antineoplastic in the palliative management of carcinoma of the gastrointestinal tract, breast, and pancreas, administered intravenously. Also used topically in the treatment of actinic keratoses.

Fluothane (floo′o-thān) trademark for a preparation of halothane.

fluotracen hydrochloride (floo″o-tra′sen) chemical name: *cis*-(±)-9,10-dihydro-*N,N*,10-trimethyl-2-(trifluoromethyl)-9-anthracenepropanamine hydrochloride; a tranquilizer and antidepressant, $C_{21}H_{24}F_3N \cdot HCl$.

fluoxetine (floo-ok′sě-tēn) chemical name: (±)-*N*-methyl-γ-[4-(trifluoromethyl)phenoxy]benzenepropanamine; an antidepressant, $C_{17}H_{18}F_3NO$.

fluoxymesterone (floo-ok″se-mes′ter-ōn) [USP] chemical name: 9-fluoro-11β,17β-dihydroxy-17-methylandrost-4-en-3-one. An androgen, $C_{20}H_{29}FO_3$, occurring as a white or practically white, crystalline powder; used in the treatment of male hypogonadism and in the palliative therapy of inoperable female breast cancer in selected patients, administered orally.

fluperamide (floo-per′ah-mīd) chemical name: 4-[4-chloro-3-(trifluoromethyl)phenyl]-4-hydroxy-*N,N*-dimethyl-α,α-diphenyl-1-piperidinebutamide; an antiperistaltic, $C_{30}H_{32}ClF_3N_2O_2$.

fluphenazine (floo-fen′ah-zēn) chemical name: 4-[3-[2-(trifluoromethyl)-10*H*-phenothiazin-10-yl]-propyl]-1-piperazineethanol. The 2-trifluoromethyl derivative of perphenazine, $C_{22}H_{26}F_3N_3OS$, the most potent of the phenothiazine tranquilizers. **f. enanthate** [USP], the enanthate ester of fluphenazine, $C_{22}H_{38}F_3N_3O_2S$, occurring as pale yellow to yellow-orange, clear to slightly turbid, viscous liquid, having the same uses as those of the hydrochloride salt, but of longer duration; administered intramuscularly and subcutaneously. **f. hydrochloride** [USP], the dihydrochloride salt of fluphenazine, $C_{22}H_{26}F_3N_3OS \cdot 2HCl$, occurring as a white or nearly white, crystalline powder; used as a tranquilizer in the treatment of manifestations of psychotic disorders, and as an antiemetic, administered orally and intramuscularly.

fluprednisolone (floo″pred-nis′o-lōn) chemical name: 6α-fluoro-11β,17,21-trihydroxypregna-1,4-diene-3,20-dione. A synthetic glucocorticoid, $C_{21}H_{27}FO_5$, occurring as a white to off-white, crystalline powder; used in the treatment of various conditions responsive to the anti-inflammatory actions of glucocorticoids, administered orally. **f. valerate,** an ester of fluprednisolone, $C_{26}H_{35}FO_6$, with actions similar to those of the base.

fluprostenol sodium (floo-pros′tě-nōl) chemical name: [1α-(*Z*),2β(1*E*,3*R**),3α,5α]-7-[3,5-dihydroxy-2-[3-hydroxy-4-[3-(trifluoromethyl)phenoxy]-1-butenyl]cyclopentyl]-5-heptenoic acid sodium salt; a prostaglandin of the F series, $C_{23}H_{28}F_3NaO_6$, used in the treatment of infertility.

fluquazone (floo′kwah-zōn) chemical name: 6-chloro-4-phenyl-1-(2,2,2-trifluoroethyl)-2(1*H*)-quinazolinone; an anti-inflammatory, $C_{16}H_{10}ClF_3N_2O$.

flurandrenolide (floor″an-dren′o-līd) [USP] chemical name: 6α-fluoro-11β,21-dihydroxy-16α,17-[(1-methylethylidine)bis(oxy)]-pregn-4-ene-3,20-dione. A glucocorticoid, $C_{24}H_{33}FO_6$, occurring as a white to off-white, fluffy, crystalline powder; used as an anti-inflammatory in the treatment of steroid-responsive dermatoses, applied topically. Called also *flurandrenolone*.

flurandrenolone (floor″an-dren′o-lōn) flurandrenolide.

flurazepam hydrochloride (floor-az′ě-pam) [USP] chemical name: 7-chloro-1-[2-(diethylamino)ethyl]-5-(2-fluorophenyl)-1,3-dihydro-2*H*-1,4-benzodiazepin-2-one dihydrochloride. A hypnotic, $C_{21}H_{23}ClFN_3O \cdot 2HCl$, occurring as an off-white to yellow, crystalline powder; administered orally.

flurbiprofen (floor-bip′-ro-fen) chemical name: (±)-2-fluoro-α-methyl-[1,1′-biphenyl]-4-acetic acid; an anti-inflammatory, $C_{15}H_{13}FO_2$, also having analgesic and antipyretic actions; used in the treatment of rheumatoid arthritis, osteoarthritis, and spondylitis.

Flurobate (floor′o-bāt) trademark for preparations of betamethasone benzoate.

flurocitabine (floo″ro-si′tah-bēn) chemical name: (2*R*-(2α,3β,-3aβ,9aβ)]-7-fluoro-2,3,3a,9a-tetrahydro-3-hydroxy-6-imino-6*H*-furo [2′,3′;4,5] oxazolo (3,2-*a*) pyrimidine-2-methanol; an antineoplastic, $C_9H_{10}FN_3O_4$.

flurogestone acetate (floor″o-jes′tōn) chemical name: 9-fluoro-11β,17-dihydroxypregn-4-ene-3,20-dione 17-acetate; a progestin, $C_{23}H_{31}FO_5$.

flurothyl (floor′o-thil) [USP] chemical name: 1,1′-oxybis[2,2,2-trifluoroethane]. A central stimulant, $C_4H_4F_6O$, occurring as a clear, colorless, volatile liquid; used as a convulsant in psychiatric disorders for which electroconvulsive therapy is usually employed, administered by inhalation.

fluroxene (floor-oks′ēn) chemical name: (2,2,2-trifluoroethoxy)ethene. A general anesthetic, $C_4H_5F_3O$, occurring as a clear, practically colorless, volatile liquid; administered by inhalation.

flush (flush) transient redness of the face and neck. See also *plethora*. **atropine f.,** flushing and dryness of the skin of the face and neck from overdosage with atropine. **breast f.,** a condition sometimes occurring in the early puerperium consisting of a tense and flushed state of the breasts with prominent veins. **carcinoid f.,** extensive blotchy red or bluish flushing on the face or trunk, often associated with diarrhea and abdominal pain and sometimes bronchospasm; it is possibly due to vasoactive kinins or other peptides associated with carcinoid tumor. **hectic f.,** a persistent or chronic flush associated with chronic debilitating disease, usually febrile, such as pulmonary tuberculosis. **histamine f.,** sudden symmetric erythema of the face and upper trunk, usually associated with throbbing headache and bounding pulse, and histaminuria; seen in urticaria pigmentosa, it may also occur a few minutes after eating fish of the scombroid family (red snapper or mahimahi) contaminated by *Proteus* during cold storage prior to cooking. **mahogany f.,** a deep red or mahogany-colored, circumscribed spot seen on one cheek in some cases of lobar pneumonia. **malar f.,** hectic flush at the malar eminence.

fluspiperone (floo-spip′er-ōn) chemical name: 1-(4-fluorophenyl)-8-[4-(4-fluorophenyl)-4-oxobutyl]-1,3,8-triazaspiro[4.5]decan-4-one; a tranquilizer, $C_{23}H_{25}F_2N_3O_2$.

fluspirilene (floo-spēr′ĭ-lēn) chemical name: 8-[4,4-bis(*p*-fluorophenyl)butyl]-1-phenyl-1,3,8-triazaspiro-[4.5]decan-4-one; a tranquilizer, $C_{29}H_{31}F_2N_3O$.

flutamide (floo′tah-mīd) chemical name: 2-methyl-*N*-[4-nitro-3-(trifluormethyl)phenyl]propanamide. A nonsteroidal antiandrogen, $C_{11}H_{11}F_3N_2O_3$; used to increase the flow of urine in benign hypertrophy of the prostate.

flutiazin (floo-ti′ah-zin) chemical name: 8-(trifluoromethyl)-phenothiazine 1-carboxylic acid; an anti- inflammatory agent for veterinary use, $C_{14}H_8F_3NO_2S$.

flutter (flut′er) a rapid vibration or pulsation. **atrial f.,** a condition of cardiac arrhythmia in which the atrial contractions are rapid (200 to 320 per minute), but regular. In many instances, a circus pathway is probably present. The ventricles are unable to respond to each atrial impulse, so that a partial block usually is present. Formerly called *auricular f.* **auricular f.,** atrial f. **diaphragmatic f.,** peculiar, wavelike fibrillations of the diagram of unknown cause; the condition may be paroxysmal or persist indefinitely. **impure f.,** atrial flutter in which the atrial rhythm is irregular. **mediastinal f.,** a condition of abnormal motility of the mediastinum during respiratory movements. **pure f.,** atrial flutter in which the atrial rhythm is regular. **ventricular f.,** a possible transition stage between ventricular tachycardia and ventricular fibrillation, the electrocardiogram showing rapid, uniform, and virtually regular oscillations, 250 or more per minute.

flutter-fibrillation (flut′er-fi-brĭ-la′shun) impure flutters that vary from moment to moment in their resemblance to flutter or fibrillation, respectively.

flux (fluks) [L. *fluxus*] 1. an excessive flow or discharge. 2. a borax-containing substance that maintains the cleanliness of metals to be united and facilitates the easy flow and attachment of solder. **bloody f.,** see *dysentery*. **celiac f.,** diarrhea accompanied by the discharge of undigested food. **hepatic f.,** bilious f. **ionic f.,** the number of mols per second passing through an area of 1 cm. oriented perpendicularly to the direction of flow of the substance. **luminous f.,** the rate of passage of radiant energy evaluated by reference to the luminous sensation produced by it. **menstrual f.,** the menses. **neutral f.,** a fusible material, usually an inorganic salt, which does not unite with the combined oxygen in the metal but merely dissolves the metal oxide (barium chloride, sodium chloride). **oxidizing f.,** a material which, when heated, gives up oxygen that may unite with base metals and form oxides (as potassium nitrate, potassium chlorate). **reducing f.,** a flux which unites with the oxygen of metallic oxides and frees the metal from such combinations.

fluxion (fluk′shun) a flowing; especially an abnormal or excessive flow of fluid to a part.

fly (fli) a dipterous, or two-winged, insect. Called also *musca*. **black f.,** a name given various individuals of the family Simuliidae. **blackbottle f.,** see *Phormia*. **bloodsucking f's,** see *Chrysops* and *Tabanus*. **blow f., bluebottle f.,** see *Calliphora*. **bot f.,** see *botfly*. **caddis f.,** a fly of the order Trichoptera; hairs and scales from these flies are a cause of allergic symptoms in susceptible persons. **cheese f.,** see *Piophila*. **deer f.,** *Chrysops discalis*. **drone f.,** *Eristalis tenax*. **dung f.,** *Sepsis violacea*. **eye f.,** any fly which attacks the eye; see *Hippelates* and *Siphunculina funicola*. **face f.,** *Musca autumnalis*. **filth f.,** *Musca domestica*. **flesh f.,** see *Sarcophaga* and *Wohlfahrtia*. **fruit f.,** see *Drosophila*. **gad f.,** see *Tabanus*. **gold f.,** *Lucilia caesar*. **green-bottle f.,** see *Lucilia* and *Phaenicia*. **heel f.,** see *Hypoderma*. **horn f.,** see *Haematobia*. **horse f.,** see *Tabanus*. **house f.,** *Musca domestica*. **hover f's,** flies, such as *Helophilus* and *Eristalis*, of the family Syrphidae. **lake f.,** see *Hexagenia bilineata*. **latrine f.,** *Fannia scalaris*. **mango f., mangrove f.,** *Chrysops dimidiata*. **moth f.,** a fly of the family Psychodidae. **motuca f.,** *Lepidoselaga lepidota*. **nose f., nostril f.,** *Oestrus ovis*. **owl f.,** a name given individuals of the family Psychodidae. **oxwarble f.,** see *Hypoderma*. **phlebotomus f.,** see *Phlebotomus*. **Russian f.,** *Lytta*. **sand f.,** see *sandfly*. **screwworm f.,** *Cochliomyia hominivorax*. **Seroot f.,** *Tabanus gra-*

tus. **snipe f.,** see *Rhagionidae*. **soldier f.,** *Hermetia illucens*, the larvae of which sometimes cause intestinal myiasis in man. **Spanish f.,** *Lytta vesicatoria*. **stable f.,** *Stomoxys calcitrans*. **tick f.,** see *Hippobosca*. **tsetse f.,** see *Glossina*. **tumbu f.,** *Cordylobia anthropophaga*. **typhoid f.** (*obs.*), *Musca domestica*. **vinegar f.,** see *Drosophila*. **warble f.,** see *Hypoderma*.

Fm chemical symbol for *fermium*.

F.M. abbreviation for L. *fi′at mistu′ra*, make a mixture.

FMN flavin mononucleotide.

focal (fo′kal) pertaining to or occupying a focus.

Fochier's abscess (fosh″e-āz′) [Alphonse *Fochier*, French gynecologist, 1845–1903] see *fixation abscess*, under *abscess*.

foci (fo′si) [L.] plural of *focus*.

focil, focile (fo′sil, fo′sĭ-le) [L. *fusillus*, a little spindle] one of the bones of the forearm or leg.

focimeter (fo-sim′ĕ-ter) an apparatus for finding the focus of a lens.

focus (fo′kus) pl. *fo′ci* [L. "fire-place"] 1. the point of convergence of light rays or of the waves of sound. 2. the chief center of a morbid process. **aplanatic f.,** that focus or point from which diverging rays pass the lens without spherical aberration. **Assmann f.,** the early exudative lesion of pulmonary tuberculosis, occurring most frequently in the subapical region; called also *Assmann's tuberculous infiltrate*. **conjugate f.,** the point at which rays that come from some definite point are brought together. **epileptogenic f.,** the area of the cerebral cortex responsible for causing epileptic seizures, as revealed in the encephalogram. **Ghon f.,** the primary parenchymal lesion of primary pulmonary tuberculosis in children; when associated with a corresponding lymph node focus, it is known as the *primary*, or *Ghon, complex*. Called also *Ghon's primary lesion* and *Ghon tubercle*. **principal foci,** points of convergence of rays parallel with the principal axis of a lens, or system: in the *eye*, (approx.) 18 mm. from the anterior nodal point, and 24 mm. from the posterior nodal point, and holding the ratio of the indices of air and vitreum (Fording). **real f.,** the point at which convergent rays intersect. **Simon's foci,** hematogenous areas in the apices of the lungs of children regarded as precursors of apical tuberculosis in later life. **virtual f.,** the point at which divergent rays would intersect if prolonged backward.

focusing (fo′kus-ing) the act of converging at a point. **isoelectric f.,** electrophoresis in which the protein mixture is subjected to an electric field in a gel medium in which a pH gradient has been established; each protein then migrates until it reaches the site (or focus) at which the pH is equal to its isoelectric point. Called also *electrofocusing*.

foe- for words beginning thus, see those beginning *fe-*.

Foerster see *Förster*.

fog (fog) a colloid system in which the dispersion medium is a gas and the disperse particles are liquid, e.g., a cloudlike mass of water droplets dispersed in air.

fogging (fog′ing) in ophthalmology, a method employed in determining the refractive error, the patient being first made artificially myopic by means of plus spheres, in order to relax all accommodation before using cylinders.

fogo (fo′go) [Port. "fire"] a name given to a skin condition in Brazil. **f. selva′gem** [Port. "wild fire"], a chronic, potentially fatal dermatosis recognized only in Brazil, and resembling severe pemphigus foliaceus; called also *Brazilian, South American*, or *wildfire pemphigus*.

foil (foil) metal in the form of an extremely thin, pliable sheet. **gold f.,** pure gold rolled into an extremely thin sheet, used in the restoration of carious or fractured teeth. **platinum f.,** pure platinum rolled into an extremely thin sheet, used as a matrix for various soldering procedures, and also in the construction of porcelain restorations, to provide internal form during their fabrication. **tin f.,** tin rolled into an extremely thin sheet, used to separate other materials, as separating the cast and denture-base material while it is being flasked and cured.

Fol. abbreviation for L. *fo′lia*, leaves.

folacin (fōl′ah-sin) folic acid.

folate (fo′lāt) a salt of folic acid; a general term for a group of substances whose molecules are made up of a form of pteroic acid conjugated with L-glutamic acid. Folates act as coenzymes that promote one-carbon transfer. They are present in natural foods, including mammalian cells.

fold (fōld) a thin, recurved margin, or doubling; called also *plica*. **alar f's,** plicae alares. **amniotic f.,** the folded edge of the amniotic membrane where it rises over and finally encloses the embryo. **aryepiglottic f.,** plica aryepiglottica. **aryepiglottic f. of Collier,** plica triangularis. **axillary f's,** the folds of skin bounding the armpit, the plica axillaris anterior, and plica axillaris posterior. **Brachet's mesolateral f.,** mesolateral f. **bulboventricular f.,** a fold between the bulbus cordis and the ventricle that disappears as the bulbus cordis is absorbed into the right ventricle. **caval f.,** a ridge that contains the superior segment of the embryonic inferior vena cava.

cecal f's, plicae cecales. **cholecystoduodenocolic f.,** an occasionally present fold of peritoneum sometimes uniting the colon, duodenum, and gallbladder. **ciliary f's,** plicae ciliares. **circular f's, circular f's of Kerckring,** plicae circulares. **conjunctival f.,** the cul-de-sac formed where the conjunctiva is reflected from the eyeball to the upper or lower eyelid; called also *palpebral f.* and *retrotarsal f.* **costocolic f.,** ligamentum phrenicolicum. **Douglas' f.,** 1. plica rectouterina. 2. linea arcuata vaginae musculi recti abdominis. **Duncan's f's,** the loose folds of peritoneum which cover the uterus immediately following delivery. **duodenojejunal f.,** plica duodenalis superior. **duodenomesocolic f.,** plica duodenalis inferior. **epicanthal f., epicanthine f.,** epicanthus (plica palpebronasalis [NA]). **epigastric f.,** plica umbilicalis lateralis, def. 1. **falciform f. of fascia lata,** margo falciformis hiatus saphenus. **fimbriated f.,** plica fimbriata. **gastric f's,** plicae gastricae. **gastropancreatic f's,** plicae gastropancreaticae. **genital f.,** genital ridge. **glossoepiglottic f's,** folds of mucous membrane extending from the base of the tongue to the epiglottis. **gluteal f.,** the crease separating the buttock from the thigh. **Guérin's f.,** a fold of mucous membrane occasionally seen in the fossa navicularis of the urethra. **Hasner's f.,** plica lacrimalis. **head f.,** a crescentic, ventral fold of the blastoderm at the future head end of the embryo. **Heister's f.,** plica spiralis. **Hensing's f.,** see under *ligament.* **horizontal f's of rectum,** plicae transversalis recti. **ileocecal f.,** plica ileocecalis. **ileocolic f.,** a crescentic fold of peritoneum forming a part of the mesentery, mesocecum, and mesocolon. **incudal f.,** plica incudis. **inferior duodenal f.,** plica duodenalis inferior. **interarticular f. of hip,** ligamentum capitis femoris. **interureteric f.,** plica interureterica. **iridial f's,** plicae iridis. **Jonnesco's f., Juvara's f.,** parietoperitoneal f. **Kerckring's f's (of small intestine),** plicae circulares. **Kohlrausch's f's,** plicae tranversales recti. **lacrimal f.,** plica lacrimalis. **f's of large intestine,** plicae semilunares coli. **longitudinal f. of duodenum,** plica longitudinalis duodeni. **mallear f. of mucous membrane of tympanum, anterior,** plica mallearis anterior tunicae mucosae cavi tympani. **mallear f. of tympanic membrane, anterior,** plica mallearis anterior membranae tympani. **mallear f. of tympanic membrane, posterior,** plica mallearis posterior membranae tympani. **mammary f.,** the primordium of the mammary gland in the early embryo; it extends from the root of the upper extremity to the inguinal fold. **Marshall's f.,** plica venae cavae sinistrae. **medullary f.,** neural f. **mesolateral f.,** the right lamella of the primitive mesentery running to the right lobe of the liver; called also *Brachet's mesolateral f.* **mesonephric f.,** mesonephric ridge. **mesouterine f.,** a fold of peritoneum supporting the uterus. **mucobuccal f.,** the cul-de-sac formed where the mucous membrane is reflected from the upper or lower jaw to the cheek. **mucolabial f.,** the line of flexure of the oral mucous membrane as it passes from the mandible or maxilla to the lip. **mucosal f.,** plica mucosa. **mucosobuccal f.,** mucobuccal f. **mucous f.,** plica mucosa. **mucous f's of rectum,** columnae anales. **nail f.,** the fold of palmar skin around the base and sides of the nail. **nasopharyngeal f.,** plica salpingopalatina. **Nélaton's f.,** a transverse fold of mucous membrane in the rectum, marking the junction of its lower and middle thirds. **neural f.,** one of the paired folds, lying one on either side of the neural plate, that form the neural tube; called also *medullary f.* **opercular f.,** a fold of tissue constituting an adhesion between the tonsil and the anterior pillar of the fauces. **palatine f's, transverse,** plicae palatinae transversae. **palmate f's,** plicae palmatae. **palpebral f.,** conjunctival f. **palpebronasal f.,** epicanthus (plica palpebronasalis [NA]). **pancreaticogastric f's,** plicae gastropancreaticae. **paraduodenal f.,** plica paraduodenalis. **parietocolic f.,** Hensing's ligament. **parietoperitoneal f.,** a fold of peritoneum in the fetus, arising at the left side of the ascending colon and attached to the parietal peritoneum at the right of the ascending colon; called also *Jonnesco's f.* and *Juvara's f.* **pharyngoepiglottic f.,** a fold of mucous membrane running backward from the epiglottis. **pituitary f's** (*obs.*), diaphragma sellae. **primitive f.,** one of the two ridges flanking the primitive groove, one on either side. **proximal nail f.,** sulcus matricis unguis. **Rathke's f's,** two fetal folds of mesoderm which unite at the median line to form Douglas' septum and to render the rectum a complete canal. **rectal f's,** plicae transversales recti. **rectouterine f.,** plica rectouterina. **rectovaginal f.,** a fold of peritoneum interposed between the rectum and vagina. **rectovesical f.,** plica rectouterina. **retrotarsal f.,** conjunctival f. **Rindfleisch's f's,** folds in the serous surface of the pericardium around the beginning of the aorta. **sacrogenital f.,** plica rectouterina. **salpingopalatine f.,** plica salpingopalatina. **salpingopharyngeal f.,** plica salpingopharyngea. **Schultze's f.,** a sickle-shaped fold of the amnion extending from the point of insertion of the cord onto the placenta to the remains of the umbilical vesicle. **semilunar f.,** plica semilunaris. **semilunar f's of colon,** plicae semilunares coli. **semilunar f. of conjunctiva,** plica semilunaris conjunctivae. **semilunar f. of transversalis fascia,** ligamentum interfoveolare. **serosal f., serous f.,** plica serosa. **sigmoid f's of**

colon, plicae semilunares coli. **spiral f.,** plica spiralis. **spiral f. of cystic duct,** plica spiralis. **stapedial f.,** plica stapedis. **sublingual f.,** plica sublingualis. **superior duodenal f.,** plica duodenalis superior. **synovial f.,** plica synovialis. **synovial f., infrapatellar, synovial f., patellar,** plica synovialis infrapatellaris. **synovial f. of hip,** ligamentum capitis femoris. **tail f.,** a crescentic, ventral fold of the blastoderm, at the future caudal end of the embryo. **transverse f's of rectum,** plicae transversales recti. **Treves' f.,** plica ileocecalis. **triangular f.,** plica triangularis. **tubal f's of uterine tube,** plicae tubariae tubae uterinae. **umbilical f., lateral,** plica umbilicalis lateralis, def. 1. **umbilical f., medial,** plica umbilicalis medialis. **umbilical f., median, umbilical f., middle,** plica umbilicalis mediana. **urogenital f.,** urogenital ridge. **vaginal f's,** rugae vaginales. **vascular cecal f.,** plica cecalis vascularis. **ventricular f.,** plica vestibularis. **Veraguth's f's** (*obs.*), an angularly distorted fold of skin on the lateral third of the upper eyelid; described by Veraguth as occurring in melancholia. **vesical f., transverse,** plica vesicalis transversa. **vestibular f.,** false vocal cord (plica vestibularis [NA]). **vestigial f. of Marshall,** plica venae cavae sinistrae. **villous f's of stomach,** plicae villosae ventriculi. **vocal f.,** true vocal cord (plica vocalis [NA]). **vocal f., false,** plica vestibularis.

folia (fo′le-ah) plural of *folium.*

foliaceous (fo″le-a′shus) [L. *folia* leaves] having, pertaining to, or resembling leaves.

folian (fo′le-an) pertaining to Folius' process; see *processus anterior mallei.*

folie (fo-le′) [Fr.] psychosis; insanity. **f. à deux** (ah-duh′), occurrence of psychosis simultaneously in two closely associated persons, one of whom is dominant and the psychogenic source of the psychosis in the second. **f. circulaire** (seer-ku-lair′), circular psychosis. **f. du doute** (du-doot′), pathologic inability to make even the most trifling decisions, an extreme obsessive-compulsive reaction. **f. du pourquoi** (du-poor-kwah′), psychopathologic constant questioning. **f. gemellaire** (zha″mě-lār′), psychosis occurring simultaneously in twins. **f. musculaire** (mus″ku-lār′), severe chorea. **f. raisonnante** (rez-un-ahnt′), the delusional form of any psychosis.

Folin's method, reagent, test (fol′inz) [Otto Knut Olof *Folin*, American physiologic chemist, 1867–1934] see under *method, reagent,* and *tests.*

folium (fo′le-um), pl. *fo′lia* [L. "leaf"] [NA] a general term for a leaflike structure, especially one of the leaflike subdivisions of the cerebellar cortex. **f. cacu′minis** (*obs.*), f. vermis. **fo′lia cerebel′li** [NA], **folia of cerebellum,** the numerous long narrow folds of the cerebellar cortex, separated by sulci and supported by white laminae; they are aggregated into the various subdivisions of the cerebellum. Called also *gyri cerebelli.* **lingual f.,** a foliate papilla of the tongue. **f. ver′mis** [NA], the part of the vermis of the cerebellum between the declive and the tuber vermis.

Folius' muscle, process (fo′le-us) [Caecilius *Folius,* anatomist of Venice, 1615–1660] see *ligamentum mallic laterale* and *processus anterior mallei.*

follicle (fol′lĭ-k'l) 1. a sac or pouchlike depression or cavity; see also *folliculus.* 2. a former name for a lymph nodule. **aggregated f's,** folliculi lymphatici aggregati. **aggregated f's of vermiform appendix,** folliculi lymphatici aggregati appendicis vermiformis. **antral f's,** folliculi ovarici vesiculosi. **atretic f.,** an ovarian follicle which has involuted. **dental f.,** the structure within the substance of the jaws enclosing the tooth before its eruption; the dental sac and its contents. **Fleischmann's f.,** an occasional follicle in the mucosa of the floor of the mouth, near the anterior border of the genioglossus muscle. **gastric f's,** 1. glandulae gastricae [propriae]. 2. folliculi lymphatici gastrici. **graafian f's,** folliculi ovarici vesiculosi. **hair f.,** one of the tubular invaginations of the epidermis that enclose the hairs, and from which the hairs grow; called also *folliculus pili* [NA]. **intestinal f's,** the intestinal glands; see *glandulae intestinales.* **lenticular f's,** folliculi lymphatici gastrici. **Lieberkühn's f's,** the intestinal glands; see *glandulae intestinales.* **lingual f's,** folliculi linguales. **lymph f.,** folliculus lymphaticus. **lymph f's of stomach,** folliculi lymphatici gastrici. **lymphatic f's, aggregated, of Peyer,** folliculi lymphatici aggregati. **lymphatic f's, laryngeal,** folliculi lymphatici laryngei. **lymphatic f's of large intestine, solitary,** folliculi lymphatici solitarii intestini crassi. **lymphatic f's of tongue,** folliculi linguales. **Montgomery's f's,** Naboth's f's. **mucous f's, nasal,** glandulae nasales. **Naboth's f's, nabothian f's,** cystlike formations caused by occlusion of the lumina of glands in the mucosa of the uterine cervix, causing them to be distended with retained secretion; called also *Montgomery's f's, Naboth's cysts, glands,* or *ovules,* and *ovula nabothi.* **ovarian f.,** the egg and its encasing cells, at any stage of its development. **ovarian f's, primary,** folliculi ovarici primarii. **ovarian f's, vesicular,** folliculi ovarici vesiculosi. **primordial f.,** an ovarian follicle consisting of an egg enclosed by a single layer of cells. **sebaceous f.,** a hair follicle supplied with a relatively large sebaceous gland, and producing a relatively insignificant hair. **secondary f's,** folliculi ovarici vesiculosi. **solitary f's,** see *folliculi lymphatici solitarii intestini crassi* and *folliculi lymphatici solitarii intestini tenuis.* **f. of Stannius,** a lymphoid unit in chicks, resembling the thymus and developing from nodules formed by proliferation of points of the epithelium in the bursa of Fabricius. **thyroid f's, f's of thyroid gland,** folliculi glandulae thyroideae. **f's of tongue,** folliculi linguales. **unilaminar f.,** primordial f.

folliclis (fol'ĭ-klis) (obs.) tuberculosis papulonecrotica.

follicular (fo-lik'u-lar) [L. *follicularis*] of or pertaining to a follicle or follicles.

folliculi (fo-lik'u-li) [L.] plural of *folliculus.*

folliculin (fŏ-lik'u-lin) estrone.

folliculitis (fŏ-lik''u-li'tis) inflammation of a follicle or follicles; used ordinarily in reference to hair follicles, but sometimes in relation to follicles of other kinds. **f. absce'dens et suffo'diens,** perifolliculitis capitis abscedens et suffodiens. **agminate f.,** inflammation of a number of follicles in one area. **f. bar'bae,** sycosis vulgaris. **f. cheloida'lis,** keloidal f. **f. decal'vans,** a rare, localized, spreading, suppurative folliculitis of unknown cause, leading to scarring, with permanent hair loss. **f. gonorrhoe'ica,** littritis caused by gonococci. **keloidal f., f. keloida'lis,** a chronic skin condition characterized by development of persistent hard follicular papules which eventually fuse, with reparative activity leading to development of typical keloidal plaques, which give the disease its name; occurring usually on the back of the neck. Called also *dermatitis papillaris capillitii* and *acne keloid.* **f. na'res per'forans,** inflammation of a hair follicle in the nose, with pustulation and destruction of the follicle, leading to extension of the process through the tissues to the external surface. **f. ulerythemato'sa reticula'ta,** a condition occurring primarily in youth, and characterized by appearance on the face of numerous closely crowded, small areas of atrophy, separated by narrow ridges, the affected area being erythematous and the skin stretched and hard. **f. variolifor'mis,** acne varioliformis.

folliculoma (fo-lik''u-lo'mah) granulosa–theca cell tumor; see under *tumor.* **f. lipidique,** a granulosa– theca cell tumor in which streamers or trabeculae of tall, columnar, lipid-laden cells are interspersed among the more characteristic collections of granulosa cells.

folliculosis (fo-lik''u-lo'sis) a disease characterized by excessive development of lymph follicles.

folliculus (fo-lik'u-lus), pl. *follic'uli*[L., dim. of *follis* a leather bag] [NA] a follicle; [NA] a general term for a very small excretory or secretory sac or gland. **follic'uli glan'dulae thyroi'deae** [NA], follicles of thyroid gland: discrete, cystlike units of the thyroid gland that are lined with cuboidal epithelium and are filled with a colloid substance; there are about 30 to each lobule. Called also *thyroid follicles.* **follic'uli lingua'les** [NA], lingual follicles: projections on the mucosa of the root of the tongue, caused by underlying nodular masses of lymphoid tissue, making up the lingual tonsil. **f. lymphat'icus,** 1. [NA] lymph follicle: a small collection of lymphoid tissue found in such places as the mucosa of the gut: called also *nodulus lymphaticus.* 2. a small transient collection of actively proliferating lymphocytes in the cortex of a lymph node, expressing the cytogenetic and defense functions of the lymphatic tissue; called also *lymphatic nodule* and *nodulus lymphaticus.* **follic'uli lymphat'ici aggrega'ti** [NA], oval elevated areas of lymphoid tissue on the mucosa of the small intestine, composed of many lymphoid follicles closely packed together; called also *noduli lymphatici aggregati* [*Peyeri*] and *Peyer's patches.* **follic'uli lymphat'ici aggrega'ti appen'dicis vermifor'mis** [NA], aggregated follicles of vermiform appendix: oval elevated areas of lymphoid tissue occupying the greater part of the submucosa of the vermiform appendix; called also *noduli aggregati processus vermiformis.* **follic'uli lymphat'ici gas'trici** [NA], lymph follicles of stomach: small lymphocytic aggregates in the interstitial tissue of the lamina propria of the stomach, especially in the pyloric region; called also *lenticular glands of stomach, lymphatic nodules of stomach,* and *noduli lymphatici gastrici.* **follic'uli lymphat'ici laryn'gei** [NA], laryngeal lymphatic follicles: lymphatic aggregations in the mucosa of the ventricle of the larynx and on the posterior surface of the epiglottis; called also *noduli lymphatici laryngei.* **follic'uli lymphat'ici liena'les** [NA], aggregations of lymphatic tissue that ensheath the arteries in the spleen; often called the *white pulp.* Called also *malpighian bodies* or *corpuscles* (*of spleen*), and *noduli lymphatici lienales* [*Malpighii*]. **follic'uli lymphat'ici rec'ti** [NA], concentrations of lymphoid tissue in the tunica mucosa of the rectum; called also *noduli lymphatici recti.* **follic'uli lymphat'ici solita'rii intesti'ni cras'si** [NA], solitary lymphatic follicles of large intestine: the areas of concentrated lymphatic tissue in the tunica mucosa of the colon; called also *noduli lymphatici solitarii intestini crassi.* **follic'-uli lymphat'ici solita'rii intesti'ni ten'uis** [NA], small lymph follicles scattered throughout the mucosa and submucosa of the small intestine; called also *noduli lymphatici solitarii intestini tenuis, solitary glands of small intestine,* and *solitary lymphatic nodules of small intestine.* **follic'uli ooph'ori**

prima'rii, folliculi ovarici primarii. **follic'uli ooph'ori vesiculo'si** [Graaf'i], folliculi ovarici vesiculosi. **follic'uli ovar'ici prima'rii** [NA], primary ovarian follicles: immature ovarian follicles, each comprising an immature ovum and the specialized epithelial cells (follicle cells) that surround it; called also *folliculi oophori primarii.* **follic'uli ovar'ici vesiculo'si** [NA], vesicular ovarian follicles: maturing ovarian follicles among whose cells fluid has begun to accumulate, leading to the formation of a single cavity or antrum and leaving the ovum eccentrically located in a hillock of follicle cells, the cumulus oophorus; called also *folliculi oophori vesiculosi* [*Graafi*], and *graafian follicles* or *vesicles.* **f. pi'li** [NA], hair follicle: one of the tubular invaginations of the epidermis that enclose the hairs, and from which the hairs grow.

Follutein (fol-lu'te-in) trademark for a preparation of chorionic gonadotropin.

Foltz's valve (fōlts'ez) [Jean Charles Eugène *Foltz,* French ophthalmologist, 1822–1876] see under *valve.*

Folvite (fōl'vīt) trademark for preparations of folic acid.

fomentation (fo''men-ta'shun) [L. *fomentatio; fomentum,* a poultice] treatment by warm and moist applications; also the substance thus applied.

fomes (fo'mēz), pl. *fo'mites* [L. "tinder"] an object, such as a book, wooden object, or an article of clothing, that is not in itself harmful, but is able to harbor pathogenic microorganisms and thus may serve as an agent of transmission of an infection; called also *fomite.*

fomite (fo'mīt) fomes.

fomites (fo'mĭ-tēz) plural of *fomes.*

fonazine mesylate (fo'nah-zēn) chemical name: 10-[2-(dimethylamino)propyl]-*N,N*-dimethylphenothiazine-2-sulfonamide monomethanesulfonate; a serotonin inhibitor, $C_{20}H_{29}N_3O_5S_3$.

Fonsecaea (fon-se-se'ah) a genus of dematiacious Fungi Imperfecti, some species of which were formerly included in the genera *Hormodendrum* and *Cladosporium.* *F. pedrosoi* and *F. compactum* are etiologic agents of chromomycosis.

fontactoscope (fon-tak'to-skōp) an instrument for measuring the radioactivity of water and gas.

Fontana's markings, spaces (fon-tah'nahz) [Felice *Fontana,* Italian naturalist and physiologist, 1720–1805] see under *marking* and *space,* and see *spatia anguli iridocornealis.*

fontanel (fon''tah-nel) fontanelle.

fontanelle (fon''tah-nel') [Fr., dim. of *fontaine* spring, filter] a soft spot, such as one of the membrane-covered spaces (*fonticuli cranii*[NA]) remaining in the incompletely ossified skull of a fetus or infant. See also *fonticulus.* **anterior f.,** fonticulus anterior. **anterolateral f.,** fonticulus sphenoidalis. **bregmatic f.,** fonticulus anterior. **Casser's f., casserian f., Casserio's f.,** fonticulus mastoideus. **cranial f's,** fonticuli cranii. **frontal f.,** fonticulus anterior. **Gerdy's f.,** a fontanelle occasionally occurring in the sagittal suture; called also *sagittal f.* **mastoid f.,** fonticulus mastoideus. **occipital f., posterior f.,** fonticulus posterior. **posterolateral f., posterotemporal f.,** fonticulus mastoideus. **quadrangular f.,** fonticulus anterior. **sagittal f.,** Gerdy's f. **sphenoidal f.,** fonticulus sphenoidalis. **triangular f.,** fonticulus posterior.

fonticuli (fon-tik'u-li) [L.] plural of *fonticulus.*

fonticulus (fon-tik'u-lus), pl. *fontic'uli* [L., dim. of *fons* fountain] [NA] fontanelle; a soft spot; one of the membrane-covered spaces remaining in the incompletely ossified skull of the fetus or infant. **f. ante'rior** [NA], anterior fontanelle: the unossified area of the skull situated at the junction of the frontal, coronal, and sagittal sutures; called also *f. frontalis* [*major*], and *frontal fontanelle.* **fontic'uli cra'nii** [NA], the membrane-covered spaces, or soft spots, remaining at the incomplete angles of the parietal and adjacent bones, until ossification of the skull is completed; called also *fontanelles.* **f. fronta'lis** [**major**], f. anterior. **f. guttu'ris,** fossa jugularis. **f. ma'jor,** f. anterior. **f. mastoi'deus** [NA], mastoid fontanelle: the unossified area of the skull at the junction of the lambdoidal, parietomastoid, and occipitomastoid sutures; called also *Casser's* or *casserian fontanelle,* and *posterolateral* or *posterotemporal fontanelle.* **f. mi'nor,** f. posterior. **f. occipita'lis, f. poste'rior** [NA], posterior fontanelle: the unossified area of the skull at the junction of the sagittal and lambdoidal sutures; called also *f. minor,* and *occipital* or *triangular fontanelle.* **f. sphenoida'lis** [NA], sphenoidal fontanelle: the unossified area at the junction of the parietal and frontal bones, the greater wing of the sphenoidal, and the squamous part of the temporal bones; called also *anterolateral fontanelle.*

food (fōōd) anything which, when taken into the body, serves to nourish or build up the tissues or to supply body heat; aliment; nutriment. **isodynamic f's,** foods which generate equal amounts of energy in heat units.

foot (foot) [L. *pes*] 1. the distal portion of the primate leg, upon which an individual stands and walks. It consists, in man, of the tarsus, metatarsus, and phalanges and the tissues encompassing them. See also *pes* and *talipes.* 2. a unit of linear measure, 1/3 yard, or 12 inches, being the equivalent of 30.48 cm. **athlete's**

f., tinea pedis. **broad f.,** metatarsus latus. **burning feet,** a deficiency disease, possibly pantothenic acid deficiency, occurring among the poor in South India and West Africa. It is marked by burning sensations in the soles and palms. **buttress f.,** a condition of periostitis or ostitis in the region of the pyramidal process of the os pedis of the horse, with fracture of the process, deformity of the hoof, and alteration of the normal angle of the joint. Called also *extensor process disease, pyramidal disease,* and *low ring-bone.* **Charcot's f.,** the deformed foot seen in tabetic arthropathy. **cleft f.,** a deformed foot in which the division between the third and fourth toes extends into the metatarsal region. **club f.,** see *talipes.* **contracted f.,** see *hoof-bound.* **crooked f.,** a condition of the horse's hoof in which one wall is concave and the opposite wall convex, giving the hoof a bent appearance; it is due to improper trimming and shoeing. **crow's f.,** one of the fine lines or creases that extend in a radial fanlike fashion from the lateral canthal regions in irregular lengths; called also *laugh line.* **dangle f., drop f.,** a condition in which the foot hangs in a plantar-flexed position, due to lesion of the peroneal nerve. **end f.,** see *end-feet.* **fescue f.,** fescue (def. 2). **flat f.,** flatfoot. **forced f.,** a painful swelling of the feet of soldiers after forced marches, due to fracture of a metatarsal bone. **Friedreich's f.,** pes cavus, with hyperextension of the toes; seen in hereditary ataxia. **fungus f.,** maduromycosis. **Hong Kong f.,** an infectious mycotic disease (dermatophytosis) of the foot occurring in China. **immersion f.,** a condition resembling trench foot occurring in persons who have spent long periods in water. **Madura f.,** maduromycosis. **march f.,** painful swelling of the forefoot, often associated with fracture of one of the metatarsal bones, following excessive foot strain. **Morand's f.,** a foot having eight toes. **Morton's f.,** see under *toe.* **mossy f.,** an infectious verrucose condition of the skin of the feet, endemic in the Amazon region of South America. **perivascular feet,** terminal expansions of the cytoplasmic processes of some astrocytes by which they are attached to blood vessels. **pricked f.,** a condition in the horse in which the sole or the frog has been punctured either in the forge or by the animal treading on a nail or some other object. **red f.,** redfoot. **reel f.,** clubfoot; see *talipes.* **rocker-bottom f.,** 1. congenital convex pes valgus, due to primary dislocation of the talonavicular joint; it may occur as an isolated primary deformity or be associated with autosomal trisomy, including trisomy 13–15 and trisomy 18; called also *rocker-bottom flatfoot.* 2. talipes equinovarus in which the foot is shaped like a rocker of a rocking-chair, occurring as a result of a transverse break in the midtarsal area; called also *rocker-bottom deformity.* **sag f.,** sagging of the arch of the foot. **shelter f.,** a swollen condition of the feet occurring among persons who spend the night in air-raid shelters. **spatula f.,** a foot in which several toes are fused together. **spread f.,** metatarsus latus. **strawberry rot f.,** dermatophilosis. **sucker f.,** a pyramidal expansion of a process of an astrocyte by which the latter is attached to a small blood vessel; called also *sucker apparatus* or *process, podium,* and *vascular foot plate.* **tabetic f.,** the flat, distorted foot seen in tabes, and due to disease of the tarsus. **taut f.,** a shortening and contraction of the calf muscles and plantar flexors of the foot, due to high-heeled shoes. **trench f.,** a condition of the feet resembling frostbite. It is due to the prolonged action of water on the skin combined with circulatory disturbance due to cold and inaction. Called also *water-bite.* **weak f.,** an early stage of flatfoot.

foot-candle (foot kan′d'l) a unit of illumination being 1 lumen per square foot or equivalent to 1.0764 milliphots. Cf. *lux.*

footdrop (foot′drop) dropping of the foot from paralysis of the anterior muscles of the leg.

foot lambert (foot lam′bert) see *lambert.*

footplate (foot′plāt) the flat portion of the stapes, which is set into the oval window on the medial wall of the middle ear. Called also *base of stapes.*

foot-pound (foot-pownd′) the work done in raising a mass of one pound the distance of one foot against gravity. Abbreviated f.p.

forage (fo-rahzh′) [Fr. "boring, drilling"] surgical creation of a V-shaped longitudinal trench in the prostate by means of electric current, thereby removing obstruction caused by its hypertrophy. The term is applied to similar cutting operations on other parts.

foramen (fo-ra′men), pl. *foram′ina* [L.] a natural opening or passage; [NA] a general term for such a passage, especially one into or through a bone. **accessory f.,** a lateral or accessory orifice, other than the main apical foramen, opening into the root canal of a tooth; called also *lateral f.* **alveolar foramina of maxilla, foram′ina alveola′ria maxil′lae** [NA], the openings of the alveolar canals at the deepest portion of the tooth sockets in the maxilla. **aortic f.,** hiatus aorticus. **apical f. of tooth, f. a′picis den′tis** [NA], an aperture at or near the apex of the root of a tooth, giving passage to the blood vessels and nerves supplying the pulp; called also *f. radicis dentis, pupal f.,* and *root f.* **auditory f., external,** meatus acusticus externus. **auditory f., internal,** porus acusticus internus. **Bartholin's f.** (*obs.*), f. obturatum. **Bichat's f.,** cisterna venae magnae cerebri. **f. of Bochdalek,** hiatus pleuroperitonealis. **Botallo's f.,** f. ovale cordis. **Bozzi's f.** (*obs.*), macula retinae.

f. cae′cum lin′guae, f. cecum linguae. **f. cae′cum medul′lae oblonga′tae,** a small triangular expansion at the lower border of the pons, formed by the termination of the anterior median fissure of the medulla oblongata; called also *f. caecum posterius, Schwalbe's f.,* and *f. of Vicq d'Azyr.* **f. cae′cum poste′rius, f. caecum of Vicq d'Azyr,** f. caecum medullae oblongatae. **caroticotympanic foramina,** canaliculi caroticotympanici. **carotid f.,** the inferior aperture of the carotid canal, giving passage to the carotid vessels. **cecal f., f. ce′cum,** f. cecum ossis frontalis. **f. cecum of frontal bone,** f. cecum ossis frontalis. **f. ce′cum lin′guae** [NA], foramen cecum of tongue: a depression on the dorsum of the tongue at the end of the median sulcus, representing the remains of the upper end of the thyroglossal duct of the embryo. **f. ce′cum os′sis fronta′lis** [NA], foramen cecum of frontal bone: a blind opening formed between the frontal crest and the crista galli; it sometimes transmits a vein from the nasal cavity to the superior sagittal sinus. Called also *cecal f.* and *f. cecum.* **f. cecum of tongue,** f. cecum linguae. **cervical f.,** f. transversarium. **condyloid f., anterior,** canalis hypoglossi. **condyloid f., posterior,** canalis condylaris. **conjugate f.,** a foramen formed by a notch in each of two opposed bones. **f. costotransversa′rium** [NA], **costotransverse f.,** the narrow space between the dorsal surface of the neck of a rib and the ventral surface of the transverse process of the corresponding vertebra. **cotyloid f.,** a passage between the margin of the acetabulum and the transverse ligament. **cribroethmoid f.,** f. ethmoidale anterius. **dental foramina,** see *foramina alveolaria maxillae* and *foramina mandibulae.* **f. diaphrag′matis [sel′lae],** the opening in the center of the diaphragm of the sella through which the infundibulum passes. **Duverney's f.,** f. epiploicum. **emissary f.,** any foramen in a cranial bone that gives passage to an emissary vein. **epiploic f., f. epiplo′icum** [NA], an opening connecting the two sacs of the peritoneum, situated below and behind the porta hepatis. **esophageal f.,** hiatus esophageus. **ethmoidal f., anterior,** f. ethmoidale anterius. **ethmoidal f., posterior,** f. ethmoidale posterius. **ethmoidal foramina,** foramina ethmoidalia. **foram′ina ethmoida′lia** [NA], ethmoidal foramina: small openings in the ethmoid bone at the junction of the medial wall with the roof of the orbit, the anterior transmitting the nasal branch of the ophthalmic nerve and the anterior ethmoid vessels, the posterior transmitting the posterior ethmoid vessels. Called also *orbital canals.* **f. ethmoida′le ante′rius** [NA], a small opening on the medial wall of the orbit, on the line of the frontoethmoidal suture, that transmits the anterior ethmoidal nerve and vessels. **f. ethmoida′le poste′rius** [NA], posterior ethmoidal foramen: a small opening on the medial wall of the orbit, on the line of the frontoethmoidal suture, that transmits the posterior ethmoidal nerve and vessels. **f. of Fallopio,** hiatus canalis nervi petrosi majoris. **Ferrein's f.,** hiatus canalis nervi petrosi majoris. **frontal f., f. fronta′le** [NA], see *incisura frontalis.* **frontoethmoidal f.,** a foramen lying on the line of the frontoethmoidal suture. **Galen's f.,** the opening of an anterior cardiac vein into the right atrium. **glandular foramina of Littre,** lacunae urethrales. **glandular f. of Morgagni, glandular f. of tongue,** f. cecum linguae. **great f.,** f. magnum. **Hartigan's f.,** a foramen said to exist in the base of the transverse process of a lumbar vertebra but seldom persisting to adult life. **Huschke's f.,** a perforation found near the inner extremity of the tympanic plate between the tympanum and the jugular fossa caused by arrest of development. **incisive f., f. incisi′vum** [NA], one of the openings in the incisive fossa of the hard palate that transmit the nasopalatine nerves. **incisor f., median,** Scarpa's f. **infraorbital f., f. infraorbita′le** [NA], the opening of the infraorbital canal on the anterior surface of the maxilla giving passage to the infraorbital nerve and vessels; called also *suborbital f.* **innominate f.,** an occasional opening in the temporal bone for passage of the small superficial petrosal nerve. **intersacral foramina,** foramina intervertebralia ossis sacri. **interventricular f., f. interventricula′re** [NA], **f. interventricula′re [Monro′i],** a communication between the lateral and the third ventricle; called also *f. of Monro.* **intervertebral f., f. intervertebra′le** [NA], the passage formed by the inferior and superior notches on the pedicles of adjacent vertebrae; it transmits a spinal nerve and vessels. **intervertebral foramina of sacrum,** foramina intervertebralia ossis sacri. **intervertebral foramina of sacrum, foram′ina intervertebra′lia os′sis sa′cri** [NA], the four short, forked tunnels in each lateral wall of the sacral canal, connecting it with the pelvic and dorsal sacral foramina; called also *intersacral canals* or *foramina.* **ischiadic f., greater,** f. ischiadicum majus. **ischiadic f., lesser,** f. ischiadicum minus. **f. ischia′dicum ma′jus** [NA], greater ischiadic foramen: a hole converted from the major sciatic notch by the sacrotuberal and sacrospinal ligaments; called also *greater sciatic f.* and *great sacrosciatic f.* **f. ischia′dicum mi′nus** [NA], lesser ischiadic foramen: a hole converted from the minor sciatic notch by the sacrotuberal and sacrospinal ligaments; called also *lesser sciatic f.* and *small sacrosciatic f.* **ischiopubic f.,** f. obturatum. **jugular f., f. jugula′re** [NA], the opening formed by the jugular notches on the temporal and occipital bones, for the transmission of various veins, arteries, and nerves. **f. of Key and Retzius,** apertura lateralis ventriculi quarti. **lacerate f., anterior,** fissura orbitalis superior. **lacerate f., middle,** f. lacerum. **lacerate f., posterior,** f. jugulare. **f. lac′e-rum** [NA], an irregular gap formed at the junction of the base of the great wing of the sphenoid bone, the tip of the petrous part of the temporal bone, and the basilar part of the occipital bone; in life its inferior aspect is filled with fibrocartilage, superior to which the internal carotid artery lies. **f. lac′erum ante′rius,** fissura orbitalis superior. **f. lac′erum me′dium,** f. lacerum. **f. lac′erum poste′rius,** f. jugulare. **lateral f.,** accessory f. **left f., inferior,** hiatus aorticus. **left f., superior,** hiatus esophageus. **f. of Luschka,** apertura lateralis ventriculi quarti. **f. of Magendie,** apertura mediana ventriculi quarti. **f. mag′num** [NA], great foramen: the large opening in the anterior and inferior part of the occipital bone, interconnecting the vertebral canal and the cranial cavity; called also *f. occipitale magnum* and *great occipital f.* **malar f.,** f. zygomaticofaciale. **f. mandib′ulae** [NA], **f. mandibula′re,** the opening on the medial surface of the ramus of the mandible, leading into the mandibular canal. **mastoid f., f. mastoi′deum** [NA], a prominent opening in the temporal bone posterior to the mastoid process and near its occipital articulation; an artery and vein usually pass through it. **maxillary f.,** hiatus maxillaris. **maxillary f., anterior,** f. mentale. **maxillary f., inferior,** f. ovale basis cranii. **maxillary f., internal,** maxillary f., posterior, f. mandibulae. **maxillary f., superior,** f. rotundum ossis sphenoidalis. **medullary f.,** f. vertebrale. **meibomian f.,** f. cecum linguae. **mental f., f. menta′le** [NA], an opening on the lateral part of the body of the mandible, opposite the second biscuspid tooth, for passage of the mental nerve and vessels. **f. of Monro,** f. interventriculare. **Mor-and′s f.,** f. cecum linguae. **Morgagni′s f., morgagnian f.,** 1. a small gap on either side, between the sternal and costal portions of the diaphragm, for the passage of the superior epigastric blood vessels and a few lymphatic vessels; called also *pleuroperitoneal f.* 2. foramen cecum linguae. 3. foramen singulare. **nasal foramina, foram′ina nasa′lia,** openings on the outer surface of each nasal bone for the transmission of blood vessels. **foram′ina nervo′sa lam′inae spira′lis,** foramina nervosa limbus laminae spiralis. **foram′ina ner-vo′sa lim′bus lam′inae spira′lis** [NA], numerous small openings in the labium limbi tympanicum for the passage of the cochlear nerves; called also *foramina nervosa laminae spiralis* and *habenulae perforatae.* **f. nutric′ium** [NA], **nutrient f.,** any one of the passages that admit the nutrient vessels to the medullary cavity of a bone. **obturator f., f. obtura′tum** [NA], the large opening between the os pubis and the ischium. **occipital f., great, occipital f., inferior,** f. magnum. **f. occipita′le mag′num,** f. magnum. **olfactory f.,** any one of the many openings of the cribriform plate of the ethmoidal bone. **optic f. of sclera,** lamina cribrosa sclerae. **optic f. of sphenoid bone, f. op′ticum os′sis sphenoida′lis,** canalis opticus. **orbitomalar f.,** f. zygomaticoorbitale. **oval f. of fetus,** fossa ovalis cordis. **oval f. of hip bone,** f. obturatum. **oval f. of sphenoid bone, f. ovale basis cranii. f. ova′le ba′sis cra′nii** [NA], an opening in the posterior part of the medial portion of the great wing of the sphenoid bone; it transmits the mandibular branch of the trigeminal nerve and some vessels. Called also *f. ovale ossis sphenoidalis* and *oval f. of sphenoid bone.* **f. ova′le cor′dis** [NA], the aperture in the septum secundum of the fetal heart that provides a communication between the atria; called also *Botallo′s f.* and *oval f. of fetus.* **f. ova′le os′sis sphenoida′lis,** f. ovale basis cranii. **f. of Pacchioni, pac-chionian f.,** f. diaphragmatis [sellae]. **palatine foramina, accessory,** foramina palatina minora. **palatine f., anterior,** f. incisivum. **palatine f., greater,** f. palatinum majus. **palatine formina, lesser,** foramina palatina minora. **palatine f., posterior,** f. palatinum majus. **foramina of palatine tonsil,** fossulae tonsillares tonsillae palatinae. **f. palati′num ma′jus** [NA], greater palatine foramen: the inferior opening of the great palatine canal, found laterally on the horizontal plate of each palatine bone opposite the root of each third molar tooth; it transmits a palatine nerve and artery. Called also *posterior palatine f., pterygopalatine f.,* and *sphenopalatine f.* **foram′ina palati′na mino′ra** [NA], lesser palatine foramina: the openings of the palatine canals behind the palatine crest and the greater palatine foramina; called also *accessory palatine foramina.* **foram′ina papilla′ria re′nis** [NA], papillary **foramina of kidney,** minute openings in the summit of each renal papilla, the orifices of the collecting tubules; called also *foveolae papillae.* **parietal f., f. parieta′le** [NA], an opening on the posterior part of the superior portion of the parietal bone near the sagittal suture, for the passage of a vein and arteriole. **pleuroperitoneal f.,** 1. hiatus pleuroperitonealis. 2. Morgagni′s f. (def. 1). **pterygopalatine f.,** f. palatinum majus. **pulpal f.,** f. apicis dentis. **quadrate f.,** f. venae cavae. **f. rad′icis den′tis,** f. apicis dentis. **Retzius′ f.,** apertura lateralis ventriculi quarti. **right f.,** f. venae cavae. **rivinian f., Rivinus′ f.,** incisura tympanica. **root f.,** f. apicis dentis. **f. rotun′dum os′sis sphenoida′lis** [NA], a round opening in the medial part of the great wing of the sphenoid bone that

transmits the maxillary branch of the trigeminal nerve; called also *superior maxillary f.* or *canal.* **sacral foramina, anterior,** foramina sacralia pelvina. **sacral foramina, dorsal,** foramina sacralia dorsalia. **sacral foramina, internal,** foramina sacralia pelvina. **sacral foramina, posterior,** foramina sacralia dorsalia. **f. of sacral canal,** hiatus sacralis. **foram′ina scara′lia anterio′ra,** foramina sacralia pelvina. **foram′ina sacra′lia dorsa′lia** [NA], dorsal sacral foramina: the eight openings (four on each side) on the dorsal surface of the sacrum for the dorsal rami of the sacral nerves; called also *foramina sacralia posteriora* and *posterior sacral foramina.* **foram′ina sacra′lia pelvi′na** [NA], the eight openings (four on each side) on the pelvic surface of the sacrum for the ventral rami of the sacral nerves. Called also *anterior sacral foramina, foramina sacralia anteriora,* and *internal sacral foramina.* **foram′ina sacra′lia posterio′ra,** foramina sacralia dorsalia. **sacrosciatic f., great,** f. ischiadicum majus. **sacrosciatic f., small,** f. ischiadicum minus. **f. of saphenous vein,** hiatus saphenus. **Scarpa′s f.,** one of the two foramina, one behind either upper medial incisor, for transmission of the nasopalatine nerves; called also *median incisor f.* **Schwalbe′s f.,** f. caecum medullae oblongatae. **sciatic f., greater,** f. ischiadicum majus. **sciatic f., lesser,** f. ischiadicum minus. **f. singula′re** [NA], the opening in the inferior vestibular area of the fundus of the internal acoustic meatus that gives passage to the nerves of the ampulla of the posterior semicircular duct; called also *Morgagni′s* or *morgagnian f.* **foramina of smallest veins of heart,** foramina venarum minimarum cordis. **Soemmering′s f.** (*obs.*), fovea centralis retinae. **spheno-palatine f.,** 1. foramen sphenopalatinum. 2. foramen palatinum majus. **f. sphenopalati′num** [NA], sphenopalatine foramen: an opening on the medial wall of the pterygopalatine fossa, interconnecting this fossa with the nasal cavity, and transmitting the sphenopalatine artery and nasal nerves. **sphenotic f.,** f. lacerum. **spinal f., f. of spinal cord,** f. vertebrale. **f. spino′sum** [NA], **spinous f.,** an opening in the great wing of the sphenoid bone, near its posterior angle, for the middle meningeal artery. **Spöndel′s f.,** a small transient foramen in the cartilaginous base of the developing skull between the ethmoid bone and the lower wings of the sphenoid. **f. of Stensen,** 1. foramen incisivum. 2. canalis incisivus. **stylomas-toid f., f. stylomastoi′deum** [NA], a foramen on the inferior part of the temporal bone between the styloid and mastoid processes, for the facial nerve and the stylomastoid artery. **suborbital f.,** f. infraorbitale. **supraorbital f., f. supraorbita′le, f. supraorbita′lis** [NA], an opening in the frontal bone in the supraorbital margin, giving passage to the supraorbital artery and nerve; it is often present as a notch (incisura frontalis) bridged only by fibrous tissue. Called also *supraorbital notch.* **suprapyriform f.,** an opening above the pyramidalis muscle through which the gluteal vessels and superior gluteal nerve pass out of the pelvis. **f. of Tarin** (*obs.*), hiatus canalis nervi petrosi majoris. **temporomalar f.,** f. zygomaticotemporale. **thebesian foramina, foram′ina thebes′ii,** foramina venarum minimarum cordis. **thyroid f.,** 1. f. thyroideum. 2. obturator f. **f. thyroi′deum** [NA], thyroid foramen: an inconstantly present opening in the upper part of the lamina of the thyroid cartilage, resulting from incomplete union of the fourth and fifth branchial cartilages. **tonsillar foramina,** see *fossulae tonsillares tonsillae palatinae* and *pharyngeae.* **f. transversa′rium** [NA], **transverse f.,** the passage in either transverse process of a cervical vertebra that, in the upper six vertebrae, transmits the vertebral vessels; it is small or may be absent in the seventh. Called also *cervical vertebral,* or *vertebroarterial f.* **vena caval f., f. ve′nae ca′vae** [NA], the opening in the respiratory diaphragm that transmits the inferior vena cava and some branches of the right vagus nerve; called also *venal caval hiatus* and *venous f.* **foram′ina vena′rum minima′rum cor′dis** [NA], foramina of smallest veins of heart: minute openings in the walls of the right atrium of the heart, through which small veins, the venae cordis minimae, empty their blood directly into the heart; called also *Vieussen′s foramina* and *thebesian foramina.* **venous f.,** f. venae cavae. **vertebral f.,** 1. foramen vertebrale. 2. foramen transversarium. **f. vertebra′le** [NA], vertebral foramen: the large opening in a vertebra formed by its body and arch; called also *medullary f.,* and *spinal f.* or *aperture.* **vertebroarterial f.,** f. transversarium. **f. of Vesalius,** an opening occasionally found medial to the foramen ovale of the sphenoid, for the passage of a vein from the cavernous sinus. **f. of Vicq d′Azyr,** f. caecum medullae oblongatae. **Vieussen′s foramina,** foramina venarum minimarum cordis. **Weitbrecht′s f.,** an opening in the capsule of the shoulder joint through which passes the synovial membrane to the bursa that lines the under surface of the subscapularis muscle. **f. of Winslow,** f. epiploicum. **zygomatic f., anterior, zygomatic f., external, zygomatic f., facial,** f. zygomaticofaciale. **zygomatic f., inferior, zygomatic f., internal, of Arnold,** f. zygomaticoorbitale. **zygomatic f., internal, of Meckel,** f. zygomaticotemporale. **zygomatic f., orbital,** f. zygomaticoorbitale. **zygomatic f., posterior,** f. zygomaticotemporale. **zygomatic f., superior,** f. zygomaticoorbitale. **zygomatic f., temporal,** f.

zygomaticotemporale. **zygomaticofacial f., f. zygomat-icofacia′le** [NA], the opening on the anterior surface of the zygomatic bone for the zygomaticofacial nerves and vessels. **zygomaticoorbital f., f. zygomaticoorbita′le** [NA], either of the two openings on the orbital surface of each zygomatic bone, which transmit branches of the zygomatic branch of the trigeminal nerve and branches of the lacrimal artery. **zygomatico-temporal f., f. zygomaticotempora′le** [NA], the opening on the temporal surface of the zygomatic bone for passage of the zygomaticotemporal nerve.

foramina (fo-ram′ĭ-nah) [L.] plural of *foramen*.

Foraminifera (fo-ram″ĭ-nif′er-ah) in some systems of classification, a class of the subphylum Sarcodina, and in others an order of the class Rhizopoda, including ameboid protozoa of the marine type, which secrete chalky, many-chambered shells with perforations through which the pseudopodia are extended for locomotion or food gathering. Accumulations of their shells on the ocean floor are gradually transformed into chalk.

foraminiferous (for″am-ĭ-nif′er-us) [*foramen* + L. *ferre* to bear] having foramina.

foraminotomy (for″am-ĭ-not′o-me) [*foramina* + Gr. *tomē* a cutting] the operation of removing the roof of intervertebral foramina, done for the relief of nerve root compression.

foraminulum (for″ah-min′u-lum), pl. *foramin′ula* [L.] a minute foramen.

foration (fo-ra′shun) [L. *forare* to bore] the act or process of trephination or boring.

force (fōrs) [L. *fortis* strong] energy, or power; that which originates or arrests motion. **catabolic f.,** energy derived from the metabolism of food. **chewing f.,** masticatory f. **electromotive f.,** the force which, by reason of differences in potential, causes a flow of electricity from one place to another, giving rise to an electric current; it is measured in volts. **extraoral f.,** force applied by orthodontic anchorage units (calvarial, occipital, or cervical) outside the oral cavity. **field f's,** hypothetical forces which have a part in the individuation processes of the early embryo. **masticatory f.,** the force applied by the muscles of mastication during the chewing of food. **nerve f., nervous f.,** in psychiatry, the amount of nervous capital or stamina a person possesses. **occlusal f.,** the force exerted on opposing teeth when the jaws are brought into approximation. **reciprocal f.,** a force applied by an orthodontic anchorage in which the resistance of one or more dental units is utilized to move one or more opposing dental units. Cf. *reciprocal anchorage.* **reserve f.,** energy above that required for normal functioning; in the heart it is the power which will take care of the additional circulatory burden imposed by bodily exertion. **rest f.,** the power of the heart necessary to maintain the circulation when the patient is at rest. **Van der Waals f's,** the relatively weak, short-range forces of attraction existing between atoms and molecules, which results in the attraction of nonpolar organic compounds to each other (hydrophobic bonding). **vital f.,** the energy which characterizes a living organism.

forceps (fōr′seps) [L.] 1. an instrument with two blades and a handle for compressing or grasping tissues in surgical operations, and for handling sterile dressings and other surgical supplies. 2. any forcipate organ or part, particularly the terminal fibers of the corpus callosum. **alligator f.,** strong toothed forceps having a double clamp. **f. ante′rior,** f. minor. **artery f.,** forceps for grasping and compressing an artery. **Asch f.,** forceps especially designed for intranasal use. **aural f.,** forceps for operations of the ear. **axis-traction f.,** specially jointed obstetrical forceps so constructed that traction may be applied in the line of the pelvic axis. **Bailey-Williamson f.,** a special obstetrical forceps used in mid- and high-forceps delivery and in breech presentations with aftercoming head. **Barton f.,** an obstetrical forceps with a hinge in one blade, which can be applied correctly to the fetal head without disturbing its relationship to the pelvic axis. **bayonet f.,** a forceps whose blades are offset from the axis of the handle. **bone f.,** forceps used for grasping bone. **Brenner f.,** a special obstetrical forceps used in breech presentations. **bulldog f.,** spring forceps for seizing an artery to arrest or prevent hemorrhage; the jaws are usually covered with rubber tubing to prevent injury to the vascular wall. **bullet f.,** a forceps for extracting bullets. **capsule f.,** forceps for removing the lens capsule in membranous cataract. **chalazion f.,** a thumb forceps with a flattened plate at the end of one arm and a matching ring on the other; it is an ophthalmologic instrument, also used for isolation of lip and cheek lesions to facilitate removal. **Chamberlen f.,** the original form of obstetrical forceps, invented by Peter Chamberlen (1560–1631), and disclosed by Hugh Chamberlen (1664–1728). **clamp f.,** 1. a forceps with an automatic lock, used for compressing arteries, the pedicle of a tumor, etc.; called also *pedicle clamp.* 2. in dentistry, forceps used to hold and open the rubber-dam clamp while it is being placed on or removed from a tooth. **clip f.,** a double-action forceps for applying wound clips; also used to designate a McKenzie forceps for applying brain clips. **Cornet′s f.,** a forceps for holding a coverglass. **DeLee f.,** a modified Simpson forceps. **dental f.,** forceps for the extraction of teeth. **disk f.,** a forceps for grasping the scleral disk in trephining the eyeball. **dressing f.,** forceps with scissor-like handles for grasping lint, drainage tubes, etc., in dressing wounds. **ear f.,** delicate forceps for extracting foreign bodies from the auditory canal. **Elliot f.,** a special obstetrical forceps used in low-forceps delivery and frank breech presentations. **epilating f.,** forceps for use in plucking out hairs. **extracting f.,** dental f. **fixation f.,** forceps for holding a part during an operation. **galea f.,** Willett f. **Garrison′s f.,** an obstetrical forceps with unfenestrated blades; called also *Luikart′s f.* **Good f.,** a special obstetrical forceps used in midforceps delivery in the anterior position. **Haig Ferguson f.,** a special obstetrical forceps used in low-forceps delivery. **Hawks-Dennen f.,** a special

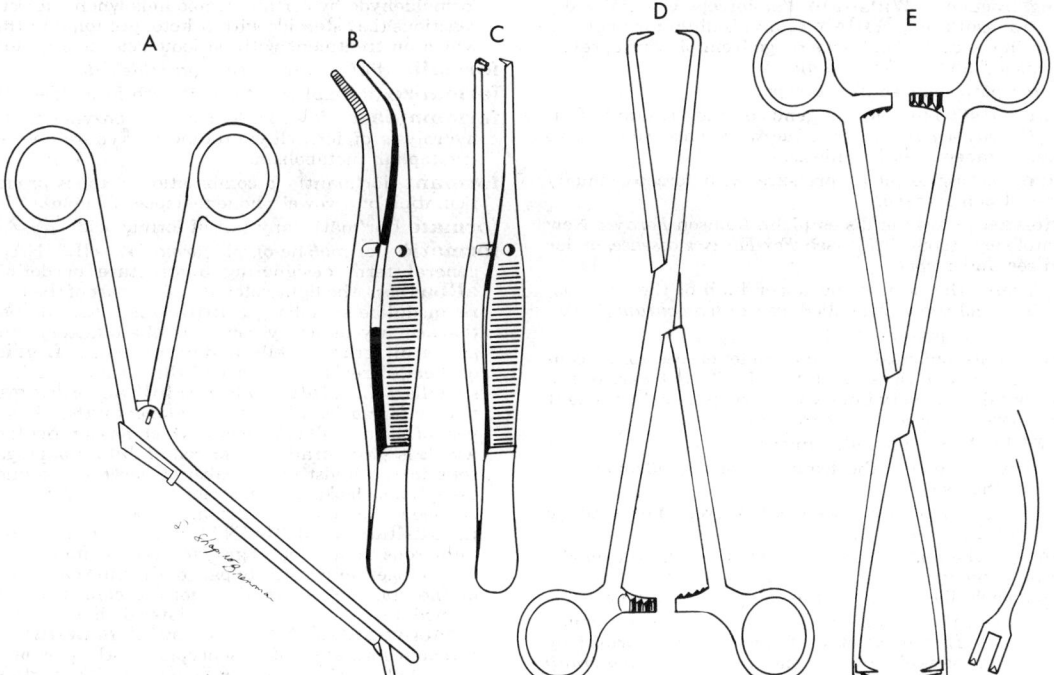

Some types of forceps: *A,* Struycken ear forceps; *B,* serrated forceps; *C,* Iris forceps, fine mouse tooth; *D,* Schroeder tenaculum forceps; *E,* Schroeder vulsellum forceps (with side view of blade).

obstetrical forceps used in midforceps delivery in the anterior position. **hemostatic f.,** forceps for controlling hemorrhage. **high f.,** see *forceps delivery, high,* under *delivery.* **Hodge's f.,** a variety of obstetrical forceps. **Kazanjian f.,** cutting forceps used for resection of the nasal dorsal hump. **Kielland's f., Kjelland's f.,** obstetrical forceps having no pelvic curve, a marked cephalic curve, and an articulation permitting a gliding movement of one blade over the other, thus allowing the blades to adapt to the sides of the fetal head when the head lies with its long diameter in the transverse diameter of the pelvis. **Knapp's f.,** forceps with roller blades, formerly used to express trachomatous granules from the conjunctiva. **Kocher's f.,** strong forceps for holding tissues during operation or for compressing bleeding tissue. **Koeberle's f.,** hemostatic f. **Laborde's f.,** forceps for grasping the tongue in Laborde's method of stimulating respiration. **Levret's f.,** modified Chamberlen forceps, curved to correspond with the curve of the parturient canal. **lithotomy f.,** forceps for removing stone from the bladder in lithotomy. **low f.,** see *forceps delivery, low,* under *delivery.* **Löwenberg's f.,** forceps for removing adenoid growths. **Luikart f.,** Garrison's f. **f. ma′jor** [NA], the terminal fibers of the corpus callosum that pass from the splenium into the occipital lobes; called also *f. posterior.* **McKenzie f.,** a forceps for applying silver clips. **mid f.,** see *midforceps delivery,* under *delivery.* **f. mi′nor** [NA], the terminal fibers of the corpus callosum that pass from the genu into the frontal lobes; called also *f. anterior.* **mosquito f.,** a small hemostatic forceps. **mouse-tooth f.,** forceps with one or more fine teeth at the tip of each blade. **obstetrical f.,** an instrument designed to extract the fetus by the head from the maternal passages without injury to it or to the mother. **Péan's f.,** a curved or straight clamp for hemostasis. **Piper f.,** a special obstetrical forceps for an aftercoming head. **point f.,** forceps used in filling root canals, which securely holds the filling cones during their placement. **f. poste′rior,** f. major. **roller f.,** forceps with a roller at the end of each blade, formerly used for compressing the granulations in trachoma; called also *trachoma f.* **rongeur f.,** a forceps designed for use in cutting bone. **sequestrum f.,** forceps with small but strong serrated jaws for removing the portions of bone forming a sequestrum. **Simpson's f.,** a form of obstetrical forceps. **speculum f.,** long slender forceps for use through a speculum. **suture f.,** forceps used to hold the needle in passing a suture; a needle holder. **Tarnier's f.,** a form of axis-traction forceps. **tenaculum f.,** forceps having a sharp hook at the end of each jaw. **thumb f.,** tissue f. **tissue f.,** forceps with one or more fine teeth at the tip of each blade, designed for handling tissues with minimal trauma during surgery; called also *thumb f.* **torsion f.,** forceps for making torsion on an artery to arrest hemorrhage. **tracheal f.,** long slender forceps for removing foreign bodies from the trachea. **trachoma f.,** roller f. **Tucker-McLean f.,** a long obstetrical forceps with a solid blade. **volsella f., vulsellum f.,** a forceps with teeth for grasping tissues and applying traction. **Walsham f's,** forceps especially designed for intranasal use. **Willett f.,** a vulsellum for applying scalp traction in the control of hemorrhage from placenta previa; called also *galea f.* and *Willet's clamp.*

forcipate (for′sĭ-pāt) shaped like forceps.

Forcipomyia (for″sĭ-po-mi′yah) a genus of midges, family Chironomidae. *F. townsen′di* and *F. u′tae* were once thought to transmit mucocutaneous leishmaniasis.

forcipressure (for′sĭ-presh-ur) pressure with forceps, chiefly for the arrest of hemorrhage.

Fordyce's disease, spot (for′dĭs-es) [John Addison *Fordyce,* New York dermatologist, 1858–1925] see *Fox-Fordyce disease,* under *disease,* and see under *spot.*

forearm (fōr′arm) the part of the upper limb of the body between the elbow and the wrist; called also *antebrachium* [NA].

forebrain (fōr′brān) prosencephalon.

foreconscious (fōr-kon′shus) 1. incapable of becoming conscious until certain conditions are fulfilled. 2. that part of the mind which contains memory impressions which may be brought into consciousness under certain conditions.

forefinger (fōr-fing′ger) the index finger.

forefoot (fōr′foot) 1. one of the front feet of a quadruped. 2. the fore part of the foot.

foregilding (fōr′gild-ing) the treatment of fresh nerve tissue with salts in histologic technique.

foregut (fōr′gut) the endodermal canal of the embryo cephalic to the junction of the yolk stalk; it gives rise to the pharynx, lung, esophagus, stomach, liver, and most of the small intestine.

forehead (fōr′hed) the part of the face above the eyes; called also *frons.* **bony f.,** the skeleton of the forehead, formed by the anterior part of the skull (frontal bone); called also *frons cranii* and *frons of cranium.*

forehead-plasty (fōr′hed-plas″te) plastic surgery of the forehead.

forekidney (fōr-kid′ne) pronephros.

Forel's commissure, decussation, field (fo-relz′) [Auguste

Henri *Forel,* Swiss psychiatrist, 1848–1931] see under *commissure, decussation,* and *field.*

forensic (fo-ren′zik) [L. *forēnsis* relating to a market place or forum] pertaining to or applied in legal proceedings.

foreplay (for′pla) the sexually stimulating, usually pleasurable play preceding intercourse.

fore-pleasure (fōr′plezh-er) sexual pleasure which precedes orgasm. Cf. *end-pleasure.*

foreskin (fōr′skin) the prepuce (preputium penis). **hooded f.,** absence of the ventral foreskin, usually associated with hypospadias.

foretop (fōr′top) the anterior portion of the mane of a horse, covering the forehead.

forewaters (fōr′wat-erz) the amniotic fluid that presents at the cervix uteri.

Forhistal (for-his′tal) trademark for preparations of dimethindene maleate.

fork (fork) a pronged instrument. **tuning f.,** a device that produces harmonic vibration when its two tines are struck; used to test hearing by air and bone conduction.

form (form) [L. *forma*] the characteristic of a structure or entity generally determined by its shape and size, or other external or visible feature. **accolé f.** (ak″o-la′), appliqué f. **appliqué f.** (ap″lĭ-ka′), the early form of *Plasmodium falciparum* which appears as a fine blue line with a chromatin dot apparently applied to the margin of an erythrocyte; called also *accolé form.* **arch f.,** the shape and contour of a dental arch. **band f's,** band cell; see under *cell.* **involution f's,** abnormal forms of bacteria arising through death of the cells and dissolution of their structure. **juvenile f.,** metamyelocyte. **L-f.,** L-phase variant; see under *variant.* **racemic f.,** see *racemate.* **retention f.,** adaptation of the form of a tooth cavity in such a way as to help maintain the filling material in the cavity. **spherical f. of occlusion,** an arrangement of teeth which places their occlusal surfaces on the surface of an imaginary sphere (usually 8 inches in diameter) with its center above the level of the teeth. **tooth f.,** the characteristic contour of a tooth, with its curves, lines, and angles, which permits the tooth to be differentiated from other teeth and its identity to be established. **young f.,** metamyelocyte.

Formad's kidney (fōr′madz) [Henry F. *Formad,* American physician, 1847–1892] see under *kidney.*

formaldehyde (fōr-mal′dĕ-hīd) a powerful disinfectant gas, HCHO, formerly used as a disinfectant for rooms, clothing, etc. A 37 per cent solution of formaldehyde gas in water (formalin) is widely used as a fixing fluid for pathologic specimens or as a preservative, and dilutions have also been used as a surgical and general antiseptic and as an astringent.

formaldehydogenic (for-mal″dĕ-hīd″o-jen′ik) [*formaldehyde* + *-genic*] producing formaldehyde; pertaining to the production of formaldehyde by certain compounds when subjected to chemical reactions (i.e., steroids with α-ketol grouping in the C-17 position which on treatment with periodic acid liberate formaldehyde).

formalin (fōr′mah-lin) see *formaldehyde.*

formalize (fōr′mal-īz) to treat with formaldehyde.

formamidase (form-am′ĭ-dās) an enzyme that catalyzes the hydrolysis of formylkynurenine to kynurenine and formate in tryptophan metabolism.

formant (fōr′mant) a combination of tones produced in the articulation of a vowel phoneme (speech sound).

formate (fōr′māt) any salt of formic acid.

formatio (for-ma′she-o), pl. *formatio′nes* [L.] [NA] formation: a general term designating a structure of definite shape. **f. al′ba** (*obs.*), the light-colored middle part of the formatio reticularis medullae spinalis. **f. bulla′ris** (*obs.*), the tissue composing the primary olfactory center in the olfactory bulb; that is, the glomeruli, granule cells, and mitral cells. **f. gris′ea** (*obs.*), the darker-colored lateral part of the formatio reticularis medullae spinalis. **f. reticula′ris medul′lae oblonga′tae** [NA], reticular formation of medulla oblongata: the phylogenetically old part of the medulla oblongata which has a reticular structure, i.e., which is structurally comprised of diffuse aggregations of nerve cells in the midst of a wealth of nerve fibers and, with certain exceptions, lacks circumscribed cell groups; it fills the spaces between the major nuclei and fiber tracts. **f. reticula′ris medul′lae spina′lis** [NA], reticular formation of spinal cord: numerous small islets of gray matter and intersecting white fibers which together constitute part of the intermediate gray substance of the spinal cord; in the thoracic cord, the formation occurs immediately dorsal to the lateral horn. **f. reticula′ris mesenceph′ali** [NA], **f. reticula′ris pedun′culi cer′ebri,** reticular formation of mesencephalon: the part of the mesencephalon that has a reticular structure like that of the medulla oblongata; it lies between the substantia nigra and the central gray matter. **f. reticula′ris pon′tis** [NA], reticular formation of pons: the part of the pars dorsalis pontis, anterior to the central gray matter, that has a structure similar to that of the reticular formation of the medulla oblongata. **f. vermicula′-**

ris (*obs.*), the tonsilla and flocculus of the cerebellum considered as one structure (Bolk).

formation (fŏr-ma′shun)   1. the process of giving shape or form; the creation of an entity, or of a structure of definite shape.   2. a structure of definite shape; see *formatio*.   **chiasma f.,** the process by which a chiasma is formed; it is the cytologic basis of genetic recombination, or crossing over.   **coffin f.,** the surrounding of dead nerve cells by satellite cells in neuronophagia.   **compromise f.,** the creation of an adjustment between a conscious intention and an unconscious opposing wish, producing the symptoms of a neurosis.   **Gothic arch f.,** Henning's sign.   **gray reticular f.,** substantia reticularis grisea medullae oblongatae.   **palisade f.,** an arrangement in cells of a glioma, the fusiform cells being arranged in compact manner pointing radially from a central area comparatively free of vessels.   **reaction f.,** the development of mental mechanisms which hold in check and repress the unconscious components of forbidden wishes.   **reticular f. of medulla oblongata,** formatio reticularis medullae oblongatae.   **reticular f. of mesencephalon,** formatio reticularis mesencephali.   **reticular f. of pons,** formatio reticularis pontis.   **reticular f. of spinal cord,** formatio reticularis medullae spinalis.   **rouleaux f.,** the aggregation of erythrocytes in structures resembling piles of coins, caused by adhesion of their flat surfaces.   **spore f.,** sporulation.   **white reticular f.,** substantia reticularis alba medullae oblongatae.

formationes (for-ma-she-o′nēz)   plural of *formatio*.

formative (fŏr′mah-tiv)   concerned in the origination and development of an organism, part, or tissue.

formboard (fŏrm′bōrd)   a board containing variously shaped cutouts into which blocks corresponding to the cutouts are to be fitted; used as a test in mental deficiency.

form-class (form-klas)   an artificial taxonomic category comparable to a class, to which organisms are provisionally assigned, as are imperfect fungi until their perfect (sexual) stages are identified. Form-classes are subdivided into form-orders, form-families, and so on.

forme (fōrm), pl. *formes* [Fr.]   form.   **f. fruste** (fōrm froost), pl. *formes frustes* [Fr. "defaced"], an atypical, especially a mild or incomplete, form, as of a disease or anomaly.   **f. tardive** (fōrm tahr-dēv′) [Fr. "late"], a late-occurring form of a disease that usually makes its appearance at an earlier age.

form-family (form-fam′ĭ-le)   see *form-class*.

formication (fōr″mĭ-ka′shun) [L. *formica* ant]   a sensation as of small insects crawling over the skin.

formiciasis (for″mĭ-si′ah-sis) [L. *formica* ant]   a condition produced by poisoning resulting from ant bites.

Formicoidea (for″mĭ-koi-de′ah)   a superfamily of ants (order Hymenoptera), some members of which may inflict painful stings.

formilase (fōr′mĭ-lās)   an enzyme that converts acetic acid into unstable formic acid.

formimino (for-mim′ĭ-no)   the group —CH=NH.

Formin (fōr′min)   trademark for preparations of methenamine.

formocortal (for-mo-kor′tal)   chemical name: 3-(2-chloroethoxy)-9-fluoro-11β,16α,17,21-tetrahydroxyl-20-oxo-pregna-3,5-diene-6-carboxaldehyde, cyclic 16,17-acetal with acetone, 21-acetate; a glucocorticoid, $C_{29}H_{38}ClFO_8$.

formol (fōr′mol)   see *formaldehyde solution*, under *solution*.

form-order (form-or′der)   see *form-class*.

formula (fŏr′mu-lah), pl. *formulas* or *formulae* [L., dim. of *forma* form]   a specific statement, using numerals and other symbols, of the composition of, or of the directions for preparing, a compound, such as a medicine, or of a procedure to follow for obtaining a desired value or result; a simplified statement, using numerals and symbols, of a single concept. See also *chemical f.*   **acoustic f.,** Brenner's f.   **Ambard's f.,** a formula for finding the urea index (*K*) in kidney disease:

$$\frac{Ur}{\sqrt{D \times \frac{70}{P}} \times \sqrt{\frac{C}{25}}} = K,$$

in which *Ur* represents the proportion of urea in the blood; *D*, the total urea for twenty-four hours in grams; *P*, the body weight of the patient in kilograms; *C*, the proportion of urea in the urine. **Arneth's f.,** an expression of the normal ratio of different types of polymorphonuclear leukocytes, depending on the number of lobes (1 to 5) that the nucleus shows, which is as follows: 1 lobe, 5 per cent; 2 lobes, 35 per cent; 3 lobes, 41 per cent; 4 lobes, 17 per cent; 5 lobes, 2 per cent.   **Arrhenius' f.,** log x = θc, in which *x* is the viscosity of the solution relative to that of the medium of suspension, *c* the percentage of volume occupied by the suspended particles, and *θ* a constant.   **Beckmann's f.,** a formula used in cryoscopy, ΔT = Km, in which Δ*T* is the difference in freezing points of the pure solvent and the solution containing a solute at molality *m*, and *K* is a constant characteristic of the particular solvent. For water, K = 1.860 deg(KgH₂O) per mole solute.   **Bernhardt's f.,** the ideal weight of an adult in kilograms equals

height in centimeters multiplied by chest circumference in centimeters divided by 240.   **Bird's f.,** the last two figures expressive of the specific gravity of urine closely represent the number of grains of solids in each ounce.   **Black's f.,** F = (W + C) – H. *W* represents the weight in pounds; *C*, the chest measurement in inches at full inspiration; and *H*, the height in inches. When *F* is over 120 a man is classed as very strong; between 110 and 120, strong; between 100 and 110, good; between 90 and 100, fair; between 80 and 90, weak; under 80, very weak. Cf. *Pignet's f.*   **Brenner's f.** (*obs.*), with the cathode in the external meatus of the ear, a loud sound is heard on closing the circuit, intensity is diminished during closure, and the sound ceases when the circuit is broken. With the anode in the meatus, no sound is heard on closing or during closure; a weak sound is heard at the break.   **Broca's f.,** the ideal weight of a full-grown man in kilograms equals the number of centimeters by which his height exceeds 1 meter.   **chemical f.,** a combination of symbols used to express the chemical constitution of a substance; in practice, different types of formulas, of varying complexity, are employed. See *empirical f., molecular f., spatial f., structural f.*   **Christison's f.,** Trapp's f.   **configurational f.,** spatial f.   **constitutional f.,** structural f.   **Demoivre's f.,** the expectation of life is equal to two thirds of the difference between the age of the person and eighty.   **dental f.,** an expression in symbols of the number and arrangement of teeth in the jaws. Letters represent the various types of teeth: I, *incisor;* C, *canine;* P, *premolar;* M, *molar.* Each letter is followed by a horizontal line. Numbers above the line represent maxillary teeth; those below, mandibular teeth. The human dental formula is $I_2^2C_1^1M_2^2 = 10$ (one side only) for deciduous teeth, and $I_2^2C_1^1P_2^2M_3^3 = 16$ (one side only) for permanent teeth.   **digital f.,** a formula expressing the relative lengths of the digits, usually 3 > 4 > 2 > 5 > 1, or 3 > 2 > 4 > 5 > 1, for the fingers, and 1 > 2 > 3 > 4 > 5, or 2 > 1 > 3 > 4 > 5, for the toes.   **Dreser's f.,** a formula comparing the molecular concentration of the urine with that of the blood, to show the work done by the kidney.   **Du Bois' f.,** the surface area, *O*, is equal to $P^{0.425} \times L^{0.725} \times 71.84$, in which *P* represents weight, and *L*, height of the body.   **Einthoven's f.,** e¹ + e³ × e². See *Einthoven's triangle*, under *triangle.*   **empirical f.,** a chemical formula which expresses the proportions of the elements present in a substance. For substances composed of discrete molecules, it expresses the relative numbers of atoms present in a molecule of the substance in the smallest whole numbers. For example, the *empirical formula* for ethane is written CH_3, whereas its actual *molecular formula* is C_2H_6.   **Fick f.,** see under *principle.*   **Florschütz's f.,** L:(2B – L), in which *L* represents body length, and *B*, circumference of abdomen. An index of 5 is normal; an index below 5 indicates the degree of overweight.   **Gale's f.,** pulse rate – pulse pressure – 111 closely represents the basal metabolic rate.   **graphic f.,** a term occasionally used to describe a "complete" structural formula, i.e., one in which every individual atom and bond is represented in the formula. The distinction is made because structural formulas are frequently written in a simplified or shortened form. See *structural f.*   **Guthrie's f.,** the ideal weight of an adult in pounds equals 110 + (5.5 × number of inches body height exceeds 5 feet).   **Haines' f.,** the product obtained by multiplying the last two digits of the number expressing its specific gravity by 1.1 (Haines' coefficient) closely represents the number of grains of solids in one fluid ounce of urine.   **Hamilton-Stewart f.,** a formula for measuring cardiac output following the rapid intravenous injection of an indicator dye: F = i/ct, in which *F* represents the blood flow in liters per minute; *i*, the injected substance in milligrams; *c*, the average dye concentration of the primary curve; and *t*, the duration of the primary curve in seconds, i.e., the time from appearance to disappearance of the dye at a fixed site if there were no recirculation of the dye.   **Häser's f.,** the product obtained by multiplying the last two digits of the number expressing its specific gravity by 2.33 (Häser's coefficient) closely represents the number of grains of solids in one liter of urine.   **Loebisch's f.,** the product obtained by multiplying the last two digits of the number expressing its specific gravity by 2.2 (Loebisch's coefficient) closely represents the number of grains of solids in one liter of urine.   **Long's f.,** the product obtained by multiplying the last two digits of the number expressing its specific gravity by 2.6 (Long's coefficient) closely represents the number of grains of solids in one liter of urine.   **McLean's f.,** a modification of Ambard's formula for finding the urea index in kidney disease:

$$\frac{\text{gm. urea per 24 hrs.} \sqrt{\text{gm. urea per L. of urine}} \times 8.96}{\text{weight in kilos} \times (\text{gm. urea per L. of blood})^2}$$

Mall's f., the age (in days) of a human embryo is equal to the square root of its length (in millimeters) from vertex to breech multiplied by 100.   **Meeh's f.,** the surface area, *O*, is equal to $K\sqrt[3]{P^2}$, in which *K* is a constant (12.3), and *P* is the weight of the body.   **molecular f.,** a chemical formula giving the number of atoms of each element present in a molecule of a substance, without indicating how they are linked.   **official f.,** one officially established by a pharmacopeia or other recognized authority.   **paretic f.,** the findings in the cerebrospinal fluid characteristic of dementia paralytica: normal or slightly increased pressure, moderate pleocytosis, moderate increase in protein, change in the colloidal gold test, and positive cerebrospinal fluid Wassermann test. **Pignet's f.,** $F = H - (C + W)$. H represents the height in centimeters; C, the chest measurement in centimeters at greatest expiration; and W, the weight in kilograms. When F is less than 10 a person is classed as very strong; between 10 and 15, strong; between 15 and 20, good; between 20 and 25, medium; between 25 and 30, weak; above 30, very weak. Cf. *Black's f.* **Poisson-Pearson f.,** a formula for calculating the percentage of error in determining the endemic index of malaria:

$$\frac{200}{n} \sqrt{\frac{2 \times (n - x)}{n}} \sqrt{1 - \frac{n - 1}{N - 1}},$$

in which N is number of children under fifteen years in the locality; n, the number examined for the spleen rate; x, the number having enlarged spleens; and x/n is the spleen rate. **projection f.,** a planar, and therefore simplified, representation of a spatial formula. **psychobiologic f.,** Meyer's term for the steps in studying and dealing with psychic disorders: What are the facts? Under what conditions do they occur? What are the factors in their working, and how do they group themselves? What are the results? How far are they modifiable? How can they be reconstructed and brought to a test? **Ranke's f.,** the number expressive of the specific gravity − 1000 × 0.52 − 5.406 closely represents the amount in grams of the albumin per liter of a serous fluid. **rational f.,** structural f. **Read's f.,** 0.75 × pulse rate + 0.75 × pulse pressure − 72 closely represents the basal metabolic rate. **Reuss' f.,** $\frac{3}{8}(S - 1000) - 2.8$, in which S is the specific gravity, closely represents the percentage of albumin present in a pathologic fluid exudate or transudate. **Rollier's f.,** a formula for gradually increasing exposure of the body to ultraviolet rays of the sun. **Runeberg's f.,** a modification of Reuss' formula in which 2.8 is replaced by 2.73 in case of a transudate and by 2.88 in case of an inflammatory exudate. **spatial f.,** a chemical formula giving the numbers of atoms of each element present in a molecule of a substance, which atom is linked to which, the types of linkages involved, and the relative positions of the atoms in space. **stereochemical f.,** spatial f. **structural f.,** a chemical formula telling how many atoms of

Structural formulas for ethyl alcohol.

each element are present in a molecule of a substance, which atom is linked to which, and the type of linkages involved; for convenience, abbreviated structural formulas are sometimes used. Called also *constitutional f., graphic f.,* and *rational f.* **Trapp's f.,** the product obtained by multiplying the last two digits of the number expressing its specific gravity by 2 (Trapp's coefficient) closely represents the number of grains of solids in one liter of urine. **Van Slyke's f.,** the urinary coefficient of various substances is equal to $D/(Bl \times \sqrt{Wt \times V})$, in which D is the daily output in grams of the substance in the urine; Bl, the grams of the same substance per liter of blood; Wt, the weight of the patient in kilograms; and V, the total volume of urine in twenty-four hours. **vertebral f.,** an expression in symbols of the number of vertebrae in each region of the spinal column; for man it is $C_7T_{12}L_5S_5Cd_4 = 33$. **Vierordt-Mesh f.,** the body surface, O, is equal to $mP_3^{\frac{2}{3}}$, in which m represents the height, and P the weight.

formulary (fŏr′mu-lār″e) a collection of recipes, formulas, and prescriptions. **National F.,** see under *N.*

formulate (fŏr′mu-lāt) 1. to state in the form of a formula. 2. to prepare in accordance with a prescribed or specified method.

formulation (fŏr″mu-la′shun) the act or product of formulating. **American Law Institute f.,** a section of the American Law Institute's Model Penal Code which states that "a person is not responsible for criminal conduct if at the time of such conduct as a result of mental disease or defect he lacks substantial capacity either to appreciate the wrongfulness of his conduct or to conform his conduct to the requirement of the law."

formyl (fŏr′mil) [L. *formic* + Gr. *hylē* matter] the radical, HCO or H·C:O—, of formic acid. **f. phenetidin,** colorless crystals, para-ethoxyformanilid, $C_2H_5O \cdot C_6H_4 \cdot NH \cdot COH$, formerly used as an antiseptic and analgesic.

formylase (form′ĭ-lās) formamidase.

formylporphyrin (for″mil-por′fĭ-rin) the form of porphyrin that in combination with iron acts as the prosthetic heme group of cytochrome *a.*

formyltransferase (for″mil-trans′fer-ās) an enzyme that catalyzes the transfer of a formyl group, as from glutamate to tetrahydrofolate.

Fornet's reaction (ring test) (fŏr-nāz′) [Walter Gustav Wilhelm *Fornet,* German physician, born 1877] see under *reaction.*

fornicate (fŏr′nĭ-kāt) 1. [L. *fornicatus* arched] shaped like an arch. 2. [L. *fornix,* a brothel] to engage in illicit sexual intercourse.

fornix (for′niks), pl. *for′nices* [L. "arch"] 1. [NA] a general term for an archlike structure or the vaultlike space created by such a structure. 2. fornix cerebri. **anterior f.,** see *f. vaginae.* **f. cer′ebri** [NA], **f. of cerebrum,** the efferent pathway of the hippocampus, projecting chiefly to the mamillary bodies and habenular nuclei; each fornix of the pathway is an arched tract that is united under the corpus callosum with the other fornix, so that together they comprise two columns, a body, and two crura. **f. conjuncti′vae infe′rior** [NA], inferior conjunctival fornix: the inferior line of reflection of the conjunctiva from the eyelid to the eyeball. **f. conjuncti′vae supe′rior** [NA], superior conjunctival fornix: the superior line of reflection of the conjunctiva from the eyelid to the eyeball; it receives the openings of the lacrimal duct. **f. pharyn′gis** [NA], **f. of pharynx,** the vault of the pharynx. **posterior f.,** see *f. vaginae.* **f. sac′ci lacrima′lis** [NA], fornix of lacrimal sac: the upper, blind extremity of the lacrimal sac. **f. vagi′nae** [NA], the recess formed between the vaginal wall and the vaginal part of the cervix; sometimes spoken of as *anterior f.* or *posterior f.,* depending on its relation to the anterior or posterior wall of the vagina; called also *fundus vaginae* or *fundus of vagina.*

Foroblique (fŏr″ob-lek′) trademark for an obliquely forward visual telescopic system used in certain cystoscopes.

Forssell's sinus (fŏr′selz) [Gösta *Forssell,* Swedish radiologist, 1876–1950] see under *sinus.*

Forssman's antigen (lipoid), syndrome (fŏrs′manz) [John *Forssman,* Swedish pathologist, 1868–1947] see under *antigen* and *syndrome.*

Forssmann (fors′man), Werner Theodor Otto. German surgeon, born 1904; co-winner, with André F. Cournand and Dickinson W. Richards, of the Nobel prize in medicine and physiology for 1956, for developing new techniques in the diagnosis and treatment of heart disease.

Förster's choroiditis (disease), photometer (fers′terz) [Carl Friedrich Richord *Förster,* German ophthalmologist, 1825–1902] see under *choroiditis,* and see *photoptometer.*

Förster's operation (fers′terz) [Otfrid *Förster,* German neurologist, 1873–1941] see under *operation.*

Förster-Penfield operation (fers′ter-pen′fĕld) [Otfrid *Förster;* Wilder Graves *Penfield,* American neurosurgeon, born 1891] see under *operation.*

Forthane (for′thān) trademark for a preparation of methylhexaneamine.

fortuitous (fŏr-tu′ĭ-tus) pertaining to or occurring by chance.

fosazepam (fos-az′ĕ-pam) chemical name: 7-chloro-1-[(dimethylphosphinyl)methyl]-1,3-dihydro-5-phenyl-2H-1,4-benzodiazepin-2-one. A benzodiazepine derivatrive, $C_{18}H_{18}ClN_2O_2P$, which has been used as a hypnotic.

fosfomycin (fos-fo-mi′sin) chemical name: (−)-(1R,2S)-(1,2-epoxypropyl)phosphonic acid; an antibiotic, $C_3H_7O_4P$, produced by *Streptomyces fradiae.*

fosfonet sodium (fos′fo-net) chemical name: phosphonoacetic acid monosodium salt monohydrate; an antiviral agent, $C_2H_3Na_2O_5P \cdot H_2O$.

Foshay's reaction, serum, test [Lee *Foshay,* American bacteriologist, born 1896] see under *reaction, serum,* and *tests.*

fospirate (fos′pĭ-rāt) chemical name: dimethyl 3,5,6-trichloro-2-pyridinyl ester; an anthelmintic for veterinary use, $C_7H_7Cl_3NO_4P$.

fossa (fos′ah), pl. *fos′sae* [L.] a trench or channel; [NA] a general term for a hollow or depressed area. **acetabular f., f. acetab′uli** [NA], a rough nonarticular area in the floor of the acetabulum above the acetabular notch. **adipose fossae,** spaces in the female breast, just beneath the skin, which contain fat. **Allen's f.** (*obs.*), a fossa on the neck of the femur. **anconal f., anconeal f.,** f. olecrani. **antecubital f.,** f. cubitalis. **f. anthel′icis** [NA], **f. of antihelix,** the depression on the medial surface of the auricle of the ear that corresponds to the anthelix on the lateral surface. **articular f. of atlas, inferior,** fovea articularis inferior atlantis. **articular f. of atlas, superior,** fovea articularis superior atlantis. **articular f. of mandible,** f. mandibularis. **articular f. for odontoid process of axis,** fovea dentis atlantis. **articular f. of temporal bone,** f. mandibularis. **f. axilla′ris** [NA], **axillary f.,** the small hollow, underneath the arm, where it joins the body at the shoulder; called also *armpit.* **Biesiadecki's f.,** f. iliacosubfascialis. **Broesike's f.,** parajejunal f. **f. caeca′lis,** a peritoneal recess at the beginning medial to and behind the cecum; it is formed by the cecal folds. **f. cani′na** [NA], **canine f.,** a wide depression on the external surface of the maxilla superolateral to the canine tooth socket; the levator anguli oris muscle arises from it. Called also *maxillary f.* **f. capitel′li,** the depression for the head of the malleus. **f. cap′itis fem′oris,** fovea capitis femoris. **f. carot′ica,** trigonum caroticum.

cerebellar f. (*obs.*), f. cranii posterior. **cerebral f.,** any one of the depressions on the floor of the cranial cavity; see *f. cranii anterior, f. cranii media,* and *f. cranii posterior.* **f. cer'ebri latera'lis [Syl'vil],** f. lateralis cerebri. **f. chor'dae duc'tus veno'si,** f. ductus venosi. **cochleariform f.,** semicanalis musculi tensoris tympani. **condylar f., f. condyla'ris** [NA], **condyloid f.,** either of two pits situated on the lateral portions of the occipital bone, one on either side of the foramen magnum, posterior to the occipital condyle; called also *f. condyloidea, postcondyloid f.,* and *posterior condyloid f.* **condyloid f., posterior,** f. condylaris. **condyloid f. of atlas,** fovea articularis superior atlantis. **condyloid f. of mandible,** f. mandibularis. **condyloid f. of temporal bone,** f. mandibularis. **f. condyloi'dea,** f. condylaris. **coronoid f. of humerus, f. coronoi'dea hu'meri** [NA], the cavity in the humerus that receives the coronoid process of the ulnar when the elbow is flexed. **f. of coronoid process,** f. coronoidea humeri. **costal f., inferior,** fovea costalis inferior. **costal f., superior,** fovea costalis superior. **costal f., transverse,** fovea costalis transversalis. **cranial f., anterior,** f. cranii anterior. **cranial f., middle,** f. cranii media. **cranial f., posterior,** f. cranii posterior. **f. cra'nii ante'rior** [NA], anterior cranial fossa: the anterior subdivision of the floor of the cranial cavity, supporting the frontal lobes of the brain, and composed of portions of three bones: the ethmoid, frontal, and sphenoid. **f. cra'nii me'dia** [NA], middle cranial fossa: the middle subdivision of the floor of the cranial cavity, supporting the temporal lobes of the brain and the pituitary gland; it is composed of the body and greater wings of the sphenoid bone and the squamous and petrous portions of the temporal bone. **f. cra'nii poste'rior** [NA], posterior cranial fossa: the posterior subdivision of the floor of the cranial cavity, lodging the cerebellum, pons, and medulla oblongata; it is formed by portions of the sphenoid, temporal, parietal, and occipital bones. **crural f.,** anulus femoralis. **cubital f.,** 1. fossa cubitalis. 2. fossa coronoidea humeri. **f. cubita'lis** [NA], cubital fossa: the depression in the anterior region of the elbow. **f. cys'tidis fel'leae,** f. vesicae felleae. **digastric f.,** 1. fossa digastrica. 2. incisura mastoidea ossis temporalis. **f. digas'trica** [NA], digastric fossa: a depression on the internal surface of the body of the mandible on each side of the symphysis to which is attached the anterior belly of the digastric muscle; called also *f. musculi biventeris,* and *digastric fovea* or *impression.* **digital f. of femur,** f. trochanterica. **digital f., inferior,** anulus femoralis. **digital f., superior,** f. inguinalis lateralis. **f. duc'tus veno'si** [NA], **f. of ductus venosus,** an impression on the posterior part of the diaphragmatic surface of the liver in the fetus, lodging the ductus venosus. **duodenal f., inferior,** recessus duodenalis inferior. **duodenal f., superior,** recessus duodenalis superior. **duodenojejunal f.,** recessus duodenalis superior. **epigastric f.,** 1. fossa epigastrica. 2. the urachal fossa. **f. epigas'trica** [NA], epigastric fossa: a fossa in the epigastric region; called also *scrobiculus cordis* and *fovea cardiaca.* **ethmoid f.,** a groove situated in the cribriform plate of the ethmoid bone; it lodges the olfactory bulb of the brain. Called also *olfactory f.* or *groove.* **f. of eustachian tube,** f. scaphoidea ossis sphenoidalis. **femoral f.,** anulus femoralis. **floccular f.,** f. subarcuata ossis temporalis. **f. of gallbladder,** f. vesicae felleae. **f. of gasserian ganglion,** impressio trigemini ossis temporalis. **Gerdy's hyoid f.,** superior carotid triangle. **f. glan'dulae lacrima'lis** [NA], fossa of lacrimal gland: a shallow depression in the lateral part of the roof of the orbit, lodging the lacrimal gland; called also *lacrimal f.* **glandular f. of frontal bone,** f. glandulae lacrimalis. **glenoid f.,** f. mandibularis. **glenoid f. of scapula,** cavitas glenoidalis. **glenoid f. of temporal bone,** f. mandibularis. **greater f. of Scarpa,** trigonum femorale. **Gruber's f.,** a diverticulum of the suprasternal space alongside of the inner end of the clavicle. **Gruber-Landzert f.,** a recess in the peritoneum in the same situation as the superior duodenal recess, but extending downward behind the duodenojejunal angle. **harderian f.,** the depression in which the harderian glands are lodged. **f. of head of femur,** fovea capitis femoris. **f. hel'icis,** scapha. **f. hemiellip'tica,** recessus ellipticus vestibuli. **f. hemisphe'rica,** recessus sphericus vestibuli. **hyaloid f., f. hyaloi'dea** [NA], a depression on the anterior surface of the vitreous body, in which the lens is lodged; called also *lenticular f. of vitreous body.* **hypogastric f.,** f. inguinalis medialis. **hypophyseal f., f. hypophys'eos, f. hypophysia'lis** [NA], a deep depression in the middle of the sella turcica of the sphenoid bone, lodging the hypophysis cerebri; called also *pituitary f.* and *sellar f.* **ileocecal f., inferior,** recessus ileocecalis inferior. **ileocecal f., superior,** recessus ileocecalis superior. **ileocolic f.,** recessus ileocecalis superior. **iliac f., f. ili'aca** [NA], a large, smooth concave area occupying much of the inner surface of the ala of the ilium, especially anteriorly; from it arises the iliacus muscle. **iliacosubfascial f., f. iliacosubfascia'lis,** an inconstant depression on the inner surface of the abdomen between the psoas muscle and the crest of the ilium; called also *Biesiadecki's f.* **f. iliopecti'nea, iliopectineal f.,** a depression between the iliopsoas and pectineus muscles in the center of the femoral triangle; called also *lesser f. of Scarpa.*

implantation f., a shallow depression at the site where the tail of a spermatozoon attaches to the head. **incisive f. of maxilla,** a slight depression on the anterior surface of the maxilla above the incisor teeth; called also *myrtiform f., f. praenasalis,* and *prenasal f.* **incudal f., f. incu'dis** [NA], **f. of incus,** a groove in the posterior wall of the tympanic cavity, lodging the short limb of the incus. **infraclavicular f.,** trigonum deltoideopectorale. **infraduodenal f.,** a recess in the peritoneum below the third portion of the duodenum. **f. infraspina'ta** [NA], **infraspinous f.,** the large, slightly concave area below the spinous process on the dorsal surface of the scapula; it is the site of origin of the infraspinatus muscle. **infratemporal f., f. infratempora'lis** [NA], the area on the side of the cranium limited superiorly by the infratemporal crest, posteriorly by the mandibular fossa, anteriorly by the infratemporal surface of the maxilla, and laterally by the zygomatic arch and part of the ramus of the mandible; called also *zygomatic f.* **inguinal f., external,** f. inguinalis lateralis. **inguinal f., internal,** f. inguinalis medialis. **inguinal f., lateral,** f. inguinalis lateralis. **inguinal f., medial, inguinal f., middle,** f. inguinalis medialis. **f. inguina'lis latera'lis** [NA], lateral inguinal fossa: the depression on the inside of the anterior abdominal wall lateral to the lateral umbilical fold; called also *fovea inguinalis lateralis* and *lateral inguinal fovea.* **f. inguina'lis media'lis** [NA], medial inguinal fossa: the depression on the inside of the anterior abdominal wall between the medial and lateral umbilical folds; called also *fovea inguinalis medialis.* **innominate f. of auricle,** cavum conchae. **intercondylar f. of femur,** f. intercondylaris femoris. **intercondylar f. of femur, anterior,** facies patellaris femoris. **intercondylar f. of tibia, anterior,** area intercondylaris anterior tibiae. **intercondylar f. of tibia, posterior,** area intercondylaris posterior tibiae. **f. intercondyla'ris fem'oris** [NA], intercondylar fossa of femur: the posterior depression between the condyles of the femur; called also *f. intercondyloidea femoris.* **f. intercondyl'ica,** intercondylaris femoris. **intercondyloid f.,** see *f. intercondylaris femoris, area intercondylaris anterior tibiae,* and *area intercondylaris posterior tibiae.* **f. intercondyloi'dea ante'rior tib'iae,** area intercondylaris anterior tibiae. **f. intercondyloi'dea fem'oris,** f. intercondylaris femoris. **f. intercondyloi'dea poste'rior tib'iae,** area intercondylaris posterior tibiae. **f. intercrura'lis,** f. interpeduncularis. **f. intermesocol'ica transver'sa,** a recess of the peritoneum in the same situation as the recessus duodenalis superior, but extending transversely. **interpeduncular f., f. interpeduncula'ris** [NA], **f. interpeduncula'ris [Tari'ni],** a depression between the two cerebral peduncles, the floor of which is the posterior perforated substance; called also *Tarin's f.* and *f. intercruralis.* **intersigmoid f.,** recessus intersigmoideus. **ischiorectal f., f. ischiorecta'lis** [NA], the potential space between the pelvic diaphragm and the skin below it; an anterior recess extends a variable distance between the pelvic and urogenital diaphragms, sometimes reaching the retropubic space. **Jobert's f.,** the fossa in the popliteal region bounded above by the adductor magnus and below by the gracilis and sartorius, best seen when the knee is bent and the thigh strongly rotated outward. **f. of Jonnesco,** the duodenojejunal fossa between the superior and inferior duodenal folds. **jugular f., f. jugula'ris,** 1. the depression at the base of the neck just above the sternum; called also *suprasternal space.* 2. jugular f. of temporal bone. **jugular f. of temporal bone, f. jugula'ris os'sis tempora'lis** [NA], a prominent depression on the inferior surface of the petrous part of the temporal bone, forming the major part of the jugular notch; it forms the anterior and lateral wall of the jugular foramen and lodges the superior bulb of the internal jugular vein. **lacrimal f.,** 1. fossa glandulae lacrimalis. 2. sulcus lacrimalis ossis lacrimalis. **f. of lacrimal gland,** f. glandulae lacrimalis. **f. of lacrimal sac,** f. sacci lacrimalis. **Landzert's f.,** recessus paraduodenalis. **lateral f. of cerebrum,** f. lateralis cerebri. **f. of lateral malleolus,** f. malleoli lateralis. **f. latera'lis cer'ebri** [NA], lateral fossa of cerebrum: a depression, in fetal life, on the lateral surface of each cerebral hemisphere at the bottom of which lies the insula; later it is closed over by the operculum, the edges of which form the lateral sulcus. Called also *f. cerebri lateralis [Sylvii]* and *f. of Sylvius.* **lenticular f., lenticular f. of vitreous body,** f. hyaloidea. **lesser f. of Scarpa,** f. iliopectinea. **f. for ligamentum teres,** fissura ligamenti teretis. **f. of little head of radius,** fovea capituli radii. **longitudinal fossae of liver, right,** fossae sagittales dextrae hepatis. **f. longitudina'lis hep'atis,** f. sagittalis sinistra hepatis. **Luschka's f.,** recessus ileocecalis superior. **Malgaigne's f.,** see *carotid triangle, superior,* under *triangle.* **f. malle'oli latera'lis** [NA], fossa of lateral malleolus: a depression on the medial aspect of the lateral malleolus behind its articular surface. **mandibular f., f. mandibula'ris** [NA], a prominent depression in the inferior surface of the squamous part of the temporal bone at the base of the zygomatic process, in which the condyloid process of the mandible rests. **mastoid f. of temporal bone,** a small triangular area between the posterior wall of the external acoustic meatus and the posterior root of the zygomatic process of the temporal bone; called also *suprameatal triangle.* **maxillary**

f., f. canina. **mesentericoparietal f.,** parajejunal f. **mesocranial f.** (obs.), f. cranii media. **mesogastric f.,** recessus duodenalis superior. **middle cranial f.,** f. cranii media. **Mohrenheim's f.,** trigonum deltoideopectorale. **f. of Morgagni,** f. navicularis urethrae. **f. mus′culi biven′teris,** f. digastrica. **mylohyoid f. of mandible,** fovea sublingualis. **myrtiform f.,** incisive f. of maxilla. **nasal f.,** the portion of the nasal cavity anterior to the middle meatus. **navicular f. of Cruveilhier,** f. scaphoidea ossis sphenoidalis. **navicular f. of male urethra,** f. navicularis urethrae. **navicular f. of sphenoid bone,** f. scaphoidea ossis sphenoidalis. **f. navicula′ris ure′thrae** [NA], **f. navicula′ris ure′thrae** [Morgag′nii], the lateral expansion of the urethra in the glans penis. **f. navicula′ris** [vestib′uli vagi′nae], f. vestibuli vaginae. **f. occipita′lis cerebra′lis** (obs.), f. lateralis cerebri. **f. olec′rani** [NA], **olecranon f.,** a depression on the posterior surface of the humerus, above the trochlea, for lodging the olecranon of the ulna when the elbow is extended. **olfactory f.,** ethmoid f. **f. of omental sac, inferior,** recessus inferior omentalis. **f. of omental sac, superior,** recessus superior omentalis. **oral f.,** stomodeum. **oval f. of heart,** f. ovalis cordis. **oval f. of thigh,** hiatus saphenus. **f. ova′lis,** recessus ellipticus vestibuli. **f. ova′lis cor′dis** [NA], oval f. of heart: a depression on the right side of the interatrial septum of the heart, representing the remains of the fetal foramen ovale. **f. ova′lis fem′oris,** hiatus saphenus. **ovarian f., f. ova′rica,** a shallow pouch on the posterior surface of the broad ligament, in which the ovary is located. **paraduodenal f.,** recessus duodenalis superior. **parajejunal f.,** a pouch of peritoneum below the lower end of the first part of the jejunum. **parietal f.,** the deepest portion of the inner surface of the parietal bone. **patellar f.,** f. hyaloidea. **patellar f. of femur,** facies patellaris femoris. **patellar f. of tibia,** area intercondylaris anterior tibiae. **perineal f.,** f. ischiorectalis. **petrosal f., f. for petrosal ganglion,** fossula petrosa. **piriform f.,** recessus piriformis. **pituitary f.,** f. hypophysialis. **f. poplit′ea** [NA], **popliteal f.,** the depression in the posterior region of the knee; called also popliteal cavity. **popliteal f. of femur,** f. intercondylaris femoris. **popliteal f. of tibia,** area intercondylaris posterior tibiae. **postcondyloid f.,** f. condylaris. **posterior f. of humerus,** f. olecrani. **f. praenasa′lis, prenasal f.,** incisive f. of maxilla. **prescapular f., prespinous f.,** a depression in the anterior surface of the spine of the scapula. **pterygoid f. of inferior maxillary bone,** fovea pterygoidea mandibulae. **pterygoid f. of sphenoid bone,** f. pterygoi′dea os′sis sphenoida′lis [NA], the posteriorly facing fossa which is formed by the divergence of the medial and lateral pterygoid plates of the sphenoid bone, and lodges the origins of the internal pterygoid muscle and tensor veli palatini muscle. **pterygomaxillary f.,** f. pterygopalatina. **f. pterygopalati′na** [NA], **pterygopalatine f.,** a small space between the front of the root of the pterygoid process of the sphenoid bone and the back of the maxilla. **radial f. of humerus, f. radia′lis hu′meri** [NA], a depression on the anterior surface of the humerus just above the capitulum. **retrocecal f.,** recessus retrocecalis. **retroduodenal f.,** a pouch of peritoneum below and behind the third portion of the duodenum. **retromandibular f., f. retromandibula′ris,** the depression posterior to the angle of the jaw, on either side, inferior to the auricle. **rhomboid f., f. rhomboi′dea** [NA], the floor of the fourth ventricle of the brain, made up of the dorsal surfaces of the medulla oblongata and pons. **Rosenmüller's f.,** recessus pharyngeus. **f. sac′ci lacrima′lis** [NA], the fossa that lodges the lacrimal sac, formed by the lacrimal sulcus of the lacrimal bone and the frontal process of the maxilla; called also lacrimal groove. **fossae sagitta′les dex′trae hep′atis,** a longitudinal fissure in the right lobe of the liver. **fossae sagitta′les hep′atis,** f. sagittalis sinistra hepatis. **f. sagitta′lis sinis′tra hep′atis,** a longitudinal fissure in the left lobe of the liver, composed of the fossa venae umbilicalis in front and the fossa ductus venosi dorsally. **scaphoid f., f. scaphoi′dea,** 1. scapha. 2. fossa triangularis auriculae. **scaphoid f. of sphenoid bone, f. scaphoi′dea os′sis sphenoida′lis** [NA], a depression on the superior part of the posterior portion of the medial plate of the pterygoid process of the sphenoid bone, giving attachment to the tensor veli palatini muscle. **f. scar′pae ma′jor,** trigonum femorale. **sellar f.,** f. hypophysialis. **semilunar f. of ulna,** incisura trochlearis ulnae. **sigmoid f.,** sulcus sinus transversi. **sigmoid f. of temporal bone,** sulcus sinus sigmoidei ossis temporalis. **sigmoid f. of ulna,** incisura trochlearis ulnae. **sigmoid f. of ulna, lesser,** incisura radialis ulnae. **sphenomaxillary f.,** f. pterygopalatina. **splenic f. of omental sac,** recessus lienalis. **f. subarcua′ta os′sis tempora′lis** [NA], **subarcuate f. of temporal bone,** a small fossa on the internal surface of the petrous part of the temporal bone just below the arcuate eminence, most prominent in the fetus. In the adult it lodges a piece of dura and transmits a small vein. **subcecal f.,** recessus ileocecalis inferior. **f. subinguina′lis,** a dpression in the anterior surface of the thigh beneath the groin. **sublingual f.,** fovea sublingualis. **submandibular f.,** fovea submandibularis. **submaxillary f.,**

fovea submandibularis. **subpyramidal f.,** a fossa on the inferior wall of the middle ear, inferior to the round window and posterior to the pyramid. **subscapular f., f. subscapula′ris** [NA], the concave ventral surface of the body of the scapula. **subsigmoid f.,** a fossa between the mesentery of the sigmoid flexure and that of the descending colon. **supraclavicular f., greater,** f. supraclavicularis major. **supraclavicular f., lesser,** f. supraclavicularis minor. **f. supraclavicula′ris ma′jor** [NA], greater supraclavicular fossa: a depression on the surface of the body, located above and behind the clavicle, lateral to the tendon of the sternocleidomastoid muscle. **f. supraclavicula′ris mi′nor** [NA], lesser supraclavicular fossa: the region of the neck in the depression behind the clavicle, about the interval between the two tendons of the sternocleidomastoid muscle; called also Zang's space. **supracondyloid f.,** a depression on the femur between the internal tuberosity and the internal supracondyloid tubercle. **supramastoid f.,** a small depression at the junction of the posterior and superior borders of the external auditory canal. **suprasphenoidal f.,** f. hypophysialis. **f. supraspina′ta** [NA], **supraspinous f.,** the deeply concave area above the spinous process on the dorsal surface of the scapula from which the supraspinous muscle takes origin. **supratonsillar f., f. supratonsilla′ris** [NA], the space between the palatoglossal and palatopharyngeal arches superior to the tonsil. **supratrochlear f., posterior,** f. olecrani. **supravesical f., f. supravesica′lis** [NA], the depression on the inside of the anterior abdominal wall between the median and the medial umbilical fold; called also fovea supravesicalis peritonaei. **sylvian f., f. of Sylvius,** 1. fossa lateralis cerebri. 2. sulcus lateralis cerebri. **Tarin's f.,** f. interpeduncularis. **temporal f.,** 1. fossa temporalis. 2. fossa cranii media. **f. tempora′lis** [NA], temporal fossa: the area on the side of the cranium outlined posteriorly and superiorly by the temporal lines, anteriorly by the frontal and zygomatic bones, laterally by the zygomatic arch, and inferiorly by the infratemporal crest. **terminal f.,** f. navicularis urethrae. **tibiofemoral f.,** a palpable space between the articular surfaces of the tibia and femur mesial (internal tibiofemoral f.) or lateral (external tibiofemoral f.) to the inferior pole of the patella. **tonsillar f., f. tonsilla′ris** [NA], the depression between the palatoglossal and palatopharyngeal arches in which the palatine tonsil is located; called also sinus tonsillaris and tonsillar sinus. **f. transversa′lis hep′atis,** porta hepatis. **f. of Treitz,** recessus duodenalis superior. **triangular f. of auricle, f. triangular′is auric′ulae** [NA], the cavity just above the concha of the ear between the crura of the anthelix. **trochanteric f., f. trochanter′ica** [NA], a deep depression on the medial surface of the greater trochanter that receives the insertion of the tendon of the obturator externus muscle. **trochlear f., f. trochlea′ris,** fovea trochlearis. **ulnar f.,** f. coronoidea humeri. **umbilical f., medial,** f. inguinalis medialis. **f. umbilica′lis hep′atis,** fissura ligamenti teretis. **urachal f.,** a depression on the inner surface of the anterior abdominal wall, between the urachus and the hypogastric artery; called also epigastric f. **f. ve′nae ca′vae,** sulcus venae cavae. **f. ve′nae umbilica′lis,** fissura ligamenti teretis. **f. vesi′cae fel′leae** [NA], the fossa on the posteroinferior surface of the liver that lodges the gallbladder; it helps separate the left and right lobes. Called also f. of gallbladder. **vestibular f., f. of vestibule of vagina, f. vestib′uli vagi′nae** [NA], the part of the vestibule between the orifice of the vagina and the frenulum of the pudendal labia; called also f. navicularis [vestibuli vaginae]. **Waldeyer's f.,** the recessus duodenalis inferior and recessus duodenalis superior considered as one space. **zygomatic f.,** f. infratemporalis.

fossae (fos′e) [L.] plural of fossa.

fossette (fos-set′) [Fr.] 1. a small depression. 2. a small and deep corneal ulcer.

fossil (fos′il) [L. fossilis to dig] any remains of an organism that has been preserved in the earth's crust.

fossula (fos′u-lah), pl. fos′sulae [L., dim. of fossa] a small fossa; [NA] a general term for a slight depression in the surface of a structure or organ. **f. of cochlear window,** f. fenestrae cochleae. **costal f., inferior,** fovea costalis inferior. **costal f., superior,** fovea costalis superior. **f. fenes′trae coch′leae** [NA], fenestra of cochlea: a depression on the medial wall of the tympanic cavity, at the bottom of which is the fenestra cochleae; called also f. of round window. **f. fenes′trae vestib′uli** [NA], fenestra of vestibule: a depression on the medial wall of the tympanic cavity, at the bottom of which is the fenestra vestibuli; called also f. of oval window and niche of oval window. **f. of oval window,** f. fenestrae vestibuli. **f. petro′sa** [NA], **petrosal f., f. of petrous ganglion,** a small depression on the under surface of the petrous portion of the temporal bone, on a small ridge separating the jugular fossa from the external carotid foramen. **f. post fenes′tram,** a connective tissue tract just behind the oval window, resembling the fissula ante fenestram, but smaller and less constant. **f. of round window,** f. fenestrae cochleae. **tonsillar fossulae of palatine tonsil,** fossulae tonsillares tonsillae palatinae. **tonsillar fossulae of pharyngeal tonsil,** fossulae tonsillares tonsillae pharyngeae. **fos′sulae tonsilla′res tonsil′lae palati′nae** [NA], tonsillar fossulae of palatine tonsil: the mouths of the tonsillar crypts of the palatine tonsils. **fos′sulae tonsilla′res tonsil′lae pharyn′geae** [NA], tonsillar fossulae of pharyngeal tonsil: the mouths of the tonsillar crypts of the pharyngeal tonsil.

fossulae (fos′u-le) [L.] plural of *fossula.*

fossulate (fos′u-lāt) marked by a small fossa; hollowed or grooved.

Foster Kennedy see *Kennedy.*

Fothergill's disease (sore throat), neuralgia, pill (foth′er-gilz) [John *Fothergill,* English physician, 1712–1780] see *scarlatina anginosa* and *trigeminal neuralgia,* under *neuralgia,* and see under *pill.*

Fothergill's operation (foth′er-gilz) [William Edward *Fothergill,* Manchester gynecologist, 1865–1926] see under *operation.*

Fouchet's test (foo-shāz′) [André *Fouchet,* French chemist, born 1894] see under *tests.*

foudroyant (foo″drah-yaw′) [Fr.] fulminant.

foulage (foo-lahzh′) [Fr. "treading, pressing of grapes"] massage in which the muscles are kneaded and pressed; called also *pétrissage.*

foulbrood (fowl′brood) a contagious disease of honeybees caused by *Bacillus alvei.*

foundation (fown-da′shun) the structure or basis on which something is built. **denture f.,** the portion of the structures and tissues of the mouth that is available to support a denture.

founder (fown′der) the crippled condition of a horse afflicted with laminitis. **chest f.,** founder accompanied by atrophy of the chest muscles. **grain f.,** a condition of indigestion or overloaded stomach in the horse due to overeating.

fourchette (foor-shet′) [Fr. "a fork-shaped object"] frenulum labiorum pudendi.

Fournier's disease, etc. (foor-ne-āz′) [Jean Alfred *Fournier,* dermatologist in Paris, 1832–1914] see under *disease, sign, tests,* and *treatment.*

fovea (fo′ve-ah), pl. *fo′veae* [L.] a pit or depression; [NA] a general term for a small pit in the surface of a structure or organ. Often used alone to indicate the central fovea of the retina. **anterior f. of humerus, greater,** fossa coronoidea humeri. **anterior f. of humerus, lesser,** fossa radialis humeri. **articular foveae for rib cartilages,** incisurae costales sterni. **articular f. of temporal bone,** fossa mandibularis. **f. articula′ris infe′rior atlan′tis** [NA], inferior articular fovea of atlas: either of the two inferior articular surfaces (facies articulares atlantis) found on the lateral masses of the atlas; called also *inferior articular facet* or *fossa of atlas.* **f. articula′ris supe′rior atlan′tis** [NA], either of the two superior articular surfaces (facies articulares superiores atlantis) found on the lateral masses of the atlas; called also *superior articular surface, facet,* or *fossa of atlas,* and *condyloid fossa of atlas.* **calcaneal f.,** sulcus calcanei. **f. cap′itis fem′oris** [NA], fovea of head of femur: a depression in the head of the femur where the ligamentum teres is attached; called also *fossa capitis femoris* and *fossa of head of femur.* **f. capit′uli ra′dii,** a shallow cup on the upper surface of the head of the radius for articulation with the capitulum of the humerus. **f. cardi′aca,** fossa epigastrica. **central f. of retina, f. centra′lis ret′inae** [NA], a tiny pit, about 1 degree wide, in the center of the macula lutea, composed of slim, elongated cones; it is the area of clearest vision, because here the layers of the retina are spread aside, permitting light to fall directly on the cones. Called also *Soemmering's foramen.* **f. of condyloid process,** f. pterygoidea mandibulae. **f. of coronoid process,** fossa coronoidea humeri. **costal f., inferior,** f. costalis inferior. **costal f., superior,** f. costalis superior. **costal f., transverse,** f. costalis transversalis. **costal foveae of sternum,** incisurae costales sterni. **f. costa′lis infe′rior** [NA], inferior costal fovea: a small facet on the lower edge of the body of a vertebra articulating with the head of a rib; called also *inferior costal fossa* or *fossula.* **f. costa′lis supe′rior** [NA], superior costal fovea: a small facet on the upper edge of the body of a vertebra articulating with the head of a rib; called also *superior costal facet, fossa,* or *fossula.* **f. costa′lis transversa′lis** [NA], transverse costal fovea: a facet on the transverse process of a vertebra for articulation with the tubercle of a rib; called also *transverse costal fossa.* **crural f.,** anulus femoralis. **dental f. of atlas, f. den′tis atlan′tis** [NA], the facet on the inner surface of the anterior arch of the atlas for the articulation of the dens of the axis. **digastric f.,** fossa digastrica. **femoral f.,** anulus femoralis. **foveae of fourth ventricle,** the inferior and superior foveae. **glandular foveae of Luschka,** foveolae granulares. **f. of head of femur,** f. capitis femoris. **f. for head of radius,** fossa radialis humeri. **f. hemiellip′tica,** recessus ellipticus vestibuli. **f. hemisphe′rica,** recessus sphericus vestibuli. **f. infe′rior** [NA], **inferior f.,** a slight depression in the sulcus limitans of the fourth ventricle, at the upper end of the trigonum nervi vagi, just caudal to the striae medullares; called also *inferior f. of sulcus limitans* and *f. of fourth ventricle.* **inferior articular f. of atlas,** f. articularis inferior atlantis. **inferior f. of floor of fourth ventricle,** f. inferior. **inguinal f., external,** fossa inguinalis lateralis. **inguinal f., internal,** fossa inguinalis

medialis. **inguinal f., lateral,** fossa inguinalis lateralis. **inguinal f., medial,** fossa inguinalis medialis. **inguinal f., middle,** fossa inguinalis medialis. **f. inguina′lis latera′lis,** fossa inguinalis lateralis. **f. inguina′lis media′lis,** fossa inguinalis medialis. **interligamentous f. of peritoneum,** fossa supravesicalis. **f. of lateral malleolus,** facies articularis malleolaris tibiae. **f. lim′bica,** a sulcus marking the lateral border of the lateral area olfactoria and gyrus hippocampi in lower mammals. **f. of little head of radius,** f. capituli radii. **malleolar f., lateral, of fibula,** facies articularis malleoli fibulae. **f. of Morgagni,** fossa navicularis urethrae. **f. nu′chae,** a depression at the nape of the neck, below the external occipital protuberance. **oblong f. of arytenoid cartilage,** f. oblonga cartilaginis arytenoideae. **f. oblon′ga cartilag′inis arytenoi′deae** [NA], oblong fovea of arytenoid cartilage: a depression on the anterolateral surface of the arytenoid cartilage, separated from the triangular pit above by the arcuate crest; called also *oblong pit of arytenoid cartilage.* **pterygoid f., f. pterygoi′dea mandib′ulae** [NA], **f. pterygoi′dea proces′sus condyloi′dei,** a depression on the inner side of the neck of the condyloid process of the mandible, for attachment of the external pterygoid muscle; called also *fovea of condyloid process,* and *pterygoid depression* or *pit.* **sublingual f., f. sublingua′lis** [NA], a depression on the inner surface of the body of the mandible, lodging a portion of the sublingual gland. **submandibular f., f. submandibula′ris** [NA], **f. submaxilla′ris,** a depression on the medial aspect of the body of the mandible, lodging a small portion of the submandibular gland; called also *submandibular* or *submaxillary fossa.* **f. supe′rior** [NA], **superior f.,** a slight depression in the sulcus limitans just rostral to the striae medullares; called also *superior f. of sulcus limitans.* **superior f. of sulcus limitans,** f. superior fossae rhomboideae. **supratrochlear f., anterior,** fossa coronoidea humeri. **supratrochlear f. of humerus,** fossa coronoidea humeri. **f. supravesica′lis peritonae′i,** fossa supravesicalis. **f. of talus,** sulcus tali. **f. of tooth of atlas,** f. dentis atlantis. **f. triangula′ris cartilag′inis arytenoi′deae** [NA], a depression on the anterolateral surface of the arytenoid cartilage, separated from the oblong pit below by the arcuate crest; called also *triangular pit of arytenoid cartilage.* **trochlear f., f. trochlea′ris** [NA], a depression on the anteromedial part of the orbital surface of the frontal bone for the attachment of the trochlea of the superior oblique muscle; it is often replaced by the trochlear spine. Called also *trochlear fossa* and *fossa trochlearis.*

foveate (fo′ve-āt) [L. *foveatus*] pitted.

foveation (fo″ve-a′shun) a pitted condition.

foveola (fo-ve′o-lah), pl. *fove′olae* [L., dim. of *fovea*] a small pit; [NA] a general term for an extremely small depression. **f. coccyg′ea** [NA], **coccygeal f.,** a dermal pit near the tip of the coccyx, indicative of the site of attachment of the embryonic neural tube to the skin; called also *postanal dimple* or *pit.* **fove′olae gas′tricae** [NA], the numerous pits in the gastric mucosa marking the openings of the gastric glands; called also *gastric pits.* **granular foveolae, fove′olae granula′res** [NA], **fove′olae granula′res [Pacchio′ni],** small pits on the internal surface of the cranial bones on either side of the groove for the superior sagittal sinus; they are occupied by the arachnoidal granulations. **fove′olae papil′lae,** foramina papillaria renis.

foveolae (fo-ve′o-le) plural of *foveola.*

foveolate (fo-ve′o-lāt) pitted.

Foville's syndrome (fo-vēlz′) [Achille Louis François *Foville,* French psychiatrist, 1831–1887] see under *syndrome.*

Fowler's incision, position (fow′lerz) [George Ryerson *Fowler,* American surgeon, 1848–1906] see under *incision* and *position.*

Fowler's solution (fow′lerz) [Thomas *Fowler,* English physician, 1736–1801] potassium arsenite solution.

Fowler-Murphy treatment [G. R. *Fowler;* John Benjamin *Murphy,* Chicago surgeon, 1857–1916] Murphy's treatment (def. 2).

fowlpox (fowl′poks) a contagious disease of domestic poultry and birds, due to a poxvirus, and marked by epithelial nodules on the unfeathered parts of the skin, especially the wattles, comb, and legs, and sometimes by membranous lesions in the respiratory passages; called also *epithelioma contagiosum.*

Fox's disease (foks′ez) [G. H. *Fox;* New York dermatologist, 1846–1937] Fox-Fordyce disease.

Fox-Fordyce disease (foks-for′dis) [G. H. *Fox;* John Addison *Fordyce,* New York dermatologist, 1858–1925] see under *disease.*

foxglove (foks′glov) see *digitalis.* **purple f.,** digitalis.

F.p. abbreviation for L. *fi′at po′tio,* let a potion be made; freezing point.

f.p. foot-pound.

F.pil. abbreviation for L. *fi′ant pil′ulae,* let pills be made.

F.R. flocculation reaction; see *Sachs-Georgi test,* under *tests.*

Fr chemical symbol for *francium.*

Fracastorius (frak″as-to′re-us) [It. Girolamo *Fracastoro*] an Italian physician, born in Verona (1483–1553), a poet, and geologist, who published in 1530 a medical poem, *Syphilis sive morbus gallicus,* in which the name syphilis was first given to the disease.

Fract. dos. abbreviation for L. *frac'ta do'si,* in divided doses.

fraction (frak'shun) in chemistry, one of the separable constituents of a substance. **filtration f.,** the portion of the plasma that is filtered through the renal glomerular membranes, calculated as the ratio of the plasma flow through both kidneys to the glomerular filtration rate per minute. **mol f.,** the ratio of the number of moles of a solute to total number of moles in the solution. **plasma f.,** the various components separated from blood plasma. **plasma protein f., human** [USP], a sterile solution of selected proteins derived from the blood plasma of adult human donors, containing 4.5 to 5.5 gm. of protein per 100 ml., of which 83 to 93 per cent is albumin, and the remainder is α- and β-globulins; used as a blood-volume supporter.

fractional (frak'shun-al) [L. *fractio* a breaking] accomplished by repeated divisions; see under *dose.*

fractionation (frak″shun-a′shun) 1. in radiology, division of the total dose of radiation into small doses administered at intervals; radiation given in this manner usually causes less biological damage than the same total dose given at one time; called also *dose fractionation.* 2. in chemistry, separation of a substance into components, as by distillation or crystallization. 3. in histology, isolation of components of living cells by differential centrifugation. **dose f.,** see *fractionation* (def. 1).

fractography (frak-tog′rah-fe) [L. *fractus* broken + Gr. *graphein* to record] a technique of photography which permits observation of jagged surfaces at high magnification.

fracture (frak'chur) [L. *fractura,* from *frangere* to break] 1. the breaking of a part, especially a bone. 2. a break or rupture in a bone. **agenetic f.,** spontaneous fracture due to imperfect osteogenesis. **apophyseal f.,** one in which a small smear fragment or a bony prominence is torn from the bone. **articular f.,** a fracture of the joint surface of a bone; called also *joint f.* **atrophic f.,** a spontaneous fracture resulting from atrophy of the bone. **avulsion f.,** an indirect fracture caused by avulsion or pull of a ligament. **Barton's f.,** fracture of the distal end of the radius into the wrist joint. **basal neck f.,** fracture of the neck of the femur at its junction with the trochanteric region. **bending f.,** an indirect fracture caused by bending of the limb. **Bennett's f.,** a fracture of the base of the first metacarpal bone running into the carpometacarpal joint and complicated by subluxation. **blow-out f.,** fracture of the orbital floor caused by a sudden increase of intraorbital pressure due to traumatic force; the orbital contents herniate into the maxillary sinus so that the inferior rectus or inferior oblique muscle may become incarcerated in the fracture site, producing diplopia on looking up. In the pure type there is disruption of the orbital floor without involvement of the orbital rim; the impure type involves the rim, i.e., there is concomitant midfacial fracture. **boxer's f.,** fracture of the metacarpal neck with volar displacement of the metacarpal head. **bucket-handle f.,** a tear in the semilunar cartilage, along the middle portion, leaving a loop of cartilage lying in the intercondylar notch. **bumper f.,** fracture of one or both legs immediately below the knee caused by an automobile bumper, often involving the tibial plateau. **bursting f.,** a comminuted fracture of the distal phalanx; called also *tuft f.* **butterfly f.,** a comminuted fracture in which there are two fragments on each side of a main fragment, somewhat resembling the wings of a butterfly. **buttonhole f.,** fracture in which the bone is perforated by a missile; called also *perforating f.* **capillary f.,** a fracture that appears in the roentgenogram as a fine hairlike line, the segments of bone not being separated; sometimes seen in fractures of the skull. **cementum f.,** the tearing of fragments of the cementum from the tooth root at the cementodentinal junction, especially that occurring in association with occlusal traumatism. **chisel f.,** oblique detachment of a piece from the head of the radius. **cleavage f.,** shelling off of cartilage with a small fragment of bone from the upper surface of the capitellum humeri (Kocher). **closed f.,** a fracture which does not produce an open wound in the skin; called also *simple f.* **Colles' f.,** fracture of the lower end of the radius in which the lower fragment is displaced posteriorly (see illustration). If the lower fragment is displaced anteriorly, it is a *reverse Colles' fracture* (Smith's fracture). **comminuted f.,** one in which the bone is splintered or crushed (see illustration). **complete f.,** one in which the bone is entirely broken across. **complicated f.,** fracture with injury of the adjacent parts. **compound f.,** open f. **compression f.,** one produced by compression; e.g., vertebral fracture. **condylar f.,** fracture of the humerus in which a small fragment including the condyle is separated from the inner or outer aspect of the bone. **congenital f.,** intrauterine f. **f. by contrecoup,** a fracture of the skull opposite to the site of impact. **deferred f.,** in the horse, one that does not separate at the time of injury because of the presence of powerful muscles or a strong covering of periosteum, but does separate when extra strain is put upon the injured part. **depressed f.,** a fracture of the skull in which a fragment is depressed. **diacondylar f.,** transcondylar f. **direct f.,** a fracture at the point of injury. **dislocation f.,** fracture of a

bone near an articulation with concomitant dislocation of that joint. **double f.,** fracture of a bone in two places; called also *segmental f.* **Dupuytren's f.,** 1. Pott's fracture. 2. (of forearm) Galeazzi's fracture. **Duverney's f.,** fracture of the ilium just below the anterior superior spine. **dyscrasic f.,** fracture due to weakening of the bone from debilitating disease. **f. en coin** (ah kwahn), a V-shaped fracture. **f. en rave** (ah rahv), a fracture in which the break is transverse at the surface, but not within. **endocrine f.,** fracture of a bone weakened by endocrine disorder, such as hyperparathyroidism. **epiphyseal f.,** fracture at the point of union of an epiphysis with the shaft of a bone. **extracapsular f.,** a fracture of the humerus or femur outside of the capsule. **fatigue f.,** a fracture attributed to the strain of prolonged walking or exercise; see *march f.* **fissure f., fissured f.,** a crack extending from a surface into, but not through, a long bone. **Galeazzi's f.,** fracture of the radius above the wrist combined with dislocation of the distal end of the ulna; called also *Dupuytren's f.* **Gosselin's f.,** a V-shaped fracture of the distal end of the tibia, extending into the ankle joint. **greenstick f.,** fracture in which one side of a bone is broken, the other being bent (see illustration); an infraction; called also *hickory-stick* or *willow f.* **grenade-thrower's f.,** fracture of the humerus caused by muscular contraction in throwing a grenade. **Guérin's f.,** Le Fort I f. **gutter f.,** a fracture of the skull in which the depression is elliptic in form. **hangman's f.,** fracture through the pedicles of the axis (C2) with or without subluxation of the second cervical vertebra on the third. **hickory-stick f.,** greenstick f. **horizontal maxillary f.,** Le Fort I f. **impacted f.,** fracture in which one fragment is firmly driven into the other. **incomplete f.,** one which does not entirely destroy the continuity of the bone. **indirect f.,** a fracture at a point distant from the site of injury. **inflammatory f.,** fracture of a bone weakened by inflammatory disease. **interperiosteal f.,** incomplete or greenstick fracture. **intra-articular f.,** a fracture of the articular surface of a bone. **intracapsular f.,** one within the capsule of a joint. **intraperiosteal f.,** a fracture without rupture of the periosteum. **intrauterine f.,** fracture of a fetal bone occurring in utero; called also *congenital f.* **joint f.,** articular fracture. **lead pipe f.,** fracture in which the cortex of the bone is slightly compressed and bulged on one side with a slight crack on the opposite side of the bone. **Le Fort's f.,** bilateral horizontal fracture of the maxilla. Le Fort fractures are classified as follows: *Le Fort I f.,* a horizontal segmented fracture of the alveolar process of the maxilla, in which the teeth are usually contained in the detached portion of the bone; called also *Guérin's f.* and *horizontal maxillary f. Le Fort II f.,* unilateral or bilateral fracture of the maxilla, in which the body of the maxilla is separated from the facial skeleton and the separated portion is pyramidal in shape; the fracture may extend through the body of the maxilla down the midline of the hard palate, through the floor of the orbit, and into the nasal cavity. Called also *pyramidal f. Le Fort III f.,* a fracture in which the entire maxilla and one or more facial bones are completely separated from the craniofacial skeleton; such fractures are almost always accompanied by multiple fractures of the facial bones. Called also *craniofacial disjunction* and *transverse facial f.* **linear f.,** a fracture extending lengthwise of the bone. **longitudinal f.,** a break in a bone extending in a longitudinal direction. **loose f.,** a fracture in which the bone is completely broken so that the broken ends have free play. **march f.,** fracture of a bone of the lower extremity, developing after repeated stresses, as seen in soldiers; called also *fatigue f.* Cf. *march foot.* **Monteggia's f.,** fracture in the proximal half of the shaft of the ulna, with dislocation of the head of the radius. Sometimes called parry fracture because it is often caused by attempts to fend off blows with the forearm. **Moore's f.,** fracture of the lower end of the radius with dislocation of the head of the ulna and imprisonment of the styloid process beneath the annular ligaments. **multiple f.,** a variety in which there are two or more lines of fracture of the same bone not communicating with each other. **neoplastic f.,** fracture due to weakening of the bone as a result of a malignant process. **neurogenic f.,** fracture due to weakening of the bone as a result of tabes, paresis, etc. **oblique f.,** fracture in which the break extends in an oblique direction. **open f.,** one in which there is an external wound leading to the break of the bone; called also *compound f.* **paratrooper f.,** fracture of the posterior articular margin of the tibia and/or of the internal or external malleolus. **parry f.,** Monteggia f. **pathologic f.,** one due to weakening of the bone structure by pathologic processes, such as neoplasia, osteomalacia, osteomyelitis, and other diseases. Called also *secondary f.* and *spontaneous f.* **perforating f.,** buttonhole f. **periarticular f.,** a fracture extending close to, but not into, a joint. **pertrochanteric f.,** fracture of the femur passing through the great trochanter. **pillion f.,** a fracture of the lower end of the femur occurring when the knee of a person riding pillion on a motorcycle is struck in a collision; it is a T-shaped fracture with displacement of the condyles behind the femoral shaft. **ping-pong f.,** an indented fracture of the skull, resembling the indentation that can be produced with the finger in a ping-pong ball; when elevated it resumes and retains its normal position. **pond f.,** fracture of the skull in which a fissure circumscribes the

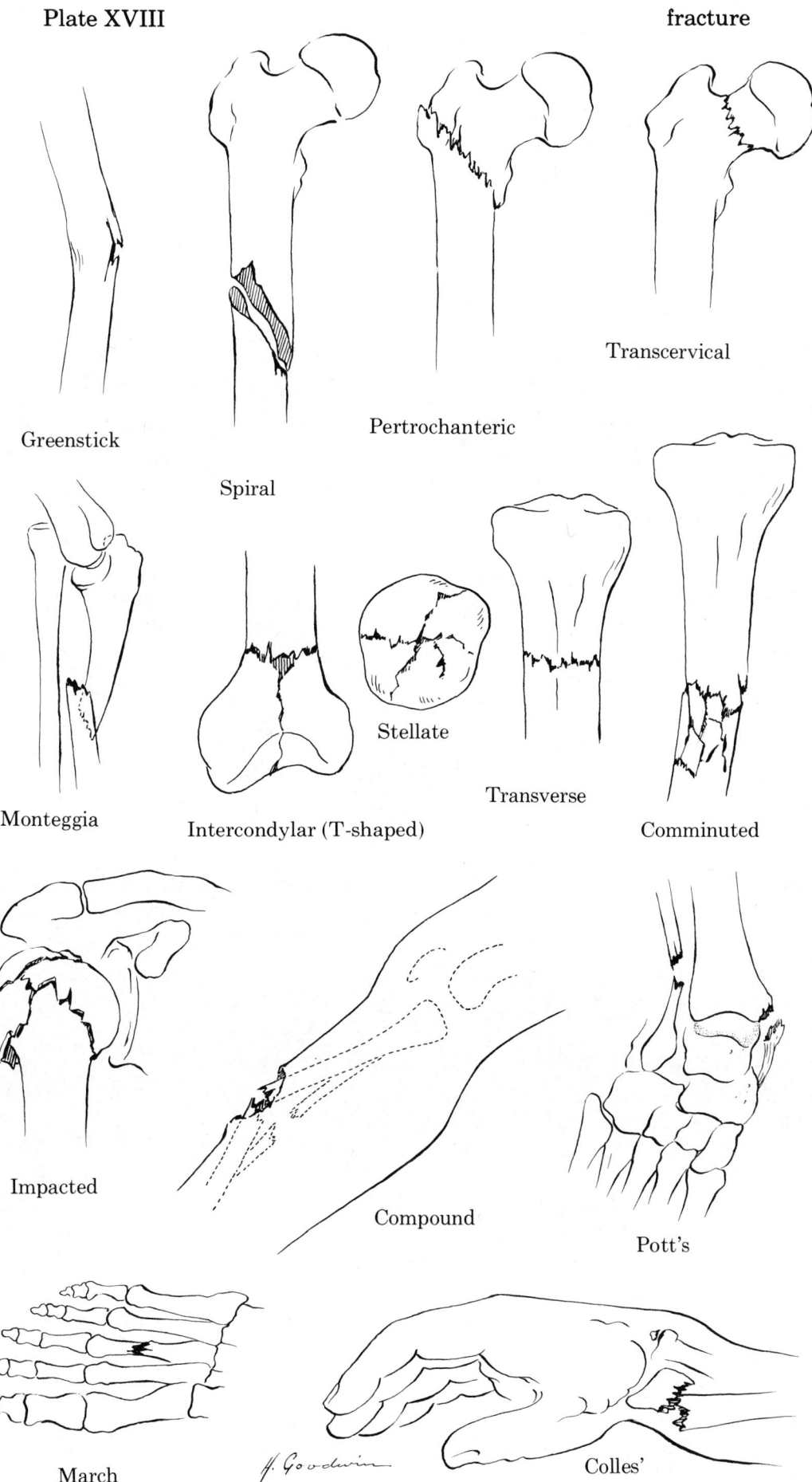

Plate XVIII

fracture

Greenstick

Pertrochanteric

Spiral

Transcervical

Monteggia

Intercondylar (T-shaped)

Stellate

Transverse

Comminuted

Impacted

Compound

Pott's

March

Colles'

VARIOUS TYPES OF FRACTURES

radiating lines, giving the depressed area a circular form.
Pott's f., fracture of the lower part of the fibula, with serious injury of the lower tibial articulation, usually a chipping off of a portion of the medial malleolus, or rupture of the medial ligament; called also *Dupuytren's f.* **pressure f.,** one caused by pressure on the bone from an adjoining tumor. **pyramidal f. (of maxilla),** Le Fort II f. **Quervain's f.,** fracture of the navicular bone together with a volar luxation of the os lunatum. **resecting f.,** a fracture in which a piece of the bone is removed by violence, as by a bullet. **secondary f.,** pathologic f. **segmental f.,** double f. **Shepherd's f.,** fracture of the astragalus, with detachment of the outer protecting edge. **silverfork f.,** fracture of the lower ends of the radius (*Colles' f.*); so called because of the shape of the deformity that it causes. **simple f.,** closed f. **simple f., complex,** a closed fracture in which there is considerable injury to adjacent soft tissues. **Skillern's f.,** complete fracture of the lower third of the radius with greenstick fracture of the lower third of the ulna. **Smith's f.,** a fracture of the lower end of the radius near its articular surface with forward displacement of the lower fragment; sometimes called *reverse Colles' fracture.* **spiral f.,** one in which the bone has been twisted apart; called also *torsion f.* **splintered f.,** a comminuted fracture in which the bone is splintered into thin, sharp fragments. **spontaneous f.,** one occurring as a result of disease of a bone or from some undiscoverable cause, and not due to trauma; called also *pathologic f.* **sprain f.,** the separation of a tendon or ligament from its insertion, taking with it a piece of bone. **sprinter's f.,** fracture of the anterior superior or of the anterior inferior spine of the ilium, a fragment of the bone being pulled off by muscular violence, as at the start of a sprint. **stellate f.,** a fracture with a central point of injury, from which radiate numerous fissures. **Stieda's f.,** fracture of the internal condyle of the femur. **subcapital f.,** fracture of a bone just below its head; especially an intracapsular fracture of the neck of the femur at the junction of the head and neck. **subcutaneous f.,** closed f. **subperiosteal f.,** a crack through a bone without alteration in its alignment or contour, the supposition being that the periosteum is not broken. **supracondylar f.,** fracture of the humerus in which the line of fracture is through the lower end of the shaft of the humerus. **torsion f.,** spiral f. **torus f.,** a fracture in which there is a localized expansion or torus of the cortex, with little or no displacement of the lower end of the bone. **transcervical f.,** fracture through the neck of the femur. **transcondylar f.,** fracture of the humerus in which the line of fracture is at the level of the condyles, transverses the fossae, and is in part within the capsule of the joint; called also *diacondylar f.* **transverse f.,** a fracture at right angles to the axis of the bone. **transverse facial f.,** Le Fort III f. **transverse maxillary f.,** a term sometimes used for horizontal maxillary fracture (Le Fort I f.). **trimalleolar f.,** fracture of the medial and lateral malleoli and the posterior tip of the tibia. **trophic f.,** one due to a trophic (nutritional) disturbance. **tuft f.,** bursting f. **Wagstaffe's f.,** separation of the internal malleolus. **willow f.,** greenstick f.

fracture-dislocation (frak′chur dis″lo-ka′shun)   a fracture of a bone near a joint, also involving dislocation.

Fraenkel (freng′kel)   see *Fränkel.*

fragiform (fraj′ĭ-form) [L. *fraga* strawberry + *forma* shaped]   shaped like a strawberry.

fragilitas (frah-jil′ĭ-tas) [L.]   fragility. **f. cri′nium,** a brittle condition of the hair. **f. os′sium,** abnormal brittleness of the bones; see *osteogenesis imperfecta.* **f. un′guium** [L. "fragility of the nails"], abnormal brittleness of the nails.

fragility (frah-jil′ĭ-te)   susceptibility, or lack of resistance, to factors capable of causing disruption of continuity or integrity. **f. of blood,** erythrocyte f. **capillary f.,** susceptibility, or lack of resistance, of capillaries to disruption under conditions of increased stress. **erythrocyte f.,** the susceptibility, or lack of resistance, of erythrocytes to hemolysis when exposed to increasingly hypotonic saline solutions (*osmotic f.*) or when subjected to mechanical trauma (*mechanical f.*). **hereditary f. of bone,** osteogenesis imperfecta. **mechanical f.,** see *erythrocyte f.* **osmotic f.,** see *erythrocyte f.*

fragilocyte (frah-jil′o-sīt)   an erythrocyte which is less than normally resistant to hypotonic saline solution.

fragilocytosis (frah-jil″o-si-to′sis)   the presence of fragilocytes in the blood.

fragment (frag′ment)   one of the small pieces into which a larger entity has been broken. **Spengler's f's,** small round bodies seen in tuberculous sputum.

fragmentation (frag″men-ta′shun)   1. a division into fragments. 2. a form of reproduction seen in certain organisms, such as flatworms, in which the body of the parent may break into several pieces, each piece then regenerating the missing parts and developing into a whole animal. **f. of myocardium,** transverse rupture of the muscle fibers of the heart.

fragmentography, mass (frag″men-tog′rah-fe)   combined gas chromatography and mass spectrometry in which quantitative analysis of the substance in question (e.g., a steriod) is based on a

determination of the abundance of certain fragments characteristic of that substance.

fraise (frāz) [Fr. "strawberry"]   a conical or hemispherical burr for cutting osteoplastic flaps or enlarging trephine openings.

frambesia (fram-be′ze-ah) [Fr. *framboise* raspberry]   yaws. **f. trop′ica,** yaws.

frambesin (fram-be′sin)   cultures of *Treponema pertenue* heated to 60° C.; used as a skin test for frambesia (yaws).

frambesioma (fram-be″ze-o′mah)   mother yaw; see under *yaw.*

framboesia (fram-be′ze-ah)   yaws.

framboesioma (fram-be″ze-o′mah)   mother yaw; see under *yaw.*

frame (frām)   a structure, usually rigid, designed for giving support to or for immobilizing a part. **Balkan f.,** a rectangular frame attached to and overhanging a bed; particularly useful in allowing bedridden patients to move more effectively and for attachment of splints. Called also *Balkan splint.* **Bradford f.,** a rectangular frame of gas pipe to which is attached a sheet of heavy canvas; used as a bed frame in tuberculosis of the spine and fracture of the thigh. **Deiters' terminal f.,** plates in the lamina reticularis uniting Deiters' phalanges with the cells of Hensen. **Foster f.,** one similar to the Stryker frame. **Hibbs' f.,** a frame used in the application of traction plaster jackets in the treatment of scoliosis. **occluding f.,** a dental articulator. **quadriplegic standing f.,** a device for supporting in the upright position a patient whose four limbs are paralyzed. **Stryker f.,** one consisting of canvas stretched on anterior and posterior frames, on which the patient can be rotated around his longitudinal axis. **trial f.,** a frame specially devised to permit easy insertion of different lenses used in correcting refractive errors of vision. **Whitman's f.,** a frame similar to Bradford's frame except that it is curved.

framework (frām′werk)   the basic structure about which something is formulated or built; as the supporting elements of a prosthesis (such as a partial denture) to which the remaining portions are attached. **scleral f.,** the larger and coarser part of the angle of the iris which is adjacent to the sclera. **uveal f.,** ligamentum pectinatum anguli iridocornealis.

Francis' disease (fran′siz) [Edward *Francis,* American physician, born 1872]   tularemia.

Francisella (fran-sĭ-sel′ah) [Edward *Francis*]   a genus of aerobic, nonmotile, gram-negative bacteria made up of very small, coccoid to ellipsoidal pleomorphic rods. **F. novi′cida,** the etiologic agent of a disease resembling tularemia in guinea pigs, hamsters, and white mice; not known to infect man. Formerly called *Pasteurella novicida.* **F. tularen′sis,** the etiologic agent of tularemia in man, being transmitted from wild animals to man by drinking water, by blood-sucking insects, or by contact; it is also the cause of a severe form of conjunctivitis known as conjunctivitis tularensis. Called also *Pasteurella tularensis.*

francium (fran′se-um)   the chemical element of atomic number 87, atomic weight 223, symbol Fr, all isotopes of which are radioactive; formerly called *virginium.*

Franco's operation (frah′ko) [Pierre *Franco,* French surgeon, 1500–1561]   suprapubic cystotomy.

franghi (fran′ge)   venereal syphilis in Syria.

Frank's operation (franks) [Rudolf *Frank,* Vienna surgeon, 1862–1913]   see under *operation.*

Franke's operation (frang′kez) [Felix *Franke,* German surgeon, born 1858]   see under *operation.*

Fränkel's sign (freng′kelz) [Albert *Fränkel,* German physician, 1848–1916]   see under *sign.*

Fränkel's speculum, test (freng′kelz) [Bernhard *Fränkel,* German laryngologist, 1836–1911]   see under *speculum* and *tests.*

Fränkel's treatment (freng′kelz) [Albert *Fränkel,* Heidelberg physician, 1864–1938]   see under *treatment.*

Frankenhäuser's ganglion (frang′ken-hoy″zerz) [Ferdinand *Frankenhäuser,* German gynecologist, died 1894]   see under *ganglion.*

Frankl-Hochwart's disease (frank′l-hoch′warts) [Lothar von *Frankl-Hochwart,* Vienna neurologist, 1862–1914]   polyneuritis cerebralis menieriformis.

Franklin glasses (frangk′lin) [Benjamin *Franklin,* American patriot, 1706–1790]   bifocal glasses.

franklinism (frangk′lin-izm) [Benjamin *Franklin*]   1. static or frictional electricity. 2. franklinization.

franklinization (frangk″lin-i-za′shun)   the therapeutic use of static electricity.

Frasera (fra′zer-ah) [after John *Fraser,* 1750–1817]   a genus of gentianaceous plants.

Fraunhofer's lines (frown′hof-erz) [Joseph von *Fraunhofer,* German optician, 1787–1826]   see under *line.*

Frazier-Spiller operation (fra′zher-spil′er) [Charles Harrison *Frazier;* William Gibson *Spiller,* American neurologist, 1863–1940]   see under *operation.*

FRC   functional residual capacity.

F.R.C.P.   Fellow of the Royal College of Physicians.

F.R.C.P.(C.) Fellow of the Royal College of Physicians of Canada.

F.R.C.P.E. Fellow of the Royal College of Physicians of Edinburgh.

F.R.C.P.(Glasg.) Fellow of the Royal College of Physicians and Surgeons of Glasgow *qua* Physician.

F.R.C.P.I. Fellow of the Royal College of Physicians in Ireland.

F.R.C.S. Fellow of the Royal College of Surgeons.

F.R.C.S.(C.) Fellow of the Royal College of Surgeons of Canada.

F.R.C.S.E. Fellow of the Royal College of Surgeons of Edinburgh.

F.R.C.S.(Glasg.) Fellow of the Royal College of Physicians and Surgeons of Glasgow *qua* Surgeon.

F.R.C.S.I. Fellow of the Royal College of Surgeons in Ireland.

F.R.C.V.S. Fellow of the Royal College of Veterinary Surgeons.

FreAmine II (fre-am′ēn) trademark for a crystalline amino acid solution for intravenous administration, containing a mixture of essential and nonessential amino acids but no peptides.

freckle (frek′l) a brownish pigmented spot on the skin due to discrete accumulation of melanin as a result of the stimulant effect of sunlight acting on clusters of melanocytes which have higher than normal tyrosinase activity. Called also *ephelis*. Cf. *lentigo*. **cold f.** (*obs.*), lentigo. **melanotic f. of Hutchinson,** a noninvasive malignant melanoma occurring most frequently on the face of women during the fourth decade, but also in both sexes at any age and on any part of the body; it may be of melanocytic rather than nevocytic origin. Called also *lentigo maligna* and *circumscribed precancerous melanosis of Dubreuilh*.

Fredet-Ramstedt operation (frĕ-da′ rahm′stet) [Pierre *Fredet*, French surgeon, 1870–1946; Conrad *Ramstedt*, German surgeon, born 1867] see under *operation*.

freemartin (fre′mar-tin) a sexually maldeveloped female calf born as a twin to a normal male calf; it is commonly sterile and intersexual as the result of male hormone reaching it through anastomosed placental vessels.

freeze-cleaving (frēz-clēv′ing) freeze-etching.

freeze-drying (frēz-dri′ing) a method of tissue preparation in which the tissue specimen is frozen and then dehydrated at low temperature in a high vacuum.

freeze-etching (frēz-ech′ing) a method used to study unfixed cells by electron microscopy, in which the object to be studied is placed in 20 per cent glycerol, frozen at –100° C., and then mounted on a chilled holder.

freeze-fracturing (frēz-frak′chur-ing) a method of preparing cells for electron-microscopical examination: a tissue specimen is frozen at –150 °C., inserted into a vaccum chamber, and fractured by a microtome; a platinum carbon replica of the exposed surfaces is made, freed of the underlying specimen, and then examined.

freeze-substitution (frēz-sub-stĭ-tu′shun) a modification of freeze-drying in which the ice within the frozen tissue is replaced by alcohol or other solvents at a very low temperature.

Frei's antigen, bubo, disease, test (frīz) [Wilhelm Siegmund *Frei*, German dermatologist, 1885–1943] see *lymphogranuloma venereum*, and see under *antigen* and *tests*.

Freiberg's infraction (fri′bergz) [Albert Henry *Freiberg*, American surgeon, 1868–1940] see under *infraction*.

fremitus (frem′ĭ-tus) [L.] a vibration perceptible on palpation. **bronchial f.,** rhonchal f. **friction f.,** the vibration caused by the rubbing together of two dry body surfaces; called also *friction rub*. **hydatid f.,** see under *thrill*. **pectoral f.,** vocal f. **pericardial f.,** a thrill of the chest wall due to the friction of the surfaces of the pericardium over each other. **pleural f.,** a palpable vibration of the wall of the thorax due to friction of the opposing surfaces of the pleura over each other. **rhonchal f.,** palpable vibrations produced by the passage of air through a large bronchial tube filled with mucus; called also *bronchial f.* **subjective f.,** a thrill felt by the patient on humming with his mouth closed. **tactile f.,** a thrill, as in the chest wall, which may be felt by a hand applied to the thorax while the patient is speaking. **tussive f.,** a thrill felt on the chest when the patient coughs. **vocal f.,** a thrill caused by speaking, and perceived by the ear of the auscultator applied to the chest; called also *pectoral f.*

frena (fre′nah) plural of *frenum*.

frenal (fre′nal) pertaining to a frenum.

French (french′) see *French scale*, under *scale*.

frenectomy (fre-nek′to-me) excision of a frenum.

Frenkel's movements (treatment) (freng-kelz′) [Heinrich S. *Frenkel*, Berlin neurologist, 1860–1931] see under *movement*.

frenoplasty (fre″no-plas′te) the correction of an abnormally attached frenum by surgically repositioning it.

frenosecretory (fre″no-se-kre′to-re) [L. *frenum* bridle + *secretory*] exercising an inhibitory or restraining power over the secretions.

frenotomy (fre-not′o-me) [L. *frenum* bridle + Gr. *tomē* a cutting] incision of a frenum or frenulum, as of the frenulum linguae in treatment of tongue-tie.

frentizole (fren′tĭ-zōl) chemical name: *N*-(6-methoxy-2-benzothiazolyl)-*N′*-phenylurea; an immunoregulator, $C_{15}H_{13}N_3O_2S$.

frenula (fren′u-lah) plural of *frenulum*.

frenuloplasty (fren′u-lo-plas″te) the correction of an abnormally attached frenulum by surgically repositioning it.

frenulum (fren′u-lum), pl. *fren′ula* [L., dim. of *frenum*] a small bridle; [NA] a general term for a small fold of integument or mucous membrane that checks, curbs, or limits the movements of an organ or part. see also *frenum*. **f. of anterior medullary velum,** f. veli medullaris superior. **f. clitor′idis** [NA], **f. of clitoris,** a fold formed by the union of the labia posterior with the clitoris; called also *crus glandis clitoridis*. **f. of ileocecal valve,** f. valvae ileocecalis. **f. of inferior lip, f. la′bii inferio′ris** [NA], the fold of mucous membrane on the inside of the middle of the lower lip, connecting the lip with the gums. **f. la′bii superio′ris** [NA], frenulum of superior lip; the fold of mucous membrane on the inside of the middle of the upper lip, connecting the lip with the gums. **f. labio′rum puden′di** [NA], frenulum of pudendal labia: the posterior union of the labia minora, anterior to the posterior commissure; called also *f. pudendi, fourchette*, and *frenum of labia*. **f. lin′guae** [NA], frenulum of tongue: the vertical fold of mucous membrane under the tongue, attaching it to the floor of the mouth; called also frenum of tongue. **f. lin′guae cerebel′li,** vincula lingulae cerebelli. **frenula of Morgagni,** see *f. valvae ileocecalis*. **f. of prepuce of penis, f. prepu′tii pe′nis** [NA], the fold on the lower surface of the glans penis that connects it with the prepuce. **f. of pudendal labia, f. puden′di,** f. labiorum pudendi. **f. of superior lip,** f. labii superioris. **f. of superior medullary velum,** f. veli medullaris superior. **f. of tongue,** f. linguae. **f. val′vae ileoceca′lis** [NA], **fren′ula val′vulae co′li,** frenulum of iliocecal valve: a fold formed by the joined extremities of the ileocecal valve, extending partly around the lumen of the colon; called also *frenula* or *frenum of Morgagni*. **f. ve′li medulla′ris anterio′ris, f. ve′li medulla′ris supe′rior** [NA], frenulum of superior medullary velum: a band that lies in the superior medullary velum at its attachment to the inferior colliculi; called also *f. of anterior medullary velum*.

frenum (fre′num), pl. *fre′na* [L. "bridle "] a restraining structure or part; see *frenulum*. **f. of labia,** frenulum labiorum pudendi. **lingual f.,** frenulum linguae. **Macdowel's f.,** a group of fibers attached to the tendon of the pectoralis muscle and strengthening the intermuscular septum. **f. of Morgagni,** frenulum valvae ileocecalis. **f. of tongue,** frenulum linguae. **f. of valve of colon,** frenulum valvae ileocecalis.

frenzy (fren′ze) [Gr. *phrenitizein* to be delirious or frantic] violent maniacal excitement.

frequency (fre′kwen-se) 1. the number of occurrences of a periodic process in a unit of time. 2. in statistics, the number of occurrences of a determinable entity per unit of time or of population. 3. the number of vibrations made by a particle or ray in one second; in electricity, the rate of oscillation or alternation in an alternating current; the number of complete cycles produced by an alternating current generator per second. **audio f.,** any frequency corresponding to a normally audible sound wave. **fusion f.,** see under *flicker*. **gene f.,** the number of loci at which a given allele is found in a given population, divided by the total number of loci at which it could occur. **high f.,** the rate of oscillation in an alternating current exceeding the rate at which muscular contraction ceases—approximately 10,000 per second. **infrasonic f.,** any frequency below the audio frequency range. **low f.,** an alternating current where frequency in cycles per second is low in reference to a certain standard, such as the pitch frequency of middle C. **recombination f.,** the frequency of crossing over of genes on homologous chromosomes, as determined by the number of recombinants divided by the total number of progeny. **subsonic f.,** infrasonic f. **supersonic f.,** ultrasonic f. **ultrasonic f.,** any frequency above the audio frequency range; see *ultrasonics*. **urinary f.,** urination at short intervals without increase in daily volume of urinary output, due to reduced bladder capacity.

Frerichs' theory (fra′riks) [Friedrich Theodor *Frerichs*, Berlin physician, 1819–1885] see under *theory*.

fressreflex (fres′re-fleks) [Ger. "eating reflex"] rhythmic sucking, chewing, and swallowing movements elicited by stroking of the lips and cheeks.

freta (fre′tah) [L.] plural of *fretum*.

fretum (fre′tum), pl. *fre′ta* [L.] a constriction, or strait. **f. hal′leri,** a constriction between the atria and ventricles of the fetal heart; called also *Haller's isthmus*.

Freud's cathartic method (froids) [Sigmund *Freud*, neurologist in Vienna, 1856–1939] see *catharsis* (def. 2).

freudian (froid′e-an) 1. pertaining to Sigmund Freud and his doctrines regarding the causes of certain nervous disorders, that they are based on the existence of unconscious sexual impressions, and that the cure of such disorders can be secured by bringing these impressions into the consciousness by psychoanalysis; the term also is applied to the theory that dreams are the expression under symbolic forms of suppressed wishes, many of which are of a sexual nature. See *unconscious* and *psychoanalysis.* 2. one who follows the teaching and theories of Sigmund Freud.

Freund adjuvant (froind) [Jules Thomas *Freund*, Hungarian-born bacteriologist in the United States, 1891–1960] see under *adjuvant.*

Freund's anomaly, operation (froindz) [Wilhelm Alexander *Freund*, German surgeon, 1833–1918] see under *anomaly* and *operation.*

Freund's reaction (froinds) [Hermann Wolfgang *Freund*, German gynecologist, 1859–1925] see under *reaction.*

Freund-Kaminer reaction (froind′kah′min-er) [Ernst *Freund,* Vienna (later London) physician, 1863–1946; Gisa *Kaminer,* Vienna physician, 1883–1941] Freund's reaction; see under *reaction.*

Frey's hairs (frīz) [Max von *Frey,* German physiologist, 1852–1932] see under *hair.*

Frey's syndrome (frīz) [Lucie *Frey,* Polish physician] auriculotemporal syndrome; see under *syndrome.*

Freyer's operation (fri′erz) [Sir Peter Johnston *Freyer,* British surgeon, 1857–1921] see under *operation.*

FRF follicle-stimulating hormone releasing factor; see *gonadotropin releasing hormone,* under *hormone.*

F.R.F.P.S.G. Fellow of the Royal Faculty of Physicians and Surgeons of Glasgow.

friable (fri′ah-b'l) [L. *friabilis*] easily pulverized or crumbled.

Fricke's bandage (frik′ez) [Johann Karl Georg *Fricke,* German surgeon, 1790–1841] see under *bandage.*

friction (frik′shun) [L. *frictio*] the act of rubbing; attrition.

Friderichsen-Waterhouse syndrome (frid″er-ik′sen-wah′ter-hows) [Carl *Friderichsen,* Danish physician, born 1886; Rupert *Waterhouse,* British physician, 1873–1958] Waterhouse-Friderichsen syndrome.

Fridericia's method (frid′er-ĭ-che-ahz) [Louis Sigurd *Fridericia,* Danish hygienist, born 1881] see under *method.*

Friedländer's bacillus, pneumobacillus, pneumonia (frēd′len-derz) [Carl *Friedländer,* German pathologist, 1847–1887] see *Klebsiella pneumoniae,* and under *pneumonia.*

Friedländer's disease (frēd′len-derz) [Carl F. *Friedländer,* German physician, born 1841] endarteritis obliterans.

Friedman's test (frēd′manz) [Maurice Harold *Friedman,* American physician, born 1903] see under *test.*

Friedman-Lapham test (frēd′man-lap′ham) [Maurice Harold *Friedman;* Maxwell Edward *Lapham,* New Orleans obstetrician, born 1899] see *Friedman's test,* under *test.*

Friedmann's vasomotor syndrome (complex) (fred′manz) [Max *Friedmann,* German neurologist, 1858–1925] see under *syndrome.*

Friedreich's ataxia (tabes), disease, foot, sign (frēd′rĭks) [Nikolaus *Friedreich,* Heidelberg physician, 1825–1882] see under *ataxia, disease, foot,* and *sign.*

friente (fre-en′te) an erythematous dermatitis once common among wood choppers and field workers, and probably caused by *Ustilago hypodytes.*

frigidity (frĭ-jid′ĭ-te) coldness; especially sexual unresponsiveness, usually applied to this state in the female. Analogous to impotence in the male.

frigolabile (frig″o-la′bīl) [L. *frigor* cold + *labilis* unstable] easily affected or destroyed by cold.

frigorific (frig″o-rif′ik) [L. *frigorificus*] producing coldness.

frigostabile (frig″o-sta′bīl) frigostable.

frigostable (frig″o-sta′bl) [L. *frigor* cold + *stabilis* firm] resistant to cold or low temperature.

frigotherapy (frig′o-ther′ah-pe) cryotherapy.

frit (frit) imperfectly fused material used as a basis for making glass, and used in the formation of porcelain teeth.

Fritsch's catheter (frich′es) [Heinrich *Fritsch,* German gynecologist, 1844–1914] Bozeman's catheter; see under *catheter.*

froe- for words beginning thus, see those beginning *fre-.*

frog (frog) 1. a tailless, leaping amphibian with a smooth skin and fully webbed feet, commonly used as a laboratory animal. 2. the band of horny substance in the middle of the sole of a horse's foot, dividing into two branches and running toward the heel in the form of a fork.

frog stay (frog sta) see *spine* (def. 3).

Fröhlich's syndrome (fra′liks) [Alfred *Fröhlich,* Vienna neurologist, 1871–1953] adiposogenital dystrophy.

Frohn's test (reagent) (frohnz) [Damianus *Frohn,* German physician, born 1843] see under *tests.*

Froin's syndrome (frow-ăn′) [Georges *Froin,* French physician, born 1874] see under *syndrome.*

frolement (frōl-maw′) [Fr.] 1. a rustling sound often heard in auscultation in disease of the pericardium. 2. a massage movement consisting of light brushing with the palm of the hand.

Froment's paper sign (fro-mahz′) [Jules *Froment,* French physician, born 1878] see under *sign.*

Frommann's lines (from′anz) [Carl *Frommann,* anatomist in Heidelberg, 1831–1892] see under *line.*

Frommel's disease, operation (from′elz) [Richard Julius Ernst *Frommel,* German gynecologist, 1854–1912] see *Chiari-Frommel syndrome,* under *syndrome,* and see under *operation.*

Frommel-Chiari syndrome (from′el-ke-ar′e) [Richard Julius Ernst *Frommel;* Johann Baptist *Chiari,* German obstetrician 1817–1854] Chiari-Frommel syndrome.

frondose (fron′dōs) [L. *frondosus* leafy] bearing fronds, or villi, as the chorion frondosum.

frons (fronz) [L. "the front, forepart"] [NA], the forehead; the region of the face above the eyes. **f. cra′nii** [NA], **f. of cranium,** the anterior extremity of the brain case; the bony forehead.

frontad (frun′tad) toward a frontal aspect.

frontal (frun′tal) [L. *frontalis*] 1. pertaining to the forehead. 2. denoting a longitudinal plane of the body; see under *plane.*

frontalis (frun-ta′lis) [L.] frontal; in official anatomical nomenclature, the term designates a relationship to the frontal or coronal plane.

frontipetal (frun-tip′ĕ-tal) [L. *frontalis* in front + *petere* to seek] directed to the front; moving in a frontal direction.

frontomalar (frun″to-ma′lar) pertaining to the frontal and malar bones.

frontomaxillary (frun″to-mak′sĭ-lār″e) pertaining to the frontal bone and the upper jaw.

frontonasal (frun″to-na′zal) pertaining to the frontal sinus and the nose.

fronto-occipital (frun″to-ok-sip′ĭ-tal) pertaining to the forehead and the occiput.

frontoparietal (frun″to-pah-ri′e-tal) pertaining to the frontal and parietal bones.

frontotemporal (frun″to-tem′po-ral) pertaining to the frontal and temporal bones.

Froriep's ganglion (fro′rēps) [August von *Froriep,* German anatomist, 1849–1917] see under *ganglion.*

Froriep's induration (fro′rēps) [Robert *Froriep,* Berlin surgeon, 1804–1861] myositis fibrosa.

Fröschel's symptom (fresh′elz) [Emil *Fröschel,* Vienna otologist, born 1884] see under *symptom.*

frost (frost) a deposit resembling that of frozen dew or vapor. **urea f.,** the appearance on the skin of salt crystals left by evaporation of the sweat in urhidrosis.

frostbite (frost′bīt) damage to tissues as the result of exposure to low environmental temperatures; called also *congelation.* **deep f.,** damage resulting from exposure to extremely low temperatures, involving not only the skin and subcutaneous tissue but also deeper tissues, sometimes leading to gangrene and loss of affected parts; it is marked by persistent ischemia, secondary thrombosis, and livid cyanosis. **superficial f.,** damage resulting from exposure to low temperatures, involving only the skin or extending to the tissue immediately beneath it; it may be manifested as simple erythema, transient anesthesia, and superficial bullae.

frottage (fro-tahzh′) [Fr. "rubbing"] 1. rubbing movement in massage; effeurage. 2. sexual gratification by rubbing against the clothing of a person of the opposite sex, especially when pressed close, as in a crowd; called also *hyphephilia.*

frotteur (fro-tur′) an individual who achieves sexual gratification by practicing frottage.

frotteurism (fro-tur′izm) frottage (def. 2).

F.R.S. Fellow of the Royal Society.

fructification (fruk″tĭ-fĭ-ka′shun) 1. the production of fruit. 2. a fruiting body. 3. a spore-bearing structure.

fructivorous (fruk-tiv′o-rus) subsisting on or eating fruits.

fructofuranose (fruk″to-fu′rah-nōs) the combining form and the more reactive form of fructose, $CH_2OH \cdot CH \cdot (CHOH)_2 \cdot CHO \cdot \cdot CH_2OH$.

β-fructofuranosidase (fruk″to-fu″rah-no′sĭ-dās) β-D-fructofuranoside fructohydrolase: an enzyme occurring in yeasts and other organisms that catalyzes the hydrolysis of sugars possessing a terminal unsubstituted β-D-fructofuranosyl residue. Reportedly absent at birth in the intestine of some animals (including man), but its level rises thereafter. Called also *invertase, invertin, saccharose,* and *sucrase.*

fructokinase (fruk″to-ki′nās) ATP:D-fructose 6-phosphotransferase: an enzyme that catalyzes the transfer of a high-energy phosphate group from a donor to D-fructose, producing D-fructose-1-phosphate; see also *kinase* (def. 1).

fructolysis (fruk-tol′ĭ-sis) the splitting up of fructose.

fructopyranose (fruk″to-pi′rah-nōs) fructose.

fructosamine (fruk″to-sa′min) an amino sugar formed by the reduction of the osazone of glucosamine.

fructosan (fruk′to-san) a hexosan, $C_6H_{10}O_5$, an anhydride of fructose; called also *levulan*.

fructosazone (fruk″to-sa′zōn) a phenyl-osazone of fructose identical with glucosazone; called also *levulosazone*.

fructose (fruk′tōs) [L. *fructus* fruit] chemical name: D-fructose. A ketohexose, $C_6H_{12}O_6$, occurring in honey and many sweet fruits and a component of many di- and polysaccharides; it is obtainable by inversion of aqueous solutions of sucrose and subsequent separation of fructose from glucose. The official preparation [USP], occurring as colorless crystals or as a white, crystalline powder, is administered intravenously as a fluid and nutrient replenisher. Called also *fructopyranose, fruit sugar*, and *levulose*. **f. diphosphate, f. 1,6-diphosphate,** the Harden-Young ester, a key intermediate in cellular glycolysis. **ferric f.,** a hematinic composed of a fructose iron complex and potassium. **f. 6-phosphate,** the Neuberg ester.

fructosemia (fruk″to-se′me-ah) the presence of fructose in the blood; seen in fructose intolerance. Called also *levulosemia*.

fructosidase (fruk-to′si-dās) β-fructofuranosidase.

fructoside (fruk-to′sīd) a compound that bears the same relation to fructose as a glucoside does to glucose.

fructosuria (fruk″to-su′re-ah) [*fructose* + Gr. *ouron* urine + *-ia*] the presence of fructose in the urine; seen in fructose intolerance. Called also *levulosuria*. **essential f.,** a benign, asymptomatic hereditary disorder of carbohydrate metabolism, transmitted as an autosomal recessive trait, caused by a defect in the hepatic enzyme fructokinase, and in which the only manifestations are fructosemia and fructosuria. See also *hereditary fructose intolerance*, under *intolerance*.

fructosyl (fruk′to-sil) a radical of fructose.

fructosyltransferase (fruk″to-sil-trans′fer-ās) an enzyme that catalyzes the transfer of a fructosyl group, as from fructan to D-glucose to form sucrose; called also *transfructosylase*.

fructovegetative (fruk″to-vej′ĕ-ta″tiv) composed of or pertaining to fruits and vegetables.

frugivorous (froo-jiv′o-rus) [L. *frux* fruit + *vorare* to eat] fructivorous; eating or subsisting on fruit.

fruit (froot) [L. *fructus*] the developed ovary of a plant, including the seed and its envelopes.

fruitarian (froo-ta′re-an) a person whose diet consists chiefly of fruits.

fruitarianism (froo-ta′re-an-izm) the use of an exclusively fruit diet.

frusemide (frus′ĕ-mīd) furosemide.

Frust. abbreviation for L. *frustilla′tim*, in small pieces.

frustration (frus-tra′shun) a condition of increased emotional tension resulting from failure to achieve sought gratifications or satisfactions, ordinarily as a result of forces outside of one's self (*external f.*), but also as a result of unconscious blocking of instinctual impulses (*internal f.*).

F.s.a. abbreviation for L. *fi′at secun′dum ar′tem*, let it be made skillfully.

FSH follicle-stimulating hormone.

FSH/LH-RH follicle-stimulating hormone and luteinizing hormone releasing hormone; see *gonadotropin releasing hormone*, under *hormone*.

FSH-RF follicle-stimulating hormone releasing factor; see under *factor*.

FSH-RH follicle stimulating hormone releasing hormone; see *gonadotropin releasing hormone*, under *hormone*.

ft. abbreviation for L. *fi′at* or *fi′ant*, let there be made, and for *foot* and *feet*.

Ft. mas. div. in pil. abbreviation for L. *fi′at mas′sa dividen′da in pil′ulae*, let a mass be made and divided into pills.

Ft. pulv. abbreviation for L. *fi′at pul′vis*, let a powder be made.

Fuadin (fu′ah-din) trademark for a preparation of stibophen.

Fuchs' coloboma, etc. (fooks) [Ernst *Fuchs*, German ophthalmologist, 1851–1930] see under *atrophy, coloboma, dimple, dystrophy,* and *syndrome*.

Fuchs' protein test [Hans J. *Fuchs*, German physician, 1873–1942] see under *tests*.

fuchsin (fook′sin) [from the pink, red, or purple flower *fuchsia*, after Leonard *Fuchs*, German botanist, 1501–1566] any of several red to purple triaminotriphenylmethane dyes. **acid f.,** a mixture of sulfonated fuchsins used in Andrade's indicator and in various complex stains; called also *acid magenta*. **basic f.,** an important histological dye, a mixture of pararosanilin, rosanilin, and magenta II. Also [USP] a mixture of rosaniline and pararosaniline hydrochlorides used as a local anti-infective. Called also *basic magenta*. **new f.,** a basic dye with staining properties much like those of basic fuchsin; it is triaminotritolylmethane chloride, or trimethyl fuchsin, $[CH_3(NH_2)\cdot C_6H_3]_2C\cdot C_6H_3(CH_3)\cdot NH_2Cl$.

fuchsinophil (fook-sin′o-fil) [*fuchsin* + Gr. *philein* to love] 1. any cell or other element readily stained with fuchsin. 2. fuchsinophilic.

fuchsinophilia (fook″sin-o-fil′e-ah) the property of staining readily with fuchsin dyes; especially the affinity of infarcted areas of the heart for acid fuchsin, which is an aid in determining diagnosis in cases of unexplained death.

fuchsinophilic (fook″sin-o-fil′ik) readily stained by fuchsin; pertaining to or characterized by fuchsinophilia.

fuchsinophilous (fook″sin-of′ĭ-lus) fuchsinophilic.

fucosan (fu′ko-san) a methylpentosan that is a constituent of the cell wall of many seaweeds, and is derived from L-fucose, or 6-deoxygalactose.

fucose (fu′kōs) an unusual monosaccharide occurring as L-fucose (6-deoxy-L-galactose) in a number of mucopolysaccharides and mucoproteins, including the blood group polysaccharides.

fucosidase (fu-ko′sĭ-dās) an enzyme that catalyzes the hydrolysis of fucoside to an alcohol and D-fucose; it occurs in two forms, α- and β-D-fucosidase. A defect in the α-form results in fucosidosis.

fucoside (fu′ko-sīd) an acetal derivative of fucose.

fucosidosis (fu″ko-si-do′sis) a hereditary neurovisceral disease, transmitted as an autosomal recessive trait, due to the absence of the enzymatic activity of α-fucosidase, and characterized by normal neurologic development during the first year of life followed by severe progressive cerebral degeneration, gradual loss of muscle strength, eventual spasticity and decorticate rigidity, emaciation, cardiomegaly with myocarditis, thick skin, excessive sweating, storage of abnormal carbohydrates and glycolipids in the liver and brain cells, and accumulation of fucose in all tissues.

fucoxanthin (fu″ko-zan′thin) [L. *fucus* rock lichen + Gr. *xanthos* yellow] the brown carotenoid found in diatoms, brown algae, and dinoflagellates.

FUDR floxuridine.

Fuerbringer (fer′bring-er) see *Fürbringer*.

fugacity (fu-gas′ĭ-te) [L. *fugacitas*, from *fugere* to flee] a measure of the escaping tendency of a substance from one phase to another phase, or from one part of a phase to another part of the same phase. The logarithm of the fugacity is proportional to the chemical potential.

-fugal (fu′gal) 1. [L., *fugare* to put to flight] a word termination implying banishing, or driving away, affixed to a stem designating the object of banishment, as *culicifugal*, driving away mosquitoes and gnats (*Culex*), or *febrifugal*, relieving or dispelling fever. 2. [L., *fugere* to flee from] a word termination implying traveling away from, affixed to a stem designating the object from which flight is made, as *centrifugal* traveling away from a center, or *corticifugal*, directed away from the cortex.

fugitive (fu′jĭ-tiv) [L. *fugitivus*] 1. wandering. 2. transient.

Fugu (fu′gu) [Jap.] a genus of Japanese puffer fish that contain a potent neurotoxin (tetrodotoxin) concentrated in the gonads and viscera, which when eaten without special cooking preparation causes generalized paralysis and in severe cases unconsciousness and death.

fugue (fūg) [L. *fuga* a flight] a dissociative reaction in which amnesia is accompanied by physical flight from customary surroundings. **epileptic f.,** a condition of clouded consciousness which may take the place of or follow an epileptic seizure.

fuguism (foo′goo-izm) [Jap. *fugu* the tetraodon fish + *-ism*] tetrodotoxism.

fuguismus (foo″goo-iz′mus) [see *fuguism*] tetrodotoxism.

fugutoxin (foo-goo-tok′sin) tetrodotoxin.

Fukala's operation (foo-kah′lahz) [Vincenz *Fukala*, Vienna ophthalmologist, 1847–1911] see under *operation*.

Fuld's test (fuldz) [Ernst *Fuld*, German internist, born 1873] see under *test*.

fulgurant (ful′gu-rant) [L. *fulgurans*, from *fulgur* lightning] coming and going like a flash of lightning.

fulgurate (ful′gu-rāt) 1. to come and go like a flash of lightning. 2. to destroy by contact with electric sparks generated by a high frequency current; see *fulguration*.

fulguration (ful″gu-ra′shun) [L. *fulgur* lightning] destruction of living tissue by electric sparks generated by a high frequency current. This may be direct or indirect. *Direct:* An insulated fulguration electrode with a metal point is connected to the uniterminal of the high frequency apparatus and a spark of electricity is allowed to impinge on the area to be treated. *Indirect:* In this procedure the patient is connected directly by a metal handle to the uniterminal and the operator utilizes an active electrode to complete an arc from the patient. **Keating-Hart's f.,** fulguration of external cancer.

fuliginous (fu-lij′ĭ-nus) [L. *fuligo* soot] sooty in color or appearance.

Fülleborn's method (fēl′ĕ-bornz) [Friedrich *Fülleborn*, German parasitologist, 1866–1933] see under *method*.

Fuller's operation [Eugene *Fuller*, New York urologist, 1858–1930] see under *operation*.

füllkörper (fēl′ker-per) [Ger., pl., "fill-bodies"] glia cells which have become degenerated; called also *filling cells*.

fulminant (ful′mĭ-nant) [L. *fulminare* to flare up] sudden, severe; occurring suddenly and with great intensity.

fulminate (ful′mĭ-nāt) to occur suddenly with great intensity.

Fulvicin (ful′vĭ-sin) trademark for a preparation of griseofulvin.

fumagillin (fu″mah-jil′in) chemical name: 2,4,6,8-decatetraenedioic acid mono[5-methoxy-4-[2-methyl-3-(3-methyl-2-butenyl)oxiranyl]-1-oxaspiro[2.5]oct-6-yl]ester. An antibiotic, $C_{26}H_{34}$-O_7, produced by *Aspergillus fumigatus.*

fumarase (fu′mah-rās) fumarate hydratase.

fumarate (fu′mar-āt) a salt of fumaric acid. In biochemistry, the term is often used interchangeably with fumaric acid (see under *acid*). **ferrous f.** [USP], a reddish orange to red-brown powder, $C_4H_2FeO_4$, slightly soluble in water; used as a hematinic in iron-deficiency anemia. **f. hydratase,** L-malate hydrolyase: an enzyme that catalyzes the equilibrium between fumaric acid (fumarate) and malic acid (malate); called also *fumarase.*

fumigacin (fu-mĭ-ga′sin) helvolic acid.

fumigant (fu′mĭ-gant) a substance used in fumigation.

fumigation (fu″mĭ-ga′shun) [L. *fumus* smoke, steam, vapor] exposure of an area or object to disinfecting fumes.

fuming (fūm′ing) [L. *fumus* smoke] smoking; emitting a visible vapor.

Fumiron (fūm′i-ron) trademark for a preparation of ferrous fumarate.

functio (funk′she-o) [L.] function. **f. lae′sa,** loss of function.

function (funk′shun) [L. *functio* a performance] the special, normal, or proper action of any part or organ. **antixenic f.,** the reactivity of living tissue to any foreign substance. **Carnot's f., carnotic f.,** the relation between the quantity of heat lost by a body and the work which can be done by it.

functional (funk′shun-al) of or pertaining to a function; affecting the functions, but not the structure; said of disturbances of function with no detectable organic cause. In chemistry, denoting the group within a molecule that participates in a chemical reaction, e.g., the —OH group of an alcohol, or the —NH_2 group of an amine.

functionalis (funk″she-o-na′lis) [L.] 1. functional. 2. stratum functionale.

functionating (funk′shun-āt-ing) in a condition of performing the proper function.

fundal (fun′dal) pertaining to a fundus.

fundament (fun′dah-ment) [L. *fundamentum*] 1. a base or foundation, such as the breech or rump. 2. the anus and parts adjacent to it.

fundamental (fun″dah-men′tal) pertaining to a base or foundation.

fundectomy (fun-dek′to-me) excision of the fundus of an organ, as the fundus of the uterus.

fundi (fun′di) [L.] plural of *fundus.*

fundic (fun′dik) pertaining to a fundus.

fundiform (fun′dĭ-form) [L. *funda* sling + *forma* form] shaped like a sling.

fundoplication (fun″do-pli-ka′shun) mobilization of the lower end of the esophagus and plication of the fundus of the stomach up around it, in treatment of peptic esophagitis to prevent reflux.

Fundulus (fun′du-lus) a genus of killifish of the order Cyprinodontidae, the common or green killifish, *F. heteroclitus,* is much used in biological research.

fundus (fun′dus), pl. *fun′di* [L.] the bottom or base of anything; [NA] a general term for the bottom or base of an organ, or the part of a hollow organ farthest from its mouth. **albinotic f.,** a fundus of the eye which permits clear visualization of the choroidal vasculature, owing to lack of pigment in the pigment epithelium and choroid. **f. albipuncta′tus,** a disorder in which gray or white mottling of the fundus of the eye is associated with night blindness; called also *Lauber's disease.* **f. of bladder,** 1. fundus vesicae urinariae. 2. apex vesicae urinariae. **f. of eye,** f. oculi. **f. flavimacula′tus,** a condition characterized by the presence of yellow to white atrophic lesions in the midperiphery or perimacular region of the fundus of the eye. **f. of gallbladder,** f. vesicae felleae. **gastric f.,** f. ventriculi. **f. of internal acoustic meatus, f. mea′tus acus′tici inter′ni** [NA], the laterally placed end or bottom of the internal acoustic meatus. **f. oc′uli,** fundus of the eye: the back portion of the interior of the eyeball, as seen by means of the ophthalmoscope. **f. of stomach,** f. ventriculi. **tessellated f., tigroid f.,** a fundus of the eye with marked exposure of the choroidal vessels due to scanty pigmentation. **f. tym′pani,** paries jugularis cavi tympani. **f. of urinary bladder,** 1. fundus vesicae urinariae. 2. apex vesicae urinariae. **f. u′teri** [NA], **f. of uterus,** the part of the uterus above the orifices of the uterine tubes. **f. of vagina, f. vagi′nae,** fornix vaginae. **f. ventric′uli** [NA], that part of the stomach to the left and above the level of the entrance of the esophagus; called also *gastric f.* and *f. of stomach.* **f. ves′icae fel′leae** [NA], the inferior, dilated portion of the gallbladder; called also *f. of gallbladder.* **f. ves′icae urina′riae** [NA], fundus of urinary bladder: the base or posterior surface of the bladder; called also *f. of bladder* and *infundibulum of urinary bladder.*

funduscope (fun′dus-skōp) [*fundus* + Gr. *skopein* to examine] an instrument for examining the fundus of the eye.

funduscopy (fun-dus′ko-pe) examination or inspection of the fundus of the eye.

fundusectomy (fun″dŭ-sek′to-me) [*fundus* + Gr. *ektomē* excision] excision of the fundus of the stomach.

fungal (fung′gal) pertaining to or caused by a fungus.

fungate (fung′gāt) to produce fungus-like growths; to grow rapidly, like a fungus.

fungemia (fun-je′me-ah) the presence of fungi in the blood stream.

fungi (fun′ji) [L.] plural of *fungus.*

Fungi Imperfecti (fun′ji im″per-fek′ti) [L., pl. "imperfect fungi"] a large heterogeneous group of fungi which have septate mycelium and in which the perfect (sexual) stage is unknown. This group includes many of the fungi that are pathogenic for animals including man and plants, among them *Candida, Cryptococcus, Histoplasma* and *Pityrosporon.* Imperfect fungi are classified in form-classes, form-orders, and so on, until their perfect stages are identified. Called also *Deuteromycetes.*

fungicidal (fun″jĭ-si′dal) [*fungus* + L. *caedere* to kill] destroying fungi.

fungicide (fun′jĭ-sīd) an agent that destroys fungi.

fungicidin (fun″jĭ-si′din) nystatin.

fungiform (fun′jĭ-form) shaped like a fungus or mushroom.

fungistasis (fun-jĭ-sta′sis) [*fungus* + Gr. *stasis* a stopping] inhibition of growth of fungi.

fungistat (fun′jĭ-stat) a substance that inhibits the growth of fungi.

fungistatic (fun″jĭ-stat′ik) inhibiting the growth of fungi.

fungisterol (fun-jis′ter-ol) a sterol, $C_{25}H_{44}O$, found in ergot and other fungi.

fungitoxic (fun″jĭ-tok′sik) exerting a toxic effect upon fungi.

fungitoxicity (fun″jĭ-tok-sis′ĭ-te) the quality of exerting a toxic effect upon fungi.

Fungizone (fun′jĭ-zōn) trademark for a preparation of amphotericin B.

fungoid (fung′goid) [*fungus* + Gr. *eidos* form] resembling a fungus, or mushroom. **chignon f.,** a nodular growth often occurring on human hair.

fungosity (fun-gos′ĭ-te) a fungoid growth or excrescence.

fungous (fung′gus) [L. *fungosus*] of the nature of, caused by, or resembling a fungus.

fungus (fung′gus), pl. *fun′gi* [L.] a general term used to denote a group of eukaryotic protists, including mushrooms, yeasts, rusts, molds, smuts, etc., which are characterized by the absence of chlorophyll and by the presence of a rigid cell wall composed of chitin, mannans, and sometimes cellulose. They are usually of simple morphological form or show some reversible cellular specialization, such as the formation of pseudoparenchymatous tissue in the fruiting body of a mushroom. The dimorphic fungi grow, according to environmental conditions, as molds or yeasts. **algae-like f.,** Phycomycetes. **alpha f.** (*obs.*), the fungus, *Trichophyton menlagrophytes* var. *quinckeanum.* **beta f.** (*obs.*), the fungus, *Trichophyton schoenleinii.* **f. of the brain,** hernia cerebri. **cerebral f., f. cere′bri,** hernia cerebri. **chignon f.,** see under *fungoid.* **club f.,** Basidiomycetes. **cutaneous f.,** dermatophyte. **fission f.,** schizomycete. **foot f.,** a fungus, such as *Madurella mycetomi,* which produces maduromycosis, or other foot infection. **gamma f.,** a strain of the fungus *Trichophyton schoenleinii.* **f. haemato′des** (*obs.*), a soft, bleeding, malignant tumor. **imperfect f.,** a fungus whose perfect (sexual) stage is unknown; Fungi Imperfecti (Deuteromycetes). **kefir fungi,** a mixture of bacteria and yeasts capable of causing lactic acid fermentation of milk of the kefir type. **mold f.,** mycelial f. **mosaic f.,** a mycelium-like intercellular deposit of cholesterol sometimes seen in scrapings from lesions thought to be fungal in origin. **mycelial f.,** any fungus that forms mycelia, in contrast to a yeast fungus; called also *mold f.* and *thread f.* **perfect f.,** a fungus for which both sexual and asexual types of spore formation are known; see *Ascomycetes, Phycomycetes,* and *Basidiomycetes.* **proper f.,** Eumycetes. **ray f.,** Actinomyces. **sac f.,** Ascomycetes. **slime f.,** Mycetozoa. **f. tes′tis,** protrusion from a scrotal sinus of a mass of granulation tissue in tuberculous epididymitis. **thread f.,** mycelial f. **true f.,** Eumycetes. **umbilical f.** (*obs.*), umbilical granuloma. **yeast f.,** any single-celled budding form of a fungus, in contrast to a mold fungus. **yeast-like f.,** single-celled budding fungi, such as yeasts.

funic (fu′nik) pertaining to the funis.

funicle (fu′nĭ-kl) funiculus.

funicular (fu-nik′u-lar) pertaining to a funiculus.

funiculi (fu-nik′u-li) plural of *funiculus.*

funiculitis (fu-nik″u-li′tis) 1. inflammation of the spermatic cord. 2. inflammation of that portion of a spinal nerve root which lies within the intervertebral canal. **endemic f.,** a disease of unknown etiology occurring chiefly in Ceylon and southern

India, marked by painful swelling of the spermatic cord, chills, nausea, and vomiting. The disease also occurs sporadically in temperate climates. **filarial f.,** secondary involvement of the spermatic cord in lymphatic filariasis.

funiculoepididymitis (fu-nik″u-lo-ep″ĭ-did″ĭ-mi′tis) inflammation of the spermatic cord and the epididymis.

funiculopexy (fu-nik′u-lo-pek″se) [L. *funiculus* cord + Gr. *pēxis* fixation] surgical fixation of the spermatic cord to the tissues in the correction of undescended testes.

funiculus (fu-nik′u-lus), pl. *funic′uli* [L.] a cord; [NA] a general term for a cordlike structure or part. **f. am′nii,** a cord of tissue by which the amnion and chorion are temporarily united in certain ruminant animals. **f. ante′rior medul′lae spina′lis** [NA], **anterior f. of spinal cord,** the white substance of the spinal cord that lies on either side between the anterior median fissure and the ventral root; called also *ventral f.* and *f. ventralis.* **cuneate f., f. cunea′tus** [Burdachi], fasciculus cuneatus medullae spinalis. **f. cunea′tus latera′lis,** a longitudinal ridge on the oblongata between the line of roots of the spinal accessory nerve and the fasciculus cuneatus. **f. cunea′tus medul′lae oblonga′tae,** fasciculus cuneatus medullae oblongatae. **dorsal f., f. dorsa′lis,** funiculus posterior medullae spinalis. **f. gra′cilis** (*obs.*), fasciculus gracilis medullae spinalis. **f. grac′ilis medul′lae oblonga′tae** (*obs.*), fasciculus gracilis medullae oblongatae. **hepatic f.,** ductus choledochus. **lateral f. of medullae oblongata, f. latera′lis medul′lae oblonga′tae** [NA], the continuation into the medulla oblongata of all the fiber tracts of the lateral funiculus of the spinal cord, with the exception of the lateral pyramidal tract. **f. latera′lis medul′lae spina′lis** [NA], lateral funiculus of spinal cord: the white substance of the spinal cord that lies on either side between the dorsal and ventral roots; called also *anterolateral column* and *lateral white commissure of spinal cord.* **ligamentous f.,** ligamentum collaterale carpi ulnare. **funic′uli medul′lae spina′lis** [NA], funiculi of spinal cord: the large bundles of fiber tracts that make up the white substance of the spinal cord. **f. poste′rior medul′lae spina′lis** [NA], **posterior f. of spinal cord,** the white substance of the spinal cord that lies on either side between the posterior median sulcus and the dorsal root; called also *dorsal f.* and *f. dorsalis.* **f. of Rolando,** fasciculus of Rolando. **f. solita′rius** (*obs.*), tractus solitarius medullae oblongatae. **f. spermat′icus** [NA], the structure that extends from the abdominal inguinal ring to the testis; called also *chorda spermatica.* See *spermatic cord.* **funiculi of spinal cord,** funiculi medullae spinalis. **f. of spinal cord, anterior,** f. anterior medullae spinalis. **f. of spinal cord, lateral,** f. lateralis medullae spinalis. **f. of spinal cord, posterior,** f. posterior medullae spinalis. **f. te′res** (*obs.*), eminentia medialis fossae rhomboideae. **f. umbilica′lis** [NA], the flexible structure connecting the umbilicus with the placenta and giving passage to the umbilical arteries and vein; called also *chorda umbilicalis* and *funis.* See *umbilical cord,* under *cord.* **ventral f., f. ventra′lis,** f. anterior medullae spinalis.

funiform (fu′nĭ-form) [L. *funis* rope + *forma* shape] resembling a rope or cord.

funis (fu′nis) [L. "cord"] any cordlike structure; particularly the umbilical cord. **f. bra′chii,** the median cephalic vein of the arm (vena mediana cephalica). **f. hippoc′ratis,** tendo calcaneus.

funnel (fun′el) a conic, hollow structure with a narrow opening at the apex, such as the vessels used in chemistry and pharmacy in filtering and for other purposes. **accessory müllerian f.,** a rudiment similar to the primordial uterine tube. **mitral f.,** the cone-shaped mitral valve seen in mitral stenosis, the orifice being at the apex of the cone. **muscular f.,** the funnel-shaped space bounded by the four straight muscles of the eye. **pial f.,** a sheath of adventitia, extended from the pia mater, loosely surrounding the blood vessels of the substance of the brain or cord. **Renver's f.,** an appliance used in treating urethral stricture. **vascular f.,** the light colored depression at the center of the disk of the retina.

F.U.O. fever of undetermined origin.

Furacin (fu′rah-sin) trademark for preparations of nitrofurazone.

Furadantin (fur″ah-dan′tin) trademark for preparations of nitrofurantoin.

furan, furane (fu′ran) a colorless liquid, CH:CH·CH:CH, from

```
|___O___|
```

wood tar.

furanose (fu′rah-nōs) a sugar in which the oxygen ring bridges carbon atoms 1 and 4 in the aldoses or carbon atoms 2 and 5 in the ketoses.

Furaspor (fur′ah-spōr) trademark for a preparation of nitrofurfuryl methyl ether; see under *ether.*

furazolidone (fu″rah-zol′ĭ-dōn) chemical name: 3-[[(5-nitro-2-furanyl)methylene]amino]-2-oxazolidinone. An antibacterial and antiprotozoal, $C_8H_7N_3O_5$, occurring as a white to slightly yellow, crystalline powder, effective against many gram-negative enteric organisms; used in the treatment of diarrhea and enteritis due to

susceptible organisms, administered orally, and (combined with nifuroxime) in bacterial, candidal, and trichomonal vaginitis, administered intravaginally.

furazolium (fūr″ah-zo′le-um) chemical name: 6,7-dihydro-3-(5-nitro-2-furyl)-5 H-imidazo [2,1-b] thiazolium; an antibacterial. **f. chloride,** the chloride salt of furazolium, $C_9H_8ClN_3O_3S$; an antibacterial. **f. tartrate,** the tartrate salt of furazolium, $C_{13}H_{13}N_3O_9S$; an antibacterial.

Fürbringer's sign, test (fer′bring-erz) [Paul *Fürbringer,* Berlin physician, 1849–1930] see under *sign* and *tests.*

furcal (fur′kal) [L. *furca* fork] shaped like a fork; forked.

furcation (fur-ka′shun) the anatomical area of a multirooted tooth where the roots divide.

furcocercous (fur″ko-ser′kus) [L. *furca* fork + Gr. *kerkos* tail] having a forked tail.

furcula (fur′ku-la) [L. "little fork"] a horseshoe-shaped ridge in the embryonic larynx, bounding the pharyngeal aperture in front and laterally.

furfuraceous (fur″fu-ra′shus) [L. *furfur* bran] fine and loose; said of scales resembling bran or dandruff.

furfural (fur′fu-ral) furfurol.

furfuran (fur′fu-ran) furan.

furfurol (fur′fu-rol) [L. *furfur* bran] an aromatic compound, CH:CH·CH:C·CHO, from the distillation of bran, sawdust, etc. It

```
|___O___|
```

causes convulsions in animals.

furibund (fu′rĭ-bund) full of fury; raging; maniacal.

furobufen (fur″o-bu′fen) chemical name: γ-oxo-2-dibenzofuran-butanoic acid; an anti-inflammatory, $C_{16}H_{12}O_4$.

furocoumarin (fu″ro-koo′mah-rin) any of a group of antifungal dyestuffs produced by certain species of plants (e.g., parsley and figs) which, on contact with skin, cause photosensitization.

furodazole (fur-o′dah-zōl) chemical name: 2-(2-furanyl)-7-methyl-1 H-imidazol hydrate; an anthelmintic, $C_{15}H_{11}N_3O_2 \cdot x$-$H_2O$.

furor (fu′ror) [L.] fury; rage. **f. epilep′ticus,** an attack of intense anger occurring in epilepsy. **f. uteri′nus,** nymphomania.

furosemide (fu-ro′sĕ-mīd) [USP] chemical name: 5-(aminosulfonyl)-4-chloro-2-[2-furanylmethyl)amino]benzoic acid. A sulfonamide, $C_{12}H_{11}ClN_2O_5S$, occurring as a white to slightly yellow, crystalline powder; used as a diuretic in the treatment of disorders in which edema is a symptom and in hypertension, administered orally, intramuscularly, and intravenously. Called also *frusemide* and *fursemide.*

Furoxone (fur-ok′sōn) trademark for preparations of furazolidone.

furrow (fur′o) a groove or trench. **atrioventricular f.,** the transverse groove marking off the atria of the heart from the ventricles. **digital f.,** any one of the transverse folds across the joints on the palmar surface of a finger. **genital f.,** a groove that appears on the genital tubercle of the fetus at the end of the second month. **gluteal f.,** the furrow which separates the buttocks; called also *intergluteal* or *natal cleft.* **Jadelot's f's,** see under *line.* **Liebermeister's f's,** depressions sometimes seen on the upper surface of the liver from pressure of the ribs, generally caused by tight garments or tight lacing of a girdle or corset. **mentolabial f.,** the hollow just above the chin. **nympholabial f.,** a groove separating the labium majus and labium minus on either side. **primitive f.,** primitive groove. **scleral f.,** sulcus sclerae. **Sibson's f.,** the lower border of the pectoralis major muscle. **skin f's,** sulci cutis.

fursalan (fur′sah-lan) chemical name: 3,5-dibromo-N-(tetrahydrofurfuryl)salicylamide; a disinfectant, $C_{12}H_{13}Br_2NO_3$.

fursemide (fur′sĕ-mīd) furosemide.

Fürstner's disease (ferst′nerz) [Carl *Fürstner,* German psychiatrist, 1848–1906] see under *disease.*

furuncle (fu′rung-k'l) [L. *furunculus*] a painful nodule formed in the skin by circumscribed inflammation of the corium and subcutaneous tissue, enclosing a central slough or "core." Furuncles are caused by staphylococci, which enter through the hair follicles, and their formation is favored by constitutional or digestive derangement and local irritation. Called also *boil* and *furunculus.*

furuncular (fu-rung′ku-lar) pertaining to or of the nature of a furuncle or boil.

furunculoid (fu-rung′ku-loid) resembling a furuncle or boil.

furunculosis (fu-rung″ku-lo′sis) 1. the persistent sequential occurrence of furuncles over a period of weeks or months. 2. the simultaneous occurrence of a number of furuncles. **f. blastomycet′ica, f. cryptococ′cica,** any systemic fungous infection in which the lesions resemble furuncles.

furunculus (fu-rung′ku-lus), pl. *furun′culi* [L.] furuncle. **f. orienta′lis** (*obs.*), cutaneous leishmaniasis.

fusaridiosis (fu″sah-rid″e-o′sis) a dermatomycosis of horses thought to be caused by the mold *Fusarium equinum* (a species now considered to be identical with *Microsporum canis*).

fusariotoxicosis (fu-sar″ĭ-o-tok″sĭ-ko'sis) a form of mycotoxicosis caused by fungi of the genus *Fusarium.*

Fusarium (fu-sa're-um) a genus of Fungi Imperfecti of the order Moniales, family Tuberculariaceae; the perfect stages of many species are included in the class Ascomycetes, order Hypocreales. Some are important pathogens of plants, and some are opportunistic infectious agents of man and animals. They have been isolated from otomycosis externa and mycotic keratitis. *F. oxysporum* and *F. solani* are frequently associated with mycotic keratitis, often destroying the eye. The *F. equinum* reported to cause a dermatomycosis of horses is probably *Microsporum canis.* **F. oxyspor'um,** a species causing banana wilt. **F. sol'anae,** a species causing potato wilt and, occasionally, mycotic keratitis of man. **F. sporotri'chiella,** a species believed to be the etiologic agent of Kashin-Beck disease.

fuscin (fu'sin) [L. *fuscus* brown] a brown pigment of the retinal epithelium.

fuse (fūz) 1. a bar, strip, or wire of easily fusible metal inserted for safety in an electric circuit; when the current increases beyond a safe strength the metal melts, thus breaking the circuit and thereby saving an apparatus from overload. 2. to join together, as the abnormal coherence of adjacent body structures.

fuseau (fĕ-zō′), pl. *fuseaux* [Fr.] a macroaleuriospore or macrocondium.

fusi (fu'si) [L.] plural of *fusus.*

fusible (fu'zĭ-b'l) susceptible of being melted or fused.

fusicellular (fu″sĭ-sel'u-lar) fusocellular.

fusidate sodium (fu'sĭ-dāt) chemical name: (17*Z*)-16β-(acetyloxy)-3α,11α-dihydroxy-29-nor-8α,9β,13α,14β-dammara-17(20),-24-diene-21-oic acid monosodium salt; an antibiotic of unspecified action, $C_{31}H_{47}NaO_4$.

fusiform (fu'zĭ-form) [L. *fusus* spindle + *forma* form] spindle shaped.

Fusiformis (fu″sĭ-for'mis) a name formerly given to the genus *Fusobacterium.* **F. necroph'orus,** *Fusobacterium necrophorum.*

fusimotor (fu″sĭ-mo'tor) denoting motor nerve fibers (of gamma motoneurons) that innervate intrafusal fibers of the muscle spindle.

fusion (fu'zhun) [L. *fusio*] 1. the act, process, or result of melting. 2. the merging or coherence of adjacent parts or bodies. 3. the coordination of the separate images of the same object in the two eyes into one. 4. the operative formation of an ankylosis or arthrodesis (*f. of joint*). **binocular f.,** see *fusion,* def. 3. **diaphyseal-epiphyseal f.,** operative establishment of bony union between the diaphysis and epiphysis, to arrest growth in length of a bone. **nerve f.,** a method of nerve anastomosis done for the purpose of inducing a regeneration which will resupply empty tracts of a nerve by new growths of fibers. **nuclear f.,** the fusion of two atomic nuclei to form a single heavier nucleus, resulting in the release of large amounts of energy. **spinal f.,** spondylosyndesis.

fusional (fu'zhun-al) marked by fusion.

Fusobacterium (fu″zo-bak-te're-um) a genus of nonsporulating obligate anaerobic filamentous bacteria occurring as normal flora in the mouth and large bowel; often found in necrotic tissue, probably as secondary invaders. Formerly called *Fusiformis.* **F. necroph'orum,** a species found in abscesses of the liver, lungs, blood, and other tissues and in chronic ulcer of the colon in man. It is also pathogenic for animals. Called also *Actinomyces necrophorus, Bacteroides funduliformis,* Schmorl's bacillus, and *Sphaerophorus necrophorus.* See also *foot rot of cattle* and *foot rot of sheep,* under *rot; necrobacillosis; calf diphtheria,* under *diphtheria,* and *Schmorl's disease,* under *disease.* **F. plau'ti-vincen'ti,** an organism found along with a spirillum (*Borrelia vincenti*) in necrotizing ulcerative gingivitis (trench mouth) and necrotizing ulcerative stomatitis. Called also *Bacteroides fusiformis.*

fusocellular (fu″so-sel'u-lar) [L. *fu'sus* spindle + *cellular*] having spindle-shaped cells.

fusospirillary (fu″so-spi'rĭ-lār″e) pertaining to or caused by fusiform bacilli and spirillae, as in necrotizing ulcerative gingivitis.

fusospirillosis (fu″so-spi″rĭ-lo'sis) necrotizing ulcerative gingivitis.

fusospirochetal (fu″so-spi″ro-ke'tal) pertaining to or caused by fusiform bacilli and spirochetes.

fusospirochetosis (fu″so-spi″ro-ke-to'sis) infection with fusiform bacilli and spirochetes.

fusostreptococcicosis (fu″so-strep″to-kok-sĭ-ko'sis) infection with fusiform bacilli and streptococci.

fustic (fus'tik) a yellow dye wood from a South American tree, *Chlorophora tinctoria.*

fustigation (fus″tĭ-ga'shun) [L. *fustigatio*] flagellation (def. 2).

fusus (fu'sus), pl. *fu'si* [L.] a spindle-like object; applied especially to minute air vesicles in a hair shaft. **cortical fusi,** the delicate air spaces appearing among the cells of the cortex as a hair grows out, produced by drying out of the fluid which fills the spaces in the living portion of the hair root. **fracture fusi,** minute rifts or ruptures observed between the keratinized cells of the cortex of a mature hair shaft which has been subjected to pressure sufficient to dissociate the cells of the particular region.

fututrix (fu-tu'triks) a female who practices tribadism.

F. vs. abbreviation for L. *fi'at venaesec'tio,* let the patient be bled.

G

G 1. symbol for *gravitational constant.* 2. symbol for *giga.* 3. gram; gingival; glucose; gonidial (colony).

g gravity; the unit of force exerted upon the body during acceleration and deceleration; gram.

g. gram (or grams).

γ the third letter of the Greek alphabet; see *gamma.* Symbol for *microgram* and *immunoglobulin.*

Ga chemical symbol for *gallium.*

GABA gamma-aminobutyric acid.

G-actin see *actin.*

gadfly (gad'fli) see *Tabanus.*

gadolinium (gad″o-lin'e-um) a rare element of atomic number 64, atomic weight 157.25, symbol Gd.

gaduhiston (gad″u-his'ton) [L. *gadus* cod + *histon*] a histone occurring in the spermatozoa of the codfish.

Gadus (ga'dus) [L.; Gr. *gados*] a genus of fishes. **G. mor'rhua,** the codfish; from its liver, cod liver oil is prepared.

Gaenslen's sign (test) (genz'lenz) [Frederick Julius *Gaenslen,* Milwaukee surgeon, 1877–1937] see under *sign.*

Gaertner see *Gärtner.*

Gaffky scale (table) (gaf'ke) [Georg Theodor August *Gaffky,* German bacteriologist, 1850–1918] see under *scale.*

Gaffkya (gaf'ke-ah) [G. T. A. *Gaffky*] a genus of microorganisms of the family Micrococcaceae, order Eubacteriales, occurring as spherical cells in tetrads, often appearing to be enclosed in a common capsule. **G. homa'ri,** a species pathogenic for lobsters but not known to occur in man. **G. tetrag'ena,** a part of the normal flora of the upper respiratory tract of man, but often pathogenic for mice and other species.

gag (gag) 1. a surgical device for holding the mouth open. 2. to retch, or strive to vomit. **Dott g.,** an instrument for keeping the mouth open during operations on the palate. **Kilner-Dott g.,** an instrument for keeping the mouth open during operations on the palate.

gage (gāj) gauge.

Gaillard-Arlt suture (ga-yahrz′) [François Lucien *Gaillard,* French physician, 1805–1869; Carl Ferdinand Ritter von *Arlt,* ophthalmologist in Vienna, 1812–1887] see under *suture.*

gain (gān) 1. an increase in amount or value; a benefit or advantage; the increase achieved by amplification of a signal. 2. to acquire, obtain, or increase. **antigen g.,** the acquisition by cells of new antigenic determinants not normally present or not normally accessible in the parent tissue. **epinosic g.,** a secondary psychic or social advantage derived from a symptom or illness, as opposed to paranosic gain. Called also *secondary g.* **paranosic g.,** the primary psychic advantage in allaying internal conflicts and preserving ego integrity, derived from neurotic illness; opposed to epinosic gain. Called also *primary g.* **primary g.,** paranosic g. **secondary g.,** epinosic g.

Gairdner's test (gārd'nerz) [Sir William Tennant *Gairdner,* Scotch physician, 1824–1907; see under *tests.*

Gaisböck's disease, syndrome (gīs'bekz) [Felix *Gaisböck,* German physician, 1868–1955] stress polycythemia.

gait (gāt) the manner or style of walking. **antalgic g.,** a limp adopted so as to avoid pain on weight-bearing structures (as in hip injuries), characterized by a very short stance phase. **ataxic g.,** an unsteady, uncoordinated walk, employing a wide base; see *tabetic g.* **cerebellar g.,** a staggering gait indicative of cerebellar disease. **Charcot's g.,** the peculiar gait seen in Friedreich's ataxia. **double step g.,** a gait in which the length and/or timing of alternate steps is noticeably different. **drag-to g.,** a gait in which the feet are dragged (rather than lifted) toward the crutches. **equine g.,** a walk accomplished mainly by flexing the hip joint; seen in crossed-leg palsy. **festinating g.,** a gait in which the patient involuntarily moves with short, accelerating steps, often on tiptoe, as seen in paralysis agitans and other nervous disorders; festination. **four-point g.,** a gait in forward motion is as follows: first one crutch and then the opposite leg, followed by the other crutch and then the other leg, and so on. **gluteal g.,** the gait characteristic of paralysis of the gluteus medius muscle, marked by a listing of the trunk toward the affected side at each step; called also *Trendelenburg g.* **heel-toe g.,** a gait in which the heel touches down first and the toes last. **helicopod g.,** a gait in which the feet describe half-circles, as in some cases of hysterical disorder. **hemiplegic g.,** a gait involving flexion of the hip because of drop-foot and circumduction of the leg. **intermittent double-step g.,** a hemiplegic gait in which there is a pause after the short step of the normal foot, or in some cases after the step of the affected foot. **Oppenheim's g.,** a gait marked by irregular oscillation of the head, limbs, and body; seen in some cases of multiple sclerosis. **scissor g.,** a gait in which one foot is passed in front of the other, producing a cross-legged progression. **spastic g.,** a walk in which the legs are held together and move in a stiff manner, the toes seeming to drag and catch. **staggering g.,** a reeling, tottering, and tipping gait in which the individual appears as if he may fall backward or lose his balance; it is associated with alcoholic and barbiturate intoxication. **steppage g.,** the gait in drop foot in which the advancing leg is lifted high in order that the toes may clear the ground. It is due to paralysis of the anterior tibial and peroneal muscles and is seen in lesions of the lower motor neuron, such as multiple neuritis, lesions of the anterior motor horn cells, and lesions of the cauda equina. **swaying g.,** cerebellar g. **swing-through g.,** a gait in which the crutches are advanced and then the legs are swung past them. **swing-to g.,** a gait in which the crutches are advanced and the legs are swung to the same point. **tabetic g.,** an ataxic gait in which the feet slap the ground; in daylight the patient can avoid some unsteadiness by watching his feet. **three-point g.,** a gait in which both crutches and the affected leg are advanced together and then the normal leg is moved forward. **Trendelenburg g.,** gluteal g. **two-point g.,** a gait in which the right foot and left crutch (or cane) are advanced together, and then the left foot and right crutch. **waddling g.,** exaggerated alternation of lateral trunk movements with an exaggerated elevation of the hip, suggesting the gait of a duck; characteristic of progressive muscular dystrophy.

galact- see *galacto-*.

galactacrasia (gal″ak-tah-kra′se-ah) [*galact-* + *a* neg. + Gr. *krasis* mixture + *-ia*] abnormal condition of the breast milk.

galactagogin (gah-lak″tah-gog′in) human placental lactogen.

galactagogue (gah-lak′tah-gog) [*galact-* + Gr. *agōgos* leading] 1. promoting the flow of milk. 2. an agent that promotes the flow of milk.

galactan (gah-lak′tan) a hemicellulose carbohydrate that yields galactose upon hydrolysis; agar is a well-known example.

galactemia (gal″ak-te′me-ah) [*galact-* + Gr. *haima* blood + *-ia*] the presence of milk in the blood.

galactic (gah-lak′tik) 1. pertaining to milk. 2. galactagogue.

galactin (gah-lak′tin) prolactin.

galactischia (gal″ak-tisk′e-ah) [*galact-* + Gr. *ischein* to suppress] suppression of the secretion of milk.

galactitol (gah-lak′tĭ-tol) dulcitol.

galacto-, galact- (gah-lak′to; gah-lakt′) [Gr. *gala, galaktos* milk] combining form denoting relationship to milk.

galactoblast (gah-lak′to-blast) [*galacto-* + Gr. *blastos* germ] a colostrum corpuscle found in the acini of the mammary gland.

galactobolic (gah-lak″to-bol′ik) of or relating to the action of neurohypophyseal peptides which contract the mammary myoepithelium and cause ejection of milk.

galactocele (gah-lak′to-sēl) [*galacto-* + Gr. *kēlē* tumor] 1. cystic enlargement of the mammary gland containing milk. 2. a hydrocele filled with a milky fluid. Called also *galactoma*.

galactocerebroside (gah-lak″to-ser′ĕ-bro-sīd) cerebroside.

galactochloral (gah-lak-to-klo′ral) a derivative, $C_8H_4Cl_3O_6$, of chloral and galactose in glossy scales; it is used as a hypnotic.

galactocrasia (gah-lak-to-kra′se-ah) galactacrasia.

galactogen (gah-lak′to-jen) a polysaccharide in the eggs of snails which yields galactose on hydrolysis.

galactogenous (gal″ak-toj′ĕ-nus) [*galacto-* + Gr. *gennan* to produce] favoring the production of milk.

galactogogue (gah-lak″to-gog) galactagogue.

galactography (gal″ak-tog′rah-fe) [*galacto-* + *-graphy*] radiography of the mammary ducts after injection of a radiopaque substance into the duct system.

galactokinase (gah-lak″to-ki′nās) ATP: D-galactose-1-phosphotransferase: an enzyme that catalyzes the transfer of a high-energy phosphate group from a donor to D-galactose, producing D-galactose-1-phosphate. See also *kinase* (def. 1).

galactolipid (gah-lak″to-lip′id) galactolipin.

galactolipin, galactolipine (gah-lak″to-li′pin) a cerebroside which yields galactose on hydrolysis; found abundantly in nervous tissue, usually as structural material. See *cerebroside*.

galactoma (gal″ak-to′mah) [*galact-* + *-oma*] galactocele.

galactometastasis (gah-lak″to-mĕ-tas′tah-sis) galactoplania.

galactometer (gal″ak-tom′ĕ-ter) [*galacto-* + Gr. *metron* measure] an instrument for measuring the specific gravity of milk.

galactopexic (gah-lak″to-pek″sik) fixing or holding galactose.

galactopexy (gah-lak′to-pek″se) the fixation of galactose by the liver.

galactophagous (gal″ak-tof′ah-gus) [*galacto-* + Gr. *phagein* to eat] feeding upon milk.

galactophlebitis (gah-lak″to-fle-bi′tis) [*galacto-* + *phlebitis*] phlegmasia alba dolens.

galactophlysis (gal″ak-tof′lĭ-sis) [*galacto-* + Gr. *phlysis* eruption] a vesicular eruption containing a milky fluid.

galactophore (gah-lak′to-for) 1. galactophorous. 2. a milk duct.

galactophoritis (gah-lak″to-fo-ri′tis) [*galacto-* + Gr. *pherein* to carry + *-itis*] inflammation of the milk ducts.

galactophorous (gal″ak-tof′o-rus) [*galacto-* + Gr. *pherein* to bear] conveying milk.

galactophygous (gal″ak-tof′ĭ-gus) [*galacto-* + Gr. *phygē* flight] arresting the milk secretion.

galactoplania (gah-lak″to-pla′ne-ah) [*galacto-* + Gr. *planē* wandering] the secretion of milk in some abnormal part; the metastasis of milk. Called also *galactometastasis*.

galactopoiesis (gah-lak″to-poi-e′sis) the production of milk by the mammary glands.

galactopoietic (gah-lak″to-poi-et′ik) [*galacto-* + Gr. *poiein* to make] 1. pertaining to, characterized by, or promoting the production of milk. 2. an agent that promotes the secretion of milk.

galactopyra (gah-lak″to-pi′rah) [*galacto-* + Gr. *pyr* fire] milk fever.

galactopyranose (gah-lak″to-pi′rah-nōs) the pyranose form of galactose, $CH_2OH \cdot CH \cdot CH \cdot (CHOH)_3 \cdot CHOH$.

galactorrhea (gah-lak″to-re′ah) [*galacto-* + Gr. *rhoia* flow] excessive or spontaneous flow of milk; persistent secretion of milk irrespective of nursing.

galactosamine (gah-lak″to-sam′in) an amino sugar, $NH_2 \cdot CH_2 \cdot C(CHOH)_4CHOH$.

galactosan (gah-lak″to-san) a polysaccharide occurring in plants, yielding galactose on hydrolysis.

galactosazone (gah-lak″to-sa′zōn) the phenylosazone of galactose, $CHOH(CHOH)_3C(:N \cdot NH \cdot C_6H_5) \cdot CH \cdot N \cdot NH \cdot C_6H_5$. It is a yellow, crystalline substance formed by treating galactose with phenylhydrazine and acetic acid. The crystals melt at 193° C. and may be used in identifying galactose.

galactoschesis (gal″ak-tos′kĕ-sis) [*galacto-* + Gr. *schesis* suppression] galactischia.

galactoscope (gah-lak′to-skōp) [*galacto-* + Gr. *skopein* to examine] a device for showing the proportion of cream in the milk.

galactose (gah-lak′tōs) an aldohexose, $CH_2OH(CHOH)_4CHO$, obtained from lactose or milk sugar by enzymatic action or by boiling with a mineral acid. It is a white crystalline substance, resembles glucose in most of its properties, but is less soluble, less sweet, and forms mucic acid when oxidized with nitric acid. D-Galactose is found in milk sugar, in the cerebrosides of the brain, in the raffinose of the sugar beet, and in many gums and seaweeds; L-galactose in flaxseed mucilage.

galactosemia (gah-lak″to-se′me-ah) a hereditary disorder of galactose metabolism occurring in two forms. The classic form, due to deficiency of the enzyme galactose-1-phosphate uridyl transferase, is marked by accumulation of galactose 1-phosphate and galactose in the tissues and by hepatomegaly, cataracts, and mental retardation, with vomiting, diarrhea, jaundice, poor weight gain, and malnutrition in early infancy. The second form, due to galactokinase deficiency, is marked only by cataract formation and accumulation of galactose in the blood and tissues. Both forms are transmitted as autosomal recessive traits.

galactosidase (gah-lak″to-si′dās) an enzyme occurring in two forms: α-*galactosidase* (melibiase) hydrolyzes the conversion of α-D-galactoside to D-galactose; β-*galactosidase* (lactase), which occurs in the kidney, liver, and intestinal mucosa, hydrolyzes the conversion of β-D-galactoside to D-galactose.

galactoside (gah-lak′to-sīd) a glycoside containing galactose.

galactosis (gal″ak-to′sis) the formation of milk by the lacteal glands.

galactostasia (gah-lak″to-sta′se-ah) galactostasis.

galactostasis (gal″ak-tos′tah-sis) [*galacto-* + Gr. *stasis* halt] 1. cessation of the milk secretion. 2. an abnormal collection of milk in the mammary glands.

galactosuria (gah-lak″to-su′re-ah) [*galactose* + Gr. *ouron* urine + *-ia*] presence of galactose in the urine.

galactotherapy (gah-lak″to-ther′ah-pe) [*galacto-* + Gr. *therapeia* treatment] 1. the treatment of suckling children by giving remedies to the mother or wet nurse. 2. milk cure. 3. (*obs.*) the hypodermic injection of the milk of a syphilitic patient for the cure of syphilis.

galactotoxin (gah-lak″to-tok′sin) [*galacto-* + Gr. *toxikon* poison] a basic substance formed in milk.

galactotoxism (gah-lak″to-tok′sizm) poisoning by milk.

galactotrophy (gal″ak-tot′ro-fe) [*galacto-* + Gr. *trophē* nutrition] feeding with milk.

galactowaldenase (gah-lak″to-wal′den-ās) UDP-glucose epimerase.

galactoxism (gal″ak-tok′sizm) galactotoxism.

galactoxismus (gah-lak″tok-siz′mus) galactotoxism.

galactozymase (gah-lak″to-zi′mās) [*galacto-* + Gr. *zymē* leaven] a starch-liquefying enzyme.

galacturia (gal″ak-tu′re-ah) [*galact-* + Gr. *ouron* urine + *-ia*] the discharge of milklike urine; chyluria.

galantamine hydrobromide (gah-lan′tah-mēn) galanthamine hydrobromide.

galanthamine hydrobromide (gah-lan′thah-mēn) the hydrobromide salt of an alkaloid, $C_{17}H_{21}NO_3 \cdot HBr$, obtained in the U.S.S.R. from the Caucasian snowdrop *Galanthus woronowii* and closely related species. It is a cholinesterase inhibitor, and is used in the U.S.S.R. in the treatment of myasthenia, myopathy, and sensory and motor dysfunction associated with disorders of the central nervous system and may be used as an antidote to nonpolarizing muscle relaxants. Called also *galantamine hydrobromide*.

gale (gahl) [Fr.] scabies.

galea (ga′le-ah) [L.] a helmet; [NA] a general term for a helmet-like structure. **g. aponeurot′ica** [NA], the aponeurotic structure of the scalp, connecting the frontal and occipital bellies of the occipitofrontalis muscle.

galeanthropy (ga″le-an′thro-pe) [Gr. *galē* cat + *anthrōpos* man] (*obs.*) a mental delusion that one has become a cat.

Galeati's glands (gal″e-ah′tēz) [Domenico Maria *Galeati*, Italian physician, 1686–1775] glandulae duodenales.

galeatus (gal″e-a′tus) [L. *galea* helmet] born with a caul.

Galeazzi's fracture, sign (gal″e-at′zēz) [Riccardo *Galeazzi*, Italian orthopedic surgeon, 1866–1952] see under the nouns.

Galen (ga′len) [Claudius (or Clarissimus) Galenus] (c. 129–199 A.D.). The celebrated Greek physician and medical writer, born at Pergamum (Asia Minor); latterly he practiced in Rome, where he became physician to the Emperor, Marcus Aurelius. Although he did not dissect the human cadaver, he made many valuable anatomical and physiological observations on animals, and his writings on these and other subjects are extensive. His influence on medicine was profound for many centuries—his teleology ("nature does nothing in vain") being particularly attractive to the medieval mind, although it was stultifying as regards advances in medical thought and practice. See also under *anastomosis*, *bandage*, and *foramen*, and see *venae cerebri internae*, and *magna*, and *ventricular laryngis*.

galenic (gah-len′ik) pertaining to the ancient system of medicine taught and practiced by Galenus, or Galen.

galenica (gah-len′ĭ-kah) galenicals.

galenicals (gah-len′ĭ-kalz) medicines prepared according to the formulas of Galen; the term is now used to denote standard preparations containing one or several organic ingredients, as contrasted with pure chemical substances.

galenics (gah-len′iks) galenicals.

galenism (ga′len-izm) Galen's system of medicine, being a blend of the humoral theory and Pythagorean number lore.

Galeodes araneoides (gal″e-o′dēz ah-ra″ne-oi′dēz) a spider-like arachnid of the Old World, with a venomous bite.

galeophilia (gal″e-o-fil′e-ah) (*obs.*) ailurophilia.

galeophobia (gal″e-o-fo′be-ah) (*obs.*) ailurophobia.

galeropia, galeropsia (gal″er-o′pe-ah, gal″er-op′se-ah) [Gr. *galeros* cheerful + *opsis* vision] exceptional clearness of vision.

gall (gawl) [L. *galla*] 1. the bile. 2. nutgall. **Aleppo g.,** nutgall. **ox g.,** see *ox bile extract*, under *extract*. **Smyrna g.,** nutgall. **wind g.,** windgall.

Gall's craniology (gawlz) [Franz Joseph *Gall*, anatomist in Vienna and Paris, 1758–1828] phrenology.

gallacetophenone (gal-as″e-to-fe′non) chemical name: 2′,3′,4′-trihydroxyacetophenone. A yellowish powder, $CH_3 \cdot CO \cdot C_6H_2(OH)_3$, used as an antiseptic.

gallamine triethiodide (gal′ah-mĭn tri″ĕ-thi′o-dīd) [USP] chemical name: 2,2′,2″-[1,2,3,-benzenetriyltris(oxy)]tris[*N*,*N*,*N*-triethyl]ethanaminium triiodide. A quaternary ammonium compound, $C_{30}H_{60}I_3N_3O_3$, occurring as a white, amorphous powder; used to induce skeletal muscle relaxation during surgery and

other procedures, such as endoscopy or intubation, administered intravenously. Called also *benzurine iodide*.

gallate (gal′āt) any salt of gallic acid.

gallbladder (gawl′blad-der) the pear-shaped reservoir for the bile on the posteroinferior surface of the liver, between the right and the quadrate lobe; from its neck, the cystic duct projects to join the common bile duct. Called also *cholecyst* and *vesica fellea* [NA]. **Courvoisier's g.,** a distended gallbladder resulting from biliary tract obstruction. **fish-scale g.,** a gallbladder with a fish-scale-like appearance due to multiple small cysts of the mucosa. **floating g.,** wandering g. **folded fundus g.,** phrygian cap. **hourglass g.,** a gallbladder in which there is an annular constriction dividing it into a wide upper and a narrower lower compartment; the anomaly may be congenital or acquired. **mobile g.,** wandering g. **sandpaper g.,** a rough state of the mucous membrane of the gallbladder caused by the presence of the cholesterin crystals. **stasis g.,** a gallbladder that contracts sluggishly in response to a fatty meal. **strawberry g.,** a gallbladder with a strawberry-like appearance, due to fine grains of cholesterin-fat material embedded in the mucosa as a result of chronic catarrhal inflammation. **wandering g.,** abnormal mobility of the fundus and body of the gallbladder.

gallein (gal′e-in) dioxyfluorescein, an aniline dye indicator which is changed in color by an alkali to red and by an acid to yellow.

Gallie transplant (gal′e) [William Edward *Gallie*, Toronto surgeon, 1882–1959] see under *transplant*.

Galli Mainini test (gal′e mi-ne′ne) [Carlos *Galli Mainini*, physician in Buenos Aires] see under *test*.

Gallionella (gal″le-o-nel′ah) [Benjamin *Gaillon*, French zoologist, 1782–1839] a genus of microorganisms of the family Caulobacteraceae, suborder Pseudomonadineae, order Pseudomonadales, occurring as stalked, kidney-shaped or rounded cells, growing only in iron-containing fresh or salt water. It includes five species, *G. ferrugin′ea*, *G. infurca′ta*, *G. ma′jor*, *G. mi′nor*, and *G. umbella′ta*.

gallipot (gal′ĭ-pot) a small pot for ointments or confections.

gallisin (gal′ĭ-sin) a substance analogous to dextrin.

gallium (gal′e-um) [L., from *Gallia* Gaul] a rare metal liquid at room temperature; atomic number, 31; atomic weight, 69.72; symbol, Ga: some of its compounds are poisonous.

gallnut (gawl′nut) nutgall.

gallon (gal′on) [L. *congius*] a measure of volume, four quarts (3785 ml.); in the United States, 231 cubic inches.

gallop (gal′op) a disordered rhythm of the heart; see under *rhythm*.

gallsickness (gawl-sik′nes) anaplasmosis.

gallstone (gawl′stōn) a concretion, usually of cholesterol, formed in the gallbladder or bile duct.

GALT gut-associated lymphoid tissue; see under *tissue*.

Galton's delta, law, whistle (gawl′tonz) [Sir Francis *Galton*, English scientist, 1822–1911] see under the nouns.

Galv. galvanic.

galvanic (gal-van′ik) 1. named for or discovered by Luigi *Galvani*, Italian physician and physiologist, 1737–1798. 2. pertaining to galvanism.

galvanism (gal′vah-nizm) [Luigi *Galvani*] 1. galvanic electricity: unidirectional electric current derived from a chemical battery. 2. the therapeutic use of direct current. **dental g.,** a physicochemical phenomenon in which two or more dissimilar metals that have been used to restore or replace missing teeth produce the flow of an electric current. In such instances the patient may experience sharp, painful shocks to the teeth, and the pulp may become hyperemic or inflamed.

galvanization (gal″vah-ni-za′shun) treatment by galvanic electricity.

galvanocautery (gal″vah-no-kaw′ter-e) cautery accomplished by application of a wire heated with a galvanic current.

galvanochemical (gal″vah-no-kem′e-kal) pertaining to the chemical action of the galvanic current.

galvanocontractility (gal″vah-no-kon″trak-til′ĭ-te) contractility in response to a galvanic stimulus.

galvanogustometer (gal″vah-no-gus-tom′ĕ-ter) an apparatus for the clinical determination of taste thresholds by the use of a galvanic current.

galvanoionization (gal″vah-no-i″on-i-za′shun) (*obs.*) iontophoresis.

galvanolysis (gal″vah-nol′ĭ-sis) [*galvanism* + Gr. *lysis* dissolution] electrolysis.

galvanometer (gal″vah-nom′ĕ-ter) [*galvanism* + Gr. *metron* measure] an instrument for measuring current by electromagnetic action. **Einthoven's g., string g., thread g.,** an apparatus for detecting very minute electric currents, consisting of a delicate thread of silvered quartz or platinum stretched between the poles of a strong magnet. The thread may be illuminated by an arc light and the shadow of the thread thrown upon a screen after being magnified by a microscope.

galvanonarcosis (gal″vah-no-nar-ko′sis) (*obs.*) electronarcosis.

galvanonervous (gal″vah-no-ner′vus) produced by application of the galvanic current to a nerve trunk.

galvanopalpation (gal″vah-no-pal-pa′shun) a method of testing the sensory and vasomotor nerves of the skin by applying a sharp-pointed anode electrode to the part of the skin to be tested, the cathode being applied to some other part of the body.

galvanosurgery (gal″vah-no-sur′jer-e) the employment of galvanic cautery in surgery.

galvanotaxis (gal″vah-no-tak′sis) the tendency of an organism to arrange itself in a medium so that its axis bears a certain relation to the direction of the current in the medium.

galvanotherapeutics, galvanotherapy (gal-vah-no-ther″-ah-pu′tiks, gal″vah-no-ther′ah-pe) the therapeutic use of galvanic current.

galvanotropism (gal″vah-not′ro-pizm) [*galvanism* + Gr. *tropos* a turn] the tendency of an organism to turn or move under the action of an electric current.

galziekte (gahl-zēk′te) [Dutch *gal* gall + *ziekte* sickness] South African name for gallsickness.

gam- see *gamo-*.

gamasid (gam′ah-sid) a mite of the Gamasides group.

Gamasidae (gah-mas′ĭ-de) former name for a family of mites of the order Acarina, the spider mites or beetle mites; they are parasitic on birds and animals. See *Gamasides group;* under *group*.

Gamasides (gah-mas′ĭ-dēz) see under *group*.

gamasoidosis (gam″ah-soi-do′sis) infestation by mites of the Gamasides group, such as the dermatitis caused by the fowl mite, *Dermanyssus*.

Gamastan (gam-as′tan) trademark for a preparation of immune human serum globulin.

Gambian horse disease, sickness (gam′be-an) [*Gambia*, a country on the west coast of Africa] see under *disease* and *sickness*.

gambir (gam′bēr) the dried aqueous, astringent extract from the leaves and twigs of *Uncaria gambier*, a rubiaceous climbing shrub of southeastern Asia, the chief constituents of which are catechin, catechutannic acid, and quercetin; formerly used as an antidiarrheal and as a gargle for sore throat. Called also *catechu* or *pale catechu*.

gamboge (gam-bōj′, gam-booj′) the yellow gum-resin from *Garcinia hanburyi* Hook. f., and other guttiferous plants of Cambodia and the East Indies; used as a drastic hydragogue cathartic. Abbreviated G.G.G. Called also *cambogia* and *gutti*.

Gambusia (gam-bu′se-ah) a genus of fish effective in destroying mosquito larvae. **G. affin′is**, a top minnow which has been introduced into every major malarious region in the world; it feeds upon the larvae of *Anopheles* mosquitoes along the surface of the water.

gamefar (gah′mĕ-fahr) pamaquine.

gametangia (gam-ĕ-tan′je-ah) plural of *gametangium*.

gametangium (gam-ĕ-tan′je-um), pl. *gametan′gia* [*gamete* + Gr. *angeion* vessel] the structure in which zygospores are developed. See *spore*.

gamete (gam′ēt) [Gr. *gametē* wife, *gametēs* husband] 1. a reproductive element; one of two cells produced by a gametocyte, male (spermatozoon) and female (ovum), whose union is necessary, in sexual reproduction, to initiate the development of a new individual. The conjugation of male and female gametes produces a zygote. 2. a male or female reproductive cell of certain Sporozoa, such as malerial plasmodia, corresponding to the spermatozoon or ovum of Metazoa, found in the gut of the host. See also *macrogamete* and *microgamete*. 3. a 1N (haploid) cell in sexual fusion.

gametic (gah-met′ik) pertaining to gametes or the primitive sexual elements.

gameto- (gam′ĕ-to) [Gr. *gametē* wife, *gametēs* husband] a combining form denoting relationship to a gamete.

gametoblast (gam′ĕ-to-blast) [*gameto-* + Gr. *blastos* germ] (*obs.*) a sporozoite.

gametocidal (gam″ĕ-to-si′dal) capable of destroying gametes or gametocytes.

gametocide (gam′ĕ-to-sīd″) [*gameto-* + L. *caedere* to kill] an agent that destroys gametes or gametocytes.

gametocinetic (gam″ĕ-to-si-net′ik) gametokinetic.

gemetocyst (gah-met′o-sist) a protective envelope surrounding a male and female gametocyte in certain Sporozoa.

gametocyte (gah-met′o-sīt) [*gameto-* + Gr. *kytos* hollow vessel] 1. an oocyte or spermatocyte; a cell that produces gametes. 2. the sexual form, male or female, of certain Sporozoa, such as malarial plasmodia, found in the erythrocytes, which may produce gametes when ingested by the secondary host. See also *macrogametocyte* and *microgametocyte*.

gametocytemia (gah-me″to-si-te′me-ah) the presence of malarial gametocytes in the blood.

gametogenesis (gam″ĕ-to-jen′ĕ-sis) [*gameto-* + Gr. *genesis* pro-

duction] the development of the male and female sex cells, or gametes.

gametogenic (gam″ĕ-to-jen′ik) producing or favoring the production of germ cells.

gametogony (gam″ĕ-tog′o-ne) 1. the development of merozoites of malarial plasmodia and other sporozoa into male and female gametes, which later fuse to form a zygote; called also *gamogony*. 2. reproduction by means of gametes.

gametoid (gam′ĕ-toid) resembling gametes or reproductive cells.

gametokinetic (gam″ĕ-to-ki-net′ik) [*gameto-* + Gr. *kinein* to move] stimulating gamete action.

gametologist (gam″ĕ-tol′o-jist) a scientist whose special study is gametology.

gametology (gam″ĕ-tol′o-je) [*gamete* + Gr. *logos* discourse] the study of gametes.

gametophagia (gam″ĕ-to-fa′je-ah) gamophagia.

gametophyte (gam′ĕ-to-fīt) [*gameto-* + Gr. *phyton* plant] the haploid or sexual stage in organisms having alternation of generations (metagenesis); it may be female (megagametophyte) or male (microgametophyte).

gametotropic (gam″ĕ-to-trop′ik) having affinity for gametes.

Gamgee tissue (gam′je) [Joseph Sampson *Gamgee*, British surgeon, 1828–1886] see under *tissue*.

gamic (gam′ik) sexual; applied to eggs which develop only after fertilization.

gamma (gam′ah) 1. the third letter in the Greek alphabet, γ; used as part of a chemical name to distinguish the third in a series of compounds or to designate the position of the third carbon atom of an aliphatic chain or the position opposite the alpha position on the naphthalene ring. 2. microgram. 3. a unit of intensity of magnetic field, $\gamma = 0.00001$ gauss. 4. a numerical expression of the degree of development of a photographic negative.

gamma benzene hexachloride (gam′ah ben″zēn hek″sah-klōr′īd) lindane.

gammacism (gam′ah-sizm) [Gr. *gamma* the letter G] the imperfect utterance of velar consonants, especially *g* and *k* sounds.

Gammacorten (gam′ah-kor″ten) trademark for a preparation of dexamethasone.

Gammagee (gam′ah-je) trademark for a preparation of immune human serum globulin.

gamma globulin see under *globulin*.

gammaglobulinopathy (gam″ah-glob″u-lin-op′ah-the) any gammopathy.

gammagram (gam′ah-gram) a graphic record of the gamma rays emitted by an object or substance.

gammagraphic (gam″ah-graf′ik) pertaining to the recording of gamma rays in the study of organs after the administration of radioactive isotopes.

gamma-lactone (gam″ah-lak′tōn) a compound having a five-membered ring structure formed by internal reaction of a carboxylic acid group with a hydroxyl group on the gamma carbon of a carbon chain.

gammaloidosis (gam″mah-loi-do′sis) amyloidosis.

gamma-pipradol (gam″ah-pip′rah-dol) azacyclonol.

gammopathy (gam-op′ah-the) an immunoproliferative disorder characterized by abnormal proliferation of the lymphoid cells producing immunoglobulins. It may be *monoclonal*, in which there is an excess of one class of heavy chain (gamma, alpha, mu, delta, or epsilon) and one type of light chain (kappa or lambda) immunoglobulin subunits produced by a single clone of cells; the monoclonal gammopathies include multiple myeloma, macroglobinemia, and heavy-chain disease. Or it may be *polyclonal*, which involves an excess of two or more classes of immunoglobulins and of both types of light chains. Polyclonal gammopathies include Hodgkin's disease and lymphatic leukemia. Called also *gammaglobulinopathy* or *immunoglobulinopathy*.

gamo-, gam- (gam′o, gam′) [Gr. *gamos* marriage] combining form denoting relationship to marriage or sexual union.

gamobium (gah-mo′be-um) [*gamo-* + Gr. *bios* life] in biology, the sexually reproducing generation in cases of metagenesis (alternation of generations). Cf. *agamobium*.

gamogenesis (gam″o-jen′ĕ-sis) [*gamo-* + Gr. *genesis* production] sexual reproduction.

gamogenetic (gam″o-jĕ-net′ik) pertaining to or exhibiting sexual reproduction.

gamogony (gam-og′o-ne) gametogony.

gamone (gam′ōn) a hypothetical substance supposed to be released by the ovum (gynogamone) and spermatozoa (androgamone) to facilitate their fusion.

gamont (gam′ont) [*gam-* + Gr. *ōn* being] 1. gametocyte. 2. either of the conjugating individuals in gregarine reproduction.

gamophagia (gam″o-fa′je-ah) [*gamo-* + Gr. *phagein* to eat] the disappearance of the male or female element in the conjugation of unicellular organisms.

gampsodactyly (gamp″so-dak′tĭ-le) [Gr. *gampsos* crooked + *dak-*

tylos digit] deformity of the toes marked by hyperextension of the first phalanx on the metatarsal and flexion of the other two phalanges; called also *clawfoot.*

Gamulin (gam′u-lin) trademark for a preparation of immune human serum globulin. **G Rh,** trademark for a preparation of Rh₀(D) immune serum globulin.

gangli- see *ganglio-.*

ganglia (gang′gle-ah) plural of *ganglion.*

ganglial (gang′gle-al) pertaining to a ganglion.

gangliated (gang′gle-āt″ed) ganglionated.

gangliectomy (gang″gle-ek′to-me) ganglionectomy.

gangliform (gang′gli-form) having the form of a ganglion.

gangliitis (gang″gle-i′tis) ganglionitis.

ganglio-, gangli- (gang′gle-o, gang′gle) [Gr. *ganglion* knot] combining form denoting relationship to a ganglion.

ganglioblast (gang′gle-o-blast″) [*ganglio-* + Gr. *blastos* germ] an embryonic cell of the cerebrospinal ganglia.

gangliocyte (gang′gle-o-sīt″) [*ganglio-* + Gr. *kytos* hollow vessel] a ganglion cell.

gangliocytoma (gang″gle-o-si-to′mah) ganglioneuroma.

ganglioform (gang′gle-o-form″) gangliform.

ganglioglioma (gang″gle-o-gli-o′mah) a glioma rich in mature neurons or ganglion cells.

ganglioglioneuroma (gang″gle-o-gli″o-nu-ro′mah) ganglioneuroma.

gangliolytic (gang″gle-o-lyt′ik) ganglioplegic.

ganglioma (gang″gle-o′mah) [*ganglio-* + *-oma*] ganglioneuroma.

ganglion (gang′gle-on), pl. *ganglia* or *ganglions* [Gr. "knot"] 1. a knot, or knotlike mass. 2. [NA] a general term for a group of nerve cell bodies located outside the central nervous system; occasionally applied to certain nuclear groups within the brain or spinal cord, e.g., basal ganglia. 3. a benign cystic tumor occur-

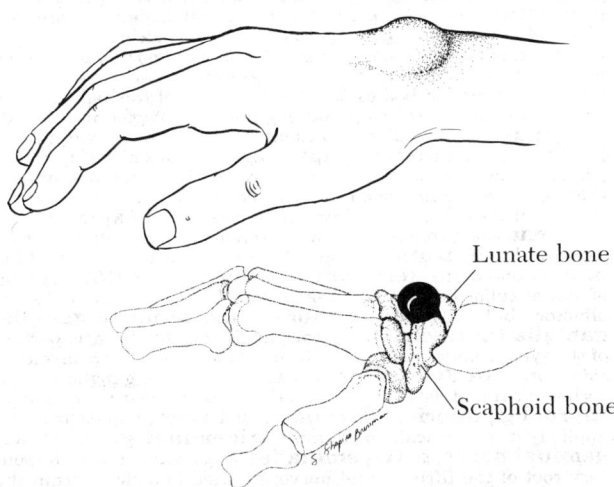

Ganglion of wrist arising from a tendon.

Lunate bone

Scaphoid bone

ring on an aponeurosis or tendon, as in the wrist or dorsum of the foot; it consists of a thin fibrous capsule enclosing a clear mucinous fluid. **accessory ganglia,** ganglia intermedia. **acousti-cofacial g.,** a ganglion of early embryonic life, a portion of which persists as the geniculate ganglion. **Acrel's g.,** a cystic tumor on an extensor tendon of the wrist. **Andersch's g.,** g. inferius nervi glossopharyngei. **anterior g. of thalamus** (*obs.*), the anterior tubercle of the thalamus. **aorticorenal g., ganglia aorticorena′lia** [NA], a more or less detached infero-lateral extension of the celiac ganglion. **Arnold's g.,** 1. ganglion oticum. 2. glomus caroticum. **auditory g.,** see *nuclei cochlearis, ventralis et dorsalis.* **Auerbach's g.,** any of the small ganglia of Auerbach's plexus. **auricular g.** (*obs.*), g. oticum. **azygous g.,** glomus coccygeum. **basal ganglia,** specific interconnected gray masses deep in the cerebral hemispheres and in the upper brainstem, including the caudate nucleus, putamen, globus pallidus, claustrum, and substantia nigra; they are involved in motor coordination. Various other subcortical nuclei and parts of the thalamus have also been considered by some to be part of the basal ganglia. Called also *basal nuclei.* **Bezold's g.,** a series of ganglion cells in the interatrial septum. **Bidder's ganglia,** ganglia on the cardiac nerves, situated at the lower end of the atrial septum. **Blandin's g.,** g. submandibulare. **Bochdalek's g., g. Bochdalek′ii,** plexus dentalis superior. **Bock's g.,** carotid g. **cardiac ganglia, gan′glia cardi′aca** [NA], ganglia of the cardiac plexus near the arterial ligament; called also *Wrisberg's g.* and *g. wrisbergi.* **carotid g.,** a ganglion of the internal carotid plexus in the cavernous sinus; called also *Bock's g.* **carotid g., inferior,** a gan-

glion of the internal carotid plexus in the lower part of the carotid canal; called also *Laumonier's g.* and *Schmiedel's g.* **carotid g., superior,** a ganglion of the internal carotid plexus in the upper part of the carotid canal. **celiac ganglia, ganglia celi′aca** [NA], two irregularly shaped ganglia, one on each crus of the diaphragm, within the celiac plexus; each contains sympathetic nerve cells and preganglionic sympathetic fibers from the greater and lesser splanchnic nerves; preganglionic parasympathetic and sensory fibers pass through the ganglia. **cephalic g.,** parasympathetic ganglia in the head, consisting of the ciliary, otic, pterygopalatine, and submandibular ganglia. **cerebrospinal ganglia,** the ganglia associated with the cranial and spinal nerves. **cervical g., inferior,** a portion of the ganglion cervicothoracicum. **cervical g., middle,** g. cervicale medium. **cervical g., superior,** g. cervicale superius. **cervical g. of uterus,** a ganglion situated near the cervix uteri; called also *Lee's g.* and *Frankenhaüser's g.* **g. cervica′le infe′rius,** a portion of the ganglion cervicothoracicum. **g. cervica′le me′dium** [NA], middle cervical ganglion: a variable ganglion, often fused with the vertebral ganglion, on the sympathetic trunk at about the level of the cricoid cartilage; its postganglionic fibers are distributed mainly to the heart, cervical region, and upper limb. Formerly called *inferior* or *superior thyroid g.* **g. cervica′le supe′rius** [NA], superior cervical ganglion: the uppermost ganglion on the sympathetic trunk, lying behind the internal carotid artery and in front of the second and third cervical vertebrae; it gives rise to postganglionic fibers to the heart via cervical cardiac nerves, to the pharyngeal plexus and thence to the larynx and pharynx, and to the head via the external and internal carotid plexuses. **cervicothoracic g., g. cervicothora′cicum** [NA], a ganglion on the sympathetic trunk at the level of the 7th cervical and 1st thoracic vertebra, anterior to the 8th cervical and 1st thoracic nerves; it has two components, the inferior cervical and first thoracic ganglia, which are usually fused, partially or completely. Its postganglionic fibers are distributed to the head and neck, heart, and upper limb. Called also *stellate g.* and *g. stellatum* [NA alternative]. **cervicouterine g.,** cervical g. of uterus. **g. cilia′re** [NA], **ciliary g.,** a parasympathetic ganglion in the posterior part of the orbit; it receives preganglionic fibers from the oculomotor nerve, and its postganglionic fibers supply the ciliary muscle and the sphincter pupillae. Sensory and postganglionic sympathetic fibers pass through the ganglion. **Cloquet's g.,** an enlargement of the nasopalatine nerve in the anterior palatine canal. **coccygeal g.,** glomus coccygeum. **cochlear g.,** ganglion spirale cochleae. **collateral ganglia,** prevertebral ganglia. **compound g.,** a cystic tumor of a tendon sheath that has been compressed into two parts by a ligament. **Corti's g.,** g. spirale partis cochlearis nervi octavi. **Darkshevich's g.** (*obs.*), Darkshevich's nucleus. **diaphragmatic ganglia** (*obs.*), ganglia phrenica. **diffuse g.,** a swelling of several adjoining tendon sheaths due to inflammatory effusion. **dorsal root g.,** spinal g. **Ehrenritter's g.,** g. superius nervi glossopharyngei. **g. extracrania′le** (*obs.*), g. inferius nervi glossopharyngei. **false g.,** an enlargement on a nerve that does not have a true ganglionic structure. **Frankenhaüser's g.,** cervical g. of uterus. **Froriep's g.,** the ganglion of the lowest occipital segment in the human embryo. **ganglia of autonomic plexuses,** ganglia plexuum autonomicrorum. **Ganser's g.,** nucleus interpeduncularis. **Gasser's g., gasserian g.,** g. trigeminale. **geniculate g., g. genic′uli ner′vi facia′lis** [NA], the sensory ganglion of the facial nerve, situated on the geniculum nervi fascialis. **g. of habenulae** (*obs.*), nucleus habenulae. **hepatic g.,** a ganglion situated near the hepatic artery. **hypogastric g.,** either of two ganglia on each side of the cervix uteri, connected with the sacral and hypogastric plexuses. **hypoglossal g.,** a ganglion of the hypoglossal nerve; rarely found in man, except in the embryo. **g. im′par** [NA], the ganglion commonly found in front of the coccyx, where the sympathetic trunks of the two sides unite. **inferior g. of glossopharyngeal nerve,** g. inferius nervi glossopharyngei. **inferior g. of vagus,** g. inferius nervi vagi. **g. infe′rius ner′vi glossopharyn′gei** [NA], inferior ganglion of glossopharyngeal nerve: the lower of two ganglia on the glossopharyngeal nerve as it passes through the jugular foramen; both contain cell bodies for the afferent fibers of the nerve. Called also *g. petrosum,* and *petrosal* or *petrous g.* **g. infe′rius ner′vi va′gi** [NA], inferior ganglion of vagus: a ganglion of the vagus nerve located just below the jugular foramen, in front of the transverse processes of the first and second cervical vertebrae; it contains cell bodies for afferent fibers of the vagus. Called also *nodose g.,* and *g. nodosum.* **inhibitory g.,** any ganglion performing an inhibitory function. **intercarotid g.** (*obs.*), glomus caroticum. **g. intercrania′le** (*obs.*), g. superius nervi glossopharyngei. **gan′glia interme′dia** [NA], **intermediate ganglia,** small groups of sympathetic nerve cells present on spinal nerves and on rami communicantes, especially in the cervical, lower thoracic, and upper lumbar regions; called also *accessory ganglia.* **interpeduncular g.** (*obs.*), nucleus interpeduncularis. **intervertebral g. of head, posterior** (*obs.*), g. superius nervi glossopharyngei. **g. intervertebra′le** (*obs.*), g. spinale. **jugular g., inferior,** g. inferius nervi glossopharyngei. **jugular g. of glos-**

sopharyngeal nerve, g. superius nervi glossopharyngei. **jugular g. of vagus nerve,** g. jugula′re ner′vi va′gi, g. superius nervi vagi. **Küttner's g.,** a large lymph node on the internal jugular vein immediately beneath the posterior belly of the digastric muscle, forming the principal lymphatic terminus of the tongue; called also *hauptganglion of Küttner.* **Langley's g.,** a collection of nerve cells in the hilus of the submaxillary gland in some animals. **Laumonier's g.,** 1. carotid g. 2. inferior carotid g. **Lee's g.,** cervical g. of the uterus. **lesser g. of Meckel,** g. submandibulare. **lingual g.** (*obs.*), g. submandibulare. **Lobstein's g.,** a ganglion on the greater splanchnic nerve above the diaphragm; probably the same as the splanchnic ganglion. **lower g. of glossopharyngeal nerve,** g. inferius nervi glossopharyngei. **lower g. of vagus nerve,** g. inferius nervi vagi. **Ludwig's g.,** a ganglion connected with the cardiac plexus and situated near the right atrium of the heart. **gan′glia lumba′lia** [NA], **lumbar ganglia,** the ganglia on the lumbar part of the sympathetic trunk, usually four or five on either side. **Luschka's g.,** glomus coccygeum. **gan′glia lymphat′ica,** lymph nodes; see *nodus lymphaticus.* **maxillary g.** (*obs.*), g. submandibulare. **Meckel's g.,** g. pterygopalatinum. **Meissner's g.,** one of the small groups of nerve cells in the submucosal (Meissner's) plexus. **mesenteric g., inferior,** g. mesentericum inferius. **mesenteric g., superior,** g. mesentericum superius. **g. mesenter′icum infe′rius** [NA], inferior mesenteric ganglion: a sympathetic ganglion in the inferior mesenteric plexus near the beginning of the inferior mesenteric artery. **g. mesenter′icum supe′rius** [NA], superior mesenteric ganglion: one or more sympathetic ganglia at the sides of, or just below, the superior mesenteric artery; commonly fused with the celiac ganglia. **g. of Müller,** g. superius nervi glossopharyngei. **nephrolumbar g.** (*obs.*), aorticorenal g. **g. ner′vi splanch′nici,** g. splanchnicum. **nodose g., g. nodo′sum,** g. inferius nervi vagi. **olfactory g.,** a mass of tissue in the embryo which develops into the olfactory nerves. **ophthalmic g.** (*obs.*), g. ciliare. **optic g., orbital g.** (*obs.*), g. ciliare. **otic g., g. o′ticum** [NA], a parasympathetic ganglion in the infratemporal fossa, medial to the mandibular nerve and just inferior to the foramen ovale: its preganglionic fibers are derived from the glossopharyngeal nerve via the lesser petrosal nerve, and its postganglionic fibers supply the parotid gland. Sensory and postganglionic sympathetic fibers pass through the ganglion. Called also *Arnold's g.* and *auricular g.* **parasympathetic ganglia,** aggregations of cell bodies of cholinergic neurons of the parasympathetic nervous system; these ganglia are located near to or within the wall of the organs being innervated. See also *cholinergic.* **pelvic ganglia, gan′glia pelvi′na** [NA], small sympathetic and parasympathetic ganglia located within the pelvic plexus. **periosteal g.,** periostitis albuminosa. **petrosal g., petrosal g., inferior, g. petro′sum, petrous g.,** g. inferius nervi glossopharyngei. **phrenic g., gan′glia phren′ica** [NA], a small sympathetic ganglion often found within the phrenic plexus at its junction with the celiac plexus. **gan′glia plex′uum autonomico′rum** [NA], **gan′glia plex′uum sympathico′rum,** ganglia of autonomic plexuses: groups of nerve cell bodies found in the autonomic plexuses, composed primarily of sympathetic postganglionic neurons; called also *ganglia of sympathetic plexuses.* **prevertebral ganglia,** sympathetic ganglia (other than those of the sympathetic trunk) in the prevertebral plexuses of the thorax and abdomen. **primary g.,** a ganglion on a tendon or aponeurosis that does not follow a local inflammation. **prostatic g.** (*obs.*), a ganglion situated on the prostate gland, and connected with the prostatic plexus. **pterygopalatine g., g. pterygopalati′num** [NA], a parasympathetic ganglion in the pterygopalatine fossa; its preganglionic fibers are derived from the facial nerve via the greater petrosal nerve and the nerve of the pterygopalatine canal. Its postganglionic fibers supply the lacrimal, nasal, and palatine glands; sensory and sympathetic fibers pass through the ganglion. Called also *Meckel's g., sphenopalatine g.,* and *g. sphenopalatinum.* **Remak's g.,** a sympathetic ganglion in the heart wall near the superior vena cava; called also *sinoatrial g.* Also, sympathetic ganglia in the diaphragmatic opening for the inferior vena cava, as well as ganglia in the gastric plexus. **renal ganglia, gan′glia rena′lia** [NA], small sympathetic ganglia within the renal plexus. **g. ret′inae,** the outer of the two subdivisions of the internal nuclear layer of the retina. **Ribes' g.,** the alleged ganglion in the termination of the internal carotid plexus around the anterior communicating artery of the brain. **sacral ganglia, gan′glia sacra′lia** [NA], the ganglia of the sacral part of the sympathetic trunk, usually three or four on either side. **Scarpa's g.,** g. vestibulare. **Schacher's g.,** g. ciliare. **Schmiedel's g.,** 1. carotid g. 2. inferior carotid g. **semilunar g.,** 1. ganglion trigeminale. 2. [pl.] ganglia celiaca. **g. semiluna′re [Gas′seri],** g. trigeminale. **sensory g.,** ganglia of the peripheral nervous system which transmit sensory impulses; also, the collective masses of nerve cell bodies in the brain subserving sensory functions. **simple g.,** a cystic tumor in a tendon sheath. **sinoatrial g.,** Remak's g. **sinus g.,** a group of nerve cells around the junction of the coronary sinus and the right atrium of the heart. **Soemmering's g.** (*obs.*), substantia ni-

gra. **solar ganglia** (*obs.*), ganglia celiaca. **sphenomaxillary g., sphenopalatine g., g. sphenopalati′num,** g. pterygopalatinum. **spinal g., g. spina′le** [NA], the ganglion found on the dorsal root of each spinal nerve, composed of the unipolar nerve cell bodies of the sensory neurons of the nerve. **spiral g., spiral g. of cochlea,** g. spirale cochleae. **spiral g. of cochlear nerve,** g. spirale partis cochlearis nervi octavi. **g. spira′le coch′leae** [NA], spiral ganglion of cochlea: the ganglion of the cochlear nerve, located within the modiolus and consisting of bipolar cells which send fibers peripherally through the foramina nervosa to the spiral organ, and centrally through the internal acoustic meatus to the cochlear nuclei of the brain stem. **g. spira′le ner′vi coch′leae, g. spira′le par′tis cochlea′ris ner′vi octa′vi** [NA], spiral ganglion of cochlear nerve: the sensory ganglion of the pars cochlearis of the eighth cranial nerve, located within the modiolus and consisting of bipolar cells which send fibers peripherally through the foramina nervosa to the spiral organ, and centrally through the internal acoustic meatus to the cochlear nuclei of the brain stem; called also *Corti's g.* **splanchnic g.,** 1. ganglion splanchnicum. 2. plexus celiacus. **g. splanch′nicum** [NA], splanchnic ganglion: a small ganglion formed on the greater splanchnic nerve near the twelfth thoracic vertebra. **stellate g.,** g. cervicothoracicum. **g. stella′tum,** NA alternative for *g. cervicothoracicum.* **submandibular g., g. submandibula′re** [NA], **g. submaxilla′re, submaxillary g.,** a parasympathetic ganglion located superior to the deep part of the submandibular gland, on the lateral surface of the hyoglossus muscle; its preganglionic fibers are derived from the facial nerve by way of the chorda tympani and lingual nerve, and its postganglionic fibers supply the submandibular and sublingual glands; sensory and postganglionic sympathetic fibers pass through the ganglion. **superior g. of glossopharyngeal nerve,** g. superius nervi glossopharyngei. **superior g. of vagus nerve,** g. superius nervi vagi. **g. supe′rius, g. supe′rius ner′vi glossopharyn′gei** [NA], superior ganglion of glossopharyngeal nerve: the upper of two ganglia on the glossopharyngeal nerve as it passes through the jugular foramen; both ganglia contain cell bodies for afferent fibers of the nerve. **g. supe′rius ner′vi va′gi** [NA], superior ganglion of vagus nerve: a small ganglion on the vagus in the jugular foramen, giving off a meningeal and an auricular branch and containing cell bodies for afferent fibers of the vagus; called also *g. jugulare nervi vagi* and *jugular g. of vagus nerve.* **suprarenal g.,** a small sympathetic ganglion in the suprarenal plexus. **sympathetic ganglia,** aggregations of cell bodies of primarily adrenergic neurons of the sympathetic nervous system; these ganglia are arranged in chainlike fashion on either side of the spinal cord. See also *adrenergic.* **ganglia of sympathetic plexuses,** ganglia plexuum autonomicorum. **ganglia of sympathetic trunk,** ganglia trunci sympathici. **synovial g.,** a myxoid cyst. **terminal g., g. termina′le** [NA], a group of nerve cells found along the terminal nerves, medial to the olfactory bulb. **gan′glia thoraca′lia, thoracic ganglia, gan′glia thora′cica** [NA], the ganglia on the thoracic portion of the sympathetic trunk, usually about eleven or twelve on either side. **g. thora′cicum pri′mum,** a portion of ganglion cervicothoracicum; it is present sometimes as a separate ganglion. **thyroid g., inferior, thyroid g., superior,** names formerly applied to g. cervicale medium. **trigeminal g., g. of trigeminal nerve, g. trigemina′le** [NA], a ganglion on the sensory root of the fifth cranial nerve, situated in a cleft within the dura mater (trigeminal cave) on the anterior surface of the petrous portion of the temporal bone, and giving off the ophthalmic and maxillary and part of the mandibular nerve; it contains the cells of origin of most of the sensory fibers of the trigeminal nerve. Called also *semilunar g.,* and *g. semilunare [Gasseri].* **Troisier's g.,** an enlarged lymph node sometimes seen above the clavicle in cases of retrosternal tumor. **gan′glia trun′ci sympath′ici** [NA], ganglia of sympathetic trunk: groups of nerve cell bodies found along each sympathetic trunk, about twenty to twenty-three on either side. **tympanic g., g. tympanicum. tympanic g. of Valentin,** a ganglion on a superior dental nerve; also, intumescentia tympanica. **g. tympan′icum** [NA], tympanic ganglion: an enlargement on the tympanic branch of the glossopharyngeal nerve. **upper g.,** g. superius nervi glossopharyngei. **vagal g., inferior,** g. inferius nervi vagi. **vagal g., superior,** g. superius nervi vagi. **Valentin's g.,** 1. intumescentia tympanica. 2. a ganglion on a superior dental nerve. **ventricular g.,** Bidder's g. **vertebral g., g. vertebra′le,** [NA], a small ganglion on one of the branches interconnecting the middle and cervicothoracic ganglia of the sympathetic trunk, in front of the vertebral artery; it contributes to the ansa subclavia and sends postganglionic fibers to the vertebral nerve and plexus and to the brachial plexus. **vestibular g., g. vestibula′re** [NA], the sensory ganglion of the pars vestibularis of the eighth cranial nerve; it is located in the superior part of the lateral end of the internal acoustic meatus and consists of bipolar cells whose peripheral processes form small nerves supplying the utricle, saccule, and semicircular canals, and whose central processes reach the vestibular nuclei of the brain stem. Called also *Scarpa's g.* **Walther's g.,** glomus coccygeum. **Wrisberg's g., g. Wrisbergi,** see *ganglia cardiaca.*

wrist g., cystic enlargement of a tendon sheath on the back of the wrist.

ganglionated (gang'gle-o-nāt-ed) provided with ganglia.

ganglionectomy (gang"gle-o-nek'to-me) [ganglio- + Gr. ektomē excision] excision of a ganglion.

ganglioneure (gang'gle-o-nūr") [ganglio- + Gr. neuron nerve] any cell of a nervous ganglion.

ganglioneuroblastoma (gang"gle-o-nu"ro-blas-to'mah) a tumor composed of ganglioneuromatous and neuroblastomatous elements.

ganglioneurofibroma (gang"gle-o-nu"ro-fi-bro'mah) ganglioneuroma.

ganglioneuroma (gang"gle-o-nu-ro'mah) a benign neoplasm composed of nerve fibers and mature ganglion cells; regarded by many as a fully differentiated neuroblastoma.

ganglionic (gang"gle-on'ik) pertaining to a ganglion.

ganglionitis (gang"gle-on-i'tis) inflammation of a ganglion. **acute posterior g.,** herpes zoster. **gasserian g.,** herpes zoster ophthalmicus.

ganglionoplegic (gang"gle-on"o-ple'jik) ganglioplegic.

ganglionostomy (gang"gle-o-nos'to-me) [ganglio- + Gr. stomoun to provide with an opening, or mouth] surgical creation of an opening into a cystic tumor on a tendon sheath or aponeurosis.

ganglioplegic (gang"gle-o-ple'jik) [ganglio- + Gr. plēgē stroke] 1. blocking transmission of impulses through the sympathetic and parasympathetic ganglia. 2. an agent that blocks the transmission of impulses through the sympathetic and parasympathetic ganglia.

ganglioside (gang'gle-o-sīd) a general designation for a member of a class of galactose-containing cerebrosides found in the tissues of the central nervous system. Gangliosides are glycolipids of the basic composition ceramide-glucose-galactose-N-acetyl neuraminic acid. **g. GM₁,** a ganglioside with the addition of an N-acetyl galactosamine and a galactose group; it accumulates in tissues in generalized gangliosidosis. **g. GM₂,** a ganglioside with the addition of N-acetyl galactosamine at the terminal; it accumulates in tissues in Tay-Sachs disease.

gangliosidoses (gang"gle-o-si-do'sēz) plural of gangliosidosis.

gangliosidosis (gang"gle-o-si-do'sis), pl. gangliosidoses. A lipid storage disorder marked by accumulation of gangliosides in tissues due to an enzyme defect. In generalized gangliosidosis, a defect of β-galactosidase results in accumulation of ganglioside GM₁ (the major monosialoganglioside); in Tay-Sachs disease, a defect of hexosaminidase A results in accumulation of ganglioside GM₂. **generalized g.,** a lipid-storage disease in which ganglioside GM₁ is stored in the tissues, due to a defect in the enzyme β-galactosidase. It is characterized principally by mental retardation, hepatomegaly, skeletal deformities, and (in about half the cases) cherry red spot. It is transmitted as an autosomal recessive trait. **GM₁ g.,** generalized g. **GM₂ g.,** Tay-Sachs disease.

gangliospore (gang'gle-o-spōr) a fungal spore developed from the swollen tip of a hypha.

gangliosympathectomy (gang"gle-o-sim"pah-thek'to-me) excision of a sympathetic ganglion.

Gangolphe's sign (gahn-golfs') [Louis Gangolphe, French surgeon] see under sign.

gangosa (gang-go'sah) [Sp. "muffled voice"] a form of treponematosis manifested as a destructive ulceration of the nose, nasopharynx, and hard palate, being one of the late lesions of yaws; called also ogo and rhinopharyngitis mutilans.

gangrene (gang'grēn) [L. gangraena; Gr. gangraina an eating sore, which ends in mortification] death of tissue, usually in considerable mass and generally associated with loss of vascular (nutritive) supply and followed by bacterial invasion and putrefaction. Cf. necrosis and necrobiosis. **anaphylactic g.,** gangrene occurring as a result of anaphylactic reaction to the injection of antigen (anaphylactogen), such as serum. **angiosclerotic g.,** dry gangrene caused by vascular sclerosis. **circumscribed g.,** gangrene that is clearly separated from normal tissue by a zone of inflammatory reaction. **cold g.,** gangrene that is not preceded by inflammation. **diabetic g.,** moist gangrene occurring in a person with diabetes; called also glycemic g. **dry g.,** necrosis occurring without subsequent bacterial decomposition, the tissues becoming dry and shriveled. **embolic g.,** that which follows the blocking of the blood supply by an embolism. **emphysematous g.,** gas g. **epidemic g.,** ergotism. **Fournier's g.,** idiopathic gangrene of the scrotum. **fulminating g.,** malignant edema. **gas g., gaseous g.,** an acute, severe, and painful condition often resulting from dirty, lacerated wounds in which the muscles and subcutaneous tissues become filled with gas and a serosanguineous exudate. The condition is due to histotoxic infection by anaerobic bacteria, among which are Clostridium perfringens, C. novyi, C. septicum (vibrion septique), C. sporogenes, and other species of Clostridium. Called also clostridial myonecrosis. **glycemic g., glykemic g.,** diabetic g. **hot g.,** gangrene which follows an inflammation. **humid g.,** moist g. **inflammatory g.,** gangrene due to acute inflammation. **mephitic g.,** gas g. **moist g.,** necrosis of tissues, with proteolytic decomposition resulting from bacterial action. **oral**

g., gangrenous stomatitis. **pressure g.,** gangrene due to pressure, as in decubitus ulcer. **primary g.,** gangrene occurring without preceding inflammation of the part. **progressive g.,** gangrene in which an effective limiting zone of inflammatory reaction does not form. **progressive bacterial synergistic g.,** a superficial spreading infection caused by the association of two organisms, neither one of which is capable of producing significant infection alone. **Raynaud's g.,** Raynaud's disease, def. 1. **secondary g.,** a form which follows a local inflammation. **senile g.,** dry gangrene affecting the extremities of the aged. **static g.,** gangrene that results from stasis of blood in a part. **symmetric g.,** gangrene of corresponding digits on both sides, due to vasomotor disturbances. **sympathetic g.,** gangrene which results from some primary condition. **thrombotic g.,** gangrene from thrombosis of an artery. **traumatic g.,** gangrene which occurs as a consequence of accidental injury. **trophic g.,** gangrene due to lesion of the trophic nerve supply of a part. **venous g.,** static g.

gangrenosis (gang"grĕ-no'sis) the development of gangrene.

gangrenous (gang'grĕ-nus) pertaining to, characterized by, or of the nature of gangrene.

ganja (gan'jah) an Asian Indian preparation of Cannabis sativa in which an infusion is made from the mature female plant tops of very carefully selected, cultivated varieties. It may also be smoked and, when incorporated into sweet meats, is known as majoon.

ganoblast (gan'o-blast) ameloblast.

Ganser's ganglion, symptom, syndrome (gan'serz) [Sigbert Joseph Maria Ganser, psychiatrist in Dresden, 1853–1931] see under symptom and syndrome, and see nucleus interpeduncularis.

Gant's clamp (gants) [Samuel Goodwin Gant, New York proctologist, 1870–1944] see under clamp.

Gant's line, operation (gants) [Frederick James Gant, English surgeon, 1825–1905] see under line and operation.

Gantanol (gan'tah-nol) trademark for preparations of sulfamethoxazole.

Gantrisin (gan'trĭ-sin) trademark for preparations of sulfisoxazole.

gap (gap) an unoccupied interval in time; an opening or hiatus. **air-bone g.,** the lag between the audiographic curves for air- and bone-conducted stimuli, as an indication of a conductive hearing loss. **auscultatory g.,** time in which sound is not heard in the auscultatory method of sphygmomanometry, occurring particularly in hypertension and in aortic stenosis. **Bochdalek's g.,** hiatus pleuroperitonealis. **chromatid g.,** a nonstaining region in a chromatid, the portions of the chromatid immediately proximal and distal to the site remaining in alignment. **interocclusal g.,** interocclusal distance; see under distance. **isochromatid g.,** a nonstaining region of the same level in two sister chromatids, the distal segments remaining in alignment with the proximal portions. **silent g.,** auscultatory g.

gapes (gāps) a disease of young fowls and turkeys caused by the gapeworm Syngamus trachea and marked by gasping and choking.

Garamycin (gar-ah-mi'sin) trademark for a preparation of gentamicin sulfate.

Garcinia (gar-sin'e-ah) a genus of guttiferous fruit trees widely cultivated in the tropics. G. hanburyi Hook. f. is the source of gamboge, G. mangostana L. of mangosteen, a delicious berry.

Gardiner-Brown's test [Alfred Gardiner-Brown, English otologist] see under tests.

Gardner's syndrome (gard'nerz) [Eldon J. Gardner] see under syndrome.

Garel's sign (gar-elz') [Jean Garel, French physician, 1852–1931] see under sign.

Garg. abbreviation for L. gargaris'mus, gargle.

gargalanesthesia (gar"g'l-an"es-the'ze-ah) absence of the tickle sense.

gargalesthesia (gar"g'l-es-the'ze-ah) the sense which perceives tickling sensations.

gargalesthetic (gar"g'l-es-thet'ik) pertaining to the tickle sense.

gargarism (gar'gar-izm) [L., Gr., gargarisma] a gargle or throat wash.

garget (gar'get) mastitis in the cow.

gargle (gar'g'l) [L. gargarisma] 1. to agitate a solution in the throat by forcing air through it so as to rinse or medicate the mucous membranes. 2. a solution used for rinsing or medicating the mouth and throat.

gargoylism (gar'goil-izm) Hurler's syndrome.

Garland's curve, triangle (gar'landz) [George Minot Garland, American physician, 1848–1926] see Ellis' line, under line, and see under triangle.

garnet (gar'net) a silicate of any combination of aluminum, cobalt, magnesium, iron, and manganese, usually coated on paper or cloth, commonly used in dentistry for polishing dentures.

Garré's osteomyelitis (disease, osteitis) (gar-āz') [Carl

Garré, Swiss surgeon, 1858–1928] sclerosing nonsuppurative osteomyelitis; see under *osteomyelitis*.

Garrod's test (gar′ods) 1. (for hematoporphyrin in urine) [Sir Archibald Edward *Garrod*, British physician, 1857–1936]. 2. (for uric acid in blood) [Alfred Baring *Garrod*, London physician, 1819–1907]. See under *tests*.

garrot (gar′ot) a form of tourniquet.

Gärtner's bacillus (gairt′nerz) [August *Gärtner*, German bacteriologist, 1848–1934] *Salmonella enteritidis*.

Gartner's cyst, duct (canal) (gart′nerz) [Hermann Treschow *Gartner*, Danish surgeon and anatomist, 1785–1827] see under *cyst*, and see *ductus epoophori longitudinales*.

Gärtner's phenomenon, tonometer (gairt′nerz) [Gustav *Gärtner*, Austrian pathologist, 1855–1937] see under *phenomenon* and *tonometer*.

Garymicin (gar″ĭ-mi′sin) trademark for a preparation of gentamicin.

gas (gas) any elastic aeriform fluid in which the molecules are separated from one another and so have free paths. **alveolar g.,** the gas in the alveoli of the lungs, where gaseous exchange with the capillary blood takes place; called also *alveolar air*. **coal g.,** a gas produced by the destructive distillation of coal and much used for domestic cooking; it is poisonous because it contains carbon monoxide. **ethyl g.,** tetraethyl lead. **expired g.,** gas expired from the lungs, especially a mixture of gas from the dead space and alveolar gas. **hemolytic g.,** arsine. **inert g.,** a gas that does not react chemically with the other constituents of a system, especially in reference to the noble gases, such as helium and argon. **lacrimator g.,** tear g. **laughing g.,** nitrous oxide. **marsh g.,** methane. **mustard g.,** dichlorodiethyl sulfide. **noble g.,** the gas elements of group VIII of the periodic table, i.e., helium, neon, argon, krypton, xenon, and radon. **olefiant g.,** ethylene. **sewer g.,** the mixture of gases and vapors from a sewer; often dangerous from the contained materials resulting from the decay of organic matter. **sneezing g.,** diphenylchlorarsine. **suffocating g.,** any of several war gases, e.g., phosgene or dephosgene oxychlor carbon, that causes intense irritation of the bronchial tubes and lungs, resulting in pulmonary edema. **sweet g.,** carbon monoxide. **tear g.,** a gas which produces severe lacrimation by irritating the conjunctivae. **vesicating g.,** dichlorodiethyl sulfide. **war g.,** any noxious gas manufactured for possible use in warfare.

gaseous (gas′e-us, gash′us) of the nature of a gas.

gasiform (gas′ĭ-form) gaseous.

Gaskell's bridge (gas′kelz) [Walter Holbrook *Gaskell*, English physiologist, 1847–1914] bundle of His.

gaskin (gas′kin) the thigh of a horse.

gasogenic (gas-o-jen′ik) producing gas.

gasometer (gas-om′ĕ-ter) a calibrated container for measuring volume of gases.

gasometric (gas″o-met′rik) pertaining to gasometry.

gasometry (gas-om′ĕ-tre) [*gas* + Gr. *metron* measure] the chemical determination of the amount of gas present in a mixture.

Gasser (gas′er), Herbert Spencer. American physiologist, 1888–1963, noted for his work on the nervous system; co-winner, with E. Joseph Erlanger, of the Nobel prize for medicine and physiology in 1944.

Gasser's ganglion (gas′erz) [Johann Laurentius *Gasser*, professor in Vienna from 1757 to 1765] ganglion trigeminale.

gasserectomy (gas″er-ek′to-me) surgical removal of the trigeminal (gasserian) ganglion.

gasserian (gas-se′re-an) named for Johann Laurentius *Gasser*, as gasserian (trigeminal) ganglion.

gaster (gas′ter) [Gr. *gastēr*] stomach.

gasteralgia (gas-ter-al′je-ah) (*obs.*) gastric colic.

gasterangiemphraxis (gas″ter-an″je-em-frak′sis) [*gaster* + Gr. *angeion* vessel + *emphraxis* obstruction] (*obs.*) obstruction of the blood vessels of the stomach.

gasteremphraxis (gas″ter-em-frak′sis) (*obs.*) 1. gasterangiemphraxis. 2. distention of the stomach.

Gasteromycetes (gas″ter-o-mi-se′tēz) a series of basidiomycetous fungi of the subclass Homobasidiomycetidae, including the puffballs and stinkhorns, in which the spores are arranged around a columella; it includes the genera *Lycoperdon*, *Calvatia*, *Geaster*, and *Phallus*.

Gasterophilus (gas″ter-of′ĭ-lus) [*gaster* + Gr. *philein* to love] a genus of dipterous insects of the family Oestridae. *G. intestinalis* is the botfly whose larva infests horses. Migration of the larva beneath the skin of their occasional human hosts may give rise to a form of creeping eruption (larva migrans). *G. hemorrhoidalis*, the nose botfly, which has orange-red terminal segments, sometimes infests man.

gastr- see *gastro-*.

gastradenitis (gas″trad-ĕ-ni′tis) [*gastr-* + Gr. *adēn* gland + *-itis*] inflammation of the stomach glands.

gastralgia (gas-tral′je-ah) [*gastr-* + *-algia*] gastric colic.

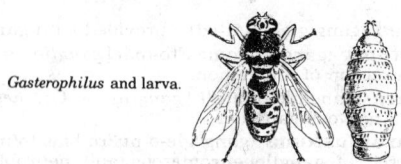

Gasterophilus and larva.

gastralgokenosis (gas-tral″go-ke-no′sis) [*gastr-* + Gr. *algos* pain + *kenōsis* emptiness] paroxysmal gastric pain when the stomach is empty, which is easily relieved by taking food.

gastramine hydrochloride (gas′trah-min) betazole hydrochloride.

gastratrophia (gas″trah-tro′fe-ah) [*gastr-* + Gr. *atrophia* atrophy] atrophic gastritis.

gastrectasia, gastrectasis (gas-trek-ta′ze-ah; gas-trek′tah-sis) [*gastr-* + Gr. *ektasis* stretching] (*obs.*) dilatation of the stomach.

gastrectomy (gas-trek′to-me) [*gastr-* + Gr. *ektomē* excision] excision of the whole (total g.) or part (subtotal g., partial g., gastric resection) of the stomach.

gastric (gas′trik) [L. *gastricus*; Gr. *gastēr* stomach] pertaining to, affecting, or originating in the stomach.

gastricsin (gas-trik′sin) a proteolytic enzyme—a hydrolase—isolated from the gastric juice. Originating from the same precursor (pepsinogen) as pepsin, it is of heavier molecular weight than pepsin, and possesses different amino acids at the N terminal.

gastrin (gas′trin) a polypeptide hormone secreted by gastrin cells of the pyloric glands, whose activity is related to the terminal tetrapeptide. It strongly stimulates secretion of gastric acid (causing contraction of the lower esophageal sphincter and modifying gastric and esophageal motility) and pepsin, and weakly stimulates secretion of pancreatic enzymes and gallbladder contraction.

gastrinoma (gas″trin-o′mah) a gastrin-secreting non–beta islet cell tumor associated with Zollinger-Ellison syndrome, usually found within the substance of the pancreas but also occurring at other sites, as in the antrum of the stomach, hilus of the spleen, and regional lymph nodes.

gastritic (gas-trit′ik) pertaining to or affected with gastritis.

gastritis (gas-tri′tis) [*gastr-* + *-itis*] inflammation of the stomach. **antral g., antrum g.,** inflammation affecting the antrum of the stomach. **atrophic g.,** chronic gastritis with atrophy of the mucous membrane and glands. **atrophic-hyperplastic g.,** a variant of atrophic gastritis in which the mucosa is of normal or even increased thickness. **catarrhal g.,** inflammation of the mucous membrane of the stomach, with hypertrophy of the membrane, secretion of an excessive quantity of mucus, and alteration of the gastric juice. The condition is marked by loss of appetite, nausea, pain, vomiting, and tympanitic distention of the stomach. **chemical g.,** inflammation caused by the ingestion of corrosive substances, with complete mucosal destruction in fatal cases; called also *corrosive g.* **chronic cystic g.,** gastritis in which the gastric and pyloric glands are dilated and lined by flattened epithelium, suggestive of a degenerative rather than an inflammatory condition. **chronic follicular g.,** an atrophic gastritis in which the size and number of lymphoid follicles in the mucosa and submucosa are greatly increased, with heavy infiltration of the entire mucosa by lymphocytes. **cirrhotic g.,** linitis plastica. **corrosive g.,** chemical g. **eosinophilic g.,** gastritis in which there is considerable edema and a heavy infiltration of all coats of the wall of the pyloric antrum by eosinophils. **erosive g.,** gastritis in which the surface epithelium is eroded, manifesting as a patchy or a diffuse lesion; exfoliative g. **exfoliative g.,** chronic gastritis in which bits of the surface of the mucous membrane are shed; erosive g. **follicular g.,** inflammation of the glands of the stomach. **giant hypertrophic g.,** excessive proliferation of the gastric mucosa, producing diffuse thickening of the stomach wall; inflammatory changes may be associated. Called also *Menetrier's disease.* **hemorrhagic g.,** erosive gastritis with bleeding. **hypertrophic g.,** gastritis with infiltration and enlargement of the glands. **phlegmonous g.,** a variety with abscesses in the stomach walls. **polypous g.,** hypertrophic gastritis with polypoid projections into the stomach. **pseudomembranous g.,** a variety in which a false membrane occurs in patches within the stomach. **radiation g.,** gastritis resulting from radiation injury. **toxic g.,** gastritis caused by the action of a poison or a corrosive agent. **zonal g.,** gastritis occurring in the vicinity of a gastric lesion, as that associated with peptic ulcer and gastric carcinoma.

gastro-, gastr- (gas′tro; gas′tr-) [Gr. *gastēr* stomach] combining form denoting relationship to the stomach.

gastroacephalus (gas″tro-a-sef′ah-lus) [*gastro-* + *a* neg. + Gr. *kephalē* head] a twin monster, the autosite bearing a headless parasite on its abdomen.

gastroadenitis (gas″tro-ad″ĕ-ni′tis) gastradenitis.

gastroadynamic (gas″tro-a″di-nam′ik) marked by an adynamic condition of the stomach.

gastroamorphus (gas″tro-a-mor′fus) [gastro- + Gr. *a* neg. + *morphē* form] a presumptive twin monster in which the parasite consists of fetal parts concealed within the abdomen of the autosite.

gastroanastomosis (gas″tro-ah-nas″to-mo′sis) gastrogastrostomy.

gastroatonia (gas″tro-ah-to′ne-ah) (obs.) atony of the stomach.

gastrocamera (gas″tro-kam′er-ah) a small camera which can be swallowed or passed down the esophagus on an appropriate instrument to photograph the inside of the stomach; it is attached to an external control box by a hollow flexible tube, and fitted with a flash lamp and inflation bulb. After the camera is inserted into the stomach, the bulb is inflated and pictures are taken as the flash lamp is triggered.

gastrocardiac (gas″tro-kar′de-ak) pertaining to the stomach and the heart.

gastrocele (gas′tro-sēl) [gastro- + Gr. *kēlē* hernia] hernial protrusion of the stomach or of a gastric pouch.

gastrochronorrhea (gas″tro-kron″o-re′ah) [gastro- + Gr. *chronos* time + *rhoia* flowing] (obs.) chronic gastric hypersecretion.

gastrocnemius (gas″trok-ne′me-us) [gastro- + Gr. *knēmē* leg] see *Table of Musculi.*

gastrocoele (gas′tro-sēl) [gastro- + Gr. *koilos* hollow] the archenteron.

gastrocolic (gas″tro-kol′ik) pertaining to or communicating with the stomach and colon, as a gastrocolic fistula.

gastrocolitis (gas″tro-ko-li′tis) [gastro- + Gr. *kolon* colon + -itis] inflammation of the stomach and colon.

gastrocoloptosis (gas″tro-ko″lop-to′sis) [gastro- + colon + Gr. *ptōsis* falling] (obs.) downward displacement of the stomach and colon.

gastrocolostomy (gas″tro-ko-los′to-me) [gastro- + Gr. *kolon* colon + *stomoun* to provide with an opening, or mouth] the creation of an artificial opening between the stomach and the colon; also, the opening so established.

gastrocolotomy (gas″tro-ko-lot′o-me) [gastro- + Gr. *kolon* colon + *tomē* a cutting] incision into the stomach and colon.

gastrocutaneous (gas″tro-ku-ta′ne-us) pertaining to the stomach and skin, or communicating with the stomach and the cutaneous surface of the body, as a gastrocutaneous fistula.

gastrodermis (gas″tro-der′mis) [gastro- + Gr. *derma* skin] the tissue lining the gut cavity of an invertebrate, which is responsible for digestion and absorption.

gastrodiaphane (gas″tro-di′ah-fān) [gastro- + Gr. *dia* through + *phainein* to show] a small electric lamp introduced into the stomach in gastrodiaphany.

gastrodiaphanoscopy (gas″tro-di-af″ah-nos′ko-pe) [gastro- + Gr. *dia* through + *phainein* to show + *skopein* to examine] gastrodiaphany.

gastrodiaphany (gas″tro-di-af′ah-ne) [gastro- + Gr. *dia* through + *phainein* to show] the exploration of the stomach by means of an electric lamp passed down the esophagus.

gastrodidymus (gas″tro-did′ĭ-mus) [gastro- + Gr. *didymos* twin] symmetrical conjoined twins joined in the abdominal region.

gastrodisciasis (gas″tro-dis-ki′ah-sis) infection caused by *Gastrodiscoides hominis.*

Gastrodiscoides (gas″tro-dis-koi′dēz) [gastro- + Gr. *diskos* disk + *eidos* form] a genus of trematodes parasitic in the intestinal tract; called also *Gastrodiscus.* **G. hom′inis,** a species common in the cecum and large intestine of pigs and occasionally in man, in Indochina, India, and Malaysia. Called also *Amphistomum hominis.*

Gastrodiscus (gas″tro-dis′kus) *Gastrodiscoides.*

gastrodisk (gas′tro-disk) the embryonic disk.

gastroduodenal (gas″tro-du″o-de′nal) pertaining to or communicating with the stomach and duodenum, as a gastroduodenal fistula.

gastroduodenectomy (gas″tro-du″o-dĕ-nek′to-me) excision of stomach and duodenum.

gastroduodenitis (gas″tro-du-od″ĕ-ni′tis) [gastro- + duodenitis] an inflammation of the stomach and duodenum.

gastroduodenoscopy (gas″tro-du″o-dĕ-nos′ko-pe) [gastro- + duodenum + Gr. *skopein* to examine] examination of the stomach and duodenum, the gastroscope usually being passed through the esophagus, occasionally through incisions in the abdominal and gastric walls if performed during operation.

gastroduodenostomy (gas″tro-du″o-dĕ-nos′to-me) [gastro- + duodenum + Gr. *stomoun* to provide with an opening, or mouth] surgical creation of an anastomosis between the stomach and the duodenum.

gastrodynia (gas″tro-din′e-ah) [gastro- + Gr. *odynē* pain] pain in the stomach.

gastroenteralgia (gas″tro-en″ter-al′je-ah) [gastro- + Gr. *enteron* intestine + -algia] pain in the stomach and intestines.

gastroenteric (gas″tro-en-ter′ik) [gastro- + Gr. *enteron* intestine] pertaining to the stomach and intestines.

gastroenteritis (gas″tro-en-ter-i′tis) [gastro- + enteritis] inflammation of the stomach and intestines. **acute infectious g.,** gastritis with acute onset, caused by various bacteria and viruses. **eosinophilic g.,** a disorder marked by infiltration of the mucosa of the small intestine by eosinophils, with edema but without vasculitis, and by eosinophilia of the peripheral blood. Symptoms, including abdominal pain, diarrhea, nausea, fever, and malabsorption, depend on the site and extent of the disorder. The stomach is also frequently involved. The disorder is commonly associated with intolerance to specific foods. See also *eosinophic granuloma* (def. 2), under *granuloma.* **g. paratypho′sa B,** gastroenteritis caused by *Salmonella paratyphi* B. **transmissible g. (T.G.E.) of swine,** a viral disease of swine occurring chiefly during the winter and characterized by severe diarrhea and acute inflammation of the gastric mucosa which may lead to ulceration and hemorrhage. The mortality rate among piglets is very high. **g. typho′sa,** a form of gastroenteritis caused by *Salmonella typhosa.*

gastroenteroanastomosis (gas″tro-en″ter-o-ah-nas″to-mo′sis) anastomosis between the stomach and small intestine in gastroenterostomy.

gastroenterocolitis (gas″tro-en″ter-o-ko-li′tis) inflammation of the stomach, small intestine, and colon.

gastroenterocolostomy (gas″tro-en″ter-o-ko-los′to-me) [gastro- + Gr. *enteron* intestine + *kolon* colon + *stomoun* to provide with an opening, or mouth] surgical creation of an opening between the stomach, intestine, and colon; also, the opening so established.

gastroenterologist (gas″tro-en″ter-ol′o-jist) a practitioner who specializes in diseases of the digestive tract.

gastroenterology (gas″tro-en″ter-ol′o-je) [gastro- + Gr. *enteron* intestine + -logy] the study of the stomach and intestines and their diseases.

gastroenteropathy (gas″tro-en″ter-op′ah-the) any disease of the stomach and intestines.

gastroenteroplasty (gas″tro-en′ter-o-plas″te) a plastic operation on the stomach and small intestine.

gastroenteroptosis (gas″tro-en″ter-op-to′sis) [gastro- + Gr. *enteron* intestine + *ptōsis* falling] downward displacement, or prolapse, of the stomach and intestines; a term based on the concept that variations in the positions of organs cause disease.

gastroenterostomy (gas″tro-en″ter-os′to-me) [gastro- + Gr. *enteron* intestine + *stomoun* to provide with an opening, or mouth] surgical creation of an artificial passage (anastomosis) between the stomach and intestines (usually the jejunum); see illustration on following page.

gastroenterotomy (gas″tro-en″ter-ot′o-me) [gastro- + Gr. *enteron* intestine + *temnein* to cut] surgical incision into the stomach and intestine.

gastroepiploic (gas″tro-ep″ĭ-plo′ik) [gastro- + Gr. *epiploon* caul] pertaining to the stomach and epiploon (omentum).

gastroesophageal (gas″tro-ĕ-sof″ah-je′al) pertaining to the stomach and esophagus, as the gastroesophageal junction.

gastroesophagitis (gas″tro-ĕ-sof″ah-ji′tis) inflammation of the stomach and esophagus.

gastroesophagostomy (gas″tro-ĕ-sof″ah-gos′to-me) surgical creation of an anastomosis between the stomach and the esophagus; done for stricture of the lower end of the esophagus.

gastrofiberscope (gas″tro-fi′ber-skōp) a fiberscope for viewing the stomach.

gastrogastrostomy (gas″tro-gas-tros′to-me) [gastro- + gastro- + Gr. *stomoun* to provide with an opening, or mouth] surgical creation of an anastomosis between the pyloric and cardiac ends of the stomach, usually performed because of hourglass contraction of the middle third of the stomach; also, the anastomosis so established.

gastrogavage (gas″tro-gah-vazh′) [gastro- + Fr. *gavage* cramming] the introduction of nutriment into the stomach by means of a tube passed through the esophagus.

gastrogenic (gas″tro-jen′ik) formed or originating in the stomach.

Gastrografin (gas″tro-graf′in) trademark for a preparation of meglumine diatrizoate.

gastrograph (gas′tro-graf) [gastro- + Gr. *graphein* to record] an apparatus for recording the motions of the stomach.

gastrohepatic (gas″tro-hĕ-pat′ik) [gastro- + Gr. *hēpar* liver] pertaining to the stomach and liver.

gastrohepatitis (gas″tro-hep-ah-ti′tis) inflammation of the stomach and liver.

gastrohydrorrhea (gas″tro-hi″dro-re′ah) [gastro- + Gr. *hydōr* water + *rhoia* flow] (obs.) the secretion by the stomach of a quantity of watery fluid deficient in hydrochloric acid and gastric enzymes.

gastrohypertonic (gas″tro-hi″per-ton′ik) marked by excessive tonicity of the stomach.

gastroileac (gas″tro-il′e-ak) pertaining to stomach and ileum.

gastroileitis (gas″tro-il-e-i′tis) inflammation of the stomach and ileum.

gastroileostomy (gas″tro-il-e-os′to-me) surgical creation of an anastomosis between the stomach and ileum; also, the anastomosis so established.

gastrointestinal (gas″tro-in-tes′tĭ-nal) [*gastro-* + *intestinal*] pertaining to or communicating with the stomach and intestine, as a gastrointestinal fistula.

gastrojejunocolic (gas″tro-jĕ-ju″no-kol′ik) pertaining to or communicating with the stomach, jejunum, and colon, as a gastrojejunocolic fistula.

gastrojejunoesophagostomy (gas″tro-jĕ-ju″no-ĕ-sof″ah-gos′-to-me) esophagojejunogastrostomosis.

gastrojejunostomy (gas″tro-jĕ-ju-nos′to-me) [*gastro-* + *jejunostomy*] surgical creation of an anastomosis between the stomach and jejunum; also, the anastomosis so established.

gastrokinesograph (gas″tro-ki-nes′o-graf) [*gastro-* + Gr. *kinēsis* motion + *graphein* to record] a device for recording the mechanical motions of the stomach.

gastrolienal (gas″tro-li′en-al) [*gastro-* + L. *lien* spleen] pertaining to the stomach and spleen.

gastrolith (gas′tro-lith) [*gastro-* + Gr. *lithos* stone] a calcareous or other concretion formed in the stomach; called also *gastric* or *stomachic calculus*.

gastrolithiasis (gas″tro-lĭ-thi′ah-sis) [*gastro-* + Gr. *lithos* stone + *-iasis*] the presence or formation of gastroliths.

gastrologist (gas-trol′o-jist) a specialist in diseases of the stomach.

gastrology (gas-trol′o-je) [*gastro-* + *-logy*] the sum of knowledge regarding the stomach.

gastrolysis (gas-trol′ĭ-sis) [*gastro-* + Gr. *lysis* loosening] surgical division of perigastric adhesions in order to mobilize the stomach.

gastromalacia (gas″tro-mah-la′she-ah) [*gastro-* + Gr. *malakia* softening] an abnormal softening or softness of the wall of the stomach; see *softening of the stomach*.

gastromegaly (gas″tro-meg′ah-le) [*gastro-* + Gr. *megas* large] enlargement of the stomach.

gastromelus (gas-trom′ĕ-lus) [*gastro-* + Gr. *melos* limb] a monster with a supernumerary leg attached to the abdomen.

gastromycosis (gas″tro-mi-ko′sis) [*gastro-* + Gr. *mykēs* fungus] a disease of the stomach caused by fungi.

gastromyotomy (gas″tro-mi-ot′o-me) [*gastro-* + Gr. *mys* muscle + *temnein* to cut] incision through the muscular coats of the stomach down to the mucosa.

gastromyxorrhea (gas″tro-mik″so-re′ah) [*gastro-* + Gr. *myxa* mucus + *rhoia* flow] excessive secretion of mucus by the stomach.

gastrone (gas′trōn) a reputed hormonal inhibitor of gastric acid secretion, extracted from gastric mucus.

gastronesteostomy (gas″tro-nes″te-os′to-me) [*gastro-* + Gr. *nēstis* jejunum + *stomoun* to provide with a mouth or opening] gastrojejunostomy.

gastropancreatitis (gas″tro-pan″kre-ah-ti′tis) inflammation of the stomach and pancreas.

gastroparalysis (gas″tro-pah-ral′ĭ-sis) paralysis of the stomach; gastric atony; gastroparesis.

gastroparesis (gas″tro-par′ĕ-sis) [*gastro-* + Gr. *paresis* paralysis] paralysis of the stomach.

gastroparietal (gas″tro-pah-ri′ĕ-tal) pertaining to the stomach and the body wall.

gastropathic (gas″tro-path′ik) pertaining to disease of the stomach.

gastropathy (gas-trop′ah-the) [*gastro-* + Gr. *pathos* disease] any disease of the stomach.

gastroperiodynia (gas″tro-per″e-o-din′e-ah) [*gastro-* + Gr. *periodos* period + *odynē* pain] periodical attacks of pain in the stomach.

gastroperitonitis (gas″tro-per″ĭ-to-ni′tis) inflammation of the stomach and peritoneum.

gastropexy (gas′tro-pek″se) [*gastro-* + Gr. *pēxis* fixation] surgical fixation of the stomach to correct displacement.

Gastrophilus (gas-trof′ĭ-lus) *Gasterophilus*.

gastrophotography (gas″tro-fo-tog′rah-fe) photography of the interior of the stomach by means of a camera either built into the distal tip of the gastroscope, or attached to the eyepiece with light being transmitted to the stomach by a fiberoptic bundle system.

gastrophotor (gas″tro-fo′tor) an instrument for gastrophotography.

gastrophrenic (gas″tro-fren′ik) [*gastro-* + Gr. *phrēn* diaphragm] pertaining to the stomach and diaphragm.

gastrophthisis (gas″tro-this′is) [*gastro-* + Gr. *phthisis* wasting] 1. hyperplasia of the gastric mucosa and submucosa, leading to thickening of the stomach walls and diminution of its cavity. 2. emaciation due to abdominal disease.

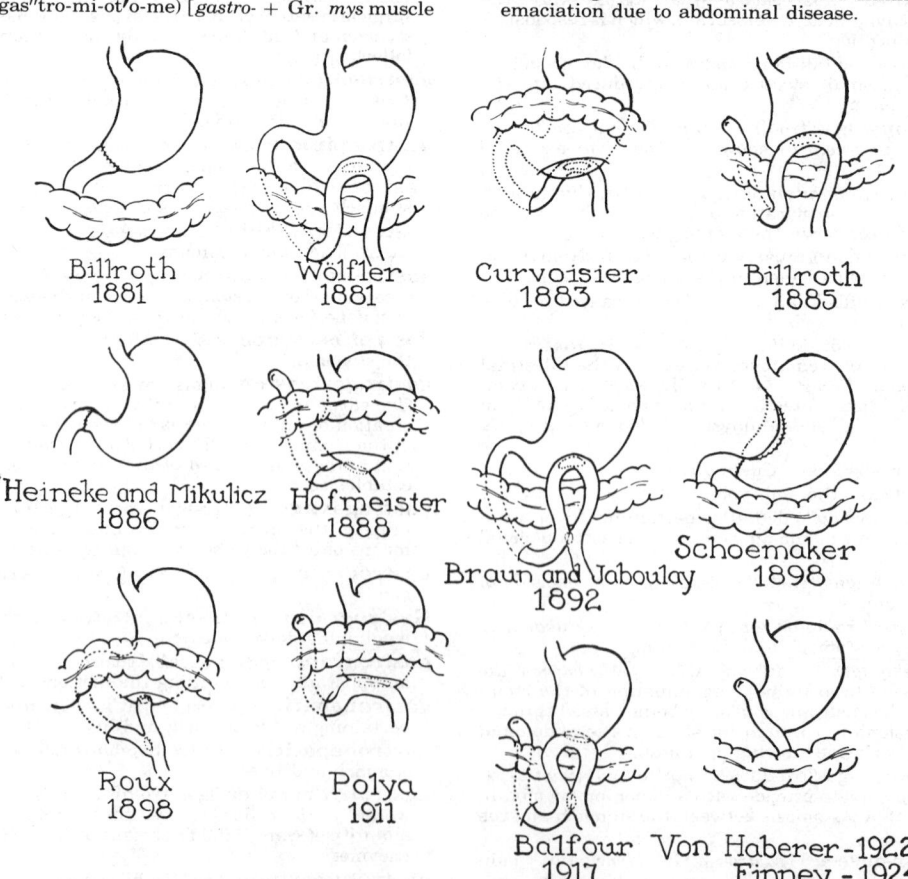

Types of gastroenterostomy.

gastroplasty (gas′tro-plas″te) [*gastro-* + Gr. *plassein* to form] plastic operation on the stomach.

gastroplegia (gas″tro-ple′je-ah) [*gastro-* + Gr. *plēgē* stroke] paralysis of the stomach.

gastroplication (gas″tro-pli-ka′shun) [*gastro-* + L. *plicare* to fold] the surgical treatment of gastric dilatation by stitching a fold in the stomach.

gastropneumonic (gas″tro-nu-mon′ik) pertaining to the stomach and lungs.

gastropod (gas′tro-pod) a mollusk of the class Gastropoda; see *snail.*

Gastropoda (gas-trop′ŏ-dah) [*gastro-* + Gr. *pous* foot] a class of mollusks embracing the snails, slugs, whelks, abalones, etc., including many species that serve as primary and intermediate hosts of pathogens.

gastroptosia (gas″tro-to′se-ah) (*obs.*) gastroptosis.

gastroptosis (gas″tro-to′sis) [*gastro-* + Gr. *ptosis* falling] downward displacement of the stomach; a term based on the outmoded concept that variation in position of abdominal organs is pathological.

gastropulmonary (gas″tro-pul′mo-nar-e) [*gastro-* + L. *pulmo* lung] pertaining to the stomach and lungs.

gastropylorectomy (gas″tro-pi″lo-rek′to-me) [*gastro-* + Gr. *pylōros* pylorus + *ektomē* excision] excision of the pyloric portion of the stomach.

gastropyloric (gas″tro-pi-lor′ik) pertaining to the stomach in its entirety and to the pylorus.

gastroradiculitis (gas″tro-rah-dik″u-li′tis) [*gastro-* + L. *radix* root + *-itis*] inflammation of the posterior roots of spinal nerves involving irritation of the sensory fibers in them which are connected with the stomach.

gastrorrhagia (gas″tro-ra′je-ah) [*gastro-* + Gr. *rhēgnynai* to break forth] hemorrhage from the stomach.

gastrorrhaphy (gas-tror′ah-fe) [*gastro-* + Gr. *rhaphē* suture] suture of a wound of the stomach.

gastrorrhea (gas″tro-re′ah) [*gastro-* + Gr. *rhoia* flow] excessive secretion of mucus or gastric juice in the stomach; gastric hypersecretion.

gastrorrhexis (gas″tro-rek′sis) [*gastro-* + Gr. *rhēxis* rupture] rupture of the stomach.

gastroschisis (gas-tros′kĭ-sis) [*gastro-* + Gr. *schisis* cleft] a congenital fissure of the abdominal wall not involving the site of insertion of the umbilical cord, and usually accompanied by protrusion of the small and part of the large intestine.

gastroscope (gas′tro-skōp) [*gastro-* + Gr. *skopein* to examine] an endoscope for inspecting the interior of the stomach. **fiber-optic g.,** a fiberscope for examining the stomach.

gastroscopic (gas″tro-skop′ik) pertaining to gastroscopy or the gastroscope.

gastroscopy (gas-tros′ko-pe) [*gastro-* + Gr. *skopein* to examine] inspection of the interior of the stomach by means of the gastroscope.

gastroselective (gas″tro-sĕ-lek′tiv) having an affinity for receptors involved in regulation of gastric activities.

gastrosia (gas-tro′se-ah) a disease of the stomach. **g. fungo′sa,** a disease of the stomach caused by fungi or molds.

gastrosis (gas-tro′sis) any disease of the stomach.

gastrospasm (gas′tro-spazm) [*gastro-* + *spasm*] spasm of the stomach.

gastrospiry (gas′tro-spi″re) [*gastro-* + L. *spirare* to breathe] aerophagia.

gastrosplenic (gas″tro-splen′ik) pertaining to the stomach and spleen.

gastrostaxis (gas″tro-stak′sis) [*gastro-* + Gr. *staxis* a dripping] the oozing of blood from the mucous membrane of the stomach; hemorrhagic gastritis.

gastrostenosis (gas″tro-stĕ-no′sis) [*gastro-* + Gr. *stenōsis* narrowing] contraction or shrinkage of the stomach.

gastrogavage (gas-tros″to-gah-vahzh′) introduction of nutriment into the stomach by means of a tube passed through a gastric fistula.

gastrostolavage (gas-tros″to-lah-vahzh′) irrigation of the stomach through a gastric fistula.

gastrostoma (gas-tros′to-mah) [*gastro-* + Gr. *stoma* mouth] a gastric fistula or a surgically created opening from the stomach through the abdominal wall.

gastrostomosis (gas-tros″to-mo′sis) gastrostomy.

gastrostomy (gas-tros′to-me) [*gastro-* + Gr. *stomoun* to provide with an opening, or mouth] surgical creation of an artificial opening into the stomach; also, the opening so established. **Beck's g.,** creation of a gastric fistula by the formation of a tube from the greater curvature of the stomach to the surface of the abdominal wall. **Witzel g.,** that in which a catheter is inserted and secured from the gastric lumen to the surface of the abdominal wall.

gastrosuccorrhea (gas″tro-suk″o-re′ah) [*gastro-* + L. *succus*

juice + Gr. *rhoia* flow] excessive and continuous secretion of gastric juice. **digestive g.,** a condition in which there is excessive secretion of gastric juice during digestion only.

gastrothoracopagus (gas″tro-tho′rah-kop′ah-gus) [*gastro-* + Gr. *thōrax* chest + *pagos* thing fixed] a double monster joined at the abdomen and thorax. **g. dipy′gus,** a double monster in which there is attached to the abdomen of the autosite a parasite consisting of the pelvis and lower extremities only; called also *dipygus parasiticus.*

gastrotome (gas″tro-tōm) a cutting instrument used in gastrotomy.

gastrotomy (gas-trot′o-me) [*gastro-* + Gr. *temnein* to cut] incision into the stomach.

gastrotonometer (gas″tro-to-nom′ĕ-ter) [*gastro-* + Gr. *tonos* tension + *metron* measure] an instrument for measuring intragastric pressure.

gastrotonometry (gas″tro-tro-nom′ĕ-tre) the measurement of intragastric pressure.

gastrotoxin (gas″tro-tok′sin) a substance that exerts a toxic effect on the stomach.

Gastrotricha (gas″tro-trik′ah) [*gastro-* + Gr. *trichos* hair] a class of very small aquatic animals of the phylum Aschelminthes, which have cilia on the ventral surface and a triradiate esophagus. In some systems of classification, they are considered to be a separate phylum.

gastrotropic (gas″tro-trop′ik) [*gastro-* + Gr. *tropos* a turning] having an affinity for or exerting a special effect upon the stomach.

gastrotympanites (gas″tro-tim″pah-ni′tēz) [*gastro-* + *tympanites*] tympanitic distention of the stomach.

gastrula (gas′troo-lah) that early embryonic stage which follows the blastula. The simplest type consists of two layers, the ectoderm and the mesentoderm, and of two cavities, one lying between the ectoderm and the entoderm; the other (the archenteron) formed by invagination so as to lie within the entoderm and having an opening (the blastopore).

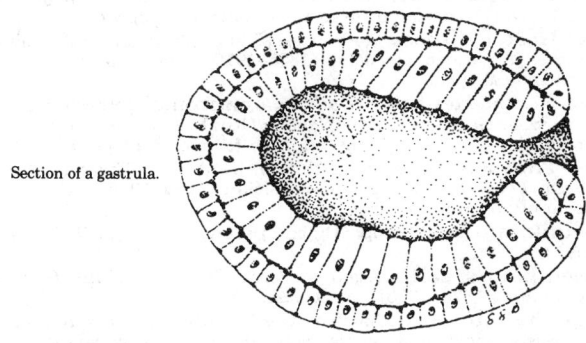

Section of a gastrula.

gastrulation (gas″troo-la′shun) the process by which a blastula becomes a gastrula or, in forms without a true blastula, the process by which three germ cell layers are acquired.

Gatch bed (gach) [Willis Dew *Gatch,* American surgeon, born 1879] see under *bed.*

gatism (ga′tizm) [Fr. *gâter* to spoil] rectal, vesical, or rectovesical incontinence.

gatophilia (gat″o-fil′e-ah) (*obs.*) ailurophilia.

gatophobia (gat″o-fo′be-ạ¹.) (*obs.*) ailurophobia.

gattine (gat′en) a form of flacherie (a disease of silkworm larvae) in which the cephalic end of affected larvae may become swollen and almost translucent; thought to be caused by a mixed infection with an unidentified virus and an enterococcus closely related to *Streptococcus faecalis.*

Gaucher's cells, disease (splenomegaly) (go-shāz′) [Phillippe Charles Ernest *Gaucher,* French physician, 1854–1918] see under *cell* and *disease.*

gauge (gāj) an instrument for determining the dimensions or caliber of anything. **Boley g.,** a watchmaker's gauge used in dentistry to measure tooth dimensions and to make other measurements important in prosthetic dentistry. **catheter g.,** a plate with graduated perforations for measuring the outside diameter of catheters.

Gaultheria (gawl-the′re-ah) [Jean François *Gaultier,* Quebec physician and botanist, 1708–1756] a genus of ericaceous plants; the leaves of *G. procumbens,* of North America, afford a fragrant volatile oil rich in methyl salicylate.

gauntlet (gawnt′let) [Fr. *gant* glove] a bandage which covers the hand and fingers like a glove.

gauss (gows) [Johann Karl F. *Gauss,* German physicist, 1777–1855] the unit of magnetic flux density; symbol *B.* In the SI system of units, it has been replaced by the *tesla.*

gaussian curve (gow′shun) [J. K. F. *Gauss*] see under *curve*.

Gauvain's fluid (go-vānz′) [Ernest Almore *Gauvain*, American dermatologist, born 1893] see under *fluid*.

gauze (gawz) a light, open-meshed fabric of muslin or similar material. Before use in surgery, it is usually sterilized and frequently impregnated with various antiseptics. **absorbable g.**, gauze made from oxidized cellulose. **absorbent g.** [USP], a well-bleached cotton cloth of plain weave, of various thread counts (20–44 per inch warp, 12–36 filling) and various weights (17.2–44.5 gm. per yard). **absorbent g., sterile,** absorbent gauze which has been sterilized and subsequently protected from contamination. **petrolatum g.** [USP], absorbent gauze saturated with white petrolatum; used as a protective covering for wounds. **zinc gelatin impregnated g.** [USP], absorbent gauze impregnated with zinc gelatin that may contain a small amount of ferric oxide.

gavage (gah-vahzh′) [Fr. "cramming"] 1. forced feeding especially through a tube passed into the stomach. 2. the therapeutic use of a very full diet; superalimentation.

Gavard's muscle (gah-vahrz′) [Hyacinthe *Gavard*, French anatomist, 1753–1802] see under *muscle*.

Gay-Lussac's law (ga″lū-sahks′) [Joseph Louis *Gay-Lussac*, French naturalist, 1778–1850] Charles' law; see under *law*.

Gaza's operation (gah′zahz) [Wilhelm von *Gaza*, German surgeon, 1883–1936] ramisection.

gaze (gaz) 1. to look in one direction for a period of time. 2. the act or state of looking steadily in one direction.

g-cal. gram calorie; see *small calorie*, under *calorie*.

Gd chemical symbol for *gadolinium*.

GDH glutamic acid dehydrogenase.

Ge chemical symbol for *germanium*.

gear (gēr) equipment. **cervical g.,** an extraoral appliance by means of which the back of the neck is used for anchorage or as a base of traction in effecting tooth movement.

Geaster (je-as′ter) a genus of basidiomycetous fungi of the order Lycoperdales, series Gasteromycetes, including the star fungi.

Gee's disease (gēz) [Samuel Jones *Gee*, London physician, 1839–1911] the infantile form of nontropical sprue.

Gee-Herter disease (ge′her′ter) [S. J. *Gee*; Christian Archibald *Herter*, American physician, 1865–1910] the infantile form of nontropical sprue.

Gee-Herter-Heubner disease, syndrome (ge′her′ter-hoib′-ner) [S. J. *Gee*; C. A. *Herter*; Johann Otto L. *Heubner*, pediatrician in Berlin, 1843–1926] the infantile form of nontropical sprue.

Gee-Thaysen disease (ge′thi′sen) [S. J. *Gee*; Thorwald Einar Hess *Thaysen*, Copenhagen physician, 1883–1936] the adult form of nontropical sprue.

geeldikkop (gēl-dik′kop) [Dutch "yellow, thick head"] tribulosis.

Gegenbaur's cell (ga′gen-bow″erz) [Carl *Gegenbaur*, German anatomist, 1826–1903] osteoblast.

gegenhalten (ga″gen-halt′en) [Ger.] an involuntary resistance to passive movement, as may occur in cerebral cortical disorders.

Geigel's reflex (gi′gelz) [Richard *Geigel*, German physician, 1859–1930] see under *reflex*.

Geiger counter, Geiger-Müller counter (gi′ger, gi′ger-mil′er) [Hans *Geiger*, German physicist in England, 1882–1945] see under *counter*.

Geissler's test (gīs′lerz) [Ernst *Geissler*, German physician in 19th century] see under *tests*.

Geissler's tube (gīs′lerz) [Heinrich *Geissler*, German inventor, 1814–1879] see under *tube*.

gel (jel) a colloid which is firm in consistency, although containing much liquid, a colloid in a gelatinous form. See *sol*. **aluminum hydroxide g.** [USP], a suspension of 3.6 to 4.4 per cent of aluminum oxide (Al$_2$O$_3$), in the form of aluminum hydroxide and hydrated oxide, used as a gastric antacid, especially in the treatment of peptic ulcer. Called also *colloidal aluminum hydroxide gel*. **aluminum hydroxide g., dried** [USP], a white, amorphous powder suitable for preparing tablets and capsules, obtained by drying aluminum hydroxide gel, and containing not less than 50 per cent aluminum oxide; used as an antacid. **aluminum carbonate g., basic,** an aqueous suspension containing the equivalent of 4.9 to 5.3 per cent aluminum oxide and not less than 2.4 per cent carbon dioxide; used as an antacid. **aluminum phosphate g.** [USP], a water suspension of aluminum phosphate and some flavoring agents; it contains 4 to 5 per cent aluminum phosphate (AlPO$_4$) and is used as a gastric antacid, especially in the treatment of gastric ulcer. **betamethasone benzoate g.** [USP], a gel containing 90 to 110 per cent of the labeled amount of betamethasone benzoate; used as a topical glucocorticoid. **corticotropin g.**, repository corticotropin injection [USP]. **fluocinonide g.** [USP], a gel containing 90 to 110 per cent of the labeled amount of fluocinonide; used as a topical glucocorticoid. **silica g.** [NF], a gel obtained by the reaction of sodium silicate with hydrochloric or sulfuric acid, and containing not less than 99 percent of silica; used as a dispersing

and suspending agent. **sodium fluoride and orthophosphoric acid g., sodium fluoride and phosphoric acid g.** [USP], a preparation containing 90 to 110 per cent of the labeled amount of fluoride ion, in an aqueous medium containing a suitable viscosity-inducing agent; used as a dental caries prophylactic, applied topically to the teeth. **tolnaftate g.** [USP], a gel containing 90 to 110 per cent of the labeled amount of tolnaftate; used as an antifungal agent. **tretinoin g.** [USP], a gel containing 90 to 130 per cent of the labeled amount of tretinoin; used as a topical keratolytic.

Gel. quav. abbreviation for L. *gelati′na qua′vis*, in any kind of jelly.

gelase (jel′ās) an enzyme that splits agar.

gelasmus (je̅-las′mus) [G. *gelasma* a laugh] hysterical laughter.

gelastic (je̅-las′tik) [Gr. *gelastos* laughable] pertaining to laughter.

gelate (jel′āt) to form a gel.

gelatification (je̅-lat″ĭ-fi-ka′shun) conversion into gelatin.

gelatigenous (jel″ah-tij′e̅-nus) producing or forming gelatin.

gelatin (jel′ah-tin) [L. *gelatina*, from *gelare* to congeal] [USP] a product obtained by partial hydrolysis of collagen derived from the skin, white connective tissue, and bones of animals; used as a suspending agent. It is also used pharmaceutically in the manufacture of capsules and suppositories, and has been suggested for intravenous use as a plasma substitute, and has been used as an adjuvant protein food. **agar g.,** nutrient bouillon solidified with gelatin and agar. **g. compound phenolized,** a mixture of gelatin, zinc oxide, glycerin, and water in phenol, used in preparing bandages (jelly bandages) for chronic ulcers and burns; especially effective in the ambulatory management of varicose ulcers. **dextrose g.,** nutrient gelatin containing dextrose. **fish g.,** fish bouillon solidified with 10 per cent of gelatin. **glucose-formate g.,** nutrient gelatin containing glucose and sodium formate. **glycerinated g.,** a preparation of gelatin and glycerin. **Japanese g.,** agar. **Kitasato's glucose-formate g.,** glucose-formate g. **lactose-litmus g.,** nutrient gelatin containing lactose and sufficient litmus solution to color the medium a deep lavender. **litmus g.,** nutrient gelatin containing sufficient litmus to give it a deep lavender color. **litmus whey g.,** litmus whey when solidified with gelatin. **meat extract g.,** meat extract bouillon solidified with gelatin. **meat infusion g.,** nutrient g. **medicated g.,** gelatin mixed with medicated substances for local application. **nutrient g.,** a culture medium consisting of nutrient bouillon solidified with 12 per cent gelatin. **silk g.,** sericin. **vegetable g.,** a gelatin-like matter obtained from vegetable tissues; see *agar*. **g. of Wharton,** Wharton's jelly. **whey g.,** whey, obtained from fresh milk which has been curdled with rennet, solidified with 10 per cent of gelatin. **wort g.,** beerwort culture medium solidified with 10 per cent of gelatin. **zinc g.** [USP], a preparation of zinc oxide, gelatin, glycerin, and purified water, applied topically as a protective.

gelatinase (je̅-lat′ĭ-nās) an enzyme that liquefies gelatin, but does not affect fibrin and egg albumin; it occurs among bacteria, molds, and yeasts.

gelatiniferous (jel″ah-tĭ-nif′er-us) [L. *gelatina* gelatin + *ferre* to bear] producing gelatin.

gelatinize (je̅-lat′ĭ-nīz) 1. to convert into gelatin. 2. to become converted into gelatin.

gelatinoid (je̅-lat′ĭ-noid) resembling gelatin.

gelatinolytic (jel″ah-tĭ-no-lit′ik) [*gelatin* + Gr. *lysis* dissolution] dissolving or splitting up gelatin.

gelatinosa (jel″ah-tĭ-no′sah) [L.] gelatinous; see entries beginning *substantia gelatinosa*, under *substantia*.

gelatinous (je̅-lat′ĭ-nus) [L. *gelatinosus*] like jelly or softened gelatin.

gelatinum (jel-ah-ti′num) [L.] gelatin. **g. glycerina′tum,** glycerinated gelatin.

gelation (je̅-la′shun) the conversion of a sol into a gel.

gelatose (jel′ah-tōs) an albumose formed by hydrolyzing gelatin by acid, alkalis, or an enzyme.

gelatum (je̅-la′tum) [L.] jelly, or gel.

geld (geld) to remove the testes, especially of the horse.

gelding (gel′ding) a castrated male animal, especially a horse.

Gelfilm (jel′film) trademark for absorbable gelatin film (q.v., under *film*).

Gelfoam (jel′fōm) trademark for an absorbable gelatin sponge.

gelidusi (ga″le-doo′se) pelidisi.

Gélineau's syndrome (zha-lĭ-no′) [Jean Baptiste Edouard *Gélineau*, French neurologist, born 1859] narcolepsy.

Gellé's test (zhel-āz′) [Marie Ernest *Gellé*, French otologist, 1834–1923] see under *tests*.

Gellhorn pessary (gel′horn) [George *Gellhorn*, St. Louis gynecologist, 1870–1936] see under *pessary*.

gelometer (jel-om′e̅-ter) a device for determining the time required for a solution to gel.

gelose (jel'ōs) agar.

gelosis (jĕ-lo'sis), pl. *gelo'ses* [L. *gelare* to freeze] a hard lump in a tissue, especially such a lump in a muscle.

gelotherapy, gelototherapy (jel"o-ther'ah-pe; jel"o-to-ther'-ah-pe) [Gr. *gelōs* laughter + *therapeia* cure] treatment of disease by provoking laughter.

gelotripsy (jel'o-trip"se) [*gelosis* + Gr. *tripsis* a rubbing] the breaking up of geloses in muscle by massage.

gelsemine (jel'sĕ-mēn) an alkaloid, $C_{20}H_{22}N_2O_2$, obtained from the roots and rhizomes of *Gelsemium sempervirens* (L.) Ait., (Loganiaceae). It acts as a mild central nervous system stimulant with toxic side effects, including double vision and muscular weakness, and may cause respiratory arrest.

Geltabs (jel'tabz) trademark for a preparation of ergocalciferol.

Gély's suture (zha-lēz') [Jules Aristide *Gély*, French surgeon, 1806–1861] see under *suture*.

gemästete (gĕ-mes'tĕ-tĕ) [Ger.] swollen or bloated: a term applied to enlarged astrocytes in the region of a degenerated area.

gemcadiol (jem"kah-di'ōl) chemical name: 2,2,9,9-tetra-methyl-1,10-decanediol; an antihyperlipidemic, $C_{14}H_{30}O_2$.

Gemella (jĕ-mel'ah) in some systems of classification, a genus of aerobic or facultatively anaerobic cocci of the family Streptoccaceae, occurring singly or in pairs with adjacent sides flattened; they are found as parasites of mammals. **G. haemoly'sans,** a species found in bronchial secretions and slime from the repiratory tract.

gemellary (jem'ĕ-lār"e) pertaining to twins.

gemellipara (jem"el-lip'ah-rah) [L. *gemelli* twins + *parere* to produce] a woman who has given birth to twins.

gemellology (gem"el-ol'o-je) [L. *gemellus* twin + *-logy*] the scientific study of twins and twinning.

geminate (jem'ĭ-nāt) [L. *geminatus*] paired; occurring in pairs.

gemination (jem-ĭ-na'shun) a doubling; in dentistry the division of a tooth bud which results in the formation of two teeth or of a double crown formed on a single root with a single pulp canal.

gemini (jem'ĭ-ni) [L.] plural of *geminus*.

geminous (jem'ĭ-nus) geminate.

geminus (jem'ĭ-nus), pl. *gem'ini* [L.] a twin. **gem'ini aequa'les,** monozygotic twins.

gemistocyte (jem-is'to-sīt) [Gr. *gemistos* laden, full + *cyte*] an astrocyte in which the cell body swells considerably, the nucleus assumes an eccentric position, and the cytoplasm is clearly visible. Called also *gemistocytic astrocyte*.

gemistocytic (jem-is"to-si'tik) composed of large round cells (gemistocytes); a term applied to astrocytomas composed of such cells.

gemma (jem'ah) [L. "bud"] a budlike body or structure.

gemmangioma (jem"an-je-o'mah) hemangioendothelioma.

gemmation (jĕ-ma'shun) [L. *gemmare* to bud] reproduction by budding, a kind of reproduction in cells in which a portion of the cell body is thrust out and then becomes separated, forming a new individual; used particularly to describe the formation of chlamydospores in fungi. See *budding*, def. 1.

gemmule (jem'ūl) [L. *gemmula*, dim. of *gemma* bud] 1. a reproductive bud; the immediate product of gemmation. 2. any one of the many little excrescences upon the dendrites of a nerve cell; called also *dendritic spine*. 3. hypothetical units assumed to be thrown off by the somatic cells, to be stored in the germ cells, and to determine the development of certain characters.

Gemonil (jem'o-nil) trademark for a preparation of metharbital.

-gen (jen') [Gr. *gennan* to produce] a word termination denoting an agent productive of the object or state indicated by the word stem to which it is affixed, as allergen (allergy), cryogen (cold), and pathogen (disease).

genal (je'nal) [L. *gena* cheek] pertaining to the cheek; buccal.

gender (jen'der) sex; the category to which an individual is assigned on the basis of sex.

gene (jēn) [Gr. *gennan* to produce] the biologic unit of heredity, self-reproducing and located at a definite position (locus) on a particular chromosome. The concept of gene is still evolving. From the standpoint of function, genes are conceived of as structural, operator, and regulator genes (see subentries). From another standpoint, they are conceived of as cistrons, mutons, and recons (see individual entries). As classically construed, the gene is approximately synonymous with cistron. **allelic g's,** genes situated at corresponding loci in a pair of chromosomes. **amorphic g.,** an amorph. **complementary g's,** two independent pairs of nonallelic genes, neither of which will produce its effect in the absence of the other; called also *reciprocal g's*. **cumulative g's,** polygenes. **derepressed g.,** in genetic theory, one that in response to an environmental demand for a particular enzyme functions to increase production of that enzyme; cf. *repressed g*. **dominant g.,** one that produces an effect (the phenotype) in the organism, regardless of the state of the corresponding allele, i.e., regardless of whether the individual is homozygous or heterozygous. **histocompatibility g.,** a gene that determines the specificity of tissue antigenicity (HLA antigens) and thus the compatibility of donor and recipient in tissue transplantation and blood transfusion; see *HLA antigens,* under *antigen*. **holandric g's,** genes in the nonhomologous region of the Y chromosome. **hologynic g's,** genes located on the X chromosome and appearing only in the female offspring. **immune response (Ir) g's,** genes of the major histocompatibility complex that govern the immune response to individual immunogens. **Ir g's,** immune response g's. **Is g's,** those genes that govern the formation of suppressor T-lymphocytes. **leaky g.,** one in which a switch in the sequence of bases in a nucleotide results in the production of a mutant protein that, because of a single amino acid replacement, has only partial enzymatic activity; a hypomorph. **lethal g.,** a gene the presence of which brings about the death of the organism, or permits its survival only under certain conditions; see also *lethal equivalent*. **modifying g's,** see under *factor*. **mutant g.,** a gene in which the loss, gain, or exchange of material has resulted in a permanent transmissible change in function. Such a gene may have become practically inactive (*amorph*), may act to antagonize or inhibit normal activity (*antimorph*), may act to increase normal activity (*hypermorph*), or may show only a slight reduction in its effectiveness (*leaky gene* or *hypomorph*). **nonstructural g's,** the operator and regulator genes, i.e., those not concerned in the formation of templates for messenger RNA. **operator g.,** in genetic theory, a gene that serves as a starting point for reading the genetic code and that, through interaction with a repressor, controls the activity of the structural genes associated with it in the operon. **pleiotropic g.,** one producing many effects in the phenotype. **recessive g.,** a gene that produces an effect in the organism only when it is transmitted by both parents, i.e., only when the individual is homozygous. **reciprocal g's,** complementary g's. **regulator g.,** in genetic theory, a gene that synthesizes repressor, a substance which, through interaction with the operator gene, switches off the activity of the structural genes associated with it in the operon. **repressed g.,** in genetic theory, one that under normal conditions does not always function to produce the maximum number of enzymes; cf. *derepressed g.* **repressor g.,** regulator g. **sex-conditioned g.,** a gene that is fully expressed in one sex only. **sex-limited g.,** a sex-linked or autosomal gene that will produce an effect in one sex only. **sex-linked g.,** a gene that is carried on the X or Y chromosome. **silent g.,** a third allele postulated to explain the complete lack of a specific enzyme activity (e.g., cholinesterase activity). **structural g.,** a gene that specifies the amino acid sequence of a polypetide chain. **sublethal g.,** a gene the presence of which handicaps or impairs the function of the organism. **supplementary g's,** two independent pairs of genes which interact in such a way that one dominant will produce its effect even in the absence of the other, but the second requires the presence of the first to be effective. **taster g.,** the gene that governs the ability to taste phenylthiourea. **wild-type g.,** the normal allele of a rare mutant gene, sometimes symbolized by +. **X-linked g.,** a gene that is carried on the X, or female sex, chromosome; generally used synonymously with sex-linked gene, since no genetic disorders have as yet been associated with genes of the Y chromosome.

geneogenous (je"ne-oj'ĕ-nus) [Gr. *genea* birth + *gennan* to produce] congenital.

genera (jen'er-ah) [L.] plural of *genus*.

general (jen'er-al) [L. *generalis*] affecting many parts or all parts of the organism; not local.

generalization (jen"er-al-i-za'shun) the phenomenon in pavlovian conditioning in which, after conditioning is established, a stimulus similar in some respect to the conditioned stimulus will also elicit the conditioned reflex.

generalize (jen'er-al-īz) to convert from a local to a general disease; to render general.

generation (jen"ĕ-ra'shun) [L. *generatio*] 1. the act or process of reproduction. 2. a class composed of all individuals removed by the same number of successive ancestors from a common predecessor, or occupying positions on the same level in a genealogical chart. **alternate g.,** the alternate reproduction by asexual and sexual means in an animal or plant species. **asexual g.,** production of a new individual (organism) not originating from the union of sexual elements (gametes); as by fission, budding, etc. **direct g.,** asexual g. **filial g., first,** all of the offspring produced by the mating of two individuals, as in a hybrid cross; symbol F_1. **filial g., second,** all of the offspring produced by the mating of two individuals of the first filial generation; symbol F_2. **nonsexual g.,** asexual g. **parental g.,** the generation with which a particular genetic study is begun; symbol P_1. **sexual g.,** production of a new individual (organism) by the union of male and female elements (gametes). **spontaneous g.,** the discredited concept of continuous generation of living organisms from nonliving matter; abiogenesis.

generative (jen'ĕ-ra"tiv) pertaining to the reproduction of the species.

generator (jen'er-a"tor) something that produces or causes to exist; a machine that converts mechanical to electrical energy. **pulse g.,** the power source for a cardiac pacemaker system, usually fueled by lithium or plutonium-238, supplying impulses to the implanted electrodes, either at a fixed rate or in some programmed pattern.

generic (jĕ-ner′ik) [L. *genus, generis* kind] 1. pertaining to a genus. 2. nonproprietary; denoting a drug name not protected by a trademark, usually descriptive of its chemical structure; sometimes called *public name.*

genesial, genesic (jĕ-ne′ze-al; jĕ-nes′ik) pertaining to generation or to origin.

genesiology (jĕ-ne″ze-ol′o-je) [*genesis* + *-logy*] the sum of what is known concerning reproduction.

genesis (jen′ĕ-sis) [Gr. *genesis* production, generation] the coming into being of anything; the process of originating. Often used as a word termination to denote the production, formation, or development of the object or state indicated by the word stem to which it is affixed, as biogenesis, gametogenesis, and pathogenesis.

genesistasis (jen″ĕ-sis′tah-sis) [*genesis* + Gr. *stasis* a stopping] interruption of the reproduction of organisms by chemotherapy so as to permit the body cells or fluids to dispose of them.

genestatic (gen″ĕ-stat′ik) tending to prevent sporulation.

genetic (jĕ-net′ik) 1. pertaining to reproduction, or to birth or origin. 2. inherited.

geneticist (jĕ-net′ĭ-sist) a specialist in genetics.

genetics (jĕ-net′iks) [Gr. *gennan* to produce] the study of heredity. **biochemical g.,** the science concerned with the chemical and physical nature of genes and the mechanism by which they control the development and maintenance of the organism. **clinical g.,** the study of the possible genetic factors influencing the occurrence of a pathologic condition. **molecular g.,** that branch of genetics concerned with the molecular structure and activities of the genetic material, including the replication of DNA, its transcription into RNA, and the translation of RNA to form proteins.

genetotrophic (jĕ-net″o-trōf′ik) pertaining to genetics and nutrition; relating to problems of nutrition which are hereditary in nature, or transmitted through the genes.

genetous (jĕ-net′us) dating from fetal life.

Geneva Convention an international agreement of 1864 whereby, among other pledges, the signatory nations pledged themselves to treat the wounded and the army medical and nursing staffs as neutrals on the field of battle.

Gengou phenomenon (zhaw-goo′) [Octave *Gengou,* French bacteriologist, 1875–1957] fixation of the complement; see under *fixation.*

genial, genian (jĕ-ni′al; jĕ-ni′an) [Gr. *geneion* chin] pertaining to the chin.

genic (jen′ik) pertaining to or caused by genes.

-genic (jen′ik) [Gr. *gennan* to produce] a word termination meaning producing, or productive of.

genicula (jĕ-nik′u-lah) [L.] plural of *geniculum.*

genicular (jĕ-nik′u-lar) pertaining to the knee.

geniculate (jĕ-nik′u-lāt) [L. *geniculatus*] bent, like a knee.

geniculum (jĕ-nik′u-lum), pl. *genic′ula* [L., dim. of *genu*] a little knee; [NA] a general term designating a sharp, kneelike bend in a small structure or organ, such as a nerve. **g. cana′lis facia′lis** [NA], **g. of facial canal,** the bend in the facial canal which lodges the geniculum nervi facialis; called also *genu of facial canal* and *knee of aqueductus fallopii.* **g. of facial nerve, g. ner′vi facia′lis** [NA], the part of the facial nerve at the lateral end of the internal acoustic meatus, where the fibers turn sharply posteroinferiorly, and where the geniculate ganglion is found; called also *external genu of facial nerve.*

genin (jen′in) aglycone.

genio- [Gr. *geneion* chin] a combining form denoting relationship to the chin. See also words beginning *mento-.*

geniocheiloplasty (je″ne-o-ki′lo-plas″te) [Gr. *geneion* chin + Gr. *cheilos* lip + *plassein* to form] plastic surgery of the chin and lip.

genioglossus (je″ne-o-glos′us) see *Table of Musculi.*

geniohyoglossus (je″ne-o-hi″o-glos′us) musculus genioglossus.

geniohyoid (je″ne-o-hi′oid) pertaining to the chin and hyoid bone.

geniohyoideus (je″ne-o-hi-oi′de-us) see *Table of Musculi.*

genioplasty (jĕ-ni′o-plas″te) [Gr. *geneion* chin + Gr. *plassein* to shape.] plastic surgery of the chin.

genital (jen′ĭ-tal) [L. *genitalis* belonging to birth] 1. pertaining to reproduction, or to the organs of generation. 2. [pl.] the reproductive organs (organa genitalia [NA]).

genitalia (jen′ĭ-ta′le-ah) [L., pl.] the reproductive organs (organa genitalia [NA]). **external g.,** see *partes genitales femininae externae* and *partes genitales masculinae externae.* **indifferent g.,** the reproductive organs of the embryo prior to the establishment of definitive sex.

genitaloid (jen′ĭ-tal-oid) [*genitalia* + Gr. *eidos* form] pertaining to the primordial sex cells, before future sexuality is distinguishable.

Female external genitalia (Bleier).

genito- (jen′ĭ-to) [L. *genitalis* belonging to birth] a combining form denoting relationship to the organs of reproduction.

genitocrural (jen″ĭ-to-kroo′ral) [*genital* + *crural*] pertaining to the genitalia and the leg.

genitofemoral (jen″ĭ-to-fem′or-al) genitocrural.

genitography (jen″ĭ-tog′rah-fe) radiography of the urogenital sinus and internal duct structures after injection of a contrast medium through the opening of the sinus.

genitoinfectious (jen″ĭ-to-in-fek′shus) venereal.

genitoplasty (jen′ĭ-to-plas″te) [*genital* + Gr. *plassein* to mold] plastic surgery on the genital organs.

genitourinary (jen″ĭ-to-u′rĭ-nar-e) pertaining to the genital and urinary organs; urogenital; urinosexual.

genius (jēn′yus) 1. distinctive character or peculiar nature. 2. superlative aptitude or ability. **g. epidem′icus,** Sydenham's theory of "epidemic constitutions," that contagious diseases are influenced by cosmic or atmospheric conditions which may change the character of and produce variations in these diseases. **g. lo′ci,** the particular susceptibility of a tissue to develop secondary tumors. **g. mor′bi,** the predominant character of a disease.

Gennari's line (band, layer, stria, stripe) (jen-nah′rēz) [Francisco *Gennari,* Italian anatomist of the 18th century] see *Baillarger's lines,* under *line.*

geno- (jen′o) [Gr. *gennan* to produce] a combining form denoting relationship to reproduction or to sex.

genoblast (jen′o-blast) [*geno-* + Gr. *blastos* germ] 1. the nucleus of the fertilized ovum. 2. a mature germ cell.

genocopy (jen′o-kop″e) an individual whose phenotype mimics that of another genotype but whose character is determined by a distinct assortment of genes; called also *genetic mimic.* Cf. *phenocopy.*

genodermatology (jen″o-der″mah-tol′o-je) that branch of dermatology which treats of hereditary skin diseases.

genodermatosis (jen″o-der-mah-to′sis) [*geno-* + *dermatosis*] a genetically determined disorder of the skin, usually generalized; if circumscribed, it is usually called *nevus.*

genome (je′nōm) [*gene* + chromos*ome*] the complete set of hereditary factors, as contained in the haploid assortment of chromosomes.

genomic (je-nom′ik) pertaining to the genome.

genophobia (jen″o-fo′be-ah) [*geno-* + Gr. *phobein* to be affrighted by + *ia*] morbid dread of sex and sexuality.

genotype (jen′o-tip) [*geno-* + Gr. *typos* type] 1. the entire genetic constitution of an individual; also, the alleles present at one or more specific loci. 2. the type species of a genus.

genotypic (jen″o-ti′pik) pertaining to or expressive of the genotype.

-genous [Gr.] a word termination signifying arising or resulting from, or produced by.

Gensoul's disease (zhan-soolz′) [Joseph *Gensoul,* French surgeon, 1797–1858] Ludwig's angina; see under *angina.*

gentamicin (jen″tah-mi′sin) an antibiotic complex isolated from the actinomycetes *Micromonospora purpurea* and *M. echinospora,* consisting of components designated A, B, C, etc. The form in medicinal use is a mixture of three fractions of the C component (C$_1$, C$_{1a}$, C$_2$); it is bactericidal for a wide range of pathogens, being highly effective against many gram-negative bacteria, especially *Pseudomonas* species, as well as some gram-positive species, especially *Staphylococcus aureus.* **g. sulfate** [USP], the sulfate salt of the antibiotic substances isolated from *Micromonospora purpurea.* It is used as an antibacterial in the treatment of infections caused by susceptible organisms involving almost all body organs and systems, especially in gram-negative bacillary infections of the urinary tract, in burns contaminated by *Pseudomomas,* sepsis, and toxemias. It is administered intramuscularly, intravenously, or applied topically to the skin, and is also applied topically to the conjunctiva in eye infections due to responsive bacteria.

gentamycin (jen″tah-mi′sin) gentamicin.

gentian (jen′shun) the dried rhizome and roots of *Gentiana lutea* L. (Gentianaceae); it has been used as a bitter tonic. It contains gentiin, gentiamarin, gentisin, gentisic acid, gentiopicrin, gentianose, and pectin. Also known as *yellow* or *pale gentian*. **g. violet** [USP], chemical name: *N*-[4-[bis[4-(dimethylamino)phenyl]-methylene]-2,5-cyclohexadiene-1-ylidene]-*N*-methylmethanaminium chloride. Hexamethylpararosaniline chloride, usually admixed with penta- and tetramethylpararosaniline chlorides, occurring as a dark green powder or greenish glistening pieces having a metallic luster. It is a dye with antibacterial, antifungal, and anthelmintic properties, applied topically in the treatment of infections of the skin and mucous membranes associated with gram-positive bacteria and molds, and administered orally in pinworm and liver fluke infections. It has been given orally, intravenously, and by transduodenal intubation in strongyloidosis.

gentianophil (jen′shan-o-fil) 1. an element staining readily with gentian violet. 2. gentianophilic.

gentianophilic (jen″shan-o-fil′ik) [*gentian* + Gr. *philein* to love] staining readily with gentian violet.

gentianophilous (jen″shan-of′ĭ-lus) gentianophilic.

gentianophobic (jen″shan-o-fo′bik) not staining readily with gentian violet.

gentianophobous (jen″shan-of′o-bus) gentianophobic.

gentianose (jen′shen-ōs) a trisaccharide, $C_{18}H_{32}O_{16}$, occurring in the rhizomes of gentian.

gentiavern (jen′shah-vern) gentian violet.

gentiopicrin (jen″she-o-pik′rin) [*gentian* + Gr. *pikros* bitter] a bitter, crystalline glycoside, $C_{16}H_{20}O_9$, from gentian root.

gentisate (jen′tĭ-sāt) a salt of gentisic acid.

Gentran (jen′tran) trademark for a preparation of dextran 70.

gentrogenin (jen″tro-jen′in) botogenin.

genu (je′nu), gen. *ge′nus*, pl. *gen′ua* [L.] [NA] 1. the knee; the site of articulation between the thigh (femur) and leg. 2. a general term used to designate any anatomical structure bent like the knee. **g. cap′sulae inter′nae** [NA], genu of internal capsule: the blunt angle formed by the union of the two limbs of the internal capsule, situated posterior to the caudate nucleus, anterior to the thalamus, and medial to the lentiform nucleus; called also *knee of internal capsule*. **g. cor′poris callo′si** [NA], **g. of corpus callosum**, the sharp ventral curve at the anterior end of the trunk of the corpus callosum. **g. extror′sum**, g. varum. **g. of facial canal**, geniculum canalis facialis. **g. of facial nerve**, properly genu nervi facialis (*internal g.*), but also applied to geniculum nervi facialis (*external g.*). **g. of facial nerve, external**, geniculum nervi facialis. **g. of facial nerve, internal**, g. nervi facialis. **g. impres′sum**, a flattening and bending of the knee joint to one side, with consequent displacement of the patella up and to the same side. **g. of internal capsule**, g. capsulae internae. **g. [inter′num] ra′dicis ner′vi facia′lis**, g. nervi facialis. **g. intror′sum**, g. valgum. **g. ner′vi facia′lis** [NA], genu of facial nerve: the bend in the fibers arising from the nucleus of the facial nerve, which produces the facial colliculus in the floor of the fourth ventricle; it is at this point that the fibers loop around the abducent nucleus. **g. recurva′tum**, hyperextension of the knee; called also *back knee*. **g. val′gum**, a deformity in which the knees are abnormally close together and the space between the ankles is increased; known also as *knock knee*. **g. va′rum**, a deformity in which the knees are abnormally separated and the lower extremities are bowed inwardly; the deformity may be in the thigh or leg, or both. Known also as *bowleg*.

genua (jen′u-ah) [L.] plural of *genu*.

genual (jen′u-al) relating to or resembling a genu.

genucubital (jen″u-ku′bĭ-tal) [L. *genu* knee + *cubitus* elbow] pertaining to the knees and elbows; see under *position*.

genufacial (jen″u-fa′shal) [L. *genu* knee + *facies* face] pertaining to the knees and face; see under *position*.

genupectoral (jen″u-pek′tor-al) [L. *genu* knee + *pectus* breast] pertaining to the knees and chest; see under *position*.

genus (je′nus), pl. *gen′era* [L.] a taxonomic category subordinate to a tribe (or subtribe) and superior to a species (or subgenus).

geny- (jen′e) [Gr. *genys* jaw] a combining form denoting relationship to the jaw.

geo- (je′o) [Gr. *gē* earth] a combining form denoting relationship to the earth, or to soil.

geobiology (je″o-bi-ol′o-je) [*geo-* + *biology*] the biology of terrestrial life.

geochemistry (je″o-kem′is-tre) [*geo-* + *chemistry*] the science concerned with study of the elements in the earth's crust and the chemical changes that occur therein.

Geocyclus (je″o-si′klus) a genus of schizomycetes with flagella-like filaments.

geode (je′ōd) [Gr. *geōdes* earthlike: so called from a fancied resemblance to a mineral geode] a dilated lymph space.

geogen (je′o-jen) an aspect of the geography or geochemistry of an area that affects organisms in it, particularly with reference to disease.

geomedicine (je″o-med′ĭ-sin) [*geo-* + *medicine*] that branch of medicine that has to do with the influence of climatic and environmental conditions on health.

geopathology (je″o-pah-thol′o-je) [*geo-* + *pathology*] the study of the peculiarities of disease in relation to topography, climate, food habits, etc., of various regions of the earth.

Geopen (je′o-pen) trademark for a preparation of carbenicillin disodium.

geophagia (je-o-fa′je-ah) [*geo-* + Gr. *phagein* to eat] the habit of eating clay or earth.

geophagism (je-of′ah-jizm) geophagia.

geophagist (je-of′ah-jist) one who eats earth habitually.

geophagy (je-of′ah-je) geophagia.

Georgi's test (ga-or′gēz) [Walter *Georgi*, German bacteriologist, 1889–1920] Sachs-Georgi test; see under *tests*.

geotaxis (je″o-tak′sis) [*geo-* + Gr. *taxis* arrangement] geotropism.

geotragia (je″o-tra′je-ah) [*geo-* + Gr. *trōgein* to chew] geophagia.

geotrichosis (je″o-tri-ko′sis) infection by *Geotrichum candidum*, which may attack the bronchi, lungs, mouth, or intestinal tract; its manifestations resemble those of candidiasis.

Geotrichum (je-ot′rĭ-kum) a genus of yeastlike imperfect fungi of the family Cryptococcaceae, order Moniliales. *G. candidum*, found in the feces and in dairy products, is the etiologic agent of geotrichosis.

geotropic (je″o-trop′ik) influenced in growth by gravity.

geotropism (je-ot′ro-pizm) [*geo-* + Gr. *tropos* a turning] a tendency of growth or movement toward or away from the earth; the influence of gravity on growth. A tendency to grow toward the earth is *positive g.*; to grow away from the earth, *negative g.*

Geraghty's test (ger′ah-tēz) [John Timothy *Geraghty*, American physician, 1876–1924] the phenolsulfonphthalein test.

geraniol (jĕ-ra′ne-ol) 1. a 10-carbon branched-chain alcohol, 2,6-dimethyl-2,6-octadien-8-ol, occurring widely in essential oils of plants. 2. a pheromone of certain species of bees, being secreted by worker bees to signal the location of food.

geratic (jĕ-rat′ik) [Gr. *gēras* old age] pertaining to old age.

geratology (jer″ah-tol′o-je) gereology.

gerbil (jer′bil) a small burrowing rodent of the genus *Gerbillus*, which is native to the more arid parts of Africa and southwestern Asia, and is capable of serving as an agent for the transmission of plague.

Gerdy's fibers, etc. (zher-dēz′) [Pierre Nicholas *Gerdy*, French physician, 1797–1856] see under *fiber, fontanelle, fossa, loop,* and *ligament*.

gereology (jer″e-ol′o-je) [Gr. *gēras* old age + *-logy*] the science which deals with old age and its phenomena.

Gerhardt's disease, sign (phenomenon), test (reaction) (ger′harts) [Carl Adolf Christian Jacob *Gerhardt*, German physician, 1833–1902] see *erythromelalgia*, and see under *sign* and *tests*.

Gerhardt's test (zher-harts′) [Charles Frédéric *Gerhardt*, French chemist, 1816–1856] see under *tests*.

Gerhardt-Semon law [Carl Adolf Christian Jacob *Gerhardt;* Sir Felix *Semon*, German laryngologist in London, 1849–1921] see under *law*.

geriatric (jer″e-at′rik) pertaining to the treatment of the aged.

geriatrician (jer″e-ah-trish′an) a specialist in geriatrics.

geriatrics (jer″e-at′riks) [Gr. *gēras* old age + *iatrikē* surgery, medicine] that branch of medicine which treats all problems peculiar to old age and the aging, including the clinical problems of senescence and senility. **dental g.,** gerodontics.

geriodontics (jer″e-o-don′tiks) gerodontics.

geriodontist (jer″e-o-don′tist) gerodontist.

geriopsychosis (jer″e-o-si-ko′sis) [Gr. *gēras* old age + *psychosis*] any one of the presenile and senile groups of mental diseases (Southard).

Gerlach's network, valve (ger′laks) [Joseph von *Gerlach*, German anatomist, 1820–1896] see under *network*, and see *valvula processus vermiformis*.

Gerlier's disease (zher-le-āz′) [Felix *Gerlier*, French physician, 1840–1914] see under *disease*.

germ (jerm) [L. *germen*] 1. a pathogenic microorganism. 2. living substance capable of developing into an organ, part, or organism as a whole; a primordium. **dental g.,** the collective tissues from which an entire tooth is formed, including the dental sac, dental organ, and dental papilla. **enamel g.,** the epithelial rudiment of the enamel organ. **hair g.,** see *hair matrix*, under *matrix*. **tooth g.,** a budlike thickening in the connective tissue of the jaw that is a primordium of a tooth. **wheat**

g., the embryo of wheat, which contains tocopherol, thiamine, riboflavin, and other vitamins.

germanin (jer′mah-nin) suramin sodium.

germanium (jer-ma′ne-um) a rare element, having the appearance of a bluish gray metalloid, atomic number 32, atomic weight 72.59; symbol, Ge.

germerine (jer′mer-ēn) a crystalline alkaloid, $C_{36}H_{57}O_{11}N$, from *Veratrum senecio*.

germicidal (jer″mĭ-si′dal) [L. *germen* germ + *caedere* to kill] lethal to pathogenic microorganisms.

germicide (jer′mĭ-sīd) an agent that kills pathogenic microorganisms.

germinal (jer′mĭ-nal) [L. *germinalis*] pertaining to or of the nature of a germ cell or the primitive stage of development.

germination (jer″mĭ-na′shun) [L. *germinatio*] the sprouting of a seed or spore or of a plant embryo.

germinative (jer′mĭ-na″tiv) [L. *germinativus*] pertaining to or causing germination.

germinoma (jer″mĭ-no′mah) a neoplasm of germ tissue (testis or ovum), e.g., a seminoma.

germitrine (jer′mĭ-trēn) an antihypertensive alkaloid isolated from green hellebore (*Veratrum viride* Ait. [Liliaceae]).

germogen (jer′mo-jen) [*germ* + Gr. *gennan* to produce] a mass of protoplasm from which reproductive cells arise.

gero-, geronto- (jer′o, jer-on′to) [Gr. *gēras* old age; *gerōn, gerontos* old man] combining form denoting relationship to old age or to the aged.

gerocomia (jer″o-ko′me-ah) [*gero-* + Gr. *komein* to care for] the care of old men; the hygiene of old age.

gerocomy (jer′o-ko″me) gerocomia.

geroderma, gerodermia (jer-o-der′mah, jer-o-der′me-ah) [*gero-* + Gr. *derma* skin] dystrophy of the skin and genitals, producing the appearance of old age (Rummo and Ferrannini, 1897). **g. osteodysplas′tica,** a condition believed to be transmitted as an X-linked recessive trait, with occasional manifestation in females, in which geroderma is associated with osseous changes, including osteoporosis and lines in the bones somewhat resembling growth rings of a tree.

gerodontia (jer-o-don′she-ah) gerodontics.

gerodontic (jer″o-don′tik) [*gero-* + Gr. *odous* tooth] 1. pertaining to changes in the dental tissues with age. 2. pertaining to the practice of gerodontics.

gerodontics (jer″o-don′tiks) the treatment of dental problems of aging persons, or those peculiar to advanced age.

gerodontist (jer″o-don′tist) a dentist who practices gerodontics.

gerodontology (jer″o-don-tol′o-je) the study of the dentition and dental problems in the aged or aging.

gerokomy (jer-o′ko-me) gerocomia.

geromarasmus (jer″o-mah-raz′mus) [*gero-* + Gr. *marasmos* a wasting] the emaciation sometimes characteristic of old age.

geromorphism (jer″o-mor′fizm) [*gero-* + Gr. *morphē* form] premature senility. **cutaneous g.,** a condition in which the skin shows at a very early age the characteristics of old age.

gerontal (jer-on′tal) pertaining to an old man or old age; senile.

gerontin (jer-on′tin) a base from the nuclei of the cells of a dog's liver, identical with spermin.

geronto- see *gero-.*

gerontologist (jer″on-tol′o-jist) a specialist in gerontology.

gerontology (jer″on-tol′o-je) [*geronto-* + *-logy*] the scientific study of the problems of aging in all their aspects—clinical, biological, historical, and sociological.

gerontophile (jer-on′to-fīl) a person who manifests gerontophilia.

gerontophilia (jer″on-to-fil′e-ah) [*geronto-* + Gr. *philein* to love] special fondness for old people.

gerontopia (jer″on-to′pe-ah) [*geronto-* + Gr. *opsis* vision] senopia.

gerontotherapeutics (jer-on″to-ther″ah-pu′-tiks) [*geronto-* + *therapeutics*] therapeutic management of aging persons designed to retard and prevent the development of many of the aspects of senescence.

gerontotherapy (jer-on″to-ther′ah-pe) gerontotherapeutics.

gerontotoxon, gerontoxon (jer-on″to-tok′son, jer-on-tok′son) [*geronto-* + Gr. *toxon* bow] the arcus senilis. **g. len′tis,** equatorial couching of the lens in the aged; no longer done.

geropsychiatry (jer″o-si-ki′ah-tre) a subspecialty of psychiatry dealing with mental illness in the elderly.

Gerota's capsule, method (ga-ro′tahz) [Dimitru *Gerota*, anatomist in Bucharest, 1867–1939] see under *capsule* and *method.*

Gerovital H3 (jer″o-vi′tal) trademark for a preparation of 2 per cent procaine hydrochloride solution with small amounts of benzoic acid, potassium metabisulfite, and disodium phosphate; it is purported to increase longevity, retard the aging process, rejuvenate the senile, and prevent or relieve various disorders, such as arthritis, arteriosclerosis, angina pectoris, etc.

Gerson-Herrmannsdorfer diet (gār′son-Har′mans-dor-fer) [Max *Gerson*; Adolph *Herrmannsdorfer*, German surgeon, born 1889] Gerson diet.

Gerstmann's syndrome (garst′manz) [Josef *Gerstmann*, Vienna neurologist, born 1887] see under *syndrome.*

gerüstmark (gĕ-rist′mark) [Ger. *Gerüst* scaffolding + *Mark* marrow] a unique, collagen-poor zone of connective tissue lying across the bone marrow adjoining the growing ends of bones; observed in scurvy.

gesarol (ges′ah-rol) chlorophenothane.

gestaclone (jes′tah-klōn) chemical name: 17β-acetyl-6-chloro-1β,1a,2β,8β,9α,10,11,12,13,14α,15,16,β-17-tetradecahydro-10β,13β-dimethyl-3*H*-dicyclopropa[1,2:16,17]cyclopenta[*a*]-phenanthren-3-one; a progestin, $C_{23}H_{27}ClO_2$.

gestagen (jes′tah-jen) any hormone with progestational activity, progesterone being the most important.

gestalt (ges-tawlt′) a whole perceptual configuration; see *gestaltism.*

gestaltism (gĕ-stawl′tizm, gĕ-shtawl′tizm) [Ger. *Gestalt* form] that theory in psychology which claims that the objects of mind, as immediately presented to direct experience, come as complete unanalyzable wholes or forms (Gestalten) which cannot be split up into parts; called also *gestalt theory.*

gestation (jes-ta′shun) [L. *gestatio*, from *gestare* to bear] the period of development of the young in viviparous animals, from the time of fertilization of the ovum until birth; see also *pregnancy.* **exterior g.,** the development of an infant after emergence from the uterus, until the time of quadrupedal locomotion, or about the age of nine months, during the period when it is in need of maternal care and might still be regarded by some as a fetus. **interior g.,** development of a fetus before birth; a term used only in contradistinction to external gestation.

gestodene (jes′to-dēn) chemical name: 13-ethyl-17α-hydroxy-18,19-dinorpregna-4,15-diene-20-yn-3-one; a progestin, $C_{21}H_{26}O_2$.

gestonorone caproate (jes-to′nor-ōn) chemical name: 17-[(1-oxohexyl)oxy]-19-norpregn-4-ene,3,20,dione hexanoate; a progestin, $C_{26}H_{38}O_4$, which has been used in the treatment of endometrial carcinoma and benign prostatic hypertrophy.

gestosis (jes-to′sis), pl. *gesto′ses* [L. *gestare* to bear] any toxemic manifestation of pregnancy.

gestrinone (jes′trĭ-nōn) chemical name: 13-ethyl-17-hydroxy-18,19-dinor-17α-pregna-4,9-11-trien-20-yn-3-one; a progestin, $C_{21}H_{24}O_2$.

G.F.R. glomerular filtration rate.

G.G.G. abbreviation for L. *gum′mi gut′tae gam′biae;* see *gamboge.*

GH growth hormone.

Ghilarducci's reaction (ge″lar-doot′shēz) [Francesco *Ghilarducci*, Italian physician, 1857–1924] see under *reaction.*

Ghon's complex, focus (primary lesion, tubercle) (gahn) [Anton *Ghon*, Prague pathologist, 1866–1936] see *primary complex,* under *complex,* and see under *focus.*

Ghon-Sachs bacillus [Anton *Ghon;* Anton *Sachs*] *Clostridium septicum.*

ghost (gōst) a faint or shadowy figure, lacking the customary substance of reality. **blood g.,** phantom corpuscle.

GH-RH growth hormone releasing hormone.

G.I. gastrointestinal; globin insulin.

Giacomini's band (jah-ko-me′nēz) [Carlo *Giacomini*, Italian anatomist, 1841–1898] see under *band.*

Giannuzzi's crescents, (bodies, cells, demilunes) (jah-noot′zēz) [Guiseppe *Giannuzzi*, Italian anatomist, 1839–1876] see under *crescent.*

giant (ji′ant) [Gr. *gigas*] a person or organism of very great size; see *gigantism.*

giantism (ji′ant-izm) 1. gigantism. 2. excessive size, as of cells or nuclei.

Giardia (je-ar′de-ah) [Alfred *Giard*, biologist in Paris, 1846–1908] a genus of flagellate protozoa of the order Polymastigida, class zoomastigophoea, found in the intestinal tract of man and of animals. **G. intestina′lis,** *G. lamblia.* **G. lamb′lia,** the species causing giardiasis in man; it is a symmetrical, pear-shaped organism with four pairs of flagella and a sucking disk by which it attaches to the mucosa of the duodenum and upper jejunum. Called also *G. intestinalis* and *Lamblia intestinalis.*

giardiasis (ji″ar-di′ah-sis) infection with *Giardia lamblia,* characterized by protracted, intermittent diarrhea with symptoms suggesting malabsorption, and by abdominal pain, distention, and flatulence; light infections are usually asymptomatic.

gibberellin (gib-ber-el′in) any of a class of phytohormones whose most striking activity is the promotion of lateral bud development in decapitated plant stems; first isolated from fungi of the genus *Gibberella.*

Gibbon's hernia (hydrocele) (gib′onz) [Q. V. *Gibbon,* American surgeon, 1813–1894] see under *hernia.*

Gibbon-Landis test (gib′on-lan′dis) [John Heysham *Gibbon,* Jr.,

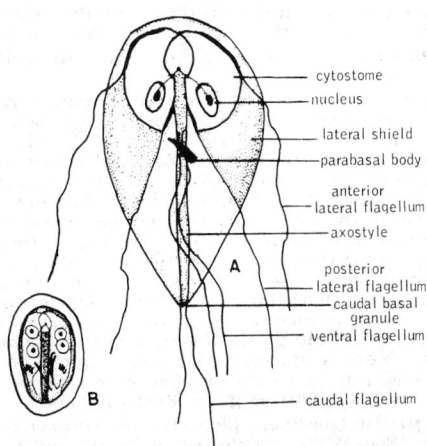

Giardia lamblia: A, trophozoite; *B*, cyst. (Cheng.)

American physician, born 1903; Eugene Markley *Landis*, American physician, born 1901]   see under *tests*.

gibbosity (gĭ-bos'ĭ-te) [L. *gibbosus* crooked]   the condition of being humped; kyphosis.

gibbous (gib'us) [L. *gibbosus*]   convex; humped; protuberant; humpbacked.

Gibbs' theorem (gibz) [Josiah Willard *Gibbs*, American physicist, 1839–1903]   see under *theorem*.

Gibbs-Donnan equilibrium (gibz-don'an) [J. W. *Gibbs;* Frederick George *Donnan*, English chemist, 1870–1956]   see under *equilibrium*.

gibbus (gib'us) [L.]   a hump.

Gibert's disease (zhe-bārz') [Camille Melchior *Gibert*, French dermatologist, 1797–1866]   pityriasis rosea.

Gibney's bandage (strapping), perispondylitis (disease) (gib'nēz) [Virgil Pendleton *Gibney*, New York surgeon, 1847–1927]   see under *bandage* and *perispondylitis*.

Gibson's murmur, rule (gib'sunz) [George Alexander *Gibson*, Edinburgh physician, 1854–1913]   see under *murmur* and *rule*.

gid (gid)   a functional and organic disease of the brain and spinal cord of domestic animals, especially a disease of sheep caused by the presence of *Coenurus cerebralis* (the larva of the dog tapeworm, *Multiceps multiceps*), and marked by unsteadiness of gait. Called also *coenurosis, staggers*, and *sturdy*.

giddiness (gid'e-nes)   dizziness.

Giemsa stain (gēm'sah) [Gustav *Giemsa*, chemist and bacteriologist in Hamburg, 1867–1948]   see *Table of Stains and Staining Methods*.

Gierke's corpuscles (gēr'kez) [Hans Paul Bernhard *Gierke*, German anatomist, 1847–1886]   see under *corpuscle*.

Gierke's disease (gēr'kez) [Edgar Otto Konrad von *Gierke*, German pathologist, 1877–1945]   glycogen storage disease, type I; see under *disease*.

Gieson (ge'son)   see *van Gieson*.

Gifford's operation, reflex, sign (gif'ordz) [Harold *Gifford*, American oculist, 1858–1929]   see under *operation, reflex,* and *sign*.

giga- (jig''ah, ji'gah) [Gr. *gigas* mighty]   a combining form designating gigantic size; used in naming units of measurement to indicate a quantity one billion (10^9) times the unit designated by the root with which it is combined.

gigantism (ji-gan'tizm; ji'gan-tizm) [Gr. *gigas* giant]   abnormal overgrowth; excessive size and stature.   **acromegalic g.,** pituitary gigantism in which the body also has the changes in the short and flat bones characteristic of acromegaly.   **cerebral g.,** gigantism in the absence of increased levels of growth hormone, attributed to a cerebral defect; infants are large, and accelerated growth continues for the first four or five years, the rate being normal thereafter. The hands and feet are large, the head large and dolicocephalic, the eyes have an antimongoloid slant, with hypertelorism. The child is clumsy, and mental retardation of varying degree is usually present. Called also *Sotos' syndrome*.   **eunuchoid g.,** gigantism in which the body shows the proportion of a eunuch and sexual deficiency.   **fetal g.,** excessive size of the fetus or newborn, as in cerebral gigantism and infants of diabetic mothers.   **hyperpituitary g.,** Launois' syndrome.   **normal g.,** gigantism in which the body proportions and sexual development are normal.   **pituitary g.,** Launois' syndrome.

giganto- (ji-gan'to) [Gr. *gigas, gigantos* huge]   a combining form meaning huge.

gigantomastia (ji-gan''to-mas'te-ah)   extreme hypertrophy of the breast.

gigantosoma (ji-gan''to-so'mah) [*giganto-* + Gr. *sōma* body]   gigantism, or great size and stature.

Gigli's operation, wire saw (jēl'yēz) [Leonardo *Gigli*, gynecologist in Florence, 1866–1908]   see under *operation* and *saw*.

gikiyami (ge''ke-yam'e)   nanukayami.

gilbert (gil'bert) [W. *Gilbert*, English physicist, 1544–1603]   the unit of magnetomotive force; symbol, *F*.

Gilbert's disease (cholemia, syndrome), sign (zhēl-bārz') [Nicolas Augustin *Gilbert*, French physician, 1858–1927]   see under *disease* and *sign*.

Gilchrist's disease, mycosis (gil'krists) [Thomas Caspar *Gilchrist*, American dermatologist, 1862–1927]   North American blastomycosis.

gildable (gil'dah-b'l)   susceptible of being colored with gold stains.

gill (gil)   1. the respiratory organ of aquatic animals, such as fish, mollusks, and many arthropods, usually a thin-walled projection from the body surface or from some part of the digestive tract whose surface is increased by filaments, lamellae, or other folds. 2. one of the thin perpendicular plates found on the underside of a mushroom cap and along which the basidia are produced.

Gill's operation (gilz) [Arthur Bruce *Gill*, American orthopedic surgeon, 1876–1965]   see under *operation*.

Gillenia (jil-le'ne-ah) [L.; after Arnold *Gill*]   a genus of rosaceous plants; the root of *G. trifoliata* and *G. stipulacea*, of North America, is mildly emetic and aperient.

Gilles de la Tourette's syndrome (disease) [Georges *Gilles de la Tourette*, French physician, 1857–1904]   see under *syndrome*.

Gillespie's operation (gil-les'pēz) [James Donaldson *Gillespie*, Scottish physician, 1823–1891]   see under *operation*.

Gilliam's operation (gil'ĭ-amz) [David Tod *Gilliam*, Columbus gynecologist, 1844–1923]   see under *operation*.

Gillies' flap (graft), operation (gil'ēz) [Sir Harold Delf *Gillies*, British plastic surgeon, 1882–1960]   see *rope flap*, under *flap*, and see under *operation*.

Gilmer's splint (gil'merz) [Thomas Lewis *Gilmer*, American oral surgeon, 1849–1931]   see under *splint*.

Gimbernat's ligament, reflex ligament (him-ber-nats') [Antonio de *Gimbernat*, Spanish surgeon and anatomist, 1734–1816]   see *ligamenta lacunare* and *ligamentum inguinale reflexum*.

ginger (jin'jer) [L. *zingiber;* Gr. *zingiberis*]   the dried rhizome of the tropical plant *Zingiber officinale*, used as a flavoring agent. It has been used in the treatment of flatulence and colic, and is used in veterinary medicine as a stimulant and carminative in atonic indigestion of horses and cattle, and in the treatment of spasmodic colic in horses.

gingiva (jin-ji'vah, jin'jĭ-vah) [L. "gum of the mouth"]   see *gingivae*.   **alveolar g.,** that portion of the gingivae which covers the alveolar process.   **areolar g.,** that portion of the gingivae which overlies the alveolar process, being bound to it by loose areolar connective tissue.   **attached g.,** the portion of the gingiva that is firm, dense, stippled, and tightly bound down to the underlying periosteum, tooth, and bone.   **buccal g.,** that portion of the gingivae which is applied to the buccal surfaces of the posterior teeth.   **cemented g.** (*obs.*), epithelial attachment of Gottlieb.   **free g.,** the portion of the gingivae that surrounds the tooth and is not directly attached to the tooth surface; called also *free gum margin*.   **interdental g.,** the soft supporting tissue that normally fills the space between two contacting teeth.   **labial g.,** that portion of the gingivae which is applied to the labial surfaces of the anterior teeth.   **lingual g.,** that portion of the gingivae which is applied to the lingual surfaces of the teeth.   **marginal g.,** the portion of the free gingiva localized at the labial, buccal, lingual, and palatal aspects of the teeth; gingival margin.   **septal g.,** that portion of the gingivae which occupies the interproximal spaces; sometimes called *gingival papillae*.

gingivae (jin-ji've, jin'jĭ-ve) [L., plural of *gingiva*] [NA]   the gums: the mucous membrane, with the supporting fibrous tissue, which overlies the crowns of unerupted teeth and encircles the necks of those that have erupted. See also under *gingiva*.

gingival (jin'jĭ-val, jin-ji'val)   pertaining to the gingivae.

gingivalgia (jin''jĭ-val'je-ah) [*gingiva* + *-algia*]   pain in the gingivae.

gingivally (jin'jĭ-val''le)   toward the gingivae.

gingivectomy (jin''jĭ-vek'to-me) [*gingiva* + Gr. *ektomē* excision]   surgical excision of all loose infected and diseased gingival tissue to eradicate periodontal infection and reduce the depth of the gingival sulcus.

gingivitis (jin''-jĭ-vi'tis) [*gingiva* + *-itis*]   inflammation involving the gingival tissue only.   **atrophic g., senile,** a condition characterized by hyperkeratinization and areas of desquamation in the gingiva.   **bismuth g.,** inflammation of the gingivae caused by local deposit of bismuth from the blood stream, after its administration for systemic disease.   **catarrhal g.,** a transitory inflammation of the gingival and/or oral mucous membranes accompanied by erythema, swelling, and occasional epithelial desquamation; usually a result of the change in the oral bacterial flora. "**cotton-roll**" **g.**, secondary infection of denuded areas of gingivae caused by adherence of epithelium to cotton rolls placed in the mouth during dental procedures. **desquamative g.**, a chronic inflammatory condition characterized by tendency of the surface epithelium of the gingivae to desquamate. **eruptive g.**, gingivitis accompanying eruption of the teeth. **fusospirochetal g.**, necrotizing ulcerative g. **g. gravida'-rum**, pregnancy g. **hemorrhagic g.**, gingivitis characterized by profuse bleeding, especially that associated with ascorbic acid deficiency. **herpetic g.**, infection of gingivae by the herpes simplex virus. **hormonal g.**, gingivitis associated with gingival enlargement, in which modification of the sex hormones, as during pregnancy and puberty, or other endocrine dysfunction, such as diabetes mellitus, may be a primary or a complicating factor. **hyperplastic g.**, gingivitis characterized by proliferation of the various tissue elements, epithelium, and connective tissue; it may be accompanied by dense infiltration of inflammatory cells. **marginal g.**, inflammation of the gingivae limited to the marginal gingiva. **marginal g., simple**, hyperemia of the gingivae with edema of the margins and gingival papillae, resulting from slight trauma or neglected dental hygiene. **marginal g., suppurative, g. margina'lis suppurati'va**, inflammation of the gingival margins, with formation of a purulent discharge. **necrotizing ulcerative g.**, trench mouth; an acute or chronic gingival infection characterized by redness and swelling, by necrosis extending from the interdental papillae along the gingival margins, and by pain, hemorrhage, a necrotic odor, and often a pseudomembrane. Called also *fusospirochetal g.* or *angina, Plaut's ulcer, Vincent's g.* or *infection, fusospirillosis, trench throat,* and *ulceromembranous g.* or *angina.* When the condition extends to other parts of the oral mucosa, with lesions involving the palate or pharynx, it is called *necrotizing ulcerative gingivostomatitis, Vincent's angina* or *stomatitis, Plaut's angina,* and *pseudomembranous angina.* **phagedenic g.**, rapidly progressive ulcerative inflammation of the gums. **pregnancy g.**, any of various gingival changes during pregnancy, ranging from gingivitis to the so-called pregnancy tumor; called also *g. gravidarum.* **scorbutic g.**, gingivitis associated with vitamin C deficiency. **streptococcal g.**, inflammation of the gingival margins caused by streptococcal infection. **ulceromembranous g.**, necrotizing ulcerative g. **Vincent's g.**, necrotizing ulcerative g.

gingivo- (jin'jĭ-vo) [L. *gingiva* gum] a combining form denoting relationship to the gingivae.

gingivoaxial (jin''jĭ-vo-ak''se-al) pertaining to or formed by the gingival and axial walls of a tooth cavity.

gingivobuccoaxial (jin''jĭ-vo-buk''ko-ak''se-al) pertaining to or formed by the gingival, buccal, and axial walls of a tooth cavity.

gingivoectomy (jin''jĭ-vo-ek''to-me) gingivectomy.

gingivoglossitis (jin''jĭ-vo-glos-si'tis) [*gingiva* + Gr. *glōssa* tongue + *-itis*] inflammation of gingivae and tongue.

gingivolabial (jin''jĭ-vo-la'be-al) pertaining to the gingivae and lips.

gingivolinguoaxial (jin''jĭ-vo-ling''gwo-ak''se-al) pertaining to or formed by the gingival, lingual, and axial walls of a tooth cavity.

gingivoplasty (jin'jĭ-vo-plas''te) [*gingivo-* + Gr. *plassein* to form] surgical modeling of the gingival margin and papillae to obtain a normal gingival contour.

gingivosis (jin''jĭ-vo'sis) [*gingivo-* + *-(o)sis*] a chronic diffuse inflammation of the gingivae, with desquamation of the papillary epithelium and mucous membrane.

gingivostomatitis (jin''jĭ-vo-sto''mah-ti'tis) inflammation involving both the gingivae and the oral mucosa. **herpetic g.**, an infection of the oral mucosa (including the gingivae) by the herpes simplex virus, characterized by redness of oral tissues, formation of multiple vesicles and painful ulcers, and fever. **necrotizing ulcerative g.**, that caused by extension to the oral mucosa of necrotizing ulcerative gingivitis, characterized by ulceration, pseudomembrane, and odor, with lesions involving the palate or pharynx as well as the oral mucosa.

ginglyform (jin'glĭ-form) ginglymoid.

ginglymoarthrodial (jin''glĭ-mo-ar-thro'de-al) partly ginglymoid and partly arthrodial.

ginglymoid (jin'glĭ-moid) [*ginglymus* + Gr. *eidos* form] resembling a ginglymus.

ginglymus (jin'glĭ-mus) [L.; Gr. *ginglymos* hinge] [NA] a type of synovial joint that allows movement in but one plane, forward and backward, as the hinge of a door; called also *ginglymoid* or *hinge joint.*

ginseng (jin'seng) [Chinese *jin-tsan* life of man] 1. any herb of the genus *Panax*, especially *P. schinseng* (Chinese ginseng) and *P. quinquefolius* (American ginseng), whose roots are used by the Chinese as a tonic, stimulant, and aphrodisiac. 2. the root of Chinese or American ginseng.

Giordano's sphincter (jor-dan'ōz) [Davide *Giordano*, Italian surgeon, born 1864] musculus sphincter ductus choledochi.

Giraldés' organ (he-ral'dās) [Joachim Albin Cardozo Cazado *Giraldés*, Portuguese surgeon in Paris, 1808–1875] paradidymis.

Girard's treatment (method) (jir-ardz') [Brig. Gen. Alfred C. *Girard*, Swiss surgeon, 1850–1916] see under *treatment.*

Girardinus (jĭ-rar'dĭ-nus) *Poecilia.* **G. poeciloi'des,** *Poecilia reticulata.*

girdle (ger'd'l) an encircling structure, or part; anything that encircles a body. Called also *cingulum* [NA]. Cf. *belt.* **Hitzig's g.**, an encircling zone of analgesia at the level of the breasts, in the area supplied by the third and sixth dorsal nerves, seen in the early stages of tabes dorsalis. **g. of inferior extremity**, pelvic g. (cingulum membri inferioris [NA]). **limbus g.**, a corneal degeneration in the form of an opaque line concentric with the limbus; called also *white limbal g. of Vogt.* **pectoral g.**, shoulder g. **pelvic g.**, the encircling bony structure supporting the lower limbs; see *cingulum membri inferioris* [NA]. **shoulder g.**, the encircling bony structure supporting the upper limbs; see *cingulum membri superioris* [NA]. **g. of superior extremity, thoracic g.**, shoulder g. (cingulum membri superioris [NA]). **Venus' g.**, mercurial plaster spread on leather or linen, once used in the treatment of syphilis; called also *balteum venereum.* **white limbal g. of Vogt,** limbus g.

Girdner's probe (gerd'nerz) [John Harvey *Girdner*, physician in New York, 1856–1933] an electric probe; see under *probe.*

gitaligenin (jĭ-tal'ĭ-jen''in) the aglycone of gitalin.

Gitaligin (jĭ-tal'ĭ-jin) trademark for a preparation of gitalin (def. 2).

gitalin (jit'ah-lin) 1. a crystalline cardiac glycoside, $C_{35}H_{56}O_{12}$, from the leaves of *Digitalis purpurea.* 2. a mixture of the digitalis glycosides gitoxin, gitaloxin, and digitoxin, having the same actions as digitalis and used like digitalis in the treatment of congestive heart failure and other cardiac disorders; administered orally. Called also *amorphous g.*

gitaloxin (jit''ah-loks'in) a cardiac glycoside from *Digitalis purpurea.*

githagism (gith'ah-jizm) poisoning by the seeds of *Agrostemma githago,* or corn cockle.

gitogenin (jit-oj'ĕ-nin) a sapogenin, $C_{27}H_{44}O_4$, from gitonin.

gitonin (jit'o-nin) a neutral saponin, $C_{50}H_{82}O_{23}$, from digitalis seed.

gitoxigenin (jĭ-tok'sĭ-jen-in) an aglycone of gitoxin, $C_{23}H_{35}O_5$.

gitoxin (jĭ-tok'sin) a cardiac glycoside, $C_{41}H_{64}O_{14}$, principally from *Digitalis purpurea* but also a constituent of *D. lanata.*

Gitterfasern (git'er-fas''ern) [Ger.] the reticular lattice fibers of the corium.

Giuffrida-Ruggieri stigma (joof-re''dah-roo''je-er'e) [Vincenzo *Giuffrida-Ruggieri*, Italian anthropologist, 1872–1922] see under *stigma.*

Givens' method (giv'enz) [Maurice Hope *Givens*, American biochemist, born 1888] see under *method.*

GIX an insecticidal compound, DFDT.

gizzard (giz'ard) the strong muscular stomach of a bird.

GL abbreviation for *greatest length*, an axis of measurement or dimension used for small flexed embryos.

Gl chemical symbol for *glucinium* (beryllium).

gl. abbreviation for L. *glan'dula* and *glan'dulae* (gland, glands).

GL 54 athomin.

glabella (glah-bel'ah) [L. *glaber* smooth] 1. the smooth area on the frontal bone between the superciliary arches. 2. the most prominent point in the midsagittal plane between the eyebrows; used as an anthropometric landmark.

glabellad (glah-bel'ad) toward the glabella.

glabellum (glah-bel'um) glabella.

glabrificin (glah-brif'ĭ-sin) [L. *glaber* smooth + *facere* to make] (*obs.*) an antibody; so called because of its property of rendering bacteria smooth or glabrous.

glabrous (gla'brus) [L. *glaber* smooth] smooth and bare.

glacial (gla'shal) [L. *glacialis*] resembling ice; vitreous; solid.

gladiate (gla'de-āt) [L. *gladius* sword] sword-shaped.

gladiolus (glah-di'o-lus) [L., dim. of *gladius* sword] corpus sterni.

gladiomanubrial (glad''e-o-mah-nu'bre-al) pertaining to gladiolus (corpus sterni) and manubrium.

glairin (glār'in) [L. *clarus* clear] (*obs.*) a gelatinous substance of bacterial origin found in the water of certain sulfur springs; called also *baregin.*

glairy (glār'e) resembling the white of an egg.

gland (gland) [L. *glans* acorn] an aggregation of cells, specialized to secrete or excrete materials not related to their ordinary metabolic needs; called also *glandula* [NA]. **absorbent g.**, lymph node. **accessory g.**, a minor mass of glandular tissue situated near or at some distance from a gland of similar structure. **acid g's**, glandulae gastricae [propriae]. **acinar g.**, acinous g. **acinotubular g.**, tubuloacinar g. **acinous g.**, a gland made up of one or more acini. **admaxillary g.**, glandula parotis accessoria. **adrenal g.**, a flattened body situated in the retroperitoneal tissues at the cranial pole of either kidney. In man, the adrenal gland is the result of fusion of two organs, recognizable

Plate XIX

gland

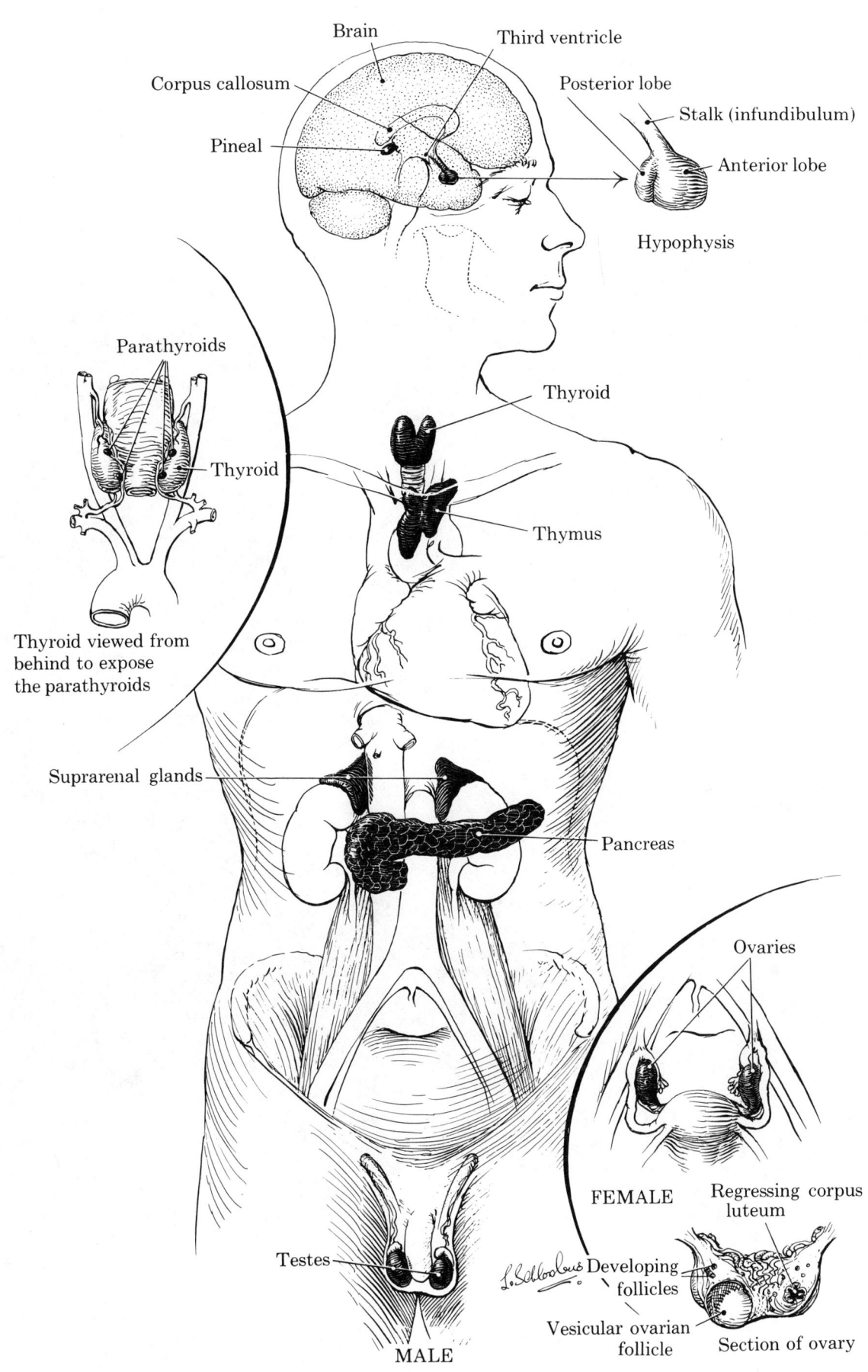

Brain

Third ventricle

Corpus callosum

Posterior lobe

Stalk (infundibulum)

Pineal

Anterior lobe

Hypophysis

Parathyroids

Thyroid

Thyroid

Thymus

Thyroid viewed from
behind to expose
the parathyroids

Suprarenal glands

Pancreas

Ovaries

FEMALE

Regressing corpus
luteum

Testes

Developing
follicles

Vesicular ovarian
follicle

Section of ovary

MALE

THE ENDOCRINE GLANDS

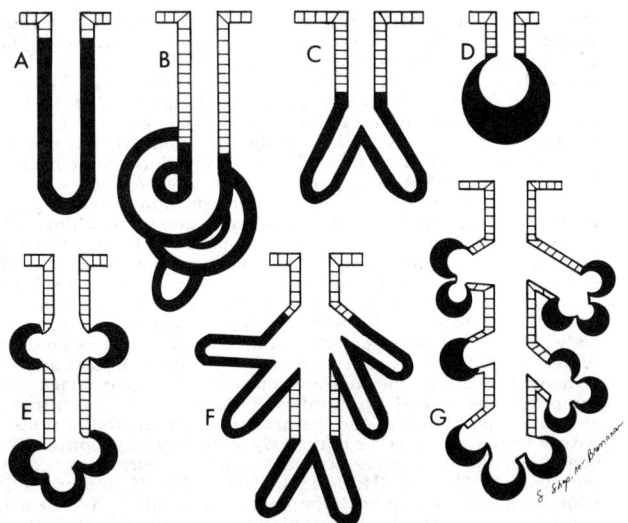

Schematic diagram of various forms of glands: *A*, simple tubular; *B*, simple coiled tubular; *C*, simple branched tubular; *D*, simple alveolar; *E*, simple branched alveolar; *F*, compound tubular; *G*, compound alveolar.

as cortex and medulla. The adrenal cortex, under control of the pituitary hormone corticotropin, elaborates steroid hormones—glucocorticoids, 17-ketosteroids, mineralocorticoids, estrogens, androgens, and progestins. The adrenal medulla elaborates the catecholamines epinephrine and norepinephrine. Called also *glandula suprarenalis* [NA] and *suprarenal g.* **adrenal g's, accessory,** accessory adrenal glandular tissue found in the abdomen or pelvis. Such tissue is usually either cortical or medullary; rarely is a true accessory adrenal gland found. Called also *glandulae suprarenales accessoriae* [NA] and *accessory suprarenal glands.* **aggregate g's, agminated g's,** folliculi lymphatici aggregati. **Albarrán's g.,** that part of the median lobe of the prostate underneath the uvula vesicae. **alveolar g.,** acinous g. **anal g.,** circumanal g's. **anteprostatic g.,** bulbourethral g. **aortic g.,** see under *body.* **apical g's of tongue,** glandulae linguales anteriores. **apocrine g.,** one the discharged secretion of which contains part of the secreting cells; see *glandulae sudoriferae.* **aporic g.,** endocrine g's. **areolar g's,** glandulae areolares. **arterial g.,** any knot of small arteries, or mass of vascular tissue, such as the glomus coccygeum. **arteriococcygeal g.,** glomus coccygeum. **arytenoid g's,** glandulae laryngeae posteriores. **Aselli's g's,** see under *pancreas.* **atribiliary g.,** adrenal g. **Avicenna's g.,** an encapsulated tumor. **axillary g's,** nodi lymphatici axillares. **Bartholin's g.,** one of the two small bodies on either side of the vaginal orifice, homologues of the bulbourethral glands in the male; called also *glandula vestibularis major* [NA]. **Bauhin's g's,** glandulae linguales anteriores. **Baumgarten's g's,** tubular glands of the conjunctiva situated on the nasal side of the eyelids. **g's of biliary mucosa,** glandulae mucosae biliosae. **Blandin's g's, Blandin and Nuhn's g's,** glandulae linguales anteriores. **blood g's, blood vessel g's,** endocrine g's. **Boerhaave's g's** (*obs.*), glandulae sudoriferae. **Bonnot's g.,** brown adipose tissue. **Bowman's g's,** glandulae olfactoriae. **brachial g's,** nodi lymphatici cubitales. **bronchial g's,** glandulae bronchiales. **Bruch's g's,** the lymph follicles of the conjunctiva of the lower lid. **Brunner's g's,** glandulae duodenales. **buccal g's,** glandulae buccales. **bulbocavernous g.,** bulbourethral g. **bulbourethral g.,** one of two glands embedded in the substance of the sphincter of the urethra, just posterior to the membranous part of the urethra; called also *Cowper's g.* and *glandula bulbourethralis* [NA]. **cardiac g's,** mucin-secreting glands at the cardiac end of the stomach surrounding the entrance of the esophagus into the stomach. **carotid g.,** glomus caroticum. **celiac g's,** lymph nodes anterior to the abdominal aorta. **ceruminous g's,** the glands in the skin of the external auditory canal that secrete the cerumen; called also *glandulae ceruminosae* [NA]. **cervical g's of uterus,** glandulae cervicales uteri. **cheek g's,** glandulae buccales. **choroid g.** (*obs.*), the choroid plexus, regarded as one of the sites of formation of the cerebrospinal fluid. **Ciaccio's g's,** glandulae lacrimales accessoriae. **ciliary g's, ciliary g's of conjunctiva,** glandulae ciliares conjunctivales. **circumanal g's,** specialized sweat and sebaceous glands situated around the anus; called also *anal g's* and *glandulae circumanales* [NA]. **Cloquet's g.,** see under *node.* **closed g.,** endocrine g's. **Cobelli's g's,** mucous glands in the mucosa of the esophagus just above the cardia. **coccygeal g.,** glomus coccygeum. **coil g.,** eccrine g. **compound g.,** one made up of a number of smaller units whose excretory ducts combine to

form ducts of progressively higher order. **conglobate g.,** a lymph node. **conglomerate g.** (*obs.*), compound g. **conjunctival g's,** glandulae conjunctivales. **Cowper's g.,** bulbourethral g. **cutaneous g's,** glands in the skin; see *glandulae cutis.* **cytogenic g.,** a term applied to the testis and the ovary because they form free living cells. **ductless g.,** one without a duct; see *endocrine g's.* **duodenal g's,** glandulae duodenales. **Duverney's g.,** bulbourethral g. **Ebner's g's,** albuminous or serous secreting glands in the posterior part of the tongue near the vallate papillae; called also *gustatory g's.* **eccrine g.,** one of the ordinary, or simple, sweat glands of the body, which is of the merocrine type; see *glandulae sudoriferae.* **Eglis' g's,** glandulae mucosae ureteris. **endocrine g's,** organs that secrete specific substances (hormones) which are released directly into the circulatory system and which influence metabolism and other body processes. The endocrine glands include the pituitary, thyroid, parathyroid, and adrenal glands, the pineal body, and the gonads. See also under *system,* and see Plate XIX. Called also *glandulae sine ductibus* [NA]. **endoepithelial g.,** intraepithelial g. **esophageal g's,** glandulae esophageae. **excretory g.,** any gland that excretes waste products from the system. **exocrine g.,** a gland which discharges its secretion through a duct opening on an internal or external surface of the body, as a lacrimal gland. Cf. *endocrine g's.* **follicular g's of tongue,** folliculi linguales. **fundic g's, fundus g's,** glandulae gastricae [propriae]. **Galeati's g's,** glandulae duodenales. **gastric g's,** the secreting glands of the stomach, including the fundic, cardiac, and pyloric glands. **gastric g's, proper,** glandulae gastricae [propriae]. **gastroepiploic g's,** nodi lymphatici gastrici [dextri et sinistri]. **g's of Gay,** glandulae circumanales. **genal g's,** glandulae buccales. **genital g.,** 1. ovary (ovarium [NA]). 2. testis. **gingival g's,** glandlike infoldings of epithelium at the junction of gingiva and tooth. **Gley's g's,** glandulae thyroideae accessoriae. **globate g.,** lymph node. **glomerate g's, glomiform g's,** glandulae glomiformes. **glossopalatine g's,** mucous glands at the posterior end of the smaller sublingual glands. **Guérin's g's,** ductus paraurethrales. **gustatory g's,** Ebner's g's. **guttural g.,** one of the mucous glands of the pharynx. **g's of Haller,** glandulae preputiales. **Harder's g's, harderian g's,** accessory lacrimal glands at the inner corner of the eye in animals that possess nictitating membranes and excrete an unctuous fluid that facilitates the movement of the third eyelid. They are rudimentary in man. **haversian g's,** villi synoviales. **hedonic g's,** glands in some of the lower animals which function during the season of sexual activity. **hemal g's,** see under *node.* **hemal lymph g's,** hemal nodes. **hematopoietic g's** (*obs.*), certain glandlike bodies which take a part in the making of the blood, such as the spleen. **hemolymph g's,** 1. hemal nodes. 2. see under *node.* **Henle's g's,** tubular glands in the conjunctiva of the eyelids. **hepatic g's,** glandulae mucosae biliosae. **heterocrine g's,** seromucous g's. **hibernating g.,** a collection of brown fatty tissue found in various regions of the body in hibernating animals; see *interscapular g.* **holocrine g.,** a gland whose discharged secretion contains entire secreting cells. **incretory g's,** endocrine g's. **intercarotid g.,** glomus caroticum. **intermediate g's,** according to some authorities, a fourth type of gastric gland (q.v.) found in a narrow region between the fundic and pyloric glands. **interscapular g.,** brown adipose tissue. **interstitial g.,** 1. (pl.) the aggregations of Leydig cells of the testis; so called because of their occurrence in clusters and their endocrine function. 2. the interstitial cells (see def. 2) of the ovary, collectively; so called because of their epithelioid appearance and presumed secretory function. **intestinal g's,** straight tubular glands in the mucous membrane of the intestines, opening, in the small intestine, between the bases of the villi, and containing argentaffin cells; called also *glandulae intestinalis* [NA]. **intraepithelial g.,** a gland situated in an epithelial layer. **intramuscular g's of tongue,** glandulae linguales anteriores. **jugular g.,** a lymph node behind the clavicular insertion of the sternomastoid muscle. **Krause's g's,** accessory lacrimal glands situated deep in the subconjunctival connective tissue, mainly in the upper fornix; called also *glandulae conjunctivales* [NA]. **labial g's of mouth,** glandulae labiales oris. **lacrimal g.,** glandula lacrimalis. **lacrimal g's, accessory,** glandulae lacrimales accessoriae. **g's of large intestine,** see *glandulae intestinales.* **large sweat g.,** an apocrine gland which usually produces an odoriferous secretion. **laryngeal g's,** glandulae laryngeae. **lenticular g's of stomach,** folliculi lymphatici gastrici. **lenticular g's of tongue,** folliculi linguales. **g's of Lieberkühn,** glandulae intestinales. **lingual g's,** glandulae linguales. **lingual g's, anterior (of Blandin and Nuhn),** glandulae linguales anteriores. **Littre's g's,** 1. glandulae preputiales. 2. glandulae urethrales urethrae masculinae. **Luschka's g.,** glomus coccygeum. **lymph g., lymphatic g.,** lymph node. **lymph g's, extraparotid,** lymph nodes overlying the parotid gland, between the superficial and deep fasciae. **malar g's,** glandulae buccales. **mammary g.,** the specialized accessory gland of the skin of female mammals that secretes milk. In the human female, it is a compound tubuloalveolar gland composed of 15 to 25 lobes arranged radially about the nipple and separated by connective and adipose tissue, each lobe having its own excretory (lactiferous) duct opening on the nipple. The lobes are subdivided into lobules, with the alveolar

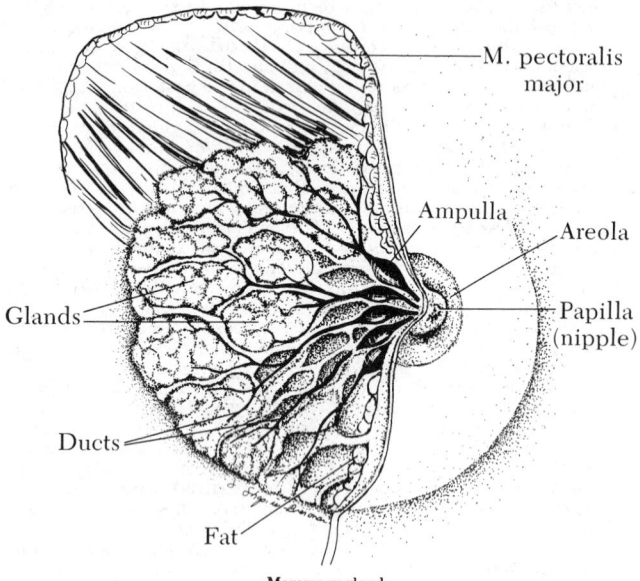

M. pectoralis major

Ampulla

Areola

Glands

Papilla (nipple)

Ducts

Fat

Mammary gland.

ducts and alveoli being the secretory portion of the gland. Called also *lactiferous gland* and *glandula mammaria* [NA]. **mammary g's, accessory,** mammae accessoriae [femininae et masculinae]. **mandibular g.,** glandula submandibularis. **Manz' g's,** glandular depressions on the borders of the eyelids. **Mehlis' g.,** gland cells surrounding the ootype of trematodes. **meibomian g's,** glandulae tarsales. **merocrine g.,** one in which the secretory cells maintain their integrity throughout the secretory cycle. **mesenteric g's,** nodi lymphatici mesenterici. **mesocolic g's,** lymph nodes in the mesentery of the colon; see *nodi lymphatici colici dextri, medii,* and *sinistri, nodi lymphatici ileocolici,* and *nodi lymphatici mesenterici inferiores.* **mixed g's,** 1. glands that have both endocrine and exocrine portions. 2. seromucous g's. **molar g's,** glandulae molares. **Moll's g's,** sweat glands that have become arrested in their development, situated obliquely in contact with and parallel to the bulbs of the eyelashes. Called also *glandulae ciliares conjunctivales* [NA]. **monoptychic g.,** a gland in which the tubules or alveoli are lined with a single layer of secreting cells. **Montgomery's g's,** glandulae areolares. **Morgagni's g's,** glandulae urethrales urethrae masculinae. **g's of mouth,** glandulae oris. **mucilaginous g's,** villi synoviales. **muciparous g.,** glandula mucosa. **mucous g.,** a gland that secretes a slimy, chemically inert material; called also *glandula mucosa* [NA]. **mucous g's, lingual,** glandulae linguales. **mucous g's of auditory tube,** glandulae tubariae. **mucous g's of duodenum,** glandulae duodenales. **mucous g's of eustachian tube,** glandulae tubariae. **multicellular g.,** one in which many cells cooperate to produce a gland complex, represented in its simplest form by a secretory sheet (q.v.) of epithelial cells. **myometrial g.,** a tissue supposed to develop in the wall of the uterus at the site of implantation of the placenta and to last until the end of pregnancy. **Naboth's g's,** Naboth's follicles. **nabothian g's,** see under *follicle.* **nasal g's,** glandulae nasales. **g. of neck,** tonsilla pharyngea. **Nuhn's g's,** glandulae linguales anteriores. **odoriferous g's of prepuce,** glandulae preputiales. **oil g's,** glandulae sebaceae. **olfactory g's,** glandulae olfactoriae. **oxyntic g's,** glandulae gastricae [propriae]. **pacchionian g's** (*obs.*), granulationes arachnoideales. **palatine g's,** glandulae palatinae. **palpebral g's,** glandulae tarsales. **pancreaticosplenic g's,** nodi lymphatici pancreaticolienales. **parafrenal g's,** glands opening near the frenum of the prepuce. **parathyroid g's,** small bodies in the region of the thyroid gland, developed from the entoderm of the branchial clefts, occurring in a variable number of pairs, commonly two (*glandula parathyroidea inferior* and *glandula parathyroidea superior* [NA]) (see inset on accompanying Plate). The parenchyma consists of masses and cords of epithelial cells, which have been divided into two main types: chief cells and oxyphil cells, but intermediate forms exist. The parathyroid glands secrete parathyroid hormone and are concerned chiefly with the metabolism of calcium and phosphorus. Called also *epithelial* or *parathyroid bodies.* **paraurethral g's,** ductus paraurethrales. **parotid g.,** the largest of the three chief, paired salivary glands; see *glandula parotis* [NA]. **parotid g., accessory,** glandula parotis accessoria. **pectoral g's,** see *nodi lymphatici axillares.* **peptic g's,** glandulae gastricae

[propriae]. **perspiratory g's** (*obs.*), glandulae sudoriferae. **Peyer's g's,** folliculi lymphatici aggregati. **pharyngeal g's,** glandulae pharyngeae. **Philip's g's,** enlarged glands above the clavicle, seen in children with tuberculosis. **pineal g.,** pineal body. **pituitary g.,** the epithelial body of dual origin located at the base of the brain in the sella turcica. It is attached by a stalk to the hypothalamus, from which it receives an important neural outflow. The pituitary gland (or *hypophysis* [NA]) is composed of two main lobes: the *adenohypophysis* (anterior lobe, lobus anterior [NA], anterior pituitary), which arises from the buccal epithelium in the embryo, and the *neurohypophysis* (posterior lobe, lobus posterior [NA], posterior pituitary), which originates in the embryo as an evagination from the floor of the diencephalon. The adenohypophysis comprises the *pars infundibularis* (or pars tuberalis), a thin cloak of cells on the anterior and lateral surfaces of the neural stalk; the *pars distalis,* the main body of the adenohypophysis; and the *pars intermedia,* an ill-defined region between the two lobes (assigned in some systems of nomenclature to the neurohypophysis). The neurohypophysis comprises the *neural stalk* (infundibulum), which is continuous with the hypothalamus, and the *neural lobe* (infundibular process, pars nervosa), which is the main body of the neurohypophysis. The adenohypophysis secretes several important hormones (growth hormone, ACTH, α-MSH, β-MSH, TSH, FSH, LH, and prolactin) which are released on stimulation of the pituitary by releasing factors secreted by the hypothalamus, and which regulate the proper functioning of the thyroid, gonads, adrenal cortex, and other endocrine organs. As a consequence, it is of vital importance to the growth, maturation, and reproduction of the individual. The neurohypophysis, formerly thought to be the source of hormones having antidiuretic and oxytocic action, is now known to serve only as a reservoir for them, releasing them as needed. Called also *glandula pituitaria* [NA alternative], *hypophysis cerebri* [NA], and *pituitary body.* **Poirier's g's,** lymph nodes on the conoid ligament at the upper border of the isthmus of the thyroid. **polyptychic g.,** a gland in which the tubules or alveoli are lined with more than one layer of secreting cells. **preen g.,** a large, compound alveolar structure present on the back of birds, above the base of the tail, which secretes an oily "water-proofing" material that the bird applies to its feathers and skin by preening. **pregnancy g's,** the glands containing female genital hormone, that is, the ovarian follicle, corpus luteum, and placenta. **prehyoid g's,** glandulae thyroidea accessoriae. **preputial g's,** glandulae preputiales. **prostate g.,** prostate. **puberty g's,** Steinach's name for the interstitial cells of Leydig in the male and the lutein cells of the ovary in the female. **pyloric g's,** glandulae pyloricae. **racemose g's,** glands composed of acini arranged like grapes on a stem. **retrolingual g.,** a rather large gland in some animals situated near the mandibular gland. **retromolar g's,** glandulae molares. **Rivinus g.,** glandula sublingualis. **Rosenmüller's g.,** 1. pars pelpebralis glandulae lacrimalis. 2. [pl.] nodi lymphatici inguinalis profundi. **saccular g.,** a gland consisting of a sac or sacs, lined with glandular epithelium. **salivary g's,** the glands of the oral cavity whose combined secretion constitutes the saliva; they include the parotid, sublingual, and submandibular glands, as well as numerous small glands in the tongue, lips, cheeks, and palate. **salivary g., abdominal,** the pancreas. **salivary g., external,** glandula parotis. **salivary g., internal,** see *glandula sublingualis* and *glandula submandibularis.* **Sandström's g's,** glandulae thyroideae accessoriae. **Schüller's g's,** diverticula of the ducts of Gartner. **sebaceous g's,** glandulae sebaceae. **sebaceous g's of conjunctiva,** glandulae sebaceae conjunctivales. **sentinel g.,** an enlarged lymph node, considered to be pathognomonic of some pathological condition elsewhere. **seromucous g.,** one that contains both serous and mucous secreting cells; called also *glandula seromucosa* [NA]. **serous g.,** a gland that secretes a watery albuminous material commonly but not always containing enzymes; called also *glandula serosa* [NA]. **Serres' g's,** pearly masses of epithelial cells near the surface of the gum of the infant. **sexual g.,** see *testis* and *ovary.* **Sigmund's g's,** the epitrochlear lymph nodes. **simple g.,** one with a nonbranching duct. **Skene's g's,** ductus paraurethrales. **g's of small intestine,** see *glandulae intestinales.* **solitary g's of large intestine,** folliculi lymphatici solitarii intestini crassi. **solitary g's of small intestine,** folliculi lymphatici solitarii intestini tenuis. **splenoid g.,** an apparently compensatory new growth that sometimes follows extirpation of the spleen. **Stahr's g.,** a lymph node situated on the facial artery. **staphyline g's,** glandulae palatinae. **subauricular g's,** nodi lymphatici retroauriculares. **sublingual g.,** the smallest of the three chief, paired salivary glands; see *glandula sublingualis* [NA]. **submandibular g., submaxillary g.,** one of the three chief, paired salivary glands; see *glandula submandibularis* [NA]. **sudoriferous g's, sudoriparous g's,** glandulae sudoriferae. **suprarenal g.,** adrenal g. **suprarenal g's, accessory,** glandulae suprarenales accessoriae. **Suzanne's g.,** a mucous gland of the mouth, beneath the alveololingual groove. **sweat g's,** glandulae sudoriferae. **synovial g's,** villi synoviales. **target g.,** a gland specifically affected by a pituitary hormone; such glands include the thyroid, adrenals, and gonads. **tarsal**

g's, tarsoconjunctival g's, glandulae tarsales. **Theile's g's,** glandlike formations in the walls of the cystic duct and in the pelvis of the gallbladder. **thymus g.,** thymus. **thyroid g.,** one of the endocrine glands, normally situated in the lower part of the front of the neck and consisting of two lobes, one on either side of the trachea and joined in front by a narrow isthmus. It secretes, stores, and liberates as neccessary the thyroid hormones (thyroxine and triiodothyronine), which require iodine for their elaboration and which are concerned in regulating the metabolic rate. It also secretes thyrocalcitonin. Called also *glandula thyroidea* [NA] and *thyroid body.* See also *thyroid.* **thyroid g's, accessory,** glandulae thyroideae accessoriae. **g's of tongue,** glandulae linguales. **tracheal g's,** glandulae tracheales. **trachoma g's,** lymphoid follicles of the conjunctiva, found chiefly near the inner canthus of the eye. **tubular g.,** any gland made up of or containing a tubule or a number of tubules. **tubuloacinar g.,** one that is both tubular and acinous. **tympanic g's,** glandulae tympanicae. **g's of Tyson,** glandulae preputiales. **unicellular g.,** a cell which performs a secretory function, as a goblet cell. **urethral g's,** see entries beginning *glandulae urethrales,* under *glandula.* **urethral g's of female urethra,** glandulae urethrales urethrae femininae. **uropygial g.,** preen g. **uterine g's,** glandulae uterinae. **utricular g's,** glandulae uterinae. **vaginal g.,** any gland occurring exceptionally in the vaginal mucous membrane. **vascular g.,** 1. glomus. 2. a hemal node. **vestibular g., greater,** glandula vestibularis major [NA]. **vestibular g's, lesser,** glandulae vestibulares minores. **Virchow's g.,** signal node. **vitelline g.,** see *vitellarium.* **vulvovaginal g.,** glandula vestibularis major. **Waldeyer's g's,** acinotubular glands in the inner skin of the attached edge of the eyelid. **Weber's g's,** the tubular mucous glands of the tongue. **g's of Wolfring,** small tubuloalveolar glands in the subconjunctival tissue above the upper border of the tarsal plate, their ducts opening on the conjunctival surface. **g's of Zeis,** modified rudimentary sebaceous glands attached directly to the follicles of the eyelashes; called also *glandulae sebaceae conjunctivales* [NA]. **Zuckerkandl's g.,** corpora paraaortica.

glanderous (glan'der-us) of the nature of or affected with glanders.

glanders (glan'derz) [L. *malleus*] a contagious disease of horses, communicable to man, and caused by the glanders bacillus, *Pseudomonas mallei.* It is marked by a purulent inflammation of mucous membranes and an eruption of nodules on the skin which coalesce and break down, forming deep ulcers, which may end in necrosis of cartilages and bones. Called also *maliasmus* and

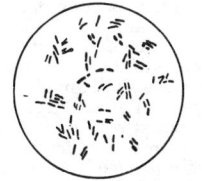

Pseudomonas mallei.

malleus; the more chronic and constitutional lymphatic form is known as *farcy.* **African g., Japanese g.,** lymphangitis epizootica.

glandes (glan'dēz) [L.] plural of *glans.*

glandilemma (glan″dĭ-lem'ah) [*gland* + Gr. *lemma* sheath] the capsule or outer envelope of a gland.

glandula (glan'du-lah), pl. *glan'dulae* [L.] [NA] a gland: an aggregation of cells, specialized to secrete or excrete materials not related to their ordinary metabolic needs. **glan'dulae areola'res** [NA], **glan'dulae areola'res [Montgomer'ii],** areolar glands: sebaceous glands of the mammary areola; called also *Montgomery's glands.* **glan'dulae bronchia'les** [NA], bronchial glands: seromucous glands in the mucosa and submucosa of the bronchial walls. **glan'dulae bucca'les** [NA], buccal glands: the serous and mucous glands on the inner surface of the cheeks. **g. bulbourethra'lis** [NA], **g. bulbourethra'lis [Cow'peri],** bulbourethral gland: either of two glands embedded in the substance of the sphincter of the male urethra, just posterior to the membranous part of the urethra; they are homologues of the greater vestibular glands in the female. Called also *Cowper's gland.* **glan'dulae cerumino'sae** [NA], ceruminous glands: the glands in the skin of the external auditory canal that secrete the cerumen. **glan'dulae cervica'les u'teri** [NA], cervical glands of uterus: compound clefts in the wall of the uterine cervix. **glan'dulae cilia'res conjunctiva'les** [NA], **glan'dulae cilia'res [Mol'li],** ciliary glands of conjunctiva: sweat glands that have become arrested in their development, situated obliquely in contact with and parallel to the bulbs of the eyelashes; called also *Moll's glands.* **glan'dulae circumana'les** [NA], circumanal glands: specialized sweat and sebaceous glands situated in an annular zone around the anus; called also *anal glands.* **g. clau'sa,** a ductless (endocrine) gland. **gland'dulae conjunctiva'les** [NA], conjunctival glands: accessory lacrimal glands situated deep in the subconjunc-

tival connective tissue, mainly in the upper fornix; called also *glandulae mucosae conjunctivae [Krausei]* and *Krause's glands.* **glan'dulae cu'tis** [NA], cutaneous glands: the glands of the skin, including the sweat glands (glandulae sudoriferae), sebaceous glands (glandulae sebaceae), and the modified sweat glands that secrete cerumen (glandulae ceruminosae). **glan'dulae duodena'les** [NA], **glan'dulae duodena'les [Brun'neri],** duodenal glands: tubuloalveolar glands in the submucous layer of the duodenum which open into the crypts of Lieberkühn; they secrete urogastrone. Called also *Brunner's glands.* **glan'dulae esophage'ae** [NA], esophageal glands: the mucous glands in the submucosa of the esophagus. **glan'dulae gas'tricae [pro'priae]** [NA], gastric glands proper: very numerous, nearly straight tubular glands located in the mucosa of the fundus and body of the stomach; they contain the cells that produce acid and pepsin. Called also *fundic glands.* **gland'dulae glomifor'mes** [NA], glomiform glands: cutaneous glomiform arteriovenous shunts found in the skin, which are called glands although they appear to be nonglandular; called also *glomerate glands.* **glan'dulae hepat'icae,** glandulae mucosae biliosae. **g. incisi'va,** a small intraoral gland in the median line of the upper jaw near the incisors. **g. intercarot'ica,** glomus caroticum. **glan'dulae intestina'les** [NA], intestinal glands: simple tubular glands in the mucous membrane of the small intestine (*intestinales intestini tenuis*), opening between the bases of the villi and containing argentaffin cells; of the large intestine (*g. intestinales intestini crassi*); and of the rectum (*g. intestinales intestini recti*). Called also *crypts, glands,* or *follicles of Lieberkühn,* and *intestinal follicles.* **glan'dulae labia'les o'ris** [NA], labial glands of the mouth: the serous and mucous glands on the inner part of the lips. **g. lacrima'lis** [NA], lacrimal gland: one of the glands that lie at the upper outer angle of the orbit and secrete the tears; they are divided into two portions, the orbital and palpebral, by the orbital fascia. **glan'dulae lacrima'les accesso'riae** [NA], accessory lacrimal glands: portions of the lacrimal gland sometimes found near the superior fornix of the conjunctiva. **g. lacrima'lis infe'rior,** pars palpebralis glandulae lacrimalis. **g. lacrima'lis supe'rior,** pars orbitalis glandulae lacrimalis. **glan'dulae laryn'geae** [NA], laryngeal glands: the mucous glands in the mucosa of the larynx. **glan'dulae laryn'geae anterio'res,** mucous glands in the anterior of the larynx. **glan'dulae laryn'geae me'diae,** mucous glands located in the arytenoepiglottic fold. **glan'dulae laryn'geae posterio'res,** mucous glands in the posterior wall of the larynx; called also *arytenoid glands.* **glan'dulae lingua'les** [NA], lingual glands: the mucous and serous glands on the surface of the tongue. **glan'dulae lingua'les anterio'res** [NA], anterior lingual glands: deeply placed mucoserous glands near the apex of the tongue. **g. mamma'ria** [NA], mammary gland: the collective glandular elements of the mamma, or breast, which secrete milk for nourishment of the young; see *mammary gland,* under *gland.* **glan'dulae mola'res** [NA], molar glands: the glands on the external aspect of the buccinator muscle, their ducts piercing it to open on the internal aspect of the cheek; called also *retromolar glands.* **g. muco'sa** [NA], mucous gland: a gland that secretes a slimy, chemically inert material. **g. muco'sae tu'bae auditi'vae,** g. tubariae. **glan'dulae muco'sae bilio'sae** [NA], glands of biliary mucosa: tubuloalveolar glands in the mucosa of the bile ducts and the neck of the gallbladder; called also *hepatic glands* and *glandulae hepaticae.* **glan'dulae muco'sae conjuncti'vae [Kraus'ei],** glandulae conjunctivales. **glan'dulae muco'sae ure'teris,** mucous glands of the ureter. **glan'dulae nasa'les** [NA], nasal glands: numerous large mucous and serous glands in the respiratory part of the nasal cavity. **glan'dulae olfacto'riae** [NA], olfactory glands: small mucous glands in the olfactory mucosa; called also *Bowman's glands.* **glan'dulae o'ris** [NA], the glands of the mouth. **glan'dulae palati'nae** [NA], palatine glands: the mucous glands on the soft palate and the posteromedial part of the hard palate; called also *staphyline glands.* **glan'dulae parathyroi'deae** [NA], small bodies in the region of the thyroid gland occurring in a variable number of pairs, commonly two, named *glandula parathyroidea superior* and *glandula parathyroidea inferior,* according to their position; see *parathyroid glands,* under *gland.* **g. paro'tis** [NA], parotid gland: the largest of the three chief, paired glands which, together with numerous small glands in the mouth, constitute the salivary glands; it is located below the zygomatic arch, below and in front of the external acoustic meatus. **g. paro'tis accesso'ria** [NA], accessory parotid gland: a more or less detached portion of the parotid gland that is frequently present. **glan'dulae pel'vis rena'lis,** mucous glands in the wall of the kidney pelvis. **glan'dulae pharyn'geae** [NA], pharyngeal glands: mucous glands beneath the tunica mucosa of the pharynx. **g. pituita'ria** [NA alternative], pituitary gland; see under *gland.* **glan'dulae preputia'les** [NA], preputial glands: small sebaceous glands of the corona of the penis and the inner surface of the prepuce, which secrete smegma; called also *Littre's crypts* or *glands.* **g. prosta'ta, g. prostat'ica,** prostate. **glan'dulae pylo'ricae** [NA], pyloric glands: the mucin-secreting glands of the pyloric part of the stomach. **glan'dulae seba'ceae** [NA], sebaceous glands: holocrine glands of the skin, secreting an oily substance, sebum, and situated in the corium. **glan′dulae seba′ceae conjunctiva′les** [NA], sebaceous glands of conjunctivae: modified rudimentary sebaceous glands attached directly to the follicles of the eyelashes; called also *glands of Zeis.* **glan′dulae seba′ceae la′bii majo′ris pudenda′lis,** sebaceous glands in the skin of the labia majora. **glan′dulae seba′ceae mam′mae,** glandulae areolares. **g. seromuco′sa** [NA], seromucous gland: a gland composed of both mucous and serous secreting cells, such as the labial glands. **g. sero′sa** [NA], serous gland: a gland that secretes a watery albuminous material, commonly but not always containing enzymes. **glan′dulae si′ne duc′tibus** [L. "glands without ducts"] [NA], the endocrine glands, including the thyroid and parathyroid glands, the pituitary gland, the adrenal gland, and the gonads; see *endocrine glands,* under *gland.* **g. sublingua′lis** [NA], sublingual gland: the smallest of the three chief, paired salivary glands, predominantly mucous in type, and draining into the oral cavity through 10 to 30 sublingual ducts; called also *Rivinus gland.* **g. submandibula′ris** [NA], **g. submaxilla′ris,** submandibular gland: one of the three chief, paired salivary glands, predominantly serous, lying partly above and partly below the posterior half of the base of the mandible. **glan′dulae sudorif′erae** [NA], sudoriferous or sweat glands: the glands that secrete sweat, situated in the corium or subcutaneous tissue, and opening by a duct on the surface of the body. They are of two types: The ordinary or *eccrine sweat glands* are unbranched, coiled, tubular glands that are distributed over almost all of the body surface, and promote cooling by evaporation of their secretion. The *apocrine sweat glands* are large, branched, specialized glands that empty into the upper portion of a hair follicle instead of directly onto the skin surface, and are found only on certain areas of the body, such as around the anus and in the axilla. Called also *sudoriparous glands.* **g. suprarena′lis** [NA], a flattened body situated in the retroperitoneal tissues at the superior pole of either kidney; see *adrenal gland,* under *gland.* **glan′dulae suprarena′les accesso′riae** [NA], accessory suprarenal gland: accessory adrenal glandular tissue found in the abdomen or pelvis. See *adrenal g., accessory,* under *gland.* **glan′dulae suprarena′les sic′cae,** desiccated adrenal glands. **glan′dulae tarsa′les** [NA], **glan′dulae tarsa′les [Meibo′mi],** tarsal glands: sebaceous follicles between the tarsi and the conjunctiva of the eyelids; called also *meibomian glands.* **g. thyroi′dea** [NA], thyroid gland: one of the endocrine glands, normally situated in the front of the lower part of the neck and consisting of two lobes, one on either side of the trachea and joined in front by a narrow isthmus. It secretes, stores, and liberates as necessary the thyroid hormones (thyroxine and triiodothyronine), which require iodine for their elaboration and are concerned in regulating the rate of metabolism. It also secretes thyrocalcitonin. Called also *thyroid body.* See also *thyroid.* **glan′dulae thyroi′deae accesso′riae** [NA], accessory thyroid glands: small exclaves of the thyroid gland that may be found any place along the course of the thyroglossal duct, as well as in the thorax. **glan′dula thyroi′dea accesso′ria suprahyoi′dea,** accessory thyroid tissue found above the hyoid bone. **glan′dulae thyroi′deae sic′cae,** desiccated thyroid glands. **glan′dulae trachea′les** [NA], tracheal glands: mucous glands in the elastic submucous coat between the cartilaginous rings and on the posterior wall of the trachea. **glan′dulae tuba′riae** [NA], mucous glands within the mucosa of the auditory tube, especially near its nasopharyngeal end; called also *glandulae mucosae tubae auditivae* and *mucous glands of auditory* or *eustachian tube.* **g. tympan′icae,** tympanic gland: a small mass situated on Jacobson's nerve in the tympanic canal. **glan′dulae urethra′les [Lit′trei],** glandulae urethrales urethrae masculinae. **glan′dulae urethra′les ure′thrae femini′nae** [NA], urethral glands of female urethra: numerous small mucous glands in the mucosa of the female urethra, some of which on either side are drained by the inconstant paraurethral ducts opening into the vestibule. **glan′dulae urethra′les ure′thrae masculi′nae** [NA], mucous glands in the wall of the male urethra; called also *Littre's glands.* **glan′dulae urethra′les ure′thrae mulie′bris,** glandulae urethrales urethrae femininae. **g. uropygia′lis,** preen gland. **glan′dulae uteri′nae** [NA], uterine glands: simple tubular glands throughout the entire thickness and extent of the endometrium, which become enlarged during the premenstrual period. **glan′dulae vesica′les ves′icae urina′riae,** mucous glands in the wall of the urinary bladder. **g. vestibula′ris ma′jor** [NA], either of two small reddish yellow bodies in the vestibular bulbs, one on each side of the vaginal orifice; they are homologues of the bulbourethral glands in the male. Called also *Bartholin's gland* and *greater vestibular gland.* **glan′dulae vestibula′res mino′res** [NA], small mucous glands opening upon the vestibular mucous membrane between the urethral and the vaginal orifice; called also *lesser vestibular glands.*

glandulae (glan′du-le) [L.] plural of *glandula.*

glandular (glan′du-lar) 1. pertaining to or of the nature of a gland. 2. pertaining to the glans penis.

glandule (glan′dūl) [L. *glandula*] a small gland.

glandulous (glan′du-lus) [L. *glandulosus*] abounding in kernels or small glands.

glans (glanz), pl. *glan′des* [L. "acorn"] [NA] a general term for a small rounded mass, or glandlike body. **g. clitor′idis** [NA], **g. of clitoris,** erectile tissue at the end of the clitoris, which is continuous with the intermediate part of the vestibular bulbs. **g. pe′nis** [NA], the cap-shaped expansion of the corpus spongiosum at the end of the penis; called also *balanus.*

Glanzmann's thrombasthenia (disease) (glahnz′manz) [Edward *Glanzmann,* Swiss pediatrician, 1887–1959] see *thrombasthenia.*

glare (glâr) a condition of discomfort in the eye and of depression of central vision produced when a bright light enters the field of vision, especially when the eye is adapted to dark. The amount of glare is directly proportional to the candle power of the light and inversely proportional to the square of the distance of the light from the eye and to its angular distance from the visual axis. *Direct g.,* when the image of the light falls on the fovea; *peripheral g.,* when it falls outside of the fovea.

glarometer (glâr-om′ĕ-ter) an instrument for measuring a person's resistance to glare from the lights of an approaching automobile.

glaserian fissure, etc. (gla-se′re-an) [named for or described by Johann Heinrich *Glaser* (Glaserius), Swiss anatomist, 1629–1675] fissura petrotympanica.

Glasgow's sign (glas′gōz) [William Carr *Glasgow,* American physician, 1845–1907] see under *sign.*

glass (glas) [L. *vit′rum*] 1. a hard, brittle, and often transparent material, usually consisting of the fused amorphous silicates of potassium or sodium, and of calcium, with silica in excess. 2. a container, usually cylindrical, made from glass. 3. (pl.) lenses worn to aid or improve vision; see *glasses, lens,* and *spectacles.* **cover g.,** a thin glass plate used to cover an object for microscopical examination. **crown g.,** a glass of low refractive index (achieved by incorporating a considerable percentage of phosphorus pentoxide); used in combination with flint glass in multielement lenses. **cupping g.,** a vessel of glass from which the air has been or can be exhausted, applied to the body for the purpose of drawing blood to the surface. **flint g.,** a highly refractive glass in which calcium has been replaced in large part by lead; used for lenses and prisms and in the manufacture of cut glass. **holvi g.,** glass more transparent than ordinary glass to ultraviolet rays. **lithium g.,** glass containing lithium, used in grenz ray x-ray tubes. **object g.,** see *objective.* **optical g.,** glass of high quality and controlled composition, used for lenses. **quartz g.,** pure fused silica, SiO_2; used for prisms, lenses, and chemical vessels (1) because its index of thermal expansion is so small that it does not crack when heated or cooled, and (2) because it transmits more ultraviolet radiation than does ordinary glass. **soluble g.,** a potassium or sodium silicate which is sometimes used in preparing immovable bandages. **test g.,** a small glass vessel, resembling a beaker, used in a chemical laboratory. **watch g.,** a relatively airtight eye shield made of metal or other substances, and having a shape similar to that of a watch crystal; used primarily to cover an exposed cornea, but may be used to guard an unaffected eye from infection from an affected eye. **water g.,** soluble g. **Wood's g.,** see under *light.*

glasses (glas′ez) spectacles; a pair of lenses arranged in a frame holding them in the proper position before the eyes, as an aid to vision. **bifocal g.,** lenses which have two different refracting powers, one for distant and one for near vision. **contact g.,** see *contact lens.* **crutch g.,** glasses which will elevate and support the upper lid of patients with ptosis. **Hallauer's g.,** glasses with grayish-green lenses which prevent the passage of blue and ultraviolet rays. **hyperbolic g.,** lenses ground with a section of a hyperbolic curve. **snow g.,** glasses with special lenses to prevent snow blindness. **sun g.,** glasses with special lenses which filter the rays of the sun. **trifocal g.,** glasses with lenses which have three different refracting powers, one for distant, one for intermediate, and one for near vision.

glassy (glas′e) like glass; hyaline or vitreous.

Glauber's salt (glow′berz) [Johann Rudolf *Glauber,* German physician and chemist, 1604–1688] sodium sulfate.

glaucarubin (glaw″kah-ru′bin) a crystalline glycoside obtained from the fruit of *Simaruba glauca* D.C. (Simorubaceae); formerly used as an amebicide.

glaucoma (glaw-ko′mah) [Gr. *glaukōma* opacity of the crystalline lens (from the dull gray gleam of the affected eye)] a group of eye diseases characterized by an increase in intraocular pressure which causes pathological changes in the optic disk and typical defects in the field of vision. **absolute g., g. absolu′tum,** the final stage of glaucoma characterized by pain in the eye and blindness. **acute congestive g.,** narrow-angle g. **air-block g.,** a form of postoperative glaucoma, resulting from blockage of the flow of aqueous by air injected inadvertently behind the iris either through the pupillary opening or through a peripheral iridectomy. **angle-closure g.,** narrow-angle g. **angle-recession g.,** glaucoma secondary to contusion injury of the eye, in which the anterior chamber is deep and the angle recedes, with exposure of the ciliary body, as seen gonioscopically, and there is blocking of the trabecular spaces. **aphakic g.,** a general term referring to glaucoma in an eye from which the lens has been removed; the glaucoma may be related to the cataract extraction or to its sequelae, or it may have existed prior to the cataract extraction. **apoplectic g.,** hemorrhagic g. **auricular g.,** that associated with increased intralabyrinthine pressure. **capsular g.,** that due to obstruction of the outlet channels of the aqueous humour. **chronic narrow-angle g.,** a form of narrow angle glaucoma without a severe congestive episode. **chronic simple g.,** open-angle g. **closed-angle g.,** narrow-angle g. **congenital g.,** infantile g. **congestive g.,** narrow-angle g. **g. consumma′tum,** g. absolutum. **Donders′ g.,** g. simplex. **enzyme g.,** a transient glaucoma developing postoperatively in patients in whom trypsin has been used in the lysis of the zonule during cataract surgery; it is usually self-limited, with no permanent damage. **hemorrhagic g.,** that which is caused by pressure from retinal hemorrhage (von Graefe). **g. im′minens,** an impending glaucoma. **infantile g.,** a form of congenital glaucoma that may be fully developed at birth, with characteristic signs (enlargement and hazing of the corneas), or it may develop at any time up to two or three years of age; these signs result from inability of the cornea and sclera to withstand the increased intraocular pressure. Called also *buphthalmos.* Cf. *juvenile g.* **inflammatory g.,** a form attended with ciliary congestion, corneal opacity, and blindness, recurring in paroxysmal attacks. **juvenile g.,** glaucoma differing from infantile glaucoma in that it occurs in older children and young adults up to 30 years of age, and there is no gross enlargement of the eyeball. **lenticular g.,** glaucoma occurring in association with congenital or traumatic dislocation of the lens, or with swelling of the lens, usually due to mechanical obstruction at the peripheral angle of the anterior chamber. **malignant g.,** glaucoma that grows rapidly worse in spite of iridectomy. **narrow-angle g.,** a form of primary glaucoma in an eye characterized by a shallow anterior chamber and a narrow angle, in which filtration is compromised as a result of the iris blocking the angle; called also *angle-closure g., closed-angle g.,* and *acute congestive g.* **neovascular g.,** a form of secondary glaucoma; glaucoma caused by neovascularization in the chamber angle. **noncongestive g.,** open-angle g. **obstructive g.,** narrow-angle g. **open-angle g.,** a form of primary glaucoma in an eye in which the angle of the anterior chamber remains open, but filtration is gradually diminished because of the tissues of the angle; called also *simple g., chronic simple g.,* and *wide-angle g.* **phakogenic g.,** glaucoma resulting from pupillary block, in turn caused by a swollen lens, with angle closure. **phakolytic g.,** glaucoma secondary to leakage of lens protein into the aqueous from a mature or more often a hypermature cataract and the subsequent ingestion of the protein by macrophages, which swell and block the trabecular spaces. It has the following characteristics: mature or hypermature cataract, open angle (often with angle recession), deep anterior chamber, uveitis, and increased intraocular pressure. **pigmentary g.,** a form of open-angle glaucoma associated with an abnormal amount of pigment dispersion in the anterior segment of the eye. **primary g.,** increased intraocular pressure occurring in an eye without previous disease; see *narrow-angle g.* and *open-angle g.* **secondary g.,** increased intraocular pressure resulting from a disease or injury, as from dislocation of the lens, tumor of the uveal tract, or hemorrhage into the anterior chamber. **simple g.,** open-angle g. **g. sim′plex,** a form with no pronounced inflammatory symptoms, but attended with progressive loss of vision. **traumatic g.,** an increase in intraocular pressure due to a nonperforating injury of the globe, resulting in vascular congestion. **vitreous-block g.,** postoperative glaucoma in which vitreous plugs the pupil, so that the aqueous, which is unable to move to the anterior chamber, forces the vitreous and iris forward, producing occlusion of the chamber angle and eventually peripheral anterior synechiae. **wide-angle g.,** open-angle g.

glaucomatous (glaw-ko′mah-tus) pertaining to or of the nature of glaucoma.

glaucosis (glaw-ko′sis) blindness caused by glaucoma.

glaucosuria (glaw″ko-su′re-ah) [Gr. *glaukos* silvery + *ouron* urine + *-ia*] indicanuria.

glaze (glāz) in dentistry, a ceramic veneer added to a porcelain restoration after it has been fired, to give a completely nonporous, glossy or semiglossy surface.

gleet (glēt) 1. a chronic form of gonorrheal urethritis. 2. a urethral discharge, especially one that is mucous or purulent. **vent g.,** cloacitis.

gleety (glēt′e) pertaining to or of the nature of gleet.

Glénard's disease (gla-narz′) [Frantz *Glénard,* French physician, 1848–1920] see *splanchnoptosis.*

glenohumeral (gle″no-hu′mer-al) pertaining to the glenoid cavity and to the humerus.

glenoid (gle′noid) [Gr. *glēnē* socket + *eidos* form] resembling a pit or socket; see *cavitas glenoidalis.*

Glenospora (gle-nos′po-rah) a former name for genus of fungi of uncertain classification, species of which have been assigned to several other genera. *G. graphii* was reported from otomycosis.

Glenosporella (gle″no-spo-rel′ah) former name for the genus *Chrysosporium.*

Gley's cells, glands (glāz) [Marcel Eugène Émile *Gley,* French physiologist, 1857–1930] see under *cell* and see *glandulae thyroidea accessoriae.*

glia (gli′ah) [Gr. "glue"] the neuroglia; also used as a word termination to denote a gluelike structure or tissue. **ameboid g.,** degenerated neuroglial cells which are rich in pale protoplasm, possess few processes, and have densely staining nuclei. **cytoplasmic g.,** enlarged neuroglial cells, rich in cytoplasm, containing vacuoles and supplied with fibrils; seen in degeneration of the spinal cord. **g. of Fañana,** a form of neuroglial cell occurring in the molecular layer of the cerebellar cortex. **fibrillary g.,** degenerated neuroglial cells containing an abundance of fibrils.

gliacyte (gli′ah-sīt) [*glia* + Gr. *kytos* hollow vessel] a cell of the neuroglia.

gliadin (gli′ah-din) [Gr. *glia* glue] an alcohol-soluble protein present in wheat and occurring in various forms (α-,β-,γ-, and W-gliadins); it contains the toxic factor associated with celiac disease.

glial (gli′al) of or pertaining to the neuroglia or glia.

gliamilide (gli-am′ĭ-lid) chemical name: *endo*-N-[2-[1-[[[[(bicyclo[2.2.1]hept-5-en-2-ylmethyl)amino]carbonyl]amino]sulfonyl]-4-piperidinyl]ethyl]-2-methoxy-3-pyridinecarboxamide; an oral hypoglycemic, $C_{23}H_{33}N_5O_5S$.

gliarase (gli′ah-rās) an aggregation of astrocytes whose cytoplasm has undergone incomplete fission.

glibenclamide (gli-ben′klah-mīd) glyburide.

glibornuride (gli-born′ūr-īd) chemical name: N-[[(3-hydroxy-4,7,7-trimethylbicyclo[2.2.1]hept-2-yl)amino]carbonyl]-4-methylbenzenesulfonamide; an orally effective hypoglycemic agent of the sulfonylurea group, $C_{18}H_{26}N_2O_4S$.

glicetanile sodium (glĭ-set′ah-nīl) chemical name: N-(5-chloro-2-methoxyphenyl)-4-[[[5-(2-methyl propyl)-2-pyrimidinyl]-amino]sulfonyl]benzeneacetamide monosodium salt; an oral hypoglycemic, $C_{23}H_{24}ClN_4NaO_4S$. Called also *glydanile sodium.*

glide (glīd) a smooth continuous movement. **mandibular g.,** the side-to-side, protrusive, and intermediate movement of the mandible occurring when the teeth or other occluding surfaces are in contact. **occlusal g.,** the movement induced by deflective tooth contact that diverts the mandible from a normal path of closure to a centric jaw relation.

gliflumide (glĭ-floo′mīd) chemical name: (−)-(S)-N-[1-(5-fluoro-2-methoxyphenyl)ethyl]-4-[[[5-(2-methylpropyl)-2-pyrimidinyl]-amino]sulfonyl]benzeneacetamide; an oral hypoglycemic, $C_{25}H_{29}FN_4O_4S$.

glio- (gli′o) [Gr. *glia* glue] a combining form denoting relationship to a gluey substance or specifically to the neuroglia.

gliobacteria (gli″o-bak-te′re-ah) [*glio-* + *bacteria*] rod-shaped schizomycetes which are surrounded by a zooglea.

glioblast (gli′o-blast) spongioblast.

glioblastoma (gli″o-blas-to′mah) [*glio-* + Gr. *blastos* germ + *-oma*] a general term for malignant forms of astrocytoma. **g. multifor′me,** an astrocytoma of Grade III or IV; it is a rapidly growing tumor, usually confined to the cerebral hemispheres and composed of a mixture of spongioblasts, astroblasts, and astrocytes. Called also *spongioblastoma multiforme* and *anaplastic astrocytoma.*

gliococcus (gli″o-kok′us) [*glio-* + Gr. *kokkos* berry] a micrococcus that forms gelatinous matter.

gliocyte (gli′o-sīt) gliacyte. **retinal g's,** Müller's fibers.

gliocytoma (gli″o-si-to′mah) glioma.

gliofibrillary (gli″o-fi′brĭ-lār-e) pertaining to fibrils of the neuroglia.

gliogenous (gli-oj′ĕ-nus) [*glio-* + Gr. *gennan* to produce] produced or formed by glial (neuroglial) cells.

glioma (gli-o′mah) [*glio-* + *-oma*] a tumor composed of tissue which represents neuroglia in any one of its stages of development. The term is sometimes extended to include all the primary intrinsic neoplasms of the brain and spinal cord, including astrocytomas, ependymomas, neurocytomas, etc. **astrocytic g.,** astrocytoma. **g. endoph′ytum,** retinoblastoma beginning in the inner layers of the retina. **ependymal g.,** a bulky, solid, rather firm but vascular tumor of the fourth ventricle. **g. exoph′ytum,** retinoblastoma beginning in the outer layers of the retina. **ganglionic g.,** a glioma that contains also ganglion cells of nearly adult type; see *neuroblastoma.* **mixed g.,** a glioma in which the cytological components are of more than one cell type, the commonest form consisting of oligodendrogliomatous foci in an otherwise typical astrocytoma. **nasal g.,** a tumorlike mass composed of ectopic neural tissue in the nasal cavity. **optic g.,** a slow-growing glioma of the optic nerve or optic chiasm heralded by visual loss, often with secondary strabismus, followed by proptosis and loss of ocular movement. **peripheral g.,** schwannoma. **g. ret′inae,** retinoblastoma. **g. sarcomato′sum,** a gliosarcoma. **telangiectatic g.,** glioma containing blood vessels.

gliomatosis (gli″o-mah-to′sis) excessive development of the neuroglia, especially of the spinal cord, in certain cases of syringomyelia.

gliomatous (gli-o′mah-tus) affected with or of the nature of glioma.

glioneuroma (gli″o-nu-ro′mah) a tumor containing both gliomatous and neuromatous elements.

gliophagia (gli″o-fa′je-ah) [glio- + Gr. phagein to eat] phagocytosis of neuroglial cells.

gliopil (gli′o-pil) [glio- + Gr. pilos felt] a dense feltwork of glial processes, as in the subependymal matrix of the ventricular system.

gliosa (gli-o′sah) (obs.) the gray matter of the spinal cord which covers the head of the dorsal horn and surrounds the central canal.

gliosarcoma (gli″o-sar-ko′mah) [glio- + sarcoma] a spindle cell glioma; see also spongioblastoma. **g. ret′inae,** retinoblastoma.

gliosis (gli-o′sis) an excess of astroglia in damaged areas of the central nervous system. **basilar g.,** gliosis affecting the brain stem, thalamus, and corpus striatum. **cerebellar g.,** gliosis affecting the cerebellum. **diffuse g.,** gliosis affecting the whole of the cerebral tissue, or widely scattered through it. **hemispheric g.,** gliosis affecting one of the cerebral hemispheres. **hypertrophic nodular g.,** a form of gliosis in which the brain is symmetrically enlarged because of hyperplasia of the neuroglial tissue. **isomorphic g.,** gliosis in which there is a regular and parallel arrangement of glial fibers. **lobar g.,** gliosis affecting a single lobe of the brain. **perivascular g.,** a form of arteriosclerosis of the cerebral vessels, marked by increase of the neuroglia about the vessels. **spinal g.,** gliosis of the spinal cord. **unilateral g.,** hemispheric gliosis.

gliosome (gli′o-sōm) [glio- + Gr. sōma body] one of the small cytoplasmic granules seen in neuroglial cells.

gliotoxin (gli″o-tok′sin) an antibiotic substance, $C_{13}H_{14}N_2O_4S_2$, obtained from several unrelated species of fungi, including species of Trichoderma, Aspergillus, and Penicillium; it is a neutral, nitrogen- and sulfur-containing compound first isolated from culture filtrates of Gliocladium (Trichoderma).

glipizide (glip′ah-zīd) chemical name: N-[2-[4-[[[(cyclohexylamino)carbonyl]amino]sulfonyl]phenyl]ethyl]-5-methylpyrazine carboxamide. An orally effective hypoglycemic, $C_{21}H_{27}N_5O_4S$, used in the treatment of diabetes mellitus in certain patients.

Gliricola (gli-rik′o-lah) a genus of biting lice. **G. porcel′li,** a biting louse found on guinea pigs.

glischrin (glis′krin) [Gr. glischros gluey] a mucin produced in urine by bacterial activity.

glischruria (glis-kroo′re-ah) [Gr. glischros gluey + ouron urine + -ia] the presence of glischrin in the urine.

glissade (glis-ād′) [Fr. "sliding"] a gliding involuntary movement of the eye in changing the point of fixation; it is a slower, smoother movement than is a saccade.

glissadic (glis-sad′ik) pertaining to a glissade.

Glisson's capsule, cirrhosis, disease, sling (glis′unz) [Francis Glisson, English physician and anatomist, 1597–1677, one of the founders of the Royal Society] see capsula fibrosa perivascularis, capsular cirrhosis, and rickets, and see under sling.

glissonitis (glis″o-ni′tis) inflammation of Glisson's capsule (capsula fibrosa perivascularis [NA].

globi (glo′bi) [L.] 1. plural of globus. 2. encapsulated globular masses containing bacilli, seen in smears of lepromatous leprosy lesions.

globidiosis (glob-bid″i-o′sis) former name for besnoitiosis.

Globidium (glo-bid′e-um) former name for Besnoitia.

globin (glo′bin) the protein constituent of hemoglobin; also any member of a group of proteins similar to the typical globin. **g. zinc insulin injection,** see under injection.

globinometer (glo″bǐ-nom′ě-ter) an instrument used in determining the proportion of oxyhemoglobin in the blood.

globoid (glo′boid) globe-shaped; spheroid.

globose (glo′bōs) [L. globus a ball] globe-shaped, spherical.

globoside (glob′o-sīd) a sphingoglycolipid containing acetylated aminosugars and simple hexoses of the general composition: ceramide-(glucose)ₘ-(galactose)ₙ-(N-acetylhexosamine)ₚ. It occurs in human serum, spleen, liver, and erythrocytes, accumulates in tissues in Sandhoff's disease, and is probably a precursor of glucocerebroside and ceramide trihexoside.

globular (glob′u-lar) 1. like a globe or globule. 2. composed of globules.

Globularia (glob″u-la′re-ah) a European shrub; G. alypum L. (Globulariaceae), a perennial herb indigenous to the Mediterranean region, is used as a purgative and for intermittent fevers.

globulariacitrin (glob″u-la″re-ah-sit′rin) rutin.

globule (glob′ūl) [L. globulus a globule] 1. a small spherical mass or body. 2. a small spherical drop of fluid or semifluid substance, e.g., a fat droplet in milk or a drop of water. 3. a little globe or pellet, as of medicine. **dentin g's,** small spherical bodies in the peripheral dentin, created by beginning calcification of the matrix about discrete foci. **Dobie's g.,** a minute stainable mass in the middle of the transparent disk of a muscle fibril.

Marchi's g's, fragments and particles of broken-up myelin which stain by Marchi's method, seen in degeneration of the spinal cord. **milk g's,** the small round masses of fat in milk which tend to separate out as cream. **Morgagni's g's,** minute opaque spheres sometimes found between the eye lens and its capsule, chiefly in cases of cataract. **myelin g's,** colorless globules resembling fat droplets and sometimes spirally marked, seen in some sputa. **polar g's,** polar bodies.

globuli (glob′u-li) [L.] plural of globulus.

globulin (glob′u-lin) [L. globulus globule] a class of proteins characterized by being insoluble in water, but soluble in saline solutions (euglobulins), or water soluble proteins (pseudoglobulins) whose other physical properties closely resemble true globulins. See serum g. **AC g., accelerator g.,** Factor V; see coagulation factors, under factor. **alpha g's,** globulins of plasma which in neutral or alkaline solutions have the greatest electrophoretic mobility, in this respect most nearly resembling the albumins. **antidiphtheritic g.,** the globulin which is the active constituent of antidiphtheritic serum. **antihemophilic g. (AHG),** Factor VIII; see coagulation factors, under factor. **antihuman g.,** precipitin for human globulin produced in nonhuman species by injection of human globulin. **anti–human g. serum** [USP], a sterile liquid preparation of serum produced by immunizing lower animals, such as rabbits or goats, with human serum or plasma or with selected human plasma proteins. It may be a general purpose reagent, containing, at a minimum, antibodies against IgG and the C3d component of complement, a reagent containing only antibodies against IgG (not heavy-chain specific), or reagents containing only antibodies specific for individual or selected components of complement or a single class of immunoglobulins (e.g., anti-IgG, heavy-chain specific). **antilymphocyte g.,** the gamma globulin fraction of antilymphocyte serum, a powerful immunosuppressant. **antitoxic g.,** the globulin which is the active constituent of an antitoxic serum. **Bence Jones g.,** see under protein. **beta g's,** globulins of plasma which have an electrophoretic mobility in neutral or alkaline solutions intermediate between that of the alpha and the gamma globulins. **corticosteroid-binding g. (CBG),** transcortin. **gamma g's,** a group of plasma globulins which, in neutral or alkaline solutions, have the slowest electrophoretic mobility and which have sites of antibody activity. See immunoglobulin. Also used, in the singular, to refer to immune g. **hepatitis B immune g.** [USP], a sterile nonpyrogenic solution consisting of globulins derived from blood plasma of human donors who have high titers of antibodies against hepatitis B surface antigen; used as a passive immunizing agent. **immune g., immune human serum g.** [USP], a sterile solution containing many antibodies normally present in adult human blood; it contains 15 to 18 gm. of protein per 100 ml., not less than 90 per cent of which is gamma globulin. Each lot is derived from an original plasma or serum pool representing venous or placental blood from at least 1000 individuals; used for passive immunization of susceptible contacts against infectious hepatitis, poliomyelitis, rubella, rubeola, and varicella, and in the treatment of gamma globulin deficiency, administered intramuscularly. Called also gamma g. and immune serum g. (human). **measles immune g.,** a sterile solution of globulins derived from the blood plasma of normal, adult human donors, which is prepared from immune serum globulin that complies, after dilution if necessary, with the measles antibody requirements of the U.S. Public Health Service. It contains not less than 10 gm. and not more than 18 gm. of protein per 100 ml., of which not less than 90 per cent is gamma globulin; used as a passive immunizing agent. **pertussis immune human g.** [USP], a sterile solution of globulins derived from the blood plasma of adult human donors immunized with pertussis vaccine, containing 10 to 18 gm. of protein per 100 ml., of which not less than 90 per cent is gamma globulin; used for the prophylaxis and treatment of pertussis, administered intramuscularly. Called also pertussis immune g. (human). **rabies immune g.** [USP], a sterile nonpyrogenic, slightly opalescent solution consisting of globulins from blood plasma or serum (negative for hepatitis B surface antigen) from adult human donors who have been immunized with rabies vaccine and have high titers of rabies antibody; used as a passive immunizing agent. **Rhₒ(D) immune human g.** [USP], a sterile solution of globulins derived from human blood plasma containing antibody to the erythrocyte factor Rhₒ(D); it contains 10 to 18 gm. of protein per 100 ml., not less than 90 per cent of which is gamma globulin. It is used to suppress formation of active Rhₒ(D) antibodies in Rhₒ(D)-negative mothers after delivery or miscarriage of a Rhₒ-(D)-positive baby or fetus when Rhₒ(D)-positive red cells enter the maternal circulation and thus to prevent erythroblastosis fetalis in the next pregnancy if the child is Rhₒ(D)-positive; administered intramuscularly. Called also Rhₒ immune g. (human), and Rhₒ (D antigen) immune g. **serum g.,** a group of proteins precipitated from plasma (or serum) by half saturation with ammonium sulfate; further fractionation of globulins into subgroups may be carried out by solubility, chromatography, electrophoresis, and ultracentrifugation. The principal groups include the α-, β-, and γ-globulins, which differ with respect to their association with lipids or carbohydrates and their content of physiologically significant features. The fractions include immunoglobulins (antibodies) in the β and γ fractions, lipoproteins in the α and β fractions, gluco- or mucoproteins, and metal-binding and metal-transporting proteins. Also present in globulin fractions are prothrombin, macroglobulin, plasminogen, euglobulin, fibrinogen, cryoglobulin, and antihemophilic globulin. **specific immune serum g.,** a sterile solution of globulins prepared from the sera of convalescent patients or those hyperimmunized to a given antigen; such preparations include measles, pertussis, mumps, tetanus, vaccinia, and Rh₀ immune globulin. **T g.,** a strong immunoglobulin band appearing in electrophoresis of horse serum after hyperimmunization; a possible subclass of IgG. **tetanus immune human g.** [USP], a sterile solution of gamma globulins derived from the blood plasma of adult human donors who have been immunized with tetanus toxoid, containing 10 to 18 gm. of protein per 100 ml., of which not less than 90 per cent is gamma globulin; used in the prophylaxis and treatment of tetanus, administered intramuscularly. Called also *tetanus immune g.* (*human*). **thyroxine-binding g.,** a plasma carrier protein that transports thyroxine in the blood. **vaccinia immune human g.** [USP], a sterile nonpyrogenic solution of globulins from the blood plasma of adult human donors who have been immunized with vaccinia virus (smallpox vaccine), containing 15 to 18 gm. of protein per ml., not less than 90 per cent of which is gamma globulin; used as a passive immunizing agent, administered intramuscularly. **g. X,** a globulin occurring in the intracellular spaces of muscle. **zoster immune g.,** specific immune globulin prepared from the plasma of those who have recovered from herpes zoster (shingles); used for prevention or treatment of varicella in susceptible or infected individuals, as those with immunodeficiency.

globulinuria (glob″u-lin-u′re-ah) [*globulin* + Gr. *ouron* urine + *-ia*] the presence of globulin in the urine.

globulose (glob′u-lōs) a proteose produced by action of pepsin on the globulins; several varieties have been described.

globulus (glob′u-lus), pl. *glob′uli* [L.] 1. the globose nucleus. 2. a pill, bolus, or spherical suppository. **glob′uli os′sei,** globules of bone tissue contained within lacunae of the calcified cartilage matrix in intrachondrial bone.

globus (glo′bus), pl. *glo′bi* [L.] 1. a sphere or ball; [NA] a general term denoting a spherical structure. 2. a subjective sensation as of a lump or mass. 3. see *globi,* def. 2. **g. abdomina′lis,** the sensation of a lump in the lower abdomen. **g. of the heel,** that portion of the wall of a horse's hoof where it curves around the heel to form the bar. **g. hyster′icus,** the subjective sensation of a lump in the throat, a condition frequently seen in hysteria. **g. ma′jor epididym′idis,** caput epididymidis. **g. mi′nor epididym′idis,** cauda epididymidis. **g. pal′lidus** [NA], the smaller and more medial part of the lentiform nucleus of the brain, separated from the putamen by the lateral medullary lamina and subdivided by the medial medullary lamina into internal and external parts; it has extensive connections with the striatum, thalamus, and mesencephalon.

glomangioma (glo-man″je-o′mah) [*glomus* + Gr. *angeion* vessel + *-oma*] a benign, often painful tumor derived from a neuromyoarterial glomus, usually occurring on the distal portions of the fingers and toes, in the skin or in deeper structures.

glomectomy (glo-mek′to-me) excision of a glomus, especially of the glomus caroticum.

glomera (glom′er-ah) [L.] plural of *glomus.*

glomerate (glom′er-āt) [L. *glomeratus* wound into a ball] crowded together into a ball.

glomerular (glo-mer′u-lar) pertaining to or of the nature of a glomerulus, especially a renal glomerulus.

glomeruli (glo-mer′u-li) [L.] plural of *glomerulus.*

glomerulitis (glo-mer″u-li′tis) inflammation of the glomeruli of the kidney, with proliferative or necrotizing changes of the endothelial or epithelial cells or thickening of the basement membrane.

glomerulonephritis (glo-mer″u-lo-ne̊-fri′tis) [*glomerulus* + *nephritis*] a variety of nephritis characterized by inflammation of the capillary loops in the glomeruli of the kidney. It occurs in acute, subacute, and chronic forms and may be secondary to hemolytic streptococcal infection. Evidence also supports possible immune or autoimmune mechanisms. **acute g.,** glomerulonephritis, typically preceded by tonsillitis or febrile pharyngitis, and characterized by proteinuria, edema, hematuria, renal failure, and hypertension. **chronic g.,** a slowly progressive glomerulonephritis generally leading to irreversible renal failure; it may be a primary disease, follow acute glomerulonephritis, or be secondary to systemic disease. Symptoms and course vary widely. **chronic lobular g.,** membranoproliferative g. **focal g.,** a condition in which only some glomeruli show inflammatory changes, others appearing normal. **focal embolic g.,** focal glomerulonephritis associated with bacterial endocarditis; see *Löhlein-Baehr lesion,* under *lesion.* **hypocomplementemic g.,** membranoproliferative g. **IgA g.,** a chronic form marked by hematuria and proteinuria and by deposits of IgA immunoglobulin in the mesangial areas of the renal glomeruli, with subsequent reactive hyperplasia of mesangial cells; called also *Berger's disease* and *IgA nephropathy.* **lobular g.,** membranoprolifer-

ative g. **lobulonodular g.,** membranoproliferative g. **malignant g.,** acute glomerulonephritis marked by a rapidly fatal course and by histological lesions in which diffuse epithelial proliferation is predominant from the outset. Principal signs are anuria, proteinuria, microscopic hematuria, and anemia. Called also *rapidly progressing g.* **membranoproliferative g., mesangiocapillary g.,** a chronic glomerulonephritis in which the glomeruli are enlarged, with marked accentuation of the lobular pattern, as a result of proliferation of mesangial cells and irregular thickening of the capillary walls which narrows the capillary lumina; it is a slowly progressive disease usually affecting older children and young adults of both sexes, with sudden onset of hematuria, proteinuria, or nephrotic syndrome. There is persistent reduction in complement levels in the serum, with deposition of activated complement components in the glomerular capillaries. Called also *chronic lobular g., hypocomplementemic g.,* and *lobular g.* **membranous g.,** a form characterized histologically by proteinaceous deposits on the glomerular capillary basement membrane or by thickening of the membrane. The clinical features are those of chronic glomerulonephritis, occasionally with transient nephrotic syndrome. **nodular g.,** membranoproliferative g. **rapidly progressing g.,** malignant g. **segmental g.,** focal glomerulonephritis in which only limited segments of affected glomeruli are diseased. **subacute g.,** persistence of acute glomerulonephritis, with or without periods of remission, which may develop into the lobular or malignant forms.

glomerulonephropathy (glo-mer″u-lo-ne̊-frop′ah-the) any noninflammatory disease of the renal glomeruli.

glomerulopathy (glo-mer″u-lop′ah-the) any disease of the renal glomeruli. **diabetic g.,** intercapillary glomerulosclerosis.

glomerulosclerosis (glo-mer″u-lo-skle-ro′sis) fibrosis and scarring which result in senescence of the renal glomeruli. **diabetic g.,** intercapillary g. **intercapillary g.,** a degenerative complication of diabetes, manifested as albuminuria, nephrotic edema, hypertension, renal insufficiency, and retinopathy.

glomerulose (glo-mer′u-lōs) glomerular.

glomerulotropin (glo-mer″u-lo-tro′pin) a substance, probably secreted by the diencephalon, capable of stimulating the zona glomerulosa of the adrenals to produce aldosterone; its rate of secretion is increased by a decreased sodium concentration.

glomerulus (glo-mer′u-lus), pl. *glomer′uli* [L., dim. of *glomus* ball] a tuft or cluster; used in anatomical nomenclature as a general term to designate such a structure, as one composed of blood vessels or nerve fibers. Often used alone to designate one of the glomeruli of the kidney (glomeruli renis [NA]). **arterial glomeruli, coccygeal,** glomus coccygeum. **glomer′uli arterio′si coch′leae** [NA], an arterial network surrounding the cochlea. **caudal glomeruli,** glomus coccygeum. **glomeruli of kidney, malpighian glomeruli,** glomeruli renis. **nonencapsulated nerve g.,** a nerve ending in the connective tissue of various organs in which the terminal branches of the nerve form spherical or elongated structures resembling glomeruli. **olfactory g.,** one of the small globular masses of dense neuropil in the olfactory bulb containing the first synapse in the olfactory pathway. **renal glomeruli, glomer′uli re′nis** [NA], globular tufts of capillaries, one projecting into the expanded end or capsule of each of the uriniferous tubules, which together with its surrounding capsule (*glomerular capsule*) constitute the renal corpuscle. Called also *glomeruli of kidney,* and *malpighian glomeruli.* See also plate accompanying *kidney.* **Ruysch's glomeruli,** glomeruli renis.

glomic (glo′mik) pertaining to or affecting a glomus.

glomoid (glo′moid) resembling a glomus.

glomus (glo′mus), pl. *glom′era* [L. "a ball"] [NA] a small, histologically recognizable body, composed primarily of fine arterioles connecting directly with veins, and possessing a rich nerve supply. **glom′era aor′tica** [NA], aortic bodies: small neurovascular structures on either side of the aorta in the region of the aortic arch; they contain chemoreceptors that play a role in reflex regulation of respiration by responding to changes in oxygen, carbon dioxide, and hydrogen ion concentration in the blood. **g. carot′icum** [NA], **carotid g., g. carotid′eum,** carotid body: a small neurovascular structure lying in the bifurcation of the right and left carotid arteries; it contains chemoreceptors that monitor the oxygen content of the blood and help to regulate respiration. **choroid g., g. choroi′deum** [NA], an enlargement of the choroid plexus of the lateral ventricle where the inferior horn joins the central part. **coccygeal g., g. coccyg′eum,** a collection of arteriovenous anastomoses formed, close to the tip of the coccyx, by the middle sacral artery; called also *Luschka's body, ganglion,* or *gland.* **cutaneous g., digital g., neuromyoarterial g.,** the total unit making up a Sucquet-Hoyer anastomosis; it is an organ located in the derma and cutaneous tissue, chiefly beneath the nails, and acting to control the circulation in the peripheral tissues. **g. intravaga′le,** an aggregation of chemoreceptors. **g. jugula′re,** an aggregation of chemoreceptors in the dome of the bulb of the jugular vein.

gloss- see *glosso-.*

glossa (glos′ah) [Gr. *glōssa*] the tongue (lingua [NA]).

glossagra (glos-sa′grah, glos′ag-rah) [*gloss-* + Gr. *agra* seizure] gouty pain of the tongue.

glossal (glos′al) pertaining to the tongue; lingual.

glossalgia (glos-sal′je-ah) [*gloss-* + *-algia*] pain in the tongue.

glossanthrax (glos-san′thraks) [*gloss-* + *anthrax*] carbuncle of the tongue.

glossectomy (glos-sek′to-me) [*gloss-* + Gr. *ektomē* excision] surgical removal of the tongue (*total g.*) or of a portion of it (*partial g.*).

Glossina (glos-si′nah) a genus of biting flies of the family Muscidae; the tsetse flies. **G. mor′sitans,** a fly of South Africa which transmits by its bite *Trypanosoma brucei*, the cause of nagana in horses; it also transmits *T. rhodesiense*, the cause of Rhodesia trypanosomiasis. **G. pallid′ipes,** a fly which trans-

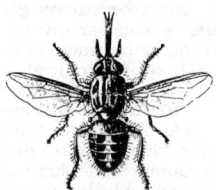

Glossina morsitans.

mits *Trypanosoma brucei.* **G. palpa′lis,** a species of Central Africa which transmits by its bite *Trypanosoma gambiense*, the organism causing African trypanosomiasis. Other species which probably transmit trypanosomes to animals and to man are: *G. brevipalpis, G. fusca, G. longipalpis, G. longipennis, G. morsitans, G. pallicera, G. pallidipes, G. swynnertoni, G. tachinoides.*

glossitis (glos-si′tis) [*gloss-* + *-itis*] inflammation of the tongue. **g. area′ta exfoliati′va,** geographic tongue. **atrophic g.,** Hunter's g. **benign migratory g.,** geographic tongue. **Hunter's g.,** a condition of the tongue seen in pernicious anemia, marked by smooth atrophy of the surface and edges. **idiopathic g.,** inflammation of the substance of the tongue and its mucous membrane. **g. mi′grans,** geographic tongue. **Moeller's g.,** chronic superficial glossitis, or glossodynia exfoliativa; an affection of the tongue sometimes extending to the cheeks and palate, affecting middle-aged people, especially women, and marked by burning pain and by red irregular patches, thinning of the papillae, and desquamation of the stratum corneum. Called also *chronic lingual papillitis.* **parasitic g., g. parasit′ica,** black tongue. **parenchymatous g.,** idiopathic g. **psychogenic g.,** glossopyrosis. **rhomboid g., median, g. rhomboi′dea media′na,** a congenital anomaly of the tongue, with a flat or slightly raised ovoid-, diamond-, or rhomboid-shaped reddish patch or plaque on the midline of the dorsal surface, immediately anterior to the circumvallate papillae.

glosso-, gloss- (glos′o, glos) [Gr. *glōssa* tongue] a combining form denoting relationship to the tongue.

glossocele (glos′o-sēl) [*glosso-* + Gr. *kēlē* tumor] swelling and protrusion of the tongue.

glossocinesthetic (glos″o-sin-es-thet′ik) glossokinesthetic.

glossocoma (glŏ-sok′o-mah) retraction of the tongue.

glossodynamometer (glos″o-di″nah-mom′ĕ-ter) [*glosso-* + *dynamometer*] an instrument for recording the power of the tongue to resist pressure.

glossodynia (glos″o-din′e-ah) [*glosso-* + Gr. *odynē* pain] pain in the tongue. **g. exfoliati′va,** Moeller's glossitis.

glossoepiglottic (glos″o-ep-ĭ-glot′ik) glossoepiglottidean.

glossoepiglottidean (glos″o-ep-ĭ-glo-tid′e-an) pertaining to the tongue and epiglottis.

glossograph (glos′o-graf) [*glosso-* + Gr. *graphein* to record] an apparatus for recording the tongue movements in speech.

glossohyal (glos″o-hi′al) [*glosso-* + *hyoid*] pertaining to the tongue and hyoid bone.

glossokinesthetic (glos″o-kin″es-thet′ik) [*glosso-* + *kinesthetic*] pertaining to the subjective perception of the movements of the tongue in speech.

glossolalia (glos″o-la′le-ah) [*glosso-* + Gr. *lalein* to babble] speech in unknown or imaginary language, as "speaking in tongues," a state observed in religious ecstasy in which the speaker (and the congregation) believes that God (or the gods) is speaking through him in celestial languages.

glossology (glŏ-sol′o-je) [*glosso-* + *-logy*] 1. the sum of knowledge regarding the tongue. 2. a treatise on nomenclature.

glossomantia (glos″o-man-ti′ah) [*glosso-* + Gr. *manteia* divination] prognosis based on the appearance of the tongue.

glossoncus (glŏ-song′kus) [*glosso-* + Gr. *onkos* mass] a swelling of the tongue.

glossopalatinus (glos″o-pal″ah-ti′nus) musculus palatoglossus.

glossopathy (glŏ-sop′ah-the) [*glosso-* + Gr. *pathos* disease] any disease of the tongue.

glossopexy (glos″o-pek′se) lip-tongue adhesion.

glossopharyngeal (glos″o-fah-rin′je-al) [*glosso-* + *pharynx*] pertaining to the tongue and pharynx.

glossopharyngeum (gos″o-fah-rin′je-um) [*glosso-* + *pharynx*] the tongue and pharynx together.

glossopharyngeus (glos″o-fah-rin′je-us) see *pars glossopharyngea musculi constrictoris pharyngis superioris.*

glossophytia (glos″o-fit′e-ah) [*glosso-* + Gr. *phyton* plant] black tongue.

glossoplasty (glos′o-plas″te) [*glosso-* + Gr. *plassein* to mold] plastic operation on the tongue.

glossoptosis (glos″op-to′sis) [*glosso-* + Gr. *ptōsis* fall] downward displacement or retraction of the tongue.

glossopyrosis (glos″o-pi-ro′sis) [*glosso-* + Gr. *pyrōsis* burning] a burning sensation in the tongue.

glossorrhaphy (glŏ-sor′ah-fe) [*glosso-* + Gr. *rhaphē* suture] suture of the tongue.

glossoscopy (glŏ-sos′ko-pe) [*glosso-* + Gr. *skopein* to examine] examination of the tongue.

glossospasm (glos′o-spazm) [*glosso-* + Gr. *spasmos* spasm] spasm of the tongue muscles.

glossosteresis (glos″o-ster-e′sis) glossectomy.

glossotilt (glos′o-tilt) [*glosso-* + Gr. *tillein* to pull] a lever which holds the tongue during one of the processes for artificial respiration.

glossotomy (glŏ-sot′o-me) [*glosso-* + Gr. *temnein* to cut] incision of the tongue.

glossotrichia (glos″o-trik′e-ah) [*glosso-* + Gr. *thrix* hair] hairy tongue.

glottal (glot′al) pertaining to the glottis.

glottic (glot′ik) 1. pertaining to the glottis. 2. pertaining to the tongue.

glottides (glot′ĭ-dēz) plural of *glottis.*

glottis (glot′is), pl. *glot′tides* [Gr. *glōttis*] [NA] the vocal apparatus of the larynx, consisting of the true vocal cords (plica vocalis) and the opening between them (rima glottidis). **false g.,** rima vestibuli. **intercartilaginous g., respiratory g.,** pars intercartilaginea rimae glottidis. **true g.,** rima glottidis.

glottitis (glŏ-ti′tis) glossitis.

glottology (glŏ-tol′o-je) glossology.

glou-glou (gloo′gloo) [Fr.] a gurgling sound produced in the stomach by various causes, such as the pressure of a girdle.

Glover's organism (gluv′erz) [T. J. *Glover*, Canadian bacteriologist, born 1887] see under *organism.*

glow (glo) incandescence; also brightness or warmth of color.

gloxazone (gloks′ah-zōn) chemical name: 2,2′-[1-(1-ethoxyethyl)-1,2-ethanediylidene]bishydrazine carbothioamide; a compound, $C_8H_{16}N_6OS_2$, used in *Anaplasma* infections in cattle.

Glu glutamic acid or glutamine.

glucagon (gloo′kah-gon) 1. a polypeptide hormone secreted by the alpha cells of the islets of Langerhans in response to hypoglycemia or to stimulation by the growth hormone of the anterior pituitary; it stimulates glycogenolysis in the liver by inducing activation of liver phosphorylase. Called also *hyperglycemic-glycogenolytic factor (HGF).* 2. [USP] the polypeptide occurring in the pancreas of these domestic mammals used for food by man, $C_{153}H_{225}N_{43}O_{49}S$, which has the property of increasing the blood glucose concentration, occurring as a fine, white or faintly colored crystalline powder; used in the form of the hydrochloride salt as an antihypoglycemic, administered parenterally. **intestinal g.,** enteroglucagon.

glucagonoma (glu″kah-gon-o′mah) a glucagon-secreting, usually malignant tumor of the alpha cells of the islets of Langerhans, which may be associated with a syndrome of dermatitis, stomatitis, elevated serum glucagon levels, abnormal glucose tolerance, weight loss, and anemia.

glucal (gloo′kal) an aldehyde derivative, $C_6H_{10}O_4$, of glucose.

glucan (gloo′kan) any polysaccharide (e.g., glycogen, starch, and cellulose) composed only of recurring units of glucose; a homopolymer of glucose.

glucase (gloo′kās) (*obs.*) an enzyme from plants and microorganisms, changing starch into dextroglucose.

glucatonia (gloo-kah-to′ne-ah) reduction of blood sugar to a point where pathologic symptoms are produced.

glucemia (gloo-se′me-ah) glycemia.

gluceptate (glu-sep′tāt) USAN contraction for glucoheptonate.

glucide (gloo′sīd) an organic substance consisting in whole or in part of carbohydrates; a general term, embracing the carbohydrates and glycosides.

glucidtemns (gloo′sid-tems) a collective name for the products produced by the digestion of starch, namely, dextrin, maltose, and glucose.

glucinium (gloo-sin′e-um) beryllium.

gluciphore (gloo′sĭ-fōr) glucophore.

gluco- (gloo′ko) [Gr. *gleukos* sweetness] a combining form denoting relationship to sweetness, or to glucose. Cf. *glyco-.*

glucocerebroside (gloo″ko-ser′ĕ-bro-sīd″) a cerebroside with a glucose sugar; it accumulates in the tissues in Gaucher's disease.

glucocinin (gloo″ko-sin′in) glucokinin.

glucocorticoid (gloo″ko-kor′tĭ-koid) 1. any of the group of corticosteroids predominantly affecting carbohydrate metabolism (promotion of gluconeogenesis, liver glycogen deposition, and elevation of blood glucose levels). They also influence fat and protein metabolism and have many other activities; e.g., they affect muscle tone and the excitation of nerve tissue and the microcirculation, increase gastric secretion, alter connective tissue response to injury, impede cartilage production, inhibit inflammatory, allergic, and immunological responses, suppress production of adrenocortical steroids and pituitary release of corticotropin, induce shrinkage of lymphatic tissue, and reduce the number of circulating lymphocytes. Some also exhibit varying degrees of mineralocorticoid activity. In man, the most important glucocorticoid is cortisol (hydrocortisone). Cf. *mineralocorticoid.* 2. of, pertaining to, or resembling a glucocorticoid.

Gluco-Ferrum (gloo″ko-fer′rum) trademark for preparations of ferrous gluconate.

glucofuranose (gloo″ko-fu′rah-nōs) a form of glucose in which carbon atoms 1 and 4 are bridged by an oxygen atom.

glucogenesis (gloo″ko-jen′ĕ-sis) the formation of glucose by the breakdown of glycogen.

glucogenic (gloo″ko-jen′ik) giving rise to or producing glucose.

glucohemia (gloo″ko-he′me-ah) glycemia.

glucokinase (gloo″ko-ki′nas) ATP:D-glucose 6-phosphotransferase. An enzyme that in the presence of ATP catalyzes the conversion of glucose to glucose 6-phosphate.

glucokinetic (gloo″ko-ki-net′ik) activating sugar so as to maintain the sugar level of the blood.

glucokinin (gloo″ko-kin′in) [*gluco-* + Gr. *kinein* to move] a hormone-like substance obtained from vegetable tissues and yeast, subcutaneous injection of which produces hypoglycemia in animals and acts on depancreatized dogs in a manner similar to insulin; called also *plant* or *vegetable insulin.*

glucolactone (gloo″ko-lak′tōn) a lactone from gluconic acid.

glucolysis (gloo-kol′ĭ-sis) glycolysis.

glucolytic (gloo″ko-lit′ik) glycolytic.

gluconate (gloo′ko-nāt) a salt of gluconic acid, containing the $HOCH_2(CHOH)_5COO-$ radical. **ferrous g.** [USP], a yellowish gray, or greenish yellow powder or granules, $C_{12}H_{22}FeO_{14} \cdot 2H_2O$, used as an iron supplement in iron-deficiency anemia; called also *iron gluconate.*

gluconeogenesis (gloo″ko-ne″o-jen′ĕ-sis) the formation of glucose from molecules that are not themselves carbohydrates, as from amino acids, lactate, and the glycerol portion of fats. Called also *glyconeogenesis.*

gluconeogenetic (gloo″ko-ne″o-jĕ-net′ik) pertaining to or involved in gluconeogenesis.

glucopenia (gloo-ko-pe′ne-ah) glycopenia.

glucophenetidin (gloo″ko-fĕ-net′ĭ-din) a derivative from paraphenetidin and dextrose, in silky white needles.

glucophore (gloo′ko-fōr) [*gluco-* + Gr. *phoros* bearing] the group of atoms in a molecule of a compound which is responsible for its sweet taste.

glucoprotein (gloo″ko-pro′te-in) glycoprotein.

glucoproteinase (gloo″ko-pro′te-in-ās) an enzyme that catalyzes the hydrolysis of glucoproteins.

glucopyranose (gloo″ko-pi′rah-nōs) a form of glucose in which carbon atoms 1 and 5 are bridged by an oxygen atom.

glucoregulation (gloo″ko-reg″u-la′shun) regulation of glucose metabolism.

glucosamine (gloo″ko-sam′ēn) chemical name: 2-amino-2-deoxy-D-glucose. An amino acid derivative of glucose, $C_6H_{13}NO_5$, obtained from mucin and chitin by hydrolysis and occurring in many polysaccharides of vertebrate tissue; called also *glycosamine.* **acetyl g.,** the structural unit of chitin.

glucosan (gloo′ko-san) an anhydro-polymer which on hydrolysis yields a hexose.

glucosazone (gloo″ko-sa′zōn) a yellow crystalline substance, $CH_2OH(CHOH)_3C(:N \cdot NH \cdot C_6H_5) \cdot CH:N \cdot NH \cdot C_6H_5$, produced by treating dextrose with phenylhydrazine and acetic acid; the crystals melt at 205° C. and may be used in the identification of glucose.

glucose (gloo′kōs) [Gr. *gleukos* sweetness; *glykys* sweet] 1. D-glucose, a monosaccharide (hexose), $C_6H_{12}O_6$, also known as *dextrose* (q.v.), found in certain foodstuffs, especially fruits, and in the normal blood of all animals. It is the end product of carbohydrate metabolism and is the chief source of energy for living organisms, its utilization being controlled by insulin. Excess glucose is converted to glycogen and stored in the liver and muscles for use as needed and, beyond that, is converted to fat and stored as adipose tissue. Glucose appears in the urine in diabetes mellitus. 2. liquid g. **Brun's g.,** a histologic clearing solution composed of glucose, distilled water, camphor, and glycerin. **gamma g.,** a very reactive form of glucose that can be isolated only as a

derivative. **liquid g.** [NF], an odorless, colorless or yellowish, thick syrupy liquid, with a sweet taste, consisting chiefly of dextrose, with dextrins, maltose, and water, and obtained by the incomplete hydrolysis of starch; used as a flavoring agent, tablet binder, and coating agent in pharamecutical preparations. It may be used as a food, often administered rectally, and has been used in the treatment of dehydration. Sometimes simply called *glucose.* **g. 1-phosphate,** an intermediate in carbohydrate metabolism, $CH_2OH \cdot CH(CHOH)_3CH \cdot O \cdot PO \cdot (OH)_2$. **g. 6-phosphate,** an intermediate in carbohydrate metabolism, $CHOH(CHOH)_3 \cdot CH \cdot CH_2O \cdot PO(OH)_2$.

glucosidase (gloo-ko′sĭ-dās) glucoside glucohydrolase: an enzyme that splits a glucoside. α-Glucosidase (maltase) occurs in the intestinal juice, and β-glucosidase (cellobiase) in the kidney, liver, and intestinal mucosa.

glucoside (gloo′ko-sīd) a glycoside in which the sugar constituent is glucose; originally the term glucoside was given to any of a variety of natural plant products containing a sugar, but it is now generally restricted to those in which the sugar is glucose. See *glycoside.*

glucosidolytic (gloo″ko-si″do-lit′ik) causing the splitting up of glucosides.

glucosin (gloo′ko-sin) any one of a group of bases derived from glucose by the action of ammonia; some are highly toxic.

glucosulfone sodium (gloo″ko-sul′fōn) chemical name: 1,1′-[sulfonylbis(4,1-phenyleneimino)]bis[1-deoxy-1-sulfo-D-glucitol]disodium salt. An antibacterial derivative of dapsone, $C_{24}H_{34}N_2Na_2O_{18}S_3$, having actions similar to those of the parent compound, occurring as white to faintly yellow, amorphous solid; used primarily as a leprostatic in the treatment of lepromatous and tuberculoid leprosy, administered intravenously.

glucosum (gloo-ko′sum) glucose.

glucosuria (gloo″ko-su′re-ah) [*glucose* + Gr. *ouron* urine + *-ia*] 1. the presence of glucose in the urine. 2. dextrosuria.

glucosyl (gloo′ko-sil) a glucose radical.

glucosyltransferase (gloo″ko-sil-trans′fer-ās) any enzyme that catalyzes the transfer of a glucosyl group, as from UDP to D-fructose to form sucrose; called also *transglucosylase.*

glucoxylose (gloo″ko-zi′lōs) a disaccharide, $C_{11}H_{20}O_{10}$, occurring in the leaves and branches of *Daviesia latifolia.*

glucurolactone (gloo″ku-ro-lak′tōn) chemical name: γ-lactone of D-glucofuranuronic acid; formerly used in treatment of arthritis, neuritis, and fibrositis.

glucuronate (gloo-ku′ro-nāt) a salt of glucuronic acid.

β-glucuronidase (gloo″ku-ron′ĭ-dās) β-D-glucuronide glucuronohydrolase: an enzyme that attacks glycosidic linkages in natural and synthetic glucuronides and has been implicated in estrogen metabolism and cell division. It occurs in the spleen, liver, and endocrine glands.

glucuronide (gloo-ku′ron-īd) any glycosidic compound of glucuronic acid; the glucuronides, which are generally inactive, constitute the major proportion of metabolites of many phenols, alcohols, and carboxylic acids.

glucuronolactone (gloo″ku-ro″no-lak′tōn) glucurolactone.

glue (gloo) an adhesive preparation in the form of impure gelatin derived from boiling certain animal substances, such as hoofs, in water.

Gluge's corpuscles (gloo′gez) [Gottlieb *Gluge*, German pathologist, 1812–1898] see under *corpuscle.*

glutamate (gloo′tah-māt) a salt of glutamic acid. In biochemistry, glutamate and glutamic acid are used interchangeably even though glutamate technically refers to the negatively charged ion.

glutaminase (gloo-tam′ĭ-nās) L-glutamine aminohydrolase: an enzyme that catalyzes the splitting of glutamine into glutamic acid and ammonia; it occurs in the liver, kidney, and brain and in bacteria and plants.

glutamine (gloo′tah-min) the monoamide of glutamic acid, $C_5H_{10}N_2O_3$, occurring in the juices of many plants and in some animal tissues; it is an important carrier of urinary ammonia and is broken down in the kidney by the enzyme glutaminase.

glutamyl (gloo′tah-mil) the univalent radical of glutamic acid.

glutaral (gloo′tah-ral) glutaraldehyde. **g. concentrate** [USP], a solution of glutaraldehyde in purified water, containing not less than 49 per cent and not more than 51 per cent by weight of glutaraldehyde; used as a disinfectant.

glutaraldehyde (gloo″tah-ral′dĕ-hīd) chemical name: pentanedial. A disinfectant, $C_5H_8O_2$, effective against vegetative gram-positive, gram-negative, and acid-fast bacteria, bacterial spores, some fungi, and viruses; used in an aqueous solution for sterilization of endoscopic equipment, thermometers, and plastic, rubber, or other non–heat-resistant equipment. It is also used topically as an anhidrotic and may be used in the treatment of warts. Glutaraldehyde is also used as a tissue fixative for light and electron microscopy because of its preservation of fine structural detail and localization of enzyme activity. Called also *glutaral.*

glutargin (gloo'tar-jin) arginine glutamate.

glutathione (gloo″tah-thi'ōn) [*glutamic acid* + Gr. *theion* sulfur] a tripeptide, γ-glutamyl-cysteinyl-glycine, HOOC·CH(NH₂)·-CH₂·CH₂·CO·NH·CH(CH₂·SH)·CO·NH·CH₂·COOH, composed of glutamic acid, cysteine, and aminoacetic acid, and isolated from animal and plant tissues. It is the coenzyme of glyoxalase and acts as a respiratory carrier of oxygen. **oxidized g.,** the precursor of reduced glutathione. Abbreviated GSSG. **reduced g.,** a tripeptide present in red cells, deficiency of which most probably predisposes erythrocytes to the oxidant and hemolytic effects of certain drugs, such as the antimalarial agents. It is functionally associated with glucose-6-phosphate dehydrogenase and reduced nicotinamide-adenine dinucleotide phosphate (NADP) in the maintenance of red cell integrity. Abbreviated GSH.

glutathionemia (gloo″tah-thi″o-ne'me-ah) the presence of glutathione in the blood.

glutathionuria (gloo″tah-thi″o-nu're-ah) the excretion of excessive amounts of glutathione in the urine.

gluteal (gloo'te-al) [Gr. *gloutos* buttock] pertaining to the buttocks.

glutelin (gloo'tĕ-lin) a simple protein, insoluble in all neutral solvents, but readily soluble in very dilute acids and alkalis and coagulable by heat; it occurs in seeds of cereals.

gluten (gloo'ten) [L. "glue"] the protein of wheat and other grains which gives to the dough its tough elastic character. **g.-casein,** a protein preparation employed in intestinal surgery to excite adhesive inflammation.

glutenin (gloo'tĕ-nin) the glutelin of wheat.

gluteofemoral (gloo″te-o-fem'or-al) [*gluteal* + *femoral*] pertaining to the buttock and thigh.

gluteoinguinal (gloo″te-o-in'gwĭ-nal) pertaining to the buttock and groin.

glutethimide (gloo-teth'ĭ-mīd) [USP] chemical name: 3-ethyl-3-phenyl-2,6-piperidinedione. A nonbarbiturate structurally related to phenobarbital, C₁₃H₁₅NO₂, occurring as a white, crystalline powder; used as a sedative and hypnotic, administered orally.

glutin (gloo'tin) 1. a viscid substance from the glutelin of wheat: gluten-casein. 2. gelatin in its soft, dissolved, or gelatinous state.

glutinous (gloo'tĭ-nus) [L. *glutinosus*] sticky; adhesive; gluey; viscid.

glutitis (gloo-ti'tis) [Gr. *gloutos* buttock + *-itis*] inflammation of the buttock.

glutolin (gloo'to-lin) an albuminoid substance found in small amounts in paraglobulin and thought to be a constant constituent of blood plasma. It is precipitated by treatment of blood plasma with magnesium sulfate.

glutoscope (gloo'to-skōp) an apparatus for observing agglutination.

glutose (gloo'tōs) an artificial glucoside that resembles glucose in many of its chemical reactions, but which seems to be inert in the body.

Gluzinski's test (gloo-zin'skēz) [Wladyslaw Antoni *Gluzinski*, a physician in Lemberg, 1856–1935] see under *tests*.

Gly glycine.

glyburide (gli'būr-īd) chemical name: 5-chloro-*N*-[2-[4-[[[(cyclohexylamino)carbonyl]amino]sulfonyl]phenyl]ethyl]-2-methoxybenzamide; an orally effective hypoglycemic agent of the sulfonylurea group, C₂₃H₂₈ClN₃O₅S. Called also *glibenclamide*.

glycal (gli'kal) an unsaturated sugar, —CH=CH—.

glycan (gli'kan) polysaccharide.

glycase (gli'kās) an enzyme that converts maltose and maltodextrin into dextrose.

glycemia (gli-se'me-ah) [Gr. *glykys* sweet + Gr. *haima* blood + *-ia*] the presence of glucose in the blood.

glycemin (gli'sĕ-min) a substance, secreted by the liver, in the blood of diabetics which has an antagonistic action toward insulin by inhibition to fixation of dextrose by erythrocytes.

glyceraldehyde (glis″er-al'de-hīd) a compound, glyceric aldehyde, CH₂OHCHOHCHO, formed by the oxidation of glycerol. **g. phosphate,** a triosephosphate which results from the decomposition of hexosephosphate in the chemistry of muscle contraction.

glycerate (glis'er-āt) a salt or ester of glyceric acid, CH₂₀H—CHOH—COOH.

glyceridase (glis'er-ĭ-dās) lipase.

glyceride (glis'er-īd) an organic acid ester of glycerol; the natural fats are glycerides of the higher fatty acids.

glycerin (glis'er-in) [L. *glycerinum*] [USP] chemical name: 1,2,3-propanetriol. A clear, colorless, syrupy liquid, C₃H₈O₃, obtained as a by-product of soap, by carbohydrate fermentation, and by propylene synthesis; administered rectally as a cathartic and orally as a diuretic to reduce intraocular pressure. It is also used as a solvent, humectant, and vehicle in various pharmaceutical preparations. See also *glycerol*.

glycerinated (glis'er-in-āt-ed) treated with or preserved in glycerin.

glycerinum (glis″er-i'num) [L.] glycerin.

glycerite (glis'er-īt) [L. *glyceritum*] a solution or mixture of a medicinal substance in glycerin; the glycerites for which official standards have been promulgated are boroglycerin, starch, and tannic acid glycerites. **boroglycerin g.,** see under *boroglycerin*. **starch g.** [NF], a preparation of starch, benzoic acid, glycerin, and purified water; used topically as an emollient; called also *glyceritum amyli*. **tannic acid g.,** a preparation of tannic acid, sodium citrate, exsiccated sodium sulfite, and glycerin, containing about 20 per cent of tannic acid; used as an astringent. Called also *glyceritum acidi tannici*.

glyceritum (glis″er-i'tum), gen. *glyceri'ti*, pl. *glyceri'ta* [L.] glycerite. **g. ac'idi tan'nici,** tannic acid glycerite. **g. am'yli,** starch glycerite. **g. boroglyceri'ni,** boro-glycerin glycerite.

glycerogel (glis'er-o-jel) a gel in which glycerin is the dispersed medium.

glycerogelatin (glis″er-o-jel'ah-tin) glycerin jelly.

glycerol (glis'er-ol) a trihydric sugar alcohol, CH₂OH·CHOH·-CH₂OH, being the alcoholic component of the fats; it is soluble in water and alcohol. Glycerol is an intermediate in the metabolism of fatty acids and serves as a phosphate acceptor. Pharmaceutical preparations are called glycerin (q.v.). **g. boroglycerite,** boroglycerin glycerite. **iodinated g.,** chemical name: 2-(1-iodoethyl)-1,3-dioxolane-4-methanol; an isomeric mixture of the iodinated dimers of glycerol, C₆H₁₁IO₃, used as an expectorant. **g. phosphate,** an intermediate in glycolysis and alcoholic fermentation, CH₂OH·CHOH·CH₂·O·PO(OH)₂.

glycerolize (glis'er-o-līz) to treat with or preserve in glycerol, as in the exposure of red blood cells to glycerol solution so that glycerol diffuses into the cells before they are frozen for preservation.

glycerophilic (glis″er-o-fil'ik) having a special affinity for glycerol.

glycerophosphatase (glis″er-o-fos'fah-tās) an enzyme which catalyzes the decomposition of glycerophosphates.

glycerophosphate (glis″er-o-fos'fāt) any salt of glycerophosphoric acid; several of them are used in nostrums together with alcohol as so-called nerve tonics. **ferric g.,** a greenish yellow powder, C₉H₂₁Fe₂O₁₈P₃, used as a tonic and in iron deficiency anemia; called also *iron glycerophosphate*.

glycerose (glis'er-ōs) a sugar formed by oxidizing glycerol; there are two glyceroses, glyceraldehyde and dihydroxyacetone.

glyceryl (glis'er-il) the trivalent radical, C₃H₅O₃, glycerol. **g. guaiacolate,** guaifenesin. **g. monostearate** [NF], a compound prepared from glycerin and stearic acid, occurring as a white waxlike solid, or white waxlike beads or flakes with a slight, pleasant, fatty odor and taste; used as an emulsifying agent. **g. triacetate,** triacetin. **g. trinitrate,** nitroglycerin.

glycidaldehyde (gli″sid-al'dĕ-hīd) a chemical used to inactivate virions in the preparation of virus vaccines.

glycide (gli'sid) glycidol.

glycidol (glis'id-ol) the oxide of hydroxypropene, isomeric with lactic aldehyde and acetol.

glycinate (gli'sin-āt) any salt of glycine (aminoacetic acid).

glycine (gli'sēn) chemical name: aminoacetic acid. A nonessential amino acid, H₂NCH₂COOH, occurring as a constituent of many proteins. It has been synthesized and is used as a gastric antacid and dietary supplement; it has also been used in the treatment of various myopathies. Glycine has also been postulated to be a neurotransmitter, inhibiting neural excitation in the central nervous system.

glycinemia (gli″sĭ-ne'me-ah) hyperglycinemia.

glycinin (glis'ĭ-nin) a globulin which constitutes 90 to 95 per cent of the protein content of soy bean.

Glyciphagus (gli-sif'ah-gus) *Glycyphagus*. **G. domes'ticus (G. pruno'rum),** *Glycyphagus domesticus*.

glyco- [Gr. *glykys* sweet] a combining form denoting relationship to sugar. Cf. *gluco-*.

glycobiarsol (gli″ko-bi-ar'sol) [USP] chemical name: [[4-(hydroxyacetyl)amino]phenyl]arsonato(1−) oxobismuth. An arsenic-and bismuth-containing compound, C₈H₉AsBiNO₆, occurring as a yellowish white to beige-pink, amorphous powder; used as an intestinal antiamebic, administered orally. It is also effective in trichomonal and candidal vaginitis and other nongonococcal vaginal infections, administered intravaginally.

glycocalix, glycocalyx (gli″ko-kal'iks) the glycoprotein and polysaccharide covering that surrounds many cells; in bacterial cells the glycocalyx forms masses of fibers which extend from the cell and by means of which the cell adheres to surfaces.

glycocholate (gli″ko-kol'āt) a salt of glycocholic acid; see *bile salts*, under *salt*.

glycocine (gli'ko-sin) aminoacetic acid.

glycoclastic (gli″ko-klas'tik) [*glyco-* + Gr. *klan* to break] glycolytic.

glycocoll (gli'ko-kol) [*glyco-* + Gr. *kolla* glue] glycine.

glycocyaminase (gli″ko-si′am″ĭ-nās) guanidinoacetate amidinohydrolase: an enzyme in the liver that hydrolyzes glycocyamine into urea and aminoacetic acid.

glycocyamine (gli″ko-si′ah-min) guanidinoacetic acid.

glycogelatin (gli″ko-jel′ah-tin) an ointment base containing glycerin and gelatin.

glycogen (gli′ko-jen) [glyco- + Gr. gennan to produce] a polysaccharide, (C₆H₁₀O₅)ₓ, the chief carbohydrate storage material in animals. It is a long-chain polymer of glucose, formed in and largely stored in the liver and to a lesser extent in muscles, being depolymerized to glucose and liberated as needed. Called also animal starch, tissue dextrin, and hepatin. **hepatic g.,** glycogen stored in the liver. **tissue g.,** glycogen stored in tissues other than the liver, especially in muscle.

glycogenase (gli′ko-jĕ-nās″) an enzyme that hydrolyzes glycogen to lower saccharides; see Cori ester, under ester.

glycogenesis (gli″ko-jen′ĕ-sis) [glyco- + genesis] 1. the formation or synthesis of glycogen. 2. the production of sugar.

glycogenetic (gli″ko-jĕ-net′ik) glycogenic.

glycogenic (gli″ko-jen′ik) pertaining to, characterized by, or promoting glycogenesis; pertaining to glycogen.

glycogenolysis (gli″ko-jĕ-nol′ĭ-sis) [glycogen + Gr. lysis dissolution] the splitting up of glycogen in the body tissues, yielding glucose.

glycogenolytic (gli″ko-jen″o-lit′ik) pertaining to, characterized by, or promoting glycogenolysis.

glycogenosis (gli″ko-jĕ-no′sis), pl. glycogenoses. Any of a group of metabolic disorders characterized by excessive storage of glycogen; for various forms, see glycogen storage disease, under disease. **generalized g.,** glycogen storage disease, type II; see under disease. **hepatorenal g.,** glycogen storage disease, type I; see under disease. **myophosphorylase deficiency g.,** glycogen storage disease, type V; see under disease.

glycogenous (gli-koj′ĕ-nus) glycogenetic.

glycogeusia (gli″ko-ju′se-ah) [glyco- + Gr. geusis taste] a condition in which there is a sweet taste in the mouth.

glycohemia (gli″ko-he′me-ah) [glyco- + Gr. haima blood + -ia] glycemia.

glycohemoglobin (gli″ko-he″mo-glo′bin) a glycosylated hemoglobin; see hemoglobin A₁c.

glycohistechia (gli″ko-his-tek′e-ah) [glyco- + Gr. histos tissue + echein to hold] the presence of an abnormally large amount of sugar in a tissue (Urbach).

glycol (gli′kol) any of a group of aliphatic dihydric alcohols, having marked hygroscopic properties and useful as solvents and plasticizers. Diethylene glycol should not be used for oral administration. **polyethylene g.,** see under P.

glycolate (gli′ko-lāt) a salt or ester of glycolic acid.

glycolipid (gli″ko-lip′id) a lipid containing carbohydrate groups, usually galactose but also glucose, inositol, or others. Phosphate may or may not be present, and glycerol or sphingosine may occur. The simplest are the glycodiacylglycerols. The glycolipids include the cerebrosides.

glycolyl (gli″ko-lil) the radical HOCH₂CO— of glycolic acid, HO·CH₂·COOH.

glycolysis (gli-kol′ĭ-sis) [glyco- + Gr. lysis solution] the anaerobic enzymatic conversion of glucose to the simpler compounds lactate or pyruvate, resulting in energy stored in the form of adenosine triphosphate (ATP), as occurs in muscle; it differs from respiration in that organic substances, rather than molecular oxygen, are used as electron acceptors.

glycolytic (gli″ko-lit′ik) pertaining to, characterized by, or promoting glycolysis.

glycometabolic (gli″ko-met-ah-bol′ik) pertaining to the metabolism of sugar.

glycometabolism (gli″ko-mĕ-tab′o-lizm) the metabolism of sugar.

glycone (gli′kōn) a glycerin suppository.

glyconeogenesis (gli″ko-ne″o-jen′ĕ-sis) [glyco- + Gr. neos new + gennan to produce] gluconeogenesis.

glyconucleoprotein (gli″ko-nu″kle-o-pro′te-in) a nucleoprotein bearing carbohydrate groups.

glycopenia (gli″ko-pe′ne-ah) [glyco- + Gr. penia poverty] a deficiency of sugar in the tissues.

glycopeptide (gli″ko-pep′tīd) any of a class of peptides that contain carbohydrates, including those that contain amino sugars.

glycopexic (gli″ko-pek′sik) pertaining to, characterized by, or promoting glycopexis.

glycopexis (gli″ko-pek′sis) [glyco- + Gr. pēxis fixation] the fixation or storing of sugar or glycogen.

Glycophagus (gli-kof′ah-gus) Glycyphagus.

glycophenol (gli″ko-fe′nol) glucide.

glycophilia (gli″ko-fil′e-ah) [glyco- + Gr. philein to love] a condition in which a very small amount of dextrose produces hyperglycemia.

glycophorin (gli″ko-for′in) a protein that projects through the thickness of the cell membrane of erythrocytes; it is attached to oligosaccharides at the outer cell membrane surface and to contractile proteins (spectrin and actin) at the cytoplasmic surface.

glycopolyuria (gli″ko-pol″e-u′re-ah) [glyco- + Gr. polys much + ouron urine + -ia] diabetes with a moderate increase of the sugar of the urine and with a marked increase of uric acid in the blood.

glycoprival (gli″ko-pri′val) [glyco- + L. privus deprived of] pertaining to or characterized by deprivation of carbohydrates.

glycoprotein (gli″ko-pro′te-in) any of a class of conjugated proteins consisting of a compound of protein with a carbohydrate group. They are distinguished by yielding in decomposition a product frequently capable of reducing alkaline solutions of cupric oxide. The glycoproteins include the mucins, the mucoids, and the chondroproteins. Glycoproteins having a very high content of polysaccharides are called proteoglycans.

glycoptyalism (gli″ko-ti′al-izm) [glyco- + Gr. ptyalon saliva] glycosialia.

glycopyrrolate (gli″ko-pir′ro-lāt) [USP] chemical name: 3-[(cyclopentylhydroxyphenylacetyl)oxy]-1,1-dimethyl pyrrolidinium bromide. A synthetic quaternary anticholinergic, C₁₉H₂₈BrNO₃, occurring as a white, crystalline powder; used in the treatment of peptic ulcer and other gastrointestinal disturbances in which hyperacidity, hypermotility, and/or spasm occur, administered orally, subcutaneously, intramuscularly, or intravenously. Called also glycopyrronium bromide.

glycopyrronium bromide (gli″ko-pir-ro′ne-um) glycopyrrolate.

glycoregulation (gli″ko-reg″u-la′shun) the control of sugar metabolism.

glycoregulatory (gli″ko-reg′u-lah-to″re) pertaining to the control of sugar metabolism.

glycorrhachia (gli″ko-ra′ke-ah) [glyco- + Gr. rhachis spine + -ia] presence of glucose in the cerebrospinal fluid.

glycorrhea (gli″ko-re′ah) [glyco- + Gr. rhoia flow] any sugary discharge, as of urine.

glycosamine (gli″ko-sam′in) glucosamine.

glycosaminoglycan (gli″kōs-am″ĭ-no-gli′kan) mucopolysaccharide, excluding its protein moiety.

glycosaminolipid (gli″kos-am″ĭ-no-lip′id) any of a class of lipids that contain amino sugars.

glycosecretory (gli″ko-se-kre′to-re) causing or concerned in the deposition of glycogen.

glycosemia (gli-ko-se′me-ah) glycemia.

glycosene (gli′ko-sēn) an anhydrosugar in which there is a double bond between two adjacent carbon atoms having hydroxyl groups in the trans position.

glycosialia (gli″ko-si-a′le-ah) [glyco- + Gr. sialon saliva + -ia] presence of glucose in the saliva.

glycosialorrhea (gli″ko-si″ah-lo-re′ah) [glyco- + Gr. sialon saliva + rhoia flow] excessive flow of saliva containing glucose.

glycosidase (gli′co-sĭ-dās) any of a large group of hydrolytic enzymes that attack glycosidic linkages. The α-glycosidases occur in the intestinal juice; the β-glycosidases in various tissues, including the liver, kidney, and spleen.

glycoside (gli′ko-sīd) any compound that contains a carbohydrate molecule (sugar), particularly any such natural product in plants, convertible, by hydrolytic cleavage, into sugar and a nonsugar component (aglycone), and named specifically for the sugar contained, as glucoside (glucose), pentoside (pentose), fructoside (fructose), etc. **cardiac g.,** any one of a group of glycosides occurring in certain plants (Digitalis, Strophanthus, Urginea, and others), which have a characteristic action on the contractile force of cardiac muscle. **cyanophoric g.,** a glycoside which on hydrolysis yields hydrocyanic acid. **sterol g.,** phytosterolin.

glycosometer (gli″ko-som′ĕ-ter) [glyco- + Gr. metron measure] an instrument used in determining the proportion of glucose in the urine.

glycosphingolipid (gli″ko-sfing″o-lip′id) a sphingolipid containing the sugar glucose or galactose.

glycostatic (gli″ko-stat′ik) tending to maintain a constant sugar level.

glycosuria (gli″ko-su′re-ah) [glyco- + Gr. ouron urine + -ia] the presence of glucose in the urine; especially the excretion of an abnormally large amount of sugar (glucose) in the urine, i.e., more than 1 gm. in 24 hours. **alimentary g.,** digestive g. **benign g.,** renal g. **digestive g.,** normal glycosuria following the ingestion of sugar. **emotional g.,** glycosuria induced by violent emotion. **epinephrine g.,** glycosuria following the injection of epinephrine. **hyperglycemic g.,** glycosuria associated with hyperglycemia. **magnesium g.,** glycosuria due to high concentration of magnesium in the blood. **nervous g.,** glycosuria produced by puncture of the fourth ventricle of the brain or by stimulation of the great splanchnic nerve. **nondiabetic g., nonhyperglycemic g., normoglycemic g., orthoglycemic g.,** renal g. **pathologic g.,** a condition in which large amounts of sugar appear in the urine for a considerable period of time. **phloridzin g., phlorhizin g.,** glycosuria following the administration of phlorhizin. **renal g.,** glycosuria occurring when there is only the normal amount of sugar in the blood, due to inherited inability of the renal tubules to reabsorb glucose completely. **toxic g.,** glycosuria produced by poisons.

glycosyl (gli′ko-sil) a radical derived from a carbohydrate.

glycosylated (gli-ko′sĭ-lāt″ed) having formed a linkage with a glycosyl group.

glycosylation (gli″ko-sĭ-la′shun) the formation of linkages with glycosyl groups.

glycosyltransferase (gli″ko-sil-trans′fer-ās) any enzyme that catalyzes the transfer of glycosyl groups from one molecule to another; the glycosyltransferases include the glucosyltransferases, fructosyltransferases, and pentosyltransferases. Called also *transglucosylase.* α**-glucan-branching g.,** α-1,4-glucan:α-1,4-glucan 6-glycosyltransferase. An enzyme that transfers part of a 1,4-glucan chain from a 4- to a 6-position, converting amylose into amylopectin. Called also *branching enzyme, Q enzyme,* and *amylo-1,4→1,6-transglucosylase.*

glycotaxis (gli″ko-tak′sis) [*glyco-* + Gr. *taxis* arrangement] the metabolic distribution of glucose to the body tissues.

glycotropic (gli″ko-trop′ik) [*glyco-* + Gr. *tropos* a turning] having an affinity for or attracting sugar; mediated by sugar; causing hyperglycemia.

glycuresis (gli″ku-re′sis) the normal increase in the glucose content of the urine which follows an ordinary carbohydrate meal.

glycuronide (gli-ku″ro-nīd) a compound formed by the union of glycuronic acid and some other substance, frequently an aromatic body.

glycuronuria (gli-ku″ro-nu′re-ah) the presence of glucuronic acid in the urine.

glycyl (glis′il) the univalent acid radical, H_2NCHC_2O, derived from aminoacetic acid.

glycylglycine (glis″il-glis′in) the simplest dipeptide, CH_2-$(NH_2)\cdot CO\cdot NH\cdot CH_2\cdot CO_2\cdot H$.

glycyltryptophan (glis″il-trip′to-fan) a dipeptide consisting of glycine and tryptophan radicals; used as a test for cancer of stomach. See under *tests.*

Glycyphagus (gli-sif′ah-gus) [Gr. *glykys* sweet + *phagein* to eat] a genus of mites. **G. domes′ticus,** the food mite; the causative agent of grocers' itch.

Glycyrrhiza (glis″ĭ-ri′zah) [Gr. *glykys* sweet + *rhiza* root] a genus of leguminous plants.

glycyrrhiza (glis″ir-ri′zah) [NF] the dried rhizome and roots of *Glycyrrhiza glabra* (Spanish licorice) or its variety *glandulifera* (Russian licorice), or of other varieties; used as a pharmaceutic necessity for the preparation of pure glycyrrhiza extract; see under *extract.* Called also *licorice, licorice root,* and *liquorid.*

glycyrrhizin (glis″ĭ-ri′zin) [L. *glycyrrhizinum*] a very sweet substance $C_{42}H_{62}O_{16}$, from glycyrrhiza; has been used in the treatment of Addison's disease.

glydanile sodium (gli′dah-nīl) glicetanile sodium.

glykemia (gli-ke′me-ah) glycemia.

glymidine sodium (gli′mĭ-dēn) chemical name: N-[5-(2-methoxyethoxy)-2-pyrimidinyl]benzene sulfonamide sodium salt; an oral hypoglycemic, $C_{13}H_{14}N_3NaO_4S$.

glyoxal (gli-ok′sal) a yellow crystalline compound, $O:HC\cdot CH:O$, prepared by the oxidation of acetaldehyde; called also *biformyl, ethanedial,* and *oxalaldehyde.*

glyoxalase (gli-ok′sah-lās) either of two enzymes: glyoxalase I is lactoyl-glutathione lyase, and glyoxalase II is hydroxyacyl-glutathione hydrolase.

glyoxalin (gli-ok′sah-lin) iminazole.

glyoxisome (gli-ok′sĭ-sōm) glyoxosome.

glyoxosome (gli-ok′so-sōm) any of the microbodies present in certain plants and microorganisms, resembling the peroxisomes of vertebrate animal cells, but having, in addition to catalase and oxidase enzymes, the enzymes of the glyoxylate cycle, a metabolic pathway involved in the conversion of fat to carbohydrate. Glyoxosomes, in association with chloroplasts, also participate in the process of photorespiration. Called also *glyoxisome.* See also *microbody* and *peroxisome,* def. 1.

glyoxylate (gli-ok′sĭ lāt) a salt of ester of glyoxylic acid.

glyphylline (gli-fil′lin) dyphylline.

Glyptocranium (glip″to-kra′ne-um) *Mastophora.* **G. gasteracanthoi′des,** *Mastophora gasteracanthoides.*

Glytheonate (gli-the′o-nāt) trademark for a preparation of theophylline sodium glycinate.

Gm [abbreviation for gamma] a genetically determined allotypic marker on the heavy chain of human IgG, inherited as a simple Mendelian trait and found on both the Fc and Fd fragments of the γ chain; over 20 allotypes are known.

gm *gram.*

G.M.C. General Medical Council (British).

Gmelin's test (ma′linz) [Leopold *Gmelin,* German physiologist, 1788–1853] see under *tests.*

GMK a preparation of green monkey kidney cells used as culture system for growing viruses, e.g., for recovering the rubella virus.

GMP guanosine monophosphate.

gnat (nat) a small dipterous insect. In England the term is applied to mosquitoes; in America to insects smaller than mosquitoes. See *Chironomidae.* **buffalo g.,** a name given various individuals of the family Simuliidae. **eye g.,** *Hippelates pusio.* **fungus g.,** a gnat whose larvae feed on fungi; see *Bradysia* and *Sciaria.* **turkey g.,** a name given various individuals of the family Simuliidae.

gnath- see *gnatho-.*

gnathalgia (nath-al′je-ah) [*gnath-* + *-algia*] pain in the jaw.

gnathic (nath′ik) pertaining to the jaw or cheek.

gnathion (nath′e-on) an anthropologic and cephalometric landmark, indicating the most outward and everted point on the profile curvature of the chin.

gnathitis (nath-i′tis) [*gnath-* + *-itis*] inflammation of the jaw.

gnatho-, gnath- (nath′o, nath) [Gr. *gnathos* jaw] a combining form denoting relationship to the jaw.

Gnathobdellidae (nath″ob-del′ĭ-de) a family of the Hirudinea, which includes leeches of the genera *Hirudo, Limnatis, Haemadipsa, Macrobdella, Theromyzon, Haemopis, Dinobdella,* and *Hirudinaria.*

gnathocephalus (nath″o-sef′ah-lus) [*gnatho-* + Gr. *kephalē* head] a monster with no head except the jaws.

gnathodynamics (nath″o-di-nam′iks) [*gnatho-* + Gr. *dynamis* power] the study of the physical forces used in mastication.

gnathodynamometer (nath″o-di″nah-mom′ĕ-ter) [*gnatho-* + *dynamometer*] an instrument for measuring the force exerted in closing the jaws; called also *occlusometer.* **bimeter g.,** a gnathodynamometer equipped with a central-bearing point of adjustable height.

gnathodynia (nath″o-din′e-ah) [*gnatho-* + *odynē* pain] pain in the jaw.

gnathography (nath-og′rah-fe) [*gnatho-* + Gr. *graphein* to record] the recording of the strength of a patient's bite by a tracing of the changes in the flow of an electric current through a bite gauge.

gnathologic (nath″o-loj′ik) relating to gnathology.

gnathology (nath-ol′o-je) a science which deals with the masticatory apparatus as a whole, including morphology, anatomy, histology, physiology, pathology, and therapeutics.

gnathoplasty (nath′o-plas″te) [*gnatho-* + Gr. *plassein* to mold] plastic surgery of the jaw or cheek.

gnathoschisis (nath-os′kĭ-sis) [*gnatho-* + Gr. *schisis* splitting] congenital cleft of the upper jaw, as in cleft palate.

gnathostatics (nath″o-stat′iks) [*gnatho-* + Gr. *statikē* the art of weighing] a method of orthodontic diagnosis based on determination of the basal and craniometric relationships between the teeth and their supporting structures.

Gnathostoma (nath-os′to-mah) [*gnatho-* + Gr. *stoma* mouth] a genus of nematode worms of the superfamily Spiruroidea, which are parasitic in cats, swine, cattle, and sometimes in man. **G. spinig′erum,** a nematode parasitic in the stomach of cats and dogs that ingest fish which contain the larvae; man acquires the larvae when he eats undercooked fish. See *gnathostomiasis.*

gnathostomatics (nath″o-sto-mat′iks) the physiology of the mouth and jaws.

gnathostomiasis (nath″o-sto-mi′ah-sis) infection with the nematode *Gnathostoma spinigerum,* acquired when undercooked fish harboring the larvae are eaten. The larvae migrate, often in the subcutaneous tissue, causing a "creeping swelling" associated with intense eosinophilia. Occasionally they migrate to deeper tissues and cause abscesses.

Gnathostomum (nath-os′to-mum) *Gnathostoma.*

gnosia (no′se-ah) the faculty of perceiving and recognizing.

gnosis (no′sis) [Gr. *gnōsis* knowledge] Edinger's term for the arousal of associative mnemonic complexes by sensory pallial impulses; one of the functions of the cerebral cortex. Cf. *praxis.*

gnotobiology (no″to-bi-ol′o-je) gnotobiotics.

gnotobiota (no″to-bi-o′tah) the specifically and entirely known microfauna and microflora of a specially reared laboratory animal.

gnotobiote (no′to-bi′ōt) a specially reared laboratory animal the microfauna and microflora of which are specifically known in their entirety.

gnotobiotic (no′to-bi-ot′ik) pertaining to a gnotobiote or to gnotobiotics. Cf. *axenic.*

gnotobiotics (no″to-bi-ot′iks) [Gr. *gnotos* known + *biota* the fauna and flora of a region] the science of rearing laboratory animals the microfauna and microflora of which are specifically known in their entirety.

gnotophoresis (no″to-for′ĕ-sis) [Gr. *gnotos* known + *phōresis* a being borne] the state of existence of an organism bearing one or more known species in intimate contact with it and no other demonstrable viable microorganisms.

gnotophoric (no''to-for'ik) pertaining to gnotophoresis.

Gn-RH gonadotropin-releasing hormone; see under *hormone*.

Goa powder (go'ah) [*Goa* a city of India] see under *powder*.

goatpox (gōt'poks) an acute, highly infectious disease of goats marked by a vesicular eruption with catarrh of the respiratory mucous membranes and caused by a poxvirus. It is less severe than sheep-pox. Called also *variola caprina*.

Godélier's law (go-da-lyāz') [Charles Pierre *Godélier*, French physician, 1813–1877] see under *law*.

Goetsch's skin reaction (test) (gech'ez) [Emil *Goetsch*, American physician, born 1883] see under *reaction*.

goiter (goi'ter) an enlargement of the thyroid gland, causing a swelling in the front part of the neck. **aberrant g.,** enlargement of an ectopic or supernumerary thyroid gland. **adenomatous g.,** enlargement of the thyroid gland caused by adenomas of the gland, or by multiple colloid nodules. **Basedow's g.,** a colloid goiter which has become hyperfunctioning after administration of iodine. **colloid g.,** a large and soft form of goiter in which the follicles of the gland are greatly distended with colloid. **congenital g.,** enlargement of the thyroid gland which is present at birth, or which results from a congenital absence of enzymes leading to inadequate production of thyroxine. **cystic g.,** an enlarged thyroid gland containing cysts formed by mucoid or colloid degeneration. **diffuse g.,** a thyroid gland which is diffusely enlarged. **diving g.,** a movable goiter located sometimes above and sometimes below the sternal notch. **endemic g.,** enlargement of the thyroid gland occurring in certain districts, particularly in the mountain regions of the Alps, Pyrenees, Carpathians, Andes, and Himalayas, and other areas where the iodine content of the normal diet is low. **exophthalmic g.,** enlargement of the thyroid gland with protrusion of the eyeballs; see *Graves' disease,* under *disease*. **fibrous g.,**

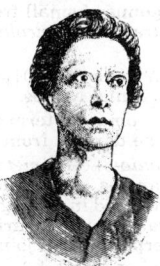

Exophthalmic goiter.

enlargement of the thyroid gland caused by hyperplasia of the capsule and stroma. **follicular g.,** parenchymatous g. **intrathoracic g.,** goiter in which a portion of the enlarged thyroid is situated in the thoracic cavity. **iodide g.,** that occurring in reaction to iodides at high concentrations, due to inhibition of iodide organification (Wolff-Chaikoff effect). **lingual g.,** an enlargement of the upper end of the original thyroglossal duct, forming a tumor at the posterior part of the dorsum of the tongue. **lymphadenoid g.,** struma lymphomatosa. **nodular g.,** an enlarged thyroid gland containing circumscribed nodules within its substance. **nontoxic g.,** that occurring sporadically and not associated with hyperthyroidism; such goiters may be either diffuse or nodular. **parenchymatous g.,** goiter marked by increase in the follicles and proliferation of the epithelium. **perivascular g.,** one which surrounds a large blood vessel. **plunging g.,** diving g. **retrovascular g.,** goiter with a process or processes behind an important blood vessel. **simple g.,** simple hyperplasia of the thyroid gland. **substernal g.,** goiter in which a portion of the enlarged gland is situated beneath the sternum. **suffocative g.,** one which causes dyspnea by pressure. **toxic g.,** Graves' disease; see under *disease*. **vascular g.,** enlargement of the thyroid gland due chiefly to dilatation of the blood vessels. **wandering g.,** diving g.

goitre (goi'ter) [Fr.] goiter.

goitrin (goi'trin) a goitrogenic substance isolated from rutabagas and turnips.

goitrogen (goi'tro-jen) a goiter-producing compound.

goitrogenic (goi-tro-jen'ik) producing goiter.

goitrogenicity (goi''tro-jĕ-nis'ĭ-te) the tendency to produce goiter.

goitrogenous (goi-troj'ĕ-nus) producing goiter.

goitrous (goi'trus) pertaining to or of the nature of goiter.

gold (gōld) a yellow metallic element occurring in masses or veins in rocks or in grains in the sand of rivers. Its symbol is Au (L. *au'rum*); atomic number, 79; atomic weight, 196.967; specific gravity, 19.32. Gold compounds are used in medicine, chiefly in arthritis, and all the compounds are poisonous. **annealed g.,** gold which has been heated in a flame to drive off any contaminating gases and increase its cohesive properties. **g. aurothio-**

sulfate, g. sodium thiosulfate. **cohesive g.,** a chemically pure gold which can be made to form a solid block when properly compacted or condensed into a tooth cavity. **colloidal g.,** a purplish suspension of minute particles of metallic gold, made by reducing a solution of bromauric acid or other acid or salt of gold, used in medicine since alchemical times. The radioactive form, made by exposure to neutrons, is used as a suspension in the pleural cavity to treat lung cancer. **crystal g., crystalline g.,** mat g. **Dutch g.,** an alloy of copper and zinc. **fibrous g.,** mat g. **mat g.,** a type of pure gold composed of flakelike crystals formed by electrodeposition. **noncohesive g.,** gold which does not weld because of a gaseous contaminant on its surface. **Nürnberg g.,** a preparation containing 2.5 per cent gold, 7.5 per cent aluminum, and 90 per cent copper. **radioactive g.,** radiogold. **g. sodium thiomalate** [USP], an odorless, fine, white to yellowish white powder with a metallic taste, $C_4H_3AuNa_2O_4S \cdot H_2O$, used in treatment of rheumatoid arthritis and nondisseminated lupus erythematosus, administered intramuscularly. Called also *sodium aurothiomalate*. **g. sodium thiosulfate,** white needle-like or prismatic small glistening crystals, $Na_3Au(S_2O_3)_2 \cdot 2H_2O$, soluble in water; used in the treatment of rheumatoid arthritis. Called also *sodium aurothiosulfate*. **g. thioglucose,** aurothioglucose.

Goldblatt's clamp, hypertension, kidney [Harry *Goldblatt*, Cleveland physician, born 1891] see under *clamp, hypertension,* and *kidney*.

Goldflam's disease (gōlt'flahmz) [Samuel *Goldflam*, Polish neurologist, 1852–1932] myasthenia gravis.

Goldflam-Erb disease (gōlt'flahm-ērb) [S. V. *Goldflam;* Wilhelm Heinrich *Erb,* German internist, 1840–1921] myasthenia gravis.

Goldscheider's percussion, test (gōld'shi-derz) [Johannes Karl August Eugen Alfred *Goldscheider,* Berlin physician, 1858–1935] see *threshold percussion,* under *percussion,* see *orthopercussion;* and see under *tests*.

Goldstein's disease, etc. (gōld'stīnz) [Hyman Isaac *Goldstein,* American physician, 1887–1954] see under *disease, hematemesis, hemoptysis,* and *sign*.

Goldstein rays (gōld'stīn) [Eugene *Goldstein,* German physicist, 1850–1930] see under *ray*.

Goldthwait's sign (symptom) (gōld'thwāts) [Joel Ernest *Goldthwait,* American orthopedic surgeon, born 1866] see under *sign*.

Golgi's complex, etc. (gol'jēz) [Camillo *Golgi,* Italian histologist, 1843–1926; co-winner, with Santiago Ramón y Cajal, of the Nobel prize for medicine and physiology in 1906 in recognition of their work on the structure of the nervous system] see under *complex, corpuscle, law, neuron, organ, Table of Stains,* and *theory*.

golgiosome (gol'je-o-sōm) mitochondrium-sized, platelike structures which make up the Golgi complex of the cell; the platelike structure consists of stacks of flattened vessels (cisternae) more commonly known as dictyosomes.

Goll's column, fasciculus (column, tract), fibers, nucleus (golz) [Friedrich *Goll,* Swiss anatomist, 1829–1903] see *fasciculus gracilis medullae spinalis,* and *nucleus gracilis,* and see under *fiber*.

Goltz's experiment, theory (gōlts'ez) [Friedrich Leopold *Goltz,* German physician, 1834–1902] see under *experiment* and *theory*.

Gombault's degeneration, neuritis (gom-bōz') [François Alexis Albert *Gombault,* French neurologist, 1844–1904] progressive hypertrophic interstitial neuropathy.

Gombault-Philippe triangle (gom-bo'fe-lēp') [F. A. A. *Gombault;* Claudius *Philippe,* French pathologist, 1866–1903] see under *triangle*.

gomitoli (go-mit'o-li) a network of capillaries in the upper infundibular stem (of the hypothalamus) that surround terminal arterioles of the superior hypophyseal arteries and that lead into portal veins to the adenohypophysis.

Gomori methods, stains [George *Gomori,* Hungarian histochemist in Chicago, 1904–1957] see *Table of Stains and Staining Methods,* under *stain*.

gomphiasis (gom-fi'ah-sis) [Gr. "tooth ache," "gnashing of the teeth"] 1. looseness of the teeth. 2. odontalgia.

gomphosis (gom-fo'sis) [Gr. *gomphōsis* a bolting together] [NA] a type of fibrous joint in which a conical process is inserted into a socket-like portion, such as the styloid process in the temporal bone, or the teeth in the dental alveoli.

gon- (gon) 1. [Gr. *gonē* seed] a combining form denoting relation to seed or to the semen. 2. [Gr. *gony* knee] a combining form denoting relationship to the knee.

gonacratia (gon''ah-kra'she-ah) [*gon-*(1) + Gr. *akrateia* incontinence] spermatorrhea.

gonad (go'nad, gon'ad) [L. *gonas,* from Gr. *gonē* seed] a gamete-producing gland; an ovary or testis. **indifferent g.,** the sexually undifferentiated gonad of the early embryo. **third g.,** the adrenal gland, so called because of the interrelationship between it and the sex glands. **streak g's,** an undeveloped gonadal structure found in the broad ligament below the fallopian tube and composed of whorled connective-tissue stroma with no germinal or secretory cells; seen most often in Turner's syndrome. Phenotypic development is female.

gonadal (go′nad-al)   pertaining to a gonad.

gonadectomize (go″nah-dek′to-mīz)   to deprive of the gonads by surgical excision.

gonadectomy (go″nah-dek′to-me) [*gonad* + Gr. *ektomē* excision] removal of an ovary or testis.

gonadial (go-nad′e-al)   pertaining to a gonad.

gonadoblastoma (gon″ah-do-blas-to′mah)   a dysgerminoma that contains all gonadal elements—germ cells, sex cord derivatives and stromal derivatives; occurring almost exclusively in abnormal gonads, most often associated with some form of gonadal dysgenesis, frequently with abnormal chromosomal karyotype.

gonadogenesis (gon″ah-do-jen′ĕ-sis) [*gonado-* + Gr. *genesis* production]   the development of the gonads in the embryo, especially the development of gonads typical of one or the other sex.

gonadoinhibitory (gon″ah-do-in-hib′ĭ-to-re)   inhibiting or preventing gonadal activity.

gonadokinetic (gon″ah-do-ki-net′ik) [*gonad* + Gr. *kinēsis* motion]   stimulating gonadal activity.

gonadopathy (gon″ah-dop′ah-the) [*gonad* + Gr. *pathos* disease] any disease of the gonads.

gonadopause (go-nad′o-paws)   the loss of gonadal activity which accompanies the aging process.

gonadorelin (go″nad-o-rel′in)   gonadotropin releasing hormone.

gonadotherapy (gon″ah-do-ther′ah-pe)   treatment by the use of hormones from the ovary or testis.

gonadotrope (go-nad′o-trōp)   1. any of the basophils (beta cells) of the adenohypophysis, the granules of which secrete follicle-stimulating hormone and luteinizing hormone. It is not yet settled whether there are two distinct cell types or whether one cell type secretes both hormones; called also *delta basophil* and *delta cell*. 2. a gonadotropic substance.

gonadotroph (go-nad′o-trōf)   gonadotrope.

gonadotrophic (gon″ah-do-tro′fik)   gonadotropic.

gonadotrophin (gon″ah-do-tro′fin)   gonadotropin.

gonadotropic (gon″ah-do-trōp′ik) [*gonad* + Gr. *tropos* a turning] stimulating the gonads; applied to hormones of the anterior pituitary which influence the gonads.

gonadotropin (gon″ah-do-tro′pin)   any hormone having a stimulating effect on the gonads. Two such hormones are secreted by the anterior pituitary: follicle-stimulating hormone and luteinizing hormone, both of which are active, but with differing effects, in the two sexes. See also *chorionic g.* **chorionic g.,** 1. the gonad-stimulating principle produced by the cytotrophoblastic cells of the placenta and excreted through the kidneys. 2. [USP] the same principle obtained from the urine of pregnant women, occurring as a white or practically white, amorphous powder; used in the treatment of certain cases of cryptorchidism and male hypogonadism, and to induce ovulation and pregnancy in certain infertile, anovulatory women, administered intramuscularly. **equine g.,** pregnant mare serum g. **human chorionic g. (HCG),** see *chorionic g.* **human menopausal g. (HMG),** menotropins. **pregnant mare serum g.,** a preparation of the follicle-stimulating substance obtained from the blood serum of pregnant mares; it has been used in the treatment of cryptorchidism, sterility, pituitary dwarfism, and other conditions in both men and women. Called also *equine g.* Abbreviated PMSG.

gonaduct (gon′ah-dukt)   the duct of a gonad; an oviduct or seminal duct.

gonagra (gon-ag′rah) [*gon-*(2) + Gr. *agra* seizure]   gout in the knee.

gonalgia (go-nal′je-ah) [*gon-*(2) + *-algia*]   pain in the knee.

gonangiectomy (gon″an-je-ek′to-me)   vasectomy.

gonarthritis (gon″ar-thri′tis) [*gon-*(2) + Gr. *arthron* joint + *-itis*] inflammation of a knee or knee joint.

gonarthrocace (gon″ar-throk′a-se) [*gon-*(2) + Gr. *arthron* joint + *kakē* evil]   white swelling of the knee, produced by tuberculous arthritis.

gonarthromeningitis (gon-ar″thro-men″in-ji′tis) [*gon-*(2) + Gr. *arthron* joint + *mēninx* membrane]   inflammation of the synovial membrane of the knee joint.

gonarthrosis (gon″ar-thro′sis)   arthritic affection of the knee joint, due to degeneration or trauma.

gonarthrotomy (gon″ar-throt′o-me) [*gon-*(2) + Gr. *arthron* joint + *temnein* to cut]   surgical incision of the knee joint.

gonatocele (go-nat′o-sēl) [*gon-*(2) + Gr. *kēlē* tumor]   tumor of the knee.

gonecyst, gonecystis (gon′ĕ-sist, gon″ĕ-sis′tis) [Gr. *gonē* seed + *kystis* bladder]   vesicula seminalis.

gonecystitis (gon″ĕ-sis-ti′tis)   inflammation of a seminal vesicle.

gonecystolith (gon″ĕ-sis′to-lith) [*gonecyst* + Gr. *lithos* stone]   a concretion in a seminal vesicle.

gonecystopyosis (gon″ĕ-sis″to-pi-o′sis) [*gonecyst* + Gr. *pyōsis* suppuration]   suppuration in a seminal vesicle.

goneitis (gon″e-i′tis) [*gon-*(2) + *-itis*]   inflammation of the knee.

gonepoiesis (gon″e-poi-e′sis) [Gr. *gonē* seed + *poiein* to make] the secretion or formation of the semen.

gonepoietic (gon″e-poi-et′ik)   pertaining to, characterized by, or promoting gonepoiesis.

Gongylonema (gon″jĭ-lo-ne′mah) [Gr. *gongylos* round + *nēma* thread]   a genus of nematodes of the superfamily Spiruroidea. **G. ingluvic′ola,** a species found in chickens. **G. neoplas′ticum,** a species occurring in the anterior portion of the digestive tract of rats. **G. pul′chrum,** a common parasite in the esophageal mucosa of sheep, goats, cattle, and pigs in the United States; it has been found in the mucosa and submucosa of the lips and mouth of man. **G. scuta′tum,** G. pulchrum.

gongylonemiasis (gon″jĭ-lo-ne-mi′ah-sis)   infection with *Gongylonema.*

gonia (go′ne-ah)   plural of *gonion.*

gonial (go′ne-al)   pertaining to the gonion.

gonidangium (gon″id-an′je-um)   a cell within which gonidia are formed.

gonidia (go-nid′e-ah)   plural of *gonidium.*

gonidiospore (go-nid′e-o-spōr)   1. a general term for a sexual spore of fungi, as one produced from an antherium. 2. a spore produced from the algal part of a lichen. See *spore.*

gonidium (go-nid′e-um), pl. *gonid′ia* [Gr. *gonē* seed]   1. the algal cell part of the thallus of a lichen. 2. a motile reproductive unit of the nitrogen-fixing bacteria *Azotobacter* and *Rhizobium.*

Gonin's operation (go-nāz′) [Jules *Gonin,* Swiss ophthalmic surgeon, 1870–1935]   see under *operation.*

gonio- (go′ne-o) [Gr. *gōnia* angle]   a combining form denoting relationship to an angle.

Goniobasis (go″ne-o-ba′sis)   a genus of small fresh-water snails. **G. sili′cula,** the host of *Troglotrema salmincola* in northwestern United States.

goniocraniometry (go″ne-o-kra″ne-om′ĕ-tre) [*gonio-* + *craniometry*]   the measurement of the cranial angles.

gonioma (gon″e-o′ma) [*gon-*(1) + *-oma*]   a term formerly applied to testicular tumors thought to be derived from sexual cells.

goniometer (go″ne-om′ĕ-ter) [*gonio-* + Gr. *metron* measure]   1. an instrument for measuring angles. 2. a plank, one end of which may be tilted to any height, used in testing for labyrinthine disease. **finger g.,** an apparatus for measuring the limits of flexion and extension of the interphalangeal joints of the fingers.

gonion (go′ne-on), pl. *go′nia* [Gr. *gōnia* angle]   a cephalometric landmark, being the most inferior, posterior, and lateral point on the external angle of the mandible.

goniophotography (go″ne-o-fo-tog′rah-fe)   photography of the angle of the anterior chamber of the eye.

Goniops (gon′e-ops)   a genus of tabanid flies.

goniopuncture (go″ne-o-punk′tūr)   a filtering operation for glaucoma, done by inserting a knife blade through clear cornea just within the limbus, across the anterior chamber, and through the opposite corneoscleral wall.

gonioscope (go′ne-o-skōp″) [*gonio-* + Gr. *skopein* to examine]   an optical instrument for examining the angle of the anterior chamber and for demonstrating ocular motility and rotation.

gonioscopy (go″ne-os′ko-pe)   examination of the angle of the anterior chamber of the eye with the gonioscope.

goniosynechia (go″ne-o-sĭ-nek′e-ah)   adhesion of the iris to the cornea at the angle of the anterior chamber of the eye.

goniotomy (go″ne-ot′o-me) [*gonio-* + Gr. *tomē* a cutting]   Barkan's operation for that type of glaucoma which is characterized by an open angle and normal depth of the anterior chamber; it consists of the opening of Schlemm's canal under direct vision secured by a contact glass.

gonitis (go-ni′tis) [*gon-*(2) + *-itis*]   inflammation of the knee. **fungous g.,** inflammation of the knee joint in which the capsule is diffusely thickened. **g. tuberculo′sa,** tuberculosis of the knee joint.

gono- (gon′o) [Gr. *gonē* seed]   a combining form denoting relationship to semen or seed.

gonoblennorrhea (gon″o-blen″o-re′ah)   gonorrheal conjunctivitis.

gonocampsis (gon″o-kamp′sis)   permanent flexion of the knee.

gonocele (gon′o-sēl)   spermatocele.

gonochorism (gon-ok′o-rizm) [*gono-* + Gr. *chōrizein* to separate]   differentiation of the gonads with normal development of the reproductive organs appropriate to the sex; the opposite of hermaphroditism.

gonococcal (gon″o-kok′al)   pertaining to gonococci.

gonococcemia (gon″o-kok-se′me-ah) [L. *gonococci* + Gr. *haima* blood + *-ia*]   the presence of gonococci in the blood.

gonococci (gon″o-kok′si) plural of *gonococcus*.

gonococcic (gon″o-kok′sik) gonococcal.

gonococcide (gon″o-kok′sīd) [*gonococcus* + L. *caedere* to kill] an agent that kills gonococci.

gonococcocide (gon″o-kok′o-sīd) [*gonococcus* + L. *caedere* to kill] gonococcide.

gonococcus (gon″o-kok′us), pl. *gonococ′ci* [*gono-* + *coccus*] an individual microorganism of the species *Neisseria gonorrhoeae*, the organism causing gonorrhea.

gonocyte (gon′o-sīt) [*gono-* + Gr. *kytos* hollow vessel] 1. the primitive reproductive cell of the embryo. 2. a secondary gamete-producing cell.

gonomery (gon-om′er-e) [*gono-* + Gr. *meros* part] the condition in which the paternal and the maternal chromosomes remain in separate groups and do not completely fuse, as occurs in certain hybrids.

gononephrotome (gon″o-nef′ro-tōm) [*gono-* + Gr. *nephros* kidney + *tomē* a section] that part of the mesoderm which develops into the reproductive and excretory organs of the embryo.

gonophage (gon′o-fāj) a bacteriophage having the gonococcus as its natural host.

gonophore (gon′o-fōr) [*gono-* + Gr. *phoros* bearing] an accessory generative organ, such as the uterine tube and uterus in the female, or spermiduct and seminal vesicle in the male.

gonorrhea (gon″o-re′ah) [*gono-* + Gr. *rhein* to flow] infection due to *Neisseria gonorrhoeae* transmitted venereally in most cases, but also by contact with infected exudates in neonatal children at birth, or by infants in households with infected inhabitants. It is marked in males by urethritis with pain and purulent discharge, but is commonly asymptomatic in females, although it may extend to produce suppurative salpingitis, oophoritis, tubo-ovarian abscess, and peritonitis. Bacteremia occurs in both sexes, resulting in cutaneous lesions, arthritis, and rarely meningitis or endocarditis.

gonorrheal (gon″o-re′al) of or pertaining to gonorrhea.

gonosome (gon′o-sōm) [*gono-* + Gr. *soma* body] former term for sex chromosome.

gonotokont (gon″o-to′kont) auxocyte.

gonotome (gon′o-tōm) [*gono-* + Gr. *tomē* a section] that part of the mesoderm which develops into the reproductive organs of the embryo.

gony- (gon′e) [Gr. *gony* knee] a combining form denoting relationship to the knee.

Gonyaulax (gon″e-aw′laks) a genus of protozoa of the order Dinoflagellata, class Phytomastigophora, found in salt, fresh, or brackish waters, and having yellow to brown chromatophores. **G. catanel′la,** a poisonous flagellate protozoon which may cause *gonyaulax poisoning* and which helps to form the destructive red tide in the ocean. See also *gonyaulax poison*, under *poison*.

gonycampsis (gon″ĭ-kamp′sis) [*gony-* + Gr. *kampsis* bending] abnormal curvature of the knee.

gonycrotesis (gon″e-kro-te′sis) [*gony-* + Gr. *krotēsis* striking] genu valgum.

gonyectyposis (gon″e-ek″tĭ-po′sis) [*gony-* + Gr. *ektypōsis* a modelling in relief] genu varum.

gonyocele (gon′e-o-sēl″) [*gony-* + Gr. *kēlē* tumor] synovitis or tuberculous arthritis of the knee.

gonyoncus (gon″e-ong′kus) [*gony-* + Gr. *onkos* bulk] tumor of the knee.

Goodell's sign (law) (good′elz) [William *Goodell*, American gynecologist, 1829–1894] see under *sign*.

Goodpasture's stain (good-pas′churs) [Ernest William *Goodpasture*, American pathologist, 1886–1960] see *Table of Stains and Staining Methods,* under *stain*.

Goodpasture's syndrome [E. W. *Goodpasture*] see under *syndrome*.

Goormaghtigh's apparatus (cells) [Norbert *Goormaghtigh,* Belgian physician, 1890–1960] juxtaglomerular cells.

Gordiacea (gor″de-a′se-ah) Nematomorpha.

Gordius (gor′de-us) [Gordian knot] a genus of the Gordiacea, the hair snakes or horsehair worms. **G. aquat′icus,** a species occasionally found as a pseudoparasite of the intestinal tract of man; its presence is the result of the accidental ingestion of infected insects. **G. medinen′sis,** *Dracunculus medinensis.* **G. robus′tus,** a species that is generally a pseudoparasite of the intestinal tract (see *G. aquaticus*), but has also been reported as invading the periorbital tissues of man.

Gordon (gor′don), Alexander (1752–1799). Scottish obstetrician who, in his *Treatise on the Epidemic Puerperal Fever of Aberdeen* (1795), first demonstrated the contagiousness of this disease.

Gordon's bodies, test (gor′donz) [Mervyn Henry *Gordon,* English physician, 1872–1953] see under *body* and *tests*.

Gordon's reflex, sign (gor′donz) [Alfred *Gordon,* American neurologist, 1874–1953] see *flexor reflex, paradoxical*, under *reflex*, and *finger phenomenon* (def. 1), under *phenomenon*.

gorget (gor′jet) a wide-grooved lithotome director.

gorondou (go-ron′doo) goundou.

Goslee tooth (goz′le) [Hart J. *Goslee,* American dentist, 1871–1930] see under *tooth*.

Gosselin's fracture (gos-laz′) [Léon Athanase *Gosselin,* French surgeon, 1815–1887] see under *fracture*.

Gossypium (gŏ-sip′e-um) [L.] a genus of tropical and subtropical malvaceous plants found in both hemispheres, including ten species, three of which (*G. barbadense, G. herbaceum,* and *G. hirsutum*) yield most of the world's cotton. The dried bark of the root of various species (cotton root bark) was formerly used as an oxytocic. See *cotton,* and see *cottonseed oil*, under *oil*.

gossypium (gŏ-sip′e-um), gen. *gossyp′ii* [L.] cotton. **g. asep′ticum, g. depura′tum, g. purifica′tum,** purified cotton.

gossypol (gos′ĭ-pol) chemical name: 2,2′-bis[8-formyl-1,6,7-trihydroxy-5-isopropyl-3-methylnaphthyl]. A poisonous yellow pigment, $C_{30}H_{30}O_8$, found in cottonseed (and named for *Gossypium*) which is detoxified by heating. Gossypol has male antifertility properties, apparently having its effects in the seminiferous tubules, where spermatozoa are produced.

GOT glutamine-oxaloacetic transaminase.

Göthlin's test (index) (get′linz) [Gustaf Fredrik *Göthlin,* Swedish physiologist, 1874–1949] see under *tests*.

Gottlieb's epithelial attachment (got′lēbz) [Bernhard *Gottlieb,* Vienna dentist, 1885–1950] see under *attachment*.

Gottstein's fibers, process (got′stīnz) [Jacob *Gottstein,* otologist in Breslau, 1832–1895] see under *fiber* and *process*.

gouge (gowj) a hollow chisel used in cutting and removing bone. **Kelley g.,** an instrument for removing cartilage grafts.

Goulard's extract, lotion, water (goo-larz′) [Thomas *Goulard,* French surgeon, 1720–1790] see *lead subacetate solution* and *diluted lead subacetate solution.*

Gouley's catheter (goo′lēz) [John Williams Severin *Gouley,* American surgeon, 1832–1920] see under *catheter*.

goundou (gōōn′doo) osteoplastic periostitis of the nose, a disease seen in natives of Central Africa and South America, marked by headache, purulent nasal discharge, and the formation of symmetrical painless swellings (bony exostoses) at the sides of the nose. It is a sequel of yaws. Called also *henpue, gundo, henpuye,* and *anakhré*.

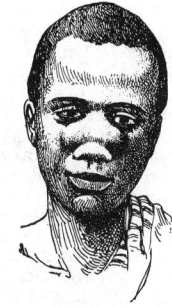

Goundou (Castellani and Chalmers).

gousiekte (goo-sek′te) [Dutch "rapid disease"] a condition in sheep marked by myocarditis, dilatation, and heart failure, caused by eating the poisonous plant *Vangueria pygmora*.

gout (gowt) [L. *gutta* a drop, because of the ancient belief that the disease was due to a "noxa" falling drop by drop into the joint] a hereditary form of arthritis characterized by an excess of uric acid in the blood (hyperuricemia) and by recurrent paroxysmal attacks of acute arthritis usually involving a single peripheral joint, followed by complete remission. The attacks result from deposition of crystals of monosodium urate in and around the joints. The hyperuricemia may be due to an increased rate of synthesis of the purine precursors of uric acid or to decreased elimination of uric acid by the kidneys, or to both. The disease, which affects chiefly men, is probably of polygenic inheritance. **abarticular g.,** that which does not affect the joints. **articular g.,** gout affecting the joints. **calcium g.,** calcinosis. **chalky g.,** tophaceous g. **irregular g.,** abarticular g. **latent g., masked g.,** lithemia without the typical features of gout. **lead g.,** gout ascribed to lead poisoning. **misplaced g.,** gout in which the arthritic symptoms have disappeared and are followed by severe constitutional disturbances; called also *Da-Costa's disease.* **oxalic g.,** oxalism. **polyarticular g.,** an atypical form of gout which attacks many joints and which resembles rheumatic fever in that an attack may last for weeks. **poor man's g.,** gout ascribed to hard work, exposure, ill feeding, and excess in the use of malt liquors. **regular g.,** articular g. **retrocedent g.,** misplaced g. **rheumatic g.,** rheumatoid arthritis. **saturnine g.,** lead g. **tophaceous g.,** gout in which there are tophi or chalky deposits of sodium urate. **visceral g.,** a disease of birds characterized by the deposition of sodium urates on the viscera.

gouty (gow′te) affected with or of the nature of gout.

Gowers' column, etc. (gow′erz) [Sir William Richard *Gowers,* celebrated English neurologist, 1845–1915] see under *column, contraction, disease, sign, solution,* and *tract,* and see *vasovagal attack,* under *attack.*

Goyrand's hernia (gwar-ahndz′) [Jean Gaspar Blaise *Goyrand,* French surgeon, 1803–1866] see under *hernia.*

G.P. general practitioner; general paresis (see *dementia paralytica*).

G6PD glucose-6-phosphate dehydrogenase.

G.P.I. general paralysis of the insane.

GPT glutamic-pyruvic transaminase.

gr. grain.

graafian follicle, vesicle (graf′e-an) [Reijnier (Regner) de *Graaf,* a celebrated Dutch physician and anatomist, 1641–1673] see *folliculi ovarici vesiculosi.*

gracile (gras′il) [L. *gracilis*] slender or delicate.

Grad. abbreviation for L. *grada′tim,* by degrees.

gradatim (gra-da′tim) [L.] gradually, by degrees.

Gradenigo's syndrome (grah-dĕ-ne′gōz) [Giuseppe *Gradenigo,* Italian physician, 1859–1926] see under *syndrome.*

gradient (gra′dē-ent) the rate of increase or decrease of a variable magnitude; also the curve which represents it. **g. of approach,** the inverse relationship between distance from a positive stimulus and the tendency to approach it. **g. of avoidance,** the inverse relationship between the distance from a negative stimulus and the tendency to withdraw from it. **density g.,** the continuous variation in density (concentration) of a solute along the height or width of a confined solution. **mitral g.,** the difference in pressure in the left atrium and the left ventricle in diastole. **systolic g.,** the difference in pressure between the left atrium and left ventricle in systole. **ventricular g.,** the net differences in ventricular electrical activity of varying duration, as determined by the algebraic sum of the electrocardiographic vectors representing the QRS and T-wave areas.

graduate (grad′u-āt) [L. *graduatus*] 1. a person who has received a degree from a university or college. 2. a measuring vessel marked by a series of lines.

graduated (grad′u-āt-ed) [L. *gradus* step] marked by a succession of lines, steps, or degrees.

Graefe's disease, knife, operation, sign (gra′fēz) [Albrecht von *Graefe,* German ophthalmologist, 1828–1870] see *ophthalmoplegia progressiva,* and see under *knife, operation,* and *sign.*

Gräfenberg's ring (graf′en-burg) [Ernest *Grafenberg,* German gynecologist in United States, 1881–1957] see under *ring.*

graft (graft) 1. any tissue or organ for implantation or transplantation. 2. to implant or transplant such tissues. See also *flap.* **accordion g.,** a full-thickness skin graft in which multiple slits have been made so that the graft may be stretched to cover a larger area. **activated g.,** a graft in which the nerves and blood supply have grown to nourish it, after a period of denervation and tenuous vascularity. **allogeneic g.,** allograft. **autochthonous g.,** autograft. **autodermic g., autoepidermic g.,** a skin graft taken from the patient's own body. **autogenous g., autologous g., autoplastic g.,** autograft. **avascular g.,** a graft of tissue in which not even transient vascularization is achieved. **Blair-Brown g.,** a split-skin graft of intermediate thickness. **bone g.,** a piece of bone taken from an animal or from some bone of the patient and used to take the place of a removed bone or bony defect. **Braun g.,** a thick skin graft. **Braun-Wangensteen g.,** implanted grafts of skin cut from a large graft. **brephoplastic g.,** the transplantation of tissue from an embryo or newborn to an adult animal. **cable g.,** a nerve graft made up of several sections of nerve in the manner of a cable. **chorioallantoic g.,** the placing of cells, tissues, or parts on the chorioallantoic membrane of the embryonic chick. **cutis g.,** dermal g. **Davis g.,** pinch g. **delayed g.,** a skin graft which is sutured back into its bed and subsequently shifted to a new recipient bed. **dermal g., dermic g.,** skin from which epidermis and subcutaneous fat have been removed; used instead of fascia in various plastic procedures. Called also *cutis g.* **diced cartilage g's,** numerous small segments of cartilage that can be packed or molded into any desired contour like wet grains of sand; used to repair faulty cartilage or bone structure. **double-end g.,** a pedicle flap or rope flap. **Douglas's g.,** sieve g. **epidermic g.,** a piece of epidermis implanted upon a raw surface; called also *Reverdin's g.* **Esser g.,** a full-thickness skin graft applied by spreading the graft over a mold of Stent preparation and suturing the graft and mold into a prepared pocket; called also *Stent's g.* **fascia g.,** a graft taken from the fascia lata or from the lumbar fascia. **fascicular g.,** a nerve graft in which the bundles of nerve fibers are approximated and sutured separately. **fat g.,** a graft of fat completely freed from its bed; used in filling depressions. **filler g.,** a graft used for the filling of defects, as the filling of a bony cyst cavity with bone chips. **free g.,** a graft of tissue completely freed from its bed, in contrast to a flap. **full-thickness g.,** a skin graft consisting of the full thickness of the skin, with little or none of the subcutaneous tissue. **gauntlet g.,** pedicle flap. **Gillies' g.,** rope flap. **hetero-**

dermic g., a skin graft taken from a donor of another species. **heterologous g., heteroplastic g.,** xenograft. **homologous g.,** allograft. **homoplastic g.,** allograft. **hyperplastic g.,** a skin graft which is in a state of active repair, as in recovery from inflammation. **implantation g.,** a graft in which small pieces of skin are embedded in granulation tissue of the same individual. **island g.,** see under *flap.* **isogeneic g., isologous g., isoplastic g.,** isograft. **jump g.,** see under *flap.* **Kiel g.,** denatured calf bone used to fill defects or restore facial contour; often used for chin and nasal augmentation. **Krause-Wolfe g.,** a graft of full thickness of the skin. **lamellar g.,** replacement of the superficial layers of an opaque cornea by a thin layer of clear cornea from a donor eye. **mucosal g.,** a graft of mucosal tissue, usually comprising the entire mucosal thickness. **nerve g.,** replacement of an area of defective nerve with a segment from a sound one. **Ollier-Thiersch g.,** a very thin skin graft in which long, broad strips of skin, consisting of the epidermis, rete, and part of the corium, are used. **omental g's,** free or attached segments of omentum used to cover suture lines following gastrointestinal or colonic surgery. **onlay bone g.,** bone used as a graft that is laid on or over cortical bone of the recipient site(s). **osseous g.,** bone g. **patch g.,** a graft of living tissue or prosthetic material used to close a vascular incision in order to enlarge the lumen of the vessel. **pedicle g.,** see under *flap.* **penetrating g.,** a full-thickness corneal transplant. **periosteal g.,** a piece of periosteum applied to a denuded area of a bone. **pinch g.,** a piece of skin about ¼ in. in diameter, obtained by elevating the skin with a needle and slicing it off with a knife; the thickness of the graft may vary, but it is always free of fat. **Reverdin g.,** epidermic g. **rope g.,** see under *flap.* **seed g.,** implantation g. **sieve g.,** a skin graft from which very small circular islands of skin are removed so that a larger denuded area can be covered, the sievelike portion being placed over one area, and the individual islands over surrounding or other denuded areas. **skin g.,** a piece of skin transplanted to replace a lost portion of the body skin surface; it may be a full-thickness, thick-split, or split-skin graft. **sleeve g.,** a graft for repairing traumatic gaps in nerves by a sleevelike extension from the distal stump which is sutured to the central stump. **split-skin g.,** a skin graft consisting of only a portion of the skin thickness. **split-thickness g.,** a graft, varying in thickness, containing only mucosal elements and no subcutaneous tissues. **sponge g.,** a bit of sponge inserted into a wound to promote the formation of granulations. **Stent g.,** Esser g. **syngeneic g.,** isograft. **thick-split g.,** a skin graft cut in small or large pieces, often including about two thirds of the full thickness of the skin. **Thiersch's g.,** Ollier-Thiersch g. **thin-split g.,** Ollier-Thiersch g. **thyroid g.,** a piece of the thyroid gland implanted in the tissues as a remedy for myxedema; no longer done. **tube g., tunnel g.,** rope flap. **valise handle g.,** a graft of the auricle of the ear. **white g.,** avascular g. **Wolfe's g., Wolfe-Krause g.,** Krause-Wolfe g.

grafting (graft′ing) the implanting or transplanting of any tissue or organ. **Mangoldt's epithelial g.,** the covering of wounds and granulating areas with epithelial tissue cut from the epidermis with a razor. **skin g.,** implantation of patches of healthy skin on a denuded area to form centers of cicatrization.

Graham's law (gra′amz) [Thomas *Graham,* English chemist, 1805–1869] see under *law.*

Graham's test (gra′amz) [Evarts Ambrose *Graham,* American surgeon, 1883–1957] see under *test.*

Graham Little syndrome (gra′am-lit′el) [Sir Ernest Gordon *Graham Little,* English physician, 1867–1950] see under *syndrome.*

Graham Steell murmur (gra′am stēl) [Graham *Steell,* English physician, 1851–1942] see under *murmur.*

Grahamella (gra″am-el′lah) a genus of the family Bartonellaceae, order Rickettsiales, made up of Bartonella-like microorganisms, and occurring as two species, *G. peromys′ci* and *G. tal′pae,* infecting deer mice and moles, respectively.

grahamellosis (gra″am-el-o′sis) infection with organisms of the genus *Grahamella.*

grain (grān) [L. *gra′num*] 1. a seed, especially of a cereal plant. 2. the twentieth part of a scruple: 0.065 gram. Abbreviated gr. **cayenne pepper g's,** brown crystals of uric acid in the urine.

grainage (grān′ij) weight in grains or parts of a grain.

gram (gram) [Fr. *gramme*] the basic unit of mass (weight) of the metric system, being the equivalent of 15.432 grains, or 0.035 ounces avoirdupois. Abbreviated gm.

-gram (gram) [Gr. *gramma* that which is written; a mark] a word termination meaning that which is written or recorded.

Gram's method, stain, solution (gramz) [Hans Christian Joachim *Gram,* Danish physician, 1853–1938] see *Table of Stains and Staining Methods,* under *stain,* and see *gram-negative* and *gram-positive.*

gram-equivalent (gram″e-kwiv′ah-lent) see under *equivalent.*

gramicidin (gram″ĭ-si′din) [USP] an antibacterial polypeptide produced by *Bacillus brevis,* which is one of the two principal components of tyrothricin, and is effective against many gram-positive organisms; it occurs as a white, or nearly white, crystalline powder, and is applied topically in pyodermic, ocular, and other localized infections due to susceptible bacteria. Called also g. D. *Gramicidin S* is a closely related substance produced by a thermophilic strain of *B. brevis;* called also *Soviet g.*

gramine (gram′in) chemical name: 3-(dimethylaminomethyl)-indole. A crystalline indole alkaloid, $C_{11}H_{14}N_2$, from barley; called also *donaxine.*

graminin (gram′ĭ-nin) a fructosan from rye flour.

graminivorous (gram″ĕ-niv′o-rus) feeding or subsisting on grass or cereal grains.

gram-ion (gram-i′on) that quantity of an ion whose weight in grams is numerically equal to the atomic weight of the ion.

grammeter (gram′me-ter) a unit of work, representing the energy expended in raising 1 gm. of weight 1 meter vertically against gravitational force. It is one thousandth of a kilogrammeter, or about 98,000 ergs.

grammole (gram′mol) gram-molecule.

gram-molecule (gram-mol′ĕ-kūl) as many grams of a substance as are numerically equal to its molecular weight. See *mole,* def. 3.

gram-negative (gram-neg′ah-tiv) losing the stain or decolorized by alcohol in Gram's method of staining, a primary characteristic of bacteria having a cell wall surface more complex in chemical composition than do the gram-positive bacteria.

gram-positive (gram-poz′ĭ-tiv) retaining the stain or resisting decolorization by alcohol in Gram's method of staining, a primary characteristic of bacteria whose cell wall is composed of peptidoglycan and teichoic acid.

grana [pl. of *granum* grain] dense green, chlorophyll-containing bodies in chloroplasts consisting of numerous, closely-packed lamellae which make them appear to be suspended in a matrix.

granatum (grah-na′tum), gen. *grana′ti* [L.] pomegranate.

Grancher's system (grahn-shāz′) [Jacques Joseph *Grancher,* French physician, 1843–1907] see *splenopneumonia,* and see under *system.*

grandiose (gran′dĭ-ōs) in psychiatry, pertaining to exaggerated belief or claims of one's importance or identity, often manifested by delusions of great wealth, power, or fame.

grandiosity (gran″de-os′ĭ-te) a condition characterized by delusions of grandeur.

grand mal (grahn mahl) see under *epilepsy.*

Grandry's corpuscles (grahn′drēz) [French anatomist of the 19th century] menisci tactus.

Granger line, sign (grān′jer) [Amedee *Granger,* New Orleans radiologist, 1879–1939] see under *line* and *sign.*

granoplasm (gran′o-plazm) granular protoplasm.

granula (gran′u-lah), pl. *gran′ulae* [L.] granule, def. 2. **g. irid′ica,** a black or brown outgrowth from the edge of the iris in horses; called also *nigroid body.*

granular (gran′u-lar) [L. *granularis*] made up of or marked by presence of granules or grains.

granulase (gran′u-lās) an enzyme thought to be present in grain and to have the power of splitting starch into achroodextrin and maltose.

granulatio (gran″u-la′she-o), pl. *granulatio′nes* [L.] [NA] a general term denoting a granule, or granular mass. **granulatio′nes arachnoidea′les** [NA], **granulatio′nes arachnoide′les [Pacchio′ni],** arachnoidal granulations: small elevations, visible to the naked eye, thought by some to be enlargements of arachnoid villi, which project into the superior sagittal sinus and associated venous lacunae and create slight depressions on the inner surface of the cranium; these granulations are the structures through which cerebrospinal fluid is reabsorbed into the blood in the venous system. Called also *arachnoid villi,* and *pacchionian bodies* or *granulations.* **granulatio′nes cerebra′les, granulatio′nes pacchio′ni,** granulationes arachnoideales.

granulation (gran″u-la′shun) [L. *granulatio*] 1. the division of hard or metallic substances into small particles. 2. the formation in wounds of small, rounded masses of tissue composed largely of capillaries and fibroblasts, often with inflammatory cells present; also a mass so formed. 3. a small, round, abnormal mass of lymphoid tissue, as on the conjunctiva of the eyelids or within the pharynx. **arachnoidal g's,** granulationes arachnoideales. **Bayle's g's,** gray tubercular nodules of the lung that have undergone fibroid degeneration. **Bright's g's,** the granulations seen in chronic interstitial nephritis. **cell g's,** small masses seen in the cytoplasm of certain cells that give the latter a characteristic appearance when stained; see the various granules, under *granule.* **exuberant g's,** excessive proliferation of granulation tissue in healing wounds. **pacchionian g's,** granulationes arachnoideales. **pyroninophlic g's,** structures seen in liver and other cells, which stain red with methyl green–pyronine by Pappenheim's stain; they are one of the early effects of carbon tetrachloride poisoning. **Reilly g's,** large azurophilic granules in the cytoplasm of polymorphonuclear leukocytes and lymphocytes, occurring in gargoylism. **Vir-**

chow's g's, granulations containing ependymal and glia fibers, found in the walls of the cerebral ventricles in general paralysis.

granulationes (gran″u-la″she-o′nēz) [L.] plural of *granulatio.*

granule (gran′ūl) [L. *granulum*] 1. a small particle or grain, as the small beadlike masses of tissue formed on the surface of wounds, or the insoluble nonmembranous particles found in cytoplasm. 2. a small pill made from sucrose. **acidophil g's,** granules staining with acid dyes, such as those of the alpha cells of the adenohypophysis; see also *carminophil*(def. 3) and *orangeophil* (def. 3). **acrosomal g.,** a large globule formed by the coalescence of proacrosomal granules, contained within a membrane-bounded *acrosomal vesicle,* which enlarges further to become the core of the acrosome of a spermatozoon. **albuminous g's,** granules seen in the cytoplasm of many normal cells; which optically disappear on the addition of acetic acid, but are not affected by ether or chloroform; called also *cytoplasmic g's.* **aleuronoid g's,** colorless myeloid colloidal bodies found in the base of pigment cells. **alpha g's,** 1. oval granules found in blood platelets; their membrane structure and the contained acid phosphatase suggest that they are lysosomes. 2. large granules in the alpha cells of the islets of Langerhans, which are insoluble in alcohol and secrete glucagon. 3. the acidophilic granules in the alpha cells of the adenohypophysis; see also *carminophil* and *orangeophil.* **Altmann's g's,** mitochondria. **amphophil g's,** granules that stain with either acid or basic dyes. **argentaffine g's,** granules which stain with silver. **azur g., azurophil g.,** a granule which stains easily with azure dyes; they are coarse reddish granules seen in many lymphocytes. **Babès-Ernst g's,** metachromatic g's. **basal g.,** basal body. **basophil g's,** granules staining with basic dyes, such as those of the beta cells of the adenohypophysis; see also *gonadotrope*(def. 3) and *thyrotrope* (def. 2). **beta g's,** 1. the granules in the beta cells of the islets of Langerhans, which secrete insulin and are soluble in alcohol. 2. basophilic granules in the beta cells of the adenohypophysis; see also *gonadotrope (def. 3)* and *thyrotrope(def. 2).* **Bollinger's g's,** 1. Bollinger's bodies. 2. small, yellowish white granules in mulberry-like masses, containing micrococci, seen in the granulation tissue of botryomycosis. **Bütschli's g's,** swellings on the bipolar rays of the amphiaster in the ovum. **carbohydrate g's,** particles of carbohydrate matter in the body fluids in the course of being assimilated. **chromatic g's, chromophilic g's,** Nissl's bodies; see under *body.* **cone g's,** the nuclei of the visual cells of the retina in its outer nuclear layer which are connected with the cones. **cortical g's,** special structures in the cortex of the ovum of many animals, which break up during fertilization and supply the material for the development of the fertilization membrane. **cytoplasmic g's,** albuminous g's. **delta g's,** fine basophilic granules occurring in the lymphocytes. **Dioscorides' g.,** a pill of lactose and gum arabic with arsenious acid. **Ehrlich's g's, Ehrlich-Heinz g's,** cell granules which stain with Ehrlich's triacid stain. **elementary g's,** hemoconia. **eosinophil g's,** granules staining with eosin. **Fauvel's g's,** peribronchitic abscesses. **fuchsinophil g's,** granules staining with fuchsin. **Fordyce's g's,** see under *spot.* **gamma g's,** a name applied to basophilic granules found in the blood, marrow, and in the tissues. **Heinz g's,** Heinz-Ehrlich bodies. **hyperchromatin g.,** azur g. **iodophil g's,** granules staining brown with iodine, seen in polymorphonuclear leukocytes in various acute infectious diseases. **juxtaglomerular g's,** stainable osmophilic secretory granules present in the juxtaglomerular cells, closely resembling zymogen granules. **kappa g.,** azur g. **keratohyalin g's,** irregularly shaped granules, representing deposits of keratohyalin on tonofibrils in the stratum granulosum epidermidis. They stain with some acid dyes and with certain basic dyes. See also *keratohyalin,* def. 1. **Kölliker's interstitial g's,** various sized granules seen in the sarcoplasm of muscle fibers. **Kretz's g's,** granules found in the liver in cirrhosis. **Langerhans' g's,** peculiar rod-shaped, membrane-bound structures with a central linear density found in the Langerhans cells of the epidermis, which resemble superficially the vermiform bodies of the Kupffer cells of the liver; called also *vermiform g's.* **Langley's g's,** granules seen in secreting serous glands. **membrane-coating g's,** granules in the uppermost cells of the stratum spinosum epidermidis, which may deposit dense material on the inner aspect of the cell membrane; they contain the enzyme acid phosphatase, and may be involved in the desquamation of the stratum corneum epidermidis. Called also *keratinosomes.* **meningeal g's,** granulationes arachnoideales. **metachromatic g's,** polymetaphosphate granules, present in many bacterial cells, which have an avidity for basic dyes and cause irregular staining of the cell; called also *Babès-Ernst bodies, corpuscles,* or *granules.* **Mezei g's** (*obs.*), spherical brownish granules seen in smears from the lesions of cutaneous actinomycosis. **Much's g's,** granules and rods found in tuberculous sputum which do not stain by the usual processes for acid-fast bacilli, but do stain with Gram stain; regarded as modified tubercle bacilli. **Neusser's g's** (*obs.*), basophil granules seen about the nuclei of leukocytes. **Nissl's g's,** Nissl's bodies. **oxyphil g's,** acidophil g's. **Paschen's g's,** see under *body.* **perichromatin g's,** granules believed to contain nucleic acid, found near the masses of nuclear chromatin in the hepatic parenchymal cells.

pigment g's, small masses of coloring matter occurring in pigment cells. **polar g's,** metachromatic g's. **proacrosomal g.,** any of the small, dense bodies found inside one of the vacuoles of the Golgi body, which fuse to form an acrosomal granule. **protein g's,** microscopically observable particles of various proteins, some anabolic and others catabolic. **rod g's,** the nuclei of rod visual cells in the outer nuclear layer of the retina which are connected with the rods. **Schrön's g.,** a small body, of doubtful origin, seen in the germinal spot of the ovum. **Schrön-Much g's,** Much's g's. **Schüffner's g's,** see under *dot.* **secretory g's,** granules in secretory cells which apparently represent material that helps to form the secretion. **seminal g's,** the small granular bodies seen in the spermatic fluid. **specific atrial g's,** membrane-bound spherical granules with a dense homogeneous interior concentrated in the core of sarcoplasm of the atrial cardiac muscle, extending in either direction from the poles of the nucleus, usually near the Golgi complex; they also may be found in limited numbers in other regions of the cell. **sphere g.,** a large granular cell or corpuscle seen in serous exudation. **sulfur g's,** peculiar granular bodies of a yellow color found in actinomycotic lesions and discharges. **thread g's,** mitochondria. **toxic g's,** basophilic cytoplasmic granules originally thought to appear in leukocytes only during infections or other toxic states, but later found to appear in the absence of systemic toxicity, probably representing developmentally anomalous lysosomes. **trichohyalin g's,** see *trichohyalin.* **vermiform g's,** Langerhans' g's. **volutin g's,** metachromatic g's. **zymogen g's,** secretory granules in certain cells, containing the precursors of enzymes that become active after they have left the cell.

granuliform (gran′u-lĭ-form) in the form of, or resembling, small grains.

granuloadipose (gran″u-lo-ad′ĭ-pōs) showing fatty degeneration which contains granules of fat.

granuloblast (gran′u-lo-blast) myeloblast.

granuloblastosis (gran″u-lo-blas-to′sis) a form of avian leukosis marked by an increase in the circulating blood of immature blood cells of the granular series; there may be infiltration of the liver or spleen.

granulocorpuscle (gran″u-lo-kor′pus′l) a small corpuscle observed in infected tissue in lymphogranuloma venereum.

granulocyte (gran′u-lo-sīt″) [*granular* + Gr. *kytos* hollow vessel] any cell containing granules, especially a leukocyte containing neutrophil, basophil, or eosinophil granules in its cytoplasm. See also *granular leukocytes,* under *leukocyte,* and *granular series,* under *series.* **band-form g.,** band cell. **segmented g.,** see under *cell.*

granulocytic (gran″u-lo-sit′ik) 1. pertaining to, characterized by, or of the nature of granulocytes. 2. pertaining to the granulocytic series; see under *series.*

granulocytopathy (gran″u-lo-si-top′ah-the) any disorder of the granular leukocytes (granulocytes).

granulocytopenia (gran″u-lo-si″to-pe′ne-ah) [*granulocyte* + Gr. *penia* poverty] agranulocytosis.

granulocytopoiesis (gran″u-lo-si″to-poi-e′sis) the production of granulocytes.

granulocytopoietic (gran″u-lo-si″to-poi-et′ik) pertaining to, characterized by, or stimulating granulocytopoiesis.

granulocytosis (gran″u-lo-si-to′sis) an abnormally large number of granulocytes in the blood.

granulofatty (gran″u-lo-fat′e) granuloadipose.

granuloma (gran″u-lo′mah) a tumor-like mass or nodule of granulation tissue, with actively growing fibroblasts and capillary buds, consisting of a collection of modified macrophages resembling epithelial cells (*epithelioid cells*), surrounded by a rim of mononuclear cells, chiefly lymphocytes and sometimes a center of giant multinucleate cells, either of the Langhans' or foreign body type; it is due to a chronic inflammatory process associated with infectious disease, such as tuberculosis (see *tubercle*), syphilis, sarcoidosis, leprosy, lymphogranuloma, etc., or with invasion by a foreign body. **amebic g.,** granulomatous lesions of the colon sometimes seen in amebiasis. **g. annula′re,** a granuloma consisting of hard, reddish nodules arranged in a circle which enlarge until they form a ring. **apical g.,** a modified type of granulation tissue containing elements of chronic inflammation located adjacent to the root apex (chronic apical periodontitis) and continuous with the periodontal ligament of a tooth which has an infected necrotic pulp; this tissue has excellent repair potential. **baln′ei,** swimming pool g. **benign g. of thyroid,** a chronic inflammation of the thyroid gland which changes it into a bulky tumor which later becomes extremely hard. **beryllium g.,** a local sarcoid-like reaction in the skin caused by the accidental implantation of a beryllium compound in abrasions or other wounds. **candida g., candidal g.,** granulomatous nodules in the form of horns or heavily crusted nodules, which develop on the scalp, face, fingers, mucous membranes, and elsewhere, in longstanding generalized candidiasis; called also *monilia,* or *monilial,* g. **central giant cell reparative g.,** see *giant cell reparative g.* **cholesterol g.,** a granulomatous lesion in which crystals of cholesterol esters are surrounded by

foreign-body giant cells in a mass of fibrotic granulation tissue. **coccidioidal g.,** coccidioidomycosis. **dental g.,** a mass of granulation tissue usually surrounded by a fibrous sac continuous with the periodontal ligament and attached to the apex of a root; it is the common result of dental caries and subsequent infection of the pulp. **Durck's g.,** malarial g. **g. endem′icum** (*obs.*), cutaneous leishmaniasis. **eosinophilic g.,** 1. a type of xanthomatosis characterized by the presence of rarefactions or cysts in one or more bones and sometimes associated with eosinophilia. 2. a disorder similar to eosinophilic gastroenteritis and characterized by localized nodular or pedunculated lesions of the gastric submucosa and muscle walls, especially of the pyloric area of the stomach, caused by infiltration of eosinophils, but without peripheral eosinophilia and allergic symptoms. It may also affect the small intestine. 3. anisakiasis. **g. fissura′tum,** a circumscribed, firm, reddish, fissured, fibrotic granuloma of the gum and buccal mucosa, occurring on an edentulous alveolar ridge and in the fold between the ridge and cheek; it is caused by an ill-fitting denture. **foreign-body g.,** a localized histiocytic skin reaction to a foreign body in the tissue, such as starch, talc, or oil. **g. fungoi′des** (*obs.*), mycosis fungoides. **g. gangraenes′cens,** a condition beginning with the formation of proliferating granulations in the nasal mucous membrane which invade the adjacent tissues and soon become gangrenous. **giant cell reparative g.,** an abnormal, benign reparative reaction to an injury, characterized by fibroplastic proliferation with numerous giant cells; the lesions occur peripherally in the soft tissue of the gingivae (giant cell epulis) and centrally in bones of the jaw. **g. glutea′le infan′tum,** a nodular dermatosis occurring on the buttocks of infants, which may be mistaken for hemangiomas or hematomas. The lesions are elevated bluish or brownwish red plaques or nodules from 1 to 3 or 4 cm. in width, containing a polymorphic cellular infiltrate with microabscesses but no suppuration, and abundant extravasation of red cells. In reported cases, treatment has been ineffective but spontaneous recovery has occurred within a few months. **Hodgkin's g.,** see under *disease.* **infectious g.,** granuloma caused by a specific microorganism, as the tubercle bacilli. **infective g.,** one due to the presence in the tissues of living agents. **g. inguina′le,** a granulomatous venereal disease characterized by deep purulent ulcerations of the skin of the external genitals, caused by *Calymmatobacterium granulomatis* and affecting especially dark-skinned people. Called also *donovanosis, fourth venereal disease, granuloma venereum, pudendal ulcer,* and *ulcerating granuloma of the pudenda.* **laryngeal g.,** a firm nodule on the larynx due to trauma, particularly from endotracheal intubation or from excessive use of the voice. **lethal midline g.,** a rare necrotizing granuloma that results in destruction of the midface and invariably in death. It is nearly always preceded by longstanding nonspecific inflammation of the nose or nasal sinuses, with purulent, often bloody discharge. It leads to extreme erosion of the nose, cheeks, hard or soft palate, and orbital cavities. **lipoid g.,** a granuloma containing lipoid cells; xanthoma. **lipophagic g.,** a granuloma attended by the loss of subcutaneous fat. **lycopodium g.,** a granulomatous lesion developing after an operation as a result of the introduction of lycopodium spores into the operative wound. **Majocchi's g.,** trichophytic g. **malarial g.,** a granulomatous lesion sometimes seen in the brain in fatal cases of cerebral malaria. **midline g.,** lethal midline g. **Mignon's eosinophilic g.,** a solitary destructive lesion affecting the skull and other bones of children and young adults. **monilia g., monilial g.,** candida g. **g. multifor′me,** a slowly progressive localized confluent papular granulomatous disease encountered so far only in Africa, clinically easily confused with tuberculoid leprosy and granuloma annulare. Necrobiosis and necrosis of collagen and elastic fibers occurs, with phagocytosis. **paracoccidioidal g.,** paracoccidioidomycosis. **peripheral giant cell reparative g.,** a pedunculated or sessile lesion of the gingivae or alveolar ridge, apparently arising from periodontal ligament or mucoperiosteum, and usually resulting from trauma, such as tooth extraction, or denture irritation. **plasma cell g.,** granuloma in which other inflammatory cells are very greatly outnumbered by plasma cells. **g. puden′di,** granuloma inguinale. **g. puden′te trop′icum,** g. inguinale. **pyogenic g., g. pyogen′icum,** a benign, solitary, dull red, soft, raised, sometimes pedunculated nodule resembling granulation tissue, found anywhere on the body, commonly intraorally, and usually occurring at the site of trauma as a response of the tissues to a nonspecific infection. It was formerly thought to be due to a botryomycotic infection and was called *botryomycosis hominis.* See also *pregnancy tumor,* under *tumor.* **reticulohistiocytic g.,** solitary reticulohistiocytoma, histologically indistinguishable from the lesions of multicentric reticulohistiocytosis (q.v.), with no systemic involvement, and occurring mainly in men. **rheumatic g's,** nodules occurring in various parts of the body in rheumatism. **g. sarcomato′des** (*obs.*), mycosis fungoides. **septic g.,** granuloma pyogenicum. **silicotic g.,** pseudotuberculoma silicoticum. **swimming pool g.,** a granulomatous lesion that complicates abrasions sustained in swimming pools, attributed to *Mycobacterium balnei (M. marinum).* It tends to heal spontaneously in a few months or years. **g. telangiectat′icum,** a form characterized by numerous dilated blood vessels. **trichophytic g., g. trichophyt′icum,** a rare form of tinea corporis, occurring chiefly on the lower legs, which is caused by *Trichophyton rubum* infecting hairs at the site of involvement. It is characterized by the development of elevated, sharply circumscribed, rather boggy granulomas, from rose red to a cyanotic hue, disseminated or arranged in chains; after persisting for three or four months the lesions are slowly absorbed, or undergo necrosis, leaving depressed scars. Called also *Majocchi's g.* and *tinea profunda.* **g. trop′icum** yaws. **ulcerating g. of the pudenda,** granuloma inguinale. **umbilical g.,** granulation tissue on the stem of the umbilical cord in newborn infants. **venereal g., g. vene′reum,** granuloma inguinale. **xanthomatous g.,** eosinophilic g. **zirconium g.,** an itchy eruption of aggregated, purple papules caused by a tuberculoid or sarcoid cutaneous reaction to zirconium salts, like those used in antiperspirants.

granulomatosis (gran″u-lo″mah-to′sis) the formation of multiple granuloma. **allergic g.,** extensive necrotizing angiitis occurring in debilitated asthmatic patients, with granulomas; called also *Churg-Strauss syndrome,* and *necrotizing angiitis with granulomata.* **g. discifor′mis chron′ica et progressi′va,** necrobiosis lipoidica. **lipophagic intestinal g.,** intestinal lipodystrophy. **lymphomatoid g.,** a systemic and visceral form of granulomatous vasculitis mimicking lymphoma and differing from its cutaneous counterpart, lymphomatoid papulosis, in that skin lesions occur in only about 30 per cent of cases; the course is highly unpredictable. **malignant g.,** Hodgkin's disease. **necrotizing respiratory g.,** Wegener's g. **g. siderot′ica,** a condition in which brownish nodules (Gamna nodules) are seen in the enlarged spleen. **Wegener's g.,** a progressive disease, characterized by granulomatous lesions of the respiratory tract, focal necrotizing arteriolitis, and, finally, widespread inflammation of all the organs of the body.

granulomatous (gran″u-lom′ah-tus) composed of granulomas.

granulomere (gran′u-lo-mēr″) the center portion of a platelet in a dry, stained blood smear, apparently filled with fine purplish red granules. Cf. *hyalomere.*

granulopenia (gran″u-lo-pe′ne-ah) agranulocytosis.

granuloplasm (gran′u-lo-plazm) endoplasm.

granuloplastic (gran″u-lo-plas′tik) [*granule* + Gr. *plassein* to form] forming granules.

granulopoiesis (gran″u-lo-poi-e′sis) [*granulocyte* + Gr. *poiein* to make] the formation of granulocytes.

granulopoietic (gran″u-lo-poi-et′ik) pertaining to or concerned in the formation of granulocytes.

granulopoietin (gran″u-lo-poi-e′tin) hypothetical substance(s) believed to serve as the humoral regulator of granulopoiesis; leukopoietin.

granulopotent (gran″u-lo-po′tent) capable of forming granules.

granulosa (gran″u-lo′sah) cumulus oophorus; see also under *cell.*

granulose (gran′u-lōs) 1. the more soluble portion of starch; see *amylose.* 2. a bacterial polysaccharide occurring as cytoplasmic granules and staining red to blue with iodine.

granulosis (gran″u-lo′sis) the formation of a mass of granules. **g. ru′bra na′si,** sweating and hyperhidrosis confined to the nose and surrounding area of the face and sometimes the chin, associated with red papules and sometimes many small vesicles; it occurs most often in children, usually clearing up at puberty. There is some evidence that an inheritable trait is involved in the etiology.

granulosity (gran″u-los′ĭ-te) a mass of granulations.

granulotherapy (gran″u-lo-ther′ah-pe) a method once used for treating infection based on the presumption that leukocytosis could be stimulated by the intravenous injection of carbon particles that would be of benefit to the infected person.

granulovacuolar (gran″u-lo-vak′u-o-lar) characterized by granules and vacuoles.

granum (gra′num) pl. *gra′na* [L.] grain; see *grana.*

grapes (grāps) 1. granulations formed in severe cases of grease in horses. 2. bovine tuberculosis.

graph (graf) [Gr. *graphein* to write, or record] a diagram or curve representing varying relationships between sets of data. Often used as a word termination denoting an instrument for writing or recording.

graphesthesia (graf″es-the′ze-ah) [Gr. *graphein* to write + *aisthēsis* perception] the sense by which are recognized figures or numbers written on the skin with a dull-pointed object.

graphic (graf′ik) [Gr. *graphein* to write] written or drawn; pertaining to representation by diagrams.

graphite (graf′ĭt) [L. *graphites,* from Gr. *graphis* a style, or writing instrument] plumbago, a form of native mineralized carbon.

graphitosis (graf″ĭ-to′sis) pneumoconiosis due to inhalation of and tissue reaction to graphite dust.

Graphium (graf′e-um) a genus of imperfect fungi which produce several cultural spore types.

grapho- (graf′o) [Gr. *graphein* to record] a combining form denoting relationship to writing or to a record.

graphoanalysis (graf″o-ah-nal′ĭ-sis) analysis of character based on handwriting.

graphocatharsis (graf″o-kah-thar′sis) a method of relieving psychic distress by writing out one's thoughts.

graphokinesthetic (graf″o-kin″es-thet′ik) [*grapho-* + Gr. *kinein* to move + *aisthēsis* perception] pertaining to the sensation aroused by the act of writing.

graphology (graf-ol′o-je) [*grapho-* + *-logy*] the study of the handwriting as a method of analyzing personality.

graphomotor (graf″o-mo′tor) [*grapho-* + *motor*] pertaining to, or affecting, the movements required in writing.

graphopathology (graf″o-pah-thol′o-je) the study of handwriting as an indication of mental or physical disorder.

graphorrhea (graf″o-re′ah) [*grapho-* + Gr. *rhoia* flow] a morbid mental condition marked by the writing of a long succession of meaningless and unconnected words.

graphoscope (graf′o-skōp) [*grapho-* + Gr. *skopein* to examine.] an instrument for treating myopia and asthenopia.

graphospasm (graf′o-spazm) [*grapho-* + Gr. *spasmos* spasm] writers' cramp.

-graphy (graf′e) [Gr. *graphein* to write, record] a word termination meaning the act of writing or recording, or a method of recording.

Grashey's aphasia (grash′ēz) [Hubert von *Grashey,* Munich psychologist, 1839–1911] see under *aphasia.*

grass (gras) any plant of the order Gramineae. Some of the grasses which by their pollen are important causes of hay fever are: Bermuda g., *Cynodon dactylon;* June g., *Poa pratensis;* Johnson g., *Sorghum halepense;* Orchard g., *Dactylis glomerata;* Redtop g., *Agrostis alba;* Sweet vernal g., *Anthoxanthum odoratum;* and Timothy g., *Phleum pratense.* **couch g.,** *Agropyron repens* (L.) Beauv. (Gramineae). **scurvy g.,** a cruciferous plant, *Cochlearia officinalis,* once used as a remedy for scurvy.

Grasset's law, phenomenon (sign) (grah-sāz′) [Joseph *Grasset,* French physician, 1849–1918] see *Landouzy-Grasset law,* under *law,* and see under *phenomenon.*

Grasset-Gaussel phenomenon (grah-sa′go-sel′) [Joseph *Grasset;* Amans *Gaussel,* French physician, 1871–1937] Grasset's phenomenon; see under *phenomenon.*

Grasset-Gaussel-Hoover sign (grah-sa′-go-sel′-hoo′ver) [Joseph *Grasset;* Amans *Gaussel;* Charles Franklin *Hoover,* American physician, 1865–1927] see under *sign.*

gratification (grat″ĭ-fĭ-ka′shun) the lowering of an emotional tension which follows the fulfillment of an instinctual aim.

Gratiola (grah-ti′o-lah) a genus of plants. **G. officina′lis,** the hedge hyssop, a scrophulariaceous plant of Europe; it is purgative, emetic, and diuretic.

Gratiolet's radiating fibers, optic radiation (grah-te″o-lāz′) [Louis Pierre *Gratiolet,* French anatomist, 1815–1865] see under *fiber,* and see *radiatio optica.*

grattage (grah-tahzh′) [Fr.] the removal of granulations (as in trachoma) by scraping or by friction with a stiff brush.

grave (grāv) [L. *gravis*] severe or serious.

gravedo (gra-ve′do) [L.] cold in the head, or nasal catarrh.

gravel (grav′el) a term applied to fairly coarse concretions of mineral salts, as from the kidneys or bladder, of smaller size than the so-called stones.

Graves' disease (grāvz) [Robert James *Graves,* Irish physician, 1796–1853] see under *disease.*

grave-wax (grāv′waks) adipocere.

gravid (grav′id) [L. *gravida* heavy, loaded] pregnant; containing developing young.

gravida (grav′ĭ-dah) a pregnant woman. Called *gravida I* or *primigravida* during the first pregnancy, *gravida II* or *secundigravida* during the second pregnancy, *gravida III* or *tertigravida* during the third pregnancy, and so on. Cf. *Para.*

gravidic (grah-vid′ik) occurring in pregnancy.

gravidism (grav′id-izm) pregnancy, or the sum of symptoms, signs, and conditions associated with it.

graviditas (grah-vid′ĭ-tas) pregnancy. **g. examnia′lis,** pregnancy in which the amnion has burst and is retracted around the insertion of the umbilical cord, but the chorion is intact. **g. exochoria′lis,** pregnancy in which the membranes have burst and shrunk, leaving the fetus in the uterus but outside of the chorion.

gravidity (grah-vid′ĭ-te) [L. *graviditas*] pregnancy; the condition of being pregnant, without regard to the outcome. Cf. *parity.*

gravidocardiac (grav″ĭ-do-kar′de-ak) [L. *gravida* + Gr. *kardia* heart] pertaining to heart disease of pregnancy.

gravidopuerperal (grav″ĭ-do-pu-er′per-al) pertaining to pregnancy and the puerperium.

gravimeter (grah-vim′ĕ-ter) [L. *gravis* heavy + *metrum* measure] an instrument for determining specific gravities.

gravimetric (grav″ĭ-met′rik) pertaining to measurement by weight; performed by weight, as gravimetric method of drug assay.

gravistatic (grav″ĭ-stat′ik) due to gravitation, as *gravistatic* pulmonary congestion.

gravitation (grav″ĭ-ta′shun) the force that tends to draw all bodies together; see *law of gravitation*.

gravitometer (grav″ĭ-tom′ĕ-ter) a balance for measuring specific gravity.

gravity (grav′ĭ-te) [L. *gravitas*] weight; tendency toward the center of the earth. **specific g.,** the weight of a substance compared with that of an equal volume of another substance taken as a standard.

Grawitz's tumor (grah′vits-ez) [Paul Albert *Grawitz*, pathologist in Greifswald, 1850–1932] see under *tumor*.

gray (gra) 1. of a hue between white and black. 2. the gray matter of the nervous system. 3. a proposed unit of absorbed radiation dose equal to 100 rads. Abbreviated Gy. **central g.,** relatively undifferentiated gray matter which retains its primitive position near the ventricles and central canal. **nervous g.** (*obs.*), Nissl's term for the unknown specific constituent of the gray matter of the nervous system. **silver g., steel g.,** nigrosin.

grease (grēs) an inflammatory swelling in a horse's leg in the region of the fetlocks and pasterns, with the formation of cracks in the skin and the excretion of oily matter.

grease-heel (grēs-hēl′) grease.

green (grēn) 1. having the color of fresh leaves or of grass. 2. a green coloring matter or dye. **acid g.,** any of several green acid dyes, generally light g. S F. **brilliant g.,** a basic dye having powerful bacteriostatic properties for gram-positive organisms; used topically as an anesthetic. **bromocresol g.** [USP], an indicator used in the determination of hydrogen ion concentration, being yellow at pH 4.0 and blue at pH 5.4. **Brunswick g.,** 1. chrome g. 2. copper arsenite. 3. copper subcarbonate. 4. copper oxychloride. **chrome g.,** chromium sesquioxide, Cr_2O_3. **diazin g. S,** Janus g. B. **ethyl g.,** brilliant g. **fast acid g. N,** light g. S F. yellowish. **Hoffman g.,** iodine g. **indocyanine g.** [USP], a tricarbocyanine dye, $C_{43}H_{47}N_2NaO_6S_2$, occurring as an olive-brown, dark green, dark blue, or black powder; used intravenously as a diagnostic aid in the determination of blood volume, cardiac output, and hepatic function. **iodine g.,** a triphenylmethane dye used as a chromatin stain. **Janus g. B,** an azo dye used supravitally for the demonstration of mitochondria. **light g., 2 G or 2 GN,** light g. S F. yellowish. **light g. N,** malachite g. **light g. S F yellowish,** an acid dye used as a plasma stain. **malachite g.,** a triphenylmethane dye used as a stain for bacteria and as an antiseptic for wounds. **malachite g. G,** brilliant g. **methyl g.,** 1. a mixture of hepta and hexa methyl-pararosaniline. 2. ethyl g. **methylene g.,** a mononitromethylene blue, interesting for its dark green metachromasia. **new solid g.,** malachite g. **Paris g.,** a double salt of copper acetate and copper meta-arsenite, $Cu(C_2H_3O_2)_2 \cdot 3Cu(AsO_2)_2$, used as an insecticide. **Schweinfurt g.,** Paris g. **solid g.,** malachite g. **Victoria g.,** malachite g.

Greene's sign (grēnz) [Charles Lyman *Greene*, American physician, 1862–1929] see under *sign*.

Greenhow's disease (grēn′howz) [Edward Headlam *Greenhow*, English physician, 1814–1888] vagabond's disease; see under *disease*.

gregaloid (greg′ah-loid) [L. *grex* flock + Gr. *eidos* form] formed by casual union of independent cells; said of a loose grouping of protozoa, including Sarcodina, which may become attached by their pseudopodia.

Gregarina (greg″ah-ri′nah) [L. *gregarius*, crowding together] a genus of sporozoa of the order Gregarinida, species of which are common parasites in the digestive tract and body cavities of insects.

gregarina (greg″ah-ri′nah), pl. *gregari′nae*. An organism of the genus *Gregarina*.

gregarine (greg′ah-rin) 1. pertaining to the Gregarinida. 2. any member of the order Gregarinida.

Gregarinida (greg″ah-ri′nĭ-dah) an order of protozoa of the subphylum Sporozoa, generally parasitic in the digestive tract and body cavities of invertebrates; it includes the genera *Gregarina*, *Monocystis*, and *Lankesteria*.

Gregory's mixture (greg′o-rēz) [James *Gregory*, Scotch physician, 1753–1821] compound powder of rhubarb; see under *powder*.

grenz rays [Ger. *Grenze*, boundary] see under *ray*.

GRF growth hormone releasing factor; see under *hormone*.

GRH growth hormone releasing hormone.

grid (grid) 1. a grating; in radiology, a device consisting essentially of a series of narrow lead strips closely spaced on their edges and separated by spacers of low density material; used to reduce the amount of scattered radiation reaching the x-ray film. 2. a chart with horizontal and perpendicular lines for plotting curves. **baby g.,** a direct reading control chart on infant growth. **focused g.,** in radiography, one in which the lead foils are placed

at an angle so that they all point toward a focus at a specified distance. **moving g.,** a grid which is moved continuously or oscillated throughout the making of a radiograph. **parallel g.,** in radiography, one in which the lead strips are oriented parallel to each other. **Potter-Bucky g.,** a grid utilizing the principle of the moving grid, with an oscillating movement. **stationary g.,** one placed in apposition to a roentgenographic film for its accentuation of detail; the grid lines will be visible on the resultant roentgenograms. **Wetzel g.,** a direct reading chart for evaluating physical fitness in terms of body build, developmental level, and basal metabolism.

grief (grēf) the normal emotional response to an external and consciously recognized loss; it is self-limited, gradually subsiding within a reasonable time.

Griesinger's disease, sign (symptom) (gre′zing-erz) [Wilhelm *Griesinger*, German neurologist, 1817–1868] see *hookworm disease*, under *disease*, and see under *sign*.

Grignard's reagent (compound) (grēn-yahrz′) [François Auguste Victor *Grignard*, French chemist, 1871–1935] see under *reagent*.

Grifulvin (grĭ-ful′vin) trademark for a preparation of griseofulvin.

Grindelia (grin-de′le-ah) [H. *Grindel*, 1776–1836] a genus of American composite-flowered plants; the leaves and flowering tops of *G. camporum*, *G. cuneifolia*, and *G. squarrosa*, of the western United States, are used as a mild expectorant.

grinding (grīnd′ing) rubbing together with force; wearing away or polishing by rubbing. See also *bruxism*. **selective g.,** the modification of the occlusal forms of teeth by grinding according to a plan. **spot g.,** occlusal equilibration.

grinding-in (grind′ing-in) the process of correcting errors in the centric and eccentric occlusions of natural or artificial teeth.

grip (grip) 1. [Fr. *grippe*] influenza. 2. a grasping or seizing. **Dabney's g.,** epidemic pleurodynia. **devil's g.,** epidemic pleurodynia.

grippal (grip′al) pertaining to grip, or influenza.

grippe (grip) influenza. **g. aurique′,** a polyneuritis sometimes resulting from the therapeutic use of gold salts. **Balkan g.,** a respiratory infection reported in the Balkans during World War II which proved to be due to *Rickettsia burneti*. See *Q fever*.

Grisactin (gris-ak′tin) trademark for a preparation of griseofulvin.

griseofulvin (gris″e-o-ful′vin) [USP] chemical name: (1′*S*-*trans*)-7-chloro-2′,4,6-trimethoxy-6′-methylspiro[benzofuran-2(3*H*),1′-[2]cyclohexene]-3,4′-dione. An antibiotic produced by *Penicillium griseofulvum* or by other means, $C_{17}H_{17}ClO_6$, occurring as a white to creamy white powder; used as an antifungal in the treatment of dermatophytic infections of the hands, feet, nails, and scalp, administered orally. Called also *Curling factor*.

griseomycin (gris″e-o-mi′sin) proactinomycin B.

Grisolle's sign (gre-zolz′) [Augustin *Grisolle*, French physician, 1811–1869] see under *sign*.

Gris-PEG (gris′peg) trademark for a preparation of griseofulvin.

Gritti's amputation (operation) (gre′tēz) [Rocco *Gritti*, surgeon in Milan, 1828–1920] see under *amputation*.

Gritti-Stokes amputation (gre′te-stōks) [Rocco *Gritti*; Sir William Stokes] see under *amputation*.

Grocco's sign (triangle, triangular dullness) (grok′ōz) [Pietro *Grocco*, physician in Florence, 1856–1916] see under *sign*.

grog (grog) navicular disease.

groin (groin) [L. *inguen*] the junctional region between the abdomen and thigh; called also *inguen* [NA].

Grönblad-Strandberg syndrome (gren′blad- strand′berg) [Ester Elizabeth *Grönblad*, Swedish ophthalmologist, born 1898; James Victor *Strandberg*, Swedish dermatologist] see under *syndrome*.

groove (grōōv) a shallow linear depression, especially one appearing during embryonic development or persisting in definitive bone or tooth substance; see also *fissure* and *sulcus*. **alveolingual g.,** the groove between the lower jaw and the tongue. **anterolateral g. of medulla,** sulcus lateralis anterior medullae oblongatae. **anterolateral g. of spinal cord,** sulcus lateralis anterior medullae spinalis. **anteromedian g. of spinal cord,** fissura mediana anterior medullae spinalis. **arterial g's,** sulci arteriosi. **atrioventricular g., auriculoventricular g.,** sulcus coronarius cordis. **basilar g.,** sulcus basilaris pontis. **basilar g. of occipital bone,** clivus ossis occipitalis. **basilar g. of sphenoid bone,** clivus ossis sphenoidalis. **bicipital g. of humerus,** sulcus intertubercularis humeri. **bicipital g., lateral,** sulcus bicipitalis lateralis. **bicipital g., medial,** sulcus bicipitalis medialis. **Blessig's g.,** a trace in the eye of the developing embryo corresponding in position with the future ora serrata retinae. **branchial g.,** an external furrow, lined with ectoderm, occurring in the embryo between two branchial arches. **buccal g.,** a developmental groove on the buccal surface of a posterior tooth. **carotid g. of sphenoid bone, cavernous g. of sphenoid bone,** sulcus caroticus ossis sphenoidalis. **costal g.,** sulcus costae. **dental g., primitive,** a groove in the border of the jaws of the embryo. **developmental g's,** fine grooves in the enamel which mark the junction of the primitive lobes of a tooth. **digastric g.,** incisura mastoidea ossis temporalis. **distobuccal g.,** the distal of the two buccal grooves ordinarily found on the mandibular first molar. **enamel g's,** the grooves bounding the enamel knot. **ethmoidal g.,** ethmoidal sulcus of nasal bone. **g. for eustachian tube,** sulcus tubae auditivae. **genital g.,** urethral g. **gingival g., free,** a shallow groove on the facial surface of the gingiva, running parallel to the margin of the gingiva at a distance of 0.5 to 1.5 mm., and usually at the level of, or somewhat apical to, the bottom of the gingival sulcus. **g. of great superficial petrosal nerve,** sulcus nervi petrosi majoris. **hamular g.,** sulcus hamuli pterygoidei. **Harrison's g.,** a horizontal depression along the lower border of the thorax, corresponding to the costal insertion of the diaphragm; seen in advanced rickets in children. **infraorbital g. of maxilla,** sulcus infraorbitalis maxillae. **interatrial g.,** a slight depression on the external surface of the heart, marking the separation of the atria. **interdental g.,** a linear, vertical depression on the surface of the interdental papillae; it functions as a sluiceway for the egress of food from the interproximal areas. **interosseous g. of calcaneus,** sulcus calcanei. **intertubercular g. of humerus,** sulcus intertubercularis humeri. **interventricular g., anterior,** sulcus interventricularis anterior. **interventricular g., posterior,** sulcus interventricularis posterior. **labial g.,** an embryonic groove produced by degeneration of the central cells of the labial lamina, which later becomes the vestibule of the oral cavity. **lacrimal g.,** fossa sacci lacrimalis. **g. of lacrimal bone,** sulcus lacrimalis ossis lacrimalis. **laryngotracheal g.,** a furrow at the caudal end of the embryonic pharynx that develops into the respiratory tract. **lateral g. for lateral sinus of occipital bone,** sulcus sinus transversi. **lateral g. for lateral sinus of parietal bone,** sulcus sinus sigmoidei ossis parietalis. **lateral g. for sigmoidal part of lateral sinus,** sulcus sinus sigmoidei ossis temporalis. **Liebermeister's g's,** developmental grooves on the surface of the liver. **lingual g.,** a developmental groove on the lingual surface of a posterior tooth. **medullary g.,** neural g. **mesiobuccal g.,** the mesial of the two buccal grooves ordinarily found on the mandibular first molar. **mesiolingual g.,** a groove over the junction of the fifth cusp on an upper molar tooth. **g. for middle temporal artery,** sulcus arteriae temporalis mediae. **musculospiral g.,** sulcus nervi radialis. **mylohyoid g. of inferior maxillary bone,** mylohyoid sulcus of mandible; see under *sulcus.* **nail g.,** a pathological linear depression of the nail plate running either lengthwise or, much more often, transversely. **nasal g., g. for nasal nerve,** ethmoidal sulcus of nasal bone. **nasolacrimal g.,** an epithelial ingrowth parallel with but medial to the nasomaxillary groove of the embryo, which marks the site of later development of the nasolacrimal duct. **nasomaxillary g.,** a furrow located between the maxillary and the lateral nasal process of the same side in the embryo. **nasopalatine g.,** a furrow on the lateral surface of the vomer for the nasopalatine nerve and vessels. **nasopharyngeal g.,** a faint line between the nasal cavity and the nasopharynx. **neural g.,** the groove produced by the invagination of the neural plate of the embryo during the process of formation of the neural tube; called also *medullary g.* **obturator g.,** sulcus obturatorius ossis pubis. **occipital g.,** sulcus arteriae occipitalis. **occlusal g's,** the developmental grooves on the occlusal surface of a posterior tooth. **olfactory g.,** ethmoid fossa. **optic g.,** sulcus chiasmatis. **palatine g., anterior,** canalis incisivus. **palatine g's of maxilla,** sulci palatini maxillae. **palatine g. of palatine bone,** sulcus palatinus major ossis palatini. **palatomaxillary g. of palatine bone,** sulcus palatinus major ossis palatini. **paraglenoid g's of hip bone,** sulci paraglenoidales ossis coxae. **paramedian g. of spinal cord, anterior** (*obs.*), sulcus intermedius anterior medullae spinalis. **paramedian g. of spinal cord, posterior** (*obs.*), sulcus intermedius posterior medullae spinalis. **posterolateral g. of spinal cord,** sulcus lateralis posterior medullae spinalis. **preauricular g's of ilium,** sulci paraglenoidales ossis coxae. **primitive g.,** a lengthwise furrow on the outer surface of the primitive streak of the embryo. **pterygopalatine g. of pterygoid plate,** sulcus pterygopalatinus processus pterygoidei. **radial g., g. for radial nerve,** sulcus nervi radialis. **sagittal g.,** a groove on the inner surface of the skull for the superior longitudinal sinus. **Sibson's g.,** a furrow sometimes seen at the lower border of the pectoralis major muscle. **sigmoid g. of temporal bone,** sulcus sinus sigmoidei ossis temporalis. **g. of small superficial petrosal nerve,** sulcus nervi petrosi minoris. **spiral g.,** sulcus nervi radialis. **subclavian g.,** a furrow along the middle of the clavicle for the subclavius muscle. **subcostal g.,** sulcus costae. **g. for superior longitudinal sinus,** sulcus sagittalis ossis parietalis. **supplemental g's,** grooves on the surface of a tooth which do not mark (as do the developmental grooves) the junction of the primitive lobes of the tooth. **g. for tibialis posticus muscle,** sulcus malleolaris tibiae. **trigeminal g.,** the embryonic structure which devel-

ops into the gasserian ganglion. **ulnar g., g. of ulnar nerve,** sulcus nervi ulnaris. **urethral g.,** the embryonic groove that becomes the penile urethra as the genital folds at each side bridge it. **venous g's,** venous sulci. **Verga's lacrimal g.,** a groove running downward from the lower orifice of the nasal duct. **vertebral g.,** the depression on each side of the spine between the spinous processes, laminae, and transverse processes; it lodges the deep back muscles.

gross (grōs) [L. *grossus* rough] coarse or large; visible to the naked eye, as gross pathology; macroscopic; taking no account of minutiae.

Gross's disease (grōs'ez) [Samuel David *Gross*, American surgeon, 1805–1884] see under *disease.*

Grossich's method (grōs'iks) [Antonio *Grossich,* surgeon in Fiume, 1849–1926] see under *method.*

Grossman's sign (grōs'manz) [Morris *Grossman,* American neurologist, born 1881] see under *sign.*

ground-glass (grownd-glas) having a filmy, hazy appearance, as in radiographs of a lung containing excess fluid.

group (grōōp) 1. an assemblage of objects having certain things in common. 2. a number of atoms forming a recognizable and usually a transferable portion of a molecule. **alcohol g.,** a combination of carbon, hydrogen, and oxygen atoms in a molecule, which is characteristic of a chemical compound known as an alcohol. There are three: —CH_2OH, the primary, =CHOH, the secondary, and ≡COH, the tertiary alcohol group. **azo g.,** a bivalent chemical group composed of two nitrogen atoms, —N:N—. **blood g.,** see *blood group,* under *B.* **coli-aerogenes g.,** a group of microorganisms which includes *Escherichia coli, Aerobacter aerogenes,* and a variety of forms intermediate between these two organisms; called also *coliform bacilli* or *coliform bacteria.* **colon-typhoid-dysentery g.,** a collective term referring to bacteria of the genera *Escherichia, Salmonella,* and *Shigella.* **complementophil g.,** in Ehrlich's side-chain theory, the group of the amboceptor by means of which it is attached to the complement. **cytophil g.,** in Ehrlich's side-chain theory, the group of the amboceptor by means of which it is anchored to the sensitive cell. **encounter g.,** a sensitivity group in which the members strive to gain emotional rather than intellectual insight with emphasis on the expression of interpersonal feelings in the group situation. **ergophore g.,** see *ergophore.* **glucophore g.,** see *glucophore.* **haptophore g.,** see *haptophore.* **heboid-paranoid g.,** a former concept of a group of mental disorders, including the juvenile insanities, dementia praecox, and paranoia. **hemorrhagic-septicemia g.,** a group of bacteria of which *Pasteurella pestis* is the type organism. **hog cholera g.,** paratyphoid-enteritidis g. **methyl g.,** a monovalent chemical group, —CH_3. **osmophore g.,** see *osmophore.* **paratyphoid-enteritidis g.,** a group of organisms of the genus *Salmonella,* causing food poisoning in man and various diseases in animals. **peptide g.,** the bivalent radical, —CO·NH—, formed by reaction between the NH_2 and COOH groups of adjacent amino acids, and by such linkage building up compounds known as di-, tri-, tetra-[etc.]peptides, depending on the number of amino acids making up the molecule. **prosthetic g.,** 1. an organic radical, nonprotein in nature, which together with a protein carrier forms an enzyme. 2. a cofactor tightly bound to an enzyme, i.e., it is an integral part of the enzyme and not readily dissociated from it. 3. a cofactor that may reversibly dissociate from the protein component of an enzyme; a coenzyme. **proteus g.,** a group of bacteria of which *Proteus vulgaris* is the type organism. **saccharide g.,** a combination of carbon, hydrogen, and oxygen atoms in a hypothetical molecule, $C_6H_{10}O_5$, the number of which in the compound determines the specific name of the polysaccharide, as di-, tri-, or tetrasaccharide. **salmonella g.,** enteric bacilli of the genus *Salmonella.* **sapophore g.,** see *sapophore.* **sensitivity g., sensitivity training g.,** a nonclinical group not intended for persons with mental illnesses or substantial emotional problems, which, in an effort to develop the assets of leadership, management, counseling, or other roles, focuses on self-awareness and understanding and on interpersonal interactions. Called also *training g.* (*T g.* or *T-g*). **T g., T-g,** sensitivity g. **sulfonic g.,** a monovalent radical, —SO_2OH. **toxophore g.,** see *toxophore.* **training g.,** sensitivity g.

grouping (grōōp'ing) the classification of individual entities according to certain common characteristics. **antigenic structural g.,** antigenic determinant; see under *determinant.* **blood g.,** the classification of blood (erythrocytes) according to the type to which it belongs; employed in determination of the suitability of blood for transfusion in a particular recipient, in cases of disputed paternity, and in certain criminal cases. See *blood group,* under *B.* **haptenic g.,** hapten.

group-specific (grōōp'spĕ-sif'ik) specific for a given group; as a blood group or certain microorganisms; said of agglutinins.

group-transfer (grōōp''trans'fer) denoting a chemical reaction, excluding oxidation and reduction, in which molecules exchange functional groups, a process catalyzed by enzymes called transferases.

Grove's cell (grōv) [Sir William Robert *Grove*, English physicist, 1811–1896] see under *cell*.

growth (grōth) 1. a normal process of increase in size of an organism as a result of accretion of tissue similar to that originally present. Cf. *differentiation.* 2. an abnormal formation, such as a tumor. 3. the proliferation of cells as in a bacterial culture. **absolute g.,** an expression of the actual increase in size of an individual, or of a particular organ or part. **accretionary g.,** increase in size resulting from increase in number of special cells by mitotic division, other more differentiated cells which perform various physiological functions having lost the ability to proliferate. **allometric g.,** the growth of different organs or parts of an organism at different rates. **appositional g.,** growth by addition at the periphery of a particular structure or part. Cf. *interstitial g.* **auxetic g.,** auxesis. **balanced g.,** a steady state condition in which every component of the cell doubles in a cell generation (time between divisions). **condylar g.,** the growth of the condyle of the temporomandibular joint, usually reflected in a downward and forward positioning of the mandible and teeth. **differential g.,** an expression of the comparison of the increases in size of dissimilar organisms, organs, or parts. **heterogonous g.,** growth of such a nature that, when it is plotted logarithmetically, it gives a straight line. **histiotypic g.,** uncontrolled growth of cells as occurs in tissue cultures. **interstitial g.,** growth occurring in the interior of parts or structures already formed. Cf. *appositional g.* **intussusceptive g.,** auxesis. **isometric g.,** the growth of different organs or parts of an organism at the same rate. **multiplicative g.,** increase in the size of an organism, organ, or part, resulting from increase in the number of cells brought about by their mitotic division, the average size of the cells remaining about the same. **new g.,** a neoplasm, or tumor. **organotypic g.,** controlled growth of cells as occurs normally in the production of organs and parts. **relative g.,** an expression of the comparison of the increases in size of similar organisms, organs, or parts.

grübelsucht (gre′bel-sōōkt) [Ger.] the drawing of overly fine distinctions (hair-splitting); worrying over trifles. Seen in obsessive-compulsive personalities.

Gruber's bougies, speculum, test (groo′berz) [Josef *Gruber*, Austrian otologist, 1827–1900] see under *bougie, speculum,* and *tests.*

Gruber's fossa, hernia, suture (groo′berz) [Wenaslaus Leopoldovich *Gruber*, Russian anatomist, 1814–1890] see under *fossa* and *hernia,* and see *fissura petrosphenooccipitalis.*

Gruber's reaction test (groo′berz) [Max von *Gruber*, bacteriologist in Munich, 1853–1927] Widal's test.

Gruber-Widal reaction, test (groo′ber-ve-dahl′) [Max von *Gruber;* Georges Fernand Isidore *Widal,* French physician, 1862–1929] Gruber's reaction.

Grubyella (groo″be-el′ah) former name for the genus *Trichophyton.*

gruel (groo′el) a thin paste or porridge made of cereal grain.

gruffs (grufs) the coarse part of a drug.

grumose, grumous (groo′mōs, groo′mus) [L. *grumus* heap] clotted or lumpy.

Grünbaum-Widal test (grēn′bowm-ve-dahl′) [A. S. *Grünbaum;* Georges Fernand Isidore *Widal,* French physician, 1862–1929] Gruber's reaction.

grundplatte (groont-plaht′tĕ) [Ger.] lamina basalis.

grutum (groo′tum) [L.] (*obs.*) milium.

Grynfelt's hernia, triangle (grin′felts) [Joseph Casimir *Grynfelt,* French surgeon, 1840–1913] see under *hernia,* and see *Lesgaft's space,* under *space.*

Grynfelt-Lesgaft triangle (grin′felt-les′gaft) [Joseph Casimir *Grynfelt;* Peter Frantsevich *Lesgaft,* Russian physician, 1837–1909] Lesgaft's space.

gryochrome (gri′o-krōm) [Gr. *gry* morsel + *chrōma* color] a nerve cell in which the stainable matter of the cell body appears as fine granules; used also adjectively.

gryphosis (gri-fo′sis) abnormal curvature; see *gryposis.*

gryposis (gri-po′sis) [Gr. *grypōsis* a crooking, hooking] abnormal curvature, as of the nails. **g. pe′nis** chordee. **g. un′guium** (*obs.*), onychogryphosis.

GSH reduced glutathione.

GSSG oxidized glutathione.

G.S.W. gunshot wound.

gt. abbreviation for L. *gut′ta,* drop.

GTH gonadotropic hormone.

GTP guanosine triphosphate.

gtt. abbreviation for L. *gut′tae,* drops.

GU genitourinary.

guaco (gwah′ko) [Spanish American] a name given to many South American plants, and especially to *Mikania guaco;* Humb. & Bonpl. (Compositae); used by certain South American natives in asthma, dyspepsia, gout, rheumatism, and skin diseases, and reportedly for snakebite.

guaiac (gwi′ak) a resin from the wood of *Guajacum officinale*

L. and *G. sanctum* L. (Zygophyllaceae), trees of Haiti and the Dominican Republic; used as a reagent in tests for occult blood and formerly in the treatment of rheumatism.

guaiacol (gwi′ah-kol) the methyl ether of pyrocatechin, a solid or a colorless oily liquid, $OH \cdot C_6H_4O \cdot CH_3$, derived from beech creosote; formerly used as an expectorant.

guaifenesin (gwi-fen′ĕ-sin) [USP] chemical name: 3-(2-methoxyphenoxy)-1,2-propanediol. The glyceryl ester of guaiacol, $C_{10}H_{14}O_4$, occurring as a white or slightly gray, crystalline powder; used as an expectorant, administered orally. Called also *glyceryl guaiacolate, guaiphenesin,* and *methphenoxydiol.*

guaiphenesin (gwi-fen′ĕ-sin) guaifenesin.

guaithylline (gwi′thĭ-lin) chemical name: theophylline compound with 3-(o-methoxyphenoxy)-1,2-propanediol; a bronchodilator and expectorant, $C_7H_8N_4O_2 \cdot C_{10}H_{14}O_4$.

guanabenz (gwan′ah-benz) chemical name: 2-[(2,6-dichlorophenyl)methylene]hydrazinecarboximidamide; an antihypertensive, $C_8H_8Cl_2N_4$.

guanacline sulfate (gwan′ah-klēn) chemical name: [2-(3,6-dihydro-4-methyl-1(2H)-pyridyl)ethyl]guanidine sulfate (1:1) dihydrate; an antihypertensive, $C_9H_{18}N_4 \cdot H_2SO_4 \cdot 2H_2O$.

guanadrel sulfate (gwan′ah-drel) chemical name: (1,4-dioxaspiro[4.5]dec-2-ylmethyl)guanidine sulfate (2:1); an antihypertensive, $(C_{10}H_{19}N_3O_2)_2 \cdot H_2SO_4$.

guanase (gwan′ās) guanine deaminase.

guancydine (gwan′sĭ-dēn) chemical name: N″-cyano-N-(1,1-dimethylpropyl) guanidine; an antihypertensive, $C_7H_{14}N_4$.

guanethidine (gwan-eth′ĭ-dēn) chemical name: [2-(hexahydro-1(2H)-azocinyl)ethyl]guanidine; an adrenergic blocking agent, $C_{10}H_{22}N_4$, which has prolonged and marked hypotensive effects. **g. monosulfate,** the monosulfate salt of guanethidine, $C_{10}H_{22}N_4 \cdot H_2SO_4$, used as an antihypertensive. **g. sulfate** [USP], the sulfate salt of guanethidine, $(C_{10}H_{22}N_4)_2 \cdot H_2SO_4$, used as an oral antihypertensive.

guanidase (gwan′ĭ-dās) an enzyme produced by several organisms, including *Aspergillus niger;* it hydrolyzes guanidine into urea and ammonia.

guanidine (gwan′ĭ-din) a poisonous base, the amidine of amino carbamic acid, $NH:C(NH_2)_2$. **g. hydrochloride,** a compound used in the treatment of myasthenia gravis.

guanidinemia (gwan′ĭ-din-e′me-ah) the presence of guanidine in the blood.

guanine (gwan′in) a white, crystalline base, 2-amino-6-oxypurine, $C_5H_5N_5O$, found in guano, fish scales, leguminous seedlings, and various animal tissues. It is a fundamental constituent of DNA and RNA, and occurs as a white deposit in the tissues of swine affected with a kind of gout. **g. nucleotide,** guanylic acid.

guanochlor sulfate (gwan′o-klor) chemical name: 2-[2-(2,6-dichlorophenoxy)ethyl]hydrazinecarboximidamide sulfate (2:1); an antihypertensive, $[C_9H_{12}Cl_2N_4O]_2 \cdot H_2SO_4$.

guanophore (gwan′o-for) [*guanine* + Gr. *phoros* bearing] a cell filled with guanine crystals which produce interference in the light and thus give the cell a silvery appearance.

guanosine (gwan′o-sin) a nucleoside, guanine riboside, $C_{10}H_{13}O_5N_5$, a major constituent of DNA and RNA; it is extracted from the leaves and unripe berries of the coffee plant and is used in biochemical research. **g. monophosphate (GMP),** a nucleotide important in metabolism and for the formation of RNA on DNA templates. **g. triphosphate (GTP),** an energy-rich compound, analogous to adenosine triphosphate (ATP), involved in several metabolic reactions, e.g., the formation of peptide bonds in protein synthesis and of an intermediate in purine synthesis.

guanoxabenz (gwahn-oks′ah-benz) chemical name: 2-[(2,6-dichlorophenyl)methylene]-N-hydroxyhydrazine carboximidamide; an antihypertensive, $C_8H_8Cl_2N_4O$.

guanoxan sulfate (gwan-oks′an) chemical name: (2,3-dihydro-1,4-benzodioxin-2-ylmethyl)guanidine; an antihypertensive, $[C_{10}H_{13}N_3O_2]_2 \cdot H_2SO_4$.

guarana (gwah-rah′nah) [Tupi-Guarani] a dried paste prepared from the seeds of *Paullinia cupana,* a tree of Brazil; used as an astringent in diarrhea.

guaranine (gwah-rah′nin) caffeine.

guard (gahrd) a protective device. **mouth g.,** an elastoplastic removable appliance, used to protect the teeth and their investing tissues in contact sports. **night g.,** an acrylic resin removable device used to stabilize the teeth and to minimize the traumatic effects of occlusal habits such as bruxism.

Guarnieri's bodies (corpuscles) (gwar″ne-er′ēz) [Guiseppi *Guarnieri,* Italian physician, 1856–1918] see under *body.*

guayule (gwi-oo′la) the Mexican rubber plant, *Parthenium argentatum,* which may produce a severe allergic dermatitis (guayule dermatitis).

gubernacular (gu″ber-nak′u-lar) pertaining to a gubernaculum.

gubernaculum (gu″ber-nak′u-lum) [L. "helm," "rudder"] something which guides. **chorda g.,** a portion of the gubernaculum testis and round ligament that develops in the body wall of the embryo. **Hunter's g.,** g. testis. **g. tes′tis** [NA], the fetal ligament attached to the lower end of the epididymis and testis and, at its other end, to the bottom of the scrotum; it is present during, and is thought to guide, the descent of the testis into the scrotum and then atrophies. Called also *Hunter's g.*

Gubler's hemiplegia, etc. (goob′lerz) [Adolphe Marie *Gubler,* French physician, 1821–1879] see under *hemiplegia, line, paralysis, sign,* and *tumor.*

Gubler-Robin typhus [A. M. *Gubler;* Albert Edouard Charles *Robin,* French physician, 1847–1928] see under *typhus.*

Gudden's commissure, law [Bernhard Alloys von *Gudden,* German neurologist, 1824–1886] see *commissurae supraorbitae,* and see under *law.*

Guelpa treatment (gwel′pah) [Guglielmo *Guelpa,* Italian physician in Paris, 1850–1930] see under *treatment.*

Guéneau de Mussy's point (ga-no′dŭ-mis-sēz′) [Noel François Odon *Guéneau de Mussy,* French physician, 1813–1885] see *de Mussy's point,* under *point.*

Guenz (gints) see *Günz.*

Guenzburg (gints′boorg) see *günzburg.*

Guérin's fold, etc. (ga-ranz′) [Alphonse François Marie *Guérin,* French surgeon, 1816–1895] see under *fold, fracture, gland, sinus,* and *valve.*

guidance (gīd′ans) 1. a guide. 2. an act of guidance. **condylar g.,** the mechanical device on a dental articulator which is intended to produce guidance in articulator movement similar to those produced by the paths of the condyles in the temporomandibular joints. **incisal g.,** the influence on mandibular movements by the contacting surfaces of the mandibular and maxillary anterior teeth.

guide (gīd) a device by which another object is led in its proper course, such as a grooved sound, or a filiform bougie over which a tunneled sound is passed, as in stricture of the urethra. **adjustable anterior g.,** an anterior guide whose superior surface may be varied to provide desired separation of dental casts in various eccentric relationships. **anterior g.,** that part of a dental articulator on which the anterior guide pin rests to maintain the vertical dimension of occlusion; it influences the degree of separation of the casts in eccentric relationships. **condylar g. inclination,** the angle of inclination of the condylar guidance mechanism of an articulator in relation to the horizontal plane of the instrument. **incisal g.,** that part of a dental articulator which maintains the incisal guide angle.

guideline (gīd′līn) any line used as a marker or indicator. **clasp g.,** survey line.

Guidi's canal (gwe′dēz) [Guido *Guidi* (L., *Vidius* (Vidus), Italian physician, 1500–1569] canalis pterygoideus.

Guillain-Barré syndrome (ge-yan′-bar-ra′) [Georges *Guillain,* French neurologist, 1876–1961; Jean Alexander *Barré,* French neurologist, born 1880] acute febrile polyneuritis.

guillotine (gil′o-tēn) [Fr.] an instrument for excising a tonsil or the uvula.

Guinard's treatment (method) (ge-narz′) [Aimé *Guinard,* French surgeon, 1856–1911] see under *treatment.*

guinea pig (gin′e pig) a small rodent, *Cavia cobaya,* used extensively for experimental work.

Guinon's disease (ge-nawz′) [Georges *Guinon,* French physician, 1859–1929] Gilles de la Tourette syndrome.

Guiteras' disease (ge-ta′ras) [Juan *Guiteras,* Cuban physician, 1852–1925] see under *disease.*

Gull's disease (gulz) [Sir William Withey *Gull,* English physician, 1816–1890] see under *disease.*

gullet (gul′et) the esophagus.

Gullstrand's slit lamp, law (gul′strandz) [Allvar *Gullstrand,* Swedish ophthalmologist, 1862–1930; winner of the Nobel prize for physiology and medicine in 1911 for his work on the dioptrics of the eye] see under *lamp* and *law.*

L-gulonolactone (gu″lo-no-lak′tōn) the immediate precursor of ascorbic acid in plants and in those animals capable of its biosynthesis; gulonolactone is itself formed from L-gulonic acid.

gulose (gu′lōs) a hexose, CH₂OH(CHOH)₄CHO, isomeric with glucose but nonfermentable.

gum (gum) [L. *gummi*] 1. a mucilaginous excretion from various plants; on hydrolysis gums yield hexoses, pentoses, and uronic acids. 2. see *gingivae.* **acaroid g.,** a resin derived from *Xanthorrhoea hastilis* and *X. arborea,* tall liliaceous plants growing in Australia. **animal g.,** a polysaccharide isolated from various proteins and tissues; possibly an impure chondroitin. **g. arabic,** acacia. **Australian g.,** wattle g. **g. benjamin, g. benzoin,** benzoin, def. 1. **blackboy g.,** acaroid g. **blue g.,** 1. eucalyptus. 2. the bluish discoloration of the gums seen in lead poisoning. **Botany Bay g.,** acaroid gum. **British g.,** dextrin. **g. camphor,** camphor. **cape g.,** a gum from *Acacia horrida.* **eucalyptus g.,** red g. **ghatti g.,** a gum from the dhava tree of India; used like acacia. **guar g.** [NF], a gum obtained from the ground endosperms of the leguminous tree *Cyamopsis tetragonolobus;* used as a tablet binder and disintegrant

in pharmaceutical preparations. **Indian g.,** karaya g. **karaya g.,** the dried gummy exudation from *Sterculia urens* or other species of *Sterculia,* which becomes gelatinous when moisture is added; used as a bulk laxative. Because of its adhesive properties, products containing karaya gum are used as dental adhesives and as skin adhesives and protective skin barriers in the fitting and care of colostomy appliances and in other conditions involving an artificial stoma. Called also *sterculia g.* **Kordofan g.,** the best variety of acacia from Kordofan and adjacent region. **mesquite g.,** a gum from *Prosopis juliflora,* of Texas; used as a substitute for acacia. **g. opium,** opium. **red g.,** an exudation from the bark of *Eucalyptus rostrata* and other species; used as an astringent in throat affections. **g. senegal,** acacia. **sterculia g.,** karaya g. **g. thus,** turpentine. **g. tragacanth,** tragacanth. **xanthan g.** [NF], a high molecular weight polysaccharide gum produced by a pure-culture fermentation of a carbohydrate with *Xanthomonas campestris,* then purified by recovery with isopropyl alcohol, dried, and milled; it contains D-glucose and D-mannose as the dominant hexose units, along with D-glucuronic acid, is prepared as the sodium, potassium, or calcium salt, and is used as a suspending agent in pharmaceutical preparations. **wattle g.,** the gum of several Australian species of *Acacia,* an excellent substitute for acacia.

gumboil (gum′boil) parulis.

gumma (gum′ah), pl. *gummas* or *gum′mata* [L. *gummi* gum] a soft, gummy tumor, such as that occurring in tertiary syphilis, made up of tissue resembling granulation tissue; syphiloma. **miliary g.,** the large gumma of syphilitic aortitis which obliterates the normal perivascular arrangement of cells. **scrofulous g.,** tuberculous g. **tuberculous g.,** a soft gummy tumor of tuberculous origin, occurring in scrofuloderma gummosa.

gummata (gum′ah-tah) plural of *gumma.*

gummate (gum′āt) an arabate.

gummatous (gum′ah-tus) of the nature of gumma.

gummi (gum′i) [L.] gum (of plants).

gummy (gum′e) resembling a gum or a gumma.

Gumprecht's shadow (goom′prekts) [Ferdinand *Gumprecht,* German physician, born 1864] see under *shadow.*

gum-resin (gum-rez′in) a concrete juice exuding from various trees. The gum-resins consist of a principle soluble in water and insoluble in alcohol, combined with a volatile oil or resin soluble in alcohol, but not in water, and include ammoniac, gamboge, myrrh, and scammony.

guncotton (gun-kot′n) pyroxylin.

gundo (goon′do) goundou.

Gunn's dots, syndrome (phenomenon) (gunz) [Robert Marcus *Gunn,* English ophthalmologist, 1850–1909] see under *dot* and *syndrome.*

Gunning's test (reaction) (gun′ingz) [Jan Willem *Gunning,* Dutch chemist, 1827–1901] see under *test.*

Gunning's splint (gun′ingz) [Thomas Brian *Gunning,* American dentist, 1813–1889] see under *splint.*

Günz's ligament (gints′ez) [Justus Gottfried *Günz,* German anatomist, 1714–1754] see under *ligament.*

Günzberg's test (gints′boorgz) [Alfred *Günzberg,* German physician, born 1861] see under *tests.*

gurgulio (gur-gu′le-o) [L. "gullet"] uvula palatina.

gurney (ger′nē) a wheeled cot used in hospitals.

Gussenbauer's operation, suture (goos′en-bow″erz) [Carl *Gussenbauer,* German surgeon, 1842–1903] see under *operation* and *suture.*

gustation (gus-ta′shun) [L. *gustatio,* from *gustare* to taste] the act of tasting or the sense of taste. **colored g.,** the association of colors with tastes.

gustatism (gus′tah-tizm) a sensation of taste produced indirectly by other than gustatory stimuli.

gustatory (gus′tah-to″re) [L. *gustatorius*] pertaining to the sense of taste.

gustin (gus′tin) a polypeptide (molecular weight, 27,000) present in saliva and containing two zinc atoms; it is apparently necessary for normal development of the taste buds.

gustometer (gus-tom′ĕ-ter) [L. *gustare* to taste + Gr. *metron* measure] an apparatus used in the quantitative determination of taste thresholds.

gustometry (gus-tom′ĕ-tre) the clinical determination of thresholds of the sense of taste.

gut (gut) 1. the intestine or bowel. 2. the primitive digestive tube, consisting of the fore-, mid-, and hindgut. 3. catgut. **blind g.,** the cecum. **postanal g.,** a temporary extension of the embryonic gut caudal to the cloaca. **preoral g.,** Seessel's pouch. **primitive g.,** archenteron. **ribbon g.,** an absorbable ribbon of the intestinal tissue of animals used for suturing where broad support is to be secured. **silkworm g.,** see *silkworm-gut,* under *S.* **tail g.,** postanal g.

Guthrie's formula (guth′rēz) [Clyde Graeme *Guthrie,* American physician, 1880–1931] see under *formula.*

Guthrie's muscle (guth'rēz) [George James *Guthrie*, English surgeon, 1785–1856] musculus sphincter urethrae.

gutta (gut'ah), pl. *gut'tae* [L.] a drop. **g. sere'na** (*obs.*), amaurosis.

guttae (gut'e) plural of *gutta*.

gutta-percha (gut"ah-per'chah) [USP] the coagulated, dried, purified latex of trees of the genera *Palaguium* and *Payena*, most commonly *Palaguium gutta;* used as a dental restoration agent and in orthopedics for fracture splints. **baseplate g.,** gutta-percha combined with fillers and coloring materials, rolled into sheets; used in dentistry for temporary restorations, filling root canals, separating teeth, and restricting gingival tissue.

Guttat. abbreviation for L. *gutta'tim*, drop by drop.

guttate (gut'āt) characterized by lesions that are drop-shaped.

guttatim (gut-ta'tim) [L.] drop by drop.

guttation (gut-ta'shun) the secretion of water by plant cells under humid conditions, an indication that the cells actively transport some materials against a concentration gradient.

guttering (gut'er-ing) the operation of cutting a gutter-like excision in a bone.

gutti (gut'i) cambogia.

gut-tie (gut'ti) 1. a twisting of the intestine of animals, causing colicky pains. 2. a condition in cattle in which a loop of intestine passes through a tear in the peritoneum and is held there, producing obstruction of the bowels.

Guttmann's sign (goot'mahnz) [Paul *Guttmann*, Berlin physician, 1834–1893] see under *sign*.

Gutt. quibusd. abbreviation for L. *gut'tis quibus'dam*, with a few drops.

guttur (gut'ur) [L.] throat.

guttural (gut'ur-al) pertaining to the throat.

gutturophony (gut"ur-of'o-ne) [*guttur* + Gr. *phōnē* voice] throaty quality of the voice.

gutturotetany (gut"ur-o-tet'ah-ne) [*guttur* + *tetany*] a guttural spasm, resulting in a kind of stutter.

Gutzeit's test (goot'zītz) [Max Adolf *Gutzeit*, Leipzig chemist, 1847–1915] see under *tests*.

Guy de Chauliac see *Chauliac*.

Guyon's amputation (operation), sign (ge-yonz') [Felix Jean Casimir *Guyon*, surgeon in Paris, 1831–1920] see under *amputation* and *sign*.

GVH graft-versus-host; see under *reaction*.

Gwathmey's oil-ether anesthesia (gwath'mēz) [James Taylor *Gwathmey*, New York surgeon, 1863–1944] see under *anesthesia*.

Gy gray, def. 3.

gymnastics (jim-nas'tiks) [Gr. *gymnastikos* pertaining to athletics] systematic muscular exercise. **ocular g.,** systematic exercise of the eye muscles in order to secure proper movement, accommodation, or fixation. **Swedish g.,** a system of exercise following a rigid pattern of carefully chosen free, active, deliberate movement, utilizing little equipment and stressing correct bodily posture. **vocal g.,** methodical exercise for the purpose of increasing the lung expansion and strengthening the voice.

Gymnema (jim-ne'mah) a genus of trees. The leaves of *G. sylvestre* R. Bv. (Asclepiadaceae), of Africa, are used to disguise the taste of unpleasant medicines. See also *gymnemic acid*, under *acid*.

gymno- (jim'no) [Gr. *gymnos* naked] a combining form meaning naked or denoting relationship to nakedness.

Gymnoascaceae (jim"no-as-ka'se-e) a family of the ascomycetous fungi, order Eurotiales, series Plectomycetes, in which the reproductive organs are in the form of naked asci. It includes the genera *Ajellomyces*, *Arthroderma*, *Gymnoascus*, and *Nannizzia*.

Gymnoascus (jim"no-as'kus) a genus of keratinophilic fungi of the family Gymnoascaceae, some species of which have been isolated from skin lesions of domestic animals and man.

gymnobacteria (jim"no-bak-te're-ah) [*gymno-* + *bacteria*] plural of *gymnobacterium*.

gymnobacterium (jim"no-bak-te're-um), pl. *gymnobacteria*. A microorganism which has no flagella.

gymnocarpous (jim"no-kar'pus) [*gymno-* + Gr. *karpos* fruit] having the hymenium, or fertile layer, exposed during spore formation; said of certain fungi.

gymnocyte (jim'no-sīt) [*gymno-* + Gr. *kytos* hollow vessel] a cell with no cell wall.

Gymnodinium (jim"no-din'e-um) a genus of protozoa of the order Dinoflagellata, class Phytomastigophora, most species of which have many colored (yellow, brown, green, or blue) chromatophores. They inhabit salt, fresh, or brackish waters and, when present in great numbers, cause the discoloration known as red tide, which may result in the death of many fish and invertebrates.

gymnoplast (jim'no-plast) [*gymno-* + Gr. *plastos* formed] a mass of protoplasm without an enclosing wall.

gymnoscopic (jim"no-skop'ik) [*gymno-* + Gr. *skopein* to examine] (*obs.*) inclined to or concerned with viewing the naked body.

gymnosophy (jim-nos'o-fe) [*gymno-* + Gr. *sophia* wisdom] (*obs.*) the cult of nakedness; nudism.

gymnosperm (jim'no-sperm) [*gymno-* + Gr. *sperma* seed] a plant in which the seeds are not enclosed in an ovary.

gymnospore (jim'no-spōr) a spore without any protective envelope.

gymnothecium (jim"no-the'se-um) the fruiting body produced by the sexual (perfect) stage of dermatophytes of the genera *Arthroderma* and *Nannizzia;* it is a loose network of mycelium through which ascospores filter and are released following maturation. Cf. *apothecium, cleistothecium,* and *perithecium.*

Gymnothorax (jim"no-tho'raks) [*gymno-* + Gr. *thōrax* chest] a genus of moray eels whose flesh is sometimes used as food.

gyn- see *gyneco-*.

gynaeco- for words beginning thus, see those beginning *gyneco-*.

gynander (jĭ-nan'der) [*gyn-* + Gr. *anēr, andros* man] 1. a hermaphrodite. 2. a masculine woman.

gynandria (jĭ-nan'dre-ah) gynandrism.

gynandrism (jĭ-nan'drizm) [*gyn-* + *andr-* + *-ism*] 1. hermaphroditism. 2. female pseudohermaphroditism.

gynandroblastoma (jĭ-nan"dro-blas-to'mah) [*gyn-* + *andro-* + *blastoma*] a rare ovarian tumor containing histological features of both arrhenoblastoma and granulosa cell tumor.

gynandroid (jĭ-nan'droid) [*gyn-* + *andr-* + Gr. *eidos* form] 1. hermaphrodite. 2. female pseudohermaphrodite.

gynandromorph (jĭ-nan'dro-morf) an individual exhibiting gynandromorphism.

gynandromorphism (jĭ-nan"dro-mor'fizm) [*gyn-* + *andro-* + Gr. *morphē* form] the presence of chromosomes of both sexes in different tissues of the body, producing a mosaic of male and female characteristics; a condition common among bees and silkworms. **bilateral g.,** bilateral hermaphroditism.

gynandromorphous (jĭ-nan"dro-mor'fus) 1. pertaining to or characterized by gynandromorphism. 2. pertaining to a gynandromorph.

gynandry (jĭ'nan-dre) gynandrism.

gynanthropia (ji"nan-thro'pe-ah) gynandrism.

gynanthropism (ji-nan'thro-pizm) gynandrism.

gynatresia (jin"ah-tre'ze-ah) [*gyn-* + *a* neg. + Gr. *trēsis* perforation] occlusion of some part of the female genital tract, especially of the vagina.

gynecic (jĭ-nes'ik) pertaining to women.

gynecium (jĭ-ne'se-um) [*gyn-* + Gr. *oikos* house] the female part of a flower; called also *pistil*.

gyneco-, gynaeco-, gyn-, gyne-, gyno- [Gr. *gynē, gynaikos* woman] a combining form denoting relationship to woman or to the female sex.

gynecogen (jin'ĕ-ko-jen) any substance (female sex hormones) which produces or stimulates female characteristics.

gynecogenic (jin"ĕ-ko-jen'ik) [*gyneco-* + Gr. *gennan* to produce] causing or producing female characteristics.

gynecography (jin"e-kog'rah-fe) roentgenography of the female reproductive tract.

gynecoid (jin'ĕ-koid) [*gyneco-* + Gr. *eidos* form] woman-like; resembling a woman.

gynecologic (gi"nĕ-ko-loj'ik, jin"ĕ-ko-loj'ik) pertaining to or affecting the female reproductive tract.

gynecological (gi"nĕ-ko-loj'ĭ-k'l, jin"ĕ-ko-loj'ĭ-k'l) pertaining to gynecology.

gynecologist (gi"nĕ-kol'o-jist, jin"ĕ-kol'o-jist) a person skilled in gynecology.

gynecology (gi"ne-kol'o-je, jin"ĕ-kol'o-je) [*gyneco-* + *-logy*] that branch of medicine which treats of diseases of the genital tract in women.

gynecomania (jin"ĕ-ko-ma'ne-ah) [*gyneco-* + Gr. *mania* madness] satyriasis.

gynecomastia (jin"ĕ-ko-mas'te-ah) [*gyneco-* + Gr. *mastos* breast] excessive development of the male mammary glands, even to the functional state. **nutritional g.,** refeeding g. **refeeding g.,** transitory enlargement of the male breast developing during rehabilitation and recovery from a state of malnutrition. **rehabilitation g.,** refeeding g.

gynecomastism (jin"ĕ-ko-mas'tizm) gynecomastia.

gynecomasty (jin'ĕ-ko-mas"te) gynecomastia.

gynecomazia (jin"ĕ-ko-ma'ze-ah) gynecomastia.

gynecopathy (jin"ĕ-kop'ah-the) [*gyneco-* + Gr. *pathos* disease] a disease peculiar to women.

gynecophoral (jin"ĕ-kof'o-ral) see under *canal*.

gynecotokology (jin"ĕ-ko-to-kol'o-je) [*gyneco-* + Gr. *tokos* birth + *-logy*] a name suggested for the combined specialities of gynecology and obstetrics.

gyneduct (jin'ĕ-dukt) [*gyne-* + *duct*] the primitive female duct; müllerian duct.

gynephilia (jin″ĕ-fil′e-ah) a morbid desire in adolescent boys to be in the company of women or girls.

gynephobia (jin″ĕ-fo′be-ah) [gyne- + Gr. phobein to be affrighted by + ia] dread of or morbid aversion to the society of women.

gyneplasty (jin′ĕ-plas″te) gynoplasty.

Gynergen (jin′ĕr-jen) trademark for preparations of ergotamine tartrate.

gynesin (jin′ĕ-sin) trigonelline.

gyno- see gyneco-.

gynogamon (ji-no-gam′ōn) a gamone released by the ovum.

gynogenesis (jin″o-jen′ĕ-sis) [gyno- + Gr. genesis production] development of an egg that is stimulated by a sperm in the absence of any participation of the sperm nucleus.

gynomerogon (jin″o-mer′o-gon) an organism developed from a fertilized ovum that contains the female pronucleus only, the cells, as a result, containing only the maternal set of chromosomes.

gynomerogone (jin″o-mer′o-gon) gynomerogon.

gynomerogony (jin″o-mĕ-rog′o-ne) [gyno- + Gr. meros part + gonos procreation] development of a portion of a fertilized ovum containing the female pronucleus only. Cf. andromerogony and merogony.

gynopathic (jin″o-path′ik) [gyno- + Gr. pathos disease] caused by or pertaining to disease of women.

gynopathy (jin-op′ah-the) any disease of women.

gynophobia (ji″no-fo′be-ah) gynephobia.

gynoplastic (ji″no-plas′tik) pertaining to gynoplastics.

gynoplastics (ji″no-plas′tiks) [gyno- + Gr. plastos formed] the plastic or reconstructive surgery of the female reproductive organs.

gynoplasty (ji′no-plas″te) plastic or reconstructive surgery of the female reproductive organs.

Gynorest (gi′no-rest) trademark for a preparation of dydrogesterone.

gypsum (jip′sum) [L.; Gr. gypsos chalk] native calcium sulfate dihydrate; when calcined, it becomes plaster of Paris, much used in making permanent dressings for fractures and in dentistry for taking dental impressions. See also calcuim sulfate.

gyrate (ji′rāt) [L. gyratus turned round] twisted in a ring or spiral shape.

gyration (ji-ra′shun) revolution in a circle or in circles.

gyre (jīr) gyrus.

gyrectomy (ji-rek′to-me) excision or resection of a cerebral gyrus, or of a portion of the cerebral cortex. **frontal g.,** topectomy.

Gyrencephala (ji″ren-sef′ah-lah) [gyrus + Gr. enkephalos brain] a group of higher mammals in which the brain is characteristically marked by convolutions. Cf. Lissencephala.

gyrencephalic (ji″ren-sĕ-fal′ik) pertaining to the Gyrencephala; having a brain marked by convolutions. Cf. lissencephalic.

gyri (ji′ri) [L.] plural of gyrus.

gyro- (ji′ro) [Gr. gyros ring or circle] a combining form meaning round or denoting relationship to a gyrus.

gyrochrome (ji′ro-krōm) [gyro- + Gr. chrōma color] a nerve cell in which the Nissl bodies have a ringlike arrangement in the cytoplasm. Cf. arkyochrome, perichrome, and stichochrome.

gyrometer (ji-rom′ĕ-ter) [gyro- + Gr. metron measure] an instrument for measuring the cerebral gyri.

Gyropus (ji′ro-pus) a genus of biting lice. **G. ova′lis,** a biting louse found on guinea pigs.

gyrose (ji′rōs) marked by curved lines or circles.

gyrospasm (ji′ro-spazm) [gyro- + Gr. spasmos spasm] rotatory spasm of the head.

gyrotrope (ji′ro-trōp) rheotrope.

gyrous (ji′rus) gyrose.

gyrus (ji′rus), pl. gy′ri [L.; Gr. gyros ring or circle] [NA] one of the tortuous elevations (convolutions) of the surface of the brain caused by infolding of the cortex; see gyri cerebri. **angular g., g. angula′ris** [NA], a convolution of the inferior parietal lobule, arching over the posterior end of the superior temporal sulcus and continuous with the middle temporal gyrus. **annectant gyri, gy′ri annecten′tes,** gyri transitivi cerebri. **gy′ri bre′ves in′sulae** [NA], short gyri of insula: the short, rostrally placed gyri on the surface of the insula; called also preinsular gyri. **Broca's g.,** see under convolution. **callosal g., g. callo′sus,** g. cinguli. **central g., anterior,** g. precentralis. **central g., posterior,** g. postcentralis. **g. centra′lis ante′rior,** g. precentralis. **g. centra′lis poste′rior,** g. postcentralis. **g. cerebel′li,** folia cerebelli. **gy′ri cere′bri** [NA], **gyri of cerebrum,** the tortuous elevations (convolutions) of the surface of the cerebral hemisphere, caused by infolding of the cortex and separated by the fissures or sulci. Many are constant enough that they have been given special names. **cingulate g., g. cin′guli** [NA], arch-shaped convolution closely related to the surface of the corpus callosum, from which it is separated by the callosal sulcus; called also callosal g. or g.

callosus. **dentate g.,** 1. gyrus dentatus (def. 1). 2. gyrus fasciolaris. **g. denta′tus,** 1. [NA], the dentate gyrus: a serrated strip of gray matter under the medial border of the hippocampus and in its depths; it is an archicortex which develops along the edge of the hippocampal fissure and which consists of molecular, granular, and polymorphic layers. Called also fascia dentata hippocampi. 2. gyrus fasciolaris. **g. fasciola′ris** [NA], a posterior and upward extension of the dentate gyrus, forming a transitional area between the dentate gyrus and the indusium griseum; called also fasciola cinerea. **g. fornica′tus,** the marginal portion of the cerebral cortex on the medial aspect of the hemisphere, including the gyrus cinguli, gyrus parahippocampalis, isthmus, and uncus; it forms a major part of the limbic system. **frontal g., ascending,** g. precentralis. **frontal g., inferior,** g. frontalis inferior. **frontal g., middle,** g. frontalis medius. **frontal g., superior,** g. frontalis superior. **g. fronta′lis infe′rior** [NA], inferior frontal gyrus: a convolution of the frontal lobe below the inferior frontal sulcus; it is divided by the anterior and ascending branches of the lateral sulcus into orbital, triangular, and opercular parts. **g. fronta′lis media′lis** [NA], the medial surface of the frontal lobe, separated from the cingulate gyrus by the cingulate sulcus, and continuous with the superior frontal gyrus above and the gyrus rectus below. **g. fronta′lis me′dius** [NA], middle frontal gyrus: a convolution of the frontal lobe between the superior and inferior frontal sulci, extending anteriorly from the precentral gyrus. **g. fronta′lis supe′rior** [NA], superior frontal gyrus: a convolution of the frontal lobe above the superior frontal sulcus, extending anteriorly from the precentral gyrus. **fusiform g., g. fusifor′mis,** a gyrus of the temporal lobe on the inferior surface of the hemisphere between the inferior temporal gyrus and the parahippocampal gyrus. It consists of a lateral and a medial part, called [NA] g. occipitotemporalis lateralis and g. occipitotemporalis medialis. **g. genic′uli,** a vestigial gyrus at the anterior end of the corpus callosum. **Heschl's g.,** gyri temporales transversi. **hippocampal g., g. hippocam′pi,** g. parahippocampalis. **infracalcarine g., g. infracalcari′nus,** g. lingualis. **gy′ri in′sulae** [NA], the gyri that are found on the surface of the insula, including the gyrus longus insulae and the gyri breves insulae. **g. lim′bicus,** gyrus fornicatus. **lingual g., g. lingua′lis** [NA], a gyrus of the occipital lobe on the inferior surface of the hemisphere, forming the inferior lip of the calcarine sulcus and, with the cuneus, the visual cortex; it is continuous anteriorly with the parahippocampal gyrus. **long g. of insula, g. lon′gus in′sulae** [NA], the long, occipitally directed gyrus on the surface of the insula. **marginal g., g. frontalis medialis. marginal g. of Turner,** g. frontalis medialis. **g. margina′lis** g. frontalis medialis. **occipital gyri, lateral,** see occipital g., inferior and occipital g., superior. **occipital g., inferior,** the lower of the two gyri separated by the lateral occipital sulcus on the lateral aspect of the occipital lobe. **occipital g., superior,** the upper of the two gyri separated by the occipital lateral sulcus on the lateral aspect of the occipital lobe. **occipitotemporal g., lateral,** g. occipitotemporalis lateralis. **occipitotemporal g., medial,** g. occipitotemporalis medialis. **g. occipitotempora′lis latera′lis** [NA], lateral occipitotemporal gyrus: the lateral portion of a gyrus (g. fusiformis) on the inferior surface of the cerebral hemisphere, separated from the medial portion by the occipitotemporal sulcus, and continuous laterally with the inferior temporal gyrus. **g. occipitotempora′lis media′lis** [NA], middle occipitotemporal gyrus: the medial portion of a gyrus (g. fusiformis) on the inferior surface of the cerebral hemisphere, separated from the lateral portion by the occipitotemporal sulcus, and from the parahippocampal gyrus by the collateral sulcus. **g. olfacto′rius latera′lis of Retzius,** limen insulae. **g. olfacto′rius media′lis,** area subcallosa. **g. olfacto′rius media′lis of Retzius,** area subcallosa. **gy′ri oper′ti** (obs.), gyri breves insulae. **orbital gyri, gy′ri orbita′les** [NA], the various irregular convolutions lateral to the olfactory sulcus on the orbital surface of the frontal lobe. **paracentral g., g. paracentra′lis,** lobulus paracentralis. **parahippocampal g., g. parahippocampa′lis** [NA], a convolution on the inferior surface of each cerebral hemisphere, lying between the hippocampal and collateral sulci; called also g. hippocampi and hippocampal g. **paraterminal g., g. paratermina′lis** [NA], a thin sheet of gray substance in front of and ventral to the genu of the corpus callosum; called also g. subcallosus and subcallosal g. **parietal g.,** any one of the convolutions into which the surface of the parietal lobe is divided. **parietal g., ascending, postcentral g., g. postcentra′lis** [NA], the convolution of the parietal lobe lying between the central and postcentral sulci; the primary sensory area of the cerebral cortex. Called also g. centralis posterior and posterior central g. **precentral g., g. precentra′lis** [NA], the convolution of the frontal lobe lying between the precentral and central sulci; the primary motor area of the cerebral cortex. Called also g. centralis anterior and anterior central g. **preinsular gyri,** gyri breves insulae. **gy′ri profun′di cer′ebri,** the deeply placed cerebral convolutions. **quadrate g.** (obs.), precuneus. **g. rec′tus** [NA], a convolution on the orbital surface of the frontal lobe, medial to the olfactory sulcus and continuous with the medial frontal gyrus on the medial surface. **short gyri of insula,** gyri breves insulae. **subcallosal g., g. subcallo′sus,** g. paraterminalis. **subcollateral g.** (obs.), the occipitotemporal gyri. **supracallosal g., g. supracallo′sus,** indusium griseum. **supramarginal g., g. supramargina′lis** [NA], the convolution of the inferior parietal lobe that curves around the upper end of the posterior branch of the lateral fissure and is continuous behind it with the superior temporal gyrus. **temporal g.,** any gyrus of the temporal lobe. **temporal g., inferior,** g. temporalis inferior. **temporal g., middle,** g. temporalis medius. **temporal g., superior,** g. temporalis superior. **temporal gyri, transverse,** gyri temporales transversi. **g. tempora′lis infe′rior** [NA], inferior temporal gyrus: the convolution of the temporal lobe lying between the inferior temporal sulcus and the lateral occipitotemporal gyrus, the two gyri being continuous at the inferolateral margin of the temporal lobe.

g. tempora′lis me′dius [NA], middle temporal gyrus: the convolution of the temporal lobe lying between the superior and the inferior temporal sulci; it is continuous posteriorly with the angular gyrus. **g. tempora′lis supe′rior** [NA], superior temporal gyrus: the convolution of the temporal lobe lying between the superior temporal sulcus and the lateral sulcus, continuous behind with the supramarginal gyrus. **gy′ri tempora′les transver′si** [NA], transverse temporal gyrus: the transverse convolutions marking the posterior extremity of the superior temporal gyrus and lying mostly in the lateral sulcus; the more marked of these, the anterior transverse temporal gyrus (Heschl's convolution), represents the cortical center for hearing. Called also *Heschl's g.* **gy′ri transiti′vi cer′ebri,** various small folds on the cerebral surface that are too inconstant to bear special names; called also *annectant gyri* and *gyri annectentes.* **uncinate g., g. uncina′tus,** uncus.

H

H chemical symbol for *hydrogen;* symbol for *henry.*

H 1. symbol for *oersted.* 2. a symbol for *Hauch,* denoting the motile or flagellate type of a microorganism, as contrasted with the O (*ohne Hauch*) or nonmotile type.

H. abbreviation for [L.] *haustus* (a draft), *horizontal,* [L.] *ho′ra* (hour), *hypermetropia,* and *Holzknecht unit.*

H⁺ symbol for *hydrogen ion.*

[H⁺] symbol for *hydrogen ion concentration.*

h symbol for *Planck's constant.*

¹H chemical symbol for *protium* (ordinary, or light, hydrogen); also written *H1, H¹,* and *hydrogen-1.* See *hydrogen.*

²H chemical symbol for *deuterium* (heavy hydrogen); also written *H2, H²,* and *hydrogen-2.* See *hydrogen.*

³H chemical symbol for *tritium;* also written *H3, H³,* and *hydrogen-3.* See under *hydrogen.*

H & E hematoxylin and eosin stain; see *Table of Stains and Staining Methods.*

HA hemadsorbent.

Ha symbol for *hahnium.*

HAA hepatitis-associated antigen.

Haab's degeneration, magnet, reflex (hahbz) [Otto *Haab,* professor of ophthalmology in Zurich, 1850–1931] see under *degeneration, magnet,* and *reflex.*

habena (hah-be′nah), pl. *habe′nae* [L. "rein"] see *habenula* (def. 2).

habenal, habenar (hah-be′nal, hah-be′nar) pertaining to the habena.

habenula (hah-ben′u-lah), pl. *haben′ulae* [L., dim. of *habena*] 1. a frenulum, or reinlike structure, such as one of a set of such structures in the cochlea. 2. [NA] a component of the epithalamus, being the small eminence on the dorsomedial eminence of the thalamus, just in front of the posterior commissure on the lateral edge of the habenular trigone; called also *pineal peduncle.* **h. arcua′ta,** the inner portion of the basilar membrane of the cochlea. **h. cona′rii,** habenula (def. 2). **Haller's h.,** vestigium processus vaginalis. **h. pectina′ta,** the outer portion of the basilar membrane of the cochlea. **haben′ulae perfora′tae,** foramina nervosa limbus laminae spiralis; see under *foramen.* **h. urethra′lis,** either of two whitish lines extending from the urinary meatus to the clitoris in girls and young women.

habenulae (hah-ben′u-le) plural of *habenula.*

habenular (hah-ben′u-lar) pertaining to the habenula.

habit (hab′it) [L. *habitus,* from *habere* to hold] 1. a fixed or constant practice established by frequent repetition. 2. predisposition or bodily temperament; see under *type.* **apoplectic h.,** habitus apoplecticus. **asthenic h.,** see under *type.* **clamping h.,** the prolonged or sustained clenching of the mandibular teeth against the maxillary teeth, a practice that may produce injury to the various elements of the stomatologic system. **drug h.,** see under *addiction.* **endothelioid h.,** a condition in which the nucleus of a cell is relatively small as compared with the cytoplasm. **full h.,** habitus apoplecticus. **glaucomatous h.,** shallowness of the anterior chamber of the eye with dilated pupil; seen in persons who have a predisposition to glaucoma. **leptosomatic h.,** a light, thin build of body. **leukocytoid h.,** endothelioid habitus. **opium h.,** opium addiction. **oral h.,** a habit that causes changes in occlusal relationships, e.g., thumb and finger sucking, tongue thrusting. **physiologic h.,** an acquired modification of behavior or response to stimulation brought about and permanently fixed by constant repetition. **pycnic h.,** a short, stocky build of body.

habitat (hab′ĭ-tat) the natural abode or home of an animal or plant species.

habituation (hah-bit″u-a′shun) 1. the gradual adaptation to a stimulus or to the environment. 2. the extinction of a condi-

tioned reflex by repetition of the conditioned stimulus; called also *negative adaptation.* 3. a condition resulting from the repeated consumption of a drug, with a desire to continue its use, but with little or no tendency to increase the dose; there may be psychic, but no physical dependence on the drug, and detrimental effects, if any, are primarily on the individual.

habitus (hab′ĭ-tus) [L. "habit"] 1. attitude (def. 1). 2. physique; see also under *habit* and *type.* **h. apoplec′ticus,** a full, heavy, thick-set body build indicating a possible tendency to apoplexy. **Buddha-like h.,** the froglike posture of the fetus due to abdominal enlargement. **h. enteroptot′icus,** the bodily conformation seen in enteroptosis, marked by a long narrow abdomen. **h. phthis′icus,** a bodily habit predisposing to pulmonary tuberculosis, marked by pallor, emaciation, poor muscular development, and small bones.

Habronema (hab″ro-ne′mah) [Gr. *habros* graceful + *nema* thread] a genus of nematode worms of the superfamily Spiruroidea, which are parasitic in the stomach of horses. The larval forms are taken up from the feces of horses by flies and the flies, swallowed by horses with their feed, transmit the larvae to the horses' stomachs. The larvae may also be transmitted to the skin of horses where they produce a dermatitis and a form of granuloma; in the conjunctiva they produce bungeye. The species are *H. megastoma, H. muscae, H. microstoma,* and *H. zebrae.*

habronemiasis (hab″ro-ne-mi′ah-sis) infection with *Habronema.* **cutaneous h.,** a disease of horses in various parts of the world, including the southern United States, Brazil, India, and the Philippines, caused by infection with larvae of *Habronema,* and characterized by cutaneous granulomas that grow in size until the skin over and around the lesions is destroyed, leaving a large raw surface. Because of the clinical similarity between cutaneous habronemiasis and hyphomycosis destruens equi, the disorders are often confused. Called also *bursautee, esponja,* and *summer sores.*

habu (hah′boo) [native name in Ryukyu Islands] an extremely venomous pit viper, *Trimeresurus flavorviridis,* inhabiting the warmer parts of East Asia, especially the Ryukyu Islands.

hachement (ash-maw′) [Fr.] a chopping or hacking stroke in massage.

Hackenbruch's experience (hah′ken-brooks) [Peter Theodor *Hackenbruch,* German surgeon, 1865–1924] (obs.) the rhombic-shaped area of anesthesia produced by the injection of a local anesthetic.

hadernkrankheit (hahd′ern-krahnk-hīt) [Ger.] a disease affecting rag-pickers, variously regarded as anthrax or malignant edema.

hae- for words beginning thus, see also those beginning *he-*.

Haeckel's law (hek′elz) [Ernst Heinrich Philipp August *Haeckel,* German naturalist, 1834–1919] see *recapitulation theory,* under *theory.*

haem (hēm) heme.

haem-, haema- see *hemo-;* for words beginning thus, see also those beginning *hem-*.

Haemadipsa (he″mah-dip′sah) [*haema-* + Gr. *dipsa* thirst] a genus of leeches, the land leeches, of the family Gnathobdellidae. **H. ceylon′ica,** a species common in Ceylon, which is annoying to man and animals because of its painful bite. **H. chilia′ni,** a species attacking horses and cattle in South America. **H. japon′ica,** a species found in Japan. **H. zeylan′dica,** a species attacking mammals in the tropical jungles of Asia.

Haemagogus (he″mah-go′gus) [*haem-* + Gr. *agōgos* leading] a genus of mosquitoes some of which transmit jungle yellow fever in tropical Central and South America.

Haemamoeba (ham″ah-me′bah) *Plasmodium.*

Haemaphysalis (hem″ah-fis′ah-lis) [Gr. *haima* blood + *physallis* bubble] a genus of ticks. **H. concin′na,** one of the vectors of *Rickettsia sibirica,* the etiologic agent of Siberian tick typhus. **H. humero'sa,** the bandicoot tick, one of the vectors of *Coxiella burneti.* **H. leach'i,** the common dog tick of South Africa; it transmits canine babesiosis. **H. leporispalus'tris,** the rabbit tick, one of the vectors of Rocky Mountain spotted fever and tularemia among wild animals. **H. puncta'ta,** a species of tick which acts as a vector of babesiosis in Southern Europe, and which has been considered the cause of tick paralysis in chickens. **H. spiniger'a,** a species occurring in the tropical forests of India that is a vector of Kyasanur Forest disease in forest workers.

haemato-   see *hemo-;* for words beginning thus, see also those beginning *hemato-.*

Haematobia (hem″ah-to′be-ah)   a genus of flies of the family Muscidae.   **H. ir'ritans,** a genus of small flies, "horn flies," which are very troublesome to cattle; called also *Lyperosia irritans* and *Siphona irritans.*

Haematopinus (hem″ah-to-pi′nus) [*haemato-* + Gr. *pinein* to drink]   a genus of sucking lice, species of which infest horses, swine, and cattle.

Haematosiphon (hem″ah-to-si′fon)   a genus of insects closely related to the genus *Cimex,* but having longer legs and a very long beak.   **H. in'dorus,** a species of southwestern United States and Mexico, which may be a serious pest of poultry and sometimes attacks man.

Haematoxylon (he″mah-tok′sĭ-lon) [*haemato-* + Gr. *xylon* wood] a genus of leguminous trees of Central America and the West Indies; the heart-wood of *H. campechianum* L. (Leguminosae), or logwood, contains tannin, hematoxylin, and resin, and is used mainly as a dye.

Haementeria (hem″en-te′re-ah)   a genus of leeches.   **H. officina'lis,** a species used for medicinal purposes in Mexico and South America.

haemo-   see *hemo-;* for words beginning thus, see also those beginning *hemo-.*

Haemobartonella (he″mo-bar″to-nel′lah)   a genus of the family Bartonellaceae, order Rickettsiales, occurring in eight species which are parasitic for various lower animals.   **H. ca'nis,** a species which infects dogs.   **H. mu'ris,** a common parasite of the laboratory rat, in which the infection is activated by splenectomy.

Haemocytozoa (hem″o-si″to-zo′ah)   Haemosporidia.

Haemodipsus (hem″o-dip′sus)   a genus of lice.   **H. ventrico'sus,** the common sucking louse of the rabbit which transmits the infective agent of tularemia from rabbit to rabbit.

Haemogregarina (hem″o-greg″ah-ri′nah)   a genus of sporozoan parasites of the order Coccidia found in the blood corpuscles of reptiles, amphibians, and some warm-blooded animals. Part of their life cycle is passed in another host, an insect, leech, or other blood-sucking invertebrate.

Haemonchus (he-mon′kus)   a genus of parasitic nematode worms of the family Trichostrongylidae.   **H. contor'tus,** the wireworm or stomach worm; a small nematode parasite of the abomasum (fourth stomach) of sheep and other ruminants, which produces weakness, wasting, and death of the infected animal; it has also been reported as having been found in man.   **H. pla'cei,** *H. contortus.*

Haemophilus (he-mof′ĭ-lus)   *Hemophilus.*

Haemophoructus (hem″o-fo-ruk′tus)   a genus of blood-sucking flies of the family Heleidae.

Haemopis (he-mo′pis)   a genus of leeches, the horse leeches, of the family Gnathobdellidae. *H. paludum* is parasitic in the nose and throat in Ceylon. *H. sanguisuga* of Europe and North Africa infests the nasal passages.

Haemoproteidae (hem″o-pro-te′ĭ-de)   a family of protozoa of the order Haemosporidia, subphylum Sporozoa, found as parasites in erythrocytes, visceral endothelial cells, leukocytes, liver cells, and other organs of vertebrate hosts. It includes the genera *Haemoproteus* and *Leukocytozoon.*

Haemoproteus (hem″o-pro′te-us)   a genus of sporozoan parasites of the family Haemoproteidae, order Haemosporidia, found in the visceral endothelial cells and erythrocytes of birds and reptiles; the sexual (perfect) stages occur in insects. *H. colum'bae* is a sluggish ameboid organism found in the red blood cells of pigeons. Its invertebrate host is a biting fly (*Pseudolynchia canariensis,* and other species of *Pseudolynchia*). Other species include: *H. danielews'kyi,* found in the crow (*Corvus cornix*), *H. noc'tuae,* found in the little owl (*Glaucidium noctuae*), and *H. pas'seris,* found in the blood of the sparrow.

haemorrhagia (hem″o-ra′je-ah) [L.]   hemorrhage.

Haemosporidia (hem″o-spo-rid′e-ah) [*haemo-* + Gr. *sporos* seed, spore]   an order of sporozoa which live parasitically in the red blood corpuscles of vertebrate animals. It includes the families Plasmodiidae, Haemoproteidae, and Babesiidae.

haemosporidia (hem″o-spo-rid′e-ah)   plural of *haemosporidium.*

haemosporidium (hem″o-spo-rid′e-um), pl. *haemosporidia.* An individual organism of the order Haemosporidia.

Haenel's symptom (ha′nelz) [Hans *Haenel,* German neurologist, 1874–1942]   see under *symptom.*

Haeser (ha′ser)   see *Häser.*

Haff disease (haf) [named for Königsberg *Haff,* a lagoon connected with the Baltic Sea, where epidemics occurred in 1924–5, 1932–3, and 1940]   see under *disease.*

hafnium (haf′ne-um) [L. *Hafniae,* Copenhagen]   a chemical element of atomic number 72 and atomic weight 178.49; symbol Hf. Discovered in a zircon, in 1923, by Coster and Hevesy of Copenhagen.

Hagedorn needle (hahg′ĕ-dorn) [Werner *Hagedorn,* German surgeon, 1831–1894]   see under *needle.*

Haglund's disease (hahg′loondz) [Sims Emil Patrik *Haglund,* Swedish orthopedist, 1870–1937]   see under *disease.*

Hagner's bag, operation (hag′nerz) [Francis Randall *Hagner,* American surgeon, 1873–1940]   see under *bag* and *operation.*

hahnemannian (hah″nĕ-man′e-an)   pertaining to Christian Friedrich Samuel *Hahnemann* (1755–1843), founder of homeopathy.

hahnemannism (hah′nĕ-man″izm)   homeopathy.

hahnium (hah′ne-um) [named for Otto *Hahn,* German physical chemist, 1879–1968]   a transuranic element of atomic number 105, atomic weight 260, symbol Ha, produced by an induced nuclear reaction.

Haidinger's brushes (hi′ding-erz) [Wilhelm von *Haidinger,* Austrian mineralogist, 1795–1871]   see under *brush.*

Haines' formula (coefficient), reagent, test (hānz′) [Walter Stanley *Haines,* Chicago chemist, 1850–1923]   see under *formula, reagent,* and *tests.*

hair (hār) [L. *pilus;* Gr. *thrix*]   a long slender filament. Applied especially to such filamentous appendages of the skin (pili [NA]), consisting of keratin; also the aggregate of such filaments, especially that of the scalp (capilli [NA]). Each hair consists of a cylindrical *shaft* and a root, which is contained in a flasklike depression (*hair follicle*) in the corium and subcutaneous tissue. The base of the root is expanded into the *hair bulb,* which rests upon and encloses the *hair papilla.*   **auditory h's,** hairlike attachments of the specialized epithelial cells of the cristae acusticae and the maculae acusticae.   **bamboo h.,** trichorrhexis nodosa.   **beaded h.,** hair marked with alternate swellings and constrictions, as seen in monilethrix.   **burrowing h.,** one which does not emerge from the skin but grows horizontally beneath its surface, exciting a foreign body papule, which may become infected. Cf. *ingrown h.*   **club h.,** a hair the root of which is surrounded by a bulbous enlargement composed of completely keratinized cells, preliminary to normal loss of the hair from the follicle; see *telogen.*   **exclamation point h.,** a hair which, when pulled out, shows atrophy and attenuation of the bulb; it is characteristic of alopecia areata.   **h's of eyebrow,** supercilia.   **Frey's h's,** stiff hairs mounted in a handle; used for testing the sensitiveness of the pressure points of the skin. **ingrown h.,** one which emerges from the skin but curves and reenters it, exciting a foreign body papule, which may become infected. Cf. *burrowing h.*   **knotted h.,** trichonodosis.   **lanugo h.,** the fine hair growing on the body of the fetus, constituting the lanugo.   **moniliform h.,** beaded h.   **h's of nose,** vibrissae.   **olfactory h's,** modified cilia that are extremely long and nonmotile, which project from the bulblike distal part of an olfactory cell (*olfactory vesicle* [def. 2]), and function as sensory receptors. Called also *olfactory cilia.*   **pubic h., h's of pubis,** pubes, def. 1.   **resting h.,** see *telogen.*   **sensory h's,** hairlike projections on the surface of sensory epithelial cells.   **stellate h.,** a hair split at the end in a starlike form.   **tactile h's,** hairs which are sensitive to touch, as the vibrissae of certain animals.   **taste h's,** short hairlike processes projecting freely into the lumen of the pit of a taste bud from the peripheral ends of the taste cells.   **terminal h.,** the coarse hair growing on various areas of the body during adult years.   **twisted h.,** a hair which at spaced intervals is twisted through an axis of 180 degrees, being abnormally flattened at the site of twisting; called also *pilus tortus.*   **vellus h.,** the downy hair growing on the body during the prepuberal years, constituting the vellus. **wooly h.,** lanugo.

hairball (hār′bawl)   trichobezoar.

haircap (hār′kap)   *Polytrichum juniperinum.*

haircast (hār′kast)   a trichobezoar filling and assuming the shape of the stomach.

halation (hal-a′shun)   indistinctness or blurring of the visual image by strong illumination coming from the same direction as the viewed object.

halazepam (hal-az′ĕ-pam)   chemical name: 7-chloro-1,3-dihydro-5-phenyl-1-(2,2,2-trifluoroethyl)-2*H*-1,4-benzodiazepin-2-one; a tranquilizer, $C_{17}H_{12}ClF_3N_2O$.

halazone (hal-ah-zōn) [USP]   chemical name: *p*-(dichlorosulfamoyl)benzoic acid. A white, crystalline powder, $C_7H_5Cl_2NO_4S$, having a chlorine-like odor; used as a disinfectant for water supplies.

halcinonide (hal-sin′o-nīd)   chemical name: 21-chloro-9-fluoro-11β-hydroxy-16α,17-[(1-methylethylidene)bis(oxy)]pregn-4-ene-

G
H

3,20-dione. A synthetic glucocorticoid, $C_{24}H_{32}ClFO_5$; used as a topical anti-inflammatory in the treatment of various steroid-responsive dermatoses.

Haldane chamber (apparatus) (hawl'dān) [John Scott *Haldane*, English physiologist, 1860–1936] see under *chamber*.

Haldol (hal'dol)   trademark for a preparation of haloperidol.

Haldrone (hal'drōn)   trademark for a preparation of paramethasone acetate.

Hales' piesimeter (hālz) [Stephen *Hales*, English physiologist, 1677–1761]   see under *piesimeter*.

half-life (haf'līf)   the time in which the radioactivity originally associated with a sample of isotopes will be reduced by one half through radioactive decay. The half-life of the remaining half will be equal to that of the original sample, and so on.   **antibody h.,** a measure of the mean survival time of antibody molecules following their formation, usually expressed as the time required to eliminate 50% of a known quantity of immunoglobulin from the animal body. Half-life varies from one immunoglobulin class to another.   **biological h.,** the time required for a living tissue, organ, or organism to eliminate one-half of a radioactive substance which has been introduced into it.   **effective h.,** the time required for the radioactivity of a radioactive nuclide to be diminished 50 per cent through the combined action of radioactive decay and biological elimination.

half-retinal (haf-ret'ĭ-nal)   pertaining to or affecting one half of the retina.

half-value   see under *layer*.

halfway house (haf'wa hous")   a residence for patients, such as mental patients, drug addicts, and alcoholics, who do not require complete hospitalization but who need an intermediate degree of care until they have again become established in the community.

halide (hal'īd)   1. haloid.   2. a binary compound of one of the halogens (fluorine, chlorine, bromine, or iodine).

hali-ichthyotoxin (hal"ĭ-ik"the-o-tok'sin)   a poisonous base of bacterial origin from stale fish.

halisteresis (hah-lis"tĕ-re'sis) [Gr. *hals* salt + *sterēsis* privation]   osteomalacia; a loss or lack of the lime salts (calcium) of bone.   **h. ce'rea,** waxy softening of the bones.

halisteretic (hah-lis"tĕ-ret'ik)   affected with or of the nature of halisteresis.

halitosis (hal-ĭ-to'sis) [L. *halitus* exhalation]   offensive breath; bad breath.

halituous (hah-lit'u-us) [L. *halitus* exhalation]   covered with moisture or vapor.

halitus (hal'ĭ-tus) [L.]   an exhalation or vapor; an expired breath.   **h. saturni'nus,** lead breath.

Hall band (hawl) [Herbert H. *Hall*, Bohemian obstetrician and gynecologist in the United States, born 1914]   see under *band*.

Hall's disease, facies, method (hawlz) [Marshall *Hall*, English physician, 1790–1857]   see *spurious hydrocephalus*, under *hydrocephalus*; see under *facies*, and see *artificial respiration*, under *respiration*.

Hall-Stone ring (hawl'ston) [Herbert H. *Hall*; Martin Lawrence *Stone*, American obstetrician and gynecologist, born 1920]   see under *ring*.

hallachrome (hal'ah-krōm)   a compound formed from dihydroxy phenylalanine by tyrosinase.

Hallauer's glasses (hal'ow-erz) [Otto *Hallauer*, Basel ophthalmologist, born 1866]   see under *glasses*.

Hallberg effect (hawl'berg) [J. Henry *Hallberg*, American radiologist]   see under *effect*.

Hallé's point (al-āz') [Adrien Joseph Marie Noël *Hallé*, French physician, born 1859]   see under *point*.

Haller's ansa, etc. (hal'erz) [Albrecht von *Haller*, Swiss physiologist, 1708–1777, the master physiologist of his time]   see under *arch, circle, cone, crypt, duct, fretum, habenula, layer, line, membrane, plexus, rete,* and *tripod*.

hallex (hal'eks), pl. *hal'lices*.   Hallux.

Hallion's test (al-yawz') [Louis *Hallion*, French physiologist, 1862–1940]   Tuffier's test.

Hallopeau's acrodermatitis (al-o-pōz') [François Henri *Hallopeau*, French dermatologist, 1842–1919]   see *acrodermatitis continua*.

hallucal (hal'u-kal)   pertaining to the hallux, or great toe.

halluces (hal'ŭ-sēs)   plural of *hallux*.

hallucination (hah-lu"sĭ-na'shun) [L. *hallucinatio;* Gr. *alyein* to wander in the mind]   a sense perception without a source in the external world; a perception of an external stimulus object in the absence of an object.   **auditory h.,** the hearing of unreal sounds.   **depressive h.,** a hallucination occurring in the course of acute depression.   **gustatory h.,** a hallucination of taste.   **haptic h.,** a tactile hallucination.   **hypnagogic h.,** a hallucination occurring between sleeping and awakening.   **lilliputian h.,** a hallucination in which things seem smaller than they actually are.   **olfactory h.,** hallucination of smell.   **reflex h.,** arousal of a secondary sensation by a sensation of a

different modality.   **stump h.,** phantom limb.   **tactile h.,** hallucination of touch.   **visual h.,** a sensation of seeing not stimulated by actual presence of the object seen.

hallucinative, hallucinatory (hah-lu'sĭ-na-tiv; hah-lu'sĭ-nah-to"re)   characterized by hallucinations.

hallucinogen (hah-lu"sĭ-no-jen") [*hallucin*ation + Gr. *gennan* to produce]   an agent which induces hallucinations.

hallucinogenesis (hah-lu"sĭ-no-jen'ĕ-sis)   the production of hallucinations.

hallucinogenetic (hah-lu"sĭ-no-jĕ-net'ik)   hallucinogenic.

hallucinogenic (hah-lu"sĭ-no-jen'ik)   producing hallucinations.

hallucinosis (hah-lu"sĭ-no'sis)   a psychosis marked by hallucinations.   **acute h., alcoholic h.,** a form of alcoholic psychosis, marked by auditory hallucinations and loose delusions of persecution.

hallucinotic (hah-lu"sĭ-not'ik)   pertaining to or characterized by hallucinosis.

hallux (hal'uks), pl. *hal'luces* [L.] [NA]   the great toe, or first digit of the foot.   **h. doloro'sa,** a painful disease of the great toe usually associated with flatfoot.   **h. flex'us,** h. rigidus.   **h. mal'leus,** hammer toe of the hallux.   **h. rig'idus,** painful flexion deformity of the great toe in which there is limitation of motion at the metatarsophalangeal joint.   **h. val'gus,** angulation of the great toe away from the midline of the body, or toward

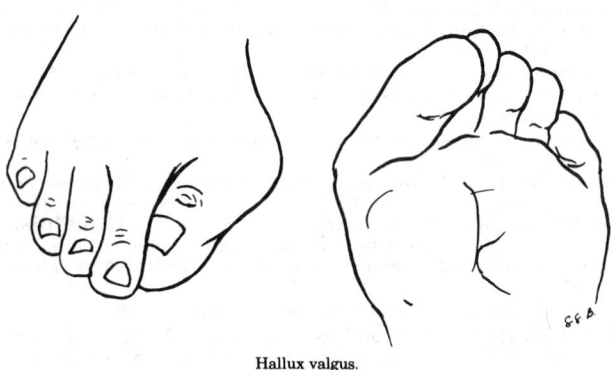

Hallux valgus.

the other toes; the great toe may ride under or over the other toes.   **h. va'rus,** angulation of the great toe toward the midline of the body, or away from the other toes.

Hallwachs effect (hal'vaks) [Franz *Hallwachs*, physiologist in Dresden, 1859–1922]   photoelectrical effect; see under *effect*.

halmatogenesis (hal"mah-to-jen'ĕ-sis) [Gr. *halma* a jump + *genesis* production]   a sudden alteration of type from one generation to another; called also *saltatory variation*.

halo (ha'lo) [L.; Gr. *halōs*]   1. a luminous or colored circle, such as the colored circle seen around a light in glaucoma.   2. a ring seen around the macula lutea in ophthalmoscopical examination.   3. the imprint of the ciliary processes upon the vitreous body.   **Fick's h.,** a colored circle appearing around a light, caused by the wearing of contact lenses; see *Fick's phenomenon*.   **h. glaucomato'sus, glaucomatous h.,** peripapillary atrophy seen in severe or chronic glaucoma.   **h. saturni'nus,** lead line.   **senile h.,** a zone of variable width surrounding the optic papilla, caused by exposure of various elements of the choroid as a result of senile atrophy of the pigmented epithelium.

halo- (hal'o) [Gr. *hals* salt]   a combining form denoting relationship to a salt.

halobacteria (hal"o-bak-te're-ah)   plural of *halobacterium*.

Halobacterium (hal"o-bak-te're-um)   a genus of halophilic microorganisms of the family Pseudomonadaceae, suborder Pseudomonadineae, order Pseudomonadales, occurring as highly pleomorphic rod-shaped cells. The halobacteria possess a purple pigment, bacteriorhodopsin (closely related to rhodopsin), which powers a system of photosynthesis. It includes five species, *H. cutiru'brum, H. halo'bium, H. marismor'tui, H. salina'rium,* and *H. trapan'icum*.

halobacterium (hal"o-bak-te're-um), pl. *halobacte'ria*.   Any member of the genus *Halobacterium*.

halodermia (hal"o-der'me-a)   any skin eruption caused by a halide.

haloduric (hal"o-du'rik) [Gr. *hals* salt + L. *durare* to endure]   capable of existing in a medium containing a high concentration of salt.

halofenate (hah"lo-fen'āt)   chemical name: 4-chloro-α-[3-(trifluoromethyl)phenoxy]benzeneacetic acid 2-(acetylamino)ethyl ester; an antihyperlipidemic and uricosuric agent, $C_{19}H_{17}ClF_3NO_4$.

Halog (hal'og)   trademark for preparations of halcinonide.

halogen (hal'o-jen, ha'lo-jen) [*halo-* + Gr. *gennan* to produce] an element of a closely related chemical family, all of which form similar (saltlike) compounds in combination with sodium and most other metals. The halogens are bromine, chlorine, fluorine, iodine, and astatine.

halogeton (hal-o-ge′ton) a small grayish brown plant introduced into the southwestern U.S. that contains soluble oxalates, which can be highly poisonous, causing respiratory difficulty and hemorrhage as well as hypocalcemia. The major species is *Halogeton glomera′tus* (Bieb.) C. A. Mey. (Polygonaceae).

haloid (hal′oid) [*halo-* + Gr. *eidos* form] saltlike; derived from or resembling a halogen.

halometer (hah-lom′ĕ-ter) [*halo-* + Gr. *metron* measure] 1. an instrument for measuring ocular halos. 2. an instrument for estimating the size of red corpuscles by measuring the diffraction halos which they produce.

halometry (hah-lom′ĕ-tre) 1. the measurement of ocular halos. 2. the measurement of the size of red blood corpuscles by utilizing the blood smear as a diffraction grating.

halopemide (hal″o-pem′id) chemical name: *N*-[2-[4-(5-chloro-2,3-dihydro-2-oxo-1*H*-benzimidazol-1-yl)-1-piperidinyl]ethyl]-4-fluorobenzamide; a tranquilizer, $C_{21}H_{22}ClFN_4O_2$.

haloperidol (hah″lo-per′ĭ-dol) [USP] chemical name: 4-[4-(4-chlorophenyl)-4-hydroxy-1-piperidinyl]-1-butanone. A tranquilizer, $C_{21}H_{23}ClFNO_2$, which also has antiemetic, hypotensive, and hypothermic actions, occurring as a white to faintly yellowish, amorphous or microcrystalline powder; used especially in the management of psychoses and for the control of the vocal utterances and tics of Gilles de la Tourette's syndrome, administered orally and intramuscularly.

halophil (hal′o-fil) a microorganism that requires a high concentration of salt for optimal growth.

halophile (hal′o-fīl) 1. halophil. 2. halophilic.

halophilic (hal″o-fil′ik) [Gr. *hals* salt + *philein* to love] pertaining to or characterized by an affinity for salt; applied to microorganisms which require a high concentration of salt for optimal growth.

halopredone acetate (hal′o-pre″don) chemical name: 17,21-bis(acetyloxy)-2-bromo-6β,9-difluoro-11β-hydroxypregna-1,4-diene-3,20-dione; a topical anti-inflammatory, $C_{25}H_{29}BrF_2O_7$.

haloprogin (hah″lo-pro′jin) chemical name: 1,2,4-trichloro-5-[(3-iodo-2-propynyl)oxy]benzene. A synthetic topical antifungal, $C_9H_4Cl_3IO$, occurring as a pale yellow, crystalline powder; used in the treatment of various forms of tinea.

halosteresis (hah-los″tĕ-re′sis) halisteresis.

Halotestin (hal″o-tes′tin) trademark for a preparation of fluoxymesterone.

Halotex (hal′o-teks) trademark for a preparation of haloprogin.

halothane (hal′o-thān) [USP] chemical name: 2-bromo-2-chloro-1,1,1-trifluoroethane. A general anesthetic, $C_2HBrClF_3$, occurring as a colorless, mobile, nonflammable, heavy liquid; administered by inhalation.

haloxon (hah-loks′on) an organophosphorus compound, $C_{14}H_{14}Cl_3O_6P$, used in veterinary medicine against intestinal nematodes.

halquinol (hal′kwin-ōl) halquinols.

halquinols (hal′kwin-ōls) a topical anti-infective compound, consisting of a mixture of 5,7-dichloro-8-quinolinol, 5-chloro-8-quinolinol, and 7-chloro-8-quinolinol in proportions resulting naturally from chlorination of 8-quinolinol; it has antiamebic, antifungal, and antibacterial actions.

Halsted's operation, suture (hal′stedz) [William Stewart *Halsted*, Baltimore surgeon, 1852–1922] see under *operation* and *suture*.

Haly Abbas see *Ali Abbas*.

halzoun (hal′zun) a disease of Syria once thought to be caused by *Fasciola hepatica* attaching itself to the pharyngeal mucous membrane, but now recognized to be more frequently the result of the presence of linguatulid larvae in the same region.

Hamamelis (ham″ah-me′lis) [Gr. *hama* together + *mēlon* apple] a genus of trees and shrubs. The leaves of *H. virginia′na* L. (Hamamelidaceae), or witch hazel, contain tannin and hamamelose.

hamamelis (ham″ah-me′lis) the dried leaves of *Hamamelis virginiana*, or witch hazel, which have been used as an astringent, and in veterinary medicine in the treatment of anal irritation of dogs.

hamamelose (ham-am′e-lōs) a natural sugar, $CH_2OH(CHOH)_2 \cdot COH(CH_2OH) \cdot COH$, from the bark of *Hamamelis virginiana*, or witch hazel.

hamarthritis (ham″ar-thri′tis) [Gr. *hama* together + *arthritis*] arthritis of all the joints at the same time.

hamartia (ham-ar′she-ah) [Gr. "defect"] a defect in tissue combination during development.

hamartial (ham-ar′she-al) pertaining to or exhibiting a hamartia.

hamarto- (ham′ar-to) [Gr. *hamartia* defect, sin] a combining form denoting relationship to a defect.

hamartoblastoma (ham-ar″to-blas-to′mah) [*hamarto-* + Gr. *blastos* germ + *-oma*] a tumor developing from a hamartoma.

hamartoma (ham″ar-to′mah) [*hamarto-* + *-oma*] a benign tumor-like nodule composed of an overgrowth of mature cells and tissues that normally occur in the affected part, but often with one element predominating.

hamartomatosis (ham″ar-to-mah-to′sis) the development of multiple hamartomas.

hamartomatous (ham″ar-to′mah-tus) pertaining to a disturbance in growth of a tissue in which the cells of a circumscribed area outstrip those of the surrounding areas.

hamartoplasia (ham″ar-to-pla′ze-ah) [*hamarto-* + Gr. *plassein* to form] overdevelopment of a tissue as a reaction to its attempts at repair.

hamate (ham′at) hooked, as the hamate bone.

hamatum (hah-ma′tum) [L. "hooked"] the os hamatum, or unciform bone.

Hamberger's schema (ham′ber-gerz) [Georg Erhard *Hamberger*, German physician, 1697–1755] see under *schema*.

Hamburger interchange (ham′boor-ger) [Hartog Jacob *Hamburger*, Dutch physiologist, 1859–1924] the ionic interchange between the corpuscles and plasma of the blood; bicarbonate passes from the erythrocytes into the plasma, and chloride ions pass from the plasma into the erythrocytes. Called also *secondary buffering*.

Hamilton's bandage, test (ham′il-tonz) [Frank Hastings *Hamilton*, American surgeon, 1813–1886] see under *bandage* and *tests*.

Hamman's disease (syndrome), sign (ham′anz) [Louis *Hamman*, American physician, 1877–1946] see under *disease* and *sign*.

Hamman-Rich syndrome (ham′an rich) [Louis *Hamman*; Arnold Rice *Rich*, American pathologist, born 1893] diffuse interstitial pulmonary fibrosis.

Hammarsten's test (ham′er-stenz) [Olof *Hammarsten*, physiologist in Upsala, 1841–1932] see under *tests*.

hammer (ham′er) 1. an instrument with a head designed for striking blows. 2. the hammer-shaped bone of the middle ear; the malleus. **Mayor's h.** (*obs.*), a metal hammer intended to be heated in boiling water and applied to the skin as a counterirritant. **Neef's h., Wagner's h.,** an instrument for the rapid opening and closing of a galvanic circuit.

Hammerschlag's method (test) (ham′er-shlahgz) [Albert *Hammerschlag*, physician in Vienna, 1863–1935] see under *method*.

Hammond's disease (ham′undz) [William Alexander *Hammond*, American neurologist, 1828–1900] athetosis.

hamster (ham′ster) a ratlike rodent, the most common of which is *Cricetus cricetus* of Europe and Western Asia, bred and used extensively as a laboratory animal. Other species are *Cricetulus larabensis*, the Chinese hamster, and *Mesocretus auratus*, the Syrian hamster.

hamstring (ham′string) one of the tendons that bound the popliteal fossa laterally and medially. **inner h.,** the tendons of the gracilis, sartorius, and two other muscles. **outer h.,** the tendon of the biceps flexor femoris.

hamular (ham′u-lar) shaped like a hook.

hamulus (ham′u-lus), pl. *ham′uli* [L. "little hook"] [NA] a general term denoting a hook-shaped process. **h. coch′leae,** h. laminae spiralis. **h. of ethmoid bone,** processus uncinatus ossis ethmoidalis. **frontal h., h. fronta′lis,** ala cristae galli. **h. of hamate bone,** h. ossis hamati. **lacrimal h., h. lacrima′lis** [NA], the hooklike process on the anterior part of the inferolateral border of the lacrimal bone, articulating with the maxilla. **h. lam′inae spira′lis** [NA], the hooklike upper end of the osseous spiral lamina. **h. os′sis hama′ti** [NA], hamulus of hamate bone: a hooklike process on the volar surface of the hamate bone, to which numerous structures are attached. **pterygoid h., h. pterygoi′deus** [NA], a hooklike process on the inferior extremity of the medial pterygoid plate of the sphenoid bone, around which the tendon of the tensor veli palatini muscle passes. **trochlear h.,** spina trochlearis.

hamycin (hah-mi′sin) an antibiotic derived from *Streptomyces pimprina*, having antifungal, antitrichomonal, and anti-inflammatory actions; it has been used topically in various fungal infections of the skin.

hand (hand) [L. *manus*] the part of the upper limb distal to the forearm: the carpus, metacarpus, and fingers together; called also *manus* [NA]. **accoucheur's h.,** obstetrician's h. **ape h.,** a hand with the thumb permanently extended. **benediction h.,** a hand in which the ring and little fingers are flexed; there is weakness of abduction and adduction of the index and middle fingers but they can be extended normally, and the thumb remains normal; seen in ulnar paralysis and syringomyelia. **claw h.,** see *clawhand*. **cleft h.,** malformation of the hand in which the division between the fingers extends into the metacarpus; also a hand in which the middle digits are absent, and the remaining fingers are abnormally large; called also *lobster-claw*

hand and *main fourché.* **club h.,** clubhand; see *talipomanus.*
dead h., an occupational disorder seen sometimes in those who use vibratory tools, and apparently caused by the multitude of concussions. The hands are painful and dark blue in color, but blanch on exposure to cold. **drop h.,** see *wristdrop.* **flat h.,** manus plana. **frozen h.,** stiffness of the hand resulting from edema accompanying trauma. **ghoul h.,** a condition in which the skin of the palm is depigmented and of a dead-white, tallow-yellow color, with blotchy areas of brownish hyperpigmentation, observed in Nigeria and thought to be associated with tertiary yaws. **Krukenberg's h.,** a forklike stump created by separating the distal ends of the ulna and radius and covering them with skin, after amputation proximal to the carpus. **lobster-claw h.,** cleft h. **Marinesco's succulent h.,** a hand marked by edema with lividity and coldness of the skin; seen in syringomyelia. **mirror h's,** a deformity in which there are two crude hands growing from a common wrist. **mitten h.,** a hand in which several fingers are fused together and have a common nail. **monkey h.,** a hand showing atrophy of the thenar muscles; called also *main en singe.* **obstetrician's h.,** the contraction of the hand in tetany; the hand is flexed at the wrist, the fingers at the metacarpophalangeal joints but extended at the interphalangeal joints, the thumb being strongly flexed into the palm. **opera-glass h.,** a pawlike hand marked by telescoping of the fingers caused by absorption of the phalanges; occurs in chronic arthritis. **phantom h.,** a paresthetic feeling as if the hand were still present after amputation. **preacher's h.,** benediction h. **skeleton h.,** a hand markedly atrophied and held in a position of extension: seen in progressive muscular atrophy; called also *main en squelette.* **spade h.,** the thick square hand of myxedema and acromegaly. **split h.,** cleft hand. **trench h.,** contracture or other incapacity of the hand from frostbite in the trenches; called also *main de tranchées.* **trident h.,** the characteristic hand of achondroplasia: the fingers are relatively of the same length, and there is a peculiar separation of the second and third fingers at the second phalangeal joint, causing the fingers to spread out. **writing h.,** a peculiar position of the hand in which the hand appears poised for writing; seen in paralysis agitans.

Hand's disease, syndrome (handz) [Alfred *Hand*, Jr., Philadelphia pediatrician, 1868–1949] Hand-Schüller-Christian disease; see under *disease.*

Hand-Schüller-Christian disease (syndrome) (hand-shil′er-kris′chan) [Alfred *Hand*; Artur *Schüller*; Henry A. *Christian*] see under *disease.*

handedness (hand′ed-nes) the preferential use in voluntary motor acts of the hand of one side. **left h.,** the preferential use in voluntary motor acts of the left hand. **right h.,** the preferential use in voluntary motor acts of the right hand.

handicap (han′dĭ-kap) any physical or mental defect or characteristic, congenital or acquired, preventing or restricting a person from participating in normal life or limiting his capacity to work.

Handley's lymphangioplasty (method) (hand′lēz) [William Sampson *Handley*, English surgeon, 1872–1962] see under *lymphangioplasty.*

handpiece (hand′pēs) that part of a dental engine which is held in the hand of the operator and which engages the bur or working point while it is being revolved.

Hanger's test (hang′erz) [Franklin M. *Hanger*, Jr., American physician, born 1894] see under *tests.*

hangnail (hang′nāl) a shred of eponychium on a proximal or lateral nail fold.

Hannover's canal (han′o-verz) [Adolph *Hannover*, Danish anatomist, 1814–1894] see under *canal.*

Hanot's cirrhosis (disease, syndrome) (an-ōz′) [Victor Charles *Hanot*, French physician, 1844–1896] 1. primary biliary cirrhosis. 2. secondary biliary cirrhosis.

Hanot-Chauffard syndrome (an-o′sho-far′) [Victor Charles *Hanot*; Anatole Marie Emile *Chauffard*, French physician, 1855–1932] see under *syndrome.*

Hansen's bacillus, disease (han′sunz) [Gerhard Henrik Armauer *Hansen*, Norwegian physician, 1841–1912] see *Mycobacterium leprae* and *leprosy.*

Hansenula (han-sen′u-lah) a genus of ascomycetous yeasts of the order Endomycetales, family Saccharomycetaceae; formerly called *Willia.* **H. anom′ala,** a nonpathogenic species commonly found in soil and in the respiratory and intestinal tracts.

Hanson's unit (han′sunz) [Adolph M. *Hanson*, American surgeon, born 1888] see under *extract* and *unit.*

haphalgesia (haf″al-je′ze-ah) [Gr. *haphē* touch + *algēsis* sense of pain + *-ia*] the sensation of pain on touching nonirritating objects or when the skin is lightly touched.

haplo- (hap′lo) [Gr. *haploos* simple, single] a combining form meaning simple or single.

haplobacteria (hap″lo-bak-te′re-ah) [*haplo-* + *bacteria*] bacteria which are not filamentous.

Haplochilus (hap″lo-ki′lus) a genus of fish. **H. pan′chax,** a small fish, called *ikan kapala timah* in Malay, which is placed in fishponds in Indonesia to eat the larvae of *Anopheles* mosquitoes.

haplodiploidy (hap″lo-dip′loi-de) the state in which males develop from unfertilized eggs and are haploid, and females develop from fertilized eggs and are diploid, as in honeybees.

haplodont (hap′lo-dont) [*haplo-* + Gr. *odous* tooth] having molar teeth without cusps or ridges.

haploid (hap′loid) [*haplo-* + Gr. *eidos* form, shape] 1. having a single set of chromosomes, as normally carried by a gamete, or having one complete set of nonhomologous chromosomes. In man, the haploid number is 23. Symbol, 1 N. Cf. *diploid* (def. 2). 2. an individual or cell having only one member of each pair of homologous chromosomes.

haploidentity (hap″lo-i-den′tĭ-te) the condition of having the same antigenic phenotype at certain specified loci; said of donor-recipient combinations in transplantation studies.

haploidy (hap′loi-de) the state of having only one member of each pair of homologous chromosomes.

haplomycosis (hap″lo-mi-ko′sis) adiospiromycosis.

haplont (hap′lont) a haploid individual.

Haplopappus (hap-lo-pap′pus) a genus of composite-flowered plants, the ingestion of which causes a disease similar to trembles.

haplopathy (hap-lop′ah-the) [*haplo-* + Gr. *pathos* disease] an uncomplicated disease.

haplophase (hap′lo-fāz) that phase in the life history of germ cells when the nuclei are haploid.

haplopia (hap-lo′pe-ah) [*haplo-* + Gr. *ōps* vision] single vision; the condition in which an object looked at is seen single and not double.

Haplorchis (hap-lor′kis) a genus of minute trematodes found in tropical areas, which are intestinal parasites of dogs, cats, and other vertebrates. **H. tai′chui,** an intestinal parasite of birds and mammals, rarely including man.

haploscope (hap′lo-skōp) [*haplo-* + Gr. *skopein* to examine] a form of stereoscope used for testing the visual axes. **mirror h.,** an instrument for making experiments, with different degrees of convergence of the visual axes.

haploscopic (hap-lo-skop′ik) pertaining to a haploscope; stereoscopic.

haplosporangin (hap″lo-spo-ran′jin) an antigen derived from the fungus *Emmonsia parva.*

Haplosporangium (hap″lo-spo-ran′je-um) *Emmonsia.*

haplotype (hap′lo-tīp) the group of alleles of linked genes contributed by either parent; the haploid genetic constitution contributed by either parent.

Hapsburg jaw, lip [*Hapsburg*, a German-Austrian royal family, including among its members many rulers of European states, such as Austria (1278–1918) and Spain (1504–1700)] see under *jaw* and *lip*; see also *hemophilia* (disease of the Hapsburgs).

hapt-, hapte- see *hapto-.*

hapten (hap′ten) a specific protein-free substance whose chemical configuration is such that it can interact with specific combining groups on an antibody, but which, unlike antigenic determinants, does not itself elicit the formation of a detectable amount of antibody. When coupled with a carrier protein, it does elicit the immune response. In humoral immunity, the antibody specificity is directed primarily to the hapten; in cell-mediated immunity, to both the hapten and the carrier protein. **group A h.,** a high-molecular-weight polysaccharide; in human blood; agglutinogen from blood group A.

haptene (hap′tēn) hapten.

haptenic (hap-ten′ik) pertaining to or caused by haptens.

haptic (hap′tik) [Gr. *haptikos* able to lay hold of] tactile.

haptics (hap′tiks) the science of touch, or the sense of contact.

haptin (hap′tin) hapten.

hapto-, hapt-, hapte- (hap′to, hapt, hap′te) [Gr. *haptein* to touch, seize upon, or hold fast] a combining form denoting relationship to touch or to seizure.

haptoglobin (hap″to-glo′bin) a group of glycoproteins in the α_2-globulin fraction of serum which share the same or similar subunits and have the common property of binding free hemoglobin. Three types, distinguished on the basis of electrophoretic patterns, are determined by the interaction of two allelic autosomal genes, Hp^1 and Hp^2. Other variants have also been described. All three types of haptoglobin consist of two kinds of polypeptide chains, termed α and β. Three different α chains and one β chain have been distinguished by electrophoresis. Haptoglobin is a heterogenous protein with a large (about 20 per cent) carbohydrate moiety.

haptometer (hap-tom′ĕ-ter) [*hapto-* + Gr. *metron* measure] an instrument for measuring sensitivity to touch.

haptophil, haptophile (hap′to-fīl) [*hapto-* + Gr. *philein* to love] having a peculiar affinity for a haptophore.

haptophore (hap′to-fōr) [*hapto-* + Gr. *phoros* bearing] in Ehrlich's side-chain theory, the specific group of the molecule of toxins, agglutinins, precipitins, opsonins, and lysins by which they become attached to their antibodies, antigens, or the receptors of cells, thus making possible their specific activity.

haptophoric (hap″to-fōr′ik) haptophorous.

haptophorous (hap-tof′o-rus) causing the combination of an antitoxin with cells; see *haptophore*.

harara (hah-rar′ah) an allergic skin reaction caused by bites of the sand fly *Phlebotomus papatasii*. It occurs in the Middle East, and is characterized by urticarial and inflammatory papules and blisters. Immunity usually follows the initial exposure. Called also *urticaria multiformis endemica*. The term is also a popular name for various types of skin eruptions.

hardening (hard′en-ing) the procedure of rendering tissue firm, so that it may be more readily cut for purposes of microscopic examination.

Harder's glands (hard′erz) [Johann Jacob *Harder*, Swiss anatomist, 1656–1711] see under *gland*.

harderian (hard′er-e-an) named for Johann Jacob *Harder*, as harderian *fossa* or *glands*.

hardness (hard′nes) 1. a quality of water produced by soluble salts of calcium and magnesium or other substances which form an insoluble curd with soap and thus interfere with its cleansing power. 2. the quality of firmness produced by cohesion of the particles composing a substance, as evidenced by its inflexibility or resistance to indentation or distortion. 3. the penetrating power of roentgen rays depending on their wavelength: the shorter the wavelength the harder the rays and the greater their penetrating power. 4. the degree of refraction of the residual gas in a glass tube: the higher the vacuum the shorter the wavelength of the resulting roentgen rays. **permanent h.,** hardness of water not removed by boiling; it is usually due to sulfates and chlorides. **temporary h.,** hardness of water removed by boiling; it is due to soluble bicarbonates, which lose CO_2 on boiling and precipitate as normal carbonates.

Hare's syndrome (hārz) [Edward Selleck *Hare*, British surgeon, 1812–1838] Pancoast's syndrome, def. 1.

harelip (hār′lip) a congenital cleft or defect in the upper lip, usually due to failure of the median nasal and maxillary processes to unite. The maxilla and palate may also be involved. **acquired h.,** a cleft of the upper lip caused by trauma. **double h.,** a cleft on either side of the upper lip as a result of bilateral failure of closure of the cleft between the median nasal and the maxillary process. **median h.,** a midline defect of the lip caused by failure of the median nasal processes to unite. **single h.,** a lateral cleft of the upper lip caused by failure of the median nasal and the maxillary process to unite.

harlequin (hahr′lĕ-kwin) a venomous snake belonging to the genus *Elaps*.

Harley's disease (har′lēz) [George *Harley*, English physician, 1829–1896] intermittent hemoglobinuria.

harmonia (har-mo′ne-ah) [L.] sutura plana.

harmony (har′mo-ne) the state of working together smoothly. **occlusal h.,** proper occlusion of the teeth occurring in various positions of the mandible. **occlusal h., functional,** such occlusion of the teeth in all positions of the mandible during mastication as will provide the greatest masticatory efficiency without imposing undue strain or trauma on the supporting tissues.

Harmonyl (har′mo-nil) trademark for preparations of deserpidine.

Harpirhynchus (har″pe-ring′kus) [Gr. *harpē* bird of prey + Gr. *rhynchos* snout] a genus of mites parasitic on birds.

harpoon (har-pōōn′) [Gr. *harpazein* to seize] an instrument for removing small pieces of living tissue for diagnostic examination.

Harrington's solution (har′ing-tonz) [Charles *Harrington*, American physician, 1856–1908] see under *solution*.

Harris' segregator (separator), suture (har′is) [Malcolm La Salle *Harris*, Chicago surgeon, 1862–1936] see under *segregator* and *suture*.

Harris' staining method (har′is) [Downey Lamar *Harris*, American pathologist, born 1875] see under *Table of Stains*.

Harris' syndrome (har′is) [Seale *Harris*, British physician, born 1870] see under *syndrome*.

Harrison antinarcotic act a Federal law, enacted March 1, 1915, which regulates the possession, sale, purchase, and prescription of habit-forming drugs, such as cocaine, morphine, opium, etc.

Harrison's groove (curve, sulcus) (har′ĭ-sunz) [Edward *Harrison*, London physician, 1766–1838] see under *groove*.

Harrower's hypothesis (har′o-erz) [Henry Robert *Harrower*, American physician, born 1883] hormone hunger.

harrowing (har′o-ing) hersage.

Hartel's treatment (method, technic) (har′telz) [Fritz *Hartel*, German surgeon] see under *treatment*.

Hartley-Krause operation (hart′le-krows) [Frank *Hartley*, New York surgeon, 1857–1913; Fedor *Krause*, German surgeon, 1857–1937] see under *operation*.

Hartmann's curet, speculum (hart′manz) [Arthur *Hartmann*, laryngologist in Berlin, 1849–1931] see under *curet* and *speculum*.

Hartmann's point, pouch, procedure (operation, colos-

tomy) (hart′manz) [Henri *Hartmann*, French surgeon, 1860–1952] See *Sudeck's critical point*, under *point*, and see under *pouch* and *procedure*.

Hartmannella (hart″man-el′ah) a genus of small amebae of the order Amoebida, class Rhizopoda. Most species are free-living, but some may be facultative parasites of the respiratory passages and central nervous system of various mammals, including man. **H. hyali′na,** a coprozoic ameba found in human feces.

hartshorn (harts′horn) 1. ammonium carbonate. 2. the horn of the stag or hart; cornu cervi.

harveian (har′ve-an) named in honor of William *Harvey*.

Harvey (har′ve), William (1578–1657). A celebrated English physician whose brilliant reasoning and innovative experiments, described in his *De motu cordis* (1628), establish him as the true discoverer of the circulation of the blood. He was also one of the first to disbelieve the doctrine of preformation of the fetus.

Häser's formula (coefficient) (ha′zerz) [Heinrich *Häser*, German physician, 1811–1884] see under *formula*.

Hashimoto's disease, struma, thyroiditis (hash″ĭ-mo′tōz) [Hakaru *Hashimoto*, Japanese surgeon, 1881–1934] struma lymphomatosa.

hashish (hash-ēsh′) [Arabic "herb"] a preparation of the unadulterated resin scraped from the flowering tops of cultivated female hemp plants, *Cannabis sativa* L. (Cannabaceae), which is smoked or chewed for its intoxicating effects. It is far more potent than marihuana. See *cannabis*. Also referred to as *charas* or *churus*.

hashishin (hash-e′shin) a person psychologically dependent on hashish.

hashishism (hash′ēsh-izm) psychological dependency on hashish.

Hasner's fold, valve (hahs′nerz) [Joseph Ritter von Artha *Hasner*, an ophthalmologist in Prague, 1819–1892] see *plica lacrimalis*.

Hassall's corpuscles (bodies) (has′alz) [Arthur Hill *Hassall*, English chemist and physician, 1817–1894] see under *corpuscle*.

Hassin's syndrome (has′inz) [George Boris *Hassin*, Russian neurologist in the United States, 1873–1951] see under *syndrome*.

Hata's phenomenon, preparation (hah′tahs) [Sahachiro *Hata*, Japanese physician, 1873–1938] see under *phenomenon* and *preparation*.

Hauch (howkh) [Ger. "breath"] See *H*.

Haudek's sign (niche) (haw′deks) [Martin *Haudek*, roentgenologist in Vienna, 1880–1931] see under *sign*.

haunch (hawnch) the hip and buttock.

hauptganglion of Küttner (howpt′gang″gle-on) Küttner's ganglion; see under *ganglion*.

Haust. abbreviation for L. *haus′tus*, a draft.

haustellum (haw-stel′lum), pl. *haustel′la* [L. from *haustus* draw up] a mouthpart of certain ectoparasites, such as bedbugs and lice, modified for piercing and sucking, consisting of a hollow tube with an eversible set of five stylets, by which the organism attaches itself to the host and through which the blood is drawn up.

haustorium (haw-stor′ĭ-um), pl. *haus′tra* [L. from *haustus* draw up] a structure of certain parasites adapted specially to penetrate the host's tissues and absorb nutrients and water.

haustra (haws′trah) plural of *haustrum*.

haustral (hos′tral) pertaining to the haustra of the colon.

haustration (hos-tra′shun) 1. the formation of a haustrum. 2. a haustrum.

haustrum (hows′trum), pl. *haus′tra* [L. *haustor* drawer] [NA] a general term denoting a recess. **haus′tra co′li** [NA], **haustra of colon,** sacculations in the wall of the colon produced by adaptation of its length to that of the tenia coli, or by the arrangement of the circular muscle fibers.

haustus (haws′tus) [L.] draft. **h. ni′ger,** black draft.

haut-mal (o-mahl′) [Fr.] grand mal; see under *epilepsy*.

HAV hepatitis A virus.

Haverhill fever (ha′ver-il) [*Haverhill*, Mass., where an epidemic occurred in 1925] see under *fever*.

Haverhillia multiformis (ha″ver-il′e-ah mul″tĭ-for′mis) the name given to a slender gram-negative streptobacillus which was found in cases of Haverhill fever; now called *Streptobacillus moniliformis*.

haversian canal (space), glands, lamella, system (ha-ver′shan) [Clopton *Havers*, English physician and anatomist, 1650–1702; known for his researches on the minute structure of bone, which were recorded in his *Osteologia nova* (1691)] see *canalis nutricius ossis* and *villi synoviales*, and see under *lamella* and *system*.

Hay's test (hāz) [Matthew *Hay*, Scotch physician, 1855–1932] see under *tests*.

Hayem's corpuscles, encephalitis, icterus (jaundice), solution (a-yawz′) [Georges *Hayem*, physician in Paris, 1841–

1933] see *platelet* and *encephalitis hyperplastica,* see *hemolytic anemia,* under *anemia,* and see under *solution.*

Hayem-Widal syndrome (a-yaw-ve′dal) [Georges *Hayem;* Georges Fernand Isidore *Widal,* French physician, 1862–1929] hemolytic anemia.

hay fever (ha fe′ver)   see under *fever.*

Haygarth's nodes (nodosites) (ha′garths) [John Haygarth, English physician, 1740–1827]   see under *node.*

Haynes' operation (hānz) [Irving Samuel *Haynes,* New York surgeon, 1861–1946]   see under *operation.*

Hazen's theorem (ha′zenz) [Allen *Hazen,* American civil engineer, born 1869]   see under *theorem.*

HB   hepatitis B.

HB$_C$ hepatitis B core (antigen); an antigen in the core of the Dane particle.

HB$_S$ hepatitis B surface (antigen); an antigen on the surface of the Dane particle.

Hb   symbol for *hemoglobin.*

HB$_c$Ag   hepatitis B core antigen.

HB$_e$Ag   e antigen.

HB$_s$Ag   hepatitis B surface antigen.

HbO$_2$ oxyhemoglobin.

H$_3$BO$_3$ boric acid.

HBr   hydrobromic acid.

HBV   hepatitis B virus.

H.C.   hospital corps.

HCG   human chorionic gonadotropin.

HCHO   formaldehyde.

HCl   hydrochloric acid.

HCN   hydrocyanic acid.

HCO$_3$ the bicarbonate radical.

H$_2$CO$_3$ carbonic acid.

HCT   hematocrit.

HD$_{50}$ a hemolyzing dose of complement that lyses 50 per cent of a suspension of sensitized red blood cells.

H.d.   abbreviation for L. *ho′ra decu′bitus,* at bedtime.

HDL   high-density lipoprotein.

HDN   hemolytic disease of the newborn; see *erythroblastosis fetalis.*

H and E   hematoxylin and eosin (stain). See *Table of Stains.*

He   chemical symbol for *helium.*

he-   for words beginning thus, see also those beginning *hae-.*

head (hed) [L. *caput;* Gr. *kephalē*] the upper, anterior, or proximal extremity of a structure or body, especially that part of an organism which contains the brain and the organs of special sense; called also *caput* [NA]. **angular h. of quadratus labii superioris muscle,** musculus levator labii superioris alaeque nasi. **articular h.,** an eminence on a bone by which it articulates with another bone. **h. of astragalus,** caput tali. **big h.,** bighead. **h. of blind colon,** cecum, def. 1. **h. of caudate nucleus,** caput nuclei caudati. **h. of condyloid process of mandible,** caput mandibulae. **coronoid h. of pronator teres muscle,** caput ulnare musculi pronatoris teretis. **deep h. of triceps brachii muscle,** caput mediale musculi tricipitis brachii. **deep h. of triceps extensor cubiti muscle,** caput mediale musculi tricipitis brachii. **drum h.,** membrana tympani. **engaged h.,** the position of the fetal head when the biparietal eminences have passed the pelvic inlet. **h. of epididymis,** caput epididymidis. **h. of femur,** caput femoris. **h. of fibula,** caput fibulae. **first h. of triceps brachii muscle,** caput longum musculi tricipitis brachii. **first h. of triceps extensor cubiti muscle,** caput longum musculi tricipitis brachii. **floating h.,** the head of the fetus when it is freely movable above the inlet of the birth canal. **great h. of adductor hallucis muscle,** caput obliquum musculi adductoris hallucis. **great h. of triceps brachii muscle,** caput laterale musculi tricipitis brachii. **great h. of triceps extensor cubiti muscle,** caput laterale musculi tricipitis brachii. **great h. of triceps femoris muscle,** musculus adductor magnus. **hot cross bun h.,** caput natiforme. **hourglass h.,** a head in which the coronal suture is depressed. **humeral h. of flexor carpi ulnaris muscle,** caput humerale musculi flexoris carpi ulnaris. **humeral h. of flexor digitorum sublimis muscle,** caput humeroulnare musculi flexoris digitorum superficialis. **humeral h. of pronator teres muscle,** caput humerale musculi pronatoris teretis. **h. of humerus,** caput humeri. **infraorbital h. of quadratus labii superioris muscle,** musculus levator labii superioris. **lateral h. of gastrocnemius muscle,** caput laterale musculi gastrocnemii. **lateral h. of triceps brachii muscle,** caput laterale musculi tricipitis brachii. **lateral h. of triceps extensor cubiti muscle,** caput laterale musculi tricipitis brachii. **little h. of humerus,** capitulum humeri. **little h. of mandible,** processus condylaris mandibulae. **little h. of metatarsal bone,** caput ossis metatarsalis. **long h. of adductor hallucis muscle,** caput obliquum musculus

adductoris hallucis. **long h. of adductor triceps muscle,** musculus adductor longus. **long h. of biceps brachii muscle,** caput longum musculi bicipitis brachii. **long h. of biceps femoris muscle,** caput longum musculi bicipitis femoris. **long h. of biceps flexor cruris muscle,** caput longum musculi bicipitis femoris. **long h. of biceps flexor cubiti muscle,** caput longum musculi bicipitis brachii. **long h. of triceps brachii muscle,** caput longum musculi tricipitis brachii. **long h. of triceps extensor cubiti muscle,** caput longum musculi tricipitis brachii. **long h. of triceps femoris muscle,** musculus adductor longus. **h. of malleus,** caput mallei. **h. of mandible,** 1. caput mandibulae. 2. processus condylaris mandibulae. **medial h. of biceps brachii muscle,** caput breve musculi bicipitis brachii. **medial h. of biceps flexor cubiti muscle,** caput breve musculi bicipitis brachii. **medial h. of gastrocnemius muscle,** caput mediale musculi gastrocnemii. **medial h. of triceps brachii muscle,** caput mediale musculi tricipitis brachii. **medial h. of triceps extensor cubiti muscle,** caput mediale musculi tricipitis brachii. **medusa h.,** caput medusae. **h. of metacarpal bone,** caput ossis metacarpalis. **h. of metatarsal bone,** caput ossis metatarsalis. **middle h. of triceps brachii muscle,** caput longum musculi tricipitis brachii. **middle h. of triceps extensor cubiti muscle,** caput longum musculi tricipitis brachii. **h. of muscle,** the end of a muscle at the site of its attachment (origin) to a bone or other fixed structure; called also *caput musculi.* **nasal h. of levator labii superioris alaeque nasi muscle,** musculus levator labii superioris alaeque nasi. **nerve h.,** discus nervi optici. **oblique h. of adductor hallucis muscle,** caput obliquum musculus adductoris hallucis. **oblique h. of adductor pollicis muscle,** caput obliquum musculi adductoris pollicis. **overriding h.,** the condition of the fetal head when it overrides the symphysis pubis instead of sinking into the pelvic cavity. **h. of pancreas,** caput pancreatis. **h. of penis,** glans penis. **h. of phalanx of fingers,** caput phalangis digitorum manus. **h. of phalanx of toes,** caput phalangis digitorum pedis. **plantar h. of flexor digitorum pedis longus muscle,** musculus quadratus plantae. **quadrate h. of flexor digitorum pedis longus muscle,** musculus quadratus plantae. **radial h. of flexor digitorum sublimis muscle,** caput radiale musculi flexoris digitorum superficialis. **radial h. of flexor digitorum superficialis muscle,** caput radiale musculi flexoris digitorum superficialis. **radial h. of humerus,** capitulum humeri. **h. of radius,** caput radii. **h. of rib,** caput costae. **saddle h.,** a head with a sunken crown. **scapular h. of triceps brachii muscle,** caput longum musculi tricipitis brachii. **scapular h. of triceps extensor cubiti muscle,** caput longum musculi tricipitis brachii. **second h. of triceps brachii muscle,** caput laterale musculi tricipitis brachii. **short h. of biceps brachii muscle,** caput breve musculi bicipitis brachii. **short h. of biceps femoris muscle,** caput breve musculi bicipitis femoris. **short h. of biceps flexor cruris muscle,** caput breve musculi bicipitis femoris. **short h. of biceps flexor cubiti muscle,** caput breve musculi bicipitis brachii. **short h. of coracoradialis muscle,** caput breve musculi bicipitis brachii. **short h. of triceps brachii muscle,** caput mediale musculi tricipitis brachii. **short h. of triceps extensor cubiti muscle,** caput mediale musculi tricipitis brachii. **short h. of triceps femoris muscle,** musculus adductor brevis. **h. of spleen,** extremitas posterior lienis. **h. of stapes,** caput stapedis. **steeple h.,** oxycephaly. **swelled h.,** bighead, def. 2. **h. of talus,** caput tali. **tower h.,** oxycephaly. **transverse h. of adductor hallucis muscle,** caput transversum musculi adductoris hallucis. **transverse h. of adductor pollicis muscle,** caput transversum musculi adductoris pollicis. **h. of ulna,** caput ulnae. **ulnar h. of flexor carpi ulnaris muscle,** caput ulnare musculi flexoris carpi ulnaris. **ulnar h. of pronator teres muscle,** caput ulnare musculi pronatoris teretis. **white h.,** witkop. **zygomatic h. of quadratus labii superioris muscle,** musculus zygomaticus minor.

Head's zones [Sir Henry *Head,* London neurologist, 1861–1940] see under *zone.*

headache (hed′āk)   pain in the head; cephalagia. **anemic h.,** headache ascribed to anemia, local or general. **bilious h.,** headache associated with gastrointestinal symptoms; usually migrainous. See *migraine.* **blind h.,** migraine. **cluster h.,** migrainous neuralgia. **congestive h.,** headache ascribed to congestion or hyperemia. **cough h.,** stabbing pain produced by the traction on pain-sensitive structures resulting from coughing or straining. **dynamite h.,** a severe headache occurring in persons handling high explosives. **functional h.,** headache due to tension or other emotional upset. **helmet h.,** pain involving the upper half of the head. **histamine h., Horton's h.,** migrainous neuralgia. **hyperemic h.,** congestive h. **lumbar puncture h.,** puncture h. **migraine h.,** see *migraine.* **miners' h.,** headache due to the gases produced by exploded nitroglycerin. **Monday morning h.,** a term sometimes applied to cases of malingering or "hangover." **organic h.,** headache due to intracranial disease or other organic disease. **postspinal h.,** puncture h. **puncture h.,** the headache and associated symptoms following puncture of the spinal canal and removal of cerebrospinal fluid. **pyrexial h.,** that due to fever. **reflex h.,** that associated with disease of some organ, as the stomach, eyes, etc.; called also *symptomatic h.* **rhinogenous h.,** headache due to nasal disease. **sick h.,** migraine. **spinal h.,** puncture h. **symptomatic h.,** reflex h. **tension h.,** a type due to prolonged overwork or emotional strain, or both, affecting especially the occipital region. **toxic h.,** headache due to systemic poisoning. **vacuum h.,** headache due to obstruction of the outlet of the frontal sinus. **vasomotor h.,** migrainous neuralgia.

headcap (hed′kap) headgear.

headgear (hed′gēr) a removable extraoral appliance used as a source of anchorage to apply force to the teeth and jaws; called also *headcap*.

headgrit (hed′grit) yellows, def. 2.

headgut (hed′gut) the foregut.

Heaf test [Frederick R. G. *Heaf*, British physician, born 1894] see *tuberculin test, Sterneedle,* under *tests.*

heal (hēl) to restore wounded parts or to make healthy; to become well or healthy.

healing (hēl′ing) a process of cure; the restoration of integrity to injured tissue. **h. by first intention,** healing in which union or restoration of continuity occurs directly without the intervention of granulations. **h. by granulation,** healing by second intention. **h. by second intention,** union by closure of a wound with granulations which form from the base and both sides toward the surface of the wound. **mental h.,** psychotherapy.

health (helth) a state of optimal physical, mental, and social well-being, and not merely the absence of disease and infirmity. **holistic h.,** a system of preventive medicine that takes into account the whole individual, his own responsibility for his well-being and the total influences—social, psychological, environmental—that affect health, including nutrition, exercise, and mental relaxation. **public h.,** the field of medicine concerned with safeguarding and improving the health of the community as a whole.

health maintenance organization (HMO) a broad term encompassing a variety of health care delivery systems utilizing group practice and providing alternatives to the fee-for-service private practice of medicine and allied health professions. They are essentially prepaid, organized systems for providing comprehensive health care within a geographic area to all persons under contract and they emphasize preventive medicine.

healthy (hel′the) pertaining to, characterized by, or promoting health.

hearing (hēr′ing) [L. *auditus*] the sense by which sounds are perceived; capacity to perceive sound. **color h.,** chromesthesia. **double disharmonic h.,** diplacusis. **monaural h.,** hearing with one ear. **visual h.,** lip reading.

hearing loss (hēr-ing los′) partial or complete loss of hearing; see also *deafness.* **Alexander's h.l.,** congenital deafness due to cochlear aplasia involving chiefly the organ of Corti and adjacent ganglion cells of the basal coil of the cochlea; a high-frequency hearing loss results. Called also *Alexander's deafness.* **conductive h.l.,** hearing loss due to a defect of the sound conducting apparatus, i.e., of the external auditory canal or middle ear. Called also *transmission h.l.* **pagetoid h.l.,** that occurring in osteitis deformans (Paget's disease) of the bones of the skull. **paradoxic h.l.,** hearing loss in which the hearing is better during loud noise. Called also *paracusia willisana.* **sensorineural h.l.,** hearing loss due to a defect in the inner ear or the acoustic nerve. **transmission h.l.** conductive h.l.

heart (hart) [L. *cor;* Gr. *kardia*] the viscus of cardiac muscle that maintains the circulation of the blood. Called also *cor* [NA]. It is divided into four cavities—two atria and two ventricles. The left atrium receives oxygenated blood from the lungs. From there the blood passes to the left ventricle, which forces it via the aorta through the arteries to supply the tissues of the body. The right atrium receives the blood after it has passed through the tissues and given up much of its oxygen. The blood then passes to the right ventricle, and then to the lungs, to be oxygenated. The major valves are four in number: the *left atrioventricular* (*bicuspid,* or *mitral*), between the left atrium and ventricle; the *right atrioventricular* (*tricuspid*), between the right atrium and ventricle; the *aortic,* at the orifice of the aorta; and the *pulmonary,* at the orifice of the pulmonary trunk. The heart tissue itself is nourished by the blood in the coronary arteries. See Plate XX. **abdominal h.,** a heart displaced into the abdominal cavity. **armored h., armour h.,** a condition marked by calcareous deposits in the pericardium. **artificial h.,** a pumping mechanism that duplicates the output, rate, and blood pressure of the natural heart. It may replace the function of the entire heart or a portion of it, and may be an intracorporeal, extracorporeal, or paracorporeal heart. **athlete's h.,** aortic incompetence due to strain in athletic exercise. **athletic h.,** hypertrophy of the heart with no disease of the valves, sometimes seen in athletes. **beer h.,** hypertrophy and dilatation of the heart attributed to excessive beer drinking; recently cobalt, as an additive in beer, has been implicated in some

instances. See also *alcoholic myocardiopathy,* under *myocardiopathy.* **beriberi h.,** heart failure from thiamine deficiency. **boat-shaped h.,** the heart of aortic regurgitation due to dilatation and hypertrophy of the left ventricle. **bony h.,** a heart or pericardium containing calcareous deposits. **booster h.,** auxiliary ventricle. **bovine h.,** cor bovinum, a greatly enlarged heart. **cervical h.,** one situated in the neck. **chaotic h.,** a heart which exhibits frequent premature systoles. **dynamite h.,** a condition occurring in workers exposed to nitroglycerin, in which the blood vessels become dilated during exposure and then, when exposure is discontinued, contract and thus reduce the blood supply to heart. **encased h.,** a heart affected with chronic constrictive pericarditis. **extracorporeal h.,** an artificial heart located outside the body and usually performing a pumping and an oxygenating function. **fat h., fatty h.,** 1. a heart affected with fatty degeneration. Called also *cor adiposum.* 2. a condition in which there is an excessive layer of fat deposited about and in the heart muscle. **fibroid h.,** a heart affected with chronic myocarditis in which fibrous tissue replaces portions of the myocardium. **flask-shaped h.,** the x-ray appearance of the heart in pericarditis with effusion. **frosted h.,** a condition in which the pericardium is thickened, giving the heart the appearance of being frosted like a cake. Cf. *hyaloserositis.* **hairy h.,** cor villosum. **hanging h.,** a condition as seen in the roentgenogram in cardioptosis, in which the heart appears as if hanging straight down from the aorta. **horizontal h.,** a counterclockwise rotation of the electrical axis (deviation to the left) of the heart; a moderate deviation (0° to −20°) is normally observed in asthenic persons with a transversely situated heart, in the obese, and in pregnant women. **hyperthyroid h.,** the heart in thyrotoxic heart disease. **hypoplastic h.,** a heart of small size. **icing h.,** frosted h. **intracorporeal h.,** an artificial heart implanted in the body. **irritable h.,** neurocirculatory asthenia. **left h.,** the left atrium and ventricle; that portion of the heart which propels the blood in systemic circulation. **lymph h.,** an organ in frogs and fishes concerned in the distribution of lymph. **mechanical h.,** artificial h. **myxedema h.,** an enlarged heart associated with hypothyroidism. **ox h.,** cor bovinum. **paracorporeal h.,** an artificial heart worn at the side of the body. **parchment h.,** see *hypoplasia of right ventricle.* **pear-shaped h.,** the x-ray appearance of the heart in combined aortic and mitral disease. **pectoral h.,** a heart situated in the front of the chest where it produces a bulging area. **pulmonary h.,** right heart. **Quain's fatty h.,** a fatty degeneration of the heart muscle. **right h.,** the right atrium and ventricle; that portion of the heart which propels the blood in the pulmonary circulation. **round h.,** the x-ray appearance of the heart in mitral stenosis and regurgitation. **sabot h.,** coeur en sabot. **soldier's h.** neurocirculatory asthenia. **systemic h.,** left heart. **tabby cat h.,** a condition of the heart in which the inner surface of the ventricular wall and the papillary muscles are streaked and spotted; seen in marked cases of fatty degeneration. Called also *thrush breast h., tiger h.,* and *tiger lily h.* **three-chambered h.,** a developmental anomaly in which the heart has a single or common ventricle with two atria emptying into it (absence of the ventricular septum), or a single or common atrium and two normal ventricles (absence of the atrial septum); called also *cor triloculare* or *trilocular h.* **thrush breast h., tiger h., tiger lily h.,** tabby cat h. **tobacco h.,** a heart showing irregularity of action attributed to excessive use of tobacco. **Traube's h.,** heart disease resulting from kidney disorder. **triatrial h.,** cor triatriatum. **trilocular h.,** three-chambered h. **vertical h.,** a clockwise rotation of the electrical axis (deviation to the right) of the heart; a moderate deviation (90° to 100°) is normally observed in asthenic persons with a vertically situated heart and in early infancy. **wandering h.,** an abnormally movable heart. **wooden-shoe h.,** coeur en sabot.

heart block (hart′blok) impairment of conduction in heart excitation; often applied specifically to atrioventricular heart block (q.v.). **arborization h.b.** (*obs.*), an intraventricular conduction defect attributed to loss of function of the distal ramifications of the bundle branches and/or Purkinje tissue. **atrioventricular h.b.,** a form in which the block occurs in the atrioventricular junctional tissue (atrioventricular node, bundle of His, or its branches); it is called *first degree h.b.* when conduction time is prolonged but all atrial beats are followed by ventricular beats; *second degree* (*partial*) *h.b.* when some, but not all, atrial beats are conducted; and *third degree* (*complete*) *h.b.* when no impulses whatsoever are conducted by the junctional tissues, owing to pathologic factors. The condition may be permanent or paroxysmal and if syncopal attacks occur, it is known as *Adams-Stokes disease.* **bundle-branch h.b.,** a form in which one ventricle is excited before the other because of absence of conduction in one of the branches of the bundle of His. **complete h.b.,** loss of conduction through the atrioventricular junctional tissue due to pathologic factors, with atrioventricular dissociation in which a sinus or atrial beat excites the atria while an idioventricular pacemaker below the site of block excites the ventricles; see also *atrioventricular h.b.* **congenital h.b.,** heart block due to defective development of junction conduction tissues of the heart; it may be associated with other cardiac anomalies. **incomplete**

h.b., second degree h.b.; see *atrioventricular h.b.* **interventricular h.b.,** bundle-branch h.b. **intraventricular h.b.,** a general term denoting an abnormal excitation pattern of the ventricles due to absence of conduction in the bundle branches or their ramifications. **Mobitz h.b.,** second degree atrioventricular heart block marked by a periodic dropped beat with a fixed P–R interval. **partial h.b.,** second degree h.b.; see *atrioventricular h.b.* **sinoatrial h.b.,** partial or complete impairment of conduction from the sinoatrial node to the atria, resulting in delay or absence of an atrial beat. **Wenckebach h.b.,** second degree atrioventricular heart block marked by a periodic dropped beat with a varying P–R interval.

heartburn (hart′bern) an esophageal symptom consisting of a retrosternal sensation of warmth or burning occurring in waves and tending to rise upward toward the neck; it may be accompanied by a reflux of fluid into the mouth (water brash). It is often associated with gastroesophageal reflux. Called also *pyrosis.*

heart failure (hart′fāl-yer) a clinical syndrome characterized by distinctive symptoms and signs resulting from disturbances in cardiac output or from increased venous pressure. Most often applied to myocardial failure with increased pressures distending the ventricle (high end-diastolic pressure [EDP]) and a cardiac output inadequate for the body's needs; often subclassified as right- or left-sided heart failure depending on whether the systemic or pulmonary veins are predominantly distended. Cf. *cardiac arrest,* under *arrest.* **acute congestive h.f.,** rapidly occurring deficiency in cardiac output marked by venocapillary congestion and hypertension and edema, usually pulmonary edema. **backward h.f.,** that produced by passive engorgement of the systemic venous system caused by a rise in distending (diastolic) pressures in the right heart. **congestive h.f.,** a clinical syndrome due to heart disease and characterized by breathlessness and abnormal sodium and water retention, resulting in edema. The congestion may occur in the lungs or in the peripheral circulation, or in both, depending on whether the heart failure is right-sided, left-sided, or general. **forward h.f.,** a concept of heart failure that emphasizes the inadequacy of cardiac output relative to body needs; edema is attributed primarily to renal retention of sodium and water, and venous distention is considered a secondary feature. **high output h.f.,** heart failure in which the cardiac output remains high, most often associated with hyperthyroidism. **left-sided h.f.,** left ventricular h.f.,** failure of adequate output by the left ventricle despite an increase in distending pressure and in end-diastolic volume, with dyspnea, orthopnea, etc.; see *heart failure.* **right-sided h.f., right ventricular h.f.,** failure of proper functioning of the right ventricle, with venous engorgement, hepatic enlargement, and subcutaneous edema; it is often combined with left-sided heart failure.

heartwater (hart-wot′er) a fatal disease of cattle, sheep, and goats, marked by fluid accumulation in the pleura, pericardium, and pleural cavity. It is caused by *Cowdria ruminantium,* which is transmitted by the ticks *Amblyomma hebraeum* and *A. variagata.*

heartworm (hart′werm) *Dirofilaria immitis.*

heat (hēt) [L. *calor;* Gr. *thermē*] 1. the sensation of an increase in temperature. 2. the energy which produces the sensation of heat. It exists in the form of molecular or atomic vibration (thermal agitation) and may be transferred by conduction through a substance, by convection by a substance, and by radiation as electromagnetic waves. 3. energy that is transferred as a consequence of a gradient in temperature. 4. estrus. **atomic h.,** the product of the atomic weight of an element and its specific heat. **conductive h.,** heat transmitted to the body by contact with a heated object, such as a hot water bag. **convective h.,** heat conveyed to the surface of the body from warm currents of water or air. **conversive h.,** heat developed in the tissues by the resistance of the tissues to the passage of high-frequency electromagnetic radiation through them. **delayed h.,** recovery heat. **dry h.,** heat that is not moist. Heated dry air is used in an apparatus such as a covered "baker," designed for the production of hyperemia. The dry air rapidly absorbs from the skin the moisture of perspiration induced in the apparatus during treatment. **initial h.,** the heat produced in muscle at the beginning of muscular contraction. Cf. *recovery h.* **latent h.,** that which apparently disappears when it is absorbed by bodies which thereby are not rendered warmer; the heat which a body may absorb without changing its temperature. **molecular h.,** the product of the molecular weight of a substance multiplied by its specific heat. **prickly h.,** miliaria rubra. **radiant h.,** heat applied to the surface of the body by rays from a source of infrared radiation, such as a heat lamp. **recovery h.,** that part of the heat developed by muscular contraction which is evolved after shortening. Cf. *initial h.* **sensible h.,** the heat which, when absorbed by a body, produces a rise in temperature. **specific h.,** the amount of heat required to raise the temperature of unit mass of a substance one degree.

Heath's operation (hēths) [Christopher *Heath,* English surgeon, 1835–1905] see under *operation.*

Heaton's operation (he′tonz) [George *Heaton,* Boston surgeon, 1808–1879] see under *operation.*

heatstroke (hēt′strōk″) see under *stroke.*

heaves (hēvz) a respiratory disturbance, most common in the Equidae, resulting from reduced elasticity in and rupture of the elastic network of the respiratory bronchioles and pulmonary alveoli and characterized by partly forced-expiration.

Hebdom. abbreviation for L. *hebdom′ada,* a week.

hebdomadal (heb-dom′ah-dal) [L. *hebdomada* a week] pertaining to the first week of life.

hebeosteotomy (heb″e-os″te-ot′o-me) *(obs.)* pubiotomy.

hebephrenia (heb″ĕ-fre′ne-ah) [Gr. *hēbē* youth + *phrēn* mind] hebephrenic schizophrenia. **grafted h.,** hebephrenia superimposed upon an already existing mental deficiency (Kraepelin).

hebephreniac (heb″ĕ-fre′ne-ak) hebephrenic.

hebephrenic (heb′ĕ-fren-ik) 1. see under *schizophrenia.* 2. an individual affected with hebephrenic schizophrenia.

Heberden's asthma, disease, nodes (signs), rheumatism (he′ber-denz) [William *Heberden,* English physician, 1710–1801] see *angina pectoris,* and see under *disease, node,* and *rheumatism.*

hebetic (hĕ-bet′ik) [Gr. *hēbētikos* youthful] pertaining to or occurring at the time of puberty.

hebetomy (he-bet′o-me) *(obs.)* pubiotomy.

hebetude (heb′ĕ-tūd) [L. *hebetudo*] apathy or dullness from any cause; in psychiatry, emotional dullness, a characteristic of schizophrenia.

hebiatrics (he″be-at′riks) ephebiatrics.

heboid (heb′oid) [Gr. *hēbē* youth + *eidos* form] the simple form of schizophrenia.

heboidophrenia (heb″oi-do-fre′ne-ah) schizophrenia marked by simple dementia; a term rarely used.

hebosteotomy (he-bos″te-ot′o-me) pubiotomy.

hebotomy (he-bot′o-me) pubiotomy.

Hebra's disease, pityriasis (he′brahs) [Ferdinand von *Hebra,* Austrian dermatologist, 1816–1880, founder of the histologic school of dermatology] see *erythema multiforme* and *dermatitis exfoliativa.*

hecatomeral (hek″ah-tom′er-al) hecatomeric.

hecatomeric (hek″ah-to-mer′ik) [Gr. *hekateron* each of two + *meros* part] having processes which divide into two, one going to each side of the spinal cord; said of certain neurons.

Hecht's phenomenon (hekts) [Adolf Franz *Hecht,* Vienna pediatrist, born 1876] Rumpel-Leede phenomenon.

Hecht's test (hekts) [Hugo *Hecht,* Prague physician, in Cleveland, born 1883] see under *tests.*

hectic (hek′tik) [L. *hecticus;* Gr. *hektikos* consumptive] associated with tuberculosis or with septic poisoning, as hectic fever.

hecto- [Fr., from Gr. *hekaton* one hundred] a combining form designating one hundred; used in naming units of measurement to indicate a quantity 100 (10²) times the unit designated by the root with which it is combined.

hectogram (hek′to-gram) a unit of mass of the metric system, being 10² grams; the equivalent of 3.527 ounces avoirdupois, or 3.215 ounces apothecaries' weight.

hectoliter (hek′to-le-ter) a unit of capacity of the metric system, being 10² liters; the equivalent of 26.4 United States or 22 Imperial gallons.

hectometer (hek-tom′ĕ-ter) a unit of linear measure of the metric system, being 10² meters, or the equivalent, roughly, of 328 feet, one inch.

H.E.D. abbreviation for German *Haut-Einheits-Dosis* (unit skin dose), a unit of roentgen-ray dosage established by Seitz and Wintz.

Hedera (hed′er-ah) a genus of climbing woody vines, including English ivy (*H. helix*).

hederiform (hed′er-ĭ-form) [L. *hedera* ivy + *forma* shape] ivy-shaped; *(obs.)* a term applied to certain nerve endings in the malpighian layer of the skin.

hedonia (he-do′ne-ah) abnormal cheerfulness.

hedonic (he-don′ik) pertaining to pleasure.

hedonics (he-don′iks) [Gr. *hēdonē* pleasure] the study of pleasurable and unpleasurable feelings.

hedonism (he′do-nizm) [Gr. *hēdonē* pleasure] devotion to pleasure; the doctrine that regards pleasure and happiness as the highest good.

hedratresia (hed″rah-tre′se-ah) [Gr. *hedra* anus + *atresia*] imperforate anus; see under *anus.*

hedrocele (hed′ro-sēl) [Gr. *hedra* anus + *kēlē* hernia] *(obs.)* hernia, or prolapse, of the intestine through the anus.

Hedulin (hed′u-lin) trademark for a preparation of phenindione.

heel (hēl) the hindmost part of the foot; called also *calx* [NA]. **anterior h.,** a triangular-shaped piece of leather fastened obliquely across the ball of the shoe just behind the heads of the metatarsal bones, the object being to support the heads, equalize the pressure, and support the anterior arch. **basketball h's,** talon noir. **big h.,** epidemic enlargement of the heel occurring

Plate XX   heart

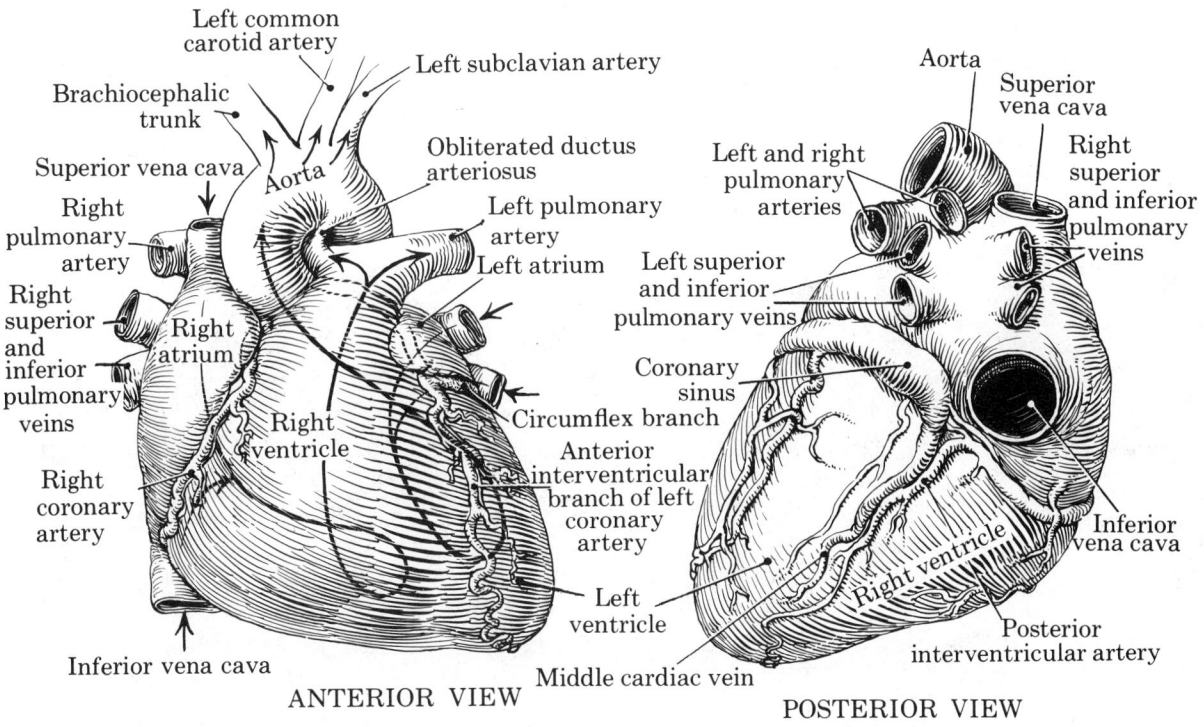

Left common
carotid artery

Brachiocephalic
trunk

Left subclavian artery

Superior vena cava

Obliterated ductus
arteriosus

Right
pulmonary
artery

Aorta

Left pulmonary
artery

Right
superior
and
inferior
pulmonary
veins

Right
atrium

Left atrium

Right
ventricle

Circumflex branch

Anterior
interventricular
branch of left
coronary
artery

Right
coronary
artery

Left
ventricle

Inferior vena cava

ANTERIOR VIEW

Aorta

Superior
vena cava

Left and right
pulmonary
arteries

Right
superior
and inferior
pulmonary
veins

Left superior
and inferior
pulmonary veins

Coronary
sinus

Right ventricle

Inferior
vena cava

Right ventricle

Posterior
interventricular artery

Middle cardiac vein

POSTERIOR VIEW

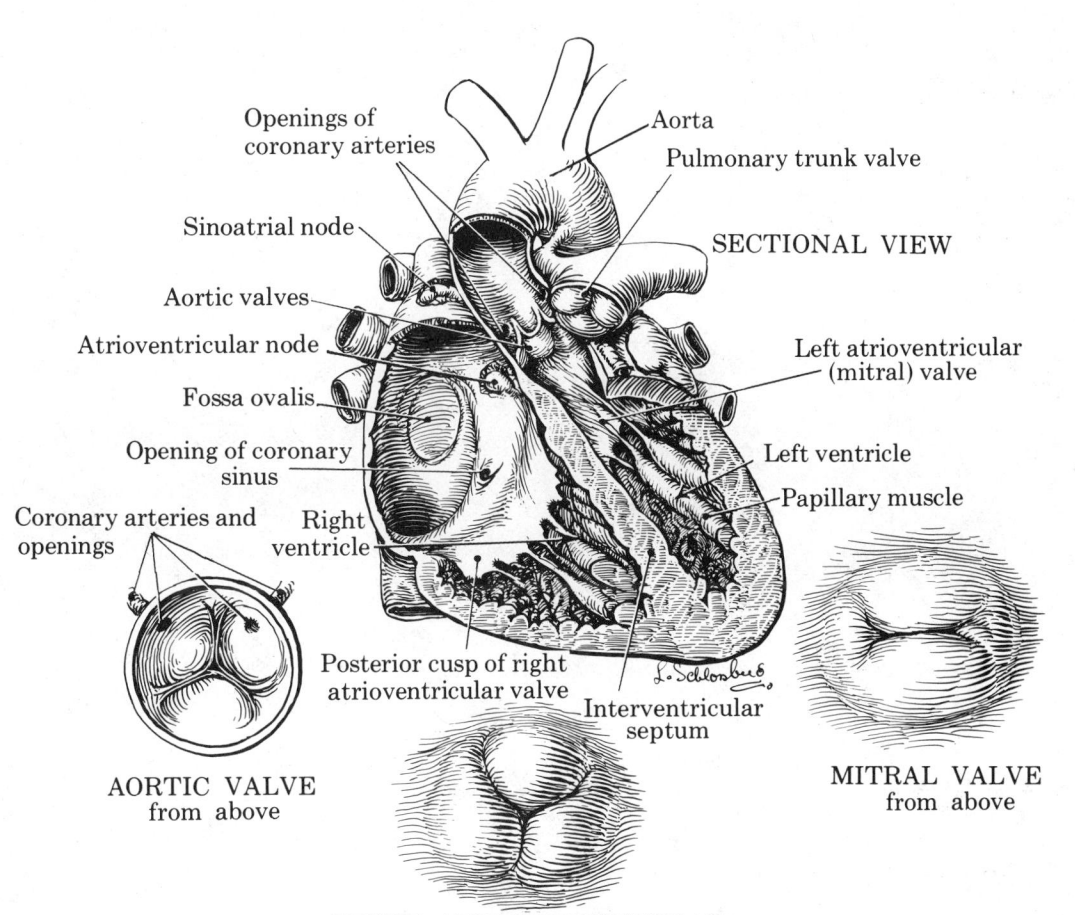

Openings of
coronary arteries

Aorta

Pulmonary trunk valve

Sinoatrial node

SECTIONAL VIEW

Aortic valves

Atrioventricular node

Left atrioventricular
(mitral) valve

Fossa ovalis

Left ventricle

Opening of coronary
sinus

Right
ventricle

Papillary muscle

Coronary arteries and
openings

Posterior cusp of right
atrioventricular valve

Interventricular
septum

L. Schlossberg

AORTIC VALVE
from above

**RIGHT ATRIOVENTRICULAR
(TRICUSPID) VALVE**   from above

MITRAL VALVE
from above

DETAILS OF STRUCTURE OF THE HEART

in parts of Africa. **contracted h.,** hoof-bound. **cracked h's,** pitted keratolysis. **gonorrheal h.,** the development of exostoses on the heel, attributed to gonorrheal infection. **painful h.,** a condition in which pain is caused by pressure on the heel. **policeman's h.,** calcanodynia in a policeman. **prominent h.,** a swelling on the back of the heel due to thickening of the periosteum of the os calcis. **Thomas h.,** a shoe correction consisting a heel $\frac{1}{2}$ in. longer and $\frac{1}{8}$–$\frac{1}{8}$ in. higher on the inside, used to bring the heel of the foot into varus and to prevent depression in the region of the head of the talus.

Heerfordt's disease (hār′forts) [Christian Frederik *Heerfordt*, Danish ophthalmologist] uveoparotid fever.

hefeflavin (hef′ĕ-fla″vin) (*obs.*) a lyochrome pigment from yeast.

hefilcon A (hĕ-fil′kon) chemical name: 2-hydroxyethyl methacrylate polymer with 1-vinyl-2-pyrrolidinone and ethylene dimethacrylate; a hydrophilic contact lens material, $(C_6H_{10}O_3)_x$ $(C_6H_9NO)_y$ $(C_{10}H_{14}O_4)_z$.

Hegar's dilator, sign (ha′garz) [Alfred *Hegar*, gynecologist in Freiburg, 1830–1914] see under *dilator* and *sign.*

Heiberg-Esmarch maneuver (hi″berg es′mark) [Jacob *Heiberg*, Norwegian surgeon, 1843–1888; Johann Friedrich August von *Esmarch*, German surgeon, 1823–1908] see under *maneuver.*

Heidenhain's cells, law, rods, stain (hi′den-hīnz) [Rudolf Peter *Heidenhain*, German physiologist, 1834–1897] see *chief cells* (def. 1) and *parietal cells*, under *cell*, and see under *law, rod,* and *stain.*

height (hīt) the vertical measurement of an object or body. **anterior facial h.,** the linear measurement along a line extending from the nasion to the menton. **apex h.,** the magnitude of the ordinates of the summated twitches of a muscle following application of electric or other stimulation. **h. of contour,** 1. a line encircling a tooth representing its greatest circumference. 2. the line encircling a tooth in a more or less horizontal plane and passing through the surface point of greatest radius. 3. the line encircling a tooth at its greatest bulge or diameter with respect to a selected path of insertion. **cusp h.,** 1. the shortest distance between the tip of a cusp of a tooth and its base plane. 2. the shortest distance between the deepest part of the central fossa of a posterior tooth and a line connecting the points of the cusps of the tooth. **posterior facial h.,** 1. a linear measure of the line perpendicular from the sella-nasion plane intersecting the mandibular plane. 2. in orthodontics, the ramus height, i.e., from condylare to gonion. **sitting h.,** sitting vertex h. **sitting suprasternal h.,** the distance from the middle of the anterior-superior border of the manubrium sterni to the surface on which the subject is seated. **sitting vertex h.,** the distance from the highest point of the head in the sagittal plane to the surface on which the subject is seated; commonly called *sitting height.* Cf. *crown-rump length.* **standing h.,** the distance from the highest point of the head in the sagittal plane to the surface on which the individual is standing, measured when the subject is not wearing shoes. Cf. *crown-heel length.*

Heilbronner's thigh (sign) (hīl′bron-erz) [Karl *Heilbronner*, Dutch physician, 1869–1914] see under *thigh.*

Heim-Kreysig sign (hīm-kri′sig) [Ernst Ludwig *Heim;* Friedrich Ludwig *Kreysig*, German physician, 1770–1839] see under *sign.*

Heimlich maneuver (hīm′lik) [Henry *Heimlich*, American physician] see under *maneuver.*

Heine's operation (hi′nez) [Leopold *Heine*, German oculist, 1870–1940] see under *operation.*

Heine-Medin disease (hi′nĕ ma′din) [Jacob von *Heine*, German physician, 1806–1879; Karl Oskar *Medin*, Swedish physician, 1847–1927] see *poliomyelitis.*

Heineke-Mikulicz pyloroplasty (operation) (hi′nĕ-kĕ mik′-u-lich) [Walter Hermann *Heineke*, German surgeon, 1834–1901; Johann von *Mikulicz*-Radecki, Polish surgeon, 1850–1905] see under *pyloroplasty.*

Heinz bodies (granules) (hīnts) [Robert *Heinz*, German pathologist, 1865–1924] Heinz-Ehrlich bodies; see under *body.*

Heinz-Ehrlich bodies (hīnts-ār′lik) [Robert *Heinz;* Paul *Ehrlich*, German bacteriologist, 1854–1915] see under *body.*

Heisrath's operation (his′raths) [Friedrich *Heisrath*, German ophthalmologist, 1850–1904] see under *operation.*

Heister's diverticulum, fold, valve (his′terz) [Lorenz *Heister*, German anatomist, 1683–1758] see *bulbus venae jugularis superior* and *plica spiralis.*

HEK human embryo kidney (cell culture).

Hektoen phenomenon (hek′tōn) [Ludvig *Hektoen*, Chicago pathologist, 1863–1951] see under *phenomenon.*

HEL human embryo lung (cell culture).

HeLa cells (he′lah) [from the name of the patient from whose carcinoma of the cervix uteri the parent carcinoma cells were isolated in 1951 at Johns Hopkins Hospital by Dr. George O. Gey] see under *cell.*

helcoid (hel′koid) [Gr. *helkos* ulcer + *eidos* form] resembling an ulcer.

helcology (hel-kol′o-je) [Gr. *helkos* ulcer + *-logy*] the scientific study of ulcers.

helcoma (hel-ko′mah) [Gr.] corneal ulcer (Hippocrates).

helcosis (hel-ko′sis) [Gr. *helkōsis*] ulceration; the formation of an ulcer.

Helcosoma tropicum (hel″ko-so′mah trop′ĭ-kum) *Leishmania tropica.*

Heleidae (hĕ-le′ĭ-de) a family of flies of the suborder Nematocerca, order Diptera, containing, among others, the four genera *Culicoides, Haemophoructus, Lasiohelea,* and *Leptoconops,* various species of which suck the blood of man, and may serve as vectors of disease. Called also *Ceratopogonidae.*

helenine (hel′ĕ-nēn) an antiviral substance produced by *Penicillium funiculosum* that is active against nucleic acid synthesis; thought to be a ribonucleoprotein.

helianthin (he-le-an′thin) methyl orange; see under *orange.*

heliation (he″le-a′shun) treatment by exposure to the sun's rays.

helical (hel′ĭ-kal) shaped like a helix.

Helicella (he″lĭ-sel′ah) a genus of snails that serves as a host of *Dicrocoelium dentriticum.*

Helicellidae (he″lĭ-sel′ĭ-de) a family of snails (suborder Stylommatophora, order Pulmonata) that serves as a host of trematodes infecting man.

helicin (hel′ĭ-sin) a glycoside formed by oxidizing salicin, which on hydrolysis yields glucose and salicylic aldehyde.

helicine (hel′ĭ-sīn) 1. of spiral form. 2. of or pertaining to a helix.

helico- (hel′ĭ-ko) [Gr. *helix* coil] a combining form denoting relationship to a coil, or to a snail (*Helix*).

helicoid (hel′ĭ-koid) [*helico-* + Gr. *eidos* form] resembling a coil or helix.

helicopepsin (hel″ĭ-ko-pep′sin) [*helico-* + *pepsin*] an enzyme resembling pepsin, from snails.

helicopod (hel′ĭ-ko-pod″) denoting a peculiar dragging gait; see under *gait.*

helicopodia (hel″ĭ-ko-po′de-ah) helicopod gait.

helicoprotein (hel″ĭ-ko-pro′te-in) [*helico-* + *protein*] a glucoprotein substance obtained from the snail, *Helix pomata.*

helicotrema (hel″ĭ-ko-tre′mah) [*helico-* + Gr. *trēma* hole] [NA] the passage of the ear that connects the scala tympani and scala vestibuli at the apex of the cochlea; called also *Breschet's* or *Scarpa's hiatus.*

heliencephalitis (he″le-en-sef″ah-li′tis) encephalitis from exposure to the sun (sunstroke).

helio- (he′le-o) [Gr. *hēlios* sun] a combining form denoting relationship to the sun.

helioaerotherapy (he″le-o-a″er-o-ther′ah-pe) [*helio-* + Gr. *aēr* air + *therapeia* treatment] treatment by exposure to the sun's rays and to fresh air.

helion (he′le-on) helium.

heliopathia (he″le-o-path′e-ah) [*helio-* + Gr. *pathos* disease] any pathological disturbance caused by sunlight.

heliosin (he″le-o′sin) a compound containing keratin and various inorganic salts.

heliosis (he″le-o′sis) [*helio-* + *-osis*] sunstroke.

heliotaxis (he″le-o-tak′sis) [*helio-* + Gr. *taxis* arrangement] phototaxis.

heliotherapy (he″le-o-ther′ah-pe) [*helio-* + *therapy*] the treatment of disease by exposing the body to the sun's rays; the therapeutic use of the sun bath.

Heliotiales (he″le-o-she-a′lēz) an order of ascomycetes (series Pyrenomycetes, subclass Euascomycetidae), some members of which are saprophytes and others are parasites of plants. It includes the genus *Sclerotinia.*

heliotrope B (he′le-o-trōp″) amethyst violet; see under *violet.*

heliotropism (he″le-ot′ro-pizm) [*helio-* + Gr. *tropē* a turn, turning] phototropism, def. 1.

helisterine (hĕ-lis′ter-in) [Gr. *helix* snail] a sterol from snails.

helium (he′le-um) [Gr. *hēlios* sun] a colorless, odorless, tasteless gas, which is not combustible and does not support combustion. It is one of the inert gaseous elements, which was first detected in the sun and is now obtained from natural gas. Symbol, He; atomic number, 2; atomic weight, 4.003. Used in medicine [USP] as a diluent for other gases, being especially useful with oxygen in the treatment of certain cases of respiratory obstruction, and as a vehicle for general anesthetics.

Helix (he′liks) a genus of gastropods that contains the common garden snails.

helix (he′liks) [Gr. "snail," "coil"] 1. a coiled structure, such as the coil of wire in an electromagnet. 2. [NA] the superior and posterior free margin of the pinna of the ear. *α-h.,* **alpha h.,** the complex structural arrangement of some protein molecules, such as keratin, in which the single polypeptide chains of proteins spiral right-handedly to form helices. Each NH group is connected to a CO group by a hydrogen bond at a distance equivalent to 3 amino acid residues; the helix makes a complete turn for each 3.6 residues. **double h., Watson-Crick h.,** a double helix, each chain of which contains information completely specifying the other chain, representing a structural formulation of the mechanism by which the genetic information in DNA reproduces itself; see *illustration.*

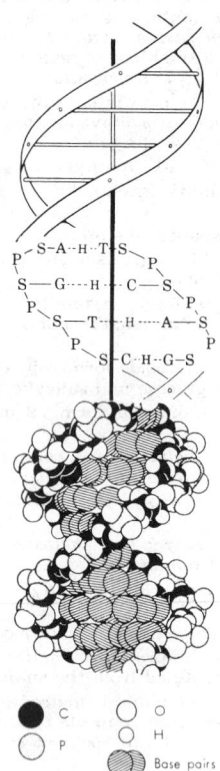

The DNA helix, representing the structure of deoxyribonucleic acid. *Upper:* as a spiral staircase. *Middle:* as an arrangement of organic molecules (A = adenine, C = cytosine, G = guanine, P = phosphate, S = sugar, T = thymine) and hydrogen bonds. *Lower:* as an arrangement of atoms of carbon, hydrogen, oxygen, and phosphorus, and base pairs as shown. (From Swanson: The Cell, Prentice-Hall, Inc., 1960.)

Hellat's sign (hel′ats) [Piotr *Hellat,* Russian otologist, 1857–1912] see under *sign.*

hellebore (hel′ĕ-bōr) [L. *helleborus;* Gr. *helleboros*] a violent gastrointestinal poison, having hydragogue, cathartic, and emmenagogue properties. **American h.,** *Veratrum viride.* **black h.,** the root of *Helleborus niger.* **green h.,** *Veratrum viride.* **white h.,** *Veratrum album.*

Hellendall's sign (hel′en-dahlz) [Hugo *Hellendall,* gynecologist in Düsseldorf, born 1872] Cullen's sign.

Heller's operation (hel′erz) [Ernst *Heller,* Leipzig surgeon, born 1877] cardiomyotomy.

Heller's test (hel′erz) [Johann Florian *Heller,* Vienna pathologist, 1813–1871] see under *tests.*

Heller-Döhle disease (hel′er-de′le) [Arnold Ludwig Gotthilf *Heller,* Kiel pathologist, 1840–1913; Karl Gottfried Paul *Döhle,* German pathologist, 1855–1928] syphilitic aortitis.

Hellin's law (hel′inz) [Dyonizy *Hellin,* Polish pathologist, 1867–1935] see under *law.*

Helmholtz's ligament, theory (helm′holtz-ez) [Hermann Ludwig Ferdinand von *Helmholtz,* German physiologist, who in 1851 invented the ophthalmoscope, 1821–1894] see under *ligament* and *theory.*

helminth (hel′minth) [Gr. *helmins* worm] a parasitic worm.

helminthagogue (hel-min′thah-gog) [*helminth* + Gr. *agōgos* leading] anthelmintic.

helminthemesis (hel″min-them′ĕ-sis) [*helminth* + Gr. *emesis* vomiting] the vomiting of worms.

helminthiasis (hel″min-thi′ah-sis) an infection with worms. **cutaneous h.,** larva migrans. **h. elas′tica,** the occurrence of elastic tumors in the groin and axilla, probably due to filariae.

helminthic (hel-min′thik) pertaining to or caused by parasitic worms.

helminthicide (hel-min′thĭ-sīd) [*helminth* + L. *caedere* to kill] vermicide.

helminthism (hel′min-thizm) the presence of worms in the body.

helminthoid (hel-min′thoid) [*helminth* + Gr. *eidos* form] wormlike.

helminthology (hel″min-thol′o-je) [*helminth* + *-logy*] the scientific study of parasitic worms.

helminthoma (hel″min-tho′mah) [*helminth* + *-oma*] a tumor caused by a parasitic worm.

helminthous (hel-min′thus) pertaining to or infected with worms.

helo- [Gr. *hēlos* nail] a combining form denoting relationship to a nail, or to a wart or callus.

Heloderma (he″lo-der′mah) [*helo-* + Gr. *derma* skin] a genus of venomous lizards of Arizona and New Mexico. *H. hor′ridum,* the Mexican beaded lizard. *H. suspec′tum,* the Gila monster.

heloma (he-lo′mah) [*helo-* + *-oma*] a corn or callosity on the hand or foot. **h. du′rum,** hard corn, the usual type occurring over joints of the toes. **h. mol′le,** a soft corn.

Helophilus (hĕ-lof′ĭ-lus) a genus of flies, hover flies, of the family Syrphidae, whose "rat-tail" maggots (larvae) may cause nasal and intestinal myiasis.

helosis (he-lo′sis) the condition of having corns.

helotomy (he-lot′o-me) [*helo-* + Gr. *temnein* to cut] the excision or, more often, the paring of corns or calluses.

Helvella (hel-vel′ah) a genus of fungi of the family Helvellaceae, the saddle fungi, species of which contain a heat-stable hemolysin. Helvellic acid is a constituent of *H. infula.* Other species, including *H. esculenta,* cause a form of mycetismus.

Helvellaceae (hel″vel-a′se-e) a family of ascomycetous fungi of the order Pezizales, series Discomycetes, some species of which are edible; it includes the genus *Helvella.*

Helweg's bundle, tract (hel′vegz) [Hans Kristian Saxtorph *Helweg,* Danish physician, 1847–1901] olivospinal tract.

hem-, hema- see *hemo-.*

hemabarometer (hem″ah-bah-rom′ĕ-ter) [*hema-* + *barometer*] an instrument for ascertaining the specific gravity of the blood.

hemachromatosis (hem″ah-kro″mah-to′sis) hemochromatosis.

hemachrome (hem′ah-krōm) hemochrome.

hemachrosis (hem″ah-kro′sis) [*hema-* + Gr. *chrōsis* coloring] (*obs.*) abnormal or excessive redness of the blood.

hemacyanin (hem″ah-si′ah-nin) hemocyanin.

hemacyte (hem′ah-sīt) hemocyte.

hemacytometer (hem″ah-si-tom′ĕ-ter) [*hema-* + Gr. *kytos* hollow vessel + Gr. *metron* measure] an instrument used in counting the blood corpuscles.

hemacytometry (hem″ah-si-tom′ĕ-tre) the counting of blood corpuscles by means of a hemacytometer.

hemacytopoiesis (hem″ah-si″to-poi-e′sis) hematopoiesis.

hemacytozoon (hem″ah-si″to-zo′on), pl. *hemacytozo′a.* (*obs.*) hemocytozoon.

hemaden (hem′ah-den) [*hem-* + Gr. *adēn* gland] an endocrine gland.

hemadenology (hem″ad-ĕ-nol′o-je) [*hem-* + Gr. *adēn* gland + *-logy*] endocrinology.

hemadostenosis (hem″ad-o-stĕ-no′sis) [Gr. *haimas* blood stream + *stenōsis* narrowing] the narrowing or obliteration of a blood vessel.

hemadsorbent (hem″ad-sor′bent) inducing or characterized by hemadsorption, as hemadsorbent viruses.

hemadsorption (hem″ad-sorp′shun) the adherence of red cells to other cells, particles, or surfaces; see under *tests.*

hemadynamometry (hem″ah-di″nah-mom′ĕ-tre) measurement of blood pressure.

hemafacient (hem″ah-fa′shent) hematopoietic.

hemafecia (hem″ah-fe′se-ah) [*hema-* + *feces*] blood in the feces.

hemagglutination (hem″ah-gloo″tĭ-na′shun) agglutination of erythrocytes, which may be caused by antibodies (see *hemagglutinin*), by certain virus particles (e.g., the viruses of influenza and mumps), or by substances such as high-molecular-weight dextrans. **passive h.,** the agglutination of erythrocytes on which antigen has been adsorbed in the presence of antiserum to that antigen. **viral h.,** the agglutination of erythrocytes (usually chicken) in the presence of hemagglutinating viruses, e.g., influenza, mumps, etc.

hemagglutinative (hem″ah-gloo′tĭ-na′tiv) pertaining to, characterized by, or causing agglutination of erythrocytes.

hemagglutinin (hem″ah-gloo′tĭ-nin) [*hem-* + *agglutinin*] an antibody that agglutinates erythrocytes, classified according to the cells which it agglutinates as *autologous* (cells of the same organism), *heterologous* (cells of individuals of other species), and *homologous* (cells of other individuals of the same species). Some hemagglutinins are effective with erythrocytes suspended in 0.85 per cent sodium chloride solution; others are ineffective unless hydrophilic colloids (e.g., albumin, fibrinogen) are added, or the erythrocytes have been treated with a proteolytic enzyme. **cold h.,** one which acts only at temperatures near 4° C. **warm h.,** one which acts only at temperatures near 37° C.

hemagonium (hem″ah-go′ne-um) [*hema-* + Gr. *gonē* seed] hemocytoblast.

hemal (he′mal) 1. pertaining to the blood or the blood vessels. 2. ventral to the spinal axis, where the heart and great vessels are located, as, e.g., the hemal arches. Cf. *neural.*

hemalexin (hem″ah-lek′sin) an alexin (complement) of the blood.

hemalum (hem-al′um) a mixture of hematoxylin and alum introduced by Mayer, widely used as a nuclear stain, especially in combination with eosin as a general oversight method. Also, any alum and hematoxylin stain. Called also *alum hematoxylin.*

hemanalysis (hem″ah-nal′ĭ-sis) [*hem-* + *analysis*] analysis or examination of the blood.

hemangiectasia (hem″an-je-ek-ta′se-ah) angiectasis.

hemangiectasis (hem″an-je-ek′tah-sis) [*hem-* + Gr. *angeion* vessel + *ektasis* dilatation] angiectasis.

hemangioameloblastoma (hĕ-man″je-o-ah-mel″o-blas-to′mah) a highly vascular ameloblastoma.

hemangioblast (hĕ-man′je-o-blast) a mesodermal cell which gives rise to both vascular endothelium and hemocytoblasts.

hemangioblastoma (hĕ-man″je-o-blas-to′mah) a capillary hemangioma of the brain consisting of proliferated blood vessel cells or angioblasts.

hemangioblastomatosis (hĕ-man″je-o-blas″to-mah-to′sis) multiple or widespread hemangioblastomas.

hemangioendothelioblastoma (hĕ-man″je-o-en″do-the″le-o-blas-to′mah) [*hem-* + Gr. *angeion* vessel + *endothelium* + Gr, *blastos* germ + *-oma*] a tumor of mesenchymal origin of which the cells tend to form endothelial cells and line blood vessels.

hemangioendothelioma (hĕ-man″je-o-en″do-the″le-o′mah) [*hemangioma* + *endothelioma*] a hemangioma in which the endothelial cells are the most prominent component. **benign h.,** a benign neoplasm of blood-vessel endothelium. **malignant h.,** hemangiosarcoma.

hemangioendotheliosarcoma (hĕ-man′je-o-en″do-the″le-o-sar-ko′mah) hemangiosarcoma.

hemangiofibroma (hĕ-man″je-o-fi-bro′mah) a hemangioma containing fibrous tissue.

hemangioma (hĕ-man″je-o′mah) [*hem-* + *angioma*] a benign tumor made up of new-formed blood vessels. Cf. *angioma* and *lymphangioma.* **ameloblastic h.,** a highly vascular ameloblastoma. **capillary h.,** nevus flammeus. **h. caverno′sum, cavernous h.,** a tumor, usually present at birth or appearing soon after, manifested as a red-blue spongy mass made up of a connective tissue framework enclosing large, cavernous,

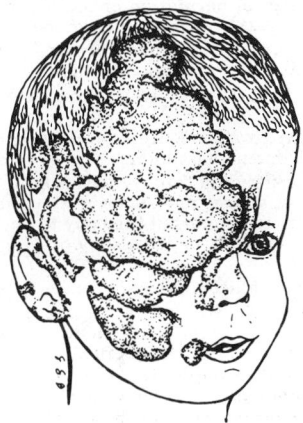

Cavernous hemangioma.

vascular spaces that are partly or entirely filled with blood. Called also *cavernous angioma, erectile tumor,* and *strawberry nevus.* **sclerosing h.,** a solidly cellular lesion (dermatofibroma or histiocytoma) purportedly developing from a hemangioma by proliferation of endothelial cells and connective tissue stroma. **strawberry h.,** a vascular nevus.

hemangiomatosis (hĕ-man″je-o-mah-to′sis) a condition in which multiple hemangiomas are developed.

hemangiopericyte (hĕ-man″je-o-per′ĭ-sīt) pericyte.

hemangiopericytoma (hĕ-man″je-o-per″ĕ-si-to′mah) a tumor composed of spindle cells with a rich vascular network, which apparently arises from pericytes. It is related to a glomus tumor but, unlike the latter, has no nerve elements.

hemangiosarcoma (hĕ-man″je-o-sar-ko′mah) a malignant tumor formed by proliferation of endothelial and fibroblastic tissue.

hemapheic (hem″ah-fe′ik) pertaining to or characterized by hemaphein.

hemaphein (hem″ah-fe′in) [*hema-* + Gr. *phaios* dusky, gray] a brown coloring matter of the blood and urine.

hemapheism (hem″ah-fe′izm) the presence of hemaphein in the urine.

hemapheresis (hem″ah-fer′ĕ-sis) [*hema-* + Gr. *aphairesis* removal] any procedure in which blood is withdrawn, a portion (plasma, leukocytes, platelets, etc.) is separated and retained, and the remainder is retransfused into the donor.

hemaphotograph (hem″ah-fo′to-graf) hemophotograph.

hemapoiesis (hem″ah-poi-e′sis) [*hema-* + Gr. *poiēsis* formation] hematopoiesis.

hemapoietic (hem″ah-poi-et′ik) hematopoietic.

hemapophysis (hem″ah-pof′ĭ-sis) [*hem-* + *apophysis*] a costal cartilage regarded as an apophysis of the hemal spine.

hemarthros (hem-ar′thros) hemarthrosis.

hemarthrosis (hem″ar-thro′sis) [*hem-* + Gr. *arthron* joint] extravasation of blood into a joint or its synovial cavity.

hemartoma (hem″ar-to′mah) hemangioma.

hemastrontium (hem″as-tron′she-um) a tissue stain prepared by adding strontium chloride to a solution of hematein and aluminum chloride in alcohol and citric acid.

hemat- see *hemo-.*

hematal (hem′ah-tal) pertaining to blood or blood vessels.

hematapostema (hem″at-ah-pos-te′mah) [*hemat-* + Gr. *apostēma* abscess] an abscess containing effused blood.

hemate (hem′āt) a compound of hematein.

hematein (hem″ah-te′in) [NF] a brownish-red, crystalline substance, $C_{16}H_{12}O_6$, derived from hematoxylin by oxidation; used as an indicator and stain.

hematemesis (hem″ah-tem′ĕ-sis) [*hemat-* + Gr. *emesis* vomiting] the vomiting of blood. **Goldstein's h.,** hematemesis due to bleeding telangiectases in the stomach.

hematencephalon (hem″at-en-sef′ah-lon) the effusion of blood into the brain.

hematherapy (hem″ah-ther′ah-pe) hemotherapy.

hemathermal (hem″ah-ther′mal) homoiothermic.

hemathermous (hem″ah-ther′mus) homoiothermic.

hemathorax (hem″ah-tho′raks) hemothorax.

hematic (he-mat′ik) 1. pertaining to or contained in blood. 2. hematinic.

hematidrosis (hem″at-i-dro′sis) [*hemat-* + Gr. *hidrōsis* sweating] the excretion of bloody sweat.

hematimeter (hem″ah-tim′ĕ-ter) hemacytometer.

hematimetry (hem″ah-tim′ĕ-tre) hemacytometry.

hematin (hem′ah-tin) 1. the hydroxide of heme formed by the oxidation of heme from the ferrous or Fe(II) to the ferric or Fe(III) state; it does not combine reversibly with oxygen. Called also *metheme.* 2. former name for *heme.*

hematinemia (hem″ah-tĭ-ne′me-ah) [*hematin* + Gr. *haima* blood + *-ia*] the presence of hematin (heme) in the blood.

hematinic (hem″ah-tin′ik) 1. pertaining to hematin. 2. an agent which improves the quality of the blood, increasing the hemoglobin level and the number of erythrocytes.

hematinogen (hem″ah-tin′o-jen) a substance that produces blood.

hematinometer (hem″ah-tin-om′ĕ-ter) hemoglobinometer.

hematinuria (hem″ah-tin-u′re-ah) [*hematin* + Gr. *ouron* urine + *-ia*] the presence of hematin (heme) in the urine.

hemato- see *hemo-.*

hematobia (hem″ah-to′be-ah) plural of *hematobium.*

hematobilia (hem″ah-to-bil′e-ah) bleeding into the biliary passages.

hematobium (hem″ah-to′be-um), pl. *hemato′bia* [*hemato-* + Gr. *bios* life] (*obs.*) any organism that lives in the blood, especially an animal microorganism.

hematoblast (hem′ah-to-blast″) hemocytoblast.

hematocatharsis (hem″ah-to-kah-thar′sis) [*hemato-* + Gr. *katharsis* purging] the ridding of the blood of toxic substances; blood lavage.

hematocele (hem′ah-to-sēl) [*hemato-* + Gr. *kēlē* tumor] an effusion of blood into a cavity, especially into the tunica vaginalis testis. **parametric h., pelvic h.,** a tumor formed by effusion of blood into Douglas' pouch. **pudendal h.,** a sanguineous tumor in a labium of the pudenda. **retrouterine h.,** parametric h. **scrotal h.,** effusion of blood into the tissues of the scrotum. **vaginal h.,** effusion of blood into the tunica vaginalis testis.

hematocelia (hem″ah-to-se′le-ah) hematocoelia.

hematocephalus (hem″ah-to-sef′ah-lus) [*hemato-* + Gr. *kephalē* head] a fetus born with its head distended with blood.

hematochezia (hem″ah-to-ke′ze-ah) [*hemato-* + Gr. *chezein* to go to stool] the passage of bloody stools.

hematochlorin (hem″ah-to-klo′rin) [*hemato-* + Gr. *chlōros* green] a green coloring matter occurring in the placenta and derived from hemoglobin.

hematochromatosis (hem″ah-to-kro″mah-to′sis) [*hemato-* + Gr. *chrōma* color] staining of tissues with blood pigment; hemochromatosis.

hematochyluria (hem″ah-to-ki-lu′re-ah) [*hemato-* + Gr. *chylos* chyle + *ouron* urine + *-ia*] the discharge of blood and chyle with the urine, due to *Wuchereria bancrofti.*

hematocoelia (hem″ah-to-se′le-ah) [*hemato-* + Gr. *koilia* cavity] effusion of blood into the peritoneal cavity.

hematocolpometra (hem″ah-to-kol″po-me′trah) [*hemato-* + Gr. *kolpos* vagina + *mētra* uterus] accumulation of menstrual blood in the vagina and uterus.

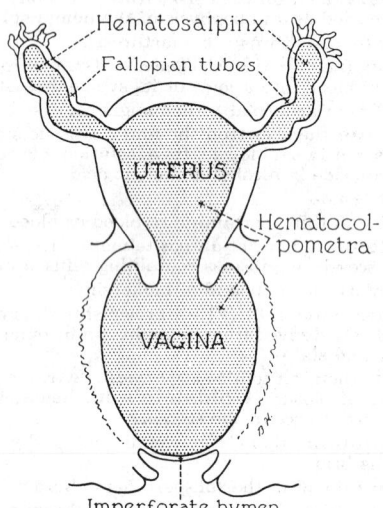

hematocolpos (hem″ah-to-kol′pos) [*hemato-* + Gr. *kolpos* vagina] an accumulation of menstrual blood in the vagina.

hematocrit (he-mat′o-krit) [*hemato-* + Gr. *krinein* to separate] the volume percentage of erythrocytes in whole blood. Originally applied to the apparatus or procedure used in its determination, but now also used to designate the result of the determination. Abbreviated HCT. **large vessel h.,** the fraction of blood, sampled from a large vessel, that is occupied by the erythrocytes as measured upon centrifugation. **whole body h.,** the fraction of the total blood volume, as measured by suitable dilution of a plasma component and an erythrocyte component, that is occupied by the erythrocytes, expressed as a percentage, showing the ratio of erythrocyte volume to total blood volume.

hematocryal (hem″ah-tok′re-al) [*hemato-* + Gr. *kryos* cold] poikilothermic.

hematocyanin (hem″ah-to-si′ah-nin) [*hemato-* + Gr. *kyanos* blue] hemocyanin.

hematocyst (hem′ah-to-sist″) [*hemato-* + Gr. *kystis* sac, bladder] an effusion of blood into the bladder or into a cyst.

hematocystis (hem″ah-to-sis′tis) hematocyst.

hematocyte (hem′ah-to-sīt) hemocyte.

hematocytoblast (hem″ah-to-si′to-blast) hemocytoblast.

hematocytolysis (hem″ah-to-si-tol′ĭ-sis) hemolysis.

hematocytometer (hem″ah-to-si-tom′ĕ-ter) hemacytometer.

hematocytopenia (hem″ah-to-si″to-pe′ne-ah) [*hematocyte* + Gr. *penia* poverty] deficiency in all the cellular elements of the blood.

hematocyturia (hem″ah-to-si-tu′re-ah) [*hematocyte* + Gr. *ouron* urine + *-ia*] the presence of red blood cells in the urine.

hematodialysis (hem″ah-to-di-al′ĭ-sis) hemodialysis.

hematoencephalic (hem″ah-to-en″sĕ-fal′ik) [*hemato-* + Gr. *enkephalos* brain] pertaining to the blood and the brain.

hematogenesis (hem″ah-to-jen′ĕ-sis) [*hemato-* + *genesis*] hematopoiesis.

hematogenic (hem″ah-to-jen′ik) 1. hematopoietic. 2. hematogenous.

hematogenous (hem″ah-toj′ĕ-nus) produced by or derived from the blood; disseminated by the circulation or through the blood stream.

hematoglobin (hem″ah-to-glo′bin) hemoglobin.

hematoglobinuria (hem″ah-to-glo-bin-u′re-ah) hemoglobinuria.

hematoglobulin (hem″ah-to-glob′u-lin) hemoglobin.

hematogone (hem′ah-to-gōn) a lymphocyte-like cell regarded as a blood cell precursor, often presenting as a naked nucleus in

the bone marrow, observed in infants and patients with pure red cell anemia, lymphocytic leukemia, and the nodular lymphomas.

hematohidrosis (hem″ah-to-hid-ro′sis) hematidrosis.

hematohistioblast (hem″ah-to-his′te-o-blast) hemohistioblast.

hematohyaloid (hem″ah-to-hi′ah-loid) [*hemato-* + *hyaloid*] the hyaline matter formed by degeneration of thrombi through conglutination of the red corpuscles or blood platelets.

hematoid (hem′ah-toid) [*hemato-* + Gr. *eidos* form] resembling blood.

hematoidin (hem-ah-toid′in) a substance which is apparently chemically identical with bilirubin but which has a different site of origin, being formed locally in the tissues from hemoglobin, particularly under conditions of reduced oxygen tension.

hematokolpos (hem″ah-to-kol′pos) hematocolpos.

hematolin (hem″ah-to′lin) a compound, $C_{68}H_{78}O_7N_8$, from heme.

hematolith (hem′ah-to-lith) (*obs.*) hemolith.

hematologist (hem″ah-tol′o-jist) a specialist in the study of the blood.

hematology (hem″ah-tol′o-je) [*hemato-* + *-logy*] that branch of medical science which treats of the morphology of the blood and blood-forming tissues.

hematolymphangioma (hem″ah-to-lim″fan-je-o′mah) [*hemato-* + L. *lympha* lymph + Gr. *angeion* vessel + *-ome*] a tumor composed of blood vessels and lymph vessels.

hematolysis (hem″ah-tol′ĭ-sis) hemolysis.

hematolytic (hem″ah-to-lit′ik) hemolytic.

hematoma (hem″ah-to′mah), pl. *hemato′mas* [*hemato-* + *-oma*] a localized collection of blood, usually clotted, in an organ, space, or tissue, due to a break in the wall of a blood vessel. **aneurysmal h.,** false aneurysm. **h. au′ris,** hematoma of the perichondrium of the ear. **epidural h.,** accumulation of blood in the epidural space, due to damage to the middle meningeal artery and producing compression of the dura mater and thus compression of the brain. Unless evacuated, it may result in herniation through the tentorium, and death. **pelvic h.,** a collection of blood in the pelvic cellular tissue. **perianal h.,** a hematoma under the perianal skin, caused by rupture of a subcutaneous vessel, the blood being kept localized by fibroelastic septa and causing much pain. **retrouterine h.,** an effusion of blood into the retrouterine connective tissue. **subdural h.,** accumulation of blood in the subdural space. In the severe *acute* form, both blood and cerebrospinal fluid enter the space as a result of laceration of the brain and a tear in the arachnoid, adding subdural compression to the direct injury to the brain. In the *chronic* form, only blood effuses into the subdural space as a result of rupture of the bridging veins, usually due to closed head injury. The effusion is a gradual process resulting, weeks after the injury, in headache, progressive stupor, and hemiparesis, followed by dilating pupil, a sign of herniation of the tentorium. **subungual h.,** an accumulation of blood under the nail plate.

hematomancy (hem′ah-to-man-se) [*hemato-* + Gr. *manteia* divination] diagnosis by examination of the blood.

hematomanometer (hem″ah-to-mah-nom′ĕter) sphygmomanometer.

hematomediastinum (hem″ah-to-me″de-as-ti′num) [*hemato-* + *mediastinum*] hemomediastinum.

hematometakinesis (hem″ah-to-met″ah-ki-ne′sis) [*hemato-* + Gr. *meta* across + *kinesis* movement] the phenomenon of the shifting of the blood from one part of the body to another, as from the skin to the internal organs; called also *borrowing-lending hemodynamic phenomenon.*

hematometer (hem″ah-tom′ĕ-ter) [*hemato-* + Gr. *metron* measure] a hemoglobinometer.

hematometra (hem″ah-to-me′trah) [*hemato-* + Gr. *mētra* uterus] an accumulation of blood in the uterus.

hematometry (hem″ah-tom′ĕ-tre) [*hemato-* + Gr. *metron* measure] measurement of the hemoglobin and estimation of the percentage of the various cells in the blood.

hematomole (he-mat′o-mōl) Breus' mole.

hematomphalocele (hem″at-om-fal′o-sēl) [*hemat-* + *omphalocele*] an umbilical hernia containing blood.

hematomphalus (hem″at-om′fah-lus) Cullen's sign; see under *sign.*

hematomycosis (hem″ah-to-mi-ko′sis) (*obs.*) fungemia.

hematomyelia (hem″ah-to-mi-e′le-ah) [*hemato-* + Gr. *myelos* marrow + *-ia*] hemorrhage into the spinal cord, usually confined to the gray substance, most often due to trauma, and marked by the sudden onset of flaccid paralysis with sensory disturbances.

hematomyelitis (hem″ah-to-mi′ĕ-li′tis) [*hemato-* + *myelitis*] acute myelitis with bloody effusion within the spinal cord.

hematomyelopore (hem″ah-to-mi′el-o-pōr″) [*hemato-* + Gr. *myelos* marrow + *poros* opening] a disease marked by the formation of canals in the spinal cord, due to hemorrhage.

hematoncometry (hem″at-on-kom′ĕ-tre) [*hemat-* + Gr. *onkos* mass + *metron* measure] measurement of blood volume.

hematonephrosis (hem″ah-to-ně-fro′sis)   presence of blood in the pelvis of the kidney.

hematonic (hem″ah-ton′ik)   a blood tonic.

hematopathology (hem″ah-to-pah-thol′o-je)   hemopathology.

hematopedesis (hem″ah-to-pě-de′sis)   hemodiapedesis.

hematopenia (hem″ah-to-pe′ne-ah) [*hemato-* + Gr. *penia* poverty]   deficiency of blood.

hematopericardium (hem″ah-to-per″ĭ-kar′de-um)   hemopericardium.

hematoperitoneum (hem″ah-to-per″ĭ-to-ne′um)   hemoperitoneum.

hematopexin (hem″ah-to-pek′sin)   hemopexin.

hematopexis (hem″ah-to-pek′sis)   hemopexis.

hematophage (hem′ah-to-fāj)   hemophagocyte.

hematophagia (hem″ah-to-fa′je-ah)   1. blood drinking.   2. the act of subsisting on the blood of another animal.   3. hemocytophagia.

hematophagocyte (hem″ah-to-fag′o-sīt)   hemophagocyte.

hematophagous (hem″ah-tof′ah-gus) [*hemato-* + Gr. *phagein* to eat]   pertaining to or characterized by hematophagia.

hematophagy (hem″ah-tof′ah-je)   hematophagia.

hematophilia (hem″ah-to-fil′e-ah)   hemophilia.

hematophyte (hem″ah-to-fīt″) [*hemato-* + Gr. *phyton* plant]   (*obs.*) any vegetable microorganism or species living in the blood.

hematophytic (hem″ah-to-fit′ik)   (*obs.*) pertaining to or caused by hematophytes.

hematopiesis (hem″ah-to-pi′ě-sis) [*hemato-* + Gr. *piesis* pressure]   blood pressure.

hematoplast (hem′ah-to-plast)   hemocytoblast.

hematoplastic (hem″ah-to-plas′tik) [*hemato-* + Gr. *plassein* to mold]   concerned in the elaboration of the blood.

hematopoiesis (hem″ah-to-poi-e′sis) [*hemato-* + Gr. *poiein* to make]   the formation and development of blood cells.   **extra-medullary h.,** the formation and development of blood cells outside the bone marrow, as in the spleen, liver, and lymph nodes.

hematopoietic (hem″ah-to-poi-et′ik) [*hemato-* + Gr. *poiein* to make]   1. pertaining to or effecting the formation of blood cells.   2. an agent that promotes the formation of blood cells.

hematopoietin (hem″ah-to-poi′e-tin)   erythropoietin.

hematoporphyria (hem″ah-to-por-fi′re-ah)   porphyria.

hematoporphyrin (hem″ah-to-por′fĭ-rin) [*hemato-* + Gr. *porphyra* purple]   chemical name: 1,3,5,8-tetramethyl-2,4-bis(α-hydroxyethyl)-6,7-dipropionic acid porphin. A dark violet, iron-free powder resulting from decomposition of hemoglobin, with the addition of HOH to the vinyl groups.

hematoporphyrinemia (hem″ah-to-por-fĭ-rin-e′me-ah)   the presence of hematoporphyrin in the blood.

hematoporphyrinism (hem″ah-to-por′fĭ-rin-izm)   a state characterized by hematoporphyrinemia and a sensitiveness to sunlight.

hematoporphyrinuria (hem″ah-to-por′fĭ-rin-u′re-ah)   the occurrence of hematoporphyrin in the urine.

Hematopota (hem″ah-top′o-tah)   *Chrysozona.*

hematorrhachis (hem-ah-tor′ah-kis) [*hemato-* + Gr. *rhachis* spine]   hematomyelia.

hematorrhea (hem″ah-to-re′ah) [*hemato-* + Gr. *rhoia* flow]   a free or copious hemorrhage.

hematosalpinx (hem″ah-to-sal′pinks)   an accumulation of blood in the uterine tube.

hematoscheocele (hem″ah-tos′ke-o-sēl″) [*hemato-* + Gr. *oscheon* scrotum + *kēlē* tumor]   a collection of blood within the scrotum.

hematoscope (hem′ah-to-skōp″) [*hemato-* + Gr. *skopein* to examine]   an instrument for the optical or spectroscopic examination of the blood.

hematoscopy (hem″ah-tos′ko-pe)   examination of the blood, as with a spectroscope.

hematosepsis (hem″ah-to-sep′sis)   septicemia.

hematoside (hem′ah-to-sīd″)   any sphingoglycolipid that contains a sialic acid component; they occur in the erythrocyte stroma and in the brain and spleen.

hematosis (hem″ah-to′sis)   (*obs.*) the formation of the blood.

hematospectrophotometer (hem″ah-to-spek″tro-fo-tom′ě-ter)   a spectrophotometer for determining the amount of hemoglobin in the blood.

hematospectroscope (hem″ah-to-spek′tro-skōp) [*hemato-* + *spectroscope*]   a spectroscope for examining thin layers of blood.

hematospectroscopy (hem″ah-to-spek-tros′ko-pe) [*hemato-* + *spectroscopy*]   the spectroscopic examination of the blood.

hematospermatocele (hem″ah-to-sper-mat′o-sēl) [*hemato-* + Gr. *sperma* seed + *kēlē* tumor]   a spermatocele containing blood.

hematospermia (hem″ah-to-sper′me-ah)   hemospermia.

hematospherinemia (hem″ah-to-sfēr″ĭ-ne′me-ah) [*hemato-* + Gr. *sphaira* sphere + *haima* blood + *-ia*]   hemoglobinemia.

hematosporidia (hem″ah-to-spo-rid′e-ah)   any member of the order Haemosporidia.

hematostatic (hem″ah-to-stat′ik) [*hemato-* + Gr. *stasis* standing]   due to or characterized by stagnation of the blood.

hematosteon (hem″ah-tos′te-on) [*hemat-* + Gr. *osteon* bone]   hemorrhage into the medullary cavity of a bone.

hematotherapy (hem″ah-to-ther′ah-pe)   hemotherapy.

hematothermal (hem″ah-to-ther′mal) [*hemato-* + Gr. *thermē* heat]   homoiothermic.

hematothorax (hem″ah-to-tho′raks)   hemothorax.

hematotoxic (hem″ah-to-tok′sik) [*hemato-* + *toxic*]   1. pertaining to hematotoxicosis.   2. poisonous to the blood and hematopoietic system.

hematotoxicosis (hem″ah-to-tok″sĭ-ko′sis)   toxic damage to the hematopoietic system.

hematotrachelos (hem″ah-to-trah-ke′los) [*hemato-* + Gr. *trachēlos* neck]   distention of the cervix of the uterus with blood, owing to atresia of the external os or of the vagina.

hematotropic (hem″ah-to-trop′ik) [*hemato-* + Gr. *tropos* a turning]   having a special affinity for or exerting a specific effect on the blood or blood cells.

hematotympanum (hem″ah-to-tim′pah-num) [*hemato-* + *tympanum*]   a hemorrhagic exudation into the midde ear.

hematoxic (hem″ah-tok′sik)   hematotoxic.

hematoxylin (hem″ah-tok′sĭ-lin)   a colorless crystalline compound, $C_{16}H_{14}O_6 + 3H_2O$, obtained by extracting logwood (*Haematoxylon campechianum*) with ether. It may be used as an indicator with a pH range of 5–6, but is mainly used in oxidized form as a stain in microscopy. See also *Table of Stains and Staining Methods.*   **alum h.,** hemalum.   **Delafield's h.,** see *Table of Stains and Staining Methods.*   **iron h.,** see *iron hematoxylin method, Heidenhain's iron hematoxylin stain,* and *Weigert's hematoxylin stain,* all in the *Table of Stains and Staining Methods.*

Hematoxylon (he″mah-tok′sĭ-lon)   *Haematoxylon.*

hematozemia (hem″ah-to-ze′me-ah) [*hemato-* + Gr. *zēmia* loss]   a gradual loss of blood.

hematozoa (hem″ah-to-zo′ah)   plural of *hematozoon.*

hematozoic (hem″ah-to-zo′ik)   pertaining to or caused by hematozoa.

hematozoon (hem″ah-to-zo′on), pl. *hematozo′a* [*hemato-* + Gr. *zōon* animal]   (*obs.*) any animal microorganism or species living in the blood.

hematuresis (hem″ah-tu-re′sis)   hematuria.

hematuria (hem″ah-tu′re-ah) [*hemat-* + Gr. *ouron* urine + *-ia*]   blood in the urine.   **endemic h.,** urinary schistosomiasis.   **enzootic bovine h.,** a disease of cattle marked by passing of blood in the urine, anemia, and debilitation.   **essential h.,** hematuria for which no cause has been determined; called also *primary h.*   **false h.,** redness of the urine due to food or drugs containing pigment.   **microscopic h.,** blood in the urine, the presence of which can be demonstrated only by the microscope.   **primary h.,** essential h.   **renal h.,** hematuria in which the blood comes from the kidney.   **urethral h.,** hematuria in which the blood comes from the urethra.   **vesical h.,** hematuria in which the blood comes from the bladder.

hemautograph (hem-aw′to-graf) [*hem-* + Gr. *autos* self + *graphein* to record]   a tracing made by an arterial blood jet.

hemautography (hem″aw-tog′rah-fe)   the recording of a hemautograph.

heme (hēm)   the nonprotein, insoluble, iron protoporphyrin constituent of hemoglobin, various other respiratory pigments and of many cells, both animal and vegetable. It is $C_{34}H_{33}O_4N_4FeOH$, an iron compound of protoporphyrin, with the iron in the ferrous, or Fe (II), state, and so constitutes the pigment portion or protein-free part of the hemoglobin molecule. It is responsible for the characteristic coloring and oxygen-carrying properties of hemoglobin. Formerly known as *hematin.*

hemendothelioma (hem″en-do-the″le-o′mah)   hemangioendothelioma.

Hementaria (he″men-ta′re-ah)   *Haementaria.*

hemeralope (hem′er-al-ōp)   a person affected with hemeralopia.

hemeralopia (hem″er-ah-lo′pe-ah) [Gr. *hēmeralops* the contrary of *nyktalops* + *ia*]   day blindness; defective vision in a bright light. The term is used in French (and incorrectly in English) to mean nyctalopia.

Hemerocampa (hem″er-o-kam′pah)   a genus of moths.   **H. leukostig′ma,** the white-marked tussock moth; in the larval stage the smaller white hairs are venomous and may produce severe urticaria.

hemerythrin (hēm″ĕ-rith′rin) [*hem-* + Gr. *erythros* red]   the coloring matter of the blood of earthworms which is contained in the plasma.

hemi- (hem′e) [Gr. *hēmi-* half] a prefix signifying one half.

hemiablepsia (hem″e-ah-blep′se-ah) hemianopia.

hemiacardius (hem″e-ah-kar′de-us) [*hemi-* + *a* neg. + Gr. *kardia* heart] one of twin fetuses in which only a part of the circulation is accomplished by its own heart.

hemiacephalus (hem″e-ah-sef′ah-lus) [*hemi-* + *a* neg. + Gr. *kephalē* head] a monster whose head lacks a brain and calvarium.

hemiacetal (hem″ĭ-as′ĕ-tal) a derivative formed by a combination of an aldehyde with an alcohol.

hemiachromatopsia (hem″e-ak″ro-mah-top′se-ah) [*hemi-* + *achromatopsia*] color blindness in one half, or in corresponding halves, of the visual field.

hemiacidrin (hem″e-as′ĭ-drin) a solution containing citric and gluconic acids, magnesium hydroxycarbonate, magnesium acid citrate, and calcium carbonate; it is capable of dissolving struvite calculi. Called also *renacidin.*

hemiageusia (hem″e-ah-gu′ze-ah) [*hemi-* + *a* neg. + Gr. *geusis* taste + *-ia*] loss or absence of the sense of taste on one side of the tongue.

hemiageustia (hem″e-ah-gūs′te-ah) hemiageusia.

hemialbumin (hem″e-al-bu′min) [*hemi-* + *albumin*] hemialbumose.

hemialbumose (hem″e-al′bu-mōs) a crystallizable product of the digestion of certain proteins; normally found in bone marrow, and occurring in the urine of osteomalacia and diphtheria.

hemialbumosuria (hem″e-al-bu″mo-su′re-ah) [*hemialbumose* + Gr. *ouron* urine + *-ia*] the presence of hemialbumose in the urine.

hemialgia (hem″e-al′je-ah) [*hemi-* + *-algia*] pain affecting one side of the body only.

hemiamaurosis (hem″e-am″aw-ro′sis) hemianopia.

hemiamblyopia (hem″e-am″ble-o′pe-ah) [*hemi-* + *amblyopia*] impairment of the visual power of one half of the retina.

hemiamyosthenia (hem″e-ah-mi″os-the′ne-ah) [*hemi-* + *a* neg. + Gr. *mys* muscle + *sthenos* strength + *-ia*] lack of muscular power on one side of the body.

hemianacusia (hem″e-an″ah-ku′ze-ah) [*hemi-* + *an* neg. + Gr. *akousia* hearing] loss of hearing in one ear only.

hemianalgesia (hem″e-an″al-je′ze-ah) [*hemi-* + *analgesia*] analgesia of one side of the body.

hemianencephaly (hem″e-an″en-sef′ah-le) [*hemi-* + Gr. *an* neg. + *enkephalos* brain] congenital absence of one side of the brain.

hemianesthesia (hem″e-an″es-the′ze-ah) anesthesia affecting only one side of the body; called also *unilateral anesthesia.* **alternate h.,** h. cruciata. **cerebral h.,** that which is due to lesion of the internal capsule of the lenticular nucleus. **crossed h.,** h. cruciata. **h. crucia′ta,** loss of sensation on one side of the face with contralateral loss of pain and temperature sense on the body, resulting from a lateral lesion in the pons or medulla, affecting both the sensory root of the trigeminal nerve and the spinothalamic tract. **mesocephalic h., pontile h.,** that which is due to disease of the pons. **spinal h.,** that which is due to a lesion of the spinal cord.

hemianopia (hem″e-ah-no′pe-ah) [*hemi-* + *an-* neg. + Gr. *ōpē* vision + *-ia*] defective vision or blindness in half of the visual field. **absolute h.,** blindness to light, color, and form, in half of the visual field. **altitudinal h.,** defective vision or blindness in a horizontal half of the visual field. **bilateral h.,** true h. **binasal h.,** heteronymous hemianopia in which the defects are in the nasal half of the field of vision in each eye. **binocular h.,** true h. **bitemporal h.,** heteronymous hemianopia in which the defects are in the temporal half of the field of vision in each eye. **h. bitempora′lis fu′gax,** transient bitemporal hemianopia. **complete h.,** hemianopia affecting an entire half of the visual field of each eye. **congruous h.,** homonymous hemianopia in which the defects in the field of vision in each eye are symmetrical in position and similar in all other respects. **crossed h.,** heteronymous h. **equilateral h.,** homonymous h. **heteronymous h.,** hemianopia affecting the nasal or the temporal half of the field of vision of each eye. **homonymous h.,** hemianopia affecting the right halves or the left halves of the visual fields of the two eyes. **horizontal h.,** altitudinal h. **incomplete h.,** hemianopia affecting less than an entire half of the visual field. **incongruous h.,** homonymous hemianopia in which the defects in the field of vision in the two eyes differ in one or more respects, as in extent or intensity. **lateral h.,** vertical h. **lower h.,** defective vision in the lower half of the visual field. **nasal h.,** defective vision or blindness in the medial vertical half of the visual field, i.e., the half nearest the nose. **quadrant h., quadrantic h.,** quadrantanopia. **relative h.,** defective vision or blindness to form or color in half of the visual field, the perception of light being retained. **temporal h.,** defective vision or blindness in the lateral vertical half of the visual field, i.e., the half nearest the temple. **true h.,** defective vision or blindness in one vertical half of each eye, usually due to a single lesion of the optic tract, at or above the level

of the chiasm. **unilateral h.,** defective vision or blindness in half of the visual field of one eye only. **uniocular h.,** unilateral h. **upper h.,** defective vision in the upper half of the visual field. **vertical h.,** defective vision or blindness in a lateral half of the visual field.

hemianopic (hem″e-ah-no′pik) pertaining to or characterized by hemianopia.

hemianopsia (hem″e-an-op′se-ah) hemianopia.

hemianoptic (hem″e-an-op′tik) hemianopic.

hemianosmia (hem″e-an-oz′me-ah) [*hemi-* + *anosmia*] loss of the sense of smell in one of the nostrils.

hemiapraxia (hem″e-ah-prak′se-ah) [*hemi-* + *apraxia*] apraxia affecting one side of the body only.

hemiarthrosis (hem″e-ar-thro′sis) [*hemi-* + *arthrosis*] a spurious synchondrosis.

Hemiascomycetidae (hem″e-as″ko-mi-se′tĭ-de) a subclass of primitive ascomycetous fungi in which the mycelium is small or lacking and the asci develop without hyphae, including the family Endomycetales.

hemiasynergia (hem″e-ah″sin-er′je-ah) [*hemi-* + *asynergia*] asynergia affecting one side of the body only.

hemiataxia (hem″e-ah-tak′se-ah) [*hemi-* + *ataxia*] ataxia affecting one side of the body only.

hemiataxy (hem″e-ah-tak′se) hemiataxia.

hemiathetosis (hem″e-ath″ĕ-to′sis) [*hemi-* + *athetosis*] athetosis affecting one side of the body only.

hemiatrophy (hem″e-at′ro-fe) [*hemi-* + *atrophy*] atrophy of one side of the body or of one half of an organ or part. **facial h.,** atrophy of one half of the face which is sometimes progressive, and is of unknown cause; called also *Romberg's disease.* **progressive lingual h.,** progressive atrophy of one lateral half of the tongue.

hemiautotroph (hem″e-aw′to-trōf) (*obs.*) a microorganism which can build up protein from inorganic nitrogen but requires organic carbon.

hemiautotrophic (hem″e-aw″to-trof′ik) [*hemi-* + *autotrophic*] (*obs.*) partly self-nourishing; a term applied to microorganisms which can build up protein from inorganic nitrogen but require organic carbon.

hemiaxial (hem″e-aks′e-al) at any oblique angle to the long axis of the body or a part.

hemiballism (hem″e-bal′izm) hemiballismus.

hemiballismus (hem″e-bal-iz′mus) [*hemi-* + Gr. *ballismos* jumping] a violent form of motor restlessness involving only one side of the body and being most marked in the upper extremity, resulting from a destructive lesion of the hypothalamic nucleus; called also *body of Luys syndrome.*

hemibladder (hem″ĭ-blad′er) a half bladder; a developmental anomaly in which the bladder is formed as two physically separated parts, each with its own ureter.

hemiblock (hem″ĭ-blok) failure in conduction of the cardiac impulse in either of the two main divisions of the left ventricular conducting system (bundle of His); it is called *left anterior hemiblock* when the anterior-superior division is interrupted and *left posterior hemiblock* when the posterior division is interrupted.

hemic (he′mik, hem′ik) [Gr. *haima* blood] pertaining to the blood.

hemicanities (hem″e-kah-nish′e-ēz) grayness of the hair on one side of the body.

hemicardia (hem″e-kar′de-ah) [*hemi-* + Gr. *kardia* heart] a congenital anomaly characterized by the presence of only half of a four-chambered heart. **h. dex′tra,** hemicardia in which the right side of the heart is present. **h. sinis′tra,** hemicardia in which the left side of the heart is present.

hemicardius (hem″e-kar′de-us) a free twin fetus whose development is greatly reduced but whose body form and various parts are still recognizable.

hemicellulase (hem″e-sel′u-lās) an enzyme that catalyzes the hydrolysis of hemicellulose.

hemicellulose (hem″e-sel′u-lōs) a general name for a group of high molecular weight carbohydrates that resemble cellulose but are more soluble and more easily decomposed. They can be extracted by dilute alkali and precipitated by dilute acid, and usually contain a hexose, a pentose, and a uronic acid.

hemicentrum (hem″e-sen′trum) [*hemi-* + *centrum*] either lateral half of a vertebral centrum.

hemicephalia (hem″e-sĕ-cfa′le-ah) [*hemi-* + Gr. *kephalē* head] congenital absence of the cerebrum.

hemicephalus (hem″e-sef′ah-lus) a monster exhibiting hemicephalia.

hemicerebrum (hem″e-ser′ĕ-brum) [*hemi-* + *cerebrum*] a cerebral hemisphere.

hemichorea (hem″e-ko-re′ah) [*hemi-* + *chorea*] chorea which affects only one side; see *Huntington's chorea,* under *chorea.*

hemichromatopsia (hem″e-kro″mah-top′se-ah) [*hemi-* + *chromatopsia*] color blindness in one half of the visual field.

hemichromosome (hem″e-kro′mo-sōm) [*hemi-* + *chromosome*] a body formed by the longitudinal division of a chromosome.

hemicolectomy (hem″e-ko-lek′to-me) [*hemi-* + *colectomy*] excision of approximately half of the colon. **left h.,** resection of the left half of the colon, from the middle of the transverse segment to the rectum. **right h.,** resection of the right half of the colon, from the ileum to the middle of the transverse segment.

hemicorporectomy (hem″e-kor″po-rek′to-me) [*hemi-* + L. *corpus* body + Gr. *ektomē* excision] surgical removal of the lower part of the body, including the bony pelvis, external genitals, and the lower part of the rectum and anus.

hemicrania (hem″e-kra′ne-ah) [*hemi-* + Gr. *kranion* skull] 1. pain or aching in one side of the head. 2. incomplete anencephaly.

hemicraniectomy (hem″e-kra″ne-ek′to-me) [*hemi-* + Gr. *kranion* skull + *ektomē* excision] Doyen's operation of sectioning the vault of the skull from before backward, near the median line, and forcing the entire side outward, thus exposing half of the brain.

hemicraniosis (hem″e-kra″ne-o′sis) a condition marked by hyperostosis on one half of the cranium or face, with cerebral involvement. The condition is believed to be due to endothelioma of the dura.

hemicraniotomy (hem″e-kra″ne-ot′o-me) [*hemi-* + Gr. *kranion* skull + *temnein* to cut] hemicraniectomy.

hemidecortication (hem″e-de-kor″tĭ-ka′shun) removal of one half of the cerebral cortex.

hemidesmosome (hem″e-des′mo-sōm) [*hemi-* + *desmosome*] a structure similar to a desmosome but representing only half of it, found on the basal surface of some epithelial cells, forming the site of attachment between the basal surface of the cell and the basement membrane. Called also *half desmosome*.

Hemidesmus (hem″e-des′mus) a genus of asclepiadaceous plants. The root of *H. in′dicus* R.Br. has been used as a demulcent, diuretic, and alterative.

hemidiaphoresis (hem″e-di″ah-fo-re′sis) [*hemi-* + *diaphoresis*] hemihyperhidrosis.

hemidiaphragm (hem″e-di′ah-fram) one half of the diaphragm.

hemidrosis (hem″ĭ-dro′sis) hemihidrosis.

hemidysergia (hem″e-dis-er′je-ah) dysergia affecting one side of the body.

hemidysesthesia (hem″e-dis″es-the′ze-ah) [*hemi-* + *dys-* + *aisthēsis* feeling] a disorder of sensation affecting one side of the body only.

hemidystrophy (hem″e-dis′tro-fe) unequal development of the two sides of the body.

hemiectromelia (hem″e-ek-tro-me′le-ah) a developmental anomaly characterized by imperfect development of the limbs of one side of the body.

hemielastin (hem″e-e-las′tin) a substance formed by the digestion or hydrolysis of elastin.

hemiencephalus (hem″e-en-sef′ah-lus) [*hemi-* + Gr. *enkephalos* brain] a fetus that lacks one cerebral hemisphere.

hemiepilepsy (hem″e-ep′ĭ-lep-se) [*hemi-* + *epilepsy*] epilepsy affecting one side of the body only.

hemifacial (hem″e-fa′shal) pertaining to or affecting one half of the face.

hemigastrectomy (hem″e-gas-trek′to-me) excision of one half of the stomach.

hemigeusia (hem″e-gu′se-ah) [*hemi-* + Gr. *geusis* taste + *-ia*] presence of taste perception on one side of the tongue only.

hemigigantism (hem″ĭ-ji′gan-tizm) overgrowth of one side of the entire body or of a portion of one side, as of the face.

hemiglossal (hem″e-glos′sal) [*hemi-* + Gr. *glōssa* tongue] affecting one side of the tongue.

hemiglossectomy (hem″e-glos-sek′to-me) [*hemi-* + Gr. *glōssa* tongue + *ektomē* excision] resection of one side of the tongue.

hemiglossitis (hem″e-glos-si′tis) [*hemi-* + Gr. *glōssa* tongue + *-itis*] inflammation involving only one side of the tongue.

hemignathia (hem″e-nath′e-ah) [*hemi-* + Gr. *gnathos* jaw + *-ia*] a developmental anomaly characterized by partial to complete lack of the lower jaw on one side.

hemihepatectomy (hem″e-hep″ah-tek′to-me) excision of half of the liver.

hemihidrosis (hem″e-hĭ-dro′sis) [*hemi-* + Gr. *hidrōs* sweat] sweating on one side of the body only.

hemihypalgesia (hem″e-hi″pal-je′ze-ah) [*hemi* + *hypalgesia*] diminished sensitiveness to pain affecting one side of the body.

hemihyperesthesia (hem″e-hi″per-es-the′ze-ah) [*hemi-* + *hyperesthesia*] abnormally increased acuteness of sensation on one side of the body.

hemihyperidrosis (hem″e-hi″per-ĭ-dro′sis) [*hemi-* + Gr. *hyper* over + *hidrōs* sweat] excessive sweating on one side of the body only; called also *hemidiaphoresis*.

hemihypermetria (hem″e-hi″per-me′tre-ah) hypermetria affecting one side of the body.

hemihyperplasia (hem″e-hi″per-pla′ze-ah) overdevelopment of one side of the body, or of one half of an organ or part, as of the cranium.

hemihypertonia (hem″e-hi″per-to′ne-ah) [*hemi-* + Gr. *hyper* over + *tonos* tension + *-ia*] increased tone of the muscles of one side, which may result in contractures; sometimes seen after a stroke. Called also *hemitonia*.

hemihypertrophy (hem″e-hi-per′tro-fe) [*hemi-* + *hypertrophy*] overgrowth of one half of the body or unilateral hypertrophy of a part. **facial h.,** hypertrophy of half of the face.

hemihypesthesia (hem″e-hi″pes-the′ze-ah) abnormally decreased acuteness of sensation on one side of the body.

hemihypoesthesia (hem″e-hi″po-es-the′ze-ah) hemihypesthesia.

hemihypometria (hem″e-hi″po-me′tre-ah) hypometria affecting one side of the body.

hemihypoplasia (hem″e-hi″po-pla′ze-ah) underdevelopment of one side of the body, or of one half of a part or organ, as of the brain.

hemihypotonia (hem″e-hi″po-to′ne-ah) [*hemi-* + Gr. *hypo* under + *tonos* tension + *-ia*] reduced muscle tone of one side of the body.

hemikaryon (hem″e-kar′e-on) [*hemi-* + Gr. *karyon* nucleus] a cell nucleus which contains the haploid number of chromosomes.

hemiketal (hem″e-ke′tal) a derivative formed by a combination of a ketone group with an alcohol.

hemilaminectomy (hem″e-lam″ĭ-nek′to-me) surgical removal of a vertebral lamina on one side only.

hemilaryngectomy (hem″e-lar″in-jek′to-me) excision of one lateral half of the larynx.

hemilateral (hem″e-lat′er-al) affecting one lateral half.

hemilesion (hem″e-le′zhun) a lesion of one side of the spinal cord only.

hemilingual (hem″e-ling′gwal) [*hemi-* + L. *lingua* tongue] affecting one side of the tongue.

hemimacroglossia (hem″e-mak″ro-glos′e-ah) enlargement of one side of the tongue.

hemimandibulectomy (hem″e-man-dib-u-lek′to-me) surgical excision of half of the mandible.

hemimelia (hem″e-me′le-ah) [*hemi-* + Gr. *melos* limb + *-ia*] a developmental anomaly characterized by absence of all or part of the distal half of a limb; see illustration under *amelia*. **fibular h.,** hemimelia of the lower limb in which the fibular side is absent. **radial h.,** hemimelia of the upper limb in which the radial side is absent. **tibial h.,** hemimelia of the lower limb, in which the tibial side is absent. **ulnar h.,** hemimelia of the upper limb, in which the ulnar side is absent.

hemimelus (hem-im′ĕ-lus) an individual exhibiting hemimelia.

hemin (he′min) [Gr. *haima* blood] the crystalline chloride of heme, $C_{34}H_{33}N_4O_4FeCl$, with the iron in the ferrous or Fe(III) state, of which Teichmann's crystals are composed.

heminephrectomy (hem″e-nĕ-frek′to-me) excision of a portion of a kidney.

heminephroureterectomy (hem″e-nef″ro-u-re″ter-ek′to-me) excision of a portion of a kidney and ureter.

hemineurasthenia (hem″e-nu″ras-the′ne-ah) neurasthenia affecting one side of the body only.

hemiobesity (hem″e-o-bēs′ĭ-te) [*hemi-* + *obesity*] obesity of one side of the body only.

hemiopalgia (hem″e-op-al′je-ah) [*hemi-* + Gr. *ōps* eye + *-algia*] pain in one side of the head and in one eye.

hemiopia (hem″e-o′pe-ah) 1. hemianopia (Plenk). 2. absence of visual power in one half of the retina.

hemiopic (hem″e-op′ik) [*hemi-* + Gr. *ōps* eye] 1. affecting one eye. 2. pertaining to hemiopia.

hemipagus (hem-ip′ah-gus) [*hemi-* + Gr. *pagos* thing fixed] twin fetuses united laterally at the thorax.

hemiparalysis (hem″e-pah-ral′ĭ-sis) hemiplegia.

hemiparanesthesia (hem″e-par″an-es-the′ze-ah) [*hemi-* + Gr. *para* below + *anesthesia*] anesthesia of the lower half of one side of the body.

hemiparaplegia (hem″e-par″ah-ple′je-ah) [*hemi-* + *paraplegia*] paralysis of the lower half of one side of the body.

hemiparesis (hem″e-par′e-sis) [*hemi-* + *paresis*] muscular weakness or partial paralysis affecting one side of the body.

hemiparesthesia (hem″e-par″es-the′ze-ah) [*hemi-* + *paresthesia*] perverted sensation on one side of the body.

hemiparetic (hem″e-pah-ret′ik) 1. pertaining to hemiparesis. 2. one affected with hemiparesis.

hemiparkinsonism (hem″e-par′kin-son-izm) parkinsonism affecting only one side of the body.

hemipelvectomy (hem″e-pel″vek′to-me) amputation of a lower limb through the sacroiliac joint.

hemipeptone (hem″e-pep′tōn) [*hemi-* + *peptone*] one of the intermediate products of pepsin digestion of protein; it is formed along with antipeptone, and differs from the latter in being convertible into amino-acids by trypsin.

hemiphalangectomy (hem″e-fal″an-jek′to-me) the excision of part of a digital phalanx.

hemipinta (hem″ĭ-pin′tah) a rare form of pinta in which the pigmentary disturbances affect only one half of the body.

hemiplacenta (hem″e-plah-sen′tah) [*hemi-* + *placenta*] an organ, composed of the chorion, yolk sac, and, usually, allantois, which puts marsupial embryos into temporary relation with the maternal uterus.

hemiplegia (hem″e-ple′je-ah) [*hemi-* + Gr. *plēgē* stroke] paralysis of one side of the body. **h. al′ternans hypoglos′sica**, hemiplegia due to lesion of the hypoglossal nerve on the side opposite the paralyzed part. **alternate h.**, that which affects a part on one side of the body and another part on the opposite side. **alternating oculomotor h.**, syndrome of Weber. **ascending h.**, ascending paralysis of one lateral half of the body. **capsular h.**, hemiplegia due to lesion of the internal capsule. **cerebral h.**, that which is due to a lesion of the brain. **contralateral h.**, hemiplegia on the side of the body opposite to the site of the brain lesion causing it. **crossed h.**, alternate h. **h. crucia′ta**, alternate h. **facial h.**, paralysis of one side of the face, the body being unaffected. **faciobrachial h.**, paralysis of one half of the face and of the arm on the same side. **faciolingual h.**, paralysis of one side of the face and tongue. **flaccid h.**, hemiplegia with loss of tone of the muscles of the paralyzed part and absence of tendon reflexes. Cf. *spastic h.* **Gubler's h.**, 1. alternate h. 2. apparent hemiplegia occurring as a symptom in hysteria. **infantile h.**, hemiplegia due to cerebral thrombosis or hemorrhage at delivery or occurring before birth. **puerperal h.**, hemiplegia of women occurring shortly after childbirth. **spastic h.**, hemiplegia marked by spasticity of the muscles of the paralyzed part and increased tendon reflexes. Cf. *flaccid h.* **spinal h.**, a form due to a lesion of the spinal cord. **Wernicke-Mann h.**, partial hemiplegia of the extremities; called also *Wernicke-Mann type.*

hemiplegic (hem″e-ple′jik) pertaining to or of the nature of hemiplegia.

hemiprostatectomy (hem″e-pros″tah-tek′to-me) removal of one lateral half of the prostate.

Hemiptera (he-mip′ter-ah) [*hemi-* + Gr. *pteron* wing] an order of insects which may be winged or wingless, including ordinary bugs and lice, characterized by having the mouth parts adapted to piercing or sucking. The families Cimicidae and Reduviidae (suborder Heteroptera) contain species of considerable medical importance.

hemipterous (he-mip′ter-us) of or pertaining to insects of the order Hemiptera.

hemipylorectomy (hem″e-pi″lor-ek′to-me) excision of half of the pylorus.

hemipyocyanin (hem″e-pi″o-si′ah-nin) an antibiotic produced by the growth of *Pseudomonas aeruginosa* which is active against *Trichophyton schoenleini* and *Candida albicans.*

hemipyonephrosis (hem″e-pi″o-ně-fro′sis) a hydronephrotic sac in a portion of the kidney; or pyonephrosis of half of a double kidney.

hemirachischisis (hem″e-rah-kis′kĭ-sis) rachischisis without prolapse of the spinal cord.

hemisacralization (hem″e-sa″kral-i-za′shun) fusion of the fifth lumbar vertebra to the first segment of the sacrum on only one side.

hemiscotosis (hem″e-sko-to′sis) hemianopia.

hemisection (hem″e-sek′shun) 1. bisection. 2. division into two equal parts.

hemiseptum (hem″e-sep′tum) either half of a septum, especially the lamina of the septum pellucidum of the brain. **h. cer′ebri**, the lateral half of the septum pellucidum of the brain.

hemisoantibody (hĕm″ĭ-so-an′tĭ-bod-e) an antibody of one individual that reacts with red blood cells of another individual of the same species.

hemisomnambulism (hem″e-som-nam′bu-lizm) somnambulism in which the subject behaves as though he were awake.

hemisomus (hem″e-so′mus) [*hemi-* + Gr. *sōma* body] an imperfectly developed fetus.

hemisotonic (hem″i-so-ton′ik) [Gr. *haima* blood + *isotonic*] having the same osmotic pressure as the blood.

hemispasm (hem′e-spazm) spasm affecting one side only.

hemisphaeria (hem″ĭ-sfe′re-ah) [L.] plural of *hemisphaerium.*

hemisphaerium (hem″ĭ-sfe′re-um) pl. *hemisphae′ria.* Hemisphere; see also *hemispherium.* **hemisphae′ria bul′bi ure′thrae**, the lateral halves of the bulb of the urethra.

hemisphere (hem′ĭ-sfēr) [*hemi-* + Gr. *sphaira* a ball or globe] half of any spherical or roughly spherical structure or organ, as the hemispheres of the brain (hemispherium [NA]). **animal h.**, the half of the mass of cells formed by cleavage of a fertilized telolecithal ovum that is nearest the animal pole. **cerebellar**

h., hemispherium cerebelli. **cerebral h.**, either of the pair of structures constituting the largest part of the brain in humans, formed by evagination of the embryonic telencephalon and separated by the fissura longitudinalis cerebri; together they comprise the cerebral cortex, centrum semiovale, basal ganglia, and rhinencephalon, and contain the lateral ventricles. The hemispheres are connected at the bottom of the fissura by the corpus callosum. Called also *hemispherium* [NA]. **dominant h.**, that cerebral hemisphere which is more concerned than the other in the integration of sensations and the control of many functions, such as the preferential use of one or the other of paired organs in voluntary movements, e.g., the left cerebral hemisphere in right-handed persons, and vice versa. However, the left hemisphere is usually dominant for speech, regardless of the handedness. **vegetal h.**, the half of the mass of cells formed by cleavage of a fertilized telolecithal ovum that is nearest the vegetal pole.

hemispherectomy (hem″ĭ-sfēr-ek′to-me) [*hemisphere* + Gr. *ektomē* excision] resection of a cerebral hemisphere.

hemispherium (hem″ĭ-sfe′re-um) pl. *hemisphe′ria* [L.] [NA] a general term denoting half of a spherical or spheroid structure. Also [NA] the cerebral hemisphere; see under *hemisphere.* **h. cerebel′li** [NA], cerebellar hemisphere: the part of the cerebellum lateral to the vermis, each hemisphere being composed of the ala lobuli centralis, lobulus quadrangularis, lobulus simplex, lobulus semilunaris superior, lobulus semilunaris inferior, lobulus biventer, tonsilla, and flocculus.

hemisphygmia (hem″ĭ-sfig′me-ah) [*hemi-* + Gr. *sphygmos* pulse] a condition in which there appears to be twice as many pulse beats as there are heart beats (pulsus bisferiens).

Hemispora stellata (hem-is′po-rah stel-la′tah) a dematiacious imperfect soil fungus reported to have been isolated from cold abscesses, periosteitis, and lesions resembling sporotrichosis.

hemispore (hem′e-spōr) a spore formed by the differentiation and division of the terminal portion of a hypha.

hemistrumectomy (hem″e-stroo-mek′to-me) hemithyroidectomy.

hemisyndrome (hem″e-sin′drōm) a syndrome indicative of a unilateral lesion of the spinal cord.

hemiterata (hem″e-ter′ah-tah) [*hemi-* + Gr. *teras* monster] a group of congenitally deformed individuals who cannot be classed as teratisms or monstrosities.

hemiteratic (hem″e-ter-at′ik) congenitally deformed, but not monstrous.

hemitetany (hem″e-tet′ah-ne) tetany limited to one side of the body.

hemithermoanesthesia (hem″e-ther″mo-an″es-the′ze-ah) absence of temperature sensation on one side of the body.

hemithorax (hem″e-tho′raks) [*hemi-* + *thorax*] one side of the chest.

hemithyroidectomy (hem″e-thi″roid-ek′to-me) excision of one lobe of the thyroid gland.

hemitomias (hem″ĭ-to′me-as) [Gr. *hēmitomias* half a eunuch] a person deprived of one testis.

hemitonia (hem″ĭ-to′ne-ah) [*hemi-* + Gr. *tonos* tension + *-ia*] hemihypertonia.

hemitoxin (hem″ĭ-tok′sin) a toxin the toxicity of which has been reduced by one half.

hemitremor (hem″e-tre′mor) tremor of one side of the body.

hemivagotony (hem″e-va-got′o-ne) hyperexcitability of the vagus nerve on one side.

hemivertebra (hem″e-ver′te-brah) 1. a developmental anomaly characterized by incomplete development of one side of a vertebra. 2. (pl., *hemiver′tebrae*) a vertebra which is incompletely developed on one side.

hemizygosity (hem″e-zi-gos′ĭ-te) the state of possessing only one of the pair of genes that influence the determination of a particular trait, as the male has no alleles on the Y chromosome for those on the X, so that his X-linked genes are expressed whether they are dominant or recessive.

hemizygote (hem″e-zi′gōt) an individual or cell exhibiting hemizygosity.

hemizygotic (hem″e-zi-got′ik) hemizygous.

hemizygous (hem″e-zi′gus) possessing only one of a pair of genes that influence the determination of a particular trait; see *hemizygosity.*

hemlock (hem′lok) 1. any fir tree of the genus *Tsuga*, especially *T. canadensis* (L.) Carr. (Pinaceae), the source of Canada pitch, of the volatile oil of hemlock, and of an astringent extract. 2. *Conium maculatum* L., or poison hemlock, a large, toxic, umbelliferous herb, which contains the poisonous alkaloid coniine; the dried, fully grown, unripe fruit has sedative, anodyne, and antispasmodic properties. 3. any of the plants of the genera Cicuta and Conium. **poison h.**, see *hemlock*, def. 2. **water h.**, *Cicuta maculata.*

hemo-, haemo-, hem-, haem-, hema-, haema-, hemat-, hemato-, haemato- (he′mo, hem, he′mah, hem′at, hem′ah-to)

[Gr. *haima, haimatos* blood] combining form denoting relationship to the blood.

hemoagglutination (he″mo-ah-gloo″tĭ-na′shun) hemagglutination.

hemoagglutinin (he″mo-ah-gloo′tĭ-nin) hemagglutinin.

hemoalkalimeter (he″mo-al″kah-lim′ĕ-ter) an instrument for ascertaining the alkalinity of the blood.

hemobilia (he″mo-bil′e-ah) hematobilia.

hemobilinuria (he″mo-bi-lin-u′re-ah)[*hemo-* + *bilin* + Gr. *ouron* urine + *-ia*] the presence of urobilin in the blood and urine.

hemoblast (he′mo-blast) hemocytoblast; see also *monophyletic theory,* under *theory.* **lymphoid h. of Pappenheim,** pronormoblast.

hemoblastosis (he″mo-blas-to′sis) (*obs.*) proliferation of the blood-forming tissues; the term includes leukosis, erythrosis, and reticuloendotheliosis.

hemocatharsis (he″mo-kah-thar′sis) hematocatharsis.

hemocatheresis (he″mo-kah-ther′ĕ-sis)[*hemo-* + Gr. *kathairesis* destruction] the destruction of blood, especially of erythrocytes.

hemocatheretic (he″mo-kath″er-et′ik) pertaining to, characterized by, or promoting hemocatheresis.

Hemoccult (he′mo-kult) trademark for a modification of the guaiac test for occult blood, in which guaiac-impregnated filter paper is used; the test is positive if the specimen turns blue.

hemocele (he′mo-sēl) hemocoelom.

hemocelom (he′mo-se′lom) hemocoelom.

hemocholecyst (he″mo-ko′le-sist) nontraumatic hemorrhage of the gallbladder.

hemocholecystitis (he″mo-ko-le-sis-ti′tis) cholecystitis with hemorrhage into the gallbladder.

hemochorial (he″mo-ko′re-al) [*hemo-* + *chorion*] denoting a type of placenta in which maternal blood comes in direct contact with the chorion.

hemochromatosis (he″mo-kro″mah-to′sis) a disorder of iron metabolism characterized by excess deposition of iron in the tissues, especially in the liver and pancreas, and by bronze pigmentation of the skin, cirrhosis, diabetes mellitus, and associated bone and joint changes. The hereditary form is called *idiopathic* (*classic*) *hemochromatosis.* The exogenous forms are observed in patients who have received transfusions and/or iron compounds over a prolonged period, resulting in iron overload. Called also *bronze* or *bronzed diabetes, iron storage disease,* and *Recklinghausen-Applebaum disease.* Cf. *hemosiderosis.*

hemochromatotic (he″mo-kro″mah-tot′ik) pertaining to or characterized by hemochromatosis.

hemochrome (he′mo-krōm) [*hemo-* + Gr. *chrōma* color] an oxygen-carrying pigment found in the blood of various animals; the hemochromes include hemoglobin, erythrocruorin, chlorocruorin, hematocyanin, and hemoerythrin.

hemochromogen (he″mo-kro′mo-jen)[*hemo-* + Gr. *chrōma* color + *gennan* to produce] a general term for a compound of heme with various proteins and other substances. **hemoglobin h.,** a hemoglobin in which the globin has been denatured.

hemochromometer (he″mo-kro-mom′ĕ-ter) [*hemo-* + Gr. *chrōma* color + *metron* measure] an instrument for making color tests of the blood to determine the proportion of hemoglobin.

hemochromometry (he″mo-kro-mom′ĕ-tre) the measurement of the quantity of hemoglobin in the blood.

hemochromoprotein (he″mo-kro″mo-pro′te-in) a colored, conjugated protein, with respiratory functions, found in the blood of animals.

hemoclasia (he″mo-kla′se-ah) the occurrence of postalimentary leukopenia; see *hemoclastic crisis,* under *crisis.*

hemoclasis (he-mok′lah-sis) [*hemo-* + Gr. *klasis* a breaking] hemolysis.

hemoclastic (he-mo-klas′tik) pertaining to, characterized by, or causing destruction or dissolution of erythrocytes; see also under *crisis.*

hemoclip (he′mo-klip) a metal clip used to ligate blood vessels.

hemocoagulin (he″mo-ko-ag′u-lin) a constituent of the venom of certain snakes which causes coagulation of the blood.

hemocoelom (he″mo-se′lom) [*hemo-* + *coelom*] 1. the part of the coelom in which the heart is developed. 2. collectively, the spaces between the cells and tissues of many invertebrates, such as most mollusks, arthropods, and tunicates, through which a bloodlike fluid (hemolymph) circulates. Sometimes spelled *hemocele* and *hemocoel.*

hemocoeloma (he″mo-se-lo′mah) [*hemo-* + *coeloma*] hemocoelom.

hemoconcentration (he″mo-kon″sen-tra′shun) decrease of the fluid content of the blood, with resulting increase in its concentration. Cf. *exemia.*

hemoconia (he″mo-ko′ne-ah) [*hemo-* + Gr. *konia* dust] small, round or dumbbell-shaped particles demonstrating brownian movement, observed in blood platelets in a wet film of blood under darkfield microscopy. Called also *blood dust* (*of Müller*) and *Müller's dust bodies.*

hemoconiosis (he″mo-ko″ne-o′sis) the presence in the blood of abnormal amounts of hemoconia.

hemocrine (he′mo-krin) having an endocrine influence in the blood.

hemocrinia (he″mo-krin′e-ah) [*hemo-* + endo*crine*] the presence of endocrine substances (hormones) in the blood.

hemocrinotherapy (he″mo-krin″o-ther′ah-pe) treatment by injection of the patient's own blood mixed with an endocrine extract.

hemocryoscopy (he″mo-kri-os′ko-pe) [*hemo-* + *cryoscopy*] cryoscopy of the blood; the ascertaining of the freezing point of the blood.

hemoculture (he′mo-kul″tūr) [*hemo-* + *culture*] a bacteriological culture of the blood.

hemocuprein (he″mo-ku′pre-in) an organic copper and protein compound isolated from erythrocytes.

hemocyanin (he″mo-si′ah-nin) [*hemo-* + Gr. *kyanos* blue] a chromoprotein occurring in the blood of mollusks and arthropods; it is a blue respiratory pigment and contains 0.17 to 0.38 per cent of copper. **keyhole-limpet h. (KLH),** the oxygen-carrying blood pigment, hemocyanin, from the "keyhole limpet" (a mollusk), frequently used as an experimental antigen in mammals; immunization with KLH is used as a test in acute myelogenous leukemia.

hemocyte (he′mo-sīt) [*hemo-* + Gr. *kytos* hollow vessel] any blood corpuscle, or formed element of the blood.

hemocytoblast (he″mo-si′to-blast) [*hemocyte* + Gr. *blastos* germ] the free stem cell from which, according to the monophyletists, by development along different lines, all the other cells of the blood are derived.

hemocytoblastoma (he″mo-si″to-blas-to′mah) a tumor containing all the cells typical of bone marrow.

hemocytocatheresis (he″mo-si″to-kah-ther′ĕ-sis) [*hemocyte* + Gr. *kathairesis* destruction] the destruction of erythrocytes.

hemocytoma (he′mo-si-to′mah) a tumor containing undifferentiated blood cells.

hemocytometer (he″mo-si-tom′ĕ-ter) hemacytometer.

hemocytophagia (he″mo-si″to-fa′je-ah) [*hemocyte* + Gr. *phagein* to devour] the ingestion and destruction of blood corpuscles by the histiocytes of the reticuloendothelial system.

hemocytophagic (he″mo-si″to-faj′ik) pertaining to or characterized by hemocytophagia.

hemocytopoiesis (he″mo-si″to-poi-e′sis) hematopoiesis.

hemocytotripsis (he″mo-si″to-trip′sis) [*hemocyte* + Gr. *tribein* to rub] the disintegration of the blood corpuscles by reason of pressure.

hemocytozoa (he″mo-si″to-zo′ah) plural of *hemocytozoon.*

hemocytozoon (he″mo-si″to-zo′on), pl. *hemocytozo′a*[*hemo-* + Gr. *kytos* hollow vessel + *zōon* animal] (*obs.*) any animal microorganism parasitic in the blood cells.

hemodia (he-mo′de-ah) [Gr. *haimōdia* condition of having the teeth on edge] (*obs.*) unusual sensitiveness of the teeth.

hemodiagnosis (he″mo-di″ag-no′sis) [*hemo-* + *diagnosis*] diagnosis by examination of the blood.

hemodialysis (he″mo-di-al′ĭ-sis) the removal of certain elements from the blood by virtue of the difference in the rates of their diffusion through a semipermeable membrane, e.g., by means of a hemodialyzer.

hemodialyzer (he″mo-di′ah-liz″er) an apparatus by which hemodialysis may be performed, blood being separated by a semipermeable membrane from a solution of such composition as to secure diffusion of certain elements out of the blood. Popularly called *artificial kidney.* **ultrafiltration h.,** one in which differences in fluid pressure bring about filtration of a protein-free fluid from the blood.

hemodiapedesis (he″mo-di″ah-pĕ-de′sis) [*hemo-* + *diapedesis*] the extravasation of blood through the skin.

hemodiastase (he″mo-di′as-tās) [*hemo-* + *diastase*] an amylolytic enzyme in the blood.

hemodilution (he″mo-di-lu′shun) increase of the fluid content of the blood with resulting decrease in concentration of its erythrocytes.

hemodynamic (he″mo-di-nam′ik) pertaining to the movements involved in the circulation of the blood.

hemodynamics (he″mo-di-nam′iks) [*hemo-* + Gr. *dynamis* power] the study of the movements of the blood and of the forces concerned therein.

hemodynamometry (he″mo-di″nah-mom′ĕ-tre) measurement of blood pressure.

hemodystrophy (he″mo-dis′tro-fe) [*hemo-* + *dys-* + Gr. *trophē* nutrition] any blood disease due to faulty blood nutrition.

hemoendothelial (he″mo-en-do-the′le-al) [*hemo-* + *endothelium*] denoting a type of placenta in which maternal blood comes in contact with the endothelium of chorionic vessels.

hemoerythrin (he″mo-e-rith′rin) [*hemo-* + Gr. *erythros* red] a red respiratory pigment found in the blood of certain worms.

Hemofil (he′mo-fil) trademark for a highly concentrated preparation of antihemophilic factor (coagulation Factor VIII).

hemofiltration (he″mo-fil-tra′shun) the removal of waste products from the blood by passing the blood through extracorporeal filters.

hemoflagellate (he″mo-flaj′ĕ-lāt) any flagellate protozoan parasite of the blood; the term includes the genera *Trypanosoma* and *Leishmania*.

hemofuscin (he″mo-fūs′in) [*hemo-* + L. *fuscus* brown] a brownish-yellow pigment that results from the decomposition of hemoglobin; it gives the urine a deep ruddy color.

hemogenesis (he″mo-jen′ĕ-sis) hematopoiesis.

hemogenic (he″mo-jen′ik) hematogenic.

hemoglobin (he″mo-glo′bin) the oxygen-carrying pigment of the erythrocytes, formed by the developing erythrocyte in bone marrow. It is a conjugated protein containing four heme groups and globin, and having the property of reversible oxygenation. A molecule of hemoglobin contains four globin polypeptide chains. They are designated α, β, γ, δ, in the adult; and each is composed of several hundred amino acids. Different types of hemoglobin are determined by the specific combination of these chains, the number of chains of the different types in the molecule being indicated by subscript numerals. For example, *hemoglobin F (fetal h.)*, which is the predominant type in the newborn, may be written as $\alpha_2^A\gamma_2^F$. *Hemoglobin A (adult h.)*, which is normally predominant in the adult is designated $\alpha_2^A\beta_2^A$ or $\alpha_2\beta_2$. Another hemoglobin, *hemoglobin A_2* (designated $\alpha_2^A\delta_2^{A2}$ or $\alpha_2^A\delta_2$), is usually present in limited minor concentrations. Many hemoglobins with differing electrophoretic mobilities and characteristics have been reported, for example, S, C, D, E, G, H, I, J, K, L, M, N, Q, Norfolk, Barts, and many others. (See also *hemoglobinopathy.*) Because refined biochemical techniques may lead to the discovery of additional hemoglobins, certain standards for nomenclature have been devised. The hemoglobin electrophoretic mobility is designated by a capital letter; if two or more hemoglobins have the same mobility, the geographic area of discovery is indicated as a subscript, for example, hemoglobin M_S, or $M_{Saskatoon}$, and hemoglobin M_M, or $M_{Milwaukee}$. To restrict the increasing use of capital letters new hemoglobins are named simply for the laboratory, hospital, or town where they were discovered, for example, hemoglobin$_{Norfolk}$. When known, the number of each amino acid substituting in each polypeptide(s) in the molecule should be indicated by the appropriate superscript numeral. Symbol *Hb*. **h. A,** normal adult hemoglobin, composed of two alpha and two beta chains, $\alpha_2^A\beta_2^A$. **h. A_{1c},** a glycosylated hemoglobin A, having a hexose attached to the N-terminal of its β-chain; its levels are increased in poorly controlled diabetics. **h. A_2,** a normal adult hemoglobin, $\alpha_2^A\delta_2$, present in small amounts, in which delta chains replace the beta chains. **Bart's h.,** an abnormal hemoglobin composed of four gamma chains having high oxygen affinity. **h. C,** a relatively common, abnormal hemoglobin in which lysine replaces glutamic acid at position six of the beta chains. It was one of the earliest hemoglobins to have its molecular abnormality defined. In the homozygous state, it produces splenomegaly, moderate or mild hemolytic anemia, recurrent jaundice, and an increased number of target cells and reticulocytes in the peripheral blood, while in the heterozygous state (*h. C trait*) anemia or disease is absent, although increased numbers of target cells are seen in the peripheral blood. **h. carbamate,** a compound of hemoglobin and CO_2, important for the transporation of CO_2 in red cells. **h. Chesapeake,** an abnormal hemoglobin in which the amino acid substitution (leucine for arginine in the alpha chain) results in a molecule so structurally abnormal that it has a high oxygen affinity. **h. D,** an abnormal hemogoblin existing in several molecular forms, all characterized by electrophoretic migration on paper or cellulose acetate at a rate identical to that of hemoglobin S, but differentiated on acid agar gel electrophoresis. The homozygous state is manifested by mild hemolytic anemia with numerous target cells in the peripheral blood, while in the heterozygous state no clinical or hematologic abnormality occurs. **deoxygenated h.,** deoxyhemoglobin. **h. E,** an abnormal hemoglobin resulting from a beta chain mutation in the hemoglobin molecule, occurring most commonly in Southeast Asia, especially Thailand. The homozygous state is manifested by mild hemolytic anemia, usually without splenomegaly, and large numbers of normochromic target cells in the peripheral blood, while in the heterozygous state no clinical or hematologic abnormality occurs. **h. F,** fetal h. **"fast" h's,** those with greater mobility on electrophoresis (in an alkaline buffer) than normal adult hemoglobin (h. A), including hemoglobin K, J, and N. **fetal h.,** the form of hemoglobin normally comprising more than half of the hemoglobin in the fetus, composed of two alpha and two gamma polypeptides ($\alpha_2^A\gamma_2^F$); it is also present in minimal amounts in adulthood and is abnormally elevated in aplastic anemia, leukemia, and certain types of thalassemia. Called also *h. F*. **glycosylated h.,** hemoglobin A_{1c}. **Gower h.,** a normal hemoglobin present in two forms, I and II, in early embryonic life, composed either entirely of epsilon chains (ϵ_4) or of two alpha and two epsilon chains ($\alpha_2\epsilon_2$) and

disappearing *in utero*. **h. Gun Hill,** an unstable hemoglobin resulting from a segmental deletion of amino acids in the beta polypeptide of the hemoglobin molecule, resulting in inability to bind heme and leading to mild hemolytic anemia. **h. H,** a rapidly migrating, abnormal hemoglobin composed of four beta chains, having a high oxygen affinity, found in a form of α-thalassemia in various ethnic groups, manifested by chronic hemolytic anemia associated with splenomegaly clinically and hypochromia, anisocytosis, and poikilocytosis of the red blood cells, with inclusion bodies detectable by supravital staining. **h. I,** an abnormal hemoglobin resulting from an amino acid substitution in the alpha chain which causes sickling in an unknown manner. **h. Lepore,** an abnormal hemoglobin having two normal alpha chains associated with two chains resulting from fusion of beta and delta chain segments. Although of considerable theoretical genetic interest, it produces only a mild anemia and, by itself, poses no special clinical problems. **h. M,** any of several hemoglobins having amino acid substitutions either in the alpha or beta chains and all associated with methemoglobinemia. **mean corpuscular h.,** see *MCH*. **muscle h.,** myoglobin. **nitric oxide h.,** a stable compound of nitric oxide and hemoglobin. **oxidized h., oxygenated h.,** oxyhemoglobin. **h. Rainier,** a hemoglobin in which histidine replaces tyrosine at position 145 in the beta chain; it has increased oxygen affinity and is associated with erythrocytosis. **reduced h.,** deoxyhemoglobin. **h. S,** the most common abnormal hemoglobin, in which valine is substituted for glutamic acid at position six of the beta chain; the heterozygous state results in sickle cell trait, the homozygous in sickle cell anemia. The delineation of the basic abnormality in molecular structure is a milestone in biochemical genetics, for it paved the way for further investigation and demonstrated that a single amino acid substitution may produce widespread, untoward clinical effects. **h. Seattle,** an abnormal hemoglobin in which glutamic acid is substituted for alanine at position 76 of the beta chain; it has decreased oxygen affinity. **"slow" h's,** those less mobile on electrophoresis (in an alkaline buffer) than normal adult hemoglobin (h. A), including hemoglobin S and D. **h. Yakima,** an abnormal hemoglobin in which histidine is substituted for aspartic acid at position 99 of the beta chain; it has increased oxygen affinity and is associated with erythrocytosis.

hemoglobinated (he″mo-glo′bin-āt-ed) containing hemoglobin.

hemoglobinemia (he″mo-glo″bĭ-ne′me-ah) [*hemoglobin* + Gr. *haima* blood] the presence of excessive hemoglobin in the plasma of the blood.

hemoglobiniferous (he″mo-glo″bĭ-nif′er-us) carrying or yielding hemoglobin.

hemoglobinocholia (he″mo-glo″bĭ-no-ko′le-ah) [*hemoglobin* + Gr. *cholē* bile + *-ia*] the occurrence of hemoglobin in the bile.

hemoglobinolysis (he″mo-glo″bĭ-nol′ĭ-sis) [*hemoglobin* + Gr. *lysis* dissolution] splitting up of hemoglobin.

hemoglobinometer (he″mo-glo″bĭ-nom′ĕ-ter) [*hemoglobin* + Gr. *metron* measure] an instrument for measuring the hemoglobin of the blood.

hemoglobinometry (he″mo-glo″bĭ-nom′ĕ-tre) the measurement of the hemoglobin of the blood.

hemoglobinopathy (he″mo-glo″bĭ-nop′ah-the) [*hemoglobin* + Gr. *pathos* disease] a hematologic disorder caused by alteration in the genetically determined molecular structure of hemoglobin, which results in a characteristic complex of clinical and laboratory abnormalities and often, but not always, overt anemia. The specific features of these hemoglobin abnormalities are related to variation of the composite globin polypeptide chains, designated α, β, γ, δ, to changes or substitutions in the sequential arrangement of the amino acids constituting these chains, or to their deletion from their appropriate place in the molecule. When analysis has revealed the site of biochemical aberration, the abnormality of the peptide chain and the number of the altered amino acid and nature of its replacement also should be indicated. For example, hemoglobin S is expressed as $\alpha_2^A\beta_2^S$, or $\alpha_2^A\beta_2^{6\,valine}$, and, more completely, hemoglobin $G_{Philadelphia}$ is expressed as $\alpha_2^G\beta_2^A$, or $\alpha_2^{6\,lysine}\beta_2^A$. If more than one hemoglobin is present, the phenotype should be designated by listing them in order of decreasing concentrations; for example, the phenotype for sickle cell trait is expressed as AS, for sickle cell anemia as SS, and for sickle cell–hemoglobin C disease as SC.

hemoglobinopepsia (he″mo-glo″bĭ-no-pep′se-ah) [*hemoglobin* + Gr. *pepsis* digestion] hemoglobinolysis.

hemoglobinophilia (he″mo-glo″bĭ-no-fil′e-ah) [*hemoglobin* + Gr. *philein* to love] the property of growing well in culture media containing hemoglobin; said of microorganisms.

hemoglobinophilic (he″mo-glo″bĭ-no-fil′ik) living on hemoglobin; in bacteriology, growing especially well in culture media containing hemoglobin.

hemoglobinous (he″mo-glo′bĭ-nus) containing hemoglobin.

hemoglobinuria (he″mo-glo″bĭ-nu′re-ah) [*hemoglobin* + Gr. *ouron* urine + *-ia*] the presence of free hemoglobin in the urine. **bacillary h.,** an infectious toxemic disease caused by *Clostridium haemolyticum*, affecting primarily cattle, occasionally sheep, and rarely dogs. In cattle, it is marked by inappetance, by cessation of rumination, lactation, and defecation, by fever, bloody diarrhea, and dark-red urine, and by anemia and hemoglobinuria. Called also *bovine h.* and *redwater disease.* **bovine h.,** 1. Texas fever. 2. bacillary h. **epidemic h.,** Winckel's disease. **intermittent h.,** hemoglobinuria occurring in isolated episodes; see *paroxysmal cold h.* and *paroxysmal nocturnal h.* **malarial h.,** blackwater fever. **march h.,** a rare form of hemoglobinuria following prolonged exercise. **paroxysmal cold h.,** a condition characterized by the sudden passage of hemoglobin in the urine following local or general exposure to cold. **paroxysmal nocturnal h.,** an uncommon, acquired paroxysmal form of hemolysis of unknown cause characterized by episodic hemoglobinuria occurring chiefly, but not always, at night, by hemosiderinuria, increased amounts of plasma hemoglobin, and a positive acid-serum (Ham) or sucrose-hemolysis test, and often associated with leukopenia or thrombocytopenia. Called also *Marchiafava-Micheli disease* or *syndrome.* **toxic h.,** that which is consequent upon the ingestion of various poisons.

hemoglobinuric (he″mo-glo″bĭ-nu′rik) pertaining to or characterized by hemoglobinuria.

hemogram (he′mo-gram) [*hemo-* + Gr. *gramma* a writing] the blood picture; a written record or a graphic representation of the differential blood count.

hemohistioblast (he″mo-his′te-o-blast″) [*hemo-* + Gr. *histos* tissue + *blastos* germ] Ferrata's name for the hypothetical stem cell of all blood cells; hence sometimes called *Ferrata's cell.* Cf. *hemocytoblast.*

hemohydraulics (he″mo-hi-draw′liks) the branch of science which deals with blood in motion; the hydraulics of the blood.

hemokinesis (he″mo-ki-ne′sis) [*hemo-* + Gr. *kinēsis* movement] the flow of blood in the body.

hemokinetic (he″mo-ki-net′ik) pertaining to or promoting the flow of blood in the body.

hemolith (he′mo-lith) [*hemo-* + Gr. *lithos* stone] (*obs.*) a concretion in the wall of a blood vessel.

hemology (he-mol′o-je) hematology.

hemolutein (he″mo-lu′te-in) a yellow pigment from the blood serum of certain animals.

hemolymph (he′mo-limf) [*hemo-* + *lymph*] 1. the blood and lymph. 2. the bloodlike fluid moving through the hemocoelom of those invertebrates (e.g., mollusks, arthropods, and tunicates) with open circulatory systems, which combines the properties of blood and lymphlike interstitial fluid.

hemolymphangioma (he″mo-lim-fan″je-o′mah) hematolymphangioma.

hemolysate (he-mol′ĭ-sāt) the product resulting from hemolysis.

hemolysin (he-mol′ĭ-sin) [*hemo-* + Gr. *lysis* dissolution] à substance which liberates hemoglobin from red blood corpuscles by interrupting their structural integrity. Hemolysins may be present naturally in the body or they may be formed therein as a result of injections of foreign red corpuscles. The hemolysin formed by the injection of blood from the same species of animal is called *isolysin* or *isohemolysin,* that by the injection from another species, a *heterolysin;* one which destroys cells of the animal's own body is an *autolysin.* Hemolysins are also produced by a variety of microorganisms. **acid h.,** one which reacts optimally at a pH below 7. **alpha h.,** a hemolysin produced by virulent human strains of streptococci that hemolyzes rabbit, sheep, cow, and goat erythrocytes but not those of man; it also destroys rabbit but not human leukocytes, and in this activity is called *Neisser-Wechsberg leukocidin.* **bacterial h.,** a toxic substance produced by bacteria and which lyses erythrocytes. **beta h.,** a staphylococcic hemolysin that hemolyzes sheep cells but only after a hot-cold lysis. **heterophile h.,** a hemolysin which has affinity for the red cells of some animal besides the one for which it is specific. **hot-cold h.,** a hemolytic toxic substance of bacterial origin that lyses erythrocytes in the cold following preliminary warm incubation. **immune h.,** a hemolysin produced by deliberate immunization of an animal with blood or blood corpuscles foreign to it, as with rabbit anti-sheep red blood cell serum (hemolysin) used in complement fixation tests.

hemolysis (he-mol′ĭ-sis) [*hemo-* + Gr. *lysis* dissolution] the liberation of hemoglobin. Hemolysis consists of the separation of the hemoglobin from the red cells and its appearance in the plasma. It may be caused by hemolysins, by chemicals, by freezing or heating, or by distilled water. **alpha h.,** the production of a zone of greenish discoloration surrounding a bacterial colony on blood-agar medium, caused by partial decomposition of hemoglobin and characteristic of pneumococci and certain streptococci. **beta h.,** the production of a clear zone immediately surrounding a bacterial colony on blood-agar medium, which is characteristic of certain pathogenic bacteria. **biologic h.,** hemolysis by lysins produced in animals and plants. **contact h.,** the hastened hemolysis of blood cells in contact with a surface. **immune h.,** the lysis by complement of erythrocytes sensitized as a consequence of interaction with specific antibody to the erythrocytes. **passive h.,** the lysis of erythrocytes on which antigen has been adsorbed in the presence of complement and antiserum

to that antigen. **siderogenous h.,** hemolytic disease accompanied by excessive iron storage, which may cause a secondary hemochromatosis, e.g., Cooley's anemia. **venom h.,** hemolysis produced by snake venom.

hemolysoid (he-mol′ĭ-soid) a hemolysin the toxophore group of which has been destroyed while the haptophore group has remained intact, enabling it to unite with the blood cell, but not to destroy it.

hemolysophilic (he″mo-li″so-fil′ik) uniting readily with hemolysin.

hemolytic (he″mo-lit′ik) pertaining to, characterized by, or producing hemolysis.

hemolyzable (he″mo-liz′ah-b'l) capable of undergoing hemolysis.

hemolyzation (he″mo-li-za′shun) the production of hemolysis.

hemolyze (he′mo-liz) to subject to or to undergo hemolysis.

hemomanometer (he″mo-mah-nom′ĕ-ter) a manometer for determining blood pressure.

hemomediastinum (he″mo-me″de-as-ti′num) an effusion of blood in the mediastinum.

hemometer (he-mom′ĕ-ter) hemoglobinometer.

hemometra (he″mo-me′trah) hematometra.

hemometry (he-mom′ĕ-tre) hematometry.

hemonephrosis (he″mo-nĕ-fro′sis) hematonephrosis.

hemo-opsonin (he″mo-op-so′nin) hemopsonin.

hemopathic (he″mo-path′ik) pertaining to disease of the blood; due to blood disorder.

hemopathology (he″mo-pah-thol′o-je) [*hemo-* + *pathology*] study of diseases of the blood.

hemopathy (he-mop′ah-the) [*hemo-* + Gr. *pathos* disease] any disease of the blood.

hemoperfusion (he″mo-per-fu′zhun) the passage of blood through an extracorporeal adsorptive system (e.g., an activated charcoal column) to remove compounds of larger molecular size (e.g., bile acids and protein-bound compounds) than can be removed by hemodialysis.

hemopericardium (he″mo-per″ĭ-kar′de-um) [*hemo-* + *pericardium*] an effusion of blood within the pericardium.

hemoperitoneum (he″mo-per″ĭ-to-ne′um) [*hemo-* + *peritoneum*] an effusion of blood in the peritoneal cavity.

hemopexin (he″mo-pek′sin) a serum glycoprotein (β_1-globulin) synthesized in the liver, which binds with free heme in the plasma and maintains it in soluble form; it also binds with certain porphyrins.

hemophage (he′mo-fāj) hemophagocyte.

hemophagocyte (he″mo-fag′o-sīt) [*hemo-* + *phagocyte*] a phagocyte which destroys blood cells.

hemophagocytosis (he″mo-fag″o-si-to′sis) hemocytophagia.

hemophil (he′mo-fil) [*hemo-* + Gr. *philein* to love] 1. thriving on blood. 2. a microorganism which grows best in media containing hemoglobin.

hemophilia (he″mo-fil′e-ah) [*hemo* + Gr. *philein* to love + *ia*] a hereditary hemorrhagic diathesis due to deficiency of coagulation Factor VIII, and characterized by spontaneous or traumatic subcutaneous and intramuscular hemorrhages; bleeding from the mouth, gums, lips, and tongue; hematuria; and hemarthroses. It affects males, being transmitted as an X-linked recessive trait. Called also *h. A, classical h.,* and *Factor VIII deficiency.* **h. A,** hemophilia due to lack of coagulation Factor VIII; see *hemophilia.* **h. B,** Factor IX deficiency; see *coagulation factors,* under *factor.* **h. C,** Factor XI deficiency; see *coagulation factors,* under *factor.* **classical h.,** hemophilia A. **h. neonato′rum,** purpura in newborn children. **vascular h.,** von Willebrand's disease.

hemophiliac (he″mo-fil′e-ak) an individual exhibiting hemophilia.

hemophilic (he-mo-fil′ik) 1. having an affinity for blood; living in blood. In bacteriology, growing especially well in culture media containing hemoglobin. 2. pertaining to or characterized by hemophilia.

hemophilioid (he″mo-fil′e-oid) [*hemophilia* + Gr. *eidos* form] resembling classical hemophilia clinically. Applied to a number of hereditary or acquired hemorrhagic disorders that are not due solely to a deficiency of blood coagulation Factor VIII. See *coagulation factors,* under *factor.*

Hemophilus (he-mof′ĭ-lus) a genus of hemophilic bacteria of the family Brucellaceae, order Eubacteriales, made up of small gram-negative rods and characterized by a nutritional requirement for the constituents of fresh blood, including hemoglobin and certain allied compounds, called X factor, and for V factor. Spelled also *Haemophilus.* **H. aegyp′tius,** an organism that is related to *H. influenzae* and is the cause of acute contagious conjunctivitis. **H. bo′vis,** *moraxella bovis.* **H. bronchisep′ticus,** *Brucella bronchiseptica.* **H. ducrey′i,** the causative agent of chancroid. **H. du′plex,** *Moraxella lacunata.* **H. hemolyt′icus,** a hemolytic form of *H. influenzae.* **H. influen′zae,** a species once thought to be the cause of epidemic influenza in man; it produces a serious form of meningitis, especially in infants. **H. parapertus′sis,** a species occasionally found in pertussis in man; called also *Bordetella parapertussis.* **H. pertus′sis,** the causative agent of pertussis in man; called also *Bordetella pertussis,* and *Bordet-Gengou bacillus.* **H. vagina′lis,** a hemophilic bacterium that causes vaginitis in women with normal ovarian function.

hemophilus (he-mof′ĭ-lus) any member of the genus *Hemophilus.* **h. of Koch-Weeks,** *Hemophilus aegyptius.* **h. of Morax-Axenfeld,** *Hemophilus duplex.*

hemophoric (he″mo-for′ik) [*hemo-* + Gr. *phoros* bearing] carrying or conveying blood.

hemophotograph (he″mo-fo′to-graf) a photograph of blood corpuscles.

hemophotometer (hem″o-fo-tom′ĕ-ter) an instrument for measuring hemoglobin in blood by photometric or color technique.

hemophthalmia, hemophthalmos, hemophthalmus (he″mof-thal′me-ah; he″mof-thal′mos; he″mof-thal′mus) [*hemo-* + Gr. *ophthalmos* eye] an extravasation of blood with the eye.

hemophthisis (he-mof′thĭ-sis) [*hemo-* + Gr. *phthisis* wasting] a term once used to indicate anemia due to insufficient nutrition of blood cells.

hemopiezometer (he″mo-pi″e-zom′ĕ-ter) [*hemo-* + Gr. *piesis* pressure + *metron* measure] any apparatus for measuring blood pressure.

hemoplastic (he″mo-plas′tik) hematoplastic.

hemopleura (he″mo-ploo′rah) hemothorax.

hemopneumopericardium (he″mo-nu″mo-per″ĭ-kar′de-um) pneumopericardium with hemorrhagic effusion.

hemopneumothorax (he″mo-nu″mo-tho′raks) pneumothorax with hemorrhagic effusion.

hemopoiesic (he″mo-poi-e′sik) hematopoietic.

hemopoiesis (he″mo-poi-e′sis) hematopoiesis.

hemopoietic (he″mo-poi-et′ik) hematopoietic.

hemopoietin (he″mo-poi-e′tin) [*hemo-* + Gr. *poein* to make] erythropoietin.

hemopoietine (he″mo-poi-e′tin) a name originally given to a substance which stimulated erythropoiesis; probably the same as erythropoietin.

hemoporphyrin (he″mo-por′fĭ-rin) a compound $C_{34}H_{38}O_4N_4$, derived from hematoporphyrin.

hemoposia (he″mo-po′ze-ah) [*hemo-* + Gr. *posis* drinking + *-ia*] the drinking of blood, as by parasites.

hemoprecipitin (he″mo-pre-sip′ĭ-tin) a blood precipitin.

hemoproctia (he″mo-prok′she-ah) [*hemo-* + Gr. *prōktos* anus] hemorrhage from the rectum.

hemoprotein (he″mo-pro′tēn) a conjugated protein containing heme as the prosthetic group.

Hemoproteus (he″mo-pro′te-us) *Haemoproteus.*

hemopsonin (he″mop-so′nin) [*hemo-* + *opsonin*] an opsonin that renders red blood cells more liable to phagocytosis; called also *hemotropin.*

hemoptic, hemoptoic (he-mop′tik; he-mop-to′ik) hemoptysic.

hemoptysic (he″mop-ti′sik) pertaining to or marked by hemoptysis.

hemoptysis (he-mop′tĭ-sis) [*hemo-* + Gr. *ptyein* to spit] the expectoration of blood or of blood-stained sputum. **cardiac h.,** hemoptysis due to heart disease and related pulmonary hypertension, as in mitral stenosis or Eisenmenger's syndrome. **endemic h.,** parasitic h. **Goldstein's h.,** hemoptysis due to bleeding telangiectases in the tracheobronchial tree. **Manson's h.,** hemoptysis due to infection of the lungs with *Paragonimus westermanii;* parasitic h. **oriental h.,** parasitic h. **parasitic h.,** a disease caused by infection of the lungs with *Paragonimus westermanii* and other lung flukes of the genus *Paragonimus.* It is marked by cough and spitting of blood and by gradual deterioration of health. Called also *endemic h., pulmonary distomatosis,* and *lung fluke disease.* **vicarious h.,** that which occurs at the time of normal menstruation; see *vicarious menstruation.*

hemopyelectasis (he″mo-pi-ĕ-lek′tah-sis) [*hemo-* + Gr. *pyelos* pelvis + *ektasis* dilatation] dilatation of the renal pelvis with an accumulation of bloody fluid.

hemopyrrol (he″mo-pir′ol) 2,3-dimethyl-4-ethylpyrrole: pyrrole produced by the drastic chemical reduction of hematoporphyrin; it was useful in solving the structure of porphyrin.

hemorrhachis (he-mor′ah-kis) hematomyelia.

hemorrhage (hem′or-ij) [*hemo-* + Gr. *rhēgnynai* to burst forth] the escape of blood from the vessels; bleeding. Small hemorrhages are classified according to size as petechiae (very small), purpura (up to 1 cm.), and ecchymoses (larger). The massive accumulation of blood within a tissue is called a hematoma. **alveolar h.,** hemorrhage from a dental alveolus. **arterial h.,** the escape of blood from an artery, e.g., ruptured aneurysm. **brain h.,** bleeding into the substance of the brain; see *stroke syndrome,* under *syndrome.* **capillary h.,** the oozing of blood from the minute vessels. **capsuloganglionic h.,** hemorrhage into the basal ganglia and internal and external capsule of the brain. **cerebral h.,** a hemorrhage into the cerebrum. See *stroke syndrome,* under *syndrome.* **concealed h.,** internal h. **dot h.,** microaneurysms of the retina, seen in diabetic retinopathy. **essential h.,** one not attributable to an established cause. **expulsive h.,** hemorrhage of the eye, breaking through both the choroid and the retina and extruding the ocular contents before it; usually occurring during the course of intraocular surgical procedure **external h.,** one in which blood escapes from the body. **extradural h.,** intracranial hemorrhage into the epidural space. **fetomaternal h.,** the leakage of fetal red blood cells into the maternal circulation. **fibrinolytic h.,** hemorrhage resulting from abnormalities in the fibrinolytic system. **flame-shaped h's,** large hemorrhagic spots in the eyeground; called also *flame spots.* **gravitating h.,** hemorrhage into the spinal canal, in which the blood settles to the lower part of the canal from the force of gravity. **intermediary h., intermediate h.,** bleeding of moderate degree. **internal h.,** hemorrhage in which the extravasated blood remains within the body. **intracerebral h.,** hemorrhage within the cerebrum; see *cerebral h.* **intracranial h.,** bleeding within the cranium, which may be extradural, subdural, subarachnoid, or cerebral. See *stroke syndrome,* under *syndrome.* **intramedullary h.,** hematomyelia. **intrapartum h.,** hemorrhage occurring during parturition. **massive h.,** loss of blood so rapid and profuse that shock supervenes unless appropriate replacement is instituted promptly. **nasal h.,** epistaxis. **parenchymatous h.,** capillary hemorrhage into the substance of an organ. **h. per rhexin,** hemorrhage from rupture of a blood vessel. **petechial h.,** hemorrhage that occurs in minute points beneath the skin. **plasma h.,** the loss of the fluid portion (plasma) of the blood. **postpartum h.,** that which occurs soon after labor or childbirth. **primary h.,** that which occurs immediately following injury. **pulmonary h.,** hemorrhage from the lungs; pneumorrhagia. **punctate h.,** spots of blood effused into the tissues from capillary hemorrhage. **recurring h.,** intermittent episodes of bleeding. **renal h.,** hemorrhage from the kidney; nephrorrhagia. **secondary h.,** bleeding which follows an accident or injury after a lapse of time. **splinter h's,** linear hemorrhages beneath the nail; when located near the base of the nail they are characteristic of subacute bacterial endocarditis. **spontaneous h.,** bleeding occurring without overt provocation. **subarachnoid h.,** intracranial hemorrhage into the subarachnoid space. **subdural h.,** cerebral hemorrhage into the subdural space; see under *hematoma,* and see *stroke syndrome,* under *syndrome.* **unavoidable h.,** that which results from the detachment of a placenta previa. **uterine h., essential,** a condition marked by hemorrhage from the uterus, and usually showing hypertrophy of the uterine mucosa and cystic disease of the ovary; called also *metropathia hemorrhagica.* **venous h.,** the escape of blood from the venous system; phleborrhagia. **vicarious h.,** the loss of blood from any area in consequence of the suppression of a bleeding in another area.

hemorrhagenic (hem″o-rah-jen′ik) [*hemorrhage* + Gr. *gennan* to produce] causing hemorrhage.

hemorrhagic (hem″o-raj′ik) pertaining to or characterized by hemorrhage; descriptive of any tissue into which bleeding has occurred.

hemorrhagin (hem″o-ra′jin) a cytolysin existing in certain venoms and poisons, such as snake venom and ricin, which is destructive to endothelial cells and blood vessels. Cf. *endotheliotoxin.*

hemorrhagiparous (hem″o-rij-ip′ah-rus) [*hemorrhage* + L. *parere* to produce] hemorrhagenic.

hemorrhea (hem-o-re′ah) hematorrhea.

hemorrheology (he″mo-re-ol′o-je) [*hemo-* + Gr. *rhoia* flow + *logos* treatise] the scientific study of the deformation and flow properties of cellular and plasmatic components of blood in macroscopic, microscopic, and submicroscopic dimensions, and the rheological properties of vessel structure with which the blood comes in direct contact.

hemorrhoid (hem′o-roid) [Gr. *haimorrhois*] a varicose dilatation of a vein of the superior or inferior hemorrhoidal plexus, resulting from a persistent increase in venous pressure. **combined h.,** mixed h. **external h.,** a varicose dilatation of a vein of the inferior hemorrhoidal plexus, situated distal to the pectinate line and covered with modified anal skin. **internal h.,** a varicose dilatation of a vein of the superior hemorrhoidal plexus, originating above the pectinate line, and covered by mucous membrane. **lingual h.,** a varicose dilatation of veins of the tongue, usually on the ventral surface. **mixed h.,** a varicose dilatation of a vein connecting the superior and inferior hemorrhoidal plexuses, forming an external and an internal hemorrhoid in continuity. **mucocutaneous h.,** mixed h. **prolapsed h.,** an internal hemorrhoid which has descended below the pectinate line and protruded outside the anal sphincter. **strangulated h.,** an internal hemorrhoid which has been prolapsed sufficiently and for long enough time for its blood supply to become occluded by the constricting action of the anal sphincter. **thrombosed h.,** one containing clotted blood.

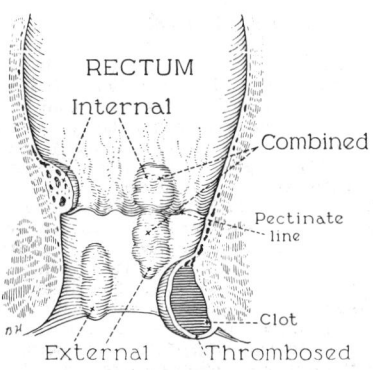

Hemorrhoids.

hemorrhoidal (hem″o-roi′dal) pertaining to, or of the nature of, hemorrhoids.

hemorrhoidectomy (hem″o-roid-ek′to-me) excision of hemorrhoids.

hemorrhoidolysis (hem″o-roid-ol′ĭ-sis) [*hemorrhoid* + Gr. *lysis* dissolution] the dissolution of hemorrhoids by chemical or electrical means.

hemosalpinx (he″mo-sal′pinks) [*hemo-* + Gr. *salpinx* tube] hematosalpinx.

hemoscope (he′mo-skōp) hematoscope.

hemosialemesis (he″mo-si″al-em′ĕ-sis) [*hemo-* + Gr. *sialon* saliva + *emesis* vomiting] the discharge of bloody saliva.

hemosiderin (he″mo-sid′er-in) [*hemo-* + Gr. *sidēros* iron] an insoluble form of storage iron in which the micelles of ferric hydroxide are so arranged as to be visible microscopically both with and without the use of specific staining methods.

hemosiderinuria (he″mo-sid″er-in-u′re-ah) the presence of hemosiderin in the urine.

hemosiderosis (he″mo-sid″er-o′sis) a focal or general increase in tissue iron stores without associated tissue damage. Cf. *hemochromatosis*. **hepatic h.,** the deposit of an abnormal quantity of hemosiderin in the liver, usually in Kupffer cells; such deposition is not associated with cirrhosis, as is hemochromatosis. **pulmonary h.,** the deposition of abnormal amounts of hemosiderin in the lungs, due to bleeding into the lung interstitium. An idiopathic form, affecting primarily children, is marked by microcytic hypochromic anemia, diffuse pulmonary infiltration, and occasionally hemoptysis; hemosiderin-laden macrophages are abundant in the lungs and may be found in the sputum.

hemosite (he′mo-sīt) (*obs.*) a blood parasite.

hemospermia (he″mo-sper′me-ah) [*hemo-* + Gr. *sperma* seed + *-ia*] the presence of blood in the semen.

Hemosporidia (he″mo-spo-rid′e-ah) Haemosporidia.

hemostasia (he″mo-sta′ze-ah) hemostasis.

hemostasis (he″mo-sta′sis, he-mos′tah-sis) [*hemo-* + Gr. *stasis* halt] 1. the arrest of bleeding, either by the physiological properties of vasoconstriction and coagulation or by surgical means. 2. interruption of the flow of blood through any vessel or to any anatomical area.

hemostat (he′mo-stat) 1. a small surgical clamp for constricting a blood vessel. 2. an agent that checks hemorrhage when properly applied to a bleeding point.

hemostatic (he″mo-stat′ik) [*hemo-* + Gr. *statikos* standing] 1. checking the flow of blood. 2. an agent that arrests the flow of blood. **capillary h.,** an agent that reduces capillary bleeding time by increasing the contractility and resistance and decreasing the permeability of the capillary wall.

hemostyptic (he″mo-stip′tik) hemostatic.

hemotherapeutics (he″mo-ther″ah-pu′tiks) hemotherapy.

hemotherapy (he″mo-ther′ah-pe) [*hemo-* + Gr. *therapeia* treatment] treatment of disease by the administration of blood or blood products, such as blood plasma.

hemothorax (he″mo-tho′raks) [*hemo-* + Gr. *thōrax* chest] a collection of blood in the pleural cavity.

hemotoxic (he″mo-tok′sik) hematotoxic.

hemotoxin (he″mo-tok′sin) an exotoxin characterized by hemolytic activity. **cobra h.,** the constituent of cobra venom which is able to lyse red blood cells of man and of various other animals without the presence of blood serum.

hemotroph (he′mo-trof) [*hemo-* + Gr. *trophē* nourishment] the sum total of the nutritive substances supplied to the embryo from the maternal blood during gestation. Cf. *histiotroph*.

hemotrophe (he′mo-trof) hemotroph.

hemotrophic (he″mo-trōf-ik) pertaining to or derived through hemotroph.

hemotropic (he″mo-trop′ik) hematotropic.

hemotropin (he-mot′ro-pin) hemopsonin.

hemotympanum (he″mo-tim′pah-num) hematotympanum.

hemoxometer (he″mok-som′ĕ-ter) [*hemo-* + *oxygen* + Gr. *metron* measure] (*obs.*) an instrument for measuring the oxygen content of the blood.

hemozoin (he″mo-zo′in) the pigment found in malarial parasites.

hemozoon (he″mo-zo′on) hematozoon.

hemuresis (hem″u-re′sis) [*hem-* + *uresis*] the voiding of bloody urine.

henbane (hen′bān) hyoscyamus.

Hench-Aldrich test (index) (hench al′drich) [Philip S. *Hench,* American physician, 1896–1965, co-winner, with E. C. Kendall and Tadeus Reichstein, of the Nobel prize for medicine and physiology in 1950 for their discoveries concerning the adrenal cortex hormones; Martha *Aldrich,* American biochemist, born 1897] see under *test.*

Henderson-Hasselbalch equation (hen′der-son-has″el-balk) [Lawrence Joseph *Henderson,* Boston chemist, 1878–1942; Karl A. *Hasselbalch,* Copenhagen scientist, 1874–1962] see under *equation.*

Henderson-Jones disease (hen′der-son-jōnz′) [Melvin Starkey *Henderson,* American orthopedic surgeon, 1883–1954; Hugh T. *Jones,* American orthopedic surgeon, born 1892] see under *disease.*

Henke's space, triangle (trigone) (hen′kēz) [Philipp Jakob Wilhelm *Henke,* German anatomist, 1834–1896] see under *space* and *triangle.*

Henle's loop, etc. (hen′lēz) [Friedrich Gustav Jakob *Henle,* German anatomist, 1809–1885, a celebrated anatomist and histologist] see under *ampulla, ansa, canal, cell, fiber, fissure, gland, layer, ligament, loop, membrane, reaction, sheath, sphincter, spine,* and *tubule.*

Henle-Coenen test (sign) (hen′le-ke′nan) [Adolf Richard *Henle,* German surgeon, born 1864; Hermann *Coenen,* German surgeon, born 1875] see under *tests.*

henna (hen′ah) the dried and powdered leaves of *Lawsonia inermis* L. (Lythraceae) and other species, which have fungicidal properties; it has been used in intestinal candidiasis, and is used as a cosmetic and hair dye.

Hennebert's sign (test) (en-bārz′) [Belgian otologist] see under *sign.*

Henoch's chorea, purpura (disease) (hen′ōks) [Edouard Heinrich *Henoch,* German pediatrist, 1820–1910] see *spasmodic tic,* under *tic,* and under *purpura.*

henogenesis (hen″o-jen′ĕ-sis) [Gr. *hen* one + *genesis* origin] ontogeny.

henpue, henpuye (hen-poo′ye) [West African] goundou.

henry (hen′re) [Joseph *Henry,* American physicist, 1797–1878] the unit of electric induction.

Henry's law (hen′rēz) [William *Henry,* English chemist, 1774–1836] see under *law.*

Henry's melanin test (reaction) [Adolf Felix Gerhard *Henry,* Istanbul pathologist, born 1894] see under *tests.*

Hensen's canal, etc. (hen′sen) [Victor *Hensen,* German anatomist and physiologist, 1835–1924] see under *body, canal, cell, disk, duct, knot, line,* and *node.*

Henshaw test (hen′shaw) [Russell *Henshaw,* New York physician] see under *tests.*

Hensing's ligament (fold) (hen′singz) [Frederich Wilhelm *Hensing,* German anatomist, 1719–1745] see under *ligament.*

hepar (he′par) [Gr. *hēpar* liver] 1. [NA] a large gland of a dark red color situated in the upper part of the abdomen on the right side; see *liver.* 2. the liver of certain animals, used in pharmaceutical preparations. 3. a liver-like or liver-colored substance. **h. adipo′sum,** fatty liver. **h. loba′tum,** a liver divided into numerous lobes by deep fissures produced by syphilis. **h. sicca′tum,** the dried and powdered liver of pigs; used as a food and medicine in organic diseases of the liver. **h. sul′furis,** sulfurated potash.

heparan sulfate (hep′ah-ram) a sulfated mucopolysaccharide structurally related to heparin; it contains alternating hexuronic acid residues (both α-L-iduronic acid and β-D-glucuronic acid) and D-glucosamine. Normally occurring in the liver, aorta, and lung, it is an accumulation product in several mucopolysaccharidoses. Called also *heparatin sulfate.*

heparin (hep′ah-rin) an acidic mucopolysaccharide composed of D-glucuronic acid and D-glucosamine, present in many tissues, especially the liver and lungs, and having potent anticoagulant properties. It is believed to act by inhibiting conversion of prothrombin to thrombin, and thus fibrinogen to fibrin. Heparin also has lipotrophic properties, promoting transfer of fat from blood to the fat depots by activation of lipoprotein lipase. **h. sodium** [USP], a mixture of active principles capable of prolonging blood clotting time, usually obtained from the lungs, intestinal mucosa, or other suitable tissues of domestic mammals used for human consumption; used in the prophylaxis and treatment of disorders in which there is excessive or undesirable clotting, such as thrombophlebitis, pulmonary embolism, and certain cardiac conditions, administered intravenously or subcutaneously.

heparinate (hep′ah-rin-āt) any salt of heparin.

heparinemia (hep″ah-rin-e′me-ah) the presence of heparin in the blood.

heparinize (hep′er-ĭ-nīz″) to treat with heparin in order to increase the clotting time of the blood.

heparitin sulfate (hep′ah-rĭ-tin) heparan sulfate.

hepat- see *hepato-*.

hepatalgia (hep″ah-tal′je-ah) [*hepat-* + Gr. *algos* pain + *-ia*] pain in the liver.

hepatargia (hep″ah-tar′je-ah) [*hepat-* + Gr. *argia* inactivity] (*obs.*) autointoxication from defective liver action.

hepatargy (hep″ah-tar′je) (*obs.*) hepatargia.

hepatatrophia (hep″ah-tah-tro′fe-ah) [*hepat-* + Gr. *atrophia* atrophy] atrophy of the liver.

hepatatrophy (hep″ah-tat′ro-fe) hepatatrophia.

hepatauxe (hep″ah-tawk′se) [*hepat-* + Gr. *auxē* increase] (*obs.*) hepatomegaly.

hepatectomize (hep″ah-tek′to-mīz) to deprive of the liver by surgical removal.

hepatectomy (hep″ah-tek′to-me) [*hepat-* + Gr. *ektomē* excision] excision of the entire (total *h.*) or of a portion (partial or subtotal *h.*) of the liver.

hepatic (hĕ-pat′ik) [L. *hepaticus;* Gr. *hēpatikos*] pertaining to the liver.

hepatico- (hĕ-pat′ĭ-ko) [Gr. *hēpatikos* of the liver] a combining form denoting relationship to a hepatic duct.

hepaticocholangiojejunostomy (hĕ-pat″ĭ-ko-ko-lan″je-o-je″ju-nos′to-me) surgical creation of a communication between the hepatic duct, another biliary duct, and the jejunum.

hepaticocholedochostomy (hĕ-pat″ĭ-ko-ko-led″o-kos′to-me) surgical anastomosis of the hepatic duct and the common bile duct.

hepaticodochotomy (hĕ-pat″ĭ-ko-do-kot′o-me) surgical incision of the hepatic duct and the common bile duct.

hepaticoduodenostomy (hĕ-pat″ĭ-ko-du″o-de-nos′to-me) surgical creation of a communication between the hepatic duct and the duodenum.

hepaticoenterostomy (hĕ-pat″ĭ-ko-en″ter-os′to-me) [*hepatico-* + Gr. *enteron* intestine + *stomoun* to provide with an opening, or mouth] surgical creation of a communication between the hepatic duct and the intestine.

hepaticogastrostomy (hĕ-pat″ĭ-ko-gas-tros′to-me) [*hepatico-* + Gr. *gastēr* stomach + *stomoun* to provide with an opening, or mouth] surgical creation of a communication between the hepatic duct and the stomach.

hepaticojejunostomy (hĕ-pat″ĭ-ko-je″ju-nos′to-me) [*hepatico-* + *jejunum* + Gr. *stomoun* to provide with an opening, or mouth] surgical creation of a communication between the hepatic duct and the jejunum.

Hepaticola (hep″ah-tik′o-lah) [*hepat-* + *colere* to inhabit] *Capillaria.*

hepaticoliasis (hĕ-pat″ĭ-ko-li′ah-sis) capillariasis.

hepaticolithotomy (hĕ-pat″ĭ-ko-lĭ-thot′o-me) incision of the hepatic duct and removal of one or more calculi.

hepaticolithotripsy (hĕ-pat″ĭ-ko-lith′o-trip-se) the operation of crushing a stone in the hepatic duct.

hepaticopulmonary (hĕ-pat″ĭ-ko-pul′mo-nar″e) pertaining to the liver and the lungs.

hepaticostomy (hĕ-pat″ĭ-kos′to-me) [*hepatico-* + Gr. *stomoun* to provide with an opening, or mouth] surgical creation of an artificial opening into the hepatic duct.

hepaticotomy (hĕ-pat″ĭ-kot′o-me) [*hepatico-* + Gr. *tomē* cutting] incision of the hepatic duct.

hepatin (hep′ah-tin) glycogen.

hepatism (hep′ah-tizm) ill health due to liver disease.

hepatitides (hep″ah-tit′ĭ-dēz) plural of *hepatitis.*

hepatitis (hep″ah-ti′tis), pl. *hepatit′ides* [*hepat-* + *-itis*] inflammation of the liver. **h. A.,** viral h. type A. **amebic h.,** invasion of liver parenchyma by trophozoites of *Entamoeba histolytica,* leading to amebic abscess. **anicteric h.,** viral hepatitis without jaundice, tending to occur chiefly in infants and young children; symptoms include mild anorexia and gastrointestinal disturbances, slight fever, and enlargement and tenderness of the liver. **h. B.,** viral h. type B. **canine virus h.,** h. contagiosa canis. **cholangiolitic h.,** inflammation of the bile ducts of the liver associated with obstructive jaundice; symptoms include progressively deepening jaundice, pruritus, dark urine, acholic stools, and a protracted course. It usually occurs in viral hepatitis. Called also *cholestatic h.* **cholestatic h.,** cholangiolitic h. **chronic active h.,** chronic persisting h. **chronic aggressive h.,** chronic persisting h. **chronic interstitial h.,** cirrhosis of the liver. **chronic persisting h.,** chronic inflammatory liver disease in which an expanding mesenchymal reaction in the portal triads progressively destroys adjacent liver cells. There is mononuclear and plasma cell infiltration of the liver

which is particularly marked adjacent to the hepatic lobules. Progressive fibrosis with nodular regeneration leads to macronodular cirrhosis. Hypergammaglobulinemia is associated with positive serological tests (LE, antinuclear, STS, and rheumatoid factor). This form of hepatitis may be a result of viral infection (some patients have positive tests for the hepatitis B antigen) and may also result from sensitivity to drugs (e.g., the laxative oxyphenisatin). Called also *chronic active* or *aggressive h.* **h. contagio′sa ca′nis,** a viral disease of dogs characterized by sore throat, fever, cough, weakness, and collapse. **enzootic h.,** Rift Valley fever. **epidemic h.,** viral h. type A. **familial h.,** hepatolenticular degeneration. **fulminant h.,** an acute fulminating form of viral hepatitis in which death is usually caused by acute yellow atrophy (q.v.) of the liver, which may cause massive destruction of large areas of the liver or of the entire organ. It is characterized by severe preicteric symptoms, the early appearance of jaundice, a sharp rise in temperature, and hemorrhages from the mucous membranes and into the skin; the liver may be tender and may decrease in size. Finally, there is confusion, drowsiness, and stuporousness, followed by coma, which deepens until death occurs. **giant cell h.,** neonatal h. **homologous serum h.,** serum h. **infectious h.,** viral h. type A. **infectious necrotic h. of sheep,** black disease. **inoculation h.,** viral h. type B. **long-incubation h.,** viral h. type B. **lupoid h.,** chronic active hepatitis, most commonly occurring in young women, characterized by the presence of LE cells in the peripheral blood. Called also *plasma cell h.* and *Kunkel's syndrome.* **MS-1 h.,** viral h. type A. **MS-2 h.,** viral h. type B. **neonatal h.,** hepatitis of uncertain etiology, occurring soon after birth; it generally tends to be chronic and is sometimes fatal. The principal characteristics include transformation of the liver cells into multinucleated giant cells, scattered throughout the lobules of the liver; prolonged persistent jaundice, leading to cirrhosis of the liver; hepatomegaly; acholic stools; bile in the urine; and low levels of urinary urobilinogen. Called also *giant cell h.* **neonatal giant cell h.,** neonatal h. **non-A, non-B h.,** a form of serum hepatitis (see *viral h. type B*) caused by a virus closely resembling hepatitis virus B. **plasma cell h.,** lupoid h. **h. seques′trans** (*obs.*), hepatitis with necrosis and disintegration of the liver tissue. **serum h.,** viral h. type B. **short-incubation h.,** viral h. type A. **suppurative h.,** inflammation of the liver attended by abscess formation. **toxipathic h.,** hepatitis caused by direct action of a poison on the liver cells. **transfusion h.,** viral h. type B. **trophopathic h.** (*obs.*), hepatitis caused by deficiency of a nutritive factor. **viral h.,** see *viral h. type A* and *viral h. type B;* a third form, caused by non-A, non-B hepatitis virus, closely resembles viral hepatitis type B. **viral h. type A,** an acute viral illness of worldwide distribution, occurring most commonly in children and young adults. It is usually transmitted by oral ingestion of infected material, but may also be transmitted parenterally (see *viral H. type B*). Although the viral agent (hepatitis virus A) has not been isolated or detected by immunological tests, transmission studies and electron microscopy indicate that patients with viral hepatitis type A excrete the infective agent in their stools for a period of weeks in the prodromal and early icteric period of illness. The incubation is short (about 15 to 50 or 60 days). The prodromal (*preicteric*) *stage* usually begins abruptly with fever, malaise, and nonspecific gastrointestinal symptoms (anorexia, nausea, upper abdominal discomfort, and vomiting); the *icteric stage* usually reaches a peak within two weeks and is characterized by jaundice, variable pruritus, dark urine, pale stool, and liver enlargement with tenderness; the *posticeteric period* refers to the period of convalescense, when malaise, tiredness, and minor abnormalities of hepatic function may persist. During the acute phase, characteristic pathological findings include necrosis of liver cells and portal and parenchymal infiltration, chiefly by mononuclear cells. Called also *h. A, epidemic h.* or *jaundice, infectious h., MS-1 h.,* and *short-incubation h.* **viral h., type B,** an acute illness caused by hepatitis B virus, formerly considered to be transmitted only by parenteral exposure (contaminated needles and administration of blood or blood products), but now known also to be transmitted by oral ingestion of contaminated material. The incubation period is long—50 to 160 or as many as 180 days. Prodromal symptoms and signs may be insidious in onset and include urticarial skin lesions and arthritis, and the acute illness tends to be more prolonged than in viral hepatitis type A; otherwise, the clinical and pathological symptoms are similar (see *viral h. type A*). Anicteric, icteric, fulminant, cholestatic, recurrent, chronic and persistent forms have been characterized. Serum antigens detected include hepatitis B surface and core antigens and e antigen, as have complete virions or Dane particles and DNA polymerase. Called also *h. B, inoculation h., long-incubation h., MS-2H., serum h., transfusion h.,* and *homologous serum h.* or *jaundice.*

hepatization (hep″ah-ti-za′shun) transformation into a liver-like mass, as the solidified state of the lung in pneumonia. **gray h.,** hepatization of the lung in which the affected tissue has a gray color. **red h.,** a form in which the affected tissue is red from excess of blood. **yellow h.,** a stage in hepatization in which the exudate is purulent.

hepatized (hep′ah-tīzd) changed into a liver-like substance.

hepato-, hepat- [Gr. *hēpar, hēpatos* liver]   combining form denoting relationship to the liver.

hepatobiliary (hep″ah-to-bil′e-ār″e)   pertaining to the liver and the bile or the biliary ducts.

hepatoblastoma (hep″ah-to-blas-to′mah)   a malignant intrahepatic tumor occurring in infants and young children and consisting chiefly of embryonic hepatic tisssue.

hepatobronchial (hep″ah-to-brong′ke-al)   pertaining to or communicating with the liver and a bronchus, as a hepatobronchial fistula.

hepatocarcinogenesis (hep″ah-to-kar″si-no-jen′ĕ-sis)   the production of carcinoma of the liver.

hepatocarcinogenic (hep″ah-to-kar″sĭ-no-jen′ik)   causing carcinoma of the liver.

hepatocarcinoma (hep″ah-to-kar″sin-o′mah)   hepatocellular carcinoma.

hepatocele (he-pat′o-sēl) [*hepato-* + Gr. *kēlē* hernia]   hernial protrusion of a part of the liver.

hepatocellular (hep″ah-to-sel′u-lar)   pertaining to or affecting liver cells.

hepatocholangeitis (hep″ah-to-ko-lan″je-i′tis)   inflammation of the liver and bile ducts.

hepatocholangiocarcinoma (hep″ah-to-ko-lan″je-o-kar″sin-o′mah)   cholangiohepatoma.

hepatocholangioduodenostomy (hep″ah-to-ko-lan″je-o-du″o-dĕ-nos′to-me)   the operation of establishing drainage of the hepatic ducts into the duodenum.

hepatocholangioenterostomy (hep″ah-to-ko-lan″je-o-en″ter-os′to-me) [*hepato-* + Gr. *cholē* bile + *angeion* vessel + *enteron* intestine + *stomoun* to provide with an opening, or mouth]   surgical creation of a communication between the hepatic duct and the intestine.

hepatocholangiogastrostomy (hep″ah-to-ko-lan″je-o-gastros′to-me)   the operation of establishing drainage of the hepatic duct into the stomach.

hepatocholangiostomy (hep″ah-to-ko-lan″je-os′to-me)   the operation of establishing drainage of the hepatic duct either through the abdominal wall (*external h.*) or into some part of the gastrointestinal tract (*internal h.*).

hepatocholangitis (hep″ah-to-ko″lan-ji′tis)   inflammation of the liver and bile ducts.

hepatocirrhosis (hep″ah-to-sĭ-ro′sis) [*hepato-* + *cirrhosis*]   cirrhosis of the liver.

hepatocolic (hep″ah-to-kol′ik)   pertaining to the liver and the colon.

hepatocuprein (hep″ah-to-koo′prin)   a soluble, bluish green copper protein present in liver tissue; it contains about 0.34 per cent copper.

hepatocystic (hep″ah-to-sis′tik)   pertaining to the liver and gallbladder.

hepatocyte (hep′ah-to-sīt)   a parenchymal liver cell.

hepatoduodenostomy (hep″ah-to-du″o-dĕ-nos′to-me) [*hepato-* + *duodenum* + Gr. *stomoun* to provide with an opening, or mouth]   the surgical creation of a communication between the liver and the duodenum.

hepatodynia (hep″ah-to-din′e-ah) [*hepato-* + Gr. *odynē* pain]   pain in the liver.

hepatodystrophy (hep″ah-to-dis′tro-fe)   acute yellow atrophy; see under *atrophy.*

hepatoenteric (hep″ah-to-en-ter′ik)   pertaining to the liver and intestine.

hepatoenterostomy (hep″ah-to-en″ter-os′to-me)   surgical creation of a communication between the liver and the intestine.

hepatoflavin (hep″ah-to-fla′vin)   riboflavin obtained from liver tissue.

hepatofugal (hep″ah-tof′u-gal) [*hepato-* + L. *fugere* to flee from]   directed or flowing away from the liver.

hepatogastric (hep″ah-to-gas′trik)   pertaining to the liver and stomach.

hepatogenic (hep″ah-to-jen′ik)   1. giving rise to or forming liver tissue. 2. hepatogenous.

hepatogenous (hep″ah-toj′ĕ-nus)   1. produced in or originating in the liver. 2. hepatogenic.

hepatoglycemia glycogenetica (hep″ah-to-gli-se′me-ah gli″ko-jĕ-net′ĭ-kah)   glycogen storage disease; see under *disease.*

hepatogram (hep′ah-to-gram″)   1. a tracing of the liver pulse in the sphygmogram. 2. a roentgenogram of the liver.

hepatography (hep″ah-tog′rah-fe) [*hepato-* + Gr. *graphein* to record]   1. a treatise on the liver. 2. the recording of a tracing of the liver pulse. 3. the making of a roentgenogram of the liver.

hepatohemia (hep″ah-to-he′me-ah) [*hepato-* + Gr. *haima* blood]   (*obs.*) congestion of the liver.

hepatoid (hep″ah-toid) [*hepato-* + Gr. *eidos* form]   resembling the liver in structure.

hepatojugular (hep″ah-to-jug′u-lar)   pertaining to the liver and jugular vein; see under *reflux.*

hepatolenticular (hep″ah-to-len-tik′u-lar)   pertaining to the liver and the lenticular nucleus.

hepatolienal (hep″ah-to-li′e-nal)   pertaining to the liver and spleen.

hepatolienography (hep″ah-to-li″ĕ-nog′rah-fe) [*hepato-* + L. *lien* spleen + Gr. *graphein* to record]   roentgenography of the liver and spleen after intravenous injection of an opaque medium.

hepatolienomegaly (hep″ah-to-li″ĕ-no-meg′ah-le)   hepatosplenomegaly.

hepatolith (hep′ah-to-lith″) [*hepato-* + Gr. *lithos* stone]   a gallstone, especially one within the liver.

hepatolithectomy (hep″ah-to-lĭ-thek′to-me) [*hepato-* + Gr. *lithos* stone + *ektomē* excision]   removal of a calculus from the liver.

hepatolithiasis (hep″ah-to-lĭ-thi′ah-sis) [*hepato-* + *lithiasis*]   the formation or presence of calculi in the intrahepatic biliary ducts.

hepatologist (hep″ah-tol′o-jist)   a specialist in hepatology.

hepatology (hep″ah-tol′o-je) [*hepato-* + *-logy*]   the study of the liver.

hepatolysin (hep″ah-tol′ĭ-sin)   a cytolysin destructive to liver cells.

hepatolysis (hep″ah-tol′ĭ-sis) [*hepato-* + Gr. *lysis* dissolution]   destruction of the liver cells.

hepatolytic (hep″ah-to-lit′ik)   pertaining to, characterized by, or causing hepatolysis.

hepatoma (hep″ah-to′mah)   a tumor of the liver, especially hepatocellular carcinoma.   **malignant h.,** hepatocellular carcinoma.

hepatomalacia (hep″ah-to-mah-la′she-ah) [*hepato-* + Gr. *malakia* softening]   softening of the liver.

hepatomegalia (hep″ah-to-mĕ-ga′le-ah) [*hepato-* + Gr. *megas* big]   hepatomegaly.   **h. glycogen′ica,** glycogen storage disease; see under *disease.*

hepatomegaly (hep″ah-to-meg′ah-le)   enlargement of the liver.   **glycogenic h.,** glycogen storage disease; see under *disease.*

hepatomelanosis (hep″ah-to-mel″ah-no′sis)   melanosis of the liver.

hepatometry (hep″ah-tom′ĕ-tre)   determination of the size of the liver.

hepatomphalocele (hep″ah-tom′fah-lo-sēl″)   omphalocele with the liver also being projected into the membranous sac outside the abdomen.

hepatomphalos (hep″ah-tom′fah-los) [*hepat-* + Gr. *omphalos* navel]   projection of the liver through the abdominal wall near the umbilicus.

hepatonephric (hep″ah-to-nef′rik)   pertaining to the liver and kidney.

hepatonephritic (hep″ah-to-nĕ-frit′ik)   pertaining to or characterized by hepatonephritis.

hepatonephritis (hep″ah-to-nĕ-fri′tis) [*hepato-* + Gr. *nephros* kidney]   a form of severe jaundice due to simultaneous inflammation of the liver and kidneys from the same cause, e.g., leptospiral infection.

hepatonephromegaly (hep″ah-to-nef″ro-meg′ah-le) [*hepato-* + Gr. *nephros* kidney + *megas* large]   enlargement of the liver and kidney.

hepatopancreas (hep″ah-to-pan′kre-as)   any of certain digestive glands of invertebrates, as the so-called liver of certain crustaceans, which secretes a fluid acting on both fats and proteins.

hepatopath (hep′ah-to-path)   a person with liver disease.

hepatopathy (hep″ah-top′ah-the) [*hepato-* + Gr. *pathos* disease]   any disease of the liver.

hepatoperitonitis (hep″ah-to-per″ĭ-to-ni′tis) [*hepato-* + *peritonitis*]   inflammation of the peritoneum covering the liver.

hepatopetal (hep″ah-top′ĕ-tal) [*hepato-* + L. *petere* to seek]   directed or flowing toward the liver.

hepatopexy (hep′ah-to-pek″se) [*hepato-* + Gr. *pēxis* fixation]   surgical fixation of the displaced liver.

hepatophage (hep′ah-to-fāj) [*hepato-* + Gr. *phagein* to eat]   a giant cell supposed to destroy the liver cells.

hepatophlebitis (hep″ah-to-flĕ-bi′tis)   inflammation of the veins of the liver.

hepatophlebography (hep″ah-to-fle-bog′rah-fe)   radiologic visualization of the outflow of the venous network of the liver performed through retrograde injection of a radiopaque solution.

hepatophlebotomy (hep″ah-to-flĕ-bot′o-me) [*hepato-* + *phlebotomy*]   the aspiration of blood from the liver.

hepatophyma (hep″ah-to-fi′mah) [*hepato-* + Gr. *phyma* growth]   (*obs.*) abscess of the liver.

hepatopleural (hep″ah-to-ploo′ral)   pertaining to the liver and the pleura, or communicating with the liver and pleural cavity, as a hepatopleural fistula.

hepatopneumonic (hep″ah-to-nu-mon′ik) [*hepato-* + Gr. *pneumonikos* of the lungs] pertaining to, affecting, or communicating with the liver and lungs; hepatopulmonary.

hepatoportal (hep″ah-to-por′tal) pertaining to the portal system of the liver.

hepatoptosis (hep″ah-to-to′sis) [*hepato-* + Gr. *ptōsis* falling] (*obs.*) dislocation of the liver; movable liver.

hepatopulmonary (hep″ah-to-pul′mo-nar″e) hepatopneumonic.

hepatorenal (hep″ah-to-re′nal) pertaining to the liver and kidneys.

hepatorrhagia (hep″ah-to-ra′je-ah) [*hepato-* + Gr. *rhēgnynai* to burst forth] hemorrhage from the liver.

hepatorrhaphy (hep″ah-tor′ah-fe) [*hepato-* + Gr. *rhaphē* suture] the suturing of the liver.

hepatorrhea (hep″ah-to-re′ah) [*hepato-* + Gr. *rhoia* flow] a morbidly excessive secretion of bile; any morbid flow from the liver.

hepatorrhexis (hep″ah-to-rek′sis) [*hepato-* + Gr. *rhēxis* rupture] rupture of the liver.

hepatoscan (hep′ah-to-skan) a surface scintiscan of the liver.

hepatoscopy (hep″ah-tos′ko-pe) [*hepato-* + Gr. *skopein* to examine] examination of the liver.

hepatosis (hep″ah-to′sis) any functional disorder of the liver. **serous h.,** veno-occlusive disease of the liver; see under *disease.*

hepatosolenotropic (hep″ah-to-so-le″no-trop′ik) [*hepato-* + Gr. *sōlēn* a channel, gutter, pipe + *tropē* a turn, turning] having an affinity for or exerting a specific effect on the cholangioles and interlobular ducts of the liver.

hepatosplenitis (hep″ah-to-splě-ni′tis) inflammation of the liver and spleen.

hepatosplenography (hep″ah-to-splě-nog′rah-fe) roentgenography of the liver and spleen.

hepatosplenomegaly (hep″ah-to-sple″no-meg′ah-le) [*hepato-* + Gr. *splēn* spleen + *megas* big] enlargement of the liver and spleen.

hepatosplenometry (hep″ah-to-splě-nom′ě-tre) determination of the size of the liver and spleen.

hepatosplenopathy (hep″ah-to-splě-nop′ah-the) any combined disorder of the liver and spleen.

hepatostomy (hep″ah-tos′to-me) [*hepato-* + Gr. *stoma* mouth] surgical creation of an opening into the liver.

hepatotherapy (hep″ah-to-ther′ah-pe) [*hepato-* + Gr. *therapeia* treatment] treatment of disease by the administration of liver or liver extract.

hepatotomy (hep″ah-tot′o-me) [*hepato-* + Gr. *tomē* a cutting] surgical incision of the liver. **transthoracic h.,** incision of the liver by resecting a rib, opening the pleural sac, and incising the diaphragm; often performed in two or three stages.

hepatotoxemia (hep″ah-to-tok-se′me-ah) [*hepato-* + *toxemia*] blood poisoning originating in the liver.

hepatotoxic (hep″ah-to-tok′sik) toxic to liver cells.

hepatotoxicity (hep″ah-to-tok-sis′ĭ-te) the quality or property of exerting a destructive or poisonous effect upon liver cells.

hepatotoxin (hep″ah-to-tok′sin) [*hepato-* + *toxin*] a toxin destructive to liver cells, especially one produced by injecting an animal with liver cells.

hepatotropic (hep″ah-to-trop′ik) [*hepato-* + Gr. *tropos* a turning] having a special affinity for or exerting a specific effect on the liver.

hepatoxic (hep″ah-tok′sik) hepatotoxic.

Hepatozoon (hep″ah-to-zo′on) [*hepato-* + Gr. *zōon* animal] a genus of sporozoan parasites of the order Coccidia, found in the red blood cells of birds and mammals. *H. canis* is transmitted to dogs by the tick *Rhipicephalus appendiculatus. H. muris,* found in the liver cells of rats, and *H. perniciosum,* found in dogs, are transmitted by the mite *Echinolaelaps echidninus.*

Hepicebrin (hep″ĭ-se′brin) trademark for a preparation of hexavitamin.

hepta,- hept- [Gr. *hepta* seven] a combining form meaning seven.

heptabarbital (hep″tah-bar′bĭ-tal) chemical name: 5-(1-cyclohepten-1-yl)-5-ethyl-2,4-6(1H,3H,5H)-pyrimidinetrione. A short-acting barbiturate, $C_{13}H_{18}N_2O_3$, occurring as a white, crystalline powder, used as a sedative and hypnotic, administered orally.

heptachromic (hep″tah-kro′mik) [*hepta-* + Gr. *chrōma* color] 1. pertaining to or exhibiting seven colors. 2. able to distinguish all seven colors of the spectrum; possessing full color vision.

heptad (hep′tad) any element having a valency of seven.

heptadactylia (hep″tah-dak-til′e-ah) heptadactyly.

heptadactylism (hep″tah-dak′tĭ-lizm) heptadactyly.

heptadactyly (hep″tah-dak′tĭ-le) [*hepta-* + Gr. *daktylos* finger] the occurrence of seven digits (fingers or toes) on one limb.

heptanal (hep′tah-nal) oenanthol.

heptapeptide (hep″tah-pep′tīd) a polypeptide containing seven amino acids.

heptaploid (hep′ta-ploid) 1. pertaining to or characterized by heptaploidy. 2. an individual or cell having seven sets of chromosomes.

heptaploidy (hep′tah-ploi″de) the state of having seven sets of chromosomes (7n).

heptargia (hep-tar′je-ah) (*obs.*) hepatargia.

heptatomic (hep″tah-tom′ik) septivalent.

heptavalent (hep-tav′ah-lent) [*hepta-* + L. *valere* to be able] septivalent.

heptoglobin (hep″to-glo′bin) a protein which is one of the fractions of blood plasma; it is said to be increased in infections, malignancy, and certain endocrine disorders.

heptoglobinemia (hep″to-glo-bĭ-ne′me-ah) abnormal increase in heptoglobin in the blood plasma.

heptose (hep′tōs) [*hept-* + *-ose*] a monosaccharide containing seven carbon atoms in a molecule.

heptosuria (hep″to-su′re-ah) presence of a heptose in the urine.

herb (erb, herb) [L. *herba*] any leafy plant without a woody stem, especially one used as a household remedy or as a flavoring. **death's h.,** belladonna leaf. **vulnerary h.,** an herb anciently regarded as healing wounds.

herbaceous (her-ba′shus) having the characters of an herb.

herbal (her′bal) a book on herbs.

herbalist (her′bal-ist) a herb doctor, or one versed in herbal lore.

Herbert's operation, pits (her′berts) [Major Herbert *Herbert,* Indian Medical Service, 1865–1942] see under *operation* and *pit.*

herbicide (her′bĭ-sīd) [L. *herba* herb + *caedere* to kill] an agent that is destructive to weeds or causes an alteration in their normal growth.

herbivore (her′bĭ-vōr) a herbivorous animal.

herbivorous (her-biv′o-rus) [L. *herba* herb + *vorare* to eat] subsisting upon plants.

Herb. recent. abbreviation for L. *herba′rium recen′tium,* of fresh herbs.

Herbst's corpuscles (herbsts) [Ernst Friedrich Gustav *Herbst,* German physician, 1803–1893] see under *corpuscle.*

hereditary (he-red′ĭ-ter-e) [L. *hereditarius*] genetically transmitted from parent to offspring.

heredity (he-red′ĭ-te) [L. *hereditas*] 1. the genetic transmission of a particular quality or trait from parent to offspring. 2. the genetic constitution of an individual. **autosomal h.,** the transmission of a quality or trait by a gene located on an autosome. **sex-linked h.,** the transmission of a quality or trait by a gene located on a sex-chromosome, for practical clinical purposes limited to transmission of a trait by a gene carried on the X chromosome. **X-linked,** sex-linked h.

heredoataxia (her″ě-do-ah-tak′se-ah) hereditary ataxia, as in Friedreich's ataxia.

heredobiologic (her″ě-do-bi″o-loj′ik) pertaining to or due to hereditary endogenic factors.

heredodegeneration (her″ě-do-de-jen″er-a′shun) a hereditary degeneration due to disease or defect of the hyaloplasm; hereditary cerebellar ataxia (Marie).

heredodiathesis (her″ě-do-di-ath′ě-sis) hereditary diathesis or predisposition.

heredofamilial (her″ě-do-fah-mil′e-al) occurring in certain families under circumstances that implicate a hereditary basis, as heredofamilial disease. The term is being discarded in favor of *familial, hereditary,* or *genetic,* whichever is more appropriate.

heredoimmunity (her″ě-do-ĭ-mu′nĭ-te) hereditary or inherited immunity.

heredoinfection (her″ě-do-in-fek′shun) germinal infection.

heredolues (her″ě-do-lu′ez) congenital syphilis.

heredoluetic (her″ě-do-lu-et′ik) pertaining to congenital syphilis.

heredopathia (her″ě-do-path′e-ah) an inherited pathological condition. **h. atac′tica polyneuritifor′mis,** Refsum's disease.

heredosyphilis (her″ě-do-sif′ĭ-lis) congenital syphilis.

heredosyphilitic (her″ě-do-sif″ĭ-lit′ik) a person affected with congenital syphilis.

heredosyphilology (her″ě-do-sif″ĭ-lol′o-je) the study of congenital syphilis.

Hérelle see *d'Hérelle.*

Herellea (hě-rel′e-ah) a genus of nonmotile, paired, gram-negative, enteric bacilli. **H. vaginic′ola,** a species that causes various nosocomial infections; called also *Acinetobacter anitratus.*

Herff's clamp (herfs) [Otto von *Herff*, Swiss gynecologist, 1856–1916] see under *clamp*.

Hering's law, etc. (her′ingz) [Carl Ewald Konstantin *Hering*, physiologist in Leipzig, 1834–1918] see under *law, test,* and *theory*.

Hering's nerve, phenomenon (her′ingz) [Heinrich Ewald *Hering*, physiologist in Cologne, 1866–1948] see *ramus sinus carotici nervi glossopharyngei,* and see under *phenomenon*.

heritability (her″ĭ-tah-bil′ĭ-te) the quality of being heritable; a measure of the extent to which a phenotype is influenced by the genotype.

heritable (her′ĭ-tah-b′l) capable of being inherited, as a genetic trait.

Hermann-Perutz reaction, test (her′man-pa′root) [Otto *Hermann*, Vienna physician; Alfred *Perutz*, Austrian dermatologist, born 1885] Perutz's reaction.

hermaphrodism (her-maf′ro-dizm) hermaphroditism.

hermaphrodite (her-maf′ro-dīt) [Gr. *hermaphroditos*] an individual exhibiting hermaphroditism (q.v.). **pseudo-h.,** see *pseudohermaphrodite*. **true h.,** an individual who has both testicular and ovarian tissue and exhibits ambiguous morphological criteria of sex; called also *true intersex*.

hermaphroditism (her-maf′ro-di-tizm″) [Gr. *hermaphroditos* a person partaking of the attributes of both sexes] originally, a state characterized by the presence of both male and female sex organs. In humans, *true hermaphroditism* is caused by anomalous differentiation of the gonads, with the presence of both ovarian and testicular tissue and of ambiguous morphologic criteria of sex. If only testicular tissue is present, but there are some female morphological criteria of sex, it is known as *male pseudohermaphroditism.* If only ovarian tissue is present, but there are some male morphological criteria of sex, it is known as *female pseudohermaphroditism.* See also *intersex* and *pseudohermaphroditism.* **bilateral h.,** that in which gonadal tissue typical of both sexes occurs on each side of the body. **dimidiate h.,** lateral h. **h. with excess,** a condition characterized by the presence of the normal organs typical of one sex with some that pertain to the opposite sex. **false h.,** pseudohermaphroditism. **lateral h.,** presence of gonadal tissue typical of one sex on one side of the body and tissue typical of the other sex on the opposite side. **protandrous h.,** the state of an organism having generative organs typical of both sexes, in which the male organs develop first, and those typical of the female sex develop later. **protogynous h.,** the state of an organism having generative organs typical of both sexes, in which the female organs develop first, and those typical of the male sex develop later. **spurious h.,** pseudohermaphroditism. **synchronous h.,** that in which the gonads of both sexes are functional at the same time. **transverse h.,** a condition in which the external genital organs are characteristic of one sex and the gonads are typical of the other. **true h.,** coexistence, in the same individual, of both ovarian and testicular tissue, with somatic characters typical of both sexes; called also *true intersex.* **unilateral h.,** presence of gonadal tissue typical of both sexes on one side and of an ovary or testis on the other.

hermaphroditismus (her-maf″ro-di-tiz′mus) hermaphroditism. **h. ve′rus,** true hermaphroditism. **h. ve′rus bilatera′lis,** bilateral hermaphroditism. **h. ve′rus latera′lis,** lateral hermaphroditism. **h. ve′rus unilatera′lis,** unilateral hermaphroditism.

Hermetia illucens (her-me′she-ah il-lu′senz) the soldier fly, the larvae of which may cause intestinal myiasis or pseudomyiasis in man.

hermetic (her-met′ik) [L. *hermeticus*] impervious to air; airtight.

hermetically (her-met′ĭ-kal-le) in an airtight manner.

hernia (her′ne-ah) [L.] the protrusion of a loop or knuckle of an organ or tissue through an abnormal opening. See Plate XXI. **abdominal h.,** hernia of some internal body structure through the abdominal wall. **acquired h.,** one brought on by lifting or by a strain or other injury. **h. adipo′sa,** fat h. **Barth's h.,** hernia of loops of intestine between the serosa of the abdominal wall and that of a persistent vitelline duct. **Béclard's h.,** femoral hernia through the saphenous opening. **Birkett's h.,** synovial h. **h. of the bladder,** hernia of a part of the bladder through any normal or other opening. **Bochdalek's h.,** congenital posterolateral diaphragmatic hernia, with extrusion of bowel and other abdominal viscera into the thorax; it is due to failure of closure of the pleuroperitoneal hiatus (foramen of Bochdalek). **cecal h.,** one that contains the cecum or a part of it. **celomic h.,** congenital protrusion of tissue through the foramen of Morgagni. **h. cere′bri,** protrusion of the brain substance through the skull, usually occurring after a brain tumor operation. **Cloquet's h.,** crural h., pectineal. **complete h.,** one in which the sac and its contents have passed through the orifice. **concealed h.,** hernia not perceptible on palpation. **congenital h.,** that which exists at birth, most commonly scrotal or umbilical. **Cooper's h.,** retroperitoneal hernia. **crural h.,** femoral h. **crural h., pectineal,** hernia within and behind the femoral vessels, the tumor resting upon the pectineus

muscle; called also *Cloquet's h.* **cystic h.,** cystocele. **diaphragmatic h.,** hernia through the diaphragm. **direct h.,** see under *inguinal h.* **diverticular h.,** the protrusion of a congenital diverticulum of the gut; called also *Littre's h.* **dry h.,** a hernia in which the sac and its contents have become intimately adherent to each other. **duodenojejunal h.,** Treitz's h. **encysted h.,** scrotal or oblique inguinal hernia in which the bowel, enveloped in its own proper sac, passes into the tunica vaginalis in such a way that the bowel has three coverings of peritoneum; called also *Hey's h.* **epigastric h.,** a hernia through the linea alba above the navel. **external h.,** see under *inguinal h.* **extrasaccular h.,** sliding h. **fat h.,** hernial protrusion of properitoneal fat through the abdominal wall; called also *h. adiposa.* **femoral h.,** hernia into the femoral canal. **foraminal h.,** hernia through the epiploic foramen. **funicular h.,** hernia of the umbilical or spermatic cord. **gastroesophageal h.,** a form of hiatal hernia in which the lower end of the esophagus and the adjacent part of the stomach herniate into the thorax. **Gibbon's h.,** hydrocele with large hernia. **gluteal h.,** femoral h. **Goyrand's h.,** inguinal hernia that does not descend into the scrotum. **Gruber's h.,** internal mesogastric hernia. **Grynfelt h.,** congenital hernia through the superior lumbar space. **Hesselbach's h.,** hernia with a diverticulum through the cribriform fascia. **Hey's h.,** encysted h. **hiatal h., hiatus h.,** protrusion of any structure through the esophageal hiatus of the diaphragm, but usually a sliding or paraesophageal hernia. **Holthouse's h.,** an inguinal hernia which has turned outward into the groin; called also *inguinocrural h.* **incarcerated h.,** hernia so occluded that it cannot be returned by manipulation; it may or may not become strangulated. Called also *irreducible h.* **incisional h.,** hernia occurring through an old abdominal incision. **incomplete h.,** one which has not passed quite through the orifice. **indirect h.,** see under *inguinal h.* **infantile h.,** oblique inguinal hernia behind the funicular process of the peritoneum. **inguinal h.,** hernia into the inguinal canal. An *indirect* inguinal hernia (*external* or *oblique* hernia) leaves the abdomen through the deep inguinal ring, and passes down obliquely through the inguinal canal, lateral to the inferior epigastric artery. A *direct* inguinal hernia (*internal* hernia) emerges between the inferior epigastric artery and the edge of the rectus muscle. **inguinocrural h.,** Holthouse's h. **inguinofemoral h.,** a combined inguinal and femoral hernia. **inguinoproperitoneal h.,** hernia that is partly inguinal and partly properitoneal; called also *Krönlein's h.* **inguinosuperficial h.,** interstitial hernia which passes through the internal inguinal ring, the inguinal canal, and the external inguinal ring, but at this point is deflected upward and outward so as to lie upon the aponeurosis of the external oblique; called also *Küster's h.* **intermuscular h., interparietal h.,** an interstitial hernia which lies between one or another of the fascial or muscular planes of the abdomen. **internal h.,** 1. a hernia which lies within the abdomen without involving the abdominal wall. 2. see under *inguinal h.* **intersigmoid h.,** hernia of the intestine through the intersigmoid fossa. **interstitial h.,** a hernia in which a knuckle of intestine lies between two layers of the abdominal wall. **h. of the iris,** protrusion of a part of the iris. **irreducible h.,** incarcerated h. **ischiatic h.,** hernia through the sacrosciatic foramen. **ischiorectal h.,** a protrusion of the abdominal viscera between fibers of the levator ani muscle; called also *perineal h.* **Krönlein's h.,** inguinoproperitoneal h. **Küster's h.,** inguinosuperficial h. **labial h.,** the protrusion of a knuckle of the gut into a labium majus. **labial h., posterior,** vaginolabial h. **Laugier's h.,** a femoral hernia perforating Gimbernat's ligament. **levator h.,** pudendal h. **Littre's h.,** diverticular h. **lumbar h.,** hernia in the loin. **mesenteric h.,** the passage of a portion of the gut through an opening in the mesentery. **mesocolic h.,** hernia into a pouch of the mesocolon. **mucosal h.,** hernia of the mucous membrane of the intestine through an opening in the muscular coat. **oblique h.,** see under *inguinal h.* **obturator h.,** protrusion through the obturator foramen. **omental h.,** a protrusion of a knuckle of omentum. **ovarian h.,** hernial protrusion of an ovary. **paraesophageal h.,** hiatal hernia in which part or almost all of the stomach protrudes through the hiatus into the thorax to the left of the esophagus, with the gastroesophageal junction remaining in place. **paraperitoneal h.,** hernia of the bladder in which only a part of the protruded bladder is covered by the peritoneum of the sac. **parasaccular h.,** sliding h. **h. par glissement** (glěs-maw′), sliding h. **parietal h.,** Richter's h. **parumbilical h.,** hernia in the region of the navel. **pectineal h.,** hernia situated beneath the pectineal fascia. **perineal h.,** ischiorectal h. **Petit's h.,** lumbar hernia in Petit's triangle. **properitoneal h.,** an interstitial hernia which is located between the parietal peritoneum and the transversalis fascia. **pudendal h.,** a hernia located in the pudendum, having passed through a rent in the levator muscle and its fascia; called also *levator h.* **h. of pulp,** protrusion of the dental pulp through the dentin wall of the pulp cavity. **pulsion h.,** a hernia produced by sudden increase of intra-abdominal pressure. **rectal h., h. in rec′to,** a hernia into the wall of the rectum. **rectovaginal h.,** rectocele. **reducible h.,** one that may be returned by manipulation.

retrocecal h., protrusion of the intestine into a pouch behind the cecum; called also *Rieux's h.* **retrograde h.,** herniation of two loops of intestine, the portion of intestine between the two loops lying within the abdominal cavity. **retroperitoneal h.,** hernia of the intestine into the superior duodenal recess. **Richter's h.,** an incarcerated or strangulated hernia in which only a portion of the circumference of the bowel wall is involved; called also *parietal h.* **Rieux's h.,** retrocecal h. **Rokitansky's h.,** protrusion of a sac of mucous membrane or of the peritoneum through separated muscular fibers of the intestine. **root h.,** finger and toe disease. **sciatic h.,** hernia through the great sacrosciatic foramen. **scrotal h.,** an inguinal hernia which has descended into the scrotum. **sliding h.,** hernia of the cecum (on the right) or the sigmoid colon (on the left) in which the wall of the viscus forms a portion of the hernial sac, the remainder of the sac being formed by the parietal peritoneum. Called also *slip h.* and *slipped h.* **sliding hiatal h.,** hiatal hernia in which the upper stomach and the cardioesophageal junction protrude upward into the posterior mediastinum; the protrusion, which may be fixed or intermittent, is partially covered by a peritoneal sac. **slip h., slipped h.,** sliding h. **spigelian h.,** abdominal hernia through the linea semilunaris. **strangulated h.,** an incarcerated hernia that is so tightly constricted as to compromise the blood supply of the hernial sac, leading to gangrene of the sac and its contents. **subpubic h.,** obturator h. **synovial h.,** protrusion of the inner lining membrane through the stratum fibrosum of a joint capsule; called also *Birkett's h.* **thyroidal h.,** obturator h. **tonsillar h.,** the extrusion of the tonsilla cerebelli through the foramen magnum. **transmesenteric h.,** protrusion of a loop of bowel through a congenital defect of the mesentery, where it may become incarcerated. **Treitz's h.,** a retroperitoneal hernia through the superior duodenal recess; called also *duodenojejunal h.* **tunicary h.,** mucosal h. **umbilical h.,** protrusion of part of the intestine at the umbilicus, the defect in the abdominal wall and protruding bowel being covered with skin and subcutaneous tissue; called also *exomphalos.* **h. u'teri inguina'le,** see *persistent müllerian duct syndrome,* under *syndrome.* **uterine h.,** hernial protrusion of the uterus. **vaginal h.,** hernia into the vagina; colpocele. **vaginal h., posterior,** downward protrusion of the pouch of Douglas, with its intestinal contents, between the posterior vaginal wall and the rectum; called also *enterocele.* **vaginolabial h.,** hernia of a viscus into the posterior end of the labium majus. **Velpeau's h.,** femoral hernia in front of the femoral vessels. **ventral h.,** hernia through the abdominal wall. **vesical h.,** protrusion of the bladder. **Von Bergmann's h.,** a small, generally intermittent form of hiatus hernia. **W h.,** retrograde h.

hernial (her′ne-al) pertaining to a hernia.

herniary (her′ne-a-re) pertaining to or associated with hernia.

herniated (her′ne-āt″ed) protruding like a hernia; enclosed in a hernia.

herniation (her″ne-a′shun) the abnormal protrusion of an organ or other body structure through a defect or natural opening in a covering membrane, muscle, or bone. **h. of intervertebral disk,** protrusion of the nucleus pulposus or annulus fibrosus of the disk, which may impinge on nerve roots. **h. of nucleus pulposus,** rupture or prolapse of the nucleus pulposus into the spinal canal. **tonsillar h.,** protrusion of the cerebellar tonsils through the foramen magnum, exerting pressure on the medulla oblongata. **transtentorial h.,** downward displacement (caudal transtentorial h.; uncal h.) of the medial structures through the tentorial notch by a supratentorial mass, exerting pressure on the underlying structures, including the brain stem. **uncal h.,** transtentorial h.

hernioappendectomy (her″ne-o-ap″en-dek′to-me) herniotomy combined with appendectomy.

hernioenterotomy (her″ne-o-en″ter-ot′o-me) herniotomy conjoined with enterotomy.

hernioid (her′ne-oid) resembling hernia.

herniolaparotomy (her″ne-o-lap″ah-rot′o-me) laparotomy for the treatment of hernia.

herniology (her″ne-ol′o-je) [*hernia* + *-logy*] the study and science of hernias.

hernioplasty (her′ne-o-plas″te) operation for the repair of hernia.

herniopuncture (her′ne-o-pungk′tūr) [*hernia* + *puncture*] surgical puncture of a hernia.

herniorrhaphy (her″ne-or′ah-fe) [*hernia* + Gr. *rhaphē* suture] surgical repair of a hernia.

herniotomy (her″ne-ot′o-me) [*hernia* + Gr. *tomē* a cutting] a cutting operation for the repair of hernia; kelotomy.

heroin (her′o-in) diacetylmorphine.

heroinism (her′o-in-izm″) addiction to the use of heroin, with its morbid effects.

heroinomania (her″o-in″o-ma′ne-ah) heroinism.

Herophilus of Chalcedon (hĕ-rof′ĭ-lus) (c. 300 B.C.) a renowned Greek physician and anatomist of Alexandria who performed dissection of the human body, and whose important

anatomical observations (e.g., on the brain, duodenum, and genitalia, and on the differentiation between nerves and blood vessels) have led many to regard him as "the Father of Anatomy."

herpangina (herp″an-ji′nah) [*herpes* + *angina*] a specific infectious disease characterized by sudden onset of fever of short duration and appearance of typical vesicular or ulcerated lesions in the faucial area or on the soft palate; caused by a coxsackievirus of the A group.

herpes (her′pēz) [L.; Gr. *herpēs*] any inflammatory skin disease characterized by the formation of small vesicles in clusters. The term was once used to denote any creeping vesicular skin disorder, including many fungal disorders, e.g., herpes circinatus (see tinea circinata) and herpes tonsurans maculosus (see pityriasis rosea), but is now usually restricted to such diseases caused by herpesviruses. When used alone, the term may refer to *herpes simplex* (dermatology) or to *herpes zoster.* **h. catarrha'lis,** h. simplex. **h. cor'neae,** herpetic inflammation involving the cornea. **h. digita'lis,** herpes simplex of the fingers. **h. facia'lis,** herpes simplex of the face. **h. febri'lis,** herpes simplex occurring as a concomitant of fever, commonly about the lips and nares; called also *fever blisters* and *cold sores.* **h. generalisa'tus,** herpetic inflammation scattered over the body. **genital h., h. genita'lis,** herpes simplex of the genitals. In women, the vesicular stage may give rise to confluent painful ulcerations and may be accompanied by neurologic symptoms. Called also *h. progenitalis.* **h. gestatio'nis,** a variant form of dermatitis herpetiformis peculiar to pregnant women, which clears upon termination of pregnancy. **h. i'ris,** erythema mulitforme in which the lesions are vesicular. **h. labia'lis,** h. febrilis. **h. menstrua'lis,** a form of herpes simplex that recurs at the menstrual period. **h. menta'lis,** herpes simplex of the submental region. **nasal h.,** an acute febrile rhinitis with eruption of vesicles around the nares and ulcerous lesions of the nasal mucous membranes, caused by a herpesvirus. **neuralgic h.,** genital herpes accompanied by rectal and vesical tenesmus and sphincteric spasms. **ocular h.,** herpes of the eye and its adnexa; see *herpetic keratoconjunctivitis.* **h. praeputia'lis,** a former name for herpes progenitalis in the male. **h. progenita'lis,** genital h. **h. recur'rens,** herpes simplex occurring in repeated attacks. **h. sim'plex,** an acute viral disease marked by groups of vesicles, each vesicle about 3 to 6 mm. in diameter, on the skin, often on the borders of the lips or the nares (*h. labialis,* cold sores), or on the genitals (*h. genitalis*). It often accompanies fever (*h. febrilis,* fever blisters), although there are other precipitating factors, such as the common cold, sunburn, skin abrasions, and emotional disturbances. Often called *herpes.* See also *Herpesvirus hominis.* **h. sim'plex recur'rens,** recurrent episodes of herpes simplex at the same site. **traumatic h.,** a self-limited cutaneous herpesvirus infection following trauma, the virus entering through burns or other wounds; the temperature rises moderately, and vesicles appear around the wound. Called also *wrestler's herpes.* **wrestler's h.,** traumatic h. **h. zos'ter,** an acute, unilateral, self-limited inflammatory disease of the cerebral ganglia and ganglia of the posterior nerve roots and peripheral nerves in a segmented distribution, caused by the virus of chickenpox. It is characterized by groups of small vesicles on inflammatory bases occurring in the cutaneous areas supplied by the affected segments and associated with neuralgic pain. Called also *acute posterior ganglionitis, shingles, zoster,* and *zona.* **h. zos'ter auricula'ris,** Ramsay Hunt syndrome, def. 1. **h. zos'ter ophthal'micus,** herpes infection involving the ophthalmic, or first division of the trigeminal nerve, characterized by a cutaneous vesicular rash on an erythematous base along the nerve path, preceded by lancinating pain. There is iridocyclitis, and corneal involvement that may lead to keratitis and corneal anesthesia. Called also *gasserian ganglionitis.* **h. zos'ter o'ticus,** Ramsay Hunt syndrome, def. 1. **h. zos'ter varicello'sus,** herpes zoster with secondary varicelliform eruption.

herpesencephalitis (her″pēz-en-sef″ah-li′tis) see under *encephalitis.*

Herpesviridae (her″pēs-vi′rĭ-de) a systematic name for the family of herpesviruses.

Herpesvirus hominis (her″pēz-vi′rus hom′ĭ-nis) the herpesvirus that causes herpes simplex; it occurs in two immunological types: Type 1 infections are primarily nongenital (e.g., herpes labialis and ocular herpes), whereas type II infections are primarily genital (herpes genitalis).

herpesvirus (her″pēz-vi′rus) any of a large group of DNA viruses found in many animal species, with a nucleocapsid about 100 mμ in diameter, composed of 162 capsomers, and sometimes enclosed in a loose membrane; the nucleic acid is a single molecule of double-stranded DNA with a molecular weight of about 100 million daltons; the viruses mature in the nucleus of the infected cell, where they induce formation of a characteristic inclusion body; some also induce formation of a cytoplasmic inclusion body. Herpesviruses are causative agents of such conditions as oral herpes simplex, genital herpes simplex, varicella, herpes zoster, cytomegalic inclusion disease in humans, and of pseudorabies and other diseases of animals. See also *herpes.*

herpetic (her-pet′ik) [L. *herpeticus*] pertaining to or of the nature of herpes; relating to or caused by herpesviruses.

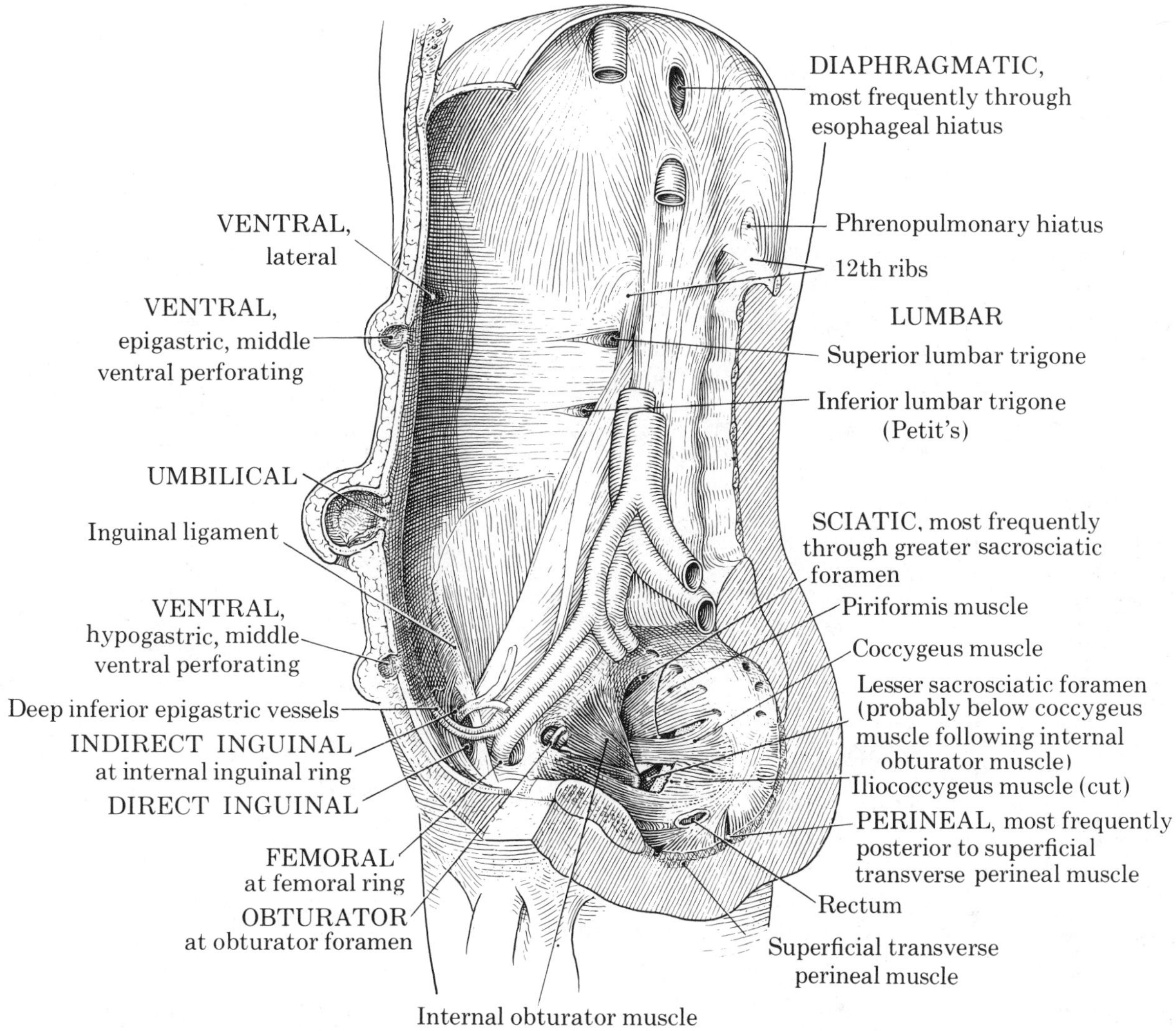

Plate XXI   hernia

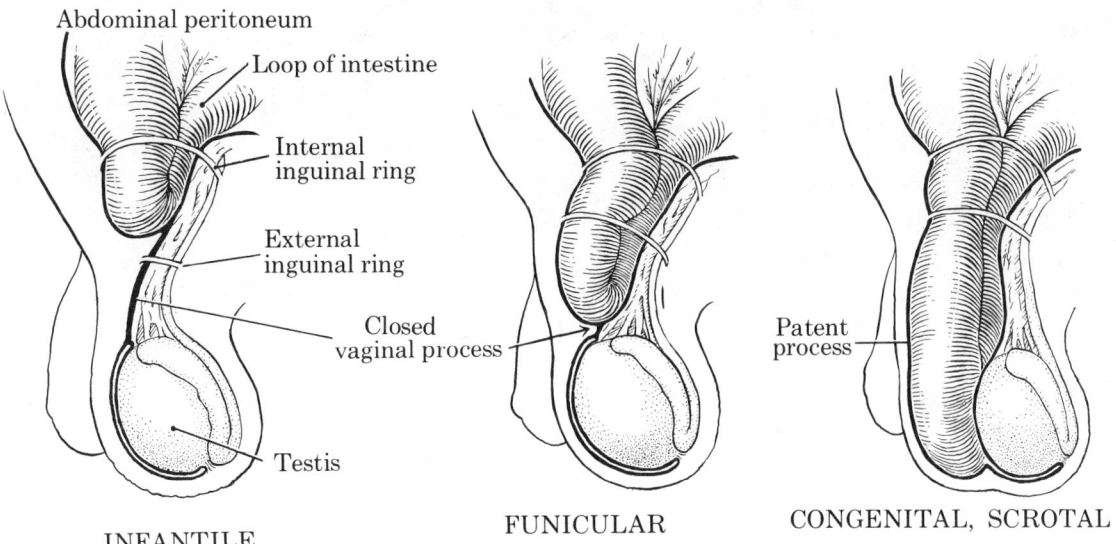

DIAPHRAGMATIC, most frequently through esophageal hiatus

VENTRAL, lateral

VENTRAL, epigastric, middle ventral perforating

Phrenopulmonary hiatus

12th ribs

LUMBAR
Superior lumbar trigone

Inferior lumbar trigone (Petit's)

UMBILICAL

Inguinal ligament

SCIATIC, most frequently through greater sacrosciatic foramen
Piriformis muscle
Coccygeus muscle
Lesser sacrosciatic foramen (probably below coccygeus muscle following internal obturator muscle)
Iliococcygeus muscle (cut)

VENTRAL, hypogastric, middle ventral perforating

Deep inferior epigastric vessels
INDIRECT INGUINAL at internal inguinal ring
DIRECT INGUINAL

PERINEAL, most frequently posterior to superficial transverse perineal muscle

FEMORAL at femoral ring
OBTURATOR at obturator foramen

Rectum

Superficial transverse perineal muscle

Internal obturator muscle

TYPES OF INTESTINAL HERNIA: ABDOMINAL AND PELVIC OPENINGS

Abdominal peritoneum
Loop of intestine
Internal inguinal ring
External inguinal ring
Closed vaginal process
Testis

Patent process

INFANTILE   FUNICULAR   CONGENITAL, SCROTAL

TYPES OF INDIRECT INGUINAL HERNIA

herpetiform (her-pet'ĭ-form) [L. *herpes* herpes + *forma* form] resembling herpes; having grouped vesicles.

herpetologist (her″pĕ-tol'o-gist) a specialist in herpetology.

herpetology (her″pĕ-tol'o-ge) the branch of zoology that specializes in the study of reptiles and amphibians.

Herpetomonas (her″pĕ-tom'o-nas) [Gr. *herpeton* creeper + *monas* monad] a genus of flagellate protozoa of the family Trypanosomatidae, order Protomastigida, found as parasites in insects, and having leptomonad, leishmanial, and crithidial stages, plus a stage that closely resembles the trypanosomes, except that it lacks an undulating membrane.

herpetophobia (her-pet″o-fo'be-ah) the morbid fear of lizards or reptiles.

Herplex (her'pleks) trademark for a preparation of idoxuridine.

Herrick's anemia (her'iks) [James Bryan *Herrick*, Chicago physician, 1861–1954] sickle cell anemia; see under *anemia*.

Herring bodies (her'ing) [Percy Theodore *Herring*, English physiologist, born 1872] see under *body*.

Herrmannsdorfer diet (her″mans-dor'fer) [Adolf *Herrmannsdorfer*, Berlin surgeon, born 1889] see *Gerson's diet*, under *diet*.

hersage (ār-sahzh′) [Fr. "combing"] surgical dissociation of the fibers of a peripheral nerve by splitting the sheath and separating the nerve, throughout the diseased area, into a ribbon of fine free fibers.

Hershey (her'she), Alfred Day. American biologist, born 1908; co-winner, with Max Delbruck and Salvador E. Luria, of the Nobel Prize in medicine and physiology for 1969, for research on the mechanism and materials of inheritance in bacteriophage.

Herter's disease (infantilism), test (her'terz) [Christian Archibald *Herter*, American physician, 1865–1910] see *infantile form of nontropical sprue*; under *sprue*, and see under *tests*.

Herter-Heubner disease (her'ter-hoib'ner) [C. A. *Herter*; Johann Otto Leonhard *Heubner*, pediatrician in Berlin, 1843–1926] the infantile form of nontropical sprue, or celiac disease.

Hertig-Rock ova (her'tig rok) [Arthur T. *Hertig*, American pathologist, born 1904; John *Rock*, American gynecologist, born 1890] see under *ovum*.

Hertwig's sheath (hert'vigz) [Richard *Hertwig*, German zoologist, 1850–1937] root sheath, def. 1.

Hertwig-Magendie phenomenon, sign (hert'vig mah-jen'de) [Richard *Hertwig*; François *Magendie*, French physiologist, 1783–1855] skew deviation.

hertz (hertz) a unit of frequency equal to one cycle per second; abbreviated Hz.

hertzian waves (rays) (hertz'e-an) [Heinrich Rudolf *Hertz*, German physicist, 1857–1894] see under *wave*.

Herxheimer's fever, fibers (spirals), reaction (herks′hīm-erz) [Karl *Herxheimer*, German dermatologist, born 1861] see under *fever* and *fiber*, and see *Jarisch-Herxheimer reaction*, under *reaction*.

Heryng's sign (her'ingz) [Teodor *Heryng*, Polish laryngologist, 1847–1925] see under *sign*.

Heschl's convolution, gyrus (hesh'l'z) [Richard L. *Heschl*, Austrian pathologist, 1824–1881] see *gyri temporales transversi*.

hesperanopia (hes″per-ah-no'pe-ah) [Gr. *hespera* evening + *an* neg. + *ops* eye] nyctalopia, def. 2.

hesperidin (hes-per'ĭ-din) chemical name: 7-[[6-*O*-(6-deoxy-α-L-mannopyranosyl)-β-D-glucopyranosyl]oxy]-2,3-dihydro-5-hydroxy-2-(3-hydroxy-4-methoxyphenyl)-H-benzopyran-4-one. A bioflavonoid, $C_{28}H_{34}O_{15}$, found in certain citrus fruits; it has been reported to reduce capillary fragility.

Hess (hes), Walter Rudolf. Swiss physiologist, born 1881, noted for research on the nervous system; co-winner, with Antonio Egas Moniz, of the Nobel prize in medicine and physiology for 1949, for his discovery of the functional organization of the interbrain as a coordinator of the activities of the internal organs.

Hesselbach's hernia, ligament, triangle (hes'el-bahks) [Franz Kaspar *Hesselbach*, German surgeon, 1759–1816] see under *hernia*, and see *ligamentum interfoveolare* and *trigonum inguinale*.

hetacillin (het″ah-sil'in) [USP] chemical name: 6-(2,2-dimethyl-5-oxo-4-phenyl-1-imidazolidinyl)-3,3-dimethyl-7-oxo-4-thia-1-azabicyclo [3.2.0] heptane-2-carboxylic acid. A semisynthetic penicillin, $C_{19}H_{23}N_3O_4S$, occurring as a white to off-white powder, which itself has no antibacterial activity, but is converted in the body to ampicillin and has actions and uses similar to those of ampicillin (q.v.); administered orally. **h. potassium** [USP], the potassium salt of hetacillin, $C_{19}H_{22}KN_3O_4S$, having antibacterial actions and uses similar to those of ampicillin; administered intravenously and intramuscularly.

hetaflur (het'ah-floor) chemical name: hexadecylamine hydrofluoride; a dental caries prophylactic, $C_{16}H_{35}N \cdot HF$.

hetastarch (het'ah-starch) a starch containing not more than 90 per cent of amylopectin, and that has been etherified so that an average of 7 to 8 of the OH groups in every 10-D-glucopyranose units of starch polymer have been converted into OCH_2CH_2OH

groups; used as a plasma volume expander, administered by infusion.

heter- see *hetero-*.

heteradelphia (het″er-ah-del'fe-ah) [*heter-* + Gr. *adelphos* brother] a joined twin monstrosity in which one fetus is much more fully developed than the other.

heteradelphus (het″er-ah-del'fus) a monster exhibiting heteradelphia.

heteradenia (het″er-ah-de'ne-ah) [*heter-* + Gr. *adēn* gland] any abnormality of the gland tissue.

heteradenic (het″er-ah-den'ik) pertaining to, affected with, or of the nature of heteradenia.

Heterakis gallinae (het″er-a'kis gah-li'ne) a nematode parasitic in the ceca of wild and domestic fowl.

heteralius (het″er-a'le-us) [*heter-* + Gr. *halios* fruitless] an extreme example of heteradelphia.

heterauxesis (het″er-awk-ze'sis) [*heter-* + Gr. *auxēsis* growth] disproportionate growth of a part in relation to another part.

heteraxial (het″er-ak'se-al) [*heter-* + *axis*] having axes of unequal length.

heterecious (het″er-e'shus) [*heter-* + Gr. *oikos* house] living upon one host in one stage or generation and upon another in the next.

heterecism (het″er-e'sizm) the state of being heterecious.

heterergic (het″er-er'jik) [*heter-* + Gr. *ergon* work] having different effects; said of two drugs one of which produces a particular effect and the other does not.

heteresthesia (het″er-es-the'ze-ah) [*heter-* + Gr. *aisthēsis* perception] variation in the degree of cutaneous sensibility on adjoining areas of the body surface.

hetero-, heter- [Gr. *heteros* other] a combining form meaning other, or denoting relationship to another.

heteroagglutination (het″er-o-ah-gloo″tĭ-na'shun) agglutination of particulate antigens (on cells or adsorbed on inert carrier particles) of one species by agglutinins derived from organisms of another species.

heteroagglutinin (het″er-o-ah-gloo'tĭ-nin) an agglutinin with reactive specificity for particulate antigen(s) in one or more species other than the species in which it originates.

heteroalbumose (het″er-o-al'bu-mōs) [*hetero-* + *albumose*] a form of hemialbumose that is not soluble in water, but is soluble in hydrochloric acid and sodium chloride solutions.

heteroalbumosuria (het″er-o-al'bu-mo-su're-ah) [*heteroalbumose* + Gr. *ouron* urine + *-ia*] the presence of heteroalbumose in the urine.

heteroallele (het″er-o-ah-lēl′) a mutation occurring in different codons of a particular cistron in homologous chromosomes.

heteroallelic (het″er-o-ah-le'lik) pertaining to a heteroallele.

heteroantibody (het″er-o-an″tĭ-bod′e) an antibody specific for antigens originating in a species other than that of the antibody producer.

heteroantigen (het″er-o-an″tĭ-jen) an antigen originating in a species different from, and therefore foreign to, the antibody producer.

heteroatom (het″er-o-at'om) any atom with a ring-shaped chemical nucleus other than the carbon atoms.

heteroauxin (het″er-o-auk'sin) a compound occurring in urine which acts as a plant growth hormone; called also *auxin B*.

Heterobasidiomycetidae (het″er-o-bah-sid″e-o-mi-se'tĭ-de) a subclass of true fungi of the Basidiomycetes, made up of the rusts and smuts, in which the basidiospores germinate by budding, repetition, or by the production of conidia, and the basidium starts as a hyphal cell with two nuclei.

Heterobilharzia (het″er-o-bil-har'ze-ah) a genus of schistosomes that parasitize mammals, including human beings. **H. america′na,** a species whose cercariae may cause a nonpatent visceral schistosomiasis in man.

heteroblastic (het″er-o-blas'tik) [*hetero-* + Gr. *blastos* germ] having origin in different kinds of tissue.

heterocaryon (het″er-o-kar'e-on) heterokaryon.

heterocellular (het″er-o-sel'u-lar) composed of cells of different kinds.

heterocentric (het″er-o-sen'trik) [*hetero-* + L. *centrum* center] made up of rays that are neither parallel nor meet in one point; said of a ray of light.

heterocephalus (het″er-o-sef'ah-lus) [*hetero-* + Gr. *kephalē* head] a monster with two unequal heads.

heterochiral (het″er-o-ki'ral) [*hetero-* + Gr. *cheir* hand] reversed as regards right and left, but otherwise the same in form and size, as the hands.

heterochromatin (het″er-o-kro'mah-tin) that state of chromatin in which it is dark-staining, genetically inactive, and tightly coiled; cf. *euchromatin*.

heterochromatinization (het″er-o-kro″mah-tin-i-za′shun) the formation of heterochromatin.

heterochromatosis (het″-o-kro″mah-to′sis)   heterochromia.

heterochromia (het″er-o-kro′me-ah) [*hetero-* + Gr. *chrōma* color + *-ia*]   diversity of color in a part or parts that should normally be of one color.   **h. i′ridis,** difference of color in the two irides, or in different areas of the same iris.

heterochromosome (het″er-o-kro′mo-sōm) [*hetero-* + *chromosome*]   a sex chromosome.

heterochromous (het″er-o-kro′mus)   marked by diversity of color; exhibiting heterochromia.

heterochron (het″er-o-krōn′)   having different or varying chronaxy.

heterochronia (het″er-o-kro′ne-ah) [*hetero-* + Gr. *chronos* time + *-ia*]   1. the formation of parts or tissues, or the occurrence of a phenomenon, at an unusual time. Cf. *synchronia* (def. 2).   2. a difference in the rate or time of occurrence between two processes. 3. difference of more than 100 per cent between the chronaxy of a muscle and that of its nerve.

heterochronic (het″er-o-kron′ik) [*hetero-* + Gr. *chronos* time] 1. pertaining to or characterized by heterochronia.   2. denoting different ages or stages of development, as between the excised organ and the implanted organ in transplantation procedures.

heterochronous (het″er-ok′ro-nus)   heterochronic.

heterochthonous (het″er-ok′tho-nus) [*hetero-* + Gr. *chthōn* a particular land or country]   originating in a region other than that in which it is found. Cf. *autochthonous*.

heterochylia (het″er-o-ki′le-ah)   the sudden varying of the gastric secretion from normal acidity to hyperacidity or anacidity.

heterocinesia (het″er-o-sĭ-ne′se-ah) [*hetero-* + Gr. *kinēsis* movement]   a condition in which the patient performs movements other than those he is instructed to perform.

heterocladic (het″er-o-klad′ik) [*hetero-* + Gr. *klados* branch] indicating an anastomosis between terminal branches from different arteries.

heterocomplement (het″er-o-kom′plĕ-ment) [*hetero-* + *complement*]   complement derived from an animal of a species different from the one which furnishes the antibody.

heterocrine (het″er-o-krin) [*hetero-* + Gr. *krinein* to separate] secreting more than one kind of matter.

heterocrisis (het″er-ok′rĭ-sis) [*hetero-* + Gr. *krisis* division]   an abnormal crisis with unusual timing and symptoms.

heterocyclic (het″er-o-sīk′lik) [*hetero-* + Gr. *kyklos* circle]   having or pertaining to a closed chain or ring formation which includes atoms of different elements.

heterocytolysin (het″er-o-si-tol′ĭ-sin)   heterolysin.

heterocytotoxin (het″er-o-si″to-tok′sin)   a toxin of one species which destroys cells from an organism of a different species.

heterocytotropic (het″er-o-si″to-trop′ik) [*hetero-* + *cyto-* + Gr. *tropos* a turning]   having an affinity for cells of different species; see under *antibody*.

Heterodera radicicola (het″er-od′er-ah rad″ĭ-sik′o-lah)   a nematode parasitic on the common root vegetables, such as radishes, carrots, turnips, potatoes, etc., as well as on celery. When infested vegetables are eaten, ova of the parasite may appear in the stools and must be distinguished from those of true parasites.

heterodermic (het″er-o-der′mik) [*hetero-* + Gr. *derma* skin] denoting a skin graft taken from an individual of another species. See *dermatoheteroplasty*.

heterodesmotic (het″er-o-des-mot′ik) [*hetero-* + Gr. *desmos* a bond]   joining dissimilar parts of the central nervous system; see under *fiber*.

heterodidymus (het″er-o-did′ĭ-mus)   heterodymus.

heterodont (het′er-o-dont) [*heter-* + Gr. *odous* tooth]   having teeth of different types, such as incisors and molars.

Heterodoxus (het″er-o-dok′sus)   a genus of insects of the order Mallophaga, the biting lice. *H. longitarsus* is parasitic on kangaroos, wallabies, and sometimes dogs in Australia. *H. spiniger* is parasitic on coyotes and wolves in the New World, and may also infest dogs.

heterodromous (het″er-od′ro-mus) [*hetero-* + Gr. *dromos* running]   moving, acting, or arranged in the opposite direction.

heterodymus (het″er-od′ĭ-mus) [*hetero-* + Gr. *didymos* twin]   a monster with a second head, neck, and thorax attached to the thorax.

heteroecious (het″er-o-e-shus)   requiring two or more hosts to complete the life cycle; said of certain fungi and insects. Cf. *autoecious*.

heteroerotism (het″er-o-er′o-tizm) [*hetero-* + Gr. *erōs* love] sexual feeling directed toward another individual. Cf. *autoerotism*.

heterofermenter (het″er-o-fer-ment′er)   a group of bacteria which produce, by fermentation, large quantities of lactic acid, along with acetic acid, ethanol, and CO_2.

heterogamete (het″er-o-gam′ēt)   a gamete of different size and structure than the one with which it unites.

heterogametic (het″er-o-gah-met′ik)   characterized by the production of gametes of different kinds, as by the production of X and Y gametes in the human male.

heterogamety (het″er-o-gam′ĕ-te)   the production of unlike gametes by an individual of one sex, as the production of X- and Y-bearing gametes by the human male.

heterogamous (het″er-og′ah-mus)   having the conjugating elements (gametes) unlike in size and structure; oogamous.

heterogamy (het″er-og′ah-me) [*hetero-* + Gr. *gamōs* marriage] reproduction resulting from the union of two cells (gametes) which differ in size and structure; oogamy.

heteroganglionic (het″er-o-gang″gle-on′ik) [*hetero-* + Gr. *ganglion* ganglion]   connecting various ganglia (of the sympathetic nervous system).

heterogeneity (het″er-o-jĕ-ne′ĭ-te)   the state or quality of being heterogeneous. In genetics, the production of identical or similar phenotypes by different genetic mechanisms. A phenotype so produced is called a genocopy or genetic mimic. **genetic h.,** the production of a specific clinical or biochemical phenotype by more than a single genotype.

heterogeneous (het″er-o-je′ne-us) [*hetero-* + Gr. *genos* kind] consisting of or composed of dissimilar elements or ingredients; not having a uniform quality throughout. In genetics, the term denotes a trait that can be produced by genes at more than one locus.

heterogenesis (het″er-o-jen′ĕ-sis) [*hetero-* + Gr. *genesis* generation]   1. alternation of generations; reproduction that differs in character in successive generations.   2. asexual generation.   3. (*obs.*) the development of a living thing from some other kind of living thing.   4. spontaneous generation.

heterogenetic (het″er-o-jĕ-net′ik)   1. pertaining to heterogenesis.   2. not arising within the organism.

heterogenic (het″er-o-jen′ik)   1. occurring in the wrong sex, as a beard upon a woman.   2. derived from a different source or species; see *xenograft*.

heterogenicity (het″er-o-jĕ-nis′ĭ-te)   heterogeneity.

heterogenote (het′er-o-je″nōt) [*hetero-* + *gene* (analogy with zygote)]   a cell which has an additional genetic fragment, different from its intact genotype; it usually results from transduction.

heterogenous (het″er-oj′ĕ-nus)   derived from a different source or species; see *xenograft*.

heteroglobulose (het″er-o-glob′u-lōs)   a heteroalbumose obtained from a globulin.

heterogony (het″er-og′ŏ-ne) [*hetero-* + Gr. *gonos* procreation] heterogenesis.

heterograft (het′er-o-graft)   xenograft.

heterography (het″er-og′rah-fe) [*hetero-* + Gr. *graphein* to record]   the writing of words other than those intended by the writer.

heterohemagglutination (het″er-o-hem″ah-gloo″tĭ-na′shun) agglutination of erythrocytes of one species by hemagglutinins derived from an individual of a different species.

heterohemagglutinin (het″er-o-hem″ah-gloo′tĭ-nin)   a hemagglutinin derived from one species that agglutinates erythrocytes of organisms of one or more other species.

heterohemolysin (het″er-o-he-mol′ĭ-sin)   1. a hemolysin occurring spontaneously in the blood of an untreated animal that will hemolyze the blood cells of an animal of another species.   2. hemolysin established in one species by deliberate immunization with blood cells of an animal of another species.

heterohexosan (het″er-o-hek′so-san)   any one of a class of heterosaccharides which contain hexose units; they are lignocellulose, pectocellulose, and lipocellulose.

heteroimmune (het″er-o-im-mūn′)   pertaining to or characterized by heteroimmunity.

heteroimmunity (het″er-o-im-mu′nĭ-te)   1. an immune state that results from the immunization of an animal belonging to one species with cells of an animal of a different species.   2. a state in which immunological response by the body to exogenous antigens, which include drugs and infectious agents, results in immunopathological changes.

heteroinfection (het″er-o-in-fek′shun)   infection from outside the organism; exogenous infection.

heteroinoculable (het″er-o-in-ok′u-lah-b'l)   susceptible of being inoculated from one individual to another.

heteroinoculation (het″er-o-in-ok″u-la′shun)   inoculation from one individual to another.

heterointoxication (het″er-o-in-tok″sĭ-ka′shun)   poisoning by material introduced from outside the body.

heterokaryon (het″er-o-kar′e-on) [*hetero-* + Gr. *karyon* nucleus] a cell or hypha containing two or more nuclei of different genetic constitutions.

heterokaryosis (het″er-o-kar″e-o′sis)   the formation of, or the state of containing, heterokaryons.

heterokeratoplasty (het″er-o-ker′ah-to-plas″te) [*hetero-* + *keratoplasty*]   grafting of corneal tissue from an individual of a species other than that of the recipient.

heterokinesis (het″er-o-ki-ne′sis) [*hetero-* + Gr. *kinēsis* motion] the differential distribution of the sex chromosomes (X and Y in humans) in the developing gametes of a heterogametic organism.

heterolactic (het″er-o-lak′tik)   bacterial fermentation which produces large quantities of lactic acid along with acetic acid, ethanol, and CO_2.

heterolalia (het″er-o-la′le-ah) [*hetero-* + Gr. *lalia* utterance] heterophasia.

heterolateral (het″er-o-lat′er-al) [*hetero-* + L. *latus* side] relating to the opposite side; contralateral.

heteroliteral (het″er-o-lit′er-al)   marked by the substitution of one letter for another in pronouncing words.

heterolith (het′er-o-lith) [*hetero-* + Gr. *lithos* stone]   an intestinal concretion not formed of mineral matter.

heterologous (het″er-ol′o-gus) [*hetero-* + Gr. *logos* due relation, proportion]   1. made up of tissue not normal to the part. 2. xenogeneic.

heterology (het″er-ol′o-je)   abnormality in structure, arrangement, or manner of formation. In chemistry, the relationship between substances of partial identity of structure but of different properties.

heterolysin (het″er-ol′ĭ-sin)   a lysin that dissolves cells of species other than the one in which it is formed, by leading to interruption of the integrity of the cell membranes; a lysin that is formed on the introduction of antigen from a different species.

heterolysis (het″er-ol′ĭ-sis) [*hetero-* + Gr. *lysis* dissolution] lysis of the cells of one species by lysin from a different species.

heterolysosome (het″er-o-li′so-sōm)   a vacuole of lysosome containing exogenous substances with digestion in progress.

heterolytic (het″er-o-lit′ik)   pertaining to or caused by heterolysis or a heterolysin.

heteromastigote (het″er-o-mas′tĭ-gōt) [*hetero-* + Gr. *mastix* lash] having several forward flagella together with one directed backward.

heteromeral (het″er-om′er-al)   heteromeric.

heteromeric (het″er-o-mer′ik) [*hetero-* + Gr. *meros* part] sending processes through one of the commissures to the white matter of the other side of the spinal cord; said of nerve cells.

heteromerous (het″er-om′er-us)   heteromeric.

heterometaplasia (het″er-o-met″ah-pla′se-ah) [*hetero-* + *metaplasia*]   development of tissue into a variety foreign to the part where it is produced.

heterometropia (het″er-o-mě-tro′pe-ah)   the state in which there is a different kind of refraction in the two eyes; antimetropia.

heteromorphic (het″er-o-mor′fik)   heteromorphous.

heteromorphosis (het″er-o-mor-fo′sis) [*hetero-* + Gr. *morphōsis* a forming]   the development, in regeneration, of an organ or structure different from the one that was lost.

heteromorphous (het″er-o-mor′fus) [*hetero-* + Gr. *morphē* form]   1. of abnormal shape or structure; differing from the type.   2. having synaptic chromosome mates which differ in size, form, or structure.

heteronephrolysine (het″er-o-ne-frol′ĭ-sin) [*hetero-* + *nephrolysine*]   (*obs.*) a nephrotoxin which acts on the cells of animals from a different species.

heteronomous (het″er-on′o-mus) [*hetero-* + Gr. *nomos* law]   1. in biology, subject to different laws of growth; specialized along different lines.   2. in psychology, subject to another will, as in hypnotism.

heteronymous (het″er-on′ĭ-mus) [*hetero-* + Gr. *onyma* name]   1. having names indicative of correlation, as male and female.   2. standing in opposite relations; see under *hemianopia.*

hetero-osteoplasty (het″er-o-os′te-o-plas″te) [*hetero-* + Gr. *osteon* bone + *plassein* to shape]   the surgical grafting in one individual of bone taken from an individual of another species.

hetero-ovular (het″er-o-ov′u-lar)   pertaining to or derived from different ova; dizygotic.

heteropagus (het″er-op′ah-gus) [*hetero-* + Gr. *pagos* thing fixed]   a twin monster in which one component (the parasite) is much smaller than and dependent on the other (the autosite).

heteropancreatism (het″er-o-pan′kre-ah-tizm)   an irregular condition of functioning on the part of the pancreas.

heteropathy (het″er-op′ah-the) [*hetero-* + Gr. *pathos* disease]   1. abnormal or morbid sensitiveness to stimuli.   2. allopathy.

heteropentosan (het″er-o-pen′to-san)   a heterosaccharide which contains pentose units, such as gums, mucilages, and pectic substances.

heterophagosome (het″er-o-fag′o-sōm) [*hetero-* + *phagosome*]   an intracytoplasmic vacuole formed by phagocytosis or pinocytosis, which becomes fused with a lysosome, subjecting its contents to enzymatic digestion. Called also *heterophagic vacuole.*

heterophagy (het″er-of′ah-je) [*hetero-* + Gr. *phagein* to eat]   the taking into a cell of exogenous material by phagocytosis or pinocytosis and the digestion of the ingested material after fusion of the newly formed vacuole with a lysosome. Cf. *autophagy.*

heterophany (het″er-of′ah-ne) [*hetero-* + Gr. *phainein* to appear]   a difference in the manifestations of the same condition.

heterophasia (het″er-o-fa′ze-ah) [*hetero-* + Gr. *phasis* speech +

-ia]   the uttering of words other than those intended by the speaker.

heterophasis (het″er-o-fa′sis)   heterophasia.

heterophemia (het″er-o-fe′me-ah) [*hetero-* + Gr. *phēmē* word] heterophasia.

heterophil (het′er-o-fil″)   1. a granular leukocyte represented by neutrophils in man but characterized in other mammals by granules which have variable sizes and staining characteristics; called also *heterophilic leukocyte.* See also *neutrophil* (def. 2).   2. heterophilic.

heterophilic (het″er-o-fil′ik) [*hetero-* + Gr. *philein* to love]   1. having affinity for antigens or antibodies other than the one for which it is specific.   2. staining with a type of stain other than the usual one.

heterophoralgia (het″er-o-fo-ral′je-ah) [*hetero-* + Gr. *phoros* bearing + *-algia*]   heterophoria associated with pain.

heterophoria (het″er-o-fo′re-ah) [*hetero-* + Gr. *pherein* to bear + *-ia*]   failure of the visual axes to remain parallel after the visual fusional stimuli have been eliminated. The various forms of heterophoria are called *phorias,* their direction being indicated by the appropriate prefix. See *cyclophoria, esophoria, exophoria, hyperphoria, hypophoria,* and *latent deviation.*

heterophoric (het″er-o-fo′rik)   pertaining to or characterized by heterophoria.

heterophosphatase (het″er-o-fos′fah-tās)   hexokinase.

heterophthalmia (het″er-of-thal′me-ah) [*hetero-* + Gr. *ophthalmos* eye + *-ia*]   difference in the direction of the axes, or in the color, of the two eyes.

heterophthalmos (het″er-of-thal′mos)   heterophthalmia.

heterophydiasis (het″er-o-fī-di′ah-sis)   heterophyiasis.

Heterophyes (het″er-of′ĭ-ēz) [*hetero-* + Gr. *phyē* stature]   a genus of minute trematode worms found in the middle third of the small intestine of man, dogs, cats, and other fish-eating mammals. *H. heterophyes* is found in Egypt, Asia, and Asia Minor. *H. katsuradai* and *H. brevicaeca* have been reported in man in Japan and the Philippines.

heterophyiasis (het″er-o-fi-i′ah-sis)   infection with trematodes of the genus *Heterophyes;* it is generally asymptomatic.

heteroplasia (het″er-o-pla′ze-ah) [*hetero-* + Gr. *plassein* to mold]   the replacement of normal by abnormal tissue; malposition of normal cells.

heteroplasm (het′er-o-plazm)   any heterologous tissue.

heteroplastic (het″er-o-plas′tik)   pertaining to heteroplasia or to heteroplasty.

heteroplastid (het″er-o-plas′tid)   a xenograft.

heteroplasty (het′er-o-plas″te) [*hetero-* + Gr. *plassein* to mold] heterotransplantation.

heteroploid (het′er-o-ploid″)   1. pertaining to or characterized by heteroploidy.   2. an individual or cell with an abnormal number of chromosomes.

heteroploidy (het′er-o-ploi″de)   the state of having an abnormal number of chromosomes.

Heteropoda (het″er-op′o-dah)   a genus of large spiders sometimes confused with tarantulas. **H. venato′ria,** a large spider found in shipments of tropical fruit, particularly bananas; its bite is painful, but not serious.

heteropodal (het″er-op′o-dal) [*hetero-* + Gr. *pous* foot]   having branches or processes of different kinds; said of nerve cells.

heteropolymeric (het″er-o-pol″e-mer′ik) [*hetero-* + *poly-* + Gr. *meros* part]   composed of dissimilar constituent building units, as a macromolecule, e.g., a protein.

heteropolysaccharide (het″er-o-pol″e-sak′ah-rīd)   any polysaccharide macromolecule containing two or more different sugars, its function varying with the nature of its residues.

heteroprosopus (het″er-o-pro′so-pus) [*hetero-* + Gr. *prosōpon* face]   janiceps.

heteroproteose (het″er-o-pro′te-ōs)   a primary proteose that is insoluble in water, but soluble in dilute salt solution.

heteropsia (het″er-op′se-ah) [*hetero-* + Gr. *opsis* vision]   unequal vision in the two eyes.

heteropsychologic (het″er-o-si″ko-loj′ik)   pertaining to ideas formed outside the individual mind.

Heteroptera (het″er-op′ter-ah) [*hetero-* + Gr. *pteron* wing]   a suborder of Hemiptera characterized by the possession of two pairs of wings, one horny, the other membranous; it includes the medically important families Cimicidae and Reduviidae.

heteroptics (het″er-op′tiks) [*hetero-* + Gr. *optikos* optic]   false or perverted vision; visual perception of objects not in the field of vision or misinterpretation of visual images.

heteropyknosis (het″er-o-pik-no′sis) [*hetero-* + Gr. *pyknōsis* condensation]   1. the quality of showing variations in density throughout.   2. a state of differential condensation observed in comparison of different chromosomes, or of different regions of the same chromosome. **negative h.,** attenuation of condensation observed in comparison of different chromosomes, or of different regions of the same chromosome. **positive h.,** accentuation of condensation observed in comparison of different chromosomes, or of different regions of the same chromosome.

heteropyknotic (het″er-o-pik-not′ik) pertaining to or characterized by heteropyknosis. **negatively h.,** showing areas of lesser condensation than normal. **positively h.,** showing areas of greater condensation than normal.

heterosaccharide (het″er-o-sak′ah-rīd) a polysaccharide containing a carbohydrate and a noncarbohydrate unit. Cf. *holosaccharide.*

heteroscope (het′er-o-skōp) [*heterophoria* + Gr. *skopein* to examine] a pair of fusion tubes so mounted as to subserve the observation of the progress of cases of heterophoria.

heteroscopy (het″er-os′ko-pe) inequality of vision in the two eyes.

heteroserotherapy (het″er-o-se′ro-ther′ah-pe) treatment of a patient by serum derived from some other individual.

heterosexual (het″er-o-seks′u-al) 1. pertaining to the opposite sex; directed toward a person of the opposite sex; the opposite of homosexual. 2. one who is sexually attracted to persons of the opposite sex.

heterosexuality (het″er-o-seks″u-al′ĭ-te) sexual desire directed toward persons of the opposite sex, as distinguished from homosexuality.

heterosis (het″er-o′sis) [Gr. *heterōsis* alteration] the condition in which the first generation hybrid shows more vigor as measured by growth, survival, and fertility, than either of the parent strains; it is believed to be caused by the dominance (or interaction) of favorable alleles not common to both parental populations. Called also *hybrid vigor.*

heterosmia (het″er-os′me-ah) [*hetero-* + Gr. *osmē* smell] a condition in which odors are incorrectly interpreted.

heterosome (het′er-o-sōm) [*hetero-* + Gr. *sōma* body] a sex chromosome.

heterospore (het′er-o-spōr) a heterosporous organism.

heterosporous (het″er-os′po-rus) [*hetero-* + Gr. *sporos* seed] having spores of two kinds, which reproduce asexually.

heterostimulation (het″er-o-stim″u-la′shun) stimulation of an animal with antigenic material originating from a different species.

heterosuggestion (het″er-o-sug-jes′chun) [*hetero-* + *suggestion*] suggestion received from another person; opposed to autosuggestion.

heterotaxia (het″er-o-tak′se-ah) [*hetero-* + Gr. *taxis* arrangement] anomalous placement or transposition of viscera or parts.

heterotaxic (het″er-o-tak′sik) affected with heterotaxia.

heterotaxis (het″er-o-tak′sis) heterotaxia.

heterotaxy (het′er-o-tak″se) heterotaxia.

heterothallic (het″er-o-thal′ik) pertaining to or exhibiting heterothallism.

heterothallism (het″er-o-thal′izm) a form of sexual reproduction in which the isogamete must fuse with a gamete formed by a cell of a different mating type, as in various algae and fungi.

heterotherapy (het″er-o-ther′ah-pe) [*hetero-* + Gr. *therapeia* treatment] treatment of disease by remedies which are antagonistic to the principal symptoms of the disease; nonspecific therapy.

heterotherm (het′er-o-therm″) an animal which exhibits heterothermy.

heterothermic (het″er-o-ther′mik) pertaining to or characterized by heterothermy.

heterothermy (het′er-o-ther″me) [*hetero-* + Gr. *thermē* heat] the exhibition of widely different body temperatures at different times or under different conditions, as certain species of birds, marsupials, or hibernating species.

heterotonia (het″er-o-to′ne-ah) [*hetero-* + Gr. *tonos* tension + *-ia*] a state characterized by variations in tension or tone.

heterotonic (het″er-o-ton′ik) pertaining to or characterized by heterotonia.

heterotopia (het″er-o-to′pe-ah) [*hetero-* + Gr. *topos* place + *-ia*] 1. displacement or misplacement of parts or organs; the presence of a tissue in an abnormal location. 2. a jumbling of sounds in words.

heterotopic (het″er-o-top′ik) occurring at an abnormal place or upon the wrong part of the body.

heterotopy (het″er-ot′o-pe) heterotopia.

heterotransplant (het″er-o-trans′plant) xenograft.

heterotransplantation (het″er-o-trans″plan-ta′shun) the operative replacement of lost or damaged parts or tissues by tissue taken from an individual of a different species (a xenograft).

heterotrichosis (het″er-o-tri-ko′sis) [*hetero-* + Gr. *trichōsis* growth of hair] growth of hair of different colors on the body. **h. supercilio′rum,** difference in color of the hairs of the two eyebrows (von Walther).

heterotrichous (het″er-ot′rĭ-kus) having irregular cilia, in size, shape, function, or distribution.

heterotroph (het′er-o-trōf″) a heterotrophic organism, such as an animal or a chlorophyll-free plant.

heterotrophia (het″er-o-tro′fe-ah) [*hetero-* + Gr. *trophē* nourishment] any disorder or fault of nutrition.

heterotrophic (het″er-o-trof′ik) [*hetero-* + Gr. *trophē* nutrition] not self-sustaining; said of organisms which require a reduced form of carbon for energy and synthesis. Cf. *autotrophic.*

heterotrophy (het″er-ot′ro-fe) 1. the state of being heterotrophic; heterotrophic nutrition. 2. heterotrophia.

heterotropia (het″er-o-tro′pe-ah) [*hetero-* + Gr. *tropē* a turn, turning + *-ia*] failure of the visual axes to remain parallel when fusion is a possibility. See *strabismus.* **comitant h., concomitant h.,** deviation of a visual axis in which the angular relation between the two visual axes remains fairly constant, whatever the position of the fixing eye. **noncomitant h.,** deviation in which the angular relation between the visual axes is not maintained. **paralytic h.,** heterotropia due to paralysis of one or more of the extraocular muscles.

heterotropy (het″er-ot′ro-pe) heterotropia.

heterotrypsin (het″er-o-trip′sin) an enzyme of the pancreatic juice.

heterotypic (het″er-o-tip′ik) pertaining to, characteristic of, or belonging to a different type.

heterotypical (het″er-o-tip′e-k'l) of a type differing from that usually or normally encountered; having characteristics peculiar to a different type; sometimes applied to the first meiotic division of the germ cells.

heterovaccine (het″er-o-vak′sēn) a vaccine made from some microorganism other than the one causing the disease for which the vaccine is used; it is one form of nonspecific therapy.

heteroxenous (het″er-ok′se-nus) [*hetero-* + Gr. *xenos* guest-friend, stranger] requiring more than one host in order to complete the life cycle; said of parasitic organisms. Cf. *monoxenous.*

heteroxeny (het″er-ok′sĕ-ne) the quality or condition of being heteroxenous.

heterozoic (het″er-o-zo′ik) [*hetero-* + Gr. *zōon* animal] pertaining to another animal or species of animal.

heterozygosis (het″er-o-zi-go′sis) the formation of a zygote by the union of gametes of unlike genetic constitution.

heterozygosity (het″er-o-zi-gos′ĭ-te) [*hetero-* + *zygosity*] the state of possessing different alleles at a given locus or loci in regard to a given character.

heterozygote (het″er-o-zi′gōt) [*hetero-* + *zygote*] an individual possessing different alleles in regard to a given character.

heterozygotic (het″er-o-zi-got′ik) heterozygous.

heterozygous (het″er-o-zi′gus) possessing different alleles at a given locus. *Doubly heterozygous:* having different alleles at each of two separate loci.

Hetrazan (het′rah-zan) trademark for preparations of diethylcarbamazine citrate.

Heublein method (hoib′lin) [Arthur Carl *Heublein,* radiologist, 1879–1932] see under *method.*

Heubner's disease (endarteritis) (hoib′nerz) [Johann Otto Leonhard *Heubner,* pediatrician in Berlin, 1843–1926] see under *disease.*

Heubner-Herter disease (hoib′ner-her′ter) [J. O. L. *Heubner;* Christian Archibald *Herter,* American physician, 1865–1910] the infantile form of nontropical sprue, or celiac disease.

heuristic (hu-ris′tik) [Gr. *heuriskein* to find out, discover] encouraging or promoting investigation; conducive to discovery.

heurteloup (her′tel-ōōp, Fr., urt-loo′) [Baron Charles Louis Stanislas *Heurteloup,* French surgeon, 1793–1864] an artificial leech, or cupping apparatus.

Heuser's membrane (hoi′zerz) [Chester *Heuser,* American embryologist, born 1885] see under *membrane.*

hex-, hexa- [Gr. *hex* six] a combining form meaning six.

hexabasic (hek″sah-ba′sik) [*hexa-* + *basic*] having six atoms replaceable by a base.

Hexa-Betalin (hek″sah-be′tah-lin) trademark for preparations of pyridoxine hydrochloride.

hexabiose (hek″sah-bi′ōs) disaccharide.

hexachlorobenzene (hek″sah-klor″o-ben′zēn) a compound, C_6Cl_6, used in organic synthesis and as a fungicide.

hexachlorocyclohexane (hek″sah-klo′ro-si″klo-hek′sān) benzene hexachloride.

hexachloroethane (hek″sah-klor″o-eth′ān) a crystal compound, CCl_3CCl_3, used against liver flukes in cattle and sheep.

hexachlorophene (hek″sah-klo′ro-fēn) [USP] chemical name: 2,2′-methylenebis-(3,4,6-trichlorophenol). An antibacterial, $C_{13}H_6$-Cl_6O_2, occurring as a white to light tan, crystalline powder, effective against gram-positive organisms; used as a topical anti-infective and detergent, mainly in soaps and dermatological preparations, and in veterinary medicine to combat flukes in ruminants.

hexachromic (hek″sah-kro′mik) [*hexa-* + Gr. *chrōma* color] 1.

pertaining to or exhibiting six colors. 2. able to distinguish only six of the seven colors of the spectrum.

hexacosane (heks-ak′o-sān) [*hexa-* + Gr. *eikosi* twenty] an aliphatic hydrocarbon, $C_{26}H_{54}$, extracted from plant waxes; called also *cerane*.

hexad (hek′sad) 1. a group or combination of six similar or related entities. 2. any element having a valency of six.

hexadactylia (hek″sah-dak-til′e-ah) hexadactyly.

hexadactylism (hek″sah-dak′tĭ-lizm) hexadactyly.

hexadactyly (hek″sah-dak′tĭ-le) [*hexa-* + Gr. *daktylos* finger + *-ia*] the occurrence of six digits (fingers or toes) on one limb.

hexadecanoate (hek″sah-dek′ah-no′āt) systematic name for palmitate, denoting that it has sixteen (*hexa* six + *deca* ten) carbon acids in a straight chain.

Hexadrol (hek′sah-drol) trademark for dexamethasone.

hexafluorenium bromide (hek″sah-flūr-en′ĭ-um) [USP] chemical name: *N,N′*-di-9*H*-fluoren-9-yl-*N,N,N′,N′*-tetramethyl-1,6-hexanediaminium dibromide. A neuromuscular blocking agent, $C_{36}H_{42}Br_2N_2$, occurring as a white, crystalline powder; used in anesthesiology to prolong and potentiate the skeletal muscle relaxing action of succinylcholine during surgery, administered intravenously.

Hexagenia bilineata (hek″sah-je′ne-ah bi-lin″e-a′tah) a mayfly of the shores of Lake Erie whose cast skins may cause asthma; called also *lake fly*.

hexahydric (hek″sah-hi′drik) containing six atoms of hydrogen.

hexahydrohematoporphyrin (hek″sah-hi″dro-hem″ah-to-por″fī-rin) one of the resulting products of the treatment of heme with alcohol and a reducing agent.

hexamer (heks′ah-mer) 1. a polymer molecule composed of six monomers. 2. a capsomer having six structural subunits.

hexamethonium (hek″sah-mĕ-tho′ne-um) chemical name: *N,N,N,N′,N′,N′*-hexamethyl-1,6-hexanediaminium; a quaternary ammonium ganglion-blocking agent, $C_{10}H_{24}N_2$. **h. bromide,** the dibromide ester of hexamethonium, $C_{12}H_{30}Br_2N_2$, having the same actions as the base; has been used as an antihypertensive, but has been largely replaced by more effective drugs. **h. chloride,** the dichloride salt of hexamethonium, $C_{12}H_{30}Cl_2N_2$, having the same actions as the base; used as an antihypertensive, administered orally and parenterally.

hexamethylated (hek″sah-meth′ĭ-lāt-ed) containing six methyl groups.

hexamethylenamine (hek″sah-meth″il-ēn-am′in) methenamine.

hexamethylendiamine (hek″sah-meth″il-ēn-di′am-in) a ptomaine, $NH_2(CH_2)_6NH_2$, from decomposing pancreas and muscle.

hexamethylpararosanilin (hek″sah-meth″il-par″ah-ro-san′ĭ-lin) see *gentian violet,* under *violet*.

hexamine (hek′sah-min) methenamine.

Hexamita (heks-am′ĭ-tah) a genus of elongate flagellate protozoa of the order Polymastigida, class Zoomastigophora, which have two anterior nuclei, six anterior flagella, and two trailing flagella. It includes free-living species as well as intestinal parasites. *H. meleagridis* causes severe enteritis in wild and domestic fowl, including turkeys, chickens, quail, and partridges. *H. muris* is found in rats, mice, hamsters, and various wild rodents, *H. salmonis* in trout and salmon, and *H. columbae* in pigeons.

hexamitiasis (heks-am″ĭ-ti′ah-sis) infection with parasites of the genus *Hexamita*.

hexamylose (heks-am′ĭ-lōs) a crystalline amylose, $(C_6H_{10}O_5)_6$.

hexane (hek′sān) *n*-hexane; an aliphatic hydrocarbon of the methane series, C_6H_{14}, obtained by distillation from petroleum, occurring as a coloress, volatile, highly flammable liquid with a characteristic odor; it is a constituent of petroleum benzin, and is used as a solvent and in spectrophotometry.

Hexanicotol (hek″sah-nik′o-tol) trademark for a preparation of inositol niacinate.

hexaploid (hek′sah-ploid) 1. pertaining to or characterized by hexaploidy. 2. an individual or cell having six sets of chromosomes.

hexaploidy (hek′sah-ploi″de) the state of having six sets of chromosomes (6 n).

Hexapoda (heks-ap′o-dah) [*hexa-* + Gr. *pous* foot] insecta.

hexatomic (hek″sah-tom′ik) [*hex-* + *atom*] 1. containing six atoms of an element, or six replaceable univalent atoms. 2. in immunology, having the power of binding six complements of different strains.

hexavaccine (hek″sah-vak′sēn) a vaccine containing six different organisms.

hexavalent (hek″sah-va′lent) having a valency of six.

Hexavibex (hek″sah-vi′beks) trademark for a preparation of pyridoxine hydrochloride.

hexavitamin (hek″sah-vi′tah-min) [NF] a preparation, in capsule or tablet form, containing vitamin A, vitamin D, ascorbic acid, thiamine hydrochloride, riboflavin, and niacinamide.

hexedine (hek′sĕ-dēn) chemical name: 2,6-bis(2-ethylhexyl)-hexahydro-7a-methyl-1*H*-imidazo[1,5-*c*]imidazole; an antibacterial, $C_{22}H_{45}N_3$.

hexenmilch (hek′sen-milkh) [Ger. "witches' milk"] a milklike secretion from the breast of a newborn infant; *witch's milk*.

hexestrol (hek-ses′trol) chemical name: 4,4′-(1,2-diethyl-1,2-ethanediyl)bisphenol. A diethylstilbestrol derivative, $C_{18}H_{22}O_2$, occurring as a white, crystalline powder, having the uses of estrogen (q.v.); administered orally and parenterally.

hexethal sodium (hek′sĕ-thal) chemical name: 5-ethyl-5-hexyl-2,4,6(1*H,3H,5H*)-pyrimidinetrione monosodium salt. A short-acting barbiturate, $C_{12}H_{19}N_2NaO_3$, used as a sedative and hypnotic.

hexetidine (heks-et′ĭ-dēn) chemical name: 1,3-bis(2-ethylhexyl)hexahydro-5-methyl-5-pyrimidinamine. An antifungal, antiprotozoal, and antibacterial agent, $C_{21}H_{45}N_3$, used mainly as a topical anti-infective in the treatment of vaginitis.

hexhydric (heks-hi′drik) containing six atoms of replaceable hydrogen.

hexobarbital (hek″so-bar′bĭ-tal) [USP] chemical name: 5-(1-cyclohexen-1-yl)-2,4,6(1*H,3H,5H*)-pyrimidinetrione. A short-acting barbiturate, $C_{12}H_{16}N_2O_3$, occurring as colorless crystals or white, crystalline powder; used as a sedative, administered orally. **h. sodium,** the sodium salt of hexobarbital, $C_{12}H_{15}N_2NaO_3$, which is a very short-acting barbiturate; used for pre- and postanesthesia sedation and hypnosis, administered orally, and for induction of short anesthesia, administered intravenously.

hexobarbitone (hek″so-bar′bĭ-tōn) hexobarbital.

hexobendine (hek″so-ben′dēn) chemical name: 3,4,5-trimethoxybenzoic acid 1,2-ethanediylbis[(methylimino)-3,1-propanediyl]ester. A vasodilator, $C_{20}H_{44}N_2O_{10}$, which has been used in the treatment of coronary insufficiency and angina of effort.

hexocyclium methylsulfate (hek″so-si′kle-um) chemical name: 4-(2-cyclohexyl-2-hydroxy-2-phenylethyl)-1,1-dimethylpiperazinium methyl sulfate (salt). A quaternary ammonium anticholinergic, $C_{21}H_{36}N_2O_5S$, occurring as a white crystalline powder, which inhibits gastric secretion and gastrointestinal motility; used especially as an adjunct in the treatment of peptic ulcer, administered orally.

hexokinase (hek″so-ki′nās) ATP:D-hexose 6-phosphotransferase. An enzyme that catalyzes the transfer of a high-energy phosphate group of a donor to D-glucose, producing D-glucose-6-phosphate. See also *kinase* (def. 1).

hexonate (hek′so-nāt) chemical name: hexamethylene-1,6-bis-(trimethylammonium) nicotinate. A ganglionic blocking agent.

hexone (hek′sōn) see under *base*.

hexosamine (hek′sōs-am″in) a nitrogenous sugar in which an amino group replaces a hydroxyl group.

hexosaminidase (heks″ōs-ah-min′ĭ-dās) an enzyme occurring in two forms that catalyzes the cleavage of hexose from ganglioside GM_2. Hexosaminidase A is deficient in Tay-Sachs disease, and hexosaminidase A and B are deficient in Sandhoff's disease. The B form also catalyzes the cleavage of globoside.

hexosan (hek′so-san) an anhydride or a polymerized form of a hexose.

hexosazone (hek″so-sa′zōn) an osazone formed from a hexose.

hexose (hek′sōs) a monosaccharide containing six carbon atoms in a molecule. **h. diphosphate,** see *Harden-Young ester,* under *ester*. **h. monophosphate,** see *hexosephosphate*.

hexosephosphatase (hek″sōs-fos′fah-tās) an enzyme that catalyzes the removal of a phosphate group from hexose phosphates.

hexosephosphate (hek″sōs-fos′fāt) an ester of glucose with phosphoric acid, which aids in the absorption of sugars and which, as the Cori, Embden, Harden-Young, Neuberg and Robison esters, is important in carbohydrate metabolism. See under *ester*.

hexosyltransferase (hek″so-sil-trans′fer-ās) any of a group of enzymes that catalyzes the transfer of a hexose group, including the glucosyltransferases; called also *transhexosylase*.

hexoxidase (heks-ok′sĭ-dās) an enzyme that catalyzes the oxidation of hexuronic (ascorbic) acid.

hexyl (hek′sil) [*hex-* + Gr. *hylē* matter] a hydrocarbon, C_6H_{13}, in many isomeric forms.

***n*-hexylamine** (hek″sil-ah′mēn) a poisonous ptomaine, CH_3-$(CH_2)_5NH_2$, from spoiled yeast and rancid cod liver oil; called also *caproylamine*.

hexylcaine hydrochloride (hek′sil-kān) [USP] chemical name: 1-cyclohexylamino-2-propanol benzoate (ester) hydrochloride. A local anesthetic, $C_{16}H_{23}NO_2 \cdot HCl$, occurring as a white powder; used for infiltration, block, and topical anesthesia.

hexylresorcinol (hek″sil-rĕ-zor′sĭ-nol) [USP] chemical name: 4-hexyl-1,3-benzenediol. An anthelmintic, $C_{12}H_{18}O_2$, occurring as white, or yellowish white, needle-shaped crystals; used in the treatment of roundworm and trematode infections, administered orally.

Hey's amputation (operation), derangement, hernia, ligament, saw (hāz) [William *Hey*, English surgeon, 1736–1819] see under *amputation, derangement,* and *saw;* see en-

cysted hernia, under *hernia;* and see *margo falciformis hiatus saphenus.*

Heymans (hay′manz), Corneille. French-Belgian physiologist, born 1892; winner of the Nobel prize for medicine and physiology in 1938 for his discovery of the role played by the sinus and aortic mechanisms in the regulation of respiration.

Heynsius' test (hīn′se-oos) [Adrian *Heynsius,* Dutch physician, 1831–1885] see under *tests.*

HF Hageman factor (coagulation Factor XII).

Hf chemical symbol of *hafnium.*

Hfr high frequency of recombination; Hfr cells are the sexual or donor (male) stage of bacteria having the F (fertility) factor in the chromosome, which enables them to transfer chromosomal material to recipient (female) bacteria not having this factor.

Hg chemical symbol for mercury (L. *hydrargyrum*).

Hgb hemoglobin.

HgCl₂ corrosive mercuric chloride.

Hg₂Cl₂ mild mercurous chloride.

HGF hyperglycemic-glycogenolytic factor (glucagon).

HGG human gammaglobulin.

HGH human (pituitary) growth hormone.

HgI₂ mercuric iodide.

Hg₂I₂ mercurous iodide.

Hg(NO₃)₂ mercuric nitrate.

HgO mercuric oxide.

Hg₂O mercurous oxide.

HHb chemical symbol for *un-ionized hemoglobin.*

H. + Hm. compound hypermetropic astigmatism.

HI hydriodic acid.

5-HIAA 5-hydroxyindoleacetic acid, a metabolic product of serotonin.

hiatal (hi-a′tal) pertaining to or affecting a hiatus.

hiation (hi-a′shun) the act of yawning.

hiatopexia, hiatopexy (hi″at-o-pek′se-ah; hi-at′o-pek″se) [*hiatus* + Gr. *pēxis* fixation] surgical fixation or repair of a genital hiatus.

hiatus (hi-a′tus) [L.] [NA] general term for a gap, cleft, or opening. **adductor h.,** h. tendineus. **h. adducto′rius,** NA alternative for *h. tendineus.* **aortic h., h. aor′ticus** [NA], the opening in the diaphragm through which the aorta and thoracic duct pass. **Breschet's h.,** helicotrema. **h. of canal for greater petrosal nerve,** h. canalis nervi petrosi majoris. **h. of canal for lesser petrosal nerve,** h. canalis nervi petrosi minoris. **h. cana′lis facia′lis, h. cana′lis ner′vi petro′si majo′ris** [NA], hiatus of canal for greater petrosal nerve: an opening in the petrous part of the temporal bone in the floor of the middle cranial fossa that transmits the greater petrosal nerve and a branch of the middle meningeal artery. **h. cana′lis ner′vi petro′si mino′ris** [NA], hiatus of canal for lesser petrosal nerve: the small, laterally placed opening on the anterior surface of the pyramid of the temporal bone that transmits the lesser petrosal nerve. **esophageal h., h. esopha′geus** [NA], the opening in the diaphragm for the passage of the esophagus and the vagus nerves. **h. of facial canal, h. of fallopian canal, h. fallo′pii, false h. of fallopian canal,** h. canalis nervi petrosi majoris. **h. femora′lis,** anulus femoralis. **h. fina′lis sacra′lis,** a cleft in the lowermost sacral vertebra. **h. for greater superficial petrosal nerve,** h. canalis nervi petrosi majoris. **h. interme′dius lumbosacra′lis,** a cleft in the region of the first sacral vertebra, considered to represent a normally delayed ossification in young subjects. **h. interos′seus,** the opening above the interosseous membrane of the forearm for the passage of the posterior interosseous vessels. **h. leuke′micus,** a condition observed in acute myeloblastic leukemia in which there are numerous myeloblasts and a number of mature neutrophils in the peripheral blood, with few or no intermediate forms; called also *hiatus leukemicus of Naegeli.* **h. lumbosacra′lis,** the gap between the arches of the fifth lumbar and first sacral vertebrae, which is greater than the space between any vertebrae at a higher level. **h. maxilla′ris** [NA], **maxillary h., h. of maxillary sinus,** a very irregular opening on the medial surface of the maxillary sinus, in the articulated skull, being largely filled by parts of several adjoining bones. **neural h.,** an opening in the neural tube during the process of closure. **h. oesophage′us,** h. esophageus. **h. pleuroperitonea′lis,** an opening in the fetal diaphragm; its failure to close leaves a congenital defect which may become a site for congenital diaphragmatic hernia. Called also *foramen of Bochdalek.* **sacral h., h. sacra′lis** [NA], the opening at the inferior end of the sacral canal formed by failure of the laminae of the fifth and sometimes the fourth sacral vertebrae to meet in the midline. **saphenous h., h. saphe′nus** [NA], the depression in the fascia lata that is bridged by the cribriform fascia and perforated by the great saphenous vein; called also *fossa ovalis femoris* and *oval fossa of thigh.* **Scarpa's h.,** helicotrema. **semilunar h., h. semiluna′ris** [NA], the deep semilunar groove anterior and inferior to the bulla of the ethmoid bone; the

anterior ethmoidal air cells, the maxillary sinus, and sometimes the frontonasal duct drain through it via the ethmoid infundibulum. **subarcuate h.,** fossa subarcuata ossis temporalis. **h. tendin′eus** [NA], the opening between the long tendon of the adductor magnus and the femur, marking the distal end of the adductor canal; called also *h. adductorius.* **tentorial h.,** incisura tentorii cerebelli. **h. tota′lis sacra′lis,** a cleft in all of the sacral vertebrae, sometimes also involving one or several of the contiguous lumbar vertebrae. **vena caval h.,** foramen venae cavae. **h. of Winslow,** foramen epiploicum.

Hibbs' frame, operation (hibz) [Russell Aubra *Hibbs,* New York surgeon, 1869–1932] see under *frame* and *operation.*

hibernation (hi″ber-na′shun) [L. *hiberna* winter] the dormant state in which certain animal species pass the winter; it is characterized by narcosis and by sharp reduction in body temperature and metabolic activity. Cf. *estivation.* **artificial h.,** a state of reduced metabolism, muscle relaxation, and a twilight sleep resembling narcosis, produced pharmacodynamically by controlled inhibition of the sympathetic nervous system and reducing the level of the homeostatic reactions of the organism.

hibernoma (hi″ber-no′mah) a rare tumor made up of large polyhedral cells with coarsely granular cytoplasm, occurring on the back or around the hips. So called because it is considered by some to be a manifestation of a vestigial fat storage organ and comparable to the dorsal fat pads of hibernating animals. See also *lipoma.*

hiccough (hik′up) hiccup.

hiccup (hik′up) an involuntary spasmodic contraction of the diaphragm, causing a beginning inspiration which is suddenly checked by closure of the glottis, causing the characteristic sound; called also *singultus.* **epidemic h.,** a condition frequently seen in epidemic encephalitis.

Hicks' sign (hiks) [John Braxton *Hicks,* English gynecologist, 1823–1897] see under *sign.*

hidebound (hid′bownd) bound down tightly to the subcutaneous tissues, said of the skin in scleroderma.

hidradenitis (hi″drad-ĕ-ni′tis) [Gr. *hidrōs* sweat + *adēn* gland + *-itis*] inflammation of a sweat gland, usually of the apocrine type. **h. axilla′ris,** hidradenitis suppurativa of the axilla. **h. suppurati′va,** a disease of the apocrine sweat glands marked by the development of one or more shotlike cutaneous nodules, which gradually enlarge to the size of a pea, and undergo softening and suppuration, with subsequent discharge; called also *hidrosadenitis axillaris* and *hidrosadenitis suppurativa.*

hidradenoid (hi-drad′ĕ-noid) resembling a sweat gland; having components resembling elements of a sweat gland.

hidradenoma (hi″drad-ĕ-no′mah) a general term for tumors of the skin the components of which resemble epithelial elements of sweat glands. Several subtypes are recognized, and these are variously designated according to histologic pattern and specific component of the sweat gland unit from which the particular tumor is thought to be derived. The tumors may be nodular (solid) or papillary. The nodular types show various histologic patterns, each of which has been given a different designation: clear cell hidradenoma, epithelioma, or carcinoma; clear cell myoepithelioma; myoepithelioma; eccrine spiradenoma; eccrine acrospiroma; and mixed tumor of the skin (chondroid syringoma). The papillary hidradenoma (also known as syringocystadenoma papilliferum) is generally found only in the vulvar or perianal region. **h. erupti′vum,** hidradenoma that develops about the time of puberty, in which the lesions appear as small, yellowish papules on the chest, limbs, and lower eyelids.

hidro- (hid′ro) [Gr. *hidrōs* sweat] a combining form denoting relation to sweat or to a sweat gland.

hidroadenoma (hid″ro-ad″ĕ-no′mah) hidradenoma.

hidrocystoma (hid″ro-sis-to′mah) [*hidro-* + *cystoma*] a retention cyst of a sweat gland.

hidrocystomatosis (hi″dro-sis″to-mah-to′sis) cystic hyperplasia of the sweat glands.

hidropoiesis (hid″ro-poi-e′sis) [*hidro-* + Gr. *poiēsis* formation] the formation and secretion of sweat.

hidropoietic (hid″ro-poi-et′ik) pertaining to, characterized by, or promoting hidropoiesis.

hidrorrhea (hid-ro-re′ah) [*hidro-* + Gr. *rhoia* flow] hyperhidrosis.

hidrosadenitis (hi″dros-ad″ĕ-ni′tis) [*hidro-* + Gr. *adēn* gland + *-itis*] hidradenitis. **h. axilla′ris,** hidradenitis suppurativa. **h. des′truens suppurati′va** (*obs.*), papulonecrotic tuberculid. **h. suppurati′va,** see under *hidradenitis.*

hidroschesis (hid-ros′kĕ-sis) [*hidro-* + Gr. *schesis* holding] anhidrosis.

hidrotic (hĭ-drot′ik, hi-drot′ik) pertaining to, characterized by, or causing sweating.

hiemal (hi′ĕ-mal) pertaining to or occurring in winter.

hier- see *hiero-.*

hieralgia (hi″er-al′je-ah) [*hier-* + *-algia*] pain in the sacrum.

hiero-, hier- (hi′er-o, hi′er) [Gr. *hiern* sacred, or sacrum] a combining form denoting relationship to the sacrum, or to religion.

hierolisthesis (hi″er-o-lis-the′sis) [*hier-* + Gr. *olisthanein* to slip] displacement of the sacrum.

Highmore's antrum, body (hi′mōrz) [Nathaniel *Highmore*, English surgeon, 1613–1685] see *sinus maxillaris* and *mediastinum testis.*

hila (hi′lah) [L.] plural of *hilum.*

hilar (hi′lar) pertaining to a hilus.

hilastic (hi-las′tik) [Gr. *hilasmos* propitiation, sacrifice] in Greek medicine, prophylactic, in the sense of diverting disease by rites of propitiation.

Hildebrandt's test (hil′de-brants) [Fritz *Hildebrandt*, German pharmacologist, born 1887] see under *tests.*

Hildenbrand's disease (hil′den-brands) [Johann Valentin von *Hildenbrand*, Austrian physician, 1763–1818] typhus.

hili (hi′li) [L.] plural of *hilus.*

hilifuge (hi′lĭ-fūj) [L. *hilus* + *fugere* to flee] radiating from the hilus of the lung; said of opacities seen on x-ray films.

hilitis (hi-li′tis) inflammation of a hilus, especially of the hilus of the lung.

Hill (hil′), Archibald Vivian. English biochemist, born 1886, noted for work on heat loss in muscle contraction; co-winner, with Otto Fritz Meyerhof, of the Nobel prize for medicine and physiology in 1922 for his discovery relating to the production of heat in muscle.

hillock (hil′ok) a small prominence or elevation. **auricular h's,** embryonic tubercles adjoining the first branchial groove that give rise to the auricle of the ear. **axon h.,** the conical expansion of an axon at its point of attachment to the body of the nerve cell. **Doyère's h.,** see under *eminence.* **germ h., germ-bearing h.,** cumulus oophorus. **seminal h.,** colliculus seminalis.

Hilton's law, line, muscle, sac (hil′tunz) [John *Hilton*, English surgeon, 1804–1878] see under *law;* see *pectinate line,* under *line;* and see *musculus aryepiglotticus* and *sacculus laryngis.*

hilum (hi′lum), pl. *hi′la* [L.]; hilus; see also entries under *hilus.*

hilus (hi′lus), pl. *hi′li* [L. "a small thing"] [NA] a general term for a depression or pit at that part of an organ where the vessels and nerves enter. Called also *hilum.* **h. glan′dulae suprarena′lis** [NA], hilus of suprarenal gland: the depression on the anterior surface of the suprarenal gland where the suprarenal vein enters the gland. **h. hep′atis,** porta hepatis. **h. of kidney,** h. renalis. **h. lie′nis** [NA], hilus of the spleen: the fissure on the gastric surface of the spleen where the vessels and nerves enter. **h. of lung,** h. pulmonis. **h. of lymph node,** h. nodi lymphatici. **h. lymphoglan′dulae,** h. nodi lymphatici. **h. no′di lymphat′ici** [NA], hilus of lymph node: the indentation on a lymph node where the arteries enter and the veins and efferent lymphatic vessels leave; called also *h. lymphoglandulae.* **h. nu′clei denta′ti** [NA], the white core of the dentate nucleus of the cerebellum. **h. nu′clei oliva′ris** [NA], hilus of olivary nucleus: the white core of the inferior olivary nucleus of the medulla oblongata, most prominent medially. **h. of olivary nucleus,** h. nuclei olivaris. **h. ova′rii** [NA], **h. of ovary,** the point on the mesovarial border of the ovary where the vessels and nerves enter. **h. pulmo′nis** [NA], hilus of the lung: the depression on the mediastinal surface of the lung where the bronchus and the blood vessels and nerves enter. **h. rena′lis** [NA], hilus of the kidney: the point on the medial margin of the kidney where the vessels, nerves, and ureter enter. **h. of spleen,** h. lienis. **h. of suprarenal gland,** h. glandulae suprarenalis.

himantosis (hi″man-to′sis) [Gr. *himantōsis,* from *himas* strap] elongation of the uvula.

hinchazon (hinch″ah-zon′) [Cuban] beriberi.

hindbrain (hīnd′brān) rhombencephalon.

Hindenlang's test (hin′den-lahngz) [Karl *Hindenlang*, German physician, 1854–1884] see under *tests.*

hindfoot (hīnd′foot) the posterior portion of the foot, comprising the region of the talus and calcaneus.

hindgut (hīnd′gut) the embryonic structure from which chiefly the colon is formed.

hind-kidney (hīnd-kid′ne) the metanephros.

Hines-Brown test (hīnz-brown) [Edgar Alphonso *Hines*, Jr., American physician, born 1906; George Elgie *Brown*, American physician, 1885–1935] see under *tests.*

hinge-bow (hinj′bo) a face-bow whose caliper ends can be adjusted to permit location of the axis of rotation of the mandible; adjustable axis face-bow.

Hinton test (hin′ton) [William Augustus *Hinton*, American bacteriologist, born 1883] see under *tests.*

HIO₃ iodic acid.

hip (hip) 1. the area of the body lateral to and including the hip joint; called also *coxa* [NA]. 2. loosely, the hip joint. **h. pointer,** contusion of the bone of the iliac crest or avulsion of muscle attachments of the iliac crest. **snapping h.,** a condition marked by a slipping around of the hip joint, sometimes with

an audible snap, due to the slipping of a tendinous band over the greater trochanter; called also *Perrin-Ferraton disease.*

hipped (hipt) having a fracture at the point of the hip; said of horses.

Hippel's disease (hip′elz) [Eugen von *Hippel*, German ophthalmologist, 1867–1939] von Hippel's disease; see under *disease.*

Hippelates (hip″ĕ-la′tēz) a genus of insects of the family Chloropidae, order Diptera. **H. fla′vipes,** the probable mechanical vector of yaws in Haiti. **H. pal′lipes,** a species that is thought to be the mechanical vector of yaws in Jamaica; called also *Oscinis pallipes.* **H. pu′sio,** the "eye gnat" of California and Florida and other southern states, which is the mechanical vector of epidemic conjunctivitis, usually of a severe, follicular type.

Hippel-Lindau disease (hip′el-lin′dow) [Eugen von *Hippel;* Arvid *Lindau*, Swedish pathologist, born 1892] von Hippel-Lindau disease; see under *disease.*

Hippeutis (hi-pu′tis) a genus of fresh-water snails. **H. canto′ri,** one of the principal intermediate hosts of the trematode *Fasciolopsis buski* in eastern China.

hippo (hip′po) ipecac.

hippo- [Gr. *hippos* horse] a combining form denoting relationship to a horse.

Hippobosca (hip-o-bos′kah) [*hippo-* + Gr. *boskein* to feed] the typical genus of the family Hippoboscidae. They are pupiparous, dipterous, parasitic insects, called winged tick flies. **H. ru′fipes,** a fly of South America whose bite transmits *Trypanosoma theileri.*

Hippoboscidae (hip″o-bos′kĭ-de) a family of parasitic flies found on bird and mammals; some have wings, others are wingless. It includes the genera *Hippobosca, Melaphagus,* and *Pseudolynchia.*

hippocampal (hip″o-kam′pal) pertaining to the hippocampus.

hippocampus (hip″o-kam′pus) [Gr. *hippokampos* sea horse] [NA] a curved elevation in the floor of the inferior horn of the lateral ventricle; interlocked with the more medially placed dentate gyrus, it consists of archipallium with three variable cell layers: the stratum oriens with polymorphic cells; a layer of double pyramids subdivided into the stratum radiatum (dendritic segment) and the stratum lucidum (cellular segment); and a layer of polymorphic cells comprising the stratum moleculare and stratum lacunosum. It is an important functional component of the limbic system and its efferent projections form the fornix. Called also *hippocampus major, Ammon's horn,* and *cornu Ammonis.* **h. ma′jor,** hippocampus. **h. mi′nor,** calcar avis. **h. nu′dus** (*obs.*), an inconstant small part of the hippocampus in the space formed by the splenial bending of the fascia dentata.

hippocoprosterol (hip″o-ko-pros′ter-ol) [*hippo-* + Gr. *kopros* dung + *sterol*] a sterol found in the feces of herbivorous animals and derived from the phytosterol of grass and other food plants, $C_{27}H_{54}O$; possibly related to coprostanol.

Hippocrates (hip-pok′rah-tēz) **of Cos** (late 5th century B.C.) the famous Greek physician who is generally regarded as the "Father of Medicine." Many of the writings of Hippocrates and his school have survived—the so-called *Corpus Hippocraticum,* but it is not certain which were written by Hippocrates himself; these writings are usually characterized by the stress laid on treatment and prognosis. An oath which appears in the body of work attributed to Hippocrates and his school, and known as the *Hippocratic oath,* has been the ethical guide of the medical profession since those days. It is as follows:

"I swear by Apollo the physician, by Æsculapius, Hygeia, and Panacea, and I take to witness all the gods, all the goddesses, to keep according to my ability and my judgment the following Oath:

"To consider dear to me as my parents him who taught me this art; to live in common with him and if necessary to share my goods with him; to look upon his children as my own brothers, to teach them this art if they so desire without fee or written promise; to impart to my sons and the sons of the master who taught me and the disciples who have enrolled themselves and have agreed to the rules of the profession, but to these alone, the precepts and the instruction. I will prescribe regimen for the good of my patients according to my ability and my judgment and never do harm to anyone. To please no one will I prescribe a deadly drug, nor give advice which may cause his death. Nor will I give a woman a pessary to procure abortion. But I will preserve the purity of my life and my art. I will not cut for stone, even for patients in whom the disease is manifest; I will leave this operation to be performed by practitioners (specialists in this art). In every house where I come I will enter only for the good of my patients, keeping myself far from all intentional ill-doing and all seduction, and especially from the pleasures of love with women or with men, be they free or slaves. All that may come to my knowledge in the exercise of my profession or outside of my profession or in daily commerce with men, which ought not to be spread abroad, I will keep secret and will never reveal. If I keep this oath faithfully, may I enjoy my life and practice my art, respected by all men and in all times; but if I swerve from it or violate it, may the reverse be my lot."

hippocratic (hip″po-krat′ik) pertaining to or described by Hippocrates of Cos, or pertaining to the school of medicine founded by him.

hippocratism (hip-pok′rah-tizm) the system of medicine attributed to Hippocrates and his school, based on imitating the processes of nature, and emphasizing treatment and prognosis.

hippocratist (hip-pok′rah-tist) a believer in or practitioner of the system of medicine attributed to Hippocrates and his school.

hippolite (hip′o-līt) hippolith.

hippolith (hip′o-lith) [*hippo-* + Gr. *lithos* stone] a bezoar, or concretion, from the alimentary tract of the horse.

hippomane (hĭ-pom′ah-ne) small, rounded, flat, amber bodies found in the allantoic fluid of various animals, especially the ungulates and ruminants.

hippomelanin (hip″o-mel′ah-nin) [*hippo-* + Gr. *melas* black] a black pigment from tumors and marrow of horses affected with melanosis.

hippostercorin (hip″o-ster′ko-rin) hippocoprosterol.

hippulin (hip′u-lin) a crystalline estrogenic steroid, $C_{18}H_{20}O_2$, with four double bonds, obtained from the urine of pregnant mares.

hippurase (hip′u-rās) hippuricase.

hippurate (hip′u-rāt) any salt of hippuric acid.

hippuria (hĭ-pu′re-ah) [*hippo-* + Gr. *ouron* urine + *-ia*] excess of hippuric acid in the urine.

hippuric (hĭ-pu′rik) [*hippo-* + Gr. *ouron* urine] derivable from the urine of horses; see under *acid*.

hippuricase (hĭ-pu′ri-kās) aminoacylase.

hippus (hip′us) [Gr. *hippos* a complaint of the eyes, such that they are always winking] abnormally exaggerated rhythmic contraction and dilation of the pupil, independent of changes in illumination or in fixation of the eyes; called also *pupillary athetosis.*

Hiprex (hi′preks) trademark for a preparation of methenamine hippurate.

hirci (hir′si) [L., plural of *hircus*] [NA] the hairs growing in the axilla.

hircin (hir′sin) [L. *hircus* goat] (obs.) ill-smelling component(s) of the suet of goats.

hircismus (hir-siz′mus) [L. *hircus* goat] the strong odor of the axillae caused by bacterial decomposition of apocrine sweat, formed only in that site.

hircus (hir′kus), pl. *hir′ci* [L. "a goat"] see *hirci.*

Hirschberg's magnet, method (hirsh′bergz) [Julius *Hirschberg,* German ophthalmologist, 1843–1925] see under *magnet* and *method.*

Hirschfeld's canals (hirsh′feldz) [I. *Hirschfeld,* American dentist] interdental canals.

Hirschfeld's disease [Felix *Hirschfeld,* German physician, born 1863] see under *disease.*

Hirschfelder's tuberculin (hirsh′fel-derz) [Joseph Oakland *Hirschfelder,* American physician, 1854–1920] oxytuberculin.

Hirschsprung's disease (hirsh′sproongz) [Harald *Hirschsprung,* a Danish physician, 1830–1916] see under *disease.*

hirsute (her′soot) [L. *hirsutus*] shaggy; having abundant or excessive hair.

hirsuties (her-soo′she-ēz) hirsutism.

hirsutism (her′soot-izm) abnormal hairiness, especially an adult male pattern of hair distribution in women. Cf. *hypertrichosis.*

hirudicidal (hĭ-roo″dĭ-si′dal) destructive to leeches.

hirudicide (hĭ-roo′dĭ-sīd) an agent that is destructive to leeches.

hirudin (hĭ-roo′din) [L. *hirudo* leech] the active principle of the secretion of the buccal glands of leeches; it has the power of preventing coagulation of the blood by acting as an antithrombin.

Hirudinaria (hir″u-dĭ-na′re-ah) a genus of leeches of the family Gnathobdella.

Hirudinea (hir″u-din′e-ah) a class of the Annelida; the leeches. It includes the genera *Haementeria, Hirudo, Hirudinaria, Haemadipsa, Limnatis, Macrobdella,* and *Haemopis.*

hirudiniasis (hir″u-dĭ-ni′ah-sis) invasion of the nose, mouth, pharynx, or larynx by leeches; attachment of leeches to the skin.

hirudinization (hĭ-roo″dĭ-ni-za′shun) [L. *hirudo* leech] 1. the process of rendering the blood noncoagulable by the injection of hirudin. 2. the application of leeches; leeching.

hirudinize (hĭ-roo′dĭ-nīz) to render the blood noncoagulable by the injection of hirudin.

Hirudo (hĭ-roo′do), pl. *hiru′dines* [L. "leech"] a genus of leeches of the family Gnathobdellidae, class Hirudinea. **H. aegyp′ti′aca,** *Limnatis nilotica.* **H. japon′ica,** the medicinal leech of Japan. **H. javan′ica,** a leech of Java, Batavia, and Burma, reported to produce internal hirudiniasis. **H. medicina′lis,** olive-gray leech formerly used extensively for therapeutic purposes. **H. quinquestria′ta,** a leech occurring in Australia. **H. sanguisor′ba,** *Haemopis sanguisuga.* **H. trocti′na,** the

common European leech, which is marked with green, orange, and black somewhat like a trout.

His histidine.

His bundle (band), disease, spindle (his′ez) [Wilhelm *His,* Jr., Swiss physician, 1863–1934] see under *bundle,* and see *trench fever,* under *fever,* and *aortic spindle* under *spindle.*

His bursa, canal (duct), space, zones [Wilhelm *His,* eminent German anatomist and embryologist, 1831–1904] see under *bursa, space,* and *zone,* and see *ductus thyroglossus.*

His-Werner disease (his′ver′ner) [William *His,* Jr.; Heinrich *Werner,* German physician, born 1874] trench fever.

Hispril (his′pril) trademark for a preparation of diphenylpyraline hydrochloride.

Hiss capsule stain (his) [Philip Hanson *Hiss,* Jr., American bacteriologist, 1869–1913] see under *Table of Stains.*

hist- see *histo-.*

Histadyl (his′tah-dil) trademark for preparations of methapyrilene.

histaffine (his-taf′in) [Gr. *histos* tissue + L. *affinis* having affinity for] 1. having affinity for tissues. 2. a substance present in the blood serum of animals affected with certain diseases that combines with certain constituents of the tissues to produce the phenomenon of complement fixation.

Histalog (his′tah-log) trademark for a preparation of betazole.

histaminase (his-tam′ĭ-nās) diamine:oxygen oxidoreductase. An enzyme that has the power of deaminating histamine; it has been used in the treatment of allergic dermatoses and intestinal intoxications. Called also *diamine oxidase.*

histamine (his′tah-mēn) chemical name: 1*H*-imidazole-4-ethanamine. A decarboxylation product of histidine, $C_5H_9N_3$, found in all body tissues, particularly in the mast cells and their related blood basophils, the highest concentration being in the lungs. It is also present in ergot and other plants and may be synthesized outside the body from histidine or citric acid. It has several functions, including (1) dilation of capillaries, which increases capillary permeability and results in a drop of blood pressure, (2) contraction of most smooth muscle tissue, including bronchial smooth muscle of the lung, (3) induction of increased gastric secretion, and (4) acceleration of the heart rate. It is also responsible for the triple response, and is implicated as a mediator of immediate hypersensitivity. On the basis of the antagonistic effects of antihistamines, it is postulated that cellular receptors of histamine are of two types: The H_1 receptors mediate the contraction of smooth muscle and the effects on capillaries; the H_2 receptors mediate the acceleration of heart rate and the promotion of gastric acid secretion. Both H_1 and H_2 receptors mediate the contraction of vascular smooth muscle. Histamine has also been postulated to be a neurotransmitter in the central nervous system. **h.₁,** the cellular receptor site for histamine responsible for the dilation of blood vessels and the contraction of smooth muscle; abbreviated H_1. **h.₂,** the cellular receptor site for histamine responsible for the stimulation of heart rate and gastric secretion; abbreviated H_2. **h. hydrochloride,** the dihydrochloride salt of histamine, $C_5H_9N_3 \cdot 2HCl$, having the same actions as the base; used as an active ingredient of several analgesic dermatological preparations. **h. phosphate** [USP], the phosphate salt of histamine, $C_5H_9N_3 \cdot 2H_3PO_4$, occurring as colorless, long prismatic crystals, having the same actions as the base; used as a diagnostic aid in testing gastric secretion, administered subcutaneously. It is also used in the diagnosis of pheochromocytoma and has been used in treating various allergic manifestations, for desensitization in cases of hypersensitivity, and in the treatment of peripheral vascular diseases, Meniere's disease, and headache.

histaminemia (his-tam″ĭ-ne′me-ah) the presence of histamine in the blood.

histaminergic (his″tah-min-er′jic) denoting those responses by histamine receptors to histamine that are blocked by histamine antagonists (e.g., cimetidine).

histaminia (his″tah-min′e-ah) a condition of shock caused by excess of histamine developed in the body or administered therapeutically.

histanoxia (his″tan-ok′se-ah) [*hist-* + *anoxia*] oxygen deprivation of the tissues due to a lessening of the blood supply.

Histaspan (his′tah span) trademark for preparations of chlorpheniramine maleate.

histic (his′tik) pertaining to or of the nature of tissue.

histidase (his′tĭ-dās) L-histidine ammonia-lyase. An enzyme of the liver that opens the imidazole ring of histidine, liberating ammonia.

histidinase (his′tĭ-dĭ-nās) histidase.

histidine (his′tĭ-din) an α-amino acid, beta-4-imidazolyl alanine, $N{:}CH \cdot NH \cdot CH{:}C \cdot CH_2CH(NH_2)COOH$, essential for optimal

growth in infants; first found as a decomposition product of the protamine of sturgeon testes (Kossel, 1896), obtainable from many proteins by the action of sulfuric acid and water. The decarboxylation of histidine results in the formation of histamine. **h.**

monohydrochloride, a crystalline substance, $C_6H_9N_3O_2 \cdot HCl$, once believed to be useful in the treatment of peptic ulcer.

histidinemia (his″tĭ-dĭ-ne′me-ah) a hereditary defect of metabolism characterized by excessive amounts of histidine in the blood and urine owing to deficient histidase activity, with consequent failure to metabolize histidine to urocanic acid. Many affected persons suffer modest mental retardation and disordered speech development. It is transmitted as an autosomal recessive trait. Called also *ahistidasia.*

histidinuria (his″tĭ-dĭ-nu′re-ah) an excess of histidine in the urine; see *histidinemia.*

histio- (his′te-o) [Gr. *histion,* diminutive of *histos* web, tissue] a combining form denoting relationship to tissue.

histioblast (his′te-o-blast″) a local histiocyte (macrophage).

histiocyte (his′te-o-sīt″) [*histio-* + Gr. *kytos* hollow vessel] macrophage. **cardiac h.,** Anitschkow's myocyte. **sea-blue h.,** a morphologically distinct, granulated histiocyte, sea-blue in color; see under *syndrome.* **wandering h's,** an active macrophage.

histiocytic (his′te-o-sit′ik) pertaining to or containing histiocytes.

histiocytoma (his″te-o-si-to′mah) [*histiocyte* + *-oma*] a tumor containing histiocytes (macrophages). **fibrous h.,** dermatofibroma. **lipoid h.,** fibroxanthoma.

histiocytomatosis (his″te-o-si-to″mah-to′sis) any generalized disorder of the reticuloendothelial system, such as xanthomatosis, Gaucher's disease, Niemann-Pick disease, lymphogranulomatosis, etc.

histiocytosis (his″te-o-si-to′sis) a condition marked by the abnormal appearance of histiocytes (macrophages) in the blood. **lipid h.,** Niemann-Pick disease. **sinus h.,** a disorder of the lymph nodes in which the distended sinuses are completely, or nearly completely, filled by histiocytes, as a result of active multiplication of the littoral cells. **h. X,** a generic term embracing eosinophilic granuloma, Letterer-Siwe disease, and Hand-Schüller-Christian disease, and indicating a shared common origin for the three entities and a common morphologic characteristic: a granulomatous infiltration composed of large histiocytes with pale eosinophilic, foamy cytoplasm and well-delimited nuclei.

histiogenic (his″te-o-jen′ik) histogenous.

histioid (his′te-oid) histoid.

histio-irritative (his″te-o-ir′ĭ-ta″tiv) [*histio-* + *irritative*] having an irritative effect on connective tissue.

histioma (his″te-o′mah) histoma.

histionic (his″te-on′ik) pertaining to or derived from a tissue.

histo-, hist- [Gr. *histos* web, tissue] a combining form denoting relationship to tissue.

histoblast (his′to-blast) [*histo-* + Gr. *blastos* germ] a tissue-forming cell.

histochemical (his″to-kem′ĭ-kal) pertaining to histochemistry or to the chemical components or activities of cells or tissues.

histochemistry (his″to-kem′is-tre) that branch of histology which deals with the identification of chemical components in cells and tissues.

histochemotherapy (his″to-ke″mo-ther′ah-pe) see *chemotherapy.*

histochromatosis (his″to-kro″mah-to′sis) [*histo-* + Gr. *chrōma* color] a general term for affections of the reticuloendothelial system, including xanthochromatosis, Gaucher's disease, and lymphogranulomatosis.

histoclastic (his″to-klas′tik) [*histo-* + Gr. *klastos* broken] breaking down tissue; said of certain cells.

histoclinical (his″to-klin′ĭ-kal) combining histological and clinical evaluation.

histocompatibility (his″to-kom-pat″ĭ-bil′ĭ-te) the quality or state of being histocompatible.

histocompatible (his″to-kom-pat″ĭ-b'l) capable of being accepted and remaining functional; said of that relationship between the genotypes of donor and host in which a graft generally will not be rejected, a relationship determined by the presence of compatible HLA antigens (see under *antigen*).

histocyte (his′to-sīt) histiocyte.

histodiagnosis (his″to-di″ag-no′sis) [*histo-* + *diagnosis*] diagnosis by microscopical examination of the tissues.

histodialysis (his″to-di-al′ĭ-sis) [*histo-* + *dialysis*] the disintegration or breaking down of tissues.

histodifferentiation (his″to-dif″er-en″she-a′shun) the acquisition of tissue characteristics by cell groups.

histofluorescence (his″to-floo″o-res′ens) fluorescence produced in the body by the administration of some substance previous to exposure to the roentgen rays.

histogenesis (his″to-jen′ĕ-sis) [*histo-* + Gr. *genesis* production] the formation or development of tissues from the undifferentiated cells of the germ layers of the embryo.

histogenetic (his″to-jĕ-net′ik) pertaining to histogenesis.

histogenous (his-toj′ĕ-nus) [*histo-* + Gr. *gennan* to produce] formed by the tissues.

histogeny (his-toj′ĕ-ne) histogenesis.

histogram (his′to-gram) [*histo* + Gr. *gramma* a drawing, picture] a diagram or graph in which the values found in a statistical study are represented by vertical bars or rectangles.

histography (his-tog′rah-fe) [*histo-* + Gr. *graphein* to write] description of the tissues.

histohematin (his″to-hem′ah-tin) [*histo-* + *hematin*] cytochrome, def. 1.

histohematogenous (his″to-hem″ah-toj′ĕ-nus) [*histo-* + Gr. *haima* blood + *gennan* to produce] formed from both the tissues and the blood.

histohydria (his″to-hi′dre-ah) the presence of an excessive amount of water in body tissue.

histohypoxia (his″to-hi-pok′se-ah) an abnormally diminished concentration of oxygen in the tissues.

histoid (his′toid) [*histo-* + Gr. *eidos* form] 1. weblike. 2. developed from but one kind of tissue. 3. like one of the tissues of the body.

histoincompatibility (his″to-in″kom-pat″ĭ-bil′ĭ-te) the quality or state of being histoincompatible.

histoincompatible (his″to-in″kom-pat″ĭ-b'l) not being accepted or remaining functional; said of that relationship between the genotypes of donor and host in which a graft generally will be rejected.

histokinesis (his″to-ki-ne′sis) [*histo-* + Gr. *kinēsis* motion] movement in the tissues of the body.

histologic, histological (his″-to-log′-ik; his″to-log′ĭ-kal) pertaining to histology.

histologist (his-tol′o-jist) one who specializes in histology.

histology (his-tol′o-je) [*histo-* + *-logy*] that department of anatomy which deals with the minute structure, composition, and function of the tissues; called also *microscopical anatomy.* **normal h.,** the histology of normal tissues. **pathologic h.,** the histology of diseased tissues; histopathology.

histolysate (his-tol′ĭ-zāt) a substance formed by histolysis.

histolysis (his-tol′ĭ-sis) [*histo-* + Gr. *lyein* to loosen] the dissolution or the breaking down of tissues.

histolytic (his″to-lit′ik) pertaining to, characterized by, or causing histolysis.

histoma (his-to′mah) [*histo-* + *-oma*] any tissue tumor, as a fibroma.

histometaplastic (his″to-met″ah-plas′tik) pertaining to, characterized by, or stimulating metaplasia of tissue.

Histomonas (his-to′mo-nas) a genus of parasitic protozoa of the order Rhizomastigida, class Zoomastigophora, found in the cecum, liver, and other tissues of turkeys, chickens, ducks, and geese. They have both an ameboid and a flagellate stage. *H. meleagridis* causes histomoniasis (blackhead) of turkeys.

histomoniasis (his″to-mo-ni′ah-sis) infection with organisms of the genus *Histomonas.* **h. of turkeys,** an infectious disease of turkeys caused by *Histomonas meleagridis,* with lesions of the intestine and liver and a dark discoloration of the comb; called also *blackhead, enterohepatitis,* and *typhlohepatitis.*

histomorphology (his″to-mor-fol′o-je) the morphology of tissues; histology.

histone (his′tōn) a simple protein containing many basic groups, soluble in water and insoluble in dilute ammonia. The globin of hemoglobin is a histone. Combined with nucleic acids they form nucleohistone, and are associated with DNA in chromatin. Some are decidedly poisonous and contain a considerable amount of phosphorus. Blood treated with histone is altered so that it coagulates with difficulty. Histone has been found in the urine in leukemia and febrile conditions. Cf. *protamine.* **h. nucleinate,** a compound of nucleic acid and histone, the characteristic constituent of lymph glands, spleen, and thymus.

histoneurology (his″to-nu-rol′o-je) [*histo-* + *neurology*] the histology of the nervous system; neurohistology.

histonomy (his-ton′o-me) [*histo-* + Gr. *nomos* law] the scientific study of tissues based on the translation, into biological terms, of quantitative laws derived from histological measurement.

histonuria (his-tōn-u′re-ah) [*histone* + Gr. *ouron* urine + *-ia*] the presence of histone in the urine.

histopathology (his″to-pah-thol′o-je) [*histo-* + *pathology*] pathologic histology.

histophysiology (his″to-fiz″e-ol′o-je) [*histo-* + *physiology*] the correlation of function with the microscopic structure of cells and tissues.

Histoplasma (his″to-plaz′mah) a genus of imperfect fungi of the family Moniliaceae, order Moniliales. **H. capsula′tum,** the etiologic agent of classic histoplasmosis, occurring as small, oval, yeastlike cells which in tissue seem to be encapsulated but are not. It grows as a mycelial fungus in the soil and as a yeast at 37° C. on agar or in tissue. Formerly called *Cryptococcus capsulatus.* **H. capsula′tum** var. **duboi′sii,** a species larger than *H. capsulatum* and *H. farciminosus,* that is the cause of the African form of histoplasmosis. **H. farcimino′sus,** the etiologic agent of lymphangitis epizootica, differing from *H. cap-*

sulatum and *H. duboisii* in having smooth macroaleuriospores in the saprophytic stage; formerly called *Blastomyces farciminosus, Leishmania farciminosa,* and *Zymonema farciminosum.*

histoplasmin (his″to-plaz′min) [USP] a sterile, standardized liquid concentrate of the soluble growth products developed by the fungus *Histoplasma capsulatum,* when grown in the mycelial phase on a synthetic medium, which contains a certified red dye; used as a dermal reactivity indicator in the diagnosis of histoplasmosis. Infection, past or present, is indicated by an area of induration of 5 mm. or larger, appearing 24 to 48 hours after injection.

histoplasmoma (his″to-plaz-mo′mah) [*Histoplasma* + Gr. -*oma* tumor] a rounded granulomatous density of the lung caused by infection with *Histoplasma capsulatum* and seen radiographically as a coin-shaped lesion.

histoplasmosis (his″to-plaz-mo′sis) infection resulting from inhalation or, infrequently, the ingestion of spores of *Histoplasma capsulatum.* Worldwide in distribution, it is particularly common in midwestern United States. The infection is asymptomatic in most cases, but in 1–5 per cent, it causes acute pneumonia, or disseminated reticuloendothelial hyperplasia with hepatosplenomegaly and anemia, or an influenza-like illness with joint effusion and erythema nodosum. Reactivated infection involves the lungs, meninges, heart, peritoneum, and adrenals in that order of frequency. It can be diagnosed by culture, or by demonstration of a rise in complement-fixing antibody titers in serum. **African h.,** a disease differentiated from the classic form of histoplasmosis by large yeast forms of *Histoplasma capsulatum* var. *duboisii* in the tissues. **ocular h.,** disseminated choroiditis resulting in scars in the periphery of the fundus near the optic nerve, and characteristic disciform macular lesions; *Histoplasma capsulatum* is strongly implicated as the causative agent.

histoplast (his′to-plast) (*obs.*) Wassermann's preparation containing extract of live staphylococcus; used locally in treatment of furuncle.

historadiography (his″to-ra″de-og′rah-fe) [*histo-* + *radiography*] roentgenography of microscopic sections of tissue.

historetention (his″to-re-ten′shun) retention of matter by the tissues.

historrhexis (his″to-rek′sis) [*histo-* + Gr. *rhēxis* rupture] breaking up of tissue; Southard's term for focal destruction of nerve tissue of noninfectious nature.

histoteliosis (his″to-tel″e-o′sis) [*histo-* + Gr. *tēle* + -*osis*] the final differentiation of cells whose fate has already been determined irreversibly.

histotherapy (his″to-ther′ah-pe) [*histo-* + *therapy*] the treatment of disease by the administration of animal tissues.

histothrombin (his″to-throm′bin) thrombin from connective tissue.

histotome (his′to-tōm) [*histo-* + Gr. *tomē* a cutting] microtome.

histotomy (his-tot′o-me) [*histo-* + Gr. *temnein* to cut] the dissection of the tissues; microtomy.

histotoxic (his″to-tok′sik) [*histo-* + Gr. *toxikon* poison] poisonous to tissue or tissues.

histotroph (his′to-trōf) [*histo-* + Gr. *trophē* nourishment] the sum total of nutritive substances supplied to the embryo in viviparous animals from sources other than the mother's blood. Cf. *hemotroph.*

histotrophic (his″to-trof′ik) 1. encouraging the formation of tissue. 2. pertaining to histotroph; with reference to nutrition through histotroph.

histotropic (his″to-trop′ik) [*histo-* + Gr. *tropos* a turning] having special affinity for tissue cells.

histozoic (his″to-zo′ik) [*histo-* + Gr. *zōē* life] living on or within the tissues; said of parasites.

histozyme (his′to-zīm) [*histo-* + Gr. *zymē* leaven] aminoacylase.

histrionic (his″tre-on′ik) pertaining to or characterized by histrionism.

histrionism (his′tre-o-nizm″) [L. *histrio* actor] the morbid or hysterical adoption of an exaggerated manner and gestures.

Hittorf's number, tube (hit′orf) [Johann Wilhelm *Hittorf,* German physicist, 1824–1914] see under *number,* and see *Crookes' tube,* under *tube.*

Hitzig's girdle, test (hits′igz) [Eduard *Hitzig,* German psychiatrist, 1838–1907] see under *girdle* and *tests.*

hives (hīvz) urticaria.

Hl symbol for *latent hyperopia.*

HLA see under *antigen.*

Hm symbol for *manifest hyperopia.*

HMG human menopausal gonadotropin.

HMO health maintenance organization.

HNO₂ nitrous acid.

HNO₃ nitric acid.

Ho chemical symbol for *holmium.*

H₂O water.

H_2O_2 hydrogen peroxide.

hoarseness (hōrs′nes) a rough or noisy quality of voice.

Hoboken's nodules, valves (ho′bo-kenz) [Nicolas von *Hoboken,* Dutch anatomist and physician, 1632–1678] see under *nodule* and *valve.*

Hoche's bandelette (hōk′ez) [Alfred Erich *Hoche,* German psychiatrist, 1865–1943] a small bundle of nerve fibers forming part of the fasciculi proprii.

Hochenegg's operation (hōk′en-egz) [Julius von *Hochenegg,* Vienna surgeon, 1859–1940] see under *operation.*

Hochsinger's phenomenon, sign (hōk′sing-erz) [Karl *Hochsinger,* Austrian pediatrician, born 1860] see under *phenomenon* and *sign.*

hock (hok) the tarsal joint or region of the tarsus in the hind leg of the horse or ox. **capped h.,** a cyst or a thickening of the skin over the point of the calcaneus in the horse. **curby h.,** a hock affected with curb. **spring h.,** stringhalt.

Hodara's disease (ho-dar′ahz) [Menahem *Hodara,* Turkish physician, died 1926] see under *disease.*

hodegetics (hod″ē-jet′iks) [Gr. *hodēgētikos* fitted for guiding] medical ethics.

Hodge's forceps, pessary, plane, etc. (hoj′ez) [Hugh Lenox *Hodge,* American gynecologist, 1796–1873] see under the nouns.

Hodgen splint (apparatus) (hoj′en) [John Thompson *Hodgen,* American surgeon, 1826–1882] see under *splint.*

Hodgkin (hoj′kin), Alan Lloyd. English physiologist, born 1914; co-winner, with John Carew Eccles and Andrew Fielding Huxley, of the Nobel prize in medicine and physiology for 1963, for discoveries concerning the ionic mechanisms involved in excitation and inhibition in the peripheral and central portions of the nerve cell membrane.

Hodgkin's cells, disease (granuloma), sarcoma (hoj′kinz) [Thomas *Hodgkin,* English physician, 1798–1866] see Sternberg-Reed cells, under *cell,* and see under *disease* and *sarcoma.*

Hodgson's disease (hoj′sonz) [Joseph *Hodgson,* English physician, 1788–1869] see under *disease.*

hodoneuromere (ho″do-nu′ro-mēr) [Gr. *hodos* path + *neuron* nerve + *meros* part] a segment of the embryonic trunk with its pair of nerves and their branches.

Hoehne's sign (ha′nez) [Ottomar *Hoehne,* German gynecologist, 1871–1932] see under *sign.*

hof [Ger. "court"] the area of the cytoplasm of a cell encircled by the concavity of the nucleus.

Hofacker-Sadler law (hof-ak′er sad′ler) [Johann Daniel *Hofacker,* German obstetrician, 1788–1828; Michael Thomas *Sadler,* English obstetrician, 1834–1923] see under *law.*

Hofbauer cells (hof′bow-er) [J. Isfred Isidore *Hofbauer,* American gynecologist, born 1878] see under *cell.*

Hoff see *van't Hoff.*

Hoffa's disease, operation (hof′az) [Albert *Hoffa,* German surgeon, 1859–1907] see under *disease,* and see *Lorenz's operation,* under *operation.*

Hoffa-Lorenz operation (hof′ah-lo′rents) [A. *Hoffa;* Adolf *Lorenz,* Austrian surgeon, 1854–1946] Lorenz's operation.

Hoffmann's anodyne, drops (hof′manz) [Friedrich *Hoffmann,* German physician, 1660–1742] see *compound ether spirit* and *ether spirit,* under *spirit.*

Hoffmann's atrophy, sign (phenomenon, reflex) [Johann *Hoffmann,* Heidelberg neurologist, 1857–1919] see *Werdnig-Hoffman paralysis,* under *paralysis,* and see under *sign.*

Hoffmann's duct [Moritz *Hoffmann,* German anatomist, 1622–1698] ductus pancreaticus.

Hoffmann-Werdnig syndrome (hof′man-verd′nig) [Johann *Hoffmann;* Guido *Werdnig,* Austrian neurologist] Werdnig-Hoffmann paralysis.

Hofmann's bacillus [Georg von *Hofmann*-Wellenhof, Austrian bacteriologist] *Corynebacterium pseudodiphtheriticum.*

Hofmann's violet [August Wilhelm von *Hofmann,* German chemist, 1818–1892] dahlia.

Hofmeister's test (hōf′mīs-terz) [Franz *Hofmeister,* German physiologic chemist, 1850–1922] see under *tests.*

Högyes's treatment (hed′yes-ez) [Endre *Högyes,* Hungarian physician, 1847–1906] see under *treatment.*

hol- see *holo-.*

holagogue (hol′ah-gog) [*hol-* + Gr. *agōgos* leading] a medicine capable of expelling all disease humors; a drastic or radical remedy.

holandric (hol-an′drik) [Gr. *holos* entire + *aner* man] inherited exclusively through the male descent; transmitted through genes located on the Y chromosome.

holarthritis (hol″ar-thri′tis) hamarthritis.

Holden's line (hōl′denz) [Luther *Holden,* English surgeon, 1815–1905] see under *line.*

holergasia (hol″er-ga′ze-ah) Meyer's term of the major psychoses; see *holergastic*.

holergastic (hol″er-gas″tik) [*hol-* + Gr. *ergon* work] Meyer's term for sweeping disorders of psychic function, i.e., major psychoses, in which the socially organized personality is deranged. Cf. *merergastic*.

holism (hōl′izm) [Gr. *holos* whole] the conception of man as a functioning whole.

holistic (ho-lis′tik) considering man as a functioning whole, or relating to the conception of man as a functioning whole; see also under *health*.

hollow (hol′o) a depressed area or concavity. **Sebileau's h.,** a depressed area beneath the tongue, formed by the oral mucosa and the sublingual glands.

hollow-back (hol′o-bak) see *lordosis*.

Holmes (hōmz), Oliver Wendell (1809–1894). Noted American physician, anatomist, and writer, whose paper *On the Contagiousness of Puerperal Fever* (1843) antedated the work of Semmelweis in its appeal for surgical cleanliness to combat this disease.

Holmes's degeneration phenomenon (sign) (hōmz) [Gordon *Holmes*, British neurologist] see under *degeneration*, and see *rebound phenomenon*, under *phenomenon*.

Holmes's operation (hōmz) [Timothy *Holmes*, English surgeon, 1825–1907] see under *operation*.

Holmes-Stewart phenomenon (hōmz-stu′art) [Gordon *Holmes*; Purves *Stewart*, London physician, 1869–1949] rebound phenomenon.

Holmgren's test (holm′grenz) [Alarik Fritniof *Holmgren*, Swedish physiologist, 1831–1897] see under *tests*.

holmium (hol′me-um) one of the rare earths; symbol, Ho; atomic number, 67; atomic weight, 164.930.

holo-, hol- [Gr. *holos* entire] a combining form meaning entire, or denoting relationship to the whole.

holoacardius (hol″o-ah-kar′de-us) [*holo-* + *a* neg. + Gr. *kardia* heart] a separate, monozygotic twin represented by a more or less shapeless and unidentifiable mass; the vascular systems of the two fetuses are connected, and the circulation is accomplished solely by the heart of the more perfect twin. **h. aceph′alus,**

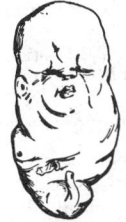 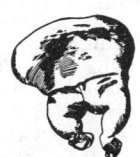

Holoacardius acormus.   Holoacardius acephalus.

an imperfectly formed free twin fetus lacking the cranial part of the body. **h. acor′mus,** an imperfectly formed free twin fetus lacking the caudal part of the body. **h. amor′phus,** an imperfectly formed free twin fetus entirely without form and recognizable parts.

holoantigen (hol″o-an′tĭ-jen) complete antigen, as opposed to hapten.

holoblastic (hol″o-blas′tik) [*holo-* + Gr. *blastos* germ] undergoing cleavage in which the entire ovum participates; dividing completely.

Holocaine (ho′lo-kān) trademark for a preparation of phenacaine hydrochloride.

holocephalic (hol″o-sĕ-fal′ik) [*holo-* + Gr. *kephalē* head] having the head entire; said of a monster.

holocrine (hol″o-krīn) [*holo-* + Gr. *krinein* to separate] wholly secretory: denoting that type of glandular secretion in which the entire secreting cell, along with its accumulated secretion, forms the secreted matter of the gland, as in the sebaceous glands. Cf. *merocrine* and *apocrine*.

holodiastolic (hol″o-di″ah-stol′ik) [*holo-* + *diastole*] pertaining to the entire diastole.

holoendemic (hol″o-en-dem′ik) [*holo-* + Gr. *endēmos* dwelling in a place] affecting practically all of the residents of a particular area.

holoenzyme (hol″o-en′zīm) the functional compound formed by the combination of an apoenzyme and its appropriate coenzyme.

hologamy (ho-log′ah-me) [*holo-* + Gr. *gamos* marriage] the condition in which the gametes are of the same size and structural type as the somatic cells.

hologastroschisis (hol″o-gas-tros′kĭ-sis) [*holo-* + Gr. *gaster* belly + *schisis* cleft] a developmental anomaly characterized by a fissure extending the entire length of the abdomen.

hologenesis (hol″o-jen′ĕ-sis) [*holo-* + Gr. *genesis* formation] the theory that man originated everywhere on earth, instead of in certain special region or regions.

hologram (hol′o-gram″) a three-dimensional image produced by holography.

holography (hol-og′raf-e) the recording of images in three-dimensional form on photographic film by exposing it to a laser beam reflected from the object under study. **acoustical h.,** holography in which sound waves reflected from an object under study are converted into light waves, which act on the emulsion of the film. The film is then exposed to a laser beam to give a three-dimensional effect.

hologynic (hol′o-jin′ik) [*holo-* + Gr. *gynē* woman] inherited exclusively through the female descent; transmitted through genes located on X chromosomes.

holomastigote (hol″o-mas″tĭ-gōt) [*holo-* + Gr. *mastix* lash] having numerous flagella scattered over the body.

holomorphosis (hol″o-mor-fo′sis) [*holo-* + Gr. *morphōsis* formation] the complete regeneration of a lost part.

holomyarial (hol″o-mi-a′re-al) a type of arrangement of the muscular system in the Nematoda. The muscle cells are small, numerous, close together, and form a band below the cuticle.

Holophyra coli (hol-of′ir-ah ko′le) *Balantidium coli*.

holophytic (hol″o-fit′ik) [*holo-* + Gr. *phyton* plant] obtaining food like a plant; said of certain protozoa. Cf. *holozoic*.

holoprosencephaly (hol″o-pros″en-sef′ah-le) failure of cleavage of the prosencephalon with a deficit in midline facial development. Cyclopia occurs in the severe form. In that due to an extra chromosome in the 13–15 group (trisomy 13–15, or trisomy D_1), there are, characteristically, low-set ears, bilateral cleft lip and palate, microcephaly, ocular anomalies, hypotelorism, mental retardation, deafness, convulsions, and ventricular septal defect. Called also *Patau's syndrome*. **familial alobar h.,** a form in which the chromosome count is normal but otherwise resembling that due to trisomy 13–15 (see *holoprosencephaly*).

holorachischisis (hol″o-rah-kis′kĭ-sis) [*holo-* + Gr. *rhachis* spinal column + *schisis* cleft] fissure of the entire spinal cord.

holosaccharide (hol″o-sak′ah-rīd) a ploysaccharide composed of sugar units only. Cf. *heterosaccharide*.

holoschisis (hol″o-ski′sis) [*holo-* + Gr. *schisis* cleft] amitosis.

Holospora (hol″o-spo′rah) [*holo-* + Gr. *sporos* seed] a genus of microorganisms of uncertain affinities which are parasitic on protozoa.

holosystolic (hol″o-sis-tol′ik) [*holo-* + *systole*] pertaining to the entire systole.

holothurin (ho″lo-thu′rin) a hemotoxic mixture of steroid glycosides obtained from holothurians, or sea cucumbers.

Holothyrus (hol″o-thi′rus) a genus of mites. The toxic secretions of *H. coccinella*, of Mauritius, may cause the death of ducks, geese, and chickens after ingestion; in humans it may produce a painful swelling of the tongue and throat.

holotonia (hol″o-to′ne-ah) [*holo-* + Gr. *tonos* tension + *-ia*] muscular spasm of the whole body.

holotonic (hol″o-ton′ik) pertaining to, characterized by, or causing holotonia.

holotopy (ho-lot′o-pe) [*holo-* + Gr. *topos* place] the position of an organ in relation to the whole body.

holotrichous (ho-lot′rĭ-kus) [*holo-* + Gr. *thrix* hair] covered uniformly with cilia.

holotype (hol′o-tīp) the type culture of a species or subspecies of microorganisms, either because it was so designated in the original description or because the original description was based on only one strain.

holozoic (hol″o-zo′ik) [*holo-* + Gr. *zōon* animal] having the nutritional characters of an animal, i.e. digesting protein. Cf. *holophytic*.

holozymase (hol″o-zi′mās) holoenzyme.

Holten's test (hol′tenz) [Cai *Holten*, Danish physician, born 1894] see under *test*.

Holth's operation (holths) [Sören *Holth*, Oslo ophthalmologist, 1863–1937] see under *operation*.

Holthouse's hernia (holt′howz-es) [Carsten *Holthouse*, English surgeon, 1810–1901] see under *hernia*.

Holzknecht's chromoradiometer, etc. (holts-knekt) [Guido *Holzknecht*, radiologist in Vienna, 1872–1931] see under *chromoradiometer, scale, space, stomach,* and *unit*.

homalocephalus (hom″ah-lo-sef′ah-lus) [Gr. *homalos* level + *kephalē* head] a person with a flat head.

homalography (hom″ah-log′rah-fe) [Gr. *homalos* level + *graphein* to write] (*obs.*) the study of anatomy by means of plane sections of the parts.

homaluria (hom″ah-lu′re-ah) [Gr. *homalos* level, even + *ourein* to make water + *-ia*] production and excretion of urine at a normal, even rate.

Homans' sign (ho′manz) [John *Homans*, American physician, 1877–1954] see under *sign*.

Homapin (ho′mah-pin) trademark for preparations of homatropine methylbromide.

homarine (hom′ah-rin) an organic nitrogen compound which is found in lobster muscle and tissues of other marine animals. It is the methyl betaine of picolinic acid, $C_5H_4N^+(CH_3)CO_2^-$.

homatropine (ho-mat′ro-pēn) chemical name: *endo*-α-hydroxybenzeneacetic acid 8-methyl-8-azabicyclo[3.2.1]oct-3-yl. The tropine ester of mandelic acid, $C_{16}H_{21}NO_3$, having anticholinergic effects similar to but weaker than those of atropine. **h. hydrobromide** [USP], the hydrobromide salt of homatropine, $C_{16}H_{21}NO_3 \cdot HBr$, occurring as white crystals or white, crystalline powder; used in ophthalmology as a cycloplegic and mydriatic, applied topically to the conjunctiva. **h. methylbromide** [USP], the 8-methyl derivative of homatropine hydrobromide, $C_{17}H_{24}BrNO_3$, occurring as a white powder; used as an antispasmodic and inhibitor of secretions, especially in gastrointestinal disorders, administered orally.

homaxial (ho-mak′se-al) having axes of the same length.

Homén′s syndrome [Ernest Alexander *Homén*, Finnish physician, 1851–1926] see under *syndrome*.

homeo-, homoeo-, homoio- (ho′me-o)[Gr. *homoios* like, resembling; always the same, unchanging] a combining form denoting sameness, similarity, or a constant, unchanging state.

homeochrome (ho′me-o-krōm″) [*homeo*- + Gr. *chrōma* color] staining with mucin stains after formol-bichromate fixation; applied to certain serous cells of the salivary glands. Cf. *tropochrome*.

homeograft (ho′me-o-graft) allograft.

homeokinesis (ho″me-o-ki-ne′sis) [*homeo*- + Gr. *kinēsis* motion] the stage of meiosis in which the daughter cells receive equal amounts and kinds of chromatin.

homeomorphous (ho″me-o-mor′fus)[*homeo*- + Gr. *morphē* form] of like form and structure.

homeo-osteoplasty (ho″me-o-os″te-o-plas′te) [*homeo*- + Gr. *osteon* bone + *plassein* to mold] the surgical implantation in an individual of a piece of a bone from an individual of the same species.

homeopath (ho′me-o-path) homeopathist.

homeopathic (ho″me-o-path′ik) pertaining to homeopathy.

homeopathist (ho″me-op′ah-thist) one who practices homeopathy.

homeopathy (ho″me-op′ah-the) [*homeo*- + Gr. *pathos* disease] a system of therapeutics founded by Samuel Hahnemann (1755–1843), in which diseases are treated by drugs which are capable of producing in healthy persons symptoms like those of the disease to be treated, the drug being administered in minute doses. Cf. *allopathy*.

homeoplasia (ho″me-o-pla′ze-ah) [*homeo*- + Gr. *plassein* to form] the formation of new tissue like that adjacent to it and normal to the part.

homeoplastic (ho″me-o-plas′tik) 1. resembling in structure the adjacent parts. 2. pertaining to, characterized by, or stimulating homeoplasia.

homeorrhesis (ho″me-o-re′sis) [*homeo*- + Gr. *rhein* to flow] the tendency to maintain a biological process, as a growth process, along a particular pathway despite the operation of factors tending to divert it.

homeosis (ho″me-o′sis) [Gr. *homoiōsis* likeness, resemblance] the formation of a body part having the characteristics normally found in a related part at a different body site.

homeostasis (ho″me-o-sta′sis) [*homeo*- + Gr. *stasis* standing] a tendency to stability in the normal body states (internal environment) of the organism. It is achieved by a system of control mechanisms activated by negative feedback; e.g., a high level of carbon dioxide in extracellular fluid triggers increased pulmonary ventilation, which in turn causes a decrease in carbon dioxide concentration. **immunologic h.,** the normal state of the adult animal in which it produces antibodies or develops cell-mediated immunity to foreign antigens but not to its own antigens.

homeostatic (ho″me-o-stat′ik) pertaining to homeostasis.

homeotherapy (ho″me-o-ther′ah-pe) [*homeo*- + Gr. *therapeia* treatment] treatment or prevention of disease with a substance similar to but not the same as the causative agent of the disease.

homeotherm (ho′me-o-therm) homoiotherm.

homeothermal (ho″me-o-ther′mal) [*homeo*- + Gr. *thermē* heat] homoiothermic.

homeotransplant (ho′me-o-trans′plant) allograft.

homeotransplantation (ho″me-o-trans″plan-ta′shun) [*homeo*- + *transplantation*] transplantation of tissues or cells from an animal of one inbred strain to a member of another within the same species, or from one individual to another of the same species, but of disparate genotype (an allograft).

homeotypic, homeotypical (ho″me-o-tip′ik; ho″me-o-tip′ĭ-k′l) [*homeo*- + Gr. *typos* type] resembling the normal or usual type.

homergic (hōm-er′jik) [*hom(o)*- + Gr. *ergon* work] having the same effect; said of two drugs each of which produces the same overt effect.

homicide (hom′ĭ-sīd) [L. *homo* man + *caedere* to kill] the taking of the life of another individual.

homiculture (hom′ĭ-kul″tūr) [L. *homo* man + *cultura* culture] positive eugenics.

homidium (ho-mid′e-um) chemical name: 3,8-diamino-5-ethyl-6-phenylphenanthredium, an effective trypanosomicide. Its bromide and chloride are used in the treatment of infections with *Trypanosoma congolense* and *T. vivax* in cattle and horses. Called also *ethidium*.

hominal (hom′ĭ-nal) [L. *homo* man] pertaining to man; pertaining to human beings.

hominid (hom′ĭ-nid) 1. pertaining to the family of humans (Hominidae). 2. a living or extinct human or humanlike type.

Hominidae (ho-min′ĭ-de) [L. *homo* man + Gr. *eidos* resemblance] a family of primates (superfamily Hominoides, suborder Anthropoidea), including both modern man (*Homo sapiens*) and fossil hominids.

homininoxious (hom″in-e-nok′shus) injurious to man.

hominoid (hom′ĭ-noid)) 1. pertaining to the Hominoidea. 2. a member of the Hominoidea.

Hominoidea (hom″ĭ-noi′de-ah) [L. *homo* man + Gr. *oeidos* likeness] a superfamily of primates (suborder Anthropoidea), including the families Pongidae (anthropoid apes) and Hominidae (man, both modern and extinct).

homme (um) [Fr.] man. **h. rouge** (um-roozh′) [Fr. "red man"], a stage in mycosis fungoides in which the red plaques become infiltrated and coalesce over a wide area of the body.

Homo (ho′mo) [L. *man*] the genus of primates (family Hominidae, superfamily Hominoides) that includes man (*H. sapiens*) and fossil hominids.

homo- [Gr. *homos* same] 1. combining form meaning the same. 2. a prefix in chemical names indicating the addition of one CH_2 group to the main compound.

homoarterenol hydrochloride (ho″mo-ar″tĕ-re′nol) nordefrin hydrochloride.

Homobasidiomycetidae (ho″mo-bah-sid″e-o-mi-se′tĭ-de) a subclass of true fungi of the Basidiomycetes, including the series Hymenomycetes and Gasteromycetes.

homobiotin (ho″mo-bi′o-tin) a homologue of biotin having an additional CH_2 group in the side chain and acting as a biotin antagonist.

homocarnosine (ho″mo-kar′no-sēn) a dipeptide consisting of γ-aminobutyric acid and histidine that is a normal constituent of the human brain.

homocentric (ho″mo-sen′trik) [*homo*- + Gr. *kentron* center] having the same center or focus.

homochronous (ho-mok′ro-nus) [*homo*- + Gr. *chronos* time] occurring at the same age in successive generations.

homocinchonine (ho″mo-sin′ko-nin) an alkaloid, $C_{19}H_{22}ON_2$, from cinchona, isomeric with cinchonine.

homocladic (ho″mo-klad′ik) [*homo*- + Gr. *klados* branch] formed between small branches of the same artery; said of such an anastomosis.

homocyclic (ho″mo-sik′lik) having or pertaining to a closed chain or ring formation which includes only atoms of the same element.

homocysteine (ho″mo-sis-te′in) a transmethylation product of methionine, $HSCH_2CH_2CHNH_2COOH$; it is an intermediate in the synthesis of cysteine.

homocystine (ho″mo-sis′tin) a synthetic alpha-alpha′-dithiobis alpha-aminobutyric acid, $[S \cdot CH_2 \cdot CH_2 \cdot CH(NH_2) \cdot COOH]_2$, which results from the demethylation of methionine. It is homologous with cystine and able to function as a source of sulfur in the body.

homocystinemia (ho″mo-sis″tin-e′me-ah) an excess of homocystine in the blood; see *homocystinuria*.

homocystinuria (ho″mo-sis″tin-u′re-ah) an inborn error of sulfur amino acid metabolism due to absence or deficiency of the liver enzyme cystathionine synthase, characterized chemically by elevated levels of methionine and homocystine in the plasma and large amounts of homocystine in the urine. Typically, the affected person is fair-skinned and blond, with mental retardation, hepatomegaly, ectopia lentis, cardiovascular disorders, and skeletal disorders, including kyphosis, scoliosis, pectus excavatum, and arachnodactyly. The clinical manifestations resemble those of Marfan's syndrome.

homocytotropic (ho″mo-si″to-trop′ik) [*homo*- + *cyto*- + Gr. *tropos* a turning] having an affinity for cells from the same species; see under *antibody*.

homodesmotic (ho″mo-des-mot′ik) [*homo*- + Gr. *desmos* bond] joining similar parts of the central nervous system; see under *fiber*.

homodont (ho′mo-dont) [*hom*- + Gr. *odous* tooth] having teeth of only one type.

homodromous (ho-mod′ro-mus) [*homo*- + Gr. *dromos* running] moving or acting in the same direction.

homoeo- see *homeo-*.

homoeosis (ho″me-o′sis) homeosis.

homoerotic (ho″mo-ĕ-rot′ik) pertaining to homoeroticism; homosexual.

homoeroticism (ho″mo-ĕ-rot′ĭ-sizm) eroticism directed toward a person of the same sex, especially when the role assumed by the affected person is passive.

homofermenter (ho″mo-fer-ment′er) an organism which ferments glucose almost exclusively to lactic acid, by way of the Embden-Meyerhof pathway.

homogamete (ho″mo-gam′ēt) one of two gametes of the same size and structure, as the X chromosome in the human female.

homogametic (ho″mo-gah-met′ik) characterized by the production of gametes of only one kind in respect to the sex chromosomes, as in the human female.

homogamous (ho-mog′ah-mus) characterized by or pertaining to homogamy.

homogamy (ho-mog′ah-me) 1. inbreeding. 2. reproduction resulting from the union of two cells (gametes) that are identical in size and structure. 3. maturation of the male (stamens) and female (pistils) gametes of a flower at the same time.

homogenate (ho-moj′ĕ-nāt) material subjected to homogenization, as tissue that is finely shredded and mixed.

homogeneity (ho″mo-jĕ-ne′ĭ-te) the state or quality of being homogeneous.

homogeneization (ho″mo-je″nĕ-i-za′shun) homogenization.

homogeneous (ho″mo-je′ne-us) [homo- + Gr. genos kind] consisting of or composed of similar elements or ingredients; of a uniform quality throughout.

homogenesis (ho″mo-jen′ĕ-sis) [homo- + Gr. genesis production] the reproduction by the same process in each generation, as contrasted with heterogenesis.

homogenetic (ho″mo-jĕ-net′ik) pertaining to or characterized by homogenesis.

homogenic (ho″mo-jen′ik) homozygous.

homogenicity (ho″mo-jĕ-nis′ĭ-te) homogeneity.

homogenization (ho-moj″ĕ-ni-za′shun) the act or process of rendering homogeneous.

homogenize (ho-moj′ĕ-nīz) to render homogeneous, or of uniform quality or consistency throughout.

homogenous (ho-moj′ĕ-nus) having a similarity of structure because of descent from a common ancestor.

homogentisuria (ho″mo-jen″tĭ-su′re-ah) the excretion of homogentisic acid in the urine, as in spontaneous alkaptonuria.

homogeny (ho-moj′ĕ-ne) homogenesis.

homoglandular (ho″mo-glan′du-lar) pertaining to the same gland.

homograft (ho′mo-graft) allograft.

homoio- see homeo-.

homoioplasia (ho″moi-o-pla′se-ah) homeoplasia.

homoiopodal (ho″moi-op′o-dal) [homoio- + Gr. pous foot] having processes of one kind only; said of nerve cells.

homoiostasis (ho″moi-os′tah-sis) homeostasis.

homoiotherm (ho-moi′o-therm) an animal which exhibits homoiothermy; a so-called warm-blooded animal, as opposed to a poikilotherm.

homoiothermal (ho″moi-o-ther′mal) homoiothermic.

homoiothermic (ho-moi′o-ther′mik) pertaining to or characterized by homoiothermy.

homoiothermism (ho″moi-o-ther′mizm) homoiothermy.

homoiothermy (ho-moi′o-ther′me) [homoio- + Gr. thermē heat] the maintenance of a constant body temperature despite changes in the environmental temperature, as in birds and mammals. Cf. poikilothermy.

homoiotoxin (ho-moi′o-tok-sin) a toxin from one individual which is toxic for other individuals of the same species.

homokeratoplasty (ho″mo-ker′ah-to-plas″te) corneal grafting with tissue derived from another individual of the same species.

homolateral (ho″mo-lat′er-al) situated on, pertaining to, or affecting the same side; ipsilateral.

homologen (ho-mol′o-jen) homologue, def. 2.

homologous (ho-mol′o-gus) [Gr. homologos agreeing, correspondent] 1. corresponding in structure, position, origin, etc., as (a) the feathers of a bird and the scales of a fish, (b) antigen and its specific antibody, (c) allelic chromosomes. Cf. analogous. 2. allogeneic.

homologue (hom′o-log) 1. any homologous organ or part; an organ similar in structure, position, and origin to another organ, as the front flippers of a seal and human hands. See analogue. 2. in chemistry, one of a series of compounds, each of which is formed from the one before it by the addition of a constant element or a constant group of elements, as in the homologous series CH_4, C_2H_6, C_3H_8, etc.; called also homologen.

homology (ho-mol′o-je) [Gr. homologia agreement] the quality of being homologous; the morphological identity of corresponding parts; structural similarity due to descent from a common form.

homolysin (ho-mol′ĭ-sin) a lysin (e.g., isohemolysin) produced by injection into the body of antigen derived from an individual of the same species.

homolysis (ho-mol′ĭ-sis) [homo- + Gr. lysis dissolution] lysis of a cell by extracts of the same type of tissue.

homomorphic (ho-mo-mor′fik) [homo- + Gr. morphē form] having chromosome mates of similar size and form during synapsis of the first meiotic division.

homomorphosis (ho″mo-mor-fo′sis) [homo- + Gr. morphōsis formation] regenerative replacement of a lost part by a similar part.

homonomous (ho-mon′o-mus) [homo- + Gr. nomos law] designating homologous serial parts, such as somites.

homonymous (ho-mon′ĭ-mus) [homo- + Gr. onoma name] 1. having the same or corresponding sound or name. 2. standing in the same relation; see under hemianopia.

homophil (ho′mo-fil) an antibody that reacts only with a specific antigen.

homophilic (ho″mo-fil′ik) [homo- + Gr. philein to love] having affinity for or reacting with a specific antigen; said of an antibody.

homoplastic (ho″mo-plas″tik) [homo- + Gr. plassein to form] 1. denoting a transplantation or grafting of tissue taken from another individual of the same species or from a member of another inbred strain of the same species. 2. denoting organs or parts, as the wings of birds and insects, that resemble one another in structure and function but not in origin or development.

homoplasty (ho′mo-plas″te) 1. operative replacement of lost parts or tissues by similar parts from another individual of the same species or from a member of another inbred strain of the same species. 2. similarity between organs or parts not due to common ancestry.

homopolysaccharide (ho″mo-pol″e-sak′ah-rīd) a polysaccharide consisting of a single recurring monosaccharide unit, as glycogen is a polymer of glucose.

homorganic (hom″or-gan′ik) [homo- + Gr. organon organ] produced by the same or by homologous organs.

homosalate (ho″mo-sal′āt) chemical name: 2-hydroxybenzoic acid 3,3,5-trimethylcyclohexyl ester; an ultraviolet sunscreen, $C_{16}H_{22}O_3$.

homosexual (ho″mo-seks′u-al) 1. pertaining to the same sex. 2. an individual who is sexually attracted toward a person of the same sex, as opposed to heterosexual.

homosexuality (ho″mo-seks″u-al′ĭ-te) [homo- + sexuality] sexual attraction toward those of the same sex. Cf. heterosexuality. **female h.,** lesbianism.

homospore (ho′mo-spōr) a homosporous organism.

homosporous (ho-mos′po-rus) [homo- + Gr. sporos seed] having spores of only one kind, which reproduce asexually.

homostimulant (ho″mo-stim′u-lant) 1. stimulating the same organ from which it is derived. 2. an extract from an organ which, on injection into the body, stimulates the same organ from which it is derived.

homostimulation (ho″mo-stim″u-la′shun) treatment by a homostimulant.

Homo-Tet (ho′mo-tet) trademark for a preparation of tetanus immune human globulin.

homothallic (hom″o-thal′ik) pertaining to or exhibiting homothallism.

homothallism (hom″o-thal′izm) a form of sexual reproduction in which the isogamete produced by one cell can fuse with another isogamete produced by the same cell, as in various algae and fungi. Cf. heterothallism.

homotherm (ho′mo-therm) homoiotherm.

homothermal (ho″mo-ther′mal) homoiothermic.

homothermic (ho″mo-ther′mik) homoiothermic.

homotonia (ho″mo-to′ne-ah) isotonia.

homotonic (ho″mo-ton′ik) isotonic.

homotopic (ho″mo-top′ik) [homo- + Gr. topos place] occurring at the same place upon the body.

homotransplant (ho″mo-trans′plant) allograft.

homotropism (ho-mot′ro-pizm) [homo- + Gr. tropos a turning] the property of cells to attract cells of a like order.

homotype (hom′o-tīp) [homo- + Gr. typos type] a part that has a reversed symmetry with its fellow of the opposite side of the body, as the hand.

homotypic (ho″mo-tip′ik) pertaining to or characteristic of a homotype.

homozoic (ho″mo-zo′ik) [homo- + Gr. zōon animal] pertaining to the same animal or same species.

homozygosis (ho″mo-zi-go′sis) the formation of a zygote by the union of gametes that possess one or more identical alleles.

homozygosity (ho″mo-zi-gos′ĭ-te) [homo- + zygosity] the state of possessing a pair of identical alleles at a given locus or loci.

homozygote (ho″mo-zi′gōt) [homo- + zygote] an individual possessing a pair of identical alleles at a given locus or loci.

homozygous (ho″mo-zi′gus) possessing a pair of identical alleles at a given locus or loci.

homunculus (ho-munk′u-lus) [L. "a little man"] 1. a dwarf without deformity or disproportion of parts. 2. the miniature human form once thought to be preformed in the sperm or ovum.

honey (hon′e) a sweet-tasting substance deposited by the honeybee, which contains between 62 and 83 per cent dextrose and fructose, and small amounts of sucrose, dextrin, and malic and acetic acids; its pH is 3.8 to 4.3.

honorarium (on″o-ra′re-um), pl. *honora′ria* [L.] a gratuity that substitutes for a professional fee.

hood (hood) a flexible covering. **tooth h.,** dental operculum.

hoof (hoof) [L. *ungula*] the hard, horny casing of the foot or ends of the digits of many animals which are, because of this feature, designated ungulates. **curved h.,** a condition in which the hoof has the wall of one side concave and the other convex. **dished h.,** a hoof which is concave from the coronet to the plantar surface. **false h.,** the hoof of an unused digit. **ribbed h., ringed h.,** a condition in which the wall of a horse's hoof is marked by ridges running parallel with the coronary margin.

hoof-bound (hoof′bound) dryness and contraction of a horse's hoof, causing lameness; called also *contracted foot* and *contracted heel.*

hook (hook) a curved instrument, usually with a sharp point, designed for holding, elevating, or exerting traction on a tissue. **blunt h.,** an instrument for exercising traction upon the fetus in certain cases of breech presentation. **Bose's h's,** small hooks used in tracheostomy. **Braun's h.,** a hook for decapitating the fetus. **Loughnane's h.,** a double-pronged hook for removing fragments of the prostate in transurethral prostatectomy. **Malgaigne's h's,** two pairs of hooks connected by a screw for approximating the pieces of a broken patella. **muscle h.,** a hook for securing and isolating an extraocular muscle; called also *squint h.* **Pajot's h.,** a hook for decapitating the fetus. **palate h., posterior,** a hook for raising the palate in rhinoscopy. **squint h.,** muscle h. **tracheostomy h.,** a hook for use in tracheostomy. **Tyrrell's h.,** a slender hook used in eye surgery.

hook-up (hook′up) the method of arranging circuits, appliances, and electrodes for a particular diagnostic or therapeutic procedure.

hookworm (hook′werm) a nematode parasitic in the intestine of man and other vertebrates; infection may cause serious illness. See also under *disease,* and see *ground itch,* under *itch.* **American h.,** *Necator americanus.* **h. of the dog,** *Ancylostoma caninum.* **European h.,** *Ancylostoma duodenale.* **h. of the rat,** *Nippostrongylus muris.* **h. of ruminants,** *Bunostomum.* **New World h.,** *Necator americanus.* **Old World h.,** *Ancylostoma duodenale.*

hoolamite (hoo′lah-mīt) a chemical detector for carbon monoxide, containing fuming sulfuric acid, iodine pentoxide, and powdered pumice; it changes from light gray to green under the influence of carbon monoxide.

hoose (hooz) a disease of sheep, cattle, goats, and swine, caused by the presence of various species of nematodes of the genera *Dictyocaulus, Metastrongylus,* and *Protostrongylus* in the bronchial tubes or in the lungs. It is marked by cough, dyspnea, anorexia, and constipation. Called also *verminous bronchitis.*

Hoover's sign (hoo′verz) [Charles Franklin *Hoover,* American physician, 1865–1927] see under *sign.*

HOP high oxygen pressure.

Hope's sign (hōps) [James *Hope,* London physician, 1801–1841] see under *sign.*

Hopkins (hop′kinz), Sir Frederick Gowland. English biologist, 1861–1947, noted for his pioneering work in vitamin research and nutritional chemistry; co-winner, with Christiaan Eijkman, of the Nobel prize in medicine and physiology in 1929.

Hopkins-Cole test (hop′kinz-kol) [Sir Frederick Gowland *Hopkins;* Sidney William *Cole,* English physiologist, born 1877] see under *tests.*

Hoplopsyllus anomalus (hop″lo-sil′us ah-nom′ah-lus) a species of flea found in the ground squirrels of western United States and transmitting plague.

Hopmann's polyp (papilloma) (hop′manz) [Carl Melchior *Hopmann,* German rhinologist, 1849–1925] see under *polyp.*

Hoppe-Seyler's test (hop″ĕ-si′lerz) [Ernst Felix Immanuel *Hoppe-Seyler,* German physiologic chemist, 1825–1895] see under *tests.*

hoquizil hydrochloride (ho′kwĭ-zil) chemical name: 2-hydroxy-2-methylpropyl 4-(6,7-dimethoxy-4-quinazolinyl)-1-piperazinecarboxylate monohydrochloride; a bronchodilator, $C_{19}H_{26}N_4O_5 \cdot HCl$.

Hor. decub. abbreviation for L. *ho′ra decu′bitus,* at bedtime.

hordein (hor′de-in) [L. *hordeum,* barley] a simple native protein from barley, a prolamine insoluble in water, but soluble in 80 per cent alcohol.

hordeolum (hor-de′o-lum) [L. "barleycorn"] a localized, purulent, inflammatory staphylococcal infection of one or more sebaceous glands (meibomian or zeisian) of the eyelids; called also *stye.* An *external hordeolum* occurs on the surface of the skin at the edge of the lid. An *internal hordeolum* is marked by swelling on the conjunctival surface of the lid.

hordeum (hor′de-um), gen. *hor′dei* [L.] barley.

horehound (hōr′hound) the labiate plant, *Marrubium vulgare* (Tourn.) L. (Labiatae), also its leaves and tops (L. *marrubium*); used as an expectorant, bitter tonic, vermifuge, and laxative.

Hor. interm. abbreviation for L. *ho′ris interme′diis,* at the intermediate hours.

horizon (hŏ-ri′zon) a numbered stage of human embryonic development defined by anatomical characteristics in order to circumvent individual uncertainties of age and variations of dimension from both natural and technical causes. Streeter outlined 23 horizons, each spanning 2 or 3 days, covering the 7-week period beginning with fertilization. **Streeter's h's,** see *horizon.*

horizontalis (hor″ĭ-zon-ta′lis) horizontal, or parallel to the plane of the horizon; [NA] a term denoting relationship to this orientation when the body is in the anatomical, i.e., the upright position.

horme (hor′ma) Monakow's term for the central source of instincts.

hormesis (hor-me′sis) [Gr. *hormēsis* rapid motion] the stimulating effect of subinhibitory concentrations of any toxic substance on any organism.

hormetic (hor-met′ik) relating to the direct motivational traits of personality, as needs, attitudes, etc.

hormic (hor′mik) [Gr. *hormē* an urge] a term applied to the theory that organic phenomena are determined by inborn instincts, tendencies, and dispositions.

hormion (hor′me-on) [Gr. *hormos* a wreath] the median anterior point of the spheno-occipital bones.

Hormocardiol (hor″mo-kar′de-ol) [*hormone* + Gr. *kardia* heart] a commercial preparation of an extract from the sinus of the frog's heart that stimulates the contraction of the frog's ventricle; used as coronary vasodilator.

Hormodendrum (hor″mo-den′drum) a former genus of Fungi Imperfecti; at present, most saprophytic species are placed in the genus *Cladosporium,* and the human pathogens, e.g., *H. pedrosoi,* in the genus *Fonsecaea.*

hormonagogue (hor-mōn′ah-gog) [*hormone* + Gr. *agōgos* leading] an agent that stimulates the production of hormones.

hormonal (hor′mo-nal) pertaining to or of the nature of a hormone.

hormone (hor′mōn) [Gr. *hormaein* to set in motion, spur on] a chemical substance, produced in the body by an organ or cells of an organ which has a specific regulatory effect on the activity of a certain organ; originally applied to substances secreted by various endocrine glands and transported in the blood stream to the target organ on which their effect was produced, the term was later applied to various substances not produced by special glands but having similar action. See also *endocrine system,* under *system.* **adaptive h.,** one, such as corticotropin or the corticoids, which is secreted during adaptation to unusual circumstances. **adenohypophyseal h.,** any hormone secreted by the adenohypophysis, including somatotropin (STH), thyrotropin (TSH), prolactin, follicle-stimulating hormone (FSH), luteinizing hormone (LH), melanocyte-stimulating hormone (MSH), and adrenocorticotropic hormone (ACTH). **adipokinetic h.,** 1. a hypothetical lipolytic hormone secreted by the pituitary gland. 2. lipolytic h. **adrenocortical h.,** any of the corticosteroids elaborated by the adrenal cortex, the major ones being the glucocorticoids and mineralocorticoids, and including some androgens, progesterone, and perhaps estrogens. See also *corticosteroid.* **adrenocorticotropic h.,** corticotropin. **adrenomedullary h's,** substances secreted by the adrenal medulla, including epinephrine and norepinephrine. **androgenic h's,** the masculinizing hormones, androsterone and testosterone. **anterior pituitary h.,** any of the several protein or polypeptide hormones secreted by the anterior lobe of the pituitary gland, including the corticotropic, growth, thyrotropic, and gonadotropic hormones. **antidiuretic h.,** a hormone secreted by the supraoptic nucleus of the hypothalamus, stored in the posterior pituitary, and released on signal by osmoreceptors in the nucleus. It has a specific effect on the epithelial cells of the distal portion of the uriniferous tubule, stimulating reabsorption of water independently of solids, and resulting in concentration of urine. It also has vasopressor activity. Called also *vasopressin.* **Aschheim-Zondek h.,** luteinizing h. **chondrotropic h.,** growth h. **chromaffin h.,** epinephrine. **chromatophorotropic h.,** intermedin. **conjugated estrogen h's,** an amorphous preparation of naturally-occurring, water-soluble, conjugated forms of mixed estrogens, chiefly sodium estrone sulfate, extracted from the urine of pregnant mares; used in estrogen hormone therapy. **corpus luteum h.,** progesterone. **cortical h.,** see *adrenocortical h.* **diabetogenic h.,** a substance in extracts of the anterior pituitary that tends to elevate the blood sugar by acting as an antagonist to insulin. It is probably not a distinct entity and its effects are probably related to those of known pituitary hormones, especially human growth hormone. **estrogenic h's,** substances capable of producing certain biological effects, the most characteristic of which are the changes which occur in mammals at estrus; the naturally occurring estrogenic hormones are β-estradiol, estrone, and estriol. **fat-mobilizing h's,** lipolytic h's. **follicle h.,** an estrogenic hormone produced by the graafian follicle. **follicle-stimulating h. (FSH),** one of the gonadotropic hormones of the anterior pituitary, which stimulates the growth and maturation of graafian follicles in the ovary, and stimulates spermatogenesis in the male. An extract from postmenopausal urine, known as human follicle-stimulating hormone or *menotropins* (q.v.), is used to induce ovulation and to promote spermatogenesis. **follicle-stimulating h., human,** 1. follicle-stimulating h. 2. menotropins. **follicle-stimulating hormone releasing h. (FSH-RH),** gonadotropin releasing h. **follicular h.,** one produced by the graafian follicle. **galactopoietic h.,** prolactin. **gastrointestinal h.,** hormones that originate in and regulate motor and secretory activity of the digestive organs, i.e., gastrin, secretin, and cholecystokinin. **gonadotropic h.,** any hormone that has an influence on the gonads. **gonadotropic h's, pituitary,** three hormones, including follicle-stimulating hormone and luteinizing hormone in mammals and prolactin in certain birds, secreted by the anterior pituitary gland which have an influence on the gonads. **gonadotropin releasing h. (Gn-RH)** a decapeptide hormone elaborated by the median eminence of the hypothalamus that stimulates the release of follicle-stimulating hormone and luteinizing hormone from the anterior lobe of the pituitary gland. A preparation of the acetate and hydrochloride salts of the same principle obtained from pigs, sheep, or other species is used in the differential diagnosis of hypothalamic, pituitary, and gonadal dysfunction. Called also *gonadorelin.* **growth h. (GH),** any substance that stimulates growth, especially one secreted by the anterior pituitary, which exerts a direct effect on protein, carbohydrate, and lipid metabolism, and controls the rate of skeletal and visceral growth. Human growth hormone (HGH) is composed of a single chain of 188 amino acids without carbohydrate substituents. Called also *somatotropin.* **growth hormone release inhibiting h.,** somatostatin. **growth hormone releasing h. (GH-RH),** see under *factor.* **human (pituitary) growth h. (HGH),** see *growth h.* **hypophysiotropic h.,** any of the hormones of the hypothalamus that stimulate or inhibit the hypophysis, including the releasing factors. **inhibiting h's,** hormones elaborated by one structure (as by the hypothalamus) that inhibit release of hormones from another structure (as from the anterior pituitary gland), e.g., *somatostatin* (growth hormone release inhibiting h.). The term is applied to substances of established clinical identity, whereas substances of unknown chemical structure are called *inhibiting factors* (see under *factor*). **inhibitory h.,** a substance that exerts a depressing influence on certain of its target organs, e.g., enterogastrone. **interstitial cell-stimulating h.,** luteinizing h.; so called because it also stimulates the Leydig (interstitial) cells of the testis. Abbreviated ICSH. **juvenile h.,** the secretion of the corpora allata which prevents metamorphosis, keeping the insect in the larval state and ensuring that the larva will molt several times and reach large size before pupating. **ketogenic h's,** lipolytic h's. **lactation h.,** prolactin. **lactogenic h.,** prolactin. **langerhansian h.,** one of the hormones secreted by the islets of Langerhans of the pancreas, including both insulin and glucagon. **lipolytic h's,** any hormone that serves to mobilize fat, i.e., to induce lipolysis, including the catecholamines, glucagon, tropic hormones of the anterior pituitary (ACTH, TSH, MSH, etc.), and growth hormone; called also *fat-mobilizing h's* and *ketogenic h's.* **local h.,** a substance with hormone-like properties, produced from blood or other body fluid precisely when and where it is needed, and usually rapidly destroyed. **luteal h.,** one secreted by the corpus luteum; see *progesterone.* **luteinizing h.,** a gonadotropic hormone of the anterior pituitary which acts with the follicle-stimulating hormone to cause ovulation of mature follicles and secretion of estrogen by thecal and granulosa cells. It is also concerned with corpus luteum formation and, in the male, stimulates the development and functional activity of Leydig (interstitial) cells. **luteinizing hormone releasing h. (LH-RH),** gonadotropin releasing h. **luteotropic h.,** luteotropin. **mammotropic h.,** prolactin. **melanocyte-stimulating h., melanophore-stimulating h.,** a peptide derived from the anterior pituitary gland in man and from the pars intermedia (hence sometimes called *intermedin*) in lower vertebrates, which influences the formation of deposition of melanin in the body and produces the color changes in the skin of amphibians, fishes, and reptiles. Abbreviated MSH. It occurs in two forms: α-MSH contains 13 amino acids and is identical in various species; β-MSH varies in size and in amino acid sequence from species to species. **neurohypophyseal h's,** the hormones that are stored and released by the neurohypophysis, i.e., oxytocin and vasopressin. **orchidic h.,** testosterone. **ovarian h.,** one secreted by the ovary, including the estrogens and gestagens. **parathyroid h.,** a polypeptide hormone secreted by the parathyroid glands, which promotes release of calcium from

bone into the extracellular fluid by activating osteoclasts and promotes increased intestinal absorption and renal tubular reabsorption of calcium, as well as increased renal excretion of phosphates. Secretion of parathyroid hormone is induced by decreased levels of calcium in the extracellular fluid. Its action is opposed by that of calcitonin. Called also *parathormone.* **placental h.,** a hormone produced by the placenta during pregnancy, including chorionic gonadotrophin, relaxin, and other substances having estrogenic, progesteronic, or adrenocorticoid activity. **placental growth h.,** human placental lactogen. **plant h.,** phytohormone. **posterior pituitary h's,** hormones derived from the posterior lobe of the pituitary, including antidiuretic hormone and oxytocin; now believed to be formed in the neuronal cells of the hypothalamic nuclei and to be stored in nerve cell endings in the posterior pituitary (neurohypophysis) for release as necessary. **progestational h.,** 1. progesterone. 2. [pl] see under *agent.* **proparathyroid h.,** an inactive precursor of parathyroid hormone; it is of larger molecular size than the active hormone. **prothoracicotropic h.,** in the development of insects, the hormone that controls secretion of ecdysone by the prothoracic glands. It is secreted by the intercerebral gland in the brain. **P.U. h.** (pregnancy urine h.), the chorionic gonadotropin found in the urine in pregnancy. **releasing h's,** hormones elaborated in one structure (as in the hypothalamus) that effect the release of hormones from another structure (as from the anterior pituitary gland); they include gonadotropin releasing hormone and thyrotropin releasing hormone. The term is applied to substances of established chemical identity, whereas substances of unknown chemical structure are called *releasing factors* (see under *factor*). **sex h's,** hormones having estrogenic (*female sex h's*) or androgenic (*male sex h's*) activity. **somatotrophic h., somatotropic h.,** growth h. **somatotropin release inhibiting h.,** somatostatin. **somatotropin releasing h. (SRH),** growth hormone releasing f. **steroid h.,** a group of biologically active organic compounds that are secreted by the adrenal cortex, testis, ovary, and placenta and which have in common a cyclopentanoperhydrophenanthrene nucleus. **testicular h., testis h.,** testosterone. **thyroid h's,** thyroxine, triiodothyronine, and calcitonin; in the singular, it refers to thyroxine and/or triiodothyronine. **thyroid-stimulating h. (TSH),** thyrotropin. **thyrotropic h.,** thyrotropin. **thyrotropin releasing h. (TRH),** a tripeptide hormone elaborated by the median eminence of the hypothalamus or obtained by synthesis, which stimulates release of thyrotropin from the anterior pituitary gland. In human subjects, it also acts as a prolactin releasing factor. A preparation is used in the diagnosis of mild hyperthyroidism and Graves' disease, and in differentiating between primary, secondary, and tertiary hypothyroidism. Called also *protirelin.*

hormonic (hor-mon′ik) hormonal.

hormonogen (hor′mon-o-jen″) prohormone.

hormonogenesis (hor″mo-no-jen′ĕ-sis) hormonopoiesis.

hormonogenic (hor″mo-no-jen′ik) hormonopoietic.

hormonology (hor″mo-nol′o-je) the science of hormones; clinical endocrinology.

hormonopexic (hor″mo-no-pek′sik) [*hormone* + Gr. *pēxis* fixation] fixing hormones.

hormonopoiesis (hor″mo-no-poi-e′sis) [*hormone* + Gr. *poiesis* a making, creation] the production of hormones.

hormonopoietic (hor″mo-no-poi-et′ik) pertaining to, characterized by, or stimulating hormonopoiesis.

hormonoprivia (hor-mōn″o-priv′e-ah) [*hormone* + L. *privus* without, deprived of] lack of hormone, or the condition produced by a deficiency of hormone in the body.

hormonosis (hor-mo-no′sis) the condition of having an excess of hormones; exogenous hormonosis is a result of therapeutic administration, as in cortisone therapy.

hormonotherapy (hor″mo-no-ther′ah-pe) treatment by the use of hormones; endocrinotherapy.

hormopoiesis (hor″mo-poi-e′sis) hormonopoiesis.

hormopoietic (hor″mo-poi-et′ik) hormonopoietic.

horn (horn) [L. *cornu*] a pointed projection such as the paired processes on the head of various animals; any structure resembling a horn in shape. Called also *cornu* [NA]. **h. of Ammon,** hippocampus. **anterior h. of lateral ventricle,** cornu anterius ventriculi lateralis. **anterior h. of spinal cord,** cornu anterius medullae spinalis. **cicatricial h.,** a hard, dry outgrowth from a cicatrix, commonly scaly and very rarely osseous. **coccygeal h.,** cornu coccygeum. **cutaneous h.,** a horny excrescence of the skin, chiefly seen on the scalp and face; called also *cornu cutaneum.* **gray h. of spinal cord, anterior,** columna anterior medullae spinalis. **gray h. of spinal cord, lateral,** columna lateralis medullae spinalis. **gray h. of spinal cord, posterior,** columna posterior medullae spinalis. **greater h. of hyoid bone,** cornu majus ossis hyoidei. **inferior h. of cerebrum,** cornu inferius ventriculi lateralis. **inferior h. of falciform margin,** cornu inferius marginis falciformis. **inferior h. of lateral ventricle,** cornu inferius ventriculi lateralis. **inferior h. of thyroid cartilage,** cornu inferius cartilaginis thyroideae. **lateral h. of hyoid**

bone, cornu majus ossis hyoidei. **lateral h. of spinal cord,** cornu laterale medullae spinalis. **lesser h. of hyoid bone,** cornu minus ossis hyoidei. **posterior h. of lateral ventricle,** cornu posterius ventriculi lateralis. **posterior h. of spinal cord,** cornu posterius medullae spinalis. **h. of pulp,** an extension of the pulp into an accentuation of the roof of the pulp chamber directly under a cusp or a developmental lobe of the tooth. **sacral h.,** cornu sacrale. **superior h. of falciform margin,** cornu superius marginis falciformis. **superior h. of hyoid bone,** cornu minus ossis hyoidei. **superior h. of thyroid cartilage,** cornu superius cartilaginis thyroideae.

Horn's sign (hornz) [C. ten *Horn*, Dutch surgeon] see under *sign*.

Horner's law, syndrome (ptosis) (hor′nerz) [Johann Friedrich *Horner*, Swiss ophthalmologist, 1831–1886] see under *law* and *syndrome*.

Horner's muscle (hor′nerz) [William Edmonds *Horner*, American anatomist, 1793–1853] pars lacrimalis musculi orbicularis oculi.

hornification (hor″nĭ-fi-ka′shun) cornification.

horny (hor′ne) having the nature and appearance of horn.

horopter (ho-rop′ter) [Gr. *horos* limit + *optēr* observer] the sum of all the points in space, the images of which fall on corresponding points of the retina. **Vieth-Müller h.,** a circle which joins the fixation point with the nodal points of the two eyes.

horopteric (hor″op-ter′ik) pertaining to a horopter.

horrida cutis (hor′ĭ-dah ku′tis) (*obs.*) cutis anserina.

horripilation (hor″ĭ-pi-la′shun) [L. *horrere* to bristle, to stand on end + *pilus* hair] erection of the fine hairs of the skin, as in cutis anserina.

horror (hor′or) [L.] dread; terror. **h. autotox′icus** [L. "fear of self poisoning"], a term coined by Ehrlich and Morgenroth in 1900 to express the refusal of a normal animal to form autoantibodies; it was believed that formation of such antibodies might result in self-destruction of the antibody producer as a result of the reaction between autoantibody and the corresponding antigen present in tissues. Now called *self-tolerance*.

horsepox (hors′poks) a mild form of poxvirus infection affecting horses, marked by a pustular eruption of the skin and sometimes of the mucosa of the mouth and nose; called also *equine smallpox*.

horse-sickness (hors-sik′nes) see *African horse sickness* and *Gambian horse sickness*, under *sickness*.

Horsley's operation, test, trephine, wax (putty) (hors′-lēz) [Sir Victor Alexander Haden *Horsley*, English surgeon, 1857–1916] see under *operation, tests, trephine,* and *wax*.

Hortega cell, method (hor-ta′gah) [Pio del Rio *Hortega*, Spanish histologist in Buenos Aires, 1882–1945] see *microglia* and under *Table of Stains*.

hortobezoar (hor″to-be-zōr′) phytobezoar.

Horton's headache, disease (arteritis, syndrome) (hōr′tunz) [Bayard Taylor *Horton*, American physician, born 1895] see *migrainous neuralgia*, under *neuralgia*, and *temporal arteritis*, under *arteritis*.

hortungskörper (hor″tungs-ker′per) [Ger., pl., "storage substances"] material deposited in body organs as one of the manifestations of aging.

H₂OsO₄ osmic acid.

Hor. un. spatio abbreviation for L. *ho′rae uni′us spa′tio*, at the end of one hour.

hospital (hos′pit-'l) [L. *hospitalium; hospes* host, guest] an institution for the treatment of the sick. "An institution suitably located, constructed, organized, managed and personneled, to supply, scientifically, economically, efficiently and unhindered, all or any recognized part of the complex requirements for the prevention, diagnosis, and treatment of physical, mental, and the medical aspect of social ills; with functioning facilities for training new workers in the many special professional, technical and economic fields essential to the discharge of its proper functions; and with adequate contacts with physicians, other hospitals, medical schools and all accredited health agencies engaged in the better health program."—Council on Medical Education. **base h.,** a hospital unit within the line of communication of the army, usually in a permanent building, designed for the reception of wounded and other patients received via field hospitals from the front, and for cases originating within the line of communication itself. **camp h.,** an immobile military unit organized and equipped for the care of the sick and wounded in camp in order to prevent immobilization of field hospitals or other mobile sanitary organizations. **closed h.,** a hospital in which only members of the staff are permitted to treat patients. **cottage h.,** a hospital consisting of a number of detached cottages. **day h.,** see *partial hospitalization*, under *hospitalization*. **evacuation h.,** a mobile advance hospital unit within the line of communication, designed to take over the functions of field hospitals when they move away with their divisions and to supplement base hospitals in their functions. **field h.,** a portable military hospital, manned by noncommissioned officers and men, located beyond the zone of conflict, 3–4 miles beyond the dressing stations, designed to shelter and care for wounded brought in by ambulance companies until they can be transported to the line of communications. **lying-in h.,** an institution for the care of obstetric patients; called also *maternity h.* **night h.,** see *partial hospitalization*, under *hospitalization*. **open h.,** 1. a mental hospital, or section of a hospital, without locked doors or other forms of physical restraint. 2. a hospital to which physicians who are not staff members may send their own patients and supervise their treatment. **teaching h.,** one that allocates a substantial part of its resources to conduct, in its own name or in association with a college or university, formal educational programs or courses of instruction that lead to granting of recognized certificates, diplomas, or degrees, or that are required for professional certification or licensure. **weekend h.,** see *partial hospitalization*, under *hospitalization*.

hospitalism (hos′pit-'l-izm″) 1. the morbid conditions due to the assembling of diseased persons in a hospital. 2. a psychoneurotic habit of attending hospital dispensaries as a patient. 3. anaclitic depression.

hospitalization (hos″pit-'l-i-za′shun) the confinement of a patient in a hospital, or the period of such confinement. **partial h.,** a psychiatric treatment program for patients who do not need full-time hospitalization, involving a special facility or an arrangement within a hospital setting to which the patient may come for treatment during the day and return home at night (*day hospital*); or return at night after a day in the community to receive treatment during the evening and to remain all night (*night hospital*); or return at the end of the week to receive treatment and remain all weekend, resuming his normal activities during the week (*weekend hospital*).

hospitalize (hos′pit-'l-īz) to place a patient in a hospital.

host (hōst) [L. *hospes*] 1. an animal or plant that harbors or nourishes another organism (parasite). 2. the recipient of an organ or other tissue transplanted from another organism (the donor). **accidental h.,** one that harbors an organism that is not ordinarily parasitic in the particular species. **alternate h.,** intermediate h. **definitive h., final h.,** the animal in which a parasite passes its adult and sexual existence. **intermediary h.,** intermediate h. **intermediate h.,** the animal in which a parasite passes its larval or nonsexual existence. **paratenic h.,** an animal acting as a substitute intermediate host of a parasite, usually having acquired the parasite by ingestion of the original host. **h. of predilection,** the host preferred by a parasite. **primary h.,** definitive h. **reservoir h.,** an animal (or species) that is infected by a parasite and which serves as a source of infection for man or another species. **secondary h.,** intermediate h. **transfer h.,** one that serves until the appropriate definitive host is reached, but is not necessary to completion of the life cycle of the parasite.

HOT human old tuberculin.

hot (hot) 1. characterized by high temperature. 2. containing dangerous radioactive material; dangerously radioactive.

Hotchkiss' operation (hoch′kis) [Lucius Wales *Hotchkiss*, American surgeon, 1860–1926] see under *operation*.

hot line (hot līn) telephone assistance for those in need of crisis intervention (q.v.), as in suicide prevention, usually available 24 hours a day, seven days a week, and staffed by nonprofessionals with mental health professionals serving as advisors or in a back-up capacity.

Hottentot bustle (hot′ten-tot) [*Hottentot*, a people of southern Africa] steatopygia.

hottentotism (hot′en-tot-izm) an exaggerated form of stuttering.

hough (hok) hock.

Houghton's test (how′tonz) [E. Mark *Houghton*, American physician, 1867–1937] see under *tests*.

Houssay animal, phenomenon (how-sāz′) [Bernardo Alberto *Houssay*, physiologist in Buenos Aires, 1887–1971; co-winner, with C. F. and G. T. Cori, of the Nobel prize in medicine and physiology for 1947 for his discovery of the role of a hormone of the anterior pituitary lobe in the metabolism of sugar.] see under *animal* and *phenomenon*.

Houston's muscle, valve (hu′stonz) [John *Houston*, Irish surgeon, 1802–1845] see under *muscle* and *valve*.

hoven (ho′ven) tympany of the stomach.

Hoverbed (hov′er-bed) trademark for a bed used for burn victims in which the entire body of the victim is supported on a stream of warm sterile air flowing upward through openings along the length of the bed.

Hovius' canal, circle, membrane, plexus (ho′ve-us) [Jacob *Hovius*, Dutch ophthalmologist, born c. 1675] see under *canal, circle,* and *plexus,* and see *entochoroidea.*

Howard's method (how′ardz) [Benjamin Douglas *Howard,* American physician, 1840–1900] see under *respiration, artificial.*

Howell's bodies, method, test (how′elz) [William Henry *Howell*, American physiologist, 1860–1945] see *Howell-Jolly bodies*, under *body*, and see under *method* and *tests*.

Howell-Jolly bodies [W. H. *Howell*; Justin Marie Jules *Jolly*, French histologist, 1870–1953] see under *body*.

Howship's lacunae (how′ships) [John *Howship*, English surgeon, 1781–1841] see *absorption lacuna*, under *lacuna*.

H.P. house physician.

Hp haptoglobin.

HPG human pituitary gonadotropin.

HPL human placental lactogen.

HPO₃ metaphosphoric acid.

H₃PO₂ hypophosphorous acid.

H₃PO₃ phosphorous acid.

H₃PO₄ orthophosphoric acid; phosphoric acid.

H₄P₂O₆ hypophosphoric acid.

H₄P₂O₇ pyrophosphoric acid.

H.S. house surgeon.

h.s. abbreviation for L. *ho′ra som′ni*, at bedtime.

H₂S hydrogen sulfide.

HSA human serum albumin.

H₂SiO₃ metasilicic acid.

H₄SiO₄ orthosilicic acid.

H₂SO₃ sulfurous acid.

H₂SO₄ sulfuric acid.

5-HT 5-hydroxytryptamine (serotonin).

Ht symbol for *total hyperopia*.

htone na (hut-to′ne-nah) a peripheral neuritis attributed to malarial origin occurring in Burma.

Hua (hu′ah) a genus of fresh-water snails. **H. ningpoen′sis,** a species of central and southern China that ingests the eggs of *Clonorchis sinensis* and in whose body the eggs hatch. **H. tou′cheana,** a first intermediate host of *Paragonimus westermani.*

Huchard's disease, sign (symptom) (e-sharz′) [Henri *Huchard*, physician in Paris, 1844–1910] see under *disease* and *sign*.

Hueck's ligament (heks) [Alexander Friedrich *Hueck*, German anatomist, 1802–1842] ligamentum pectinatum anguli iridocornealis.

Huët-Pelger nuclear anomaly (hew′et-pel′ger) [G. J. *Huët*, Dutch physician, born 1879; Karel *Pelger*, Dutch physician, 1885–1931] see *Pelger-Huët nuclear anomaly*, under *anomaly*.

Hueter's bandage, etc. (he′terz) [Karl *Hueter*, German surgeon, 1838–1882] see under *bandage, line, maneuver,* and *sign.*

Huggins operation, test (hug′inz) [Charles Brenton *Huggins*, Canadian-born surgeon in the United States, born 1901; co-winner, with Francis Peyton Rous, of the Nobel prize in medicine and physiology for 1966, for his discoveries concerning hormonal treatment of cancer of the prostate] see under *operation* and *tests.*

Hughes' reflex (hūz) [Charles Hamilton *Hughes*, American neurologist, 1839–1916] virile reflex, def. 2.

Huguenin's edema (e-gen-az′) [Gustave *Huguenin*, Swiss psychiatrist, 1841–1920] see under *edema.*

Huguier's canal, etc. (e-ge-āz′) [Pierre Charles *Huguier*, French surgeon, 1804–1873] see under *canal, circle,* and *sinus.*

Huhner test (hoon′er) [Max *Huhner*, New York urologist, 1873–1947] see under *tests.*

hum (hum) an indistinct, low, prolonged sound. **venous h.,** a continuous blowing, singing, or humming murmur heard on auscultation over the right jugular vein in the sitting or erect position; it is an innocent sign that is obliterated on assumption of the recumbent position or on exerting pressure over the vein. Called also *bruit de diable* and *humming-top murmur.*

Human's sign (hu′manz) [J. U. *Human*, London physician] chin-retraction sign.

Humatin (hu′mah-tin) trademark for preparations of paromomycin sulfate.

humectant (hu-mek′tant) [L. *humectus*, from *humectare* to be moist] 1. moistening. 2. a moistening or diluent substance.

humectation (hu″mek-ta′shun) the act of moistening.

humeral (hu′mer-al) [L. *humeralis*] of or pertaining to the humerus.

humeri (hu′mer-i) [L.] plural of *humerus.*

humeroradial (hu″mer-o-ra′de-al) pertaining to the humerus and the radius.

humeroscapular (hu″mer-o-skap′u-lar) pertaining to the humerus and the scapula.

humeroulnar (hu″mer-o-ul′nar) pertaining to the humerus and the ulna.

humerus (hu′mer-us), pl. *hu′meri* [L.] [NA] the bone that extends from the shoulder to the elbow articulating proximally with the scapula and distally with the radius and ulna; see Plate accompanying *skeleton*. **h. va′rus,** a bent humerus.

humidifier (hu-mid′ĭ-fi″er) an apparatus for controlling humidity by adding to the content of moisture in the air of a room.

humidity (hu-mid′ĭ-te) [L. *humiditas*] the degree of moisture, especially of that in the air. **absolute h.,** the actual amount of vapor in the atmosphere expressed in grains per cubit foot. **relative h.,** the percentage of moisture in the air as compared to the amount necessary to cause saturation, which is taken as 100.

humin (hu′min) 1. humic acid. 2. the dark amorphous material which is formed during the acid hydrolysis of a protein, chiefly from tryptophan.

humor (hu′mor), pl. *humors, humo′res* [L. "a liquid"] a fluid or semifluid substance; used in anatomical nomenclature to designate certain fluid materials in the body. See also *humoralism.* **aqueous h., h. aquo′sus** [NA], the fluid produced in the eye, occupying the anterior and posterior chambers, and diffusing out of the eye into the blood; regarded as the lymph of the eye, its composition varies from that of lymph in the body generally. Called also *aqueous* and *hydatoid.* **h. cristalli′nus, crystalline h.,** 1. the crystalline lens. 2. the vitreous body. **ocular h.,** one of the humors of the eye—the aqueous or vitreous. **plasmoid h.,** aqueous or vitreous humor containing an abnormally high amount of protein; formed after trauma or inflammation, it has a cloudy appearance and the proteins tend to coalesce. **vitreous h.,** 1. corpus vitreum. 2. humor vitreus. **h. vit′reus** [NA], the vitreous humor: the watery substance, resembling aqueous humor, contained within the interstices of the stroma in the vitreous body.

humoral (hu′mor-al) pertaining to the humors of the body. See also under *theory.*

humoralism (hu′mor-al-izm″) the obsolete doctrine that all diseases arise from some change of the humors; see *humoral theory,* under *theory.*

humorism (hu′mor-izm) humoralism.

Humorsol (hu′mor-sol) trademark for a solution of demecarium bromide.

humpback (hump′bak) kyphosis.

Humphry's ligament (hum′frēz) [Sir George Murray *Humphry*, English anatomist, 1820–1896] ligamenta meniscofemorale anterius.

humus (hu′mus) [L.] a dark mold of decayed vegetable material, used therapeutically in certain forms of the mud bath.

hunchback (hunch′bak) 1. kyphosis. 2. an individual characterized by a rounded deformity of the back, or kyphosis.

hunger (hung′ger) a craving, as for food. **air h.,** a distressing dyspnea occurring in paroxysms; called also *Kussmaul's* or *Kussmaul-Kien respiration.* **calcium h.,** a condition due to calcium defect, marked by severe headache during and after menstruation. **chlorine h.,** a desire for salt due to deficiency of chlorine in the blood. **hormone h.,** deficiency in the supply to any organ of the specific hormone on which its proper functioning depends.

Hunner's ulcer (hun′erz) [Guy LeRoy *Hunner*, American surgeon, born 1868] see under *ulcer.*

Hunt's atrophy, etc. (huntz) [James Ramsay *Hunt*, American neurologist, 1872–1937] see under *atrophy* and *phenomenon;* see *dyssynergia cerebellaris myoclonica;* and see *Ramsay Hunt syndrome,* under *syndrome.*

Hunt's method, reaction (test) [Reid *Hunt,* American pharmacologist, 1870–1948] see under *method* and *reaction.*

Hunter's canal, gubernaculum, operation (hunt′erz) [John *Hunter,* Scottish anatomist and surgeon, 1728–1793] see *canalis adductorius* and *gubernaculum testis,* and see under *operation.*

Hunter's glossitis [William *Hunter,* English physician, 1861–1937] see under *glossitis.*

Hunter's ligament, line [William *Hunter,* Scottish anatomist, 1718–1783, brother of John Hunter] see *ligamentum teres uteri* and *linea alba.*

hunterian (hun-te′re-an) named for or described by John Hunter, as hunterian chancre (hard chancre).

Huntington's chorea (disease) (hunt′ing-tunz) [George *Huntington,* American physician, 1850–1916] see under *chorea.*

Huppert's test (hoōp′erts) [Hugo *Huppert,* Bohemian physician, 1832–1904] see under *tests.*

Hurler's syndrome (disease) (hoor′lerz) [Gertrud *Hurler,* Austrian pediatrician] see under *syndrome.*

Hürthle cells, cell tumor (her′tel) [Karl *Hürthle,* German histologist, born 1860] see under *cell* and *tumor.*

Hurtley's test (hert′lēz) [William Holdsworth *Hurtley,* English scientist, 1867–1936] see under *tests.*

Huschke's canal, foramen, ligaments, valve (hoosh′kez) [Emil *Huschke,* German anatomist, 1797–1858] see under *canal* and *foramen,* and see *plicae gastropancreaticae* and *plica lacrimalis,* under *plica.*

husk (husk) hoose.

Hutchinson's disease, etc. (huch′in-sunz) [Sir Jonathan

Hutchinson, English surgeon, 1828–1913] see under *disease, facies, mask, patch, pupil, sign, tooth,* and *triad.*

Hutchinson-Gilford disease, syndrome (huch′in-sun-gil′-ford) [Sir Jonathan *Hutchinson;* Hastings *Gilford,* English physician, 1861–1941] progeria.

hutchinsonian (huch″in-so′ne-an) named for or described by Sir Jonathan Hutchinson.

Hutchison type (syndrome) (huch′ĭ-son) [Sir Robert *Hutchison,* English pediatrician, 1871–1960] see under *type.*

Hu-Tet (hu′tet) trademark for a preparation of tetanus immune human globulin.

Hutinel's disease (e-tin-elz′) [Victor Henri *Hutinel,* pediatrician in Paris, 1849–1933] see under *disease.*

Huxley (huks′le), Andrew Fielding. English physiologist, born 1917; co-winner, with John Carew Eccles and Alan Lloyd Hodgkin, of the Nobel prize in medicine and physiology for 1963, for discoveries concerning the ionic mechanism involved in excitation and inhibition in peripheral and central parts of the nerve cell membrane.

Huxley's layer (membrane) (huks′lēz) [Thomas Henry *Huxley,* English physiologist and naturalist, 1825–1895] see under *layer.*

huygenian (hi-jen′e-an) named for Christian *Huygens* (or Huyghens), a Dutch physicist, 1629–1695; see under *eyepiece.*

HVL half-value layer.

Hy. hyperopia.

hyal (hi′al) hyoid.

hyal- see *hyalo-.*

hyalin (hi′ah-lin) [Gr. *hyalos* glass] 1. a translucent albuminoid substance, one of the products of amyloid degeneration. 2. a substance composing the walls of hydatid cysts. **hematogenous h.,** hematohyaloid.

hyaline (hi′ah-lĭn) [Gr. *hyalos* glass] glassy and transparent or nearly so; see also under *membrane.*

hyalinization (hi″ah-lin″ĭ-za′shun) conversion into a substance resembling glass.

hyalinosis (hi″ah-lin-o′sis) hyaline degeneration. **h. cu′tis et muco′sae,** lipoid proteinosis.

hyalinuria (hi″ah-lin-u′re-ah) the discharge of hyalin in the urine, usually in the form of casts composed of protein in an acid pH.

hyalitis (hi″ah-li′tis) 1. inflammation of a hyaloid membrane (membrana vitrea). 2. inflammation of the vitreous body; vitreocapsulitis. **asteroid h.,** see under *hyalosis.* **h. puncta′ta,** inflammation of the vitreous body marked by the formation of small opacities. **h. suppurati′va,** a purulent inflammation of the vitreous body.

hyalo-, hyal- [Gr. *hyalos* glass] a combining form denoting resemblance to glass.

hyalogen (hi-al′o-jen) [*hyalo-* + Gr. *gennan* to produce] an albuminous substance occurring in cartilage, the vitreous body, etc., and convertible into hyalin.

hyaloid (hi′ah-loid) [*hyal-* + Gr. *eidos* form] resembling glass.

hyaloidin (hi″ah-loid′in) a carbohydrate radical from mucoproteins; it resembles chondroitin, but contains no sulfuric acid.

hyaloiditis (hi″ah-loi-di′tis) hyalitis.

hyalomere (hi′ah-lo-mēr″) [*hyalo-* + Gr. *meros* part] a zone of homogeneous or finely fibrillar pale blue cytoplasm surrounding the central granular portion (granulomere) of a platelet in a dry, stained blood smear. Cf. *granulomere.*

hyalomitome (hi″ah-lo-mit′ōm) hyaloplasm, def. 1.

Hyalomma (hi″ah-lom′ah) [*hyal-* + Gr. *omma* eye] a genus of ticks. *H. anatol′icum* is a cattle tick of Africa, India, and southern Europe, which may transmit Uzbekistan hemorrhagic fever and a Near Eastern variety of equine encephalomyelitis. *H. margina′tum* transmits Crimean hemorrhagic fever. *H. maurita′nicum* transmits *Theileria parva,* a protozoan parasite that causes many deaths in cattle in northern Africa.

hyalomucoid (hi″ah-lo-mu′koid) the mucoid of the vitreous body.

hyalonyxis (hi″ah-lo-nik′sis) [*hyalo-* + Gr. *nyxis* pricking] the act of puncturing the vitreous body.

hyalophagia (hi″ah-lo-fa′je-ah) [*hyalo-* + Gr. *phagein* to eat] the eating of glass.

hyalophagy (hi″ah-lof′ah-je) hyalophagia.

hyaloplasm (hi′ah-lo-plazm″) [*hyalo-* + Gr. *plasma* anything formed] 1. the more fluid, finely granular substance of the cytoplasm of cells; called also *paraplasm, interfilar mass, interfilar substance, interfibrillar substance of Flemming, paramitome, enchylema,* and *cytolymph.* 2. axoplasm. **nuclear h.,** karyolymph.

hyaloserositis (hi″ah-lo-se″ro-si′tis) [*hyalo-* + *serum* + *-itis*] a form of inflammation of serous membranes marked by hyalinization of the serous exudate into a pearly investment of the organ concerned. Cf. *frosted heart* and *perihepatitis chronica hyperplastica.* **progressive multiple h.,** Concato's disease.

hyalosis (hi″ah-lo′sis) degenerative changes in the vitreous humor. **asteroid h.,** a usually unilateral condition of the eye, most frequently seen in older men, characterized by the presence of spherical or star-shaped, calcium-containing opacities in the vitreous humor, which, when illuminated under an examining light, appear to sparkle; vision is usually unaffected. Called also *asteroid hyalitis* and *Benson's disease.*

hyalosome (hi-al′o-sōm) [*hyalo-* + Gr. *sōma* body] a structure resembling the nucleolus of a cell, but staining only slightly.

hyalotome (hi-al′o-tōm) hyaloplasm.

hyalurate (hi″ah-lu′rāt) a salt or ester of hyaluronic acid.

hyaluronate (hi″ah-lu′ro-nāt) a salt or ester of hyaluronic acid.

hyaluronidase (hi″ah-lu-ron′ĭ-dās) hyaluronate glycanohydrolase: an enzyme that catalyzes the hydrolysis of hyaluronic acid, the cement substance of the tissues. It is found in leeches, in snake and spider venom, in testes, and in malignant tissues, and is produced by a variety of pathogenic bacteria, enabling them to spread through the host's tissues. A pharmaceutical preparation suitable for injection [NF], which is a sterile, dry, soluble, enzyme product prepared from mammalian testes and capable of hydrolyzing mucopolysaccharides of the type of hyaluronic acid, is used to aid absorption and dispersion of other injected drugs and fluids, for hypodermoclysis, and for improving resorption of radiopaque media. Called also *Duran-Reynals factor, invasin,* and *diffusion* or *spreading factor.*

Hyazyme (hi′ah-zīm) trademark for a preparation of hyaluronidase for injection.

hybenzate (hi-ben′zāt) USAN contraction for *o*-(4-hydroxybenzoyl)benzoate.

hybrid (hi′brid) [L. *hybrida* mongrel] an animal or plant produced from parents different in kind, such as parents belonging to two different strains, varieties, or species. **false h.,** an individual produced by a form of gynogenesis in which the foreign spermatozoon enters the ovum, activates it to cell division, but does not fuse with the egg nucleus.

hybridism (hi′brid-izm) 1. the state of being a hybrid. 2. the production of hybrids.

hybridity (hi-brid′ĭ-te) the state of being a hybrid.

hybridization (hi″brid-i-za′shun) 1. the act or process of producing hybrids. In molecular genetics, the creation of RNA-DNA hybrids by annealing a radioactively labeled RNA fraction with denatured DNA, so that the RNA becomes associated with the complementary DNA. 2. the technique of fusing somatic cells of different species or of inserting foreign DNA into a bacterial plastid. 3. in chemistry, a procedure whereby orbitals of intermediate energy and desired directional character are constructed by taking an appropriate linear combination of atomic orbitals e.g., sp³ hybrid orbitals are formed from one s and three p orbitals.

hybridoma (hi″brĭ-do′mah) a cell culture consisting of a clone of fused (hybrid) cells of different kinds, e.g., mouse lymphocytes and myeloma cells. A spleen cell producing antibody against a specific antigenic determinant may be rendered "immortal" by fusing it with a tumor cell, with the aid of a surface-altering agent such as polyethylene glycol. The resulting hybrid will proliferate into a clone of cells producing homogeneous monoclonal antibody of a single specificity.

hycanthone (hi-kan′thōn) chemical name: 1-[[2-(diethylamino)ethyl]amino]-4-(hydroxymethyl)-9*H*-thioxanthen-9-one. A more active and less toxic metabolite of the antischistosomal drug lucanthone, $C_{20}H_{24}N_2O_2S$, highly effective against *Schistosoma haematobium* and *S. mansoni.* **h. mesylate,** the mesylate salt of hycanthone, $C_{20}H_{24}N_2O_2S \cdot CH_3SO_3H$, having the same actions as the base; administered intramuscularly.

hyclate (hi′klāt) USAN contraction for monohydrochloride hemiethanolate hemihydrate.

Hycodan (hi′ko-dan) trademark for preparations of hydrocodone bitartrate.

hydantoin (hi-dan′to-in) a crystalline base derivable from allantoin, $CO \cdot NH \cdot CH_2 \cdot CO \cdot NH.$

hydantoinate (hi″dan-to′in-āt) any salt of hydantoin.

hydathode (hi′dah-thōd) a water-secreting structure found on the edges and tips and leaves of many plants.

hydatid (hi′dah-tid) [L. *hydatis,* a drop of water] 1. a hydatid cyst. 2. any cystlike structure; see under *mole.* **alveolar h's,** see *hydatid disease, alveolar,* under *disease.* **h. of Morgagni,** a cystlike remnant of the müllerian duct attached to a testis or to the oviduct; see *appendix testis* and *appendices vesiculosi epoophori.* Called also *morgagnian cyst.* **sessile h.,** appendix testis. **Virchow's h.,** alveolar hydatid disease.

hydatidiform (hi″dah-tid′ĭ-form) resembling a hydatid cyst; see under *mole.*

hydatidosis (hi″dah-tĭ-do′sis) hydatid disease; infection with *Echinococcus.*

hydatidostomy (hi″dah-tĭ-dos′to-me) [*hydatid* + Gr. *stoma* mouth] incision and drainage of a hydatid cyst.

hydatiduria (hi″dah-tĭ-du′re-ah) the excretion of hydatid material in the urine.

Hydatigena (hi″dah-tij′en-ah) *Taenia.*

hydatism (hi′dah-tizm) [Gr. *hydatis* water] the sound caused by the presence of fluid in a cavity.

hydatoid (hi′dah-toid) 1. the aqueous humor. 2. the hyaloid membrane (membrana vitrea [NA]). 3. pertaining to the aqueous humor.

Hydeltra (hi-del′trah) trademark for preparations of prednisolone.

Hydergine (hi′der-jin) trademark for a mixture of equal parts of dihydroergocornine, dihydroergocristine, and dihydrocryptine, in the form of methansulfonate salts, used as a vasodilator for the treatment of peripheral vascular disease.

hydnocarpate (hid-no-kar′pāt) a salt of hydnocarpic acid.

Hydnocarpus (hid″no-kar′pus) a genus of Indomalayan trees. *H. wightiana* Blume and *H. anthelmintica* Pierre (Flacourtiaceae) are sources of chaulmoogra oil.

hydr- see *hydro-.*

hydracetin (hi-dras′ĕ-tin) acetylphenylhydrazine.

hydracid (hi-dras′id) 1. haloid acid. 2. binary acid.

hydradenitis (hi″drad-ĕ-ni′tis) hidradenitis.

hydradenoma (hi″drad-ĕ-no′mah) hidradenoma.

hydraeroperitoneum (hi-dra″ĕ-ro-per″ĭ-to-ne′um) [*hydr-* + Gr. *aēr* air + *peritoneum*] a collection of watery fluid and gas in the peritoneal cavity.

hydragogue (hi′drah-gog) [*hydr-* + Gr. *agōgos* leading] 1. producing watery discharge, especially from the bowels. 2. a cathartic which causes watery purgation.

hydralazine hydrochloride (hi-dral′ah-zēn) [USP] chemical name: 1-hydrazinophthalazine hydrochloride. An antihypertensive, $C_8H_8N_4 \cdot HCl$, occurring as a white crystalline powder; administered orally, intramuscularly, or intravenously.

hydramine (hi′drah-min) an amine derived from a glycol in which one hydroxyl is replaced by an amino group.

hydramnion (hi-dram′ne-on) hydramnios.

hydramnios (hi-dram′ne-os) [*hydr-* + *amnion*] excess of amniotic fluid.

hydranencephaly (hi″dran-en-sef′ah-le) complete or almost complete absence of the cerebral hemispheres, the space they normally occupy being filled with cerebrospinal fluid.

Hydrangea (hi-dran′je-ah) a genus of saxifragaceous trees and shrubs. A glycoside from the dried rhizome and roots of *H. arborescens* L. (Saxifragaceae) was formerly used as a diuretic. Called also *seven barks.*

hydrangiography (hi-dran″je-og′rah-fe) [*hydr-* + Gr. *angeion* vessel + *graphein* to write] 1. a description of the lymphatic vessels. 2. lymphangiography.

hydrangiology (hi-dran″je-ol′o-je) [*hydr-* + Gr. *angeion* vessel + *-logy*] lymphangiology.

hydrangiotomy (hi-dran″je-ot′o-me) [*hydr-* + Gr. *angeion* vessel + *tomē* a cutting] lymphangiotomy.

hydrargyri (hi-drar′jĭ-ri) genitive of L. *hydrargyrum*, mercury. **h. bichlo′ridum**, mercury bichloride. **h. chlo′ridum corrosi′vum**, mercury bichloride. **h. iodi′dum fla′vum**, mercurous iodide, yellow. **h. iodi′dum ru′brum**, mercuric iodide, red. **h. ox′idum fla′vum**, mercuric oxide, yellow. **h. sali′cylas**, mercuric salicylate.

hydrargyria, hydrargyrism (hi″drar-jir′e-ah; hi-drar′jĭ-rizm) mercury poisoning; see under *poisoning.*

hydrargyromania (hi-drar′jĭ-ro-ma′ne-ah) mental disorder due to mercury poisoning.

hydrargyrorelapsing (hi-drar″jĭ-ro-re-laps′ing) relapsing after apparently successful mercurial treatment.

hydrargyrosis (hi-drar″jĭ-ro′sis) mercury poisoning; see under *poisoning.*

hydrargyrum (hi-drar′jĭ-rum), gen. *hydrar′gyri* [L. "liquid silver"] mercury. **h. ammonia′tum**, ammoniated mercury. **h. chlo′ridum mi′te**, calomel. **h. olea′tum**, mercury oleate.

hydrarthrodial (hi″drar-thro′de-al) pertaining to hydrarthrosis.

hydrarthrosis (hi″drar-thro′sis) [*hydr-* + Gr. *arthron* joint + *-osis*] an accumulation of watery fluid in the cavity of a joint. **intermittent h.**, serous effusion into a joint occurring periodically.

hydrase (hi′drās) hydratase.

hydratase (hi′drah-tās) any enzyme (hydro-lyase) that catalyzes the hydration or dehydration of C—O linkages. Formerly called *hydrase.*

hydrate (hi′drāt) [L. *hydras*] 1. any compound of a radical with H_2O. 2. any salt or other compound that contains water of crystallization.

hydrated (hi′drāt-ed) [L. *hydratus*] combined with water; forming a hydrate or a hydroxide.

hydration (hi-dra′shun) 1. the act of combining or causing to

combine with water. 2. the condition of being combined with water.

hydraulics (hi-draw′liks) [*hydr-* + Gr. *aulos* pipe] the branch of physics which treats of the action of liquids under physical laws.

hydrazine (hi′drah-zin) a colorless, gaseous diamine, H_2N--NH_2; also any member of a group of its substitution derivatives. Called also *diamide.*

hydrazinolysis (hi″drah-zin-ol′ĭ-sis) cleavage of the peptide bonds of a peptide by hydrazine, with the C-terminal residue appearing as a free amino acid.

hydrazone (hi-drah-zōn) a compound formed from an aldehyde or ketone by the action of phenylhydrazine.

Hydrea (hi-dre′ah) trademark for a preparation of hydroxyurea.

hydremia (hi-dre′me-ah) [*hydr-* + Gr. *haima* blood] excess of water in the blood; a condition in which the proportion of the serum in the blood to the corpuscles is excessive.

hydrencephalocele (hi″dren-sef′ah-lo-sēl) [*hydr-* + *encephalocele*] encephalocystocele.

hydrencephalomeningocele (hi″dren-sef″ah-lo-mĕ-ning′go-sēl) hernial protrusion through a cranial defect of the meninges containing cerebrospinal fluid and brain substance.

hydrencephalus (hi″dren-sef′ah-lus) hydrocephalus.

hydrencephaly (hi″dren-sef′ah-le) hydrocephalus.

hydrepigastrium (hi″drep-ĭ-gas′tre-um) [*hydr-* + *epigastrium*] a collection of watery fluid between the peritoneum and the abdominal wall.

hydriatric (hi″dre-at′rik) [*hydr-* + Gr. *iatikos, iatrikos* healing] pertaining to hydrotherapy.

hydriatrics (hi″dre-at′riks) hydrotherapy.

hydric (hi′drik) pertaining to or combined with hydrogen; containing replaceable hydrogen.

hydride (hi′drīd) [Gr. *hydōr* water] any compound of hydrogen with an element or radical.

hydrindicuria (hi″drin-dĭ-ku′re-ah) the presence in the urine of indoles related to both tryptophan and phenylalanine.

hydrion (hi-dri′on) hydrogen ion.

hydro-, hydr- [Gr. *hydōr* water] combining form denoting relationship to water or to hydrogen.

hydroa (hid-ro′ah) a vesicular eruption attended with intense itching and burning, occurring on surfaces of the skin exposed to sunlight; it usually affects prepubertal boys, and tends to recur each summer. Some consider it to be associated with erythropoietic protoporphyria. The eruption in *h. aestiva′le* is polymorphic, whereas *h. vaccinifor′me*, which is considered by some to be a severe form of hydroa aestivale, is marked by the formation of umbilicated bullae that heal with scarring.

hydroadipsia (hi″dro-ah-dip′se-ah) [*hydro-* + *a* neg. + Gr. *dipsa* thirst] absence of thirst for water.

hydroappendix (hi″dro-ah-pen′diks) distention of the vermiform appendix with a watery fluid.

Hydrobiidae (hi″dro-be′ĭ-de) a family of snails (order Mesogastropoda) that includes the subfamilies Hydrobiinae and Buliminae, which are intermediate hosts of various species of parasitic flukes.

Hydrobiinae (hi″dro-be′ĭ-ne) a subfamily of snails (family Hydrobiidae, order Mesogastropoda) that includes the genus *Oncomelania*, the intermediate host of *Schistosoma japonicum.*

hydrobilirubin (hi″dro-bil″ĭ-roo′bin) [*hydro-* + *bilirubin*] a brownish-red pigment, $C_{32}H_{40}N_4O_7$, derivable from bilirubin by reduction. It is believed to be identical with stercobilin and urobilin.

hydroblepharon (hi″dro-blef′ah-ron) [*hydro-* + Gr. *blepharon* eyelid] edema of the eyelids.

hydrobromide (hi″dro-bro′mīd) an addition salt of hydrobromic acid. Cf. *hydrochloride.*

Hydrocal (hi′dro-kal) trademark for an artificial stone (a gypsum product) used in dentistry.

hydrocalycosis (hi″dro-kal″ĭ-ko′sis) [*hydro-* + *calyx* + *-osis*] a usually asymptomatic cystic dilatation of a major renal calix, lined by transitional epithelium and due to obstruction of the infundibulum.

hydrocalyx (hi″dro-kal′iks) a cyst in the renal cortex caused by obstruction at the infundibulum; the entire calyx dilates to form the cyst wall.

hydrocarbarism (hi″dro-kar′bar-izm) hydrocarbonism.

hydrocarbon (hi″dro-kar′bon) an organic compound that contains carbon and hydrogen only. The hydrocarbons are divided into *alicyclic, aliphatic,* and *aromatic* hydrocarbons, according to the arrangement of the atoms and the chemical properties of the compounds. **alicyclic h.,** a hydrocarbon that has cyclic structure and aliphatic properties. **aliphatic h.,** a hydrocarbon in which no carbon atoms are joined to form a ring. **aromatic h.,** a hydrocarbon that has cyclic structure and a closed conjugated system of double bonds that gives it the characteristic chemical properties of the parent aromatic hydrocarbon, benzene

(C_6H_6); other typical aromatic hydrocarbons are toluene (C_7H_8), naphthalene ($C_{10}H_8$), anthracene ($C_{14}H_{10}$), and phenanthrene ($C_{14}H_{10}$). **carcinogenic h.,** a condensed nuclear aromatic hydrocarbon that tends to cause cancer when applied to the skin or when otherwise administered. **cyclic h.,** one of a series of hydrocarbons having the general formula C_nH_{2n}, the carbon atoms being thought of as having a closed ring structure. **saturated h.,** a hydrocarbon that has the maximum number of hydrogen atoms for a given carbon structure, such as methane, ethane, propane, cyclopropane, and the butanes. **unsaturated h.,** an aliphatic or alicyclic hydrocarbon that has less than the maximum number of hydrogen atoms for a given carbon structure, such as ethylene, acetylene, propylene, cyclohexene, and the butanes.

hydrocarbonism (hi″dro-kar′bon-izm) poisoning by hydrocarbons.

hydrocardia (hi″dro-kar′de-ah) hydropericardium.

hydrocele (hi′dro-sēl) [*hydro-* + Gr. *kēlē* tumor] a circumscribed collection of fluid, especially a collection of fluid in the tunica vaginalis of the testicle or along the spermatic cord.

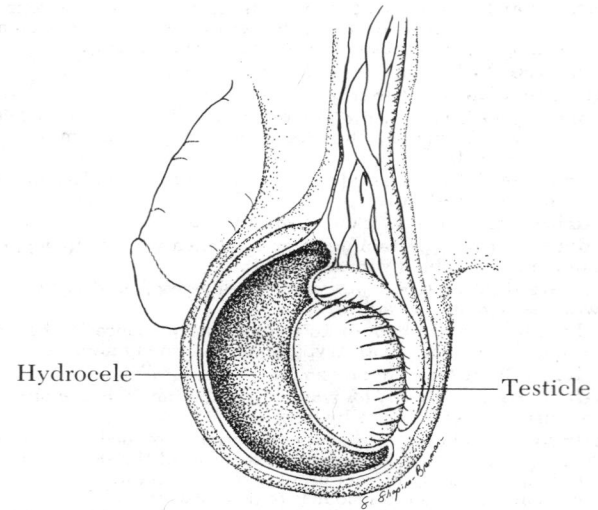

Hydrocele — — Testicle

cervical h., a serous dilatation of a persistent cervical duct, or sometimes of a deep cervical lymph space; called also *h. colli* and *Maunoir's h.* **chylous h.,** a form in which the fluid is milky in appearance. **h. col′li,** cervical h. **communicating h.,** hydrocele in which the processus vaginalis testis is patent. **congenital h.,** hydrocele in the unobliterated canal between the peritoneal cavity and that of the tunica vaginalis. **diffused h.,** a collection of fluid diffused in the loose connective tissue of the spermatic cord. **Dupuytren's h.,** bilocular hydrocele of the tunica vaginalis testis. **encysted h.,** one which occurs in cysts outside the cavity of the tunica vaginalis testis. **h. fem′inae,** an affection of the round ligament of the female resembling ordinary hydrocele. **funicular h.,** hydrocele of the tunica vaginalis of the spermatic cord in a space closed toward the testis and open toward the peritoneal cavity. **Gibbon's h.,** see under *hernia.* **hernial h.,** distention of the hernial sac with a fluid. **Maunoir's h.,** cervical hydrocele. **h. mulie′-bris** (*obs.*), a watery dilatation of the canal of Nuck; called also *Nuck's h.* **h. of neck,** cervical h. **Nuck's h.** (*obs.*), h. muliebris. **h. rena′lis,** a condition in which the renal capsule forms part of a cyst wall so that the kidney is partially or almost wholly surrounded by the cyst; although often found after trauma in adults, such a cyst is of congenital origin. **scrotal h.,** a circumscribed collection of fluid in the scrotum. **h. spina′lis,** spina bifida.

hydrocelectomy (hi″dro-se-lek′to-me) [*hydrocele* + Gr. *ektomē* excision] excision of a hydrocele.

hydrocenosis (hi″dro-se-no′sis) [*hydro-* + Gr. *kenōsis* emptying] removal of dropsical fluid.

hydrocephalic (hi″dro-sĕ-fal′ik) pertaining to or affected with hydrocephalus.

hydrocephalocele (hi″dro-sef′ah-lo-sēl″) encephalocystocele.

hydrocephaloid (hi″dro-sef′ah-loid) 1. resembling hydrocephalus. 2. see under *disease.*

hydrocephalus (hi-dro-sef′ah-lus) [*hydro-* + Gr. *kephalē* head] a condition marked by dilatation of the cerebral ventricles, most often occurring secondarily to obstruction of the cerebrospinal fluid pathways (see *ventricular block,* under *block*), and accompanied by an accumulation of cerebrospinal fluid within the skull; the fluid is usually under increased pressure, but occasionally may be normal or nearly so. It is typically characterized by enlargement of the head, prominence of the forehead, brain atrophy, mental deterioration, and convulsions, and may be congenital or

acquired, and be of sudden onset (*acute h.*) or be slowly progressive (*chronic* or *primary h.*). **communicating h.,** hydrocephalus in which there is no obstruction in the ventricular system, and cerebrospinal fluid passes readily out of the brain into the spinal canal, but is not absorbed. **h. ex vac′uo,** a compensatory replacement by cerebrospinal fluid of the volume of tissue lost in atrophy of the brain. **noncommunicating h.,** obstructive h. **normal-pressure h., normal-pressure occult h.,** dementia, ataxia, and urinary incontinence with pneumoencephalographic evidence of hydrocephalus, i.e., with enlarged ventricles associated with inadequacy of the subarachnoid spaces, but with normal cerebrospinal fluid pressure; occurring in middle-aged and older persons. Called also *occult normal-pressure h.* **obstructive h.,** hydrocephalus due to ventricular block (q.v.); called also *noncommunicating h.* **occult normal-pressure h.,** normal-pressure h. **otitic h.,** acute hydrocephalus caused by spread of the inflammation of otitis media to the cranial cavity. **secondary h.,** hydrocephalus resulting from meningitis.

hydrocephaly (hi″dro-sef′ah-le) hydrocephalus.

hydrochloride (hi″dro-klo′rīd) an addition salt of hydrochloric acid, for instance with quinine. The hydrochloric acid adds on in such a way that the valence of the basic nitrogen is changed from three to five. In a sense the alkaloid hydrochlorides may be looked on as derivatives of ammonium chloride:

$$\begin{array}{c} H \\ H-N \\ H \end{array} \begin{array}{c} H \\ Cl \end{array}$$

hydrochlorothiazide (hi″dro-klo″ro-thi′ah-zīd) [USP] chemical name: 6-chloro-3,4-dihydro-2*H*-1,2,4-benzothiadiazine-7-sulfonamide-1,1-dioxide. An orally effective diuretic and antihypertensive, $C_7H_8ClN_3 \cdot O_4S_2$, occurring as a white or nearly white, crystalline powder.

hydrocholecystis (hi″dro-ko″le-sis′tis) [*hydro-* + Gr. *cholē* bile + *kystis* bladder] distention of the gallbladder with watery fluid; hydrops of the gallbladder.

hydrocholeresis (hi″dro-ko″lĕ-re′sis) [*hydro-* + Gr. *cholē* bile + *hairesis* a taking] choleresis characterized by increase in water output, or induction of the excretion of bile relatively low in specific gravity, viscosity, and total solid content.

hydrocholeretic (hi″dro-ko″lĕ-ret′ik) pertaining to, characterized by, or producing hydrocholeresis.

hydrocholesterol (hi″dro-ko-les′ter-ol) a reduced form of cholesterol.

hydrocinchonidine (hi″dro-sin-kon′ĭ-din) an alkaloid, $C_{19}H_{24}ON_2$, isomeric with cinchonine.

hydrocirsocele (hi″dro-sir′so-sēl) [*hydro-* + *cirsocele*] hydrocele combined with varicocele.

hydrocodone bitartrate (hi″dro-ko′dōn) [USP] a semisynthetic product of codeine, $C_{18}H_{21}NO_3 \cdot C_4H_6O_6 \cdot 2\frac{1}{2}H_2O$, occurring as a fine, white, crystalline powder, having narcotic analgesic effects similar to but more active than those of codeine; used as an antitussive, administered orally. Called also *dihydrocodeinone bitartrate.*

hydrocollidine (hi″dro-kol′ĭ-din) [*hydro-* + *collidine*] a poisonous oily ptomaine, $C_8H_{13}N$, from nicotine, decayed flesh, and stale fish.

hydrocolloid (hi″dro-kol′loid) [*hydro-* + *colloid*] a colloid system in which water is the dispersion medium. **irreversible h.,** a hydrocolloid which can be converted from the sol to the gel condition but cannot be reverted to a sol by any simple means. **reversible h.,** a hydrocolloid which can be reverted from the gel to the sol condition by increase in temperature.

hydrocolpos (hi″dro-kol′pos) [*hydro-* + Gr. *kolpos* vagina] a collection of watery fluid in the vagina.

hydroconion (hi″dro-ko′ne-on) [*hydro-* + Gr. *konis* dust] an atomizer or vaporizer for throwing liquids in a fine spray.

hydrocortamate hydrochloride (hi″dro-kor′tah-māt) chemical name: cortisol 21-ester with *N,N*-diethylglycine hydrochloride. A synthetic glucocorticoid, $C_{27}H_{41}NO_6 \cdot HCl$, used topically as an anti-inflammatory in the treatment of steroid-responsive dermatoses.

hydrocortisone (hi″dro-kor′tĭ-sōn) chemical name: 11β,-17α,21-trihydroxypregn-4-ene-3,20-dione. The major glucocorticoid, $C_{21}H_{30}O_5$, elaborated by the human adrenal cortex (or *cortisol,* as it is usually referred to by biochemists), or the same substance produced synthetically; it has life-maintaining properties and also has appreciable mineralocorticoid activity. The official preparation [USP] and its salts are used in the treatment of inflammations, allergies, pruritus, collagen diseases (rheumatoid arthritis, lupus erythematosus, etc.), some neoplasms, acute or chronic adrenocortical deficiency, severe status asthmaticus, and shock. **h. acetate** [USP], an ester of hydrocortisone, $C_{23}H_{32}O_6$, occurring as a white to practically white, crystalline powder, having actions and uses similar to those of the base; administered by intra-articular or soft-tissue injection or applied topically to the skin or conjunctiva. **h. cyclopentylpropionate, h. cypionate** [USP], an ester of hydrocortisone, $C_{29}H_{42}O_6$, occurring as a white to practically white, crystalline powder, having actions and uses similar to those of the base; administered orally. **h. hemisuccinate** [USP], an ester of hydrocortisone, $C_{25}H_{34}O_8$, having actions and uses similar to those of the base. **h. sodium phosphate** [USP], a water-soluble ester of hydrocortisone, $C_{21}H_{29}Na_2O_8P$, occurring as a white to light yellow powder, having actions and uses similar to those of the base; administered intravenously or intramuscularly, especially for adrenocortical insufficiency. **h. sodium succinate** [USP], a water-soluble ester of hydrocortisone, $C_{25}H_{33}NaO_8$, occurring as a white or nearly white crystalline powder, having actions and uses similar to those of the base; administered intravenously or intramuscularly, especially for acute adrenocortical insufficiency. **h. valerate,** an ester of hydrocortisone, $C_{26}H_{38}O_6$, having actions similar to those of the base.

Hydrocortone (hi″dro-kor′tōn) trademark for preparations of hydrocortisone.

hydrocyanism (hi″dro-si′an-izm) poisoning with hydrocyanic acid.

hydrocyst (hi′dro-sist) [hydro- + Gr. kystis sac, bladder] a cyst with watery contents.

hydrocystadenoma (hi″dro-sis″tad-ĕ-no′mah) papillary hidradenoma; see hidradenoma.

hydrodiascope (hi″dro-di′ah-skōp) [hydro- + Gr. dia through + skopein to see] an instrument used in the treatment of astigmatism.

hydrodictiotomy (hi″dro-dik″te-ot′o-me) an operation for displacement of the retina (R. Secondi).

hydrodiffusion (hi″dro-dĭ-fu′zhun) diffusion in an aqueous medium.

hydrodipsia (hi″dro-dip′se-ah) thirst for water.

hydrodipsomania (hi″dro-dip″so-ma′ne-ah) an epileptic condition characterized by attacks of insatiable thirst.

hydrodiuresis (hi″dro-di′u-re′sis) [hydro- + diuresis] copious secretion of urine of low specific gravity.

Hydrodiuril (hi″dro-di′u-ril) trademark for a preparation of hydrochlorothiazide.

hydrodynamics (hi″dro-di-nam′iks) [hydro- + dynamics] that branch of the science of mechanics which treats of the movement of fluids and of solids contained in fluids.

hydroelectric (hi″dro-e-lek′trik) pertaining to water and electricity.

hydroencephalocele (hi″dro-en-sef′ah-lo-sēl) encephalocystocele.

hydroflumethiazide (hi″dro-floo″mĕ-thi′ah-zīd) [USP] chemical name: 3,4-dihydro-6-(trifluoromethyl)-2H-1,2,4-benzothiadiazine-7-sulfonamide 1,1-dioxide. An antihypertensive and diuretic, $C_8H_8F_3N_3O_4S_2$, occurring as a white to cream-colored, finely divided, crystalline powder; administered orally.

hydrogel (hi′dro-jel) a gel that has water as its dispersion medium.

hydrogen (hi′dro-jen) [hydro- + Gr. gennan to produce] the lightest element, an odorless, tasteless, colorless gas that is inflammable and explosive when mixed with air. It is found in water and in almost all organic compounds. Its ion is the active constituent of all acids in the water system. Its symbol is H; atomic number, 1; atomic weight, 1.00797; specific gravity, 0.069. Hydrogen exists in three isotopes: ordinary, or light, hydrogen is the mass 1 isotope, also called protium; heavy hydrogen is the mass 2 isotope, also called deuterium; mass 3 isotope is tritium. **arseniuretted h.,** see under arsine. **h. cyanide,** an extremely poisonous colorless liquid or gas, HCN, used as a rodenticide and insecticide, its toxic effect being due to its inhibition of the oxidation of cytochrome, resulting in suppression of cellular respiration; it can cause tachypnea, dyspnea, paralysis, and respiratory arrest. Called also hydrocyanic acid. **h. disulfide,** an ill-smelling liquid, H_2S_2. **heavy h.,** see hydrogen. **light h.,** see hydrogen. **h. monoxide,** water, H_2O. **ordinary h.,** see hydrogen. **h. peroxide,** a strongly disinfectant cleansing and bleaching liquid, H_2O_2, used in dilute solution in water, mainly as a wash or spray. **h. selenide,** a poisonous gas, H_2Se; its inhalation causes an obstinate coryza and destroys the sense of smell. **h. sulfide,** an offensive and poisonous gas, H_2S, used as a chemical reagent; called also hydrosulfuric or sulfhydric acid. **sulfuretted h.,** h. sulfide.

hydrogenase (hi′dro-jen-ās) hydrogen: ferredoxin oxidoreductase. An enzyme that catalyzes the reduction of various substances by means of molecular hydrogen. **fumaric h.,** a yellow enzyme that catalyzes the reduction of fumaric acid to succinic acid.

hydrogenate (hi′dro-jen-āt″) to cause to combine with hydrogen; to reduce with hydrogen.

hydrogenize (hi′dro-jen-īz) hydrogenate.

hydrogenlyase (hi″dro-jen-li′ās) an adaptive enzyme formed by many strains of Escherichia coli that catalyzes the breakdown of formic acid to carbon dioxide and hydrogen.

hydrogenoid (hi-droj′ĕ-noid) a homeopathic term denoting a constitution or temperament that will not tolerate much moisture.

Hydrogenomonas (hi-dro″jĕ-no-mo′nas) a genus of schizomy-

cetes of the family Methanomonadaceae, suborder Pseudomonadinae, order Pseudomonadales, occurring as facultative chemoautotrophic, short, rod-shaped cells obtaining energy from the oxidation of hydrogen. It includes four species, H. fa′cilis, H. fla′va, H. panto′tropha, and H. vit′rea.

hydrogymnastic (hi″dro-jim-nas′tik) pertaining to exercises performed in the water.

hydrogymnastics (hi″dro-jim-nas′tiks) therapeutic exercise performed in water.

hydrohematonephrosis (hi″dro-hem″ah-to-nĕ-fro′sis) [hydro- + Gr. haima blood + nephros kidney] distention of the pelvis of the kidney with an accumulation of bloody urine.

hydrohepatosis (hi″dro-hep″ah-to′sis) [hydro- + Gr. hēpar liver] a condition in which there is a collection of watery fluid in the liver.

hydrohymenitis (hi″dro-hi″men-i′tis) [hydro- + Gr. hymēn membrane + -itis] inflammation of a serous membrane.

hydrokinesitherapy (hi″dro-ki-ne″sĭ-ther′ah-pe) [hydro- + Gr. kinēsis movement + therapeia treatment] treatment by underwater exercise.

hydrokinetic (hi″dro-ki-net′ik) relating to the movement of water or other fluid, as in a whirlpool bath.

hydrokinetics (hi″dro-ki-net′iks) [hydro- + Gr. kinēsis motion] that branch of mechanics which treats of fluids in motion.

hydrokollag (hi″dro-kol′ag) a suspension of finely particulate graphite, used in experimental study of ciliary action and lymphatic drainage.

hydrol (hi′drol) a final mother liquor obtained in the manufacture of glucose from cornstarch.

hydrolabile (hi″dro-la′bil) having a tendency to lose weight under carbohydrate or salt restriction or following infections or gastrointestinal disease. Cf. hydrostabile.

hydrolability (hi″dro-lah-bil′ĭ-te) [hydro- + L. labilis liable to change] a condition in which tissue fluids tend to vary in quantity.

hydrolase (hi′dro-lās) one of the six main groups of enzymes, comprising those that catalyze the hydrolytic cleavage of a compound, such as esters, peptides, glycosides, and amides. **acetoacetylglutathione h.,** an enzyme that catalyzes the hydrolysis of acetoacetylglutathione to acetoacetate and glutathione. **acetyl-CoA h.,** an enzyme that catalyzes the hydrolysis of acetyl-CoA to CoA and acetate; called also acetyl-CoA deacylase. **acid h's,** a collective term for the enzymes of lysosomes. **formyl-CoA h.,** an enzyme that catalyzes the hydrolysis of formyl-CoA to CoA and formate. **guanosine h.,** an enzyme that catalyzes the conversion of guanosine into guanine and sugar. **hydroxyacylglutathione h.,** an enzyme that catalyzes the hydrolysis of S-2-hydroxyacylglutathione to glutathione and a 2-hydroxyacid anion; called also glyoxalase II. **3-hydroxyisobutyryl-CoA h.,** an enzyme that catalyzes the hydrolysis of 3-hydroxyisobutyryl-CoA to CoA and 3-hydroxyisobutyrate. **hydroxymethylglutaryl-CoA h.,** an enzyme that catalyzes the hydrolysis of 3-hydroxy-3-methylglutaryl-CoA to CoA and 3-hydroxy-3-methylglutarate. **palmitoyl-CoA h.,** an enzyme that catalyzes the hydrolysis of palmitoyl CoA to CoA and palmitate. **succinyl-CoA h.,** an enzyme that catalyzes the hydrolysis of succinyl-CoA to CoA and succinate.

hydrology (hi-drol′o-je) [hydro- + -logy] the sum of knowledge regarding water and its uses.

Hydrolose (hi′dro-lōs) trademark for a preparation of methylcellulose.

hydro-lyase (hi″dro-li′ās) any lyase that removes water from a compound.

hydrolymph (hi′dro-limf) [hydro- + lymph] the thin, watery nutritive fluid of certain of the lower animals.

hydrolysate (hi-drol′ĭ-zāt) a compound produced by hydrolysis. **protein h.,** a mixture of amino acids prepared by splitting a protein with acid, alkali, or enzyme. Such preparations provide the nutritive equivalent of the original material (casein, lactalbumin, fibrin, etc.) in the form of its constituent amino acids; used in special diets or for patients unable to take the ordinary food proteins.

hydrolysis (hi-drol′ĭ-sis) pl. hydrol′yses [hydro- + Gr. lysis dissolution] the splitting of a compound into fragments by the addition of water, the hydroxyl group being incorporated in one fragment, and the hydrogen atom in the other.

hydrolyst (hi′dro-list) an agent that promotes hydrolysis.

hydrolyte (hi′dro-līt) a substance undergoing hydrolysis.

hydrolytic (hi-dro-lit′ik) pertaining to, characterized by, or promoting hydrolysis.

hydrolyze (hi′dro-līz) to subject to hydrolysis.

hydroma (hi-dro′mah) hygroma.

hydromassage (hi″dro-mah-sahzh′) massage by means of moving water.

hydromeningitis (hi″dro-men″in-ji′tis) [hydro- + meningitis] meningitis with serous effusion.

hydromeningocele (hi″dro-mĕ-ning′go-sēl) [hydro- + Gr.

mēninx membrane + *kēlē* hernia] protrusion of the meninges through a defect in the skull or spine, forming a sac containing cerebrospinal fluid.

hydrometer (hi-drom′ĕ-ter) [*hydro-* + Gr. *metron* measure] an instrument for determining the specific gravities of a fluid.

hydrometra (hi″dro-me′trah) [*hydro-* + Gr. *mētra* uterus] a collection of watery fluid in the uterus.

hydrometric (hi″dro-met′rik) pertaining to hydrometry.

hydrometrocolpos (hi″dro-me″tro-kol′pos) [*hydro-* + Gr. *mētra* uterus + *kolpos* vagina] a collection of watery fluid in the uterus and vagina.

hydrometry (hi-drom′ĕ-tre) the measurement of the specific gravity of a fluid by means of the hydrometer.

hydromicrocephaly (hi″dro-mi″kro-sef′ah-le) microcephaly with an abnormal amount of cerebrospinal fluid.

hydromorphone (hi″dro-mor′fōn) chemical name: 4,5α-epoxy-3-hydroxy-17-methyl-methylmorphinan-6-one. A morphine alkaloid, $C_{17}H_{19}NO_3$, occurring as a fine, white or practically white, crystalline powder, having narcotic analgesic effects similar to but greater and of shorter duration than those of morphine; administered as the sulfate salt by subcutaneous injection. **h. hydrochloride** [USP], the hydrochloride salt of hydromorphone, $C_{17}H_{19}NO_3 \cdot HCl$, having the same actions as the base; administered orally and subcutaneously. Called also *dihydromorphinone hydrochloride*.

Hydromox (hi′dro-moks) trademark for preparations of quinethazone.

hydromphalus (hi-drom′fah-lus) [*hydro-* + Gr. *omphalos* navel] a cystic accumulation of watery fluid at the umbilicus.

hydromyelia (hi″dro-mi-e′le-ah) a pathologic condition characterized by accumulation of fluid in the enlarged central canal of the spinal cord.

hydromyelocele (hi″dro-mi-el′o-sēl) [*hydro-* + *myelocele*] hydromyelomeningocele.

hydromyelomeningocele (hi″dro-mi″ĕ-lo-mĕ-ning′go-sēl) [*hydro-* + Gr. *myelos* marrow + *mēninx* membrane + *kēlē* hernia] a defect of the spine marked by protrusion of the membranes and tissue of the spinal cord, forming a fluid-filled sac.

hydromyoma (hi″dro-mi-o′mah) [*hydro-* + *myoma*] uterine leiomyoma with cystic degeneration.

hydronaphthylamine (hi″dro-naf″thil-am′in) a powerfully mydriatic substance, $C_{10}H_{11}NH_2$.

hydronephrosis (hi″dro-nĕ-fro′sis) [*hydro-* + Gr. *nephros* kidney] distention of the pelvis and calices of the kidney with urine, as a result of obstruction of the ureter, with accompanying atrophy of the parenchyma of the organ. **closed h.,** a permanent condition, resulting from complete obstruction of the ureter. **open h.,** an intermittent condition, resulting from sporadic or incomplete obstruction of the ureter.

hydronephrotic (hi″dro-nĕ-frot′ik) pertaining to or characterized by hydronephrosis.

hydronium (hi-dro′ne-um) the hydrated proton, H_3O^+; it is the form in which the proton (hydrogen ion, H^+) exists in aqueous solution, a combination of H^+ and H_2O.

Hydronol (hi′dro-nol) trademark for a preparation of isosorbide.

hydropancreatosis (hi″dro-pan″kre-ah-to′sis) the accumulation of watery fluid in the pancreas.

hydroparotitis (hi″dro-par″o-ti′tis) distention of the parotid gland with watery fluid.

hydropathic (hi″dro-path′ik) pertaining to hydropathy.

hydropathy (hi-drop′ah-the) [*hydro-* + Gr. *pathos* disease] (*obs.*) treatment of disease by the application of water; particularly a system of treatment which professes to cure all diseases by the use of water; water cure.

hydropenia (hi″dro-pe′ne-ah) [*hydro-* + Gr. *penia* poverty] deficiency of water in the body.

hydropenic (hi″dro-pe′nik) relating to hydropenia.

hydropericarditis (hi″dro-per″ĭ-kar-di′tis) pericarditis attended with a watery effusion in the pericardial sac.

hydropericardium (hi″dro-per″ĭ-kar′de-um) [*hydro-* + *pericardium*] abnormal accumulation of serous fluid in the pericardial cavity.

hydroperinephrosis (hi″dro-per″ĭ-nĕ-fro′sis) [*hydro-* + Gr. *peri* around + *nephros* kidney + *-osis*] a collection of fluid in the retroperitoneal connective tissue and opening into the pelvis of the kidney.

hydroperion (hi″dro-per′e-on) [*hydro-* + Gr. *peri* around + *ōon* egg] the fluid between the capsular and parietal decidua.

hydroperitoneum (hi″dro-per″ĭ-to-ne′um) [*hydro-* + *peritoneum*] ascites, or abnormal accumulation of fluid in the peritoneal cavity.

hydroperitonia (hi″dro-per″ĭ-to′ne-ah) ascites.

hydropexia (hi″dro-pek′se-ah) hydropexis.

hydropexic (hi″dro-pek′sik) [*hydro-* + Gr. *pēxis* fixation] fixing or holding water; pertaining to the holding of water.

hydropexis (hi″dro-pek′sis) the fixation or holding of water.

hydrophagocytosis (hi″dro-fag″o-si-to′sis) [*hydro-* + *phagocytosis*] the absorption by macrophages of plasma surrounding them; called also *Lewis' phenomenon*.

hydrophil (hi′dro-fil) hydrophilic.

hydrophilia (hi-dro-fil′e-ah) [*hydro-* + Gr. *philein* to love + *-ia*] the property of absorbing water.

hydrophilic (hi″dro-fil′ik) readily absorbing moisture; hygroscopic; having strongly polar groups that readily interact with water.

hydrophilism (hi-drof′ĭ-lizm) hydrophilia.

hydrophilous (hi-drof′ĭ-lus) hydrophilic.

Hydrophiodae (hi-drof′ĭ-o-de) a family of venomous sea snakes of the Indo-Pacific region, characterized by an oarlike tail and immovable hollow fangs. See table accompanying *snake*.

hydrophobia (hi″dro-fo′be-ah) [*hydro-* + Gr. *phobein* to be affrighted by + *-ia*] rabies. **paralytic h.,** see under *rabies*.

hydrophobic (hi″dro-fo′bik) 1. pertaining to or affected with hydrophobia (rabies). 2. not readily absorbing water, or being adversely affected by water, as a hydrophobic colloid. 3. lacking polar groups and, therefore, insoluble in water.

hydrophorograph (hi″dro-fo′ro-graf) [*hydro-* + Gr. *phora* a being borne, or carried along + *graphein* to record] an instrument for measuring and recording the pressure and/or flow of a fluid, especially the flow of urine or the pressure of the spinal fluid.

hydrophthalmia (hi″drof-thal′me-ah) hydrophthalmos; buphthalmos.

hydrophthalmos (hi″drof-thal′mos) [*hydro-* + Gr. *ophthalmos* eye] a form of glaucoma characterized by marked enlargement and distention of the fibrous coats of the eye; buphthalmos. **h. ante′rior,** that which affects the anterior portion of the eyeball only. **h. poste′rior,** that affecting the posterior part of the eyeball only. **h. tota′lis,** that which affects the entire eyeball.

hydrophthalmus (hi″drof-thal′mus) hydrophthalmos; buphthalmos.

hydrophysometra (hi″dro-fi″so-me′trah) [*hydro-* + *physometra*] physohydrometra.

hydrophyte (hi′dro-fīt) [Gr. *hydrō* water + *phyton* plant] a plant adapted to grow in a very wet environment, either completely aquatic or rooted in water or mud but with stems and leaves above the water.

hydropic (hi-drop′ik) [L. *hydropicus;* Gr. *hydrōpikos*] pertaining to or affected with dropsy.

hydropigenous (hi″dro-pij′ĕ-nus) causing dropsy.

hydroplasma (hi″dro-plaz′mah) [*hydro-* + Gr. *plasma* something formed] the watery or liquid part of the protoplasm.

hydropneumatosis (hi″dro-nu″mah-to′sis) [*hydro-* + Gr. *pneumatōsis* inflation] a collection of fluid and gas within the tissues.

hydropneumogony (hi″dro-nu-mo′go-ne) [*hydro-* + Gr. *pneuma* air + *gony* knee] the injection of air into a joint with a view to obtaining information with regard to the presence of effusion in the joint.

hydropneumopericardium (hi″dro-nu″mo-per″ĭ-kar′de-um) [*hydro-* + Gr. *pneuma* air + *pericardium*] a collection of watery fluid and gas within the pericardium.

hydropneumoperitoneum (hi″dro-nu″mo-per″ĭ-to-ne′um) [*hydro-* + Gr. *pneuma* air + *peritoneum*] a collection of watery fluid and gas in the peritoneal cavity.

hydropneumothorax (hi″dro-nu″mo-tho′raks) [*hydro-* + Gr. *pneuma* air + *thōrax* chest] a collection of fluid and gas within the pleural cavity.

hydroponics (hi″dro-pon′iks) the soil-less cultivation of plants on liquid media containing the necessary nutrient.

hydropotherapy (hi″dro-po-ther′ah-pe) [Gr. *hydrōps* dropsy + *therapeia* treatment] the therapeutic injection of ascitic fluid.

hydrops (hi′drops) [L.; Gr. *hydrōps*] the abnormal accumulation of serous fluid in the tissues or in a body cavity; called also *dropsy*. **h. abdom′inis,** ascites. **h. ad mat′ulam,** polyuria. **h. am′nii,** hydramnios. **h. an′tri,** effusion of serous fluid into the maxillary sinus. **h. artic′uli,** hydrarthrosis. **endolymphatic h.,** an accumulation of endolymph in the inner ear resulting in deafness and tinnitus, and sometimes vertigo (Meniere's disease); called also *labyrinthine h*. **fetal h., h. feta′lis,** gross edema of the entire body, associated with severe anemia, occurring in erythroblastosis fetalis. **h. follic′uli,** accumulation of fluid in the graafian follicle, forming a large solitary follicular cyst. **h. hypos′trophos,** angioneurotic edema. **h. labyrin′thi, labyrinthine h.,** endolymphatic h. **h. pericar′dii,** hydropericardium. **h. spu′rius,** pseudomyxoma peritonaei. **h. tu′bae,** hydrosalpinx. **h. tu′bae prof′luens,** a condition in which the abdominal opening of the uterine tube becomes closed, and the tube may reach enormous proportions as it fills with serum; peristaltic action of the tube causes colicky pain, until the fluid escapes through the uterine opening. Called also *intermittent hydrosalpinx*.

hydropyonephrosis (hi″dro-pi″o-ně-fro′sis) [*hydro*- + Gr. *pyon* pus + *nephros* kidney + *-osis*] the accumulation of urine and pus in the pelvis of the kidney.

hydroquinone (hi″dro-kwin′ōn) [USP] chemical name: 1,4-benzenediol. A depigmenting agent, $C_6H_6O_2$, occurring as fine white needles; applied topically to the skin.

hydrorachis (hi-dror′ah-kis) [*hydro*- + Gr. *rhachis* spine] a collection of water in the vertebral canal.

hydrorachitis (hi″dro-rah-ki′tis) [*hydro*- + Gr. *rhachis* spine + *-itis*] inflammation within the vertebral canal, attended with a watery effusion.

hydrorrhea (hi″dro-re′ah) [*hydro*- + Gr. *rhoia* flow] a copious watery discharge. **h. gravida′rum,** a periodic or intermittent discharge of clear, yellowish, or bloody fluid from the uterus, caused by escape of amniotic fluid or resulting from decidual metritis. **nasal h.,** watery discharge from the nose.

hydrosalpinx (hi″dro-sal′pinks) [*hydro*- + Gr. *salpinx* trumpet] a collection of watery fluid in a uterine tube, occurring as the end-stage of pyosalpinx. **h. follicula′ris,** hydrosalpinx in which there is no central cystic cavity, the lumen being broken up into compartments as the result of fusion of the tubal plicae. **intermittent h.,** hydrops tubae profluens. **h. sim′plex,** hydrosalpinx characterized by excessive distention and thinning of the wall of the uterine tube, the plicae being few and widely separated.

hydrosarcocele (hi″dro-sar′ko-sēl) [*hydro*- + *sarcocele*] combined hydrocele and sarcocele.

hydroscheocele (hi-dros′ke-o-sēl″) [*hydro*- + Gr. *oscheon* scrotum + *kēlē* hernia] a scrotal hernia containing a collection of serous fluid.

hydroscope (hi″dro-skōp) [*hydro*- + Gr. *skopein* to examine] an instrument for detecting the presence of water.

hydrosol (hi′dro-sol) a sol in which the continuous phase (dispersion medium) is water.

hydrosoluble (hi″dro-sol′u-b'l) soluble in water.

hydrosphygmograph (hi″dro-sfig′mo-graf) [*hydro*- + Gr. *sphygmos* pulse + *graphein* to record] a sphygmograph with water for an index.

hydrospirometer (hi″dro-spi-rom″ě-ter) [*hydro*- + L. *spirare* to breathe + Gr. *metron* measure] a spirometer in which a column of water serves as an index.

hydrostabile (hi″dro-sta′bil) preserving a stable weight under diet restrictions or gastrointestinal disease. Cf. *hydrolabile.*

hydrostat (hi′dro-stat) [*hydro*- + Gr. *histanai* to halt] a device by which the height of fluid in a container (column or reservoir) is regulated.

hydrostatic (hi″dro-stat′ik) [*hydro*- + Gr. *statikos* standing] pertaining to a liquid in a state of equilibrium; see under *pressure.*

hydrostatics (hi″dro-stat′iks) the science of liquids in a state of rest or equilibrium and of the pressures they exert.

hydrosynthesis (hi″dro-sin′the-sis) a chemical reaction in which water is formed.

hydrosyringomyelia (hi″dro-sǐ-ring″go-mi-e′le-ah) [*hydro*- + Gr. *syrinx* tube + *myelos* marrow] coexistence of hydromyelia and syringomyelia.

Hydrotaea (hi″dro-te′ah) a genus of flies. **H. meteor′ica,** a species which attacks the eyes and nostrils of man and animals.

hydrotaxis (hi″dro-tak′sis) [*hydro*- + Gr. *taxis* arrangement] an orientation movement of motile organisms or cells in response to stimulation by water or moisture.

hydrotherapeutics (hi″dro-ther″ah-pu′tiks) hydrotherapy.

hydrotherapy (hi″dro-ther′ah-pe) [*hydro*- + Gr. *therapeia* service done to the sick] the application of water in any form, either internally or externally, in the treatment of disease.

hydrothermic (hi″dro-ther′mik) relating to the temperature effects of water, as in hot baths.

hydrothionammonemia (hi″dro-thi″o-nam″o-ne′me-ah) [*hydro*- + Gr. *theion* sulfur + *ammonium* + *haima* blood] the occurrence of ammonium hydrosulfide in the blood.

hydrothionemia (hi″dro-thi″o-ne′me-ah) [*hydro*- + Gr. *theion* sulfur + *haima* blood] the presence of hydrogen sulfide in the blood.

hydrothionuria (hi″dro-thi″o-nu′re-ah) [*hydro*- + Gr. *theion* sulfur + *ouron* urine + *-ia*] the presence of hydrogen sulfide in the urine.

hydrothorax (hi″dro-tho′raks) [*hydro*- + Gr. *thorax* chest] a collection of watery fluid in the pleural cavity; pleural effusion with transudate. **chylous h.,** the presence of chyle in the thoracic cavity, due to obstruction of or rupture of the thoracic duct.

hydrotomy (hi-drot′o-me) [*hydro*- + Gr. *tomē* a cutting] the dissection or separation of parts by the forcible injection of water.

hydrotropism (hi-drot′ro-pizm) [*hydro*- + Gr. *tropē* a turn, turning] a growth response of a nonmotile organism elicited by the presence of water or moisture.

hydrotubation (hi″dro-too-ba′shun) a method of maintaining patency of the uterine tube, in which hydrocortisone in saline solution is introduced into the tube followed by chymotrypsin in saline solution.

hydroureter (hi″dro-u-re′ter) abnormal distention of the ureter with urine or with a watery fluid, due to obstruction from any cause; cf. *megaloureter.*

hydroureterosis (hi″dro-u-re″ter-o′sis) hydroureter.

hydrouria (hi″dro-u′re-ah) [*hydro*- + Gr. *ouron* urine + *-ia*] hydruria.

hydrous (hi′drus) containing water.

hydrovarium (hi″dro-va′re-um) [*hydro*- + L. *ovarium* ovary] a collection of serous fluid in an ovary.

hydroxide (hi-drok′sīd) any compound of hydroxyl radical (OH), or of hydroxide ion, OH^-, with another radical or atom. **ferric h.,** the hydrated oxide of iron, $Fe(OH)_3$, a reddish brown substance, formerly used as an antidote in arsenic poisoning. Called also *iron hydroxide.*

hydroxocobalamin (hi-drok″so-ko-bal′ah-min) [USP] chemical name: cobinamide dihydroxide, dihydrogen phosphate (ester), mono(inner salt),3′-ester with 5,6-dimethyl-1-α-D-ribofuranosylbenzimidazole. An analogue of cyanocobalamin, $C_{62}H_{89}CoN_{13}O_{15}P$, in which the cyanide ion is replaced with a hydroxyl ion, occurring as dark red crystals or as a red crystalline powder; it possesses exceptionally long-acting hematopoietic activity. Called also *vitamin B_{12b}.*

hydroxy- (hi-drok′se) a chemical prefix indicating presence of the univalent radical OH.

hydroxyacetanilide (hi-drok″se-as″ě-tan′ǐ-lid) acetaminophen.

hydroxyamphetamine hydrobromide (hi-drok″se-am-fet′ah-mēn) [USP] chemical name: 4-(2-aminopropyl)phenol hydrobromide. An adrenergic, $C_9H_{13}NO \cdot HBr$, occurring as a white, crystalline powder; used as a mydriatic, applied topically to the conjunctiva. It is also used topically as a nasal decongestant and orally as a pressor agent in the treatment of heart block, carotid sinus syndrome, and postural hypotension.

hydroxyapatite (hi-drok″se-ap′ah-tīt) an inorganic compound, $Ca_{10}(PO_4)_6(OH)_2$, found in the matrix of bone and the teeth, which gives rigidity to these structures.

hydroxybenzene (hi-drok″se-ben′zēn) phenol.

hydroxychloroquine sulfate (hi-drok″se-klo′ro-kwin) [USP] chemical name: 7-chloro-4-{4-[ethyl(2-hydroxyethyl)amino]-1-methylbutylamino}-quinoline sulfate. A quinoline derivative, $C_{18}H_{26}ClN_3O \cdot H_2SO_4$, occurring as a white or nearly white, crystalline powder; used as an antimalarial and as a lupus erythematosus suppressant, administered orally. It has also been used in the treatment of rheumatoid arthritis and symptomatic cases of giardiasis.

25-hydroxycholecalciferol (hi-drok″se-ko″le-kal-sif′ě-rol) a metabolically activated form of vitamin D (cholecalciferol), which is synthesized in the liver. It is the precursor of 1,25-dihydroxycholecalciferol. Called also *calcidiol* and *calcifediole.*

17-hydroxycorticosteroid (hi-drok″se-kor″tǐ-ko-ste′roid) any adrenocorticosteroid with a dihydroxyacetone side chain, including hydrocortisone (cortisol) and 11-deoxycortisone. Called also *Porter-Silber chromogen.*

17-hydroxycorticosterone (hi-drok″se-kor″tǐ-ko-ster′ōn) hydrocortisone.

hydroxydione sodium succinate (hi-drok″se-di′ōn) chemical name: 21-(3-carboxy-1-oxopropoxy)-5β-pregnane-3,20-dione sodium succinate. A steroid, $C_{25}H_{35}NaO_6$, used as a general anesthetic, administered intravenously.

25-hydroxyergocalciferol (hi″drok-se-er″go-kal-sif′ě-rol) an activated form of vitamin D (ergocalciferol) synthesized in the liver.

hydroxyestrin benzoate (hi-drok″se-es′trin) estradiol benzoate.

hydroxyl (hi-drok′sil) the univalent radical OH.

hydroxylase (hi-drok′sǐ-lās) any of a group of enzymes (oxidoreductases) bringing about the coupled oxidation of two donors, with incorporation of oxygen into one of the donors. **aryl 4-h.,** an enzyme catalyzing aniline and reduced NADP to 4-hydroxyaniline and NADP. **cholesterol 20-h.,** an enzyme that catalyzes the change of cholesterol and reduced NADP to 20-β-hydroxycholesterol and NADP. **dopamine h.,** an enzyme that catalyzes the change of 3,4-dihydroxyphenylethylamine and ascorbate to norepinephrine and dehydroascorbate. **estradiol 6-β-h.,** an enzyme that catalyzes the change of estradiol and reduced NADP to 6-β-hydroxyestradiol and NADP. **estriol 2-h.,** an enzyme that catalyzes the change of estriol and reduced NAD(P) to 2-hydroxyestriol and NAD(P). **p-hydroxyphenylpyruvate h.,** an enzyme that catalyzes the change of p-hydroxyphenylpyruvate and ascorbate to homogentisate, dehydroascorbate, and carbon dioxide. **imidazoleacetate h.,** an enzyme that catalyzes the change of imidazoleacetate and reduced NAD to imidazoloneacetate and NAD. **kynurenate h.,** an enzyme catalyzing the change of kynurenate and reduced NADP to kynurenate 7,8-dihydrodiol and NADP. **kynurenine 3-h.,**

an enzyme catalyzing the change of L-kynurenine and reduced NADP to 3-hydroxy-L-kynurenine and NADP. **phenylalanine h.,** an enzyme that catalyzes the change of L-phenylalanine and tetrahydropteridine to L-tyrosine and dihydropteridine; called also *phenylalaninase.* **squalene h.,** an enzyme catalyzing the change of squalene and reduced NADP to lanosterol and NADP; called also *squalene oxydocyclase.* **steroid β-h.,** an enzyme that catalyzes the change of a steroid and reduced NADP to a β-hydroxysteroid and NADP.

hydroxylysine (hi″drok-sil′ĭ-sin) one of the alpha amino acids, $NH_2 \cdot CH_2 \cdot CHOH(CH_2)_2 \cdot CH(NH_2) \cdot COOH$.

hydroxymethyltransferase (hi-drok″se-meth″il-trans′fer-ās) an enzyme that catalyzes the transfer of a hydroxymethyl group, as from L-serine to tetrahydrofolate.

hydroxynervone (hi-drok″se-ner′vōn) a cerebroside occurring in brain tissue.

hydroxyphenamate (hi-drok″se-fen′ah-māt) chemical name: 2-phenyl-1,2-butanediol-1-carbamate; a minor tranquilizer, $C_{11}H_{15}NO_3$, formerly used in the treatment of anxiety and tension.

hydroxyphenylethylamine (hi-drok″se-phen″il- eth″il-am′in) tyramine.

hydroxyprogesterone capraote (hi-drok″se-pro-jes′ter-ōn) [USP] chemical name: 17α-[(1-oxohexyl)oxy]pregna-4-ene-3,20-dione. A synthetic progestin, $C_{27}H_{40}O_4$, occurring as a white or creamy white, crystalline powder; used in the treatment of functional uterine bleeding, abnormalities of the menstrual cycle, threatened abortion, and uterine cancer, administered intramuscularly. Called also *h. hexanoate.*

hydroxyproline (hi-drok″se-pro′lin) an amino acid, gamma-hydroxy-alpha-pyrrolidin-carboxylic acid, produced in the digestion or hydrolytic decomposition of proteins, especially of collagens.

hydroxyprolinemia (hi-drok″se-pro″len-e′me-ah) a disorder of amino acid metabolism characterized by an excess of free hydroxyproline in the plasma and urine, due to a defect in the enzyme hydroxyproline oxidase; it may be associated with mental retardation.

hydroxypropyl methylcellulose (hi-drok″sĭ-pro′pil) chemical name: cellulose 2-hydroxypropyl methyl ether. The propylene glycol ether of methylcellulose, occurring as a white to slightly off-white, fibrous or granular powder, and supplied in differing degrees of viscosity; used as a suspending and viscosity-increasing agent and tablet excipient in pharmaceutical preparations, and applied topically to the conjunctiva to protect the cornea during certain ophthalmic procedures and to lubricate the cornea.

17-hydroxysteroid (hi-drok″se-ste′roid) an excretion product of adrenocorticosteroids.

hydroxystilbamidine isethionate (hi-drok″se-stil-bam′ĭ-dēn) [USP] chemical name: 4-[2-[4-(aminoiminomethyl)phenyl]ethenyl]-3-hydroxybenzenecarboximidamide bis(2-hydroxyethanesulfonate) (salt). An antifungal and antiprotozoal, $C_{16}H_{16}N_4O \cdot 2C_2H_6O_4S$, occurring as a fine, yellow, crystalline powder; used as an antileishmanial, administered by intramuscular or intravenous infusion. It has also been used in the treatment of some fungal infections, such as North American blastomycosis.

hydroxytetracycline (hi-drok″se-tet″rah-si′klēn) oxytetracycline.

5-hydroxytryptamine (hi-drok″se-trip′tah-mēn) serotonin.

hydroxyurea (hi-drok″se-u-re′ah) [USP] an antineoplastic agent, $CH_4N_2O_2$, occurring as a white to off-white powder; used in the treatment of melanoma, resistant chronic myelocytic leukemia, and recurrent, metastatic, or inoperable ovarian carcinoma, administered orally. It is an inhibitor of ribonucleotide reductase.

hydroxyvaline (hi-drok″se-val′in) an amino acid obtained by protein hydrolysis.

hydroxyzine (hi-drok′sĭ-zēn) chemical name: 2-[2-[4-[(4-chlorophenyl)phenylmethyl]-1-piperazinyl]ethoxy]ethanol. A synthetic drug, $C_{21}H_{27}ClN_2O_2$, with central nervous system depressant, antispasmodic, antihistaminic, and antifibrillatory actions. **h. hydrochloride** [USP], the dihydrochloride salt of hydroxyzine, $C_{21}H_{27}ClN_2O_2 \cdot 2HCl$, occurring as white powder; used in the treatment of anxiety, tension, and agitation in conditions of emotional stress, in acute and chronic urticaria and other manifestations of allergic dermatoses, as an antiemetic, and as pre- and postoperative sedative, administered orally or intramuscularly. **h. pamoate** [USP], the pamoate salt of hydroxyzine, $C_{21}H_{27}ClN_2O_2 \cdot C_{23}H_{16}O_6$, occurring as light yellow powder, having the actions and uses of the hydrochloride salt; administered orally.

Hydrozoa (hi″dro-zo′ah) [Gr. *Hydra* a mythical nine-headed monster + *zoon* animal] a class of coelenterates that usually possess colonial branching polyps and small medusae, including the genus *Physalia* (Portuguese man-of-war).

hydrozoan (hi″dro-zo′an) an individual of the class Hydrozoa.

hydruria (hi-droo′re-ah) [*hydr-* + Gr. *ouron* urine + *-ia*] excretion of urine of low osmolality or specific gravity.

hydruric (hi-droo′rik) characterized by hydruria.

hyenanchin (hi″ĕ-nan′kin) a poisonous substance, $C_{15}H_{18}O_7$,

from the outer envelopes of the fruit of *Hyaenanche globosa*, of South Africa. It somewhat resembles strychnine in its action.

Hygeia (hi-je′ah) [Gr. *Hygieia*] the goddess of health, one of the daughters of Æsculapius, the mythical god of healing, who assisted in the rites at the early temples of healing.

hygeiolatry (hi″je-ol′ah-tre) [Gr. *Hygieia* + *latreia* servitude] (*obs.*) excessive attention to one's own health.

hygeiophrontis (hi″je-o-fron′tis) anxious concern about one's own health; hypochondriasis.

hygeiophrontistic (hi″je-o-fron-tis′tik) pertaining to or characterized by hygeiophrontis.

hygieist (hi-je′ist) hygienist.

hygiene (hi′jēn) [Gr. *hygieia* health] the science of health and of its preservation. **industrial h.,** that branch of preventive medicine which is concerned with the protection of health of the industrial population. **mental h.,** the science which deals with the development of healthy mental and emotional reactions and habits; psychophylaxis. **oral h.,** the proper care of the mouth and teeth for the maintenance of health and the prevention of disease. **radiation h.,** the science of practices involved in human protection from radiation injury. **sex h.,** that department of hygiene which deals with sex, sexual conduct, and personal sex hygiene as these are related to individual and community health. **social h.,** that department of hygiene which deals with the promotion of sexual health, embracing personal sex hygiene, healthy marriage and family relations, and sex education. The term is sometimes used as a euphemism for venereal disease control.

hygienic (hi″je-en′ik) pertaining to hygiene, or conducive to health.

hygienics (hi″je-en′iks) a system of principles for promoting health; hygiene.

hygienism (hi-je′en-izm) devotion to the observance of hygienic rules.

hygienist (hi-je′nist, hi′je-en″ist) a specialist in hygiene. **dental h.,** an auxiliary member of the dental profession who has been trained in the art of removing calcareous deposits and stains from the surfaces of the teeth and in providing additional services and information on the prevention of oral disease; such persons are employed in private dental offices or are active in school or public health programs.

hygienization (hi″je-en″i-za′shun) the establishment of hygienic conditions.

hygieology (hi″je-ol′o-je) [Gr. *hygieia* health + *-logy*] the complete science upon which the arts of hygiene and sanitation are based.

hygiogenesis (hi″je-o-jen′ĕ-sis) [Gr. *hygiēs* healthy + *gennan* to produce] the mechanism of the processes which lead to maintenance of health.

hygiology (hi″je-ol′o-je) hygieology.

hygrechema (hi″grĕ-ke′mah) an auscultation sound caused by the presence of water.

hygric (hi′grik) [Gr. *hygros* moist] pertaining or relating to moisture.

hygro- [Gr. *hygros* moist] a combining form meaning moist or denoting relationship to moisture.

hygroblepharic (hi″gro-blĕ-far′ik) [*hygro-* + Gr. *blepharon* eyelid] denoting an excessive watery condition of the eyelids.

hygroma (hi-gro′mah), pl. *hygro′mas* or *hygro′mata* [*hygro-* + *-oma*] a sac, cyst, or bursa distended with a fluid. **h. col′li,** a watery tumor of the neck. **cystic h., h. cys′ticum,** cystic lymphangioma. **Fleischmann's h.,** enlargement of a bursa in the floor of the mouth, to the outer side of the genioglossus muscle. **h. praepatella′re,** housemaid's knee. **subdural h.,** a collection of fluid in the subdural space resulting from liquefaction of a subdural hematoma; see under *hematoma.*

hygromatous (hi-gro′mah-tus) pertaining to or of the nature of hygroma.

hygrometer (hi-grom′ĕ-ter) [*hygro-* + Gr. *metron* measure] an instrument for measuring the moisture of the atmosphere. **hair h., Saussure's h.,** a hygrometer whose action is determined by the elongation and contraction of a hair under the influence of moisture.

hygrometric (hi″gro-met′rik) pertaining to hygrometry.

hygrometry (hi-grom′ĕ-tre) [*hygro-* + Gr. *metron* measure] the measurement of the proportion of moisture in the air.

hygromycin (hi″gro-mi′sin) an antibiotic, $C_{23}H_{29}NO_{12}$, produced by *Streptomyces hygroscopicus* and *S. noboritoensis;* called also *hygromycin A.* **h. B,** an anthelmintic, $C_{15}H_{28}O_{10}$, used in swine.

hygroscopic (hi″gro-skop′ik) taking up and retaining moisture readily.

Hygroton (hi′gro-ton) trademark for a preparation of chlorthalidone.

Hykinone (hi′kin-ōn) trademark for a preparation of menadione sodium bisulfite.

hyl- see *hylo-.*

hyla (hi'lah) (*obs.*) a lateral extension of the aqueduct of Sylvius (aqueductus cerebri).

hyle (hi'le) [Gr. *hylē* matter] the theoretical primitive substance from which all matter was once thought to be composed. See *protyl*.

hyle- see *hylo-*.

Hylemyia (hi''lĕ-mi'ah) a genus of flies, the larvae of which infest vegetables and may be swallowed if the latter are eaten raw. *H. anti'qua*, onion root maggot. *H. bras'sicae*, the cabbage root maggot.

hylergography (hi''ler-gog'rah-fe) [Gr. *hylē* matter + *ergon* work + *graphein* to write] a recording of the effect of environmental materials on a cell.

hylic (hi'lik) [Gr. *hylē* matter] composed of matter; a term applied by Adami to the pulp tissues of the embryo.

hylo-, hyl-, hyle- [Gr. *hylē* matter] combining form denoting relationship to matter (material or substance). Cf. *-yl*.

hylogenesis (hi''lo-jen'ĕ-sis) [*hylo-* + Gr. *genesis* formation] the formation of matter.

hylogeny (hi-loj'ĕ-ne) hylogenesis.

hylology (hi-lol'o-je) [*hylo-* + *-logy*] the study of elementary or crude materials.

hylopathism (hi-lop'ah-thizm) [*hylo-* + Gr. *pathos* disease] the obsolete doctrine that disease is due to changes in the constitution of matter.

hylopathist (hi-lop'ah-thist) (*obs.*) a believer in the theory of hylopathism.

hylotropic (hi''lo-trop'ik) pertaining to or characterized by hylotropy.

hylotropy (hi-lot'ro-pe) [Gr. *hylē* matter + *tropē* a turn, turning] the ability of a substance to change from one physical form to another (e.g., solid to liquid, liquid to gas) without change in chemical composition; change of phase.

hylozoism (hi-lo'zo-izm) [*hylo-* + Gr. *zōon* animal] the doctrine that all matter in the universe is alive.

hymecromone (hi''mĕ-kro'mōn) chemical name: 7-hydroxy-4-methyl-2*H*-1-benzopyran-2-one; a choleretic and biliary antispasmodic, $C_{10}H_8O_3$.

hymen (hi'men) [Gr. *hymēn* membrane] [NA] the membranous fold which partially or wholly occludes the external orifice of the vagina. **annular h.**, circular g. **h. bifenestra'tus, h. bifo'ris**, a hymen with two openings side by side and a broad septum between them. **circular h.**, a hymen with a circular opening. **cribriform h.**, a hymen pierced by many small perforations. **denticular h.**, a hymen with an opening which has serrate edges. **falciform h.**, a sickle-shaped hymen. **fenestrated h.**, cribriform h. **imperforate h.**, one which completely closes the vaginal orifice. **infundibuliform h.**, a hymen that has a central opening with sloping sides. **lunar h.**, a moon-shaped hymen. **septate h., h. sep'tus**, a hymen in which the opening is divided by a narrow septum. **h. subsep'tus**, a hymen in which the opening is partially filled by a septum growing out of one wall, but not reaching the other.

hymenal (hi'men-al) pertaining to the hymen.

hymenectomy (hi''men-ek'to-me) [Gr. *hymēn* membrane, hymen + *ektomē* excision] excision of the hymen.

hymenitis (hi''men-i'tis) [Gr. *hymēn* membrane + *-itis*] inflammation of the hymen.

hymenium (hi-me'ne-um) [*dim.* of Gr. *hymēn* membrane] the fertile, or spore-forming, surface of a fungus, which is composed of hyphae lining the fruiting body.

hymenolepiasis (hi''mĕ-no-lep-i'ah-sis) infection with *Hymenolepis*.

Hymenolepididae (hi''men-o-lep'ĭ-di-de) a family of small to medium-sized tapeworms of the order Cyclophyllidea, subclass Cestoda, which parasitizes birds and mammals, including man. *Hymenolepis* is the genus of medical importance.

Hymenolepis (hi''mĕ-nol'ĕ-pis) [Gr. *hymēn* membrane + *lepis* rind] a genus of tapeworms of the family Hymenolepididae. **H. diminu'ta**, a tapeworm of rats and mice, occasionally found in man. **H. frater'na**, the rodent form of *H. nana*; often called *H. nana* var. *fraterna*. **H. lanceola'ta**, *Drepanidotaenia lanceolata*. **H. na'na**, the dwarf tapeworm, a species about 7 to 80 mm. long that is parasitic in rats, mice, and man, especially children. Infected persons are usually asymptomatic, but in massive infection symptoms may include dizziness, abdominal pain, diarrhea, insomnia, convulsions, etc. **H. na'na** var. **frater'na**, *H. fraterna*.

hymenology (hi''men-ol'o-je) [Gr. *hymēn* membrane + *-logy*] the sum of what is known regarding the membranes.

Hymenomycetes (hi''mĕ-no-mi-se'tēz) a series of fungi of the subclass Homobasidiomycetes, class Basidiomycetes, including the orders Polyporales and Agaricales.

Hymenoptera (hi''men-op'ter-ah) [Gr. *hymēn* membrane + *pteron* wing] an order of insects usually having two pairs of well developed membranous wings, as the bees, wasps, ants, etc.

hymenopteran (hi''men-op'ter-an) any insect of the order Hymenoptera.

hymenopterism (hi''men-op'ter-izm) poisoning by the stings or bites of insects of the order Hymenoptera, as of a bee or wasp.

hymenorrhaphy (hi''men-or'ah-fe) [Gr. *hymēn* hymen + *rhaphē* seam] the closure of the vagina by sutures at the hymen.

hymenotomy (hi''men-ot'o-me) [Gr. *hymēn* membrane + *temnein* to cut] surgical incision of the hymen.

hyobasioglossus (hi''o-ba''se-o-glos'us) the basal part of the hyoglossus muscle.

hyodeoxycholaneresis (hi''o-de-ok''se-ko''lah-ner'ĕ-sis) [*hyodeoxycholic* acid + Gr. *hairesis* a taking] (*obs.*) increase in the output or elimination of hyodeoxycholic acid in the bile. Cf. *cholaneresis*.

hyoepiglottic (hi''o-ep''ĭ-glot'ik) pertaining to the hyoid bone and the epiglottis.

hyoepiglottidean (hi''o-ep''ĭ-glo-tid'e-an) hyoepiglottic.

hyoglossal (hi''o-glos'al) [hyoid bone + Gr. *glōssa* tongue] pertaining to the hyoid bone and the tongue or to the hyoglossal muscle.

hyoid (hi'oid) [Gr. *hyoeides* U-shaped] 1. shaped like the Greek letter upsilon (υ). 2. pertaining to the hyoid bone.

hyoscine (hi'o-sin) [L. *hyoscina*] scopolamine.

hyoscyamine (hi''o-si'ah-min) [USP] chemical name: [3(*S*)-endo]-α-(hydroxymethyl)benzeneacetic acid 8-methyl-8-azabicyclo[3.2.1]oct-3-yl ester. An anticholinergic alkaloid, $C_{17}H_{23}NO_3$, derived from *Hyoscyamus niger*, *Atropa belladonna*, and other solanaceous plants, occurring as a white, crystalline powder; it is the levorotatory component of racemic atropine with actions and uses similar to those of atropine but with more potent central and peripheral effects. It is administered orally or parenterally. **h. hydrobromide** [USP], a salt of hyoscyamine, $C_{17}H_{23}NO_3$·HBr, occurring as white crystals or as a crystalline powder, having actions and uses similar to those of atropine, administered orally or parenterally. **h. sulfate** [USP], a salt of hyoscyamine, $(C_{17}H_{23}NO_3)_2$·H_2SO_4·$2H_2O$, occurring as white crystals or as a crystalline powder, having actions and uses similar to those of atropine, administered orally or parenterally.

Hyoscyamus (hi''o-si'ah-mus) [L.; Gr. *hys* swine + *kyamos* bean] a genus of annual or biennial solanaceous plants; the leaves, seeds, flowers, and tops of *H. ni'ger* L. contain the anticholinergic alkaloids hyoscyamine and scopolamine.

hyoscyamus (hi''o-si'ah-mus) the dried leaf of *Hyoscyamus niger* L., with or without its stem and top, which contains the anticholinergic alkaloids hyoscyamine and scopolamine; formerly used as a smooth muscle relaxant and to produce parasympathetic blockade. Called also *henbane* and *black henbane*.

Hyostrongylus rubidus (hi''o-stron'jĭ-lus roo'bĭ-dus) a small red nematode worm found in the stomach of pigs.

hyothyroid (hi''o-thi'roid) pertaining to the hyoid bone and the thyroid cartilage.

hypacidemia (hi-pas''ĭ-de'me-ah) [Gr. *hypo* under + *acid* + *haima* blood] deficiency of an acid in the blood.

hypacusia (hi''pah-ku'ze-ah) hypoacusis.

hypacusis (hi''pah-ku'sis) [Gr. *hypo* under + *akousis* hearing] hypoacusis.

hypadrenia (hi''pah-dre'ne-ah) Addison's disease.

hypalbuminemia (hi''pal-bu''mĭ-ne'me-ah) hypoalbuminemia.

hypalgesia (hi''pal-je'ze-ah) [Gr. *hypo* under + *algēsis* pain] diminished sensitiveness to pain.

hypalgesic (hi''pal-je'sik) pertaining to, characterized by, or producing hypalgesia.

hypalgetic (hi''pal-jet'ik) hypalgesic.

hypalgia (hi-pal'je-ah) hypalgesia.

hypamnion (hi-pam'ne-on) hypamnios.

hypamnios (hi-pam'ne-os) [Gr. *hypo* under + *amnion*] deficiency of the amniotic fluid.

hypanakinesia (hi-pan''ah-ki-ne'ze-ah) [Gr. *hypo* under + *anakinēsis* exercise + *-ia*] hypokinesia.

hypanakinesis (hi-pan''ah-ki-ne'sis) hypokinesia.

hypaphorine (hi-paf'o-rin) a crystalline alkaloid, $C_{14}H_{18}N_2O_2$, obtained from *Erythrina americana* Mill., and other members of the leguminosae; it is a convulsive poisonous alkaloid.

Hypaque (hi'pāk) trademark for preparations of diatrizoate meglumine and diatrizoate sodium.

hyparterial (hi''par-te're-al) [Gr. *hypo* under + *artēria* artery] beneath an artery, applied especially to the bronchi which are so situated.

hypaxial (hi-pak'se-al) ventral to the long axis of the body.

hypazoturia (hi''paz''o-tu're-ah) [Gr. *hypo* under + *azoturia*] excretion of urine of low nitrogen concentration.

hypencephalon (hi''pen-sef'ah-lon) [Gr. *hypo* under + *enkephalos* brain] (*obs.*) the mesencephalon, pons, and medulla.

hypenchyme (hi'pen-kīm) the primitive embryonic tissue formed in the cavity of the archenteron.

hyper- [Gr. *hyper* above] a prefix signifying above, beyond, or excessive. See also words beginning *super-*.

hyperabsorption (hi″per-ab-sorp′shun) increased intestinal absorption of a substance.

hyperacanthosis (hi″per-ak″an-tho′sis) [*hyper-* + Gr. *akantha* prickle + *-osis*] acanthosis.

hyperacid (hi″per-as′id) [*hyper-* + L. *acidus* sour] abnormally or excessively acid.

hyperacidaminuria (hi″per-as″id-am″ĭ-nu′re-ah) excess of amino acids in the urine.

hyperacidity (hi″per-ah-sid′ĭ-te) an excessive degree of acidity. **gastric h.,** hyperchlorhydria.

hyperacousia (hi″per-ah-koo′ze-ah) hyperacusis.

hyperactive (hi″per-ak′tiv) pertaining to or characterized by hyperactivity; hyperkinetic. See also *hyperkinetic syndrome,* under *syndrome.*

hyperactivity (hi″per-ak-tiv′ĭ-te) abnormally increased activity. Developmental hyperactivity of children is characterized by constant motion—exploring, experimenting, etc.—and usually accompanied by distractibility and low tolerance for frustration. It usually abates during adolescence. Hyperactivity may also result from brain damage and psychoses. Called also *hyperkinesia.*

hyperacusia (hi″per-ah-ku′ze-ah) hyperacusis.

hyperacusis (hi″per-ah-ku′sis) [*hyper-* + Gr. *akousis* hearing] an exceptionally acute sense of hearing, the hearing threshold being unusually low. The term has been used to denote a painful sensitiveness to sounds, but there is no necessary relationship between the threshold of hearing and that of discomfort.

hyperacute (hi″per-ah-kūt′) extremely acute.

hyperadenosis (hi″per-ad″ĕ-no′sis) [*hyper-* + Gr. *adēn* gland + *-osis*] a condition characterized by enlargement of the glands.

hyperadiposis (hi″per-ad″ĭ-po′sis) [*hyper-* + *adiposis*] extreme adiposity or fatness.

hyperadiposity (hi″per-ad″ĭ-pos′ĭ-te) hyperadiposis.

hyperadrenalemia (hi″per-ah-dre″nal-e′me-ah) the presence of an abnormally increased amount of adrenal secretion in the blood.

hyperadrenalism (hi″per-ah-dre′nal-izm) abnormally increased secretory activity of the adrenal gland.

hyperadrenia (hi″per-ah-dre′ne-ah) hyperadrenalism.

hyperadrenocorticism (hi″per-ah-dre″no-kor′tĭ-sizm) a condition characterized by abnormally increased functional activity of the cortex of the adrenal gland. See *Cushing's syndrome* (def. 1), under *syndrome.*

hyperaffective (hi″per-af-fek′tiv) pertaining to or characterized by hyperaffectivity.

hyperaffectivity (hi″per-af″fek-tiv′ĭ-te) abnormally increased sensibility to mild superficial stimuli; the quality of abnormally heightened emotional reactivity.

hyperakusis (hi″per-ah-koo′sis) hyperacusis.

hyperalbuminemia (hi″per-al-bu″mĭ-ne′me-ah) an abnormally high albumin content of the blood.

hyperalbuminosis (hi″per-al-bu″mĭ-no′sis) a condition characterized by presence of an excess of albuminoids.

hyperaldosteronemia (hi″per-al″do-stēr″ōn-e′me-ah) abnormal increase in the level of aldosterone in the blood.

hyperaldosteronism (hi″per-al″do-ster′ōn-izm) aldosteronism.

hyperaldosteronuria (hi″per-al″do-stēr″ōn-u′re-ah) the presence of excessive amounts of aldosterone in the urine.

hyperalgesia (hi″per-al-je′ze-ah) [*hyper-* + Gr. *algēsis* pain] excessive sensitiveness or sensibility to pain. **auditory h.,** the condition in which slight noises cause pain. **muscular h.,** the condition in which slight exertion causes great pain.

hyperalgesic (hi″per-al-je′sik) pertaining to or characterized by hyperalgesia.

hyperalgetic (hi″per-al-jet′ik) hyperalgesic.

hyperalgia (hi-per-al′je-ah) [*hyper-* + *-algia*] hyperalgesia.

hyperalimentation (hi″per-al″ĭ-men-ta′shun) the ingestion or administration of a greater than optimal amount of nutrients. **parenteral h.,** the intravenous administration of the total nutrient requirements of the patient with gastrointestinal dysfunction, accomplished via a central venous catheter, usually inserted in the superior vena cava. Called also *total parenteral nutrition* and *total parenteral alimentation.*

hyperalimentosis (hi″per-al″ĭ-men-to′sis) disease due to excess in eating.

hyperalkalescence (hi″per-al″kah-les′ens) an excess of alkalinity.

hyperalkalinity (hi″per-al″kah-lin′ĭ-te) excessive alkalinity.

hyperallantoinuria (hi″per-ah-lan″to-in-u′re-ah) an excess of allantoin in the urine.

hyperalonemia (hi″per-al″o-ne′me-ah) [*hyper-* + Gr. *hals* salt + *haima* blood] excess of salts in the blood.

hyperalphalipoproteinemia (hi″per-al″fah-lip″o-pro″te-in-

e′me-ah) the presence of abnormally high levels of α-lipoproteins in the serum.

hyperaminoacidemia (hi″per-am″ĭ-no-as″ĭ-de′me-ah) presence of amino acids in the blood in excess of the normal amount.

hyperammonemia (hi″per-am″mo-ne′me-ah) elevated levels of ammonia or its compounds in the blood. A congenital form occurs in two types: *Type 1,* due to deficiency of carbamoyl phosphate synthetase, is marked by vomiting, lethargy, and flaccidity and by elevated plasma and urinary levels of glycine. *Type 2,* due to deficiency of ornithine transcarbamylase, is marked by vomiting, lethargy, coma, and hepatomegaly. Symptoms are aggravated by protein ingestion. Hyperammonemia may also occur in other nongenetic diseases, as in severe liver disease. Called also *ammonemia.*

hyperammoniemia (hi″per-ah-mo″ne-e′me-ah) hyperammonemia.

hyperammonuria (hi″per-am″mo-nu′re-ah) increased excretion of ammonia in the urine.

hyperamylasemia (hi″per-am″il-ās-e′me-ah) abnormally high elevation of amylase in the blood serum.

hyperanacinesia (hi″per-an″ah-si-ne′ze-ah) hyperkinesia.

hyperanakinesia (hi″per-an″ah-ki-ne′ze-ah) [*hyper-* + Gr. *anakinēsis* exercise + *-ia*] hyperkinesia.

hyperandrogenism (hi″per-an′dro-jen-izm) a state characterized or caused by an excessive secretion of androgens.

hyperaphia (hi″per-a′fe-ah) [*hyper-* + Gr. *haphē* touch] tactile hyperesthesia.

hyperaphic (hi″per-af′ik) pertaining to or characterized by hyperaphia (tactile hyperesthesia).

hyperarousal (hi″per-ah-row′sal) a state of increased psychological and physiological tension marked by such effects as reduced tolerance to pain, insomnia, fatigue, accentuation of personality traits, etc.

hyperazotemia (hi″per-az″o-te′me-ah) [*hyper-* + *azotemia*] an excess of nitrogenous matter, usually urea, in the blood.

hyperazoturia (hi″per-az″o-tu′re-ah) presence of an excessive amount of nitrogenous matter in the urine.

hyperbaric (hi″per-bār′ik) [*hyper-* + Gr. *baros* weight] characterized by greater than normal pressure or weight; applied to gases under greater than atmospheric pressure, as hyperbaric oxygen, or to a solution of greater specific gravity than another taken as a standard of reference.

hyperbarism (hi″per-bar′izm) the condition resulting from exposure to ambient gas pressure or atmospheric pressures that exceed the pressure within body tissues, fluids, and cavities.

hyperbasophilic (hi″per-bas″o-fil′ik) staining intensely with basic dyes.

hyperbetalipoproteinemia (hi″per-ba″tah-lip″o-pro″te-in-e′me-ah) increased accumulation of β-lipoproteins in the blood. **familial h.,** familial hyperlipoproteinemia, type IIa.

hyperbicarbonatemia (hi″per-bi-kar″bo-nāt-e′me-ah) the presence of an excessive amount of bicarbonate in the blood.

hyperbilirubinemia (hi″per-bil″ĭ-roo″bĭ-ne′me-ah) excessive concentrations of bilirubin in the blood, which may lead to jaundice; the hyperbilirubinemias are classified as conjugated or unconjugated, according to the predominant form of bilirubin in the blood. **congenital h.,** Crigler-Najjar syndrome. **conjugated h.,** that due to defective excretion of conjugated bilirubin by the liver cells or to anatomic obstruction to bile flow within the liver or in the extrahepatic bile duct system, it includes Dubin-Johnson syndrome and Rotor's syndrome. **constitutional h.,** Gilbert's disease. **neonatal h.,** a mild, transient, "physiological" hyperbilirubinemia of the unconjugated type occurring in the normal neonate; a transient familial form also occurs, with onset of jaundice within four days after birth, which may lead to kernicterus. **unconjugated h.,** that due to excessive bilirubin production (hemolysis), to defective clearance of bilirubin from the blood by the liver, or to defective conjugation by the liver; it includes hemolytic states, Crigler-Najjar syndrome, Gilbert's syndrome, and neonatal hyperbilirubinemia.

hyperblastosis (hi″per-blas-to′sis) [*hyper-* + Gr. *blastos* germ] an overgrowth of some specific tissue.

hyperbrachycephalic (hi″per-brak″e-sĕ-fal′ik) having a cephalic index of 85.5 or more.

hyperbrachycephaly (hi″per-brak″e-sef′ah-le) the condition of being hyperbrachycephalic.

hyperbradykininemia (hi″per-brad″ĕ-ki″nin-e′me-ah) elevated levels of bradykinin in the blood, marked by a feeling of warmth, flushing, wheezing, or nausea.

hyperbradykininism (hi″per-brad″ĕ-ki′nin-izm) a syndrome characterized by high plasma levels of bradykinin, in which standing produces a fall in systolic blood pressure, an increase in diastolic pressure and heart rate, and a purplish discoloration and ecchymoses over the legs.

hyperbulia (hi″per-bu′le-ah) [*hyper-* + Gr. *boulē* will] morbid development of the will; excessive wilfulness.

hypercalcemia (hi″per-kal-se′me-ah) [*hyper-* + *calcium* + Gr.

haima blood] an excess of calcium in the blood; manifestations include fatigability, muscle weakness, depression, anorexia, nausea, and constipation. **idiopathic h.,** a condition of infants, associated with vitamin D intoxication, and characterized by elevated serum calcium levels and increased density of the skeleton, with mental deterioration progressing to idiocy, and nephrocalcinosis causing chronic uremia.

hypercalcinemia (hi″per-kal″sĭ-ne′me-ah) hypercalcemia.

hypercalcinuria (hi″per-kal″sĭ-nu′re-ah) hypercalciuria.

hypercalcipexy (hi″per-kal′sĭ-pek″se) excessive fixation of calcium.

hypercalciuria (hi″per-kal″sĭ-u′re-ah) excess of calcium in the urine.

hypercapnia (hi″per-kap′ne-ah) [*hyper-* + Gr. *kapnos* smoke] excess of carbon dioxide in the blood.

hypercapnic (hi″per-kap′nik) pertaining to or characterized by hypercapnia.

hypercarbia (hi″per-kar′be-ah) hypercapnia.

hypercarotenemia (hi″per-kar″o-tēn-e′me-ah) an excess of carotene in the blood.

hypercarotinemia (hi″per-kar″o-tĭ-ne′me-ah) hypercarotenemia.

hypercatabolic (hi″per-kat″ah-bol′ik) pertaining to, characterized by, or causing hypercatabolism.

hypercatabolism (hi″per-kah-tab′o-lizm) abnormally increased catabolism.

hypercatharsis (hi″per-kah-thar′sis) [*hyper-* + Gr. *katharsis* purge] excessive purgation.

hypercathartic (hi″per-kah-thar′tik) [*hyper-* + Gr. *kathartikos* purgative] excessively cathartic.

hypercellular (hi″per-sel′u-lar) pertaining to or characterized by hypercellularity.

hypercellularity (hi″per-sel″u-lār′ĭ-te) a state characterized by an abnormal increase in the number of cells present, as in bone marrow.

hypercementosis (hi″per-se″men-to′sis) excessive development of secondary cementum on the surfaces of tooth roots.

hypercenesthesia (hi″per-se″nes-the′ze-ah) [*hyper-* + *cenesthesia*] (obs.) a feeling of exaggerated well being, as seen in general paralysis and sometimes in mania.

hyperchloremia (hi″per-klo-re′me-ah) an excess of chloride in the blood.

hyperchloremic (hi″per-klo-re′mik) pertaining to or characterized by hyperchloremia.

hyperchlorhydria (hi″per-klōr-hi′dre-ah) excessive secretion of hydrochloric acid by the stomach cells.

hyperchloridation (hi″per-klo″ri-da′shun) the administration of an excess of sodium chloride.

hyperchloruration (hi″per-klōr′u-ra′shun) an excess of chlorides in the body.

hyperchloruria (hi″per-klōr-u′re-ah) excess of chlorides in the urine.

hypercholesteremia (hi″per-ko-les″ter-e′me-ah) hypercholesterolemia.

hypercholesteremic (hi″per-ko-les′ter-e″mik) hypercholesterolemic.

hypercholesterinemia (hi″per-ko-les″ter-in-e′me-ah) hypercholesterolemia.

hypercholesterolemia (hi″per-ko-les″ter-ol-e′me-ah) [*hyper-* + *cholesterol* + Gr. *haima* blood + *-ia*] excess of cholesterol in the blood. **familial h.,** familial hyperlipoproteinemia, type IIa.

hypercholesterolemic (hi″per-ko-les″ter-ol-e′mik) pertaining to, characterized by, or tending to produce hypercholesterolemia.

hypercholesterolia (hi″per-ko-les″ter-ol′e-ah) abnormally high cholesterol content of the bile.

hypercholia (hi″per-ko′le-ah) [*hyper-* + Gr. *cholē* bile + *-ia*] excessive secretion of bile.

hyperchondroplasia (hi″per-kon″dro-pla′se-ah) excessive development of cartilage.

hyperchromaffinism (hi″per-kro-maf′ĭ-nizm) a condition caused by excessive secretion of chromaffin in the body, marked by paroxysms of arterial hypertension.

hyperchromasia (hi″per-kro-ma′se-ah) hyperchromatism.

hyperchromatic (hi″per-kro-mat′ik) 1. staining more intensely than is normal. 2. pertaining to or marked by hyperchromatism.

hyperchromatin (hi″per-kro′mah-tin) the part of the chromatin that stains with blue aniline dyes.

hyperchromatism (hi″per-kro′mah-tizm) [*hyper-* + Gr. *chrōma* color] excessive pigmentation, especially a form of degeneration of a cell nucleus in which it becomes filled with particles of pigment, or chromatin.

hyperchromatopsia (hi″per-kro″mah-top′se-ah) [*hyper-* + Gr.

chrōma color + *opsis* vision] a condition in which all objects appear colored.

hyperchromatosis (hi″per-kro″mah-to′sis) 1. increased staining capacity. 2. hyperchromatism.

hyperchromemia (hi″per-kro-me′me-ah) [*hyper-* + Gr. *chrōma* color + *haima* blood + *-ia*] a high color index of the blood.

hyperchromia (hi″per-kro′me-ah) hyperchromatism.

hyperchromic (hi″per-kro′mik) highly or excessively stained or colored.

hyperchylia (hi″per-ki′le-ah) excessive secretion of gastric juice.

hyperchylomicronemia (hi″per-ki″lo-mi″kro-ne′me-ah) the presence in the blood of an excessive number of particles of fat (chylomicrons); see *familial hyperlipoproteinemia, type I,* under *hyperlipoproteinemia.* **familial h.,** familial hyperlipoproteinemia, type I.

hypercoagulability (hi″per-ko-ag″u-lah-bil′ĭ-te) the state of being more readily coagulated than normal.

hypercoagulable (hi″per-ko-ag′u-lah-bl) characterized by abnormally increased coagulability.

hypercoria (hi″per-ko′re-ah) hyperkoria.

hypercorticalism (hi″per-kor′tĭ-kal-izm) hyperadrenocorticism.

hypercorticism (hi″per-kor′tĭ-sizm) hyperadrenocorticism.

hypercortisolism (hi″per-kor′tĭ-sōl″izm) a complex of symptoms and signs due to excessive production or administration of hydrocortisone; hyperadrenocorticism.

hypercreatinemia (hi″per-kre″ah-tĭ-ne′me-ah) an abnormality of creatine metabolism in skeletal muscle, a common feature of thyrotoxicosis.

hypercrine (hi″per-krin′) due to endocrine hyperfunction.

hypercrinemia (hi″per-krin-e′me-ah) hypercrinism.

hypercrinia (hi″per-krin′e-ah) hypercrinism.

hypercrinism (hi″per-kri′nizm) [*hyper-* + Gr. *krinein* to separate] the bodily state caused by excessive secretion of any endocrine gland.

hypercrisia (hi″per-kris′e-ah) hypercrinism.

hypercryalgesia (hi″per-kri″al-je′ze-ah) [*hyper-* + Gr. *kryos* cold + *algēsis* pain] excessive sensitiveness to cold.

hypercryesthesia (hi″per-kri″es-the′ze-ah) [*hyper-* + Gr. *kryos* cold + *aisthēsis* perception] hypercryalgesia.

hypercupremia (hi″per-ku-pre′me-ah) an excess of copper in the blood.

hypercupriuria (hi″per-ku″pre-u′re-ah) an excess of copper in the urine.

hypercyanotic (hi″per-si″ah-not′ik) extremely cyanotic.

hypercyesis (hi″per-si-e′sis) [*hyper-* + Gr. *kyēsis* gestation] superfetation.

hypercythemia (hi″per-si-the′me-ah) [*hyper-* + Gr. *kytos* hollow vessel + *haima* blood + *-ia*] abnormal increase in the number of erythrocytes in the blood.

hypercytochromia (hi″per-si″to-kro′me-ah) [*hyper-* + Gr. *kytos* hollow vessel + *chrōma* color] increased staining capacity of a blood cell.

hypercytosis (hi″per-si-to′sis) [*hyper-* + Gr. *kytos* hollow vessel + *-osis*] a condition characterized by an abnormally increased number of cells, especially of leukocytes.

hyperdactylia (hi″per-dak-til′e-ah) hyperdactyly.

hyperdactylism (hi″per-dak′tĭ-lizm) hyperdactyly.

hyperdactyly (hi-per-dak′tĭ-le) [*hyper-* + Gr. *daktylos* finger] the presence of more than the normal number of fingers or toes.

hyperdicrotic (hi″per-di-krot′ik) [*hyper-* + *dicrotic*] exhibiting marked dicrotism.

hyperdicrotism (hi″per-dik′ro-tizm) [*hyper-* + *dicrotism*] the quality of being hyperdicrotic; extreme dicrotism.

hyperdiploid (hi′per-dip″loid) polyploid.

hyperdiploidy (hi′per-dip″loi-de) polyploidy.

hyperdipsia (hi″per-dip′se-ah) [*hyper-* + Gr. *dipsa* thirst + *-ia*] intense thirst of relatively brief duration.

hyperdistention (hi″per-dis-ten′shun) excessive distention.

hyperdiuresis (hi″per-di″u-re′sis) [*hyper-* + *diuresis*] excessive excretion of urine.

hyperdontia (hi″per-don′she-ah) a condition characterized by the presence of supernumerary teeth.

hyperdynamia (hi″per-di-na′me-ah) [*hyper-* + Gr. *dynamis* force] excessive muscular activity. **h. u′teri,** excessive uterine contractions in labor.

hyperdynamic (hi″per-di-nam′ik) pertaining to or characterized by hyperdynamia.

hypereccrisia (hi″per-ek-kris′e-ah) [*hyper-* + Gr. *ekkrisis* excretion + *-ia*] a state characterized by abnormally increased excretion.

hypereccrisis (hi″per-ek′krĭ-sis) hypereccrisia.

hypereccritic (hi-per-ek-krit′ik) pertaining to or exhibiting hypereccrisia.

hyperechema (hi″per-e-ke′mah) [*hyper-* + Gr. *ēchēma* sound] exaggeration of auditory sensations.

hyperelectrolytemia (hi-per-e-lek″tro-li-te′me-ah) an abnormally high concentration of electrolytes in the blood.

hyperemesis (hi″per-em′ĕ-sis) [*hyper-* + Gr. *emesis* vomiting] excessive vomiting. **h. gravida′rum,** pernicious vomiting of pregnancy. **h. lacten′tium,** excessive vomiting of nursing babies.

hyperemetic (hi″per-e-met′ik) characterized by excessive vomiting.

hyperemia (hi″per-e′me-ah) [*hyper-* + Gr. *haima* blood + *-ia*] an excess of blood in a part; engorgement. **active h.,** excess of blood in a part due to local or general relaxation of the arterioles. **arterial h.,** active h. **Bier's passive h.,** the induction of venous congestion by applying a thin rubber band, for the treatment of joint affections and inflammatory conditions. **collateral h.,** increased flow of blood through collateral vessels when the flow through the main artery is arrested. **constriction h.,** Bier's passive h. **fluxionary h.,** active h. **leptomeningeal h.,** congestion of the pia-arachnoid. **passive h.,** an excess of blood in a part resulting from obstruction to its outflow from the area. **reactive h.,** an excess of blood in a part following restoration of its temporarily arrested flow. **stauungs h.,** Bier's passive h. **venous h.,** passive h.

hyperemic (hi″per-e′mik) marked by hyperemia.

hyperemization (hi″per-e″mi-za′shun) the production of hyperemia, especially when employed for therapeutic purposes.

hyperemotivity (hi″per-e″mo-tiv′ĭ-te) hyperaffectivity.

hyperencephalus (hi″per-en-sef′ah-lus) [*hyper-* + Gr. *enkephalos* brain] a monster with the cranial vault absent and the brain exposed.

hyperendemic (hi″per-en-dem′ik) present in a community at all times and with a high rate of incidence.

hyperendocrinia (hi″per-en″do-krin′e-ah) hyperendocrinism.

hyperendocrinism (hi″per-en-dok′rĭ-nizm) [*hyper-* + Gr. *endon* within + *krinein* to separate] abnormally increased activity of an endocrine organ.

hyperendocrisia (hi″per-en″do-kris′e-ah) hyperendocrinism.

hyperenergia (hi″per-en-er′je-ah) excessive energy or activity.

hypereosinophilia (hi″per-e″o-sin-o-fil′e-ah) excessive eosinophilia.

hyperephidrosis (hi″per-ef′ĭ-dro′sis) [*hyper-* + Gr. *epi* upon + *hidrōs* sweat] (*obs.*) hyperhidrosis.

hyperepinephrinemia (hi″per-ep′ĭ-nef″rĭ-ne′me-ah) [*hyper-* + *epinephrine* + Gr. *haima* blood] an excess of epinephrine in the blood.

hyperepinephry (hi″per-ep′ĭ-nef′re) excessive secretion of epinephrine by the adrenal gland.

hyperequilibrium (hi″per-e″kwĭ-lib′re-um) an excessive tendency to vertigo.

hypererethism (hi″per-er′ĕ-thizm) extreme irritability.

hyperergasia (hi″per-er-ga′se-ah) [*hyper-* + Gr. *ergon* work] abnormally increased functional activity.

hyperergia (hi″per-er′je-ah) 1. hyperergasia. 2. hyperergy.

hyperergic (hi″per-er′jik) 1. more energetic than normal. 2. pertaining to or characterized by hyperergy.

hyperergy (hi′per-er″je) [*hyper-* + *allergy*] hypersensitivity to allergens; extreme allergy.

hypererythrocythemia (hi″per-ĕ-rith″ro-si-the′me-ah) hypercythemia.

hyperesophoria (hi″per-es″o-fo′re-ah) [*hyper-* + Gr. *esō* inward + *phorein* to bear] a tendency of the visual axis to deviate upward and inward.

hyperesthesia (hi″per-es-the′ze-ah) [*hyper-* + Gr. *aisthēsis* sensation + *-ia*] increased sensitivity to stimulation. **acoustic h., auditory h.,** hyperacusis. **cerebral h.,** that due to a cerebral lesion. **gustatory h.,** hypergeusesthesia. **muscular h.,** muscular oversensitivity to pain or fatigue. **olfactory h.,** hyperosmia. **oneiric h.,** increase of sensitivity or of pain during sleep and dreams. **optic h.,** abnormal sensitivity of the eye to light. **sexual h.,** abnormal increase of the sexual impulse. **tactile h.,** excessive tactile sensibility; called also *hyperaphia* and *hyperpselaphesia.*

hyperesthetic (hi″per-es-thet′ik) pertaining to or characterized by hyperesthesia.

hyperestrinemia (hi″per-es-trĭ-ne′me-ah) hyperestrogenemia.

hyperestrinism (hi″per-es′trin-izm) a condition due to excessive secretion of estrin and characterized by functional uterine bleeding (menometrorrhagia).

hyperestrogenemia (hi″per-es″tro-jĕ-ne′me-ah) an excessive amount of estrogens in the blood.

hyperestrogenism (hi″per-es′tro-jen-izm″) a state characterized or caused by excessive secretion of estrogen.

hyperestrogenosis (hi″per-es″tro-jĕ-no′sis) an abnormally elevated level of estrogens in the body.

hypereuryopia (hi″per-u″re-o′pe-ah) [*hyper-* + Gr. *eurys* wide + *ōps* eye + *-ia*] abnormally wide opening of the eyes.

hyperevolutism (hi″per-e-vol′u-tizm) a condition characterized by development in excess of the normal.

hyperexcretory (hi″per-eks′kre-to-re) marked by excessive secretion.

hyperexophoria (hi″per-ek″so-fo′re-ah) [*hyper-* + Gr. *exō* outward + *phorein* to bear + *-ia*] a tendency of the visual axis to deviate upward and outward.

hyperexplexia (hi″per-eks-pleks′e-ah) a congenital condition of exaggerated startle reactions with hypertonia, hypokinesia, and brisk cerebral bulbar reflexes at birth.

hyperextension (hi″per-ek-sten′shun) extreme or excessive extension of a limb or part.

hyperferremia (hi″per-fer-re′me-ah) an excess of iron in the blood.

hyperferremic (hi″per-fer-re′mik) pertaining to or characterized by hyperferremia.

hyperferricemia (hi″per-fer″ĭ-se′me-ah) hyperferremia.

hyperfibrinogenemia (hi″per-fi-brin″o-jĕ-ne′me-ah) an excess of fibrinogen in the blood.

hyperflexion (hi″per-flek′shun) forcible overflexion of a limb or part.

hyperfolliculinemia (hi″per-fo-lik″u-li-ne′me-ah) the presence of an excessive amount of estrogen in the blood.

hyperfolliculinism (hi″per-fo-lik″u-lin-izm) any condition caused by the presence in the body of excessive quantities of estrogen.

hyperfolliculinuria (hi″per-fo-lik″u-lĭ-nu′re-ah) the presence of an excessive amount of estrogen in the urine.

hyperfunctioning (hi″per-funk′shun-ing) excessive functioning of an organ.

hypergalactia (hi″per-gah-lak′she-ah) [*hyper-* + Gr. *gala* milk] excessive secretion of milk.

hypergalactosis (hi″per-gal″ak-to′sis) hypergalactia.

hypergalactous (hi″per-gah-lak′tus) pertaining to, characterized by, or causing hypergalactia.

hypergammaglobulinemia (hi″per-gam″ah-glob″u-lĭ-ne′me-ah) an excess of gamma globulins in the blood; it is seen frequently in chronic infectious diseases. **monoclonal h.,** an excess of homogeneous immunoglobulin molecules of a single specificity in the blood following the proliferation of a clone of immunoglobulin-producing cells. **polyclonal h.,** an excess of several classes of immunogammaglobulin in the blood.

hypergasia (hip″er-ga′se-ah) hypoergasia.

hypergastrinemia (hi″per-gas′trin-e′me-ah) the presence of an excess of gastrin in the blood.

hypergenesis (hi″per-jen′ĕ-sis) [*hyper-* + Gr. *genesis* development] excessive development, hypertrophy, or redundancy.

hypergenetic (hi″per-jĕ-net′ik) pertaining to or characterized by hypergenesis.

hypergenitalism (hi″per-jen′ĭ-tal-izm) hypergonadism.

hypergeusesthesia (hi″per-gūs″es-the′ze-ah) [*hyper-* + Gr. *geusis* taste + *aisthēsis* perception + *-ia*] excessive or abnormal acuteness of the sense of taste.

hypergeusia (hi″per-gu′se-ah) hypergeusesthesia.

hypergia (hi-per′je-ah) 1. hypoergasia. 2. diminished sensitivity in allergy.

hypergigantosoma (hi″per-ji-gan″to-so′mah) [*hyper-* + Gr. *gigas* giant + *sōma* body] excessive tallness, or gigantism.

hyperglandular (hi″per-glan′du-lar) marked by abnormally increased glandular activity.

hyperglobulinemia (hi″per-glob″u-lĭ-ne′me-ah) abnormally high globulin content of the blood.

hyperglucagonemia (hi″per-gloo″kah-gŏn-e′me-ah) abnormally high levels of glucagon in the blood.

hyperglycemia (hi″per-gli-se′me-ah) [*hyper-* + Gr. *glykys* sweet + *haima* blood + *-ia*] abnormally increased content of sugar in the blood.

hyperglycemic (hi″per-gli-se′mik) 1. pertaining to, characterized by, or causing hyperglycemia. 2. an agent that causes an increase in the level of glucose in the blood.

hyperglyceridemia (hi″per-glis″er-ĭ-de′me-ah) an excess of glycerides, usually triglycerides, in the blood.

hyperglyceridemic (hi″per-glis″er-ĭ-de′mik) pertaining to, characterized by, or producing hyperglyceridemia.

hyperglycinemia (hi″per-gli″sĭ-ne′me-ah) a hereditary congenital disorder involving excessive glycine in the blood. One form is accompanied by episodic vomiting, lethargy, dehydration, ketosis, and intolerance of protein in the diet, with hyperglycinuria, hypogammaglobulinemia, neutropenia, increased susceptibility to infection, thrombocytopenia, and periodic purpura; it leads to developmental retardation. A second form is characterized by lethargy, weak cry, generalized hypotonia, absence of reflexes, intolerance of glycine in the diet, and periodic myoclonic jerks, in the absence of vomiting, ketosis, neutropenia, and thrombocytopenia. Both forms are transmitted as autosomal recessive traits.

hyperglycinuria (hi″per-gli″sĭ-nu′re-ah) an excess of glycine in the urine; see *hyperglycinemia.*

hyperglycistia (hi″per-gli-sis′te-ah) [*hyper-* + Gr. *glykys* sweet + *histos* tissue] excess of sugar in the bodily tissues.

hyperglycodermia (hi″per-gli″ko-der′me-ah) [*hyper-* + Gr. *glykys* sweet + *derma* skin + *-ia*] the presence of an excessive amount of sugar in the skin.

hyperglycogenolysis (hi″per-gli″ko-jen-ol′ĭ-sis) excessive splitting up of glycogen, resulting in an excess of dextrose in the body.

hyperglycoplasmia (hi″per-gli″ko-plaz′me-ah) the presence of a greater amount than normal of sugar in the blood plasma.

hyperglycorrhachia (hi″per-gli″ko-ra′ke-ah) [*hyper-* + Gr. *glykys* sweet + *rhachis* spine] the presence of a greater than normal concentration of glucose in the cerebrospinal fluid.

hyperglycosemia (hi″per-gli″ko-se′me-ah) hyperglycemia.

hyperglycosuria (hi″per-gli″ko-su′re-ah) [*hyper-* + *glycosuria*] extreme glycosuria.

hyperglycystia (hi″per-gli-sis′te-ah) hyperglycistia.

hyperglykemia (hi″per-gli-ke′me-ah) hyperglycemia.

hypergnosia (hi″per-no′se-ah) [*hyper-* + Gr. *gnōsis* knowledge] a paranoic condition marked by distortion of perception with a tendency to project psychic conflicts to the environment.

hypergonadism (hi″per-go′nad-izm) a condition resulting from or characterized by abnormally increased functional activity of the gonads, with excessive growth and precocious sexual development.

hyperguanidinemia (hi″per-gwan″ĭ-dĭ-ne′me-ah) the presence of an excess of guanidine in the blood.

hyperhedonia (hi″per-hĕ-do′ne-ah) [*hyper-* + Gr. *hēdonē* pleasure] morbid increase of the feeling of pleasure in agreeable acts.

hyperhedonism (hi″per-he′do-nizm) hyperhedonia.

hyperhemoglobinemia (hi″per-he″mo-glo″bĭ-ne′me-ah) the presence of an excessive amount of hemoglobin in the blood.

hyperheparinemia (hi″per-hep″ah-rĭ-ne′me-ah) the presence of an excessive amount of heparin in the blood.

hyperhepatia (hi″per-he-pat′e-ah) [*hyper-* + Gr. *hēpar* liver] hyperfunction of the liver.

hyperhidrosis (hi″per-hi-dro′sis) [*hyper-* + Gr. *hidrōsis* sweating] excessive perspiration. **h. unilatera′lis,** excessive sweating on one side of the body only.

hyperhidrotic (hi″per-hi-drot′ik) pertaining to, characterized by, or causing hyperhidrosis.

hyperhormonal (hi-per-hōr′mo-nal) excessive in hormone activity; due to hormone excess.

hyperhormonic (hi″per-hōr-mon′ik) hyperhormonal.

hyperhormonism (hi″per-hōr′mōn-izm) endocrine hyperfunction.

hyperhydration (hi″per-hi-dra′shun) a state of excessive water content of the body.

hyperhydrochloria (hi″per-hi-dro-klo′re-ah) hyperchlorhydria.

hyperhydrochloridia (hi″per-hi-dro-klo-rid′e-ah) hyperchlorhydria.

hyperhypophysism (hi″per-hi-pof′ĭ-sizm) hyperpituitarism.

hyperidrosis (hi″per-i-dro′sis) hyperhidrosis.

hyperimmune (hi″per-im-mūn′) possessing very large quantities of specific antibodies in the serum.

hyperimmunity (hi″per-ĭ-mu′nĭ-te) a degree of immunity greater than is usually found under similar circumstances.

hyperimmunization (hi″per-im″u-ni-za′shun) the practice of establishing a heightened state of actively acquired immunity by the administration of repeated (booster) doses of antigen, or of passively acquired immunity by the injection of hyperimmune gamma globulin.

hyperimmunoglobulinemia (hi″per-im′u-no-glob″u-lin-e′me-ah) abnormally high levels of immunoglobulins in the serum. **h. E,** extremely high levels of IgE in the serum, associated with cutaneous anergy and deficient antibody response, as occurs in Job's syndrome.

hyperinflation (hi″per-in-fla′shun) excessive inflation or expansion, as of the lungs; overinflation.

hyperingestion (hi″per-in-jes′chun) ingestion of a greater than optimal amount of nutrients.

hyperinsulinar (hi″per-in′su-lin-ar) pertaining to or characterized by excessive secretion of insulin.

hyperinsulinemia (hi″per-in″su-lĭ-ne′me-ah) the presence of an excessive amount of insulin in the blood.

hyperinsulinism (hi″per-in′su-lin-izm″) 1. excessive secretion

of insulin by the pancreas, resulting in hypoglycemia. 2. insulin shock.

hyperinterrenal (hi″per-in″ter-re′nal) pertaining to or resulting from overactivity of the adrenal glands.

hyperinterrenopathy (hi″per-in″ter-re-nop′ah-the) [*hyper-* + *interrenal* + Gr. *pathos* disease] any disease due to overactivity of the adrenal glands, as hyperadrenocorticism and Cushing's syndrome.

hyperinvolution (hi″per-in″vo-lu′shun) superinvolution.

hyperiodemia (hi″per-i″o-de′me-ah) the presence of an excessive amount of iodine in the blood.

hyperirritability (hi″per-ir″ĭ-tah-bil′ĭ-te) pathological responsiveness to slight stimuli.

hyperisotonia (hi″per-i″so-to′ne-ah) [*hyper-* + Gr. *isos* equal + *tonos* tension] marked equality of tone or of tonicity.

hyperisotonic (hi″per-i″so-ton′ik) [*hyper-* + Gr. *isos* equal + *tonos* tension, or tone] hypotonic; denoting a solution that contains more than 0.45 per cent sodium chloride, in which erythrocytes become crenated as a consequence of exosmosis.

hyperkalemia (hi″per-kah-le′me-ah) abnormally high potassium concentration in the blood, most often due to defective renal excretion. It is characterized clinically by electrocardiographic abnormalities (elevated T waves and depressed P waves, and eventually by atrial asystole). In severe cases, weakness and flaccid paralysis may occur. Called also *hyperpotassemia.*

hyperkaliemia (hi″per-kal″e-e′me-ah) hyperkalemia.

hyperkeratinization (hi″per-ker″ah-tin″i-za′shun) [*hyper-* + *keratinization*] the excessive development or retention of keratin by the epidermis.

hyperkeratosis (hi″per-ker″ah-to′sis) [*hyper-* + Gr. *keras* horn] 1. hypertrophy of the corneous layer of the skin, or any disease characterized by it; called also *acanthokeratodermia.* 2. hypertrophy of the cornea. 3. a skin disease of cattle marked by inflammation and thickening of the horny layer, and caused by the ingestion of grease containing high levels of chlorinated hydrocarbons. Once thought to be caused by a virus, it was called *x disease.* Called also *perkeratosis.* **h. congenita′lis palma′ris et planta′ris,** keratosis palmaris et plantaris. **epidermolytic h.,** a hereditary disease transmitted as an autosomal dominant trait, characterized by hyperkeratosis, blisters, and erythema. At birth, the skin is completely covered by thick, horny, armor-like scales, which are soon shed, leaving a raw surface on which the scales re-form. Formerly called *bullous congenital ichthyosiform erythroderma.* **h. follicula′ris et parafollicula′ris in cu′tem pen′etrans,** hyperkeratosis follicularis in cutem penetrans. **h. follicula′ris in cu′tem pen′etrans,** a very rare follicular disease characterized by keratotic pegs, which are usually discrete but may form circinate patches; they develop in the hair follicles and eccrine ducts, penetrating the epidermis and extending down into the corium, where they cause a foreign-body reaction and pain. Called also *hyperkeratosis penetrans, hyperkeratosis follicularis et parafollicularis in cutem penetrans,* and *Kyrle's disease.* **h. follicula′ris veg′etans,** keratosis follicularis. **h. in cu′tem pen′etrans,** h. follicularis in cutem penetrans. **h. lacuna′ris,** a condition in which the tonsillar crypts contain hard, firmly attached masses. **h. pen′etrans,** hyperkeratosis follicularis in cutem penetrans. **h. subungua′lis,** hyperkeratosis affecting the nail beds.

hyperketonemia (hi″per-ke″to-ne′me-ah) an abnormally increased concentration of ketone bodies in the blood.

hyperketonuria (hi″per-ke″to-nu′re-ah) the presence of an excessive quantity of ketone in the urine.

hyperketosis (hi″per-ke-to′sis) the formation of an excess of ketone.

hyperkinemia (hi″per-ki-ne′me-ah) [*hyper-* + Gr. *kinein* move + *haima* blood + *-ia*] abnormally high cardiac output (blood circulation) when at rest and supine, as in the hyperkinetic syndrome.

hyperkinemic (hi″per-ki-ne′mik) 1. increasing blood flow through a tissue. 2. an agent which increases the flow of blood through a tissue area.

hyperkinesia (hi″per-ki-ne′ze-ah) [*hyper-* + Gr. *kinēsis* motion + *-ia*] abnormally increased motor function or activity; hyperactivity. See *hyperkinetic syndrome,* under *syndrome.* **professional h.,** occupation neurosis.

hyperkinesis (hi″per-ki-ne′sis) hyperkinesia.

hyperkinetic (hi″per-ki-net′ik) pertaining to or characterized by hyperkinesia; hyperactive. See *hyperkinetic syndrome,* under *syndrome.*

hyperkoria (hi″per-ko′re-ah) [*hyper-* + Gr. *koros* satiety + *-ia*] an early sense of satiety.

hyperlactacidemia (hi″per-lakt″as-ĭ-de′me-ah) an excessive amount of lactic acid in the blood.

hyperlactation (hi″per-lak-ta′shun) lactation in greater than normal amount or for a longer than usual period.

hyperlecithinemia (hi″per-les″ĭ-thĭ-ne′me-ah) excess of lecithin in the blood.

hyperlethal (hi″per-le′thal) more than sufficient to cause death.

hyperleukocytosis (hi″per-lu″ko-si-to′sis) [*hyper-* + *leukocyte* + *-osis*] an abnormally excessive increase in the number of leukocytes in the blood.

hyperleydigism (hi″per-li′dig-izm) overactivity of Leydig's cells.

hyperlipemia (hi″per-li-pe′me-ah) [*hyper-* + Gr. *lipos* fat + *haima* blood + *-ia*] elevated concentration of triglycerides in the plasma. See also *hyperlipoproteinemia.* **carbohydrate-induced h.,** hyperlipoproteinemia, type IV. **fat-induced h.,** hyperlipoproteinemia, type I.

hyperlipidemia (hi″per-lip″ĭ-de′me-ah) [*hyper-* + *lipid* + Gr. *haima* blood + *-ia*] a general term for elevated concentrations of any or all of the lipids in the plasma, including hyperlipoproteinemia, hypercholesterolemia, etc.

hyperlipoidemia (hi″per-li″poi-de′me-ah) hyperlipemia.

hyperlipoproteinemia (hi″per-lip″o-pro″te-in-e′me-ah) an excess of lipoproteins in the blood, due to a disorder of lipoprotein metabolism, and occurring as an acquired or familial condition. **acquired h.,** hyperlipoproteinemia occurring secondarily to some other disorder, such as hypothyroidism, nephrotic syndrome, or hypoadrenocorticism, or as a result of environmental factors, including diet. **familial h.,** any of a group of inherited disorders of lipoprotein metabolism, classified into five major phenotypes based on clinical features, enzymatic abnormalities, and serum lipoprotein electrophoretic patterns. *Type I,* transmitted as a recessive trait, is caused by deficient activity of lipoprotein lipase with resultant inability to dispose of dietary triglycerides (in chylomicrons); it may be manifested by repeated bouts of abdominal pain and vomiting, recurrent acute pancreatitis, eruptive xanthomas, hepatosplenomegaly, and lipemia retinalis. Called also *Bürger-Grütz syndrome, fat-induced hyperlipemia,* and *familial hyperchylomicronemia. Type II,* in which the nature of the biochemical defect is unknown, is transmitted as a dominant trait with evidence of occurrence of both homozygous and heterozygous forms; it may be characterized by tendinous and tuberous xanthomas, xanthelasmas, early onset of corneal arcus, and accelerated atherosclerosis, especially of the coronary arteries. Two subtypes have been described: *Type IIa* characterized by increased levels of low-density lipoproteins and normal levels of very low-density lipoproteins (called also *familial hyperbetalipoproteinemia* and *familial hypercholesterolemia*); and *Type IIb,* characterized by elevated levels of both low-density and very low-density lipoproteins. *Type III,* in which the mode of inheritance and biochemical abnormality are uncertain, is characterized by accumulation of abnormal β-lipoproteins resembling pre-betalipoproteins, and may be manifested by planar xanthomas and less often by tendinous xanthomas and premature coronary and peripheral atherosclerosis; called also *broad-beta disease* and *familial dysbetalipoproteinemia. Type IV,* in which the nature of the mode of inheritance and biochemical abnormality are uncertain, is characterized by elevated serum levels of endogenously synthesized triglycerides, and may be manifested by increased incidence of vascular disease, abnormal glucose tolerance, and family history of diabetes mellitus. Called also *carbohydrate-induced hyperlipemia* and *familial hyperprebetalipoproteinemia. Type V,* in which the nature of the mode of inheritance and biochemical abnormality are uncertain, is characterized by accumulation of very low-density lipoproteins and chylomicrons in the blood and may be accompanied by diabetes mellitus, eruptive xanthomas, and recurrent acute pancreatitis. Called also *mixed hyperlipemia.* **mixed h.,** familial h., type V.

hyperliposis (hi″per-lĭ-po′sis) an excess of fat in the blood serum or tissues.

hyperlithemia (hi″per-lĭ-the′me-ah) presence in the blood of a high concentration of lithium.

hyperlithic (hi″per-lith′ik) pertaining to or characterized by an excess of lithic (uric) acid.

hyperlithuria (hi″per-lith-u′re-ah) excess of lithic (uric) acid in the urine.

hyperlordosis (hi″per-lor-do′sis) extremely marked lordosis.

hyperlucency (hi″per-lu′sen-se) excessive radiolucency.

hyperluteinization (hi″per-lu″te-in-i-za′shun) excessive luteinization of the cystic follicles of the ovary.

hyperlutemia (hi″per-lu-te′me-ah) an increased amount of luteal hormone (progesterone) in the blood.

hyperlysinemia (hi″per-li″sēn-e′me-ah) an inborn error of amino acid metabolism characterized by elevated levels of lysine in the blood and marked by vomiting, spasticity, coma, and mental retardation; symptoms are related to protein intake.

hypermagnesemia (hi″per-mag″ně-se′me-ah) an abnormally large magnesium content of the blood plasma; manifestations include lethargy, weakness, electrocardiographic abnormalities and, as levels increase, loss of deep tendon reflexes, somnolence, and coma.

hypermania (hi″per-ma′ne-ah) intense mania with overwhelming tensions and marked disorientation.

hypermastia (hi″per-mas′te-ah) [*hyper-* + Gr. *mastos* breast] 1. the presence of one or more supernumerary mammary glands. 2. hypertrophy of the mammary gland.

hypermature (hi″per-mah-tūr) past the stage of maturity.

hypermegasoma (hi″per-meg″ah-so′mah) [*hyper-* + Gr. *megas* great + *sōma* body] excessive tallness and size; gigantism.

hypermelanotic (hi″per-mel″ah-not′ik) characterized by an excessive deposit of melanin.

hypermenorrhea (hi″per-men″o-re′ah) [*hyper-* + Gr. *mēn* month + *rhein* to flow] excessive uterine bleeding occurring at regular intervals, the period of flow being of usual duration.

hypermesosoma (hi″per-mes″o-so′mah) [*hyper-* + Gr. *mesos* middle + *sōma* body] a stature somewhat exceeding the ordinary.

hypermetabolic (hi″per-met″ah-bol′ik) exhibiting an increased metabolic rate.

hypermetabolism (hi″per-mě-tab′o-lizm) abnormally increased utilizaton of material by the body; increased metabolism. **extrathyroidal h.,** abnormally elevated basal metabolism unassociated with thyroid disease.

hypermetamorphosis (hi″per-met″ah-mor′fo-sis) too rapid drift of thought activity, leading to mental distraction and confusion, and forming a chief element in mania; excessive attentiveness to visual stimuli, as in the Klüver-Bucy syndrome.

hypermetaplasia (hi″per-met″ah-pla′se-ah) abnormally increased metaplasia.

hypermetria (hi″per-me′tre-ah) [Gr. "a passing all measure, overflow"] a condition in which voluntary muscular movement overreaches the intended goal.

hypermetrope (hi″per-mě-trōp′) hyperope.

hypermetropia (hi″per-me-tro′pe-ah) [*hyper-* + Gr. *metron* measure + *ōps* eye + *-ia*] hyperopia.

hypermicrosoma (hi″per-mi″kro-so′mah) [*hyper-* + Gr. *mikros* small + *sōma* body] extreme smallness of body; marked dwarfishness.

hypermimia (hi″per-mim′e-ah) [*hyper-* + Gr. *mimia* representation by means of art] excessive use of gestures when speaking.

hypermineralization (hi″per-min″er-al-i-za′shun) the presence of an excess of mineral elements in the body.

hypermnesia (hi″perm-ne′ze-ah) [*hyper-* + Gr. *mnēmē* memory] excessive crowding or unusual clarity of memory images.

hypermnesic (hi″perm-ne′sik) 1. pertaining to or characterized by hypermnesia. 2. marked by excessive mental activity.

hypermodal (hi″per-mo′dal) in statistics, relating to the values or items located to the right of the mode in a variations curve.

hypermorph (hi′per-morf) [*hyper-* + Gr. *morphē* form] 1. a person who is tall but of low sitting height, with bony and narrow arms and legs, slender body, narrow nose, shoulders, thorax, and lips. Cf. *hypomorph* (def. 1) and *mesomorph* (def. 2). 2. in genetics, a mutant gene characterized by an increase in the activity it influences. Cf. *hypomorph* (def. 2).

hypermotility (hi″per-mo-til′ĭ-te) excessive or abnormally increased motility, as of the gastrointestinal tract.

hypermyotonia (hi″per-mi″o-to′ne-ah) [*hyper-* + Gr. *mys* muscle + *tonos* tension + *-ia*] excess of muscular tonicity.

hypermyotrophy (hi″per-mi-ot′ro-fe) [*hyper-* + Gr. *mys* muscle + *trophē* nourishment] excessive development of the muscular tissue.

hypernanosoma (hi″per-na″no-so′mah) [*hyper-* + Gr. *nanos* dwarf + *sōma* body] a very short but not absolutely dwarfish stature.

hypernasality (hi″per-na-zal′ĭ-te) a quality of voice in which the emission of air through the nose is excessive due to velopharyngeal incompetence; it causes deterioration of intelligibility of speech.

hypernatremia (hi″per-nah-tre′me-ah) [*hyper-* + L. *natron* sodium + Gr. *haima* blood + *-ia*] excessive amount of sodium in the blood.

hypernatremic (hi″per-na-tre′mik) pertaining to, characterized by, or causing hypernatremia.

hypernatronemia (hi″per-nat″ro-ne′me-ah) hypernatremia.

hypernea (hi″per-ne′ah) hypernoia.

hyperneocytosis (hi″per-ne″o-si-to′sis) [*hyper-* + Gr. *neos* new + *kytos* hollow vessel + *-osis*] leukocytosis in which an excessive number of immature forms of leukocytes are present.

hypernephritis (hi″per-ně-fri′tis) inflammation of the adrenal gland.

hypernephroid (hi″per-nef′roid) resembling the adrenal gland.

hypernephroma (hi″per-ně-fro′mah) [*hyper-* + Gr. *nephros* kidney + *-oma*] renal cell carcinoma whose structure resembles that of the cortical tissue of the adrenal gland. See also *Grawitz's tumor,* under *tumor.*

hyperneurotization (hi″per-nu-rot″i-za′shun) [*hyper-* + Gr. *neuron* nerve] the implantation of a foreign motor nerve into a muscle possessing its normal innervation in order to increase the energy force of the muscle.

hypernitremia (hi″per-ni-tre′me-ah) [*hyper-* + *nitrogen* + Gr. *haima* blood] excessive nitrogen in the blood.

hypernoia (hi″per-noi′ah) [*hyper-* + Gr. *nous* mind] excessive mental activity.

hypernomic (hi″per-nom′ik) [*hyper-* + Gr. *nomos* law] above the law; unrestrained; excessive.

hypernormal (hi″per-nor′mal) in excess of what is normal.

hypernutrition (hi″per-nu-trish′un) overfeeding and its ill effects.

hyperontomorph (hi″per-on′to-morf) [*hyper-* + Gr. *ōn* being + *morphē* form] a person with a tendency to hyperthyroidism.

hyperonychia (hi″per-o-nik′e-ah) [*hyper-* + Gr. *onyx* nail + *-ia*] onychauxis.

hyperonychosis (hi″per-on″e-ko′sis) onychauxis.

hyperope (hi′per-ōp) an individual exhibiting hyperopia.

hyperopia (hi″per-o′pe-ah) [*hyper-* + Gr. *ōps* eye + *-ia*] that error of refraction in which rays of light entering the eye parallel to the optic axis are brought to a focus behind the retina, as a result of the eyeball being too short from front to back. Called also *farsightedness* (because the near point is more distant than it is in emmetropia with an equal amplitude of accommodation) and *hypermetropia*. **absolute h.**, that amount of hyperopia which cannot be corrected by accommodation. **axial h.**, that which is due to shortness of the anteroposterior axis of the eye. **curvature h.**, hyperopia due to insufficient convexity of the refracting surfaces. **facultative h.**, that amount of hyperopia which can be entirely corrected by the ciliary muscle, i.e., by the effort of accommodation; called also *relative h.* **index h.**, hyperopia caused by deficient refractive power in the media of the eye. **latent h.**, that part of the total hyperopia corrected by the physiologic tone of the ciliary muscle and revealed only when that muscle is paralyzed by the use of a drug, such as atropine. **manifest h.**, that part of the total hyperopia not corrected by the physiologic tone of the ciliary muscle and revealed with cycloplegic examination. **relative h.**, facultative h. **total h.**, the sum of manifest and latent hyperopia combined.

hyperopic (hi″per-o′pik) pertaining to or exhibiting hyperopia; farsighted.

hyperorchidism (hi″per-or′ki-dizm) [*hyper-* + Gr. *orchis* testicle] abnormally increased functional activity of the testes.

hyperorexia (hi″per-o-rek′se-ah) [*hyper-* + Gr. *orexis* appetite + *-ia*] an abnormally increased appetite.

hyperorthocytosis (hi″per-or″tho-si-to′sis) [*hyper-* + Gr. *orthos* straight + *kytos* hollow vessel + *-osis*] leukocytosis in which the proportion of the various forms of leukocytes is normal.

hyperosmia (hi″per-oz′me-ah) [*hyper-* + Gr. *osmē* smell] abnormally increased sensitiveness to odors.

hyperosmolality (hi″per-os″mo-lal′ĭ-te) an increase in the osmolality of the body fluids.

hyperosmolarity (hi″per-oz″mo-lar′i-te) abnormally increased osmolar concentration.

hyperosmotic (hi″per-os-mot′ik) 1. producing or caused by abnormally rapid osmosis. 2. containing a higher concentration of osmotically active components than a standard solution.

hyperosphresia (hi″per-os-fre′ze-ah) [*hyper-* + Gr. *osphrēsis* smell + *-ia*] hyperosmia.

hyperosteogeny (hi″per-os″te-oj′ĕ-ne) [*hyper-* + Gr. *osteon* bone + *gennan* to produce] excessive development of bone.

hyperostosis (hi″per-os-to′sis) [*hyper-* + Gr. *osteon* bone + *-osis*] hypertrophy of bone; exostosis. **h. cortica′lis generalisa′ta**, a hereditary disorder, transmitted as an autosomal recessive trait, characterized principally by osteosclerosis of the skull, mandible, clavicles, ribs, and diaphyses of long bones, associated with elevated blood alkaline phosphatase; beginning during puberty, it sometimes leads to optic atrophy and perceptive deafness owing to nerve pressure exerted by thickening of the base of the skull. Called also *hyperphosphatasemia tarda* and *van Buchem's syndrome*. **h. cra′nii**, hyperostosis involving the cranial bones. **flowing h.**, melorheostasis. **h. fronta′lis inter′na**, thickening of the inner table of the frontal bone, which may be associated with hypertrichosis and obesity; it most commonly affects women near menopause. Called also *Morel's syndrome; Morgagni's disease, hyperostosis*, or *syndrome; Morgagni-Stewart-Morel syndrome*; and *Stewart-Morel syndrome*. **infantile cortical h.**, a disease of young infants characterized by soft tissue swellings over the affected bones, fever, and irritability, and marked by periods of remission and exacerbation; called also *Caffey's disease*. **Morgagni's h.**, h. frontalis interna. **senile ankylosing h. of spine**, a disorder of the elderly characterized by large osteophytes that bridge vertebrae and, in association with calcified ligaments, may resemble ankylosing spondylitis.

hyperostotic (hi″per-os-tot′ik) pertaining to or exhibiting hyperostosis.

hyperovaria (hi″per-o-va′re-ah) [*hyper-* + L. *ovarium* ovary] sexual precocity in girls due to excessive ovarian secretion.

hyperovarianism (hi″per-o-va′re-an-izm) hyperovaria.

hyperovarism (hi″per-o′vah-rizm) hyperovaria.

hyperoxaluria (hi″per-ok″sah-lu′re-ah) the excretion of an excessive amount of oxalate in the urine; high concentrations of oxalates in the urine may lead to the formation of urinary calculi. Called also *oxaluria*. **enteric h.**, a form occurring after extensive resection or disease of the ileum and resulting from excessive absorption of oxalate from the colon, with formation of calcium oxalate calculi in the urinary tract. **primary h.**, a genetic disorder characterized by urinary excretion of large amounts of oxalate, with nephrolithiasis, nephrocalcinosis, early onset of renal failure, and often a generalized deposit of calcium oxalate (oxalosis), resulting from a defect in glyoxalate metabolism. The disorder occurs in two types: Type 1, hyperoxaluria accompanied by glycolic aciduria, is due to a defect of the enzyme soluble α-ketoglutarate: glyoxylate carboligase. Type 2, hyperoxaluria with D-glyceric aciduria, is due to a defect of the enzyme glyoxalate reductase. Both types are autosomal recessive traits.

hyperoxemia (hi″per-ok-se′me-ah) [*hyper-* + Gr. *oxys* sharp + *haima* blood] excessive acidity of the blood.

hyperoxia (hi″per-ok′se-ah) an excess of oxygen in the system, resulting from exposure to high oxygen concentrations, especially to hyperbaric pressures of oxygen.

hyperoxic (hi″per-ok′sik) pertaining to or characterized by hyperoxia.

hyperoxidation (hi″per-ok″sĭ-da′shun) excessive oxidation.

hyperpallesthesia (hi″per-pal″es-the′ze-ah) [*hyper-* + *pallesthesia*] abnormally increased sensibility to vibrations.

hyperpancreorrhea (hi″per-pan″kre-o-re′ah) excessive secretion from the pancreas.

hyperparasite (hi″per-par′ah-sīt) [*hyper-* + *parasite*] a parasite that preys on a parasite. **second degree h.**, a parasite that preys on a hyperparasite.

hyperparasitic (hi″per-par-ah-sit′ik) living parasitically upon a parasite; biparasitic.

hyperparasitism (hi″per-par′ah-si″tizm) infestation with a hyperparasite.

hyperparathyroidism (hi″per-par″ah-thi′roid-izm) abnormally increased activity of the parathyroid glands, which may be primary or secondary. *Primary hyperparathyroidism* is associated with neoplasia (chiefly adenomas) or hyperplasia. The excess of parathyroid hormone leads to alteration in function of cells of bone, renal tubules, and gastrointestinal mucosa. It may result in kidney stones and calcium deposits in the renal tubules; in generalized decalcification of bone (osteoporosis), resulting in pain and tenderness of bones and spontaneous fractures; and in hypercalcemia, leading to muscular weakness and gastrointestinal symptoms such as anorexia, nausea, vomiting, and abdominal pains. *Secondary hyperparathyroidism* occurs when the serum calcium tends to fall below normal, as in chronic renal disease, vitamin-D deficiency, etc. *Tertiary hyperparathyroidism* refers to that due to a parathyroid adenoma arising from secondary hyperplasia caused by chronic renal failure.

hyperparotidism (hi″per-pah-rot′ĭ-dizm) excessive activity of the parotid gland.

hyperpathia (hi″per-path′e-ah) abnormally exaggerated subjective response to painful stimuli.

hyperpepsia (hi″per-pep′se-ah) [*hyper-* + Gr. *pepsis* digestion] impairment of digestion, due to hyperchlorhydria.

hyperpepsinemia (hi″per-pep″sĭ-ne′me-ah) an abnormally high level of pepsin in the blood.

hyperpepsinia (hi″per-pep-sin′e-ah) abnormally profuse secretion of pepsin in the stomach.

hyperpepsinuria (hi″per-pep″sĭ-nu′re-ah) an abnormally high level of pepsin in the urine.

hyperperistalsis (hi″per-per″ĭ-stal′sis) excessively active peristalsis.

hyperpermeability (hi″per-per″me-ah-bil′ĭ-te) undue or abnormal permeability, as of a cell membrane or a vessel wall.

hyperpexia (hi″per-pek′se-ah) [*hyper-* + Gr. *pēxis* fixation + *-ia*] fixation of an excessive amount of a substance by a tissue.

hyperpexy (hi″per-pek′se) hyperpexia.

hyperphagia (hi″per-fa′je-ah) [*hyper-* + Gr. *phagein* to eat] ingestion of a greater than optimal quantity of food.

hyperphalangia (hi″per-fah-lan′je-ah) presence of more than the normal number of phalanges in the longitudinal axis of a digit.

hyperphalangism (hi″per-fah-lan′jizm) hyperphalangia.

hyperphasia (hi″per-fa′ze-ah) [*hyper-* + Gr. *phasis* speech] excessive talkativeness.

hyperphenylalaninemia (hi″per-fen″il-al″ah-nĭ-ne′me-ah) an excess of phenylalanine in the blood, as in phenylketonuria.

hyperphonesis (hi″per-fo-ne′sis) [*hyper-* + Gr. *phōnēsis* sounding] an increase in intensity of the vocal sound in auscultation, or of the percussion note.

hyperphonia (hi″per-fo′ne-ah) [*hyper-* + Gr. *phōnē* voice] excessively energetic phonation, as in stuttering.

hyperphoria (hi″per-fo′re-ah) [*hyper-* + Gr. *phorein* to bear] a form of heterophoria in which there is permanent upward deviation of the visual axis of an eye after the visual fusional stimulus has been eliminated.

hyperphosphatasemia (hi″per-fos″fah-ta-se′me-ah) high levels of alkaline phosphatase in the blood; see *hyperphosphatasia*. **h. tar′da,** hyperostosis corticalis generalisata.

hyperphosphatasia (hi″per-fos″fah-ta′ze-ah) a hereditary condition marked by abnormally high alkaline phosphatase levels in the serum and by macrocranium, short neck and thorax, lateral bowing of the femurs, and anterior bowing of the tibias; transmitted as an autosomal recessive trait. Called also *juvenile Paget's disease*.

hyperphosphatemia (hi″per-fos″fah-te′me-ah) an excessive amount of phosphates in the blood; it is usually asymptomatic.

hyperphosphaturia (hi″per-fos″fah-tu′re-ah) an excessive amount of phosphates in the urine.

hyperphosphoremia (hi″per-fos″fo-re′me-ah) an excessive amount of phosphorus compounds in the blood.

hyperphrenia (hi″per-fre′ne-ah) [*hyper-* + Gr. *phrēn* mind] 1. great mental excitement. 2. excessive mental activity.

hyperpiesia (hi″per-pi-e′se-ah) (*obs.*) abnormally high blood pressure occurring independently of any discoverable organic disease.

hyperpiesis (hi″per-pi′e-sis) [*hyper-* + Gr. *piesis* pressure] (*obs.*) abnormally high pressure, as elevated blood pressure.

hyperpietic (hi″per-pi-et′ik) pertaining to, characterized by, or causing hyperpiesis.

hyperpigmentation (hi″per-pig″men-ta′shun) abnormally increased pigmentation.

hyperpinealism (hi″per-pi′ne-al-izm) abnormally increased activity of the pineal body.

hyperpituitarism (hi″per-pĭ-tu′ĭ-tah-rizm″) a condition due to pathologically increased activity of the pituitary gland, either of (1) the basophilic cells (**basophilic h.**) which results in basophil adenoma causing compression of the pituitary (see *hypopituitarism*); or (2) of the eosinophilic cells (**eosinophilic h.**) which produces overgrowth, acromegaly and gigantism, or true hyperpituitarism.

hyperplasia (hi″per-pla′ze-ah) [*hyper-* + Gr. *plasis* formation] the abnormal multiplication or increase in the number of normal cells in normal arrangement in a tissue. Cf. *hypertrophy*. **adrenal cortical h.,** hyperplasia of adrenal cortical cells, as in adrenogenital syndrome and Cushing's syndrome. **angiolymphoid h.,** solitary or multiple cutaneous tumors consisting of mature and immature vascular structures intermingled with a copious infiltrate of lymphocytes, histiocytes, eosinophils, and mast cells; lymphoid follicles may occur. **cementum h.,** hypercementosis. **chronic perforating h. of pulp,** internal resorption of a tooth. **congenital adrenal h.,** adrenogenital syndrome. **congenital virilizing adrenal h.,** adrenogenital syndrome. **endometrial h., h. endome′trii,** abnormal overgrowth of the endometrium. **giant follicular h.,** a disorder of the lymph nodes, generally confined to the cervical lymph nodes, which may simulate follicular lymphoma, but cytologically the follicles contain both macrophages and lymphoblasts. **gingival h.,** a general term for gross increase in size of gingival tissues, localized or diffuse, and resulting from a number of conditions. See also *gingival fibromatosis*, under *fibromatosis*. **inflammatory h.,** hyperplasia brought about by inflammation. **juxtaglomerular cell h.,** a syndrome in which hypertrophy and hyperplasia of juxtaglomerular cells produces hypokalemic alkalosis and hyperaldosteronism; it is characterized by absence of hypertension in the presence of markedly increased plasma renin concentrations, and by insensitivity to the pressor effects of angiotensin. It usually affects children and is perhaps hereditary, and may be associated with other anomalies, such as mental retardation and short stature. Called also *Bartter's syndrome*. **lipoid h.,** increased formation of lipoid-containing cells. **neoplastic h.,** hyperplasia brought about by a new growth. **ovarian stromal h.,** thecomatosis. **polar h.,** excessive development at either extremity of the embryo, producing a monster either with two heads or with three or more lower limbs. **pseudoepitheliomatous h.,** a benign, advanced epithelial hypertrophy. **Swiss-cheese h.,** hyperplasia of a tissue which on section shows openings as in Swiss cheese.

hyperplasmia (hi″per-plaz′me-ah) [*hyper-* + *plasma*] 1. excess in the proportion of blood plasm to corpuscles. 2. abnormally large size of erythrocytes through the absorption of plasma.

hyperplastic (hi″per-plas′tik) pertaining to or characterized by hyperplasia.

hyperploid (hi′per-ploid) [*hyper-* + *-ploid*] 1. having more than the typical number of chromosomes in unbalanced sets, as in Down's syndrome. 2. an individual or cell having more than the typical number of chromosomes in unbalanced sets.

hyperploidy (hi′per-ploi′de) the state of being hyperploid. Cf. *aneuploidy*.

hyperpnea (hi″perp-ne′ah) [*hyper-* + Gr. *pnoia* breath] abnormal increase in the depth and rate of the respiratory movements.

hyperpneic (hi″perp-ne′ik) pertaining to or characterized by hyperpnea.

hyperpolarization (hi″per-po″lar-i-za′shun) any increase in the amount of electrical charge separated by the cell membrane and hence in the strength of the transmembrane potential.

hyperpolypeptidemia (hi″per-pol″e-pep″tĭ-de′me-ah) excess of polypeptides in the blood.

hyperponesis (hi″per-po-ne′sis) [*hyper-* + Gr. *ponesis* toil, exertion] dysponesis in which there is excessive action-potential output from the motor and premotor areas of the cortex.

hyperponetic (hi″per-po-net′ik) pertaining to or characterized by hyperponesis.

hyperposia (hi″per-po′ze-ah) [*hyper-* + Gr. *posis* drinking + *-ia*] abnormally increased ingestion of fluids for relatively brief periods. Cf. *polyposia*.

hyperpostpituitary (hi″per-pōst″pĭ-tu′ĭ-ter″e) pertaining to excess of posterior pituitary hormones.

hyperpotassemia (hi″per-pot″ah-se′me-ah) excess of potassium in the blood. See *hyperkalemia*.

hyperpragic (hi″per-praj′ik) characterized by excessive mental activity.

hyperpraxia (hi″per-prak′se-ah) [*hyper-* + Gr. *praxis* exercise] abnormal mental activity.

hyperprebetalipoproteinemia (hi″per-pre-ba″tah-lip″o-pro″te-in-e′me-ah) an excess of prebetalipoproteins (very low-density lipoproteins) in the blood; see *hyperlipoproteinemia*, type IV. Called also *prebetalipoproteinemia*. **familial h.,** familial hyperlipoproteinemia, type IV.

hyperpresbyopia (hi″per-pres″be-o′pe-ah) excessive presbyopia.

hyperproinsulinemia (hi″per-pro-in″su-lin-e′me-ah) elevated levels of proinsulin or proinsulin-like material in the blood.

hyperprolactinemia (hi″per-pro-lak″tin-e′me-ah) increased levels of prolactin in the blood, which, in women, is associated with infertility and may lead to galactorrhea, and, in men, has been reported to cause impotence; often but not invariably associated with microadenoma of the anterior pituitary.

hyperprolactinemic (hi″per-pro-lak′tĭ-ne′mik) pertaining to, characterized by, or affected by hyperprolactinemia.

hyperprolanemia (hi″per-pro″lah-ne′me-ah) an excessive amount of prolan A in the blood.

hyperprolinemia (hi″per-pro″lĭ-ne′me-ah) a disorder of amino acid metabolism characterized by an excess of proline in the body fluids. It occurs in two types, both of which are probably benign. *Type I* is caused by a defect in the oxidation of proline to pyrroline carboxylate. *Type II* involves a defect in the oxidation of pyrroline carboxylate and is characterized by a greater degree of hyperprolinemia and by urinary excretion of pyrroline carboxylate.

hyperprosexia (hi″per-pro-sek′se-ah) [*hyper-* + Gr. *prosechein* to heed] a condition in which the mind is occupied by one idea to the exclusion of others.

hyperproteinemia (hi″per-pro″te-in-e′me-ah) [*hyper-* + *protein* + Gr. *haima* blood + *-ia*] the presence of an abnormally high amount of protein in the blood; see also *hyperlipoproteinemia*.

hyperproteosis (hi″per-pro″te-o′sis) a condition caused by an excess of protein in the diet.

hyperpselaphesia (hi″per-psel″ah-fe′ze-ah) [*hyper-* + Gr. *psēlaphēsis* touch + *-ia*] tactile hyperesthesia.

hyperpsychosis (hi″per-si-ko′sis) [*hyper-* + Gr. *psyche* soul] exaggeration of mental activity with abnormal rapidity of the flow of thought.

hyperptyalism (hi″per-ti′al-izm) [*hyper-* + Gr. *ptyalon* spittle] ptyalism.

hyperpyremia (hi″per-pi-re′me-ah) [*hyper-* + Gr. *pyreia* fuel + *haima* blood + *-ia*] excess of unoxidized carbonaceous matter in the blood.

hyperpyretic (hi″per-pi-ret′ik) pertaining to, exhibiting, or causing hyperpyrexia.

hyperpyrexia (hi″per-pi-rek′se-ah) [*hyper-* + Gr. *pyressein* to be feverish] a highly elevated body temperature. **malignant h.,** see under *hyperthermia*.

hyperpyrexial (hi″per-pi-rek′se-al) pertaining to hyperpyrexia.

hyperreactive (hi″per-re-ak′tiv) pertaining to or characterized by a greater than normal response to stimuli.

hyperreflexia (hi″per-re-flek′se-ah) [*hyper-* + *reflex* + *-ia*] exaggeration of reflexes. **autonomic h.,** paroxysmal hypertension, bradycardia, sweating of the forehead, severe headache, and gooseflesh due to distention of the bladder and rectum; it is associated with lesions above the outflow of the splanchnic nerves.

hyperreninemia (hi″per-re″nin-e′me-ah) a condition of elevated levels of renin in the blood, which may lead to aldosteronism and hypertension.

hyperreninemic (hi″per-re″nin-e′mik) producing or characterized by hyperreninemia.

hyperresonance (hi″per-rez′o-nans) an exaggerated resonance.

hypersalemia (hi″per-sal-e′me-ah) abnormally increased content of salt in the blood.

hypersaline (hi″per-sa′lin) excessively saline: a term applied to treatment by the administration of large doses of sodium chloride.

hypersalivation (hi″per-sal″ĭ-va′shun) ptyalism.

hypersarcosinemia (hi″per-sar″ko-sēn-e′me-ah) an inborn error of metabolism due to a defect of sarcosine dehydrogenase and marked by elevated levels of sarcosine in the blood.

hypersecretion (hi″per-se-kre′shun) excessive secretion. **gastric h.,** hyperchlorhydria.

hypersegmentation (hi″per-seg″men-ta′shun) the appearance of being divided into multiple segments or lobes. **hereditary h. of neutrophils,** a hereditary condition in which the neutrophils are multilobed; called also *Undritz anomaly.*

hypersensibility (hi″per-sen″sĭ-bil′ĭ-te) excessive sensibility or sensitivity to a substance or stimulus.

hypersensitive (hi″per-sen′sĭ-tiv) 1. exhibiting abnormally increased sensitivity. 2. having the specific or general ability to react with characteristic signs and symptoms to the application or contact with certain substances (allergens) in amounts innocuous to normal (nonsensitized) individuals. See *hypersensitivity.*

hypersensitivity (hi″per-sen′sĭ-tiv″ĭ-te) a state of altered reactivity in which the body reacts with an exaggerated response to a foreign agent. Hypersensitivity reactions are pathologic processes induced by immune responses and may be classified as immediate or delayed, or as: *type I,* the immediate hypersensitivity reactions (e.g., anaphylaxis); *type II,* in which injury is produced by antibody against tissue antigens (e.g., nephrotoxic nephritis); *type III,* in which injury is produced by antigen-antibody complex, especially by soluble complexes formed by slight antigen excess (e.g., Arthus reaction and serum sickness); and *type IV,* the delayed hypersensitivity reactions (e.g., contact dermatitis). **contact h.,** a type IV hypersensitive reaction of the skin produced by contact with a chemical substance having the properties of an antigen or hapten; it includes contact dermatitis. **delayed h.,** a slowly developing increase in cell-mediated (T-lymphocyte) immune response to a specific antigen; it is involved in the graft rejection phenomenon, autoimmune disease, and contact dermatitis, as well as in antimicrobial immunity. **immediate h.,** antibody-mediated hypersensitivity characterized by release of mediators (e.g., histamine and eosinophilchemotactic factor) from reagin-sensitized mast cells, causing increased vascular permeability, edema, and smooth muscle contraction. It includes anaphylaxis and atopy. The ability to react in this way can be transferred to another individual by injection of serum.

hypersensitization (hi″per-sen″sĭ-ti-za′shun) the process of rendering or the condition of being abnormally sensitive. See *hypersensitivity* and *anaphylaxis.*

hyperserotonemia (hi″per-se″ro-to-ne′me-ah) an elevation of the serum serotonin level.

hypersialosis (hi″per-si″ah-lo′sis) ptyalism.

hyperskeocytosis (hi″per-ske″o-si-to′sis) [*hyper-* + Gr. *skaios* left + *kytos* hollow vessel + *-osis*] hyperneocytosis.

hypersomatatropism (hi″per-so-mat″ah-trop′izm) increased secretion of growth hormone.

hypersomia (hi″per-so′me-ah) [*hyper-* + Gr. *sōma* body] gigantism.

hypersomnia (hi″per-som′ne-ah) [*hyper-* + L. *somnus* sleep] uncontrollable drowsiness; pathologically excessive sleep.

hypersphyxia (hi″per-sfik′se-ah) [*hyper-* + Gr. *sphyxis* pulse + *-ia*] increased activity of the circulation with increased blood pressure.

hypersplenia (hi″per-sple′ne-ah) hypersplenism.

hypersplenism (hi″per-splen′izm) a condition characterized by exaggeration of the suggested inhibitory or destructive functions of the spleen, resulting in deficiency of the peripheral blood elements, singly or in combination, hypercellularity of the bone marrow, and usually, but not always, splenomegaly.

hyperspongiosis (hi-per-spon″je-o′sis) proliferation of the substantia spongiosa ossium.

Hyperstat (hi′per-stat) trademark for a preparation of diazoxide.

hypersteatosis (hi″per-ste-ah-to′sis) seborrhea.

hyperstereoroentgenography (hi″per-ste″re-o-rent″gen-og′rah-fe) stereoroentgenography with great distance between the homologous points.

hyperstereoskiagraphy (hi″per-ste″re-o-ski-ag′rah-fe) hyperstereoroentgenography.

hypersthenia (hi″per-sthe′ne-ah) [*hyper-* + Gr. *sthenos* strength] great strength or tonicity.

hypersthenic (hi″per-sthen′ik) pertaining to or characterized by hypersthenia.

hypersthenuria (hi″per-sthĕ-nu′re-ah) [*hyper-* + Gr. *sthenos* strength + *ouron* urine + *-ia*] increased osmolality of the urine.

hypersuprarenalemia (hi″per-su″prah-re″nal-e′me-ah) hyperadrenalemia.

hypersuprarenalism (hi″per-su″prah-re′nal-izm) hyperadrenalism.

hypersusceptibility (hi″per-sŭ-sep″tĭ-bil′ĭ-te) a condition of abnormally increased susceptibility to poisons, infective agents, or agents which in the normal individual are entirely innocuous. See also *anaphylaxis.*

hypersympathicotonus (hi″per-sim-path″ĕ-ko-to′nus) an increased tone of the sympathetic nervous system.

hypertarachia (hi″per-tah-rak′e-ah) [*hyper-* + Gr. *tarachē* confusion] extreme irritability of the nervous system.

hypertelorism (hi″per-te″lor-izm) [*hyper-* + Gr. *tēlouros* distant] 1. abnormally increased distance between two organs or parts. 2. ocular h. **ocular h., orbital h.,** a condition characterized by abnormal increase in the interorbital distance, often associated with cleidocranial or craniofacial dysostosis, and occasionally accompanied by mental deficiency.

Hypertensin (hi″per-ten′sin) trademark for a preparation of angiotensin amide.

hypertensinase (hi″per-ten′sin-ās) angiotensinase.

hypertensinogen (hi″per-ten-sin′o-jen) angiotensinogen.

hypertension (hi″per-ten′shun) [*hyper-* + *tension*] persistently high arterial blood pressure. Various criteria for its threshold have been suggested, ranging from 140 mm. Hg systolic and 90 mm. Hg diastolic to as high as 200 mm. Hg systolic and 110 mm. Hg diastolic. Hypertension may have no known cause (*essential* or *idopathic h.*) or be associated with other primary diseases (*secondary h.*); see also *blood pressure,* under *pressure.* **accelerated h.,** progressive hypertension marked by the funduscopic vascular changes of malignant hypertension but without papilledema. **adrenal h.,** hypertension associated with an adrenal tumor that secretes mineral corticosteroids, e.g., hyperaldosteronism. **benign h.,** chronic hypertension of relatively mild degree; it may develop into malignant hypertension. **benign intracranial h.,** pseudotumor cerebri. **borderline h.,** a condition in which the arterial blood pressure is sometimes within the normotensive range and sometimes within the hypertensive range; called also *labile h.* **essential h.,** hypertension occurring without discoverable organic cause; called also *primary h.* and *idiopathic h.* **Goldblatt h.,** see under *kidney.* **idiopathic h.,** essential h. **intracranial h.,** a syndrome of increased intracranial pressure and papilledema with no focal neurologic signs and with normal-sized cerebral ventricles. **labile h.,** borderline h. **low-renin h.,** essential hypertension associated with low levels of plasma-renin concentration or low renin activity. **malignant h.,** a severe hypertensive state with poor prognosis; it is characterized by papilledema of the ocular fundus with vascular exudative and hemorrhagic lesions, medial thickening of small arteries and arterioles, and left ventricular hypertrophy. Diastolic pressures as high as 130 mm. Hg or more are commonly present. **neuromuscular h.,** a condition of hyperexcitability and hyperirritability of reflex response; called also *anxiety tension state.* **ocular h.,** persistently elevated intraocular pressure in the absence of any other signs of glaucoma; it may or may not progress to chronic simple glaucoma. **pale h.,** malignant h. **portal h.,** abnormally increased blood pressure in the portal venous system, a frequent complication of cirrhosis of the liver. **primary h.,** essential h. **pulmonary h.,** increased pressure (above 30 mm. Hg systolic and 12 mm. Hg diastolic) within the pulmonary circulation. **red h.,** benign h. **renal h.,** hypertension due to or associated with renal disease with a factor of parenchymal ischemia. **renovascular h.,** hypertension due to occlusive disease of the renal arteries. **secondary h.,** hypertension due to or associated with a variety of primary diseases, such as renal disorders, disorders of the central nervous system, endocrine diseases, and vascular diseases. **splenoportal h.,** obstruction of the splenic venous system resulting in enlargement of the liver and manifestation of ascites and other evidence of portal cirrhosis. **symptomatic h.,** secondary h. **systemic venous h.,** elevation of systemic venous pressure, usually detected by inspection of the jugular veins. **vascular h.,** hypertension.

hypertensive (hi″per-ten′siv) 1. characterized by or causing increased tension or pressure, as abnormally high blood pressure. 2. a person with abnormally high blood pressure.

hypertensor (hi″per-ten′sor) a pressor agent.

Hyper-Tet (hip′per-tet) trademark for a preparation of tetanus immune human globulin.

hypertetraploid (hi″per-tet″rah-ploid) having more than the tetraploid number of chromosomes in unbalanced sets (4n + x).

hyperthecosis (hi″per-the-ko′sis) hyperplasia with excessive luteinization of the cells of the inner stromal layer, the theca interna, of the ovary; it may be associated with hirsutism and amenorrhea.

hyperthelia (hi″per-the′le-ah) [*hyper-* + Gr. *thēlē* nipple] the presence of supernumerary nipples.

hyperthermal (hi″per-ther′mal) marked by abnormally high temperature.

hyperthermalgesia (hi″per-ther″mal-je′ze-ah) [*hyper-* + Gr. *thermē* heat + *algēsis* pain] abnormally increased sensitivity to heat.

hyperthermesthesia (hi″per-ther″mes-the′ze-ah) [*hyper-* + Gr. *thermē* heat + *aisthēsis* perception + *-ia*] increased sensibility for heat.

hyperthermia (hi″per-ther′me-ah) [*hyper-* + Gr. *thermē* heat + *-ia*] abnormally high body temperature, especially that induced for therapeutic purposes. **h. of anesthesia,** malignant h. **malignant h.,** an autosomal dominantly inherited condition, occurring in patients undergoing general anesthesia, and causing a sudden, rapid rise in body temperature, associated with signs of increased muscle metabolism, such as tachycardia, tachypnea, sweating, and cyanosis, and, usually, muscle rigidity. Called also *h. of anesthesia* and *malignant hyperpyrexia.*

hyperthermoesthesia (hi″per-ther″mo-es-the′ze-ah) hyperthermesthesia.

hyperthermy (hi″per-ther′me) hyperthermia.

hyperthrombinemia (hi″per-throm″bĭ-ne′me-ah) abnormally high thrombin content of the blood.

hyperthymergasia (hi″per-thi″mer-ga′ze-ah) [*hyper-* + Gr. *thymos* spirit + *ergon* work] Meyer's term for overactivity of mood, marked by excitement, agitation, elation, and exaggerated self-feeling.

hyperthymergastic (hi″per-thi″mer-gas′tik) pertaining to or characterized by hyperthymergasia.

hyperthymia (hi″per-thi′me-ah) [*hyper-* + Gr. *thymos* spirit + *-ia*] excessive emotionalism.

hyperthymic (hi″per-thi′mik) marked by hyperthymia.

hyperthymism (hi″per-thi′mizm) a condition attributed to excessive activity of the thymus gland.

hyperthyrea (hi″per-thi′re-ah) hyperthyroidism.

hyperthyreosis (hi″per-thi″re-o′sis) hyperthyroidism.

hyperthyroid (hi″per-thi′roid) marked by or due to hyperthyroidism.

hyperthyroidism (hi″per-thi′roi-dizm) excessive functional activity of the thyroid gland, characterized by increased basal metabolism, goiter, and disturbances in the autonomic nervous system and in creatine metabolism. This term is sometimes used to refer to *Graves' disease.* **masked h.,** hyperactivity of the thyroid gland without the classic symptoms but manifested by symptoms restricted to a single system, as by cardiovascular symptoms.

hyperthyroidosis (hi″per-thi″roi-do′sis) hyperthyroidism.

hyperthyroxinemia (hi″per-thi-rok″sĭ-ne′me-ah) excess of thyroxine in the blood.

hypertonia (hi″per-to′ne-ah) [*hyper-* + Gr. *tonos* tension] a condition of excessive tone of the skeletal muscles; increased resistance of muscle to passive stretching. **h. oc′uli,** high intraocular pressure; see *glaucoma.* **h. polycythae′mica,** increased blood pressure associated with polycythemia.

hypertonic (hi″per-ton′ik) a biological term denoting a solution which when bathing body cells causes a net flow of water across the semipermeable cell membrane out of the cell. Also, denoting a solution having a greater tonicity than another solution, e.g., the blood, with which it is compared.

hypertonicity (hi″per-to-nis′ĭ-te) the state or quality of being hypertonic.

hypertonus (hi″per-to′nus) hypertonia.

hypertoxic (hi″per-tok′sik) excessively toxic.

hypertoxicity (hi″per-tok-sis′ĭ-te) the state or quality of being excessively toxic.

hypertrichosis (hi″per-trik-o′sis) [*hyper-* + Gr. *thrix* hair + *-osis*] excessive growth of hair, especially a localized or generalized excessive growth. Cf. *hirsutism.* **h. pin′nae au′ris,** an abnormally excessive growth of hair on the pinna of the ear, a trait which is thought to be transmitted by a gene on the Y chromosome.

hypertriglyceridemia (hi″per-tri-glis″er-i-de′me-ah) an excess of triglycerides in the blood; an inherited form occurs in familial hyperlipoproteinemia, types IIb and IV.

hypertriploid (hi″per-trip′loid) having more than the triploid number of chromosomes in unbalanced sets (3n + x).

hypertrophia (hi″per-tro′fe-ah) hypertrophy.

hypertrophic (hi″per-trof′ik) pertaining to or marked by hypertrophy.

hypertrophy (hi-per′tro-fe) [*hyper-* + Gr. *trophē* nutrition] the enlargement or overgrowth of an organ or part due to an increase in size of its constituent cells. Cf. *hyperplasia.* **adaptive h.,** increase in size in response to changed conditions, as, for example, increased thickness of the walls of a hollow organ when the outflow is obstructed. **Billroth h.,** idiopathic benign hypertrophy of the pylorus. **compensatory h.,** that which results from an increased workload due to some physical defect, as of the left ventricle of the heart due to hypertension. **complementary h.,** increase in size of the remaining part of an organ to take the place of a portion which has been lost. **concentric h.,** in-

creased thickness of the walls of an organ, with no enlargement and with diminished capacity. **eccentric h.,** hypertrophy of a hollow organ, with dilatation of its cavity. **false h.,** enlargement due to an increase in only one constituent element of an organ or part, more commonly the stroma. **functional h.,** hypertrophy of an organ or part caused by its increased activity. **hemifacial h.,** overgrowth of one side of the face. **Marie's h.,** enlargement of the soft parts of the joints resulting from periostitis. **numeric h.,** that which is due to an increased number of structural elements. **physiologic h.,** temporary increase in the size of an organ produced by physiologic activity, as in the female breast during pregnancy and lactation. **pseudomuscular h.,** pseudohypertrophic muscular dystrophy. **quantitative h.,** hyperplasia. **simple h.,** that which is due to a simple increase of the number of structural elements. **true h.,** enlargement due to an increase of all the component elements of an organ or part. **unilateral h.,** overgrowth of one side of the entire body or of a portion of one side, as of the face. **ventricular h.,** hypertrophy of the myocardium of a ventricle. **vicarious h.,** hypertrophy of an organ in consequence of the failure of another organ of allied function.

hypertropia (hi″per-tro′pe-ah) [*hyper-* + Gr. *trepein* to turn] strabismus in which there is permanent upward deviation of the visual axis of an eye.

Hypertussis (hi″per-tus′sis) trademark for a preparation of pertussis immune human globulin.

hyperuresis (hi″per-u-re′sis) polyuria.

hyperuricacidemia (hi″per-u″rik-as″ĭ-de′me-ah) hyperuricemia.

hyperuricaciduria (hi″per-u″rik-as″ĭ-du′re-ah) hyperuricuria.

hyperuricemia (hi″per-u″rĭ-se′me-ah) excess of uric acid in the blood; it is a prerequisite for the development of gout and may lead to renal disease.

hyperuricemic (hi″per-u″rĭ-se′mik) pertaining to or characterized by hyperuricemia.

hyperuricuria (hi″per-u″rik-u′re-ah) excess of uric acid in the urine.

hypervaccination (hi″per-vak″sĭ-na′shun) the subsequent inoculation (one or more times) of a previously immunized animal with enough vaccine to enable it to afford a serum protective to other animals.

hypervalinemia (hi″per-val″ĭ-ne′me-ah) an inborn error of metabolism, possibly due to a defect in valine transamination, characterized by elevated levels of valine in the plasma and urine and by failure to thrive; it may occur alone or with elevated levels of other amino acids, as in maple syrup urine disease. Called also *valinemia.*

hypervascular (hi″per-vas′ku-lar) extremely vascular.

hypervegetative (hi″per-vej″ĕ-ta′tiv) [*hyper-* + L. *vegetativus* plant-fashion] denoting a constitutional body type in which the visceral, nutritional functions predominate.

hyperventilation (hi″per-ven″tĭ-la′shun) 1. a state in which there is an increased amount of air entering the pulmonary alveoli (increased alveolar ventilation), resulting in reduction of carbon dioxide tension and eventually leading to alkalosis. 2. abnormally prolonged, rapid, and deep breathing, frequently used as a test procedure in epilepsy and tetany.

hyperviscosity (hi″per-vis-kos′ĭ-te) excessive viscosity, as of the blood; see also under *syndrome.*

hypervitaminosis (hi″per-vi″tah-mĭ-no′sis) a condition due to ingestion of an excess of one or more vitamins; called also *supervitaminosis.* **h. A,** a symptom complex resulting from ingestion of excessive amounts of vitamin A, with skin pigmentation, generalized pruritus, changes in the horny structures of the skin, and loss of hair; serum levels of vitamin A usually are elevated to more than 100 mg. per 100 ml. **h. D,** a symptom complex resulting from ingestion of excessive amounts of vitamin D, with weakness, fatigue, loss of weight, and other symptoms.

hypervitaminotic (hi″per-vi″tah-mĭ-not′ik) pertaining to or characterized by hypervitaminosis.

hypervolemia (hi″per-vo-le′me-ah) [*hyper-* + *volume* + Gr. *haima* blood + *-ia*] abnormal increase in the volume of circulating fluid (plasma) in the body.

hypervolemic (hi″per-vo-le′mik) pertaining to or characterized by hypervolemia.

hypervolia (hi″per-vo′le-ah) augmented water content or volume of a given compartment, e.g., as of a cell.

hypesthesia (hip″es-the′ze-ah) hypoesthesia.

hypha (hi′fah), pl. *hy′phae* [L.] one of the filaments or threads composing the mycelium of a fungus.

hyphae (hi′fe) [L.] plural of *hypha.*

hyphal (hi′ful) pertaining to a hypha.

hyphedonia (hip″hĕ-do′ne-ah) [*hypo-* + Gr. *hēdonē* pleasure + *-ia*] morbid diminution of the feeling of pleasure in acts that normally give pleasure.

hyphema (hi-fe′mah) [Gr. *hyphaimos* suffused with blood,

blood-shot; especially of the eyes] hemorrhage within the anterior chamber of the eye. Called also *hyphemia.*

hyphemia (hi-fe′me-ah) [*hypo-* + Gr. *haima* blood + *-ia*] 1. (*obs.*) oligemia. 2. hyphema.

hyphephilia (hif″e-fil′e-ah) [Gr. *hyphē* web + *philein* to love] sexual gratification by contact with fabrics, such as velvet, silk, etc.

hyphidrosis (hīp″hid-ro′sis) [*hypo-* + Gr. *hidrōs* sweat + *-osis*] too scanty perspiration.

Hyphomicrobiaceae (hi‴fo-mi-kro′be-a′se-e) a family of Schizomycetes (order Hyphomicrobiales), made up of cells attached to one another by a slender filament, daughter cells arising from such filaments or from one growing out of the pole of a mature cell. It includes two genera, *Hyphomicrobium* and *Rhodomicrobium.*

Hyphomicrobiales (hi‴fo-mi-kro′be-a′lēz) an order of Schizomycetes, made up of ovoid, ellipsoidal, spherical, or pyriform cells which commonly occur in aggregates but may occur singly or in pairs, and which multiply by budding or by budding and longitudinal fission. It includes two families, Hyphomicrobiaceae and Pasteuriaceae.

Hyphomicrobium (hi‴fo-mi-kro′be-um) a genus of microorganisms of the family Hyphomicrobiaceae, order Hyphomicrobiales, made up of ovoid cells growing in a dense clump from which filaments radiate outward. The type species is *H. vulga′re.*

Hyphomyces (hi-fo-mi′sēz) a genus of phycomycetous fungi the members of which do not sporulate; they appear to be related to the genus *Mortierella* (order Mucorales, family Mucoraceae). **H. des′truens,** the etiologic agent of hyphomycosis destruens equi.

hyphomycete (hi‴fo-mi-sēt) any individual organism of the Hyphomycetes, an imperfect mold in contrast to an imperfect yeast.

Hyphomycetes (hi‴fo-mi-se′tēz) [pl., Gr. *hyphē* web + Gr. *mykēs* fungus] the mycelial (hyphal) fungi, i.e., molds, of the Fungi Imperfecti (Deuteromycetes).

hyphomycetic (hi‴fo-mi-set′ik) (*obs.*) due to the presence of mold, or mycelial, fungi.

hyphomycetoma (hi‴fo-mi‴se-to′mah) (*obs.*) a tumor caused by hyphomycetes (imperfect fungi).

hyphomycosis (hi‴fo-mi-ko′sis) 1. infection with fungi of the genus *Hyphomyces.* 2. (*obs.*) infection with hyphomycetes (imperfect fungi). **h. des′truens e′qui,** a disease of horses and mules in India, Indonesia, Europe, and southern United States, caused by *Hyphomyces destruens;* it is marked by the formation of subcutaneous abscesses that enlarge until the skin over and around the lesions is destroyed, leaving large raw surfaces. Because of the clinical similarity between hyphomycosis destruens equi and cutaneous habronemiasis, the disorders are often confused.

hyphylline (hi-fil′in) dyphylline.

hypisotonic (hīp″i-so-ton′ik) less than isotonic.

hypnagogic (hip″nah-goj′ik) 1. producing sleep. 2. occurring just before sleep; said of dreams.

hypnagogue (hip′nah-gog) [*hypno-* + Gr. *agōgos* leading] 1. hypnotic; pertaining to drowsiness. 2. an agent that induces sleep or drowsiness.

hypnalgia (hip-nal′je-ah) [*hypno-* + Gr. *algos* pain + *-ia*] pain that occurs during sleep.

hypnesthesia (hip″nes-the′ze-ah) [*hypno-* + Gr. *aisthēsis* perception + *-ia*] (*obs.*) sleepiness.

hypnic (hip′nik) [Gr. *hypnikos*] inducing or pertaining to sleep.

hypno- [Gr. *hypnos* sleep] a combining form denoting relationship to sleep.

hypnoanalysis (hip″no-ah-nal′ĭ-sis) [*hypno-* + *analysis*] a method of psychotherapy in which psychoanalysis is employed in conjunction with hypnosis.

hypnoanesthesia (hip″no-an″es-the′ze-ah) induction of the anesthetic state by hypnosis.

hypnobatia (hip″no-ba′she-ah) [*hypno-* + Gr. *bainein* to walk] (*obs.*) somnambulism; def. 1.

hypnocinematograph (hip″no-sin″ĕ-mat′o-graf) [*hypno-* + Gr. *kinēma* movement + *graphein* to record] an apparatus for recording the movements made by a sleeping person.

hypnocyst (hip′no-sist) [*hypno-* + *cyst*] a quiescent cyst.

hypnodontia (hip″no-don′she-ah) hypnodontics.

hypnodontics (hip″no-don′tiks) [*hypnosis* + Gr. *odous* tooth] the application of controlled suggestion and hypnosis in the practice of dentistry.

hypnogenetic (hip″no-jĕ-net′ik) hypnogenic.

hypnogenic (hip″no-jen′ik) [*hypno-* + Gr. *gennan* to produce] inducing sleep or a hypnotic state.

hypnogenous (hip-noj′ĕ-nus) hypnogenic.

hypnoid (hip′noid) resembling hypnosis or the hypnotic state.

hypnoidal (hip-noi′dal) pertaining to a state resembling hypnosis.

hypnoidization (hip″noi-di-za′shun) the production of light hypnosis or of the hypnoid state.

hypnolepsy (hip′no-lep″se) [*hypno-* + Gr. *lēpsis* seizure] narcolepsy.

hypnology (hip-nol′o-je) [*hypno-* + *-logy*] the sum of what is known regarding sleep and hypnotism.

hypnonarcoanalysis (hip″no-nar″ko-ah-nal′ĭ-sis) psychoanalysis with the patient hypnotized and narcotized with a sedative drug.

hypnonarcosis (hip″no-nar-ko′sis) light hypnosis combined with narcosis.

hypnopedia (hip″no-pe′de-ah) [*hypno-* + *paideia* education] sleep learning; learning during sleep, as by listening to recordings.

hypnopompic (hip″no-pom′pik) [*hypno-* + Gr. *pompē* a sending away, a sending home] persisting after sleep; applied to visions or dreams that persist prior to complete awakening.

hypnosia (hip-no′ze-ah) uncontrollable drowsiness.

hypnosis (hip-no′sis) an artificially induced passive state in which there is increased amenability and responsiveness to suggestions and commands, provided that these do not conflict seriously with the subject's own conscious or unconscious wishes.

hypnosophy (hip-nos′o-fe) [*hypno-* + Gr. *sophia* wisdom] the study of sleep and its phenomena.

hypnotherapy (hip″no-ther′ah-pe) [*hypno-* + Gr. *therapeia* treatment] the use of hypnosis in the treatment of disease.

hypnotic (hip-not′ik) [Gr. *hypnōtikos*] 1. inducing sleep. 2. pertaining to or of the nature of hypnotism. 3. a drug that acts to induce sleep.

hypnotism (hip′no-tizm) 1. the method or practice of inducing hypnosis. 2. hypnosis.

hypnotist (hip′no-tist) one who induces hypnosis.

hypnotization (hip″no-ti-za′shun) the induction of hypnosis.

hypnotize (hip′no-tiz) to put into a state of hypnosis.

hypnotoxin (hip″no-tok′sin) 1. a toxin that is supposed to accumulate during the waking hours, until finally it is sufficient to inhibit the activity of the cortical cells and thus induce sleep. 2. a toxic substance derived from the tentacles of *Physalia,* the Portuguese man-of-war, characteristically causing a central nervous system depression, affecting both motor and sensory elements.

hypo (hi′po) 1. a popular designation for a hypodermic inoculation or syringe. 2. a contraction for sodium thiosulfate, used as a photographic fixing agent.

hypo- [Gr. *hypo* under] a prefix signifying beneath, under, or deficient. In chemistry, it denotes that the principal element in the compound is combined in its lowest state of valence.

hypoacidity (hi″po-ah-sid′ĭ-te) deficiency of acid; lack of normal acidity.

hypoactive (hi″po-ak′tiv) pertaining to or characterized by hypoactivity.

hypoactivity (hi″po-ak-tiv′ĭ-te) abnormally diminished activity, as of peristalsis.

hypoacusis (hi″po-ah-ku′sis) [*hypo-* + Gr. *akousis* hearing] slightly diminished auditory sensitivity, with hearing threshold levels above the normal limit so that the impairment is measureable in decibels.

hypoadenia (hi″po-ah-de′ne-ah) [*hypo-* + Gr. *adēn* gland + *-ia*] abnormally diminished glandular activity.

hypoadrenalemia (hi″po-ah-dre′nal-e′me-ah) the presence of an abnormally decreased amount of adrenal secretion in the blood.

hypoadrenalism (hi″po-ah-dre′nal-izm) abnormally diminished activity of the adrenal gland, as in Addison's disease.

hypoadrenia (hi″po-ah-dre′ne-ah) hypoadrenalism.

hypoadrenocorticism (hi″po-ah-dre″no-kor′tĭ-sizm) abnormally diminished secretion of the adrenal cortex; see *Addison's disease.*

hypoaffective (hi″po-af-fek′tiv) pertaining to or characterized by hypoaffectivity.

hypoaffectivity (hi″po-af″fek-tiv′ĭ-te) abnormally diminished sensibility to superficial stimuli; the quality of abnormally decreased emotional reactivity.

hypoalbuminemia (hi″po-al-bu′mĭn-e′me-ah) an abnormally low albumin content of the blood.

hypoalbuminosis (hi″po-al-bu″mĭ-no′sis) a condition characterized by an abnormally low level of albumin.

hypoaldosteronemia (hi″po-al″do-stēr′o-ne′me-ah) an abnormally low level of aldosterone in the blood.

hypoaldosteronism (hi″po-al″do-stēr′ōn-izm) a deficiency of aldosterone in the body, usually associated with hypoadrenalism, and characterized by hypotension and a tendency to excrete excessive salt. **isolated h.,** a rare endocrine disorder characterized by reduced or absent aldosterone production, with normal production of all other adrenal steroids.

hypoaldosteronuria (hi″po-al″do-stēr″o-nu′re-ah) presence of an abnormally low level of aldosterone in the urine.

hypoalgesia (hi″po-al-je′se-ah) hypalgesia.

hypoalimentation (hi″po-al″ĭ-men-ta′shun) insufficient nourishment.

hypoalkaline (hi″po-al′kah-lin) less alkaline than normal.

hypoalkalinity (hi″po-al″kah-lin′ĭ-te) the state of being less alkaline than normal.

hypoalonemia (hi″po-al′o-ne′me-ah) [hypo- + Gr. hals salt + haima blood + -ia] a deficiency of salts in the blood.

hypoaminoacidemia (hi″po-am″ĭ-no-as″ĭ-de′me-ah) the presence of less than the normal amount of amino acids in the blood.

hypoandrogenism (hi″po-an-dro′jen-izm) deficiency of androgen.

hypoazoturia (hi″po-az″o-tu′re-ah) [hypo- + L. azotum nitrogen + Gr. ouron urine + -ia] diminished excretion of nitrogenous material in the urine.

hypobaric (hi″po-bār′ik) [hypo- + Gr. baros weight] characterized by less than normal pressure or weight; applied to gases under less than atmospheric pressure or to a solution of lower specific gravity than another taken as a standard of reference. See under solution.

hypobarism (hi″po-bar′izm) the condition resulting from exposure to ambient gas pressure or atmospheric pressures that are below those within body tissues, fluids, cavities.

hypobaropathy (hi″po-bār-op′ah-the) [hypo- + Gr. baros pressure + pathos disease] the disturbances experienced in high altitudes due to reduced air pressure; see high-altitude sickness and mountain sickness, under sickness.

hypobasophilism (hi″po-ba-sof′ĭ-lizm) hypopituitarism.

hypobetalipoproteinemia (hi″po-ba″tah-lip″o-pro″te-in-e′me-ah) the presence of abnormally low levels of β-lipoprotein in the serum, as in debilitating diseases and malabsorption syndromes.

hypobilirubinemia (hi″po-bil″ĭ-ru″bĭ-ne′me-ah) abnormal diminution of bilirubin in the blood.

hypoblast (hi′po-blast) [hypo- + Gr. blastos germ] entoderm.

hypoblastic (hi″po-blas′tik) entodermic.

hypobranchial (hi″po-brang′ke-al) [hypo- + Gr. branchia gills] located beneath the branchial arches.

hypobromite (hi″po-bro′mīt) any salt of hypobromous acid.

hypobulia (hi″po-bu′le-ah) [hypo- + Gr. boulē will + -ia] (obs.) abnormal feebleness of the will.

hypocalcemia (hi″po-kal-se′me-ah) [hypo- + calcium + Gr. haima blood + -ia] reduction of the blood calcium below normal; manifestations include hyperactive deep tendon reflexes, Chvostek's sign, muscle and abdominal cramps, and carpopedal spasm.

hypocalcia (hi″po-kal′se-ah) deficiency of calcium.

hypocalcification (hi″po-kal″sĭ-fĭ-ka′shun) diminished calcification. **enamel h.,** a dental defect in which the enamel is soft and undercalcified, although normal in quantity and histological features. See also amelogenesis imperfecta.

hypocalcipectic (hi″po-kal″sĭ-pek′tik) pertaining to or characterized by hypocalcipexy.

hypocalcipexy (hi″po-kal′sĭ-pek″se) deficient calcium fixation.

hypocalciuria (hi″po-kal″se-u′re-ah) an abnormally diminished amount of calcium in the urine.

hypocapnia (hi″po-kap′ne-ah) [hypo- + Gr. kapnos smoke + -ia] deficiency of carbon dioxide in the blood, resulting from hyperventilation and eventually leading to alkalosis.

hypocapnic (hi″po-kap′nik) pertaining to or characterized by hypocapnia.

hypocarbia (hi″po-kar′be-ah) hypocapnia.

hypocellular (hi″po-sel′u-lar) pertaining to or characterized by hypocellularity.

hypocellularity (hi″po-sel″u-lār′ĭ-te) a state of abnormal decrease in the number of cells present, as in bone marrow.

hypocelom (hi″po-se′lom) hypocoelom.

hypocenesthesia (hi″po-sen″es-the′ze-ah) [hypo- + cenesthesia] (obs.) lack of the normal sense of well being, as seen in hypochondria.

hypocenter (hi″po-sen′ter) the spot immediately beneath the exact site of explosion of an atomic bomb.

hypochloremia (hi″po-klo-re′me-ah) an abnormally diminished level of chloride in the blood.

hypochloremic (hi″po-klo-re′mik) pertaining to or characterized by hypochloremia.

hypochlorhydria (hi″po-klor-hi′dre-ah) [hypo- + Gr. chlōros green + hydōr water + -ia] deficiency of hydrochloric acid in the gastric juice. Cf. achlorhydria.

hypochloridation (hi″po-klo″rĭ-da′shun) chloride deficiency in the system.

hypochloridemia (hi″po-klo″rid-e′me-ah) hypochloremia.

hypochlorite (hi″po-klo′rīt) [hypo- + Gr. chlōros green] any salt of hypochlorous acid; used as a medicinal agent, particularly as a diluted solution of sodium hypochlorite. See sodium hypochlorite solution, diluted, under solution.

hypochlorization (hi″po-klo″ri-za′shun) reduction of the amount of sodium chloride in the diet.

hypochloruria (hi″po-klo-ru′re-ah) [hypo- + chloride + Gr. ouron urine + -ia] deficiency of chlorides in the urine.

hypocholesteremia (hi″po-ko-les″tĕ-re′me-ah) hypocholesterolemia.

hypocholesteremic (hi″po-ko-les″tĕ-re′mik) hypocholesterolemic.

hypocholesterinemia (hi″po-ko-les″ter-ĭ-ne′me-ah) hypocholesterolemia.

hypocholesterolemia (hi″po-ko-les″ter-o-le′me-ah) an abnormally diminished amount of cholesterol in the blood.

hypocholesterolemic (hi″po-ko-les″ter-o-le′mik) pertaining to, characterized by, or producing hypocholesterolemia.

hypocholia (hi-po-ko′le-ah) oligocholia.

hypocholuria (hi″po-ko-lu′re-ah) abnormal reduction in the amount of bile in the urine.

hypochondria (hi″po-kon′dre-ah) 1. plural of hypochondrium. 2. hypochondriasis.

hypochondriac (hi″po-kon′dre-ak) 1. pertaining to the hypochondrium or to hypochondriasis. 2. a person affected with hypochondriasis.

hypochondriacal (hi″po-kon-dri′ah-kal) affected with hypochondriasis.

hypochondriasis (hi″po-kon-dri′ah-sis) [so called because the hypochondrium, and especially the spleen, was supposed to be the seat of this disorder] morbid anxiety about one's health, often associated with numerous and varying symptoms which cannot be attributed to organic disease; called also hypochondria.

hypochondrium (hi″po-kon′dre-um), pl. hypochon′dria [hypo- + Gr. chondros cartilage] regio hypochondriaca [dextra et sinistra].

hypochordal (hi″po-kor′dal) situated ventral to the notochord.

hypochromasia (hi″po-kro-ma′ze-ah) [hypo- + Gr. chrōma color] 1. the condition of staining less intensely than normal. 2. decrease of hemoglobin in the erythrocytes so that they are abnormally pale in color.

hypochromatic (hi″po-kro-mat′ik) containing an abnormally small number of chromosomes; marked by hypochromatism.

hypochromatism (hi″po-kro′mah-tizm) [hypo- + chromatin] abnormally deficient pigmentation, especially deficiency of the chromatin in a cell nucleus.

hypochromatosis (hi″po-kro″mah-to′sis) the gradual fading and disappearance of the nucleus (the chromatin) of a cell.

hypochromemia (hi″po-kro-me′me-ah) [hypo- + Gr. chrōma color + haima blood + -ia] a condition in which the blood has an abnormally low color index. **idiopathic h.,** idiopathic hypochromic anemia.

hypochromia (hi″po-kro′me-ah) [hypo- + Gr. chrōma color + -ia] 1. abnormal decrease in the hemoglobin content of the erythrocytes. 2. hypochromatism.

hypochromic (hi″po-kro′mik) pertaining to or marked by hypochromia.

hypochromotrichia (hi″po-kro″mo-trik′e-ah) abnormally reduced pigmentation of the hair.

hypochrosis (hi″po-kro′sis) [hypo- + Gr. chrōma color + -osis] anemia in which there is an abnormally small amount of hemoglobin in the blood.

hypochylia (hi″po-ki′le-ah) [hypo- + Gr. chylos chyle + -ia] deficiency of chyle.

hypocinesia (hi″po-si-ne′ze-ah) hypokinesia.

hypocinesis (hi″po-si-ne′sis) hypokinesia.

hypocist (hi′po-sist) hypocistis.

hypocistis (hi″po-sis′tis) the juice and extract of various species of the parasitic herb Cytinus, as of C. hypocistis of southern Europe: astringent.

hypocitremia (hi″po-sĭ-tre′me-ah) [hypo- + citric acid + Gr. haima blood + -ia] abnormally low content of citric acid in the blood.

hypocitruria (hi″po-sĭ-troo′re-ah) [hypo- + citric acid + Gr. ouron urine + -ia] excretion of urine containing an abnormally small amount of citric acid.

hypocoagulability (hi″po-ko-ag′u-lah-bil′ĭ-te) the state of being less readily coagulated than normal.

hypocoagulable (hi″po-ko-ag′u-lah-bl) characterized by abnormally decreased coagulability.

hypocoelom (hi″po-se′lom) [hypo- + Gr. koilōma hollow] the ventral portion of the coelom of any embryonic vertebrate.

hypocolasia (hi″po-ko-la′ze-ah) hypokolasia.

hypocomplementemia (hi″po-kom″plĕ-men-te′me-ah) diminution of complement levels in the blood.

hypocomplementemic (hi″po-kom″plĕ-men-te′mik) denoting or involving lowered levels of complement in the blood.

hypocondylar (hi″po-kon′dĭ-lar) below a condyle.

hypocone (hi′po-kōn) [*hypo-* + Gr. *kōnos* cone] the distolingual cusp of an upper molar tooth.

hypoconid (hi″po-ko′nid) the distobuccal cusp of a lower molar tooth.

hypoconulid (hi″po-kon′u-lid) the distal, or fifth, cusp of a lower molar tooth; usually found on the mandibular first molar.

hypocorticalism (hi″po-kor′tĭ-kal-izm) hypoadrenocorticism.

hypocorticism (hi″po-kor′tĭ-sizm) hypoadrenocorticism.

hypocotyl (hi″po-kot′il) [*hypo-* + *kotyle* hollow] the part of the axis of a plant embryo or seedling below the point of attachment of the cotyledon and from which the radicle, or primary root, grows.

Hypocreales (hi″po-kre-a′les) a family of ascomycetous fungi.

hypocrine (hi′po-krin) due to endocrine hypofunction.

hypocrinia (hi″po-krin′e-ah) hypocrinism.

hypocrinism (hi″po-kri′nism) [*hypo-* + Gr. *krinein* to secrete] a bodily state due to deficient secretion of any endocrine gland.

hypocupremia (hi″po-ku-pre′me-ah) an abnormally diminished concentration of copper in the blood.

hypocyclosis (hi″po-si-klo′sis) [*hypo-* + Gr. *kyklos* circle + *-osis*] insufficiency of accommodation due either to undue rigidity of the crystalline lens (*lenticular h.*) or to weakness of the ciliary muscle (*ciliary h.*).

hypocystotomy (hi″po-sis-tot′o-me) [*hypo-* + *cystotomy*] the surgical opening of the urinary bladder through the perineum.

hypocythemia (hi″po-si-the′me-ah) [*hypo-* + Gr. *kytos* cell + *haima* blood + *-ia*] deficiency in the number of erythrocytes in the blood.

hypocytosis (hi″po-si-to′sis) [*hypo-* + *-cyte* + *-osis*] defect or scantiness of corpuscles in the blood.

hypodactyly (hi″po-dak′tĭ-le) the presence of less than the normal number of fingers or toes.

hypoderm (hi′po-derm) [*hypo-* + Gr. *derma* skin] a vague expression used loosely to mean either the panniculus adiposus or the region where the panniculus and the dermis intermingle.

Hypoderma (hi″po-der′mah) [*hypo-* + Gr. *derma* skin] a genus of ox-warble flies or heel flies of the family Oestridae whose larvae cause a creeping eruption in man and cattle. **H. bo′vis,** a species whose larvae infest cattle, seriously damaging the hide and interfering with the nutrition of the animal; it sometimes causes a creeping eruption in man. **H. linea′tum,** an ox-warble fly of cattle in the United States.

hypodermatic (hi″po-der-mat′ik) hypodermic.

hypodermatoclysis (hi″po-der-mah-tok′lĭ-sis) hypodermoclysis.

hypodermatomy (hi″po-der-mat′o-me) [*hypo-* + Gr. *derma* skin + *temnein* to cut] incision of the subcutaneous tissue.

hypodermiasis (hi″po-der-mi′ah-sis) infection by *Hypoderma;* see *larva migrans.*

hypodermic (hi″po-der′mik) [*hypo-* + Gr. *derma* skin] applied or administered beneath the skin.

hypodermis (hi″po-der′mis) [*hypo-* + Gr. *derma* skin] 1. tela subcutanea. 2. the outer cellular layer of the body of invertebrates which secretes the cuticular exoskeleton.

hypodermoclysis (hi″po-der-mok′lĭ-sis) [*hypo-* + Gr. *derma* skin + *klyzein* to wash out] introduction into the subcutaneous tissues of fluids, especially physiologic sodium chloride solution, to replace inadequate intake or loss of water and salt during illness or operation.

hypodermolithiasis (hi″po-der′mo-lĭ-thi′ah-sis) [*hypo-* + Gr. *derma* skin + *lithos* stone + *-iasis*] the formation or presence of subcutaneous calcareous nodes.

hypodiaphragmatic (hi″po-di′ah-frag-mat′ik) below the diaphragm.

hypodiploid (hi′po-dip″loid) 1. pertaining to or characterized by hypodiploidy. 2. an individual or cell with less than the diploid number of chromosomes.

hypodiploidy (hi′po-dip″loi-de) the state of having less than the diploid number of chromosomes (< 2n).

hypodipsia (hi″po-dip′se-ah) [*hypo-* + Gr. *dipsa* thirst + *-ia*] abnormally diminished thirst. See *subliminal thirst,* under *thirst.*

hypodontia (hi″po-don′she-ah) partial anodontia.

hypodynamia (hi″po-di-na′me-ah) [*hypo-* + Gr. *dynamis* force] diminished power. **h. cor′dis,** diminished cardiac power.

hypodynamic (hi″po-di-nam′ik) pertaining to poor ventricular contractility.

hypoeccrisia (hi″po-ek-kris′e-ah) [*hypo-* + Gr. *ekkrisis* excretion + *-ia*] a state characterized by abnormally diminished excretion.

hypoeccrisis (hi″po-ek′krĭ-sis) hypoeccrisia.

hypoeccritic (hi″po-ek-krit′ik) pertaining to or characterized by hypoeccrisia.

hypoechoic (hi″po-ĕ-ko′ik) in ultrasonography, giving off few echoes; said of tissues or structures that reflect relatively few of the ultrasound waves directed at them.

hypoelectrolytemia (hi″po-e-lek″tro-lī-te′me-ah) abnormally decreased electrolyte content of the blood.

hypoemotivity (hi″po-e″mo-tiv′ĭ-te) hypoaffectivity.

hypoendocrinia (hi″po-en″do-krin′e-ah) hypoendocrinism.

hypoendocrinism (hi″po-en-dok′rĭ-nizm) [*hypo-* + Gr. *endon* within + *krinein* to secrete] abnormally decreased activity of an endocrine gland.

hypoendocrisia (hi″po-en″do-kris′e-ah) hypoendocrinism.

hypoeosinophilia (hi″po-e″o-sin″o-fil′e-ah) eosinopenia.

hypoepinephrinemia (hi″po-ep″ĭ-nef″rĭ-ne′me-ah) an abnormally low level of epinephrine in the blood.

hypoequilibrium (hi″po-e″kwĭ-lib′re-um) unusual freedom from tendency to vertigo.

hypoergasia (hi″po-er-ga′se-ah) [*hypo-* + Gr. *ergon* work] abnormally decreased functional activity.

hypoergia (hi″po-er′je-ah) 1. hypoergasia. 2. hyposensitivity to allergens.

hypoergic (hi″po-er′jik) 1. less energetic than normal. 2. pertaining to or characterized by hypoergy.

hypoergy (hi″po-er′je) abnormally diminished reactivity.

hypoesophoria (hi″po-es″o-fo′re-ah) a tendency of the visual axis to deviate downward and medially when fusion is prevented.

hypoesthesia (hi″po-es-the′ze-ah) [*hypo-* + Gr. *aisthēsis* sensation + *-ia*] abnormally decreased sensitivity to stimulation. **acoustic h., auditory h.,** hypoacusis. **gustatory h.,** hypogeusesthesia. **olfactory h.,** hyposmia. **tactile h.,** hypopselaphesia.

hypoesthetic (hi″po-es-thet′ik) pertaining to or characterized by hypoesthesia.

hypoestrinemia (hi″po-es″trĭ-ne′me-ah) hypoestrogenemia.

hypoestrogenemia (hi″po-es″tro-jĕ-ne′me-ah) an abnormally diminished amount of estrogen in the blood, as in the menopause.

hypoevolutism (hi″po-e-vol′u-tizm) a condition characterized by abnormally retarded development.

hypoexophoria (hi″po-ek″so-fo′re-ah) a tendency of the visual axis to deviate downward and laterally when fusion is prevented.

hypoferremia (hi″po-fĕ-re′me-ah) deficiency of iron in the blood.

hypoferrism (hi″po-fer′izm) [*hypo-* + L. *ferrum* iron] deficiency of iron in the system.

hypofertile (hi″po-fer′til) having a diminished reproductive capacity.

hypofertility (hi″po-fer-til′ĭ-te) diminished reproductive capacity.

hypofibrinogenemia (hi″po-fi-brin″o-jĕ-ne′me-ah) abnormally low fibrinogen content of the blood.

hypofunction (hi″po-funk′shun) diminished function.

hypogalactia (hi″po-gah-lak′she-ah) deficiency of milk secretion.

hypogalactous (hi″po-gah-lak′tus) [*hypo-* + Gr. *gala* milk] producing a deficient secretion of milk.

hypogammaglobulinemia (hi″po-gam″ah-glob″u-lĭ-ne′me-ah) an immunological deficiency state characterized by an abnormally low level of generally all classes of gamma globulin in the blood. A physiologic temporary form occurs in normal infants at about three months of age. When prolonged to 18 months of age or more, it is called *transient hypogammaglobulinemia.* See also *agammaglobulinemia.* **acquired h.,** that which becomes manifest after early childhood. *Primary acquired h.* is an immunoglobulin deficiency state, without thymus abnormalities, that affects adults of either sex between the ages of 30 and 50 years. All classes of immunoglobulins are lacking, with overall levels of approximately 10–200 mg./100 ml. *Secondary acquired h.* is a form, without thymus abnormalities, in which there occurs profound diminution in normal immunoglobulin production, resulting in complications attributable to antibody deficiency. **common variable i.,** see under *immunodeficiency.* **congenital h.,** a genetic immunodeficiency state without thymus involvement, which occurs as an X-linked recessive (Bruton type), as an autosomal recessive, and as a sporadic form. It is usually recognized at 4 to 6 months of age, when maternal immunoglobulin has virtually disappeared from the circulation. All classes of immunoglobulin are lacking, with overall levels lying below 50 mg./100 ml. Delayed sensitivity responsiveness is usually unimpaired. There is an extraordinary susceptibility to infection with encapsulated pyogenic organisms (pneumococcus, hemophilus, streptococcus, etc.). **physiologic h.,** a temporary form seen in the normal infant at about three months of age; when the condition is prolonged it is called *transient h.* **primary h., secondary h.,** see *acquired h.* **transient h.,** see *physiologic h.*

hypoganglionosis (hi″po-gang″gle-o-no′sis) deficiency in the number of myenteric ganglion cells in the distal segment of the large bowel, resulting in constipation; it is a variant of congenital megacolon.

hypogastric (hi″po-gas′trik) [L. *hypogastricus*] 1. situated below the stomach. 2. pertaining to the hypogastrium. 3. pertaining to the internal iliac artery.

hypogastrium (hi″po-gas′tre-um) [*hypo-* + Gr. *gastēr* stomach] regio pubica.

hypogastropagus (hi″po-gas-trop′ah-gus) [*hypo* + Gr. *gastēr* belly + *pagos* thing fixed] conjoined twins united at the hypogastric region.

hypogastroschisis (hi″po-gas-tros′kĭ-sis) [*hypo-* + Gr. *gastēr* belly + *schisis* cleft] a developmental anomaly in which an abdominal fissure is restricted to the hypogastric region.

hypogenesis (hi″po-jen′ĕ-sis) [*hypo-* + Gr. *genesis* production] defective embryonic growth or development. **polar h.,** defective development at either extremity of the embryo, resulting in deformity.

hypogenetic (hi″po-jĕ-net′ik) pertaining to or characterized by hypogenesis.

hypogenitalism (hi″po-jen′ĭ-tal-izm″) hypogonadism.

hypogeusesthesia (hi″po-gūs″es-the′ze-ah) [*hypo-* + Gr. *geusis* taste + *aisthēsis* perception + *-ia*] abnormally diminished acuteness of the sense of taste.

hypogeusia (hi″po-gu′ze-ah) hypogeusesthesia.

hypoglandular (hi″po-glan′du-lar) marked by abnormally decreased glandular activity.

hypoglossal (hi″po-glos′al) [*hypo-* + Gr. *glōssa* tongue] situated under the tongue.

hypoglottis (hi″po-glot′is) [*hypo-* + Gr. *glōssa* tongue] 1. the under side or part of the tongue. 2. ranula.

hypoglucagonemia (hi″po-gloo″kah-gon-e′me-ah) abnormally reduced levels of glucagon in the blood.

hypoglycemia (hi″po-gli-se′me-ah) [*hypo-* + Gr. *glykys* sweet + *haima* blood + *-ia*] an abnormally diminished content of glucose in the blood, which may lead to tremulousness, cold sweat, piloerection, hypothermia, and headache, accompanied by confusion, hallucinations, bizarre behavior, and ultimately, convulsions and coma. **factitial h., factitious h.,** apparently spontaneous hypoglycemia in a diabetic, which is in fact caused by the surreptitious injection of insulin. **fasting h.,** hypoglycemia occurring in the fasting state, i.e., after the glucose contents of the intestine have been absorbed; it occurs in such conditions as in insulinoma, glycogen storage disease, starvation, malabsorption, hypopituitarism, and adrenocortical insufficiency. **leucine-induced h.,** familial infantile hypoglycemia induced by ingestion of leucine, which causes an exaggerated release of insulin in susceptible persons; it is transmitted as an autosomal recessive trait. **mixed h.,** hypoglycemia occurring during the fasting state, and following the ingestion of carbohydrate; it occurs in hypoglycemia of infancy, anterior pituitary and adrenocortical insufficiency, and tumors of the islet cells of the pancreas. **reactive h.,** hypoglycemia occurring after the ingestion of carbohydrate, with an excessive release of insulin.

hypoglycemic (hi″po-gli-se′mik) 1. pertaining to, characterized by, or producing hypoglycemia. 2. an agent that acts to lower the level of glucose in the blood.

hypoglycemosis (hi″po-gli″sĕ-mo′sis) an abnormally diminished content of glucose in the blood and tissues; see *hypoglycemia.*

hypoglycin, hypoglycine (hi″po-gli′sin; hi″po-gli′sēn) a hypoglycemic principle occurring in two forms (A and B), from the fruit and seed of the akee tree; it inhibits hepatic gluconeogenesis.

hypoglycogenolysis (hi″po-gli″ko-jen-ol′ĭ-sis) depressed glycogenolysis.

hypoglycorrhachia (hi″po-gli″ko-ra′ke-ah) [*hypo-* + Gr. *glykys* sweet + *rhachis* spine + *-ia*] less than the normal content of glucose in the cerebrospinal fluid; usually indicative of meningeal infection.

hypognathous (hi-pog′nah-thus) 1. having a protruding lower jaw. 2. of the nature of a hypognathus.

hypognathus (hi-pog′nah-thus) [*hypo-* + Gr. *gnathos* jaw] a parasitic monster attached to the lower jaw of the autosite.

hypogonadia (hi″po-go-nad′e-ah) hypogonadism.

hypogonadism (hi″po-go′nad-izm) a condition resulting from or characterized by abnormally decreased functional activity of the gonads, with retardation of growth and sexual development. **hypogonadotropic h.,** that due to failure to secrete gonadotropins. **primary h.,** that due to defective development or function of the gonads. **secondary h.,** hypogonadotropic h.

hypogonadotropic (hi″po-gon″ah-do-trop′ik) relating to or caused by deficiency of gonadotropin.

hypogranulocytosis (hi″po-gran″u-lo-si-to′sis) reduction in the number of granular leukocytes in the blood. Cf. *agranulocytosis.*

hypohepatia (hi″po-he-pat′e-ah) [*hypo-* + Gr. *hēpar* liver] deficient functioning of the liver.

hypohidrosis (hi″po-hi-dro′sis) [*hypo-* + Gr. *hidrōsis* sweating] abnormally diminished perspiration.

hypohidrotic (hi″po-hĭ-drot′ik) pertaining to, characterized by, or causing hypohidrosis.

hypohormonal (hi″po-hōr′mo-nal) deficient in hormone; due to hormone deficiency.

hypohormonic (hi″po-hōr-mon′ik) hypohormonal.

hypohormonism (hi-po-hor′mōn-izm) endocrine hypofunction.

hypohydration (hi″po-hi-dra′shun) a state of decreased water content of the body; dehydration.

hypohydrochloria (hi″po-hi″dro-klo′re-ah) hypochlorhydria.

hypohypnotic (hi″po-hip-not′ik) marked by light sleep or hypnosis.

hypohypophysism (hi″po-hi-pof′ĭ-sizm) hypopituitarism.

hypoidrosis (hi″po-id-ro′sis) hypohidrosis.

hypoimmunity (hi″po-ĭ-mu′nĭ-te) lowered immunity.

hypoinsulinemia (hi″po-in″su-lĭ-ne′me-ah) a deficiency of insulin in the blood.

hypoinsulinism (hi″po-in′su-lin-izm″) deficient secretion of insulin by the pancreas, resulting in hyperglycemia.

hypoiodidism (hi″po-i-o′dĭ-dizm) [*hypo-* + *iodide* + *-ism*] deficiency of iodide in the body.

hypoisotonic (hi″po-i″so-ton′ik) less than isotonic; said of a solution having a lesser osmotic power than another.

hypokalemia (hi″po-ka-le′me-ah) abnormally low potassium concentration in the blood; it may result from potassium loss by renal secretion or by the gastrointestinal route, as by vomiting or diarrhea. It may be manifested clinically by neuromuscular disorders ranging from weakness to paralysis, by electrocardiographic abnormalities (depression of the T wave and elevation of the U wave), by renal disease, and by gastrointestinal disorders.

hypokalemic (hi″po-ka-le′mik) 1. pertaining to or characterized by hypokalemia. 2. an agent that acts to lower the potassium content of the blood.

hypokaliemia (hi″po-kal″e-e′me-ah) hypokalemia.

hypokinemia (hi″po-ki-ne′me-ah) [*hypo-* + Gr. *kinein* to move + *haima* blood + *-ia*] subnormal cardiac output.

hypokinesia (hi″po-ki-ne′ze-ah) [*hypo-* + Gr. *kinēsis* motion + *-ia*] abnormally decreased mobility; abnormally decreased motor function or activity, having multiple causes.

hypokinesis (hi″po-ki-ne′sis) hypokinesia.

hypokinetic (hi″po-ki-net′ik) pertaining to or characterized by hypokinesia.

hypolactasia (hi″po-lak-ta′ze-ah) deficiency of lactase activity in the intestines.

hypokolasia (hi″po-ko-la′ze-ah) [*hypo-* + Gr. *kolazein* to curtail, to correct + *-ia*] (obs.) functional weakness of the inhibiting mechanism.

hypolarynx (hi″po-lar′inks) the infraglottic compartment of the larynx from the true vocal cords to the first tracheal ring.

hypolemmal (hi″po-lem′al) [*hypo-* + Gr. *lemma* sheath] located beneath a sheath, as the end-plates of motor nerves under the sarcolemma of muscle.

hypolethal (hi″po-le′thal) not sufficient to cause death.

hypoleydigism (hi″po-li′dig-izm) abnormally diminished functional activity of Leydig's interstitial cells.

hypolipemia (hi″po-li-pe′me-ah) an abnormally decreased amount of fat in the blood.

hypolipidemic (hi″po-lip″ĭ-de′mik) promoting the reduction of lipid concentrations in the serum.

hypolipoproteinemia (hi″po-lip″o-pro″te-in-e′me-ah) the presence of abnormally low levels of lipoproteins in the serum, as in hypobetalipoproteinemia and Tangier disease.

hypoliposis (hi″po-li-po′sis) a deficiency of lipids in the blood or tissues. Lipids are transported in the blood as lipoproteins; see *hypolipoproteinemia.*

hypolutemia (hi″po-lu-te′me-ah) a decreased amount of luteal hormone (progesterone) in the blood.

hypolymphemia (hi″po-lim-fe′me-ah) [*hypo-* + *lymph* + Gr. *haima* blood + *-ia*] abnormal deficiency in the proportion of lymphocytes in the blood.

hypomagnesemia (hi″po-mag″nĕ-se′me-ah) an abnormally low magnesium content of the blood plasma, manifested chiefly by neuromuscular hyperirritability. It may result from malabsorption, dehydration, alcoholism, or renal disease.

hypomania (hi″po-ma′ne-ah) [*hypo-* + Gr. *mania* madness] mania of a moderate type.

hypomaniac (hi″po-ma′ne-ak) a person affected with hypomania.

hypomanic (hi″po-ma′nik) pertaining to or resembling hypomania.

hypomastia (hi-po-mas′te-ah) [*hypo-* + Gr. *mastos* breast + *-ia*] abnormal smallness of the mammary glands.

hypomazia (hi″po-ma′ze-ah) hypomastia.

hypomegasoma (hi″po-meg″ah-so′mah) [*hypo-* + Gr. *megas* great + *sōma* body] tallness; tall stature.

hypomelancholia (hi″po-mel″an-ko′le-ah) [*hypo-* + Gr. *melancholia* melancholia] melancholia with but slight mental disorder.

hypomelanism (hi″po-mel′ah-nizm) a condition in which production of melanin is limited and insufficient for protection against sunlight. **dominant oculocutaneous h.,** a hereditary syndrome transmitted as an autosomal dominant trait, which resembles a partial form of albinism in most respects; it is marked by translucency of the irises on transillumination, and greatly increased sensitivity to ultraviolet radiation in the 290–320 mm. range, with production of erythema and some dyskeratosis.

hypomelanosis (hi″po-mel″ah-no′sis) [*hypo-* + *melanosis*] diminution in supply of melanin in the skin; also sometimes used to denote localized absence of melanin. See also *hypomelanism*. **idiopathic guttate h.,** a common, slowly progressive, symmetrical eruption of sharply defined, depigmented macules of irregular shape up to 6 to 8 mm. in diameter, appearing on the extensor surfaces of the forearms and on the shins of adults.

hypomenorrhea (hi″po-men″o-re′ah) [*hypo-* + Gr. *mēn* month + *rhein* to flow] uterine bleeding of less than the normal amount occurring at regular intervals, the period of flow being of the same or less than usual duration.

hypomere (hi′po-mēr) 1. the ventrolateral portion of a myotome, innervated by an anterior ramus of a spinal nerve. 2. the lateral plate of mesoderm that develops into the walls of the body cavities.

hypomesosoma (hi″po-mes″o-so′mah) [*hypo-* + Gr. *mesos* middle + *sōma* body] a stature somewhat below the medium.

hypometabolic (hi″po-met″ah-bol′ik) pertaining to hypometabolism.

hypometabolism (hi″po-mĕ-tab′o-lizm) [*hypo-* + *metabolism*] abnormally decreased utilization of any substance by the body in metabolism; low metabolic rate.

hypometria (hi″po-me′tre-ah) ["a deficiency"; by analogy with Gr. *eumetria, hypermetria*] a condition in which voluntary muscular movement falls short of reaching the intended goal.

hypomicron (hi″po-mi′kron) submicron.

hypomicrosoma (hi″po-mi-kro-so′mah) [*hypo-* + Gr. *mikros* small + Gr. *sōma* body] the very smallest normal stature.

hypomineralization (hi″po-min″er-al-i-za′shun) deficiency of mineral elements in the body.

hypomnesis (hi″pom-ne′sis) [*hypo-* + Gr. *mnēmē* memory] defective memory.

hypomodal (hi″po-mo′dal) in statistics, relating to the values or items located to the left of the mode in a variations curve.

hypomorph (hi′po-morf) [*hypo-* + Gr. *morphē* form] 1. a person who is short in standing height as compared with his sitting height. Cf. *hypermorph* (def. 1), and *mesomorph* (def. 2). 2. in genetics, a mutant gene that shows only a partial reduction in the activity it influences. Cf. *hypermorph* (def. 2).

hypomorphic (hi″po-mor′fik) pertaining to a hypomorph.

hypomotility (hi″po-mo-til′ĭ-te) deficient movement in any part.

hypomyotonia (hi″po-mi″o-to′ne-ah) [*hypo-* + Gr. *mys* muscle + *tonos* tension + *-ia*] deficient muscular tonicity.

hypomyxia (hi″po-mik′se-ah) [*hypo-* + Gr. *myxa* mucus + *-ia*] decreased secretion of mucus.

hyponanosoma (hi″po-na″no-so′mah) [*hypo-* + Gr. *nanos* dwarf + *sōma* body] the extreme of dwarfishness, or nanism.

hyponasality (hi″po-na-zal′ĭ-te) a quality of voice in which there is a complete lack of nasal emission of air and nasal resonance, so that the speaker sounds as if he has a cold. Called also *denasality*.

hyponatremia (hi″po-nah-tre′me-ah) deficiency of sodium in the blood; salt depletion. **depletional h.,** that in which there is a low level of sodium and of body fluids (dehydration). **dilutional h.,** that in which there is a low level of serum sodium but a high level of body sodium and body fluids (edema). **hyperlipemic h.,** apparent hyponatremia (when expressed per unit of plasma) due to a high concentration of lipids combined with proteins in the blood plasma.

hyponatruria (hi″po-nah-troo′re-ah) an abnormally low level of sodium in the urine.

hyponea (hi″po-ne′ah) hyponoia.

hyponeocytosis (hi″po-ne″o-si-to′sis) [*hypo-* + Gr. *neos* new + *-cyte* + *-osis*] leukopenia with immature forms of leukocytes present in the blood.

hyponitremia (hi″po-ni-tre′me-ah) a low level of nitrogen in the blood, sometimes associated with protein malnutrition.

hyponoia (hi″po-noi′ah) [*hypo-* + Gr. *nous* mind + *-ia*] sluggish mental activity.

hyponoic (hi″po-no′ik) arising from early formed but unconscious processes (Kretschmer).

hyponychial (hi″po-nik′e-al) subungual; beneath a nail.

hyponychium (hi″po-nik′e-um) [*hypo-* + Gr. *onyx* nail] [NA] the thickened epidermis underneath the free distal end of the nail.

hyponychon (hi-pon′ĭ-kon) [*hypo-* + Gr. *onyx* nail] ecchymosis beneath the nail.

hypo-orchidia (hi″po-or-kid′e-ah) defective endocrine activity of the testes.

hypo-orchidism (hi″po-or′ki-dizm) defective activity of the testes.

hypo-orthocytosis (hi″po-or″tho-si-to′sis) [*hypo-* + Gr. *orthos* regular + *-cyte* + *-osis*] leukopenia in which the proportion of the various forms of leukocytes is normal.

hypo-osmolality (hi″po-os″mo-lal′ĭ-te) a decrease in the osmolality of the body fluids.

hypo-ovaria (hi″po-o-va′re-ah) defective endocrine activity of the ovaries.

hypo-ovarianism (hi″po-o-va′re-an-izm) hypo-ovaria.

hypopallesthesia (hi″po-pal″es-the′ze-ah) [*hypo-* + *pallesthesia*] abnormally decreased sensibility to vibrations.

hypopancreatism (hi″po-pan′kre-ah-tizm″) diminished pancreatic activity.

hypopancreorrhea (hi″po-pan″kre-o-re′ah) abnormally diminished secretion from the pancreas.

hypoparathyreosis (hi″po-par″ah-thi′re-o′sis) hypoparathyroidism.

hypoparathyroidism (hi″po-par″ah-thi′roid-izm) the condition produced by greatly reduced function of the parathyroids or by the removal of those bodies. The lack of parathyroid hormone leads to a fall in plasma calcium level—which may result in increased neuromuscular excitability and, ultimately, tetany—followed by a rise in plasma phosphate level, resulting in a decrease in bone resorption and consequent density of bone. There may also be dermatologic, ophthalmologic (cataracts), psychiatric, and dental symptoms.

hypopepsia (hi″po-pep′se-ah) [*hypo-* + Gr. *pepsis* digestion + *-ia*] impairment of digestion, due to hypochlorhydria.

hypopepsinia (hi″po-pep-sin′e-ah) deficiency in the pepsin secretion of the stomach.

hypoperfusion (hi″po-per-fu′zhun) decreased blood flow through an organ, as in circulatory shock; if prolonged it may result in permanent cellular dysfunction and death.

hypoperistalsis (hi″po-per″ĭ-stal′sis) abnormally sluggish peristalsis.

hypopexia (hi″po-pek′se-ah) [*hypo-* + Gr. *pēxis* fixation + *-ia*] the fixation by a tissue of a deficient amount of a substance.

hypopexy (hi′po-pek″se) hypopexia.

hypophalangism (hi″po-fah-lan′jizm) less than the usual number of phalanges of a finger or toe.

hypophamine (hi-pof′ah-min) the substance once thought to be the active principle of the posterior lobe of the pituitary gland. **alpha h.,** oxytocin. **beta h.,** vasopressin.

hypopharyngeal (hi″po-fah-rin′je-al) pertaining to the hypopharynx.

hypopharyngoscope (hi″po-fah-ring′go-skōp) an instrument for inspecting the lower part of the pharynx.

hypopharyngoscopy (hi″po-far″in-gos′ko-pe) examination of the lower part of the pharynx.

hypopharynx (hi″po-far′inks) that division of the pharynx which lies below the upper edge of the epiglottis and opens into the larynx and esophagus.

hypophonesis (hi″po-fo-ne′sis) [*hypo-* + Gr. *phōnēsis* sounding] diminished intensity of the sound in auscultation or percussion.

hypophonia (hi″po-fo′ne-ah) [*hypo-* + Gr. *phōnē* voice + *-ia*] defective speech due to lack of phonation and resulting in whispering.

hypophoria (hi″po-fo′re-ah) [*hypo-* + Gr. *phorein* to bear + *-ia*] heterophoria in which there is downward deviation of the visual axis of an eye when visual fusional stimuli are eliminated. When both eyes are affected, it is called *cataphoria*.

hypophosphatasia (hi″po-fos″fah-ta′ze-ah) an inborn error of metabolism with a genetic basis, characterized by lowered phosphatase activity of the serum, due, apparently, to lack of alkaline phosphatase in the cells, and resulting in defective rebuilding and mineralization of bone, and always marked by excretion of phosphoethanolamine in the urine. The disorder is most severe when it occurs in the first six months of life, with marked demineralization of bone and, commonly, craniostenosis, exophthalmos, and brain damage, death usually occurring within a year. In older infants and children, the bone disease resembles rickets, and there is early loss of teeth. In adults, it may take the form of osteomalacia or be asymptomatic.

hypophosphate (hi″po-fos′fāt) a salt of hypophosphoric acid.

hypophosphatemia (hi″po-fos″fah-te′me-ah) an abnormally decreased amount of phosphates in the blood; manifestations include hemolysis, lassitude, weakness, and convulsions. It may be found in hyperparathyroidism, rickets, osteomalacia, and several renal tubular abnormalities, including the Fanconi syndrome. **familial h.,** a hereditary disorder of phosphate metabolism, transmitted as a sex-linked trait, which may be associated with vitamin D–resistant rickets (q.v.).

hypophosphatemic (hi″po-phos″fah-te′mik) pertaining to or characterized by hypophosphatemia.

hypophosphaturia (hi″po-fos″fah-tu′re-ah) an abnormally decreased amount of phosphate in the urine.

hypophosphite (hi″po-fos′fīt) any salt of hypophosphorous acid.

hypophosphoremia (hi″po-fos″fo-re′me-ah) hypophosphatemia.

hypophrenia (hi″po-fre′ne-ah) [hypo- + Gr. phrēn mind + -ia] mental retardation.

hypophrenic (hi″po-fren′ik) [hypo- + Gr. phrēn diaphragm, mind] 1. below the diaphragm. 2. mentally retarded.

hypophrenium (hi″po-fre′ne-um) a peritoneal space between the diaphragm and the transverse colon.

hypophrenosis (hi″po-fre-no′sis) Southard's term for feeble-mindedness, including idiocy, imbecility, moronity, and subnormality.

hypophyseal (hi″po-fiz′e-al) pertaining to a hypophysis, especially to the hypophysis cerebri, or pituitary gland.

hypophysectomize (hi″po-fiz-ek′to-mīz) to remove the hypophysis, or pituitary gland.

hypophysectomy (hi-pof″ĭ-sek′to-me) [hypophysis + Gr. ektomē excision] surgical removal of the hypophysis, or pituitary gland.

hypophyseoportal (hi″po-fiz″e-o-por′tal) pertaining to the portal system of the pituitary gland; see under system.

hypophyseoprivic (hi″po-fiz″e-o-priv′ik) pertaining to deficiency of hormone secretion by the hypophysis (pituitary gland).

hypophyseotropic (hi″po-fiz″e-o-trop′ik) acting on the hypophysis (pituitary gland), as a hypophyseotropic hormone.

hypophysial (hi″po-fiz′e-al) hypophyseal.

hypophysiectomy (hi″po-fiz″e-ek′to-me) hypophysectomy.

hypophysioprivic (hi″po-fiz″e-o-priv′ik) hypophyseoprivic.

hypophysiotropic (hi″po-fiz″e-o-trop′ik) hypophyseotropic.

hypophysis (hi-pof″ĭ-sis) [hypo- + Gr. phyein to grow] [NA] the pituitary gland (see under gland), an epithelial body of dual origin located at the base of the brain in the sella turcica. **h. cer′e-bri,** see pituitary gland, under gland. **pharyngeal h.,** a mass in the pharyngeal wall with structure similar to that of the hypophysis. **h. sic′ca,** posterior pituitary.

hypophysitis (hi-pof″ĭ-si′tis) inflammation of the hypophysis.

hypophysoma (hi-pof″ĭ-zo′mah) a tumor of the hypophysis.

hypophysoprivic (hi-pof″ĭ-zo-pri′vik) hypophyseoprivic.

hypopiesia (hi-po-pi-e′se-ah) abnormally low blood pressure occurring independently of any discoverable organic disease.

hypopiesis (hi″po-pi-e′sis) [hypo- + Gr. piesis pressure] abnormally low pressure, as abnormally low blood pressure.

hypopietic (hi″po-pi-et′ik) pertaining to, characterized by, or causing hypopiesis.

hypopigmentation (hi″po-pig″men-ta′shun) abnormally diminished pigmentation, as distinct from complete loss of pigment.

hypopigmenter (hi″po-pig-men′ter) an agent that reduces pigmentation of the skin; a bleach.

hypopinealism (hi″po-pin′e-al-izm″) defective functional activity of the pineal body.

hypopituitarism (hi″po-pĭ-tu′ĭ-tah-rizm″) diminution or cessation of the pituitary function due to surgical removal of the pituitary gland, to ablation by irradiation, or to spontaneous causes, as in chromophobe adenoma or postpartum necrosis (Sheehan's syndrome). It leads to hormonal deficiency—varying with the degree of dysfunction—of the following: (a) gonadotropins, with consequent regression of secondary sex characteristics and decrease in libido; (b) somatotropin, which in children results in pituitary dwarfism; (c) thyrotropin (see hypothyroidism); (d) corticotropin, resulting in symptoms similar to those in hypoadrenalism.

hypoplasia (hi″po-pla′ze-ah) [hypo- + Gr. plasis formation + -ia] incomplete development or underdevelopment of an organ or tissue; it is less severe in degree than aplasia. **cartilage-hair h.,** a form of dwarfism among Amish people, inherited as an autosomal recessive trait and associated with multiple skeletal abnormalities and sparse, short, fine, brittle, light-colored hair. **enamel h.,** incomplete or defective development of the enamel of the teeth; it occurs in a hereditary form, as in amelogenesis imperfecta, usually affecting both the deciduous and permanent teeth and generally involving only the enamel, or in an environmental form due to various factors, e.g., vitamin deficiency, exanthematous diseases, congenital syphilis, fluorosis, and local injury or trauma. **h. of mesenchyme,** osteogenesis imperfecta. **oligomeganephronic renal h.,** oligomeganephronia. **h. of right ventricle,** a defective development of the right ventricular myocardium, which may be paper-thin (parchment heart); there may be right-sided heart failure. **Turner's h.,** see under tooth.

hypoplastic (hi″po-plas′tik) marked by hypoplasia.

hypoplasty (hi″po-plas″te) hypoplasia.

hypoploid (hi′po-ploid) the aneuploid condition in which there is less than the normal diploid number of chromosomes, e.g., 45 chromosomes in man, the 2n−1 state.

hypopnea (hi″po-ne′ah) [hypo- + Gr. pnoia breath] abnormal decrease in the depth and rate of the respiratory movements.

hypopneic (hi″po-ne′ik) pertaining to or characterized by hypopnea.

hypoponesis (hi″po-po-ne′sis) [hypo- + Gr. ponēsis toil, exertion] dysponesis in which there is insufficient action-potential output from the motor and premotor areas of the cortex.

hypoporosis (hi″po-po-ro′sis) [hypo- + Gr. pōros callus + -osis] deficient formation of callus after fracture.

hypoposia (hi″po-po′ze-ah) [hypo- + Gr. posis drinking + -ia] abnormally diminished ingestion of fluids.

hypopotassemia (hi″po-po″tah-se′me-ah) hypokalemia.

hypopotassemic (hi″po-po″tah-se′mik) hypokalemic.

hypopotentia (hi″po-po-ten′she-ah) [hypo- + L. potentia power] a condition of diminished power, especially of diminished electrical activity of the cerebral cortex.

hypopraxia (hi″po-prak′se-ah) [hypo- + Gr. praxis action + -ia] abnormally diminished activity.

hypoprolanemia (hi″po-pro″lah-ne′me-ah) (obs.) a lessened amount of prolan A in the blood.

hypoprosody (hi″po-pros′o-de) diminution of the normal variation of stress, pitch, and rhythm of speech.

hypoproteinemia (hi″po-pro″tĭ-ne′me-ah) abnormal decrease in the amount of protein in the blood, sometimes resulting in edema and fluid accumulation in serous cavities. **prehepatic h.,** hypoproteinemia occurring as a result of prolonged ingestion of faulty low-protein diet.

hypoproteinia (hi″po-pro″tēn′e-ah) a subnormal protein status of the body.

hypoproteinic (hi″po-pro″tēn′ik) pertaining to or characterized by hypoproteinia.

hypoproteinosis (hi″po-pro″tĭ-no′sis) deficiency of proteins or protein foods.

hypoprothrombinemia (hi″po-pro-throm″bĭ-ne′me-ah) deficiency of prothrombin (coagulation Factor II) in the blood; called also Factor II deficiency.

hypopselaphesia (hi″pop-sel″ah-fe′ze-ah) [hypo- + Gr. psēlaphēsis touch + -ia] diminution or dullness of the tactile sense; tactile hypoesthesia.

hypopsychosis (hi″po-si-ko′sis) [hypo- + Gr. psychē mind, soul + -osis] diminution of the function of thought; blunting of the thought processes.

hypopteronosis cystica (hi″po-ter-on′o-sis sis″tĭ-kah) [hypo- + Gr. pteron feather] a condition observed in birds, known commonly as "lumps," in which a cyst forms when the growth of the feather shaft is confined within the follicle.

hypoptyalism (hi″pop-ti′al-izm) [hypo- + Gr. ptyalon spittle] abnormally decreased secretion of saliva, as in xerostomia.

hypopus (hi-po′pus) a stage in the development of the grain mites (Acaridae) between the first and the second nymph stages.

hypopyon (hi-po′pe-on) [hypo- + Gr. pyon pus] an accumulation of pus in the anterior chamber of the eye.

hyporeactive (hi″po-re-ak′tiv) pertaining to or characterized by a less than normal response to stimuli.

hyporeflexia (hi″po-re-flek′se-ah) weakening of the reflexes.

hyporeninemia (hi″po-re′nin-e′me-ah) low levels of renin in the blood.

hyporeninemic (hi″po-re′nin-e′mik) characterized by low levels of renin in the blood.

hyporrhea (hi″po-re′ah) [hypo- + Gr. rhoia flow] slight hemorrhage.

hyposalemia (hi″po-sah-le′me-ah) [hypo- + L. sal salt + Gr. haima blood + -ia] abnormally decreased concentration of salt in the blood.

hyposalivation (hi″po-sal″ĭ-va′shun) hypoptyalism.

hyposarca (hi″po-sar′kah) anasarca.

hyposcheotomy (hi-pos″ke-ot′o-me) [hypo- + Gr. oscheon scrotum + tomē cut] puncture of a testicular hydrocele at the lower portion of the tunica vaginalis.

hyposcleral (hi″po-skle′ral) under the sclerotic coat of the eye.

hyposecretion (hi″po-se-kre′shun) diminished secretion as of a gland.

hyposensitive (hi″po-sen′sĭ-tiv) 1. exhibiting abnormally decreased sensitivity. 2. having the specific or general ability to react to a specific allergen reduced by repeated and gradually increasing doses of the offending substance.

hyposensitivity (hi″po-sens″ĭ-tiv′te) the condition of being hyposensitive.

hyposensitization (hi″po-sen″sĭ-ti-za′shun) the act or process of making hyposensitive; desensitization.

hyposexuality (hi″po-seks″u-al′ĭ-te) deficiency in sexuality.

hyposiagonarthritis (hi″po-si-ag″on-ar-thri′tis) inflammation of the temporomandibular joint.

hyposialadenitis (hi″po-si″al-ad″ĕ-ni′tis) [*hypo-* + Gr. *sialon* saliva + *adēn* gland + *-itis*] inflammation of the submaxillary salivary gland.

hyposialosis (hi″po-si″ah-lo′sis) hypoptyalism.

hyposkeocytosis (hi″po-ske″o-si-to′sis) [*hypo-* + Gr. *skaios* left + *-cyte* + *-osis*] hyponeocytosis.

hyposmia (hi-poz′me-ah) [*hypo-* + Gr. *osmē* smell + *-ia*] abnormally decreased sensitivity to odors.

hyposmolarity (hi-poz″mo-lar′i-te) abnormally decreased osmolar concentration.

hyposmosis (hi″pos-mo′sis) decreased speed of osmosis.

hyposomatotropism (hi″po-so″mat-o-tro′pizm) a condition of deficient secretion of somatotropin (growth hormone) or of inadequate secretion of somatotropin, resulting in short stature.

hyposomia (hi″po-so′me-ah) [*hypo-* + Gr. *sōma* body + *-ia*] inadequate bodily development.

hyposomnia (hi″po-som′ne-ah) insomnia.

hypospadia (hi″po-spa′de-ah) hypospadias.

hypospadiac (hi″po-spa′de-ak) a person affected with hypospadias.

hypospadias (hi″po-spa′de-as) [*hypo-* + Gr. *spadōn* a rent] a developmental anomaly in the male in which the urethra opens on the underside of the penis or on the perineum. **balanic h., balanitic h.,** the commonest type of hypospadias, in which the urethral orifice opens at the site of the frenum, which may be rudimentary or absent; the normal site of the urinary meatus is represented on the glans penis as a blind pit. Called also *glandular h.* **female h.,** a developmental anomaly in the female in which the urethra opens into the vagina. **glandular h.,** balanic h. **penile h.,** hypospadias in which the urethral opening lies between the glandular sulcus and the junction of the penis and scrotum. **penoscrotal h.,** hypospadias in which the urethral orifice is at the junction of the penis and scrotum; it may be associated with congenital chordee. **perineal h.,** hypospadias with anomalous development of the genitalia, the rudimentary penis often being engulfed by an overlying bifid scrotum. The extreme form is called *pseudovaginal h.* **pseudovaginal h.,** see *perineal h.*

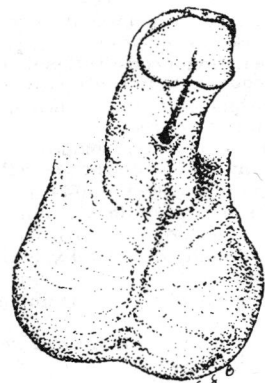

Hypospadias with chordee.

hyposphresia (hi″pos-fre′ze-ah) [*hypo-* + Gr. *osphrēsis* smell + *-ia*] hyposmia.

hyposplenism (hi″po-splen′izm) a condition characterized by diminished functioning of the spleen, resulting in an increase in peripheral blood elements.

hypostasis (hi-pos′tah-sis) [*hypo-* + Gr. *stasis* halt] poor or stagnant circulation in a dependent part of the body or organ, as in venous insufficiency.

hypostatic (hi″po-stat′ik) 1. pertaining to, caused by, or associated with hypostasis. 2. abnormally static; said of certain inherited traits which are liable to be suppressed by other traits.

hyposteatolysis (hi″po-ste″ah-tol′ĭ-sis) inadequate hydrolysis of fats during ingestion.

hyposteatosis (hi″po-ste″ah-to′sis) deficient secretion of sebum.

hyposthenia (hi″pos-the′ne-ah) [*hypo-* + Gr. *sthenos* strength + *-ia*] an enfeebled state; weakness.

hyposthentiant (hi″pos-the′ne-ant) reducing the strength; debilitant.

hyposthenic (hi″pos-then′ik) pertaining to or characterized by hyposthenia.

hyposthenuria (hi″pos-thĕ-nu′re-ah) a condition characterized by inability to form urine of high specific gravity. **tubu-**

lar h., hyposthenuria occurring as a result of injury to the epithelial cells of the renal tubules.

hypostomia (hi″po-sto′me-ah) [*hypo-* + Gr. *stōma* mouth + *-ia*] a developmental anomaly characterized by abnormal smallness of the mouth, the slit being vertical instead of horizontal.

hypostosis (hip″os-to′sis) [*hypo-* + Gr. *osteon* bone + *-osis*] deficient development of bone.

hypostypsis (hi″po-stip′sis) [*hypo-* + Gr. *stypsis* contraction] moderate astringency.

hypostyptic (hi″po-stip′tik) moderately or mildly styptic.

hyposulfite (hi″po-sul′fit) sodium thiosulfate.

hyposuprarenalemia (hi″po-su″prah-re″nal-e′me-ah) hypoadrenalemia.

hyposuprarenalism (hi″po-su″prah-re′nal-izm) hypoadrenalism.

hyposympathicotonus (hi″po-sim-path″ĭ-ko-to′nus) a decreased tone of the sympathetic nervous system.

hyposynergia (hi″po-sĭ-ner′je-ah) [*hypo-* + *synergia*] defective coordination.

hyposystole (hi″po-sis′to-le) [*hypo-* + *systole*] (*obs.*) abnormal diminution of the systole.

hypotaxia (hi″po-tak′se-ah) [*hypo-* + Gr. *taxis* arrangement + *-ia*] a condition of diminished control over the will and actions, such as occurs in the first stage of hypnotism.

hypotelorism (hi″po-tel′o-rizm) [*hypo-* + Gr. *tēlouros* distant] abnormally decreased distance between two organs or parts. **ocular h., orbital h.,** a condition characterized by abnormal decrease in the intraorbital distance, consistently present in trigonocephaly.

hypotension (hi″po-ten′shun) abnormally low blood pressure; seen in shock but not necessarily indicative of it. See also *blood pressure,* under *pressure.* **chronic orthostatic h., chronic idiopathic orthostatic h., idiopathic orthostatic h.,** Shy-Drager syndrome. **orthostatic h.,** a fall in blood pressure associated with dizziness, syncope, and blurred vision occurring upon standing or when standing motionless in a fixed position; it can be acquired or idiopathic, transient or chronic, and occur alone or secondary to a disorder of the central nervous system, such as the Shy-Drager syndrome (see under *syndrome*). Called also *postural o.* and *postural syncope.* **postural h.,** orthostatic h. **vascular h.,** severe hypotension from dilatation of the blood vessels.

hypotensive (hi″po-ten′siv) 1. characterized by or causing diminished tension or pressure, as abnormally low blood pressure. 2. a person with abnormally low blood pressure.

hypotensor (hi″po-ten′sor) a substance that lowers the blood pressure; a hypotensive agent.

hypotetraploid (hi″po-tet′rah-ploid) having fewer than the tetraploid number of chromosomes in unbalanced sets (4n−x).

hypothalamic (hi″po-thah-lam′ik) of or involving the hypothalamus.

hypothalamotomy (hi″po-thal″ah-mot′o-me) [*hypothalamus* + Gr. *temnein* to cut] production of lesions in the posterolateral part of the hypothalamus; done in the treatment of psychotic disorders.

hypothalamus (hi″po-thal′ah-mus) [NA] the portion of the diencephalon which forms the floor and part of the lateral wall of the third ventricle. Anatomically, it includes the optic chiasm, mamillary bodies, tuber cinereum, infundibulum, and hypophysis, but for physiological purposes the hypophysis is considered a distinct structure. The hypothalamic nuclei comprise that part of the corticodiencephalic mechanisms which activates, controls, and integrates the peripheral autonomic mechanisms, endocrine activity, and many somatic functions, e.g., a general regulation of water balance, body temperature, sleep, and food intake, and the development of secondary sex characteristics. The hypothalamus secretes vasopressin and oxytocin, which are stored in the pituitary, as well as many releasing factors (hypophyseotropic hormones) by means of which it exerts control over functions of the adenohypophysis portion of the pituitary gland.

hypothenar (hi-poth′ĕ-nar) [*hypo-* + Gr. *thenar* palm] 1. [NA] the fleshy eminence on the palm along the ulnar margin. 2. relating to this eminence.

hypothermal (hi″po-ther′mal) [*hypo-* + Gr. *thermē* heat] pertaining to or characterized by reduced body temperature.

hypothermia (hi″po-ther′me-ah) [*hypo-* + Gr. *thermē* heat + *-ia*] a low body temperature, as that due to exposure in cold weather or a state of low temperature of the body induced as a means of decreasing metabolism of tissues and thereby the need for oxygen, as used in various surgical procedures, especially on the heart, or in an excised organ being preserved for transplantation. **endogenous h.,** abnormally reduced body temperature resulting from physiologic causes, due to dysfunction of the central nervous system or of the endocrine system.

hypothermic (hi″po-ther′mik) pertaining to or exhibiting reduced body temperature, pertaining to hypothermia.

hypothermy (hi″po-ther′me) hypothermia.

hypothesis (hi-poth'ĕ-sis) a supposition that appears to explain a group of phenomena and is assumed as a basis of reasoning and experimentation. See also *theory*. **biogenic amine h.,** the hypothesis that certain biogenic amines, especially dopamine, norepinephrine, and serotonin, play a role in the pathogenesis of affective disorders. **cardionector h.,** the hypothesis that there are two pacemakers or cardionectors in the heart; one, the atrionector, controls the atria, and the other, the ventriculonector, controls the ventricles. **Gad's h.,** the arterial and portal venous communications in the portal canal meet at an acute angle, leaving a wedge-shaped valve between them at their junction. **gate h.,** gate theory. **Harrower's h.,** hormone hunger; see under *hunger*. **insular h.,** the hypothesis that diabetes mellitus is due to disordered function of the islands of Langerhans in the pancreas. **jelly roll h.,** a theory explaining the formation of nerve myelin, which states that it consists of successive layers of the plasma membrane of a Schwann cell wrapped spirally around the axon in a jelly roll fashion. **lattice h.,** a theory of the nature of the antigen-antibody reaction which postulates reaction between multivalent antigen and divalent antibody to give an antigen-antibody complex of a lattice-like structure. **Lyon h.,** all X chromosomes in a cell in excess of one are inactivated (in the form of sex chromatin) on a random basis in all mammalian cells at an early stage of embryogenesis. In effect, then, the normal human female is a mosaic for heterozygous X-linked genes, since the paternal X chromosome is inactivated in some cells and the maternal one in the remainder. **Makeham's h.,** the assumption that death is due to two co-existing causes: (1) chance, which is constant; (2) inability to withstand destruction, which progresses geometrically. **one gene–one enzyme h.,** the concept that each gene directly determines a unique enzyme specificity, thereby controlling enzyme synthesis and other chemical reactions. **Semon-Hering h.,** mnemic theory. **sliding-filament h.,** the stretching of individual muscle fibers raises the number of tension-developing bridges that can be formed between the sliding contractile protein elements (actin and myosin) and thus augments the force of the next muscle contraction. **Starling's h.,** the direction and rate of fluid transfer between blood plasma in the capillary and fluid in the tissue spaces depend on the hydrostatic pressure on each side of the capillary wall, on the osmotic pressure of protein in plasma and in tissue fluid, and on the properties of the capillary wall as a filtering membrane. **unitarian h.,** the theory that antibody is a single species of modified serum globulin regardless of the overt consequences of its reaction with homologous antigen, e.g., agglutination, precipitation, complement fixation, etc. **Woods-Fildes h.** (*obs.*), that the sulfonamides tend to replace para-aminobenzoic acid, which is an essential metabolite for certain bacteria.

hypothrepsia (hi"po-threp'se-ah) malnutrition.

hypothrombinemia (hi"po-throm"bĭ-ne'me-ah) a deficiency of thrombin in the blood.

hypothymergasia (hi"po-thi"mer-ga'se-ah) [*hypo-* + Gr. *thymos* spirit + *ergon* work + *-ia*] Meyer's term for underactivity of mood, marked by depression, stupor, sadness, and anxiety.

hypothymergastic (hi"po-thi"mer-gas'tik) pertaining to or characterized by hypothymergasia.

hypothymia (hi"po-thi'me-ah) [*hypo-* + Gr. *thymos* spirit + *-ia*] abnormal diminution of emotional tone; diminution of feeling tone.

hypothymic (hi"po-thi'mik) marked by hypothymia.

hypothymism (hi"po-thi'mizm) abnormally deficient thymus activity.

hypothyrea (hi"po-thi're-ah) hypothyroidism.

hypothyreosis (hi"po-thi"re-o'sis) hypothyroidism.

hypothyroid (hi"po-thi'roid) marked by or due to hypothyroidism.

hypothyroidation (hi"po-thi"roi-da'shun) the induction of hypothyroidism.

hypothyroidea (hi"po-thi-roi'de-ah) hypothyroidism.

hypothyroidism (hi"po-thi'roid-izm) deficiency of thyroid activity. In adults, it is most common in women and is characterized by decrease in basal metabolic rate, tiredness and lethargy, sensitivity to cold, and menstrual disturbances. If untreated, it progresses to full-blown myxedema. In infants, severe hypothyroidism leads to cretinism. In juveniles, the manifestations are intermediate, with less severe mental and developmental retardation and only mild symptoms of the adult form.

hypothyrosis (hi"po-thi-ro'sis) hypothyroidism.

hypotonia (hi"po-to'ne-ah) [*hypo-* + Gr. *tonos* tone + *-ia*] a condition of diminished tone of the skeletal muscles; diminished resistance of muscles to passive stretching. **benign congenital h.,** a condition marked by signs of weakness and floppiness in babies, due to nonprogressive weakness of skeletal muscles from birth. **h. oc'uli,** low intraocular pressure.

hypotonic (hi-po-ton'ik) a biological term denoting a solution which, when bathing body cells, causes a net flow of water across the semipermeable cell membrane into the cell. Also, denoting a solution having less tonicity than another solution, e.g., the blood, with which it is compared.

hypotonicity (hi"po-to-nis'ĭ-te) the state or quality of being hypotonic.

hypotonus (hi-pot'o-nus) hypotonia.

hypotony (hi-pot'o-ne) hypotonia.

hypotoxicity (hi"po-tok-sis'ĭ-te) [*hypo-* + Gr. *toxikon* poison] the state or quality of possessing mitigated or diminished toxicity.

Hypotricha (hi"po-trik'ah) a suborder of ciliate protozoa of the Spirotricha.

hypotrichiasis (hi"po-trĭ-ki'ah-sis) congenital alopecia.

hypotrichosis (hi"po-trĭ-ko'sis) [*hypo-* + Gr. *thrix* hair + *-osis*] presence of less than the normal amount of hair.

hypotrichous (hi-po'trĭk-us) [*hypo-* + Gr. *thrix* hair] having no cilia on the dorsal surface; said of certain ciliates.

hypotriploid (hi"po-trip'loid) having fewer than the triploid number of chromosomes in unbalanced sets (3n–x).

hypotrophy (hi-pot'ro-fe) [*hypo-* + Gr. *trophē* nutrition] abiotrophy.

hypotropia (hi"po-tro'pe-ah) [*hypo-* + Gr. *tropos* a turning + *-ia*] strabismus in which there is permanent downward deviation of the visual axis of an eye.

hypotryptophanic (hi"po-trip-to-fan'ik) caused by deficiency of tryptophan in the diet.

hypotympanotomy (hi"po-tim"pah-not'o-me) surgical opening of the hypotympanum.

hypotympanum (hi"po-tim'pah-num) a space in the middle ear, below the lower edge of the sulcus tympanicus.

hypouremia (hi"po-u-re'me-ah) an abnormally low level of urea in the blood.

hypouresis (hi"po-u-re'sis) oligourea.

hypouricemia (hi"po-u"rĭ-se'me-ah) deficiency of uric acid in the blood, along with xanthinuria, due to deficiency of xanthine oxidase, the enzyme required for conversion of hypoxanthine to xanthine and of xanthine to uric acid.

hypouricuria (hi"po-u"rĭ-ku're-ah) deficiency of uric acid in the urine.

hypourocrinia (hi"po-u"ro-krin'e-ah) [*hypo-* + Gr. *ouron* urine + *krinein* to secrete + *-ia*] deficient secretion of urine.

hypovaria (hi"po-va're-ah) hypo-ovaria.

hypovarianism (hi"po-va're-an-izm) hypo-ovaria.

hypovegetative (hi"po-vej'ĕ-ta'tiv) [*hypo-* + L. *vegetativus* plant-fashion] denoting a constitutional body type in which somatic systems predominate in contrast to visceral organs.

hypovenosity (hi"po-ve-nos'ĭ-te) incomplete development of the venous system in any area.

hypoventilation (hi"po-ven"tĭ-la'shun) a state in which there is a reduced amount of air entering the pulmonary alveoli.

hypovitaminosis (hi"po-vi"tah-min-o'sis) a condition due to a deficiency of one or more essential vitamins; see specific vitamins.

hypovolemia (hi"po-vo-le'me-ah) [*hypo-* + *volume* + Gr. *haima* blood + *-ia*] abnormally decreased volume of circulating fluid [plasma] in the body.

hypovolemic (hi"po-vo-le'mik) pertaining to or characterized by hypovolemia.

hypovolia (hi"po-vo'le-ah) diminished water content or volume, as of extracellular fluid.

hypoxanthine (hi"po-zan'thēn) 6-oxypurine, a purine base, $C_5H_4N_4O$, being an intermediate product of uric acid synthesis, formed from adenylic acid and itself a precursor of xanthine.

hypoxemia (hi"pok-se'me-ah) [*hypo-* + *oxygen* + Gr. *haima* blood + *-ia*] deficient oxygenation of the blood; hypoxia.

hypoxia (hi-pok'se-ah) reduction of oxygen supply to tissue below physiological levels despite adequate perfusion of the tissue by blood. Cf. *anoxia*. **anemic h.,** hypoxia due to reduction of the oxygen-carrying capacity of the blood as a result of a decrease in the total hemoglobin or an alteration of the hemoglobin constituents. **histotoxic h.,** that due to impaired utilization of oxygen by tissues, as in cyanide poisoning. **hypoxic h.,** that due to insufficient oxygen reaching the blood, as at decreased barometric pressures at high altitudes. **stagnant h.,** that due to failure to transport sufficient oxygen because of inadequate blood flow, as in heart failure.

hypoxic (hi-pok'sik) pertaining to or characterized by hypoxia.

hypoxidosis (hi-pok"sĭ-do'sis) impaired cell function due to reduced supply of oxygen.

HypRho-D (hip'ro) trademark for a preparation of Rh₀(D) immune serum globulin.

hypsarhythmia (hip"sah-rith'me-ah) see *hypsarrhythmia*.

hypsarrhythmia (hip"sah-rith'me-ah) [Gr. *hypsi* high + *arrhythmos* unrhythmical + *-ia*] Gibbs' term for an electroencephalographic abnormality sometimes observed in infants, with random, high-voltage slow waves and spikes that arise from multiple foci and spread to all cortical areas. The disorder is usually characterized by spasms or quivering spells (myoclonus), and is commonly associated with mental retardation.

hypsi- (hip′se) [Gr. *hypsi* high] a combining form meaning high.

hypsibrachycephalic (hip″se-brak″e-sĕ-fal′ik) [*hypsi-* + Gr. *brachys* broad + *kephalē* head] having the head broad and high.

hypsicephalic (hip″se-sĕ-fal′ik) [*hypsi-* + Gr. *kephalē* head] having a vertical index over 75.

hypsicephaly (hip″se-sef′ah-le) oxycephaly.

hypsiconchous (hip″se-kong′kus) [*hypsi-* + Gr. *konchē* shell] having an orbital index over 85.

hypsiloid (hip′sĭ-loid) [Gr. *hypsiloeidēs* in the shape of an T] shaped like the Greek letter T, capital upsilon. Cf. *hyoid.*

hypsistaphylia (hip″sĭ-stah-fil′e-ah) [*hypsi-* + Gr. *staphylē* uvula + *-ia*] highness and narrowness of the palate.

hypsistenocephalic (hip″se-sten″o-sĕ-fal′ik) [*hypsi-* + Gr. *stenos* narrow + *kephalē* head] having a high, curved vertex, cheek bones prominent, and jaws prognathic.

hypso- (hip′so) [Gr. *hypsos* height] a combining form denoting relationship to height.

hypsocephalous (hip″so-sef′ah-lus) [*hypso-* + Gr. *kephalē* head] having a high vertex; having a breadth-height index of the head of over 75.

hypsochrome (hip′so-krōm) [*hypso-* + Gr. *chrōma* color] an atom or group whose introduction into a compound shifts the compound's absorption maximum to a shorter wavelength; cf. *bathochrome.*

hypsochromy (hip″so-kro′me) a shift of the absorption band toward higher frequencies (shorter wavelengths), with lightening of color.

hypsodont (hip′so-dont) [*hypso-* + Gr. *odous* tooth] having prism-shaped teeth with high crowns, as in many herbivorous mammals.

hypsokinesis (hip″so-ki-ne′sis) [*hypso-* + Gr. *kinēsis* motion] a backward swaying, retropulsion, or falling when in erect posture, seen in cases of paralysis agitans and other forms of the amyostatic syndrome.

hypsonosus (hip-so′no-sus) [*hypso-* + Gr. *nosos* disease] mountain sickness; balloon sickness.

hypsotherapy (hip″so-ther′ah-pe) [*hypso-* + *therapy*] the therapeutic use of high altitude.

hypurgia (hi-pur′je-ah) [L.; Gr. *hypourgiai* medical services] the sum of the minor or subsidiary factors that make for recovery in any particular case.

hyrtenal (her′tĭ-nal) a terpene aldehyde, $(CH_3)_2C:C_6H_7 \cdot CHO$, from the tropical tree *Hernandia peltata.*

Hyrtl's loop (anastomosis), recess, sphincter (hēr′tlz) [Jozsef *Hyrtl,* eminent anatomist at Prague and Vienna, 1810–1894] see under *loop* and *sphincter,* and see *recessus epitympanicus.*

hysteralgia (his″tĕ-ral′je-ah) [*hystero-* + *-algia*] metralgia or metrodynia.

hysteratresia (his″ter-ah-tre′ze-ah) atresia of the uterus.

hysterectomy (his″tĕ-rek′to-me) [*hystero-* + Gr. *ektomē* excision] the operation of excising the uterus, performed either through the abdominal wall (*abdominal h.*) or through the vagina (*vaginal h.*). **abdominal h.,** excision of the uterus through an incision in the abdominal wall. **cesarean h.,** cesarean section followed by removal of the uterus. **chemical h.,** destruction of the endometrium by means of caustic chemicals. **complete h.,** total h. **partial h.,** subtotal h. **radical h.,** 1. Wertheim's operation (def. 1). 2. Schauta's operation. **subtotal h.,** hysterectomy in which the cervix is left in place. **supracervical h., supravaginal h.,** subtotal h. **total h.,** hysterectomy in which the uterus and cervix are completely excised; called also *panhysterectomy.* **vaginal h.,** excision of the uterus through the vagina.

hysteresis (his″tĕ-re′sis) [Gr. *hysterēsis* a lagging behind] a time lag in the occurrence of two associated phenomena, as between cause and effect. **protoplasmic h.,** a postulated cause of cell senescence: the colloidal state of the protoplasm is altered, becoming less dispersed, with loss of water and electrical charge.

hystereurynter (his″ter-u-rin′ter) [*hystero-* + Gr. *eurynein* to widen] an instrument for dilating the os uteri: a metreurynter.

hystereurysis (his″ter-u-rĭ-sis) dilatation of the os uteri.

hysteria (his-tēr′e-ah) [Gr. *hystera* uterus + *-ia*] a psychoneurosis, the symptoms of which are based on conversion and which is characterized by lack of control over acts and emotions, by morbid self-consciousness, by anxiety, by exaggeration of the effect of sensory impressions, and by simulation of various disorders. Symptoms may take the form of hyperesthesia; pain and tenderness in the region of the ovaries, spine, and head; anesthesia and other sensory disturbances; choking sensation; dimness of vision; paralysis; tonic spasms; convulsions; retention of urine; vasomotor disturbances; fever, hallucinations, and catalepsy. **anxiety h.,** hysteria showing conversion phenomena with recurring attacks of anxiety. **canine h.,** fright disease. **conver-**

sion h., see *hysterical neurosis,* under *neurosis.* **dissociative h.,** see *hysterical neurosis,* under *neurosis.* **fixation h.,** hysteria in which the symptoms are based on those of an organic disease, as the persistence of a nervous cough after pertussis. **h. ma′jor,** hysteria characterized by the sudden onset of dream states, stupors, and paralyses (described by Charcot). **h. mi′-nor,** hysteria with mild convulsions in which consciousness is not lost. **monosymptomatic h.,** hysteria which manifests itself by one symptom only.

hysteriac (his-tēr′e-ak) a person affected with hysteria.

hysteric (his-ter′ik) pertaining to or characterized by hysteria.

hysterical (his-ter′ĭ-kal) characterized by hysteria.

hystericism (his-ter′ĭ-sizm) a tendency toward hysteria.

hysterics (his-ter′iks) popular term for an uncontrollable emotional outburst.

hysteriform (his-ter′ĭ-form) having the appearance of hysteria.

hysterism (his′ter-izm) hysteria.

hystero- [Gr. *hystera* uterus] a combining form denoting relationship to the uterus, or to hysteria; see also *metro-.*

hysterobubonocele (his″ter-o-bu-bon′o-sēl) an inguinal hernia containing the uterus.

hysterocarcinoma (his″ter-o-kar″sĭ-no′mah) endometrial carcinoma.

hysterocatalepsy (his″ter-o-kat′ah-lep″se) hysteria with cataleptic symptoms.

hysterocele (his′ter-o-sēl″) [*hystero-* + Gr. *kēlē* hernia] hernia of the uterus.

hysterocleisis (his″ter-o-kli′sis) [*hystero-* + Gr. *kleisis* closure] surgical closure of the os uteri.

hysterocolpectomy (his″ter-o-kol-pek′to-me) [*hystero-* + Gr. *kolpos* vagina + *ektomē* excision] surgical removal of the uterus and vagina.

hysterocolposcope (his″ter-o-kol′po-skōp) [*hystero-* + Gr. *kolpos* vagina + *skopein* to examine] an electrically lighted device for viewing the interior of the uterus.

hysterocystic (his″ter-o-sis′tik) pertaining to the uterus and the bladder.

hysterocystocleisis (his″ter-o-sis″to-kli′sis) [*hystero-* + Gr. *kystis* bladder + *kleisis* closure] the operation of turning the cervix uteri into the bladder and suturing it; done for the relief of vesicouterovaginal fistula or for ureterouterine fistula. Called also *Bozeman's operation.*

hysterocystopexy (his″ter-o-sis′to-pek″se) [*hystero-* + Gr. *kystis* bladder + *pēxis* fixation] ventrovesicofixation.

hysterodynia (his″ter-o-din′e-ah) [*hystero-* + Gr. *odynē* pain] metralgia or metrodynia.

hysteroepilepsy (his″ter-o-ep′ĭ-lep″se) a severe type of hysteria with convulsions simulating those of epilepsy. At first there occur loss of consciousness and spasms, followed by a stage of violent spasmodic movements and mental disturbance, and finally a condition marked by delirium, erotic symptoms, etc.

hysteroepileptogenic (his″ter-o-ep″ĭ-lep″to-jen′ik) [*hysteroepilepsy* + Gr. *gennan* to produce] producing hysteroepilepsy.

hysteroerotic (his″ter-o-ĕ-rot′ik) pertaining to eroticism in hysteria.

hysterogenic (his″ter-o-jen′ik) [*hystero-* + Gr. *gennan* to produce] causing hysterical phenomena or symptoms.

hysterogram (his′ter-o-gram) a roentgenogram of the uterus.

hysterograph (his′ter-o-graf) [*hystero-* + Gr. *graphein* to record] an apparatus for measuring the strength of uterine contractions in labor.

hysterography (his″tĕ-rog′rah-fe) [*hystero-* + Gr. *graphein* to record] 1. graphic recording of the strength of uterine contractions in labor. 2. roentgenography of the uterus after instillation of a contrast medium. Called also *metrography* and *uterography.*

hysteroid (his′ter-oid) [*hystero-* + Gr. *eidos* form] resembling hysteria.

hysterolaparotomy (his″ter-o-lap″ah-rot′o-me) [*hystero-* + Gr. *lapara* flank + *tomē* a cutting] incision of the uterus through the abdominal wall.

hysterolith (his′ter-o-lith″) [*hystero-* + Gr. *lithos* stone] a uterine calculus.

hysterology (his″tĕ-rol′o-je) [*hystero-* + *-logy*] the sum of what is known regarding the uterus.

hysterolysis (his″tĕ-rol′ĭ-sis) [*hystero-* + Gr. *lysis* dissolution] the operation of loosening the uterus from its attachments or adhesions.

hysteromania (his″ter-o-ma′ne-ah) [*hystero-* + Gr. *mania* madness] 1. hysterical mania. 2. nymphomania.

hysterometer (his″tĕ-rom′ĕ-ter) [*hystero-* + Gr. *metron* measure] an instrument for measuring the uterus.

hysterometry (his″tĕ-rom′ĕ-tre) [*hystero-* + Gr. *metron* measure] the measurement of the dimensions of the uterus.

hysteromyoma (his″ter-o-mi-o′mah) uterine leiomyoma.

hysteromyomectomy (his″ter-o-mi″o-mek′to-me) [*hystero-* + *myoma* + Gr. *ektomē* excision] excision of a uterine leiomyoma.

hysteromyotomy (his″ter-o-mi-ot′o-me) [*hystero-* + Gr. *mys* muscle + *tomē* a cutting] incision of the uterus for the purpose of removing a solid tumor.

hysteronarcolepsy (his″ter-o-nar′ko-lep″se) narcolepsy caused by hysteria.

hysteroneurasthenia (his″ter-o-nu″ras-the′ne-ah) neurasthenia occurring in association with hysteria.

hysteropathy (his″tĕ-rop′ah-the) [*hystero-* + Gr. *pathos* disease] any uterine disease or disorder.

hysterope (his′ter-ōp) a person affected with hysteropia.

hysteropexia (his″ter-o-pek′se-ah) hysteropexy.

hysteropexy (his″ter-o-pek-se) [*hystero-* + Gr. *pēxis* fixation] the fixation of a displaced uterus by a surgical operation. It may be done by ventrofixation, shortening of the round ligaments, shortening of the sacrouterine ligaments, shortening of the endopelvic fascia (Manchester type operation). It is distinguished as *abdominal* or *vaginal*, according as the uterus is fastened to the abdominal wall or to the vagina.

hysteropia (his″ter-o′pe-ah) [*hystero-* + Gr. *ōps* eye] hysteric disorder of the vision.

hysteroptosia (his″ter-op-to′ze-ah) metroptosis.

hysteroptosis (his″ter-op-to′sis) metroptosis.

hysterorrhaphy (his-ter-or′ah-fe) [*hystero-* + Gr. *rhaphē* suture] 1. hysteropexy. 2. the operation of suturing of the lacerated uterus.

hysterorrhexis (his″ter-o-rek′sis) metrorrhexis.

hysterosalpingectomy (his″ter-o-sal″pin-jek′to-me) [*hystero-* + Gr. *salpinx* tube + *ektomē* excision] excision of the uterus and uterine tubes.

hysterosalpingography (his″ter-o-sal″ping-gog′rah-fe) [*hystero-* + Gr. *salpinx* tube + *graphein* to record] roentgenography of the uterus and uterine tubes after the injection of opaque material. Called also *uterosalpingography, uterotubography, hysterotubography, metrosalpingography, metrotubography.*

hysterosalpingo-oophorectomy (his″ter-o-sal-ping″go-o″of-o-rek′to-me) excision of the uterus, uterine tubes, and ovaries.

hysterosalpingostomy (his″ter-o-sal″ping-gos′to-me) [*hystero-* + Gr. *salpinx* tube + *stomoun* to provide with an opening, or mouth] the operation of forming an anastomosis between the uterus and the distal portion of the uterine tube after excision of a strictured or obstructed portion of the tube.

hysteroscope (his′ter-o-skōp″) [*hystero-* + Gr. *skopein* to examine] an endoscope used in direct visual examination of the canal of the uterine cervix and the cavity of the uterus.

hysteroscopy (his″ter-os′ko-pe) inspection of the uterus.

hysterospasm (his′ter-o-spazm″) spasm of the uterus.

hysterostat (his′ter-o-stat) [*hystero-* + Gr. *statikos* stopping] a mechanical intrauterine device for holding sealed sources of ionizing radiation (radium, cesium-137, etc.) in order to give planned patterns of irradiation.

hysterostomatocleisis (his″ter-o-sto″mah-to-kli′sis) [*hystero-* + Gr. *stoma* mouth + *kleisis* closure] an operation for vesicovaginal fistula consisting of closure of the cervical canal and conversion of the vesical and uterine cavities into one common cavity by means of an opening between them.

hysterostomatome (his″ter-o-sto′mah-tōm) a knife used in hysterostomatomy.

hysterostomatomy (his″ter-o-sto-mat′o-me) [*hystero-* + Gr. *stoma* mouth + *temnein* to cut] incision of the os or cervix uteri. See *Dührssen's incision,* under *incision.*

hysterosyphilis (his″ter-o-sif′ĭ-lis) a hysterical neurosis due to syphilitic disease.

hysterotabetism (his″ter-o-ta′bĕ-tizm) combined hysteria and tabes.

hysterothermometry (his″ter-o-ther-mom′ĕ-tre) uterothermometry.

hysterotome (his″ter-o-tōm) [*hystero-* + Gr. *tomē* a cutting] an instrument for incising the uterus.

hysterotomy (his″ter-ot′o-me) [*hystero-* + Gr. *temnein* to cut] incision of the uterus. **abdominal h.,** incision of the uterus through the wall of the abdomen. **vaginal h.,** incision of the uterus through the vagina.

hysterotrachelectasia (his″ter-o-tra″kel-ek-ta′se-ah) surgical dilation of the cervix and uterus.

hysterotrachelectomy (his″ter-o-tra″kel-ek′to-me) amputation of the cervix uteri; trachelectomy.

hysterotracheloplasty (his″ter-o-tra″kel-o-plas″te) plastic repair of the cervix uteri; tracheloplasty.

hysterotrachelorrhaphy (his″ter-o-tra″kel-or′ah-fe) [*hystero-* + Gr. *trachelos* neck + *rhaphē* suture] the operation of suturing the cervix uteri.

hysterotrachelotomy (his″ter-o-tra″kel-ot′o-me) [*hystero-* + Gr. *trachelos* neck + *tomē* a cutting] incision of the cervix uteri.

hysterotraumatic (his″ter-o-traw-mat′ik) [*hystero-* + Gr. *trauma* wound] pertaining to or associated with hysterotraumatism.

hysterotraumatism (his″ter-o-traw′mah-tizm) hysteric symptoms following traumatism.

hysterotubography (his″ter-o-tu-bog′rah-fe) hysterosalpingography.

hysterovagino-enterocele (his″ter-o-vaj″ĭ-no-en′ter-o-sēl) [*hystero-* + *vagina* + Gr. *enteron* intestine + *kēlē* hernia] hernia containing the uterus, vagina, and intestine.

Hytakerol (hi-tak′er-ol) trademark for preparations of dihydrotachysterol.

Hyzyd (hiz′id) trademark for a preparation of isoniazid.

Hz hertz.

I

I chemical symbol for *iodine.*

131I, I 131 chemical symbol for the radioactive isotope of iodine of atomic mass 131 and a half-life of 8.07 days; formerly written I^{131}.

132I, I 132 chemical symbol for the radioactive isotope of iodine of atomic mass 132 and a half-life of 2.4 hours; formerly written I^{132}.

i. optically inactive; said of chemical substances incapable of rotating the plane of polarized light.

I.A. impedance angle.

-ia a word termination indicating state or condition.

IAEA International Atomic Energy Agency.

I.A.G.P. International Association of Geographic Pathology.

I.A.G.U.S. International Association of Genito-Urinary Surgeons.

iamatology (i″am-ah-tol′o-je) [Gr. *iama, iamatos* remedy + *-logy*] the study or science of remedies.

I.A.M.M. International Association of Medical Museums.

ianthinopsia (i-an″thĭ-nop′se-ah) [Gr. *ianthinos* violet + *opsis* vision] violet vision; a condition in which objects seem to be violet colored.

I.A.P.B. International Association for Prevention of Blindness.

I.A.P.P. International Association for Preventive Pediatrics.

-iasis (i′ah-sis) a word termination meaning a process or the condition resulting therefrom, particularly a morbid condition. See *-sis.*

iathergy (i-ath′er-je) [Gr. *iathēnai* to have been cured + *ergon* work] the state of immunity existing in an immunized individual in whom the tuberculin skin sensitivity has been abolished by specific desensitization.

iatraliptic (i″ah-trah-lip′tik) [Gr. *iatreia* cure + *aleiphein* to anoint] pertaining to the application of remedies by inunction and friction.

iatraliptics (i″ah-trah-lip′tiks) treatment by inunction and friction.

iatrarchy (i′ah-trar″ke) [Gr. *iatros* physician + *archē* rule] government by physicians.

iatreusiology (i″ah-troo″se-ol′o-je) [Gr. *iatreusis* treatment + *-logy*] the science of treatment; therapeutics.

iatreusis (i″ah-troo′sis) [Gr.] treatment.

iatric (i-at′rik) [Gr. *iatrikos*] pertaining to medicine or to a physician.

iatro- [Gr. *iatros* physician] a combining form denoting relationship to a physician or to medicine.

Iatrobdella (i″at-ro-del′ah) (obs.) *Hirudo.*

iatrochemical (i-at″ro-kem′ĕ-kal) pertaining to iatrochemistry.

iatrochemist (i-at″ro-kem′ist) a person belonging to the school of iatrochemistry.

iatrochemistry (i-at″ro-kem′is-tre) [*iatro-* + *chemistry*] the name of a school of medicine of the 17th century, which espoused the theory that all the phenomena of life and disease are based on chemical action.

iatrogenesis (i-at″ro-jen′ĕ-sis) [*iatro-* + Gr. *genesis* production] the creation of additional problems or complications resulting from treatment by a physician or surgeon.

iatrogenic (i-at″ro-jen′ik) [*iatro-* + Gr. *gennan* to produce] resulting from the activity of physicians. Originally applied to disorders induced in the patient by autosuggestion based on the physician's examination, manner, or discussion, the term is now applied to any adverse condition in a patient occurring as the result of treatment by a physician or surgeon.

iatrology (i″ah-trol′o-je) [*iatro-* + *-logy*] the science of medicine.

iatromathematical (i-at″ro-math″ĕ-mat′ĭ-kal) iatrophysical.

iatromechanical (i-at″ro-mĕ-kan′ĭ-kal) iatrophysical.

iatrophysical (i-at″ro-fiz′ĭ-kal) the name of a school of medicine in the 17th century which held that all the phenomena of life and disease are based on the laws of physics.

iatrophysicist (i-at″ro-fiz′ĭ-sist) a person belonging to the iatrophysical school.

iatrophysics (i-at″ro-fiz′iks) [*iatro-* + Gr. *physikos* natural]. 1. the physics of medicine or of medical and surgical treatment. 2. the treatment of diseases by physical or mechanical means; physiatrics.

iatrotechnics (i-at″ro-tek′niks) [*iatro-* + Gr. *technē* art] the techniques of medical and surgical practice.

iatrotechnique (i-at″ro-tek-nēk′) iatrotechnics.

I.B. inclusion body.

Ibn Rushd see *Averroes*.

Ibn Sinā see *Avicenna*.

Ibn Zuhr see *Avenzoar*.

ibogaine (i-bo′gah-ēn) an alkaloid, $C_{20}H_{26}N_2O$, from the root of *Tabernanthe iboga* Baill. (Apocynaceae) that has antidepressant and euphoric properties; it is isomeric with tabernanthine.

ibufenac (i-bu′fĕ-nak) chemical name: 4-(2-methylpropyl)benzeneacetic acid; an analgesic and anti-inflammatory, $C_{13}H_{18}O_2$, formerly used in the treatment of rheumatic conditions.

ibuprofen (i-bu′pro-fen) chemical name: α-methyl-4-(2-methylpropyl)benzeneacetic acid. An anti-inflammatory agent, $C_{13}H_{18}O_2$, also having analgesic and antipyretic actions; used in the treatment of rheumatoid arthritis and osteoarthritis, administered orally.

IC inspiratory capacity; irritable colon.

ICD International Classification of Diseases (of the World Health Organization); intrauterine contraceptive device.

ice (īs) any of the six solid forms of water; but usually the common low-density form melting at 0° C. at 1 atmosphere. **Dry I.,** trademark for carbon dioxide snow.

Iceland disease (īs′land) benign myalgic encephalomyelitis.

Iceland moss (īs′land maws′) see under *moss*.

ichnogram (ik′no-gram) [Gr. *ichnos* a footprint + *gramma* mark] a footprint, in ink on paper.

ichor (i′kor) [Gr. *ichōr*] a thin, serous, or sanious fluid from a sore or wound.

ichoremia (i″kor-e′me-ah) [*ichor* + Gr. *haima* blood + *-ia*] septicemia.

ichoroid (i′ko-roid) [*ichor* + Gr. *eidos* form] resembling ichor or pus.

ichorous (i′kor-us) of the nature of a serum or ichor.

ichorrhea (i-ko-re′ah) [*ichor* + Gr. *rhoia* flow] a copious discharge of ichorous fluid or sanies.

ichorrhemia (i″ko-re′me-ah) [*ichor* + Gr. *haima* blood + *-ia*] septicemia.

ichthammol (ik′tham-mol) [USP] a reddish brown to brownish black viscous fluid, with a strong, characteristic odor, obtained by the destructive distillation of certain bituminous schists, sulfonation of the distillate, and neutralization of the product with ammonia; used as a local skin anti-infective. Called also *ammonium ichthyosulfonate* and *ammonium sulfoichthyolate*.

ichthyism (ik′the-izm) ichthyismus.

ichthyismus (ik″the-iz′mus) [Gr. *ichthys* fish] ichthyotoxism.

ichthyo- (ik′the-o) [Gr. *ichthys* fish] a combining form denoting relationship to fish.

ichthyoacanthotoxin (ik″the-o-ah-kan″tho-tok′sin) [*ichthyo-* + Gr. *akantha* thorn + *toxikon* poison] the venom secreted by venomous fishes, in connection with stings, spines, or "teeth."

ichthyoacanthotoxism (ik″the-o-ah-kan″tho-tok′sizm) intoxication resulting from injuries produced by the stings, spines, or "teeth" of venomous fishes.

ichthyocolla (ik″the-o-kol′ah) [*ichthyo-* + Gr. *kolla* glue] a form of gelatin prepared from the swimming-bladders of the Russian sturgeon, *Acipenser huso;* used as an adhesive and clarifying agent. Called also *isinglass*.

ichthyohemotoxin (ik″the-o-he″mo-tok′sin) [*ichthyo-* + Gr. *haima* blood + *toxikon* poison] a toxic substance found in the blood of certain fish.

ichthyohemotoxism (ik″the-o-he″mo-tok′sizm) intoxication

caused by the ingestion of ichthyohemotoxin, characterized by gastrointestinal and neurological disturbances.

ichthyoid (ik′the-oid) [*ichthyo-* + Gr. *eidos* form] resembling a fish; shaped like a fish.

Ichthyol (ik′the-ol) trademark for a preparation of ichthammol.

ichthyology (ik″the-ol′o-je) that branch of zoology specializing in study of fishes.

ichthyolsulfonate (ik″the-ol-sul′fo-nāt) a salt of ichthyolsulfonic acid, a derivative of ichthammol.

ichthyootoxin (ik″the-o″o-tok′sin) [*ichthyo-* + Gr. *ōon* egg + *toxikon* poison] a toxic substance derived from the roe of certain fish; see also *ichthyootoxism*.

ichthyootoxism (ik″the-o″o-tok′sizm) intoxication caused by the ingestion of toxic fish roe, characterized by gastrointestinal and neurological disturbances.

ichthyophagia (ik″the-o-fa′je-ah) [*ichthyo-* + Gr. *phagein* to eat + *-ia*] the practice of subsisting on fish.

ichthyophagous (ik″the-of′ah-gus) eating or subsisting on fish.

Ichthyophthirius multifiliis (ik″the-o-thir′e-us mul″ti-fil′e-is) a ciliate protozoon of the subclass Euciliatia that produces lesions in the skin of fresh-water fish, often resulting in death.

ichthyosarcotoxin (ik″the-o-sar″ko-tok′sin) [*ichthyo-* + Gr. *sarx, sarkos* flesh + *toxikon* poison] the poison found in the flesh of poisonous fishes, excluding toxins which may result from bacterial contamination.

ichthyosarcotoxism (ik″the-o-sar″ko-tok′sizm) fish poisoning; intoxication characterized by various gastrointestinal and neurological disturbances, resulting from the ingestion of the flesh of poisonous fishes, excluding ordinary bacterial food poisoning. See, for example, *ciguatera, elasmobranch, gymnothorax,* and *scombroid poisoning,* under *poisoning.*

ichthyosiform (ik″the-o′sĭ-form) resembling ichthyosis.

ichthyosis (ik″the-o′sis) [*ichthyo-* + *-osis*] any of several generalized skin disorders characterized by dryness, roughness, and scaliness, due to hypertrophy of the horny layer, occurring as a result of excessive production or excessive retention of keratin, or a molecular defect in the keratin. Commonly used alone to refer to *i. vulgaris.* **i. congen′ita,** lamella exfoliation of the newborn (see under *exfoliation*). **i. feta′lis,** lamellar exfoliation of the newborn (see under *exfoliation*). **i. hys′trix, i. hys′trix gra′vior,** a rare form of epidermolytic hyperkeratosis, characterized by generalized, dark brown, linear verrucoid ridges somewhat like *porcupine skin.* The linear verrucous lesions of ichthyosis hystrix must be differentiated from linear verrucous nevi. **lamellar i.,** a hereditary disease transmitted as an autosomal recessive trait, present at birth or soon thereafter, and characterized by diffuse erythema and large, quadrilateral, grayish brown scales; it may be associated with small stature, oligophrenia, spastic paralysis, hypoplasia of the genitals, hypotrichia, and shortened life-span. Formerly called *nonbullous congenital ichthyosiform erythroderma.* **lamellar i. of the newborn,** see under *exfoliation.* **linear i.,** linear verrucous epidermal nevus. **i. lin′guae,** leukoplakia. **nacreous i.** (*obs.*), a form marked by pearly scales. **i. palma′ris, i. palma′ris et planta′ris, i. planta′ris,** keratosis palmaris et plantaris. **i. sauroder′ma,** lamellar exfoliation of the newborn persisting into childhood, in which the skin is covered with thick plates somewhat like the skin of a crocodile; called also *alligator* or *crocodile skin.* **i. sim′plex,** i. vulgaris. **i. u′teri,** a condition marked by the transformation of the columnar epithelium of the endometrium into stratified squamous epithelium. **i. vulga′ris,** a hereditary form of ichthyosis transmitted as an autosomal dominant or sex-linked recessive trait. The *autosomal dominant form* usually appears after three months of age and rarely involves the flexural surfaces. The *sex-linked form* may be present at birth or appear shortly thereafter, and is marked by large, thick, dry scales on the neck, scalp, ears, face, and flexures of the antecubital, popliteal, and axillary fossae. Called also *i. simplex.*

ichthyotic (ik″the-ot′ik) pertaining to or characterized by ichthyosis.

ichthyotoxic (ik″the-o-tok′sik) caused by the toxic principle of fish.

ichthyotoxicology (ik″the-o-tok″sĭ-kol′o-je) [*ichthyo-* + Gr. *toxikon* poison + *-logy*] the science of poisons derived from certain fish, their cause, detection, and effects, and the treatment of conditions produced by them.

ichthyotoxicum (ik″the-o-tok′sĭ-kum) [*ichthyo-* + Gr. *toxikon* poison] an obsolete term proposed (1889) to designate a toxic substance found in eel serum.

ichthyotoxin (ik″the-o-tok′sin) [*ichthyo-* + *toxin*] a general term applied to any type of toxic substance derived from fish.

ichthyotoxism (ik″the-o-tok′sizm) [*ichthyo-* + *toxin* + *-ism*] a general term applied to intoxication caused by any toxic substance derived from fish.

I.C.N. International Council of Nurses.

I.C.R.P. International Commission on Radiological Protection.

I.C.R.U. International Commission on Radiological Units and Measurements.

I.C.S. International College of Surgeons.

ICSH interstitial cell–stimulating hormone (luteinizing hormone).

I.C.T. inflammation of connective tissue; insulin coma therapy.

ictal (ik′tal) [L. *ictus* stroke] pertaining to, characterized by, or caused by a stroke or an acute epileptic seizure.

icterepatitis (ik″ter-ep″ah-ti′tis) icterohepatitis.

icteric (ik-ter′ik) pertaining to or affected with jaundice.

icteritious (ik″ter-ish′us) icteric.

ictero- [L. *icterus;* Gr. *ikteros*] a combining form meaning affected with or pertaining to jaundice.

icteroanemia (ik″ter-o-ah-ne′me-ah) a disease marked by the development of icterus and anemia, with splenic enlargement, urobilinuria, and a hemolysis associated with fragility of the red blood corpuscles. Called also *hemolytic icteroanemia* and *Widal's syndrome.*

icterogenic (ik″ter-o-jen′ik) [*icterus* + Gr. *gennan* to produce] causing icterus.

icterogenicity (ik″ter-o-jĕ-nis′ĭ-te) ability to cause icterus.

icterohematuria (ik″ter-o-hem″ah-tu′re-ah) jaundice associated with hematuria. **i. of sheep,** a form caused by *Babesia ovis,* which is transmitted by *Rhipicephalus bursa.*

icterohematuric (ik″ter-o-hem″ah-tu′rik) pertaining to icterohematuria; marked by jaundice and hematuria.

icterohemoglobinuria (ik″ter-o-he″mo-glo″bĭ-nu′re-ah) combined jaundice and hemoglobinuria.

icterohepatitis (ik″ter-o-hep″ah-ti′tis) inflammation of the liver with marked jaundice.

icteroid (ik′ter-oid) [*icterus* + Gr. *eidos* form] resembling jaundice.

icterus (ik′ter-us) [L.; Gr. *ikteros*] jaundice. **i. castren′sis gra′vis** (*obs.*), leptospiral jaundice. **chronic familial i.,** hereditary spherocytosis. **congenital familial i.,** hereditary spherocytosis. **congenital hemolytic i.,** hereditary spherocytosis. **epidemic catarrhal i.,** a mild form of leptospiral jaundice. **i. gra′vis,** acute yellow atrophy; see under *atrophy.* **i. gra′vis neonato′rum,** severe jaundice in the newborn, usually a form of isoimmunization with Rh factor; called also *erythroleukoblastosis.* See also *kernicterus.* **i. infectio′sus,** leptospiral jaundice. **i. me′las** ["black jaundice"] (*obs.*), Winckel's disease. **i. neonato′rum,** the jaundice sometimes seen in newborn children. **nuclear i.,** kernicterus. **i. prae′cox,** mild jaundice developing within the first 24 hours of life (before physiologic jaundice normally occurs), due to incompatibility of the ABO blood group system between mother and infant; it usually clears rapidly and spontaneously, only occasionally resulting in hemolytic disease. **spirochetal i.,** leptospiral jaundice. **i. typhoi′des,** acute yellow atrophy; see under *atrophy.*

ictus (ik′tus), pl. *ic′tus* [L. "stroke"] a seizure, stroke, blow, or sudden attack; see also *seizure.* **i. cor′dis,** the heart beat. **i. epilep′ticus,** an epileptic attack. **i. immunisato′rius,** the injection of a large quantity of bacteria, toxin, or other antigen for the purpose of inducing the formation of a large quantity of antibody. **i. paralyt′icus,** a paralytic stroke. **i. san′guinis,** stroke due to cerebral hemorrhage. **i. so′lis,** a sunstroke.

ICU intensive care unit.

ID intradermal; inside diameter.

I.D. infective dose.

ID₅₀ median infective dose, being that amount of pathogenic microorganisms which will produce infection in 50 per cent of the test subjects.

Id. abbreviation for L. *i′dem,* the same.

id (id) [Gr. *idios* own, peculiar] 1. Freud's term for the self-preservative tendencies and the instincts as a totality; the true unconscious. It is the reservoir of instinctive impulses and is dominated by the pleasure principle. 2. a rash associated with but remote from the main lesion of the disease, and considered to be an allergic reaction following cutaneous sensitization to the causative agent of the disease. Often used as a word termination in combination with a root representing the causative factor, as syphilid, dermatophytid, etc. 3. see *biophore.*

-id (id) 1. [Gr. *eidos* form, shape] a word termination meaning having the shape of, or resembling. 2. see *id,* def. 2.

idant (i′dant) see *biophore.*

-ide a suffix signifying a binary chemical compound, such as a chloride, sulfide, or carbide.

Ide test (reaction) [Sobei *Ide;* Tamao *Ide,* physicians in Tokyo] see under *tests.*

idea (i-de′ah) [Gr. "form"] a mental impression or conception. **autochthonous i.,** an idea which comes into the mind in some unaccountable way, independently of trains of thought, and which is strange, but cannot be accounted for by a hallucination. **compulsive i.,** an idea which intrudes, recurs, and persists despite reason and will, and which impels toward some inappropri-ate act. **dominant i.,** a morbid or other impression that controls or colors every action and thought. **fixed i.,** a morbid impression or belief which stays in the mind and cannot be changed by reason; called also *idée fixe.* **hyperquantivalent i.** (*obs.*), an idea which has become of the utmost importance to the patient, absorbing his thought, and excluding anything which might tend to discredit its truth. **imperative i.,** compulsive i. **i. of reference, referential i.,** the assumption by a patient that the words and actions of others refer to himself or the projection of the causes of his own imaginary difficulties upon someone else; called also *delusion of reference.*

ideal (i-de′al) having some relation to ideas, impressions, or imaginations. **ego i.,** the standard of perfection unconsciously created by an individual for himself.

idealization (i-de″al-i-za′shun) a conscious or unconscious mental mechanism in which the individual overestimates an admired aspect or attribute of another person.

ideation (i″de-a′shun) the distinct mental presentation of objects.

ideational (i″de-a′shun-al) relating to ideation or the formation of objects and images in the mind.

idée (e-da′) [Fr.] idea. **i. fixe** (e-da′fēks′), fixed idea.

identification (i-den″tĭ-fi-ka′shun) a mental mechanism of the unconscious by which the ego attaches or transfers to itself qualities or properties belonging to other persons or objects. **cosmic i.,** identification of one's self with the universe, as in schizophrenic delusions of omnipotence.

identity (i-den′tĭ-te) the aggregate of characteristics by which an individual is recognized by himself and others. **core gender i.,** gender i. **ego i.,** a sense of unity and continuity of one's own personality. **gender i.,** a person's concept of himself as being male and masculine or female and feminine, or ambivalent, usually based on the physical characteristics, parental attitudes and expectations, and psychological and social pressures to which the individual is subjected. It is the private experience of gender role. Cf. *gender role,* under *role.*

ideodynamism (i-de″o-di′nah-mizm) [*idea* + Gr. *dynamis* power] the stimulation, through the cerebral cells, by an idea, of those nerve fibers which are to realize that idea.

ideogenetic (i″de-o-jĕ-net′ik) induced by or related to vague sense impressions rather than organized images.

ideogenous (i″de-oj′ĕ-nus) ideogenetic.

ideoglandular (i″de-o-glan′du-lar) arousing glandular activity as a result of some recollection or thought.

ideokinetic (i-de″o-ki-net′ik) ideomotor.

ideology (i″de-ol′o-je, id″e-ol′o-je) [Gr. *idea* + *-logy*] 1. the science of the development of ideas. 2. the body of ideas characteristic of an individual or of a social unit.

ideometabolic (i″de-o-met-ah-bol′ik) producing metabolic activity as a result of mental action, normal or other.

ideometabolism (i″de-o-mĕ-tab′o-lizm) metabolism produced by mental influence.

ideomotion (i″de-o-mo′shun) motion or muscular action which is neither reflex nor volitional, but is induced by some dominant idea.

ideomotor (i″de-o-mo′tor) aroused by an idea or thought; said of involuntary motion so aroused.

ideomuscular (i″de-o-mus′ku-lar) producing involuntary muscular action as a result of some ideation, memory, or hallucination.

ideophrenia (i″de-o-fre′ne-ah) a morbid mental state characterized by marked perversion of ideas.

ideophrenic (i″de-o-fren′ik) pertaining to or exhibiting ideophrenia.

ideoplastia (i″de-o-plas′te-ah) [*idea* + Gr. *plassein* to form] (*obs.*) the passive inert condition of a patient under complete hypnosis in which he is capable of receiving suggestions of ideas from the hypnotist.

ideovascular (i″de-o-vas′ku-lar) producing vascular change as a result of some ideation, memory, or hallucination.

idio- (id′e-o) [Gr. *idios* own, peculiar] a combining form denoting relationship to self or to one's own, or to something separate and distinct.

idioagglutinin (id″e-o-ah-gloo′tĭ-nin) [*idio-* + *agglutinin*] an agglutinin that originates independently of any transfer or artifical means in the animal in which it is formed.

idioblapsis (id″e-o-blap′sis) [*idio-* + Gr. *blapsis* a harming, damage] Coca's name for a nonreaginic food allergy in which (1) the hereditary influence controlling it is independent of atopic inheritance, (2) allergic antibodies are not demonstrable, (3) many symptoms are not represented in the atopic group, and (4) the allergic reaction practically always causes acceleration of the pulse.

idioblaptic (id″e-o-blap′tik) [*idio-* + Gr. *blastikos* hurtful] pertaining to or characterized by idioblapsis.

idioblast (id′e-o-blast) [*idio-* + Gr. *blastos* germ] any one of the hypothetical ultimate units of a cell; a biophore.

idiochromatin (id″e-o-kro′mah-tin) [*idio-* + *chromatin*] chromatin concerned in reproduction; the chromatin bearing the ids (see *biophore*).

idiochromidia (id″e-o-kro-mid′e-ah) [*idio-* + . *chromidia*] that part of the chromidia or extranuclear chromatin which takes part in the reproduction of the cell. Cf. *trophochromidia*.

idiochromosome (id″e-o-kro′mo-sōm) any sex chromosome.

idiocrasy (id″e-ok′rah-se) idiosyncrasy.

idiocratic (id″e-o-krat′ik) idiosyncratic.

idiocy (id′e-o-se) severe mental retardation; a former category of mental retardation, which comprised individuals having an IQ of less than 25. See *mental retardation*, under *retardation*. Cf. *imbecility* and *moronity*. **absolute i.,** profound i. **amaurotic familial i.,** former name for cerebral sphingolipidosis; see under *sphingolipidosis*. **athetosic i.,** athetosis. **Aztec i.,** microcephalic i. **cretinoid i.,** cretinism. **developmental i.,** severe mental retardation due to arrest of brain development. **eclamptic i.,** severe mental retardation associated with convulsions. **epileptic i.,** severe mental retardation combined with epilepsy. **erethistic i.,** severe mental retardation associated with activity and restlessness. **genetous i.,** severe mental retardation dating from fetal life. **hemiplegic i.,** severe mental retardation combined with hemiplegia. **hydrocephalic i.,** severe mental retardation combined with chronic hydrocephalus. **intrasocial i.,** severe mental retardation in which the patient is capable of performing some regular occupation. **Kalmuk i.,** mongolian i. **microcephalic i.,** severe mental retardation associated with microcephaly; called also *Aztec i.* or *type,* and *bird's head type.* **mongolian i.,** a name formerly applied to the marked mental retardation associated with *Down's syndrome;* called also *Kalmuck (Kalmuk) i.* or *type.* **moral i.,** an absence of moral sense. **paralytic i.,** severe mental retardation combined with paralysis. **paraplegic i.,** severe mental retardation associated with paraplegia. **plagiocephalic i.,** severe mental retardation associated with plagiocephaly. **profound i.,** the severest form of mental retardation, usually associated with small size and physical abnormality; called also *absolute i.* **scaphocephalic i.,** severe mental retardation associated with scaphocephaly. **sensorial i.,** severe mental retardation associated with early loss of any of the special senses. **spastic amaurotic axonal i.,** infantile neuroaxonal dystrophy. **torpid i.,** severe mental retardation associated with inactivity and dullness. **traumatic i.,** severe mental retardation that results from an injury received at birth or in infancy. **xerodermic i.,** DeSanctis-Cacchione syndrome.

idiogamist (id″e-og′ah-mist) [*idio-* + Gr. *gamos* marriage] (*obs.*) a person who is capable of coitus with only one particular woman, or with only a few selected ones, being impotent with all others.

idiogenesis (id″e-o-jen′ĕ-sis) [*idio-* + Gr. *genesis* production] the spontaneous origin of disease.

idioglossia (id″e-o-glos′e-ah) [*idio-* + Gr. *glōssa* tongue + *-ia*] imperfect articulation, with the utterance of meaningless vocal sounds.

idioglottic (id″e-o-glot′ik) pertaining to idioglossia.

idiogram (id′e-o-gram″) [*idio-* + *-gram*] a diagrammatic representation of a chromosome complement, based on measurement of the chromosomes of a number of cells. Cf. *karyotype*.

idioheteroagglutinin (id″e-o-het″er-o-ah-gloo′tĭ-nin) [*idio-* + Gr. *heteros* other + *agglutinin*] a heteroagglutinin normally present in the blood.

idioheterolysin (id″e-o-het-er-ol′ĭ-sin) a heterolysin normally present in the blood.

idiohypnotism (id″e-o-hip′no-tizm) [*idio-* + *hypnotism*] spontaneous or self-induced hypnotism.

idio-imbecile (id″e-o-im′bĕ-sil) a grade of mental deficiency between idiot and imbecile.

idioisoagglutinin (id″e-o-i″so-ah-gloo′tĭ-nin) an isoagglutinin normally present in the blood, and not produced artificially.

idioisolysin (id″e-o-i-sol′ĭ-sin) a lysin normally present which lyses the cells of other members of the same species as the animal in which it is formed.

idiolalia (id″e-o-la′le-ah) a condition marked by the use of invented language.

idiolog (id′e-o-log) a word that has meaning only to the user.

idiologism (id″e-ol′o-jizm) the utterance of words that are meaningless to anyone but the speaker.

idiolysin (id″e-ol′ĭ-sin) [*idio-* + *lysin*] a lysin, normally present in the blood and not produced by artificial means, that lyses the cells of the animal in which it is formed.

idiomere (id′e-o-mēr) chromomere (def. 1).

idiomuscular (id″e-o-mus′ku-lar) [*idio-* + L. *musculus* muscle] pertaining to the muscular tissue apart from any nerve stimulus; a term applied to certain muscular contractions which occur in degenerated muscles only.

idioneurosis (id″e-o-nu-ro′sis) [*idio-* + Gr. *neuron* nerve] (*obs.*) any neurosis arising from the nerves themselves; an idiopathic neurosis.

idiopathetic (id″e-o-pah-thet′ik) idiopathic.

idiopathic (id″e-o-path′ik) of the nature of an idiopathy; self-originated; of unknown causation.

idiopathy (id″e-op′ah-the) [*idio-* + Gr. *pathos* disease] a morbid state of spontaneous origin; one neither sympathetic nor traumatic. **toxic i.,** any one of a group of diseases due to hypersensitivity to particular proteins, and including asthma, hay fever, urticaria, angioneurotic edema, and some forms of eczema and gastrointestinal disorder.

idiophore (id′e-o-fōr) [*idio-* + Gr. *pherein* to bear] the (theoretical) primary form of living cell substance.

idioplasm (id′e-o-plazm″) [*idio-* + Gr. *plasma* anything formed] germ plasm.

idiopsychologic (id″e-o-si″ko-loj′ik) pertaining to ideas formed within one's own mind.

idioreflex (id″e-o-re′fleks) [*idio-* + *reflex*] a reflex brought about by a cause within the same organ.

idioretinal (id″e-o-ret′ĭ-nal) pertaining to the retina alone; a term applied to a visual sensation occurring without any visual stimulus.

idiosome (id′e-o-sōm″) [*idio-* + Gr. *sōma* body] 1. a supposed ultimate element of living matter. 2. the centrosome of a spermatocyte, together with surrounding Golgi apparatus and mitochondria.

idiospasm (id′e-o-spazm) a spasm of a limited area or region.

idiosyncrasy (id″e-o-sin′krah-se) [*idio-* + Gr. *synkrasis* mixture] 1. a habit or quality of body or mind peculiar to any individual. 2. an abnormal susceptibility to some drug, protein, or other agent which is peculiar to the individual.

idiosyncratic (id″e-o-sin-krat′ik) pertaining to or characterized by idiosyncrasy.

idiot (id′e-ot) [Gr. *idiōtēs* one in private station, ignoramus] a person without intellect and understanding; a former name for a mentally retarded person of the lowest order, i.e., having an IQ of less than 25. See *mental retardation*, under *retardation*. Cf. *imbecile* and *moron*. **erethistic i.,** see under *idiocy*. **mongolian i.,** former name for a person affected with Down's syndrome. **profound i.,** see under *idiocy*. **i.-savant** (e-joo′sah-vaht) [Fr. "learned idiot"], a person who is severely mentally retarded in some respects, yet has a particular mental faculty that is developed to an unusually high degree, as memory, mathematics, or music. **torpid i.,** see under *idiocy*.

idiotope (id′ĭ-o-tōp″) a site on the variable portion of an antibody molecule that can be recognized by a combining site of other antibodies.

idiotopy (id′e-o-top″e) [*idio-* + Gr. *topos* place] the position and relation of the parts of an organ among themselves.

idiotoxin (id″e-o-tok′sin) allergen; atopen; an antigen that elicits an allergic reaction.

idiotrophic (id″e-o-trof′ik) [*idio-* + Gr. *trophē* nutrition] capable of selecting its own nourishment.

idiotropic (id″e-o-trop′ik) [*idio-* + Gr. *tropos* a turning] a term applied to the type of personality which is satisfied with its own inner intellectual and emotional experiences.

idiot-savant see under *idiot*.

idiotype (id′e-o-tīp) an antigenic determinant present on and characteristic of a certain antibody molecule, usually located in the variable (combining site) region. Idiotypic markers or determinants distinguish among antibody molecules, even those of the same isotype and allotype.

idiovariation (id″e-o-var″e-a′shun) a mutation or change in the germ plasm, the cause of which is unknown.

idioventricular (id″e-o-ven-trik′u-lar) relating to or affecting the cardiac ventricle alone, as idioventricular rhythm.

idiozome (id′e-o-zōm) idiosome.

iditol (i′dĭ-tol) a hexahydric alcohol, $CH_2OH(CHOH)_4CH_2OH$, a reduction product of the hexose known as idose.

idose (i′dōs) an aldohexose.

idoxuridine (i-doks-ur′ĭ-dēn) [USP] chemical name: 2′-deoxy-5-iodouridine. An analog of pyrimidine, $C_9H_{11}IN_2O_5$, occurring as a white crystalline powder, which inhibits viral DNA synthesis; used as an antiviral agent in the treatment of herpes simplex keratitis, applied topically to the conjunctiva. Abbreviated IDU.

IDU idoxuridine.

IE immunoelectrophoresis.

I.E. abbreviation for Ger. *immunitäts Einheit* (immunizing unit); see *antitoxin unit*, under *unit*.

I-em-hotep Imhotep.

ifosfamide (i-fos′fah-mīd) chemical name: *N*,3-bis(2-chloroethyl)tetrahydro-2*H*-1,3,2-oxazaphosphorin-2-amine 2-oxide; an antineoplastic, $C_7H_{15}Cl_2N_2O_2P$.

Ig immunoglobulin of any of the five classes: IgA, IgD, IgE, IgG, or IgM; see *immunoglobulin*.

ignatia (ig-na′she-ah) [L.] the poisonous dried ripe seed of *Strychnos ignatii;* it contains several alkaloids, the principal ones being strychnine and brucine, and has been used as a bitter tonic.

igniextirpation (ig″ne-eks″ter-pa′shun) [L. *ignis* fire + *extirpatio* extirpation] the excision of an organ by hot cautery.

ignioperation (ig″ne-op″er-a′shun) [L. *ignis* fire + *operation*] an operation performed by use of hot cautery.

ignipuncture (ig′ne-punk″tūr) [L. *ignis* fire + *punctura* puncture] therapeutic puncture with hot needles.

ignis (ig′nis) [L.] fire. **i. inferna′lis** ["infernal fire"], ergotism.

ignisation (ig″ni-za′shun) [L. *ignis* fire] hyperthermia produced by exposure to artificial sources of heat.

ignotine (ig′no-tin) carnosine.

IgT a hypothetical antigen receptor on T cell surfaces.

I.H. infectious hepatitis.

II-para secundipara.

III-para tertipara.

I.K. abbreviation for Ger. *immunekörper*, immune bodies. See *tuberculin*, and *Spengler's immune bodies*, under *body*.

Il chemical symbol for *illinium*, former name for promethium.

I.L.A. International Leprosy Association.

Ile isoleucine.

ileac (il′e-ak) 1. of the nature of ileus. 2. pertaining to the ileum.

ileadelphus (il″e-ah-del′fus) iliopagus.

ileal (il′e-al) pertaining to the ileum.

ileectomy (il″e-ek′to-me) [*ileum* + Gr. *ektomē* excision] surgical removal of the ileum.

ileitis (il″e-i′tis) inflammation of the ileum. **distal i.,** Crohn's disease affecting the ileum. **regional i., terminal i.,** Crohn's disease affecting the ileum.

ileo- (il′e-o) [L. *ileum*] a combining form denoting relationship to the ileum.

ileocecal (il″e-o-se′kal) pertaining to the ileum and cecum.

ileocecostomy (il″e-o-se-kos′to-me) surgical creation of an opening between the ileum and the cecum; also, the opening so established.

ileocecum (il″e-o-se′kum) the ileum and cecum considered as one organ.

ileocolic (il″e-o-kol′ik) pertaining to the ileum and colon.

ileocolitis (il″e-o-ko-li′tis) inflammation of the ileum and colon. **tuberculous i.,** tuberculous inflammation of the ileum and colon. **i. ulcero′sa chron′ica,** a chronic form characterized by fever, rapid pulse, anemia, diarrhea and right iliac pain.

ileocolonic (il″e-o-ko-lon′ik) ileocolic.

ileocolostomy (il″e-o-ko-los′to-me) [*ileo-* + *colon* + Gr. *stoma* mouth] surgical creation of an opening between the ileum and colon; also, the opening so established.

ileocolotomy (il″e-o-ko-lot′o-me) [*ileo-* + *colon* + Gr. *temnein* to cut] surgical incision of the ileum and colon.

ileocystoplasty (il″e-o-sis′to-plas″te) [*ileo-* + Gr. *kystis* bladder + *plassein* to form] surgical reconstruction of the bladder, incorporating an isolated loop of the ileum as part of the bladder wall.

ileocystostomy (il″e-o-sis-tos′to-me) surgical creation of an opening between the urinary bladder and ileum.

ileoileostomy (il″e-o-il″e-os′to-me) [*ileo-* + *ileo-* + Gr. *stoma* mouth] surgical creation of an opening between two parts of the ileum; also, the opening so established.

ileoproctostomy (il″e-o-prok-tos′to-me) [*ileo-* + Gr. *prōktos* rectum + *stoma* mouth] anastomosis of the ileum and rectum.

ileorectal (il″e-o-rek′tal) pertaining to or communicating with the ileum and rectum, as an ileorectal fistula.

ileorectostomy (il″e-o-rek-tos′to-me) ileoproctostomy.

ileorrhaphy (il″e-or′ah-fe) [*ileo-* + Gr. *rhaphē* suture] operative repair of the ileum.

ileosigmoid (il″e-o-sig′moid) pertaining to the ileum and the sigmoid.

ileosigmoidostomy (il″e-o-sig″moi-dos′to-me) [*ileo-* + *sigmoid flexure* + Gr. *stoma* mouth] surgical creation of an opening between the ileum and the sigmoid colon; also, the opening so established.

ileostomy (il″e-os′to-me) [*ileo-* + Gr. *stoma* mouth] surgical creation of an opening into the ileum, usually by establishing an ileal stoma on the abdominal wall.

ileotomy (il″e-ot′o-me) [*ileo-* + Gr. *temnein* to cut] incision of the ileum.

ileotransversostomy (il″e-o-trans″vers-os′to-me) surgical creation of an opening between the ileum and the transverse colon.

Iletin (il′ĕ-tin) trademark for a preparation of insulin for injection. **Lente I.,** trademark for a preparation of insulin zinc suspension; see under *suspension*. **NPH I.,** trademark for a preparation of insulin isophane suspension; see under *suspension*. **Semilente I.,** trademark for a preparation of prompt-acting insulin zinc suspension; see under *suspension*. **Ultralente I.,** trademark for a preparation of extended-action zinc insulin suspension; see under *suspension*.

ileum (il′e-um) [L.] [NA] the distal portion of the small intestine, extending from the jejunum to the cecum; called also *intestinum ileum*. **duplex i.,** congenital duplication of the ileum.

ileus (il′e-us) [L; Gr. *eileos*, from *eilein* to roll up] obstruction of the intestines. **adynamic i.,** ileus resulting from inhibition of bowel motility, which may be produced by numerous causes, most frequently by peritonitis. **dynamic i., hyperdynamic i.,** spastic i. **mechanical i.,** ileus due to mechanical causes, such as hernia, adhesions, volvulus, etc. **meconium i.,** ileus in the newborn due to blocking of the bowel with thick meconium; a manifestation of fibrocystic disease (mucoviscidosis). **occlusive i.,** mechanical i. **paralytic i., i. paralyt′icus,** adynamic i. **spastic i.,** ileus due to persistent contracture of a bowel segment; see *Ogilvie's syndrome*, under *syndrome*. **i. subpar′ta,** ileus due to pressure of the gravid uterus on the pelvic colon.

Ilex (i′leks) a genus of aquifoliaceous shrubs and tree, including the hollies. *I. verticillata*. (L.) Gray (*Prinos verticillatus*), the black alder, or winterberry, has a tonic and astringent bark.

ilia (il′e-ah) plural of *ilium*.

iliac (il′e-ak) [L. *iliacus*] pertaining to the ilium.

iliadelphus (il″e-ah-del′fus) iliopagus.

ilicin (il′ĭ-sin) a bitter antiperiodic compound derived from holly, *Ilex aquifolium*.

Ilidar (il′ĭ-dar) trademark for a preparation of azapetine phosphate.

ilio- (il′e-o) [L. *ilium*] a combining form denoting relationship to the ilium or flank.

iliococcygeal (il″e-o-kok-sij′e-al) pertaining to the ilium and coccyx.

iliocolotomy (il″e-o-ko-lot′o-me) surgical incision of the colon in the iliac region.

iliocostal (il″e-o-kos′tal) [*ilio-* + L. *costa* rib] connecting or pertaining to the ilium and ribs.

iliofemoral (il″e-o-fem′or-al) pertaining to the ilium and femur.

iliofemoroplasty (il″e-o-fem′or-o-plas″te) operative fusion of a tuberculous hip joint by splitting the great trochanter from the shaft of the femur and inserting into the fissure a flap of bone bent down from the lateral surface of the ilium.

iliohypogastric (il″e-o-hi″po-gas′trik) pertaining to the ilium and hypogastrium.

ilioinguinal (il″e-o-in′gwĭ-nal) pertaining to the iliac and inguinal regions.

iliolumbar (il″e-o-lum′ber) pertaining to the iliac and lumbar regions, or to the flank and loin.

iliolumbocostoabdominal (il″e-o-lum″bo-kos″to-ab-dom′ĭ-nal) pertaining to the iliac, lumbar, costal, and abdominal regions.

iliometer (il″e-om′ĕ-ter) [*iliac* spines + Gr. *metron* measure] an instrument for determining the relative heights of the iliac spines and their relative distance from the center of the spinal column.

iliopagus (il″e-op′ah-gus) [*ilio-* + Gr. *pagos* thing fixed] symmetrical conjoined twins united in the iliac region.

iliopectineal (il″e-o-pek-tin′e-al) pertaining to the ilium and pubes.

iliopelvic (il″e-o-pel′vik) pertaining to the iliac region or muscle and to the pelvis.

iliopsoas (il″e-o-so′as) see *Table of Musculi*.

iliopubic (il″e-o-pu′bik) iliopectineal.

iliosacral (il″e-o-sa′kral) pertaining to the ilium and the sacrum.

iliosciatic (il″e-o-si-at′ik) pertaining to the ilium and the ischium.

iliospinal (il″e-o-spi′nal) pertaining to the ilium and the spinal column.

iliothoracopagus (il″e-o-tho″rah-kop′ah-gus) [*ilium* + Gr. *thōrax* chest + *pagos* thing fixed] symmetrical conjoined twins fused from the pelvis to the thorax.

iliotibial (il″e-o-tib′e-al) pertaining to or extending between the ilium and tibia.

iliotrochanteric (il″e-o-tro-kan-ter′ik) pertaining to the ilium and a trochanter.

ilioxiphopagus (il″e-o-zi-fop′ah-gus) symmetrical conjoined twins fused from the pelvis to the xiphoid process.

ilium (il′e-um), pl. *il′ia* [L.] the expansive superior portion of the hip bone (os coxae); it is a separate bone in early life. See illustration accompanying *skeleton*. Called also *os ilium* [NA].

ill (il) 1. not well; sick. 2. a disease or disorder. **föhn i.,** the headache, weariness, and depression reported to be felt when the föhn (a special wind from the south in Central Europe) blows. **joint i.,** navel i. **leg i.,** foot rot; see under *rot*. **louping i.,** encephalomyelitis primarily affecting sheep in Great Britain and Ireland, caused by a virus which is transmitted by the tick, *Ixodes ricinus*. **navel i.,** generalized septicemia affecting foals, lambs, and calves, usually characterized by omphalophlebitis and the formation of abscesses in the joints resulting in polyarthritis; it is due to infection through the open navel by various organisms, including species of *Staphylococcus, Streptococcus, Shigella, Escherichia,* and *Pasteurella,* and has a high mortality rate. Called also *joint i.* **quarter i.,** blackleg. **thorter i.,** gid.

illacrimation (il″ak-rĭ-ma′shun) epiphora.

illaqueation (il″ak-we-a′shun) [L. *illaqueare* to ensnare] the cure of an ingrowing eyelash by drawing it out with a loop.

Illicium (il-is′e-um) [L.] a genus of magnoliaceous trees and shrubs whose fruit, Chinese anise, is the source of anise oil. The leaves of *I. religiosum,* or sikimi, are the source of sikimin.

illinition (il-ĭ-nish′un) [L. *illinire* to smear] the application of an ointment or liniment with rubbing.

illinium (il-lin′e-um) [University of *Illinois*] former name of the element *promethium.*

illness (il′ness) a condition marked by pronounced deviation from the normal healthy state; sickness. **compressed-air i.,** decompression sickness. **emotional i.,** mental disorder. **functional i.,** a disorder having no clearly defined physical cause or structural change, i.e., having no detectable organic basis; called also *functional disorder.* **high-altitude i.,** see under *sickness.* **manic-depressive i.,** see under *psychosis.* **mental i.,** see under *disorder.* **psychosomatic i.,** an illness in which the manifestations are mainly physical with at least a partial emotional basis; see also *psychophysiological disorder,* under *disorder.* **radiation i.,** see under *sickness.*

illumination (ĭ-lu″mĭ-na′shun) [L. *illuminatio*] the lighting up of a part, cavity, organ, or object for inspection. The degree of illumination at any point of a surface is the density of the luminous flux at that point. **axial i.,** the transmission or reflection of light along the axis of a microscope. **central i.,** axial i. **contact i.,** illumination of the eye by means of an instrument which is pressed directly to the cornea and conjunctiva. **critical i.,** the focusing of light precisely upon an object inspected. **darkfield i., dark-ground i.,** the throwing of peripheral rays of light upon a microscopical object from the side, the center rays being blocked out: the object appears bright upon a dark background. See under *microscope,* and see *ultramicroscope.* **direct i.,** the throwing of light upon a microscopical object from above or from the direction of observation. **focal i.,** the throwing of light upon the focus of a lens or mirror. **Köhler i.,** an improved method of illumination by adjustment of the substage Abbe condenser, for obtaining the best image detail in microscopical work. **lateral i., oblique i.,** illumination in which the object is illuminated by oblique light. **through i.,** the tranmission of light through an object, or from the direction opposite to that of observation.

illuminator (ĭ-lu″mĭ-na′tor) the source of light for viewing an object. **Abbe's i.,** see under *condenser.*

illuminism (ĭ-lu′min-izm) a state marked by delusions of communication with supernatural beings.

illusion (ĭ-lu′zhun) [L. *illusio*] a false or misinterpreted sensory impression; a false interpretation of a real sensory image. Cf. *delusion.* **Kuhnt's i.,** similar intervals seem smaller in the temporal field than in the nasal field of a single eye. **passive i.,** an illusion determined by the nature of the sense organs and the environment, as double vision of a single object.

illusional (ĭ-lu″zhun-al) pertaining to or characterized by illusions.

illutation (il″u-ta′shun) [L. *in* in + *lutum* mud] treatment by mud baths.

Ilopan (il′o-pan) trademark for a preparation of dexpanthenol.

Ilosone (il′o-sōn) trademark for a preparation of erythromycin estolate.

Ilotycin (i″lo-ti′sin) trademark for preparations of erythromycin.

Ilozyme (il′o-zīm) trademark for a preparation of pancrelipase.

I.M. intramuscularly (by intramuscular injection).

im- 1. a prefix, replacing *in-* before words beginning with *b, m, p.* 2. a prefix in chemical names indicating the bivalent group >NH.

I.M.A. Industrial Medical Association.

ima (i′mah) [L.] lowest.

imafen hydrochloride (im′ah-fen) chemical name: 2,3,5,6-tetrahydro-5-phenyl-1*H*-imidazo[1,2-*a*]imidazole monohydrochloride; an antidepressant, $C_{11}H_{13}N_3 \cdot HCl$.

image (im′ij) [L. *imago*] a picture or conception with more or less likeness to an objective reality. See also *imaging.* **accidental i.,** after-image. **acoustic i.,** a concept corresponding to something heard. **auditory i.,** acoustic i. **body i.,** a three-dimensional concept of one's self, recorded in the cortex by the perception of ever-changing postures of the body, and constantly changing with them. **direct i., erect i.,** virtual i. **eidetic i.,** an unusually vivid, elaborate, and exact mental image formed in response to a visual stimulus, which may be part of a fantasy or a memory. **false i.,** the one formed by the deviating eye in strabismus. **heteronymous i.,** the two images seen when the eyes are focused on a point beyond the object.

homonymous i., the two images seen when the eyes are focused on a point nearer than the object. **incidental i.,** the impression of an image which remains on the retina after the object has been removed. **inverted i.,** real i. **memory i.,** a sensation or sense perception as it is pictured in the memory. **mental i.,** any concept corresponding to an object appreciated by the senses. **mirror i.,** 1. the image of light made visible by the reflecting surface of the cornea and lens when illuminated through the slit lamp. 2. an identical reproduction of an object except for transposition of right and left relations, as appears in the reflection of an object in a mirror. **motor i.,** the organized cerebral model of the possible movements of the body. **negative i.,** after-image. **ocular i.,** visual i. **optical i.,** one formed by the reflection of refraction of rays of light. **Purkinje i's, Purkinje-Sanson mirror i's,** reflected images formed on the anterior surface of the cornea and the anterior and posterior surfaces of the crystalline lens. The images on the two anterior surfaces are virtual and noninverted, and the image on the posterior surface is real and inverted. Useful in the study of the movement of the lens surfaces in accommodation and, formerly, in the evaluation of cataract. **radioisotope i.,** a quasi-pictorial representation of the distribution of radioactive materials in the body. **real i.,** one formed where the emanating rays are collected, in which the object is pictured as being inverted. **retinal i.,** the representation formed upon the retina of an object seen. **Sanson's i's,** Purkinje i's. **sensory i.,** a representation formed by means of one or more of the sense organs. **specular i.,** mirror i., def. 1. **tactile i.,** a mental concept corresponding to an object perceived by the sense of touch. **virtual i.,** a picture from projected light rays that are intercepted before focusing, as by a plane mirror. **visual i.,** a mental concept corresponding to an object perceived by the sense of sight.

imagines (ĭ-maj′ĭ-nēz) [L.] plural of *imago.*

imaging (im′ah-jing) the production of clarity, contrast, and detail in images, especially in radiological and ultrasound images. **electrostatic i.,** a method of visualizing deep structures of the body, in which an electron beam, rather than x-rays, is passed through the patient and the emerging beam (unabsorbed electrons) strikes an electrostatically charged vacuum-packed plate, dissipating the charge according to the strength of the beam. A record (e.g., a film) is then made from the plate.

imago (ĭ-ma′go), pl. *ima′goes,* or *imag′ines* [L.] 1. the final or adult stage of an insect. Cf. *larva, pupa.* 2. in psychoanalysis, a childhood memory or fantasy of a loved person that remains in adult life.

imagocide (ĭ-ma′go-sīd) [*imago* + L. *caedere* to kill] an agent that destroys adult insects, especially adult mosquitoes.

imapunga (im-ah-pung′ah) a disease occurring to a limited extent among African cattle; closely related in pathology to African horse sickness.

imbalance (im-bal′ans) lack of balance, especially lack of balance between muscles, as in weakness of ocular muscles. **autonomic i.,** autonomic ataxia; any disturbance of the autonomic nervous system. **sympathetic i.,** vagotonia. **vasomotor i.,** autonomic i.

imbecile (im′bĕ-sil) 1. defective mentally. 2. a former name for a mentally retarded person of the second lowest order, i.e., having an IQ of 25 to 49. See *mental retardation,* under *retardation.* Cf. *idiot* and *moron.* **moral i.,** one affected with moral imbecility; previously called *amoralis.*

imbecility (im″bĕ-sil′ĭ-te) [L. *imbecillitas*] mental retardation; a former category of mental retardation comprising individuals having an IQ of 25 to 49. See *mental retardation,* under *retardation.* Cf. *idiocy* and *moronity.* **moral i.,** moral insanity in which the moral sense is stunted; previously called *amoralia.* **phenylpyruvic i.,** phenylketonuria.

imbed (im-bed′) embed; see *embedding.*

imbibition (im″bĭ-bish′un) [L. *imbibere* to drink] 1. the absorption of a liquid. 2. insudation. **hemoglobin i.,** absorption by the tissue of free hemoglobin.

imbricated (im′brĭ-kāt″ed) [L. *imbricatus; imbrex* tile] overlapping like tiles or shingles.

imbrication (im″brĭ-ka′shun) the overlapping of apposing surfaces, like shingles on a roof.

ImD$_{50}$ the immunizing dose of vaccine or antigen sufficient to protect 50% of the animals in a particular test group.

Imhoff tank (im′hof) [Karl *Imhoff,* German sanitarian, born 1876] digestion tank; see under *tank.*

Imhotep (im′ho-tep) (c. 2600 B.C.) an Egyptian physician of the third dynasty (founded by Zoser) who was later worshiped as a healing god. He is the first physician whose name is known.

imidamine (im″id-am′in) antazoline.

imidazole (im″id-az′ōl) a base,

$$\text{HC—N} \quad \underset{\text{HC—N}}{\overset{\|}{}} \quad \overset{\text{H}}{\underset{}{\text{>CH,}}}$$

found combined with alanine in histidine.

imidazolylethylamine (im″id-az″o-lil-eth″il-am′in)   histamine.

imide (im′id)   any compound containing the bivalent group, > NH, to which are attached only acid radicals.

imido- (ĭ-me′do)   a prefix denoting the presence in a compound of the bivalent group > NH attached to two acid radicals.

imidocarb hydrochloride (ĭ-mid′o-karb)   chemical name: N,N'-bis[3-(4,5-dihydro-1H-imidazol-2-yl)phenyl] urea dihydrochloride; an antiprotozoal effective against *Babesia*, $C_{19}H_{20}N_6 \cdot O \cdot 2HCl$.

imidogen (ĭ-me′do-jen)   the bivalent radical > NH.

iminazole (im″in-az′ōl)   imidazole.

imino- (ĭ-me′no)   a prefix used to denote the presence of the bivalent group > NH attached to nonacid radicals.

iminoglycinuria (ĭ-me″no-gli″sin-u′re-ah)   a benign hereditary disorder of renal tubular reabsorption of glycine and imino acids (proline and hydroxyproline), marked by excessive levels of all three substances in the urine.

iminourea (ĭ-me″no-u-re′ah)   guanidine.

imipramine hydrochloride (ĭ-mip′rah-mēn) [USP]   chemical name: 10,11-dihydro-N,N-dimethyl-5H-dibenz[b,f]azepine-5-propanamine monohydrochloride. A tricyclic antidepressant, $C_{19}H_{24}N_2 \cdot HCl$, occurring as a white to off-white, crystalline powder; used especially in the treatment of endogenous depression and in childhood enuresis, administered orally.

Imlach's fat plug (im′laks) [Francis *Imlach*, Scottish physician, 1819–1891]   see under *plug*.

immature (im″ah-tūr′) [L. *in* not + *maturus* mature]   unripe or not fully developed.

immediate (ĭ-me′de-it) [L. *in* not + *mediatus* mediate]   direct; with nothing intervening; occurring without delay.

immedicable (ĭ-med′ĭ-kah-b'l) [L. *immedicabilis*]   beyond the hope of cure.

immersion (ĭ-mer′shun) [L. *immersio*]   1. the placing or plunging of a body into a liquid. 2. the use of the microscope with the object and object glass both covered with a liquid. **homogeneous i.,** the employment in microscopy of nearly the same refractive power as the cover glass. **oil i.,** the covering of the microscopical objective and the object with oil. **water i.,** the covering of the microscopical objective and the object with water.

immiscible (ĭ-mis′ĭ-b'l)   not susceptible to being mixed.

immobility (im″mo-bil′ĭ-te)   1. the state of being immovable. 2. chronic hydrocephalus of cattle.

immobilization (im-mo′bil-i-za′shun)   the act of rendering immovable, as by a cast or splint.

immobilize (im-mo′bil-īz) [L. *in* not + *mobilis* movable]   to render incapable of being moved, as by a cast or splint.

Immu-G (im′u-je)   trademark for a preparation of immune globulin.

immune (ĭ-mūn′) [L. *immunis* free, exempt]   1. being highly resistant to a disease because of the formation of humoral antibodies or the development of cellular immunity, or both, or as a result of some other mechanism, as interferon activity in viral infections. 2. characterized by the development of humoral antibodies or cellular immunity, or both, following antigenic challenge. 3. produced in response to antigenic challenge, as immune serum globulin. 4. an immune individual.

immunifacient (ĭ-mu″nĭ-fa′shent)   producing immunity; said of diseases, such as diphtheria and typhoid, which for a time after infection produce immunity against themselves.

immunifaction (ĭ-mu″nĭ-fak′shun)   immunization.

immunisin (ĭ-mu′nĭ-zin)   antibody.

immunity (ĭ-mu′nĭ-te) [L. *immunitas*]   1. the condition of being immune; security against a particular disease; nonsusceptibility to the invasive or pathogenic effects of foreign microorganisms or to the toxic effect of antigenic substances. Called also *functional* or *protective i.* See also *active i., nonspecific i.,* and *passive i.* 2. heightened responsiveness to antigenic challenge that leads to more rapid binding or elimination of antigen than in the nonimmune state; it includes both humoral and cell-mediated immunity. 3. the capacity to distinguish foreign material from self, and to neutralize, eliminate, or metabolize that which is foreign by the physiologic mechanisms of the immune response. **acquired i.,** specific immunity attributable to the presence of antibody and to a heightened reactivity of antibody-forming cells, specifically immune lymphoid cells (responsible for the cell-mediated immunity), and of phagocytic cells, following prior exposure to an infectious agent or its antigens, or passive transfer of antibody or immune lymphoid cells; called also *adaptive i.* **active i.,** acquired immunity attributable to the presence of antibody or of immune lymphoid cells formed in response to antigenic stimulus. **actual i.,** active i. **adoptive i.,** passive immunity of the cell-mediated type conferred by the administration of sensitized lymphocytes from an immune donor. **antibacterial i.,** immunity against the action of bacteria, i.e., the ability to resist infection by bacteria. **antiblastic i.,** immunity due to forces antagonistic to the growth of the microorganism in the body of the

host organism. **antitoxic i.,** immunity against toxins, attributable to the presence of specific antitoxin(s) in the immune individual. **antiviral i.,** immunity against viruses. **artificial i.,** acquired (active or passive) immunity produced by deliberate exposure to an antigen, as in vaccination. **athreptic i.,** an obsolete concept attributing immunity to exhaustion of bacterial foodstuffs from the growth medium. **bacteriolytic i.,** antibacterial immunity attributable to the lytic action of sera. **cell-mediated i., cellular i.,** specific acquired immunity in which the role of small lymphocytes of thymic origin (T-lymphocytes) is predominant; it is responsible for resistance to infectious diseases caused by certain bacteria, fungi, and viruses, certain aspects of resistance to cancer, delayed hypersensitivity reactions, certain autoimmune diseases, and allograft rejection, and plays a role in certain allergies. **community i.,** herd i. **congenital i.,** the immunity which an individual possesses at birth. **cross i.,** immunity produced by inoculation with an agent (e.g., a bacterium or virus) that is different from, but closely related to, the agent causing the disease. **familial i.,** genetic i. **genetic i.,** innate i. **herd i.,** the resistance of a group to attack by a disease because of the immunity of a large proportion of the members and the consequent lessening of the likelihood of an affected individual coming into contact with a susceptible individual. **humoral i.,** acquired immunity in which the role of circulating antibodies (immunoglobulins) is predominant; these antibodies are products of B-lymphocytes and plasma cells. **infection i.,** resistance to infection by reason of an already existing infection by the same or an antigenically related microorganism. **inherent i.,** innate i. **inherited i.,** innate i. **innate i.,** immunity based on the genetic constitution of the individual; natural immunity. Called also *genetic i., inherent i.,* and *inherited i.* **intrauterine i.,** passive immunity acquired by the fetus as a consequence of the passage of maternal IgG antibodies from an immune mother through the placenta into the fetal circulation. **local i.,** immunity manifested predominantly in a restricted anatomical region or type of tissue; antibodies of the class termed secretory or exocrine IgA account for many manifestations of local immunity. **maternal i.,** passively transferred humoral immunity from the mother to the offspring, across the placenta before birth in primates, from the colostrum in ungulates via the intestines, and from the egg yolk in birds. **maturation i.,** increase in resistance to disease that comes with development to maturity. **mixed i.,** passive immunity succeeded by active immunity as a consequence of serovaccination. **native i.,** nonspecific immunity due to the genetic endowment of the host. **natural i.,** the capacity of the normal (not specifically immunized) animal to respond immunologically; immunity inherited or acquired passively *in utero* or through the maternal milk, or acquired actively by clinical or subclinical infection. **nonspecific i.,** immunity arising from the sum of immune responses that do not involve antigenic stimulation of antibody formation or cell-mediated immunity; it includes lysozyme and interferon activity, phagocytosis, the inflammatory response, and chemical and physical barriers to infection. **nutritional i.,** immunity postulated to result from the withholding by host cells of an essential nutrilite (e.g., iron) from invading pathogens. **opsonic i.,** immunity due to the presence of opsonins. **passive i.,** acquired immunity produced by the administration of preformed antibody or specifically sensitized lymphoid cells. **phagocytic i.,** immunity attributable to the activity of phagocytes in the engulfment and destruction of the agents producing disease. **placental i.,** intrauterine i. **postoncolytic i.,** immunity to tumor development following regression of a previously existing tumor. **preemptive i.,** interference phenomenon, def. 2. **Profeta's i.,** the alleged immunity against syphilitic infection possessed by some children of syphilitic parents. **racial i.,** genetically determined resistance that all or most of the members of a race manifest toward a certain infection. **residual i.,** immunity which remains for varying periods after the complete disappearance of the infection. **species i.,** resistance of members of a particular species to a disease; immunity enjoyed by members of a particular species and determined by their genetic constitution. **specific i.,** immunity against a particular disease, e.g., scarlet fever, or against a particular antigen. **sterile i.,** that in which the immune response results in complete removal of the infectious agent from the host, or in removal to the point that the agent is no longer detectable in the host. **tissue i.,** local i. **toxin-antitoxin i.,** an active antitoxic immunity produced by injecting subcutaneously a nearly neutral mixture of diphtheria toxin and antitoxin.

immunization (im″u-ni-za′shun)   the process of rendering a subject immune, or of becoming immune. **active i.,** stimulation with a specific antigen to induce an immune response. **collateral i.,** inoculation with an organism other than the one causing an existing infection. **isopathic i.,** active i. **occult i.,** immunization produced in some unknown, spontaneous way. **passive i.,** the conferral of specific immune reactivity on previously nonimmune individuals by the administration of sensitized lymphoid cells or serum from immune individuals. **Rh i., rhesus i.,** see under *sensitization*. **side-to-side i.,** an immunization method in which the antigen is injected into one side of the body and the corresponding antibody into the other side.

immunizator (im″u-ni-za′tor) that which renders immune.

immunize (im′u-nīz) to render immune.

immunoabsorbent (im″u-no-sor′bent) immunosorbent.

immunoadjuvant (im″u-no-aj′e-vent) a nonspecific stimulator of the immune response, e.g., BCG vaccine or Freund's complete and incomplete adjuvants.

immunoadsorbent (im″u-no-ad-sor′bent) a preparation of antigen attached to an insoluble support, or antigen in an insoluble form, which adsorbs homologous antibodies from a serum sample or other immunoglobulin mixture. Specific antibody may later be collected by elution from the immunoadsorbent material.

immunoassay (im″u-no-as′sa) quantitative determination of antigenic substances (e.g., hormones, drugs, vitamins, etc.) by serological means, as by immunofluorescent techniques, radioimmunoassay, etc.

immunobiology (im″u-no-bi-ol′o-je) that branch of biology dealing with immunologic effects on such phenomena as infectious disease, growth and development, recognition phenomena, hypersensitivity, heredity, aging, cancer, and transplantation.

immunoblast (im″u-no-blast′) lymphoblast.

immunoblastic (im″u-no-blas′tik) pertaining to or involving the stem cells (immunoblasts) of lymphoid tissue.

immunocatalysis (im″u-no-kah-tal′ĭ-sis) the concept that enzyme substrate and specifically inhibitive reaction products have their respective counterparts in antigen, their antibody precursors, and specific antibodies.

immunochemistry (im″u-no-kem′is-tre) that branch of biological science concerned with the physical chemical basis of immune phenomena and their interactions.

immunochemotherapy (im″u-no-ke″mo-ther′ah-pe) a combination of immunotherapy and chemotherapy.

immunocompetence (im″u-no-kom′pĕ-tens) the ability or capacity to develop an immune response (i.e., antibody production and/or cell-mediated immunity) following exposure to antigen; called also *immunologic competence.*

immunocompetent (im″u-no-kom′pĕ-tent) exhibiting immunocompetence.

immunocomplex (im″u-no-kom′pleks) antibody combined with its specific antigen; deposition of immunocomplexes that fix complement in tissues may lead to inflammation and tissue injury, as in immune complex glomerulonephritis.

immunocompromised (im″m-no-kom′pro-mizd) having the immune response attenuated by administration of immunosuppressive drugs, by irradiation, by malnutrition, and by some disease processes (e.g., cancer).

immunoconglutinin (im″u-no-kon-gloo′tin) antibody formed against complement components that are part of an antigen-antibody complex, especially C̄3.

immunocyte (im″u-no-sīt′) a cell of the lymphoid series which can react with antigen to produce antibody or to become active in cell-mediated immunity or delayed hypersensitivity reactions; called also *immunologically competent cell.*

immunocytoadherence (im″u-no-si″to-ad-hēr′ens) the aggregation of red cells to form rosettes around lymphocytes with surface immunoglobulins.

immunocytochemistry (im″u-no-si″to-kem′is-tre) immunochemistry applied to the study of intracellular activities.

immunodeficiency (im″u-no-dĕ-fish′en-se) a deficiency in immune response, either in that mediated by humoral antibody or in that mediated by immune lymphoid cells. **combined i.,** deficiency of lymphoid cells that mediate both humoral (B-lymphocytes) and cellular (T-lymphocytes) immunity. **common variable i.,** hypogammaglobulinemia of late onset marked by increased incidence of recurrent pyogenic infections especially pneumococcal pneumonia; cellular immune dysfunction occurs in some individuals. Called also *common variable hypogammaglobulinemia.* **severe combined i.,** see under *disease.*

immunodepression (im″u-no-dĕ-presh′un) immunosuppression.

immunodepressive (im″u-no-dĕ-pres′iv) immunosuppressive.

immunodermatology (im″u-no-der″mah-tol′o-je) the study of immunologic phenomena as they affect skin disorders and their treatment or prophylaxis.

immunodiagnosis (im″u-no-di″ag-no′sis) diagnosis based on blood serum reactions to antigens; serodiagnosis.

immunodiffusion (im″u-no-dĭ-fu′zhun) the diffusion of antigen and antibody from separate reservoirs to form decreasing concentration gradients in hydrophilic gels.

immunodominance (im″u-no-dom′ĭ-nans) the degree to which a subunit of an antigenic determinant is involved in binding or reacting with specific antibody.

immunodominant (im″u-no-dom′ĭ-nant) denoting the subunits of the antigenic determinant group that most influence the specificity of the induced antibodies.

immunoelectrophoresis (ĭ-mu″no-e-lek″tro-fo-re′sis) counterimmunoelectrophoresis. **counter i.,** counterimmunoelectrophoresis; see under *C.* **reverse i.,** a procedure identical to counterimmunoelectrophoresis, with the positions of the antigen and antibody being interchanged. **rocket i.,** that in which antigen is electrophoresed from a well through a layer of agar gel containing antiserum; cone-shaped (rocket) areas of precipitate are formed by each antigen-antibody system in the antibody layer. **two-dimensional i.,** a technique for separation and semiquantitation of a mixture of antigens in which a solution of antigens in gel is separated in one direction on the basis of electrophoretic mobilities and then in a direction at right angles to the first by further electrophoresis into a sheet of agar containing antibodies.

immunoenhancement (im″mu-no-en-hans′ment) the process of increasing of the level of immune response by various specific and nonspecific means.

immunoferritin (im″u-no-fer′ĭ-tin) an antibody labeled with ferritin; when combined with antigen, the antigenic determinant sites are visible under the electron microscope.

immunofiltration (im″u-no-fil-tra′shun) the extraction of antibodies in pure form by subjection of serum to insoluble specific antigen, the antigen then being removed from the antibody by treatment with soluble carriers. Called also *electrosyneresis.* **analytical i.,** a technique for revealing the presence of specific antigens in a solution contaminated with cross-reacting antigens; the cross-reacting antigens are "filtered" out by use of an antiserum reagent (heterologous) that contains antibodies against the cross-reacting antigens but not against the homologous specific antigens. **preparative i.,** an immunochemical technique for the isolation and characterization of cancer-distinctive proteins developed by G. I. Abelev; unwanted antigens are precipitated out or slowed down by antibodies during electrophoresis while the desired antigens continue to move at an uninterrupted rate. The antibodies used are those against normal constituents known by previous immunoanalysis to contaminate the solution of tumor proteins.

immunofluorescence (im″u-no-floo′o-res′ens) a method of determining the location of antigen (or antibody) in tissue by the pattern of fluorescence resulting when the tissue is exposed to the specific antibody (or antigen) labeled with a fluorochrome. **direct i.,** immunofluorescence. **indirect i.,** that in which two sets of antibodies are used, the first set being specific for the target protein and the second, which is labeled with a fluorescent chemical group, being specific for the first antibody.

immunogen (im′u-no-jen) any substance that is capable of eliciting an immune response, as opposed to a tolerogen.

immunogenetic (ĭ-mu″no-jĕ-net′ik) pertaining to or concerned with the interrelations of immune reactions and genetic constitution, as in the study of blood groups or tissue antigens.

immunogenetics (im″u-no-jĕ-net′iks) [*immuno-* + *genetics*] originally, the study of genetic variation by immunological methods; now also includes the study of genetic factors that control the immune response of the individual and the transmission of those factors from generation to generation.

immunogenic (im″u-no-jen′ik) producing immunity; evoking an immune response.

immunogenicity (im″u-no-jĕ-nis′ĭ-te) the property that endows a substance with the capacity to provoke an immune response, or the degree to which a substance possesses this property.

immunoglobulin (im″u-no-glob′u-lin) a protein of animal origin endowed with known antibody activity, synthesized by lymphocytes and plasma cells. Immunoglobulins function as specific antibodies and are responsible for the humoral aspects of immunity. They are found in the serum and in other body fluids and tissues, including the urine, spinal fluid, lymph nodes, spleen, etc. Molecularly, each immunoglobulin is made up of two light chains and two heavy chains, this basic four-chain unit being repeated in the higher molecular weight forms, as in the pentameric IgM molecule. There are five antigenically different kinds of heavy chains, which form the basis of the five classes of immunoglobulins (IgA, IgD, IgE, IgG, IgM; see Table on following page). In addition there are two types of light chains, designated κ and λ, which are common to all five classes, although an individual immunoglobulin molecule has either κ or λ chains, not both. Symbol Ig or γ. **exocrine i's,** secretory i's. **secretory i's,** IgA immunoglobulins in which two IgA molecules are linked by a polypeptide (secretory piece) and by a J chain; they are present in nonvascular fluids, as in intestinal secretions, saliva, bile, respiratory tract secretions, synovial fluid, etc. Called also *exocrine i's.*

immunoglobulinopathy (im″mu-no-glob″u-lin-op′ah-the) gammopathy.

immunohematology (ĭ-mu″no-hem″ah-tol′o-je) that branch of hematology which studies antigen-antibody reactions and analogous phenomena as they relate to the pathogenesis and clinical manifestations of blood disorders.

immunoheterogeneity (im″u-no-het″er-o-jĕ-ne-ĭ-te) the quality of being immunoheterogeneous.

immunoheterogeneous (im″u-no-het″er-o-je′ne-us) occurring in two or more immunoreactive forms.

immunohistochemical (im″u-no-his″to-kem′ĭ-kal) denoting the application of antigen-antibody interactions to histochemical techniques, as in the use of immunofluorescence.

HUMAN IMMUNOGLOBULIN CLASSES: SOME PHYSICAL AND BIOLOGIC PROPERTIES

CLASS	MEAN SERUM CONCENTRATION (mg/100 ml)	MOLECULAR WEIGHT	$S_{20.w}$	MEAN SURVIVAL T/2 (days)	BIOLOGIC FUNCTION	HEAVY CHAIN DESIGNATION	NO. OF SUBCLASSES
γG or IgG	1240	150,000	7	23	1. Fix complement 2. Cross placenta 3. Heterocytotropic antibody	γ	4
γA or IgA	280	170,000	7, 10, 14	6	1. Secretory antibody	α	2
γM or IgM	120	890,000	19	5	1. Fix complement 2. Efficient agglutination	μ	1
γD or IgD	3	150,000	7	2.8	1. Lymphocyte surface receptor	δ	2
γE or IgE	.03	196,000	8	1.5	1. Reaginic antibody 2. Homocytotropic antibody	ε	1

From Bellanti: Immunology.

immunohistofluorescence (im″u-no-his-to-floo″o-res′ens) histofluorescence accomplished by injection of antibody labeled with fluorochrome.

immunoincompetent (im″u-no-in-kom′pĕ-tent) lacking the ability or capacity to develop an immune response to antigenic challenge.

immunologic, immunological (im″u-no-loj′ik im″u-no-loj′-ĕ-kal) pertaining to immunology.

immunologist (im″u-nol′o-jist) a person who makes a special study of immunology.

immunology (im″u-nol′o-je) that branch of biomedical science concerned with the response of the organism to antigenic challenge, the recognition of self from not self, and all the biological (*in vivo*), serological (*in vitro*), and physical chemical aspects of immune phenomena.

immunomodulation (im″u-no-mod″u-la′shun) adjustment of the immune response to a desired level, as in immunopotentiation, immunosuppression, or induction of immunologic tolerance.

immunoparasitology (im″u-no-par″ah-si-tol′o-je) immunology as applied to the interaction of animal parasites and their hosts.

immunoparesis (im″u-no-pah-re′sis) inadequate immune response to an infectious agent.

immunopathogenesis (im″u-no-path″o-jen′ĕ-sis) a process in which the course of a disease is altered or affected by an immune response (either the cellular [T-cell] or humoral [B-cell] response) or by the products of an immune reaction, such as the antigen-antibody-complement complexes deposited in renal glomeruli.

immunopathologic (im″u-no-path″o-loj′ik) pertaining to immunopathology.

immunopathology (im″u-no-pah-thol′o-je) 1. that branch of biomedical science concerned with immune reactions associated with disease, whether the reactions be beneficial, without effect, or harmful. 2. the structural and functional manifestations associated with immune responses to disease.

immunophysiology (im″u-no-fiz″e-ol′o-je) the physiology of immunological processes.

immunopotency (im″u-no-po′ten-se) the immunogenic capacity of an individual antigenic determinant on an antigen molecule to initiate antibody synthesis.

immunopotentiation (im″u-no-po-ten″she-a′shun) 1. the restoration or enhancement of inefficient immune response mechanisms by administration of biologically active substances. 2. accentuation of the response to an immunogen, in a normal individual, by another substance, factor, or specific treatment.

immunopotentiator (im″u-no-po-ten′she-a-tor) an agent, e.g., a vaccine, that on injection induces a generalized immune response.

immunoprecipitation (im″u-no-pre-sip″ĭ-ta′shun) precipitation resulting from interaction of specific antibody and antigen.

immunoproliferative (im″u-no-pro-lif′er-ah-tiv) characterized by the proliferation of lymphoid cells producing immunoglobulins, as in immunoproliferative disorders, including the gammopathies.

immunoprophylaxis (im″u-no-pro″fĭ-lak′sis) the prevention of disease by the use of vaccines or therapeutic antisera.

immunoprotein (im″u-no-pro′te-in) immunoglobulin.

immunoradiometric (im″u-no-ra″de-o-met′rik) denoting an immunoassay technique in which the substance to be measured combines directly with radioactively labeled antibody.

immunoradiometry (im″u-no-ra″de-om′ĕ-tre) the use of radiolabelled antibody (in the place of radiolabelled antigen) in radioimmunoassay techniques.

immunoreaction (ĭ-mu″no-re-ak′shun) the reaction that takes place between an antigen and its antibody or between an antigen and an immunocyte sensitized to it.

immunoreactive (im″u-no-re-ak′tiv) exhibiting immunoreaction.

immunoregulation (im″u-no-reg″u-la′shun) the control of specific immune responses and interactions between B- and T-lymphocytes and macrophages.

immunoresponsiveness (im″u-no-re-spon′siv-ness) the capacity to react immunologically.

immunoselection (im″u-no-sĕ-lek′shun) the survival of certain cell lines attributable to their having the least surface antigenicity and thus the least susceptibility to antibody and/or immune lymphoid cells.

immunosenescence (im″u-no-sĕ-nes′ens) the weakening and atrophy of the immune system with advancing age.

immunosorbent (im″u-no-sor′bent) an insoluble support for antigen or antibody used to absorb homologous antibodies or antigens, respectively, from a mixture; the antibodies or antigens so removed may then be eluted in pure form. See also *absorption method*, under *method*. Called also *immunoabsorbent*.

immunostimulant (im″u-no-stim′u-lant) 1. stimulating an immune response. 2. an agent that stimulates the immune response.

immunostimulating (im″u-no-stim′u-la″ting) enhancing the immune response.

immunostimulation (im″u-no-stim″u-la′shun) stimulation of an immune response, e.g., by use of BCG vaccine.

immunosuppressant (im″u-no-su-pres-ant) immunosuppressive.

immunosuppression (im″u-no-su-presh′un) the prevention or diminution of the immune response, as by irradiation or by administration of antimetabolites, antilymphocyte serum, or specific antibody; called also *immunodepression*.

immunosuppressive (im″u-no-su-pres′iv) 1. pertaining to or inducing immunosuppression. 2. an agent that induces immunosuppression.

immunosurgery (ĭ-mu″no-ser′jer-e) the employment of specific immune therapy in surgical practice.

immunosurveillance (im″u-no-ser-va′lens) a term used to denote the monitoring function of the immune system in recognizing and reacting against (i.e., rapidly destroying) newly developed aberrant cells arising by somatic mutation and containing new antigens, e.g., malignant cells; thought to be done by the cell-mediated portion of the immune system.

immunosympathectomy (im″u-no-sim″pah-thek′to-me) destruction of the sympathetic ganglia by intravenous injection into newborn animals of an antiserum to a protein essential to the life of sympathetic nerve cells.

immunotherapy (ĭ-mu″no-ther′ah-pe) passive immunization of an individual by administration of preformed antibodies (serum or gamma globulin) actively produced in another individual; by

Plate XXII   immunoglobulin

MOLECULAR STRUCTURE OF IMMUNOGLOBULINS

THE FIVE CLASSES

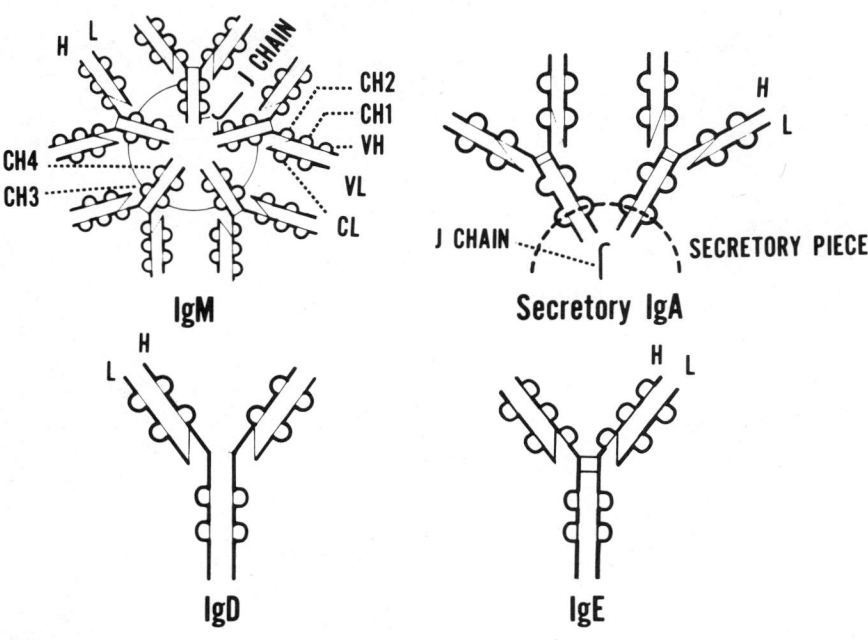

STRUCTURE OF IMMUNOGLOBULIN G & A SUBCLASSES

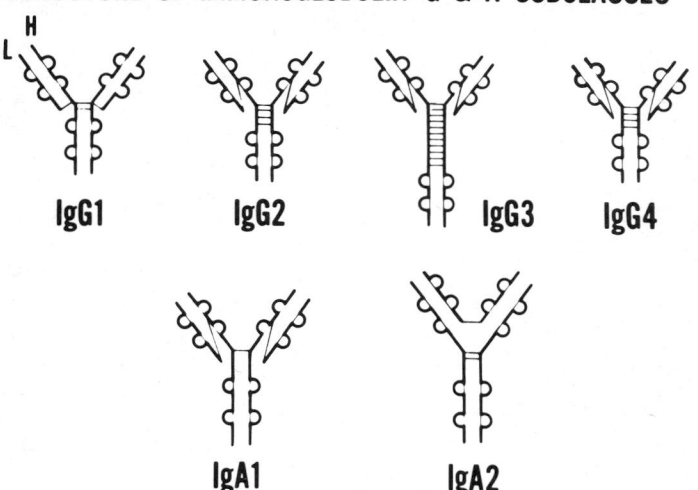

Schematic representation of the basic four polypeptide chain, monomeric unit structure of immunoglobulin molecules. Heavy (H) chains determine *class*. Those in IgG are gamma, in IgM are mu, in IgA are alpha, in IgD are delta, and in IgE are epsilon. The two *types* of light (L) chains (kappa and lambda) are shared in common by all five immunoglobulin classes, although only one *type* is present in any individual molecule. Both heavy and light chains have looped structures referred to as domains or regions. Heavy chains possess one variable (VH) (wherein the antigen-binding site resides) and three constant (CH1, CH2, CH3) regions, with the exception of IgM and IgE which contain one variable (VH) and four constant regions (CH1, CH2, CH3, CH4). Light chains contain one variable (VL) and one constant (CL) region each. The heavy and light chains are fastened together by disulfide bonds as well as noncovalent forces. The disulfide bonds differ in number at the *hinge* (inter H chain) region according to immunoglobulin subclass. Antigen-binding sites are located in the variable (amino-terminus) regions of each immunoglobulin monomer. IgM and dimeric or multimeric IgA molecules have J chains which are associated with the ability of these molecules to form polymers. Secretory IgA contains a secretory piece made by epithelial cells and believed to protect the molecule from enzymatic cleavage in the hinge region. Serum IgA2 has no heavy to light chain disulfide bonds, whereas IgA1 has a classic structure.

extension, the term has come to include the use of immunopotentiators, replacement of immunocompetent lymphoid tissue (e.g., bone marrow or thymus), etc.

immunotoxin (im″u-no-tok′sin) any antitoxin.

immunotransfusion (ĭ-mu″no-trans-fu′zhun) transfusion of blood from donors previously immunized by the bacteria infecting the patient, or from the specific infection or of blood from persons recently recovered from the specific infection.

immunotropic (im″u-no-trop′ik) tending to enhance immune response mechanisms.

immunprotein (ĭ-mūn-pro′te-in) immunoglobulin.

Imodium (ĭ-mo′de-um) trademark for a preparation of loperamide hydrochloride.

IMPA incisal mandibular plane angle.

impact (im′pakt) [L. *impactus*] a sudden and forcible collision.

impacted (im-pakt′ed) [L. *impactus*] driven firmly in; closely or firmly lodged in position, as an impacted tooth.

impaction (im-pak′shun) [L. *impactio*] the condition of being firmly lodged or wedged. In obstetrics, the indentation of any fetal parts of one twin onto the surface of its co-twin, so that the simultaneous partial engagement of both twins is permitted. **ceruminal i.,** an accumulation of cerumen in the external auditory canal. **dental i.,** the condition in which a tooth is embedded in the alveolus so that its eruption is prevented, or is locked in position by bone, restoration, or surfaces of adjacent teeth, preventing either its normal occlusion or its routine removal. **fecal i.,** a collection of putty-like or hardened feces in the rectum or sigmoid.

impalpable (im-pal′pah-b'l) [L. *in* not + *palpare* to feel] impossible of being detected by touch; extremely fine, or small.

impaludation (im″pal-u-da′shun) the application of malariotherapy.

impar (im′par) [L. "unequal"] [NA] a general anatomical term meaning unpaired; having no fellow; azygous.

imparidigitate (im-par″ĭ-dij′ĭ-tāt) [L. *impar* unequal + *digitus* finger] perissodactylous.

impatency (im-pa′ten-se) the condition of being closed or obstructed.

impatent (im-pa′tent) not open; closed or obstructed.

impedance (im-pēd′ans) the opposition to the flow of an alternating current, which is the vector sum of ohmic resistance plus additional resistance, if any, due to induction, to capacity, or to both. Its symbol is Z. The resistance due to the inductive and condenser characteristics of a circuit is called reactance. In mechanics, the resistance to an applied force. **acoustic i.,** an expression of the opposition to passage of sound waves, being a function of the density and elasticity of a substance.

imperative (im-per′ah-tiv) [L. *imperativus*] dominant; not subject to control by the will.

imperception (im″per-sep′shun) defective power of perception.

imperforate (im-per′fo-rāt) [L. *imperforatus*] not open; abnormally closed, as imperforate anus.

imperforation (im-per″fo-ra′shun) the state of being abnormally closed.

imperialine (im-pe′re-al-in) a crystalline alkaloid, $C_{27}H_{43}NO_3$, from the bulbs of the liliaceous plant *Fritillaria imperialis.*

imperious (im-per′e-us) overruling or compulsive; said of acts or motions that are not under control of the will.

impermeable (im-per′me-ah-b'l) [L. *in* not + *per* through + *meare* to move] not permitting passage, as of fluid.

impervious (im-per′ve-us) [L. *impervius*] impenetrable; not affording a passage.

impetiginization (im″pe-tij″ĭ-ni-za′shun) the development of impetigo upon an area previously affected with some other skin disease.

impetiginous (im″pe-tij′ĭ-nus) [L. *impetiginosus*] pertaining to or of the nature of impetigo.

impetigo (im″pĕ-ti′go) [L.] a streptococcal or staphylococcal infection of the skin characterized by fragile, grouped, pinhead-sized vesicles or pustules that become confluent and rupture early, forming rapidly enlarging and spreading erosions with bright yellow crusts that are attached in the center and have elevated margins. Called also *i. contagiosa.* **Bockhart's i.,** a superficial folliculitis, usually caused by *Staphylococcus aureus,* marked by the formation of small purulent pustules at the orifices of the pilosebaceous glands, and affecting especially the scalp and the extremities. Called also *superficial pustular perifolliculitis.* **i. bullo′sa, bullous i.,** a staphylococcal skin infection, occurring in infants and children, or rarely in sweaty flexures of adults, and characterized by rapid formation of fragile bullae up to 2 or 3 cm. in diameter, which break early and heal centrally, leaving crusted arcuate or annular erosions. Called also *i. contagiosa bullosa, i. neonatorum,* and *pemphigus neonatorum.* **chronic symmetric i.,** pityriasis alba. **i. circina′ta,** impetigo of bullous (staphylococcal) type, in which several lesions may become confluent or in which a large bulla ruptures, leaving circinate, raw, often crusted lesions. **i. contagio′sa,** impetigo. **i. contagio′sa**

bullo′sa, i. bullosa. **i. herpetifor′mis,** a very rare, acute, potentially fatal disorder affecting the skin and mucous membranes, characterized by groups of small, symmetrically ringed pustules that sometimes coalesce, associated with severe constitutional symptoms, including continuous and intermittent fever, chills, vomiting, diarrhea, and sometimes delirium; it is usually seen in women during the last trimester of pregnancy, but men and nonpregnant women have been affected. **i. neonato′rum,** i. bullosa. **i. pityroi′des,** pityriasis alba. **i. sic′ca,** pityriasis alba. **staphylococcal i., staphylococcic i.,** bullous i. **i. vulga′ris,** i. contagiosa.

impf-malaria (impf′mah-la″re-ah) [Ger.] malaria produced by injection of infectious material; see *induced malaria,* under *malaria,* and see *malariotherapy.*

impilation (im″pi-la′shun) rouleau formation; see under *formation.*

Implacentalia (im″plas-en-ta′le-ah) in former classifications, a division of the class Mammalia, comprising the mammals that do not have a placenta, such as the monotremes.

implant[1] (im-plant′) to insert or to graft (as tissue, or an inert or radioactive material) into the intact tissues or a body cavity of the recipient.

implant[2] (im′plant) material (e.g., tissue, inert material, or radioactive material) inserted or grafted into the body. **dental i.,** an alloplastic material placed into or onto a jawbone to support a crown(s). **endometrial i's,** fragments of endometrial mucosa transferred through the oviducts and implanted on the uterus, ovaries, or pelvic peritoneum. **endo-osseous i.,** an artificial tooth of variable form inserted into the alveolar bone and protruding through the mucosa to provide support on which a restoration can be placed. **magnetic i.,** a tissue-tolerated, magnetized metal placed within the bone to aid in denture retention; a similar magnet is placed in the overlying denture to complete the field. **subperiosteal i.,** a metal appliance made to conform to the shape of a bone and placed on its surface beneath the periosteum, with lugs protruding through the mucosa to support an overlying denture.

implantation (im″plan-ta′shun) [L. *in* into + *plantare* to set] 1. attachment of the blastocyst to the epithelial lining of the uterus, its penetration through the epithelium, and, in humans, its embedding in the compact layer of the endometrium, occurring six or seven days after fertilization of the ovum. 2. the insertion of an organ or tissue, such as skin, nerve, or tendon, in a new site in the body. 3. the insertion or grafting into the body of biological, living, inert, or radioactive material. **central i.,** superficial i. **circumferential i.,** superficial i. **eccentric i.,** embedding of the blastocyst within a recess of the uterine cavity. **filigree i.,** the insertion of a network of silver or other metallic mesh in the abdominal wall for the purpose of closing a large hernial defect. **hypodermic i.,** the placing of a medicine in the subcutaneous tissue. **interstitial i.,** complete embedding of a blastocyst within the endometrium. **nerve i.,** the operation of inserting and attaching a nerve into the sheath of another nerve. **parenchymatous i.,** the introduction of therapeutic material into the substance of a tumor. **periosteal i.,** the operation of inserting a normal tendon into the periosteum of a bone at the insertion of a paralyzed tendon to take the place of the latter. **silk i.,** the operation of restoring a paralyzed tendon by implanting strands of sterile silk so that they will stimulate the formation of fascial sheaths along the line of the paralyzed tendon; called also *Lange's operation.* **superficial i.,** embedding of the blastocyst so that the blastocyst, and later the chorionic sac, comes to occupy the uterine cavity. **teratic i.,** the partial blending of an imperfect with a nearly perfect fetus.

implantodontics (im″plan-to-don′tiks) that branch of dentistry that deals with implanting alloplastic materials into or onto the jaw bones to support overlying dental appliances.

implantodontist (im″plan-to-don′tist) a dentist who specializes in implantodontics.

implantology (im″plan-tol′o-je) the science dealing with implants.

implosion (im-plo′zhun) in behavior therapy, a form of desensitization for the treatment of phobias and related disorders; the patient is repeatedly exposed, in imagination or real life, to emotionally distressing stimuli while the therapist makes verbal interpretation of the psychological meaning of the stimuli in order to intensify the patient's emotional arousal. Cf. *flooding* and *systematic desensitization.* The term *implosion* has also been used synonymously with *flooding.*

impotence (im′po-tens) [L. *in* not + *potentia* power] lack of power, chiefly of copulative power in the male due to failure to initiate an erection or to maintain an erection until ejaculation. It may be *atonic,* due to paralysis of the motor nerves (nervi erigentes) without evidence of lesion of the central nervous system; *paretic,* due to lesion in the central nervous system, particularly in the spinal cord; *psychic,* dependent on mental complex; *symptomatic,* due to some other disorder, such as injury to nerves in the perineal region, by virtue of which the sensory portion of the erection reflex arc is interrupted.

impotency (im′po-ten″se) impotence.

impotentia (im″po-ten′she-ah) [L.] impotence. **i. coeun′di,** inability of the male to perform the sexual act. **i. erigen′di,** inability to have an erection of the penis. **i. generan′di,** inability to reproduce.

impregnate (im-preg′nāt) [L. *impregnare*] 1. to render pregnant; to fertilize. 2. to saturate or charge with.

impregnation (im″preg-na′shun) [L. *impregnatio*] 1. the act of fecundation or of rendering pregnant. 2. the process or act of saturation; a saturated condition.

impressio (im-pres′se-o), pl. *impressio′nes* [L.] an impression, indentation, or concavity; [NA] a general term for an indentation produced in the surface of one organ by pressure exerted by another. **i. cardi′aca hep′atis** [NA], cardiac impression of the liver: a depression on the superior part of the diaphragmatic surface of the liver, corresponding to the position of the heart. **i. cardi′aca pulmo′nis** [NA], cardiac impression of the lung: the indentation on the medial surface of either lung produced by the heart and pericardium. **i. col′ica hep′atis** [NA], colic impression of the liver: a variable concavity in the right lobe of the liver, where it is in contact with the right flexure of the colon. **impressio′nes digita′tae** [NA], digitate or digital impressions: poorly defined depressions on the inner surface of the cranium, corresponding to the gyri of the brain. **i. duodena′les hep′atis** [NA], duodenal impression of the liver: a concavity on the right lobe of the liver where it is in contact with the descending part of the duodenum. **i. esopha′gea hep′atis** [NA], esophageal impression of the liver: a concavity on the left lobe of the liver corresponding to the position of the abdominal part of the esophagus; called also *i. oesophagea hepatis*. **i. gas′trica hep′atis** [NA], gastric impression of the liver: a large concavity in the left lobe of the liver where it is in contact with the anterior surface of the stomach. **i. gas′trica re′nis,** a concavity on the anterior surface of the left kidney where it is in contact with the stomach. **i. hepat′ica re′nis,** an impression on the anterior surface of the left kidney where it is in contact with the liver. **i. ligamen′ti costoclavicula′ris** [NA], impression of the costoclavicular ligament: the point on the inferior surface of the clavicle where the costoclavicular ligament is attached; called also *tuberositas costalis claviculae* and *costal tuberosity of clavicle*. **i. meningea′lis,** see *foveolae granulares*. **i. muscula′ris re′nis,** a depression on the posterior surface of the kidney where it is in contact with the psoas muscle. **i. oesopha′gea hep′atis,** i. esophagea hepatis. **i. petro′sa pal′lii,** a shallow groove on the base of the brain corresponding to the superior angle of the petrous portion of the temporal bone. **i. rena′lis hep′atis** [NA], renal impression of the liver: the concavity on the right lobe of the liver where it is in contact with the right kidney. **i. suprarena′lis hep′atis** [NA], suprarenal impression of the liver: a small concavity on the right lobe of the liver, superior to the renal impression, caused by contact with the right suprarenal gland. **i. trigem′ini os′sis tempora′lis** [NA], trigeminal impression of the temporal bone: the shallow impression in the floor of the middle cranial fossa on the petrous part of the temporal bone, lodging the semilunar ganglion of the trigeminal nerve.

impression (im-presh′un) [L. *impressio*] 1. a slight indentation or depression; see *impressio*. 2. a negative copy or counterpart of some object made by bringing into contact with the object, with varying degrees of pressure, some plastic material which later becomes solidified, as a dental impression. 3. an effect produced upon the mind, body, or senses by some external stimulus, or agent. **anatomic i.,** an impression of the form of a dental arch or portion thereof that records the structures in a passive or unstrained form, making possible a static relationship of a prosthesis produced from such an impression. **angular i. for gasserian ganglion,** impressio trigemini ossis temporalis. **basilar i.,** a developmental deformity of the occipital bone and upper end of the cervical spine, in which the latter appears to have pushed the floor of the occipital bone upward; called also *platybasia* and *basilar invagination*. **bridge i.,** an impression made for the purpose of constructing or assembling a fixed restoration, fixed partial denture, or bridge. **cardiac i.,** an impression made by the heart on another organ; see *impressio cardiaca hepatis* and *impressio cardiaca pulmonis*. **cardiac i. of liver,** impressio cardiaca hepatis. **cardiac i. of lung,** impressio cardiaca pulmonis. **cleft palate i.,** a negative mold made of a cleft palate, to facilitate construction of a prosthetic appliance. **colic i. of liver,** impressio colica hepatis. **complete denture i.,** 1. one made of the entire edentulous arch of the maxilla or mandible, for the purpose of construction of a complete denture. 2. a negative registration of the entire denture-bearing, stabilizing area of the maxilla or mandible. 3. a negative registration of the entire denture foundation and border seal areas of the edentulous mouth. **i. of costoclavicular ligament,** impressio ligamenti costoclavicularis. **deltoid i. of humerus,** tuberositas deltoidea humeri. **dental i.,** an impression of the jaw and/or teeth made in some plastic substance, such as plaster of Paris, special waxes, modeling compound, zinc oxide paste, reversible colloids, rubber, or alginate materials, which is later filled in with plaster of Paris to produce a facsimile of the oral structures present. **digastric i.,** fossa digastrica. **digital i′s, digitate i′s,** impressiones digitatae.

direct bone i., one made of the denuded jaw bone, for the purpose of constructing an implant denture. **duodenal i. of liver,** impressio duodenalis hepatis. **esophageal i. of liver,** impressio esophagea hepatis. **final i.,** one used for making the master cast for a dental prosthesis. **gastric i.,** an impression made by the stomach on another organ; see *impressio gastrica hepatis* and *impressio gastrica renis*. **gastric i. of liver,** impressio gastrica hepatis. **hydrocolloid i.,** a denture impression made of a hydrocolloid material. **lower i.,** mandibular i. **mandibular i.,** an impression of the mandibular jaw and related tissues and dental structures. **maxillary i.,** an impression of the maxillary jaw and related tissues and dental structures; called also *upper i.* **meningeal i.,** see *foveolae granulares*. **mercaptan i.,** a dental impression made of mercaptan (polysulfide), a rubber base elastic material. **partial denture i.,** one made of part or all of a partially edentulous arch for the purpose of constructing a partial denture. **preliminary i., primary i.,** one which is made for the purpose of diagnosis or for the construction of a tray. **renal i. of liver,** impressio renalis hepatis. **rhomboid i. of clavicle,** impressio ligamenti costoclavicularis. **sectional i.,** a dental impression that is made in sections. **suprarenal i. of liver,** impressio suprarenalis hepatis. **trigeminal i. of temporal bone,** impressio trigemini ossis temporalis. **upper i.,** maxillary i.

impressiones (im-pres″e-o′nēz) [L.] plural of *impressio*.

imprinting (im′print-ing) a species-specific, rapid kind of learning during a critical period of early life in which social attachment and identification are established.

improcreant (im-pro′kre-ant) unable to procreate; infertile.

impuberal (im-pu′ber-al) lacking pubic hairs; not yet having reached puberty.

impuberism (im-pu′ber-izm) the condition of not having reached puberty.

impulse (im′puls) 1. a sudden pushing force. 2. a sudden uncontrollable determination to act. 3. a nerve impulse. **apex i., apical i.,** a cardiac impulse usually caused by left ventricular contraction and characterized by a relatively localized outward movement beginning synchronously with the first heart sound. **cardiac i.,** 1. the palpable or recorded movement of the chest wall caused by the heartbeat. 2. excitation wave; see under *wave*. **episternal i.,** an aortic impulse felt at the episternal (suprasternal) notch. **irresistible i.,** an urge to act that is impossible to resist; see also under *tests*. **left parasternal i′s,** cardiac impulses categorized according to their location along the upper, mid, or lower left sternal border. An *upper left parasternal impulse* is usually caused by a systolic expansion of a dilated pulmonary artery; a *mid* to *lower left parasternal impulse* usually occurs as a result of a right ventricular contraction, and is characterized by an outward movement beginning synchronously with the first heart sound, but is sometimes caused by mitral incompetence. **nerve i., neural i.,** the electrochemical process propagated along nerve fibers. **right parasternal i′s,** cardiac impulses categorized according to their location along the upper, mid, or lower right sternal border.

impulsion (im-pul′shun) an abnormal impulse to perform certain acts, usually of a disagreeable nature. **wandering i.,** fugue.

imu (e′moo) a disorder endemic among the Ainu of Japan, marked by a mental state that renders the patient liable to attacks of psychomotor disorder precipitated by some emotional shock.

Imuran (im′u-ran) trademark for a preparation of azathioprine.

IMViC, imvic a mnemonic indicating the tests used in classifying coliform bacteria, namely indole, methyl red, Voges-Proskauer, and citrate.

In chemical symbol for *indium*.

in- [L. *in* in, into] 1. a prefix signifying in, within, or into. 2. an intensive prefix. 3. [L. *in* not] a negative or privative prefix.

I.N.A. International Neurological Association.

inacidity (in″ah-sid′ĭ-te) anacidity.

inaction (in-ak′shun) [L. *in* not + *actio* act] imperfect response to a normal stimulus.

inactivate (in-ak′tĭ-vāt) to render inactive; to destroy the activity of.

inactivation (in-ak″tĭ-va′shun) the destruction of biological activity, as of a virus, by the action of heat or other physical or chemical means. **i. of the complement,** the destruction of activity of the complement, usually produced by heating serum to 56° C. for 30 minutes. **heat i.,** the inactivation of C1 and C2 components of complement and of factor B of the alternative pathway by heating in a water bath to 56°C for 20 minutes.

inactose (in-ak′tōs) an optically inactive plant sugar.

inadequacy (in-ad′ĕ-kwah-se) [L. *in* not + *adaequare* to make equal] inability to perform an allotted function; insufficiency; incompetence.

inagglutinable (in-ah-gloo′tĭ-nah-b′l) not agglutinable.

inalimental (in″al-ĭ-men′tal) [L. *in* not + *alimentum* food] not nutritious; not serviceable as food.

inanimate (in-an′ĭ-māt) [L. *in* not + *animatus* alive] 1. without life. 2. lacking in animation.

inanition (in″ah-nish′un) [L. *inanis* empty] a condition characterized by marked weakness, extreme weight loss, and a decrease in metabolism resulting from prolonged (usually weeks to months) and severe insufficiency of food.

inappetence (in-ap′ĕ-tens) [L. *in* not + *appetere* to desire] lack of desire or appetite.

Inapsine (in-ap′sēn) trademark for a preparation of droperidol.

inarticulate (in″ar-tik′u-lāt) [L. *in* not + *articulatus* joined] not having joints; disjointed; not uttered like articulate speech.

in articulo mortis (in ar-tik′u-lo mor′tis) [L.] at the very point of death.

inassimilable (in″ah-sim′ĭ-lah-b'l) [L. *in* not + *assimilable*] not susceptible of being utilized as nutriment.

inaxon (in-ak′son) [Gr. *is, inos* fiber + *axōn* axis] a nerve cell whose axon breaks up into terminal filaments at a considerable distance from the cell. Cf. *dendraxon.*

inborn (in′born) congenitally formed or acquired during intrauterine life; see also *inborn error,* under *metabolism.*

inbreeding (in′brēd-ing) the mating of closely related individuals, or of individuals having closely similar genetic constitutions.

incallosal (in″kah-lo′sal) characterized by absence of the corpus callosum, and usually associated with mental retardation.

incandescent (in″kan-des′ent) [L. *incandescens* glowing] glowing with heat and light; emitting light on being heated.

incarcerated (in-kar′ser-āt″ed) [L. *incarceratus* imprisoned] imprisoned; constricted; subjected to incarceration.

incarceration (in-kar″ser-a′shun) [L. *in* in + *carcer* prison] unnatural retention or confinement of a part, as may occur in hernia.

incarnatio (in″kar-na′she-o) [L. *incarnare* to invest in flesh] ingrowth. **i. un′guis,** unguis incarnatus; ingrowth of a toenail; ingrown toenail.

incarnative (in-kar′nah-tiv) [L. *incarnare* to invest in flesh] 1. promoting the formation of granulations. 2. an agent that promotes granulations.

incasement (in-kās′ment) the act of surrounding or state of being surrounded, as with a case. See *preformation.*

incendiarism (in-sen′de-ar-izm) a criminal tendency to set fires. Cf. *pyromania.*

incertae sedis (in-ser′te se′dis) [L.] of uncertain position; said of taxa that are of uncertain classification.

incest (in′sest) sexual intercourse or other sexual activity between persons so closely related that marriage between them is legally or culturally prohibited.

inch (inch) a unit of linear measure, one-twelfth of a foot, or one thirty-sixth of a yard, being the equivalent of 2.54 cm.

inchacao (in-chah-kah′o) [Brazilian] beriberi.

incidence (in′sĭ-dens) [L. *incidere* (*in* + *cadere*), to occur, to happen] an expression of the rate at which a certain event occurs, as the number of new cases of a specific disease occurring during a certain period. Cf. *prevalence.*

incident (in′sĭ-dent) [L. *incidens* falling upon] 1. falling or striking upon, as incident radiation. 2. (*obs.*) afferent.

incineration (in-sin″ĕ-ra′shun) [L. *in* into + *cineres* ashes] the act of burning to ashes; cremation.

incipient (in-sip′e-ent) beginning to exist; coming into existence.

incisal (in-si′zal) cutting.

incised (in-sīzd′) [L. *incisus*] cut; made by cutting.

incision (in-sizh′un) [L. *incidere* (*in* + *caedere*), to cut open, to cut through] 1. a cut, or a wound produced by cutting with a sharp instrument. 2. the act of cutting. **Auvray i.,** an incision for splenectomy: the usual incision is made along the outer border of the left rectus muscle up to the costal cartilages, and then extended upward and posteriorly over the lower ribs to the level of the eighth interspace. **Bar's i.** (*obs.*), an incision for cesarean section made in the midline of the abdomen above the umbilicus, the uterus being incised longitudinally. **Battle's i., Battle-Jalaguier-Kammerer i.,** a procedure consisting of a vertical abdominal incision through the skin and superficial fascia, vertical division of the anterior layer of the rectal sheath, with retraction of the rectus muscle medialward, and vertical division of the posterior layer of the sheath nearer the median line, together with the subserous areolar tissue and peritoneum. **Bergmann's i.,** an incision for exposing the kidney, made from the outer border of the erector spinae at the level of the twelfth rib, toward the junction of the outer and middle third of Poupart's ligament. **Bevan's i.,** one for exposing the gallbladder; see illustration. **celiotomy i.,** an incision made through the abdominal wall to give access to the peritoneal cavity. **Chernez i.,** an abdominal incision in the surgical approach to the female reproductive organs. **confirmatory i.,** an incision into a tumor, an organ, or the peritoneal cavity, made for the purpose of confirming a diagnosis. **crucial i.,** a cross-shaped incision. **Deaver's i.** (*for appendicitis*), incision through the anterior

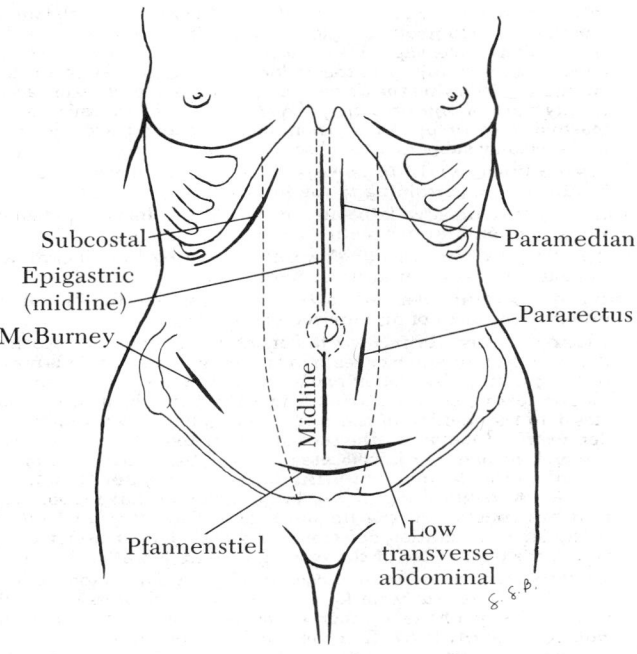

Various abdominal incisions.

sheath of the right rectus muscle, the muscle then being retracted medially. **Dührssen's i's,** incisions made in the cervix uteri to facilitate delivery; hysterostomatomy. **Fergusson's i.,** an incision for excision of the upper jaw; it runs along the junction of the nose with the cheek, around the ala of the nose to the median line, and descends to bisect the upper lip. **Fowler's angular i.,** an incision for anterolateral abdominal section. **hockey stick i.,** one shaped like a hockey stick, often used for operation on the biliary tract; see also *Meyer's hockey stick i.* **Kehr's i.,** an abdominal incision for exposing a wide field; it extends from the xiphoid cartilage to the umbilicus in the median line, then around the umbilicus, and again vertically in a caudad direction, often to the pubis. **Kocher's i.,** an incision for exposure of the gallbladder, 10 cm. long, parallel with and 4 cm. below the right costal margin. **Küstner's i.,** a semilunar abdominal incision convex distalward, through the suprapubic fat, following one of the natural folds of the skin; the upper flap is detached from the aponeurosis of the external oblique, and then the usual incision is made parallel to the rectus muscle. **Langenbeck's i.,** an abdominal incision through the linea semilunaris parallel to the fibers of the rectus abdominis muscle; often done in operations on the spleen, colon, tail of pancreas, and occasionally the kidney. **lateral rectus i.,** see illustration. **Longuet's i.,** see under *operation.* **Maylard i.,** an abdominal incision in the surgical approach to the female reproductive organs. **McArthur's i.,** a vertical upper incision through the rectus muscle, with transverse division of the posterior sheath and peritoneum. **McBurney's i.,** an abdominal incision parallel to the fibers of the external oblique muscle, about one-third the distance along a line from the anterior superior iliac spine to the umbilicus, half the incision being above and the remainder below this point. The skin and subcutaneous fat are incised down to the external oblique, the fibers of which are split; the underlying internal oblique and transversus abdominalis are then split and separated. **median i.,** one in the midline of the body; see illustration. **Meyer's hockey stick i.,** one for entering the lower abdomen through the anterior wall, partly by intramuscular separation, partly by transverse division of muscle, forming an incision shaped somewhat like a hockey stick. **Nagamatsu i.,** in renal surgery, an extrapleural retroperitoneal dorsolumbar approach to the kidney that provides an osteoplastic flap of the lower rib cage. **paramedian i.,** see illustration. **paravaginal i.,** incision of the vagina and perineum in order to secure enlargement of the vulvovaginal outlet, and thereby permit easy access to the vagina in cancer operations, and, rarely, to facilitate childbirth; called also *Schuchardt's i.* and *vaginoperineotomy.* **Perthes' i.** (for exposure of the gallbladder), a vertical right rectus incision from ensiform to umbilicus, extending laterally at the lower end across the rectus to the costal margin. **Pfannenstiel's i.,** a curved abdominal incision, the convexity being directed downward, just above the symphysis, passing through skin, superficial fascia, and aponeurosis, exposing the pyramidalis and rectus muscles, which are separated from each other in the midline, the peritoneum then being opened vertically. See illustration. **relief i.,** one made to relieve tension in tissue. **Schuchardt's i.,** paravaginal i. **Vischer's lumboiliac i.,** separation of the muscular and tendinous fibers of the abdominal muscles of the lumboiliac region, just above the center of the iliac crest, in their cleavage lines, without transverse division of the muscle fibers or injury to the abdominal nerves. **Warren's i.,** an incision following the thoracomammary fold, permitting access to any part of the breast. **Wilde's i.,** (*obs.*) exposure of the mastoid process by an incision behind the auricle, done for postauricular subperiosteal abscess in mastoiditis.

incisive (in-si'siv) [L. *incisivus*] 1. having the power or quality of cutting. 2. pertaining to the incisor teeth.

incisolabial (in-si″zo-la'be-al) denoting the incisal and labial surfaces of an anterior tooth.

incisolingual (in-si″zo-ling'gwahl) denoting the incisal and lingual surfaces of an anterior tooth.

incisoproximal (in-si″zo-prok'sĭ-mal) denoting the incisal and proximal surfaces of an anterior tooth.

incisor (in-si'zer) [L. *incidere* to cut into] 1. adapted for cutting. 2. any of the four anterior teeth in either jaw; a tooth that is mesial to the canines. See under *tooth*. **central i., first i.,** the two incisor teeth (see under *tooth*) in each jaw which are located closer to the midline of the body. **Hutchinson's i's,** see under *tooth*. **lateral i.,** the second incisor tooth on either side of the midline of either jaw, located distal to the central incisor and mesial to the canine. **medial i.,** central i. **second i.,** lateral i. **shovel-shaped i's,** large upper medial incisor teeth that are concave on the lingual side; called also *hawk-bill i's*. **winged i.,** a rotation deformity of a maxillary incisor tooth in which the distal edge of the tooth protrudes labially.

incisura (in-si-su'rah), pl. *incisu'rae* [L.] a cut, notch, or incision; [NA] a general term for an indention or depression, chiefly on the edge of a bone or other structure. Called also *incisure* and *notch*. **i. acetab'uli** [NA], incisure of acetabulum: a notch in the inferior portion of the lunate surface of the acetabulum. **i. angula'ris ventric'uli** [NA], the lowest point on the lesser curvature of the stomach, marking the junction of the cranial two-thirds and caudal one-third of the stomach; called also *gastric notch*. **i. ante'rior au'ris** [NA], anterior incisure of the ear: a depression between the crus of the helix and the tragus; called also *auricular notch*. **i. ap'icis cor'dis** [NA], incisure of apex of the heart: a slight notch found at the site where the anterior and posterior interventricular sulci become continuous and cross the right margin of the heart. **i. cardi'aca pulmo'nis sinis'-tri** [NA], cardiac incisure of left lung: a notch in the anterior border of the left lung; called also *cardiac notch of left lung*. **i. cardi'aca ventric'uli** [NA], cardiac incisure of the stomach: a notch at the junction of the esophagus and the greater curvature of the stomach; called also *cardiac notch of stomach*. **incisu'rae cartilag'inis mea'tus acus'tici** [NA], two vertical fissures in the anterior part of the cartilage of the external acoustic meatus; called also *Santorini's fissures*. **i. cerebel'li ante'rior,** a wide notch on the anterior surface of the cerebellum, occupied by the inferior colliculi and superior cerebellar peduncles; called also *anterior cerebellar notch*. **i. cerebel'li poste'rior,** a notch between the cerebellar hemispheres posteriorly, containing the falx cerebelli; called also *posterior cerebellar notch*. **i. clavicula'ris ster'ni** [NA], clavicular incisure of the sternum: an oval surface on each side of the cranial border of the manubrium, where it articulates with the clavicle; called also *clavicular notch of sternum*. **incisu'rae costa'les ster'ni** [NA], costal incisures of the sternum: the facets on the sternum, seven on each lateral edge, for articulation with the costal cartilages; called also *costal notches of sternum*. **i. ethmoida'lis os'sis fronta'lis** [NA], ethmoidal incisure of frontal bone: a space between the orbital parts of the frontal bone, in which the ethmoid bone is lodged; called also *ethmoid notch of frontal bone*. **i. fastig'ii** [NA], a transverse furrow on the ventricular surface of the cerebellar lamina of the developing cerebellum. **i. fibula'ris tib'iae** [NA], fibular incisure of tibia: a depression on the lateral surface of the lower end of the tibia, which articulates with the lower end of the fibula; called also *fibular notch*. **i. fronta'lis** [NA], frontal incisure: a notch located in the supraorbital margin of the frontal bone medial to the supraorbital notch or foramen, for transmission of branches of the supraorbital nerve and vessels; frequently converted into a foramen (foramen frontalis) by a bridge of osseous tissue; called also *frontal notch*. **i. interarytenoi'dea laryn'gis** [NA], interarytenoid incisure of larynx: the posterior portion of the aditus laryngis between the two arytenoid cartilages; called also *interarytenoid notch*. **i. interloba'ris hep'atis,** i. ligamenti teretis. **i. interloba'ris pulmo'nis,** an incisure separating adjacent lobes of a lung; see *fissura obliqua pulmonis* and *fissura horizontalis pulmonis dextri*. **i. intertrag'ica** [NA], the intertragic incisure: the notch at the lower part of the pinna of the ear between the tragus and the antitragus; called also *intertragic notch*. **i. ischiad'ica ma'jor** [NA], greater ischiadic incisure: the large notch on the posterior border of the hip bone, where the posterior borders of the ilium and the ischium become continuous; called also *greater ischiadic* or *sciatic notch*. **i. ischiad'ica mi'nor** [NA], lesser ischiadic incisure: the notch on the posterior border of the ischium just inferior to the ischiadic spine; called also *lesser ischiadic* or *sciatic notch*. **i. jugula'-**

ris os'sis occipita'lis [NA], jugular incisure of occipital bone: a notch on the anterior surface of the jugular process of the occipital bone, forming the posterior wall of the jugular foramen; called also *jugular notch of occipital bone*. **i. jugula'ris os'sis tempora'lis** [NA], jugular incisure of temporal bone: a prominent depression on the inferior surface of the petrous part of the temporal bone. It forms the anterior and lateral wall of the jugular foramen and lodges the superior bulb of the internal jugular vein in its lateral part and the glossopharyngeal, vagus, and accessory nerves in its medial part; called also *jugular notch of temporal bone*. **i. jugula'ris ster'ni** [NA], jugular incisure of sternum: the notch on the upper border of the sternum between the clavicular notches; called also *jugular notch of sternum*. **i. lacrima'lis maxil'lae** [NA], lacrimal incisure of maxilla: an indentation on the posterior border of the frontal process of the maxilla, that lodges the lacrimal sac; called also *lacrimal notch of maxilla*. **i. ligamen'ti te'retis** [NA], a notch in the inferior border of the liver, occupied by the ligamentum teres in the adult; called also *i. umbilicalis, umbilical notch* or *incisure*, and *notch of the ligamentum teres*. **i. man-dib'ulae** [NA], incisure of mandible: a deep notch on the upper edge of the ramus of the mandible between the condyle and the coronoid process; called also *mandibular notch*. **i. mas-toi'dea os'sis tempora'lis** [NA], mastoid incisure of temporal bone: a deep groove on the medial surface of the mastoid process of the temporal bone, which gives origin to the posterior belly of the digastric muscle; called also *mastoid notch*. **i. nasa'lis maxil'lae** [NA], nasal incisure of maxilla: the large notch in the anterior border of the maxilla that forms the lateral and inferior margins of the anterior nasal aperture; called also *nasal notch of maxilla*. **i. pancre'atis** [NA], a notch at the junction of the left half of the head of the pancreas and the neck of the pancreas; called also *pancreatic notch*. **i. parieta'lis os'sis tempora'lis** [NA], parietal incisure of temporal bone: the notch found on the upper margin of the temporal bone where the squamous and parietomastoid sutures meet; called also *parietal notch of temporal bone*. **i. perone'a tib'iae,** i. fibularis tibiae. **i. preoccipita'lis** [NA], preoccipital incisure: a notch near the posterior end of the inferolateral border of the cerebral hemisphere. A line joining it to the parietooccipital sulcus serves to delineate the parietal and temporal lobes from the occipital lobe; called also *preoccipital notch*. **i. radia'lis ul'nae** [NA], radial incisure of ulna: the cavity on the outer side of the coronoid process, articulating with the rim of the head of the radius; called also *radial notch (of ulna)*. **i. Rivi'ni,** i. tympanica [Rivini]. **i. Santori'ni,** 1. incisura anterior auris. 2. see *incisurae carti-laginis meatus acustici*. **i. scap'ulae** [NA], incisure of scapula: a notch, converted into a foramen by a ligament, on the upper border of the scapula at the base of the coracoid process; called also *scapular notch*. **i. semiluna'ris tib'iae,** i. fibularis tibiae. **i. semiluna'ris ul'nae,** i. trochlearis ulnae. **i. sphenopalati'na os'sis palati'ni** [NA], sphenopalatine incisure of palatine bone: a notch between the oribital and sphenoid processes of the palatine bone; it is converted into a foramen by the under surface of the sphenoid bone; called also *sphenopalatine notch of palatine bone*. **i. supraorbita'lis** [NA], supraorbital incisure: a palpable notch in the frontal bone at the junction of the medial one-third and lateral two-thirds of the supraorbital margin, for transmission of the supraorbital nerve and vessels to the forehead. In life it is bridged by fibrous tissue, which is sometimes ossified, forming a bony aperture (foramen supraorbitalis). Called also *supraorbital notch*. **i. tempora'lis,** a slight fissure between the uncus of the parahippocampal gyrus and the apex of the temporal lobe. **i. tento'rii cerebel'li** [NA], incisure of tentorium of cerebellum: an opening at the anterior part of the cerebellum, formed by the free, internal border of the tentorium and the dorsum sellae of the sphenoid, and occupied chiefly by the mesencephalon; called also *tentorial notch*. **i. termina'lis au'ris** [NA], terminal incisure of the ear: a deep notch separating the lamina tragi and cartilage of the external acoustic meatus from the main auricular cartilage. **i. thyroi'-dea infe'rior** [NA], inferior thyroid incisure: a notch at the lower part of the anterior border of the thyroid cartilage; called also *inferior thyroid notch*. **i. thyroi'dea supe'rior** [NA], superior thyroid incisure: a deep notch in the upper portion of the anterior border of the thyroid cartilage; called also *superior thyroid notch*. **i. trag'ica,** i. intertragica. **i. trochlea'ris ul'nae** [NA], a large concavity on the anterior surface at the proximal end of the ulna, formed by the olecranon and coronoid processes, for articulation with the trochlea of the humerus; called also *i. semilunaris ulnae* and *trochlear notch of ulna*. **i. tym-pan'ica [Rivi'ni]** [NA], tympanic notch: a defect in the upper portion of the tympanic part of the temporal bone, between the greater and lesser tympanic spines, which is filled in by the pars flaccida of the tympanic membrane. **i. ulna'ris ra'dii** [NA], ulnar incisure of radius: a concavity on the medial side of the distal extremity of the radius, articulating with the head of the ulna; called also *ulnar notch (of radius)*. **i. umbilica'lis,** i. ligamenti teretis. **i. vertebra'lis infe'rior** [NA], inferior vertebral incisure: the indentation found below each pedicle of a vertebra which, with the indentation located above the pedicle of the vertebra below, forms the intervertebral foramen; called also *inferior vertebral notch.* **i. vertebra′lis supe′rior** [NA], superior vertebral incisure: the indentation found above each pedicle of a vertebra which, with the indentation located below the corresponding pedicle of the vertebra above, forms the intervertebral foramen; called also *superior vertebral notch.*

incisurae (in″si-su′re) [L.] plural of *incisura.*

incisure (in-si′zhūr) a cut, notch, or incision; called also *incisura* [NA]. **i. of acetabulum,** incisura acetabuli. **i. of apex of heart,** incisura apicis cordis. **i. of calcaneus,** sulcus tendinis musculi flexoris hallucis longi calcanei. **cardiac i. of left lung,** incisura cardiaca pulmonis sinistra. **cardiac i. of stomach,** incisura cardiaca ventriculi. **clavicular i. of sternum,** incisura clavicularis sterni. **costal i's of sternum,** incisurae costales sterni. **cotyloid i.,** incisura acetabuli. **digastric i. of temporal bone,** incisura mastoidea ossis temporalis. **i. of ear, anterior,** incisura anterior auris. **i. of ear, terminal,** incisura terminalis auris. **ethmoidal i. of frontal bone,** incisura ethmoidalis ossis frontalis. **falciform i. of fascia lata,** margo falciformis hiatus saphenus. **fibular i. of tibia,** incisura fibularis tibiae. **frontal i.,** incisura frontalis. **humeral i. of ulna,** incisura trochlearis ulnae. **iliac i., lesser,** incisura ischiadica minor. **interarytenoid i. of larynx,** incisura interarytenoidea laryngis. **interclavicular i.,** incisura jugularis sterni. **intertragic i.,** incisura intertragica. **ischiadic i., greater,** incisura ischiadica major. **ischiadic i., lesser,** incisura ischiadica minor. **jugular i. of occipital bone,** incisura jugularis ossis occipitalis. **jugular i. of sternum,** incisura jugularis sterni. **jugular i. of temporal bone,** incisura jugularis ossis temporalis. **lacrimal i. of maxilla,** incisura lacrimalis maxillae. **i's of Lantermann, i's of Lantermann-Schmidt,** channels of cytoplasm in the myelin sheath of neurons that lead back to the Schwann cell body; they appear as oblique lines or slashes in the sheath. Called also *Lantermann's clefts* and *Schmidt-Lantermann i's.* **lateral i. of sternum,** incisura clavicularis sterni. **i. of mandible,** incisura mandibulae. **mastoid i. of temporal bone,** incisura mastoidea ossis temporalis. **maxillary i., inferior,** margo lacrimalis maxillae. **nasal i. of frontal bone,** margo nasalis ossis frontalis. **nasal i. of maxilla,** incisura nasalis maxillae. **obturator i. of pubic bone,** sulcus obturatorius ossis pubis. **palatine i.,** fissura pterygoidea. **palatine i. of Henle,** incisura sphenopalatina ossis palatini. **parietal i. of temporal bone,** incisura parietalis ossis temporalis. **patellar i. of femur,** facies patellaris femoris. **peroneal i. of tibia,** incisura fibularis tibiae. **popliteal i.,** fossa intercondylaris femoris. **preoccipital i.,** incisura preoccipitalis. **pterygoid i.,** fissura pterygoidea. **radial i. of ulna,** incisura radialis ulnae. **Rivinus' i.,** incisura tympanica [Rivini]. **i. of scapula,** incisura scapulae. **Schmidt-Lanterman i's,** i's of Lanterman. **semilunar i.,** incisura scapulae. **semilunar i., greater, of ulna,** incisura trochlearis ulnae. **semilunar i., lesser, of ulna,** incisura radialis ulnae. **semilunar i. of mandible,** incisura mandibulae. **semilunar i. of radius,** incisura ulnaris radii. **semilunar i. of scapula,** incisura scapulae. **semilunar i. of sternum,** incisura clavicularis sterni. **semilunar i. of sternum, superior,** incisura jugularis sterni. **semilunar i. of tibia,** incisura fibularis tibiae. **semilunar i. of ulna,** incisura trochlearis ulnae. **sigmoid i. of mandible,** incisura mandibulae. **sigmoid i. of ulna,** incisura trochlearis ulnae. **sphenopalatine i. of palatine bone,** incisura sphenopalatina ossis palatini. **sternal i.,** incisura jugularis sterni. **supraorbital i.,** incisura supraorbitalis. **suprascapular i.,** incisura scapulae. **i. of talus,** sulcus tendinis musculi flexoris hallucis longi tali. **i. of tentorium of cerebellum,** incisura tentorii cerebelli. **thoracic i.,** angulus infrasternalis thoracis. **thyroid i., inferior,** incisura thyroidea inferior. **thyroid i., superior,** incisura thyroidea superior. **trochlear i. of ulna,** incisura trochlearis ulnae. **ulnar i. of radius,** incisura ulnaris radii. **umbilical i.,** incisura ligamenti teretis. **vertebral i., greater, vertebral i., inferior,** incisura vertebralis inferior. **vertebral i., lesser, vertebral i., superior,** incisura vertebralis superior.

incitant (in-sīt′ant) an inciting or causative agent, as one that causes infectious disease or induces an allergic reaction.

incitogram (in-si′to-gram) the neural conditions which organize and initiate efferent impulses.

inclinatio (in″kli-na′she-o), pl. *inclinatio′nes* [L.] inclination. **i. pel′vis** [NA], pelvic inclination: the angle between the plane of the superior aperture of the minor pelvis and the horizontal plane, when the body is in the erect position; called also *pelvic incline.*

inclination (in″kli-na′shun) [L. *inclinatio* a leaning] a sloping or leaning; the angle of slope from a particular line or plane of reference. Applied especially in dentistry to the deviation of a tooth from the vertical and also to cusp slopes on the occlusal surfaces or other surfaces of a tooth. **condylar guidance i., condylar guide i.,** the angle of inclination of the condylar guidance to an accepted horizontal plane. **lateral condylar i.,** the direction of the lateral condyle path. **lingual i.,** deviation of a tooth from the vertical, in the direction of the tongue. **pelvic i., i. of pelvis,** inclinatio pelvis.

inclinationes (in″kli-na″she-o′nēz) plural of *inclinatio.*

incline (in′klīn) inclination. **pelvic i., i. of pelvis,** inclinatio pelvis.

inclinometer (in″kli-nom′ĕ-ter) an instrument for determining the ocular diameter.

inclusion (in-klu′zhun) [L. *inclusio*] 1. the act of enclosing or condition of being enclosed. 2. anything that is enclosed; often used alone to refer to cell inclusions. **cell i.,** a usually lifeless, often temporary, constituent of the cytoplasm of a cell, such as an accumulation of proteins, fats, carbohydrates, pigments, secretory granules, crystals, or other insoluble components. **dental i.,** 1. a tooth so surrounded with bony material that it is unable to erupt. 2. a cyst of oral soft tissue or bone. **fetal i.,** a partially developed embryo enclosed within the body of its twin. **Guarnieri's i's,** see under *body.* **intranuclear i's,** inclusion bodies. **leukocyte i's,** Döhle's inclusion bodies. **Walthard's i's,** see under *islet.*

incoagulability (in″ko-ag″u-lah-bil′ĭ-te) the state of being incapable of coagulation.

incoagulable (in″ko-ag′u-lah-b'l) not susceptible to coagulation.

incoherent (in″ko-hēr′ent) [L. *in* not + *cohaerere* to cling together] without proper sequence; incongruous.

incompatibility (in″kom-pat″ĭ-bil′ĭ-te) the quality of being incompatible. See also *histoincompatibility.* **chemical i.,** the quality of not being miscible with another given substance without a chemical change. **physiologic i.,** the quality of not being administrable with another given remedy on account of their antagonistic pharmacologic effects. **therapeutic i.,** opposition in therapeutic effect between two or more medicines.

incompatible (in″kom-pat′ĭ-b'l) [L. *incompatibilis*] not suitable for combination or simultaneous administration; mutually repellent. See also *histoincompatible.*

incompetence (in-kom′pe-tens) [L. *in* not + *competens* sufficient] 1. physical or mental inadequacy or insufficiency. 2. the legal status of a person determined by the court to be unable to manage his own affairs. **aortic i.,** see under *regurgitation.* **i. of the cardiac valves,** see *valvular regurgitation,* under *regurgitation.* **ileocecal i.,** inability of the ileocecal valve to prevent the flow of material from the colon to the ileum. **relative i.,** inadequate closure of a cardiac valve associated with dilatation of the corresponding ventricle of the heart. **valvular i.,** see *valvular regurgitation,* under *regurgitation.*

incompetency (in-kom′pe-ten″se) incompetence.

incompetent (in-kom′pe-tent) 1. lacking competence; unable to perform the required functions. 2. an individual who is unable to perform the required functions of everyday living. 3. a person determined by the court to be unable to manage his own affairs.

incompressible (in″kom-pres′ĭ-b'l) not susceptible of being squeezed together.

incontinence (in-kon′tĭ-nens) [L. *incontinentia*] 1. inability to control excretory functions, as defecation (fecal i.) or urination (urinary i.). 2. immoderation or excess. **active i.,** incontinence in which the bowels or bladder are emptied involuntarily, but at regular intervals and in the normal way. **fecal i., i. of the feces,** failure of voluntary control of the anal sphincters, with involuntary passage of feces and flatus. **intermittent i.,** loss of control of the urine on a sudden movement or on pressure on the bladder, due to interruption of the voluntary path above the lumbar center. **overflow i.,** urinary incontinence due to pressure of retained urine in the bladder after the bladder has contracted to its limits, with dribbling of urine; called also *paradoxical i.* **paradoxical i.,** overflow i. **paralytic i.,** fecal and urinary incontinence caused by relaxation of the sphincters from destruction of the lumbar centers. **passive i.,** incontinence of urine in which the bladder is full and cannot be emptied in the normal way, but the urine dribbles away from mere pressure. **rectal i.,** fecal i. **stress i.,** involuntary discharge of urine due to anatomic displacement which exerts an opening pull on the bladder orifice, as in straining or coughing. **urinary i., i. of urine,** failure of voluntary control of the vesical and urethral sphincters, with constant or frequent involuntary passage of urine.

incontinent (in-kon′tĭ-nent) 1. unable to control excretory functions; see *incontinence.* 2. immoderate.

incontinentia (in-kon″tĭ-nen′she-ah) [L.] incontinence. **i. al′vi,** fecal incontinence. **i. pigmen′ti,** a hereditary disorder occurring almost exclusively in females, in which early vesicular and later verrucous and bizarrely pigmented skin lesions are associated with developmental defects of the eyes, bones, and central nervous system. Called also *Bloch-Sulzberger syndrome.* **i. uri′nae,** urinary incontinence. **i. vul′vae** (*obs.*), flatus vaginalis.

incoordination (in″ko-or″dĭ-na′shun) [L. *in* not + *coordination*] lack of the normal adjustment of muscular motions; failure of organs to work harmoniously.

incorporation (in-kor′po-ra′shun) [L. *in* into + *corpus* body] 1. the union of one substance with another, or with others, in a composite mass. 2. the unconscious mental mechanism in which attitudes of another person are taken into the mind of an individual, following the model of oral ingestion and swallowing.

incostapedial (ing″ko-sta-pe′de-al) pertaining to the incus and stapes.

increment (in′kre-ment) [L. *incrementum*] addition, or increase; the amount by which a given quantity or value is increased. **absolute i.,** the exact amount by which anything is increased. **relative i.,** the amount by which anything is increased, in relation to the original size or volume.

incretion (in-kre′shun) (*obs.*) an internal secretion; a hormone.

incretodiagnosis (in-kre″to-di″ag-no′sis) diagnosis of disease of internal secretions (endocrine disease).

incretogenous (in″kre-toj′ĕ-nus) caused by an internal secretion (hormone).

incretology (in″kre-tol′o-je) [*incretion* + *-logy*] endocrinology.

incretopathy (in″kre-top′ah-the) [*incretion* + Gr. *pathos* disease] any disease of internal secretions (endocrine disease).

incretory (in′kre-to-re) pertaining to internal secretion; endocrine.

incretotherapy (in-kre″to-ther′ah-pe) treatment by the administration of hormones.

incross (in′kros) the mating of individuals homozygous for the same gene.

incrustation (in″krus-ta′shun) [L. *in* on + *crusta* crust] 1. the formation of a crust. 2. a crust, scale, or scab.

incubate (in′ku-bāt) [L. *incubare* to lie in or on; to watch over jealously] 1. to place in an optimal situation for development, as by provision of the proper temperature and humidity for the growth of living cells, such as ova, microorganisms, or tissue cells. 2. to maintain a culture or a reaction mixture at a fixed temperature. 3. material which has been incubated.

incubation (in″ku-ba′shun) [L. *incubatio*] 1. the induction of development, as (*a*) the development of an infectious disease from the entrance of the pathogen to the appearance of clinical symptoms (see also under *period* and cf. *decubation*); (*b*) the development of disease-producing microorganisms in an intermediate or in the ultimate host; or (*c*) the development of microorganisms or other cells in appropriate media. 2. the development of the embryo in the eggs of oviparous animals. 3. in Greek medicine, the rite of sleeping in the Æsculapian temples, medical advice being rendered in a dream, or by the priests, if patients waked.

incubator (in′ku-ba-ter) 1. an apparatus for maintaining a premature infant in an environment of proper temperature and humidity. 2. an apparatus for maintaining a constant and suitable temperature for the development of eggs, cultures of microorganisms, or other living cells.

incubus (in′ku-bus) [L.] 1. a nightmare. 2. a heavy mental burden.

incudal (ing′ku-dal) [L. *incus* anvil] pertaining to the incus.

incudectomy (ing″ku-dek′to-me) [L. *incus* anvil + Gr. *ektome* excision] surgical removal of the incus.

incudiform (ing-ku′dĭ-form) anvil-shaped.

incudomalleal (ing″ku-do-mal′e-al) pertaining to the incus and malleus.

incudostapedial (ing″ku-do-sta-pe′de-al) pertaining to the incus and stapes.

incurable (in-ku′rah-b'l) not susceptible of being cured.

incurvation (in″kur-va′shun) [L. *incurvare* to bend in] a condition of being bent in.

incus (ing′kus) [L. "anvil"] [NA] the middle of the three ossicles of the ear, which, with the stapes and malleus, serves to conduct vibrations from the tympanic membrane to the inner ear. See Plate accompanying *ear.* Called also *anvil.*

incyclophoria (in-si″klo-fo′re-ah) cyclophoria in which the upper pole of the vertical axis of the eye deviates toward the midline of the face, or toward the nose; called also *negative* or *minus cyclophoria.* Cf. *excyclophoria.*

incyclotropia (in-si″klo-tro′pe-ah) cyclotropia in which the upper pole of the vertical axis of the eye deviates toward the midline of the face, or toward the nose; called also *negative* or *minus cyclotropia.*

in d. abbreviation for L. *in di′es,* daily.

indanedione (in″dān-di′ōn) any of a group of synthetic anticoagulants derived from 1,3-indanedione, including phenindione, chemically different from the coumarin (q.v.) drugs but similar to them in structure and actions, i.e., they impair the hepatic synthesis of the vitamin K–dependent coagulation factors (prothrombin, Factors VII, IX, and X).

Indecidua (in″de-sid′u-ah) a division of the class Mammalia, comprising the mammals without a decidua, including whales and ungulates.

indenization (in-den″i-za′shun) innidiation.

indentation (in″den-ta′shun) [L. *indentatio; dens* tooth] 1. a condition of being notched; a notch, pit, or depression. 2. the act of indenting, as with the finger.

Inderal (in′der-al) trademark for a preparation of propranolol hydrochloride.

index (in′deks), pl. *indexes* or *in′dices* [L.] 1. [NA] the second digit of the hand, or forefinger; the finger adjacent to the thumb. 2. an expression of the ratio of one dimension of an object to another dimension, or of one measurable value to another, usually determined by multiplying the smaller value by 100 and dividing by the larger value. 3. a formula based on measurable values to express a value incapable of precise determination. 4. a core or mold used in dentistry to record or maintain the relative position of a tooth or teeth to one another and/or to a cast, to ensure reproduction in the dental prosthesis of their original position. **ACH i.,** an index for nutritional condition of children based on measurements of arm girth, chest depth, and hip width. **air velocity i.** (*obs.*), the ratio between the maximal breathing capacity and the vital capacity. **altitudinal i.,** the relation of the cranial height to the cranial length; called also *height i.* and *length-height i.* **alveolar i.,** gnathic i. **antibacterial i.,** in competitive inhibition, the minimal value of the ratio of inhibitor to metabolite just sufficient to prevent the growth of the organism. **antitryptic i.,** a number representing the increased viscosity of a solution of casein treated with trypsin to which the blood serum of a cancer patient has been added, as compared with the viscosity after the same procedure in which the blood serum is normal. **Arneth i.,** see under *formula.* **auricular i.,** the relation of the width to the height of the auricle of the ear. **auriculoparietal i.,** the ratio of the breadth of the skull between the auricular points to its greatest breadth. **auriculovertical i.,** the ratio of the height of the skull above the auricular point to its greatest height. **Ayala i.,** see under *quotient.* **baric i.,** 100 times the body weight divided by the cube of the stature. **basilar i.,** the ratio of the distance between the basion and the alveolar point to the total length of the skull. **Becker-Lennhoff i.,** Lennhoff's i. **biochemical racial i.,** the ratio of the percentage of persons having agglutinogen A in their erythrocytes to the percentage having agglutinogen B, or the ratio of persons of blood group II to those of blood group III. **body build i.,** body weight divided by the square of the stature. **Bouchard's i.** (of adiposity or emaciation), the weight in kilograms divided by the height in decimeters; in a normal adult male each decimeter of height weighs 4200 gm. **brachial i.,** 100 times the length of the forearm divided by the length of the upper arm. **Broders' i.,** an index of malignancy based on the fact that the more undifferentiated or embryonic the cells of a tumor, the more malignant is the tumor. Grade 1 contains one fourth undifferentiated cells; Grade 2, one half undifferentiated cells; Grade 3, three fourths undifferentiated cells; Grade 4, all cells undifferentiated. **Brugsch i.,** chest circumference × 100 divided by body length. **calcium i.,** the relative amount of calcium in the blood compared with that in a 1:6000 solution of calcium oxide. **cardiac i.,** the minute cardiac output per square meter of body surface; a normal average is 2.8 liters. **cardiothoracic i.,** the size of the heart in relation to the size of the chest, being the greatest transverse diameter of the heart shadow as compared with the greatest transverse diameter of the chest shadow on radioscopy. **I.-Catalogue,** Index-Catalogue of the Library of the Surgeon General's Office, published from 1880 to 1950; replaced by Current List of Medical Literature published to 1959; in 1960 replaced by Index Medicus. **centromeric i.,** the ratio of the length of the shorter arm of a mitotic chromosome to the total length of the chromosome. **cephalic i.,** 100 times the maximal head breadth divided by the maximal head length. **cephalo-orbital i.,** 100 times the capacity of the cranium divided by the capacity of the two orbits. **cephalorhachidian i.,** cerebrospinal i. **cephalospinal i.,** the ratio of the area of the foramen magnum in square meters and the cranial capacity in cubic centimeters. **cerebral i.,** the ratio of the greatest transverse to the greatest anteroposterior diameter of the cranial cavity. **cerebrospinal i.,** the figure obtained by multiplying the final cerebrospinal pressure by the quantity of fluid withdrawn in spinal puncture and then dividing by the initial pressure. **chemotherapeutic i.,** therapeutic i. **color i.,** an outmoded concept for an expression of the relative amount of hemoglobin contained in a red blood corpuscle compared with that of a normal individual of the patient's age and sex; divide the percentage of hemoglobin by the percentage of erythrocytes. **Colour I.,** a publication of the Society of Dyers and Colourists and the American Association of Textile Chemists and Colorists containing an extensive list of dyes and dye intermediates. Each chemically distinct compound is identified by a specific number, the C.I. number, avoiding the confusion of trivial names used for dyes in the dye industry. **coronofrontal i.,** the ratio of the greatest frontal to the greatest coronal breadth of the head. **cranial i.,** 100 times the maximal breadth of the skull divided by its length. **Cumulated I. Medicus,** an annual publication of the National Library of Medicine, comprising the twelve monthly issues of the Index Medicus. **degenerative i.,** 1. an index indicating the accumulation of granules (possibly toxic) in the cytoplasm. 2. an index introduced by Schilling, reflecting the increased number of neutrophilic leukocytes with narrow, deeply staining nuclei in the peripheral blood. The process of maturation of these cells supposedly is arrested. **dental i.,** the result obtained by multiplying the dental length by 100 and dividing by the length of the basinasal line. **effective temperature i.,** an index indicating the warmth due to air temperature, air movement, and humidity. **empathic i.,** the degree of empathy felt by one person toward another. **endemic i.,** the percentage of persons in any locality affected with an endemic disease. **facial i.,** the relation of the length of the face to its width, obtained by multiplying by 100 the bizygomatic width and dividing the product by the distance from the ophryon to the alveolar point. **femorohumeral i.,** 100 times the length of the upper arm divided by the length of the thigh. **Flower's i.,** dental i. **forearm-hand i.,** 100 times the length of the hand divided by the length of the forearm. **Fourmentin's thoracic i.,** the number obtained by multiplying the transverse diameter of the thorax by 100 and dividing by the anteroposterior diameter. **generation i.,** the number that shows the rate of increase from generation to generation; in the binary division of bacteria, if all survive the rate will be 2; if some die the rate will be less. **gnathic i.,** the degree of prominence of the jaws; the distance from the basion to the front of the jaw expressed as a percentage of the distance from the basion to the midpoint of the nasal suture. **habitus i.,** 100 times the sum of the chest girth and the abdominal girth divided by the stature. **hair i.,** the figure obtained by dividing the least diameter of the cross section of a hair by its greatest diameter and multiplying by 100; a high index indicates an approximately round shape; a low index indicates an ovoid cross section. **hand i.,** 100 times the breadth of the hand divided by the length of the hand. **hematopneic i.,** a figure denoting the intensity of blood oxygenation. **hemophagocytic i.,** the relative phagocytic power of leukocytes in the presence of serum; called also *opsonocytophagic i.* **hemorenal i., hemorenal salt i.,** the ratio of the amount of inorganic salts in the urine to that in the blood, obtained by dividing the electric resistance of the blood by that of the urine. **Hench-Aldrich i.,** see under *test.* **icteric i., icterus i.,** a figure expressing the amount of bilirubin in the blood, determined by comparing the color of the blood serum with an arbitrary standard potassium dichromate solution; indicative of liver function. **intermembral i.,** 100 times the length of the entire arm divided by the length of the entire leg. **juxtaglomerular i.,** semiquantitative estimation of the degree of granulation of juxtaglomerular cells obtained by a counting method and expressed as a ratio to the number of glomeruli. **Kaup i.,** weight divided by the length of the body squared. **length-breadth i.,** the breadth of the skull expressed as a percentage of its length. **length-height i.,** the height of the skull expressed as a percentage of its length. **Lennhoff's i.,** the number obtained by dividing 100 times the distance from the sternal notch to the symphysis pubis by the greatest circumference of the abdomen. **leukopenic i.,** in food allergies, if ingestion of the suspected food is followed within 1½ hours by a significant fall (1000 or more) in the total leukocyte count, allergic hypersensitivity to that food is indicated. Cf. *hemoclastic crisis,* under *crisis.* **Livi's i.,** $100 \times \sqrt[3]{P \cdot 6}$, in which P = body weight in grams × body length in centimeters. **lower leg-foot i.,** 100 times the length of the foot divided by the length of the lower leg. **Macdonald i.,** the proportion of children with enlarged spleen that also show malarial parasites by microscopical examination. **McLean's i.,** see under *formula.* **maxilloalveolar i.,** 100 times the distance between the two most lateral points on the surface of the alveolar margins, usually opposite the middle of the second molar teeth, divided by the maxilloalveolar length. **I. Medicus,** a monthly publication of the National Library of Medicine in which the world's leading biomedical literature is indexed by author and subject; see also *Cumulated I. Medicus.* **metacarpal i.,** the average of the figures obtained by dividing the lengths of the right second, third, fourth, and fifth metacarpal bones by their respective breadths at the exact midpoint; stated to range normally between 5.4 and 7.9. A value above 8.4 is diagnostic of arachnodactyly. **mitotic i.,** the ratio of the number of cells in a population undergoing mitosis to the number not undergoing mitosis. **morphological i.,** the volume of the trunk divided by the length of the limbs. **morphologic face i.,** 100 times the distance from the nasion to the gnathion divided by the bizygomatic breadth. **nasal i.,** 100 times the maximal breadth of the nasal aperture divided by the nasion-nasospinale height. **nucleoplasmic i.,** the relation of the size of the nucleus of a cell to that of the cytoplasm, expressed numerically by the quotient of the nuclear volume divided by the difference between the volume of the cell and the nuclear volume. **obesity i.,** body weight divided by body volume. **opsonic i.,** a measure of opsonic activity determined by the ratio of the number of microorganisms phagocytized by normal leukocytes in the presence of serum from an individual infected by the microorganism, to the number phagocytized in serum from a normal individual. **opsonocytophagic i.,** hemophagocytic i. **orbital i. (of Broca),** 100 times the height of the opening of the orbit, divided by its width. **palatal i., palatine i., palatomaxillary i.,** 100 times the maximal palatal breadth divided by the maximal palatal length. **parasite i.,** the percentage of individuals in a population whose blood smears show the presence of malarial parasites. **phagocytic i.,** 1. the average number

of bacteria ingested per leukocyte of a patient's blood. 2. (*of Arneth*) the proportion in the blood of multinuclear neutrophil leukocytes with nuclei having three or more lobes. **physiognomonic upper face i.,** 100 times the distance from the nasion to the stomion divided by the bizygomatic breadth. **Pignet i.,** see under *formula.* **Pirquet's i.** (of nutritional status), multiply the weight in grams by 10, divide this product by the sitting height in centimeters and extract the cube root of this quotient. A result lower than 0.945 indicates faulty nutrition. See also *pelidisi.* **ponderal i.,** an index of body mass determined by dividing the height in inches by the cube root of the weight in pounds. **Quarterly Cumulative I. Medicus,** a former publication of the American Medical Association, in which was indexed most of the medical literature in the world; replaced by Cumulated I. Medicus. **radiohumeral i.,** 100 times the maximal length of the radius divided by the maximal length of the humerus. **refractive i.,** the refractive power of a medium compared with that of air, which is assumed to be 1. Symbol n, or n_D. **refractive i., absolute,** an expression of the ratio of the velocity of light in air to its velocity in a specific substance. **refractive i., relative,** an expression of the ratio of the absolute refractive indexes of two different optically dense substances. **Röhrer's i.** (of the state of nutrition), multiply the weight in grams by 100 and divide the product by the cube of the height in centimeters. **sacral i.,** 100 times the breadth of the sacrum, divided by the length. **salivary urea i.,** see *Hench-Aldrich test,* under *tests.* **short increment sensitivity i. (SISI),** a hearing test in which tones of 1 to 5dB increments in intensity and lasting 0.5 seconds are superimposed on a continuous (carrier) tone of the same frequency at random intervals, the carrier tone being 20 decibels above the speech reception threshold. **spleen i.,** the percentage of individuals in the population having enlarged spleens; used in malaria surveys. **splenometric i.,** an index of the amount of malarial infection; obtained by multiplying the spleen rate by the average enlarged spleen. **staphylo-opsonic i.,** the opsonic index in staphylococcic infection, estimated by using *Staphylococcus aureus* as the test microorganism. **therapeutic i.,** originally, the ratio of the maximum tolerated dose to the minimum curative dose; now defined, so as to account for variability of individual response, as the ratio of the median lethal dose (LD_{50}) to the median effective dose (ED_{50}). It is used in assessing the safety of a drug. Called also *chemotherapeutic i.* **thoracic i.,** the ratio of the anteroposterior diameter of the thorax to the transverse diameter. **tibiofemoral i.,** 100 times the length of the lower leg divided by the length of the thigh. **tibioradial i.,** 100 times the length of the forearm divided by the length of the lower leg. **trunk i.,** 100 times the bi-acromial breadth divided by the sitting suprasternale height. **tuberculo-opsonic i.,** the opsonic index in tuberculous infection, estimated by using *Mycobacterium tuberculosis* as the test microorganism. **ureosecretory i.,** see *Ambard's formula,* under *formula.* **uricolytic i.,** the percentage of uric acid oxidized to allantoin before being secreted. **vertical i.,** 100 times the height of the skull divided by the length. **vital i.,** the ratio of births to deaths within a given time in a population; called also *birth-death ratio.* **xanthoproteic i.,** see *Mulder's test* (def. 2), under *tests.* **zygomaticoauricular i.,** the ratio between the zygomatic and auricular diameters of the skull.

indican (in'dĭ-kan) 1. a yellow indoxyl glycoside, $C_6H_4 \cdot NH \cdot CH:C \cdot O \cdot C_6H_{11}O_5$, from plants that yield indigo. On hydrolysis it yields glucose and indoxyl. 2. potassium indoxyl sulfate, $C_6H_4 \cdot NH \cdot CH \cdot CO \cdot SO_2 \cdot OK$, formed by decomposition of trytophan in the intestines, absorbed, conjugated, and excreted in the urine.

indicanemia (in″dĭ-kan-e′me-ah) [*indican* + Gr. *haima* blood + *-ia*] the presence of indican in the blood.

indicanmeter (in″dĭ-kan-me′ter) an instrument for estimating the amount of indican in the urine.

indicanorachia (in″dĭ-kan-o-ra′ke-ah) the presence of indican in the spinal fluid.

indicant (in′dĭ-kant) 1. indicating. 2. a symptom which indicates the true diagnosis or treatment.

indicanuria (in″dĭ-kan-u′re-ah) [*indican* + Gr. *ouron* urine + *-ia*] the presence in the urine of indican in excessive quantity.

indicarmine (in″dĭ-kar′min) indigotindisulfonate sodium.

indicatio (in″dĭ-ka′she-o) [L.] indication. **i. causa′lis,** an indication as to the treatment of a disease afforded by its cause. **i. curati′va, i. mor′bi,** an indication as to treatment afforded by the nature of the morbid processes observed. **i. symptomat′ica,** an indication as to disease afforded by the symptoms that may arise.

indication (in″dĭ-ka′shun) [L. *indicatio*] a sign or circumstance which points to or shows the cause, pathology, treatment, or issue of an attack of disease; that which points out; that which serves as a guide or warning.

indicator (in′dĭ-ka″ter) [L.] 1. the index finger (index [NA]). 2. the extensor muscle of the index finger (musculus extensor indicis [NA]). 3. any substance which, when added in small quantities, shows the appearance or disappearance of a chemical individual by a conspicuous change of color or the attainment of a certain pH. **anaerobic i.,** a dilute solution of methylene blue is decolorized in the absence of oxygen. **Andrade's i.,** a solution of acid fuchsin in water, decolorized to a yellow color by sodium hydrate solution, and added to sugar bouillon culture medium. An acid-producing organism cultivated on this bouillon turns the medium magenta red. **complex i.,** in psychoanalysis, anything that discloses or indicates the working of a complex. **dew point i.,** an instrument for measuring relative humidity or moisture content of a gas by measuring its dew point. **radioactive i.,** see under *tracer*. **redox i.,** a pigment which indicates by a change of color the change in pH. **Schneider's i.,** an index designed to reflect cardiovascular fitness, based mainly on heart rate during and after mild exercise.

indicophose (in'dĭ-ko"fōz) an indigo-colored phose.

Indiella (in"de-el'ah) former name for the genus *Madurella*.

indifférence (ahn-de"fa-rahns') [Fr.] indifference. **belle i.** (bel"ahn-de"fa-rahns') [Fr. "beautiful indifference"], a complacent attitude toward their condition and symptoms shown by hysterical patients.

indifferent (in-dif'er-ent) [L. *indifferens*] not tending one way or another; neutral; having no preponderating affinity.

indigenous (in-dij'ĕ-nus) [L. *indigenus*] native, or not exotic; native to a particular place or country.

indigestible (in"di-jes'tĭ-b'l) [*in*- neg. + *digestible*] not susceptible of being digested.

indigestion (in"di-jes'chun) lack or failure of digestion; commonly used to denote vague abdominal discomfort after meals. **acid i.,** hyperchlorhydria. **fat i.,** inability to digest fat; steatorrhea. **gastric i.,** indigestion taking place in or due to some disorder of the stomach. **intestinal i.,** imperfect performance of the digestive function of the intestine. **nervous i.,** nervous dyspepsia. **sugar i.,** defective ability to digest sugar, resulting in fermentative diarrhea.

indigitation (in-dij"ĭ-ta'shun) [L. *in* into + *digitus* finger] intussusception (def. 1), or invagination.

indiglucin (in"dĭ-gloo'sin) a sweet substance obtained together with indigo on the decomposition of plant indican.

indigo (in'dĭ-go) [Gr. *Indikon* Indian dye] a blue dyeing material from various leguminous and other plants (*Indigofera tinctoria*, etc.), being the aglycone of indican; also made synthetically. It is sometimes found in the sweat and the urine, where it is derived from urinary indican (indoxyl sulfate).

indigogen (in'dĭ-go-jen) a crystalline principle from indigo.

indigopurpurine (in"dĭ-go-pur'pu-rin) a purple pigment occasionally found in the urine.

indigotin (in"dĭ-go'tin) a neutral, tasteless, dark blue powder, $C_{16}H_{10}N_2O_2$, the principal ingredient of commercial indigo; called also *indigo blue*.

indigotindisulfonate sodium (in"dĭ-go"tin-di-sul'fo-nāt) [USP] chemical name: 2-(1,3-dihydro-3-oxo-5-sulfo-2*H*-indol-2-ylidene)-2,3-dihydro-3-oxo-1*H*-indole-5-sulfonic acid disodium salt. A dye, $C_{16}H_8N_2Na_2O_8S$, occurring as a dusky, purplish blue powder or blue granules; used as a diagnostic aid for determining renal function, administered intravenously. Called also *indigo carmine*, *indicarmine*, and *soluble indigo blue*.

indirect (in"di-rekt') [L. *indirectus*] 1. not immediate or straight. 2. acting through an intermediary agent.

indirubin (in"di-roo'bin) a red pigment occasionally found in the urine.

indirubinuria (in"di-roo"bin-u're-ah) the presence of indirubin in the urine.

indiscriminate (in"dis-krim'ĭ-nāt) [L. *in* not + *discrimen* distinction] affecting various parts without distinction.

indisposition (in"dis-po-zish'un) the condition of being slightly ill; a slight illness.

indium (in'de-um) [L. *indicum* indigo] a metallic element; atomic number, 49; atomic weight, 114.82; symbol, In; named from its blue line in the spectrum. It is used in semiconductor research and in bearing alloys.

individuation (in"dĭ-vid"u-a'shun) 1. the process of developing individual characteristics. 2. differential regional activity in the embryo occurring in response to organizer influence.

Indocin (in'do-sin) trademark for a preparation of indomethacin.

Indoklon (in-dok'lon) trademark for a preparation of flurothyl. See also under *therapy*.

indolaceturia (in"do-las"ĕ-tu're-ah) the presence of indolacetic acid in the urine; excessive amounts of 5-OH-indoleacetic acid, the urinary metabolite of serotonin, may be excreted when carcinoid tumors are present.

indole (in'dōl) a compound, $C_6H_4CH:CH\cdot NH$, obtained from

coal tar and indigo, and produced by the decomposition of tryptophan in the intestines. It is also found in cultures of the spirillum of cholera (*Vibrio cholerae*) and other bacteria; a color test for its production is used in classifying enteric bacteria. It is responsible in part for the peculiar odor of the feces. In cases of

intestinal obstruction, it accumulates in the intestine and is found in large quantities in the urine in conjugated form.

indolent (in'do-lent) [L. *in* not + *dolens* painful] causing little pain, as an *indolent* tumor; slow growing, as an indolent lesion.

indologenous (in"do-loj'ĕ-nus) [*indole* + Gr. *gennan* to produce] causing the formation of indole.

indoluria (in"dōl-u're-ah) the presence of indole in the urine.

indomethacin (in"do-meth'ah-sin) [USP] chemical name: 1-(4-chlorobenzoyll)-5-methoxy-2-methyl-1*H*-indole-3-acetic acid. A nonsteroidal anti-inflammatory agent, $C_{19}H_{16}ClNO_4$, which also has antipyretic and analgesic properties, occurring as a pale yellow to yellow-tan powder; used in the treatment of rheumatoid arthritis, rheumatoid spondylitis, osteoarthritis of the hip, and acute gouty arthritis in selected patients, administered orally.

indophenol (in"do-fe'nol) any one of a series of dyes which are nitrogen derivatives of quinone.

indophenolase (in"do-fe'nōl-ās) (obs.) cytochrome oxidase.

indophenol-oxidase (in"do-fe"nol-ok'sĭ-dās) cytochrome oxidase.

indoprofen (in"do-pro'fen) chemical name: 2-(1,3-dihydro-1-oxo-2*H*-isoindol-2-yl)-α-methylbenzeneacetic acid; an analgesic and anti-inflammatory, $C_{17}H_{15}NO_3$.

indoramin (in-dor'ah-min) chemical name: *N*-[1-[2-(1*H*-indol-3-yl)ethyl]-4-piperidyl]benzamide; an antihypertensive, $C_{22}H_{25}N_3O$.

indoxyl (in-dok'sil) [Gr. *indikon* indigo + *oxys* sharp] an oxidation product of indole, $C_6H_4\cdot C(OH):CH\cdot NH$, formed by decomposition from tryptophan, and excreted in the urine as indican (potassium indoxyl sulfate).

indoxylemia (in-dok"sil-e'me-ah) [*indoxyl* + Gr. *haima* blood + *-ia*] the presence of indoxyl in the blood.

indoxyl-sulfate (in-dok'sil-sul'fāt) a compound found in the urine in some cases in which great putrefactive changes are occurring in the intestine.

indoxyluria (in"dok-sil-u're-ah) [*indoxyl* + Gr. *ouron* urine + *-ia*] the presence of an excess of indoxyl in the urine.

indriline hydrochloride (in'drĭ-lēn) chemical name: *N,N*-dimethyl-1-phenyl-1*H*-inden-1-ethylamine hydrochloride; a central nervous system stimulant, $C_{19}H_{21}N\cdot HCl$.

induced (in-dūst') [L. *inducere* to lead in] 1. produced artificially. 2. produced by induction.

inducer (in-dūs'er) something that induces. In biosynthesis, a compound that induces the synthesis of a specific enzyme or sequence of enzymes, by antagonizing the action of the corresponding repressor, or by some other mechanism.

inductance (in-duk'tans) that property of a circuit by virtue of which a magnetic field is associated with the circuit when the circuit is carrying current. The unit of inductance, or "self-induction," is the henry.

induction (in-duk'shun) [L. *inductio*] 1. the act or process of inducing or causing to occur, especially the production of a specific morphogenetic effect in the developing embryo through the influence of evocators or organizers, or the production of anesthesia or unconsciousness by use of appropriate agents. 2. the appearance of an electric current or of magnetic properties in a body because of the presence of another electric current or magnetic field nearby. **autonomous i.,** induction in which the inductor forms no part of the portion produced. **complementary i.,** induction in which the inductor forms a part of the portion produced. **somatic i.,** the production of new characters through the influence of the soma on the germ cells. **Spemann's i.,** the stimulating and directing effect shown by certain tissues on neighboring tissues or parts in early development of the embryo. **spinal i.,** that process by which one reflex lowers the threshold of another reflex which otherwise cannot be penetrated.

inductogram (in-duk'to-gram) roentgenogram.

inductor (in-duk'ter) a tissue elaborating a chemical substance which acts to determine the growth and differentiation of embryonic parts. Cf. *activator* (def. 2) and *organizer*.

inductorium (in"duk-to're-um) an apparatus for generating currents of induced electricity; as in physiological experiments.

inductotherm (in-duk'to-therm) an apparatus for producing high body temperature by electric induction.

inductothermy (in-duk'to-ther"me) the production of artificial fever by electric induction.

indulin (in'du-lĭn) a coal tar dye, used as a histologic stain.

indulinophil (in"du-lin'o-fil) 1. an element easily stainable with indulin. 2. indulinophilic.

indulinophilic (in"du-lin-o-fil'ik) [*indulin* + Gr. *philein* to love] stainable with indulin.

indurated (in'du-rāt"ed) [L. *indurare* to harden] hardened; rendered hard.

induration (in"du-ra'shun) [L. *induratio*] 1. the quality of being hard; the process of hardening. 2. an abnormally hard spot or place. **black i.,** the hardening and pigmentation of lung tissue seen in pneumonia. **brawny i.,** inflammatory hardening and thickening of tissues. **brown i.,** 1. a deposit of altered blood pigment in the lung in pneumonia. 2. marked increase of the connective tissue of the lung and excessive pigmentation, due to long-continued congestion from valvular heart disease or to anthracosis. **cyanotic i.,** a congested, dense, and purple state of the kidney in which the blood current is slowed and the transudation of fluid through the glomeruli is impeded. **fibroid i.,** cirrhosis. **Froriep's i.,** myositis fibrosa. **granular i.,** cirrhosis. **gray i.,** an induration of lung tissue in or after pneumonia, without pigmentation. **laminate i.,** a thin layer of round-cell infiltration of the corium in chancre. **parchment i.,** laminate i. **penile i.,** Peyronie's disease. **phlebitic i.,** chronic edema of the lower third of the leg with inflammation and thrombosis of the superficial veins, leading to induration of the skin and subcutaneous tissue and a constricting band of fibrosis; called also *indurated cellulitis.* **plastic i.,** sclerosis of the corpora cavernosa of the penis. **red i.,** interstitial pneumonia in which the lung is red and congested.

indurative (in′du-ra″tiv) pertaining to or marked by induration.

indusium griseum (in-du′ze-um gris′e-um) [L.] [NA] a thin layer of gray substance on the dorsal aspect of the corpus callosum; called also *supracallosal gyrus* and *gyrus supracallosus.*

-ine a suffix indicating an alkaloid, an organic base, or a halogen.

inebriant (in-e′bre-ant) [L. *inebriare* to make drunk] 1. an inebriating agent. 2. inebriating.

inebriation (in-e″bre-a′shun) [L. *inebriatio*] the condition of being drunk.

inebriety (in″ĕ-bri′ĕ-te) [L. *in* intensive + *ebrietas* drunkenness] habitual drunkenness.

inelastic (in″e-las′tik) lacking elasticity.

Inermicapsifer (in-er″mĭ-kap′sĭ-fer) a genus of tapeworms, family Linstowiidae, parasitic in hyraxes and rodents in Africa; *I. arvicanthidis* has been found in humans in Cuba and Central America.

inert (in-ert′) having no action; not reacting with other elements, as inert gases.

inertia (in-er′she-ah) [L.] inactivity; inability to move spontaneously. **colonic i.,** weak muscular activity of the colon, leading to distention of the organ and constipation. **i. u′teri,** sluggishness of the uterine contractions during labor.

in extremis (in ek-stre′mis) [L. "at the end"] at the point of death.

Inf. abbreviation for L. *infun′de,* pour in.

infancy (in′fan-se) the early period of life; see *infant.*

infant (in′fant) [L. *infans; in* neg. + *fans* speaking] a young child; considered to designate the human young from birth or from the termination of the newborn period (the first four weeks of life) to the time of assumption of erect posture (12 to 14 months); it is regarded by some to extend to the end of the first 24 months. **floppy i.,** see under *syndrome.* **immature i.,** one weighing 500 to 999 grams (17 ounces to 2.2 pounds) at birth, usually before the twenty-eighth week of gestation, and having an extremely poor chance of survival. **mature i.,** one weighing 2500 grams (5.5 pounds) or more at birth, usually at or near full term, and having an optimum chance of survival. **newborn i.,** the human young during the first two to four weeks after birth. **postmature i., post-term i.,** an infant born at any time after the beginning of the forty-second week (288 days) of gestation. **premature i.,** one usually born after the twenty-seventh week and before full term, and arbitrarily defined as an infant weighing 1000 to 2499 grams (2.2 to 5.5 lbs.) at birth, having poor to good chance of survival, depending on the weight. In countries where adults are smaller than in the United States, the upper limit is 2250 grams (5 lbs.). Other criteria such as crown-heel length (less than 47 cm.) and occipitofrontal diameter (less than 11.5 cm.) have also been used. **preterm i.,** an infant born at any time before the thirty-seventh completed week (259 days) of gestation. **term i.,** an infant born anytime from the beginning of the thirty-eighth week (260 days) to the end of the forty-first week (287 days) of gestation.

infanticide (in-fan′tĭ-sīd) [L. *infans* infant + *caedere* to kill] the taking of the life of an infant.

infanticulture (in-fan′tĭ-kul″tūr) puericulture.

infantile (in′fan-tīl) [L. *infantilis*] pertaining to an infant or to infancy.

infantilism (in′fan-tĭ-lizm″, in-fan′tĭ-lizm) a condition in which the characters of childhood persist into adult life; it is marked by mental retardation, underdevelopment of the sexual organs, and often, but not always, by dwarfism. Cf. *progeria.* **Brissaud's i.,** infantile myxedema. **cachetic i.,** infantilism due to chronic infection or poisoning. **celiac i.,** infantilism resulting from the infantile form of nontropical sprue (celiac disease); see under *sprue.* **dysthyroidal i.,** infantilism due to defective thyroid activity. **hepatic i.,** infantilism associated with hepatic cirrhosis. **Herter's i.,** the infantile form of nontropical sprue; see under *sprue.* **hypophyseal i.,** a type of dwarfism, with retention of infantile characteristics, due to undersecretion of the growth hormone and the gonadotropic hormones of the anterior pituitary gland (adenohypophysis); called also *pituitary infantilism, pituitary dwarfism, Levi-Lorain dwarfism, Paltauf's dwarfism, ateleiosis.* **intestinal i.,** the infantile form of nontropical sprue; see under *sprue.* **Levi-Lorain i., Lorain's i.,** hypophyseal i. **lymphatic i.,** infantilism associated with lymphatism. **myxedematous i.,** cretinism. **pancreatic i.,** a form caused by defective pancreatic action. **partial i.,** arrested development of a single part or tissue. **pituitary i.,** hypophyseal i. **regressive i.,** reversion to an infantile state after body growth has been completed. **renal i.,** renal osteodystrophy. **reversive i.,** regressive i. **sex i.,** continuance of the prepuberal sex characters and behavior beyond the usual age of puberty. **sexual i.,** retardation of sexual development, as in adiposogenital dystrophy. **symptomatic i.,** infantilism due to general defective development of tissues. **tardy i.,** regressive i. **toxemic i.** (*obs.*), the infantile form of nontropical sprue; see under *sprue.* **universal i.,** general dwarfishness in stature with absence of the secondary sexual characteristics.

infantorium (in″fan-to′re-um) a hospital for the newborn and young infants.

infarct (in′farkt) [L. *infarctus*] an area of coagulation necrosis in a tissue due to local ischemia resulting from obstruction of circulation to the area, most commonly by a thrombus or embolus. See under *infarction.* **anemic i.,** an area of necrosis in a tissue produced by sudden arrest of circulation in a vessel; called also *pale i.* and *white i.* **bilirubin i's,** masses of crystals of bilirubin in the pyramids of the kidneys, especially in the newborn. **bland i.,** an uninfected infarct. **bone i.,** an area of bone tissue which has become necrotic as a result of loss of its arterial blood supply. **Brewer's i's,** dark-red, wedge-shaped areas, resembling infarcts, seen on section of a kidney in pyelonephritis. **calcareous i.,** a deposit of calcium salt in the tissues. **cystic i.,** an infarct enclosed in a membrane. **embolic i.,** one caused by an embolus. **hemorrhagic i.,** an infarct that is red in color owing to the oozing of red corpuscles into the dead area; called also *red i.* **pale i.,** anemic i. **red i.,** hemorrhagic i. **septic i.,** one in which the tissues have been invaded by pathogenic organisms. **thrombotic i.,** one caused by a thrombus. **uric acid i.,** a deposit of uric acid crystals in the renal tubules of the newborn. **white i.,** anemic i.

infarctectomy (in″fark-tek′to-me) surgical removal of an infarct.

infarction (in-fark′shun) [L. *infarcire* to stuff in] 1. the formation of an infarct. 2. an infarct. **anterior myocardial i.,** infarction localized to the left ventricular free wall between the interventricular groove and the lateral margin of the anterior papillary muscle; it is characterized electrocardiographically by abnormal Q waves in V_3 or V_4. **anteroinferior myocardial i.,** one involving features of both anterior and inferior myocardial infarction. **anterolateral myocardial i.,** one involving features of both anterior and lateral myocardial infarction. **anteroseptal myocardial i.,** one involving features of both anterior and septal infarction. **atrial i.,** the formation of an infarct in a cardiac atrium, which may be due to coronary artery occlusion, periarteritis nodosa, obliterating endarteritis of the small branches of coronary arteries, or other conditions. **cardiac i.,** myocardial i. **cerebral i.,** an ischemic condition of the brain, producing a persistent focal neurological deficit in the area of distribution of one of the cerebral arteries. **Freiberg's i.,** Köhler's bone disease, def. 2. **inferior myocardial i.,** one localized in the region between the lateral border of the posterior papillary muscle and the posterior septum; it is characterized electrocardiographically by abnormal Q waves in lead II, III, or aV_F. **inferolateral myocardial i.,** one involving features of both inferior and lateral myocardial infarctions. **intestinal i.,** occlusion of an artery or arteriole in the wall of the intestine, resulting in the formation of an area of coagulation necrosis. **lateral myocardial i.,** infarction in the region between the lateral margin of the anterior papillary muscle and the lateral margin of the posterior papillary muscle; it is marked electrocardiographically by abnormal Q waves in V_5 or V_6. **mesenteric i.,** coagulation necrosis of the intestines due to a decrease in blood flow in the mesenteric vasculature; it may be caused by occlusion of the mesenteric arteries or by cardiogenic abnormalities or hypovolemia (*nonocclusive mesenteric i.*). **myocardial i.,** gross necrosis of the myocardium, as a result of interruption of the blood supply to the area, as in coronary thrombosis. **posterior myocardial i.,** one localized in the basal third of the posteroinferior heart wall; it is characterized electrocardiographically by abnormal R waves in V_1 or V_2. **pulmonary i.,** localized necrosis of lung tissue caused by obstruction of the arterial blood supply, most often due to pulmonary embolism. Clinical manifestations range from the nonexistent to pleuritic chest pain, dyspnea, hemoptysis, and tachycardia. **septal myocardial i.,** one localized to the interventricular septum and characterized electrocardiographically by abnormal Q waves in V_1 or V_2. **transmural myocardial i.,** one involving the entire thickness of the heart wall.

infaust (in′fowst) [L. *infaustus* unlucky] unfavorable.

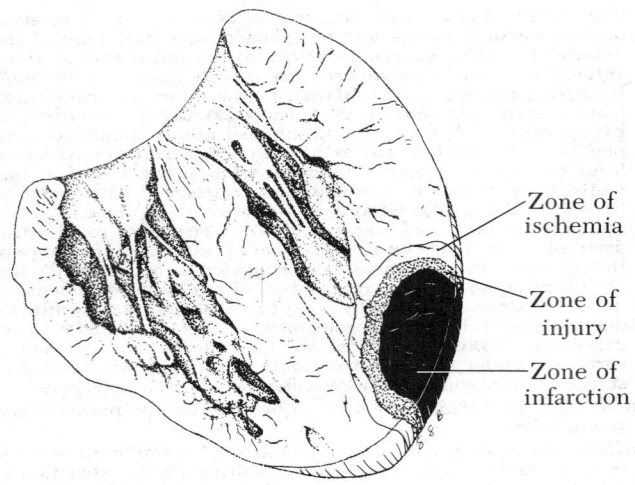

Zone of
ischemia

Zone of
injury

Zone of
infarction

Myocardial infarction shown in cross-section of heart (ventricles only).

infectible (in-fek′tĭ-b′l) capable of being infected.

infection (in-fek′shun) 1. invasion and multiplication of micro-organisms in body tissues, which may be clinically inapparent or result in local cellular injury due to competitive metabolism, toxins, intracellular replication, or antigen-antibody response. The immunological response may be transient or prolonged, and consists of a cellular response (delayed hypersensitivity) or the production of specific (immunoglobulin) antibody to the components of the infecting organism or its toxins. 2. an infectious disease. Cf. *infestation*. **aerial i.,** airborne i. **agonal i.,** terminal i. **airborne i.,** infection by inhalation of organisms suspended in air on water droplets or dust particles. **apical i.,** infection situated at the apex of the root of a tooth. **autochthonous i.,** a infection due to organisms present in the environment, as on a hospital ward. **contact i.,** direct i. **cross i.,** infection transmitted between individuals infected with different pathogenic microorganisms. **cryptogenic i.,** infection whose pathogenesis is unclear or undefinable, as salmonella arteritis with no preceding salmonella infection elsewhere. **diaplacental i.,** infection acquired through the placenta. **direct i.,** infection produced by direct contact with another person. **droplet i.,** infection due to inhalation of respiratory pathogens suspended on liquid particles 10 micra in diameter or less exhaled by someone already infected, whether as a carrier or with symptomatic disease. **dustborne i.,** infection by pathogens which have become affixed to particles of dust and are transmitted by that means. **ectogenous i.,** exogenous i. **endogenous i.,** infection due to reactivation of organisms present in a dormant focus, as occurs in tuberculosis, histoplasmosis, coccidioidomycosis, etc. **exogenous i.,** infection caused by organisms not normally present in the body but which have gained entrance from the environment. **focal i.,** infection confined to a single organ or tissue; certain focal infections, as in the tonsillar crypts, periodontal tissues, and the prostatic bed, are a source of systemic disease as a result of blood-stream dissemination of the offending pathogen. **germinal i.,** transmission of infection to the child by means of the ovum or sperm of the parent. **herd i.,** an epidemiological term for an infection in any large group. **inapparent i.,** subclinical i. **indirect i.,** infection transmitted by water, food, or other means of conveyance. **latent i.,** a phase during the course of some established infections during which the pathogenic microorganisms are dormant and manifestations of disease that may have been recognizable earlier are no longer detectable, as in latent syphilis. **mass i.,** infection produced by a large number of pathogenic organisms in the circulation. **mixed i.,** infection of an organ or tissue by more than one microorganism, as in wound infections, abscesses, pneumonia, and rarely meningitis and endocarditis; mixtures of every type occur, e.g., bacterial and viral, bacterial and fungal, and protozoan and viral. **phytogenic i.,** infection caused by plant organisms. **pyogenic i.,** an infection caused by pus-producing organisms. *Staphylococcus aureus* and *Streptococcus pyogenes* are customarily implied, although many other species of bacteria and fungi and some viruses are capable of evoking a polymorphonuclear inflammatory response. **Rachmat i.,** Sumatra jaundice. **retrograde i.,** an infection that ascends a duct or tube against the flow of secretions or excretions, as in the urinary tract. **Salinem i.,** a form of leptospirosis occurring in Salinem and caused by *Leptospira pyrogenes*; called also *Salinem fever*. **secondary i.,** infection by a microorganism following an infection by another kind of microorganism. **silent i.,** subclinical i. **subclinical i.,** infection associated with no detectable symptoms but caused by microorganisms capable of producing easily recognizable diseases, such as poliomyelitis or mumps; it is detected by the production of

antibody, or by delayed hypersensitivity exhibited in skin test reaction to such antigens as tuberculoprotein. **terminal i.,** an acute infection occurring near the end of a disease and frequently causing death. **Vincent's i.,** acute necrotizing ulcerative gingivitis. **water-borne i.,** infection caused by microorganisms which may be transmitted through water and acquired through ingestion, bathing, or other means. **zoogenic i.,** infection caused by animal organisms, such as protozoa and helminths. Cf. *phytogenic i.*

infectiosity (in-fek″she-os′ĭ-te) the degree of infectiousness of a microorganism.

infectious (in-fek′shus) caused by or capable of being communicated by infection; infective.

infectiousness (in-fek′shus-nes) the state or quality of being infectious.

infective (in-fek′tiv) [L. *infectivus*] infectious; capable of producing infection; pertaining to or characterized by the presence of pathogens.

infectivity (in″fek-tiv′ĭ-te) infectiousness.

infecundity (in″fe-kun′dĭ-te) [L. *infecunditas*] sterility or barrenness.

inferent (in′fer-ent) afferent.

inferior (in-fēr′e-or) [L. "lower"; neut. *inferius*] situated below, or directed downward; [NA] a term used in reference to the lower surface of an organ or other structure, or to the lower of two (or more) similar structures.

inferolateral (in″fer-o-lat′er-al) [L. *inferus* low + *latus* side] situated below and to one side.

inferomedian (in″fer-o-me′de-an) [L. *inferus* low + *medius* middle] situated in the middle of the under side.

inferoposterior (in″fer-o-pos-tēr′e-or) situated below and behind.

infertile (in′fer-til) not fertile; exhibiting infertility.

infertilitas (in″fer-til′ĭ-tas) [L.] infertility.

infertility (in″fer-til′ĭ-te) [L. *in* not + *fertilis* fruitful, prolific] diminished or absent capacity to produce offspring; the term does not denote complete inability to produce offspring as does *sterility*. Called also *relative sterility*. **primary i.,** infertility occurring in patients who have never conceived. **secondary i.,** infertility occurring in patients who have previously conceived.

infestation (in-fes-ta′shun) parasitic attack or subsistence on the skin and its appendages, as by insects, mites, or ticks; sometimes used to denote parasitic invasion of the tissues or organs, as by helminths. Cf. *infection*.

infibulation (in-fib-u-la′shun) [L. *infibulare* to buckle together] the act of buckling, or fastening as if with buckles, especially the ancient practice of fastening of the prepuce or labia majora with clasps or stitches to prevent copulation; called also *pharaonic circumcision*.

infiltrate (in-fil′trāt) 1. to penetrate the interstices of a tissue or substance. 2. material deposited by infiltration. **Assmann's tuberculous i.,** see under *focus*.

infiltration (in″fil-tra′shun) [L. *in* into + *filtration*] the diffusion or accumulation in a tissue or cells of substances not normal to it or in amounts in excess of the normal. Also, the material so accumulated. Cf. *degeneration*. **adipose i.,** fatty i. **calcareous i.,** a deposit of lime and magnesium salts in the tissues. **calcium i.,** a deposit of calcium salts within the tissues of the body. **cellular i.,** the migration and accumulation of cells within the tissues. **epituberculous i.,** a collateral hyperemia and inflammatory infiltration surrounding a tuberculous focus. **fatty i.,** 1. a deposit of fat in the tissues, especially between the cells. 2. the presence of fat vacuoles in the cytoplasm of cells, as occurs in fatty change in the liver, myocardium, and kidneys. **gelatinous i.,** gray i. **glycogen i.,** abnormal accumulations of glycogen within the cytoplasm of cells, as occurs in diabetes mellitus and the glycogen storagen diseases. **gray i.,** a condition of the lungs in acute tuberculosis in which, after death, they assume a gray appearance; called also *gelatinous i.* **inflammatory i.,** that formed by an inflammatory exudation penetrating the interstices of a tissue. **lymphocytic i. of skin,** an abnormal accumulation of lymphocytes in the skin, characterized by asymptomatic, pink to reddish brown, flat, discoid papules which enlarge to form well-defined, slightly elevated, firm, erythematous plaques with a smooth surface and no follicular plugging; the lesions most frequently occur on the face, neck, and upper back of men, and persist for years. **paraneural i.,** paraneural anesthesia. **sanguineous i.,** infiltration with extravasated blood. **serous i.,** the abnormal presence of lymph in a tissue. **tuberculous i.,** the formation of a group or of groups of tuberculous cells and bacilli in a tissue. **urinous i.,** extravasation of urine into a tissue.

infirm (in-firm′) [L. *infirmis*; *in* not + *firmus* strong] weak; feeble, as from disease or old age.

infirmary (in-fir′mah-re) [L. *infirmarium*] a hospital or place where sick or infirm persons are maintained or treated; commonly used to denote a space or a building set aside for the care of members of a group or community; a dispensary.

infirmity (in-fir′mĭ-te) [L. *infirmitas*] 1. a feeble or weak state of the body or mind. 2. a disease or condition producing weakness.

inflammagen (in-flam′ah-jen) an irritant that elicits both edema and the cellular response of inflammation. Cf. *edemagen*.

inflammation (in″flah-ma′shun) [L. *inflammatio; inflammare* to set on fire] a localized protective response elicited by injury or destruction of tissues, which serves to destroy, dilute, or wall off (sequester) both the injurious agent and the injured tissue. It is characterized in the acute form by the classical signs of pain (dolor), heat (calor), redness (rubor), swelling (tumor), and loss of function (functio laesa). Histologically, it involves a complex series of events, including dilatation of arterioles, capillaries, and venules, with increased permeability and blood flow; exudation of fluids, including plasma proteins; and leukocytic migration into the inflammatory focus. **acute i.,** inflammation, usually of sudden onset, characterized by the classical signs (see *inflammation*), in which the vascular and exudative processes predominate. **adhesive i.,** that which promotes the adhesion of contiguous surfaces. **atrophic i.,** a form which results in atrophy and deformity. **catarrhal i.,** a form which affects principally a mucous surface, and which is marked by a copious discharge of mucus and epithelial debris. **chronic i.,** inflammation of slow progress and marked chiefly by the formation of new connective tissue; it may be a continuation of an acute form or a prolonged low-grade form, and usually causes permanent tissue damage. **cirrhotic i.,** atrophic i. **croupous i.,** a fibrinous inflammation leading to the formation of a false membrane. **diffuse i.,** one that is both interstitial and parenchymatous or is spread over a large area. **disseminated i.,** one that has a number of distinct foci. **exudative i.,** one in which the prominent feature is an exudate. **fibrinous i.,** one that is characterized by an exudate of coagulated fibrin. **fibroid i.,** atrophic i. **focal i.,** one that is confined to a single spot or to a few limited spots. **granulomatous i.,** an inflammation, usually chronic, characterized by the formation of granulomas; see also *granuloma*. **hyperplastic i.,** one which leads to the formation of new connective tissue fibers. **hypertrophic i.,** inflammation marked by increase in the size of the elements composing the affected tissue. **interstitial i.,** one that primarily affects the stroma of an organ. **metastatic i.,** one that is reproduced in a distant part by the conveyance of infectious material through the blood vessels and lymph organs. **necrotic i.,** inflammation attended by death of the affected tissue. **obliterative i.,** inflammation of the lining membrane of a cavity or vessel, producing adhesions between the surfaces and consequent obliteration of the lumen. **parenchymatous i.,** one that primarily affects the essential tissue elements of an organ. **plastic i., productive i., proliferous i.,** hyperplastic i. **pseudomembranous i.,** an acute inflammatory response to a powerful necrotizing toxin, such as the diptheria toxin, characterized by the formation on a mucosal surface, most often in the pharynx, larynx, respiratory passages, and intestinal tract, of a false membrane composed of precipitated fibrin, necrotic epithelium, and inflammatory white cells. **purulent i.,** suppurative i. **sclerosing i.,** atrophic i. **seroplastic i.,** inflammation accompanied by both serous and plastic exudation. **serous i.,** one which produces an exudation of serum. **simple i.,** that in which there is no flow of pus or other product of inflammation. **specific i.,** one that is due to a particular microorganism. **subacute i.,** a condition intermediate between chronic and acute inflammation, exhibiting some of the characteristics of each. **suppurative i.,** one characterized by the formation of pus. **toxic i.,** one that is caused by a poison, such as a bacterial product. **traumatic i.,** one that is caused by an injury. **ulcerative i.,** that in which necrosis on or near the surface leads to loss of tissue and creation of a local defect (ulcer).

inflammatory (in-flam′ah-to″re) pertaining to or characterized by inflammation.

inflation (in-fla′shun) [L. *in* into + *flare* to blow] 1. distention with air, gas, or a fluid. 2. the act of distending with air or with a gas.

inflator (in-fla′tor) an instrument for inflating any organ for therapeutic or diagnostic purposes.

inflection, inflexion (in-flek′shun) [L. *inflexio; in* in + *flectere* to bend] the act of bending inward or state of being bent inward, as of a limb.

inflorescence (in″flo-res′ens) the structure or arrangement of the flowers of a plant.

influenza (in″flu-en′zah) [Ital. "influenza"] an acute viral infection involving the respiratory tract, occurring in isolated cases, in epidemics, or in pandemics striking many continents simultaneously or in sequence. It is marked by inflammation of the nasal mucosa, the pharynx, and conjunctiva, and by headache and severe, often generalized myalgia. Fever, chills, and prostration are common. Involvement of the myocardium and of the central nervous system occur infrequently. A necrotizing bronchitis and interstitial pneumonia are prominent features of severe influenza and account for the susceptibility of patients to secondary bacterial pneumonia due to *Streptococcus pneumoniae, Haemophilus influenzae,* and *Staphylococcus aureus.* The incubation period is one to three days and the disease ordinarily lasts for three to ten days. Influenza is caused by a number of serologically distinct strains of virus, designated A (with many subgroups), B, and C. See *influenza virus,* under *virus.* **i. A,** the most common variety of influenza caused by the type A strain of influenza virus; epidemics of this form occur at two- to three-year intervals. The causative strain is subject to wide variations in antigenic type, called antigenic shift, and outbreaks of influenza A caused by such antigenic types have been called *Asian i., Spanish i., Russian i.,* and so on. See *influenza virus,* under *virus.* **Asian i.,** a pandemic of influenza A occurring in 1957, thought to originate in China. **avian i.,** Newcastle disease. **i. B,** a variety of influenza caused by the type B strain of influenza virus; epidemics of this form occur at four- to five-year intervals. See *influenza virus,* under *virus.* **i. C,** a variety of influenza occurring sporadically and caused by the type C strain of influenza virus. See *influenza virus,* under *virus.* **endemic i.,** a disease resembling epidemic influenza, but less severe in character, occurring during the winter season; called also *influenza nostras.* **epidemic i.,** influenza occurring in localized outbreaks. **equine i.,** horse i. **feline i.,** a name loosely applied to any of a group of highly contagious viral infections of the respiratory tract in cats. **Hong Kong i.,** a pandemic of influenza A occurring in 1968, thought to originate in Hong Kong. **horse i.,** a highly contagious respiratory disease in horses which is caused by a virus. **intestinal i.,** popular name for an acute, transient diarrheal disease apparently of infectious origin. **laryngeal i.,** influenza in horses in which pharyngitis is the chief symptom. **i. lymphat′ica,** infectious mononucleosis. **i. nos′tras,** endemic influenza. **pandemic i.,** influenza occurring in waves that spread widely over the world at irregular intervals. **Russian i.,** a pandemic of influenza A occurring in 1978, thought to originate in the U.S.S.R. **Spanish i.,** a name given to the acute influenza-like disease, a pandemic of which passed over Europe and America during the summer and autumn of 1918. **summer i. of Italy,** phlebotomus fever. **swine i.,** a highly contagious disease of hogs caused by simultaneous infection with *Hemophilus influenzae* and a virus.

influenzal (in″flu-en′zal) pertaining to influenza.

infolding (in-fōld′ing) 1. the folding inward of a layer of tissue, as in the formation of the neural tube in the embryo. 2. the enclosing of redundant tissue by suturing together the walls of the organ on either side of it.

informosome (in-for′mo-sōm) a name suggested for the combination of mRNA and protein found in the cytoplasm of eukaryotic cells.

infra- (in′frah) [L. *infra* beneath] a prefix meaning situated, formed, or occurring beneath the element indicated by the word stem to which it is affixed.

infra-axillary (in″frah-ak′sĭ-lār″e) below the axilla.

infrabulge (in′frah-bulj) the surfaces of a tooth gingival to the height of contour, or sloping cervically; cf. *suprabulge.*

infraclass (in′frah-klas) a taxonomic category sometimes established, subordinate to a subclass and superior to an order.

infraclavicular (in″frah-klah-vik′u-lar) beneath a clavicle.

infraclusion (in″frah-kloo′zhun) the condition in which the occluding surface of a tooth does not reach the normal occlusal plane and is out of contact with the opposing tooth.

infraconstrictor (in″frah-kon-strik′tor) the inferior constrictor of the pharynx.

infracortical (in″frah-kor′tĭ-kal) beneath the cortex, as of the brain.

infracostal (in″frah-kos′tal) [*infra-* + L. *costa* rib] below a rib or below the ribs.

infracotyloid (in″frah-kot′ĭ-loid) beneath the cotyloid cavity or acetabulum.

infraction (in-frak′shun) [L. *in* into + *frac′tio* break] incomplete fracture of a bone without displacement of the fragments. **Freiberg's i.,** osteochondrosis of the head of the second metatarsal bone.

infradentale (in″frah-den-ta′le) a cephalometric landmark, being the highest anterior point on the gingiva between the mandibular medial (central) incisors.

infradian (in″frah-de′an, in-fra′de-an) [*infra-* + L. *dies* day] pertaining to a period of more than 24 hours; applied to the rhythmic repetition of certain phenomena in living organisms occurring in cycles of more than a day (infradian rhythm). Cf. *circadian* and *ultradian.*

infradiaphragmatic (in″frah-di″ah-frag-mat′ik) below the diaphragm.

infraduction (in″frah-duk′shun) the turning downward of a part, especially of the eye.

infraglenoid (in″frah-gle′noid) below the fossa of the glenoid cavity.

infraglottic (in″frah-glot′ik) below the glottis.

infrahyoid (in″frah-hi′oid) below the hyoid bone.

inframamillary (in″frah-mam′ĭ-lār″e) below the nipple.

inframammary (in″frah-mam′ah-re)   below the mammary gland.

inframandibular (in″frah-man-dib′u-lar)   beneath the lower jaw.

inframarginal (in″frah-mar′jĭ-nal)   situated below a margin or border.

inframaxillary (in″frah-mak′sĭ-lār″e)   beneath the upper jaw (maxilla).

infranuclear (in″frah-nu′kle-ar)   below a nucleus.

infraocclusion (in″frah-ŏ-kloo′zhun)   infraclusion.

infraorbital (in″frah-or′bĭ-tal)   lying under or on the floor of the orbit.

infrapatellar (in″frah-pah-tel′ar)   below the patella.

infraplacement (in″frah-plās′ment)   infraclusion.

infrapsychic (in″frah-si′kik)   below the psychic level; automatic.

infrared (in-frah-red′)   denoting thermal radiation of wavelength greater than that of the red end of the visible spectrum, between the red waves and the radio waves, having wavelengths between 0.75 and 1000 μm. Infrared rays emanating from tissues are the basis of thermography. **far i., long-wave i.,** infrared radiation of the longest wavelength, i.e., furthest from the visible spectrum (wavelength about 3.0 to 1000 μm.). **near i., short-wave i.,** infrared radiation of the shortest wavelength, i.e., closest to the visible spectrum (wavelength about 0.75 to 3.0 μm.).

infrascapular (in″frah-skap′u-lar)   beneath the scapula.

infrasonic (in″frah-son′ik)   below the frequency range of the waves normally perceived as sound by the human ear.

infraspinous (in″frah-spi′nus)   beneath the spine of the scapula.

infrasternal (in″frah-ster′nal)   below the sternum.

infratemporal (in″frah-tem′po-ral)   below the temporal fossa.

infratentorial (in″frah-ten-to′re-al)   beneath the tentorium of the cerebellum.

infratonsillar (in″frah-ton′sĭ-lar)   below the faucial tonsil.

infratracheal (in″frah-tra′ke-al)   beneath the trachea.

infratrochlear (in″frah-trok′le-ar)   beneath the trochlea.

infratubal (in″frah-tu′bal)   beneath a tube.

infraturbinal (in″frah-tur′bĭ-nal)   the inferior turbinate bone.

infraumbilical (in″frah-um-bil′ĭ-kal)   beneath the umbilicus.

infraversion (in″frah-ver′zhun) [infra- + version]   1. downward deviation of an eye.   2. infraclusion.

infriction (in-frik′shun) [L. in on + frictio rubbing]   the rubbing of medicaments into the skin.

infundibula (in″fun-dib′u-lah) [L.]   plural of infundibulum.

infundibular (in″fun-dib′u-lar)   of the nature of or resembling an infundibulum.

infundibulectomy (in″fun-dib″u-lek′to-me)   excision of the infundibulum of the heart.   **Brock's i.,** resection of the interior portion of the hypertrophied outflow tract of the right ventricle to assist in relief of pulmonary stenosis in tetralogy of Fallot.

infundibuliform (in″fun-dib′u-lĭ-form″) [L. infundibulum funnel + forma form]   shaped like a funnel.

infundibuloma (in″fun-dib-u-lo′mah)   a tumor of the infundibulum hypothalami.

infundibulopelvic (in″fun-dib″u-lo-pel′vik)   pertaining to an infundibulum and a pelvis, as of the kidney.

infundibulum (in″fun-dib′u-lum), pl. infundib′ula [L. "funnel"]   1. a funnel-shaped passage; [NA] a general term for such a structure. Often used alone to refer to the infundibulum hypothalami and to the median eminence (of the hypothalamus).   2. NA alternative for conus arteriosus.   **crural i., i. crura′le,** canalis femoralis.   **ethmoidal i. of cavity of nose, i.** ethmoidale cavi nasi.   **ethmoidal i. of ethmoid bone,** infundibulum ethmoidale ossis ethmoidalis.   **i. ethmoida′le ca′vi na′si** [NA], a passage connecting the cavity of the nose with the anterior ethmoidal cells and the frontal sinus.   **i. ethmoida′le os′sis ethmoida′lis** [NA], a variable sinuous passage extending upward from the middle nasal meatus through the ethmoidal labyrinth, communicating with the anterior ethmoidal cells and often with the frontal sinus.   **i. of fallopian tube,** i. tubae uterinae.   **i. of heart,** conus arteriosus.   **i. hypothal′ami** [NA], a hollow, funnel-shaped mass in front of the tuber cinereum, which extends to the posterior lobe of the pituitary gland. Called also hypophyseal stalk.   **infundibula of kidney,** calices renales minores.   **i. na′si, i. of nose,** 1. infundibulum ethmoidale cavi nasi.   2. infundibulum ethmoidale ossis ethmoidalis.   **i. pulmo′nis, i. pulmo′num,** any of the ductuli alveolares.   **infundib′ula re′num,** calices renales minores.   **i. tu′bae uteri′nae** [NA], infundibulum of uterine tube: the funnel-like dilation at the distal end of the uterine tube.   **i. of urinary bladder,** fundus vesicae urinariae.   **i. of uterine tube,** i. tubae uterinae.

infusible (in-fu′zĭ-b'l)   incapable of being melted.

infusion (in-fu′zhun)   1. [L. infusio; from in into + fundere to pour] the steeping of a substance in water for obtaining its proximate principles.   2. [L. infusum, gen. infusi] the product of the process of steeping a drug for the extraction of its medicinal principles.   3. the therapeutic introduction of a fluid other than blood, as saline solution, into a vein. NOTE—An infusion flows in by gravity, an injection is forced in by a syringe, an instillation is dropped in, an insufflation is blown in, and an infection slips in unnoticed.   **amniotic fluid i.,** a complication of labor in which rupture of the uterine venous sinuses permits the entrance of amniotic fluid into the maternal circulation.   **cold i.,** the product of steeping a drug in cold water.   **meat i.** (for bacteriological use), fresh lean meat free from fat is ground and extracted with water; the mixture is infused overnight in the refrigerator, gradually raised to the boiling point, and filtered.   **saline i.,** introduction, either subcutaneously or intravenously, of saline solution.

infusodecoction (in-fu″so-de-kok′shun)   a mixture of the infusion and the decoction of a substance.

Infusoria (in″fu-so′re-ah) [L. pl., so called because found in infusions, after exposure to air]   1. Ciliophora.   2. a group of protozoa found in foul water and infusions of decaying organic matter.

infusoriotoxin (in″fu-so″re-o-tok′sin)   a toxin destructive to Infusoria (Ciliophora).

infusum (in-fu′sum) [L.]   an infusion, def. 2.

ingesta (in-jes′tah) [L. pl., in into + gerere to carry]   food and drink taken into the stomach.

ingestant (in-jes′tant)   a substance that is or may be taken into the body by way of the mouth, or through the digestive system.

ingestion (in-jes′chun)   the act of taking food, medicines, etc., into the body, by mouth.

ingestive (in-jes′tiv)   pertaining to or affecting an ingestion.

ingluvies (in-gloo′ve-ēz) [L.]   1. the craw or crop of birds.   2. the first stomach (rumen) of ruminant animals.

Ingrassia's process (apophysis), wings (in-grah′se-ahs) [Giovanni Filippo Ingrassia, Italian anatomist, 1510–1580]   see ala minor ossis sphenoidalis, and see wings of sphenoid bone, under wing.

ingravescent (in″grah-ves′ent) [L. in upon + gravesci to grow heavy]   gradually increasing in severity.

ingrowth (in′grōth)   an inward growth; something that grows inward or into.   **epithelial i.,** a complication of intraocular surgery, most often cataract extraction, or of penetrating wounds of the cornea where wound healing is poor, in which epithelium proliferates through the wound into the anterior chamber, causing obstruction of the trabecula, and sometimes pupillary block, resulting in glaucoma. Called also epithelial downgrowth.

inguen (ing′gwen), pl. in′guina [L.] [NA]   the groin; the junctural region between the abdomen and thigh.

inguina (ing′gwĭ-nah) [L.]   plural of inguen.

inguinal (ing′gwĭ-nal) [L. inguinalis]   pertaining to the inguen, or groin.

inguinoabdominal (ing″gwĭ-no-ab-dom′ĭ-nal)   pertaining to the groin and the abdomen.

inguinocrural (ing″gwĭ-no-kroo′ral)   pertaining to the groin and the thigh.

inguinodynia (ing″gwĭ-no-din′e-ah)   pain in the groin, a common symptom of hysteria.

inguinolabial (ing″gwĭ-no-la′be-al)   pertaining to the groin and labium.

inguinoscrotal (ing″gwĭ-no-skro′tal)   pertaining to the groin and the scrotum.

INH   trademark (from isonicotine hydrazine) for preparations of isoniazid.

inhalant (in-ha′lant)   a substance that is or may be taken into the body by way of the nose and trachea, or through the respiratory system.   **antifoaming i.,** an agent inhaled as a vapor to prevent the formation of foam in the respiratory passages of a patient with pulmonary edema.

inhalation (in″hah-la′shun) [L. inhalatio]   1. the drawing of air or other substances into the lungs; see also under anesthesia and therapy.   2. any drug or solution of drugs administered (as by means of nebulizers or aerosols) by the nasal or oral respiratory route for local or system effect.   **isoproterenol sulfate i.** [USP], a solution of isoproterenol hydrochloride in purified water made isotonic by the addition of sodium chloride; used as a bronchodilator administered by inhalation as an aerosol.

inhale (in-hāl′) [L. inhalare]   to take into the lungs by breathing.

inhaler (in-ha′ler)   1. an apparatus for administering vapor or volatilized remedies or anesthetics by inhalation.   2. an apparatus to prevent dust, smoke, noxious gases, or the like from entering the lungs, or to enable a person with affected lungs to breathe cold or damp air with less danger and discomfort.   **Allis′ i.,** an apparatus for administering ether, chloroform, or other highly volatile liquid anesthetics by the drop method.   **ether i.,** an apparatus for administering the vapor of ether as an anesthetic.   **H. H. i.,** an oxygen inhaler used in treating gassed patients;

named from the inventors, Henderson and Haggard. **Junker i.**, a bottle-like inhaler formerly used for administration of chloroform (1867).

inherent (in-hēr′ent) [L. *inhaerens* sticking fast] implanted by nature; intrinsic; innate.

inheritance (in-her′ĭ-tans) 1. the acquisition of characters or qualities by transmission from parent to offspring. 2. that which is transmitted from parent to offspring. **alternative i.**, inheritance in which the characters are inherited from one parent. **amphigonous i.**, inheritance of characteristics from both parents. **biparental i.**, amphigonous i. **blending i.**, inheritance in which the characters of mother and father seem to blend in the offspring. **complemental i.**, inheritance of characters dependent on the presence of two independent pairs of nonallelic genes (complementary genes), both of which must be present before a given character can be expressed. **crisscross i.**, inheritance by offspring of characters from the parent of the opposite sex. **cytoplasmic i.**, transmission of characters dependent on self-perpetuating elements not nuclear in origin. **dominant i.**, see under *gene*. **duplex i.**, amphigonous i. **holandric i.**, inheritance carried only by males, as by genes on the Y chromosome. **hologynic i.**, inheritance carried only by females, as by genes on the X chromosome. **homochronous i.**, the inheritance of characteristics which appear in the offspring at the same age as they appeared in the parent. **homotropic i.**, the alleged inheritance of acquired characteristics. **intermediate i.**, inheritance in which the phenotype of the heterozygote falls between that of either homozygote. **maternal i.**, the transmission of characters that are dependent on peculiarities of the egg cytoplasm produced, in turn, by nuclear genes. **mendelian i.**, see *Mendel's law*, under *law*. **monofactorial i.**, the acquisition of a characteristic or quality, the transmission of which depends on a single gene. **multifactorial i.**, the acquisition of a characteristic or quality, the manifestation of which is subject to modification by a number of genes. **polygenic i.**, inheritance of quantitative characters, such as skin color, height, and intelligence in humans, which is dependent on the cumulative action of several or many different genes (polygenes or multiple factors), each of which produces a slight effect on the total condition; called also *quantitative i.* **quantitative i.**, polygenic i. **quasidominant i.**, inheritance in which there is direct transmission, generation to generation, of a recessive trait in populations in which the gene is frequent or inbreeding is intense; thus, although it is produced by the mating of a recessive homozygote with a heterozygote, the proportion of affected offspring resembles that in dominant inheritance. **recessive i.**, see under *gene*. **sex-linked i.**, see under *gene*. **supplemental i.**, inheritance of characters dependent on the presence of two independent pairs of nonallelic genes (supplementary genes) that interact in such a way that one gene supplements the action of the second gene. **unit i.**, inheritance in which the characters of the parents, instead of blending in the offspring, may reappear unchanged in a later generation.

inhibin (in-hib′in) a postulated nonsteroid testicular factor, believed to be a peptide, elaborated by the seminiferous tubules and thought to inhibit pituitary production of follicle-stimulating hormone.

inhibit (in-hib′it) to retard, arrest, or restrain.

inhibition (in″hĭ-bish′un) [L. *inhibere* to restrain; *in* in + *habere* to have] arrest or restraint of a process. In psychiatry, the unconscious restraining of an instinctual drive, as of the sex drive (by impotence or frigidity). **allosteric i.**, a form of enzyme inhibition; see under *site*. **competitive i.**, inhibition of enzyme activity in which the inhibitor (substrate analogue) competes with the substrate for binding sites on the enzymes; such inhibition is reversible, since it can be overcome by increasing the substrate concentration. Called also *selective i.* **contact i.**, the inhibition of cell division and cell motility in normal animal cells when in close contact with each other. **endproduct i.**, inhibition of an activity resulting from the effect of the endproduct of a biosynthetic process on an earlier step in the process. Called also *feedback i.* **enzyme i.**, inhibition of enzyme activity, as in competitive or endproduct inhibition. **false feedback i.**, inhibition of the initial steps of a process by an analogue of the endproduct of the specific process; see *endproduct i.* **feedback i.**, endproduct i. **noncompetitive i.**, inhibition of enzyme activity by inhibitors that combine with the enzyme on a site other than that utilized by the substrate; such inhibition may be irreversible. **proactive i.**, the interference of earlier learning in the retention of new learning; cf. *retroactive i.* **reciprocal i.**, the inhibition of one group of muscles on excitation of their antagonists, a phenomenon resulting from reciprocal innervation (q.v.). **reflex i.**, a condition in which a negative response is evoked by a stimulus. **retroactive i.**, the interference of new learning in the recall of earlier learning; cf. *proactive i.* **selective i.**, competitive i. **uncompetitive i.**, inhibition of enzyme activity in which the inhibitor combines with the enzyme and with the enzyme-substrate complex. **Wedensky i.**, a partial block to conduction in a nerve may transmit impulses at low frequencies but not at higher frequencies.

inhibitive (in-hib′ĭ-tiv) inhibitory.

inhibitor (in-hib′ĭ-tor) 1. any substance that interferes with a chemical reaction, growth, or other biological activity. 2. a chemical substance that acts to inhibit, or hold in check, the action of a tissue organizer or the growth of microorganisms. 3. a mechanical device for curing mouth breathing. **aldosterone i.**, an agent that blocks the action of aldosterone on the renal tubules. **cholesterol i.**, an agent that suppresses the production of cholesterol or decreases the level of cholesterol in the blood. **cholinesterase i.**, an agent that inhibits the action of cholinesterase. **mitotic i.**, a substance that slows or arrests the process of mitosis, e.g., colchicine.

inhibitory (in-hib′ĭ-tor″e) [L. *inhibere* to restrain] restraining or arresting any process; effecting a stay or arrest, partial or complete.

inhibitrope (in-hib′ĭ-trōp) one in whom certain stimuli tend to produce arrest of function.

inhomogeneity (in-ho″mo-jĕ-ne′ĭ-te) lack of normal homogeneity.

inhomogeneous (in″ho-mo-je′ne-us) lacking homogeneity.

iniac (in′e-ak) pertaining to the inion.

iniad (in′e-ad) toward the inion.

inial (in′e-al) iniac.

iniencephalus (in″e-en-sef′ah-lus) a fetus exhibiting iniencephaly.

iniencephaly (in″e-en-sef′ah-le) [Gr. *inion* occiput + *enkephalos* brain] a developmental anomaly characterized by enlargement of the foramen magnum, and absence of the laminal and spinal processes of the cervical, dorsal, and sometimes lumbar vertebrae, with vertebrae reduced in number and irregularly fused, the brain and much of the cord occupying a single cavity.

inio- (in′e-o) [Gr. *inion* occiput] a combining form denoting relationship to the occiput.

iniodymus (in″e-od′ĭ-mus) [*inio-* + Gr. *didymos* twin] iniopagus.

inion (in′e-on) [Gr. "the back of the head"] [NA] the most prominent point of the external occipital protuberance.

iniopagus (in″e-op′ah-gus) [*inio-* + Gr. *pagos* thing fixed] conjoined symmetrical twins fused at the occiput.

iniops (in′e-ops) [*inio-* + Gr. *ōps* eye] a double-faced monster with the posterior face incomplete.

initial (ĭ-nish′al) [L. *initialis*, from *initium* beginning] pertaining to the very first stage of any process.

initis (in-i′tis) [Gr. *is, inos* fiber] inflammation of the substance of a muscle.

injectable (in-jek′tah-b'l) 1. capable of being injected. 2. a substance that may be injected.

injected (in-jekt′ed) 1. introduced by injection. 2. congested.

injectio (in-jek′she-o), pl. *injectio′nes* [L., from *in* into + *jacere* to throw] injection.

injection (in-jek′shun) [L. *injectio*] 1. the act of forcing a liquid into a part, as into the subcutaneous tissues, the vascular tree, or an organ. Cf. *infusion* (def. 3). 2. a substance so forced or administered. Officially, in pharmacy, a solution of a medicament suitable for injection. See also under specific substances. 3. the condition of being injected; congestion. **adrenal cortex i.**, a preparation containing a mixture of the endocrine principles derived from the cortex of adrenal glands; formerly used in treatment of adrenal insufficiency. **anatomical i.**, an injection into the vessels or organs of the cadaver, designed to facilitate dissection or demonstration. **Brown-Séquard i.**, injection of testicular extract. **circumcorneal i.**, dilatation of the ciliary and conjunctival blood vessels close to the limbus, and diminishing toward the periphery. **coarse i.**, an anatomical injection that fills only the larger vessels. **dextrose i.**, a sterile solution of dextrose in water for injection; used as a fluid and nutrient replenisher. **endermic i.**, intracutaneous i. **epifascial i.**, one made upon the surface of a fascia, particularly the fascia lata. **ethiodized oil i.** [USP], see under *oil*. **exciting i.**, sensitizing i. **fine i.**, an anatomical injection that fills even the smallest vessels. **fructose i.**, a sterile solution of fructose in water, used as a fluid and nutrient replenisher. **gaseous i.**, injection of gas or air for therapeutic purposes as in collapse therapy; for diagnostic purposes, as in ventriculography; or for facilitating anatomical demonstrations. **gelatin i.**, a preservative injection of which gelatin is the base. **hypodermic i.**, an injection made into the subcutaneous tissues; called also *subcutaneous i.* **intracutaneous i.**, intradermal i., intradermic i., one made into the corium or substance of the skin. **intramuscular i.**, an injection into the substance of a muscle. **intrathecal i.**, injection of a substance through the theca of the spinal cord into the subarachnoid space. **intravascular i.**, an injection made into a vessel. **intravenous i.**, an injection made into a vein. **iodinated I 125 albumin i.** [USP], a sterile, buffered isotonic solution containing not less than 10 mg. of radioiodinated normal human albumin per liter, and adjusted to provide not more than 1 millicurie of radioactivity per milliliter, used as a diagnostic aid in determining blood volume and cardiac output. **iodinated I 131 albumin i.** [USP], a sterile aqueous suspension of albumin human iodinated with ^{131}I and denatured to produce aggregates of controlled particle size; each ml. contains 300 µg to 3.0 mg. of aggregated albumin with specific activity of 200 microcuries to 1.2 millicuries per mg. **iron dextran i.** [USP], a sterile colloidal solution of ferric hydroxide in complex with partially hydrolyzed dextran of low molecular weight, in water for injection; used as a hematinic. **iron sorbitex i.** [USP], a sterile solution of a complex of iron, sorbitol, and citric acid that is stabilized with the aid of dextrin and an excess of sorbitol; used as an hematinic. **jet i.**, injection of a drug in solution through the intact skin by an extremely fine jet of the solution under high pressure. **opacifying i.**, the injection of a radiopaque substance into the vessels or into some body cavity for diagnostic radiological study. **oxytocin i.** [USP], a sterile solution in water of an oxytocic principle prepared by synthesis or obtained from the posterior lobe of the pituitary gland of domestic animals that are used for food by man; used to stimulate contraction of smooth muscle, particularly the pregnant uterus. **paraperiosteal i.**, the production of local anesthesia by deposition of a local anesthetic solution close to the periosteum; the solution is then free to diffuse through the cortical bony plate and anesthetize the larger terminal nerve fibers. **parathyroid i.** [USP], a sterile solution of water-soluble principles of the parathyroid glands, administered intramuscularly to maintain the level of calcium in the blood; called also *parathyroid extract*. **parenchymatous i.**, one made into the substance of an organ. **posterior pituitary i.** [NF], a sterile solution in water of the principles from the posterior lobe of the pituitary of domestic animals that are used for food by man; used as an oxytocic, in the treatment of diabetes insipidus, and to stimulate intestinal peristalsis. **preparatory i.**, sensitizing i. **preservative i.**, an injection that serves to protect a cadaver or specimen from decay. **protamine sulfate i.** [USP], a sterile isotonic solution prepared from the sperm or from the mature testes of fish belonging to the genus *Oncorhynchus, Salmo,* or *Trutta;* used to counteract the action of heparin. **protein hydrolysate i.** [USP], a sterile solution of amino acids and short-chain peptides, used as a fluid and nutrient replenisher. **Ringer's i.** [USP], a sterile solution of sodium chloride, potassium chloride, and calcium chloride in water for injection, given as a fluid and electrolyte replenisher by intravenous infusion. **Ringer's i., lactated** [USP], a sterile solution of calcium chloride, potassium chloride, sodium chloride, and sodium lactate in water for injection, given as a fluid and electrolyte replenisher by intravenous infusion. **Schlösser i.**, see under *treatment*. **sclerosing i.**, the injection into a blood vessel of material (e.g., sodium citrate) which will tend to obliterate the vessel; used in varicose veins, angioma, etc. **sensitizing i.**, the first injection of sensitizing antigen. **sodium chloride i.** [USP], a sterile isotonic solution of sodium chloride in water for injection, used as a fluid and electrolyte replenisher and as an irrigating solution. It is also used as a vehicle for the injection of medications. **sodium pertechnetate Tc 99m i.** [USP], a sterile solution containing radioactive technetium (^{99m}Tc) in the form of sodium pertechnetate and sufficient sodium chloride to make the solution isotonic. **sodium radiochromate i.**, sodium chromate Cr 51 i. **subcutaneous i.**, hypodermic i. **technetium Tc 99m albumin aggregated i.** [USP], see under *technetium*. **vasopressin i.** [USP], a sterile solution in water for injection of the water-soluble, pressor principle of the posterior lobe of the pituitary of healthy domestic animals that are used as food by man; used as an antidiuretic.

injector (in-jek'tor) [L. *injicere* to inject] an instrument used in making injections.

injury (in'ju-re) [L. *injuria; in* not + *jus* right] harm or hurt; a wound or maim. Usually applied to damage inflicted to the body by an external force. **birth i.**, impairment of body function or structure due to adverse influences to which the infant has been subjected at birth. **blast i.**, see *blast*, def. 3. **deceleration i.**, an injury sustained by sudden deceleration in the movement of the body, as in a motor vehicle accident; the brain is especially liable to such trauma. **egg-white i.**, biotin deficiency; see *biotin*. **Goyrand's i.**, pulled elbow. **steering-wheel i.**, injury to the chest and sometimes contusion of the heart in motorists, caused by being thrown forward against the steering wheel. **whiplash i.**, a nonspecific term applied to injury to the spine and spinal cord at the junction of the fourth and fifth cervical vertebrae, occurring as the result of rapid acceleration or deceleration of the body. Because of their greater mobility, the four upper vertebrae act as the lash, and the lower three act as the handle of the whip.

inlay (in'la) material laid into a defect in tissue. In dentistry, a filling that is made outside the tooth to correspond with the form of a cavity and then cemented into the tooth. **cast i.**, gold i. **epithelial i.**, a method of securing epithelialization of an unhealed deep wound. A mold of the wound cavity is taken and covered with a Thiersch graft of epidermis, the whole being inserted into the wound cavity, and the edges then approximated with sutures. The mold is removed after ten days, leaving the cavity completely epithelialized. Called also *Esser's operation.* See also under *onlay*. **gold i.**, one made of gold or of a gold alloy. **porcelain i.**, an inlay made of porcelain.

inlet (in'let) an avenue of ingress. **pelvic i.**, the superior aperture of the minor pelvis, bounded by the crest and pecten of the pubic bones, the arcuate lines of the ilia, and the anterior margin of the base of the sacrum; called also *apertura pelvis superior* [NA].

I.N.N. International Nonproprietary Names, the nonproprietary designation recommended by the World Health Organization for any pharmaceutical preparation. Such names are selected according to general principles set forth by the World Health Organization, and lists are published periodically in the *WHO Chronicle*.

innate (in'nāt) [L. *in* in + *nasci* to be born] inborn; hereditary; congenital.

innervation (in"er-va'shun) [L. *in* into + *nervus* nerve] 1. the distribution or supply of nerves to a part. 2. the supply of nervous energy or of nerve stimulus sent to a part. **double i.**, innervation of a structure by two kinds of nerve fibers, e.g., sympathetic and parasympathetic. **reciprocal i.**, the innervation of muscles around the joints, where the motor centers are so connected in pairs that when one is excited the center of the corresponding antagonist is inhibited.

innidiation (ĭ-nid"e-a'shun) [L. *in* into + *nidus* nest] the development of cells in a part to which they have been carried by metastasis; called also *colonization* and *indenization*.

innocent (in'o-sent) [L. *innocens; in* not + *nocere* to harm] not malignant, benign; not tending of its own nature to a fatal issue.

innocuous (ĭ-nok'u-us) harmless.

innominatal (ĭ-nom"ĭ-na'tal) pertaining to the innominate (brachiocephalic) artery or to the innominate (hip) bone.

innominate (ĭ-nom'ĭ-nāt) [L. *innominatus* nameless; *in* not + *nomen* name] not having a name; nameless. The term has been applied to certain structures better identified by their descriptive names, as the innominate (brachiocephalic) artery and the innominate (hip) bone.

Innovar (in'o-var) a trademark for a preparation of droperidol and fentanyl citrate in a 50:1 ratio; used as a neuroleptanalgesic.

innoxious (ĭ-nok'shus) [L. *in* not + *noxius* harmful] not injurious; not hurtful.

innutrition (in"nu-trish'un) want of nutrition.

ino- (in'o) [Gr. *is, inos* fiber] a combining form denoting relationship to a fiber, or fibrous material.

inoblast (in'o-blast) [*ino-* + Gr. *blastos* germ] any connective tissue cell in the formative stage.

inoccipitia (in-ok"sĭ-pit'e-ah) absence or deficiency of the occipital lobe of the brain.

inochondritis (in"o-kon-dri'tis) [*ino-* + Gr. *chondros* cartilage + *-itis*] inflammation of a fibrocartilage.

inocula (in-ok'u-lah) [L.] plural of *inoculum*.

inoculability (ĭ-nok"u-lah-bil'ĭ-te) the quality or state of being inoculable.

inoculable (ĭ-nok'u-lah-b'l) 1. susceptible of being inoculated; transmissible by inoculation. 2. not immune against a disease transmissible by inoculation.

inoculate (ĭ-nok'u-lāt) to communicate a disease by inserting its etiologic agent; to implant microbes or infective materials in or on culture media; to introduce immune serum, vaccines of various kinds, and other antigenic materials for preventive, curative, or experimental purposes.

inoculation (ĭ-nok"u-la'shun) [L. *inoculatio,* from *in* into + *oculus* bud] introduction of microorganisms, infective material, serum, and other substances into tissues of living plants and animals, or culture media; introduction of a disease agent, e.g., vaccine virus, into a healthy individual to produce a mild form of the disease followed by immunity. **curative i.**, the injection of a preparation (e.g., a biological preparation such as antiserum) for curative purposes. **protective i.**, the injection of a biological preparation, e.g., a vaccine or an antiserum, to protect against a disease; vaccination against a disease.

inoculum (ĭ-nok'u-lum), pl. *inoc'ula* [L.] the substance used in inoculation.

inocyte (in'o-sīt) [*ino-* + *-cyte*] a cell of fibrous tissue.

inogen (in'o-jen) [*ino-* + Gr. *gennan* to produce] a hypothetical substance of the muscular tissue, the sudden breaking up of which was once supposed to cause muscular contraction.

inogenesis (in"o-jen'ĕ-sis) the formation of fibrous tissue.

inogenous (in-oj'ĕ-nus) produced from or producing fibrous tissue.

inoglia (in-og'le-ah) [*ino-* + Gr. *glia* glue] fibroglia.

inohymenitis (in"o-hi"mĕ-ni'tis) [*ino-* + Gr. *hymēn* membrane + *-itis*] inflammation of any fibrous membrane.

inolith (in'o-lith) [*ino-* + Gr. *lithos* stone] a fibrous concretion.

inomyositis (in"o-mi"o-si'tis) fibromyositis.

inoperable (in-op'er-ah-b'l) not suitable to be operated upon.

inophragma (in"o-frag'mah) [*ino-* + Gr. *phragmos* a fencing in] ground membrane; a name given to the Z band and M band (q.v. under *band*) because they continue uninterruptedly as transverse membranes through all the adjoining fibrils of a muscle fiber. See *mesophragma* and *telophragma*.

inorganic (in″or-gan′ik) [*in-* not + *organic*] 1. having no organs. 2. not of organic origin. 3. pertaining to substances not of organic origin. 4. in chemistry, denoting substances not derived from hydrocarbons.

inosclerosis (in″o-skle-ro′sis) [*ino-* + Gr. *skleros* hard] sclerosis or induration by increase of fibrous tissue.

inoscopy (in-os′ko-pe) [*ino-* + Gr. *skopein* to examine] the diagnosis of disease by artificial digestion and examination of the fibers or fibrinous matter of the sputum, blood, effusions, etc.

inosculate (in-os′ku-lāt) [L. *in* into + *osculum* little mouth] to unite or communicate by means of small openings or anastomoses.

inosculation (in-os″ku-la′shun) the establishment of communication, by means of small openings or anastomoses, applied especially to establishment of such communication between already existing blood vessels or other tubular structures that come in contact.

inose (in′ōs) inositol.

inosemia (in″o-se′me-ah) [*ino-* + Gr. *haima* blood + *-ia*] 1. an excess of fibrin in the blood. 2. the presence of inose (inositol) in the blood.

inosinate (in-o′sĭ-nāt) a salt of inosinic acid.

inosine (in′o-sin) a nucleoside, $C_{10}H_{12}O_5N_4$, resulting from the cleavage of inosinic acid or from deamination of adenosine; it is a compound of hypoxanthine and ribose. **i. monophosphate,** inosinic acid; see under *acid*.

inosite (in′o-sīt) inositol.

inositis (in″o-si′tis) [*ino-* + *-itis*] inflammation of fibrous tissue.

inositol (in-o′sĭ-tol) 1. any of the stereoisomeric forms of inositol, especially *myo*-inositol (see def. 2). 2. chemical name: *myo*-inositol. A sugar-like vitamin of the B complex, $C_6H_{12}O_6$, which is found in many plant and animal tissues and has been synthesized. It is concerned in the growth of yeast, promotes growth of several species of bacteria, and is curative of mouse alopecia, and may have lipotrophic activity; called also *antialopecia factor* and *meso-inositol*. **i. niacinate,** a peripheral vasodilator, $C_{42}H_{30}N_6O_{12}$.

inositoluria (in″o-si″tol-u′re-ah) inosituria.

inosituria (in″o-si-tu′re-ah) [*inosite* + Gr. *ouron* urine + *-ia*] the occurrence of inositol in the urine, as in diabetes inositus; called also *inosuria*.

inostosis (in″os-to′sis) the re-formation of bony tissue to replace such tissue which has been destroyed.

inosuria (in″o-su′re-ah) 1. an excess of fibrin in the urine. 2. inosituria.

inotagma (in″o-tag′mah) [*ino-* + Gr. *tagma* arrangement] a linear arrangement of the contractile structural elements of a muscle cell.

inotropic (in″o-trop′ik) [*ino-* + Gr. *trepein* to turn or influence] affecting the force or energy of muscular contractions. **negatively i.,** weakening the force of muscular contraction. **positively i.,** increasing the strength of muscular contraction.

inotropism (in-ot′ro-pizm) the quality of influencing the contractility of muscle fibers.

in ovo (in o′vo) [L.] in the egg; referring specifically to various experimental procedures involving the use of chick embryos.

inquest (in′kwest) [L. *in* into + *quaerere* to seek] a legal inquiry before a coroner or medical examiner, and usually a jury, into the manner of a death.

inquiline (in′kwĭ-līn) [L. *inquilinus* a lodger] an organism that lives within the body of another, but does not derive its nourishment from the host.

inructation (in″ruk-ta′shun) abnormal and noisy swallowing of air.

insalivation (in″sal-ĭ-va′shun) [L. *in* in + *saliva* spittle] the saturation of the food with saliva in mastication.

insalubrious (in″sah-lu′bre-us) not salubrious; not conducive to health.

insane (in-sān′) [L. *in* not + *sanus* sound] mentally deranged. See *insanity*.

insanitary (in-san′ĭ-ter-e) not in a good sanitary condition; not conducive to good health; unclean.

insanity (in-san′ĭ-te) [L. *insanitas*, from *in* not + *sanus* sound] mental derangement or disorder. The term is a social and legal rather than a medical one, and indicates a condition which renders the affected person unfit to enjoy liberty of action because of the unreliability of his behavior with concomitant danger to himself and others. **affective i.,** affective psychosis. **alcoholic i.,** alcoholic psychosis. **alternating i.,** manic-depressive psychosis. **anticipatory i.,** that which appears in a patient at an earlier age than that at which it attacked the parent. **choreic i.,** Huntington's chorea. **circular i.,** see under *psychosis*. **climacteric i.,** involutional melancholia. **communicated i.,** folie à deux. **compound i.,** the concurrence of two or more forms of insanity. **compulsive i.,** insanity in which the patient is completely dominated by impulse or obsessions.

consecutive i., that which follows some neurosis or other disease. **cyclic i.,** circular psychosis. **doubting i.,** insanity characterized by morbid doubt, suspicion, and indecision. **emotional i.,** affective psychosis. **homicidal i.,** insanity marked by a desire to take human life. **homochronous i.,** that which appears in the patient at the same age at which it appeared in the patient's father or mother. **hysteric i.,** anxiety hysteria. **impulsive i.,** a compelling tendency to acts of violence. **manic-depressive i.,** manic-depressive psychosis. **moral i.,** that which is marked by impairment of the moral sense, as in moral idiocy and moral imbecility; called also *moral oligophrenia, pathomania,* and *Ray's mania.* **perceptional i.,** a form marked by hallucinations and illusions. **periodic i.,** that which recurs at regular intervals. **polyneuritic i.,** Korsakoff's psychosis. **primary i.,** any insanity not known to be consequent upon some previous attack or disease. **puerperal i.,** see under *psychosis*. **recurrent i.,** mental aberration with lucid intervals. **senile i.,** senile psychosis. **simultaneous i.,** folie à deux. **toxic i.,** toxic psychosis.

inscriptio (in-skrip′she-o), pl. *inscriptio′nes* [L., from *in* upon + *scribere* to write] inscription. **i. tendin′ea,** intersectio tendinea. **inscriptio′nes tendin′eae mus′culi rec′ti abdom′inis,** intersectiones tendineae musculi recti abdominis.

inscription (in-skrip′shun) [L. *inscriptio*] 1. a mark, or line. 2. that part of a prescription which contains the names and amounts of the ingredients. **tendinous i.,** intersectio tendinea. **tendinous i's of rectus abdominis muscle,** intersectiones tendineae musculi recti abdominis.

inscriptiones (in-skrip″she-o′nēz) [L.] plural of *inscriptio*.

insect (in′sekt) any individual of the class Insecta.

Insecta (in-sek′tah) [L. from *in* + *sectum* cut] a class of the Arthropoda whose members are characterized by division into three parts: head, thorax, and abdomen; there are three orders of medical interest, Hemiptera, Diptera, and Siphonaptera.

insectarium (in″sek-ta′re-um) a place for breeding and raising insects.

insecticide (in-sek′tĭ-sīd) [L. *insectum* insect + *caedere* to kill] any substance selectively poisonous to insects.

insectifuge (in-sek′tĭ-fūj) [*insect* + L. *fugare* to put to flight] a preparation that repels insects.

Insectivora (in″sek-tiv′o-rah) [*insect* + L. *vorare* to devour] an order of small, terrestrial mammals, including moles, shrews, etc., which feed primarily on invertebrates, especially on insects.

insectivore (in-sek′tĭ-vōr) an individual of the order Insectivora.

insectivorous (in″sek-tiv′o-rus) subsisting on insects.

insemination (in-sem″ĭ-na′shun) [L. *inseminatus* sown, from *in* into + *semen* seed] the deposit of seminal fluid within the vagina or cervix. **artificial i.,** introduction of semen into the vagina or cervix by artificial means. **donor i., heterologous i.,** artificial insemination in which the semen used is that of a man other than the woman's husband; called also A.I.D. **homologous i.,** artificial insemination in which the husband's semen is used; called also A.I.H.

insenescence (in″sĕ-nes′ens) the process of growing old.

insensible (in-sen′sĭ-b'l) [L. *in* not + *sensibilis* appreciable] 1. not appreciable by or perceptible to the senses. 2. devoid of consciousness or of sensibility.

insert (in′sert) 1. to implant. 2. something that is implanted. **intramucosal i.,** a nonreactive metal device affixed to the tissue-borne surface of a denture that offers added retentive qualities to the denture; it consists of a base, a cervix, and a head.

insertio (in-ser′she-o) [L.] insertion. **i. velamento′sa,** velamentous insertion.

insertion (in-ser′shun) [L. *insertio*, from *in* into + *serere* to join] 1. the act of implanting, or the condition of being implanted. 2. the place of attachment, as of a muscle to the bone which it moves. **parasol i.,** insertion of the umbilical cord in the placenta, in which the vessels of the cord separate before they join the placenta and resemble the ribs of a parasol. **velamentous i.,** attachment of the umbilical cord to the membranes, with the vessels coursing for a long or short distance between the amnion and the chorion to the body of the placenta.

insheathed (in-shēthd′) enclosed within a sheath.

insidious (in-sid′e-us) [L. *insidiosus* deceitful, treacherous] coming on in a stealthy manner; of gradual and subtle development.

insight (in′sīt) 1. in psychiatry, the patient's awareness of his illness, ranging from partial recognition that his symptoms are abnormal to more thorough understanding of the origin, nature, and mechanisms of his attitudes and behavior; self-understanding. 2. in problem solving, the sudden perception of the appropriate relationships of things that results in a solution.

in situ (in si′tu) [L.] in the natural or normal place; confined to the site of origin without invasion of neighboring tissues.

insolation (in″so-la′shun) [L. *insolare* to expose to the sun; *in* in + *sol* sun] 1. treatment by exposure to the sun's rays; the sun bath. 2. sunstroke. **asphyxial i.,** sunstroke with low temperature, cold skin, and feeble pulse. **hyperpyrexial i.,** thermic fever with very high temperature, coma, and congested skin.

insoluble (in-sol′u-b′l) [L. *insolubilis,* from *in* not + *solvere* to dissolve] not susceptible of being dissolved.

insomnia (in-som′ne-ah) [L. *in* not + *somnus* sleep + *-ia*] inability to sleep; abnormal wakefulness.

insomniac (in-som′ne-ak) an individual exhibiting insomnia.

insomnic (in-som′nik) characterized by insomnia; unable to sleep.

insonate (in-so′nāt) to expose to ultrasound waves.

insorption (in-sorp′shun) the movement of a substance into the blood; said of such movement from the contents of the gastrointestinal tract into the circulating blood.

inspection (in-spek′shun) [L. *inspectio, inspicere* to behold] examination by the eye.

inspectionism (in-spek′shun-izm) voyeurism.

inspersion (in-sper′zhun) [L. *inspersio; in* upon + *spargere* to sprinkle] the act of sprinkling, as with a powder.

inspirate (in′spĭ-rāt) inhaled gas (or air).

inspiration (in″spĭ-ra′shun) [L. *inspirare,* from *in* in + *spirare* to breathe] the act of drawing air into the lungs.

inspirator (in′spĭ-ra″tor) [L.] (*obs.*) a form of inhaler or respirator.

inspiratory (in-spi′rah-to″re) pertaining to or subserving inspiration.

inspirium (in-spi′re-um) [L.] an inspiration.

inspirometer (in″spi-rom′ĕ-ter) [*inspire* + Gr. *metron* measure] an apparatus for measuring the amount of air inspired.

inspissated (in-spis′āt-ed) [L. *inspissatus,* from *in* intensive + *spissare* to thicken] being thickened, dried, or rendered less fluid.

inspissation (in″spis-sa′shun) [L. *inspissatio*] 1. the act or process of rendering dry or thick by the evaporation of readily vaporizable parts. 2. the condition of being rendered less thin by evaporation.

inspissator (in-spis′a-tor) an apparatus for inspissating fluids, such as blood serum.

instar (in′stahr) [L. "a form"] any stage of an arthropod between molts.

instep (in′step) the dorsal part of the arch of the foot.

instillation (in″stil-la′shun) [L. *instillatio,* from *in* into + *stillare* to drop] administration of a liquid drop by drop.

instillator (in′stil-la″tor) an instrument for performing instillations.

instinct (in′stinkt) [L. *instinctus; in* on + *stinguere* to prick] a complex of unlearned responses that is characteristic of species. **death i.,** in psychoanalysis, the latent instinctive impulse toward death, a controversial concept in Freud's later work. **ego i.,** any instinct that is not sexual, particularly the self-preservative instincts. **herd i.,** the instinct or urge to be one of a group and to conform to the standards of that group in conduct and opinion. **mother i.,** the complex behavior in a mother which accomplishes the care of the young; whether such an instinct exists at the human level is uncertain.

instinctive (in-stink′tiv) of the nature of an instinct; performed apparently without the exercise of the reason.

institutes (in′stĭ-tūts) [L. *institutum* established regulation] established or fundamental principles. **i. of medicine,** the fundamental principles of medical science; especially physiology, pathology, and the kindred branches of medical education.

instrument (in′stroo-ment) [L. *instrumentum; instruere* to furnish] any tool, appliance, or apparatus. **Feleky's i.,** one used for massaging the prostate.

instrumental (in″stroo-men′tal) pertaining to or performed by instruments.

instrumentarium (in″stroo-men-ta′re-um) the instruments or equipment required for any particular operation or purpose; the physical adjuncts with which a physician combats disease.

instrumentation (in″stroo-men-ta′shun) the use of instruments; work performed with instruments.

insuccation (in″sŭ-ka′shun) [L. *insuccare* to soak in; *in* into + *succus* juice] the thorough soaking of a drug before preparing an extract from it.

insudation (in″su-da′shun) [*in-* + L. *sudare* to sweat] 1. the accumulation, as in the kidney or the arterial (intimal) wall, of substances derived from the blood. 2. the substance so accumulated.

insufficiency (in″sŭ-fish′en-se) [L. *insufficientia,* from *in* not + *sufficiens* sufficient] the condition of being insufficient or inadequate to the performance of the allotted duty. **active i.,** the inability of a muscle to act owing to the abnormal (or other) approximation of its insertion to its origin. **adrenal i.,** hypoadrenalism. **aortic i.,** see under *regurgitation.* **capsular i.,** hypoadrenalism. **cardiac i.,** insufficiency of the heart muscle; see also *heart failure.* **coronary i.,** decrease in flow of blood

through the coronary blood vessels. **i. of the externi,** insufficient power in the externi muscles of the eye, so that they are overbalanced by the interni, producing esophoria. **i. of the eyelids,** a condition in which the eyes are closed only by a conscious effort. **gastric i., gastromotor i.,** inability of the stomach to empty itself; myasthenia gastrica. **hepatic i.,** inability of the liver properly to perform its functions. **ileocecal i.,** inability of the ileocecal valve to prevent backflow of contents from the cecum into the ileum. **i. of the interni,** insufficient power in the interni muscles of the eye, so that they are overbalanced by the externi, producing exophoria. **mitral i.,** see under *regurgitation.* **muscular i.,** the inability of a muscle to do its normal work by a normal contraction. **myocardial i.,** insufficiency of the heart muscle; see also *heart failure.* **parathyroid i.,** hypoparathyroidism. **placental i.,** inability of the placenta to properly perform its functions, which compromises the fetal environment so that the fetus is in jeopardy. **pulmonary i.,** see *pulmonic regurgitation,* under *regurgitation.* **renal i.,** a state of disordered function of the kidneys verifiable by quantitative tests. See also *renal failure,* under *failure.* **thyroid i.,** hypothyroidism. **tricuspid i.,** see under *regurgitation.* **uterine i.,** weakness of the contractile power of the uterus, due to muscular atony. **i. of the valves, valvular i.,** see under *regurgitation.* **velopharyngeal i.,** failure of closure of the velopharyngeal portal, due to cleft palate, muscular dysfunction, etc., resulting in defective speech. **venous i.,** inadequacy of the venous valves and impairment of venous return (venous stasis) from the legs, often with edema and sometimes with stasis ulcers at the ankle. **vertebrobasilar i.,** transient ischemia of the brain stem and cerebellum due to stenosis of the vertebral or basilar artery, resulting in attacks of such symptoms as vertigo, diplopia, nystagmus, muscle weakness, and dysarthria.

insufficientia (in″sŭ-fish″e-en′she-ah) [L.] insufficiency.

insufflation (in″sŭ-fla′shun) [L. *in* into + *sufflatio* a blowing up] 1. the act of blowing a powder, vapor, gas, or air into a body cavity. Cf. *infusion* (def. 3). 2. finely powdered or liquid drugs carried into the respiratory passages by such devices as aerosols. **cranial i.,** the forcing of air into the subdural space and the cerebral ventricles. **endotracheal i.,** introduction of air into the trachea through a tube passed into the larynx; employed to inflate the lungs during intrathoracic operations. **i. of the lungs,** the act of blowing air into the lungs for the purpose of artificial respiration. **perirenal i.,** the injection of air around the kidneys for the purpose of roentgen visualization of the adrenal glands. **presacral i.,** the injection of gas, usually carbon dioxide, around the kidneys through a needle inserted into the retrorectal space for the purpose of roentgen visualization of the entire retroperitoneal space, with delineation of renal and adrenal areas. **tubal i.,** see *Rubin's test,* under *test.*

insufflator (in′sŭ-fla″tor) an instrument used in performing insufflation.

insula (in′su-lah), pl. *in′sulae* [L. "island"] [NA] a triangular area of the cerebral cortex which forms the floor of the lateral cerebral fossa; it is covered over and hidden from view by the juxtaposition of the opercula, which thus forms the lateral sulcus. Called also *insula* or *island of Reil.* **insulae of Peyer,** folliculi lymphatici aggregati. **i. of Reil, i. Rei′lii,** insula.

insulae (in′su-le) [L.] plural of *insula.*

insular (in′su-lar) pertaining to an island, especially to the insula or to the islands of Langerhans.

insularine (in′su-lar-in) a yellow amorphous alkaloid, $C_{37}H_{38}O_6N_2$, from *Cissampelos insularis.*

insular-pancreatotropic (in″su-lar-pan″kre-ah-to-trop′ik) having affinity for or a stimulating action on the islands of Langerhans in the pancreas.

insulation (in″sŭ-la′shun) [L. *insulare* to make an island of] 1. the surrounding of a space or body with material designed to prevent the entrance or escape of radiant or electrical energy. 2. the material so used.

insulator (in′su-la″tor) any substance or appliance of such nonconducting properties that it can be used to secure insulation.

insulin (in′su-lin) [L. *insula* island (of the pancreas) + *-in*] a double-chain protein hormone formed from proinsulin in the beta cells of the pancreatic islets of Langerhans. The major fuel-regulating hormone in humans, it is secreted into the blood in response to a rise in concentration of glucose in the blood and also to a rise in amino acid concentration. Insulin promotes the storage of glucose in the liver, skeletal muscle, and adipose tissue, promotes the uptake of amino acids by skeletal muscle, increases protein synthesis, accelerates lipid synthesis, and inhibits lipolysis and gluconeogenesis. A sterile solution of this hypoglycemic principle of the pancreas (regular insulin), prepared in accordance with USP standards, containing 40, 80, 100, and 500 USP insulin units per milliliter, and suitable for intravenous and intramuscular injection, is used in the treatment of diabetes mellitus. **dalanated i.,** an insulin derivative prepared by the removal of the C-terminal alanine from the B chain of insulin. **globin i.,** a combination of insulin with the globin of erythrocytes; in rapidity of onset and duration of action it seems to be midway between insulin and protamine zinc insulin. **globin zinc i.,**

an intermediate-acting insulin consisting of insulin modified by the addition of zinc chloride and globin, the latter obtained from beef blood. The USP preparation, suitable for injection, contains 40, 80, or 100 USP insulin units per ml.; administered subcutaneously in the treatment of diabetes mellitus. **isophane i.,** see under *suspension.* **i. lente,** insulin zinc suspension; see under *suspension.* **neutral i.,** a neutral, buffered solution of insulin obtained from pigs. **NPH i.,** isophane insulin suspension; see under *suspension.* **plant i.,** glucokinin. **protamine i., i. protaminate,** insulin precipitated from a solution of insulin hydrochloride with a monoprotamine compound and suitably buffered; it is more slowly absorbed than ordinary insulin and its action is correspondingly prolonged. **protamine zinc i.,** see under *suspension.* **regular i.,** the active principle of the pancreas of slaughterhouse animals (cattle or swine), used in sterile acidified solution. See *insulin.* **semilente i.,** prompt-acting insulin suspension. **i. tannate,** a salt of insulin claimed to have certain advantages over regular insulin. **three-to-one i.,** a combination of regular insulin and protamine zinc insulin, having the activity of three parts of the former and one part of the latter. **ultralente i.,** extended-action insulin suspension. **vegetable i.,** glucokinin. **zinc-protamine i.,** protamine zinc insulin suspension; see under *suspension.*

insulinase (in′su-lin-ās) an enzyme previously reported in body tissues that destroys or inactivates insulin; this effect is probably due to several nonspecific proteases.

insuline (in′su-līn) insulin.

insulinemia (in″su-lĭ-ne′me-ah) [*insulin* + Gr. *haima* blood + *-ia*] the presence of insulin in the blood.

insulinlipodystrophy (in″su-lin-li″po-dis′tro-fe) the local disappearance of fat in diabetic patients on insulin treatment.

insulinogenesis (in″su-lin-o-jen′ĕ-sis) the formation and release of insulin by the islands of Langerhans.

insulinogenic (in″su-lin″o-jen′ik) pertaining to, characterized by, or promoting insulinogenesis.

insulinoid (in′su-lin-oid″) 1. resembling insulin. 2. any substance with hypoglycemic properties like those of insulin.

insulinoma (in″su-lin-o′mah) a tumor of the beta cells of the islets of Langerhans; although usually benign, such tumors are among the most important causes of hypoglycemia.

insulinopenic (in″su-lin-o-pe′nik) diminishing, or pertaining to a decrease in, the level of circulating insulin; said of most forms of diabetes mellitus characterized by clear-cut deficiency of insulin production.

insulism (in′su-lizm) hyperinsulinism.

insulitis (in′su-li′tis) cellular infiltration of the islands of Langerhans, possibly in response to invasion by an infectious agent.

insulogenic (in″su-lo-jen′ik) insulinogenic.

insuloma (in″su-lo′mah) [L. *insula* island (of Langerhans) + *-oma*] insulinoma.

insulopathic (in″su-lo-path′ik) pertaining to, or due to, abnormal insulin secretion.

insultus (in-sul′tus) [L.] an attack.

insusceptibility (in″sŭ-sep″tĭ-bil′ĭ-te) the quality of not being susceptible; immunity.

intake (in-tāk′) the substances, or the quantities thereof, taken in and utilized by the body. **caloric i.,** the food ingested or otherwise taken into the body. **fluid i.,** the fluid taken into the body by drinking or parenterally.

Intal (in′tal) trademark for a preparation of cromolyn sodium.

integration (in″tĕ-gra′shun) 1. assimilation; anabolic action or activity. 2. the combining of different acts so that they cooperate toward a common end; coordination. 3. assimilation into the personality, as of knowledge and experience, as reflected in distinctive behavior patterns. 4. in bacterial genetics, assimilation of genetic material from one bacterium (donor) into the chromosome of another (recipient). **biological i.,** the acquisition of functional coordination during embryonic development through humoral and nervous influences. **primary i.,** the recognition by a child that his body is a unit apart from the environment; it is probably not achieved before the second half of the first year of life. **secondary i.,** the sublimation of the separate elements of the early sexual instinct into the mature psychosexual personality.

integrator (in′tĕ-gra″tor) an instrument for measuring body surfaces.

integument (in-teg′u-ment) [L. *integumentum*] a covering or investment; the skin. **common i.,** the covering of the body, or skin; see *integumentum commune.*

integumentary (in-teg-u-men′tar-e) 1. pertaining to or composed of skin. 2. serving as a covering, like the skin.

integumentum (in-teg″u-men′tum) [L., from *in* on + *tegere* to cover] [NA] a general term denoting a covering, or investment. **i. commu′ne** [NA], common integument: the covering of the body, or skin, including its various layers and the accessory structures (hair, nails, and skin glands, including the breast, or mammary gland).

in tela (in te′lah) [L.] in tissue; relating especially to stained histological preparations.

intellect (in′te-lekt) [L. *intellectus,* from *intelligere* to understand] the mind, thinking faculty, or understanding.

intellection (in″te-lek′shun) the objectively appreciable evaluation of relationships by the mind.

intellectualization (in″tĕ-lek″chu-al-ĭ-za′shun) the mental process in which reasoning is used as a defense against confronting unconscious conflict and its stressful emotions.

intelligence (in-tel′ĭ-jens) [L. *intelligere* to understand] the ability to comprehend or understand; see also under *quotient.*

intemperance (in-tem′per-ans) [L. *in* not + *temperare* to moderate] excess or lack of self-control in respect of food and drink; immoderate indulgence in the use of alcoholic drinks.

intensification (in-ten″sĭ-fi-ka′shun) [L. *intensus* intense + *facere* to make] 1. the act of making anything intense. 2. the process of becoming intense.

intensimeter (in″ten-sim′ĕ-ter) Fürstenau's device for measuring the intensity of roentgen rays; it is based on the variation of electric resistance of a selenium cell under influence of irradiation at different intensities.

intensionometer (in-ten″se-o-nom′ĕ-ter) an ionometric instrument for measuring the intensity of roentgen rays. Two series of plates, separated by an air gap that serves as the dielectric, are connected to opposite terminals in a closed chamber. An electric circuit is completed when the air becomes ionized by the roentgen rays, and the difference in electric potential is registered by deflection of a galvanometer needle.

intensity (in-ten′sĭ-te) [L. *intensus* intense; *in* on + *tendere* to stretch] the condition or quality of being intense; a high degree of tension, activity, or energy. **i. of electric field,** the force exerted on a unit charge in an electric field. **luminous i.,** the light-giving power of a source of light. Cf. *candle power.* **i. of roentgen rays,** the roentgen-ray energy passing per unit time through unit area normal to the direction of propagation.

intensive (in-ten′siv) [L. *in* on + *tendere* to stretch] of great force or intensity; see also *intensive care unit,* under *unit.*

intention (in-ten′shun) [L. *intentio,* from *in* upon + *tendere* to stretch] a manner of healing; see under *healing.*

inter- (in′ter) [L. *inter* between] a prefix meaning situated, formed, or occurring between elements indicated by the word stem to which it is affixed.

interaccessory (in″ter-ak-ses′o-re) connecting the accessory processes of the vertebrae.

interacinar (in″ter-as′ĭ-nar) situated between acini.

interacinous (in″ter-as′ĭ-nus) interacinar.

interaction (in″ter-ak′shun) the quality, state, or process of (two or more things) acting on each other. **drug i.,** the action of one drug upon the effectiveness or toxicity of another (or others).

interagglutination (in″ter-ah-gloo-tĭ-na′shun) agglutination of one kind of cell by agglutinins against a nearly related kind (i.e., by crossreacting agglutinins).

interalveolar (in″ter-al-ve′o-lar) between alveoli.

interangular (in″ter-ang′gu-lar) situated or occurring between two or more angles.

interannular (in″ter-an′u-lar) [*inter-* + L. *annulus* ring] situated between two rings or constrictions.

interarticular (in″ter-ar-tik′u-lar) [*inter-* + L. *articulus* joint] situated between articular surfaces.

interarytenoid (in″ter-ar′e-te′noid) between the arytenoid cartilages.

interatrial (in″ter-a′tre-al) situated between the atria of the heart.

interauricular (in″ter-aw-rik′u-lar) interatrial.

interbrain (in′ter-brān) 1. thalamencephalon. 2. diencephalon.

intercalary (in-ter′kah-ler″e) [L. *intercalarius; inter-* + *calare* to call] inserted or placed between; interposed.

intercalate (in-ter′kah-lāt) [L. *intercalatus*] to insert between.

intercalation (in-ter″kah-la′shun) a speech neurosis in which a word or sound is interposed between words or phrases.

intercalatum (in″ter-kah-la′tum) (*obs.*) substantia nigra.

intercanalicular (in″ter-kan″ah-lik′u-lar) between canaliculi.

intercapillary (in″ter-kap′ĭ-lār-e) among or between capillaries.

intercarotic (in″ter-kah-rot′ik) between the carotid arteries.

intercarotid (in″ter-kah-rot′id) intercarotic.

intercarpal (in″ter-kar′pal) between the carpal bones.

intercartilaginous (in″ter-kar″tĭ-laj′ĭ-nus) connecting or situated between two or more cartilages.

intercavernous (in″ter-kav′er-nus) between two cavities.

intercellular (in″ter-sel′u-lar) situated between the cells of any structure.

intercentral (in″ter-sen′tral) situated between or connecting two or more nerve centers.

intercerebral (in″ter-ser′ĕ-bral) connecting or situated between the two cerebral hemispheres.

interchondral (in″ter-kon′dral) intercartilaginous.

intercilium (in″ter-sil′e-um) [*inter-* + L. *cilium* eyelash] the space between the eyebrows.

interclavicular (in″ter-klah-vik′u-lar) [*inter-* + L. *clavicula* clavicle] situated between the clavicles.

interclinoid (in″ter-kli′noid) pertaining to or passing between the clinoid processes.

intercoccygeal (in″ter-kok-sij′e-al) situated between the segments of the coccyx.

intercolumnar (in″ter-ko-lum′nar) [*inter-* + L. *columna* column] situated between columns or pillars.

intercondylar (in″ter-kon′dĭ-lar) situated between two condyles.

intercondyloid (in″ter-kon′dĭ-loid) intercondylar.

intercondylous (in″ter-kon′dĭ-lus) intercondylar.

intercostal (in″ter-kos′tal) [*inter-* + L. *costa* rib] situated between the ribs.

intercostohumeral (in″ter-kos-to-hu′mer-al) pertaining to an intercostal space and the humerus.

intercourse (in′ter-kōrs) [L. *intercursus* running between] mutual exchange. **sexual i.,** coitus.

intercricothyrotomy (in″ter-kri″ko-thi-rot′o-me) [*inter-* + *cricothyroid* + Gr. *temnein* to cut] incision of the larynx through the cricothyroid membrane; inferior laryngotomy.

intercristal (in″ter-kris′tal) between two crests.

intercritical (in″ter-krit′ĭ-kal) denoting the period between attacks, as of gout.

intercross (in′ter-kros) the mating of individuals heterozygous for the same gene.

intercrural (in″ter-kru′ral) between two crura.

intercurrent (in″ter-kur′ent) [L. *intercurrens,* from *inter-* + *currere* to run] breaking into and modifying the course of an already existing disease.

intercuspation (in″ter-kus-pa′shun) the fitting together of the cusps of opposing teeth in occlusion.

intercusping (in″ter-kusp′ing) the occlusion of the cusps of the teeth of one jaw with the depressions in the teeth of the other jaw.

intercutaneomucous (in″ter-ku-ta″ne-o-mu′kus) mucocutaneous.

interdeferential (in″ter-def″er-en′shal) between the two ductus deferentes.

interdental (in″ter-den′tal) [*inter-* + L. *dens* tooth] situated between the proximal surfaces of adjacent teeth in the same dental arch. Cf. *interocclusal.*

interdentium (in″ter-den′she-um) the interproximal space; see under *space.*

interdigit (in″ter-dij′it) the space between any two contiguous fingers or toes.

interdigital (in″ter-dij′ĭ-tal) [*inter-* + L. *digitus* finger] situated between two adjacent fingers or toes.

interdigitate (in″ter-dij′ĭ-tāt) [*inter-* + L. *digitus* finger] to interlock and interrelate, as the fingers of clasped hands.

interdigitation (in″ter-dij″ĭ-ta′shun) [*inter-* + L. *digitus* digit] 1. an interlocking of parts by finger-like processes. 2. any one of a set of finger-like processes. 3. in density, intercuspation.

interface (in′ter-fās) in chemistry, the surface of separation or boundary between two phases of a heterogeneous system. **dineric i.,** the interface between two immiscible liquids.

interfacial (in″ter-fa′shal) pertaining to an interface.

interfascicular (in″ter-fah-sik′u-lar) [*inter-* + L. *fasciculus* bundle] situated between fasciculi.

interfeminium (in″ter-fĕ-min′e-um) [L.] (*obs.*) the space between the thighs, or the inside of the thighs.

interfemoral (in″ter-fem′o-ral) between the thighs.

interfemus (in″ter-fe′mus) [L.] interfeminium.

interference (in″ter-fēr′ens) [*inter-* + L. *ferire* to strike] 1. a merging of two waves of light or of sound, producing in the first instance darkness, in the other, silence. 2. an interplay of two intrinsic pacemakers in the heart, one or the other dominating the rhythm; see also *interference dissociation,* under *dissociation.* 3. in dentistry, any premature contact point along the occlusal surface of the teeth that prevents maximum contact, function, and proper alignment in full occlusion.

interfering (in″ter-fēr′ing) brushing; the striking or rubbing of the fetlock of a horse by the opposite foot.

interferometer (in″ter-fēr-om′ĕ-ter) an instrument for measuring lengths or movements by means of the phenomena caused by the interference of two rays of light, or of sound (acoustic i.).

interferometry (in″ter-fēr-om′ĕ-tre) the use of the interferometer for measuring distances or movements.

interferon (in″ter-fēr′on) a class of small soluble proteins produced and released by cells invaded by virus, which induce in noninfected cells the formation of an antiviral protein that inhibits viral multiplication; although not virus-specific, interferons are more effective in animal cells of the same species that produced them. Type I, or classical, interferon is produced by leukocytes, as well as nonlymphoid cells, in response to virus infection. Interferon production may alo be induced by certain bacteria, rickettsiae, etc., and by specifically sensitized lymphocytes following interaction with specific antigen or antigen-antibody complex. The latter form, known as *Type II* or *immune interferon,* is capable of affecting antibody production and cell-mediated immunity.

interfibrillar (in″ter-fi′bril-ar) [*inter-* + L. *fibrilla* small fiber] between or among fibrils.

interfibrillary (in″ter-fi′brĭ-lār″e) interfibrillar.

interfibrous (in″ter-fi′brus) between fibers.

interfilamentous (in″ter-fil″ah-men′tus) between filaments.

interfilar (in″ter-fi′lar) [*inter-* + L. *filum* thread] between or among the fibrils of a reticulum.

interfrontal (in″ter-fron′tal) between the halves of the frontal bone.

interfurca (in″ter-fur′kah), pl. *interfur′cae* [*inter-* + L. *furca* fork] the area lying between and at the base of divided tooth roots.

interfurcae (in″ter-fur′se) [L.] plural of *interfurca.*

interganglionic (in″ter-gang″gle-on′ik) [*inter-* + *ganglion*] between ganglia.

intergemmal (in″ter-jem′al) [*inter-* + L. *gemma* bud] between taste buds or other buds.

intergenic (in″ter-jen′ik) occurring between two genes.

interglobular (in″ter-glob′u-lar) [*inter-* + L. *globulus* globule.] between or among globules, as of the dentin.

intergluteal (in″ter-gloo′te-al) between the buttocks.

intergonial (in″ter-go′ne-al) between the tips of the two angles of the mandible.

intergrade (in′ter-grād) [*inter-* + L. *gradus* a step] a step or stage between two other stages. **sex i.,** an individual showing characteristics between the typical male and female condition. See *intersex* and *hermaphroditism.*

intergranular (in″ter-gran′u-lar) between the granule cells of the brain.

intergyral (in″ter-ji′ral) between cerebral gyri or convolutions.

interhemicerebral (in″ter-hem″ĭ-ser′ĕ-bral) intercerebral.

interhemispheric (in″ter-hem″ĭ-sfer′ik) intercerebral.

interictal (in″ter-ik′tal) occurring between attacks or paroxysms.

interior (in-tēr′e-or) [L. "inner"; neut. *interius*] 1. situated inside; inward. 2. an inner part or cavity.

interischiadic (in″ter-is″ke-ad′ik) between the two ischia.

interkinesis (in″ter-ki-ne′sis) [*inter-* + Gr. *kinēsis* motion] a period intervening between the first and second divisions in meiosis, similar to the interphase in mitosis.

interlabial (in″ter-la′be-al) [*inter-* + L. *labium* lip] between the lips, or between any two labia.

interlamellar (in″ter-lah-mel′ar) [*inter-* + L. *lamella* layer] situated between lamellae.

interligamentary (in″ter-lig″ah-men′tah-re) between or among ligaments.

interligamentous (in″ter-lig″ah-men′tus) interligamentary.

interlobar (in″ter-lo′bar) [*inter-* + L. *lobus* lobe] situated or occurring between lobes.

interlobitis (in″ter-lo-bi′tis) interlobular pleurisy.

interlobular (in″ter-lob′u-lar) [*inter-* + L. *lobulus* lobule] situated or occurring between lobules.

interlocking (in″ter-lok′ing) a complication of labor in twin births in which the inferior surface of the chin of one twin is hooked to that of its co-twin above or below the pelvic inlet. When this condition occurs in the true pelvis, it is called *compaction.*

intermalleolar (in″ter-mah-le′o-lar) between the malleoli.

intermamillary (in″ter-mam′ĭ-lār″e) between the nipples.

intermammary (in″ter-mam′ah-re) between the breasts.

intermarriage (in″ter-mar′ij) [*inter-* + L. *maritare* to wed] 1. the marriage of persons related by blood or consanguinity. 2. the marriage of persons of different races.

intermaxilla (in″ter-mak-sil′ah) the intermaxillary bone.

intermaxillary (in″ter-mak′sĭ-lār″e) situated between the two maxillae.

intermediary (in″ter-me′de-ār″e) [*inter-* + L. *medius* middle] 1. performed or occurring in a median stage; neither early nor late; intermediate. 2. an intermediate stage.

intermediate (in″ter-me′de-it) [*inter-* + L. *medius* middle] 1. placed between; intervening; resembling, in part, each of two extremes. 2. a substance formed in a chemical process that is essential to the formation of the end product of the process.

intermedin (in″ter-me′din) melanocyte-stimulating hormone; so called because in amphibia, reptiles, and fish, it is secreted by the pars intermedia of the pituitary gland.

intermediolateral (in″ter-me″de-o-lat′er-al) both intermediate and lateral.

intermedius (in″ter-me′de-us) intermediate; [NA] a term denoting the middle of three structures, one of which is situated closer to and the other farther from the midline of the body or part.

intermembranous (in″ter-mem′brah-nus) situated or occurring between membranes.

intermeningeal (in″ter-mĕ-nin′je-al) situated or occurring between the meninges.

intermenstrual (in″ter-men′stroo-al) [*inter-* + *menstrual*] occurring between the menstrual periods.

intermenstruum (in″ter-men′stroo-um) the interval between two menstrual periods.

intermetacarpal (in″ter-met″ah-kar′pal) [*inter-* + *metacarpal*] situated between the metacarpal bones.

intermetameric (in″ter-met″ah-mer′ik) between two metameres.

intermetatarsal (in″ter-met″ah-tar′sal) situated or occurring between the metatarsal bones.

intermission (in″ter-mish′un) [L. *intermissio; inter* between + *mittere* to send] an interval; a period of temporary cessation, as between two occurrences or paroxysms.

intermitotic (in″ter-mi-tot′ik) pertaining to or occurring during the interval between successive mitoses.

intermittent (in″ter-mit′ent) [L. *intermittens; inter* between + *mittere* to send] occurring at separated intervals; having periods of cessation of activity.

intermolecular (in″ter-mo-lek′u-lar) between molecules.

intermural (in-ter-mu′ral) [*inter-* + L. *murus* wall] situated between the walls of an organ or organs.

intermuscular (in″ter-mus′ku-lar) situated between muscles.

intern (in′tern) 1. [Fr. *interne*] a graduate of a medical or dental school serving and residing in a hospital preparatory to being licensed to practice medicine or dentistry. Cf. *resident.* 2. [Fr. *interner*] to confine within certain geographical or physical boundaries.

internal (in-ter′nal) [L. *internus*] situated or occurring within or on the inside; many anatomical structures formerly called internal are now correctly termed medial.

internalization (in-ter″nal-ĭ-za′shun) the mental process whereby certain attributes, attitudes, or standards of others are unconsciously taken as one's own.

internarial (in″ter-na′re-al) [*inter-* + L. *nares* nostrils] situated between the nares.

internasal (in″ter-na′zal) situated between the nasal bones.

internatal (in″ter-na′tal) [*inter-* + L. *nates* buttocks] between the buttocks or gluteal prominences.

internation (in″ter-na′shun) the act of confining within certain physical boundaries, as the confinement of a mental patient.

International Nonproprietary Names see *I.N.N.*

interne (in-tern′) [Fr.] intern.

interneuron (in″ter-nu′ron) any neuron, in a chain of neurons, which is situated between the primary afferent (sensory) neuron and the final motoneuron. Also, any neuron whose processes are entirely confined within a specific area, as within the olfactory lobe, and which synapse with neurons extending into that area.

internist (in-ter′nist) a physician who specializes in the diagnosis and medical, as opposed to surgical and obstetrical, treatment of diseases of adults.

internodal (in″ter-no′dal) between two nodes.

internode (in′ter-nōd) [*inter-* + L. *nodus* knot] a space between two nodes. **i. of Ranvier,** the segment of a nerve fiber between two nodes of Ranvier.

internodular (in″ter-nod′u-lar) between two nodules.

internship (in′tern-ship) the position or term of service of an intern in a hospital.

internuclear (in″ter-nu′kle-ar) 1. pertaining to or affecting structures between nuclei, as internuclear ophthalmoplegia. 2. between the nuclear layers of the retina.

internuncial (in″ter-nun′she-al) [L. *internuncius* a go-between] serving as a medium of communication between nerve cells or centers; see *interneuron.*

internus (in-ter′nus) internal; [NA] a term denoting something situated nearer to the center of an organ or a cavity.

interocclusal (in″ter-ŏ-kloo′zal) situated between the occlusal surfaces of opposing teeth in the two dental arches, as the interocclusal rest space. Cf. *interdental.*

interoceptive (in′ter-o-sep′tiv) Sherrington's term for the internal surface field of distribution of receptor organs; see *receptor* (def. 3), exteroceptive, and *proprioceptive.*

interoceptor (in″ter-o-sep′tor) any one of the sensory nerve terminals which are located in and transmit impulses from the viscera; see *receptor* (def. 3), *exteroceptor,* and *proprioceptor.*

interofection (in″ter-o-fek′shun) the responses of the body to changes in the internal environment of the body effected by the sympathetic system.

interofective (in″ter-o-fek′tiv) affecting the interior of the organism; a term applied by Cannon to the autonomic nervous system.

interogestate (in″ter-o-jes′tāt) 1. developing within the uterus. 2. the fetus during gestation.

interoinferiorly (in″ter-o-in-fēr′e-or″le) inwardly and in a downward position or direction.

interolivary (in″ter-ol′ĭ-vār″e) situated between the olivary bodies of the brain.

interorbital (in″ter-or′bĭ-tal) [*inter-* + L. *orbita* orbit] situated between the orbits.

interosseal (in″ter-os′e-al) [*inter-* + L. *os* bone] 1. situated between bones. 2. pertaining to the interossei muscles.

interosseous (in″ter-os′e-us) [L. *interosseus; inter* between + *os* bone] between bones.

interpalpebral (in″ter-pal′pe-bral) between the eyelids.

interpandemic (in″ter-pan-dem′ik) denoting outbreaks of an infectious disease (e.g., influenza) occurring between major pandemics of the same disease.

interparietal (in″ter-pah-ri′ĕ-tal) [*inter-* + L. *paries* wall] 1. intermural. 2. situated between the parietal bones.

interparoxysmal (in″ter-par″ok-siz′mal) occurring between paroxysms.

interpediculate (in″ter-pĕ-dik′u-lāt) between the pedicles of a vertebra, as interpediculate distance.

interpeduncular (in″ter-pĕ-dunk′u-lar) [*inter-* + L. *pedunculus* peduncle] situated between two peduncles, as between two cerebellar peduncles.

interphalangeal (in″ter-fah-lan′je-al) [*inter-* + *phalangeal*] situated between two contiguous phalanges.

interphase (in′ter-fāz) the interval between two successive cell divisions, during which the chromosomes are not individually distinguishable and the normal physiological processes proceed. Formerly called *resting phase.*

interphyletic (in″ter-fi-let′ik) [*inter-* + *phyletic*] intermediate in form between two types of cell.

interpial (in″ter-pi′al) situated between the two layers of the pia mater.

interplant (in′ter-plant) [*inter-* + L. *plantare* to set] an embryonic part isolated by transference to an indifferent environment provided by another embryo.

interpleural (in″ter-ploor′al) between two layers of the pleura, as between the visceral and the parietal pleura.

interpolar (in″ter-po′lar) [*inter-* + L. *polus* pole] situated between two poles.

interpolation (in-ter″po-la′shun) 1. surgical implantation of tissue. 2. the determination of intermediate values in a series on the basis of observed values.

interposition (in″ter-po-zish′un) the act of placing between; the condition of being interposed.

interpositum (in″ter-poz′i-tum) [L.] interposed; see under *velum.*

interpretation (in-ter″prĕ-ta′shun) in psychotherapy, the therapist's explanation of the latent or hidden meanings of what the patient says, does, or experiences, in terms which are understandable to him.

interprotometamere (in″ter-pro″to-met′ah-mēr) [*inter-* + Gr. *prōtos* first + *meta* across + *meros* part] the structure between the primary segments of the embryo.

interproximal (in″ter-prok′sĭ-mal) between adjoining surfaces, as the space between adjacent teeth.

interpubic (in″ter-pu′bik) [*inter-* + L. *pubes*] between the pubic bones.

interpupillary (in″ter-pu′pĭ-lar″e) between the pupils.

interradial (in″ter-ra′de-al) situated between rays.

interrenal (in″ter-re′nal) [*inter-* + *renal*] between the kidneys.

interrupted (in″ter-rupt′ed) [L. *interruptus; inter* between + *ruptus* broken] not continuous; marked by intermissions or breaches of continuity.

interscapilium (in″ter-skah-pil′e-um) [L.] the space between the scapulae.

interscapular (in″ter-skap′u-lar) [*inter-* + L. *scapula* shoulder blade] situated between the scapulae.

interscapulum (in″ter-skap′u-lum) the interscapilium.

intersciatic (in″ter-si-at′ik) between the two ischia.

intersectio (in″ter-sek′she-o) pl. *intersectio′nes* [L., from *inter* between + *secare* to cut] [NA] a general term denoting a cutting across, or between; a site at which one structure cuts across another. **i. tendin′ea,** tendinous intersection: a fibrous band that crosses the belly of a muscle and more or less completely divides it into two parts; called also *inscriptio tendinea.* **intersectio′nes tendin′eae mus′culi rec′ti abdom′inis** [NA], tendinous intersections of rectus abdominis muscle: three or more fibrous bands that cross the front of the rectus abdominis muscle, fusing with the anterior layer of its sheath; called also *inscriptiones tendineae musculi recti abdominis.*

intersection (in″ter-sek′shun) a site at which one structure cuts across another. **tendinous i.,** intersectio tendinea.

intersectiones (in″ter-sek″she-o′nēz) [L.] plural of *intersectio.*

intersegment (in″ter-seg′ment) 1. any one of a series of segments, like the angiotomes, etc. 2. a metamere.

intersegmental (in″ter-seg-men′tal) between segments.

interseptal (in″ter-sep′tal) between two septa.

interseptum (in″ter-sep′tum) [L.] the diaphragm.

intersex (in′ter-seks) 1. intersexuality. 2. an individual who shows intermingling, in varying degrees, of the characters of each sex, including physical form, reproductive organs, and sexual behavior. See also *hermaphrodite* and *pseudohermaphrodite.* **female i.,** a female pseudohermaphrodite: an individual who shows one or more contradictions of the morphological criteria of sex but who has only female gonadal tissue and shows sex chromatin in the somatic cells. **male i.,** a male pseudohermaphrodite: an individual who shows one or more contradictions of the morphological criteria of sex but who has only male gonadal tissue and shows no sex chromatin in the somatic cells. **true i.,** a true hermaphrodite: an individual who shows one or more contradictions of the morphological criteria of sex and possesses both male and female gonadal tissue; the chromatin test may be either positive or negative.

intersexual (in″ter-seks′u-al) pertaining to or characterized by intersexuality.

intersexuality (in″ter-seks″u-al′ĭ-te) the intermingling, in varying degrees, of the characters of each sex, including physical form, reproductive organs, and sexual behavior, in one individual, as a result of some flaw in embryonic development. See also *intersex, hermaphroditism,* and *pseudohermaphroditism.*

interspace (in′ter-spās) a space between two similar structures. **dineric i.,** the surface between two liquid phases.

interspinal (in-ter-spi′nal) between two spinous processes.

interspinous (in″ter-spi′nus) interspinal.

intersternal (in″ter-ster′nal) between parts of the sternum.

interstice (in-ter′stis) [L. *interstitium*] a small interval, space, or gap in a tissue or structure.

interstitial (in″ter-stish′al) [L. *interstitialis; inter* between + *sistere* to set] pertaining to or situated between parts or in the interspaces of a tissue.

interstitium (in″ter-stish′ĭ-um) [L.] 1. interstice. 2. interstial tissue.

intertarsal (in″ter-tar′sal) situated between the tarsal bones.

intertransverse (in″ter-trans-vers′) [*inter-* + L. *transversus* turned across] situated between or connecting the transverse processes of the vertebrae.

intertriginous (in″ter-trij′ĭ-nus) affected with or of the nature of intertrigo.

intertrigo (in″ter-tri′go) [*inter-* + L. *terere* to rub] superficial dermatitis occurring on apposed surfaces of the skin, as the creases of the neck, folds of the groin and armpit, and beneath pendulous breasts; it is characterized by erythema, maceration, burning, itching, and sometimes erosions, fissures, and exudations. It is caused by moisture, warmth, friction, sweat retention, and infectious agents; obesity is a predisposing factor. **i. labia′lis,** perlèche.

intertrochanteric (in″ter-tro″kan-ter′ik) [*inter-* + *trochanter*] situated in or pertaining to the space between the greater and the lesser trochanter.

intertubercular (in″ter-tu-ber′ku-lar) between tubercles.

intertubular (in″ter-tu′bu-lar) [*inter-* + L. *tubulus* tubule] situated between or among tubules.

interureteral (in″ter-u-re′ter-al) interureteric.

interureteric (in″ter-u″rĕ-ter′ik) [*inter-* + *ureter*] situated between the ureters.

intervaginal (in″ter-vaj′ĭ-nal) situated between sheaths.

interval (in′ter-val) [*inter-* + L. *vallum* rampart] the space between two objects or parts; the lapse of time between two recurrences or paroxysms. **atrioventricular i.,** the P–R interval; the time between atrial and ventricular systole. **auriculoventricular i.,** atrioventricular i. **cardioarterial i.,** the time between the apex beat and arterial pulsation; abbreviated c.-a. i. **focal i.,** the distance from the anterior to the posterior focal point; called also *Sturm's i.* **lucid i.,** a brief period of remission of symptoms in a psychosis. **postsphygmic i.,** see under *period.* **P–R i.,** the portion of the electrocardiogram between the onset of the P wave (atrial activity) and the QRS complex (ventricular activity). **presphygmic i.,** see under *period.* **QRST i., Q–T i.,** the duration of ventricular electrical activity. **Sturm's i.,** focal i.

intervalvular (in″ter-val′vu-lar) between valves.

intervascular (in″ter-vas′ku-lar) between blood vessels.

intervention (in″ter-ven′shun) the act or fact of interfering so

as to modify. **crisis i.,** 1. an immediate, short-term, psychotherapeutic approach, the goal of which is to help resolve a personal crisis within the individual's immediate environment. 2. the procedures involved in responding to an emergency.

interventricular (in″ter-ven-trik′u-lar) [*inter-* + L. *ventriculum* ventricle] situated between ventricles.

intervertebral (in″ter-ver′tĕ-bral) [*inter-* + *vertebra*] situated between two contiguous vertebrae; see under *disk.*

intervillous (in″ter-vil′us) [*inter-* + L. *villus* tuft] situated between or among villi.

intestinal (in-tes′tĭ-nal) [L. *intestinalis*] pertaining to the intestine.

intestine (in-tes′tin) [L. *intesti′nus* inward, internal; Gr. *enteron*] the portion of the alimentary canal extending from the pyloric opening of the stomach to the anus; called also *bowel* and *gut.* See *intestinum.* **blind i.,** cecum, def. 1. **empty i.,** jejunum. **iced i.,** peritonitis chronica fibrosa encapsulans. **jejunoileal i.,** intestinum tenue mesenteriale. **large i.,** the distal portion of the intestine; see *intestinum crassum* [NA]. **mesenterial i.,** intestinum tenue mesenteriale. **segmented i.,** colon. **small i.,** the proximal portion of the intestine; see *intestinum tenue* [NA]. **straight i.,** rectum.

intestino-intestinal (in-tes′tĭ-no-in-tes′tĭ-nal) pertaining to two different portions of the intestine, as the intestino-intestinal reflex.

intestinum (in″tes-ti′num) pl. *intesti′na* [L., from *intestinus* inward, internal] intestine: the portion of the alimentary canal extending from the pyloric opening of the stomach to the anus: it is a membranous tube, comprising the intestinum tenue and the intestinum crassum, whose function is to complete the processes of digestion, to provide the body (through absorption) with water, electrolytes, and nutrients, and to move along and store fecal wastes until they are expelled. **i. cae′cum,** cecum, def. 1. **i. cras′sum** [NA], the large intestine: the distal portion of the intestine, about five feet long, extending from its junction with the small intestine to the anus; it comprises the cecum, colon, rectum, and anal canal. **i. il′eum,** ileum. **i. jeju′num,** jejunum. **i. rec′tum,** rectum. **i. ten′ue** [NA], the small intestine: the proximal portion of the intestine, smaller in caliber than the large intestine, and about twenty feet long, extending from the pylorus to the cecum; it comprises the duodenum, jejunum, and ileum. **i. ten′ue mesenteria′le** the portion of the small intestine which has a mesentery, comprising the jejunum and ileum.

intima (in′tĭ-mah) [L.] [NA] a general term denoting an innermost structure; see *tunica intima vasorum.*

intimal (in′tĭ-mal) pertaining to the inner layer of the blood vessels (tunica intima vasorum).

intimitis (in″tĭ-mi′tis) inflammation of the tunica intima of an artery or vein.

Intocostrin (in″to-kos′trin) trademark for a preparation of tubocurarine chloride.

intolerance (in-tol′er-ans) [L. *in* not + *tolerare* to bear] inability to withstand or consume. **alcoholic i.,** 1. the inability to take alcohol without going on to excess. 2. an excessive response to a small amount of alcohol. **drug i.,** the state of reacting to the normal pharmacologic doses of a drug with the symptoms of overdosage. **hereditary fructose i.,** a hereditary disorder of metabolism transmitted as an autosomal recessive trait, involving deficient activity of the hepatic enzyme fructose-1-phosphate aldolase; it occurs in infants soon after the introduction of fructose in the diet, and is characterized by hypoglycemia and its clinical manifestations, associated with various other symptoms, including fructosuria, fructosemia, anorexia, vomiting, failure to thrive, jaundice, splenomegaly, and an aversion to fructose-containing foods. If the condition is left untreated, death may occur. See also *essential fructosuria,* under *fructosuria.*

intorsion (in-tor′shun) [L. *in* toward + *torsio* twisting] tilting of the upper part of the vertical meridian of the eye toward the midline of the face.

intorter (in′tor-ter) an internal rotator.

intoxication (in-tok″sĭ-ka′shun) [L. *in* intensive + Gr. *toxikon* poison] 1. poisoning; the state of being poisoned. 2. the condition produced by excessive use of an alcohol, especially ethanol. **acid i.,** acidosis of a severe grade. **alkaline i.,** alkalosis of a severe grade. **anaphylactic i.,** anaphylactic shock. **bongkrek i.,** poisoning from bongkrek, a native Javanese dish, prepared by means of molds from copra press cake. When the fermentation process is faulty, severe poisoning occurs, with vomiting, profuse perspiration, muscle cramps, and coma. Called also *tempeh poisoning.* **intestinal i.,** autointoxication. **roentgen i.,** radiation sickness. **serum i.,** a condition of temporary intoxication which sometimes follows the injection of serum; see *serum sickness,* under *sickness.* **water i.,** the condition induced by the undue retention of water with sodium depletion; it is marked by lethargy, nausea, vomiting, and mild mental aberrations, and in severe cases by convulsions and coma.

intra- (in′trah) [L. *intra* within] a prefix meaning situated, formed, or occurring within the element indicated by the word stem to which it is affixed.

intra-abdominal (in″trah-ab-dom′ĭ-nal)　within the abdomen.

intra-acinous (in″trah-as′ĭ-nus)　within an acinus.

intra-appendicular (in″trah-ap′en-dik′u-lar)　within the appendix.

intra-arachnoid (in″trah-ah-rak′noid)　within or underneath the arachnoid.

intra-arterial (in″trah-ar-te′re-al)　within an artery or arteries.

intra-articular (in″trah-ar-tik′u-lar) [*intra-* + L. *articulus* joint]　within a joint.

intra-atomic (in″trah-ah-tom′ik)　within an atom.

intra-atrial (in″trah-a′tre-al)　within an atrium.

intra-aural (in″trah-aw′ral)　within the ear.

intra-auricular (in″trah-aw-rik′u-lar)　intra-atrial.

intrabronchial (in″trah-brong′ke-al)　situated or occurring within a bronchus.

intrabuccal (in″trah-buk′al)　within the mouth or within the cheek.

intracanalicular (in″trah-kan″ah-lik′u-lar)　within canaliculi.

intracapsular (in″trah-kap′su-lar)　within a capsule.

intracardiac (in″trah-kar′de-ak)　within the heart.

intracarpal (in″trah-kar′pal)　within the wrist.

intracartilaginous (in″trah-kar″tĭ-laj′ĭ-nus)　within a cartilage; endochondral.

intracavitary (in″trah-kav′ĭ-tār″e)　within a cavity, as that of the cervix or of the uterus.

intracelial (in″trah-se′le-al)　within one of the body cavities.

intracellular (in″trah-sel′u-lar) [*intra-* + L. *cellula* cell]　situated or occurring within a cell or cells.

intracephalic (in″trah-sĕ-fal′ik)　within the brain.

intracerebellar (in″trah-ser″ĕ-bel′ar)　situated within the cerebellum.

intracerebral (in″trah-ser′ĕ-bral)　situated within the cerebrum.

intracervical (in″trah-ser′vĕ-kal)　situated within the canal of the cervix uteri.

intrachondral (in″trah-kon′dral)　endochondral.

intrachondrial (in″trah-kon′dre-al)　endochondral.

intrachordal (in″trah-kor′dal)　within the notochord.

intracisternal (in″trah-sis-ter′nal)　within a cistern, especially the cisterna cerebellomedularis.

intracolic (in″trah-kol′ik)　within the colon.

intracordal (in″trah-kor′dal) [*intra-* + L. *cor* heart]　within the heart.

intracorporal (in″trah-kor′po-ral)　intracorporeal.

intracorporeal (in″trah-kor-po′re-al)　situated or occurring within the body.

intracorpuscular (in″trah-kor-pus′ku-lar)　occurring within corpuscles.

intracostal (in″trah-kos′tal)　on the inner surface of the rib.

intracranial (in″trah-kra′ne-al)　situated within the cranium.

intracrureus (in″trah-kroo-re′us)　the internal part of the musculus vastus intermedius.

intractable (in-trak′tah-b'l)　resistant to cure, relief, or control.

intracutaneous (in″trah-ku-ta′ne-us)　within the skin.

intracystic (in″trah-sis′tik)　within a cyst.

intracytoplasmic (in″trah-si′to-plaz′mik)　within the cytoplasm of a cell.

intrad (in′trad) [*intra-* + *-ad*]　(obs.) within; inward in situation or direction.

intradermal (in″trah-der′mal)　within the dermis.

intradermoreaction (in″trah-der″mo-re-ak′shun)　intradermal reaction.

intraductal (in″trah-duk′tal)　situated or occurring within the duct of a gland.

intraduodenal (in″trah-du″o-de′nal)　within the duodenum.

intradural (in″trah-du′ral)　within or beneath the dura.

intraepidermal (in″trah-ep″ĭ-der′mal)　within the epidermis.

intraepiphyseal (in″trah-ep″ĭ-fiz′e-al)　within an epiphysis.

intraepithelial (in″trah-ep″ĭ-the′le-al)　situated among the cells of the epithelium.

intraerythrocytic (in″trah-ĕ-rith″ro-sit′ik)　located or occurring within the erythrocyte.

intrafascicular (in″trah-fah-sik′u-lar)　within a fascicle.

intrafat (in″trah-fat′)　situated in or introduced into fatty tissue, as the subcutaneous tissue.

intrafetation (in″trah-fe-ta′shun)　the development of a fetus within another fetus.

intrafilar (in″trah-fi′lar) [*intra-* + L. *filum* thread]　situated within a reticulum.

intrafissural (in″trah-fish′u-ral)　within a cerebral fissure.

intrafistular (in″trah-fis′tu-lar)　within a fistula.

intrafollicular (in″trah-fo-lik′u-lar)　within a follicle.

intrafusal (in″trah-fu′zal) [*intra-* + L. *fusus* spindle]　pertaining to the striated fibers within a muscle spindle.

intragalvanization (in″trah-gal″van-i-za′shun)　the galvanization of the inner surface of any organ.

intragastric (in″trah-gas′trik)　situated or occurring within the stomach.

intragemmal (in″trah-jem′al) [*intra-* + L. *gemma* bud]　situated within a bud, as a taste bud.

intragenic (in″trah-jen′ik)　within a gene.

intraglandular (in″trah-glan′du-lar)　within a gland.

intraglobular (in″trah-glob′u-lar)　within a globe or globule, as within an erythrocyte.

intragyral (in″trah-ji′ral)　within a cerebral gyrus.

intrahepatic (in″trah-hĕ-pat′ik)　within the liver.

intrahyoid (in″trah-hi′oid)　within the hyoid bone.

intraictal (in″trah-ik′tal)　occurring during an attack or seizure.

intraintestinal (in″trah-in-tes′tĭ-nal)　within the intestine.

intrajugular (in″trah-jug′u-lar)　within the jugular foramen, process, or vein.

intralamellar (in″trah-lah-mel′ar)　within lamellae.

intralaryngeal (in″trah-lah-rin′je-al)　within the larynx.

intralesional (in″trah-le′zhun-al)　occurring in or introduced directly into a localized lesion.

intraleukocytic (in″trah-lu″ko-si′tik)　within a leukocyte.

intraligamentous (in″trah-lig″ah-men′tus)　within a ligament.

intralingual (in″trah-ling′gwal)　within the tongue.

Intralipid (in″trah-lip′id)　trademark for an intravenous fat emulsion containing 10 per cent soybean oil stablized with egg-yolk phospholipids; used to prevent or correct deficiency of essential fatty acids and to provide calories in high density form during total parenteral nutrition.

intralobar (in″trah-lo′bar)　within a lobe.

intralobular (in″trah-lob′u-lar)　within a lobule.

intralocular (in″trah-lok′u-lar)　within the loculi of a structure.

intraluminal (in″trah-lu′mĭ-nal)　within the lumen of a tube, as of a blood vessel.

intramammary (in″trah-mam′ah-re)　within the breast.

intramarginal (in″trah-mar′jĭ-nal)　within a margin.

intramastoiditis (in″trah-mas″toi-di′tis)　inflammation of the mastoid antrum and cells of the mastoid process.

intramatrical (in″trah-mat′re-kal)　within a matrix.

intramedullary (in″trah-med′u-lār″e)　1. within the spinal cord.　2. within the medulla oblongata.　3. within the marrow cavity of a bone.

intramembranous (in″trah-mem′brah-nus)　within a membrane.

intrameningeal (in″trah-mĕ-nin′je-al)　within the meninges.

intramolecular (in″trah-mo-lek′u-lar)　within the molecule.

intramural (in″trah-mu′ral) [*intra-* + L. *murus* wall]　within the wall of an organ.

intramuscular (in″trah-mus′ku-lar) [*intra-* + L. *musculus* muscle]　within the substance of a muscle.

intramyocardial (in″trah-mi′o-kar′de-al)　within the myocardium.

intranarial (in″trah-na′re-al)　within the nares.

intranasal (in″trah-na′zal) [*intra-* + L. *nasus* nose]　within the nose.

intranatal (in″trah-na′tal)　occurring during birth.

intraneural (in″trah-nu′ral)　within or into a nerve.

intranuclear (in″trah-nu′kle-ar)　within a nucleus, as a cell nucleus.

intraocular (in″trah-ok′u-lar) [*intra-* + L. *oculus* eye]　within the eye.

intraoperative (in″trah-op′er-a″tiv)　occurring during the course of a surgical operation.

intraoral (in″trah-o′ral)　within the mouth.

intraorbital (in″trah-or′bĭ-tal) [*intra-* + L. *orbita* orbit]　within the orbit.

intraosseous (in″trah-os′e-us)　within a bone.

intraosteal (in″trah-os′te-al)　intraosseous.

intraovarian (in″trah-o-va′re-an)　within the ovary.

intraovular (in″trah-o′vu-lar)　within an ovum.

intraparenchymatous (in″trah-par″en-kim′ah-tus)　within the parenchyma of an organ.

intraparietal (in″trah-pah-ri′ĕ-tal) [*intra-* + L. *paries* wall]　1. intramural.　2. situated in the parietal region of the brain.

intrapartum (in″trah-par′tum)　occurring during childbirth, or during delivery.

intrapelvic (in″trah-pel′vik)　within the pelvis.

intrapericardial (in″trah-per″ĭ-kar′de-al) within the pericardium.

intraperineal (in″trah-per″ĭ-ne′al) within the tissues of the perineum.

intraperitoneal (in″trah-per″ĭ-to-ne′al) within the peritoneal cavity.

intrapial (in″trah-pe′al) within or beneath the pia mater.

intraplacental (in″trah-plah-sen′tal) within the placenta.

intrapleural (in″trah-ploor′al) within the pleura.

intrapontine (in″trah-pon′tīn) [*intra-* + L. *pons*] within the substance of the pons.

intraprostatic (in″trah-pros-tat′ik) within the prostate gland.

intraprotoplasmic (in″trah-pro″to-plaz′mik) within the protoplasm.

intrapsychic (in-trah-si′kik) occurring inside the mind; taking place within the mind.

intrapsychical (in″trah-si′ke-kal) intrapsychic.

intrapulmonary (in″trah-pul′mo-ner″e) situated in the substance of the lung.

intrapyretic (in″trah-pi-ret′ik) [*intra-* + Gr. *pyretos* fever] during the stage of fever.

intrarachidian (in″trah-rah-kid′e-an) intraspinal.

intrarectal (in″trah-rek′tal) within the rectum.

intrarenal (in″trah-re′nal) within the kidney.

intraretinal (in″trah-ret′ĭ-nal) within the retina.

intrascleral (in″trah-skle′ral) within the sclera.

intrascrotal (in″trah-skro′tal) within the scrotum.

intrasellar (in″trah-sel′ar) within the sella turcica.

intraserous (in″trah-se′rus) within the blood serum.

intraspinal (in″trah-spi′nal) situated or occurring within the vertebral column.

intrasplenic (in″trah-sple′nik) within the spleen.

intrasternal (in″trah-ster′nal) within the sternum.

intrastitial (in″trah-stish′al) within the cells or fibers of a tissue.

intrastromal (in″trah-stro′mal) within the stroma of an organ.

intrasynovial (in″trah-sĭ-no′ve-al) within the synovial cavity of a joint.

intratarsal (in″trah-tar′sal) within or on the inner side of the tarsus.

intratesticular (in″trah-tes-tik′u-lar) within the testis.

intrathecal (in″trah-the′kal) within a sheath; see also under *injection*.

intrathenar (in″trah-the′nar) situated between the thenar and hypothenar eminences.

intrathoracic (in″trah-tho-ras′ik) endothoracic.

intratonsillar (in″trah-ton′sĭ-lar) within a tonsil.

intratrabecular (in″trah-trah-bek′u-lar) within a trabecula.

intratracheal (in″trah-tra′ke-al) endotracheal.

intratubal (in″trah-tu′bal) situated or occurring within a tube, especially within a uterine tube.

intratubular (in″trah-tu′bu-lar) within the tubules of an organ.

intratympanic (in″trah-tim-pan′ik) within the tympanic cavity.

intraureteral (in″trah-u-re′ter-al) within the ureter.

intraurethral (in″trah-u-re′thral) within the urethra.

intrauterine (in″trah-u′ter-in) within the uterus.

intravaginal (in″trah-vaj′ĭ-nal) within the vagina.

intravasation (in-trav″ah-za′shun) the entrance of foreign material into a blood vessel.

intravascular (in″trah-vas′ku-lar) [*intra-* + L. *vasculum* vessel] within a vessel or vessels.

intravenation (in″trah-ve-na′shun) the entrance or injection of foreign matter into a vein.

intravenous (in″trah-ve′nus) within a vein or veins.

intraventricular (in″trah-ven-trik′u-lar) within a ventricle.

intraversion (in″trah-ver′zhun) (*obs.*) unusual narrowness of the dental arch.

intravertebral (in″trah-ver′te-bral) intraspinal.

intravesical (in″trah-ves′e-kal) [*intra-* + L. *vesica* bladder] situated within the bladder.

intravillous (in″trah-vil′us) situated within a villus.

intravital (in″trah-vi′tal) occurring during life.

intra vitam (in′trah vi′tam) [L.] during life.

intravitelline (in″trah-vi-tel′in) within the vitellus or yolk.

intravitreous (in″trah-vit′re-us) into or within the vitreous.

intrazole (in′trah-zōl) chemical name: 1-(4 chlorobenzoyl)-3-(1*H*-tetrazol-5-yimethyl)-1*H*-indole; an anti-inflammatory, C₁₇-H₁₂ClN₅O.

intrinsic (in-trin′sik) [L. *intrinsecus* situated on the inside] situated entirely within or pertaining exclusively to a part.

intriptyline hydrochloride (in-trip′tĭ-lēn) chemical name: 4-(5*H*-dibenzo[*a,d*]cyclohepten-5-ylidene)-*N,N*-dimethyl-2-butynylamine hydrochloride; an antidepressant, C₂₁H₁₉N·HCl.

intro- (in′tro) [L. *intro* within] a prefix meaning into or within.

introducer (in″tro-du′ser) an intubator.

introfier (in′tro-fi″er) a liquid which has the property of lowering the interfacial tension of emulsions.

introflexion (in″tro-flek′shun) a bending inward.

introgastric (in″tro-gas′trik) [*intro-* + Gr. *gastēr* stomach] conveyed or leading into the stomach.

introitus (in-tro′ĭ-tus), pl. *intro′itus* [L., from *intro* within + *ire* to go] [NA] a general term for the entrance to a cavity or space. **i. oesoph′agi,** the entrance into the esophagus. **i. pel′vis,** apertura pelvis superior. **i. vagi′nae,** ostium vaginae.

introjection (in″tro-jek′shun) [*intro-* + L. *jacere* to throw] a mental operation by which a person appropriates an occurrence or characteristic and makes it a part of himself, or turns against himself the hostility felt toward another.

intromission (in″tro-mish′un) [*intro-* + L. *mittere* to send] the insertion of one part or instrument into another.

Intropin (in′tro-pin) trademark for a preparation of dopamine hydrochloride.

introrsus (in-tror′sus) [L.] turned in.

introspection (in″tro-spek′shun) [*intro-* + L. *spicere* to look] the contemplation or observation of one's own thoughts and feelings; self-analysis.

introsusception (in″tro-sus-sep′shun) [*intro-* + L. *suscipere* to receive] intussusception.

introversion (in″tro-ver′shun) [*intro-* + L. *versio* a turning] 1. the turning outside in, more or less completely, of an organ. 2. a turning inward of the libido, so that interest does not move toward an object, but turns inward to the self.

introvert (in′tro-vert) 1. a person whose libido is turned inward upon himself. 2. to turn one's interest toward one's self.

intubate (in′tu-bāt) to treat by intubation.

intubation (in″tu-ba′shun) [L. *in* into + *tuba* tube] the insertion of a tube into a body canal or hollow organ, as into the trachea or stomach. **endotracheal i.,** insertion of a tube into the trachea for administration of anesthesia, maintenance of an airway, aspiration of secretions, ventilation of the lungs, or prevention of entrance of foreign material into the tracheobronchial tree. **nasal i.,** insertion of a tube into the respiratory or gastrointestinal tract through the nose. **nasotracheal i.,** insertion of a tube through the nose into the trachea to serve as an airway. **oral i.,** insertion of a tube into the respiratory or gastrointestinal tract through the mouth. **orotracheal i.,** insertion of a tube through the mouth into the trachea to serve as an airway.

intubationist (in-tu-ba′shun-ist) one who performs an intubation.

intubator (in′tu-ba-tor) an instrument used in intubation.

intumesce (in-tu-mes′) to swell up.

intumescence (in-tu-mes′ens) [L. *intumescentia*] 1. a swelling, normal or abnormal. 2. the process of swelling.

intumescent (in-tu-mes′ent) [L. *intumescens*] swelling or becoming swollen.

intumescentia (in-tu-mĕ-sen′she-ah), pl. *intumescen′tiae* [L.] [NA] a general term for an enlargement or swelling. **i. cervica′lis** [NA], the enlargement of the cervical spinal cord, at the level of attachment of the nerves to the upper limbs. **i. lumba′lis** [NA], the enlargement of the lumbar spinal cord, at the level of attachment of the nerves to the lower limbs. **i. tympan′ica,** an enlargement on the tympanic branch of the glossopharyngeal nerve.

intussusception (in″tus-sus-sep′shun) [L. *intus* within + *suscipere* to receive] a receiving within; specifically: (1) the prolapse of one part of the intestine into the lumen of an immediately adjoining part (Treves, 1899). There are four varieties: *colic,* involving segments of the large intestine; *enteric,* involving only the small intestine; *ileocecal,* in which the ileocecal valve prolapses into the cecum, drawing the ileum along with it; and *ileocolic,* in which the ileum prolapses through the ileocecal valve

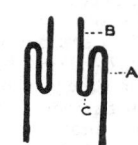

Schema for an intussusception: *A,* intussuscipiens; *B,* entering layer, *C,* intussusceptum (Stevens).

into the colon. (2) In physiology, the reception into an organism of matter, such as food, and its transformation into new protoplasm. **agonic i., postmortem i.,** intussusception occurring in the death agony. **retrograde i.,** the invagination of a distal part of the bowel into a proximal part.

intussusceptum (in″tus-sus-sep′tum) [L.] the portion of intestine that has been invaginated within another part in intussusception.

intussuscipiens (in″tus-sus-sip′e-ens) [L.] the portion of intestine into which another portion has invaginated in intussusception.

Inula (in′u-lah) [L.] a genus of composite flowers. *I. helenium* L. yields alantic acid. Its rhizome contains inulin. The root has numerous uses in folk medicine.

inulase (in′u-lās) β-2,1-fructan fructanohydrolase, an enzyme occurring in *Aspergillus niger, Pencillium glaucum, Saccharomyces fragilis,* and other fungi, and in higher plants, which changes inulin into fructose with one D-glucose molecule per molecule of inulin.

inulin (in′u-lin) a vegetable starch, $(C_6H_{10}O_5)_4$, an indigestible polysaccharide occurring in the rhizome of certain plants (Compositae). It is a polymer of fructofuranose, yields fructose on hydrolysis, and is used in a test for determining renal function.

inulinase (in′u-lin-ās) inulase.

inuloid (in′u-loid) a colorless compound, $C_6H_{10}O_5$, resembling inulin, but more soluble.

inunction (in-ungk′shun) [L. *in* into + *unguere* to anoint] 1. the act of anointing or of applying an ointment with friction. 2. an ointment made with lanolin as a menstruum.

inunctum (in-ungk′tum) inunction, def. 2. **i. men′tholis compos′itum,** compound menthol ointment.

in utero (in u′ter-o) [L.] within the uterus.

InV [abbreviation of a patient's name] an allotypic antigenic site on the constant region of κ chains of human immunoglobulins; three allotypes are known.

invaccination (in-vak″sĭ-na′shun) inadvertent inoculation during vaccination with organisms other than those prepared for the vaccine.

in vacuo (in vak′u-o) [L.] in a vacuum.

invaginate (in-vaj′ĭ-nāt) to infold one portion of a structure within another portion.

invagination (in-vaj″ĭ-na′shun) [L. *invaginatio,* from *in* within + *vagina* sheath] 1. the state of being or the process of becoming invaginated. 2. in embryology, a process by which (*a*) one region of a hollow, single-walled, spherical blastula caves in to form and line a new cavity in the now cup-shaped, double-walled gastrula, or (*b*) an ever-deepening pit develops into a diverticulum or tube from the surface into the tissues below. 3. intussusception. **basilar i.,** basilar impression.

invalid (in′vah-lid) [L. *invalidus; in* not + *validus* strong] 1. not well and strong. 2. a person who is disabled by illness or infirmity.

invasin (in-va′zin) hyaluronidase.

invasion (in-va′zhun) [L. *invasio; in* into + *vadere* to go] 1. the attack or onset of a disease. 2. the simple harmless entrance of bacteria into the body or their deposition in the tissues, as distinguished from infection. 3. the infiltration and active destruction of surrounding tissue, a characteristic of malignant tumors.

invasive (in-va′siv) 1. having the quality of invasiveness. 2. involving puncture or incision of the skin or insertion of an instrument or foreign material into the body; said of diagnostic techniques.

invasiveness (in-va′siv-nes) 1. the ability of a microorganism to enter the body and to spread more or less widely throughout the tissues; the organism may or may not cause an infection or a disease. See *hyaluronidase.* 2. the ability to infiltrate and actively destroy surrounding tissue; said of malignant tumors.

invermination (in-ver″mĭ-na′shun) infestation of the body by vermin.

Inversine (in-ver′sēn) trademark for a preparation of mecamylamine hydrochloride.

inversion (in-ver′zhun) [L. *inversio; in* into + *vertere* to turn] a turning inward, inside out, upside down, or other reversal of the normal relation of a part. In psychiatry, the condition of being a sexual invert; homosexuality. In genetics, a chromosomal aberration caused by the inverted reunion of the middle segment after breakage of a chromosome at two points, resulting in a change in sequence of genes or nucleotides; e.g., the sequence *abcdefg* may be inverted to *abfedcg.* **carbohydrate i.,** hydrolysis of disaccharides or polysaccharides to monosaccharides. **chromosome i.,** see under *aberration.* **sexual i.,** homosexuality. **thermic i.,** the state in which the body temperature is highest in the morning. **i. of uterus,** a turning of the uterus inside out, whereby the fundus is forced through the cervix and protrudes into or outside of the vagina. **visceral i.,** the more or less complete right and left transposition of the viscera; see *situs inversus viscerum.*

inversus (in-ver′sus) [L.; *in* into + *vertere* to turn] opposite to, or inverted from, the normal; see *situs inversus viscerum.*

invert (in′vert) a person whose sexual interests and impulses are directed toward a person of the same sex; a homosexual.

invertase (in-ver′tās) β-fructofuranosidase.

Invertebrata (in-ver″tĕ-bra′tah) a former division of the animal kingdom, including all forms that have no spinal column.

invertebrate (in-ver′tĕ-brāt) 1. any animal that has no spinal column; a nonvertebrate animal. 2. having no spinal column.

invertin (in-ver′tin) β-fructofuranosidase.

invertor (in-ver′tor) a muscle that turns a part inward.

invertose (in′ver-tōs) invert sugar, a levorotatory mixture of glucose and fructose obtained by the hydrolysis of dextrorotary sucrose.

invest (in′vest) to surround, envelop, or embed in an investment material.

investing (in-vest′ing) the process of entirely or partly covering or enveloping an object, such as a denture, tooth, wax form, crown, etc., with a refractory investment material before curing, soldering, or casting. **vacuum i.,** making a mold around a pattern in a vacuum, done to avoid trapping air in the investing material; the investing of a pattern within a vacuum.

investment (in-vest′ment) the material in which a denture, tooth, crown, or pattern for a dental restoration is enclosed before curing, soldering, or casting, or the process of enclosing it in such material.

inveterate (in-vet′er-āt) [L. *inveteratus; in* intensive + *vetus* old] chronic and confirmed; long established and of difficult cure.

inviscation (in″vis-ka′shun) [L. *in* among + *viscum* slime] the mixing of the food with the mucous secretion of the mouth in mastication.

in vitro (in ve′tro) [L.] within a glass; observable in a test tube; in an artificial environment.

in vivo (in ve′vo) [L.] within the living body.

involucre (in′vo-lu″ker) an involucrum.

involucrum (in″vo-lu′krum), pl. *involu′cra* [L.; *in* in + *volvere* to wrap] a covering or sheath, such as contains the sequestrum of a necrosed bone.

involuntary (in-vol′un-ter″e) [L. *involuntarius; in* against + *voluntas* will] performed independently of the will; contravolitional.

involuntomotory (in-vol″un-to-mo′tor-e) pertaining to motion that is not voluntary.

involute (in′vo-lūt) [L. *in* into + *volvere* to roll] 1. to return to normal size after enlargement. 2. to regress; to change to an earlier or to a more primitive condition. See *involution.*

involution (in″vo-lu′shun) [L. *involutio; in* into + *volvere* to roll] 1. a rolling or turning inward. 2. one of the movements involved in the gastrulation of many animals. 3. a retrograde change of the entire body or in a particular organ, as the retrograde changes in the female genital organs that result in normal size after delivery. 4. the progressive degeneration occurring naturally with advancing age, resulting in shriveling of organs or tissues. **senile i.,** the progressive degeneration that occurs naturally with advancing age, resulting in the shriveling of organs or tissues.

involutional (in″vo-lu′shun-al) pertaining to, due to, or occurring in involution.

Io chemical symbol for *ionium.*

iocarmate meglumine (i″o-kar′māt) chemical name: 3,3′-[(1,6-dioxo-1,6-hexanediyl)diimino]bis[2,4,6-triiodo-5-[(methylamino)carbonyl]benzoic acid compound with 1-deoxy-1-(methylamino)-D-glucitol (1:2). The meglumine salt of iocarmic acid, $C_{24}H_{20}I_6N_4O_8 \cdot 2C_7H_{17}NO_5$, used as a radiopaque medium in lumbosacral radiculography, cerebral ventriculography, and knee arthrography.

iodamide (i-o′dah-mīd) chemical name: 3-(acetylamino)-5-[(acetylamino)methyl]-2,4,6-triiodobenzoic acid; a diagnostic radiopaque medium, $C_{12}H_{11}I_3N_2O_4$.

Iodamoeba (i″o-dah-me′bah) a genus of amebas of the order Amoebida, class Rhizopoda, having a large vesicular nucleus that contains a large endosome surrounded by globular granules; found in the intestine of man and other mammals. The cysts, which are usually uninucleate, contain a conspicuous glycogen vacuole. **I. bütsch′lii.** a species of nonpathogenic amebas found in the human intestinal tract; the cysts (formerly called iodine cysts) usually contain a large glycogen mass which stains intensely with iodine. Called also *I. williamsi.* **I. su′is,** a species morphologically indistinguishable from *I. bütschlii,* but found in pigs. **I. wil′liamsi,** *I. bütschlii.*

iodate (i′o-dāt) any salt of iodic acid.

iod-Basedow (i-ōd-bas′ĕ-dow) jodbasedow.

iodemia (i″o-de′me-ah) [*iodine* + Gr. *haima* blood + *-ia*] the presence of iodides in the blood.

iodide (i′o-dīd) any binary compound of iodine: a compound of iodine with an element or radical. Iodide inhibits the release of thyroid hormone from the thyroid gland. **ferrous i.,** reddish to grayish-black masses, FeI_2, formerly used in chronic tuberculosis and now used as a catalyst; called also *iron iodide.*

iodimetry (i″o-dim′ĕ-tre) [*iodine* + Gr. *metron* measure] 1. the estimation of the quantity of iodine in a mixture or compound. 2. in quantitative analysis, the procedure used to determine an oxidizing agent consisting of the quantitative oxidation of potassium iodide to free iodine, and then titration with sodium thiosulfate.

iodinate (i-o′dĭ-nāt) to combine or compound with iodine.

iodination (i″o-din-a′shun) the incorporation or addition of iodine in a compound.

iodine (i′o-din) [Gr. *ioeides* violet-like, from the color of its vapor] 1. a halogen element of a peculiar odor and acrid taste; symbol, I; atomic number, 53; atomic weight, 126.904. It is a nonmetallic element, occurring in heavy, grayish black plates or granules. Iodine is essential in nutrition, being especially necessary for the synthesis of thyroid hormones (thyroxine and triiodothyronine), which regulate the metabolic rate in all cells. 2. [USP] a preparation of iodine used as a topical anti-infective (see also under *solution*). Iodine, usually in the form of iodides, is used in the treatment of hyperthyroidism. **butanol-extractable i.,** iodine that can be separated from the plasma proteins by extraction with certain organic solvents, such as butanol; it serves as a measure of thyroid hormone levels in the blood. Abbreviated BEI. **imidecyl i.,** a topical anti-infective compound, consisting of a mixture of 2-alkyl-(C_7H_{15} to $C_{17}H_{35}$)-1-(carboxymethyl)-1-(2-hydroxyethyl)-2-imidazolinium chloride; 3,6,9,12,15,18,21,24,27,30,-33,36,39-tridecaoxadopentacontan-1-ol; and iodine. **povidone i.,** see *povidone-iodine*. **protein-bound i.,** iodine firmly bound to protein in the body serum, determination of which constitutes one test of thyroid function. **radioactive i.,** radioiodine.

iodinophil (i″o-din′o-fil) [*iodine* + Gr. *philein* to love] 1. any cell or other element readily stainable with iodine. 2. iodinophilous.

iodinophilous (i″o-din-of′ĭ-lus) readily stainable with iodine.

iodipamide (i″o-dip′ah-mīd) [USP] chemical name: 3,3′-[(1,6-dioxo-1,6-hexanediyl)diimino]bis[2,4,6-triiodobenzoic acid]; a radiopaque medium, $C_{20}H_{14}I_6N_2O_6$, used as the meglumine and sodium salts. **i. meglumine, i. methylglucamine** [USP], the meglumine salt of iodipamide, $(C_7H_{17}NO_5)_2 \cdot C_{20}H_{14}I_4N_2O_6$; used as a radiopaque medium in cholangiography and cholecystography, administered intravenously. **i. sodium,** the sodium salt of iodipamide, $C_{20}H_{12}I_6N_2Na_2O_6$, used as a radiopaque medium in cholangiography and cholecystography, administered intravenously.

iodism (i′o-dizm) chronic poisoning by iodine or iodine compounds; it is marked by coryza, ptyalism, frontal headache, emaciation, weakness, and eruptions on the skin.

iodize (i′o-dīz) to impregnate with iodine or to put under its influence; to incorporate iodine or one of its compounds.

iodobrassid (i″o-do-bras′sid) chemical name: ethyl diiodobrassidate; used in iodide therapy and as a radiopaque medium.

iodochlorhydroxyquin (i-o″do-klōr″hi-drok′se-kwin) [USP] chemical name: 5-chloro-7-iodo-8-quinolinol. An antiamebic, antibacterial, and antifungal agent with antieczematic and antipruritic properties, C_9H_5ClINO, occurring as a voluminous, spongy, yellowish white to brownish yellow powder. It is used in the treatment of amebic dysentery, and as a local anti-infective in a wide range of dermatoses, including all types of eczema, and in vaginitis due to *Trichomonas vaginalis, Candida albicans, Trichophyton,* or mixed bacteria; administered orally, topically, or intravaginally. Called also *clinoquinol.*

iodocholesterol (i-o″do-ko-les′ter-ol) a radioisotope, ^{131}I-19-iodocholesterol, used in visualization of the adrenal glands by the photoscintillation scanner.

iododerma (i-o″do-der′mah) [*iodine* + Gr. *derma* skin] any skin eruption or lesion resulting from iodism.

iodoform (i-o′do-form) [*iodine* + *formyl*] chemical name: triiodomethane. A greenish yellow powder or crystals, CHI_3, having a strong, penetrating odor, containing about 96 per cent of iodine, and soluble in chloroform and ether and somewhat in alcohol and water: used as a topical anti-infective, applied to the skin.

iodoformism (i′o-do-form″izm) poisoning by iodoform.

iodoformum (i″o-do-for′mum) iodoform.

iodogenic (i″o-do-jen′ik) [*iodine* + Gr. *gennan* to produce] yielding or producing iodine.

iodoglobulin (i″o-do-glob′u-lin) an iodine-containing globulin (protein).

iodohippurate sodium (i-o″do-hip′u-rāt) chemical name: *o*-iodohippurate sodium. An iodine-containing compound, C_9H_7-$INNaO_3$, administered orally, intravenously, or by retrograde injection into the bladder as a radiopaque medium in pyelography. When labeled with radioactive iodine 131, it may be used as a diagnostic aid in determination of renal function.

iodolography (i″o-do-log′rah-fe) roentgenologic visualization of an organ or part after the injection into it of iodized oil.

iodomethamate sodium (i-o″do-meth′ah-māt) chemical name: 1,4-dihydro-3,5-diiodo-1-methyl-4-oxo-2,6-pyridinedicar-

boxylic acid disodium salt. A radiopaque medium, $C_8H_3I_2NNaO_5$, used in urography.

iodometric (i″o-do-met′rik) pertaining to iodometry.

iodometry (i″o-dom′ĕ-tre) [*iodine* + Gr. *metron* measure] estimation of the quantity of a chemical by titration with iodine.

iodophenol (i″o-do-fe′nol) 1. a mono-iodophenol, $OH \cdot C_6H_5I$. 2. a preparation of iodine, phenol, and glycerin: antiseptic.

iodophil (i′o-do-fil) iodinophil.

iodophilia (i″o-do-fil′e-ah) [*iodine* + Gr. *philein* to love + *-ia*] the reaction shown by leukocytes in certain conditions when treated with iodine or iodides. Normal leukocytes are colored bright yellow, but in certain pathologic conditions, as toxemia and severe anemia, the polymorphonuclears show diffuse brownish coloration. When the staining affects the leukocytes themselves, it is termed *intracellular;* when only the particles around the leukocytes are affected, it is *extracellular.*

iodophor (i-o′do-fōr) a compound consisting of iodine combined with a carrier, such as polyvinylpyrrolidone, used in veterinary medicine as a preoperative skin disinfectant.

iodophthalein sodium (i-o″do-thal′e-in) chemical name: disodium salt of tetraiodophenolphthalein; used as a radiopaque medium in cholecystography.

iodopsin (i″o-dop′sin) [Gr. *iōdes* violet colored + *opsis* vision] a photosensitive violet retinal pigment found in the retinal cones of some animals and important for color vision; called also *visual violet.*

iodopyracet (i-o″do-pi′rah-set) chemical name: 3,5-diiodo-4-oxo-1(4*H*)-pyridineacetic acid compound with 2,2′-iminodiethanol (1:1). A radiopaque medium, $C_{11}H_{16}I_2N_2O_5$, used especially in urography; administered intravenously or intramuscularly.

iodoquinol (i-o″do-kwin′ol) [USP] chemical name: 5,7-diiodo-8-quinolinol. An amebicide, $C_{15}H_{13}I_2NO_4$, occurring as a light yellowish to tan, microcrystalline powder; used in the treatment of intestinal amebiasis, administered orally, and in *Trichomonas vaginalis* vaginitis, administered intravaginally. It has also been used topically in fungal and bacterial skin infections and in seborrheic dermatitis. Called also *diiodohydroxyquin.*

iodosulfate (i″o-do-sul′fāt) a combination of a base with iodine and sulfuric acid.

iodotherapy (i″o-do-ther′ah-pe) [*iodine* + Gr. *therapeia* treatment] treatment with iodine or the iodides.

iodothyroglobulin (i″o-do-thi″ro-glob′u-lin) thyroglobulin.

iodothyronine (i″o-do-thi″ro-nēn) a nonspecific term for iodinated thyronines, including the thyroid hormones triiodothyronine and tetraiodothyronine (thyroxine).

iodotyrosine (i″o-do-ti′ro-sēn) any iodinated derivative of tyrosine.

iodoventriculography (i″o-do-ven-trik″u-log′rah-fe) ventriculography with iodine contrast medium.

iodovolatilization (i″o-do-vol″ah-til-i-za′shun) the liberation of free iodine by living epidermal cells in the iodogenic layer of certain brown algae or kelp. It accumulates in the algae as potassium iodide and has been used as a commercial source of iodine.

iodum (i-o′dum), gen. *io′di* [L.] iodine.

ioduria (i″o-du′re-ah) the presence of iodides in the urine.

ion (i′on) [Gr. *iōn* going] an atom or radical having a charge of positive (cation) or negative (anion) electricity owing to the loss (positive) or gain (negative) of one or more electrons. Substances that form ions are called electrolytes. See *ionic theory,* under *theory.* **dipolar i.,** zwitterion. **gram i.,** the weight in grams of an ion numerically equal to the atomic or molecular weight of the ion. **hydrogen i.,** the nucleus of the hydrogen atom or a hydrogen atom that has lost its electron, H^+; it bears a positive charge equivalent to the negative charge of the electron and is called a proton. **hydronium i.,** the hydrated form, H_3O^+, in which the proton (hydrogen ion, H^+) exists in aqueous solution; a combination of H^+ and H_2O.

Ionamin (i-o′nah-min) trademark for a preparation of phentermine.

ionic (i-on′ik) pertaining to an ion or to ions.

ionium (i-o′ne-um) [*ion*] a radioactive isotope of thorium, of atomic weight 230.5; it emits both alpha and gamma rays.

ionization (i″on-i-za′shun) 1. the dissociation of a substance in solution into ions. 2. iontophoresis. **avalanche i.,** the multiplicative process in which a single charged particle, accelerated by a strong electric field, produces additional charged particles through collision with neutral gas molecules; called also *Townsend i.* **Townsend i.,** avalanche i.

ionize (i′on-īz) to separate into ions.

ionocolorimeter (i″o-no-kol″or-im′ĕ-ter) an apparatus for measuring the ionic acidity of a solution.

ionogen (i-on′o-jen) [*ion* + Gr. *gennan* to form] a substance that can be ionized.

ionogenic (i-on″o-jen′ik) forming or supplying ions.

ionometer (i″o-nom′ĕ-ter) an instrument for the measurement of the intensity or quantity of radiation from an ionizing radiation source.

ionometry (i″o-nom′ĕ-tre) roentgenometry.

ionone (i′on-ōn) [Gr. *ion* violet] an odoriferous derivative of orris root, $C_{13}H_{20}O$, prepared commercially from citral and used as a perfume.

ionophore (i′on-o-fōr″) any molecule, as of a drug, that increases the permeability of cell membranes to a specific ion.

ionophose (i′o-no-fōz) [Gr. *ion* violet + *phose*] a violet phose.

ionoscope (i-on′o-skōp) an instrument for detecting alkaline or acid impurity in nitrous oxide.

ionosphere (i-on′o-sfēr) the region of the atmosphere characterized by the formation of ions by the action of solar radiations upon the atmospheric constituents.

ionotherapy (i″o-no-ther′ah-pe) 1. [*ion* + *therapy*] iontophoresis. 2. [Gr. *ion* violet + *therapy*] treatment by means of ultraviolet rays.

ion-protein (i-on-pro′te-in) a protein molecule combined with an inorganic ion.

iontherapy (i″on-ther′ah-pe) iontophoresis.

iontophoresis (i-on″to-fo-re′sis) the introduction by means of the electric current, of ions of soluble salts into the tissues of the body, often for therapeutic purposes; a form of electro-osmosis. Called also *iontherapy*.

iontophoretic (i-on″to-fo-ret′ik) pertaining to iontophoresis.

iontoquantimeter (i-on″to-quan-tim′ĕ-ter) [*ion* + *quantimeter*] ionometer.

iontoradeometer (i-on″to-ra″de-om′ĕ-ter) ionometer.

IOP intraocular pressure.

iophendylate (i″o-fen′dĭ-lāt) [USP] chemical name: iodo-ι-methylbenzene decanoic acid. A radiopaque medium, $C_{19}H_{29}IO_2$, occurring as a colorless to pale yellow, viscous liquid; used in myelography, administered intrathecally or by special injection.

iopydol (i-o-pi′dōl) chemical name: 1-(2,3-dihydroxypropyl)-3,5-diiodo-4(1*H*)-pyridinone; a radiopaque medium for bronchography, $C_8H_9I_2NO_3$.

iopydone (i-o-pi′dōn) chemical name: 3,5-diiodo-4(1*H*)-pyridinone; a radiopaque medium for bronchography, $C_5H_3I_2NO$.

iosulamide meglumine (i″o-sul′ah-mīd) chemical name: 3,3′-[sulfonylbis[(1-oxo-3,1-propanediyl)imino]]bis[5-(acetylethyl-amino)-2,4,6-triiodobenzoic acid] compound with 1-deoxy-1-(methylamino)-D-glucitol(1:1); a radiopaque medium, $C_{28}H_{28}I_6N_4O_{10}$·$C_7H_{17}NO_5$.

iotacism (i-o′tah-sizm) [Gr. *iōta* letter I] excessive use of the sound of the Greek letter iota (English e, as in be) in speaking.

iothalamate (i-o-thal′ah-māt) any salt of iothalamic acid.
i. meglumine, a radiopaque medium, $C_{18}H_{26}I_3N_2O_9$, available in solution, consisting of iothalamic acid in water for injection, prepared with the aid of meglumine; used intra-arterially in cerebral angiography and peripheral arteriography and intravenously in excretory urography and peripheral pyelography. **i. sodium,** a radiopaque medium, $(C_{11}H_8I_3N_2NaO_4)$, available in solution, consisting of iothalamic acid in water for injection, prepared with the aid of sodium hydroxide; used intra-arterially or intravenously in angiocardiography and aortography.

iothiouracil (i″o-thi″o-u′rah-sil) chemical name: 5-iodo-2-thiouracil; a thyroid inhibitor.

I.P. intraperitoneally; isoelectric point.

I.P.A.A. International Psychoanalytical Association.

I-para primipara.

ipecac (ip′ĕ-kak) [USP] the dried rhizome and roots of *Cephaelis ipecacuanha* (Brotero) Rich. (Rubiaceae) (Rio or Brazilian i.) or of *C. acuminata* Karsten (Cartagena, Nicaragua, or Panama i.). Originally introduced as a remedy for dysentery, it has been replaced by its alkaloid emetine for that purpose, and is now used in syrup as an emetic, particularly in cases of poisoning. It also has expectorant properties. **powdered i.** [USP] ipecac reduced to a very fine powder; used in the preparation of ipecac syrup.

ipodate (i′po-dāt) 3-[[(dimethylamino)methylene]amino]-2,4,-6-triiodobenzenepropanoic acid, $C_{12}H_{13}I_3N_2O_2$. **i. calcium** [USP], the calcium salt of ipodate, $C_{24}H_{24}CaI_6N_4O_4$, occurring as a white to off-white, fine, crystalline powder; used as a radiopaque medium in cholecystography, administered orally. **i. sodium** [USP], the sodium salt of ipodate, $C_{12}H_{12}I_3N_2O_2$, occurring as a white to off-white fine, crystalline powder; used as a radiopaque medium in cholecystography, administered orally.

ipomea (i″po-me′ah) the dried root of *Ipomoea orizabensis*, used as a cathartic; called also *Mexican scammony* and *orizaba jalap root*.

Ipomoea (i″po-me′ah) a genus of herbs and shrubs of the family Convolvulaceae, comprising some 300 species. Some species, e.g., *I. orizabensis* Ledenois, contain cathartic resins; others, e.g., *I. violacea* L., possess psychotomimetic indole alkaloids, such as lysergic acid amide.

IPPB intermittent positive pressure breathing; see under *breathing*.

Ipral (ip′ral) trademark for preparations of probarbital.

ipratropium bromide (ĭ-prah-tro′pe-um) chemical name: (+)-(*endo,syn*)-3-(3-hydroxy-1-oxo-2-phenylpropoxy)-8-methyl-8-(1-methylethyl)-8-azoniabicyclo[3,2,1]octane bromide; a bronchodilator, $C_{20}H_{30}BrNO_3$.

iprindole (ĭ-prin′dōl) chemical name: 6,7,8,9,10,11-hexahydro-*N,N*-dimethyl-5*H*-cyloöct[*b*]indole-5-propanamine; an antidepressant, $C_{19}H_{28}N_2$.

iproniazid (i″pro-ni′ah-zid) chemical name: 4-pyridinecarboxylic acid 2-(1-methylethyl)hydrazine; a monoamine oxidase inhibitor, antidepressant, and antitubercular, $C_9H_{13}N_3O$.

ipronidazole (i-pro-nīd′ah-zōl) chemical name: 1-methyl-2-(1-methylethyl)-5-nitro-1*H*-imidazole; an antiprotozoal, $C_7H_{11}N_3O_2$, effective against *Histomonas*.

iproxamine hydrochloride (ĭ-proks′ah-mēn) chemical name: 4-[2-(dimethylamino)ethoxy]-2-methyl-5-(1-methylethyl)-phenyl 1-methylethyl ester hydrochloride; a vasodilator, $C_{18}H_{29}NO_4$·HCl.

ipsation (ip-sa′shun) [L. *ipse* himself] masturbation.

ipsi- [L. *ipse* self] a combining form meaning the same.

ipsilateral (ip″sĭ-lat′er-al) [L. *ipse* self + *latus* side] situated on, pertaining to, or affecting the same side, as opposed to contralateral.

ipsism (ip′sizm) masturbation.

IPSP inhibitory postsynaptic potential.

I.Q. intelligence quotient; see under *quotient*.

Ir chemical symbol for *iridium*.

irascibility (ĭ-ras″ĭ-bil′ĭ-te) [L. *irascibilis* ill tempered] morbid irritability and quickness of temper.

IRC inspiratory reserve capacity.

Ircon (ir′kon) trademark for a preparation of ferrous fumarate.

irid- see *irido-*.

iridal (i′rĭ-dal) iridic.

iridalgia (i″rĭ-dal′je-ah) pain in the iris.

iridauxesis (ir″id-awk-se′sis) [*irid-* + Gr. *auxēsis* increase] thickening of the iris.

iridectasis (ir″ĭ-dek′tah-sis) [*irid-* + Gr. *iktasis* dilatation] dilatation of the iris, or pupil of the eye.

iridectome (ir″ĭ-dek′tōm) [*irid-* + Gr. *ektemnein* to cut out] a cutting instrument for use in iridectomy.

iridectomesodialysis (ir″ĭ-dek″to-me″so-di-al′ĭ-sis) [*irid-* + Gr. *ektomē* excision + *mesos* middle + *dialysis* loosening] excision and separation of adhesions around the inner edge of the iris.

iridectomize (ir″ĭ-dek′to-mīz) to remove part of the iris by excision.

iridectomy (ir″ĭ-dek′to-me) [*irid-* + Gr. *ektomē* excision] surgical excision of part of the iris; called also *corectomy*. **optic i., optical i.,** excision of part of the iris as a means of enlarging an abnormally small pupil and improving vision. **peripheral i.,** surgical excision of a peripheral portion of the iris. **preliminary i., preparatory i.,** iridectomy performed prior to removal of the lens in cataract surgery. **sector i.,** surgical excision of a portion of the iris extending from the pupil through the peripheral iris. **stenopeic i.,** excision of a small part of the iris, with preservation of the sphincter. **therapeutic i.,** iridectomy performed for the cure of disease of the eye.

iridectopia (ir″ĭ-dek-to′pe-ah) [*irid-* + Gr. *ektopos* displaced + *-ia*] displacement of the iris of the eye.

iridectropium (ir″ĭ-dek-tro′pe-um) ectropion uveae.

iridemia (ir″ĭ-de′me-ah) [*irid-* + Gr. *haima* blood + *-ia*] hemorrhage from the iris.

iridencleisis (ir″ĭ-den-kli′sis) [*irid-* + Gr. *enklein* to lock in] the surgical creation of a permanent drain by incarceration of a slip of the iris within a corneal or limbal incision to act as a wick through which the aqueous is filtered from the anterior chamber to the subconjunctival tissues; done to reduce intraocular pressure.

iridentropium (ir″ĭ-den-tro′pe-um) entropion uveae.

irideremia (ir″ĭ-der-e′me-ah) [*irid-* + Gr. *erēmia* want of, absence] congenital absence of the iris.

irides (ir′ĭ-dēz) [Gr.] plural of *iris*.

iridescence (ir″ĭ-des′ens) [L. *iridescere* to gleam like a rainbow] the condition of gleaming with bright and changing colors.

iridescent (ir″ĭ-des′ent) [L. *iridescens*] gleaming with bright colors like those of the rainbow.

iridesis (i-rid′ĕ-sis) [*iris* + Gr. *desis* a binding] the operation of repositioning the pupil by bringing a sector of the iris through a corneal or limbal incision and fixing the sector with a suture.

iridiagnosis (i″rĭ-di-ag-no′sis) iridodiagnosis.

iridial (i-rid′e-al) iridic.

iridian (i-rid′e-an) iridic.

iridic (i-rid′ik) pertaining to the iris.

iridium (ĭ-rid′e-um, i-rid′e-um) [L. *iris* rainbow, from the tints of its salts] a very hard white metal; symbol, Ir; atomic number, 77; atomic weight, 192.2.

iridization (ir″ĭ-di-za′shun) the subjective perception of iridescent halos about lights, occurring in glaucoma.

irido-, irid- [Gr. *iris, iridos* rainbow, colored circle] combining form denoting relationship to the iris of the eye, or to a colored circle.

iridoavulsion (ir″ĭ-do-ah-vul′shun) complete tearing away of the iris from its periphery.

iridocapsulitis (ir″ĭ-do-kap-su-li′tis) inflammation of the iris and the capsule of the lens.

iridocele (i-rid′o-sēl) [*irido-* + Gr. *kēlē* hernia] hernial protrusion of a part of the iris through the cornea.

iridochoroiditis (ir″ĭ-do-ko″roi-di′tis) inflammation of the iris and the choroid.

iridocoloboma (ir″ĭ-do-kol″o-bo′mah) [*irido-* + Gr. *kolobōma* mutilation] congenital fissure or coloboma of the iris.

iridoconstrictor (ir″ĭ-do-kon-strik′tor) a muscle element or an agent which acts to constrict the pupil of the eye.

iridocorneosclerectomy (ir″ĭ-do-kor″ne-o-skle-rek′to-me) surgical excision of a portion of the iris, cornea, and sclera for glaucoma.

iridocyclectomy (ir″ĭ-do-si-klek′to-me) [*irido-* + Gr. *kyklos* circle + *ektomē* excision] surgical removal of a portion of the iris and of the ciliary body.

iridocyclitis (ir″ĭ-do-si-kli′tis) [*irido-* + Gr. *kyklos* circle + *-itis*] inflammation of the iris and of the ciliary body; anterior uveitis. **heterochromic i.,** unilateral low-grade iridocyclitis, leading to depigmentation of the iris of the affected eye; called also *heterochromic uveitis.*

iridocyclochoroiditis (ir″ĭ-do-si″klo-ko″roi-di′tis) [*irido-* + Gr. *kyklos* circle + *choroiditis*] inflammation of the iris, ciliary body, and choroid coat.

iridocystectomy (ir″ĭ-do-sis-tek′to-me) an operation to establish an artificial pupil in an eye in which the iris adheres to the residual lens capsule, accomplished by excising a portion of the iris and lens capsule through a corneal incision.

iridocyte (i-rid′o-sīt) [*irido-* + *-cyte*] one of the cells in the scales of fishes that contains crystals of guanine capable of producing iridescence.

iridodesis (ir″ĭ-dod′ĕ-sis) iridesis.

iridodiagnosis (ir″ĭ-do-di″ag-no′sis) diagnosis of disease by the appearance of the iris, its color, markings, changes, etc.

iridodialysis (ir″ĭ-do-di-al′ĭ-sis) [*irido-* + Gr. *dialysis* loosening] 1. coredialysis. 2. the separation or loosening of the iris from its attachment. 3. division or splitting of the iris (traumatic, or surgical), producing more than one pupil.

iridodiastasis (ir″ĭdo-di-as′tah-sis) a defect of the peripheral border of the iris, but not affecting the pupillary margin, producing the clinical appearance of more than one pupil.

iridodilator (ir″ĭ-do-di-la′tor) 1. the dilator muscle of the pupil. 2. an agent which acts to dilate the pupil of the eye.

iridodonesis (ir″ĭ-do-do-ne′sis) [*irido-* + Gr. *donēsis* tremor] abnormal tremulousness of the iris on movements of the eye, occurring in subluxation of the lens, depriving the iris of this support.

iridokeratitis (ir″ĭ-do-ker″ah-ti′tis) [*irido-* + Gr. *keras* horn, cornea + *-itis*] inflammation of the iris and cornea.

iridokinesia (ir″ĭ-do-ki-ne′ze-ah) iridokinesis.

iridokinesis (ir″ĭ-do-ki-ne′sis) [*irido-* + Gr. *kinēsis* movement] the contraction and expansion of the iris.

iridokinetic (ir″ĭ-do-ki-net′ik) pertaining to iridokinesis.

iridoleptynsis (ir″ĭ-do-lep-tin′sis) [*iris* + Gr. *leptynsis* attenuation] thinning or atrophy of the iris.

iridology (ir″ĭ-dol′o-je) [*irido-* + *-logy*] the study of the iris, particularly of its color, markings, changes, etc., as associated with disease.

iridolysis (ir″ĭ-dol′ĭ-sis) [*irido-* + Gr. *lysis* a loosening] the surgical release of adhesions of the iris.

iridomalacia (ir″ĭ-do-mah-la′she-ah) [*irido-* + Gr. *malakia* softness] softening of the iris.

iridomesodialysis (ir″ĭ-do-me″so-di-al′ĭ-sis) [*irido-* + Gr. *mesos* middle + *dialysis* loosening] surgical loosening of adhesions around the inner edge of the iris.

iridomotor (ir″ĭ-do-mo′tor) pertaining to movements of the iris; affecting contraction or dilation of the pupil of the eye.

iridoncus (ir″ĭ-dong′kus) [*irid-* + Gr. *onkos* bulk] tumor or swelling of the iris.

iridoparalysis (ir″ĭ-do-pah-ral′ĭ-sis) iridoplegia.

iridopathy (ir″ĭ-dop′ah-the) [*irido-* + Gr. *pathos* disease] disease of the iris.

iridoperiphakitis (ir″ĭ-do-per″e-fa-ki′tis) [*irido-* + Gr. *peri* around + *phakos* lens] inflammation of the capsule of the crystalline lens.

iridoplegia (ir″ĭ-do-ple′je-ah) [*iris* + Gr. *plēgē* stroke + *-ia*] paralysis of the sphincter of the iris, with lack of contraction or dilation of the pupil. **accommodation i.,** failure of the pupil to contract when an accommodative effort is made. **complete**

i., paralysis of the sphincter of the pupil, with failure to react to any stimulus. **reflex i.,** failure of the pupil to contract under the influence of light or when skin is stimulated. **sympathetic i.,** failure of the pupil to dilate when the skin is stimulated.

iridoptosis (ir″ĭ-dop-to′sis) [*irido-* + Gr. *ptōsis* falling] prolapse of the iris.

iridopupillary (ir″ĭ-do-pu′pĭ-ler″e) pertaining to the iris and the pupil.

iridorhexis (ir″ĭ-do-rek′sis) [*irido-* + Gr. *rhēxis* rupture] 1. rupture of the iris. 2. the tearing away of the iris.

iridoschisis (ir″ĭ-dos′kĭ-sis) splitting of the mesodermal stroma of the iris into two layers so that the anterior section separates and disintegrates into fibrils, the unattached ends of which float freely in the anterior chamber.

iridosclerotomy (ir″ĭ-do-skle-rot′o-me) [*irido-* + *sclera* + Gr. *tomē* a cutting] incision of the sclera and of the edge of the iris in treatment of glaucoma.

iridosteresis (ir″ĭ-do-ste-re′sis) [*irido-* + Gr. *sterēsis* loss] the removal of part or all of the iris.

iridotasis (ir″ĭ-dot′ah-sis) [*irido-* + Gr. *tasis* stretching] the operation of stretching the iris in treatment of glaucoma.

iridotomy (ir″ĭ-dot′o-me) [*irido-* + Gr. *tomē* a cutting] incision of the iris, as in creating an artificial pupil.

iridovirus (ir″ĭ-do-vi′rus) any of a group of large, morphologically similar DNA viruses, which infect the larvae of various insects, giving an iridescent appearance to the infected insect; called also *iridescent virus.*

I.R.I.S. International Research Information Service.

Iris (i′ris) a genus of perennial iridaceous herbs. The roots of several species, *I. florentina* L., *I. germanica* L., and *I. pallida* L., are the source of orris. *I. versicolor* L. (blue flag), a plant indigenous to America, is the source of a substance formerly used as a purgative, emetic, and diuretic. Some species, e.g., *I. missouriensis* Nutt., have been reported to be poisonous to livestock due to an irritant principle in the leaves and rootstalks that causes gastroenteritis.

iris (i′ris), pl. *ir′ides* [Gr. "rainbow," "halo"] 1. [NA] the circular pigmented membrane behind the cornea, perforated by the pupil; the most anterior portion of the vascular tunic of the eye, it is made up of a flat bar of circular muscular fibers surrounding the pupil, a thin layer of smooth muscle fibers by which the pupil is dilated, thus regulating the amount of light entering the eye, and posteriorly two layers of pigmented epithelial cells. 2. the rhizome of *Iris versicolor,* formerly used as a purgative, emetic, and diuretic. **i. bombé,** a condition in which the iris is bowed forward by the collection of aqueous humor between the iris and lens

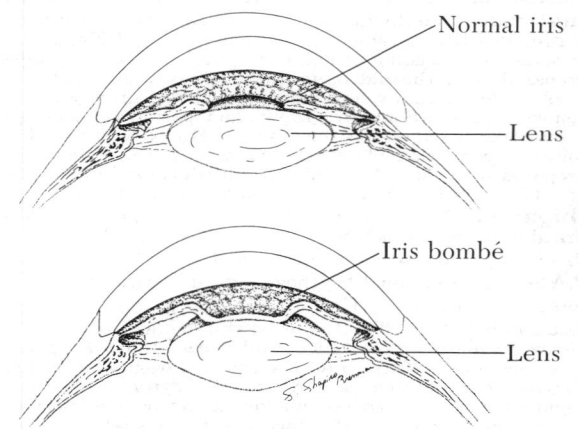

Normal iris contrasted with iris bombé.

in total posterior synechia. **Florentine i.,** 1. *Iris florentina* L. 2. orris. **tremulous i.,** one characterized by abnormal tremulousness; see *iridodonesis.* **umbrella i.,** i. bombé.

irisin (i′rĭ-sin) a fructose polysaccharide, $(C_6H_{10}O_5)_n$, from *Iris pseudo-acorus;* it is an aperient and cholagogue.

irisopsia (i″ris-op′se-ah) [Gr. *iris* rainbow + *opsis* vision] a visual defect in which objects appear surrounded by rings of colored light.

iritic (i-rit′ik) pertaining to or of the nature of iritis.

iritis (i-ri′tis) [*iris* + *-itis*] inflammation of the iris, usually marked by pain, congestion in the ciliary region, photophobia, contraction of the pupil, and discoloration of the iris. **i. catamenia′lis,** iritis recurring before each menstrual period. **diabetic i.,** iritis marked by the deposit of glycogen in diabetic patients. **follicular i.,** iritis marked by multiple small nodules the size of a pinhead. **gouty i.,** painful iritis occurring in gouty patients; uratic iritis. **i. papulo′sa,** iritis with papules in the iris; usually syphilitic. **plastic i.,** a variety in which the exudate consists of fibrinous matter which forms new tissue. **purulent i.**, iritis in which the exudate is purulent. **serous i.**, iritis in which the exudate consists of serum. **spongy i.**, iritis with a fibrinous exudate, forming a spongy mass in the anterior chamber. **sympathetic i.**, iritis occurring in sympathetic ophthalmoplegia. **uratic i.**, gouty i.

iritoectomy (i″rĭ-to-ek′to-me) [iris + Gr. ektomē excision] surgical excision of deposits of after-cataract on the iris, together with iridectomy, to form an artificial pupil.

iritomy (i-rit′o-me) iridotomy.

irium (ir′e-um) sodium lauryl sulfate.

iron (i′ern) [A. S. iren; L. ferrum] a metallic element found in certain minerals, in nearly all soils, and in mineral waters: atomic number 26; atomic weight, 55.847; specific gravity, 7.85–7.88; symbol, Fe. Iron is an essential constituent of hemoglobin, cytochrome, and other components of respiratory enzyme systems. Its chief functions are in the transport of oxygen to tissues (hemoglobin) and in cellular oxidation mechanisms. Depletion of iron stores may result in iron-deficiency anemia (see under *anemia*). Iron is used to build up the blood in anemia. The compounds of iron are astringent and styptic. **i. acetate,** a compound, $Fe(C_2H_3O_2)_3$, used as an astringent. **alcoholized i.,** pulverized i. **i. and ammonium citrate,** see *ferric ammonium citrate,* under *ammonium.* **i. and ammonium sulfate,** see *ferric* and *ferrous ammonium sulfates,* under *ammonium.* **i. and ammonium tartrate,** see *ferric ammonium tartrate,* under *ammonium.* **i. arsenate,** ferrous arsenate. **i. arsenite,** ferric arsenite. **available i.,** that portion of iron in the food which can be separated from the total iron content by digestive processes. **i. carbonate,** ferrous carbonate. **i. chloride,** either of the binary compounds $FeCl_2$ or $FeCl_3$. **i. choline citrate,** ferrocholinate. **i. citrate,** ferric citrate. **i. citrate green,** a complex ferric ammonium citrate used for intramuscular and subcutaneous injection. **dialyzed i.,** an aqueous solution of ferric oxychloride prepared by dialysis. **i. gluconate,** ferrous gluconate. **i. glycerophosphate,** ferric glycerophosphate. **i. hydroxide,** ferric hydroxide. **i. iodide,** ferrous iodide. **i. iodobehanate,** an amorphous, reddish brown powder, formerly used in scrofula, chlorosis, rickets, etc. **i. magnesium sulfate,** a greenish white powder, $FeSO_4 \cdot MgSO_4 + 7H_2O$, used in anemia. **i. protosulfate,** ferrous sulfate. **Quevenne's i.,** reduced iron. **radioactive i.,** radioiron. **reduced i.,** finely powdered metallic iron obtained by precipitation with hydrogen from a solution of any soluble salt of iron. **i. sorbitex,** a hematinic preparation consisting of a sterile colloidal solution of a complex of trivalent iron, sorbitol, and citric acid, stabilized with dextrin and sorbitol. **i. subcarbonate,** an amorphous, brownish powder, consisting mainly of iron hydroxide. **i. subsulfate,** ferric subsulfate. **i. succinate,** a green-gray substance said to be useful in cholelithiasis. **i. sulfate,** ferrous sulfate.

irotomy (i-rot′o-me) iridotomy.

irradiate (ĭ-ra′de-āt) 1. to treat with roentgen rays or other form of radioactivity. 2. to apply ionizing radiation for therapeutic or diagnostic purposes.

irradiation (i-ra″de-a′shun) [L. in into + radiare to emit rays] 1. treatment by photons, electrons, neutrons, or other ionizing radiations. 2. the dispersion of nervous impulse beyond the normal path of conduction. 3. the application of rays, such as ultraviolet rays, to a substance to increase its vitamin efficiency. 4. a phenomenon in which, owing to the difference in the illumination of the field of vision, objects appear to be much larger than they really are. **interstitial i.,** therapeutic irradiation by the insertion into tissues of radioactive sources in fluid form, e.g., colloidal radioactive gold (^{198}Au), or in solid form, e.g., metallic needles or seeds. **Medinger-Craver i.** (obs.), whole-body i. **ultraviolet blood i.,** a treatment involving removal of blood from a patient, exposing it to ultraviolet light, and returning it to the patient's circulation; abbreviated UBI. **whole-body i.,** exposure of the entire body to ionizing radiation from external radiation sources.

irreducible (ir″re-dūs′ĭ-b'l) not susceptible to reduction, as a fracture, dislocation, or chemical substance.

irregular (ir-reg′u-lar) [L. in not + regula rule] not in conformity with the rule of nature; not recurring at regular intervals.

irregularity (ir-reg″u-lar′ĭ-te) the quality of not conforming with the rule of nature, or of not occurring at regular intervals. **i. of pulse,** arrhythmia.

irreinoculability (ir″re-in-ok″u-lah-bil′ĭ-te) immunity due to the effects of a previous inoculation beyond the possibility of successful reinoculation.

irrespirable (ir″re-spīr′ah-b'l) not possible of being breathed, or not possible of being breathed with safety.

irreversibility (ir″re-ver″sĭ-bil′ĭ-te) the quality of being incapable of being reversed. **i. of conduction,** the principle that the pathway for every reflex permits passage of the nerve impulse in one direction only.

irreversible (ir″re-ver′sĭ-b'l) incapable of being reversed.

irrigate (ir′ĭ-gāt) to wash out, as a wound; lavage.

irrigation (ir″ĭ-ga′shun) [L. irrigatio; in into + rigare to carry water] 1. washing by a stream of water or other fluid; see also *lavage.* 2. a liquid used for irrigation. **acetic acid i.** [USP], a sterile aqueous solution, containing, in each 100 ml., 237.5 to 262.5 mg. of glacial acetic acid; used to irrigate the bladder in the treatment of urinary infections with cystitis. **aminoacetic acid i.** [USP], a sterile aqueous solution, containing 95 to 105 per cent of the labeled amount of aminoacetic acid; used to irrigate body cavities. **continuous i.,** the maintenance of a constant stream of water over an inflamed surface. **mediate i.,** the passing of a stream of hot or cold water through a flexible tube coiled around a part. **Ringer's i.** [USP], a sterile solution containing, in each 100 ml., 820–900 mg. of sodium chloride, 25–35 mg. of potassium chloride, and 30–36 mg. of calcium chloride in water for injection; used as a topical physiological salt solution. Called also *Ringer's mixture* and *Ringer's solution.* **sodium chloride i.** [USP], a sterile aqueous solution, containing 0.85 to 0.95 per cent of sodium chloride; used to irrigate wounds and body cavities and as an enema to flush the colon and promote evacuation. Called also *sodium chloride solution.*

irrigator (ir′ĭ-ga″tor) [L. "waterer"] an apparatus for performing irrigation.

irrigoradioscopy (ir″ĭ-go-ra″de-os′ko-pe) roentgenoscopy of the intestines during the introduction of a contrast enema.

irrigoscopy (ir″ĭ-gos′ko-pe) irrigoradioscopy.

irritability (ir″ĭ-tah-bil′ĭ-te) [L. irritabilitas, from irritare to tease] 1. the quality of being irritable, or of responding to stimuli. 2. abnormal responsiveness to slight stimuli. **i. of the bladder,** a condition in which the presence of a small amount of urine in the bladder produces a desire to urinate. **chemical i.,** responsiveness to a stimulus that acts by producing a chemical change in the tissues. **electric i.,** responsiveness of nerve or muscle to the stimulus of an electric current passed through it. **faradic i.,** the property of responding by muscular contraction to faradic current. **galvanic i.,** the property of muscle by which it responds to a galvanic current. **mechanical i.,** responsiveness to a mechanical stimulus. **muscular i.,** the normal contractile quality of muscular tissue. **myotatic i.,** the power of a muscle to contract in response to stretching. **nervous i.,** 1. the ability of a nerve to transmit impulses. 2. morbid excitability of the nervous system. **specific i.,** see under *law.* **i. of the stomach,** a condition of the stomach in which vomiting is caused by normal amounts of digestible food. **tactile i.,** a condition of cells that repels foreign particles; negative chemotaxis.

irritable (ir′ĭ-tah-b'l) [L. irritabilis; irritare to tease] 1. capable of reacting to a stimulus. 2. abnormally sensitive to a stimulus.

irritant (ir′ĭ-tant) [L. irritans] 1. giving rise to irritation. 2. an agent that produces irritation. **primary i.,** an agent that produces irritation, especially of the skin, on the first exposure to it.

irritation (ir″ĭ-ta′shun) [L. irritatio] 1. the act of stimulating. 2. a state of overexcitation and undue sensitivity. **cerebral i.,** the second stage of brain concussion. **direct i.,** irritation due to direct stimulation of a part. **functional i.,** that which is attended with functional derangement without organic lesion; also overexcitability due to excessive functional activity.

irritative (ir′ĭ-ta″tiv) dependent on or caused by irritation.

Irukandji sting (ir″u-kan′je) [Irukandji, an aboriginal tribe in the vicinity of Cairns, Queensland, Australia] see under *sting.*

IRV inspiratory reserve volume.

I.S. intercostal space.

I.S.A. Instrument Society of America.

Isambert's disease (e-zahm-bārz′) [Emile Isambert, French physician, 1827–1876] see under *disease.*

isamoxole (i″sah-moks′ōl) chemical name: N-butyl-2-methyl-N-(4-methyl-2-oxazolyl)propanamide; an antiasthmatic, $C_{12}H_{20}N_2O_2$.

isatin (i′sah-tin) a crystalline compound, $C_8H_5O_2N$, in the form of yellowish red crystals, soluble in alcohol and ether, slightly soluble in water: used as a reagent.

isauxesis (is″awk-se′sis) [Gr. isos equal + auxēsis increase] growth of a part or parts at the same rate as the growth of the whole.

ischemia (is-ke′me-ah) [Gr. ischein to supress + haima blood + -ia] deficiency of blood in a part, due to functional constriction or actual obstruction of a blood vessel. **myocardial i.,** deficiency of blood supply to the heart muscle, due to obstruction or constriction of the coronary arteries. **i. ret′inae,** anemia of the retina (Graefe).

ischemic (is-kem′ik) pertaining to, or affected with, ischemia.

ischesis (is-ke′sis) [Gr. ischein to supress] retention or suppression of a discharge.

ischia (is′ke-ah) [L.] plural of *ischium.*

ischiac (is′ke-ak) ischiatic.

ischiadelphus (is″ke-ah-del′fus) [ischio- + Gr. adelphos brother] ischiodidymus.

ischiadic (is″ke-ad′ik) ischiatic.

ischial (is′ke-al) ischiatic.

ischialgia (is″ke-al′je-ah) [*ischio-* + *-algia*] pain in the pelvis (ischium).

ischias (is′ke-as) ischialgia.

ischiatic (is″ke-at′ik) [L. *ischiaticus*] pertaining to the ischium or to the haunch.

ischidrosis (is″kid-ro′sis) [Gr. *ischein* to suppress + *hidrōs* sweat + *-osis*] anhidrosis.

ischiectomy (is″ke-ek′to-me) surgical removal or excision of part of the hip.

ischio- (is′ke-o) [Gr. *ischion* hip] a combining form denoting relationship to the ischium, or to the hip.

ischioanal (is″ke-o-a′nal) [*ischio-* + *anus*] pertaining to ischium and anus.

ischiobulbar (is″ke-o-bul′bar) [*ischio-* + L. *bulbus* bulb] pertaining to the ischium and the bulb of the urethra.

ischiocapsular (is″ke-o-kap′su-lar) [*ischio-* + L. *capsula* capsule] pertaining to the ischium and the capsular ligament of the hip joint.

ischiocele (is′ke-o-sēl″) [*ischio-* + Gr. *kēlē* hernia] hernia through the sacrosciatic notch.

ischiococcygeal (is″ke-o-kok-sij′e-al) pertaining to the ischium and coccyx.

ischiococcygeus (is″ke-o-kok-sij′e-us) [*ischio-* + Gr. *kokkyx* coccyx] 1. musculus coccygeus. 2. the posterior part of the levator ani.

ischiodidymus (is″ke-o-did′ĭ-mus) [*ischio-* + Gr. *didymos* twin] symmetrical conjoined twins united at the pelvis.

ischiodymia (is″ke-o-dim′e-ah) [*ischio-* + Gr. *didymos* twin + *-ia*] the condition of symmetrical conjoined twins united at the pelvis.

ischiodynia (is″ke-o-din′e-ah) [*ischio-* + Gr. *odynē* pain] ischialgia.

ischiofemoral (is″ke-o-fem′o-ral) [*ischio-* + *femur*] pertaining to the ischium and femur.

ischiofibular (is″ke-o-fib′u-lar) pertaining to the ischium and the fibula.

ischiohebotomy (is″ke-o-he-bot′o-me) [*ischio-* + Gr. *hēbē* pubes + *temnein* to cut] the operation of dividing the ischiopubic ramus and the ascending ramus of the pubes.

ischiomelus (is″ke-om′ĕ-lus) [*ischio-* + Gr. *melos* limb] a monster with an extra limb attached at the base of the spine.

ischionitis (is″ke-o-ni′tis) inflammation of the tuberosity of the ischium.

ischiopagia (is″ke-o-pa′je-ah) the condition exhibited by an ischiopagus.

ischiopagus (is-ke-op′ah-gus) [*ischio-* + Gr. *pagos* thing fixed] conjoined twins fused at the ischia, the axes of the two bodies extending in a straight line but in opposite directions.

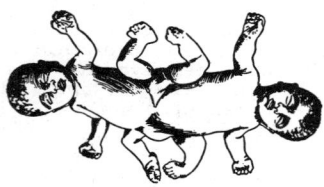

Ischiopagus.

ischiopagy (is″ke-op′ah-je) ischiopagia.

ischiopubic (is″ke-o-pu′bik) pertaining to the ischium and pubis.

ischiorectal (is″ke-o-rek′tal) pertaining to the ischium and rectum.

ischiosacral (is″ke-o-sa′kral) pertaining to the ischium and sacrum.

ischiothoracopagus (is″ke-o-tho″rah-kop′ah-gus) iliothoracopagus.

ischiovaginal (is″ke-o-vaj′ĭ-nal) pertaining to the ischium and vagina.

ischiovertebral (is″ke-o-ver′te-bral) pertaining to the ischium and the vertebral column.

ischium (is′ke-um), pl. *is′chia* [L.; Gr. *ischion* hip] the inferior dorsal part of the hip bone; it is a separate bone in early life. See illustration accompanying *skeleton*. Called also *os ischii* [NA].

ischo- (is′ko) [Gr. *ischein* to suppress] a combining form meaning suppressed, or denoting relationship to suppression.

ischogyria (is″ko-ji′re-ah) [*ischo-* + *gyrus*] a condition in which the cerebral convolutions have a jagged appearance, as in bulbar sclerosis.

ischuretic (is″ku-ret′ik) pertaining to ischuria.

ischuria (is-ku′re-ah) [*ischo-* + Gr. *ouron* urine + *-ia*] suppression or retention of the urine. **i. paradox′a,** a condition in which the bladder is overdistended with urine, although the patient continues to urinate. **i. spas′tica,** ischuria caused by spasm of the sphincter urinae.

I.S.C.P. International Society of Comparative Pathology.

iseiconia (īs″i-ko′ne-ah) iso-iconia.

iseiconic (īs″i-kon′ik) iso-iconic.

iseikonia (īs″i-ko′ne-ah) iso-iconia.

isethionate (is″-eth-i′o-nāt) USAN contraction for 2-hydroxy-ethanesulfonate.

I.S.G.E. International Society of Gastro-Enterology.

I.S.H. International Society of Hematology.

Ishihara's test (ish″ĭ-hah′rahz) [Shinobu *Ishihara,* Japanese ophthalmologist, born 1879] see under *tests.*

isinglass (i′sin-glas) ichthyocolla. **Japanese i.,** agar.

island (i′land) a cluster of cells or an isolated piece of tissue. See also *islet.* **blood i's,** aggregations of mesenchyme cells in the angioblast of the early embryo, which develop into vascular endothelium and blood corpuscles. **i's of Calleja,** discrete collections of pyramidal and polymorphic cells in the caudal part of the anterior perforated substance (olfactory tubercle). **cartilage i's,** see *intrachondrial bone,* under *bone.* **i's of Langerhans,** islets of Langerhans. **olfactory i's,** i's of Calleja. **i's of pancreas,** islets of Langerhans. **Pander's i's,** reddish yellow cords of corpuscular matter in the splanchnopleure of the embryo which develop into blood and blood vessels. **i. of Reil,** insula.

islet (i′let) a cluster of cells or an isolated piece of tissue; see also *island.* **blood i's,** see under *island.* **Calleja's i's,** see under *island.* **i's of Langerhans,** irregular microscopic structures scattered throughout the pancreas and comprising its endocrine portion. In man, they are composed of at least three types of cells, the *alpha cells,* which secrete the hyperglycemic factor glucagon; the *beta cells,* which are the most abundant and secrete insulin, and the *delta cells,* which secrete somatostatin. Degeneration of the beta cells, whose secretion (insulin) is important in carbohydrate metabolism, is one of the causes of diabetes mellitus. Called also *islands of Langerhans* and *islets* or *islands of pancreas.* **i's of pancreas,** i's of Langerhans. **Walthard's i's,** microscopic inclusions of the germinal epithelium of the ovary, found either in contact with the serosal covering or just below it; they have been implicated in the development of Brenner tumors. Called also *Walthard's cell rests* or *inclusions.*

-ism (iz′m) [Gr. *-izō* + *-mos*] a word termination meaning state, condition, or fact of being, or the process or result of an action.

I.S.M. International Society of Microbiologists.

Ismelin (is′me-lin) trademark for a preparation of guanethidine sulfate.

iso- (i′so) [Gr. *isos* equal] a prefix or combining form meaning equal, alike, or the same. In immunology, it indicates *from* a genetically identical individual (as an isograft) or existing in alternate forms in the same species (as an isoantigen).

I.S.O. International Standards Organization.

isoadrenocorticism (i″so-ah-dre″no-kōr′tĭ-sizm) the normal state of secretion of the cells of the adrenal cortex, as distinguished from hypo- or hyperadrenocorticism.

isoagglutination (i″so-ah-gloo″tĭ-na′shun) agglutination of cells from members of a species by agglutinins originating in genetically dissimilar members of the same species.

isoagglutinin (i″so-ah-gloo′tĭ-nin) an agglutinin from members of a species that agglutinates cells of genetically different members of the same species.

isoallele (i″so-ah-lēl′) an allelic gene that is considered as being normal but can be distinguished from another allele by its differing phenotypic expression when in combination with a dominant mutant allele.

isoalloxazine (i″so-ah-lok′sah-zēn) an isomer of alloxazine from which riboflavins and other flavins are derived.

isoamyl nitrite (i″so-am′il ni-trīt) amyl nitrite.

isoamylamine (i″so-am″il-am′in) a liquid ptomaine, $(CH_3)_2$-CHCH_2CH_2NH_2, obtainable from stale yeast, cod liver oil, and other sources, especially the distillation of horn with potassium hydroxide. Leucine by the loss of CO_2 becomes isoamylamine.

isoamylase (i″so-am′ĭ-lās) 1. any of the several isoenzymes of α-amylase. 2. a hydrolase that catalyzes the hydrolysis of 1,6-α-glucosidic branch linkages in glycogen and amylopectin, and their β-limit dextrans.

isoanaphylaxis (i″so-an″ah-fĭ-lak′sis) anaphylaxis produced by the administration of serum from the same species, as in man by the administration of human serum.

isoandrosterone (i″so-an-dro′stēr-ōn) epiandrosterone.

isoantibody (i-so-an′tĭ-bod″e) an antibody produced by one individual that reacts with antigens (isoantigens) of another individual of the same species; called also *alloantibody.*

isoantigen (i″so-an′tĭ-jen) an antigen that exists in alternative (allelic) forms in a species, and thus induces an immune response when one form is transferred (as by blood transfusion or tissue graft) to members of the species who lack it. Typical isoantigens are the blood group antigens. Called also *alloantigen.* **H i.,** an antigen of the ABO blood group system.

isobar (i′so-bar) [*iso-* + Gr. *baros* weight] 1. one of two or more chemical species with the same atomic weight but different atomic numbers.   2. a line on a map or chart depicting the boundaries of an area of constant atmospheric pressure.

isobaric (i″so-bār′ik) [iso- + Gr. *baros* weight]   see under *solution*.

isobody (i′so-bod″e)   isoantibody.

isobolism (i-sob′o-lizm) [iso- + Gr. *ballein* to throw]   the tendency of motor nerve fibers to undergo maximal excitation on stimulation.

isobornyl thiocyanoacetate (i″so-bor′nil thi″o-si″ah-no-as′e-tāt)   chemical name: terpinyl thiocyanoacetate; used as a pediculicide.

isobucaine hydrochloride (i″so-bu′kān) [USP]   chemical name: 2-methyl-2-[(2-methylpropyl)amino]-1-propanol benzoate (ester) hydrochloride. A local anesthetic, $C_{15}H_{23}NO_2 \cdot HCl$, occurring as a white, crystalline solid; used in combination with epinephrine in dentistry.

isobutamben (i″so-bu-tam′ben)   chemical name: 4-aminobenzoic acid 2-methylpropyl ester; a topical anesthetic, $C_{11}H_{15}NO_2$.

isobutanol (i″so-bu′tah-nol″)   isobutyl alcohol.

isocaloric (i″so-kah-lo′rik)   containing or providing the same number of calories; equicaloric.

isocarboxazid (i″so-kar-bok′sah-zid) [USP]   chemical name: 5-methyl-3-isoxazolecarboxylic acid 2-(phenylmethyl)hydrazide. A monoamine oxidase inhibitor, $C_{12}H_{13}N_3O_2$, occurring as a white or nearly white, crystalline powder; used as an antidepressant, administered orally.

isocarveol (i″so-kar′ve-ol)   pinocarveol.

isocellobiose (i″so-sel″o-bi′ōs)   a disaccharide once considered to be formed in the degradation of cellulose; now recognized as a mixture of cellobiose with oligosaccharides.

isocellular (i″so-sel′u-lar) [iso- + L. *cellula* cell]   composed of cells of the same kind and size.

isocholesterin (i″so-ko-les′ter-in)   isocholesterol.

isocholesterol (i″so-ko-les′ter-ol)   a compound found with cholesterol in wool; apparently a mixture of C_{30} trimethyl cholestanes.

isochromatic (i″so-kro-mat′ik) [iso- + Gr. *chrōma* color]   of the same color throughout.

isochromatophil (i″so-kro-mat′o-fil) [iso- + Gr. *chrōma* color + *philein* to love]   staining equally well with the same dye.

isochromosome (i″so-kro′mo-sōm)   an abnormal chromosome having a median centromere and two identical arms, formed by the transverse, rather than the normal longitudinal, splitting of a replicating chromosome.

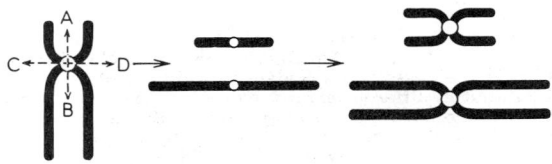

Isochromosomes. Formation by division of the submedian centromere in plane C–D instead of plane A–B, as normally occurs, resulting in formation of two abnormal metacentric chromosomes, each containing duplication of the chromosomal material of one arm and no material of the other arm of the original chromosome. (Thompson and Thompson.)

isochron (i′so-kron)   having equal chronaxy.

isochronal (i-sok′ro-nal)   isochronous.

isochronia (i-so-kro′ne-ah)   1. a condition of correspondence between processes with respect to their time, rate, or frequency. 2. the condition of having the same chronaxy as between a muscle and its nerve.

isochronic (i″so-kron′ik)   isochronous.

isochronism (i-sok′ro-nizm)   isochronia.

isochronous (i-sok′ro-nus) [iso- + Gr. *chronos* time]   performed in equal times; said of motions and vibrations occurring at the same time and being equal in duration.

isochroous (i-sok′ro-us) [iso- + Gr. *chroa* color]   isochromatic.

isocitrate (i″so-sit′rāt)   a salt of isocitric acid; in biochemistry, the term is often used interchangeably with isocitric acid (see under *acid*).

isocoagulase (i″so-ko-ag′u-lās)   a term designating collectively the antigenic types of coagulase.

isocolloid (i-so-kol′oid)   a colloid having the same composition in both phases—the disperse phase and the dispersion medium.

isocomplement (i″so-kom′plĕ-ment)   complement from the same individual (or from one of the same species) who supplies the antibody.

isocomplementophilic (i″so-kom″plĕ-men-to-fil′ik)   having affinity for isocomplements.

isoconazole (i″so-ko′nah-zōl)   chemical name: 1-[2-(2,4-dichloro-

phenyl)-2-[(2,6-dichlorophenyl)methoxyethyl]-1*H*-imidazole; an antibacterial and antifungal, $C_{18}H_{14}Cl_4N_2O$.

isocoria (i″so-ko′re-ah) [iso- + Gr. *korē* pupil]   equality in size of the two pupils.

isocortex (i″so-kor′teks)   neopallium.

isocreatinine (i″so-kre-at′ĭ-nin)   a base similar to creatinine reported to have been found in the muscle of fish.

Isocrin (i′so-krin)   trademark for a preparation of oxyphenisatin acetate.

isocyanide (i″so-si′ah-nīd)   one of a class of organic cyanides characterized by their disagreeable odor and formed by heating silver cyanide with alkyl iodides; called also *carbylamine*.

isocyclic (i″so-si′klik) [iso- + Gr. *kyklos* circle]   homocyclic.

isocytolysine (i″so-si-tol′ĭ-sin) [iso- + *cytolysine*]   a cytolysine that acts on the cells of animals of the same species as that from which it is derived.

isocytosis (i″so-si-to′sis) [iso- + -*cyte* + -*osis*]   equality of the size of cells, especially red blood corpuscles.

isocytotoxin (i″so-si″to-tok′sin)   a cytotoxin that is toxic for homologous cells of the same species.

isodactylism (i-so-dak′til-izm) [iso- + Gr. *daktylos* finger + -*ism*]   a condition in which the fingers are of relatively even length.

isodesmosine (i″so-des′mo-sēn)   one of two unusual amino acids found in elastin, the other being desmosine.

isodiagnosis (i″so-di″ag-no′sis)   diagnosis of a condition by inoculation of a susceptible animal with blood from a patient suspected of having an inapparent infection.

isodiametric (i″so-di″ah-met′rik) [iso- + Gr. *dia* through + *metron* measure]   having the same diameter in all directions.

isodispersoid (i″so-dis-per′soid)   isocolloid.

isodontic (i″so-don′tik) [iso- + Gr. *odous* tooth]   having all the teeth of the same size and shape.

isodose (i′so-dōs)   a radiation dose of equal intensity to more than one body area; see also under *curve*.

isodulcite (i″so-dul′sīt)   rhamnose.

isodynamic (i″so-di-nam′ik) [iso- + Gr. *dynamis* power]   exhibiting equal force or power.

isodynamogenic (i″so-di-nam″o-jen′ik) [iso- + Gr. *dynamis* power + *gennan* to produce]   producing equal force or power.

isoeffect (i″so-ĕ-fekt′)   an effect midway between two reference points; see under *line*.

isoelectric (i″so-e-lek′trik) [iso- + *electric*]   showing no variation in electric potential.

isoenergetic (i″so-en″er-jet′ik)   exhibiting equal energy.

isoenzyme (i″so-en′zīm)   isozyme.   **Regan i.** a tumor-associated antigen identical to placental alkaline phosphatase.

isoetharine (i-so-eth′ah-rēn)   chemical name: 4-[(1-hydroxy-2-[(1-methylethyl)amino]-butyl]-1,2-benzenediol. An adrenergic, $C_{13}H_{21}NO_3$, used as a bronchodilator in the treatment of bronchial asthma and bronchospasm, administered by inhalation. Its hydrochloride and mesylate salts are prepared in conformance with USP standards.

isoflupredone acetate (i″so-floo″pre-dōn)   chemical name: 21-(acetyloxy)-9-fluoro-11β,17-dihydroxypregna-1,4-diene-3,20-dione; an anti-inflammatory, $C_{23}H_{29}FO_6$.

isoflurane (i″se-flur′ān)   chemical name: 2-chloro-2-(difluoromethoxy)-1,1,1-trifluoroethane; an inhalation anesthetic, $C_3H_2Cl-F_5O$.

isoflurophate (i″so-floo′ro-fāt) [USP]   chemical name: bis(1-methylethyl)ester phosphorofluoridic acid. A cholinergic, $C_6H_{14}-FO_3P$, occurring as a clear, colorless to faintly yellow liquid with an extremely irritating vapor; used as a miotic, applied topically to the conjunctiva in the treatment of glaucoma.

isogame (i-sog′ah-me)   isogamy.

isogamete (i″so-gam′ēt)   a gamete of the same size as the gamete with which it unites.

isogametic (i″so-gah-met′ik)   characterized by the production of gametes of the same size.

isogamety (i″so-gam′e-te)   production by an individual of one sex of gametes identical with respect to the sex chromosome.

isogamous (i-sog′ah-mus)   having the conjugating elements (gametes) similar.

isogamy (i-sog′ah-me) [iso- + Gr. *gamos* marriage]   reproduction resulting from the union of two cells (gametes) that are identical in size and structure, as occurs in protozoa.

isogeneic (i″so-jĕ-ne′ik)   syngeneic.

isogeneric (i″so-jĕ-ner′ik)   of the same kind; pertaining to or obtained from individuals of the same genus.

isogenesis (i″so-jen′ĕ-sis) [iso- + Gr. *genesis* production]   similarity in the processes of development.

isogenous (i-soj′ĕ-nus)   developed from the same cell.

isograft (i′so-graft)   a graft between genetically identical individuals. Typically, isografts are grafts between identical twins, between animals of a single highly inbred strain, or between the

F_1 hybrid produced by crossing inbred strains. Called also *isogeneic graft*, and *syngraft*.

isohemagglutination (i″so-hem″ah-gloo″tĭ-na′shun) agglutination of erythrocytes caused by a hemagglutinin from another individual of the same species.

isohemagglutinin (i″so-hem″ah-gloo′tĭ-nin) a hemagglutinin that agglutinates the erythrocytes of other individuals of the same species.

isohemolysin (i″so-he-mol′ĭ-sin) [*iso-* + *hemolysin*] a hemolysin that acts on the blood of animals of the same species as that from which it is derived.

isohemolysis (i″so-he-mol′ĭ-sis) hemolysis of the blood corpuscles of an animal by the lysins in serum from another animal of the same species.

isohemolytic (i″so-he″mo-lit′ik) pertaining to or characterized by isohemolysis.

isohydric (i″so-hi′drik) a term applied to the series or cycle of chemical reactions in the erythrocyte in which carbon dioxide is taken up and oxygen released without the production of an excess of hydrogen.

iso-iconia (i″so-i-ko′ne-ah) [*iso-* + Gr. *eikōn* image] a condition in which the image of an object is the same in both eyes.

iso-iconic (i″so-i-kon′ik) marked by iso-iconia.

isoimmunization (i″so-im″u-ni-za′shun) development of antibodies against an antigen derived from a genetically dissimilar individual of the same species; see also *isoantigen*. **Rh i.,** the development of agglutinins against Rhesus (Rh) blood group antigens in an Rh-negative person in response to transfusion of Rh-positive blood, which may lead to transfusion reactions, or in an Rh-negative woman pregnant with an Rh-positive fetus, which may lead to development of erythroblastosis fetalis in a subsequent pregnancy. The D antigen of erythrocytes stimulates an immune response that leads to these two reactions more commonly than do other Rh blood group antigens.

isokreatinin (i″so-kre-at′ĭ-nin) a ptomaine from decaying fish, crystallizable in a yellow powder, $C_4H_7N_3O$.

isolactose (i″so-lak′tōs) a disaccharide formed by the action of lactase on glucose and galactose.

isolate (i′so-lāt) 1. to separate from other persons, materials, or objects. 2. a population that has been obtained by isolation, such as living organisms (bacteria or other cells) obtained in pure culture, or (higher organisms) separated by geographical, genetic, ecological, or social barriers which prevent their interbreeding with other individuals beyond those barriers, and are thus differentiated from others of their kind by the accumulation of new characteristics.

isolation (i″so-la′shun) the process of isolating, or the state of being isolated, such as (*a*) the physiologic separation of a part, as by tissue culture or by interposition of inert material; (*b*) the chemical extraction of an unknown substance in pure form from a tissue; (*c*) the separation from contact with others of patients having a communicable disease; (*d*) the successive propagation of a growth of microorganisms until a pure culture is obtained; or (*e*) an unconscious mental mechanism in which there is defensive failure to connect behavior with motives, or contradictory attitudes and behavior with each other.

isolator (i″so-la′tor) anything that isolates. **surgical i.,** a large, clear, plastic bag with man-sized pockets that is attached to the patient's body during surgical procedures to prevent contamination by infective agents; the pockets, in which the nurses and surgeons stand, have plastic helmets, earphones and microphones for communication, and closed sleeves leading into the bag through which the surgeons work.

isolecithal (i″so-les′ĭ-thal) [*iso-* + *lekithos* yolk] having yolk evenly distributed throughout the cytoplasm of the ovum.

isoleucine (i″so-lu′sin) an amino acid, ethylmethyl-alpha-aminopropionic acid, $CH_3(C_2H_5)\cdot CHCH(NH_2)\cdot COOH$, produced by the hydrolysis of fibrin and other proteins; essential for optimal growth in infants and for nitrogen equilibrium in human adults.

isoleukoagglutinin (i″so-lu″ko-ah-glu′tĭ-nin) see *leukoagglutinin.*

isologous (i-sol′o-gus) characterized by an identical genotype; see *isograft.*

isolysin (i-sol′ĭ-sin) a lysin that acts on the cells of animals of the same species as that from which it is derived.

isolysis (i-sol′ĭ-sis) lysis of cells by isolysins.

isolytic (i″so-lit′ik) pertaining to isolysis.

isomaltase (i″so-mawl′tās) an enzyme of the intestinal mucosa that catalyzes the splitting of isomaltose.

isomaltose (i″so-mawl′tōs) an isomeric form of maltose formed by treating glucose with strong acids or by the action of maltase on glucose; it occurs in beer, urine, blood, honey, liver, and other natural substances. Called also *brachiose* and *dextrinose.*

isomastigote (i″so-mas′tĭ-gōt) [*iso-* + Gr. *mastix* lash] having two equal and similar flagella at the anterior pole.

isomer (i′so-mer) [*iso-* + Gr. *meros* part] any compound exhibit-

ing, or capable of exhibiting, isomerism. An isomer may be structural or stereochemical; see *isomerism.*

isomerase (i-som′er-ās) a major class of enzymes comprising those that catalyze the process of isomerization, such as the interconversion of aldoses and ketoses, or the shift of a double bond, e.g., 3-ketosteroid-Δ^4,Δ^5-isomerase. **arabinose i.,** an enzyme that catalyzes the aldose-ketose interconversion of arabinose to ribulose. **arabinosephosphate i.,** an enzyme that catalyzes the aldose-ketose interconversion of D-arabinose-5-phosphate to D-ribulose-5-phosphate. **acetylglucosaminephosphate i.,** an enzyme that catalyzes the aldose-ketose interconversion of 2-acetamido-2-deoxy-D-glucose-6-phosphate and $2H_2O$ to D-fructose-6-phosphate, ammonia, and acetate. **erythrose i.,** an enzyme which catalyzes the aldose-ketose interconversion of D-erythrose to D-erythrulose. **glucosaminephosphate i.,** an enzyme that catalyzes the aldose-ketose interconversion of 2-amino-2-deoxy-D-glucose-6-phosphate and water to D-fructose-6-phosphate and ammonia. **glucosephosphate i.,** an enzyme found in muscle extract which catalyzes an equilibrium between glucose 6-phosphate and fructose 6-phosphate; called also *phosphohexoisomerase.* **glucuronate i.,** an enzyme that catalyzes the aldose-ketose interconversion of D-glucuronate to D-fructuronate; called also *uronic i.* **isopentenylpyrophosphate i.,** an enzyme that catalyzes the migration of a double bond in the conversion of dimethylallyl pyrophosphate to isopentenyl pyrophosphate. **L-rhamnose i.,** an enzyme that catalyzes the aldose-ketose interconversion of L-rhamnose to L-rhamnulose. **maleate i.,** an enzyme that catalyzes the *cis-trans* conversion of maleate to fumarate. **maleylacetoacetate i.,** an enzyme of the liver that catalyzes the *cis-trans* conversion of 4-maleylacetoacetate to 4-fumarylacetoacetate. **maleylpyruvate i.,** an enzyme that catalyzes the *cis-trans* conversion of 3-maleylpyruvate to 3-fumarylpyruvate. **mannose i.,** an enzyme that catalyzes the aldose-ketose interconversion of D-mannose to D-fructose. **mannosephosphate i.,** an enzyme that catalyzes the aldose-ketose interconversion of D-mannose-6-phosphate to D-fructose-6-phosphate. **retinal i., retinene i.,** an enzyme of the retina that catalyzes the *cis-trans* conversion of all-*trans*-retinal to 11-*cis*-retinal. **ribosephosphate i.,** an enzyme of the liver that catalyzes the aldose-ketose interconversion of D-ribose-5-phosphate to D-ribulose-5-phosphate. **triosephosphate i.,** an enzyme that catalyzes the aldose-ketose interconversion of D-glyceraldehyde 3-phosphate to dihydroxyacetone phosphate. **uronic i.,** glucuronate i. **vinylacetyl-CoA i.,** an enzyme that catalyzes the migration of a double bond in the conversion of vinylacetyl-CoA to crotonyl-CoA. **xylose i.,** an enzyme that catalyzes the aldose-ketose interconversion of D-xylose to D-xylulose.

isomeric (i″so-mer′ik) pertaining to or exhibiting isomerism.

isomeride (i-som′er-īd) isomer.

isomerism (i-som′ĕ-rizm) [*iso-* + Gr. *meros* part] the possession by two or more distinct compounds of the same molecular formula, each molecule possessing an identical number of atoms of each element, but in different arrangement. Isomerism is divided into two broad classifications: *structural isomerism* and *stereochemical isomerism,* or *stereoisomerism.* **chain i.,** a type of structural isomerism in which the compounds differ in regard to the linkages

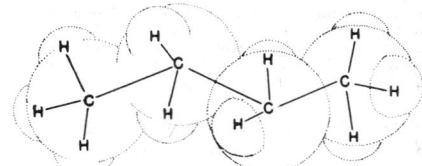

Normal butane

Isobutane

Chain isomerism (Luder, Vernon, and Zuffanti).

in the basic chain of carbon atoms; see illustration. **dynamic i.,** tautomerism. **functional group i.,** a type of structural isomerism dependent upon the presence of different functional groups, such compounds being of distinct chemical types, e.g., ethyl alcohol, C_2H_5OH, and dimethyl ether, CH_3OCH_3. **geo-**

metric i., a type of stereoisomerism usually described as being dependent upon some form of restricted rotation, enabling the component parts of the molecule to occupy different spatial positions. Thus, *cis-* and *trans-*dichloroethylene are said to be geometric isomers, the isomerism resulting from the lack of freedom of rotation about the double bond. In the case of *cis-* and *trans-*decalin, however, the rigidity of the fused ring structure is responsible for the isomerism. **nuclear i.,** chain i. **optical i.,** a type of stereoisomerism in which an appreciable number of molecules exhibit any of the following effects on polarized light: the isomers (*a*) rotate the plane of polarization to the *same* degree in *opposite* directions (enantiomorphism), (*b*) rotate the plane of polarization to a *different* degree in either the same direction or in opposite directions, or (*c*) have no effect on the plane because of so-called internal compensation (diastereoisomerism). **position i.,** a type of structural isomerism in which the position occupied by an atom or group differs with reference to the same fundamental carbon chain; for example, *n*-propyl chloride, CH_3-CH_2CH_2Cl, and isopropyl chloride, $CH_3CHClCH_3$. **spatial i.,** stereoisomerism. **stereochemical i.,** stereoisomerism. **structural i.,** the possession by two or more compounds of the same molecular formula but of different structural formulas, the linkages of the atoms being different, in contrast to stereoisomerism, in which the structural arrangements of the atoms are the same. **substitution i.,** position i.

isomerization (i-som″er-i-za′shun) the process whereby any isomer, whether structural or stereochemical, is converted into another, usually requiring special conditions of temperature, pressure, or catalysts.

isometheptene hydrochloride (i″so-meth′ep-tēn) chemical name: *N*,1,5-trimethyl-4-hexenylamine hydrochloride. An adrenergic, $C_9H_{20}ClN$, used as an antispasmodic for the urinary and gastrointestinal tracts and as a vasodilator in the treatment of migraine; administered intramuscularly.

isometric (i″so-met′rik) [*iso-* + Gr. *metron* measure] 1. maintaining, or pertaining to, the same measure or length; of equal dimensions. 2. not isotonic.

isometropia (i″so-mĕ-tro′pe-ah) [*iso-* + Gr. *metron* measure + *ōps* eye] equality in the refraction of the two eyes.

isometry (i-som′ĕ-tre) equality of dimension.

isomicrogamete (i″so-mi″kro-gam′ēt) [*iso-* + *microgamete*] a protozoan sexual cell or gamete of a small size, but equal in size to the gamete with which it conjugates.

isomorphic (i″so-mor′fik) isomorphous.

isomorphism (i″so-mor′fizm) [*iso-* + Gr. *morphē* form] the quality of being isomorphous.

isomorphous (i″so-mor′fus) [*iso-* + Gr. *morphē* form] having the same form. In genetics, denoting genotypes of polyploid organisms which produce similar gametes even though containing genes in different combinations on homologous chromosomes.

isomuscarine (i″so-mus′kah-rin) a basic substance formed by oxidizing choline; it is isomeric with muscarine, but has different physiologic properties.

isomylamine hydrochloride (i″so-mil′ah-mēn) chemical name: 1-(3-methylbutyl)-cyclohexanecarboxylic acid 2-(diethylamino)ethyl ester hydrochloride; a smooth muscle relaxant, C_{18}-$H_{35}NO_2 \cdot HCl$.

isonaphthol (i″so-naf′thol) betanaphthol.

isonephrotoxin (i″so-nef″ro-tok′sin) [*iso-* + *nephrotoxin*] a nephrotoxin which acts on cells of the animals of the same species from which it is derived.

isoniazid (i″so-ni′ah-zid) [USP] chemical name: 4-pyridinecarboxylic acid hydrazide. An antibacterial, $C_6H_7N_3O$, occurring as colorless or white crystals or white, crystalline powder; used as a tuberculostatic, administered orally and intramuscularly.

isonicotinoylhydrazine (i″so-nik″o-tin″o-il-hi′drah-zēn) isoniazid.

isonicotinylhydrazine (i″so-nik″o-tin″il-hi′drah-zēn) isoniazid.

isonipecaine (i″so-nip′e-kān) meperidine hydrochloride.

isonitril (i″so-ni′tril) isocyanide.

iso-oncotic (i″so-on-kot′ik) having the same oncotic pressure.

iso-osmotic (i″so-oz-mot′ik) isosmotic.

Isopaque (i″so-pāk′) trademark for preparations of metrizoate sodium.

Isoparorchis trisimilitubis (i″so-par-or′kis tri-sim″ĭ-li-tu′bis) a fluke, commonly parasitic in the air bladder of fish in India and China and sometimes found in man.

isopathy (i-sop′ah-the) [*iso-* + Gr. *pathos* disease] the treatment of disease by means of products of the disease or with material from the organ affected, e.g., smallpox by giving minute doses of variolous matter, disease of the liver by giving extract of liver, etc.

isopatin (i-sop′ah-tin) an immunizing agent of animal origin which gives no biuret reaction and yet is active in small amounts.

isophagy (i-sof′ah-je) [*iso-* + Gr. *phagein* to eat] autolysis.

isophan (i′so-fan) [*iso-* + Gr. *phainein* to show] a hybrid which

looks like other hybrids, but yet has a different germinal constitution.

isophenolization (i″so-fe″nol-i-za′shun) the injection of isophenol to produce paralysis or destruction of a sympathetic nerve.

isophoria (i″so-fo′re-ah) [*iso-* + Gr. *phoros* bearing + *-ia*] equality in the tension of the vertical muscles of each eye; absence of hyperphoria and of hypophoria.

isophotometer (i″so-fo-tom′ĕ-ter) a device for analysis of radiographs and other filmed images.

Isophrin (i′so-frin) trademark for a preparation of phenylephrine hydrochloride.

isopia (i-so′pe-ah) [*iso-* + Gr. *ōps* vision] equality of vision in the two eyes.

isoplassont (i″so-plas′ont) [*iso-* + Gr. *plassein* to form] either of two things which have certain features in common.

isoplastic (i″so-plas′tik) [*iso-* + *plastic*] taken from another animal of the same species or from another inbred strain within the same species; said of tissue transplants or grafts.

isoprecipitin (i″so-pre-sip′ĭ-tin) a precipitin that is active against antigens of animals of the same species (but of dissimilar genetic makeup) as the animal in which it is formed.

isopregnenone (i″so-preg′ne-nōn) dydrogesterone.

isoprenaline (i″so-pren′ah-lēn) isoproterenol.

isoprene (i′so-prēn) the basic building unit of terpenes, C_5H_8.

isopropamide iodide (i″so-pro′pah-mīd) [USP] chemical name: γ-(aminocarbonyl)-*N*-methyl-*N*,*N*-bis(1-methylethyl)-γ-phenylbenzenepropanaminium iodide. A long-acting quaternary anticholinergic, $C_{23}H_{33}IN_2O$, used in the treatment of peptic ulcer and other gastrointestinal disorders marked by hyperacidity and hypermotility, administered orally.

isopropanol (i″so-pro′pah-nol) isopropyl alcohol.

isopropyl (i″so-pro′pil) the univalent radical, $(CH_3)_2CH$. **i. alcohol, i. rubbing alcohol,** see under *alcohol.* **i. meprobamate,** carisoprodol. **i. myristate** [NF], a compound of isopropyl alcohol and saturated high molecular weight fatty acids, principally myristic acid, occurring as a clear, oily liquid; used as an emollient in pharmaceutical preparations.

isopropylarterenol (i″so-pro″pil-ar″tĕ-re′nol) isoproterenol.

isopropyl-benzanthracene (i″so-pro″pil-benz-an′thrah-sēn) a carcinogenic hydrocarbon, 6-isopropyl 1:2-benzanthracene.

isoproterenol (i″so-pro″tĕ-re′nol) chemical name: 4-[1-hydroxy-2-[(1-methylethyl)amino]ethyl]-1,2-benzenediol. A synthetic adrenergic, $C_{11}H_{17}NO_3$, derived from norepinephrine, having powerful bronchodilator and cardiac stimulant actions. **i. hydrochloride** [USP], the hydrochloride salt of isoproterenol, $C_{11}H_{17}NO_3 \cdot HCl$, occurring as a white to practically white, crystalline powder; used chiefly as a bronchodilator in the treatment of bronchial asthma, administered by oral inhalation, sublingually, and parenterally. It may also be used in the management of shock, treatment and prevention of cardiac standstill and arrhythmias, and treatment of bronchospasm during anesthesia. **i. sulfate** [USP], the sulfate salt of isoproterenol, $(C_{11}H_{17}NO_3)_2 \cdot H_2$-$SO_4 \cdot 2H_2O$, having the appearance, actions, and uses as the hydrochloride salt; administered by oral inhalation.

isopter (i-sop′ter) [*iso-* + Gr. *opter* observer] a line depicting the area in the field of vision in which the visual acuity is the same.

isopyknic (i″so-pik′nik) [*iso-* + Gr. *pyknos* thick] of equal density or thickness; see under *centrifugation.*

isopyknosis (i″so-pik-no′sis) [*iso-* + Gr. *pyknōsis* condensation] the state of being of uniform density; applied especially to a state of uniform condensation observed in comparison of different chromosomes, or of different regions of the same chromosome.

isopyknotic (i″so-pik-not′ik) pertaining to or characterized by isopyknosis.

Isordil (i′sor-dil) trademark for preparations of isosorbide dinitrate.

isorhodeose (i″so-ro′de-ōs) a sugar, *d*-glucomethylose or 6-deoxy-D-glucose, $CH_3(CHOH)_4CHO$, from cinchona bark.

isoriboflavin (i″so-ri″bo-fla′vin) a compound, dichlororibityl isoalloxazine, which can produce riboflavin deficiency.

isorrhea (i″so-re′ah) [*iso-* + Gr. *rhein* to flow] the maintenance of a relatively constant body fluid volume and composition; water and solute intake is balanced by an equivalent output of the substances from the body.

isorrheic (i″so-re′ik) pertaining to or characterized by isorrhea.

isorrhopic (i″so-rop′ik) [*iso-* + Gr. *rhopē* momentum] of equal value.

isorubin (i″so-ru′bin) new fuchsin.

isoscope (i′so-skōp) [*iso-* + Gr. *skopein* to examine] an apparatus for observing the changes of position of the horizontal and vertical lines in the movements of the eyeball.

isosensitization (i″so-sen″sĭ-ti-za′shun) allosensitization.

isoserine (i″so-se′rin) a compound, $CH_2NH_2 \cdot CHOH \cdot COOH$, isomeric with serine.

isoserotherapy (i″so-se″ro-ther′ah-pe) treatment by use of an isoserum.

isoserum (i″so-se′rum) [*iso-* + *serum*] a serum obtained from a person who has had the same disease as the patient who is being treated.

isosexual (i″so-seks′u-al) [*iso-* + *sexual*] pertaining to or characteristic of the same sex.

isosmotic (i″sos-mot′ik) having the same osmotic pressure.

isosmoticity (i″sos-mo-tis′ĭ-te) the state or quality of being isosmotic.

isosorbide (i″so-sor′bĭd) chemical name: 1,4:3,6-dianhydro-D-glucitol. An osmotic diuretic, $C_6H_{10}O_4$, used to rapidly reduce intraocular pressure in glaucoma. **i. dinitrate,** the dinitric acid ester of isosorbide, $C_6H_8N_2O_8$, occurring as a white, crystalline powder, having coronary and peripheral vasodilating properties; used in the treatment of coronary insufficiency and angina pectoris, administered sublingually and orally.

isospermotoxin (i″so-sper″mo-tok′sin) a cytotoxic antibody that destroys spermatozoa; it is developed in the blood after the injection of spermatozoa of the same species as that in which it is formed.

Isospora (i-sos′po-rah) [*iso-* + Gr. *sporos* spore] a genus of sporozoan parasites, order Coccidia, characterized by two sporoblasts, each containing four sporozoites in the oocyst, and found in birds, amphibians, reptiles, and mammals, including man. **I. bel′li,** a species that parasitizes the small intestine of man; infection (coccidiosis) is usually asymptomatic but may result in a severe watery mucous diarrhea. **I. bigem′ina,** a form found in dogs and cats, closely resembling *I. hominis;* called also *Coccidium bigeminum.* **I. fe′lis,** a species causing intestinal coccidiosis in cats. **I. hom′inis,** a species causing coccidiosis in man; called also *Coccidium hominis.* **I. laca′zei,** a species causing intestinal coccidiosis in passerine birds. **I. rivol′ta,** a species causing intestinal coccidiosis in dogs and cats.

isospore (i′so-spōr) [*iso-* + Gr. *sporos* spore] 1. an isogamete of organisms that reproduce by spores. 2. an asexual spore produced by a homosporous organism.

isosporiasis (i-sos″po-ri′ah-sis) infection with *Isospora.*

isosporous (i-sos′po-rus) having isospores.

isostere (i′so-stēr) a substance which stands in the same place as or in place of another compound owing to similarity in structure, configuration, or other molecular parameters. See *competitive inhibition,* under *inhibition.*

isosthenuria (i″sos-thĕ-nu′re-ah) [*iso-* + Gr. *sthenos* strength + *ouron* urine + *-ia*] the excretion of urine with the same osmolality as that of plasma.

isostimulation (i″so-stim″u-la′shun) stimulation of an animal with antigenic material originating from other animals of the same species.

isothebaine (i″so-the′ba-in) chemical name: 1-hydroxy-2-11-dimethoxyaporphine. An alkaloid, $C_{19}H_{21}O_3N$, from *Papaver orientalis.*

isotherapy (i″so-ther′ah-pe) [*iso-* + Gr. *therapeia* treatment] isopathy.

isotherm (i′so-therm) a line on a map or chart depicting the boundaries of an area in which the temperature is the same.

isothermal (i″so-ther′mal) [*iso-* + Gr. *thermē* heat] isothermic.

isothermic (i″so-ther′mik) having the same temperature.

isothermognosis (i″so-ther″mo-no′sis) [*iso-* + Gr. *thermē* heat + *gnōsis* recognition] disordered sense perception in which pain, cold, and heat stimuli are all perceived as heat.

isothiazine hydrochloride (i″so-thi′ah-zēn) ethopropazine hydrochloride.

isothiocyanate (i″so-thi″o-si′ah-nāt) a salt of isothiocyanic acid. **allyl i.,** a compound, $C_3H_5\cdot NCS$, found in oil of mustard. **butyl i.,** a compound, $CH_3\cdot CH(CH_3)CH_2NCS$, found in horseradish and used as an intermediate pesticide, herbicide, and pharmaceutical. **phenyl-ethyl i.,** a compound, $CH_3\cdot CH(C_6H_5)NCS$, found in oil of mignonette.

isothipendyl (i″so-thi′pen-dil) chemical name: 10-(2-dimethyl-amino-2-methylethyl)-10*H*-pyrido[3,2-*b*][1,4]benzothiazine. A compound, $C_{16}H_{19}N_3S$, used as an antihistaminic.

isotone (i′so-tōn) one of several nuclides having the same number of neutrons, but differing in the number of protons in their nuclei.

isotonia (i″so-to′ne-ah) [*iso-* + Gr. *tonos* tone] 1. a condition of equal tone, tension, or activity. 2. equality of osmotic pressure between two elements of a solution or between two different solutions.

isotonic (i″so-ton′ik) [*iso-* + Gr. *tonos* tone] a biological term denoting a solution in which body cells can be bathed without a net flow of water across the semipermeable cell membrane. Also, denoting a solution having the same tonicity as some other solution with which it is compared, such as physiologic salt solution and the blood serum.

isotonicity (i″so-to-nis′ĭ-te) the quality of being isotonic.

isotope (i′so-tōp) [*iso-* + Gr. *topos* place] a chemical element having the same atomic number as another (i.e., the same number of nuclear protons) but possessing a different atomic mass (i.e., a

different number of nuclear neutrons). **radioactive i.,** radioisotope. **stable i.,** an isotope that does not transmute into another element with emission of corpuscular or electromagnetic radiations.

isotopology (i″so-to-pol′o-je) the scientific study of isotopes, and of their uses and applications.

isotoxic (i″so-tok′sik) pertaining to an isotoxin.

isotoxin (i″so-tok′sin) [*iso-* + *toxin*] a toxin that is poisonous to other animals of the same species.

isotransplant (i″so-trans′plant) [*iso-* + *transplant*] isograft.

isotransplantation (i″so-trans″plan-ta′shun) the transplanting of an isograft.

isotretinoin (i″so-tret′ĭ-noin) a synthetic form of retinoic acid (13-*cis*-retinoic acid) used orally to clear cystic and conglobate acne.

Isotricha (i-sot′rĭ-kah) a genus of ciliate parasites. *I. intestinalis* and *I. prostoma* are found in the stomachs of cattle.

isotrimorphism (i″so-tri-mor′fizm) [*iso-* + Gr. *treis* three + *morphē* form] isomorphism between the three forms of two trimorphous substances.

isotrimorphous (i″so-tri-mor′fus) pertaining to or characterized by isotrimorphism.

isotron (i′so-tron) an apparatus for separating isotopes electromagnetically.

isotropic (i″so-trop′ik) [*iso-* + Gr. *tropos* a turning] 1. similar in all directions with respect to a property, as in a cubic crystal or a piece of glass. 2. being singly refractive.

isotropy (i-sot′ro-pe) the quality or condition of being isotropic.

isotypical (i″so-tip′ĭ-kal) [*iso-* + *typical*] of the same type.

isouretin (i″so-u-re′tin) formamidoxim, $NH_2CH{:}NOH$, a compound isomeric with urea.

isovalericacidemia (i″so-vah-ler″ik-as″ĭ-de″me-ah) isovaleric acidemia.

isoxepac (i-soks′ĕ-pak) chemical name: 6,11-dihydro-11-oxo-dibenz[*b,e*]-oxepin-2-acetic acid; an anti-inflammatory, $C_{16}H_{12}O_4$.

isoxicam (i-soks′ĭ-kam) chemical name: 4-hydroxy-2-methyl-*N*-(5-methyl-3-isoxazolyl)-2*H*-1,2-benzothiazine-3-carboxamide 1,1-dioxide; an anti-inflammatory, $C_{14}H_{13}N_3O_5S$.

isoxsuprine hydrochloride (i-sok′su-prēn) [USP] chemical name: 4-hydroxy-α-[1-[(1-methyl-2-phenoxyethyl)amino]ethyl]-benzenemethanol hydrochloride. An adrenergic $C_{18}H_{23}NO_3\cdot HCl$, occurring as a white, crystalline powder; used as a vasodilator in the treatment of cerebral vascular insufficiency and of peripheral vascular diseases such as arteriosclerosis obliterans, thromboangiitis obliterans, and Raynaud's disease. It is administered orally or intramuscularly.

isozyme (i′so-zīm) one of the multiple forms in which an enzyme may exist in a different species, the various forms differing chemically, physically, and/or immunologically, but catalyzing the same reaction although with different affinities for the substrate. For example, lactate dehydrogenase may exist in five different forms arising from different tetramer combinations of its two subunits. Called also *isoenzyme.*

issue (is′u) a discharge of pus, blood, or other matter; a suppurating lesion emitting such a discharge.

isthmectomy (is-mek′to-me) [*isthmus* + Gr. *ektomē* excision] excision of an isthmus, particularly the isthmus of the thyroid gland affected with goiter.

isthmi (is′mi) plural of *isthmus.*

isthmian (is′me-an) isthmic.

isthmic (is-mik) pertaining to an isthmus.

isthmitis (is-mi′tis) inflammation of the isthmus of the fauces.

isthmoparalysis (is″mo-pah-ral′ĭ-sis) isthmoplegia.

isthmoplegia (is″mo-ple′je-ah) [*isthmus* + Gr. *plēgē* stroke] paralysis of the isthmus faucium.

isthmospasm (is′mo-spazm″) spasm of an isthmus, as of the isthmus of a uterine tube or of the fauces.

isthmus (is′mus), pl. *isth′mi* [Gr. *isthmos*] a narrow connection between two larger bodies or parts; [NA] a general term for such a connecting structure or region. **anterior i. of fauces,** i. faucium. **i. of aorta, i. aor′tae** [NA], **aortic i.,** a narrowed portion of the aorta, especially noticeable in the fetus, at the point where the ductus arteriosus is attached. **i. of auditory tube,** i. tubae auditivae. **i. of cartilage of auricle, i. cartilag′inis au′ris** [NA], a bridge of cartilage connecting the cartilage of the external acoustic meatus with the main part of the cartilage of the auricle of the external ear. **i. of cingulate gyrus,** i. gyri cinguli. **i. of eustachian tube,** i. tubae auditivae. **i. of fallopian tube,** i. tubae uterinae. **i. of fauces, i. fau′cium** [NA], the constricted aperture between the cavity of the mouth and the pharynx. **i. glan′dulae thyroi′deae** [NA], isthmus of thyroid gland: the band of tissue connecting the lobes of the thyroid gland. **i. gy′ri cin′guli** [NA], **i. gy′ri fornica′ti,** isthmus of cingulate gyrus: the constricted portion of the cingulate gyrus, connecting with the parahippocampal gyrus in the region of the splenium of the corpus callosum. **Haller's i.,** fretum halleri. **i. of His,** i. rhombencephali. **Krönig's i.,** a narrow, ribbon-like area of resonance extending over the shoulder and connecting the larger areas of resonance on the chest and back, overlying the apex of the lung (Krönig's fields). **i. of limbic lobe,** i. gyri cinguli. **oropharyngeal i., pharyngo-oral i.,** i. faucium. **i. prosta′tae** [NA], **i. of prostate,** the commissure on the base of the prostate, between the right and the left lateral lobe. **i. rhombenceph′ali** [NA], **i. of rhombencephalon,** a narrow segment of the brain in the fetus, forming the plane of separation between the rhombencephalon and the cerebrum; called also *i. of His.* **i. of thyroid gland,** i. glandulae thyroideae. **i. tu′bae auditi′vae** [NA], isthmus of auditory tube: the narrowest part of the auditory tube, at the junction of the pars ossea and the pars cartilaginea of the tube. **i. tu′bae uteri′nae** [NA], the narrow part of the uterine tube at its junction with the uterus. **i. ure′thrae,** a constricted part of the urethra, at the junction of the cavernous with the membranous urethra. **i. u′teri** [NA], **i. of uterus,** the constricted part of the uterus between the cervix and the body. **i. of Vieussens,** limbus fossae ovalis.

I.S.U. International Society of Urology.

Isuprel (i′su-prel) trademark for a preparation of isoproterenol.

isuria (i-su′re-ah) [Gr. *isos* equal + *ouron* urine + *-ia*] excretion of urine at a uniform rate.

I.T.A. International Tuberculosis Association.

Itard's catheter (e-tarz′) [Jean Marie Gaspard *Itard,* French otologist, 1774–1838] see under *catheter.*

Itard-Cholewa sign (e-tar′ ko-la′vah) [J. M. G. *Itard;* Erasmus Rudolph *Cholewa,* German physician, born 1845] see under *sign.*

itate (i′tāt) a substance in milk which oxidizes nitrite to nitrate.

itch (ich) 1. a skin disorder marked by itching. 2. (*obs.*) scabies. **Aujesky's i.,** pseudorabies. **bakers′ i.,** any of several inflammatory dermatoses of the hands, especially chronic monilial paronychia, occurring with special frequency in bakers. **barbers′ i.,** 1. tinea barbae. 2. sycosis vulgaris. **barley i.,** grain i. **Caripito i.,** a condition accompanied by rash and itching, developing in seamen visiting the harbor of Caripito (on the San Juan river, in Venezuela), caused by dust or hairs from the wings of moths. **clam diggers′ i.,** swimmers′ i. **copra i.,** a dermatitis affecting those who unload coconuts, caused by the mite *Tyrophagus castellani.* **Cuban i.,** variola minor. **dew i.,** ground i. **dhobie i.,** allergic contact dermatitis caused by catechols in the marking fluid (bhilawanol oil) used on laundry by the native washermen (dhobie) of India. **grain i.,** a dermatitis accompanied by itching, caused by a mite, *Pyemotes ventricosus,* which preys on the larvae of a certain insect which lives on straw, grain, and other plants. The dermatitis affects chiefly persons (grain harvesters, threshers, packers, etc.) who work with the host plants, and sometimes those who handle packaged cereals infested with weevils. Called also *acarodermatitis urticarioides* and *straw-mattress dermatitis.* **grocers′ i.,** a vesicular dermatitis caused by *Glycyphagus domesticus,* found in stored hides, dried fruits, and grain, or *Tyrophagus castellanei* or *T. longior,* found in copra and cheese, respectively. **ground i.,** the itching eruption caused by the entrance into the skin of the larvae of *Necator americanus* or *Ancylostoma duodenale* (see *hookworm disease,* under *disease*). Called also *uncinarial dermatitis.* **jock i.,** tinea cruris. **mad i.,** pseudorabies. **Malabar i.,** tinea imbricata. **mattress i., millers′ i.,** grain i. **miners′ i.,** ground i. **Philippine i.,** variola minor. **seven-year i.,** scabies. **straw i.,** grain i. **swimmers′ i.,** an itching dermatitis caused by penetration of the skin by larval forms (cercaria) of schistosomes; it occurs in bathers in waters infested with these organisms. Called also *clam diggers′ i., cutaneous schistosomiasis,* and *schistosome* or *swimmer's dermatitis.* **winter i.,** an itching of the skin occurring in cold weather, unassociated with structural lesions; called also *pruritus hiemalis.*

itching (ich′ing) an unpleasant cutaneous sensation that provokes the desire to scratch or rub the skin. A symptom in various skin diseases, it may also occur idiopathically. Called also *pruritus.*

iter (i′ter) [L.] a way or tubular passage. **i. ad infundib′ulum,** the passage from the third ventricle of the brain to the infundibulum. **i. chordae anterius,** an opening in the anterior part of the middle ear for exit of the chorda tympani nerve from the tympanic cavity; called also *Huguier's canal.* **i. chordae posterius,** an opening in the posterior part of the middle ear for entrance of the chorda tympani nerve into the tympanic cavity. **i. den′tium,** the area through which a permanent tooth makes its appearance. **i. e ter′tio ad quar′tum ventric′ulum,** aqueductus cerebri. **i. of Sylvius,** aqueductus cerebri.

iteral (i′ter-al) pertaining to an iter.

iteroparity (it″er-o-par′ĭ-te) [L. *iterare* to repeat + *parere* to bear] the state, in an individual organism, of reproducing repeatedly, or more than once in a lifetime.

iteroparous (it″er-op′ah-rus) reproducing more than once in a lifetime.

-ites [Gr. *-itēs,* a masculine termination agreeing with *hydrops* dropsy (understood)—e.g., tympanites, the windy dropsy] a word termination indicating dropsy of the part denoted by the word stem to which it is attached.

ithycyphos (ith″e-si′fōs) ithyokyphosis.

ithylordosis (ith″e-lor-do′sis) [Gr. *ithys* straight + *lordōsis* bending forward] lordosis without any lateral curvature.

ithyokyphosis (ith″e-o-ki-fo′sis) [Gr. *ithys* straight + *kyphos* humped + *-osis*] backward projection of the spinal column.

-itides plural form of *-itis.*

-itis, pl. *-it′ides* [*-itis,* a feminine adjectival termination agreeing with Gr. *nosos* (understood)—e.g., neuritis = Gr. *hē neuritis nosos,* the disease of the nerves, which soon becomes the inflammatory disease] a word termination denoting inflammation of the part indicated by the word stem to which it is attached.

Ito-Reenstierna test (e′to rēn-ster′nah) [Hayazo *Ito,* Japanese pathologist, born 1865; John *Reenstierna,* Swedish dermatologist, born 1882] see under *tests.*

ITP idiopathic thrombocytopenic purpura.

Itrumil (it′roo-mil) trademark for a preparation of iothiouracil.

I.U. immunizing unit; international unit.

IUCD intrauterine contraceptive device.

IUD intrauterine contraceptive device.

I.V. intravenously (by intravenous injection).

ivory (i′vo-re) [L. *ebur, eburneus*] 1. the bonelike substance (modified dentin) of the tusks of elephants or of such large mammals as the walrus. 2. dentin (dentinum [NA]).

I.V.T. intravenous transfusion.

Ivy's method (i′vēz) [Andrew Conway *Ivy,* Chicago, physiologist, born 1893] see *bleeding time,* under *time.*

Iwanoff's (Iwanow's) cysts (e-wan′ofs) [Wladimir P. *Iwanoff* (Iwanow), Russian ophthalmologist, born 1861] see *Blessig's cysts,* under *cyst.*

Ixodes (iks-o′dēz) [Gr. *ixōdes* like bird-lime] a genus of ticks that are parasitic on man and other animals. **I. bicor′nis,** *Rhipicentor bicornis.* **I. canisu′ga,** the British dog tick, a species commonly infesting dogs in Britain; also found in Western Europe and North America. **I. cavipal′pus,** an African tick that infests monkeys and children. **I. fre′quens,** a species that infests cattle, horses, and man in Japan. **I. hexag′onus,** a species that infests wild and domestic carnivores in Europe and Africa. **I. holocy′clus,** a tick, particularly of marsupials, but which causes a tick paralysis in young cattle in New South Wales, and may be the vector of North Queensland tick typhus. **I. pacif′icus,** a common deer and cattle tick of California, which may bite man, and is thought to be a possible vector of tularemia. **I. persulca′tus,** the taiga tick, vector of Russian spring-summer encephalitis. **I. pilo′sus,** a species infesting many animals in South Africa; formerly thought to cause paralysis in sheep. **I. pu′tus,** a species that infests the nests of many marine birds. **I. ra′sus,** a species that attacks a variety of insectivores, rodents, ungulates, carnivores, and occasionally man and other primates in Africa. **I. rici′nus,** the castor bean tick, which is parasitic on cattle, sheep, and wild animals, and transmits the agents of gallsickness, malignant jaundice in dogs, tularemia, louping ill, and Russian spring-summer encephalitis. **I. rubicun′dus,** a species that may cause a tick paralysis in sheep, goats, and cattle in West Africa. A single human case has been reported. **I. scapula′ris,** the black-legged tick of the Eastern United States, which may inflict a painful bite in man. **I. spinipal′pus,** a species that infests rabbits and squirrels in British Columbia, and may transmit Powassan virus.

ixodiasis (iks″o-di′ah-sis) any disease or lesion due to the bite of ticks; infestation with ticks.

ixodic (ik-sod′ik) caused by ticks.

Ixodidae (iks-od′ĭ-de) a family of the superfamily Ixodoidea, comprising the hard ticks, distinguished from the soft-bodied ticks (Argasidae) by the presence of a scutum. It includes the following genera: *Amblyomma, Anocentor, Aponomma, Boophilus, Dermacentor, Haemaphysalis, Hyalomma, Ixodes, Margaropus, Rhipicentor,* and *Rhipicephalus.*

Ixodides (iks-od′ĭ-dēz) the ticks, a suborder of Acarina, including the superfamily Ixodoidea, which comprises the families Ixodidae, or hard ticks, and Argasidae, or soft ticks.

Ixodiphagus (iks″o-dif′ah-gus) a genus of hymenopterans. **I. caucur′tei,** a hymenopteran parasite of ticks of the family Ixodidae.

ixodism (iks′o-dizm) ixodiasis.

Ixodoidea (iks″o-doi′de-ah) a superfamily of the suborder Ixodides, which embraces the families Argasidae, or soft ticks, and Ixodidae, or hard ticks.

Izar's reagent (i′zarz) [Guido *Izar,* Italian pathologist, born 1883] see under *reagent.*

-ize [Gr. *-izō*] a word termination denoting subjection to the specific action or treatment indicated by the stem to which it is affixed, as *adrenalectomize, thyroidectomize,* etc.

J

J symbol for *Joule's equivalent*.

jaagsiekte, jaagziekte (yahg-sēk'tĕ; yahg-zēk'tĕ) [Afrikaans *jag* hunt + *siekte* sickness] a chronic progressive pneumonia of sheep marked by adenomatosis of the alveolar epithelium. Spelled also *jagsiekte* and *jagziekte*.

Jaboulay's amputation (operation), button (zhah″boo-lāz') [Mathieu *Jaboulay*, French surgeon, 1860–1913] see *interpelvi-abdominal amputation*, and see under *button*.

Jaccoud's fever, sign (zhah-kōoz') [Sigismond *Jaccoud*, French physician, 1830–1913] see under *fever* and *sign*.

jacket (jak'et) an enveloping structure or garment, especially a covering for the trunk or for the upper part of the body; see also under *crown*. **Minerva j.,** a plaster-of-Paris jacket reaching from the crest of the ilia to the chin, for fracture of the vertebrae. **plaster-of-Paris j.,** a casing of plaster of Paris enveloping the body for the purpose of correcting deformities. **porcelain j.,** a jacket crown of porcelain. **Sayre's j.,** a plaster-of-Paris jacket used as a support for the spinal column. **strait j.,** see *straitjacket*. **Willock's respiratory j.,** a sort of jacket once used to strengthen the movements of respiration in emphysema of the lungs.

jackscrew (jak'skroo) a device operated by means of a screw in a threaded socket, used in orthodontics to expand the dental arch and move individual teeth.

Jackson's law, etc. (jak'sunz) [John Hughlings *Jackson*, London neurologist, 1835–1911] see under *law, rule, sign,* and *syndrome*.

Jackson's membrane (veil) [Jabez North *Jackson*, surgeon in Kansas City, 1868–1935] see under *membrane*.

Jackson's safety triangle, sign [Chevalier *Jackson*, American laryngologist, 1865–1958] see under *triangle*, and see *asthmatoid wheeze*, under *wheeze*.

Jackson's sign [James *Jackson*, Jr., Boston physician, 1810–1834] see under *sign*, def. 3.

jacksonian epilepsy (jak-so'ne-an) [John Hughlings *Jackson*] see under *epilepsy*.

Jacob (zhah-kob'), François. French biologist, born 1920; cowinner with André Michael Lwoff and Jacques Lucien Monod, of the Nobel prize in medicine and physiology for 1965, for discoveries concerning the genetic control of enzymes and virus synthesis.

Jacob's membrane, ulcer (ja'kubz) [Arthur *Jacob*, Irish ophthalmologist, 1790–1874] see *layer of rods and cones*, under *layer*, and see under *ulcer*.

Jacobaeus operation (yah″ko-ba'us) [Hans Christian *Jacobaeus*, Swedish surgeon, 1879–1937] see under *operation*.

jacobine (ja'ko-bin) a poisonous alkaloid, $C_{18}H_{25}O_6N$, from the composite-flowered plant *Senecio jacobea*; it may cause necrosis of the liver.

Jacobson's anastomosis, etc. (ja'kub-sunz) [Ludwig Levin *Jacobson*, Danish anatomist, 1783–1843] see under *anastomosis, canal, cartilage, nerve, organ, plexus,* and *sulcus*.

Jacobson's retinitis [Julius *Jacobson*, German ophthalmologist, 1828–1889] syphilitic retinitis.

Jacobsthal's test (yak'obz-talz) [Erwin Wolfgang Jakob *Jacobsthal*, Hamburg bacteriologist, born 1879] see under *tests*.

Jacquet's dermatitis (erythema) (zhak-āz') [Leonard Marie Lucien *Jacquet*, French dermatologist, 1860–1914] diaper dermatitis.

jactatio (jak-ta'she-o) [L.] jactitation. **j. cap'itis noctur'na,** rhythmic rolling of the head of a child just before falling asleep.

jactation (jak-ta'shun) jactitation.

jactitation (jak″tĭ-ta'shun) [L. *jactitatio; jactitare* to toss] the tossing to and fro of a patient in acute disease.

jaculiferous (jak″u-lif'er-us) [L. *jaculum* dart + *ferre* to bear] bearing prickles.

Jadassohn's macular atrophy, sebaceous nevus, test (yah'das-ōnz) [Josef *Jadassohn*, German dermatologist in Bern, 1863–1936] see *anetoderma*, see under *nevus*, and see *irrigation test*, under *tests*.

Jadelot's lines (furrows) (zhad-lōz') [Jean François Nicolas *Jadelot*, physician in Paris, 1791–1830] see under *line*.

Jaeger's test types (ya'gerz) [Edward *Jaeger* von Jastthal, Austrian oculist, 1818–1884] see under *test types*.

Jaffé's reaction, test (zhah-fāz') [Max *Jaffé*, German physiologic chemist, 1841–1911] see under *reaction* and *tests*.

jagsiekte, jagziekte (yahg-sēk'tĕ; yahg-zēk'tĕ) jaagsiekte.

Jakob's disease (yak'obz) [Alfons Maria *Jakob*, German psychiatrist, 1884–1931] Creutzfeldt-Jakob syndrome.

Jakob-Creutzfeldt disease (yak'ob-kroits'felt) [Alfons Maria

Jakob; Hans Gerhard *Creutzfeldt*, German psychiatrist, 1885–1964] Creutzfeldt-Jakob disease.

Jaksch's anemia (disease), test (yaksh) [Rudolf von *Jaksch*, physician in Prague, 1855–1947] see *anemia pseudoleukemica infantum*, and see under *tests*.

jalap (jal'ap) [Sp. *jalapa*, from *Jalapa*, a city of Mexico] the dried tuberous root of *Exogonium purga* (Hayne) Lindl. Convolvulaceae; its resins possess cathartic properties.

Janet's disease, test (zhah-nāz') [Pierre Marie Felix *Janet*, French physician, 1859–1947] see *psychasthenia*, and see under *tests*.

Janeway's pills (jān'wāz) [Edward Gamaliel *Janeway*, American physician, 1841–1911] see under *pill*.

Janeway's sphygmomanometer, spots (jān'wāz) [Theodore Caldwell *Janeway*, American physician, 1872–1917] see under *sphygmomanometer* and *spot*.

janiceps (jan'ĭ-seps) [L. *Janus* a two-faced god + *caput* head] a double monster with one head and two opposite faces. **j. asym'metros,** a janiceps with one imperfect and one more complete face. **j. parasit'icus,** a double monster in which there is partial duplication of the head in the frontal plane.

Janin's tetanus (zhah-naz') [Joseph *Janin*, French physician, born 1864] kopf-tetanus.

Janošík's embryo (yan'o-siks) [Jan *Janošík*, Prague anatomist, 1856–1927] see under *embryo*.

Jansen's disease, test [W. Murk *Jansen*, Dutch orthopedic surgeon, 1867–1935] see *metaphyseal dysostosis*, under *dysostosis*, and see under *tests*.

Jansen's operation (yan'senz) [Albert *Jansen*, German otologist, 1859–1933] see under *operation*.

Jansky's classification (jan'skēz) [Jan *Jansky*, Czech psychiatrist, 1873–1921] see under *classification*.

Janthinosoma (jan″thĭ-no-so'mah) a genus of mosquitoes; it is often considered to be a subgenus of the genus *Psorophora*. **J. lut'zi,** a species which transports the eggs of botflies (*Dermatobia*) glued to its abdomen. **J. postica'ta,** a species which also transports the eggs of the botfly.

Jaquet's apparatus (zhah-kāz') [Alfred *Jaquet*, Swiss pharmacologist, 1865–1937] see under *apparatus*.

jar (jar) a wide-mouthed, glass or earthenware container. **bell j.,** a glass vessel, closed at top, open at bottom, used in laboratory vacuum experiments. **Leyden j.,** a glass jar partially covered inside and out with tinfoil or other metal, used as a condenser or collector of electricity.

jararaca (jah″rah-rak'ah) a venomous pit viper, *Bothrops jararaca*, of tropical and southern South America.

Jarcho's pressometer (jahr'kōz) [Julius *Jarcho*, New York obstetrician, born 1882] see under *pressometer*.

jargon (jar'gon) the technical or specialized language used in a profession or other field of activity.

jargonaphasia (jar″gon-ah-fa'ze-ah) a speech defect in which several words are run into one.

Jarisch-Herxheimer reaction (yah'rish-herks'hīm-er) [Adolf *Jarisch*, Austrian dermatologist, 1850–1902; Karl *Herxheimer*, German dermatologist, 1861–1944] see under *reaction*.

Jarjavay's muscle (zhar'zah-vaz) [Jean François *Jarjavay*, French physician, 1815–1868] see under *muscle*.

Jarotzky's (Jarotsky's) treatment (yar-ot'skēz) [Alexander *Jarotzky*, Moscow physician, born 1866] see under *treatment*.

Jarvis' operation (jahr'vis) [William Chapman *Jarvis*, New York laryngologist, 1855–1895] see under *operation*.

Jatropha (jat'ro-fah) [Gr. *iatros* physician + *trophē* nourishment] a genus of tropical euphorbiaceous plants. Various species possess purgative, stomachic, febrifuge, and astringent properties. Common to Mexico and South America. *J. curcas* L. and *J. multifida* L. (physic nut) produce seeds containing a purgative oil and a potentially toxic phytotoxin.

jaundice (jawn'dis) [Fr. *jaunisse*, from *jaune* yellow] a syndrome characterized by hyperbilirubinemia and deposition of bile pigment in the skin, mucous membranes and sclera with resulting yellow appearance of the patient; called also *icterus*. **acholuric j.,** jaundice without bilirubinuria, associated with elevated unconjugated bilirubin that is not excreted by the kidney; seen in hemolytic disease and other forms of unconjugated hyperbilirubinemia. **acholuric familial j.,** hereditary spherocytosis. **anhepatic j., anhepatogenous j.,** yellow appearance of the skin and mucous membranes not caused by liver disease. **black j.,** Winckel's disease. **breast milk j.,** elevated unconjugated bilirubin in some breast-fed infants due to the presence of 5-β-pregnane-3-α-20-β-dial, which inhibits glucuronyl transferase conjugating activity. **Budd's j.,** acute yellow atrophy of the liver; see under *atrophy*. **catarrhal j.** (obs.), infectious hepatitis. **cholestatic j.,** jaundice resulting from an abnormality in the flow of bile, usually accompanied by elevation of serum alkaline phosphatase, retention of bile salts (with resulting pruritus) and varying hypercholesterolemia. The cholestasis may be *extrahepatic,* due to obstruction caused by a stone, stricture, or neoplasm, or *intrahepatic,* which may be due to liver cell disease (e.g., hepatitis), or altered permeability and/or obstruction of the intrahepatic biliary system (as in drug reactions or hepatic infiltrative disease). **chronic acholuric j.,** hereditary spherocytosis. **Crigler-Najjar j.,** see under *syndrome.* **epidemic j.,** viral hepatitis type A. **familial acholuric j.,** hereditary spherocytosis. **febrile j.,** leptospiral j. **hemolytic j.,** hemolytic anemia. **hemorrhagic j.,** leptospiral j. **hepatocellular j.,** jaundice caused by injury to or disease of the liver cells. **hepatogenic j., hepatogenous j.,** that which is due to some disease or disorder of the liver. **homologous serum j., human serum j.,** viral hepatitis type B. **infectious j., infective j.,** 1. infectious hepatitis. 2. leptospiral j. **latent j.,** hyperbilirubinemia without yellow staining of the tissues. **leptospiral j.,** a severe form of leptospirosis characterized by fever, jaundice, myalgia, and occasionally by meningitis and nephritis. Called also *Weil's disease, infectious spirochetal jaundice, icterogenic spirochetosis, spirochetosis icterohaemorrhagica, leptospirosis icterohaemorrhagica,* and *Fiedler's disease.* **malignant j.,** acute yellow atrophy of the liver; see under *atrophy.* **malignant j. of dogs,** canine piroplasmosis. **mechanical j.,** obstructive j. **j. of the newborn,** icterus neonatorum. **nonhemolytic j.,** jaundice caused by an abnormality in the metabolism of bilirubin, and resulting in an excessive accumulation of unconjugated bilirubin in the blood. The various forms include *Crigler-Najjar syndrome, Dubin-Johnson syndrome, Gilbert's disease, physiologic jaundice of newborn, hyperbilirubinemia of premature infant,* and *Rotor's syndrome.* **nonhemolytic j., congenital,** Crigler-Najjar syndrome. **nonhemolytic j., congenital familial,** Crigler-Najjar syndrome. **nuclear j.,** kernicterus. **obstructive j.,** that which is due to an impediment to the flow of the bile from the liver cells to the duodenum. **occult j.** (*obs.*), latent j. **physiologic j.,** mild icterus neonatorum lasting the first few days after birth. **picric acid j.,** jaundice due to picric acid poisoning; seen in munition workers and in malingering soldiers who deliberately ingest picric acid. **post-arsphenamine j.,** jaundice following the administration of arsphenamine. **regurgitation j.,** jaundice attributed to escape of bile from the bile canaliculi into the blood stream and marked by urobilinogen in the urine. **retention j.,** a form of jaundice due to inability of the liver to dispose of the bilirubin provided by the circulating blood. **Schmorl's j.,** kernicterus. **spirochetal j.,** leptospiral j. **Sumatra j.,** a form of leptospirosis endemic in Sumatra, caused by *Leptospira* serotypes and presumed to be similar to Hasami fever and nanukayami. Called also *Rachmat infection.* **toxemic j., toxic j.,** jaundice produced by poisons, such as phosphorus, arseniuretted hydrogen, picric acid, snake venom, etc.

Javal's ophthalmometer (zhah-valz′) [Louis Emile *Javal,* French oculist, 1839–1907] see *ophthalmometer.*

jaw (jaw) either of the two bony structures (mandible and maxilla) in the head of vertebrates, bearing the teeth (in dentate species) and enabling carnivores to seize their prey and others to bite and chew food. **bird-beak j.,** the condition produced by protrusion of the upper jaw; called also *parrot j.* **big j.,** actinomycosis in cattle. **cleft j.,** a deformity of the jaw due to unilateral or bilateral failure of union of the median nasal and maxillary processes in the anterior palatal region, leaving a cleft or clefts through the alveolus. **crackling j.,** noise (crepitation) in the normal or diseased joint associated with jaw movement. **drop j.,** the paralytic stage of rabies in a dog, in which the jaw drops. **Hapsburg j.,** a mandibular prognathous jaw, often accompanied by a thick overdeveloped lower lip (Hapsburg lip), as seen in many members of the Hapsburg family. **lower j.,** mandibula. **lumpy j.,** actinomycosis in cattle. **parrot j.,** bird-beak j. **phossy j.,** phosphonecrosis. **pig j.,** an abnormal protrusion of the upper jaw of the horse, with hypertrophy of the teeth. **pipe j.,** a painful condition of the jaws caused by carrying a tobacco pipe in the mouth. **rubber j.,** a softened condition of the jaw in animals, caused by resorption and replacement of the bone by fibrous tissue, occurring in association with renal osteodystrophy; osteoporosis. **upper j.,** maxilla.

Jaworski's corpuscles (bodies), test (yah-wor′skēz) [Walery *Jaworski,* Polish physician, 1849–1924] see under *corpuscle* and *tests.*

Jeanselme's nodules (zhah-selmz′) [Antoine Edouard *Jeanselme,* French dermatologist, 1858–1935] see under *nodule.*

jecorize (jek′o-rīz) [L. *jecur* liver] to impart to a food the therapeutical qualities of cod liver oil, as by treating milk with ultraviolet ray.

Jectofer (jek′to-fer) trademark for a preparation of iron sorbitex.

jecur (je′kur) [L.] liver.

Jeddah ulcer (jed′ah) [*Jeddah,* a town of Arabia] cutaneous leishmaniasis.

Jeffersonia (jef″er-so′ne-ah) [named for T. *Jefferson,* 1743–1826] a genus of berberidaceous herbs. The root of *J. diphylla* (L.) Pers., of North America, is tonic, diuretic, and expectorant; emetic in large doses.

Jefron (jef′ron) trademark for a preparation of polyferoxe.

jejunal (jĕ-joo′nal) pertaining to the jejunum.

jejunectomy (jĕ″joo-nek′to-me) [*jejuno-* + Gr. *ektomē* excision] excision of the jejunum.

jejunitis (jĕ″joo-ni′tis) inflammation of the jejunum.

jejuno- [L. *jejunum* empty] a combining form denoting relationship to the jejunum.

jejunocecostomy (jĕ-joo″no-se-kos′to-me) [*jejuno-* + *cecum* + Gr. *stoma* opening] the operation of forming an anastomosis between the jejunum and cecum; also, the anastomosis so established.

jejunocolostomy (jĕ-joo″no-ko-los′to-me) [*jejuno-* + *colon* + Gr. *stoma* mouth] the formation of an anastomosis between the jejunum and the colon; also, the anastomosis so formed.

jejunoileal (jĕ-joo″no-il′e-al) pertaining to the jejunum and ileum; connecting the proximal jejunum with the distal ileum.

jejunoileitis (jĕ-joo″no-il″e-i′tis) inflammation of the jejunum and ileum together.

jejunoileostomy (jĕ-joo″no-il″e-os′to-me) [*jejuno-* + *ileum* + Gr. *stoma* mouth] the formation of an anastomosis between the proximal jejunum and the terminal ileum; also, the stoma so created.

jejunojejunostomy (jĕ-joo″no-jĕ″joo-nos′to-me) the operative formation of an anastomosis between two portions of the jejunum; also, the union so established.

jejunorrhaphy (jĕ″joo-nor′ah-fe) [*jejuno-* + Gr. *rhaphē* suture] operative repair of the jejunum.

jejunostomy (jĕ″joo-nos′to-me) [*jejuno-* + Gr. *stomoun* to provide with an opening, or mouth] the surgical creation of a permanent opening between the jejunum and the surface of the abdominal wall; also, the opening so established.

jejunotomy (jĕ″joo-not′o-me) [*jejuno-* + Gr. *temnein* to cut] surgical incision of the jejunum.

jejunum (jĕ-joo′num) [L. "empty"] [NA] that portion of the small intestine which extends from the duodenum to the ileum; called also *intestinum jejunum.*

Jellinek's sign (symptom) (yel′ĭ-neks) [Stefan *Jellinek,* physician in Vienna, born 1871] see under *sign.*

jelly (jel′e) [L. *gelatina*] a soft substance which is coherent, tremulous, and more or less translucent; generally, a colloidal semisolid mass. **cardiac j.,** a gelatinous substance present between the endothelium and myocardium of the embryonic heart, that transforms into the connective tissue of the endocardium. **contraceptive j.,** a nongreasy jelly for introduction into the vagina to prevent conception. **cyclomethycaine sulfate j.** [USP], a preparation containing 90 to 110 per cent of the labeled amount of cyclomethycaine sulfate in a water-soluble, viscous base; used as a local anesthetic, applied topically. **enamel j.,** stellate reticulum. **glycerin j.** [NF], a compound of gelatin, arsenic trioxide, and glycerin, used as a reagent; called also *glycerogelatin.* **lidocaine hydrochloride j.** [USP], a preparation containing 95 to 105 per cent of the labeled amount of lidocaine hydrochloride in a suitable, water-soluble, sterile, viscous base; used as a local anesthetic, applied topically to the mucous membranes. **mineral j.,** petrolatum. **petroleum j.,** petrolatum. **pramoxine hydrochloride j.** [USP], a preparation containing 94 to 106 per cent of the labeled amount of pramoxine hydrochloride; used as a local anesthetic, applied topically. **Wharton's j.,** the soft, jelly-like, homogeneous intercellular substance of the umbilical cord; it gives the reaction for mucin and contains thin collagenous fibers which increase in number with the age of the fetus.

Jendrassik's maneuver (yen-drah′siks) [Ernst *Jendrassik,* physician in Budapest, 1858–1921] see under *maneuver.*

Jenner (jen′er), Edward. An English physician (1749–1823), who developed the process of producing immunity to smallpox by inoculation (vaccination) with cowpox (vaccinia) vaccine.

Jenner's stain (jen′erz) [Louis Leopold *Jenner,* London physician, 1866–1904] see *Table of Stains and Staining Methods.*

jennerian (jen-ne′re-an) named for Edward *Jenner.*

jennerization (jen″er-i-za′shun) production of immunity to a disease by inoculation of an attenuated form of the virus producing the disease.

Jensen's classification (yen′senz) [Orla *Jensen,* Danish physiologic chemist] see under *classification.*

Jensen's sarcoma (tumor), (yen′senz) [Carl Oluf *Jensen,* Danish veterinary pathologist, 1864–1934] see under *sarcoma.*

jerk (jerk) a sudden reflex or involuntary movement. **Achilles j., ankle j.,** triceps surae j. **biceps j.,** biceps reflex. **crossed j.,** adduction of the leg when attempt is made to elicit the quadriceps jerk on the opposite side. **elbow j.,** involuntary flexion of the elbow on striking the tendon of the biceps or triceps muscle. **jaw j.,** jaw reflex. **knee j.,** quadriceps j.

quadriceps j., a twitchlike contraction of the quadriceps muscle, elicited by sharply tapping the patellar ligament; called also *knee j.* **tendon j.,** see under *reflex*. **triceps surae j.,** a twitchlike contraction of the triceps surae muscle, elicited by sharply tapping the muscle or the Achilles tendon; called also *ankle j.*

Jesionek lamp (yes-e′o-nek) [Albert *Jesionek,* Giessen dermatologist, 1870–1935] see under *lamp.*

jessur (jes′er) native Bengal name for Russell's viper.

Jesu Haly see *Ali ben Iza.*

Jewett nail (joo′et) [Eugene Lyon *Jewett,* American surgeon, born 1900] see under *nail.*

jhin jhinia (jin jin′e-ah) an epidemic condition, perhaps a neuromimesis, first noticed in 1935 in Calcutta. It is characterized by a tingling sensation in the sole of one or both feet, especially in the great toe, and often by a feeling of pressure in the head and by trembling of the whole body.

jigger (jig′ger) chigoe.

Jobert's fossa, (zho-bārz′) [Antoine Joseph *Jobert* de Lamballe, French surgeon, 1799–1867] see under *fossa.*

Jocasta complex (jo-kas′tah) see under *complex.*

Jochmann's test (yōk′manz) [Georg *Jochmann,* Berlin internist, 1874–1915] 1. Müller-Jochmann test. 2. antitrypsin test. See under *tests.*

jodbasedow (i″od-bas′e-do) iodine-induced hyperthyroidism.

Joest's bodies (yests) [Ernst *Joest,* Dresden veterinary pathologist, 1873–1926] see under *body.*

Joffroy's reflex, sign (zhof-rwhahz′) [Alexis *Joffroy,* French physician, 1844–1908] see under *reflex* and *sign.*

Johne's bacillus, disease (yo′nez) [Heinrich Albert *Johne,* German pathologist, 1839–1910] see *Mycobacterium paratuberculosis* and under *disease.*

johnin (yo′nin) a filtrate of cultures of Johne's bacillus (*Mycobacterium paratuberculosis*), similar to tuberculin, used to produce a skin reaction (johnin reaction) in testing cattle for Johne's disease.

Johnson's test (john′sonz) [Sir George *Johnson,* English physician, 1818–1896] see under *tests.*

Johnson-Stevens disease (john′son-ste′venz) [Frank Chambliss *Johnson,* 1894–1934; Albert Mason *Stevens,* 1884–1945, American pediatricians] Stevens-Johnson syndrome.

joint (joint) [L. *junctio* a joining, connection] an articulation: the place of union or junction between two or more bones of the skeleton, especially a junction that admits of more or less motion of one or more bones. See also *articulatio* and *junctura.* For English names of specific joints not included here, see under *articulation.* **amphidiarthrodial j.,** amphidiarthrosis. **ankle j.,** articulatio talocruralis. **arthrodial j.,** plane j. **ball-and-socket j.,** spheroidal j. **biaxial j.,** one permitting movement in two of the assumed three mutually perpendicular axes, or having two degrees of freedom, as the ellipsoidal joint. **bilocular j.,** a joint in which the synovial cavity is divided into two compartments by an interarticular cartilage, as the temporomandibular joint. **bleeders' j.,** hemorrhage into a joint in persons of a hemorrhagic diathesis. **Brodie's j.,** hysteric j. **Budin's j.,** a band of cartilage seen at birth between the squamous and the two condylar portions of the occipital bone. **cartilaginous j.,** one in which the components are connected by cartilage; called also *junctura cartilaginea* [NA]. **Charcot's j.,** neuropathic arthropathy. **Chopart's j.,** articulatio tarsi transversa. **Clutton's j.,** painless symmetrical hydrarthrosis, especially of the knee joints, seen in hereditary syphilis. **cochlear j.,** a form of hinge joint which permits of some rotation or lateral motion, as the knee joint. **coffin j.,** the second interphalangeal joint of the foot of a horse. **composite j., compound j.,** a joint in which several bones articulate; articulatio composita [NA]. **condyloid j.,** one in which an ovoid head of one bone moves in an elliptical cavity of another, permitting all movements except axial rotation, as the metacarpophalangeal joints; articulatio condylaris [NA]. **Cruveilhier's j.,** articulatio atlantooccipitalis. **diarthrodial j.,** synovial j. **dry j.,** one affected with chronic villous arthritis. **elbow j.,** the joint between the arm and forearm; see *articulatio cubiti* [NA]. **ellipsoidal j.,** a biaxial joint resembling a ball-and-socket joint, but with the articulating surfaces much longer in one direction than in the direction at right angles, the circumference of the joint thus resembling an ellipse, as the radiocarpal joint; articulatio ellipsoidea [NA]. **enarthrodial j.,** spheroidal j. **facet j's,** the articulations of the vertebral column. **false j.,** pseudarthrosis. **fibrocartilaginous j.,** one in which the participating elements are united by fibrocartilage, usually separated from the bones by thin plates of hyaline cartilage; called also *symphysis.* **fibrous j.,** one in which the components are connected by fibrous tissue; see *junctura fibrosa* [NA]. **flail j.,** one showing abnormal mobility. **freely movable j.,** synovial j. **fringe j.,**

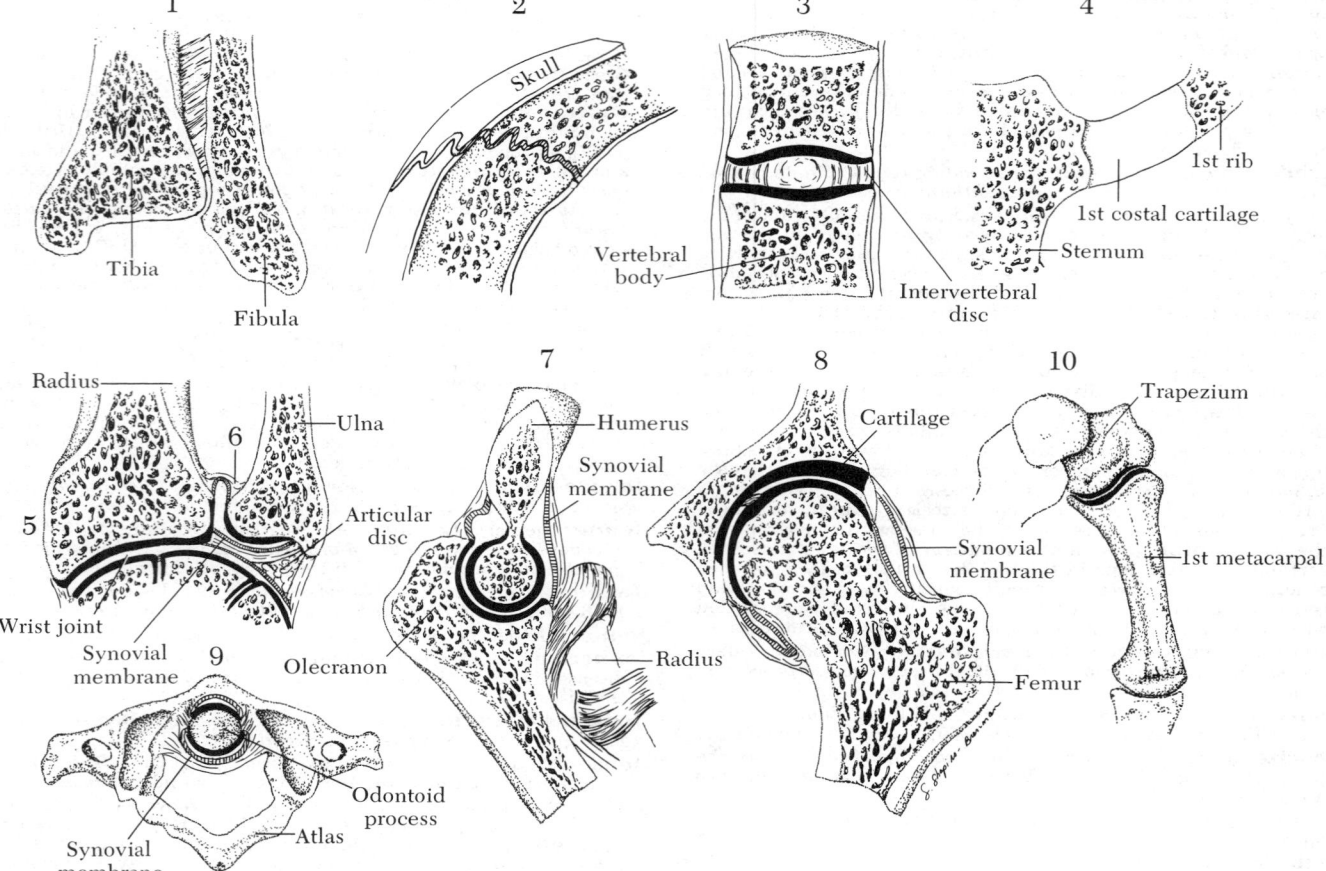

Various kinds of joints: *Fibrous*—1. syndesmosis (tibiofibular). 2. suture (skull). *Cartilaginous*—3. symphysis (vertebral bodies). 4. synchondrosis (1st rib and sternum). *Synovial*—5. condyloid (wrist). 6. gliding (radioulnar). 7. Hinge or ginglymus (elbow). 8. Bell and socket (hip). 9. Pivot (atlantoaxial). 10. Saddle (carpometacarpal of thumb).

one affected with chronic villous arthritis. **ginglymoid j.,** ginglymus. **gliding j.,** plane j. **hemophilic j.,** bleeders' j. **hinge j.,** ginglymus. **hip j.,** the joint formed at the head of the femur and the acetabulum of the hip bone; called also *articulatio coxae* [NA] and *articulation of the hip.* Loosely called hip. **hysteric j.,** a condition which resembles arthritis but is of psychic origin. **immovable j.,** fibrous j. **intercarpal j's,** the articulations between the carpal bones; called also *articulationes intercarpeae* [NA]. **irritable j.,** a joint subject to attacks of inflammation without discoverable cause. **knee j.,** the compound joint between the femur, patella, and tibia; see *articulatio genus* [NA]. **ligamentous j.,** syndesmosis. **Lisfranc's j.,** see *articulationes tarsometatarseae,* under *articulatio.* **j's of Luschka,** a series of jointlike structures at the lateral edges of the vertebral bodies from vertebra C3 to T1, forming small spurlike lips at the upper surface, covered with cartilage, and containing a capsule filled with fluid. They are considered by some to be true diarthrodial joints, and by others to be degenerative spaces of the intervertebral disks filled with extracellular fluid and lined by a membrane formed by fibrocytes. They are frequent sites of spur formation. **midcarpal j.,** the joint between the scaphoid, lunate, and cuneiform bones and the second row of the carpal bones; called also *articulatio mediocarpea* [NA]. **mixed j.,** one combining features of different types of joints. **multiaxial j.,** spheroidal j. **open j.,** a veterinary term for a joint in which the surface of the bones is exposed, as a result of inflammation and sloughing of the tissues. **peg-and-socket j.,** gomphosis. **pivot j.,** a uniaxial joint in which one bone pivots within a bony or an osseoligamentous ring; articulatio trochoidea [NA]. **plane j.,** a type of synovial joint in which the opposed surfaces are flat or only slightly curved; called also *articulatio plana* [NA], *gliding j.,* and *arthrodial j.* **polyaxial j.,** spheroidal j. **rotary j.,** pivot j. **sacrococcygeal j.,** junctura sacrococcygea. **saddle j.,** a joint having two saddle-shaped surfaces at right angles to each other; articulatio sellaris [NA]. **scapuloclavicular j.,** articulatio acromioclavicularis. **sellar j.,** saddle j. **shoulder j.,** articulatio humeri. **simple j.,** a joint in which only two bones articulate; articulatio simplex [NA]. **socket j. of tooth,** gomphosis. **spheroidal j.,** a type of synovial joint in which a spheroidal surface on one bone ("ball") moves within a concavity ("socket") on the other bone, as in the hip joint. Called also *articulatio spheroidea* [NA] and *ball-and-socket j.* **spiral j.,** cochlear j. **stifle j.,** the articulation in quadrupeds corresponding with the knee joint of man, consisting actually of two joints, that between the femur and tibia, and that between the femur and patella. **synarthrodial j.,** fibrous j. **synovial j.,** a special form of articulation permitting more or less free movement; see *junctura*

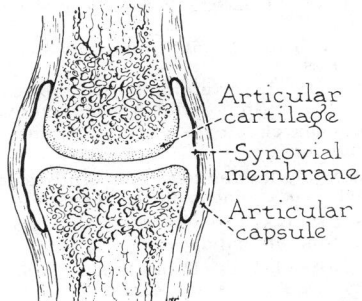

Section of synovial joint (King and Showers).

synovialis [NA]. See illustration. **tarsal j., transverse,** articulatio tarsi transversa. **through j.,** synovial j. **trochoid j.,** pivot j. **uniaxial j.,** one permitting movement in only one of the assumed three mutually perpendicular axes, or having only one degree of freedom, as a hinge joint and the interphalangeal joints. **unilocular j.,** a synovial joint having only one cavity. **von Gies j.,** a chronic syphilitic chondro-osteoarthritis.

Jolles' test (yol′ez) [Adolf *Jolles,* Austrian chemist, born 1863] see under *tests.*

Jolly's bodies (zho-lēz′) [Justin Marie Jules *Jolly,* French histologist, 1870–1953] Howell-Jolly bodies; see under *body.*

Jolly's reaction (yo′lēz) [Friedrich *Jolly,* German neurologist, 1844–1904] see under *reaction.*

Jonas' symptom (yo′nas) [Siegfried *Jonas,* Austrian physician, born 1874] see under *symptom.*

Jones' albumosuria, cylinder, protein (jōnz) see *Bence Jones.*

Jones' nasal splint (jōnz) [John *Jones,* American surgeon, 1729–1791] see under *splint.*

Jones' position (jōnz) [Sir Robert *Jones,* English surgeon, 1858–1933] see under *position.*

Jonnesco's fold, fossa, operation (jo-nes′kŏz) [Thoma *Jonnesco,* Rumanian surgeon, 1860–1926] see *parietoperitoneal fold,* under *fold,* see *recessus duodenalis superior,* and see *sympathectomy.*

Jonston's arc [Johns *Jonston,* Polish physician, 1603–1675] alopecia areata.

josamycin (jo″sah-mi′sin) an antibiotic of unspecified action, $C_{42}H_{69}NO_{15}$.

joule (jōōl) [James Prescott *Joule,* English physicist, 1818–1889] the SI unit of energy and heat, being the work done by a force of 1 newton acting over a distance of 1 meter.

Joule's equivalent (jōōlz) [James Prescott *Joule,* English physicist, 1818–1889] see under *equivalent.*

Jourdain's disease (zhoor-daz′) [Anselme Louis Bernard Berdrillet *Jourdain,* French surgeon, 1734–1816] see under *disease.*

juccuya (ŭ-koo′yah) the ulcerative type of cutaneous leishmaniasis.

juga (joo′gah) [L.] plural of *jugum.*

jugal (joo′gal) [L. *jugalis; jugum* yoke] 1. connecting like a yoke. 2. pertaining to the cheek.

jugale (joo-ga′le) the jugal point; see under *point.*

jugate (joo′gāt) 1. locked together. 2. marked by ridges.

Juglans (joo′glans) [L. "Jove's nut," walnut] a genus of juglandaceous trees; the walnuts. Certain species yield juglone, and *J. cinerea* L. (butternut tree) yields juglans and juglandic acid. The dried inner bark of *J. cinerea* was formerly used as a mild laxative.

juglans (joo′glans) the root bark of *Juglans cinerea,* the butternut tree, formerly used as a mild laxative.

juglone (jug′lōn) chemical name: 5-hydroxy-1,4-naphthoquinone. An antibiotic substance, $C_{10}H_6O_3$, derived from the leaves of certain species of *Juglans* and from walnut shells, which has antihemorrhagic properties and is active against certain fungi.

jugomaxillary (joo″go-mak′sĭ-lār″e) pertaining to the zygomatic bone and the maxilla.

jugular (jug′u-lar) [L. *jugularis: jugulum* neck] 1. pertaining to the neck. 2. a jugular vein.

jugulation (jug″u-la′shun) [L. *jugulare* to cut the throat of] the sudden and rapid arrest of disease by therapeutical measures.

jugum (joo′gum), pl. *ju′ga* [L. "a yoke"] [NA] a general term for a depression or ridge connecting two structures. **alveola′ria mandib′ulae** [NA], depressions on the anterior surface of the alveolar process of the mandible, between the ridges caused by the roots of the incisor teeth. **ju′ga alveola′ria maxil′lae** [NA], the depressions on the anterior surface of the alveolar process of the maxilla, between the ridges caused by the roots of the incisor teeth. **ju′ga cerebra′lia os′sium cra′nii,** cerebral ridges of cranial bones: variable ridges on the inner surface of the cranium, corresponding to the sulci of the brain. **j. pe′nis,** a forceps for compressing the penis. **j. sphenoida′le** [NA], the portion of the body of the sphenoid bone that connects the lesser wings.

juice (jōōs′) [L. *jus* broth] any fluid from an animal or plant tissue; see also *succus.* **appetite j.,** gastric juice secreted during eating and varying in character with the appetite for the food which is being eaten. **cancer j.,** a milky juice obtained from cancerous tissue, and containing cancer cells. **cherry j.,** liquid expressed from the fresh ripe fruit of *Prunus cerasus* L. (Rosaceae) used as an ingredient in preparing flavored vehicles for pharmaceuticals and liqueurs. **gastric j.,** succus gastricus. **intestinal j.,** succus entericus. **pancreatic j.,** succus pancreaticus. **press j.,** liquid obtained by submitting finely ground tissue to great pressure. **raspberry j.,** the liquid expressed from the fresh ripe fruit of varieties of *Rubus idaeus* L. (European red raspberry) or *Rubus strigosus* Michx. (American red raspberry); used in a syrup as a flavored vehicle for drugs.

Jukes family (jooks) see under *family.*

julep (joo′lep) [L. *julapium*] a sweetened alcoholic drink or cordial of various kinds.

jumentous (joo-men′tus) [L. *jumentum,* a beast of burden] having a strong animal odor.

jumping (jump′ing) Gilles de la Tourette's syndrome.

jumping the bite correction of cross-bite.

junction (junk′shun) the place of meeting or of coming together, as of two different organs or types of tissue; see also *joint* and *junctura.* **adherent j.,** zonula adherens. **amelodentinal j.,** dentinoenamel j. **cardioesophageal j.,** esophagogastric j. **cementodentinal j.,** dentinocemental j. **cementoenamel j.,** the line at which the cementum covering the root of a tooth and the enamel covering its crown meet, designated anatomically as the cervical line. **dentinocemental j.,** the plane of meeting between the dentin and cementum on the root of a tooth. **dentinoenamel j.,** the plane of meeting between the dentin and enamel on the crown of a tooth. **dermoepidermal j.,** the plane of meeting between the dermis and epidermis. **esophagogastric j.,** the site of transition from the stratified squamous epithelium of the esophagus to the simple columnar epithelium of the cardia of the stomach; called also *cardioesophageal j.* and *gastroesophageal j.* **fibromuscular j.**, a junction between the muscular elements of the wall of the corpus uteri and the fibrous tissue of the cervix. **gap j.**, a narrowed portion (about 3µm.) of the intercellular space which contains channels (about 2µm. in diameter) linking adjacent cells and through which pass ions, most sugars, amino acids, nucleotides, vitamins, hormones, and cyclic AMP. In electrically excitable tissues, these gap junctions serve to transmit electrical impulses via ionic currents and are known as *electronic synapses;* they are present in such tissues as myocardial tissue. Called also *nexus.* **gastroesophageal j.**, esophagogastric j. **ileocecal j.**, the junction of the ileum and cecum, located at the lower right side of the abdomen and fixed to the posterior abdominal wall. **intermediate j.**, zonula adherens. **manubriogladiolar j.**, synchondrosis sternalis. **mucocutaneous j.**, the site of transition between skin and mucous membrane. **mucogingival j.**, a variable, grossly indistinct but histologically distinct, line marking the separation of the gingival tissue from that of the oral mucosa. **myoneural j.**, the site of apposition (a chemical synapse) between a nerve fiber and the motor endplate of the skeletal muscle which it innervates; the axon terminals of the excited fiber release acetylcholine, which diffuses across the synaptic cleft and becomes transiently bound to receptors of the motor endplate, where it causes electrical changes that result in propagation of an action potential, which in turn induces contraction of the muscle fiber. Called also *neuromuscular j.* **neuromuscular j.**, myoneural j. **occluding j.**, zonula occludens. **osseous j's**, the sites of union of different bones; called also *articulationes* [NA]. **sclerocorneal j.**, the junction between the sclera and the cornea, marked on the outer surface of the eyeball by a slight furrow. **tendinous j's**, conexus intertendineus. **tight j.**, an intercellular junction at which adjacent plasma membranes are joined tightly together by interlinked rows of integral membrane proteins, which create a seal impermeable to intercellular passage of molecules. **ureteropelvic j.**, junction of the ureter and the kidney at the pelvis of the kidney. **ureterovesical j.**, the junction of the bladder and ureter; called also *ureterotrigonal complex.*

junctional (junk′shun-al)   pertaining to a junction.

junctura (junk-tu′rah), pl. *junctu′rae* [L. "a joining"]   a general term used in anatomical nomenclature to designate the site of union between different structures; see also *articulatio* and *joint.* **j. cartilagin′ea** [NA], cartilaginous joint: a form of articulation in which the union of the bony elements is by intervening cartilage; it includes synchondrosis and symphysis. Called also *amphiarthrosis.* **junctu′rae cin′guli mem′bri inferio′-ris** [NA], the articulations of the girdle of the inferior member, i.e., the sacroiliac articulation and the symphysis pubica. **junctu′rae cin′guli mem′bri superio′ris** [NA], the articulations of the girdle of the superior member, i.e., the acromioclavicular and sternoclavicular articulations. **junctu′rae colum′nae vertebra′lis, thora′cis, et cra′nii** [NA], the articulations of the vertebral column, thorax, and cranium. **j. fibro′sa** [NA], fibrous joint: a form of articulation in which the union of the bony elements is by continuous intervening fibrous connective tissue; it includes suture, syndesmosis, and gomphosis. Called also *synarthrosis.* **j. lumbosacra′lis** [NA], the articulation between the sacrum and lumbar vertebrae. **junctu′rae mem′bri inferio′ris li′beri** [NA], the articulations of the free inferior member, i.e., of the thigh, leg, and foot. **junctu′rae mem′bri superio′ris li′beri** [NA], the articulations of the free superior member, i.e., of the arm, forearm, and hand. **j. os′sium**, a joint; see also *articulatio.* **junctu′rae os′sium**, NA alternative for *articulationes;* see *articulatio.* **juncturae os′sium cin′guli extremita′tis pelvi′nae**, juncturae cinguli membri inferioris. **junctu′rae os′sium cin′guli extremita′tis thora′cicae**, juncturae cinguli membri superioris. **j. sacrococcyg′ea** [NA], sacrococcygeal joint: the articulation between the coccyx and the sacrum; called also *symphysis sacrococcygea.* **j. synovia′lis** [NA], synovial joint: a specialized form of articulation permitting more or less free movement, the union of the bony elements being surrounded by an articular capsule enclosing a cavity lined by synovial membrane; called also *diarthrosis.* See illustration under *joint.* **junctu′rae ten′dinum**, conexus intertendineus. **juncturae zygapophysea′les** [NA], the articulations between the articular processes of the vertebrae.

juncturae (junk-tu′re) [L.]   plural of *junctura.*

Jung (yoong), Carl Gustav.   Swiss psychiatrist (1875–1961), founder of the school of analytic psychology, which postulates a collective unconscious of mankind.

Jung's method (yoongz) [Carl Gustav *Jung,* Swiss psychiatrist, 1875–1961]   analytic psychology.

Jung's muscle (yoongz) [Karl Gustav *Jung,* Swiss anatomist, 1794–1864]   musculus pyramidalis auriculae.

Jungbluth's vasa propria (vessels) (yoong′bloots) [Hermann *Jungbluth,* German physician]   see *vasa propria of Jungbluth,* under *vas.*

Jüngling's disease (yeng′lingz) [Otto *Jüngling,* German surgeon, 1884–1944]   sarcoidosis.

juniper (joo′nĭ-per)   1. any of the trees or shrubs of the genus *Juniperus.* 2. the dried ripe fruit of *Juniperus communis* L., or common juniper tree, formerly used as a diuretic; the fruit is used for flavoring certain alcoholic beverages. Called also *juniper berries.*

Juniperus (joo-nip′er-us)   a genus of coniferous trees and shrubs of the family Cupressaceae, including *J. communis* L., the juniper tree, and *J. sabina* L., the evergreen shrub or savin.

junk (junk)   oakum, formerly used in surgical dressings.

Junker inhaler (apparatus, bottle) (junk′er) [Ferdinand Ethelbert *Junker,* English physician of 19th century]   see under *inhaler.*

Junod's boot (zhoo-nōz′) [Victor Theodor *Junod,* French physician, 1809–1881]   see under *boot.*

jurisprudence (joor″is-proo′dens) [L. *juris prudentia* knowledge of law]   the scientific study or application of the principles of law and justice. **dental j.**, the application of the principles of law and justice as they relate to the practice of dentistry. **medical j.**, the application of the principles of law and justice as they relate to the practice of medicine and the relations of physicians to each other and to society in general; called also *forensic medicine.*

jury-mast (joor′e-mast)   an upright bar used in supporting the head in cases of tuberculosis of the spine (Pott's disease).

juscul.   abbreviation for L. *jus′culum,* soup or broth.

jusculum (jus′ku-lum) [L.]   soup or broth.

justo major (jus′to ma′jor)   see *pelvis aequabiliter justo major.*

justo minor (jus′to mi′nor)   see *pelvis aequabiliter justo minor.*

Justus' test (joos′toos) [J. *Justus,* Hungarian dermatologist]   see under *tests.*

jute (jōōt)   the fibers of tropical herbs or undershrubs of *Corchorus capsularis* L. (Tiliaceae), formerly used in surgical dressings.

juvantia (joo-van′she-ah) [L. pl.]   adjuvant and palliative medicines or appliances.

juvenile (joo′vě-nīl)   1. pertaining to youth or childhood; young or immature. 2. a youth or child; a young animal.

juxta- [L. *juxta* near, close by]   a combining form meaning situated near or adjoining.

juxta-articular (juks″tah-ar-tik′u-lar) [L. *juxta* near + *articulus* joint]   situated near a joint or in the region of a joint.

juxtaepiphyseal (juks″tah-ep-ĭ-fiz′e-al) [*juxta-* + *epiphysis*]   near to or adjoining an epiphysis.

juxtaglomerular (juks″tah-glo-mer′u-lar) [*juxta-* + *glomerulus*]   near to or adjoining a glomerulus of the kidney, as juxtaglomerular cells.

juxtangina (juks-tan′jĭ-nah) [L. "almost quinsy"]   inflammation involving the muscles of the pharynx.

juxtaposition (juks″tah-po-zish′un) [*juxta-* + L. *positio* place]   apposition.

juxtapyloric (juks″tah-pi-lor′ik) [*juxta-* + *pylorus*]   situated near the pylorus or the pyloric part of the stomach (see *pars pylorica ventriculi).*

juxtaspinal (juks-tah-spi′nal) [*juxta-* + *spine*]   close to the spinal column.

juxtavesical (juks″tah-ves′ĭ-kal) [*juxta-* + *vesical*]   situated near or adjoining the urinary bladder.

K

K chemical symbol for *potassium* [L. *kalium*].

K. cathode; Kelvin.

k symbol for *constant*.

κ symbol for *magnetic susceptibility*.

Ka. kathode (cathode).

kabure (kah-boo′re) a skin disease in Japan, probably caused by the burrowing of the cercariae of *Schistosoma japonica* in the skin.

Kabyle leprosy (kah-bīl′) [named for a tribe of Berbers of Algeria and Tunisia] see under *leprosy*.

Kader's operation (kah′ders) [Bronislaw *Kader*, Polish surgeon, 1863–1937] see under *operation*.

Kaes' feltwork, line (kiz) [Theodor *Kaes*, German neurologist, 1852–1913] see under *feltwork* and *line*.

Kaes-Bekhterev layer [Theodor *Kaes*; Vladimir Mikhailovich *Bekhterev*, Russian neurologist, 1857–1927] Bekhterev's layer.

Kafka's test (reaction) (kaf′kaz) [Victor *Kafka*, German physician, 1881–1955] see under *tests*.

Kafocin (ka-fo′sin) trademark for a preparation of cephaloglycin.

Kahlbaum's disease (kahl′bowmz) [Karl Ludwig *Kahlbaum*, German physician, 1828–1899] catatonic schizophrenia.

Kahler's disease, law (kah′lerz) [Otto *Kahler*, Austrian physician, 1849–1893] see *multiple myeloma*, and see under *law*.

Kahn's test (kahnz) [Reuben Leon *Kahn*, American bacteriologist, born 1887] see under *tests*, def. 1.

kahweol (kah′we-ol) [Turkish *galweh* coffee] a white crystalline lipid which forms the principal part of the unsaponifiable fraction of coffee.

kaif (kif) [Arabic] dreamy tranquillity from the use of drugs.

kaino- see *ceno-* (def. 1).

kaiserling (ki′zer-ling) 1. Kaiserling's solution. 2. a specimen preserved in Kaiserling's solution.

Kaiserling's method, solution (fixative) (ki′zer-lings) [Karl *Kaiserling*, German pathologist, 1869–1942] see under *method* and *solution*.

kak- for words beginning thus, see also those beginning *cac-*.

kakergasia (kak-er-ga′se-ah) cacergasia.

kakesthesia (kak-es-the′ze-ah) cacesthesia.

kakidrosis (kak-i-dro′sis) [Gr. *kakos* bad + *hidrōs* perspiration + *-osis*] an extremely disagreeable odor of the sweat.

kakke (kahk′ka) [Japanese] beriberi.

kakodyl (kak′o-dil) cacodyl.

kakosmia (kak-oz′me-ah) [Gr. *kakos* bad + *osmē* smell + *-ia*] cacosmia.

kakotrophy (kak-ot′ro-fe) cacotrophy.

kala-azar (kah′lah ah-zar′) [Hindi, "black fever"] an infectious disease with a high fatality rate, occurring along the Mediterranean shore, in West Africa, Mesopotamia, southern Russia, India, North China, South and Central America, and Mexico. It is marked by fever, progressive anemia, wasting, enlargement of the spleen and liver, and dropsy, and is caused by the parasite *Leishmania donovani*, which infects the reticuloendothelial cells, especially of the spleen and liver. It is transmitted to man by the bites of various sandflies of the genus *Phlebotomus*, except in the New World where the main vector is believed to be *Lutzomyia longipalpis*. Called also *febrile tropical splenomegaly, visceral leishmaniasis, Leishman's anemia, Assam fever, Dumdum fever, cachectic fever,* and *black fever* or *sickness*. **canine k.-a.,** Mediterranean k. **infantile k.-a.,** Mediterranean k. **Mediterranean k.-a.,** a form affecting infants, chiefly in countries bordering on the Mediterranean, formerly ascribed to *Leishmania infantum*, which is now regarded as identical with *L. donovani*; called also *canine* or *infantile k.-a.*

kaladana (kal-ah-da′nah) the dried seeds of *Ipomoea nil* L.; used in India and China for its purgative and anthelmintic properties.

kalafungin (kah-lah-fun′jin) an antifungal antibiotic substance produced by *Streptomyces tanashiensis* strain *kala*.

kalagua (kah-lah′gwah) a drug used in South America in the treatment of tuberculosis.

kalemia (kah-le′me-ah) [L. *kalium* potassium + Gr. *haima* blood + *-ia*] the presence of potassium in the blood; see *hyperkalemia*.

kali (ka′li, kah′le) [Ger.] potash. **k. arsenico′sum,** potassium arsenite solution; see under *solution*.

kaliemia (ka-le-e′me-ah) kalemia.

kaligenous (ka-lij′e-nus) [*kalium* + Gr. *gennan* to produce] producing potash.

kalimeter (kah-lim′ĕ-ter) alkalimeter.

kaliopenia (ka″le-o-pe′ne-ah) [L. *kalium* potassium + Gr. *penia* poverty] hypokalemia.

kaliopenic (ka″le-o-pe′nik) pertaining to, characterized by, or producing kaliopenia.

kalium (ka′le-um) [L.] potassium.

kaliuresis (ka″le-u-re′sis) [L. *kalium* potassium + Gr. *ourēsis* a making water] the excretion of potassium in the urine.

kaliuretic (ka″le-u-ret′ik) 1. pertaining to, characterized by, or promoting kaliuresis. 2. an agent that promotes kaliuresis.

kallak (kal′ak) [Eskimo for disease of the skin] a pustular dermatitis occurring in the Eskimos.

kallidin (kal′lĭ-din) a type of kinin liberated by the action of kallikrein on a globulin of blood plasma. Two forms have been identified: *kallidin I* is the same as bradykinin; *kallidin II* is a decapeptide composed of bradykinin with an N-terminal lysine added.

Kallikak family (kal′ĭ-kak) [Gr. *kallos* beauty + *kakos* bad] see under *family*.

kallikrein (kal″lĭ-kre′in) any of a group of peptide hydrolases of the subgroup serine proteinases present in blood plasma and in various glands, such as the pancreas and salivary glands, as well as in urine and lymph. Their major action is the liberation of polypeptides called kinins (bradykinin and kallidin) from kininogens of the plasma α-2-globulins. Called also *kininogenin* and *kininogenase*.

kallikreinogen (kal″lĭ-kri′no-jin) the inactive precursor of kallikrein, which is normally present in blood; its conversion into kallikrein may be triggered by a variety of physical or chemical changes. For example, the Hageman factor activates plasma kallikreinogen.

Kalmia (kal′me-ah) a genus of ericaceous shrubs, the leaves of which have been used in syphilis, diarrhea, and chronic inflammatory disorders, and are thought to possess cardiac and sedative properties; *K. latifolia* L. (mountain laurel) and other related species yield the poisonous principle andromedotoxin.

Kalmuk idiocy (kal′mook) [*Kalmuk*, a Mongolian people in Asia and Russia] severe mental retardation associated with Down's syndrome.

kaluresis (kal″u-re′sis) kaliuresis.

kaluretic (kal″u-ret′ik) kaliuretic.

kalymana-bacterium (kal″ĭ-ma′na bak-te′re-um) a Brazilian term for *Donovania granulomatis*, the organism causing granuloma inguinale.

kamala (kam′ah-lah) the glands and hairs of the capsules of *Mallotus philippinensis* Muell.-Arg. (Euphorbiaceae), an East Indian shrub; it has been used as a purgative and is used in veterinary medicine as a teniacide. Called also *rottlera*.

Kaminer's reaction (kam′ĭ-ner) [Gisa *Kaminer*, Vienna physician, 1883–1941] Freund's reaction.

kanamycin (kan″ah-mi′sin) chemical name: *O*-3-amino-3-deoxy-α-D-glucopyranosyl-(1→6)-*O*-[6-amino-6-deoxy-α-D-glucopyranosyl-(1→4)]-2-deoxy-D-streptamine. A water-soluble antibiotic derived from *Streptomyces kanamyceticus*, first isolated in Japan in 1957; it is effective against some gram-positive, many gram-negative, and some acid-fast bacteria. **k. sulfate** [USP], the sulfate salt of kanamycin, $C_{18}H_{36}N_4O_{11} \cdot H_2SO_4$, occurring as a white, crystalline powder; used especially in the treatment of infections due to gram-negative bacteria, such as *Klebsiella*, *Aerobacter*, some *Proteus* species, *Serratia*, an *Escherichia coli*, and has been used in the treatment of pulmonary tuberculosis, administered orally, intramuscularly, and intravenously.

Kanavel's sign (kan-a′velz) [Allen Buchner *Kanavel*, Chicago surgeon, 1874–1938] see under *sign*.

kangaroo (kang″gah-roo′) a marsupial mammal of Australasia; a tendon is derived from its tail that is valued as a ligature.

kansasii (kan-sas′e-in) a product prepared from *Mycobacterium kansasii*, comparable to tuberculin, used in a cutaneous test of hypersensitivity.

Kantrex (kan′treks) trademark for preparations of kanamycin.

kanyemba (kan″e-em′bah) an acute rectitis of unknown cause, reported from South America and Northern Rhodesia.

Kaochlor (ka′o-klōr) trademark for a preparation of potassium chloride.

kaodzera (kah″od-ze′rah) Rhodesian trypanosomiasis.

kaolin (ka′o-lin) [USP] a native hydrated aluminum silicate, powdered and freed from gritty particles by elutriation. A soft white or yellowish white powder with a claylike taste, used as an adsorbent and in kaolin mixture with pectin. Called also *argilla*, *bolus alba*, and *China clay*.

kaolinosis (ka″o-lin-o′sis) pneumoconiosis caused by inhaling particles of kaolin.

Kaon (ka′on)   trademark for preparations of potassium gluconate.

Kaplan's test (kap′lanz) [David M. *Kaplan*, New York physician, born 1870]   see under *tests.*

Kaposi's sarcoma, varicelliform eruption (kap′o-sēz) [Moritz *Kaposi* (Moritz Kaposi Kohn), Austrian dermatologist, 1837–1902]   see under *eruption* and *sarcoma.*

Kappadione (kap″pah-di′ōn)   trademark for a preparation of menadiol sodium diphosphate.

Kappeler's maneuver (kap′ĕ-lerz) [Otto *Kappeler*, German surgeon, 1841–1909]   see under *maneuver.*

kaps-   for words beginning thus, see those beginning *caps-.*

kara-kurt (kah′rah-koort″)   the venomous Russian spider *Latrodectus lugubris.*

karaya (kar′a-ah)   see under *gum.*

Karell's diet, treatment (cure) (kah′relz) [Philip *Karell*, Russian physician, 1806–1886]   see under *diet* and *treatment.*

Karroo syndrome (kah-roo′) [*Karroo*, region of South Africa]   see under *syndrome.*

Kartagener's syndrome (triad) (kar-tag′ĕ-nerz) [Manes *Kartagener*, German physician]   see under *syndrome.*

Karyamoebina falcata (kar″e-am-ĕ-bi′nah fal-ka′tah)   *Entamoeba histolytica.*

karyapsis (kar″e-ap′sis) [*karyo-* + Gr. *hapsis* joining]   union of nuclei in a conjugating cell.

karyenchyma (kar″e-en′kĭ-mah) [*karyo-* + Gr. *enchymos* juicy]   karyolymph.

karyo- (kar′e-o) [Gr. *karyon* nucleus, or nut]   a combining form denoting relationship to a nucleus; see also words beginning *caryo-.*

karyochromatophil (kar″e-o-kro-mat′o-fil) [*karyo-* + Gr. *chrōma* color + *philein* to love]   having a stainable nucleus.

karyochrome (kar′e-o-krōm″) [*karyo-* + Gr. *chrōma* color]   a nerve cell the nucleus of which is deeply stainable, while the body is not; its nucleus is larger than that of a cytochrome, and there are varieties designated by Greek letters.

karyochylema (kar″e-o-ki-le′mah)   karyolymph.

karyoclasis (kar″e-ok′lah-sis)   karyoklasis.

karyoclastic (kar″e-o-klas′tik)   karyoklastic.

karyocyte (kar″e-o-sīt) [*karyo-* + *-cyte*]   a nucleated cell.

karyogamic (kar″e-o-gam′ik) [*karyo-* + Gr. *gamos* marriage]   pertaining to or characterized by union of nuclei.

karyogamy (kar″e-og′ah-me) [*karyo-* + Gr. *gamos* marriage]   cell conjugation with union of nuclei.

karyogen (kar′e-o-jen″) [*karyo-* + Gr. *gennan* to produce]   an organic iron compound found in certain cell nuclei, especially the head of the spermatozoon.

karyogenesis (kar″e-o-jen′ĕ-sis) [*karyo-* + Gr. *genesis* production]   the development of the nucleus of a cell.

karyogenic (kar″e-o-jen′ik)   forming the nucleus of a cell; pertaining to karyogenesis.

karyogonad (kar″e-o-go′nad) [*karyo-* + Gr. *gonē* seed]   micronucleus, def. 1.

karyokinesis (kar″e-o-ki-ne′sis) [*karyo-* + Gr. *kinesis* motion]   the phenomena involved in division of the nucleus, usually an early stage in the process of cell division, or mitosis. **asymmetrical k.,** mitosis in which the chromosomes divide unequally and into dissimilar masses. **hyperchromatic k.,** mitosis in which the number of chromosomes is abnormally large. **hypochromatic k.,** mitosis in which the number of chromosomes is abnormally small.

karyokinetic (kar″e-o-ki-net′ik)   pertaining to or of the nature of karyokinesis.

karyoklasis (kar″e-ok′lah-sis) [*karyo-* + Gr. *klasis* breaking]   the breaking down of the cell nucleus or nuclear membrane.

karyoklastic (kar″e-o-klas′tik)   1. breaking down cell nuclei. 2. arresting mitosis.

karyolobic (kar″e-o-lo′bik)   having a lobe-shaped nucleus.

karyology (kar″e-ol′o-je) [*karyo-* + *-logy*]   the branch of cytology which deals with the cell nucleus.

karyolymph (kar′e-o-limf″) [*karyo-* + *lymph*]   the liquid part of a cell nucleus, as contrasted with the chromatin and linin.

karyolysis (kar″e-ol′ĭ-sis) [*karyo-* + Gr. *lysis* dissolution]   a form of necrobiosis in which the nucleus of a cell swells and gradually loses its chromatin.

Karyolysus lacertarum (kar-e-ol′ĭ-sus las-er-ta′rum) [*karyo-* + Gr. *lyein* to loose]   a coccidian parasite from the blood of lizards.

karyolytic (kar″e-o-lit′ik)   producing or pertaining to karyolysis; destroying cell nuclei.

karyomegaly (kar″e-o-meg′ah-le) [*karyo-* + Gr. *megalē* great]   abnormal enlargement of the nucleus of a cell, not caused by polyploidy.

karyomere (kar′e-o-mēr″)   1. chromomere (def. 1). 2. a vesicle containing only a small portion of the typical nucleus, usually following abnormal mitosis.

karyometry (kar″e-om′ĕ-tre) [*karyo-* + Gr. *metron* measure]   measurement of a cell nucleus.

karyomicrosome (kar″e-o-mi′kro-sōm) [*karyo-* + *microsome*]   nucleomicrosome.

karyomit (kar′e-o-mit) [*karyo-* + Gr. *mitos* thread]   a chromatin thread of the nuclear network.

karyomitome (kar″e-om′ĭ-tōm)   the nuclear chromatin network.

karyomitosis (kar″e-o-mi-to′sis)   division of the nucleus of a cell preceding mitosis.

karyomitotic (kar″e-o-mi-tot′ik)   pertaining to karyomitosis.

karyomorphism (kar″e-o-mor′fizm) [*karyo-* + Gr. *morphē* form]   the shape of a cell nucleus.

karyon (kar′e-on) [Gr. *karyon* nucleus]   the nucleus of a cell.

karyophage (kar′e-o-fāj″) [*karyo-* + Gr. *phagein* to eat]   a protozoon that exercises phagocytic action on the nucleus of the cell it infects.

karyoplasm (kar′e-o-plazm″) [*karyo-* + Gr. *plasma* plasm]   the nucleoplasm, or protoplasm of the nucleus of a cell.

karyoplasmic (kar″e-o-plaz′mik)   pertaining to karyoplasm.

karyoplast (kar′e-o-plast)   the nucleus of a cell.

karyoplastin (kar″e-o-plas′tin)   the substance of a mitotic spindle; the parachromatin.

karyopyknosis (kar″e-o-pik-no′sis)   shrinkage of a cell nucleus, with condensation of the chromatin into a solid, structureless mass or masses.

karyopyknotic (kar″e-o-pik-not′ik)   pertaining to, characterized by, or causing karyopyknosis.

karyoreticulum (kar″e-o-re-tik′u-lum) [*karyo-* + *reticulum*]   the fibrillar part of the karyoplasm as distinguished from the fluid part of karyolymph.

karyorrhectic (kar″e-o-rek′tik)   pertaining to, characterized by, or causing karyorrhexis.

karyorrhexis (kar″e-o-rek′sis) [*karyo-* + Gr. *rhēxis* a breaking]   rupture of the cell nucleus in which the chromatin disintegrates into formless granules which are extruded from the cell.

karyosome (kar′e-o-sōm″) [*karyo-* + Gr. *sōma* body]   any of the condensed irregular clumps of chromatin dispersed in the chromatin network of a cell; called also *net knot, false nucleolus, chromatin nucleolus, chromatin reservoir,* and *chromocenter.*

karyospherical (kar″e-o-sfer′ĕ-kal)   possessing a spherical nucleus.

karyostasis (kar″e-os′tah-sis) [*karyo-* + Gr. *stasis* halt]   the so-called resting stage of the nucleus between mitotic divisions.

karyota (kar″e-o′tah)   nucleated cells.

karyotheca (kar″e-o-the′kah) [*karyo-* + Gr. *thēkē* sheath]   nuclear membrane.

karyotin (kar′e-o-tin)   chromatin.

karyotype (kar′e-o-tīp) [*karyo-* + *type*]   the chromosomal constitution of the nucleus of a cell; by extension, the photomicrograph of chromosomes arranged according to the Denver classification. Cf. *idiogram,* and see illustration accompanying *chromosome.*

karyotypic (kar″e-o-tip′ik)   pertaining to or representative of the karyotype.

karyozoic (kar″e-o-zo′ik) [*karyo-* + Gr. *zōon* animal]   existing in or inhabiting the nuclei of cells, as do certain protozoa.

kasai (kah-si′)   a syndrome occurring in the Congo, characterized by anemia, depigmentation of the skin, and edema, all of which may be secondary to iron deficiency.

kasal (ka′sal)   chemical name: basic sodium aluminum phosphate; a food additive, $Na_8Al_2(OH)_2(PO_4)_4$, with about 30 per cent dibasic sodium phosphate.

kat   symbol for katal.

kat-, kata- [Gr. *kata* down]   prefix meaning down, against. For words beginning thus, see also those beginning *cat-, cata-.*

katachromasis (kat″ah-kro′mah-sis)   the process by which the daughter chromosomes reconstruct the daughter nuclei.

katadidymus (kat″ah-did′ĭ-mus) [*kata-* + Gr. *didymos* twin]   a twin monster divided above, but single toward the podalic pole (monstra duplicia katadidyma—Förster).

katal (kat′al)   a unit of measurement proposed to express activities of all catalysts, including enzymes, being that amount of a catalyst, such as an enzyme, which catalyzes a reaction rate of 1 mole of substrate per second. Symbol kat.

katalase (kat′ah-lās)   catalase.

kataphylaxis (kat″ah-fi-lak′sis)   the transport of phylactic agents to the site of infection.

katathermometer (kat″ah-ther-mom′ĕ-ter)   a pair of alcoholic thermometers, one with a dry bulb and one with a wet bulb. They are heated to 110° F., exposed to the air, and the time noted that it takes each bulb to fall from 100° to 90° F. From this the temperature as it affects the body can be deduced.

Katayama (kat′ah-yah′mah)   *Oncomelania.*

Katayama disease (kat″ah-yah′mah) [*Katayama*, a genus of snails] schistosomiasis japonica.

Katayama's test (kat″ah-yah′mahz) [Kunika *Katayama*, Japanese physician, 1856–1931] see under *tests*.

katechin (kat′e-chin) Blum's term for a blood constituent which has an antithyroid effect; called also *Blum substance*.

katharometer (kath″ah-rom′ĕ-ter) an instrument for electrometric determination of basal metabolic rates.

kathepsin (kah-thep′sin) cathepsin.

kathisophobia (kath″i-so-fo′be-ah) akathisia.

katholysis (kah-thol′ĭ-sis) electrolysis with the cathode needle.

katine (ka′tin) an alkaloid, d-norpseudoephedrine, $C_9H_{13}NO$, from *Catha edulis* Forsk. (Celastraceae); it acts on the nervous system like cocaine, but has no local anesthetic properties, and is used as an appetite depressant and mild euphoriant. The leaves are used as tea and masticatory in Ethiopia, East and South Africa, and Yemen.

kation (kat′e-on) cation.

katolysis (kah-tol′ĭ-sis) [Gr. *katō* below + *lysis* dissolution] the incomplete or intermediate conversion of complex chemical bodies into simpler compounds; applied especially to digestive processes.

katophoria (kat″o-for′re-ah) katotropia.

katotropia (kat″o-tro′pe-ah) [Gr. *katō* below + *trepein* to turn] deviation of the visual axes below the object looked at; called also *katophoria*.

Katz formula [Johann Rudolf *Katz*, German colloid chemist, 1880–1938] see under *formula*.

katzenjammer (kats′en-yam′er) [Ger.] the symptoms of headache, nausea, possibly cerebral edema, and functional neuritis, following ingestion of alcohol; hangover.

Kay Ciel (ka′sēl) trademark for preparations of potassium chloride.

Kayexalate (ka-ek′sah-lāt) trademark for a preparation of sodium polystyrene sulfonate.

Kayser's disease (ki′zers) [Bernhard *Kayser*, German ophthalmologist, 1869–1954] hepatolenticular degeneration.

Kayser-Fleischer ring (ki′zer flīsh′er) [Bernhard *Kayser*; Bruno *Fleischer*, Munich physician, 1848–1904] see under *ring*.

KBr Potassium bromide.

kc. kilocycle.

KC₂H₃O₂ potassium acetate.

KCl potassium chloride.

KClO₃ potassium chlorate.

K₂CO₃ potassium carbonate.

kc.p.s. kilocycles per second.

KCT kathodal (cathodal) closing tetanus.

Keating-Hart's fulguration (method, treatment) (ke′ting-harts) [Walter Valentine de *Keating-Hart*, French physician, 1870–1922] see *fulguration*.

kebocephaly (keb″o-sef′ah-le) cebocephaly.

ked (ked) the sheep tick, *Melophagus ovinus*.

Keegan's operation (ke′ganz) [Denis Francis *Keegan*, English surgeon, 1840–1920] see under *operation*.

keel (kēl) a septicemic enteritis of ducklings caused by *Salmonella anatum*.

Keeley cure (ke′le) [Leslie E. *Keeley*, American physician, 1834–1900] see *cure*.

Keen's operation, sign (kēnz) [William Williams *Keen*, Philadelphia surgeon, 1837–1932] see *omphalectomy*, and see under *sign*.

Keflex (kef′leks) trademark for a preparation of cephalexin.

Keflin (kef′lin) trademark for a preparation of cephalothin sodium.

Kefzol (kef′zōl) trademark for a preparation of cefazolin sodium.

Kehr's incision, operation (kārz) [Hans *Kehr*, German surgeon, 1862–1916] see under *incision* and *operation*.

Kehrer's reflex (kār′erz) [Ferdinand *Kehrer*, German neurologist, born 1883] see under *reflex*.

keirospasm (ki′ro-spazm) [Gr. *keirein* to shear + *spasm*] an occupational neurosis affecting barbers, characterized by spasmodic contraction of the muscles of the fingers, hand, and forearm.

Keith's bundle, node (kēths) [Sir Arthur *Keith*, London anatomist, 1866–1955] see under *bundle*, and see *sinoatrial node*, under *node*.

Keith's low ionic diet [Norman M. *Keith*, American physician, born 1885] see under *diet*.

Keith-Flack node [Sir Arthur *Keith*; Martin William *Flack*, physiologist in London, 1882–1931] sinoatrial node.

kelectome (ke′lek-tōm) [Gr. *kēlē* tumor + *ektomē* excision] a device used in removing specimens of tissue from tumors.

Kelene (kel′ēn) trademark for a preparation of ethyl chloride.

Kelling's test (kel′ings) [Georg *Kelling*, German physician, born 1866] see under *tests*.

Kelly's operation (kel′ēz) [Joseph Dominic *Kelly*, otolaryngologist in New York, born 1888] arytenoidopexy.

Kelly's operation, sign, speculum (kel′ēz) [Howard Atwood *Kelly*, American surgeon, 1858–1943] see under *operation* (def. 1), *sign*, and *speculum*.

keloid (ke′loid) [Gr. *kēlē* tumor + *eidos* form] a sharply elevated, irregularly-shaped, progressively enlarging scar due to the formation of excessive amounts of collagen in the corium during connective tissue repair. **acne k.**, keloidal folliculitis. **Addison's k.**, morphea. **Alibert's k., cicatricial k., false k.** (*obs.*), a growth resembling a true keloid, but resulting from hypertrophy of a cicatrix. **k. of gums**, fibromatosis gingivae.

kelosomus (ke-lo-so′mus) celosomus.

kelotomy (ke-lot′o-me) [Gr. *kēlē* a rupture + *temnein* to cut] herniotomy.

kelp (kelp) any of various large brown marine algae of the genus *Laminaria*, which are widely used as food in the Orient, and are the source of alginates.

kelvin (kel′vin) [after Lord *Kelvin*] the SI unit of thermodynamic temperature equal to 1/273.15 of the absolute temperature of the triple point of water. See also *absolute temperature*, under *temperature*, and *Kelvin scale*, under *scale*. Abbreviated K.

Kelvin scale (kel′vin) [Lord *Kelvin* (William Thompson), British physicist, 1824–1907] see under *scale*.

Kemadrin (kem′ah-drin) trademark for a preparation of procyclidine hydrochloride.

Kempner diet (kemp′ner) [Walter *Kempner*, American physician, born 1903] see under *diet*.

Kenacort (ken′ah-kort) trademark for preparations of triamcinolone.

Kenalog (ken′ah-log) trademark for preparations of triamcinolone acetonide.

Kendall's method (ken′dahlz) [Edward Calvin *Kendall*, American chemist, 1886–1972, noted for his work on hormones, especially the adrenal steroids; co-winner, with P. S. Hench and T. Reichstein, of the Nobel prize for physiology and medicine in 1950] see under *method*.

Kennedy's syndrome (ken′ĕ-dēz) [Foster *Kennedy*, New York neurologist, 1884–1952] see under *syndrome*.

Kenny's treatment (method) (ken′e) [Sister Elizabeth *Kenny* of Brisbane, Australia, later in U.S.A., 1886–1952] see under *treatment*.

keno- [Gr. *kenos* empty] a combining form denoting empty; see also words beginning *ceno-*.

kenotoxin (ke′no-tok-sin) [*keno-* + *toxin*] the toxin of fatigue; produced in muscle by muscular contractions.

Kent's bundle (kents) [Albert Frank Stanley *Kent*, English physiologist, 1863–1958] see under *bundle*.

Kent-His bundle [A. F. S. *Kent*; Wilhelm *His*, Jr.] bundle of His.

kentrokinesis (ken″tro-ki-ne′sis) centrokinesia.

kentrokinetic (ken″tro-ki-net′ik) centrokinetic.

kephal- for words beginning thus, see those beginning *cephal-*.

Kepone (ke′pōn) trademark for a polychlorinated ketone, $C_{10}Cl_{10}O$, used as an insecticide; workers exposed to this nonbiodegradable compound have suffered neurologic symptoms, such as tremors and slurred speech.

Kerandel's sign (symptom) (ker″an-delz′) [Jean François *Kerandel*, French colonial physician, 1873–1934] see under *sign*.

keraphyllocele (ker″ah-fil′o-sēl) [Gr. *keras* horn + *phyllon* leaf + *kēlē* tumor] keratoma, def. 2.

kerasin (ker′ah-sin) a cerebroside, $C_{48}H_{93}O_8N$, obtained from brain tissue; it yields galactose, sphingosine, and lignoceric acid on hydrolysis.

keratalgia (ker″ah-tal′je-ah) [*kerato-* + *-algia*] pain in the cornea.

keratan sulfate (ker′ah-tan) a sulfated mucopolysaccharide, including *keratan sulfate I* and *keratan sulfate II*, which contain N-acetyl glucosamine and galactose instead of uronic acid; II also contains D-acetylgalactosamine. Keratan sulfate is an important component of the proteoglycan of cartilage and occurs in the cornea and the nucleus pulposus. It is also an accumulation product in Morquio's syndrome. Called also *keratosulfate*.

keratectasia (ker″ah-tek-ta′ze-ah) [*kerato-* + Gr. *ektasis* extension] protrusion of a thinned, scarred cornea; called also *corneal ectasia*.

keratectomy (ker″ah-tek′to-me) [*kerato-* + Gr. *ektomē* excision] excision of a portion of the cornea, usually done for anterior staphyloma.

keratic (ker-at′ik) 1. pertaining to keratin. 2. pertaining to the cornea.

keratin (ker′ah-tin) a scleroprotein which is the principal constituent of epidermis, hair, nails, horny tissues, and the organic matrix of the enamel of the teeth. It is a very insoluble protein, contains high amounts of sulfur as cystine, and also yields tyrosine and leucine on decomposition. Its solution in glacial acetic acid or ammonia is sometimes used in coating pills when the latter are desired to pass through the stomach unchanged. **false k.,** pseudokeratin.

keratinase (ker′ah-tĭ-nās) a proteolytic enzyme that hydrolyzes keratin; one form occurs in the intestinal secretion of larva of the clothes moth and aids in the breakdown of wool keratin.

keratinization (ker″ah-tin″ĭ-za′shun) the development of or conversion into keratin.

keratinize (ker′ah-tin-īz) to make, or become, keratinous.

keratinocyte (kĕ-rat′ĭ-no-sīt) the epidermal cell which synthesizes keratin; constituting 95 per cent of the epidermal cells and, with the melanocyte, forming the binary cell system of the epidermis. In its various successive stages it is known as basal cell, prickle cell, and granular cell. Called also *malpighian cell.*

keratinoid (ker′ah-tin-oid) a form of keratin-coated tablet not soluble in the stomach, but readily soluble in the intestine.

keratinosome (kĕ-rat′ĭ-no-sōm″) a cellular membrane-coating granule.

keratinous (ke-rat′ĭ-nus) containing or of the nature of keratin.

keratitis (ker″ah-ti′tis) [*kerato-* + *-itis*] inflammation of the cornea. **acne rosacea k.,** a severe keratitis associated with acne rosacea of the cornea and eyelids. **actinic k.,** a form due to the action of ultraviolet light. **aerosol k.,** keratitis following direct exposure of the eye to chemical sprays from aerosol cans, including hair spray, insecticides, etc. **alphabet k.,** striate k. **k. arbores′cens,** dendriform k. **artificial silk k.,** keratitis occurring among workers in artificial silk manufacture; it is marked by blurring of vision with the appearance of haloes around lights. **band k., band-shaped k., k. bandelette,** ribbon-like k. **k. bullo′sa,** the formation of large or small bullae or blebs upon the cornea. **deep k.,** interstitial k. **dendriform k., dendritic k.,** herpetic keratitis resulting in a branching ulceration of the cornea. **desiccation k.,** lagophthalmic k. **Dimmer′s k.,** k. nummularis. **disciform k., k. discifor′mis,** keratitis with the formation of a round or oval, disklike opacity of the cornea. **exposure k.,** lagophthalmic k. **fascicular k.,** keratitis attended by the formation of a band of blood vessels. **k. filamento′sa,** keratitis with twisted filaments of mucoid material on the surface of the cornea. **furrow k.,** dendriform k. **herpetic k.,** 1. keratitis, commonly with dendritic ulceration (*dendriform* or *dendritic k.*), due to infection with herpes simplex virus. 2. keratitis occurring in herpes zoster ophthalmicus. **hypopyon k.,** suppurative keratitis associated with purulent infiltration and hypopyon; see *ulcus serpens corneae.* **interstitial k.,** a chronic variety of keratitis with deep deposits in the substance of the cornea, which becomes hazy throughout and has a ground-glass appearance (Sichel, 1837). The disease is associated with congenital syphilis, and occurs in children before the fifteenth year. Called also *parenchymatous k., deep k.,* and *k. profunda.* **lagophthalmic k.,** that which accompanies lagophthalmos; it is due to exposure of the eyeball to the air. **lattice k.,** bilateral hereditary dystrophy of the cornea with the formation of interwoven filamentous lesions. **marginal k.,** phlyctenular keratitis in which the papules are arranged around the margin of the cornea. **metaherpetic k.,** keratitis occurring as a result of recurrent herpesvirus infection of the cornea, characterized by shallow ulceration of an anesthetic cornea, accompanied by parenchymatous infiltration and often by persistent iridocyclitis and secondary glaucoma; called also *metaherpes.* **mycotic k.,** keratomycosis. **neuroparalytic k.,** keratitis characterized by dryness and fissuring of the corneal epithelium as a result of an injury to the trifacial nerve which prevents proper closing of the eyelids; called also *trophic k.* **neurotrophic k.,** keratitis due to loss of corneal sensation. **k. nummula′ris,** a slowly developing benign type of keratitis marked by corneal deposits forming circular areas with sharply defined edges surrounded by a halo of less dense character; called also *Dimmer′s k.* **parenchymatous k.,** interstitial k. **k. petrif′icans,** keratitis with calcareous changes. **phlyctenular k.,** see under *keratoconjunctivitis.* **k. profun′da,** interstitial k. **k. puncta′ta, punctate k.,** an old term for the formation of cellular and fibrinous deposits (keratic precipitates) on the posterior surface of the cornea, occurring after injury or iridocyclitis and giving an appearance of fine drops of dew. **k. puncta′ta subepithelia′lis,** a form with gray areas on the cornea under Bowman′s membrane, with an intact superficial epithelium. **k. pustulifor′mis profun′da,** a painful keratitis marked by deep-seated yellow intracorneal spots, hypopyon, and purulent iritis. **k. ramifica′ta superficia′lis,** a disease of the tropics marked by superficial loss of the epithelium of the cornea. **reaper′s k.,** suppurative keratitis due to the wounding of the cornea by the awn of some grain, as barley. **reticular k.,** familial degeneration of the cornea with reticular areas. **ribbon-like k.,** the formation of a transverse film on the cornea. **rosacea k.,** acne rosacea k. **sclerosing k.,** keratitis associated with scleritis, leading to hyperplasia. **scrofulus k.,** phlyctenular keratitis. **secondary k.,** keratitis due to disease of some other part of the eye. **serpiginous k.,** ulcus serpens corneae. **k. sic′ca,** keratoconjunctivitis sicca. **striate k.,** keratitis marked by parallel and intersect-

ing lines on the corneal epithelium; called also *alphabet k.* **suppurative k.,** keratitis attended with, or assoiated with, suppuration. **trachomatous k.,** pannus trachomatosus. **trophic k.,** neuroparalytic k. **vascular k.,** keratitis accompanied by the formation of blood vessels beneath the conjunctiva and outer layers of the cornea. **vesicular k.,** keratitis with the development of small vesicles on the surface. **xerotic k.,** dryness of the cornea; a condition that precedes keratomalacia. **zonular k.,** ribbon-like k.

kerato- (ker′ah-to) [Gr. *keras* horn, cornea] a combining form denoting relationship to the cornea, or to horny tissue.

keratoacanthoma (ker″ah-to-ak″an-tho′mah) [*kerato-* + *acanthoma*] a rapidly growing papular lesion, with a crater filled with a keratin plug, which reaches maximum size and then resolves spontaneously within four to six months from onset. Prior to involution it is often difficult and sometimes impossible to distinguish sharply from shallowly invasive squamous cell carcinoma. **multiple k.,** the occurrence of several to many keratoacanthomas, identical to the solitary type, usually affecting the face, trunk, or genitalia; a familial type has been reported. Called also *multiple self-healing squamous epithelioma.*

keratoangioma (ker″ah-to-an″je-o′mah) (*obs.*) angiokeratoma.

keratocele (ker′ah-to-sēl″) [*kerato-* + Gr. *kēlē* hernia] hernia of the innermost layer of the cornea (Descemet′s membrane).

keratocentesis (ker″ah-to-sen-te′sis) [*kerato-* + Gr. *kentēsis* puncture] aqueous paracentesis.

keratoconjunctivitis (ker″ah-to-kon-junk″tĭ-vi′tis) inflammation of the cornea and conjunctiva. **epidemic k.,** a highly infectious disease characterized by relatively little ocular exudate, development of round subepithelial corneal opacities in association with the keratitis, and often swelling of regional lymph nodes; systemic symptoms, especially headache, may also be present. Adenovirus type 8 has been repeatedly isolated from patients with the disease. **epizootic k.,** a keratoconjunctivitis of cattle, caused by *Moraxella bovis* and characterized by discharge and clouding or destruction of the cornea. **flash k.,** keratoconjunctivitis caused by exposure to a welding arc or other source of ultraviolet rays. **phlyctenular k.,** a form marked by the formation of a small, gray, circumscribed lesion, or phlyctenule, at the corneal limbus; it has been associated with malnutrition, tuberculosis, and staphylococcus sensitivity. Called also *phlyctenular keratitis, phlyctenular ophthalmia,* and *strumous ophthalmia.* See also *phlyctenulosis.* **shipyard k.,** epidemic k. **k. sic′ca,** a condition marked by hyperemia of the conjunctiva, lacrimal deficiency, thickening of the corneal epithelium, itching and burning of the eye, and often reduced visual acuity. **viral k.,** epidemic k.

keratoconus (ker″ah-to-ko′nus) [*kerato-* + Gr. *kōnos* cone] a noninflammatory, usually bilateral protrusion of the cornea, the apex being displaced downward and nasally. It occurs most commonly in females at about puberty. The cause is unknown, but hereditary factors may play a role. Called also *conical cornea.*

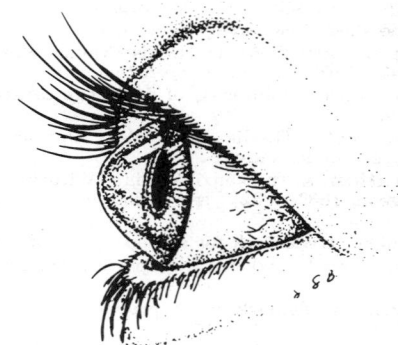

Keratoconus.

keratocyte (ker′ah-to-sīt) [*kerato-* + Gr. *kytos* cell] one of the flattened connective tissue cells between the lamellae of fibrous tissue composing the cornea, with branching processes that intercommunicate with those of other cells.

keratoderma (ker″ah-to-der′mah) [*kerato-* + Gr. *derma* skin] 1. a horny skin or covering. 2. the cornea. 3. hypertrophy of the horny layer of the skin. **k. blennorrha′gicum,** pustular psoriasis associated with gonorrhea, as in Reiter′s disease. **k. climacter′icum, endocrine k.,** circumscribed hyperkeratosis of the palms and soles, occurring in menopausal women. **k. palma′re et planta′re, symmetric k.,** keratosis palmaris et plantaris.

keratodermatocele (ker″ah-to-der′mah-to-sēl) [*kerato-* + *dermato-* + Gr. *kēlē* hernia] keratocele.

keratodermia (ker″ah-to-der′me-ah) [*kerato-* + Gr. *derma* skin + *-ia*] keratoderma. **k. blennorrha′gica,** keratoderma blennorrhagicum. **k. excen′trica** (*obs.*), porokeratosis. **k. palma′ris et planta′ris**, keratosis palmaris et plantaris. **k. planta′ris sulca′ta**, pitted keratolysis.

keratoectasia (ker″ah-to-ek-ta′ze-ah) kerectasis.

keratogenesis (ker″ah-to-jen′ĕ-sis) the formation or production of horny material.

keratogenetic (ker″ah-to-jĕ-net′ik) pertaining to keratogenesis.

keratogenous (ker″ah-toj′ĕ-nus) [*kerato-* + Gr. *gennan* to produce] giving rise to a growth of horny material.

keratoglobus (ker″ah-to-glo′bus) [*kerato-* + L. *globus* globe] a rare bilateral condition in which the cornea is enlarged and globular in shape.

keratohelcosis (ker″ah-to-hel-ko′sis) [*kerato-* + Gr. *helkōsis* ulceration] ulceration of the cornea.

keratohemia (ker″ah-to-he′me-ah) [*kerato-* + Gr. *haima* blood + *-ia*] the presence of deposits of blood in the cornea.

keratohyalin (ker″ah-to-hi′ah-lin) 1. a substance in the granules in the granular layer of the epidermis, the origin and chemistry of which are unclear, but which may be involved in the process of keratinization. See also *keratohyaline granules*, under *granule*. 2. a substance found in granules in the Hassall corpuscles of the thymus.

keratohyaline (ker″ah-to-hi′ah-līn) 1. both horny and hyaline. 2. pertaining to keratohyalin or to the keratohyalin granules or the keratohyaline layer (stratum granulosum epidermidis). 3. keratohyalin.

keratoid (ker′ah-toid) [*kerato-* + Gr. *eidos* form] resembling horn or corneal tissue.

keratoiditis (ker″ah-toi-di′tis) keratitis.

keratoiridocyclitis (ker″ah-to-ir″ĭ-do-sik-li′tis) inflammation of the cornea, iris, and ciliary body.

keratoiridoscope (ker″ah-to-i-rid′o-skōp) [*kerato-* + Gr. *iris* iris + *skopein* to examine] a form of compound microscope for examining the eye.

keratoiritis (ker″ah-to-i-ri′tis) [*kerato-* + Gr. *iris* iris + *-itis*] inflammation of the cornea and iris. **hypopyon k.**, hypopyon keratitis.

keratoleptynsis (ker″ah-to-lep-tin′sis) [*kerato-* + Gr. *leptynsis* attenuation] removal of the anterior portion of the cornea and covering of the denuded area with bulbar conjunctiva.

keratoleukoma (ker″ah-to-lu-ko′mah) [*kerato-* + *leukoma*] a white opacity of the cornea.

keratolysis (ker″ah-tol′ĭ-sis) [*kerato-* + Gr. *lysis* dissolution] softening and dissolution or peeling of the horny layer of the epidermis. **k. neonato′rum** (*obs.*), dermatitis exfoliativa neonatorum. **pitted k., k. planta′re sulca′tum**, a tropical disease marked by thickening and deep fissuring of the skin of the soles, particularly the anterior region of the heels, which occurs during the rainy season and clears up during the dry season; called also *chaluni, cracked heels, keratodermia plantare sulcatum*, and *keratoma plantare sulcatum*.

keratolytic (ker″ah-to-lit′ik) 1. pertaining to, characterized by, or producing keratolysis. 2. an agent that promotes keratolysis.

keratoma (ker″ah-to′mah), pl. *keratomas* or *kerato′mata* [*kerato-* + *-oma*] 1. keratosis. 2. a horny tumor on the inner surface of the wall of a horse's hoof; called also *keraphyllocele*. **k. diffu′sum** (*obs.*), ichthyosis congenita. **k. palma′re et planta′re**, keratosis palmaris et plantaris. **k. planta′re sulca′tum**, pitted keratolysis. **k. seni′le**, actinic keratosis.

keratomalacia (ker″ah-to-mah-la′she-ah) [*kerato-* + Gr. *malakia* softness] a usually bilateral condition associated with vitamin A deficiency. It begins with xerotic spots (Bitôt's spots) on the conjunctiva, while the cornea becomes xerotic and insensitive (xerotic keratitis); the haze increases until finally the entire cornea becomes soft, and colliquative necrosis occurs.

keratomata (ker″ah-to′mah-tah) plural of *keratoma*.

keratome (ker′ah-tōm) [*kerato-* + Gr. *temnein* to cut] a knife for incising the cornea.

keratometer (ker″ah-tom′ĕ-ter) [*kerato-* + Gr. *metron* measure] an instrument for measuring the curves of the cornea.

keratometric (ker″ah-to-met′rik) pertaining to keratometry, or to measurements made with a keratometer.

keratometry (ker″ah-tom′ĕ-tre) the measurement of the cornea.

keratomileusis (ker″ah-to-mĭ-loo′sis) keratoplasty in which a slice of the patient's cornea is removed, shaped to the desired curvature on a lathe after freezing, and then sutured back on the remaining cornea to correct optical error.

keratomycosis (ker″ah-to-mi-ko′sis) [*kerato-* + Gr. *mykēs* fungus + *-osis*] fungous infection of the cornea. **k. lin′guae**, black tongue.

keratonosis (ker″ah-to-no′sis) (*obs.*) any anomaly in the horny structure of the epidermis.

keratonosus (ker″ah-ton′o-sus) [*kerato-* + Gr. *nosos* disease] any disease of the cornea.

keratonyxis (ker″ah-to-nik′sis) [*kerato-* + Gr. *nyssein* to puncture] aqueous paracentesis.

keratopathy (ker″ah-top′ah-the) a noninflammatory disease of the cornea. **band k., band-shaped k.**, a degenerative condition in which a gray band develops axially from the limbus at the level of Bowman's membrane into the exposed part of the cornea in the palpebral aperture.

keratophakia (ker″ah-to-fa′ke-ah) [*kerato-* + Gr. *phakos* lentil, lens] a form of keratoplasty in which a slice of donor's cornea is shaped to a desired curvature and inserted between layers of the recipient's cornea to change its curvature.

keratoplasty (ker′ah-to-plas″te) [*kerato-* + Gr. *plassein* to form] plastic surgery of the cornea; corneal grafting. **optic k.**, transplantation of corneal material to replace scar tissue which interferes with vision. **refractive k.**, that in which a section of cornea is removed from the patient or a donor, shaped to the desired curvature, and inserted either between (keratophakia) layers of or on (keratomileusis) the patient's cornea to change its curvature and correct optical errors. **tectonic k.**, transplantation of corneal material to replace tissue which has been lost.

keratoprotein (ker″ah-to-pro′te-in) [*kerato-* + *protein*] the protein of the horny tissues of the body, such as the hair, nails, and epidermis.

keratorhexis, keratorrhexis (ker″ah-to-rek′sis) [*kerato-* + Gr. *rhēxis* rupture] rupture of the cornea.

keratoscleritis (ker″ah-to-skle-ri′tis) inflammation of the cornea and sclera.

keratoscope (ker′ah-to-skōp″) [*kerato-* + Gr. *skopein* to examine] an instrument for examining the cornea.

keratoscopy (ker″ah-tos′ko-pe) the examination of the cornea; more especially the study of the reflections of light from its anterior surface.

keratosis (ker″ah-to′sis), pl. *kerato′ses* [*kerato-* + *-osis*] any horny growth, such as a wart or callosity, usually either an actinic keratosis or a seborrheic keratosis. **actinic k.**, a sharply outlined, red or skin-colored, flat or elevated, verrucous or keratotic growth, which may develop into a cutaneous horn, and may give rise to a squamous cell carcinoma; it usually affects the middle-aged or elderly, especially those of fair complexion, and is caused by excessive exposure to the sun. Called also *solar k;* formerly called *keratoma senile* and *senile k.* **arsenic k., arsenical k.**, a precancerous condition manifested by multiple horny growths, usually on the palms and soles and occasionally on other areas; it is caused by the ingestion of arsenic for medicinal purposes. **k. blennorrha′gica**, keratoderma blennorrhagicum. **k. diffu′sa feta′lis** (*obs.*), lamellar exfoliation of the newborn (see under *exfoliation*). **k. follicula′ris**, a rare hereditary condition manifested by areas of crusting, itching, verrucous papular growths, usually occurring symmetrically on the trunk, axillae, neck, face, scalp, and retroauricular areas; called also *Darier's disease*. **k. follicula′ris conta′giosa** (*obs.*), a rare form of cornification of the skin, thought to be of a contagious nature. **gonorrheal k.**, keratoderma blennorrhagicum. **k. labia′lis** (*obs.*), a condition marked by indurated keratinized patches on the mucosa of the lips. **k. lin′guae**, leukoplakia. **k. obtu′rans**, a condition characterized by a mass of epidermic scales and cerumen obstructing the external auditory meatus. **k. palma′ris et planta′ris**, a congenital, hereditary condition characterized by thickening of the stratum corneum of the skin of the palms and soles, sometimes with painful lesions resulting from the formation of fissures. It is often associated with other anomalies, including alopecia, vitiligo, acanthosis nigricans, ichthyosis, clubbed fingers, and mental retardation; some cases have been associated with cancer of the esophagus. Most varieties are transmitted as an autosomal dominant trait. **k. pharyn′gea**, a condition characterized by projection of numerous white horny masses from the tonsils and from the orifices of the lymph follicles in the wall of the pharynx. **k. pila′ris**, a condition in which hyperkeratosis is limited to the hair follicles, usually on the extensor surfaces of the thighs and arms, but occurring anywhere, with discrete follicular papules which re-form after removal. **k. puncta′ta**, a form of hyperkeratosis in which the lesions are localized in multiple points on the palms and soles; it is transmitted as an autosomal dominant. **roentgen k.**, premalignant keratotic lesions occurring at the site of severe chronic radiodermatitis. **seborrheic k., k. seborrhe′ica**, a benign, noninvasive tumor of epidermal origin, characterized by hyperplasia of the keratinocytes, ordinarily developing in middle life in the form of numerous yellow or brown, sharply marginated, oval, raised lesions; called also *seborrheic wart, verruca senilis, basal cell acanthoma*, and *basal cell papilloma*. **senile k., k. seni′lis**, actinic k. **solar k.**, actinic k. **stucco k.**, a condition marked by multiple focal keratin-accumulating lesions, usually on the ankles and feet of elderly men who have dry skin; it is thought by many to be a form of seborrheic keratosis notably lacking in cysts or pseudocysts, but others believe it to be a distinctive keratosis very similar to tar keratosis. **k. suprafollicula′ris** (*obs.*), k. pilaris. **tar k.**, a keratosis caused by exposure to tar, in which keratotic foci develop, sometimes followed by the formation of keratoacanthomas or intraepidermal, squamous, or basal cell carcinoma.

keratosulfate (ker″ah-to-sul′fāt) keratan sulfate.

keratotic (ker″ah-tot′ik) pertaining to, characterized by, or promoting keratosis.

keratotome (ker-at′o-tōm) keratome.

keratotomy (ker″ah-tot′o-me) [Gr. *keras* cornea + *temnein* to cut] surgical incision of the cornea. **delimiting k.,** incision of the cornea in ulcus serpens by a cut tangential to the advancing border of the ulcer and made to emerge at a corresponding point in the other side. **radial k.,** an operation in which a series of incisions is made in the cornea from its outer edge toward its center in spoke-like fashion; done to flatten the cornea and thus to correct myopia.

keratotorus (ker″ah-to-to′rus) [*kerato*- + L. *torus* a protuberance] a vaultlike protrusion of the cornea.

keraunoneurosis (kĕ-raw″no-nu-ro′sis) [Gr. *keraunos* lightning + *neurosis*] a neurosis due to electric shock.

Kerckring's folds (valves), ossicles (kerk′ringz) [Theodorus *Kerckring*, Dutch anatomist, 1640–1693] see under *plicae circulares*, and see under *ossicle*.

kerectasis (ke-rek′tah-sis) [Gr. *keras* cornea + *ektasis* distention] a uniform bulging or protrusion of the cornea.

kerectomy (ke-rek′to-me) [Gr. *keras* cornea + *ektomē* excision] surgical removal of a part of the cornea.

kerion (ke′re-on) [Gr. *kērion* honeycomb] a nodular, boggy, exudative, circumscribed tumefaction which is covered with pustules, occurring in association with tinea infections, usually tinea barbae and tinea capitis. **k. cel′si, Celsus' k.** (*obs.*), kerion.

keritherapy (ker″ĭ-ther′ah-pe) [Gr. *kēros* wax + *therapeia* treatment] 1. treatment by baths of liquid paraffin. 2. treatment of extensive burns with paraffin solutions.

kerma (ker′mah) [*k*inetic *e*nergy *r*eleased in *ma*terial + *a*] a unit of quantity that represents the kinetic energy transferred to charged particles by the uncharged particles per unit mass of the irradiated medium.

kermes (ker′mēz) [Arabic, Persian] the *Coccus ilicis,* an insect found on the leaves of various oaks, chiefly on *Quercus coccifera* (kermes-oak). It furnishes a red pigment which is used as a dyestuff.

kernel (ker′nel) that part of an atom left after removal of the valence electrons.

kernicterus (ker-nik′ter-us) [Ger. "nuclear jaundice"] a condition with severe neural symptoms, associated with high levels of bilirubin in the blood. It is characterized by deep yellow staining of the basal nuclei, globus pallidus, putamen, and caudate nucleus, as well as the cerebellar and bulbar nuclei, and gray substance of the cerebrum, and is accompanied by widespread destructive changes. It is commonly a sequela of icterus gravis neonatorum. Called also *bilirubin encephalopathy.*

Kernig's sign (ker′nigz) [Vladimir Mikhailovich *Kernig,* Russian physician, 1840–1917] see under *sign.*

keroid (ker′oid) [Gr. *keroeidēs* hornlike] 1. resembling horn. 2. resembling the cornea.

Kerona pediculus (kĕ-ro′nah pe-dik′u-lus) a ciliate protozoon of the suborder Hypotricha that lives as a commensal.

kerosene, kerosine (ker′o-sēn) a colorless volatile liquid distilled from petroleum; it is used as a reagent and in insecticides.

kerotherapy (ker′o-ther′ah-pe) keritherapy.

kerril (ker′il) a venomous sea snake, *Kerilia jerdoni,* of the Indian Ocean.

Ketaject (ket′ah-jekt) trademark for a preparation of ketamine hydrochloride.

ketal (ke′tal) a derivative formed by a combination of a ketone with an alcohol.

Ketalar (ket′ah-lar) trademark for a preparation of ketamine hydrochloride.

ketamine hydrochloride (kēt′ah-mēn) [USP] chemical name: 2-(2-chlorophenyl)-2-(methylamino)cyclohexanone hydrochloride. A rapid-acting general anesthetic, $C_{13}H_{16}ClNO \cdot HCl$, occurring as a white, crystalline powder; administered intramuscularly and intravenously.

ketazocine (ke-ta′zo-sēn) chemical name: (2α,6α,11S*)-3-(cyclopropylmethyl)3,4,5,6-tetrahydro-8-hydroxy-6,11-dimethyl-2,6-methano-3-benzazocin-1(2*H*)-one; an analgesic, $C_{18}H_{23}NO_2$.

ketazolam (ke-ta′zo-lam) chemical name: 11-chloro-8,12b-dihydro-2,8-dimethyl-12b-phenyl-4*H*[1,3]oxazino[3,2-*d*]-[1,4]benzodiazepine; a minor tranquilizer, $C_{20}H_{17}ClN_2O_3$.

keten (ke′ten) ketene.

ketene (ke′tēn) a colorless gas of penetrating odor, carbomethane, $H_2C:CO$; also any one of several derivatives from it. It combines with water to form acetic acid.

kethoxal (ke-thoks′al) chemical name: 3-ethoxy-1,1-dihydroxy-2-butanone; an antiviral agent, $C_6H_{12}O_4$.

ketimine (ke′tĭ-min) a compound in which the oxygen of a ketone is replaced by the imino group.

ketipramine fumarate (ke-tip′rah-mēn) chemical name: 5-

[3-(dimethylamino)propyl]-5,11-dihydro-10*H*-dibenz[*b,f*]azepin-10-one fumarate (1:1); an antidepressant, $C_{19}H_{22}N_2O \cdot C_4H_4O_4$.

keto- a prefix which denotes possession of the carbonyl group, :C:O, in a structure in which the other two bonds to carbon are attached to hydrocarbon moieties.

keto-acid (ke″to-as′id) see under *acid.*

ketoacid-lyase (ke″to-as″id-li′ās) a lyase that catalyzes the removal of keto acid, as from citrate to form acetate and oxaloacetate.

ketoacidosis (ke″to-ah″sĭ-do′sis) acidosis accompanied by the accumulation of ketone bodies (ketosis) in the body tissues and fluids, as in diabetic acidosis.

ketoaciduria (ke″to-as″ĭ-du′re-ah) the presence of keto acids in the urine. **branched-chain k.,** maple syrup urine disease.

keto-aldehyde (ke″to-al′de-hīd) see under *aldehyde.*

ketoaminoacidemia (ke″to-ah-me″no-as″ĭ-de′me-ah) maple syrup urine disease.

ketoconazole (ke″to-kon′ah-zōl) a broad-spectrum antifungal agent, given orally, that has been reported effective in the treatment of a variety of extensive, chronic cutaneous fungal infections.

Keto-Diastix (ke″to-di′ah-stiks) trademark for a reagent strip designed for the determination of ketones and glucose in urine.

ketogenesis (ke″to-jen′ĕ-sis) [*ketone* + Gr. *genesis* production] the production of ketone (acetone) bodies.

ketogenetic (ke″to-je-net′ik) forming ketone bodies.

ketogenic (ke″to-jen′ik) forming or capable of being converted into ketone bodies. Metabolic sources are fatty acids and some of the amino acids of protein.

α-ketoglutarate (ke″to-gloo′tah-rāt) a salt of α-ketoglutaric acid; in biochemistry, the term is often used interchangeably with α-ketoglutaric acid (see under *acid*).

ketoheptose (ke″to-hep′tōs) a ketone sugar containing seven carbon atoms: $C_7H_{14}O_7$.

ketohexose (ke″to-hek′sōs) a hexose which contains a ketone group. Cf. *aldohexose.*

ketohydroxyestratriene (ke″to-hi-drok″se-es′trah-tri″ēn) estrone.

ketohydroxyestrin (ke″to-hi-drok″se-es′trin) estrone.

ketol (ke′tol) a ketonic alcohol.

ketolysis (ke-tol′ĭ-sis) [*ketone* + Gr. *lysis* dissolution] the cleavage of ketone bodies.

ketolytic (ke″to-lit′ik) pertaining to, characterized by, or promoting ketolysis.

ketone (ke′tōn) any of a large class of organic compounds containing the carbonyl group, C═O, whose carbon atom is joined to two other carbon atoms, that is, with the carbonyl group occurring within the carbon chain. See also under *body.* **dimethyl k.,** acetone.

ketonemia (ke″to-ne′me-ah) [*ketone* + Gr. *haima* blood + *-ia*] an excess of ketone bodies in the blood, as in starvation and diabetes mellitus.

ketonic (ke-to′nik) pertaining to or developed from a ketone.

ketonization (ke″to-ni-za′shun) conversion into a ketone.

ketonuria (ke″to-nu′re-ah) [*ketone* + Gr. *ouron* urine + *-ia*] ketone bodies in the urine, as in diabetes mellitus.

ketonurine (ke″tōn-u′rin) the urine excreted after administration of a ketogenic diet.

ketoplasia (ke″to-pla′se-ah) the formation of ketone bodies.

ketoplastic (ke″to-plas′tik) [*ketone* + Gr. *plassein* to form] pertaining to, characterized by, or promoting the formation of ketone bodies.

ketopregnene (ke″to-preg′nēn) a progestational agent isolated from human placentas and corpora lutea in two forms, Δ⁴-3-ketopregnene-20(α)-ol and Δ⁴-3-ketopregnene-20(β)-ol.

ketoprofen (ke″to pro′fen) chemical name: *m*-benzoylhydratropic acid. An anti-inflammatory, antipyretic, and analgesic, $C_{16}H_{14}O_3$, used in the treatment of rheumatoid arthritis, osteoarthritis, and ankylosing spondylitis.

β-ketoreductase (ke″to-re-duk′tās) L-3-hydroxyacyl-CoA:NAD oxidoreductase: an enzyme in liver, muscle, kidney, heart, and other tissues which, with NADH as coenzyme, reduces acetoacetyl-CoA (reversibly) to β-hydroxybutyryl-CoA.

ketose (ke′tōs) a ketone derivative of a polyatomic alcohol (any sugar which contains a ketone group).

ketoside (ke′to-sīd) any glycoside which yields a ketose on hydrolysis.

ketosis (ke-to′sis) a condition characterized by an abnormally elevated concentration of ketone bodies in the body tissues and fluids; it is a complication of diabetes mellitus and starvation.

ketosteroid (ke-to′ste-roid) a steroid that possesses ketone groups on functional carbon atoms. The 17-ketosteroids have a ketone group on the 17th carbon atom. They are found in the urine of normal men and women and in excess in certain adrenal cortex and ovarian tumors. The principal ketosteroids are androsterone, epiandrosterone, etiocholanolone, dehydroisoandrosterone, and estrone.

ketosuria (ke″to-su′re-ah) the presence of ketose in the urine.

keto-tetrahydrophenanthrene (ke″to-tet″rah-hi′dro-fe-nan′thrēn) 1-keto-1,2,3,4-tetrahydrophenanthrene, a carcinogenic substance.

ketotetrose (ke″to-tet′rōs) a ketose that contains 4 carbon atoms.

ketotic (ke-tot′ik) pertaining to, characterized by, or causing ketosis.

ketourine (ke″to-u′rin) ketonurine.

ketoxime (ke-tok′sīm) the oxime derivative of a ketone.

kev. abbreviation for *kilo* (1000) *electron volts;* the equivalent of 3.82 × 10⁻¹⁷ gram calories, or 1.6 × 10⁻⁹ ergs.

key (ke) 1. an instrument for opening a lock, or a device for making or breaking an electric circuit; by extension, any tool for revealing specific information. **torquing k.,** an orthodontic instrument used to facilitate the engaging of rectangular arch wires into the edgewise brackets.

keynote (ke′nōt) in homeopathy, the characteristic property of a drug which indicates its use in treating a similar symptom of disease.

Key-Retzius connective tissue sheath, foramen (ke′ ret′ze-us) [Ernst Axel Henrik *Key,* Swedish physician, 1832–1901; Magnus Gustaf *Retzius,* Swedish histologist, 1842–1919] see *connective tissue sheath of Key and Retzius,* under *sheath,* and see *apertura lateralis ventriculi quarti.*

kg. kilogram.

kg.-cal. kilogram-calorie; see *large calorie,* under *calorie.*

kg.-m. kilogram-meter.

KHCO₃ potassium bicarbonate.

khellin (kel′in) chemical name: 4,9-dimethoxy-7-methyl-5*H*-furo[3,2-*g*][1]benzopyran-5-one. An active principle, C₁₄H₁₂O₅, from the fruit of *Ammi visnaga* Lam., an umbelliferous plant of Eastern Mediterranean regions; an antihypertensive and vasodilator.

KI potassium iodide.

kibe (kīb) (*obs.*) chilblain.

kibisitome (ki-bis′ĭ-tōm) [Gr. *kibisis* pouch + *tomē* a cut] cystitome.

kidinga pepo (kid-in′gah pe′po) [″cramplike pains″] a disease of Zanzibar, probably the same as dengue.

kidney (kid′ne) [L. *ren;* Gr. *nephros*] either of the two organs in the lumbar region that filter the blood, excreting the end-products of body metabolism in the form of urine, and regulating the concentrations of hydrogen, sodium, potassium, phosphate, and other ions in the extracellular fluid. Called also *ren* [NA]. Each kidney is about four inches long, two inches wide, and one inch thick, and weighs from four to six ounces. The kidney is of characteristic shape, and presents a notch on the inner, concave, border, known as the *hilus,* which communicates with the cavity or sinus of the kidney and through which the vessels, nerves, and ureter pass. The kidney consists of a *cortex* and a *medulla.* The medullary substance forms pyramids, whose bases are in the cortex and whose apices, which are called *papillae,* project into the calices of the kidney. The renal pyramids number from 10 to 15. The parenchyma of each kidney is composed of about one million *renal tubules* (nephrons, the functional unit of the kidney), held together by a little connective tissue. Each tubule begins blindly in a renal corpuscle, consisting of a glomerulus and its capsule, situated within the cortex. After a neck or constriction below the capsule, it becomes the proximal convoluted tubule, Henle's loop, distal convoluted tubule, arched collecting tubule, and then the straight collecting tubule, which opens at the apex of a renal papilla. The straight collecting tubules converge as they descend, forming groups in the center, known as *medullary rays.* See Plate XXIII. **abdominal k.,** an ectopic kidney situated above the iliac crest with the hilus adjacent to the second lumbar vertebra. **amyloid k.,** one marked by deposition of amyloid, usually concentrated in small blood vessels and capillaries; called also *Rokitansky's k.* **arteriosclerotic k.,** one characterized by sclerotic changes of intrarenal arteries and large arterioles. **artificial k.,** a popular name for an extracorporeal device employed to remove from the blood, while being circulated outside the body, elements which are usually excreted in the urine; see *hemodialyzer.* Intracorporeal artificial kidneys are under development, in which intestinal or pulmonary tissue is used as the filtration membrane. **atrophic k.,** one is diminished in size because of inadequate circulation and/or loss of nephrons. **cake k.,** a solid, irregularly lobed organ of bizarre shape, usually situated in the pelvis toward the midline, developed as result of fusion of the two renal anlagen. **cicatricial k.,** a shriveled, irregular, and scarred kidney, resulting from suppurative pyelonephritis. **clump k.,** cake k. **congested k.,** large red k. **contracted k.,** an atrophic kidney which may be scarred and granular. **crush k.,** lower nephron nephrosis. **cyanotic k.,** passive congestion of the kidney. **cystic k.,** a kidney contain-

ing one or more cysts. **definite k.,** metanephros. **disk k.,** a disk-shaped organ produced by fusion of both poles of the contralateral kidney anlagen. **doughnut k.,** an anomalous organ resulting from bipolar fusion of the renal anlagen before rotation begins, both kidneys being on the same level. **fatty k.,** a kidney affected with fatty degeneration. **flea-bitten k.,** a kidney which has small, randomly scattered petechiae on its surface, sometimes seen in bacterial endocarditis. **floating k.,** hypermobile k. **Formad's k.,** an enlarged and deformed kidney, sometimes seen in chronic alcoholism. **fused k.,** a single anomalous organ developed as a result of fusion of the renal anlagen. **Goldblatt k.,** one in which the blood flow is obstructed, resulting in renal hypertension. **head k.,** pronephros. **hind k.,** metanephros. **horseshoe k.,** an anomalous organ developed as a result of fusion of the corresponding poles of the renal anlagen. **hypermobile k.,** one that is freely movable. **lardaceous k.,** amyloid k. **large red k.,** a congested, edematous kidney which may result from inflammation, impaired venous circulation, or urinary obstruction; called also *congested k.* **lumbar k.,** an ectopic kidney situated opposite the sacral promontory in the iliac fossa, anterior to the iliac vessels. **lump k.,** cake k. **medullary sponge k.,** sponge k. **middle k.,** mesonephros. **mortar k.,** putty k. **movable k.,** hypermobile k. **mural k.,** a kidney located in a pocket of peritoneum in the abdominal wall. **myelin k.,** a kidney infiltrated with myelin, producing minute whitish specks or streaks on its surface. **pelvic k.,** an ectopic kidney situated opposite the sacrum and below the aortic bifurcation. **polycystic k.,** see *polycystic disease of the kidneys,* under *disease.* **primordial k.,** pronephros. **putty k.,** one containing caseous material trapped by stricture of the ureter by tuberculous granulations in renal tuberculosis. **Rokitansky's k.,** amyloid k. **Rose-Bradford k.,** a form of fibrotic kidney of inflammatory origin found in young subjects. **sacciform k.,** a distended kidney; nephrectasia. **sigmoid k.,** a deformed and fused kidney, the upper pole of one kidney being fused with the lower pole of the other. **sponge k.,** a rare congenital condition, anatomically characterized by multiple small cystic dilatations of the collecting tubules of the medullary portion of the renal pyramids, giving the organ a spongy, porous feeling and appearance. It is usually asymptomatic, but there may be calculus formation within the cysts, hematuria, renal colic, or recurrent renal infection. **supernumerary k.,** a kidney in addition to the two usually present, developed as the result of splitting of the nephrogenic blastema, or from separate metanephric blastemas into which partially or completely reduplicated ureteral stalks enter to form separate capsulated kidneys. In some cases the separation of the reduplicated organ is incomplete (*fused supernumerary k.*). **thoracic k.,** an ectopic kidney that partially or completely protrudes above the diaphragm into the posterior mediastinum. **wandering k.,** hypermobile k. **waxy k.,** amyloid k.

Kielland's (Kjelland) forceps (kel′andz) [Christian *Kielland,* Norwegian obstetrician and gynecologist, 1871–1941] see under *forceps.*

Kienböck atrophy, etc. (kēn′bek) [Robert *Kienböck,* Austrian roentgenologist, 1871–1953] see under *atrophy, disease, dislocation,* and *phenomenon.*

Kienböck-Adamson points (kēn′bek-ad′am-son) [Robert *Kienböck;* Horatio George *Adamson,* London dermatologist, 1865–1955] see under *point.*

Kiernan's spaces (kēr′nanz) [Francis *Kiernan,* English physician, 1800–1874] see under *space.*

Kiesselbach's area (space) (ke′sel-bahks) [Wilhelm *Kiesselbach,* German laryngologist, 1839–1902] see under *area.*

kiestein (ki-es′te-in) kyestein.

kil (kil) a white, sticky, soapy clay from the Black Sea region; when sterilized, it is employed as an ointment base for use in skin diseases.

Kilian's line (kil′e-anz) [Hermann Friedrich *Kilian,* German gynecologist, 1800–1863] see under *line.*

killeen (kil′lēn) chondrus.

Killian's operation (kil′e-anz) [Gustav *Killian,* German laryngologist, 1860–1921] see under *operation.*

Killian's test (kil′e-anz) [John Allen *Killian,* biochemist in New York, born 1891] see under *tests.*

kilo- [Fr., from Gr. *chilioi* thousand] a combining form used in naming units of measurement to indicate a quantity one thousand (10³) times the unit designated by the root with which it is combined.

kilocalorie (kil′o-kal″o-re) large calorie; see under *calorie.*

kilocycle (kil′o-si″kl) a unit of 1000 (10³) cycles, e.g., 1000 cycles per second, applied to the frequency of electromagnetic waves. Abbreviated kc.

kilogram (kil′o-gram) a unit of mass (weight) of the metric system, being 1000 (10³) grams, or the equivalent of 2.204623 pounds avoirdupois and of 2.679229 pounds apothecaries' weight. Abbreviated kg.

kilogram-meter (kil′o-gram-me′ter) a unit of work, representing the energy required to raise 1 kg. of weight 1 meter vertically against gravitational force, equivalent to about 7.2 foot-pounds and equal to 1000 gram-meters. Abbreviated kg.-m.

kilohertz (kil′o-hertz) one thousand (10^3) hertz (cycles per second). Abbreviated kHz.

kiloliter (kil′o-le″ter) [Fr. *kilolitre*] a unit of capacity of the metric system, being 1000 (10^3) liters, or the equivalent of 264.18 gallons. Abbreviated kl.

kilomegacycle (kil″o-meg′ah-si″kl) a unit of 1000 (10^3) megacycles (10^9 cycles), e.g., 1000 megacycles per second, applied to the frequency of electromagnetic waves. Abbreviated kMc.

kilometer (kil′o-me″ter, kĭ-lom′ĕ-ter) [Fr. *kilométre*] a unit of linear measurement of the metric system, being 1000 (10^3) meters, or the equivalent of 3280.83 feet, or about five-eighths of a mile. Abbreviated km.

kilonem (kil′o-nem) [*kilo-* + *nem*] a unit of nutritive value, the equivalent of 667 calories; see also *nem.*

kilounit (kil″o-u′nit) a quantity equivalent to one thousand (10^3) units.

kilovolt (kil′o-vōlt) a unit of electrical pressure or electromotive force, being 1000 (10^3) volts. Abbreviated kv.

kilurane (kil′u-rān) a unit of radioactivity, being 1000 (10^3) uranium units.

Kimberley horse disease (kim′ber-le) [Kimberley, a district in northeastern Western Australia] see under *disease.*

Kimmelstiel-Wilson syndrome (kim′el-stēl wil′son) [Paul *Kimmelstiel,* German pathologist in the United States, born 1900; Clifford *Wilson,* English physician, born 1906] intercapillary glomerulosclerosis.

Kimpton-Brown tube (kimp′ton brown′) [Arthur Ronald *Kimpton,* Boston surgeon] see under *tube.*

kimputu (kēm-poo′too) [African] relapsing fever.

kinanesthesia (kin″an-es-the″ze-ah) [Gr. *kinēsis* motion + *anesthesia*] loss of power of perceiving the sensation of movement, due to derangement of deep sensibility.

kinase (ki′nās) 1. a subclass of the transferases, comprising the enzymes that catalyze the transfer of a high-energy group of a donor, usually adenosine triphosphate, to some acceptor, and variously named, according to the acceptor, as *creatine kinase, fructokinase, galactokinase, hexokinase,* etc. Called also *phosphokinase, phosphotransferase,* and *transphosphorylase.* 2. an enzyme that activates a zymogen, variously named, according to its source, as *enterokinase, staphylokinase,* and *streptokinase.* **acetate k.,** ATP:acetate phosphotransferase: an enzyme that catalyzes the transfer of a phosphate group from ATP to acetate; called also *acetokinase.* **acetol k.,** an enzyme that transfers a phosphate group from ATP to hydroxyacetone. **adenosine k.,** an enzyme of the liver and kidney that catalyzes the transfer of a phosphate group from ATP to form adenosine phosphate. **adenylate k.,** ATP:AMP phosphotransferase: a heat-stable enzyme of skeletal muscle, heart, brain, and liver that activates the yeast hexokinase system, thus making possible the transfer of phosphate from ADP to fructose or glucose. Called also *myokinase.* **aspartate k.,** an enzyme that catalyzes the transfer of a phospho group from ATP to aspartate to form phosphoaspartate. **bacterial k.,** 1. a kinase of bacterial origin. 2. an enzyme of bacterial origin that activates a precursor (plasminogen) of a plasma protease (plasmin). **carbamate k.,** an enzyme of the liver that catalyzes the transfer of a phosphate group from ATP associated with ammonia and carbon dioxide, to form ADP and carbamoylphosphate. **creatine k.,** ATP:creatine phosphotransferase. An enzyme that catalyzes the transfer of a high-energy phosphate group from ATP to creatine, producing phosphocreatine and ADP; widely distributed in tissues, including muscle and brain. **glycerol k.,** an enzyme of the liver and kidney that catalyzes the transfer of a phosphate group from ATP to form ADP and L-glycerol-3-phosphate. **insulin k.,** an enzyme assumed to exist in the liver which activates insulin; possibly equatable with the peptidase which catalyzes pro-insulin to insulin conversion. **mevalonate k.,** an enzyme occurring in the liver and in yeast that catalyzes the transfer of a phosphate group from ATP to form ADP and 5-phosphomevalonate. **nucleoside monophosphate k.,** an enzyme of the liver that catalyzes the transfer of a phosphate group from ATP to form ADP and a nucleoside diphosphate. **phosphoglycerate k.,** ATP:3-phospho-D-glycerate 1-phosphotransferase. An enzyme that reversibly catalyzes the transfer of a high-energy phosphate group from ATP to D-3-phosphoglycerate, producing D-1,3-diphosphoglycerate, one of the enzymatic steps in glycolysis. **phosphomevalonate k.,** an enzyme occurring in yeast that catalyzes the transfer of a phosphate group from ATP to form ADP and 5-pyrophosphomevalonate. **protein k.,** any protein that catalyzes the transfer of a phosphate group from ATP to form a phosphoprotein. **pyruvate k.,** an enzyme occurring in all tissues of the body that catalyzes the transfer of a phosphate group from ATP to form ADP and phosphoenolpyruvate. **tissue k.,** fibrinokinase.

kine- see *kinesio-.* For words beginning thus, see also words beginning *cine-.*

kinematics (kin″ĕ-mat′iks) [Gr. *kinēma* motion] that phase of mechanics which deals with the possible motions of a material body.

kinematograph (kin″ĕ-mat′o-graf) [Gr. *kinēma* motion + *graphein* to record] an instrument for exhibiting pictures of objects in motion; it is of considerable service in diagnosis.

kinemia (ki-ne′me-ah) cardiac output; see under *output.*

kinemic (ki-ne′mik) [*kine-* + Gr. *haima* blood] pertaining to kinemia.

kineplastics (kin″ĕ-plas′tiks) kineplasty.

kineplasty (kin′ĕ-plas″te) [Gr. *kinein* to move + *plassein* to form] plastic amputation; amputation in which the stump is so formed as to be utilized for motor purposes.

kinesalgia (kin″ĕ-sal′je-ah) [*kinesio-* + *-algia*] pain on muscular exertion.

kinescope (kin′ĕ-skōp) [*kine-* + Gr. *skopein* to examine] an instrument for measuring ocular refraction, in which the patient observes a fixed object through a slit in a moving disk.

kinesia (ki-ne′se-ah) kinetosis.

kinesialgia (ki-ne′se-al′je-ah) kinesalgia.

kinesiatrics (ki-ne″se-at′riks) [*kinesio-* + Gr. *iatrikē* surgery, medicine] kinesitherapy.

kinesics (ki-ne′siks) the study of body movement as a part of the process of communication.

kinesi-esthesiometer (ki-ne″se-es-the″ze-om′ĕ-ter) [*kinesio-* + Gr. *aisthēsis* perception + *metron* measure] an instrument for estimating or measuring the sense of motion.

kinesimeter (kin″ĕ-sim′ĕ-ter) [*kinesio-* + Gr. *metron* measure] 1. an instrument for the quantitative measurement of movements. 2. an instrument for exploring the surface of the body to test cutaneous sensibility.

kinesio-, kine- [Gr. *kinēsis* movement] a combining form denoting relationship to movement.

kinesiodic (ki-ne″se-od′ik) kinesodic.

kinesiology (ki-ne″se-ol′o-je) [*kinesio-* + *-logy*] the sum of what is known regarding human motion; the study of motion of the human body.

kinesiometer (ki-ne″se-om′ĕ-ter) kinesimeter.

kinesioneurosis (ki-ne″se-o-nu-ro′sis) [*kinesio-* + *neurosis*] a functional nervous disorder characterized by motor disturbances, such as spasms or tics.

kinesiotherapy (ki-ne″se-o-ther′ah-pe) kinesitherapy.

kinesis (ki-ne′sis) [Gr.] 1. movement, e.g., the activity of an organism in response to a stimulus; the direction of the response is not controlled by the direction of the stimulus (in contrast to a taxis). 2. a word termination denoting movement or motion, e.g., cytokinesis.

kinesitherapy (ki-ne″sĕ-ther′ah-pe) [*kinesio-* + Gr. *therapeia* cure] the treatment of disease by movements or exercise.

kinesodic (kin″ĕ-sod′ik) [*kinesio-* + Gr. *hodos* way] conducting or pertaining to the conduction of motor impulses.

kinesthesia (kin″es-the″ze-ah) [*kine-* + Gr. *aisthēsis* perception + *-ia*] the sense by which movement, weight, position, etc., are perceived; commonly used to refer specifically to the perception of changes in the angles of joints.

kinesthesiometer (kin″es-the″ze-om′ĕ-ter) [*kinesthesia* + Gr. *metron* measure] an instrument for testing kinesthesia.

kinesthesis (kin″es-the′sis) kinesthesia.

kinesthetic (kin″es-thet′ik) pertaining to kinesthesia or the muscular sense.

kinetia (ki-ne′te-ah) kinetosis.

kinetic (kĭ-net′ik) [Gr. *kinētikos*] pertaining to or producing motion.

kineticist (ki-net′ĭ-sist) a specialist in kinetics.

kinetics (kĭ-net′iks, ki-net′iks) [Gr. *kinētikos* of or for putting in motion] the branch of dynamics that pertains to the turnover, or rate of change, of a specific factor (e.g., erythrocytes— erythrokinetics, leukocytes— leukokinetics, or iron—ferrokinetics), commonly expressed as units of amount per unit time. **chemical k.,** the study of the rates and mechanisms of chemical reactions.

kinetin (ki-ne′tin) a highly potent plant-growth factor, 6-furfurylaminopurine, which promotes cytokinesis in tobacco callus tissue.

kinetism (kin′ĕ-tizm) the ability to perform or initiate muscular action.

kineto- [Gr. *kinētos* movable] a combining form meaning movable.

kinetocardiogram (ki-ne″to-kar′de-o-gram) the graphic record obtained by kinetocardiography; called also *precordial cardiogram.*

kinetocardiography (ki-ne″to-kar′de-og′rah-fe) the technique of graphically recording the slow vibrations of the anterior chest wall in the region of the heart, the vibrations representing the absolute motion of the heart at a given point on the chest.

Plate XXIII

kidney

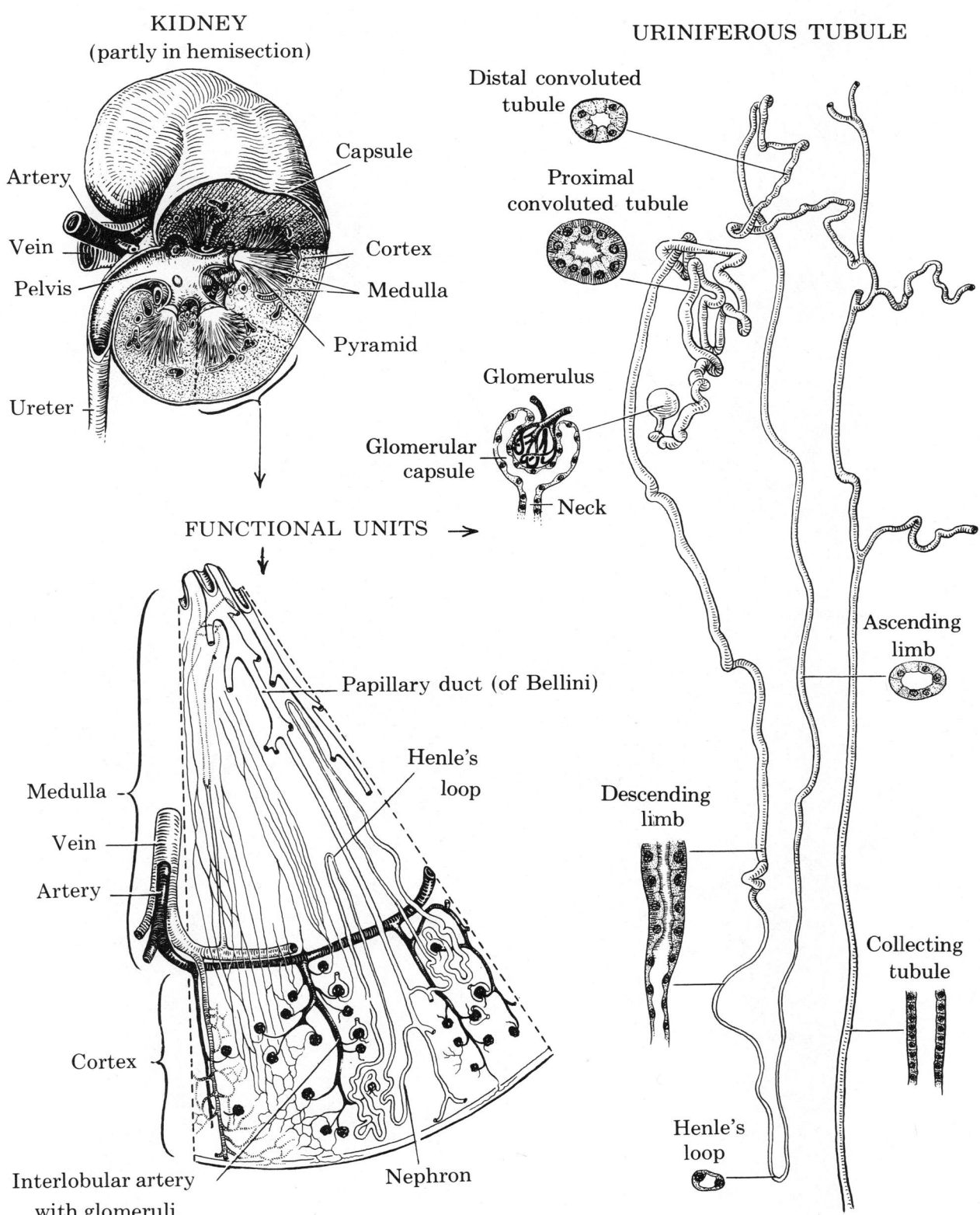

KIDNEY
(partly in hemisection)

URINIFEROUS TUBULE

Artery

Vein

Pelvis

Ureter

Capsule

Cortex

Medulla

Pyramid

Distal convoluted
tubule

Proximal
convoluted tubule

Glomerulus

Glomerular
capsule

Neck

FUNCTIONAL UNITS →

Medulla

Vein

Artery

Papillary duct (of Bellini)

Henle's
loop

Ascending
limb

Descending
limb

Collecting
tubule

Cortex

Interlobular artery
with glomeruli

Nephron

Henle's
loop

DETAILS OF STRUCTURE OF THE KIDNEY

kinetochore (ki-ne′to-kōr) [*kineto-* + Gr. *chora* space] centromere.

kinetocyte (ki-ne′to-sīt) [*kineto-* + *-cyte*] a term once applied to one of the round or oval bodies about the size of a blood platelet, as forming a fourth element in the blood, where they move actively among the corpuscles; called also *Edelmann's cell.*

kinetogenic (ki-ne″to-jen′ik) [*kineto-* + Gr. *gennan* to produce] causing or producing movement.

kinetographic (ki-ne″to-graf′ik) [*kineto-* + Gr. *graphein* to record] recording graphically the movements of parts and features.

kinetonucleus (ki-ne″to-nu′kle-us) [*kineto-* + *nucleus*] kinetoplast.

kinetoplasm (ki-ne′to-plazm) [*kineto-* + Gr. *plasma* something formed] the most highly contractile portion of the cytoplasm of a cell; the energy plasm: the term is applied to the chromatophilic elements in the nervous tissue.

kinetoplast (ki-ne′to-plast) [*kineto-* + Gr. *plassein* to form] a structure associated with the basal body in many protozoa, primarily the Mastigophora; it is rich in DNA, and, like the basal body, it replicates independently.

kinetoscope (ki-ne′to-skōp) [*kineto-* + Gr. *skopein* to examine] an apparatus designed to make serial photographs depicting body motions.

kinetoscopy (ki″nĕ-tos′ko-pe) serial photography which exhibits the motions of the limbs or features; used in diagnosis of disorders of gait and in the study of muscle action.

kinetoses (ki″ne-to′sēz) [Gr.] plural of *kinetosis.*

kinetosis (ki″ne-to′sis), pl. *kineto′ses* [*kineto-* + *-osis*] any disorder caused by unaccustomed motion; see *motion sickness.*

kinetosome (ki-ne′to-sōm) [*kineto-* + Gr. *sōma* body] basal corpuscle.

kinetotherapy (ki-ne″to-ther′ah-pe) kinesitherapy.

King unit (king) [Earl J. *King,* Toronto biochemist, born 1901] see under *unit.*

kingdom (king′dum) [Anglosaxon *cyningdom*] classically, one of the three categories into which natural objects are usually classified: the *animal kingdom,* including all animals; the *plant kingdom,* including all plants; and the *mineral kingdom,* including all objects and substance without life. A fourth kingdom, the *Protista,* includes all single-celled organisms.

kinin (ki′nin) any of a group of endogenous peptides that cause vasodilation, increase vascular permeability, cause hypotension, and induce contraction of smooth muscle. **venom k.,** a peptide found in the venom of insects. **wasp k.,** a potent, pain-provoking peptide present in wasp venom.

kininase II (ki′nin-ās) an enzyme that catalyzes the cleavage of C-terminal peptides from substrates, including bradykinin and angiotension I (converting it to angiotensin II).

kininogen (ki′nin-o-jen″) an α_2-globulin of plasma that is a precursor of the kinins.

kink (kink′) a bend or twist. **ileal k., Lane's k.,** the term once applied to sharp twists in the distal ileum caused by Lane's bands; such twists were thought to result in chronic partial obstruction of the ileum.

kino (ki′no) the dried juice of *Pterocarpus marsupium* Roxb. (Leguminosae), of southern Asia, and of various other trees; it has been used as an astringent because of its high content of kinotannic acid.

kino- [Gr. *kinein* to move] a combining form denoting relationship to movement.

kinocentrum (ki″no-sen′trum) centrosome.

kinocilia (ki″no-sil′e-ah) [L.] plural of *kinocilium.*

kinocilium (ki″no-sil′e-um), pl. *kinocil′ia.* A motile, protoplasmic filament on the free surface of a cell. Cf. *stereocilium.*

kinohapt (ki′no-hapt) [*kino-* + Gr. *haptein* to touch] an esthesiometer for making several tactile stimulations at definite intervals or space.

kinology (ki-nol′o-je) kinesiology.

kinomometer (ki″no-mom′ĕ-ter) [*kino-* + Gr. *metron* measure] an instrument for estimating the degree of motion in fingers and wrist.

kinoplasm (ki′no-plazm) [*kino-* + Gr. *plasma* plasm] (*obs.*) Strasburger's name for a distinct type of protoplasm that tends to form fibrillar structures and is mechanically active.

kinoplastic (ki″no-plas′tik) pertaining to kinoplasm.

Kinorhyncha (kin″o-rin′kah) [*kino-* + Gr. *rhynchos* snout] a class of small marine animals of the phylum Aschelminthes, which have a cuticle divided into segments and a retractible spiny head. In some systems of classification, they are considered to be a separate phylum.

kinosphere (ki′no-sfēr) [*kino-* + *sphere*] aster.

kinotoxin (ki″no-tok′sin) [*kino-* + *toxin*] a fatigue toxin.

kinovin (kin-o′vin) quinovin.

kinship (kin′ship) a group of individuals of varying degrees of descent from a common ancestor.

kiono- (ki′on-o) for words beginning thus, see those beginning *ciono-.*

kiotome (ki′o-tōm) [Gr. *kiōn* column + *temnein* to cut] a knife for amputating the uvula.

kiotomy (ki-ot′o-me) the use of the kiotome; amputation of the uvula.

Kirchner's diverticulum (kērk′nerz) [Wilhelm *Kirchner,* Würzburg otologist, 1849–1936] see under *diverticulum.*

Kirk's amputation (kirks) [Major General Norman Thomas *Kirk,* former Surgeon General of U.S. Army, 1888–1960] see under *amputation.*

Kirmisson's operation (kēr″me-sawz′) [Edouard *Kirmisson,* French surgeon, 1848–1927] see under *operation.*

Kirschner wire (kērsh′ner) [Martin *Kirschner,* German surgeon, 1879–1942] see under *wire.*

Kirstein's method (ker′stīnz) [Alfred *Kirstein,* German physician, 1863–1922] see under *method.*

Kisch's reflex (kish′ez) [Bruno *Kisch,* Austrian physiologist, born 1891] Kehrer's reflex.

kitasamycin (kit″ah-sah-mi′sin) an antibiotic substance produced by *Streptomyces kitasatoensis,* active against most grampositive and some gram-negative bacteria, as well as certain other pathogenic microorganisms. Called also *leucomycin.*

Kitasato's filter (ke-tah-sah′tōz) [Shibasaburo *Kitasato,* Japanese bacteriologist, 1852–1931] see under *filter.*

kitol (ki′tol) [Gr. *kētos* sea monster, big fish] a substance from whale oil which yields vitamin A on heating.

Kittel's treatment (kit′elz) [M. J. *Kittel,* German physician] see under *treatment.*

k.j. knee jerk.

Kjeldahl's method (test) (kel′dahlz) [Johan Gustav Christoffer *Kjeldahl,* Danish chemist, 1849–1900] see under *method.*

Kjelland (kel′land) see *Kielland.*

kl. klang; kiloliter.

Klapp's creeping treatment (klaps) [Rudolf *Klapp,* surgeon in Berlin, 1873–1949] see under *treatment.*

Klebs-Löffler bacillus (klebz′ lef′ler) [T.A.E. *Klebs,* Friederich A. J. *Löffler,* German bacteriologist, 1852–1915] *Corynebacterium diphtheriae.*

Klebsiella (kleb″se-el′lah) [T.A.E. *Klebs*] a genus of microorganisms of the tribe Escherichieae, family Enterobacteriaceae, order Eubacteriales, made up of plump short rods with rounded ends, usually occurring singly, and frequently found in the respiratory or intestinal tract in man. **K. friedlän′deri,** *K. pneumoniae.* **K. ozae′nae,** an organism isolated from patients with ozena and also from patients with atrophic rhinitis. **K. pneumo′niae,** an organism closely similar to *Aerobacter aerogenes;* it is the etiologic agent of Friedländer pneumonia and other infections of the respiratory tract. Called also *Friedländer's bacillus* or *pneumobacillus, K. friedländeri,* and formerly *Bacillus pneumoniae.* **K. rhinoscleroma′tis,** an organism isolated

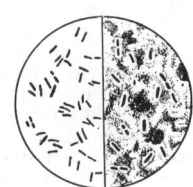

Klebsiella pneumoniae.

from the nasal secretions of patients with rhinoscleroma.

kleeblattschädel (kla″blat-sha′del) [Ger.] cloverleaf skull; a congenital anomaly in which there is intrauterine synostosis of multiple or all cranial sutures. See under *syndrome.*

Klemm's tetanus (klemz) [Paul *Klemm,* surgeon in Riga, 1861–1921] kopf-tetanus.

Klemperer's tuberculin (klem′per-erz) [Felix (1866–1932) and Georg (1865–1946) *Klemperer,* Berlin physicians] see under *tuberculin.*

klepto- (klep′to) [Gr. *kleptein* to steal] combining form denoting relationship to theft or stealing.

kleptolagnia (klep″to-lag′ne-ah) [*klepto-* + *lagneia* lust] sexual gratification produced by theft.

kleptomania (klep″to-ma′ne-ah) [*klepto-* + Gr. *mania* madness] an uncontrollable impulse to steal, the objects taken usually having a symbolic value of which the subject is unconscious, rather than an intrinsic value.

kleptomaniac (klep″to-ma′ne-ak) an individual exhibiting kleptomania.

Klieg eye (klēg) [named from *Kliegl,* the manufacturer of electric lamps used in moving picture making] see under *eye.*

Klimow's test (klim′ofs) [Ivan Alex. *Klimow,* Russian physician, born 1865] see under *tests.*

Kline's test (klīn) [Benjamin S. *Kline*, American pathologist, born 1886] see under *tests*.

Klinefelter's syndrome (klīn′fel-terz) [Harry Fitch *Klinefelter*, Jr., American physician, born 1912] see under *syndrome*.

Klippel's disease (klĭ-pelz′) [Maurice *Klippel*, French neurologist, 1858–1942] arthritic general pseudoparalysis.

Klippel-Feil sign, syndrome (klĭ-pel′fīl) [Maurice *Klippel*; André *Feil*, French physician, born 1884] see under *sign* and *syndrome*.

kliseometer (klis″e-om′ĕ-ter) cliseometer.

Kloeckera (kle′ker-ah) a genus of ascomycetous yeasts of the family Saccharomycetaceae. **K. apicula′tus,** a species from fermenting fruit; its oval cells are joined at the ends. Called also *Saccharomyces apiculatus.*

Klumpke's paralysis (kloomp′kez) [Madame A. *Klumpke* Dejerine, Parisian neurologist, 1859–1927, wife of Joseph Jules Dejerine] see under *paralysis*.

Klumpke-Dejerine paralysis, syndrome (kloomp′kĕ-dezh″er-ēn′) [Madame A. *Klumpke* Dejerine; Joseph Jules *Dejerine*, French neurologist, 1849–1917] Klumpke's paralysis.

km. kilometer.

kMc. kilomegacycle.

kMc.p.s. kilomegacycles per second.

KMnO₄ potassium permanganate.

Knapp's forceps, operation, streaks (striae) (naps) [Herman Jakob *Knapp*, New York ophthalmologist, 1832–1911] see under *forceps, operation,* and *streak*.

Knapp's test (knaps) [Karl *Knapp*, German chemist] see under *tests*.

kneading (nēd′ing) a movement in massage consisting of grasping and pressing of muscles.

knee (ne) 1. the site of articulation between the thigh (femur) and leg; called also *genu* [NA]. 2. any structure bent like the knee. **k. of aquaeduc′tus fallo′pii,** geniculum canalis facialis. **back k.,** genu recurvatum. **beat k.,** a subcutaneous cellulitis over the kneecap. **big k.,** 1. bursitis over the knee in cattle. 2. a tumor of the bony parts of the knee joint in horses. **Brodie's k.,** a chronic synovitis of the knee joint in which the affected parts acquire a soft and pulpy consistency. **capped k.,** distention of the synovial bursa over the knee joint of horses or cattle. **football k.,** a swollen, relaxed, somewhat tender condition of the knee seen in football players. **hooped k.,** the presence of exostoses in the knee of a horse. **housemaid's k.,** inflammation of the bursa in front of the patella, with fluid accumulating within it. **in k.,** genu valgum. **k. of internal capsule,** genu capsulae internae. **knock k.,** genu valgum. **locked k.,** inability to extend the leg fully as a result of tear of the medial semilunar cartilage. **out k.,** genu varum, or bowleg. **rugby k.,** Schlatter's disease. **septic k.,** a suppurating knee joint. **sprung k.,** forward bending of the knee of a horse, due to shortening of the flexor tendons. **trick k.,** popular term for a knee joint susceptible to locking in position, most often due to longitudinal splitting of the medial meniscus.

knee-gall (ne′gawl) distension of the carpal sheath at the back of the knee joint in the horse.

kneippism (nīp′izm) [Rev. Father Sebastian *Kneipp*, 1821–1897, who introduced the practice] a system of hydrotherapy involving applications of cold water, as cold bathing, walking barefoot in the morning dew, etc.

Knemidokoptes (ne″mĭ-do-kop′tēz) a genus of mites. *K. gallinae,* the depluming mite, causes depluming of fowls. *K. mu′tans* causes scaly legs in fowl and cage birds.

knife (nīf) a cutting instrument of various shapes and sizes. **Beer's k.,** a knife with a triangle-shaped blade, formerly used in operations for cataract and for excising staphyloma of the cornea. **Blair k.,** a knife with a long sharp blade used to cut skin grafts. **buck k.,** a knife with spear-shaped cutting points, used for interdental incision during gingivectomy. **button k.,** a small knife used for the cutting of cartilage. **cataract k.,** a knife for cutting the cornea in operations for cataract. **cautery k.,** a knife connected with an electric battery, so that the tissues may be seared while being cut, in order to prevent bleeding. **electric k., endotherm k.,** a knife-shaped electrode or steel needle which cuts by causing dissolution of tissue when activated by a high-frequency current. **Goldman-Fox k.,** any of various surgical instruments designed for the incision and contouring of gingival tissue. **Graefe's k.,** a slender knife used in linear extraction of cataract. **hernia k.,** herniotome. **Humby k.,** a knife with a roller attached, used for cutting skin grafts of varying thickness; the distance between the roller and the blade of the knife can be varied by means of a calibration device. **Kirkland k.,** a heart-shaped knife, sharp on all edges, used for primary gingivectomy incision. **Liston's knives,** long-bladed amputation knives. **Merrifield's k.,** a knife with a long narrow triangular blade in a shank, used for gingivectomy incisions. **Ramsbotham's sickle k.,** a sickle-shaped knife used for intrauterine decapitation of a fetus.

knismogenic (nis″mo-jen′ik) [Gr. *knismos* tickling + *gennan* to produce] producing a tickling sensation.

knitting (nit′ing) the physiological process of repair of a fractured bone.

KNO₃ potassium nitrate.

knob (nob) a bulbous mass or protuberance. **surfers' k's,** see under *nodule.* **synaptic k's,** end-feet.

knock (nok) a sound as of a blow against a firm surface. **pericardial k.,** a clear, metallic clicking sound heard over the precordium in certain cases of penetrating chest wounds in the neighborhood of the pericardium; ascribed to emphysema of the mediastinal connective tissue or to free air in the interstitial connective tissue of the lung. Cf. *clicking pneumothorax,* under *pneumothorax.*

knock-knee (nok′ne) genu valgum.

Knoepfelmacher's butter meal (knep′fel-mahk′erz) [Wilhelm *Knoepfelmacher*, pediatrist in Vienna, born 1866] see under *meal.*

knokkelkoorts (nok′el-koorts) [Dutch "knuckle fever"] dengue in the Netherlands East Indies.

knot (not) 1. an intertwining of the ends or parts of one or more threads, sutures, or strips of cloth so they cannot easily be

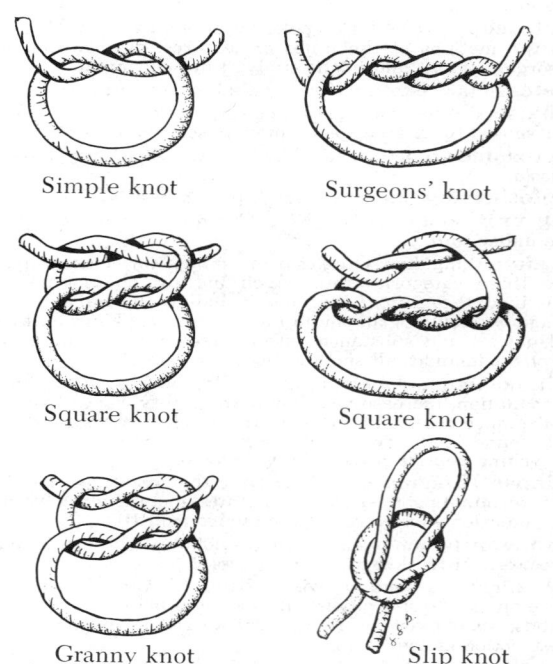

Simple knot   Surgeons' knot

Square knot   Square knot

Granny knot   Slip knot

separated. 2. in anatomy, a knoblike swelling or protuberance, as a node. **clove-hitch k.,** a knot consisting of two contiguous loops that are applied around an object, the ends of the cord being toward each other; used for making traction on a part for the reduction of dislocations. **double k.,** friction k. **enamel k.,** a small dense group of epithelial cells in the stellate reticulum of a developing tooth, which disappears before enamel formation begins. **false k.,** 1. a local bulge on the umbilical cord caused by protuberant vessels. Cf. *true k.* 2. granny k. **friction k.,** a knot in which the ends of the cord are twisted twice around each other before being tied. **granny k.,** a double knot in the second loop of which the end of one cord is over, and the other under, its fellow, so that the loops do not lie in the same line. **Hensen's k.,** primitive k. **net k.,** karyosome. **primitive k.,** a mass of cells at the cranial end of the primitive streak, related to the organization of an embryo. **protochordal k.,** primitive k. **reef k.,** a double knot in which the free ends of the second knot lie in the same plane as the ends of the first knot; called also *square k.* **sailor's k., square k.,** reef k. **stay k.,** a knot made with two or more ligatures, each being tied with the first half of a reef knot; then all the ends of one side are taken in one hand, and all the ends on the other side in the other hand, and tied as if they formed one single thread. **surfers' k's,** see under *nodule.* **surgeons' k., surgical k.,** a knot in which the thread is passed twice through the first loop. **syncytial k's,** protuberances of syncytium along the chorionic villi. **true k.,** a simple knot produced in the looped umbilical cord during pregnancy. Cf. *false k.*

knuckle (nuk′'l) the dorsal aspect of any phalangeal joint, especially of the metacarpophalangeal joints of the flexed fingers. By extension sometimes applied to any anatomical structure of similar appearance, such as an extruded loop of intestine in hernia. **aortic k.,** the hump or knuckle formed by the aortic arch as seen in radiographs in anteroposterior projections.

knuckling (nuk′ling) a condition in which the fetlock joint of a horse is pushed upward and forward, due to shortening of the tendons behind.

Kobelt's tubes, tubules (ko′belts) [George Ludwig *Kobelt*, German physician, 1804–1857] see under *tube* and *tubule*.

Kober's test (ko′berz) [Philip Adolph *Kober*, American chemist, born 1884] see under *tests*.

Kobert's test (ko′bärts) [Eduard Rudolf *Kobert*, German chemist, 1854–1918] see under *tests*.

KOC kathodal (cathodal) opening contraction.

Koch's bacillus, etc. (kōks) [Robert *Koch*, German bacteriologist, 1843–1910, the discoverer of the tubercle bacillus; winner of the Nobel prize for medicine in 1905] see under *bacillus, phenomenon, postulate, reaction,* and *tuberculin.*

Koch's node (kōks) [Walter *Koch*, German surgeon, born 1880] atrioventricular node.

Koch-Weeks bacillus (hemophilus) (kōk-wēks) [Robert *Koch*; John Elmer *Weeks*, New York ophthalmologist, 1853–1949] *Hemophilus aegyptius.*

Kocher's forceps, operation, reflex (kōk′erz) [Emil Theodor *Kocher*, Swiss surgeon, 1841–1917, the first surgeon to excise the thyroid gland; winner of the Nobel prize for medicine in 1909] see under *forceps, operation,* and *reflex.*

kocherization (kōk″er-i-za′shun) operative reflexion of a flap of the duodenum for exposure of the ampulla of the common bile duct.

Kocks' operation (kōks) [Joseph *Kocks*, German surgeon, 1846–1916] see under *operation.*

Koeberlé's forceps (ke″ber-lāz′) [Eugène *Koeberlé*, French surgeon, 1828–1915] hemostatic forceps.

Koenecke's reaction, test (ke-nek′ez) see under *tests.*

Kogoj's pustule (ko-goiz) [Franjo *Kogoj*, Yugoslavian physician, born 1894] see *spongiform pustule of Kogoj,* under *pustule.*

KOH potassium hydroxide.

koha (ko′hah) a Japanese drug derived from cyanine; given intravenously it is said to stimulate the formation of leukocytes and of new tissue and thus hasten wound healing.

Köhler's bone disease (ka′lerz) [Alban *Köhler*, German physician, 1874–1947] see under *disease.*

Kohlrausch's folds (valves) (kōl′rowsh-ez) [Otto Ludwig Bernhard *Kohlrausch*, German physician, 1811–1854] plicae transversales recti.

Kohn's pores (kōnz) [Hans *Kohn*, German pathologist, born 1866] interalveolar pores; see under *pore.*

Kohnstamm's phenomenon (kōn′stahmz) [Oscar Felix *Kohnstamm*, German physician, 1871–1917] after-movement.

koilo- [Gr. *koilos* hollow] a combining form meaning hollow or concave.

koilonychia (koi″lo-nik′e-ah) [*koilo-* + *onyx* nail + *-ia*] dystrophy of the fingernails, sometimes associated with iron deficiency anemia, in which they are thin and concave, with the edges raised; called also *spoon nail.*

koilorrhachic (koi″lo-rak′ik) [*koilo* + Gr. *rhachis* spine] having a vertebral column in which the lumbar curvature is concave anteriorly. Cf. *kyphosis, kyrtorrhachic,* and *orthorrhachic.*

koilosternia (koi″lo-ster′ne-ah) [*koilo-* + *sternum* + *-ia*] funnel chest.

koino- see *ceno-.*

koinonia (koi-no′ne-ah) [Gr. *koinōnia* community] associated or common action, as of like cells in the same tissue.

koinotropy (koi-not′ro-pe) interest in social or public relationships; identification with the public interest.

koktigen (kok′tĭ-jen) [L. *coctus* cooked + Gr. *gennan* to produce] a vaccine made by boiling salt solution emulsion of an organism.

Kolantyl (ko-lan′til) trademark for a preparation of alumina and magnesia.

Kölliker's column, etc. (kel′ĭ-kerz) [Rudolf Abert von *Kölliker*, eminent Swiss anatomist, histologist, and zoologist, professor at Zurich and Würzburg, 1817–1905] see under *column, granule, membrane,* and *nucleus.*

Kollmann's dilator (kol′manz) [Arthur *Kollmann*, Leipzig urologist, born 1858] see under *dilator.*

Kolmer's test (kōl′merz) [John A. *Kolmer*, American pathologist, 1886–1962] see under *tests.*

kolp- for words beginning thus, see those beginning *colp-.*

kolypeptic (ko″le-pep′tik) [Gr. *kōlyein* to hinder + *peptikos* peptic] hindering or checking digestion.

kolytic (ko-lit′ik) Hunt's term for the inhibitory temperament, marked by calmness, self-control, with a tendency to passivity of mind and body. Cf. *erethitic.*

Konakion (kon″ah-ki′on) trademark for a preparation of phytonadione (vitamin K₁).

Kondoleon's operation (kon-do′le-onz) [Emmerich (Emmanuel)

Kondoleon, surgeon in Athens, 1879–1939] see under *operation.*

König's operation, syndrome (ken′igz) [Franz *König*, German surgeon, 1832–1910] see under *operation* and *syndrome.*

König's rods (ken′igz) [Charles Joseph *König*, German otologist, born 1868] see under *rod.*

konimeter (ko-nim′ĕ-ter) konometer.

koniocortex (ko″ne-o-kor′teks) [Gr. *konis* dust + *cortex*] the granular cortex of sensory areas of the brain.

koniology (ko″ne-ol′o-je) coniology.

konometer (ko-nom′ĕ-ter) [Gr. *konis* dust + *metron* measure] an apparatus for counting the number of dust particles in the air.

Konsyl (kon′sil) a brand of psyllium hydrophilic muciloid.

koomis (koo′mis) koumiss.

kopf-tetanus (kopf-tet′ah-nus) [Ger. *Kopf* head + *tetanus*] cerebral tetanus.

kophemia (ko-fe′me-ah) [Gr. *kōphos* deaf] word deafness.

kopiopia (ko″pe-o′pe-ah) copiopia.

Koplik's spots (sign) (kop′liks) [Henry *Koplik*, New York pediatrician, 1858–1927] see under *spot.*

Kopp's asthma (kops) [Johann Heinrich *Kopp*, German physician, 1777–1858] thymic asthma.

kopr-, kopro- for words beginning thus, see also those beginning *copr-, copro-.*

kopratin (kop′rah-tin) [Gr. *kopros* dung] the chemical substance which produces the so-called pyridine-hemochromogen spectrum in the pyridine test for blood. It is produced from alpha-hematin by putrefaction.

koprosterin (kop″ro-ste′rin) coprostanol.

Korányi's auscultation (percussion), sign (ko-ran′yēz) [Baron *Korányi*, Hungarian physician, 1828–1913] see under *auscultation* and *sign.*

Korányi's treatment (ko-ran′yēz) [Baron Alexander von *Korányi* (Sandor), Hungarian physician, 1866–1944] see under *treatment.*

Korányi-Grocco triangle (ko-ran′ye-grok′o) [Baron F. von *Korányi;* Pietro *Grocco*, physician in Florence, 1857–1916] see *Grocco's sign* (def. 1), under *sign.*

Kornberg (korn′berg), Arthur. United States physician and biochemist, born 1918; co-winner, with Severo Ochoa, of the Nobel prize in medicine and physiology for 1959, for work in the discovery of enzymes for producing nucleic acids artificially.

koro (ko′ro) a phobia seen chiefly in the Far East and Southeast Asia consisting of anxiety and the fear that the penis will retract into the abdomen and cause death. Called also *coro.*

koronion (ko-ro′ne-on), pl. *koro′nia* [Gr. *korōnē* crow, crown] coronion.

koroscopy (ko-ros′ko-pe) retinoscopy.

Korotkoff's method, sounds, test (ko-rot′kofs) [Nicolai Sergeevich *Korotkoff*, Russian physician, born 1874] see under the nouns.

Korsakoff's (Korsakov's) psychosis (disease, syndrome) (kor-sak′ofs) [Sergei Sergeevich *Korsakoff*, Russian neurologist, 1854–1900] see under *psychosis.*

Körte-Ballance operation (kēr′te-bal′ans) [Werner *Körte*, Berlin surgeon, 1853–1937; Sir Charles Alfred *Ballance*, British surgeon, 1856–1936] see under *operation.*

kosam (ko′sam) a small evergreen shrub, *Brucea sumatrana* Roxb. (Simaroubaceae), of southeastern Asia and Australia, whose seeds are sometimes used locally in the treatment of diarrhea, dysentery, and uterine hemorrhage.

Koshevnikoff's (Koschewnikow's, Kozhevnikov's) disease, epilepsy (ko-shev′ne-kofs) [Alexei Jakovlevich *Koshevnikoff*, Russian neurologist, 1836–1902] epilepsia partialis continua.

Kossel's test (kos′elz) [Albrecht *Kossel*, German physiologist, 1853–1927; winner of the Nobel prize for physiology and medicine in 1910, for his contributions to the chemistry of the cell through works on proteins, including the nucleic substances] see under *tests.*

Köster's nodule (kes′terz) [Karl *Köster*, German pathologist, 1843–1904] see under *nodule.*

Kottmann's test (reaction) (kot′manz) [K. *Kottmann*, German physician, 1877–1952] see under *tests.*

koumiss (koo′mis) [Tartarian] a fermented alcoholic drink prepared from cow's milk; originally from mare's milk by the Tartars. **kefir k.,** milk fermented with kefir fungi.

Kovalevsky's canal (ko″val-ev′skēz) [Alexander Onufrievich *Kovalevsky*, Russian embryologist, 1840–1901] neurenteric canal.

Kowarsky's test (ko-var′skēz) [Albert *Kowarsky*, physician in Berlin] see under *tests.*

Koyter's muscle (koi′terz) [Volcherus *Koyter*, Dutch anatomist, 1534–1600] musculus corrugator supercilii.

K.P. keratitic precipitates; see *keratitis punctata,* under *keratitis.*

K₃PO₄ normal ortho- or tribasic potassium phosphate.

Kr chemical symbol for *krypton*.

Krabbe's disease (leukodystrophy) (krab′ēz) [Knud H. *Krabbe*, Danish neurologist, 1885–1961] see under *disease*.

Kraepelin's classification (kra′pa-linz) [Emil *Kraepelin*, Munich psychiatrist, 1856–1926] see under *classification*.

krait (krāt) an extremely venomous elapid snake of the genus *Bungarus;* see table accompanying *snake*.

Krameria (krah-me′re-ah) [J. G. H. and W. H. *Kramer*, German botanists] a genus of leguminous shrubs and herbs. The dried roots of *K. triandra* R. et P., or Peruvian rhatany, and of *K. argentea* Mart., or Brazilian rhatany, were formerly used as an astringent because of their high content of krameric acid.

Kraske's operation (kras′kēz) [Paul *Kraske*, German surgeon, 1851–1930] see under *operation*.

kratom (krah′tom) a masticatory containing the leaves of *Mitragyna speciosa* Korth. (Rubiaceae), which is chewed in Thailand.

kratometer (kra-tom′ĕ-ter) a prism-refracting instrument for use in orthoptic training.

krauomania (kraw″o-ma′ne-ah) a tic marked by rhythmic movements, such as balancing, head rotation, etc.

kraurosis (kraw-ro′sis) [Gr. *krauros* brittle] a dry, shriveled condition of a part, especially of the vulva (see *k. vulvae*). **k. pe′nis,** balanitis xerotica obliterans. **k. vul′vae,** an atrophic disease affecting the female external genitalia, most often of older women, resulting in drying and shriveling of the parts, and marked by leukoplakic patches on the mucosa, itching, dyspareunia, dysuria, and soreness. It occurs most commonly as a result of lichen sclerosus et atrophicus of the vulva, but may be associated with other types of genital atrophy. Called also *leukokraurosis, leukoplakic vulvitis,* and *Breisky's disease.*

Krause's bulbs, etc. (krow′zez) [Wilhelm Johann Friedrich *Krause*, German anatomist, 1833–1910] see under *bulb, corpuscle, line, membrane,* and *suture.*

Krause's ligament, valve (krow′zez) [Karl Friedrich Theodor *Krause*, German anatomist, 1797–1868] see *ligamentum transversum perinei,* and see *Béraud's valve,* under *valve.*

Krause's operation (krow′zez) [Fedor Victor *Krause*, German surgeon, 1857–1937] see under *operation.*

Krause-Wolfe graft (krowz-wolf) [Fedor *Krause;* John Reissberg *Wolfe*, Scotch ophthalmologist, 1824–1904] see under *graft.*

kreatin (kre′ah-tin) creatine.

krebiozen (krĕ-bi′o-zen) a substance identified as creatine by the Food and Drug Administration, isolated from the blood of horses injected with *Actinomyces bovis,* claimed to be effective in the treatment of cancer; its sale is banned in the United States.

Krebs cycle (krebz) [Sir Hans Adolf *Krebs*, German biochemist in England, 1900–1981; co-winner, with F. A. Lipmann, of the Nobel prize for medicine and physiology in 1953 for discovery of the tricarboxylic acid cycle] tricarboxylic acid cycle; see under *cycle.*

Krebs' leukocyte index (krebz) [Carl *Krebs*, Copenhagen pathologist, born 1892] see under *index.*

kreo- for words beginning thus, see also those beginning *creo-.*

kreotoxicon (kre″o-tok′sĭ-kon) the substance in poisonous meat that produces the toxic symptoms; see *meat poisoning,* under *poisoning.*

kreotoxin (kre″o-tok′sin) any basic poison generated in a flesh food by a plant microorganism; see *meat poisoning,* under *poisoning.*

kreotoxism (kre″o-tok′sizm) [Gr. *kreas* meat + *toxikon* poison] meat poisoning; see under *poisoning.*

kresofuchsin (kres″o-fook′sin) a blue-gray powder used as a stain in histology; its aqueous solution is red, the alcoholic solution blue.

kresol (kres′ol) cresol.

Kretschmann's space (krech′mahnz) [Friedrich *Kretschmann,* German otologist, 1858–1934] see under *space.*

Kretschmer types (krech′mer) [Ernst *Kretschmer,* German psychiatrist, 1888–1964] see under *type.*

Kretz's granules, paradox (krets′ez) [Richard *Kretz,* German pathologist, 1865–1920] see under *granule* and *paradox.*

Kreysig's sign (kri′zigs) [Friedrich Ludwig *Kreysig,* physician in Dresden, 1770–1839] Heim-Kreysig sign; see under *sign.*

krimpsiekte (krimp-zēk′te) a disease of cattle in South Africa caused by poisoning with the plant *Cotyledon wallachii.*

krinin (krin′in) crinin.

Krishaber's disease (krēs″hab-ārz′) [Maurice *Krishaber,* Hungarian physician in France, 1836–1883] see under *disease.*

Kristeller's method (expression, technique) (kris′tel-er) [Samuel *Kristeller,* Berlin gynecologist, 1820–1900] see under *method.*

Krogh (krōg), August. Danish physiologist, 1874–1949, noted for his research on the capillaries; winner of the Nobel prize for medicine and physiology in 1920.

Kromayer's burn, lamp (kro′mi-erz) [Ernst Ludwig Franz *Kromayer,* German dermatologist, 1862–1933] see under *burn* and *lamp.*

Krompecher's carcinoma, tumor (krōm′pek-erz) [Edmund *Krompecher,* pathologist in Budapest, 1870–1926] rodent ulcer; see under *ulcer.*

kromskop (krōm′skōp) [German, from Gr. *chrōma* color + *skopein* to examine] an apparatus used for color photography of pathological specimens.

Kronecker's center, puncture (kro′nek-erz) [Karl Hugo *Kronecker,* Swiss pathologist, 1839–1914] see under *center* and *puncture.*

Krönig's field (area), isthmus (kra′nigz) [Georg *Krönig,* physician in Berlin, 1856–1911] see under *field* and *isthmus.*

Krönlein's hernia, operation (krān′linz) [Rudolf Ulrich *Krönlein,* surgeon in Zurich, 1847–1910] see *inguinoproperitoneal hernia,* under *hernia,* and see under *operation.*

Krukenberg's hand (arm) (kroo′ken-bergz) [Hermann *Krukenberg,* German surgeon, born 1863] see under *hand.*

Krukenberg's spindle, tumor (kroo′ken-bergz) [Friedrich Ernst *Krukenberg,* German pathologist, born 1871] see under *spindle* and *tumor.*

Krukenberg's veins (kroo′ken-bergz) [Adolph *Krukenberg,* German anatomist, 1816–1877] venae centrales hepatis.

Kruse's brush (kroo′zez) [Walther *Kruse,* German bacteriologist, 1864–1943] see under *brush.*

kryoscopy (kri-os′ko-pe) cryoscopy.

krypto- (krip′to) for words beginning thus, see also these beginning *crypto-.*

krypton (krip′ton) [Gr. *kryptos* hidden] an inert gaseous chemical element found in the atmosphere; atomic number, 36; atomic weight, 83.80; symbol, Kr.

KSC kathodal (cathodal) closing contraction.

K₂SO₄ potassium sulfate.

KST kathodal (cathodal) closing tetanus.

K.U.B. kidney, ureter, and bladder.

kubisagari, kubisgari (koo-bis″ah-gah′re, koo′bis-gah′re) a form of Gerlier's disease (paralytic vertigo) endemic in Japan (Gerlier-Nakano, 1884).

Kuhlmann's test (kool′manz) [Frederick *Kuhlmann,* American psychologist, 1876–1941] see under *tests.*

Kuhn's mask (kōōnz) [Ernst *Kuhn,* Prussian physician, 1873–1920] see under *mask.*

Kuhn's tube (kōōnz) [Franz *Kuhn,* Berlin surgeon, 1866–1929] see under *tube.*

Kühne's methylene blue (ke′nez) [Heinrich *Kühne,* German histologist] see *methylene blue.*

Kühne's muscular phenomenon, terminal plates, spindle (ke′nez) [Wilhelm Friedrich (Willy) *Kühne,* German physiologist, 1837–1900] see *Porret's phenomenon,* under *phenomenon,* see under *plate,* and see *muscle spindle,* under *spindle.*

Kuhnt's illusion (kōōnts) [Hermann *Kuhnt,* German ophthalmologist, 1850–1925] see under *illusion.*

kukuruku (koo″koo-roo′koo) a disease of the Kukuruka division of Nigeria of unknown etiology, marked by fever and jaundice; clinically and pathologically it resembles yellow fever.

Kulchitsky's cells (kool-chits′kēz) [Nicolai K. *Kulchitsky,* Russian histologist, 1856–1925] see under *cell.*

Kulenkampff's anesthesia (koo′len-kahmpfs) [Dietrich *Kulenkampff,* German surgeon, born 1880] see under *anesthesia.*

Külz's cast (cylinder), test (kiltsez) [Rudolph Eduard *Külz,* German physician, 1845–1895] see *coma casts,* under *cast,* and see under *tests.*

kumiss (koo′mis) koumiss.

Kümmell's disease (spondylitis) (kim′elz) [Hermann *Kümmell,* surgeon in Hamburg, 1852–1937] see under *disease.*

Kümmell-Verneuil disease (kim′el-ver″na′e) [Hermann *Kümmell;* Aristide August Stanislas *Verneuil,* French surgeon, 1823–1895] Kümmell's disease.

kumyss (koo′mis) koumiss.

Küntscher nail (kint′sher) [Gerhard *Küntscher,* German surgeon, born 1902] see under *nail.*

Kupffer's cells (koop′ferz) [Karl Wilhelm von *Kupffer,* German anatomist, 1829–1902] see under *cell.*

kupramite (ku′prah-mīt) a gas mask adsorbent for ammonia fumes.

Kupressoff's center (koo-pres′ofs) [Ivan *Kupressoff,* Russian physician of the 19th century] micturition center; see under *center.*

Kurloff's (Kurlov's) bodies (koor′lofs) [Mikhail Georgievich *Kurloff,* Russian physician, 1859–1932] see under *body.*

Kurthia (kur′the-ah) [Heinrich *Kurth,* German bacteriologist, 1860–1901] a genus of microorganisms of the family Brevibacteriaceae, order Eubacteriales, made up of long rods with rounded ends, found in decomposing material. It includes three species, *K. besson'ii, K. varia'bilis,* and *K. zop'fii.*

kuru (koo'roo) a chronic, progressive, uniformly fatal nervous system disorder caused by a slow virus and transmissible to subhuman primates. It is found only among the Fore and neighboring peoples of New Guinea and is thought to be associated with cannibalism. The chief symptoms are truncal and limb ataxia, a shivering-like tremor, and dysarthria, but strabismus and extrapyramidal symptoms may also be found. Pathologically, the brain shows the changes of the spongiform encephalopathies: neuronal loss, astrogliosis, and status spongiosus; amyloid plaques are also present in about two thirds of the cases.

Kurunegala ulcer (koo''roo-na-gah'lah) [the name of a district in Ceylon] pyosis tropica.

Küss' experiment (kes) [Emil *Küss,* German physiologist, 1815–1871] see under *experiment.*

Kussmaul's aphasia, etc. (koos'mowlz) [Adolph *Kussmaul,* German physician, 1822–1902] see under *aphasia, disease, paralysis, pulse, respiration,* and *sign.*

Kussmaul-Kien respiration (koos'mowl-kēn) [Adolf *Kussmaul;* Alphonse M. J. *Kien,* German physician] air hunger; see under *hunger.*

Kussmaul-Landry paralysis (koos'mowl-lan'dre) [Adolf *Kussmaul;* Jean Baptiste Octave *Landry,* French physician, 1826–1865] acute febrile polyneuritis.

Kussmaul-Maier disease (koos'mowl-mi'er) [Adolf *Kussmaul;* Rudolf *Maier,* German physician, 1824–1888] periarteritis nodosa.

Küstner's law, sign (kist'nerz) [Otto Ernst *Küstner,* gynecologist in Breslau, 1850–1931] see under *law* and *sign.*

Kutrol (ku'trol) trademark for a preparation of urogastrone.

kuttarosome (kut-tar'o-sōm) [Gr. *kyttaros* cell of a honeycomb + *soma* body] a structure at the neck of a retinal cone composed of a series of parallel bars.

kv. kilovolt.

kvp. kilovolt peak.

kw. kilowatt.

kwashiorkor (kwash-e-or'kor) [local name in Gold Coast, Africa, "displaced child"] a syndrome produced by severe protein deficiency, characterized by retarded growth, changes in skin and hair pigment, edema, and pathologic changes in the liver, including fatty infiltration, necrosis, and fibrosis. Other findings are peevish mental apathy, atrophy of the pancreas, gastrointestinal disorders, anemia, low serum albumin, and dermatoses. The skin may exhibit darkened, thickened patches on limbs and back which may desquamate, leaving pink, almost raw surfaces of a pellagroid appearance. First reported from Africa, kwashiorkor is now known to occur throughout the world, but mainly in the tropics and subtropics, and is now considered to be related to marasmus. **marasmic k.,** a condition in which there is deficiency of both calories and protein, with severe tissue wasting, loss of subcutaneous fat, and usually dehydration.

kwaski see under *shakes.*

Kwell (kwel) trademark for preparations of lindane.

kw.-hr. kilowatt-hour.

kyano- for words beginning thus, see also those beginning *cyano-.*

kyanophane (ki'ah-no-fān) [Gr. *kyanos* blue + *phainein* to appear] a supposed bluish pigment from the oil globules of the retinal cones.

kyestein (ki-es'te-in) a film sometimes seen on stale urine, formerly thought a sign of pregnancy.

kyllosis (kil-lo'sis) [Gr. *kyllōsis* a crippling] clubfoot, or other deformity of the foot.

kymatism (ki'mah-tizm) myokymia.

kymocyclograph (ki''mo-si'klo-graf) an apparatus for recording movement.

kymogram (ki'mo-gram) a tracing or other graphic record made by a kymograph.

kymograph (ki'mo-graf) [Gr. *kyma* wave + *graphein* to record] an instrument for recording variations or undulations, arterial or other.

kymography (ki-mog'rah-fe) the use of the kymograph. **roentgen k.,** roentgenkymography.

kymotrichous (ki''mo-trik'us) [Gr. *kyma* wave + *thrix* hair] having wavy hair.

Kynex (ki'neks) trademark for preparations of sulfamethoxypyridazine.

kynocephalus (ki''no-sef'ah-lus) [Gr. *kyōn* dog + *kephalē* head] a human fetus with a head resembling that of a dog.

kynurenin (kin''u-re'nin) kynurenine.

kynurenine (ki''nu-ren'in) [Gr. *kyon* dog + L. *ren* kidney] a crystalline nitrogenous base, first isolated from dog urine; $NH_2C_6H_4CO \cdot CH_2CH(NH_2)COOH$ (3-anthraniloylalanine), a metabolite of tryptophan found in microorganisms and in the urine of normal animals, and a precursor of kynurenic acid. It is also an intermediate in the conversion of tryptophan to niacin, a member of the vitamin B complex.

kyogenic (ki''o-jen'ik) [Gr. *kyēsis* pregnancy + *gennan* to produce] pregnancy producing: a term used by Wiesner to describe the anterior pituitary hormone which stimulates the corpora lutea to secrete progestin.

kyphos (ki'fos) [Gr. "a hump"] the convex prominence of the spine in kyphosis.

kyphoscoliosis (ki''fo-sko''le-o'sis) [*kyphosis* + *scoliosis*] backward and lateral curvature of the spinal column, as in vertebral osteochondrosis (Scheuermann's disease).

kyphosis (ki-fo'sis) [Gr. *kyphōsis* humpback] abnormally increased convexity in the curvature of the thoracic spine as viewed from the side; hunchback. Cf. *lordosis* and *scoliosis.* **k. dorsa'lis juveni'lis, juvenile k., Scheuermann's k.,** see *osteochondrosis.*

kyphotic (ki-fot'ik) affected with or pertaining to kyphosis.

kyphotone (ki'fo-tōn) [Gr. *kyphos* a hump + *tonos* brace] an apparatus for reducing deformity in Pott's disease.

kyrin (ki'rin) a peptide obtained by Siegfried by the partial hydrolysis of proteins and assumed to be a fundamental protein unit.

kyrtorrhachic (ker''to-rak'ik) [Gr. *kyrtos* curved, convex + *rhachis* spine] having a vertebral column in which the lumbar curvature is convex anteriorly. Cf. *koilorrhachic* and *orthorrhachic.*

kysth-, kystho- [Gr. *kysthos* vagina] a combining form formerly used to designate reference to the vagina; for words beginning thus, see those beginning *colpo-.*

kyto- [Gr. *kytos* hollow vessel] for words beginning thus, see those beginning *cyto-.*

L

L. 1. an abbreviation for *Latin, Lactobacillus, left, light sense, libra* (pound, balance), *liter, length, limes* (boundary), *lumbar* (in vertebral formulas), and *coefficient of induction.* 2. Ehrlich's symbol for *lethal* (fatal).

L₀ Ehrlich's symbol for *limes nul,* i.e., a toxin-antitoxin mixture which is completely neutralized and therefore will not kill an animal.

L+ Ehrlich's symbol for *limes tod,* i.e, a toxin-antitoxin mixture which contains one fatal dose in excess and which will kill the experimental animal.

L- (el-) chemical prefix (small capital) which specifies that the substance corresponds in configuration to the standard substance L-glyceraldehyde, i.e., belongs to the same configurational family. In carbohydrate nomenclature, the symbol refers to the configurational family of the *highest numbered* asymmetric carbon atom, as in L-rhamnose. In amino acid nomenclature, under rules adopted in 1947, the symbol refers to the configurational family to which the *lowest numbered* asymmetric carbon atom, i.e., the 2-carbon atom or α-carbon atom, belongs, as in L-threonine. This prefix does not indicate direction of rotation, as does *l-.* Opposed to D-.

L$_g$- (el-sub-je) see L-; this chemical prefix (with the subscript *g*) is occasionally used to emphasize that the rules of carbohydrate nomenclature are being employed. The subscript refers to the standard monosaccharide, glyceraldehyde. Opposed to D$_g$-.

L$_s$- (el-sub-es) see L-; this chemical prefix (with the subscript *s*) is used where needed in amino acid nomenclature to avoid possible confusion with carbohydrate nomenclature, as in L$_s$-threonine. The subscript refers to the standard amino acid, serine. Opposed to D$_s$-.

l. liter.

l- (el) 1. chemical abbreviation for *levo-* (i.e., left or counterclockwise) with reference to the direction in which the plane of polarized light is rotated when passed through a solution of the substance or through the substance itself if a liquid; opposed to *d-* (*dextro-*). Cf. L-. 2. when used with one of the additional symbols (+) or (−), especially in amino acid nomenclature in the literature from 1923 until 1947 or a little later, the prefix refers to the configurational family to which the 2-carbon atom or α-carbon atom of the amino acid belongs, and the actual direction of the rotation in a specified solvent is indicated by the plus or minus sign, as in *l*(+)-alanine; opposed to *d*(−)- or *d*(+)-, as in *d*(−)-alanine or *d*(+)-cystine.

λ lambda, the eleventh letter of the Greek alphabet; symbol for *decay constant.*

La chemical symbol for *lanthanum*.

L. & A. light and accommodation (reaction of pupils).

lab [Ger.] rennin.

Labarraque's solution (lab″ah-raks′) [Antoine Germain *Labarraque*, French chemist, 1777–1850] see under *solution*.

Labbé's triangle, vein (lab-āz′) [Léon *Labbé*, French surgeon, 1832–1916] see under *triangle*, and see *vena anastomatica superior*.

label (la′b'l) something that identifies; an identifying mark, tag, etc. **radioactive l.,** radioactive isotopes introduced into tissue to identify the role of the normal element in metabolism.

labetalol hydrochloride (lah-bet′ah-lōl) chemical name: 2-hydroxy-5-[1-hydroxy-2-[(1-methyl-3-phenylpropyl)amino] ethyl]-benzamide monohydrochloride; a beta-adrenergic blocking agent with some alpha-adrenergic blocking activity, $C_{19}H_{24}N_2O_3 \cdot HCl$.

labia (la′be-ah) [L.] plural of *labium*.

labial (la′be-al) [L. *labialis*] pertaining to a lip, or labium.

labialism (la′be-ah-lizm″) defective speech, with use of labial sounds.

labially (la′be-al-e) toward the lips.

labichorea (la″be-ko-re′ah) labiochorea.

Labidognatha (lab″ĭ-dog′nah-thah) a suborder of spiders (order Araneae), including the medically important families, Theridiidae and Loxoscelidae.

labile (la′bīl) [L. *labilis* unstable, from *labi* to glide] 1. gliding; moving from point to point over the surface; unstable; fluctuating. 2. chemically unstable. **heat l.,** thermolabile.

lability (lah-bil′ĭ-te) the quality of being labile. In psychiatry, emotional instability; a tendency to show alternating states of gaiety and somberness.

labio- (la′be-o) [L. *labium* lip] a combining form denoting relationship to a lip, especially to the lips of the mouth.

labioalveolar (la″be-o-al-ve′o-lar) 1. pertaining to the lip and dental alveoli. 2. pertaining to the labial side of a dental alveolus.

labiocervical (la″be-o-ser′vĭ-kal) 1. pertaining to the labial surface of the neck of an anterior tooth. 2. labiogingival.

labiochorea (la″be-o-ko-re′ah) [L. *labium* lip + *chorea*] a choreic stiffening of the lips in speech, with stammering.

labioclination (la″be-o-kli-na′shun) deviation of an anterior tooth from the vertical, in the direction of the lips.

labiodental (la″be-o-den′tal) pertaining to the lips and teeth.

labiogingival (la″be-o-jin′jĭ-val) pertaining to or formed by the labial and gingival walls of a tooth cavity.

labioglossolaryngeal (la″be-o-glos″o-lah-rin′je-al) [L. *labium* lip + Gr. *glōssa* tongue + *larynx*] pertaining to the lips, tongue, and larynx.

labioglossopharyngeal (la″be-o-glos″o-fah-rin′je-al) pertaining to the lips, tongue, and pharynx.

labiograph (la′be-o-graf″) [L. *labium* lip + Gr. *graphein* to record] an instrument for recording the motions of the lips in speaking.

labioincisal (la″be-o-in-si′zal) pertaining to or formed by the labial and incisal surfaces of a tooth.

labiolingual (la″be-o-ling′gwal) 1. pertaining to the lips and the tongue. 2. pertaining to the labial and lingual surfaces of an anterior tooth.

labiologic (la″be-o-loj′ik) pertaining to labiology.

labiology (la″be-ol′o-je) the study of the movements of the lips in speaking and singing.

labiomental (la″be-o-men′tal) pertaining to the lip and chin.

labiomycosis (la″be-o-mi-ko′sis) [L. *labium* lip + Gr. *mykēs* fungus] any disease of the lips due to a fungus, such as perlèche and thrush.

labionasal (la″be-o-na′zal) pertaining to the lip and nose.

labiopalatine (la″be-o-pal′ah-tin) pertaining to the lip and palate.

labioplacement (la″be-o-plās′ment) displacement of a tooth toward the lip.

labioplasty (la′be-o-plas″te) [L. *labium* lip + Gr. *plassein* to mold] cheiloplasty.

labiotenaculum (la″be-o-te-nak′u-lum) [L. *labium* lip + *tenaculum*] an instrument for holding the lip.

labioversion (la″be-o-ver′zhun) displacement of a tooth labially from the line of occlusion.

labium (la′be-um), pl. *la′bia* [L.] a fleshy border or edge; used in anatomical nomenclature as a general term to designate such a structure. In the plural, often used alone to designate the *labia majora* and *minora pudendi*. Called also *lip*. See also *limbus* and *margo*. **l. ante′rius orific′ii exter′ni u′teri,** l. anterius ostii uteri. **l. ante′rius os′tii pharyn′gei tu′bae auditi′vae,** the anterior lip of the pharyngeal opening of the auditory tube. **l. ante′rius os′tii u′teri** [NA], anterior lip of ostium of uterus: the anterior projection of the cervix into the vagina; it is shorter and thicker than the posterior lip. Called also *l. anterius orificii externi uteri*. **l. cer′ebri,** an edge of a deep

sulcus, e.g., the lips of the calcarine sulcus. **l. exter′num cris′tae ili′acae** [NA], the outer margin or external lip of the iliac crest. **l. infe′rius o′ris** [NA], the lower lip: the fleshy margin of the inferior border of the mouth. **l. infe′rius val′vulae co′li,** the inferior lip of the valve between the ileum and cecum. **l. inter′num cris′tae ili′acae** [NA], the inner margin or internal lip of the iliac crest. **l. latera′le lin′eae as′perae fem′oris** [NA], lateral lip of linea aspera of femur: the outer part of the linea aspera, which becomes continuous with the gluteal tuberosity, and ends at the greater trochanter. **l. lim′bi tympan′icum lam′inae spira′lis** [NA], the tympanic lip of the limb of the spiral lamina: the lower border of the internal spiral sulcus, formed by the lower extremity of the limbus laminae spiralis; called also *l. tympanicum laminae spiralis*. **l. lim′bi vestibula′re lam′inae spira′lis** [NA], the vestibular lip of the limb of the spiral lamina: the upper border of the internal spiral sulcus, formed by the upper extremity of the limbus laminae spiralis; called also *l. vestibulare laminae spiralis*. **l. ma′jus puden′di** [NA], pl. *la′bia majo′ra puden′di*, the greater lip of the pudendum: an elongated fold running downward and backward from the mons pubis in the female, one on either side of the median pudendal cleft. **l. mandibula′re,** l. inferius oris. **l. maxilla′re,** l. superius oris. **l. media′le lin′eae as′perae fem′oris** [NA], medial lip of linea aspera of the femur: the inner part of the linea aspera, which becomes continuous with the intertrochanteric line. **l. mi′nus puden′di** [NA], pl. *la′bia mino′ra puden′di*, lesser lip of the pudendum: a small fold of skin located on either side, between the labium majus and the opening of the vagina. **la′bia o′ris** [NA], the lips: the fleshy upper and lower margins of the mouth. **l. poste′rius orific′ii exter′ni u′teri,** l. posterius ostii uteri. **l. poste′rius os′tii pharyn′gei tu′bae auditi′vae,** the posterior lip of the pharyngeal opening of the auditory tube. **l. poste′rius os′tii u′teri** [NA], posterior lip of ostium of the uterus: the posterior projection of the cervix into the vagina; called also *l. posterius orificii externi uteri*. **l. supe′rius o′ris** [NA], the upper lip: the fleshy margin of the superior border of the mouth. **l. supe′rius val′vulae co′li,** the superior lip of the valve between the ileum and cecum. **l. tympan′icum lam′inae spira′lis,** l. limbi tympanicum laminae spiralis. **l. ure′thrae,** either lateral margin of the external urinary meatus. **l. vestibula′re lam′inae spira′lis,** l. limbi vestibulare laminae spiralis. **l. voca′le,** a projection at each side of the rima glottidis.

labor (la′bor) [L. "work"] the function of the female organism by which the product of conception is expelled from the uterus through the vagina to the outside world. Labor may be divided into three stages: The first (the stage of dilatation) begins with the onset of regular uterine contractions and ends when the os is completely dilated and flush with the vagina, thus completing the birth canal. The second stage (stage of expulsion) extends from the end of the first stage until the expulsion of the infant is completed. The third stage (placental stage) extends from the expulsion of the child until the placenta and membranes are expelled and contraction of the uterus is completed. Called also *accouchement*, *childbirth*, *confinement*, *delivery*, *parturition*, and *travail*. See also *labor pains*, under *pain*. **artificial l.,** induced l. **atonic l.,** labor protracted because of atony of the uterus. **complicated l.,** labor in which cephalopelvic disproportion, hemorrhage, or some other untoward event occurs. **delayed l.,** postponed l. **dry l.,** labor in which the amniotic fluid escapes before the onset of uterine contractions. **false l.,** see *false pains*. **immature l.,** labor taking place between the sixteenth and the twenty-eighth week of pregnancy. **induced l.,** labor brought on by mechanical or other extraneous means, usually by the intravenous injection of oxytocin. **instrumental l.,** labor in which birth of the baby is facilitated by the use of instruments. **mimetic l.,** see *false pains*. **missed l.,** retention of a dead fetus in the uterus beyond the period of normal gestation. **multiple l.,** labor in which two or more infants are born. **obstructed l.,** labor hindered by some mechanical obstruction, such as a contraction in some region of the parturient canal or a tumor. **postmature l., postponed l.,** labor occurring two weeks or more after the expected date of confinement. **precipitate l.,** labor which occurs with undue rapidity. **premature l.,** expulsion of a viable infant before the normal end of gestation, usually applied to interruption of pregnancy between the twenty-eighth and the thirty-seventh week. **premature l., habitual,** delivery occurring in at least three successive pregnancies at about the same stage of development and prior to completion of the full gestation period. **prolonged l., protracted l.,** labor prolonged beyond the ordinary 18 hour limit. **spontaneous l.,** labor in which no artificial aid is required.

laboratorian (lab″o-rah-to′re-an) a person who devotes himself to laboratory work, as distinguished from a clinician.

laboratory (lab′o-rah-to″re) [L. *laboratorium*] a place equipped for performing experimental work or investigative procedures, for the preparation of drugs, chemicals, etc. **clinical l.,** a laboratory for examination of materials derived from the human body for the purpose of providing information on diagnosis, prevention, or treatment of disease.

Laborde's forceps, method, sign (test) (lah-bordz′) [Jean Baptiste Vincent *Laborde*, French physician, 1830–1903] see under *forceps* and *method*, and see *Cloquet's needle sign*, under *sign*.

labra (la′brah) [L.] plural of *labrum*.

labrale (lah-bra′le) an anthropometric landmark on the border of the lip. **l. infe′rius**, the lowest point, in the midsagittal plane, on the vermilion border of the lower lip. **l. supe′rius**, the highest point, in the midsagittal plane, on the vermilion border of the upper lip.

labrocyte (lab′ro-sīt) [Gr. *labros* greedy + *-cyte*] a mast cell.

labrum (la′brum), pl. *la′bra* [L.] [NA] a general term for an edge, brim, or lip. **l. acetabula′re** [NA], acetabular lip: a ring of fibrocartilage attached to the rim of the acetabulum of the hip bone, increasing the depth of the cavity; called also *l. glenoidale articulationis coxae*. **l. glenoida′le** [NA], glenoid lip: a ring of fibrocartilage attached to the rim of the glenoid cavity of the scapula, increasing the depth of the cavity; called also *l. glenoidale articulationis humeri*. **l. glenoida′le articulati-o′nis cox′ae**, l. acetabulare. **l. glenoida′le articulati-o′nis hu′meri**, l. glenoidale.

laburine (lah-bu′rĭ-nēn) cytisine.

labyrinth (lab′ĭ-rinth) [Gr. *labyrinthos*] a system of intercommunicating cavities or canals, especially that constituting the internal ear (auris internus [NA]). **acoustic l.**, cochlea, def. 2. **bony l.**, the bony part of the internal ear; called also *labyrinthus osseus* [NA] or *osseus l.* **cortical l.**, a network of tubules and blood vessels in the cortex of the kidney. **endolymphatic l.**, labyrinthus membranaceus. **l. of ethmoid, ethmoidal l.**, labyrinthus ethmoidalis. **Ludwig's l's**, spaces between Bertin's columns and the cortical arches. **membranous l.**, a system of communicating epithelial sacs and ducts within the bony labyrinth; see *labyrinthus membranaceus* [NA]. **nonacoustic l.**, statokinetic l. **olfactory l.**, labyrinthus ethmoidalis. **osseous l.**, bony l. **perilymphatic l.**, spatium perilymphaticum. **statokinetic l.**, the vestibule and semicircular canals; called also *nonacoustic l.*

labyrinthectomy (lab′ĭ-rin-thek′to-me) [*labyrinth* + Gr. *ektomē* excision] excision of the labyrinth of the ear.

labyrinthi (lab″ĭ-rin′thi) [L.] plural of *labyrinthus*.

labyrinthine (lab″ĭ-rin′thīn) pertaining to a labyrinth.

labyrinthitis (lab″ĭ-rin-thi′tis) inflammation of the labyrinth; otitis interna. **circumscribed l.**, that due to erosion of the bony wall of a semicircular canal with exposure of the membranous labyrinth.

labyrinthodont (lab″ĭ-rin′tho-dont) [Gr. *labyrinthos* labyrinth + *odontos* tooth] an extinct amphibian in which the enamel of the tooth was completely invaginated into the dentin; labyrinthodonts were the first terrestrial vertebrates and the ancestors of modern amphibian and reptiles.

labyrinthotomy (lab″ĭ-rin-thot′o-me) [*labyrinth* + Gr. *temnein* to cut] surgical incision into the labyrinth.

labyrinthus (lab″ĭ-rin′thus), pl. *labyrin′thi* [L.; Gr. *labyrinthos*] 1. [NA] a general term for a system of intercommunicating cavities or canals. 2. the internal or inner ear (auris interna [NA]). Called also *labyrinth*. **l. ethmoida′lis** [NA], the ethmoidal labyrinth: either of the paired lateral masses of the ethmoid bone, consisting of numerous thin-walled cellular cavities, the ethmoidal cells. **l. membrana′ceus** [NA], the membranous labyrinth: a system of communicating epithelial sacs and ducts, including the endolymphatic duct, utricle, saccule, and semicircular ducts, lodged within the bony labyrinth and containing endolymph. **l. os′seus** [NA], the bony part of the internal ear; the bony or osseous labyrinth.

lac (lak), pl. *lac′ta*, gen. *lac′tis* [L.] 1. milk. 2. any milklike medicinal preparation. 3. a resinous material collected from various tropical trees, secreted by an insect, *Laccifer lacca* Kerr (Coccidae), and used in the preparation of shellac. **l. femini′num**, the secretion of the human mammary gland. **l. fermen′tum**, koumiss. **l. sulfu′ris**, precipitated sulfur. **l. vacci′num**, cow's milk. **l. virgina′le** ["virgin's milk"], a strained liquor of litharge; an ancient remedial wash, variously prepared, but not entirely obsolete.

laccase (lak′ās) *p*-diphenol oxidase.

Laccifer (lak′sĭ-fer) a genus of insects, including *L. lacca* Kerr (Coccidae), which is the source of lac and shellac.

lacerable (las′er-ah-b'l) capable of becoming lacerated.

lacerated (las′er-āt″ed) [L. *lacerare* to tear] torn; mangled; wounded by a jagged instrument.

laceration (las″er-a′shun) [L. *laceratio*] 1. the act of tearing. 2. a torn, ragged, mangled wound.

lacertofulvin (lah-ser″to-ful′vin) [L. *lacertus* lizard + *fulvus* yellow] a yellow coloring matter from the skin of certain reptiles.

lacertus (lah-ser′tus) [L., "lizard," because of a fancied resemblance] [NA] a general term for certain fibrous attachments of muscles. **l. cor′dis**, see *trabeculae carneae cordis*. **l. fibro′sus mus′culi bicip′itis bra′chii**, aponeurosis musculi bicipitalis brachii. **l. me′dius Weitbrech′tii, l. me′di-**

us Wrisber′gii, ligamentum longitudinale anterius. **l. mus′culi rec′ti latera′lis bul′bi** [NA], the check ligament of the lateral rectus muscle, which is attached to the lateral palpebral ligament.

Lachesis (lak′ĕ-sis) [L.; Gr. *Lachesis* one of the three Fates] a genus of venomous snakes of Central and South America. *L. mu′ta* is the bushmaster, or suruçucu.

lachry- (lak′re) for words beginning thus, see those beginning *lacri-*.

lacinia (lah-sin′e-ah) [L. "fringe"] (*obs.*) fimbria, def. 1.

lacmus (lak′mus) [Ger. *Lackmus*] litmus.

lacrima (lak′rĭ-mah), pl. *lacrimae* [L.] see *tears*.

lacrimae (lak′rĭ-me) [L.] plural of *lacrima;* the watery secretion of the lacrimal glands. See *tears*.

lacrimal (lak′rĭ-mal) [L. *lacrimalis; lacrima* tear] pertaining to the tears.

lacrimalin (lak-rim′ah-lin) a substance obtained from the secretion of the lacrimal gland, said to have induced a flow of tears.

lacrimase (lak′rĭ-mās) an enzyme obtained from the secretion of the lacrimal gland; possibly identical to lysozyme.

lacrimation (lak″rĭ-ma′shun) [L. *lacrimatio*] the secretion and discharge of tears.

lacrimator (lak′rĭ-ma″tor) a substance which increases the flow of tears, such as certain gases.

lacrimatory (lak′rĭ-mah-to″re) causing a flow of tears.

lacrimonasal (lak″rĭ-mo-na′zal) pertaining to the lacrimal sac and the nose.

lacrimotome (lak′rĭ-mo-tōm) a knife for incising the lacrimal sac or duct.

lacrimotomy (lak″rĭ-mot′o-me) [L. *lacrima* tear + Gr. *tomē* a cutting] incision of the lacrimal sac or duct.

lactacidemia (lak-tas″ĭ-de′me-ah) [*lactic acid* + Gr. *haima* blood + *-ia*] an excess of lactic acid in the blood, as after violent exercise.

lactacidin (lak-tas′ĭ-din) a food preservative composed of lactic and salicylic acids.

lactacidogen (lak″tah-sid′o-jen) [*lactic acid* + Gr. *gennan* to produce] a term used by Embden to designate the hexose phosphate precursor of lactic acid in muscle contraction.

lactaciduria (lak-tas″ĭ-du′re-ah) [*lactic acid* + Gr. *ouron* urine + *-ia*] the presence of lactic acid in the urine.

lactagogue (lak′tah-gog) [L. *lac* milk + Gr. *agōgos* leading] galactagogue.

lactalbumin (lak″tal-bu′min) an albumin found in milk and resembling serum albumin.

lactam (lak′tam) a cyclic amide formed from aminocarboxylic acids by the elimination of water. They are isomeric with lactims, which are enol forms of lactams.

$$
\begin{array}{cc}
-\mathrm{C}{=}\mathrm{O} & -\mathrm{C}-\mathrm{OH} \\
| & \| \\
-\mathrm{NH} & -\mathrm{N} \\
\text{lactam} & \text{lactim}
\end{array}
$$

β-lactamase (ba″tah-lak′tah-mās) either of two enzymes: β-lactamase I is penicillinase; β-lactamase II is cephalosporinase.

lactamide (lak-tam′id) the amide of lactic acid, $CH_3CHOH{\cdot}{\cdot}CONH_2$.

Lactarius (lak-ta′re-us) a genus of fungi of the order Agaricales, series Homobasidiomycetidae, having white spores, and including both edible and poisonous species. When they are cut or broken, a white or milk-like substance is discharged. *L. delicio′sus*, an edible species, is the source of lactaroviolin.

lactaroviolin (lak″tah-ro-vi′o-lin) chemical name: 1-formyl-4-methyl-7-isopropenylazalone. A pigment, $C_{15}H_{14}O$, isolated from the fungus *Lactarius deliciosus*.

lactase (lak′tās) β-galactosidase.

lactate (lak′tāt) 1. any salt of lactic acid. In biochemistry, the terms lactate and lactic acid are used interchangeably, even though lactate technically refers to the negatively charged ion. 2. to secrete milk. **ferrous l.**, greenish white crystals or powder, $Fe(C_3H_5O_3)_2$, used orally as a hematinic. **lactic acid l.**, a substance formed by concentration by the boiling of lactic acid; used in the preparation of sodium lactate (def. 2).

lactation (lak-ta′shun) [L. *lactatio*, from *lactare* to suckle] 1. the secretion of milk. 2. the period of the secretion of milk. 3. suckling.

lactational (lak-ta′shun-al) pertaining to lactation.

lacteal (lak′te-al) [L. *lacteus* milky] 1. pertaining to milk. 2. any of the intestinal lymphatics that transport chyle; so called because during absorption they are white from absorbed fat. Called also *chyliferous vessels* and *lacteal vessels*.

lactenin (lak′tĕ-nin) a bacteriostatic substance in milk.

lactescence (lak-tes′ens) [L. *lactescere* to become milky] resemblance to milk; milkiness.

lactic (lak′tik) pertaining to milk; see also under *acid*.

lacticemia (lak″tĭ-se′me-ah) the presence of lactic acid in the blood.

lactiferous (lak-tif′er-us) [L. *lac* milk + *ferre* to bear] producing or conveying milk.

lactifuge (lak′tĭ-fūj) [L. *lac* milk + *fugare* to expel] 1. checking or stopping the secretion of milk. 2. an agent that checks the secretion of milk.

lactigenous (lak-tij′ĕ-nus) [L. *lac* milk + Gr. *gennan* to produce] producing or secreting milk.

lactigerous (lak-tij′er-us) [L. *lac* milk + *gerere* to carry] lactiferous.

lactim (lak′tim) see under *lactam*.

lactimorbus (lak″tĭ-mor′bus) [L. *lac* milk + *morbus* disease] milk sickness.

lactin (lak′tin) lactose, or milk sugar.

lactinated (lak′tĭ-nāt″ed) prepared with lactose.

lactivorous (lak-tiv′o-rus) [L. *lac* milk + *vorare* to devour] feeding or subsisting upon milk.

lacto- (lak′to) [L. *lac, lactis* milk] a combining form denoting relationship to milk.

Lactobacillaceae (lak″to-bas″il-la′se-e) a family of Schizomycetes (order Eubacteriales), made up of long or short rods or cocci which divide in one plane only, producing chains or tetrads. It includes two tribes, *Lactobacilleae* and *Streptococceae*. Formerly called *Lactobacteriaceae*.

Lactobacilleae (lak″to-bah-sil′e-e) a tribe of microorganisms of the family Lactobacillaceae, order Eubacteriales, made up of straight or curved rods occurring usually singly or in chains, but sometimes in filaments. It includes five genera, *Catenabacte′rium, Cillobacte′rium, Eubacte′rium, Lactobacil′lus,* and *Ramibacte′-rium*.

lactobacilli (lak″to-bah-sil′li) plural of *lactobacillus*.

lactobacillin (lak″to-bah-sil′in) a preparation of lactic acid bacteria to be added to milk to cause lactic acid fermentation.

Lactobacillus (lak″to-bah-sil′lus) a genus of microorganisms of the tribe Lactobacilleae, family Lactobacillaceae, order Eubacteriales, occurring as large gram-positive, anaerobic or microaerophilic bacilli, some of which are considered to be etiologically related to dental caries but are otherwise nonpathogenic. They are separable into 15 species falling into two groups, the homofermentative group producing only lactic acid, and the heterofermentative group producing other end-products of fermentation. **L. acidoph′ilus,** a homofermentative lactobacillus producing the fermented product, acidophilus milk. **L. bif′idus,** a homofermentative lactobacillus predominating in the intestinal flora of breast-fed infants. **L. bulgar′icus,** a homofermentative lactobacillus producing the fermented product known as Bulgarian or bulgaricus milk.

lactobacillus (lak″to-bah-sil′us), pl. *lactobacil′li*. An organism of the genus *Lactobacillus*. **l. of Boas-Oppler,** see under *bacillus*.

Lactobacteriaceae (lak″to-bak-te″re-a′se-e) a former name of a family of Schizomycetes now called *Lactobacillaceae*.

lactobutyrometer (lak″to-bu″tĭ-rom′ĕ-ter) [*lacto-* + *butyrometer*] an instrument for measuring the proportion of cream in milk.

lactocele (lak′to-sēl) galactocele.

lactochrome (lak′to-krōm) [*lacto-* + Gr. *chrōma* color] riboflavin.

lactoconium (lak-to-ko′ne-um) [*lacto-* + Gr. *konis* dust] one of the small particles, of unknown nature, seen with the ultramicroscope in the milk of animals.

lactocrit (lak′to-krit) [*lacto-* + Gr. *krites* judge] an instrument for estimating the amount of fat in milk.

lactodensimeter (lak″to-den-sim′ĕ-ter) lactometer.

lactofarinaceous (lak″to-far″ĭ-na′shus) composed of milk and farinaceous foods; said of a diet.

lactoferrin (lak′to-fer″in) an iron-binding protein found in neutrophils and secretions (milk, tears, saliva, bile, etc.), having bactericidal activity and acting as an inhibitor of colony formation by granulocytes and macrophages.

lactoflavin (lak′to-fla″vin) [*lacto-* + L. *flavus* yellow] riboflavin.

lactogen (lak′to-jen) any substance that enhances lactation, the principal one being prolactin. **human placental l.,** a polypeptide hormone secreted by the placenta that disappears from the circulation immediately after delivery. It has lactogenic, luteotropic, and growth-promoting activity, is immunologically similar to human growth hormone, and inhibits maternal insulin activity during pregnancy. Called also *human somatomammotropin* and *placental growth hormone*. Abbreviated HPL.

lactogenesis (lak″to-jen′ĕ-sis) the establishment of milk secretion in the mammary glands.

lactogenic (lak″to-jen′ik) stimulating the production of milk.

lactoglobulin (lak″to-glob′u-lin) a globulin occurring in milk.

immune l's, antibodies (immunoglobulins) occurring in the colostrum of animals.

lactometer (lak-tom′ĕ-ter) [*lacto-* + Gr. *metron* measure] an instrument for ascertaining the specific gravity of milk.

lactone (lak′tōn) 1. an aromatic liquid, $C_{10}H_8O_4$, prepared by distillation from lactic acid. 2. tablets containing lactic acid bacteria; used in preparing buttermilk. 3. a cyclic organic compound in which the chain is closed by ester formation between a carboxyl and a hydroxyl group in the same molecule.

lacto-ovovegetarian (lak″to-o″vo-vej″ĕ-ta′re-an) a vegetarian who includes eggs and dairy products in his diet.

lactophenin (lak″to-fe′nin) a bitter, crystalline powder, C_6H_4- $(OC_2H_5) \cdot NH \cdot CO \cdot CH(OH)CH_3$, derived from phenetidin and lactic acid, soluble in 500 parts of cold and in 55 parts of boiling water; formerly used as an analgesic and antipyretic.

lactophosphate (lak″to-fos′fāt) [*lacto-* + L. *phosphas* phosphate] any salt of lactic and phosphoric acids.

lactoprecipitin (lak″to-pre-sip′ĭ-tin) a precipitin which will precipitate the casein of milk in his diet.

lactoprotein (lak″to-pro′te-in) a protein derived from milk.

lactorrhea (lak″to-re′ah) galactorrhea.

lactosazone (lak″to-sa′zōn) the phenylosazone of lactose. It is a yellow crystalline substance made by treating lactose with phenylhydrazine and acetic acid. The crystals melt at 200° C. and may be used in identifying lactose.

lactoscope (lak′to-skōp) [*lacto-* + Gr. *skopein* to examine] a device showing the proportion of cream in milk.

lactose (lak′tōs) [L. *saccharum lactis*] [USP] 4-*O*-β-D-galactopyranosyl-D-glucose. A white crystalline sugar (disaccharide), $C_{12}H_{22}O_{11}$, obtained from milk which on hydrolysis with acids or certain enzymes yields glucose and galactose; used as a tablet and capsule diluent. It is also used as an osmotic laxative and diuretic, and in infant feeding formulas. Lactose, a constituent of milk, is not tolerated in many persons after weaning, owing to reduced lactase activity. Called also *lactin* and *milk sugar*. **beta l.,** a disaccharide obtained by allowing a solution of lactose to crystallize above 93.5° C.; it is sweeter and more soluble than lactose.

lactoserum (lak″to-se′rum) the serum of an animal into which has been injected milk from another animal. Lactoprecipitins in the serum precipitate the casein of milk from an animal of the same species as that from which the milk was taken.

lactoside (lak″to-sīd) a compound of glucose and galactose.

lactosidosis (lak″to-si-do′sis), pl. *lactosido′ses*. The accumulation of lactoside in tissues. **ceramide l.,** a sphingolipidosis in which ceramide lactoside accumulates in neural and visceral tissues owing to a deficiency of a β-galactosidase; it is characterized by psychomotor deterioration and visceromegaly and by macrocytic anemia, leukopenia, and thrombocytopenia. Called also *ceramide lactoside lipidosis* and *lactosyl ceramidosis*.

lactosum (lak-to′sum) lactose.

lactosuria (lak″to-su′re-ah) [*lactose* + Gr. *ouron* urine + *-ia*] the presence of lactose in the urine, observed frequently during lactation.

lactotherapy (lak″to-ther′ah-pe) [*lacto-* + *therapy*] treatment by milk diet.

lactotoxin (lak″to-tok′sin) a toxic substance formed in milk.

lactotrope (lak′to-trōp) an acidophilic cell of the anterior pituitary that secretes prolactin; called also *mammotrope*.

lactotroph (lak′to-trōf) lactotrope.

lactotrophin, lactotropin (lak″to-tro′fin; lak″to-tro′pin) prolactin.

lactovegetarian (lak″to-vej″ĕ-ta′re-an) 1. pertaining to, consisting of, or subsisting on milk (or other dairy products) and vegetables. 2. a vegetarian who uses dairy products in addition to vegetables in his diet.

Lactuca (lak-tu′kah) [L.] a genus of composite-flowered plants, including *L. sati′va* L., common lettuce, and *L. viro′sa* L., the inspissated juice of which was formerly used as a sedative and hypnotic.

lactulose (lak′tū-lōs) chemical name: 4-*O*-β-D-galactopyranosyl-D-fructose. A synthetic disaccharide, $C_{12}H_{22}O_{11}$, used as a cathartic and to enhance excretion or formation of ammonia in the treatment of portosystemic encephalopathy, including the stages of hepatic precoma and coma.

lacuna (lah-ku′nah), pl. *lacu′nae* [L.] 1. a small pit or hollow cavity; [NA] a general term for such a compartment within or between other body structures. Called also *lake*. 2. a defect or gap, as in the field of vision (scotoma). **absorption l.,** a pit or groove in developing bone that is undergoing resorption, frequently found to contain osteoclasts; called also *Howship's l.* **air l.,** a cavity filled with air, such as those occurring in the hairs. **Blessig's l.,** see *Blessig's cysts.* **blood l.,** any one of the blood-filled spaces in the trophoblast of the embryo that serve hemotrophic nutrition. **bone l.,** a small cavity within the bone matrix containing an osteocyte and from which slender canaliculi radiate and penetrate the adjacent lamellae to anastomose with the canaliculi of neighboring lacunae, thus forming a system of cavities interconnected by minute canals. Called also *osseous l.* **cartilage l.,** any of the small cavities within the cartilage matrix, containing a chondrocyte, or cartilage cell. **cerebral lacunae,** small areas of cerebral ischemic infarction resulting from occlusion of branches of the middle cerebral, posterior cerebral, and basilar arteries; seen in association with hypertension and arteriosclerosis. **great l. of urethra,** fossa navicularis urethrae. **Howship's l.,** absorption l. **intervillous l.,** one of the blood spaces of the placenta in which the fetal villi are found; called also *trophoblastic l.* **lateral lacunae, lacu′nae latera′les** [NA], venous meshworks within the dura mater on either side of the superior sagittal sinus; arachnoidal granulations project into them. **l. mag′na,** fossa navicularis urethrae. **lacunae of Morgagni,** lacunae urethrales in the male urethra. **lacu′nae Morga′gnii ure′thrae mulie′bris,** glandulae urethrales urethrae femininae. **l. of muscles, l. musculo′rum** [NA], a compartment beneath the inguinal ligament for the passage of the iliopsoas muscle and femoral nerve, separated from the lacuna vasorum by the iliopectineal arch. **osseous l.,** bone l. **parasinoidal l's,** lacunae laterales. **l. pharyn′gis,** a depression at the pharyngeal end of the auditory tube. **trophoblastic l.,** intervillous l. **lacunae of urethra, urethral lacunae,** lacunae urethrales. **urethral lacunae of Morgagni,** lacunae urethrales in the male urethra. **lacu′nae urethra′les** [NA], urethral lacunae: numerous small depressions or pits in the mucous membrane of the urethra, with their openings usually directed distally. Some contain openings of ducts of the urethral glands. **l. vaso′rum** [NA], **l. of vessels,** a space for the passage of the femoral vessels into the thigh, separated from the lacuna musculorum by the iliopectineal arch.

lacunae (lah-ku′ne) [L.] plural of *lacuna.*

lacunar (lah-ku′nar) pertaining to or containing lacunae; of the nature of a lacuna.

lacune (lah-kūn′) lacuna.

lacunule (lah-ku′nūl) [L. *lacunula*] a small lacuna.

lacus (la′kus), pl. *la′cus* [L.] lake. **l. lacrima′lis** [NA], lacrimal lake: the triangular space at the medial angle of the eye, where the tears collect.

Ladd-Franklin theory (lad-frangk′lin) [Christine *Ladd-Franklin*, Baltimore physician, 1847–1930] see under *theory.*

Ladendorff's test (lah′den-dorfs) [August *Ladendorff*, German physician of the 19th century] see under *tests.*

Ladin's sign (la′dinz) [Louis Julius *Ladin*, American gynecologist, born 1862] see under *sign.*

lae- for words beginning thus, see also those beginning *le-.*

Laelaps (le′laps) *Echinolaelaps.*

Laennec's catarrh, etc. (la″en-neks′) [René Théophile Hyacinthe *Laennec*, distinguished French physician and inventor of the stethoscope, 1781–1826] see under *catarrh, cirrhosis, disease, pearl, sign,* and *thrombus.*

Laetrile (la′ĕ-tril) trademark for *l*-mandelonitrile-β-glucuronic acid, derived by hydrolysis of amygdalin and oxidation of the resulting *l*-mandelonitrile-β-glucoside; it is alleged to have antineoplastic properties. The term is sometimes used interchangeably with *amygdalin.*

laeve (le′vĕ) [L. *levis* smooth] nonvillous, as the *chorion laeve.*

laevo- (le′vo) for words beginning thus, see those beginning *levo-.*

Lafora's bodies, disease, sign (lah-fo′rahz) [Gonzalo Rodríguez *Lafora*, Spanish physician, born 1887] see under *body* and *sign,* and see *myoclonus epilepsy,* under *epilepsy.*

Lag. abbreviation for L. *lage′na,* a flask.

lag (lag) 1. the period of time elapsing between the application of a stimulus and the resulting reaction. 2. the early period following a bacterial inoculation into a culture medium, in which growth or cell division is slow; called also *lag phase.* **nitrogen l.,** the time that elapses after the administration of a protein before there appears in the urine an amount of nitrogen equivalent to that administered.

lagena (lah-je′nah) [L. "flask"] 1. a part of the upper extremity of the ductus cochlearis. 2. the curved, flask-shaped organ of hearing in vertebrates lower than mammals.

lageniform (lah-jen′ĭ-form) [L. *lagena* flask + *form*] flask-shaped.

lagnesis (lag-ne′sis) [Gr. *lagneia* salaciousness] (*obs.*) erotomania.

lagnosis (lag-no′sis) [Gr. *lagnos* salacious, lustful] (*obs.*) excessive sexual desire, especially in the male; satyriasis.

Lagochilascaris minor (lag″o-ki-las′kah-ris mi′nor) a nematode worm found in subcutaneous abscesses of man in Trinidad and Surinam.

lagophthalmos (lag″of-thal′mos) [Gr. *lagōs* hare + *ophthalmos* eye] a condition in which the eye cannot be completely closed.

lagophthalmus (lag″of-thal′mus) lagophthalmos.

Lagrange's operation (lah-grah′zez) [Pierre Félix *Lagrange,* French ophthalmologist, 1857–1928] sclerectoiridectomy.

la grippe (lah grip′) [Fr.] influenza.

laiose (li′ōs) a pale yellow substance, $C_6H_{12}O_6$, found in the urine in diabetes mellitus; it is nonfermentable and levorotatory.

lake (lāk) [L. *lacus*] 1. to undergo separation of hemoglobin from the erythrocytes, a phenomenon sometimes occurring in blood. 2. a circumscribed collection of fluid in a hollow or depressed area. See also *lacuna.* **lacrimal l.,** lacus lacrimalis. **marginal l's,** discontinuous venous lacunae, relatively free of villi, near the edge of the placenta, formed by merging of the marginal portions of the intervillous space with the subchorial lake. Called also *marginal sinus,* because it was thought to be circumferentially continuous and important for placental drainage. **subchorial l.,** the portion of the placenta, relatively free of villi, just beneath the chorionic plate; at the edge of the placenta it becomes continuous with irregular channels to form the marginal lakes. Called also *subchorial space.*

Lake's pigment (lāks′) [Richard *Lake,* English otorhinolaryngologist, 1861–1949] see under *pigment.*

laliatry (lah-li′ah-tre) [Gr. *lalia* talking + *iatria* therapy] the study and treatment of disorders of speech.

lallation (lah-la′shun) [L. *lallatio*] a babbling, infantile form of speech.

Lallemand's bodies (lal-mahz′) [Claude François *Lallemand,* French surgeon, 1790–1854] Bence Jones cylinders.

lalo- (lal′o) [Gr. *lalein* to babble, speak] a combining form denoting relationship to speech, or babbling.

lalognosis (lal″og-no′sis) [*lalo-* + Gr. *gnōsis* knowledge] the understanding of speech.

laloneurosis (lal″o-nu-ro′sis) [*lalo-* + *neurosis*] (*obs.*) any nervous speech disorder.

lalopathology (lal″o-pah-thol′o-je) [*lalo-* + *pathology*] the branch of medicine which deals with disorders of speech.

lalopathy (lah-lop′ah-the) [*lalo-* + Gr. *pathos* illness] any disorder of speech.

laloplegia (lal″o-ple′je-ah) [*lalo-* + Gr. *plēgē* stroke] paralysis of the organs of speech.

lalorrhea (lal″o-re′ah) [*lalo-* + Gr. *rhoia* flow] an abnormal or excessive flow of words.

Lalouette's pyramid (lal″oo-ets′) [Pierre *Lalouette,* French physician, 1711–1792] see under *pyramid.*

Lamarck's theory (lah-marks′) [Jean Baptiste Pierre Antoine Monet de *Lamarck,* French naturalist, 1744–1829] see under *theory.*

lambda (lam′dah) [the eleventh letter of the Greek alphabet, Λ or λ] the point at the site of the posterior fontanel where the lambdoid and sagittal sutures meet.

lambdacism, lambdacismus (lam′dah-sizm; lam-dah-siz′mus) [Gr. *lambdakismos*] 1. the substitution of *l* for *r* in speaking. 2. inability to utter correctly the sound of *l.*

lambdoid (lam′doid) [Gr. *lambda* + *eidos* form] shaped like the Greek letter Λ or λ.

lambert (lam′bert) [Johann Heinrich *Lambert,* German mathematician and physicist, 1728–1777] a unit of brightness, being the brightness of a perfect diffuser emitting one lumen per square centimeter. The unit generally used is one one-thousandth of this and is called a *millilambert.* When the area chosen is one square foot the unit is called a *foot lambert.*

Lambert's cosine law (lam′berts) [Johann Heinrich *Lambert*] see under *law.*

Lambert's treatment (lam′berts) [Alexander *Lambert,* American physician, 1861–1939] see under *treatment.*

Lamblia (lam′ble-ah) [Vilem Dusan *Lambl,* Bohemian physician, 1824–1895] *Giardia.* **L. intestina′lis,** *Giardia lamblia.*

lambliasis, lambliosis (lam-bli′ah-sis; lam-ble-o′sis) infection with *Giardia lamblia.*

Lambotte's treatment (lam-bots′) [Albin *Lambotte,* Belgian surgeon] see under *treatment.*

lame (lām) incapable of normal locomotion; deviation from the normal gait.

lame foliacée (lam′fol-yă-sā′) [Fr. *lame* plate, lamina; *foliacée* foliaceous] the whorled or concentrically laminated connective tissue structures contained in some nevi; called also *foliate lamina.*

lamel (lam′el) lamella, def. 2.

lamella (lah-mel′ah), pl. *lamel′lae* [L., dim. of *lamina*] 1. a thin leaf or plate, as of bone. 2. a medicated disk or wafer prepared from gelatin, glycerin, and distilled water, and containing a small quantity of an alkaloid, to be inserted under the eyelid. **annulate lamel′lae,** cytoplasmic organelles which consist of parallel arrays of cisternae exhibiting small annuli or circular fenestrae at very regular intervals along their length. **articular l.,** the layer of bone to which an articular cartilage is attached. **basic l.,** circumferential l. **circumferential l.,** one of the layers of bone that underlie the periosteum (*external circumferential l.*) and endosteum (*internal circumferential l.*); called also *basic l.* **concentric l.,** haversian l. **cornoid l.,** a horny plug of parakeratotic tissue penetrating the epidermis; seen in porokeratosis of Mibelli. **enamel lamellae,** imperfectly calcified areas of enamel which usually extend from the outer surface through the entire thickness of the enamel and which are visible only in thin sections under the microscope. **endosteal l.,** one of the bony plates lying beneath the endosteum. **ground l.,** interstitial l. **haversian l.,** one of the concentric bony plates surrounding a haversian canal. **intermediate l.,** interstitial l. **interstitial l.,** one of the bony plates that fill in between the haversian systems; called also *ground l.* or *intermediate l.* **osseous l.,** any one of the thin plates into which bone can be divided. **periosteal l., peripheral l.,** the layer of bone lying next to the periosteum. **posterior border l. of Fuchs,** the fibrillar layer of the dilator muscle of the iris; called also *Henle's membrane.* **triangular l.,** the area above the roof of the third ventricle of the brain occupied by the velum interpositum. **vitreous l.,** lamina basalis.

lamellae (lah-mel′e) [L.] plural of *lamella.*

lamellar (lah-mel′ar) pertaining to or resembling lamellae.

lamellasome (lah-mel′ah-sōm) [*lamella* + Gr. *sōma* body] an intracytoplasmic membranous inclusion consisting of a series of invaginated lamellae enclosed by a common membrane. Such structures appear to be confined to unicellular blue-green algae.

lamelliform (lah-mel′ĭ-form) resembling lamellae.

lamellipodia (lah-mel″ĭ-po′de-ah), sing. *lamellipodium* [*lamella* + Gr. *pous* foot + *-ia*] delicate sheetlike extensions of cytoplasm which form transient adhesions with the cell substrate and wave gently, enabling the cell to move along the substrate.

lamellipodium (lah-mel″ĭ-po′de-um) singular of lamellipodia.

lamina (lam′ĭ-nah), pl. *lam′inae* [L.] a thin flat plate, or layer; [NA] a general term for such a structure, or a layer of a composite structure. The term is often used alone to mean the lamina arcus vertebrae. **l. affix′a** [NA], the narrow strip of ependyma overlying the thalamostriate vein and stria terminalis in the central part of the lateral ventricle. **alar l., l. ala′ris** [NA], either of the pair of longitudinal zones of the embryonic neural tube dorsal to the sulcus limitans, from which are developed the dorsal gray columns of the spinal cord and the sensory centers of the brain; called also *alar plate.* **lam′inae al′bae cerebel′li** [NA], white laminae of the cerebellum: the core of white substance that supports a folium of the cerebellar cortex; called also *laminae medullares cerebelli.* **anterior limiting l., l. limitans anterior corneae. l. ante′rior vagi′nae mus′culi rec′ti abdo′minis** [NA], the portion of its sheath lying anterior to the rectus abdominis muscle, formed by aponeuroses of the internal and external oblique above the arcuate line and by the aponeuroses of the internal oblique and transversus, below the arcuate line. **l. ar′cus ver′tebrae** [NA], lamina of the vertebral arch: either of the pair of broad plates of bone flaring out from the pedicles of the vertebral arches and fusing together at the midline to complete the dorsal part of the arch and provide a base for the spinous process. **basal l., l. basalis. basal l. of choroid, l.** basalis choroideae. **basal l. of ciliary body, l.** basalis corporis ciliaris. **l. basa′lis** [NA], the basal lamina: either of the pair of longitudinal zones of the embryonic neural tube ventral to the sulcus limitans, from which are developed the ventral gray columns of the spinal cord and the motor centers of the brain; called also *basal plate.* **l. basa′lis chorioi′deae,** basalis choroideae. **l. basa′lis choroi′deae** [NA], basal lamina of the choroid: the transparent inner layer of the choroid, in contact with the pigmented layer of the retina. Called also *Bruch's layer* or *membrane,* and *l. vitrea.* **l. basa′lis cor′poris cilia′ris** [NA], basal lamina of the ciliary body: the innermost layer of the ciliary body, continuous with the basal lamina of the choroid. **l. basila′ris duc′tus cochlea′ris** [NA], the wall of the cochlear duct, which separates it from the scala tympani; the spiral organ lies against it. Called also *basilar membrane of cochlear duct.* **Bowman's l.,** l. limitans anterior corneae. **l. cartilag′inis cricoi′deae** [NA], lamina of cricoid cartilage: the broad posterior part of the cricoid cartilage. **l. cartilag′inis latera′lis tu′bae auditi′vae** [NA], lateral lamina of cartilage of auditory tube: the smaller of the two laminae that compose the tubal cartilage; it lies in the lateral wall of the auditory tube. **l. cartilag′inis media′lis tu′bae auditi′vae** [NA], medial lamina of cartilage of auditory tube: the larger of the two laminae that compose the tubal cartilage; it lies in the medial wall of the auditory tube. **l. cartilag′inis thyroi′deae [dex′tra et sinis′tra]** [NA], lamina of thyroid cartilage: either of the broad plates that form the sides (right and left) of the thyroid cartilage, converging anteriorly to meet at the midline. **l. choriocapilla′ris,** l. choroidocapillaris. **l. chorioi′dea epithelia′lis thal′ami,** the ependyma lining the superior surface of the thalamus. **l. chorioi′dea epithelia′lis ventric′uli latera′lis,** the ependyma lining the lateral ventricle of the cerebrum. **l. chorioi′dea epithelia′lis ventric′uli quar′ti,** the ependyma lining the roof of the fourth ventricle of the cerebrum. **l. choroidocapilla′ris** [NA], the inner layer of the choroid, composed of a single-layered network of small capillaries; called also *choriocapillaris l.* **l. cine′rea termina′lis** (*obs.*), l. terminalis hypothalami. **cribriform l.,** fascia cribrosa. **cribriform l. of ethmoid bone,** lamina cribrosa ossis ethmoidalis. **cribriform l. of transverse fascia,** septum femorale. **l.**

cribro′sa os′sis ethmoida′lis [NA], cribriform lamina of ethmoid bone: the horizontal plate of the ethmoid bone that forms the roof of the nasal cavity; it is perforated by many foramina for the passage of the olfactory nerves. Called also *cribriform plate of ethmoid bone.* **l. cribro′sa scle′rae,** the perforated portion of the sclera through which pass the axons of the ganglion cells of the retina; called also *optic foramen of sclera.* **l. of cricoid cartilage,** l. cartilaginis cricoideae. **dental l.,** a thickened epithelial band along the margin of the gum, in the embryo, from which the enamel organs are developed. **dental l., lateral,** a perpendicular layer of cells connecting the developing tooth germ to the dental lamina. **l. denta′lis,** dental l. **l. denta′ta,** labium limbi vestibulare laminae spiralis. **dentogingival l.,** dental l. **descending l. of sphenoid bone,** processus pterygoideus ossis sphenoidalis. **l. du′ra,** a thin layer of compact bone that covers the alveolar bone of the jaws and lines the sockets of the teeth. In dental radiographs, it appears as a thin radiopaque line, and in the tooth sockets it is separated from the images of teeth by the radiolucent image of the periodontal membrane. **elastic l., external,** external elastic membrane. **elastic l. internal,** internal elastic membrane. **l. elas′tica ante′rior [Bow′mani],** l. limitans anterior corneae. **l. elas′tica poste′rior [Demour′si, Descem′eti],** l. limitans posterior corneae. **episcleral l., l. episclera′lis** [NA], loose connective and elastic tissue covering the sclera and anteriorly connecting it with the conjunctiva. **epithelial l., l. epithelia′lis** [NA], the layer of ependymal cells covering the choroid plexus. **l. exter′na os′sium cra′nii** [NA], outer plate of cranial bone: the outer compact layer of bone of the flat bones of the head; called also *outer table of bones of skull.* **external l. of peritoneum,** peritoneum parietale. **external l. of pterygoid process,** l. lateralis processus pterygoidei. **l. fibrocartilagin′ea interpu′bica,** discus interpubicus. **foliate l.,** lame foliacée. **l. fus′ca scle′rae** [NA], a thin layer of loose, pigmented connective tissue on the inner surface of the sclera, connecting it with the choroid. **l. horizonta′lis os′sis palati′ni** [NA], horizontal plate of palatine bone: the horizontal part of the palatine bone, forming the posterior part of the hard palate. **inferior l. of sphenoid bone,** processus pterygoideus ossis sphenoidalis. **l. inter′na os′sium cra′nii** [NA], inner plate of cranial bone: the inner compact layer of bone of the flat bones of the head; called also *inner table of bones of skull.* **internal l. of pterygoid process,** l. medialis processus pterygoidei. **interpubic l., fibrocartilaginous,** discus interpubicus. **labial l.,** the ectodermal plate that on splitting separates lip from gum, thus forming the labial groove. **labiodental l.,** the thickened ectodermal band from which the dental and labial laminae develop. **labiogingival l.,** labial l. **lateral l. of cartilage of auditory tube,** l. cartilaginis lateralis tubae auditivae. **lateral l. of pterygoid process,** l. lateralis processus pterygoidei. **l. latera′lis cartilag′inus tu′bae auditi′vae,** l. cartilaginis lateralis tubae auditivae. **l. latera′lis proces′sus pterygoi′dei** [NA], lateral lamina of the pterygoid process: either of a pair of bony plates projecting downward from the roots of the greater wings of the sphenoid bone and forming the medial wall of the ipsilateral infratemporal fossa; called also *lateral plate of pterygoid process.* **l. lim′itans ante′rior cor′neae** [NA], anterior limiting lamina: a thin layer of the cornea beneath the outer layer of stratified epithelium, composed of condensed stroma, between it and the substantia propria; called also *l. elastica anterior [Bowmani]* and *Bowman's membrane.* **l. lim′itans poste′rior cor′neae** [NA], posterior limiting lamina: a thin hyaline membrane between the substantia propria and the endothelial layer of the cornea; called also *l. elastica posterior [Demoursi, Descemeti]* and *Descemet's membrane.* **limiting l., anterior,** l. limitans anterior corneae. **limiting l., posterior,** l. limitans posterior corneae. **medial l. of cartilage of auditory tube,** l. cartilaginis medialis tubae auditivae. **medial l. of pterygoid process,** l. medialis processus pterygoidei. **l. media′lis cartilag′inis tu′bae auditi′vae,** l. cartilaginis medialis tubae auditivae. **l. media′lis proces′sus pterygoi′dei** [NA], medial lamina of pterygoid process: either of a pair of bony plates projecting downward from the roots of the greater wings of the sphenoid bone and forming the lateral boundary of the ipsilateral posterior aperture of the nasal cavity and the most posterior part of the lateral wall of the nasal cavity. Called also *medial plate of pterygoid process.* **lami′nae mediastina′les,** the mediastinal layers of the pleura. **lam′inae medulla′res cerebel′li,** laminae albae cerebelli. **l. medulla′ris latera′lis cor′poris stria′ti** [NA], lateral medullary lamina: a layer of fibers running through the globus pallidus and dividing it into a lateral and a medial part. **l. medulla′ris media′lis cor′poris stria′ti** [NA], medial medullary lamina: a layer of fibers separating the putamen from the globus pallidus. **lam′inae medulla′res thal′ami** [NA], medullary layers of the thalamus: bands of white matter in the thalami. Two such bands occur in each thalamus; the lateral medullary lamina covers the lateral aspect of the thalamus, and the medial medullary lamina, with its associated intralaminar nuclei, separates the medial and lateral thalamic nuclei. **l. medulla′ris transver′sa cor′poris quadrigem′ini,** stratum album profundum corporis quadrigemini. **medullary l., lateral,** l. medullaris lateralis. **medullary l., medial,** l. medullaris medialis. **medullary laminae of thalamus,** laminae medullares thalami. **l. membrana′cea tu′bae auditi′vae** [NA], **membranous l. of auditory tube,** the connective tissue lamina that supports the inferior and lateral parts of the auditory tube. **l. mesenter′ii pro′pria,** the proper layer of the mesentery. **l. modi′oli** [NA], a bony plate extending upward toward the cupula as a continuation of the modiolus and of the bony spiral lamina of the cochlea. **l. muscula′ris muco′sae** [NA], the thin layer of smooth muscle fibers usually found as a part of the tunica mucosa mucosa deep to the lamina propria mucosae. **l. muscula′ris muco′sae co′li** [NA], the muscular layer of the tunica mucosa of the colon. **l. muscula′ris muco′sae esoph′agi** [NA], the muscular layer of the tunica mucosa of the esophagus. **l. muscula′ris muco′sae intesti′ni cras′si** [NA], the muscular layer of the tunica mucosa of the large intestine. **l. muscula′ris muco′sae intesti′ni rec′ti,** l. muscularis mucosae recti. **l. muscula′ris muco′sae intesti′ni ten′uis** [NA], the muscular layer of the tunica mucosa of the small intestine. **l. muscula′ris muco′sae rec′ti** [NA], the muscular layer of the tunica mucosa of the rectum. **l. muscula′ris muco′sae ventric′uli** [NA], the muscular layer of the tunica mucosa of the stomach. **orbital l., l. orbita′lis os′sis ethmoida′lis** [NA], a thin plate of bone laterally bounding the ethmoid labyrinth on either side and forming part of the medial wall of the orbit; called also *l. papyracea.* **palatine l. of maxilla,** processus palatinus maxillae. **l. papyra′cea,** l. orbitalis ossis ethmoidalis. **l. parieta′lis pericar′dii** [NA], the parietal layer of the serous pericardium; it lines the fibrous pericardium. **l. parieta′lis tu′nicae vagina′lis pro′priae tes′tis, l. parieta′lis tu′nicae vagina′lis tes′tis** [NA], parietal layer of tunica vaginalis of testis: the outer layer of the tunica vaginalis of the testis, separated from the visceral layer by a cavity. **periclaustral l.,** capsula extrema. **perpendicular l. of ethmoid bone,** l. perpendicularis ossis ethmoidalis. **l. perpendicula′ris os′sis ethmoida′lis** [NA], perpendicular lamina of ethmoid bone: a thin bony plate that descends from the inferior surface of the cribriform plate of the ethmoid bone and participates in forming the nasal septum; called also *perpendicular plate of ethmoid bone.* **l. perpendicula′ris os′sis palati′ni** [NA], the flat, vertical, bony plate that extends superiorly on either side from the palatine bone; it is surmounted by the orbital and sphenoidal processes. Called also *pars perpendicularis ossis palatini* and *perpendicular plate of palatine bone.* **posterior limiting l.,** l. limitans posterior corneae. **l. poste′rior vagi′nae mus′culi rec′ti abdo′minis** [NA], the portion of its sheath lying posterior to the rectus abdominis muscle, formed by the transversus abdominis and its aponeurosis at the level of the xiphoid process; below the xiphoid process, to the arcuate line, it is formed by the aponeuroses of the internal oblique and the transversus. **l. pretrachea′lis fas′ciae cervica′lis** [NA], the layer of the cervical fascia that is anterior to the trachea. **l. prevertebra′lis fas′ciae cervica′lis** [NA], the prevertebral fascia: the layer of the cervical fascia that is anterior to the vertebrae; called also *fascia praevertebralis.* **l. profun′da fas′ciae tempora′lis** [NA], the deep portion of the fascia investing the temporal muscle. **l. profun′da mus′culi levato′ris pal′pebrae superio′ris** [NA], the deeper of the two layers of the levator palpebrae superioris muscle. **proper l. of mesentery,** lamina mesenterii propria. **l. pro′pria membra′nae tym′pani,** the middle fibrous basis of the tympanic membrane, attached, except anterosuperiorly, to the tympanic plate of the temporal bone. **l. pro′pria muco′sae** [NA], proper mucous membrane: the connective tissue coat of a mucous membrane just deep to the epithelium and basement membrane. **l. quadrigem′ina,** l. tecti mesencephali. **l. reticula′ris,** the perforated hyaline membrane which covers the organ of Corti. **rostral l., l. rostra′lis,** the thin terminal part of the rostrum of the corpus callosum passing down in front of the anterior commissure to the anterior perforated substance and the paraterminal gyrus. **l. sep′ti pellu′cidi** [NA], **l. of septum pellucidum,** either of the thin, vertical sheets, separated by a cleftlike space, which constitute the septum pellucidum. **spiral l., bony,** l. spiralis ossea. **spiral l., secondary,** l. spiralis secundaria. **l. spira′lis os′sea** [NA], bony spiral lamina: a double plate of bone winding spirally around the modiolus and dividing the spiral canal of the cochlea incompletely into two parts, the scala tympani and the scala vestibuli; called also *spiral plate.* **l. spira′lis secunda′ria** [NA], secondary spiral lamina: a bony projection on the outer wall of the osseous spiral lamina in the lower part of the first turn of the cochlea. **submucous l. of stomach,** tela submucosa ventriculi. **l. superficia′lis fas′ciae cervica′lis** [NA], the layer of the cervical fascia that lies deep to the skin. **l. superficia′lis fas′ciae tempora′lis** [NA], the superficial portion of the fascia investing the temporal muscle. **l. superficia′lis mus′culi levato′ris palpe′brae superio′ris** [NA], the superficial of the two layers of the levator palpebrae superioris muscle. **l. suprachorioi′dea, suprachoroid l., l. suprachoroi′dea** [NA], the outermost layer of the choroid, which connects it with the sclera; called also *suprachoroid layer.* **l. supra-**

neuropor′ica, the part of lamina terminalis caudal to the anterior neuropore of the embryo; it cannot be delimited accurately in human embryos. **tectal l. of mesencephalon, l. tec′ti mesenceph′ali** [NA], the layer of mingled gray and white substance, in the tectum of the mesencephalon, from which arise the superior and inferior colliculi; called also *quadrigeminal plate.* **terminal l. of hypothalamus, l. termina′lis hypothal′ami** [NA], a thin plate derived from the telencephalon extending upward from the optic chiasm and preoptic recess, and forming the anterior wall of the third ventricle of the cerebrum; called also *terminal plate.* **l. of thyroid cartilage,** l. cartilaginis thyroideae [dextra et sinistra]. **l. tra′gi** [NA], l. **tra′gica,** the longitudinal curved lamina of cartilage in the tragus of the auricle, at the beginning of the cartilaginous portion of the external acoustic meatus. **ungual laminae,** cristae matricis unguis. **vascular l. of choroid,** l. vasculosa choroideae. **vascular l. of stomach,** tela submucosa ventriculi. **l. vasculo′sa chorioi′deae, l. vasculo′sa choroi′deae** [NA], vascular lamina of choroid: the layer of the choroid between the suprachoroid and choriocapillary layers, containing the largest blood vessels; called also *Haller's membrane.* **l. of verte-bra, l. of vertebral arch,** l. arcus vertebrae. **l. viscera′-lis pericar′dii** [NA], visceral layer of pericardium: the inner layer of the serous pericardium; it is in contact with the heart and the roots of the great vessels; called also *epicardium* [NA alternative], and *visceral pericardium.* **l. viscera′lis tu′nicae vagina′lis pro′priae tes′tis, l. viscera′lis tu′nicae vagina′lis tes′tis** [NA], visceral layer of tunica vaginalis of testis: the inner part of the tunica vaginalis of the testis, firmly attached to the testis and epididymis. **l. vit′rea,** l. basalis choroideae. **vitreal l., vitreous l.,** Bruch's membrane. **white laminae of cerebellum,** laminae albae cerebelli.

laminae (lam′ĭ-ne) [L.] plural of *lamina.*

laminagram (lam′ĭ-nah-gram) a roentgenogram of a selected layer of the body made by body-section roentgenography.

laminagraph (lam′ĭ-nah-graf) an x-ray machine for making roentgenograms of a layer of tissue at a selected depth.

laminagraphy (lam″ĭ-nag′rah-fe) [L. *lamina* layer + Gr. *graphein* to record] see *body section roentgenography,* under *roentgenography.*

laminar (lam′ĭ-nar) [L. *laminaris*] made up of, or arranged in, laminae.

Laminaria (lam″ĭ-na′re-ah) a genus of seaweeds, the kelps, various species of which are used as sources of alginates; see *laminarin.* The dried stems of *L. digitata* are used to dilate the uterine cervix in induced abortion.

laminarin (lam″ĭ-na′rin) a polysaccharide from seaweed (*Laminaria*) consisting essentially of β-D-glucose residues. **l. sulfate,** the sulfated form, having antilipemic and anticoagulant properties.

laminarinase (lah″mĭ-na′rĭ-nās) β-1,3(4)-glucan glucanohydrolase. An enzyme that catalyzes the hydrolysis of laminarin and lichenin to glucose; called also *lichenase.*

laminated (lam′ĭ-nāt″ed) made up of thin layers or laminae; disposed in laminae or layers.

lamination (lam″ĭ-na′shun) a laminated structure or arrangement.

laminectomy (lam″ĭ-nek′to-me) [L. *lamina* layer + Gr. *ektomē* excision] excision of the posterior arch of a vertebra.

laminitis (lam″ĭ-ni′tis) inflammation of a lamina, and especially of the laminae of a horse's foot; see *founder.*

laminogram (lam′ĭ-no-gram) laminagram.

laminography (lam″ĭ-nog′rah-fe) laminagraphy; see *body section roentgenography,* under *roentgenography.*

laminotomy (lam″ĭ-not′o-me) [*lamina* + Gr. *tomē* a cutting] the operation of dividing the lamina of a vertebra.

lamp (lamp) an apparatus for furnishing heat or light. **annealing l.,** an alcohol lamp for heating and purifying gold leaf to be used for filling tooth cavities. **arc l.,** a source of light consisting of gaseous particles from the electrodes of an electric arc which are raised to a temperature of incandescence by an electric current. **Birch-Hirschfeld l.,** a lamp for light treatment in eye diseases. **carbon arc l.,** a lamp that produces an intense white light from an electric arc between carbon rods; used in artificial light therapy. **cold quartz mercury vapor l.,** an ultraviolet radiation lamp having a low vapor pressure, low amperage, high voltage, and a glow discharge; more than 95 per cent of its emission is in the resonance emission line of mercury vapor at 254 mμ. **diagnostic l.,** a light used for observing subtle shadings in weak fluorescence, for external body examinations, observations of tissue fluorescence, identification of vulvar fluorescence, chromatography, etc. **Eldridge-Green l.,** an arrangement of lights for testing color vision. **Finsen l.,** a carbon arc lamp operating at 50 volts and 50 amperes so constructed that radiation is concentrated on an area 1 inch square; a water-cooled quartz system is used to remove caloric radiation and a compression quartz piece to dehematize the skin. **Finsen-Reya l.,** a modification of the Finsen lamp in which the electrodes are placed at right angles to each other. **Gull-**

strand's slit l., one embodying a diaphragm containing a slitlike opening, by means of which a narrow flat beam of intense light may be projected into the eye. It gives intense illumination so that microscopic study may be made of the conjunctiva, cornea, iris, lens, and vitreous, the special feature being that it illuminates a section through the substance of these structures. Called also *slit-lamp biomicroscope.* **Jesionek l.,** a light for giving artificial sunlight baths. **Kromayer's l.,** a small water-cooled mercury vapor lamp with a quartz window that produces ultraviolet radiation. **Lortet l.,** an electric lamp used in Finsen light treatment. **mercury vapor l.,** a lamp in which the arc is struck in mercury and is enclosed in a quartz burner; used in light therapy. There are two types, the air-cooled and water-cooled (*Kromayer's l*). **mignon l.** (min′yun), a minute electric light used in cystoscopy, etc. **quartz l.,** a mercury vacuum lamp made of melted quartz glass embedded in a running water-bath, used for applying ultraviolet light treatment. **Simpson l.,** see under *light.* **slit l.,** Gullstrand's slit l. **tungsten arc l.,** an electric arc lamp having tungsten electrodes; it has been used in the treatment of acne, alopecia, etc. **ultraviolet l.,** one which produces ultraviolet rays. **Wood's l.,** see under *light.*

lampas (lam′pas) a swelling and hardening of the mucosa of the hard palate, immediately behind the upper incisors in horses; called also *palatitis.*

Lamprocystis (lam″pro-sis′tis) a genus of microorganisms of the family Thiorhodaceae, suborder Rhodobacteriineae, order Pseudomonadales, made up of spherical to ovoid cells embedded in a common gelatinous capsule. The type species is *L. roseopersici′na.*

lamprophonia (lam″pro-fo′ne-ah) [Gr. *lampros* clear + *phōnē* voice + *-ia*] clearness of voice.

lamprophonic (lam″pro-fon′ik) pertaining to or characterized by lamprophonia.

Lamus (la′mus) a former genus name of predatory insects of the family Reduviidae now placed under the genera *Panstrongylus* and *Triatoma.*

lamziekte (lam′zēk-te) [Dutch "lame-sickness"] a disease of cattle in South Africa secondary to bovine osteophagia; the cattle chew putrefying bones and thus absorb the toxin of *Clostridium botulinum.*

lana (lan′ah), pl. and gen. *lan′ae* [L.] wool.

lanatoside C (lah-nat′o-sīd) [NF] an easily absorbed and stable glycoside, $C_{49}H_{76}O_{20}$, obtained from the leaves of *Digitalis lanata*. It occurs as colorless or white, odorless crystals or powder, and is used as a cardiotonic where digitalis is recommended.

lanaurin (lan′aw-rin) a pyrrole pigment found in the sweat and urine of sheep which may color the wool yellow.

lance (lans) [L. *lancea*] 1. lancet. 2. to cut or incise with a lancet.

Lancefield classification (lans′fēld) [Rebecca Craighill *Lancefield*, New York bacteriologist, born 1895] see under *classification.*

lanceolate (lan′se-o-lāt) shaped like a lance.

Lancereaux's diabetes (lahn″ser-ōz′) [Étienne *Lancereaux*, physician in Paris, 1829–1910] see under *diabetes.*

lancet (lan′set) [L. *lancea* lance] a small pointed and two-edged surgical knife. **abscess l.,** a wide-bladed lancet with one convex and one concave edge. **acne l.,** a form with a narrow blade for puncturing the papules of acne. **gingival l.,** a knife for incising the gingivae. **gum l.,** gingival l. **laryngeal l.,** a delicate knife for operations within the larynx; it is operated through a cannula. **spring l.,** one the blade of which is held by a spring.

Lancet coefficient (lan′set) [*The Lancet*, a British medical periodical] see under *coefficient.*

lancinating (lan′sĭ-nāt″ing) [L. *lancinans*] tearing, darting, or sharply cutting; see under *pain.*

Lancisi's nerves, stria (lan-che′sēz) [Giovanni Maria *Lancisi*, Italian physician, 1654–1720] see *stria longitudinalis lateralis corporis callosi* and *stria longitudinalis medialis corporis callosi.*

Landau's color test (reaction) (lahn′dowz) [Leopold *Landau*, German surgeon, 1848–1920] see under *tests.*

landmark (land′mark) a readily recognizable anatomical structure used as a point of reference in establishing the location of another structure or in determining certain measurements.

Landolt's bodies (lahn-dolts′) [Edmond *Landolt*, ophthalmologist in Paris, 1846–1926] see under *body.*

Landouzy's disease, dystrophy (type) (lan-doo′zēz) [Louis Théophile Joseph *Landouzy*, French physician, 1845–1917] see *leptospiral jaundice*, under *jaundice*, and see *Landouzy-Dejerine dystrophy*, under *dystrophy.*

Landouzy-Dejerine dystrophy (atrophy, type) (lan-doo′ze-deh″zher-ēn′) [L. T. J. *Landouzy*; Joseph Jules *Dejerine*, French neurologist, 1849– 1917] see under *dystrophy.*

Landouzy-Grasset law (lan-doo′ze-gras-sa′) [L. T. J. *Landouzy*; Joseph *Grasset*, French physician, 1849– 1918] see under *law.*

Landry's paralysis (disease, palsy, syndrome) (lan-drēz′) [Jean Baptiste Octave *Landry*, French physician, 1826–1865] acute febrile polyneuritis.

Landsteiner (land′sti-ner) Karl. Austrian pathologist and immunologist in the United States, 1868–1943, winner of the Nobel prize for physiology and medicine in 1930 for his discovery of the human blood groups.

Landström's muscle (lahnd′stremz) [John *Landström*, Swedish surgeon, 1869–1910] see under *muscle.*

Lane's band, disease, kink, operation, plates (lānz) [Sir William Arbuthnot *Lane*, English surgeon, 1856–1943] see under the *nouns.*

Langdon Down's disease (lang′don downz) [John *Langdon Down*, British physician, 1828–1896] Down's syndrome.

Lange's operation (lahng′ez) [Fritz *Lange*, German orthopedist, born 1864] silk implantation; see under *implantation.*

Lange's solution, test (reaction) (lahng′ez) [Carl *Lange*, German physician, born 1883] see under *solution*, and see *colloidal gold test*, under *tests.*

Langenbeck's amputation, incision, etc. (lahng′en-beks) [Bernhard Rudolf Konrad von *Langenbeck*, German surgeon, 1810–1887] see under *amputation, flap, incision,* and *triangle.*

Langer's axillary arch, lines, muscle (lang′erz) [Carl Ritter von Edenberg von *Langer*, Austrian anatomist, 1819–1887] see under *arch* and *muscle*, and see *cleavage lines*, under *line.*

Langerhans' cells (corpuscles), islets (islands), layer (lahng′er-hanz) [Paul *Langerhans*, German pathologist, 1847–1888] see under *cell* and *islet*, and see *stratum granulosum epidermidis.*

Langhans' cells, layer, stria (lahng′hahnz) [Theodor *Langhans*, German pathologist, 1839–1915] see under *cell*, and see *cytotrophoblast.*

Langley's ganglion, granules, nerves (lang′lēz) [John Newport *Langley*, English physiologist, 1852–1925] see under *ganglion* and *granule*, and see *pilonidal nerves*, under *nerve.*

laniary (lan′e-a″re) [L. *laniare* to tear to pieces] suitable for lacerating, or tearing to pieces; said of canine teeth.

Lankesterella ranarum (lan-kes″ter-el′ah rah-na′rum) [Sir Edwin Ray *Lankester*, British zoologist, 1847–1930] a coccidian parasite of the red blood cells of the frog.

Lankesteria culicis (lan″kes-te′re-ah ku′lĭ-sis) a gregarine sporozoon parasitic in the gut of the mosquito *Aedes aegypti.*

lanolin (lan′o-lin) [L. *lanolinum; lana* wool + *oleum* oil] [USP] the purified fatlike substance from the wool of sheep, *Ovis aries,* occurring as a yellowish white mass and mixed with 25 to 30 per cent of water; used as a water-in-oil ointment base. **anhydrous l.** [USP], lanolin that contains not more than 0.25 per cent of water, used as an absorbent ointment base.

lanosterol (lah-nos′ter-ol) a triterpenic sterol, $C_{30}H_{50}O$, formed from squalene; it is the parent steroid in animals, being itself converted in several steps to cholesterol.

Lanoxin (lah-nok′sin) trademark for preparations of digoxin.

Lantermann's incisures (clefts) (lahn″ter-mahnz′) [A.J. *Lantermann*, American anatomist in Strassburg, 19th century] see under *incisure.*

Lantermann-Schmidt incisures (lahn″ter-mahn′-schmit′) [A. J. Lantermann; Henry D. *Schmidt*, American anatomist, 1823–1888] incisures of Lantermann.

lanthanic (lan′than-ik) [Gr. *lanthanein* to escape notice, to be concealed] symptom-free; said of a symptomless disease that is undetected, or detected by accident.

lanthanin (lan′thah-nin) oxychromatin.

lanthanum (lan′thah-num) [Gr. *lanthanein* to be concealed] a rare metallic element; symbol, La; atomic number, 57; atomic weight, 138.91.

lanuginous (lah-nu′jĭ-nus) [L. *lanuginosus*] covered with lanugo.

lanugo (lah-nu′go) [L.] [NA] the fine hair on the body of the fetus; called also *down* and *wooly hair.*

lanum (la′num) [L. *lana* wool] lanolin.

Lanz's operation, point (lahnts) [Otto *Lanz*, surgeon in Amsterdam, 1865–1935] see under *operation* and *point.*

L.A.O. Licentiate in Obstetric Science.

LAP lyophilized anterior pituitary (tissue).

lapactic (lah-pak′tik) [Gr. *lapaktikos, lapassein* to discharge] pertaining to or effecting a removal; purgative; laxative.

laparectomy (lap″ah-rek′to-me) [*laparo-* + Gr. *ektomē* excision] excision of a portion or of portions of the abdominal wall; performed for the purpose of overcoming laxity of the walls and to gain support.

laparo- (lap′ah-ro) [Gr. *lapara* flank] a combining form denoting relationship to the loin or flank. Sometimes used loosely in reference to the abdomen.

laparocele (lap′ah-ro-sēl) ventral hernia.

laparocholecystotomy (lap″ah-ro-ko″le-sis-tot′o-me) [*laparo-*

+ Gr. *cholē* bile + *kystis* bladder + *tomē* a cutting] incision of the gallbladder through an abdominal section; cholecystotomy.

laparocolectomy (lap″ah-ro-ko-lek′to-me) [*laparo-* + Gr. *kolon* colon + *ektomē* excision] colectomy.

laparocolostomy (lap″ah-ro-ko-los′to-me) [*laparo-* + Gr. *kolon* colon + *stomoun* to provide with an opening, or mouth] ′ surgical creation of a permanent opening into the colon by an incision in the anterolateral wall of the abdomen; colostomy.

laparocolotomy (lap″ah-ro-ko-lot′o-me) [*laparo-* + Gr. *kolon* colon + *tomē* a cutting] colotomy through the abdominal wall.

laparocystectomy (lap″ah-ro-sis-tek′to-me) [*laparo-* + Gr. *kystis* cyst + *ektomē* excision] removal of a cyst by an abdominal incision.

laparocystidotomy (lap″ah-ro-sis″tĭ-dot′o-me) [*laparo-* + Gr. *kystis* bladder + *tomē* a cutting] incision into the bladder through the abdominal wall just above the pubes.

laparocystotomy (lap″ah-ro-sis-tot′o-me) [*laparo-* + Gr. *kystis* bladder + *tomē* a cutting] 1. the removal of an extrauterine fetus, the sac being allowed to remain. 2. laparotomy with removal of the contents of a cyst.

laparoenterostomy (lap″ah-ro-en″ter-os′to-me) [*laparo-* + Gr. *enteron* intestine + *stomoun* to provide with an opening, or mouth] surgical creation of an artificial opening into the intestine through the abdominal wall.

laparoenterotomy (lap″ah-ro-en″ter-ot′o-me) [*laparo-* + Gr. *enteron* intestine + *tomē* a cutting] laparotomy with incision into the intestine.

laparogastroscopy (lap″ah-ro-gas-tros′ko-pe) [*laparo-* + *gastroscopy*] examination of the interior of the stomach through an abdominal incision.

laparogastrostomy (lap″ah-ro-gas-tros′to-me) [*laparo-* + Gr. *gastēr* stomach + *stomoun* to provide with an opening, or mouth] surgical creation of a permanent gastric fistula through the abdominal wall.

laparogastrotomy (lap″ah-ro-gas-trot′o-me) [*laparo-* + Gr. *gastēr* stomach + *tomē* a cutting] incision into the stomach through the abdominal wall.

laparohepatotomy (lap″ah-ro-hep″ah-tot′o-me) [*laparo-* + *hepatotomy*] incision of the liver through the abdominal wall.

laparohysterectomy (lap″ah-ro-his″ter-ek′to-me) [*laparo-* + Gr. *hystera* uterus + *ektomē* excision] removal of the uterus through an opening in the abdominal wall.

laparohystero-oophorectomy (lap″ah-ro-his″ter-o-o″of-ŏ-rek′to-me) [*laparo-* + Gr. *hystera* uterus + *oophorectomy*] laparotomy with removal of the uterus and ovaries.

laparohysterosalpingo-oophorectomy (lap″ah-ro-his″ter-o-sal-ping″go-o″of-ŏ-rek′to-me) removal of the uterus, uterine tubes, and ovaries through an abdominal incision.

laparohysterotomy (lap″ah-ro-his″ter-ot′o-me) [*laparo-* + Gr. *hystera* uterus + *tomē* a cutting] laparotomy with incision of the uterus.

laparoileotomy (lap″ah-ro-il″e-ot′o-me) [*laparo-* + *ileum* + Gr. *tomē* a cutting] laparotomy with incision of the ileum.

laparomonodidymus (lap″ah-ro-mon″o-did′ĭ-mus) [*laparo-* + Gr. *monos* single + *didymos* twin] a monster, double above but single below the pelvis.

laparomyitis (lap″ah-ro-mi-i′tis) [*laparo-* + Gr. *mys* muscle + *-itis*] inflammation of the abdominal or lumbar muscles.

laparomyomectomy (lap″ah-ro-mi″o-mek′to-me) [*laparo-* + Gr. *mys* muscle + *ektomē* excision] the removal of a myoma by an abdominal incision.

laparonephrectomy (lap″ah-ro-ně-frek′to-me) [*laparo-* + Gr. *nephros* kidney + *ektomē* excision] removal of a kidney by an incision in the loin.

laparorrhaphy (lap-ah-ror′ah-fe) [*laparo-* + Gr. *rhaphē* suture] suturation of the abdominal wall.

laparosalpingectomy (lap″ah-ro-sal″pin-jek′to-me) [*laparo-* + Gr. *salpinx* tube + *ektomē* excision] removal of a uterine tube through an abdominal incision.

laparosalpingo-oophorectomy (lap″ah-ro-sal- ping″go-o″of-ŏ-rek′to-me) removal of a uterine tube and ovary through an abdominal incision.

laparosalpingotomy (lap″ah-ro-sal″pin-got′o-me) [*laparo-* + Gr. *salpinx* tube + *tomē* a cutting] incision of a uterine tube through an abdominal incision.

laparoscope (lap′ah-ro-skōp″) an instrument comparable to an endoscope by means of which the peritoneal cavity can be inspected; peritoneoscope.

laparoscopy (lap″ah-ros′ko-pe) [*laparo-* + Gr. *skopein* to examine] examination of the interior of the abdomen by means of a laparoscope.

laparosplenectomy (lap″ah-ro-sple-nek′to-me) [*laparo-* + Gr. *splēn* spleen + *ektomē* excision] laparotomy with excision of the spleen.

laparosplenotomy (lap″ah-ro-sple-not′o-me) [*laparo-* + Gr. *splēn* spleen + *tomē* a cutting] the operation of making an in-

cision in the flank to gain access to the spleen, usually for the purpose of draining a cyst or abscess of the spleen.

laparotomaphilia (lap″ah-rot″o-mah-fil′e-ah) [*laparotomy* + Gr. *philein* to love + *-ia*] Munchausen's syndrome (q.v.) in which the patient desires abdominal surgery.

laparotome (lap′ah-ro-tōm) a knife used in laparotomy.

laparotomy (lap-ah-rot′o-me) [*laparo-* + Gr. *tomē* a cutting] surgical incision through the flank; less correctly, but more generally, abdominal section at any point.

laparotyphlotomy (lap″ah-ro-tif-lot′o-me) [*laparo-* + Gr. *typhlon* cecum + *tomē* a cutting] incision into the cecum through the flank.

Lapicque's constant, law (lah-pēks′) [Louis *Lapicque*, French physiologist, 1866–1952] see under *constant* and *law.*

lapinization (lap″in-i-za′shun) [Fr. *lapin* rabbit] passage of a virus through rabbits as a means of modifying its characteristics.

lapinize (lap′in-īz) to attenuate (as a virus or vaccine) by serial passage through rabbits.

lapis (la′pis, lap′is) [L.] stone. **l. al′bus,** the native silicofluoride of calcium. **l. calamina′ris,** calamine. **l. imperia′lis, l. inferna′lis, l. luna′ris,** silver nitrate.

lapsus (lap′sus) [L., from *labi* to slip or fall] 1. an error, or slip, thought to be revealing of an unconscious wish or association. 2. falling or dropping of a part; ptosis. **l. cal′ami,** an unconsciously motivated slip of the pen. **l. lin′guae,** an unconsciously motivated slip of the tongue. **l. memo′riae,** an unconsciously motivated lapse of memory.

lapyrium chloride (lah-pēr′e-um) chemical name: 1-[2-oxo-2-[[2-[(1-oxododecyl)oxy]ethyl]amino]ethyl]pyridinium chloride. A surfactant, $C_{21}H_{35}ClN_2O_3$, used in pharmaceutic preparations.

Larat's treatment (lah-raz′) [Jules Louis François Adrien *Larat*, French physician, born 1857] see under *treatment.*

lard (lard) [L. *lardum*] the purified internal fat of the abdomen of the hog. **benzoinated l.,** a preparation of lard containing 1 per cent benzoin; used as a vehicle for medicinal agents and in ointments. Called also *adeps benzoinatus.*

lardacein (lar-da′se-in) a protein found in tissues affected with amyloid degeneration. It is characterized by being insoluble in nearly all reagents, not acted upon by the gastric juice, and not readily subject to putrefaction. It gives a brown color with iodine and sulfuric acid.

lardaceous (lar-da′shus) 1. resembling lard. 2. containing lardacein.

Lardennois' button (lar″den-wahz′) [Henri *Lardennois*, French surgeon, born 1872] see under *button.*

Largon (lar′gon) trademark for a preparation of propiomazine hydrochloride.

larithmics (lah-rith′miks) [Gr. *laos* people + *arithmos* number] the study which deals with population in its quantitative aspects.

Larix (la′riks) [L.] a genus of coniferous trees, the larches. The astringent bark of *L. europaea* D.C. (Pinaceae) has been used in skin diseases and in pectoral complaints.

larixin (la-rik′sin) azaric acid.

larkspur (lark′spur) the dried ripe seeds of *Delphinium ajacis* L. (Ranunculaceae), used medically as a pediculicide. Listed as poisonous plant due to its content of alkaloids, including delphinine. Called also *staggerweed.*

Larodopa (lar″o-do′pah) trademark for preparations of levodopa.

Larotid (lar′o-tid) trademark for preparations of amoxicillin.

Larrey's amputation (operation), bandage, cleft, spaces (lar-rāz′) [Dominique Jean (Baron de) *Larrey*, French surgeon, 1766–1842; the greatest military surgeon of his time, serving in the Napoleonic wars] see under *amputation, bandage,* and *space,* and see *trigonum sternocostale.*

Larsen's disease, Larsen-Johansson disease (lar′senz; lar′sen-yo-han′son) [Christian Magnus Falsen Sinding *Larsen*; Sven *Johansson*, Swedish surgeon, born 1880] see under *disease.*

larva (lar′vah), pl. *lar′vae* [L.] an independent, motile, sometimes feeding, developmental stage in the life history of an animal. Cf. *imago* (def. 1) and *pupa.* **l. cur′rens,** a variant of larva migrans caused by *Strongyloides stercoralis,* in which progression of the linear lesion is as rapid as 10 cm. in an hour, instead of a few centimeters a day, as is usual with lesions due to *Ancylostoma brasiliense.* **l. mi′grans,** a disease marked by a thin, red, bizarrely convoluted, papular or vesicular line of eruption that gradually extends at one end while fading at the other. It is most often due to the presence of larvae of the cat and dog hookworm, *Ancylostoma braziliense,* which burrow beneath the skin, but cannot complete their migration to the gut; called also *creeping eruption.* The term is also applied to similar lesions caused by larvae of botflies of the genus *Gasterophilus* (cutaneous or dermal myiasis), nematodes of the genus *Gnathostoma* (creeping disease), larvae of filaria of the genus *Dirofilaria* (dirofilariasis), larvae of *Hypoderma linearis* (hypodermiasis or ox-warble disease), and larvae of other species. **l. mi′grans, ocular,** infection of the eye with larvae of roundworms (*Toxocara canis* or *T. cati*), which may lodge in the choroid or retina or migrate to the vitreous; on the death of the larvae, a granulomatous inflammation occurs, the lesion varying from a translucent elevation of the retina, to massive retinal detachment and pseudoglioma. Called also *human toxocariasis*. **l. migrans, visceral,** a condition caused by prolonged migration of larvae of nematodes in human tissues other than skin, characterized by persistent hypereosinophilia, hepatomegaly, and frequently by pneumonitis; commonly caused by *Toxocara canis* or *T. cati*, which do not complete their life cycle in man. See also *l. migrans, ocular*. **rat-tailed l.,** see *Eristalis tenax*.

larvaceous (lar-va′shus) larvate.

larvae (lar′ve) [L.] plural of *larva*.

larval (lar′val) 1. pertaining to larvae. 2. larvate.

larvate (lar′vāt) [L. *larva* mask] masked; concealed: said of a disease or a symptom of disease.

larvicide (lar′vĭ-sīd) [*larva* + L. *caedere* to kill] an agent destructive to insect larvae. **Panama l.,** a mixture of crude carbolic acid, rosin, and caustic soda, heated to a uniform dark colored soap; formerly used in Panama to kill *Anopheles* larvae.

larviphagic (lar′vĭ-fa′jik) larvivorous.

larviposition (lar″vĭ-po-zish′un) the act of depositing larvae (living maggots) in the tissues of a host.

larvivorous (lar-viv′o-rus) [*larva* + L. *vorare* to eat] feeding on or consuming larvae; said especially of fish which ingest mosquito larvae.

laryngalgia (lar″in-gal′je-ah) [*laryngo-* + *-algia*] pain in the larynx.

laryngeal (lah-rin′je-al) of or pertaining to the larynx.

laryngect (lar′in-jekt″) laryngectomee.

laryngectomee (lar″in-jek′to-me) a person whose larynx has been removed.

laryngectomy (lar″in-jek′to-me) [*laryngo-* + Gr. *ektomē* excision] extirpation of the larynx.

laryngendoscope (lar″in-jen′do-skōp) [*laryngo-* + Gr. *endon* within + *skopein* to examine] an instrument for viewing the interior of the larynx.

laryngismal (lar″in-jiz′mal) pertaining to laryngismus.

laryngismus (lar″in-jiz′mus) [L.; Gr. *laryngismos* a whooping] spasm of the larynx. **l. paralyt′icus,** roaring. **l. strid′-ulus,** a condition marked by sudden laryngeal spasm, with a crowing inspiration and the development of cyanosis. It occurs in laryngeal inflammations and as an independent disease, especially in connection with rickets. Called also *Miller's* or *Wichmann's asthma*.

laryngitic (lar″in-jit′ik) pertaining to laryngitis.

laryngitis (lar″in-ji′tis) inflammation of the larynx, a condition attended with dryness and soreness of the throat, hoarseness, cough, and dysphagia. **acute catarrhal l.,** a form characterized by aphonia or hoarseness, pain and dryness of the throat, dyspnea, a wheezy cough, and more or less fever. **atrophic l.,** an extreme form of chronic catarrhal laryngitis. **chronic catarrhal l.,** a form of laryngitis due to recurring inflammation or more frequently a sequela of acute catarrhal laryngitis, characterized by atrophy of the glands of the mucous membrane. See also *l. sicca*. **croupous l.,** a condition occurring chiefly in infants or small children and characterized by a resonant barking cough, hoarseness, and stridor. Infection, allergy, a foreign body, or new growths may be the cause. Laryngeal diphtheria was once a common cause but is now relatively rare. **diphtheritic l.,** laryngitis caused by diphtheria; diphtheritic croup. **membranous l.,** laryngitis attended with the formation of a false membrane. **necrotic l.,** calf diphtheria. **phlegmonous l.,** a usually fatal complication of erysipelas, smallpox, etc. attended with submucous suppuration and edema. **l. sic′ca,** chronic laryngitis in which the usual secretions are gluelike; it often accompanies atrophic rhinitis. **l. stridulo′sa,** laryngismus stridulus. **subglottic l.,** inflammation of the under surface of the vocal cords. **syphilitic l.,** a chronic form due to syphilitic involvement of the larynx. **tuberculous l.,** a chronic form due to tuberculous ulceration of the larynx. **vestibular l.,** viral laryngitis in which edema forms a ring outlining the vestibule of the larynx.

laryngo- (lah-ring′go) [Gr. *larynx* larynx] a combining form denoting relationship to the larynx.

laryngocele (lah-ring′go-sēl) [*laryngo-* + Gr. *kēlē* hernia] a congenital anomalous air sac communicating with the cavity of the larynx, which may become manifest as an enlargement seen as a tumor-like lesion on the outside of the neck; the enlargement is increased by intralaryngeal pressure, as from coughing. **ventricular l., l. ventricula′ris,** congenital dilatation or herniation of the sacculus or appendix of the laryngeal ventricle.

laryngocentesis (lah-ring″go-sen-te′sis) [*laryngo-* + Gr. *kentēsis* puncture] surgical puncture of the larynx.

laryngofission (lah-ring″go-fish′un) laryngofissure.

laryngofissure (lah-ring″go-fish′ūr) the operation of opening

the larynx by a median incision through the thyroid cartilage, for the removal of cancer of the larynx; median laryngotomy.

laryngogram (lah-ring′go-gram) a roentgenogram of the larynx.

laryngography (lar″ing-gog′rah-fe) [*laryngo-* + Gr. *graphein* to record] 1. the description of the larynx. 2. roentgenography of the larynx after instillation of a radiopaque substance into it.

laryngohypopharynx (lah-ring″go-hi′po-far′inks) the posterior wall of the hypopharynx, the piriform sinus, and areas adjacent to the larynx, considered together.

laryngology (lar″ing-gol′o-je) [*laryngo-* + *-logy*] that branch of medicine which has to do with the throat, pharynx, larynx, nasopharynx, and tracheobronchial tree.

laryngomalacia (lah-ring″go-mah-la′she-ah) [*laryngo-* + Gr. *malakia* softness] flaccidity of the epiglottis and aryepiglottic folds, as in congenital laryngeal stridor.

laryngometry (lar″ing-gom′ĕ-tre) [*laryngo-* + Gr. *metron* measure] measurement of the larynx.

laryngoparalysis (lah-ring″go-pah-ral′ĭ-sis) [*laryngo-* + *paralysis*] paralysis of the larynx.

laryngopathy (lar″ing-gop′ah-the) [*laryngo-* + Gr. *pathos* disease] any disorder of the larynx.

laryngopharyngeal (lah-ring″go-fah-rin′je-al) pertaining to the larynx and pharynx.

laryngopharyngectomy (lah-ring″go-far″in-jek′to-me) excision of the larynx and pharynx.

laryngopharyngeus (lah-ring″go-fah-rin′je-us) the inferior constrictor of the pharynx.

laryngopharyngitis (lah-ring″go-far″in-ji′tis) inflammation of the larynx and pharynx.

laryngopharynx (lah-ring″go-far′inks) [*laryngo-* + *pharynx*] the portion of the pharynx which lies below the upper edge of the epiglottis and opens into the larynx and esophagus (pars laryngea pharyngis [NA]).

laryngophony (lar″ing-gof′o-ne) [*laryngo-* + Gr. *phōnē* voice] the vocal sound as heard in auscultation of the larynx.

laryngophthisis (lar″ing-gof′thĭ-sis) [*laryngo-* + Gr. *phthisis* phthisis] tuberculosis of the larynx.

laryngoplasty (lah-ring″go-plas′te) [*laryngo-* + Gr. *plassein* to mold] plastic surgery of the larynx.

laryngoplegia (lar″ing-go-ple′je-ah) [*laryngo-* + Gr. *plēgē* stroke + *-ia*] paralysis of the larynx.

laryngoptosis (lah-ring″go-to′sis) [*laryngo-* + Gr. *ptōsis* fall] a lowering and mobilization of the larynx as sometimes seen in the aged.

laryngopyocele (lah-ring″go-pi′o-sēl) a laryngocele containing pus.

laryngorhinology (lah-ring″go-ri-nol′o-je) [*laryngo-* + Gr. *rhis* nose + *-logy*] the sum of what is known regarding the larynx and nose and their diseases.

laryngorrhagia (lar″ing-go-ra′je-ah) [*laryngo-* + Gr. *rhēgnynai* to break] hemorrhage from the larynx.

laryngorrhaphy (lar″ing-gor′ah-fe) [*laryngo-* + Gr. *rhaphē* suture] the operation of suturing the larynx.

laryngorrhea (lar″ing-go-re′ah) [*laryngo-* + Gr. *rhoia* flow] excessive secretion of mucus whenever the voice is used.

laryngoscleroma (lah-ring″go-skle-ro′mah) [*laryngo-* + *scleroma*] scleroma of the larynx.

laryngoscope (lah-ring″go-skōp) [*laryngo-* + Gr. *skopein* to examine] an endoscope for use in direct visual examination of the larynx.

laryngoscopic (lar″ing-go-skop′ik) pertaining to laryngoscopy.

laryngoscopist (lar″ing-gos′ko-pist) an expert in laryngoscopy.

laryngoscopy (lar″ing-gos′ko-pe) [*laryngo-* + Gr. *skopein* to examine] examination of the interior of the larynx, especially that performed with the laryngoscope (*direct laryngoscopy*). **direct l.,** direct visual examination of the interior of the larynx performed with a speculum or with a laryngoscope. **indirect l.,** examination of the interior of the larynx by observation of the reflection of it in a laryngeal mirror. **mirror l.,** indirect l. **suspension l.,** examination of the larynx performed with a direct laryngoscope suspended so as to leave both hands of the examiner free.

laryngospasm (lah-ring′go-spazm) [*laryngo-* + Gr. *spasmos* spasm] spasmodic closure of the larynx.

laryngostasis (lar″ing-gos′tah-sis) [*laryngo-* + Gr. *stasis* stoppage] croup.

laryngostat (lah-ring′go-stat) an appliance for holding a source of radioactive material within the larynx.

laryngostenosis (lah-ring″go-stĕ-no′sis) [*laryngo-* + Gr. *stenōsis* contracture] narrowing or stricture of the larynx.

laryngostomy (lar″ing-gos′to-me) [*laryngo-* + Gr. *stomoun* to provide with an opening, or mouth] surgical creation of an artificial opening into the larynx.

laryngostroboscope (lar″ing-go-strob′o-skōp) [*laryngo-* + Gr. *strophos* whirl + *skopein* to examine] an apparatus for observing the intralaryngeal phenomena with a stroboscopic light.

laryngotome (lah-ring′go-tōm) an instrument used in incising the larynx.

laryngotomy (lar″ing-got′o-me) [*laryngo-* + Gr. *tomē* a cutting] surgical incision of the larynx. **complete l.,** the longitudinal slitting of the entire larynx. **inferior l.,** incision of the larynx through the cricothyroid membrane. **median l.,** incision of the larynx through the thyroid cartilage; laryngofissure. **superior l., subhyoid l.,** incision of the larynx through the thyrohyoid membrane. **thyrohyoid l.,** subhyoid l.

laryngotracheal (lah-ring″go-tra′ke-al) pertaining to the larynx and trachea.

laryngotracheitis (lah-ring″go-tra″ke-i′tis) inflammation of the larynx and trachea. **avian l., infectious l.,** a viral disease of poultry characterized by respiratory distress, gasping, and expectoration of bloody exudate.

laryngotracheobronchitis (lah-ring″go-tra″ke-o-brong-ki′tis) inflammation of the larynx, trachea, and bronchi; the acute form is the most common cause of croup.

laryngotracheobronchoscopy (lah-ring″go-tra″ke-o-bronkos′ko-pe) endoscopic examination of the larynx, trachea, and bronchi.

laryngotracheoscopy (lah-ring″go-tra″ke-os′ko-pe) peroral laryngoscopy and tracheoscopy.

laryngotracheotomy (lah-ring″go-tra″ke-ot′o-me) [*laryngo-* + *tracheotomy*] incision of the larynx and trachea.

laryngovestibulitis (lah-ring″go-ves-tib″u-li′tis) inflammation of the vestibule of the larynx.

laryngoxerosis (lah-ring″go-ze-ro′sis) [*laryngo-* + Gr. *xērōsis* a drying up] dryness of the larynx.

larynx (lar′inks), pl. *laryn′ges* [Gr. "the upper part of the windpipe"] [NA] the musculocartilaginous structure, lined with mucous membrane, connected to the superior part of the trachea and to the pharynx inferior to the tongue and the hyoid bone; the essential sphincter guarding the entrance into the trachea and functioning secondarily as the organ of voice. It is formed by nine cartilages—the thyroid, cricoid, epiglottis, two arytenoid, two corniculate, and two cuneiform cartilages, connected by ligaments. **artificial l.,** an electromechanical device which, when activated, produces sounds used in speech, by simulating laryngeal activity, and thus enables a laryngectomized person to converse.

lasalocid (lah-sal′o-sid) chemical name: 6-[7*R*-[5*S*-ethyl-5-(5*R*-ethyltetrahydro-5-hydroxy-6*S*-methyl-2*H*-pyran-2*R*-yl)tetrahydro-3*H*-methyl-2*S*-furanyl]-4*S*-hydroxy-3*R*,5*S*-dimethyl-6-oxononyl]-2-hydroxy-3-methylbenzoic acid; a coccidiostat for use in poultry, $C_{34}H_{54}O_8$.

lasanum (las′ah-num) [L. "a night commode"] an obstetric chair.

lascivia (lah-siv′e-ah) [L. "wantonness"] (*obs.*) satyriasis.

Lasègue's disease, sign (syndrome) (lah-sāgz′) [Ernest Charles *Lasègue*, French physician, 1816–1883] see under *disease* and *sign.*

laser (la′zer) [*l*ight *a*mplification by *s*timulated *e*mission of *r*adiation] a device which transforms light of various frequencies into an extremely intense, small, and nearly nondivergent beam of monochromatic radiation in the visible region with all the waves in phase. Capable of mobilizing immense heat and power when focused at close range, it is used as a tool in surgical procedures, in diagnosis, and in physiologic studies.

Lasiohelea (las″e-o-he′le-ah) a genus of blood-sucking flies of the family Heleidae.

Lasix (la′siks) trademark for preparations of furosemide.

Lassar's paste, betanaphthol paste, plain zinc paste (las′arz) [Oskar *Lassar*, German dermatologist, 1849–1907] see under *paste.*

lassitude (las′ĭ-tūd) [L. *lassitudo* weariness] weakness; exhaustion.

latah (lah′tah) a mental disorder seen chiefly among the Malays and other people of Southeast Asia, characterized by hypersuggestibility, echolalia, echopraxis, coprolalia, disorganization, and automatic obedience.

Lat. dol. abbreviation for L. *late′ri dolen′ti,* to the painful side.

latebra (lat′ĕ-brah) [L. "hiding place"] a flask-shaped mass of white yolk extending from the blastodisk to the center of eggs such as those of birds.

latency (la′ten-se) a state of seeming inactivity, as that occurring between the instant of stimulation and the beginning of response; see also under *period.*

latent (la′tent) [L. *latens* hidden] concealed; not manifest; potential.

latentiation (la-ten″she-a′shun) the process of making latent; in pharmacology, the chemical modification of a biologically active compound to affect its absorption, distribution, etc., the modified compound being transformed after administration to the active compound by biological processes.

laterad (lat′er-ad) toward a side or a lateral aspect.

lateral (lat′er-al) [L. *lateralis*] 1. denoting a position farther from the median plane or midline of the body or of a structure. 2. pertaining to a side.

lateralis (lat″er-a′lis) lateral; [NA] a term denoting a structure situated farther from the midplane of the body.

laterality (lat″er-al′ĭ-te) a relationship to one side, such as a tendency, in voluntary motor acts, to use preferentially the organs (hand, foot, ear, eye) of the same side. **crossed l.,** the preferential use, in voluntary motor acts, of contralateral members of the different pairs of organs, as the right eye and the left hand. **dominant l.,** the preferential use, in voluntary motor acts, of ipsilateral members of the different pairs of organs, as the right ear, eye, hand, and leg (dextrality) or of the left ear, eye, hand, and leg (sinistrality).

latericeous (lat″er-ish′us) lateritious.

lateritious (lat″er-ish′us) [L. *lateritius; later* brick] resembling brick dust.

latero- (lat′er-o) [L. *latus* side] a combining form denoting relationship to the side.

lateroabdominal (lat″er-o-ab-dom′ĭ-nal) pertaining to the side and the abdomen.

laterodeviation (lat″er-o-de″ve-a′shun) deviation or slight displacement to one side.

lateroduction (lat″er-o-duk′shun) [*latero-* + L. *ducere* to draw] movement of an eye to either side.

lateroflexion (lat″er-o-flek′shun) flexion to either side.

lateroposition (lat″er-o-po-zish′un) displacement to one side.

lateropulsion (lat″er-o-pul′shun) [*latero-* + L. *pellere* to drive] an involuntary tendency to go to one side while walking.

laterotorsion (lat″er-o-tor′shun) [*latero-* + L. *torquere* to turn] twisting of the vertical meridian of the eye to the right or to the left.

lateroversion (lat″er-o-ver′shun) [*latero-* + *version*] a turning to one side, as of the uterus.

latex (la′teks) [L. "fluid"] a viscid, milky juice secreted by some seed plants.

latexed (lat-eksd′) (*obs.*) bent to one side.

latexion (la-tek′shun) (*obs.*) lateral flexion.

Latham's circle (la′thamz) [Peter Mere *Latham,* English physician, 1789–1875] see under *circle.*

lathyrism (lath′ĭ-rizm) a morbid condition resulting from ingestion of the seeds of leguminous plants of the genus *Lathyrus,* which includes many kinds of peas; it is characterized by spastic paraplegia, pain, hyperesthesia, and paresthesia. Cf. *lupinosis* and *osteolathyrism.*

lathyritic (lath″ĭ-rit′ik) pertaining to or characterized by lathyrism.

lathyrogen (lath′ĭ-ro-jen) any agent that causes lathyrism.

lathyrogenic (lath″ĭ-ro-jen′ik) capable of producing the symptoms characteristic of lathyrism.

latissimus (lah-tis′ĭ-mus) [L.] widest; [NA] a general term denoting a broad structure, as a muscle.

latrodectism (lat″ro-dek′tizm) [*Latrodectus* + -*ism*] intoxication caused by venom of spiders of the genus *Latrodectus.*

Latrodectus (lat″ro-dek′tus) [L. *latro* robber + Gr. *daknein* to bite] a genus of poisonous spiders. *L. mac′tans,* a species found in the United States, is commonly known as the "black widow." Its bite may cause severe symptoms or even death. *L. bisho′pi* is found in southern Florida; *L. curarien′sis* in Brazil and Argentina; *L. geomet′ricus* in California and southern Florida; *L. hassel′tii* in New Zealand; *L. lugu′bris,* (kara-kurt) in Russia; *L. macula′tus* in South Africa; *L. malmigniat′tus* in Europe; and *L. tredecimgutta′tus* in Southern Europe and Asiatic Russia.

LATS long-acting thyroid stimulator.

lattice (lat′is) a framework of regularly placed, intersecting narrow strips, such as the geometrical arrangement of the atoms in a crystal as shown by x-ray analysis.

latus (la′tus) [L.] 1. broad, wide 2. [NA] the side; flank.

laudable (law′dah-bl) [L. *laudabilis*] commendable; healthy; see under *pus.*

laudanum (law′dah-num) opium tincture.

laugh (laf) 1. an act or paroxysm of laughter. 2. to indulge in laughter. **canine l., sardonic l.,** risus sardonicus.

laughter (laf′ter) a series of spasmodic and partly involuntary expirations with inarticulate vocalization, normally indicative of merriment, often a hysteric manifestation or a reflex result of tickling. **compulsive l., forced l., obsessive l.,** hearty laughter for which there is no occasion; a symptom in schizophrenia.

Laugier's hernia, sign (lo″zhe-āz′) [Stanislas *Laugier,* French surgeon, 1799–1872] see under *hernia* and *sign.*

Laumonier's ganglion (lo-mon″e-āz′) [Jean Baptiste Philippe Nicolas Réné *Laumonier,* French surgeon, 1749–1818] 1. carotid ganglion. 2. inferior carotid ganglion.

Launois-Cléret syndrome (lo-nwah′kla-rah′) [Pierre-Emile *Launois*, French physician, 1856–1914; M. *Cléret*] Fröhlich's syndrome.

Laurence-Biedl syndrome (law′rens-be′del) [John Zachariah *Laurence*, British ophthalmologist, 1830–1874; Arthur *Biedl*, Prague endocrinologist, 1869–1933] see under *syndrome*.

Laurence-Moon-Biedl syndrome [J. Z. *Laurence*; R. C. *Moon*; A. *Biedl*] Laurence-Biedl syndrome.

laureth 9 (law′reth) a spermaticide and surfactant consisting of a mixture of polyethylene glycol monododecyl ethers averaging about 9 ethylene oxide groups per molecule.

laurocerasus (law″ro-ser′ah-sus) [L. *laurus* laurel + *cerasus* cherry] the European cherry laurel, an evergreen cherry tree, *Prunus laurocerasus*.

Lauth's canal, sinus (lowts) [Ernst Alexander *Lauth*, Strasbourg physiologist, 1803–1837] sinus venosus sclerae.

Lauth's ligament (lowts) [Thomas *Lauth*, Strasbourg anatomist and surgeon, 1758–1826] ligamentum transversum atlantis.

Lauth's violet (lawths) [Charles *Lauth*, English chemist, 1836–1913] thionine hydrochloride.

lavage (lah-vahzh′) [Fr.] 1. the irrigation or washing out of an organ, such as the stomach or bowel. 2. to wash out, or irrigate. **l. of the blood, blood l.,** the washing out of toxic matters from the blood by injecting serum into the veins. **ether l.,** see *Souligoux-Morestin method*, under *method*. **gastric l.,** lavage of the stomach. **intestinal l.,** dialysis by instillation and withdrawal of a rinsing fluid in the intestine for the removal, through the intestinal mucosa, of elements which are not being excreted by the kidneys. **peritoneal l.,** dialysis by instillation and withdrawal of a rinsing fluid in the peritoneal cavity. **pleural l.,** irrigation of the pleural cavity. **systemic l.,** lavage of the blood.

Lavandula (lah-van′du-lah) [L.] a genus of labiate plants; lavenders. The flowers of *L. officinalis* Chaix (*L. vera* DC.), Labiatae, contain a volatile oil used in fumigation, perfumery, moth repellant, and occasionally as a carminative.

lavation (la-va′shun) [L. *lavatio*] lavage.

Lavdovski's nucleoid (lav-dov′skēz) [Mikhail Dormidontovich *Lavdovski*, Russian histologist, 1846–1903] centrosome.

Lavema (lah-ve′mah) trademark for preparations of oxyphenisatin.

lavement (lāv′ment) lavage.

Laveran's bodies, corpuscles (lav-ranz′) [Charles Louis Alphonse *Laveran*, French physician, 1845–1922, noted for discovery of the parasite causing malaria; winner of the Nobel prize for medicine in 1907] see *Plasmodium*.

Laverania (lav″er-a′ne-ah) [C. L. A. *Laveran*] a name formerly applied to the malarial parasite, *Plasmodium falciparum*.

laveur (lah-vur′) [Fr.] an instrument for performing lavage or irrigation.

law (law) a uniform or constant fact or principle. **Allen's paradoxic l.,** whereas in normal individuals the more sugar is given the more is utilized, the reverse is true in diabetics. **all-or-none l.,** see *all or none*. **Ambard's l's** (*obs.*), 1. with the urinary urea concentration constant, the output of urea varies directly as the square of the concentration of the blood urea. 2. with the blood urea concentration constant, the output of urea varies inversely as the square root of the urinary concentration. **Angström's l.,** the wavelengths of the light absorbed by a substance are the same as those given off by it when luminous. **l. of anticipation,** Mott's l. of anticipation. **Aran's l.,** fractures of the base of the skull (except those by contrecoup) result from injuries to the vault, the fractures extending by radiation along the line of shortest circle. **Arndt's l., Arndt-Schulz l.,** weak stimuli increase physiologic activity and very strong stimuli inhibit or abolish activity. **l's of articulation,** a set of rules to be followed in arranging teeth to produce a balanced articulation. **l. of avalanche,** hypothetical law assumed by Ramón y Cajal, that multiple sensations may be aroused in the brain by a simple sensation at the periphery. **l. of average localization,** visceral pain is most accurately localized in the least mobile viscus. **Avogadro's l.,** equal volumes of all perfect gases at the same temperature and pressure contain the same number of molecules or, in the case of monatomic gases, of atoms. **Babinski's l.,** the law of voltaic vertigo that a normal subject inclines to the side of the positive pole; one with disease of the labyrinth falls to the side to which he tends to incline spontaneously. If the labyrinth is destroyed, then there is no reaction. **Baer's l.,** those more general features that are common to all the members of a group of animals are developed in the embryo earlier than the more special features that distinguish the various members of the group. This concept is the predecessor of the recapitulation theory. **Barfurth's l.,** the axis of the tissue in a regenerating structure is at first perpendicular to the cut. **Baruch's l.,** when the temperature of the water used in a bath is above or below that of the skin the effect is stimulating; when both temperatures are the same the effect is sedative. **Bastian's l., Bastian-Bruns l.,** if there is a complete transverse lesion in the spinal cord cephalad to the lumbar enlargement, the

tendon reflexes of the lower extremities are abolished. **Baumès's l.,** Colles' l. **Beer's l.,** the absorption of light by a solution is a function of the concentration of the solute and the absorption depth of the solution. **Behring's l.,** the blood and serum of an immunized person, when transferred to another subject, will render the latter immune. **Bell's l., Bell-Magendie l.,** the anterior roots of the spinal nerves are motor roots, and the posterior are sensory. **Bergonié-Tribondeau l.,** the sensitivity of cells to radiation varies directly with the reproductive capacity of the cells and inversely with their degree of differentiation. **biogenetic l.,** ontogeny recapitulates phylogeny; see *recapitulation theory*, under *theory*. **Boudin's l.,** there is antagonism between malaria and tuberculosis. **Bowditch's l.,** 1. see *all-or-none* 2. nerves cannot be tired out by stimulation. **Boyle's l.,** at a constant temperature the volume of a perfect gas varies inversely as the pressure, and the pressure varies inversely as the volume. **Breton's l.,** there is a parabolic relation between stimulus and just noticeable difference, expressed by the formula $S = (R/C)^{\frac{1}{2}}$. **Buhl-Dittrich l.,** the supposed principle that in every case of acute miliary tuberculosis there exists within the body at least one old focus of caseation. **Bunge's l.,** the secreting cells of the mammary gland in the dog, cat, and rabbit take from the blood plasma mineral salts in the exact proportion in which they are needed for developing and building up the offspring. **Bunsen-Roscoe l.,** the photochemical effect produced is equal to the product of the intensity of the illumination and the duration of exposure. **Camerer's l.,** children of the same weight have the same food requirements regardless of their ages. **Charles' l.,** at a constant pressure the volume of a given mass of perfect gas varies directly with the absolute temperature. **Colles' l.,** a child that is affected with congenital syphilis, its mother showing no signs of the disease, will not infect its mother (1837). **Colles-Baumès l.,** Colles' l. **Collin's l.,** in infants and children, if after removal of a neoplasm, metastasis or recurrence does not occur for a period equivalent to the age of the patient plus nine months, the possibility of such occurrence is slight. **l. of conservation of energy,** in any given system the amount of energy is constant; energy is neither created nor destroyed, but only transformed from one form to another. **l. of conservation of matter,** in any chemical reaction atoms are neither created nor destroyed but simply change partners. **l. of contrary innervation,** Meltzer's l. **Cope's l.,** genera with little specialization originate many types of organisms; highly specialized genera produce but few biological variations. **Coulomb's l.,** the force of attraction or repulsion between two electrified bodies is proportional directly to the quantities of electric charge, and inversely as the square of their distance apart. **Courvoisier's l.,** when the common bile duct is obstructed by a stone, dilatation of the gallbladder is rare; when the duct is obstructed in some other way, dilatation is common. **Coutard's l.,** in radiotherapy, the point of origin of a mucous membrane tumor is the last site to heal following irradiation. **Curie's l.,** all substances may be rendered radioactive by the influence of the emanations of radium, and substances thus influenced hold their radioactivity longer when inclosed in some material through which the emanations cannot pass. **Cushing's l.,** increase of intracranial tension causes increase of blood pressure to a point slightly above the pressure exerted against the medulla. **Dalton's l.,** the pressure exerted by a mixture of nonreacting gases is equal to the sum of the partial pressures of the separate components. **Dalton-Henry l.,** when a fluid absorbs a mixture of gases, it will absorb as much of each gas as it would have absorbed of either gas separately. **l. of definite proportions,** any compound always contains the same kind of elements in the same proportions; called also *Proust's l*. **l. of denervation,** denervation of a structure increases its sensitivity to chemical stimulation. **Descartes' l.,** the sine of the angle of incidence bears a constant relation to the sine of the angle of refraction for two given media. **Desmarres' l.,** when the visual axes are crossed the images are uncrossed; when the axes are uncrossed (diverging) the images are crossed. Useful in determining presence of esophoria and exophoria, and esotropia and exotropia. **l. of diffusion,** any process set up in the nerve centers affects the organism throughout by a process of diffused motion. **Dollo's l.,** phyletic development is irreversible, i.e., reversion to an ancestral peculiarity (atavism) is impossible. **Donders' l.,** the rotation of the eye around the line of sight is not voluntary; when attention is fixed upon a remote object, the amount of rotation is determined entirely by the angular distance of the object from the median plane and from the horizon. **Draper's l.,** only the rays that are absorbed by a photochemical substance will produce a chemical change in it. **DuBois-Reymond's l.,** it is the variation of current density, and not the absolute value of current density at any given moment, that acts as a stimulus to a muscle or motor nerve. **Dulong and Petit's l.,** the atoms of all elements have exactly the same capacity for heat. **Edinger's l.,** a gradual increase in the function of the neuron causes at first increased growth, but if irregular and excessive, then it leads to atrophy and degeneration. **Einstein-Starck l.** (of photochemical equivalence), according to the quantum theory, quanta of light are absorbed at random during irradiation; the absorption of one quantum of light by a molecule (or atom) produces only one activated molecule (or atom). **Einthoven l.**, if electrocardiograms are taken simultaneously with the three leads, at any given instant the potential in lead II is equal to the sum of the potentials in leads I and III. **Elliott's l.**, the activity of epinephrine is due to a stimulation of the endings of the sympathetic nerve. **Ewald's l.**, nystagmus resulting from endolymph currents in a semicircular canal is in a direction parallel with the plane of that canal and opposite to the current, and in the horizontal canals the amount of ocular motor impulse derived from the canals whose hair cells are bent toward the utricle is twice as great as from the other (short end); but in the vertical canals the reverse is true. **l. of excitation,** a motor nerve responds by the contraction of its muscle to the alterations of the strength of an electric current and not to its absolute strength. **l. of facilitation,** when an impulse has passed once through a certain set of neurons to the exclusion of others, it will tend to take the same course on a future occasion, and each time it traverses this path the resistance in the path will be smaller. See also *facilitation* (def. 2). **Faget's l.**, in yellow fever, contrary to the normal relationship, a falling pulse rate is associated with a constant temperature, or a constant pulse rate with a rising temperature. **Fajans' l.**, the product left after the emission of alpha rays has a valance less by two than that of the parent radioactive substance; the product left after the emission of beta rays has a valence greater by one than that of the parent radioactive substance. **Faraday's l.**, in electrolysis the amount of an ion liberated in any given time is proportional to the strength of the current. **Farr's l.**, "subsidence is a property of all zymotic diseases"; the gradually diminishing increase of incidence in an epidemic disease, by virtue of which the epidemic curve first ascends rapidly, then more slowly to a maximum, with a descent more rapid than the ascent. **l. of fatigue (Houghton's),** when the same muscle or group of muscles is kept in constant action until fatigue sets in, the total work done, multiplied by the rate of work, is constant. **Fechner's l.**, the intensity of a sensation produced by a varying stimulus varies directly as the logarithm of that stimulus. **Ferry-Porter l.**, critical fusion frequency is directly proportional to the logarithm of the light intensity. **Fick's first l. of diffusion,** a substance will diffuse through an area at a rate which is dependent upon the difference in concentration of the substance at two given points. **Fildes' l.**, the presence of syphilitic reagin in the blood of the newborn is diagnostic, not of syphilis in the infant but of syphilis in the mother. **first l. of thermodynamics,** see *l's of thermodynamics.* **Fitz's l.** (*obs.*), acute pancreatitis is to be suspected when a previously healthy person is suddenly affected with violent epigastric pain, vomiting, and collapse, followed inside of twenty-four hours by epigastric swelling, tympanites, or resistance, with slight elevation of temperature. **Flatau's l.**, the greater the length of the fibers of the spinal cord, the closer are they situated to the periphery. **Flechsig's myelogenetic l.**, myelogenetic l. **Flint's l.**, the ontogeny of an organ is the phylogeny of its blood supply. **Flourens' l.**, stimulation of the semicircular canal causes nystagmus in the plane of that canal. **Froriep's l.**, the skull is developed by the annexation of true vertebrae, the head growing at the expense of the neck. **Galton's l.**, each parent contributes, on an average, one fourth, or $(0.5)^2$, of an individual's heritage, each grandparent one sixteenth, or $(0.5)^4$, each great-grandparent one sixty-fourth, or $(0.5)^6$, etc., the occupier of each ancestral place in the *n*th degree, whatever the value of *n*, contributing $(0.5)^{2n}$ of the heritage. **Galton's l. of regression,** average parents tend to produce average children; minus parents tend to produce minus children; plus parents tend to produce plus children; but the offspring of extreme parents, whether plus or minus, inherit the parental peculiarities in a less marked degree than the latter were manifested in the parents themselves. **Gay-Lussac's l.**, Charles' l. **Gerhardt-Semon l.**, various peripheral and central lesions affecting the recurrent laryngeal nerve cause the vocal cord to assume a position between abduction and adduction, the paralysis of the parts being incomplete. **Giraud-Teulon l.**, binocular retinal images are formed at the intersection of the primary and secondary axes of projection. **Godélier's l.**, tuberculosis of the peritoneum is invariably associated with tuberculosis of the pleura. **Golgi's l.**, the severity of a malarial attack depends upon the number of parasites in the blood. **Gompertz's l.**, there is a quantitative relation between the probability of death from a given disease and age. **Goodell's l.**, see under *sign.* **Graham's l.**, the rate of diffusion of a gas through porous membranes is in inverse ratio to the square root of their density. **Grasset's l.**, Landouzy-Grasset l. **l. of gravitation,** all bodies attract each other with a force that is directly proportional to their masses and inversely proportional to the square of their distance apart; called also *Newton's l.* **Grotthus' l.**, only those rays of ultraviolet light that are absorbed produce a chemical effect. **Gudden's l.**, the degeneration of the proximal end of a divided nerve is cellulipetal. **Guldberg and Waage's l.**, the velocity of a chemical reaction is proportional to the active masses of the reacting substances; called also *l. of mass action* and *mass l.* **Gull-Toynbee l.**, in otitis media, the lateral sinus and cerebellum are liable to involvement in mastoid disease, and the cerebrum may be attacked when the roof of the tympanum becomes carious. **Gullstrand's l.**, in strabismus, if the patient is made to turn his head while fixing a distant object and the corneal reflex of either eye moves in the direction in which the head is turning, then the movement is toward the weaker muscle. **Gunn's l.**, in treating a dislocation, the limb must be placed in the same position as at the time of injury and force exerted on the displaced bone in the reverse direction to that which caused the dislocation. **Haeckel's l.**, ontogeny recapitulates phylogeny; see *recapitulation theory,* under *theory.* **Hanau's l's of articulation,** a set of purely physical laws that must be observed in the formation of the masticatory surfaces of natural dentition or dentures, to assure establishment or production of balanced articulation. **Hardy-Weinberg l.**, the proportions of the three genotypes determined by two alleles (A and a) occurring with a frequency of p and q, respectively, in a randomly mating population will remain constant from one generation to the next: $AA = p^2$, $Aa = 2\ pq$, $aa = q^2$. Mutation, selection, migration, and genetic drift can disturb this equilibrium. **l. of the heart,** the energy set free at each contraction of the heart is a simple function of the length of the fibers composing its muscular walls (Starling). **Heidenhain's l.**, glandular secretion always involves change in the structure of the gland. **Hellin's l., Hellin-Zeleny l.**, one in about 89 pregnancies ends in the birth of twins; one in 89×89, or 7921, of triplets; one in $89 \times 89 \times 89$, or 704,969, of quadruplets. **Henry's l.**, the solubility of a gas in a liquid solution is proportional to the partial pressure of the gas. **Hering's l.**, 1. the principle of bilateral ocular innervation; equal innervation is sent to the muscles of the two eyes so that one eye is never moved independently of the other. 2. the clearness or purity of any conception or sensation depends on the proportion existing between its intensity and the sum total of the intensities of all the simultaneous conceptions and sensations. **Heyman's l.**, the threshold value of a visual stimulus is increased in proportion to the strength of the inhibitory stimulus. **Hilton's l.**, a nerve trunk which supplies the muscles of any given joint also supplies the muscles which move the joint and the skin over the insertions of such muscles. **Hoff's l.**, van't Hoff's l. **Hoorweg's l.**, there is a duration of electric discharge above which time is not a factor, and a duration of discharge below which the time is a factor, in the provocation of neuromuscular response. **Horner's l.**, ordinary color blindness is transmitted from males to males through normal females. **l. of independent assortment,** the members of gene pairs segregate independently during meiosis. **l. of initial value,** Wilder's l. of initial value. **l. of the intestines** (*obs.*), the presence of a bolus in the intestine induces contraction above and inhibition below the stimulus, thereby producing a progression of the intestinal contents (Starling). **l. of inverse square,** the intensity of radiation is inversely proportional to the square of the distance between the point of source and the irradiated surface. **l. of isochronism,** a nerve and its innervated muscle have identical chronaxie values. **isodynamic l.**, in the production of heat in the body the different foodstuffs are interchangeable in accordance with their heat-producing values. **l. of isolated conduction,** the wave of change or nervous impulse which passes through a neuron is never communicated to other neurons except at the terminals. **Jackson's l.**, the nerve functions that are latest developed are the earliest to be destroyed. **Kahler's l.**, the ascending branches of the posterior roots of the spinal nerves pass within the cord in succession from the root zone toward the mesial plane. **Knapp's l.**, there should be no difference in retinal image size in the correction of spherical axial anisometropia, provided that the lenses are placed at the anterior focal point of the eye. **Koch's l.**, see *Koch's postulates,* under *postulate.* **Küstner's l.**, if an ovarian tumor is left-sided, torsion of its pedicle takes place toward the right; if right-sided, toward the left. **Lambert's cosine l.**, the intensity of radiation on an absorbing surface varies as the cosine of the angle of incidence for parallel rays. **Landouzy-Grasset l.**, in lesion of one cerebral hemisphere the head is turned to the side of the brain lesion if there is paralysis, and to that of the affected muscles if there is spasticity. **Lapicque's l.**, the chronaxy is inversely proportional to the diameter of the nerve fiber. **Laplace's l.**, in hemodynamics, the pressure produced in the ventricles depends not only on the tension developed by the cardiac ventricular muscle in contraction but also on the size and shape of the heart. **Leopold's l.**, when the placenta is inserted upon the posterior wall of the uterus, the oviducts assume directions converging upon the anterior wall; but when the insertion is on the anterior wall during recumbency, the tubes turn backward and become parallel to the axis of the body. **Levret's l.**, the insertion of the cord is marginal in placenta previa. **Listing's l.**, when the eyeball is moved from a resting position, the rotational angle in the second position is the same as if the eye were turned about a fixed axis perpendicular to the first and second position of the visual line. **Lossen's l.**, hemophiliac males do not transmit the condition to their offspring. **Louis' l.**, 1. pulmonary tuberculosis generally begins in the left lung. 2. tuberculosis of any part is attended by localization in the lungs. **Magendie's l.**, Bell's l. **malthusian l.**, the hypothesis that population tends to outrun the means available to sustain it. **Marey's l.**, as the blood pressure rises, the pulse rate slows. **Mariotte's l.,** Boyle's l. **l. of mass action, mass l.,** Guldberg and Waage's l. **Maxwell-Boltzmann distribution l.,** a method for calculating the relative number of molecules in a given population which possess a given amount of energy. **Meltzer's l.** (*of contrary innervation*), all living functions are continually controlled by two opposing forces: augmentation or action on the one hand, and inhibition on the other. **Mendel's l., mendelian l.,** in the inheritance of certain traits or characters, the offspring are not intermediate in character between the parents but inherit from one or the other parent in this respect. For example, if a pea plant with the factor tallness (TT) is mated with one with the factor shortness (SS) then some of the offspring will inherit TT, some TS, and some SS in the ratio: TT, 2TS, SS. The TT's are homozygous (pure) tall, the SS's are homozygous short, and the TS's are heterozygous. Which parent the TS ones resemble will depend on whether T or S is dominant. The TT's mated with TT's breed pure as do the SS's with SS's. The TS's mated with TS's again produce TT's, TS's and SS's in the same ratio as above. TS's mated with TT's or SS's give the same combinations but in a different ratio. Today, Mendel's law is usually expressed as the *law of independent assortment* (q.v.) and the *law of segregation* (q.v.). **Mendeléeff's l.,** periodic l. **Metchnikoff's (Mechnikov's) l.,** whenever the body is attacked by bacteria, the polymorphonuclear leukocytes and the large mononuclear leukocytes quickly become protective phagocytes. **Meyer's l.,** the internal structure of fully developed normal bone represents the lines of greatest pressure or traction and affords the greatest possible resistance with the least possible amount of material. **Michaelis-Menten l.,** a method for determining the rate of enzymatic reaction in relation to the concentration of the substrate. **Minot's l.,** organisms age fastest when young. **Mott's l. of anticipation,** when the children of the insane become insane they do so at a much earlier age than did their parents. Contemporary evidence indicates that this law does not hold true. **Müller's l.,** l. of specific irritability. **Müller-Haeckel l.,** biogenetic l. **l. of multiple variants,** any variation from the normal in the bones of the hand or foot is always multiple. **myelogenetic l.** (of Flechsig), the myelination of the nerve fibers of the developing brain takes place in a definite sequence so that fibers belonging to particular functional systems mature at the same time. **Naegeli's l.,** a disease in which eosinophils are present in one-half normal, normal, or increased numbers cannot be typhoid; and the appearance of even a few of such cells must incite caution in the diagnosis. **Nernst's l.,** the current required to stimulate muscle action varies as the square root of its frequency. **Neumann's l.,** the molecular heat in compounds of analogous constitution is always the same. **Newland's l.,** a forerunner of the periodic law, in which the chemical elements, arranged in order of their atomic weights, showed a repetition of properties in octaves. **Newton's l.,** l. of gravitation. **Nysten's l.,** rigor mortis affects first the muscles of mastication, next those of the face and neck, then those of the upper trunk and arms, and last of all those of the legs and feet. **Ohm's l.,** the strength of an electric current varies directly as the electromotive force, and inversely as the resistance. **Ollier's l.,** in the case of two parallel bones which are joined at their extremities by ligaments, arrest of growth in one of them involves growth disturbance in the other. **Pajot's l.,** a solid body contained within another body having smooth walls will tend to conform to the shape of those walls; this law governs the rotating movements of the fetus during labor. **Pascal's l.,** pressure applied to a liquid at any point is transmitted equally in all directions. **periodic l.,** if the elements are arranged in the sequence of their atomic numbers, they fall into distinctive periods of 2, 8, 8, 18, 18, and 32 elements; see also *periodic table,* under *table.* Called also *Mendeléeff's l.* **Petit's l.,** Dulong and Petit's l. **Pfeiffer's l.,** the blood serum of an animal immunized against a disease will, when introduced into the body of another (susceptible) animal, protect the recipient by destroying the bacteria causing that disease. See also under *phenomenon.* **Pflüger's l.,** a nerve tract is stimulated when catelectrotonus develops or anelectrotonus disappears, but not under the reverse conditions. **Poiseuille's l.,** the volume flow in a tube is (*a*) directly proportional to the pressure drop along the length of the tube and to the fourth power of the radius of the tube, and (*b*) is inversely proportional to the length of the tube and to the viscosity of the fluid. **Prévost's l.,** in a lateral cerebral lesion the head is turned toward the side involved. **Profeta's l.,** the apparently nonsyphilitic child born of syphilitic parents is immune. **Proust's l.,** l. of definite proportions. **psychophysical l.,** Weber-Fechner l. **Raoult's l.,** 1. (*for freezing points*) the depression of the freezing point for the same type of electrolyte dissolved in a given solvent is proportional to the molecular concentration of the solute. 2. (*for vapor pressures*) (*a*) the vapor pressure of a volatile substance from a liquid solution is equal to the mole fraction of that substance times its vapor pressure in the pure state. (*b*) when a nonvolatile nonelectrolyte is dissolved in a solvent the decrease in vapor pressure of that solvent is equal to the mole fraction of the solute times the vapor pressure of the pure solvent. **l. of reciprocal proportions,** two chemical elements that unite with a third element do so in proportions that are multiples of those in which they unite with each other. **l. of referred pain,** referred pain only arises from irritation of nerves which are sensitive to those stimuli that produce pain when applied to the surface of the body. **l. of refraction,** rays of light passing from a rarer to a denser medium are deflected toward a perpendicular to the surface of incidence, whereas rays passing from a denser to a rarer medium are deflected away from the perpendicular. **l. of refreshment,** the refreshment of a laboring muscle depends on the rate of supply of arterial blood. **l. of regression,** Galton's l. of regression. **l. of relativity,** simultaneous and successive sensations modify each other. **Ricco's l.,** the relation between intensity and area of illumination: intensity times area equals constant. **Ritter's l.,** both the opening and the closing of an electric current produce stimulation in a nerve. **Ritter-Valli l.,** the primary increase and secondary loss of irritability in a nerve, produced by a section which separates from the nerve center, travel in a peripheral direction. **Rosa's l.,** the possibilities of phyletic variation in an organism decrease in proportion to the extent of its development. **Rubner's l.,** 1. (*law of constant energy consumption*) the rapidity of growth is proportional to the intensity of the metabolic process. 2. (*law of constant growth quotient*) the same fractional part of the entire energy is utilized for growth; this fractional part is called the "growth quotient." **Schroeder van der Kolk's l.,** the sensory fibers of a mixed nerve are distributed to the parts moved by muscles which are stimulated by the motor fibers of the same nerve. **Schütz's l., Schütz-Borissov l.,** the velocity of enzyme action is directly proportional to the square root of its concentration: an empirical observation applied to crude preparations of pepsin and a few other proteases, and explained by the presence of an inhibitor in equilibrium with the enzyme. **second l. of thermodynamics,** see *l's of thermodynamics.* **l. of segregation,** in each generation the ratio of (*a*) pure dominants, (*b*) dominants giving descendants in the proportion of three dominants to one recessive, and (*c*) pure recessives is 1 : 2 : 1. This ratio follows from the fact that the two alleles of a gene cannot be a part of a single gamete, but must segregate to different gametes (see *meiosis*). **Semon's l., Semon-Rosenbach l.,** in progressive organic diseases of the motor laryngeal nerves, the abductors of the vocal cords (posterior cricoarytenoids) are the first, and occasionally the only, muscles affected. **Sherrington's l.,** 1. every posterior spinal nerve root supplies a special region of the skin, although fibers from adjacent spinal segments may invade such a region. 2. when a muscle receives a nerve impulse to contract, its antagonist receives simultaneously an impulse to relax (see *reciprocal innervation*). **l. of similars,** see *homeopathy.* **l. of sines,** the sine of the angle of incidence is equal to the sine of the angle of reflection multiplied by a constant quantity. **Snell's l.,** Descartes' l. **Spallanzani's l.,** the law that regeneration is more complete in younger individuals than in older ones. **l. of specific irritability,** every sensory nerve reacts to one form of stimulus and gives rise to one form of sensation only, though if under abnormal conditions it be excited by other forms of stimuli, the sensation evoked will be the same. Called also *Müller's l.* **Starling's l.,** 1. the heart output per beat is directly proportional to the diastolic filling. 2. see *l. of the heart.* 3. see *l. of the intestines.* **Stokes' l.,** a muscle situated above an inflamed membrane is often affected with paralysis. **surface l.,** at constant temperature, the heat production, heat loss, and oxygen consumption in an animal are inversely proportional to the free surface or to the square of a linear dimension. **Talbot's l.,** when complete fusion occurs and the sensation is uniform, the intensity is the same as would occur were the same amount of light spread uniformly over the disk. **Teevan's l.,** fractures of bones occur in the line of extension, and not in the line of compression. **l's of thermodynamics,** *Zeroth law:* two systems in thermal equilibrium with a third system are in thermal equilibrium with each other. *First law:* energy is conserved in any process; i.e., the energy gained (or lost) by a system is exactly equal to the energy lost (or gained) by the surroundings. *Second law:* there is always an increase in entropy in any naturally occurring (spontaneous) process. *Third law:* absolute zero is unattainable. **third l. of thermodynamics,** see *l's of thermodynamics.* **Toynbee's l.,** in cases of brain disease due to otitis, the cerebellum and lateral sinuses are affected from the mastoid, and the cerebrum from the tympanic roof. **Valli-Ritter l.,** see Ritter-Valli l. **van der Kolk's l.,** Schroeder van der Kolk's l. **van't Hoff's l.,** 1. many substances in solution exert an osmotic pressure equal to the gas pressure that they would exert if their molecules were in a gaseous state and occupied a volume equal to that of the solution under the same conditions of temperature and pressure. 2. van't Hoff's rule; see under *rule.* **Virchow's l.,** the cell elements of tumors are derived from normal and preexisting tissue cells. **Vulpian's l.,** when a portion of the brain is destroyed, the functions of that part are carried on by the remaining parts. **Waller's l., wallerian l.,** if the sensory fibers of the root of a spinal nerve be divided on the central side of the ganglion, the fibers on the peripheral side of the cut do not degenerate; while those that remain connected with the cord degenerate. **Walton's l.,** l. of reciprocal proportions. **Weber's l.,** the variation of stimulus which causes the smallest appreciable change in sensation maintains an approximately fixed ratio to the whole stimulus. **Weber-Fechner l.,** for a sensation to increase by equal amounts (arithmetical progression), the stimulus must increase by geometrical progression; called also *psychophysical l.* **Weigert's l.,** loss or destruction of elements in the organic world is apt to be followed by overproduction of such elements in the reparative process. **Wilder's l. of initial value,** the more intense the function of a vegetative organ, the weaker its capacity for being excited by stimuli and the stronger its reaction to depressing factors; with extremely high or low initial value, there is marked tendency to paradoxic reactions (reversal of direction of reaction). **Wolff's l.,** a bone, normal or abnormal, develops the structure most suited to resist the forces acting upon it. **Wundt-Lamansky l.,** the line of vision in moving through a vertical plane parallel to the frontal plane moves in straight lines in the vertical and horizontal directions, but in curved paths in all other movements. **zeroth l. of thermodynamics,** see *l's of thermodynamics.* **Zeune's l.,** the proportion of cases of blindness is less in the Temperate than in the Frigid Zone, and increases in the Torrid Zone as the equator is approached.

lawrencium (law-ren′se-um) [Ernest Orlando *Lawrence,* American physicist, 1901–1958; builder of the first cyclotron for the production of high-energy particles, and winner of the Nobel prize for physics in 1939] the chemical element of atomic number 103, atomic weight 257, symbol Lw; produced in 1961 by bombardment of californium isotopes of mass 250, 251, and 252.

Lawson Tait see *Tait.*

lawsone (law′sōn) 2-hydroxy-1,4-naphthoquinone, $C_{10}H_6O_3$, a principle isolated from the leaves of *Lawsonia inermis* L. (Lythraceae), used as a topical sunscreen agent.

Lawsonia (law-so′ne-ah) a genus of tropical Old World shrubs, including *L. inermis,* the source of lawsone and of henna.

laxation (lak-sa′shun) defecation.

laxative (lak′sah-tiv) [L. *laxativus*] 1. aperient; mildly cathartic. 2. an agent that acts to promote evacuation of the bowel; a cathartic or purgative. **bulk l.,** an agent that acts to promote evacuation of the bowel by increasing the volume of the feces.

laxator (lak-sa′tor) [L. *laxare* to unloose or relax] that which slackens or relaxes. **l. tym′pani ma′jor,** ligamentum mallei anterius. **l. tym′pani mi′nor,** ligamentum mallei laterale.

layer (la′er) a sheetlike mass of tissue of nearly uniform thickness, several of which may be superimposed, one above another, as in the epidermis; called also *lamina* and *stratum.* **abscission l.,** a special layer or zone of thin-walled cells, loosely joined together, extending across the base of the petiole, thus weakening the base of the leaf, permitting the leaf to fall. **adamantine l.,** enamelum. **ambiguous l.,** the second layer of the cerebral cortex, counting from without; named from the indefinite shapes of many of its cells. **ameloblastic l.,** the inner layer of cells of the enamel organ, created by its invagination, which forms the enamel prisms. **bacillary l.,** l. of rods and cones. **Baillarger's l.,** see under *line.* **basal l.,** 1. lamina basalis choroideae. 2. stratum basale epidermidis. **basal l. of epidermis,** stratum basale epidermidis. **basement l.,** see under *membrane.* **Bekhterev's l.,** a layer of fibers in the external granular layer of the cerebral cortex. **Bernard's glandular l.,** a layer of cells which line the acini of the pancreas. **blastodermic l.,** germ l. **Bowman's l.,** lamina limitans anterior corneae. **Bruch's l.,** lamina basalis choroideae. **cerebral l.,** a term applied to the fifth to ninth layers of the retina. **Chievitz l.,** a transient fiber layer separating the inner and outer neuroblastic layers of the optic cup. **choriocapillary l.,** lamina choroidocapillaris. **circular l. of drumhead,** stratum circulare membranae tympani. **circular l. of muscular tunic of colon,** stratum circulare tunicae muscularis coli. **circular l. of muscular tunic of rectum,** stratum circulare tunicae muscularis recti. **circular l. of muscular tunic of small intestine,** stratum circulare tunicae muscularis intestini tenuis. **circular l. of muscular tunic of stomach,** stratum circulare tunicae muscularis ventriculi. **circular l. of tympanic membrane,** stratum circulare membranae tympani. **claustral l.** (*obs.*), claustrum. **clear l. of epidermis,** stratum lucidum epidermidis. **columnar l.,** 1. layer of rods and cones. 2. mantle layer. **compact l.,** stratum compactum. **cortical l.,** the cortex of an organ, as of the brain or kidney. **cutaneous l. of tympanic membrane,** stratum cutaneum membranae tympani. **cuticular l.,** a striate border of modified cytoplasm at the free end of some columnar cells. **deep l. of triangular ligament,** fascia diaphragmatis urogenitalis superior. **Dobie's l.,** Z band; see under *band.* **enamel l.,** the outermost layer of cells of the enamel organ. **ependymal l.,** the innermost layer of the wall of the primitive neural tube, bounding the central canal, which differentiates regionally into the roof plate and the floor plate. **epitrichial l.,** the most superficial layer of the epidermis of the embryo. **fibrous l. of articular capsule,** membrana fibrosa capsulae articularis. **Floegel's l.,** a granular layer in each transparent lateral disk of a muscle fibril. **functional l.,** stratum functionale. **ganglion cell l.,** a layer of the retina, situated between the inner molecular layer and the stratum opticum, or nerve fiber layer, consisting essentially of the ganglion

cells of the retina, and containing also the fibers of Müller, neuroglia, and branches of the retinal vessels. **ganglionic l. of cerebellum,** stratum gangliosum cerebelli. **ganglionic l. of optic nerve,** stratum ganglionare nervi optici. **ganglionic l. of retina,** stratum ganglionare retinae. **Gennari's l.,** see *Baillarger's lines,* under *line.* **germ l.,** one of the three primary layers of cells of the embryo (ectoderm, entoderm, or mesoderm), from which the tissues and organs develop. **germinative l., germinative l. of epidermis,** 1. stratum germinativum epidermidis [Malpighii]. 2. stratum basale epidermidis. **germinative l. of nail,** stratum germinativum unguis. **granular l. of cerebellum,** stratum granulosum cerebelli. **granular l. of epidermis,** stratum granulosum epidermidis. **granular l. of follicle of ovary,** stratum granulosum folliculi ovarii vesiculosi. **granular l. of Tomes,** a layer formed by a series of areas of imperfectly calcified dentin, found immediately under the dentinocemental junction. **granule l.,** stratum granulosum cerebelli. **gray l. of superior colliculus,** stratum griseum colliculi superioris. **half-value l.,** the thickness of a given substance which, when introduced in the path of a given beam of rays, will reduce its intensity to one half of the initial value; called also *half-value thickness.* Abbreviated *HVL.* **Haller's l.,** that portion of the vascular layer of the choroid which is made up of large vessels. **Henle's l.,** the outer layer of cells of the inner root sheath of a hair follicle, lying between the outer root sheath and Huxley's layer. **Henle's fiber l.,** the outer plexiform layer in the region of the macula retinae; see also *entoretina.* **horny l. of epidermis,** stratum corneum epidermidis. **horny l. of nail,** stratum corneum unguis. **Huxley's l.,** a layer of the inner root sheath of a hair follicle, lying between Henle's layer and the inner sheath cuticle. **inferior l. of pelvic diaphragm,** fascia diaphragmatis pelvis inferior. **Kaes-Bekhterev's l.,** Bekhterev's l. **keratohyaline l.,** stratum granulosum epidermidis. **Langerhans' l.,** stratum granulosum epidermidis. **Langhans' l.,** cytotrophoblast. **longitudinal l. of muscular tunic of colon,** stratum longitudinale tunicae muscularis coli. **longitudinal l. of muscular tunic of rectum,** stratum longitudinale tunicae muscularis recti. **longitudinal l. of muscular tunic of small intestine,** stratum longitudinale tunicae muscularis intestini tenuis. **longitudinal l. of muscular tunic of stomach,** stratum longitudinale tunicae muscularis ventriculi. **malpighian l.,** stratum germinativum epidermidis [Malpighii]. **mantle l.,** middle layer of the wall of the primitive neural tube, containing primitive nerve cells and later forming the gray substance of the central nervous system. **marginal l.,** the outermost layer of the wall of the primitive neural tube, a fibrous mesh into which the nerve fibers later grow, forming the white substance of the central nervous system. **medullary l's of optic thalamus, internal** (*obs.*), laminae medullares thalami. **Meynert's l.,** the layer of pyramidal cells in the cortex of the cerebrum. **molecular l. of cerebellum,** stratum moleculare cerebelli. **molecular l., inner,** plexiform l., inner. **molecular l., outer,** plexiform l., outer. **mucous l.,** stratum germinativum epidermidis [Malpighii]. **mucous l. of tympanic membrane,** stratum mucosum membranae tympani. **muscular l. of fallopian tube,** tunica muscularis tubae uterinae. **muscular l. of stomach, inner,** stratum circulare tunicae muscularis ventriculi. **nerve fiber l.,** a layer of the retina, situated between the ganglion cell layer and the internal limiting membrane, consisting essentially of the axons of the ganglion cells which pass through the lamina cribrosa to form the optic nerve. **nervous l.,** all of the retina except the pigment layer; the inner layer of the optic cup. **neuroepidermal l.,** ectoderm. **neuroepithelial l. of retina,** stratum neuroepitheliale retinae. **Nitabuch's l.,** see under *stria.* **nuclear l. of cerebellum,** stratum granulosum cerebelli. **nuclear l., inner,** a layer of the retina, situated between the outer and inner molecular layers, consisting essentially of the sensory bipolar cells. **nuclear l., outer,** a layer of the retina, situated between the external limiting membrane and the outer molecular layer, consisting essentially of the rod and cone granules (nuclei). **odontoblastic l.,** the epithelioid layer of odontoblasts in contact with the dentin of teeth; the layer of cells lines the pulp cavities, remaining functional after maturation of a tooth. **Ollier's l., osteogenetic l.,** the innermost layer of the periosteum. **palisade l.,** the basal layer of the mucous membrane layer of the tympanic membrane. **Pander's l.,** the splanchnopleural layer of the mesoblast. **papillary l. of corium,** stratum papillare corii. **parietal l. of pelvic fascia,** fascia diaphragmatis pelvis superior. **parietal l. of tunica vaginalis of testis,** lamina parietalis tunicae vaginalis testis. **peripheral l.,** the outer portion of the molecular layer of the cerebral cortex. **perpendicular l. of ethmoid bone,** lamina perpendicularis ossis ethmoidalis. **pigmented l. of ciliary body,** stratum pigmenti corporis ciliaris. **pigmented l. of eyeball,** stratum pigmenti bulbi oculi. **pigmented l. of iris,** stratum pigmenti iridis. **pigmented l. of retina,** stratum pigmenti retinae. **plexiform l., inner,** the inner plexiform layer of the retina, between the inner nuclear layer and the ganglion cell layer, consisting primarily of the arborization of the axons of the bipolar cells with the dendrites of the ganglion cells.

Called also *inner molecular l.* **plexiform l., outer,** the outer plexiform layer of the retina, between the outer nuclear layer and the inner nuclear layer, consisting essentially of the arborization of the axons of the rod and cone granules with the dendrites of the bipolar cells. Called also *outer molecular l.* **prickle-cell l.,** the layer of the skin between the granular layer and the basal layer, characterized by the presence of prickle cells; called also *stratum spinosum epidermidis* [NA]. **Purkinje l.,** the layer of Purkinje cells in the cerebellar cortex, between the superficial molecular layer and the subjacent granular layer. **radiate l. of tympanic membrane,** stratum radiatum membranae tympani. **Rauber's l.,** the most external of the three layers of cells which form the blastodisc in the young embryo; called also *blastodermic ectoderm* and *primitive ectoderm.* **reticular l. of corium,** stratum reticulare corii. **l. of rods and cones,** a layer of the retina, situated immediately beneath the pigment epithelium, between it and the external limiting membrane, comprising the sensitive elements of the retina, the cones, containing a visual pigment, iodopsin, and the rods, containing visual purple, or rhodopsin. **Rohr's l.,** see under *stria.* **Sattler's l.,** that portion of the vascular layer of the choroid which is made up of medium-sized vessels. **sclerotogenous l., skeletogenous l.,** the layer of mesoderm cells surrounding the notochord of the embryo and developing into the axial skeleton. **second half-value l.,** the additional thickness of material needed to reduce a radiation beam from one half to one fourth of its original exposure rate. **somatic l.,** the external layer of the lateral mesoderm after the coelomic split occurs; the inner component of somatopleure of the embryo. **spinous l. of epidermis,** stratum spinosum epidermidis. **splanchnic l.,** the internal layer of the lateral mesoderm after the coelomic split occurs; the component of splanchnopleure outside the entoderm of the embryo. **spongy l.,** stratum spongiosum. **subcallosal l.,** the layer of nerve fibers on the lower side of the corpus callosum. **subendocardial l.,** the layer of loose fibrous tissue uniting the endocardium and myocardium. **subendothelial l.,** a middle, fibrous layer of the tunica intima of typical blood vessels, located between the endothelium and internal elastic membrane. **subepicardial l.,** the layer of loose connective tissue uniting the epicardium and myocardium. **submantle l.,** a layer of interglobular dentin usually situated just below the cover (mantle) dentin. **submucous l.,** tela submucosa. **submucous l. of bladder,** tela submucosa vesicae urinariae. **submucous l. of colon,** tela submucosa coli. **submucous l. of esophagus,** tela submucosa esophagi. **submucous l. of pharynx,** tela submucosa pharyngis. **submucous l. of small intestine,** tela submucosa intestini tenuis. **submucous l. of stomach,** tela submucosa ventriculi. **subodontoblastic l.,** Weil's basal l. **subpapillary l.,** the layer of the corium immediately underlying the layer containing the dermal papillae. **subserous l.,** tela subserosa. **subserous l. of peritoneum,** tela subserosa peritonei. **superficial l. of fascia of perineum,** fascia perinei superficialis. **superficial l. of triangular ligament,** fascia diaphragmatis urogenitalis inferior. **superior l. of pelvic diaphragm,** fascia diaphragmatis pelvis superior. **suprachorioid l.,** lamina suprachoroidea. **synovial l. of articular capsule,** membrana synovialis capsulae articularis. **Tomes' granular l.,** granular l. of Tomes. **trophic l.,** the entoderm. **Unna's l** (*obs.*), stratum granulosum epidermidis. **vegetative l.,** the entoderm. **vertical l. of ethmoid bone,** lamina perpendicularis ossis ethmoidalis. **visceral l. of pelvic fascia,** fascia pelvis visceralis. **visceral l. of pericardium,** lamina visceralis pericardii. **visceral l. of tunica vaginalis of testis,** lamina visceralis tunicae vaginalis testis. **Waldeyer's l.,** the vascular layer of the ovary. **Weil's basal l.,** a clear layer relatively free of cells, just inside of the layer of odontoblasts of the tooth pulp, made up of delicate fibrils of connective tissue communicating with the processes of odontoblasts. **white l's of cerebellum,** laminae albae cerebelli. **Zeissel's l.,** a layer in the stomach wall between the tunica muscularis mucosae and the tela submucosa. **zonal l. of quadrigeminal body,** stratum zonale corporis quadrigemini. **zonal l. of thalamus,** stratum zonale thalami.

lazar (laz'ar) [*Lazarus,* the leper of the Bible] (*obs.*) 1. leper; leprosy patient. 2. of or pertaining to leprosy, as lazar house (leprosarium).

lazaretto (laz″ah-ret'o) 1. a hospital for contagious diseases. 2. a quarantine station.

lb. abbreviation for L. *li′bra,* pound.

LBF *lactobacillus bulgaricus* factor.

L.Ch. Licentiate in Surgery.

LD lethal dose; (perception of) light difference.

LD₅₀ median lethal dose; a dose that is lethal for 50 per cent of the test subjects.

L.D.A. left dorso-anterior (position of the fetus).

LDH lactate dehydrogenase.

LDL low-density lipoproteins.

L-dopa see *dopa.*

L.D.P. left dorsoposterior (position of the fetus).

L.D.S. Licentiate in Dental Surgery.

LE lupus erythematosus; see also under *cell.*

leaching (lēch'ing) lixiviation.

lead¹ (led) [L. *plumbum*] a soft, grayish blue metal with poisonous salts; symbol, Pb; atomic number, 82; atomic weight, 207.19. See also under *poisoning.* **l. acetate** [USP], colorless crystals, masses, or granules, $Pb(C_2H_3O_2)_2 \cdot 3H_2O$, used as a reagent and astringent. **l. arsenate,** a mixture of arsenate of soda and acetate of lead, $PbHAsO_4$, in water, used as an insecticide, and in veterinary medicine to kill tapeworms. **black l.,** graphite. **l. chloride,** a compound, $PbCl_2$, used as a reagent and pigment. **l. chromate,** a lemon-yellow powder, $PbCrO_4$, used in stains; called also *chrome yellow.* **l. monoxide,** a binary compound, PbO, called *litharge* when crystalline and *massicot* when amorphous; used as a reagent. **l. nitrate,** a sweetish crystalline agent, $Pb(NO_3)_2$, used as a reagent. **l. oleate,** a white powder, $Pb(C_{18}H_{33}O_2)_2$, used in varnishes. **l. oxide,** see *l. monoxide* and *l. tetroxide.* **radioactive l.,** radiolead. **red l.,** lead tetroxide. **l. selinide,** a compound, PbSe, occurring as gray crystals. **l. subacetate,** a basic acetate of lead. **sugar of l.,** l. acetate. **tetra-ethyl l.,** a highly poisonous organic lead compound, $Pb(C_2H_5)_4$, used as an antiknock agent in internal combustion motors; it can be absorbed through the skin and may cause mental symptoms and death. Called also *ethyl gas.* **l. tetroxide,** a red powder, Pb_3O_4, which may be used like the monoxide. **white l.,** a basic lead carbonate.

lead² (lēd) any of the conductors connected to the electrocardiograph. Also any of the records made by the electrocardiograph, varying with the part of the body from which the current is led off. It is customary to use three peripheral leads; lead I, right arm and left arm; lead II, right arm and left leg; lead III, left arm and left leg; and at least six leads from the precordial region. Called also *derivation.* **aV_F l.,** a unipolar lead in which the positive lead is on the left leg. **aV_L l.,** a unipolar lead in which the positive terminal is on the left arm. **aV_R l.,** a unipolar lead in which the positive terminal is on the right arm. **bipolar l.,** an array involving two electrodes placed at different body sites. **esophageal l.,** one attached to an electrode inserted within the esophagus. **limb l's,** any of the three leads customarily used in electrocardiography. **precordial l's,** leads in which one electrode is placed on the chest and the other is connected to one or more extremities. Such leads are indicated as follows: CR = chest + right arm; CL = chest + left arm; CF = chest and left leg; V = chest + junction of leads from right and left arms and left leg (sometimes called *Wilson l's*). Subscript numbers 1 to 6 indicate at which points on the chest the lead is taken. **unipolar l.,** an

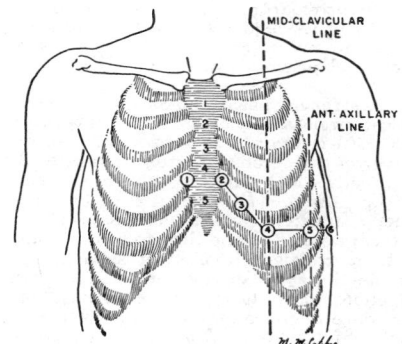

Precordial leads (Graybiel and White).

array of two electrodes, only one of which transmits potential variation. **V l's,** precordial leads further designated by a subscript numeral (V₁ to V₆) according to the position along the intercostal spaces. **Wilson's l's,** see *precordial l's.*

leaflet (lēf'let) a structure resembling a small leaf, especially a cusp of a heart valve.

leakage (lēk-ij) the escape of fluid from a vessel or other container.

learning (ler'ning) a relatively long-lasting adaptive behavioral change occurring as a result of experience. **insight l.,** the highest form of learning, characterized by the ability to evaluate and combine previous experiences to solve a problem or achieve a desired goal. **latent l.,** that which occurs without reinforcement, becoming apparent only when a reinforcement or reward is introduced.

leash (lēsh) a bundle of cordlike structures, as nerves, blood vessels, fibers, etc.

leben (leb'en) [Arabic] a ferment drink of Egypt made from the milk of cows, buffaloes, and goats.

Leber's congenital amaurosis, etc. (la-berz') [Theodor *Leber,* German ophthalmologist, 1840–1917] see under *amaurosis, atrophy, corpuscle, disease,* and *plexus.*

Lebistes (lĕ-bis′tēz) a genus of small fish, the guppy. **L. reticula′tus,** a species of top-feeding minnows, commonly known as "millions," cultivated in the Barbados to eliminate mosquito larvae.

Leboyer method (technique) (lĕ-boi-ya′) [Frederick *Leboyer*, French obstetrician] see under *method.*

lecanopagus (lek″an-op′ah-gus) [Gr. *lekanē* basin + *pagos* thing fixed] symmetrical conjoined twins fused at the pelvis.

Lecat's gulf (lĕ-kahz′) [Claude Nicolas *Lecat*, French surgeon, 1700–1768] the hollow of the bulbous portion of the urethra.

leche de higuerón (la′cha da ēg″a-ron′) [Sp. milk of fig] the sap or latex of wild fig trees e.g, *Ficus anthelmintica* Mart. (Moraceae), of Central and South America, used as a vermifuge.

lechopyra (lek″o-pi′rah) [Gr. *lechō* parturient woman + *pyr* fever] puerperal fever.

lecithal (les′ĭ-thal) [Gr. *lekithos* yolk] having a yolk. Used as a word termination, affixed to a word stem descriptive of the state of the yolk substance, as *centrolecithal, isolecithal,* etc. See also entries under *ovum.*

lecithalbumin (les″ĭ-thal′bu-min) a compound of albumin and lecithin, found in the stomach, liver, kidney, lungs, and spleen.

lecithid (les′ĭ-thid) a compound of lecithin with venom hemolysin. **cobra l.,** a hemolytic compound formed by cobra toxin and the lecithin of the blood.

lecithin (les′ĭ-thin) [Gr. *lekithos* yolk of egg] any of a group of phosphoglycerides consisting of esters of glycerol with two molecules of long-chain aliphatic acids and one of phosphoric acid, the latter being esterified with the alcohol group of choline. Lecithins are found in animal tissues, especially in nerve tissue, the liver, semen, egg yolk, and in smaller amounts in bile and blood, and are major constituents of cell membranes. They differ from each other in the nature of their long-chain acyl groups. Called also *phosphatidylcholine.*

lecithinase (les′ĭ-thin-ās) a group of enzymes (lecithinase A to D) now known as phospholipase (q.v.). **cobra l.,** phospholipase A, one of the constituents of cobra venom, in part responsible for its hemolytic effect.

lecithinemia (les″ĭ-thĭ-ne′me-ah) the presence of lecithin in the blood.

lecitho- (les′ĭ-tho) [Gr. *lekithos* yolk] a combining form denoting relationship to the yolk of an egg or ovum.

lecithoblast (les′ĭ-tho-blast″) [*lecitho-* + Gr. *blastos* germ] the primitive entoderm of a two-layered blastodisc.

lecithoprotein (les″ĭ-tho-pro′te-in) a compound of the protein molecule with a lecithin; lecithoproteins occur in all cells.

lecithovitellin (les″ĭ-tho-vi-tel′in) a suspension of egg yolk in a solution of sodium chloride; it reacts with the toxin of *Clostridium welchii* to produce a precipitate or an opacity.

Leclanché's cell (lĕ″klan-shāz′) [Georges *Leclanché,* French physicist, 1839–1882] see under *cell.*

lectin (lek′tin) any of a group of hemagglutinating proteins found primarily in plant seeds, which bind specifically to the branching sugar molecules of glycoproteins and glycolipids on the surface of cells. Certain lectins selectively cause agglutination of erythrocytes of certain blood groups and of malignant cells but not their normal counterparts; others stimulate the proliferation of lymphocytes.

lectotype (lek′to-tīp) in bacteriology, a type culture taken from a group of organisms for which the original investigator did not designate a type; this type is seldom used.

ledbänder (led′ben-der) [Ger.] Büngner's bands; see under *band.*

Le Dentu's suture (lĕ-den-tūz′) [Jean François-Auguste *Le Dentu,* Paris surgeon, 1841–1926] see under *suture.*

Lederberg (led′er-berg), Joshua. United States biochemist, born 1925; co-winner, with George Wells Beadle and Edward Lawrie Tatum, of the Nobel prize in medicine and physiology for 1958, for work in genetics and heredity.

Ledercillin (led″er-sil′lin) trademark for preparations of penicillin G procaine.

Lederer's anemia (disease) (led′er-erz) [Max *Lederer,* Brooklyn pathologist, 1885–1952] see under *anemia.*

Leduc's current (lĕ-dooks′) [Stéphane Armand Nicolas *Leduc,* French physicist, 1853–1939] see under *current.*

Lee's ganglion (lēz) [Robert *Lee,* English physician, 1793–1877] cervical ganglion of the uterus; see under *ganglion.*

leech (lēch) [L. *hirudo*] 1. any of the annelids of the class Hirudinea, especially *Hirudo medicinalis.* Some species, the bloodsuckers, may become temporarily parasitic upon animals, including man. Leeches were formerly used extensively for drawing blood. See also *hirudin* and *leeching* (def. 1). 2. to apply leeches. 3. (*obs.*) a physician. **American l.,** *Macrobdella decora.* **artificial l.,** an apparatus for drawing blood by artificial suction. **Heurteloup's l.,** an artificial leech. **horse l.,** see *Limnatis* and *Haemopis.* **land l.,** *Haemadipsa.* **medicinal l.,** *Hirudo medicinalis.*

leeching (lēch′ing) the application of a leech for the withdrawal of blood; formerly used extensively in the treatment of various disorders; called also *hirudinization.*

Leeuwenhoekia australiensis (lu″en-ho′ke-ah aus-tra″le-en′sis) [Antonj van *Leeuwenhoek,* Dutch microscopist, 1632–1723] a mite found at Sydney, New South Wales, which may cause great irritation by burrowing in the skin.

left-handed (left-han′ded) using the left hand preferentially, or more skillfully than the right, in voluntary motor acts. See also *laterality.*

leg (leg) the lower limb, especially the part from knee to foot; called also *crus* [NA]. **Anglesey l.,** a form of jointed artificial leg; named from a marquis of Anglesey. **badger l.,** inequality in the length of the legs. **baker l.,** genu valgum. **bandy l.,** genu varum. **Barbados l.,** elephantiasis of the leg. **bayonet l.,** uncorrected backward displacement of the bones of the leg at the knee, followed by ankylosis at the joint. **black l.,** symptomatic anthrax. **bow l.,** genu varum. **deck l's,** edema of the lower legs, occurring in ship passengers in tropical zones. **elephant l.,** elephantiasis. **milk l.,** phlegmasia alba dolens. **red l.,** a fatal septicemia in frogs apparently caused by *Proteus hydrophilus.* **restless l's,** a condition characterized by a disagreeable, creeping, irritating sensation deep inside both legs, usually between the knee and the ankle. The subject can obtain relief only by walking about or keeping his legs moving. **rider's l.,** strain of the adductor muscles of the thigh in horseback riders. **scaly l.,** an enlarged and encrusted condition of the legs in fowls caused by sarcoptic mites of the genus *Knemidokoptes.* **scissor l.,** deformity with crossing of the legs in walking, due to spasticity of adductor muscles of the thighs. **tennis l.,** the condition resulting from a sudden tear at the musculotendinous junction of the medial belly of the gastrocnemius muscle, usually occurring in older persons participating in tennis and other sports activities. **tropical l's,** deck l's. **white l.,** phlegmasia alba dolens.

Legal's disease, test (la-galz′) [Emmo *Legal,* German physician, 1859–1922] see under *disease* and *tests.*

Legg's disease (legz) [Arthur Thornton *Legg,* Boston surgeon, 1874–1939] osteochondritis of the capitular epiphysis of the femur; see *osteochondrosis.*

Legg-Calvé-Perthes disease (leg′-kal-va′-per′tez) [Arthur T. *Legg;* Jacques *Calvé,* French orthopedist, 1875–1954; Georg Clemens *Perthes,* German surgeon, 1869–1927] osteochondritis of the capitular epiphysis of the femur; see *osteochondrosis.*

leghemoglobin (leg″he-mo-glo′bin) a pigment found in leguminous root nodules.

Legionella pneumophila (le″jun-el′ah nu-mof′ĭ-lah) the provisional name for a species of gram-negative, rod-shaped bacteria which require both cysteine and iron for growth; it is the causative agent of legionnaires' disease and Pontiac fever and occurs in several different immunologic forms.

legionellosis (le″jun-el-o′sis) disease caused by infection with *Legionella pneumophila,* including legionnaires' disease and Pontiac fever.

legume (leg′ūm) the pod or fruit of a leguminous plant, such as peas and beans.

legumelin (leg′u-me′lin) an albumin from lentils, beans, and other leguminous seeds.

legumin (lĕ-gu′min) [L. *legumen* pulse] a globulin from the seeds of various plants, chiefly of the order *Leguminosae.*

leguminivorous (lĕ-gu″mĭ-niv′o-rus) feeding on legumes (beans and peas).

leiasthenia (li″as-the′ne-ah) [*leio-* + *asthenia*] asthenia of smooth muscle.

Leichtenstern's encephalitis (type), sign (phenomenon) (līk′ten-sternz) [Otto Michael *Leichtenstern,* German physician, 1845–1900] see *hemorrhagic encephalitis,* under *encephalitis,* and see under *sign.*

Leiner's disease, test (li′nerz) [Karl *Leiner,* Austrian pediatrician, 1871–1930] see *erythroderma desquamativum,* and see under *tests.*

leio- (li′o) [Gr. *leios* smooth] a combining form meaning smooth.

leiodermia (li″o-der′me-ah) [*leio-* + Gr. *derma* skin] abnormal glossiness and smoothness of the skin.

leiodystonia (li″o-dis-to′ne-ah) [*leio-* + *dystonia*] dystonia of smooth muscle.

Leiognathus bacoti (li-og′nah-thus bah-ko′te) *Ornithonyssus bacoti.*

leiomyoblastoma (li″o-mi″o-blas-to′mah) epithelioid leiomyoma.

leiomyofibroma (li″o-mi″o-fi-bro′mah) a leiomyoma in which there is a prominent fibromatous component.

leiomyoma (li″o-mi-o′mah) [*leio-* + Gr. *mys* muscle + *-oma*] a benign tumor derived from smooth muscle, most commonly of the uterus; called also *fibroid.* **bizarre l.,** epithelioid l. **l. cu′tis,** a neoplasm characterized by numerous tender, red nodules, 2 to 10 mm. in diameter, consisting of masses of smooth muscle cells derived from the arrector pili muscles. **epithelioid l.,** a relatively rare smooth muscle tumor, usually of the stomach, in which the cells are polygonal rather than spindle-shaped; called also *bizarre l.* and *leiomyoblastoma.* **l. u'teri,** a leiomyoma of the uterus, usually occurring in the third and fourth decades, characterized by the development, most commonly within the myometrium, of multiple, sharply circumscribed, uncapsulated, gray-white tumors, which are firm, usually round, and show a whorled pattern on cut section; called also *fibromyoma uteri, myoma previum,* and, colloquially, *fibroids.* **vascular l.,** a tumor consisting of a coil of blood vessels surrounded by a network of muscular fibers.

leiomyosarcoma (li″o-mi″o-sar-ko′mah) a sarcoma containing large spindle cells of smooth muscle, most commonly of the uterus or retroperitoneal region.

leiotrichous (li-ah′tri-kus″) [*leio-* + Gr. *thrix* hair] having smooth, straight hair.

leipo- (lip′o) for words beginning thus, see those beginning *lipo-*.

Leishman's anemia, etc. (lēsh′manz) [Sir William Boog *Leishman,* English army surgeon, 1865–1926] see under *anemia, cell, nodule,* and *Table of Stains.*

Leishman-Donovan bodies (lēsh′man-don′o-van) [Sir William B. *Leishman;* Charles *Donovan,* Irish physician in Sanitary Service in India, 1863–1951] see under *body.*

Leishmania (lēsh-ma′ne-ah) [Sir William B. *Leishman*] a genus of parasitic protozoa of the family Trypanosomatidae, order Protomastigida, found chiefly in the reticuloendothelial cells of the skin or viscera of vertebrates. The organisms have only two stages in their life cycle: a leptomonad stage, usually spent in the intestine of an insect host, and the typical leishmanial form, developing in a vertebrate host. The leptomonad stage is elongate and possesses a free flagellum, whereas the leishmanial stage is round or oval and has no free flagellum. **L. aethio′pica,** the name given to the etiologic agent of diffuse cutaneous leishmaniasis in Ethiopia and Kenya. **L. brasilien′sis, L. brazilien′sis,** a form infecting man, dogs, and monkeys; it is morphologically identical with *L. donovani* and is the cause of mucocutaneous leishmaniasis. **L. brasilien′sis guyanen′sis,** a subspecies of *L. brasiliensis* that is the etiologic agent of pian bois, a form of cutaneous leishmaniasis of the New World. **L. cani′num,** *L. donovani.* **L. donova′ni,** a species infecting man, dogs, cats, sheep, and cattle; it is the cause of visceral leishmaniasis, or kala-azar. Called also *L. infantum.* **L. enriet′tii,** a species causing an infection in guinea pigs. **L. farcimino′sa,** former name for *Histoplasma farciminosus.* **L. infan′tum,** *L. donovani.* **L. mexica′na,** a species that is the etiologic agent of chiclero ulcer, a form of cutaneous leishmaniasis of the New World. **L. nilot′ica,** *L. tropica.* **L. peruvia′na,** a species that is the etiologic agent of uta, a form of cutaneous leishmaniasis of the New World; considered by some to be a subspecies of *L. brasiliensis.* **L. pifa′noi** the name given to the etiologic agent of diffuse cutaneous leishmaniasis in Venezuela. **L. trop′ica,** a species morphologically identical with *L. donovani* and having a similar life history. It has been divided into two subspecies: *L. tropica major,* the cause of the rural form of cutaneous leishmaniasis of the Old World, and *L. tropica minor,* the cause of the urban form.

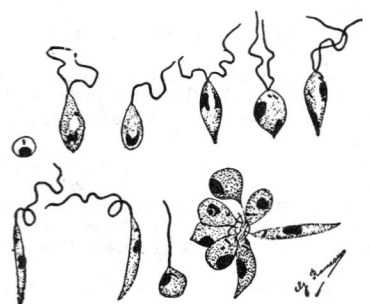

Leishmanial and leptomonad forms of *Leishmania tropica* (Ch. Nicolle).

leishmania (lēsh-măn′ē-ăh) 1. any organism of the genus *Leishmania.* 2. any individual of the family Trypanosomatidae when exhibiting the typical leishmanial (amastigote) form during its life cycle.

leishmanial (lēsh-măn′ē-ăl) 1. pertaining to or caused by leishmanias. 2. denoting a morphologic stage in the development of certain hemoflagellates; see *amastigote.*

leishmaniasis (lēsh″mah-ni′ah-sis) infection caused by *Leishmania.* **American l., l. america′na,** mucocutaneous l. **anergic l., anergic cutaneous l.,** diffuse cutaneous l. **Brazilian l.,** mucocutaneous l. **canine l.,** a disease of dogs and children in the Mediterranean region caused by *L. donovani.* In young children the onset is acute with fatalities occurring in untreated cases. Clinically it may very closely resemble congestive splenomegaly. Leukopenia is a prominent feature and agranulocytosis may supervene, with secondary infection and cancrum oris resulting. **l. cuta′nea diffu′sa,** diffuse cutaneous l. **cuta-**

neous l., dermal l., an endemic disease characterized by the development on the exposed parts of the body of a papule, single or multiple, which develops into a nodule and breaks down to form an ulcer with a granulation tissue base and a surrounding zone of inflammation. The disease has been divided into Old World and New World forms. The Old World form is caused by one of the subspecies of *Leishmania tropica,* transmitted by sandflies, usually of the genus *Phlebotomus,* and occurs throughout the Mediterranean region, North Africa, parts of India and China, Middle East, and Soviet Asia. It has been subdivided into two distinct types according to clinical manifestations and epidemiology: an acute, rapidly evolving *rural* (humid, moist, wet) form, caused by *L. tropica major,* with rodents acting as the reservoir host, and having an incubation period of a few weeks to a few months and a duration of up to six months; and an *urban* (dry) form, caused by *L. tropica minor* with both dogs and man acting as reservoir hosts, and having an incubation period of many months to over a year and a duration of many months. The Old World form of the disease has received many names, according to its locality of occurrence, as oriental sore, Aleppo boil, Delhi sore, Penjdeh sore, Natal sore, Bagdad sore, Biskra button, Lahore sore, Kandahar sore, furunculosis orientalis, oriental button, tropical ulcer, etc. The New World form occurs throughout Central and South America with the exception of Chile and Argentina, and is characterized by lesions that develop and heal similarly to those of the Old World form, but tend to be less nodular and more ulcerative and destructive; it is caused by *L. mexicana* or *L. braziliensis,* or their subspecies. Many varieties of cutaneous leishmaniasis of the New World exist, including *mucocutaneous leishmaniasis, chicle* or *chiclero ulcer, uta,* and *pian bois,* which differ as to etiologic agent, vector, distribution, pathology, epidemiology, and clinical course and manifestations. **diffuse cutaneous l., disseminated cutaneous l.,** a rare, chronic form of generalized cutaneous leishmaniasis, occurring in Central and South America, especially Venezuela and Brazil and in India, Sudan, Ethiopia, and Kenya, in which a primary lesion spreads locally to other parts of the skin, producing lesions resembling those of lepromatous leprosy; in Venezuela, the etiologic agent has been called *Leishmania pifanoi* and, in Ethiopia and Kenya, *L. aethiopica.* Called also *l. cutanea diffusa* and *l. tegmentaria diffusa.* **infantile l.,** Mediterranean kala-azar. **lupoid l.,** l. recidivans. **Mexican cutaneous l.,** chiclero ulcer. **mucocutaneous l., naso-oral l., nasopharyngeal l.,** an endemic, zoonotic forest disease, a form of cutaneous leishmaniasis of the New World, found widely distributed in Central and South America, except Chile and Argentina, caused by *Leishmania brasiliensis,* and transmitted by sandflies, usually of the genus *Lutzomyia;* it is characterized by the presence of primary cutaneous lesions which spread locally to the mucous membranes of the nose, mouth, and pharynx and which ulcerate and cause widespread destruction of tissue with marked deformity. Called also *l. americana,* American l., Brazilian l., and espundia. **New World l.,** see *cutaneous l.* **Old World l.,** see *cutaneous l.* **post–kala-azar dermal l.,** a condition sometimes occurring in India one to two years after treatment of or spontaneous recovery from kala-azar, or in Africa as the disease subsides. The early lesions are hypopigmented or erythematous macules on the face and sometimes on the arms, legs, and trunk; on the face, the lesions become nodular or papular, closely resembling lepromatous leprosy. Thinning of the epidermis over a nodular granulomatous lesion sometimes occurs after inadequate drug therapy of kala-azar. **l. recid′ivans,** a relapsing form of cutaneous leishmaniasis of the Old World, resembling tuberculosis of the skin, in which the ulcer heals incompletely, scarring centrally but spreading peripherally, or heals and recrudesces at the edge of the scar; it may last for many years. Called also *lupoid l.* **rural l.,** see *cutaneous l.* (of Old World). **l. tegmenta′ria diffu′sa,** diffuse cutaneous l. **urban l.,** see *cutaneous l.* (of Old World). **visceral l.,** kala-azar.

leishmanicidal (lēsh″man-ĭ-si′dal) destructive to *Leishmania.*

leishmanid (lēsh′man-id) the early cutaneous nodule of cutaneous leishmaniasis.

leishmaniosis (lēsh″man-e-o′sis) leishmaniasis.

leishmanoid (lēsh′mah-noid) an eruption of whitish patches along with nodules and papules following partially cured kala-azar; called also *dermal leishmanoid.*

leistungskern (līs′toongs-kern) [Ger.] the functional part or active center of a cell.

Lelaps (le′laps) *Echinolaelaps.* **L. echidni′nus,** *Echinolaelaps echidninus.*

Leloir's disease (lēl-warz′) [Henri Camille *Leloir,* French dermatologist, 1855–1896] discoid lupus erythematosus.

lema (le′mah) [Gr. *lēmē*] sebum palpebrale.

Lembert's suture (lah-bārz′) [Antoine *Lembert,* French surgeon, 1802–1851] see under *suture.*

lemic (le′mik) [Gr. *loimos* plague] pertaining to an epidemic disease, as the plague.

lemma (lem′ah) [Gr. "rind," "husk"] a collective term for the egg membranes (primary, secondary, and tertiary). Also used as a word termination denoting a sheath, as the neurilemma and oolemma.

lemmoblast (lem′o-blast) a primitive or immature lemmocyte.

lemmoblastic (lem″o-blas′tik) forming or developing into neurilemma tissue.

lemmocyte (lem′o-sīt) [Gr. *lemma* husk + *-cyte*] a cell derived from the neural crest and developing into a neurilemma cell.

lemnisci (lem-nis′si) plural of *lemniscus*.

lemniscus (lem-nis′kus) pl. *lemnis′ci* [L.; Gr. *lēmniskos* fillet] a ribbon or band; [NA] a general term for a band or bundle of fibers in the central nervous system. **acoustic l., l. acus′ticus** (*obs.*), l. lateralis. **lateral l., l. latera′lis** [NA], a tract of longitudinal fibers extending upward through the lateral part of the tegmental substance of the pons, formed chiefly by fibers arising from the opposite cochlear nuclei and the trapezoid body, and ascending to terminate in the inferior colliculus and medial geniculate body. **medial l., l. media′lis** [NA], a tract arising from the internal arcuate fibers of the nuclei gracilis and cuneatus, and crossing to the opposite side in the lower part of medulla oblongata to ascend, first between the two olives, and then through the pars dorsalis pontis just dorsal to the pontine nuclei; it continues through the tegmentum of the midbrain and ends in the ventral posterior part of the thalamus. Each lemniscus carries sensory impulses from the opposite side of the body. Called also *sensory l.* or *l. sensitivus*. **optic l.**, tractus opticus. **l. sensiti′vus, sensory l.,** l. medialis. **spinal l., l. spina′lis** [NA], the part of each spinothalamic tract within the pons and mesencephalon, forming a diffuse bundle between the medial and lateral lemnisci. It carries pain, temperature, and tactile impulses from the opposite side of the body and ends in the ventral posterior part of the thalamus. **trigeminal l., l. trigemina′lis** [NA], fibers conveying sensory impulses from the trigeminal nuclei to the ventral posterior part of the opposite thalamus; they ascend intermingled with the spinal lemniscus and adjacent medial lemniscus.

lemography (le-mog′rah-fe) [Gr. *loimos* plague + *graphein* to write] a treatise on the plague or other epidemic disease.

lemology (le-mol′o-je) [Gr. *loimos* plague + *-logy*] the science of contagious and epidemic diseases, especially the plague.

lemon (lem′un) the fruit of *Citrus limon* (Linné) Burmann filius (Rutaceae); the peel contains a volatile oil used as a flavoring agent, and the fruit contains citric and ascorbic acids.

lemoparalysis (le″mo-pah-ral′ĭ-sis) [Gr. *laimos* gullet + *paralysis*] paralysis of the esophagus.

lemostenosis (lem″o-stĕ-no′sis) [Gr. *laimos* gullet + *stenōsis* narrowing] stenosis of the esophagus.

Lemuroidea (lem″u-roi′de-ah) a suborder of Primates, consisting of the lemurs, animals resembling monkeys but having, usually, a sharp, foxlike muzzle and a tail which is usually long and furry, but never prehensile.

Lenard rays (len-ard′) [Philipp *Lenard*, Hungarian physicist, 1862–1947] see under *ray*.

Lenetran (len′ĕ-tran) trademark for a preparation of mephenoxalone.

length (length) an expression of the longest dimension of an object, or of the measurement between the two ends. **arch l.,** the amount of space available for the permanent teeth as measured from the mesial aspect of the first molar on one side to the mesial aspect of the first molar on the opposite side along an imaginary line of the dental arch. **basialveolar l.,** the distance from the basion to the lower end of the intermaxillary suture. **basinasal l.,** the distance from the basion to the center of the suture between the frontal and nasal bones. **crown-heel l.,** an expression of measurement from the crown of the head to the heel in embryos, fetuses, and infants; the equivalent of *standing height* in older individuals. **crown-rump l.,** an expression of measurement from the crown of the head to the breech in embryos, fetuses, and infants; the equivalent of *sitting vertex height* in older individuals. **focal l.,** the distance between a lens and an object from which all rays of light are brought to a focus. **foot l.,** a heel-toe measurement useful in estimating the age of fetuses because the foot dimensions are less subject to artifacts of curvature and shrinkage than is the fetus as a whole. **greatest l.,** a dimension used to express the size of very young embryos that have not yet developed the structures permitting measurement of crown-rump length. **sitting l.,** the distance from the crown of the head to the coccyx. **stem l.,** the distance from the vertex to a line joining the ischial tuberosities. **wave l.,** see *wavelength*.

leniceps (len′ĭ-seps) [L. *lenis* mild + *capere* to seize] a short-handled obstetric forceps.

leniquinsin (len″ĭ-kwin′sin) chemical name: *N*-[(3,4-dimethoxyphenyl)methylene]-6,7-dimethoxy-4-quinolinamine; an antihypertensive, $C_{20}H_{20}N_2O_4$.

lenitive (len′ĭ-tiv) [L. *lenire* to soothe] 1. demulcent or soothing. 2. a demulcent remedy.

Lennander's operation (len-an′derz) [Karl Gustav *Lennander*, Swedish surgeon, 1857–1908] see under *operation*.

Lennhoff's index, sign (len′hofs) [Rudolf *Lennhoff*, German physician, 1866–1933] see under *index* and *sign*.

Lennox syndrome [William Gordon *Lennox*, American neurologist, born 1884] see under *syndrome*.

lenperone (len′per-ōn) chemical name: 4-[4-(4-fluorobenzoyl)-1-piperidinyl]-1-(4-fluorophenyl)-1-butanone; a tranquilizer, $C_{22}H_{23}F_2NO_2$.

lens (lenz) [L. "lentil"] 1. a piece of glass or other transparent substance so shaped as to converge or scatter the rays of light, especially the glass used in appropriate frames or other instruments to increase the visual acuity of the human eye. See also *glasses* and *spectacles*. 2. [NA] the transparent biconvex body of the eye situated between the posterior chamber and the vitreous body, constituting part of the refracting mechanism of the eye. See *eye*. Called also *l. crystallina* or *crystalline l.* **achromatic l.,**

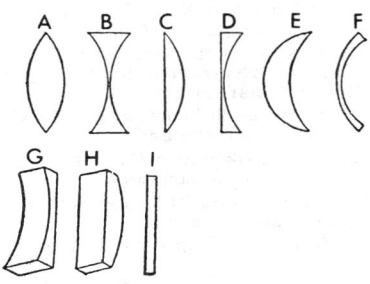

Lenses: *A–F*, Spherical lenses: *A*, biconvex; *B*, biconcave; *C*, planoconvex; *D*, planoconcave; *E*, concavoconvex; *F*, convexoconcave; *G, H*, cylindrical lenses, concave and convex; *I*, ordinary flat lens.

one corrected for chromatic aberration. **acrylic l.,** a plastic lens used to replace the crystalline lens after cataract surgery. **adherent l.,** contact l. **aplanatic l.,** one that serves to correct spherical aberration. **apochromatic l.,** one corrected for chromatic and spherical aberration. **biconcave l.,** a lens that has both surfaces concave. **biconvex l.,** a lens that has both surfaces convex. **bicylindrical l.,** one that has both surfaces cylindrical. **bifocal l.,** a lens made up of two segments with different refractive powers, ordinarily with the upper for far and the lower segment for near vision; see under *glasses*. **bispherical l.,** one that is spherical on both sides. **Brücke l.,** a combination of a double convex and double concave lens so arranged as to give considerable working distance. **cataract l.,** a powerful lens for glasses to be used after cataract operation. **compound l.,** a lens made up of two or more segments. **concave l.,** a lens with one or both (biconcave) surfaces curved like a section of the interior of a hollow sphere; it diverges the rays of light. Called also *diverging l.* and *minus l.* **concavoconcave l.,** biconcave l. **concavoconvex l.,** one that has one concave surface and one convex surface; a converging meniscus lens. Called also *positive meniscus.* **contact l.,** a curved shell of glass or plastic applied directly over the globe or cornea to correct refractive errors. **converging l., convex l.,** a lens curved like a section of the exterior of a hollow sphere; it brings light to a focus. Called also *plus l.* **convexoconcave l.,** one that has one convex and one concave surface; a diverging meniscus lens. Called also *negative meniscus.* **Coquille plano l.,** one that is +8D on one side and −8D on the other. **Crookes' l.,** one made from glass rendered opaque to ultraviolet and infrared rays but transparent to visible light. **crossed l.,** one with front and back surfaces of different curvatures. **l. crystallina, crystalline l.,** the lens of the eye; see *lens*, def. 2. **cylindrical l.,** one that is a section of a cylinder cut parallel to its axis, with one surface plane and the other concave or convex. **decentered l.,** one in which the optical axis does not pass through the center. **dispersing l.,** an incorrect name for *concave l.* (diverging l.). **diverging l.,** concave l. **immersion l.,** see under *objective*. **iseikonic l.,** one that is used to correct aniseikonia; such lenses affect the focus of the rays entering the eye and also the magnification of the images formed on the retina. **meniscus l.,** a lens that has one spherical convex and one spherical concave surface; see *concavoconvex l.* and *convexoconcave l.* **meter l.,** a converging lens with a focal length of one meter and a refracting power of one diopter. **minus l.,** concave l. **omnifocal l.,** a lens the power of which increases continuously and regularly in a downward direction, thereby avoiding the discontinuity in field and power which is apparent in bifocal and trifocal lenses. **orthoscopic l.,** one that gives a very flat and undistorted field of vision. **periscopic l.,** one with a 1.25D base curve. **planoconcave l.,** a lens with one plane and one concave side. **planoconvex l.,** a lens with one plane and one convex side. **plus l.,** convex l. **punktal l.,** a toric lens which is corrected for astigmatism over the entire field of vision. **retroscopic l.,** one tilted inward at the top. **spherical l.,** one that is a segment of a sphere. **toric l.,** a meniscus lens with a cylindrical curve ground on the spherical surface of one side. **trial l.,** any one of a set of lenses used in testing the vision. **trifocal l.,** a lens made up of three segments with different refractive powers, ordinarily with the upper for distant, the middle for intermediate, and the lower for near vision; see *trifocal glasses,* under *glasses.*

lensometer (lenz-om′ĕ-ter) a device for measuring the optical characteristics of lenses.

lentectomize (len-tek′to-mīz) to remove the crystalline lens by surgical excision.

lentectomy (len-tek′to-me) [*lens* + Gr. *ektomē* excision] surgical excision of the crystalline lens.

lenticel (len′tĭ-sel) a lens-shaped gland, especially one of those at the base of the tongue.

lenticonus (len″tĭ-ko′nus) [*lens* + L. *conus* cone] a conical protrusion of the substance of the crystalline lens, covered by capsule or connective tissue, occurring more frequently on the posterior surface, and usually affecting only one eye.

lenticula (len-tik′u-lah) [L.] the lenticular nucleus.

lenticular (len-tik′u-lar) [L. *lenticularis*] 1. pertaining to or shaped like a lens. 2. pertaining to the crystalline lens. 3. pertaining to the lenticular nucleus.

lenticulo-optic (len-tik″u-lo-op′tik) pertaining to the lenticular nucleus and the optic thalamus.

lenticulostriate (len-tik″u-lo-stri′āt) pertaining to the lenticular nucleus and the corpus striatum.

lenticulothalamic (len-tik″u-lo-thah-lam′ik) relating to the lenticular nucleus and the thalamus.

lentiform (len′tĭ-form) shaped like a lens; see also under *nucleus.*

lentigines (len-tij′ĭ-nēz) [L.] plural of *lentigo.*

lentiginosis (len-tij″ĭ-no′sis) the presence of multiple lentigines. **progressive cardiomyopathic l.,** multiple symmetrical lentigines, hypertrophic obstructive cardiomyopathy, and retarded growth, sometimes with mental retardation.

lentiginous (len-tij′ĭ-nus) characterized by multiple lentigines; pertaining to or of the nature of a lentigo.

lentiglobus (len″tĭ-glo′bus) [*lens* + L. *globus* sphere] an exaggerated curvature of the crystalline lens, producing a spherical bulging on its anterior surface.

lentigo (len-ti′go), pl. *lentig′ines* [L. "freckle"] a round or oval, flat, brown, pigmented spot on the skin due to increased deposition of melanin and associated with an increased number of melanocytes at the epidermodermal junction. Cf. *freckle.* **l. malig′na, malignant l.,** melanotic freckle of Hutchinson; see under *freckle.*

lentitis (len-ti′tis) phakitis.

lentivirus (len″tĭ-vi′rus) any of a group of retroviruses, including those that cause maedi and visna in sheep.

lentoptosis (len″to-to′sis) [*lens* + Gr. *ptōsis* falling] phacocele.

lentula (len′chu-lah) a flexible, loosely spiraled, wirelike, rotating instrument, usually mounted in a dental handpiece, used to force sealer cement or paste into the root canal.

Leo's test (la′ōz) [Hans *Leo,* German physician, 1854–1927] see under *tests.*

Leonicenus (le-on″ĭ-se′nus) [It. Niccolò Leoniceno] (1428–1524). Professor of medicine at Padua, Bologna, and Ferrara; renowned for translating Hippocrates and Galen from Greek into Latin, for an early (1497) work on syphilis, and for a controversial book (1492) in which he courageously corrected many of the errors (particularly botanical) in Pliny's famous *Historia naturalis.*

Leonides (le-on′ĭ-dēz) (2nd–3rd century A.D.) a Greek surgeon who flourished in Rome, and whose writings are cited by Aëtius.

leontiasis (le″on-ti′ah-sis) [Gr. *leōn* lion] the leonine facies of lepromatous leprosy, due to nodular invasion of the subcutaneous tissue of the face, giving it a vaguely leonine appearance. **l. os′sea, l. os′sium,** bilateral and symmetrical hypertrophy of the bones of the face and cranium, giving it a vaguely leonine appearance; called also *megalocephaly.*

Leontodon (le-on′to-don) [Gr. *leōn* lion + *odous* tooth] *Taraxacum.*

Leopold's law (la′o-poldz) [Christian Gerhard *Leopold,* German physician, 1846–1911] see under *law.*

leotropic (le″o-trop′ik) [Gr. *laios* left + *tropos* a turning] running spirally from right to left. Cf. *dexiotropic.*

leper (lep′er) a person afflicted with leprosy; a term now in disfavor.

lepidic (lĕ-pid′ik) [Gr. *lepis* scale] 1. pertaining to scales. 2. pertaining to embryonic layers.

lepido- (lep′ĭ-do) [Gr. *lepis* flake or scale] a combining form meaning flake or scale.

lepidoma (lep″ĭ-do′mah) [*lepido-* + *-oma*] (*obs.*) a tumor derived from lepidic tissue; an endothelioma or a mesothelioma. **endothelial l.** (*obs.*), an endothelioma of the blood vessels or lymphatics.

Lepidophyton (lep″ĭ-dof′ĭ-ton) [*lepido-* + Gr. *phyton* plant] former name for *Trichophyton concentricum.*

Lepidoptera (lep″ĭ-dop′ter-ah) [*lepido-* + Gr. *pteron* wing] an order of insects including the butterflies and moths.

lepidosis (lep″ĭ-do′sis) [*lepido-* + *-osis*] (*obs.*) any scaly eruption.

lepocyte (lep′o-sīt) [Gr. *lepos* rind + *-cyte*] any nucleated cell having a cell wall.

lepothrix (lep′o-thriks) [Gr. *lepos* scale + *thrix* hair] trichomycosis axillaris.

lepra (lep′rah) [Gr. *lepra* the leprosy, which makes the skin scaly] leprosy; (prior to the mid 19th century) psoriasis. See also under *reaction.* **l. manchada,** lazarine leprosy.

leprechaunism (lep′rĕ-kon″izm) an exceedingly rare and lethal familial condition marked by slow development both physically and mentally, by elfin facies (wide-set eyes and low-set ears, with hirsutism), as suggested by the name, and by severe endocrine disorders, as indicated by enlargement of the clitoris and breasts in females and of the phallus in males. Called also *Donohue's syndrome.*

leprid (lep′rid) cutaneous lesion or lesions of tuberculoid leprosy, being hypopigmented or erythematous macules or plaques showing no evidence of *Mycobacterium leprae* by ordinary methods of examination. Cf. *leproma.*

lepride (lep′rēd) leprid.

leprologist (lep-rol′o-jist) a physician experienced in the study and treatment of leprosy.

leprology (lep-rol′o-je) the study of leprosy.

leproma (lep-ro′mah) a superficial granulomatous nodule rich in *Mycobacterium leprae,* and the characteristic lesion of lepromatous leprosy. Cf. *leprid.*

lepromatous (lep-ro′mah-tus) pertaining to lepromas; see *lepromatous leprosy,* under *leprosy.*

lepromin (lep′ro-min) a repeatedly boiled, autoclaved, gauze-filtered suspension of finely triturated lepromatous tissue and leprosy bacilli, used in the skin test for tissue resistance to leprosy; called also *Mitsuda antigen.* See also under *tests.*

leprosarium (lep″ro-sa′re-um) [L.] a hospital or colony for the treatment and isolation of leprosy patients.

leprosary (lep′ro-sār″e) [L. *leprosa′rium*] leprosarium.

leprostatic (lep″ro-stat′ik) 1. inhibiting the growth of *Mycobacterium leprae.* 2. an agent that inhibits the growth of *Mycobacterium leprae.*

leprosy (lep′ro-se) [Gr. *lepros* scaly, scabby, rough] a chronic communicable disease, caused by a specific microorganism, *Mycobacterium leprae,* which produces various granulomatous lesions in the skin, the mucous membranes, and the peripheral nervous system. Two principal or polar types are recognized: lepromatous and tuberculoid. A combination of these types is called *borderline* or *dimorphous leprosy.* Called also *lepra, elephantiasis graecorum,* and *Hansen's disease.* **anesthetic l.,** former term for tuberculoid leprosy. **borderline l.,** a form of leprosy that is transitional between the tuberculoid and lepromatous forms; called also *dimorphous l.* **cutaneous l.,** lepromatous l. **dimorphous l.,** borderline l. **indeterminate l.,** leprosy in which hypopigmented macules of uncharacteristic histology occur; it may develop into the lepromatous, tuberculoid, or borderline type. **Kabyle l.,** a congenital disease affecting Kabyles, members of a tribe of Berbers of Algeria and Tunisia; it is probably tertiary syphilis. **lazarine l.,** a pure diffuse variant of lepromatous leprosy in which lepromas are absent but the entire integument may become infiltrated and localized gangrenous macules may occur; it is rarely seen outside Costa Rica and western Mexico. Loosely used to refer to bullous or ulcerating manifestations of leprosy. Called also *lepra manchada, spotted leprosy,* and *Lucio leprosy.* **lepromatous l.,** that polar form of leprosy characterized by the presence of lepromas and invariably by the presence of *Mycobacterium leprae* in abundance from the onset; nerve damage occurs very slowly, usually symmetrically, and the skin reaction to lepromin is negative. It is the only form which may regularly serve as a source of infection to others, until treatment is begun. **Lucio l.,** lazarine l. **macular l., maculoanesthetic l.,** tuberculoid leprosy with hypopigmented, anesthetic, macular skin lesions. **mixed l.,** obsolete term for a supposed combination of lepromatous and tuberculoid leprosy; actually a combination of skin and nerve lesions. As originally used, it included both lepromatous and tuberculoid cases. **murine l.,** a progressive infection of rats caused by *Mycobacterium leprae murium,* much used as a laboratory model for the evaluation of antimycobacterial drugs; called also *rat l.* **neural l.,** tuberculoid l. **nodular l.,** lepromatous l. **rat l.,** murine l. **reactional l.,** the condition observed during any of the recurring episodes of acute exacerbation of leprosy (accompanied in the lepromatous form by fever and, often, erythema multiforme) which may punctuate the course of either polar form of the disease. **spotted l.,** lazarine l. **trophoneurotic l.,** tuberculoid leprosy in which the visible lesions result entirely from the effects of denervation of tissue in the course of the disease, rather than from the leprosy infection itself. **tuberculoid l.,** that polar type of leprosy (known formerly as neural or maculoanesthetic l.) in which, as a result of high cell-mediated resistance to the infection, *Mycobacterium leprae* are few or lacking by ordinary methods of examination, and nerve damage occurs very early, so that all skin lesions are denervated from the start, often with dissociation of sensation. The cutaneous reaction to injected lepromin is positive, and the patient is rarely a source of infection to others. **water-buffalo l.,** a chronic disease of water buffaloes caused by the acid-fast bacillus *Mycobacterium leprae bubalorum.*

leprotic (lep-rot′ik) pertaining to or affected with leprosy.

leprous (lep′rus) [L. *leprosus*] afflicted with leprosy.

leptandra (lep-tan′drah) [Gr. *leptos* thin + *anēr* anther] the rhizome and rootlets of *Veronica virginica* (L.) Farw. (Scrophulariaceae), used as a cathartic.

leptazol (lep′tah-zol) pentylenetetrazol.

lepto- (lep′to) [Gr. *leptos* slender] a combining form meaning slender, thin, or delicate.

leptocephalic (lep″to-sĕ-fal′ik) characterized by leptocephaly.

leptocephalous (lep″to-sef′ah-lus) leptocephalic.

leptocephalus (lep″to-sef′ah-lus) [*lepto-* + Gr. *kephalē* head] a person with an abnormally tall, narrow skull.

leptocephaly (lep″to-sef′ah-le) abnormal tallness and narrowness of the skull.

leptochroa (lep-to-kro′ah) [*lepto-* + Gr. *chroa* skin] (*obs.*) abnormal delicacy of skin.

leptochromatic (lep″to-kro-mat′ik) [*lepto-* + *chromatin*] having a fine chromatin network.

Leptocimex (lep″to-si′meks) *Cimex*. **L. boue′ti,** *Cimex boueti.*

Leptoconops (lep″to-ko′nops) a genus of blood-sucking flies of the family Heleidae.

leptocyte (lep′to-sīt) [*lepto-* + Gr. *kytos* cell] an erythrocyte characterized by a hemoglobinated peripheral border, surrounding a clear area containing a "bull's-eye" center of pigment, as seen in thalassemia.

leptocytosis (lep″to-si-to′sis) the presence of leptocytes in the blood.

leptodactylous (lep″to-dak′tĭ-lus) [*lepto-* + Gr. *daktylos* finger] possessing slender digits.

leptodactyly (lep″to-dak′tĭ-le) abnormal slenderness of the digits.

Leptodera pellio (lep-to′der-ah pel′e-o) *Rhabditis pellio.*

leptodermic (lep″to-der′mik) [*lepto-* + Gr. *derma* skin] (*obs.*) thin skinned.

leptodontous (lep″to-don′tus) [*lepto-* + Gr. *odous* tooth] having slender teeth.

leptomeningeal (lep″to-mĕ-nin′je-al) pertaining to the leptomeninges.

leptomeninges (lep″to-mĕ-nin′jēz), sing. *leptomen′inx* [*lepto-* + *meninges*] the pia mater and arachnoid considered together as one functional unit; the pia-arachnoid.

leptomeningioma (lep″to-me-nin″je-o′mah) a tumor of the leptomeninges.

leptomeningitis (lep″to-men″in-ji′tis) [*leptomeninx* + *-itis*] inflammation of the pia and arachnoid of the brain or spinal cord. Leptomeningitis is variously qualified as acute, basilar, cerebrospinal, chronic, epidemic, external, infantile, intracranial, purulent, nonpurulent, serous, tuberculous, etc. Cf. *pachymeningitis.* **l. inter′na,** inflammation of the pia mater. **sarcomatous l.,** diffuse sarcomatous infiltration of the pia mater.

leptomeningopathy (lep″to-men″in-gop′ah-the) [*leptomeninges* + Gr. *pathos* disease] any disease of the leptomeninges.

leptomeninx (lep″to-men′inks) [*lepto-* + Gr. *mēninx* membrane] singular of leptomeninges.

Leptomitus (lep-tom′ĭ-tus) former name for the genus *Absidia.*

leptomonad (lep″to-mo′nad) 1. pertaining to the genus *Leptomonas.* 2. denoting a morphologic stage in the development of certain protozoa of the family Trypanosomatidae; see *promastigote.* 3. any individual of the family Trypanosomatidae when exhibiting the typical leptomonad (promastigote) form during its life cycle.

Leptomonas (lep″to-mo′nas) a genus of parasitic protozoa of the family Trypanosomatidae, order Protomastigida, found in the digestive tract of various insects, and characterized by having an elongate body with a relatively large nucleus near the center and a long thin flagellum arising from a blepharoplast and kinetoplast near the anterior end. During their life cycle, the organisms lose the flagellum, round up into typical amastigote (leishmanial) forms, and become cysts; when the cysts are ingested by the next host, they escape, develop another flagellum, and attain the adult form.

leptomonas (lep″to-mo′nas) 1. any organism of the genus *Leptomonas.* 2. leptomonad (def. 3).

leptonema (lep″to-ne′mah) [*lepto-* + Gr. *nēma* thread] a presynaptic stage of meiosis in which the chromatin is in the form of fine spireme threads.

leptonomorphology (lep″to-no-mor-fol′o-je) the morphology of membranes.

leptopellic (lep″to-pel′ik) [*lepto-* + Gr. *pella* bowl] having a narrow pelvis.

leptophonia (lep″to-fo′ne-ah) [*lepto-* + Gr. *phōnē* voice] weakness or feebleness of the voice.

leptophonic (lep″to-fon′ik) pertaining to or characterized by leptophonia.

leptoprosope (lep-top′ro-sōp) an individual exhibiting leptoprosopia.

leptoprosopia (lep″to-pro-so′pe-ah) [*lepto-* + Gr. *prosōpon* face + *-ia*] narrowness of the face, with slender features, round, open orbits, long nose, narrow nostrils, and small mouth.

leptoprosopic (lep″to-pro-so′pik) pertaining to or characterized by leptoprosopia.

Leptopsylla (lep″to-sil′ah) a genus of fleas. **L. mus′culi,** *L. segnis.* **L. seg′nis,** the common flea of the mouse and rat, being the vector of plague; called also *Ctenopsyllus segnis* and *L. musculi.*

leptorrhine (lep′to-rīn) [*lepto-* + Gr. *rhis* nose] having a nasal index below 48.

leptoscope (lep′to-skōp) [*lepto-* + Gr. *skopein* to examine] an optical apparatus for measuring the thickness of the plasma membrane of a cell.

leptosomatic (lep″to-so-mat′ik) [*lepto-* + Gr. *sōma* body] having a light, thin body.

leptosome (lep′to-sōm) a person with a slender light physique.

Leptospira (lep″to-spi′rah) [*lepto-* + Gr. *speira* coil] a genus of microorganisms of the family Treponemataceae, order Spirochaetales, made up of finely coiled organisms 6 to 20 μ long, the spirals measuring 0.3 μ in depth and 0.5 μ in amplitude with hooked ends. They have been separated into antigenic varieties or serotypes given species status, but it is now proposed that all serotypes be placed in the single species *L. interrogans.* The organisms are pathogenic for man and other mammals, and usually occur in rodent reservoirs of infection. **L. austra′lis,** the etiologic agent of Mossman fever in Queensland, Australia. **L. autumna′lis,** the etiologic agent of Hasami fever in Japan, pretibial fever in the United States, and Sumatra jaundice. **L. bata′viae,** a species found in naturally occurring infections in rats and field mice; it causes leptospiral infections in Southeast Asia, Japan, and Europe. **L. biflex′a,** a name used in the United States and Great Britain to designate a nonpathogenic saprophytic species resembling *L. icterohemorrhagiae.* In Germany, it is called *Spirochaeta pseudoicterogenes.* It has been suggested that this name be used to include all the nonpathogenic leptospires. See *L. interrogans.* **L. canico′la,** the etiologic agent of Stuttgart disease. **L. grippotypho′sa,** the etiologic agent of leptospiral jaundice, harvest fever, and Schlammfieber in western Europe, and probably of Andaman A fever in the Netherlands East Indies. **L. heb′domidis,** the etiologic agent of nanukayami (seven-day fever) in Japan; the field vole, *Microtus montebelli* is the probable host. **L. hy′os,** an etiologic agent of swineherd's disease. **L. icterohaemorrha′giae,** the etiologic agent of leptospiral jaundice (Weil's disease) in man and yellows in dogs. **L. inter′rogans,** the proposed single species of *Leptospira,* containing all serotypes, including the interrogans complex, which comprises all pathogenic strains (over 120 serotypes), and the biflexa complex, which contains mainly saprophytic strains with no known hosts. **L. pomo′na,** an etiologic agent of swineherd's disease, swine and bovine leptospirosis, and Pomona fever. **L. pyrog′enes,** the etiologic agent of Salinem infection.

leptospira (lep″to-spi′rah) an individual organism belonging to the genus *Leptospira.*

leptospiral (lep″to-spi′ral) of, pertaining to, or caused by leptospiras.

leptospire (lep′to-spīr) an individual organism belonging to the genus *Leptospira.*

leptospirosis (lep″to-spi-ro′sis) infection by *Leptospira.* The infections are transmitted to man from dogs, swine, and rodents or by contact with contaminated water, as in swamps, canals, or ponds. All pathogenic leptospiral species (or serotypes) are probably capable of causing any of the clinical syndromes, including lymphocytic meningitis, hepatitis, and nephritis, separately or in combinations. Epidemics of meningitis, of febrile disease, or of hepatitis have been named for the regions in which they occurred or for the leptospiral species, implying a specific relationship between a species and a single clinical syndrome. **anicteric l., benign l. benign l.,** leptospirosis characterized by the absence of jaundice and by a milder course and symptoms than those in the more severe forms. Marked meningism may occur, and a skin rash may be an outstanding feature. Called also *anicteric l.* and *seven-day fever.* **bovine l., l. of cattle,** a disease of cattle caused primarily by *Leptospira pomona* and marked by fever, icterus, and anemia, especially in calves. Pregnant animals may abort, and lactating animals may develop mastitis. **canine l.,** see *Stuttgart disease,* under *disease,* and see *yellows.* **equine l.,** a disease caused by several serotypes of *Leptospira* and characterized by fever, icterus, and depression. Recurrent iridocyclitis and abortion are also associated. **l. icterohemorrha′gica,**

leptospiral jaundice. **swine l.,** a disease of swine most commonly caused by *Leptospira pomona*. In the acute form, occurring in young pigs, it is marked by fever, icterus, hemorrhages, and death. It may cause abortion in pregnant sows. Transmitted to man, it causes swineherd's disease.

leptospiruria (lep″to-spir-u′re-ah) [*lepto-* Gr. *ouron* urine + ia] excretion of *Leptospira* in the urine, due to their invasion of the renal tubules.

leptostaphyline (lep″to-staf′ĭ-lin) [*lepto-* + Gr. *staphylē* bunch of grapes, uvula] having a palatal index of 79.9 or less.

leptotene (lep′to-tēn) [*lepto-* + Gr. *tainia* ribbon] the stage of meiosis in which the chromosomes are slender, like threads. See *meiosis*.

leptothricosis (lep″to-thri-ko′sis) leptotrichosis.

Leptothrix (lep′to-thriks) [*lepto-* + Gr. *thrix* hair] a genus of microorganisms of the family Chlamydobacteriaceae, order Chlamydobacteriales, made up of attached or unattached, straight or spirally twisted trichomes, with a sheath originally thin and colorless but later becoming thicker and yellow or brown, with the deposition of ferric hydroxide. Widely distributed and usually found in fresh water, it includes thirteen species: *L. bucca′lis, L. discoph′ora, L. echin′ata, L. epiphyt′ica, L. lopho′lea, L. ma′jor, L. ochra′cea, L. pseudovacuola′ta, L. side′ropous, L. sku′jae, L. therma′lis, L. volu′bilis,* and *L. winograd′skii*.

leptothrix (lep′to-thriks) any microorganism of the genus *Leptothrix*.

leptotrichosis (lep″to-trĭ-ko′sis) infection with any species of *Leptothrix*. **l. conjuncti′vae,** Parinaud's oculoglandular syndrome caused by a leptothrix.

Leptotrombidium (lep″to-trom-bid′e-um) a subgenus of *Trombicula*.

Leptus (lep′tus) [L.] a name for the larval form of mites of the genus *Trombicula* and the subgenus *Eutrombicula*. **L. akamu′shi,** *Trombicula akamushi*. **L. ir′ritans,** *Eutrombicula irritans*.

Lerch's percussion [Otto *Lerch*, physician in New Orleans, born 1894] drop percussion.

leresis (ler-e′sis) [Gr. *lērēsis*] agitated or senile loquacity or garrulousness.

lergotrile (ler′go-trīl) chemical name: 2-chloro-6-methylergoline-8-acetonitrile; a prolactin inhibitor, $C_{17}H_{18}ClN_3$. **l. mesylate,** the monomethanesulfonate salt of lergotrile, $C_{17}H_{18}Cl-N_3 \cdot CH_4O_3S$, which has been used as an antiparkinsonian agent.

Leri's sign (la′rēz) [André *Leri*, French physician, 1875–1930] see under *sign*.

Leriche's disease, syndrome (lĕ-rēsh′ez) [René *Leriche*, French surgeon, 1879–1955] see *post-traumatic osteoporosis,* under *osteoporosis,* and see under *syndrome*.

Leritine (ler′ĭ-tin) trademark for preparations of anileridine.

Lermoyez's syndrome (ler″moi-yāz′) [Marcel *Lermoyez*, French otolaryngologist, 1858–1929] see under *syndrome*.

l.e.s. local excitatory state.

lesbian (lez′be-an) [Gr. *Lesbios* of Lesbos, an island off the west coast of Asia Minor, the home of the poetess Sappho and her followers] 1. pertaining to homosexuality between females. 2. a female homosexual.

lesbianism (lez′be-ah-nizm) homosexuality between women; called also *sapphism*.

Lesch-Nyhan syndrome [Michael *Lesch*, American physician, born 1939; William L. *Nyhan*, Jr., American physician, born 1926] see under *syndrome*.

Lesgaft's space (triangle) (les′gafts) [Petr Frantsevich *Lesgaft*, Russian physician, 1837–1909] see under *space*.

lesion (le′zhun) [L. *laesio; laedere* to hurt] any pathological or traumatic discontinuity of tissue or loss of function of a part. **Armanni-Ebstein l.,** vacuolization of the renal tubular epithelium in the region of the loop of Henle and the convoluted tubules in diabetes, due to glycogen deposition. **Baehr-Löhlein l.,** Löhlein-Baehr l. **birds' nest l.,** crescentic thickenings or pockets resembling secondary valve structures, below the aortic valve. **Blumenthal l.,** a proliferative vascular lesion in the smaller arteries in diabetics. **Bracht-Wächter l.,** focal collections of lymphocytic and mononuclear cells in the myocardium. **central l.,** any lesion of the central nervous system. **coin l.,** a rounded coinlike tumor. **Councilman l.,** see under *body*. **Duret's l.,** effusion of blood in the region of the fourth ventricle of the cerebrum as a result of slight injury. **Ebstein's l.,** hyaline degeneration and insular necrosis of epithelial cells of the renal tubules in diabetes mellitus. **Ghon's primary l.,** Ghon focus. **gross l.,** a lesion that is visible to the naked eye. **herpetiform l. of Cole,** a vesicle which develops within a few days after venereal exposure to lymphogranuloma venereum. It occurs on the penis, within the urethra, in the anal region, on the labia, within the vagina, or in the cervix. It bursts to form a shallow grayish chancre. **histologic l.,** a microscopic lesion. **impaction l.,** an osteopathic term for a lesion of any spinal joint in which there is present abnormal thickening of the intervertebral disk with approximation of all the bony parts. **indis-**

criminate l., a lesion affecting different distinct parts or systems of the body. **initial syphilitic l.,** chancre, def. 1. **irritative l.,** one that stimulates the functions of the part where it is situated. **Janeway l.,** a small erythematous or hemorrhagic lesion, usually on the palms or soles, in bacterial endocarditis. **local l.,** one in the nervous system giving origin to distinctive local symptoms. **Löhlein-Baehr l.,** a focal glomerular lesion of necrosis and hyalinization occurring in bacterial endocarditis; the process has been described as focal embolic glomerulonephritis. **molecular l.,** a lesion not visible even with the aid of a microscope. **onion scale l.,** the concentric circumvascular fibrosis often found in the spleen and lymph nodes in systemic lupus erythematosus. **organic l.,** structural l. **partial l.,** one that involves only a part of an organ or of the diameter of a conducting tract. **peripheral l.,** a lesion of the nerve endings. **precancerous l.,** a lesion in a tissue in which the cells are likely to become malignant. **primary l.,** the original lesion manifesting a disease, such as chancre in syphilis or tuberculous chancre. **ring-wall l.,** multiple small ring hemorrhages which simulate proliferation of a glial ring; seen in pernicious anemia. **structural l.,** one that produces an obvious change in a tissue. **systemic l.,** one limited to a system or set of organs with a common function. **total l.,** one involving the whole of an organ or of the diameter of a conducting tract. **trophic l.,** a lesion manifested by a disturbance in the nutrition of a part. **wire-loop l.,** thickened capillary walls of some parts of a glomerular tuft in disseminated lupus erythematosus.

lesocupethy (les″o-ku′peh-the) [*learning, society, culture,* and *personality theory*] a term suggested by Murdock to embrace the unified psychological and social sciences.

Lesser's test (les′erz) [Fritz *Lesser*, Berlin dermatologist, born 1873] see under *tests*.

LET linear energy transfer: the energy dissipation of ionizing radiation over a given linear distance. Highly penetrating radiations, such as gamma rays, cause very low ion concentration and thus have a relatively low LET, beta particles and x-rays have an intermediate LET, and alpha particles have a relatively high LET.

let-down (let′down) the transport of milk from the alveoli of the breast to the ducts; called also *milk l.* See also under *reflex*.

lethal (le′thal) [L. *lethalis,* from *lethum* death] deadly; fatal. See under *dose, equivalent, factor, gene,* etc.

lethality (le-thal′ĭ-te) the ratio of deaths from a given disease to existing cases of that disease.

lethargus (le-thar′gus) [Gr. *lēthargos* lethargic, forgetful] African trypanosomiasis.

lethargy (leth′ar-je) [Gr. *lēthargia* drowsiness] a condition of drowsiness or indifference. **African l.,** African trypanosomiasis. **hysteric l.,** the sleep stage of hypnosis. **induced l.,** hypnotic trance. **lucid l.,** loss of will power with consequent inability to act, although intellectually conscious.

lethe (le′the) [Gr. *lēthē* forgetfulness] amnesia; complete loss of memory.

letheral (le′ther-al) pertaining to lethe.

lethologica (leth-o-loj′ĭ-kah) [Gr. *lēthē* forgetfulness + *logos* word] (*obs.*) inability to remember the proper word.

letimide hydrochloride (let′ĭ-mīd) chemical name: 3-[2-(diethylamino)ethyl]-2*H*-1,3-benzoxazine-2,4-(3*H*)-dione monohydrochloride; an analgesic, $C_{14}H_{18}N_2O_3 \cdot HCl$.

Letter (let′er) trademark for a preparation of levothyroxine sodium.

Letterer-Siwe disease (let′ter-er si′we) [Erich *Letterer,* German physician, born 1895; Sture August *Siwe,* German physician, born 1897] see under *disease*.

Leu leucine.

leucemia (loo-se′me-ah) leukemia.

leucine (loo′sin) [Gr. *leukos* white] chemical name: 2-amino-4-methylpentanoic acid. An amino acid, $C_6H_{13}NO_2$, or α-aminoisocaproic acid, essential for optimal growth in infants and for nitrogen equilibrium in human adults. It is obtained by the digestion or hydrolytic cleavage of protein.

leucinethylester (loo″sin-eth″il-es′ter) an oily liquid, $(CH_3)_2$-$CH \cdot CH_2CH(NH_2) \cdot CO_2 \cdot C_2H_5$.

leucinimide (loo″sin-im′id) the anhydride of leucine, $C_{12}H_{22}$-N_2O_2, a diketopiperazine; it may be produced by evaporation of leucine solutions.

leucinosis (loo″sĭ-no′sis) any condition in which leucine appears in the urine.

leucinuria (loo″sin-u′re-ah) [*leucine* + Gr. *ouron* urine + *-ia*] the presence of leucine in the urine.

leucismus (loo-siz′mus) [Gr. *leukos* white + *-izō* + *-mos*] a state of whiteness. **l. pilo′rum,** blaze.

leuco- [Gr. *leukos* white] a combining form meaning white; see also words beginning *leuko-*.

leucocyte (loo′ko-sīt) leukocyte.

leucocytosis (loo″ko-si-to′sis) leukocytosis.

Leucocytozoon (loo″ko-si″to-zo′on) [*leuco-* + *cyto-* + Gr. *zoon* animal] a genus of sporozoan parasites of the family Haemoproteidae, order Haemosporidia, found primarily in birds, and transmitted by the blackfly (*Simulium*) or by other dipterans. The schizogonic stages are found in endothelial cells of the liver, kidney, and spleen; the gametocytes are found in erythrocytes. **L. ana′tis,** a species found in ducks. **L. an′seris,** a species found in geese. **L. maclean′i,** a species found in the common pheasant (*Phasianus colchicus*). **L. pal′lidum,** see *Ross' bodies,* under *body.* **L. sakharof′fi,** a species found in the crow (*Corvus cornix*). **L. smith′i,** a species found in the domestic turkey (*Meleagris gallopavo*).

leucofluorescein (loo″ko-floo″o-res′e-in) fluorescin, produced from fluorescein by reduction with zinc powder in an acid medium.

Leucoium (loo-ko′ĭ-um) [L.; Gr. *leukos* white + *ion* violet] a genus of old world amaryllidaceous plants. *L. aesti′vum* and *L. ver′num* (called snowflake) are common in garden culture: emetic and poisonous.

leucon (loo′kon) leukon.

leucomycin (loo″ko-mi′sin) kitasamycin.

Leuconostoc (loo″ko-nos′tok) a genus of nonpathogenic, grampositive, saprophytic, facultative anaerobes assigned in some systems of classification to the tribe Streptococceae, family Lactobacillus; in other classifications, assigned to the family Streptoccaceae. They are spherical but often lenticular, nonmotile cells, some species of which form dextran. **L. citro′vorum, L. cremor′is,** a species found in milk and dairy products. **L. dextra′nicum,** a dextran-forming species found on fruit and vegetables and in milk and dairy products. **L. lac′tis,** a species found in milk and dairy products. **L. mesenteroi′des,** a dextran-forming species found in slimy sugar solutions, on fruit and vegetables, and in milk and dairy products. **L. oenos′,** a species found in wine.

leucopterin (loo-kop′ter-in) chemical name: 2-amino-4,6,7-pteridinediol. A colorless pigment, $C_6H_5N_5O_3$, isolated from butterfly wings, especially white wings, and also from xanthopterin by oxidation. See *pterin.*

leucosin (loo′ko-sin) an albumin found in the cereal grains.

leucotomy (loo-kot′o-me) leukotomy.

Leucotrichaceae (loo″ko-trĭ-ka′se-e) a family of schizomycetes (order Beggiatoales), made up of short cylindrical cells occurring in long trichomes, found in fresh and salt water containing decomposing algae. It includes a single genus, *Leucothrix.* These microorganisms resemble the blue-green algae but do not contain photosynthetic pigments.

leucovorin (loo″ko-vo′rin) folinic acid. **l. calcium** [USP], the calcium salt of folinic acid, $C_{20}H_{21}CaN_7O_7 \cdot 5H_2O$, occurring as a yellowish white or yellow powder; used as an antidote for folic acid antagonists, e.g., methotrexate, when there is need to reverse the toxic effects of the latter and in the treatment of megaloblastic anemias due to folic acid deficiency, administered intramuscularly.

Leudet's tinnitus (bruit, sign) (led-āz′) [Théodor Emile *Leudet,* physician at Rouen, 1825–1887] see under *tinnitus.*

leukapheresis (loo″kah-fĕ-re′sis) [*leuk*ocyte + Gr. *aphairesis* removal] the selective separation and removal of leukocytes from withdrawn blood, the remainder of the blood then being retransfused into the donor.

leukemia (loo-ke′me-ah) [Gr. *leukos* white + *haima* blood + *-ia*] a progressive, malignant disease of the blood-forming organs, characterized by distorted proliferation and development of leukocytes and their precursors in the blood and bone marrow. Leukemia is classified clinically on the basis of (1) the duration and character of the disease—*acute* or *chronic;* (2) the type of cell involved—*myeloid* (*myelogenous*), *lymphoid* (*lymphogenous*), or *monocytic;* (3) increase or nonincrease in the number of abnormal cells in the blood—*leukemic* or *aleukemic* (*subleukemic*). **acute promyelocytic l.,** promyelocytic l. **aleukemic l., aleukocythemic l.,** leukemia in which the total white blood cell count in the peripheral blood is either normal or below normal; it may be lymphocytic, monocytic, or myelogenous. **basophilic l.,** a disorder resembling acute or chronic leukemia in which the basophilic leukocytes predominate. **blast cell l.,** stem cell l. **chronic granulocytic l., chronic myelocytic l.,** a form of leukemia occurring mainly between the age of 25 and 60, usually associated with a unique chromosomal abnormality, in which the major clinical manifestations of malaise, hepatosplenomegaly, anemia, and leukocytosis are related to abnormal, excessive, unrestrained overgrowth of granulocytes in the bone marrow. **l. cu′tis,** involvement of the skin in leukemia, with tumor-like lesions. See *leukemid.* **embryonal l.,** stem cell l. **eosinophilic l.,** a form of leukemia in which the eosinophil is the predominating cell. Although resembling chronic myelocytic leukemia in many ways, this form may follow an acute course despite the absence of predominantly blast forms in the peripheral blood. **l. of fowls,** an infectious disease of the hematopoietic organs of fowls with atrophy of the bone marrow and changes in the viscera. **granulocytic l.,** myelocytic l. **Gross' l.,** a transmissible murine leukemia, first transmitted to newborn C3H mice by inoculation of filtrate of leukemic tissue from AK2 mice, thus demonstrating its viral etiology.

hairy-cell l., leukemic reticuloendotheliosis. **hemoblastic l., hemocytoblastic l.,** stem cell l. **histiocytic l.,** acute monocytic l. **leukopenic l.,** aleukemic l. **lymphatic l., lymphoblastic l., lymphocytic l., lymphogenous l., lymphoid l.,** leukemia associated with hyperplasia and overactivity of the lymphoid tissue, in which the leukocytes are lymphocytes or lymphoblasts. **lymphosarcoma cell l.,** a form of leukemia characterized by large numbers of lymphosarcoma cells in the peripheral blood; depending on the degree of bone marrow involvement, it may be a variant of lymphosarcoma. **mast cell l.,** a type of leukemia characterized by the presence of overwhelming numbers of tissue mast cells in the peripheral blood. **megakaryocytic l.,** hemorrhagic thrombocythemia. **micromyeloblastic l.,** a form of granulocytic leukemia in which the immature, nucleoli-containing cells are small and are distinguishable from lymphocytes only by supravital staining. **monocytic l.,** leukemia in which the predominating leukocytes are identified as monocytes. The disease is generally divided into two main categories: the Naegeli type, in which many of the cells resemble myeloblasts, or cells of the myeloid series; and the Schilling type, in which the cells more truly resemble monocytes or histiocytes. **myeloblastic l.,** leukemia in which myeloblasts predominate. **myelocytic l., myelogenous l., myeloid granulocytic l.,** leukemia arising from myeloid tissue in which the granular, polymorphonuclear leukocytes and their precursors predominate. **myelomonocytic l.,** the Naegeli type of monocytic leukemia in which the predominate leukocytes resemble cells of the myeloid series. **Naegeli l.,** see *monocytic l.* **plasma cell l.,** leukemia in which the predominating cell in the peripheral blood is the plasma cell; whether this is a distinct form of leukemia or a phase of multiple myeloma remains moot. **plasmacytic l.,** plasma cell l. **promyelocytic l.,** a subvariety of acute granulocytic leukemia in which the predominant cells are promyelocytes, rather than myeloblasts, often associated with abnormal bleeding secondary to thrombocytopenia, hypofibrinogenemia, and decreased levels of Factor V. **Rieder cell l.,** a form of myeloblastic leukemia in which the blood contains asynchronously developed cells with immature cytoplasm and a lobulated, indented, comparatively more mature nucleus. **Schilling's l.,** see *monocytic l.* **stem cell l.,** a form of leukemia in which the predominating cell is so immature and primitive that its classification becomes exceedingly difficult. Called also *embryonal l., hemoblastic l., hemocytoblastic l.,* and *undifferentiated cell l.* **subleukemic l.,** aleukemic l. **undifferentiated cell l.,** stem cell l.

leukemic (loo-ke′mik) pertaining to or affected with leukemia.

leukemid (loo-ke′mid) any of the polymorphic skin eruptions associated with leukemia; clinically, they may be nonspecific, i.e., papular, macular, purpuric, etc., but histopathologically they may represent true leukemic infiltrations.

leukemogen (loo-ke′mo-jen) any substance that causes or produces leukemia.

leukemogenesis (loo-ke″mo-jen′ĕ-sis) the induction of or development of leukemia.

leukemogenic (loo-ke″mo-jen′ik) causing leukemia.

leukemoid (loo-ke′moid) [*leukemia* + Gr. *eidos* form] characterized by blood and sometimes clinical findings resembling true leukemia to such a degree that initial differentiation between the process causing the observed alterations and leukemia becomes extremely difficult.

leukencephalitis (look″en-sef″ah-li′tis) [*leuko-* + *encephalitis*] inflammation of the white matter of the brain.

Leukeran (loo′ker-an) trademark for a preparation of chlorambucil.

leukexosis (loo″kek-so′sis) an aggregation of dead leukocytes in one of the channels of the body.

leukin (loo′kin) 1. a relatively thermostabile lytic substance that can be extracted from polymorphonuclear leukocytes and that attacks particularly *Bacillus anthracis* and other spore-bearing aerobes. Called also *leukocytic alexin* and *leukocytic endolysin.* 2. leucine.

leuko- [Gr. *leukos* white] a combining form meaning white, or denoting relationship to a white corpuscle, or leukocyte.

leukoagglutinin (loo″ko-ah-gloo′tĭ-nin) an agglutinin directed against leukocytes. *Isoleukoagglutinins* are isoantibodies directed against the leukocytes of some but not all members of a species. Isoimmunization with these, as when incompatible blood is received by transfusion or placental transfer, may lead to disease. *Autoleukoagglutinins* are autoantibodies associated with leukopenia.

leukoblast (loo′ko-blast) [*leuko-* + Gr. *blastos* germ] an immature granular leukocyte. **granular l.,** promyelocyte.

leukoblastosis (loo″ko-blas-to′sis) a general term for proliferation of leukocytes, including myelosis and lymphadenosis.

leukocidin (loo″ko-si′din) [*leuk*ocyte + L. *caedere* to kill] a substance produced by some pathogenic bacteria that is toxic to polymorphonuclear leukocytes, killing the cells with or without lysis. **Neisser-Wechsberg l.,** a leukocidin produced by staphylococci that destroys rabbit but not human leukocytes; it is identical with alpha hemolysin. **Panton-Valentine (P-V) l.,** a leukocidin produced by staphylococci that destroys human and rabbit leukocytes.

leukocoria (loo″ko-ko′re-ah) leukokoria.

leukocrit (loo′ko-krit) [leuko- + Gr. krinein to separate] the volume percentage of leukocytes in whole blood.

leukocytal (loo″ko-si′tal) leukocytic.

leukocyte (loo′ko-sīt) [leuko- + Gr. kytos cell] 1. any colorless, ameboid cell mass. 2. white blood cell or corpuscle. The varieties of leukocytes may be classified into two main groups: granular l's and nongranular l's (see below). **agranular l's,** nongranular l's. **basophilic l.,** basophil, def. 2. **endothelial l.,** Mallory's name for the large wandering cells of the circulating blood and the tissues which have notable phagocytic properties; see endotheliocyte. **eosinophilic l.,** eosinophil. **granular l's (granulocytes),** leukocytes with abundant granules in the cytoplasm, which are divided into three groups: (1) Neutrophils, cells with fine neutrophilic granules in the cytoplasm and an irregular lobed nucleus; see neutrophil (def. 1). (2) Eosinophils, cells with coarse eosinophilic granules in the cytoplasm and a bilobed nucleus; see eosinophil. (3) Basophils, cells with coarse basophilic granules in the cytoplasm and a bent nucleus that is partially constricted into two lobes; see basophil (def. 2). See also granulocytic series, under series. **heterophilic l's,** heterophil, def. 1. See also neutrophil, def. 1. **hyaline l.,** monocyte. **lymphoid l's,** nongranular l's. **mast l.,** a name sometimes used to designate the circulating blood basophil, which is morphologically and histogenetically different from the tissue mast cell. **motile l.,** a leukocyte that has the power of ameboid movement. **neutrophilic l.,** neutrophil, def. 1. **nongranular l's,** leukocytes without specific granules in their cytoplasm, including the lymphocytes and monocytes. Called also agranular l's and lymphoid l's. **nonmotile l.,** a leukocyte without the power of ameboid movement. **polymorphonuclear l.,** any of the fully developed, segmented cells of the granulocytic series, especially a neutrophil, whose nuclei contain three or more lobes joined by filamentous connections. See neutrophil, def. 1. **polynuclear neutrophilic l.,** neutrophil, def. 1. **transitional l.,** former name for monocyte. **Türk's irritation l.,** Türk's cell; see under cell.

leukocythemia (loo″ko-si-the′me-ah) [leuko- + -cyte + Gr. haima blood + -ia] leukemia.

leukocytic (loo″ko-sit′ik) pertaining to leukocytes.

leukocytoblast (loo″ko-si′to-blast) [leukocyte + Gr. blastos germ] leukoblast.

leukocytogenesis (loo″ko-si″to-jen′ĕ-sis) [leukocyte + Gr. genesis production] the formation of leukocytes.

leukocytoid (loo′ko-si″toid) [leukocyte + Gr. eidos form] resembling a leukocyte.

leukocytology (loo″ko-si-tol′o-je) the study of leukocytes.

leukocytolysin (loo″ko-si-tol′ĭ-sin) a lysin that leads to disruption of leukocytes.

leukocytolysis (loo″ko-si-tol′ĭ-sis) [leukocyte + Gr. lysis dissolution] the breaking down or destruction of leukocytes. **venom l.,** destruction of leukocytes with snake venom.

leukocytolytic (loo″ko-si″to-lit′ik) 1. pertaining to, characterized by, or causing leukocytolysis. 2. an agent that causes leukocytolysis.

leukocytoma (loo″ko-si-to′mah) [leukocyte + -oma] a tumorlike mass of leukocytes.

leukocytopenia (loo″ko-si″to-pe′ne-ah) [leukocyte + Gr. penia poverty] leukopenia.

leukocytophagy (loo″ko-si-tof′ah-je) [leukocyte + Gr. phagein to devour] the ingestion and destruction of leukocytes by histiocytes of the reticuloendothelial system.

leukocytoplania (loo″ko-si″to-pla′ne-ah) [leukocyte + Gr. planē wandering] the wandering of leukocytes or their passage through a membrane.

leukocytopoiesis (loo″ko-si″to-poi-e′sis) [leukocyte + Gr. poiein to make] the production of leukocytes.

leukocytosis (loo″ko-si-to′sis) a transient increase in the number of leukocytes in the blood, resulting from various causes, as hemorrhage, fever, infection, inflammation, etc. **absolute l.,** increase in the total number of leukocytes in the blood. **agonal l.,** leukocytosis occurring just before death. **basophilic l.,** increase of the basophilic leukocytes in the blood. **mononuclear l.,** mononucleosis. **neutrophilic l.,** an increase in the number of polymorphonuclear neutrophil leukocytes in the blood. **pathologic l.,** that occurring as the result of some morbid condition, such as infection or trauma. **physiologic l.,** that caused by factors other than disease or trauma. **pure l.,** increase of the polymorphonuclear leukocytes of the blood. **relative l.,** increase in the proportion of any variety of leukocytes in the blood, without increase of the total number of leukocytes. **terminal l.,** agonal l. **toxic l.,** leukocytosis occurring in intoxication with blood poisons.

leukocytotactic (loo″ko-si″to-tak′tik) pertaining to or marked by leukotaxis.

leukocytotaxis (loo″ko-si″to-tak′sis) leukotaxis.

leukocytotherapy (loo″ko-si″to-ther′ah-pe) treatment by the administration of leukocytes.

leukocytotoxicity (loo″ko-si″to-tok-sis′ĭ-te) lymphocytotoxicity.

leukocytotoxin (loo″ko-si″to-tok′sin) a toxin that destroys leukocytes.

leukocytotropic (loo″ko-si″to-trop′ik) having a selective affinity for leukocytes.

Leukocytozoon (loo″ko-si″to-zo′on) Leucocytozoon.

leukocyturia (loo″ko-si-tu′re-ah) [leukocyte + Gr. ouron urine + -ia] the discharge of leukocytes in the urine.

leukoderivative (loo″ko-de-riv′ah-tiv) any white derivative from a pigment or coloring matter.

leukoderma (loo″ko-der′mah) [leuko- + Gr. derma skin] an acquired type of localized loss of melanin pigmentation of the skin, differing from vitiligo only in that the cause may be more or less apparent. **l. acquisi′tum centrif′ugum,** halo nevus. **l. col′li,** syphilitic l. **syphilitic l.,** indistinct coarsely mottled hypopigmentation, usually on the sides of the neck, occurring in late secondary syphilis; called also collar of pearls and l. colli.

leukodermatous (loo″ko-der′mah-tus) pertaining to or characterized by leukoderma.

leukodermia (loo″ko-der′me-ah) leukoderma.

leukodermic (loo″ko-der′mik) leukodermatous.

leukodextrin (loo″ko-deks′trin) an intermediate compound formed in the transformation of starch into sugar; achroodextrin.

leukodystrophy (loo″ko-dis′tro-fe) disturbance of the white substance of the brain. See leukoencephalopathy. **globoid l., globoid cell l.,** Krabbe's disease. **hereditary cerebral l.,** familial centrolobar sclerosis. **Krabbe's l.,** see under disease. **metachromatic l.,** a form of leukoencephalopathy transmitted as an autosomal recessive trait, characterized by an accumulation of a sphingolipid (sulfatide) in neural and non-neural tissues, with a diffuse loss of myelin in the central nervous system. The infantile form usually begins in the second year of life, most commonly before the thirtieth month, with blindness, motor disturbances, rigidity, mental deterioration, and sometimes convulsions; called also Greenfield's disease and diffuse cerebral sclerosis. The adult form begins after 16 years of age, usually with psychiatric disturbances that progress to dementia; the motor and posture disturbances appear late in the course of this form. A juvenile form with an onset between four and ten years of age has also been observed. Called also metachromatic leukoencephalopathy, metachromatic leukoencephaly, and sulfatide lipidosis. **spongiform l.,** Canavan's disease. **sudanophilic l.,** familial centrolobar sclerosis.

leukoedema (loo″ko-e-de′mah) an abnormality of the buccal mucosa, resembling early leukoplakia, consisting of an increase in thickness of the epithelium, with intracellular edema of the spinous or malpighian layer.

leukoencephalitis (loo″ko-en-sef″ah-li′tis) [leuko- + Gr. enkephalos brain + -itis] 1. inflammation of the white substance of the brain. 2. forage poisoning; a noncontagious disease of horses, the lesion of which is softening of the white matter of the brain. It is marked by drowsiness, dimmed vision, unsteady gait, and paralysis of the throat. **acute hemorrhagic l.,** a fatal postinfection or allergic encephalopathy with a fulminating course, characterized by necrosis of the walls of the blood vessels, particularly the venules, resulting in multiple petechial hemorrhages in the white matter of the brain. **l. periaxia′lis concentri′ca,** Baló's disease. **van Bogaert's sclerosing l.,** subacute sclerosing panencephalitis.

leukoencephalopathy (loo″ko-en-sef″ah-lop′ah-the) any of a group of diseases affecting the white matter of the brain, especially of the cerebral hemispheres, and occurring as a rule in infants and children. The term leukodystrophy is used to denote such disorders due to defect in the formation and maintenance of myelin in infants and children. **metachromatic l.,** see under leukodystrophy. **multifocal progressive l.,** progressive multifocal l. **progressive multifocal l.,** a generally fatal disease probably of viral origin, in which the demyelination is usually found in the white matter but may rarely be seen in the brain stem and cerebellum. It occurs secondary to various neoplastic diseases, including lymphosarcoma and lymphatic or myeloid leukemia. Called also multifocal progressive l. **subacute sclerosing l.,** subacute sclerosing panencephalitis.

leukoencephaly (loo″ko-en-sef′ah-le) leukoencephalopathy. **metachromatic l.,** see under leukodystrophy.

leukoerythroblastosis (loo″ko-ĕ-rith″ro-blas-to′sis) an anemic condition associated with space-occupying lesions (myelophthisis) of the bone marrow and characterized by a variable number of immature erythroid and myeloid cells in the circulation; called also leukoerythroblastic anemia, and myelopathic or myelophthisic anemia.

leukogram (loo′ko-gram) a diagram or tabulation representing the leukocytes of a specimen of blood.

leukokeratosis (loo″ko-ker″ah-to′sis) [*leuko-* + *keratosis*] leukoplakia.

leukokinesis (loo″ko-ki-ne′sis) the movement of the leukocytes within the circulatory system.

leukokinetic (loo″ko-ki-net′ik) pertaining to leukokinesis.

leukokinetics (loo″ko-ki-net′iks) [*leukocyte* + Gr. *kinētikos* of or for putting in motion] the quantitative, dynamic study of *in vivo* production, circulation, and destruction of leukocytes.

leukokoria (loo″ko-ko′re-ah) [*leuko-* + Gr. *korē* pupil + *-ia*] a condition characterized by appearance of a whitish reflex or mass in the pupillary area back of the lens.

leukokraurosis (loo″ko-kraw-ro′sis) kraurosis vulvae.

leukolymphosarcoma (loo″ko-lim″fo-sar-ko′mah) lymphosarcoma cell leukemia.

leukolysin (loo-kol′ĭ-sin) leukocytolysin.

leukolysis (loo-kol′ĭ-sis) leukocytolysis.

leukolytic (loo-ko-lit′ik) leukocytolytic.

leukoma (loo-ko′mah) [Gr. *leukōma* whiteness] 1. a dense white opacity of the cornea. 2. leukoplakia buccalis. **l. adhae′rens,** a white tumor of the cornea enclosing a prolapsed adherent iris.

leukomaine (loo′ko-mān) [Gr. *leukōma* whiteness] any one of a large group of basic substances resembling alkaloids, normally present in the tissues, which are products of metabolism and are probably excrementitious. Some of them may become toxic, and many are physiologically active.

leukomainemia (loo″ko-mān-e′me-ah) [*leukomaine* + Gr. *haima* blood + *-ia*] excess of leukomaines in the blood.

leukomainic (loo″ko-mān′ik) pertaining to, caused by, or characterized by a leukomaine.

leukomatous (loo-ko′mah-tus) affected with or of the nature of leukoma.

leukomonocyte (loo″ko-mon′o-sīt) [*leuko-* + Gr. *monos* single + *-cyte*] a lymphocyte.

leukomyelitis (loo″ko-mi″ĕ-li′tis) [*leuko-* + Gr. *myelos* marrow + *-itis*] inflammation of the white substance of the spinal cord.

leukomyelopathy (loo″ko-mi″ĕ-lop′ah-the) [*leuko-* + Gr. *myelos* marrow + *pathos* disease] any disease of the white substance of the spinal cord.

leukomyoma (loo″ko-mi-o′mah) lipomyoma.

leukon (loo′kon) a general term once applied to the circulating leukocytes and the cells from which they arise; it is the counterpart of erythron and thrombon.

leukonecrosis (loo″ko-nĕ-kro′sis) [*leuko-* + Gr. *nekrōsis* necrosis] gangrene resulting in the formation of a white slough.

leukonychia (loo″ko-nik′e-ah) [*leuko-* + Gr. *onyx* nail + *-ia*] a whitish discoloration of the nails of unknown cause; it may rarely be total, but is usually partial. Exceptionally, it may occur in transverse streaks (*l. striata*) or bands.

leukopathia (loo″ko-path′e-ah) [*leuko-* + Gr. *pathos* illness] leukoderma. **l. puncta′ta reticula′ris symmet′rica,** an eruption of depigmented macules on the forearms and shins of adults; probably identical with idiopathic guttate hypomelanosis. **l. un′guium,** leukonychia.

leukopathy (loo-kop′ah-the) leukopathia. **symmetric progressive l.,** an eruption of depigmented macules on the forearms and shins of adults; probably identical with idiopathic guttate hypomelanosis.

leukopedesis (loo″ko-pĕ-de′sis) [*leukocyte* + Gr. *pēdan* to leap] the outward passage of leukocytes through intact vessels walls; leukocytic diapedesis.

leukopenia (loo″ko-pe′ne-ah) [*leukocyte* + Gr. *penia* poverty] reduction in the number of leukocytes in the blood, the count being 5000 per cu. mm. or less. **basophil l., basophilic l.,** abnormal reduction in the number of basophil leukocytes in the blood. **congenital l.,** congenital neutropenia. **malignant l., pernicious l.,** agranulocytosis.

leukopenic (loo″ko-pe′nik) pertaining to, characterized by, or causing leukopenia.

leukophagocytosis (loo″ko-fag″o-si-to′sis) leukocytophagy.

leukophyl (loo′ko-fil) leukophyll.

leukophyll (lu′ko-fil) [*leuko-* + Gr. *phyllon* leaf] a colorless substance in plant tissues which becomes converted into protochlorophyll.

leukophyte (loo′ko-fīt) an alga containing no chlorophyll, i.e., a colorless alga.

leukoplakia (loo″ko-pla′ke-ah) [*leuko-* + Gr. *plax* plate + *-ia*] a disease marked by the development upon the mucous membrane of the cheeks (*l. buccalis*), gums, or tongue (*l. lingualis*) of white, thickened patches which cannot be rubbed off and which sometimes show a tendency to fissure. It is common in smokers and sometimes becomes malignant. Called also *leukokeratosis, leukoma, smokers' tongue, smokers' patches, psoriasis buccalis, psoriasis linguae,* and *ichthyosis linguae.* **l. pe′nis,** balanitis xerotica obliterans. **l. vul′vae,** a sometimes precancerous condition in which there are hypertrophic grayish white infiltrated

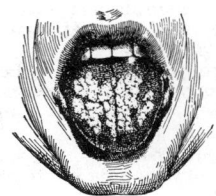

Leukoplakia of the tongue (Homans).

patches on the vulvar mucosa, characterized chiefly by intense pruritus, although erosion, ulceration, and fissuring are common. When associated with atrophic changes, it is known as *kraurosis vulvae* or *lichen sclerosus et atrophicus.*

leukoplasia (loo″ko-pla′ze-ah) leukoplakia.

leukoplast (loo′ko-plast) leukoplastid.

leukoplastid (loo″ko-plas′tid) [*leuko-* + Gr. *plassein* to form] a colorless granule of the plant cells from which the starch-producing elements are formed.

leukopoiesis (loo″ko-poi-e′sis) production of leukocytes.

leukopoietic (loo″ko-poi-et′ik) [*leukocyte* + Gr. *poiein* to make] forming or producing leukocytes.

leukopoietin (loo″ko-poi-e′tin) a hypothetical substance(s) believed to serve as the humoral regulator of leukopoiesis; granulopoietin.

leukoprecipitin (loo″ko-pre-sip′ĭ-tin) a precipitin specific for leukocyte antigens.

leukoprophylaxis (loo″ko-pro″fĭ-lak′sis) the increase by artificial means of the number of leukocytes in the blood in order to secure immunity to surgical infection.

leukopsin (loo-kop′sin) [*leuko-* + Gr. *ōps* eye] visual white; the colorless matter into which rhodopsin is changed by exposure to white light. It is reconvertible into rhodopsin under proper conditions.

leukorrhagia (loo″ko-ra′je-ah) [*leuko-* + Gr. *rhēgnynai* to break forth] profuse leukorrhea.

leukorrhea (loo″ko-re′ah) [*leuko-* + Gr. *rhoia* flow] a whitish, viscid discharge from the vagina and uterine cavity. **menstrual l., periodic l.,** leukorrhea in place of or along with the menses.

leukorrheal (loo″ko-re′al) pertaining to or marked by leukorrhea.

leukosarcoma (loo″ko-sar-ko′mah) [*leuko-* + *sarcoma*] the development of a leukemic blood picture in patients originally having a well-differentiated, lymphocytic type of malignant lymphoma. The circulating cells contain an ovoid nucleus and nucleoli, and are morphologically different from the mature-type lymphocyte seen in chronic lymphocytic leukemia.

leukosarcomatosis (loo″ko-sar-ko″mah-to′sis) a condition marked by the development of multiple sarcomas composed of leukemic cells.

leukoscope (loo′ko-skōp) [*leuko-* + Gr. *skopein* to examine] an instrument of Helmholtz's, modified by A. König, for testing color blindness.

leukosis (loo-ko′sis), pl. *leuko′ses.* Proliferation of leukocyte-forming tissue, including myelosis and lymphadenosis. Such proliferation forms the basis of leukemia. **acute l.,** see *Marek's disease,* under *disease.* **avian l.,** a group of transmissible, virus-induced diseases of chickens, characterized by proliferation of immature erythroid, myeloid, or lymphoid cells. Leukemic forms include erythroblastosis and myelosis and, rarely, lymphoblastic leukemia. Solid tumors in visceral organs are seen in cases of lymphoid leukosis, erythroblastosis, and myelocytomatosis. All of the causative viruses are related, and some induce "related neoplasms," such as sarcomas, hemangiomas, nephroblastomas, hepatocarcinomas, and osteopetrosis, a condition marked by thickening of the diaphyses of the long bones. These conditions are now classified as belonging to the leukosis sarcoma group, but were once included, along with Marek's disease, in the avian leukosis complex. Called also, according to the form taken, *avian lymphomatosis, osteopetrosis gallinarum,* and *visceral lymphomatosis.* **avian l. complex,** see *avian l.* **fowl l.,** avian l. **lymphoid l.,** a form of leukosis involving chiefly the lymphocytes. **myeloblastic l.,** a form involving chiefly the myeloblasts. **myelocytic l.,** a form involving chiefly the myelocytes. **skin l.,** see *Marek's disease,* under *disease.*

leukotactic (loo″ko-tak′tik) pertaining to leukotaxis; having the power of attracting leukocytes.

leukotaxin (loo″ko-tak′sin) leukotaxine.

leukotaxine (loo″ko-tak′sin) a crystalline nitrogenous polypeptide that appears when tissue is injured, that can be recovered from inflammatory exudates, and that promotes leukocytosis and increases capillary permeability and the diapedesis of leukocytes.

leukotaxis (loo″ko-tak′sis) [*leuko-* + Gr. *taxis* arrangement] the cytotaxis of leukocytes; the tendency of leukocytes to collect in regions of injury and inflammation; see also *leukotaxine.*

leukotherapy (loo″ko-ther′ah-pe) [*leuko-* + Gr. *therapeia* treatment] treatment by the administration of leukocytes. **preventive l.,** leukoprophylaxis.

Leukothrix (loo′ko-thriks) a genus of Schizomycetes of the order Beggiatoales, family Leukotrichaceae.

leukothrombin (loo″ko-throm′bin) a fibrin factor formed by leukocytes in the blood.

leukotome (loo′ko-tōm) [*leuko-* + Gr. *tomē* a cut] a cannula through which a loop of wire is passed to perform the operation of leukotomy or lobotomy.

leukotomy (loo-kot′o-me) the operation of cutting the white matter in the oval center of the frontal lobe of the brain; prefrontal lobotomy. **transorbital l.,** leukotomy performed by way of the orbital plate.

leukotoxic (loo″ko-tok′sik) destructive to leukocytes.

leukotoxicity (loo″ko-tok-sis′ĭ-te) the quality of having a toxic or deleterious effect on leukocytes.

leukotoxin (loo″ko-tok′sin) [*leukocyte* + *toxin*] a cytotoxin destructive to the leukocytes.

Leukotrichaceae (loo″ko-tri·ka′se-e) a family of Schizomycetes, order Beggiatoales.

leukotrichia (loo″ko-trik′e-ah) [*leuko-* + Gr. *thrix* hair + *-ia*] whiteness of the hair, in a circumscribed area.

leukourobilin (loo″ko-u-ro-bi′lin) [*leuko-* + *urobilin*] a colorless decomposition product of urobilin.

leukovirus (loo″ko-vi′rus) any of a group of morphologically similar, ether-sensitive, RNA viruses causing leukemia and tumors in animals; the group includes avian leukosis virus, Rous sarcoma virus, and murine leukemia virus.

Leunbach's paste (loi″en-bakhs′) [Jonathan Høegh *Leunbach*, Danish physician, born 1884] see under *paste*.

Levaditi's stain (lev″ah-de′tēz) [Constantin *Levaditi*, Roumanian bacteriologist in Paris, 1874–1928] see *Table of Stains*.

levallorphan tartrate (lev″al-lor′fan) [USP] chemical name: 17-allylmorphinan-3-ol[R-(R^*,R^*)]-2,3-dihydroxybutanedioate (1:1) (salt). An analogue of levorphanol, $C_{19}H_{25}NO \cdot C_4H_6O_6$, occurring as a white to practically white, crystalline powder, which acts as an antagonist to analgesic narcotics; used in the treatment of respiratory depression produced by narcotic analgesics, administered parenterally.

levamfetamine (le″vam-fet′ah-mēn) chemical name: (−)-α-methylbenzeneethanamine. The levorotatory form of amphetamine, $C_9H_{13}N$, having actions similar to the racemic form but less potent than the racemic or dextrorotatory (dextroamphetamine) forms. See *amphetamine*, def. 1. Spelled also *levamphetamine*. **l. succinate,** the succinate salt of levamfetamine, $C_9H_{13}N \cdot C_4H_6O_4$, used in the treatment of narcolepsy, hyperkinetic behavior disorders, and as an anorexic agent in the treatment of obesity; administered orally.

levamisole hydrochloride (le-vam′ĭ-sōl) chemical name: (*S*)-2,3,5,6-tetrahydro-6-phenylimidazo[2,1-*b*]thiazole monohydrochloride. An oral imidazole used as an anthelmintic, $C_{11}H_{12}N_2S \cdot HCl$, effective against roundworms, hookworms, and strongyloids. It is also an immunopotentiator and has been used (investigatively) to stimulate the immune response in cancer.

levamphetamine (le″vam-fet′ah-mēn) levamfetamine.

levan (lev′an) a hexosan from various grasses which on hydrolysis yields levulose.

levansucrase (lev″an-su′krās) β-2,6-fructan:D-glucose 6-fructosyltransferase: a bacterial enzyme that converts sucrose into fructan (levan) and glucose.

levarterenol (lev″ar-tĕ-re′nol) the levorotatory isomer of norepinephrine (q.v.), a much more potent pressor agent than the natural dextrorotatory isomer. **l. bitartrate,** norepinephrine bitartrate.

levator (le-va′tor), pl. *levato′res* [L. *levare* to raise] 1. [NA] a muscle for elevating the organ or structure into which it is inserted; see entries beginning *musculus levator*, in *Table of Musculi*. 2. a surgical instrument used to raise depressed osseous fragments in fractures of the skull and other bones.

levatores (lev″ah-to′rēz) [L.] plural of *levator*.

level (lev′el) 1. relative position, rank, or concentration. 2. a cerebrospinal center for combining or integrating impulses; the first level is spinal, the second is brainstem, the third is cortical. 3. in psychology, the sphere in which a tendency shows itself toward consciousness and adult activity. **isoelectric l.,** the level of recorded resting potential of a cell; the baseline of the electrocardiogram.

Lévi's syndrome (la′vez) [E. Léopold *Lévi*, Paris endocrinologist, 1868–1933] see under *syndrome*.

levicellular (lev″ĭ-sel′u-lar) [L. *levis* smooth + *cellula* cell] smooth celled.

levidulinose (le-vid′u-lin-ōs) a naturally occurring trisaccharide found in manna; on hydrolysis it yields one molecule of glucose and two molecules of mannose.

levigation (lev″ĭ-ga′shun) [L. *levigare* to render smooth] the grinding into a powder of a hard or moistened substance.

Levin's tube (lĕ-vinz′) [Abraham Louis *Levin*, New Orleans physician, 1880–1940] see under *tube*.

levitation (lev″ĭ-ta′shun) [L. *levis* light] 1. a hallucinatory sensation of floating or rising in the air. 2. a support system for severe burn victims, consisting of a bed in the form of an inflatable chamber containing numerous outlets through which humidified, warm, sterile air is released at a pressure sufficient to raise the patient so that he is supported in a sterile air environment.

levo- (le′vo) [L. *laevus* left] 1. a combining form meaning left, to the left. 2. a chemical prefix, for which the symbol (−) is frequently substituted, used to emphasize that the substance is the levorotatory enantiomorph, whether the configurational family is known or not. This practice avoids possible confusion with the occasional erroneous use of *l-* standing alone to designate the configurational family to which the substance belongs. Opposed to *dextro-*.

levocardia (le″vo-kar′de-ah) [*levo-* + Gr. *kardia* heart] a term denoting the normal position of the heart, used when other viscera are transposed; cf. *dextrocardia*. **isolated l.,** levocardia associated with transposition (situs inversus) of the abdominal viscera, congenital structural anomaly of the heart, and sometimes with absence of the spleen. **mixed l.,** corrected transposition of the great vessels; see under *transposition*.

levocardiogram (le″vo-kar′de-o-gram) [*levo-* + *cardiogram*] a rarely used term denoting that part of the normal electrocardiogram representing electric activity or depolarization potentials of the left ventricle.

levoclination (le″vo-kli-na′shun) [*levo-* + L. *clinatus* leaning] rotation of the upper poles of the vertical meridians of the two eyes to the left. Cf. *dextroclination*.

levocycloduction (le″vo-si″klo-duk′shun) levoduction.

levodopa (le″vo-do′pah) [USP] chemical name: 3-hydroxy-L-tyrosine. The levorotatory isomer of dopa, $C_9H_{11}NO_4$, occurring as a white to off-white crystalline powder; used as an antiparkinsonian agent, administered orally. See *dopa*.

Levo-Dromoran (le″vo-dro′mo-ran) trademark for preparations of levorphanol tartrate.

levoduction (le″vo-duk′shun) movement of either eye to the left.

levofuraltadone (le″vo-fūr-al′tah-dōn) chemical name: (−)-5-(4-morpholinylmethyl)-3-[[(5-nitro-2-furanyl)methylene]amino]-2-oxazolidinone; an antibacterial and antiprotozoal, $C_{13}H_{16}N_4O_6$.

levogram (lev′o-gram) [*levo-* + Gr. *graphein* to record] a rarely used term denoting electrocardiographic tracing showing left axis deviation, indicative of left ventricular hypertrophy.

levogyral (le″vo-ji′ral) [*levo-* + L. *gyrare* to turn] levorotatory.

levogyration (le″vo-ji-ra′shun) levorotation.

Levoid (le′void) trademark for a preparation of levothyroxine sodium.

levomepromazine (le″vo-mĕ-pro′mah-zēn) methotrimeprazine.

levomethadyl acetate (le″vo-meth′ah-dil) chemical name: (−)-β-[2-(dimethylamino)propyl]-α-ethyl-β-phenylbenzeneethanol acetate (ester). A narcotic analgesic, $C_{23}H_{31}NO_2$, used in the treatment of heroin addiction.

levonordefrin (le″vo-nor′dĕ-frin) [USP] chemical name: (−)-4-(2-amino-1-hydroxypropyl)-1,2 benzenediol. An adrenergic, $C_9H_{13}NO_3$, the levo isomer of nordefrin, occurring as a white to buff-colored, crystalline powder; used as a vasoconstrictor in solutions of local anesthetics, especially in dentistry.

Levophed (lev′o-fed) trademark for a preparation of norepinephrine bitartrate.

Levoprome (le′vo-prōm) trademark for a preparation of methotrimeprazine.

levopropoxyphene napsylate (le″vo-pro-pok′sĕ-fēn nap′sĭ-lāt) [USP] chemical name: [R-(R^*,S^*)]-α-(2-(dimethylamino)-1-methylethyl]-α-phenylbenzenethanol propanoate (ester) compound with 2-naphthalenesulphonic acid (1:1) monohydrate. The napsylate salt of the levo isomer of propoxyphen, $C_{22}H_{29}NO_2 \cdot C_{10}H_8O_3S \cdot H_2O$, occurring as a white powder; used as an antitussive, administered orally.

levopropylcillin potassium (le″vo-pro″pil-sil′in) chemical name: potassium 3,3-dimethyl-7-oxo-6-(−)-(2-phenoxybutyramido)-4-thia-1-azabicyclo[3.2.0]heptane-2-carboxylate; an antibacterial, $C_{18}H_{21}KN_2O_5S$, effective against gram-positive organism. Called also *propicillin*.

levorotary (le″vo-ro′tah-re) levorotatory.

levorotation (le″vo-ro-ta′shun) a turning to the left.

levorotatory (le″vo-ro′tah-to′re) [*levo-* + L. *rotare* to turn] turning the plane of polarization of polarized light to the left.

levorphanol (lēv-or′fah-nol) see *sodium levothyroxine*, under *sodium*.

levorphanol tartrate (le-vor′fah-nōl) [USP] chemical name: 17-methylmorphinan-3-ol [R-(R^*,R^*)]-2,3-dihydroxybutanedioate (1:1) (salt) dihydrate. A synthetic narcotic analgesic, $C_{17}H_{23}NO \cdot C_4H_6O_6 \cdot 2H_2O$, occurring as a white, crystalline powder; administered orally and subcutaneously.

levosin (le′vo-sin) a starch occurring in wheat flour, rye, bran, and stubble.

levothyroxine sodium (le″vo-thi-rok′sēn) [USP] chemical name: O-(4-hydroxy-3,5-diiodophenyl)-3,5-diiodo-L-tyrosine monosodium salt hydrate. The monosodium salt of the levo isomer of the thyroid hormone thyroxine, $C_{15}H_{10}I_4NNa_4 \cdot xH_2O$, occurring as a light yellow to buff-colored, hygroscopic powder; used for replacement therapy in reduced or absent thyroid function, administered orally.

levotorsion (le″vo-tor′shun) levoclination.

levoversion (le″vo-ver′zhun) an act of turning to the left; in ophthalmology, movement of the eyes to the left.

levoxadrol hydrochloride (le-voks′ah-drōl) chemical name: (–)-2-(2,2-diphenyl-1,3-dioxolan-4-yl)piperidine hydrochloride; a local anesthetic and smooth muscle relaxant, $C_{20}H_{23}NO_2 \cdot HCl$.

Levret's forceps, law, etc. (lev-rāz′) [André *Levret*, French accoucheur, 1703–1780] see under the nouns.

Levugen (lev′u-jen) trademark for a preparation of fructose.

levulan (lev′u-lan) fructosan.

levulin (lev′u-lin) a starchlike compound, $C_6H_{10}O_5$, occurring in certain plant tubers.

levulosan (lev″u-lo′san) fructosan, a fructose (fructofuranose) polysaccharide, e.g., inulin.

levulosazone (lev″u-lo′sa-zōn) fructosazone.

levulose (lev′u-lōs) [L. *laevus* left + *-ose*] fructose.

levulosemia (lev″u-lo-se′me-ah) [*levulose* + Gr. *haima* blood + *-ia*] fructosemia.

levulosuria (lev″u-lo-su′re-ah) [*levulose* + Gr. *ouron* urine + *-ia*] fructosuria.

levurid (lev′u-rid) a generalized allergic dermatitis ("id") caused by infection at a remote site with *Candida* or *Cryptococcus.*

levuride (lev′u-rid) levurid.

lewisite (lu′ĭ-sīt) [named for W. Lee *Lewis*, American chemist, 1879–1943] chemical name: dichloro(2-chlorovinyl)arsine. A lethal war gas, $AsCl_2CH:CHCl$. It is a vesicant, lacrimator, and lung irritant.

Lewisohn's method (lu′ĭ-sonz) [Richard *Lewisohn*, New York surgeon, born 1875] see under *method.*

Leyden's ataxia, crystals, disease (li′denz) [Ernst Victor von *Leyden*, German physician, 1832–1910] see *pseudotabes*, see *Charcot-Leyden crystals*, under *crystal*, and see under *disease.*

Leyden jar (li′den) see under *jar.*

Leyden-Moebius dystrophy, type (li′den-me′be-us) [E. V. von *Leyden*; Paul Julius *Moebius*, German neurologist, 1853–1907] limb-girdle muscular dystrophy.

Leydig's cells, cylinders, duct (li′digz) [Franz von *Leydig*, German anatomist, 1821–1908] see under *cell* and *cylinder*, and see *ductus mesonephricus.*

leydigarche (li″dig-ar′ke) [*Leydig* cells + Gr. *archē* beginning] the establishment or beginning of gonadal function in the male.

Lf limit flocculation; see *Lf unit*, under *unit.*

L.F.A. left fronto-anterior (left mento-anterior, a position of the fetus).

L.F.D. least fatal dose (of a toxin).

L-form L-phase variant; see under *variant.*

L.F.P. left frontoposterior (left mentoposterior, a position of the fetus).

L.F.P.S. Licentiate of the Faculty of Physicians and Surgeons.

L.F.T. left frontotransverse (left mentotransverse, a position of the fetus).

LGH lactogenic hormone.

LH luteinizing hormone.

Lhermitte's sign (lār′mits) [Jean *Lhermitte*, Paris neurologist, 1877–1959] see under *sign.*

LH-RH luteinizing hormone releasing hormone; see *gonadotropin releasing hormone*, under *hormone.*

Li chemical symbol for *lithium.*

LIA leukemia-associated inhibitory activity; see under *activity.*

Lib. abbreviation for L. *li′bra*, a pound.

liberomotor (lib″er-o-mo′tor) [L. *liber* free + *motor* mover] pertaining to voluntary and conscious movements or actions.

libidinal (lĭ-bid′ĭ-nal) pertaining to or of the nature of libido; erotic.

libidinous (lĭ-bid′ĭ-nus) [L. *libidinosus*] lustful or salacious.

libido (lĭ-be′do, lĭ-bi′do), pl. *libid′ines* [L.] 1. sexual desire. 2. the energy derived from the primitive impulses. In psychoanalysis the term is applied to the motive power of the sex life; in freudian psychology to psychic energy in general. **bisexual l.,** the fixation of the sexual impulse on both masculine and feminine. **ego l.,** self-love; narcissism.

Libman-Sacks disease (syndrome) (lib′man-saks′) [Emanuel *Libman*, New York physician, 1872–1946; Benjamin *Sacks*, New York physician] atypical verrucous endocarditis.

LiBr lithium bromide.

libra (li′brah) [L.] 1. pound. 2. balance.

Librium (lib′re-um) trademark for preparations of chlordiazepoxide hydrochloride.

lice (līs) plural of *louse.*

license (li′sens) [L. *licere* to be permitted] a permit to perform acts which without it would be illegal.

licentiate (li-sen′she-āt) [L. *licentia* license] one holding a license from an authorized agency entitling him to practice a particular profession.

lichen (li′ken) [Gr. *leichēn* a tree-moss] 1. any of the many thallophytic plants formed by mutualistic combination of an alga and a fungus, the algal component being a green or blue-green alga, and the fungal usually an ascomycete. 2. a name applied to many different kinds of papular skin diseases in which the lesions are typically small, firm papules that are usually set very close together, the specific type being indicated by a modifying term. **l. amyloido′sus,** a lichenoid skin eruption, most often of the shins, characterized by localized cutaneous amyloidosis; called also *lichinoid amyloidosis.* **l. chron′icus sim′plex,** l. simplex chronicus. **l. cor′neus hypertro′phicus,** a papular skin eruption of thickened and horny lesions. **l. fibromucinoido′sus,** l. myxedematosus. **l. myxedemato′sus,** a condition characterized by abnormal amounts of acid mucopolysaccharides (mucinosis) in the intersticies of the cutis, as well as in vessels of many organs, and a widespread eruption of asymptomatic soft, pale-red or yellowish papules 2 to 3 mm. in diameter, which do not coalesce. Although the condition resembles myxedema, it is not associated with thyroid dysfunction. **l. nit′idus,** a rare skin eruption consisting of numerous, pinhead-sized, pale, flat, sharply marginated, glistening, exquisitely discrete papules, scarcely raised above the level of the skin; called also *Pinkus' disease.* **l. obtus′us cor′neus,** a papular eruption of thickened, blunt lesions; probably identical with prurigo nodularis. **l. pila′ris,** l. spinulosus. **l. planopila′ris,** a variant of lichen planus characterized by formation, around the hair follicles, of acuminate horny papules, in addition to the typical lesions of ordinary lichen planus; in its full-blown form there is also loss of hair from the scalp and other regions of the body. **l. pla′nus,** an inflammatory skin disease with wide, flat, violaceous, itchy, polygonal papules having a characteristic sheen, occurring in circumscribed patches, and often very persistent. The hair follicles and nails may become involved, and the buccal mucosa may be affected. The etiology is unknown but an emotional basis is suspected. **l. pla′nus, acute bullous,** a variety of lichen planus in which the dermal infiltrate produces subepidermal clefts that become frank blisters; binding of complement to the basement membrane may be the fundamental lesion. **l. pla′nus, hypertrophic, l. pla′nus hypertroph′icus,** lichen planus in which there is marked acanthosis and a great increase in the thickness of the granular layer of the epidermis, with a particularly heavy lymphocytic infiltration immediately under the epidermis, and a verrucous surface. **l. ru′ber monilifor′mis,** a variant of lichen simplex chronicus, the supposed beaded arrangement of papules being the prominent alveolar pattern of the skin between the deepened furrows. **l. ru′ber pla′nus,** l. planus. **l. sclero′sus et atroph′icus,** a chronic, atrophic skin disease characterized by white, angular, flat, well-defined, indurated papules with an erythematous halo and follicular, black, keratotic plugs. It is the most common cause of kraurosis vulvae in females and balanitis xerotica obliterans in males. Called also *white-spot disease* and *Csillag's disease.* **l. scrofuloso′rum, l. scrofulo′sus,** an eruption of minute reddish lichenoid follicular papules, occurring in children or young adults with tuberculosis, as a result of hematogenous dissemination of bacilli in a person with strong tuberculin sensitivity. **l. sim′plex chron′icus,** a skin disease of psychogenic origin, marked by a pruritic discrete or, more often, confluent lichenoid papular eruption, usually confined to a localized area, especially the anogenital region, back of the neck, knee, ankle, or elbow flexures, or dorsum of the hands and feet; called also *circumscribed* or *localized neurodermatitis, neurodermatitis circumscripta, lichen Vidal*, and *Vidal's disease.* **l. spinulo′sus,** a condition in which there is a horn or spine in the center of each hair follicle; called also *l. pilaris.* **l. stria′tus,** a condition characterized by an otherwise asymptomatic linear lichenoid papular eruption, usually occurring in children, almost always along the line separating the lumbar from the sacral neuromeres or the cervical from the thoracic neuromeres and clearing spontaneously after about 6 to 18 months. **l. trop′icus,** miliaria rubra. **l. urtica′tus,** papular urticaria. **l. Vidal,** l. simplex chronicus.

lichenase (li′ken-ās) laminarinase.

lichenification (li-ken″ĭ-fi-ka′shun) thickening of the epidermis, with exaggeration of its normal markings so that the striae form a criss-cross pattern, enclosing flat-topped, shiny, smooth quadrilateral facets between them. It is caused by scratching and rubbing in excess of what the normal pain threshold would permit, usually in persons predisposed by inheritance of the atopic diathesis.

licheniformin (li-ken″ĭ-form′in) a group of antibiotic substances (licheniformin A, B, and C) isolated from *Bacillus subtilis*, resembling subtilin in their properties.

lichenin (li′kĕ-nin) a starchy demulcent polysaccharide, $(C_6H_{10}-O_5)_n$, which yields glucose on hydrolysis. It occurs abundantly in Iceland moss, *Cetraria islandica*. Called also *lichen starch* and *moss starch*.

lichenization (li″ken-i-za′shun) (*obs.*) the development of patches of lichen.

lichenoid (li′ken-oid) [*lichen* + Gr. *eidos* form] resembling the skin lesions designated as lichen.

Lichtheim's aphasia, etc. (likt′hīmz) [Ludwig *Lichtheim*, German physician, 1845–1928] see under *aphasia, disease, plaque, sign, syndrome,* and *tests.*

Lichtheimia (lik-thi′me-ah) former name for the genus *Absidia.*

Lic.Med. Licentiate in Medicine.

Li₂CO₃ lithium carbonate.

licorice (lik′o-ris) glycyrrhiza.

lid (lid) an eyelid. **granular l's,** trachoma, def. 1. **tucked l. of Collier,** a retraction of the upper eyelid in cases of ophthalmoplegia due to a supranuclear lesion in the brain stem.

Lida-Mantle (li″dah-man′t'l) trademark for a preparation of lidocaine.

Liddel and Sherrington reflex [Edward George Tandy *Liddel*, British physiologist, born 1895; Sir Charles Scott *Sherrington*, English physiologist, 1857–1952] stretch reflex.

Lidex (li′deks) trademark for preparations of fluocinonide.

lidocaine (li′do-kān) [USP] chemical name: 2-(diethylamino)-*N*-(2,6-dimethylphenyl)acetamide. A drug, $C_{14}H_{22}N_2O$, having anesthetic, sedative, analgesic, anticonvulsant, and cardiac depressant activities, occurring as a white or slightly yellow, crystalline powder; used as a local anesthetic, applied topically to the skin and mucous membranes. **l. hydrochloride** [USP], the monohydrated monohydrochloride salt of lidocaine, $C_{14}H_{22}N_2$-$O \cdot HCl \cdot H_2O$, occurring as a white, crystalline powder; used as a cardiac antiarrhythmic, administered intravenously, and to produce local anesthesia by infiltration injection and epidural and peripheral nerve block.

lidofenin (li″do-fen′in) chemical name: *N*-(carboxymethyl)-*N*-[2-[(2,6-dimethylphenyl)amino]-2-oxoethyl]glycine; a diagnostic aid for determination of hepatic function, $C_{14}H_{18}N_2O_5$.

lidofilcon (li″do-fil′kon) chemical name: 1-ethenyl-2-pyrrolidinone polymer with methyl 2-methyl-2-propenoate, 2-propenyl 2-methyl-2-propenoate, and 1,2-ethanediyl bis(2-methyl-2-propenoate); either of two hydrophilic contact lens materials, $(C_6H_9NO)_w(C_5H_8O_2)_x(C_7H_{10}O_2)_y(C_{10}H_{14}O_4)_z$, one of which contains 70 per cent water (*lidofilcon A*), and the other 85 per cent water (*lidofilcon B*).

lidoflazine (li-do-fla′zēn) chemical name: 4-[4,4-bis-(4-fluorophenyl)butyl]-*N*-(2,6-dimethylphenyl)-1-piperazineacetamide; a coronary vasodilator, $C_{30}H_{35}F_2N_2O$.

lie (li) the situation of the long axis of the fetus with respect to that of the mother; see *presentation.* **transverse l.,** the situation of the fetus during labor when the long axis of its body crosses the long axis of the maternal body. The shoulder usually presents first, but the arm, trunk, or any other part of the trunk may be the first to appear. Called also *torso, transverse,* or *trunk presentation.* See table of Positions of the Fetus in Various Presentations, under *position.*

Lieben's test (reaction) (le′benz) [Adolf *Lieben*, Austrian chemist, 1836–1914] see under *tests.*

Lieberkühn's ampulla, crypts, follicles, glands (le′ber-kēnz) [Johann Nathaniel *Lieberkühn*, German anatomist, 1711–1756] see under *ampulla,* and see *glandulae intestinales.*

Liebermann's test (le′ber-mahnz) [Leo von Szentlörincz *Liebermann,* Hungarian physician, 1852–1926] see under *tests.*

Liebermeister's furrows, grooves, rule (le′ber-mis″terz) [Carl von *Liebermeister,* German physician, 1833–1901] see under *furrow, groove,* and *rule.*

Liebig's test, theory (le′bigz) [Baron Justus von *Liebig,* German chemist, 1803–1873] see under *tests* and *theory.*

lien (li′en) [L.] [NA] the spleen: a large glandlike but ductless organ situated in the upper part of the abdomen; see *spleen.* **l. accesso′rius** [NA], a connected or detached outlying portion, or exclave, of the spleen; called also *accessory spleen.* **l. mo′bilis,** floating spleen.

lienal (li-e′nal) pertaining to the spleen; splenic.

lienculus (li-en′ku-lus) an accessory spleen (lien accessorius [NA].

lienectomy (li″ĕ-nek′to-me) splenectomy.

lienitis (li″ĕ-ni′tis) splenitis.

lieno- (li-e′no) [L. *lien* spleen] a combining form denoting relationship to the spleen.

lienocele (li-e′no-sēl) splenocele.

lienography (li″e-nog′rah-fe) splenography.

lienomalacia (li-e″no-mah-la′she-ah) splenomalacia.

lienomedullary (li-e″no-med′u-la″re) splenomedullary.

lienomyelogenous (li-e″no-mi″ĕ-loj′ĕ-nus) splenomyelogenous.

lienomyelomalacia (li-e″no-mi″ĕ-lo-mah-la′she-ah) splenomyelomalacia.

lienopancreatic (li-e″no-pan″kre-at′ik) splenopancreatic.

lienopathy (li″e-nop′ah-the) splenopathy.

lienorenal (li-e″no-re′nal) pertaining to the spleen and the kidney.

lienotoxin (li-e″no-tok′sin) [*lieno-* + *toxin*] splenotoxin.

lienteric (li″en-ter′ik) affected by or of the nature of a lientery.

lientery (li′en-ter″e) [Gr. *leienteria; leios* smooth + *enteron* intestine] diarrhea in which the stools contain undigested food.

lienunculus (li″en-ung′ku-lus) a detached mass or exclave of splenic tissue; an accessory spleen.

Liepmann's apraxia (lēp′manz) [Hugo Carl *Liepmann,* Berlin neurologist, 1863–1925] see under *apraxia.*

Liesegang's phenomenon (striae, waves) (le′zĕ-gahng) [Ralph Eduard *Liesegang,* German chemist, 1869–1947] see under *phenomenon.*

Lieutaud's triangle (body), uvula (luette) (lu-toz′) [Joseph *Lieutaud,* French physician, 1703–1780] see *trigonum vesicae* and *uvula vesicae.*

LIF left iliac fossa; leukocyte inhibitory factor.

life (līf) [L. *vita;* Gr. *bios* or *zōe*] the aggregate of vital phenomena; a certain peculiar stimulated condition of organized matter; that obscure principle whereby organized beings are peculiarly endowed with certain powers and functions not associated with inorganic matter. Generally, living things share, in varying degrees, the following characteristics: organization, irritability, movement, growth, reproduction, and adaptation. **animal l.,** vegetative life conjoined with the employment of the senses and with spontaneous movements. **intellectual l., mental l., psychic l.,** that which is attended by conscious exercise of feelings, impulses, and will, and by reason. **intrauterine l., uterine l.,** the period of life spent in the uterus; i.e., embryonic and fetal life. **vegetative l.,** that which is manifested in automatic acts requisite for the maintenance of the individual and the propagation of the species.

lifibrate (lĭ-fi′brāt) chemical name: bis(4-chlorophenoxy)acetic acid 1-methyl-4-piperidinyl ester; an antihyperlipidemic, $C_{20}H_{21}-Cl_2NO_4$.

lig. ligament; ligamentum.

ligament (lig′ah-ment) 1. a band of fibrous tissue that connects bones or cartilages, serving to support and strengthen joints; see *ligamentum.* 2. a double layer of peritoneum extending from one visceral organ to another. 3. cordlike remnants of fetal tubular structures that are nonfunctional after birth. **accessory l.,** any ligament that strengthens or supports another. **accessory l's, volar,** ligamenta palmaria. **accessory l's of digits of hand,** ligamenta palmaria. **accessory l. of Henle, lateral,** ligamentum laterale articulationis temporomandibularis. **accessory l. of Henle, medial,** ligamentum sphenomandibulare. **accessory l. of humerus,** ligamentum coracohumerale. **accessory l's of metacarpophalangeal joints,** ligamenta collateralia articulationum metacarpophalangearum. **acromioclavicular l.,** ligamentum acromioclaviculare. **acromiocoracoid l.,** ligamentum coracoacromiale. **adipose l. of knee (of Cruveilhier),** plica synovialis infrapatellaris. **alar l's,** ligamenta alaria. **alar l's of knee,** plicae alares. **alveolodental l.,** periodontal l. **annular l., dorsal common,** retinaculum extensorum manus. **annular l., inferior,** ligamentum arcuatum pubis. **annular l., internal,** retinaculum musculorum flexorum pedis. **annular l., tracheal,** ligamenta anularia trachealia. **annular l. of ankle, external,** retinaculum musculorum peroneorum superius. **annular l. of ankle, internal,** retinaculum musculorum flexorum pedis. **annular l. of base of stapes,** ligamentum anulare stapedis. **annular l. of carpus, posterior,** retinaculum extensorum manus. **annular l's of digits of foot,** see *pars anularis vaginae fibrosae digitorum pedis.* **annular l's of digits of hand,** see *pars anularis vaginae fibrosae digitorum manus.* **annular l. of femur,** zona orbicularis articulationis coxae. **annular l. of finger,** pars anularis vaginae fibrosae digitorum manus. **annular l. of malleolus, external,** retinaculum musculorum extensorum pedis inferius. **annular l. of malleolus, internal,** retinaculum musculorum flexorum pedis. **annular l. of radius,** ligamentum anulare radii. **annular l. of stapes,** ligamentum anulare stapedis. **annular l. of tarsus, anterior,** retinaculum musculorum extensorum pedis inferius. **annular l's of tendon sheaths of fingers,** see *pars anularis vaginae fibrosae digitorum manus.* **annular l. of wrist, dorsal posterior,** retinaculum extensorum manus. **anococcygeal l.,** ligamentum anococcygeum. **anterior l. of colon,** tenia omentalis. **anterior l. of head of fibula,** ligamentum capitis fibulae anterius. **anterior l. of head of rib,** ligamentum capitis costae radiatum. **anterior l. of malleus,** ligamentum mallei anterius. **anterior l. of neck of rib,** ante-

Plate XXIV   ligament

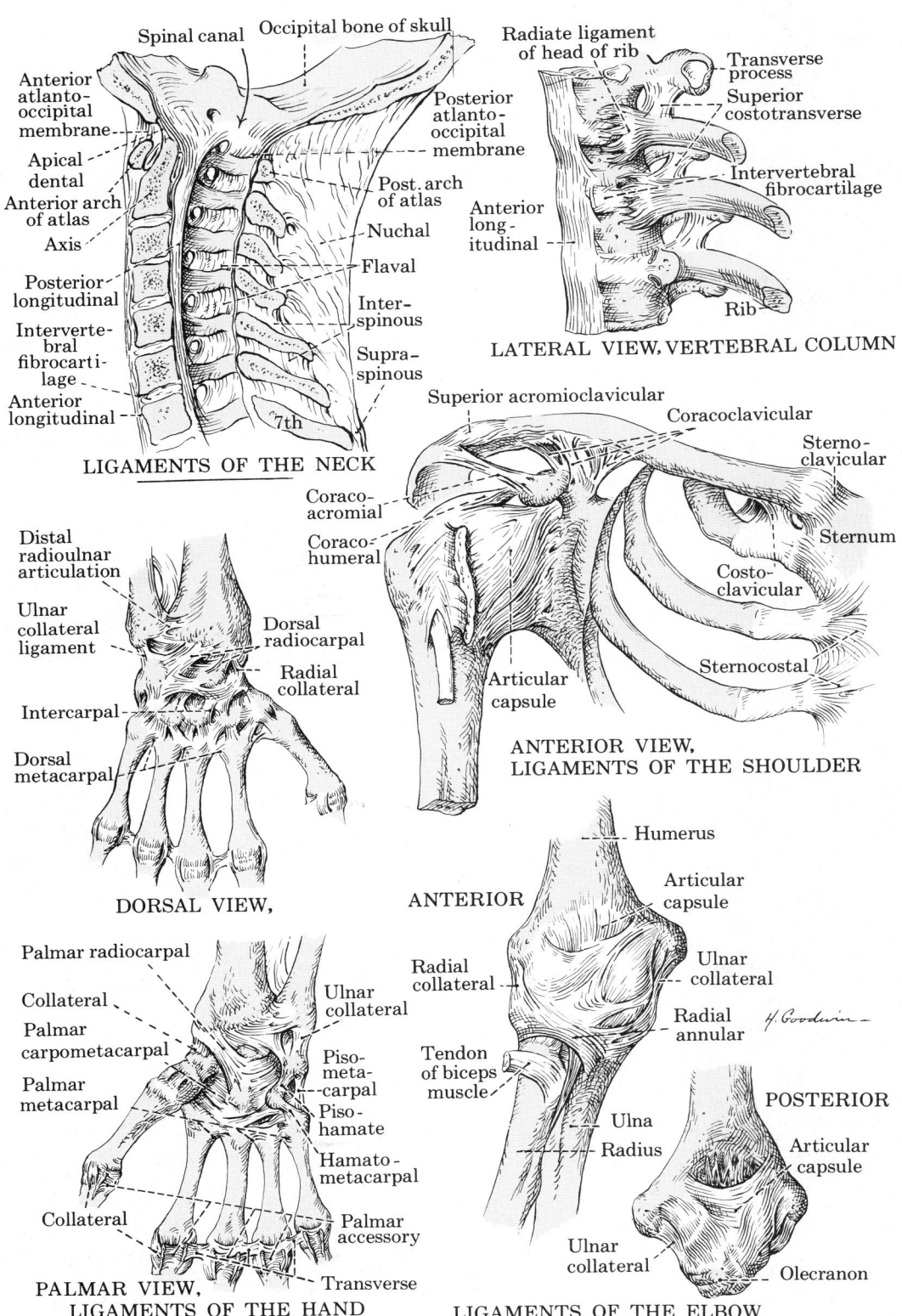

Spinal canal   Occipital bone of skull

Anterior atlanto-occipital membrane

Apical dental

Anterior arch of atlas

Axis

Posterior longitudinal

Intervertebral fibrocartilage

Anterior longitudinal

Posterior atlanto-occipital membrane

Post. arch of atlas

Nuchal

Flaval

Interspinous

Supraspinous

7th

LIGAMENTS OF THE NECK

Radiate ligament of head of rib

Transverse process

Superior costotransverse

Anterior longitudinal

Intervertebral fibrocartilage

Rib

LATERAL VIEW, VERTEBRAL COLUMN

Distal radioulnar articulation

Ulnar collateral ligament

Intercarpal

Dorsal metacarpal

Dorsal radiocarpal

Radial collateral

DORSAL VIEW,

Superior acromioclavicular

Coracoacromial

Coracohumeral

Articular capsule

Coracoclavicular

Sternoclavicular

Sternum

Costoclavicular

Sternocostal

ANTERIOR VIEW, LIGAMENTS OF THE SHOULDER

Palmar radiocarpal

Collateral

Palmar carpometacarpal

Palmar metacarpal

Collateral

PALMAR VIEW, LIGAMENTS OF THE HAND

Ulnar collateral

Pisometacarpal

Pisohamate

Hamatometacarpal

Palmar accessory

Transverse

ANTERIOR

Radial collateral

Tendon of biceps muscle

Humerus

Articular capsule

Ulnar collateral

Radial annular

H. Goodwin

Ulna

Radius

POSTERIOR

Articular capsule

Ulnar collateral

Olecranon

LIGAMENTS OF THE ELBOW

ARTICULAR LIGAMENTS

Plate XXV   ligament

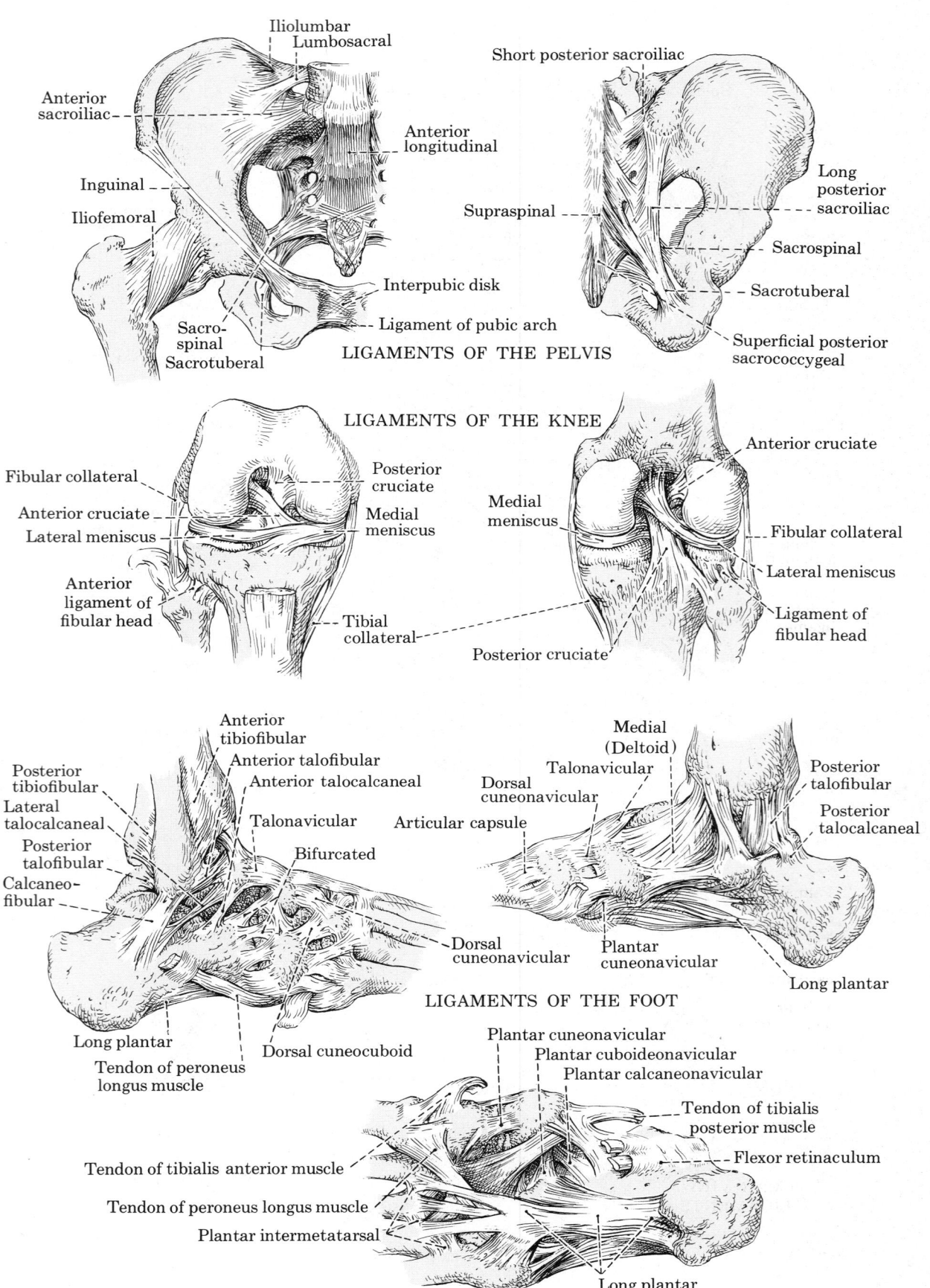

Iliolumbar
Lumbosacral
Short posterior sacroiliac
Anterior sacroiliac
Anterior longitudinal
Long posterior sacroiliac
Inguinal
Supraspinal
Iliofemoral
Sacrospinal
Sacrotuberal
Interpubic disk
Sacro-spinal
Sacrotuberal
Ligament of pubic arch
Superficial posterior sacrococcygeal

LIGAMENTS OF THE PELVIS

LIGAMENTS OF THE KNEE

Fibular collateral
Posterior cruciate
Anterior cruciate
Medial meniscus
Lateral meniscus
Anterior cruciate
Medial meniscus
Fibular collateral
Lateral meniscus
Anterior ligament of fibular head
Ligament of fibular head
Tibial collateral
Posterior cruciate

Anterior tibiofibular
Anterior talofibular
Anterior talocalcaneal
Posterior tibiofibular
Medial (Deltoid)
Talonavicular
Lateral talocalcaneal
Talonavicular
Dorsal cuneonavicular
Posterior talofibular
Posterior talofibular
Articular capsule
Posterior talocalcaneal
Calcaneo-fibular
Bifurcated
Dorsal cuneonavicular
Plantar cuneonavicular
Long plantar
Long plantar
Dorsal cuneocuboid
Tendon of peroneus longus muscle

LIGAMENTS OF THE FOOT

Plantar cuneonavicular
Plantar cuboideonavicular
Plantar calcaneonavicular
Tendon of tibialis posterior muscle
Tendon of tibialis anterior muscle
Flexor retinaculum
Tendon of peroneus longus muscle
Plantar intermetatarsal
Long plantar

ARTICULAR LIGAMENTS

rior portion of ligamentum costotransversarium superius. **anterior l. of radiocarpal joint,** ligamentum radiocarpeum palmare. **l. of antibrachium (of Weitbrecht),** chorda obliqua membranae interosseae antebrachii. **apical dental l., apical odontoid l.,** ligamentum apicis dentis axis. **appendiculo-ovarian l.,** a fold of peritoneum extending between the appendix and the broad ligament of the uterus. **Arantius' l.,** ligamentum venosum. **arcuate l.,** ligamentum flavum. **arcuate l., lateral,** ligamentum arcuatum laterale. **arcuate l., medial,** ligamentum arcuatum mediale. **arcuate l., median,** l. arcuatum medianum. **arcuate l., pubic,** ligamentum arcuatum pubis. **arcuate l. of diaphragm, external,** ligamentum arcuatum laterale. **arcuate l. of diaphragm, internal,** ligamentum arcuatum mediale. **arcuate l. of diaphragm, lateral,** ligamentum arcuatum laterale. **arcuate l. of knee,** ligamentum popliteum arcuatum. **arcuate l. of pubis, inferior,** ligamentum arcuatum pubis. **Arnold's l.,** ligamentum incudis superius. **articular l. of vertebrae,** capsula articularis articulationum vertebrarum. **arytenoepiglottic l.,** plica aryepiglottica. **atlantooccipital l., anterior, atlantooccipital l., deep,** membrana atlantooccipitalis anterior. **atlantooccipital l., posterior,** membrana atlantooccipitalis posterior. **l's of auditory ossicles,** ligamenta ossiculorum auditus. **l's of auricle of external ear,** ligamenta auricularia. **auricular l., anterior,** ligamentum auriculare anterius. **auricular l., posterior,** ligamentum auriculare posterius. **auricular l., superior,** ligamentum auriculare superius. **Barkow's l.,** the anterior and posterior parts of the elbow joint capsule. **Bellini's l.,** a band passing as part of the capsule of the hip joint to the greater trochanter. **Bérard's l.,** the suspensory ligament of the pericardium, extending to the third and fourth thoracic vertebrae. **Berry's l.,** ligamentum thyrohyoideum. **Bertin's l.,** ligamentum iliofemorale. **Bichat's l.,** the lower bundle of the dorsal sacroiliac ligament. **bifurcate l.,** ligamentum bifurcatum. **bifurcate l's, deep,** ligamenta metatarsea plantaria. **bifurcate l's of Arnold, deep,** ligamenta tarsometatarsea plantaria. **Bigelow's l.,** ligamentum iliofemorale. **bigeminate l's of Arnold,** ligamenta tarsometatarsea dorsalia. **l. of Botallo,** ligamentum arteriosum. **Bourgery's l.,** ligamentum popliteum obliquum. **brachiocubital l.,** ligamentum collaterale ulnare. **brachioradial l.,** ligamentum collaterale radiale. **broad l. of liver,** ligamentum falciforme hepatis. **broad l. of lung,** ligamentum pulmonale. **broad l. of uterus,** the peritoneal fold that supports the uterus on either side; called also *ligamentum latum uteri* [NA]. **Brodie's l.,** the transverse humeral ligament. **Burns' l.,** margo falciformis hiatus saphenus. **calcaneocuboid l.,** ligamentum calcaneocuboideum. **calcaneocuboid l., plantar,** ligamentum calcaneocuboideum plantare. **calcaneofibular l.,** ligamentum calcaneofibulare. **calcaneonavicular l.,** ligamentum calcaneonaviculare. **calcaneonavicular l., dorsal,** ligamentum calcaneonaviculare dorsale. **calcaneonavicular l., plantar,** ligamentum calcaneonaviculare plantare. **calcaneotibial l.,** pars tibiocalcanea ligamenti medialis. **Caldani's l.,** a band passing from the inner border of the coracoid process to the lower border of the clavicle, the first rib, and the tendon of the subclavius. **Campbell's l.,** suspensory l. of axilla. **Camper's l.,** diaphragma urogenitale. **canthal l's,** see *ligamentum palpebrale mediale* and *raphe palpebralis lateralis*. **capitular l., volar,** ligamentum metacarpeum transversum profundum. **capsular l.,** capsula articularis. **capsular l., internal,** ligamentum capitis femoris. **capsular l., pelviprostatic,** fascia prostatae. **Carcassonne's l.,** ligamentum puboprostaticum. **cardinal l.,** part of a thickening of the visceral pelvic fascia beside the cervix and vagina, passing laterally to merge with the upper fascia of the pelvic diaphragm; called also *lateral cervical l.* **carpal l., dorsal,** see *ligamenta intercarpea dorsalia*. **carpal l., oblique accessory,** ligamentum radiocarpeum palmare. **carpal l., radiate,** ligamentum carpi radiatum. **carpal l., ulnar,** ligamentum collaterale carpi ulnare. **carpometacarpal l's, anterior,** ligamenta carpometacarpea palmaria. **carpometacarpal l's, dorsal,** ligamenta carpometacarpea dorsalia. **carpometacarpal l's, oblique palmar,** ligamenta carpometacarpea palmaria. **carpometacarpal l's, palmar,** ligamenta metacarpea palmaria. **carpometacarpal l's, posterior,** ligamenta carpometacarpea dorsalia. **carpometacarpal l's, volar,** ligamenta carpometacarpea palmaria. **Casser's l., casserian l.,** ligamentum mallei laterale. **caudal l. of common integument,** retinaculum caudale. **cervical l., anterior,** membrana tectoria. **cervical l., lateral,** cardinal l. **cervical l., posterior,** ligamentum nuchae. **cervical l. of sinus tarsi,** a strong band behind the bifurcate ligament, extending upward to the neck of the talus. **cervicobasilar l.,** membrana tectoria. **check l's of axis,** ligamenta alaria. **chondrosternal l., interarticular,** ligamentum sternocostale intraarticulare. **chondroxiphoid l's,** ligamenta costoxiphoidea. **l. of Civinini,** ligamentum pterygospinale. **Clado's l.,** an occasional peritoneal fold connecting the infundibulopelvic ligament and the mesoappendix. **clavicular l., external capsular,** ligamentum acromioclaviculare. **Cloquet's**

l., vestigium processus vaginalis. **coccygeal l., superior,** ligamentum iliofemorale. **collateral l., fibular,** ligamentum collaterale fibulare. **collateral l., radial,** ligamentum collaterale radiale. **collateral l., radial carpal,** ligamenta collaterale carpi radiale. **collateral l., tibial,** ligamentum collaterale tibiale. **collateral l., ulnar,** ligamentum collaterale ulnare. **collateral l., ulnar carpal,** ligamenta collaterale carpi ulnare. **collateral l. of carpus, radial,** ligamentum collaterale carpi radiale. **collateral l. of carpus, ulnar,** ligamentum collaterale carpi ulnare. **collateral l's of interphalangeal articulations of foot,** ligamenta collateralia articulationum interphalangearum pedis. **collateral l's of interphalangeal articulations of hand,** ligamenta collateralia articulationum interphalangearum manus. **collateral l's of joints of fingers,** ligamenta collateralia articulationum interphalangearum manus. **collateral l's of joints of toes,** ligamenta collateralia articulationum interphalangearum pedis. **collateral l's of metacarpophalangeal articulations,** ligamenta collateralia articulationum metacarpophalangearum. **collateral l's of metatarsophalangeal articulations,** ligamenta collateralia articulationum metatarsophalangearum. **Colles' l.,** ligamentum inguinale reflexum. **l's of colon,** teniae coli. **common l. of knee (of Weber),** ligamentum transversum genus. **common l. of wrist joint, deep,** ligamentum collaterale carpi radiale. **conoid l.,** ligamentum conoideum. **Cooper's l.,** ligamentum pectineale. **Cooper's suspensory l's,** ligamenta suspensoria mammae. **coracoacromial l.,** ligamentum coracoacromiale. **coracocapsular l's,** ligamenta cinguli extremitatis superioris. **coracoclavicular l.,** ligamentum coracoclaviculare. **coracoclavicular l., external,** ligamentum trapezoideum. **coracoclavicular l., internal,** ligamentum conoideum. **coracohumeral l.,** ligamentum coracohumerale. **coracoid l. of scapula,** ligamentum transversum scapulae superius. **cordiform l. of diaphragm,** centrum tendineum. **coronary l. of liver,** ligamentum coronarium hepatis. **coronary l. of radius,** ligamentum anulare radii. **costocentral l., anterior,** ligamentum capitis costae radiatum. **costocentral l., interarticular,** ligamentum capitis costae intraarticulare. **costoclavicular l.,** ligamentum costoclaviculare. **costocolic l.,** ligamentum phrenicolicum. **costocoracoid l.,** ligamentum transversum scapulae superius. **costopericardiac l.,** a band of connective tissue joining the upper costosternal articulation with the pericardium. **costosternal l's, radiate,** ligamenta sternocostalia radiata. **costotransverse l.,** ligamentum costotransversarium. **costotransverse l., anterior,** ligamentum costotransversarium superius. **costotransverse l., lateral,** ligamentum costotransversarium laterale. **costotransverse l., posterior,** ligamentum costotransversarium superius. **costotransverse l., superior,** ligamentum costotransversarium superius. **costotransverse l. of Krause, posterior,** ligamentum costotransversarium laterale. **costovertebral l.,** ligamentum capitis costae radiatum. **costoxiphoid l's,** ligamenta costoxiphoidea. **cotyloid l.,** labrum acetabulare. **Cowper's l.,** fascia pectinea. **cricoarytenoid l., posterior,** ligamentum cricoarytenoideum posterius. **cricopharyngeal l., cricosantorinian l.,** ligamentum cricopharyngeum. **cricothyroarytenoid l.,** conus elasticus laryngis. **cricothyroid l.,** ligamentum cricothyroideum. **cricotracheal l.,** ligamentum cricotracheale. **crucial l's of fingers,** see *pars cruciformis vaginae fibrosae digitorum manus*. **crucial l. of foot,** retinaculum musculorum extensorum pedis inferius. **cruciate l. of atlas,** ligamentum cruciforme atlantis. **cruciate l's of fingers,** see *pars cruciformis vaginae fibrosae digitorum manus*. **cruciate l's of knee,** ligamenta cruciata genus. **cruciate l. of knee, anterior,** ligamentum cruciatum anterius genus. **cruciate l. of knee, posterior,** ligamentum cruciatum posterius genus. **cruciate l. of leg,** retinaculum musculorum extensorum pedis inferius. **cruciate l's of toes,** see *pars cruciformis vaginae fibrosae digitorum pedis*. **cruciform l. of atlas,** ligamentum cruciforme atlantis. **crural l.,** ligamentum inguinale. **Cruveilhier's l's,** ligamenta palmaria. **cubitoradial l.,** chorda obliqua membranae interosseae antibrachii. **cubitoulnar l.,** ligamentum collaterale ulnare. **cuboideometatarsal l's, short,** ligamenta tarsometatarsea plantaria. **cuboideonavicular l., dorsal,** ligamentum cuboideonaviculare dorsale. **cuboideonavicular l., oblique,** ligamentum cuboideonaviculare plantare. **cuboideonavicular l., plantar,** ligamentum cuboideonaviculare plantare. **cubonavicular l.,** ligamentum cuboideonaviculare plantare. **cuboscaphoid l., plantar,** ligamentum cuboideonaviculare plantare. **cuneocuboid l., dorsal,** ligamentum cuneocuboideum dorsale. **cuneocuboid l., interosseous,** ligamentum cuneocuboideum interosseum. **cuneocuboid l., plantar,** ligamentum cuneocuboidum plantare. **cuneometatarsal l's, interosseous,** ligamenta cuneometatarsea interossea. **cuneonavicular l's, dorsal,** ligamenta cuneonavicularia dorsalia. **cuneonavicular l's, plantar,** ligamenta cuneonavicularia plantaria. **cutaneophalangeal l's,** connecting fibers from the sides of the phalanges near the joints to the skin. **cysticoduodenal l.,** an anomalous fold of peritoneum extending between the gallbladder and the duodenum. **deep l's of tarsus**, ligamenta tarsi profunda. **deltoid l. of ankle**, ligamentum mediale. **deltoid l. of elbow**, ligamentum collaterale ulnare. **dentate l. of spinal cord, denticulate l.**, ligamentum denticulatum. **Denucé's l.**, a short, wide band connecting the radius and the ulna at the wrist. **diaphragmatic l.**, the involuting urogenital ridge that becomes the suspensory ligament of the ovary. **dorsal l's, carpal**, ligamenta intercarpea dorsalia. **dorsal l's, talonavicular**, ligamentum talonaviculare. **dorsal l's of bases of metacarpal bones**, ligamenta metacarpea dorsalia. **dorsal l's of bases of metatarsal bones**, ligamenta metatarsea dorsalia. **dorsal l. of radiocarpal joint**, ligamentum radiocarpeum dorsale. **dorsal l's of tarsus**, ligamenta tarsi dorsalia. **dorsal l. of wrist**, retinaculum extensorum manus. **Douglas' l.**, plica rectouterina. **duodenohepatic l.**, ligamentum hepatoduodenale. **duodenorenal l.**, ligamentum duodenorenale. **epihyal l.**, ligamentum stylohyoideum. **external l's of Barkow, plantar**, ligamenta intercuneiformia plantaria. **external l. of mandibular articulation**, ligamentum laterale articulationis temporomandibularis. **external l. of neck of rib**, ligamentum costotransversarium posterius. **fabellofibular l.**, an occasional ligament apparently replacing the short lateral ligament when the fabella is present; it originates directly from the fabella, passes between the condylar portions of the plantaris and lateral gastrocnemius muscles, and is attached to the apex of the fibula. **falciform l.**, processus falciformis ligamenti sacrotuberosi. **falciform l. of liver**, ligamentum falciforme hepatis. **fallopian l., l. of Fallopius**, ligamentum inguinale. **false l.**, 1. any suspensory ligament that is a peritoneal fold and not of true ligamentous structure. 2. a peritoneal connection between the vertex and sides of the bladder and the walls of the pelvis. **Ferrein's l.**, the thick external part of the capsule of the temporomandibular joint. **fibrous l., anterior**, ligamentum sternoclaviculare anterius. **fibrous l. posterior**, ligamentum sternoclaviculare posterius. **flaval l.**, ligamentum flavum. **Flood's l.**, the superior glenohumeral ligament. **fundiform l. of penis**, ligamentum fundiforme penis. **gastrocolic l.**, ligamentum gastrocolicum. **gastrohepatic l.**, ligamentum hepatogastricum. **gastrolienal l.**, ligamentum gastrolienale. **gastropancreatic l's of Huschke**, plicae gastropancreaticae. **gastrophrenic l.**, ligamentum gastrophrenicum. **gastrosplenic l.**, ligamentum gastrolienale. **genitoinguinal l.**, ligamentum genitoinguinale. **Gerdy's l.**, suspensory l. of axilla. **Gimbernat's l.**, ligamentum lacunare. **l's of girdle of inferior extremity**, ligamenta cinguli extremitatis inferioris. **l's of girdle of superior extremity**, ligamenta cinguli extremitatis superioris. **glenohumeral l's**, ligamenta glenohumeralia. **glenoid l's of Cruveilhier**, ligamenta plantaria articulationum metatarsophalangearum. **glenoid l. of humerus, glenoid l. of Macalister**, labrum glenoidale. **glenoid l. of mandibular fossa**, a ring of fibrocartilage connected with the rim of the mandibular fossa. **Günz's l.**, part of the obturator membrane. **hamatometacarpal l.**, fibers connecting the hamulus of the hamate bone with the base of the fifth metacarpal bone. **l. of head of femur**, ligamentum capitis femoris. **Helmholtz's l.**, that part of the anterior ligament of the malleus which is attached to the greater tympanic spine. **l's of Helvetius**, ligamenta pylori. **Henle's l.**, falx inguinalis. **Hensing's l.**, a small serous fold from the upper end of the descending colon to the abdominal wall. **hepatic l's**, folds of peritoneum extending from the liver to adjacent structures. **hepatocolic l.**, ligamentum hepatocolicum. **hepatocystocolic l.**, a hepatocolic ligament arising from the gallbladder. **hepatoduodenal l.**, ligamentum hepatoduodenale. **hepatogastric l.**, ligamentum hepatogastricum. **hepatogastroduodenal l.**, omentum minus. **hepatorenal l.**, ligamentum hepatorenale. **hepatoumbilical l.**, ligamentum teres hepatis. **Hesselbach's l.**, ligamentum interfoveolare. **Hey's l.**, margo falciformis hiatus saphenus. **Hueck's l.**, ligamentum pectinatum anguli iridocornealis. **Humphry's l.**, ligamentum meniscofemorale anterius. **Hunter's l.**, ligamentum teres uteri. **Huschke's l's**, plicae gastropancreaticae. **hyaloideocapsular l.**, the tissue connecting the vitreous body to the peripheral zone of the lens capsule. **hyoepiglottic l.**, ligamentum hyoepiglotticum. **iliocostal l.**, ligamentum lumbocostale. **iliofemoral l.**, ligamentum iliofemorale. **iliolumbar l.**, ligamentum iliolumbale. **iliopectineal l.**, arcus iliopectineus. **iliopubic l.**, ligamentum inguinale. **iliosacral l's, anterior**, ligamenta sacroiliaca ventralia. **iliosacral l's, interosseous**, ligamenta sacroiliaca interossea. **iliosacral l., long**, ligamentum sacroiliaca dorsalia. **iliotibial l. of Maissiat**, tractus iliotibialis. **iliotrochanteric l.**, a portion of the articular capsule of the hip joint. **inferior l. of epididymis**, ligamentum epididymidis inferius. **inferior l. of neck of rib**, posterior portion of ligamentum costotransversarium posterius. **inferior l. of neck of rib of Henle**, ligamentum costotransversarium. **inferior l. of tubercle of rib**, ligamentum costotransversarium laterale. **infundibulopelvic l.**, ligamentum suspensorium ovarii. **inguinal l.**, ligamentum inguinale. **inguinal l., anterior**, crus mediale an-

uli inguinalis superficialis. **inguinal l., external**, ligamentum inguinale. **inguinal l., internal**, 1. ligamentum inguinale reflexum. 2. crus mediale anuli inguinalis superficialis. **inguinal l., posterior**, ligamentum interfoveolare. **inguinal l., reflex**, ligamentum inguinale reflexum. **inguinal l. of Blumberg**, ligamentum interfoveolare. **inguinal l. of Cooper**, ligamentum pectineale. **interarticular l.**, any ligament situated within the capsule of a joint. **interarticular l. of articulation of humerus**, caput longum musculi bicipitis brachii. **interarticular l. of head of rib**, ligamentum capitis costae intraarticulare. **interarticular l. of hip joint**, ligamentum capitis femoris. **intercarpal l's, dorsal**, ligamenta intercarpea dorsalia. **intercarpal l's, interosseous**, ligamenta intercarpea interossea. **intercarpal l's, palmar**, ligamenta intercarpea palmaria. **intercarpal l's, volar**, ligamenta intercarpea palmaria. **interclavicular l.**, ligamentum interclaviculare. **intercostal l's, external**, see *membrana intercostalis externa*. **intercostal l's, internal**, see *membrana intercostalis interna*. **intercuneiform l's, dorsal**, ligamenta intercuneiformia dorsalia. **intercuneiform l's, interosseous**, ligamenta intercuneiformia interossea. **intercuneiform l's, plantar**, ligamenta intercuneiformia plantaria. **interfoveolar l.**, ligamentum interfoveolare. **intermaxillary l.**, raphe pterygomandibularis. **intermetacarpal l's, anterior, intermetacarpal l's, distal**, see *ligamentum metacarpeum transversum profundum*. **intermetacarpal l's, dorsal**, ligamenta metacarpea dorsalia. **intermetacarpal l's, interosseous**, ligamenta metacarpea interossea. **intermetacarpal l's, palmar**, ligamenta metacarpea palmaria. **intermetacarpal l's, proximal, anterior**, ligamentametacarpea palmaria. **intermetacarpal l's, proximal, posterior**, ligamenta metacarpea dorsalia. **intermetacarpal l's, transverse, dorsal**, ligamenta metacarpea dorsalia. **intermetacarpal l's, transverse, volar**, ligamenta metacarpea palmaria. **intermetatarsal l's, interosseous**, ligamenta metatarsea interossea. **intermetatarsal l's, plantar, distal**, see *ligamentum metatarseum transversum profundum*. **intermetatarsal l's, proximal, dorsal**, ligamenta metatarsea dorsalia. **intermetatarsal l's, proximal, plantar**, ligamenta metatarsea plantaria. **intermetatarsal l's, transverse, dorsal**, ligamenta metatarsea dorsalia. **intermetatarsal l's, transverse, plantar**, ligamenta metatarsea plantaria. **intermuscular l., fibular**, septum intermusculare anterius cruris. **intermuscular l. of arm, external**, septum intermusculare brachii laterale. **intermuscular l. of arm, internal**, septum intermusculare brachii mediale. **intermuscular l. of arm, lateral**, septum intermusculare brachii laterale. **intermuscular l. of arm, medial**, septum intermusculare brachii mediale. **intermuscular l. of thigh, external**, septum intermusculare femoris laterale. **intermuscular l. of thigh, lateral**, septum intermusculare femoris laterale. **intermuscular l. of thigh, medial**, septum intermusculare femoris mediale. **internal l. of neck of rib**, ligamentum costotransversarium superius. **interosseous l., radioulnar**, membrana interossea antebrachii. **interosseous l's, transverse metacarpal**, ligamenta metacarpea interossea. **interosseous l's of Barkow, internal**, ligamenta intercuneiformia plantaria. **interosseous l's of bases of metacarpal bones**, ligamenta metacarpea interossea. **interosseous l's of bases of metatarsal bones**, ligamenta metatarsea interossea. **interosseous l. of Cruveilhier, costovertebral**, ligamentum capitis costae intraarticulare. **interosseous l. of Cruveilhier, transversocostal**, ligamentum costotransversarium. **interosseous l's of knee**, ligamenta cruciata genus. **interosseous l. of leg**, membrana interossea cruris. **interosseous l. of pubis**, discus interpubicus. **interosseous l. of pubis (of Winslow)**, ligamentum transversum perinei. **interosseous l's of tarsus**, ligamenta tarsi interossea. **interprocess l.**, a ligament that connects two processes on the same bone. **interpubic l.**, discus interpubicus. **interspinal l., interspinous l.**, ligamentum interspinale. **intertarsal l's, dorsal**, ligamenta tarsi dorsalia. **intertarsal l's, interosseous**, ligamenta tarsi interossea. **intertarsal l's, plantar**, ligamenta tarsi plantaria. **intertransverse l.**, ligamentum intertransversarium. **interureteral l.**, plica interureterica. **intervertebral l.**, 1. either of the two longitudinal ligaments of the vertebrae (ligamentum longitudinale anterius and ligamentum longitudinale posterius). 2. one of the disci intervertebrales. **intraarticular l. of head of rib**, ligamentum capitis costae intraarticulare. **ischiocapsular l., ischiofemoral l.**, ligamentum ischiofemorale. **ischioprostatic l.**, diaphragma urogenitale. **ischiosacral l's**, see *ligamentum sacrospinale* and *ligamentum sacrotuberale*. **Krause's l.**, ligamentum transversum perinei. **laciniate l.**, retinaculum musculorum flexorum pedis. **laciniate l., external**, retinaculum musculorum peroneorum superius. **lacunar l., lacunar l. of Gimbernat**, ligamentum lacunare. **lambdoid l.**, retinaculum musculorum extensorum pedis inferius. **lateral l. of carpus, radial**, ligamentum collaterale carpi radiale. **lateral l. of carpus, ulnar**, ligamentum collaterale carpi ulnare. **lateral l. of colon**, tenia omentalis. **lateral l's of**

joints of fingers, ligamenta collateralia articulationum interphalangearum manus. **lateral l's of joints of toes,** ligamenta collateralia articulationum interphalangearum pedis. **lateral l. of knee,** ligamentum collaterale fibulare. **lateral l's of liver,** see *ligamentum triangulare dextrum hepatis* and *ligamentum triangulare sinistrum hepatis.* **lateral l. of malleus,** ligamentum mallei laterale. **lateral meniscofemoral l.,** ligamentum meniscofemorale posterius. **lateral l's of metacarpophalangeal joints,** ligamenta collateralia articulationum metacarpophalangearum. **lateral l's of metatarsophalangeal joints,** ligamenta collateralia articulationum metatarsophalangearum. **lateral l. of temporomandibular articulation,** ligamentum laterale articulationis temporomandibularis. **lateral l. of temporomandibular joint, external,** ligamentum laterale articulationis temporomandibularis. **lateral l. of temporomandibular joint, internal,** ligamentum sphenomandibulare. **lateral l. of wrist joint, external,** ligamentum collaterale carpi radiale. **lateral l. of wrist joint, internal,** ligamentum collaterale carpi ulnare. **Lauth's l.,** ligamentum transversum atlantis. **l. of left superior vena cava,** plica venae cavae sinistrae. **lienophrenic l.,** ligamentum phrenicolienale. **lienorenal l.,** a fold of peritoneum connecting the spleen and the left kidney. **Lisfranc's l.,** a fibrous band running from the lower external surface of the medial cuneiform bone to the internal surface of the base of the second metatarsal bone. **Lockwood's l.,** the thickened area of contact between Tenon's capsule and the sheaths of the inferior rectus and inferior oblique muscles. **longitudinal l., anterior,** ligamentum longitudinale anterius. **longitudinal l., posterior,** ligamentum longitudinale posterius. **longitudinal l. of abdomen,** linea alba. **lumbocostal l.,** ligamentum lumbocostale. **l's of Luschka,** ligamenta sternopericardiaca. **Mackenrodt's l.,** plica rectouterina. **l. of Maissiat,** tractus iliotibialis. **Mauchart's l's,** ligamenta alaria. **maxillary l., lateral,** ligamentum laterale articulationis temporomandibularis. **maxillary l., middle,** ligamentum sphenomandibulare. **l. of Mayer,** ligamentum carpi radiatum. **Meckel's l.,** Meckel's band. **medial l.,** ligamentum mediale. **medial l. of elbow joint,** ligamentum collaterale ulnare. **medial l. of wrist,** ligamentum collaterale carpi ulnare. **meniscofemoral l., anterior,** ligamentum meniscofemorale anterius. **meniscofemoral l., posterior,** ligamentum meniscofemorale posterius. **mesocolic l. of colon,** tenia mesocolica. **metacarpal l's, dorsal,** ligamenta metacarpea dorsalia. **metacarpal l's, interosseous,** ligamenta metacarpea interossea. **metacarpal l's, palmar,** ligamenta metacarpea palmaria. **metacarpal l's, transverse, deep,** ligamenta metacarpeum transversum profundum. **metacarpal l., transverse, superficial,** ligamentum metacarpeum transversum superficiale. **metacarpophalangeal l's, anterior, metacarpophalangeal l's, palmar,** ligamenta palmaria. **metatarsal l., anterior,** ligamentum metatarseum transversum profundum. **metatarsal l's, dorsal,** ligamenta metatarsea dorsalia. **metatarsal l's, interosseus,** ligamenta metatarsea interossea. **metatarsal l's, lateral,** ligamenta metacarpea interossea. **metatarsal l's, lateral proper (of Weber), metatarsal l's, lateral (of Weitbrecht),** ligamenta metatarsea interossea. **metatarsal l's, plantar,** ligamenta metatarsea plantaria. **metatarsal l., plantar, anterior,** ligamentum metatarseum transversum profundum. **metatarsal l., transverse, deep,** ligamentum metatarseum transversum profundum. **metatarsal l., transverse, interosseous,** ligamenta metatarsea interossea. **metatarsal l., transverse, superficial,** ligamentum metatarseum transversum superficiale. **metatarsophalangeal l's, inferior,** ligamenta plantaria articulationum metatarsophalangearum. **metatarsophalangeal l's, plantar,** ligamenta plantaria articulationum metatarsophalangearum. **middle l. of neck of rib,** ligamentum costotransversarium. **mucous l.,** plica synovialis. **l. of nape,** ligamentum nuchae. **navicularicuneiform l's, plantar,** ligamenta cuneonavicularia plantaria. **nephrocolic l.,** fasciculi from the fatty capsule of the kidney passing down on the right side to the posterior wall of the ascending colon and on the left side to the posterior wall of the descending colon. **nuchal l.,** ligamentum nuchae. **oblique l. of Cooper, oblique l. of forearm,** chorda obliqua membranae interosseae antebrachii. **oblique l's of knee,** ligamenta cruciata genus. **oblique l. of knee, posterior,** ligamentum popliteum obliquum. **oblique l. of scapula,** ligamentum transversum scapulae superius. **oblique l. of superior radioulnar joint,** chorda obliqua membranae interosseae antebrachii. **obturator l., atlantooccipital,** membrana atlantooccipitalis anterior. **obturator l. of atlas,** see *membrana atlantooccipitalis anterior* and *posterior.* **obturator l. of pelvis,** membrana obturatoria. **occipitoaxial l.,** membrana tectoria. **occipitoodontoid l's,** ligamenta alaria. **odontoid l., middle,** ligamentum apicis dentis axis. **odontoid l's of axis,** ligamenta alaria. **orbicular l. of radius,** ligamentum anulare radii. **ovarian l.,** ligamentum ovarii proprium. **palmar l's,** 1. ligamenta palmaria. 2. see *aponeurosis palmaris.* **palmar l., transverse, deep,** ligamenta metacarpeum transversum pro-

fundum. **palmar l. of carpus,** ligamentum carpi radiatum. **palmar l. of radiocarpal joint,** ligamentum radiocarpeum palmare. **palpebral l., medial,** ligamentum palpebrale mediale. **patellar l.,** ligamentum patellae. **patellar l., internal,** retinaculum patellae mediale. **patellar l., lateral,** retinaculum patellae laterale. **pectinate l. of iridocorneal angle,** ligamentum pectinatum anguli iridocornealis. **pectineal l.,** ligamentum pectineale. **pelvic l., posterior, great,** ligamentum sacrotuberale. **pelvic l., posterior, short,** ligamentum sacrospinale. **pelvic l., transverse,** ligamentum transversum perinei. **l's of pelvic girdle,** ligamenta cinguli extremitatis inferioris. **pelviprostatic l., basal,** fascia prostatae. **perineal l., transverse,** ligamentum transversum perinei. **perineal l. of Carcassone,** ligamentum transversum perinei. **periodontal l.,** the connective tissue structure that surrounds the roots of the teeth and holds them in the dental alveoli. See also *periodontium.* **Petit's l.,** uterosacral l. **Pétrequin's l.,** the anterior thickened portion of the temporomaxillary capsule. **petrosphenoid l.,** 1. synchondrosis sphenopetrosa. 2. synchondrosis sphenooccipitalis. **petrosphenoid l., anterior,** synchondrosis sphenopetrosa. **pharyngeal l., pharyngeal l., middle,** raphe pharyngis. **phrenicocolic l.,** ligamentum phrenicocolicum. **phrenicolienal l., phrenicosplenic l.,** ligamentum phrenicolienale. **phrenocolic l.,** ligamentum phrenicocolicum. **pisimetacarpal l.,** ligamentum pisometacarpeum. **pisohamate l.,** ligamentum pisohamatum. **pisometacarpal l.,** ligamentum pisometacarpeum. **pisouncinform l., pisouncinate l.,** ligamentum pisohamatum. **plantar l's,** ligamenta plantaria articulationum metatarsophalangearum. **plantar l., long,** ligamentum plantare longum. **plantar l's of bases of metatarsal bones,** ligamenta metatarsea plantaria. **plantar l's of little heads of metacarpal bones,** see *ligamentum metacarpeum transverum profundum.* **plantar l. of second metatarsal bone,** see *ligamenta tarsometatarsea plantaria.* **plantar l. of tarsus,** ligamentum tarsi plantaria. **popliteal l., arcuate,** ligamentum popliteum arcuatum. **popliteal l., external,** retinaculum ligamenti arcuati. **popliteal l., oblique,** ligamentum popliteum obliquum. **posterior l. of head of fibula,** ligamentum capitis fibulae posterius. **posterior l. of incus,** ligamentum incudis posterius. **posterior l. of pinna,** ligamentum auriculare posterius. **posterior l. of radiocarpal joint,** ligamentum radiocarpeum dorsale. **Poupart's l.,** ligamentum inguinale. **preurethral l. of Waldeyer,** ligamentum transversum perinei. **prismatic l. of Weitbrecht,** ligamentum capitis femoris. **proper l's of costal cartilages,** see *membrana intercostalis externa.* **pterygomandibular l.,** raphe pterygomandibularis. **pterygomaxillary l.,** raphe pterygomandibularis. **pterygospinal l.,** ligamentum pterygospinale. **pubic l., inferior,** 1. ligamentum arcuatum pubis. 2. ligamentum suspensorium ovarii. **pubic l., superior,** ligamentum pubicum superius. **pubic l. of Cowper,** ligamentum inguinale. **pubic l. of Cruveilhier, anterior,** discus interpubicus. **pubocapsular l.,** ligamentum pubofemorale. **pubofemoral l.,** ligamentum pubofemorale. **puboischiadic l. of prostate gland,** fascia diaphragmatis urogenitalis superior. **pubaprostatic l.,** ligamentum puboprostaticum. **puborectal l.,** 1. ligamentum puboprostaticum. 2. ligamentum pubovesicale. **pubovesical l.,** ligamentum pubovesicale. **pulmonary l.,** ligamentum pulmonale. **quadrate l.,** ligamentum quadratum. **radial l., lateral,** ligamentum collaterale carpi radiale. **radial l. of cubitocarpal articulation,** ligamentum collaterale carpi radiale. **radiate l.,** ligamentum capitis costae radiatum. **radiate l., lateral,** ligamentum collaterale carpi ulnare. **radiate l. of carpus,** ligamentum carpi radiatum. **radiate l. of head of rib,** ligamentum capitis costae radiatum. **radiate l. of Mayer,** ligamentum carpi radiatum. **radiocarpal l., anterior,** ligamentum radiocarpeum palmare. **radiocarpal l., dorsal,** ligamentum radiocarpeum dorsale. **radiocarpal l., palmar,** ligamentum radiocarpeum palmare. **radiocarpal l., volar,** ligamentum radiocarpeum palmare. **rectouterine l.,** musculus rectouterinus. **reflex l. of Gimbernat,** ligamentum inguinale reflexum. **reinforcing l's,** ligaments that serve to reinforce joint capsules. **rhomboid l. of clavicle,** ligamentum costoclaviculare. **rhomboid l. of wrist,** ligamentum radiocarpeum dorsale. **ring l. of hip joint,** zona orbicularis articulationis coxae. **Robert's l.,** ligamentum meniscofemorale posterius. **round l. of acetabulum,** ligamentum capitis femoris. **round l. of Cloquet,** ligamentum capitis costae intraarticulare. **round l. of femur,** ligamentum capitis femoris. **round l. of forearm,** chorda obliqua membranae interosseae antebrachii. **round l. of uterus,** ligamentum teres uteri. **sacciform l.,** capsula articularis radioulnaris distalis. **sacrococcygeal l., dorsal, deep,** ligamentum sacrococcygeum dorsale profundum. **sacrococcygeal l., dorsal, superficial,** ligamentum sacrococcygeum dorsale superficiale. **sacrococcygeal l., lateral,** ligamentum sacrococcygeum laterale. **sacrococcygeal l., ventral,** ligamentum sacrococcygeum ventrale. **sacroiliac l's, anterior,** ligamenta sacroiliaca ventralia. **sacroiliac l's, dorsal,** ligamenta sacroiliaca dorsalia. **sacroiliac l's,**

interosseous, ligamenta sacroiliaca interossea. **sacroiliac l., posterior, long, sacroiliac l., posterior, short,** see *ligamenta sacroiliaca dorsalia.* **sacroiliac l's, ventral,** ligamenta sacroiliaca ventralia. **sacrosciatic l., anterior,** ligamentum sacrospinale. **sacrosciatic l., great,** ligamentum sacrotuberale. **sacrosciatic l., internal,** ligamentum sacrospinale. **sacrosciatic l., least,** ligamentum sacrospinale. **sacrospinal l., sacrospinous l.,** ligamentum sacrospinale. **sacrotuberal l., sacrotuberous l.,** ligamentum sacrotuberale. **salpingopharyngeal l.,** plica salpingopharyngea. **Santorini's l.,** ligamentum cricopharyngeum. **Sappey's l.,** the thicker posterior part of the capsule of the temporomandibular joint. **scaphocuneiform l's, plantar,** ligamenta cuneonavicularia plantaria. **l. of Scarpa,** cornu superius marginis falciformis. **Schlemm's l's,** two ligamentous bands strengthening the capsule of the shoulder joint. **scrotal l. of testis,** gubernaculum testis. **serous l.,** ligamentum serosum. **short lateral l.,** a knee ligament attached to the lowest part of the lateral femoral condyle and extending beyond the dorsum of the semilunar cartilage to the apex of the fibula. See also *fabellofibular l.* **short plantar l.,** ligamenta calcaneocuboideum plantare. **l's of shoulder girdle,** ligamenta cinguli extremitatis superioris. **sphenoidal l., external,** ligamentum intercuneiformia plantaria. **sphenoideotarsal l's,** ligamenta tarsometatarsea plantaria. **sphenomandibular l.,** ligamentum sphenomandibulare. **spinoglenoid l.,** ligamentum transversum scapulae inferius. **spinosacral l.,** ligamentum sacrospinale. **spiral l. of cochlea,** ligamentum spirale cochleae. **splenogastric l.,** ligamentum gastrolienale. **splenophrenic l.,** ligamentum phrenicolienale. **spring l.,** ligamentum calcaneonaviculare plantare. **stapedial l.,** l. anulare stapedis. **stellate l., anterior,** ligamentum capitis costae radiatum. **sternoclavicular l., anterior,** ligamentum sternoclaviculare anterius. **sternoclavicular l., posterior,** ligamentum sternoclaviculare posterius. **sternocostal l's,** ligamenta sternocostalia radiata. **sternocostal l., interarticular, sternocostal l., intraarticular,** ligamentum sternocostale intraarticulare. **sternocostal l's, radiate,** ligamenta sternocostalia radiata. **sternopericardiac l's,** ligamenta sternopericardiaca. **stylohyoid l.,** ligamentum stylohyoideum. **stylomandibular l., stylomaxillary l., stylomylohyoid l.,** ligamentum stylomandibulare. **subflaval l.,** ligamentum flavum. **subpublic l.,** ligamentum arcuatum pubis. **superficial l. of carpus,** 1. ligamentum radiocarpeum dorsale. 2. ligamentum radiocarpeum palmare. **superior l. of epididymis,** ligamentum epididymidis superius. **superior l. of hip,** ligamentum iliofemorale. **superior l. of incus,** ligamentum incudis superius. **superior l. of malleus,** ligamentum mallei superius. **superior l. of neck of rib, anterior,** the anterior part of the superior costotransverse ligament. **superior l. of neck of rib, external,** the posterior part of the superior costotransverse ligament. **superior l. of pinna,** ligamentum auriculare superius. **suprascapular l.,** ligamentum transversum scapulae superius. **supraspinal l., supraspinous l.,** ligamentum supraspinale. **suspensory l., marsupial,** plica synovialis infrapatellaris. **suspensory l. of axilla,** a layer ascending from the axillary fascia and ensheathing the pectoralis minor muscle; so called because traction by it, when the arm is abducted, produces the hollow of the armpit. Called also *Campbell's l.* and *Gerdy's l.* **suspensory l. of axis,** ligamentum apicis dentis. **suspensory l. of bladder,** plica umbilicalis mediana. **suspensory l's of breast,** ligamenta suspensoria mammae. **suspensory l. of clitoris,** ligamentum suspensorium clitoridis. **suspensory l. of humerus,** ligamentum coracohumerale. **suspensory l. of lens,** zonula ciliaris. **suspensory l. of liver,** ligamentum falciforme hepatis. **suspensory l's of mammary gland,** ligamenta suspensoria mammae. **suspensory l. of ovary,** ligamentum suspensorium ovarii. **suspensory l. of penis,** ligamentum suspensorium penis. **suspensory l. of spleen,** ligamentum phrenicolienale. **sutural l.,** a band of fibrous tissue between the opposed bones of a suture or immovable joint. **synovial l.,** a large synovial fold. **synovial l. of hip,** ligamentum capitis femoris. **talocalcaneal l., anterior,** ligamentum talocalcaneum anterius. **talocalcaneal l., interosseous,** ligamentum talocalcaneum interosseum. **talocalcaneal l., lateral,** ligamentum talocalcaneum laterale. **talocalcaneal l., medial,** ligamentum talocalcaneum mediale. **talocalcaneal l., posterior,** ligamentum talocalcaneum posterius. **talofibular l., anterior,** ligamentum talofibulare anterius. **talofibular l., posterior,** ligamentum talofibulare posterius. **talonavicular l.,** ligamentum talonaviculare. **talotibial l., anterior,** pars tibiotalaris anterior ligamenti medialis. **talotibial l., posterior,** pars tibiotalaris posterior ligamenti medialis. **tarsal l., anterior,** retinaculum musculorum extensorum pedis inferius. **tarsometatarsal l's, dorsal,** ligamenta tarsometatarsea dorsalia. **tarsometatarsal l's, planter,** ligamenta tarsometatarsea plantaria. **temporomandibular l.,** ligamentum laterale articulationis temporomandibularis. **tendinotrochanteric l.,** a portion of the capsule of the hip joint. **tensor l.,** musculus tensor tympani. **Teutleben's l's,** lateral folds joining the

pericardium and diaphragm. **thyroepiglottic l.,** ligamentum thyroepiglotticum. **thyrohyoid l.,** ligamentum thyrohyoideum. **thyrohyoid l., median,** ligamentum thyrohyoideum medianum. **tibiofibular l.,** syndesmosis tibiofibularis. **tibiofibular l., anterior,** ligamentum tibiofibulare anterius. **tibiofibular l., posterior,** ligamentum tibiofibulare posterius. **tibionavicular l.,** pars tibionavicularis ligamenti medialis. **Toynbee's l.,** musculus tensor tympani. **transverse l. of acetabulum,** ligamentum transversum acetabuli. **transverse l. of atlas,** ligamentum transversum atlantis. **transverse l. of carpus,** retinaculum flexorum manus. **transverse l. of knee,** ligamentum transversum genus. **transverse l. of leg,** retinaculum musculorum extensorum pedis superius. **transverse l's of little heads of metacarpal bones,** see *ligamentum metacarpeum transversum profundum.* **transverse l's of little heads of metatarsal bones,** see *ligamentum metatarseum transversum profundum.* **transverse l. of little head of rib,** ligamentum capitis costae intraarticulare. **transverse l. of pelvis,** ligamentum transversum perinei. **transverse l. of scapula, inferior,** ligamentum transversum scapulae inferius. **transverse l. of scapula, superior,** ligamentum transversum scapulae superius. **transverse l. of tibia,** retinaculum musculorum extensorum pedis superius. **transverse l. of wrist,** retinaculum flexorum manus. **transverse l's of wrist, dorsal,** ligamenta intercarpea dorsalia. **transverse humeral l.,** a band of fibers bridging the intertubercular groove of the humerus and holding the tendon of the biceps muscle in the groove; called also *Brodie's l.* **transversocostal l., superior,** ligamentum costotransversarium superius. **trapezoid l.,** ligamentum trapezoideum. **l. of Treitz,** musculus suspensorius duodeni. **triangular l. of abdomen,** ligamentum inguinale reflexum. **triangular l. of Colles,** fascia diaphragmatis urogenitalis superior. **triangular l. of linea alba,** adminiculum lineae albae. **triangular l. of liver, left,** ligamentum triangulare sinistrum hepatis. **triangular l. of liver, right,** ligamentum triangulare dextrum hepatis. **triangular l. of pubis, anterior,** ligamentum arcuatum pubis. **triangular l. of scapula,** ligamentum transversum scapulae inferius. **triangular l. of thigh,** ligamentum inguinale reflexum. **triangular l. of urethra,** ligamentum puboprostaticum. **trigeminate l's of Arnold,** ligamenta tarsometatarsea dorsalia. **triquetral l.,** 1. ligamentum cricoarytenoideum posterius. 2. ligamentum coracoacromiale. **triquetral l. of foot,** ligamentum calcaneofibulare. **triquetral l. of scapula,** ligamentum transversum scapulae inferius. **trochlear l.,** ligamentum metacarpeum transversum profundum. **trochlear l's of foot,** ligamenta plantaria articulationum metatarsophalangearum. **trochlear l's of hand,** ligamenta palmaria. **trochlear l's of little heads of metacarpal bones,** see *ligamenta metacarpeum transversum profundum.* **true l. of bladder, anterior,** 1. ligamentum puboprostaticum. 2. ligamentum pubovesicale. **tuberososacral l.,** ligamentum sacrotuberale. **tubopharyngeal l. of Rauber,** plica salpingopharyngea. **Tuffier's inferior l.,** that part of the mesentery which is connected with the wall of the iliac fossa. **ulnar l., lateral, ulnar l. of carpus,** ligamentum collaterale carpi ulnare. **ulnocarpal l., palmar,** ligamentum ulnocarpeum palmare. **umbilical l., lateral,** ligamentum umbilicale mediale. **umbilical l., medial,** ligamentum umbilicale mediale. **umbilical l., median, umbilical l., middle,** ligamentum umbilicale medianum. **utero-ovarian l.,** ligamentum ovarii proprium. **uteropelvic l's,** expansions of muscular tissue in the broad ligament of the uterus, radiating from the fascia over the obturator internus to the side of the uterus and the vagina. **uterosacral l.,** a part of the thickening of the visceral pelvic fascia beside the cervix and vagina, passing posteriorly in the rectouterine fold to attach to the front of the sacrum; called also *Petit's l.* **vaginal l.,** ligamentum vaginale. **vaginal l's of fingers,** vaginae fibrosae digitorum manus. **vaginal l's of toes,** vaginae fibrosae digitorum pedis. **l. of vaginal sheaths,** ligamentum vaginale. **l's of vaginal sheaths of fingers,** vaginae fibrosae digitorum manus. **l's of vaginal sheaths of toes,** vaginae fibrosae digitorum pedis. **l's of Valsalva,** ligamenta auricularia. **venous l. of liver,** ligamentum venosum. **ventricular l. of larynx,** ligamentum vestibulare. **vertebropleural l.,** membrana suprapleuralis. **l. of Vesalius,** ligamentum inguinale. **vesical l., lateral,** ligamentum umbilicale mediale. **vesicopubic l.,** ligamentum pubovesicale. **vesicoumbilical l.,** ligamentum umbilicale mediale. **vesicouterine l.,** a ligament that extends from the anterior aspect of the uterus to the bladder. **vestibular l.,** ligamentum vestibulare. **vocal l.,** ligamentum vocale. **volar l's of bases of metacarpal bones,** ligamenta metacarpea palmaria. **volar l. of carpus, proper,** retinaculum flexorum manus. **volar l's of carpus, transverse, deep,** ligamenta metacarpea palmaria. **volar l's of little heads of metacarpal bones,** see *ligamentum metacarpeum transversum profundum.* **volar l. of wrist, anterior,** retinaculum flexorum manus. **Walther's oblique l.,** ligamentum talofibulare posterius. **Weitbrecht's l.,** chorda obliqua membranae interosseae antebrachii. **Winslow's l.,** ligamentum popliteum obliquum. **Wrisberg's l.,** ligamentum meniscofemorale posterius. **xiphicostal l's of Macalister, xiphoid l's,** ligamenta costoxiphoidea. **Y l.,** ligamentum iliofemorale. **yellow l.,** ligamentum flavum. **Zinn's l.,** anulus tendineus communis. **zonal l. of thigh,** zona orbicularis articulationis coxae.

ligamenta (lig″ah-men′tah) [L.] plural of *ligamentum;* and see *Table of Ligamenta.*

ligamentopexis (lig″ah-men″to-pek′sis) [*ligament* + Gr. *pēxis* fixation] ligamentopexy.

ligamentopexy (lig″ah-men″to-pek′se) ventrosuspension by shortening or suturing the round ligaments of the uterus.

ligamentous (lig″ah-men′tus) pertaining to or of the nature of a ligament.

ligamentum (lig″ah-men′tum), pl. *ligamen′ta* [L. "a bandage," from *ligare* to bind] [NA] a ligament: a band of tissue that connects bones or supports viscera. Some ligaments are distinct fibrous structures; some are folds of fascia or of indurated peritoneum; still others are relics of fetal organs. For names of specific structures, see *Table of Ligamenta.*

TABLE OF LIGAMENTA

Descriptions are given on NA terms, and include anglicized names of specific ligaments.

ligamen′ta accesso′ria planta′ria, ligamenta plantaria articulationum metatarsophalangearum.

ligamen′ta accesso′ria vola′ria, ligamenta palmaria.

l. acromioclavicula′re [NA], acromioclavicular ligament: a dense band that joins the superior surface of the acromion and the acromial extremity of the clavicle together, and strengthens the superior part of the articular capsule.

ligamen′ta ala′ria [NA], alar ligaments: two strong bands that pass from the posterolateral part of the tip of the dens of the axis upward and laterally to the condyles of the occipital bone; they limit rotation of the head.

l. annula′re ba′seos stape′dis, l. anulare stapedis.

ligamen′ta annula′ria digito′rum ma′nus, see *pars anularis vaginae fibrosae digitorum manus.*

ligamen′ta annula′ria digito′rum pe′dis, see *pars anularis vaginae fibrosae digitorum pedis.*

l. annula′re ra′dii, l. anulare radii.

ligamen′ta annula′ria [trachea′lia], ligamenta anularia trachealia.

l. anococcyg′eum [NA], anococcygeal ligament: a fibrous band connecting the posterior fibers of the sphincter of the anus to the coccyx.

l. anula′re ra′dii [NA], annular ligament of radius: a strong fibrous band that encircles the head of the radius and holds it in position; it is attached the the anterior and posterior margins of the radial notch of the ulna, forming, with the notch, a complete ring. Called also *l. annulare radii.*

l. anula′re stape′dis [NA], annular ligament of stapes: a ring of fibrous tissue that attaches the base of the stapes to the fenestra vestibuli of the inner ear; called also *l. annulare baseos stapedis.*

ligamen′ta anula′ria trachea′lia [NA], tracheal annular ligaments: circular horizontal ligaments that join the tracheal cartilages together; called also *ligamenta annularia[trachealia]* and *tracheal annular ligaments.*

l. a′picis den′tis ax′is [NA], apical dental ligament: a cord of tissue extending from the tip of the dens of the axis to the occipital bone, near the anterior margin of the foramen magnum; it is usually delicate, but is sometimes well developed. Called also *l. apicis dentis epistrophei.*

l. a′picis den′tis epistro′phei, l. apicis dentis axis.

l. arcua′tum latera′le [NA], lateral arcuate ligament: the ligamentous arch, formed by the fascia of the quadratus lumborum muscle, constituting part of the lumbar portion of the diaphragm; called also *arcus lumbocostalis lateralis [Halleri].*

l. arcua′tum media′le [NA], medial arcuate ligament: the ligamentous arch, formed by the fascia of the psoas muscle, constituting part of the lumbar portion of the diaphragm; called also *arcus lumbocostalis medialis [Halleri].*

l. arcua′tum media′num [NA], median arcuate ligament: the ligamentous arch across the front of the aorta, interconnecting the crura of the diaphragm; called also *median arcuate ligament.*

l. arcua′tum pu′bis [NA], arcuate ligament of pubis: a thick archlike band of fibers situated along the inferior margin of the symphysis pubis. Its fibers are attached to the medial borders of the inferior rami of the pubic bones and thus it rounds out and forms the summit of the pubic arch. Called also *inferior pubic ligament.*

l. arterio′sum [NA], a short, thick, strong fibromuscular cord extending from the pulmonary artery to the arch of the aorta; it is the remains of the ductus arteriosus. Called also *l. arteriosum arteriae pulmonalis* and *ligament of Botallo.*

l. arterio′sum arte′riae pulmona′lis, l. arteriosum.

ligamen′ta auricula′ria [NA], ligaments of auricle: the three ligaments, anterior, superior, and posterior, that help attach the auricle to the side of the head; called also *ligaments of Valsalva.*

ligamen′ta auricula′ria [Valsal′vae], ligamenta auricularia.

l. auricula′re ante′rius [NA], anterior auricular ligament: the auricular ligament that passes from the helix and tragus to the zygoma.

l. auricula′re ante′rius [Valsal′vae], l. auriculare anterius.

l. auricula′re poste′rius [NA], posterior auricular ligament: the auricular ligament that passes from the eminence of the concha to the mastoid part of the temporal bone.

l. auricula′re poste′rius [Valsal′vae], l. auriculare posterius.

l. auricula′re supe′rius [NA], superior auricular ligament: the auricular ligament that passes from the spine of the helix to the superior margin of the bony external acoustic meatus.

l. auricula′re supe′rius [Valsal′vae], l. auriculare superius.

ligamen′ta ba′sium [os′sium metacarpa′lium] dorsa′lia, ligamenta metacarpea dorsalia.

ligamenta ba′sium [os′sium metacarpa′lium] interos′sea, ligamenta metacarpea interossea.

ligamen′ta ba′sium [os′sium metacarpa′lium] vola′ria, ligamenta metacarpea palmaria.

ligamen′ta ba′sium [os′sium metatarsa′lium] dorsa′lia, ligamenta metatarsea dorsalia.

ligamen′ta ba′sium [os′sium metatarsa′lium] interos′sea, ligamenta metatarsea interossea.

ligamen′ta ba′sium [os′sium metatarsa′lium] planta′ria, ligamenta metatarsea plantaria.

l. bifurca′tum [NA], bifurate ligament: a Y-shaped ligament on the dorsum of the foot, comprising the calcaneonavicular and calcaneocuboid ligaments.

l. calcaneocuboi′deum [NA], calcaneocuboid ligament: the band of fibers connecting the superior surface of the calcaneus and the dorsal surface of the cuboid bone; called also *pars calcaneocuboidea ligamenti bifurcati.*

l. calcaneocuboi′deum planta′re [NA], plantar calcaneocuboid ligament: a short, wide, strong band connecting the plantar surfaces of the calcaneus and the cuboid bone; called also *short plantar ligament.*

l. calcaneofibula′re [NA], calcaneofibular ligament: a band of fibers arising from the lateral surface of the lateral malleolus of the fibula just anterior to the apex and passing inferiorly and posteriorly to be attached to the lateral surface of the calcaneus.

l. calcaneonavicula′re [NA], calcaneonavicular ligament: the band of fibers connecting the superior surface of the calcaneus and the lateral surface of the navicular bone; called also *pars calcaneonavicularis ligamenti bifurcati.*

l. calcaneonavicula′re dorsa′le, dorsal calcaneonavicular ligament: the dorsal portion of the calcaneonavicular part of the bifurcate ligament, connecting the dorsal surfaces of the calcaneus and the navicular bone.

l. calcaneonavicula′re planta′re [NA], plantar calcaneonavicular ligament: a broad, thick band passing from the anterior margin of the sustentaculum tali to the plantar surface of the navicular bone; it bears on its deep surface a fibrocartilage that helps to support the head of the talus.

l. calcaneotibia′le, pars tibiocalcanea ligamenti medialis.

l. cap′itis cos′tae intraarticula′re [NA], interarticular ligament of head of rib: a horizontal band of fibers attached to the crest separating the two articular facets on the head of the rib, and to the intervertebral disk, thus dividing the joint of the head of the rib into two cavities. It is lacking in the joints of the first, tenth, eleventh, and twelfth ribs. Called also *l. capituli costae interarticulare.*

l. cap′itis cos′tae radia′tum [NA], radiate ligament of head of rib: fibers that from their attachement on the ventral surface of the head of a rib radiate medially, in a fanlike manner, to attach to the two adjacent vertebrae and to the intervertebral disk between them; called also *l. capituli costae radiatum.*

l. cap′itis fem′oris [NA], ligament of head of femur: a curved triangular or V-shaped fibrous band, attached by its apex to the anterosuperior part of the fovea of the head of the femur and by its base to the sides of the acetabular notch and the intervening transverse ligament of the acetabulum. Called also *l. teres femoris* and *round ligament of femur.*

l. cap′itis fib′ulae ante′rius [NA], anterior ligament of head of fibula: a band of fibers that passes obliquely superiorly from the anterior part of the head of the fibula to the lateral condyle of the tibia.

l. cap′itis fib′ulae poste′rius [NA], posterior ligament of head of fibula: a band of fibers that passes obliquely superiorly from the posterior part of the head of the fibula to the lateral condyle of the tibia.

l. capit′uli cos′tae interarticula′re, l. capitis costae intraarticulare.

l. capit′uli cos′tae radia′tum, l. capitis costae radiatum.

ligamen′ta capit′uli fib′ulae, see *l. capitis fibulae anterius* and *l. capitis fibulae posterius.*

ligamen′ta capitulo′rum [os′sium metacarpa′lium] transver′sa, see *l. metacarpeum transversum profundum.*

ligamen′ta capitulo′rum [os′sium metatarsa′lium] transver′sa, see *l. metatarseum transversum profundum.*

l. car′pi dorsa′le, retinaculum extensorum manus.

l. car′pi radia′tum [NA], radiate carpal ligament: a group of about seven fibrous bands which diverge in all directions on the palmar surface of the mediocarpal joint; the majority radiate from the capitate to the scaphoid, lunate, and triquetral bones.

l. car′pi transver′sum, retinaculum flexorum manus.

l. car′pi vola′re, transverse reinforcing fibers in the antebrachial fascia over the palmar surface of the wrist.

ligamen′ta carpometacar′pea dorsa′lia [NA], dorsal carpometacarpal ligaments: a series of bands on the dorsal surface of the carpometacarpal articulations, joining the carpal bones to the bases of the second to fifth metacarpals. The second metacarpal bone is thus joined to the trapezium, trapezoid, and capitate, the third to the capitate, the fourth to the capitate and hamate, and the fifth to the hamate.

ligamen′ta carpometacar′pea palma′ria [NA], palmar carpometacarpal ligaments: a series of bands on the palmar surface of the carpometacarpal articulations, joining the carpal bones to the second to fifth metacarpals. The second metacarpal bone is thus joined to the trapezium, the third to the trapezium, capitate, and hamate, the fourth to the hamate, and the fifth to the hamate. Called also *ligamenta carpometacarpea volaria* and *volar carpometacarpal ligaments.*

ligamen′ta carpometacar′pea vola′ria, ligamenta carpometacarpea palmaria.

l. cauda′le integumen′ti commu′nis, retinaculum caudale.

l. ceratocricoi′deum ante′rius, a fibrous band that extends from the anterior surface of the tip of the inferior cornu of the thyroid cartilage forward and downward and is attached to the side of the arch of the cricoid cartilage.

ligamen′ta ceratocricoi′dea latera′lia, fibrous bands that extend downward and back from the tip of the inferior cornu of the thyroid cartilage and are attached to the lower, lateral, outer surface of the lamina of the cricoid cartilage.

ligamen′ta ceratocricoi′dea posterio′ra, fibrous bands that extend from the posterior surface of the inferior cornu of the thyroid cartilage near its tip upward, backward, and medially, and are attached to the superior lateral margin of the lamina of the cricoid cartilage.

ligamen′ta cin′guli extremita′tis inferio′ris, ligaments of the pelvic girdle, including (intrinsic) the iliolumbar, sacrotuberous, and sacrospinous ligaments and the superior and arcuate ligaments of the symphysis pubis, and (extrinsic) those of the sacroiliac and hip joints.

ligamen′ta cin′guli extremita′tis superio′ris, ligaments of the shoulder girdle, including (intrinsic) the coracoacromial and the inferior and superior transverse scapular ligaments and (extrinsic) those of the sternoclavicular articulation.

ligamen′ta collatera′lia articulatio′num digito′rum ma′nus, ligamenta collateralia articulationum interphalangearum manus.

ligamen′ta collatera′lia articulatio′num digito′rum pe′dis, ligamenta collateralia articulationum interphalangearum pedis.

ligamen′ta collatera′lia articulatio′num interphalangea′rum ma′nus [NA], collateral ligaments of interphalangeal articulations of hand: massive fibrous bands on each side of the interphalangeal joints of the fingers; they are placed diagonally, the proximal ends being near the dorsal, and the distal ends near the palmar margins of the digits. Called also *ligamenta collateralia articulationum digitorum manus.*

ligamen′ta collatera′lia articulatio′num interphalangea′rum pe′dis [NA], collateral ligaments of interphalangeal articulations of foot: fibrous bands, one on either side of each of the interphalangeal joints of the toes; Called also *ligamenta collateralia articulationum digitorum pedis.*

ligamen′ta collatera′lia articulatio′num metacarpophalangea′rum [NA], collateral ligaments of metacarpophalangeal articulations: massive, strong fibrous bands on either side of each metacarpophalangeal joint, holding the two bones involved in each joint firmly together.

ligamen′ta collatera′lia articulatio′num metatarsophalangea′rum [NA], collateral ligaments of metatarsophalangeal articulations: strong fibrous bands on either side of each metatarsophalangeal joint, holding the two bones involved in each joint firmly together.

l. collatera′le car′pi radia′le [NA], radial carpal collateral ligament: a short, thick band that passes from the tip of the styloid process of the radius to attach to the scaphoid bone.

l. collatera′le car′pi ulna′re [NA], ulnar carpal collateral ligament: a strong fibrous band that passes from the tip of the styloid

process of the ulna and is attached to the triquetral and pisiform bones.

l. collatera′le fibula′re [NA], collateral fibular ligament: a strong, round fibrous cord on the lateral side of the knee joint, entirely independent of the capsule of the knee joint; it is attached superiorly to the posterior part of the lateral epicondyle of the femur and inferiorly to the lateral side of the head of the fibula just in front of the styloid process.

l. collatera′le radia′le [NA], collateral radial ligament: a large bundle of fibers arising from the lateral epicondyle of the humerus and fanning out to be attached to the lateral side of the annular ligament of the radius.

l. collatera′le tibia′le [NA], collateral tibial ligament: a broad, flat, longitudinal band on the medial side of the knee joint; it is attached superiorly to the medial epicondyle of the femur, inferiorly to the medial surface of the body of the tibia, and in between to the medial meniscus.

l. collatera′le ulna′re [NA], collateral ulnar ligament: a triangular bundle of fibers attached proximally to the medial epicondyle of the humerus, distally to the coronoid process of the ulna and the medial surface of the olecranon, and to a ridge running between the two.

l. col′li cos′tae, l. costotransversarium.

ligamen′ta colum′nae vertebra′lis et cra′nii, ligaments of the vertebral column and cranium.

l. conoi′deum [NA], conoid ligament: the conical, posteromedial portion of the coracoclavicular ligament, attached inferiorly by its tip to the base of the coracoid process of the scapula and superiorly by its base to the inferior surface of the clavicle.

l. coracoacromia′le [NA], coracoacromial ligament: one of three intrinsic ligaments of the scapula, a strong broad triangular band that is attached by its base to the lateral border of the coracoid process and by its tip to the summit of the acromion just in front of the articular facet for the clavicle.

l. coracoclavicula′re [NA], coracoclavicular ligament: a strong band that joins the coracoid process of the scapula and the acromial extremity of the clavicle; it is divided into two parts, the trapezoid and conoid ligaments.

l. coracohumera′le [NA], coracohumeral ligament: a broad band that arises from the lateral border of the coracoid process of the scapula and passes downward and laterally to be attached to the major tubercle of the humerus.

l. corona′rium hep′atis [NA], coronary ligament of the liver: the line of reflection of the peritoneum from the diaphragmatic surface of the liver to the under surface of the diaphragm.

l. costoclavicula′re [NA], costoclavicular ligament: a short, powerful ligament that extends from the superior margin of the first costal cartilage to the inferior surface at the sternal end of the clavicle.

l. costotransversa′rium [NA], costotransverse ligament: short fibers that connect the dorsal surface of the neck of a rib with the anterior surface of the transverse process of the corresponding vertebra; called also *l. colli costae.*

l. costotransversa′rium ante′rius, anterior portion of ligamentum costotransversarium superius.

l. costotransversa′rium latera′le [NA], lateral costotransverse ligament: a fibrous band that passes transversely from the posterior surface of the tip of a transverse process of a vertebra to the nonarticular part of the tubercle of the corresponding rib; called also *l. tuberculi costae.*

l. costotransversa′rium poste′rius, posterior portion of ligamentum costotransversarium superius.

l. costotransversa′rium supe′rius [NA], superior costotransverse ligament: a strong band of fibers ascending from the crest of the neck of a rib to the transverse process of the vertebra above; it may be divided into a stronger anterior portion and a weaker posterior portion. It is lacking for the first rib.

ligamen′ta costoxiphoi′dea [NA], costoxiphoid ligaments: inconstant strandlike bands that pass obliquely from the anterior surface of the seventh and sometimes from the sixth costal cartilage to the anterior surface of the xiphoid process of the sternum. Some bands may also be present on the posterior surface.

l. cricoarytenoi′deum poste′rius [NA], posterior cricoarytenoid cartilage: the ligament extending from the lamina of the cricoid cartilage to the medial surface of the base and muscular process of the arytenoid cartilage.

l. cricopharyn′geum [NA], cricopharyngeal ligament: a ligament extending from the cricoid lamina to the midline of the pharynx.

l. cricothyreoi′deum [me′dium], l. cricothyroideum.

l. cricothyroi′deum [NA], cricothyroid ligament: a flat band of white fibrous tissue extending from the inferior thyroid notch down to the arcus of the cricoid cartilage, thus forming the conus elasticus; called also *l. cricothyreoideum [medium].*

l. cricotrachea′le [NA], cricotracheal ligament: a narrow fibrous ring that connects the lower margin of the cricoid cartilage with the upper tracheal cartilage; it is continuous posteriorly with the membranous wall of the trachea.

l. crucia′tum ante′rius ge′nu, l. cruciatum anterius genus.

l. crucia′tum ante′rius ge′nus [NA], anterior cruciate ligament of knee: a strong band that arises from the posteromedial portion of the lateral condyle of the femur, passes anteriorly and inferiorly between the condyles, and is attached to the depression in front of the intercondylar eminence of the tibia. Called also *l. cruciatum anterius genu.*

l. crucia′tum atlan′tis, l. cruciforme atlantis.

l. crucia′tum cru′ris, retinaculum musculorum extensorum pedis inferius.

ligamen′ta crucia′ta digito′rum ma′nus, see *pars cruciformis vaginae fibrosae digitorum manus.*

ligamen′ta crucia′ta digito′rum pe′dis, see *pars cruciformis vaginae fibrosae digitorum pedis.*

ligamen′ta crucia′ta ge′nu, ligamenta cruciata genus.

ligamen′ta crucia′ta ge′nus [NA], cruciate ligaments of knee: strong, thick bundles situated in the knee joint between the condyles of the femur, which together form a somewhat cross-shaped structure; called also *ligamenta cruciata genu.* See *l. cruciatum anterius genus* and *l. cruciatum posterius genus.*

l. crucia′tum poste′rius ge′nu, cruciatum posterius genus.

l. crucia′tum poste′rius ge′nus [NA], posterior cruciate ligament of knee: a strong band that arises from the anterolateral surface of the medial condyle of the femur, passes posteriorly and inferiorly between the condyles, and is inserted into the posterior intercondylar area of the tibia. Called also *l. cruciatum posterius genu.*

l. crucifor′me atlan′tis [NA], cruciform ligament of atlas: a ligament in the form of a cross, of which the transverse ligament of the atlas forms the horizontal bar, and the longitudinal fascicles the vertical bar of the cross; called also *l. cruciatum atlantis.*

l. cuboideonavicula′re dorsa′le [NA], dorsal cuboideonavicular ligament: a fibrous bundle connecting the dorsal surfaces of the cuboid and navicular bones.

l. cuboideonavicula′re planta′re [NA], plantar cuboideonavicular ligament: a fibrous band connecting the plantar surfaces of the cuboid and navicular bones.

l. cuneocuboi′deum dorsa′le [NA], dorsal cuneocuboid ligament: fibers connecting the dorsal surfaces of the cuboid and lateral cuneiform bones.

l. cuneocuboi′deum interos′seum [NA], interosseous cuneocuboid ligament: fibers connecting the central portions of the adjacent surfaces of the cuboid and lateral cuneiform bones, between the articular surfaces.

l. cuneocuboi′deum planta′re [NA], plantar cuneocuboid ligament: a band of fibers connecting the plantar surfaces of the cuboid and lateral cuneiform bones.

ligamen′ta cuneometatar′sea interos′sea [NA], interosseous cuneometatarsal ligaments: fibrous bands that join the adjacent surfaces of the cuneiform and the metatarsal bones.

ligamen′ta cuneonavicula′ria dorsa′lia [NA], dorsal cuneonavicular ligaments: bands that join the dorsal surface of the navicular bone to the dorsal surfaces of the three cuneiform bones; called also *ligamenta navicularicuneiformia dorsalia.*

ligamen′ta cuneonavicula′ria planta′ria [NA], plantar cuneonavicular ligaments: bands that join the plantar surface of the navicular bone to the adjacent plantar surfaces of the three cuneiform bones; called also *ligamenta navicularicuneiformia plantaria.*

l. deltoi′deum, NA alternative for *l. mediale.*

l. denticula′tum [NA], denticulate ligament: a fold of pia mater of the spinal cord, beginning in a longitudinal line along the spinal cord between the lines of attachment of the anterior and posterior roots. The lateral edge is scalloped and has about 21 pointed processes that extend laterally and fuse with the arachnoid and dura mater. Called also *dentate ligament of spinal cord.*

l. duodenorena′le, duodenorenal ligament: a fold of peritoneum that passes from the duodenum to the right kidney.

l. epididym′idis infe′rius [NA], inferior ligament of epididymis: a strand of fibrous tissue, covered with a reflection of the tunica vaginalis, which connects the lower end of the body of the epididymis with the testis.

l. epididym′idis supe′rius [NA], superior ligament of epididymis: a strand of fibrous tissue, covered with a reflection of the tunica vaginalis, which connects the upper end of the body of the epididymis with the testis.

ligamen′ta extracapsula′ria [NA], ligaments of a joint capsule that are outside the capsule.

l. falcifor′me hep′atis [NA], falciform ligament of the liver: a sickle-shaped sagittal fold of peritoneum that helps to attach the liver to the diaphragm, separates the right and left lobes of the liver, and extends from the coronary ligament of the liver behind to the umbilicus in front; called also *broad ligament of liver.*

ligamen′ta fla′va, plural of *l. flavum.*

l. fla′vum [NA], any of a series of bands of yellow elastic tissue attached to and extending between the ventral portions of the laminae of two adjacent vertebrae, from the junction of the axis and the third cervical vertebra to the junction of the fifth lumbar vertebra and the sacrum. They assist in maintaining or regaining the erect position and serve to close in the spaces between the arches. Called also *arcuate, flaval,* and *yellow ligament.*

l. fundifor′me pe′nis [NA], fundiform ligament of penis: a broad elastic band of fascial fibers that arises from the linea alba and from the fibrae intercrurales just above the symphysis pubis and then passes down to the penis, where it divides and passes around the penis and on into the scrotum.

l. gastrocol′icum [NA], gastrocolic ligament: a peritoneal fold, part of the greater omentum, that extends from the greater curvature of the stomach to the transverse colon.

l. gastroliena′le [NA], gastrosplenic ligament: a peritoneal fold extending from the greater curvature of the stomach to the hilus of the spleen and containing blood vessels, nerves, and lymph nodes.

l. gastrophren′icum [NA], gastrophrenic ligament: a fold of peritoneum continuous with the gastrosplenic ligament, extending from right under surface of the diaphragm to the cardiac part of the stomach.

l. genitoinguina′le [NA], genitoinguinal ligament: the embryonic precursor of the gubernaculum testis.

ligamen′ta glenohumera′lia [NA], glenohumeral ligaments: bands, usually three in number, on the inner surface of the articular capsule of the humerus, attached to the margin of the glenoid cavity and to the anatomical neck of the humerus.

l. hepatocol′icum [NA], hepatocolic ligament: an occasional fold of peritoneum, an extension of the lesser omentum to the right, passing from the lower surface of the liver near the gallbladder to the right colic flexure.

l. hepatoduodena′le [NA], hepatoduodenal ligament: a peritoneal fold that passes from the porta hepatis to the superior portion of the duodenum. It is continuous on the left with the gastrohepatic ligament, and on the right it forms one of the borders of the epiploic foramen. It contains the hepatic artery, portal vein, bile duct, nerves, and lymphatics.

l. hepatogas′tricum [NA], hepatogastric ligament: a peritoneal fold, part of the lesser omentum, that passes from the under surface of the liver to the lesser curvature of the stomach.

l. hepatorena′le [NA], hepatorenal ligament: a fold of peritoneum that passes from the back part of the lower surface of the liver to the front of the right kidney and forms the right margin of the epiploic foramen.

l. hyoepiglot′ticum [NA], hyoepiglottic ligament: a triangular elastic band with its base attached to the upper border of the body of the hyoid bone and its tip to the anterosuperior surface of the epiglottis.

l. hyothyreoi′deum latera′le, l. thyrohyoideum.

l. hyothyreoi′deum me′dium, l. thyrohyoideum medianum.

l. iliofemora′le [NA], iliofemoral ligament: a very strong triangular or inverted Y-shaped band that covers the anterior and superior portions of the hip joint. It arises by its apex from the lower part of the anterior inferior iliac spine and is inserted by its base into the intertrochanteric line of the femur.

l. iliolumba′le [NA], iliolumbar ligament: a strong band that passes from the transverse processes of the fourth and fifth lumbar vertebrae to the internal lip of the adjacent portion of the iliac crest.

l. incu′dis poste′rius [NA], posterior ligament of incus: a fibrous band by which the cartilaginous tip of the short crus of the incus is fixed to the fossa incudis.

l. incu′dis supe′rius [NA], superior ligament of incus: a fibrous band that passes from the body of the incus to the roof of the tympanic cavity just back of the superior ligament of the malleus.

l. inguina′le [NA], inguinal ligament: a fibrous band running from the anterior superior spine of the ilium to the spine of the pubis.

l. inguina′le [Poupar′ti], l. inguinale.

l. inguina′le reflex′um [NA], reflex inguinal ligament: a triangular band of fibers arising from the lacunar ligament and the pubic bone and passing diagonally upward and medially behind the superficial abdominal ring and in front of the inguinal aponeurotic falx to the linea alba.

l. inguina′le reflex′um [Colle′si], l. inguinale reflexum.

ligamen′ta intercar′pea dorsa′lia [NA], dorsal intercarpal ligaments: several bands that extend transversely across the dorsal surfaces of the carpal bones, connecting various ones together.

ligamen′ta intercar′pea interos′sea [NA], interosseous intercarpal ligaments: short fibrous bands that join the adjacent surfaces of the various carpal bones.

ligamen′ta intercar′pea palma′ria [NA], palmar intercarpal ligaments: several bands that extend transversely across the palmar surfaces of the carpal bones, connecting various ones together; called also *ligamenta intercarpea volaria* and *volar intercarpal ligaments.*

ligamen′ta intercar′pea vola′ria, ligamenta intercarpea palmaria.

l. interclavicula′re [NA], interclavicular ligament: a flattened band that passes from the superior surface of the sternal end of one clavicle across the superior margin of the sternum to the same position on the other clavicle.

ligamen′ta intercosta′lia, see *membrana intercostalis externa* and *membrana intercostalis interna.*

ligamen′ta intercosta′lia exter′na, see *membrana intercostalis externa.*

ligamen′ta intercosta′lia inter′na, see *membrana intercostalis interna.*

ligamen′ta intercuneifor′mia dorsa′lia [NA], dorsal intercuneiform ligaments: fibrous bands connecting the dorsal surfaces of the three cuneiform bones.

ligamen′ta intercuneifor′mia interos′sea [NA], interosseous intercuneiform ligaments: short fibrous bands that join the adjacent surfaces of the medial and intermediate, and the intermediate and lateral, cuneiform bones.

ligamen′ta intercuneifor′mia planta′ria [NA], plantar intercuneiform ligaments: fibrous bands that join the plantar surfaces of the cuneiform bones.

l. interfoveola′re [NA], interfoveolar ligament: a thickening in the transversalis fascia on the medial side of the deep inguinal ring; it is connected above to the transversus muscle and below to the inguinal ligament.

l. interfoveola′re [Hesselba′chi], l. interfoveolare.

l. interspina′le [NA], interspinal ligament: any of several fine fibrous membranes that extend from one vertebral spinous process to the next. They extend obliquely from the yellow ligaments ventrally to the supraspinous ligament dorsally, and contain white fibrous and yellow elastic tissue. They are poorly developed or lacking in the cervical region.

ligamen′ta interspina′lia, see *l. interspinale.*

ligamen′ta intertransversa′ria, see *l. intertransversarium.*

l. intertransversa′rium [NA], intertransverse ligament: any of several poorly developed fibrous bands that extend from one vertebral transverse process to the next. They consist of fine membranes in the lumbar region and of small cords in the thoracic region, and are lacking in the cervical region.

ligamen′ta intracapsula′ria [NA], ligaments within a joint capsule.

l. ischiocapsula′re, l. ischiofemorale.

l. ischiofemora′le [NA], ischiofemoral ligament: a broad triangular band on the posterior surface of the hip joint. Its base is attached to the ischium posterior and inferior to the acetabulum; its fibers pass superiorly, laterally, and anteriorly across the capsule, bend over the neck, and in part are inserted into the inner side of the trochanteric fossa of the femur and in part blend into the zona orbicularis. Called also *l. ischiocapsulare* and *ischiocapsular ligament.*

l. lacinia′tum, retinaculum musculorum flexorum pedis.

l. lacuna′re [NA], lacunar ligament: a small triangular membrane with its base just medial to the femoral ring; one side is attached to the inguinal ligament and the other to the pectineal line of the pubis.

l. lacuna′re [Gimberna′ti], l. lacunare.

l. latera′le articulatio′nis temporomandibula′ris [NA], lateral ligament of temporomandibular articulation: a strong triangular fibrous band that is attached superiorly by its base to the zygomatic process of the temporal bone, passes down on the lateral side of the joint in contact with the capsule, and is inserted by its apex into the lateral and posterior surfaces of the neck of the condyloid process of the mandible. Called also *l. temporomandibulare* and *temporomandibular ligament.*

l. la′tum u′teri [NA], broad ligament of uterus: a broad fold of peritoneum extending from the side of the uterus to the wall of the pelvis; it is divided into the mesometrium, mesosalpinx, and mesovarium.

l. lienorena′le, NA alternative for *l. phrenicolienale.*

l. longitudina′le ante′rius [NA], anterior longitudinal ligament: a single long, fibrous band in the midline, attached to the ventral surfaces of the bodies of the vertebrae; it extends from the occipital bone and the anterior tubercle of the atlas down to the sacrum.

l. longitudina′le poste′rius [NA], posterior longitudinal ligament: a single mid-line fibrous band attached to the dorsal surfaces of the bodies of the vertebrae, extending from the occipital bone to the coccyx.

l. lumbocosta′le [NA], lumbocostal ligament: a strong fascial band that passes from the twelfth rib to the tips of the transverse processes of the first and second lumbar vertebrae.

l. mal′lei ante′rius [NA], anterior ligament of malleus: a fibrous band that extends from the neck of the malleus just above the anterior process to the anterior wall of the tympanic cavity close to the petrotympanic fissure. Some of the fibers pass through the fissure to the spina angularis of the sphenoid bone.

l. mal′lei latera′le [NA], lateral ligament of malleus: a triangular fibrous band that passes from the posterior portion of the incisura tympanica to the head or neck of the malleus.

l. mal′lei supe′rius [NA], superior ligament of malleus: a delicate fibrous strand passing from the roof of the tympanic cavity to the head of the malleus.

l. malle′oli latera′lis ante′rius, l. tibiofibulare anterius.

l. malle′oli latera′lis poste′rius, l. tibiofibulare posterius.

l. media′le [NA], medial ligament: a large fan-shaped ligament on the medial side of the ankle, passing from the medial malleolus of the tibia down onto the tarsal bones. It comprises four parts: pars tibionavicularis, pars tibiocalcanea, pars tibiotalaris anterior, and pars tibiotalaris posterior. Called also *l. deltoideum* [NA alternative] and *deltoid ligament of ankle.*

l. meniscofemora′le ante′rius [NA], anterior meniscofemoral ligament: a small fibrous band of the knee joint, attached to the posterior area of the lateral meniscus and passing superiorly and medially, anterior to the posterior cruciate ligament, to attach to the anterior cruciate ligament.

l. meniscofemora′le poste′rius [NA], posterior meniscofemoral ligament: a small fibrous band of the knee joint, attached to the posterior area of the lateral meniscus and passing superiorly and medially, posterior to the posterior cruciate ligament, to the medial condyle of the femur.

ligamen′ta metacar′pea dorsa′lia [NA], dorsal metacarpal ligaments: bands that interconnect the bases of the second to fifth metacarpal bones by passing transversely from bone to bone on their dorsal surfaces; called also *ligamenta basium* [*ossium metacarpalium*] *dorsalia.*

ligamen′ta metacar′pea interos′sea [NA], interosseous metacarpal ligaments: short, strong fibrous bands situated between the adjacent surfaces of the bases of the second to fifth metacarpal bones, just distal to the articular surfaces; called also *ligamenta basium* [*ossium metacarpalium*] *interossea.*

ligamen′ta metacar′pea palma′ria [NA], palmar metacarpal ligaments: bands that interconnect the bases of the second to fifth metacarpal bones by passing transversely from bone to bone on their palmar surfaces; called also *ligamenta basium* [*ossium metacarpalium*] *volaria.*

l. metacar′peum transver′sum profun′dum [NA], deep transverse metacarpal ligament: a narrow fibrous band that extends across and is attached to the palmar surfaces of the heads of the second to fifth metacarpal bones, joining them together. Called also *ligamenta capitulorum* [*ossium metacarpalium*] *transversa.*

l. metacar′peum transver′sum superficia′le [NA], superficial transverse metacarpal ligament: transverse fibers occupying the intervals between the diverging longitudinal bands of the palmar aponeurosis.

ligamen′ta metatar′sea dorsa′lia [NA], dorsal metatarsal ligaments: light transverse bands on the dorsal surfaces of the bases of the second to fifth metatarsal bones, similar to the corresponding ligaments on the metacarpal bones; called also *ligamenta basium* [*ossium metatarsalium*] *dorsalia.*

ligamen′ta metatar′sea interos′sea [NA], interosseous metatarsal ligaments: bands between the bases of the second to fifth metatarsal bones, similar to the corresponding ligaments of the hand; called also *ligamenta basium* [*ossium metatarsalium*] *interossea.*

ligamen′ta metatar′sea planta′ria [NA], plantar metatarsal ligaments: strong transverse bands on the plantar surfaces of the bases of the second to fifth metatarsal bones; called also *ligamenta basium* [*ossium metatarsalium*] *plantaria.*

l. metatar′seum transver′sum profun′dum [NA], deep transverse metatarsal ligament: a narrow fibrous band that extends across, is attached to the plantar surfaces of, and thus joins together the heads of all the metatarsal bones; called also *ligamenta capitulorum* [*ossium metatarsalium*] *transversa.*

l. metatar′seum transver′sum superficia′le [NA], superficial transverse metatarsal ligament: fibers that lie in the superficial fascia of the sole of the foot beneath the heads of the metatarsal bones.

ligamen′ta navicularicuneifor′mia dorsa′lia, ligamenta cuneonavicularia dorsalia.

ligamen′ta navicularicuneifor′mia planta′ria, ligamenta cuneonavicularia plantaria.

l. nu′chae [NA], nuchal ligament: a broad, fibrous, roughly triangular sagittal septum in the back of the neck, separating the right and left sides. It extends from the tips of the spinous processes of all the cervical vertebrae to attach to the entire length of the external occipital crest. Caudally it is continuous with the supraspinous ligament.

ligamen′ta ossiculo′rum audi′tus [NA], ligaments of auditory ossicles: the ligaments of the auditory ossicles, comprising the anterior, lateral, and superior ligaments of the malleus, the posterior and superior ligaments of the incus, and the annular ligament of the stapes.

l. ova′rii pro′prium [NA], ovarian ligament: a musculofibrous cord in the broad ligament, joining the ovary to the upper part of the lateral margin of the uterus just below the attachment of the uterine tube; called also *utero-ovarian ligament.*

ligamen′ta palma′ria [NA], palmar ligaments: thick, dense fibrocartilaginous plates on the palmar surfaces of the metacarpophalangeal articulations, between the collateral ligaments. They are firmly connected to the bases of the proximal phalanges but only loosely connected to the metacarpal bones. Called also *ligamenta accessoria volaria* and *volar accessory ligaments.*

l. palpebra′le latera′le [NA], lateral palpebral ligament: a ligament that anchors the lateral end of the superior and inferior tarsal plates to the margin of the orbit; called also *canthal ligament.*

l. palpebra′le media′le [NA], medial palpebral ligament: fibrous bands that connect the medial ends of the tarsi to the bones of the orbit, an anterior bundle passing in front of the lacrimal sac and being attached to the frontal process of the maxilla, and a posterior bundle passing behind the lacrimal sac and being attached to the posterior crest of the lacrimal bone.

l. patel′lae [NA], patellar ligament: the continuation of the central portion of the tendon of the quadriceps femoris muscle distal to the patella; it extends from the patella to the tuberosity of the tibia.

l. pectina′tum an′guli iridocornea′lis [NA], pectinate ligament of iridocorneal angle: a few poorly developed fibers found in the iridocorneal angle, interconnecting the cornea, iris, and ciliary muscle; called also *l. pectinatum iridis.*

l. pectina′tum i′ridis, l. pectinatum anguli iridocornealis.

l. pectinea′le [NA], pectineal ligament: a strong aponeurotic lateral continuation of the lacunar ligament along the pectineal line of the pubis; called also *Cooper's ligament* and *inguinal ligament of Cooper*.

l. phrenicocol'icum [NA], phrenicocolic ligament: a peritoneal fold that passes from the left colic flexure to the adjacent costal portion of the diaphragm.

l. phrenicoliena'le [NA], phrenicosplenic ligament: a peritoneal fold that passes from the diaphragm to the concave surface of the spleen; called also *l. lienorenale* [NA alternative].

l. pisohama'tum [NA], pisohamate ligament: a fibrous band extending from the pisiform bone to the hook of the hamate bone.

l. pisometacar'peum [NA], pisometacarpal ligament: a fibrous band extending from the pisiform bone to the bases of the fifth, usually the fourth, and sometimes the third metacarpal bone.

ligamen'ta planta'ria articulatio'num metatarsophalangea'rum [NA], thick, dense bands situated on the plantar surfaces of the metatarsophalangeal articulations between the collateral ligaments; called also *ligamenta accessoria plantaria*.

l. planta're lon'gum [NA], long plantar ligament: the longest ligament of the foot, arising from the lower surface of the calcaneus as far back as the lateral and the medial processes, passing forward over the tendon of the peroneus longus, and inserting into the bases of the second through fifth metatarsal bones.

l. poplite'um arcua'tum [NA], arcuate popliteal ligament: a band of variable and ill-defined fibers at the posterolateral part of the knee joint; it is attached inferiorly to the apex of the head of the fibula, arches superiorly and medially over the popliteal tendon, and merges with the articular capsule. Called also *popliteal arch* and *arcuate ligament of knee*.

l. poplite'um obli'quum [NA], oblique popliteal ligament: a broad band of fibers that arises from the medial condyle of the tibia, merges more or less with the tendon of the semimembranosus, and passes obliquely across the back of the knee joint to the lateral epicondyle of the femur. It contains large openings for the passage of vessels and nerves.

l. pterygospina'le [NA], pterygospinal ligament: a band of fibers extending from the upper part of the superior border of the lateral pterygoid plate to the spine of the sphenoid bone; called also *l. pterygospinosum*.

l. pterygospino'sum, l. pterygospinale.

l. pu'bicum supe'rius [NA], superior pubic ligament: fibers that pass transversely across the superior margin of the symphysis pubis; attached to the bones and to the interpubic disk, they extend laterally as far as the pubic tubercle.

l. pubocapsula're, l. pubofemorale.

l. pubofemora'le [NA], pubofemoral ligament: a band that arises from the entire length of the obturator crest of the pubic bone and passes laterally and inferiorly to merge into the capsule of the hip joint, some fibers reaching to the lower part of the neck of the femur. Called also *l. pubocapsulare*.

l. puboprostat'icum [NA], puboprostatic ligament: a thickening of the superior fascia of the pelvic diaphragm in the male that, laterally, extends from the prostate to the tendinous arch of the pelvic fascia and, medially, is a forward continuation of the tendinous arch to the pubis.

l. puboprostat'icum latera'le, lateral extension of ligamentum puboprostaticum.

l. puboprostat'icum me'dium, medial extension of ligamentum puboprostaticum.

l. pubovesica'le [NA], pubovesical ligament: a thickening of the superior fascia of the pelvic diaphragm in the female that, laterally, extends from the neck of the bladder to the tendinous arch of the pelvic fascia and, medially, is a forward continuation of the tendinous arch to the pubis.

l. pubovesica'le latera'le, lateral extension of ligamentum pubovesicale.

l. pubovesica'le me'dium, medial extension of ligamentum pubovesicale.

l. pulmona'le [NA], pulmonary ligament: a vertical pleural fold that extends from the hilus down to the base on the medial surface of the lung, forming the posterior boundary of the impressio cardiaca; called also *broad ligament of lung*.

ligamen'ta pylo'ri, thickened bands of the longitudinal muscular layer of the stomach situated on the anterior and the posterior surfaces of the antrum pyloricum.

l. quadra'tum [NA], quadrate ligament: a fibrous bundle connecting the distal margin of the radial notch of the ulna to the neck of the radius.

l. radiocar'peum dorsa'le [NA], dorsal radiocarpal ligament: a fibrous band that passes obliquely from the posterior border of the distal extremity of the radius to the dorsal surfaces of the proximal row of carpal bones, especially the triquetral and lunate, and to the dorsal intercarpal ligaments.

l. radiocar'peum palma're [NA], palmar radiocarpal ligament: several bundles of fibers that pass obliquely from the styloid process and the distal anterior margin of the radius to the lunate, triquetral, capitate, and hamate bones; called also *l. radiocarpeum volare* and *volar radiocarpal ligament*.

l. radiocar'peum vola're, l. radiocarpeum palmare.

l. sacrococcyg'eum ante'rius, l. sacrococcygeum ventrale.

l. sacrococcyg'eum dorsa'le profun'dum [NA], deep dorsal sacrococcygeal ligament: the terminal portion of the posterior longitudinal ligament of the vertebral column; it helps to unite the dorsal surfaces of the fifth sacral and the coccygeal vertebrae. Called also *l. sacrococcygeum posterius profundum*.

l. sacrococcyg'eum dorsa'le superficia'le [NA], superficial dorsal sacrococcygeal ligament: a fibrous band continuous with the supraspinous ligament of the vertebral column; attached cranially to the margin of the sacral hiatus, and diverging as it passes caudally to attach to the dorsal surface of the coccyx. Called also *l. sacrococcygeum posterius superficiale*.

l. sacrococcyg'eum latera'le [NA], lateral sacrococcygeal ligament: a fibrous band, homologous with the intertransverse ligaments, that passes from the transverse process of the first coccygeal vertebra to the lower lateral angle of the sacrum, thus helping to complete the foramen of the fifth sacral nerve.

l. sacrococcyg'eum poste'rius profun'dum, l. sacrococcygeum dorsale profundum.

l. sacrococcyg'eum poste'rius superficia'le, l. sacrococcygeum dorsale superficiale.

l. sacrococcyg'eum ventra'le [NA], ventral sacrococcygeal ligament: a flat band, homologous with the anterior longitudinal ligament of the vertebral column, that passes from the lower part of the sacrum over onto the anterior part of the coccyx; called also *l. sacrococcygeum anterius*.

ligamen'ta sacroili'aca anterio'ra, ligamenta sacroiliaca ventralia.

ligamen'ta sacroili'aca dorsa'lia [NA], dorsal sacroiliac ligaments: numerous strong bands that pass from the tuberosity of the ilium and the posterior inferior and posterior superior iliac spines to the intermediate sacral crest and adjacent areas of the sacrum.

ligamen'ta sacroili'aca interos'sea [NA], interosseous sacroiliac ligaments: numerous short, strong bundles connecting the tuberosities and adjacent surfaces of the sacrum and the ilium.

l. sacroili'acum poste'rius bre've, see *ligamenta sacroiliaca dorsalia*.

l. sacroili'acum poste'rius lon'gum, see *ligamenta sacroiliaca dorsalia*.

ligamen'ta sacroili'aca ventra'lia [NA], ventral sacroiliac ligaments: numerous thin fibrous bands passing from the ventral margin of the auricular surface of the sacrum to the adjacent portions of the ilium; called also *ligamenta sacroiliaca anteriora* and *anterior sacroiliac ligaments*.

l. sacrospina'le [NA], sacrospinal ligament: a deep, thin triangular band, attached by its apex to the spine of the ischium and by its base to the lateral margins of the sacrum and the coccyx; called also *l. sacrospinosum*.

l. sacrospino'sum, l. sacrospinale.

l. sacrotubera'le [NA], sacrotuberal ligament: a large, flat band that is attached below to the ischial tuberosity, spreads out as it ascends, and is attached to the lateral margins of the sacrum and the coccyx and to the posterior inferior iliac spine; called also *l. sacrotuberosum*.

l. sacrotubero'sum, l. sacrotuberale.

l. sero'sum, serous ligament: a fold of peritoneum or other serous membrane that helps to hold an organ or part in position and transmits blood vessels and nerves.

l. sphenomandibula're [NA], sphenomandibular ligament: a thin aponeurotic band that extends from the angular spine of the sphenoid bone downward medial to the temporomandibular articulation and attaches to the lingula of the mandible.

l. spira'le coch'leae [NA], spiral ligament of cochlea: the thickened outer or centrifugal portion of the periosteum of the cochlear duct, forming a spiral band to which the basal membrane is attached.

l. sternoclavicula're, see *l. sternoclaviculare anterius* and *l. sternoclaviculare posterius*.

l. sternoclavicula're ante'rius [NA], anterior sternoclavicular ligament: a thick reinforcing band on the anterior portion of the articular capsule of the sternoclavicular articulation. It is attached superiorly to the anterior and superior parts of the sternal extremity of the clavicle and inferiorly to the anterior surface of the manubrium of the sternum.

l. sternoclavicula're poste'rius [NA], posterior sternoclavicular ligament: a thick reinforcing band on the posterior portion of the articular capsule of the sternoclavicular articulation. It is attached superiorly to the posterior and superior parts of the sternal extremity of the clavicle and inferiorly to the posterior surface of the manubrium of the sternum.

l. sternocosta'le interarticula're, l. sternocostale intraarticulare.

l. sternocosta'le intraarticula're [NA], intra-articular sternocostal ligament: a horizontal fibrocartilaginous plate in the center of the second sternocostal joint, which joins the tip of the costal cartilage to the fibrous junction between the manubrium and the body of the sternum, and thus divides the joint into two parts. Called also *l. sternocostale interarticulare*.

ligamen'ta sternocosta'lia radia'ta [NA], radiate sternocostal ligaments: fibrous bands attached to the sternal end of a costal cartilage, radiating from there out onto the ventral part of the sternum.

ligamen'ta sternopericardi'aca [NA], sternopericardiac ligaments: two (superior and inferior) or more fibrous bands that attach the pericardium to the dorsal surface of the sternum.

l. stylohyoi'deum [NA], stylohyoid ligament: a vertical fibroelastic aponeurotic cord attached above to the tip of the styloid process of the temporal bone and below to the lesser horn of the hyoid bone.

l. stylomandibula're [NA], stylomandibular ligament: an aponeurotic band attached superiorly to the tip of the styloid process of the temporal bone and inferiorly to the angle and posterior margin of the ramus of the mandible.

l. supraspina'le [NA], supraspinal ligament: a single long, vertical fibrous band passing over and attached to the tips of the spinous processes of the vertebrae from the seventh cervical to the sacrum; it is continuous above with the ligamentum nuchae.

l. suspenso'rium clitor'idis [NA], suspensory ligament of clitoris: a strong fibrous band that comes from the external deep investing fascia and attaches the root of the clitoris to the linea alba, symphysis pubis, and arcuate pubic ligament.

ligamen'ta suspenso'ria mam'mae [NA], suspensory ligaments of mammary gland: fibrous processes, extending from the corpus mammae to the corium, homologous with the retinacula cutis of other regions of the body.

l. suspenso'rium ova'rii [NA], suspensory ligament of ovary: the portion of the broad ligament lateral to and above the ovary; it contains the ovarian vessels and nerves and passes upward over the iliac vessels.

l. suspenso'rium pe'nis [NA], suspensory ligament of penis: a strong fibrous band that comes from the external deep investing fascia and attaches the root of the penis to the linea alba, symphysis pubis, and arcuate pubic ligament.

l. talocalca'neum ante'rius, anterior talocalcaneal ligament: a fibrous band passing from the front and lateral surface of the neck of the talus to the superior surface of the calcaneus; it forms the posterior border of the sinus tarsi.

l. talocalca'neum interos'seum [NA], interosseous talocalcaneal ligament: fibrous bands in the sinus tarsi, passing between the opposed surfaces of the calcaneus and the talus.

l. talocalca'neum latera'le [NA], lateral talocalcaneal ligament: a fibrous band passing from the lateral surface of the talus to that of the calcaneus.

l. talocalca'neum media'le [NA], medial talocalcaneal ligament: a fibrous band connecting the medial tubercle of the talus with the sustentaculum tali of the calcaneus.

l. talocalca'neum poste'rius, posterior talocalcaneal ligament: a fibrous band connecting the processus posterior tali with the upper and medial part of the calcaneus.

l. talofibula're ante'rius [NA], anterior talofibular ligament: one or more fibrous bands that pass from the anterior surface of the lateral malleolus of the fibula to the anterior margin of the lateral articular surface of the talus.

l. talofibula're poste'rius [NA], posterior talofibular ligament: a strong fibrous horizontal band passing from the posteromedial face of the lateral malleolus of the fibula to the area of the posterior process of the talus.

l. talonavicula're [NA], talonavicular ligament: a broad, thin fibrous band passing from the dorsal and lateral surfaces of the neck of the talus to the dorsal surface of the navicular bone; called also *l. talonaviculare* [*dorsale*] and *talonavicular dorsal ligament.*

l. talonavicula're [dorsa'le], l. talonaviculare.

l. talotibia'le ante'rius, pars tibiotalaris anterior ligamenti medialis.

l. talotibia'le poste'rius, pars tibiotalaris posterior ligamenti medialis.

ligamen'ta tar'si dorsa'lia [NA], dorsal ligaments of tarsus: including the bifurcate, the dorsal cuboideonavicular, cuneocuboid, cuneonavicular, and intercuneiform, and the talonavicular ligaments; called also *dorsal intertarsal ligaments.*

ligamen'ta tar'si interos'sea [NA], interosseous ligaments of the tarsus, including the interosseous cuneocuboid, intercuneiform, talocalcaneal ligaments.

ligamen'ta tar'si planta'ria [NA], plantar ligaments of tarsus: the inferior ligaments of the foot, comprising the long plantar and the plantar calcaneocuboid, calcaneonavicular, cuneonavicular, cuboideonavicular, intercuneiform, and cuneocuboid ligaments.

ligamen'ta tar'si profun'da, the deep ligaments of the tarsus.

ligamen'ta tarsometatar'sea dorsa'lia [NA], dorsal tarsometatarsal ligaments: fibrous bands passing from the dorsal surfaces of the bases of the metatarsal bones to the dorsal surfaces of the cuboid and the three cuneiform bones.

ligamen'ta tarsometatar'sea planta'ria [NA], plantar tarsometatarsal ligaments: fibrous bands passing from the plantar surfaces of the bases of the metatarsal bones to the plantar surfaces of the cuboid and the three cuneiform bones.

l. temporomandibula're, l. laterale articulationis temporomandibularis.

l. te'res fem'oris, l. capitis femoris.

l. te'res hep'atis [NA], a fibrous cord, the remains of the left umbilical vein, extending from the porta hepatis, where it is attached to the left branch of the portal vein, out through the fissure of the ligamentum teres and the falciform ligament to the umbilicus.

l. te'res u'teri [NA], round ligament of uterus: a fibromuscular band in the female that is attached to the uterus near the attachment of the uterine tube, passing then along the broad ligament, out through the inguinal ring, and into the labium majus.

l. thyreoepiglot'ticum, l. thyroepiglotticum.

l. thyroepiglot'ticum [NA], thyroepiglottic ligament: a fibrous band that attaches the petiolus of the epiglottis to the thyroid cartilage just below the superior notch; called also *l. thyreoepiglotticum.*

l. thyrohyoi'deum [NA], thyrohyoid ligament: a round elastic cord that forms the posterior margin of the thyrohyoid membrane; it extends from the tip of the superior horn of the thyroid cartilage upward to the tip of the greater horn of the hyoid bone. Called also *l. hyothyreoideum laterale* and *Berry's ligament.*

l. thyrohyoi'deum media'num [NA], median thyrohyoid ligament: the central, thicker portion of the thyrohyoid membrane; its broader upper part is attached to the body of the hyoid bone and its narrow lower end to the superior incisure of the thyroid cartilage. Called also *l. hyothyreoideum medium.*

l. tibiofibula're ante'rius [NA], anterior tibiofibular ligament: a flat triangular band that passes diagonally, inferiorly, and laterally from the anterior portion of the lateral surface of the distal end of the tibia to the anterior surface of the distal end of the fibula; called also *l. malleoli lateralis anterius.*

l. tibiofibula're poste'rius [NA], posterior tibiofibular ligament: a fibrous band that passes diagonally, inferiorly, and laterally from the posterior surface of the distal end of the tibia to the adjacent posterior surface of the distal end of the fibula; called also *l. malleoli lateralis posterius.*

l. tibionavicula're, pars tibionavicularis ligamenti medialis.

l. transver'sum acetab'uli [NA], transverse ligament of acetabulum: a fibrous band continuous with the acetabular lip of the hip joint, which bridges the acetabular notch and converts it into a foramen.

l. transver'sum atlan'tis [NA], transverse ligament of atlas: the strong horizontal portion of the cruciform ligament of the atlas. It is attached at each end to the lateral masses of the atlas and curves posteriorly around the dens of the axis. It thus divides the atlantal ring into a smaller anterior division for the dens and a larger posterior division for the spinal cord and related structures. Called also *Lauth's ligament.*

l. transver'sum cru'ris, retinaculum musculorum extensorum pedis superius.

l. transver'sum ge'nu, l. transversum genus.

l. transver'sum ge'nus [NA], transverse ligament of knee: a more or less distinct bundle of fibers in the knee joint, joining together the anterior convex margin of the lateral meniscus and the anterior concave margin or anterior end of the medial meniscus; called also *l. transversum genu.*

l. transver'sum pel'vis, l. transversum perinei.

l. transver'sum perine'i [NA], transverse perineal ligament: the strengthened fused portion of the superior and inferior fasciae of the urogenital diaphragm at the anterior border of the diaphragm; called also *l. transversum pelvis* and *transverse pelvic ligament.*

l. transver'sum scap'ulae infe'rius [NA], inferior transverse ligament of scapula: one of three intrinsic ligaments of the scapula, composed of more or less distinct fascial fibers that pass from the lateral border of the spine of the scapula to the adjacent margin of the glenoid cavity, thus converting the notch at the base of the spine into a foramen for the passage of the suprascapular vessels and nerves to the infraspinous fossa.

l. transver'sum scap'ulae supe'rius [NA], superior transverse ligament of scapula: one of three intrinsic ligaments of the scapula, a band of fibers that bridges the scapular notch, thus forming a foramen for the passage of the suprascapular nerve. One end is attached to the base of the coracoid process, the other end to the medial border of the scapular notch.

l. trapezoi'deum [NA], trapezoid ligament: a broad, flat band forming the anterolateral portion of the coracoclavicular ligament; it is attached inferiorly to the superior surface of the coracoid process of the scapula and superiorly to the oblique ridge on the inferior surface of the clavicle.

l. triangula're dex'trum hep'atis [NA], right triangular ligament of liver: the pointed right extremity of the coronary ligament of the liver where the superior and the inferior layer join in their attachment to the diaphragm.

l. triangula're sinis'trum hep'atis [NA], left triangular ligament of liver: a triangular extension of the left extremity of the coronary ligament, which helps to attach the left lobe of the liver to the diaphragm.

l. tuber'culi cos'tae, l. costotransversarium laterale.

l. ulnocar'peum palma're [NA], palmar ulnocarpal ligament: bundles of fibers that pass from the styloid process of the ulna to the carpal bones.

l. umbilica'le latera'le, former NA term for *l. umbilicale mediale.*

l. umbilica'le media'le [NA], a fibrous cord, the remains of the obliterated umbilical artery, which is situated in and produces the lateral umbilical fold. Called also *obliterated hypogastric artery, lateral umbilical ligament, l. umbilicale laterale,* and *medial umbilical ligament.*

l. umbilica'le media'num [NA], median umbilical ligament: a fibrous cord, the remains of the partially obliterated urachus, that extends from the bladder to the umbilicus; it is situated in and produces the median umbilical fold. Called also *l. umbilicale medium* and *middle umbilical ligament.*

l. umbilica′le me′dium, l. umbilicale medianum.

l. vagina′le, vinculum tendinum.

ligamen′ta vagina′lia digito′rum ma′nus, vaginae fibrosae digitorum manus.

ligamen′ta vagina′lia digito′rum pedis, vaginae fibrosae digitorum pedis.

l. ve′nae ca′vae sinis′trae, plica venae cavae sinistrae.

l. veno′sum [NA], venous ligament of liver: a fibrous cord, the remains of the fetal ductus venosus, lying in the fissura ligamenti venosi.

l. veno′sum [Aran′tii], l. venosum.

l. ventricula′re, l. vestibulare.

l. vestibula′re [NA], vestibular ligament: the membrane that extends from the thyroid cartilage in front to the anterolateral surface of the arytenoid cartilage behind; it lies within the vestibular fold, above the vocal ligament. Called also *l. ventriculare* and *ventricular ligament of larynx.*

l. voca′le [NA], vocal ligament: the elastic tissue membrane that extends from the thyroid cartilage in front to the vocal process of the arytenoid cartilage behind; it lies within the vocal fold, below the vestibular ligament.

---

ligand (li′gand, lig′and) [L. *ligare* to tie or bind] an organic molecule that donates the necessary electrons to form coordinate covalent bonds with metallic ions, as oxygen is bound to the central iron atom of hemoglobin. The term is also used to indicate any ion or molecule that reacts to form a complex with another molecule, frequently a macromolecule, as an antigen-antibody complex.

ligase (li′gās, lig′ās) any of a class of enzymes that catalyze the joining together of two molecules coupled with the breakdown of a pyrophosphate bond in ATP or a similar triphosphate. Called also *synthetase* (q.v.).

ligate (li′gāt) to tie or bind with a ligature.

ligation (li-ga′shun) [L. *ligatio*] the application of a ligature. **Barron l.,** treatment of hemorrhoids by binding them with rubber ligatures so that the ligated portion sloughs away within several days. **pole l.,** ligation of both poles of the thyroid gland for the purpose of limiting the amount of blood to and from the gland; employed in Basedow's disease. **teeth l.,** 1. the binding together of teeth with wire for stabilization and immobilization following traumatic injury. 2. the tying of arch wires into orthodontic brackets. **tubal l.,** sterilization of the female by constricting the uterine tubes by means of ligatures; the tubes may, in addition, be severed or crushed.

ligature (lig′ah-chūr) [L. *ligatura*] 1. any substance, such as catgut, cotton, silk, or wire, used to tie a vessel or strangulate a part. 2. in orthodontics, a string or wire used to fasten a tooth to an orthodontic appliance or to another tooth. **chain l.,** a kind of interlocking ligature used in typing pedicles in several places, a long thread being carried through the pedicle in several places. **elastic l.,** a band of caoutchouc used to strangulate hemorrhoids and pedunculated growths. **Erichsen's l.** (*obs.*), a double thread of white and black for ligating nevi. **interlacing l., interlocking l.,** a continuous suture in which the loops interlock. **kangaroo l.,** a prepared tendon from a kangaroo's tail; used as a ligature. **lateral l.,** a ligature so applied as to check, but not to interrupt, the distal blood flow. **occluding l.,** a ligature that occludes the blood supply to distal tissue. **provisional l.,** one applied at the beginning of an operation, but removed before its termination. **soluble l.,** a ligature of prepared animal membrane which is subsequently absorbed, the time of absorption depending upon the method of preparation and the size of the ligature. **suboccluding l.,** a ligature that obstructs the main blood supply, but leaves unimpaired a portion of tissue capable of establishing capillary anastomosis. **terminal l.,** a ligature applied to the transected end of a vessel. **thread-elastic l.,** an elastic thread used for various force applications in orthodontic therapy.

ligg. ligaments, or ligamenta.

light (līt) the electromagnetic radiation having a velocity of about 3×10^{10} cm. (186,284 miles) per second, and the vibrations in space being at right angles to the direction of transmission. Frequently construed as limited to the range of wavelength between 3900 and 7700 angstroms, which provides the stimulus for the subjective sensation of sight, but sometimes considered as including part of the ultraviolet and infrared ranges as well. **actinic l.,** light rays capable of producing chemical effects. **axial l., central l.,** light whose rays are parallel to each other and to the optic axis. **coherent l.,** light of a single frequency that travels in intense, nearly perfect, parallel rays without appreciable divergence. **cold l.,** a light transmitted through a quartz or plastic structure to dissipate the heat. The lamp may be applied directly to the skin and is used for transillumination of the tissues for cancer diagnosis. **l. difference,** the difference between the two eyes in their sensitivity to light; often abbreviated L.D. **diffused l.,** that which has been scattered by reflection and refraction. **Finsen l.,** light consisting principally of the violet and ultraviolet rays given off by a Finsen lamp; used in the treatment of lupus and similar diseases. **idioretinal l.,** sensation of light that occurs in the complete absence of the electromagnetic waves that ordinarily stimulate the sensation. **infrared l.,** see under *ray*. **intrinsic l.** (of the retina), the dim light always present in the visual field. **Landeker-Steinberg l.,** a light that emits a spectrum similar to that of the sun except that the ultraviolet waves are eliminated; used therapeutically. **l. minimum,** the smallest degree of light perceived by the eye; often abbreviated L.M. **Minin l.,** a therapeutic lamp for the administration of violet and ultraviolet light.

monochromatic l., one of the colors of the spectrum into which light is divided by a prism. **neon l.,** a light that contains no ultraviolet and no infrared rays. **oblique l.,** the light that falls obliquely on a surface. **polarized l.,** light the vibrations of which are made over one plane or in circles or ellipses. **reflected l.,** light whose rays have been turned back from an illuminated surface. **refracted l.,** light whose rays have been bent out of their original course by passing through a transparent membrane. **Simpson l.,** an electric arc light with electrodes of tungstate of iron and manganese; formerly used in the treatment of skin lesions. **transmitted l.,** light the rays of which have passed through an object. **Tyndall l.,** the light that is reflected or dispersed by particles suspended in a gas or liquid; see *Tyndall phenomenon*, under *phenomenon*. **ultraviolet l.,** see under *ray*. **white l.,** that produced by a mixture of all wavelengths of electromagnetic energy perceptible as light. **Wood's l.,** ultraviolet radiation from a mercury-vapor source, transmitted through a nickel-oxide filter (Wood's filter or glass), which holds back all but a few violet rays of the visible spectrum and passes ultraviolet wavelengths of about 365 nm.; much used in the diagnosis of fungus infections of the scalp and erythrasma, and also to reveal the presence of porphyrins and fluorescent minerals.

lightening (līt′en-ing) the sensation of decreased abdominal distention produced by the descent of the uterus into the pelvic cavity, occurring from two to three weeks before labor begins.

ligneous (lig′ne-us) woody; having a wooden feeling.

Lignières' test (reaction) (lēn-yārz′) [José *Lignières*, physician in Buenos Aires, 1868–1933] see under *tests*.

lignin (lig′nin) a polysaccharide which in connection with cellulose forms the cell wall of plants and thus of wood.

lignocaine (lig′no-kān) lidocaine.

lignocellulose (lig″no-sel′u-lōs) a heterohexosan composed of lignin and cellulose, and forming the cell walls of woody plants.

lignum (lig′num), gen. *lig′ni* [L.] wood. **l. sanc′tum, l. vi′tae,** the heartwood of *Guajacum officinale* Linne or of *G. sanctum* Linne.

ligroin, ligroine (lig′ro-in) a petroleum fraction similar in nature to (and sometimes used synonymously with) petroleum benzin; it is used as an organic solvent. Called also *naphtha*.

ligula, ligule (lig′u-lah, lig′ūl) [L. "strap"] (*obs.*) tenia ventriculi quarti.

Lilienthal's probe (lil′e-en-thalz″) [Howard *Lilienthal*, surgeon in New York, 1861–1946] see under *probe*.

limb (lim) 1. one of the paired appendages of the body used in locomotion or grasping. In man, an arm or a leg with all its component parts; called also *membrum* [NA] and, formerly, *extremitas*. In embryology, the limbs are divided into four main parts: the *zonoskeleton*, comprising the scapula and clavicle (as a unit) and the hip bone; the *stylopodium*, comprising the humerus and femur; the *zygopodium*, comprising the radius and ulna and the tibia and fibula; and the *autopodium*, comprising the hand and the foot. 2. a structure or part resembling an arm or leg. **anacrotic l.,** the ascending portion of a tracing of the pulse wave obtained by the manometer or the sphygmograph. **l's of anthelix,** crura anthelicis; see under *crus*. **catacrotic l.,** the descending portion of a tracing of the pulse wave obtained by the manometer or the sphygmograph. **l. of incus, long,** crus longum incudis. **l. of incus, short,** crus breve incudis. **l. of internal capsule, anterior,** crus anterius capsulae internae. **l. of internal capsule, posterior,** crus posterius capsulae internae. **pectoral l.,** the arm (membrum superius), or a homologous part. **pelvic l.,** the leg (membrum inferius), or a homologous part. **phantom l.,** the sensation, after amputation of a limb, that the absent part is still present; there may also be paresthesias, transient aches, and intermittent or continuous pain perceived as originating in the absent limb. **l. of stapes, anterior,** crus anterius stapedis. **l. of stapes, posterior,** crus posterius stapedis. **thoracic l.,** pectoral l.

limbal (lim′bal) limbic; occurring at the junction of the cornea and conjunctiva.

limberneck (lim′ber-nek) a disease of fowl resulting from ingestion of food contaminated with *Clostridium botulinum*, and characterized by a flaccid paralysis which gives the condition its name.

limbi (lim′bi) [L.] plural of *limbus*.

limbic (lim′bik) pertaining to a limbus, or margin; forming a border around; see under *system*.

Limbitrol (lim′bĭ-trol) trademark for a combination of amitriptyline and chlordiazepoxide.

limbus (lim′bus), pl. *lim′bi* [L.] a border, hem, fringe; [NA] a general term for the border of certain structures. See also *labium* and *margo*. **alveolar l. of mandible,** arcus alveolaris mandibulae. **alveolar l. of maxilla,** arcus alveolaris maxillae. **l. alveola′ris mandib′ulae,** arcus alveolaris mandibulae. **l. alveola′ris maxil′lae,** arcus alveolaris maxillae. **l. angulo′sus,** linea obliqua cartilaginis thyroideae. **l. chorioi′deus** (*obs.*), that part of the embryonic gyrus fornicatus which forms, in the adult, the choroid plexus of the lateral ventricle. **l. conjuncti′vae,** 1. l. corneae. 2. anulus conjunctivae. **l. of cornea, l. cor′neae,** the periphery of the cornea where it joins the sclera. **l. cortica′lis** (*obs.*), the part of the embryonic gyrus which forms, in the adult, the subiculum, dentate gyrus, and indusium griseum. **l. foram′inis ova′lis** [NA], the border of the foramen ovale. **l. fos′sae ova′lis** [NA], **l. fos′sae ova′lis [Vieussen′ii],** the prominent rounded margin of the fossa ovalis cordis. **l. lam′inae spira′lis os′seae** [NA], the thickened periosteum of the osseous spiral lamina at the attachment of the vestibular membrane. **l. lu′teus ret′inae,** macula retinae. **l. medulla′ris** (*obs.*), the part of the embryonic gyrus fornicatus which forms, in the adult, the fimbria of the hippocampus and the fornix. **l. membra′nae tym′pani,** 1. the thickened margin of the tympanic membrane attached to the tympanic sulcus. 2. anulus fibrocartilagineus membranae tympani. **lim′bi palpebra′les anterio′res** [NA], the rounded anterior edges of the free margin of the eyelids, from which the eyelashes arise. **lim′bi palpebra′les posterio′res** [NA], the sharp posterior edges of the free margin of the eyelids, closely applied to the eyeball. **spiral l.,** l. laminae spiralis osseae. **l. of Vieussens,** l. fossae ovalis.

lime (līm) [L. *calx*] 1. calcium oxide. 2. [USP] a pharmaceutical preparation containing not less than 95 per cent of calcium oxide; used as a pharmaceutical necessity. 3. the acid fruit of *Citrus aurantifolia;* its juice, which contains ascorbic acid, is antiscorbutic and refrigerant. **l. arsenate,** a solution of white arsenic and sal soda in water, used as an insecticide. **barium hydroxide l.,** a mixture of barium hydroxide octahydrate and calcium hydroxide used as a carbon dioxide absorbant in the administration of anesthetic gases and oxygen. **chlorinated l.,** a white or grayish white powder used as a bleaching agent and disinfectant and, formerly, as a topical germicide. **slaked l.,** calcium hydroxide. **soda l.,** a mixture of calcium oxide and sodium hydroxide. **sulfurated l.,** see *calx sulfurata*.

limen (li′men), pl. *lim′ina* [L.] threshold, as of a stimulus; [NA] a general term for the beginning point, boundary, or threshold of a structure. **l. of insula, l. in′sulae** [NA], the point at which the cortex of the insula is continuous, on the inferior surface of the cerebral hemisphere, with the cortex of the frontal lobe. **l. na′si** [NA], the ridge at the junction of the lateral nasal cartilage and the lateral crus of the greater alar cartilage, marking the boundary between the vestibule of the nose and the nasal cavity proper. **l. of twoness,** the distance between two points of contact on the skin necessary for their recognition as giving rise to separate stimuli.

limina (lim′ĭ-nah) [L.] plural of *limen*.

liminal (lim′ĭ-nal) [L. *limen* threshold] barely appreciable to the senses; pertaining to a threshold.

liminometer (lim″ĭ-nom′ĕ-ter) [*limen* + Gr. *metron* measure] an instrument for measuring the strength of stimulus applied over a tendon and determining the reflex threshold.

limit (lim′it) [L. *limes* boundary] a boundary, as one that confines. **Anstie's l.,** see under *rule*. **assimilation l.,** the amount of carbohydrate that an organism can metabolize without causing glycosuria; called also *saturation limit*. **audibility l.,** the extremes of frequency beyond which the human ear perceives no sound: lower limit, 8 Hz; upper, 20,000 Hz. **elastic l.,** the extent to which elastic material may be deformed without impairing its ability to return to original dimensions. **l. of flocculation,** a term used in expressing the strength of toxin, toxoid, and antitoxin; see *Lf dose*, under *dose*. **l. of perception,** the minimum visual angle below which perception is impossible: an object to be perceived must subtend a visual angle of four or five minutes, thus making its image on the retina about the size of a retinal cone of 3.3–3.6 microns in diameter. **quantum l.,** minimum wavelength. **saturation l.,** assimilation l.

limitans (lim′ĭ-tanz) [L.] limiting; see *membrana limitans*.

limitation (lim-ĭ-ta′shun) circumscription; the act of limiting, or state of being limited. **eccentric l.,** a circumscribed condition of the visual field, more pronounced at some parts of the periphery than at others. **genetic l.,** the necessity that all cells react in accordance with the standards of the particular species to which they belong.

limitrophic (lim″ĭ-trof′ik) controlling nutrition.

Limnatis (lim-na′tis) the land leeches, a genus of the family Gnathobdellidae, class Hirudinea. **L. nilot′ica,** a species of North Africa, middle Europe, and the Near East, where they are commonly used for drawing blood. They sometimes become lodged in the nasal passages, larynx and pharynx of mammals, and when present in large numbers may cause anemia and asphyxia. Called also *Hirudo aegyptiaca*.

limo (li′mo), gen. *limo′nis* [L.] lemon.

limonene (lim′o-nēn) an essential oil found in the peel of oranges and lemons; it is a terpene, $C_3H_5 \cdot C_6H_8 \cdot CH_3$.

limonis (li-mo′nis) [L.] genitive of *limo*, lemon.

limonite (lim′o-nīt) hydrous ferric oxide, $2Fe_2O \cdot 3H_2O$, an ore of iron.

limophthisis (li-mof′thĭ-sis) [Gr. *limos* hunger + *phthisis* wasting] wasting from lack of food or starvation.

limosis (li-mo′sis) [Gr. *limos* hunger] abnormal or morbid hunger.

limotherapy (li″mo-ther′ah-pe) [Gr. *limos* hunger + *therapeia* cure] hunger cure, the treatment of disease by fasting or by a meager diet. Formerly used in an attempt to treat a variety of diseases, e.g., syphilis and cancer; now used in the treatment of obesity.

Linacre (lin′ah-ker), Thomas (1460–1524). A noted English physician and classicist, who was physician to Henry VIII and the first president of the Royal College of Physicians of London. He was also renowned for his translations of Greek classics (e.g., Galen) into Latin.

linamarin (lin″ah-mah′rin) a bitter glycoside, $C_{10}H_{17}O_6N$, found in flax, *Linum usitatissimum* L. (Linaceae) and the lima bean, *Phaseolus limensis* Macf. (Leguminosae). Called also *phaseolunatin*.

Lincocin (lin-ko′sin) trademark for a preparation of lincomycin hydrochloride.

lincomycin (lin″ko-mi′sin) chemical name: (2S-*trans*)-methyl-6,8-dideoxy-6-[[(1-methyl-4-propyl-2-pyrrolidinyl)carbonyl]amino]-1-thio-D-*erythro*-α-D-*galacto*-octopyranoside. An antibiotic, $C_{18}H_{34}N_2O_6S$, primarily a gram-positive specific antibacterial, produced by a variant of *Streptomyces lincolnesis*. **l. hydrochloride** [USP], the monohydrated monohydrochloride salt of lincomycin, $C_{18}H_{34}N_2O_6S \cdot HCl \cdot H_2O$, occurring as a white or practically white, crystalline powder; used as an antibacterial, mainly in the treatment of infections due to susceptible strains of streptococci, pneumococci, and staphylococci, administered intramuscularly and intravenously.

lincture (lingk′tūr) an electuary.

linctus (lingk′tus) [L. "a licking"] an electuary.

lindane (lin′dān) [USP] chemical name: 1α,2α,3β,4α,5α,6β-hexachlorocyclohexane. The gamma isomer of benzene hexachloride, $C_6H_6Cl_6$, occurring as a white, crystalline powder; an insecticide more potent than chlorophenothane (DDT), it is used as a pediculicide and scabicide, applied topically to the skin. Called also *gamma benzene hexachloride*.

Lindau's disease (lin′dowz) [Arvid *Lindau*, Swedish pathologist, born 1892] von Hippel-Lindau disease.

Lindau-von Hippel disease (lin′dow-von hip′el) [Arvid *Lindau;* Eugen *von Hippel*, German ophthalmologist, 1867–1939] von Hippel-Lindau disease.

Lindbergh pump [Charles A. *Lindbergh*, American aviator, born 1902] see under *pump*.

Lindemann's cannula, method (lin′dĕ-manz) [August *Lindemann*, German surgeon, born 1880] see under *cannula* and *method*.

line (līn) [L. *lin′ea*] a stripe, streak, mark, or narrow ridge; often an imaginary line connecting different anatomical landmarks. Called also *linea* [NA]. **abdominal l.,** any line upon the surface of the abdomen, such as one indicating the boundary of a muscle. **absorption l's,** dark lines in the spectrum due to absorption of light by the substance (usually an incandescent gas or vapor) through which the light has passed. Cf. *absorption bands*, under *band*. **accretion l's,** incremental l's. **adrenal l.,** Sergent's white adrenal l. **alveolar l.,** a line from the nasion to the prosthion (alveolar point). **alveolobasilar l.,** a line from the basion to the prosthion (alveolar point). **alveolonasal l.,** a line from the prosthion (alveolar point) to the nasion. **l. of Amici,** Z band; see under *band*. **angular l.,** an irregular jagged line dividing the anterior surface of the iris into two regions. **anococcygeal l., white,** ligamentum anococcygeum. **anocutaneous l.,** pectinate l. **arcuate l. of ilium,** linea arcuata ossis ilii. **arcuate l. of occipital bone, external superior,** linea nuchae superior. **arcuate l. of occipital bone, highest,** linea nuchae suprema. **arcuate l. of occipital bone, inferior,** linea nuchae inferior. **arcuate l. of occipital bone, superior,** linea nuchae superior. **arcuate l. of occipital bone, supreme,** linea nuchae suprema. **arcuate l. of pelvis,** linea terminalis pelvis. **arcuate l. of sheath of rectus abdominis muscle,** linea arcuata vaginae musculi recti abdominis. **atropic l.,** one normal to the place of the axes of rotation of the eye. **auriculobregmatic l.,** a line from the auricular point to the bregma. **axillary l.,** linea axillaris. **Baillarger's l's,** two bands of white fibers seen on section of the cerebral cortex, running parallel to the surface of the cortex, and distinguished as *inner* (lying in the internal granular layer) and *outer* (lying in the granular layer). In the area striata only the outer line is visible and here it is known as the *l.* or *stripe of Gennari.* In agranular cortex, both lines tend to be absent. **base l.,** 1. one from the infraorbital ridge to the external auditory meatus and the middle line of the occiput. 2. a known quantity or a set of known quantities used as a reference point in evaluating similar data. **base-apex l.,** a line perpendicular to the edge of a prism and bisecting the refracting angle of the prism. **basinasal l.,** one from the basion to the nasion. **basiobregmatic l.,** one from the basion to the bregma. **Baudelocque's l.,** see under *diameter.* **Beau's l's,** transverse furrows occurring on the fingernails, usually a sign of systemic disease, but also due to trauma, coronary occlusion, hypercalcemia, skin disease, etc. **biauricular l.,** a line passing over the vertex from one auditory meatus to the other. **bi-iliac l.,** one joining the most prominent points of the two iliac crests. **bismuth l.,** a thin blue-black line along the gingival margin in bismuth poisoning, especially in persons with poor oral hygiene; cf. *lead l.* **Blaschko's l's,** the pattern of lines separating skin surface areas supplied by individual peripheral nerves. **blood l.,** a line of direct descent through several generations. **blue l.,** see *bismuth l.* and *lead l.* **Borsieri's l.,** see under *sign.* **Brödel's white l.,** a longitudinal white line on the anterior surface of the kidney near the convex border. **Brücke's l's,** broad bands alternating with Z bands in the fibrils of the striated muscles. **Bryant's l.,** 1. the vertical side of the iliofemoral triangle. 2. a test line for detecting shortening of the femur. **Burton's l.,** lead l. **calcification l's,** incremental l's. **cell l.,** a group of animal cells derived from a primary culture at the time of first subculture; it is considered to be an *established cell line* when it demonstrates the potential for indefinite subculture *in vitro.* **cement l.,** a name applied to a line, visible in microscopical examination of bone in cross section, marking the boundary of an osteon (haversian system). **cervical l.,** an anatomical landmark determined by the junction of the enamel- and the cementum-covered portions of a tooth (the cementoenamel junction); the dividing line between the crown and root portions of a tooth. **Chaussier's l.,** the median raphe of the corpus callosum. **Chiene's l's,** a set of lines established to aid in localizing the cerebral centers. **Clapton's l.,** a green line on the gums in copper poisoning. **clavicular l.,** one following the course of the clavicles. **cleavage l's,** linear clefts in the skin indicative of direction of the fibers. The cleavage lines, which correspond closely to the crease lines of the skin, assume a characteristic pattern in each part of the body but vary with body configuration. Called also *Langer's lines.* **Conradi's l.,** a line from the base of the xiphoid process to the point on the chest at which the apex beat is felt, indicating the upper limit of percussion dullness of the left lobe of the liver. **contour l's,** l's of Owen. **copper l.,** a greenish or red line at the border of the gums in copper poisoning. **Correra's l.,** a line in the roentgenogram of the chest, around the outline of the thorax, and bounding the lung fields. **Corrigan's l.,** a purplish line observed on the gums in copper poisoning. **costoarticular l.,** a line from the sternoclavicular joint to a point on the eleventh rib. **costoclavicular l.,** linea parasternalis. **costophrenic septal l's,** see *Kerley's l's.* **cricoclavicular l.,** a line from the cricoid cartilage of the larynx to the point at which the upward projection of the anterior axillary line intersects the clavicle. **cruciate l.,** eminentia cruciformis. **curved l. of ilium,** linea arcuata ossis ilii. **curved l. of ilium, inferior,** linea glutea inferior. **curved l. of ilium, middle,** linea glutea anterior. **curved l. of ilium, superior,** linea glutea posterior. **curved l. of occipital bone, highest,** linea nuchae suprema. **curved l. of occipital bone, inferior,** linea nuchae inferior. **curved l. of occipital bone, superior,** linea nuchae superior. **curved l. of occipital bone, supreme,** linea nuchae suprema. **Czermak's l's,** spatia interglobularia; see under *spatium.* **Daubenton's l.,** a line from the opisthion to the basion. **dentate l.,** pectinate l. **De Salle's l.,** nasal l. **Dobie's l.,** Z band; see under *band.* **l. of Douglas,** linea arcuata vaginae musculi recti abdominis. **Duhot's l.,** a line from the superior iliac spine to the apex of the sacrum. **dynamic l's,** lines on the face, e.g., laugh lines and frown lines, which develop as a result of repetitious right-angled pull on the skin by the muscles of expression; they are considered a sign of aging. **Eberth's l's,** microscopic broken or scalariform lines at the junction of the cardiac muscle cells. **ectental l.,** the line of junction between the ectoderm and entoderm. **l's of election,** l's of expression. **Ellis' l., Ellis-Garland l.,** an S-shaped line on the chest, showing the upper border of pleuritic effusions. **embryonic l.,** the primitive streak in the center of the germinal area. **epiphyseal l.,** 1. linea epiphysialis. 2. a strip of lesser density apparent in the roentgenogram of a long bone, representing the noncalcified portion of the cartilaginous growth plate between the epiphysis and the diaphysis. **established cell l.** see *cell l.* **l's of expression,** the natural skin lines and creases of the face and neck, which are the preferred lines of incision in facial and cervical surgery; called also *l's of election.* **facial l.,** a straight line connecting the nasion and pogonion. **Farre's white l.,** the boundary of the insertion of the mesovarium at the hilus of the ovary. **Feiss' l.,** a line from the medial malleolus to the plantar surface of the first metatarsophalangeal joint. **l. of fixation,** a straight line extending through the center of rotation of the eye to the object of vision. **focal l., anterior,** a line whose direction is perpendicular to the meridian of greatest curvature of a refracting surface. **focal l., posterior,** a line whose direction is perpendicular to the meridian of least curvature of a refracting surface. **Fraunhofer's l's,** dark lines of the solar spectrum. **Frommann's l's,** transverse marks on the axon of a medullated nerve fiber, rendered visible by silver nitrate. **fulcrum l.,** the imaginary axis around which a removable partial denture tends to rotate. **fulcrum l., retentive,** an imaginary line connecting the retentive points of clasp arms on retaining teeth adjacent to mucosa-borne denture bases, around which a denture tends to rotate when subjected to such forces as the pull of sticky foods. **fulcrum l., stabilizing,** an imaginary line connecting occlusal rests, around which a denture tends to rotate during mastication. **Gant's l.,** one described on the femur below the greater trochanter, for service as a guide in surgical operations. **genal l.,** one of Jadelot's lines, extending from the nasal line near the mouth toward the malar bone. **l. of Gennari,** see *Baillarger's l's.* **gingival l.,** 1. a line determined by the level to which the gingiva extends on a tooth; although it tends to follow the curvature of the cervical line, the two rarely coincide. 2. any linear mark visible on the surface of the gingiva, such as the discoloration resulting from the ingestion of lead (lead l.). **gluteal l., anterior,** linea glutea anterior. **gluteal l., inferior,** linea glutea inferior. **gluteal l., posterior,** linea glutea posterior. **Gottinger's l.,** a line along the upper border of the zygomatic arch. **Granger l.,** a curved line seen in the roentgenograms of skulls, indicating the position of the optic groove. **Gubler's l.,** a line connecting the apparent origins of the roots of the fifth nerve. **gum l.,** gingival l. (def. 1.). **Haller's l.,** fissura mediana anterior medullae spinalis. **Hampton l.,** a significant roentgenologic characteristic associated with the niche of the typical benign gastric ulcer in profile. **Harris l's,** lines of retarded growth seen radiographically at the epiphyses of long bones. **heave l.,** a groove appearing along the costal arch coincidental with forced contraction of the abdominal muscles following the normal passive expiratory movement in an animal with heaves. **Helmholtz's l.,** a line perpendicular to the plane of the axis of rotation of the eyes. **Hensen's l.,** M band; see under *band.* **Hilton's white l.,** pectinate l. **Holden's l.,** a sulcus below the inguinal fold, crossing the capsule of the hip joint. **hot l.,** see under *H.* **Hudson's l., Hudson-Stähli l.,** pigmented line of the cornea; a linear horizontal brown mark located at about the junction of the middle and lower thirds of the cornea but not reaching the limbus, seen in the normal corneas of 16 per cent of aged individuals. Called also *Stähli's pigment l.* and *superficial l. of the cornea.* **Hueter's l.,** a straight line connecting the medial epicondyle of the humerus with the top of the olecranon when the arm is extended. **Hunter's l.,** linea alba. **iliopectineal l.,** linea arcuata ossis illii. **incremental l's of Ebner, incremental l's of Owen,** l's of Owen. **infracostal l.,** one connecting the lower borders of the tenth costal cartilages. **infrascapular l.,** a horizontal line at the level of the inferior angles of the scapulae. **intercondylar l., intercondyloid l.,** linea intercondylaris femoris. **intermediate l. of iliac crest,** linea intermedia cristae iliacae. **interspinal l.,** a line on the abdomen connecting the two anterior superior iliac spines. **intertrochanteric l., intertrochanteric l., anterior,** linea intertrochanterica. **intertrochanteric l., posterior,** crista intertrochanterica. **intertuberal l.,** a line drawn between the prominences of the frontal bone. **intertubercular l.,** an imaginary line drawn transversely across the abdomen at the level of the iliac crests. **intraperiod l's,** see *period l's.* **isoeffect l's,** in radiotherapy, lines on a rectangular graph representing doses of radiation having tumoricidal effects and those having complicating necrotic effects in normal tissues. **isothermal l's,** lines on a map or chart indicating areas of uniform temperature. **Jadelot's l's,** lines of the face in young children, described as being indicative of specific types of disease; the genal, labial, nasal, and oculozygomatic lines. Called also *Jadelot's furrows.* **K l's, L l's, M l's, N l's, O l's, P l's,** groups of lines in a roentgen-ray spectrum, determined by the stability level to which the replacement electron "drops"; the K lines come from the level nearest the nucleus of the atom and have the shortest wavelength. **l. of Kaes,** a thin layer of fibers in the external granular layer of the cerebral cortex. **Kerley's l's,** horizontal linear densities 1 to 2.5 cm. long on chest roentgenograms; they are arranged in stepladder fashion and are believed to represent widening of the interlobular septa, as by edema (in mitral stenosis) or fibrosis (in silicosis). When peripherally situated, particularly at the base of the lungs, they are called *Kerley's B l's,* or *costophrenic septal lines.* When centrally situated, they are called *Kerley's A l's.* **Kilian's l.,** a prominent line on the promontory of the sacrum. **Krause's l.,** Z band; see under *band.* **L l's,** see under *K l's.* **labial l.,** one of Jadelot's lines, extending laterally from the angle of the mouth; said to indicate disease of the lungs. **Langer's l's,** cleavage l's. **lead l.,** a gray or bluish black line at the gingival margin in lead poisoning, seen especially in patients with poor oral hygiene; it is similar to the bismuth line, but is somewhat more diffuse. Called also *blue l.* and *Burton's line* or *sign.* **lip l.,** a line at the level to which the margin of either lip extends on the teeth. **lip l., high,** the highest level on the teeth or gingival tissue reached by the upper lip in normal function or during a broad smile. **lip l., low,** the lowest level on the teeth reached by the lower lip in normal function or during a broad smile. **lower lung l.,** a horizontal line in roentgenograms of the upper part of the abdomen, running from the lateral chest wall toward the first lumbar vertebra on each side, and representing the lower posterior boundary of the pleural cavity. **M l's,** see *K l's.* **magnetic l's of force,** lines indicating direction of force in a magnetic field. **major dense l's, major period l's,** see *period l's.* **mamillary l.,** linea mamillaris. **mammary l.,** milk line. **median l.,** an imaginary vertical line on the body surface, dividing the surface equally into right and left sides. **median l., anterior,** linea mediana anterior. **median l., posterior,** linea mediana posterior. **Mees' l's,** transverse white lines on the fingernails, as in chronic arsenic poisoning and sometimes in leprosy. **mesenteric l.,** see *mesenteric triangle,* under *triangle.* **Meyer's l.,** the axial line of the big toe which if extended passes through the center of the heel if shoes have never been worn. **midaxillary l.,** linea axillaris. **midclavicular l.,** linea mamillaris. **middle l. of scrotum,** raphe scroti. **midspinal l.,** a perpendicular line down the middle of the vertebral column. **midsternal l.,** a line passing through the middle of the sternum from the cricoid cartilage to the xiphoid. **milk l.,** a ridge of thickened epithelium from axilla to groin in the mammalian embryo along which nipples and mammary glands develop, all but one subsequently disappearing in the human. Called also *mammary l.* and *mammary ridge.* **Monro's l.,** one from the umbilicus to the anterior superior spine of the ilium. **Monro-Richter l.,** one from the umbilicus to the left anterior superior iliac spine. **Morgan's l.,** a secondary crease in the lower eyelids in atopic dermatitis; called also *Dennie's sign.* **Moyer's l.,** a line from the middle of the body of the third sacral vertebra to a point midway between the anterior superior iliac spines. **muscular l's of scapula,** lineae musculares scapulae. **mylohyoid l. of mandible, mylohyoidean l.,** linea mylohyoidea mandibulae. **N l's,** see under *K l's.* **nasal l.,** one of Jadelot's lines, extending from the ala nasi in a semicircle around the mouth. **nasobasilar l.,** a line through the basion and nasal point. **nasolabial l.,** a line extending from the ala nasi to the angle of the mouth. **Nélaton's l.,** a line from the anterior superior spine of the ilium to the most prominent part of the tuberosity of the ischium. **neonatal l.,** a line in the enamel and dentin of a tooth at a position corresponding to the surface of enamel and dentin present at the time of birth. **nigra l.,** linea nigra. **nipple l.,** linea mamillaris. **nuchal l., highest,** linea nuchae suprema. **nuchal l., inferior,** linea nuchae inferior. **nuchal l., median, nuchal l., middle,** crista occipitalis externa. **nuchal l., superior,** linea nuchae superior. **nuchal l., supreme,** linea nuchae suprema. **O l's,** see under *K l's.* **oblique l.,** one which follows an oblique course; see terms beginning *linea obliqua.* **oblique l. of femur,** linea intertrochanterica. **oblique l. of fibula,** 1. crista medialis fibulae. 2. margo anterior fibulae. **oblique l. of mandible,** linea obliqua mandibulae. **oblique l. of mandible, internal,** linea mylohyoidea mandibulae. **oblique l. of thyroid cartilage,** linea obliqua cartilaginis thyroideae. **oblique l. of tibia,** linea musculi solei. **l. of occlusion,** Angle's term for "the line with which, in form and position according to type, the teeth must be in harmony if in normal occlusion"; the line of contact between the maxillary and mandibular teeth when the jaws are closed. **oculozygomatic l.,** one of Jadelot's lines, extending outward from the medial canthus toward the zygoma; said to be a sign of some disorder of the nervous system. **Ogston's l.,** a line from the tubercle of the femur to the intercondylar notch. **omphalospinous l.,** a line on the abdomen connecting the umbilicus and the anterior superior spine of the ilium; a guide to the location of McBurney's point. **orthostatic l's,** natural furrows on the neck, due to physiologic skin excess required at certain areas for the purpose of flexion and extension. **Ouchterlony l.,** in immunodiffusion, a line of antigen-antibody precipitate formed in agar gel. **l's of Owen,** curvilinear lines resembling the growth rings of a tree on transverse section, demarcating layers of interglobular spaces in the deeper parts of the dentin of the crown of a tooth; they are caused by incomplete calcification of the dentin. Called also *incremental l's of Owen.* **P l's,** see under *K l's.* **papillary l.,** linea mamillaris. **parasternal l.,** linea parasternalis. **Pastia's l's,** see under *sign.* **pectinate l.,** a sinuous line following the level of the anal valves and crossing the bases of the columns between them, marking the junction of the zone of the anal canal lined with stratified squamous epithelium and the zone lined with columnar epithelium; called also *anocutaneous l.,* and *dentate l.* or *margin.* **pectineal l.,** 1. linea pectinea femoris. 2. pecten ossis pubis. **pelvic pain l.,** an imaginary line beneath which pain impulses from the bladder neck, prostate, urethra, uterine cervix, and the lower end of the colon are conducted. **period l's,** a series of

light and dark lines occurring in a concentric, repeating pattern in mature myelin: the darker lines (*major dense l's*) represent the apposition of the inner, cytoplasmic surfaces of the Schwann cell plasma membrane; the lighter lines (*intraperiod l's*) bisect the spaces between the darker lines, and represent the apposition of the outer surfaces of the membrane. **Pickerill's imbrication l's,** horizontal lines on the surface of tooth enamel. **pigmented l. of the cornea,** Hudson's l. **Poirier's l.,** a line running from the nasofrontal angle to a point just above the lambda. **popliteal l. of femur,** linea intercondylaris femoris. **popliteal l. of tibia,** linea musculi solei. **Poupart's l.,** an imaginary line on the surface of the abdomen, passing perpendicularly through the midpoint of Poupart's ligament. **precentral l.,** a line on the head, extending from a point midway between the inion and glabella downward and forward. **primitive l.,** primitive streak. **pupillary l.,** pupillary axis. **quadrate l.,** a slight ridge sometimes seen passing vertically downward from the middle of the intertrochanteric crest on the posterior surface of the femur. **recessional l's,** lines or markings on the teeth due to the recession, in the formative period of the teeth, of the soft tissue which gives place to the dentin. **Reid's base l.,** base l. (def. 1). **Retzius' l's,** incremental l's. **Robson's l.,** an imaginary line drawn from the nipple to the umbilicus. **Rolando's l.,** a line on the head marking the position of the fissure of Rolando beneath. **Roser's l.,** Nélaton's l. **rough l. of femur,** linea aspera femoris. **Salter's l's,** l's of Owen. **scapular l.,** linea scapularis. **Schoemaker's l.,** one connecting the point of the trochanter with the anterior superior iliac spine; the extension of this line normally runs above the umbilicus, but runs below the umbilicus when the trochanter is higher than normal. **Schreger's l's,** bands of Schreger. **Schwalbe's l.,** see under *ring.* **semicircular l's, supreme,** linea nuchae suprema. **semicircular l. of Douglas,** linea arcuata vaginae musculi recti abdominis. **semicircular l. of frontal bone,** linea temporalis ossis frontalis. **semicircular l. of occipital bone, highest,** linea nuchae suprema. **semicircular l. of occipital bone, middle,** linea nuchae superior. **semicircular l. of occipital bone, superior,** linea nuchae superior. **semicircular l. of parietal bone, inferior,** linea temporalis inferior ossis parietalis. **semicircular l. of parietal bone, superior,** linea temporalis superior ossis parietalis. **semilunar l.,** linea semilunaris. **Sergent's white adrenal l.,** a white line on the abdomen caused by drawing the finger nail across it; seen in cases of deficient adrenal activity. **Shenton's l.,** a curved line seen in the roentgenogram of the normal hip joint, formed by the top of the obturator foramen. **l. of sight,** a straight line from the center of the pupil to the object viewed. **simian l.,** see under *crease.* **Skinner's l.,** Shenton's l. **soleal l. of tibia,** linea musculi solei. **Spieghel's l., spigelian l., Spigelius' l.,** linea semilunaris. **spiral l. of femur,** linea intertrochanterica. **Stähli's l., Stähli's pigment l.,** Hudson's l. **sternal l., sternal l., lateral,** linea sternalis. **subcostal l.,** a transverse line on the surface of the abdomen at the level of the lower edge of the tenth costal cartilage. **subscapular l's,** lineae musculares scapulae. **superficial l. of the cornea,** Hudson's l. **supraorbital l.,** a line across the forehead, just above the root of the external angular process of the frontal bone. **survey l.,** 1. the line indicating the height of a tooth after the cast has been positioned according to the chosen path of insertion. 2. a line produced on a cast of a tooth by a surveyor scriber, marking the greatest height of contour in relation to the chosen path of insertion of the restoration. 3. a line drawn on a tooth or teeth by means of a surveyor for the purpose of determining the positions of the various parts of a clasp or clasps. Called also *clasp guideline.* **Sydney l.,** see under *crease.* **sylvian l.,** a line on the head extending from the external angular process of the frontal bone to a point three fourths of an inch below the most prominent point of the parietal bone. It coincides with the direction of the fissure of Sylvius. **temporal l., inferior,** linea temporalis inferior ossis parietalis. **temporal l., superior,** linea temporalis superior ossis parietalis. **temporal l. of frontal bone,** linea temporalis ossis frontalis. **temporal l. of parietal bone, inferior,** linea temporalis inferior ossis parietalis. **temporal l. of parietal bone, superior,** linea temporalis superior ossis parietalis. **terminal l. of pelvis,** linea terminalis pelvis. **Thompson's l.,** a red line observed on the gingivae in pulmonary tuberculosis. **thyroid red l.,** an erythematous line produced by irritation of the skin on the front of the neck and upper part of the chest in patients with hyperthyroidism. **Topinard's l.,** a line between the glabella and the mental point. **transverse l's of sacral bone, transverse l. of sacrum,** lineae transversae ossis sacri. **trapezoid l.,** linea trapezoidea. **triradiate l's,** the stars of the embryonic lens. **Trümmerfeld l.,** a zone of metaphyseal degeneration sometimes seen in the bones in infantile scurvy. **Ullmann's l.,** in cases of spondylolisthesis, a line extended upward at a right angle from the anterior edge of the first sacral vertebra to the superior surface of the sacrum will pass through the last lumbar vertebra. **umbilicoiliac l.,** a line from the umbilicus to the anterior superior spine of the ilium. **l. of Venus,** the principal transverse line on the palmar surface of the wrist. **vibrating l.,** a functional line marking the anatomical boundary between the movable and immovable tissues of the palate. **Virchow's l.,** a line from the root of the nose to the lambda. **visual l.,** axis opticus. **Voigt's l's,** a dorsoventral pigmented line of demarcation on the skin, usually extending bilaterally and symmetrically for about 10 cm., along the lateral edge of the biceps muscle; seen in 20 to 26 per cent of blacks and rarely in whites. Called also *Futcher l's.* **Wagner's l.,** a thin whitish line at the junction of the epiphysis and diaphysis of a bone, formed by preliminary calcification. **white l.,** linea alba. **white adrenal l.,** Sergent's white adrenal l. **white l. of ischiococcygeal muscle,** ligamentum anococcygeum. **white l. of pelvic fascia,** arcus tendineus fasciae pelvis. **white l. of pelvis,** arcus tendineus musculi levatoris ani. **white l. of pharynx,** raphe pharyngis. **Wrisberg's l's,** a set of filaments connecting the motor and sensory roots of the trigeminal nerve. **Z l.,** Z band. **l's of Zahn,** laminations visible in antemortem blood clots, caused by alternating layers of gray-white fibrin interspersed with narrow zones of apparent red-blue clot. **Zöllner's l's,** a set of lines of peculiar arrangement designed to be used as an ocular test.

linea (lin′e-ah), pl. *lin′eae* [L.] a stripe, streak, mark, or narrow ridge; [NA] a general term for a streak or narrow ridge on the surface of some structure. Called also *line.* **l. al′ba** [NA], **l. al′ba abdom′inis,** white line: the tendinous median line on the anterior abdominal wall between the two rectus muscles, formed by the decussating fibers of the aponeuroses of the three flat abdominal muscles. **l. al′ba cervica′lis,** the blending of the fascial sheaths of the sternothyroid and sternohyoid muscles in the median plane of the neck. **lin′eae albican′tes,** see *striae atrophicae.* **l. arcua′ta os′sis il′ii** [NA], arcuate line of ilium: the iliac portion of the terminal line, limiting the ala of the ilium inferiorly on its medial surface. **l. arcua′ta vagi′nae mus′culi rec′ti abdom′inis** [NA], arcuate line of sheath of rectus abdominis muscle: a crescentic line marking the termination of the posterior layer of the sheath of the rectus abdominis muscle, just below the level of the iliac crest; called also *l. semicircularis* [*Douglasi*] and *semicircular line of Douglas.* **l. as′pera fem′oris** [NA], rough line of femur: a roughened longitudinal line with two lips, on the posterior surface of the shaft of the femur; it gives attachment to various muscles. **lin′eae atroph′icae,** striae atrophicae. **l. axilla′ris** [NA], axillary line: an imaginary vertical line passing through the middle of the axilla, dividing the body into an anterior and a posterior portion. **l. epiphysia′lis** [NA], epiphyseal line: a line on the surface of an adult long bone marking the site of junction of the epiphysis and diaphysis. **l. glu′tea ante′rior** [NA], anterior gluteal line: the middle of three rough curved lines on the gluteal surface of the ala of the ilium; it begins from the iliac crest about an inch posterior to the anterior superior iliac spine and arches more or less posteriorly to the greater sciatic notch. **l. glu′tea infe′rior** [NA], inferior gluteal line: a rough curved line, often indistinct, on the gluteal surface of the ala of the ilium; it runs from the notch between the anterior superior and anterior inferior iliac spines posteriorly to the anterior part of the greater sciatic notch. **l. glu′tea poste′rior** [NA], posterior gluteal line: a rough curved line on the gluteal surface of the ala of the ilium; it begins from the iliac crest about two inches anterior to the posterior superior iliac spine and runs downward to the greater sciatic notch. **l. iliopectin′ea,** l. arcuata ossis ilii. **l. innomina′ta,** l. terminalis pelvis. **l. intercondyla′ris fem′oris** [NA], **l. intercondyloi′dea fem′oris,** intercondylar line: a transverse ridge separating the floor of the intercondylar fossa from the popliteal surface of the femur, and giving attachment to the posterior portion of the capsular ligament of the knee. **l. interme′dia cris′tae ili′acae** [NA], intermediate line of iliac crest: the area between the inner and outer lips of the iliac crest. **l. intertrochanter′ica** [NA], intertrochanteric line: a line running obliquely downward and medially from the tubercle of the femur, winding around the medial side of the body of the bone. **l. intertrochanter′ica poste′rior,** crista intertrochanterica. **l. mamilla′ris** [NA], mamillary line: an imaginary vertical line on the anterior surface of the body, passing through the center of the nipple; called also *l. medioclavicularis* [NA alternative] and *midclavicular line.* **l. media′na ante′rior** [NA], anterior median line: an imaginary vertical line on the anterior surface of the body, dividing the surface equally into right and left sides. **l. media′na poste′rior** [NA], posterior median line: an imaginary vertical line on the posterior surface of the body, dividing the surface equally into right and left sides. **l. medioclavicula′ris,** NA alternative for *l. mamillaris.* **l. mensa′lis,** any one of the lines on the palm caused by flexion of the middle, ring, and little fingers. **lin′eae muscula′res scap′ulae,** muscular lines of scapula: low ridges on the costal surface of the scapula, marking the site of attachment of muscle fibers. **l. mus′culi sol′ei** [NA], soleal line of tibia: a line extending from the fibular facet downward and inward across the posterior surface of the tibia, giving attachment to fibers of the soleus muscle; called also *l. poplitea tibiae* and *popliteal line of tibia.* **l. mylohyoi′dea mandib′ulae** [NA], mylohyoid line of mandible: a ridge on the inner surface of the mandible from the base of the symphysis to the ascending ramus behind the last molar tooth; it affords

attachment to the mylohyoid muscle and superior constrictor of the pharynx. **l. ni′gra,** a name given the tendinous mesial line of the abdomen (l. alba) when it has become pigmented in pregnancy. **l. nu′chae infe′rior** [NA], inferior nuchal line: the lowest of the three nuchal lines found on the outer surface of the occipital bone, extending laterally from the middle of the external occipital crest to the jugular process. **l. nu′chae supe′rior** [NA], superior nuchal line: a curved line on the outer surface of the occipital bone, extending from the external occipital protuberance toward the lateral angle, and giving attachment medially to the trapezius muscle and laterally to the sternocleidomastoid muscle. **l. nu′chae supre′ma** [NA], highest or supreme nuchal line: a sometimes indistinct line arching upward from the external occipital protuberance and running toward the lateral angle of the occipital bone: the epicranial aponeurosis attaches to it. **l. obli′qua cartilag′inis thyroi′deae** [NA], oblique line of thyroid cartilage: a line on the external surface of the lamina of the thyroid cartilage, extending between the two thyroid tubercles. **l. obli′qua fib′ulae,** crista medialis fibulae. **l. obli′qua mandib′ulae** [NA], oblique line of mandible: a ridge on the external surface of the body of the mandible extending from the mental tubercle to the anterior border of the ascending ramus on either side. **l. obli′qua tib′iae,** l. musculi solei. **l. parasterna′lis,** parasternal line: an imaginary line on the anterior surface of the body midway between the mamillary line and the border of the sternum. **l. pectin′ea fem′oris** [NA], pectineal line: a line running down the posterior surface of the shaft of the femur, giving attachment to the pectineus muscle. **l. poplite′a tib′iae,** l. musculi solei. **l. scapula′ris** [NA], scapular line; an imaginary vertical line on the posterior surface of the body, passing through the inferior angle of the scapula. **l. semicircula′ris [Doug′lasi],** l. arcuata vaginae musculi recti abdominis. **l. semiluna′ris** [NA], **l. semiluna′ris [Spige′li],** semilunar line: a curved line along the lateral border of each rectus abdominis muscle, corresponding to the meeting of the aponeuroses of the internal oblique and transverse abdominal muscles; called also *Spieghel's line* and *Spigelius' line.* **l. spira′lis,** l. intertrochanterica. **l. splen′dens, Macal′ister,** the sheath for the anterior spinal artery formed by the pia mater in the fissura mediana anterior medullae spinalis. **l. sterna′lis,** sternal line: an imaginary verticle line on the ventral surface of the body, corresponding to the lateral border of the sternum. **l. tempora′lis infe′rior os′sis parieta′lis** [NA], inferior temporal line of parietal bone: a curved line on the external surface of the parietal bone, marking the limit of attachment of the temporal muscle. **l. tempora′lis os′sis fronta′lis** [NA], temporal line of frontal bone: a ridge extending upward and backward from the zygomatic process of the frontal bone, dividing into superior and inferior parts that are continuous with corresponding lines on the parietal bone, and giving attachment to the temporal fascia. **l. tempora′lis supe′rior os′sis parieta′lis** [NA], superior temporal line of parietal bone: a curved line on the external surface of the parietal bone, above and parallel to the inferior temporal line, giving attachment to the temporal fascia. **l. termina′lis pel′vis** [NA], terminal line of pelvis: a line on the inner surface of either pelvic bone, extending from the sacroiliac joint to the iliopubic eminence anteriorly, and marking the plane separating the false from the true pelvis. **lin′eae transver′sae os′sis sa′cri** [NA], transverse lines of sacrum: four transverse ridges on the pelvic surface of the sacrum, running between the pairs of pelvic sacral foramina, marking the positions of the former intervertebral disks. **l. trapezoi′dea** [NA], trapezoid line: a ridge extending anterolaterally from the conoid tubercle on the inferior surface of the clavicle, giving attachment to the trapezoid portion of the coracoclavicular ligament. **l. vi′sus,** an imaginary line from the fovea centralis of the retina to the point of fixation of the eye. **l. vita′lis** [L. "line of life"], a line on the palm curving around the thenar eminence.

lineae (lin′e-e) [L.] plural of *linea.*

lineage (lin′e-ij) [L. *linea* line] descent traced down from or back to a common ancestor. **cell l.,** the developmental history of cells as traced from the first division of the original cell or cells.

linear (lin′e-ar) [L. *linearis*] pertaining to or resembling a line.

liner (lin′er) material applied to the inside of the walls of a cavity or container, for protection or insulation of the surface. **cavity l.,** a substance, e.g., a varnish, applied to the tooth surface exposed by caries, to protect the dentin and insulate the pulp and to enhance the initial seal of the restoration.

lingua (ling′gwah), pl. *lin′guae* [L. "tongue"] [NA], the tongue: the movable, muscular organ on the floor of the mouth, subserving the special sense of taste and aiding in mastication, deglutition, and the articulation of sound; called also *glossa.* See *tongue.* **l. dissect′ta,** geographic tongue. **l. fistura′ta,** fissured tongue. **l. frena′ta,** tonguetie. **l. geograph′ica,** geographic tongue. **l. ni′gra,** black tongue. **l. plica′ta,** fissured tongue. **l. scrota′lis,** fissured tongue. **l. villo′sa ni′gra,** black tongue.

linguae (ling′gwe) [L.] plural of *lingua.*

lingual (ling′gwal) [L. *lingualis*] pertaining to or toward the tongue; glossal.

linguale (ling-gwa′le) the point at the upper end of the symphysis of the lower jaw on its lingual surface.

lingualis (ling-gwa′lis), pl. *lingua′les* [L.] relating to the tongue.

lingually (ling′qwal-le) toward the tongue.

Linguatula (ling-gwat′u-lah) the tongueworms, a genus of the family Linguatulidae, order Porocephalidae, which, in the adult form, inhabit the frontal, nasal, and maxillary sinuses of animals, sometimes including man. Their larval form (known as *Pentastoma* and *Porocephalus*) infests the digestive organs and lungs. See *halzoun.* **L. rhina′ria,** *L. serrata.* **L. serra′ta,** a spe-

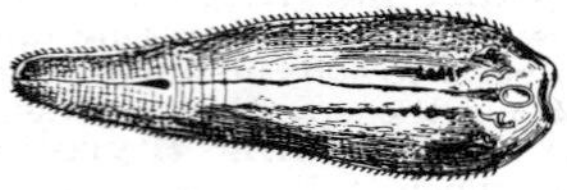

Linguatula, larval form (Mitchell).

cies whose adult forms are found in the frontal sinuses and nasal passages of canines and felines. Eggs, passed in the nasal discharges of infected animals, may be ingested by cattle, sheep, rabbits, or occasionally man, and on hatching, bore through the intestinal wall and finally become encysted in the viscera.

linguatuliasis (ling-gwat″u-li′ah-sis) invasion of the body by *Linguatula.*

linguatulid (ling-gwat′u-lid) any member of the family Linguatulidae.

Linguatulidae (lin-gwah-tu′lĭ-de) a family of endoparasitic wormlike arthropods of the order Porocephalida, class Pentastomida, having flattened bodies. Adults are usually found in the nasal passages of felines and canines, and the larvae are found in the viscera of a variety of mammals, including man. It includes the genus *Linguatula.*

linguatulosis (ling-gwat″u-lo′sis) linguatuliasis.

linguiform (ling′gwĭ-form) tongue-shaped.

lingula (ling′gu-lah), pl. *lin′gulae* [L., dim. of *lingua*] [NA] a general term for a small tongue-like structure. **l. cerebel′li** [NA], **l. of cerebellum,** the most ventral part of the vermis of the cerebellum, where the superior medullary velum attaches. **l. of left lung,** l. pulmonis sinistri. **l. of lower jaw,** l. mandibulae. **l. of mandible, l. mandib′ulae** [NA], the sharp medial boundary of the mandibular foramen, to which is attached the sphenomandibular ligament. **l. pulmo′nis sinis′tri** [NA], lingula of left lung: a projection from the lower portion of the upper lobe of the left lung, just beneath the cardiac notch, between the cardiac impression and the inferior margin. **l. of sphenoid, sphenoidal l., l. of sphenoida′lis** [NA], a slender ridge of bone on the lateral margin of the carotid sulcus, projecting backward between the body and great wing of the sphenoid bone.

lingulae (ling′gu-le) [L.] plural of *lingula.*

lingular (ling′gu-lar) pertaining to a lingula.

lingulectomy (ling″gu-lek′to-me) excision of the lingula of the upper lobe of the left lung.

linguo- [L. *lingua* tongue] a combining form denoting relationship to the tongue.

linguoaxial (ling″gwo-ak′se-al) pertaining to or formed by the lingual and axial walls of a tooth cavity.

linguocervical (ling″gwo-ser′vĭ-kal) 1. pertaining to the lingual surface of the neck of a tooth. 2. linguogingival.

linguoclination (ling″gwo-kli-na′shun) lingual inclination.

linguoclusion (ling″gwo-kloo′zhun) lingual occlusion.

linguodental (ling″gwo-den′tal) pertaining to the tongue and the teeth.

linguodistal (ling″gwo-dis′tal) pertaining to or formed by the lingual and distal surfaces of a tooth, or the lingual and distal walls of a tooth cavity.

linguogingival (ling″gwo-jin′jĭ-val) pertaining to the tongue and gingiva; pertaining to or formed by the lingual and gingival walls of a tooth cavity.

linguoincisal (ling″gwo-in-si′zal) pertaining to or formed by the lingual and incisal surfaces of a tooth.

linguomesial (ling″gwo-me′ze-al) pertaining to or formed by the lingual and mesial surfaces of a tooth, or the lingual and mesial walls of a tooth cavity.

linguo-occlusal (ling″gwo-ŏ-kloo′zal) pertaining to or formed by the lingual and occlusal surfaces of a tooth.

linguopapillitis (ling″gwo-pap″ĭ-li′tis) [L. *lingua* tongue + *papillitis*] inflammation or ulceration of the papillae of the edges of the tongue.

linguoplacement (ling′gwo-plās″ment) [L. *lingua* tongue + *displacement*] lingual placement.

linguopulpal (ling″gwo-pul′pal) pertaining to or formed by the lingual and pulpal walls of a tooth cavity.

linguoversion (ling″gwo-ver′zhun) displacement of a tooth lingually from the line of occlusion.

liniment (lin′ĭ-ment) [L. *linimentum; linere* to smear] an oily liquid preparation to be used on the skin. **camphor l.,** a preparation of camphor and cottonseed oil used as a local irritant to the skin. **camphor and soap l.,** a preparation of green soap, camphor, rosemary oil, alcohol, and purified water, used as a local irritant to the skin. **chloroform l.,** a preparation of chloroform with camphor and soap liniment used as a local irritant to the skin. **medicinal soft soap l.,** green soap tincture.

linimentum (lin″ĭ-men′tum) [L.] liniment. **l. cam′phorae,** camphor liniment. **l. cam′phorae et sapo′nis,** camphor and soap liniment. **l. chlorofor′mi,** chloroform liniment. **l. sapo′nis mol′lis,** green soap tincture.

linin (li′nin) [L. *linum* thread] the faintly staining substance composing the fine, netlike threads found in the nucleus of a cell, where it bears the chromatin in the form of granules. Cf. *achromatin.*

linitis (lĭ-ni′tis) [Gr. *linon* thread + *-itis*] inflammation of the gastric cellular tissue. **l. plas′tica,** diffuse fibrous proliferation of the submucous connective tissue of the stomach, resulting in thickening and fibrosis so that the organ is constricted, inelastic, and rigid (like a leather bottle). It is almost always a manifestation of adenocarcinoma but is also seen in benign conditions such as gastric syphilis. Called also *Brinton's disease, gastric sclerosis, cirrhosis of the stomach, cirrhotic gastritis,* and *leather bottle stomach.*

linkage (lingk′ij) 1. the connection between different atoms in a chemical compound, or the symbol representing it in structural formulas; see also *bond.* 2. in genetics, the association of genes having loci on the same chromosome, which results in the tendency of a group of such nonallelic genes to be associated in inheritance. 3. in psychology, the connection between a stimulus and its response.

linked (linkt) in genetics, referring to characters which are united so as invariably to be inherited together. See also *X-linked,* under *gene.*

Linodil (lin′o-dil) trademark for a preparation of inositol niacinate.

Linognathus (lin-og′nah-thus) a genus of insects of the order Anoplura, sucking lice. *L. peda′lis* infests sheep. *L. seto′sus* the dog, *L. sten′opis* the goat. *L. vitu′li* is the long-nosed louse of the ox.

linolein (lin-o′le-in) [L. *linum* flax + *oleum* oil] a neutral fat from linseed oil; the triglyceride of linoleic acid.

linseed (lin′sēd) the dried ripe seed of *Linum usitatissimum* L. (Linaceae), used as a topical demulcent and emollient; called also *flaxseed* and *linum.*

Linser's method (lin′serz) [Paul *Linser,* German dermatologist, born 1871] see under *method.*

Linstowiidae (lin-sto-wi′ĭ-de) a family of medium-sized or small tapeworms of the order Cyclophyllidea, subclass Cestoda, which parasitize birds, reptiles, and mammals, including man; medically important genera are *Oochoristica* and *Inermicapsifer.*

lint (lint) [L. *linteum,* from *linum,* flax] an absorbent surgical dressing material once made by scraping or picking apart old woven linen, but now a specially finished fabric woven in sheets; called also *patent l.* or *sheet l.*

lintin (lin′tin) a loose fabric of prepared absorbent cotton used in dressing wounds.

lintine (lin′tēn) cotton lint from which the oil has been removed.

linum (li′num) [L. "flax"] linseed.

lio- (li′o) for words beginning thus, see also those beginning *leio-*.

Li_2O lithium oxide.

LiOH lithium hydroxide.

Lioresal (li-ōr′ĕ-sal) trademark for a preparation of baclofen.

liothyronine (li″o-thi′ro-nēn) chemical name: *O*-(4-hydroxy-3-iodophenyl)-3,5-diiodo-L-tyrosine. The synthetic levo isomer of the thyroid hormone triiodothyronine, $C_{15}H_{12}I_3NO_4$, which is more potent and has a more rapid action than thyroxine. **l. sodium** [USP], the monosodium salt of liothyronine, $C_{15}H_{11}I_3$-NNa O_4, occurring as a light tan, crystalline powder; used for thyroid replacement or supplementation in hypothyroidism and simple (nontoxic) goiter, administered orally.

liotrix (li′o-triks) a mixture of liothyronine sodium and levothyroxine sodium in a ratio of 1:4 in terms of weight; used for replacement therapy in conditions in which there is deficient production of thyroid hormones, administered orally.

lip (lip) 1. either the upper or lower fleshy margin of the mouth, together called *labia oris* [NA]. 2. a marginal part; called also *labium.* **acetabular l.,** labrum acetabulare. **anterior l. of cervix of uterus,** labium anterius ostii uteri. **anterior l. of ostium of uterus,** labium anterius ostii uteri. **anterior l. of pharyngeal opening of auditory tube,** labium anterius ostii pharyngei tubae auditivae. **cleft l.,** harelip. **double l.,** redundancy of the submucous tissue and mucous membrane of the lip on either side of the median line. **external l. of iliac crest,** labium externum cristae iliacae. **external l. of linea aspera of femur,** labium laterale lineae asperae femoris. **fibrocartilaginous l. of acetabulum,** labrum acetabulare. **glenoid l.,** labrum glenoidale. **gle-**

noid l. of articulation of hip, labrum acetabulare. **glenoid l. of articulation of humerus,** labrum glenoidale. **greater l. of pudendum,** labium majus pudendi. **Hapsburg l.,** a thick overdeveloped lower lip that often accompanies a Hapsburg jaw. **inferior l.,** the lower lip (labium inferius oris [NA]). **inferior l. of ileocecal valve,** labium inferius valvulae coli. **internal l. of iliac crest,** labium internum cristae iliacae. **lateral l. of linea aspera of femur,** labium laterale lineae asperae femoris. **lesser l. of pudendum,** labium minus pudendi. **lower l.,** labium inferius oris. **medial l. of linea aspera of femur,** labium mediale lineae asperae femoris. **posterior l. of cervix of uterus,** labium posterius ostii uteri. **posterior l. of ostium of uterus,** labius posterius ostii uterus. **posterior l. of pharyngeal opening of auditory tube,** labium posterius ostii pharyngei tubae auditivae. **rhombic l.,** the lateral boundary of the rhombencephalon during embryonic life. **superior l.,** the upper lip (labium superius oris [NA]). **superior l. of ileocecal valve,** labium superius valvulae coli. **tympanic l. of limb of spiral lamina,** labium tympanicum limbi laminae spiralis. **upper l.,** labium superius oris. **vestibular l. of limb of spiral lamina,** labium vestibulare limbi laminae spiralis.

lipacidemia (lip″as-ĭ-de′me-ah) [lipo- + L. acidus acid + Gr. haima blood + -ia] the presence of an excess of fatty acids in the blood, as in diabetes mellitus.

lipaciduria (lip″as-ĭ-du′re-ah) [lipo- + L. acidus acid + Gr. ouron urine + -ia] the presence of fatty acids in the urine.

liparocele (lip-ar′o-sēl) [Gr. liparos oily + kēlē tumor] a fatty scrotal tumor; also a hernia containing fatty material.

liparodyspnea (lip″ah-ro-disp′ne-ah) the dyspnea of the obese.

liparoid (lip′ah-roid) fatty; resembling fat.

liparomphalus (lip″ah-rom′fah-lus) [Gr. liparos oily + omphalos navel] (obs.) a lipoma of the umbilicus.

lipase (lip′ās, lī′pās) [Gr. lipos fat + -ase] glycerol-ester hydrolase; any of a group of widely occurring enzymes that catalyze the hydrolysis of ester linkages between the fatty acids and glycerol of the triglycerides and phospholipids. They occur in milk, the pancreas, adipose tissue, the stomach, and other tissues. **lipoprotein l.,** an esterase that catalyzes the hydrolysis of the constituent triglycerides of chylomicrons to form free fatty acid anions and glycerol. **pancreatic l.,** steapsin.

lipasic (li-pa′sik) 1. pertaining to lipase. 2. lipolytic.

lipasuria (lip″ās-u′re-ah) the presence of lipase in the urine.

lipectomy (lĭ-pek′to-me) [lipo- + Gr. ektomē excision] the excision of a mass of subcutaneous adipose tissue, as from the abdominal wall; called also adipectomy.

lipedema (lip″ĕ-de′mah) [lipo- + edema] an accumulation of excess fat and fluid in subcutaneous tissues.

lipemia (lĭ-pe′me-ah) [lipo- + Gr. haima blood + -ia] an excess of fat or lipid in the blood; hypercholesterolemia; hyperlipemia. **alimentary l.,** that which occurs after the ingestion of food. **l. retina′lis,** a high level of lipids in the blood, manifested by a milky appearance of the veins and arteries of the retina.

lipese (lip′ēs) an early term used to describe an enzyme that brings about the synthesis of fats.

lipid (lip′id) any of a heterogeneous group of fats and fatlike substances characterized by being water-insoluble and being extractable by nonpolar (or fat) solvents such as alcohol, ether, chloroform, benzene, etc. All contain as a major constituent aliphatic hydrocarbons. The lipids, which are easily stored in the body, serve as a source of fuel, are an important constituent of cell structure, and serve other biological functions. Lipids may be considered to include fatty acids, neutral fats, waxes, and steroids. Compound lipids comprise the glycolipids, lipoproteins, and phospholipids.

lipidase (lip′ĭ-dās) a general term for an enzyme that catalyzes the splitting up of lipids.

lipide (lip′īd) lipid.

lipidemia (lip″ĭ-de′me-ah) hyperlipidemia.

lipidic (lip-id′ik) pertaining to or containing lipids.

lipidol (lip′ĭ-dol) a lipid alcohol; an aliphatic fatty alcohol.

lipidolysis (lip″ĭ-dol′ĭ-sis) the splitting up of lipids.

lipidolytic (lip″ĭ-do-lit′ik) pertaining to, characterized by, or causing lipidolysis.

lipidosis (lip″ĭ-do′sis) a general term for disorders of cellular lipid metabolism involving abnormal accumulations of lipids. The lipidoses include Hand-Schüller-Christian disease, Niemann-Pick disease, Tay-Sachs disease, and Gaucher's disease. **ceramide lactoside l.,** ceramide lactosidosis. **cerebroside l.,** cerebrosidosis. **hereditary dystopic l.,** angiokeratoma corporis diffusum. **sphingomyelin l.,** Niemann-Pick disease. **sulfatide l.,** metachromatic leukodystrophy.

lipidtemns (lip′id-temz) a collective name for the products formed by the digestion of fats, namely, glycerin and fatty acids.

lipiduria (lip″ĭ-du′re-ah) [lipid + Gr. ouron urine + -ia] the presence of lipids in the urine.

lipin (lip′in) [Gr. lipos fat] lipid.

Lipiodol (lip-i′o-dol) trademark for iodized oil used as a contrast medium.

Lipmann (lip′man), Fritz Albert. German biochemist in America, born 1899; co-winner, with Hans Adolph Krebs, of the Nobel prize in medicine and physiology for 1953 for his discovery of coenzyme A and its importance in intermediary metabolism.

lipo- (lip′o) [Gr. lipos fat] a combining form denoting relationship to fat or to lipids.

lipoadenoma (lip″o-ad′ĕ-no-mah) lipomatosis of the parenchyma of a gland.

lipoarthritis (lip″o-ar-thri′tis) [lipo- + arthritis] inflammation of the fatty tissue of a joint.

lipoatrophy (li″po-at′ro-fe) 1. focal atrophy of subcutaneous fat at the sites of insulin injections. 2. lipodystrophy.

lipoblast (lip′o-blast) [lipo- + Gr. blastos germ] a specialized connective tissue cell which develops into a fat cell.

lipoblastoma (lip″o-blas-to′mah) [lipo- + Gr. blastos germ + -oma] a benign fatty tumor composed of a mixture of embryonal lipoblastic cells in a myxoid stroma and mature fat cells; the tumor cells are arranged in lobules and occur most often in children.

lipocaic (lip″o-ka′ik) [lipo- + Gr. kaiein to burn] a substance extracted from the pancreas which reputedly prevents the deposition of fat in the livers of animals after pancreatectomy and after other surgical procedures.

lipocardiac (lip″o-kar′de-ak) [lipo- + Gr. kardia heart] relating to a fatty heart.

lipocatabolic (lip″o-kat″ah-bol′ik) pertaining to or effecting the destructive metabolism of fat.

lipocele (lip′o-sēl) [lipo- + Gr. kēlē tumor] adipocele.

lipocellulose (lip″o-sel′u-lōs) a heterohexosan composed of lipids and cellulose.

lipoceratous (lip″o-ser′ah-tus) adipoceratous.

lipocere (lip′o-sēr) [lipo- + L. cera wax] adipocere.

lipochondria (lip″o-kon′dre-ah) [lipo- + Gr. chondrion granule] lipid-containing inclusions in the cytoplasm of amphibian eggs.

lipochondrodystrophy (lip″o-kon″dro-dis′tro-fe) [lipo- + Gr. chondros cartilage + dystrophy] Hurler's syndrome.

lipochondroma (lip″o-kon-dro′mah) [lipo- + Gr. chondros cartilage + -oma] a tumor composed of mature lipomatous and cartilaginous elements; such lesions are now generally called benign mesenchymoma.

lipochrome (lip′o-krōm) [lipo- + Gr. chrōma color] any one of a group of fat-soluble hydrocarbon pigments, such as carotin, xanthophyll, lutein, chromophane, and the natural coloring material of butter, egg yolk, and yellow corn. They are also known as carotenoids.

lipochromemia (lip″o-kro-me′me-ah) [lipochrome + Gr. haima blood + -ia] the presence of an excess of lipochrome in the blood.

lipochromogen (lip″o-kro′mo-jen) a substance that becomes converted into lipochrome.

lipoclasis (lĭ-pok′lah-sis) [lipo- + Gr. klasis breaking] lipolysis.

lipoclastic (lip″o-klas′tik) [lipo- + Gr. klastikos breaking up] lipolytic.

lipocorticoid (lip″o-kor′tĭ-koid) a corticoid effective in causing deposition of fat, especially in the liver.

lipocyanine (lip″o-si′ah-nin) [lipo- + Gr. kyanos blue] a blue pigment resulting from the action of strong sulfuric acid on lipochrome.

lipocyte (lip′o-sīt) [lipo- + -cyte] a fat cell.

lipodieresis (lip″o-di-er′ĕ-sis) [lipo- + Gr. diairesis a taking] the splitting up or the decomposition of fat.

lipodieretic (lip″o-di-er-et′ik) pertaining to, characterized by, or causing lipodieresis.

lipodystrophia (lip″o-dis-tro′fe-ah) lipodystrophy. **l. intestina′lis,** intestinal lipodystrophy. **l. progressi′va,** a disease characterized by the progressive and symmetrical disappearance of subcutaneous fat from the parts above the pelvis, facial emaciation, and abnormal accumulation of fat about the thighs and buttocks. Called also lipodystrophy.

lipodystrophy (lip″o-dis′tro-fe) [lipo- + Gr. dystrophia dystrophy] 1. any disturbance of fat metabolism. 2. lipodystrophia progressiva. **congenital generalized l.,** a hereditary condition characterized by the virtual absence of subcutaneous adipose tissue, macrosomia (thick skin, large hands and feet, muscular hypertrophy, heavy bones), visceromegaly (heart, kidneys, spleen, and liver), hypertrichosis, acanthosis nigricans, and reduced glucose tolerance in the presence of high insulin levels; it is transmitted as an autosomal recessive trait. **inferior l.,** lipodystrophy of the lower limbs. **insulin l.,** a local reduction of the subcutaneous fat in a region repeatedly injected with insulin. **intestinal l.,** a disease marked by diarrhea with fatty stools, arthritis, emaciation, and loss of strength, and attended with deposit of fat in the intestinal lymphatic tissue; called also Whipple's disease and lipophagia granulomatosis. **progressive l.,** lipodystrophia progressiva.

lipoferous (lĭ-pof′er-us) [lipo- + L. ferre to carry] 1. carrying fat. 2. sudanophil.

lipofibroma (lip″o-fi-bro′mah) a lipoma containing areas of fibrosis.

lipofuscin (lip″o-fus′sin) any one of a class of fatty pigments formed by the solution of a pigment in fat. Cf. lipochrome.

lipofuscinosis (lip″o-fu″sin-o′sis) any disorder due to abnormal storage of lipofuscins. **neuronal ceroid l.,** a group of hereditary autosomal recessive diseases characterized by the accumulation in neurons and other tissues of lipopigments (ceroid and lipofuscin); clinically there is central nervous deterioration, optic atrophy, macular degeneration, retinitis pigmentosa, and seizures.

lipogenesis (lip″o-jen′ĕ-sis) [lipo- + genesis] the formation of fat; the transformation of nonfat food materials into body fat.

lipogenetic (lip″o-jĕ-net′ik) lipogenic.

lipogenic (lip″o-jen′ik) forming, producing, or caused by fat.

lipogenous (lĭ-poj′ĕ-nus) [lipo- + Gr. gennan to produce] producing fatness.

lipogranuloma (lip″o-gran-u-lo′mah) [lipo- + granuloma] a nodule of lipoid material; a foreign body inflammation of adipose tissue containing granulation tissue and oil cysts.

lipogranulomatosis (lip″o-gran″u-lo-mah-to′sis) a condition of faulty lipid metabolism in which yellow nodules of lipoid matter are deposited in the skin and mucosae, giving rise to granulomatous reactions. **Farber's l.,** see under syndrome.

lipohemarthrosis (lip″o-hem″ar-thro′sis) [lipo- + Gr. haima blood + arthron joint + -osis] the presence of fat-containing blood in a joint, with intra-articular fracture.

lipohemia (lip″o-he′me-ah) lipemia.

Lipo-Hepin (lip″o-hep′in) trademark for a preparation of heparin sodium.

lipohistiodieresis (lip″o-his″te-o-di-er′ĕ-sis) the disappearance of stored fat from body tissue.

lipohyalin (lip″o-hi′ah-lin) the lipid deposited in the beta cells of the pancreas in association with hyalinization in diabetes.

lipoid (lip′oid) [lipo- + Gr. eidos form] 1. fatlike; resembling fat; adipoid. 2. lipid. **acetone-insoluble l's,** lipids, consisting largely of lecithins, precipitated from an ethereal extract of dried ox heart by adding an excess of acetone; used as an antigen in the Wassermann test after being brought into solution in a mixture of 1 part of ether and 9 parts of methanol. **anisotropic l.,** a lipid having doubly refractive properties. **Forssman's l.,** Forssman's antigen.

lipoidal (lip-oi′dal) fatlike; resembling fat.

lipoidemia (lip″oi-de′me-ah) lipemia.

lipoidic (lĭ-poi′dik) fatlike; resembling fat.

lipoidolytic (lĭ-poi″do-lit′ik) lipidolytic.

lipoidosis (lip″oi-do′sis) a disturbance of lipid metabolism with abnormal deposit of lipids in the cells. **arterial l.,** atherosclerosis. **cerebroside l.,** Gaucher's disease. **cholesterol l.,** Hand-Schüller-Christian disease. **l. cu′tis et muco′sae,** lipoid proteinosis. **phosphatide l.,** Niemann-Pick disease. **renal l.,** lipid nephrosis.

lipoidproteinosis (lip″oid-pro″te-in-o′sis) a familial disease occurring in the course of latent diabetes, marked by yellowish nodules on the skin and mucosae, keratotic lesions on the extremities, and hoarseness due to faulty lipid metabolism.

lipoidsiderosis (lip″oid-sid-ĕ-ro′sis) the deposit of iron pigment in lipids.

lipoiduria (lip″oi-du′re-ah) lipiduria.

lipolipoidosis (lip″o-lip″oi-do′sis) the presence of lipoids and neutral fats in the cells.

Lipo-Lutin (li″po-lu′tin) trademark for preparations of progesterone.

lipolysis (lĭ-pol′ĭ-sis) [lipo- + Gr. lysis dissolution] the decomposition or splitting up of fat; called also adipolysis.

lipolytic (lip″o-lit′ik) pertaining to, characterized by, or causing lipolysis; adipolytic.

lipoma (lĭ-po′mah) [lipo- + -oma] a benign tumor usually composed of mature fat cells. At times the tumor may be composed partly or entirely of fetal fat cells (hibernoma). **l. annula′re col′li,** Madelung's neck. **l. arbores′cens,** a lipoma within a joint having a treelike form. **l. capsula′re,** a fatty tumor due to increase of the fat in the capsule of an organ. **l. caverno′sum,** angiolipoma. **diffuse l.,** diffuse lipomatosis. **l. diffu′sum re′nis,** lipomatous nephritis. **l. doloro′sa,** see nodular circumscribed lipomatosis, under lipomatosis. **fat cell l., fetal,** hibernoma. **l. fibro′sum,** a lipoma in which there are areas of fibrosis. **intradural l.,** lipoma with components within or beneath the dura mater of the spine or sacrum. **l. myxomato′des,** a lipomyxoma. **nevoid l.** (obs.), angiolipoma. **l. ossif′icans,** an ossified lipoma. **l. petrif′icans** (obs.), a calcified lipoma. **l. petrif′icum ossif′icans** (obs.), an ossified lipoma. **l. sarcomato′des,** liposarcoma. **telangiectatic l., l. telangiecto′des,** angiolipoma.

lipomatoid (lĭ-po′mah-toid) resembling a lipoma.

lipomatosis (lip″o-mah-to′sis) a condition characterized by abnormal localized, or tumor-like, accumulations of fat in the tissues. **l. atroph′icans,** localized accumulations of fat in certain tissues, associated with emaciation of the rest of the body; see also lipodystrophia progressiva. **congenital l. of pancreas,** Schwachman-Diamond syndrome. **diffuse l.,** abnormal increase of subcutaneous fat in the parts above the pelvis, usually in males. **l. doloro′sa,** lipomatosis in which the adipose de-

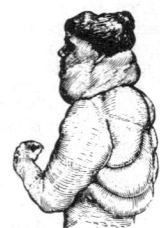

Diffuse lipomatosis (Babcock).

posits are tender or painful. **l. gigan′tea,** a form in which the adipose deposits form large masses. **nodular circumscribed l.,** the formation of multiple circumscribed or encapsulated lipomas which may be distributed symmetrically (multiple symmetrical lipomatosis) or haphazardly or which may form a collar around the neck (Madelung's neck). At times they may be painful (lipoma, or lipomatosis, dolorosa). **renal l., l. re′nis, replacement l. of kidney,** partial replacement of the renal parenchyma (usually an atrophic or hydronephrotic kidney) by adipose tissue. **symmetrical l.,** see nodular circumscribed l.

lipomatous (lĭ-po′mah-tus) affected with, or of the nature of, lipoma.

lipomeningocele (lip″o-mĕ-ning′go-sēl) meningocele associated with an overlying lipoma, in spina bifida.

lipomeria (li″po-me′re-ah) [Gr. leipein to leave + meros a part] monstrosity consisting of the congenital absence of a limb.

lipometabolic (lip″o-met″ah-bol′ik) pertaining to metabolism of fat.

lipometabolism (lip″o-mĕ-tab′o-lizm) [lipo- + metabolism] the metabolism of fat; utilization of fat.

lipomicron (lip″o-mi′kron) a microscopic fat particle in the blood.

lipomucopolysaccharidosis (lip″o-mu″ko-pol″e-sak-ah-rĭ-do′-sis) mucolipidosis I.

lipomyohemangioma (lip″o-mi″o-hĕ-man″je-o′mah) a hamartoma composed of adipose, muscle, and vascular tissue.

lipomyoma (lip″o-mi-o′mah) a benign mesenchymoma composed of leiomyomatous and lipomatous tissues.

lipomyxoma (lip″o-miks-o′mah) a myxoma containing fatty elements.

liponephrosis (lip″o-nĕ-fro′sis) lipid nephrosis.

liponeurocyte (lip″o-nu′ro-sīt) the name given by Cramer to cells found in the pituitary body of rats.

Liponyssus (lip″o-nis′us) [lipo- + Gr. nyssein to pierce] former name for Ornithonyssus. **L. baco′ti,** Ornithonyssus bacoti. **L. bur′sa,** Ornithonyssus buarsa. **L. sylvia′rum,** Ornithonyssus sylviarum.

lipopathy (lĭ-pop′ah-the) [lipo + pathy] any disorder of lipid metabolism.

lipopectic (lip″o-pek′tik) pertaining to, characterized by, or causing lipopexia.

lipopenia (lip″o-pe′ne-ah) [lipo- + Gr. penia poverty] deficiency of lipids in the body.

lipopenic (lip″o-pe′nik) pertaining to, characterized by, or causing lipopenia.

lipopeptid (lip″o-pep′tid) a poorly defined group of fat-like substances composed of amino acids and fatty acids.

lipopexia (lip″o-pek′se-ah) [lipo- + Gr. pēxis fixation] the accumulation of fat in the tissues.

lipopexic (lip″o-pek′sik) lipopectic.

lipophage (lip′o-fāj) a cell that ingests or absorbs fat.

lipophagia (lip″o-fa′je-ah) lipophagy. **l. granulomato′sis,** intestinal lipodystrophy.

lipophagic (lip″o-fa′jik) [lipo- + Gr. phagein to eat] pertaining to, characterized by, or causing lipophagy; lipolytic.

lipophagy (lĭ-pof′ah-je) the absorption of fat; lipolysis.

lipophanerosis (lip″o-fan″ĕ-ro′sis) the process by which invisible fat in certain cells becomes detectable as small droplets.

lipophil (lip′o-fil) an element that has an affinity for fat.

lipophilia (lip″o-fil′e-ah) [lipo- + Gr. philein to love + -ia] 1. affinity for fat. 2. a tendency of the obese for fat fixation.

lipophilic (lip″o-fil′ik) having an affinity for fat; pertaining to or characterized by lipophilia.

lipophore (lip′o-fōr) [lipo- + Gr. *phoros* bearing] a pigment cell containing a lipochrome pigment; chromatophore.

lipopolysaccharide (lip″o-pol″e-sak′ah-rīd) a molecule or compound in which lipids and polysaccharides are linked, as in cell membranes.

lipoprotein (lip″o-pro′te-in) a combination of a lipid and protein, possessing the general properties (e.g., solubility) of proteins. Practically all of the lipids of the plasma are present as lipoprotein complexes, α- and β-lipoproteins being distinguished by electrophoresis. The β-lipoproteins transport more of the total plasma cholesterol, contain a higher concentration of both free and esterified cholesterol, and have a higher cholesterol/phospholipid ratio than α-lipoproteins. Cf. *proteolipid.* **high-density l. (HDL),** a plasma lipoprotein containing high levels of protein, little triglycerides, moderate levels of phospholipids, and relatively little cholesterol. **low-density l. (LDL),** a plasma lipoprotein containing a low percentage of triglycerides, moderate levels of phospholipids, high levels of cholesterol, and moderate levels of protein. **very low-density l. (VLDL),** a plasma lipoprotein containing high concentrations of triglycerides, moderate concentrations of both phospholipids and cholesterol, and little protein. Called also *prebetalipoprotein.*

lipoproteinemia (lip″o-pro″te-in-e′me-ah) the presence of excessive lipoproteins in the blood.

lipoproteinosis (lip″o-pro″te-in-o′sis) lipoid proteinosis.

liporhodin (lip″o-ro′din) [lipo- + Gr. *rhodon* rose] a red lipochrome.

liposarcoma (lip″o-sar-ko′mah) [lipo- + *sarcoma*] a malignant tumor derived from primitive or embryonal lipoblastic cells which exhibit varying degrees of lipoblastic and/or lipomatous differentiation.

liposis (lĭ-po′sis) [Gr. *lipos* fat + -*osis*] lipomatosis.

liposoluble (lip″o-sol′u-b'l) [lipo- + *soluble*] soluble in fats.

liposome (lip′o-sōm) [lipo- + Gr. *sōma* body] a spherical particle in an aqueous medium, formed by a lipid bilayer enclosing an aqueous compartment.

lipostomy (li-pos′to-me) [Gr. *leipein* to fail + *stoma* mouth] congenital smallness or absence of the mouth.

Liposyn (lip′o-sin) trademark for an intravenous fat emulsion containing 10 per cent safflower oil stabilized with egg phospholipids; used to prevent deficiency of essential fatty acids during prolonged total parenteral nutrition.

lipothymia (li″po-thi′me-ah) [Gr. *leipein* to fail + *thymos* mind] a feeling of faintness; syncope.

lipotrophic (lip″o-trof′ik) pertaining to, characterized by, or causing lipotrophy.

lipotrophy (lĭ-pot′ro-fe) [lipo- + Gr. *trophē* nutrition] increase of bodily fat.

lipotropic (lip″o-trop′ik) 1. acting on fat metabolism by hastening the removal of or decreasing the deposit of fat in the liver. 2. an agent that has such effects.

β-lipotropin (lip″o-tro′pin) a polypeptide synthesized by cells of the adenohypophysis which promotes the mobilization of fat and the darkening of the skin by stimulation of melanocytes. It also contains two sequences of amino acid residues identified as β-endorphin and methionine enkephalin.

lipotropism (lĭ-pot′ro-pizm) the condition of being lipotropic.

lipotropy (lĭ-pot′ro-pe) [lipo- + Gr. *tropē* a turning] lipotropism.

lipotuberculin (lip″o-tu-ber′ku-lin) a preparation of tuberculin that includes the fatty fraction of *Mycobacterium tuberculosis* in solution or emulsion.

lipovaccine (lip″o-vak′sēn) [lipo- + *vaccine*] a vaccine prepared by suspending microorganisms in vegetable oil for the purpose of delaying absorption of the antigenic substances.

lipovitellin (lip″o-vi-tel′in) a lipoprotein found in the yolk of eggs.

lipoxanthine (lip″o-zan′thin) [lipo- + Gr. *xanthos* yellow] a yellow lipochrome.

lipoxidase (lĭ-pok′sĭ-dās) lipoxygenase.

lipoxygenase (lĭ-poks′ĭ-jĕ-nās) linoleate:oxygen oxidoreductase. An enzyme that catalyzes the addition of molecular oxygen to the double bonds of polyunsaturated fatty acids, to form a peroxide of the acid. Obtained from plants. Called also *lipoxidase.*

lipoxysm (lip-oks′izm) [Gr. *lipos* fat + *oxys* sharp, acid] poisoning by oleic acid.

lippa (lip′ah) blepharitis ciliaris.

lipping (lip′ing) 1. a wedge-shaped shadow in the roentgenogram of chondrosarcoma between the cortex and the elevated periosteum. 2. the development of a bony overgrowth in osteoarthritis.

lippitude (lip′ĭ-tūd) [L. *lippitudo; lippus* bleareyed] blepharitis ciliaris.

Lipschütz bodies, cell, ulcer (disease) (lip′shitz) [Benjamin *Lipschütz,* Austrian dermatologist, 1878–1931] see under *body,* and see *centrocyte* and *ulcus vulvae acutum.*

lipsotrichia (lip″so-trik′e-ah) [Gr. *leipein* to leave + *thrix* hair] trichomadesis.

lipuria (lĭ-pu′re-ah) [Gr. *lipos* fat + *ouron* urine + -*ia*] the presence of oil or fat in the urine.

lipuric (lĭ-pu′rik) pertaining to or characterized by lipuria.

Liq. abbreviation for *liquor.*

Liquaemin (lik′wah-min) trademark for preparations of sodium heparin.

Liquamar (lik′wah-mar) trademark for a preparation of phenprocoumon.

liquefacient (lik″wĕ-fa′shent) [L. *liquefaciens*] having the quality to convert a solid material into a liquid, producing liquefaction.

liquefaction (lik″wĕ-fak′shun) [L. *liquefactio; liquere* to flow + *facere* to make] the conversion of a material into a liquid form.

liquefactive (lik″wĕ-fak′tiv) pertaining to, characterized by, or causing liquefaction.

liquescent (lik-wes′ent) [L. *liquescere* to become liquid] tending to become liquid; becoming liquid.

liquid (lik′wid) [L. *liquidus; liquere* to flow] 1. a substance that flows readily in its natural state. 2. flowing readily; neither solid nor gaseous. See also *fluid, liquor, mixture,* and *solution.* **Declat's l.,** a solution of carbolate of ammonia for external and internal use in cholera. **Müller's l.,** see under *fluid.* **Pasteur's l.,** see under *solution.*

liquiform (lik′wĕ-form) resembling a liquid.

Liquiprin (lik′wĭ-prin) trademark for a preparation of acetaminophen.

liquogel (lik′wo-jel) a gel which after melting gives a sol of low viscosity. Cf. *viscogel.*

liquor (lik′er, li′kwor), pl. *liquors, liquo′res* [L.]. 1. a liquid, especially an aqueous solution containing a medicinal substance. 2. a general term used in anatomical nomenclature for certain fluids of the body. See also *fluid, liquid,* and *solution.* **l. am′nii,** amniotic fluid. **l. cerebrospina′lis** [NA], cerebrospinal fluid (CSF): the fluid contained within the four ventricles of the brain, the subarachnoid space, and the central canal of the spinal cord; formed by choroid plexuses and brain parenchyma, it circulates through the ventricles into the subarachnoid space and is absorbed into the venous system. **l. cho′rii,** a fluid which separates the amnion from the chorion in the early stages of gestation. **l. cotun′nii,** perilymph (perilympha [NA]). **l. enter′icus,** succus entericus. **l. follic′uli,** follicular fluid: an albuminous fluid in the vesicular ovarian follicle surrounding the ovum. **l. gas′tricus,** succus gastricus. **Morgagni's l.** (*obs.*), a fluid between the eye lens and its capsule. **mother l.,** the liquid from which any substance has been separated by crystallization. **l. pancreat′icus,** succus pancreaticus. **l. pericar′dii,** pericardial fluid: a fluid found in small amount in the potential space between the parietal and visceral laminae of the serous pericardium. **l. prostat′icus,** succus prostaticus. **l. pu′ris,** the fluid portion of pus. **l. san′guinis,** the fluid portion of the blood; the blood plasma. **l. of Scarpa, l. scar′pae,** endolymph (endolympha [NA]). **l. sem′inis,** the fluid portion of the semen.

liquores (li-kwo′rēz) [L.] plural of *liquor.*

liquorice (lik′er-is) see *Glycyrrhiza.*

liquorrhea (li″kwo-re′ah) [L. *liquor* liquid + Gr. *rhoia* flow] an excessive discharge of any body fluid, e.g., liquorrhea nasalis.

Lirugen (li′ru-jen) trademark for a preparation of live attenuated measles virus vaccine.

Lisacort (lis′ah-kort) trademark for a preparation of prednisone.

Lisfranc's amputation, etc. (lis-frahnks′) [Jacques *Lisfranc,* French surgeon, 1790–1847] see under *amputation, joint, ligament,* and *tubercle.*

Lissauer's marginal zone, paralysis, tract (column) (lis′ow-erz) [Heinrich *Lissauer,* German neurologist, 1861–1891] see under *paralysis* and *zone,* and see *tractus dorsolateralis.*

Lissencephala (lis″en-sef′ah-lah) [Gr. *lissos* smooth + *enkephalos* brain] a group of placental mammals in which the brain is characteristically smooth or is marked by few convolutions, as bats, rodents, etc. Cf. *Gyrencephala.*

lissencephalia (lis″en-sĕ-fa′le-ah) agyria.

lissencephalic (lis″en-sĕ-fal′ik) 1. pertaining to the Lissencephala. 2. having cerebral hemispheres without or with only shallow convolutions, the normal appearance of the brain of many animals (e.g., bats, rodents). Cf. *gyrencephalic.* 3. agyric.

lissencephaly (lis″sen-sef′ah-le) agyria.

lissive (lis′iv) [Gr. *lissos* smooth] relieving muscle spasm without interfering with function.

Lister (lis′ter), Baron Joseph (1827–1912). English surgeon whose publication in 1867 of the principles of antiseptic surgery made "clean" operations a reality, and catalyzed the development of modern surgery.

Listerella (lis″ter-el′ah) *Listeria.*

listerellosis (lis″ter-el-lo′sis) listeriosis.

Listeria (lis-ter′e-ah) [Baron Joseph *Lister*] a genus of microorganisms of the family Corynebacteriaceae, order Eubacteriales, made up of coccoid to bacillary gram-positive microorganisms apparently occurring primarily in lower animals, in which it produces septicemic or encephalomyelitic disease in sporadic or epizootic form. It infects man to produce an upper respiratory disease, with angina, lymphadenitis, and conjunctivitis, or a septicemic disease which may be transmitted transplacentally in pregnant women, or it may assume an encephalitic form. Human disease is often, but not invariably, associated with a monocytosis. There is a single species, *L. monocytog′enes.*

listerial (lis-ter′e-al) pertaining to or caused by organisms of the genus *Listeria.*

listeriosis (lis-ter″e-o′sis) a sporadic disease of animals and occasionally of man caused by *Listeria monocytogenes;* nervous signs are common in ruminants, and necrosis of the liver in monogastric animals. Because affected animals tend to move in circles, it is also known as *circling disease.*

listerism (lis′ter-izm) the principles and practice of antiseptic and aseptic surgery.

Listing's law, plane (lis′tingz) [Johann Benedict *Listing,* German physiologist, 1808–1882] see under *law* and *plane.*

Liston's forceps, knives, operation (lis′tonz) [Robert *Liston,* Scottish surgeon in London, 1794–1847] see under *forceps, knife,* and *operation.*

liter (le′ter, li′ter) [Fr. *litre*] a unit of volume in the metric system, equal to 1000 cubic centimeters, or 1 cubic decimeter, or to 1.0567 quarts liquid measure. Abbreviated l or L.

lithagogectasia (lith″ah-go″jek-ta′se-ah) [*litho-* + Gr. *agōgos* leading + *ektasis* stretching] lithectasy.

lithagogue (lith′ah-gog) [*litho-* + Gr. *agōgos* leading] 1. expelling calculi. 2. a remedy that promotes the expulsion of calculi.

Lithane (lith′ān) trademark for a preparation of lithium carbonate.

lithangiuria (lith″an-je-u′re-ah) [*litho-* + Gr. *angeion* vessel + *ouron* urine + *-ia*] calculous disease of the urinary tract.

litharge (lith′arj) [Gr. *lithargyros; lithos* stone + *argyros* silver] see *lead monoxide.*

lithate (lith′āt) a urate.

lithecbole (lith-ek′bo-le) [*litho-* + Gr. *ekbolē* expulsion] expulsion of a calculus.

lithectasy (lǐ-thek′tah-se) [*litho-* + Gr. *ektasis* stretching] the extraction of calculi through the mechanically dilated urethra.

lithectomy (lǐ-thek′to-me) lithotomy.

lithemia (lǐ-the′me-ah) [*lithic acid* + Gr. *haima* blood + *-ia*] excess of lithic or uric acid and the urates in the blood; it is due to imperfect metabolism of the nitrogenous elements.

lithemic (lǐ-the′mik) pertaining to, affected with, or of the nature of lithemia.

lithia (lith′e-ah) see *lithium.*

lithiasic (lith″e-as′ik) pertaining to lithiasis.

lithiasis (lǐ-thi′ah-sis) [*litho-* + *-iasis*] 1. a condition characterized by the formation of calculi and concretions. Called also *calculosis.* **appendicular l.,** a condition in which the lumen of the vermiform appendix becomes obstructed with calculi; it is said to run in families, and to be akin to gout and rheumatism. **l. conjuncti′vae,** a condition marked by the formation of white, calcareous concretions in the acini of the meibomian glands. **pancreatic l.,** the presence of calcium concretions in the pancreas, usually associated with pancreatic exocrine (digestive enzymes) and endocrine (insulin) insufficiency, with steatorrhea, weight loss, and diabetes mellitus.

lithic (lith′ik) 1. pertaining to calculus. 2. pertaining to lithium.

lithium (lith′e-um) [Gr. *lithos* stone] a white metal; atomic number, 3; atomic weight, 6.939; symbol, Li; its oxide, lithia, Li_2O, is alkaline; its salts are solvents of uric acid to a certain extent in the test tube: based on this, it was formerly erroneously thought to be indicated in gout and rheumatic conditions. Lithium salts (lithium carbonate) are used in treating the manic phase of manic-depressive disorders. **l. benzoate,** a salt, $C_6H_5 \cdot CO \cdot O \cdot Li$, in a white powder or in scales. **l. bromide,** a white, deliquescent, slightly bitter granular powder, $LiBr \cdot H_2O$, formerly used as a central nervous system depressant. **l. cacodylate,** a salt, $(CH_3)_2AsOLi$, formerly used as an arsenical remedy in gouty and rheumatic conditions and in anemia. **l. caffeine sulfonate,** a salt formerly used in gout and rheumatism and as a diuretic. **l. carbonate** [USP], chemical name: carbonic acid dilithium salt. A white, granular powder, Li_2CO_3, used in the treatment of acute manic states and in the prophylaxis of recurrent affective disorders manifested by depression or mania only, or those in which both mania and depression occur occasionally, administered orally. **l. citrate,** a white crystalline powder, $C_6H_5O_7Li_3 + 4H_2O$. **l. dithiosalicylate,** an amorphous salt formerly used in the treatment of gout and rheumatism. **l. formate,** s salt in colorless needles, $HCOOLi + H_2O$, formerly used in gout and rheumatism. **l. glycerophosphate,** a white powder, $C_3H_5(OH)_2 \cdot PO_2(OLi)_2$, formerly used as a nerve

tonic and antilithic. **l. iodate,** a salt, $LiIO_3$, formerly used in gouty and renal disorders. **l. salicylate,** a white crystalline powder, $OH \cdot C_6H_4 \cdot COOLi$, once used in rheumatism.

litho- (lith′o) [Gr. *lithos* stone] a combining form denoting relationship to stone or to a calculus.

lithocenosis (lith″o-sě-no′sis) [*litho-* + Gr. *kenōsis* evacuation] the removal from the bladder of the fragments of calculi that have been crushed.

lithoclast (lith′o-klast) [*litho-* + Gr. *klan* to crush] a lithotrite, or stone-crushing forceps, of various forms.

lithoclysmia (lith″o-kliz′me-ah) [*litho-* + Gr. *klysma* clyster] treatment of calculus by injecting solvent liquids into the bladder.

lithocystotomy (lith″o-sis-tot′o-me) [*litho-* + Gr. *kystis* bladder + *temnein* to cut] a cutting operation for removing a stone from the bladder.

lithodialysis (lith″o-di-al′ǐ-sis) [*litho-* + Gr. *dialyein* to dissolve] 1. the solution of calculi in the bladder by injected solvents. 2. the crushing of a calculus in the bladder.

lithogenesis (lith″o-jen′ě-sis) [*litho-* + Gr. *gennan* to produce] the formation of calculi.

lithogenic (lith″o-jen′ik) promoting the formation of calculi.

lithogenous (lǐ-thoj′ě-nus) producing or causing the formation of calculi.

lithokelyphopedion (lith″o-kel″ǐ-fo-pe′de-on) [*litho-* + Gr. *kelyphos* sheath + *paidion* child] a lithopedion in which both the fetus and the membranes are petrified.

lithokelyphos (lith″o-kel′ǐ-fos) [*litho-* + Gr. *kelyphos* sheath] a dead fetus in which the fetal membranes are calcified.

lithokonion (lith″o-ko′ne-on) [*litho-* + Gr. *konios* dusty] an instrument for pulverizing calculi in the bladder.

litholabe (lith′o-lab) [*litho-* + Gr. *lambanein* to hold] an instrument for holding a vesical calculus in the operation for its removal.

litholapaxy (lǐ-thol′ah-pak″se) [*litho-* + Gr. *lapaxis* evacuation] the crushing of a calculus in the bladder, followed at once by the washing out of the fragments; called also *lithotripsy.* **Bigelow's l.,** the crushing of a stone by a special kind of lithotrite and the removal of the fragments by another apparatus.

lithology (lǐ-thol′o-je) [*litho-* + *-logy*] the sum of what is known regarding calculi and their treatment.

litholysis (lǐ-thol′ǐ-sis) [*litho-* + Gr. *lysis* dissolution] the solution of calculi in the bladder.

litholyte (lith′o-līt) [*litho-* + Gr. *lysis* dissolution] an instrument used in injecting solvents of calculi into the bladder.

litholytic (lith″o-lit′ik) 1. dissolving stones or calculi. 2. an agent that dissolves calculi.

lithometer (lǐ-thom′ě-ter) [*litho-* + Gr. *metron* measure] an instrument for measuring calculi.

lithomoscus (lith″o-mos′kus) [*litho-* + Gr. *moschos* calf] lithopedion in cattle.

lithomyl (lith′o-mil) [*litho-* + Gr. *mylē* mill] an instrument for crushing a stone in the bladder.

lithonephria (lith″o-nef′re-ah) [*litho-* + Gr. *nephros* kidney] any disease condition due to the presence of calculi in the kidney.

lithonephritis (lith″o-ně-fri′tis) [*litho-* + *nephritis*] inflammation of the kidney due to irritation of calculi.

lithonephrotomy (lith″o-ně-frot′o-me) [*litho-* + Gr. *nephros* kidney + *tomē* a cutting] the operative removal of a renal calculus.

lithontriptic (lith″on-trip′tik) lithotriptic.

lithopedion (lith″o-pe′de-on) [L. *lithopaedium;* from Gr. *lithos* stone + *paidion* child] a dead fetus that has become stony or pertrified *in utero;* calcified fetus.

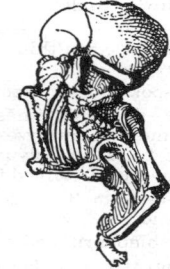

Lithopedion (Arey).

lithophone (lith′o-fōn) [*litho-* + Gr. *phōnē* sound] a device for indicating the presence of a calculus by the sound which the latter emits when struck.

lithoscope (lith′o-skōp) [*litho-* + Gr. *skopein* to examine] an instrument for examining calculi in the bladder.

lithotome (lith′o-tōm) a knife for performing lithotomy.

lithotomist (lǐ-thot′o-mist) one who performs a lithotomy.

lithotomy (lĭ-thot′o-me) [*litho-* + Gr. *tomē* a cutting] incision of a duct or organ, especially of the bladder, for removal of stone. **bilateral l.**, one performed by a transverse incision across the perineum. **high l.**, suprapubic l. **lateral l.**, one in which the incision is before the rectum and to one side of the raphe. **marian l.**, **median l.**, one in which the incision is made on the raphe of the perineum anterior to the anus. **mediolateral l.**, a combination of the median and lateral operations. **perineal l.**, that in which the incision is made in the perineum. **prerectal l.**, marian l. **rectal l.**, **rectovesical l.**, one performed by an incision within the dilated rectum. **suprapubic l.**, one performed by an incision above the pubes. **vaginal l.**, **vesicovaginal l.**, one performed by an incision within the vagina.

lithotony (lĭ-thot′o-ne) [*litho-* + Gr. *teinein* to stretch] the creation of an artificial bladder fistula which is dilated to allow the extraction of a stone.

lithotresis (lith″o-tre′sis) [*litho-* + Gr. *trēsis* a boring] the drilling or boring of holes in a calculus.

lithotripsy (lith′o-trip″se) [*litho-* + Gr. *tribein* to rub] litholapaxy.

lithotriptic (lith′o-trip′tik) pertaining to or producing lithotripsy.

lithotriptor (lith′o-trip″tor) an instrument for crushing calculi in the bladder.

lithotriptoscope (lith″o-trip′to-skōp) an instrument for performing lithotriptoscopy.

lithotriptoscopy (lith″o-trip-tos′ko-pe) [*litho-* + Gr. *tripsis* a crushing + *skopein* to examine] the crushing of a vesical calculus under direct visual control.

lithotrite (lith′o-trīt) [*litho-* + Gr. *tribein* to rub] an instrument for crushing a stone in the bladder.

lithotrity (lĭ-thot′rĭ-te) the crushing of a vesical calculus within the bladder by means of the lithotrite.

lithotroph (lith′o-trōf) [*litho-* + Gr. *trophē* nutrition] a microorganism that lives in and obtains energy from the oxidation of inorganic materials. The group includes the sulfur, nitrifying, and perhaps also the iron bacteria. Formerly called *inorgoxydant*.

lithotrophic (lith″o-trof′ik) pertaining to a lithotroph.

lithous (lith′us) [Gr. *lithos* stone] pertaining to or of the nature of a calculus.

lithoxiduria (lith″ok-sĭ-du′re-ah) [*litho-* + *oxide* + Gr. *ouron* urine + *-ia*] xanthinuria.

lithuresis (lith″u-re′sis) [*litho-* + Gr. *ourēsis* urination] the passage of gravel through the urethra with the urine.

lithureteria (lith″u-rĕ-te′re-ah) [*litho-* + Gr. *ourētēr* ureter] calculous disease of the ureter.

litmocidin (lit″mo-si′din) a toxic antibiotic substance obtained from *Nocardia cyaneus*. It is an anthocyanidine derivative and is bacteriostatic and bactericidal for cocci, *Vibrio cholerae*, and tubercle bacilli in vitro. It is a red indicator pigment (acid—red; alkali—blue).

litmus (lit′mus) a pigment prepared from *Rocella tinctoria* and other lichens, used as a test for acidity and alkalinity. It has a pH range of 4.5 to 8.3. Crude fractions are *azolitmin, erythrolitmin* and *erythrolein*. The principal chemically-defined component is a polymer of 7-hydroxy-2-phenoxazone.

Litomosoides carinii (lit″o-mo-soi′dēz kah-rin′e-i) a filarial worm found in the pleural and peritoneal cavities of the cotton rat, *Sigmodon hispidus*.

litre (le′ter) [Fr.] liter.

Litten's diaphragm phenomenon (sign) (lit′enz) [Moritz *Litten*, German physician, 1845–1907] see under *phenomenon*.

litter (lit′er) 1. a stretcher for transporting the sick or wounded. 2. the offspring produced at one birth by a multiparous animal.

Little's area (lit′elz) [James Laurence *Little*, American surgeon, 1836–1885] see *Kiesselbach's area* under *area*.

Little's disease (lit′elz) [William John *Little*, English physician, 1810–1894] see under *disease*.

Littre's crypts, glands, hernia, operation (le′trz) [Alexis *Littre*, French surgeon, 1658–1725] see *glandulae preputiales* and *glandulae urethrales urethrae masculinae*; see *diverticular hernia*, under *hernia*; and see under *operation*.

littritis (lit-tri′tis) inflammation of the urethral (Littre's) glands.

Litzmann's obliquity (litz′manz) [Karl Konrad Theodor *Litzmann*, German gynecologist, 1815–1890] see under *obliquity*.

livedo (lĭ-ve′do) [L.] a discolored spot or patch on the skin, commonly due to passive congestion; commonly used alone to refer to *l. reticularis*. **l. annula′ris**, **l. racemo′sa**, l. reticularis. **l. reticula′ris**, a peripheral vascular condition characterized by a reddish blue netlike mottling of the skin of the extremities; called also *asphyxia reticularis, l. annularis* and *l. racemosa*. **l. reticula′ris idiopath′ica**, a reticulated mottling of the skin occurring at first on exposure of the skin to cold, but later often becoming persistent. **l. reticula′ris symptomat′ica**, mottling of the skin due to some demonstrable cause, often to polyarteritis nodosa. **l. telangiectat′ica**, permanent mottling of the skin due to anomaly of the capillaries of the skin.

livedoid (liv′e-doid) pertaining to or resembling livedo.

liver (liv′er) [L. *jecur*; Gr. *hēpar*] 1. a large gland of a dark-red color situated in the upper part of the abdomen on the right side. Called also *hepar*[NA]. Its domed upper surface fits closely against and is adherent to the inferior surface of the right diaphragmatic dome, and it has a double blood supply from the hepatic artery and the portal vein. It comprises thousands of minute lobules (lobuli hepatitis), the functional units of the liver (see also *liver acinus*, under *acinus*, and *portal lobule*, under *lobule*). Its manifold functions include the storage and filtration of blood, the secretion of bile, the excretion of bilirubin and other substances formed elsewhere in the body, and numerous metabolic functions, including the conversion of sugars into glycogen, which it stores. It is essential to life. 2. the same gland of certain animals sometimes used as food or from which pharmaceutical products are prepared. **albuminoid l.**, **amyloid l.**, a liver which is the seat of an albuminoid or amyloid degeneration; called also *waxy l.* **biliary cirrhotic l.**, one in which the bile ducts are clogged and distended, the substance of the organ being inflamed; due to biliary cirrhosis. **brimstone l.**, an enlarged liver of a deep-yellow color, seen in some cases of congenital syphilis. **bronze l.**, the bronze-colored liver seen in malaria, which results from deposition of malarial pigment (q.v.). **cirrhotic l.**, one that is the site of cirrhosis. **degraded l.**, a human liver divided into many lobes. **fatty l.**, one affected with fatty infiltration. **fatty l. of Brahmin children**, a term used for kwashiorkor in India. **floating l.**, wandering l. **foamy l.**, a liver seen post mortem, marked by the presence of numerous gas bubbles. **frosted l.**, perihepatitis chronica hyperplastica. **hobnail l.**, a liver whose surface is marked by nail-like points from cirrhosis. **icing l.**, perihepatitis chronica hyperplastica. **infantile l.**, biliary cirrhosis of children; see under *cirrhosis*. **iron l.**, the condition of the liver in hepatic siderosis. **lardaceous l.**, albuminoid l. **nutmeg l.**, one presenting a mottled appearance when cut. **pigmented l.**, one containing pigment, usually a result of malaria and melanemia, or the Dubin-Johnson syndrome. **polycystic l.**, congenital cystic disease of the liver. **sago l.**, one affected with amyloid degeneration, the acini resembling boiled sago grains, i.e., translucent granules 2 or 3 mm. in diameter. **stasis l.**, the liver in stasis cirrhosis. **sugar-icing l.**, perihepatitis chronica hyperplastica. **wandering l.**, a displaced and movable liver. **waxy l.**, albuminoid l.

livetin (li′vĕ-tin) a protein found in yolk of egg.

Livi's index (le′vēz) [Rodolfo *Livi*, Italian physician, 1856–1920] see under *index*.

livid (liv′id) [L. *lividus*, lead-colored] discolored, as from the effects of contusion or congestion; black and blue.

lividity (lĭ-vid′ĭ-te) [L. *lividitas*] the quality of being livid; discoloration, as of dependent parts, by the gravitation of the blood. **postmortem l.**, livor mortis.

Livierato's sign (le″ve-er-at′ōz) [Panagino *Livierato*, Italian physician, 1860–1936] see under *sign*.

Livingston's triangle (liv′ing-stunz) [Edward Meakin *Livingston*, American surgeon, born 1895] see under *triangle*.

livor (li′vor), pl. *livo′res* [L.] discoloration. **l. mor′tis**, discoloration appearing on dependent parts of the body after death, as a result of cessation of circulation, stagnation of blood, and settling of the blood by gravity; called also *postmortem lividity*.

Lixaminol (liks-am′ĭ-nol) trademark for preparations of aminophylline.

lixiviation (liks″iv-e-a′shun) [L. *lixivia* lye] the separation of soluble from insoluble matter by dissolving out the soluble matter and drawing off the solution; called also *leaching*.

lixivium (liks-iv′e-um) [L.] any alkaline filtrate obtained by leaching ashes or other similar powdered substance; lye.

Lizars' operation (li′zarz) [John *Lizars*, Edinburgh surgeon, 1787(?)–1860] see under *operation*.

L.K.Q.C.P.I. Licentiate of the King and Queen's College of Physicians of Ireland.

L.L.L. left lower lobe (of the lung).

L.M. Licentiate in Midwifery; light minimum; linguomesial.

L.M.A. left mentoanterior (position of the fetus).

LMF leukocyte mitogenic factor.

L.M.P. left mentoposterior (position of the fetus); last menstrual period.

L.M.R.C.P. Licentiate in Midwifery of the Royal College of Physicians.

L.M.S. Licentiate in Medicine and Surgery.

L.M.S.S.A. Licentiate in Medicine and Surgery of the Society of Apothecaries.

L.M.T. left mentotransverse (position of the fetus).

LNPF lymph node permeability factor.

L.O.A. left occipito-anterior (position of the fetus).

Loa (lo′ah) [a native word in Angola, West Africa] a genus of filarial nematodes. **L. lo′a**, a threadlike worm of West Africa,

1–2 inches long, that inhabits the subcutaneous connective tissue of the body, which it traverses freely. It is seen especially about the orbit and even under the conjunctiva. It causes itching and occasionally edematous swellings (Calabar swellings). The immature forms or microfilariae are diurnal, being found in the peripheral circulation in greatest concentrations during the day. Flies of the genus *Chrysops* are the intermediate hosts and vectors. Formerly called *Filaria loa.*

load (lōd) the quantity of a measurable entity borne, by an object or organism, such as the work (*work l.*) required of an individual, or the body content, as of water, salt, or heat, especially as it varies from normal. **occlusal l.,** the total force exerted on the teeth through the occlusal surfaces during mastication.

loading (lōd′ing) administering sufficient quantities of a substance to test the subject's ability to metabolize it, as in the histidine loading test.

loaiasis (lo″ah-i′ah-sis) loiasis.

lobar (lo′ber) of, pertaining to, or affecting a lobe.

lobate (lo′bāt) [L. *lobatus*] provided with lobes, or disposed in lobes.

lobation (lo-ba′shun) the formation of lobes; the state of having lobes. **renal l.,** the appearance on x-ray films of small notches along the surface of the kidney, indicating the location of renal lobes.

lobe (lōb) [L. *lobus*; Gr. *lobos*] 1. a more or less well-defined portion of any organ, especially of the brain, lungs, and glands. Lobes are demarcated by fissures, sulci, connective tissue, and by their shape. 2. one of the main divisions of the crown of a tooth, developmentally representing a center of calcification. **anterior l. of hypophysis, anterior l. of pituitary gland,** lobus anterior hypophyseos. **appendicular l.,** Riedel's l. **azygos l.,** a small accessory or anomalous lobe situated at the apex of the right lung. **caudate l. of cerebrum** (*obs.*), insula. **caudate l. of liver,** lobus caudatus. **l's of cerebrum,** lobi cerebri. **crescentic l. of cerebellum, inferior,** lobulus semilunaris inferior. **crescentic l. of cerebellum, superior,** lobulus semilunaris superior. **cuneate l.,** cuneus. **digastric l.,** lobulus biventer. **flocculonodular l.,** the archicerebellum: the phylogenetically oldest portion of the cerebellum consisting of a node and two flocculi; it receives direct and secondary vestibular fibers and projects chiefly to the vestibular nuclei and reticular formation. **frontal l.,** the anterior portion of the pallium; see *lobus frontalis.* **hepatic l's,** the lobes of the liver, designated the right and left and the caudate and quadrate; see *lobus caudatus, lobus hepatis dexter* and *sinister,* and *lobus quadratus hepatis.* **lateral l's of prostate gland,** see *lobus prostatae [dexter et sinister].* **limbic l.,** gyrus fornicatus. **linguiform l.,** Riedel's l. **l's of liver,** hepatic l's. **l. of liver, left,** lobus hepatis sinister. **l. of liver, right,** lobus hepatis dexter. **l's of lung,** see *lung.* **l's of mammary gland,** lobi glandulae mammariae. **median l. of prostate,** l. medius prostatae. **neural l.,** see *pituitary gland,* under *gland.* **occipital l.,** the posterior portion of the cerebral hemisphere; see *lobus occipitalis.* **olfactory l.,** lobus olfactorius. **optic l's,** corpora quadrigemina. **parietal l.,** the upper central lobe of the pallium; see *lobus parietalis.* **piriform l.,** the piriform area (q.v.); in lower mammals, the lateral exposed portion of the olfactory cerebral cortex. **polyalveolar l.,** a congenital disorder characterized in early infancy by the presence of far more than the normal number of alveoli in a lobe of the lungs; thereafter, normal multiplication of alveoli does not take place and they become enlarged, i.e., emphysematous. **posterior l. of hypophysis, posterior l. of pituitary gland,** lobus posterior hypophyseos. **prefrontal l.,** the part of the frontal lobe of the brain anterior to the ascending convolution. **l's of prostate,** see *lobus prostatae [dexter et sinister].* **pulmonary l's,** see *lung.* **pyriform l.,** piriform l. **pyramidal l. of thyroid gland,** lobus pyramidalis glandulae thyroideae. **quadrangular l. of cerebellum,** lobulus quadrangularis cerebelli. **quadrate l. of cerebral hemisphere,** precuneus. **quadrate l. of liver,** lobus quadratus hepatis. **renal l's,** lobi renales. **Riedel's l.,** an anomalous tongue-shaped mass of tissue projecting from the right lobe of the liver. **semilunar l., inferior,** lobulus semilunaris inferior. **semilunar l., superior,** lobulus semilunaris superior. **spigelian l.,** lobus caudatus. **temporal l.,** the lower lateral lobe of the cerebral hemisphere; see *lobus temporalis.* **temporosphenoidal l. of cerebral hemisphere** (*obs.*), lobus temporalis. **l's of thymus,** see *lobus thymi [dexter et sinister].* **l's of thyroid gland,** see *lobus glandulae thyroideae [dexter et sinister].* **vagal l.,** visceral l. **vermiform l.** (*obs.*), vermis cerebelli. **visceral l.,** the visceral sensory area of fishes.

lobectomy (lo-bek′to-me) [Gr. *lobos* lobe + *ektomē* excision] excision of a lobe, as of the thyroid, liver, brain, or lung. See also *lobotomy.*

lobelia (lo-be′le-ah) the dried leaves and tops of *Lobelia inflata* L. (Campanulaceae), an herb with properties resembling those of nicotine.

lobeline (lob′e-lin) alpha-lobeline, $C_{22}H_{27}NO_2$, the principal alkaloid of *Lobelia inflata,* an annual herb of eastern United States

and Canada, formerly used to restore normal respiration in asphyxia due to traumatic shock. Currently used in certain anti-smoking preparations.

lobendazole (lo-ben′dah-zōl) chemical name: 1*H*-benzimidazol-2-yl-carbamic acid ethyl ester; a veterinary anthelmintic, $C_{10}H_{11}N_3O_2$.

lobi (lo′bi) [L.] plural of *lobus.*

lobite (lo′bīt) limited to a definite lobe.

lobitis (lo-bi′tis) inflammation of a lobe, especially of a lobe of the lung.

Loboa loboi (lo-bo′ah lo′boi) an as yet uncultured yeast that is the causative agent of keloidal blastomycosis.

lobopod (lo′bo-pod″) lobopodium.

lobopodia (lo″bo-po′de-ah) plural of *lobopodium.*

lobopodium (lo″bo-po′de-um), pl. *lobopo′dia* [Gr. *lobos* lobe + *pous* foot] a blunt pseudopodium composed of both ectoplasm and endoplasm, or of endoplasm alone. Cf. *axopodium, filopodium,* and *rhizopodium.*

lobotomy (lo-bot′o-me) incision into a lobe; in psychosurgery, surgical incision of all the fibers of a lobe of the brain. **frontal l., prefrontal l.,** an operation in which, through holes drilled in the skull, the white matter of the frontal lobe is incised with a leukotome passed through a cannula; called also *leukotomy.* **transorbital l.,** see under *leukotomy.*

Lobstein's disease (syndrome), ganglion (lōb′stīnz) [Johann Friedrich Georg Christian Martin *Lobstein,* surgeon in Strasbourg, 1777–1835] see *osteogenesis imperfecta,* and see under *ganglion.*

lobular (lob′u-lar) [L. *lobularis*] of or pertaining to a lobule.

lobulated (lob′u-lāt″ed) made up of or divided into lobules.

lobulation (lob″u-la′shun) the process of becoming or the state of being lobulated. **portal l.,** in the liver, the lobulated pattern of surviving tissue and the areas in which the tissue has been destroyed after occlusion of the hepatic vein.

lobule (lob′ūl) a small lobe; see *lobulus.* **anterior l. of pituitary gland,** lobus anterior hypophyseos. **l. of auricle,** lobulus auriculae. **biventral l.,** lobulus biventer. **central l. of cerebellum,** lobulus centralis cerebelli. **cortical l's of kidney,** lobuli corticales renis. **l's of epididymis,** lobuli epididymidis. **falciform l.** (*obs.*), cuneus. **fusiform l.** (*obs.*), polus temporalis. **hepatic l's,** lobuli hepatis. **l's of lung,** segmenta bronchopulmonalia. **l's of mammary gland,** lobuli glandulae mammariae. **paracentral l.,** lobulus paracentralis. **parietal l., inferior,** lobulus parietalis inferior. **parietal l., superior,** lobulus parietalis superior. **portal l.,** a polygonal mass of liver tissue, larger than a liver acinus, containing portions of three adjacent hepatic lobules, and having a portal vein at its center and a central vein peripherally at each corner. **primary l. of lung,** the anatomical and functional unit of the lung; distal to a terminal bronchiole, it consists of respiratory bronchioles, two or more alveolar ducts, atria, alveolar sacs, and alveoli. See Plate XLVI. **pulmonary l's,** segmenta bronchopulmonalia. **quadrangular l. of cerebellum,** lobulus quadrangularis cerebelli. **respiratory l.,** primary l. of lung. **secondary l. of lung,** an anatomical subdivision of a pulmonary segment, consisting of several branching primary lobules. **semilunar l., inferior,** lobulus semilunaris inferior. **semilunar l., superior,** lobulus semilunaris superior. **l's of testis,** lobuli testis. **l's of thymus,** lobuli thymi. **l's of thyroid gland,** lobuli glandulae thyroideae.

lobulette (lob″u-let′) [Fr.] (*obs.*) 1. a minute lobule. 2. any one of the primary divisions of a lobule.

lobuli (lob′u-li) [L.] plural of *lobulus.*

lobulose (lob′u-lōs) divided into lobules.

lobulous (lob′u-lus) lobulose.

lobulus (lob′u-lus), pl. *lob′uli* [L., dim of *lobus*] a lobule, or small lobe; [NA] a general term for a small lobe or one of the primary divisions of a lobe. **l. auric′ulae** [NA], lobule of auricle: the inferior, dependent part of the auricle below the antitragus, which contains fibrous and fatty tissue but no cartilage. **l. biven′ter** [NA], biventral lobule: a lobule on the inferior surface of the hemisphere of the cerebellum situated between the tonsilla of the cerebellum and the inferior semilunar lobule; called also *digastric l.* **l. centra′lis cerebel′li** [NA], central lobule of cerebellum: the portion of the vermis between the lingula and the culmen, resting on the lingula and the anterior medullary velum. **lob′uli cortica′les re′nis** [NA], cortical lobules of kidney: more or less distinctly marked small polygonal areas on the surface of a kidney; each area corresponds to a medullary ray together with its attached renal corpuscles and tubules. **lob′uli epididym′idis** [NA], lobules of epididymis: the wedge-shaped parts of the head of the epididymis, each comprising a single efferent ductule of the testis; called also *coni epididymidis* [NA alternative]. **lob′uli glan′dulae mam′ma′riae** [NA], lobules of mammary gland: the smaller subdivisions that make up a lobe of the mammary gland, each drained by a single branch of a lactiferous duct. Called also *lobuli mammae.* See *mammary gland,* under *gland.* **lob′uli glan′dulae**

thyroi′deae [NA], lobules of thyroid gland: irregular areas on the surface of the thyroid gland produced by entrance into the gland of fibrous trabeculae from the sheath. **lob′uli hep′a-tis** [NA], hepatic lobules: the small vascular units comprising the substance of the liver, each of which is polygonal in shape with a central vein at its center and portal canals peripherally at the corners. See also *liver acinus*, under *acinus*. **lob′uli mam′-mae**, lobuli glandulae mammariae. **l. paracentra′lis** [NA], paracentral lobule: a lobe on the medial surface of the cerebral hemisphere, continuous with the precentral and postcentral gyri of the frontal and parietal lobes, and limited below by the cingulate sulcus; it is comprised of motor and sensory cortex, chiefly for the lower limb. **l. parieta′lis infe′rior** [NA], inferior parietal lobule: the lobule that forms the posterior part of the lateral portion of the parietal lobe of the cerebrum. It lies below the intraparietal sulcus, above the posterior ramus of the lateral cerebral fissure, and behind the postcentral sulcus. It includes the supramarginal and the angular gyri. In the dominant hemisphere, it is concerned with language mechanisms. **l. parieta′lis supe′rior** [NA], superior parietal lobule: the posterior part of the upper portion of the parietal lobe of the brain; it lies behind the postcentral sulcus, in front of the parietooccipital fissure, and above the intraparietal sulcus. It comprises association areas concerned with general sensory functions. **lob′uli pulmo′num**, segmenta bronchopulmonalia. **l. quadran-gula′ris cerebel′li** [NA], quadrangular lobule of cerebellum: the part of the hemisphere of the cerebellum continuous with the culmen and declive of the vermis. Sometimes used to refer to only that part of the hemisphere continuous with the culmen. **l. semiluna′ris infe′rior** [NA], inferior semilunar lobule: that part of the hemisphere of the cerebellum continuous with the tuber vermis. Called also *inferior crescentic lobe of cerebellum* and, in comparative anatomy, *crus II*. **l. semiluna′ris supe′rior** [NA], superior semilunar lobule: that part of the hemisphere of the cerebellum continuous with the folium vermis. Called also *superior crescentic lobe of cerebellum* and, in comparative anatomy, *crus I*. **l. sim′plex** [NA], that part of the cerebellar hemisphere which is continuous with the declive of the vermis. **lob′uli tes′tis** [NA], lobules of testis: the pyramidal subdivisions of the testicular substance, each with its base against the albuginea and its apex at the mediastinum, and composed largely of tubuli seminiferi. **lob′uli thy′mi** [NA], lobules of thymus: the smaller subdivisions of the lobes of the thymus gland, separated by fibrous trabeculae.

lobus (lo′bus), pl. *lo′bi* [L.] a lobe; a more or less well defined portion of any organ; [NA] a general term for such subdivisions, especially of the brain, lungs, and various glands, demarcated by fissures, sulci, or connective tissue septa. **l. ante′rior hypo-phys′eos** [NA], the anterior lobe of the pituitary gland (hypophysis), which arises from the buccal epithelium in the embryo; called also *adenohypophysis* [NA alternative]. See discussion under *pituitary gland*. **l. cauda′tus** [NA], **l. cauda′tus [Spige′-li]**, caudate lobe of liver: a small lobe of the liver bounded on the right by the inferior vena cava, which separates it from the right lobe, and on the left by the attachment of the gastrohepatic ligament, which separates it from the left lobe. **lo′bi cer′e-bri** [NA], lobes of cerebrum: the well defined areas of the pallium, demarcated by fissures, sulci, and arbitrary lines, including the frontal, temporal, parietal, and occipital lobes. See Plate accompanying *brain*. **l. fronta′lis** [NA], frontal lobe: the anterior portion of the cerebral hemisphere, extending from the frontal pole to the sulcus centralis. **lo′bi glan′dulae mamma′riae** [NA], lobes of mammary gland: the major subdivisions of the secreting portion of the mammary gland, each drained by a single lactiferous duct and further subdivided into lobules (lobuli glandulae mammariae). See *mammary gland*, under *gland*. Called also *lobi mammae*. **l. glan′dulae thyroi′deae [dex′ter et sinis′ter]** [NA], lobe of thyroid gland: either of the lobes (right or left) of the thyroid gland, closely applied to either side of the trachea, cricoid cartilage, and thyroid cartilage. **l. hep′atis dex′ter** [NA], right lobe of liver: the largest of the four lobes of the liver. Anteriorly, it is separated from the left lobe by the falciform ligament. Posteroinferiorly, it is separated from the caudate lobe by the inferior vena cava and from the quadrate lobe by the gallbladder. Used in the broad sense, the term includes the caudate and quadrate lobes. **l. hep′atis sinis′ter** [NA], left lobe of liver: the smaller of the two main lobes of the liver. Anteriorly, it is separated from the right lobe by the falciform ligament. Posteroinferiorly, it is separated from the caudate and quadrate lobes by the attachment of the gastrohepatic ligament and the ligamentum teres. **l. infe′rior pulmo′nis** [NA], the inferior lobe of either lung. **lo′bi mam′mae**, lobi glandulae mammariae. **l. me′dius prosta′tae** [NA], median lobe of prostate: a normal enlargement of the isthmus of the prostate that sometimes occurs. **l. me′dius pulmo′nis dex′tri** [NA], the middle lobe of the right lung. **l. occipita′lis** [NA], occipital lobe: the posterior portion of the cerebral hemisphere, extending from the posterior pole to the parieto-occipital fissure on the medial surface, but continuous with the parietal lobe on the lateral surface. **l. olfacto′rius**, olfactory lobe: a term applied to the olfactory apparatus on the lower surface of the frontal lobe of the brain. It consists of the olfactory bulb, tract, and trigone.

l. parieta′lis [NA], parietal lobe: the upper central lobe of the cerebral hemisphere, separated from the temporal lobe below by the lateral sulcus, but continuous at the posterior end of that sulcus, and separated from the frontal lobe in front by the central sulcus. Behind, it is continuous with the occipital lobe on the lateral surface, but separated from it by the parieto-occipital sulcus on the medial surface. **lo′bi placen′tae**, distinct areas on the uterine surface of the placenta, demarcated by the connective tissue septa. **l. poste′rior hypophys′eos** [NA], the posterior lobe of the pituitary gland (hypophysis), which originates in the embryo as an evagination from the floor of the diencephalon; called also *neurohypophysis* [NA alternative]. See discussion under *pituitary gland*. **l. prosta′tae [dex′ter et sinis′ter]** [NA], lobe of prostate: either of the paired halves (right and left) of the prostate, separated by a more or less distinct median sulcus; called also *lateral lobes of prostate gland*. **l. pyramida′lis glan′dulae thyroi′deae** [NA], pyramidal lobe of the thyroid gland: an occasional third lobe of the thyroid gland which extends upward from the isthmus across the thyroid cartilage to the hyoid bone; it is the remains of the thyroid stalk of the fetus. **l. quadra′tus hep′atis** [NA], quadrate lobe of liver: a small lobe of the liver bounded on the right by the gallbladder, which separates it from the right lobe, and on the left by the ligamentum teres, which separates it from the left lobe. **lo′bi rena′les** [NA], renal lobes: the units of the kidney, each consisting of a pyramid and its surrounding cortical substance; the division of the kidney into lobes is more distinctly marked in some animals and in infants than in the human adult. **l. spige′lii**, l. caudatus. **l. supe′rior pulmo′nis** [NA], the superior lobe of either lung. **l. tempora′lis** [NA], temporal lobe: the lower lateral lobe of the cerebral hemisphere, lying below the posterior ramus of the lateral sulcus, lateral to the collateral sulcus, and merging behind with the occipital lobe. **l. thy′mi [dex′ter et sinis′ter]** [NA], lobe of thymus: either of the two chief parts (right or left) of the thymus, which meet in the midline. **l. va′gi**, visceral lobe.

local (lo′kal) [L. *localis*] restricted to or pertaining to one spot or part; not general.

localization (lo″kah-li-za′shun) 1. the determination of the site or place of any process or lesion. 2. restriction to a circumscribed or limited area. 3. prelocalization. **cerebral l.**, the determination of the situation of the various centers of the brain; also the limitation of the various cerebral faculties to a particular center or organ of the brain. **elective l.**, selective l. **germinal l.**, the location on a blastoderm of prospective organs; see *fate map*, under *map*. **selective l.**, the tendency of a microorganism to infect a specific variety of tissue.

localized (lo′kal-īzd) not general; restricted to a limited region or to one or more spots.

localizer (lo′kal-īz″er) an instrument for locating solid particles in the eyeball by means of the roentgen ray, as the Berman localizer, Roper-Hall localizer, and Wildgen-Reck localizer.

locator (lo′ka-ter) an instrument or apparatus by which the location of an object is determined. **abutment l.**, a thin resin base made on a diagnostic denture cast into which holes have been cut to predetermine locations of the cuspids and molars. **Berman-Moorhead l.**, an instrument for locating metallic fragments embedded in body tissues. **electroacoustic l.**, an apparatus that amplifies into an audible click the contact of a probe with a solid object; used in locating foreign objects within the body.

Loc. dol. abbreviation for L. *lo′co dolen′ti*, to the painful spot.

lochia (lo′ke-ah) [Gr. *lochia*] the vaginal discharge that takes place during the first week or two after childbirth. **l. al′ba**, the final vaginal discharge after childbirth, when the amount of blood is decreased and the leukocytes are increased. **l. cruen′ta**, l. rubra. **l. purulen′ta**, l. alba. **l. ru′bra**, the vaginal discharge of almost pure blood immediately after childbirth. **l. sanguinolen′ta**, the thick, maroon-colored vaginal discharge occurring a few days after childbirth. **l. sero′sa**, the serous vaginal discharge occurring about four or five days after childbirth.

lochial (lo′ke-al) pertaining to the lochia.

lochiocolpos (lo″ke-o-kol′pos) [*lochia* + Gr. *kolpos* vagina] distention of the vagina by retained lochia.

lochiocyte (lo′ke-o-sīt″) [*lochia* + *-cyte*] one of the characteristic decidual cells of the lochia.

lochiometra (lo″ke-o-me′trah) [*lochia* + Gr. *mētra* uterus] distention of the uterus by retained lochia.

lochiometritis (lo″ke-o-me-tri′tis) [*lochia* + *metritis*] puerperal metritis.

lochiorrhagia (lo″ke-o-ra′je-ah) [*lochia* + Gr. *rhēgnynai* to burst forth] lochiorrhea.

lochiorrhea (lo″ke-o-re′ah) [*lochia* + Gr. *rhoia* flow] an abnormally profuse discharge of lochia.

lochioschesis (lo″ke-os′kĕ-sis) [*lochia* + Gr. *schesis* retention] retention of the lochia; lochiostasis.

lochiostasis (lo″ke-os′tah-sis) [*lochia* + Gr. *stasis* halt] retention of the lochia; lochioschesis.

lochometritis (lo″ko-me-tri′tis) [Gr. *lochos* childbirth + *metritis*] puerperal metritis.

loci (lo′si) [L.] plural of *locus.*

Locke's solution (fluid) (loks) [Frank Spiller *Locke,* British physician] see under *solution.*

lockjaw (lok′jaw) 1. tetanus. 2. trismus.

Lockwood's ligament (lok′woodz) [Charles Barrett *Lockwood,* English surgeon, 1856–1914] see under *ligament.*

loco (lo′ko) [Sp. "insane"] 1. a name of various leguminous plants of the genera *Astragalus, Hosackia, Sophora,* and *Oxytropis,* poisonous to horses, cattle, and sheep in certain arid regions because of the selenium they contain. 2. locoism. 3. an animal affected with locoism.

locoism (lo′ko-izm) a disease of horses, cattle, and sheep caused by poisoning by loco and marked by locomotor disturbances, trembling, depression, and, in pregnant animals, absorption. Called also *loco disease* and *loco poisoning.*

locomotion (lo″ko-mo′shun) [L. *locus* place + *movere* to move] movement or the ability to move from one place to another. **brachial l.,** brachiation.

locomotive (lo″ko-mo′tiv) pertaining to locomotion.

locomotor (lo″ko-mo′tor) of or pertaining to locomotion; pertaining to or affecting the locomotive apparatus of the body. See under *ataxia.*

locomotorial (lo″ko-mo-to′re-al) pertaining to the locomotorium.

locomotorium (lo″ko-mo-to′re-um) the locomotive apparatus of the body.

locomotory (lo″ko-mo′tor-e) pertaining to locomotion.

Locorten (lo-kor′ten) trademark for a preparation of flumethasone pivalate.

locular (lok′u-lar) pertaining to a loculus.

loculate (lok′u-lāt) divided into loculi.

loculi (lok′u-li) [L.] plural of *loculus.*

Loculoascomycetidae (lok″u-lo-as″ko-mi-se′tī-de) a subclass of ascomycetous fungi, including the order Myriangiales.

loculus (lok′u-lus), pl. *loc′uli* [L.] 1. a small space or cavity. 2. a local enlargement of the uterus in some mammals, containing an embryo.

locum (lo′kum) [L.] place. **l. ten′ens, l. ten′ent,** a practitioner who temporarily takes the place of another.

locus (lo′kus), pl. *lo′ci* [L.] place; [NA] a general term for a site in the body. In genetics, the specific site of a gene on a chromosome. **l. ceru′leus** [NA], a pigmented eminence in the superior angle of the floor of the fourth ventricle of the brain. **l. cine′reus,** l. ceruleus. **complex l.,** one in which recombination can occur at more than one site. **l. ferrugin′eus,** l. ceruleus. **H-2 l.,** the major histocompatibility locus of the mouse, having more than twenty alleles coding for at least thirty-three alloantigenic specificities; believed to be composed of two gene clusters, H-2k and H-2D, the H-2k being closest to the centromere. **heteromorphic l.,** a locus that exists in two or more allelic forms. **l. mino′ris resisten′tiae,** a site of lessened resistance; an area, structure, or organ offering little resistance to invasion by microorganisms and/or their toxins. **l. ni′ger** (*obs.*), substantia nigra. **l. perfora′tus an′ticus** (*obs.*), substantia perforata anterior. **l. perfora′tus pos′ticus** (*obs.*), substantia perforata posterior. **l. ru′ber,** nucleus ruber.

lodoxamide tromethamine (lo-dok′sah-mīd) chemical name: 2,2′-[(2-chloro-5-cyano-1,3-phenylene)diimino]bis[2-oxoacetic acid] compound with 2-amino-2-(hydroxymethyl)-1,3-propanediol (1:2); an antiasthmatic and antiallergic, $C_{11}H_6ClN_3O_6 \cdot 2C_4H_{11}NO_3$.

Loeb's deciduoma, reaction (lēb) [Leo *Loeb,* American pathologist, born 1869] see under *deciduoma* and *reaction.*

Loefflerella (lef″ler-el′ah) former name for a genus of schizomycetes, species of which are now assigned to *Pseudomonas.*

loemology (le-mol′o-je) [Gr. *loimos* plague + *-logy*] lemology.

loempe (lem′pe) beriberi.

Loevit's cell (le′fits) [Moritz *Loevit,* Prague pathologist, 1851–1918] erythroblast.

Loewi's test (reaction, symptom) (la′vēz) [Otto *Loewi,* German pharmacologist in the United States, 1873–1961; co-winner in 1936, with Sir Henry Hallett Dale, of the Nobel prize for physiology and medicine, for their work on the chemical transmission of nerve impulses] see under *tests.*

Löffler's agar (culture medium) blood serum, stain (lef′lerz) [Friederich August Johannes *Löffler,* German bacteriologist, 1852–1915] see under *agar, blood serum,* and *Table of Stains.*

Löffler's endocarditis (disease), syndrome (eosinophilia, pneumonia, (lef′lerz) [Wilhelm *Löffler,* Swiss physician] see under *endocarditis* and *syndrome.*

löffleria (lef-le′re-ah) [F.A.J. *Löffler*] a condition in which the diphtheria bacillus is present without the ordinary symptoms of diphtheria.

logadectomy (log″ah-dek′to-me) [Gr. *logades* the whites of the eyes + *ektomē* excision] excision of a portion of the conjunctiva.

logaditis (log″ah-di′tis) [Gr. *logades* the whites of the eyes + *-itis*] inflammation of the sclera.

logagnosia (log″ag-no′ze-ah) [*logo-* + *a* neg. + Gr. *gnōsis* knowledge] aphasia, alogia, or other central word defect.

logagraphia (log″ah-graf′e-ah) [*logo-* + *a* neg. + Gr. *graphein* to write] inability to express ideas in writing.

logamnesia (log″am-ne′ze-ah) [*logo-* + Gr. *amnēsia* forgetfulness] receptive aphasia.

logaphasia (log″ah-fa′ze-ah) [*logo-* + *aphasia*] expressive aphasia.

logasthenia (log″as-the′ne-ah) [*logo-* + *asthenia*] disturbance of that faculty of the mind which deals with the comprehension of speech.

logo- (log′o) [Gr. *logos* word] a combining form denoting relationship to words or speech.

logoclonia (log″o-klon′e-ah) [*logo-* + Gr. *klonos* tumult + *-ia*] spasmodic repetition of end syllables of words; logoklony.

logogram (log′o-gram) the graphic record of the symptoms and signs exhibited by a specific patient, charted by means of the logoscope.

logoklony (log′o-klon″e) logoclonia.

logokophosis (log″o-ko-fo′sis) [*logo-* + Gr. *kōphōsis* deafness] word deafness; inability to comprehend spoken language.

logomania (log″o-ma′ne-ah) [*logo-* + Gr. *mania* madness] overtalkativeness.

logoneurosis (log″o-nu-ro′sis) [*logo-* + *neurosis*] (*obs.*) any neurosis with disorder of the speech.

logopathy (log-op′ah-the) [*logo-* + Gr. *pathos* illness] any disorder of speech arising from derangement of the central nervous system.

logopedia (log″o-pe′de-ah) logopedics.

logopedics (log-o-pe′diks) [*logo-* + ortho*pedics*] the science dealing with the study and treatment of speech defects.

logoplegia (log″o-ple′je-ah) [*logo-* + Gr. *plēgē* stroke] paralysis of the speech organs.

logorrhea (log″o-re′ah) [*logo-* + Gr. *rhoia* flow] excessive or abnormal volubility.

logoscope (log′o-skōp) [Gr. *logos* a thought, idea, or word + *skopein* to regard or view] a device, in slide-rule form, designed to facilitate identification of the diseases in which certain signs and symptoms occur.

logoscopy (lo-gos′ko-pe) the use of a logoscope for determining the differential diagnostic possibilities in a patient exhibiting certain signs and symptoms.

logospasm (log′o-spazm) [*logo-* + Gr. *spasmos* spasm] the spasmodic utterance of words.

-logy [Gr. *logos* word, reason] a word termination meaning the science or study of, or a treatise on, the subject designated by the stem to which it is affixed.

Löhlein's diameter (la′linz) [Hermann Christian Adolf *Löhlein,* German gynecologist, 1847–1901] see under *diameter.*

Lohnstein's saccharimeter (lōn′stīnz) [Theodor *Lohnstein,* German physician, 1866–1918] see under *saccharimeter.*

loiasis (lo-i′ah-sis) the state of being infected with nematodes of the genus *Loa.*

loimic (loi′mik) [Gr. *loimos* plague] lemic.

loimographia (loi″mo-gra′fe-ah) [Gr. *loimos* plague + *graphein* to write] lemography.

loimology (loi-mol′o-je) lemology.

loin (loin) the part of the back between the thorax and the pelvis; called also *lumbus* [NA].

Lombardi's sign (lom-bar′dēz) [Antonio *Lombardi,* physician in Naples] see under *sign.*

lometraline hydrochloride (lo-met′rah-lēn) chemical name: 8-chloro-1,2,3,4-tetrahydro-5-methoxy-*N,N*-dimethyl-1-naphthalenamine hydrochloride; a tranquilizer and antiparkinsonian agent, $C_{13}H_{18}ClNO \cdot HCl$.

lomofungin (lo-mo-fun′jin) chemical name: 6-formyl-4,7,9-trihydroxy-1-phenazinecarboxylic acid methyl ester; an antifungal antibiotic derived from *Streptomyces lomondensis* var. *lomondensis.*

lomosome (lo′mo-sōm) [Gr. *lōma* hem, fringe + *sōma* body] a sponge-like structure in fungi contiguous with the hyphal wall as revealed by the electron microscope.

Lomotil (lo′mo-til) trademark for preparations of diphenoxylate hydrochloride and atropine.

lomustine (lo-mus′tēn) chemical name: *N*-(2-chloroethyl-*N′*-cyclohexyl-*N*-nitrosourea. An antineoplastic, $C_9H_{16}ClN_3O_2$, having actions similar to those of the alkylating agents; used in conjunction with other agents as palliative therapy in the treatment of Hodgkin's disease and brain tumors, administered orally. Code name: CCNU.

Lonchocarpus (lon″ko-kar′pus) a genus of leguminous tropical trees and shrubs which furnish rotenone.

Long's formula (coefficient) (longz) [John Harper *Long*, American physician, 1856–1927] see under *formula*.

longevity (lon-jev′ĭ-te) [L. *longus* long + *aevum* age] the condition or quality of being long lived.

longilineal (lon″jĭ-lin′e-al) built along long, narrow lines; dolichomorphic.

longimanous (lon″jĭ-man′us) [L. *longus* long + *manus* hand] having long hands.

longipedate (lon″jĭ-pe′dāt) [L. *longus* long + *pes* foot] having long feet.

longiradiate (lon″jĭ-ra′de-āt) having long radiations; a term applied to certain neuroglial cells.

longissimus (lon-jis′ĭ-mus) [L.] longest; [NA] a general term denoting a long structure, as a muscle.

longitudinal (lon″jĭ-tu′dĭ-nal) [L. *longitudo* length] lengthwise; parallel to the long axis of the body or an organ.

longitudinalis (lon″jĭ-tu″dĭ-na′lis) [L.] lengthwise; [NA] a term denoting a structure that is parallel to the long axis of the body or an organ.

longitypical (lon″jĭ-tip′ĭ-kal) longilineal; dolichomorphic.

longsightedness (long-sīt′ed-nes) hyperopia.

longus (long′gus) [L.] long; [NA] a general term denoting a long structure, as a muscle.

loop (loōp) a turn or sharp curve in a cordlike structure; see also *ansa*. **capillary l's,** minute endothelial tubes that carry blood in the papillae of the skin. **closed l.,** a system in which the input to one or more of the subsystems is affected by its own output. **Gerdy's interauricular l.,** a small muscular bundle in the interatrial septum of the heart. **Henle's l.,** a U-shaped turn in the medullary portion of a renal tubule, with a descending limb from the proximal convoluted tubule and an ascending limb to the distal convoluted tubule; see also *kidney*. **l. of hypoglossal nerve,** ansa cervicalis. **Hyrtl's l.,** an occasional looplike anastomosis between the right and left hypoglossal nerves in the geniohyoid muscle. **lenticular l.,** ansa lenticularis. **Meyer's l.,** one formed by some of the fibers of the optic radiation as they loop around the inferior horn of the lateral ventricle before turning posteriorly. **open l.,** a system on which an input alters the output, but the output has no effect on the input. Cf. *closed l.* **peduncular l.,** ansa peduncularis. **platinum l.,** a loop of platinum or other suitable wire mounted in a handle for use in transferring microorganisms to other culture media. **l's of spinal nerves,** ansae nervorum spinalium. **Stoerck's l.,** the primitive loop in the embryonic uriniferous tubule which develops into a Henle loop and a portion of the proximal convoluted tubule. **subclavian l.,** ansa subclavia. **ventricular l.,** the early, U-shaped loop of the embryonic heart. **l. of Vieussens,** ansa subclavia.

loopful (loōp′ful) the quantity of liquid that can be held within the loop of platinum wire used in transferring microorganisms to other culture media.

loosening (lu′sen-ing) in psychiatry, a disorder of thinking in which association of ideas become so shortened, fragmented, and disturbed as to lack logical relationship; often seen in schizophrenia.

L.O.P. left occipitoposterior (position of the fetus).

loperamide hydrochloride (lo-per′ah-mīd) chemical name: 4-(4-chlorophenyl)-4-hydroxy-*N,N*-dimethyl-α,α-diphenyl-1-piperidinebutanamide monohydrochloride. An antiperistaltic, $C_{29}H_{33}$ $ClN_2O_2 \cdot HCl$, which exerts a direct effect on the muscles of the intestinal wall; used in the treatment of acute nonspecific diarrhea and chronic diarrhea associated with inflammatory bowel disease and to reduce the volume of discharge from ileostomies. It is administered orally.

lophodont (lof′o-dont) [Gr. *lophos* ridge + *odous* tooth] having cheek teeth on which the cusps have become connected to form ridges, as in elephants and some rodents.

Lophophora (lo-fof′o-rah) a genus of Mexican cacti. **L. williamʹsii,** a species whose flowering heads (mescal buttons) are the source of peyote and mescaline.

lophophorine (lo-fof′o-rin) a poisonous alkaloid, $C_{13}H_{17}NO_3$, from *Lophophora williamsii*, having effects similar to those of mescaline.

Lophotrichea (lo″fo-trik′e-ah) a group of bacteria, including those forms which have a tuft of cilia at one pole.

lophotrichous (lo-fot′rĭ-kus) [Gr. *lophos* ridge, tuft + *thrix* hair] having two or more flagella at one end; said of a bacterial cell. See *flagellum*.

Lopressor (lo-pres′or) trademark for preparations of metoprolol tartrate.

Lorain's infantilism (disease, type) (lo-rān′) [Paul Joseph *Lorain*, Paris physician, 1827–1875] hypophyseal infantilism.

lorajmine hydrochloride (lor-aj′mēn) chemical name: 17-(chloroacetate)ajmalan-17*R*,21α-diol monohydrochloride; a cardiac depressant with antiarrhythmic action, $C_{22}H_{27}ClN_2O_3 \cdot HCl$.

lorazepam (lor-ah′zĕ-pam) chemical name: 7-chloro-5-(2-chlorophenyl)-1,3-dihydro-3-hydroxy-2*H*-1,4-benzodiazepin-2-one. A benzodiazepine derivative, $C_{15}H_{10}Cl_2N_2O_2$, occurring as a nearly white powder; used as an antianxiety agent, administered orally.

lorbamate (lor-bah′māt) chemical name: 2-(hydroxymethyl)-2-methylpentyl cyclopropanecarbamate carbamate (ester); a muscle relaxant, $C_{12}H_{22}N_2O_4$.

lorcainide hydrochloride (lor-ka′nīd) chemical name: *N*-(4-chlorophenyl)-*N*-[1-(1-methylethyl)-4-piperidinyl] benzeneacetamide monohydrochloride; an antiarrhythmic cardiac depressant, $C_{22}H_{27}ClN_2O \cdot HCl$.

lordoscoliosis (lor″do-sko″le-o′sis) [*lordosis* + *scoliosis*] lordosis complicated with scoliosis.

lordosis (lor-do′sis) [Gr. *lordosis*] the anterior concavity in the curvature of the lumbar and cervical spine as viewed from the side. The term is used to refer to abnormally increased curvature (hollow back, saddle back, swayback) and to the normal curvature (normal lordosis). Cf. *kyphosis* and *scoliosis*.

lordotic (lor-dot′ik) pertaining to or characterized by lordosis.

Lorenz (lo-renz′), Konrad Z. Vienna zoologist, born 1903; cowinner, with Karl von Frisch and Nikolaas Tinbergen, of the Nobel prize in medicine and physiology for 1973, for his pioneer work in ethology, particularly on imprinting and aggression.

Lorenz's operation, osteotomy, sign (lo′rents-ez) [Adolf *Lorenz*, Austrian surgeon, 1854–1946] see under *operation, osteotomy*, and *sign*.

Loreta's operation (lo-re′tahz) [Pietro *Loreta*, Italian surgeon, 1831–1889] see under *operation*.

Lorfan (lor′fan) trademark for preparations of levallorphan tartrate.

Loridine (lor′ĭ-dēn) trademark for a preparation of cephaloridine.

Lossen's rule (law) (los′enz) [Herman Friedrich *Lossen*, Heidelberg surgeon, 1842–1909] see under *rule*.

L.O.T. left occipitotransverse (position of the fetus).

Lot. abbreviation for L. *lo′tio*, lotion.

lota (lo′tah) pinta.

lotio (lo′she-o) [L.] lotion. **l. adstrin′gens,** a mixture of sulfuric acid, alcohol, and oil of turpentine. **l. al′ba, l. sulfura′ta,** white lotion.

Lotioblanc (lo″she-o-blangk′) trademark for a preparation of white lotion.

lotion (lo′shun) [L. *lotio*] a liquid suspension or dispersion for external application to the body. **Abercrombie's l.** (*obs.*), an infusion of tobacco. **amphotericin B l.** [USP], a lotion containing 90 to 125 per cent of the labeled amount of amphotericin B and conforming to FDA regulations for antibiotics; used as a topical antifungal. **benzyl benzoate l.** [USP], a watery solution of benzyl benzoate, triethanolamine, and oleic acid; used as a topical scabicide. **benzyl benzoate-chlorophenothane-benzocaine l.,** a watery solution of benzyl benzoate, chlorophenothane, benzocaine, and polysorbate 80; used as a scabicide and pediculicide, applied topically. **betamethasone dipropionate l.** [USP], a lotion containing 90 to 110 per cent of the labeled amount of betamethasone; used as a topical glucocorticoid. **betamethasone valerate l.** [USP], a preparation containing betamethasone valerate equivalent to 95 to 115 per cent of the labeled amount of betamethasone; used as an anti-inflammatory glucocorticoid. **calamine l.** [USP], a preparation of calamine with zinc oxide, glycerin, bentonite magma, and calcium hydroxide solution, used topically as a protectant. **calamine l., phenolated** [USP], a mixture of calamine lotion and liquefied phenol, used topically as a protectant. **dimethisoquin hydrochloride l.** [USP], a preparation containing 90 to 115 per cent of the labeled amount of dimethisoquin hydrochloride; used as a local anesthetic to relieve pain, itching, and burning of the skin. **flurandrenolide l.** [USP], a lotion containing 90 to 110 per cent of the labeled amount of flurandrenolide; used as a topical glucocorticoid. **gamma benzene hexachloride l.,** lindane l. **Goulard's l.,** diluted lead subacetate solution. **hydrocortisone l.** [USP], a preparation containing 90 to 110 per cent of the labeled amount hydroxycortisone; used as a topical anti-inflammatory in steroid-responsive dermatoses. **lindane l.** [USP], a preparation containing 90 to 110 per cent of the labeled amount of gamma benzene hexachloride in a suitable aqueous vehicle; used as a pediculicide and scabicide, applied topically to the skin. Called also *gamma benzene hexachloride l.* **methylbenzethonium chloride l.** [USP], an emulsion containing 0.067 per cent methylbenzethonium chloride; used as a local anti-infective, applied topically to the genitalia, rectum, thighs, and intertriginous areas in the treatment of ammonia dermatitis and in the treatment and prevention of dermatoses caused by contact with urine, feces, and perspiration. **nystatin l.** [USP], a lotion containing 90 to 140 per cent of the labeled amount of nystatin and conforming to FDA regulations for antibiotics; used as a topical antifungal. **selenium sulfide l.** [USP], an aqueous, stabilized suspension containing 90 to 110 per cent of the labeled amount of selenium sulfide; used as a topical antifungal in the treatment of tinea versicolor, as a topical keratolytic, and applied to the scalp to control seborrheic dermatitis and dandruff. **white l.** [USP], a preparation of zinc sulfate, sulfurated potash, and purified water, used as a topical astringent and protectant; called also *lotio alba.*

Lotrimin (lo-trim′in) trademark for preparation of clotrimazole.

Lotusate (lo′tŭ-sāt) trademark for a preparation of talbutal.

louchettes (loo-shets′) [Fr.] a kind of goggles formerly worn for the correction of strabismus.

Louis's angle, law (loo-ēz′) [Pierre Charles Alexandre *Louis*, French physician, 1787–1872; the founder of medical statistics] see *angulus sterni*, and see under *law.*

loupe (loop) [Fr.] a convex lens for magnifying or for concentrating light upon an object. **corneal l.,** a magnifying lens, properly mounted, for examining the cornea of the eye.

louse (lows), pl. *lice* [L. *pediculus*] a general name for various parasitic insects; the true lice, which infest mammals, belong to the order Anoplura. Species parasitic upon man are *Pediculus humanus capitis,* the head louse; *P. humanus corporis,* the body or clothes louse; and *Phthirus pubis,* the crab louse, which lives in the hair upon the pubes and other hairy areas of the body, such as the eyelashes, eyebrows, and axillae. The causal organisms of typhus, relapsing fever, trench fever, and possibly plague are transmitted by the bite of lice. **biting l.,** Mallophaga. **body l.,** *Pediculus humanus corporis.* **chicken l.,** *Dermanyssus gallinae.* **clothes l.,** *Pediculus humanus corporis.* **crab l.,** *Phthirus pubis.* **goat l.,** *Linognathus stenopis.* **head l.,** *Pediculus humanus capitis.* **horse l.,** *Trichodectes pilosus.* **pubic l.,** *Phthirus pubis.* **sucking l.,** Anoplura.

lousicide (lows′ĭ-sīd) pediculicide.

Löwe's ring (la′vez) [Karl Friedrich *Löwe*, German optician, born 1874] see under *ring.*

Lowe's syndrome (disease) (lōz) [Charles Upton *Lowe*, American pediatrician, born 1921] oculocerebrorenal syndrome.

Löwenberg's canal, forceps, scala (la′ven-bergz) [Benjamin Benno *Löwenberg*, otologist in Vienna and Paris, born 1836] see under *canal* and *forceps,* and see *ductus cochlearis.*

Löwenstein's culture medium (la′ven-stīnz) [Ernst *Löwenstein,* Vienna pathologist, born 1878] see under *culture medium.*

Löwenthal's tract (la′ven-talz) [Wilhelm *Löwenthal,* German physician, 1850–1894] see under *tractus tectospinalis.*

Lower's rings, tubercle (lo′erz) [Richard *Lower,* English anatomist, 1631–1691] see under *anuli fibrosi cordis* and *tuberculum intervenosum.*

Löwitt's bodies, lymphocytes (la′vits) [Moritz *Löwitt,* German physician, 1851–1918] lymphogonia.

Lowman balance board (lo′man) [Charles LeRoy *Lowman,* American orthopedic surgeon, born 1879] an isosceles triangle board on which the patient walks with feet in supination; for correction of flatfeet.

Lowy's test (lo′ēz) [Otto *Lowy,* American pathologist, born 1879] see under *tests.*

loxapine (loks′ah-pēn) chemical name: 2-chloro-11-(4-methyl-1-piperazinyl)dibenz[*b,f*][1,4]oxazepine; a tricyclic antipsychotic agent, $C_{18}H_{18}ClN_3O$. **l. succinate,** the succinate salt of loxapine, $C_{18}H_{18}ClN_3O \cdot C_4H_6O_4$, used in the treatment of schizophrenia, administered orally.

loxarthron (loks-ar′thron) [Gr. *loxos* oblique + *arthron* joint] an oblique deformity of a joint without luxation.

loxarthrosis (loks″ar-thro′sis) loxarthron.

loxia (lok′se-ah) torticollis.

Loxitane (loks′ĭ-tān) trademark for preparations of loxaprine succinate.

loxophthalmus (loks″of-thal′mus) [Gr. *loxos* oblique + *opthalmos* eye] strabismus.

Loxosceles (loks-os′sĕ-lēz) a genus of six-eyed spiders of the family Loxoscelidae. **L. lae′ta,** the brown spider, which is the causative agent of loxoscelism in Central South America. **L. reclu′sa,** the brown recluse spider, which causes loxoscelism in North America.

Loxoscelidae (loks″os-sel′ĭ-de) a family of spiders (suborder Labidognatha), the false hackled band spinners, which includes the genus *Loxosceles.*

loxoscelism (lok-sos′sĕ-lizm) a morbid condition resulting from the bite of the brown spider, *Loxosceles laeta,* or the (brown) recluse spider, *L. reclusa,* beginning with a painful erythematous vesicle and progressing to a gangrenous slough of the affected area; first recognized in South America, a few cases have been diagnosed in North America. **viscerocutaneous l.,** a sometimes fatal condition resulting from the bite of the brown spider, with fever and hematuria occurring, in addition to the local reaction.

loxotomy (lok-sot′o-me) [Gr. *loxos* oblique + *temnein* to cut] oval amputation.

Loxotrema ovatum (lok″so-tre′mah o-va′tum) *Metagonimus yokogawai.*

lozenge (loz′enj) [Fr.] 1. a medicated tablet or disk; a troche. 2. a triangular area of tissue marked for excision in plastic surgery.

L.P.F. leukocytosis-promoting factor.

L.P.N. licensed practical nurse.

L.R.C.P. Licentiate of the Royal College of Physicians.

L.R.C.P.&S.I. Licentiate of the Royal College of Physicians and Surgeons, Ireland.

L.R.C.S. Licentiate of the Royal College of Surgeons.

L.R.C.S.E. Licentiate of the Royal College of Surgeons, Edinburgh.

LRF luteinizing hormone releasing factor; see *gonadorelin.*

L.S.A. left sacroanterior (position of the fetus); Licentiate of Society of Apothecaries.

L.Sc.A. left scapulo-anterior (position of the fetus).

L.Sc.P. left scapuloposterior (position of the fetus).

LSD lysergic acid diethylamide; see *lysergide.*

L.S.P. left sacroposterior (position of the fetus).

L.S.T. left sacrotransverse (position of the fetus).

LT lymphotoxin.

LTF lymphocyte transforming factor.

LTH luteotropic hormone (lactogenic hormone).

Lu chemical symbol for *lutetium.*

Lubarsch's crystals (loo′barsh-ez) [Otto *Lubarsch,* German pathologist, 1860–1933] see under *crystal.*

lubb (lub) a syllable used to represent, or mimic, the first sound of the heart in auscultation. See *lubb-dupp.*

lubb-dupp (lub-dup′) syllables used to represent the combination of the first and second heart sounds. See *lubb* and *dupp.*

Luc's operation (luks) [Henri *Luc,* French laryngologist, 1855–1925] Caldwell-Luc operation.

Lucae's probe (loo′kāz) [August *Lucae,* otologist in Berlin, 1835–1911] see under *probe.*

lucanthone hydrochloride (loo-kan′thōn) chemical name: 1-[[2-(diethylamino)ethyl]amino]-4-methyl-9*H*-thioxanthen-9-one monohydrochloride. An antischistosomal, $C_{20}H_{24}N_2OS \cdot HCl$, occurring as a yellowish orange powder; administered orally.

Lucas' sign (loo′kas) [Richard Clement *Lucas,* English physician, 1846–1915] see under *sign.*

Lucatello's sign (loo″kah-tel′ōz) [Luigi *Lucatello,* Italian physician, 1863–1926] see under *sign.*

Luciani's triad (loo″che-an′ēz) [Luigi *Luciani,* Italian physiologist, 1842–1919] see under *triad.*

lucid (loo′sid) [L. *lucidus* clear] clear; not obscure; as, *lucid* interval.

lucidification (loo-sid″ĭ-fi-ka′shun) [L. *lucidus* clear + *facere* to make] the clearing up of the protoplasm of cells.

lucidity (loo-sid′ĭ-te) the quality or state of having a clear mind; clearness of the mind.

luciferase (loo-sif′er-ās) [L. *lux* light + *ferre* to bear + *-ase*] an enzyme, of which there are many forms, that catalyzes the bioluminescent reaction in certain animals capable of luminescence. The substrate is luciferin; ATP and molecular oxygen are required for the complete reaction. The color of light emitted is determined by the form of the enzyme.

luciferin (loo-sif′er-in) a heterocyclic phenol which can be reduced and oxidized. It exists in many forms and is present in certain animals capable of bioluminescence; when acted upon by luciferase, in the presence of ATP and molecular oxygen, it produces light.

lucifugal (loo-sif′u-gal) [L. *lux* light + *fugere* to flee from] avoiding, or being repelled by, bright light.

Lucilia (loo-sil′e-ah) the greenbottle flies, a genus of the family Calliphoridae that have a blue or green metallic iridescence. **L. cae′sar,** the common "gold fly" which ordinarily breeds in meat or carrion; its larvae have been found in the intestine and in myiasis of the skin. **L. cupri′na,** *Phaenicia cuprina.* **L.**

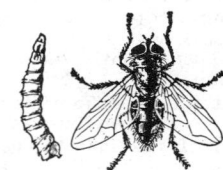

Larva and adult of *Lucilia caesar.*

illus′tris, a species which usually deposits its eggs in carcasses, but is sometimes found in the wool of sheep. **L. regi′na,** *Phormia regina.* **L. serica′ta,** *Phaenicia sericata.*

lucipetal (loo-sip′ĭ-tal) [L. *lux* light + *petere* to seek] seeking, or being attracted to, bright light.

lucium (loo′se-um) a supposed chemical element discovered in 1896, later found to be a mixture of rare earth metals.

Lücke's test (lik′ez) [George Albert *Lücke*, German surgeon, 1829–1894] see under *tests*.

lückenschädel (lik′en-sha″del) [Ger.] a condition marked by defective calcification of the skull bones, combined with meningocele or encephalocele.

lucotherapy (loo″ko-ther′ah-pe) [L. *lux* light + *therapy*] the treatment of disease by rays of light.

Ludloff's sign (lood′lawfs) [Karl *Ludloff*, surgeon in Breslau, born 1864] see under *sign*.

Ludwig's angina (lood′vigz) [Wilhelm Friedrich von *Ludwig*, German surgeon, 1790–1865] see under *angina*.

Ludwig's angle (lood′vigz) [Daniel *Ludwig*, German anatomist, 1625–1680] angulus sterni.

Ludwig's ganglion, theory (lood′vigz) [Karl Friedrich Wilhelm *Ludwig*, eminent German physiologist, 1816–1895, one of the greatest teachers of physiology of all time] see under *ganglion* and *theory*.

Luer's syringe (loo′erz) [German instrument maker in Paris, died 1883] see under *syringe*.

lues (loo′ez) [L. "a plague"] syphilis. **l. hep′atis,** syphilis of the liver. **l. nervo′sa,** syphilis with marked nervous lesions. **l. tar′da,** late syphilis. **l. vene′rea,** syphilis.

luetic (loo-et′ik) syphilitic.

luetin (loo′ĕ-tin) an extract of a killed culture of several strains of *Treponema pallidum,* used in the skin test for syphilis. See *Noguchi's luetin reaction* under *reaction*.

luette (loo-et′) [Fr.] uvula. **Lieutaud's l.,** uvula vesicae.

lug (lug) the part of a dental casting that projects. **retention l.,** a piece of metal soldered either to an orthodontic band or to an artificial crown to create greater undercut for retention of a dental prosthesis.

Lugol's caustic, solution (loo-golz′) [Jean Guillaume Auguste *Lugol*, physician in Paris, 1786–1851] see under *caustic,* and see *iodine solution, strong,* under *solution*.

L.U.L. left upper lobe (of lungs).

lumbago (lum-ba′go) [L. *lumbus* loin] pain in the lumbar region. **ischemic l.,** pain in the lower back and buttock(s) due to vascular insufficiency, as in terminal aortic occlusion.

lumbar (lum′ber) pertaining to the loins, the part of the back between the thorax and the pelvis.

lumbarization (lum″ber-i-za′shun) a condition in which the first segment of the sacrum is not fused with the second, so that there is one additional articulated vertebra and the sacrum consists of only four segments.

lumbo- [L. *lumbus*] a combining form denoting relationship to the loins.

lumboabdominal (lum″bo-ab-dom′ĭ-nal) pertaining to the loins and abdomen.

lumbocolostomy (lum″bo-ko-los′to-me) [L. *lumbus* loin + *colostomy*] the operation of forming a permanent opening into the colon by an incision through the lumbar region.

lumbocolotomy (lum″bo-ko-lot′o-me) [L. *lumbus* loin + *colotomy*] an incision into the colon through the loin.

lumbocostal (lum″bo-kos′tal) [L. *lumbus* loin + *costa* rib] pertaining to the loin and ribs.

lumbocrural (lum″bo-kroo′ral) pertaining to or affecting the lumbar and crural regions.

lumbodorsal (lum″bo-dor′sal) pertaining to the lumbar and dorsal regions.

lumbodynia (lum″bo-din′e-ah) [L. *lumbus* loin + Gr. *odyne* pain] lumbago.

lumboiliac (lum″bo-il′e-ak) pertaining to the loin and ilium.

lumboinguinal (lum″bo-ing′gwĭ-nal) pertaining to the loins and the groin.

lumbosacral (lum″bo-sa′kral) pertaining to the loins and sacrum.

lumbrical (lum′brĭ-kal) 1. of the earthworms or related annelids. 2. a muscle of the hand; see *musculi lumbricales*.

lumbrici (lum-bri′se) [L.] plural of *lumbricus*.

lumbricide (lum′brĭ-sīd) [*lumbricus* + L. *caedere* to kill] an agent that destroys lumbrici (ascarides).

lumbricoid (lum′brĭ-koid) [*lumbricus* + Gr. *eidos* form] resembling the earthworm; designating the ascaris.

lumbricosis (lum″brĭ-ko′sis) the condition of being infected with lumbrici (ascarides).

Lumbricus (lum-bri′kus) [L. "earthworm"] a genus of annelids, including the earthworm, *L. terres′tris,* which may act as the host of *Metastrongylus elongatus,* the intermediate host of the virus causing swine influenza.

lumbricus (lum-bri′kus), pl. *lumbri′ci* [L.] 1. the ascaris. 2. an earthworm.

lumbus (lum′bus) [L.] [NA] the part of the back between the thorax and the pelvis; called also *loin*.

lumen (loo′men), pl. *lu′mina* [L. "light"] 1. the cavity or channel within a tube or tubular organ. 2. the unit of light flux: it is the

flux emitted in a unit solid angle by a uniform point source of one candela. Called also *meter candle.* **residual l.,** the remains of Rathke's pouch located between the pars distalis and pars intermedia of the pituitary gland.

lumichrome (loo′mĭ-krōm) chemical name: 7,8-dimethylalloxazine. A product, $C_{12}H_{10}N_4O_2$, of the irradiation decomposition of riboflavin.

lumiflavin (loo″mĭ-fla′vin) chemical name: 7,8,10-trimethylisoalloxazine. A product, $C_{13}H_{12}N_4O_2$, of the luminiferous decomposition of riboflavin.

lumina (loo′min-ah) plural of *lumen*.

Luminal (loo′mĭ-nal) trademark for preparations of phenobarbital.

luminal (loo′mĭ-nal) pertaining to the lumen of a tubular structure.

luminescence (loo″mĭ-nes′ens) the property of giving off light without showing a corresponding degree of heat.

luminiferous (loo″mĭ-nif′er-us) [L. *lumen* light + *ferre* to bear] conveying light or propagating those vibrations which constitute light.

luminophore (loo′mĭ-no-fōr″) [L. *lumen* light + Gr. *phoros* bearing] a chemical group that gives the property of luminescence to organic compounds.

luminous (loo′mĭ-nus) emitting or reflecting light; glowing with light.

lumirhodopsin (loo″mĭ-ro-dop′sin) a partially split combination of all-*trans* retinal and scotopsin, occurring as rhodopsin if exposed to light.

lumps (lumps) hypopteronosis cystica.

Lumsden's center (lumz′denz) [Thomas William *Lumsden,* British physician, 1874–1953] pneumotaxic center.

lunacy (loo′nah-se) [L. *luna* moon] insanity; so named because it was supposed to be sometimes due to or affected by the influence of the moon.

lunar (loo′nar) [L. *lunaris; luna* moon, also silver] 1. pertaining to the moon. 2. pertaining to or containing silver, as lunar caustic (silver nitrate).

lunare (loo-na′re) the lunate bone (os lunatum [NA]).

lunate (loo′nāt) [L. *luna* moon] moon-shaped, or crescentic; see *os lunatum*.

lunatic (loo′nah-tik) [L. *lunaticus;* from *luna* moon] a mentally deranged person.

lunatomalacia (loo-na″to-mah-la′she-ah) osteochondrosis of the semilunar (carpal lunate) bone; see *Kienböck's disease* (def. 1), under *disease*.

Lundvall's blood crisis (loond′valz) [Halvar *Lundvall,* Swedish neurologist] see under *crisis*.

lung (lung) [L. *pulmo;* Gr. *pneumon* or *pleumon*] the organ of respiration; called also *pulmo* [NA]. Either of the pair of organs that effect the aeration of the blood. The lungs occupy the lateral cavities of the chest, separated from each other by the heart and mediastinal structures. The right lung is composed of superior, middle, and inferior lobes, and the left, of superior and inferior lobes. Each lobe is subdivided into two to five bronchopulmonary segments which are separated by connective tissue septa. Pulmonary disorders may be confined to, or localized in, one or more of these segments. Each lung consists of an external serous coat (the visceral layer of the pleura), subserous areolar tissue, and lung parenchyma. The latter is made up of lobules, which are bound together by connective tissue. A primary lobule consists of a terminal bronchiole, respiratory bronchioles, and alveolar ducts, which communicate with many alveoli, each alveolus being surrounded by a network of capillary blood vessels. It is between the alveoli and capillaries that gas exchange takes place. See Plates XXVI and XLIX. **arc-welder l.,** siderosis (def. 1). **artificial l.,** oxygenator. **bird-breeder's l.,** pigeon-breeder's l. **black l.,** pneumoconiosis of coal workers. **brown l.,** byssinosis. **cardiac l.,** chronic congestion of the lung due to mitral stenosis or left ventricular failure; microscopic examination shows evidence of recurring edema, heart failure cells, and vascular changes. **coalminer's l.,** pneumoconiosis of coal workers. **drowned l.,** airless lung, the air passages being filled with exudate. The volume occupied by a drained lung (or lobe) is usually greater than normal, whereas in atelectasis it is less than normal. **eosinophilic l.,** tropical eosinophilia. **farmer's l.,** a morbid condition caused by inhalation of moldy hay dust, characterized by breathlessness with cyanosis or with a dry cough, anorexia, and weight loss; called also *thresher's l.* and *harvester's l.* **fibroid l.,** a lung affected with chronic fibrosis. **harvester's l.,** farmer's l. **honeycomb l.,** the appearance of multiple small radiolucent shadows on the lung x-ray, representing dilatations of the smaller, less rigid airways or multiple small cysts or cavities. **hyperlucent l.,** unilateral emphysema. **iron l.,** a popular name for the Drinker respirator. **masons' l.,** a lung affected with pneumoconiosis due to the inhalation of dusts associated with this occupation. **miners' l.,** pneumoconiosis of coal workers. **pigeon-breeder's l.,** a respiratory disorder caused by an acquired hypersensitivity to bird excreta following intimate contact with birds; symptoms include chills, fever, and cough. Pulmonary fibrosis may result. Called also *bird-breeder's l.* **shock l.,** adult respiratory distress syndrome. **silo-filler's l.,** a rare form of acute bronchitis affecting individuals who inhale high levels of nitrogen oxides, particularly the dioxide, while working in freshly filled silos. **thresher's l.,** farmer's l. **trench l.,** a condition observed in the trenches in World War I, characterized by attacks of rapid breathing. **vanishing l.,** in emphysema, conversion of the lungs into a delicate, fine network of remaining blood vessels among which no alveolar walls survive. **wet l.,** accumulation of fluid in the lungs; pulmonary edema. **white l.,** pneumonia alba.

lungmotor (lung′mo-tor) an apparatus for forcing air or air and oxygen into the lungs.

lungworm (lung′werm) a parasitic worm that invades the lungs, e.g., the trematode *Paragonimus westermani* in man, the nematode *Metastrongylus elongatus* in hogs, etc.

lunula (loo′nu-lah), pl. *lu′nulae* [L., dim. of *luna* moon] [NA] a general term for a small crescentic or moon-shaped area. **lunulae of aortic valves,** lunulae valvularum semilunarium aortae. **l. of nail,** l. unguis. **lunulae of pulmonary trunk valves,** lunulae valvularum semilunarium trunci pulmonalis. **l. of scapula,** incisura scapulae. **lunulae of semilunar valves,** lunulae valvularum semilunarium. **lunulae of semilunar valves of aorta,** lunulae valvularum semilunarium aortae. **l. un′guis** [NA], lunula of the nail: the crescentic white area at the base of the nail on a finger or toe. **lu′nulae valvula′rum semilunarium aor′tae** [NA], lunulae of semilunar valves of aorta: small thinned areas in the cusps of the valve of the aorta, one located on each side of the nodule of each cusp, between the free margin and the most peripheral segment of the cusp. **lu′nulae valvula′rum semiluna′rium trunci pulmonalis** [NA], lunulae of semilunar valves of pulmonary trunk: small thinned areas in the cusps of the valve of the pulmonary trunk, one located on each side of the nodule of each cusp, close to the free margin and the most peripheral segment of the cusp. **lu′nulae valvula′rum semiluna′rium arte′riae pulmona′lis,** lunulae valvularum semilunarium trunci pulmonalis.

lunulae (loo′nu-le) [L.] plural of *lunula.*

lupeose (loo′pe-ōs) a tetrasaccharide from the seeds of herbs of the genus *Lupinus.*

lupia (loo′pe-ah) an old term for encysted tumor of the eyelids (Himley).

lupiform (loo′pĭ-form) [L. *lupus* + *forma* form] 1. resembling lupus. 2. resembling a wen.

lupinosis (loo″-pĭ-no′sis) a morbid often fatal condition affecting domestic animals, including cattle, sheep, goats, and horses, due to the ingestion of seeds of leguminous herbs of the genus *Lupinus,* and characterized chiefly by acute atrophy of the liver. Cf. *lathyrism.*

lupoid (loo′poid) 1. pertaining to lupus vulgaris. 2. a variant of sarcoidosis marked by small papular lesions.

lupus (loo′pus) [L. "wolf" or "pike"] a name originally given to a destructive type of skin condition, implying "a local degeneration, strumous in its origin, essentially chronic in its character, and 'attended with more or less hypertrophy, with absorption, and with ulceration'. As one or other of these characters is most marked, . . . a special name [is applied]," e.g., lupus erythematosus, lupus tuberculosus. Although the term is frequently used alone to designate lupus vulgaris and sometimes lupus erythematosus, without a modifier it has no specific meaning. **chilblain l.,** l. pernio, def. 2. **drug-induced l.,** a syndrome closely resembling systemic lupus erythematosus, precipitated by prolonged use of various drugs, most commonly hydralazine, isoniazid, various anticonvulsants, and procainamide. **l. erythemato′sus,** an inflammatory dermatitis; see *l. erythematosus, discoid,* and *l. erythematosus, systemic.* **l. erythemato′sus, discoid, l. erythemato′sus discoi′des,** a chronic, superficial inflammation of the skin, marked by red macules up to 3 or 4 cm. in width, and covered with scanty adherent scales, which extend into patulous follicles, which fall off, leaving scars. The lesions typically form a butterfly pattern over the bridge of the nose and cheeks, but other areas may be involved. Clinical variants include *l. erythematosus hypertrophicus, l. erythematosus profundus,* and *l. tumidus.* **l. erythemato′sus, systemic (SLE),** a generalized connective tissue disorder, affecting mainly middle-aged women, ranging from mild to fulminating, and characterized by skin eruptions similar to those seen in discoid lupus erythematosus, arthralgia, arthritis, leukopenia, anemia, visceral lesions (including renal involvement, pericarditis, and pleurisy), neurologic manifestations, lymphadenopathy, fever, and other constitutional symptoms. Typically, there are many abnormal immunologic phenomena, including hypergammaglobulinemia and hypocomplementemia, deposition of antigen-antibody complexes, and the presence of antinuclear antibodies and LE cells. **l. erythemato′sus hypertroph′icus, l. erythemato′sus hypertroph′icus et profun′dus,** a rare form of discoid lupus erythematosus, occurring chiefly on the lower face, especially the lower lip with extension to the vermilion border and sides of the mouth and chin, in which great thickening of the skin in conjunction with scarring produces an almost warty plaque, with deep involvement of the corium. **l. erythemato′sus profun′dus,** a variant of discoid or systemic lupus erythematosus, in which deep brawny indurations or subcutaneous nodules occur under normal or, less often, involved skin; the overlying skin may be erythematous, atrophic and ulcerated and on healing may leave a depressed scar. **l. erythemato′sus tu′midus,** a variant of discoid or systemic lupus erythematosus in which the lesions consist of raised reddish purple or brown plaques, which may resemble erysipelas or cellulitis. **l. exul′cerans,** a variant of lupus vulgaris in which the lesions break down to produce deep, indolent ulcers. **hydralazine l.,** see under *syndrome.* **l. hypertroph′icus,** 1. a variant of lupus vulgaris in which the lesions consist of a warty vegetative growth, often crusted or slightly exudative, usually occurring on moist areas near body orifices. 2. l. erythematosus hypertrophicus. **laryngeal l.,** infection of the larynx and epiglottis in lupus vulgaris. **l. milia′ris dissemina′tus fa′ciei,** lupus characterized by multiple, discrete, superficial nodules 2 to 3 mm. in diameter on the face, particularly on the eyelids, upper lip, chin, and nares; the lesions are considered by some to be tuberculids. **l. nephritis,** see under *nephritis.* **l. per′nio,** 1. a condition marked by soft, violaceous skin lesions on the cheeks, forehead, nose, ears, and digits, frequently associated with bone cysts; it may be the first manifestation of sarcoidosis or occur in the chronic stage of the disease. The term is sometimes used as a synonym of sarcoidosis. 2. a form of discoid lupus erythematosus aggravated by cold, initially resembling chilblains, in which the lesions consist of erythematous infiltrated patches on the exposed areas of the body, such as the face, nose, ears, and hands, especially the knuckles of the fingers; called also *chilblain l.* **l. pla′nus,** a variant of lupus vulgaris in which the lesions are smooth flat patches composed of reddish brown nodules. **l. tu′midus,** 1. a variant of lupus vulgaris in which the lesions consist of localized, soft edematous patches somewhat resembling keloids. 2. l. erythematosus tumidus. **l. vulga′ris,** the most common and severe form of tuberculosis of the skin, most often affecting the face, characterized by the formation of reddish brown (apple-jelly colored) patches of nodules in the corium, which progressively spread peripherally, with central atrophy, causing ulceration and scarring and destruction of cartilage in involved sites. Clinical variants of the disease include *lupus exulcerans, lupus hypertrophicus, lupus planus,* and *lupus tumidus.* **warty l.,** tuberculosis verrucosa cutis.

Luria (loor′i-ah), Salvador Edward. Italian biologist in the United States, born 1912; co-winner, with Max Delbruck and Alfred D. Hershey, of the Nobel Prize in medicine and physiology for 1969, for research on the mechanisms and materials of inheritance in bacteriophage.

Luride (loo′rīd) trademark for a preparation sodium fluoride.

Luschka's crypts, etc. (lush′kahz) [Hubert von *Luschka,* celebrated German anatomist, 1820–1875] see under *bursa, crypt, duct, gland, muscle,* etc.

lusus (loo′sus) [L.] a game, sport. **l. natu′rae,** a sport, a minor congenital anomaly; see *mutation* (def. 2) and *theory of mutation.*

luteal (loo′te-al) pertaining to or having the properties of the corpus luteum or its active principle.

lutecium (loo-te′she-um) lutetium.

luteectomy (loo″te-ek′to-me) excision of the corpus luteum.

lutein (loo′te-in) [L. *luteus* yellow] 1. a yellow pigment, or lipochrome, $C_{48}H_{56}O_2$, from the corpus luteum, from fat cells, and from the yolk of eggs. It is closely related to xanthophyll. 2. any lipochrome. **serum l.,** a lipochrome found in blood serum.

luteinic (loo″te-in′ik) 1. pertaining to lutein or to the corpus luteum. 2. pertaining to luteinization.

luteinization (loo″te-in″i-za′shun) the process by which a postovulatory ovarian follicle transforms into a corpus luteum through vascularization, follicular cell hypertrophy, and lipid accumulation, the latter in some species giving the yellow color indicated by the term.

Lutembacher's syndrome (complex, disease) (loo′tembak″erz) [René *Lutembacher,* French physician, born 1884] see under *syndrome.*

luteohormone (loo″te-o-hor′mōn) progesterone.

luteoid (loo′te-oid) [*luteum* + Gr. *eidos* form] a substance simulating the hormone activity of the corpus luteum.

luteoma (loo″te-o′mah) 1. a granulosa-theca cell tumor in which there has been luteinization of the cells. 2. nodular hyperplasia of ovarian lutein cells sometimes occurring in the last trimester of pregnancy; it may be unilateral or bilateral. Called also *l. of pregnancy* or *pregnancy l.*

luteose (loo″te-ōs) a neutral polysaccharide present in luteic acid.

luteotrope (loo′te-o-trōp) mammotrope.

luteotrophic (loo″te-o-trof′ik) luteotropic.

luteotrophin (loo″te-o-tro′fin) luteotropin.

luteotropic (loo″te-o-trop′ik) stimulating the formation of the corpus luteum; see *luteotropin.*

lung

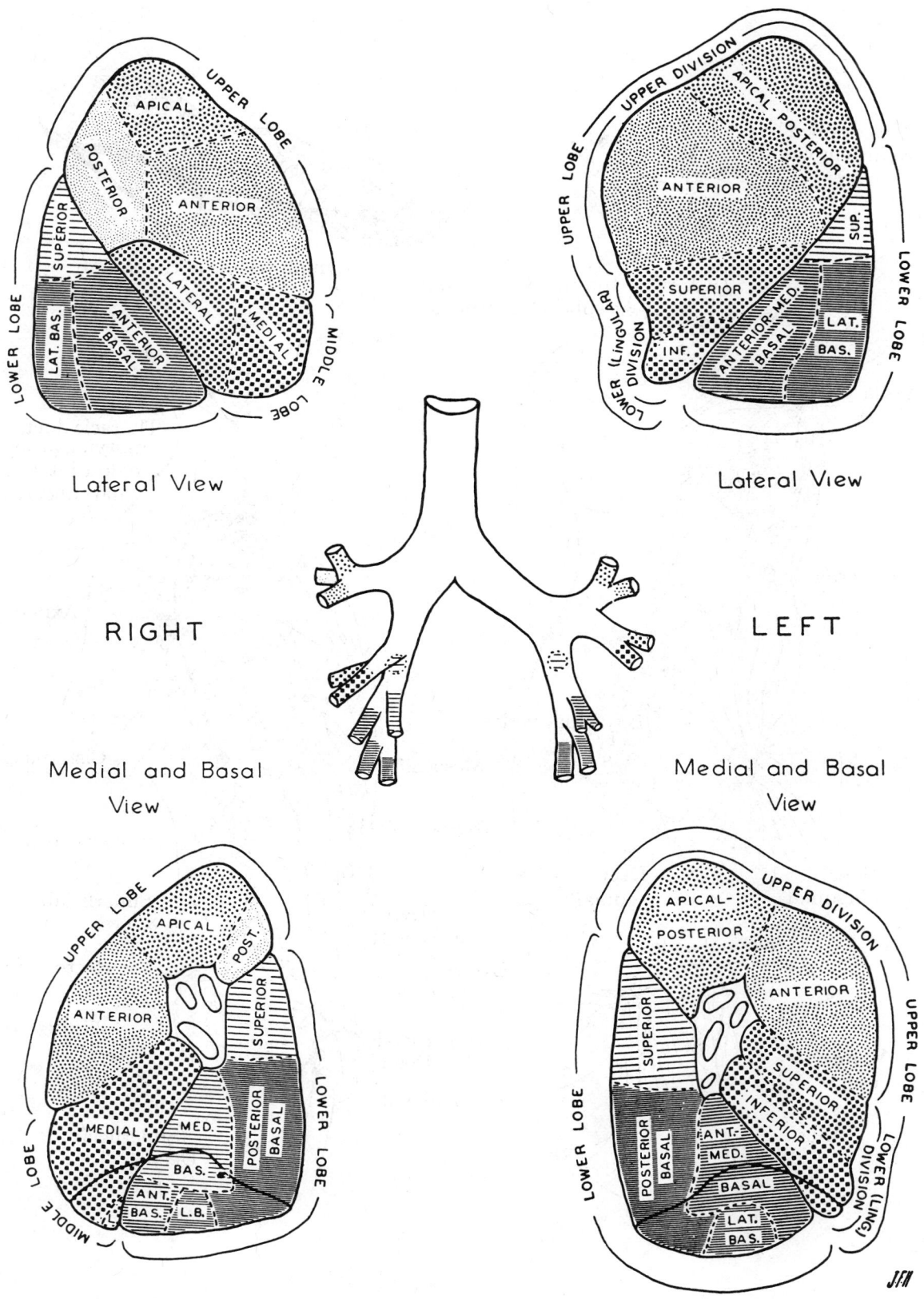

Lateral View

Lateral View

RIGHT

LEFT

Medial and Basal
View

Medial and Basal
View

PULMONARY SEGMENTS

Tracheobronchial branching correlated with subdivision of the lungs. Each bronchus is marked the same as the segment it branches out to supply, and should be designated by the same name. The terminology used is that suggested by Jackson and Huber (Diseases of the Chest, volume 9, 1943).

Plate XXVII   lymph

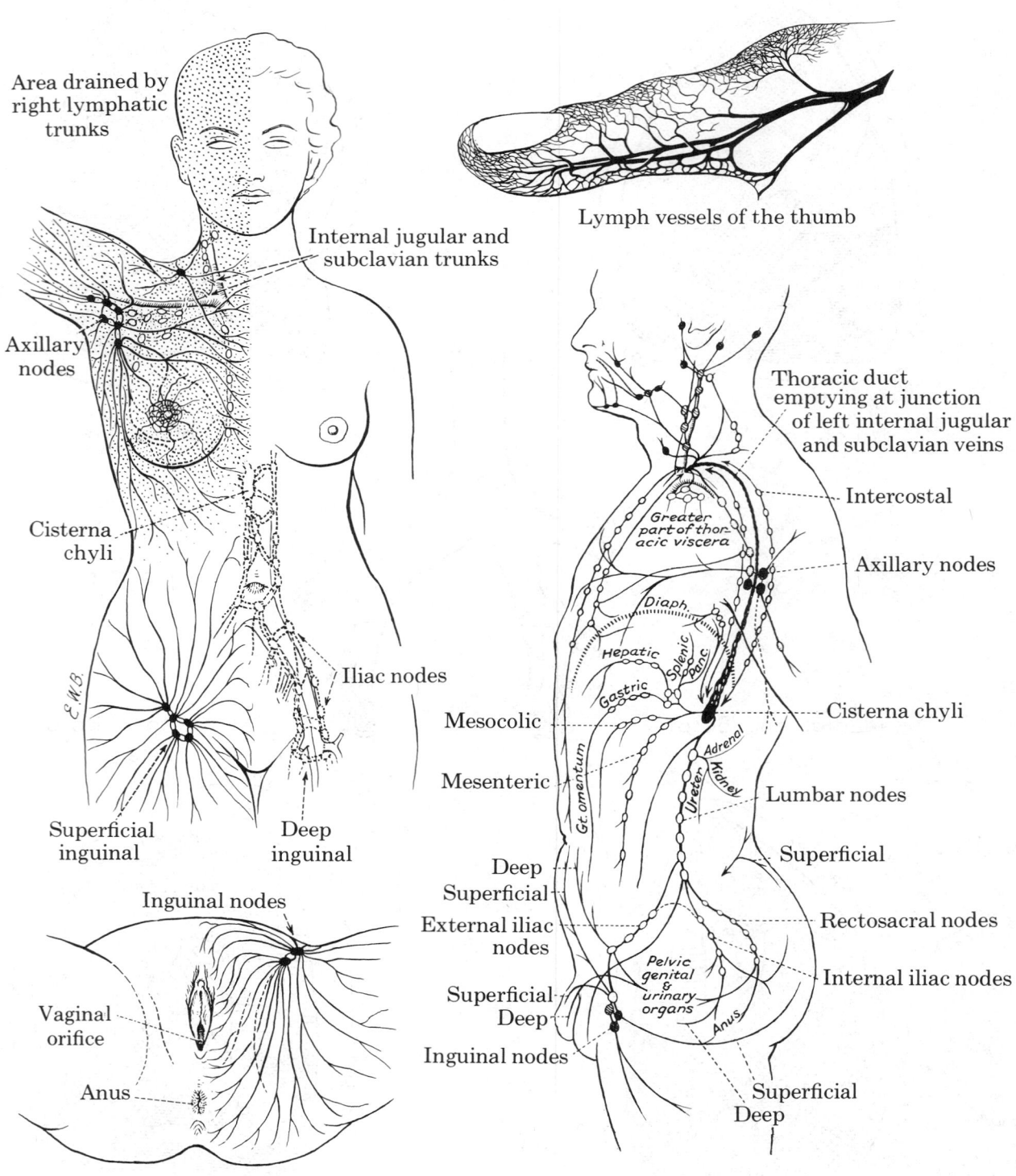

Area drained by right lymphatic trunks

Internal jugular and subclavian trunks

Axillary nodes

Cisterna chyli

Iliac nodes

Superficial inguinal

Deep inguinal

Lymph vessels of the thumb

Thoracic duct emptying at junction of left internal jugular and subclavian veins

Intercostal

Greater part of thoracic viscera

Axillary nodes

Diaph.

Hepatic

Splenic

Panc.

Gastric

Cisterna chyli

Mesocolic

Adrenal

Kidney

Ureter

Lumbar nodes

Mesenteric

Gt. omentum

Superficial

Deep
Superficial

Rectosacral nodes

External iliac nodes

Pelvic genital & urinary organs

Anus

Internal iliac nodes

Superficial
Deep

Inguinal nodes

Superficial
Deep

Inguinal nodes

Vaginal orifice

Anus

**DIAGRAMMATIC REPRESENTATION OF LYMPHATIC DRAINAGE
OF VARIOUS PARTS OF THE BODY**

luteotropin (loo″te-o-tro′pin) a hormone of the anterior pituitary gland which stimulates formation of the corpus luteum; identical with prolactin. Called also *luteotropic hormone.*

lutetium (loo-te′she-um) the chemical element, atomic number 71, atomic weight 174.97, symbol Lu.

Lutrexin (loo-trek′sin) trademark for a preparation of lututrin.

Lutromone (loo′tro-mōn) trademark for a preparation of progesterone.

lututrin (loo′tu-trin) a protein or polypeptide substance obtained from the corpus luteum of sow ovaries by a process of salting out followed by dialysis; used as a uterine relaxant in treatment of functional dysmenorrhea.

Lutzomyia (loot″zo-mi′ah) a genus of sandflies of the family Psychodidae, the females of which suck blood. **L. andu′zei,** a species that transmits pian bois (forest yaws) in the Guyanas, Brazil, and Venezuela. **L. flaviscutella′ta,** a species that is a vector of *Leishmania mexicana;* sometimes used as a synonym of *L. olmeca.* **L. longipal′pis,** a species believed to transmit kala-azar in South America. **L. nogu′chu,** *Phlebotomus noguchii.* **L. olme′ca,** a species that is the vector of *Leishmania mexicana* in Brazil; sometimes used as a synonym of *L. flaviscutellata.* **L. peruen′sis,** a species that transmits uta in the Peruvian Andes. **L. verruca′rum,** a species that transmits uta in the Peruvian Andes.

lux (luks) [L. "light"] in SI, the metric unit of illumination, being one lumen per square meter; called also *meter candle.* Cf. *foot-candle.*

luxatio (luk-sa′she-o) [L.] dislocation. **l. cox′ae congen′ita,** congenital dislocation of the hip. **l. erec′ta,** dislocation of the shoulder so that the arm stands straight up above the head. **l. imperfec′ta,** a sprain. **l. perinea′lis,** a form of dislocation of the hip in which the head of the femur lies in the perineum.

luxation (luk-sa′shun) [L. *luxatio*] dislocation. **Malgaigne's l.,** pulled elbow.

luxuriant (luk-su′re-ant) growing freely or excessively.

luxus (luks′us) [L.] excess; see under *consumption* and *heart.*

Luys' body, body syndrome, nucleus (loo-ēz′) [Jules Bernard *Luys,* French physician, 1828–1897] see *pituitary gland,* under *gland,* see *body of Luys syndrome,* under *syndrome,* and see *nucleus subthalamicus.*

Luys' segregator (separator) (loo-ēz′) [Georges *Luys,* French physician, 1870–1953] see under *segregator.*

luz (looz) [Hebrew] a bone, located in the spinal column, from which, according to the Talmudists, the body is restored at the resurrection.

L.V.H. left ventricular hypertrophy.

L.V.N. licensed vocational nurse.

Lwoff (lwauf), André Michael. French microbiologist and virologist, born 1902; co-winner, with François Jacob and Jacques Lucien Monod, of the Nobel prize in medicine and physiology for 1965, for discoveries concerning the genetic control of enzymes and virus synthesis.

Ly any T-cell antigen that serves as a basis for grouping T-lymphocytes into classes on the basis of function.

lyase (li′ās) any of a class of enzymes that remove groups from their substrates (other than by hydrolysis), leaving double bonds, or that conversely add groups to double bonds. They include decarboxylases, carboxylases, aldolases, synthetases, hydratases, and dehydratases. **N-acetylneuraminate l.,** an enzyme that catalyzes the conversion of N-acetylneuraminate to 2-acetamido-2-deoxy-D-mannose and pyruvate. **adenylosuccinate l.,** one that catalyzes the conversion of adenylosuccinate to fumarate and AMP. **alginate l.,** one that catalyzes the elimination of 4,5-D-mannuronate residues from alginate, thus bringing about depolymerization. **S-alkylcysteine l.,** one that catalyzes the conversion of S-methyl-L-cysteine to pyruvate, ammonia, and methyl mercaptan. **alliin l.,** a pyridoxal-phosphate protein that catalyzes the conversion of S-alkyl-L-cysteinesulfoxide to 2-aminoacrylate and an alkyl sulfenate. **argininosuccinate l.,** one that catalyzes the conversion of L-argininosuccinate to fumarate and L-arginine. **chondroitin sulfate l.,** an enzyme that catalyzes the elimination of 4,5-D-glucuronate residues, thus bringing about depolymerization. **citrate l.,** one that catalyzes the conversion of citrate to acetate and oxaloacetate. **hyaluronate l.,** one that catalyzes the conversion of hyaluronate to n-3(β-D-gluco-4,5-en-urono)-2-acetamido-2-deoxy-D-glucose. **hydroxymethylglutaryl-CoA l.,** one that catalyzes the conversion of 3-hydroxy-3-methylglutaryl-CoA to acetyl-CoA and acetoacetate. **hydroxynitrile l.,** an enzyme (flavoprotein) that catalyzes the conversion of mandelonitrile to benzaldehyde and hydrocyanic acid. **isocitrate l.,** an enzyme that catalyzes the conversion of isocitrate to succinate and glyoxylate. **lactoyl-glutathione l.,** an enzyme occurring in the liver, kidney, and muscle that catalyzes the change of methylglyoxal to lactic acid by the addition of water; called also *glyoxalase I.* **pectate l.,** an enzyme that catalyzes the elimination of 4,5-D-galacturonate residues from pectate, thus bringing about depolymerization. **polyglucuronide l.,** an enzyme that catalyzes the elimination of 4,5-D-glucuronate residues from polysaccha-rides containing 1,4-linked D-glucuronate, thus bringing about depolymerization.

lycanthropy (li-kan′thro-pe) [Gr. *lykos* wolf + *anthrōpos* man] a delusion in which the patient believes himself a wolf.

lycetamine (li-se′tah-mēn) chemical name: (S)-2,6-diamino-N-hexadecylhexanamide; a topical antimicrobiol, $C_{22}H_{47}N_3O$.

Lychnis githago (lik′is gith-a′go) *Agrostemma githago.*

lycine (li′sin) betaine.

lycomania (li″ko-ma′ne-ah) lycanthropy.

lycopene (li′ko-pēn) the red carotinoid pigment, $C_{40}H_{56}$, of tomatoes and various berries and fruits.

lycopenemia (li″ko-pĕ-ne′me-ah) a variant of carotenemia resulting from the prolonged and excessive ingestion of tomato juice, which contains lycopene.

Lycoperdales (li″ko-per-da′lēs) the puffballs, an order of fungi of the series Gasteromycetes, class Basidiomycetes, including the genera *Calvatia, Lycoperdon,* and *Geaster.*

Lycoperdon (li″ko-per′don) [Gr. *lykos* wolf + *perdesthai* to break wind] a genus of fungi of the order Lycoperdales, class Basidiomycetes; the puffballs. In folk medicine, the dust (spores) is puffed and inhaled to treat nosebleeds.

lycoperdonosis (li″ko-per″do-no′sis) a respiratory disease caused by the inhalation of many spores from mature *Lycoperdon* mushrooms.

Lycopodium (li″ko-po′de-um) [Gr. *lykos* wolf + *pous* foot] a genus of club-mosses which yield lycopodium.

lycopodium (li″ko-po′de-um) a light dry powder formed by the yellow inflammable sporules of *Lycopodium clavatum, L. saururus,* and other species; formerly used as a dusting and absorbent powder, and as a coating for pills. The spores are uniform in size and for this reason are used as a measuring unit in microscopy.

lycorexia (li″ko-rek′se-ah) [Gr. *lykos* wolf + *orexis* appetite] ravenous, wolfish hunger.

lycorine (lik′o-rin) an alkaloid having emetic properties, from the bulbs of the plant *Lycoris radiata;* identical with narcissine.

Lycoris (lik′ŏ-ris) a genus of poisonous, amaryllidaceous plants of China and Japan. *L. radia′ta* Herb. is the source of sekisanine; the bulbs, which contain lycorine, are used in Chinese medicine as an expectorant and emetic.

Lycosa tarentula (li-ko′sah tah-ren′tu-lah) the European tarantula.

lydimycin (lid″ĭ-mi′sin) chemical name: 5-(hexahydro-2-oxo-1 H-thieno[3,4-d]imidazol-4-yl)pentenoic acid; an antifungal antibiotic produced by *Streptomyces lydicus,* $C_{10}H_{14}N_2O_3S$.

lye (li) an alkaline percolate from wood ashes; lixivium. Household lye is a crude mixture of sodium hydroxide with some sodium carbonate.

lying-in (li″ing-in′) 1. puerperal. 2. the puerperium.

Lymnaea (lim-ne′ah) a genus of pond snails. *L. ollula* and *L. bulimoides* serve as first intermediate hosts of *Fasciola hepatica;* other species are the hosts of schistosome flukes that cause schistosome dermatitis.

lymph (limf) [L. *lympha* water] 1. a transparent, slightly yellow liquid of alkaline reaction, found in the lymphatic vessels and derived from the tissue fluids. It is occasionally of a light-rose color from the presence of red blood corpuscles, and is often opalescent from particles of fat. Under the microscope, lymph is seen to consist of a liquid portion and of cells, most of which are lymphocytes. Lymph is collected from all parts of the body and returned to the blood via the lymphatic system. Called also *lympha* [NA]. See Plate XXVII. 2. any clear, watery fluid resembling true lymph. **animal l.,** vaccine or other lymph from an animal. **aplastic l.,** lymph that contains an excess of leukocytes and does not tend to become organized; called also *corpuscular l.* **bovine l.,** vaccine lymph from the cow. **calf l.,** lymph for vaccination or other lymph obtained from calves. **corpuscular l.,** aplastic l. **croupous l.,** inflammatory lymph that tends to the formation of a false membrane. **euplastic l., fibrinous l.,** that which tends to coagulate and become organized. **glycerinated l.,** vaccine virus mixed with glycerin in order to destroy any bacteria. **humanized l.,** material containing vaccinia virus collected from vaccinial vesicles of humans. **inflammatory l.,** the lymph produced by inflammation, as in a wound. **intercellular l.,** lymph occupying the intercellular spaces of tissues. **intravascular l.,** the lymph of the lymph vessels. **Koch's l.,** see *New* and *Old tuberculin,* under *tuberculin.* **plastic l.,** inflammatory lymph that has a tendency to become organized. **tissue l.,** lymph derived from the tissues and not from the blood. **vaccine l., vaccinia l.,** material containing vaccinia virus collected from vaccinial vesicles of calves; used for active immunization against smallpox.

lymph- see *lympho-.*

lympha (lim′fah) [L. "water"] [NA] the fluid found in the lymphatic vessels; see *lymph.*

lymphaden (lim′fah-den) [*lymph-* + Gr. *adēn* gland] a lymph node.

lymphadenectasis (lim-fad"ĕ-nek'tah-sis) [*lymph-* + Gr. *adēn* gland + *ektasis* distention] enlargement of a lymph node.

lymphadenectomy (lim-fad"ĕ-nek'to-me) [*lymphaden* + Gr. *ektomē* excision] surgical excision of one or more lymph nodes.

lymphadenhypertrophy (lim-fad"en-hi-per'tro-fe) [*lymphaden* + *hypertrophy*] hypertrophy of a lymph node.

lymphadenia (lim"fah-de'ne-ah) [*lymphaden* + *-ia*] hypertrophy of the lymph nodes. **l. os'sea** (*obs.*), multiple myeloma.

lymphadenitis (lim-fad"ĕ-ni'tis) [*lymph-* + Gr. *adēn* gland + *-itis*] inflammation of lymph nodes. **caseous l.,** inflammation of the lymph nodes associated with tuberculosis of some other part, but showing no tubercle bacilli in the lymphatics. **mesenteric l.,** a condition clinically resembling acute appendicitis, in which there is inflammation of the mesenteric lymph nodes receiving lymph from the intestine. A septal form, which is frequently fatal, and a milder form, which is self-limited, are caused by *Yersinia* (*Pasteurella*) *pseudotuberculosis*. Called also *mesenteric adenitis*. **nonbacterial regional l.,** cat-scratch disease. **paratuberculous l.,** caseous l. **regional l.,** cat-scratch disease. **tuberculoid l.,** inflammation of the lymph nodes similar to that in tuberculosis lymphadenitis; it may be caused by such disorders as sarcoidosis, regional enteritis, leprosy, syphilis, and several fungal infections. **tuberculous l.,** tuberculosis of the lymph nodes, involving most often the cervical and mediastinal nodes, due to lymphatic spread from a primary pulmonary infection or to hematogenous dissemination. Affected nodes may suppurate, with formation of draining sinuses. Primary infection of the cervical lymph nodes, once a common disorder, was known as scrofula. Called also *tuberculous lymphadenopathy*.

lymphadenocele (lim-fad'ĕ-no-sēl") a cyst of a lymph node; called also *adenolymphocele*.

lymphadenocyst (lim-fad'ĕ-no-sist") a degenerated lymph node caused by occlusion of its incoming lymph vessels. By dilatation of the lymph sinuses it becomes a fine-meshed network.

lymphadenogram (lim-fad'ĕ-no-gram") a roentgenogram of lymph nodes.

lymphadenography (lim-fad"ĕ-nog'rah-fe) roentgenographic visualization of the lymph nodes, following injection of radiopaque material into a lymphatic vessel.

lymphadenoid (lim-fad'ĕ-noid) [*lymph-* + Gr. *adēn* gland + *eidos* form] resembling the tissue of lymph nodes; lymphadenoid tissue includes the spleen, bone marrow, tonsils, and the lymphatic tissue of the organs and mucous membranes.

lymphadenoleukopoiesis (lim-fad"ĕ-no-lu"ko-poi-e'sis) the production of leukocytes by the lymphadenoid tissue.

lymphadenoma (lim"fad-ĕ-no'mah) hyperplasia of the lymphadenoid tissue; lymphoma. **malignant l.** (*obs.*), malignant lymphoma. **multiple l.,** (*obs.*), Hodgkin's disease.

lymphadenomatosis (lim-fad"ĕ-no-mah-to'sis) (*obs.*) generalized malignant lymphoma. **general l. of bones** (*obs.*), multiple myeloma.

lymphadenopathy (lim-fad"ĕ-nop'ah-the) [*lymphaden* + Gr. *pathos* disease] disease of the lymph nodes. **angioimmunoblastic l.,** immunoblastic l. **dermatopathic l.,** regional lymph node enlargement associated with melanoderma and various diseases in which erythroderma is chronically present, e.g., exfoliative dermatitis and generalized neurodermatitis; called also *lipomelanotic reticulosis*. **giant follicular l.,** see under *lymphoma*. **immunoblastic l.,** a hyperimmune disorder resembling Hodgkin's disease, characterized by fever, night sweats, weight loss, maculopapular rash, malaise, and generalized lymphadenopathy, and by proliferation of arborizing small vessels, prominent immunoblastic proliferation, hepatosplenomegaly, polyclonal hypergammaglobulinemia, mild hemolytic anemia and leukocytosis, and deposition of an amorphous interstitial material. Called also *angioimmunoblastic l.* **tuberculous l.,** see under *lymphadenitis*.

lymphadenosis (lim-fad"ĕ-no'sis) [*lymphaden* + *-osis*] hypertrophy or proliferation of lymphoid tissue. **acute l.,** infectious mononucleosis. **l. aleuce'mica parasita'ria,** East Coast fever. **aleukemic l.,** a disease marked by diffuse generalized hyperplasia of the lymphadenoid system (lymph glands, spleen, bone marrow, tonsils, and other lymphatic tissues), but without leukemia; see also *pseudoleukemia* and *lymphosarcoma*. **l. benig'na cu'tis,** a benign inflammatory hyperplasia of lymphocytes in the skin, often in follicular arrangement, principally occurring on the face or ears of young adults in the form of solitary or disseminated yellowish brown to bluish red nodules that may progressively enlarge but usually involute spontaneously after a few months or years. Called also *lymphocytoma cutis*, *Bäfverstedt's syndrome*, and *Spiegler-Fendt sarcoid*.

lymphadenotomy (lim-fad"ĕ-not'o-me) incision of a lymph node.

lymphadenovarix (lim-fad"ĕ-no-va'riks) enlargement of the lymph nodes from the pressure of dilated lymph vessels.

lymphagogue (lim'fah-gog) an agent that promotes the production of lymph.

lymphangeitis (lim"fan-je-i'tis) lymphangitis.

lymphangial (lim-fan'je-al) pertaining to a lymphatic vessel.

lymphangiectasia (lim-fan"je-ek-ta'ze-ah) lymphangiectasis. **intestinal l.,** dilatation of the intestinal lymphatic system, particularly the lacteals in the intestinal villi, characterized by protein-losing enteropathy, steatorrhea, and lymphopenia. It may be congenital, due to abnormality of the lymphatic system (as in Milroy's disease), or acquired, due to involvement of the major intestinal lymphatic ducts by inflammatory processes or neoplasm, or to increased lymphatic pressure, as in valvular heart disease and constrictive pericarditis.

lymphangiectasis (lim-fan"je-ek'tah-sis) [*lymph-* + Gr. *angeion* vessel + *ektasis* distention] dilatation of the lymphatic vessels. **cystic l.,** cystic lymphangioma.

lymphangiectatic (lim-fan"je-ek-tat'ik) pertaining to or marked by lymphangiectasis.

lymphangiectodes (lim-fan"je-ek-to'dēz) (*obs.*) lymphangioma circumscriptum.

lymphangiectomy (lim-fan"je-ek'to-me) excision of one or more lymphatic vessels.

lymphangiitis (lim-fan"je-i'tis) lymphangitis.

lymphangioadenography (lym-fan"je-o-ad"ĕ-nog'rah-fe) lymphography.

lymphangioendothelioblastoma (lim-fan"je-o-en"do-the"le-o-blas-to'mah) (*obs.*) lymphangioendothelioma.

lymphangioendothelioma (lim-fan"je-o-en"do-the-le-o'mah) lymphangioma in which the endothelial cells are the dominant component.

lymphangiofibroma (lim-fan" je-o-fi-bro' mah) a fibrosing lymphangioma.

lymphangiogram (lim-fan"je-o-gram) a roentgenogram of the lymphatic vessels.

lymphangiography (lim-fan"je-og'rah-fe) roentgenography of the lymphatic vessels following the injection of contrast medium. **pedal l.,** radiography of the lymphatic channels of the lower extremity after injection of contrast medium into the first and second interdigital spaces of the foot.

lymphangiology (lim-fan"je-ol'o-je) [*lymph-* + Gr. *angeion* vessel + *-logy*] the branch of anatomy relating to the lymphatic vessels.

lymphangioma (lim-fan"je-o'mah) a tumor composed of new-formed lymph spaces and channels; called also *angioma lymphaticum*. **l. capsula're varico'sum** (*obs.*), lymphangioma circumscriptum. **l. caverno'sum,** dilatation of the lymphatic vessels resulting in cavities filled with lymph; called also *cavernosa lymphaticum*. **cavernous l.,** l. cavernosum. **l. circumscrip'tum,** a skin lesion of early life marked by the development of groups, a few centimeters in diameter, of yellow to red vesicles, connected with the lymphatic vessels. **cystic l., l. cys'ticum,** a cystic growth occurring almost exclusively in the neck or groin and more commonly in children than in adults, and thought to originate from some anomaly in development of the primitive lymphatic spaces. The symptoms are largely the result of compression of adjoining structures by the mass. **fissural l.,** simple or cavernous lymphangiomas at the site of fetal fissures. **l. sim'plex,** dilatation of a lymph vessel over a circumscribed area. **l. tubero'sum mul'tiplex** (*obs.*), a skin disease marked by the development of groups of papules or tubercles resembling and believed to be lymphangioma. **l. xanthelasmoi'deum** (*obs.*), lymphangioma circumscriptum marked by formation on the skin of yellow or brownish patches.

lymphangiomyomatosis (lim-fan"je-o-mi"o-mah-to'sis) a progressive disorder of women of child-bearing age, marked by nodular and diffuse interstitial proliferation of smooth muscle in the lungs, lymph nodes, and thoracic duct.

lymphangiophlebitis (lim-fan"je-o-flĕ-bi'tis) inflammation of the lymph vessels and veins.

lymphangioplasty (lim-fan'je-o-plas"te) [*lymph-* + Gr. *angeion* vessel + *plassein* to form] operative restoration or replacement of lymph vessels that have been destroyed. **Handley's l.,** treatment of elephantiasis by means of drains made of long cotton and silk threads inserted into the tissues; called also *Handley's method*.

lymphangiosarcoma (lim-fan"je-o-sar-ko'mah) a malignant tumor of lymphatic vessels, usually arising in a limb that is the site of chronic lymphedema.

lymphangiotomy (lim-fan"je-ot'o-me) [*lymph-* + Gr. *angeion* vessel + *temnein* to cut] incision into a lymphatic vessel, usually performed for cannulation prior to lymphangiography.

lymphangitis (lim"fan-ji'tis) inflammation of a lymphatic vessel or vessels. Acute lymphangitis may result from spread of bacterial infection (most commonly beta-hemolytic streptococci) into the lymphatics, manifested by painful subcutaneous red streaks along the course of the vessels. **l. carcinomato'sa,** a pseudoinflammatory lesion of the lymphatic vessels of the peritoneum, with edema of the area and proliferation of fibrous tissues around the vessels, due to the infiltration of cancer cells from peritoneal tumors. **l. epizoot'ica,** a chronic contagious disease of horses caused by a yeast fungus, *Histoplasma farciminosus*, and marked by purulent inflammation of the subcutaneous lymphatic vessels and of the regional lymph glands. Called also *pseudofarcy, blastomycosis farciminosus, cryptococcus farcy, lymphosporidiosis, African glanders, Japanese glanders, Japanese farcy, Neapolitan farcy.* **gummatous l.,** cladiosis. **ulcerative l.,** a chronic contagious disease of horses and other equines, characterized by inflammation of the lymph vessels and a tendency toward ulceration of the skin over the parts affected; called also *ulcerative cellulitis.* **l. ulcero′sa pseudofarcino′sa,** a disease of horses resembling glanders, and due to a bacillus closely resembling the glanders bacillus, *Actinobacillus mallei;* called also *pseudoglanders.*

lymphapheresis (lim″fah-fer′ĕ-sis) lymphocytapheresis.

lymphatic (lim-fat′ik) [L. *lymphaticus*] 1. pertaining to lymph or a lymph vessel; by extension, the term is used alone to designate a lymphatic vessel or, in the plural, to designate the lymphatic system. 2. of a sluggish or phlegmatic temperament.

lymphaticostomy (lim-fat″ĭ-kos′to-me) [*lymphatic* + Gr. *stomoun* to provide with an opening, or mouth] surgical creation of an opening into a lymphatic duct, usually the thoracic duct.

lymphatism (lim′fah-tizm) 1. a morbid state due to excessive production or growth of lymphoid tissues, resulting in impaired development and lowered vitality; called also *lymphotoxemia, lymphoidotoxemia,* and *status lymphaticus.* 2. the lymphatic temperament; a slow or sluggish habit.

lymphatitis (lim″fah-ti′tis) inflammation of some part of the lymphatic system.

lymphatogenous (lim″fah-toj′ĕ-nus) produced by or derived from the lymph; disseminated by the lymph circulation or through the lymph channels.

lymphatology (lim″fah-tol′o-je) the study of the lymph and lymphatic system.

lymphatolysin (lim″fah-tol′ĭ-sin) a lysin that acts on lymphatic tissue.

lymphatolysis (lim″fah-tol′ĭ-sis) [*lymphatic* + Gr. *lysis* dissolution] the destruction or solution of lymphatic tissue.

lymphatolytic (lim″fah-to-lit′ik) [*lymphatic* + Gr. *lysis* dissolution] destroying lymphatic tissue.

lymphatome (lim′fah-tōm) lymphotome.

lymphectasia (lim″fek-ta′ze-ah) [*lymph-* + Gr. *ektasis* distention] distention with lymph.

lymphedema (lim″fe-de′mah) [*lymph-* + *edema*] chronic unilateral or bilateral edema of the extremities due to accumulation of interstitial fluid as a result of stasis of lymph, which is secondary to obstruction of lymph vessels or disorders of the lymph nodes. **congenital l.,** Milroy's disease. **l. prae′cox,** primarily of young females, characterized by puffiness and swelling of the lower limbs, and occurring at or near puberty. **l. tar′da,** lymphedema of late onset, after 35 years of age.

lymphendothelioma (lim″fen-do-the′le-o′mah) (*obs.*), lymphangioendothelioma.

lymphenteritis (lim″fen-ter-i′tis) enteritis with serous infiltration.

lymphepithelioma (limf″ep-ĭ-the′le-o′mah) lymphoepithelioma.

lymphization (lim″fi-za′shun) the formation of lymph.

lymphnoditis (limf″no-di′tis) inflammation of a lymph node; lymphadenitis.

lympho-, lymph- [L. *lympha* water] a combining form denoting relationship to lymph, lymphoid tissue, lymphatics, or lymphocytes.

lymphoblast (lim′fo-blast) [*lympho-* + Gr. *blastos* germ] the immature, nucleolated precursor of the mature lymphocyte.

lymphoblastic (lim″fo-blas′tik) pertaining to a lymphoblast.

lymphoblastoma (lim″fo-blas-to′mah) poorly differentiated lymphocytic malignant lymphoma.

lymphoblastomatosis (lim″fo-blas″to-mah-to′sis) the condition produced by the presence of lymphoblastomas.

lymphoblastomatous (lim″fo-blas-to′mah-tus) of the nature of or characterized by lymphoblastoma.

lymphoblastomid (lim″fo-blas-to′mid) any specific cutaneous lesion of lymphoblastoma.

lymphoblastosis (lim″fo-blas-to′sis) excess of lymphoblasts in the blood. **acute benign l.,** former term for infectious mononucleosis.

lymphocele (lim′fo-sēl) [*lympho-* + Gr. *kēlē* tumor] (*obs.*) cystic lymphangioma.

lymphocerastism (lim″fo-se-ras′tizm) [*lympho-* + Gr. *kerastos* mixed] the formation of lymphoid cells.

lymphocinesia (lim″fo-si-ne′ze-ah) [*lympho-* + Gr. *kinēsis* motion] lymphokinesis.

lymphocyst (lim′fo-sist) (*obs.*) cystic lymphangioma.

lymphocytapheresis (lim″fo-si″tah-fer′ĕ-sis) [*lymphocyte* + Gr. *aphairesis* removal] the selective removal of lymphocytes from withdrawn blood, which is then retransfused into the donor. Called also *lymphapheresis.*

lymphocyte (lim′fo-sīt) [*lympho-* + *-cyte*] a mononuclear leukocyte 7μ to 20μ in diameter, with a deeply staining nucleus containing dense chromatin, and a pale-blue–staining cytoplasm. It is chiefly a product of lymphoid tissue and participates in humoral and cell-mediated immunity. See also *lymphocytic series,* under *series.* **activated l.,** one that has reacted immunologically on exposure to antigen or to a mitogen, such as phytohemagglutinin. **B-l's,** "bursa-equivalent" lymphocytes, i.e., lymphocytes that are thymus-independent, migrating to the tissues without passing through or being influenced by the thymus; they are analogous to the avian lymphocytes governed by the bursa of Fabricius. Humans have no discrete bursa and the exact location of B-lymphocyte production is not known, but gut-associated lymphoid tissue, fetal liver, and bone marrow are considered to be the primary sites of origin of B-lymphocytes, being designated bursal equivalent tissue. B-lymphocytes play a major role in humoral immunity; on stimulation by antigen, they mature into plasma cells that synthesize humoral antibody. Called also *B cells.* Cf. *T-l's.* **"bursa-equivalent" l's,** B-l's. **killer l's,** see under *cell.* **null l's,** see under *cell.* **Rieder's l.,** a lymphocyte having a nucleus which is lobed and twisted; seen in chronic lymphocytic lymphemia. **T-l's,** thymus-dependent lymphocytes, i.e., lymphocytes that either pass through the thymus or are influenced by it on their way to the tissues; they can suppress or assist the stimulation of antibody production in B-lymphocytes in the presence of antigen, and can kill such cells as tumor and transplant tissue cells. They act directly or by elaboration of lymphokines, are largely responsible for cell-mediated immunity, and have the property of anamnestic response. Several subsets of T-lymphocytes are recognized on the basis of surface markers and function. Called also *T cells.* Cf. *B-l's.* **thymus-dependent l's,** T-l's. **thymus-independent l's,** B-l's. **transformed l's,** blastlike cells occurring as a result of stimulation *in vitro* by nonspecific mitogens or by specific antigens; they are increased in size, have abundant cytoplasm, and their nucleoli are visible.

lymphocytic (lim″fo-sit′ik) pertaining to, characterized by, or of the nature of lymphocytes; see also under *series.*

lymphocytoblast (lim″fo-si′to-blast) lymphoblast.

lymphocytoma (lim″fo-si-to′mah) [*lymphocyte* + *-oma*] well-differentiated lymphocytic malignant lymphoma. **l. cu′tis,** lymphadenosis benigna cutis.

lymphocytomatosis (lim″fo-si″to-mah-to′sis) the condition produced by the presence of lymphocytomas.

lymphocytomatous (lim″fo-si-to′mah-tus) of the nature of or characterized by lymphocytoma.

lymphocytopenia (lim″fo-si″to-pe′ne-ah) reduction in the number of lymphocytes in the blood.

lymphocytopheresis (lim″fo-si″to-fer′ĕ-sis) lymphocytapheresis.

lymphocytopoiesis (lim″fo-si″to-poi-e′sis) [*lymphocyte* + Gr. *poiein* to make] the development of lymphocytes.

lymphocytopoietic (lim″fo-si″to-poi-et′ik) pertaining to or characterized by lymphocytopoiesis.

lymphocytorrhexis (lim″fo-si″to-rek′sis) the rupturing or bursting of lymphocytes.

lymphocytosis (lim″fo-si-to′sis) excess of normal lymphocytes in the blood or in any effusion. **acute infectious l.,** an acute, benign infectious disease of children characterized by an excess of normal small lymphocytes in the blood without lymphadenopathy or splenomegaly, and with varying degrees of clinical expression and constitutional response; called also *Carl Smith disease.*

lymphocytotic (lim″fo-si-tot′ik) pertaining to lymphocytosis.

lymphocytotoxicity (lim″fo-si″to-tok-sis′ĭ-te) the quality or capability of lyzing lymphocytes, as in procedures in which lymphocytes having a specific cell surface antigen are lyzed when incubated with antiserum and complement. Called also *leukocytotoxicity.*

lymphocytotoxin (lim″fo-si″to-tok′sin) a toxin that has a specific destructive action on lymphocytes.

lymphodermia (lim″fo-der′me-ah) [*lympho-* + Gr. *derma* skin] (*obs.*) any disease of the lymphatics of the skin.

lymphoduct (lim′fo-dukt) a lymphatic vessel.

lymphoepithelioma (lim″fo-ep″ĭ-the′le-o′mah) a pleomorphic, poorly differentiated (transitional cell) carcinoma arising from modified epithelium overlying the lymphoid tissue of the nasopharynx; it has a high frequency among young adults of Oriental extraction. Called also *lymphoepithelial carcinoma, Schmincke tumor,* and *Regaud tumor.*

lymphoganglin (lim″fo-gang′glin) a hypothetical hormone from lymph nodes.

lymphogenesis (lim″fo-jen′ĕ-sis) the production of lymph.

lymphogenous (lim-foj′ĕ-nus) [*lympho-* + Gr. *gennan* to produce] 1. producing lymph. 2. produced from lymph or in the lymphatics.

lymphoglandula (lim″fo-glan′du-lah), pl. *lymphoglan′dulae.* Lymph node (*nodus lymphaticus* [NA]).

lymphogram (lim'fo-gram) a roentgenogram of the lymphatic vessels and lymph nodes.

lymphogranuloma (lim″fo-gran″u-lo′mah) Hodgkin's disease. **l. benig′num** (*obs.*), sarcoidosis. **l. inguina′le**, l. venereum. **l. malig′num,** Hodgkin's disease. **Schaumann's benign l.** (*obs.*), sarcoidosis. **l. vene′reum,** an infectious disease of venereal origin caused by a strain of *Chlamydia* and marked initially by a primary transient ulcerative lesion of the genitals, followed by regional lymph node hypertrophy; in later stages, lymphatic obstruction may result in elephantiasis of the external genitalia, while scarring accounts for strictures of the rectum. Called also *lymphogranuloma inguinale, lymphopathia venereum, poradenitis nostras, Frei's disease, Nicolas-Favre disease, fifth venereal disease, climatic bubo, tropical bubo,* etc.

lymphogranulomatosis (lim″fo-gran″u-lo-mah-to′sis) 1. infectious granuloma of the lymphatic system. 2. a term used by continental writers as a synonym for Hodgkin's disease. See also *pseudoleukemia*. **benign l.,** sarcoidosis. **l. cu′tis,** the cutaneous manifestation of Hodgkin's disease. **l. inguina′lis,** lymphogranuloma venereum. **l. malig′na,** Hodgkin's disease.

lymphography (lim-fog′rah-fe) roentgenography of the lymphatic channels and lymph nodes, following injection of radiopaque material in a lymphatic vessel.

lymphohistiocytic (lim″fo-his″te-o-sit′ik) involving lymphocytes and histiocytes.

lymphohistioplasmacytic (lim″fo-his″te-o-plas″mah-sit′ik) involving lymphocytes, histiocytes, and plasmacytes.

lymphoid (lim′foid) [*lymph* + Gr. *eidos* form] resembling or pertaining to lymph or tissue of the lymphoid system.

lymphoidectomy (lim″foi-dek′to-me) excision of lymphoid tissue, such as adenoids and tonsils.

lymphoidocyte (lim-foi′do-sīt) an embryonic cell considered by some to be the stem cell for all types of blood cells; hemocytoblast.

lymphoidotoxemia (lim-foi″do-tok-se′me-ah) lymphatism (def. 1).

lymphokentric (lim″fo-ken′trik)[*lympho-* + Gr. *kentron* a stimulant] stimulating the formation of lymphoid cells. Cf. *myelokentric*.

lymphokine (lim′fo-kīn) [*lympho-* + Gr. *kinēsis* movement] a general term for soluble protein mediators released by sensitized lymphocytes on contact with antigen and which play a role in macrophage activation, lymphocyte transformation, and cell-mediated immunity.

lymphokinesis (lim″fo-ki-ne′sis) [*lympho-* + Gr. *kinēsis* movement] 1. the movement of the endolymph in the semicircular canals. 2. the circulation of lymph in the body.

lymphology (lim-fol′o-je) [*lympho-* + *-logy*] the study of the lymphatic system.

lympholytic (lim″fo-lit′ik) causing destruction of lymphocytes.

lymphoma (lim-fo′mah) a general term applied to any neoplastic disorder of the lymphoid tissue, including Hodgkin's disease. Benign lymphoma is rare; the term *lymphoma* often is used alone to denote malignant lymphoma. Recent classifications of malignant lymphomas are based on the predominant cell type and its degree of differentiation; the various categories may be subdivided into nodular and diffuse types depending on the predominant pattern of cell arrangement. **African l.,** Burkitt's l. **Burkitt's l.,** a form of undifferentiated malignant lymphoma, usually found in central Africa, but also reported from other areas, and manifested most often as a large osteolytic lesion in the jaw or as an abdominal mass. The Epstein-Barr virus, a herpesvirus, has been isolated from Burkitt's lymphoma, and has been implicated as a causative agent. Called also *Burkitt's tumor* and *Africian l.* **clasmocytic l.,** histiocytic malignant l. **giant follicular l.,** nodular well differentiated lymphocytic malignant lymphoma, so called because its microscopic appearance is characterized by multiple, proliferative, follicle-like nodules which disturb the normal architecture of the lymph nodes. Called also *giant follicular lymphadenopathy*, and *Brill-Symmers* or *Symmers' disease*. **granulomatous l.,** Hodgkin's disease. **lymphoblastic l.,** poorly differentiated lymphocytic malignant l. **lymphocytic l.,** see *malignant l., well-differentiated lymphocytic* and *poorly-differentiated lymphocytic*. **malignant l.,** see *lymphoma*. **malignant l., histiocytic,** a form in which the predominant cell is the primitive mesenchymal element or one which has differentiated into the identifiable reticulum cell; called also *reticulum cell sarcoma* and *clasmocytic l*. **malignant l., mixed cell,** a form that contains proliferations of both histiocytes and lymphocytes. **malignant l., poorly differentiated lymphocytic,** a form in which the predominant cell is morphologically similar to the lymphoblast and contains a fine nuclear chromatin structure with one or more nucleoli; called also *lymphoblastoma, lymphoblastic l.,* and *lymphoblastic lymphosarcoma.* **malignant l., undifferentiated,** a form in which relatively large stem cells with large nuclei, pale, scanty cytoplasm, and indistinct borders are predominant; called also *stem cell l.* and *reticulosarcoma.* **malignant l., well-differentiated lymphocytic,** a form in which the predominant cell is the

mature lymphocyte; called also *lymphocytoma, lymphocytic l.,* and *lymphocytic lymphosarcoma.* **stem cell l.,** malignant l., undifferentiated.

lymphomatoid (lim-fo′mah-toid) resembling lymphoma.

lymphomatosis (lim″fo-mah-to′sis) the development of multiple lymphomas in various parts of the body. **avian l., l. of fowl,** avian leukosis involving chiefly the lymphocytes. **l. granulomato′sa** (*obs.*), Hodgkin's disease. **neural l.,** see *Marek's disease*, under *disease*. **ocular l.,** see *Marek's disease*, under *disease*. **visceral l.,** see *avian leukosis*, under *leukosis*.

lymphomatous (lim-fo′mah-tus) pertaining to or of the nature of lymphoma.

lymphomyeloma (lim″fo-mi-ě-lo′mah) (*obs.*) multiple myeloma.

lymphomyxoma (lim″fo-mik-so′mah) any benign growth consisting of adenoid tissue.

lymphonodi (lim″fo-no′di) [L.] plural of *lymphonodus*.

lymphonodus (lim″fo-no′dus), pl. *lymphono′di* [*lympho-* + L. *nodis* a knot] NA alternative for *nodus lymphaticus*.

lymphopathia (lim″fo-path′e-ah) lymphopathy. **l. vene′reum,** lymphogranuloma venereum.

lymphopathy (lim-fop′ah-the) [*lympho-* + Gr. *pathos* disease] any disease of the lymphatic system. **ataxic l.,** a sudden swelling of the lymph nodes sometimes accompanying the pain crises of locomotor ataxia.

lymphopenia (lim-fo-pe′ne-ah) [*lymphocyte* + Gr. *penia* poverty] decrease in the proportion of lymphocytes in the blood.

lymphoplasm (lim′fo-plazm) spongioplasm, def. 1.

lymphoplasty (lim′fo-plas″te) lymphangioplasty.

lymphopoiesis (lim″fo-poi-e′sis) [*lympho-* + Gr. *poiein* to make] 1. the development of lymphatic tissue. 2. lymphocytopoiesis.

lymphopoietic (lim″fo-poi-et′ik) pertaining to, characterized by, or causing lymphopoiesis.

lymphoproliferative (lim″fo-pro-lif′er-ah-tiv) pertaining to or characterized by proliferation of lymphoid tissue; see under *syndrome*.

lymphoreticular (lim″fo-rě-tik′u-lar) pertaining to the reticuloendothelial cells of the lymph nodes.

lymphoreticulosis (lim″fo-re-tik″u-lo′sis) proliferation of the reticuloendothelial cells of the lymph glands. **benign l.,** cat-scratch fever.

lymphorrhage (lim′fo-rij) an accumulation of lymphocytes in a muscle.

lymphorrhagia (lim″fo-ra′je-ah) [*lympho-* + Gr. *rhegnynai* to break out] lymphorrhea.

lymphorrhea (lim″fo-re′ah) [*lympho-* + Gr. *rhoia* flow] a flow of lymph from cut or ruptured lymph vessels.

lymphorrhoid (limf′o-roid) a localized dilatation of a perianal lymph channel, resembling a hemorrhoid; sometimes occurring in lymphogranuloma venereum.

lymphosarcoma (lim″fo-sar-ko′mah) a general term applied to malignant neoplastic disorders of lymphoid tissue, but not including Hodgkin's disease. See *lymphoma*. **fascicular l.,** sclerosing l. **lymphoblastic l.,** poorly differentiated lymphocytic malignant lymphoma. **lymphocytic l.,** well-differentiated lymphocytic malignant lymphoma. **sclerosing l.,** a form occurring mainly in childhood, in which the tumor has a fine collagenous stroma and the lymphocytes are arranged in serried rows between the fibers, often giving the tumor a distinctive whorled pattern.

lymphosarcomatosis (lim″fo-sar″ko-mah-to′sis) a condition characterized by the presence of multiple lesions of lymphosarcoma.

lymphosporidiosis (lim″fo-spo-rid″e-o′sis) lymphangitis epizootica.

lymphostasis (lim-fos′tah-sis) [*lympho-* + Gr. *stasis* standing] stoppage of the lymph flow.

lymphotaxis (lim″fo-tak′sis) [*lymphocyte* + Gr. *taxis* arrangement] the property of attracting or repulsing lymphocytes.

lymphotism (lim′fo-tizm) a disordered state associated with the development of adenoid tissue.

lymphotome (lim′fo-tōm) [*lympho-* + Gr. *tomē* a cut] an instrument for excising accumulations of lymphoid tissue.

lymphotoxemia (lim″fo-tok-se′me-ah) toxemia due to excess of lymphoid material or lymphoid tissue, as in rickets, Graves' disease, enlarged thymus, etc.

lymphotoxin (lim″fo-tok′sin) a chemical mediator released by sensitized lymphocytes and involved in target-cell injury and inhibition of cell division.

lymphotrophy (lim-fot′ro-fe) [*lympho-* + Gr. *trephein* to nourish] the attractive energy of cells for lymph.

lymphous (lim′fus) pertaining to or containing lymph.

lymph-vascular (limf-vas′ku-lar) pertaining to or containing lymphatic vessels.

Lynchia maura (lin′ke-ah maw′rah) *Pseudolynchia canariensis.*

Lynen (li'nen), Feodor. German biochemist, born 1911; co-winner, with Konrad Bloch, of the Nobel prize for medicine and physiology in 1964, for investigations in biosynthesis of fatty acids and cholesterol.

lynestrenol (lin-es'trĕ-nōl) chemical name: 19-nor-17α-pregn-4-en-20-yn-17-ol; a progestin, $C_{20}H_{28}O$.

Lynoral (lin'or-al) trademark for a preparation of ethinyl estradiol.

lyo- (li'o) [Gr. *lyein* to dissolve] combining form meaning dissolved.

lyochrome (li'o-krōm) [*lyo-* + Gr. *chrōma* color] flavin.

lyogel (li'o-jel) [*lyo-* + *gel*] a gel containing much liquid. Cf. *xerogel*.

Lyon hypothesis (li'on) [Mary L. *Lyon*, British geneticist] see under *hypothesis*.

Lyon method, test (li'on) [Bethuel Boyd Vincent *Lyon*, American physician, 1880–1953] Meltzer-Lyon test; see under *tests*.

lyonization (li″on-i-za'shun) [after Mary L. *Lyon*] the process by which or the condition in which all X chromosomes of the cells in excess of one are inactivated on a random basis.

lyonized (li'o-nīzd) [after Mary L. *Lyon*] denoting the inactivated X chromosome in a cell, according to the Lyon hypothesis.

lyophil (li'o-fil) a lyophilic substance; a material that readily goes into solution.

lyophile (li'o-fīl) 1. lyophil. 2. lyophilic.

lyophilic (li″o-fil'ik) [*lyo-* + Gr. *philein* to love] having an affinity for solution; designating a colloid system in which the solvent and the dispersed particles mutually attract each other and which is quite stable.

lyophilization (li-of″ĭ-li-za'shun) the creation of a stable preparation of a biological substance (blood plasma, serum, etc.), by rapid freezing and dehydration of the frozen product under high vacuum.

lyophilize (li-of'ĭ-līz) to subject to lyophilization.

lyophilizer (li-of'ĭ-li-zer) an instrument used in lyophilization; a freeze dryer.

lyophobe (li'o-fōb) [*lyo-* + *phobia*] a lyophobic substance; a material that does not readily go into or tends to separate out from solution.

lyophobic (li″o-fo'bik) [*lyo-* + Gr. *phobein* to fear] not having an affinity for solution; designating a colloid system in which no attraction exists between the solvent and the dispersed particles and which is unstable.

lyosol (li'o-sol) a sol in which the dispersion medium is a liquid.

lyosorption (li″o-sorp'shun) the selective adsorption of the solvent portion of a solution.

lyotropic (li″o-trop'ik) [*lyo-* + Gr. *tropos* a turning] entering easily into solution; readily soluble.

Lyperosia irritans (li″per-o'se-ah ir'ĭ-tans) *Haematobia irritans*.

Lyponyssus (li″po-nis'us) a genus of mites which sometimes attack man. *L. baco'ti* live normally on rats, *L. bur'sae* on birds.

lypressin (li-pres'in) chemical name: 8-L-lysine vasopressin. A form of vasopressin that contains lysine, $C_{46}H_{65}N_{13}O_{12}S$, as that from pigs. A synthetic preparation is used as an antidiuretic and vasoconstrictor in the treatment of diabetes insipidus due to deficiency of endogenous posterior pituitary antidiuretic hormone (vasopressin), administered by intranasal spray. See also *argipressin*.

lyra (li'rah) [L., Gr. "a stringed instrument resembling the lute"] a name applied to certain anatomical structures because of their fancied resemblance to a lute. **l. Da'vidis** (*obs.*), commissura fornicis.

lyre (līr) lyra. **l. of David** (*obs.*), commissura fornicis.

Lys lysine.

lysate (li'sāt) 1. the material formed by the lysis of cells. 2. a medicinal preparation obtained from an animal organ by means of artificial digestion.

lysatin (lis'ah-tin) a principle derived from casein by Drechsel, later shown to be a mixture of lysine and arginine.

lyse (līz) 1. to cause or produce disintegration of a compound, substance, or cell. 2. to undergo lysis.

lysergide (li'ser-jīd) chemical name: N,N-diethyllysergamide. A hallucinogenic compound, $C_{20}H_{25}N_3O$, derived from lysergic acid; it has been used experimentally in the study and treatment of mental disorders. The substance has also been found to be antagonistic to serotonin in its action on smooth muscle. The side effects include bizarre behavior and, reportedly, psychosis and chromosomal damage. Called also *LSD* and *lysergic acid diethylamide*.

lysidin (lis'ĭ-din) a red crystalline body, methylglyoxalidin, $CH_2 \cdot NH \cdot C(CH_3):N \cdot CH_2$; also its yellowish or pinkish, soapy, 50 per cent solution: used as a solvent for uric acid. **l. bitartrate**, a soluble, white, crystalline powder, of one third the solvent power of pure lysidin.

lysimeter (li-sim'ĕ-ter) [Gr. *lysis* dissolution + *metron* measure] an apparatus for determining the solubilities of substances.

lysin (li'sin) [Gr. *lyein* to dissolve] an antibody, such as an alpha lysin, which has the power of causing dissolution of cells. The term includes hemolysin, bacteriolysin, cytolysin, etc. **beta l.**, a naturally occurring and relatively thermostabile bactericidal serum constituent of certain animals that is not inactivated by a temperature of 56–60° C. for 30–40 minutes. **Dubos' l.** (*obs.*), tyrothricin. **immune l.**, a cytolytic antibody that interacts with cellular antigen to mediate lysis of the cell by complement. **sperm l.**, a general term for the enzymatic substances of spermatozoa which dissolve egg membranes and permit penetration; these lysins are thought to be produced by the acrosome.

lysine (li'sēn) an amino acid, $NH_2(CH_2)_4 \cdot CH(NH_2) \cdot COOH$, or α-ε-diaminocaproic acid, a hydrolytic product of protein first isolated from casein (Drechsel, 1889); essential for optimal growth in infants and for maintenance of nitrogen equilibrium in human adults.

lysinogen (li-sin'o-jen) [*lysin* + Gr. *gennan* to produce] an antigenic substance capable of inducing the formation of lysins.

lysinogenesis (li″sin-o-jen'ĕ-sis) the production or formation of lysins.

lysinosis (lis″ĭ-no'sis) [Gr. *lyein* to dissolve + *is, inos* fiber + *-osis*] lung disease due to inhaling cotton fibers, as in mills; lyssinosis.

lysis (li'sis) [Gr. "dissolution; a loosing, setting free, releasing"] 1. destruction, as of cells by a specific lysin. 2. decomposition, as of a chemical compound by a specific agent. 3. mobilization of an organ by division of restraining adhesions. 4. the gradual abatement of the symptoms of a disease; cf. *crisis*, def. 1. **hot-cold l.**, lysis that occurs only if the material is incubated as usual and then allowed to stand overnight at room temperature.

lyso- (li'so) [Gr. *lysis* dissolution] a combining form, indicating lysis or dissolution.

lysobacteria (li″so-bak-te're-ah) (*obs.*) bacteria that are able to dissolve other bacteria, both alive and dead.

lysocephalin (li″so-sef'ah-lin) a cephalin from which a fatty acid radical has been removed, as by the action of cobra venom.

lysocythin (li″so-si'thin) a substance formed by combination between an animal poison and the body tissues and having a cytolytic action.

Lysodren (li'so-dren) trademark for a preparation of mitotane.

lysogen (li'so-jen) [*lysin* + Gr. *gennan* to produce] an antigen that elicits the formation of a lytic antibody; called also *lysinogen*.

lysogenesis (li″so-jen'ĕ-sis) 1. the production of lysis or lysins. 2. lysogenicity.

lysogenic (li-so-jen'ik) [*lysin* + Gr. *gennan* to produce] 1. producing lysins or causing lysis. 2. pertaining to lysogenicity.

lysogenicity (li″so-jĕ-nis'ĭ-te) [*lyso-* + Gr. *gennan* to produce + *-ity* condition] 1. the ability to produce lysins or cause lysis. 2. the potentiality of a bacterium to produce phage. 3. the specific association of the phage genome, the prophage, with the bacterial genome in such a way that only a few, if any, phage genes are transcribed.

lysogeny (li-soj'e-ne) lysogenicity.

lysokinase (li″so-ki'nās) a general term for substances of the fibrinolytic system that activate the plasma proactivators.

lysolecithin (li″so-les'ĭ-thin) a lecithin from which the α' (i.e., terminal) fatty acid radical has been removed, as by the action of phospholipase A; it has strong hemolytic properties and occurs in trace amounts in the pancreas.

lysophosphatide (li″so-fos'fah-tīd) a phosphatide from which one molecule of fatty acid has been split off, as by the action of cobra venom.

lysosomal (li″so-so'mal) of or pertaining to a lysosome.

lysosome (li'so-sōm) [*lyso-* + Gr. *sōma* body] one of the minute bodies seen with the electron microscope in many types of cells, containing various hydrolytic enzymes and normally involved in the process of localized intracellular digestion. Injury to a lysosome is followed by release into the cell of the enzymes, which may damage the cell and give rise to wasting and other pathologic aspects of certain diseases, as in muscular dystrophy. **primary l.**, one that has not yet been engaged in digestive activities. **secondary l.**, a primary (or another secondary) lysosome that has fused with a phagosome (or pinosome), bringing hydrolases in contact with the ingested material and resulting in digestion of the material. See also *autophagy* (def. 2) and *heterophagy*.

lysostaphin (li-so-staf'in) an antibacterial enzyme produced by *Staphylococcus staphylolyticus*; it is specifically active against staphylococci.

lysostripping (li″so-strip'ing) the phenomenon in which antigens of the cell membrane, in the presence of excess antibody, gather over one pole of the cell and are then phagocytized by the cell, so that the cell membrane is "stripped" of that particular antigen.

lysotype (li'so-tīp) [*lyso-* + *type*] phage type.

lysozym (li'so-zīm) lysozyme.

lysozyme (li'so-zim) [Gr. *lysis* dissolution + *zymē* leaven] mucopeptide *N*-acetylmuramylhydrolase: a crystalline, basic enzyme which is present in saliva, tears, egg white, and many animal fluids and which functions as an antibacterial agent, especially effective in lysing *Micrococcus lysodeikticus*. Other bacteria, e.g., *Escherichia coli* and *Salmonella typhosa*, as well as chitin are attacked to a lesser extent. Called also *mucopeptide glucohydrolase* and *muramidase*.

lysozymuria (li″so-zi-mu′re-ah)   urinary excretion of elevated levels of lysozyme.

lyssa (lis′ah) [Gr. "frenzy"; "*the worm* under the tongue of dogs, removed because of the belief that it caused rabies"]   1. rabies. 2. septum linguae.

lyssic (lis′ik)   pertaining to rabies.

lysso- (lis′o) [Gr. *lyssa* frenzy]   a combining form denoting relationship to rabies.

lyssodexis (lis″o-dek′sis) [*lysso-* + Gr. *dexis* a bite]   the bite of a rabid dog.

lyssoid (lis′oid) [*lysso-* + Gr. *eidos* form]   resembling rabies.

lyssophobia (lis″o-fo′be-ah) [*lysso-* + *phobia*]   morbid dread of rabies, with symptoms simulating those of that disease.

Lyster tube (lis′ter) [William J. L. *Lyster*, U. S. Army surgeon, 1869–1947]   see under *tube*.

lyterian (li-te′re-an)   indicative of the approach of lysis.

lytic (lit′ik)   1. pertaining to lysis or to a lysin.   2. producing lysis.   3. a word termination denoting lysis of the substance indicated by the stem to which it is affixed.

Lytta (lit′ah)   a genus of blister beetles; called also *Russian fly*. **L. vesicato′ria**, a species of beetles known as Spanish fly, or blister bug; it is the source of cantharidin. Called also *Cantharis vesicatoria*.

lytta (lit′ah)   rabies.

lyxose (lik′sōs)   an aldopentose, CH₂OH·(CHOH)₃·CHO.

lyze (līz)   lyse.

M

M   1. symbol for *molar* (solution); the expressions M/10, M/100, etc., denote the strength of a solution in comparison with the molar, as tenth molar, hundredth molar, etc.   2. symbol for *mega*.

M.   abbreviation for L. *mil, mille*, thousand; *misce*, mix; *mistura*, mixture; *macerare*, macerate; and for *maximal, meter, minim, muscle, myopia*, and *mucoid* colony (see under *colony*).

m.   meter.

μ   mu, the twelfth letter of the Greek alphabet; symbol for *micron*. See also *mu*.

M.A.   mental age; meter angle; Master of Arts.

Ma   symbol for *masurium;* now called *technetium*.

ma.   milliampere.

M.A.B.   British abbreviation for *Metropolitan Asylums Board*.

M.A.C.   maximum allowable concentration (of poisons encountered in industry, etc.).

Mac.   abbreviation for L. *macerare*, macerate.

Macaca (mah-kak′ah)   a genus of Old World monkeys. **M. cynomul′gus**, a species of South American monkeys, much used as laboratory animals. **M. mulat′ta**, a species of monkeys widely used in physiological research.

macaja, macaya (mah-kah′yah)   a fixed oil obtained from the fruit of the palm tree, *Acrocomia sclerocarpa*.

McBurney's incision, etc. (mak-ber′ne) [Charles *McBurney*, New York surgeon, 1845–1913]   see under *incision, operation, point*, and *sign*.

McCarthy's reflex (mah-kar′thēz) [Daniel J. *McCarthy*, American neurologist, 1874–1958]   see under *reflex*.

MacConkey's agar, broth (mah-kon′kēz) [Alfred Theodore *MacConkey*, English bacteriologist, 1861–1931]   see under *culture medium*.

Mace (mās)   trademark for an aerosol mixture of organic lacrimators.

macerate (mas′er-āt)   to soften by wetting or soaking; see *maceration*.

maceration (mas″er-a′shun) [L. *maceratio*]   the softening of a solid by soaking. In histology, the softening of a tissue by soaking, especially in acids, until the connective tissue fibers are so dissolved that the tissue components can be teased apart. In obstetrics, the degenerative changes with discoloration and softening of tissues, and eventual disintegration, of a fetus retained in the uterus after its death.

macerative (mas′er-a″tiv)   characterized by maceration.

Macewen's operation, sign, triangle (mak-u′enz) [Sir William *Macewen*, surgeon in Glasgow, 1848–1924]   see under *operation* and *sign*, and see *suprameatal triangle*, under *triangle*.

McGinn-White sign (mak-gin′hwit) [Sylvester *McGinn*, American cardiologist, born 1904; Paul Dudley *White*, American cardiologist, born 1886]   see under *sign*.

Machaon (mak′ah-on)   the older of two brothers, the younger being Podalirius, who were the sons of Aesculapius and, according to legend, were the chief medical officers attached to the Greek forces during the Trojan war.

Mache unit (mah′keh) [Heinrich *Mache*, Austrian physicist, born 1876]   see under *unit*.

machine (mah-shēn′) [L. *machina*]   a contrivance or apparatus for the production, conversion, or transmission of some form of energy or force. **heart-lung m.,** a combination blood pump (artificial heart) and blood oxygenator (artificial lung) used in open-heart surgery. **Holtz m.,** an apparatus for developing static electricity. **Van de Graaff m.,** an electrostatic gener-

ator of high voltage. **Wimshurst m.,** a machine for the development of static current.

macho (mah′cho)   (*obs.*) the tubercle type of cutaneous leishmaniasis.

Macht's test (makts) [David Israel *Macht*, American pharmacologist, born 1882]   see under *tests*.

macies (ma′she-ēz) [L.]   wasting.

macintosh (mak′in-tosh) [Charles *Macintosh*, Scottish chemist, 1766–1843, the inventor]   cloth made waterproof by treating with a solution of India-rubber; once used for surgical dressings.

macis (ma′sis) [L.]   mace.

Mackenrodt's ligament, operation (mahk′en-rōts) [Alwin Karl *Mackenrodt*, German gynecologist, 1859–1925]   see *plica rectouterina*, and see under *operation*.

Mackenzie's disease (mah-ken′zēz) [Sir James *Mackenzie*, Scottish physician, 1853–1925]   see *x disease* (def. 1), under *disease*.

Mackenzie's syndrome (mah-ken′zēz) [Sir Stephen *Mackenzie*, London physician, 1844–1909]   see under *syndrome*.

Maclagan's thymol turbidity test (mak-lahg′anz) [Noel Francis *Maclagan*, English pathologist, born 1904]   see *thymol turbidity test*, under *tests*.

McLean's formula (index) (mak-lānz′) [Franklin C. *McLean*, American physiologist, born 1888]   see under *formula*.

MacLean-Maxwell disease (mak-lān′ maks′-wel) [Charles Murray *MacLean*, physician in West Africa; James Laidlaw *Maxwell*, English physician in Formosa]   see under *disease*.

Macleod (mak-lowd′), John James Rickard.   Scottish physiologist, 1876–1935; co-winner, with Sir Frederick Grant Banting, of the Nobel prize for medicine and physiology in 1923, for their discovery of insulin.

MacLeod's capsular rheumatism (mak-lowdz′) [Roderick *MacLeod*, Scottish physician, 1795–1852]   see under *rheumatism*.

MacMunn's test (mak-munz′) [Charles Alexander *MacMunn*, British pathologist, 1852–1911]   see under *tests*.

McNaughten   see *M'Naghten*.

McPheeters' treatment (mak-fe′terz) [Herman Oscar *McPheeters*, American surgeon, born 1891]   see under *treatment*.

MacQuarrie's test (mah-kwor′ēz) [F. W. *MacQuarrie*, American psychologist]   see under *tests*.

Macracanthorhynchus (mak″rah-kan″tho-ring′kus)   a genus of acanthocephalans. **M. hirudina′ceus**, a species parasitic in swine in the United States; formerly called *Echinorhynchus gigas* and *E. hominis*.

macradenous (mak-rad′ĕ-nus) [*macro-* + Gr. *adēn* gland]   having large glands.

macrencephalia (mak-ren′sĕ-fa′le-ah)   macrencephaly.

macrencephaly (mak″ren-sef′ah-le) [*macro-* + Gr. *enkephalos* brain]   overgrowth of the brain.

macro- [Gr. *makros* large, or long]   a combining form meaning large, or of abnormal size or length.

macroaggregate (mak″ro-ag′re-gāt)   an unusually large aggregate of a substance.

macroaleuriospore (mak″ro-ah-lu′re-o-spōr)   a large, usually multicellular, aleuriospore; sometimes used interchangeably with macroconidium.

macroamylase (mak″ro-am′ĭ-lās)   a homogeneous molecular complex in which normal serum amylase may be bound to a variety of specific binding proteins, probably immunoglobulins, forming a complex too large for renal excretion; although not correlated with specific disease states, it may be suspected in hyperamylasemia or pancreatitis when urinary amylase levels are not raised concomitantly with serum levels.

macroamylasemia (mak″ro-am″il-ah-se′me-ah) the presence of macroamylase in the blood.

macroamylasemic (mak″ro-am″il-ah-se′mik) pertaining to or characterized by macroamylasemia.

macroanalysis (m k″ro-ah-nal′ĭ-sis) chemical analysis using 0.1 to 0.2 gm. of the substance under study.

Macrobdella (mak″ro-del′ah) a genus of leeches of the family Gnathobdellidae. **M. deco′ra,** the American leech, a small species widely distributed in United States and Canada, which is sometimes used in drawing blood.

macrobiota (mak″ro-bi-o′tah) the macroscopic living organisms of a region; the combined macroflora and macrofauna of a region.

macrobiotic (mak″ro-bi-ot′ik) pertaining to the macrobiota, or to macroscopic living organisms.

macroblast (mak′ro-blast) [macro- + Gr. blastos germ] an abnormally large nucleated red blood cell; a large young normoblast with megaloblastic features. **m. of Naegeli,** proerythroblast.

macroblepharia (mak″ro-blĕ-fa′re-ah) [macro- + Gr. blepharon eyelid] abnormal largeness of the eyelid.

macrobrachia (mak″ro-bra′ke-ah) [macro- + Gr. brachiōn arm] abnormal size or length of the arms.

macrocardius (mak″ro-kar′de-us) [macro- + Gr. kardia heart] a monster with an extremely large heart.

macrocephalia (mak″ro-sĕ-fa′le-ah) macrocephaly.

macrocephalic (mak″ro-se-fal′ik) macrocephalous.

macrocephalous (mak″ro-sef′ah-lus) having an excessively large head.

macrocephalus (mak″ro-sef′ah-lus) megalocephaly.

macrocephaly (mak″ro-sef′ah-le) [macro- + Gr. kephalē head] excessive size of the head.

macrocheilia (mak″ro-ki′le-ah) [macro- + Gr. cheilos lip + -ia] excessive size of the lips.

macrocheiria (mak″ro-ki′re-ah) [macro- + Gr. cheir hand + -ia] excessive size of the hands.

macrochemical (mak″ro-kem′ĕ-kal) pertaining to macrochemistry.

macrochemistry (mak″ro-kem′is-tre) [macro- + chemistry] chemistry in which the reactions may be seen with the naked eye. Cf. microchemistry.

macrochilia (mak″ro-ki′le-ah) macrocheilia.

macrochiria (mak″ro-ki′re-ah) macrocheiria.

macroclitoris (mak″ro-klit′o-ris) hypertrophy of the clitoris.

macrocnemia (mak″rok-ne′me-ah) [macro- + Gr. knēmē shin + -ia] a condition in which the legs are abnormally large below the knee.

macrocolon (mak″ro-ko′lon) megacolon.

macroconidium (mak″ro-ko-nid′e-um), pl. macroconidia [macro- + conidium] a large, frequently multicelled conidium or exospore; sometimes used interchangeably with macroaleuriospore; see spore.

macrocornea (mak″ro-kor′ne-ah) [macro- + cornea] megalocornea.

macrocrania (mak″ro-kra′ne-ah) abnormal increase in the size of the skull, the facial area being disproportionately small in comparison.

macrocyst (mak′ro-sist) [macro- + cyst] a large cyst.

macrocytase (mak″ro-si′tās) a term once used to describe the proteolytic activity of macrophages.

macrocyte (mak′ro-sīt) [macro- + -cyte] an abnormally large erythrocyte, i.e., one from 10 to 12 microns in diameter. Cf. megalocyte and gigantocyte.

macrocytic (mak″ro-sit′ik) pertaining to macrocytes.

macrocythemia (mak″ro-si-the′me-ah) [macrocyte + Gr. haima blood + -ia] a condition in which the erythrocytes are larger than normal.

macrocytosis (mak″ro-si-to′sis) macrocythemia.

macrodactylia (mak″ro-dak-til′e-ah) macrodactyly.

macrodactyly (mak″ro-dak′tĭ-le) [macro- + Gr. daktylos finger] abnormal largeness of the fingers and toes.

Macrodantin (mak″ro-dan′tin) trademark for a preparation of nitrofurantoin.

macrodont (mak′ro-dont) macrodontic.

macrodontia (mak″ro-don′she-ah) [macro- + Gr. odous tooth] abnormal increase in size of the teeth; it may affect a single tooth, or all of them (generalized macrodontia), and be true or only relative.

macrodontic (mak″ro-don′tik) pertaining to or characterized by macrodontia.

macrodontism (mak″ro-don′tizm) macrodontia.

macrodystrophia (mak″ro-dis-tro′fe-ah) [macro- + dys- + trophē nutrition] overgrowth of a part. **m. lipomato′sa**

progressi′va, partial gigantism associated with tumor-like overgrowth of adipose tissue.

macroelement (mak″ro-el′ĕ-ment) a chemical element, such as sodium or potassium, that is essential in nutrition and is distributed throughout the tissues in relatively large amounts, as opposed to trace elements.

macroencephaly (mak″ro-en-sef′ah-le) macrencephaly.

macroerythroblast (mak″ro-ĕ-rith′ro-blast) macroblast.

macroesthesia (mak″ro-es-the′ze-ah) [macro- + Gr. aisthēsis perception + -ia] a sensory impression that all things are larger than they really are.

macrofauna (mak″ro-faw′nah) the animal life, visible to the naked eye, which is present in or characteristic of a special location.

macroflora (mak″ro-flo′rah) the plant life, visible to the naked eye, which is present in or characteristic of a special location.

macrogamete (mak″ro-gam′et) [macro- + Gr. gametē wife] the larger, less active female gamete in anisogamy, which is fertilized by the smaller male gamete (microgamete).

macrogametocyte (mak″ro-gah-me′to-sīt) [macro- + Gr. gametē wife + -cyte] 1. a cell that produce macrogametes. 2. the female gametocyte of certain Sporozoa, such as malarial plasmodia, which matures into a macrogamete.

macrogastria (mak″ro-gas′tre-ah) [macro- + Gr. gastēr stomach + -ia] (obs.) dilatation of the stomach.

macrogenesy (mak″ro-jen′ĕ-se) [macro- + Gr. genesis production] gigantism.

macrogenia (mak″ro-jen′e-ah) [macro- + Gr. genys jaw] overdevelopment of the chin area.

macrogenitosomia (mak″ro-jen′ĭ-to-so′me-ah) [macro- + genito- + Gr. sōma body + -ia] excessive bodily development, with unusual enlargement of the genital organs. **m. pre′cox,** excessive bodily development, with marked enlargement of the genital organs, occurring at an unusually early age.

macrogingivae (mak″ro-jin-ji′ve) fibromatosis gingivae.

macroglia (mak-rog′le-ah) neuroglial cells of ectodermal origin, i.e., the astrocytes and oligodendrocytes considered together. Originally, the term was used synonymously with astroglia.

macroglobulin (mak″ro-glob′u-lin) a globulin of high molecular weight, in the 1,000,000 category, with sedimentation constants of 19S, as determined by ultracentrifugation; it has many of the characteristics of IgM. It is observed in the blood in a number of diseases, but mainly in various proliferative disturbances affecting the lymphoid, plasma cell, and reticuloendothelial systems.

macroglobulinemia (mak″ro-glob″u-lĭ-ne′me-ah) [macroglobulin + Gr. haima blood + -ia] a condition characterized by increase in macroglobulins in the blood. **Waldenström's m.,** a rare, progressive syndrome of the reticuloendothelial system first described by J. Waldenström, observed particularly in males past age 50, and associated with the presence of (monoclonal) IgM paraprotein, adenopathy, hepatomegaly, splenomegaly, hemorrhagic phenomena, anemia, and lymphocytosis and plasmacytosis of the bone marrow.

macroglossia (mak″ro-glos′e-ah) [macro- + Gr. glōssa tongue + -ia] excessive size of the tongue.

macrognathia (mak″ro-na′the-ah) [macro- + Gr. gnathos jaw + -ia] enlargement of the jaw.

macrogol (mak′ro-gol) solid and liquid polyethylene glycols, used as ointment bases and available in a wide range of degrees of solidity designated by numbers, the higher the harder.

macrographia (mak″ro-gra′fe-ah) macrography.

macrography (mak-rog′rah-fe) [macro- + Gr. graphein to write] the formation in writing of letters that are larger than the normal writing of the individual.

macrogyria (mak″ro-ji′re-ah) [macro- + gyrus] moderate reduction in the number of sulci of the cerebrum, sometimes with increase in the brain substance, resulting in excessive size of the gyri.

macrolabia (mak″ro-la′be-ah) [macro- + L. labium lip] macrocheilia.

macrolecithal (mak″ro-les′ĭ-thal) [macro- + Gr. lekithos yolk] having a large amount of yolk; see under ovum.

macroleukoblast (mak″ro-lu′ko-blast) a large leukoblast.

macrolide (mak′ro-līd) a macrolide antibiotic; see under antibiotic.

macrolymphocyte (mak″ro-lim′fo-sīt) a large lymphocyte.

macrolymphocytosis (mak-ro-lim″fo-si-to′sis) the presence of an increased number of large lymphocytes.

macromania (mak″ro-ma′ne-ah) [macro- + Gr. mania madness] 1. delusive belief that external objects or one's own members are larger than they really are. 2. megalomania; delusions of grandeur.

macromastia (mak″ro-mas′te-ah) [macro- + Gr. mastos breast + -ia] oversize of the breasts or mammae.

macromazia (mak″ro-ma′ze-ah) [*macro-* + Gr. *mazos* breast + *-ia*] macromastia.

macromelia (mak″ro-me′le-ah) enlargement of one or more limbs.

macromelus (mak-rom′e-lus) [*macro-* + Gr. *melos* limb] a fetus with abnormally large or long limbs.

macromere (mak′ro-mēr) [*macro-* + Gr. *meros* part] one of the large blastomeres formed by unequal cleavage of a fertilized ovum, located in the vegetal hemisphere and dividing less rapidly than the micromeres of the animal hemisphere.

macromethod (mak′ro-meth″od) a chemical method in which the substance to be analyzed is used in customary (not minute) quantity. Cf. *micromethod.*

macromimia (mak″ro-mim′e-ah) excessive or exaggerated mimicry.

macromolecular (mak″ro-mo-lek′u-lar) having large molecules; pertaining to macromolecules.

macromolecule (mak″ro-mol′ĕ-kūl) a very large molecule having a polymeric chain structure, as in proteins, polysaccharides, and other natural and synthetic polymers.

macromonocyte (mak″ro-mon′o-sīt) a very large monocyte.

macromyeloblast (mak″ro-mi′ĕ-lo-blast) a large myeloblast.

macronodular (mak″ro-nod′u-lar) characterized by large nodules.

macronormoblast (mak″ro-nor′mo-blast) a very large nucleated red blood corpuscle; macroblast.

macronucleus (mak″ro-nu′kle-us) [*macro-* + *nucleus*] in ciliate protozoa, the larger of two types of nucleus in each cell, which governs cell metabolism and growth. Called also *trophic nucleus* or *trophonucleus.* Cf. *micronucleus,* def. 1.

macronychia (mak″ro-nik′e-ah) [*macro-* + Gr. *onyx* nail + *-ia*] abnormal length of the finger nails.

macropathology (mak″ro-pah-thol′o-je) [*macro-* + *pathology*] the nonmicroscopical pathologic account of any disease or organ.

macrophage (mak′ro-fāj) [*macro-* + Gr. *phagein* to eat] any of the large, mononuclear highly phagocytic cells with a small, oval, sometimes indented nucleus and inconspicuous nucleoli, occurring in the walls of blood vessels (adventitial cells) and in loose connective tissue (histiocytes, phagocytic reticular cells). Derived from monocytes, they are components of the reticuloendothelial system and are usually immobile (fixed macrophages, resting wandering cells), but when stimulated by inflammation become actively mobile (free macrophages, wandering histiocytes). Macrophages also interact with B- and T-lymphocytes to facilitate antibody production. **alveolar m's,** rounded, granular, mononuclear phagocytes within the alveoli of the lungs that ingest inhaled particulate matter; called also *alveolar phagocytes* and *dust cells.* **armed m's,** those capable of inducing cytotoxicity as a consequence of antigen-binding by cytophilic antibodies on their surfaces or by factors derived from T-lymphocytes. **fixed m.,** a quiescent phagocyte, such as the histiocyte of loose connective tissue or those lining the sinuses of the liver, spleen, lymph nodes, and bone marrow. **free m.,** an ameboid phagocyte present at the site of inflammation; called also *polyblast* and *inflammatory macrophage.* **inflammatory m.,** free m.

macrophagocyte (mak″ro-fag′o-sīt) a phagocyte of relatively large size.

macrophagus (mak-krof′ah-gus) macrophage.

macrophallus (mak″ro-fal′us) [*macro-* + Gr. *phallos* penis] abnormal largeness of the penis.

macrophthalmia (mak″rof-thal′me-ah) [*macro-* + Gr. *ophthalmos* eye + *-ia*] abnormal enlargement of the eyeball.

macrophthalmous (mak″rof-thal′mus) having abnormally large eyes.

macropia (mah-kro′pe-ah) [*macro-* + Gr. *ōps* eye] macropsia.

macroplasia (mak″ro-pla′ze-ah) [*macro-* + Gr. *plasis* forming + *-ia*] excessive growth of a part or tissue.

macroplastia (mak″ro-plas′te-ah) macroplasia.

macropodia (mak″ro-po′de-ah) [*macro-* + Gr. *pous* foot + *-ia*] excessive size of the feet.

macropolycyte (mak″ro-pol′e-sīt) a hypersegmented polymorphonuclear leukocyte of greater than normal size. Cf. *polycyte.*

macropromyelocyte (mak″ro-pro-mi′ĕ-lo-sīt) a very large promyelocyte.

macroprosopia (mak″ro-pro-so′pe-ah) [*macro-* + Gr. *prosōpon* face + *-ia*] excessive size of the face.

macropsia (mah-krop′se-ah) [*macro-* + Gr. *opsis* vision + *-ia*] a disturbance of vision in which objects are seen as larger than they actually are.

macrorhinia (mak″ro-rin′e-ah) [*macro-* + Gr. *rhis* nose + *-ia*] excessive size of the nose.

macroscelia (mak″ro-se′le-ah) [*macro-* + Gr. *skelos* leg + *-ia*] excessive size of the legs.

macroscopic (mak″ro-skop′ik) [*macro-* + Gr. *skopein* to examine] visible with the unaided eye or without the microscope.

macroscopical (mak″ro-skop′e-kal) 1. pertaining to macroscopy. 2. macroscopic.

macroscopy (mah-kros′ko-pe) examination with the naked eye.

macrosigmoid (mak″ro-sig′moid) [*macro-* + *sigmoid*] abnormal enlargement of the sigmoid.

macrosis (mah-kro′sis) [*macro-* + *-osis*] increase in size.

macrosmatic (mak″ros-mat′ik) [*macro-* + Gr. *osmasthai* to smell] having the sense of smell strongly or acutely developed.

macrosomatia (mak″ro-so-ma′she-ah) [*macro-* + Gr. *sōma* body] great bodily size. **m. adipo′sa congen′ita,** an obese type of premature development probably dependent on hyperfunction of the adrenal cortex.

macrosplanchnic (mak″ro-splank′nik) [*macro-* + Gr. *splanchnon* viscus] having large viscera: a term applied to that type of body constitution in which the horizontal diameters are excessively developed as compared with the vertical ones. Cf. *microsplanchnic* and *pyknic.*

macrospore (mak′ro-spōr) [*macro-* + Gr. *sporos* seed] 1. the larger spore form when spores of two sizes are present, as in certain fungi and protozoa. 2. megaspore.

macrostereognosia (mak″ro-ste″re-o-no′se-ah) [*macro-* + Gr. *stereos* solid + *gnōsis* knowledge + *-ia*] abnormality of perception in which objects felt seem larger than they really are.

macrostomia (mak″ro-sto′me-ah) [*macro-* + Gr. *stoma* mouth + *-ia*] greatly exaggerated width of the mouth, resulting from failure of union of the maxillary and mandibular processes, with extension of the oral orifice toward the ear. The defect may be unilateral or bilateral.

macrostructural (mak″ro-struk′tūr-al) pertaining to gross structure.

macrotia (mak-ro′she-ah) [*macro-* + Gr. *ous* ear] abnormal enlargement of the pinna of the ear.

macrotome (mak′ro-tōm) [*macro-* + Gr. *tomē* cut] an apparatus for cutting large sections of tissue for anatomical study.

macrotooth (mak′ro-tōōth), pl. *macroteeth.* An abnormally large tooth.

macula (mak′u-lah), pl. *mac′ulae* [L.]. 1. a stain, spot, or thickening; [NA] a general term for an area distinguishable by color or otherwise from its surroundings. Often used alone to refer to the macula retinae. 2. a macule: a discolored spot on the skin that is not elevated above the surface. 3. a moderately dense scar of the cornea that can be seen without special optical aids, appreciated as a gray spot intermediate between a nebula and a leukoma. **acoustic maculae, mac′ulae acus′ticae,** see *m. sacculi* and *m. utriculi.* **m. acus′tica sac′culi,** m. sacculi. **m. acus′tica utric′uli,** m. utriculi. **m. adher′ens,** desmosome. **mac′ulae al′bidae,** white spots sometimes seen after death on the serous layer of the peritoneum. **mac′ulae atroph′icae,** white patches resembling scars formed on the skin by atrophy. **mac′ulae caeru′leae,** faint grayish blue spots, less than 1 cm. in diameter, sometimes occurring peripheral to the axillae or groins in patients with pediculosis corporis or pubis, caused by a substance in louse saliva that converts bilirubin to biliverdin; called also *taches bleuâtres.* **cerebral m.,** tache cérébrale. **m. commu′nis,** a thickened area on the wall of the otic vesicle that divides into the macula sacculi and macula utriculi. **m. cor′neae,** a circumscribed opacity of the cornea. **mac′ulae cribro′sae** [NA], see *m. cribrosa inferior, m. cribrosa media,* and *m. cribrosa superior.* **m. cribro′sa infe′rior** [NA], the perforated area on the wall of the vestibule through which branches of the vestibulocochlear nerve pass to the posterior semicircular canal. **m. cribro′sa me′dia** [NA], the perforated area on the vestibular wall through which branches of the vestibulocochlear nerve pass to the sacculus. **m. cribro′sa supe′rior** [NA], the perforated area on the vestibular wall through which branches of the vestibulocochlear nerve pass to the utricle and to the anterior and lateral semicircular canals. **m. den′sa,** a zone of compact, heavily nucleated cells, located in the distal renal tubule where it makes contact with the vascular pole of the glomerulus, and closely associated anatomically with the juxtaglomerular cells of the afferent arteriole. **false m.,** the extramacular point on the retina of a squinting eye which receives the same light stimulus as the macula of the fixing eye. **m. fla′va laryn′gis,** a yellowish nodule visible at one end of a vocal cord. **m. fla′va ret′inae,** m. retinae. **m. follic′uli,** the point on the surface of a vesicular ovarian follicle where rupture occurs. **m. germinati′va,** germinal area. **m. gonorrhoe′ica,** the red inflamed orifice of the duct of Bartholin's gland in gonorrheal vulvitis; called also *Saenger's m.* **mac′ulae lac′teae,** maculae albidae. **m. lu′tea ret′inae,** m. retinae. **maculae of membranous labyrinth,** see *m. sacculi* and *m. utriculi.* **mongolian m.,** see under *spot.* **m. ret′inae** [NA], an irregular yellowish depression on the retina, about 3 degrees wide, lateral to and slightly below the optic disk; it is the site of absorption of short wavelengths of light, and it is thought that its variation in size, shape, and coloring may be related to variant types of color vision. Called also *m. lutea retinae.* **m. sac′culi** [NA], a thickening in the wall of the saccule where the epithelium contains hair cells that are stimulated by linear acceleration and deceleration and gravity. The *m. sacculi* and *m. utriculi* together are called *maculae acusticae* or *acoustic maculae*. **Saenger's m.,** m. gonorrhoeica. **m. sola'ris** (*obs.*), a freckle. **mac'ulae tendin'eae,** maculae albidae. **m. utric'uli** [NA], a thickening in the wall of the utricle where the epithelium contains hair cells that are stimulated by linear acceleration and deceleration and gravity. The *macula sacculi* and the *macula utriculi* together are called *maculae acusticae* or *acoustic maculae*.

maculae (mak'u-le) [L.] plural of *macula*.

macular (mak'u-lar) pertaining to or characterized by the presence of macules; pertaining to the macula retinae.

maculate (mak'u-lāt) [L. *maculatus* spotted] macular.

macule (mak'ūl) a macula.

maculocerebral (mak"u-lo-ser'e-bral) pertaining to the macula retinae and the brain.

maculopapular (mak"u-lo-pap'u-lar) both macular and papular, as an eruption consisting of both macules and papules; sometimes erroneously used to designate a papule that is only slightly elevated.

maculovesicular (mak"u-lo-vě-sik'u-lar) both macular and vesicular.

MacWilliam's test (mak-wil'yamz) [John Alexander *MacWilliam*, British physician, 1857–1937] see under *tests*.

mad (mad) 1. insane. 2. rabid.

madarosis (mad"ah-ro'sis) [Gr. *madaros* bald] loss of the eylashes or eyebrows.

madder (mad'er) the root of *Rubia tinctoria* L. (Rubiaceae) affording a red dye, mainly alizarin and purpurin.

Maddox prism, rods (mad'oks) [Ernest Edmund *Maddox*, English ophthalmologist, 1860–1933] see under *prism* and *rod*.

Madelung's deformity, etc. [Otto Wilhelm *Madelung*, surgeon in Strasbourg, 1846–1926] see under *deformity, disease,* and *neck*.

Madurella (mad"u-rel'ah) a genus of imperfect fungi of the family Dematiaceae. *M. gris'ea* and *M. myceto'mi* are etiologic agents of maduromycosis.

maduromycosis (mah-du"ro-mi-ko'sis) a chronic disease caused by a variety of fungi (e.g., *Madurella mycetomi*) or actinomycetes (e.g., *Nocardia brasiliensis, Streptomyces madurae,* and others), affecting the foot, hands, legs, or other parts, including the internal organs. The most common form is that of the foot, known as *Madura foot*. Following infection through a penetrating wound, the deep tissues become necrosed, sinuses form, and there is marked swelling of the part, in which nodules and vesicles develop. Sinuses discharge pus and penetrate into the bone. The pus contains red, black, or yellow granules which are composed of mycelial filaments of the infecting organism.

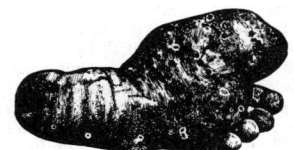

Maduromycosis.

maedi (mi'theh) a chronic progressive pulmonary disease of sheep in Iceland, caused by a virus.

mafenide (maf'en-īd) chemical name: 4-(aminomethyl)benzenesulfonamide. An antibacterial homologue of sulfanilamide, $C_7H_{10}N_2O_2S$, active against many gram-positive and gram-negative organisms. **m. acetate** [USP], the monoacetate salt of mafenide, $C_7H_{10}N_2O_2S \cdot C_2H_4O_2$, occurring as a white, crystalline powder, having the same antibacterial activity as the base; used as a topical anti-infective for adjunctive therapy of patients with second- and third-degree burns. **m. hydrochloride,** the hydrochloride salt of mafenide, $C_7H_{10}N_2O_2S \cdot HCl$, having antibacterial activity similar to that of the acetate salt; used as a topical anti-infective.

Maffucci's syndrome (mah-fu'chēz) [Angelo *Maffucci*, Italian physician, 1845–1903] see under *syndrome*.

mafilcon A (mah-fil'kon) chemical name: 2-methyl-2-propenoic acid 2-hydroxyethyl ester polymer with pentyl 2-methyl-2-propenoate, ethenyl acetate, ethenyl propanoate, and 3-hydroxy-2-naphthalenyl 2-methyl-2-propenoate; a hydrophilic contact lens material, $(C_6H_{10}O_3)_v(C_9H_{16}O_2)_w(C_4H_6O_2)_x(C_5H_8O_2)_y(C_{14}H_{12}-O_3)_z$.

Mag. abbreviation for L. *mag'nus,* large.

magaldrate (mag'al-drāt) [USP] chemical name: aluminum magnesium hydroxide. A chemical combination of aluminum hydroxide and magnesium hydroxide, corresponding approximately to the formula $Al_2H_{14}Mg_4O_{14} \cdot 2H_2O$; used as an oral antacid.

Magan (mag'an) trademark for magnesium salicylate.

mageiric (mah-ji'rik) [Gr. *mageirikos* relating to cookery] pertaining to cookery or dietetics.

magenblase (mah"gen-blah'zě) [Ger. "stomach bubble"] in the radiograph of the stomach, a dark area above the light shadow of the opaque meal, marking a collection of gas in the upper part of the stomach.

Magendie's foramen, etc. (ma-jen'dēz) [François *Magendie,* French physiologist, 1783–1855; the pioneer of experimental physiology in France] see under *foramen, law, phenomenon, solution,* and *space.*

Magendie-Hertwig sign (ma-jen'de-hert'vig) [François *Magendie;* Richard *Hertwig,* German zoologist, 1850–1937] skew deviation.

magenstrasse (mah"gen-stras'sě) [Ger. "stomach street"] canalis ventriculi.

magenta (mah-jen'tah) basic fuchsin. **acid m.,** acid fuchsin. **basic m.,** basic fuchsin. **m. O,** pararosanilin. **m. I,** rosanilin. **m. II,** triaminoditolyphenylmethane chloride, a component of basic fuchsin. **m. III,** new fuchsin.

magersucht (mah'ger-sookt) [Ger.] pathologic leanness.

maggot (mag'ot) a soft-bodied larva of an insect, especially a form living in decaying flesh. The living maggots of the greenbottle fly (*Phaenicia sericata*) and the blackbottle fly (*Phormia regina*) have been used in the treatment of osteomyelitis and other suppurative infections in order to clear away dead tissue and promote healing, this latter effect being due to the allantoin in the secretions of the maggots. **Congo floor m.,** *Auchmeromyia luteola.* **rat-tail m.,** a maggot of a hover-fly of the genera *Eristalis* and *Helophilus;* they cause intestinal and nasal myiasis. **sheep m.,** the maggot of *Phaenicia sericata* and other species of the family Calliphoridae, which invade the tissue of sheep in the British Isles and elsewhere.

magistery (maj'is-ter"e) [L. *magisterium; magister* master] a precipitate; any subtle or masterly preparation.

magistral (maj'is-tral) [L. *magister* master] pertaining to a master; applied to medicines that are prepared in accordance with a physician's prescription.

Magitot's disease (mazh"ĭ-tōz') [Emile *Magitot,* French dentist, 1833–1897] see under *disease.*

magma (mag'mah) [Gr. *massein* to knead] 1. a suspension of finely divided material in a small amount of water. 2. a thin, pastelike substance composed of organic material. **bentonite m.** [NF], a preparation of bentonite and purified water used as a suspending agent. **bismuth m.,** milk of bismuth. **dihydroxyaluminum aminoacetate m.** [USP], a white viscous suspension of dihydroxyaluminum aminoacetate in water, yielding an amount of aluminum oxide equivalent to between 28.5 and 35.0 per cent of the labeled amount of dihydroxyaluminum aminoacetate; used as a gastric antacid. **magnesia m.,** milk of magnesia; see under *milk.* **m. reticula're,** a mesenchymal reticulum within the early chorionic sac.

Magnacort (mag'nah-kort) trademark for a preparation of hydrocortamate.

Magnan's movement, symptom (sign) (mag'nanz) [Valentin Jacques Joseph *Magnan,* alienist in Paris, 1835–1916] see under *movement* and *symptom.*

magnesemia (mag"nes-e'me-ah) the presence of an excess of magnesium in the blood.

magnesia (mag-ne'zhe-ah) [the name of a district in ancient Lydia] magnesium oxide. **m. al'ba,** magnesium carbonate. **m. calcina'ta,** magnesium oxide. **m. carbonata'da,** magnesium carbonate. **citrate of m.,** magnesium citrate. **milk of m.,** see under *milk.* **m. us'ta,** magnesium oxide.

magnesite (mag-ne'sīt) native magnesium carbonate, $MgCO_3$; used like plaster of Paris in splints and dressings.

magnesium (mag-ne'ze-um), gen. *magne'sii* [L.] a light, silvery, metallic element; symbol, Mg; atomic number, 12; atomic weight, 24.312; specific gravity, 1.74. Its salts are essential in nutrition, being required for the activity of many enzymes, especially those concerned with oxidative phosphorylation. It is a component of both intra- and extracellular fluids and is excreted in the urine and feces. The serum level is approximately 2 mEq/liter. Deficiency causes irritability of the nervous system with tetany, vasodilation, convulsions, tremors, depression, and psychotic behavior. **m. aluminum silicate** [NF], a colloidal montmorillonoid saponite, in which magnesium has substantially replaced aluminum in the crystal lattice. It is available in Types IA, IB, IC, IIA, IIIA, and IIIB, which differ in viscosity and ratio of aluminum content to magnesium content. Used as a suspending agent for pharmaceuticals. **m. carbonate** [USP], a basic hydrated magnesium carbonate containing the equivalent of 40 to 43.5 per cent of magnesium oxide, used as an antacid. **m. chloride** [USP], colorless, deliquescent flakes or crystals, $MgCl_2 \cdot 6H_2O$, used as an electrolyte replenisher and as a pharmaceutic necessity for hemodialysis and peritoneal dialysis fluids. **m. citrate,** a white, odorless crystalline powder or granules, $Mg_3(C_6H_5O_7)_2 \cdot 14H_2O$, used in solution as a mild cathartic; called also *citrate of magnesia.* **m. hydroxide** [USP], a bulky white powder, $Mg(OH)_2$, used as an antacid and cathartic. **m. oxide** [USP], a bulky (*light m. oxide*) or relatively dense (*heavy m. oxide*) white powder, containing, after ignition, at least 96 per cent of MgO;

used as a sorbent in pharmaceutical preparations, and as an antacid and laxative. **m. peroxide,** a white powder, MgO_2, insoluble in water, but gradually decomposed with the liberation of oxygen; used as an antacid. **m. phosphate** [USP], a bulky, white powder, $Mg_3(PO_4)_2 \cdot 5H_2O$, used as an antacid. **m. salicylate,** the magnesium salt of salicylic acid, used as an antiarthritic. **m. stearate** [NF], a compound of magnesium with varying proportions of stearic and palmitic acids, used as a tablet lubricant in pharmaceutical preparations. **m. sulfate** [USP], small, colorless crystals, usually needle-like, $MgSO_4 \cdot 7H_2O$, used as an anticonvulsant and electrolyte replenisher, administered intramuscularly and intravenously. It is also used as a cathartic and as a local anti-inflammatory. Called also *Epsom salt.* **m. sulfate, exsiccated,** hydrated magnesium sulfate the weight of which has been reduced 25 per cent by drying at 100° C.: an aperient. **m. trisilicate** [USP], a compound of magnesium oxide and silicon dioxide with varying proportions of water, used as a pharmaceutic necessity and antacid.

magnet (mag′net) [L. *magnes;* Gr. *magnēs* magnet] a lodestone; native iron oxide that attracts iron; also a bar of steel or iron that attracts iron and has magnetic polarity. **Grüning's m.,** one made up of a number of steel rods; used in removing metal particles from the eye. **Haab's m.,** a powerful magnet for extracting foreign metallic bodies from the eye. **Hirschberg's m.,** an electromagnet for removing particles of iron from the eye. **permanent m.,** one with permanent magnetic qualities. **temporary m.,** a substance that possesses magnetic properties only during the passage of an electric current or when a permanent magnet is near it.

magnetic (mag-net′ik) pertaining to, derived from, or having the properties of a magnet.

magnetism (mag′nĕ-tizm) magnetic attraction or repulsion. **animal m.,** a hypothetical force or power alleged by Mesmer to be transmitted to his subjects undergoing therapeutic hypnosis. Cf. *mesmerism.*

magnetization (mag″net-i-za′shun) the act or process of rendering an object or substance magnetic.

magnetocardiograph (mag-ne″to-kar′de-o-graf) a cardiograph that generates electrical signals proportional to magnetic pulses emanating from electrical activity in the heart.

magnetoconstriction (mag-ne″to-kon-strik′shun) a change in the dimensions of a body produced by the application of a magnetic field.

magnetoelectricity (mag-ne″to-e″lek-tris′ĭ-te) electricity induced by means of a magnet.

magnetoencephalograph (mag-ne″to-en-sef′ah-lo-graf) an instrument for recording magnetic signals proportional to electroencephalographic waves emanating from electrical activity in the brain.

magnetoinduction (mag-ne″to-in-duk′shun) magnetic induction.

magnetology (mag″nĕ-tol′o-je) that branch of physics which treats of magnetics.

magnetometer (mag″nĕ-tom′ĕ-ter) [*magnetic* + Gr. *metron* measure] an apparatus for measuring magnetic forces.

magneton (mag′nĕ-ton) an ultimate elemental magnetic particle.

magnetotherapy (mag-ne″to-ther′ah-pe) the treatment of disease by magnets or by magnetism.

magnetron (mag′nĕ-tron) an electric vacuum tube for generating extremely short electromagnetic waves (microwaves).

magnetropism (mag-net′ro-pizm) [*magnet* + Gr. *tropē* a turn, turning] a growth response in a nonmotile organism under the influence of a magnet.

magnicellular (mag″nĭ-sel′u-lar) composed of large cells, as opposed to parvicellular.

magnification (mag″nĭ-fi-ka′shun) [L. *magnificatio; magnus* great + *facere* to make] 1. apparent increase in size as under the microscope. 2. the process of making something appear larger, as by use of lenses. 3. the ratio of apparent (image) size to real size.

magnify (mag′nĭ-fi) [L. *magnus* great + *facere* to make] to cause to appear larger by the use of lenses or suitable mirrors.

magnocellular (mag″no-sel′u-lar) magnicellular.

Magnolia (mag-no′le-ah) [after Pierre *Magnol,* 1638–1715] a genus of magnoliaceous trees.

magnolia (mag-no′le-ah) the bitter aromatic bark of *Magnolia acuminata* L., *M. glauca* L., and *M. tripetala* (Magnoliaceae), once used as a diaphoretic and antifebrile in southern United States.

magnum (mag′num) [L.] great; the os magnum (os capitatum [NA]).

mahamari (mah″hah-mah′re) the native name for a form of plague occurring in the southern slopes of the Himalayas.

Maher's disease (ma′herz) [James J. E. *Maher,* New York physician, 1857–1931] paracolpitis.

Mahler's sign (mah′lerz) [Richard A. *Mahler,* German obstetrician] see under *sign.*

ma huang (mah hoo-ang′) the native name for various species of *Ephedra,* including *E. sinica* Stapf., *E. equisetina* Bunge, and *E. vulgaris,* whose stems and leaves furnish ephedrine.

Maier's sinus (mi′erz) [Rudolf *Maier,* German physician 1824–1888] see under *sinus.*

maim (mām) 1. to disable by a wound; to dismember by violence. 2. a dismemberment or disablement effected by violence.

Maimonides (mi-mon′ĭ-dēz) (1135–1204) Rabbi Moses ben Maimon, called the greatest Jew after Moses, a native of Spain who later practiced medicine in Morocco and Egypt. A prayer attributed to him is considered to rank beside the oath of Hippocrates as an ethical guide to the medical profession.

main (mān) [Fr.] hand. **m. d'accoucheur** (mān″dak-oo-shuhr′), obstetrician's hand; see under *hand.* **m. de tranchées** (mān″dŭ-tran-sha′), trench hand. **m. en crochet** (ma″nong-kro-sha′), a permanently flexed condition of the third and fourth fingers. **m. en griffe** (ma″nong-grif′), clawhand. **m. en lorgnette** (ma″nong-lor-nyet′), opera-glass hand. **m. en pince** (ma″nong-pins′), cleft hand. **m. en singe** (ma″nong-sēnzh′), monkey hand. **m. en squelette** (ma″nong-skel-et′), skeleton hand. **m. fourché** (mān″foor-sha′), cleft hand. **m. succulente** (mān″suk-u-lent′), see *Marinesco's succulent hand,* under *hand.*

Mainini (mi-ne′ne) see *Galli Mainini.*

maise (māz) [L. *mais* maize] Indian corn; a cereal grain, the seed of *Zea mays.*

maisin (ma′zin) a protein found in the seeds of maize.

maisonneuve (ma″zo-nev′) Maisonneuve's urethrotome.

Maisonneuve's amputation, bandage, urethrotome (ma″zo-nevz′) [Jules Germain François *Maisonneuve,* French surgeon, 1809–1897] see under *amputation, bandage,* and *urethrotome.*

Maissiat's band (ligament, tract) (ma″se-ahz′) [Jacques Henri *Maissiat,* French anatomist, 1805–1878] tractus iliotibialis.

maizenate (ma′zen-āt) any salt of maizenic acid.

Majocchi's disease (purpura) (mah-yok′ēz) [Domenico *Majocchi,* Italian physician, 1849–1929] purpura annularis telangiectodes.

majoon (mah-joon′) see *ganja.*

makro- (mak′ro) for words thus beginning, see those beginning *macro-.*

mal (mahl) [Fr.; L. *malum* ill] disease. **m. de caderas,** a disease of horses, mules, and dogs in South America, characterized by weakness, especially of the hind quarters, and a staggering, swinging gait. It is caused by *Trypanosoma equinum* (now considered to be identical with *T. evansi*), which is transmitted by tabanid flies and by vampire bats (*Desmodus rotundus*). **m. de Cayenne,** elephantiasis. **m. comitial,** epilepsy. **grand m.,** see under *epilepsy.* **haut m.,** grand mal epilepsy. **m. de Meleda,** symmetrical keratosis of the palms and soles associated with an ichthyotic thickening of the wrists and ankles, a hereditary congenital disorder occurring endemically in the island of Meleda, off the coast of Dalmatia. It is transmitted as an autosomal dominant. **m. de mer,** seasickness. **m. morado,** a dermatitis caused by infection with *Onchocerca volvulus.* **m. perforant,** perforating ulcer of the foot. **petit m.,** see under *epilepsy.* **m. del pinto,** pinta. **m. rouge,** a syndrome occurring after inhalation or ingestion of calcium cyanamide followed by drinking an alcoholic beverage, marked by intense flushing, rapid pulse and pounding heart, panting respiration, and perception of the taste and smell of acetaldehyde in the exhaled breath, which may be followed by nausea, vomiting, and a precipitous fall in blood pressure; the extent and severity of the symptoms depend on the amount of calcium cyanamide and alcohol in the system. The reactions are due to the inhibition by calcium cyanamide of one or more of the enzymes required for oxidation of acetaldehyde formed from alcohol, resulting in the accumulation of acetaldehyde and the altered vascular reaction to it. A similar syndrome, also due to accumulation of acetaldehyde, occurs on ingestion of disulfiram followed by drinking an alcoholic beverage, but in addition there is impaired taste, unpleasant breath and perspiration, and lessened sexual potency.

mala (ma′lah) [L.] 1. NA alternative for *bucca,* or cheek. 2. the cheek bone.

malabsorption (mal″ab-sorp′shun) impaired intestinal absorption of nutrients; see also under *syndrome.*

Malacarne's pyramid, space (antrum) (mal″ah-kar′nāz) [Michele Vincenzo Giacintos *Malacarne,* Italian surgeon, 1744–1816] see *substantia perforata posterior,* and see under *pyramid.*

malacia (mah-la′she-ah) [Gr. *malakia*] 1. the morbid softening or softness of a part or tissue. Also used with combining forms to denote specific conditions, as *osteomalacia.* 2. craving for highly spiced food and dishes, as pickles, salads, mustard, etc. **metaplastic m.,** osteitis fibrosa cystica. **myeloplastic m.,** osteogenesis imperfecta. **porotic m.,** softening accompanied by proliferation of connective tissue. **m. traumat′ica,** Kienböck's disease (def. 2.).

malacic (mah-la'sik)   marked by malacia or morbid softness.

malaco- [Gr. *malakos* soft]   a combining form meaning a condition of abnormal softness.

malacoma (mal"ah-ko'mah) [*malaco-* + *-oma*]   a morbidly soft part or spot.

malacoplakia (mal"ah-ko-pla'ke-ah) [*malaco-* + Gr. *plax* plaque]   the formation of soft patches on the mucous membrane of a hollow organ.   **m. vesi'cae,** a soft, yellowish, fungus-like growth on the mucous membrane of the bladder and ureters.

malacosarcosis (mal"ah-ko-sar-ko'sis) [*malaco-* + Gr. *sarx* flesh]   softness of muscular tissue.

malacosis (mal"ah-ko'sis)   malacia.

malacosteon (mal"ah-kos'te-on) [*malaco-* + Gr. *osteon* bone]   osteomalacia.

malacotic (mal"ah-kot'ik)   inclined to malacia; soft; said of teeth.

malactic (mah-lak'tik)   1. softening; emollient.   2. an emollient medicine.

maladie (mal"ah-de') [Fr.]   a disease.   **m. bleue,** morbus caeruleus.   **m. de Capdepont,** dentinogenesis imperfecta.   **m. des jambes** (da-zhamb'), a disease of rice growers in Louisiana, probably beriberi.   **m. de Nicolas et Favre,** lymphogranuloma venereum.   **m. de plongeurs** (duh-plon-zher'), inflammation and ulceration in divers in the Mediterranean caused by the stings of sea anemones.   **m. de Roger,** Roger's disease.   **m. du sommeil** (du-so-ma'e), African trypanosomiasis.   **m. des tics,** Gilles de la Tourette syndrome.

maladjustment (mal"ad-just'ment)   in psychiatry, defective adaptation to environment, marked by anxiety, depression, and irritability.

malady (mal'ah-de) [Fr. *maladie*]   any disease or illness.

malagma (mah-lag'mah) [Gr.]   an emollient or cataplasm.

malaise (mal-āz') [Fr.]   a vague feeling of bodily discomfort.

malakoplakia (mal"ah-ko-pla'ke-ah)   malacoplakia.

malalignment (mal"ah-līn'ment)   displacement out of line, especially displacement of the teeth from their normal relation to the line of the dental arch.

malalinement (mal"ah-līn'ment)   malalignment.

malar (ma'lar) [L. *mala* cheek]   pertaining to the cheek or cheek bone.

malaria (mah-la're-ah) [It. "bad air"]   an infectious febrile disease caused by protozoa of the genus *Plasmodium*, which are parasitic in the red blood cells, and are transmitted by the bites of infected mosquitoes of the genus *Anopheles*. The disease is characterized by attacks of chills, fever, and sweating, occurring at intervals which depend on the time required for development of a new generation of parasites in the body. After recovery from the acute attack, the disease has a tendency to become chronic, with occasional relapses.   **algid m.,** falciparum malaria characterized by peripheral vascular failure, with coldness of the skin, prostration, and extensive involvement of the vessels of the gastrointestinal tract and other abdominal viscera.   **benign tertian m.,** vivax m.   **bilious remittent m.,** a pernicious form of falciparum malaria characterized by severe nausea, continual vomiting, high remittent fever, and jaundice appearing about the second day after onset.   **bovine m.,** Texas fever.   **cerebral m.,** falciparum malaria with delirium or coma, as a result of localization of parasites (parasitic thrombus) in the brain.   **cold m.,** algid m.   **m. comato'sa,** cerebral malaria characterized by coma.   **dysenteric m.,** falciparum malaria characterized by bloody diarrhea.   **estivoautumnal m.,** former name for falciparum malaria when it was endemic in the United States.   **falciparum m.,** the most serious form of malaria, caused by *Plasmodium falciparum*, characterized by severe constitutional symptoms and sometimes causing death.   **gastric m.,** falciparum malaria in which there is continual vomiting.   **hemolytic m.,** blackwater fever.   **hemorrhagic m.,** falciparum malaria in which hemorrhage is a prominent symptom.   **induced m.,** malaria that is purposely produced by introduction of the causative parasites, as sometimes used in treating neurosyphilis.   **malignant tertian m.,** falciparum m.   **ovale m.,** a mild disease caused by infection with *Plasmodium ovale*, usually characterized by a few regularly recurring tertian febrile paroxysms, beginning with a feeling of chilliness or cold shivers rather than the rigors typical of vivax malaria, and tending to end in spontaneous recovery.   **pernicious m.,** falciparum m.   **quartan m.,** that in which the febrile paroxysms occur every 72 hours, or every fourth day counting the day of occurrence as the first day of each cycle; it is caused by *Plasmodium malariae*, which requires 72 hours for completion of each asexual cycle in the crythrocyte.   **quotidian m.,** that in which the febrile paroxysms occur daily, due to simultaneous infection with two broods of *Plasmodium vivax*, which complete their 42- to 47-hour cycle on alternate days. See *vivax m.*   **subtertian m.,** falciparum m.   **tertian m.,** that in which the febrile paroxysms occur every 42 to 47 hours, or every third day counting the day of occurrence as the first day of the cycle. See *vivax m.*   **therapeutic m.,** induced m.   **vivax m.,** malaria caused by *Plasmodium vivax*, the form most common and most likely to recur; the febrile paroxysms commonly occur every other day (tertian m.), but may occur daily (quotidian m.), if there are two broods of parasites segmenting on alternate days.

malariacidal (mah-la"re-ah-si'dal)   destructive to malarial plasmodia; plasmodicidal.

malarial (mah-la're-al)   pertaining or due to malaria.

malariatherapy (mah-la"re-ah-ther'ah-pe)   malariotherapy.

malariologist (mah-la"re-ol'o-jist)   a person versed in or engaged in the study of malaria.

malariology (mah-la"re-ol'o-je) [*malaria* + *-logy*]   the study of malaria.

malariometry (mah-la"re-om'ĕ-tre)   the employment of quantitative methods in the study of malaria.

malariotherapy (mah-la"re-o-ther'ah-pe)   treatment of dementia paralytica by infecting the patient with malarial parasites, usually the parasite of tertian malaria (*Plasmodium vivax*) or of quartan malaria (*P. malariae*).

malarious (mah-la're-us)   pertaining to or marked by the presence of malaria.

malaris (mah-la'ris) [L.]   malar.

Malassez's disease, rests (mal"ah-sāz') [Louis Charles *Malassez*, physiologist in Paris, 1842–1909]   see under *disease* and *rest*.

Malassezia (mal"ah-se'ze-ah) [Louis Charles *Malassez*] *Pityrosporon*.   **M. furfur, M. macfadyani, M. tropica,** *Pityrosporon orbiculare*.

malassimilation (mal"ah-sim"ĭ-la'shun) [L. *malus* ill + *assimilatio* a rendering like]   1. imperfect, faulty, or disordered assimilation.   2. the inability of the gastrointestinal tract to transport to the body fluids one or more ingested nutrients, whether due to faulty digestion (maldigestion) or to impaired intestinal mucosal transport (malabsorption).

malate (ma'lāt)   any salt of malic acid; in biochemistry, the term is often used interchangeably with malic acid (see under *acid*).

malathion (mal"ah-thi'on)   chemical name: O,O-dimethyl-S-(1,2-dicarboxyethyl)dithiophosphate. An organophosphorus compound used as an insecticide.

malaxate (mal'ak-sāt)   to knead, as in making pills.

malaxation (mal"ak-sa'shun) [Gr. *malaxis* a softening]   an act of kneading.

Malcotran (mal'ko-tran)   trademark for a preparation of homatropine methylbromide.

maldevelopment (mal"de-vel'op-ment)   abnormal growth or development.

maldigestion (mal"di-jes'chun)   impaired digestion.

male (māl)   1. an organism of the sex that begets young or that produces spermatozoa.   2. masculine.

maleate (mal'e-āt)   any salt or ester of maleic acid.

malemission (mal"e-mish'un)   failure of the semen to be discharged from the urinary meatus in coitus.

Malerba's test (mah-ler'bahz) [Pasquale *Malerba*, Italian physician, 1849–1917]   see under *tests*.

maleruption (mal"ĕ-rup'shun)   faulty eruption of a tooth, so that it is out of its normal position.

malethamer (mal-eth'ah-mer)   a high weight copolymer of ethylene with maleic anhydride, cross-linked with 1 to 2 per cent, by weight, of vinyl crotonate; an antiperistalic agent.

malformation (mal"for-ma'shun) [L. *malus* evil + *formatio* a forming]   defective or abnormal formation; deformity; an anatomical aberration, especially one acquired during development.   **Arnold-Chiari m.,** see under *deformity*.

malfunction (mal-funk'shun)   dysfunction.

Malgaigne's amputation, etc. (mal-gānz') [Joseph François *Malgaigne*, French surgeon, 1806–1865]   see under *amputation, hook, luxation, pad,* and *triangle*.

maliasmus (mal"e-as'mus)   glanders, or farcy.

malignancy (mah-lig'nan-se) [L. *malignare* to act maliciously]   a tendency to progress in virulence; the quality of being malignant.

malignant (mah-lig'nant) [L. *malignans* acting maliciously]   tending to become progressively worse and to result in death. Having the properties of anaplasia, invasion, and metastasis; said of tumors.

malignin (mah-lig'nin)   a protein fragment present in the serum of patients with malignant glial tumors.

malignogram (mah-lig'no-gram)   a systematic arrangement of numerical values assigned to the various factors in cases of carcinoma.

mali-mali (mah"le-mah'le)   a form of saltatory spasm endemic in the Philippines.

malingerer (mah-ling'ger-er) [Fr. *malingre* sickly]   an individual who is guilty of malingering.

malingering (mah-ling'ger-ing)   the willful, deliberate, and fraudulent feigning or exaggeration of the symptoms of illness or injury, done for the purpose of a consciously desired end.

malinterdigitation (mal″in-ter-dij″i-ta′shun) failure of interdigitation of parts which are normally so related.

Mall's formula (mahlz) [Franklin Paine *Mall*, Baltimore anatomist, 1862–1917] see under *formula*.

malleability (mal″e-ah-bil′i-te) the quality of being malleable.

malleable (mal′e-ah-b'l) [L. *malleare* to hammer] susceptible of being beaten out into a thin plate.

malleal (mal′e-al) mallear.

mallear (mal′e-ar) pertaining to a malleus (def. 1).

malleation (mal″e-a′shun) [L. *malleare* to hammer] sharp and swift muscular twitching of the hands.

mallein (mal′e-in) [L. *malleus* glanders] a fluid from cultures of the glanders bacillus or an extract of the bacillus, which causes a rise of temperature when injected into an animal affected with glanders.

malleoidosis (mal″e-oi-do′sis) melioidosis.

malleoincudal (mal″e-o-ing′ku-dal) pertaining to the malleus and incus.

malleolar (mal-e′o-lar) pertaining to a malleolus.

malleoli (mal-le′o-li) [L.] plural of *malleolus*.

malleolus (mal-le′o-lus), pl. *malle′oli* [L., dim. of *malleus* hammer] a rounded process, such as the protuberance on either side of the ankle joint; [NA], a general term for such a process. **external m., m. exter′nus,** m. lateralis. **m. fib′ulae, fibular m.,** m. lateralis fibulae. **inner m., internal m., m. inter′nus,** m. medialis. **lateral m.,** m. lateralis. **lateral m. of fibula,** m. lateralis fibulae. **m. latera′lis** [NA], lateral malleolus: the rounded protuberance on the lateral surface of the ankle joint, produced by the m. lateralis fibulae. **m. latera′lis fib′ulae** [NA], lateral malleolus of fibula: the process at the outer side of the lower end of the fibula, forming, with the malleolus medialis tibiae, the mortise in which the talus articulates. **medial m.,** m. medialis. **medial m. of tibia,** m. medialis tibiae. **m. media′lis** [NA], medial malleolus: the rounded protuberance on the medial surface of the ankle joint, produced by the m. medialis tibiae. **m. media′lis tib′iae** [NA], medial malleolus of tibia: the process at the inner side of the lower end of the tibia, forming, with the malleolus lateralis fibulae, the mortise in which the talus articulates. **outer m.,** m. lateralis. **radial m., m. radia′lis,** processus styloideus radii. **m. tib′iae, tibial m.,** m. medialis tibiae. **ulnar m., m. ulna′ris,** processus styloideus ulnae.

Malleomyces (mal″e-o-mi′sēz) [L. *malleus* glanders + Gr. *mykēs* fungus] a name formerly given a genus of schizomycetes (order Eubacteriales). **M. mal′lei,** Pseudomonas mallei. **M. pseudomal′lei, M. whitmo′ri,** Pseudomonas pseudomallei.

malleotomy (mal″e-ot′o-me) [*malleus* + Gr. *tomē* a cutting] 1. the operation of dividing the malleus in cases of ankylosis of the ossicles of the middle ear. 2. the operation of separating the malleoli by dividing the ligaments which hold them together.

malleus (mal′e-us) [L. "hammer"] 1. [NA] the largest of the auditory ossicles, and the one attached to the membrana tympani; its club-shaped head articulates with the incus. Called also *hammer*. See Plate accompanying *ear*. 2. glanders.

mallochorion (mal″o-ko′re-on) [Gr. *mallos* wool + *chorion*] the primitive chorion; so called because of its villi.

Mallophaga (mal-of′ah-gah) [Gr. *mallos* wool + *phagein* to eat] an order of biting lice, the bird lice, which feed on the feathers and hair of birds and which may attack man and other mammals. It includes the genera Damalinia, Felicola, Heterodoxus, and Trichodectes. Cf. *Anoplura*.

Mallory's bodies, stain (mal′o-rēz) [Frank Burr *Mallory*, pathologist in Boston, 1862–1941] see under *body*, and see *Table of Stains*.

mallow (mal′o) [L. *malva*] any plant of the genus *Malva*. The flowers and leaves of *M. sylvestris* L. and *M. rotundifolia* L. (malvaceae) are demulcent and emollient, and are used in Asia and India for these properties.

malnutrition (mal″nu-trish′un) any disorder of nutrition; it may be due to unbalanced or insufficient diet or to defective assimilation or utilization of foods. **malignant m.,** kwashiorkor. **protein m.,** kwashiorkor.

malocclusion (mal″o-kloo′zhun) such malposition and contact of the maxillary and mandibular teeth as to interfere with the highest efficiency during the excursive movements of the jaw that are essential for mastication; originally classified by Angle into four major groups, depending on the anteroposterior jaw relationship as indicated by interdigitation of the first molar teeth, but Class IV is not used (see table). **closed-bite m.,** see *closed bite*, under *bite*. **open-bite m.,** see *open bite*, under *bite*.

malonal (mal′o-nal) (obs.) barbital.

malonyl (mal′o-nil) the divalent radical, OCCH₂CO.

Malpighi's pyramids, vesicles (mal-pig′ēz) [Marcello *Malpighi*, Italian anatomist, 1628–1694] see *pyramides renales* and *alveoli pulmonis*.

ANGLE'S CLASSIFICATION OF MALOCCLUSION

Class I (Neutroclusion). Normal anteroposterior relationship of the jaws, as indicated by correct interdigitation of maxillary and mandibular molars, but with crowding and rotation of teeth elsewhere, i.e., a dental dysplasia or an arch length deficiency.

Class II (Distoclusion). The lower dental arch is posterior to the upper in one or both lateral segments; the lower first molar is distal to the upper first molar.
  Division 1. Bilaterally distal with narrow maxillary arch and protruding upper incisors.
  Subdivision, unilaterally distal with other characteristics the same.
  Division 2. Bilaterally distal with normal or square-shaped maxillary arch, retruded maxillary central incisors, labially malposed maxillary lateral incisors, and an excessive overbite.
  Subdivision. Unilaterally distal with other characteristics the same.

Class III (Mesioclusion). The lower arch is anterior to the upper in one or both lateral segments; lower first molar is mesial to upper first molar.
  Division. Mandibular incisors are usually in anterior crossbite.
  Subdivision. Unilaterally mesial, with other characteristics the same.

Class IV. The occlusal relations of the dental arches present the peculiar condition of being in distal occlusion upon one lateral half, and in mesial occlusion upon the other half of the mouth.

malpighian bodies, etc. (mal-pig′i-an) [Marcello Malpighi, Italian anatomist, 1628–1694] see under *body, capsule, cell, corpuscle, glomerulus, layer, rete, stigma,* and *tuft*.

malposed (mal-pōzd′) not in the normal position.

malposition (mal″po-zish′un) [L. *malus* bad + *positio* placement] abnormal or anomalous position.

malpractice (mal-prak′tis) [L. *mal* bad + *practice*] improper or injurious practice; unskillful and faulty medical or surgical treatment.

malpraxis (mal-prak′sis) malpractice.

malpresentation (mal″prez-en-ta′shun) a faulty or abnormal fetal presentation.

malrotation (mal″ro-ta′shun) abnormal or pathologic rotation, as of the vertebral column; failure of normal rotation of an organ, as of the gut, during embryological development.

malt (mawlt) [L. *maltum*] grain, for the most part barley, which has been soaked, made to germinate, and then dried; it contains dextrin, maltose, and diastase. It is nutritive and digestant, aiding in the digestion of starchy foods, and is used in tuberculosis, cholera infantum, and other wasting diseases.

maltase (mawl′tās) α-glucosidase. See *glucosidase*.

malthusian law (mal-thu′se-an) [Rev. Thomas Robert *Malthus*, English economist, 1766–1834] see under *law*.

maltobiose (mawl″to-bi′ōs) maltose.

maltodextrin (mawl″to-dek′strin) a dextrin convertible into maltose.

maltoflavin (mawl″to-fla′vin) a flavin or lyochrome malt.

maltol (mawl′tol) a compound, 3-hydroxy-2-methyl-4-pyrone, CH·CH·CO·C(OH):C(CH₃).
|_____O_____|

maltosazone (mawl″to-sa′zōn) the phenylosazone of maltose, a yellow crystalline substance formed by treating maltose with phenyl hydrazine and acetic acid; the crystals melt at 205° C. and may be used in identifying maltose.

maltose (mawl′tōs) 4-*O*-[α-D-glucopyranosyl]-D-glucopyranose: a white crystalline disaccharide formed when starch is hydrolyzed by amylase; used as a nutrient and sweetener. Called also *maltobiose*.

maltoside (mawl′to-sīd) acetal of maltose, formed by condensation of an anomeric hydroxyl group with an alcohol; a compound homologous with a glucoside, but in which the sugar is maltose instead of glucose.

maltosuria (mawl″to-su′re-ah) the presence of maltose in the urine.

maltotriose (mawl″to-tri′ōs) a sugar consisting of three glucose molecules, resulting from the action of amylase on starch or glycogen.

maltum (mal′tum) [L.] malt.

malturned (mal-turnd′) turned abnormally; said of teeth twisted on their central axes.

Malucidin (mal″u-si′din) trademark for a yeast extract which has abortifacient activity in the dog, cat, and sheep.

malum (ma′lum) [L.] evil or disease. **m. articulo′rum seni′lis,** a painful, degenerative state of a joint, occurring as a result of aging. **m. cox′ae,** hip-joint disease. **m. cox′ae seni′lis,** osteoarthritis of the hip joint. **m. malan′num** ["evil year disease"], the name given during the Middle Ages to a carbunculus or gangrenous eruption affecting the jaws of man or animals, possibly anthrax or glanders. **m. per′forans pe′-dis,** perforating ulcer of the foot. **m. seni′le,** a variety of osteoarthritis peculiar to aged persons; see *morbus coxae senilis.* **m. vene′reum,** syphilis. **m. vertebra′le suboccipita′le,** tuberculosis of the atlas and axis.

malunion (mal-ūn′yon)   union of the fragments of a fractured bone in a faulty position.

Malva (mal′vah) [L.]   see *mallow.*

malvaria (mal-va′re-ah) [L. *malva* mallow + *-ia*] a term suggested by Hoffer and Osmond for a condition characterized by the presence of mauve factor (a substance that, on paper chromatography, gives a mauve color) in the urine; it has been reported in schizophrenia.

Maly's test (mah′lēz) [Richard Leo *Maly,* Austrian chemist, 1839–1894] see under *tests.*

mamanpian (mah-mahn′′pe-ahn′) [Fr. *maman* mother + *pian* yaw] mother yaw.

mamba (mam′bah)   an extremely venomous elapid tree snake of the genus *Dendroaspis.*

mamelon (mam′ĕ-lon) [Fr. "nipple"] 1. one of three tubercles sometimes present on the cutting edge of an incisor tooth. 2. the nipple-like elevation in the umbilicus, considered to be the remains of the solid lower part of the umbilical cord which contained the umbilical arteries and urachus.

mamelonated (mam′ĕ-lon-āt′′ed) (obs.) mamillated.

mamelonation (mam′′ĕ-lo-na′shun) (obs.) mamillation.

mamilla (mah-mil′ah), pl. *mamil′lae* [L., dim. of *mamma,* a breast, teat] 1. the nipple (papilla mammae [NA]). 2. any nipple-like structure. Written also *mammilla.*

mamillae (mah-mil′le) [L.]   plural of *mamilla.*

mamillaria (mam′′il-la′re-a)   miliaria profunda.

mamillary (mam′ĭ-ler′′e) [L. *mamilla,* dim. of *mamma,* a breast, teat] pertaining to or resembling a nipple.

mamillated (mam′′ĭ-lāt′ed)   having nipple-like projections.

mamillation (mam′′il-la′shun) 1. the condition of being mamillated. 2. a nipple-like elevation or projection.

mamilliform (mah-mil′ĭ-form) [*mamilla* + L. *forma* form] shaped like a nipple.

mamilliplasty (mah-mil′ĭ-plas′′te)   theleplasty.

mamillitis (mam′′ĭ-li′tis) [*mamilla* + *-itis*] inflammation of the mamilla, or nipple; thelitis.

mamma (mam′ah), pl. *mam′mae* [L.] [NA] the breast: the modified cutaneous, glandular structure on the anterior aspect of the thorax that contains, in the female, the elements that secrete milk for nourishment of the young. See *mammary gland,* under *gland.* **mam′mae accesso′riae [femini′nae et masculi′nae] [NA], accessory mammae,** mammary glands present in excess of the normal number, generally found along the line of the embryonic mammary crest; called also *accessory mammary glands.* **m. areola′ta,** a condition of the breast in which there is bulging of the areola of the nipple. **m. masculi′na [NA],** the rudimentary mammary gland of the male; called also *m. virilis.* **supernumerary mammae,** mammae accessoriae [femininae et masculinae]. **m. vir′ilis,** m. masculina.

mammae (mam′e) [L.]   plural of *mamma.*

mammal (mam′al)   an individual belonging to the class Mammalia.

mammalgia (mah-mal′je-ah)   mastalgia.

Mammalia (mah-ma′le-ah) a class of warm-blooded vertebrate animals, including all that possess hair and suckle their young.

mammalogy (mah-mal′o-je) [*mammal* + *-logy*] the study of mammals.

mammaplasty (mam′ah-plas′′te) [L. *mamma* + Gr. *plassein* to shape, form] plastic reconstruction of the breast, as may be performed to augment or reduce its size. **Aries-Pitanguy m.,** an operation to reduce mild to moderate macromastia. **augmentation m.,** plastic reconstruction of the breast, with increase of its volume by insertion of an autogenous or prosthetic material.

mammary (mam′er-e) [L. *mammarius*] pertaining to the mamma, or breast.

mammatrope (mam′ah-trōp)   mammotrope.

mammectomy (mah-mek′to-me) [*mamma* + Gr. *ektomē* excision] excision of the breast; mastectomy.

mammiform (mam′ĭ-form) [*mamma* + L. *forma* form] shaped like the mamma, or breast.

mammilla (mah-mil′ah)   mamilla.

Mammillaria (mam′′il-la′re-ah) a genus of cacti which have numerous sharp spines capable of inflicting painful wounds.

mammillary (mam′ĭ-ler′′e)   mamillary.

mammillated (mam′ĭ-lāt′ed)   mamillated.

mammillation (mam′′ĭ-la′shun)   mamillation.

mammilliform (mah-mil′ĭ-form)   mamilliform.

mammillitis (mam′′ĭ-li′tis)   mamillitis.

mammiplasia (mam′′ĭ-pla′ze-ah)   mammoplasia.

mammitis (mam-i′tis)   mastitis.

mammo- [Gr. *mammē,* Gr., L. *mamma* the mother's breast] a combining form denoting relationship to the breast, or mammary gland; see also words beginning *masto-* and *mazo-.*

mammogen (mam′o-jen)   any compound that promotes breast development.

mammogenesis (mam′′mo-jen′ĕ-sis) the development of the mammary glands to the functional state.

mammogram (mam′o-gram)   a roentgenogram of the breast.

mammography (mam-og′rah-fe)   roentgenography of the mammary gland.

mammoplasia (mam′′mo-pla′ze-ah) [*mammo-* + Gr. *plasis* formation + *-ia*] the development of breast tissue; called also *mastoplasia.* **adolescent m.,** the development of breast tissue at adolescence, applied especially to the development and later regression which occurs in males during puberty.

mammoplasty (mam′o-plas′′te) [*mammo-* + Gr. *plassein* to shape, form] plastic reconstruction of the breast, as may be done to augment or reduce its size.

mammose (mah-mōs′) [L. *mammosus*] 1. having large breasts, or mammae. 2. mamillated.

mammotomy (mam-mot′o-me)   mastotomy.

mammotrope (mam′o-trōp) one of the acidophils (alpha cells) of the adenohypophysis that stain with an affinity for azocarmine and erythrosin, and are thought to secrete prolactin or luteotropin. Called also *luteotrope* and *prolactin cell.*

mammotropic (mam′′-o-trop′ik) [*mammo-* + Gr. *tropikos* inclined] having affinity for or a stimulating effect on the mammary gland.

mammotropin (mah-mot′ro-pin) the lactogenic hormone, prolactin.

Man.   abbreviation for L. *manip′ulus,* a handful.

manaca (man′ah-kah) the Brazilian plant, *Brunfelsia (Franciscea) hopeana* Benth. (Solanaceae); formerly used in the treatment of syphilis and rheumatism.

manchette (man-chet′) [Fr. "a cuff"] a temporary band around the neck of a spermatozoon.

manchineel (man′′kĭ-nēl′) the *Hippomane mancinella,* a tree of tropical America; it contains a caustic poisonous sap or juice.

mancinism (man′si-nizm) [L. *mancus* crippled] left-handedness.

mandama (man-dam′ah)   the native name for phrynoderma.

Mandelamine (man′′del-ah′mēn) trademark for a preparation of methenamine mandelate.

mandelate (man′del-āt) any salt of mandelic acid; *ammonium mandelate* and *calcium mandelate* are used as urinary anti-infectives.

mandible (man′dĭ-b'l) the bone of the lower jaw; see *mandibula.*

mandibula (man-dib′u-lah), pl. *mandib′ulae* [L.] [NA] the mandible: the horseshoe-shaped bone forming the lower jaw; the largest and strongest bone of the face, presenting a body and a pair of rami, which articulate with the skull at the temporomandibular joints.

mandibulae (man-dib′u-le) [L.]   plural of *mandibula.*

mandibular (man-dib′u-lar)   pertaining to the lower jaw bone, or mandible.

mandibulopharyngeal (man-dib′′u-lo-fah-rin′je-al) pertaining to the mandible and the pharynx.

Mandragora (man-drag′o-rah) [L.] a genus of solanaceous plants. *M. officinarum* L. (Solanaceae), the true European or oriental mandrake, has the general properties of belladonna, and was formerly used as a narcotic and sedative. It contains the alkaloids mandragorine, hyoscyamine, and scopolamine.

mandrake (man′drāk)   see *Mandragora.*

mandrel (man′drel) the shaft on which a dental tool is held in the dental handpiece, for rotation by the dental engine.

mandril (man′dril)   mandrel.

mandrin (man′drin)   a stilet or guide for a catheter.

maneuver (mah-noo′ver) any dextrous proceeding; applied especially to procedures employed by the obstetrician in manual delivery of an infant. See also entries under *method, technique,* etc. **Adson's m.,** see under *tests.* **Allen m.,** with the forearm flexed at a right angle, the arm is extended horizontally and rotated externally at the shoulder, the head being rotated to the contralateral shoulder; obliteration of the radial pulse suggests scalenus anticus syndrome. **Bracht's m.** (for breech presentation), the breech is allowed to spontaneously deliver up to the umbilicus. The body and extended legs are held together with both hands maintaining the upward and anterior rotation of the fetal body. When the anterior rotation is nearly complete, the fetal body is held against the mother's symphysis. Maintenance of this position leads to spontaneous completion of delivery. **Brandt-Andrews m.,** a method of expressing the placenta from the uterus in the third stage of labor: the left hand grasps the umbilical cord while the right is placed on the maternal abdomen with the fingers over the anterior uterine surface. The right hand is gently pressed backward and slightly upward as the left applies gentle traction on the cord. **Chassard-Lapiné m.,** the patient sits and bends forward as far as possible. The roentgen rays, directed from above, penetrate the spine and outline the sigmoid loops in a transverse projection. **Credé's m.,** see under *method.* **DeLee's m.,** an obstetrical method of changing a face presentation to a brow presentation. **Engel-Lysholm m.,** a radiologic method of determining the size of the retrogastric organs or masses: the patient takes effervescent powders to fill his stomach with carbon dioxide, and assumes a prone position; a lateral view of the abdomen with a horizontal beam, and a posteroanterior projection with a vertical beam are made. **forward-bending m.,** a method of detecting retraction signs in neoplastic changes in the mammae; the patient bends forward from the waist with chin held up and arms extended toward the examiner. If retraction is present, an asymmetry in the breast is seen. **Fowler m.,** a test for tight intrinsic muscles in ulnar deviation of the digits: in rheumatoid arthritis a heavy, taut ulnar band is demonstrated when the digit is held in its normal axial relationship. **Halstead m.,** while the examiner exerts downward traction on the upper limb to be tested, the subject rotates his head toward the contralateral shoulder; obliteration of the radial pulse is suggestive of scalenus anticus syndrome. **Heiberg-Esmarch m.** (*obs.*), a pushing forward by the anesthetist of the patient's lower jaw in order to prevent the tongue from slipping backward. **Heimlich m.,** a method of dislodging food or other material from the throat of a choking victim: after wrapping the arms around the victim and allowing his upper torso to hang forward, make a fist with one hand and grasp it with the other; with both hands placed against the victim's abdomen slightly above the navel and below the rib cage, forcefully press into the abdomen with a quick upward thrust. If the victim is sitting, stand behind him and perform the same procedure, and if he is prone or unconscious, turn him on his back, kneel astride the torso, place both hands at the location on the victim's abdomen as described above and press forcefully with a sharp upward thrust. The maneuver may be repeated several times if necessary. **Hodge m.,** pressing up on the sinciput of the fetus during the labor pains, to increase flexion and thus assist rotation. **Hoguet's m.,** withdrawing the sac from beneath the deep epigastric vessels in hernioplasty. **Hueter's m.,** downward and forward pressure on the patient's tongue by the left forefinger of the physician during introduction of a stomach tube. **Jendrassik's m.,** a procedure for emphasizing the patellar reflex: the patient hooks his hands together by the flexed fingers and pulls apart as hard as he can. **Kappeler's m.** (*obs.*), a drawing forward of the patient's lower jaw by the anesthetist. **Leopold's m's,** four maneuvers in palpating the abdomen for ascertaining the position and presentation of the fetus. **Lovset's m.,** extraction of the arms in breech birth by clockwise and counterclockwise rotation of the fetus, after it has been expelled up to the umbilicus. **McDonald m.,** measurement of the contour of the abdomen from the upper margin of the symphysis pubis to the uterine fundus to calculate the duration of pregnancy. **Mauriceau m.,** a method of delivering the after-coming head in cases of breech presentation. **Müller's m.,** an inspiratory effort with a closed glottis after expiration, used during fluoroscopic examination to cause a negative intrathoracic pressure which is helpful in recognizing esophageal varices, and distinguishing vascular from nonvascular structures. **Müller-Hillis m.,** procedures for ascertaining the relation between the size of the fetal head and the pelvis of the mother. **Munro Kerr m.,** a maneuver for ascertaining the proportion between the head of the fetus and the pelvis of the mother. **Nägeli's m.,** upward traction on the patient's head applied with one hand under the occiput and the other under the jaw, for cure of nosebleed. **Pajot's m.,** for forceps traction along the axis of superior strait; one hand over the lock of the forceps pulls downward towards the floor, while the other hand applies horizontal traction. **Phalen's m.** (for detection of carpal tunnel syndrome), the size of the carpal tunnel is reduced by holding the affected hand with the wrist fully flexed or extended for 30 to 60 seconds, or by placing a sphygmomanometer cuff on the involved arm and inflating to a point between diastolic and systolic pressure for 30 to 60 seconds. **Pinard's m.,** a method of bringing down the foot in breech extraction. **Prague m.,** a method in breech presentation of engaging the head by bringing down the breech and making traction on the head with the finger, which is hooked over the nape of the neck. **Ritgen m.,** delivery of the fetal head by lifting the head upward and forward through the vulva, between pains, by pressing with the tips of the fingers upon the perineum behind the anus. **Saxtorph's m.,** Pajot's m. **Scanzoni m.,** a method of forceps rotation of the fetal head in the posterior position of the occiput. **Schatz's m.,** an obstetrical method of changing a face presentation into a brow presentation. **Schreiber's m.,** rubbing of the inner side of the upper part of the thigh while testing for patellar reflex. **Toynbee m.,** pinching the nostrils and swallowing; if the auditory tube is patent, the tympanic membrane will retract medially. **Valsalva's m.,** 1. forcible

exhalation effort against a closed glottis; the resultant increase in intrathoracic pressure interferes with venous return to the heart. 2. forcible exhalation effort against occluded nostrils and a closed mouth; the increased pressure in the eustachian tube and middle ear causes the tympanic membrane to move outward. **Van Hoorn's m.,** a maneuver like the Prague maneuver, with the addition of pressure on the fetal forehead from outside. **Wigand's m.,** see under *version.*

manganese (man'gah-nēs) [L. *manganum, manganesium*] a metal resembling iron; symbol, Mn; atomic number, 25; atomic weight, 54.938; specific gravity, 7.2. Manganous salts occur in body tissue in very small amounts and act as an activator of liver arginase and other enzymes. See also *manganese poisoning,* under *poisoning.* **m. butyrate,** a red powder, $(CH_3CH_2CH_2COO)_2$-Mn, formerly used in treatment of some skin diseases. **m. glycerophosphate,** a white or pinkish white powder, C_3H_7Mn-O_6P, formerly used as a hematinic and nerve tonic. **m. hypophosphite,** a pink, granular or crystalline powder, $Mn(H_2$-$PO_2)_2 \cdot H_2O$, used as a nutrient and dietary supplement and formerly as a hematinic. **m. sulfate,** a salt, $MnSO_4 + 4H_2O$, used in veterinary medicine in the prevention of perosis in poultry.

manganic (man-gan'ik) pertaining to manganese as a trivalent element.

manganism (man'gah-nizm) manganese poisoning; see under *poisoning.*

manganous (man'gah-nus) pertaining to manganese as a divalent element.

manganum (man'gah-num) [L.] manganese.

mange (mānj) a communicable skin disease of domestic animals, due to various mites, including *Chorioptes, Demodex, Notoedres, Psoroptes, Sarcoptes,* etc. **demodectic m., follicular m.,** an often intractable form of mange caused by infestation with mites of the genus *Demodex.* **psoroptic m.,** mange caused by species of the genus *Psoroptes.* **sarcoptic m.,** mange due to infestation with mites of the genus *Sarcoptes,* which burrow into the skin. **Texas m.** (*obs.*), grain itch.

Mangoldt's epithelial grafting (mahn'gōlts) [Heinrich von *Mangoldt,* Dresden surgeon, 1860–1909] see under *grafting.*

mangosteen (man'gos-tēn) the pericarp of the fruit of *Garcinia mangostana* L. (Guttiferaceae); astringent.

mangostin (man'gos-tin) a yellow, crystalline, xanthone type of pigment, $C_{23}H_{24}O_6$, from mangosteen rind.

mania (ma'ne-ah) [Gr. "madness"] 1. a phase of mental disorder characterized by an expansive emotional state, elation, hyperirritability, overtalkativeness or flight of ideas, and increased motor activity; specifically, the manic type of manic-depressive psychosis. 2. as a combining form, it signifies obsessive preoccupation with something, as in *dipsomania, erotomania, tomomania,* etc. **acute hallucinatory m.,** Ganser's syndrome. **akinetic m.,** marked emotional exaltation with decreased psychomotor activity. **m. àpotu,** delirium tremens. **Bell's m.,** acute delirium. **dancing m.,** a disorder characterized by uncontrolled dancing. **doubting m.,** folie de doute. **epileptic m.,** mania with attacks of violence following, preceding, or replacing an epileptic attack. **hysterical m.,** mania as one of the concomitants of a hysterical condition. **periodical m.,** a condition in which maniacal attacks of varying duration follow one another at more or less regular intervals. **puerperal m.,** the manic reaction that sometimes follows childbirth. **Ray's m.,** so-called moral insanity. **reasoning m.,** simple mania with active but perverted ideation. **religious m.,** mania with abnormal or perverted religious impulses. **transitory m.,** severe frenzied mania the attacks of which are of short duration. **unproductive m.,** a condition in which the behavior is that of mania, but the patient's thinking and speech are repressed.

maniac (ma'ne-ak) [L. *maniacus*] one who is affected with mania.

maniacal (mah-ni'ah-kal) affected with mania.

manic (ma'nik) pertaining to or affected with mania.

manic-depressive (ma'nik-de-pres'iv) alternating between attacks of mania and depression; see under *psychosis.*

manikin (man'ĭ-kin) a model of the body, with movable members and parts, used to illustrate anatomy, or for the teaching of nursing and obstetrics, or certain surgical procedures, such as the removal of foreign bodies by bronchoscopy.

maniloquism (mah-nil'o-kwizm) [L. *manus* hand + *loqui* speak] dactylology.

maniluvium (man'ĭ-lu've-um) a hand bath.

Manip. abbreviation for L. *manip'ulus,* a handful.

maniphalanx (man''ĭ-fa'lanks) [L. *manus* hand + *phalanx*] a phalanx of the hand.

manipulation (mah-nip''u-la'shun) [L. *manipulare* to handle] skillful or dextrous treatment by the hand. In physical therapy, the forceful passive movement of a joint beyond its active limit of motion. **conjoined m.,** manipulation with both hands.

manipulus (mah-nip'u-lus) [L.] handful.

Mann's sign (manz) [John Dixon *Mann,* English physician, 1840–1912] see under *sign.*

Mann-Bollman fistula (man-bol′man) [Frank Charles *Mann,* American physiologist and surgeon, 1887–1962; Jesse Louis *Bollman,* American physiologist, born 1896] see under *fistula.*

Mann-Williamson ulcer (man′wil′yam-son) [Frank C. *Mann;* Carl S. *Williamson,* American surgeon, 1896–1952] see under *ulcer.*

manna (man′ah) [L.] the dried saccharine exudation from the flowering ash tree, *Fraxinus ornus* L. (Oleaceae); its chief constituents are mannitol, mucilage, and sugar, and it has been used as a laxative.

mannan (man′an) a hard, white, insoluble polysaccharide, $(C_6H_{10}O_5)_n$, which yields mannose on hydrolysis; it is found in the vegetable ivory nut, *Phytelephas macrocarpa,* and other plants.

mannans (man′anz) a complex polysaccharide containing mannose $(C_6H_{12}O_6)$ and other moieties, frequently found in the cell walls of fungi, particularly yeasts.

mannerism (man′er-izm) a stereotyped movement or habit peculiar to a given individual.

manninotriose (man″ĭ-no-tri′ōs) a trisaccharide, $C_{18}H_{32}O_{16}$, from ash manna, which on hydrolysis yields two molecules of galactose and one of glucose.

mannitan (man′ĭ-tan) a modified form of mannitol, having an internal ring formation in the molecule and which tends to revert to mannitol.

mannite (man′īt) mannitol.

mannitol (man′ĭ-tol) a sugar alcohol, $HOCH_2(CHOH)_4CH_2OH$, widely distributed in plants and fungi, and obtained from manna and seaweeds. A preparation [USP] containing between 98 and 102 per cent of mannitol, calculated on a dry basis, is used intravenously as a diuretic. It is also used in diagnostic tests of kidney function. Called also *mannite.* **m. hexanitrate,** a compound formed by the nitration of mannitol; used as a vasodilator, mainly in urinary insufficiency.

mannitose (man′ĭ-tōs) mannose.

Mannkopf's sign (symptom) (mahn′kopfs) [Emil Wilhelm *Mannkopf,* German physician, 1836–1918] see under *sign.*

Mannkopf-Rumpf sign (mahn′kopf-roompf) [E. W. *Mannkopf;* Heinrich Theodore *Rumpf,* German physician, born 1851] Mannkopf's sign.

mannocarolose (man″o-kar′o-lōs) a polysaccharide made up of D-mannose units and formed by the growth of *Penicillium charlesii* on culture media containing glucose.

mannohydrazone (man″o-hi′drah-zōn) the phenylhydrazone of mannose. It consists of colorless platelike crystals which melt at 195° C. and may be used in identifying mannose.

mannoketoheptose (man″o-ke″to-hep′tōs) a natural sugar, $CH_2OH\cdot CO(CHOH)_4\cdot CH_2OH$, found in the avocado, *Persea americana* mill.

mannopyranose (man″o-pi′rah-nōs) mannose in cyclic hemiacetal form.

mannosan (man′o-san) mannan.

mannose (man′ōs) a monosaccharide, $CH_2OH\cdot (CHOH)_4\cdot CHO$: an aldohexose sugar produced by the oxidation of mannitol, similar to dextrose in general properties and conveniently prepared by hydrolyzing the vegetable ivory nut.

mannosidase (man′o-sĭ-dās) an enzyme, a glycoside hydrolase that catalyzes the hydrolysis of mannoside to an alcohol and D-mannose. The two forms, α- and β-mannosidase, react with α-D- and β-D-mannoside, respectively.

mannoside (man′o-sīd) a glycoside of mannose.

mannosidosis (man′ōs-ĭ-do′sis) an inborn error of metabolism marked by a defect in α-mannosidase activity that results in lysosomal accumulation of mannose-rich substrates; clinically, there are coarse facial features, upper respiratory congestion and infections, profound mental retardation, hepatosplenomegaly, cataracts, radiographic signs of dyostosis multiplex, and gibbus deformity. A much milder clinical form also occurs. It is thought to be an autosomal recessive trait.

mannosidostreptomycin (man″o-si″do-strep″to-mi′sin) a natural compound of streptomycin joined glycosidically to D-mannose.

mannosocellulose (man-o″so-sel′u-lōs) a variety of polysaccharide from coffee; it is changed by hydrolysis into mannose and dextrose.

Manoiloff's (Manoilov's) reaction (man-oi′lofs) [E. O. *Manoiloff,* Russian physician, born 1867] see under *reaction.*

manometer (mah-nom′ĕ-ter) [Gr. *manos* thin + *metron* measure] an instrument for measuring the pressure or tension of liquids or gases, as the blood, etc. **aneroid m.,** a device that measures pressure by means of an elastic container as compared to that of a vacuum, a true total-pressure-measuring instrument.

manometric (man″o-met′rik) 1. pertaining to or ascertained by the manometer. 2. varying with the pressure.

manoptoscope (man-op′to-skōp) [L. *manus* hand + Gr. *optos* seen + *skopein* to examine] an apparatus for detecting ocular dominance.

manoscopy (man-os′ko-pe) the measurement of the density of gases.

Man. pr. abbreviation for L. *ma′ne pri′mo,* early in the morning.

manquea (mahn-ka′ah) actinobacillosis of young cattle in South America, marked by the formation of abscesses upon the legs.

mansa (man′sah) the root or rhizome of *Anemonopsis californica* Hook. and Arn. (syn. *Houttuynia californica* Benth. and Hook.), Saururaceae. A perennial herbaceous plant indigenous to southwestern United States and adjacent Mexico, where it is locally used to relieve colds and indigestion, and to purify the blood.

Manson's hemoptysis, schistosomiasis (disease) (man′sonz) [Sir Patrick *Manson,* British physician, 1844–1922] see under *hemoptysis* and *schistosomiasis.*

Mansonella ozzardi (man″so-nel′ah o-zar′de) a filarial nematode parasite found in the mesentery and visceral fat of man in Panama, Yucatan, Guyana, Surinam, and Argentina.

mansonelliasis (man″so-nel-i′ah-sis) infection with *Mansonella ozzardi*; it is generally asymptomatic.

Mansonia (man-so′ne-ah) a genus of mosquitoes, several species of which transmit *Brugia malayi.* Some species may also transmit viruses such as those causing equine encephalomyelitis.

Mansonioides (man-so-ne-oi′-dēz) a subgenus of *Mansonia.* **M. annulif′era,** the chief vector of *Wuchereria malayi* in India.

mantle (man′t′l) [L. *mantellum* cloak] an enveloping cover or layer. **brain m.,** pallium. **chordomesodermal m.,** a continuous epithelial sheet composed of notochordal and mesodermal material during gastrulation. **myoepicardial m.,** a layer of visceral mesoderm in the early embryo, surrounding the endocardial tube and developing into the myocardium and epicardium.

Mantoux conversion, reversion, test (reaction) (man-too′) [Charles *Mantoux,* French physician, 1877–1947] see under *conversion, reversion,* and *tests.*

mantra (man′trah) a Sanskrit syllable or word repeated over and over again in the technique of transcendental meditation.

manual (man′u-al) [L. *manualis; manus* hand] of or pertaining to the hand; performed by the hand or hands.

manubria (mah-nu′bre-ah) [L.] plural of *manubrium.*

manubrium (mah-nu′bre-um), pl. *manu′bria* [L.] [NA] a general term for a handle-like structure or part; often used alone to designate the manubrium sterni. **m. mal′lei** [NA], **m. of malleus,** the largest process of the malleus; it is attached to the middle layer of the tympanic membrane and has the tendon of the tensor tympani muscle attached to it. **m. ster′ni** [NA], **m. of sternum,** the cranial portion of the sternum, which articulates with the clavicles and the first two pairs of ribs; called also *presternum.*

manudynamometer (man″u-di″nah-mom′ĕ-ter) [L. *manus* hand + Gr. *dynamis* force + *metron* measure] an apparatus for measuring the force of the thrust of an instrument.

manus (ma′nus), pl. *ma′nus* [L.] [NA], the hand: the distal portion of the arm, including the carpus, metacarpus, and fingers. **m. ca′va,** a hand deformed by a deep hollowing of the palm. **m. exten′sa,** backward deviation of the hand. **m. flex′a,** forward deviation of the hand. **m. pla′na,** flattening of the arch formed normally by the proximal row of the carpal bones; flat hand. **m. superexten′sa,** manus extensa. **m. val′ga,** clubhand marked by deflection of the hand toward the radial side; Madelung's deformity. **m. va′ra,** clubhand marked by deflection of the hand to the ulnar side.

manyplies (men′ĭ-plīz″) omasum.

Manz's glands (mahnts′ez) [Wilhelm *Manz,* German ophthalmologist, 1833–1911] see under *gland.*

manzanita (man″zah-ne′ta) [Sp., dim. of *manzana* apple] a small shrub or tree *Arctostaphylos manzanita* Parry (Ericaceae), found in the western part of the United states; the leaves are used by the local Indians as a medicinal tea, astringent, tonic, and diuretic.

Manzullo's test (man-zul′ōz) [Alfredo *Manzullo,* Buenos Aires physician] see *tellurite test,* under *tests.*

MAO monoamine oxidase.

Maolate (ma′o-lāt) trademark for a preparation of chlorphenesin carbamate.

map (map′) a two-dimensional graphic representation of arrangement in space. **fate m.,** a plan of a blastula or early gastrula stage of an embryo showing areas of prospective significance in normal development. **genetic m.,** a graphic representation of the linear arrangement of genes on a chromosome, their relative distance from one another being given in map units (see under *unit*). **linkage m.,** a graphic representation of the relative positions of, and distances between, genes on the same chromosome.

mapping (map′ing) the locating of the relative position of genes on a chromosome.

maprotiline (mah-pro′tĭ-lēn) chemical name: *N*-methyl - 9, 10 - ethanoanthracene - 9 (10*H*)-propylamine; an antidepressant, $C_{20}H_{23}N$.

Marañón's sign (reaction), syndrome (mar-ahn′yonz) [Gregorio *Marañón*, Spanish physician, 1888– 1960] see under *sign* and *syndrome*.

Maranta (mah-ran′tah) [after B. *Maranta*, physician in Venosa, died 1554] a genus of tropical herbs; the roots of several species afford a starch used as a dusting powder and demulcent.

marantic (mah-ran′tik) [Gr. *marantikos* wasting away] marasmic.

marasmatic (mar″az-mat′ik) marasmic.

marasmic (mah-raz′mik) pertaining to or characterized by marasmus.

marasmoid (mah-raz′moid) [Gr. *marasmos* a dying away + *eidos* form] resembling marasmus.

marasmus (mah-raz′mus) [Gr. *marasmos* a dying away] a form of protein-calorie malnutrition chiefly occurring during the first year of life, characterized by growth retardation and progressive wasting of subcutaneous fat and muscle, but usually with retention of the appetite and mental alertness. Infectious diseases may be precipitating factors. Marasmus is now considered to be related to kwashiorkor. Called also *infantile atrophy, athrepsia, pedatrophy,* and *decomposition* (Finkelstein), *m. infantilis,* and *m. lactanium.* **enzootic m.,** a condition of malnutrition in domestic herbivorous animals due to a deficiency of one or more of the trace elements, especially cobalt and copper. It is marked by progressive emaciation, severe anemia, and finally prostration; similar conditions are *bush sickness* in New Zealand, *pine* or *pining* in Scotland, and *salt sickness* in Florida. **nutritional m.,** marasmic kwashiorkor.

marble (mar′bl) [L. *marmor*] native crystalline calcium carbonate occurring as a rock.

marbleization (mar″bel-i-za′shun) the state of being veined like marble.

marc (mark) [Fr.] the residue left after maceration of substances used in the preparation of various drugs.

Marcaine (mar-kān′) trademark for a preparation of bupivacaine hydrochloride.

march (march) in neurology, the progression of epileptic activity through the motor cortex, as in jacksonian epilepsy.

Marchand's adrenals (organs) (mar′shandz) [Felix Jacob *Marchand*, German pathologist, 1846–1928] see under *adrenal,* and see *adventitial cell,* under *cell.*

marche à petits pas (marsh-ah-pte′pah) [Fr.] a gait in which the patient takes very short steps: seen in cerebral arteriosclerotic rigidity.

Marchi's balls, etc. (mar′kēz) [Vittorio *Marchi,* Italian physician, 1851–1908] see under *ball, globule, reaction, Table of Stains,* and *tract.*

Marchiafava-Bignami disease (mar″ke-ah-fah′vah-bēn-yah′me) [Ettore *Marchiafava,* Italian pathologist, 1847–1935; Amico *Bignami,* Italian pathologist, 1862–1929] see under *disease.*

Marchiafava-Micheli disease, syndrome (mar″ke-ah-fah′-vah-me-ka′le) [Ettore *Marchiafava;* F. *Micheli,* Italian clinician] paroxysmal nocturnal hemoglobinuria.

marcid (mar′sid) [L. *marcere* to waste away] wasting away.

marcov (mar′kov) [L. *marcere* to waste away] marasmus.

Marcus Gunn (mar′kus gun) see *Gunn.*

marcy (mar′se) a filtrable agent associated with an afebrile type of viral diarrhea.

Maréchal's test (mar″a-shalz′) [Louis Eugène *Maréchal,* French physician] see under *tests.*

Maréchal-Rosin test (mar″a-shal′-ro′zen) [L. E. *Maréchal;* Heinrich *Rosin,* Berlin physician, born 1863] Maréchal's test.

marennin (mah-ren′in) a green pigment from the oysters of Marennes, in France; derived from the chlorophyll of a microorganism that infests them.

Marezine (mar′ē-zēn) trademark for a preparation of cyclizine hydrochloride.

Marfan's puncture (epigastric puncture, method) sign, syndrome (mar-fahnz′) [Bernard-Jean Antonin *Marfan,* French pediatrician, 1858–1942] see under *puncture, sign* and *syndrome.*

marfanoid (mar′fan-oid) having the characteristic symptoms of Marfan's syndrome.

margarid (mar′gar-id) pearl-like.

margarine (mar′jar-in) [Gr. *margaron* pearl] 1. a food product containing 80 per cent of fat, manufactured primarily from refined cottonseed and soybean oils— sources of vitamin E and essential fatty acids—and fortified to supply a minimum of 15,000 U.S.P. units of vitamin A per pound; called also *oleomargarine.* 2. a (theoretical) trimargarate of propenyl.

margaritoma (mar″gar-ĭ-to′mah) cholesteatoma.

margarone (mar′gar-on) palmitone.

Margaropus (mar-gar′o-pus) a genus of ticks of the family Ixodidae. **M. annula′tus,** *Boophilus annulatus.* **M. winthem′i,** the beady-legged winter horse tick, a species found on horses and other large herbivores in South Africa.

margin (mar′jin) an edge or border, such as the boundary of an organ or other anatomic structure; called also *margo* [NA]. **alveolar m. of mandible,** arcus alveolaris mandibulae. **alveolar m. of maxilla,** arcus alveolaris maxillae. **axillary m. of scapula,** margo lateralis scapulae. **cartilaginous m. of acetabulum,** labrum acetabulare. **ciliary m. of iris,** margo ciliaris iridis. **convex m. of testis,** margo anterior testis. **coronal m. of frontal bone,** margo parietalis ossis frontalis. **coronal m. of parietal bone,** margo frontalis ossis parietalis. **crenate m. of spleen, cristate m. of spleen,** margo superior lienis. **dentate m.,** pectinate line. **falciform m. of fascia lata, falciform m. of saphenus hiatus,** margo falciformis hiatus saphenus. **falciform m. of white line of pelvic fascia,** arcus tendineus fasciae pelvis. **m. of fibula, anterior,** margo anterior fibulae. **m. of fibula, posterior,** margo posterior fibulae. **m. of foot, fibular, m. of foot, lateral,** margo lateralis pedis. **m. of foot, medial,** margo medialis pedis. **free gingival m.,** the localized tissue surrounding the tooth, forming the gingival crest; it maintains the gingival crevice and is free of attachment; free gum margin. **free m. of eyelid,** the conjunctival-lined portion of each eyelid, about 1 mm. broad, overlying the eyeball; the anterior border of each bears the eyelashes, and the posterior border is closely applied to the eyeball. **free m. of ovary,** margo liber ovarii. **free gum m.,** free gingival m. **frontal m. of parietal bone,** margo frontalis ossis parietalis. **gingival m., gum m.,** the border of the gingiva surrounding, but unattached to, the substance of the teeth; the crest of the free gingiva. **m. of humerus, lateral,** margo lateralis humeri. **m. of humerus, medial,** margo medialis humeri. **m. incisa′lis** [NA], the occlusal margin of an incisor tooth. **m. infe′rior cer′ebri** [NA], the inferior lateral margin of the cerebral hemisphere; called also *m. inferolateralis cerebri.* **infraorbital m. of maxilla,** margo infraorbitalis maxillae. **infraorbital m. of orbit,** margo infraorbitalis orbitae. **interosseous m. of fibula,** margo interosseus fibulae. **interosseous m. of tibia,** margo interosseus tibiae. **m. of kidney, lateral,** margo lateralis renis. **m. of kidney, medial,** margo medialis renis. **lacrimal m. of maxilla,** margo lacrimalis maxillae. **lambdoid m. of occipital bone,** margo lambdoideus squamae occipitalis. **lambdoid m. of parietal bone,** margo occipitalis ossis parietalis. **m. of lung, anterior,** margo anterior pulmonis. **m. of lung, inferior,** margo inferior pulmonis. **malar m.,** margo zygomaticus alae majoris. **mamillary m.,** margo mastoideus squamae occipitalis. **mastoid m. of occipital bone,** margo mastoideus squamae occipitalis. **mastoid m. of parietal bone,** angulus mastoideus ossis parietalis. **mesovarial m. of ovary,** margo mesovaricus ovarii. **m. of nail, free,** margo liber unguis. **m. of nail, hidden,** margo occultus unguis. **m. of nail, lateral,** margo lateralis unguis. **nasal m. of frontal bone,** margo nasalis ossis frontalis. **obtuse m. of spleen,** margo inferior lienis. **occipital m. of parietal bone,** margo occipitalis ossis parietalis. **occipital m. of temporal bone,** margo occipitalis ossis temporalis. **m. of pancreas, superior,** margo superior pancreatis. **parietal m. of frontal bone,** margo parietalis ossis frontalis. **parietal m. of great wing of sphenoid bone,** margo parietalis alae majoris. **parietal m. of occipital bone,** margo lambdoideus squamae occipitalis. **parietal m. of parietal bone,** margo sagittalis ossis parietalis. **parietal m. of temporal bone,** margo parietalis ossis temporalis. **m. of parietal bone, anterior, m. of parietal bone, frontal,** margo frontalis ossis parietalis. **m. of parietal bone, sagittal, m. of parietal bone, superior,** margo sagittalis ossis parietalis. **parietofrontal m. of great wing of sphenoid bone,** margo frontalis alae majoris. **pupillary m. of iris,** margo pupillaris iridis. **radial m's of fingers,** facies laterales digitorum manus. **radial m. of forearm,** margo lateralis antebrachii. **m. of radius, dorsal,** margo posterior radii. **m. of scapula, anterior,** margo lateralis scapulae. **m. of scapula, external,** margo lateralis scapulae. **m. of scapula, lateral,** margo lateralis scapulae. **m. of scapula, superior,** margo superior scapulae. **sphenoidal m. of parietal bone,** angulus sphenoidalis ossis parietalis. **sphenoidal m. of temporal bone,** margo sphenoidalis ossis temporalis. **sphenotemporal m. of parietal bone,** margo squamosus ossis parietalis. **m. of spleen, anterior, m. of spleen, superior,** margo superior lienis. **squamous m. of great wing of sphenoid bone,** margo squamosus alae majoris. **squamous m. of parietal bone,** margo squamosus ossis parietalis. **straight m. of testis,** margo posterior testis. **supraorbital m. of frontal bone,** margo supraorbitalis ossis frontalis. **supraorbital m. of orbit,** margo supraorbitalis orbitae. **m. of suprarenal gland, inferior,** facies renalis glandulae suprarenalis. **m. of suprarenal gland, medial,** margo medialis glandulae suprarenalis. **m. of suprarenal gland, superior,** margo superior glandulae suprarenalis. **temporal m. of parietal**

bone, margo squamosus ossis parietalis. **m. of testis, anterior, m. of testis, external,** margo anterior testis. **m. of testis, internal, m. of testis, posterior,** margo posterior testis. **m. of tibia, anterior,** margo anterior tibiae. **m. of tibia, medial,** margo medialis tibiae. **tibial m. of foot,** margo medialis pedis. **m. of tongue, m. of tongue, lateral,** margo linguae. **m. of ulna, anterior,** margo anterior ulnae. **m. of ulna, dorsal, m. of ulna, posterior,** margo posterior ulnae. **ulnar m's of fingers,** facies mediales digitorum manus. **ulnar m. of forearm,** margo medialis antebrachii. **m. of uterus, lateral,** margo uteri [dexter et sinister]. **vertebral m. of scapula,** margo medialis scapulae. **volar m. of radius,** margo anterior radii. **volar m. of ulna,** margo anterior ulnae. **zygomatic m. of great wing of sphenoid bone,** margo zygomaticus alae majoris.

marginal (mar′jĭ-nal) [L. *marginalis; margo* margin] pertaining to a margin or border.

margination (mar″jĭ-na′shun) accumulation and adhesion of leukocytes to the epithelial cells of blood vessel walls at the site of injury in the early stages of inflammation.

margines (mar′jĭ-nēz) [L.] plural of *margo*.

marginoplasty (mar-jin′o-plas-te) [L. *margo* margin + Gr. *plassein* to mold] surgical restoration of a border, as of the eyelid.

margo (mar′go), pl. *mar′gines* [L.] a margin, edge, or border; [NA] a general term for the edge of a structure. See also *labium* and *limbus*. **m. alveola′ris,** see *arcus alveolaris mandibulae* and *arcus alveolaris maxillae*. **m. ante′rior fib′ulae** [NA], anterior margin of fibula: the anterolateral border of the body of the fibula; called also *crista anterior fibulae* and *anterior crest of fibula*. **m. ante′rior hep′atis,** m. inferior hepatis. **m. ante′rior lie′nis,** m. superior lienis. **m. ante′rior pancrea′tis** [NA], the anterior margin of the pancreas, which bounds the anterior and inferior surfaces; called also *anterior border of pancreas*. **m. ante′rior pulmo′nis** [NA], anterior margin of lung: the ventral border of either lung, which descends from behind the sternum, a little to the left of the midline, and curves laterally to meet the inferior margin. **m. ante′rior ra′dii** [NA], the edge of the radius that runs obliquely between the radial tuberosity and the styloid process; called also *m. volaris radii, volar margin of radius*, and *anterior border of radius*. **m. ante′rior tes′tis** [NA], anterior margin of testis: the rounded free border of the testis. **m. ante′rior tib′iae** [NA], anterior margin of tibia: the prominent anteromedial margin of the body of the tibia, separating the medial and lateral surfaces; called also *crista anterior tibiae* and *anterior border of tibia*. **m. ante′rior ul′nae** [NA], anterior margin of ulna: the volar border of the ulna, separating the medial and posterior surfaces; called also *m. volaris ulnae* and *volar margin of ulna*. **m. axilla′ris scap′ulae,** m. lateralis scapulae. **m. cilia′ris i′ridis** [NA], ciliary margin of iris: the outer border of the iris, where it is continuous with the ciliary body. **m. dex′ter cor′dis** [NA]; the curved right margin of the heart, which runs from the apex toward the right, marking the junction of the sternocostal and diaphragmatic surfaces of the heart; the inferior portion, especially, tends to be a sharp edge. Called also *right border of heart*. **m. dorsa′lis ra′dii,** m. posterior radii. **m. dorsa′lis ul′nae,** m. posterior ulnae. **m. falcifor′mis fas′ciae la′tae,** m. falciformis hiatus saphenus. **m. falcifor′mis hia′tus saphe′nus** [NA], falciform margin of saphenous hiatus: the lateral margin of the saphenous hiatus; called also *m. falciformis fasciae latae*. **m. fibula′ris pe′dis,** NA alternative for *m. lateralis pedis*. **m. fronta′lis a′lae mag′nae,** m. frontalis alae majoris. **m. fronta′lis a′lae majo′ris** [NA], frontal margin of great wing of sphenoid bone: a roughened area on the great wing of the sphenoid bone where it articulates with the frontal bone; it is situated at the upper lateral margin of the orbital surface of the great wing where this meets the cerebral and temporal surfaces. Called also *m. frontalis alae magnae*. **m. fronta′lis os′sis parieta′lis** [NA], frontal margin of parietal bone: the edge of the parietal bone that articulates with the frontal bone along the coronal suture. **m. infe′rior hep′atis** [NA], the anteroinferior edge of the liver, separating the anterior and the visceral surface; called also *m. anterior hepatis* and *inferior border of liver*. **m. infe′rior lie′nis** [NA], a straight margin of the spleen somewhat less prominent than the superior margin, separating the renal surface from the diaphragmatic surface; called also *m. posterior lienis* and *inferior border of spleen*. **m. infe′rior pancrea′tis** [NA], the inferior margin of the pancreas, which bounds the inferior and posterior surfaces; called also *m. posterior pancreatis*. **m. infe′rior pulmo′nis** [NA], inferior margin of lung: the border of the lung that extends in a curve behind the sixth costal cartilage, the upper margin of the eighth rib in the axillary line, the ninth or tenth rib in the scapular line, and passes medially to the eleventh costovertebral joint. **m. inferolatera′lis cer′ebri,** NA alternative for *m. inferior cerebri*. **m. inferomedia′lis cer′ebri,** NA alternative for *m. medialis cerebri*. **m. infraglenoida′lis tib′iae,** the margin of bone that forms the circumference of the condyles of the tibia just inferior to the facies articularis superior. **m. infraorbita′lis maxil′lae** [NA], infraorbital margin of maxilla: the short rounded edge of the maxilla where the orbital surface becomes continuous with the anterior surface. **m. infraorbita′lis or′bitae** [NA], infraorbital margin of orbit: the inferior edge of the entrance to the orbit, formed by the infraorbital process of the zygomatic bone and the infraorbital margin of the maxilla. **m. interos′seus fib′ulae** [NA], a prominent ridge medial to the anterior border of the fibula, connected with a similar ridge on the tibia by a strong, wide fibrous sheet, the interosseous membrane; called also *crista interossea fibulae* and *interosseous border, crest,* or *ridge of fibula*. **m. interos′seus ra′dii** [NA], the prominent medial border of the radius, connected with a similar ridge on the ulna by a strong, wide fibrous sheet, the interossesous membrane; called also *crista interossea radii* and *interosseous border, crest,* or *ridge of radius*. **m. interos′seus tib′iae** [NA], interosseous margin of tibia: the prominent lateral border of the body of the tibia, which separates the posterior and lateral surfaces and gives attachment to the interosseous membrane; called also *crista interossea tibiae* and *interosseous border, crest,* or *ridge of tibia*. **m. interos′seus ul′nae** [NA], the prominent lateral border of the ulna, connected with a similar ridge on the radius by the interosseous membrane; called also *crista interossea ulnae* and *interosseous border, crest,* or *ridge of ulna*. **m. lacrima′lis maxil′lae** [NA], lacrimal margin of maxilla: the posterior border of the frontal process of the maxilla where it articulates with the lacrimal bone; called also *lacrimal border of maxilla*. **m. lambdoi′deus squa′mae occipita′lis** [NA], lambdoid margin of occipital bone: the edge of the occipital bone that extends from the lateral angle to the superior angle, articulating with the parietal bone to help form the lambdoid suture; called also *parietal margin of occipital bone*. **m. latera′lis antebra′chii** [NA], the lateral, or radial, border of the forearm; called also *m. radialis antebrachii* [NA alternative]. **mar′gines latera′les digito′rum pe′dis,** facies laterales digitorum pedis. **m. latera′lis hu′meri** [NA], lateral margin of humerus: the edge of the humerus that extends from posteroinferior part of the greater tubercle to the lateral epicondyle; called also *lateral angle* or *border of humerus*. **m. latera′lis [lin′guae],** m. linguae. **m. latera′lis pe′dis** [NA], the lateral, or fibular, border of the foot; called also *m. fibularis pedis* [NA alternative]. **m. latera′lis re′nis** [NA], lateral margin of kidney: the convex narrow border of the kidney. **m. latera′lis scap′ulae** [NA], lateral margin of scapula: the thick edge of the scapula, extending from the inferior margin of the glenoid cavity to the inferior angle; called also *m. axillaris scapulae* and *lateral border of scapula*. **m. latera′lis un′guis** [NA], lateral margin of nail: the edge on either side of the nail. **m. latera′lis u′teri,** m. uteri [dexter et sinister]. **m. li′ber ova′rii** [NA], free margin of ovary: the broad, convex border of the ovary, opposite the mesovarial margin. **m. li′ber un′guis** [NA], the overhanging, distal, free edge of the nail. **m. lin′guae** [NA], margin of tongue: the lateral border of the body of the tongue; called also *m. lateralis* [*linguae*]. **m. mastoi′deus squa′mae occipita′lis** [NA], mastoid margin of occipital bone: the edge of the occipital bone that extends from the jugular process to the lateral angle, articulating with the part of the temporal bone that bears the mastoid process. **m. media′lis antebra′chii** [NA], the medial, or ulnar, border of the forearm; called also *m. ulnaris antebrachii* [NA alternative]. **m. media′lis cer′ebri** [NA], inferior medial margin of the cerebral hemisphere; called also *m. inferomedialis cerebri*. **mar′gines media′les digito′rum pe′dis,** facies mediales digitorum pedis. **m. media′lis glan′dulae suprarena′lis** [NA], medial margin of suprarenal gland: the medial border, which with the superior border divides the anterior from the posterior surface. **m. media′lis hu′meri** [NA], medial margin of humerus: the edge of the humerus that begins at the lesser tubercle above and continues downward to the medial epicondyle; called also *medial angle* or *border of humerus*. **m. media′lis pe′dis** [NA], the medial, or tibial, border of the foot; called also *m. tibialis pedis* [NA alternative]. **m. media′lis re′nis** [NA], medial margin of kidney: the concave border of the kidney, which contains the hilus. **m. media′lis scap′ulae** [NA], the thin edge of the scapula extending from the superior to the inferior angle; called also *m. vertebralis scapulae* and *vertebral border* or *margin of scapula*. **m. media′lis tib′iae** [NA], medial margin of tibia: the border that extends between the medial condyle and medial malleolus of the tibia, separating the medial and posterior surfaces; called also *medial angle* or *border of tibia*. **m. mesova′ricus ova′rii** [NA], mesovarial margin of ovary: the border of the ovary that is attached to the broad ligament by means of the mesovarium. **m. nasa′lis os′sis fronta′lis** [NA], nasal margin of frontal bone: the articular surface, on each nasal part of the frontal bone, that articulates with the nasal bones and with the frontal processes of the maxilla. **m. na′si,** the lower, free, margin of the ala nasi and septum nasi that surrounds the external naris. **m. occipita′lis os′sis parieta′lis** [NA], occipital margin of parietal bone: the edge of the parietal bone that articulates with the occipital bone at the lambdoid suture. **m. occipita′lis os′sis tempora′lis** [NA], occipital margin of temporal bone: the border of the petrous part of the temporal bone that articulates with the occipital bone along the occipitomastoid suture. **m. occul′tus un′guis** [NA], the proximal, buried edge of the nail. **m. pal′pebrae,** see *free margin of eyelid*.

m. parieta′lis a′lae majo′ris [NA], parietal margin of great wing of sphenoid bone: the superior extremity of the squamous margin of the great wing of the sphenoid bone where it articulates with the parietal bone; called also *angulus parietalis ossis sphenoidalis.* **m. parieta′lis os′sis fronta′lis** [NA], parietal margin of frontal bone: the posterior border of the frontal bone, semicircular in shape, which articulates with the parietal bones. **m. parieta′lis os′sis tempora′lis** [NA], parietal margin of temporal bone: the superior border of the squamous part of the temporal bone where it articulates with the parietal bone; called also *m. parietalis squamae temporalis.* **m. parieta′lis squa′mae tempora′lis,** m. parietalis ossis temporalis. **m. pe′dis latera′lis,** m. lateralis pedis. **m. pe′dis media′lis,** m. medialis pedis. **m. poste′rior fib′ulae** [NA], posterior margin of fibula: the posterolateral margin of the body of the fibula; called also *crista lateralis fibulae* and *posterior border* or *crest of fibula.* **m. poste′rior lie′nis,** m. inferior lienis. **m. poste′rior pancrea′tis,** m. inferior pancreatis. **m. poste′rior ra′dii** [NA], the edge of the radius that extends from the posterior part of the radial tuberosity to the middle tubercle; called also *m. dorsalis radii,* and *dorsal margin* or *posterior border of radius.* **m. poste′rior tes′tis** [NA], posterior margin of testis: the border of the testis that is attached to the epididymis and the lower end of the ductus deferens; called also *dorsum of testis.* **m. poste′rior ul′nae** [NA], posterior margin of ulna: the dorsal border of the ulna, separating the posterior and medial surfaces; called also *m. dorsalis ulnae.* **m. pupilla′ris i′ridis** [NA], pupillary margin of iris: the inner edge of the iris, surrounding the pupil. **m. radia′lis antebra′chii,** NA alternative for *m. lateralis antebrachii.* **m. radia′lis antibra′chii,** m. lateralis antebrachii. **mar′gines radia′les digito′rum ma′nus,** facies laterales digitorum manus. **m. radia′lis hu′meri,** m. lateralis humeri. **m. sagitta′lis os′sis parieta′lis** [NA], sagittal margin of parietal bone: the edge of the parietal bone that articulates with the other parietal bone along the sagittal suture; called also *parietal* or *superior margin of parietal bone.* **m. sphenoida′lis os′sis tempora′lis** [NA], sphenoidal margin of temporal bone: the anterior border of the temporal bone, articulating with the great wing of the sphenoid bone; called also *m. sphenoidalis squamae temporalis.* **m. sphenoida′lis squa′mae tempora′lis,** m. sphenoidalis ossis temporalis. **m. squamo′sus a′lae mag′nae,** m. squamosus alae majoris. **m. squamo′sus a′lae majo′ris** [NA], squamous margin of great wing of sphenoid bone: the border of the great wing of the sphenoid bone that articulates with he squama of the temporal bone; called also *m. squamosus alae magnae.* **m. squamo′sus os′sis parieta′lis** [NA], squamous margin of parietal bone: the inferior edge of the parietal bone, which articulates with the sphenoid and temporal bones along the squamous suture. **m. supe′rior cer′ebri** [NA], the superior medial margin of the cerebral hemisphere; called also *m. superomedialis cerebri.* **m. supe′rior glan′dulae suprarena′lis** [NA], the superior margin or border of the suprarenal gland, which with the medial border divides the anterior from the posterior surface. **m. supe′rior lie′nis** [NA], superior margin of spleen: a somewhat sharp, convex line, sometimes serrated, between the gastric and diaphragmatic surfaces of the spleen; called also *m. anterior lienis* and *superior border of spleen.* **m. supe′rior pancre′atis** [NA], the superior border of the pancreas, which bounds the anterior and posterior surfaces. **m. supe′rior scap′ulae** [NA], superior margin of scapula: the thin, short edge of the scapula, extending from the superior angle to the coracoid process; called also *superior border of scapula.* **m. superomedia′lis cer′ebri,** NA alternative for *m. superior cerebri.* **m. supraorbita′lis or′bitae** [NA], supraorbital margin of orbit: the superior edge of the entrance to the orbit, formed by the supraorbital margin of the frontal bone. **m. supraorbita′lis os′sis fronta′lis** [NA], supraorbital margin of frontal bone: the antero-inferior edge of the frontal bone, bending down laterally to the zygomatic bone and medially to the frontal process of the maxilla; it marks the junction between the squama and the orbital portion of the bone. **m. tibia′lis pe′dis,** NA alternative for *m. medialis pedis.* **m. ulna′ris antebra′chii,** NA alternative for *m. medialis antebrachii.* **m. ulna′ris antibra′chii,** m. medialis antebrachii. **mar′gines ulna′res digito′rum ma′nus,** facies mediales digitorum manus. **m. ulna′ris hu′meri,** m. medialis humeri. **m. u′teri [dex′ter et sini′s′ter]** [NA], lateral margin of uterus: either border of the uterus (right and left) at the upper portion of which the uterine tube is attached; called also *m. lateralis uteri.* **m. vertebra′lis scap′ulae,** m. medialis scapulae. **m. vola′ris ra′dii,** m. anterior radii. **m. vola′ris ul′nae,** m. anterior ulnae. **m. zygomat′icus a′lae mag′nae,** m. zygomaticus alae majoris. **m. zygomat′icus a′lae majo′ris** [NA], zygomatic margin of great wing of sphenoid bone: the border on the great wing of the sphenoid bone that separates its temporal and orbital surfaces and articulates with the zygomatic bone; called also *m. zygomaticus alae magnae.*

mariahuana, mariajuana (mah-re-ah-wah′nah) marihuana.

mariculture (mar″ĭ-kul′chur) [L. *mare* sea + culture] the cultivation of sea life to provide nutrients.

Marie's ataxia, etc. (mahrēz′) [Pierre *Marie,* French physician, 1853–1940] see under *ataxia, disease, hypertrophy, sign,* and *syndrome.*

Marie-Bamberger disease (mah-re′-bahm′ber-ger)[Pierre *Marie;* Eugen *Bamberger,* Austrian physician, 1858–1921] hypertrophic pulmonary osteoarthropathy.

Marie-Strümpell disease, syndrome (mah-re′ strim′pel) [Pierre *Marie;* Adolf von *Strümpell,* physician in Leipzig, 1853–1925] rheumatoid spondylitis.

Marie-Tooth disease (mah-re′-tooth′) [Pierre *Marie;* Howard Henry *Tooth,* English physician, 1856–1926] progressive neuropathic (peroneal) muscular atrophy.

mariguana (mar″ĭ-hwah′nah) marihuana.

marihuana (mar″ĭ-hwan′ah) [Portuguese] a crude preparation of the leaves and flowering tops of (male or female plants) *Cannabis sativa* L. (Cannabaceae), usually employed in cigarets and inhaled as smoke for its euphoric properties. See *cannabis.*

marijuana (mar″ĭ-hwah′nah) marihuana.

Marinesco's succulent hand (sign) (mar″ĭ-nes′kōz) [Georges *Marinesco,* Roumanian neurologist, 1863–1938] see under *hand.*

marinobufagin (mar″ĭ-no-bu′fah-jin) a cardiac poison, $C_{24}H_{32}O_5$, from the skin of the toad, *Bufo marinus.*

marinotherapy (mar″ĭ-no-ther′ah-pe) treatment by residence at the seashore.

Mariotte's experiment, law, spot (mar″e-ots′) [Edme *Mariotte,* French physicist, 1620–1684] see under *experiment,* and see *Boyle's law,* under *law,* and *blind spot,* under *spot.*

mariposia (mar″ĭ-po′ze-ah) [L. *mare* the sea + Gr. *posis* drinking + -ia] thalassoposia.

marisca (mah-ris′kah), pl. *maris′cae* [L. *marisca* a large fig] a hemorrhoid.

mariscal (mah-ris′kal) hemorrhoidal.

marital (mar′ĭ-tal) of or pertaining to marriage.

maritonucleus (mar″ĭ-to-nu′kle-us) [L. *maritus* married + *nucleus*] the nucleus of the ovum after the sperm cell has entered it.

Marjolin's ulcer (mar″zho-lanz′) [Jean Nicolas *Marjolin,* French surgeon 1780–1850] see under *ulcer.*

mark (mark) a spot, blemish, or other circumscribed area visible on a surface, particularly on the skin or mucous membrane. **beauty m.,** a small pigmented nevus, particularly on the cheek, said to enhance the appearance. **birth m.,** see *birthmark.* **pock m.,** see *pockmark.* **Pohl's m.,** a limited thinning of the shaft of a hair, usually accompanied by interruption of the medulla; it is usually a sign of systemic disease, but may be due to trauma, coronary occlusion, skin disease, or the therapeutic administration of a single substantial dose of an antimetabolite, such as methotrexate or cyclophosphamide. **port-wine m.,** nevus flammeus. **raspberry m., strawberry m.,** cavernous hemangioma.

marker (mark′er) something that identifies or that is used to identify. **genetic m.,** a genetic polymorphism with a simple mode of inheritance occurring with different frequencies in different populations, and therefore useful in family studies, studies of the distribution of genes in populations, and linkage analysis.

marking (mark′ing) a conspicuous line or spot visible on a surface. **Fontana's m's,** minute transverse folds seen on a divided nerve trunk.

Marlow's test (mar′lōz) [Frank William *Marlow,* Syracuse ophthalmologist, 1858–1942] see under *tests.*

marma (mar′mah) the ancient Indian name for a place or region of vital importance in the body which, if injured, results in serious consequences or death.

marmoration (mar″mo-ra′shun) [L. *marmor* marble] marbleization.

marmoreal (mar-mo′re-al) resembling marble, as bone in osteopetrosis.

marmot (mar′mot) any of several large terrestrial animals of the squirrel family, members of the genera *Marmota* and *Arctomys,* found in the Northern Hemisphere, such as the hoary marmot, yellow-bellied marmot, and woodchuck or ground-hog of North America and the tarbagan of Asia; they may be natural reservoirs of the plague.

Marplan (mar′plan) trademark for a preparation of isocarboxazid.

Marriott's method (mar′e-ots) [William McKim *Marriott,* American physician, 1885–1936] see under *method.*

marrow (mar′o) the soft organic material that fills the cavities of the bones (see *medulla ossium*); called also *medulla.* **bone m.,** medulla ossium. **bone m., red,** medulla ossium rubra. **bone m., yellow,** medulla ossium flava. **depressed m.,** bone marrow exhibiting decreased hematopoietic activity. **fat m.,** medulla ossium flava. **gelatinous m.,** bone marrow that has lost its blood cells and its fat and has acquired a gelatinous appearance. **red m.,** medulla ossium rubra. **spinal m.,** the spinal cord (medulla spinalis [NA]). **yellow m.,** medulla ossium flava.

marrowbrain (mar′o-brān) the myelencephalon; def. 1.

mars (marz) [L.] iron.

Marsden's paste (marz′denz) [Alexander Edwin *Marsden*, London surgeon, 1832–1902] see under *paste.*

Marsh's disease (marsh′ez) [Sir Henry *Marsh*, Irish physician, 1790–1860] Graves' disease.

Marsh's test (marsh′ez) [James *Marsh*, English chemist, 1789–1846] see under *tests.*

Marshall's fold, vein (mar′shalz) [John *Marshall*, English anatomist, 1818–1891] see *plica venae cavae sinistrae* and *vena obliqua atrii sinistri.*

Marshall Hall see *Hall.*

marsupia (mar-su′pe-ah) [L.] plural of *marsupium.*

marsupial (mar-su′pe-al) [L. *marsupium* a pouch] a member of the order Marsupialia.

Marsupialia (mar-su″pe-a′le-ah) an order of the class Mammalia characterized by the possession of an abdominal pouch, or marsupium, in which the young, which are born in a very underdeveloped state, are carried and nourished until their development is complete. It includes the opossums, kangaroos, wallabies, koala bears, and wombats. In some systems of classification, it is considered to be an order of the infraclass or subclass Metatheria, class Mammalia.

marsupialization (mar-su″pe-al-i-za′shun) [L. *marsupium* pouch] the creation of a pouch; applied especially to surgical exteriorization of a cyst by resection of the anterior wall and suture of the cut edges of the remaining cyst to the adjacent edges of the skin, thereby establishing a pouch of what was formerly an enclosed cyst.

marsupium (mar-su′pe-um), pl. *marsu′pia* [L. "a pouch"] 1. the scrotum. 2. an external abdominal pouch or fold of skin for carrying the young; it contains the mammary glands and occurs in marsupials and the spiny anteaters. Also a similar structure for carrying eggs and/or the young, as in the male sea horse. **marsu′pia patella′ris,** plicae alares.

martial (mar′shal) [L. *martialis; mars* iron] containing iron; ferruginous or chalybeate.

Martin's bandage, disease, operation, etc. (mar′tinz) [Henry Austin *Martin,* American surgeon, 1824–1884] see under the nouns.

Martinotti's cells (mar″tĭ-not′ez) [Giovanni *Martinotti,* Bologna pathologist, 1857–1928] see under *cell.*

masc. mass concentration.

maschaladenitis (mas″kal-ad″ĕ-ni′tis) [Gr. *maschalē* armpit + *adēn* gland + *-itis*] inflammation of the glands of the axilla.

maschaloncus (mas″kal-ong′kus) a tumor of the axilla.

masculation (mas″ku-la′shun) the development of male characteristics.

masculine (mas′ku-lin) [L. *masculinus*] pertaining to the male sex, or possessing qualities normally characteristic of the male.

masculinity (mas″ku-lin′ĭ-te) the possession of masculine qualities.

masculinization (mas″ku-lin-i-za′shun) the normal induction or development of male sex characters in the male. Also, the induction or development of male secondary sex characters in the female. Called also *virilization.*

masculinize (mas″ku-lĭ-nīz″) to produce male characteristics (virilism) in a female.

masculinovoblastoma (mas″ku-lin-o″vo-blas-to′mah) lipoid cell tumor of ovary; see under *tumor.*

masculonucleus (mas″ku-lo-nu′kle-us) arsenoblast.

maser (ma′zer) [*m*icrowave *a*mplification by *s*timulated *e*mission of *r*adiation] a device which produces an extremely intense, small, and nearly nondivergent beam of monochromatic radiation in the microwave region with all waves in phase.

mask (mask) [Fr. *masque*] 1. to cover or conceal, as the masking of the nature of a disorder by the presence of unrelated signs, symptoms, organisms, etc. In audiometry, to obscure or diminish a sound by the presence of another sound of different frequency. 2. an appliance for shading, protecting, or medicating the face. 3. in dentistry, to camouflage metal parts of a prosthesis by covering with opaque material. **BLB m.,** an oxygen-breathing mask for use at high altitudes; it has a combined inspiratory and expiratory valve and a bag for rebreathing (Boothby, Lovelace, Bulbulian). It has also been used for clinical administration of oxygen. **Curschmann's m.,** a mask formerly used for inhaling turpentine vapors. **death m.,** a plaster cast of the face of a dead person. **ecchymotic m.,** cyanotic discoloration of the head and neck as a result of traumatic asphyxia. **full-face m.,** a device used in anesthesia to confine the gas to be delivered through the mask into the respiratory tract through the nose or mouth. **Hutchinson's m.,** a sensation as if the skin of the face were compressed by a mask; often a symptom of tabes dorsalis. **Kuhn's m.,** a mask worn over the nose and mouth, which, by obstructing the respiration, was reported to produce

artificial hyperemia of the pulmonary tissues; formerly used in treating pulmonary tuberculosis. **meter m.,** an oxygen-breathing mask designed to provide fixed percentage admixtures of air and oxygen. **Parkinson's m.,** see under *facies.* **m. of pregnancy,** see *melasma.* **tabetic m.,** Hutchinson's m. **Wanscher's m.,** a mask for ether anesthesia.

masochism (mas′o-kizm) [Leopold von Sacher-*Masoch,* an Austrian novelist, 1836–1895] a form of sexual perversion in which cruel or humiliating treatment gives sexual gratification to the recipient.

masochist (mas′o-kist) one who is given to masochism.

Mas. pil. abbreviation for L. *mas′sa pilula′rum,* pill mass.

mass (mas) [L. *massa*] 1. a lump or body made up of cohering particles; see also *massa.* 2. a cohesive mixture suitable for being made up into pills. 3. that characteristic of matter which gives it inertia. The mass of a hypothetical atom of atomic weight 1.000 (a dalton) is 1.648×10^{-24} gm., and the mass of any other atom may be found by multiplying this number by the atomic weight of the atom. **achromatic m.,** the nonstaining portion of the karyokinetic figure. **appendiceal m., appendix m.,** a palpable mass in the right iliac fossa or right loin due to acute appendicitis, usually with abscess secondary to rupture; occasionally caused by adherent omentum and intestine. **atomic m.,** the mass of a neutral atom of a nuclide, usually expressed in atomic mass units (amu). **blue m.,** mercury m. **body cell m.,** the total weight of the cells of the body, including the cell nucleus, cytoplasm, water, salt, protein, and surrounding membrane, but excluding extracellular water and extracellular solids such as collagen, elastin, and bone matrix, constituting in essence the total mass of oxygen-utilizing, carbohydrate-burning, and energy-exchanging cells of the body; regarded as proportional to total exchangeable potassium in the body. **electronic m.,** the mass of a negative electron when moving at moderate velocity; it is 8.999×10^{-28} gm. **ferrous carbonate m.,** a soft, dark greenish gray substance containing 36 to 41 per cent of ferrous carbonate; used in anemia. **fibrillar m. of Flemming,** spongioplasm, def. 1. **injection m.,** a suspension or solution, usually colored, injected into blood vessels or other tissue spaces to permit their demonstration on dissection or sectioning. **inner cell m.,** an aggregation of cells at one pole of the blastocyst, which is destined to form the embryo proper. **intermediate m.,** adhesio interthalamica. **intermediate cell m.,** nephrotome. **lateral m. of atlas,** massa lateralis atlantis. **lateral m's of ethmoid bone,** see *labyrinthus ethmoidalis.* **lateral m. of sacrum,** pars lateralis ossis sacri. **lateral m. of vertebrae,** pediculus arcus vertebrae. **lean body m.,** that part of the body including all its components except neutral storage lipid; in essence, the fat-free mass of the body. **mercury m.,** a mixture of mercury oleate, mercury, honey, glycerin, glycyrrhiza, and althea, containing 31–35 per cent of mercury; used in the treatment of pediculosis pubis. Called also *massa hydrargyri,* blue mass, and *blue pill.* **pill m., pilular m.,** a drug mass of the proper consistency for being made into pills. **Priestley's m.,** a green or brownish substance sometimes seen upon the canine and incisor teeth, caused by chromogenic microorganisms. **Stent's m.,** a plastic resinous material which sets into a very hard substance; used in surgery for making molds shaped to keep grafts in place. See also *stent.* **tigroid m's,** Nissl's bodies. **Vallet's m.,** ferrous carbonate m. **ventrolateral m.,** that portion of the primitive lateral mass of the embryo from which are developed the abdominal, thoracic, and anterior cervical muscles.

massa (mas′ah), pl. *mas′sae* [L.] a unified lump or mass of material; [NA] a general term for an accumulation of cells or cohesive tissue. Called also *mass.* **m. fer′ri carbona′tis,** ferrous carbonate mass. **m. hydrar′gyri,** mercury mass. **m. innomina′ta,** paradidymis. **m. interme′dia,** adhesio interthalamica. **m. latera′lis atlan′tis** [NA], lateral mass of atlas: the thickened lateral portion of the atlas to which the arches are attached and which bears the articulating surfaces and the transverse process. **mas′sae latera′les os′sis ethmoida′lis,** see *labyrinthus ethmoidalis.* **m. latera′lis os′sis sa′cri,** pars lateralis ossis sacri. **m. latera′lis ver′tebrae,** pediculus arcus vertebrae. **m. mol′lis** (obs.), adhesio interthalamica.

massae (mas′se) [L.] plural of *massa.*

massage (mah-sahzh′) [Fr.; Gr. *massein* to knead] the systematic therapeutical friction, stroking, and kneading of the body. **auditory m.,** massage of the drum membrane. **cardiac m.,** rhythmic compression of the heart by pressure applied manually over the sternum (closed cardiac massage) or directly to the heart through an opening in the chest wall (open cardiac massage); done to reinstate and maintain circulation. **Cederschiöld's m.,** massage by making rhythmic pressure over the parts. **douche m.,** massage combined with the application of a douche. **electrovibratory m.,** massage by means of an electric vibrator. **heart m.,** cardiac m. **hydropneumatic m.,** massage by means of air forced through a tube at the end of which is a chamber containing water, the water chamber being applied to the part to be massaged. **tremolo m.,** a variety of mechanical massage. **vapor m.,** treatment of a lung cavity by a medicated and nebulized vapor under interrupted pressure. **vibratory m.**, massage by rapidly repeated light percussion with a vibrating hammer or sound.

Masselon's spectacles (mas″ĕ-lawz′) [Miche Julien *Masselon*, French ophthalmologist, 1844–1917] see under *spectacles*.

Masset's test (mas-āz′) [Alfred Auguste *Masset*, French physician, born 1870] see under *tests*.

masseter (mas-se′ter) [Gr. *masētēr* chewer] see *musculus masseter*.

masseteric (mas″e-ter′ik) pertaining to the masseter muscle.

masseur (mah-ser′) [Fr.] 1. a man who performs massage. 2. an instrument for performing massage.

masseuse (mah-suhz′) [Fr.] a woman who performs massage.

massicot (mas′ĭ-kot) lead monoxide, PbO.

massive (mas′iv) having a solid bulky form; heavy; in a mass; complete.

Masson stain (mas-on) [C. L. Pierre *Masson*, Montreal pathologist, born 1880] see *Table of Stains*.

massotherapy (mas″o-ther′ah-pe) [Gr. *massein* to knead + *therapy*] the treatment of disease by massage.

MAST acronym for Military Anti-Shock Trousers, inflatable trousers used to induce autotransfusion of blood from the lower to the upper part of the body.

mast- see *masto-*.

mastadenitis (mas″tad-ĕ-ni′tis) [*mast-* + Gr. *adēn* gland + *-itis*] inflammation of the mammary gland; mastitis.

mastadenoma (mas″tad-ĕ-no′mah) [*mast-* + Gr. *adēn* gland + *-oma*] tumor of the breast.

mastalgia (mas-tal′je-ah) [*mast-* + *-algia*] pain in the mammary gland.

mastatrophia (mas″tah-tro′fe-ah) mastatrophy.

mastatrophy (mas-tat′ro-fe) [*mast-* + *atrophy*] atrophy of the mammary gland.

mastauxe (mas-tawk′se) [*mast-* + Gr. *auxē* increase] enlargement of the breast.

mastectomy (mas-tek′to-me) [*mast-* + Gr. *ektomē* excision] excision of the breast; mammectomy. **Halsted radical m.**, removal of the breast, pectoral muscles, axillary lymph nodes, and associated skin and subcutaneous tissue in breast cancer. **modified radical m.**, total mastectomy with axial node dissection, but leaving the pectoral muscles intact. **subcutaneous m.**, excision of breast tissue with preservation of overlying skin, nipple, and areola so that breast form may be reconstructed. **Willy Meyer radical m.**, an operation basically similar to Halsted's radical mastectomy but differing in certain technical details.

Master "2-step" exercise test (mas′ter) [Arthur M. *Master*, American physician, born 1895] see under *tests*.

Masterone (mas′tĕ-rōn) trademark for a preparation of diomostanolone propionate.

masthelcosis (mas″thel-ko′sis) [*mast-* + Gr. *helkōsis* ulceration] ulceration of the breast or mammary gland.

mastic (mas′tik) [L. *mastiche*; Gr. *mastichē*] a yellowish, hard, resinous exudation obtained from the shrub *Pistacia lentiscus* L. (Anacardiaceae), indigenous to the Mediterranean Islands, especially Chios. It is widely used in Greece as characteristically flavored chewing gum base, and contains about 2 per cent volatile oil and several resin acids. Used in tooth cements as dental liner and in plasters, lacquers, and incense, and pharmaceutically in enteric coatings for tablets.

mastication (mas″tĭ-ka′shun) [L. *masticare* to chew] the process of chewing food in preparation for swallowing and digestion.

masticatory (mas′tĭ-kah-to″re) 1. subserving or pertaining to mastication; affecting the muscles of mastication. 2. a remedy to be chewed but not swallowed.

mastiche (mas′tĭ-kĕ) [L.] mastic.

Mastigophora (mas″tĭ-gof′o-rah) [Gr. *mastix* whip + *pherein* to bear] a subphylum of Protozoa comprising those having one or more flagella throughout most of the life cycle, and a simple, centrally located nucleus. Most are free-living, but many are parasitic in both invertebrates and vertebrates, including man. It includes two classes, Phytomastigophora and Zoomastigophora. Called also *Flagellata* and *Euflagellata*.

mastigophoran (mas″tĭ-gof′o-ran) any individual of the subphylum Mastigophora.

mastigophorous (mas″tĭ-gof′o-rus) of or pertaining to the subphylum Mastigophora.

mastigote (mas′tĭ-gōt) any organism of the subphylum Mastigophora.

mastitis (mas-ti′tis) [*mast-* + *-itis*] inflammation of the mammary gland, or breast. **chronic cystic m.**, cystic disease of breast; see under *disease*. **gargantuan m.**, pathologic enlargement of the breasts to a tremendous size. **glandular m.**, parenchymatous m. **interstitial m.**, inflammation of the stroma of the mammary gland. **m. neonato′rum**, a general term applied to an abnormal condition of the breast of the newborn, such as hypertrophy, engorgement and secretion, or inflammation, with or without suppuration. **parenchymatous m.**, inflammation of the secreting elements of the mammary gland. **periductal m.**, inflammation of tissues about the ducts of the mammary gland. **phlegmonous m.**, inflammation of the breast leading to abscess formation. **plasma cell m.**, a morbid condition of the breast characterized by infiltration of the breast stroma with plasma cells and proliferation of the cells lining the ducts, thought by some to be the end-stage of mammary duct ectasia. **puerperal m.**, a form of mastitis occurring after delivery. **retromammary m.**, **submammary m.**, paramastitis. **stagnation m.**, a local engorgement affecting one or more lobules of the breast and forming a painful lump in the organ; it occurs during early lactation. Called also *caked breast*. **suppurative m.**, pyogenic infection of the breast.

masto-, mast- [Gr. *mastos* breast] a combining form denoting relationship to the breast or to the mastoid process; see also words beginning *mammo-*.

mastocarcinoma (mas″to-kar″sĭ-no′mah) [*masto-* + *carcinoma*] carcinoma of the breast.

mastoccipital (mas″tok-sip′ĭ-tal) masto-occipital.

mastochondroma (mas″to-kon-dro′mah) [*masto-* + *chondroma*] a chondroma of the breast.

mastochondrosis (mas″to-kon-dro′sis) mastochondroma.

mastocyte (mas′to-sīt) [Ger. *Mast* food + *-cyte*] a mast cell.

mastocytoma (mas″to-si-to′mah) a mast cell tumor; see under *tumor*. **solitary m.**, a solid focal aggregation of mast cells, which may be the first manifestation of juvenile urticaria pigmentosa.

mastocytosis (mas″to-si-to′sis) an accumulation, either local or systemic, of mast cells in the tissues; when widespread in the skin it is known as *urticaria pigmentosa*. **diffuse cutaneous m.**, a rare variety of urticaria pigmentosa with diffuse cutaneous involvement, causing leathery thickening of the entire skin, sometimes with an orange color. **systemic m.**, a stationary or progressive form of adult urticaria pigmentosa in which the mast cells infiltrate the skin and such organs as the lymph nodes, bone, blood, spleen, and liver; called also *systemic mast cell disease*.

mastodynia (mas″to-din′e-ah) [*masto-* + Gr. *odynē* pain] pain in the breast.

mastogram (mas′to-gram) a roentgenogram of the breast.

mastography (mas-tog′rah-fe) [*masto-* + Gr. *graphein* to write] roentgenography of the breast.

mastoid (mas′toid) [Gr. *mastos* breast + *eidos* form] 1. breast shaped. 2. the mastoid process of the temporal bone. 3. pertaining to the mastoid process.

mastoidal (mas-toi′dal) pertaining to the mastoid process of the temporal bone.

mastoidale (mas″toi-da′le) the lowest point of the mastoid process.

mastoidalgia (mas″toi-dal′je-ah) [*mastoid* + *-algia*] pain in the mastoid region.

mastoidea (mas″toi-de-ah) pars mastoideus ossis temporalis.

mastoidectomy (mas″toi-dek′to-me) [*mastoid* + Gr. *ektomē* excision] excision of the mastoid cells or the mastoid process of the temporal bone.

mastoideocentesis (mas-toi″de-o-sen-te′sis) [*mastoid* + Gr. *kentēsis* puncture] paracentesis of the mastoid cells.

mastoideum (mas-toi′de-um) pars mastoideus ossis temporalis.

mastoiditis (mas″toi-di′tis) inflammation of the mastoid antrum and cells. **Bezold's m.**, a form in which the pus has escaped into the digastric groove and deep to the head of the sternocleidomastoid muscle. **m. exter′na**, inflammation of the periosteum of the mastoid process. **m. inter′na**, inflammation of the cells of the mastoid. **sclerosing m.**, mastoiditis attended with hardening and condensation of the bone. **silent m.**, a progressive destructive mastoiditis with mild systemic and local manifestations.

mastoidotomy (mas″toi-dot′o-me) [*mastoid* + Gr. *temnein* to cut] surgical incision of the mastoid process of the temporal bone.

mastoidotympanectomy (mas-toi″do-tim″pah-nek′to-me) radical mastoidectomy.

mastomenia (mas″to-me′ne-ah) [*masto-* + Gr. *mēniaia* the menses] vicarious menstruation from the breast.

mastoncus (mas-tong′kus) [*masto-* + Gr. *onkos* bulk] a tumor of the breast or mammary gland.

masto-occipital (mas″to-ok-sip′ĭ-tal) pertaining to the mastoid process and the occipital bone.

mastoparietal (mas″to-pah-ri′ĕ-tal) [*mastoid* + *parietal*] pertaining to the mastoid process and the parietal bone.

mastopathia (mas″to-path′e-ah) mastopathy. **m. cys′tica**, a morbid condition of the mammary gland, with the formation of cysts.

mastopathy (mas-top′ah-the) [*masto-* + Gr. *pathos* disease] disease of the mammary gland. **cystic m.**, mastopathia cystica.

mastopexy (mas′to-pek-se) [*masto-* + Gr. *pēxis* fixation.] mammaplasty performed to correct a pendulous breast.

Mastophora (mas-tof′o-rah) a genus of spiders; called also *Glyptocranium.* **M. gasteracanthoi′des,** the venomous cat-headed spider of Peru, Chile, and Argentina that has been shown to cause necrotic spot among vineyard workers.

mastoplasia (mas″to-pla′ze-ah) mammoplasia.

mastoplastia (mas″to-plas′te-ah) [*masto-* + Gr. *plassein* to form] hyperplasia of breast tissue.

mastoplasty (mas′to-plas″te) mammaplasty.

mastoptosis (mas″to-to′sis) [*masto-* + Gr. *ptōsis* fall] pendulous breasts.

mastorrhagia (mas″to-ra′je-ah) [*masto-* + Gr. *rhegnynai* to burst forth] hemorrhage from the mammary gland.

mastoscirrhus (mas″to-skir′us) [*masto-* + Gr. *skirros* hardness] hardening, or scirrhus, of the mammary gland.

mastosis (mas-to′sis), pl. *masto′ses* [*mast-* + *-osis*] a general term for pathologic changes in the breast of a degenerative and productive type characterized by enlargement and by the presence of painful nodular tumefactions.

mastosquamous (mas-to-skwa′mus) pertaining to or affecting the mastoid and squama of the temporal bone.

mastostomy (mas-tos′to-me) [*masto-* + Gr. *stomoun* to provide with an opening, or mouth] incision of the breast for drainage.

mastotic (mas-tot′ik) characterized by mastosis.

mastotomy (mas-tot′o-me) [*masto-* + Gr. *tomē* a cutting] surgical incision of a breast.

masturbation (mas″tur-ba′shun) [L. *manus* hand + *stuprare* to rape] production of orgasm by self-manipulation of the genitals.

Matas' band, operation, test (mat′as) [Rudolph *Matas*, surgeon in New Orleans, 1860–1957] see under *band*, see *endoaneurysmorrhaphy*, and see *tourniquet test* (def. 2), under *tests*.

matching (mach′ing) comparison for the purpose of selecting objects having similar or identical characteristics. In transplantation immunology, a method of measuring the degree of tissue compatibility between two individuals, done by such tests as the mixed leukocyte culture test. **m. of blood,** the procedure of comparing the blood of a contemplated donor with that of the patient (recipient) to ascertain whether their bloods belong to the same group. **cross m.,** determination of the compatibility of the blood of a donor and that of a recipient before transfusion by placing cells of the donor in the recipient's serum and cells of the recipient in the donor's serum. Absence of agglutination, hemolysis, and cytotoxicity indicates that the two blood specimens are compatible.

maté (mah-ta′) [Spanish American] the dried leaves of *Ilex paraguensis* St. Hil., Aquifoliaceae, a tree grown throughout Brazil, Uruguay, Paraguay, and Argentina as a source of tea. Its several synonyms include, yerba maté, Bartholomew's tea, Paraguay tea, and Jesuit's tea. It contains caffein and tannins, and has been used as a tonic, diuretic, stomachic, stimulant, and laxative (large doses).

Mátéfy test (reaction) (mah-ta′fe) [László *Mátéfy*, Hungarian physician, born 1889] see under *tests*.

mater (ma′ter) [L.] mother. **dura m.** ["hard mother"], see *dura mater.* **pia m.** ["tender mother"], see *pia mater.*

materia (mah-te′re-ah), pl. *mate′riae* [L.] matter, or substance; see also *materies.* **m. al′ba,** whitish deposits on the teeth, composed of mucus and epithelial cells containing bacteria and filamentous organisms. **m. den′tica,** that branch of study which deals with medicinal substances used in the practice of dentistry. **m. med′ica,** that branch of medical study which deals with drugs, their sources, preparations, and uses; pharmacology. **M. Med′ica Pu′ra,** Hahnemann's work giving the result of his provings of sixty-one drugs; it forms the basis of the homeopathic materia medica. **m. pec′cans,** materies peccans.

material (mah-te′re-al) substance or elements from which a concept may be formulated, or an object constructed. **base m.,** any substance that may be used in making the base for an artifical denture, such as acrylic resin, metal, polystyrene, etc. **cross-reacting m.,** a protein produced by a mutant cistron that reacts antigenically with antibody against the unaltered protein. Abbreviated CRM. **genetic m.,** material transmitted from an organism to those of succeeding generations and responsible for the features characteristic of the species, as well as for the heritable difference between individuals of the species. **impression m.,** any substance that may be used in making an impression of the teeth and other structures of the mouth, such as plaster of paris, alginates, rubber compounds, etc. **tissue equivalent m.,** a material whose absorbing and scattering properties for a given radiation simulate as closely as possible those of a given biological tissue, such as bone, fat, or muscle. Water, for example, is usually the best tissue equivalent material for muscle and soft tissue.

materies (mah-te′re-ēz) [L.] substance; see also *materia.* **m. mor′bi** [L. "substance of disease"], the element or principle which

causes a disease. **m. pec′cans** [L. "offending substance"], the principle that causes the pathologic changes occurring in disease.

maternal (mah-ter′nal) [L. *maternus; mater* mother] pertaining to the mother.

maternity (mah-ter′nĭ-te) [L. *mater* mother] 1. motherhood. 2. a lying-in hospital.

maternohemotherapy (mah-ter″no-he″mo-ther′ah-pe) [*maternal* + *hemotherapy*] injection of infants with blood from their mothers, formerly used in an attempt to transfer immunity to such diseases as measles and poliomyelitis from mother to child.

Mathieu's disease (mat′e-ūz′) [Albert *Mathieu*, physician in Paris, 1855–1917] leptospiral jaundice.

matico (mah-te′ko) the leaves of *Piper elongatum* Vahl. (*P. angustifolium* R. and P.), Piperaceae, a shrub of South and Central America; formerly used as an astringent and hemostatic. It contains volatile oil, maticin, tannin, and mucilage.

mating (māt′ing) [Ger. *mat* companion] pairing of individuals of the opposite sex, especially for reproduction. **assortative m.,** the mating of individuals with others of similar qualities or constitutions, as intelligence or stature. Called also *nonrandom mating.* **assorted m.,** assortive m. **assortive m.,** assortative m. **backcross m.,** the mating of a heterozygote and a recessive homozygote; useful in revealing, through the phenotypes of the offspring, the genotype of the heterozygous parent. **nonrandom m.,** assortative m. **random m.,** the mating of individuals without regard to any similarity between them.

matiniose (mah″tin-e-o′se) a Fijian word for yaws, which was once heavily endemic there.

matlazahuatl (mat-lahz″ah-waht′l) a form of typhus endemic in Mexico.

matrass (mat′ras) a glass vessel with a long neck used for treating dry substances in chemical procedures.

matrical (mat′rĭ-kal) of or relating to a matrix.

Matricaria (mat″rĭ-ka′re-ah) [L.] the dried flower heads of the composit plant *Matricaria chamomilla* L. It contains volatile oil, anthemic acid, tannin, and matricarin. Used as a counterirritant externally and as a carminative internally in the form of a tea. Also known as *chamomile tea.*

matrices (ma′trĭ-sēz) plural of *matrix.*

matricial (ma-trish′al) matrical.

matriclinous (mat″rĭ-kli′nus) matroclinous.

matrilineal (ma″trĭ-lin′e-al) [L. *mater* mother + *linea* line] descended through the female line.

matrix (ma′triks), pl. *ma′trices* [L.] 1. the intercellular substance of a tissue, as bone matrix, or the tissue from which a structure develops, as hair or nail matrix. 2. a metal band used to provide proper form to a dental restoration, such as amalgam in a prepared cavity. **amalgam m.,** matrix band. **bone m.,** the intercellular substance of bone, consisting of osteocollagenous fibers embedded in an amorphous ground substance and inorganic salts. **capsular m.,** territorial m. **cartilage m.,** the intercellular substance of cartilage, consisting of cells and extracellular fibers embedded in an amorphous ground substance; see also *interterritorial m.* and *territorial m.* **cytoplasmic m.,** the aggregating factor of the basic molecular fabric which ties together the ribosomes, RNA, proteins, small molecules, and water in the cytoplasm. **fluid m.,** Cannon's term for blood and lymph which bathe the cells of the body; see *homeostasis.* **functional m.,** the contiguous and motivating soft tissue organs and tissues in the growth of the craniofacial complex. **hair m.,** the epidermic root of the hair follicle. **interterritorial m.,** a paler-staining region located among the darker territorial matrices. **mitochondrial m.,** the dense substance, generally homogeneous but sometimes finely filamentous or granulated, found in the inner chamber (intercristal space) of mitochondria. **nail m.,** m. unguis. **sarcoplasmic m.,** the liquid substance which fills muscle cells; it contains the soluble enzymes of the cell. **territorial m.,** basophilic material surrounding groups of cartilage cells. **m. un′guis** [NA], the nail matrix: the tissue upon which the deep aspect of the nail rests; called also *nail bed.* The term is also used to denote the proximal portion of the nail bed from which growth chiefly proceeds.

matroclinous (mat″ro-kli′nus) [Gr. *mētēr* mother + *klinein* to incline] inheriting or inherited from the mother; possessing characters inherited from the mother.

matrocliny (mat″ro-kli′ne) the state of being matroclinous.

matt (mat) a term applied to a macroscopic morphology of bacterial colonies that are dull and slightly granular, i.e., neither smooth and glistening nor rough.

matter (mat′er) 1. substance; anything that occupies space. 2. pus. **gelatinous m.,** substantia gelatinosa; see entries beginning thus, under *substantia.* **gray m. of nervous system,** substantia grisea. **radiant m.,** matter in a condition of extreme tenuity or ultragaseous state; gas exhausted to about one millionth of its original density, so that it has lost its original properties and has acquired new, particularly luminous, ones. **white m. of nervous system,** substantia alba.

Matulane (mat′u-lān) trademark for a preparation of procarbazine hydrochloride.

maturant (mach′u-rant) an agent that promotes suppuration.

maturate (mach′u-rāt) 1. to mature. 2. to suppurate.

maturation (mach″u-ra′shun) [L. *maturatio; maturus* ripe] 1. the stage or process of becoming mature or fully developed. The attainment of emotional and intellectual maturity. In biology, a process of cell division during which the number of chromosomes in the germ cells is reduced to one half the number characteristic of the species. 2. suppuration.

mature (mah-chur) [L. *maturus*] 1. to develop to maturity; to ripen. 2. fully developed; ripe.

maturity (mah-chur′rĭ-te) the period of attainment of maximal development.

Matut. abbreviation for L. *matuti′nus*, in the morning.

matutinal (mah-tu′tĭ-nal) [L. *matutinalis*] pertaining to or occurring in the morning.

matzoon (mat-zūn′) [Armenian] a fermented milk preparation similar to yogurt, originally prepared in Asia Minor.

Mauchart's ligament (mow′karts) [Burkhard David *Mauchart*, German anatomist, 1696–1751] ligamenta aloria.

Maumené's test (mōm-nāz′) [Edme Jules *Maumené*, French chemist, born 1818] see under *tests*.

Maunoir's hydrocele (mo′nwarz) [Jean Pierre *Maunoir*, French surgeon, 1768–1861] cervical hydrocele.

Maurer's dots (clefts, spots, stippling) (mow′rerz) [Georg *Maurer*, German physician in Sumatra] see under *dot*.

Mauriac's syndrome (mo″re-aks′) [Pierre *Mauriac*, French surgeon] see under *syndrome*.

Mauriceau's lance, maneuver (mo′re-sōz) [François *Mauriceau*, French obstetrician, 1637–1709] see under *lance* and *maneuver*.

Mauthner's cell, fiber, membrane (sheath), test (mowt′-nerz) [Ludwig *Mauthner*, Austrian ophthalmologist, 1840–1894] see under *cell, fiber*, and *tests*, and see *axolemma*.

mauvein (mo′ve-in) aniline purple, a violet dye, $C_{27}H_{24}N_4$, used as an indicator, with a pH range of −0.1 to 2.9, being yellow at −0.1 and crimson at 2.9.

Maxcy's disease (mak′sēz) [Kenneth Fuller *Maxcy*, American bacteriologist, born 1889] see under *disease*.

Maxibolin (mak-sĭb′o-lin) trademark for a preparation of ethylestrenol.

maxilla (mak-sil′ah), pl. *maxil′las, maxil′lae* [L.] [NA] the irregularly shaped bone that with its fellow forms the upper jaw; it assists in the formation of the orbit, the nasal cavity, and the palate, and lodges the upper teeth. **inferior m.,** mandible (mandibula [NA]).

maxillae (mak-sil′e) [L.] plural of *maxilla*.

maxillary (mak′sĭ-ler″e) [L. *maxillaris*] pertaining to the maxilla.

maxillectomy (mak″sĭ-lek′to-me) surgical removal of the maxilla.

maxillitis (mak″sĭ-li′tis) inflammation of the maxilla.

maxillodental (mak-sil″o-den′tal) pertaining to the maxilla and the maxillary teeth.

maxilloethmoidectomy (mak″sil-o-eth″moi-dek′to-me) excision of the portion of the maxilla surrounding the maxillary sinus and of the cribriform plate and anterior ethmoid cells.

maxillofacial (mak-sil″o-fa′shal) pertaining to the maxilla and the face.

maxillojugal (mak-sil″o-ju′gal) pertaining to the maxilla and the cheek.

maxillolabial (mak-sil″o-la′be-al) pertaining to the maxilla and the lip.

maxillomandibular (mak-sil″o-man-dib′u-lar) pertaining to the maxilla and the mandible.

maxillopalatine (mak-sil″o-pal′ah-tīn) pertaining to the maxilla and the palatine bone.

maxillopharyngeal (mak-sil″o-fah-rin′je-al) pertaining to the maxilla and the pharynx.

maxillotomy (mak″sĭ-lot′o-me) surgical sectioning of the maxilla which allows movement of all or a part of the maxilla into the desired position.

maxima (mak′sĭ-mah) [L.] plural of *maximum*.

maximal (mak′sĭ-mal) the greatest possible, allowable, or appreciable; the reverse of *minimal*.

maximum (mak′sĭ-mum), pl. *max′ima* [L. "greatest"] 1. the greatest possible or actual effect or quantity. 2. the acme of a disease or process. 3. largest; utmost. 4. Pirquet's term for the greatest quantity of food which the organism can digest. **tubular m.,** the highest rate in milligrams per minute at which the renal tubules can transfer a substance either from the tubular luminal fluid to the interstitial fluid or from the interstitial fluid to the tubular luminal fluid. Abbreviated T_m.

Maxipen (mak′sĭ-pen) trademark for a preparation of phenethicillin potassium.

Maxitate (mak′sĭ-tāt) trademark for preparations of mannitol hexanitrate.

maxwell (maks′wel) [James Clerk *Maxwell*, British physicist, 1831–1879] the unit of magnetic flux; replaced in SI by the *weber*.

Maxwell's ring, spot (maks′welz) [Patrick William *Maxwell*, Irish ophthalmologist, 1856–1917] see under *ring*, and see *macula retinae*.

Maydl's operation (ma′delz) [Karel *Maydl*, Bohemian surgeon, 1853–1903] see under *operation*.

mayer (ma′er) [Julius Robert von *Mayer*, German physicist, 1814–1878] a unit of heat capacity; it is the capacity of a body that is warmed one degree centigrade by one joule. Abbreviated *my*.

Mayer's hemalum, muchematein (ma′erz) [Paul *Mayer*, German-Italian scientist, 1848–1923] see *Table of Stains*.

Mayer's test (reagent) (ma′erz) [Ferdinand F. *Mayer*, American pharmaceutical chemist of the 19th century] see under *tests*.

mayfly (ma′fli) an insect of the order Ephimeroptera with two, or sometimes one, pair of triangular membranous wings. See *Hexagenia bilineata*.

Mayo's operation, sign (ma′ōz) [William James (1861–1939) and Charles Horace (1865–1939) *Mayo*, American surgeons] see under *operation* and *sign*.

Mayo Robson see *Robson*.

Mayor's hammer, scarf [Mathias Louis *Mayor*, Swiss surgeon, 1776–1846] see under *hammer* and *scarf*.

maytansine (ma-tan′sēn) an antineoplastic derived from species of *Maytenus*, a genus of tropical American shrubs and trees, $C_{34}H_{46}ClN_3O_{10}$.

maza (maz′ah) [Gr. "a barley cake"] the placenta, def. 1.

maze (māz) a complicated system of intersecting paths used in intelligence tests and in demonstrating learning in experimental animals.

mazic (ma′zik) relating to the placenta; placental.

mazindol (ma′zin-dōl) chemical name: 5-(4-chlorophenyl)-2,5-dihydro-3H-imidazo[2,1-a]isoindol-5-ol. An adrenergic, $C_{16}H_{13}ClN_2O$, having amphetamine-like actions; used as an anorexic in the short-term treatment of exogenous obesity, administered orally.

mazo- [Gr. *mazos* breast] a combining form denoting relationship to the breast; see also words beginning *mammo-* and *masto-*.

mazodynia (ma″zo-din′e-ah) mastodynia.

mazopexy (ma′zo-pek″se) mastopexy.

mazoplasia (ma″zo-pla′se-ah) [*mazo-* + Gr. *plassein* to form] degenerative epithelial hyperplasia of the mammary acini.

mazun (ma′zun) a fermented milk preparation made in Armenia from buffalos' or goats' milk.

Mazzini's test (mah-ze′nēz) [L. Y. *Mazzini*, American scientist] see under *tests*.

Mazzoni's corpuscle (mad-zo′nēz) [*Vittorio Mazzoni*, Italian physician] see under *corpuscle*.

M.B. abbreviation for L. *Medici′nae Baccalau′reus*, Bachelor of Medicine.

m.b. abbreviation for L. *mis′ce be′ne*, mix well.

MBP an antigen prepared from *Brucella melitensis*, *B. bovis* and *B. suis*, formerly used in the treatment of brucellosis.

MBSA methylated bovine serum albumin, a commonly employed immunogen in experimental immunology.

mbundu (em-boon′doo) a West African poison made from roots of trees of genus *Strychnos*.

M.C. abbreviation for L. *Magis′ter Chirur′giae*, Master of Surgery, and for *Medical Corps*.

Mc. megacurie; megacycle.

mc. millicurie.

μC microcurie.

μc. microcurie.

mcg. microgram.

MCH mean corpuscular hemoglobin, an expression of the average hemoglobin content of a single cell in micromicrograms, obtained by multiplying the hemoglobin in grams by ten and dividing by the number of red cells (in millions).

mc.h. millicurie-hour.

mc-h millicurie-hour.

μc.h. microcurie-hour.

MCHC mean corpuscular hemoglobin concentration, an expression of the average hemoglobin concentration in per cent, obtained by multiplying the hemoglobin in grams by 100 and dividing by the hematocrit determination.

MCHg mean corpuscular hemoglobin.

mc-hr millicurie-hour.

μC hr. microcurie-hour.

mcoul millicoulomb.

μcoul microcoulomb.

Mc.p.s. megacycles per second.

M.C.S.P. Member of the Chartered Society of Physiotherapists (Brit.).

MCT mean circulation time.

MCV 1. mean corpuscular volume, an expression of the average volume of individual red cells in cubic microns, obtained by multiplying the hematocrit determination by ten and dividing by the number of red cells (in millions). 2. mean clinical value, a number obtained by assigning a numerical value to the response as noted in a number of patients receiving a specific treatment, adding these numbers, and dividing by the number of patients treated.

Md chemical symbol for *mendelevium*.

M.D. abbreviation for L. *Medici'nae Doc'tor*, Doctor of Medicine.

M.D.A. motor discriminative acuity; [L.] mento-dextra anterior (right mento-anterior, a position of the fetus).

M.D.P. [L.] *mento-dextra posterior* (right mentoposterior, a position of the fetus).

M.D.T. [L.] *mento-dextra transversa* (right mentotransverse, a position of the fetus).

Me chemical symbol for *methyl*, or CH_3.

meal (mēl) 1. a portion of food or foods taken at some particular and usually stated or fixed time. Often given with the specific purpose of aiding diagnostic examination. See also *test meal* (under *T*). 2. a coarsely ground substance, prepared from various grains. **bismuth m.**, an opaque meal in which some preparation of bismuth is the opaque constituent. **Boyden m.**, a test meal for the study of gallbladder evacuation in cholecystographic studies, consisting of 3 egg yolks, 3 teaspoonfuls of powdered whole milk, and 1 dessertspoonful of sugar with a drop of vanilla, with water slowly added up to make 200 ml. **butter m.**, a concentrated food containing butter, milk, flour, and sugar. **Knoepfelmacher's butter m.**, a preparation of milk, flour, butter, and sugar, used in child feeding. **liver m.**, a mixture of desiccated beef liver, malted milk, and powdered cinnamon; used for liver diet. **opaque m.**, a light meal, sometimes a glass of buttermilk, which contains some substance opaque to the roentgen rays, so that the outline of the stomach and the intestinal tract can be determined by roentgenography or roentgenoscopy. **Oslo m.** [Carl Schiotz of *Oslo*], a meal for school children consisting of a third of a liter of unskimmed milk, whole-meal bread with margarine and goat's-milk cheese, half an orange, half an apple, and a raw carrot. **retention m.**, a form of test meal which is retained, a specimen of the stomach contents being removed from time to time for analysis. **test m.**, see *test meal*, under *T*.

mean (mēn) an average; a numerical value intermediate between two extremes. In statistical methods, the abscissa of the center of gravity of the variables or of the frequency polygon. **arithmetical m.**, the arithmetical average. **geometrical m.**, the antilogarithm of the arithmetical mean of the logarithm of a series of values.

measles (me'zelz) 1. a highly contagious viral infection involving primarily the respiratory tract and reticuloendothelial tissues. Called also *rubeola*. A prodrome of three to five days duration begins about eight days after inhalation of the virus in droplets derived from a person in the prodromal or early eruptive phase of the infection. Coryza, cervical lymphadenitis, Koplik's spots, palpebral conjunctivitis, photophobia, myalgia, malaise, and a harassing cough with steadily mounting fever precede the skin eruption. The skin becomes covered with red papules that appear behind the ears and on the face before spreading rapidly down the trunk and onto the arms and legs. The papules are discrete but gradually become more confluent. The lesions flatten, turn brown, and slowly desquamate on about the sixth day, when the temperature has returned to normal. It may be complicated by bacterial pneumonia, otitis media, and by a demyelinating encephalitis. Fatalities are due to the severity of measles itself, or to the bacterial or immunological complications. 2. cysticercal disease of domestic animals. **atypical m.**, a form of natural measles infection affecting those who previously received killed measles virus vaccine, characterized by fever, headache, myalgia, abdominal symptoms, and cough, followed by a maculopapular rash that begins on the wrist and ankles, then spreads to the palms, soles, and trunk before fading. There is peripheral edema, pneumonitis and, often, pleural effusion. The disease may be confused with meningococcemia or rickettsial diseases. **bastard m.**, rubella. **black m.**, a severe form in which the eruption is very dark and petechial. **confluent m.**, measles in which the lesions of the eruption coalesce. **German m.**, rubella. **hemorrhagic m.**, black m. **pork m.**, a condition in which pork is infected with the *Cysticercus cellulosae*.

measly (me'zle) containing cysticerci.

measure (mezh'er) [L. *mensuura*] 1. to determine the extent or quantity of a substance. 2. a specific extent or quantity of a substance. 3. a graduated scale by which the dimensions or mass of an object or substance may be determined. See *tables of weights and measures*, under *weight*.

meatal (me-a'tal) pertaining to a meatus.

meatome (me'ah-tōm) meatotome.

meatometer (me"ah-tom'ĕ-ter) [L. *meatus* passage + *metrum* measure] an instrument for measuring a meatus.

meatorrhaphy (me"ah-tor'ah-fe) [L. *meatus* + Gr. *rhaphē* suture] suture of the cut end of the urethra to the glans penis after incision for enlarging the meatus.

meatoscope (me-at'o-skōp) [L. *meatus* meatus + Gr. *skopein* to examine] a speculum for examining the urinary meatus.

meatoscopy (me"ah-tos'ko-pe) the inspection of any meatus, especially the urinary meatus or the vesical orifice of a ureter. **ureteral m.,** cystoscopic inspection of the vesical orifice of a ureter.

meatotome (me-at'o-tōm) an instrument for performing meatotomy.

meatotomy (me"ah-tot'o-me) [L. *meatus* passage + Gr. *temnein* to cut] incision of the urinary meatus in order to enlarge it.

meatus (mea'tus), pl. *meat'tus* [L., "a way, path, course"] an opening or passage; [NA] a general term for an opening or passageway in the body. **acoustic m., external,** m. acusticus externus. **acoustic m., external, bony,** meatus acusticus externus osseus. **acoustic m., external cartilaginous,** m. acusticus externus cartilagineus. **acoustic m., internal,** m. acusticus internus. **acoustic m., internal, bony,** m. acusticus internus osseus. **m. acus'ticus exter'nus** [NA], external acoustic meatus: the passage of the external ear leading to the tympanic membrane; called also *external auditory m.* **m. acus'ticus exter'nus cartilagin'eus** [NA], cartilaginous external acoustic meatus: the cartilaginous part of the external acoustic meatus, found lateral to the bony part. **m. acus'ticus exter'nus os'seus** [NA], bony external acoustic meatus: the opening in the external surface of the temporal bone, posterior to the condyle of the mandible and anterior to the mastoid air cells. **m. acus'ticus inter'nus** [NA], internal acoustic meatus: the passage through which the facial, intermediate, and vestibulocochlear nerves and the labyrinthine artery pass. **m. acus'ticus inter'nus os'seus** [NA], bony internal acoustic meatus: the opening on the posterior surface of the petrous part of the temporal bone through which the facial, intermediate, and vestibulocochlear nerves, and the labyrinthine artery pass. **m. audito'rius exter'nus** [NA], m. acusticus externus. **m. audito'rius exter'nus cartilagin'eus,** m. acusticus externus cartilagineus. **m. audito'rius exter'nus os'seus,** m. acusticus externus osseus. **m. audito'rius inter'nus,** m. acusticus internus. **m. audito'rius inter'nus os'seus,** m. acusticus internus osseus. **auditory m., external,** m. acusticus externus. **auditory m., external, bony,** m. acusticus externus osseus. **auditory m., external, cartilaginous,** m. acusticus externus cartilagineus. **auditory m., internal,** m. acusticus internus. **auditory m., internal, bony,** m. acusticus internus osseus. **m. con'chae ethmoturbina'lis mino'ris,** m. nasi superior. **m. con'chae maxilloturbina'lis,** m. nasi inferior. **m. con'chae turbina'lis majo'ris,** m. nasi superior. **fish-mouth m.,** a red, swollen, and everted urinary meatus seen in the first stage of acute gonorrhea. **nasal m., common, bony,** m. nasi communis osseus. **nasal m., inferior,** m. nasi inferior. **nasal m., inferior, bony,** m. nasi inferior osseus. **nasal m., middle,** m. nasi medius. **nasal m., middle, bony,** m. nasi medius osseus. **nasal m., superior,** m. nasi superior. **nasal m., superior, bony,** m. nasi superior osseus. **m. na'si commu'nis,** common meatus of nose: the anterior space on either side of the nasal septum into which the three meatuses open. **m. na'si commun'nis os'seus,** bony common meatus of nose: the space on either side of the nasal septum bounded by the bones of the cranium. **m. na'si infe'rior** [NA], inferior meatus of nose: the space beneath the inferior nasal concha, into which the nasolacrimal duct opens. **m. na'si infe'rior os'seus** [NA], bony inferior meatus of nose: the opening in the cranium overhung by the inferior bony nasal concha. **m. na'si me'dius** [NA], middle meatus of nose: the space beneath the middle nasal concha, with which the anterior ethmoidal cells and frontal and maxillary sinuses communicate. **m. na'si me'dius os'seus** [NA], bony middle meatus of nose: the opening in the cranium overhung by the middle bony nasal concha. **m. na'si supe'rior** [NA], superior meatus of nose: the narrow cavity below the superior nasal concha, with which the posterior ethmoidal cells communicate. **m. na'si supe'rior os'seus** [NA], bony superior meatus of nose: the slender, channel-like opening in the cranium inferior to the superior bony nasal concha. **nasopharyngeal m.,** m. nasopharyngeus. **nasopharyngeal m., bony,** m. nasopharyngeus osseus. **m. nasopharyn'geus** [NA], nasopharyngeal meatus: the part of the nasal cavity coinciding with the bony nasopharyngeal cavity. **m. nasopharyn'geus os'seus** [NA], bony nasopharyngeal meatus: the opening in the cranium between the posterior edges of the middle and inferior bony nasal conchae and the choanae. **m's of nose,** see *m. nasi communis, m. nasi inferior, m. nasi medius,* and *m. nasi superior.* **m. of nose, bony, common,** m. nasi communis osseus. **m. of nose, common,** m. nasi communis. **m. of nose, inferior,** m. nasi inferior. **m. of nose, inferior, bony,** m. nasi inferior osseus. **m. of nose, middle,**

m. nasi medius. **m. of nose, middle, osseous,** m. nasi medius osseus. **m. of nose, superior,** m. nasi superior. **m. of nose, superior, osseous,** m. nasi superior osseus. **m. urina′rius, urinary m.,** the external urethral orifice: the opening of the urethra on the body surface through which urine is discharged. See *ostium urethrae externa feminina* and *ostium urethrae externum masculinae.*

Mebaral (meb′ah-ral) trademark for a preparation of mephobarbital.

mebendazole (me-ben′dah-zōl) [USP] chemical name: (5-benzoyl-1*H*-benzimidazol-2-yl)carbamic acid methyl ester. An anthelmintic, $C_{16}H_{13}N_3O_3$, used in the treatment of trichuriasis, enterobiasis, ascariasis, and hookworm disease, administered orally.

mebeverine hydrochloride (mĕ-bev′er-ēn) chemical name: 4-[ethyl(*p*-methoxy-α-methylphenethyl)amino]butyl veratrate hydrochloride; a smooth muscle relaxant, $C_{25}H_{35}NO_5 \cdot HCl$.

mebutamate (mĕ-bu′tah-māt) chemical name: 2-methyl-2-(1-methylpropyl)-1,3-propanediol dicarbamate. A mildly tranquilizing, antihypertensive agent, $C_{10}H_{20}N_2O_4$, occurring as a white, crystalline powder; used alone or in conjunction with diuretics and other hypotensive drugs, administered orally.

mecamine (mek′ah-min) mecamylamine.

mecamylamine hydrochloride (mek″ah-mil′ah-min) [USP] chemical name: *N*,2,3,3-tetramethylbicyclo[2.2.1]heptan-2-amine hydrochloride. A ganglionic-blocking agent, $C_{11}H_{21}N \cdot HCl$, occurring as a white, crystalline powder; used as an antihypertensive, usually in the treatment of moderate to severe hypertension, administered orally.

mechanical (me-kan′ĭ-kal) [Gr. *mēchanikos*] 1. pertaining to or accomplished by mechanical or physical forces. 2. performed by means of some artificial mechanism.

mechanicoreceptor (me-kan″ĭ-ko-re-sep′tor) mechanoreceptor.

mechanicotherapeutics, mechanicotherapy (me-kan″ĭ-ko-ther″ah-pu′tiks, me-kan″ĭ-ko-ther′ah-pe) mechanotherapy.

mechanics (me-kan′iks) the science dealing with the motions of material bodies, including kinematics, dynamics, and statics. **animal m.,** biomechanics. **body m.,** the application of kinesiology to use of the body in daily life activities and to the prevention and correction of problems related to posture. **developmental m.,** embryological mechanisms as revealed mainly by experimentation.

mechanism (mek′ah-nizm) [Gr. *mēchanē* machine] 1. a machine or machine-like structure. 2. the manner of combination of parts, processes, etc., which subserve a common function. 3. the theory that the phenomena of life are based on the same physical and chemical laws which operate in the inorganic world; opposed to *vitalism.* **countercurrent m.,** the renal mechanism by which urine is concentrated; it is dependent upon the anatomical arrangement of the loops of Henle and the vasa recta. **defense m.,** a mental mechanism by which psychic tension is diminished, e.g., repression, denial, overcompensation, rationalization, etc. Called also *escape m.* **Douglas' m.,** see under *method.* **Duncan m.,** expulsion of the placenta with the maternal, or rough, surface appearing at the vulva. **escape m.,** defense m. **Frank-Starling m.,** the ventricular response to an increase in either volume load or pressure load by diastolic distention and increased energy release. **m. of labor,** the factors involved in the expulsion of the fetus, placenta, and membranes through the birth canal in labor. **mental m.,** 1. the organization of mental operations. 2. an unconscious and indirect manner of gratifying a repressed desire. **neutralizing m.,** a mental mechanism which neutralizes the manifest content of a dream. **oculogyric m.,** the series of nerve centers concerned in movements of the eye. **outgoing m.,** the apparatus by which words are uttered or ideas expressed, as in speech, writing, or in the use of expressive gestures. **ping-pong m.,** a process in which one substrate reacts with an enzyme and dissociates into one product, leaving a functional group attached to the enzyme; in a second reaction, the modified enzyme transfers the attached functional group to a second substrate, forming a second product and releasing the enzyme in its original form. **re-entrant m.,** see *re-entry.* **somatic m.,** the structures and organs through which the somatic activities of the body are performed. **splanchnic m.,** the structures and organs through which the visceral activities of the body are performed.

mechanist (mek′ah-nist) one who believes that all phenomena relating to life are based on physical and chemical properties only.

mechano- [Gr. *mēchanē* machine] a combining form meaning mechanical or denoting relationship to a machine.

mechanocyte (mek′ah-no-sīt″) [*mechano-* + *-cyte*] fibroblast.

mechanogymnastics (mek″ah-no-jim-nas′tiks) gymnastics carried out by means of mechanical apparatus, such as the Zander apparatus.

mechanology (mek″ah-nol′o-je) [*mechano-* + *-logy*] the science of mechanics.

mechanoreceptor (mek″ah-no-re-sep′tor) a receptor that is excited by mechanical pressures or distortions, as those responding to sound, touch, and muscular contractions.

mechanotherapy (mek″ah-no-ther′ah-pe) [*mechano-* + Gr. *therapeia* treatment] the use of mechanical apparatus in the treatment of disease or its results, especially as an aid in performing therapeutic exercises.

mechanothermy (mek″ah-no-ther′me) [*mechano-* + Gr. *thermē* heat] therapeutic heat produced by massage, exercise, etc.

mechlorethamine hydrochloride (mek″lōr-eth′ah-mēn) [USP] chemical name: 2-chloro-*N*-(2-chloroethyl)-*N*-methylethanamine hydrochloride. A cytotoxic alkylating agent, $C_5H_{11}Cl_2N \cdot HCl$, the first of the nitrogen mustards, having immunosuppressive properties as well as cytotoxic activities, occurring as a white, crystalline powder; used as an antineoplastic in many types of malignancies, especially in the treatment of Hodgkin's disease. Called also *nitrogen mustard.*

Mechnikov (mech′nĭ-kov″) see *Metchnikoff.*

mecism (me′sizm) [Gr. *mēkos* length] abnormal lengthening of a part.

mecistocephalic (me-sis″to-sĕ-fal′ik) [Gr. *mēkistos* tallest + *kephalē* head] having a cephalic index less than 71.

mecistocephalous (me-sis″to-sef′ah-lus) mecistocephalic.

Mecistocirrhus (me-sis″to-sir′us) a genus of nematode parasites found in the fourth stomach of ruminants. **M. digita′tus,** a species found in various ruminants, and in man and swine; called also *Strongylus gibsoni.*

Meckel's band (ligament), cavity (space), ganglion (mek′elz) [Johann Friedrich *Meckel* (the elder), Berlin anatomist, 1714–1774] see under *band,* and see *cavum trigeminale, ganglion pterygopalatinum,* and *ganglion submandibulare.*

Meckel's cartilage (rod), diverticulum, plane, syndrome (mek′elz) [Johann Friedrich *Meckel* (the younger) (grandson of J. F. Meckel, the elder), anatomist in Halle, 1781–1833] see under *cartilage, diverticulum, plane,* and *syndrome.*

meckelectomy (mek″el-ek′to-me) [*Meckel's ganglion* + Gr. *ektomē* excision] surgical removal of Meckel's lesser (the submandibular) ganglion.

meclizine hydrochloride (mek′lĭ-zēn) [USP] chemical name: 1-[(4-chlorophenyl)phenylmethyl]-4-[(3-methylphenyl)methyl]piperazine dihydrochloride monohydrate. An antihistamine, $C_{25}H_{27}ClN_2 \cdot 2HCl \cdot H_2O$, occurring as a white or slightly yellowish, crystalline powder; used as an antiemetic in the management of nausea, vomiting, and dizziness associated with motion sickness, administered orally. Called also *parachloramine.*

meclocycline (mek-lo-si′klēn) chemical name: 7-chloro-4-(dimethylamino)-1,4,4a,5,5a-6,11,12a-octahydro-3,5,10,12,12a-pentahydroxy-6-methylene-1,11-dioxo-2-naphthacenecarboxamide; an antibiotic of unspecified action, $C_{22}H_{21}ClN_2O_8$.

mecloqualone (mĕ-klo-kwah′lōn) chemical name: 3-(2-chlorophenyl)-2-methyl-4(3*H*)-quinazolinone; a sedative and hypnotic, $C_{15}H_{11}ClN_2O$.

mecobalamine (me″ko-bal′ah-min) a naturally occurring hematopoietic vitamin found in the blood, $C_{63}H_{91}CoN_{13}O_{14}P$, closely related to cyanocobalamin, in which the cyano radical has been replaced by a methyl radical.

mecocephalic (me″ko-sĕ-fal′ik) [Gr. *mēkos* length + Gr. *kephalē* head] dolichocephalic.

meconate (mek′o-nāt) [Gr. *mēkōn* poppy + *-ate*] any salt of meconic acid.

meconiorrhea (mĕ-ko″ne-o-re′ah) [*meconium* + Gr. *rhoia* flow] excessive discharge of meconium.

meconium (mĕ-ko′ne-um) [L.; Gr. *mēkōnion*] 1. a dark green mucilaginous material in the intestine of the full term fetus, being a mixture of the secretions of the intestinal glands and some amniotic fluid. 2. opium.

mecrylate (mĕ-kri′lāt) chemical name: 2-cyano-2-propenoic acid methyl ester; a tissue adhesive for use in surgery, $C_5H_5NO_2$.

mecystasis (mĕ-sis′tah-sis) [Gr. *mēkynein* to lengthen + *stasis* a setting] a state in which a muscle fiber is relatively increased in length, resists stretch, contracts, and relaxes, and manifests the same tension as before elongation.

M.E.D. minimal effective dose; minimal erythema dose.

Medawar (med′ah-war), Peter B. English biologist, born 1915; co-winner, with Macfarlane Burnet, of the Nobel prize in medicine and physiology for 1960, for the theoretical solution to the problem of transplanting tissues and vital organs from one animal to another.

medazepam hydrochloride (mĕ-daz′ĕ-pam) chemical name: 7-chloro-2,3-dihydro-1-methyl-5-phenyl-1*H*-1,4-benzodiazepine monohydrochloride; a minor tranquilizer, $C_{16}H_{15}ClN_2 \cdot HCl$.

Medex [Fr. *médecin extension* extension of the physician] a program that recruits former military medics for training and practice as physician assistants; abbreviated Mx.

medi (mi′theh) maedi.

media (me′de-ah) [L.] 1. plural of *medium.* 2. middle; see *tunica media.*

mediad (me′de-ad) [L. *medium* middle + *ad* toward] toward a median line or plane.

medial (me′de-al) [L. *medialis*] 1. pertaining to the middle;

closer to the median plane or the midline of a body or structure. 2. pertaining to the middle layer of structures.

medialecithal (me″de-ah-les′ĭ-thal) [*media-* + Gr. *lekithos* yolk] possessing a medium amount of yolk; see under *ovum*.

medialis (me″de-a′lis) medial; [NA] a general term denoting a structure situated nearer to the median plane or the midline of a body or structure.

median (me′de-an) [L. *medianus*] 1. situated in the median plane or in the midline of a body or structure. 2. the perpendicular line which divides the area of a frequency curve into two equal halves.

medianus (me″de-a′nus) [L.] median, or situated in the middle; [NA] a general term denoting structures lying in the median plane, that is, in the plane dividing the body into right and left halves.

mediaometer (me″de-ah-om′ĕ-ter) [*media* + Gr. *metron* measure] an instrument for detecting and measuring refractive errors of the dioptric mediums.

mediastina (me″de-as-ti′nah) [L.] plural of *mediastinum*.

mediastinal (me″de-as-ti′nal) [L. *mediastinalis*] of or pertaining to the mediastinum.

mediastinitis (me″de-as″tĭ-ni′tis) inflammation of the mediastinum. **fibrous m., indurative m.,** an exuberant inflammatory sclerogenic process of infectious, rheumatic, hemorrhagic, or undetermined origin, which may be associated with fibrous pericarditis and with inflammatory fibrous masses in other parts of the body; it is often accompanied by obstruction of mediastinal structures, especially the superior vena cava, and, less often, the tracheobronchial tree, the esophagus, and other structures.

mediastinography (me″de-as″tĭ-nog′rah-fe) roentgenography of the mediastinum.

mediastinogram (me″de-as-ti′no-gram) a roentgenogram of the mediastinum.

mediastinopericarditis (me″de-as″tĭ-no-per″ĭ-kar-di′tis) adhesive pericarditis in which the adhesions extend from the pericardium to the mediastinum. See also *adhesive pericarditis*, under *pericarditis*.

mediastinoscope (me″de-ah-sti′no-skōp) a specially designed endoscope used in mediastinoscopy.

mediastinoscopic (me″de-as″tĭ-no-skop′ik) pertaining to the mediastinoscopy or to mediastinoscopy.

mediastinoscopy (me″de-as″tĭ-nos′ko-pe) examination of the mediastinum by means of an endoscope inserted through an anterior midline incision just above the thoracic inlet, permitting direct inspection and biopsy of tissue in the anterior superior mediastinum.

mediastinotomy (me″de-as″ti-not′o-me) [*mediastinum* + Gr. *tomē* a cutting] the operation of cutting into the mediastinum. Performed from the front, it is *anterior* or *cervical m.;* from the back, *posterior* or *dorsal m.*

mediastinum (me″de-as-ti′num), pl. *mediasti′na* [L.] 1. a median septum or partition. 2. [NA] the mass of tissues and organs separating the two lungs, between the sternum in front and the vertebral column behind, and from the thoracic inlet above to the diaphragm below. It contains the heart and its large vessels, the trachea, esophagus, thymus, lymph nodes, and other structures and tissues, and is divided into anterior, middle, posterior, and superior regions. Called also *septum mediastinale* or *mediastinal septum.* **anterior m., m. ante′rius** [NA], the division of the mediastinum bounded behind by the pericardium, in front by the sternum, and on each side by the pleura. It contains loose areolar tissue, lymphatic vessels, the internal thoracic vessels of the left side, and the origins of the sternohyoid, sternothyroid, and triangularis sterni muscles. Called also *cavum mediastinale anterius* or *anterior mediastinal cavity*. **m. cerebel′li** (*obs.*), falx cerebelli. **m. cer′ebri** (*obs.*), falx cerebri. **m. me′dium** [NA], **middle m.,** the division of the mediastinum containing the heart enclosed in its pericardium, the ascending aorta, the superior vena cava, the bifurcation of the trachea, the pulmonary arteries and veins, the phrenic nerves, a large portion of the roots of the lungs, and the arch of the azygos vein. **posterior m., m. poste′rius** [NA], the division of the mediastinum bounded behind by the vertebral column, in front by the pericardium, and on each side by the pleurae. It contains the descending aorta, the greater and lesser azygos veins, the superior intercostal vein, the thoracic duct, the esophagus, the vagus nerves, and the great splanchnic nerves. Caled also *cavum mediastinale posterius* or *posterior mediastinal cavity*. **superior m., m. supe′rius** [NA], the division of the mediastinum extending from the pericardium to the root of the neck, and containing the esophagus and the trachea behind, the thymus or its remains in front, and the great vessels related to the heart and pericardium in between. **m. tes′tis** [NA], the partial septum of the testis, formed near its posterior border by fibrous tissue which is continuous with the tunica albuginea; called also *body of Highmore*.

mediastinus (me″de-as-ti′nus) [L.] an assistant physician or surgeon.

mediate (me′de-it) indirect; accomplished by the aid of an intervening medium.

mediation (me″de-a′shun) the act of interposing or serving as an intermediary. **chemical m.,** the concept that excitation in passing from a pre- to a postsynaptic neural element undergoes a necessary chemical step.

mediator (me′de-a″tor) an object or substance by which something is mediated, such as (1) a structure of the nervous system that transmits impulses eliciting a specific response; (2) a chemical substance (transmitter substance) that induces activity in an excitable tissue, such as nerve or muscle; or (3) a substance released from cells as the result of the interaction of antigen with antibody or by the action of antigen with a sensitized lymphocyte.

medicable (med′ĭ-kah-bl) subject to treatment with reasonable expectation of cure.

medical (med′ĭ-kal) pertaining to medicine or to the treatment of diseases; pertaining to medicine as opposed to surgery.

medicament (med′ĭ-kah-ment, mĕ-dik′ah-ment) [L. *medicamentum*] a medicinal substance or agent.

medicamentosus (med″ĭ-kah-men-to′sus) [L.] medicamentous.

medicamentous (med″ĭ-kah-men′tus) pertaining to, used in, or caused by a drug or drugs.

Medicare (med′ĭ-kār) a program administered by the Social Security Administration which provides medical care for the aged.

medicaster (med′ĭ-kas″ter) a pretender to medical skill; a charlatan or quack.

medicate (med′ĭ-kāt) [L. *medicatus*] to impregnate or imbue with a medicinal substance.

medicated (med′ĭ-kāt″ed) imbued with a medicinal substance.

medication (med″ĭ-ka′shun) [L. *medicatio*] 1. impregnation with a medicine. 2. the administration of remedies. 3. a medicament. **conservative m.,** treatment aimed to build up the vital powers of the patient. **dialytic m.,** treatment by the internal use of artificial mineral waters, i.e., dilute aqueous solutions of salts. **hypodermatic m.,** the introduction of remedial agents beneath the skin. **ionic m.,** iontophoresis. **sublingual m.,** the administration of medicine by placing it beneath the tongue. **substitutive m.,** medication for the purpose of causing an acute nonspecific inflammation to overcome a specific one. **transduodenal m.,** the administration of medicine through a duodenal tube into the intestines without soiling the stomach.

medicator (med′ĭ-ka″tor) an instrument for carrying medicines into a cavity of the body; an applicator.

medicephalic (me″de-sĕ-fal′ik) median cephalic; see under *vein*.

medicinal (me-dis′ĭ-nal) [L. *medicinalis*] 1. having healing qualities. 2. pertaining to a medicine or to healing.

medicine (med′ĭ-sin) [L. *medicina*] 1. any drug or remedy. 2. the art and science of the diagnosis and treatment of disease and the maintenance of health. 3. the treatment of disease by nonsurgical means. **aviation m.,** that branch of medicine which has to do with the physiological, medical, psychological, and epidemiological problems involved in aviation. **clinical m.,** 1. the study of disease by direct examination of the living patient. 2. the last two years of the usual curriculum in a medical college. **comparative m.,** the study of phenomena basic to the diseases of all species. **compound m.,** a medicine containing a mixture of several drugs. **domestic m.,** the home treatment of disorders without the advice of a physician. **dosimetric m.,** the practice of administering medicines by an exact and determinate system of doses. **emergency m.,** that specialty which deals with acutely ill or injured patients who require immediate medical treatment. **environmental m.,** that which considers the effects of the environment on man, including rapid population growth, changes and extremes in temperature, alterations in atmospheric pressure, water and air pollution, radiation, travel, etc. **experimental m.,** the study of disease based on experimentation in animals. **family m.,** see under *practice*. **folk m.,** the use of home remedies and procedures as handed down by tradition. **forensic m.,** the application of medical knowledge to questions of law; medical jurisprudence; called also *legal m*. **galenic m.,** an absolute system of practice based upon the teachings of Galen. **geriatric m.,** geriatrics. **group m.,** the practice of medicine by a group of physicians, usually representing various specialties, who are associated together for the cooperative diagnosis, treatment, and prevention of disease. Called also *group practice*. **hermetic m.,** spagyric m. **holistic m.,** a system of medicine which considers man as an integrated whole, or as a functioning unit. **hyperbaric m.,** the treatment of disease in an environment of higher than atmospheric pressure. **Indian m.,** a North American form of quackery alleged to be derived from the aboriginals. **internal m.,** that branch of medicine dealing especially with the diagnosis and medical treatment of diseases and disorders of the internal structures of the human body. **ionic m.,** treatment by electrochemical means, as by cataphoresis and iontophoresis. **laboratory animal m.,** that specialty of veterinary medicine which deals with the diagnosis, treatment, and prevention of disease in animals used as subjects in biomedical activities. **legal m.,** forensic m. **mental m.,** psychiatry. **neo-hippocratic m.,** neo-hippocratism. **nuclear m.,** that branch of medicine concerned with the use of radionuclides in the diagnosis and treatment of disease. **patent m.,** a drug or remedy protected by a trademark, available without prescription. **physical m.,** physiatrics. **preclinical m.,** 1. medical practice devoted to keeping the well well and preventing or postponing the development of clinical conditions in the near sick; preventive medicine. 2. the first two years of the usual curriculum in a medical college. **preventive m.,** that branch of study and practice which aims at the prevention of disease. **proprietary m.,** a drug or remedy to which the manufacturing pharmaceutical house has exclusive (proprietary) rights, and which is marketed usually under a name that is registered as a trademark. **psychologic m.,** medicine in its relation to mental diseases. **psychosomatic m.,** a system of medicine which aims at discovering the exact nature of the relationship of the emotions and bodily function, affirming the principle that the mind and body are one; the simultaneous application of physiologic and psychologic technics in the study and treatment of illness. **rational m.,** practice of medicine based upon actual knowledge; opposed to *empiricism.* **social m.,** phases of preventive medicine and the care of the sick which concern the community as a whole or large groups of persons rather than the individual. **socialized m.,** a system of medical care regulated and controlled by the government, in which the government assumes responsibility for providing for the health needs and hospital care of the entire population, at no direct cost or at a nominal fee to the individual, by means of subsidies obtained by taxation. Called also *state m.* **space m.,** that branch of aviation medicine concerned solely with conditions to be encountered by man in space. **spagyric m.** (*obs.*), semialchemistic system of practice established by Paracelsus (1493–1541). **sports m.,** the field of medicine concerned with injuries sustained in athletic endeavors, including their prevention, diagnosis, treatment, etc. **state m.,** socialized m. **static m.,** practice of medicine based on the varying relations of administration of food, excretion, and body weight. **suggestive m.,** treatment of disease by suggestion or hypnosis. **tropical m.,** medical science as applied to diseases occurring primarily in tropical and subtropical countries. **veterinary m.,** the science of treatment of the diseases of animals.

medicochirurgic (med″ĭ-ko-ki-rur′jik) pertaining to medicine and surgery.

medicodental (med″ĭ-ko-den′tal) pertaining to both medicine and dentistry.

medicolegal (med″ĭ-ko-le′gal) pertaining to medicine and law, or to forensic medicine.

medicomechanical (med″ĭ-ko-me-kan′ĭ-kal) both medicinal and mechanical.

medicophysics (med″ĭ-ko-fiz′iks) physics as applied to medicine.

medicopsychological (med″ĭ-ko-si″ko-loj′ĭ-kal) pertaining to medicopsychology.

medicopsychology (med″ĭ-ko-si-kol′o-je) the science of medicine in its relations with the mind or with mental diseases.

medicosocial (med″ĭ-ko-so′shal) having both medical and social aspects, as, for example, the prevention and treatment of venereal disease.

medicotopographical (med″ĭ-ko-to″po-graf′ĭ-kal) pertaining to topography in its relation to disease.

medicozoological (med″ĭ-ko-zo-o-loj′ĭ-kal) pertaining to zoology in its relation to medicine.

medicus (med′ĭ-kus), pl. *med′ici* [L.] physician.

medifrontal (me″dĭ-fron′tal) median and frontal; pertaining to the middle of the forehead.

Medin's disease (ma′dēnz) [Oskar *Medin,* Swedish physician, 1847–1928] see *poliomyelitis.*

mediocarpal (me″de-o-kar′pal) midcarpal.

mediooccipital (me″de-ok-sip′ĭ-tal) midoccipital.

mediolateral (me″do-o-lat′er-al) [L. *medius* middle + *lateralis* lateral] pertaining to the middle and to one side.

medionecrosis (me″de-o-ne-kro′sis) necrosis of the tunica media of a blood vessel, often leading to its rupture. **m. of aorta,** Erdheim's cystic medial necrosis.

mediotarsal (me″de-o-tar′sal) [L. *medius* middle + *tarsus*] pertaining to the middle of the tarsus.

mediscalenus (me″de-skah-le′nus) musculus scalenus medius.

medisect (me′dĭ-sekt) [L. *medius* middle + *secare* to cut] to divide or dissect medially.

meditation (med″ĭ-ta′shun) the act of reflecting upon or contemplating; an exercise in contemplation. **transcendental m.,** a technique for attaining a state of physical relaxation and psychological calm by the regular practice of a relaxation procedure which entails the repetition of a mantra.

medium (me′de-um), pl. *mediums* or *me′dia* [L. "middle"] 1. means. 2. a substance which transmits impulses. 3. a substance used in the culture of bacteria; see *culture medium,* under C. 4. a preparation used in treating histologic specimens. **Bruns' glucose m.,** a mixture of distilled water, glucose, glycerin, and camphorated spirit, used for mounting fresh tissue specimens.

clearing m., a substance used for rendering histologic specimens transparent. **contrast m.,** a radiopaque substance used to facilitate roentgen visualization of internal structures of the body. **culture m.,** a substance used to support the growth of microorganisms or other cells; see *culture medium,* under C. **dioptric media,** refracting media. **disperse m., dispersion m., dispersive m.,** the continuous or external portion of a colloid system in which the particles of the disperse phase are distributed; it is analogous to the solvent in a true solution. Cf. *disperse phase.* **mounting m.,** mountant. **nutrient m.,** a culture medium to which certain nutrient materials have been added. **radiopaque m.,** a substance that may be injected into a cavity or region to increase its density in x-ray examination and thereby aid in diagnosis. **refracting media,** the transparent tissues and fluids in the eye through which light rays pass and by which they are refracted and brought to a focus on the retina; the structures include the cornea, aqueous humor, crystalline lens, and vitreous body. Called also *dioptric media.* **separating m.,** any substance which facilitates separation, such as a coating used upon a surface which serves to prevent adherence to it of another surface; used in dentistry on impressions to facilitate removal of the cast. **Wickersheimer's m.,** see under *fluid.*

medius (me′de-us) [L.] in the middle; [NA] a term used in reference to a structure lying between two other structures that are anterior and posterior, superior and inferior, or internal and external in position.

MEDLARS (med′larz) [*MED*ical *L*iterature *A*nalysis and *R*etrieval *S*ystem] a computerized bibliographic system of the National Library of Medicine, from which the Index Medicus is produced.

MEDLINE (med′lin) [from *MEDLARS* on-*line*] a computerized bibliographic retrieval system, an on-line segment of MEDLARS.

medorrhea (med″o-re′ah) [Gr. *mēdea* genitals + *rhoia* flow] a urethral discharge.

medrogestone (med-ro-jes′tōn) chemial name: 6,17-dimethyl-pregna-4,6-diene-3,20-dione; a progestin, $C_{23}H_{32}O_2$.

Medrol (med′rol) trademark for preparations of methylprednisolone.

medronate disodium (med′ro-nāt) methylenebisphosphonic acid disodium dihydrogen salt; a pharmaceutic aid, $CH_4Na_2O_6P_2$.

medroxyprogesterone acetate (med-rok″se-pro-jes′ter-ōn) [USP] chemical name: 6(α)-17-(acetyloxy)-6-methyl-pregna-4-ene-3,20-dione. A progestin, $C_{24}H_{34}O_4$, occurring as a white to off-white, crystalline powder; used in the treatment of endometriosis, uterine cancer, habitual and threatened abortion, and menstrual disorders, administered orally or intramuscularly. It has been used in contraceptive products.

medrysone (med′rĭ-sōn) chemical name: 11β-hydroxy-6α-methylpregn-4-ene-3,20-dione. A synthetic glucocorticoid, $C_{22}H_{32}O_3$, occurring as a white to off-white, crystalline powder; used as an anti-flammatory in allergic and inflammatory eye conditions, such as episcleritis, allergic and vernal conjunctivitis, applied topically to the conjunctiva.

medulla (mĕ-dul′ah), pl. *medul′lae* [L.] the inmost part; [NA] a general term for the inmost portion of an organ or structure. Called also *marrow.* **adrenal m.,** m. glandulae suprarenalis. **m. of bone,** m. ossium. **m. glan′dulae suprarena′lis** [NA], suprarenal medulla: the inner, reddish brown, soft part of the suprarenal gland; it synthesizes, stores, and releases catecholamines. Called also *substantia medullaris, glandulae suprarenalis* and *adrenal medulla.* **m. of kidney,** m. renis. **m. of lymph node,** m. nodi lymphatici. **m. neph′rica,** m. renis. **m. no′di lymphat′ici** [NA], medulla of lymph node: the central part of a lymph node, comprising cords and sinuses; called also *substantia medullaris lymphoglandulae.* **m. oblonga′ta** [NA], the truncated cone of nerve tissue continuous above with the pons and below with the spinal cord; it lies anterior to the cerebellum, and the upper part of its posterior surface forms the floor of the lower part of the fourth ventricle; it contains ascending and descending tracts, and important collections of nerve cells that deal with vital functions, such as respiration, circulation, and special senses. It is derived (developed) from the myelencephalon of the embryo. See also *brain stem,* under B. **m. os′sium,** bone marrow: the soft material filling the cavities of the bones, made up of a meshwork of connective tissue containing branching fibers, the meshes being filled with marrow cells, which consist variously of fat cells, large nucleated cells or myelocytes, and giant cells called megakaryocytes. See *m. ossium flava* and *rubra.* **m. os′sium fla′va** [NA], yellow bone marrow: ordinary bone marrow of the kind in which the fat cells predominate. **m. os′sium ru′bra** [NA], red bone marrow: marrow of developing bone, of the ribs, vertebrae, and many of the smaller bones; it is the site of production of erythrocytes and granular leukocytes. **m. re′nis** [NA], medulla of kidney: the inner part of the substance of the kidney, composed chiefly of collecting elements and loops of Henle, organized grossly into pyramids; called also *substantia medullaris renis.* **spinal m., m. spina′lis** [NA], the spinal cord; see under *cord.* **suprarenal m., m. of suprarenal gland,** m. glandulae suprarenalis. **m. of thymus,** the central portion of each lobule of the thymus; it contains many more reticular cells and far fewer lymphocytes than does the surrounding cortex.

medullae (mě-dul′e) [L.] plural of *medulla*.

medullary (med′u-lār″e) [L. *medullaris*] pertaining to the marrow or to any medulla; resembling marrow.

medullated (med′u-lāt″ed) myelinated.

medullation (med″u-la′shun) the formation of a medulla or marrow; especially the formation of the medullary sheath around a nerve fiber.

medullectomy (med″u-lek′to-me) [L. *medulla* marrow + Gr. *ektomē* excision] excision of the medulla of an organ, as of the adrenal gland.

medulliadrenal (mě-dul″ĭ-ah-dre′nal) medulloadrenal.

medullitis (med″u-li′tis) 1. osteomyelitis. 2. myelitis.

medullization (med″u-li-za′shun) the enlargement of the haversian canals in rarefying osteitis, followed by their conversion into marrow channels; also the replacement of bone by marrow cells.

medulloadrenal (me-dul″o-ah-dre′nal) pertaining to the adrenal medulla.

medulloarthritis (me-dul″o-ar-thri′tis) [L. *medulla* marrow + *arthritis*] inflammation of the marrow spaces of the articular extremities of bones.

medulloblast (mě-dul′o-blast) an undifferentiated cell of the embryonic medullary (neural) tube which may develop into either a neuroblast or a spongioblast.

medulloblastoma (mě-dul″o-blas-to′mah) a cerebellar tumor composed of undifferentiated neuroepithelial cells; it is highly radiosensitive.

medulloencephalic (mě-dul″o-en″sě-fal′ik) myeloencephalic.

medulloepithelioma (mě-dul″o-ep″ĭ-the″le-o′-mah) a rare tumor of the brain composed of primitive neuroepithelial cells lining the tubular spaces.

medulloid (med′u-loid) [*medulla* + Gr. *eidos* form] an adrenergic substance with a hormonal activity simulating that of the adrenal medulla.

medullosuprarenoma (mě-dul″o-su″prah-re-no′mah) pheochromocytoma.

medullotherapy (mě-dul″o-ther′ah-pe) Pasteur's preventive treatment of rabies with emulsions of fixed virus in rabbit spinal cord.

medusa (mě-doo-sah) [Gr. *Medusa* one of the three mythological gorgons] a jellyfish; a free-swimming, umbrella-shaped form in the life cycle of certain cnidarians.

medusocongestin (mě-du″so-kon-jes′tin) a toxic substance derived from the tentacles of the jelly fish, *Rhizostoma cuvieri*, which, when injected into laboratory animals, causes intense congestion of the splanchnic vessels; believed to be identical with congestin.

mefenorex hydrochloride (mě-fen′o-reks) chemical name: *N*-(3-chloropropyl)-α-methylphenethylamine hydrochloride; an anorexic, $C_{12}H_{18}ClN \cdot HCl$.

mefexamide (mě-feks′ah-mīd) chemical name: *N*-[2-(diethylamino)ethyl]-2-(4-methoxyphenoxy)acetamide; a central nervous system stimulant, $C_{15}H_{24}N_2O_3$.

mefloquine (mef′lo-kwin) chemical name: (±)-(*R**,*S**)-α-2-piperidinyl-2,8-bis(trifluoromethyl)quinolinemethanol. An antimalarial, $C_{17}H_{16}F_6N_2O$, which has been used in the treatment of drug-resistant falciparum malaria.

mefruside (mef′roo-sīd) chemical name: 4-chloro-*N*¹-methyl-*N*¹-(tetrahydro-2-methylfurfuryl)-*m*-benzenedisulfonamide; a diuretic, $C_{13}H_{19}ClN_2O_5S_2$.

MEG see *magnetoencephalograph*.

mega- [Gr. *megas* big, great] a combining form designating great size; see also words beginning *megalo-*. Used in naming units of measurement to indicate a quantity one million (10^6) times the unit designated by the root with which it is combined.

megabladder (meg″ah-blad′er) a condition marked by permanent overdistention of the bladder.

megacalycosis (meg″ah-kal″ĭ-ko′sis) [*mega-* + *calyx* + *-osis*] nonobstructive dilatation of the renal calices due to malformation of the renal papillae.

megacardia (meg″ah-kar′de-ah) [*mega-* + Gr. *kardia* heart] cardiomegaly.

megacaryoblast (meg″ah-kar′e-o-blast″) megakaryoblast.

megacaryocyte (meg″ah-kar′e-o-sīt″) megakaryocyte.

Megace (mě-gās′) trademark for a preparation of megestrol acetate.

megacecum (meg″ah-se′kum) [*mega-* + *cecum*] a cecum which is abnormally large.

megacephalic (meg″ah-sě-fal′ik) megalocephalic.

megacephalous (meg″ah-sef′ah-lus) megalocephalic.

megacephaly (meg″ah-sef′ah-le) megalocephaly.

megacholedochus (meg″ah-ko-led′o-kus) abnormal dilatation of the common bile duct.

megacolon (meg″ah-ko′lon) abnormally large or dilated colon; the condition may be congenital or acquired, acute or chronic. **acquired m., acquired functional m.,** colonic enlargement associated with chronic constipation; it may be due to faulty bowel habits and is particularly common in mentally retarded children and adults with chronic mental illness. Called also *idiopathic m.* **acute m.,** toxic m. **aganglionic m.,** congenital m. **congenital m., m. congen′itum,** megacolon due to congenital absence of myenteric ganglion cells in a distal segment of the large bowel. The resultant loss of motor function in this segment causes massive hypertrophic dilatation of the normal proximal colon; the aganglionic segment usually remains narrowed, but may dilate passively. The condition appears soon after birth, is commoner in males, and causes extreme constipation, abdominal distention, sometimes vomiting, and, when severe, growth retardation. Called also *Hirschsprung's disease, aganglionic m.,* and *pelvirectal achalasia.* **idiopathic m.,** acquired m. **toxic m.,** acute dilatation of the colon associated with amebic or ulcerative colitis; the dilatation may precede perforation of the colon. Called also *acute m.*

megacurie (meg″ah-ku′re) a unit of radioactivity, being one million (10^6) curies; abbreviated Mc.

megacycle (meg″ah-si″k′l) a unit of one million (10^6) cycles, e.g., 1,000,000 cycles per second, applied to the frequency of electromagnetic waves; abbreviated Mc.

megacystis (meg″ah-sis′tis) megalocystis.

megadont (meg′ah-dont) [*mega-* + Gr. *odous* tooth] having a dental index above 44.

megadontia (meg″ah-don′she-ah) macrodontia.

megadontic (meg″ah-don′tik) macrodontic.

megadontism (meg″ah-don′tizm) the state of having abnormally large teeth, or a dental index above 44.

megaduodenum (meg″ah-du″o-de′num) abnormally large or dilated duodenum; it may be congenital or acquired, as in intestinal scleroderma, and is usually due to a disorder of motor function.

megadyne (meg′ah-dīn″) [*mega-* + *dyne*] a million (10^6) dynes.

megaesophagus (meg″ah-ĕ-sof′ah-gus) see *achalasia*.

megagamete (meg″ah-gam′ēt) (obs.) macrogamete.

megagametophyte (meg″ah-gah-me′to-fīt) [*mega-* + Gr. *gametē* wife + *phyton* plant] the female gametophyte in heterosporous plants, developed from the megaspore.

megahertz (meg′ah-hertz) one million (10^6) hertz (cycles per second). Abbreviated MHz.

megakaryoblast (meg″ah-kar′e-o-blast) the earliest cytologically identifiable precursor in the thrombocytic series, which matures to form the promegakaryocyte.

megakaryocyte (meg″ah-kar′e-o-sīt) [*mega-* + Gr. *karyon* nucleus + *-cyte*] the giant cell of bone marrow, a large cell with a greatly lobulated nucleus; mature blood platelets are released from its cytoplasm.

megakaryocytopoiesis (meg″ah-kar″e-o-sīt″o-poi-e′sis) [*megakaryocyte* + Gr. *poiesis* a making] the production of megakaryocytes.

megakaryocytosis (meg″ah-kar″e-o-si-to′sis) the presence of megakaryocytes in the blood or of excessive numbers in the bone marrow.

megalakria (meg″ah-lak′re-ah) [*megalo-* + Gr. *akron* extremity] acromegaly.

megalecithal (meg″ah-les′ĭ-thal) [*mega-* + Gr. *lekithos* yolk] macrolecithal.

megalencephalon (meg″al-en-sef′ah-lon) [*megalo-* + Gr. *enkephalos* brain] an abnormally large brain.

megalencephaly (meg″al-en-sef′ah-le) macrencephaly.

megalgia (meg-al′je-ah) [Gr. *megas* large + *-algia*] severe pain, as in muscular rheumatism.

megalo- [Gr. *megas, megale* big, great] a combining form designating great size; see also words beginning *mega-*.

megaloblast (meg′ah-lo-blast″) [*megalo-* + Gr. *blastos* germ] a large, nucleated, immature progenitor of an abnormal red blood cell series, sequentially following the promegaloblast in development and retaining some of its features; megaloblasts correspond to normoblasts of the normal red cell maturation series and are correspondingly classified as basophilic, polychromatic, and orthochromatic. **m. of Sabin,** pronormoblast.

megaloblastoid (meg″ah-lo-blas′toid) resembling a megaloblast.

megalobulbus (meg″ah-lo-bul′bus) enlargement of the duodenal cap in the roentgenogram.

megalocardia (meg″ah-lo-kar′de-ah) [*megalo-* + Gr. *kardia* heart] cardiomegaly.

megalocaryocyte (meg″ah-lo-kar′e-o-sīt) megakaryocyte.

megalocephalia (meg″ah-lo-sě-fa′le-ah) megalocephaly.

megalocephalic (meg″ah-lo-sě-fal′ik) pertaining to or characterized by megalocephaly.

megalocephaly (meg″ah-lo-sef′ah-le) [*megalo-* + Gr. *kephalē* head]   1. unusually large size of the head.   2. progressive enlargement of the bones of the head, face, and neck; leontiasis ossea.

megaloceros (meg″ah-los′ĕ-rus) [*megalo-* + *keras* horn]   a monster having projections from the forehead resembling horns.

megalocheiria (meg″ah-lo-ki′re-ah) [*megalo-* + Gr. *cheir* hand + *-ia*]   abnormal largeness of the hands.

megaloclitoris (meg″ah-lo-kli′to-ris)   hypertrophy of the clitoris.

megalocornea (meg″ah-lo-kor′ne-ah) [*megalo-* + *cornea*]   a usually bilateral developmental anomaly of the cornea, which is of abnormal size at birth, sometimes reaching a diameter of more than 18 mm. in the adult. It may be inherited as an X-linked recessive or as an autosomal dominant trait. Called also *macrocornea.*

megalocystis (meg″ah-lo-sis′tis) [*megalo-* + Gr. *kystis* bladder]   an abnormally enlarged bladder.

megalocyte (meg′ah-lo-sīt″) [*megalo-* + *-cyte*]   an extremely large erythrocyte, i.e., one measuring 12 to 25 microns in diameter.

megalocytosis (meg″ah-lo-si-to′sis)   macrocythemia.

megalodactylia (meg″ah-lo-dak-til′e-ah)   megalodactyly.

megalodactylism (meg″ah-lo-dak′tĭ-lizm)   megalodactyly.

megalodactylous (meg″ah-lo-dak′tĭ-lus)   exhibiting megalodactyly.

megalodactyly (meg″ah-lo-dak′tĭ-le) [*megalo-* + Gr. *daktylos* finger]   abnormal largeness of fingers or toes.

megalodontia (meg″ah-lo-don′she-ah)   macrodontia.

megaloenteron (meg″ah-lo-en′ter-on) [*megalo-* + Gr. *enteron* intestine]   (*obs.*) enteromegaly.

megaloesophagus (meg″ah-lo-ĕ-sof′ah-gus)   see *achalasia.*

megalogastria (meg″ah-lo-gas′tre-ah) [*megalo-* + Gr. *gastēr* stomach + *-ia*]   enlargement or abnormally large size of the stomach.

megaloglossia (meg″ah-lo-glos′e-ah) [*megalo-* + Gr. *glōssa* tongue + *-ia*]   macroglossia.

megalographia, megalography (meg″ah-lo-gra′fe-ah; meg″-ah-log′rah-fe)   macrography.

megalohepatia (meg″ah-lo-he-pat′e-ah) [*megalo-* + Gr. *hēpar* liver + *-ia*]   hepatomegaly.

megalokaryocyte (meg″ah-lo-kar′e-o-sīt″)   megakaryocyte.

megalomania (meg″ah-lo-ma′ne-ah) [*megalo-* + Gr. *mania* madness]   unreasonable conviction of one's own extreme greatness, goodness, or power; the ideas in megalomania are known as *delusions of grandeur.*

megalomaniac (meg″ah-lo-ma′ne-ak)   an individual exhibiting megalomania.

megalomelia (meg″ah-lo-me′le-ah) [*megalo-* + Gr. *melos* limb + *-ia*]   abnormal largeness of the limbs.

megalomicin potassium phosphate (meg″ah-lo-mi′sin)   chemical name: megalomicin A compound with potassium dihydrogen phosphate; an antibiotic of unspecified action, $C_{44}H_{80}N_2O_{15}·2KH_2PO_4$.

megalonychia (meg″ah-lo-nik′e-ah)   the condition of having unusually large nails.

megalopenis (meg″ah-lo-pe′nis)   excessive size of the penis.

megalophthalmos (meg″ah-lof-thal′mos) [*megalo-* + Gr. *ophthalmos* eye]   abnormally large size of the eyes. **anterior m.,** megalocornea.

megalophthalmus (meg″ah-lof-thal′mus)   megalophthalmos.

megalopia (meg″ah-lo′pe-ah) [*megalo-* + Gr. *ōps* + *-ia*]   abnormal enlargement of the eyes.

megalopodia (meg″ah-lo-po′de-ah) [*megalo-* + Gr. *pous* foot + *-ia*]   excessive size of the feet.

megalopsia (meg″ah-lop′se-ah) [*megalo-* + Gr. *opsis* vision + *-ia*]   macropsia.

Megalopyge (meg″ah-lo-pij′e)   a genus of hairy moths whose larvae (caterpillars) have stinging hairs. **M. opercula′ris,** a species whose hairs pierce the skin and cause caterpillar hair poisoning (flannel moth dermatitis).

megaloscope (meg′ah-lo-skōp″) [*megalo-* + Gr. *skopein* to examine]   a large magnifying lens; a magnifying speculum or mirror.

megalosplanchnic (meg″ah-lo-splank′nik)   (*obs.*) having abnormally large viscera.

megalosplenia (meg″ah-lo-sple′ne-ah) [*megalo-* + Gr. *splen* spleen + *-ia*]   splenomegaly.

megalospore (meg′ah-lo-spōr″)   a macrospore.

Megalosporon (meg″ah-los′po-ron) [*megalo-* + Gr. *sporos* seed]   a former genus of fungi made up of large-spored dermatophytes (Sabouraud, 1903). *M. ec′tothrix* included those that form arthrospores on the outside of the hair shaft, and *M. en′dothrix* included those that form arthrospores within the hair shaft. Now included in *Trichophyton.*

megalosporon (meg″ah-los′po-ron), pl. *megalos′pora.*   An organism of the genus *Megalosporon.*

megalosyndactyly (meg″ah-lo-sin-dak′tĭ-le) [*megalo-* + *syndac-*

tyly]   a condition in which the digits are very large and more or less completely grown together.

megalothymus (meg″ah-lo-thi′mus)   an enlarged thymus.

megaloureter (meg″ah-lo-u-re′ter) [*megalo-* + *ureter*]   congenital ureteral dilatation without demonstrable cause; called also *congenital* or *primary m., megaureter, primary ureteral atony,* and *ureteral neuromuscular dysplasia.* Cf. *hydroureter.* **congenital m., primary m.,** megaloureter. **reflux m.,** dilatation of the ureter associated with vesicoureteral reflux.

-megaly [Gr. *megaleios* magnificent, *megalē* great]   a word termination indicating enlargement of the structure signified by the root to which it is attached, as splenomegaly.

meganucleus (meg″ah-nu′kle-us)   (*obs.*) macronucleus.

megaprosopous (meg″ah-pros′o-pus) [*mega-* + Gr. *prosōpon* face]   having a large face.

megarectum (meg-ah-rek′tum)   a greatly dilated rectum.

Megarhinini (meg″a-rhi′ni-ne)   a tribe of tropical non-bloodsucking mosquitoes; they fly by day, feed on flowers, and are usually highly colored. Their large larvae are predaceous and have been used to control the breeding of bloodsucking mosquitoes.

Megarhinus (meg″ah-ri′nus)   a genus of large, showy, but harmless mosquitoes of tropical and subtropical countries.

Megaselia (meg″ah-se′le-ah)   a genus of flies the larvae of which may cause myiasis in man. *M. scalaris* and *M. rufipes* cause wound myiasis, and *M. scalaris* may also cause intestinal myiasis.

megaseme (meg′ah-sēm) [*mega-* + Gr. *sēma* sign]   having an orbital index of 89 or more.

megasigmoid (meg″ah-sig′moid) [*mega-* + *sigmoid*]   an enormously dilated sigmoid.

megasoma (meg″ah-so′mah) [*mega-* + Gr. *sōma* body]   great size and stature, not amounting to gigantism.

megasporangium (meg″ah-spo-ran′je-um), pl. *megasporan′gia* [*mega-* + Gr. *sporos* seed + *angeion* vessel]   the sporangium in which megaspores develop.

megaspore (meg′ah-spōr) [*mega-* + Gr. *sporos* seed]   1. macrospore.   2. macroconidium.   3. one of four haploid spores, usually larger than the microspore, formed in the megasporangium from a megaspore mother cell, and from which the megagametophyte, or female gametophyte, develops.

Megatrichophyton (meg″ah-tri″ko-fi′ton)   a former genus made up of some large-spored dermatophytes (as *M. equi′num* and *M. megni′ni*); now considered synonymous with *Trichophyton.*

megaunit (meg′ah-u″nit)   a quantity one million (10^6) times that of a standard unit.

megaureter (meg″ah-u-re′ter)   megaloureter.

megavitamin (meg″ah-vi′tah-min)   a dose of vitamin(s) vastly exceeding the amount recommended for nutritional balance.

megavolt (meg′ah-vōlt) [*mega-* + *volt*]   a million (10^6) volts.

megavoltage (meg″ah-vol′tij)   in ionizing radiation therapy, voltage greater than 1 megavolt. Cf. *supervoltage.*

megestrol acetate (mĕ-jes′trōl)   chemical name: 17-(acetyloxy)-6-methyl-16-methylene-pregna-4,6-diene-3,20-dione. A synthetic progestin, $C_{25}H_{32}O_4$, occurring as a white, crystalline powder; used as an antineoplastic in adjunctive or palliative management of recurrent or metastatic endometrial carcinoma, administered orally.

Megimide (meg′ĭ-mīd)   trademark for a preparation of bemegride.

Méglin's point (ma-glanz′) [J. A. *Méglin,* French physician, 1756–1824]   see under *point.*

meglumine (meg′lu-mēn) [USP]   chemical name: 1-deoxy-1-(methylamino)-*D*- glucitol. A crystalline base, $C_7H_{17}NO_5$, occurring as white to faintly yellowish white, crystals or powder; used in the preparation of certain radiopaque media. Called also *methylglucamine.* See also under *diatrizoate* and *iodipamide.* **m. diatrizoate,** a salt of 3,5-diacetamido-2,4,6-triiodobenzoic acid, $C_{18}H_{26}I_3N_3O_9$, occurring as a clear, colorless to pale yellow, slightly viscous liquid; used as a diagnostic radiopaque medium for intravascular use in angiocardiography and excretory urography. **m. iodipamide,** a salt of iodipamide, occurring as a clear, colorless to pale yellow, slightly viscous liquid; used as a diagnostic radiopaque medium in cholecystography. Called also *methylglucamine iodipamide.* **m. iothalamate,** a salt of iodothalamic acid, $C_{18}H_{26}I_3N_3O_9$, occurring as a clear, colorless to pale yellow, slightly viscous liquid; used as a diagnostic radiopaque medium for intravascular use in cerebral angiography, excretory urography, and peripheral arteriography.

meglutol (meg′lu-tōl)   chemical name: 3-hydroxy-3-methyl pentanedioic acid; an antihyperlipoproteinemic, $C_6H_{10}O_5$.

megohm (meg′ōm) [*mega-* + *ohm*]   a million (10^6) ohms.

megophthalmos (meg-of-thal′mos) [*mega-* + Gr. *ophthalmos* eye]   buphthalmos; hydrophthalmos.

megrim (me′grim)   migraine.

mehlnährschaden (māl″nahr-shad′en) [Ger.]   a nutritional deficiency syndrome similar to kwashiorkor, due to inadequate protein intake and overabundance of carbohydrate; the clinical characteristics include growth failure, preservation of subcutane-

Meiosis (only two of the 23 human chromosome pairs are shown, the chromosomes from one parent in black, from the other parent in outline). FIRST MEIOTIC DIVISION: *A, leptotene*—first appearance of chromosomes as thin threads; *B, zygotene*—pairing (synapsis) of chromosomes; *C, pachytene*—chromosomal thickening and shortening, the individual chromatids becoming visible; *D, diplotene*—longitudinal separation of chromatids, the centromere remaining intact and a chiasma being formed (NOTE: prophase includes *A* to *D* plus diakinesis [not shown]); *E. metaphase*—movement of chromosomes into the equatorial plane; *F, anaphase*—separation of pairs, one member going to each pole; *G, telophase*—cell division, each of the two daughter cells being haploid. SECOND MEIOTIC DIVISION: *prophase* (not shown)—chromosomes become visible; *H, metaphase*—movement of chromosomes into equatorial plane; *I, anaphase*—division of centromeres, the chromatids going to opposite poles; *J, telophase*—cell division, each daughter cell being haploid. (Thompson and Thompson.)

ous fat with wasting of muscle, edema, and psychomotor abnormalities.

meibomian cyst, foramen, glands, stye (mi-bo′me-an) [Heinrich *Meibom*, German anatomist, 1638–1700] see *chalazion, foramen cecum linguae,* and *glandulae tarsales,* and see under *stye.*

meibomianitis (mi-bo″me-ah-ni′tis) inflammation of the meibomian glands.

meibomitis (mi″bo-mi′tis) meibomianitis.

Meige's disease (mehzh′ez) [Henri *Meige*, French physician, 1866–1940] Milroy's disease.

Meigs' capillaries, test (megz) [Arthur V. *Meigs*, Philadelphia physician, 1850–1912] see under *capillary* and *tests.*

Meigs' syndrome (megz) [Joe Vincent *Meigs*, American surgeon, 1892–1963] see under *syndrome.*

Meinicke test (reaction) (mi′nĭ-ke) [Ernst *Meinicke*, German physician, 1878–1945] see under *tests.*

meio- [Gr. *meiōn* smaller] a combining form denoting decrease in size or number; see also words beginning *mio-.*

meiogenic (mi″o-jen′ik) [Gr. *meiosis* + *gennan* to produce] promoting or causing meiosis.

meiosis (mi-o′sis) [Gr. *meiōsis* diminution] a special method of cell division, occurring in maturation of the sex cells, by means of which each daughter nucleus receives half the number of chromosomes characteristic of the somatic cells of the species. See illustration. Cf. *mitosis.*

meiotic (mi-ot′ik) pertaining to, characteristic of, or characterized by meiosis.

Meirowsky phenomenon (mi-rof′ske) [Emil *Meirowsky*, German-American dermatologist, 1876–1960] see under *phenomenon.*

Meissner's corpuscles, ganglion, plexus (mīs′nerz) [Georg *Meissner*, German physiologist, 1829–1905] see *corpuscula tactus, plexus submucosus,* and under *ganglion.*

mel (mel) [L.] 1. honey. 2. a compound of honey with some medicinal agent.

melagra (mel-ag′rah) [Gr. *melos* limb + *agra* seizure] muscular pain in the extremities.

melalgia (mel-al′je-ah) [Gr. *melos* limb + *-algia*] pain in the limbs.

melancholia (mel″an-ko′le-ah) [*melano-* + Gr. *cholē* bile + *-ia*] a depressed and unhappy emotional state with abnormal inhibition of mental and bodily activity. **acute m.,** an acute form of melancholia marked in, addition to the usual symptoms, by loss of appetite, emaciation, insomnia, and subnormal temperature. **affective m.,** melancholia corresponding to the depressive phase of manic-depressive psychosis. **m. agita′ta, agitated m.,** agitated depression. **m. atton′ita,** stuporous m. **m. with delirium,** melancholia with distressing delusions and hallucinations. **m. hypochondri′aca,** extreme hypochondriasis. **involutional m.,** a major affected disorder occurring during involution, and marked by agitation, worry, anxiety, somatic preoccupation, severe insomnia, and sometimes paranoid reactions; formerly thought to be associated with the climacteric. Called also *involutional psychosis.* **recurrent m.,** a condition in which attacks of melancholia follow one another at more or less regular intervals. **m. religio′sa,** the delusion of one's own personal damnation. **m. simplex,** a mild form with neither delusions nor great excitement. **stuporous m.,** a form in which the patient lies motionless and silent, with fixed eyes and indifference to surroundings; there are sometimes hallucinations.

melancholiac (mel″an-ko′le-ak) 1. affected with melancholia. 2. a person affected with melancholia.

melanemesis (mel″ah-nem′ĕ-sis) [*melano-* + Gr. *emein* to vomit] black vomit.

melanemia (mel″ah-ne′me-ah) [*melano-* + Gr. *haima* blood + *-ia*] the presence of black, pigmentary masses in the blood, as in hemochromatosis.

Melania (mĕ-la′ne-ah) a generic name formerly applied to smaller fresh water operculate snails, now classified under a number of genera of the family Melaniidae (Thiaridae).

melanicterus (mel″ah-nik′ter-us) Winckel's disease.

melaniferous (mel″ah-nif′er-us) [*melanin* + L. *ferre* to bear] containing melanin or other black pigment.

melanin (mel′ah-nin) [Gr. *melas* black] the dark amorphous pigment of the skin, hair, and various tumors, of the choroid coat of the eye and the substantia nigra of the brain. It is produced by polymerization of oxidation products of tyrosine and dihydroxyphenyl compounds, and contains carbon, hydrogen, nitrogen, oxygen, and often sulfur. **artificial m., factitious m.,** a compound resembling melanin, formed when a protein is heated in strong hydrochloric acid; called also *melanoid*.

melanism (mel′ah-nizm) excessive pigmentation or blackening of the integuments or tissues, usually of genetic origin; melanosis. **industrial m.,** the gradual darkening of populations of organisms living in soot-darkened habitats due to the selective pressure of predators, the darker individuals tending to survive as the conspicuous individuals are eaten, thus favoring the genotype that darkens their color. The peppered moth, *Biston betularia*, has undergone this change. **metallic m.,** argyria.

melanistic (mel″ah-nis′tik) characterized by melanism.

melano- [Gr. *melas* black] a combining form meaning black, or denoting relation to melanin.

melanoacanthoma (mel″a-no-ak″an-tho′ma) a rare, benign, shallowly invasive papilloma composed of basal cell–like keratinocytes pervaded with highly dendritic, deeply pigmented melanocytes.

melanoameloblastoma (mel″ah-no-ah-mel″o-blas-to′mah) melanotic neuroectodermal tumor.

melanoblast (mel′ah-no-blast″, mĕ-lan′o-blast) [*melano-* + Gr. *blastos* germ] a cell originating from the neural crest that differentiates into a melanocyte.

melanoblastoma (mel″ah-no-blas-to′mah) melanotic neuroectodermal tumor.

melanoblastosis (mel″ah-no-blas-to′sis) a condition characterized by the presence of melanoblasts.

melanocarcinoma (mel″ah-no-kar″sĭ-no′mah) [*melano-* + *carcinoma*] malignant melanoma.

melanocyte (mel′ah-no-sīt, mĕ-lan′o-sīt) any of the dendritic clear cells of the epidermis that synthesize tyrosinase and, within their melanosomes, the pigment melanin; the melanosomes are then transferred from melanocytes to keratinocytes. **dendritic m.,** those having cytoplasmic projections laden with melanosomes to be transferred to keratinocytes.

melanocytic (mel″ah-no-sit′ik) pertaining to or composed of melanocytes.

melanocytoma (mel″ah-no-si-to′mah) a neoplasm or hamartoma composed of melanocytes. **compound m.,** juvenile melanoma. **dermal m.,** 1. blue nevus. 2. cellular blue nevus.

melanoderm (mel′ah-no-derm) a person belonging to one of the black races.

melanoderma (mel″ah-no-der′mah) [*melano-* + Gr. *derma* skin] an abnormally increased amount of melanin in the skin, due either to an increase in the production of melanin by the melanocytes normally present or to an increase in the number of melanocytes, with production of hyperpigmented patches. **parasitic m.,** vagabonds' disease. **senile m.,** pigmentation of the skin in the aged.

melanodermatitis (mel″ah-no-der″mah-ti′tis) dermatitis associated with an increased deposit of melanin in the skin. **m. tox′ica lichenoi′des,** a condition occurring in persons exposed, usually occupationally, to tars and subsequently to sunlight; marked by pruritus and the appearance of lichenoid papules, hyperpigmentation, and telangiectasia.

melanodermic (mel″ah-no-der′mik) having a dark skin.

melanoepithelioma (mel″ah-no-ep″ĭ-the-le-o′mah) malignant melanoma.

melanoflocculation (mel″ah-no-flok″u-la′shun) a flocculation test for malaria, performed with a melanin antigen; see *Henry's test,* under *tests.*

melanogen (mĕ-lan′o-jen) [*melanin* + Gr. *gennan* to produce] a colorless chromogen, convertible into melanin, which may occur in the urine in certain diseases.

melanogenesis (mel″ah-no-jen′ĕ-sis) the production of melanin.

melanogenic (mel″ah-no-jen′ik) causing the production of melanin.

melanoglossia (mel″ah-no-glos′e-ah) [*melano-* + Gr. *glōssa* tongue] black tongue.

melanoid (mel′ah-noid) [*melano-* + Gr. *eidos* form] 1. resembling melanin; of a dark color. 2. a material resembling melanin. See *artificial melanin.*

Melanolestes (mel″ah-no-les′tēz) a genus of insects. **M. pic′ipes,** the "black corsair" or "kissing bug"; its bite much resembles the sting of a wasp, but it is often much more serious.

melanoleukoderma (mel″ah-no-lu″ko-der′mah) [*melano-* + Gr. *leukos* white + *derma* skin] a mottled appearance of the skin, as in chronic arsenic poisoning. **m. col′li,** syphilitic leukoderma about the neck.

melanoma (mel″ah-no′mah) [*melano-* + *-oma*] a tumor made up of melanin-pigmented cells. When used alone, the term refers to malignant melanoma. **amelanotic m.,** an unpigmented malignant melanoma. **Cloudman's m. S91,** a firm, black subcutaneous tumor originally found at the base of the tail of a female DBA mouse, and proven to be transplantable to, and invariably metastatic in, other DBA mice and BALB/c mice. **Harding-Passey m.,** a transplantable, nonmetastasizing melanoma originally found on the ear of a brown mouse. **juvenile m.,** a benign, elevated, firm, pink to purplish red papule, perhaps with a slightly scaly surface, which usually occurs on the face, especially on the cheeks, and most commonly originates before puberty. Histologically, the lesion suggests and has been mistaken for malignant melanoma. Called also *compound melanocytoma, spindle cell nevus,* and *Spitz nevus.* **malignant m.,** a malignant tumor, usually developing from a nevus and consisting of black masses of cells with a marked tendency to metastasis. Called also *melanocarcinoma, melanoepithelioma, melanosarcoma, melanoscirrhus,* etc. **subungual m.,** melanotic whitlow.

melanomatosis (mel″ah-no″mah-to′sis) the formation of melanomas in various parts of the body.

melanomatous (mel″ah-no′mah-tus) characterized by or pertaining to melanoma.

melanonychia (mel″ah-no-nik′e-ah) [*melano-* + Gr. *onyx* nail + *-ia*] blackening of the nail by melanin pigmentation.

melanophage (mel′ah-no-fāj″) a histiocyte laden with phagocytosed melanin.

melanophore (mel′ah-no-fōr″) [*melano-* + Gr. *phoros* bearing] a pigment cell containing melanin, especially such a cell in fishes, amphibians, and reptiles. Cf. *chromatophore.*

melanophorin (mel″ah-nof′o-rin) a principle thought to stimulate melanophores.

melanoplakia (mel″ah-no-pla′ke-ah) [*melano-* + Gr. *plax* plate + *-ia*] the formation of melanin-pigmented patches on the oral mucous membrane.

melanoprecipitation (mel″ah-no-pre-sip″ĭ-ta′shun) the precipitation of melanin pigment; used as a test for malaria.

melanoptysis (mel″ah-nop′tĭ-sis) [*melano-* + Gr. *ptyein* to spit] the expectoration of black sputum, as in anthracosis.

melanosarcoma (mel″ah-no-sar-ko′mah) [*melano-* + *sarcoma*] malignant melanoma.

melanosarcomatosis (mel″ah-no-sar-ko″mah-to′sis) melanomatosis.

melanoscirrhus (mel″ah-no-skir′us) [*melano-* + *scirrhus*] malignant melanoma.

melanosis (mel″ah-no′sis) [*melano-* + *-osis*] 1. melanism; a condition characterized by abnormal pigmentary deposits. 2. disorder of pigment metabolism. **circumscribed precancerous m. of Dubreuilh,** melanotic freckle of Hutchinson; see under *freckle.* **m. co′li,** a condition in which the mucous membrane of the colon is black or dark brown due to the presence of pigment-laden macrophages within the lamina propria. The pigment is not true melanin. **m. oc′uli,** a usually congenital condition in which there is a diffuse increase in pigmentation of the uveal tract and often of the more superficial ocular tissues. **Riehl's m.,** a rare pigmentary affection of the skin of the face marked by itching, reddening, desquamation, and a spotty brown pigmentation. **m. scle′rae,** congenital flecks of pigmentation in the sclera. **tar m.,** a diffuse mottled pigmentation of the skin due to contact with tar or pitch.

melanosome (mel′ah-no-sōm″) any of the granules within the melanocytes that contain tyrosinase and synthesize melanin; they are transferred from the melanocytes to keratinocytes.

melanotic (mel″ah-not′ik) pertaining to or characterized by the presence of melanin.

melanotrichia (mel″ah-no-trik′e-ah) [*melano-* + Gr. *thrix* hair + *-ia*] abnormal hyperpigmentation of the hair. **m. lin′guae,** black tongue.

melanotroph (mel′ah-no-trōf″) a pituitary cell that elaborates melanocyte-stimulating hormone (MSH).

melanotropic (mel″ah-no-trop′ik) [*melanin* + Gr. *tropikos* turning] having an affinity for melanin; influencing the deposit of melanin.

melanthin (mel-an′thin) an amorphous and poisonous glycoside, or saponin, $C_{20}H_{33}O_7$, from the seeds of *Nigella sativa.*

melanuresis (mel″an-u-re′sis) melanuria.

melanuria (mel″an-u′re-ah) [*melano-* + Gr. *ouron* urine + *-ia*] the excretion of darkly stained urine or of urine which turns dark on standing.

melanuric (mel″an-u′rik) pertaining to or marked by melanuria.

melanurin (mel″an-u′rin) a black substance from morbid urine in certain rare cases.

melarsoprol (mel-ar′so-prōl) chemical name: 2-[4-[(4,6-diamino-1,3,5-triazin-2-yl)amino]phenyl]-1,3,2-dithiarsolane-4-methanol. An antiprotozoal effective against *Trypanosoma*, $C_{12}H_{15}AsN_6$-OS_2, occurring as a cream-colored powder; used in the treatment of advanced cases of African trypanosomiasis, administered intravenously.

melasma (mě-laz′mah) [Gr. *melas* black] a condition in which blotchy, brown macules from one to several centimeters in diameter occur typically on the cheeks, temples, and forehead. It often appears during pregnancy (*m. gravidarum*), the macules sometimes becoming confluent ("mask of pregnancy"), and at menopause, but is most frequently seen in those taking oral contraceptives. Occasionally, the condition occurs in the absence of such factors, and infrequently in men. Called also *chloasma*. **m. addison′nii,** Addison's disease. **m. gravida′rum,** melasma occurring during pregnancy; see *melasma*. Called also *chloasma gravidarum* and *chloasma uterina*. **m. suprarena′le,** Addison's disease.

melatonin (mel″ah-to′nin) 5-methoxy-*N*-acetyl tryptamine, a hormone synthesized by the pineal gland, which produces marked lightening of dermal pigmentation in amphibians by stimulating the aggregation of melanosomes in melanophores, and inhibits gonad development and influences estrus in mammals. It is secreted at a rate inversely dependent on environmental lighting, being synthesized and released in response to norepinephrine, whose rate of release, in turn, declines when light activates retinal photoreceptors.

Meleda disease (mě′la-dah) [*Meleda*, a small island off the Dalmatian coast, where the condition is prevalent, because of intermarriage within the small population] mal de Meleda.

melena (mě-le′nah) [Gr. *melaina*, feminine of Gr. *melas* black] 1. the passage of dark, pitchy, and grumous stools stained with blood pigments or with altered blood. 2. black vomit. **m. neonato′rum,** melena of the newborn, due to the extravasation of blood into the alimentary canal. **m. spu′ria,** melena in nurslings in which the blood comes from the fissured nipple of the nursing mother. **m. ve′ra,** true melena.

melenemesis (mel″ě-nem′ě-sis) [Gr. *melaina* black + *emesis* vomiting] (*obs.*) black vomit.

melengestrol acetate (mel-en-jes′trōl) chemical name: 17-hydroxy-6-methyl-16-methylenepregna-4,6-diene-3,20-dione acetate; a progestin and antineoplastic, $C_{25}H_{32}O_4$.

melenic (mě-le′nik) marked by melena.

meletin (mel′ě-tin) quercetin.

melezitose (mě-lez′ĭ-tōs) a trisaccharide, $C_{18}H_{32}O_{16}$, from manna, from the sap of poplars and conifers, which on hydrolysis yields glucose and turanose.

meli- [Gr. *meli* honey] combining form meaning sweet, or denoting a relationship to honey.

melibiase (mel″ĭ-bi′ās) α-galactosidase.

melibiose (mel″ĭ-bi′ōs) chemical name: 6-*O*-α-D-galactopyranosyl-D-glucose. A disaccharide obtained from melitose. On hydrolysis it yields galactose and dextrose.

melicera, meliceris (mel″ĭ-se′rah; mel″ĭ-se′ris) [Gr. *meli* honey + *kēros* wax] 1. a cyst filled with honey-like substance. 2. viscid, syrupy.

melicitose (mě-lis′ĭ-tōs) melezitose.

melilotoxin (mel″ĭ-lo-tok′sin) bishydroxycoumarin.

melioidosis (me″le-oi-do′sis) [Gr. *melis* a distemper of asses + *eidos* resemblance] an infectious disease of rodents transmissible to man, caused by *Pseudomonas pseudomallei* and occurring in India, Malay states, and Indonesia. The human disease is characterized in some by a chronic granulomatous pneumonia or a chronic extrapulmonary form with multiple abscess formation, and in others by a fulminant septicemia with a high mortality rate despite antibiotic therapy. Formerly called *Whitmore's disease*.

Melissa (mě-lis′ah) [Gr. "bee"] a genus of labiate plants. The tops and leaves of *M. officina′lis*, containing tannin and an essential oil, are a cooling stimulant and diaphoretic. Called also *blue, lemon,* or *sweet balm*.

melissotherapy (mě-lis″o-ther′ah-pe) [Gr. *melissa* bee + *therapeia* medical treatment] treatment with bee venom; called also *apiotherapy*.

melitensis (mel″ĭ-ten′sis) brucellosis.

melitin (mel′ĭ-tin) a preparation of soluble antigen of *Brucella melitensis*.

melitis (mě-li′tis) [Gr. *mēlon* cheek + *-itis*] inflammation of the cheek.

melitococcus (mel-ĭ-to-kok′us) (*obs.*) *Brucella melitensis*.

melitoptyalism (mel″ĭ-to-ti′ah-lizm) [*meli-* + Gr. *ptyalon* saliva + *-ism*] the secretion of saliva containing glucose.

melitoptyalon (mel″ĭ-to-ti′ah-lon) glucose occurring in the saliva.

melitose (mel′ĭ-tōs) a crystalline sugar from cottonseed meal and Australian manna, which is obtained from various species of *Eucalyptus*. It is a trisaccharide, $C_{18}H_{32}O_{16}$ + $5H_2O$, which on hydrolysis yields dextrose, fructose, and galactose. Called also *raffinose* and *melitriose*.

melitracen hydrochloride (mel″ĭ-tra′sen) chemical name: 3-(10,10-dimethyl-9(10*H*)-anthracenylidene)-*N,N*-dimethyl-1-propanamine hydrochloride; a tricyclic antidepressant, $C_{21}H_{25} \cdot N$-HCl.

melitriose (mě-lit′ri-ōs) melitose.

Melittangium (mel″ĭ-tan′je-um) [*meli-* + Gr. *angeion* vessel] a genus of bacteria occurring in manure.

melituria (mel″ĭ-tu′re-ah) [*meli-* + Gr. *ouron* urine + *-ia*] the presence of any sugar in the urine. **m. inosi′ta,** inosituria.

melituric (mel″ĭ-tu′rik) pertaining to or affected with melituria.

melizame (mel′ĭ-zām) chemical name: 3-(1*H*-tetrazol-5-yloxy)-phenol; a sweetener, $C_7H_6N_4O_2$.

melizitose (mě-liz′ĭ-tōs) melezitose.

Mellaril (mel′ah-ril) trademark for preparations of thioridazine hydrochloride.

mellitum (mě-li′tum), pl. *melli′ti* [L.] a pharmaceutical preparation made with honey.

mellituria (mel″ĭ-tu′re-ah) melituria.

melodidymus (mel″o-did′ĭ-mus) [Gr. *melos* limb + *didymos* twin] an individual with a supernumerary limb.

melomelus (mě-lom′e-lus) [Gr. *melos* limb + *melos* limb] a monster with normal limbs and rudimentary supernumerary limbs.

meloncus (mě-long′kus) [Gr. *mēlon* cheek + *onkus* bulk] tumor of the cheek.

melonoplasty (mě-lon′o-plas″te) meloplasty.

Melophagus (mě-lof′ah-gus) a genus of wingless flies of the family Hippoboscidae. **M. ovi′nus,** a species that is a common ectoparasite of sheep and goats; although not a true tick, it is known as the sheep tick, or sheep ked.

meloplasty (mel′o-plas″te) [Gr. *mēlon* cheek + *plassein* to form] plastic surgery of the cheek.

melorheostosis (mel″o-re″os-to′sis) [Gr. *melos* limb + *rhein* to flow + *osteon* bone] a form of osteosclerosis or hyperostosis extending in a linear track through one of the long bones of an extremity, and consisting of proliferated ivory-like new bone. Called also *m. leri*. See *rheostosis*.

melosalgia (mel″o-sal′je-ah) [Gr. *melos* limb + *-algia*] pain in the lower limbs.

meloschisis (mě-los′kĭ-sis) macrostomia.

melotia (mě-lo′she-ah) [Gr. *mēlon* cheek + *ous* ear + *-ia*] a developmental anomaly characterized by displacement of the ear onto the cheek.

Melotte's metal (mel-ots′) [George W. *Melotte*, American dentist, 1835–1915] see under *metal*.

melotus (mělo′tus) an individual exhibiting melotia.

melphalan (mel′fah-lan) [USP] chemical name: 4-[bis(2-chloroethyl)amino]-L-phenylalanine. A cytotoxic alkylating agent that is the phenylalanine derivative of nitrogen mustard, $C_{13}H_{18}Cl_2N_2O_2$, occurring as an off-white to buff powder; used as an antineoplastic, especially in the treatment of multiple myeloma, administered orally.

Meltzer's law, method (anesthesia) (melt′serz) [Samuel James *Meltzer*, American physiologist, 1851–1920] see under *law* and *method*.

Meltzer-Lyon test (method) (melt′ser li′on) [S. J. *Meltzer*; B. B. Vincent *Lyon*, Philadelphia physician, 1880–1953] see under *tests*.

MEM macrophage electrophoretic mobility (test).

member (mem′ber) [L. *membrum*] 1. a part of the body distinct from the rest in function or position. 2. a limb. See also *membrum*.

memberment (mem′ber-ment) the manner of arrangement of parts in a body.

membra (mem′brah) plural of *membrum*.

membrana (mem-brah′nah), pl. *membra′nae* [L.] a membrane, or thin skin; [NA] a general term for a thin layer of tissue covering a surface, lining a cavity, or dividing a space or organ. **m. abdom′inis,** peritoneum. **m. adamanti′na,** cuticula dentis. **m. adventi′tia,** 1. tunica adventitia. 2. decidua capsularis. 3. a membrane not normal to the part; adventitious membrane. **m. agni′na,** amnion. **m. atlantooccipita′lis ante′rior** [NA], anterior atlanto-occipital membrane: a single midline ligamentous structure that passes from the anterior arch of the atlas to the anterior margin of the foramen magnum, and corresponds in position with the anterior longitudinal ligament of the vertebral column. **m. atlantooccipita'lis poste'rior** [NA], posterior atlanto-occipital membrane: a single midline ligamentous structure that passes from the posterior arch of the atlas to the posterior margin of the foramen magnum, and corresponds in position with the ligamenta flava. **m. basa'lis duc'tus semicircula'ris** [NA], basal membrane of semicircular duct: the basement membrane underlying the epithelium of a semicircular duct. **m. basila'ris duc'tus cochlea'ris**, lamina basilaris ductus cochlearis. **m. cadu'ca**, see *membranae deciduae*. **m. capsula'ris**, capsula articularis. **m. choriocapilla'ris**, lamina choroidocapillaris. **membra'nae decid'uae** [NA], decidual or deciduous membranes: the endometrium of the pregnant uterus, all of which, except the deepest layer, is shed at parturition. See subentries under *decidua*. **m. elas'tica laryn'gis**, m. fibroelastica laryngis. **m. epipapilla'ris**, an abnormal fibrous membrane on the optic disk. **m. fibroelas'tica laryn'gis** [NA], fibroelastic membrane of larynx: the fibroelastic layer beneath the mucous coat of the larynx, comprising the quadrangular membrane and the conus elasticus; called also *m. elastica laryngis*. **m. fibro'sa cap'sulae articula'ris** [NA], fibrous membrane of articular capsule: the outer of the two layers of the articular capsule of a synovial joint, composed of dense white fibrous tissue; called also *stratum fibrosum capsulae articularis*. **m. flac'cida**, pars flaccida membranae tympani. **m. fus'ca**, lamina fusca sclerae. **m. germinati'va**, blastoderm. **m. granulo'sa**, layers of cuboidal epithelial cells at the periphery of an ovarian follicle and surrounding the antrum or fluid-filled cavity. **m. granulo'sa exter'na**, the external granular layer of the retina. **m. granulo'sa inter'na**, the internal granular layer of the retina. **m. hyaloi'dea**, m. vitrea. **m. hyothyreoi'dea**, m. thyrohyoidea. **m. intercosta'lis exter'na** [NA], external intercostal membrane: any of the aponeurotic bands parallel with, and perhaps replacing, the fibers of the external intercostal muscles in the spaces between the costal cartilages, from the ventral tips of the ribs medially to the sternum; called also *ligamenta intercostalia externa*. **m. intercosta'lis inter'na** [NA], internal intercostal membrane: any of the aponeurotic bands parallel with, and perhaps replacing, the fibers of the internal intercostal muscles in the spaces between the ribs, from the angles of the ribs medially to the vertebral column; called also *ligamenta intercostalia interna*. **m. interos'sea antebra'chii** [NA], **m. interos'sea antibra'chii**, interosseous membrane of forearm: a thin fibrous sheet that connects the bodies of the radius and ulna, passing from the interosseous margin of the radius to that of the ulna. **m. interos'sea cru'ris** [NA], interosseous membrane of leg: a thin aponeurotic lamina attached to the interosseous margins of the tibia and fibula, deficient for a short distance at the proximal end of the bones; it separates the muscles on the anterior and posterior parts of the leg. **m. lim'itans**, 1. one of the limiting membranes of the retina; see *external* and *internal limiting membrane* (def. 1), under *membrane*. 2. the limiting membrane of glia fibrils and perivascular feet separating the neural parenchyma from the pia and blood vessels. **m. muco'sa na'si**, tunica mucosa nasi. **m. muco'sa ves'icae fel'leae**, tunica mucosa vesicae felleae. **m. nic'titans**, 1. plica semilunaris conjunctivae. 2. nictitating membrane. **m. obtura'ria** [NA], obturator membrane: a strong membrane that fills the obturator foramen except superiorly at the obturator groove, where a deficiency is left, the obturator canal. **m. obtura'ria** [stape'dis], m. stapedis. **m. obtura'trix**, m. obturatoria. **m. orbita'lis musculo'sa**, a system of smooth muscles deep in the orbit. **m. perfora'ta**, a term sometimes used to designate the first appearance of dentin in the fetus, manifested as a thick limiting line between the ameloblasts and odontoblasts. **m. perine'i**, NA alternative for *fascia diaphragmatis urogenitalis inferior*. **m. pituito'sa**, tunica mucosa nasi. **m. pro'pria**, lamina propria mucosae. **m. pro'pria duc'tus semicircula'ris** [NA], proper membrane of semicircular duct: the outer, loose, connective tissue layer of a semicircular duct. **m. pupilla'ris** [NA], pupillary membrane: a mesodermal layer attached to the rim or front of the iris during embryonic development, sometimes persisting in the adult. **m. quadrangula'ris** [NA], quadrangular membrane: the upper part of the fibroelastic membrane of the larynx. **m. reticula'ris duc'tus cochlea'ris** [NA], **m. reticula'ta**, reticular membrane: a netlike membrane over the spiral organ; the free ends of the outer hair cells pass through its apertures. **m. ruyschia'na**, lamina choridocapillaris. **m. saccifor'mis**, the synovial membrane of the inferior radioulnar articulation. **m. sero'sa**, 1. tunica serosa. 2. the chorion. **m. seroti'na**, decidua basalis. **m. spira'lis duc'tus cochlea'ris**, NA alternative for *paries tympanicus ductus cochlearis*. **m. stape'dis** [NA], stapedial membrane: a membrane filling the arch formed by the crura and base of the stapes; called also *m. obturatoria* [*stapedis*]. **m. statoconi'orum macula'rum** [NA], statoconic membrane of maculae: the gelatinous membrane surmounting the maculae, containing the statoconia, and having special sensory hairs projecting into it. **m. ster'ni** [NA], sternal membrane: the thick fibrous membrane that envelopes the sternum; it is formed by the intermingling of fibers of the radiate sternocostal ligaments, the periosteum, and the tendinous origin of the pectoralis

major. **m. succin'gens**, the pleura. **m. suprapleura'lis** [NA], suprapleural membrane: the strengthened portion of the endothoracic fascia attached to the inner part of the first rib and the transverse process of the seventh cervical vertebra. **m. synovia'lis cap'sulae articula'ris** [NA], synovial membrane of articular capsule: the inner of the two layers of the articular capsule of a synovial joint, composed of loose connective tissue and having a free smooth surface that lines the joint cavity. It secretes the synovial fluid. Called also *stratum synoviale capsulae articularis*. **m. tecto'ria** [NA], tectorial membrane: a strong fibrous band connected cranially with the basilar part of the occipital bone and caudally with the dorsal surface of the bodies of the second and third cervical vertebrae. It is actually the cranial prolongation of the deeper portion of the posterior longitudinal ligament of the vertebral column. **m. tecto'ria duc'tus cochlea'ris** [NA], tectorial membrane of cochlear duct: a delicate gelatinous mass resting on the spiral organ of the ear and connected with the hairs of the hair cells; called also *Corti's membrane*. **m. ten'sa**, pars tensa membranae tympani. **m. thyrohyoi'dea** [NA], thyrohyoid membrane: a broad fibroelastic sheet attached above to the upper margin of the posterior surface of the hyoid bone and below to the upper border of the thyroid cartilage; called also *m. hyothyreoidea*. **m. tym'pani** [NA], tympanic membrane: the obliquely placed, thin membranous partition between the external acoustic meatus and the tympanic cavity. The greater portion, the pars tensa, is attached by a fibrocartilaginous ring to the tympanic plate of the temporal bone; the much smaller, triangular portion, the pars flaccida, is situated anterosuperiorly between the two mallear folds. Called also *drumhead* and, loosely, *eardrum*. **m. tym'pani secunda'ria** [NA], secondary tympanic membrane: the membrane that closes in the fenestra cochlearis; called also *Scarpa's membrane*. **m. versic'olor of Fielding**, tapetum, def. 2. **m. vestibula'ris** [NA alternative], **m. vestibula'ris** [Reiss'neri], paries vestibularis ductus cochlearis. **m. vi'brans**, pars tensa membranae tympani. **m. vitelli'na**, vitelline membrane. **m. vit'rea** [NA], vitreous membrane: a delicate boundary layer investing the vitreous body of the eye; called also *m. hyaloidea* or *hyaloid membrane*.

membranaceous (mem"brah-na'shus) [L. *membranaceus*] of the nature of a membrane.

membranae (mem-bra'ne) [L.] plural of *membrana*.

membranate (mem'brah-nāt) having the character of a membrane.

membrane (mem'brān) a thin layer of tissue which covers a surface, lines a cavity, or divides a space or organ; see also *membrana*. **abdominal m.**, peritoneum. **accidental m.**, false m. **adamantine m.**, cuticula dentis. **adventitious m.**, a membrane not normal to the part. **alveolocapillary m.**, an exquisitely thin tissue barrier, the mechanism for gas exchange between alveolar air and capillary blood in the lung. **alveolodental m.**, periodontium. **anal m.**, cloacal m. **animal m.**, a thin membranous diaphragm, as of bladder, used as a dialyzer. **aponeurotic m.**, aponeurosis. **arachnoid m.**, arachnoidea. **Ascherson's m.**, the covering of casein enclosing the milk globules. **asphyxial m.**, hyaline m. (def. 2); so called because of its interference with gaseous exchange in the lungs. **atlanto-occipital m., anterior**, membrana atlanto-occipitalis anterior. **atlanto-occipital m., posterior**, membrana atlantooccipitalis posterior. **Baer's m.**, chromicized pig's bladder, used as a dressing over cut bone surfaces. **basal m. of semicircular duct**, membrana basalis ductus semicircularis. **basement m.**, the delicate layer of extracellular condensation of mucopolysaccharides and proteins underlying the epithelium of mucous membranes and secreting glands. **basilar m. of cochlear duct**, lamina basilaris ductus cochlearis. **Bichat's m.**, Henle's fenestrated m. **birth m's**, the amnion and chorion. **Bowman's m.**, a thin layer of the cornea composed of condensed stroma, between the outer layer of stratified epithelium and the substantia propria; called also *lamina limitans anterior corneae* [NA]. **Bruch's m.**, lamina basalis choroideae. **Brunn's m.**, the epithelium of the olfactory region of the nose. **bucconasal m.**, oronasal m. **buccopharyngeal m.**, 1. fascia pharyngobasilaris. 2. oropharyngeal m. **capsular m.**, capsula articularis. **capsulopupillary m.**, membrana pupillaris. **cell m.**, plasma m. **chorioallantoic m.**, chorioallantois. **chromatic m.**, a continuous layer of chromatin substance situated on the internal surface of a nuclear membrane. **cloacal m.**, the thin, temporary barrier between the hindgut and the exterior, formed by the outer and inner germ layers of the embryo; called also *anal m.* and *anal plate*. **complex m.**, a membrane made up of several layers differing in structure. **compound m.**, a membrane, like that of the tympanum, made up of two distinct layers. **Corti's m.**, membrana tectoria ductus cochlearis. **costocoracoid m.**, fascia clavipectoralis. **cribriform m.**, fascia cribrosa. **cricothyroid m.**, cricovocal m., conus elasticus laryngis. **croupous m.**, a false membrane formed in true croup. **cyclitic m.**, a false membrane which sometimes covers the vitreous body in cyclitis. **Debove's m.**, the delicate layer between the epithelium and the tunica propria of the bronchial, tracheal, and intestinal mucous membranes. **decidual m's, deciduous**

m's, membranae deciduae. **Demours' m.** (obs.), lamina limitans posterior corneae. **dentinoenamel m.,** a continuous thin membrane laid down by ameloblasts adjoining the basement membrane separating them from the dentin in an early developing tooth. **Descemet's m.,** a thin hyaline membrane between the substantia propria and the endothelial layer of the cornea; called also *lamina limitans posterior corneae* [NA]. **diphtheritic m.,** a false membrane characteristic of diphtheria and resulting from coagulation necrosis. **drum m.,** membrana tympani. **Duddell's m.** (obs.), lamina limitans posterior corneae. **egg m.,** any of several investments surrounding the ovum or egg: if derived from the ovum itself, as the vitelline membrane, it is *primary;* if from the follicular cells, as the zona pellucida, it is secondary; if from the oviduct, as the albumen around rabbit's egg or the albumen and shell of hen's egg, it is *tertiary.* Called also *egg envelope* and, collectively, *lemma.* **elastic m.,** a variety of membrane composed largely of elastic fibers. **elastic m., external,** a fenestrated elastic membrane that constitutes the innermost component of the tunica adventitia of arteries. **elastic m., internal,** a fenestrated elastic membrane that constitutes the outermost component of the tunica intima of arteries. **enamel m.,** 1. cuticula dentis. 2. the inner layer of cells within the enamel organ of the dental germ in the fetus; called also *Hannover's intermediate m.* **endoneural m.,** neurilemma. **exocoelomic m.,** Heuser's m. **extraembryonic m's,** the trophoblastic parts of the conceptus that support the embryo or fetus by attachment, mechanical protection, endocrine action, and the mediation of chemical exchange with the maternal circulation. They include the yolk sac, allantois, amnion, umbilical cord, and chorion, including the placenta. To these, some would add the maternal component, the decidua. Called also *fetal m's.* **false m.,** a morbid pellicle or skinlike layer resembling an organized and living membrane, but made up of coagulated fibrin with bacteria and leukocytes, such as may be formed on mucous membranes in diphtheria. **fenestrated m.,** one of the multiply-perforated elastic sheets of the tunica intima and tunica media of arteries. **fertilization m.,** a strong membrane formed around the fertilized ovum in some species of animals by adhesion of part of the contents of the cortical granules to the inner surface of the vitelline membrane; it prevents the entry of additional spermatozoa. **fetal m's,** extraembryonic m's. **fibroelastic m. of larynx,** membrana fibroelastica laryngis. **fibrous m. of articular capsule,** membrana fibrosa capsulae articularis. **Fielding's m.,** tapetum, def. 2. **germinal m.,** blastoderm. **glassy m.,** 1. the basement membrane of a vesicular ovarian follicle which in cross-section appears as a distinct brilliant line and which persists in the ovary long after its follicle has degenerated. Called also *m. of Slavianski.* 2. lamina basalis choroideae. 3. hyaline m., def. 1. **glomerular m.,** the membrane covering a glomerular capillary. **gradocol m's,** thin membranes made of colloidion or similar substances and graded as to porosity; used in ultrafiltration and sometimes to estimate the diameters of viruses. **ground m.,** inophragma. **Haller's m.,** lamina vasculosa choroideae. **Hannover's intermediate m.,** enamel m., def. 2. **haptogen m.,** the membrane of protein matter formerly believed to enclose milk globules. **Held's limiting m.,** blood-brain barrier. **Henle's m.,** 1. posterior border lamella of Fuchs; see under *lamella.* 2. formerly, the lamina basalis choroideae. **Henle's elastic m.,** a fenestrated layer between the outer and middle tunics of certain arteries. **Henle's fenestrated m.,** a subendothelial fibroelastic fenestrated layer in the tunica intima of an artery; called also *Bichat's m.* **Heuser's m.,** a delicate sac of mesoblastic tissue that develops as a lining of the blastocyst or chorionic cavity just after implantation, forms the exocoelomic cavity, and quickly disappears; called also *exocoelomic membrane.* **Hovius' m.** (obs.), the entochoroidea. **Huxley's m.,** the cellular membrane of the root sheath and proximal end of a hair. **hyaline m.,** 1. the membrane between the outer root sheath and the inner fibrous layer of a hair follicle. 2. a layer of eosinophilic hyaline material lining the alveoli, alveolar ducts, and bronchioles, found at autopsy in infants who have died of respiratory distress syndrome of the newborn. Called also *asphyxial membrane* and *vernix membrane.* See *respiratory distress syndrome,* under *syndrome.* **hyaloid m.,** membrana vitrea. **hymenal m.,** hymen. **hyoglossal m.,** a fibrous lamina connecting the under surface of the tongue with the hyoid bone. **hyothyroid m.,** membrana thyrohyoidea. **intercostal m., external,** membrana intercostalis externa. **intercostal m., internal,** membrana intercostalis interna. **interosseous m., radioulnar, interosseous m. of forearm,** membrana interossea antebrachii. **interosseous m. of leg,** membrana interossea cruris. **interspinal m's,** see *ligamentum interspinale.* **intersutural m.,** the pericranium lying between the cranial sutures. **ion-selective m.,** a membrane that is more permeable to particular types of ions than to other types, e.g., K⁺-selective glass membrane. Many biological membranes exhibit ion-selective behavior. **Jackson's m.,** a delicate curtain or web of adhesions (regarded by some as a sheet of peritoneum) which may extend from the lateral abdominal wall to the cecum, covering the cecum and producing obstruction of the bowel; called also *Jackson's veil.* **Jacob's m.,** layer of rods and cones. **keratoge-**

nous m., matrix unguis. **Kölliker's m.,** membrana reticularis ductus cochlearis. **Krause's m.,** Z band; see under *band.* **ligamentous m.,** membrana tectoria. **limiting m.,** a membrane which constitutes the border of some tissue or structure. **limiting m., external,** 1. a thin fenestrated sheet in the retina, through which extend the visual rods and cones. 2. a membrane investing the external surface of the embryonic neural tube. **limiting m., internal,** 1. the innermost layer of the retina. 2. a membrane lining the internal surface of the embryonic neural tube. **Mauthner's m.,** axolemma. **medullary m.,** endosteum. **mucocutaneous m.,** a membrane that is partly mucous and partly cutaneous, like that of the tympanum. **mucous m.,** tunica mucosa. **mucous m., proper,** lamina propria mucosae. **mucous m. of colon,** tunica mucosa coli. **mucous m. of esophagus,** tunica mucosa esophagi. **mucous m. of gallbladder,** tunica mucosa vesicae felleae. **mucous m. of mouth,** tunica mucosa oris. **mucous m. of pharynx,** tunica mucosa pharyngis. **mucous m. of rectum,** tunica mucosa recti. **mucous m. of small intestine,** tunica mucosa intestini tenuis. **mucous m. of stomach,** tunica mucosa ventriculi. **mucous m. of tongue,** tunica mucosa linguae. **mucous m. of ureter,** tunica mucosa ureteris. **mucous m. of urinary bladder,** tunica mucosa vesicae urinariae. **Nasmyth's m.,** primary (enamel) cuticle. **nictitating m.,** a transparent fold of skin lying deep to the other eyelids at the mesial side, which may be drawn over the front of the eyeball; the so-called third eyelid, found in reptiles and birds generally and in many mammals. **nuclear m.,** 1. either of the membranes, inner and outer, comprising the nuclear envelope. 2. nuclear envelope. **oblique m. of forearm,** chorda obliqua membrana interosseae antebrachii. **obturator m.,** membrana obturatoria. **obturator m. of atlas, anterior,** membrana atlantooccipitalis anterior. **obturator m. of atlas, posterior,** membrana atlantooccipitalis posterior. **obturator m. of larynx,** membrana thyrohyoidea. **occipitoaxial m., long,** membrana tectoria. **olfactory m.,** the olfactory portion of the mucous membrane lining the nasal fossa. **oral m.,** fascia pharyngobasilaris. **oronasal m.,** a thin epithelial plate separating the nasal pits from the oral cavity of the embryo. **oropharyngeal m.,** a transient embryonic septum at the cranial limit of the foregut, in the depths of the stomodeum; called also *buccopharyngeal m.* **otolithic m.,** membrana statoconiorum macularum. **ovular m.,** vitelline m. **palatine m.,** the membrane covering the roof of the mouth. **pericolic m., pericolonic m.,** occasional bands of peritoneum extending between the abdominal wall and the serosa of the colon. **peridental m.,** periodontium. **perineal m.,** fascia diaphragmatis urogenitalis inferior. **periodontal m.,** periodontal ligament. **periorbital m.,** periorbita. **pharyngeal m., pharyngobasilar m.,** fascia pharyngobasilaris. **pituitary m. of nose,** tunica mucosa nasi. **placental m.,** the semipermeable membrane that separates the fetal from the maternal blood in the placenta. In the human (hemochorial) placenta, it is composed of fetal vascular endothelium, cytotrophoblast, and syncytium, and it becomes thinner as pregnancy progresses. Called also *placental barrier.* **plasma m.,** the structure enveloping a cell, enclosing the cytoplasm, and forming a selective permeability barrier; it consists of lipids, proteins, and some carbohydrates, the lipids thought to form a bilayer in which integral proteins are embedded to varying degrees. Called also *cell m., cytoplasmic m.,* and *plasmalemma.* **platelet demarcation m.,** a more or less tridimensional system of paired membranes that serve to partition the megakaryocyte cytoplasm, each partition containing azurophilic granules and representing a future blood platelet. **pleuropericardial m.,** a membrane in the embryo separating the heart and the lung sac. **pleuroperitoneal m.,** a membrane in the embryo separating the pleural cavity from the peritoneal cavity and developing into a part of the diaphragm. **proligerous m.,** cumulus oophorus. **proper m. of semicircular duct,** membrana propria ductus semicircularis. **prophylactic m.,** pyophylactic m. **pseudoserous m.,** a membrane resembling serous membrane, but differing from it in structure. **pulmonary hyaline m.,** hyaline membrane, def. 2. **pupillary m.,** membrana pupillaris. **purpurogenous m.,** the pigment epithelium of the eye. **pyogenic m.,** a membrane which produces pus. **pyophylactic m.,** a fibrinous membrane lining a pus cavity and tending to prevent reabsorption of injurious materials. **quadrangular m.,** membrana quadrangularis. **Ranvier's m.,** Rénaut's layer. **Reichert's m.** (obs.), lamina limitans anterior corneae. **Reissner's m.,** paries vestibularis ductus cochlearis. **reticular m., reticulated m.,** membrana reticularis ductus cochlearis. **Ruysch's m., ruyschian m.,** lamina choroidocapillaris. **Scarpa's m.,** membrana tympani secundaria. **schneiderian m.,** tunica mucosa nasi. **Schwann's m.,** neurilemma. **semipermeable m.,** a membrane that permits the passage of a solvent, such as water, but prevents the passage of the dissolved substance, or solute. **serous m.,** tunica serosa. **shell m.,** a double fibrous layer lining the shell of the egg of some animals, such as birds. **Shrapnell's m.,** pars flaccida membranae tympani. **m. of Slavianski,** glassy m., def. 1. **slit m.,** one of the exceedingly thin membranes that bridge the slit pores between adjacent pedicels of the podocytes of the renal glomerulus, and close the pores at their bases. **spiral m. of cochlear duct,** membrana spiralis ductus cochlearis. **stapedial m.,** membrana stapedis. **statoconic m. of maculae,** membrana statoconiorum macularum. **sternal m., m. of sternum,** membrana sterni. **striated m.,** see *zona pellucida,* def. 1. **subenamel m.,** a membrane said to exist between the enamel of a tooth and the stellate reticulum. **subepithelial m.,** basement membrane. **submucous m.,** tela submucosa. **submucous m. of stomach,** tela submucosa ventriculi. **suprapleural m.,** membrana suprapleuralis. **synaptic m.,** the layer separating the neuroplasm of an axon from that of the body of the nerve cell with which it makes synapsis. **synovial m. of articular capsule,** membrana synovialis capsulae articularis. **tarsal m.,** orbital septum. **tectorial m.,** membrana tectoria. **tectorial m. of cochlear duct,** membrana tectoria ductus cochlearis. **tendinous m.,** aponeurosis. **Tenon's m.,** vagina bulbi. **thyreohyoid m.,** membrana thyrohyoidea. **Traube's m.,** a film of potassium ions formed at the plane of contact of the two liquids, when a solution of potassium ferrocyanide is brought into contact with a solution of a copper salt. **tympanic m.,** the membrane separating the middle from the external ear; see *membrana tympani.* **tympanic m., secondary,** membrana tympani secundaria. **undulating m.,** a protoplasmic membrane running like a fin along the body of certain protozoa; its margin is formed by a flagellum which may continue free beyond the undulating membrane. **unit m.,** the trilaminar structure of the plasma membrane as seen under the electron microscope and postulated to be the same for the membranes of all cells, the cell nucleus, and organelles (mitochondria, etc.). **vascular m. of viscera,** tela submucosa. **vernix m.,** hyaline m. (def. 3); so called because it was originally thought to be the result of aspiration of vernix by the fetus *in utero.* **vestibular m. of cochlear duct,** paries vestibularis ductus cochlearis. **virginal m.,** hymen. **vitelline m.,** the cytoplasmic, noncellular membrane surrounding the eggs of various animals, especially the membrane enveloping the yolk of telolecithal eggs. **vitreous m.,** 1. membrana vitrea. 2. lamina basalis choroidea. 3. lamina limitans posterior corneae. 4. hyaline membrane (def. 1). **Volkmann's m.,** a thin, yellowish membrane, studded with miliary tubercles, lining the fibrous wall of a tubercular abscess. **Wachendorf's m.,** 1. membrana pupillaris. 2. plasma m. **yolk m.,** vitelline m. **Zinn's m.,** zonula ciliaris.

membranectomy (mem″brah-nek′to-me) excision of a membrane.

membranelle (mem″brah-nel′) a small membrane composed of cilia, seen in ciliate organisms.

membraniform (mem-bra′nĭ-form) resembling a membrane.

membranin (mem′brah-nin) a preparation made from the cell wall and/or cell membrane of yeast cells.

membranocartilaginous (mem″brah-no-kar″tĭ-laj′ĭ-nus) 1. developed in both membrane and cartilage. 2. partly cartilaginous and partly membranous.

membranoid (mem′brah-noid) resembling a membrane.

membranolysis (mem″brän-ol′ĭ-sis) disruption of a cell membrane.

membranous (mem′brah-nus) [L. *membranosus*] pertaining to or of the nature of a membrane.

membrum (mem′brum) pl. *mem′bra* [L.] a limb, or member, of the body; [NA] a general term for one of the limbs, that is, the upper (arm, forearm, hand), or lower (thigh, leg, foot). Called also *extremitas* (pl. *extremitates*) or *extremity.* **m. infe′rius** [NA], the lower limb of the body (thigh, leg, and foot); called also *extremitas inferior.* **m. mulie′bre,** clitoris. **m. supe′rius** [NA], the upper limb of the body (arm, forearm, and hand); called also *extremitas superior.* **m. viri′le,** penis.

memory (mem′o-re) [L. *memoria*] that mental faculty by which sensations, impressions, and ideas are recalled. **anterograde m.,** a memory serviceable for events long past, but not able to acquire new recollections. **coast m.,** tropical amnesia. **eye m.,** visual memory. **immunologic m.,** the capacity of the immune system to respond more rapidly and strongly to subsequent antigenic challenge than to the first exposure. **kinesthetic m.,** the memory of movements in the limbs and other parts of the body. **long-term m.,** memory that is retained over long periods of time. **screen m.,** a consciously tolerable memory serving as a "screen" for another memory that may be disturbing or emotionally painful if recalled. **short-term m.,** memory that is lost within a brief period (seconds, minutes, or longer) unless reinforced. **visual m.,** memory for visual impressions.

memotine hydrochloride (mem′o-tēn) chemical name: 3,4-dihydro-1-[(4-methoxyphenoxy)methyl] isoquinoline hydrochloride; an antiviral agent, $C_{17}H_{17}NO_2 \cdot HCl$.

menacme (mĕ-nak′me) [Gr. *mēn* month + *akmē* top] 1. the height of menstrual activity. 2. that period of a woman's life which is marked by menstrual activity.

menadiol sodium diphosphate (men″ah-di′ol) [USP] chemical name: 2-methyl-1,4-naphthalenediol bis(dihydrogen phos-

phate) tetrasodium salt hexahydrate. A synthetic, water-soluble derivative of menadione (vitamin K₃) to which it is converted in the body, $C_{11}H_8N_4O_8P_2 \cdot 6H_2O$, occurring as a white to pink powder, and used as a prothrombinogenic vitamin for the same purposes as menadione (q.v.); administered orally, intravenously, and subcutaneously.

menadione (men″ah-di′ōn) [USP] chemical name: 2-methyl-1,4-naphthalenedione. A synthetic, oil-soluble vitamin K derivative, $C_{11}H_8O_2$, occurring as a bright yellow, crystalline powder; used as a source of vitamin K in the treatment of hemorrhagic conditions associated with hypoprothrominemia, such as obstructive jaundice, biliary fistula, sprue, celiac disease, and ulcerative colitis, and after prolonged use of salicylates, administered orally and intramuscularly. Called also *menaphthone* and *vitamin K₃.* **m. sodium bisulfite** [USP], a water-soluble derivative of menadione, $C_{11}H_9NaO_5S \cdot 3H_2O$, occurring as a white crystalline powder, having the same actions and uses as menadione; administered intravenously, and subcutaneously, and sometimes orally and intramuscularly.

Menagen (men′ah-jen) trademark for a preparation of estrone.

menalgia (men-al′je-ah) [Gr. *mēn* month + *-algia*] pain accompanying menstruation.

menaphthone (men-af′thōn) menadione.

menaquinone (men″ah-kwin′ōn) any of a series of compounds in which the phytyl side chain of phytonadione (vitamin K₁) is replaced by a side chain of prenyl units and which have vitamin K activity; they are synthesized, in particular, by gram-positive bacteria. Called also *farnoquinone* and *vitamin K₂.*

menarchal (mĕ-nar′kal) pertaining to menarche.

menarche (mĕ-nar′ke) [Gr. *mēn* month + *archē* beginning] the establishment or beginning of the menstrual function.

menarcheal, menarchial (mĕ-nar′ke-al) pertaining to or characterized by the establishment of the menstrual function (menarche).

Mendel's law (men′delz) [Gregor Johann *Mendel,* 1822–1884, Austrian monk and naturalist] see under *law.*

Mendel's reflex [Kurt *Mendel,* German neurologist, 1874–1946] see under *reflex.*

Mendel's test [Felix *Mendel,* German physician, 1862–1912] see *Mantoux test,* under *tests.*

Mendel-Bekhterev reflex, sign (men′del-bek- ter′yev) [Kurt *Mendel;* V. M. *Bekhterev,* Russian neurologist, 1857–1927] see under *reflex* and *sign.*

Mendeléeff's (Mendeleev's) law, test (men″dĕ-la′efs) [Dimitri Ivanovich *Mendeléeff,* Russian chemist, 1834–1907] see *periodic law,* under *law,* and see under *tests.*

mendelevium (men″dĕ-le′ve-um) [Dimitri Ivanovich *Mendeléeff*] the radioactive chemical element of atomic number 101, atomic weight 256, symbol Md, originally discovered in debris from a thermonuclear explosion in 1952.

mendelian (men-de′le-an) named for Gregor Johann *Mendel;* see under *character,* and see *Mendel's law,* under *law.*

mendelism (men′del-izm) see *mendelian characters,* under *character,* and *Mendel's law,* under *law.*

mendelizing (men′del-iz″ing) exhibiting the simple patterns of inheritance of various contrasting traits elaborated by Gregor Mendel; see *Mendel's laws,* under *law.*

Mendelsohn's test (men′del-sōnz) [Martin Alfred *Mendelsohn,* German physician, 1860–1930] see under *tests.*

Menest (men′est) trademark for a preparation of esterified estrogens.

Ménétrier's disease (mān″a-tre-ārz′) [Pierre *Ménétrier,* French physician, 1859–1935] giant hypertrophic gastritis.

Menformon (men′for-mon) trademark for a preparation of estrone.

Menge's pessary (meng′gez) [Karl *Menge,* Heidelberg gynecologist, 1864–1945] see under *pessary.*

menhidrosis (men″hid-ro′sis) [Gr. *mēn* month + *hidrōs* sweat] a form of vicarious menstruation consisting of monthly discharge of sweat, sometimes bloody.

menidrosis (men″id-ro′sis) menhidrosis.

Meniere's disease (syndrome) (men″e-ārz′) [Prosper *Meniere,* French physician, 1799–1862. The spelling *Meniere* appears on his birth certificate, *Ménière* and *Méníère* on his works. *Ménière* was the choice of his son] see under *disease.*

meningeal (mĕ-nin′je-al) of or pertaining to the meninges.

meningematoma (mĕ-nin″jem-ah-to′mah) hematoma of the dura mater.

meningeocortical (mĕ-nin″je-o-kor′tĭ-kal) of or pertaining to the meninges and cortex of the brain.

meningeoma (mĕ-nin″je-o′mah) meningioma.

meningeorrhaphy (mĕ-nin″je-or′ah-fe) [Gr. *mēninx* membrane + *rhaphē* suture] suture of the meninges.

meninges (mĕ-nin′jēz) [Gr., pl. of *mēninx* membrane] [NA] the three membranes that envelop the brain and spinal cord: the dura mater, pia mater, and arachnoid.

meninghematoma (mĕ-ninj″hem-ah-to′mah) meningematoma.

meningina (men″in-ji′nah) (*obs.*) pia-arachnoid.

meninginitis (men″in-jin-i′tis) inflammation of the meningina (pia-arachnoid); leptomeningitis.

meningioma (mĕ-nin″je-o′mah) [*meninges* + *-oma* tumor] a hard, slow-growing, usually vascular tumor which occurs mainly along the meningeal vessels and superior longitudinal sinus, invading the dura and skull and leading to erosion and thinning of the skull. **angioblastic m.,** angioblastoma.

meningiomatosis (mĕ-nin″je-o″mah-to′sis) a condition characterized by the formation of multiple meningiomas.

meningism (mĕ-nin′jizm) 1. the symptoms and signs of meningeal irritation associated with acute febrile illness or dehydration without actual infection of the meninges. Called also *Duprés disease* or *syndrome*. 2. a hysterical simulation of meningitis.

meningismus (men″in-jis′mus) meningism.

meningitic (men″in-jit′ik) pertaining to or of the nature of meningitis.

meningitides (men″in-jit′ĭ-dēz) plural of *meningitis*.

meningitis (men″in-ji′tis), pl. *meningit′ides* [Gr. *mēninx* membrane + *-itis*] inflammation of the meninges. When it affects the dura mater, the disease is termed *pachymeningitis;* when the arachnoid and pia mater are involved, it is called *leptomeningitis,* or meningitis proper. **acute aseptic m.,** aseptic m. **African m.,** see under *trypanosomiasis*. **amebic m.,** an acute meningoencephalitis caused by invasion of the central nervous system by one of the normally free-living species of *Acanthamoeba, Hartmanella,* or *Naegleria*. **aseptic m.,** the name given to a mild form of meningitis, most cases of which are caused by viruses; see *viral m*. **m. of the base, basilar m.,** that which affects the meninges at the base of the brain. **benign lymphocytic m.,** viral m. **m. carcinomato′sa,** a misnomer for the condition of widespread carcinomatous infiltration of the meninges; the condition is not inflammatory. **cerebral m.,** inflammation of the meninges of the brain. **cerebrospinal m.,** an inflammation of the membranes of the brain and spinal cord; it may be caused by many different organisms. Abbreviated C.S.M. **eosinophilic m.,** meningitis resulting from infection with *Angiostrongylus cantonensis,* characterized by an increase in lymphocytes and a high percentage of eosinophils in the cerebrospinal fluid; called also *eosinophilic meningoencephalitis*. **epidemic cerebrospinal m.,** an acute infectious disease attended by seropurulent inflammation of the membranes of the brain and spinal cord, and due to infection by the *Neisseria meningitidis*. The disease appears usually in epidemics, and the symptoms are those of acute cerebral and spinal meningitis, in addition to which there is usually an eruption of erythematous, herpetic, or hemorrhagic spots upon the skin. The fulminating or malignant form is known as *Waterhouse-Friderichsen syndrome*. Called also *cerebrospinal fever* and *meningococcic m*. **external m.,** pachymeningitis externa. **gummatous m.,** meningitis during the tertiary stage of syphilis in which there are many small gummata in the membranes. **internal m.,** pachymeningitis interna. **lymphocytic m.,** viral m. **meningococcal m.,** epidemic cerebrospinal m. **Mollaret's m.,** recurrent febrile attacks, malaise, headache, and meningeal signs accompanied by a marked polymorphonuclear inflammatory reaction in the cerebrospinal fluid. **mumps m.,** an aseptic meningitis secondary to mumps. **m. necrotox′ica reacti′va,** a condition marked by areas of focal cerebral softening with symptoms and signs of meningeal irritation suggesting primary inflammatory changes of the cerebral cortex. **occlusive m.,** leptomeningitis of children which leads to the closure of the lateral and median apertures of the fourth ventricle. **m. ossif′icans,** ossification of the cerebral meninges. **otitic m.,** a form that sometimes complicates an attack of otitis media. **parameningococcus m.,** meningitis caused by parameningococcus. **posterior m.,** meningitis of the cerebellar region. **purulent m.,** that which is suppurative. **Quincke's m.,** acute aseptic meningitis. **septicemic m.,** that which is due to septic blood poisoning. **m. sero′sa,** serous m. **m. sero′sa circumscrip′ta,** meningitis giving rise to cystic accumulations of serous fluid which cause symptoms of tumors. **m. sero′sa circumscrip′ta cys′tica,** chronic meningitis with cyst formation. **serous m.,** meningitis with serous exudation into the ventricles and subarachnoid spaces and slight to moderate changes in the spinal fluid. **simple m.,** that in which there is an exudate of fibrin and serum. **spinal m.,** inflammation of the meninges of the spinal cord. **sterile m.,** meningitis in which there is no infection, e.g., that caused by injection of contrast medium to myelography. **m. sympath′ica,** a condition of the cerebrospinal fluid caused by inflammation in the neighborhood of the meninges. It is marked by increase in the pressure of the fluid and increase in its albumin and cellular content. The fluid is sterile and there may be symptoms of meningitis. **torula m., torular m.,** meningitis due to infection with *Cryptococcus neoformans* (*Torula histolytica*). **tubercular m., tuberculous m.,** a severe meningitis caused by *Mycobacterium tuberculosis*. **viral m.,** meningitis due to various viruses, such as the coxsackieviruses, mumps virus, and the virus of lymphocytic choriomenin-

gitis, characterized by malaise, fever, headache, nausea, cerebrospinal fluid pleocytosis (principally lymphocytic), abdominal pain, stiffness of the neck and back, and a short uncomplicated course. Called also *aseptic m., acute aseptic m., benign lymphocytic m.,* and *lymphocytic m*.

meningo- [Gr. *mēninx* membrane] a combining form denoting relationship to the membranes covering the brain and/or spinal cord, or to other membrane.

meningoarteritis (mĕ-ning″go-ar″ter-i′tis) inflammation of the meningeal arteries.

meningoblastoma (mĕ-ning″go-blas-to′mah) primary malignant melanoma of the meninges.

meningocele (mĕ-ning′go-sēl) [*meningo-* + Gr. *kēlē* hernia] hernial protrusion of the meninges through a defect in the skull (*cranial m.*) or vertebral column (*spinal m.*). **spurious m.,** Billroth's disease, def. 1.

meningocephalitis (mĕ-ning″go-sef″ah-li′tis) meningoencephalitis.

meningocerebritis (mĕ-ning″go-ser″ĕ-bri′tis) [*meningo-* + *cerebritis*] meningoencephalitis.

meningococcemia (mĕ-ning″go-kok-se′me-ah) invasion of the blood stream by meningococci. **acute fulminating m.,** Waterhouse-Friderichsen syndrome.

meningococci (mĕ-ning″go-kok′si) plural of *meningococcus*.

meningococcidal (mĕ-ning″go-kok-si′dal) [*meningococcus* + L. *caedere* to kill] destroying meningococci.

meningococcin (mĕ-ning″go-kok′sin) an antigenic material precipitated from saline suspensions of the meningococcus by means of alcohol. It is applied as a skin test (intradermal) in the detection of meningococcus carriers.

meningococcosis (mĕ-ning″go-kok-ko′sis) infection caused by meningococci.

meningococcus (mĕ-ning″go-kok′us), pl. *meningococ′ci* [*meningo-* + Gr. *kokkos* berry] an individual organism of the species *Neisseria meningitidis*.

meningocortical (mĕ-ning″go-kor′tĭ-kal) pertaining to or affecting the meninges and cortex of the brain.

meningocyte (mĕ-ning′go-sīt) a histiocyte of the meninges.

meningoencephalitis (mĕ-ning″go-en-sef″ah-li′tis) [*meningo-* + Gr. *enkephalos* brain + *-itis*] inflammation of the brain and meninges. **chronic m.,** dementia paralytica. Called also *encephalomeningitis*. **eosinophilic m.,** eosinophilic meningitis. **mumps m.,** a usually benign form seen in children, caused by the mumps virus, and characterized by fever, vomiting, nuchal rigidity, lethargy, parotitis, headache, convulsions, abdominal pain, diarrhea, and delirium. **primary amebic m.,** a highly fatal form of meningoencephalitis, most often caused by free-living amebas of the genus *Naegleria,* and usually acquired by swimming in fresh water inhabited by large numbers of the amebas. It is characterized by a rapidly deteriorating course and death in three to five days. **syphilitic m.,** dementia paralytica.

meningoencephalocele (mĕ-ning″go-en-sef′ah-lo-sēl″) [*meningo-* + Gr. *enkephalos* brain + *kēlē* hernia] hernial protrusion of the meninges and brain substance through a defect in the skull. Called also *encephalomeningocele*.

meningoencephalomyelitis (mĕ-ning″go-en-sef″ah-lo-mi″ĕ-li′tis) [*meningo-* + Gr. *enkephalos* brain + *myelos* marrow + *-itis*] inflammation of the meninges, brain, and spinal cord.

meningoencephalomyelopathy (mĕ-ning″go-en-sef″ah-lo-mi″ĕ-lop′ah-the) disease involving the meninges, brain, and spinal cord.

meningoencephalopathy (mĕ-ning″go-en-sef″ah-lop′ah-the) noninflammatory disease of the cerebral meninges and the brain. Called also *encephalomeningopathy*.

meningofibroblastoma (mĕ-ning″go-fi″bro-blas-to′mah) meningioma.

meningogenic (mĕ-ning″go-jen′ik) [*meningo-* + Gr. *gennan* to produce] arising in the meninges.

meningoma (men″in-go′mah) meningioma.

meningomalacia (mĕ-ning″go-mah-la′she-ah) [*meningo-* + Gr. *malakia* softness] softening of a membrane.

meningomyelitis (mĕ-ning″go-mi″ĕ-li′tis) [*meningo-* + Gr. *myelos* marrow + *-itis*] inflammation of the spinal cord and its membranes.

meningomyelocele (mĕ-ning″go-mi″ĕ-lo-sēl″) [*meningo-* + Gr. *myelos* marrow + *kēlē* hernia] hernial protrusion of a part of the meninges and substance of the spinal cord through a defect in the vertebral column. See illustration on following page.

meningomyeloencephalitis (mĕ-ning″go-mi″ĕ-lo-en-sef″ah-li′tis) inflammation of the meninges, spinal cord, and the brain.

meningomyeloradiculitis (mĕ-ning″go-mi″ĕ-lo-rah-dik″u-li′tis) inflammation of the meninges, spinal cord, and roots of the spinal nerves.

meningo-osteophlebitis (mĕ-ning″go-os″te-o-fle-bi′tis) [*meningo-* + Gr. *osteon* bone + *phleps* vein + *-itis*] periostitis with inflammation of the veins of a bone.

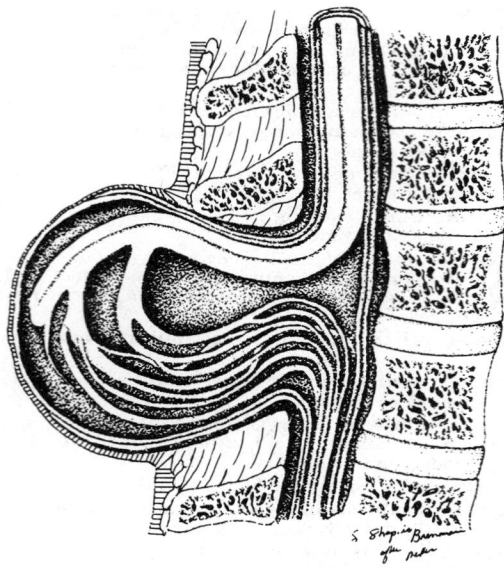

Meningomyelocele (after Netter, from Ciba Collection).

meningopathy (men″in-gop′ah-the) [*meningo-* + Gr. *pathos* disease] any disease of the meninges.

meningopneumonitis (mĕ-ning″go-nu-mo-ni′tis) a disease produced in experimental animals by the injection of the etiologic agent of psittacosis (*Chlamydia psittaci*), and marked by acute meningitis and pneumonitis.

meningorachidian (mĕ-ning″go-rah-kid′e-an) [*meningo-* + Gr. *rhachis* spine] pertaining to the spinal cord and its membranes.

meningoradicular (mĕ-ning″go-rah-dik′u-lar) [*meningo-* + L. *radix* root] pertaining to the meninges and the roots of the cranial and spinal nerves.

meningoradiculitis (mĕ-ning″go-rah-dik″u-li′tis) inflammation of the meninges and roots of the spinal nerves.

meningorecurrence (mĕ-ning″go-re-kur′ens) syphilitic meningitis induced in a syphilitic patient by antisyphilitic treatment.

meningorrhagia (mĕ-ning″go-ra′je-ah) [*meningo-* + Gr. *rhēgnynai* to break] hemorrhage from the cerebral or spinal membranes.

meningorrhea (mĕ-ning″go-re′ah) [*meningo-* + Gr. *rhoia* flow] effusion of blood between or upon the meninges.

meningosis (men″in-go′sis) the membranous attachment of bones to each other.

meningothelioma (mĕ-ning″go-the″le-o′mah) meningioma.

meningovascular (mĕ-ning″go-vas′ku-lar) pertaining to the blood vessels of the meninges.

meninguria (men″in-gu′re-ah) [*meningo-* + Gr. *ouron* urine + *-ia*] the occurrence of membranous shreds in the urine.

meninx (me′ninks), pl. **menin′ges** [Gr. *mēninx* membrane] a membrane; especially one of the three membranes enveloping the brain and spinal cord. **m. fibro′sa** (*obs.*), the dura mater. **m. sero′sa** (*obs.*), the arachnoidea. **m. ten′uis** (*obs.*), the pia-arachnoid. **m. vasculo′sa** (*obs.*), the pia mater.

meniscal (mĕ-nis′kal) of or pertaining to a meniscus.

meniscectomy (men″ĭ-sek′to-me) excision of an intra-articular meniscus, as in the knee joint.

menischesis (men″ĭ-ske′sis) menoschesis.

menisci (men-is′si) plural of *meniscus.*

meniscitis (men″ĭ-si′tis) inflammation of a meniscus of the knee joint.

meniscocyte (mĕ-nis′ko-sīt) [Gr. *mēniskos* crescent + *-cyte*] a sickle cell.

meniscocytosis (mĕ-nis″ko-si-to′sis) sickle cell anemia, see under *anemia.*

meniscosynovial (mĕ-nis″ko-sin-o′ve-al) pertaining to a meniscus and the synovial membrane.

meniscus (mĕ-nis′kus), pl. **menis′ci** [L.; Gr. *mēniskos*, crescent] 1. a crescent-shaped structure appearing at the surface of a liquid column, as in a pipet or buret, made concave or convex by the influence of capillarity. 2. [NA] a general term for a crescent-shaped structure of the body. Often used alone to designate one of the crescent-shaped disks of fibrocartilage attached to the superior articular surface of the tibia. **m. of acromioclavicular joint,** discus articularis articulationis acromioclavicularis. **articular m., m. articula′ris** [NA], a pad, commonly a wedge-shaped crescent of fibrocartilage or dense fibrous tissue,

found in some synovial joints; one side forms a marginal attachment at the articular capsule and the other two sides extend into the joint, ending in a free edge. **converging m.,** a concavoconvex lens. **discoid m., discoid lateral m.,** a semilunar lateral meniscus of the knee that has been transformed into a thickened, irregular discoid mass as a result of excess motion of the meniscus, which in turn results from congenital absence of attachment of the posterior horn of the meniscus to the tibial plateau. The excess motion also causes a clicking sound on flexion and extension of the knee. Occasionally, a discoid medial meniscus is observed. Called also *congenital discoid meniscus.* **diverging m.,** a convexoconcave lens. **m. of inferior radioulnar joint,** discus articularis articulationis radioulnaris distalis. **joint m.,** articular m. **Kuhnt's m.,** the lining of the physiologic cup of the optic disk, composed of a thick accumulation of neuroglia. **lateral m. of knee joint, m. latera′lis articulatio′nis ge′nus** [NA], a crescent-shaped disk of fibrocartilage, but nearly circular in form, attached to the lateral margin of the superior articular surface of the tibia; called also *m. lateralis articulationis genu.* **medial m. of knee joint, m. media′lis articulatio′nis ge′nus** [NA], a crescent-shaped disk of fibrocartilage attached to the medial margin of the superior articular surface of the tibia; called also *m. medialis articulationis genu.* **negative m.,** a convexoconcave lens. **positive m.,** a concavoconvex lens. **m. of sternoclavicular joint,** discus articularis articulationis sternoclavicularis. **tactile menisci, menis′ci tac′tus** [NA], small, cup-shaped, tactile nerve endings within the skin, many of which are formed by branches of a single nerve fiber, and each of which is in contact with a single, modified epithelial cell; they are found in the deep epidermis, in hair follicles, and in the hard palate, and function as touch receptors. Called also *Grandy's corpuscles, Grandy-Merkel corpuscles, tactile disks, Merkel's cells, corpuscles,* or *disks,* and *Merkel's tactile cells.* **m. of temporomaxillary joint,** discus articularis articulationis temporomandibularis.

menispermine (men″ĭ-sper′min) a crystalline alkaloid, C$_{18}$H$_{24}$N$_2$O$_2$, from *Anamirta cocculus* L. Wight & Arn. (Menispermaceae).

Menispermum (men″ĭ-sper′mum) [Gr. *mēnē* moon + *sperma* seed] a genus of plants. The rhizome and roots of *M. canadense* L. (Menispermaceae) (moonseed, or yellow parilla) are tonic and alterative. Because this vine, including the leaves and fruits, resemble a grapevine, children have ingested the fruits and been poisoned, sometimes fatally.

meno- [Gr. *mēn* month; *mēniaia* the menses] a combining form denoting relationship to the menses.

menolipsis (men″o-lip′sis) temporary cessation of the menses.

menometrorrhagia (men″o-met″ro-ra′je-ah) excessive uterine bleeding occurring both during the menses and at irregular intervals.

menopausal (men″o-paw′zal) pertaining to or associated with the menopause.

menopause (men′o-pawz) [*meno-* + Gr. *pausis* cessation] cessation of menstruation in the human female, occurring usually between the age of 48 and 50. See also *climacteric.* **artificial m.,** cessation of menstruation produced by artificial means, such as surgical operation or irradiation. **m. prae′cox,** premature failure of ovulation, possibly due to primary germ cell deficiency, acquired refractoriness to pituitary gonadotropin, or autoimmunization.

menoplania (men″o-pla′ne-ah) [*meno-* + Gr. *planē* deviation] metastasis or aberration of the menses; vicarious menstruation.

menorrhagia (men″o-ra′je-ah) [*meno-* + Gr. *rhēgnynai* to burst forth] excessive uterine bleeding occurring at the regular intervals of menstruation, the period of flow being of greater than usual duration.

menorrhalgia (men″o-ral′je-ah) [*menorrhea* + *-algia*] dysmenorrhea.

menorrhea (men″o-re′ah) [*meno-* + Gr. *rhoia* flow] 1. the normal discharge of the menses. 2. too free or profuse menstruation.

menorrheal (men″o-re′al) pertaining to menorrhea.

menoschesis (mĕ-nos′kĕ-sis, men″o-ske′sis) [*meno-* + Gr. *schesis* retention] retention of the menses.

menostasia (men″o-sta′ze-ah) menostasis.

menostaxis (men″o-stak′sis) [*meno-* + Gr. *staxis* a dropping, dripping] excessively prolonged menstruation.

menotropins (men″o-tro′pins) [USP] an extract of human postmenopausal urine containing both follicle-stimulating hormone and luteinizing hormone. In females, it has the property of stimulating growth and maturation of ovarian follicles. In males, it has the properties of maintaining and stimulating testicular interstitial cells (Leydig tissue) related to testosterone production and of being responsible for full development and maturation of spermatozoa in the seminiferous tubules. Called also *human follicle-stimulating hormone* and *human menopausal gonadotropin.*

menses (men′sēz) [L., pl. of *mensis* month] the monthly flow of blood from the genital tract of women; see *menstruation.*

menstrual (men'stroo-al) [L. *menstrualis*] pertaining to the menses.

menstruant (men'stroo-ant) a person who is menstruating or is capable of menstruating.

menstruate (men'stroo-āt) [L. *menstruare*] to discharge blood from the genital tract at monthly intervals; see *menstruation*.

menstruation (men'stroo-a'shun) the cyclic, physiologic discharge through the vagina of blood and muscosal tissues from the nonpregnant uterus; it is under hormonal control and normally recurs, usually at approximately four-week intervals, in the absence of pregnancy during the reproductive period (puberty through menopause) of the female of the human and a few species of primates. It is the culmination of the menstrual cycle; see illustration accompanying *cycle*. **anovular m., anovulatory m.,** periodic uterine bleeding without preceding ovulation. **delayed m.,** menstruation the first appearance of which is delayed beyond the sixteenth year. **difficult m.,** dysmenorrhea. **infrequent m.,** menstruation occurring less frequently than normal. **nonovulational m.,** anovular m. **profuse m.,** menstruation marked by excessive flow. **regurgitant m.,** a back flow through the uterine tubes by which epithelial cells and other materials may be discharged through the tubal ostia and deposited on the ovaries and adjacent organs, as in endometriosis. **retrograde m.,** regurgitant m. **scanty m.,** menstruation marked by abnormally slight flow. **supplementary m.,** menstrual discharge from the uterus and also from some other part. **suppressed m.,** failure of the menstrual flow to appear. **vicarious m.,** discharge of blood from an extragenital source at the time a menstrual period is normally expected; thought to result from generally increased capillary permeability related to the menstrual cycle.

menstruous (men'stroo-us) pertaining to menstruation.

menstruum (men'stroo-um) [L. *menstruus* menstruous: it was long believed that the menstrual fluid had a peculiar solvent quality] a solvent medium. **Pitkin m.,** a medium for the administration of heparin, consisting of a mixture of gelatin, dextrose, glacial acetic acid, and water.

mensual (men'su-al) [L. *mensis* month] monthly.

mensuration (men"su-ra'shun) [L. *mensuratio; mensura* measure] the act or process of measuring.

mentagrophyton (men"tah-grof'ĭ-ton) [L. *mentagra* sycosis + Gr. *phyton* plant] a former name for the fungus, *Trichophyton mentagrophytes*, the cause of sycosis barbae and other skin and nail infections.

mental (men'tal) 1. [L. *mens* mind] pertaining to the mind; psychic. 2. [L. *mentum* chin] pertaining to the chin.

mentalis (men-ta'lis) [L.] relating to the chin.

mentality (men-tal'ĭ-te) the mental power or activity.

mentation (men-ta'shun) mental activity.

Mentha (men'thah) [L.] a genus of labiate plants, the mints. **M. canaden'sis,** wild mint. **M. cardia'ca,** Scotch spearmint; see *spearmint*. **M. piperi'ta,** peppermint. **M. pule'gium,** true, or European, pennyroyal. **M. spica'ta, M. vir'idis,** common spearmint.

menthol (men'thol) [USP] chemical name: 5-methyl-2-(1-methylethyl)cyclohexanol. An alcohol, $C_{10}H_{20}O$, obtained from diverse mint oils or prepared synthetically, occurring as colorless, hexagonal crystals, usually needle-like, or in fused masses, or crystalline powder; it may be levorotatory (*l*-menthol), from natural or synthetic sources, or racemic (*dl*-menthol). It is used as a topical antipruritic, and in inhalers for treatment of upper respiratory disorders or added to water for inhalation in acute bronchitis. Called also *peppermint camphor*.

menthyl (men'thil) the monovalent radical, $C_{10}H_{19}$.

menticide (men'tĭ-sīd) [L. *mens* mind + *caedere* to kill] brainwashing.

mentimeter (men-tim'ĕ-ter) [L. *mens* mind + Gr. *metron* measure] a method or means of measuring mental capacity.

mento- [L. *mentum* chin] a combining form denoting relationship to the chin. See also words beginning *genio-*.

mentoanterior (men"to-an-te're-or) [*mento-* + *anterior*] see under *position*.

mentolabial (men"to-la'be-al) [*mento-* + L. *labium* lip] pertaining to the chin and lip.

menton (men'ton) an anthropologic and cephalometric landmark, indicating the most inferior point on the midline contour of the chin on a lateral jaw projection.

mentoplasty (men'to-plas"te) [*mento-* + Gr. *plassein* to form] plastic surgery of the chin; surgical correction of deformities and defects of the chin.

mentoposterior (men"to-pos-te're-or) [*mento-* + *posterior*] see under *position*.

mentotransverse (men"to-trans-vers') [*mento-* + *transverse*] see under *position*.

mentula (men'tu-lah) [L.] penis.

mentulagra (men"tu-lag'rah) [L. *mentula* penis + Gr. *agra* seizure] 1. priapism. 2. chordee.

mentulate (men'tu-lāt) having a large penis.

mentum (men'tum) [L.] [NA] the chin.

Menyanthes (men"e-an'thēz) [perhaps from Gr. *mēn* month + *anthos* flower] a genus of gentianaceous plants. *M. trifolia'ta* L., or buckbean, is a bitter tonic and has febrifuge properties, and has been used as an emergency food, beer additive, and tea substitute.

meobentine sulfate (me"o-ben'tēn) chemical name: *N*-[(4-methoxyphenyl)methyl]-*N'*,*N''*-dimethylguanidine sulfate (2:1); an antiarrhythmic cardiac depressant, $(C_{11}H_{17}N_3O_2)\cdot H_2SO_4$.

Meonine (me'o-nīn) trademark for a preparation of racemethionine.

mepacrine hydrochloride (mep'ah-krin) quinacrine hydrochloride.

meparfynol (mĕ-par'fĭ-nōl) chemical name: 3-methyl-1-pentyn-3-ol. A sedative and hypnotic, $C_6H_{10}O$, administered orally. Called also *methylparafynol* and *methylpentynal*.

mepartricin (mĕ-par'trĭ-sin) an antifungal and antiprotozoal; it is a methyl ester of partricin (q.v.), used chiefly in the treatment of vaginal and cutaneous candidiasis, applied topically.

mepazine acetate (mep'ah-zēn) chemical name: 10-[(1-methyl-3-piperidinyl)methyl]-10*H*-phenothiazine acetate. A tranquilizer, $C_{19}H_{22}N_2S$, used mainly in the treatment of tension and anxiety states, but also used as a pre- or postoperative sedative; administered orally or intramuscularly.

mepenzolate bromide (mĕ-pen'zo-lāt) [USP] chemical name: 3-[(hydroxydiphenylacetyl)oxy]-1,1-dimethylpiperidinium bromide. An oral anticholinergic, $C_{21}H_{26}BrNO_3$, occurring as a white or light cream-colored powder; used mainly in disorders in which hypermotility of the colon is a feature.

meperidine hydrochloride (mĕ-per'ĭ-dēn) [USP] chemical name: 1-methyl-4-phenyl-4-piperidinecarboxylic acid ethyl ester. A synthetic narcotic analgesic, $C_{15}H_{21}NO_2\cdot HCl$, occurring as a fine, white, crystalline powder, used as a preanesthetic medication, postoperative sedative, obstetric analgesic, and when a relatively short duration of analgesia is desired; administered orally in tablets or intramuscularly or subcutaneously. Abuse of this drug may lead to dependence. Called also *isonipecaine* and *pethidine hydrochloride*.

mephenamine (mĕ-fen'ah-mēn) orphenadrine.

mephenesin (mĕ-fen'ĕ-sin) chemical name: 3-(2-methylphenoxy)-1,2-propanediol. A skeletal muscle relaxant, $C_{10}H_{14}O_3$, occurring as a white crystalline powder; administered orally.

mephenoxalone (mef"en-ok'sah-lōn) chemical name: 5-[(*o*-methoxyphenoxy)methyl]-2-oxazolidinone; a mild tranquilizer and skeletal muscle relaxant, $C_{11}H_{13}NO_4$.

mephentermine sulfate (mĕ-fen'ter-mēn) [NF] chemical name: *N,α,α*-trimethylbenzeneethanamine sulfate (2:1). An adrenergic, $(C_{11}H_{17}N)_2\cdot H_2SO_4$, occurring as white crystals or as a crystalline powder; used for its vasopressor effects in the treatment of certain hypotensive states, administered orally, intramuscularly, and intravenously. It is also applied topically to the nasal mucosa as a decongestant.

mephenytoin (mĕ-fen'ĭ-to-in) [USP] chemical name: 5-ethyl-3-methyl-5-phenyl-2,4-imidazolidinedione. An anticonvulsant, $C_{12}H_{14}N_2O_2$, occurring as a white, crystalline powder; used for the control of grand mal, focal, jacksonian, and psychomotor epileptic seizures that are refractory to other drugs, administered orally.

mephitic (mĕ-fit'ik) [L. *mephiticus; mephitis* foul exhalation] emitting a foul odor.

mephitis (mĕ-fi'tis) [L.] a foul exhalation.

mephobarbital (mef"o-bar'bĭ-tal) [USP] chemical name: 5-ethyl-1-methyl-5-phenyl-2,4,6(1*H*,3*H*,5*H*)-pyrimidinetrione. A long-acting barbiturate, $C_{13}H_{14}N_2O_3$, occurring as a white, crystalline powder; used as a sedative in the treatment of anxiety, tension, and apprehension and as an anticonvulsant in grand mal and petit mal epilepsy, administered orally.

Mephyton (mef'ĭ-ton) trademark for preparations of phytonadione (vitamin K_1).

mepivacaine hydrochloride (mĕ-piv'ah-kān) [USP] chemical name: *N*-(2,6-dimethylphenyl)-1-methyl-2-piperidinecarboxamide monohydrochloride. An analogue of lidocaine, $C_{15}H_{22}N_2O\cdot HCl$, occurring as a white, crystalline solid; used to produce local anesthesia by infiltration injection, peripheral nerve block, and epidural block.

Meprane (me'prān) trademark for preparations of promethestrol dipropionate.

meprednisone (mĕ-pred'nĭ-sōn) [USP] chemical name: 17α,21-dihydroxy-16β-methyl-pregna-1,4-diene-3,11,20-trione. A synthetic glucocorticoid, $C_{22}H_{28}O_5$, occurring as a white to creamy white powder; used in the treatment of inflammatory, allergic, rheumatic, and other corticosteroid-responsive diseases, such as certain endocrine, respiratory, neoplastic, and collagen diseases, administered orally.

meprobamate (mĕ-pro'bah-māt, mep'ro-bam'āt) [USP] chemical name: 2-methyl-2-propyl-1,3-propanediol. A carbamate derivative, $C_9H_{18}N_2O_4$, occurring as a white powder, having tranquilizing, muscle relaxant, and anticonvulsant actions. It is used as an oral sedative for the relief of anxiety and tension, as an adjunct in the treatment of conditions in which anxiety and tension are manifested, and to promote sleep in anxious tense patients; it is also used in musculoskeletal disorders and as an anticonvulsant in petit mal epilepsy. An intramuscular injection is used as adjunctive therapy in tetanus. **isopropyl m.,** carisoprodol.

Meprospan (mĕ-pro'span) trademark for a preparation of meprobamate.

Meprotabs (mĕ-pro'tabs) trademark for a preparation of meprobamate.

meprylcaine hydrochloride (mep'ril-kān) [USP] chemical name: 2-methyl-2-(propylamino)-1-propanol benzoate (ester) hydrochloride. A local anesthetic, $C_{14}H_{21}NO_2 \cdot HCl$, occurring as a white, crystalline powder; used for infiltration and nerve block anesthesia.

mepyramine maleate (me-pir'ah-mēn) pyrilamine maleate.

mepyrapone (mĕ-pi'rah-pōn) metyrapone.

mEq. milliequivalent.

meq. milliequivalent.

mequidox (mek'wi-doks) chemical name: 3-methyl-2-quinoxalinemethanol 1,4-dioxide; an antibacterial, $C_{10}H_{10}N_2O_3$.

mer- see *mero-*.

meralgia (me-ral'je-ah) [*mero-* (2) + *-algia*] pain in the thigh. **m. paresthet'ica,** a disease marked by paresthesia, pain, and numbness in the outer surface of the thigh, in the region supplied by the lateral femoral cutaneous nerve, due to entrapment of the nerve at the inguinal ligament. Called also *Bernhardt's disturbance of sensation.*

meralluride (mer-al'u-rīd) chemical name: [3-[[[(3-carboxy-1-oxopropyl)amino]carbonyl]amino]-2-methoxypropyl](1,2,3,6-tetrahydro-1,3-dimethyl-2,6-dioxo-7*H*-pyrin-7-yl)mercury. A mercurial diuretic, $C_{16}H_{22}HgN_6O_7$, occurring as a white to slightly yellow powder; used in the treatment of edema secondary to such conditions as congestive heart failure, nephrosis, and the ascites of liver disease, administered intramuscularly and subcutaneously.

merbromin (mer-bro'min) chemical name: (2',7'-dibromo-3',6'-dihydroxy-3-oxospiro[isobenzofuran-1(3*H*),9'[9*H*]xanthene]-4'-yl)-hydroxomercury disodium salt; a topical antibacterial, $C_{20}H_8Br_2$-$HgNa_2O_6$.

mercaptan (mer-kap'tan) [L. *mercurium captans* seizing or combining with mercury] any compound containing the —SH group bound to carbon.

mercaptide (mer-kap'tid) a compound derived from a mercaptan, with a metal replacing the sulfur hydrogen radical.

mercaptoethanol (mer-kap"to-eth'ah-nol) a reducing agent, $HS \cdot CH_2CH_2 \cdot OH$, that may attack disulfide bonds in proteins, reducing them to sulfhydryl groups, often destroying their physiological activity; e.g., they may inhibit mitosis.

mercaptol (mer-kap'tol) a compound formed from a ketone by introducing two thio-alkyl groups in place of the bivalent oxygen.

mercaptomerin sodium (mer-kap"to-mer'in) [USP] chemical name: [3-[[(3-carboxy-2,2,3-trimethylcyclopentyl)carbonyl]amino]-2-methoxypropyl](mercaptoacetato-*S*) disodium salt. An organomercurial diuretic, $C_{16}H_{25}HgNNa_2O_6S$, occurring as a white, hygroscopic powder or amorphous solid, having a characteristic honeycomb structure; used in the treatment of edema secondary to such conditions as heart disease, nephrosis, and the ascites of liver disease, administered intramuscularly and subcutaneously.

mercaptopurine (mer-kap"to-pu'rēn) [USP] chemical name: 6*H*-purine-6-thione monohydrate. An analogue of hypoxanthine and adenine that is a purine (adenine) antagonist, $C_5H_4N_4S$, interfering with DNA synthesis; occurring as a yellow crystalline powder, it is used as an antineoplastic, primarily in the treatment of acute leukemia, administered orally. It also has immunosuppressive properties.

Mercier's bar (valve), catheter (mer-se-āz') [Louis Auguste *Mercier,* French urologist, 1811–1882] see *plica interureterica,* and under *catheter.*

mercocresols (mer'ko-kre'solz) a combination of cresol derivatives and an organic mercury, used for its germicidal, fungicidal, and bacteriostatic properties.

Mercuhydrin (mer"ku-hi'drin) trademark for preparations of meralluride.

mercupurin (mer-ku'pu-rin) former name for mercurophylline.

mercuramide (mer-kūr'ah-mīd) mersalyl.

mercurammonium (mer-ku"rah-mo'ne-um) a precipitate produced when ammonium hydroxide is added to a solution of a mercuric salt. **m. chloride,** ammoniated mercury.

mercurial (mer-ku're-al) [L. *mercurialis*] 1. pertaining to mercury. 2. a preparation of mercury.

Mercurialis (mer-ku"re-a'lis) a genus of slender herbs of Europe. *M. an'nua* L. (Euphorbiaceae), French mercury, was formerly used as a diuretic and antisyphilitic.

mercurialism (mer-ku're-al-izm") mercury poisoning; see under *poisoning.*

mercurialization (mer-ku"re-al-i-za'shun) the act or process of putting under the influence of mercury.

mercurialized (mer-ku're-al-īzd) treated with mercury; containing mercury.

mercuric (mer-ku'ric) pertaining to mercury as a bivalent element. **m. benzoate,** a white, crystalline, tasteless salt, $(C_6H_5 \cdot CO \cdot O)_2Hg + H_2O$, formerly used in the treatment of syphilis. **m. chloride,** mercury bichloride. **m. cyanide,** a very poisonous salt, $Hg(CN)_2$, formerly used in the treatment of syphilis. **m. iodide, red,** mercury biniodide, HgI_2; formerly used as an antibacterial agent. **m. oxide, yellow,** a yellow to orange-yellow, heavy, impalpable powder, HgO, used as a local anti-infective in ophthalmology. Called also *Pagenstecher's ointment.* **m. oxycyanide,** a white crystalline powder, $Hg(CN)_2 \cdot HgO$, formerly used as an antiseptic and antisyphilitic. **m. salicylate,** a white, tasteless powder, $(OH \cdot C_6H_4 \cdot CO_2)_2Hg$, insoluble in water and alcohol, formerly used in the treatment of syphilis.

Mercurochrome (mer-ku'ro-krōm) trademark for preparations of merbromin.

mercurophylline (mer"ku-ro-fil'lin) a mixture of the sodium salt of 3-[[3-(hydroxymercuri)-2-methoxypropyl]-carbamoyl]-1,2,2-trimethyl($\pm$)cyclopentane carboxylic acid and theophylline in molecular proportions, used as a mercurial diuretic. Formerly called *mercupurin.*

mercurous (mer'ku-rus) pertaining to mercury as a monovalent element. **m. chloride,** calomel. **m. iodide, yellow,** a bright yellow insoluble amorphous powder, HgI; formerly used in the treatment of syphilis.

mercury (mer'ku-re) [L. *mercurius,* or *hydrargyrum*] a metallic element, liquid at ordinary temperatures; quicksilver. Its symbol is Hg; atomic number, 80; atomic weight, 200.59; specific gravity, 13.546. It is insoluble in ordinary solvents, being only partially soluble in boiling hydrochloric acid. It may be dissolved, however, in nitric acid. Mercury forms two sets of compounds—*mercurous,* in which a single atom of mercury combines with a monovalent radical, and *mercuric,* in which a single atom of mercury combines with a bivalent radical. Mercury and its salts have been employed therapeutically as purgatives; as alteratives in chronic inflammations; as antisyphilitics, intestinal antiseptics, disinfectants, and astringents. They are absorbed by the skin and mucous membranes, causing chronic mercury poisoning (see under *poisoning*). Because of toxicity, the use of mercurials is diminishing. The mercuric salts are more soluble and irritant than the mercurous. See also under *mercuric* and *mercurous.* **ammoniated m.** [USP], a topical anti-infective, $HgNH_2Cl$, occurring in white, pulverulent pieces or as a white amorphous powder. **m. bichloride,** an extremely poisonous compound, $HgCl_2$, occurring as odorless, heavy, colorless crystals, as crystalline masses, or as a white powder: formerly used in the treatment of syphilis and now as a disinfectant. Called also *mercuric chloride.* **m. with chalk,** metallic mercury rubbed up with chalk and honey until the particles are very small; used in pediculosis pubis. **m. chloride, mild,** calomel. **French m.,** *Mercurialis annua.* **m. oleate,** a mixture of yellow mercuric oxide and oleic acid: applied locally in parasitic skin diseases. **m. perchloride,** m. bichloride. **m. salicylate,** a basic salt, $Hg \cdot C_6H_3(OH) \cdot COOH$, containing 54 to 59 per cent of mercury; formerly used in syphilis.

Mercuzanthin (mer"ku-zan'thin) trademark for a preparation of mercurophylline.

merergasia (mer-er-ga'se-ah) see *merergastic.*

merergastic (mer"er-gas'tik) [*mero-* (1) + *ergon* work] Meyer's term for "part disorders," the simplest type of disorder of psychic function, characterized by emotional instability and anxiety (psychoneuroses or neuroses). Cf. *holergastic.*

merethoxylline procaine (mer"ĕ-thok'sĭ-lēn) a combination of the organomercurial merethoxylline (dehydro-2-[*N*-(3'-hydroxymercuri-2'-methoxyethoxy)propylcarbamny]phenoxyacetic acid) with theophylline and procaine; used in the treatment of edema secondary to such conditions as congestive heart failure and nephrotic syndrome, administered intramuscularly and subcutaneously.

meridian (mĕ-rid'e-an) an imaginary line on the surface of a spherical body; see also *meridianus.* **m. of cornea,** an imaginary line marking the intersection with its surface of an antero-posterior plane passing through the apex of the cornea. **m's of eyeball,** meridiani bulbi oculi.

meridiani (mĕ-rid"e-a'ni) [L.] plural of *meridianus.*

meridianus (mĕ-rid"e-a'nus), pl. *meridia'ni* [L., from *medius* middle + *dies* day] an imaginary line on the surface of a spherical body, marking the intersection with the surface of a plane passing through its axis. Called also *meridian.* **meridia'ni bul'bi oc'uli** [NA], meridians of eyeball: imaginary lines encircling the eyeball, marking the intersection with its surface of planes passing through its anteroposterior axis.

meridional (mĕ-rid'e-o-nal) pertaining to a meridian or made along a meridian; as, *meridional* section.

merisis (mer'ĭ-sis) growth in size due to cell division.

merism (mer'izm) [Gr. *meros* a part] the repetition of parts in an organism so as to form a regular pattern.

meristem (mer′ĭ-stem) [Gr. *merizein* to divide] the undifferentiated embryonic tissue of plants.

meristematic (mer″ĭ-stĕ-mat′ik) pertaining to or composed of meristem.

meristic (mer-is′tik) [Gr. *meristikos* fit for dividing] pertaining to or possessing merism; symmetrical; having symmetrically arranged parts.

meristoma (mer″ĭ-sto′mah) [*meristem* + *-oma*] a tumor of meristem.

Merkel's cells (corpuscles, disks, tactile cells) (mer′kelz) [Friedrich Sigmund *Merkel*, German anatomist, 1845–1919] menisci tactus.

Merkel's filtrum, muscle (mer′kelz) [Karl Ludwig *Merkel*, German anatomist, 1812–1876] see *filtrum ventriculi* and *musculus ceratocricoideus.*

Merkel-Ranvier cells (mer′kel-rahn-ve-a′) [F. S. *Merkel*; Louis Antoine *Ranvier*, French pathologist, 1835–1922] see *Merkel's cells*, under *cell.*

mermithid (mer′mĭ-thid) pertaining to or of the family Mermithidae.

Mermithidae (mer-mith′ĭ-de) a family of nematodes of the superfamily Mermithoidea; the cabbage snakes.

Mermithoidea (mer″mith-oi′de-ah) a superfamily of aphasmids including the cabbage snakes (family Mermithidae), the larvae of which may accidentally occur in the human digestive tract as contaminants of food or water.

mero- 1. [Gr. *meros* part] a combining form meaning part. 2. [Gr. *mēros* thigh] a combining form denoting relationship to the thigh.

meroacrania (mer″o-ah-kra′ne-ah) [*mero-*(1) + *a* neg. + Gr. *kranion* skull] congenital absence of part of the cranium.

meroblastic (mer″o-blas′tik) [*mero-*(1) + Gr. *blastos* germ] undergoing cleavage in which only part of the ovum participates; partially dividing.

merocele (me′ro-sēl) [*mero-*(2) + *kēlē* hernia] (*obs.*) femoral hernia.

merocoxalgia (me″ro-kok-sal′je-ah) [*mero-*(2) + L. *coxa* hip + *-algia*] pain in the thigh and hip.

merocrine (me′o-krīn) [*mero-*(1) + Gr. *krinein* to separate] partly secreting; denoting that type of glandular secretion in which the secreting cell remains intact throughout the process of formation and discharge of the secretory products; as in the salivary and pancreatic glands. Cf. *apocrine* and *holocrine.*

merocyte (mer′o-sīt) [*mero-*(1) + *-cyte*] supernumerary sperm nucleus in the ovum in cases of polyspermy.

merodiastolic (mer″o-di-ah-stol′ik) [*mero-*(1) + *diastole*] pertaining to a part of the diastole.

meroergasia (mer″o-er-ga′se-ah) see *merergastic.*

merogamy (mĕ-rog′ah-me) microgamy.

merogastrula (mer″o-gas′troo-lah) the gastrula of a meroblastic ovum.

merogenesis (mer″o-jen′ĕ-sis) [*mero-*(1) + Gr. *genesis* production] cleavage of an ovum.

merogenetic (mer″o-jĕ-net′ik) pertaining to merogenesis.

merogenic (mer″o-jen′ik) pertaining to or producing segmentation.

merogonic (mer″o-gon′ik) pertaining to or resulting from merogony.

merogony (mĕ-rog′o-ne) [*mero-*(1) + Gr. *gonos* procreation] the development of a portion only of an ovum; see *andromerogony* and *gynomerogony.* **diploid m.,** development of a portion of an ovum containing the fused male and female pronuclei. **parthenogenetic m.,** development, as a result of artificial stimulation, of a part of an ovum containing the nucleus.

merology (mĕ-rol′o-je) [*mero-*(1) + *-logy*] (*obs.*) that part of anatomy which deals with elementary tissues.

meromelia (mer″-o-me′le-ah) [*mero-*(1) + *melos* limb + *-ia*] a general term denoting congenital absence of any part of a limb (as in adactyly, hemimelia, and phocomelia), as opposed to amelia, or absence of the entire limb.

meromicrosomia (mer″o-mi″kro-so′me-ah) [*mero-*(1) + *microsomia*] unusual smallness of some part of the body.

meromorphosis (mer″-o-mor-fo′sis) [*mero-*(1) + Gr. *morphōsis* a shaping, bringing into shape] incomplete restoration or regeneration of a lost part.

meromyarial, meromyarian (mer″o-mi-a′re-al; mer″o-mi-a′re-an) [*mero-*(1) + Gr. *mys* muscle] designating a type of nematode musculature in which there are only a few muscle cells in a given area, the cells being platymyarial in type.

meromyosin (mer″o-mi′o-sin) a fragment of the myosin molecule isolated by treatment with proteolytic enzymes; there are two types, heavy (H-meromyosin) and light (L-meromyosin). *L-Meromyosin* makes up the major part of the rodlike backbone of the molecule; *H-meromyosin* contains the subfragment responsible for the ATP-ase activity of myosin.

meronecrobiosis (me″ro-nek″ro-bi-o′sis) meronecrosis.

meronecrosis (me″ro-nĕ-kro′sis) [*mero-*(1) + *necrosis*] cellular necrosis.

meropia (mĕ-ro′pe-ah) [*mero-*(1) + Gr. *ōps* vision + *-ia*] partial blindness.

merorachischisis (me″ro-rah-kis′kĭ-sis) [*mero-*(1) + Gr. *rhachis* spine + *schisis* fissure] fissure of a part of the spinal cord.

meroscope (me′ro-skōp) (*obs.*) an instrument for performing meroscopy.

meroscopy (mĕ-ros′ko-pe) [*mero-*(1) + Gr. *skopein* to examine] (*obs.*) fractional auscultation of the heart; dissociated auscultation of various parts of the cardiac cycle.

merosmia (mĕ-ros′me-ah) [*mero-*(1) + Gr. *osmē* smell + *-ia*] a disorder of the sense of smell in which certain odors are not perceived.

merostotic (mer″os-tot′ik) [*mero-*(1) + L. *os* bone] pertaining to or affecting only a part of a bone.

merotomy (mĕ-rot′o-me) [*mero-*(1) + Gr. *temnein* to cut] dissection into segments, especially the dissection of a cell.

merozoite (mer″o-zo′ĭt) [*mero-*(1) + Gr. *zōon* animal] one of the organisms formed by multiple fission (schizogony) of a sporozoite within the body of the host during the asexual phase of reproduction of malarial plasmodia and other sporozoa; merozoites differentiate into male and female gametes, which fuse to form the zygote (gametogony).

merozygote (mer″o-zi′gōt) [*mero-*(1) + Gr. *zygōtos* yolked together] the partially diploid bacterial zygote that results from the transfer of a portion of the genetic information of a donor cell to the total genetic information of the recipient.

Merphenyl (mer′fen-il) trademark for preparations of phenylmercuric compounds.

mersalyl (mer′sah-lil) chemical name: [3-[[2-(carboxymethoxy)-benzoyl]amino]-2-methoxypropyl]hydroxymercury monosodium salt. A mercurial diuretic, $C_{13}H_{16}HgNNaO_6$, used in combination with theophylline in the treatment of edema secondary to such conditions as cardiorenal diseases, nephrosis, and hepatic cirrhosis, administered intramuscularly and intravenously.

Merseburg triad (mār′zeh-boorg) [*Merseburg*, a town in Germany] see under *triad.*

Merthiolate (mer-thi′o-lāt) trademark for preparations of thimerosal.

Merulius (mĕ-roo′le-us) a genus of fungi of the class Basidiomycetes, order Polyporales. *M. lac′rymans* is the cause of "dry rot" of wood.

merycism (mer′ĭ-sizm) [Gr. *mērykismos* chewing the cud] rumination.

merycismus (mer″ĭ-siz′mus) merycism.

Merzbacher-Pelizaeus disease (merz′bak-er-pa″le-zi′us) [Ludwig *Merzbacher*, German physician in Buenos Aires, born 1875; Friedrich *Pelizaeus*, German neurologist, born 1850] familial centrolobar sclerosis.

mesad (me′sad) toward the median line or plane; mesiad.

mesal (me′sal) [Gr. *mesos* middle] mesial.

mesangial (mes-an′je-al) of or pertaining to the mesangium.

mesangiocapillary (mes-an″je-o-kap′ĭ-lar″e) pertaining to or affecting the mesangium and the associated capillaries.

mesangium (mes-an′je-um) the thin membrane which helps to support the capillary loops in a renal glomerulus.

Mesantoin (mĕ-san′to-in) trademark for a preparation of mephenytoin.

mesaortitis (mes″a-or-ti′tis) [*meso-* + *aortitis*] (*obs.*) inflammation of the middle coat of the aorta.

mesaraic (mes″ah-ra′ik) [*meso-* + Gr. *mesaraion* the mesentery] mesenteric.

mesarteritis (mes″ar-ter-i′tis) [*meso-* + Gr. *artēria* artery + *-itis*] inflammation of the middle coat of an artery. **Mönckeberg's m.,** see under *arteriosclerosis.*

mesaticephalic (mes-at″ĭ-se-fal′ik) [Gr. *mesatos* medium + *kephalē* head] mesocephalic.

mesatikerkic (mes-at″ĭ-ker′kik) [Gr. *mesatos* medium + *kerkis* the radius of the arm] having a radiohumeral index of 75–80.

mesatipellic (mes-at″ĭ-pel′ik) [Gr. *mesatos* medium + *pella* bowl] having a transverse diameter of the pelvic inlet almost the same as that of the true conjugated diameter.

mesatipelvic (mes-at″ĭ-pel′vik) mesatipellic.

mesaxon (mes-ak′son) a pair of parallel membranes marking the line of edge-to-edge contact of the sheath cell (Schwann cell) encircling the axon.

mescal (mes-kahl′) [Mex.] 1. *Lophophora williamsii* (Lemaire) Coult. (Cactaceae). 2. a liquor distilled from pulque, a fermented drink obtained from the juice of species of *Agave* in Mexico and Central America.

mescaline (mes′kah-lin) a poisonous alkaloid, 3,4,5-trimethoxyphenylethylamine, $(CH_3 \cdot O)_3 C_6H_2 \cdot CH_2 \cdot CH_2 \cdot NH_2$, in the form of a colorless alkaline oil from the flowering heads (mescal buttons) of *Lophophora williamsii* (Lemaire) Coult. (Cactaceae). It produces an intoxication with delusions of color and music.

mescalism (mes′kah-lizm)   intoxication caused by mescal buttons or mescaline.

mesectic (mes-ek′tik) [mes- + Gr. *echein* to hold]   (obs.) taking up (by the blood) a normal amount of oxygen at a given PO_2, i.e., having a normal dissociation curve.

meseclazone (mĕ-sek′lah-zōn)   chemical name: 7-chloro-3,3a-dihydro-2-methyl-2*H*,9*H*-isoxazolo[3,2-*b*][1,3]benzoxacine-9-one; an anti-inflammatory, $C_{11}H_{10}ClNO_3$.

mesectoblast (mes-ek′to-blast)   ectomesoblast.

mesectoderm (mĕ-sek′to-derm)   embryonic migratory cells, derived from the neural crest of the head, that contribute to the formation of the meninges and become pigment cells.

mesencephal (mes-en′sĕ-fal)   mesencephalon.

mesencephalic (mes-en″sĕ-fal′ik)   pertaining to the mesencephalon.

mesencephalitis (mes″en-sef″ah-li′tis)   inflammation of the mesencephalon.

mesencephalohypophyseal (mes″en-sef″ah-lo-hi-po-fiz′e-al)   pertaining to the mesencephalon and the pituitary gland (hypophysis).

mesencephalon (mes″en-sef′ah-lon) [meso- + Gr. *enkephalos* brain]   1. [NA] the part of the brain developed from the middle of the three primary vesicles of the embryonic neural tube; it comprises the tectum and the cerebral peduncles; see Plate accompanying *brain*. See also *brain stem*, under B.   2. the middle of the three primary brain vesicles in the embryo, lying between the prosencephalon and the rhombencephalon. Called also *midbrain*.

mesencephalotomy (mes″en-sef″ah-lot′o-me) [mesencephalon + Gr. *tomē* a cutting]   surgical production of lesions in the midbrain, especially in the pain-conducting pathways for the relief of intractable pain.

mesenchyma (mĕ-seng′kĭ-mah) [meso- + Gr. *enchyma* infusion]   the meshwork of embryonic connective tissue in the mesoderm from which are formed the connective tissues of the body, and also the blood vessels and lymphatic vessels.

mesenchymal (mĕ-seng′kĭ-mal)   pertaining to the mesenchyma.

mesenchyme (mes′eng-kīm)   mesenchyma.

mesenchymoma (mes″en-ki-mo′mah)   a mixed mesenchymal tumor composed of two or more cellular elements not commonly associated, not counting fibrous tissue as one of the elements. **benign m.,** a benign tumor composed of two or more clearly recognizable mesenchymal elements in addition to fibrous tissue. **malignant m.,** a sarcoma composed of two or more cellular elements (excluding fibrous tissue); a mixed cell sarcoma.

mesenterectomy (mes″en-tĕ-rek′to-me) [mesentery + Gr. *ektomē* excision]   resection of the mesentery.

mesenteric (mes″en-ter′ik) [Gr. *mesenterikos*]   pertaining to the mesentery.

mesenteriolum (mĕ-sen″ter-i′o-lum)   a small mesentery. **m. appen′dicis vermifor′mis, m. proces′sus vermifor′-mis,** mesoappendix.

mesenteriopexy (mes″en-ter′e-o-pek″se) [mesentery + Gr. *pēxis* fixation]   fixation or suspension of a torn mesentery.

mesenteriorrhaphy (mes″en-ter″e-or′ah-fe) [mesentery + Gr. *rhaphē* suture]   suture or repair of the mesentery.

mesenteriplication (mes″en-ter″e-pli-ka′shun) [mesentery + L. *plicare* to fold]   shortening the mesentery by plication.

mesenteritis (mes″en-tĕ-ri′tis)   inflammation of the mesentery. **retractile m.,** inflammation of the mesentery producing thickening, sclerosis, and retraction, and occasionally resulting in distortion of intestinal loops.

mesenterium (mes″en-te′re-um) [NA]   the mesentery: the peritoneal fold attaching the small intestine to the posterior abdominal wall. **m. commu′ne, m. dorsa′le commu′ne** [NA], dorsal common mesentery: the primitive embryonic mesentery, a double-layered median partition formed by association of the splanchnic mesoderm with the entoderm, extending from the roof of the coelom toward the midventral wall, and dividing the coelom into halves; it contains the primitive gut, and encloses the heart, lungs, and liver as they develop.

mesenteron (mes-en′ter-on) [meso- + Gr. *enteron* intestine]   the midgut.

mesentery (mes′en-ter″e)   a membranous fold attaching various organs to the body wall. Commonly used with specific reference to the peritoneal fold attaching the small intestine to the dorsal body wall. Called also *mesenterium* [NA]. **m. of ascending part of colon,** mesocolon ascendens. **caval m.,** a ridge, at the right of the embryonic mesogastrium, in which develops a hepatic segment of the inferior vena cava. **common m., common m., dorsal,** mesenterium dorsale commune. **m. of descending part of colon,** mesocolon descendens. **dorsal m.,** mesenterium dorsale commune. **primitive m.,** mesenterium dorsale commune. **m. of rectum,** mesorectum. **m. of sigmoid colon,** mesocolon sigmoideum. **m. of transverse part of colon,** mesocolon transversum. **ventral m.,** the embryonic mesentery attaching the duodenal

region of the early intestine to the ventral body wall. **m. of vermiform appendix,** mesoappendix.

mesentoderm (mĕ-sen′to-derm)   the inner layer of an amphibian gastrula not yet separated into mesoderm and entoderm.

mesentomere (mes-en′to-mēr)   a blastomere not yet divided into mesomeres and entomeres.

mesentorrhaphy (mes″en-tor′ah-fe) [mesentery + Gr. *rhaphē* suture]   suture or repair of the mesentery.

mesepithelium (mes″ep-ĭ-the′le-um)   mesothelium.

MeSH (mesh)   *M*edical *S*ubject *H*eadings, a thesaurus published by the National Library of Medicine for use in MEDLARS.

mesiad (me′ze-ad)   toward the middle; mesad.

mesial (me′ze-al)   nearer the center line of the dental arch.

mesially (me′ze-al″e)   toward the median line.

mesien (me′ze-en)   pertaining to the mesion.

mesiobuccal (me″ze-o-buk′kal)   pertaining to or formed by the mesial and buccal surfaces of a tooth, or the mesial and buccal walls of a tooth cavity.

mesiobucco-occlusal (me″ze-o-buk″ko-ŏ-kloo′zal)   pertaining to or formed by the mesial, buccal, and occlusal surfaces of a tooth.

mesiobuccopulpal (me″ze-o-buk″ko-pul′pal)   pertaining to or formed by the mesial, buccal, and pulpal walls of a tooth cavity.

mesiocervical (me″ze-o-ser′vĭ-kal)   1. pertaining to the mesial surface of the neck of a tooth.   2. mesiogingival.

mesioclination (me″ze-o-kli-na′shun)   deviation of a tooth from the vertical, in the direction of the tooth next mesial (anterior) to it in the dental arch.

mesioclusion (me″ze-o-kloo′zhun)   a malrelation of the dental arches in which the mandibular arch is in an anterior position in relation to the maxillary arch (prognathism); called also *anteroclusion*.

mesiodens (me′ze-o-denz), pl. *mesioden′tes*.   A small supernumerary tooth with a cone-shaped crown and a short root, occurring singly or paired, and generally situated palatally between the maxillary central incisors.

mesiodentes (me″ze-o-den′tēz)   plural of *mesiodens*.

mesiodistal (me″ze-o-dis′tal)   pertaining to the mesial and distal surfaces of a tooth.

mesiogingival (me″ze-o-jin′jĭ-val)   pertaining to or formed by the mesial and gingival walls of a tooth cavity.

mesioincisodistal (me″ze-o-in-si″so-dis′tal)   pertaining to the mesial, incisal, and distal surfaces of an anterior tooth.

mesiolabial (me″ze-o-la′be-al)   pertaining to or formed by the mesial and labial surfaces of a tooth, or the mesial and labial walls of a tooth cavity.

mesiolabioincisal (me″ze-o-la″be-o-in-si′zal)   pertaining to or formed by the mesial, labial, and incisal surfaces of a tooth.

mesiolingual (me″ze-o-ling′gwal)   pertaining to or formed by the mesial and lingual surfaces of a tooth, or the mesial and lingual walls of a tooth cavity.

mesiolinguoincisal (me″ze-o-ling″gwo-in-si′zal)   pertaining to or formed by the mesial, lingual, and incisal surfaces of a tooth.

mesiolinguo-occlusal (me″ze-o-ling″gwo-ŏ-kloo′zal)   pertaining to or formed by the mesial, lingual, and occlusal surfaces of a tooth.

mesiolinguopulpal (me″ze-o-ling″gwo-pul′pal)   pertaining to or formed by the mesial, lingual, and pulpal walls of a tooth cavity.

mesion (me′se-on) [Gr. *mesos* middle]   the plane that divides the body into right and left symmetric halves.

mesio-occlusal (me″ze-o-ŏ-kloo′zal)   pertaining to or formed by the mesial and occlusal surfaces of a tooth, or the mesial and occlusal walls of a tooth cavity.

mesio-occlusion (me″ze-o-ŏ-kloo′zhun)   mesioclusion.

mesio-occlusodistal (me″ze-o-ŏ-kloo″so-dis′tal)   pertaining to the mesial, occlusal, and distal surfaces of a posterior tooth.

mesiopulpal (me″ze-o-pul′pal)   pertaining to or formed by the mesial and pulpal walls of a tooth cavity.

mesiopulpolabial (me″ze-o-pul″po-la′be-al)   pertaining to or formed by the mesial, pulpal, and labial walls of a tooth cavity.

mesiopulpolingual (me″ze-o-pul″po-ling′gwal)   pertaining to or formed by the mesial, pulpal, and lingual walls of a tooth cavity.

mesioversion (me″ze-o-ver′zhun)   the condition of a tooth which is nearer than normal to the median line of the face along the dental arch.

mesiris (mes-i′ris) [meso- + *iris*]   the middle layer of the iris.

mesitylene (mes-it′ĭ-lēn)   symmetric trimethylbenzene, $C_6H_3(CH_3)_3$, from coal tar.

Mesmer (mes′mer), Franz (Friedrick) Anton.   An Austrian (1733–1815), who first demonstrated hypnotism in Vienna in about 1775. See *animal magnetism,* under *magnetism,* and see *mesmerism*.

mesmerism (mes′mer-izm) [after Franz A. *Mesmer*, 1733–1815]   1. the use of animal magnetism and hypnotism as practiced by Mesmer.   2. hypnotism.

meso- [Gr. *mesos* middle] 1. a prefix signifying "middle, " either situated in the middle or intermediate. 2. in chemistry, a prefix signifying inactive or without effect on polarized light.

meso-aortitis (mes″o-a″or-ti′tis) inflammation of the middle coat of the aorta. **m. syphilit′ica**, inflammation of the middle coat of the aorta due to syphilis.

mesoappendicitis (mes″o-ah-pen″dĭ-si′tis) inflammation of the mesoappendix.

mesoappendix (mes″o-ah-pen′diks) [*meso-* + *appendix*] [NA] the peritoneal fold attaching the appendix to the mesentery of the ileum; called also *mesenteriolum processus vermiformis*.

mesoarial (mes″o-a′re-al) pertaining to the mesovarium.

mesoarium (mes″o-a′re-um) mesovarium.

mesobacteria (mes″o-bak-te′re-ah) plural of *mesobacterium*.

mesobacterium (mes″o-bak-te′re-um), pl. *mesobacte′ria*. A rod-shaped microorganism of medium size.

mesobilin (mes″o-bi′lin) a compound, $C_{33}H_{42}O_6N_4$, occurring in the urine as a derivative of bilirubin via enterohepatic circulation.

mesobilirubin (mes″o-bil″ĭ-roo′bin) a compound, $C_{33}H_{44}O_6N_4$, formed by the reduction of bilirubin.

mesobilirubinogen (mes″o-bil″ĭ-roo-bin′o-jen) a reduced form of bilirubin, formed in the intestine, which on oxidation forms stercobilin.

mesobiliviolin (mes″o-bil″ĭ-vi′o-lin) an oxidation product of mesobilirubinogen and of stercobilinogen.

mesoblast (mes′o-blast) [*meso-* + Gr. *blastos* germ] mesoderm, especially in the early stages.

mesoblastema (mes″o-blas-te′mah) the cells composing the mesoblast.

mesoblastic (mes″o-blas′tik) pertaining to or derived from the mesoblast.

mesobronchitis (mes″o-brong-ki′tis) [*meso-* + *bronchitis*] inflammation of the middle coat of the bronchi.

mesocardia (mes″o-kar′de-ah) [*meso-* + Gr. *kardia* heart] atypical location of the heart with the apex in the middle line of the thorax.

mesocardium (mes″o-kar′de-um) [*meso-* + Gr. *kardia* heart] that part of the embryonic mesentery which connects the embryonic heart with the body wall in front and the foregut behind. **arterial m.**, that part of the pericardium which encloses the aorta and pulmonary artery. **dorsal m.**, the temporary dorsal mesentery of the heart in the embryo; its site is represented by the transverse sinus of the pericardium. **lateral m.**, pulmonary ridge. **venous m.**, that part of the pericardium which encloses the venae cavae and pulmonary veins. **ventral m.**, a mesentery attaching the heart to the ventral body wall; it is scarcely represented in human development.

mesocarpal (mes″o-kar′pal) midcarpal.

mesocecal (mes″o-se′kal) pertaining to the mesocecum.

mesocecum (mes″o-se′kum) [*meso-* + *cecum*] the occasionally occurring mesentery of the cecum.

mesocele (mes′o-sēl) [*meso-* + Gr. *koilia* hollow] (*obs.*) aqueductus cerebri.

mesocephalic (mes″o-sĕ-fal′ik) 1. pertaining to the mesocephalon. 2. having a cephalic index between 76.0 and 80.9.

mesocephalon (mes″o-sef′ah-lon) mesencephalon.

Mesocestoides (mes″o-ses-toi′dēz) a genus of tapeworms of the family Mesocestoididae, whose larvae are often found in the coelom or peritoneum of dogs, cats, mice, snakes, and other vertebrates; the adult form is found in the intestines of carnivorous animals, including man, dogs, cats, racoons, and meat-eating birds.

Mesocestoididae (mes″o-ses-toi′dĭ-de) a family of medium-sized to large tapeworms of the order Cyclophyllidea, subclass Cestoda, which parasitize carnivorous birds and mammals. *Mesocestoides* is the type genus.

mesochondrium (mes″o-kon′dre-um) [*meso-* + Gr. *chondros* cartilage] the matrix in which are embedded the cellular elements of hyaline cartilage.

mesochoroidea (mes″o-ko-roi′de-ah) the middle coat of the choroid.

mesococci (mes″o-kok′si) plural of *mesococcus*.

mesococcus (mes″o-kok′us), pl. *mesococ′ci*. A spherical microorganism of medium size.

mesocoelia (mes″o-se′le-ah) (*obs.*) aqueductus cerebri.

mesocolic (mes″o-kol′ik) pertaining to the mesocolon.

mesocolon (mes″o-ko′lon) [*meso-* + Gr. *kolon* colon] [NA] the process of the peritoneum by which the colon is attached to the posterior abdominal wall. It is divided into ascending, transverse, descending, and sigmoid or pelvic portions, according to the segment of the colon to which it gives attachment. **m. ascen′dens** [NA], ascending m., the peritoneum attaching the ascending colon to the posterior abdominal wall, usually obliterated when the ascending colon becomes retroperitoneal. **m. descen′dens** [NA], descending m., the peritoneum attaching the descending colon to the posterior abdominal wall; it is usually

absent because the descending colon is ordinarily retroperitoneal. **iliac m.**, m. sigmoideum. **left m.**, m. descendens. **pelvic m.**, m. sigmoideum. **right m.**, m. ascendens. **sigmoid m., m. sigmoi′deum** [NA], the peritoneum attaching the sigmoid colon to the posterior abdominal wall; called also *pelvic m.* **transverse m., m. transver′sum** [NA], the peritoneum attaching the transverse colon to the posterior abdominal wall.

mesocolopexy (mes″o-ko′lo-pek″se) [*mesocolon* + Gr. *pēxis* fixation] suspension or fixation of the mesocolon.

mesocoloplication (mes″o-ko″lo-pli-ka′shun) [*mesocolon* + *plication*] plication of the mesocolon to limit its mobility.

mesocord (mes′o-kord) an umbilical cord adherent to the placenta by a connecting fold of the amnion; more correctly, the connecting fold itself.

mesocornea (mes″o-kor′ne-ah) substantia propria corneae.

mesocranic (mes″o-kra′nik) having a cranial index between 75.0 and 79.9.

mesocuneiform (mes″o-ku′ne-ĭ-form) os cuneiforme intermedius.

mesocyst (mes′o-sist) [*meso-* + Gr. *kystis* bladder] the layer of peritoneum attaching the gallbladder to the liver.

mesocytoma (mes″o-si-to′mah) [*mesocyte* + *-oma*] a connective tissue tumor.

mesoderm (mes′o-derm) [*meso-* + Gr. *derma* skin] the middle layer of the three primary germ layers of the embryo, lying between the ectoderm and the entoderm. From it are derived the connective tissue, bone and cartilage, muscle, blood and blood vessels, lymphatics and lymphoid organs, notochord, pleura, pericardium, peritoneum, kidney, and gonads. Cf. *ectoderm* and *entoderm*. **extraembryonic m.**, that located outside the embryo and belonging to fetal accessory organs. **gastral m.**, that infolded with the entoderm during gastrulation. **head m.**, loose mesoderm, cranial to the somites. **lateral m.**, the lateral sheets of mesoderm within which the embryonic coelom arises. **paraxial m.**, that lying alongside the notochord and neural tube. **peristomal m.**, that derived from the ventral lip of the blastopore or from the primitive streak. **somatic m.**, the outer of the two layers into which the embryonic mesoderm divides; associated with ectoderm to constitute the somatopleure. **splanchnic m.**, the inner of the two layers into which the embryonic mesoderm divides; associated with entoderm to constitute splanchnopleure.

mesodermal (mes″o-der′mal) pertaining to or derived from the mesoderm.

mesodermic (mes″o-der′mik) pertaining to the mesoderm.

mesodermopath (mes″o-der′mo-path) [*mesoderm* + Gr. *pathos* disease] (*obs.*) a person who is constitutionally susceptible to diseases of the tissues derived from embryonic mesoderm, such as heart and kidneys, arteries and veins, joints and muscles.

mesodiastolic (mes″o-di″ah-stol′ik) [*meso-* + *diastole*] pertaining to the middle of the diastole.

mesodont (mes′o-dont) [*meso-* + Gr. *odous* tooth] having a dental index between 42 and 44.

mesodontic (mes″o-don′tik) having medium sized teeth.

mesodontism (mes″o-don′tizm) the state of having medium sized teeth, or a dental index between 42 and 44.

mesoduodenal (mes″o-du″o-de′nal) pertaining to the mesoduodenum.

mesoduodenum (mes″o-du″o-de′num) [*meso-* + *duodenum*] the mesenteric fold which in early fetal life encloses the duodenum.

mesoepididymis (mes″o-ep″ĭ-did′ĭ-mis) a fold of tunica vaginalis that sometimes connects the epididymis with the testicle.

mesoesophagus (mes″o-ĕ-sof′ah-gus) the portion of the primitive mesentery which encloses the developing esophagus.

mesogaster (mes″o-gas′ter) [*meso-* + Gr. *gastēr* belly] mesogastrium.

mesogastric (mes″o-gas′trik) pertaining to the mesogastrium.

mesogastrium (mes″o-gas′tre-um) [*meso-* + Gr. *gastēr* belly] [NA] the portion of the primitive mesentery which encloses the stomach, and from which the greater omentum is developed.

mesoglea (mes″o-gle′ah) [*meso-* + Gr. *gloia* glue] the layer between the epidermis and gastrodermis of coelenterates.

mesoglia (mĕ-sog′le-ah) 1. microglia. 2. oligodendroglia.

mesoglioma (mes″o-gli-o′mah) a tumor of the mesoglia; a microglioma or oligodendroglioma.

mesogluteal (mes″o-gloo′te-al) pertaining to the gluteus medius muscle.

mesogluteus (mes″o-gloo′te-us) musculus gluteus medius.

mesognathic (mes″og-na′thik) mesognathous.

mesognathous (mĕ-sog′nah-thus) having a gnathic index between 98 and 103.

Mesogonimus (mes″o-gon′ĭ-mus) a former name for a genus of flukes, certain species of which are now included in the genera *Paragonimus* and *Heterophyes*. **M. heteroph′yes**, *Heterophyes heterophyes*.

mesohemin (mes″o-he′min) a reduced form of hemin, $C_{34}H_{36}O_4N_4FeCl$.

mesohyloma (mes″o-hi-lo′mah) [meso- + Gr. hylē matter + -oma] mesothelioma.

mesohypoblast (mes″o-hi′po-blast) mesentoderm.

mesoileum (mes″o-il′e-um) the mesentery of the ileum.

***meso*-inositol** (mes″o-in-o′sĭ-tol) inositol, def. 2.

mesojejunum (mes″o-je-ju′num) the mesentery of the jejunum.

mesolecithal (mes″o-les′ĭ-thal) [meso- + Gr. lekithos yolk.] possessing a moderate amount of yolk.

mesology (mĕ-sol′o-je) ecology.

mesomelic (mes″o-mel′ik) [meso- + Gr. melus limb] pertaining to the midportion of the arm or leg.

mesomere (mes′o-mēr) [meso- + Gr. meros part] 1. a blastomere of size intermediate between a macromere and a micromere. 2. a midzone of the mesoderm between the epimere and hypomere.

mesomeric (mes″o-mer′ik) exhibiting mesomerism.

mesomerism (mĕ-som′er-izm) the existence of organic chemical structures differing only in the position of electons, rather than atoms. For example, the two Kekulé structures for benzene. Such a molecule does not possess one electronic structure part of the time and another structure the rest of the time; the actual electronic state of the molecule is at all times intermediate to the two extremes.

mesometrium (mes″o-me′tre-um) [meso- + Gr. mētra uterus] 1. [NA] the portion of the broad ligament below the mesovarium, composed of the layers of peritoneum that separate to enclose the uterus. 2. the tunica muscularis uteri, or myometrium.

mesomorph (mes′o-morf) [meso- + Gr. morphē form] 1. an individual having a type of body build in which tissues derived from the mesoderm predominate. There is relative preponderance of muscle, bone, and connective tissue, usually with heavy, hard physique of rectangular outline. This somatotype is classified between the ectomorph and the endomorph. 2. a well-proportioned individual, as contrasted to a hypermorph (def. 1) and a hypomorph (def. 1).

mesomorphic (mes″o-mor′fik) pertaining to or characteristic of a mesomorph.

mesomorphy (mes′o-mor″fe) [meso- + Gr. morphē form] the condition of being a mesomorph.

mesomucinase (mes″o-mu′sĭ-nās) a testicular mucinolytic enzyme that may play a role in fertilization.

mesomula (mĕ-som′u-lah) an early stage of the embryo, when it consists of an epithelial ectoderm and entoderm enclosing a mass of mesenchyma.

meson (mes′on, me′zon) [Gr. mesos middle] 1. mesion. 2. a subatomic, short-lived particle of a mass less than that of a proton but more than that of an electron, carrying either a positive or a negative electric charge; called also mesotron.

mesonasal (mes″o-na′zal) situated in the middle of the nose.

mesonephric (mes″o-nef′rik) pertaining to the mesonephros.

mesonephroi (mes″o-nef′roi) plural of mesonephros.

mesonephroma (mes″o-ne-fro′mah) a rare malignant tumor of the female genital tract, most often the ovary, formerly considered to be derived from mesonephric rests (Schiller). Two varieties are recognized: (1) clear cell carcinoma, so called because of its histologic resemblance to renal cell carcinoma, and now considered to be of müllerian duct derivation, and (2) an embryonal tumor, variously called infantile embryonal carcinoma, endodermal sinus tumor, and yolk sac tumor, occurring chiefly in children. The latter variety may also arise in the testis.

mesonephron (mes″o-nef′ron) mesonephros.

mesonephros (mes″o-nef′ros), pl. mesoneph′roi [meso- + Gr. nephros kidney] [NA] the excretory organ of the embryo, arising caudad to the pronephric rudiments or the pronephros and using its duct. The mesonephros consists of a long tube in the lower part of the body cavity, running parallel with the spinal axis and joined at right angles by a row of twisting tubes. Called also corpus Wolffi and wolffian body.

meso-omentum (mes″o-o-men′tum) the fold by which the omentum is attached to the abdominal wall.

meso-ontomorph (mes″o-on′to-morf) [meso- + Gr. ōn being + morphē form] a person of stocky build.

mesopallium (mes″o-pal′e-um) [meso- + L. pallium cloak] paleopallium.

mesopexy (mes′o-pek″se) mesenteriopexy.

mesophile (mes′o-fīl) an organism which grows best at temperatures between 20° and 45° C.

mesophilic (mes″o-fil′ik) [meso- + Gr. philein to love] fond of moderate temperature; said of bacteria which develop best at temperatures between 20° and 45° C. Cf. psychrophilic and thermophilic.

mesophlebitis (mes″o-fle-bi′tis) inflammation of the middle coat of a vein.

mesophragma (mes″o-frag′mah) [meso- + Gr. phragmos a fenc-

ing in] a name given to the M band. Cf. inophragma, and Z band, under band.

mesophryon (mĕ-sof′re-on) [meso- + Gr. ophrys eyebrow] the glabella or its central point.

mesophyll (mes′o-fil) [meso- + Gr. phyllon leaf] the tissue of the inner part of a leaf.

mesopia (mes-o′pe-ah) the condition of having mesopic vision.

mesopic (mes-op′ik) [meso- + Gr. ōpsis sight] pertaining to vision at intermediate levels of illumination, e.g., at twilight.

Mesopin (mes′o-pin) trademark for a preparation of homatropine methylbromide.

mesopneumon (mes″o-nu′mon) [meso- + Gr. pneumon lung] the union of the two layers of the pleura at the hilus of the lung.

mesopneumonium (mes″o-nu-mo′ne-um) (obs.) mesopneumon.

mesoporphyrin (mes″o-por′fĭ-rin) a crystalline iron-free porphyrin, $C_{34}H_{38}O_4N_4$, from heme obtained by a process of reduction.

mesoprosopic (mes″o-pro-sop′ik) [meso- + Gr. prosōpon face] having a face of moderate width.

mesopsychic (mes″o-si′kik) pertaining to the middle period of mental development.

mesopulmonum (mes″o-pul-mo′num) the portion of the embryonic mesentery that encloses the laterally expanding lung.

mesorachischisis (mes″o-rah-kis′kĭ-sis) [meso- + rachischisis] partial rachischisis; partial fissure of the spinal cord.

mesorchial (mĕ-sor′ke-al) pertaining to the mesorchium.

mesorchium (mes-or′ke-um) [meso- + Gr. orchis testis] [NA] the portion of the primitive mesentery that encloses the fetal testis, represented in the adult by a fold between the testis and epididymis.

mesorectum (mes″o-rek′tum) [meso- + rectum] the fold of peritoneum connecting the upper portion of the rectum with the sacrum.

mesoretina (mes″o-ret′ĭ-nah) [meso- + retina] the middle layer of the retina.

mesoridazine (mes″o-rid′ah-zēn) chemical name: 10-[2-(1-methyl-2-piperidinyl)ethyl]-2-(methylsulfinyl)-10H-phenothiazine; a metabolite of thioridazine, $C_{21}H_{26}N_2OS_2$. **m. besylate** [USP], **m. benzenesulfonate,** the besylate salt of mesoridazine, $C_{21}H_{26}N_2OS_2 \cdot C_6H_6O_3S$, occurring as a white to pale yellowish powder; an antipsycotic agent, used in the treatment of alcoholism, schizophrenia, psychoneurotic manifestations, and behavioral problems in mental deficiency and chronic brain syndrome, administered orally and intramuscularly.

mesoropter (mes″o-rop′ter) [meso- + Gr. horos boundary + Gr. optēr observer] the normal position of the eyes with their muscles at rest.

mesorrhaphy (mes-or′ah-fe) mesenteriorrhaphy.

mesorrhine (mes′o-rin) [meso- + Gr. rhis nose] having a nasal index between 48 and 53.

mesosalpinx (mes″o-sal′pinks) [meso- + Gr. salpinx tube] [NA] the part of the broad ligament of the uterus above the mesovarium, composed of layers that enclose the uterine tube.

mesoscapula (mes″o-skap′u-lah) spina scapula.

mesoseme (mes′o-sēm) [meso- + Gr. sēma sign] having an orbital index between 83 and 89.

mesosigmoid (mes″o-sig′moid) the peritoneal fold by which the sigmoid flexure is attached to the posterior abdominal wall.

mesosigmoiditis (mes″o-sig″moi-di′tis) inflammation of the mesosigmoid.

mesosigmoidopexy (mes″o-sig-moi′do-pek″se) [mesosigmoid + Gr. pēxis fixation] suspension or fixation of the mesosigmoid in the treatment of prolapse of the rectum.

mesoskelic (mes″o-skel′ik) [meso- + Gr. skelos leg] having legs of normal length.

mesosoma (mes″o-so′mah) [meso- + Gr. sōma body] medium stature.

mesosomatous (mes″o-so′mah-tus) having medium stature.

mesosome (mes′o-sōm) [meso- + Gr. sōma body] an invagination of the cell membrane occurring in certain bacteria. Various mesosomes are associated with DNA replication and with protein secretion.

mesostaphyline (mes″o-staf′ĭ-lin) having a palatal index between 80.0 and 84.9.

mesostenium (mes″o-ste′ne-um) mesenterium.

mesosternum (mes″o-ster′num) [meso- + Gr. sternon sternum] the corpus sterni.

mesostroma (mes″o-stro′mah) the embryonic fibrillar tissue analogous to the vitreous, which develops into Bowman's and Descemet's membranes.

mesosyphilis (mes″o-sif′ĭ-lis) secondary syphilis.

mesosystolic (mes″o-sis-tol′ik) [meso- + Gr. systolē systole] pertaining to the middle of the systole.

mesotarsal (mes″o-tar′sal) midtarsal.

mesotendineum (mes″o-ten-din′e-um) [NA] the delicate connective tissue sheath attaching a tendon to its fibrous sheath.

mesotendon (mes″o-ten′don) mesotendineum.

mesotenon (mes″o-ten′on) mesotendineum.

mesothelial (mes″o-the′le-al) pertaining to the mesothelium.

mesothelioma (mes″o-the″le-o′mah) a malignant tumor derived from mesothelial tissue (peritoneum, pleura, pericardium); it appears as broad sheets of cells, with some regions containing spindle-shaped, sarcoma-like cells and other regions showing adenomatous patterns. Pleural mesotheliomas have been linked to exposure to asbestos.

mesothelium (mes″o-the′le-um) [meso- + epithelium] [NA] the layer of flat cells, derived from the mesoderm, which lines the coelom or body cavity of the embryo. In the adult, it forms the simple squamous epithelium which covers all true serous membranes (peritoneum, pericardium, pleura).

mesothenar (mes-oth′e-nar) [meso- + Gr. thenar palm] musculus adductor pollicis.

mesothorium (mes″o-tho′re-um) a disintegration product of thorium, intermediate between thorium and radiothorium and isotopic with radium. It has radioactive properties and has been used in the treatment of cancer.

mesotron (mes′o-tron) meson, def. 2.

mesotropic (mes″o-trop′ik) situated in the middle of a cavity, as the abdomen.

mesotympanum (mes″o-tim′pah-num) the portion of the middle ear medial to the tympanic membrane.

mesouranic (mes″o-u-ran′ik) mesuranic.

mesovarium (mes″o-va′re-um) [NA] the portion of the broad ligament of the uterus between the mesometrium and mesosalpinx, which is drawn out to enclose and hold the ovary in place.

Mesozoa (mes″o-zo′ah) [meso- + Gr. zōon animal] a small group of tiny parasites whose relationships to the Protozoa and Metazoa are uncertain.

mesterolone (mes-ter′o-lōn) chemical name: 17β-hydroxy-1α-methyl-5α-androstan-3-one; an androgen, $C_{20}H_{32}O_2$, with actions and uses similar to those of testosterone.

Mestinon (mes′tǐ-non) trademark for preparations of pyridostigmine bromide.

mestranol (mes′trah-nōl) [USP] chemical name: 3-methyoxy-19-nor-17α- pregna-1,3,5(10)-triene -20-yne-17α-ol. The 3-methyl ether of ethinyl estradiol, $C_{21}H_{26}O_2$, occurring as a white to creamy white, crystalline powder; used as the estrogen component of several progestin-estrogen oral contraceptives.

mesuprine hydrochloride (mes′ǔ-prēn) chemical name: 2′-hydroxy-5′-[1-hydroxy-2-[p-methoxyphenethyl)amino]propyl]-methanesulfonanilide monohydrochloride; a vasodilator and smooth muscle relaxant, $C_{19}H_{26}N_2O_5S \cdot HCl$.

mesuranic (mes″u-ran′ik) [meso- + Gr. ouranos palate] having a maxilloalveolar index between 110.0 and 114.9.

mesylate (mes′ǐ-lāt) USAN contraction for methanesulfonate.

Met methionine.

met (met) a unit of measurement of heat production by the body: the metabolic heat produced by a resting-sitting subject, being 50 kilogram calories per square meter of body surface per hour.

meta- [Gr. meta after, beyond, over] a prefix indicating (1) change, transformation, or exchange; (2) after or next; (3) the 1,3 position in derivatives of benzene.

meta-arthritic (met″ah-ar-thrit′ik) occurring as a consequence or result of arthritis.

metabasis (mě-tab′ah-sis) [meta- + Gr. bainein to go] 1. a change in the manifestations or course of a disease. 2. metastasis, or change in the site of a morbid process from one region of the body to another.

metabiosis (met″ah-bi-o′sis) [meta- + Gr. biōsis way of life] the dependence of one organism upon another for its existence; commensalism.

metabolic (met″ah-bol′ik) pertaining to or of the nature of metabolism.

metabolimeter (met″ah-bo-lim′ě-ter) [metabolism + Gr. metron measure] an apparatus for measuring basal metabolism.

metabolimetry (met″ah-bo-lim′ě-tre) the measurement of basal metabolism.

metabolism (mě-tab′o-lizm) [Gr. metaballein to turn about, change, alter] the sum of all the physical and chemical processes by which living organized substance is produced and maintained (anabolism), and also the transformation by which energy is made available for the uses of the organism (catabolism). **ammonotelic m.,** that in which ammonia is the final product of nitrogen metabolism. **basal m.,** the minimal energy expended for the maintenance of respiration, circulation, peristalsis, muscle tonus, body temperature, glandular activity, and the other vegetative functions of the body. The rate of basal metabolism (basal metabolic rate) is measured by means of a calorimeter, in a subject at absolute rest, 14 to 18 hours after eating, and is expressed in calories per hour per square meter of body surface.

endogenous m., metabolism of the proteins of the body tissues. **energy m.,** the metabolic processes by which energy is released. **excess m. of exercise,** the amount by which the oxygen consumed or the carbon dioxide eliminated during exercise and recovery exceeds the corresponding amounts during sleep. **exogenous m.,** metabolism of ingested foodstuffs. **inborn error of m.,** a genetically determined biochemical disorder in which a specific enzyme defect produces a metabolic block that may have pathologic consequences at birth (e.g., phenylketonuria) or in later life (e.g., diabetes mellitus); called also enzymopathy and genetotrophic disease. **intermediary m.,** the various chemical reactions involved in the transformation of food molecules into essential cellular building blocks. **ureotelic m.,** that in which urea is the final product of nitrogen metabolism. **uricotelic m.,** that in which uric acid is the final product of nitrogen metabolism.

metabolite (mě-tab′o-līt) any substance produced by metabolism or by a metabolic process. **essential m.,** a necessary constituent of normal metabolic processes.

metabolizable (mě-tab′o-liz″ah-b′l) capable of being transformed by metabolism.

metabolon (mě-tab′o-lon) a form of matter having only a temporary existence, formed during the conversion of one material to another, as during radioactive decay.

metabromsalan (met″ah-brom′sah-lan) chemical name: 3,5-dibromo-2-hydroxy-N-phenylbenzamide. A disinfectant with antibacterial and antifungal activities, $C_{13}H_9Br_2NO_2$, used mainly in medicated soaps.

metabutethamine hydrochloride (met″ah-bu-teth′ah-min) chemical name: 2-[(2-methylpropyl)amino]ethanol 3-aminobenzoate(ester) monohydrochloride. A local anesthetic, $C_{13}H_{21}ClN_2O_2 \cdot HCl$, occurring as a white crystalline solid; used in dentistry to produce infiltration and nerve block anesthesia.

metabutoxycaine hydrochloride (met″ah-bu-tok′se-kān) chemical name: 3-amino-2-butoxybenzoic acid 2-diethylaminoethyl ester hydrochloride. A local anesthetic, $C_{17}H_{28}N_2O_3 \cdot HCl$, used in dentistry.

metacarpal (met″ah-kar′pal) 1. pertaining to the metacarpus. 2. a bone of the metacarpus.

metacarpectomy (met″ah-kar-pek′to-me) excision or resection of a metacarpal bone.

metacarpophalangeal (met″ah-kar″po-fah-lan′je-al) pertaining to the metacarpus and phalanges.

metacarpus (met″ah-kar′pus) [meta- + Gr. karpos wrist] [NA] the part of the hand between the wrist and the fingers, its skeleton being five cylindric bones (metacarpals) extending from the carpus to the phalanges.

metacele (met′ah-sēl) metacoele.

metacentric (met″ah-sen′trik) having the centromere near the middle, so that the arms of the replicating chromosome are approximately equal in length. Cf. acrocentric and submetacentric.

metacercaria (met″ah-ser-ka′re-ah), pl. metacerca′riae. The encysted resting or maturing stage of a trematode parasite in the tissues of an intermediate host (mollusks, aquatic arthropods, fishes, or amphibia) or on vegetation. The metacercaria may be the infective or transfer stage to man and other animals.

metacercariae (met″ah-ser-ka′re-e) plural of metacercaria.

metachemical (met″ah-kem′ĭ-kal) beyond the bounds of chemistry.

metachromasia (met″ah-kro-ma′ze-ah) [meta- + Gr. chrōma color] 1. a condition in which tissues do not stain true with a given stain. 2. staining in which the same stain colors different tissues in different tints. 3. the change of color produced by staining.

metachromatic (met″ah-kro-mat′ik) [meta- + Gr. chrōmatikos relating to color] staining differently with the same dye; said of tissues in which different elements take on different colors when a certain dye is applied. By extension, said of dyes by which different tissues are stained differently.

metachromatin (met″ah-kro′mah-tin) the basophil element in chromatin.

metachromatism (met″ah-kro′mah-tizm.) metachromasia.

metachromatophil (met″ah-kro-mat′o-fil) a cell that does not stain in the usual manner with a given stain.

metachromia (met″ah-kro′me-ah) metachromasia.

metachromic (met″ah-kro′mik) metachromatic.

metachromophil (met-ah-kro′mo-fil) [meta- + Gr. chrōma color + philein to love] staining in an abnormal manner with a given stain.

metachromophile (met″ah-kro′mo-fīl) metachromophil.

metachromosome (met″ah-kro′mo-sōm) one of two small chromosomes which conjugate only in the last phase of the spermatocyte division.

metachronous (mě-tak′ro-nus) [meta- + Gr. chronos time] occurring at different times.

metachrosis (met″ah-kro′sis) [meta- + Gr. chrōsis coloring] change of color in animals.

metachysis (mĕ-tak′ĭ-sis) [meta- + Gr. chysis effusion] the transfusion of blood.

metacinesis (met″ah-si-ne′sis) [meta- + Gr. kinēsis motion] the separation of daughter stars (asters) from each other in mitosis.

metacoele (met′ah-sēl) [meta- + Gr. koilia hollow] 1. (obs.) that cavity of the metencephalon which, with the epicoele, makes up the fourth ventricle. 2. metacoeloma.

metacoeloma (met″ah-se-lo′mah) that part of the embryonic coelom which develops into the pleuroperitoneal cavity.

metacone (met′ah-kōn) [meta- + Gr. kōnos cone] the distobuccal cusp of an upper molar tooth.

metaconid (met″ah-kon′id) the mesiolingual cusp of a lower molar tooth.

metaconule (met″ah-kon′ūl) the distal intermediate cusp of an upper molar tooth in lower animals.

metacortandracin (met″ah-kor-tan′drah-sin) prednisone.

metacortandralone (met″ah-kor-tan′drah-lōn) prednisolone.

metacresol (met″ah-kre′sol) one of the three isomeric forms of cresol, and the most strongly antiseptic of the group. **m. acetate,** a compound that has been used in fungus infections. **m. purple, m. sulfonphthalein,** a triphenylmethane compound which is a brilliant indicator, being red at pH 1.2, blue at pH 2.8, yellow at pH 7.4, and purple at pH 9.0.

metacyesis (met″ah-si-e′sis) [meta- + Gr. kyēsis pregnancy] extrauterine pregnancy.

metaduodenum (met″ah-du″o-de′num) the portion of the duodenum distal to the duodenal papilla, developed embryonically from the midgut.

metagaster (met″ah-gas′ter) [meta- + Gr. gastēr belly] the permanent intestinal canal of the embryo.

metagastrula (met″ah-gas′troo-lah) [meta- + gastrula] a gastrula with a cleavage differing from that of the standard type.

metagelatin (met″ah-jel′ah-tin) a substance produced by treating gelatin with oxalic acid.

metagenesis (met″ah-jen′ĕ-sis) [meta- + genesis] alternation of generations; alternation in regular sequence of asexual with sexual methods of reproduction in the same species, as in certain fungi.

metagglutinin (met″ah-gloo′tĭ-nin) partial agglutinin.

metaglobulin (met″ah-glob′u-lin) a fibrogenous substance occurring in cell protoplasm; fibrinogen.

metagonimiasis (met″ah-go″nĭ-mi′ah-sis) infection with Metagonimus.

Metagonimus (met″ah-gon′ĭ-mus) [meta- + Gr. gonimos productive] a genus of trematodes. **M. ova′tus,** M. yokogawai. **M. yokoga′wai,** an intestinal trematode found in the small intestine of man and mammals in Japan, China, Indonesia, Balkans, and Israel.

metagrippal (met″ah-grip′al) occurring as a result of influenza (grippe).

metahemoglobin (met″ah-he″mo-glo′bin) methemoglobin.

metaherpes (met″ah-her′pēz) metaherpetic keratitis.

Metahydrin (met″ah-hi′drin) trademark for a preparation of trichlormethiazide.

metaicteric (met″ah-ik-ter′ik) occurring after jaundice.

metainfective (met″ah-in-fek′tiv) occurring after an infection; a term applied to a febrile state occurring during convalescence from an infectious disease.

metakinesis (met″ah-ki-ne′sis) 1. metacinesis. 2. Lloyd Morgan's term for the hypothetical property possessed by all types of life of being endowed with something which is not consciousness, but which has the potentiality of developing into consciousness. 3. metaphase.

metal (met′l) [L. metallum; Gr. metallon] any element marked by luster, malleability, ductility, and conductivity of electricity and heat and which will ionize positively in solution. **alkali m.,** one of a group of monovalent metals including lithium, sodium, potassium, rubidium, and cesium. **alkaline earth m's,** a group of grayish white, malleable metals that are easily oxidized in air, comprising beryllium, magnesium, calcium, strontium, barium, and radium. **Babbitt m.,** an alloy of tin, copper, and antimony; sometimes used in dentistry. **bell m.,** an alloy of copper and tin. **colloidal m.,** a colloidal solution of a metal; see electrosol. **fusible m.,** an alloy that melts at a relatively low temperature, as at or around the boiling point of water. Bismuth, lead, and tin are usually the principal constituents. **Melotte's m.,** a rather soft alloy consisting of bismuth, lead, and tin, sometimes used in dentistry; called also Newton's alloy. **Wood's m.,** a metal used in making casts of blood vessels: bismuth, 50 per cent; lead, 25 per cent; tin, 12.5 per cent; cadmium, 12.5 per cent.

metalbumin (met-al-bu′min) [meta- + albumin] pseudomucin.

metaldehyde (met-al′de-hīd) a crystalline body, a polymer of acetaldehyde, $(CH_3 \cdot CHO)_3$, formerly used as an antiseptic.

metallaxis (met″ah-lak′sis) [Gr. "exchange," "interchange"] the

transformation or building over of an organ by pathologic processes.

metallergy (met-al′er-je) a condition in which an allergic state, produced by specific sensitization, predisposes the organism to react to other antigens with the same clinical manifestations as the original reaction.

metallesthesia (met″al-es-the′ze-ah) [metal + Gr. aisthēsis perception + -ia] the recognition of metals by the sense of touch.

metallic (me-tal′ik) pertaining to or made of metal.

metallization (met″l-i-za′shun) impregnation with metals.

metallized (met″l-īzd) treated with metals.

metallocyanide (me-tal″o-si′ah-nīd) a compound of cyanogen with a metal.

metalloenzyme (mĕ-tal″o-en′zīm) an enzyme containing tightly bound metal atoms as an integral part of its structure, e.g., carboxypeptidase and the cytochromes.

metalloflavoprotein (mĕ-tal″o-fla″vo-pro′te-in) any metalloprotein, e.g., xanthine oxidase, that functions as a dehydrogenase, catalyzing the oxidation of a substrate by a mechanism that involves the reduction of a prosthetic group, a derivative of riboflavin.

metalloid (met′l-oid) [metal + Gr. eidos form] 1. any element with both metallic and nonmetallic properties, as silicon, boron, or arsenic. 2. any metallic element that has not all the characters of a typical metal. 3. resembling a metal.

metallophilic (mĕ-tal″o-fil′ik) having an affinity for metal-containing stains; said of cells.

metalloplastic (me-tal″o-plas′tik) pertaining to the plastic use of metals.

metalloporphyrin (me-tal″o-por′fĭ-rin) a combination of a metal with porphyrin, e.g., heme (iron) and turacin (copper).

metalloscopy (met″l-os′ko-pe) [metal + Gr. skopein to examine] observation of the effects of applying metal to the body.

metallotherapy (me-tal″o-ther′ah-pe) [metal + Gr. therapeuein to heal] the treatment of disease by applying metals to the skin.

metallurgy (met′l-ur″je) [metal + Gr. ergon work] the science and art of using metals.

metal-sol (met′l-sol″) a colloidal solution of a metal.

metamer (met′ah-mer) a compound exhibiting, or capable of exhibiting, metamerism.

metamere (met′ah-mēr) [meta- + Gr. meros part] one of a series of homologous segments of the body of an animal. In genetic theory, one of a varying number of common repeating units that make up the repressor segment of a chromosomal locus, the actual number of metameres in a given locus being proportional to the degree of repression of the trait in question.

metameric (met″ah-mer′ik) pertaining to or characterized by metamerism.

metamerism (me-tam′er-ism) 1. a type of structural isomerism in which different radicals of the same chemical type are attached to the same polyvalent element and yet give rise to compounds possessing identical molecular formulas. For example, diethylamine, $(C_2H_5)_2NH$, and methyl propylamine, $CH_3NHC_3H_7$. The term metamerism is seldom used, such compounds being called simply structural isomers of the same chemical type. 2. arrangement into metameres by the serial repetition of a structural pattern. Cf. antimere.

Metamine (met′ah-mēn) trademark for preparations of trolnitrate phosphate.

metamorphopsia (met″ah-mor-fop′se-ah) [meta- + Gr. morphē form + opsis sight] a disturbance of vision in which objects are seen as distorted in shape. **m. va′rians,** metamorphopsia in which the outline of the object seems to change as it is being viewed.

metamorphosis (met″ah-mor′fo-sis) [meta- + Gr. morphōsis a shaping, bringing into shape] change of shape or structure, particularly a transition from one developmental stage to another, as from larva to adult form. **fatty m.,** any normal or pathologic transformation of fat, including fatty infiltration and fatty degeneration. **ovulational m.,** the developmental changes which occur during ovulation. **platelet m.,** viscous m. **retrograde m., retrogressive m.,** degeneration; more often a retrograde metabolic change. **revisionary m.,** cataplasia. **structural m.,** viscous m. **tissue m.,** any change in tissues, either normal or pathologic. **viscous m.,** the progressive and irreversible aggregation and fusion of blood platelets during the process of coagulation; called also structural m. and platelet m.

metamorphotic (met″ah-mor-fot′ik) pertaining to or characterized by metamorphosis.

Metamucil (met″ah-mu′sil) trademark for a preparation of psyllium hydrophilic mucilloid.

metamyelocyte (met″ah-mi′ĕ-lo-sīt″) a precursor in the granulocytic series, being a cell intermediate in development between a promyelocyte and the mature, segmented (polymorphonuclear), granular leukocyte, and having an indented (juvenile) nucleus. Called also juvenile cell or form, and young form.

Metandren (mĕ-tan′dren) trademark for preparations of methyltestosterone.

metanephric (met″ah-nef′rik) of or pertaining to the metanephros.

metanephrine (met″ah-nef′rin) chemical name: α-(methylaminomethyl vanillyl alcohol(3-methylepinephrine): a metabolite of epinephrine excreted in the urine and found in certain tissues.

metanephrogenic (met″ah-nef″ro-jen′ik) [*meta-* + Gr. *nephros* kidney + *gennan* to produce] capable of giving rise to the metanephros.

metanephroi (met″ah-nef′roi) plural of *metanephros.*

metanephron (met″ah-nef′ron) metanephros.

metanephros (met″ah-nef′ros), pl. *metaneph′roi* [*meta-* + Gr. *nephros*, kidney] the permanent embryonic kidney, which develops later than and caudal to the mesonephros, from the mesonephric duct and nephrogenic cord.

metaneutrophil (met″ah-nu′tro-fil) [*meta-* + *neutrophil*] staining abnormally with neutral stains.

metanucleus (met″ah-nu′kle-us) [*meta-* + *nucleus*] the egg nucleus during the maturative period.

metapeptone (met″ah-pep′tōn) [*meta-* + *peptone*] a digestive product between dyspeptone and parapeptone.

metaphase (met′ah-fāz) [*meta-* + *phase*] the second stage of cell division (mitosis or meiosis), during which the contracted chromosomes, each consisting of two chromatids, are arranged in the equatorial plane of the spindle prior to separation. See *meiosis* and *mitosis.*

Metaphedrin (met″ah-fed′rin) trademark for a preparation of nitromersol and ephedrine.

Metaphen (met′ah-fen) trademark for preparations of nitromersol.

metaphrenia (met″ah-fre′ne-ah) [*meta-* + Gr. *phrēn* mind] a term introduced by Staercke for the mental condition in which the interests are withdrawn from the family or group and directed to personal gain or aggrandisement.

metaphrenon (met″ah-fre′non) [Gr. "the part behind the midriff"] (*obs.*) the back, especially the region about the kidneys.

metaphyseal (met″ah-fiz′e-al) pertaining to or of the nature of a metaphysis.

metaphyses (me-taf′ĭ-sēz) plural of *metaphysis.*

metaphysial (met″ah-fiz′e-al) metaphyseal.

metaphysis (me-taf′ĭ-sis), pl. *metaph′yses* [*meta-* + Gr. *phyein* to grow] the wider part at the extremity of the shaft of a long bone, adjacent to the epiphyseal disk. During development it contains the growth zone and consists of spongy bone; in the adult it is continuous with the epiphysis.

metaphysitis (met″ah-fis-i′tis) inflammation of the metaphysis of a long bone.

metaplasia (met″ah-pla′ze-ah) [*meta-* + Gr. *plassein* to form] the change in the type of adult cells in a tissue to a form which is not normal for that tissue. **myeloid m.,** the occurrence of myeloid tissue in extramedullary sites; specifically, a syndrome characterized by splenomegaly, anemia, the presence of nucleated erythrocytes and immature granulocytes in the circulating blood, and extramedullary hematopoiesis in the liver and spleen. The primary form is also known as *agnogenic myeloid metaplasia, myelosclerosis,* and *myelofibrosis.* The secondary or symptomatic form may be associated with various diseases, including carcinomatosis, tuberculosis, leukemia, and polycythemia vera. **myeloid m., agnogenic,** a condition characterized by foci of extramedullary hematopoiesis, splenomegaly, immature red and white cells in the peripheral blood, and mild to moderate anemia; it is grouped by some hematologists with the myeloproliferative disorders. Called also *aleukemic* or *nonleukemic myelosis,* and *leukoerythroblastic anemia.* **pseudopyloric m.,** gastric metaplasia in which the gastric glands disappear and are replaced by tubules that closely resemble normal pyloric glands. **m. of pulp,** a state of the pulp tissue of a tooth in which it has deteriorated from its power of dentin formation to the condition of connective tissue. **squamous m.,** the transformation of pseudostratified ciliated epithelium into stratified squamous epithelium, as occurs in certain pathologic conditions or may be produced experimentally.

metaplasis (mĕ-tap′lah-sis) the stage in which the organism has attained completed growth.

metaplasm (met′ah-plazm) [*meta-* + Gr. *plasma* something formed] deuteroplasm.

metaplastic (met″ah-plas′tik) 1. pertaining to or characterized by metaplasia. 2. formed by or of the nature of metaplasm (deutoplasm).

metaplexus (met″ah-plek′sus) (*obs.*) the choroid plexus of the fourth ventricle of the brain.

metapneumonic (met″ah-nu-mon′ik) [*meta-* + *pneumonia*] succeeding or following pneumonia.

metapodialia (met″ah-po′de-a′le-ah) [*meta-* + Gr. *pous* foot] a collective term for the bones of the metacarpus and metatarsus.

metapophysis (met″ah-pof′ĭ-sis) [*meta-* + *apophysis*] the mamillary process on the superior articular or prearticular processes of certain vertebrae.

metapore (met′ah-pōr) (*obs.*) apertura mediana ventriculi quarti.

Metaprel (met′ah-prel) trademark for preparations of metaproterenol sulfate.

metaproterenol sulfate (met″ah-pro-ter′ĕ-nōl) chemical name: 5-[1-hydroxy-2-[(1-methylethyl)amino]ethyl]-1,3-benzenediol sulfate (2:1) salt. A β-adrenergic, $(C_{11}H_{17}NO_3)_2H_2 \cdot SO_4$, similar in chemical structure to isoproterenol but having longer lasting effects; used as a bronchodilator in the treatment of bronchial asthma and for reversible bronchospasm associated with bronchitis and emphysema, administered orally and by inhalation.

metapsyche (met″ah-si′ke) [*meta-* + Gr. *psychē* soul] (*obs.*) the metencephalon.

metapsychics (met″ah-si′kiks) [*meta-* + Gr. *psychē* soul] the science which deals with psychic phenomena that are beyond the realm of consciousness; parapsychology.

metapsychology (met″ah-si-kol′o-je) a term applied to various philosophical theories about mental functions and mental "structures" which are justifiable on logical grounds but not verifiable by experiment or observation; in psychoanalysis such theories concern the topography (id, ego, superego) and economics (quantities of psychic energy or excitation) of mental processes.

metapyrone (met-ah-pi′rōn) metyrapone.

metaraminol (met″ah-ram′ĭ-nol) [USP] chemical name: α-(1-aminoethyl)-3-hydroxybenzenemethanol[R-(R*,R*)]-2,3-dihydroxybutanedioate (1:1) (salt). An adrenergic with potent vasopressor activity, $C_9H_{13}NO_2 \cdot C_4H_6O_6$; used especially for the prevention and treatment of acute hypotensive states occurring with spinal anesthesia and for adjunctive therapy of hypotension due to hemorrhage, reactions to medications, surgical complication, and shock associated with brain damage due to trauma or tumor, administered intramuscularly and intravenously.

metarchon (met-ar′kon) an agent which, without being toxic, so changes the behavior of a pest that its persistence is diminished, e.g., a confusing sex attractant.

metargon (met-ar′gon) a name given an isotope of argon, atomic weight 38.

metarhodopsin (met″ah-ro-dop′sin) an intermediate compound that is formed as rhodopsin absorbs light and eventually dissociates to opsin and *trans*-retinal; see *retinal,* def. 2.

metarteriole (met″ar-te′re-ōl) an arterial capillary.

metarubricyte (met″ah-roo′brĭ-sīt) orthochromatic normoblast.

metasomatome (met″ah-so′mah-tōm) one of the constrictions between successive protovertebrae.

metastable (met′ah-sta″b'l) 1. a condition differing from stable in that, although the substance is stable in small perturbations, it can be transformed to a more stable condition by relatively large perturbations. 2. subject to inevitable change or destruction eventually, but apparently stable owing to slowness of change.

metastasectomy (mĕ-tas″tah-sek′to-me) surgical excision of metastases.

metastases (mĕ-tas′tah-sēz) plural of *metastasis* (def. 2).

metastasis (mĕ-tas′tah-sis) [*meta-* + Gr. *stasis* stand] 1. the transfer of disease from one organ or part to another not directly connected with it. It may be due either to the transfer of pathogenic microorganisms (e.g., tubercle bacilli) or to transfer of cells, as in malignant tumors. The capacity to metastasize is a characteristic of all malignant tumors. 2. Pl. *metastases.* A growth of pathogenic microorganisms or of abnormal cells distant from the site primarily involved by the morbid process. **biochemical m.,** the transportation from the point of production and the deposition in previously normal tissues of abnormal or pathologically produced biochemical substances which bring about immunological or other changes in the tissues. **calcareous m.,** the formation of bone salts in the kidneys and elsewhere in softening of bone. **contact m.,** transfer from one surface to another with which the former is in contact. **crossed m.,** passage of material from the venous to the arterial circulation without going through the lungs. **direct m.,** metastasis in the direction of the blood or lymph stream. **implantation m.,** metastasis brought about by transfer of tumor cells by fluid and their implantation in a distant location. **paradoxical m., retrograde m.,** metastasis taking place in a direction opposite to that of the blood stream. **transplantation m.,** metastasis from one tissue to another.

metastasize (me-tas′tah-sīz) to form new foci of disease in a distant part by metastasis.

metastatic (met″ah-stat′ik) pertaining to or of the nature of metastasis.

metasternum (met″ah-ster′num) [*meta-* + Gr. *sternon* sternum] processus xiphoideus.

Metastrongylidae (met″ah-stron-jil′e-de) a family of nematodes of the superfamily Strongyloidea, comprising the lungworms; it includes the genera *Metastrongylus* and *Angiostrongylus*.

Metastrongylus (met″ah-stron′jĭ-lus) a genus of parasitic nematodes of the family Metastrongylidae. *M. elonga′tus,* a species found in the lungs of hogs, is a host of the swine influenza virus.

metasynapsis (met″ah-sĭ-nap′sis) end-to-end union of the chromosomes in synapsis.

metasyncrisis (met″ah-sin′krĭ-sis) the elimination of waste or morbid matter.

metasyndesis (met″ah-sin-de′sis) metasynapsis.

metasyphilis (met″ah-sif′ĭ-lis) [*meta-* + *syphilis*] 1. congenital syphilis with general degeneration but without syphilids. 2. parasyphilis.

metasyphilitic (met″ah-sif″ĭ-lit′ik) 1. following or resulting from syphilis. 2. pertaining to hereditary syphilis.

metatarsal (met″ah-tar′sal) 1. pertaining to the metatarsus. 2. a bone of the metatarsus.

metatarsalgia (met″ah-tar-sal′je-ah) [*meta-* + Gr. *tarsos* tarsus + *-algia*] pain and tenderness in the metatarsal region.

metatarsectomy (met″ah-tar-sek′to-me) excision or resection of the metatarsus.

metatarsophalangeal (met″ah-tar″so-fah-lan′je-al) pertaining to the metatarsus and the phalanges of the toes.

metatarsus (met″ah-tar′sus) [*meta-* + Gr. *tarsos* tarsus] [NA] the part of the foot between the tarsus and the toes, its skeleton being the five long bones (the metatarsals) extending from the tarsus to the phalanges. **m. adductoca′vus,** a deformity of the foot in which metatarsus adductus is associated with pes cavus. **m. adductova′rus,** a deformity of the foot in which metatarsus adductus is associated with metatarsus varus. **m. adduc′tus,** a congenital deformity of the foot in which the fore part of the foot deviates toward the midline. **m. atav′icus,** abnormal shortness of the first metatarsal bone. **m. brev′is,** a condition in which the first metatarsal bone is shorter than normal and often abducted. **m. la′tus,** a broadened foot due to spreading of the anterior part of the foot resulting from separation of the heads of the metatarsal bones from each other; called also *broad foot* and *spread foot.* **m. pri′mus va′rus,** angulation of the first metatarsal bone toward the midline of the body, producing an angle sometimes of 20 degrees or more between its base and that of the second metatarsal bone. **m. va′rus,** a congenital deformity of the foot in which its inner border is off the ground with the sole turned inward, the patient walking on the outer border of the foot.

metathalamus (met″ah-thal′ah-mus) [NA] the part of the diencephalon composed of the medial and lateral geniculate bodies; often considered to be part of the thalamus.

Metatheria (met″ah-the′rĭ-ah) [*meta-* + Gr. *thērion* beast, animal] in some systems of classification, a subclass of the Mammalia and in others an infraclass of the subclass Theria, including the pouched mammals or marsupials.

metatherian (met″ah-the′ri-an) any member of the Metatheria.

metathesis (mĕ-tath′ĕ-sis) [*meta-* + Gr. *thesis* placement] 1. the artificial transfer of a morbid process. 2. a chemical reaction in which an element or radical in one compound exchanges places with another element or radical in another compound.

metathetic (met″ah-thet′ik) pertaining to or of the nature of metathesis.

metathrombin (met″ah-throm′bin) [*meta-* + *thrombin*] the inactive combination of thrombin and antithrombin.

metatroph (met′ah-trōf) a metatrophic organism.

metatrophia (met-ah-tro′fe-ah) 1. atrophy from malnutrition. 2. a change in diet.

metatrophic (met-ah-trof′ik) utilizing organic matter for food. Cf. *paratrophic.*

metatrophy (met-at′ro-fe) [*meta-* + Gr. *trophē* nutrition] 1. the state of being metatrophic; metatrophic nutrition. 2. metatrophia.

metatypic (met″ah-tip′ik) metatypical.

metatypical (met″ah-tip′e-kal) composed of the elements of the tissue on which it develops, but having those elements arranged in an atypical manner; said of tumors.

metavanadate (met″ah-van′ah-dāt) any salt of vanadic acid. **sodium m.,** a highly poisonous salt, $NaVO_3 \cdot 4H_2O$.

metaxalone (mĕ-taks′ah-lōn) chemical name: 5-[(3,5-dimethylphenoxy)methyl]-2-oxazolidinone. A smooth muscle relaxant, $C_{12}H_{15}NO_3$, used in the treatment of painful musculoskeletal conditions, administered orally.

metaxenia (met″ah-ze′ne-ah) an improper term for ectogony.

metaxeny (me-tak′sĕ-ne) metoxeny.

Metazoa (met″ah-zo′ah) [*meta-* + Gr. *zōon* animal] that division of the animal kingdom which embraces all multicellular animals whose cells become differentiated to form tissues. It includes all animals except Protozoa.

metazoa (met″ah-zo′ah) plural of *metazoon.*

metazoal (met″ah-zo′al) 1. belonging to the Metazoa. 2. pertaining to or caused by metazoa.

metazoan (met″ah-zo′an) 1. pertaining to metazoa; metazoal. 2. a metazoon.

metazonal (met″ah-zo′nal) situated after or below a sclerozone.

metazoon (met″ah-zo′on), pl. *metazo′a.* An individual of the Metazoa.

Metchnikoff's law, theory (mech′nĭ-kof) [Elie *Metchnikoff* (Ilia Ilich *Mechnikov*), a Russian zoologist in Paris, 1845–1916; discoverer of phagocytes and phagocytosis, co-winner, with Paul Ehrlich, of the Nobel prize for medicine and physiology in 1908] see under *law* and *theory.*

metecious (me-te′shus) [*meta-* + Gr. *oikos* house] heterecious.

metencephal (met-en′se-fal) the metencephalon.

metencephalic (met-en″sĕ-fal′ik) pertaining to the metencephalon.

metencephalon (met″en-sef′ah-lon) [*meta-* + Gr. *enkephalos* brain] 1. [NA] the anterior portion of the rhombencephalon, comprising the cerebellum and the pons; see Plate accompanying *brain.* 2. the anterior of the two brain vesicles formed by specialization of the rhombencephalon in the developing embryo. Called also *afterbrain* and *epencephalon.*

metencephalospinal (met″en-sef″ah-lo-spi′nal) pertaining to the metencephalon (cerebellum) and the spinal cord.

meteorism (me′te-ŏ-rizm″) [Gr. *meteōrizein* to raise up] tympanites; the presence of gas in the abdomen or intestine.

meteorology (me′te-o-rol′o-je) [Gr. *meteōros* high in the air + *-logy*] the science of the atmosphere and its phenomena; the science of the weather.

meteoropathology (me″te-ĕ-ro-pah-thol′o-je) the pathology of conditions caused by atmospheric conditions.

meteoropathy (me″te-ĕ-rop′ah-the) [Gr. *meteōros* high in the air + *pathos* disease] any disorder due to conditions of climate.

meteororesistant (me″te-ĕ-ro-re-zis′tant) comparatively insensitive to weather conditions.

meteorosensitive (me″te-ĕ-ro-sen′si-tiv) abnormally sensitive to weather conditions.

meteorotropic (me″te-ĕ-ro-trop′ik) responding to influence by meteorological factors; pertaining to or characterized by meteorotropism.

meteorotropism (me″te-ĕ-rot′ro-pizm) the response to influence by meteorological factors noted in certain biological events, such as sudden death, attacks of angina, joint pain, insomnia, and traffic accidents.

metepencephalon (met″ep-en-sef′ah-lon) [*meta-* + *epi-* + Gr. *enkephalos* brain] myelencephalon.

meter (me′ter) [Gr. *metron* measure; Fr. *mètre*] 1. the basic unit of linear measure in the metric system, approximately equivalent to 39.37 inches; formerly established as the length of a bar of an alloy of platinum and iridium preserved in a vault at the International Bureau of Weights and Measures, near Paris. Although its dimension is unchanged, it is now defined in terms of the wavelength of a certain line in the spectrum of krypton. Abbreviated m. 2. an apparatus devised to measure the quantity of anything passing through it, such as of a gas, amperes of electric current, etc. **dosage m.,** dosimeter. **flicker m.,** flicker photometer. **light m.,** an instrument for measuring light in foot candles. **peak flow m.,** an instrument for measuring the flow of air in the early part of forced expiration. **rate m.,** a radiation detector whose output is proportional to instantaneous radiation intensity (rate of radioactive emissions).

-meter [Gr. *metron* measure] a word termination designating relationship to measurement, or denoting especially an instrument used in measuring.

metergasis (met″er-ga′sis) [*meta-* + Gr. *ergon* work] change of function.

metestrum (mĕ-tes′trum) metestrus.

metestrus (mĕ-tes′trus) [*meta-* + L. *oestrus*] the period of subsiding follicular function or rest following estrus in female mammals.

metformin (met-for′min) chemical name: 1,1-dimethylbiguanide; an oral hypoglycemic, $C_4H_{11}N_5$.

methacholine (meth″ah-ko′lēn) chemical name: 2-(acetyloxy)-*N,N,N*-trimethyl-1-propanaminium. A powerful cholinergic, $C_8H_{18}NO_2$, with actions similar to those of acetylcholine. **m. bromide,** the bromide salt of methacholine, $C_8H_{18}BrNO_2$, occurring as a white, crystalline powder, having actions and uses similar to those of the chloride salt; administered orally. **m. chloride** [USP], the chloride salt of methacholine, $C_8H_{18}ClNO_2$, occurring as colorless or white crystals or as a white, crystalline powder; used as a cholinergic, especially in the treatment of Raynaud's disease, scleroderma, vascular spasm due to cold, and chronic varicose ulcers, administered orally, subcutaneously, and by iontophoresis. Called also *acetyl-betamethylcholine chloride.*

methacrylate (meth-ak′rĭ-lāt″) an acrylic resin widely used in denture bases and as an adhesive for joint prostheses; see also *methyl methacrylate.*

methacycline (meth″ah-si′klēn) chemical name: 4 S-dimethylamino-1,4α,4aα,5α,5aα,6,11,12aα-octahydro-3,5,10,12,12a-pentahydroxy-6-methylene-1,11-dioxo-2-naphthacencarboxamide. A semisynthetic broad-spectrum antibiotic of the tetracycline group, $C_{22}H_{22}N_2O_8$, derived from oxytetracycline. **m. hydrochloride** [USP], the monohydrochloride salt of methacycline, $C_{22}H_{22}$-$N_2O_8 \cdot HCl$, occurring as a yellow to dark yellow crystalline powder; used as an antibacterial, administered orally.

methadone hydrochloride (meth′ah-don) [USP] chemical name: 6-(dimethylamino)-4,4-diphenyl-3-hepanone hydrochloride. A synthetic narcotic, $C_{21}H_{27}NO \cdot HCl$, occurring as colorless crystals or white, crystalline powder, possessing pharmacologic actions similar to those of morphine and heroin and almost equal addiction liability; used as an analgesic and as a narcotic abstinence syndrome suppressant in the treatment of heroin addiction (see also *narcotic blockade*, under *blockade*), administered orally, intramuscularly, and subcutaneously.

methadyl acetate (meth′ah-dil) chemical name: β-[2-(dimethylamino)propyl]-α-ethyl-β-phenylbenzeneethanol; a narcotic analgesic, $C_{23}H_{31}NO_2$. Called also *acetylmethadol*.

methallenestril (meth″al-ĕ-nes′tril) chemical name: β-ethyl-6-methoxy-α,α-dimethyl-2-naphthalenepropionic acid. A synthetic, nonsteroidal, orally effective, estrogenic drug, $C_{18}H_{22}O_3$, occurring as a white, crystalline powder, having uses similar to those of estrogen (q.v.).

methallibure (meth-al′ĭ-būr) chemical name: 1-methyl-6-(1-methylallyl)-2,5-dithiobiurea. A substance, $C_7H_{14}N_4S_2$, used as an anterior pituitary activator in swine.

methamphetamine (meth″am-fet′ah-mēn) chemical name: (S)-N,α-dimethylbenzeneethanamine. A sympathomimetic amine of the amphetamine group, $C_{10}H_{15}N$. Abuse of this drug may lead to dependence; see *amphetamine*, def. 1. **m. hydrochloride,** white crystals or white, crystalline powder, $C_{10}H_{15}N \cdot HCl$, used chiefly for its central stimulant effects in the treatment of mental depression, psychopathic states, narcolepsy, and exogenous obesity, and for its calming effects in hyperkinetic children. It also has pressor effects and is used in various hypotension states, especially in regional and spinal anesthesia and after ganglionic blockade.

methandriol (meth-an′dre-ol) chemical name: 17α-methyl-5-androstene-3β,17β-diol; an anabolic agent.

methandrostenolone (meth-an″dro-sten′o-lōn) [NF] chemical name: 17β-hydroxy-17α-methylandrosta-1,4-dien-3-one. An androgen, $C_{20}H_{28}O_2$, occurring as white to off-white crystals or crystalline powder; used especially in the adjunctive treatment of senile and postmenopausal osteoporosis and in selected cases of pituitary dwarfism, administered orally.

methane (meth′ān) a colorless, odorless, inflammable gas, CH_4, produced by decomposition of organic matter, which may explode when mixed with air or oxygen; it is the first member of a homologous series of saturated hydrocarbons, including butane, ethane, hexane, pentane, and propane. Called also *marsh gas*.

Methanobacterium (meth″ah-no-bak-te′re-um) a genus of microorganisms of the family Spirillaceae, suborder Pseudomonadineae, order Pseudomonadales, made up of long, slightly curved, slender rods with rounded ends, containing deeply staining granules. They are anaerobes that derive energy by reduction of CO_2 to methane. The genus includes four species, *C. flaves′cens, C. ful′vus, C. ochra′ceus,* and *C. vulga′ris.*

Methanococcus (meth″ah-no-kok′kus) a genus of microorganisms of the family Micrococcaceae, order Eubacteriales, made up of gram-variable spherical cells which are chemoheterotrophic and saprophytic; they are strict anaerobes that derive energy from the formation of methane from H_2,CO_2, and formate.

methanogen (meth′ah-no-jen″) an anaerobic microorganism that grows in the presence of carbon dioxide and produces methane gas. Methanogens are found in the stomach of cows, in swamp mud, and other environments in which oxygen is not present.

methanogenic (meth″ah-no-jen′ik) producing methane.

methanol (meth′ah-nol) [USP] a clear, colorless, flammable liquid, CH_3OH, with characteristic odor, miscible with alcohol, ether, and water; used as a solvent.

methanolysis (meth″ah-nol′ĭ-sis) alcoholysis of methyl alcohol.

Methanomonadaceae (meth″ah-no-mo″nah-da′se-e) a family of Schizomycetes (order Pseudomonadales, suborder Pseudomonadineae), found in soil and water, and deriving energy from oxidation of simple carbon compounds. It includes three genera, *Carboxydomonas, Hydrogenomonas,* and *Methanomonas.*

Methanomonas (meth″ah-no-mo′nas) a genus of microorganisms of the family Methanomonadaceae, suborder Pseudomonadineae, order Pseudomonadales, occurring as monotrichous cells obtaining energy from the oxidation of methane to CO_2 and H_2O. The type species is *M. methan′ica.*

methantheline bromide (mĕ-than′thĕ-lēn) [USP] chemical name: N,N-diethyl-N-methyl-2-[(9 H-xanthene-9-ylcarbonyl)oxy]-ethanaminium bromide. A quaternary ammonium anticholinergic, $C_{21}H_{26}BrNO_3$, occurring as a white or nearly white powder; used in conditions requiring inhibition of gastrointestinal and genitourinary motility, in hyperhidrosis, or in control of normal

sweating. *Sterile methantheline* is prepared in conformance with USP specifications.

methapyrilene (meth″ah-pīr′ĭ-lēn) chemical name: N,N-dimethyl-N′-2-pyridinyl-N′-(2-thienylmethyl)-1,2-ethanediamine. An antihistaminic, $C_{14}H_{19}N_3S$, which also has moderate sedative action. **m. fumarate** [USP], the fumarate salt of methapyrilene, $(C_{14}H_{19}N_3S)_2 \cdot 3C_4H_4O_4$, occurring as a white, crystalline powder, having actions and uses similar to those of the hydrochloride salt; administered orally. **m. hydrochloride** [USP], the monohydrochloride salt of methapyrilene, $C_{14}H_{19}N_3S \cdot HCl$, occurring as a white, crystalline powder, having the same actions as the base; used in the treatment of allergic manifestations, nausea and vomiting of pregnancy. and insomnia, administered orally.

methaqualone (mĕ-thah′kwah-lōn) [USP] chemical name: 2-methyl-3-(2-methylphenyl)-4(3 H)-quinazolinone. A hypnotic and sedative, $C_{16}H_{14}N_2O$, occurring as a white, crystalline powder; administered orally. **m. hydrochloride** [USP], the monhydrochloride salt of methaqualone, $C_{16}H_{14}N_2O \cdot HCl$, having the same appearance, actions, uses, and route of administration as the base.

metharbital (mĕ-thar′bĭ-tal) [USP] chemical name: 5,5-diethyl-1-methyl-2,4,6(1 H,3 H,5 H)pyrimidinetrione. A barbital derivative, $C_9H_{14}N_2O_3$, occurring as a white to nearly white, crystalline powder; used as an anticonvulsant for the control of grand mal, petit mal, myoclonic, and mixed types of epileptic seizures, administered orally.

methazolamide (meth″ah-zo′lah-mīd) [USP] chemical name: N-[5-(aminosulfonyl)-3-methyl-1,3,4-thiadiazol-2(3 H)-ylidene]acetamide. A carbonic anhydrase inhibitor, $C_5H_8N_4O_3S_2$, occurring as a white or faintly yellow, crystalline powder; used chiefly to reduce intraocular pressure in the treatment of glaucoma, administered orally.

methdilazine (meth-di′lah-zēn) [USP] chemical name: 10-[(1-methyl-3-pyrrolidinyl)methyl]-10 H-phenothiazine. An antihistaminic, $C_{18}H_{20}N_2S$, occurring as a light tan, crystalline powder; used as an antipruritic in dermatoses of various origins, administered in chewable tablets. **m. hydrochloride** [USP], the monohydrochloride salt of methdilazine, $C_{18}H_{20}N_2S \cdot HCl$, having the same appearance, actions, and uses as the base; administered orally.

methectic (mĕ-thek′tik) [Gr. *methektikos* participating] denoting participation of the various strata of intelligence.

methemalbumin (met″hem-al-bu′min) a brownish pigment formed by the binding of albumin with the ferric complex of protoporphyrins (heme), occurring only when the serum has been depleted of unsaturated haptoglobin; it is indicative of intravascular hemolysis. Formerly called *pseudomethemoglobin.*

methemalbuminemia (met″hem-al-bu″min-e′me-ah) the presence of methemalbumin in the blood.

metheme (met′hēm) heme.

methemoglobin (met-he′mo-glo′bin) a compound formed from hemoglobin by oxidation of the ferrous to the ferric state with essentially ionic bonds. A small amount of methemoglobin is present in the blood normally, but injury or toxic agents convert a larger proportion of hemoglobin into methemoglobin, which does not function reversibly as an oxygen carrier.

methemoglobinemia (met″he-mo-glo″bi-ne′me-ah) [*methemoglobin* + Gr. *haima* blood + *-ia*] the presence of methemoglobin in the blood, resulting in cyanosis. It may be drug-induced or be due to a defect in the enzyme NADH methemoglobin reductase (an autosomal recessive trait) or to an abnormality in hemoglobin M (an autosomal dominant trait).

methemoglobinemic (met″he-mo-glo″bĭ-ne′mik) 1. pertaining to or causing methemoglobinemia. 2. an agent that causes methemoglobinemia.

methemoglobinuria (met″he-mo-glo-bi-nu′re-ah) [*methemoglobin* + Gr. *ouron* urine + *-ia*] the occurrence of methemoglobin in the urine.

methenamine (meth-en′ah-mēn) [USP] chemical name: 1,3,5,7-tetraazatricyclo[3.3.1.1³,⁷]decane. Colorless, lustrous crystals or a white crystalline powder, $C_6H_{12}N_4$, used as a urinary antibacterial, administered orally. **m. hippurate,** a compound of methenamine and hippuric acid, $C_6H_{12}N_4 \cdot C_9H_9NO_3$, used orally as a urinary antibacterial. **m. mandelate** [USP], a salt of methenamine and mandelic acid, $C_{14}H_{20}N_4O_3$, occurring as a white crystalline powder; used orally as a urinary antibacterial.

methenolone (mĕ-then′o-lōn) chemical name: 17β-hydroxy-1α-methyl-5α-androst-1-en-3-one; an anabolic steroid, $C_{20}H_{30}O_2$. **m. acetate,** an ester of methenolone $C_{22}H_{32}O_3$; an anabolic steroid. **m. enanthate,** an ester of methenolone, $C_{27}H_{42}O_3$; an anabolic steroid.

Methergine (meth′er-jin) trademark for preparations of methylergonovine maleate.

methestrol diproprionate (meth′es-trol) promethestrol diproprionate.

methetoin (mĕ-thet′o-in) chemical name: 5-ethyl-1-methyl-5-phenyl-2,4-imidazolidinedione; an anticonvulsant, $C_{12}H_{14}N_2O_2$, which has been used in the treatment of epilepsy.

methexenyl (meth-ek′se-nyl) hexobarbital.

methicillin sodium (meth″ĭ-sil″in) [USP] chemical name: 6-(2,6-dimethoxybenzamido)-3,3-dimethyl-7-oxo-4-thia-1-azabicyclo[3.2.0]heptane-2-carboxylic acid sodium salt. A semisynthetic penicillin, $C_{17}H_{19}N_2NaO_6S$, occurring as a fine, white, crystalline powder; used intravenously or intramuscularly as an antibacterial in resistant staphylococcal infections. Called also *dimethoxyphenyl penicillin sodium*.

methilepsia (meth″il-ep′se-ah) methomania.

methimazole (meth-im′ah-zōl) [USP] chemical name: 1,3-dihydro-1-methyl-2H-imidazole-2-thione. A thyroid inhibitor, $C_4H_6N_2S$, occurring as a pale buff, crystalline powder; used in the treatment of hyperthyroidism, administered orally. Called also *thiamazole*.

methiodal sodium (meth-i′o-dal) [USP] chemical name: iodomethanesulfonic acid sodium salt. An iodine containing compound, CH_2INaO_3S, occurring as white, crystalline powder; used as a radiopaque medium in urography, administered intravenously.

methionine (mĕ-thi′o-nin) 1. a naturally occurring amino acid, $C_5H_{11}NO_2S$, which is an essential component of the diet, furnishing both methyl groups and sulfur necessary for normal metabolism. 2. racemethionine.

methisazone (mĕ-this′ah-zōn) chemical name: 2-(1,2-dihydro-1-methyl-2-oxo-3H-indol-3-ylidene)hydrazinecarbothioamide. An antiviral agent, $C_{10}H_{10}N_4OS$, which has been used to provide short-term protection against smallpox and the severe complications of vaccination.

Methium (meth′e-um) trademark for preparations of hexamethonium chloride.

methixene hydrochloride (mĕ-thiks′ēn) chemical name: 1-methyl-3-(9H-thioxanthen-9-yl-methyl)piperidine hydrochloride monohydrate. An anticholinergic, $C_{20}H_{23}NS \cdot HCl \cdot H_2O$, occurring as a white, crystalline powder, having a direct spasmolytic effect on smooth muscle; used in the treatment of gastrointestinal hypermotility and spasm associated with functional bowel disease, administered orally.

methocarbamol (meth″o-kar′bah-mol) [USP] chemical name: 3-(2-methoxyphenoxy)-1,2-propanediol 1-carbamate. A skeletal muscle relaxant, $C_{11}H_{15}NO_5$, occurring as a white powder; administered orally, intramuscularly, and intravenously.

Methocel (meth′o-sel) trademark for a preparation of methylcellulose.

method (meth′ud) [Gr. *methodos*] the manner of performing any act or operation; a procedure or technique. See also under *maneuver, stains, tests, treatment,* etc. **Abbe's string m.,** string method treatment. **Abbott's m.,** treatment of scoliosis by lateral pulling and counterpulling on the spinal column by means of wide bandages and pads until the deformity is overcorrected, and then applying a plaster jacket to produce pressure, counterpressure, and fixation of the spine in its corrected position. **A.B.C. (alum, blood, clay) m.,** a method of deodorizing and precipitating sludge by the addition of alum, charcoal (or some other material), and clay to the raw sewage. **absorption m.,** the separate and selective removal of agglutinins from specific immune sera by the addition of homologous particulate antigen(s) (e.g., bacterial cells or red blood cells) to the immune sera, or by the passage of specific immune sera through columns containing antigen on an insoluble support (immunosorbent) with which the homologous antibody combines and is thereby removed from the serum. **acetoacetic acid, m's for,** see *Folin and Hart's m., Scott and Wilson's m.,* and *Van Slyke and Palmer's m.,* and see *acetoacetic acid test,* under *tests.* **acetone, m's for,** see *Folin's m.* (1,2), *Folin and Hart's m., Messinger and Huppert's m., Shaffer and Marriott's m.,* and *Scott and Wilson's m.,* and see *acetone test,* under *tests.* **Achard-Castaigne m.,** the methylene blue test. **acid hematin m.** (*for hemoglobin*): dilute the blood in tenth normal HCl and compare the color with a standard heme solution or glass standards. **Addis m.,** see under *count* and *tests.* **Adelmann's m.,** forcible flexion of an extremity to control arterial hemorrhage, a procedure used only in extreme emergencies as first aid. **adrenaline, m. for,** see *epinephrine, m. for.* **Ahlfeld's m.,** hand disinfection with hot water and alcohol. **albumin in urine, m's for,** see *Esbach's m., Folin's m.* (12), *Folin and Denis' m.* (1), *Folin's gravimetric m., Kwilecki's m., Scherer's m.,* and *turbidity m.,* and see *albumin test,* under *tests.* **alkali reserve, m's for,** see *Fridericia's m., Marriott's m., Van Slyke and Cullen's m.* (1), and *Van Slyke and Fitz's m. allantoin, m's for,* see *Folin's m.* (15), *Plimmer and Skelton's m., Wiechowski and Handorsky's m.* **Altmann-Gersh m.,** a method of preparing tissue for histologic study by freeze drying. **amino-acid nitrogen, m's for,** see *nitrogen, amino-acid, m's for.* **ammonia nitrogen, m's for,** see *nitrogen, ammonia, m's for.* **arch bar m.,** a method of establishing intermaxillary fixation: available teeth are ligated to arch bars and orthodontic rubber bands are used between the two arches to bring the teeth into occlusion. **Arnold and Gunning's m.** (*for total nitrogen*), a modified form of the Kjeldahl process for urine. **Aronson's m.,** volatilizing formaldehyde gas from the solid polymer, trioxymethylene, by heat. **Asken-**

stedt's m. (Parker's modification) (*for indican*): precipitate the urine with solid mercuric chloride; oxidize the indican to indigo with Obermeyer's reagent; shake out with chloroform and compare the blue color with a standard solution of indigo. **Austin and Van Slyke's m.** (*for chlorides in whole blood*): lake the blood with distilled water, precipitate the proteins with picric acid, and then proceed as in McLean and Van Slyke's method for chlorides in oxalated plasma. **Autenrieth and Funk's m.** (*for cholesterol*): boil the blood or serum to saponify the fats; extract with chloroform and evaporate the chloroform; make a Liebermann-Burchard test on the residue and compare it with a standard solution of cholesterol. **autoclave m.,** see *Clark-Collip m.* (2). **Baer's m.,** prevention of the re-forming of adhesions by the injection of sterilized oil into an ankylosed joint. **Bang's m.,** 1. estimation of the quantities of the sugar, albumin, urea, etc., in the blood by examination of a few drops only, collected on blotting paper. 2. (*for dextrose*): to an excess of the boiling reagent (an alkaline solution of copper thiocyanate), add the urine and titrate the excess of copper thiocyanate with hydroxylamine sulfate. 3. (*a micromethod for dextrose*): boil the urine with an excess of the reagent ($KHCO_3$, 160 gm.; K_2CO_3, 100 gm.; KCl, 66 gm.; $CuSO_4 \cdot 5H_2O$, 4.4 gm.; and water to 1 liter) and titrate excess of CuCl with a solution of iodine, using starch as an indicator. **Baréty's m.,** an extension method for treating hip disease and fracture of the thigh. **Barger's m.,** a method for determining osmotic pressure from vapor pressure. **Barraquer's m.,** phacoerysis. **Bence Jones protein, m. for,** see *Folin and Denis' m.* (2). **Benedict's m.,** 1. (*for dextrose*): titrate the sugar in the urine with the following reagent: $CuSO_4$ (crystals), 18 gm.; Na_2CO_3 (crystals), 200 gm.; sodium citrate, 200 gm.; potassium thiocyanate, 125 gm.; potassium ferrocyanide, 5 per cent solution, 5 ml.; water to make 1 liter. 2. (*for total sulfur*): add the reagent (crystallized copper nitrate, 200 gm.; sodium chlorate, 50 gm.; water to make 1 liter) to the urine and evaporate to dryness, ignite, take up in dilute hydrochloric acid, precipitate with $BaCl_2$, filter, dry, and weigh. 3. (*for urea*): the urea is hydrolyzed to ammonium carbonate by heating with $KHSO_4$ and $ZnSO_4$, made alkaline, distilled into standard sulfuric acid, and the excess acid titrated. 4. (*for uric acid in blood*): the same as *Benedict and Franke's m. for uric acid in urine.* **Benedict and Denis' m.** (*for total sulfur*): mix the urine with the reagent [$Cu(NO_3)_2$, 25 gm.; NaCl, 25 gm.; NH_4NO_3, 10 gm.; and water 100 ml.] and evaporate to dryness, ignite, dissolve in 10 per cent hydrochloric acid, and test for inorganic sulfates by Folin's method (6) (q.v.). **Benedict and Franke's m.** (*for uric acid in urine*): to the diluted urine add sodium cyanide and the arsenophosphotungstic acid reagent; the blue color produced is compared with a standard uric acid solution. **Benedict and Hitchcock's m.** (*for uric acid*): precipitate the uric acid with an ammoniacal silver-magnesium solution (3 per cent silver lactate solution, 70 ml.; magnesia mixture, 30 ml.; concentrated ammonium hydroxide, 100 ml.). Dissolve the precipitate with potassium cyanide and add uric acid reagent (boil 100 gm. of sodium tungstate and 80 ml. of 85 per cent phosphoric acid in 750 ml. of water for two hours and make up to 1 liter) and sodium carbonate solution. Compare in colorimeter with a known uric acid standard. **Benedict and Leche's m.** (*for inorganic phosphate in blood*): the method is the same as that of Fiske and Subbarow except that the reducing agent is a hydroquinone-sulfite mixture instead of amino-naphthol-sulfonic acid. **Benedict and Murlin's m.** (*for amino-acid nitrogen by formal titration*): add phosphotungstic acid to the urine to precipitate ammonia and other basic substances, neutralize to litmus, add solution of formaldehyde, and titrate with tenth normal sodium hydroxide. **Benedict and Osterberg's m.** (*for sugar in normal urine*): treat the urine with picric acid, sodium carbonate, and acetone; compare the red color produced with a standard solution of sugar. **Benedict and Theis' m.,** 1. (*for lipoid phosphorus*): oxidize the lipoid phosphorus to phosphoric acid with a mixture of concentrated nitric and sulfuric acids and then proceed as with inorganic phosphates. 2. (*for phenols in blood*): to 10 ml. of blood filtrate add 1 ml. of 1 per cent gum acacia solution, 1 ml. of 50 per cent sodium acetate solution, 1 ml. of the diazotized nitroaniline reagent, mix and after one minute add 2 ml. of a 20 per cent sodium carbonate solution. Compare the orange color with a standard phenol solution containing 0.025 mg. of phenol in 10 ml. **Bergeim's m.** (*for indole in feces*): make the feces alkaline and distil off phenols. Make distillate acid with H_2SO_4 and redistil to leave NH_3 in residue. To the second distillate add beta-naphtha-quinone sodium monosulfonate and alkali. Extract the blue color with chloroform and compare it with that of a standard solution of indole similarly treated. **Berger's m.,** suture of transverse fracture of the patella. **Bergonié's m.,** see under *treatment.* **Bertrand's m.** (*for glucose*): boil the urine with alkaline copper sulfate solution, filter, dissolve the precipitate in an acid solution of ferric sulfate, and titrate with potassium permanganate. **beta-hydroxybutyric acid, m's for,** see *Black's m.* and *Van Slyke and Palmer's m.* **Bethea's m.,** see under *sign.* **bile pigments, m's for,** see *Meulengracht's m., Wallace and Diamond's m.,* and see under *tests.* **Bivine's m.,** treatment of strychnine poisoning by administration of chloral hydrate. **Black's m.** (*for beta-hydroxybutyric acid*): evaporate the urine to a small volume, acidify, add plaster of Paris to form a coarse meal, extract the beta-hydroxybutyric acid with ether in a Soxhlet apparatus, evaporate to dryness, take up in water, and determine the amount by a polariscope. **Blanchard's m.,** see under *treatment.* **Bloor's m.,** 1. (*for lipoid phosphorus*), see *Benedict and Theis' m.* (1). 2. (*for cholesterol*): extract the cholesterol from whole blood with hot alcohol-ether. Dry, extract with chloroform, and determine by the Liebermann-Burchardt reaction. **Bloor, Pelkan, and Allen's m.** (*for fatty acids and cholesterol*): extract the lipoids by an alcohol-ether mixture, saponify, extract the cholesterol with chloroform and the soaps with hot alcohol. The cholesterol is then determined colorimetrically and the fatty acids nephelometrically. **Bock and Benedict's m.** (*for total nitrogen*): it is similar to Folin and Farmer's method, except that the ammonia is distilled instead of aerated over into the acid. **Bogg's m.** (*for protein in milk*): this is a modification of Esbach's method for protein in urine; the protein being precipitated with Bogg's reagent instead of with picric acid. **Brandt's m.** (*obs.*), deep massage of the fallopian tubes for expression of the pus in pyosalpinx. **Brandt-Andrews m.,** see under *maneuver.* **Brehmer's m.,** see under *treatment.* **Breslau's m.,** volatilizing formaldehyde from dilute (8 per cent) solutions to prevent polymerization. **brine flotation m.** (*for concentration of ova*): suspend a portion of the stool in a saturated solution of sodium chloride; let it stand for a time and collect the ova from the surface. **Brunn's m.,** see *Breslau's m.* **Brunninghausen's m.,** dilatation of the cervix for the introduction of premature labor. **calcium, m's for,** see *Clark-Collip's m.* (1), *Corley and Denis' m., Kramer and Tisdall's m.* (2), *Lyman's m., McCrudden's m.,* and *Shohl and Pedley's m.,* and see under *tests.* **caliper m.,** a method for approximating fat content in the body by measuring the thickness of folds of the skin at stated areas of the body by means of specially designed calipers. **Callahan's m.,** a method in which the root canal of a tooth is first flooded with a chloroform-rosin solution and then gutta-percha is dissolved in this solution; called also *chloropercha m.* **carbon dioxide, m. for,** see *Fridericia's m.* and *Van Slyke and Cullen's m.* (1). **Carrel's m.,** 1. a method of end-to-end suture of blood vessels. 2. see under *treatment.* 3. a method of determining when to make secondary closure of wounds. A loop of material is taken from the wound, spread on a slide, stained, and the number of bacteria counted. **casein, m. for,** saturate the milk with magnesium sulfate, filter, wash, determine the nitrogen by the Kjeldahl method, and multiply the result by 6.37; see also *Hart's m.,* and see *casein test,* under *tests.* **Castaneda's m.** (*for rickettsiae in smears*): (1) a thin smear is made in a phosphate buffer (pH 7.6) and air-dried, (2) stained with methylene blue solution for 3 minutes, (3) counterstained with safranine solution, and (4) washed, blotted, and dried. Rickettsiae appear pale blue; cell nuclei and protoplasm are red. **cathartic m.,** a method of treating psychoneuroses by enabling the patient, through properly directed questions, to bring to full consciousness the vague and unformed dread from which he has been suffering. **Cathelin's m.,** introduction of anesthetics into the epidural space through the sacrococcygeal ligament. **Chandler's m.** (*for fibrinogen*): precipitate the fibrinogen with calcium chloride, centrifugalize, and determine the nitrogen in the clot. **Chaput's m.,** treatment of osteomyelitis by scraping the cavity and inserting fat taken from the thigh or abdomen. **Chervin's m.,** see under *treatment.* **Chick-Martin m.,** testing the germicidal value of disinfectants for water supplies; it is applied in the presence of 3 per cent of human feces and for a fixed period of thirty minutes. **chlorides, m's for,** see *Austin and Van Slyke's m., Dehn and Clark's m., McLean and Van Slyke's m., Mohr's m., Volhard and Arnold's m., Volhard and Harvey's m.,* and *Whitehorn's m.* **chloropercha m.,** Callahan's m. **cholesterol, m's for,** see *Autenrieth and Funk's m., Bloor's m.* (2), *Bloor, Pelkan, and Allen m.,* and *Myers and Wardell's m.,* and see under *tests.* **Ciaccio's m.,** treatment of tissue for the purpose of rendering visible the intracellular lipoids; they are fixed with acid chromate solution and stained with sudan III. **Clark-Collip m.,** 1. (*for calcium in serum*): dilute the serum and add ammonium oxalate; wash the precipitate, dissolve with sulfuric acid, and titrate with potassium permanganate. 2. (*for urea in blood*): to 5 ml. of blood filtrate add 1 ml. of NH_4Cl and heat in autoclave at 150 C. for ten minutes. Make alkaline, distil into acid, and titrate, using methyl red as indicator. **Clausen's m.,** 1. (*for lactic acid in blood*): remove the glucose by adding copper sulfate and calcium hydroxide, filter, and proceed with filtrate as in Clausen's method for lactic acid in urine. 2. (*for lactic acid in urine*): extract the lactic acid from the urine with ether, convert it into acetaldehyde by treatment with sulfuric acid, add sodium bisulfite, and titrate with standard iodine solution. **closed-plaster m.,** treatment of wounds, compound fractures, and osteomyelitis by enclosing the limb in an immobilizing plaster cast. See *Orr treatment* and *Trueta treatment,* under *treatment.* **Converse m.,** reconstruction of the ear lobe by raising a flap of skin below the auricle with a superior base about one third larger than the proposed lobe; a full-thickness skin graft covers the defect at the site of the flap except for the last third of the medial aspect of the pedicle. **Corley and Denis m.** (*for calcium in tissues*): if there is only a small amount of organic material, it may be removed by washing, aided by nitric acid. With more organic material, add 5 volumes of tenth normal sodium hydroxide and heat in autoclave at 180° C. for two hours. Precipitate as oxalate, dissolve in sulfuric acid, and titrate with potassium permanganate. **Corning's m.,** spinal anesthesia, def. 1. **Corri's m.** (*for lactic acid in tissues*): precipitate the protein with $HgCl_2$, remove the mercury from the filtrate with H_2S, and determine lactic acid by Clausen's method. **Couette m.,** a method for measuring viscosity by calculating the rate of movement of an inner cylinder separated from an outer cylinder by a thin layer of the fluid whose viscosity is being tested. **Coutard's m.,** a method of x-ray irradiation by protracted and fractionated dosage. **creatine, m's for,** see *Folin's m.* (7,8), *Folin, Benedict, and Myers' m., Folin and Wu's m.* (2), and *Meyer's m.* **creatinine, m's for,** see *Folin's m.* (9), *Folin and Wu's m.* (1,2), and *Shaffer's m.,* and see under *tests.* **Credé's m.,** 1. method of expressing the placenta by forcing the uterus down into the pelvis and at the same time squeezing the uterus from all sides so that its contents are expelled. 2. a similar method for expressing urine from the bladder, especially in paralytic bladder. 3. the placing of a drop of 2 per cent solution of silver nitrate in each eye of a newborn child for the prevention of ophthalmia neonatorum. **Cronin m.,** an operation to correct a flat nasal tip with short columella by using bilateral flaps of skin elevated in the floor of the nostrils. **crystallizing oxyhemoglobin, m. for,** see *Reichert's m.* **cubicle m.,** the treatment of patients with contagious disease by placing each patient in one of the cubicle-like compartments into which the ward is divided. **Cuignet's m.,** skiametry. **cup plate m.,** see *ring test* (def. 1), under *tests.* **Dakin-Carrel m.,** Carrel's treatment; see under *treatment.* **Defer's m.,** treatment of hydrocele by evacuation and cauterization of the sac with silver nitrate. **Dehn and Clark's m.** (*for chlorides*): oxidize any interfering organic matter with sodium peroxide and then proceed with Volhard and Arnold's method. **Delore's m.,** manual osteoclasis for correcting genu valgum. **Demme's m.,** treatment of hydrocele by injection of iodine. **Denis' m.** (*for magnesium in serum*): remove the calcium by the Clark-Collip method, precipitate as magnesium ammonium phosphate, dissolve the precipitate in tenth normal HCl, reduce it with amino-naphthol-sulfonic acid, and compare the blue color with a standard solution of ammonium magnesium phosphate in 0.1 per cent HCl. **Denis and Leche's m.** (*for total sulfate*): add acid and autoclave to decompose protein, then precipitate with barium chloride, dry, and weigh. **Denman's m.,** see under *evolution.* **dextrose, m's for,** see *glucose (dextrose), m's for.* **diacetic acid, m's for,** see *acetoacetic acid, m's for.* **Dickinson m.,** a method of controlling postpartum hemorrhage: the entire uterus is grasped through the abdominal wall, lifted out of the pelvis, and compressed against the spinal column. **direct m.,** in ophthalmoscopy, that in which the ophthalmoscope is held close to the eye examined and an erect virtual image is obtained of the fundus. **direct aeration m.** (*for urea in blood*), see *Myers' m.* **direct centrifugal flotation m.,** Lane m. **Domagk's m.** (*for demonstration of reticuloendothelial cells*): a culture of gram-positive staphylococci in physiologic salt solution is injected into the femoral vein of a rat which is then killed in fifteen to thirty minutes. In formalin-fixed sections stained by cresyl violet or by Gram's stain followed by alum-carmine, Kupffer's cells and other cells of the reticuloendothelial system stand out strikingly. **Douglas' m.,** spontaneous evolution of the fetus from transverse lie: an arm prolapses, the head is arrested above the pelvic inlet and rotates to the pubis, the chest, abdomen, and breech rotate downward, and then the legs, the other arm, and lastly the head appear. **Dubois' m.,** a method of psychotherapy involving explanation to the patient of his condition and the securing of the patient's cooperation in his treatment. **Duke's m.,** see *bleeding time,* under *time.* **Duncan's m.,** autotherapy, def. 3. **Duplay's m.,** reconstruction of the glandular urethra in hypospadias by using a buried skin strip. **Eggleston's m.,** a method of administering digitalis leaf. **Eicken's m.,** examination of the hypopharynx, with the cricoid cartilage drawn forward. **Ellerman-Erlandsen m.,** tuberculin titer test. **Ellinger's m.** (*for indican*): precipitate the urine with basic lead acetate and filter. To the filtrate add Obermayer's reagent. Shake out the indigo with chloroform, evaporate off the chloroform, and titrate the residue with potassium permanganate. **epinephrine, m. for,** see *Folin, Cannon, and Denis' m.* See also *epinephrine test,* under *tests.* **Epstein's m.** (*for dextrose*): a modification of the Lewis and Benedict method, making it possible to make the test with very little blood. **Esbach's m.** (*for albumin in urine*): precipitate the protein with picric acid, let precipitate settle in a graduated tube, and read the result. **ethereal sulfates, m's for,** see *sulfates, ethereal, m's for.* **Fahraeus m.,** a method for determining the rate of sedimentation of erythrocytes. **fatty acids, m. for,** see *Bloor, Pelkan, and Allen m.* **Faust's m.,** a method of diagnosing helminth and protozoan infections by centrifugation of washed feces with zinc sulfate of a specific gravity of 1.180, after which eggs and protozoan cysts may be removed from the supernatant layer. **fibrinogen, m. for,** see *Chandler's m.* **Fichera's m.,** see under *treatment.* **Fick m.,** see under *principle.* **Finikoff's m.** (*obs.*), see under *treatment.* **Fishberg's m.,** one for determining specific gravity of the urine, which serves as a concentration test of renal function. **Fiske's m.** (*for total fixed base*): remove phosphates with ferric chloride, convert fixed bases into sulfates by heating in H_2SO_4, ignite, take up in water, precipitate sulfates as benzidine sulfate, and titrate with alkali. **Fiske and Subbarow's m.,** 1. (*for acid-soluble phosphorus in blood*): destroy organic matter by heating with sulfuric and nitric acids, precipitate the phosphates as magnesium ammonium phosphate, and reduce the precipitate with para-amino-naphthol-sulfonic acid. Compare the blue color with a standard phosphate solution. 2. (*for inorganic phosphates*): the phosphates are precipitated as ammonium phosphomolybdate. This is then reduced by para-amino-naphthol-sulfonic acid and the blue color compared colorimetrically with a standard solution. **Fitz Gerald m.,** zone therapy. **fixed base, m. for,** see *Fiske's m.* **flash m.,** a method of pasteurizing milk whereby the milk is brought up to a temperature of 178° F. and chilled at once. Cf. *holding m.* **flotation m.,** any method for separating cysts and ova from the heavier component of the stool and which depends upon the use of a solution intermediate in density between the parasitic material (which floats) and the bulk of the feces (which remains as sediment after centrifugation). **Folin's m.,** 1. (*for acetone*): aerate the acetone from the urine over into an alkaline hypo-iodite solution of known strength. The acetone is thus changed to iodoform and the excess of iodine is titrated with a standard thiosulfate solution, using starch as an indicator. 2. (*for acetone*): micromethod. Aerate the acetone over into a solution of sodium bisulfite and then determine the amount of nephelometric comparison with a standard acetone solution using Scott and Wilson's reagent. 3. (*for amino acids in blood*): make 10 ml. of protein-free blood filtrate slightly alkaline to phenolphthalein. Add 2 ml. of beta-naphthaquinone solution and place in the dark. The next day add 2 ml. of acetic acid-acetate solution and 2 ml. of 4 per cent thiosulfate solution. Dilute to 25 ml. and compare the blue color with a standard amino-acid solution similarly treated. 4. (*for amino-acid nitrogen in blood*): treat the urine with permutit to remove the ammonia and then with beta-naphtha-quinone sulfonic acid. The red color is compared with a standard amino acid solution. 5. (*for ammonia nitrogen*): sodium carbonate is added to the urine to free the ammonia, which is aerated into standard acid and titrated. 6. (*for blood sugar*): to 2 ml. of neutral protein-free blood filtrate, add 2 ml. of the Folin copper solution and heat in boiling water bath ten minutes. Cool and add 2 ml. of acid molybdate reagent. Dilute to 25 ml. mark and compare the blue color with a standard glucose solution similarly treated. 7. (*for creatine*): precipitate the proteins of the blood with picric acid and filter. To the filtrate add sodium hydroxide and compare color with a standard solution of creatine. 8. (*for creatine in urine*): change creatine into creatinine by heating at 90° C. for three hours in the presence of third normal HCl. Determine creatinine by picric acid and alkali and deduct the preformed creatinine. 9. (*for creatinine in urine*): to the urine add picric acid and sodium hydroxide and compare the red color with a half normal solution of potassium bichromate. 10. (*for ethereal sulfates*): remove the inorganic sulfates with barium chloride and then the conjugated sulfates after hydrolyzing with boiling dilute hydrochloric acid. 11. (*for inorganic sulfates*): acidify the urine with hydrochloric acid, precipitate with barium chloride, filter, dry, ignite, and weigh. 12. (*for protein in urine*): add acetic acid and heat, wash, dry, and weigh the precipitate. 13. (*for total acidity*): add potassium oxalate to the urine to precipitate the calcium which should otherwise precipitate at the neutral point, and titrate with tenth normal sodium hydroxide, using phenolphthalein as an indicator. 14. (*for total sulfates*): boil the urine for thirty minutes with dilute hydrochloric acid, precipitate with barium chloride, filter, dry, ignite, and weigh. 15. (*for urea and allantoin*): decompose the urea by heating with magnesium chloride and hydrochloric acid, distil off the ammonia, and titrate. **Folin's gravimetric m.** (*for protein in urine*): precipitate the protein by heat and acetic acid; centrifugalize, wash, dry, and weigh the precipitate. **Folin and Bell's m.** (*for ammonia in urine*), see *permutit m.* **Folin, Benedict and Myers' m.** (*for creatine in urine*): to 20 ml. of urine add 20 ml. of normal HCl and autoclave at 120° C. for one half hour. Neutralize, add picric acid and alkali, and compare the color with a standard solution of potassium bichromate. **Folin and Berglund's m.** (*for sugar in normal urine*): remove interfering substances by shaking the urine with Lloyd's alkaloidal reagent and then proceed as in the Folin-Wu method. **Folin, Cannon, and Denis' m.** (*for epinephrine*): add Folin's uric acid phosphotungstic reagent and sodium carbonate to the unknown and estimate amount by comparison of blue color with a standard uric acid solution similarly treated. **Folin and Denis' m.,** 1. (*for albumin*): precipitate the albumin with sulfosalicylic acid and compare the turbidity with that of a standard protein solution; called also *turbidity m.* 2. (*for Bence Jones protein*): coagulate the Bence Jones protein at 60° C., centrifugalize, wash, precipitate with 50 per cent alcohol, dry, and weigh. 3. (*for nitrogen in urine*): destroy the organic matter in the diluted urine with the phosphoric-sulfuric acid-copper sulfate mixture, add Nessler's reagent, and compare it with a standard ammonia solution. 4. (*for nonprotein nitrogen*): it is much the same as Folin and Wu's method except that the proteins are removed with

methyl alcohol and zinc chloride. The alcohol is boiled off and the nitrogen changed into ammonia and nesslerized in the usual way. 5. (*for phenols*): precipitate interfering substances by adding acid silver lactate solution and colloidal iron. To 20 ml. of the filtrate add 5 ml. of the phosphotungstic phosphomolybdic acid reagent and 15 ml. of a saturated solution of sodium carbonate and compare the blue color, etc. 6. (*for urea*): the same as the method of Folin and Pettibone except that the urine is diluted twenty to one hundred times to prevent sugar from interfering with the test. 7. (*for uric acid in blood*): remove the proteins by boiling acetic acid and then proceed with Benedict and Hitchcock's method. **Folin and Farmer's m.** (*for total nitrogen*): a modified microchemical Kjeldahl method for urine. Decompose the nitrogenous bodies with sulfuric acid as usual, add alkali, aerate the ammonia over into standard acid, nesslerize, and compare with a standard solution of ammonium sulfate. **Folin and Flander's m.** (*for hippuric acid*): 100 ml. of the urine is evaporated to dryness with 10 ml. of 5 per cent sodium hydroxide. Hydrolyze the residue with nitric acid, shake out the benzoic acid with chloroform, and titrate it with tenth normal sodium alcoholate, using phenolphthalein as indicator. **Folin and Hart's m.** (*for acetone and acetoacetic acid*): determine the acetone by Folin's method, then heat the urine with hydrochloric acid to change acetoacetic acid to acetone, and determine again. **Folin and Macallum's m.** (*for ammonia nitrogen*): to the urine add potassium carbonate and potassium oxalate, aerate the ammonia over into standard acid, nesslerize, and compare with a standard solution of ammonium sulfate. **Folin, McEllroy, and Peck's m.** (*for dextrose in urine*): mix 5 ml. of an acidified 5.9 per cent copper sulfate solution, 1 ml. of 20 per cent sodium carbonate solution and then add 4 to 5 gm. of phosphate-thiocyanate mixture. Heat and add enough urine to produce a sudden turbidity after not more than five seconds of boiling; 25 mg. of glucose will reduce the 5 ml. of copper solution. **Folin and Peck's m.** (*for dextrose*): to the boiling copper solution of Folin and McEllroy run in urine until the color changes from green to yellow. **Folin and Pettibone's m.** (*for urea*): microchemical. The urea is decomposed by heating with potassium acetate and acetic acid, the ammonia is liberated by sodium hydroxide, aerated over into standard acid, and nesslerized. **Folin and Shaffer's m.** (*for uric acid*): phosphates and certain organic substances are first precipitated by an acetic acid solution of ammonium sulfate and uranium acetate. The uric acid is then precipitated as ammonium urate and the amount determined by titration with potassium permanganate. **Folin and Wright's m.** (*for nitrogen in urine*): a simplified macro-Kjeldahl method in which the digestion is brought about by a mixture of phosphoric and sulfuric acids aided by ferric chloride, and the liberated ammonia is distilled without the use of a condenser. **Folin and Wu's m.,** 1. (*for creatinine*): the color produced by the unknown (protein-free blood filtrate or urine) in an alkaline solution of picric acid is compared in a colorimeter with the color produced by a known solution of creatinine or with a standard solution of potassium bichromate. 2. (*for creatine plus creatinine*): the creatine of a protein-free blood filtrate is changed to creatinine by heating with dilute HCl in an autoclave, and the creatinine thus produced together with the preformed is determined colorimetrically after adding an alkaline picrate solution. 3. (*for glucose*): the protein-free blood filtrate is boiled with a dilute alkaline copper tartrate solution, the cuprous oxide is dissolved by adding a phosphomolybdic-phosphoric acid solution, and the blue color produced is compared with the color from sugar solutions of known strength. 4. (*nonprotein nitrogen*): the total nonprotein nitrogen in the protein-free blood filtrate is determined by setting free the nitrogen as ammonia by the Kjeldahl process, nesslerizing this ammonia, and comparing with a standard. 5. (*for protein-free blood filtrate*): lake the blood with distilled water, add sodium tungstate and sulfuric acid, and filter. 6. (*for urea*): change the urea to ammonia by means of urease, and nesslerize. 7. (*for uric acid*): uric acid is precipitated from the protein-free blood filtrate or from urine by silver lactate, treated with phosphotungstic acid, and the blue color compared with the color produced by known amounts of uric acid. **Folin and Youngburg's m.** (*for urea in urine*): the ammonia is removed from the urine by permutit, the urea is changed to ammonium carbonate by urease, and nesslerized directly. **m's for (volatilizing)** formaldehyde gas, see *Aronson's m., Breslau's m., lime m., Schlossmann's m.,* and *Trillat's m.* **formol titration, m's of,** see *Benedict and Murlin's m., Malfatti's m.,* and *Sörensen's m.* **Freiburg m.,** twilight sleep; see under *sleep.* **Freud's cathartic m.,** catharsis, def. 2. **Frey and Gigon's m.** (*for amino-acid nitrogen*): a modified form of Sörensen's method in that the ammonia is aspirated off after adding the barium hydroxide. **Fridericia's m.** (*for alveolar carbon dioxide tension*): the carbon dioxide is absorbed into a solution of potassium hydroxide and the decrease in volume read in percentage in a special apparatus. **Fülleborn's m.** (*for ova in stools*): grind 1 gm. of stool and mix with 20 ml. of a saturated solution of sodium chloride. Allow to stand one hour or more, then float coverglasses on the surface and transfer them, without draining, to slides. **gasometric m.** (*for urea*), see *Stehle's m.* **Gerota's m.,** injection of the lymphatics with a dye, such as prussian blue, which is soluble in chloroform or ether, but not in water. **Gilmer m.** (*of establishing intermaxillary fixation*): a wire ligature is passed about the necks of all available teeth and twisted until the wire is tight about the teeth. The teeth are placed in occlusion and the wires are twisted, one upper to one lower wire. **Girard's m.**, see under *treatment*. **Givens' m.** (*for peptic activity*): varying amounts of diluted gastric juice are added to a series of tubes containing pea globulin, the mixtures are incubated, and the amount of digestion noted. **glucose (dextrose), m's for,** see *Bang's m., Benedict's m.* (1), *Benedict and Osterberg's m., Bertrand's m., Epstein's m., Folin's m.* (6), *Folin and Berglund's m., Folin, McElroy, and Peck's m., Folin and Peck's m., Folin and Wu's m.* (3), *Hagedorn and Jensen's m., Lewis and Benedict's m., Peter's m., Power and Wilder's m., Stammer's m.,* and *Sumner's m.* See also *dextrose test*, under *tests*. **gold number m.**, colloidal gold test. **Gram's m.,** see *Table of Stains*, under *stain*. **Greenwald's m.** (*for nonprotein nitrogen*): the proteins are precipitated by trichloracetic acid, the filtrate is decomposed by sulfuric acid as in the Kjeldahl method, the ammonia is distilled off and the amount titrated with tenth normal sodium hydroxide. **Greenwald and Lewman's m.** (*for titratable alkali of blood*): the protein of the blood is precipitated with an excess of picric acid. Both the free and the total picric acid in the filtrate are then determined. The difference represents the picric acid which is combined with the bases of the blood. **Griffith's m.** (*for hippuric acid*): extract the hippuric acid with ether. Distil off the ether and destroy urea in the residue with sodium hypobromite solution. Determine the nitrogen in the residue by the Kjeldahl method. **Gross's m.** (*for tryptic activity*): add increasing amounts of a trypsin solution to a series of tubes of pure, fat-free casein which have been heated to 40° C. Incubate at 40° C. for fifteen minutes. Test by adding a few drops of acetic acid (dilute) to each tube. A precipitate on acidification indicates that digestion is incomplete or lacking; no precipitate indicates digestion. **Grossich's m.**, the use of tincture of iodine as an antiseptic in surgical operations. **guanidine, m's for,** see *Pfiffner and Myers' m., Weber's m.* **Guinard's m.,** see under *treatment*. **Hagedorn and Jensen's m.** (*for sugar in blood*): precipitate the protein with zinc hydroxide. Heat the filtrate with potassium ferricyanide solution and determine the amount of ferricyanide reduced by adding an iodide solution and titrating the iodine set free with sodium thiosulfate. **Hahn's m.**, a method of performing pylorodiosis in which the anterior gastric wall is invaginated with the fingers, which are then thrust through the pyloric canal. Cf. *Loreta's m.* **Hall's m.** (*for total purine nitrogen*): remove phosphates by means of magnesia mixture and precipitate the purine bodies in a specially graduated tube by means of silver nitrate and ammonium hydroxide. After twenty-four hours read the volume of the purine precipitate. **Hamilton's m.** (*in postpartum hemorrhage*): compress the uterus between a fist in the vagina and a hand pressing down the abdominal wall. **Hammerschlag's m.** (*for specific gravity of blood*): prepare a mixture of benzene and chloroform of about 1.050 specific gravity. Into this let fall a drop of blood and add benzene or chloroform until the drop neither rises nor sinks. Then take the specific gravity of the mixture. **Handley's m.,** see under *lymphangioplasty*. **Hart's m.** (*for casein in milk*): precipitate the casein from the diluted milk, filter, wash, and redissolve in excess of tenth normal potassium hydroxide, and titrate remaining alkali with tenth normal HCl. The difference is casein. **Hartel's m.,** see under *treatment*. **Heintz's m.** (*for uric acid*): precipitate the urine by adding hydrochloric acid, filter off the crystals, wash, dry, and weigh. **hemoglobin, m's for,** see *acid hematin m., Dare's m.,* and *Sahli's m.*, and see under *tests*. **Henriques and Sörensen's m.** (*for amino-acid nitrogen by solution of formaldehyde titration*), see *Sörensen's m.* **Herter and Foster's m.** (*for indole in feces, modified by Bergeim*): make the feces alkaline and distil. Make the distillate acid and distil again. To the second distillate add beta-naphtha-quinone sodium monosulfonate and alkali. Extract the blue color with chloroform and compare it with a standard solution of indole containing 0.1 mg. of indole per milliliter. **Heublein m.,** ionizing irradiation of the whole body with low-dose increments protracted for ten to twenty hours per day over several days. **hippuric acid, m's for,** see *Folin and Flander's m., Griffith's m.,* and *Roaf's m.*, and see under *tests*. **Hirschberg's m.,** measurement of the deviation of a strabismic eye by observing the reflection of a candle from the cornea. **Hodgen's m.,** treatment of traumatic tetanus by large doses of Fowler's solution. **holding m.,** a method of pasteurizing milk whereby the milk is heated to 65° C. and kept at that temperature for thirty to forty-five minutes. Cf. *flash m.* **Howard's m.** (*of artificial respiration*): the patient is placed on his back, hands under his head, with a cushion so placed that his head is lower than his abdomen. Manual rhythmical pressure is then applied upward and inward against the lower lateral parts of the chest. **Howell's m.** (*for clotting time of blood*): place 5 ml. of blood in a 21-mm. test tube with suitable precautions. Tilt the tube every two minutes and note time of clotting. **Hunt's m.** (*for the activity of thyroid products*): mice on a cracker diet are fed varying amounts of the thyroid product for ten days. They are then injected with 0.4 mg. of acetonitrile per gram of body weight. If the product is active, the treated mice

usually live, whereas untreated mice are killed in two hours by 1.2 mg. per gram of body weight. **Hunter and Given's m.** (*for uric acid and purine bases*): precipitate and decompose the precipitate as in the Krueger-Schmidt method. Determine the uric acid in an aliquot part and in the remainder destroy the uric acid by oxidation and determine the purine bases as in the Krueger-Schmidt method. **hydrogen ion concentration, m. for,** see *Levy, Rowntree, and Marriott's m.* **indican, m's for,** see *Askenstedt's m.* and *Ellinger's m.*, and see under *tests*. **indole, m's for,** see *Bergeim's m.* and *Herter-Foster m.*, and see under *tests*. **inorganic phosphates, m. for,** see *phosphates, inorganic, m. for.* **inorganic sulfates, m's for,** see *sulfates, inorganic, m's for.* **iodine, m's for,** see specific methods, including *Kendall's m., Leipert's m.* **iron, m's for,** see *Walker's m., Wolter's m.,* and *Wong's m.*, and see under *tests*. **Ivy's m.,** see *bleeding time*, under *time*. **Japanese m.,** a method for fixing paraffin sections to glass slides with the use of Mayer's albumin. **Johnson's modification m.,** a modification of the Callahan method of filling root canals, in which the main canal is filled with a central core of solid gutta-percha. **Kaiserling's m.,** a procedure for preserving the natural colors in museum preparations, employing formaldehyde and potassium acetate. **Karr's m.** (*for urea in blood*): change the urea to ammonium carbonate by means of urease, nesslerize directly, and compare the color with that of a standard urea solution similarly treated. **Keating-Hart's m.,** see under *fulguration*. **Kendall's m.** (*for iodine in thyroid tissue*): oxidize the organic matter by fusion in KNO_3 and strong KOH. Acidify, oxidize with bromine, add an excess of KI, and titrate the liberated iodine with sodium thiosulfate. **Kenny's m.,** see under *treatment*. **Kety-Schmidt m.,** a method of measuring perfusion flow of blood through brain tissue. **Kirstein's m.,** inspection of the larynx without a laryngoscope by having the patient incline his head far back and depressing the tongue. **Kjeldahl's m.** (1883), a method of determining the amount of nitrogen in an organic compound. It consists in heating the material to be analyzed with strong sulfuric acid. The nitrogen is thereby converted to ammonia, which is distilled off and caught in tenth normal solution of sulfuric acid. By titration the amount of ammonia is determined, and from this the amount of nitrogen is estimated. **Klüver-Barrera m.,** a histologic staining method in which myelin sheaths are stained blue-green and the cells purple. **Koch and McMeekin's m.** (*for total nitrogen*): destroy organic matter with sulfuric acid and hydrogen peroxide, and nesslerize the resulting solution directly. **Korotkoff's m.,** the auscultatory method of determining blood pressure. **Kramer and Gittleman's m.** (*for sodium in serum*): dry and ash the serum. Take it up in 0.1 per cent HCl and make slightly alkaline with KOH. Precipitate with the pyroantimonate reagent and alcohol, dissolve precipitate in strong HCl, add potassium iodide, and titrate with sodium thiosulfate. **Kramer and Tisdall's m.,** 1. (*for potassium in serum*): precipitate with sodium cobaltinitrite reagent, treat precipitate with acid permanganate solution, then with sodium oxalate, and titrate with standard permanganate. 2. (*for calcium in serum*): precipitate the calcium as oxalate. Wash, dissolve, and titrate with potassium permanganate. **Kristeller's m.,** a method of expelling the fetus in labor. The fetal head should be in the vulva and the abdomen must be sufficiently relaxed so that the assistant may grasp the fundus. The grip on the fundus is made by the fingers of the two hands parallel behind and the thumb in front, the line of force being in the direction of the axis of the inlet. The expression should be done in one or two sustained efforts. **Krogh's m.** (*for urea*): the urea is oxidized by sodium hypobromite to carbon dioxide and nitrogen in an alkaline solution which absorbs the carbon dioxide. The remaining nitrogen is then measured. **Krueger and Schmidt's m.** (*for uric acid and purine bases*): precipitate the uric acid with copper sulfate, decompose the precipitate with sodium sulfite, acidify, concentrate, and let uric acid crystals separate. Determine the nitrogen in them by the Kjeldahl method. Reprecipitate the purine bases with copper sulfate, filter, wash, and determine the nitrogen in the precipitate by the Kjeldahl method. **Kwilecki's m.** (*for albumin*): 10 drops of a 10 per cent solution of ferric chloride are added to the urine before proceeding with the regular method of Esbach. **Laborde's m.,** the making of rhythmical traction movements on the tongue in order to stimulate the respiratory center in asphyxiation. **lactalbumin, m. for,** remove casein from the milk with magnesium sulfate, add Alman's reagent to the filtrate, determine the nitrogen in the precipitate by the Kjeldahl method, and multiply the result by 6.37. **lactic acid, m's for,** see specific methods, including *Clausen's m.* (1), (2), *Corri's m., von Furth and Charnass' m.* See also *lactic acid test*, under *tests*. **Lamaze m.,** a psychoprophylactic method of preparing for delivery, involving education of the prospective mother in the physiology of pregnancy and parturition and in techniques (e.g., breathing exercises and bearing down) to ease delivery. **Lane m.,** a method of diagnosing hookworm infection by centrifugation of 1 ml. of washed feces mixed with brine, the tube being covered with a cover slip on which the eggs can be counted. Called also *direct centrifugal flotation method,* or *D.C.F.* **lateral condensation m.,** multiple cone m. **Leboyer m.,** a method of delivery of the infant based upon the theory that the violence associated with birth causes emotional trauma to the infant and that this trauma will affect the child's personality and throughout his life. The concepts of this method emphasize that the delivery should be gentle and controlled, without unnecessary intervention; the infant should be handled gently, with the head, neck, and sacrum supported; the infant should not be overstimulated and be allowed to breath spontaneously, without painful stimuli, such as spanking. Called also *Leboyer technique*. **Leipert's m.** (*for iodine in blood*): destroy organic matter with chromic-sulfuric acid. Reduce iodic acid to free iodine with arsenous acid, distil off the iodine, and titrate. **Levy, Rowntree, and Marriott's m.** (*for hydrogen ion concentration of blood*): dialyze the blood through a collodion tube against neutral physiologic salt solution; then match the color produced by phenolsulfonphthalein in the dialysate and in solution of known hydrogen ion concentration. **Lewis and Benedict's m.** (*for dextrose*): the proteins of the blood are precipitated by means of picric acid, sodium carbonate is added, and the color of the picramic acid solution is compared with that of a standard glucose solution. **Lewisohn's m.** (*obs.*), a method of indirect transfusion by adding sodium citrate to the blood. **lime m.**, a method of generating or volatilizing formaldehyde gas. Forty per cent formaldehyde, containing 10 per cent of sulfuric acid, is poured over quicklime in a suitable container; 1½ to 2 pounds of lime should be used for each pint of the solution. **Lindemann's m.** (*for transfusion*): one needle cannula is placed in a vein of the donor's arm and another in the arm of the patient. Syringes are filled from the donor and emptied into the recipient through the cannulas. The method is now obsolete. **Linser's m.**, treatment of varicose veins by the injection of corrosive mercuric chloride. **Loreta's m.**, pylorodiosis performed by inserting the fingers through a gastrostomy incision. Cf. *Hahn's m.* **Lorthiore's m.**, radical cure of hernia by dissection and extirpation of the sac without opening the inguinal canal. **Lovset's m.**, see under *maneuver*. **Lyman's m.** (*for calcium*): precipitate the calcium from the protein-free blood filtrate or from urine as calcium oxalate, redissolve in dilute acid and reprecipitate as calcium ricinate, and determine the amount nephelometrically. **Lyon's m.**, Meltzer-Lyon test; see under *tests*. **McCrudden's m.** (*for calcium and magnesium*): make 200 ml. of urine faintly acid to litmus, add 10 ml. of concentrated hydrochloric acid, precipitate with oxalic acid, filter, ignite, and weigh as calcium oxide, or filter and titrate the precipitate with potassium permanganate. This gives the calcium. For the magnesium, add to the filtrate from the calcium, nitric acid, evaporate to dryness, and heat until the residue fuses. Take up in water, add sodium acid phosphate and ammonia, filter, wash, ignite, and weigh as the pyrophosphate. **Maclachlan m.**, a method of conditioning liquid sludge by the application of sulfur dioxide gas. **McLean and Van Slyke's m.** (*for chlorides*): precipitate the chlorides from oxalated plasma with an excess of silver nitrate and titrate the excess with potassium iodide and starch. **magnesium, m's for**, see *Denis' m.* and *McCrudden's m.* **Malfatti's m.** (*for ammonia nitrogen by solution of formaldehyde titration*): add potassium oxalate to the urine and make neutral to phenolphthalein with tenth normal sodium hydroxide; add the neutral solution of formaldehyde and titrate again. **Marfan's m.**, epigastric puncture. **Marriott's m.** (*for alkali reserve*): the patient rebreathes the air in a bag until its carbon dioxide tension is virtually that of venous blood. This air is then bubbled through a standard bicarbonate solution until the solution is saturated and the color produced is compared with standard color tubes. **Marshall's m.** (*for urea*): the urea is changed into ammonium carbonate by the enzyme urease and the ammonia titrated with tenth normal hydrochloric acid, using methyl orange, as indicator. **Meltzer's m.**, insufflation through an endotracheal tube of air containing an anesthetic vapor; employed in thoracic surgery. **Meltzer-Lyon m.**, see *Meltzer-Lyon test*, under *tests*. **Messinger and Huppert's m.** (*for acetone*): the same as the method of Folin and Hart except that the acetone is distilled instead of aspirated. **Mett's m.** (*for peptic activity*), see *Nirenstein and Schiff's m.* **Meulengracht's m.** (*for bile pigment in serum*): the serum is diluted until the yellow color corresponds to that of a standard potassium bichromate solution. **Meyer's m.** (*for creatine*): a modification of Folin and Benedict's method in that the creatine is changed into creatinine after adding hydrochloric acid by digesting in an autoclave. **Minkowski's m.**, same as *Naunyn-Minkowski m.* **Moerner-Sjöqvist m.**, see *Sjöqvist m.* **Mohr's m.** (*for chlorides*): oxidize interfering organic matter by igniting with potassium nitrate. To the solution of the ash add potassium chromate, and titrate with standard silver nitrate until the red silver chromate appears. **Monias and Shapiro's m.**, convert the indican into indigolignon and compare with a standard. **Morestin's m.**, see under *operation*. **Morison's (Rutherford) m.**, an obsolete method of treating wounds by opening up and mechanical cleansing of the wound, sponging with alcohol, and the application to the raw surfaces of a thin layer of a paste consisting of 1 part of bismuth subnitrate, 2 parts of iodoform, and enough liquid paraffin to make a soft paste. This paste is known as bismuth iodoform paraffin paste or Morison's paste, or in vernacular in the British Isles as bipp or B.I.P. The wound is then

sutured without drainage. **multiple cone m.**, a method of filling root canals in which the main portion of each canal is filled with a well-fitting primary gutta-percha cone or silver point in conjunction with sealer cement or paste, and the remaining canal space is packed with auxiliary gutta-percha cones. A root canal spreader (condenser) is used to force gutta-percha into the canal laterally for condensation and to create space for auxiliary gutta-percha points. Called also *lateral condensation m.* **Murphy m.**, 1. suture of an artery by invaginating the ends over a cylinder in two pieces which can then be removed. 2. continuous proctoclysis; the continuous administration per rectum of saline solution, drop by drop, from an elevated reservoir. Called also *Murphy drip*. 3. see *Murphy treatment* (def. 2), under *treatment*. **Myers' m.** (*for urea in blood*): change the urea to ammonium carbonate by the action of urease, aerate off the ammonia into an acid solution, and nesslerize; called also *direct aeration m.* **Myers and Wardell's m.** (*for cholestrol*): dry the blood on plaster of Paris and extract the cholesterol with chloroform. Add acetic anhydride and sulfuric acid and compare the color with that of a standard solution of cholesterol similarly treated. **Nägeli's m.**, see under *maneuver*. **Naunyn-Minkowski m.**, palpation of the kidney after first dilating the colon with gas. **Neumann's m.**, local anesthesia for surgery on the ear by the subperiosteal injection of a solution of cocaine and epinephrine. **Nikiforoff's m.**, a method of fixing blood films by placing them for from five to fifteen minutes in absolute alcohol, pure ether, or equal parts of alcohol and ether. **Nimeh's m.**, a method of determining the size of liver and spleen, based on measurements made on flat films of the hepatic and splenic regions taken separately without any preparation or after retroperitoneal insufflation of carbon dioxide gas. The ventricle diameter is the index of the size of the liver, the broad diameter that of the spleen. **Nirenstein and Schiff's m.** (*for peptic activity*): Mett's tubes are placed in the solution to be tested and incubated for twenty-four hours. The length of the column digested at each end is then determined. **nitrogen, amino acid, m's for**, see *Benedict and Murlin's m.*, *Folin's m.* (4), *Frey and Gignon's m.*, *Sörensen's m.*, *Van Slyke's m.*, and *Van Slyke and Meyer's m.* **nitrogen, ammonia, m's for**, see *Folin's m.* (5), *Folin and Macallum's m.*, *Malfatti's m.*, and *permutit m.*, and see under *tests*. **nitrogen, nonprotein, m's for**, see *Folin and Denis' m.* (4), *Folin and Wu's m.* (4), and *Greenwald's m.* **nitrogen, purine, m. for**, see *Hall's m.* **nitrogen, total, m's for**, see *Arnold and Gunning's m.*, *Bock and Benedict's m.*, *Folin and Denis' m.* (3), *Folin and Farmer's m.*, *Folin and Wright's m.*, *Koch and McMeekin's m.*, *Taylor and Hulton's m.* **Oberst's m.**, local anesthesia produced by injecting saline solution or distilled water into the subcutaneous connective tissue. **Ogata's m.**, a method of stimulating respiration by stroking the chest. **Ogino-Knaus m.**, the rhythm method of birth control. **Ombrédanne m.**, a reconstruction of the urethra in hypospadias, in which a flap is raised in a direction proximal to the urethral opening and rotated distally so that its most proximal point lies at the glans. **optical density m.**, the measuring of growth rates of cells by taking the optical density or turbidity of a dense population and comparing this with optical densities of known dilutions of the sample. **Orr m.**, see under *treatment*. **Orsi-Brocco m.**, palpatory percussion of the heart. **Osborne and Folin's m.** (*for total sulfur in urine*): destroy the organic matter in the concentrated urine and oxidize the sulfur by fusing with sodium peroxide. Precipitate with barium chloride, wash, dry, ignite, and weigh. **ova concentration, m. for**, see *brine flotation m.* **oxalic acid, m. for**, see *Salkowski, Autenrieth, and Barth's m.* **Pajot's m.**, decapitation of the fetus with Pajot's hook. **panoptic m.**, see *Giemsa's staining method*, in Table of Stains. **Pap's silver m.**, a method for demonstrating reticulum. **Parker's m.** (*for indican*), see *Askenstedt's m.* **Pasteur's m.** (*obs.*), 1. (*for Bacillus anthracis*): a method of attenuating bacteria by growing them at a temperature higher than body temperature, usually 42° to 43° C. 2. (*for the preparation of rabies vaccine*): the spinal cords of rabbits infected with rabies (fixed virus) are removed aseptically, dried, and emulsified. **Pavlov's m.**, study of the changes in the salivary reflex produced by psychic influence. See also *conditioned response*, under *response*, and see *conditioning*. **Payr's m.**, the use of absorbable cylinders of magnesium for performing suture of blood vessels. **peptic activity, m's for**, see specific methods, including *Given's m.*, *Nirenstein and Schiff's m.* **permutit m.** (*for ammonia in urine*): add permutit to the urine and shake for five minutes. Wash the permutit ammonia compound several times, add sodium hydroxide, and nesslerize. Compare the color with a standard solution of ammonium sulfate. Called also *Folin and Bell's m.* **Peter's m.** (*for dextrose*): boil the unknown in an excess of the reagent, filter off the reduced copper, and titrate the filtrate with potassium iodide and standard thiosulfate solution. **Pfiffner and Myers' m.** (*for guanidine in blood*): a colorimetric method by the use of an alkaline nitroprusside-ferricyanide reagent. **phenol, m's for**, see *Benedict and Theis' m.* (2), *Folin and Denis' m.* (5), *Tisdall's m.* See also *phenol test*, under *tests*. **phosphates, inorganic, m's for**, see *Benedict and Leche's m.*, *Fiske and Subbarow's m.* (2). **phosphorus, m. for**, see *uranium acetate m.* **phosphorus, acid-solu-**

ble, m. for, see *Fiske and Subbarow's m.* (1). **phosphorus, lipoid, m. for,** see *Benedict and Theis' m.* (1). **Pickrell's m.,** see under *spray*. **Plimmer and Skelton's m.** (*for allantoin*): determine the urea and allantoin by Folin's method (15), and the urea alone by Marshall's urease method. The difference is allantoin. **point source m.,** a method of intracavitary irradiation of the bladder wall utilizing a small point source of radiation at the center of a Foley catheter bag inflated with a radiopaque solution containing methylene blue or indigo carmine. **potassium, m. for,** see *Kramer and Tisdall's m.* (1). **Power and Wilder's m.** (*for glucose in urine*): remove interfering substances with mercuric sulfate. To the filtrate add alkaline ferricyanide; heat for ten minutes, cool, and add KI and an acid zinc sulfate solution. Titrate the liberated iodine with standard thiosulfate solution. **Price-Jones m.,** see under *curve*. **probit m.,** a method of calculating a 50 per cent end-point by interpolation, as in plotting the probit of percentage death against the logarithm of the dose to determine the median lethal dose. **Prochownick's m.,** artificial respiration for asphyxia of the newborn by compression of the child's chest while his head is allowed to hang backward. **protein in milk, m. for,** see *Bogg's m.* **protein in urine, m's for,** see *albumin in urine, m's for.* **protein-free blood filtrate, m's for,** see *Folin's m.* (6), *Folin and Denis' m.* (5), and *Folin and Wu's m.* (5). **Purdy's m.,** the use of the centrifuge for the determination of the quantity of albumin, chlorides, sulfates, etc. **purine bodies, m's for,** see *Hunter and Given's m., Krueger and Schmidt's m., Salkowski's m., Salkowski and Arnstein's m.,* and *Welker's m.,* and see under *tests*. **purine, nitrogen, m. for,** see *nitrogen, purine, m. for.* **Purmann's m.,** extirpation of the aneurysmal sac in aneurysm. **radioactive balloon m.,** a method of intracavitary irradiation of the bladder wall utilizing a Foley catheter bag filled with a radioactive solution. **Raiziss and Dubin's m.** (*for ethereal and inorganic sulfates*): oxidize the urine by Benedict's method, precipitate the sulfate with benzidine hydrochloride, as in the method of Rosenheim and Drummond, and titrate with tenth normal potassium permanganate. **Reed and Muench m.,** a method of calculating a 50 per cent end-point by interpolation, as in plotting the logarithm of the dose against the logarithm of accumulated deaths to determine the median lethal dose. **Rehfuss' m.,** see under *tests*. **retrofilling m.,** a method of filling the root canal of a tooth, particularly the apical portion, from the apex of the root, which has been surgically exposed. **Reverdin's m.,** epidermic graft. **rhythm m.,** a method of preventing conception by restricting coitus to the so-called safe period, avoiding the days just before and after the expected time of ovulation. **Ritchie's formol-ether m.,** a method whereby feces, fixed in a formol-saline solution, is extracted with ether to remove fatty materials, and the washed sediment examined for protozoan cysts and helminth ova. **Ritgen's m.,** see under *maneuver*. **Roaf's m.** (*for the preparation of hippuric acid*): add 125 gm. of ammonium sulfate and 7.5 gm. of concentrated sulfuric acid to 500 ml. of urine of a horse. Hippuric acid will crystallize out. **Romanovsky's (Romanowsky's) m.,** see *Table of Stains*. **Rosenheim and Drummond's m.** (*for ethereal and inorganic sulfates*): precipitate the sulfates with benzidine hydrochloride and titrate the acid in the benzidine sulfate with tenth normal potassium hydroxide. **Ruhemann's uricometer m.** (*for uric acid*): urine is added in a specially graduated tube to a mixture of carbon bisulfide and iodine solution until the carbon bisulfide is decolorized. **Sahli's m.** (*for estimation of hemoglobin*): convert the hemoglobin into acid hematin by adding HCl and compare the color with a standard color scale. **Salkowski's m.** (*for purine bodies and uric acid*): precipitate as silver magnesium salts, decompose the precipitate with hydrogen sulfide, precipitate uric acid by means of sulfuric acid, and the purine bodies as silver salts. **Salkowski and Arnstein's m.** (*for purines*): precipitate the urine with magnesia mixture and to the filtrate add 3 per cent ammoniacal silver nitrate solution. Wash the precipitate and determine the nitrogen in it by the Kjeldahl method. The uric acid nitrogen is separately determined and deducted. **Salkowski, Autenrieth and Barth's m.** (*for oxalic acid*): precipitate the oxalic acid by means of calcium chloride. Dissolve the precipitate in hydrochloric acid, extract the oxalic acid with ether, and reprecipitate it as calcium oxalate. **Satterthwaite's m.,** artificial respiration produced by alternating pressure and relaxation upon the abdomen. **Scherer's m.** (*for proteins*): precipitate the protein by boiling with dilute acetic acid, wash, dry, and weigh. **Schlösser's m.,** see *Schlösser's treatment,* under *treatment*. **Schlossmann's m.,** to prevent polymerization, 10 per cent of glycerin is added to formaldehyde before it is volatilized by heat. **Schüller's m.,** a method of performing artificial respiration by rhythmic raisings of the thorax by means of the fingers hooked under the ribs. **Schweninger's m.,** reduction of obesity by the restriction of fluids in the diet. **Scott and Wilson's m.** (*for acetone and acetoacetic acid*): distil the acetone into an alkaline solution of basic mercuric cyanide, filter, and titrate the precipitate with potassium thiocyanate. **sectional m.,** a method of filling root canals of teeth in which preselected gutta-percha cones are cut into 2 to 3 mm. segments and the canal is filled with these segments in sequential order. **Shaffer's**

m. (*for creatinine*): Folin's method (9), adapted to very dilute solutions. **Shaffer-Hartmann m.,** a chemical method for determining glucose levels in the blood, utilizing a cupric reagent incorporating potassium iodate and iodide and based on the amount of iodate reduced by the cuprous oxide to iodide, and thus on the amount of reducing sugars present. **Shaffer and Marriott's m.** (*for acetone bodies*): precipitate the urine with basic lead acetate and ammonia. Distil off the acetone (acetone and diacetic acid). Oxidize the residue with potassium bichromate and distil again (beta-hydroxybutyric acid). Titrate the distillates with standard iodine and thiosulfate solutions. **Shohl and Pedley's m.** (*for calcium in urine*): oxidize the urine with ammonium persulfate, precipitate the calcium as oxalate, add H_2SO_4 to the precipitate, and titrate with potassium permanganate. **Siffert m.,** a method for computing the volume of the gallbladder by tracing the gallbladder shadow on transparent paper and comparing it with a standard. **single cone m.,** a method of filling the root canal of a tooth with a single, well-fitting gutta-percha cone or silver point in conjunction with a sealer cement or paste. **Sippy m.,** see under *treatment*. **Sjöqvist's m.,** quantitative estimation of the urea in the urine by means of a baryta mixture. **Sluder's m.,** see under *operation*. **Smellie's m.,** delivery of the after-coming head with the body of the child resting on the forearm of the obstetrician. **sodium, m. for,** see *Kramer and Gittleman's m.* **Somogyi m.,** 1. (*for blood glucose*): a modification of the Shaffer-Hartmann method in which the cuprous oxide reduces an arsenomolybdate reagent, yielding a more stable end product. 2. (*for amylase activity*): a method based on the disappearance of the blue color given by iodine and amylose (linear fraction of starch) after amylase in serum, urine, etc., is allowed to act on starch. **Sörensen's m.** (*for amino acids by solution of formaldehyde titration*): titrate the urine for total acidity using phenolphthalein as indicator, add fresh solution of formaldehyde (15 ml. of formalin, 30 ml. of water, and sufficient sodium to make it faintly alkaline to phenolphthalein), and titrate again. **Souligoux-Morestin m.,** the use of ether lavage of the peritoneal cavity in acute infections of the abdominal and pelvic viscera. **specific gravity, m. for,** see *Hammerschlag's m.* and *Fishberg's m.,* and see under *tests*. **split cast m.,** 1. a procedure for placing indexed casts on a dental articulator to facilitate their removal and replacement on the instrument. 2. the procedure of checking the ability of a dental articulator to receive or be adjusted to a maxillomandibular relation record. **Stammer's m.** (*for glucose in blood*): precipitate blood proteins by boiling with acid sodium sulfate and treatment with dialyzed iron. In a test tube place 20 ml. of blood filtrate, 2 drops of a 20 per cent solution of sodium hydroxide and 1 ml. of a 0.0075 per cent solution of methylene blue. Boil until the blue color is discharged. The length of time required indicates the amount of sugar present. Time is counted from the beginning of vigorous boiling: thirty-seven seconds indicates 0.3 per cent sugar; sixty seconds, 0.225 per cent; one minute twenty-five seconds, 0.175 per cent; one minute fifty-five seconds, 0.125 per cent; and two minutes forty-five seconds, 0.075 per cent. **Stas-Otto m.,** a method of separating alkaloids and similar amino compounds. **Stehle's m.** (*for urea*): decompose the urea in a Van Slyke pipet by sodium hypobromite and measure the nitrogen; called also *gastrometric m.* **Steinach's m.,** see *Steinach's operation,* under *operation*. **Stockholm and Koch's m.** (*for total sulfur in biological material*): the material is disintegrated by heating in strong sodium hydroxide, then oxidized with 30 per cent H_2O_2, and then with nitric acid, and bromine. Precipitate the sulfuric acid with barium, wash, dry, ignite, and weigh. **sugar, m's for,** see *glucose (dextrose), m's for.* **sulfates, ethereal, m's for,** see *Folin's m.* (10), *Raiziss and Dubin's m.,* and *Rosenheim and Drummond's m.* **sulfates, inorganic, m's for,** see *Folin's m.* (11), *Raiziss and Dubin's m.,* and *Rosenheim and Drummond's m.* **sulfur, total, m's for,** see *Benedict's m.* (2), *Benedict and Denis' m., Denis and Leche's m., Folin's m.* (14), *Osborne and Folin's m.,* and *Stockholm and Koch's m.* **Sumner's m.** (*for sugar in urine*): heat 1 ml. of urine and 3 ml. of Sumner's dinitrosalicylic acid reagent, dilute to 25 ml. and compare the color with that of a standard sugar solution similarly treated. **suspension m.,** a method of intracavitary irradiation of the bladder wall by instilling a radioactive solution or suspension directly into the bladder by means of a catheter. **Taylor and Hulton's m.** (*for total nitrogen*): similar to Folin and Farmer's method except that small amounts of sulfuric acid are used and the ammonia is nesslerized in the original tube without being aerated over into acid. **Thane's m.,** a method of locating the fissure of Rolando. Its upper end is about one-half inch behind the middle of a line uniting the inion and the glabella, and its lower end about one-quarter inch above and one and one-quarter inches behind the external angular process of the frontal bone. **Thézac-Porsmeur m.,** heliotherapy of suppurating wounds by concentrating the sun's rays on the part by means of a large double convex lens mounted on a cylinder of canvas three feet long. **thyroid activity, m. for,** see *Hunt's m.,* and see *thyroid function tests,* under *tests*. **Tisdall's m.** (*for phenols in urine*): extract the phenolic substances from the urine with ether and then shake them from the ether with 10 per cent NaOH. Neutralize and proceed as in the Folin and Denis method (5). **total acidity,**

m. for, see *Folin's m.* (13). **total fixed base, m. for,** see *Fiske's m.* **total nitrogen, m. for,** see *nitrogen, total, m. for.* **total sulfur, m. for,** see *sulfur, total, m. for.* **Tracy and Welker's m.** (*for deproteinizing urine*): a method depending on the use of aluminum hydroxide cream. **Trillat's m.,** volatilization of formaldehyde in an autoclave under pressure to prevent polymerization. **Trueta m.,** see under *treatment.* **tryptic activity, m. for,** see *Gross's m.* **Tswett's m.,** chromatography. **Tuffier's m.** (*obs.*), see *spinal anesthesia* (def. 1), under *anesthesia.* **turbidity m.** (*for albumin*), see *Folin and Denis' m.* (1). **uranium acetate m.** (*for phosphorus*): add sodium acetate and acetic acid to the urine, heat to boiling, and titrate with a special uranium acetate solution. **urea, m's for,** see *Benedict's m.* (3), *Clark and Collip's m.* (2), *Folin's m.* (15), *Folin and Denis' m.* (6), *Folin and Pettibone's m., Folin and Wu's m.* (6), *Folin and Youngsburg's m., Karr's m., Krogh's m., Marshall's m., Myers' m., Sjöqvist's m., Stehle's m.,* and *Van Slyke and Cullen's m.* (2). See also *urea test,* under *tests.* **urease m's,** see *Marshall's m.* and *Van Slyke and Cullen's m.* (2), and see under *tests.* **uric acid, m's for,** see *Benedict and Franke's m., Benedict and Hitchcock's m., Folin and Denis' m.* (7), *Folin and Shaffer's m., Folin and Wu's m.* (7), *Heintz's m., Hunter and Given's m., Krueger and Schmidt's m., Ruhemann's m.,* and *Salkowski's m.* See also *uric acid test,* under *tests.* **urobilinogen, m. for,** see *Wallace and Diamond's m.,* and see *urobilin test,* under *tests.* **van Gehuchten's m.,** fixing of a histologic tissue in a mixture of glacial acetic acid 10 parts, chloroform 30 parts, and alcohol 60 parts. **Van Slyke's m.** (*for amino-nitrogen*): the unknown is treated with nitrous acid in a special apparatus and the nitrogen liberated is measured. **Van Slyke and Cullen's m.,** 1. (*for the carbon dioxide in blood,* or *for the alkali reserve of blood*): freshly prepared oxalated plasma is brought into equilibrium with the carbon dioxide of expired air, acid is then added to a measured amount of the blood, the carbon dioxide is pumped out and measured. 2. (*for urea*): the urea is changed into ammonium carbonate by means of the enzyme urease, the ammonia is aerated over into standard acid, and the excess titrated. **Van Slyke and Fitz's m.** (*for alkali reserve*): collect the urine for a two-hour period between meals; note amount and determine the ammonia and the titratable acid by Folin's methods. The plasma carbon dioxide capacity (C) may be calculated from the formula $C = 80 - 5\sqrt{D} \div W$, where D = rate of excretion per twenty-four hours, and W = body weight in kilograms. **Van Slyke and Meyer's m.** (*for amino-acid nitrogen*): precipitate the proteins of the blood by means of alcohol and then proceed by Van Slyke's nitrous acid method. **Van Slyke and Palmer's m.** (*for organic acids in urine*): remove carbonates and phosphates and titrate with acid from the turning point for phenolphthalein to the turning point for tropeolin OO. **Volhard and Arnold's m.** (*for chlorides*): acidify the urine with nitric acid and add a known amount of silver nitrate. Titrate excess of silver nitrate with ammonium sulfocyanate, using ferric thiocyanate as indicator. **Volhard and Harvey's m.** (*for chlorides*): similar to the method of Volhard and Arnold except that the silver chloride is not filtered out, the excess of silver nitrate being titrated in the original mixture. **von Fürth and Charnass' m.** (*for lactic acid in blood*): remove the glucose and convert the lactic acid into acetaldehyde by permanganate. Combine the aldehyde with sodium bisulfite and determine the bound sulfite iodometrically. **Walker's m.** (*for iron in foods*): ignite sample, cool, and dissolve in dilute HNO_3. Filter, oxidize, filtrate with H_2O_2, add potassium thiocyanate, and compare color with standard iron solution, similarly treated. **Wallace and Diamond's m.** (*for urobilinogen*): add Ehrlich's aldehyde reagent to a series of dilutions of the urine, note the highest dilution which shows a faint pink coloration, and express the result in terms of this dilution. **Wallhauser and Whitehead's m.,** the use of autogenous gland filtrate in the treatment of Hodgkin's disease. **Wardill four-flap m.,** a method of cleft palate repair using four flaps. **Waring's m.,** a method of sewage disposal by subsurface irrigation; called also *Waring's system.* **Watson's m.** (*for the induction of labor*): the successive administration of castor oil, quinine, and pituitrin. **Weber's m.** (*for guanidine*): a colorimetric method based on the reaction of guanidine with an alkaline nitro-prusside-ferricyanide reagent. **Welcker's m.,** determination of the total blood volume by bleeding and then washing out the blood vessels. **Welker's m.** (*for purine bodies*): remove the phosphates with magnesia mixture, then precipitate the purine bodies with silver nitrate and ammonium hydroxide. Determine nitrogen in the precipitate by Kjeldahl's method. **Welker and Marsh's m.** (*for clarifying milk*): a method using aluminum hydroxide. **Westergren m.** (*for erythrocyte sedimentation rate*): 4.5 ml. of venous blood is mixed thoroughly with 0.5 ml. of a 3.8 per cent solution of sodium citrate; a narrow-bore (2.5 mm.) tube calibrated downward from zero to 200 is then filled with the mixture to the zero mark and placed securely in a rack in an exactly vertical position. The level of red cells is read in millimeters in exactly 60 minutes. **Whipple's m.,** the use of liver in pernicious anemia. **Whitehorn's m.** (*for chlorides in blood*): to the protein-free blood filtrate add nitric acid, then heat, and add an excess of silver nitrate. Titrate excess silver with thiocyanate, using ferric ammonium sulfate as indicator. **Wiechowski**

and Handorsky's m. (*for allantoin*): precipitate the urine with phosphotungstic acid, with lead acetate, and with silver acetate to remove chlorides, ammonia, and basic substances. Then add sodium acetate and 0.5 per cent mercuric acetate to precipitate the allantoin, which may be weighed, submitted to a Kjeldahl, or titrated with ammonium thiocyanate. **Wintrobe and Landsberg's m.** (*for the sedimentation rate of red blood cells*): determine the amount of sedimentation after one hour, then centrifuge and measure the volume of the packed red cells. Correct the first reading by the second by means of a table. **Wolter's m.** (*for iron*): add nitric acid to urine, evaporate to dryness, ignite, oxidize the iron with hydrogen peroxide, add potassium iodide and starch, and titrate excess of iodine with one-hundredth normal thiosulfate. **Wright's m.,** treatment of wounds by irrigating first with hypertonic salt solution and then with isotonic salt solution. Vaccines may be used as adjuvants. Finally the wound is closed. **Wynn m.,** a procedure for repair of bilateral cleft lips by means of a long, narrow triangular flap. **Ziehl-Neelsen's m.,** see *acid-fast stain* in *Table of Stains.* **Zsigmondy's gold number m.,** colloidal gold test.

methodism (meth′ŏ-dizm) the system of the Methodist school of medicine.

Methodist (meth′ŏ-dist) 1. an ancient sect or school, which based the practice of medicine on a few simple rules and theories. This school, influenced by Asclepiades, was founded (c. 50 B.C.) by Themison of Laodicea. The Methodists believed that disease is caused either by a narrowing of the internal pores of the body (*status strictus*) or by their excessive relaxation (*status laxus*). Such extreme simplification of the nature of disease is discernible as late as the 18th century, for example, in the so-called Brunonian system (John Brown, 1735–1788). 2. A believer in or practitioner of the Methodist theory of medicine.

methodology (meth″ŏ-dol′o-je) the science of method; the science which deals with the principles of procedure in research and study.

methohexital (meth″o-hek′sĭ-tal) [USP] chemical name: (±)-1-methyl-5-(1-methyl-2-pentynyl)-5-(2-propenyl)-2, 4, 6(1*H,* 3*H,* 5*H*)-pyrimidinetrione. An ultrashort-acting barbiturate, $C_{14}H_{18}$-N_2O_3, occurring as a white to faintly yellowish white, crystalline powder; used as a pharmaceutic necessary in the preparation of the sodium salt for injection. **m. sodium** [USP], the monosodium salt of methohexital, $C_{14}H_{17}N_2NaO_3$, occurring as a white to off-white hygroscopic powder; used as a general anesthetic, administered intravenously.

methomania (meth″o-ma′ne-ah) [Gr. *methē* drunkenness + *mania* madness] morbid desire for alcoholic beverages.

methopholine (meth″o-fo′lēn) chemical name: 1-(*p*-chlorophenethyl)-1,2,3,4-tetrahydro-6,7-dimethoxy-2-methylisoquinoline; an analgesic, $C_{20}H_{24}ClNO$.

methopromazine maleate (meth″o-pro′mah-zēn) methoxypromazine maleate.

methotrexate (meth″o-trek′sāt) [USP] chemical name: *N*-[4-[[(2,4-diamino-6-pteridinyl)methyl]methylamino]benzoyl]-L-glutamic acid. A folic acid antagonist, $C_{20}H_{22}N_8O_5$, occurring as an orange-brown, crystalline powder; used as an antineoplastic agent in the treatment of acute and subacute lymphocytic and meningeal leukemia, gestational choriocarcinoma, chorioadenoma destruens, hydatidiform mole, and advanced stages of lymphosarcoma, and as an antipsoriatic agent, administered orally and intramuscularly. It has also been used as an immunosuppressive agent in immunologically mediated disorders.

methotrimeprazine (meth″o-tri-mep′rah-zēn) [USP] chemical name: (−)-2-methoxy-*N,N*β-trimethyl-10*H*-phenothiazine-10-propanamine. An analgesic, $C_{19}H_{24}N_2OS$, occurring as a fine, white, crystalline powder; administered intramuscularly. Called also *levomepromazine.*

methoxamine hydrochloride (mě-thok′sah-mēn) chemical name: α-(1-aminoethyl)-2,5-dimethoxybenzenemethanol hydrochloride. An adrenergic, $C_{11}H_{17}NO_3 \cdot HCl$, occurring as colorless or white, platelike crystals or white, crystalline powder; used for its vasopressor effect to support, restore, or maintain blood pressure during anesthesia and in the treatment of paroxysmal supraventricular tachycardia, administered intramuscularly and intravenously.

methoxsalen (mě-thok′sah-len) [USP] chemical name: 9-methoxy-7*H*-furo[3,2-g][1]benzopyran-7-one. A psoralen found in *Amni majus* and other plants, $C_{12}H_8O_4$, occurring as white to cream-colored fluffy, needle-like crystals; used orally and topically in conjunction with exposure to ultraviolet light to facilitate repigmentation in idiopathic vitiligo, and to produce a phototoxic reaction in psoriasis. It is also used as a suntan accelerator and sun protectant.

methoxychlor (mě-thok′se-klor) chemical name: 1,1′-(2,2,2-trichloroethylidene)bis[4-methoxybenzene]. A chlorinated hydrocarbon insecticide, $C_{16}H_{15}Cl_3O_2$, effective against mosquito larvae and houseflies.

methoxyflurane (mě-thok″se-floo′rān) [USP] chemical name: 2,2-dichloro-1,1-difluoro-1-methoxyethane. A general anesthetic with analgestic action, $C_3H_4Cl_2F_2O$, occurring as a clear, colorless, mobile liquid; administered by inhalation.

methoxyl (mĕ-thok′sil) the chemical group, $CH_3 \cdot O—$.

methoxyphenamine hydrochloride (mĕ-thok″se-fen′ah-mēn) [USP] chemical name: 2-methoxy-N,α-dimethybenzene-ethanamine hydrochloride. An adrenergic, $C_{11}H_{17}NO \cdot HCl$, occurring as a white to off-white, crystalline powder; used mainly as a bronchodilator in the treatment of bronchial asthma, administered orally.

methoxypromazine maleate (mĕ-thok″se-pro′mah-zēn) chemical name: 2-methoxy-N,N-dimethyl-10H-phenothiazine-10-propanamine maleate; a central depressant, $C_{22}H_{26}N_2O_5S$. Called also *methopromazine maleate*.

8-methoxypsoralen (mĕ-thok″se-sor′ah-len) methoxsalen.

methphenoxydiol (meth″fen-ok″sĭ-di′ol) guaifenesin.

methscopolamine bromide (meth″sko-pol′ah-mēn) [USP] chemical name: [7(S)-(1α,2β,4β,5α,7β)]-7-(3-hydroxy-1-oxo-2-phenylpropoxy)-9,9-dimethyl-3-oxa-9-azoniatricyclo[3.3.1.0²,⁴]nonane bromide. An anticholinergic, the quaternary ammonium derivative of scopolamine hydrobromide, $C_{18}H_{24}BrNO_4$, occurring as white crystals or as a white, crystalline powder, it has an inhibitory effect on gastric secretion and gastrointestinal motility and is used as an adjunct for the treatment of peptic ulcer and gastric disorders associated with spasm, hyperacidity, and hypermotility, administered orally, subcutaneously, and intramuscularly. Called also *scopolamine methylbromide*.

methsuximide (meth-suk′sĭ-mīd) [USP] chemical name: 1,3-dimethyl-3-phenyl-2,5-pyrrolidinedione. An anticonvulsant, $C_{12}H_{13}NO_2$, occurring as a white to grayish white, crystalline powder; used in the treatment of petit mal and psychomotor epilepsy, administered orally.

methyclothiazide (meth″ĭ-klo-thi′ah-zīd) [USP] chemical name: 6-chloro-3-(chloromethyl)-3,4-dihydro-2-methyl-2H-1,2,4-benzothiadiazine-7-sulfonamide 1,1-dioxide. An orally effective diuretic and antihypertensive drug, $C_9H_{11}Cl_2N_3O_4S_2$, occurring as a white or practically white, crystalline powder; used in the treatment of hypertension and in edema associated with congestive heart failure, hepatic cirrhosis, chronic renal disease, pregnancy, premenstrual syndrome, obesity, and corticosteroid and estrogen therapy.

methyl (meth′il) [Gr. *methy* wine + *hylē* wood] the chemical group or radical $CH_3—$, sometimes abbreviated Me. **m. amylketone,** a volatile oil, $C_5H_{11} \cdot CO \cdot CH_3$, found in oil of cloves. **m. anthranilate,** chemical name: methyl 2-aminobenzoate. A volatile oil $NH_2 \cdot C_6H_4 \cdot CO \cdot O \cdot CH_3$, the odoriferous constituent or neroli oil, bergamot, jasmine, and other essential oils. **m. benzene,** toluene. **m. chloride,** the hydrochloric acid ester of methyl alcohol, CH_3Cl. When converted by pressure from gas into liquid, it can be used in spray form as a local anesthetic. **m. cyanide,** acetonitrile. **m. ethyl-maleicimid,** a substituted pyrrole, $C_2H_5(C \cdot CO \cdot NH \cdot CO)CCH_3$, obtained from hemoglobin and from chlorophyl. **m. ethyl-pyrrole,** a substituted pyrrole, $CH_3(C:CH \cdot NH:CH:C)C_2H_5$, obtained from, and probably a constituent of, bilirubin. **m. eugenol,** a volatile oil, $C_3H_5 \cdot C_6H_3(OCH_3)_2$, found in oil of bay. **m. heptenone,** a volatile oil, $C_8H_{16}O$, found in lemon-grass oil. **m. hydride,** methane. **m. hydroxy-furfurol,** the furfural, $CH_3 \cdot C:CH \cdot C(OH):C \cdot CHO$, produced from the hexose in Molisch's test and which produces the color. **m. iodide,** a colorless or brownish liquid, CH_3I, used as a local anesthetic and formerly as a vesicant. **m. isobutyl ketone** [NF], chemical name: 4-methyl-2-pentanone. A transparent, colorless, mobile, volatile liquid, $C_6H_{12}O$; used as an alcohol denaturant in pharmaceutical preparations. **m. methacrylate,** a plastic material, a resin, $C_5H_8O_2$, used in dentistry and as the basis for an acrylic bone cement in orthopedic surgery, as in total hip replacement. **m. salicylate** [NF], chemical name: 2-hydroxybenzoic acid methyl ester. A colorless, yellowish, or reddish liquid, $C_8H_8O_3$, produced synthetically or obtained by maceration and subsequent distillation with steam from the leaves of *Gaultheria procumbens* or from the bark of *Betula lenta;* used as a flavor in pharmaceutic preparations, and topically in liniments, ointments, and lotions as a counterirritant to relieve pain in rheumatic conditions, lumbago, and sciatica. It is a common cause of salicytate poisoning in children. Called also *betula oil, gaultheria oil, sweet birch oil,* and *wintergreen* oil. **m. sulfonate,** a crystalline, noncaustic, and nonpoisonous antiseptic. **m. telluride,** a gas, $(CH_3)_2Te$, of penetrating odor found in excreta of animals after feeding with telluric and tellurious acids.

methylal (meth′ĭ-lal) a colorless liquid, $CH_2(OCH_3)_2$, used as a hypnotic and anesthetic and like formaldehyde in certain chemical reactions.

methylamine (meth″il-am′in) a gaseous ptomaine CH_3NH_2, from decaying fish and from comma-bacillus cultures.

methylarsinate (meth″il-ar′si-nāt) a salt of methylarsinic acid.

methylate (meth′ĭ-lāt) 1. a compound of methyl alcohol and a base. 2. to add methyl group to a substance.

methylated (meth″ĭ-lāt-ed) containing or combined with a methyl group.

methylation (meth″ĭ-la′shun) treatment with reagent to add a methyl group to a compound.

methylatropine nitrate (meth″il-at′ro-pēn) chemical name: endo-(+)-3-(3-hydroxy-1-oxo-2-phenylpropoxy)-8,8-dimethyl-8-azoniabicyclo[3.2.1] octane nitrate (salt). A quaternary ammonium derivative of atropine, $C_{18}H_{26}N_2O_6$, having the same actions and uses as atropine (q.v.), but with much less effect on the central nervous system and with strong ganglionic blocking activity. Called also *atropine methonitrate* and *atropine methylnitrate*.

methylaurin (meth″il-aw′rin) a substance, $C_{23}H_{16}O_3$, derivable from aurin.

methylbenzethonium chloride (meth″il-ben″zĕ-tho′ne-um) [USP] chemical name: N,N-dimethyl-N-[2-[2-[methyl-4-(1,1,3,3-tetramethylbutyl)phenoxy]ethoxy]ethyl]benzenemethanaminium chloride monohydrate. A disinfectant quaternary compound, $C_{28}H_{44}ClNO_2 \cdot H_2O$, occurring as white crystals, which is bacteriostatic for urea-splitting organisms that may cause ammonia dermatitis. It is applied topically to areas of the skin coming in contact with urine, feces, or perspiration, and is used in a rinse for diapers, bed linen, and undergarments of incontinent adults and children.

methylcellulose (meth″il-sel′u-lōs) [USP] a methyl ether of cellulose, occurring as a white, fibrous powder or granules, supplied in differing degrees of viscosity; used as a suspending and viscosity-increasing agent and tablet excipient in pharmaceutical preparations, administered orally as a cathartic, and applied topically to the conjunctiva to protect the cornea during certain ophthalmic procedures and to lubricate the cornea. **hydroxypropyl m.,** see under *H.*

methylchloroformate (meth″il-klo″ro-for′māt) a lacrimatory gas, $ClCOOCH_3$, used as a warning agent in fumigations with hydrocyanic acid.

methylcholanthrene (meth″il-ko-lan′thrēn) a carcinogenic hydrocarbon, $C_{21}H_{16}$, from deoxycholic acid, cholic acid, and cholesterol.

methylcreosol (meth″il-kre′o-sol) a phenol, $C_9H_{12}O_2$, obtainable from wood tar creosote.

methylcytosine (meth″il-si′to-sin) a pyrimidine occurring in deoxyribonucleic acid.

methyldichlorarsin (meth″il-di″klor-ar′sin) a lethal and vesicating war gas, CH_3AsCl_2.

methyldihydromorphinone (meth″il-di-hi″dro-mor′fĭ-nōn) metopon (def. 2).

methyldopa (meth″il-do′pah) [USP] chemical name: 3-hydroxy-α-methyl-L-tyrosine. An orally effective antihypertensive, $C_{10}H_{13}NO_4 1\frac{1}{2}H_2O$, occurring as a white to yellowish white, fine powder.

methyldopate hydrochloride (meth″il-do′pāt) [USP] chemical name: 3-hydroxy-α-methyl-L-tyrosine ethyl ester hydrochloride. The ethyl ester hydrochloride of methyldopa, $C_{12}H_{17}NO_4 \cdot HCl$, occurring as a white to practically white, crystalline powder; used as an antihypertensive, administered by intravenous infusion.

methylene (meth″ĭ-lēn) the bivalent hydrocarbon radical, CH_2. **m. bichloride,** 1. see *m. chloride.* 2. a mixture of methyl alcohol and chloroform formerly used as an anesthetic agent. **m. blue,** see under *blue.* **m. chloride, m. dichloride,** a volatile anesthetic liquid, CH_2Cl_2, resembling chloroform, formerly used as an anesthetic in minor operations.

methylenophil (meth″ĭ-len′o-fil) 1. an element easily stainable with methylene blue. 2. methylenophilous.

methylenophilous (meth″il-en-of′ĭ-lus) [*methylene* + Gr. *philein* to love] stainable with methylene blue.

methylergonovine maleate (meth″il-er″go-no′vēn) [USP] chemical name: 9,10-didehydro-N-[1-(hydroxymethyl)propyl]-6-methylergoline-8β(S)-carboxamide (Z)-2-butenedioate (1:1) (salt). An oxytocic, $C_{20}H_{25}N_3O_2 \cdot C_4H_4O_4$, occurring as a white to pinkish tan, microcrystalline powder; used especially to prevent or combat postpartum hemorrhage and atony, administered orally, intramuscularly, and intravenously.

methylglucamine (meth″il-gloo′kah-mīn) 1. a compound prepared from D-glucose and methylamine, used in the synthesis of pharmaceuticals. 2. meglumine.

methylglyoxalase (meth″il-gli-oks′ah-lās) an enzyme that catalyzes the change of methylglyoxal to lactic acid.

methylglyoxalidin (meth″il-gli″oks-al′ĭ-din) lysidin.

methylguanidine (meth″il-gwan′ĭ-din) a poisonous ptomaine, $NH \cdot C(NH)_2NH \cdot CH_3$, from spoiled fish, etc.

methylhexamine (meth″il-heks′ah-mēn) methylhexaneamine.

methylhexaneamine (meth″il-hek-sān′ah-min) chemical name: 1,3-dimethylamylamine. A colorless to pale yellow liquid, $C_7H_{17}N$, readily soluble in alcohol, used for its sympathomimetic action in nasal congestion. Called also *methyhexamine.*

methylhydantoin (meth″il-hi-dan′to-in) a crystalline compound, $CH_3 \cdot N \cdot CO \cdot NH \cdot CO \cdot CH_2$, found in fresh meat, and formed by the decomposition of creatine.

methylic (mĕ-thil′ik) containing methyl.

methylindol (meth″il-in′dōl) skatole.

methylmelubrin (meth″il-mel′u-brin) dipyrone.

methylmercaptan (meth″il-mer-kap′tan) a gas, methyl hydrosulfide, CH$_3$·SH, formed in the intestines by the decomposition of proteins; said to impart to the urine the odor noticed after eating asparagus, and to the breath the characterisic odor of fetor hepatis.

methylmorphine (meth″il-mor′fēn) codeine.

methylparaben (meth″il-par′ah-ben) [NF] chemical name: 4-hydroxybenzoic acid methyl ester. An antifungal agent, C$_8$H$_8$O$_3$, occurring as small, colorless crystals, or white, crystalline powder; used as a preservative in pharmaceutical preparations.

methylparafynol (meth″il-par′ah-fi′nol) meparfynol.

methylpentynol (meth″il-pen′tĭ-nol) meparfynol.

methylphenidate hydrochloride (meth″il-fen′ĭ-dāt) [USP] chemical name: (R*,R*)-(+)-α-phenyl-2-piperidineacetic acid methyl ester hydrochloride. A central stimulant, C$_{14}$H$_{19}$NO$_2$·HCl, occurring as a white, fine, crystalline powder; used in the treatment of hyperkinetic children, various types of depression, and narcolepsy, administered orally.

methylphenyl levulosazone (meth″il-fen′il lev″u-lo′sa-zōn) the methyl-phenyl-osazone of levulose, CH$_2$OH(CHOH)$_4$C[:N·N-(CH$_3$)·C$_6$H$_5$]·CHCH·NHN(CH$_3$)·C$_6$H$_5$:, homologous with glucosazone.

methylphenylhydrazine (meth″il-fe″nil-hi′drah-zin) a reagent, C$_6$H$_5$N(CH$_3$)NH$_2$, by which ketoses can be distinguished from aldoses, as the former yield osazones, the latter, hydrazines.

methylprednisolone (meth″il-pred′nĭ-so-lōn) [USP] chemical name: 11β,17, 21-trihydroxy-6α-methylpregna-1,4-diene. A synthetic glucocorticoid derived from prednisolone, C$_{22}$H$_{30}$O$_5$, with slightly greater anti-inflammatory activity and slightly less sodium-retaining activity than prednisolone; occurring as a white to practically white, crystalline powder, it is administered orally in the treatment of various conditions responsive to the anti-inflammatory actions of glucocorticoids, including rheumatoid arthritis and other collagen diseases, allergic conditions, and certain inflammatory eye diseases, and in acquired hemolytic anemias, lymphoma, and leukemia. **m. acetate** [USP], the 21-acetate ester of methylprednisolone, C$_{24}$H$_{32}$O$_6$, occurring as a white or practically white, crystalline powder, having actions and uses similar to those of the base; administered by enema, intra-articular, intramuscular, intralesional, or intracutaneous injection, and applied topically. **m. hemisuccinate** [USP], the hemisuccinate salt of methylprednisolone, C$_{26}$H$_{34}$O$_8$, occurring as a white or nearly white hygroscopic solid, having actions and uses similar to those of the base. **m. sodium phosphate,** the 21-phosphate disodium salt of methylprednisolone, C$_{22}$H$_{29}$Na$_2$O$_8$P, having actions similar to those of the base. **m. sodium succinate** [USP], the 21-succinate sodium salt of methylprednisolone, C$_{26}$-H$_{33}$NaO$_8$, occurring as a white or nearly white, amorphous solid, having actions and uses similar to those of the base; used chiefly for short-term emergency treatment, administered by intramuscular or intravenous injection.

methylpurine (meth″il-pu′rin) see under *purine*.

methylpyrapone (meth″il-pi′rah-pōn) metyrapone.

methylpyridine (meth″il-pi′ri-din) a basic substance, C$_5$H$_4$-(CH$_3$)N, oxidized in the body to pyridine-carboxylic acid.

methylquinoline (meth″il-kwin′o-lin) an oily basic substance, C$_9$H$_6$N·CH$_3$, from the secretion of the skunk.

methylrosaniline chloride (meth″il-ro-zan′i-lin) gentian violet; see under *violet*.

methyltestosterone (meth″il-tes-tos′ter-ōn) [USP] chemical name: 17β-hydroxy-17α-methylandrost-4-en-3-one. A synthetic androgen derived from cholesterol, C$_{20}$H$_{30}$O$_2$, occurring as white or creamy white crystals or crystalline powder, having actions similar to those of testosterone (q.v.); used as replacement therapy for androgen deficiency in males, in the palliation of certain inoperable mammary cancers, and to prevent postpartum breast pain and engorgement in the non-nursing mother, administered orally or sublingually.

methyltheobromine (meth″il-the″o-bro′mēn) caffeine.

methylthionine chloride (meth″il-thi′o-nin) methylene blue.

methylthiouracil (meth″il-thi″o-u′rah-sil) [USP] chemical name: 2,3-dihydro-6-methyl-2-thioxo-4(1H)-pyrimidinone. A thyroid suppressant, C$_5$H$_6$N$_2$OS, occurring as a white, crystalline powder; used in the treatment of hyperthyroidism, especially to prepare patients for thyroid surgery and to maintain those who are poor surgical risks, administered orally. Abbreviated MTU.

methyltransferase (meth″il-trans′fer-ās) any enzyme that catalyzes transmethylation, for example, the transfer of methyl groups from methionine (S-adenosylmethionine) to nicotinamide to form N-methylnicotinamide, to guanidinoacetic acid to form creatine, or to methylated bases of nucleic acids. Called also *transmethylase*.

methyluramine (meth″il-u-ram′in) methylguanidine.

methylxanthine (meth″il-zan′thin) any of the methylated derivatives of xanthine, including caffeine, theobromine, and theophylline and their derivatives.

methynodiol diacetate (mĕ-thin″o-di′ōl) chemical name: 11β-methyl-19-norpregn-4-en-20-yne-3β,17α-diol; a progestin, C$_{25}$H$_{34}$O$_4$.

methyprylon (meth″ĭ-pri′lon) [USP] chemical name: 3,3-diethyl-5-methyl-2,4-piperidinedione. A hypnotic, C$_{10}$H$_{17}$NO$_2$, occurring as a white, or nearly white, crystalline powder; administered orally.

methysergide (meth″ĭ-ser′jīd) chemical name: 9,10-didehydro-N-[1-(hydroxymethyl)propyl]-1,6-dimethylergoline-8-β-carboxamide. A potent serotonin antagonist, C$_{21}$H$_{27}$N$_3$O$_2$, having direct vasoconstrictor effects. **m. maleate** [USP], the maleate salt of methysergide, C$_{21}$H$_{27}$N$_3$O$_2$·C$_4$H$_4$O$_4$, occurring as a white to yellowish white or reddish white, crystalline powder, having the same actions as the base; used as an analgesic in the treatment of vascular (migraine) headache in certain patients, administered orally.

metiamide (mĕ-ti′ah-mīd) chemical name: N-methyl-N′-[2-[[(5-methyl-1H-imidazol-4-yl)methyl]thio]ethyl]thiourea; a histamine H$_2$-antagonist, C$_9$H$_{16}$N$_4$S$_2$.

metiapine (mĕ-ti′ah-pēn) chemical name: 2-methyl-11-(4-methyl-1-piperazinyl)dibenzo[b,f][1,4]thiazepine; a tranquilizer, C$_{19}$H$_{21}$N$_3$S, which has been used in the treatment of schizophrenia.

Meticortelone (met″ĭ-kor′tĕ-lōn) trademark for preparations of prednisolone.

Meticorten (met″ĭ-kor′ten) trademark for a preparation of prednisone.

metizoline hydrochloride (mĕ-tiz′o-lēn) chemical name: 4,5-dihydro-2-[(2-methylbenzo[b]thien-3-yl)methyl]-1H-imidazole monohydrochloride; an adrenergic with vasoconstrictor effects, C$_{13}$H$_{14}$N$_2$S·HCl.

metmyoglobin (met-mi″o-glo′bin) a compound formed from myoglobin by oxidation of the ferrous to the ferric state.

metoclopramide hydrochloride (met″o-klo′prah-mīd) chemical name: 4-amino-5-chloro-N-[2-(diethylamino)ethyl]-o-anisamide monohydrochloride; an antiemetic, C$_{14}$H$_{22}$ClN$_3$O$_2$·HCl.

metocurine iodide (met″o-ku′rēn) [USP] chemical name: 6,6′,6′,12′-tetramethoxy-2,2,2′,2′-tetramethyltubocuraranium diiodide. A skeletal muscle relaxant, C$_{40}$H$_{48}$I$_2$N$_2$O$_6$, occurring as a white or nearly white, crystalline powder; administered intravenously. Called also *dimethyl tubocurarine iodide*.

metoestrum (met-es′trum) metestrus.

metoestrus (met-es′trus) metestrus.

metogest (met′o-jest) chemical name: 17β-hydroxy-16,16-dimethylestr-4-en-3-one; a hormone, C$_{20}$H$_{30}$O$_2$.

Metol (me′tol) trademark for a photographic developer, N-methyl-p-aminophenol sulfate, CH$_3$NHC$_6$H$_4$OH·H$_2$SO$_4$, which sometimes is the cause of a dermatitis in those who use it.

metolazone (mĕ-tōl′ah-zōn) chemical name: 7-chloro-1,2,3,4-tetrahydro-2-methyl-3-(2-methylphenyl)-4-oxo-6-quinazolinesulfonamide. A diuretic, saluretic, and antihypertensive, C$_{16}$H$_{16}$-ClN$_3$O$_3$S, used in the treatment of mild to moderate hypertension and edema associated with congestive heart failure and renal disease, administered orally.

metonymy (mĕ-ton′ĭ-me) [*meta-* + Gr. *onyma* name] disorder of thinking in which the patient uses, instead of the correct term, a poor approximation to it.

metopagus (mĕ-top′ah-gus) metopopagus.

metopic (me-top′ik) pertaining to the forehead; frontal.

metopimazine (met″o-pim′ah-zēn) chemical name: 1-[3-[2-(methylsulfonyl)phenothiazin-10-yl]propyl]isonipecotamide; an antiemetic, C$_{22}$H$_{27}$N$_3$O$_3$S$_2$.

metopion (mĕ-to′pe-on) glabella.

Metopirone (met″o-pi′rōn) trademark for preparations of metyrapone.

metopism (met′o-pizm) the persistence of the frontal suture.

metopo- [Gr. *metōpon* forehead] a combining form denoting relationship to the forehead.

metopodynia (met″o-po-din′e-ah) [*metopo-* + Gr. *odynē* pain] frontal headache.

metopon (mĕ-to′pon) 1. [Gr. *metōpon* forehead] (*obs.*) the anterior portion of the frontal lobe of the brain. 2. a morphine derivative, methyldihydromorphinone hydrochloride, used to relieve pain.

metopopagus (met″o-pop′ah-gus) [*metopo-* + Gr. *pagos* thing fixed] a craniopagus in which the fusion is in the region of the forehead.

metoposcopy (met″o-pos′ko-pe) [*metopo-* + Gr. *skopein* to examine] the analysis of character based on shape of the forehead.

metoprine (met′o-prēn) chemical name: 5-(3,4-dichlorophenyl)-6-methyl-2,4-pyrimidinediamine; an antineoplastic, C$_{11}$H$_{10}$Cl$_2$N$_4$.

metoprolol (mĕ-to′pro-lōl) chemical name: 1-[4-(2-methoxyethyl)phenyl]-3-[(1-methylethyl)amino-2-propanol; an antiadrenergic, $C_{15}H_{25}NO_3$, which is chiefly a beta$_1$ blocker. Used orally in the treatment of hypertension.

Metorchis (met-or'kis) [*meta-* + Gr. *orchis* testicle] *Pseudamphistomum.*

metoserpate hydrochloride (met"o-ser'pāt) chemical name: methyl 11,17α,18α-trimethoxy-3β,20α-yohimban-16β-carboxylate monohydrochloride; a veterinary sedative, $C_{24}H_{32}N_2O_5 \cdot HCl$.

metoxenous (mě-tok'sě-nus) [*meta-* + Gr. *xenos* host] requiring two hosts for the full cycle of existence; said of certain parasites.

metoxeny (mě-tok'sě-ne) the condition of being metoxenous.

metra (me'trah) [Gr. *metra* womb] the uterus, or womb.

metra- see *metro-.*

metralgia (mě-tral'je-ah) [*metra-* + *-algia*] pain in the uterus; metrodynia.

metraterm (me'trah-term) [*metra-* + L. *terminus* boundary] the external opening of the uterus in some tapeworms (Diphyllobothriidae).

metratonia (me"trah-to'ne-ah) [*metra-* + Gr. *atonia* atony] uterine atony.

metratrophia (me"trah-tro'fe-ah) [*metra-* + Gr. *atrophia* atrophy] uterine atrophy.

Metrazol (met'rah-zol) trademark for preparations of pentylenetetrazol. See also under therapy.

metre (me'ter) meter.

metrechoscopy (met"rě-kos'ko-pe) [Gr. *metron* measure + *ēchō* sound + *skopein* to examine] combined mensuration, auscultation, and inspection.

metrectasia (me"trek-ta'se-ah) [*metra-* + Gr. *ektasis* extension] dilatation of the nonpregnant uterus.

metrectomy (mě-trek'to-me) [*metra-* + Gr. *ektomē* excision] hysterectomy.

metrectopia (me"trek-to'pe-ah) [*metra-* + Gr. *ektopos* displaced + *-ia*] uterine displacement.

Metreton (met'rě-ton) trademark for a preparation of prednisolone sodium phosphate.

metreurynter (me"troo-rin'ter) [*metra-* + Gr. *eurynein* to stretch] an inflatable bag for dilating the cervical canal of the uterus.

metreurysis (me-troo'ri-sis) dilatation of the uterine cervix with the metreurynter.

metria (me'tre-ah) any inflammatory condition of the uterus during the puerperium.

metric (met'rik) [Gr. *metron* measure] 1. pertaining to measures based on the meter; see *Table of Weights and Measures.* 2. having the meter as a basis.

metrifonate (met"ri-fo'nāt) chemical name: (2,2,2-trichloro-1-hydroxyethyl)phosphoric acid dimethyl ester. An organophosphorus insecticide, $C_4H_8Cl_3O_4P$, used externally as a topical ectoparasiticide and internally as a veterinary anthelmintic. Called also *trichlorfon.*

metriocephalic (met"re-o-sě-fal'ik) [Gr. *metrios* moderate + *kephalē* head] having a skull with a vertical index between 72 and 77.

metriphonate (met"ri-fo'nāt) metrifonate.

metritis (mě-tri'tis) [*metra-* + *-itis*] inflammation of the uterus. Several varieties are named, according to the part of the organ affected—cervical, corporeal, interstitial, and parenchymatous. **m. dis'secans, dissecting m.,** metritis characterized by the passage of fragments or large masses of the necrotic uterine wall.

puerperal m., infection of the uterus of the puerperal woman.

metrizamide (mě-triz'ah-mīd) chemical name: 2-[[3-(acetylamino)-5-(acetylmethylamino)-2,4,6-triiodobenzoyl]amino]-2-deoxy-D-glucose. A radiopaque medium, $C_{18}H_{22}I_3N_3O_8$, used in lumbar myelography; it is water-soluble and is absorbed into the blood stream from the cerebrospinal fluid.

metrizoate sodium (met-ri-zo'āt) chemical name: 3-acetamido-2,4,6-triiodo-5-(*N*-methylacetamido)benzoate; a diagnostic radiopaque medium, $C_{12}H_{10}I_3N_2NaO_4$.

metro-, metra- [Gr. *metra* uterus] a combining form denoting relationship to the uterus. See also *hystero-,* and words beginning thus.

metrocarcinoma (me"tro-kar"si-no'mah) endometrial carcinoma.

metrocele (me'tro-sēl) [*metro-* + Gr. *kēlē* hernia] hernia of the uterus; hysterocele.

metrocolpocele (me"tro-kol'po-sēl) [*metro-* + Gr. *kolpos* vagina + *kēlē* hernia] hernia of the uterus and the vagina.

metrocystosis (me"tro-sis-to'sis) formation of cysts in the uterus.

metrocyte (me'tro-sīt) [Gr. *mētēr* mother + *-cyte*] a mother cell.

metrodynia (me"tro-din'e-ah) [*metro-* + Gr. *odynē* pain] pain in the uterus; metralgia.

metroendometritis (me"tro-en"do-me-tri'tis) combined inflammation of the uterus and its mucous membranes.

metrofibroma (me"tro-fi-bro'mah) [*metro-* + *fibroma*] leiomyoma of the uterus.

metrogenous (mě-troj'ě-nus) derived from the uterus.

metrography (mě-trog'rah-fe) hysterography.

metroleukorrhea (me"tro-lu"ko-re'ah) leukorrhea of uterine origin.

metrology (mě-trol'o-je) [Gr. *metron* measure + *-logy*] the science which deals with measurement.

metrolymphangitis (me"tro-limf"an-ji'tis) inflammation of the uterine lymphatic vessels.

metromalacia (me"tro-mah-la'she-ah) [*metro-* + Gr. *malakia* softness] abnormal softening of the uterus.

metromalacoma (me"tro-mal-ah-ko'mah) metromalacia.

metromenorrhagia (me"tro-men"o-ra'je-ah) metrorrhagia combined with menorrhagia.

metronidazole (me"tro-ni'dah-zōl) [USP] chemical name: 2-methyl-5-nitro-1*H*-imidazole-1-ethanol. An antitrichomonal and antiamebic, $C_6H_9N_3O_3$, occurring as white to pale yellow crystals or crystalline powder; administered orally and intravaginally in *Trichomonas vaginalis* infection in females and orally in male trichomoniasis, and administered orally in intestinal and extraintestinal amebiasis. It is also effective against infections with *Giardia lamblia* and obligate anaerobic bacteria.

metronoscope (mě-tron'o-skōp) an instrument for giving exercises in rhythmic reading to correct poorly coordinated ocular movements.

metroparalysis (me"tro-pah-ral'i-sis) paralysis of the uterus.

metropathia (me"tro-path'e-ah) metropathy. **m. hemorrha'gica,** essential uterine hemorrhage.

MULTIPLES AND SUBMULTIPLES OF THE METRIC SYSTEM

MULTIPLES AND SUBMULTIPLES	PREFIX	PRONUNCIATION	SYMBOL
$1,000,000,000,000 = 10^{12}$	tera	ter'a	T
$1,000,000,000 = 10^9$	giga	ji'ga	G
$1,000,000 = 10^6$	mega	meg'a	M
$1,000 = 10^3$	kilo	kil'o	k
$100 = 10^2$	hecto	hek'to	h
$10 = 10$	deka	dek'a	dk
[The unit = one]			
$0.1 = 10^{-1}$	deci	des'i	d
$0.01 = 10^{-2}$	centi	sen'ti	c
$0.001 = 10^{-3}$	milli	mil'i	m
$0.000\ 001 = 10^{-6}$	micro	mi'kro	μ
$0.000\ 000\ 001 = 10^{-9}$	nano	nan'o	n
$0.000\ 000\ 000\ 001 = 10^{-12}$	pico	pe'co	p
$0.000\ 000\ 000\ 000\ 001 = 10^{-15}$	femto	fem'to	f
$0.000\ 000\ 000\ 000\ 000\ 001 = 10^{-18}$	atto	at'to	a

International Committee on Weights and Measures, 1962. From Style Manual for Biological Journals.

metropathic (me″tro-path′ik) pertaining to or characterized by uterine disorder.

metropathy (mĕ-trop′ah-the) [metro- + Gr. *pathos* suffering] any uterine disease or disorder. **syncytiotrophoblastic m.,** syncytial endometritis.

metroperitoneal (me″tro-per″ĭ-to-ne′al) pertaining to the uterus and peritoneum, or communicating with the uterine and peritoneal cavities, as a metroperitoneal fistula.

metroperitonitis (me″tro-per″ĭ-to-ni′tis) [metro- + *peritonitis*] inflammation of the peritoneum about the uterus, or peritonitis resulting from infection after metritis.

metrophlebitis (me″tro-fle-bi′tis) [metro- + Gr. *phleps* vein + -*itis*] inflammation of the veins of the uterus.

Metropine (met′ro-pin) trademark for preparations of methylatropine nitrate.

metroplasty (me″tro-plas′te) reconstructive surgery on the uterus.

metropolis (me-trop′o-lis) [Gr. *mētropolis* mother-state, as opposed to her colonies] the area in which a particular species of organisms commonly occurs.

metroptosis (me″tro-to′sis) [metro- + Gr. *ptōsis* falling] downward displacement, or prolapse of the uterus.

metrorrhagia (me″tro-ra′je-ah) [metro- + Gr. *rhēgnynai* to burst out] uterine bleeding, usually of normal amount, occurring at completely irregular intervals, the period of flow sometimes being prolonged. **m. myopath′ica,** uterine hemorrhage due to insufficient contraction of uterine muscles after parturition.

metrorrhea (me″tro-re′ah) [metro- + Gr. *rhoia* flow] a free or abnormal uterine discharge.

metrorrhexis (me″tro-rek′sis) [metro- + Gr. *rhēxis* rupture] rupture of the uterus.

metrosalpingitis (me″tro-sal″pin-ji′tis) [metro- + Gr. *salpinx* tube + -*itis*] inflammation of the uterus and oviducts.

metrosalpingography (me″tro-sal″ping-gog′rah-fe) hysterosalpingography.

metroscope (me′tro-skōp) hysteroscope.

metrostasis (mĕ-tros′tah-sis) [Gr. *metron* measure + *stasis* a setting] a state in which the length of a muscle fiber is relatively fixed, and at which length it contracts and relaxes.

metrostaxis (me″tro-stak′sis) [metro- + Gr. *staxis* a dripping] a slight but persistent escape of blood from the uterus.

metrostenosis (me″tro-ste-no′sis) [metro- + Gr. *stenosis* contraction] contraction or stenosis of the cavity of the uterus, as in Asherman's syndrome.

metrotherapy (met″ro-ther′ah-pe) [Gr. *metron* measure + *therapeia* treatment] treatment by measurement, i.e., by demonstrating to the patient his improvement by means of accurate measurements of the increase in the voluntary movements of an impaired joint.

metrotomy (mĕ-trot′o-me) (*obs.*) hysterotomy.

metrotoxin (me″tro-tok′sin) a substance from the pregnant uterus which is thought to exert an inhibitory action on ovarian function.

metrotubography (me″tro-tu-bog′rah-fe) hysterosalpingography.

-metry [Gr. *metrein* to measure] a word termination meaning the act of measuring, or the measurement of, the object measured being indicated by the stem to which it is affixed, as *hemoglobinometry.*

M. et sig. abbreviation for L. *mi′sce et sig′na,* mix and write a label.

Mett's method, test tubes (mets) [Emil Ludwig Paul *Mett,* German physician of the 19th century] see *Nirenstein and Schiff's method,* under *method,* and see under *tests,* and *tube.*

Metubine (mĕ-tu′bin) trademark for a preparation of metocurine iodide.

meturedepa (met″ūr-ĕ-dē′pah) chemical name: ethyl[bis(2,2-dimethyl-1-aziridinyl)phosphinyl]carbamate; an antineoplastic, $C_{11}H_{22}N_3O_3P$.

Metycaine (met′ĭ-kān) trademark for preparations of piperocaine.

metyrapone (mĕ-tēr′ah-pōn) [USP] chemical name: 2-methyl-1,2-di-3-pyridyl-1-propanone. A synthetic compound, $C_{14}H_{14}N_2O$, that selectively inhibits the enzyme (steroid 11β-hydroxylase) involved in the biosynthesis of corticosteroids, particularly cortisol; occurring as a white to light amber, fine, crystalline powder, it is used as a diagnostic aid for determination of hypothalamicopituitary-adrenocortical reserve, administered orally. Called also *mepyrapone, metapyrone,* and *methylpyrapone.* **m. tartrate,** the tartrate salt of metyrapone, $C_{14}H_{14}N_2O·2C_4H_6O_6$, used for the same purpose as the base; administered by intravenous infusion.

metyrosine (mĕ-ti′ro-sēn) chemical name: (–)-α-methyl-L-tyrosine; an antihypertensive, $C_{10}H_{13}NO_3$.

Meulengracht's diet, method (moi′len-grakts) [Einar *Meulen-*

---

gracht, Danish internist, born 1887] see under *diet* and *method.*

Mev. million electron volts; the equivalent of $3.82 × 10^{-14}$ small calories, or $1.6 × 10^{-6}$ ergs.

mevalonate (mĕ-val′o-nāt) a salt or dissociated form of mevalonic acid, a precursor of squalene, cholesterol, and coenzyme Q in plants and animals and of carotenoids and rubber in plants.

mexrenoate potassium (meks-ren′o-āt) chemical name: 17-hydroxy-3-oxo-17α-pregn-4-ene-7α,21-dicarboxylic acid 7-methyl ester monopotassium salt dihydrate; an aldosterone antagonist, $C_{24}H_{33}KO_6·2H_2O$.

Meyer's disease (mi′erz) [Hans Wilhelm *Meyer,* Danish physician, 1824–1895] see under *disease.*

Meyer's line, organ, sinus (mi′erz) [Georg Hermann von *Meyer,* anatomist in Zürich, 1815–1892] see under *line, organ,* and *sinus.*

Meyerhof (mi′er-hof″), Otto Fritz. German physiologist, 1884–1951, noted for his work on the metabolism of muscles; co-winner, with Archibald Vivian Hill, of the Nobel prize for medicine and physiology in 1922.

Meynert's bundle, etc. (mi′nerts) [Theodor Herman *Meynert,* professor of neurology and psychiatry at Vienna, 1833–1892] see under *bundle, cell, commissure, fasciculus,* and *tract.*

Meynet's nodes (ma-nāz′) [Paul Claude Hyacinthe *Meynet,* French physician, 1831–1892] see under *node.*

mezereon (me-ze′re-on) mezereum.

mezereum (me-ze′re-um) [L.] the dried bark of *Daphne mezereum* L. (Thymelaeaceae), a shrub of Europe; formerly used as a diaphoretic, diuretic, and stimulant. It has long been recognized as a poisonous plant, particularly through ingestion of its berries. The plant parts are acrid and produce vesication when rubbed on the skin.

mezlocillin (mez″lo-sil′in) an antibiotic of unspecified action, $C_{21}H_{25}N_5O_8S_2$.

μf. microfarad.

M.F.D. minimum fatal dose.

M. flac. abbreviation for L. *membra′na flac′cida* (pars flaccida membranae tympani [NA]).

M. ft. abbreviation for L. *mistu′ra fi′at,* let a mixture be made.

Mg chemical symbol for *magnesium.*

mg. milligram.

mγ milligamma (millimicrogram, micromilligram, or nanogram).

μg. microgram.

μγ microgamma (micromicrogram, or picogram).

MgCl₂ magnesium chloride.

mgm abbreviation for milligram.

MgO magnesium oxide.

MgSO₄ magnesium sulfate.

MHC major histocompatibility complex.

M.H.D. minimum hemolytic dose.

mHg millimeters of mercury.

mho (mo) [*ohm* spelled backwards] siemens.

miana (mi-an′ah) a relapsing fever found throughout Iran, and apparently in Syria, Cyprus, Libya, Israel, and Jordan.

Mianeh bug [the city of *Mianeh,* Iran] see under *bug.*

mianserin hydrochloride (me-an′ser-in) chemical name: 1,2,3,4,10,14b-hexahydro-2-methyldibenzo[c,f]pyrazino[1,2-a]azepine monohydrochloride; a serotonin inhibitor and antihistaminic, $C_{18}H_{20}N_2·HCl$.

miasm (mi′azm) miasma.

miasma (mi-az′mah) [Gr. "defilement, pollution"] a supposed noxious emanation from the soil or earth, alleged to be the cause of diseases endemic in certain areas, such as malaria, before the true cause became known. See *tellurism.*

miasmatic (mi″az-mat′ik) pertaining to or caused by miasma.

Mibelli's porokeratosis (me-bel′ez) [Vittorio *Mibelli,* Italian dermatologist, 1860–1910] porokeratosis.

mibolerone (mi-bōl′er-ōn) chemical name: 17β-hydroxy-7α,17-dimethylester-4-en-3-one; an androgenic and anabolic agent, $C_{20}H_{30}O_2$.

mica (mi′kah) [L.] 1. a crumb or grain; a small particle. 2. a group of complex aluminum silicate compounds, some of which can produce pulmonary fibrosis if inhaled in finely divided form in high concentrations over a prolonged period.

micaceous (mi-ka′shus) pertaining to or resembling mica; occurring in silvery gray flakes.

MicaTin (mi′kah-tin) trademark for preparations of miconazole nitrate.

mication (mi-ka′shun) any quick motion, such as winking.

micatosis (mi″kah-to′sis) pneumoconiosis due to inhalation of and tissue reaction to mica particles.

micella (mi-sel′ah) see *micelle.*

micelle (mi-sel′) a colloid particle formed by an aggregation of small molecules.

Michaelis's rhomboid (me-ka′lēz) [Gustav Adolf *Michaelis*, Kiel gynecologist, 1798–1848] see under *rhomboid*.

miconazole nitrate (mĭ-kon′ah-zōl) chemical name: 1-[2-(2,4-dichlorophenyl)-2-[(2,4-dichlorophenyl) methoxy] ethyl]-1*H*-imidazole mononitrate. A synthetic antifungal agent, $C_{18}H_{14}Cl_4N_2$-$O \cdot HNO_3$, used topically in the treatment of tinea pedis, tinea cruris, and tinea corpora due to *Trichophyton rubrum*, T. *mentagrophytes*, and *Epidermophyton floccosum;* of cutaneous candidiasis, and of tinea versicolor; and intravaginally in the treatment of vulvovaginal candidiasis.

micr- see *micro-*.

micra (mi′krah) plural of *micron*.

micranatomy (mi″kran-at′o-me) [*micro-* + *anatomy*] microscopical anatomy; histology.

micrangiopathy (mi″kran-je-op′ah-the) (*obs.*) microangiopathy.

micrangium (mi-kran′je-um) a capillary.

micranthine (mi-kran′thin) a crystalline alkaloid, $C_{34}H_{32}N_2$-O_6, from bark of the tree *Daphnandra micrantha* (Tul.) Benth. (Monimiaceae).

micrencephalia (mi″kren-sĕ-fa′le-ah) micrencephaly.

micrencephalon (mi″kren-sef′ah-lon) [*micr-* + Gr. *enkephalos* brain] 1. a small brain. 2. (*obs.*) the cerebellum.

micrencephalous (mi″kren-sef′ah-lus) having a small brain.

micrencephaly (mi″kren-sef′ah-le) [*micr-* + Gr. *enkephalos* brain] abnormal smallness of the brain.

micrergy (mi′krer-je) micrurgy.

micro-, micr- [Gr. *mikros* small] combining form designating small size; used in naming units of measurement to indicate one-millionth (10^{-6}) of the unit designated by the root with which it is combined.

microabscess (mi″kro-ab′ses) a very small, localized collection of pus. **Munro m.,** a minute collection of neutrophilic polymorphonuclear leukocytes lying immediately below the horny layer or just within the upper portion of the malpighian layer of the epidermis; seen in psoriasis. **Pautrier m.,** a collection of hyperchromatic mononuclear cells within the epidermis, characterizing malignant lymphoma of the skin, particularly mycosis fungoides.

microadenoma (mi″kro-ad″ĕ-no′mah) an adenoma, as of the anterior pituitary gland, less than 10 mm. in diameter.

microadenopathy (mi″kro-ad″ĕ-nop′ah-the) [*micro-* + Gr. *adēn* gland + *pathos* disease] disease of the small lymphatics.

microaerophile (mi″kro-a′er-o-fīl) a microaerophilic microorganism.

microaerophilic (mi″kro-a′er-o-fil″ik) [*micro-* + *aero-* + Gr. *philein* to love] requiring oxygen for growth but at lower concentration than is present in the atmosphere; said of bacteria.

microaerophilous (mi″kro-a″er-of′ĭ-lus) microaerophilic.

microaerotonometer (mi″kro-a″er-o-to-nom′ĕ-ter) an instrument for measuring the volume of gases in the blood.

microaggregate (mi″kro-ag′rĕ-gat) a microscopic collection of particles, as of platelets, leukocytes, and fibrin that occurs in stored blood.

microaleuriospore (mi″kro-ah-lu′re-o-spōr) a small aleuriospore; sometimes used interchangeably with microcondium.

microammeter (mi″kro-am′ĕ-ter) an instrument for measuring currents in the microampere range.

microanalysis (mi″kro-ah-nal′ĭ-sis) [*micro-* + *analysis*] the chemical analysis of minute quantities of material.

microanastomosis (mi″kro-an-as″to-mo′sis) anastomosis between very small tubular structures.

microanatomy (mi″kro-ah-nat′o-me) histology, especially organology.

microaneurysm (mi″kro-an′u-rizm) a microscopic aneurysm, a characteristic feature of thrombotic purpura.

microangiopathic (mi″kro-an″je-o-path′ik) pertaining to or characterized by microangiopathy.

microangiopathy (mi″kro-an″je-op′ah-the) [*micro-* + Gr. *angeion* vessel + *pathos* disease] disease of the small blood vessels. **diabetic m.,** the presence of generalized basement membrane thickening of capillaries throughout many vascular beds, occurring in diabetics. **thrombotic m.,** the formation of thrombi in the arterioles and capillaries; see *thrombotic thrombocytopenic purpura*, under *purpura*.

microangioscopy (mi″kro-an″je-os′ko-pe) capillaroscopy.

microbacteria (mi″kro-bak-te′re-ah) [L.] plural of *microbacterium*.

Microbacterium (mi″kro-bak-te′re-um) a genus of microorganisms of the family Corynebacteriaceae, order Eubacteriales, made up of gram-positive rods found in dairy products and characterized by relatively high resistance to heat. **M. fla′vum,** an aerobic species occurring predominantly in dairy products and producing lactic acid without gas in carbohydrate fermentation. **M. lac′ticum,** an aerobic species occurring in the intestinal tract and producing lactic acid without gas in carbohydrate fermentation.

microbacterium (mi″kro-bak-te′re-um), pl. *microbacte′ria* [L.] 1. an organism belonging to the genus Microbacterium. 2. a microorganism.

microbalance (mi″kro-bal″ans) a balance for measuring minute changes in weight.

microbar (mi′kro-bahr) a unit of pressure, being one-millionth (10^{-6}) bar.

microbe (mi′krōb) [*micro-* + Gr. *bios* life] a minute living organism, a microphyte or microzoon; applied especially to those minute forms of life which are capable of causing disease in animals, including bacteria, protozoa, and fungi.

microbemia (mi″kro-be′me-ah) (*obs.*) microbiemia.

microbial (mi-kro′be-al) of or pertaining to or caused by microbes.

microbian (mi-kro′be-an) 1. pertaining to or of the nature of a microbe. 2. a microbe.

microbic (mi-kro′bik) microbial.

microbicidal (mi-kro′bĭ-si′dal) [*microbe* + L. *caedere* to kill] destructive to microbes.

microbicide (mi-kro′bĭ-sīd) [*microbe* + L. *caedere* to kill] an agent that destroys microbes.

microbid (mi′kro-bid) (*obs.*) any skin lesion due to allergy to a microorganism or its products.

microbiemia (mi″kro-bi-e′me-ah) (*obs.*) the presence of microbes in the blood; bacillemia; septicemia.

microbioassay (mi″kro-bi′o-as′a) determination of the active power of a nutrient or other factor by noting its effect upon the growth of a microorganism, as compared with the effect of a standard preparation.

microbiological (mi″kro-bi′o-loj′ĭ-kal) pertaining to microbiology.

microbiologist (mi″kro-bi-ol′o-jist) one specializing in microbiology.

microbiology (mi″kro-bi-ol′o-je) [*micro-* + Gr. *bios* life + *-logy*] the science which deals with the study of microorganisms, including bacteria, fungi, viruses, and pathogenic protozoa.

microbiophotometer (mi″kro-bi″o-fo-tom′ĕ-ter) an instrument for measuring the growth of bacterial cultures by the turbidity of the medium.

microbiota (mi″kro-bi-o′tah) the microscopic living organisms of a region; the combined microflora and microfauna of a region.

microbiotic (mi″kro-bi-ot′ik) pertaining to the microbiota, or to microscopic living organisms.

microblast (mi′kro-blast) [*micro-* + Gr. *blastos* germ] an erythroblast of small size, i.e., 5μ or less in diameter.

microblepharia (mi″kro-blĕ-fa′re-ah) [*micro-* + Gr. *blepharon* eyelid + *-ia*] a developmental anomaly characterized by abnormal shortness of the vertical dimensions of the eyelids.

microblepharism (mi″kro-blef′ah-rizm) microblepharia.

microblepharon (mi″kro-blef′ah-ron) an abnormally small eyelid.

microblephary (mi″kro-blef′ah-re) microblepharia.

microbody (mi″kro-bod′e) 1. any of the membrane-bound, ovoid or spherical, granular cytoplasmic particles containing enzymes and other substances, which originate in the endoplasmic reticulum of vertebrate liver and kidney cells and other cells, and in protozoa, yeast, and many cell types of higher plants. Two types of microbodies are *peroxisomes* (found in vertebrates) and *glyoxysomes* (found in plants and microorganisms). 2. peroxisome.

microbrachia (mi″kro-bra′ke-ah) [*micro-* + Gr. *brachiōn* arm] abnormal smallness of the arms.

microbrachius (mi″kro-bra′ke-us) [*micro-* + Gr. *brachiōn* arm] a fetus with preternaturally small arms.

microbrenner (mi″kro-bren′er) [*micro-* + Ger. *Brenner* burner] a needle-pointed electric cautery.

microburet (mi″kro-bu-ret′) a buret with a capacity of the order of 0.1 to 10 ml., with graduated intervals of 0.001 to 0.02 ml.

microcalix (mi″kro-kal′iks) a very small renal calix arising by caliceal branching, usually at the side of a calix of normal size. Written also *microcalyx*.

microcalorie (mi″kro-kal′o-re) the heat required to raise 1 ml. of distilled water from 0 to 1° C.

microcalory (mi″kro-kal′o-re) microcalorie.

microcalyx (mi″kro-kal′iks) microcalix.

microcardia (mi″kro-kar′de-ah) [*micro-* + Gr. *kardia* heart] smallness of the heart.

microcaulia (mi″kro-kaw′le-ah) [*micro-* + Gr. *kaulos* penis] abnormal smallness of the penis.

microcentrum (mi″kro-sen′trum) [*micro-* + Gr. *kentron* center] centrosome.

microcephalia (mi″kro-sĕ-fa′le-ah) microcephaly.

microcephalic (mi″kro-sĕ-fal′ik) pertaining to or exhibiting microcephaly.

microcephalism (mi″kro-sef′ah-lizm) microcephaly.

microcephalous (mi″kro-sef′ah-lus) microcephalic.

microcephalus (mi″kro-sef′ah-lus) an individual with a very small head.

microcephaly (mi″kro-sef′ah-le) [micro- + Gr. kephalē head] abnormal smallness of the head, usually associated with mental retardation.

microcheilia (mi″kro-ki′le-ah) [micro- + Gr. cheilos lip] abnormal smallness of the lips.

microcheiria (mi″kro-ki′re-ah) [micro- + Gr. cheir hand + -ia] abnormal smallness of the hands, as a result of hypoplasia of all the skeletal elements.

microchemical (mi″kro-kem′ĭ-kal) pertaining to microchemistry.

microchemistry (mi″kro-kem′is-tre) [micro- + chemistry] the study of chemical reactions using quantities invisible to the naked eye; chemistry which deals with minute quantities (a few milligrams) of substances, using apparatus of small size. Cf. macrochemistry.

microcinematography (mi″kro-sin″ĕ-mah-tog′rah-fe) the making of moving picture photographs of microscopic subjects.

microcirculation (mi″kro-sir″ku-la′shun) the flow of blood in the entire system of finer vessels (100 microns or less in diameter) of the body (the microvasculature).

microclimate (mi″kro-kli′mit) the immediate climatic environment, as that of a vector insect.

microclyster (mi″kro-klis′ter) [micro- + clyster] a rectal injection of a small amount of substance.

microcnemia (mi″kro-ne′me-ah) [micro- + Gr. knēmē tibia] abnormal shortness of the lower leg.

Micrococcaceae (mi″kro-kok-ka′se-e) [micro- + Gr. kokkos berry] in some systems of classification, a family of gram-positive, aerobic or facultatively anaerobic bacteria of the order Eubacteriales, made up of spherical cells dividing primarily in two or three planes, and sometimes remaining in contact after division, and including the genera Gaffkya, Methanococcus, Micrococcus, Peptococcus, Sarcina, and Staphylococcus. In other systems of classification, it includes the genera Micrococcus, Planococcus, and Staphylococcus.

micrococci (mi″kro-kok′si) plural of micrococcus.

Micrococcus (mi″kro-kok′us) a genus of microorganisms of the family Micrococcaceae, order Eubacteriales, spherical, gram-positive cells, usually occurring in irregular masses, saprophytic and nonpathogenic forms found in soil, water, etc. Sixteen species have been recognized.

micrococcus (mi″kro-kok′us) 1. an organism of the genus Micrococcus. 2. a spherical microorganism of extremely small size.

microcolon (mi″kro-ko′lon) an abnormally small colon.

microcolony (mi′kro-kol″o-ne) a microscopical colony of bacteria.

microconcentration (mi″kro-kon″-sentra′shun) a minute amount of solute, less than 0.05 per cent of the solution.

microconidia (mi″kro-ko-nid′e-ah) plural of microconidium.

microconidium (mi″kro-ko-nid′e-um), pl. microconid′ia. a small, usually single-celled conidium or exospore; sometimes used interchangeably with microaleuriospore; see spore.

microcoria (mi″kro-ko′re-ah) [micro- + Gr. korē pupil] smallness of the pupil.

microcornea (mi″kro-kor′ne-ah) [micro- + cornea] a usually bilateral developmental anomaly, in which the cornea is unusually small (less than 11 mm. after one year of age), due to arrest of development. It may be associated with other ocular abnormalities, such as microphthalmia, hydrophthalmia, multiple defects of the anterior chamber, cataract, and glaucoma, and may be inherited as an X-linked recessive or as an autosomal dominant trait.

microcoulomb (mi″kro-koo′lom) a unit of quantity of current electricity, being one one-millionth (10⁻⁶) of a coulomb. Abbreviated μcoul.

microcrania (mi″kro-kra′ne-ah) abnormal smallness of the skull, the cranial cavity being reduced in all diameters, and the facial area being disproportionately large in comparison.

microcrith (mi′kro-krith) [micro- + crith] (obs.) the weight of one atom of hydrogen.

microcrystal (mi′kro-kris′tal) an extremely minute crystal.

microcrystalline (mi″kro-kris′tal-īn) [micro- + crystalline] made up of minute crystals.

microcurie (mi′kro-ku′re) a unit of radioactivity, being one one-millionth (10⁻⁶) curie, or the quantity of radioactive material in which the number of nuclear disintegrations is 3.7 × 10⁴ per second. Abbreviated μC.

microcurie-hour (mi′kro-ku″re-owr″) a unit of exposure equivalent to that obtained by exposure for one hour to radioactive material disintegrating at the rate of 3.7 × 10⁴ atoms per second. Abbreviated μC hr.

Microcyclus (mi″kro-si′klus) a genus of microorganisms of the family Spirillaceae, suborder Pseudomonadineae, order Pseudomonadales, made up of nonmotile, small, slightly curved rods which during growth form a closed ring. The type species is M. aqua′ticus.

microcyst (mi′kro-sist) [micro- + Gr. kystis sac, bladder] a very small cyst.

microcystometer (mi″kro-sis-tom′ĕ-ter) a small portable cystometer.

microcytase (mi″kro-si′tās) a cytase formed by microphages and capable of dissolving bacteria.

microcyte (mi′kro-sīt) [micro- + -cyte] an abnormally small erythrocyte, i.e., one 5 microns or less in diameter.

microcythemia (mi″kro-si-the′me-ah) [microcyte + Gr. haima blood + -ia] a condition in which the erythrocytes are smaller than normal.

microcytosis (mi″kro-si-to′sis) microcythemia.

microcytotoxicity (mi″kro-si″to-tok-sis′ĭ-te) the capability of lyzing or damaging cells as detected in procedures (e.g., lymphocytotoxicity procedures) using extremely minute amounts of material, viz., target cells, antibody, and complement.

microdactylia (mi″kro-dak-til′e-ah) microdactyly.

microdactyly (mi″kro-dak′tĭ-le) [micro- + Gr. daktylos finger] abnormal smallness of the digits.

microdensitometer (mi″kro-dens″ĭ-tom′ĕ-ter) an instrument used in spectroscopy to measure lines in a spectrum by light transmission measurement.

microdentism (mi″kro-den′tizm) microdontia.

microdermatome (mi″kro-der′mah-tōm) an instrument for cutting very thin skin sections.

microdetermination (mi″kro-de-ter″mĭ-na′shun) a chemical examination in which minute quantities of the substance to be examined are used.

microdissection (mi″kro-di-sek′shun) dissection of tissue or cells under the microscope.

microdont (mi′kro-dont) [micro- + Gr. odous tooth] having a dental index below 42.

microdontia (mi″kro-don′she-ah) abnormal smallness of the teeth; it may affect a single tooth, or all of them (generalized m.), and be true or only relative.

microdontic (mi″kro-don′tik) pertaining to or characterized by microdontia.

microdontism (mi″kro-don′tizm) microdontia.

microdosage (mi′kro-do″sij) dosage in small quantities.

microdose (mi′kro-dōs) a very small dose.

microdrepanocytic (mi″kro-drep″ah-no-sit′ik) containing microcytic and drepanocytic elements, as in sickle cell–thalassemia disease.

microdrepanocytosis (mi″kro-drep″ah-no-si-to′sis) sickle cell–thalassemia disease.

microecology (mi″kro-ĕ-kol′o-je) the branch of ecology of parasites concerned with the relationships of the organisms and the environment provided by the hosts.

microecosystem (mi″kro-e″ko-sis′tem) a miniature ecological system, occurring naturally or produced in the laboratory for experimental purposes.

microelectrophoresis (mi″kro-e-lek″tro-fo-re′sis) electrophoresis in which migrating particles are observed by light microscopy; submicroscopic particles such as viruses are made visible by aggregation or are adsorbed onto carriers such as collodion particles or finely ground glass.

microelectrophoretic (mi″kro-ĕ-lek″tro-fo-ret′ik) pertaining to microelectrophoresis.

microembolus (mi″kro-em′bo-lus), pl. microem′boli. an embolus of microscopic size.

microencephaly (mi″kro-en-sef′ah-le) micrencephaly.

microenvironment (mi″kro-en-vi′ron-ment) the environment at the microscopic or cellular level.

microerythrocyte (mi″kro-ĕ-rith′ro-sīt) microcyte.

microestimation (mi″kro-es″tĭ-ma′shun) microdetermination.

microfarad (mi″kro-far′ad) a unit of electrical capacity, being one one-millionth of a farad (10⁻⁶ f.); abbreviated μf.

microfauna (mi″kro-faw′nah) the animal life, visible only under the microscope, which is present in or characteristic of a special location.

microfibril (mi″kro-fi′bril) an extremely small fibril.

microfilament (mi″kro-fil′ah-ment) any of the submicroscopic filaments composed chiefly of actin, found in the cytoplasmic matrix of almost all cells, often in close association with the microtubules; they are believed by some to have a supportive and cytoskeletal function and/or to mediate movement of the cell and of the organelles within it.

microfilaremia (mi″kro-fil″ah-re′me-ah) the presence of microfilariae in the circulating blood.

microfilaria (mi″kro-fi-la′re-ah) the prelarval stage of Filarioidea in the blood of man and in the tissues of the vector. This term is sometimes incorrectly used as a genus name and is then spelled

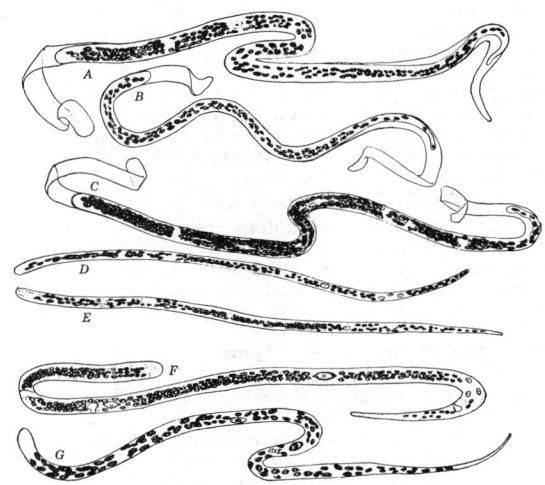

Microfilariae of (A) *Wuchereria bancrofti*, 270 × 8.5 μ; (B) *Brugia malayi*, 200 × 6 μ; (C) *Loa loa*, 275 × 7 μ; (D) *Acanthocheilonema perstans*, 200 × 4.5 μ; (E) *Mansonella ozzardi*, 205 × 5 μ; (F) *Onchocerca volvulus*, 320 × 7.5 μ; (G) *Dirofilaria immitis*, 300 × 6 μ. A, B, and C have sheaths covering the body. (Cheng.)

with a capital M. **m. bancrof′ti**, the microfilaria of *Wuchereria bancrofti*. **m. diur′na**, the microfilaria of *Loa loa*. **m. lo′a**, the microfilaria of *Loa loa*. **m. streptocer′ca**, the microfilaria of *Dipetalonema streptocerca*, found in the subcutaneous tissues. **m. vol′vulus**, the prelarval form of *Onchocerca volvulus*, found in skin snips taken from infected persons.

microfilm (mi′kro-film) 1. a trade term for 16- or 35-millimeter film to be used in high-speed automatic machines for the photographic reproduction, in greatly reduced size, of books, documents, forms, or other record files. 2. to photographically reproduce, in greatly reduced size, on film specially designed for the purpose.

microflora (mi″kro-flo′rah) the plant life, visible only under the microscope, which is present in or characteristic of a special location.

microfluorometry (mi″kro-floo″or-om′ĕ-tre) cytophotometry.

microgamete (mi″kro-gam′ēt) [*micro-* + Gr. *gametēs* spouse] the smaller, actively motile male gamete which fertilizes the macrogamete in anisogamy.

microgametocyte (mi″kro-gah-me′to-sīt) [*micro-* + Gr. *gametēs* spouse + *-cyte*] 1. a cell that produces microgametes. 2. the male gametocyte of certain Sporozoa, such as malarial plasmodia.

microgametophyte (mi″kro-gah-me′to-fīt) [*micro-* + Gr. *gametēs* husband + *phyton* plant] the male gametophyte in heterosporous plants, developed from the microspore.

microgamma (mi″kro-gam′mah) picogram.

microgamy (mi-krog′ah-me) conjugation or fusion when the gametes are smaller than the somatic cells.

microgastria (mi″kro-gas′tre-ah) [*micro-* + Gr. *gastēr* stomach + *-ia*] congenital smallness of the stomach.

microgenesis (mi″kro-jen′ĕ-sis) [*micro-* + Gr. *genesis* production] abnormally small development of a part.

microgenia (mi″kro-jen′e-ah) [*micro-* + Gr. *genys* jaw] underdevelopment of the mental symphysis of the mandible, resulting in an extremely small chin; a similar appearance is caused by malocclusion with excessive prominence of the alveolar structures.

microgenitalism (mi″kro-jen′ĭ-tal-izm) [*micro-* + *genitalism*] smallness of the external genitals.

microglia (mi-krog′le-ah) the small, non-neural, interstitial cells of mesodermal origin that form part of the supporting structure of the central nervous system. They are of various forms and may have slender branched processes. They are migratory and act as phagocytes to waste products of nerve tissue. Called also *Hortega cells*, *gitter cells*, *mesoglia*, and *microgliocytes*.

microgliacyte (mi-krog′le-ah-sīt) microgliocyte.

microglial (mi-krog′le-al) of or pertaining to the microglia.

microgliocyte (mi-krog′le-o-sīt) [*microglia* + *-cyte*] the early cell which develops into a microglial cell.

microglioma (mi″kro-gli-o′mah) a tumor composed of microglial cells.

microgliomatosis (mi″kro-gli′o-mah-to′sis) a condition characterized by the formation of tumors containing microglia; called also *reticulum cell sarcoma of the brain*.

microglobulin (mi″kro-glob′u-lin) any globulin, or any fragment of a globulin, of low molecular weight.

microglossia (mi″kro-glos′e-ah) [*micro-* + Gr. *glōssa* tongue + *-ia*] undersize of the tongue.

micrognathia (mi″kro-na′the-ah) [*micro-* + Gr. *gnathos* jaw + *-ia*] unusual or undue smallness of the jaws.

microgonioscope (mi″kro-go′ne-o-skōp) [*micro-* + Gr. *gōnia* angle + *skopein* to examine] an instrument for observing and measuring the angles of the anterior chamber of the eye; used in examining the eye in glaucoma.

microgram (mi′kro-gram) a unit of mass (weight) of the metric system, being one-millionth of a gram (10^{-6} gm.), or one one-thousandth of a milligram (10^{-3} mg.). Abbreviated μg. or mcg. Symbol γ.

micrograph (mi′kro-graf) 1. an instrument for recording extremely minute movements. It acts by making a greatly magnified record on a photographic film of the minute motions of a diaphragm. 2. the photograph of a minute object or specimen (tissue, etc.) as seen through a microscope. **electron m.**, the photograph of an object through an electron microscope.

micrography (mi-krog′rah-fe) [*micro-* + Gr. *graphein* to write] 1. an account of microscopic objects. 2. examination with the microscope.

microgyri (mi″kro-ji′ri) plural of *microgyrus*.

microgyria (mi″kro-jir′e-ah) [*micro-* + Gr. *gyros* + *-ia*] polymicrogyria.

microgyrus (mi″kro-ji′rus), pl. *microgy′ri* [*micro-* + *gyrus*] an abnormally small, malformed convolution of the brain.

microhematocrit (mi″kro-he-mat′o-krit) the rapid determination of packed cell volume of erythrocytes of an extremely small quantity of blood, by use of a capillary tube and a high speed centrifuge.

microhepatia (mi″kro-he-pat′e-ah) [*micro-* + Gr. *hēpar* liver] smallness of the liver.

microhistology (mi″kro-his-tol′o-je) [*micro-* + *histology*] microscopical histology.

microhm (mi′krōm) [*micro-* + *ohm*] one-millionth part of an ohm.

microincineration (mi″kro-in-sin″er-a′shun) the incineration of minute specimens of tissue or other substance, for identification from the ash of the elements composing it.

microinfarct (mi″kro-in′farkt) a very small infarct due to obstruction of circulation in capillaries, arterioles, or small arteries.

microinjector (mi″kro-in-jek′tor) an instrument for infusion of very small amounts of fluids or drugs into animals or humans.

microinvasion (mi″kro-in-va′zhun) microscopic extension of malignant cells into adjacent tissue in carcinoma in situ.

microinvasive (mi″kro-in-va′siv) exhibiting or pertaining to microinvasion.

microkinematography (mi″kro-kin″ĕ-mah-tog′rah-fe) [*micro-* + Gr. *kinēma* movement + *graphein* to write] the making of moving pictures of microscopic objects.

microlecithal (mi″kro-les′ĭ-thal) [*micro-* + Gr. *lekithos* yolk] containing little yolk.

microlentia (mi″kro-len′she-ah) microphakia.

microlesion (mi″kro-le′zhun) a minute lesion.

microleukoblast (mi″kro-lu′ko-blast) myeloblast.

microliter (mi′kro-le″ter) [Fr. *microlitre*; *micro-* + *liter*] a thousandth part of a milliliter or a millionth part of a liter. Usually abbreviated μl.

microlith (mi′kro-lith) [*micro-* + Gr. *lithos* stone] a minute concretion or calculus.

microlithiasis (mi″kro-lĭ-thi′ah-sis) [*micro-* + *lithiasis*] the formation of minute concretions in an organ. **m. alveola′ris pulmo′num, pulmonary alveolar m.,** a condition caused by deposition in the alveoli of the lungs of minute calculi, which appear roentgenographically as fine, sandlike mottling.

microlymphoidocyte (mi″kro-lim-foi′do-sīt) a small, nongranular, immature lymphoidocyte.

micromandible (mi″kro-man′dĭ-b'l) extreme smallness of the mandible.

micromanipulation (mi″kro-mah-nip″u-la′shun) the performance of surgery, injections, dissections, etc., by means of micromanipulators.

micromanipulator (mi″kro-mah-nip′u-la″tor) an attachment to a microscope for manipulating tiny instruments used in examination and dissection of minute objects under the microscope.

micromanometer (mi″kro-man-om′ĕ-ter) an apparatus for indicating gas or vapor pressure from a very small sample, as of blood, fluid, etc.

micromanometric (mi″kro-man″o-met′rik) relating to gas or vapor pressure from very small samples, as of blood, fluid, etc.

micromastia (mi″kro-mas′te-ah) abnormal smallness of the mamma.

micromaxilla (mi″kro-mak-sil′ah) extreme smallness of the maxilla.

micromazia (mi″kro-ma′ze-ah) [*micro-* + Gr. *mazos* breast] micromastia.

micromegalopsia (mi″kro-meg″ah-lop′se-ah) [*micro-* + Gr. *megas* large + *opsis* vision] the condition in which objects appear too small or too large or too small and too large by turns.

micromelia (mi″kro-me′le-ah) [*micro-* + Gr. *melos* limb + *-ia*] a developmental anomaly characterized by abnormal smallness or shortness of the limbs.

micromelus (mi-krom′e-lus) an individual exhibiting micromelia.

micromere (mi′kro-mēr) [*micro-* + Gr. *meros* part] one of the small blastomeres formed by unequal cleavage of a fertilized ovum, located in the animal hemisphere and dividing more rapidly than the macromeres of the vegetal hemisphere.

micrometabolism (mi″kro-mĕ-tab′o-lism) metabolism as studied by micromethods.

micrometastasis (mi″kro-mĕtas′tah-sis) the spread of cancer cells from the primary tumor to distant sites, where they form microscopic secondary tumors.

micrometeorology (mi″kro-me″te-er-ol′o-je) that branch of meteorology dealing with the effects on living organisms of the extra-organic aspects of the physical environment within a few inches of the surface of the earth.

micrometer[1] (mi-krom′ĕ-ter) [*micro-* + Gr. *metron* measure] an instrument for measuring objects seen through the microscope. **diffraction m.,** halometer. **eyepiece m.,** a micrometer that is used in connection with the eyepiece of a microscope. **filar m.,** an eyepiece micrometer in which the micrometer screw acts upon a slide carrying a movable wire: one revolution of the screw moves the wire 1 mm. across the field. **ocular m.,** eyepiece m. **stage m.,** a micrometer fastened to the stage of a microscope.

micrometer[2] (mi′kro-me″ter) one-millionth (10^{-6}) of a meter; abbreviated μm. Called also *micron*.

micromethod (mi″kro-meth′od) any technique involving use of exceedingly small quantities of material. Cf. *macromethod.*

micrometry (mi-krom′e-tre) the measurement of microscopic objects.

micromicro- a prefix used in naming units of measurement to indicate one-millionth of one-millionth (10^{-12}) of the unit designated by the root with which it is combined. Now supplanted by the prefix *pico-.*

micromicrocurie (mi″kro-mi″kro-ku′re) one-millionth (10^{-6}) microcurie, or 10^{-12} curie. Abbreviated μμC. Called also *picocurie.*

micromicrogram (mi″kro-mi″kro-gram) one-millionth (10^{-6}) microgram, or 10^{-12} gram. Abbreviated μμg. Called also *picogram.*

micromicron (mi″kro-mi′kron) a unit of linear measure in the metric system, being 10^{-6} micron, 10^{-9} millimeter, or 10^{-12} meter. Abbreviated μμ.

micromilligram (mi″kro-mil′ĭ-gram) a unit of mass (weight) in the metric system, being 10^{-6} milligram, or 10^{-9} gram. Abbreviated μmg. Called also *nanogram.*

micromillimeter (mi″kro-mil′ĭ-me″ter) a unit of linear measure in the metric system, being 10^{-6} millimeter. Abbreviated μmm. Called also *nanometer.*

micromolecular (mi″kro-mo-lek′u-lar) composed of small molecules.

Micromonospora (mi″kro-mo-nos′po-rah) [*micro-* + Gr. *monos* single + *sporos* seed] a genus of microorganisms of the family Streptomycetaceae, order Actinomycetales, made up of saprophytic forms occurring in soil and water.

micromonosporin (mi″kro-mo-nos′po-rin) an antibiotic substance produced by cultures of *Micromonospora,* which is active against gram-positive bacteria.

Micromyces (mi-krom′ĭ-sēz) [*micro-* + Gr. *mykēs* fungus] *Streptothrix.*

micromyelia (mi″kro-mi-e′le-ah) [*micro-* + Gr. *myelos* marrow + *-ia*] abnormal smallness of the spinal cord.

micromyeloblast (mi″kro-mi′ĕ-lo-blast) a small, immature myelocyte, observed in micromyeloblastic leukemia.

micromyelolymphocyte (mi″kro-mi″ĕ-lo-lim′fo-sit) micromyeloblast.

micron (mi′kron), pl. *mi′crons, mi′cra* [Gr. *mikros* small] a unit of linear measure in the metric system, being 10^{-3} millimeter, or 10^{-6} meter. Abbreviated μ.

microneedle (mi″kro-ne′d′l) a fine glass needle for use in micrurgy.

microneurosurgery (mi″kro-nu″ro-ser′jer-e) surgery conducted under high magnification with miniaturized instruments on microscopic vessels and structures of the nervous system.

micronize (mi′kro-nīz) [Gr. *micron* a small thing] to reduce to a fine powder; to reduce to particles a micron in diameter.

micronodular (mi″kro-nod′u-lar) marked by the presence of small nodules.

micronormoblast (mi″kro-nor′mo-blast) an abnormal red cell precursor in which there has been defective hemoglobin synthesis, characterized by a narrow rim of cytoplasm and a rather overdeveloped, pyknotic nucleus.

micronucleus (mi″kro-nu′kle-us) [*micro-* + *nucleus*] 1. in ciliate protozoa, the smaller of two types of nucleus in each cell, which functions in sexual reproduction. Cf. *macronucleus.* 2. a small nucleus. 3. the nucleolus.

micronutrient (mi″kro-nu′tre-ent) any essential dietary element required only in small quantities, e.g., trace minerals.

micronychia (mi″kro-nik′e-ah) [*micr-* + Gr. *onyx* nail] abnormal smallness of the nails of fingers or toes.

micronychosis (mi″kro-nik-o′sis) micronychia.

micro-orchidia (mi″kro-or-kid′e-ah) microrchidia.

microorganic (mi″kro-or-gan′ik) pertaining to a microorganism.

microorganism (mi″kro-or′gan-izm) [*micro-* + *organism*] a minute living organism, usually microscopic. Those of medical interest are bacteria, rickettsiae, viruses, molds, yeasts, and protozoa.

microorganismal (mi″kro-or″gan-iz′mal) pertaining to microorganisms.

microparasite (mi″kro-par′ah-sīt) a parasitic microorganism.

micropathology (mi″kro-pah-thol′o-je) [*micro-* + *pathology*] 1. the sum of what is known regarding minute pathologic changes. 2. the pathology of diseases caused by microorganisms.

micropenis (mi″kro-pe′nis) microphallus.

microperfusion (mi″kro-per-fu′zhun) perfusion of a minute amount of a substance.

microphage (mi′kro-fāj) [*micro-* + Gr. *phagein* to eat] a phagocyte of small size; an actively motile, neutrophilic leukocyte capable of phagocytosis.

microphagocyte (mi″kro-fag′o-sīt) [*micro-* + *phagocyte*] microphage.

microphakia (mi″kro-fa′ke-ah) [*micro-* + Gr. *phakos* lens + *-ia*] abnormal smallness of the crystalline lens.

microphallus (mi″kro-fal′us) [*micro-* + Gr. *phallos* penis] abnormal smallness of the penis.

microphone (mi′kro-fōn) a device for converting an acoustic signal into an electric signal for purposes of amplification or transmission. **cardiac catheter-m.,** phonocatheter.

microphonic (mi″kro-fon′ik) 1. serving to amplify sound. 2. cochlear m's. **cochlear m's,** the electrical potentials generated in the hair cells of the organ of Corti in response to acoustic stimulation; called also *cochlear potentials.*

microphotograph (mi″kro-fo′to-graf) [*micro-* + *photograph*] a photograph of small size. Cf. *photomicrograph.*

microphthalmia (mi″krof-thal′me-ah) [*micro-* + Gr. *ophthalmos* eye + *-ia*] microphthalmos.

microphthalmos (mi″krof-thal′mus) [*micro-* + Gr. *ophthalmos* eye] abnormal smallness in all dimensions of one or both eyes; in the absence of other ocular defects, it is called *pure microphthalmos* or *nanophthalmos.*

microphthalmoscope (mi″krof-thal′mo-skōp) an instrument for performing fundus microscopy.

microphthalmus (mi″krof-thal′mus) 1. microphthalmos. 2. a person affected with microphthalmos.

microphysics (mi″kro-fiz′iks) [*micro-* + *physics*] the science which deals with the ultimate structure of matter, i.e., with molecules, atoms, and electrons.

microphyte (mi′kro-fīt) [*micro-* + Gr. *phyton* plant] a microscopic vegetable organism. Cf. *microzoon.*

microphytic (mi″kro-fit′ik) (*obs.*) pertaining to or caused by microphytes.

micropia (mi-kro′pe-ah) micropsia.

micropinocytosis (mi″kro-pi″no-si-to′sis) the taking up into a cell of specific macromolecules by invagination of the plasma membrane which is then pinched off, resulting in small vesicles in the cytoplasm.

micropipet (mi″kro-pi-pet′) a pipet for handling small quantities of liquids (up to 1 ml.).

micropituicyte (mi″kro-pi-tu′ĭ-sīt) see *pituicyte.*

microplasia (mi″kro-pla′ze-ah) [*micro-* + Gr. *plassein* to form] dwarfism.

microplating (mi′kro-plāt″) the use of minute amounts of material in the plating of microorganisms.

microplethysmography (mi″kro-pleth″is-mog′rah-fe) [*micro-* + Gr. *plēthysmos* increase + *graphein* to record] the recording of minute changes in the size of a part as produced by the circulation of blood in it.

micropodia (mi″kro-po′de-ah) [*micro-* + Gr. *pous* foot] abnormal smallness of the feet.

micropolariscope (mi″kro-po-lar′ĭ-skōp) a microscope with a polariscope attached.

micropolygyria (mi″kro-pol″e-ji′re-ah) polymicrogyria.

microprecipitation (mi″kro-pre-sip″ĭ-ta′shun) precipitation with a minute amount (½ to 1 drop or less) of reagent observed under the microscope.

micropredation (mi″kro-pre-da′shun) the derivation by an organism of elements essential for its existence from larger organisms of other species which it does not destroy.

micropredator (mi″kro-pred′ah-tor) [*micro-* + L. *praedator* a plunderer, pillager] an organism, e.g., the mosquito, that derives elements essential for its existence from other species of organisms, larger than itself, without causing their destruction.

microprobe (mi′kro-prōb) a minute probe, as one used in microsurgery. **laser m.,** a laser beam utilized to vaporize a minute area of tissue, as in a biopsy specimen, which is then subjected to emission spectrography.

microprojection (mi″kro-pro-jek′shun) [*micro-* + *projection*] the throwing of the image of a microscopic object on a screen.

microprojector (mi″kro-pro-jek′tor) a projector that fits the viewing stage of a microscope and enlarges the image on an illuminated viewing screen.

microprosopus (mi″kro-pro-so′pus) [*micro-* + Gr. *prosōpon* face] a fetus with a small or undeveloped face.

micropsia (mi-krop′se-ah) [*micro-* + Gr. *opsis* vision + *-ia*] a condition in which objects are seen as smaller than they actually are.

microptic (mi-krop′tik) pertaining to or affected with micropsia.

micropuncture (mi″kro-punk′chur) the creation of minute openings by piercing.

micropus (mi-kro′pus) [*micro-* + Gr. *pous* foot] a person with abnormally small feet.

micropyle (mi′kro-pīl) [*micro-* + Gr. *pylē* gate] 1. an opening through which the spermatozoon enters the ovum of certain animals, including some sporozoa and arthropods. 2. a minute opening at the base of the ovule of a seed plant through which the pollen grains enter.

microradiogram (mi″kro-ra′de-o-gram) a picture produced by microradiography.

microradiography (mi″kro-ra″de-og′rah-fe) [*micro-* + *radiography*] a process by which an x-ray shadow image (radiograph) of a small or very thin object is produced on fine-grained photographic film under conditions which permit subsequent microscopic examination or enlargement of the radiograph at linear magnifications of up to several hundred and with a resolution approaching the resolving power of the photographic emulsion (about 1000 lines per millimeter).

microrchidia (mi″kror-kid′e-ah) [*micro-* + Gr. *orchis* testicle + *-ia*] abnormal smallness of the testicle.

microrefractometer (mi″kro-re″frak-tom′ĕ-ter) a refractometer for the discovery of variations in the minute structures, e.g., in blood corpuscles.

microrespirometer (mi″kro-res″pĭ-rom′ĕ-ter) an apparatus for investigating the oxygen utilization of isolated tissues.

microrhinia (mi″kro-rin′e-ah) [*micro-* + Gr. *rhis* nose] abnormal smallness of the nose.

microroentgen (mi″kro-rent′gen) [*micro-* + *roentgen*] one millionth of a roentgen; abbreviated μR.

microscelous (mi-kros′kĕ-lus) [*micro-* + Gr. *skelos* leg] short-legged.

Microscilla (mi″kro-sil′ah) a genus of schizomycetes of the family Vitreoscillaceae.

microscler (mi′kro-sklēr) dolichomorphic.

microscope (mi′kro-skōp) [*micro-* + Gr. *skopein* to view] an instrument used to obtain an enlarged image of small objects and reveal details of structure not otherwise distinguishable. **acoustic m.,** one in which very high frequency sound waves (close to one billion cycles per second [one gigahertz]) are focused on the object and the reflected beam is processed electronically and stored for display on a television screen. **beta ray m.,** one which reveals emission of beta particles from a microscopic specimen by means of a scintillator. **binocular m.,** a microscope which has two eyepieces, making possible simultaneous viewing with both eyes. **capillary m.,** an instrument for giving an enlarged image of capillaries, often used for viewing the capillaries of the nail bed. **centrifuge m.,** a microscope built into a high-speed centrifuge, by which a magnified image of a specimen undergoing centrifugal force may be produced. **comparison m.,** an instrument which permits simultaneous viewing of parts of images of two separate specimens, involving two microscopes bridged together with a comparison eyepiece, or one microscope with two body tubes and lens systems. **compound m.,** one that consists of two lens systems, one above the other, in which the image formed by the system nearer the object (objective) is further magnified by the system nearer the eye (eyepiece). **corneal m.,** a specially designed instrument with lens of high magnifying power, for observing minute changes in the cornea and iris. **darkfield m.,** one with a central stop in the condenser, permitting diversion of the light rays and illumination of the object from the side, so that the details appear light against a dark background. See also *ultramicroscope.* **electron m.,** one in which an electron beam, instead of light, forms an image for viewing on a fluorescent screen, or for photography. **epic m.,** see *epimicroscope.* **fluorescence m.,** one used for the examination of specimens stained with fluorochromes or fluorochrome complexes, e.g., a fluorescein-labeled antibody, which fluoresces in ultraviolet light. **Greenough m.** (*obs.*), a binocular, biobjective, stereoscopic instrument giving a low-power erect image. **hypodermic m.,** a combination of a fiberoptic probe (housed in a hypodermic needle) and a microscope for examining cell structure in tissue and muscle without a cutaneous incision. **infrared m.,** one in which radiation of 800 mμ or longer wavelength is used as the image-forming energy. **integrating m.,** one in which a special mechanical stage permits recording of the sizes of the components of the specimen. **interference m.,** a microscope for observing the same kind of refractile detail as that observed with the phase microscope, but utilizing two separate beams of light which are sent through the specimen and combined with each other in the image plane. **ion m.,** an electron microscope modified to use ions (e.g., of lithium), instead of electrons. **laser m.,** see *laser microprobe.* **light m.,** one in which the specimen is viewed under visible light. **opaque m.,** one with vertical illumination or with the condenser built around the objective (epimicroscope) for viewing opaque specimens. **operating m.,** a specially designed instrument employed in the performance of delicate surgical procedures, as in operations on the middle ear, on small blood vessels, or in some operations on a vocal cord. **Oto-m.,** see *Oto-microscope.* **phase m., phase-contrast m.,** a microscope which alters the phase relationships of the light passing through and that passing around the object, the contrast permitting visualization of the object without the necessity for staining or other special preparation. **polarizing m.,** one equipped with a polarizer, analyzer, and means for measurement of the alteration of the polarized light by the specimen. **polarizing m., rectified,** a polarizing microscope corrected for depolarization from curved lens surfaces so that full apertures can be used. **projection x-ray m.,** a microscope using soft x-radiation for high resolution; the images may be photographed or observed directly on a fluorescent viewing screen. **reflecting m.,** one which utilizes mirrors instead of lenses to form the image. **Rheinberg m.,** a darkfield microscope in which the condenser is modified by having a colored instead of an opaque stop, with the annulus in a complementary color. **scanning m., scanning electron m.,** an electron microscope in which a beam of electrons scans over a specimen point by point and builds up an image on the fluorescent screen of a cathode ray tube. **schlieren m.,** one in which light is deviated by the insertion of one or two diaphragms in the optical system, to reveal differences in refractive index in a specimen. **simple m.,** one which consists of a single lens; a magnifying glass. **slit lamp m.,** a corneal microscope with a special attachment that permits examination of the endothelium on the posterior surface of the cornea. **stereoscopic m.,** a binocular biobjective microscope, or a binocular monobjective microscope modified to give a three-dimensional view of the specimen. **stroboscopic m.,** one which utilizes flashing illumination, permitting analysis of motion in the specimen. **trinocular m.,** a binocular microscope with a third eyepiece tube for photomicrography or other use. **ultra-m.,** see *ultramicroscope.* **ultrasonic m.,** one which utilizes the reflection of ultrasonic or mechanical vibration to reveal the detail of the specimen. **ultraviolet m.,** a microscope which utilizes reflecting optics or quartz and other ultraviolet-transmitting lenses, with radiation of less than 400 mμ wavelength as the image-forming energy. **x-ray m.,** one in which a beam of x-rays is used instead of light, the image usually being reproduced on film.

microscopic (mi″kro-skop′ik) of extremely small size; visible only by the aid of the microscope.

microscopical (mi″kro-skop′e-k′l) 1. pertaining to microscopy. 2. microscopic.

microscopist (mi-kros′ko-pist) a person skilled in using the microscope.

microscopy (mi-kros′ko-pe) [*micro-* + Gr. *skopein* to examine] examination under or observation by means of the microscope. **clinical m.,** employment of the microscope in making clinical diagnoses. **electron m.,** examination by means of the electron microscope. **fluorescence m.,** microscopy of natural fluorescent materials or of specimens stained with fluorochromes, which emit light when exposed to blue or ultraviolet light. **fundus m.,** examination of the fundus of the eye with an instrument which combines a corneal microscope with an ophthalmoscope. **immunofluorescent m.,** fluorescent microscopy in which antigens are identified by exposing them to homologous antibodies labeled with a fluorescent tracer. **television m.,** projection on a television screen of the image obtained by use of a flying spot, or scanning, microscope, or by use of a television camera over a microscope.

microsecond (mi'kro-sek"und) one-millionth of a second; abbreviated μsec.

microsection (mi"kro-sek'shun) an extremely thin section for examination with the microscope.

microseme (mi'kro-sēm) [*micro-* + Gr. *sēma* sign] having an orbital index of 83 or less.

Microsiphonales (mi"kro-si"fo-na'lēz) see *Trichomycetes*.

microslide (mi'kro-slīd) the slide on which objects for microscopical examination are mounted.

microsmatic (mi"kros-mat'ik) [*micro-* + Gr. *osmasthai* to smell] having the sense of smell, but of relatively feeble development, as in man.

microsoma (mi"kro-so'mah) [*micro-* + Gr. *sōma* body] a very short but not dwarfish stature.

microsomal (mi"kro-so'mal) of or pertaining to microsomes.

microsomatia (mi"kro-so-ma'she-ah) microsomia.

microsome (mi'kro-sōm) [*micro-* + Gr. *sōma* body] any of the vesicular fragments of endoplasmic reticulum formed after disruption and centrifugation of cells.

microsomia (mi"kro-so'me-ah) [*micro-* + Gr. *sōma* body + *-ia*] an undersized state of the body. **m. feta'lis,** abnormally small size of the fetus.

microspectrophotometer (mi"kro-spek"tro-fo-tom'ĕ-ter) a system combining a microscope with a spectrophotometer.

microspectroscope (mi"kro-spek'tro-skōp) [*micro-* + *spectroscope*] a spectroscope to be used in connection with a microscope for the examination of the spectra of microscopic objects.

microsphere (mi-kro-sfēr') centrosome.

microspherocyte (mi"kro-sfe'ro-sīt) spherocyte.

microspherocytosis (mi"kro-sfe"ro-si-to'sis) spherocytosis.

microspherolith (mi"kro-sfēr'o-lith) a particle resembling a miniature gallstone in the bile.

microsphygmia (mi-kro-sfig'me-ah) [*micro-* + Gr. *sphygmos* pulse + *-ia*] a pulse that is difficult to perceive by the finger.

microsphygmy (mi"kro-sfig'me) microsphygmia.

microsphyxia (mi"kro-sfik'se-ah) (*obs.*) microsphygmia.

Microspira (mi"kro-spi'rah) [*micro-* + Gr. *speira* coil] a genus name used in early classifications for a group of small, spiral-shaped microorganisms.

Microspironema (mi"kro-spi"ro-ne'mah) [*micro-* + Gr. *speira* coil + *nema* thread] a genus name once proposed for organisms now included in the genus *Treponema*.

microsplanchnic (mi"kro-splank'nik) having the abdominal portion of the body relatively smaller than the thoracic; a term applied to a type of bodily constitution in which the vertical diameters are excessively developed as compared with the horizontal ones. Cf. *macrosplanchnic* and *pyknic*.

microsplanchnous (mi"kro-splank'nus) microsplanchnic.

microsplenia (mi"kro-sple'ne-ah) [*micro-* + Gr. *splēn* spleen + *-ia*] smallness of the spleen.

microsplenic (mi"kro-sple'nik) marked by smallness of the spleen.

microsporangia (mi"kro-spo-ran'je-ah) plural of microsporangium.

microsporangium (mi"kro-spo-ran'je-um), pl. *microsporan'gia* [*micro-* + Gr. *sporos* seed + *angeion* vessel] the sporangium in which microspores develop.

microspore (mi"kro-spōr) [*micro-* + Gr. *sporos* seed] 1. the smaller spore form when spores of two sizes are present, as in certain fungi and protozoa. 2. in heterogenous plants, one of four haploid spores, usually smaller than the megaspore, formed in the microspangium from a microspore mother cell, and from which the microgametophyte, or male gametophyte, develops. See also *pollen*.

microsporid (mi-kros'po-rid) a secondary skin eruption which is an expression of hypersensitivity to *Microsporum* infection, and occurring in an area remote from the site of infection.

Microsporidia (mi"kro-spo-rid'e-a) [*micro-* + *sporidium*] an order of sporozoa having small spores and usually one polar capsule, generally found as parasites of arthropods and fishes but also found in other hosts. It includes the genus *Nosema*.

microsporidian (mi"kro-spo-rid'e-an) any protozoon of the order Microsporidia.

Microsporon (mi-kros'po-ron) *Microsporum*.

microsporosis (mi"kro-spo-ro'sis) a ringworm infection caused by one of the fungi of the genus *Microsporum*.

Microsporum (mi-kros'po-rum) [*micro* + Gr. *sporos* seed] a genus of small-spored ectothrix ringworm fungi (dermatophytes) of the Fungi Imperfecti, order Moniliales, family Moniliaceae, which cause various diseases of the skin and hair. As the perfect (sexual) stages are identified, they are classified in the genus *Nannizzia*. Called also *Microsporon*. Besides the species listed below, *M. cook'ei, M. distor'tum,* and *M. na'num* are pathogenic but have been isolated from man only rarely. **M. audoui'ni,** the most common cause of prepuberal tinea capitis in Europe and of about half the cases in the United States. **M. ca'nis,** a

common cause of ringworm in cats and dogs; often transmitted to children, in whom it causes tinea capitis and tinea corporis. It is also probably the cause of a dermatomycosis in horses. **M. feli'neum,** *M. canis.* **M. ful'vum,** a geophilic species sometimes contracted from soil, which causes tinea corporis or tinea capitis. **M. fur'fur,** *Pityrosporon orbiculare.* **M. gyp'seum,** a species commonly found in soil; it is a common cause of tinea capitis and tinea corporis in South America, and less frequently in other parts of the world. **M. lano'sum,** *M. canis.*

microstat (mi'kro-stat) the stage and finder of a microscope.

microsthenic (mi"kro-sthen'ik) [*micro-* + Gr. *sthenos* strength] having feeble muscular power.

Microstix-3 (mi"kro-stiks) trademark for a reagent strip with a chemical test area for recognition of nitrite in urine, which turns pink on contact with nitrite, and two culture areas for semiquantification of bacterial growth after 18–24 hours of incubation; one culture area supports both gram-negative and gram-positive organisms, the other, only gram-negative organisms.

microstomia (mi"kro-sto'me-ah) [*micro-* + Gr. *stoma* mouth + *-ia*] a congenital defect in which the mouth is unusually small.

microstrabismus (mi"kro-strah-biz'mus) [*micro-* + Gr. *strabismos* a squinting] strabismus of such slight degree that the deviation is undetectable by the usual methods.

microsurgery (mi'kro-ser"jer-e) dissection of minute structures under the microscope by means of instruments held in the hand, as in microsurgery of the ear and larynx.

microsyringe (mi"kro-sēr'inj) a syringe fitted with a screw-thread micrometer head for the accurate control of minute measurements.

Microtatobiotes (mi"kro-ta"to-bi-o'tēz) [Gr. *mikrotatos* smallest + *biōtes* one must live] a proposed taxonomic class comprising the orders Rickettsiales and Virales.

microtechnic (mi"kro-tek'nik) micrology.

microthelia (mi"kro-the'le-ah) [*micro-* + Gr. *thēlē* nipple + *-ia*] unusual smallness of the nipples.

microthrombosis (mi"kro-throm-bo'sis) presence of many small thrombi in the capillaries and other small blood vessels of various organs of the body.

microthrombus (mi"kro-throm'bus), pl. *microthrom'bi* [*micro-* + Gr. *thrombos* clot] a small thrombus located in a capillary or other small blood vessel.

microtia (mi-kro'she-ah) [*micro-* + Gr. *ous* ear + *-ia*] gross hypoplasia or aplasia of the pinna of the ear, with a blind or absent external auditory meatus.

microtiter (mi"kro-ti'ter) a titer of minute quantity.

microtome (mi'kro-tōm) [*micro-* + Gr. *tomē* a cut] an instrument for cutting thin slices of tissue for microscopical study. **freezing m.,** a microtome for cutting frozen sections. **rocking m.,** a microtome in which the specimen is held in the end of a lever which passes up and down over a stationary knife. **rotary m.,** one in which a wheel action is translated into a back-and-forth movement of the specimen being sectioned. **sliding m.,** one in which the specimen being sectioned is made to slide on a tract.

microtomy (mi-krot'o-me) [*micro-* + Gr. *temnein* to cut] the cutting of thin sections; called also *histotomy*.

microtonometer (mi"kro-to-nom'ĕ-ter) a small tonometer for measuring the oxygen and carbon dioxide tension in arterial blood.

microtransfusion (mi"kro-trans-fu'zhun) introduction into the circulation of a small quantity of blood of another individual, as sometimes occurs with transplacental passage of a small amount of fetal blood into the maternal circulation.

microtrauma (mi"kro-traw'mah) a slight trauma or lesion; a microscopic lesion.

Microtrombidium akamushi (mi"kro-trom-bid'e-um ak"-ah-moo'she) *Trombicula akamushi*.

microtropia (mi"kro-tro'pe-ah) microstrabismus.

microtubule (mi"kro-tu'būl) any of the slender, tubular structures composed chiefly of tubulin, found in the cytoplasmic ground substance of nearly all cells; they are involved in maintenance of cell shape and in the movements of organelles and inclusions, and form the spindle fibers of mitosis. In cilia and flagella, they are constantly arranged with two single microtubules in the center and nine pairs of doublets arrayed around the central two.

Microtus (mi-kro'tus) [*micro-* + Gr. *ous, ōtos,* ear] a genus of small rodents distributed throughout the Arctic land areas, commonly called voles or meadow mice. **M. montebel'li,** the field vole, which is probably the host of *Leptospira hebdomidis,* the etiologic agent of nanukayami.

microtus (mi-kro'tus) an individual exhibiting microtia.

microunit (mi'kro-u"nit) one-millionth (10^{-6}) of a standard unit; abbreviated μU.

microvascular (mi"kro-vas'ku-lar) pertaining to the microvasculature.

microvasculature (mi"kro-vas'ku-lah-tūr) the portion of the vasculature of the body comprising the finer vessels, sometimes described as including all vessels with an internal diameter of 100 microns or less.

microvilli (mi″kro-vil′i) [pl. of L. *microvillus* a tuft of hair] minute cylindrical processes on the free surface of a cell, especially cells of the proximal convolution in a renal tubule and of the intestinal epithelium, which increase the surface size of the cell; see also *brush border,* under *border.*

microvillus (mi″kro-vil′us) a minute process or protrusion from the free surface of a cell; see *microvilli.*

microviscosimeter (mi″kro-vis″ko-sim′ĕ-ter) a viscosimeter for measuring the viscosity of blood plasma, using a small quantity of blood.

microvivisection (mi″kro-viv″ĭ-sek′shun) microdissection.

microvolt (mi″kro-volt) [*micro-* + *volt*] one-millionth of a volt. Abbreviated μv.

microvoltometer (mi″kro-vōl-tom′ĕ-ter) an instrument for detecting minute changes of electric potential in the body.

microwatt (mi′kro-wat) [*micro-* + *watt*] one-millionth of a watt; abbreviated μw.

microwave (mi′kro-wāv) a wave typical of electromagnetic radiation between far infrared and radio waves, generally regarded as extending from 300,000 to 100 megacycles (wavelength of 1 mm. to 30 cm.).

microxycyte (mi-krok′sĭ-sīt) [*micro-* + Gr. *oxys* sharp, acid + *-cyte*] any finely granular oxyphil cell.

microxyphil (mi-krok′sĭ-fil) microxycyte.

microzoa (mi″kro-zo′ah) plural of *microzoon.*

microzoaria (mi″kro-zo-a′re-ah) [*micro-* + Gr. *zōon* animal] a general term for all microorganisms.

microzoon (mi″kro-zo′on), pl. *microzo′a* [*micro-* + Gr. *zōon* animal] a microscopic animal organism. Cf. *microphyte.*

micrurgic (mi-krur′jik) pertaining to micrurgy.

micrurgy (mi′krur-je) [*micro-* + Gr. *ergon* work] micromanipulative technic in the field of a microscope. See *micromanipulator.*

Micrurus (mi-kroo′rus) a genus of venomous elapid snakes. *M. ful′vius* is the coral, or harlequin, snake. Called also *Elaps.* See table accompanying *snake.*

miction (mik′shun) urination.

micturate (mik′tu-rāt) urinate.

micturition (mik″tu-rish′un) [L. *micturire* to urinate] the passage of urine; urination.

M.I.D. minimum infective dose.

midaflur (mi′dah-floor) chemical name: 4-amino-2,2,5,5-tetrakis(trifluoromethyl)-3-imidazoline; a sedative, $C_7H_3F_{12}N_3$.

midaxilla (mid″ak-sil′ah) the center of the axilla.

midbody (mid′bod-e) 1. a body or a mass of granules developed in the equatorial region of the spindle during the anaphase of mitosis. 2. the middle region of the trunk.

midbrain (mid′brān) mesencephalon.

midcarpal (mid-kar′pal) between the two rows of bones of the carpus.

Middeldorpf's triangle (splint) (mid″l-dorpfs) [Albrecht Theodor *Middeldorpf,* Breslau surgeon, 1824–1868] see under *triangle.*

middlepiece (mid″l-pēs) the portion of a spermatozoon between its head and flagellum.

midfoot (mid′foot) the middle portion of the foot, comprising the region of the navicular, cuboid, and cuneiform bones.

midfrontal (mid-fron′tal) pertaining to the middle of the forehead.

midge (mij) a small dipterous insect of the family Chironomidae; many species give painful bites, and some are vectors of *Mansonella ozzardi* and *Dipetalonema perstans.* **owl m.,** *Phlebotomus.*

midget (mij′et) a normal dwarf; an individual who is undersized but perfectly formed.

midgetism (mij′ĕ-tizm) the condition of being a midget.

midgut (mid′gut) the region of the embryonic digestive tube into which the yolk sac opens; ahead of it is the foregut and caudal to it is the hindgut.

Midicel (mid′ĭ-sel) trademark for a preparation of sulfamethoxypyridazine.

midoccipital (mid″ok-sip′ĭ-tal) pertaining to or located in the middle of the occiput.

midpain (mid′pān) intermenstrual pain.

midperiphery (mid″pĕ-rif′er-e) the middle zone of the fundus.

midpiece (mid′pēs) in early immunological theory, the euglobulin fraction of guinea pig serum, which corresponded to component C1 of complement.

midplane (mid′plān) the median plane of a bilateral structure.

midriff (mid′rif) the diaphragm (diaphragma [NA]); the middle

region of the torso; the region between the lower border of the breast and the waistline.

midsection (mid-sek′shun) a cut through the middle of any organ or part.

midsternum (mid-ster′num) mesosternum.

midtarsal (mid-tar′sal) between the two rows of bones of the tarsus.

midtegmentum (mid″teg-men′tum) the median or central part of the tegmentum.

midwife (mid′wīf) an individual who practices midwifery; see *nurse-midwife.*

midwifery (mid′wi-fer-e) the practice of assisting in childbirth. See *nurse-midwife* and *obstetrics.*

Mierzejewski effect (mēr″ze-yef′ske) [Jan Lucian *Mierzejewski,* Polish neurologist and psychiatrist, 1839–1908] see under *effect.*

Miescher's corpuscles, tubules (tubes) (me′sherz) [Johann Friedrich *Miescher,* Swiss pathologist, 1811–1887] see *Rainey's corpuscles,* under *corpuscle,* and see under *tubule.*

Miescheria (me-she′re-ah) [J. F. *Miescher*] *Sarcocystis.*

MIF melanocyte-stimulating hormone inhibiting factor; migration inhibiting factor. See under *factor.*

migraine (mi′grān, me′grān) [Fr., from Gr. *hemikrania* an affection of half of the head] an often familial symptom complex of periodic attacks of vascular headache, usually temporal and unilateral in onset, commonly associated with irritability, nausea, vomiting, constipation or diarrhea, and often photophobia; attacks are preceded by constriction of the cranial arteries, usually with resultant prodromal sensory (especially ocular) symptoms, and commence with the vasodilation that follows. **abdominal m.,** migraine in which abdominal symptoms (nausea and vomiting) are prominent. **acute confusional m.,** a rare variant of classical migraine occurring in children, marked by attacks of confusion and disorientation, with agitation manifested as a mixture of apprehension and combativeness; headache may not appear at first but always develops eventually. **fulgurating m.,** violent migraine developing abruptly. **hemiplegic m.,** migraine associated with varying degrees of transient hemiplegia or hemiparesis. **ophthalmic m.,** migraine accompanied by amblyopia or other visual disturbance. **ophthalmoplegic m.,** periodic migraine accompanied by ophthalmoplegia.

migraineur (me″grān-er′) [Fr.] a person who suffers from migraine.

migrainoid (mi′grah-noid) [*migraine* + Gr. *eidos* form] resembling migraine.

migrainous (mi′gra-nus) resembling, or of the nature of migraine.

migrateur (me″grah-ter′) [Fr.] a person with an obsession to wander.

migration (mi-gra′shun) [L. *migratio*] 1. an apparently spontaneous change of place, as of symptoms. 2. the movement of leukocytes through the walls of the vessels: diapedesis. **anodic m.,** the migration of a negatively charged particle toward the positive pole in an electrical field. **cathodic m.,** the migration of a positively charged particle toward the negative pole in an electric field. **external m.,** the passage of an ovum from the ovary to the oviduct of the opposite side without passing through the uterus. **internal m.,** the passing of an ovum from an ovary into the uterus in the normal way, followed by its entry into the opposite oviduct or, in animals with separate uterine horns, into the opposite horn. **m. of leukocytes,** the passage of white corpuscles through the wall of a vessel; diapedesis. **m. of ovum,** 1. the passage of the ovum into the uterine tube after its discharge from the ovary. 2. the passage of the ovum through the reproductive tract and through the uterine epithelium into the stroma. **retrograde m.,** the passage into the upper urinary tract of foreign bodies introduced through the urethra. **tooth m.,** the normal physiological drift of a tooth. **transperitoneal m.,** external migration.

Migula's classification (me′goo-lahz) [Walter *Migula,* German naturalist, born 1863] see under *classification.*

Mikedimide (mi-ked′ĭ-mīd) trademark for a preparation of bemegride.

mikro- for words beginning thus, see those beginning *micro-.*

Mikulicz's cells, etc. (mik′u-lich″ez) [Johann von *Mikulicz*-Radecki, Polish surgeon, 1850–1905] see under *angle, cell, clamp, disease, drain, pad, pyloroplasty,* and *syndrome.*

mil (mil) contraction of *milliliter.*

milammeter (mil-am′ĕ-ter) milliammeter.

mildew (mil′du) vernacular term for any fungus growing on vegetable or other material; also the condition caused by such a fungus. *Downy* or *powdery mildew* refers to ascomycetous fungi of the *Erysiphe* (order Erysiphales) that cause disease of grapes and other plants.

milenperone (mĭ-len′pĕ-rōn) chemical name: 5-chloro-1-[3-[4-(4-fluorobenzoyl)-1-piperidinyl]propyl]-1,3-dihydro-2*H*-benzimidazol-2-one; a tranquilizer, $C_{22}H_{23}ClFN_3O_2$.

Miles' operation (mīlz) [William Ernest *Miles*, British surgeon, 1869–1947] see under *operation*.

milfoil (mil′foil) see *Achillea*.

milia (mil′e-ah) [L.] plural of *milium*. **m. neonato′rum,** white, evanescent, pinhead-sized papules which occur on the face and less often the trunk of the newborn infant and disappear within a few weeks; they are keratin cysts filled with keratinous debris, located superficially in the pilosebaceous follicles.

Milian's erythema, sign (mēl-yahz′) [Gaston Auguste *Milian*, French dermatologist, 1871–1945] see under *erythema* and *sign*.

miliaria (mil″e-a′re-ah) [L. *milium* millet] a syndrome of cutaneous changes associated with sweat retention and extravasation of sweat occurring at different levels in the skin; when used alone, it refers to *m. rubra*. **m. al′ba,** m. crystallina. **m. crystalli′na,** miliaria in which the sweat escapes in or just beneath the stratum corneum, producing noninflammatory vesicles which, because of the thinness of the layer covering them, have the appearance of clear droplets. Called also *m. alba* and *sudamina*. **m. profun′da,** miliaria in which the sweat escapes into the middermis, producing nonpruritic, inflammatory papules which change in size with the sweating response of the patient; usually occurring only as a late sequel to recurrent severe generalized miliaria rubra, and, when extensive, leading to heat intolerance, as in tropical anhidrotic asthenia. Called also *mamillaria*. **m. ru′bra,** a condition resulting from obstruction to the ducts of the sweat glands, probably caused in part by prolonged maceration of the skin surface; the sweat escapes into the epidermis, producing pruritic erythematous papulovesicles. The severity of the symptoms fluctuates with the heat load of the individual. Called also *prickly heat*.

miliary (mil′e-a-re) [L. *miliaris* like a millet seed] 1. resembling a millet seed. 2. characterized by the formation of lesions resembling millet seeds, as in miliary tuberculosis.

Milibis (mil′ĭ-bis) trademark for preparations of glycobiarsol.

milieu (me-lyuh′) [Fr.] surroundings: environment. **m. extérieur** (me-lyuh′ eks-ta″re-ur′), the external environment. **m. intérieur** (me-lyuh′ an-ta″re-ur′) [Fr. "interior environment"], Claude Bernard's term for the blood and lymph which bathe the cells of the body.

milipertine (mil-ĭ-per′tēn) chemical name: 5,6 - dimethoxy-3 - [2 - [4 - (*o*-methoxyphenyl) - 1 - piperazinyl]ethyl]-2-methylindole; a tranquilizer, $C_{24}H_{31}N_3O_3$.

milium (mil′e-um), pl. *mil′ia* [L. "millet seed"] a tiny, spheroidal, white epithelial cyst lying superficially within the skin, usually of the face, containing lamellated keratin and often associated with vellus hair follicles; milia commonly occur in large numbers and are found especially over the eyelids, cheeks, and forehead. Popularly called *whitehead*. **colloid m.,** a small, firm, translucent, yellowish papule in the corium which is the seat of colloid degeneration. The papules develop gradually and spread over the skin, usually of the face and back of the hands, most often in persons long exposed to strong sunlight. Called also *colloid pseudomilium, hyaloma,* and *Wagner's disease*.

milk (milk) [L. *lac*] 1. the fluid secretion of the mammary gland forming the natural food of young mammals. 2. any whitish milklike substance, e.g., coconut milk or plant latex. 3. a liquid (emulsion or suspension) resembling the secretion of the mammary gland. **acidophilus m.,** milk fermented with cultures of *Lactobacillus acidophilus*; used in gastrointestinal disorders in attempts to modify the bacterial flora of the intestinal tract. **adapted m.,** milk especially modified so as to adapt it to the child's digestive capacity. **after-m.,** the stripping, or last, milk taken at any one milking. **albumin m.,** specially prepared milk, poor in lactose and salts and rich in casein and fat. **m. of bismuth** [USP], a suspension of bismuth hydroxide and bismuth subcarbonate in water, yielding between 5.2 and 5.8 per cent of bismuth trioxide; used as an astringent and antacid. Called also *bismuth magma*. **bitter m.,** milk that is bitter in taste when first drawn because of bitter herbs in the feed or that later becomes bitter from the growth of certain microorganisms. **blue m.,** milk made blue in color by the action of bacteria, usually *Pseudomonas syncyanea*. **Budd m., buddeized m.** (obs.), milk sterilized by adding hydrogen dioxide and heating, so as to decompose the dioxide and liberate the oxygen. **Bulgarian m., bulgaricus m.,** milk fermented with cultures of *Lactobacillus bulgaricus*. **cancer m.,** a viscid opaque granular fluid which may be scraped from the surface of a carcinoma which has undergone fatty degeneration. **casein m.,** a prepared milk containing very little salts and sugars and a large amount of fat and casein. **certified m.,** milk whose purity is certified by a committee of physicians or a medical milk commission. **citric acid m.,** milk prepared by adding 4 gm. of dehydrated citric acid to a quart of milk. **condensed m.,** milk which has been partly evaporated and sweetened with sugar. **diabetic m.,** milk containing a small percentage of lactose. **dialyzed m.,** milk from which the sugar has been abstracted by being passed by dialysis through a parchment membrane. **evaporated m.,** milk prepared by evaporation of half its water content. **fat m.,** modified milk that contains as much or more fat than human

milk. **fore-m.,** 1. the first milk taken at any one milking. 2. colostrum. **fortified m.,** milk made more nutritious by the addition of cream or white of egg; also vitamin D m. **grade A m.,** milk which may contain not more than 30,000 bacteria per milliliter as delivered. **grade B m.,** milk which may contain not more than 100,000 bacteria per milliliter. **homogenized m.,** milk so treated that the fats become intimately combined with the general body of the milk, the emulsified particles of fat being made so minute that the cream does not separate. **hydrochloric acid m.,** acid milk prepared by adding 5 ml. of tenth normal hydrochloric acid to 100 ml. of cow's milk. **laboratory m.,** milk prepared according to a special formula. **lemon juice m.,** acid milk prepared by adding ¾ oz. (22 ml.) of lemon juice to 1 quart of cow's milk. **litmus m.,** a bacterial culture medium consisting of milk and litmus as an indicator, used for the culture of lactic-acid bacteria and *Clostridium*. **m. of magnesia** [USP], a suspension of 7.0 to 8.5 per cent of magnesium hydroxide used as an antacid and cathartic; called also *magnesia magma*. **metallized m.,** milk in which metals (copper, iron, magnesium) are dissolved; used to produce regeneration of hemoglobin. **modified m.,** milk in which the constituents have been made to correspond in amount to the composition of human milk. **perhydrase m.,** milk to which hydrogen dioxide has been added. **protein m.,** a modified milk preparation having a relatively low content of carbohydrate and fat and a relatively high protein content. **purple m.,** a culture medium consisting of skim milk and bromcresol purple, used like litmus milk for the culture of bacteria to determine acid production, and coagulation and proteolysis of casein. **red m.,** milk made red by blood, eating of madder root, or the growth of *Erythrobacillus prodigiosus* or other microorganisms. **ropy m.,** milk which has become viscid so that it can be drawn out into threads. It is usually caused by the growth of *Alcaligenes viscolactis* and is eaten as a delicacy in Norway. **Schloss m.,** a modified milk containing the same proportion of salts and fat as human milk. **skimmed m.,** milk from which the cream has been removed. **soft curd m.,** milk the curd of which has been rendered soft and homogeneous by boiling, by the addition of cream or by the addition of sodium citrate. **sour m.,** milk containing lactic acid, produced by the action of lactic acid bacteria. **m. of sulfur,** precipitated sulfur. **uterine m.,** a white milky substance in the gravid uterus of some species, presumably for nourishment of the embryo. **uviol m.,** milk sterilized by the action of ultraviolet rays. **vegetable m.,** synthetic milk made out of vegetables. **vinegar m.,** acid milk prepared by adding vinegar to cow's milk. **virgin's m.,** lac virginale. **vitamin D m.,** cow's milk to which vitamin D has been added either by direct addition, by exposure to ultraviolet light, or by feeding irradiated yeast to the cows. **witch's m.,** milk secreted in the breast of the newborn child; hexenmilch. **yeast m.,** milk from cows which have been fed on irradiated yeast; it has antirachitic potency.

milking (milk′ing) the pressing out of the contents of a tubular part, such as the urethra, by running the finger along it.

milk-leg (milk′leg) postpartum iliofemoral thrombophlebitis.

Milkman's syndrome (milk′manz) [Louis Arthur *Milkman*, American roentgenologist, 1895–1951] see under *syndrome*.

milkpox (milk′poks) variola minor.

milk sick (milk′sik) poisoning by white snake root, *Eupatorium urticaefolium*.

Millar's asthma (mil′arz) [John *Millar*, British physician, 1733–1805] laryngismus stridulus.

Millard's test (mil′ards) [Henry B. *Millard*, American physician, 1832–1893] see under *tests*.

Millard-Gubler syndrome (paralysis) (me-yar′-goob′ler) [Auguste L. J. *Millard*, French physician, 1830–1915; Adolphe Marie *Gubler*, French physician, 1821–1879] see under *syndrome*.

Miller-Abbott tube [T. Grier *Miller*, Philadelphia physician, born 1886; William Osler *Abbott*, Philadelphia physician, 1902–1943] see under *tube*.

milli- [L. *mille* thousand] a prefix used in naming units of measurement to indicate one one-thousandth (10^{-3}) of the unit designated by the root with which it is combined.

milliammeter (mil″e-am′ĕ-ter) an ammeter which registers a current in milliamperes.

milliampere (mil″e-am′pēr) [Fr.] one-thousandth of an ampere; abbreviated ma.

milliampere-minute (mil″e-am″pēr-min′ut) a unit of electrical quantity equivalent to that delivered by one milliampere in one minute.

milliamperemeter (mil″e-am-pēr′me-ter) milliammeter.

millibar (mil″ĭ-bar) one-thousandth part of a bar.

millicoulomb (mil″ĭ-koo′lom) a unit of quantity of current electricity, being one one-thousandth (10^{-3}) of a coulomb; abbreviated mcoul.

millicurie (mil″ĭ-ku′re) a unit of radioactivity, being one one-thousandth (10^{-3}) curie, or the quantity of radioactive material in which the number of nuclear disintegrations is 3.7×10^7 per second; abbreviated mc.

millicurie-hour (mil″ĭ-ku′re-owr″) a unit of dose equivalent to that obtained by exposure for one hour to radioactive material disintegrating at the rate of 3.7×10^7 atoms per second; abbreviated mc.h.

milliequivalent (mil″ĭ-e-kwiv′ah-lent) the number of grams of a solute contained in one milliliter of a normal solution; abbreviated mEq.

milligamma (mil″ĭ-gam′mah) nanogram; abbreviated $\mu\gamma$.

milligram (mil″ĭ-gram) [*milli-* + *gram*] a unit of mass (weight) in the metric system, being 10^{-3} gram, or the equivalent of 0.015432 grains; abbreviated mg.

Millikan rays (mil′ĭ-kan) [Robert Andrews *Millikan*, American physicist, 1868–1953] cosmic rays.

millilambert (mil″ĭ-lam′bert) one-thousandth of a lambert.

milliliter (mil′ĭ-le″ter) [*milli-* + *liter*] a unit of volume in the metric system, being one one-thousandth (10^{-3}) liter, or the equivalent of 0.033815 of a fluid ounce; abbreviated ml.

millimeter (mil′ĭ-me-ter) a unit of linear measure of the metric system, being one one-thousandth (10^{-3}) meter, or about 0.03937 inch; abbreviated mm.

millimicro- a prefix used in naming units of measurement to indicate one-thousandth of one-millionth (10^{-9}) of the unit designated by the root with which it is combined; now supplanted by the prefix *nano-*.

millimicrocurie (mil″ĭ-mi″kro-ku′re) one-thousandth (10^{-3}) microcurie, or 10^{-9} curie; abbreviated mμc. Called also *nanocurie*.

millimicrogram (mil″ĭ-mi″kro-gram) one-thousandth (10^{-3}) microgram, or 10^{-9} gram; abbreviated mμg. Called also *nanogram*.

millimicrometer (mil″lĭ-mi-krom′ĕ-ter) nanoliter.

millimicron (mil″ĭ-mi′kron) a unit of linear measure in the metric system, being 10^{-3} micron, 10^{-6} millimeter, or 10^{-9} meter; abbreviated mμ.

millimole (mil″ĭ-mōl) one-thousandth part of a mole (def. 3); abbreviated mM.

millimu (mil″ĭ-mu) millimicron.

milling-in (mil′ing-in) the correction of disharmonies of occlusion of natural or artificial teeth by modification of their occlusal surfaces by abrasives while they are rubbed together in the mouth or on the articulator.

millinormal (mil″ĭ-nor′mal) having a concentration one-thousandth of normal; abbreviated mN.

millions (mil′yunz) a name applied to various small fish that devour mosquito larvae; see *Lebistes reticulatus*.

milliosmol, milliosmole (mil″ĭ-os′mōl) one-thousandth of an osmol; the unit of osmotic pressure equal to one-thousandth gram molecular weight of a substance divided by the number of particles or ions into which a substance dissociates in one liter of solution. Abbreviated mOsm.

millipede (mil″ĭ-pēd) a more or less cylindrical arthropod of the order Chilognatha, class Diplopoda, characterized by having two pairs of short legs on most of its body segments; millipedes may have from 13 to almost 200 pairs of legs.

milliphot (mil′e-fot) the practical unit of illumination being 0.001 phot and approximately one foot candle.

millirad (mil′ĭ-rad) a unit of absorbed radiation dose, 10^{-3} rad; abbreviated mrad.

milliroentgen (mil′ĭ-rent″gen) a unit of dose equal to one-thousandth (10^{-3}) roentgen; abbreviated mr.

millisecond (mil″ĭ-sek′ond) one-thousandth of a second; abbreviated msec.

milliunit (mil′ĭ-u″nit) one-thousandth (10^{-3}) of a standard unit; abbreviated mU.

millivolt (mil′ĭ-vōlt) one-thousandth of a volt; abbreviated mv.

Millon's test (reaction, reagent) (mil′onz) [Auguste N. E. *Millon*, French chemist, 1812–1867] see under *tests*.

Mills' disease (milz) [Charles Karsner *Mills*, Philadelphia neurologist, 1845–1931] ascending hemiplegia.

Mills-Reincke phenomenon (milz-rīn′kĕ) [Hiram F. *Mills*, American engineer; J. J. *Reincke*, German physician] see under *phenomenon*.

Milontin (mi-lon′tin) trademark for preparations of phensuximide.

Milpath (mil′path) trademark for a preparation of meprobamate and tridihexethyl chloride.

milphae (mil′fe) [Gr. *milphai*] the falling out of the hair of the eyelids.

milphosis (mil-fo′sis) [Gr. *milphōsis*] milphae.

Milroy's disease (edema) (mil′roys) [William Forsyth *Milroy*, American physician, 1855–1942] see under *disease*.

Milton's edema (mil′tonz) [John Laws *Milton*, dermatologist in London, 1820–1898] angioneurotic edema.

Miltown (mil′town) trademark for a preparation of meprobamate.

milzbrand (milts′brahnt) [Ger.] anthrax.

Mima (me′mah) a genus of nonmotile, paired, gram-negative, enteric bacilli, causing a variety of nosocomial infections, including meningitis, pneumonia, urinary tract infections, etc. Called also *Acinetobacter lwoffi*.

mimbane hydrochloride (mim′bān) chemical name: 1-methylyohimbane monohydrochloride; an analgesic, $C_{20}H_{26}H_2 \cdot HCl$.

mimesis (mi-me′sis) [Gr. *mimēsis* imitation] the simulation of one disease or bodily process by another.

mimetic (mi-met′ik) [Gr. *mimētikos*] marked by simulation of another bodily process or disease. Also used as a word termination indicating simulation of a function, process, etc., designated by the root to which it is affixed, as *sympathomimetic*.

mimic (mim′ik) mimetic. **genetic m.,** genocopy.

mimicry (mim′ĭk-re′) [Gr. *mimos* to imitate] an adaptation for survival in which an organism takes on a resemblance to some other organism or a nonliving object.

mimmation (mi-ma′shun) the habitual insertion of the "m" sound in speech in places where it does not belong.

mimosis (mi-mo′sis) mimesis.

min. abbreviation for L. *min′imum*, a minim.

Minamata disease (min″ah-mah′tah) [*Minamata* Bay, Japan] see under *disease*.

Mincard (min′kard) trademark for a preparation of aminometradine.

mind (mīnd) [L. *mens*; Gr. *psychē*] the faculty, or function of the brain, by which an individual becomes aware of his surroundings and of their distribution in space and time, and by which he experiences feelings, emotions, and desires, and is able to attend, to remember, to reason, and to decide.

Mindererus, spirit of (min-der-e′rus) [Raymund *Minderer*, German physician, 1570(?)–1621] ammonium acetate solution.

mineral (min′er-al) [L. *minerale*] a nonorganic homogeneous solid substance, usually a constituent of the earth's crust.

mineralocorticoid (min″er-al-o-kor′tĭ-koid) 1. any of the group of corticosteroids, principally aldosterone, predominantly involved in the regulation of electrolyte and water balance through their effect on ion transport in epithelial cells of the renal tubules, resulting in retention of sodium and loss of potassium; some also possess varying degrees of glucocorticoid activity. Cf. *glucocorticoid*. 2. of, pertaining to, or resembling a mineralocorticoid.

mingin (min′jin) a nitrogenous compound, $C_{13}H_{18}N_2O_2$, found in small amounts in the urine.

mini- [*mini*ature] a combining form denoting something smaller than the usual thing of its kind.

minify (min′ĭ-fi) [L. *minus* less] to render less; to diminish. The opposite of magnify.

minilaparotomy (min″e-lap″ah-rot′o-me) [*mini-* + *laparotomy*] a small (about 5 mm.) upper abdominal incision for liver biopsy or open transhepatic cholangiography, or a small (1 to 4 cm.) incision just above the pubic hairline for sterilization by tubal occlusion, the uterine tubes being brought into the operative field by a uterine manipulator.

Mini-Lix (min′ĭ-liks) trademark for a preparation of aminophylline.

minim (min′im) [L. *minimum* least] a unit of capacity (liquid measure), being one-sixtieth part of a fluid dram, or the equivalent of 0.0616 milliliter.

minima (min′ĭ-mah) [L.] plural of *minimum*.

minimal (min′ĭ-mal) [L. *minimus* least] smallest or least; the smallest possible.

minimum (min′ĭ-mum), pl. *min′ima* [L. "smallest"] the smallest amount or lowest limit. **m. audib′ile,** auditory threshold. **m. cognoscib′ile,** the threshold of visual recognition of complicated shapes or contours. **m. legib′ile,** the threshold of visible recognition of form, as of test letters or numbers. **light m.,** the minimum intensity of light which is visually perceptible in completely darkened surroundings; called also *liminal value*. **m. sensib′ile,** threshold of consciousness. **m. separab′ile,** the least distance that two objects may be apart and still be distinguished as two. **m. visib′ile,** light m.

Minin light (min′in) [A. V. *Minin*, Russian surgeon] see under *light*.

minium (min′e-um) [L.] lead tetroxide.

Minkowski's figure, method (min-kov′skēz) [Oskar *Minkowski*, Lithuanian physician in Wiesbaden, 1858–1931] see under *figure*, and see *Naunyn-Minkowski method*, under *method*.

Minkowski-Chauffard syndrome (min-kov′ske-sho-far′) [Oskar Minkowski; Anatole-Marie-Emile *Chauffard*, French physician, 1855–1932] hereditary spherocytosis.

Minocin (mĭ-no′sin) trademark for preparations of minocycline hydrochloride.

minocycline (mĭ-no-si′klēn) chemical name: 4S,7-bis(dimethylamino)-1,4α,4aα,5,5aα,6,11,12aα-octahydro-3,10,12,12a-tetrahydroxy-1,11-dioxo-2-naphthacenecarboxamide; a semisynthetic broad-spectrum antibiotic of the tetracycline group, $C_{23}H_{27}N_3O_7$. **m. hydrochloride** [USP], the monohydrochloride salt of minocycline, $C_{23}H_{27}N_3O_7 \cdot HCl$, occurring as a yellow, crystalline powder; used in the treatment of a wide variety of infections due to tetracycline-susceptible bacteria and to some tetracycline-resistant organisms, especially staphylococci, administered orally and intravenously.

Minor's disease, sign (me′norz) [Lazar Salomonovich *Minor*, Russian neurologist, 1855–1942] see under *disease* and *sign*.

Minot-Murphy diet, treatment (mi′nut-mur′fe) [George Richards *Minot*, American physician, 1885–1950, and William Parry *Murphy*, American physician, born 1892, co-winners, with George Hoyt Whipple, of the Nobel prize for medicine and physiology in 1934, for their work on pernicious anemia] see under *treatment*.

minoxidil (mĭ-noks′ĭ-dil) chemical name: 6-(1-piperidinyl)-2,4-pyrimidinediamine 3-oxide; a potent, long-acting orally effective vasodilator, $C_9H_{15}N_5O$, acting primarily on arterioles, used as an antihypertensive.

mint (mint) see *Mentha*. **mountain m.,** a plant of the genus *Pycnanthemum*. **wild m.,** a fragrant North American plant, *Mentha canadensis*, L. (Labiatae), resembling pennyroyal in its odor and other properties. It is the source of an essential oil with a lemon-like odor used in perfumery.

Mintezol (min′tĕ-zol) trademark for a preparation of thiabendazole.

minuthesis (min-u′thĕ-sis) [Gr. *minuthēsis* a wasting] a decrease in the psychophysical sensitivity of a sense organ due to continuous stimulation of that organ; fatigue.

M.I.O. minimal identifiable odor.

mio- [Gr. *meiōn* smaller] a combining form meaning less; see also words beginning *meio-*.

miocardia (mi″o-kar′de-ah) [*mio-* + Gr. *kardia* heart] the contraction of the heart; systole.

Miochol (mi′o-kol) trademark for a preparation of acetylcholine chloride.

miodidymus (mi″o-did′ĭ-mus) [*mio-* + Gr. *didymos* twin] a fetus with two heads joined at the occiputs.

miolecithal (mi″o-les′ĭ-thal) [*mio-* + Gr. *lekithos* yolk] containing little yolk.

mionectic (mi″o-nek′tik) [Gr. *meionektikos* disposed to take too little] (*obs.*) taking up (by the blood) less than a normal amount of oxygen at a given P_{O_2}, i.e., the dissociation curve shifts to the right. Cf. *mesectic* and *pleonectic*.

miophone (mi′o-fōn) [*mio-* + Gr. *phōnē* sound] a microphone for testing the muscles.

miopragia (mi″o-pra′je-ah) [*mio-* + Gr. *prassein* to perform] decreased functional activity.

miopus (mi′o-pus) [*mio-* + Gr. *ōps* face] a monster with two fused heads, one face being rudimentary.

miosis (mi-o′sis) [Gr. *meiōsis* diminution] 1. contraction of the pupil. 2. meiosis. 3. that stage of disease during which the intensity of the symptoms diminishes. **irritative m.,** spastic miosis. **paralytic m.,** miosis due to paralysis of the dilator of the iris. **spastic m.,** miosis due to spasm of the sphincter pupillae. **spinal m.,** miosis occurring in spinal diseases.

miostagmin (mi″o-stag′min) [*mio-* + Gr. *stagma* drop] a hypothetical substance in the blood serum of infected animals which combines with antigen to lower the surface tension of the mixture.

miotic (mi-ot′ik) 1. pertaining to, characterized by, or producing miosis (def. 1). 2. an agent that causes the pupil to contract. 3. meiotic.

miracidia (mi-rah-sid′e-ah) plural of *miracidium*.

miracidium (mi-rah-sid′e-um), pl. *miracid′ia* [Gr. *meirakidion* a boy, lad, stripling] the first stage larva of a trematode which undergoes further development in the body of a snail.

miraculin (mir-ak′u-lin) a glycoprotein from the fruit of the tropical plant *Synsepalum dulcificum* which, after it is tasted, is able to change the perception of the taste of acids from sour to sweet.

Miradon (mir′ah-don) trademark for a preparation of anisindione.

mire (mēr) [Fr.; L. *mirari* to look at] one of the figures on the arm of an opthalmometer whose images are reflected on the cornea. The measurement of their variations measures the amount of corneal astigmatism.

mirincamycin hydrochloride (mir-in′kah-mi″sin) chemical name: methyl 7-chloro-6,7,8-trideoxy-6-[[4-pentyl-2-pyrrolidinyl)-carbonyl]amino]-1-thio-α-*threo*-α-D-*galacto*-octapyranoside(2*S-cis*)-mixture with methyl 7-chloro-6,7,8-trideoxy-6-[[(*trans*-4-pentyl-2(*S*)-pyrrolidinyl)carbonyl]amino]-1-thio-L-*threo*-α-D-*galacto*-octapyranoside monohydrochloride; an antibacterial and antimalarial, $C_{19}H_{35}ClN_2O_5S \cdot HCl$.

mirror (mir′or) [Fr. *miroir*] a polished surface that reflects sufficient light to yield images of objects in front of it. **concave m.,** one with a concave reflecting surface. **convex m.,** one with a convex reflecting surface. **dental m.,** mouth m.

frontal m., head m., a circular mirror strapped to the head of the examiner, used to reflect light into a cavity, especially in connection with nasal, pharyngeal, and laryngeal examinations and to some extent in surgery of these organs. **Glatzel m.,** a flat plate of cold metal held horizontally below and in front of the nose. The patch of moisture deposited on its polished surface indicates the relative functional patency of the two sides of the nose. **mouth m.,** a small mirror attached at an angle to a handle, for use in dentistry. **nasographic m.,** Glatzel m. **plane m.,** one with a flat reflecting surface. **van Helmont's m.,** centrum tendineum.

miryachit (mir-e′ah-chit) [Russ.] a variety of saltatory spasm, or jumping disease, prevalent in Siberia.

mis-action (mis-ak′shun) any accidental act, lapse of memory, or slip of the tongue, attributed to lack of normal repression of the ego, as in sleep or fatigue.

misanthropia, misanthropy (mis″an-thro′pe-ah; mis-an′-thro-pe) [*miso-* + Gr. *anthrōpos* man + -*ia*] hatred of mankind.

miscarriage (mis-kar′ij) loss of the products of conception from the uterus before the fetus is viable; spontaneous abortion.

misce (mis′e) [L.] mix.

miscegenation (mis″ĕ-jĕ-na′shun) [L. *miscere* to mix + *genus* race] the intermarriage or cohabitation of persons of different races, or the interbreeding of races.

miscible (mis′ĭ-b'l) susceptible of being mixed.

miserere mei (miz″er-a′re ma′e) [L. "have mercy on me"] 1. volvulus. 2. intestinal colic.

miso- (mis′o) [Gr. *misos* hatred felt against] a combining form meaning hatred of.

misogamy (mĭ-sog′ah-me) [*miso-* + Gr. *gamos* marriage] morbid aversion to marriage.

misogyny (mĭ-soj′ĭ-ne) [*miso-* + Gr. *gynē* woman] aversion to women.

misonidazole (mi″so-nid′ah-zōl) chemical name: α-(methoxymethyl)-2-nitro-1*H*-imidazole-1-ethanol; an antitrichomonal antiprotozoal, $C_7H_{11}N_3O_4$.

missexual (mis-seks′u-al) pertaining to an abnormal sexual balance, on the theory that every person is a mixture of male and female elements in varying degrees.

mist. abbreviation for L. *mistu′ra*, a mixture.

mistletoe (mis″'l-to) any of several related parasitic shrubs of the family Loranthaceae that grow on various trees, such as the apple and other deciduous trees, including *Viscum album* L. (*European m.*) and *Phorandendron flavescens* (Pursh.) Nutt. (*American m.*), preparations of which were formerly used for their oxytocic, emmenagogic, cardiac stimulant, and vasodilator properties. Toxic principles in mistletoe include pressor amines, beta-phenylethylamine, and tyramine, and it is the source of the glutinous principle viscin.

mistura (mis-tu′rah) [L.] mixture. **m. cre′tae,** chalk mixture. **m. glycyrrhi′zae compos′ita,** brown mixture. **m. oleobalsam′ica,** oleobalsamic mixture: alcoholic solution of balsam of Peru with aromatic oils and flavoring; used as a skin stimulant. **m. pectora′lis,** expectorant or pectoral mixture: ammonium carbonate 1.75 per cent, fluid extract of senega and squill each 3.5 per cent, camphorated tincture of opium 17.5 per cent, water, and syrup of tolu.

MIT monoiodotyrosine.

Mit. abbreviation for L. *mit′te*, send.

mitapsis (mit-ap′sis) [*mito-* + Gr. *hapsis* joining] the fusion of the chromatin granules in the final stage of cell conjugation.

Mitchell's disease, treatment (mich′elz) [Silas Weir *Mitchell*, Philadelphia neurologist, 1829–1914] see *erythromelalgia*, and see *Weir Mitchell's treatment*, under *treatment*.

mitchella (mich-el′ah) [John *Mitchell*, American botanist, 18th century] a creeping perennial herb, *Mitchella repens*, L. (Rubiaceae), squaw vine, partridge berry, deerberry, of the U.S. and Canada; used for its diuretic, astringent, and antidiarrheal properties, and formerly as a uterine tonic.

mite (mīt) any arthropod of the order Acarina except the ticks. The mites are minute animals, related to the spiders, usually having transparent or semitransparent bodies; they may be parasitic on man and domestic animals, producing various irritations of the skin (acariasis). Mites important to human and veterinary medicine are *Acarapis, Acarus, Allodermanyssus, Chorioptes, Demodex, Dermanyssus, Eutrombicular, Glycyphagus, Knemidokoptes, Neoschoengastia, Notoedres, Ornithonyssus, Otodectes, Pediculoides, Pneumonyssus, Psoroptes, Rhizoglyphus, Sarcoptes, Tetranychus, Trombicula, Tyrophagus*. **auricular m.,** see *Otodectes*. **beetle m.,** see *Gamasidae*. **bird m., chicken m.,** *Dermanyssus gallinae*. **burrowing m.** see *Sarcoptes*. **cheese m.,** *Tyrophagus longior*. **clover m.,** *Bryobia praetiosa*. **coolie-itch m.,** *Rhizoglyphus parasiticus*. **copra m.,** *Tyrophagus castellani*. **depluming m.,** *Knemidokoptes gallinae*. **face m.,** *Demodex folliculorum*. **flour m.,** *Tyrophagus farinae*. **follicle m.,** see *Demodex*. **food m.,** *Glycyphagus domesticus*. **fowl m.,** see *Dermanyssus*. **hair follicle m.,** *Demodex folliculorum*. **harvest m.,** see *chigger*.

house dust m., *Dermatophagoides pteronyssimus.* **itch m.,** see *Notoedres* and *Sarcoptes.* **kedani m.,** *Trombicula akamushi.* **louse m.,** *Pyemotes.* **mange m.,** see *Sarcoptes scabiei* and *mange.* **meal m.,** *Tyrophagus.* **mouse m.,** *Allodermanyssus sanguineus.* **mower's m.,** see *chigger.* **Northern fowl m.,** *Ornithonyssus sylviarum.* **onion m.,** *Acarus rhyzoglypticus hyacinthi.* **poultry m.,** *Dermanyssus gallinae.* **rat m.,** see *Ornithonyssus.* **red m.,** see *chigger.* **scab m.,** see *Psoroptes.* **spider m.,** see *Gamasidae.* **spinning m.,** *Bryobia praetiosa.* **straw m.,** *Pyemotes.* **tropical fowl m.,** *Ornithonyssus bursa.* **tropical rat m.,** *Ornithonyssus bacoti.*

mitella (mi-tel′ah) [L.] an arm sling.

Mithracin (mith′rah-sin) trademark for a preparation of mithramycin.

mithramycin (mith″rah-mi′sin) [USP] an antineoplastic antibiotic, $C_{52}H_{72}O_{24}$, produced by *Streptomyces argillaceus, S. tanashienis,* and *S. plicatus,* occurring as a yellow, crystalline powder; used in the treatment of certain inoperable testicular malignancies, administered by intravenous infusion. It has also been used in the symptomatic treatment of hypercalcemia and hypercalciuria associated with various advanced neoplasms.

mithridatism (mith′rĭ-da″tizm) [after *Mithridates,* died 63 B.C., king of Pontus, who reportedly took poisons so as to become immunized against them] the acquisition of immunity to the effects of a poison by ingestion of gradually increasing amounts of it.

miticidal (mi″tĭ-si′dal) destructive to mites.

miticide (mi′tĭ-sīd) an agent that is destructive to mites.

mitigate (mit′ĭ-gāt) [L. *mitigara* to soften] to moderate; to render milder.

mitis (mi′tis) [L.] mild.

mito- [Gr. *mitos* thread] a combining form meaning threadlike, or denoting relationship to a thread.

mitocarcin (mi″to-kar′sin) an antineoplastic antibiotic derived from *Streptomyces* species.

mitochondria (mi″to-kon′dre-ah, mit″o-kon′dre-ah), pl. of *mitochondrion* [*mito-* + Gr. *chondrion* granule] small spherical to rod-shaped components (organelles) found in the cytoplasm of cells, enclosed in a double membrane, with an internal membrane space between the two units, the inner one infolded into the interior of the organelle as a series of projections (cristae). They are the principal sites of the generation of energy (in the form of ion gradients and adenosine triphosphate [ATP] synthesis) resulting from the oxidation of foodstuffs, and they contain the enzymes of the Krebs and fatty acid cycles and the respiratory pathway. Mitochondria also contain RNA and DNA, by means of which they can independently replicate and code for the synthesis of some of their proteins. Called also *chondriosomes.*

mitochondrial (mi″to-kon′dre-al) of or pertaining to mitochondria.

mitochondrion (mi″to-kon′dre-on) singular of *mitochondria.*

mitocromin (mi″to-kro′min) an antineoplastic antibiotic produced by *Streptomyces viridochromogenes.*

mitogen (mi′to-jen) a substance that induces mitosis and cell transformation, especially lymphocyte transformation (q.v.). See also *lymphocyte transforming factor,* under *factor.*

mitogenesia (mit″o-jĕ-ne′se-ah) mitogenesis.

mitogenesis (mi″to-jen′ĕ-sis) [*mitosis* + Gr. *genesis* production] the production, or causation, of mitosis in or transformation of a cell.

mitogenetic (mi″to-jĕ-net′ik) pertaining to, inducing, or characterized by mitogenesis.

mitogenic (mi″to-jen′ik) causing or inducing mitosis or cell transformation.

mitokinetic (mit″o-ki-net′ik) [*mito-* + Gr. *kinēsis* motion] a term applied to the force existing in the kinoplasm of a cell which produces the achromatic spindle in karyokinesis.

mitomalcin (mi″to-mal′sin) an antineoplastic antibiotic produced by *Streptomyces malayensis.*

mitome (mi′tōm) a thready network of the protoplasm of a cell; the more solid portion of cell protoplasm.

mitomycin (mi″to-mi′sin) 1. any of a complex of three chemically related antineoplastic antibiotics with antitumor activity (designated A, B, and C), isolated from cultures of the soil bacterium *Streptomyces caespitosus,* which interfere with DNA synthesis (and thus with mitosis) by cross-linking, without markedly affecting RNA synthesis or protein synthesis. The C component is the most potent member of the complex (see def. 2). 2. [USP] mitomycin C: chemical name: 6-amino-8-[[(aminocarbonyl)oxy]methyl]-1a*R*-(1aα,8β,8aα,8bα)-hexahydro-8a-methoxy-5-methylazirino[2′,3′:3,4]pyrrolo[1,2-*a*]indole-4,7-dione. The component of the mitomycin complex with the most potent and effective antitumor activity, $C_{15}H_{18}N_4O_5$; used as adjunct therapy in adenocarcinoma of the stomach and pancreas, administered intravenously.

mitoplasm (mit′o-plazm) [*mito-* + Gr. *plassein* to form] the chromatic substance of a cell nucleus.

mitoschisis (mĭ-tos′kĭ-sis) [*mito-* + Gr. *schisis* split] karyokinesis.

mitoses (mi-to′sēz) plural of *mitosis.*

mitosin (mit′o-sin) a hormone producing mitosis or follicular maturation.

mitosis (mi-to′sis), pl. *mito′ses* [*mito-* + *-osis*] a method of indirect division of a cell, consisting of a complex of various processes, by means of which the two daughter nuclei normally receive identical complements of the number of chromosomes characteristic of the somatic cells of the species. Mitosis, the process by which the body grows and replaces cells, is divided into four phases. 1. *Prophase:* Formation of paired chromosomes; disappearance of nuclear membrane; appearance of the achromatic spindle; formation of polar bodies. 2. *Metaphase:* Arrangement of chromosomes in the equatorial plane of the central spindle to form the monaster. Chromosomes separate into exactly similar halves. 3. *Anaphase:* The two groups of daughter chromosomes separate and move along the fibers of the central spindle, each toward one of the

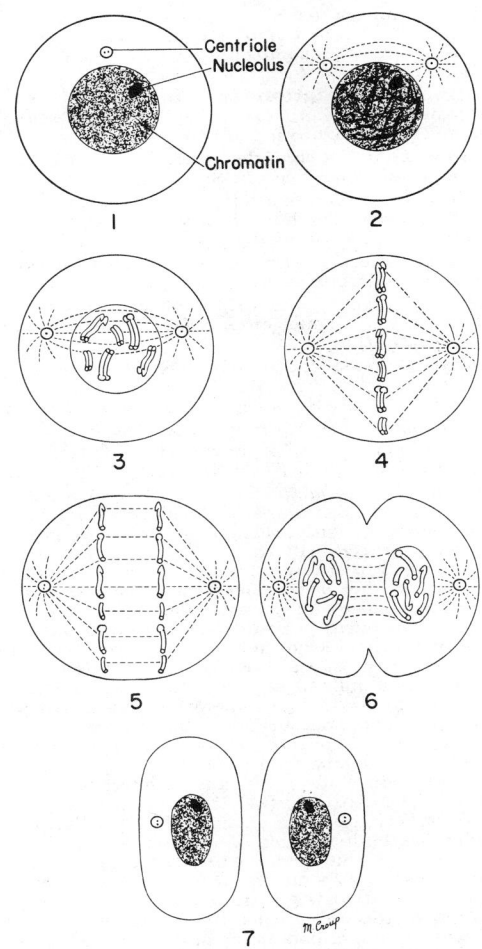

Mitosis shown as occurring in a cell of a hypothetical animal with a diploid chromosome number of six (haploid number three); one pair of chromosomes is short, one pair is long and hooked, and one pair is long and knobbed. *1,* Resting stage. *2,* Early prophase: centriole divided and chromosomes appearing. *3,* Later prophase: centrioles at poles, chromosomes shortened and visibly doubled. *4,* Metaphase: chromosomes arranged on equator of spindle. *5,* Anaphase: chromosomes migrating toward poles. *6,* Telophase: nuclear membranes formed; chromosomes elongating; cytoplasmic divisions beginning. *7,* Daughter cells: resting phase. (Villee.)

asters, forming the diaster. 4. *Telophase:* The daughter chromosomes resolve themselves into a reticulum and the daughter nuclei are formed; the cytoplasm divides, forming two complete daughter cells. NOTE: The term *mitosis* is used interchangeably with cell division, but strictly speaking it refers to nuclear division, whereas *cytokinesis* refers to division of the cytoplasm. In some cells, as in many fungi and the fertilized eggs of many insects, nuclear division occurs within the cell unaccompanied by division of the cytoplasm and formation of daughter cells. Cf. *meiosis.* **heterotypic m.,** mitosis in which the halves of bivalent chromosomes move away from each other toward the poles, as occurs in the first, or reductional, division of meiosis. **homeotypic m.,** the ordinary type of cell division in mitosis, as occurs also in the second, or equational, division of meiosis. **multicentric m.,** pluripolar m. **pathologic m.,** atypical, asymmetrical mitosis indicative of malignancy. **pluripolar m.,** cell division that results in the formation of more than two daughter cells.

mitosome (mit′o-sōm) [*mito-* + Gr. *sōma* body] a body formed from the spindle fibers of the preceding mitosis; a spindle remnant.

mitosper (mi′to-sper) an antineoplastic substance derived from *Aspergillus glaucus.*

mitospore (mi′to-spōr) an asexual spore, so called because it is produced by mitosis; when motile it is called a *zoospore.*

mitotane (mi′to-tān) [USP] chemical name: 1-chloro-2-[2,2-dichloro-1-(4-chlorophenyl)ethyl]benzene. An antineoplastic, C_{14}-$H_{10}Cl_4$, occurring as a white crystalline powder; used for the treatment of inoperable adrenocortical carcinoma of both functional and nonfunctional types, administered orally.

mitotic (mi-tot′ik) pertaining to mitosis.

mitral (mi′tral) 1. shaped somewhat like a miter. 2. pertaining to the mitral or bicuspid valve.

mitralism (mi′tral-izm) a tendency toward the development of mitral lesions in the heart.

mitralization (mi″tral-i-za′shun) straightening of the left border and prominence of the pulmonary salient of the cardiac shadow, a configuration commonly seen roentgenographically in mitral stenosis.

Mitsuda antigen, reaction, test (mit′su-dah) [Kensuke *Mitsuda,* Japanese physician, born 1876] see *lepromin,* see under *reaction,* and see *lepromin test,* under *tests.*

mittelschmerz (mit′el-shmārts) [Ger. *mittel* mid, middle, + *ʼschmerz* pain, suffering] intermenstrual pain.

mittor (mit′or) [L. *mittere* to send] any one of the terminals of a neuron which gives off an impulse or stimulus to the ceptors of an adjoining neuron; see *neuromittor.*

mixed (mikst) affecting various parts at once; showing two or more different characteristics.

mixidine (mik′sĭ-dēn) chemical name: 3,4-dimethoxy-*N*-(1-methyl-2-pyrrolidinylidene)benzeneethanamine; a coronary vasodilator, $C_{15}H_{22}N_2O_2.$

mixoscopia (miks″o-sko′pe-ah) [Gr. *mixis* intercourse + *skopein* to examine] sexual perversion in which gratification is obtained by the sight of others engaged in sexual intercourse.

mixoscopy (miks-os′ko-pe) mixoscopia.

mixotrophic (mik″so-trof′ik) having the nutritional characters of both animals and plants.

mixture (miks′tūr) [L. *mixtura, mistura*] a combination of different drugs or ingredients, as a fluid resulting from mixing a fluid with other fluids, or with solids, or a suspension of a solid in a liquid. See also under *mistura.* **A.C.E. m.,** a mixture of alcohol, chloroform, and ether. **Agazotti's m.,** a mixture of oxygen and carbon dioxide, formerly used for aviation sickness. **Aldrich m.,** a 1 per cent aqueous solution of gentian violet for the treatment of burns. **Bagot's m.,** a local anesthetic mixture of cocaine hydrochloride and spartein sulfate, in boiled water. **Biedert's cream m.,** a food for young infants, containing cream, water, and milk sugar. **brown m.,** a mixture containing glycyrrhiza fluidextract, antimony potassium tartrate, paregoric, alcohol, glycerin, and purified water; used as an expectorant. Formerly called *compound opium* and *glycyrrhiza mixture.* **Castellani's m.,** a mixture for treating yaws, containing tartar emetic, sodium salicylate, potassium iodide, sodium bicarbonate, and water. **Chabaud's m.,** a fixative mixture containing alcohol, phenol, formalin, and acetic acid. **chalk m.,** prepared chalk, with bentonite magma, cinnamon water, and saccharin sodium; used as an antacid. **expectorant m.,** see *mistura pectoralis.* **Gregory's m.,** compound powder of rhubarb; see under *powder.* **Gunning's m.,** a mixture used in estimating the nitrogen in the urine, consisting of 15 ml. of concentrated sulfuric acid, 10 gm. of potassium sulfate, and 0.5 gm. of copper sulfate. **kaolin m. with pectin** [NF], a preparation containing kaolin, pectin, powdered tragacanth, benzoic acid, saccharin sodium, glycerin, and peppermint oil in purified water; used as an adsorbent and demulcent. **Mayer's glycerin-albumin m.,** a mixture of equal parts of white of egg and glycerin, with a little camphor or phenol, for affixing paraffin sections to slides. **oleobalsamic m.,** see *mistura oleobalsamica.* **opium and glycyrrhiza m., compound,** former name for *brown mixture.* **pectoral m.,** mistura pectoralis. **racemic m.,** racemate. **Ringer's m.,** see under *irrigation.* **T.-A. m.,** see *toxin-antitoxin.* **Tellyesniczky's m.,** see under *fluid.* **toxin-antitoxin m.,** see *toxin-antitoxin.* **triple dye-soap m.,** equal parts of triple dye and soap solution (sapo molis diluted with three parts of water), used as a pliable coagulum for burns. **Vincent's m.,** a powder composed of an intimate mixture of sodium hypochlorite and boric acid; used as a wound dressing.

Miyagawanella (mi″yah-ga″wah-nel′ah) [Yoneji *Miyagawa,* Japanese bacteriologist, born 1885] a former genus of organisms now assigned to the genus *Chlamydia.* The species making up the genus (and the diseases associated with them) are now assigned as follows: *M. lymphogranulomato′sis* (lymphogranuloma venereum) and *M. bronchopneumo′niae* (mouse pneumonitis) are assigned to *Chlamydia trachomatis.* And the species *M. bo′vis* (calf enteritis), *M. fe′lis* (feline pneumonitis), *M. illi′nii* (pneumonitis), *M. louisia′-*

nae (Louisiana pneumonitis), *M. opos′sumi* (oppossum encephalitis), *M. ornitho′sis* (ornithosis), *M. o′vis* (enzootic abortion of ewes), *M. pe′coris* (sporadic bovine encephalomyelitis), *M. pneumo′niae* (human pneumonitis), and *M. psit′taci* (psittacosis) are assigned to the single species *Chlamydia psittaci.*

MK monkey lung (cell culture).

M.K.S. abbreviation for *meter-kilogram-second* system, a system of measurements in which the units are based on the meter as the unit of length, the kilogram as the unit of mass, and the second as the unit of time.

M.L. Licentiate in Medicine.

ml. milliliter.

M.L.A. abbreviation for L. *mento-laeva anterior* (left mentoanterior, a position of the fetus), and for *Medical Library Association.*

M.L.D. 1. median lethal dose. 2. minimum lethal dose.

M.L.P. abbreviation for L. *mento-laeva posterior* (left mentoposterior, a position of the fetus).

M.L.T. abbreviation for L. *mento-laeva transversa* (left mentotransverse, a position of the fetus).

M.M. mucous membranes.

mM. millimole.

mm. millimeter; muscles.

MMPI Minnesota Multiphasic Personality Inventory.

mm.p.p. millimeters partial pressure (partial pressure expressed in millimeters of mercury).

mμ millimicron.

mμc. millimicrocurie (nanocurie).

mμg. millimicrogram (nanogram).

μl. microliter.

μmg. micromilligram.

μmm. micromillimeter.

$\mu\mu$ micromicron.

$\mu\mu$c. micromicrocurie (picocurie).

$\mu\mu$g. micromicrogram (picogram).

Mn chemical symbol for *manganese.*

mN millinormal.

M'Naghten (McNaughten) rule (mik-naw′ten) [from *M'Naghten,* a person who in 1843 was acquitted by a British court of murder on the ground of insanity] see under *rule.*

mnemic (ne′mik) mnemonic.

mnemism (ne′mizm) mnemic theory.

mnemonic (ne-mon′ik) [Gr. *mnēmonikos* pertaining to memory] pertaining to, characterized by, or promoting recollection, or memory.

mnemonics (ne-mon′iks) the cultivation or improvement of memory by special methods or techniques.

mnemotechnics (ne″mo-tek′niks) mnemonics.

M.O. Medical Officer.

Mo chemical symbol for *molybdenum.*

Moban (mo′ban) trademark for a preparation of molindone hydrochloride.

mobility (mo-bil′ĭ-te) [L. *mobilitas*] 1. capability of movement, of being moved, or of flowing freely. 2. rate of movement of a charged particle in an applied electric field. **electrophoretic m.,** the velocity of a charged particle per unit of potential gradient in electrophoresis.

mobilization (mo″bĭ-li-za′shun) the process of making a fixed or ankylosed part movable. **stapes m.,** surgical correction of immobility of the stapes, in treatment of deafness.

mobilometer (mo″bil-om′ě-ter) an instrument for measuring the consistency of liquids such as oil, cream, liquid foods, etc.

Möbius' disease, sign, syndrome (me′be-us) [Paul Julius *Möbius,* German neurologist, 1853–1907] see under *disease, sign,* and *syndrome.*

moccasin (mok′ah-sin) a common name applied to several species of snakes, but usually denoting the venomous semiaquatic pit viper *Agkistrodon piscivorus,* or water moccasin, less frequently *A. contortrix,* or Highland moccasin. See table accompanying *snake.*

mocezuelo (mo″se-zwa′lo) [Mexican] trismus neonatorum.

mock-up (mok′up) a full-sized model of an apparatus or other equipment constructed out of substitute materials, used in instruction or for study and improvement of design.

modality (mo-dal′ĭ-te) 1. a homeopathic term signifying a condition which modifies drug action; a condition under which symptoms develop, becoming better or worse. 2. a method of application of, or the employment of, any therapeutic agent; limited usually to physical agents. 3. a specific sensory entity, such as taste.

mode (mōd) in statistics, the value or item in a variations curve which shows the maximum frequency of occurrence.

model (mod′el) something that represents something else, as a model for diagnostic or anatomical study. In dentistry, a cast. **animal m.,** any condition found in an animal that is of value in studying a biological phenomenon, e.g., a pathological mechanism of an animal disorder useful in studying human disease.

moderator (mod′er-a-tor) in nuclear chemistry and physics, a substance, such as graphite or beryllium, used to cut down the flux of subatomic particles or radiation by absorption of the same.

Moderil (mod′er-il) trademark for a preparation of rescinnamine.

modification (mod″ĭ-fi-ka′shun) the process or result of changing the form or characteristics of an object or substance. **behavior m.**, see under *therapy*. **racemic m.**, see *racemate*.

modifier (mod′ĭ-fi-er) something that alters or changes; in the plural, modifying factors (polygenes).

modioliform (mo″de-o′lĭ-form) shaped like the hub of a wheel.

modiolus (mo-di′o-lus) [L. "nave," "hub"] [NA] the central pillar or columella of the cochlea; called also *columella cochleae*.

Mod. praesc. abbreviation for L. *mo′do praescrip′to*, in the way directed.

modulating (mod″u-lāt′ing) in psychology, a form of facial deceit in which an individual modifies his facial expressions so as to show more or less of an emotion than is being experienced.

modulation (mod″u-la′shun) [L. *modulare* to measure] the normal capacity of cell adaptability to its environment. **antigenic m.**, the alteration of antigenic determinants in a living cell surface membrane following interaction with antibody.

modulator (mod″u-la′tor) a specific inductor that brings out characteristics peculiar to a definite region.

Moe plate (mo) [John H. *Moe*, American surgeon, born 1905] see under *plate*.

Moebius see *Möbius*.

Moeller's glossitis (me′lerz) [Julius Otto Ludwig *Moeller*, German surgeon, 1819–1887] see under *glossitis*.

Moeller's reaction (me′lerz) [Alfred *Moeller*, German bacteriologist, born 1868] rhinoreaction.

Moeller-Barlow disease (me′ler-bar′lo) [J. O. L. *Moeller*; Sir Thomas *Barlow*, London physician, 1845–1945] see under *disease*.

Moenckeberg (menk′ĕ-berg) see *Mönckeberg*.

Moentjang tina the Malay term in Indonesia for intoxication caused by the use in food of oil obtained from the fruit of the tropical tree *Hernandia sonora* L. (Hernandiaceae). Ordinarily the oil is used only in lamps.

Moerner-Sjöqvist method, test (mer′ner-syek′vist) [Carl Thore *Moerner*, Swedish physician, 1864–1917; John August *Sjöqvist*, Swedish physician, 1863–1934] see *Sjöqvist method*, under *method*.

mogi- [Gr. *mogis* with difficulty] a combining form meaning difficult, or with difficulty.

mogiarthria (moj-e-ar′thre-ah) [*mogi-* + Gr. *arthroun* to utter distinctly + *-ia*] a form of dysarthria in which there is defective coordination of the muscles involved.

mogilalia (moj-e-la′le-ah) [*mogi-* + *lalia* chatter] difficulty in speech; stuttering.

mogiphonia (moj-e-fo′ne-ah) [*mogi-* + Gr. *phōnē* voice] difficulty in making vocal sounds.

M.O.H. Medical Officer of Health.

Mohr's test (mōrz) [Francis *Mohr*, American pharmaceutical chemist] see under *tests*.

Mohrenheim's fossa (mo′ren-hīmz) [Baron Joseph Jacob Freiherr von *Mohrenheim*, Austrian surgeon, died 1799] trigonum deltoideopectorale.

moiety (moi′ĕ-te) [Fr. *moitié*, from L. *medietas*, *medius*, middle] any equal part; a half; also any part or portion. **carbohydrate m.**, a carbohydrate-derived portion of the structure of a molecule. **corrin m.**, a complex ring system in the vitamin B₁₂ molecule, closely related to the porphyrins of the cytochromes.

moist (moist) somewhat wet; damp.

mol (mol) mole, def. 3.

molal (mo′lal) containing one mole of solute per kilogram of solvent. NOTE: *molal* refers to the weight of the solvent, *molar* to the volume of solvent.

molality (mo-lal′ĭ-te) the number of moles of a solute per kilogram of pure solvent. NOTE: *Molality* refers to the weight of the solvent, *molarity* to the volume of the solvent.

molar (mo′lar) 1. [L. *moles* mass] pertaining to a mass; not molecular. 2. [L. *molaris* to do with grinding] adapted for grinding; see under *tooth*. 3. a posterior tooth which is used for grinding food and which acts as a major jaw support in the dental arch; see under *tooth*. 4. containing one mole of solute per liter of solution; cf. *molal*. **impacted m.**, a molar tooth that is prevented from erupting, or from taking its place in normal occlusion. **Moon's m's**, see under *tooth*. **mulberry m.**, a malformed first molar tooth with irregular crown, the enamel apparently consisting of an agglomerate mass of globules; usually seen in congenital syphilis. **sixth-year m.**, one of the permanent first molar teeth, so called because it usually erupts at the age of 6 years immediately posterior to the last molar of the deciduous

dentition. **third m.**, dens serotinus. **twelfth-year m.**, one of the permanent second molar teeth, so called because it usually erupts at the age of 12 years.

molariform (mo-lar′ĭ-form) shaped like a molar tooth.

molarity (mol-ar′ĭ-te) the number of moles of a solute per liter of solution. Cf. *molality*.

molasses (mo-las′ez) [L. *mellaceus* like honey] a thick, sweet syrup, the residue left after crystallization of sugar; treacle. **sugar-house m.**, that which is left after the refining of sugar. **West India m.**, a variety obtained in making raw sugar.

molc. molar concentration.

mold (mōld) 1. any of a large group of parasitic and saprophytic fungi that cause mold or moldiness and that exist as multicellular filamentous colonies; also, the deposit or growth produced by such fungi. The dimorphic fungi exist, according to environmental conditions, as molds or unicellular (yeast) forms. The common molds are *Mucor*, *Penicillium*, *Rhizopus*, and *Aspergillus*. See accompanying Plate XXVIII. 2. a form in which an object is given shape, or cast. 3. a term used in dentistry to specify the shape of an artificial tooth. **slime m.**, a fungus-like microorganism considered by some to be a protozoon and by others to be a fungus; see *Mycetozoida*. Called also *slime animal*. **white m.**, white or slightly woolly patches which form on the surface of meat in cold storage and other products due to the growth of various species of fungi.

molding (mōld′ing) 1. the creation of shape, or fashioning of an object. 2. the shaping of the fetal head in adjustment to the size and shape of the birth canal. **border m.**, the shaping of dental impression material by the manipulation or action of the tissues and structures adjacent to the borders of an impression. **compression m.**, the pressing or squeezing together of a plastic dental material to form a shape in a mold. **injection m.**, the fashioning of an object by forcing a plastic material into a closed mold through appropriate openings. **tissue m.**, border m.

mole (mōl) [L. *moles* a shapeless mass] 1. a fleshy mass or tumor formed in the uterus by the degeneration or abortive development of an ovum. 2. a nevocytic nevus; the term is also used to designate a pigmented fleshy growth, and is applied loosely to any blemish of the skin. 3. that amount of a substance (in a system) that contains as many elementary entities (atoms, ions, molecules, or radicals) as there are carbon atoms in 12 grams of carbon-12 (¹²C), or that amount of a chemical compound whose mass in grams is equivalent to its formula mass (see *gram-molecule*, and see *gram molecular weight*, under *weight*. A mole is considered to be equal to 6.023×10^{23} (Avogadro's number) elementary entities. Abbreviated mol. **blood m.**, a mass in the uterus made up of blood clots, the placenta, and fetal membranes retained after fetal death. **Breus' m.**, a malformation of the ovum consisting of tuberous subchorional hematoma of the decidua; called also *hematomole*. **cystic m.**, hydatidiform m. **false m.**, an intrauterine mass formed from a polyp or neoplasm. **fleshy m.**, 1. a blood mole which has assumed a fleshlike appearance. 2. one formed by a dead ovum in the uterus. **gram m.**, mole, def. 3. **hairy m.**, hairy nevus. **hydatid m.**, hydatidiform m., an abnormal pregnancy resulting from a pathologic ovum, with proliferation of the epithelial covering of the chorionic villi and dissolution and cystic cavitation of the avascular stroma of the villi. It results in a mass of cysts resembling a bunch of grapes. Called also *cystic* or *vesicular m.* **invasive m.**, **malignant m.**, **metastasizing m.**, chorioadenoma destruens. **pigmented m.**, see under *nevus*. **stone m.**, a mole which has undergone a calcareous degeneration. **true m.**, a mole which represents the degenerated ovum itself. **tubal m.**, the mass of blood clot and chorionic villi found after death of the conceptus in a tubal pregnancy. **vesicular m.**, hydatidiform m.

molecular (mo-lek′u-lar) of, pertaining to, or composed of molecules.

molecule (mol′ĕ-kūl) [L. *molecula* little mass] a very small mass of matter; the smallest amount of a substance which can exist alone; an aggregation of atoms; specifically, a chemical combination of two or more atoms which form a specific chemical substance. To break up the molecule into its constituent atoms is to change its character. The number and kind of atoms in a molecule vary with the compound. **diatomic m.**, one containing two atoms. **hexatomic m.**, one containing six atoms. **monatomic m.**, one which consists of a single atom. **nonpolar m.**, a molecule in which the electrical potential is symmetrically distributed over the molecule. **polar m.**, a molecule in which the electrical potential is not symmetrically distributed. **tetratomic m.**, a molecule made up of four atoms. **triatomic m.**, one composed of three atoms.

molilalia (mol″ĭ-la′le-ah) mogilalia.

molimen (mo-li′men), pl. *molim′ina* [L. "effort"] a laborious effort made for the performance of any normal body function, especially that manifested by a variety of mild but unpleasant symptoms preceding or accompanying the menstrual period; when such symptoms are severe, the condition is known as premenstrual tension.

molimina (mo-lim′ĭ-nah) plural of *molimen*.

molindone hydrochloride (mo-lin′dōn) chemical name: 3-

ethyl-1,5,6,7-tetrahydro-2-methyl-5-(4-morpholinylmethyl)-4*H*-indol-4-one monohydrochloride. A sedative and tranquilizer, $C_{16}H_{24}N_2O_2 \cdot HCl$, occurring as a white, crystalline powder; used in the management of schizophrenia, administered orally.

Mol-Iron (mōl-i′ron)   trademark for preparations of ferrous sulfate.

Molisch's test (reaction) (mol′ish-ez) [Hans *Molisch*, chemist in Vienna, 1856–1937]   see under *tests*.

Moll's glands (molz) [Jacob Antonius *Moll*, Dutch ophthalmologist, 1832–1914]   glandulae ciliaris conjunctivales.

mollescuse (mol-les′kūs) [L. *mollis* soft]   softening.

Mollicutes (mol″ĭ-ku′tēz) [L. *mollis* soft + *cutis* skin]   in some systems of classification, a class of microorganisms of the kingdom Procaryotae that includes prokaryotes lacking a true cell wall, therefore they are considered to be unrelated to the bacteria (see *Bacteria*). The class comprises the smallest living organisms, the members occurring as pleomorphic, coccoid, or filamentous cells with a tendency to produce myceloid structures, which are bounded by a triple-layered pliable membrane. It consists of a single order, the Mycoplasmatales.

mollin (mol′in)   a glycerinated soft soap with excess of fats, used as a vehicle for medicines to be applied externally.

mollities (mo-lish′e-ēz) [L.]   softness; abnormal softening. **m. os′sium,** osteomalacia. **m. un′guium** (*obs.*), abnormal softness of the nails.

mollusc (mol′usk)   mollusk.

Mollusca (mŏ-lus′kah) [L. *molluscus* soft]   a phylum of animals containing snails, slugs, mussels, oysters, clams, octopuses, nautiluses, squids, cuttlefish, etc.

molluscacidal (mŏ-lusk″ah-si′dal)   destructive to snails and other mollusks.

molluscacide (mŏ-lusk′ah-sīd)   an agent that will destroy snails and other mollusks.

molluscicide (mŏ-lus′sĭ-sīd)   molluscacide.

molluscous (mŏ-lus′kus)   pertaining to molluscum.

molluscum (mŏ-lus′kum) [L. *molluscus* soft]   the name given to various skin diseases characterized by the formation of soft rounded cutaneous tumors; when used alone it refers to *m. contagiosum*. **m. contagio′sum,** a skin disease caused by a virus and marked by the formation of firm, rounded, translucent, crateriform papules containing caseous matter and peculiar capsulated bodies (molluscous bodies). The papules are very chronic in their course, and are without general symptoms.

mollusk (mol′usk)   any member of the phylum Mollusca.

Moloney test (mo-lo′ne) [Peter J. *Moloney*, Canadian immunochemist, born 1891]   see under *tests*.

molting (mōlt′ing)   ecdysis.

molugram (mol′u-gram)   a gram-molecule.

Mol. wt.   molecular weight.

molybdate (mo-lib′dāt)   any salt of molybdic acid; some are used as tests, especially for the detection of heavy metal ions.

molybdenosis (mo-lib″dĕ-no′sis)   chronic molybdenum poisoning; see under *poisoning*.

molybdenum (mo-lib′dĕ-num) [Gr. *molybdos* lead]   a hard, silvery-white, metallic element; symbol, Mo; atomic number, 42; atomic weight, 95.94; specific gravity, 10.2. It is an essential trace element, being a component of the enzymes xanthine oxidase, aldehyde oxidase, and nitrate reductase. See also under *poisoning*.

molybdic (mo-lib′dik)   containing molybdenum as a hexavalent element.

molybdoprotein (mo-lib″do-pro′te-in)   an enzyme containing molybdenum (q.v.).

molybdous (mo-lib′dus)   containing molybdenum as a tetravalent element.

momentum (mo-men′tum) [L.]   the quantity of motion; the product of mass by velocity.

monacid (mon-as′id)   containing one atom of hydrogen that is replaceable by a base; said of a salt or of an alcohol.

monad (mon′ad) [Gr. *monas* a unit]   1. a single-celled protozoon or a single-celled coccus.   2. a univalent radical or element.   3. in meiosis, one member of a tetrad.

Monadidae (mon-ad′ĭ-de)   an order of protozoa of the class Zoomastigophora, subphylum Mastigophora, including the genus *Monas*.

monadin (mon′ah-din)   any microorganism or species belonging to the Monadina.

Monadina (mon″ah-di′nah)   in former classifications, a group of organisms including the orders Phytomonadina and Protomonadina.

Monakow's syndrome, theory, tract (bundle, fasciculus) (mon-ah′kovz) [Constantin von *Monakow*, neurologist in Zurich, 1853–1930]   see under *syndrome*, and see *diaschisis* and *tractus rubrospinalis*.

Monaldi's drainage (mo-nal′dēz) [V. *Monaldi*, Italian physician]   see under *drainage*.

monamide (mon-am′id)   monoamide.

monamine (mon-am′in)   monoamine.

monaminergic (mon-am″in-er′jik)   monoaminergic.

monangle (mon′ang-g′l)   having only one angle; Black's term for a dental instrument having only one angulation in the shank connecting the handle, or shaft, with the working portion of the instrument, known as the blade, or nib.

Monarda (mo-nar′dah)   American horsemint; wildbergamot. The leaves of *Monarda punctata* L. (Labiatae). A herbaceous plant found throughout the midwest and northeast United States and formerly used for its carminative and aromatic stimulant properties.

monarthric (mon-ar′thrik)   pertaining to or affecting a single joint.

monarthritis (mon″ar-thri′tis) [*mono-* + *arthritis*]   inflammation of a single joint.   **m. defor′mans,** arthritis deformans of a single joint.

monarticular (mon″ar-tik′u-lar)   monarthric.

Monas (mo′nas) [Gr. *monas* monad]   a genus of minute, solitary, free-swimming, flagellate protozoa of the family Monadidae, order Protomonadina.

monaster (mon-as′ter) [*mono-* + Gr. *astēr* star]   the single star-shaped figure at the end of the prophase in mitosis.

monathetosis (mon″ath-ĕ-to′sis) [*mono-* + *athetosis*]   athetosis of one limb.

monatomic (mon″ah-tom′ik) [*mono-* + Gr. *atomos* indivisible]   1. univalent.   2. monobasic.   3. consisting of monatomic molecules.

monauchenos (mon-awk′ĕ-nus)   a dicephalic monster with one neck.

monaural (mon-aw′ral)   pertaining to one ear.

monavalent (mon-av′ah-lent)   monovalent.

monavitaminosis (mon″ah-vi″tah-min-o′sis)   a deficiency disease in which only one vitamin is lacking in the diet.

monaxon (mon-ak′son) [*mono-* + Gr. *axōn* axis]   a neuron possessing only one axon.

monaxonic (mon″ak-son′ik)   having one axon.

Mönckeberg's arteriosclerosis, calcification, degeneration, mesarteritis, sclerosis (menk′e-bergz) [Johann Georg *Mönckeberg*, pathologist at Bonn, 1877–1925]   see under *arteriosclerosis*.

Mondeville (mon″dĕ-ve′yuh), Henri de (1260–1320)   a distinguished French surgeon—surgeon to Philip the Fair and Louis X—who wrote a surgical text (the first French one) containing many observations (e.g., on wound healing) that were far ahead of the times.

Mondonesi reflex (mon″do-na′ze) [Filippo *Mondonesi*, Italian physician]   bulbomimic reflex.

Mondor's disease (mon′dorz) [Henri *Mondor*, French surgeon, 1885–1962]   see under *disease*.

monecious (mon-e′shus)   monoecious.

monensin (mo-nen′sin)   an antibacterial, antifungal, and antiprotozoal antibiotic, $C_{36}H_{62}O_{11}$, produced by *Streptomyces cinnamonensis*, which has been used in veterinary medicine.

moner (mo′ner)   a non-nucleated mass of protoplasm.

Monera (mo-ne′rah) [Gr. *monērēs* single]   in some classifications, a kingdom comprising the unicellular prokaryotes, i.e., bacteria and blue-green algae, (see also *Procaryotae*), and in other classifications, also including viruses and rickettsiae.

monerula (mo-ner′u-lah), pl. *moner′ulae* [Gr. *monērēs* single]   an impregnated ovum with as yet no cleavage nucleus.

monesia (mo-ne′ze-ah) [L.]   an extract from monesia bark, the product of *Chrysophyllum glyciphloeum*, Casar. (Sapotaceae), a tree of Brazil; it is astringent and stomachic, and contains saponins, tannins, and glycyrrhizin.

monesthetic (mon″es-thet′ik) [Gr. *monos* single + *aisthēsis* perception]   pertaining to or affecting a single sense or sensation.

monestrous (mon-es′trus)   completing only one estrous cycle in each sexual season.

Monge's (mon′gez) [Carlos *Monge*, pathologist in Lima, Peru, born 1884]   chronic mountain sickness.

mongolian (mon-go′le-an) [see *mongolism*]   pertaining to, resembling, or belonging to the Mongols; a term formerly applied to defects characteristic of Down's syndrome.

mongolism (mon′go-lizm) [*Mongol*, a member of one of the chief ethnological divisions of Asiatic peoples]   Down's syndrome; so called because of facial characteristics typical of this condition. **translocation m.,** mongolism in which, although there are the normal 46 chromosomes, the genetic material of chromosome 21 is triplicated within each somatic cell instead of duplicated, as is normal.

mongoloid (mon′go-loid) [see *mongolism*]   1. pertaining to or resembling the Mongols.   2. an individual with Down's syndrome.

Moniezia (mon″ĭ-e′ze-ah)   a genus (family Anoplocephalidae) of tapeworms of cattle, goats, and sheep.

Plate XXVIII molds

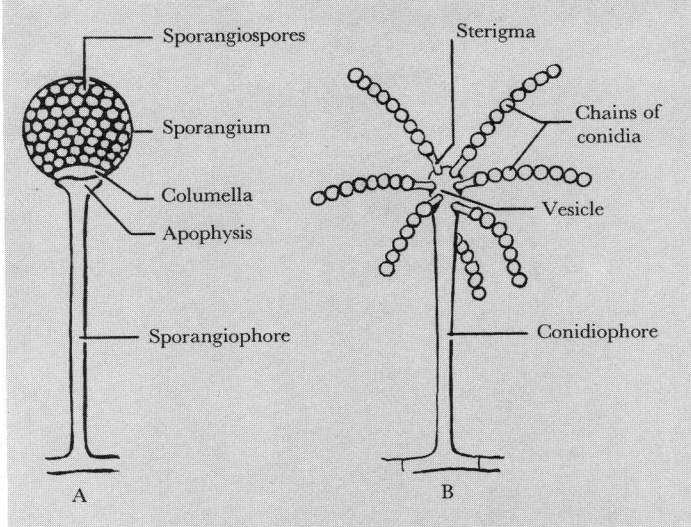

Fruiting bodies of Rhizopus (A) and Aspergillus (B). (Carpenter: Microbiology.)

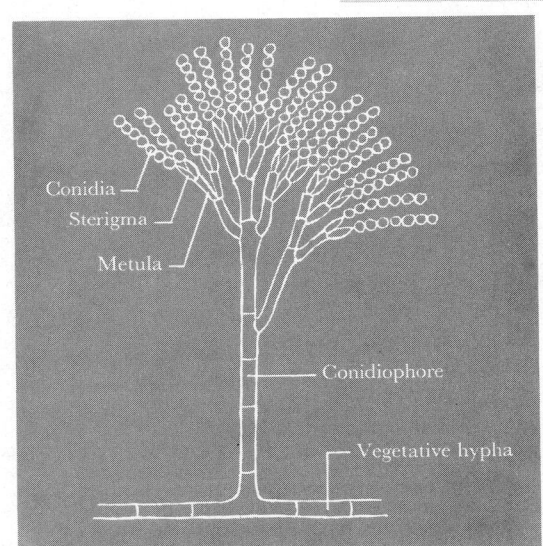

Drawing of *Penicillium*, showing the brushlike appearance of the parallel chains of conidia characteristic of this genus. (Carpenter: Microbiology.)

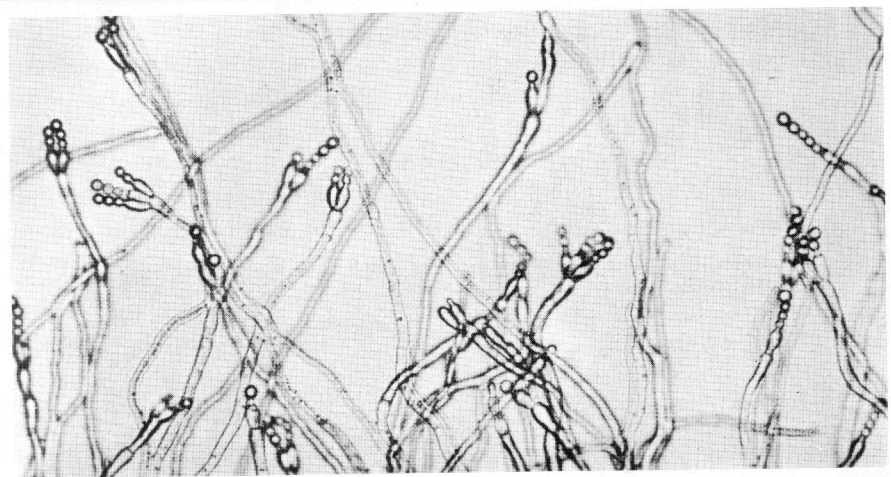

Photomicrograph of a *Penicillium*, showing twisted, branching hyphae and a few chains of conidia. (Courtesy of The Abbott Laboratories, North Chicago, Ill.)

CHARACTERISTIC STRUCTURES OF COMMON MOLDS

monilated (mon′il-āt″ed) moniliform.

monilethrix (mo-nil′e-thriks) [L. *monile* necklace + Gr. *thrix* hair] a disease condition, inherited as an autosomal dominant trait, in which the hairs exhibit marked multiple constrictions, with a beading effect, and are very brittle, rarely reaching an inch in length before breaking.

Monilia (mo-nil′e-ah) [L. *monile* necklace] 1. a former name for a genus of fungi now called *Candida*. 2. a genus of imperfect fungi of the family Moniliaceae, order Moniliales; its perfect (sexual) stage is *Sclerotinia*.

Moniliaceae (mo-nil″e-a′se-e) a family of colorless or light-colored imperfect fungi of the order Moniliales, which includes the genera *Histoplasma, Blastomyces, Sporothrix, Trichophyton, Coccidioides, Aspergillus, Trichoderma, Verticillium, Trichothecium* and *Penicillium*.

monilial (mo-nil′e-al) pertaining to or caused by *Monilia*.

Moniliales (mo-nil″e-a′lēz) an order of imperfect fungi whose conidia are usually borne directly on undifferentiated mycelia, and including the families Cryptococcaceae, Moniliaceae, Dematiaceae, and Tuberculariaceae. Formerly called *Conidiosporales.*

moniliasis (mon-ĭ-li′ah-sis) an infection caused by *Monilia*. See *candidiasis.*

moniliform (mo-nil′ĭ-form) [L. *monile* necklace + *forma* form] shaped like a necklace or string of beads.

Moniliformis (mo-nil″ĭ-for′mis) a genus of acanthocephalans. *M. monilifor′mis* (formerly *Echinorhynchus moniliformis*) is a parasite of rats, mice, and dogs, and a facultative parasite in man.

moniliid (mo-nil′e-id) candidid.

moniliosis (mo-nil″e-o′sis) candidiosis.

Monistat (mo′nĭ-stat) trademark for a preparation of miconazole nitrate.

monitor (mon′ĭ-tor) [L. "one who reminds," from *monere* to remind, admonish] 1. to check constantly on a state or condition, as on the vital signs of a patient under anesthesia and undergoing surgery, or to determine the amount of exposure to radiation. 2. an apparatus used to observe or record such physiological signs as respiration, pulse, and blood pressure in an anesthetized patient or one undergoing surgical or other procedures.

monium (mo′ne-um) [Gr. *monos* single] (*obs.*) a name given an earth metal discovered in 1898, later found to be a mixture of rare earth metals.

Moniz (mo′nēz), Antonio Egas. Portugese neurosurgeon 1874–1955, noted for the development of cerebral angiography and the introduction of prefrontal lobotomy; co-winner, with Walter Rudolf Hess, of the Nobel prize for medicine and physiology in 1949.

monkey paw (mon′ke-paw) a condition in which the thumb lies in adduction and extension and cannot be opposed so as to touch the tips of the other fingers, owing to weakness of the opposing muscles of the thumb, as in lesion of the median nerve.

monkeypox (mon′ke-poks) a mild disease resembling smallpox, occurring in laboratory monkeys, and caused by a virus related to the smallpox virus. Several human cases have been reported in West Africa.

Monneret's pulse (mon-rāz′) [Jules Auguste Edward *Monneret*, physician in Paris, 1810–1868] see under *pulse*.

mono- [Gr. *monos* single] a combining form denoting one or single; limited to one part; in chemistry, combined with one atom.

monoamide (mon″o-am′īd) an amide containing one amide group.

monoamine (mon″o-am′ēn) an amine molecule containing one amino group, e.g., serotonin, dopamine, and norepinephrine.

monoaminergic (mon″o-am″in-er′jik) of or pertaining to neurons that secrete the monoamine neurotransmitters dopamine, norepinephrine, and serotonin.

monoaminodiphosphatide (mon″o-am″ĭ-no-di-fos′fah-tīd) a phosphatide containing 1 atom of nitrogen and 2 of phosphorus to the molecule.

monoaminomonophosphatide (mon″o-am″ĭ-no-mon″o-fos′-fah-tīd) a phosphatide containing 1 atom of nitrogen and 1 of phosphorus to the molecule.

monoamniotic (mon″o-am″ne-ot′ik) having or developing within a single amniotic cavity; said of monozygotic twins.

monoanesthesia (mon″o-an″es-the′ze-ah) [*mono-* + *anesthesia*] anesthesia of a single part or organ.

monoarticular (mon″o-ar-tik′u-lar) monarthric.

monobacillary (mon″o-bas′ĭ-lār″e) caused by or containing a single species of bacillus.

monobacterial (mon″o-bak-te′re-al) monobacillary.

monobasic (mon″o-ba′sik) [*mono-* + Gr. *basis* base] having but one base; a term applied to an acid having only one replaceable atom of hydrogen and therefore yielding only one series of salts, as HCl.

monobenzone (mon″o-ben′zōn) [USP] chemical name: 4-(phenylmethoxy)phenol. A melanin-inhibiting agent, $C_{13}H_{12}O_2$, occur-ring as a white, crystalline powder; used as a depigmenting agent, applied topically to the skin.

monoblast (mon′o-blast) [*mono-* + Gr. *blastos* germ] the earliest precursor in the monocytic series, which matures to develop into the promonocyte; monoblasts have a fine chromatin structure and nucleoli are usually visible. They are not normally seen in the bone marrow or peripheral blood, but may be seen in monocytic anemia.

monoblastoma (mon″o-blas-to′mah) a neoplasm containing monoblasts and monocytes.

monoblepsia (mon″o-blep′se-ah) [*mono-* + Gr. *blepsis* sight + *-ia*] 1. a condition of the vision in which it is more distinct when only one eye is used. 2. a variety of color blindness in which only one color is perceived.

monobrachia (mon″o-bra′ke-ah) [*mono-* + Gr. *brachion* arm + *-ia*] a developmental anomaly characterized by the presence of a single arm.

monobrachius (mon″o-bra′ke-us) an individual exhibiting monobrachia.

monobromated (mon″o-bro′māt-ed) [L. *monobromatus*] having a single atom of bromine in each molecule.

monobromophenol (mon″o-bro′mo-fe′nol) a violet-colored liquid, $OH \cdot C_6H_4Br$, of penetrating odor, soluble in water, alcohol, and ether, formerly used as an external antiseptic.

monocalcic (mon″o-kal′sik) containing one atom of calcium in the molecule.

monocardian (mon-o-kar′de-an) [*mono-* + Gr. *kardia* heart] possessing a heart with a single atrium and ventricle, as that of a shark.

monocelled (mon′o-seld) [*mono-* + *cell*] unicellular; consisting of a single cell.

monocellular (mon″o-sel′u-lar) unicellular.

monocephalus (mon″o-sef′ah-lus) [*mono-* + Gr. *kephalē* head] a monster with one head but with some duplication of its parts. **m. tet′rapus dibra′chius,** a monster with one head, two arms, and partial or complete duplication of the pelvis, with four legs, the pair belonging to one member often being fused in a single limb. **m. tri′pus dibra′chius,** a monster with one head, two arms, and partial duplication of the pelvis, with a median third leg or leg rudiment.

monochlorothymol (mon″o-klo″ro-thi′mol) chlorothymol.

monochord (mon′o-kord) [*mono-* + Gr. *chordē* cord] (*obs.*) an instrument for testing upper tone audition. It consists of a long steel or silver wire fastened at the ends and having an intermediate movable clamp. The tone is produced by longitudinal friction. Called also *Schultze's monochord*.

monochorea (mon″o-ko-re′ah) [*mono-* + *chorea*] chorea affecting but one limb.

monochorial (mon″o-ko′re-al) monochorionic.

monochorionic (mon″o-ko″re-on′ik) [*mono-* + *chorionic*] having or developing in a common chorionic sac; said of monozygotic twins.

monochroic (mon″o-kro′ik) [*mono-* + Gr. *chroa* color] having only one color; monochromatic.

monochromasy (mon″o-kro′mah-se) blindness to all colors but one: color blindness, in which all colors are seen as one color.

monochromat (mon″o-kro′mat) a person affected by monochromatism; called also *achromat*.

monochromatic (mon″o-kro-mat′ik) [*mono-* + Gr. *chrōma* color] 1. existing in or having only one color. 2. pertaining to or affected by monochromatism. 3. staining with only one dye at a time. Cf. *polychromatic*.

monochromatism (mon″o-kro′mah-tizm) complete color blindness; inability to discriminate hues, all colors of the spectrum appearing as neutral grays with varying shades of light and dark. Called also *achromatism, achromatopia,* and *achromotopsia*. **cone m.,** that in which there is some cone function and normal visual acuity and which is not associated with nystagmus and photophobia. **rod m.,** that in which there is complete absence of cone function and which is accompanied by poor vision, photophobia, and nystagmus.

monochromatophil (mon″o-kro-mat′o-fil) [*mono-* + Gr. *chrōma* color + *philein* to love] 1. stainable with only one kind of stain. 2. any cell or other element that will take only one stain.

monochromophilic (mon″o-kro″mo-fil′ik) stainable with only one kind of stain.

monoclinic (mon″o-klin′ik) [*mono-* + Gr. *klinein* to incline] a term applied to crystals in which the vertical axis is inclined to one lateral axis, but is at right angles to the other.

monoclonal (mon″o-klōn′al) derived from a single cell; pertaining to a single clone.

monocontaminated (mon″o-kon-tam′ĭ-nāt″ed) infected by a single species of microorganism, or by a single type of contaminating agent; see *monoxenic*.

monocontamination (mon″o-kon-tam″ĭ-na′shun) experimental infection of a previously germ-free animal by a single infectious agent.

monocorditis (mon″o-kōr-di′tis) inflammation of one vocal cord.

monocranius (mon″o-kra′ne-us) [*mono-* + Gr. *kranion* cranium] monocephalus.

monocrotic (mon″o-krot′ik) characterized by monocrotism.

monocrotism (mo-nok′ro-tizm) [*mono-* + Gr. *krotos* beat] a simple pulse wave contour having neither an anacrotic nor a dicrotic notch.

monocular (mon-ok′u-lar) [*mono-* + L. *oculus* eye] 1. pertaining to or having but one eye. 2. having but one eyepiece, as in a microscope.

monoculus (mon-ok′u-lus) [*mono-* + L. *oculus* eye] 1. a bandage for covering one eye. 2. a cyclops.

monocyclic (mon″o-si′klik) pertaining to one cycle. In chemistry, having a molecular structure containing only one ring.

monocyesis (mon″o-si-e′sis) [*mono-* + Gr. *kyēsis* pregnancy] pregnancy with a single fetus.

Monocystis (mon″o-sis′tis) [*mono-* + Gr. *kystis* sac, bladder] a genus of sporozoa of the order Gregarinidia, species of which are parasitic in the seminal vesicles of the earthworm.

monocyte (mon′o-sīt) [*mono-* + *-cyte*] a mononuclear phagocytic leukocyte, 13μ to 25μ in diameter, with an ovoid or kidney-shaped nucleus, containing lacey, linear chromatin, and abundant gray-blue cytoplasm filled with fine, reddish and azurophilic granules. Formed in the bone marrow from the promonocyte, monocytes are transported to tissues, as of the lung and liver, where they develop into macrophages. Formerly called *large mononuclear leukocyte,* and *hyaline* or *transitional leukocyte.* See also *monocytic series,* under *series.*

monocytic (mon″o-sit′ik) 1. pertaining to, characterized by, or of the nature of monocytes. 2. pertaining to the monocytic series; see under *series.*

monocytoid (mon″o-si′toid) resembling a monocyte.

monocytopenia (mon″o-si″to-pe′ne-ah) [*monocyte* + Gr. *penia* poverty] abnormal decrease in the proportion of monocytes in the blood.

monocytopoiesis (mon″o-si″to-poi-e′sis) [*monocyte* + Gr. *poiein* to make] the formation of monocytes.

monocytosis (mon″o-si-to′sis) increase in the proportion of monocytes in the blood.

Monod (mŏ-no′), Jacques Lucien. French biochemist, born 1910; co-winner with François Jacob and André Michael Lwoff, of the Nobel prize in medicine and physiology for 1965, for discoveries concerning the genetic control of enzymes and virus synthesis.

monodactylia (mon″o-dak-til′e-ah) monodactyly.

monodactylism (mon-o-dak′til-izm) monodactyly.

monodactyly (mon″o-dak′tĭ-le) [*mono-* + Gr. *daktylos* finger] a developmental anomaly characterized by the presence of only one digit on a hand or foot.

monodal (mon-o′dal) [*mono-* + Gr. *hodos* road] having connection with one terminal of a resonator or of a grounded solenoid, so that the patient is a capacitor for entrance and exit of high frequency currents.

monodermoma (mon″o-der-mo′mah) a tumor that has developed from one germinal layer.

monodiplopia (mon″o-dĭ-plo′pe-ah) [*mono-* + Gr. *diploos* double + *ōps* eye + *-ia*] double vision in one eye only.

Monodontus (mon″o-don′tus) *Bunostomum.*

Monodral bromide (mon′o-dral) trademark for preparations of penthienate bromide.

monoecious (mon-e′shus) [*mono-* + Gr. *oikos* house] having reproductive organs typical of both sexes in a single individual.

monoethanolamine (mon″o-eth″ah-nōl′ah-mēn) chemical name: 2-aminoethanol. An amino alcohol, C_2H_7NO, found in cephalins and phospholipids, and derived metabolically by decarboxylation of serine. The official preparation [NF], occurring as a clear, colorless, moderately viscous liquid, is used as a surfactant in pharmaceutical preparations. A combination of monoethanolamine and oleic acid (known as *ethanolamine oleate*) has been used as a sclerosing agent in the injection treatment of varicose veins. Called also *colamine* and *ethanolamine.*

monofilm (mon′o-film) a monomolecular layer transferred to a prepared plate.

monogametic (mon″o-gah-met′ik) [*mono-* + *gamete*] having only one kind of gamete with respect to the sex chromosomes, as the human female.

monogamy (mo-nog′ah-me) [*mono-* + Gr. *gamos* marriage] marriage to a single spouse.

monoganglial (mon″o-gang′gle-al) affecting a single ganglion.

monogastric (mon″o-gas′trik) [*mono-* + Gr. *gaster* stomach] having but one belly or stomach.

monogen (mon′o-jen) 1. a univalent chemical element which combines in only one proportion. 2. an antiserum produced by the use of one antigen (i.e., immunogen).

monogenesis (mon″o-jen′ĕ-sis) [*mono-* + Gr. *genesis* production]

1. the production of only male or female offspring. 2. the theory that all things develop from a single cell.

monogenic (mon-o-jen′ik) pertaining to or influenced by a single gene.

monogerminal (mon″o-jer′mĭ-nal) monozygotic.

monoglyceride (mon″o-glis′er-īd) a compound consisting of one molecule of fatty acid esterified to glycerol.

monogonia (mon″o-go′ne-ah) plural of *monogonium.*

monogonium (mon″o-go′ne-um), pl. *monogo′nia.* (*obs.*) any of the asexual forms of the malarial parasite as it occurs in the blood; these forms produce the febrile attacks. Cf. *schizont.*

monograph (mon′o-graf) [*mono-* + Gr. *graphein* to write] an essay or treatise on one subject.

monohybrid (mon″o-hi′brid) the offspring of parents differing in one character.

monohydrated (mon″o-hi′drāt-ed) united with a single molecule of water or a single hydroxyl group.

monohydric (mon″o-hi′drik) containing one atom of replaceable hydrogen.

monoinfection (mon″o-in-fek′shun) infection with a single kind of organism.

monoiodotyrosine (mon″o-i-o″do-ti′ro-sēn) an iodinated amino acid that is an intermediate in the synthesis of thyroxine and triiodothyronine. Abbreviated MIT.

monokaryon (mon″o-ka′re-on) [*mono-* + Gr. *karyon* kernel] a growth stage in the mycelium of fungi, especially Basidiomycetes, in which each cell has one haploid nucleus.

monokaryote (mon″o-kar′e-ōt) a cell having one haploid nucleus.

monokaryotic (mon″o-kar″e-ot′ik) pertaining to the monokaryon or to a monokaryote.

monoketoheptose (mon″o-ke″to-hep′tōs) a natural sugar, $CH_2OH \cdot CO(CHOH)_4 \cdot CH_2OH$, found in the avocado, *Persea gratissima.*

monolayer (mon″o-la′er) pertaining to or consisting of a single layer, such as a monolayer sheet of cells in cultures used in studies of viruses.

monolene (mon′o-lēn) a clear white, oily hydrocarbon.

monolepsis (mon″o-lep′sis) [*mono-* + Gr. *lēpsis* a taking] the transmission to the offspring of the characters of one parent, to the exclusion of those of the other.

monolocular (mon″o-lok′u-lar) [*mono-* + L. *loculus* cell] having but one cavity or compartment, as a cyst.

monomania (mon″o-ma′ne-ah) [*mono-* + Gr. *mania* madness] psychosis on a single subject or class of subjects. **emotional m.,** monomania with respect to one or a few related emotions. **intellectual m.,** a monomania with respect to one or a few related delusions.

monomaxillary (mon″o-mak′sĭ-ler″e) affecting one jaw.

monomelic (mon″o-mel′ik) [*mono-* + Gr. *melos* limb] affecting one limb.

monomer (mon′o-mer) a simple molecule of a compound of relatively low molecular weight; a substance consisting of simple unrepeated structural units, but capable of reaction to form a dimer, trimer, polymer, etc. **fibrin m.,** the material resulting from the highly specific and orderly cleavage of fibrinogen by thrombin; through polymerization, these monomers form macromolecular fibrin.

monomeric (mon″o-mer′ik) [*mono-* + Gr. *meros* part] pertaining to, made up of, or affecting a single segment, as distinguished from dimeric, polymeric, etc. In genetics, determined by a gene or genes at a single locus either in the heterozygous or homozygous state.

monometallic (mon″o-mĕ-tal′ik) having one atom of a metal in the molecule.

monomicrobic (mon″o-mi-kro′bik) characterized by the presence of a single species of microbe.

monomolecular (mon″o-mo-lek′u-lar) pertaining to or involving one molecule.

monomoria (mon″o-mo′re-ah) [*mono-* + Gr. *mōria* silliness, folly] monomania.

monomorphic (mon″o-mor′fik) [*mono-* + Gr. *morphē* form] existing in only one form; maintaining the same form throughout all stages of development.

monomorphism (mon″o-mor′fizm) the quality or condition of being monomorphic.

monomorphous (mon″o-mor′fus) composed of lesions all of the same age, form, and shape, as a monomorphous eruption, such as variola.

monomphalus (mon-om′fah-lus) [*mono-* + Gr. *omphalos* navel] a double monster joined at the navel.

monomyoplegia (mon″o-mi′o-ple′je-ah) [*mono-* + Gr. *mys* muscle + *plēgē* stroke] paralysis restricted to a single muscle.

monomyositis (mon″o-mi″o-si′tis) [*mono-* + *myositis*] a myositis of the biceps muscle occurring periodically.

Mononchus (mon-ong′kus) a genus of nematodes living in fresh water or moist soil, reportedly found in human urine, probably representing a case of spurious parasitosis.

mononephrous (mon″o-nef′rus) [*mono-* + Gr. *nephros* kidney] affecting one kidney only.

mononeural (mon″o-nu′ral) pertaining to or receiving branches from a single nerve.

mononeuric (mon″o-nu′rik) [*mono-* + Gr. *neuron* nerve] having only one neuron.

mononeuritis (mon″o-nu-ri′tis) [*mono-* + Gr. *neuron* nerve + *-itis*] disease of a single nerve. **m. mul′tiplex,** simultaneous disease of several peripheral nerves.

mononeuropathy (mon″o-nu-rop′ah-thē) disease affecting a single nerve. **cranial m.,** disease of one of the cranial nerves, as the seventh cranial nerve in Bell's palsy.

mononoea (mon″o-ne′ah) [*mono-* + Gr. *nous* mind] mental concentration on a single subject.

monont (mon′ont) (*obs.*) schizont.

mononuclear (mon″o-nu′kle-ar) [*mono-* + *nucleus*] 1. having but one nucleus; mononucleate; uninucleated. 2. a cell having a single nucleus, especially a monocyte of the blood or tissues.

mononucleate (mon″o-nu′kle-āt) having a single nucleus; mononuclear.

mononucleosis (mon″o-nu″kle-o′sis) the presence of an abnormally large number of mononuclear leukocytes (monocytes) in the blood. **cytomegalovirus (CMV) m.,** see *infectious m.* **infectious m.,** an acute infectious disease caused by the Epstein-Barr virus, and characterized by fever, malaise, sore throat, hepatic dysfunction, lymphadenopathy, hepatosplenomegaly, atypical lymphocytes (resembling monocytes) in the peripheral blood, and high titers of agglutinins against sheep cells (heterophile titer). A marked asthenia persists throughout the course of the disease and the convalescent period. A similar syndrome has been associated with primary cytomegalovirus infection. Called also *glandular fever, acute benign lymphoblastosis, acute epidemic lymphadenosis, monocytic angina,* and *acute infectious adenitis.* **post-transfusion m.,** postperfusion syndrome.

mononucleotide (mon″o-nu′kle-o-tīd″) a product obtained by the digestion or hydrolytic decomposition of nucleic acid. It is a compound of phosphoric acid and a pentoside. The latter is a combination of a pentose (ribose or 2-deoxyribose) with one of the following bases: guanine, adenine, cytosine, uracil, or thymine.

mono-osteitic (mon″o-os″te-it′ik) denoting a type of osteitis which affects a single bone.

mono-ovular (mon″o-ov′u-lar) monovular.

monoparesis (mon″o-pah-re′sis) [*mono-* + Gr. *paresis* slackening of strength, paralysis] paresis of a single limb.

monoparesthesia (mon″o-par″es-the′ze-ah) [*mono-* + *paresthesia*] paresthesia of a single limb.

monopathy (mo-nop′ah-the) [*mono-* + Gr. *pathos* disease] a disease affecting a single part.

monopenia (mon″o-pe′ne-ah) monocytopenia.

monophagia (mon″o-fa′je-ah) [*mono-* + Gr. *phagein* to eat + *-ia*] 1. desire for one kind of food only. 2. the eating of only one meal a day.

monophagism (mo-nof′ah-jizm) monophagia.

monophasia (mon″o-fa′ze-ah) [*mono-* + Gr. *phasis* speaking] aphasia with ability to utter but one word or phrase.

monophasic (mon″o-fa′zik) exhibiting only one phase or variation. Cf. *diphasic, triphasic.*

monophosphate (mon″o-fos′fāt) a salt containing a single phosphate radical.

monophthalmus (mon″of-thal′mus) [*mono-* + Gr. *ophthalmos* eye] a cyclops.

monophyletic (mon″o-fi-let′ik) [*mono-* + Gr. *phylē* tribe] arising or descended from a single cell type.

monophyletism (mon″o-fi′lĕ-tizm) monophyletic theory; see under *theory.*

monophyletist (mon″o-fi′lĕ-tist) an adherent of the monophyletic theory, as in blood origin.

monophyodont (mon″o-fi′o-dont) [*mono-* + Gr. *phyein* to grow + *odous* tooth] having only one set of teeth, and those permanent.

monopia (mon-o′pe-ah) [*mono-* + Gr. *ops* eye + *-ia*] cyclopia.

monoplasmatic (mon″o-plaz-mat′ik) [*mono-* + Gr. *plasma* plasm] made up of a single substance.

monoplast (mon′o-plast) [*mono-* + Gr. *plastos* formed] a single constituent cell.

monoplegia (mon″o-ple′je-ah) [*mono-* + Gr. *plēgē* stroke] paralysis of a limb.

monoplegic (mon″o-ple′jik) pertaining to or characterized by monoplegia.

monopodia (mon″o-po′de-ah) [*mono-* + Gr. *pous* foot + *-ia*] a type of symmelia characterized by the presence of one median foot.

monopodial (mon″o-po′de-al) pertaining to or characterized by monopodia; having a single median foot.

monopoiesis (mon″o-poi-e′sis) the development of monocytes.

monopolar (mon″o-po″lar) monoterminal.

monops (mon′ops) [*mono-* + Gr. *ōps* eye] cyclops.

monopsychosis (mon″o-si-ko′sis) monomania.

Monopsyllus (mon″o-sil′us) [*mono-* + Gr. *psylla* flea] a genus of fleas. **M. ani′sus,** the common rat flea of Japan and North China.

monoptychial (mon″o-ti′ke-al) [*mono-* + Gr. *ptychē* fold] arranged in a single layer; said of glands whose cells are arranged on the basement membrane in a single layer. Cf. *polyptychial.*

monopus (mon′o-pus) [*mono-* + Gr. *pous* foot] a fetus having but a single foot or leg.

monorchia (mon-or′ke-ah) monorchism.

monorchid (mon-or′kid) an individual exhibiting monorchism.

monorchidic (mon″or-kid′ik) [*mono-* + Gr. *orchis* testicle] pertaining to or characterized by monorchism; having but one descended testicle.

monorchidism (mon-or′kid-izm) monorchism.

monorchis (mon-or′kis) monorchid.

monorchism (mon′or-kizm) the condition of having only one testis in the scrotum.

Monorchotrema (mon-or″ko-tre′mah) [*mono-* + Gr. *orchis* testicle + *trēma* aperture] a genus of heterophyid flukes found in birds and mammals in the Middle East and Taiwan, and characterized by having only a single testis. They have as invertebrate host an operculate snail, and as first vertebrate host an edible fish.

monorecidive (mon″o-res″ĭ-dēv′) chancre redux.

monorhinic (mon″o-rin′ik) pertaining to or possessing one nasal cavity.

monosaccharide (mon″o-sak′ah-rīd) a simple sugar; a carbohydrate which cannot be decomposed by hydrolysis. The monosaccharides are colorless crystalline substances, with a sweet taste and have the same general formula CH_2O. They are classified according to the number of carbon atoms in the chain into diose ($C_2H_4O_2$), triose ($C_3H_6O_3$), tetrose ($C_4H_8O_4$), pentose ($C_5H_{10}O_5$), hexose ($C_6H_{12}O_6$), and heptose ($C_7H_{14}O_7$). Those containing an aldehyde group are termed *aldoses;* those with a ketone group *ketoses.*

monosaccharose (mon″o-sak′ah-rōs) monosaccharide.

monose (mon′ōs) a monosaccharide.

monosexual (mon″o-sek′su-al) showing the traits of one sex only.

monosodium glutamate (mon″o-so′de-um glu′tah-māt) sodium glutamate.

monosome (mon′o-sōm) 1. the unpaired sex chromosome; called also *unpaired allosome.* 2. the single chromosome present in monosomy.

monosomic (mon″o-so′mik) pertaining to or characterized by monosomy.

monosomy (mon′o-so″me) the absence of one chromosome of a homologous pair in the complement of an otherwise diploid cell (2n−1), as seen in the XO aberration in Turner's syndrome.

monospasm (mon′o-spazm) [*mono-* + *spasm*] spasm of a single limb or part. Different varieties are distinguished according to the part affected or to the site of the causal lesion; as, brachial, facial, lateral, peripheral, etc.

monospecific (mon″o-spĕ-sif′ik) having an effect only on a particular kind of cell or tissue, or reacting with a single antigen, as a monospecific antiserum.

monospermy (mon′o-sper″me) [*mono-* + Gr. *sperma* seed] fertilization in which only one spermatozoon enters the ovum.

Monosporium (mon″o-spo′re-um) a genus of imperfect fungi, family Moniliaceae, order Moniliales; its perfect (sexual) stage is *Allescheria.* **M. apiosper′mum,** one of the causative organisms of maduromycosis; its perfect stage is *Allescheria boydii.*

Monostoma (mon″o-sto′mah) [Gr. *monos* single + *stoma* mouth] *Paramphistomum.*

Monostomum (mon″o-sto′mum) *Paramphistomum.*

monostotic (mon″os-tot′ik) [*mono-* + Gr. *osteon* bone] pertaining to or affecting a single bone.

monostratal (mon″o-stra′tal) pertaining to a single layer or stratum.

monostratified (mon″o-strat′ĭ-fīd) disposed in a single layer or stratum.

monosubstituted (mon″o-sub′stĭ-tūt″ed) having only one atom in the molecule replaced.

monosymptom (mon″o-simp′tom) [*mono-* + *symptom*] a symptom occurring singly.

monosymptomatic (mon″o-simp″to-mat′ik) expressed by a single symptom.

monosynaptic (mon″o-sĭ-nap′tik) pertaining to or relayed through only one synapse.

monosyphilid, monosyphilide (mon″o-sif′ĭ-lid) [*mono-* + *syphilid*] showing only a single syphilitic lesion.

monoterminal (mon″o-ter′mĭ-nal) the use of one terminal

only in giving treatments, the ground acting as the second terminal.

monothermia (mon″o-ther′me-ah) [*mono-* + Gr. *thermē* heat] a condition in which the temperature of the body remains the same throughout the day.

monothetic (mon″o-thet′ik) [*mono-* + Gr. *thetikos* fit for placing] denoting a taxonomic group classified on the basis of a single character, as opposed to polythetic.

monothioglycerol (mon″o-thi″o glis′er-ol) [NF] chemical name: 3-mercapto-1,2-propanediol. A clear, colorless, moderately viscous liquid, C_2H_7NO, used as a preservative in pharmaceutical preparations.

monotic (mon-o′tik) [*mono-* + Gr. *ous* ear] affecting, pertaining to, or possessing a single ear.

monotocous (mo-not′o-kus) [*mono-* + Gr. *tokos* birth] giving birth to but one offspring at a time.

Monotremata (mon″o-tre′mah-tah) the lowest order of mammals, including animals which lay eggs similar to those of reptiles, and nourish their young by a mammary gland which has no nipple, in a shallow pouch developed only during lactation. The only living representatives are the spiny anteater and duck-billed platypus. In some systems of classification, considered to be an order of subclass Prototheria, class Mammalia.

monotreme (mon′o-trēm) a member of the order Monotremata.

Monotricha (mo-not′rĭ-kah) a group of bacteria including those forms which have one polar flagellum.

monotrichic (mon″o-trik′ik) monotrichous.

monotrichous (mo-not′rĭ-kus) [*mono-* + Gr. *thrix* hair] having a single polar flagellum; said of a bacterial cell. See *flagellum*.

monotropic (mon″o-trop′ik) [*mono-* + Gr. *tropos* a turning] affecting only one particular species of bacterium or one variety of tissue. Cf. *polytropic*.

monoureide (mon″o-u′re-id) see *ureide*.

monovalent (mon″o-va′lent) 1. having a valency or potency of one. 2. denoting an antibody capable of combining with only one antigenic specificity, or an antigen capable of combining with only one antibody specificity.

monovular (mon-ov′u-lar) pertaining to or derived from a single ovum.

monovulatory (mon-ov′u-lah-to″re) ordinarily discharging only one ovum in one ovarian cycle.

monoxenic (mon″o-zen′ik) [*mono-* + Gr. *xenos* a guest-friend, stranger] associated with a single species of microorganisms; said of otherwise germ-free animals contaminated by a single type of organism.

monoxenous (mo-nok′sĕ-nus) requiring only one host in order to complete the life cycle; said of certain parasitic organisms. Cf. *heteroxenous*.

monoxeny (mo-nok′sĕ-ne) [*mono-* + Gr. *xenos* host] the quality or condition of being monoxenous.

monoxide (mon-ok′sīd) an oxide containing but one atom of oxygen; vernacularly applied to carbon monoxide.

monoxygenase (mon-oks′ĭ-jen-ās) an oxidative enzyme that transfers only one atom of oxygen to each substrate molecule.

monozygosity (mon″o-zi-gos′ĭ-te) the state of developing from one zygote.

monozygotic (mon″o-zi-got′ik) pertaining to or derived from one fertilized ovum (zygote), as identical twins.

monozygous (mon″o-zi′gus) monozygotic.

Monro's bursa, foramen, line, sulcus (fissure) (mon-roz′) [Alexander *Monro* (Secundus), Scottish anatomist and surgeon, 1733–1817] see *bursa intratendinea, foramen interventriculare,* and *sulcus hypothalamicus,* and see under *line*.

Monro-Richter line (mon-ro′ rik′ter) [Alexander *Monro;* August Gottlieb *Richter,* surgeon in Göttingen, 1742–1812] see under *line*.

mons (monz), pl. *mon′tes* [L. "mountain"] [NA] a general term for an elevation, or eminence. **m. pu′bis** [NA], the rounded fleshy prominence over the symphysis pubis. **m. ure′teris,** a papilla-like elevation of the mucosa of the bladder at its junction with the ureter. **m. ven′eris,** m. pubis.

Monsonia (mon-so′ne-ah) a genus of African and Asiatic geraniaceous plants. Some of the species are used in medicine as astringents and for dysentery.

monster (mon′ster) [L. *monstrum*] a fetus or infant with such pronounced developmental anomalies as to be grotesque and usually nonviable. Called also *teras*. **acardiac m.,** acardius. **acraniate m.,** a fetus lacking cranium and a brain as such. **autositic m.,** one capable of independent life, the circulation of which supplies nutrition to a parasitic monster. **celosomian m.,** a celosomus. **compound m.,** one which shows some duplication of body parts. **cyclopic m.,** a cyclops. **diaxial m.,** one which shows duplication of the body axis. **double m.,** one arising from a single ovum but with duplication or doubling of head, trunk, or limbs; see *anadidymus, anakatadidymus,* and *katadidymus.* **emmenic m.,** an infant that menstruates.

endocymic m., one which is retained in the uterus and forms the basis of a dermoid tumor. **Gila m.,** a venomous lizard, *Heloderma suspectum,* found especially in Arizona and New Mexico. **hair m.,** one with a heavy hair-coat. **monoaxial m.,** a monster which has a single body axis. **parasitic m.,** an imperfect fetus unable to exist alone and attached to or deriving its nutrition from the circulation of another, more perfectly developed fetus. **polysomatous m.,** a monster consisting of multiple components, each of which shows some of the characteristics of a separate individual. **single m.,** one with a single body but with a defect, malformation, or displacement, or an enlargement or duplication of an organ; see *monstrum.* **sirenoform m.,** a sirenomelus. **triplet m.,** a monster with triplication of body parts. **twin m.,** double m.

monstra (mon′strah) [L.] plural of *monstrum.*

monstricide (mon′strĭ-sīd) [*monster* + L. *caedere* to kill] destruction of a fetal monster.

monstrosity (mon-stros′ĭ-te) [L. *monstrositas*] 1. great congenital deformity. 2. a monster or teratism.

monstrum (mon′strum), pl. *mon′stra* [L.] a monster. **m. abun′dans,** m. per excessum. **m. defic′iens,** m. per defectum. **m. per defec′tum,** a single monster in which all or part of an organ is missing. **m. per exces′sum,** a single monster in which an organ is enlarged or duplicated. **m. per fab′ricam alie′nam,** a single monster in which an organ is wrongly formed or displaced. **m. sirenofor′me,** a sirenomelus.

Monteggia's dislocation, fracture (mon-tej′ahz) [Giovanni Battista *Monteggia,* Italian surgeon, 1762–1815] see under *dislocation* and *fracture.*

Montgomery's cups, follicles, glands, tubercles (mont-gom′er-ēz) [William Fetherstone *Montgomery,* Irish obstetrician, 1797–1859] see under *cup* and *tubercle,* and see *Naboth's follicle,* under *follicle,* and *glandulae areolares.*

monticulus (mon-tik′u-lus), pl. *montic′uli* [L.] a small eminence. **m. cerebel′li,** the projecting or central part of the superior vermis.

mood (mood) the emotional state of an individual, e.g., elation or depression. **pure m.,** a mood which is not directed toward an object, such as anxiety, depression, or happiness.

Moon's teeth (molars) (moonz) [Henry *Moon,* 19th century English surgeon] see under *tooth.*

Moore's fracture (moorz) [Edward Mott *Moore,* American surgeon, 1814–1902] see under *fracture.*

Moore's syndrome (moorz) [Matthew T. *Moore,* American neuropsychiatrist, born 1901] abdominal epilepsy.

Moore's test (moorz) [John *Moore,* English physician of the 19th century] see under *tests.*

Mooren's ulcer (moor′enz) [Albert *Mooren,* German oculist, 1828–1899] see under *ulcer.*

Moorhead foreign body locator (moor′hed) [John J. *Moorhead,* New York surgeon, born 1874] Berman-Moorhead locator.

Moots-McKesson ratio (moots′mak-ke′son) [Charles W. *Moots,* American physician, 1869–1933; Elmer Isaac *McKesson,* American physician, 1881–1935] see under *ratio.*

MOPP a regimen of mechlorethamine, Oncovin (vincristine), procarbazine, and prednisone, used in cancer chemotherapy.

morament (mōr-am′ent) (*obs.*) a feebleminded person without moral sense.

moramentia (mōr″ah-men′she-ah) (*obs.*) the condition of being feebleminded and without moral sense.

Morand's foot, foramen, spur (mor-ahnz′) [Sauveur François *Morand,* French surgeon, 1697–1773] see under *foot,* and see *foramen cecum* and *calcar avis.*

morantel tartrate (mo-ran′tel) chemical name: (*E*)-1,4,5,6-tetrahydro-1-methyl-2-[2-(3-methyl-2-thienyl)ethenyl]pyrimidine[*R*-(*R**,*R**)]-2,3-dihydroxybutanedioate (1:1); an anthelmintic, $C_{12}H_{16}N_2S \cdot C_4H_6O_6$, which has been used in veterinary medicine.

Morax-Axenfeld conjunctivitis, diplococcus (bacillus, hemophilus) (mōr′aks ak′sen-felt″) [Victor *Morax,* ophthalmologist in Paris, 1866–1935; Theodor *Axenfeld,* German ophthalmologist, 1867–1930] see under *conjunctivitis,* and see *Hemophilus duplex.*

Moraxella (mo″rak-sel′ah) [Victor *Morax*] in some classifications, a genus of microorganisms of the family Brucellaceae, order Eubacteriales, made up of gram-negative, nonmotile, short, rod-shaped cells occasionally occurring singly, and found as parasites and pathogens in warm-blooded animals. **M. bo′vis,** the etiologic agent of epizootic keratoconjunctivitis in cattle; called also *Hemophilus bovis.* **M. lacuna′ta,** the etiologic agent of a chronic or acute blepharoconjunctivitis in man; called also *Hemophilus duplex.* **M. liquefa′ciens,** a strain of *M. lacunata* found in association with conjunctivitis in man. Classified as *M. lacunata* subsp. *liquefaciens.*

morbid (mor′bid) [L. *morbidus* sick] 1. pertaining to, affected with, or inducing disease; diseased. 2. unhealthy or unwholesome, as a morbid desire or fear.

morbidity (mor-bid′ĭ-te) 1. the condition of being diseased or morbid. 2. the sick rate; the ratio of sick to well persons in a community.

morbidostatic (mor″bĭ-do-stat′ik) checking morbidity; inhibiting the progression of morbid changes, or disease.

morbific (mor-bif′ik) [L. *morbificus; morbus* sickness + *facere* to make] causing disease.

morbigenous (mor-bij′ĕ-nus) producing disease.

morbilli (mor-bil′i) [L.] measles.

morbilliform (mor-bil′ĭ-form) [L. *morbilli* measles + *forma* shape] like measles; resembling the eruption of measles.

morbillous (mor-bil′us) pertaining to measles.

morbus (mor′bus) [L.] disease. **m. addiso′nii,** Addison's disease. **m. apoplectifor′mis,** Meniere's disease. **m. cadu′-cus,** epilepsy. **m. caeru′leus,** the cyanotic group of congenital heart disease, with venous-arterial shunt. **m. comitia′lis,** epilepsy. **m. cox′ae seni′lis,** hip-joint disease of aged people. **m. coxa′rius,** hip-joint disease. **m. divin′us,** epilepsy. **m. dormiti′vus,** African trypanosomiasis. **m. ele′phas,** elephantiasis. **m. gal′licus,** syphilis. **m. hercu′leus,** epilepsy. **m. mise′riae,** any disease due to want and neglect. **m. mor′sus mu′ris,** rat-bite fever. **m. nau′ticus, m. navit′icus,** seasickness. **m. pediculo′sus,** infestation with lice. **m. sa′cer,** epilepsy. **m. seni′lis,** rheumatoid arthritis. **m. strangulato′rius,** diphtheria. **m. vagabon′dus,** vagabond's disease. **m. virgin′eus,** chlorosis. **m. werlho′fii** [Werlhof's disease], (obs.) idiopathic thrombocytopenic purpura.

M.O.R.C. Medical Officers Reserve Corps.

morcellation (mor″sel-a′shun) [Fr. *morcellement*] the division of solid tissue (as a tumor) into pieces, followed by its removal piecemeal.

morcellement (mor″sel-maw′) morcellation.

mordant (mor′dant) [L. *mordere* to bite] 1. a substance capable of intensifying or deepening the reaction of a specimen to a stain; the chief mordants are alum, aniline, oil, and phenol. 2. to subject to the action of a mordant preliminary to staining.

Mor. dict. abbreviation for L. *mo′re dic′to,* in the manner directed.

Morel ear, syndrome (mo′rel) [Benoît Augustin *Morel,* French alienist, 1809–1873] see under *ear,* and see *hyperostosis frontalis interna.*

Morel-Kraepelin disease (mo-rel′ kra′pĕ-lin) [B. A. *Morel;* Emil *Kraepelin,* German psychiatrist, 1856–1926] schizophrenia.

Morelli's test (reaction) (mo-rel′ēz) [F. *Morelli,* Italian physician, died 1918] see under *tests.*

mores (mo′rēz) [L., pl. of *mos,* "manners"] the traditions and habits which are generally regarded as conducive to social welfare.

Moreschi's phenomenon (mo-res′kēz) [Carlo *Moreschi,* Italian pathologist, 1876–1921] fixation of complement; see under *fixation.*

Morestin's operation (method) (mor″es-taz′) [Hippolyte *Morestin,* French surgeon, 1869–1919] see under *operation.*

Moretti's test (mo-ret′ēz) [E. *Moretti,* physician in Milan] see under *tests.*

Morgagni's appendix, etc. (mor-gahn′yēz) [Giovanni Battista *Morgagni,* Italian anatomist and pathologist, 1682–1771; professor at Padua, and the founder of pathological anatomy, whose superb clinicopathological reports were published in 1761 under the title *De sedibus et causis morborum* ("The Seats and Causes of Disease")] see under *appendix, caruncle, column, crypt,* etc.

Morgagni-Adams-Stokes syndrome [Giovanni Battista *Morgagni;* Robert *Adams,* Irish physician, 1791–1875; William *Stokes,* Irish physician, 1804–1878] Adams-Stokes disease.

Morgan (mor′gan), Thomas Hunt. American biologist, 1866–1945, noted for his discoveries concerning the hereditary functions of the chromosomes; winner of the Nobel prize for medicine in 1933.

morgan [from T. H. *Morgan*] a unit of map distance on a chromosome in which the mean number of recombinations is unity. In a centimorgan the probability of recombination is 1 per cent.

Morgan's bacillus (mor′ganz) [Harry de Reimer *Morgan,* British physician, died 1931] *Proteus morgani.*

morgue (morg) [Fr.] a place where dead bodies may be temporarily kept, for identification or until claimed for burial.

moria (mo′re-ah) [Gr. *mōria* folly] dementia or fatuity. In psychiatry, a morbid tendency to joke.

moribund (mor′ĭ-bund) [L. *moribundus*] in a dying state.

Moringa (mo-rin′gah) a genus of plants. **M. pterygosper′-ma,** an East Indian plant, the sajina or horseradish tree, the nuts of which yield an oil that was once used in the treatment of rheumatism and dyspepsia. It is the source of pterygospermin, an antibiotic.

Morison's method (paste), pouch (mor′ĭ-sunz) [James Rutherford *Morison,* British surgeon, 1853–1939] see under *method* and *pouch.*

Morita therapy (mo-re′tah) [Shomei *Morita,* Japanese physician] see under *therapy.*

Moritz reaction, test (mo′rits) [Friedrich Heinrich Ludwig *Moritz,* German physician, 1861–1938] Rivalta's reaction.

Mörner's body, reagent, test (mer′nerz) [Carl Axel Hampus *Mörner,* Stockholm chemist, 1854–1917] see under *reagent* and *tests,* and see *nucleoalbumin,* and *nitroprusside test* (def. 1), under *tests.*

Mornidine (mor′nĭ-dēn) trademark for preparations of pipamazine.

Moro's reaction (test), embrace reflex (mo′rōz) [Ernst *Moro,* pediatrist in Heidelberg, 1874–1951] see under *reaction* and *reflex.*

moron (mo′ron) [Gr. *mōros* stupid] in a former classification, a mentally retarded person with an IQ of 50 to 69. See *mental retardation.* Cf. *idiot* and *imbecile.*

moronism (mo′ron-izm) moronity.

moronity (mo-ron′ĭ-te) the condition of being a moron.

morosis (mo-ro′sis) moronity.

-morph [Gr. *morphē* form] a word termination denoting relationship to form or shape, such as an individual possessing a certain form, indicated by the preceding root, as *mesomorph.*

morphallactic (mor″fah-lak′tik) pertaining to or characterized by morphallaxis.

morphallaxis (mor″fah-lak′sis) [Gr. *morphē* form + *allaxis* exchange] the renewal of lost tissue or a part by reorganization of the remaining part of the body of an animal.

morphea (mor-fe′ah) [Gr. *morphē* form] a condition in which there is connective tissue replacement of the skin and sometimes of the subcutaneous tissues, marked by the formation of ivory white or pinkish patches, bands, or lines that are sometimes bordered by a purplish areola. The lesions are firm, but not hard, and are usually depressed; they may remain localized or may involute, leaving atrophy and scarring. Called also *circumscribed* or *localized scleroderma.* Cf. *systemic scleroderma.* **m. gut-ta′ta, guttate m.,** a form marked by the formation of multiple, white, shiny, beadlike spots, which may be surrounded by a thin pinkish or purplish border; called also *white-spot disease.* **linear m., m. linea′ris,** see under *scleroderma.*

morpheme (mor′fēm) a meaningful unit of sound.

morphia (mor′fe-ah) morphine.

morphina, pl. and gen. *morphi′nae* [L.] morphine.

morphine (mor′fēn) [L. *morphina, morphinum*] chemical name: 7,8-didehydro-4,5-epoxy-17-methylmorphinan-3,6-diol. The principal and most active narcotic alkaloid of opium (q.v.), $C_{17}H_{19}NO_3$, occurring as a white, crystalline powder or as white, acicular crystals, and having powerful analgesic action and some central stimulant action. In the United States, it is usually used in the form of the sulfate salt, while in Germany and Great Britain, the hydrochloride salt is usually preferred. Abuse of morphine and its salts leads to dependence. **dimethyl m.,** thebaine. **m. hy-drochloride,** the trihydrate hydrochloride salt of morphine, $C_{17}H_{19}NO_3 \cdot HCl \cdot 3H_2O$, occurring as colorless, silky crystals or crystalline powder, having the same actions as the base; used as a narcotic analgesic, usually administered orally. It is the form usually preferred in Germany and Great Britain. **m. sulfate** [USP], the pentahydrate sulfate salt of morphine, $(C_{17}H_{19}NO_3)_2 \cdot H_2SO_4 \cdot 5H_2O$, occurring as white, feathery, silky crystals, cubical masses or crystals, or white, crystalline powder, and having the same actions as the base; used as a narcotic analgesic, administered parenterally. It is the form usually preferred in the United States.

morphinic (mor-fin′ik) pertaining to morphine.

morphinism (mor′fin-izm) a morbid state due to the habitual misuse of morphine; also morphine addiction.

morphinist (mor′fin-ist) a morphine addict.

morphinistic (mor″fi-nis′tik) pertaining to or characteristic of morphinism.

morphinium (mor-fin′e-um) [L.] morphine. **m. sulfate,** morphine sulfate.

morphinization (mor″fin-i-za′shun) subjection to the influence of morphine.

morphinomania (mor″fin-o-ma′ne-ah) 1. morphine addiction. 2. psychosis due to the misuse of morphine.

morphiomania (mor″fe-o-ma′ne-ah) morphinomania.

morphium (mor′fe-um) morphine.

morpho- [Gr. *morphē* form] a combining form denoting relationship to form.

morphodifferentiation (mor″fo-dif″er-en″she-a′shun) the arrangement of formative cells in the development of tissues or organs, which leads to production of the ultimate shape of the structure.

morphoea (mor-fe′ah) morphea.

morphogen (mor′fo-jen) a diffusible substance in embryonic tissue postulated to form a concentration gradient that influences morphogenesis.

morphogenesia (mor″fo-jĕ-ne′se-ah) morphogenesis.

morphogenesis (mor″fo-jen′ĕ-sis) [Gr. *morphē* form + *gennan* to produce] the evolution and development of form, as the development of the shape of a particular organ or part of the body, or the development undergone by individuals who attain the type to which the majority of the individuals of the species approximate.

morphogenetic (mor″fo-jĕ-net′ik) producing growth; producing form or shape.

morphogeny (mor-foj′ĕ-ne) morphogenesis.

morphography (mor-fog′rah-fe) [*morpho-* + Gr. *graphein* to write] a description of organized beings, with special reference to their forms and structure.

morphological (mor″fo-loj′ĭ-kal) pertaining to morphology.

morphology (mor-fol′o-je) [*morpho-* + *-logy*] the science of the forms and structure of organisms; the form and structure of a particular organism, organ, or part.

morpholysis (mor-fol′ĭ-sis) [*morpho-* + Gr. *lysis* dissolution] destruction of form.

morphometry (mor-fom′ĕ-tre) [*morpho-* + Gr. *metron* measure] the measurement of the forms of organisms.

morphon (mor′fon) [Gr. *morphōn* forming] an individual organism or structural unit.

morphophyly (mor-fof′ĭ-le) [*morpho-* + Gr. *phylon* tribe] the branch of phylogenesis dealing with the evolutionary development of form.

morphophysics (mor″fo-fiz′iks) the study of the physical and chemical causes of development.

morphoplasm (mor′fo-plazm) [*morpho-* + Gr. *plasma* anything formed] the substance of the cellular reticulum.

morphosis (mor-fo′sis) [Gr. *morphōsis* a shaping, bringing into shape] the process of formation of a part or organ.

morphotic (mor-fot′ik) pertaining to morphosis or formation; concerned in a formative process.

-morphous [Gr. *morphē* form, shape] a word termination indicating the manner of shape or form.

morpio, morpion (mor′pe-o, mor′pe-on), pl. *morpio′nes* [L.] the crab louse, *Phthirus pubis*.

Morquio's syndrome (disease) (mor-ke′ōz) [Louis *Morquio*, pediatrician in Montevideo, 1867–1935] see under *syndrome*.

Morquio-Ullrich disease (mor-ke′o-ool′rik) [Louis *Morquio*; Otto *Ullrich*, German physician, 1894–1957] Morquio's syndrome.

morrhua (mor′u-ah) [L.] the codfish, *Gadus morrhua*, which furnishes cod liver oil.

morrhuate (mor′u-āt) a salt of morrhuic acid. **m. sodium** [NF], the sodium salts of the fatty acids of cod liver oil; used as a sclerosing agent, especially for the treatment of varicose veins and hemorrhoids, injected in solution into varicosities.

morrhuin (mor′u-in) [L. *morrhua* codfish] a thick oily ptomaine, $C_{19}H_{27}N_3$, from some samples of cod liver oil.

mors (morz) [L.] death. **m. thy′mica,** sudden death allegedly occurring in thymic asthma and lymphatism (def. 2).

morsal (mor′sal) [L. *morsus* bite] taking part in mastication; a term applied to the masticating surface of a bicuspid or molar.

Mor. sol. abbreviation for L. *mo′re sol′ito*, in the usual way.

morsulus (mor′su-lus) [L., dim. of *morsus* bite] a troche.

morsus (mor′sus) [L.] bite; sting. **m. diab′oli,** the fimbriae at the ovarian extremity of an oviduct. **m. huma′nus,** a bite by a human being.

mortal (mor′tal) [L. *mortalis*] 1. subject to death, or destined to die. 2. fatal; causing or terminating in death.

mortality (mor-tal′ĭ-te) 1. the quality of being mortal. 2. the *death rate*; see under *rate*. 3. in life insurance, the ratio of deaths that take place to expected deaths. **actual m.,** the number of deaths in 1,000,000 insured lives, over a period of 100 years. **annual actual m.,** the number of deaths per 100 insured lives. **perinatal m.,** the death rate of infants about the time of birth, often considered as including stillbirths and deaths in the first week of life. **tabular m.,** the expected death rate per 1000 insured persons as shown in the mortality table.

mortalogram (mor-tal′o-gram) a graphic presentation, in grid form, of crude and age-standardized mortality rates and the numerical distribution of deaths for a given cause according to the time period, age, and sex, and the median age at death.

mortar (mor′tar) [L. *mortarium*] a bell-shaped or urn-shaped vessel of glass, iron, porcelain, or other material, in which drugs are beaten, crushed, or ground with a pestle.

mortician (mor-tish′an) [L. *mors* death] an undertaker; a person trained to care for the dead.

Mortierella (mor-te-ah-rel′ah) a genus of phycomycetous fungi of the order Mucorales, family Mucoraceae, species of which have been isolated from lesions of mucormycosis.

mortification (mor″tĭ-fi-ka′shun) gangrene or sphacelus; molar death.

mortinatality (mor″tĭ-na-tal′ĭ-te) [L. *mors* death + *natus* birth] natimortality.

mortisemblant (mor″tĭ-sem′blant) apparently dead.

Morton's cough (mor′tunz) [Richard *Morton*, English physician, 1637–1698] see under *cough*.

Morton's current (mor′tunz) [William James *Morton*, American neurologist, 1846–1920] see under *current*.

Morton's toe (disease, foot, neuralgia), test (mor′tunz) [Thomas George *Morton*, Philadelphia surgeon, 1835–1903] see under *toe* and *tests*.

mortuary (mor′tu-a″re) [L. *mortuarium* tomb] 1. pertaining to death. 2. a place where dead bodies are kept until burial or cremation.

morula (mor′u-lah) [L. *morus* mulberry] the solid mass of blastomeres formed by cleavage of a fertilized ovum.

morular (mor′u-lar) 1. pertaining to a morula. 2. resembling a mulberry.

morulation (mor″u-la′shun) the process of formation of the morula.

moruloid (mor′u-loid) [L. *morus* mulberry + Gr. *eidos* form] 1. shaped like a mulberry. 2. a bacterial colony in the form of a mulberry-like mass.

Morvan's chorea, disease, syndrome (mor′vanz) [Augustin Marie *Morvan*, French physician, 1819–1897] see under *chorea*, *disease*, and *syndrome*.

mosaic (mo-za′ik) [Gr. *mouseion*; L. *opus musivum*] a pattern made of numerous small pieces fitted together. (1) *Genetics:* an individual having two or more cell lines that are karotypically or genotypically distinct and are derived from a single zygote. Cf. *chimera*. (2) *Embryology:* the condition in the fertilized eggs of some species, such as the sea urchin, whereby the cells of early stages have developed cytoplasm which determines the parts that are to develop. (3) *Plant pathology:* a viral disease characterized by mottling of the foliage.

mosaicism (mo-za′ĭ-sizm) in genetics, the presence in an individual of two or more cell lines that are karyotypically or genotypically distinct and are derived from a single zygote. Cf. *chimerism*. **erythrocyte m.,** the mixture of two blood types in each of nonidentical twins as a result of anastomosis of placental blood vessels. **gonadal m.,** mosaicism that results from mutation early in embryogenesis so that some of the germ cells are mutants. Offspring of a gonadal mosaic for a dominate trait can show the trait although it is not manifested in the parent.

Moschcowitz's disease, test (sign) (mos′ko-witz) [Eli *Moschcowitz*, American physician, born 1879] see *febrile pleiochromic anemia*, under *anemia*, and *thrombotic thrombopenic purpura*, under *purpura*, and see under *tests*.

Moschcowitz's operation (mos′ko-witz) [Alexis Victor *Moschcowitz*, American surgeon, 1865–1933] see under *operation*.

Mosenthal's test (mo′zen-thalz) [Herman Otto *Mosenthal*, American physician, 1878–1954] see under *tests*.

Moser's serum (mo′zerz) [Paul *Moser*, pediatrician in Vienna, 1865–1924] see under *serum*.

Mosetig-Moorhof bone wax (filling) (mōs-et′ig-mōr′hof) [Albert von *Mosetig-Moorhof*, German surgeon, 1838–1907] see under *wax*.

Mosler's diabetes (mos′lerz) [Karl Friedrich *Mosler*, German physician, 1831–1911] see under *diabetes*.

mOsm milliosmol.

mosquito (mos-ke′to), pl. *mosquitoes* [Sp. "little fly"] a popular name for gnatlike, bloodsucking and venomous insects of the family Culicidae and of various genera, chiefly *Culex, Aedes, Anopheles, Mansonia, Haemagogus, Psorophora, Theobaldia* and *Chagasia*. **anautogenous m.,** a mosquito that requires a blood meal in the adult stage for the production of viable eggs. **arygamous m.,** a mosquito that requires large or outdoor spaces for breeding. **autogenous m.,** a mosquito that can produce viable eggs without a blood meal. **house m.,** see *Culex pipiens* and *C. quinquefasciatus*. **steyogamous m.,** a mosquito that can breed in captivity in limited spaces. **tiger m.,** *Aedes aegypti*.

mosquitocidal (mos-ke″to-si′dal) destructive to mosquitoes.

mosquitocide (mos-ke′to-sīd) [*mosquito* + L. *caedere* to kill] an agent that is destructive to mosquitoes.

moss (mos) 1. any plant or species of the cryptogamic class *Musci*. 2. material composed of or derived from a plant of the cryptogamic class *Musci*. **Ceylon m.,** a red seaweed, *Gracilaria lichenoides* (L.) Harv. (Gracilariaceae); one of the sources of agar, and also used for food. In China, it is considered to be a pectoral and antidysenteric. **Iceland m.,** *Cetraria*, def. 2. **Irish m.,** juniper m., *Polytrichum juniperinum*. **pearl m., salt rock m.,** chondrus.

Moss' classification (mos′ez) [William Lorenzo *Moss*, American physician, born 1876] see under *classification*.

Mosse's syndrome (mos′ez) [Max *Mosse*, Berlin physician, born 1873] see under *syndrome*.

Mosso's ergograph, sphygmomanometer (mos′ōz) [Angelo *Mosso*, Italian physiologist, 1846–1910] see under *ergograph* and *sphygmomanometer*.

Motais' operation (mo-tāz′) [Ernest *Motais*, French ophthalmologist, 1845–1913] see under *operation*.

moth (mawth) a lepidopterous insect. **brown-tail m.,** *Euproctis chrysorrhoea.* **flannel m.,** see *Megalopyge.* **io m.,** *Automeris io.* **meal m.,** *Asopia farinalis.* **tussock m.,** *Hemerocampa leucostigma.*

mother (muth′er) [L. *mater*] the female parent. Also, something from which another thing is derived, as a *mother cell.* **Colles' m.,** the apparently normal mother of a syphilitic child. **m. of vinegar,** *Acetobacter aceti.*

motile (mo′til; mōt′l; mo′tīl) having spontaneous but not conscious or volitional movement.

motilin (mo-til′in) a polypeptide hormone (2700 daltons, 22 amino acids) secreted by the enterochromaffin cells of the gut; it causes increased motility of several portions of the gut and stimulates pepsin secretion. In human beings, its release is stimulated by the presence of acid and fat in the duodenum; the physiologic role of the hormone in gastrointestinal function is not yet known.

motility (mo-til′ĭ-te) the ability to move spontaneously.

motivation (mo″tĭ-va′shun) in psychology, any of the forces that regulate behavior directed toward satisfying needs or achieving goals.

motive (mo′tiv) in psychology, any state that affects an individual's goal-directed behavior. **achievement m.,** the desire to achieve for the sake of achievement per se. **aroused m.,** one that is actively influencing behavior, or that can be inferred from actual behavior.

motoceptor (mo′to-sep″tor) any muscle sense receptor.

motofacient (mo″to-fa′shent) producing motion; a term applied to that phase of muscular activity by which the muscle produces actual motion, in contradistinction to the *nonmotofacient* phase in which the muscle is contracting without producing motion.

motoneuron (mo″to-nu′ron) motor neuron; a neuron possessing a motor function; an efferent neuron conveying motor impulses. **alpha m's,** neurons of the anterior spinal cord that give rise to the alpha fibers which innervate the skeletal muscle fibers. **gamma m's,** neurons of the anterior spinal cord that give rise to the gamma (fusimotor) fibers which innervate intrafusal fibers of the muscle spindle. **heteronymous m's,** those supplying muscles other than the one from which the afferent impulses originate. **homonymous m's,** those supplying the muscle from which the afferent impulses originate. **lower m's,** peripheral neurons whose cell bodies lie in the ventral gray columns of the spinal cord and whose terminations are in skeletal muscles. **peripheral m's,** neurons in a peripheral reflex arc that receive impulses from interneurons and transmit them to voluntary muscles. **upper m's,** neurons in the cerebral cortex that conduct impulses from the motor cortex to motor nuclei of the cerebral nerves or to the ventral gray columns of the spinal cord.

motor (mo′tor) [L.] 1. a muscle, nerve, or center that effects or produces movement. 2. producing or subserving motion. **m. oc″uli** (*obs.*), the third cranial nerve (nervus oculomotorius [NA]). **plastic m.,** the tissues of an amputation stump used to secure motion in an artificial limb.

motorgraphic (mo″tor-graf′ik) kinetographic.

motorial (mo-to′re-al) pertaining to motion or to a motorium.

motoricity (mo″tor-is′ĭ-te) the faculty of performing movement; power of movement.

motorium (mo-to′re-um) [L.] 1. a motor center. 2. the motor apparatus of the body. 3. in psychology, the mental functions that direct purposeful activities.

motorius (mo-to′re-us) [L.] a motor nerve.

motorogerminative (mo″tor-o-jer′mĭ-na-tiv) developing into the muscles; said of portions of the mesoderm.

motorpathy (mo-tor′path-the) [*motor* + Gr. *pathos* disease] treatment of disease by gymnastics.

Motrin (mo′trin) trademark for a preparation of ibuprofen.

Mott's law of anticipation (motz) [Sir Fredrick Walker *Mott*, English neurologist, 1853–1926] see under *law.*

mottling (mot′ling) a condition of spotting with patches of color.

mouche (mōōsh), pl. *mouches* [Fr.] a speck, or fly. **mouches volantes** (mōōsh vo-lahnt′), muscae volitantes.

moulage (moo-lahzh′) [Fr. "molding"] the making of molds or models in wax or plaster, as of a structure or a lesion; also such a mold or model.

mould (mōld) see *mold.*

moulding (mōld′ing) molding.

mounding (mownd′ing) the rising in a lump of a wasting muscle when struck; called also *myoedema.*

mount (mownt) to prepare specimens and slides for study.

mountant (mownt′ant) a medium, such as natural resins, polymers, or glycerol, in which objects are embedded for study, especially with the microscope; called also *mounting medium.*

mounting (mownt′ing) 1. the preparation of specimens and slides for study. The chief media used in mounting large specimens are alcohol and glycerin jelly; for microscopic objects on a slide, Canada balsam and glycerin. 2. attachment, in the laboratory, of the maxillary and/or mandibular cast to an articulator. **split cast m.,** 1. a dental cast with key grooves on its base, mounted on an articulator for the purpose of easy removal and accurate replacement. Split remounting metal plates may be used instead of grooves in casts. 2. a means for testing the accuracy of articulator adjustment.

mouse (mows) 1. a small rodent belonging to the genus *Mus,* frequently used as an experimental animal. 2. a small weight, or movable structure. **C.F.W. m.** (cancer-*free white* mouse), one of a strain of mice bred for use in cancer research laboratories. **joint m.,** one of the portions of the fringes in the synovial membrane of joints in osteoarthritis which are changed into cartilage and become free in the joints. Cf. *arthrolith* and *arthrophyte.* **nude m., nu nu m.,** a mouse with congenital absence of the thymus, associated with a striking deficiency of T-lymphocytes and with hairlessness. **NZB (New Zealand black) m.,** an inbred mouse that develops an autoimmune disease that closely resembles systemic lupus erythematosus in man. **peritoneal m.,** a free body in the peritoneal cavity, probably representing a small mass of omentum or epiploic appendage which has twisted off and become coated with fibrin, and sometimes appearing as a soft density on the roentgenogram. **pleural m.,** a fibrinous body sometimes seen by x-ray of the chest in the pleural space.

mousepox (mows′poks) infectious ectromelia.

mouth (mowth) [L. *os, oris*] an opening or aperture. Specifically, the anterior or proximal opening of the alimentary canal, which is bounded anteriorly by the lips and which contains the tongue and teeth. Called also *os* [NA]. **Ceylon sore m.,** tropical sprue. **denture sore m.,** 1. trauma or inflammation of the oral mucous membranes caused by ill-fitting dentures, hypersensitivity to the chemical components of dentures, and/or proliferation of microorganisms with subsequent infection. **dry m.,** xerostomia. **glass-blowers' m.,** swelling of the parotid gland in glass-blowers, a parotid pneumatocele. **parrot m.,** retraction of the lower jaw in the horse. **rubber sore m.** (*obs.*), denture sore m. **tapir m.,** a condition in which the mouth has something of the appearance of that of a tapir, the orbicular oris muscle being atrophied, and the lips thickened and separated; seen in Landouzy-Dejerine dystrophy. **trench m.,** necrotizing ulcerative gingivitis. **white m.,** thrush, def. 1.

mouthwash (mowth′wosh) a solution for rinsing the mouth, e.g., the official [NF] preparation of potassium bicarbonate, sodium borate, thymol, eucalyptol, methyl salicylate, amaranth solution, alcohol, glycerin, and purified water.

movement (mōōv′ment) 1. an act of moving; motion. 2. an act of defecation. **active m.,** voluntary movement produced by the person's own muscles, as opposed to passive m. **ameboid m.,** the movement of an ameba or leukocyte by virtue of the flow of cytoplasm, resulting in the protrusion of a pseudopodium, or a movement similar to it. **angular m.,** a movement which changes the angle between two bones. **associated m.,** a movement of parts which act together, as of the eyes. **automatic m.,** a movement originating within the organism, but not by an act of the will. **Bennett m.,** the lateral shift of the mandibular condyles and articular disks in the direction of the working bite as the lower jaw swings in preparation for mastication. **border m.,** any extreme compass of mandibular movement limited by bone, ligaments, or soft tissues; usually applied to horizontal mandibular movements. **border tissue m's,** movements produced by action of the muscles and other tissues adjoining the borders of a denture. **brownian m., Brownian-Zsigmondy m., brunonian m.,** the dancing motion of minute particles suspended in a liquid, due to thermal agitation. **choreic m's, choreiform m's,** irregular, jerky movements of muscles or groups of muscles. **ciliary m.,** the lashing motion of cilia occurring in certain of the tissues. **circus m.,** 1. a peculiar circular gait; an involuntary rolling or tumbling movement, the result of lesions of the brain and basal nerve centers. 2. a re-entrant mechanism of the excitatory wave in the atrium of the heart; a "circular" path characterized by a gap between the excitatory and refractory tissue, usually resulting in conduction to the ventricle of only a fraction of the impulses. A circus movement is one mechanism of atrial flutter. See also *re-entry.* **contralateral associated m.,** a movement on the paralyzed side in hemiplegia associated with active movement of the corresponding part on the unaffected side. **dystonic m.,** a large slow, amplified athetoid movement. **euglenoid m.,** a wormlike writhing movement resulting from local expansion and contraction of the body, seen in flagellates with thin pellicles and very plastic bodies, as in some species of the genus *Euglena* and other protozoa. **excessive m.,** hyperkinesia. **excursive m's,** those movements performed by the mandible in mastication; see *lateral, protrusive,* and *retrusive excursion,* under *excursion.* **fetal m.,** that of a fetus in the uterus usually observable at about 18 weeks in a primigravida and at about 16 weeks in a multipara. **forced m.,** a movement caused by an injury to a motor center or a conducting path. **Frenkel's m's,** a series of movements of precision to be performed by ataxic patients for the purpose of restoring lost coordination. **hinge m.,** movement occurring in a single plane, as that occurring in opening or closing of the mouth. **index m.,** a movement of the cephalic part of a body about the fixed caudal part. **intermediary m's,** all movements of which the mandible is capable between the extreme lateral, protrusive, and retrusive positions. **jaw m.,** mandibular m. **Magnan's m.,** forward and backward movement of the tongue when it is drawn out; observed in dementia paralytica. Called also *trombone tremor of tongue.* **mandibular m.,** any movement of which the mandible is capable. **mandibular m., free,** any unhampered movement of the mandible. **mandibular m's, functional,** those movements of the mandible which occur in the performance of some function, as mastication, swallowing, articulation of vocal sounds, and yawning. **masticatory m's,** those movements of the mandible occurring in the mastication of food. **molecular m.,** brownian m. **morphogenetic m.,** a flowing of cell groups concerned with the formation of germ layers or of organ primordia. **nastic m.,** a response of a plant to external stimuli that is independent of the direction from which the stimuli come; some of the so-called sleep movements are nastic movements. **nucleopetal m.,** the movement of a male pronucleus toward the female pronucleus in the fertilized ovum. **opening m.,** that movement of the mandible by which the distance between the anterior teeth of the mandible and maxilla is increased. **opening m., posterior,** the opening movement of the mandible about the terminal hinge axis. **passive m.,** any movement of the body effected by a force entirely outside of the organism; see *passive exercise.* **pendular m.,** one of the movements of the small intestine in digestion, consisting of a gentle swinging to and fro of the different loops; these movements are ascribed to rhythmical contractions of the longitudinal muscles. See also *segmentation m.* **rapid eye m. (REM),** see *REM sleep,* under *sleep.* **reflex m.,** an involuntary stereotyped movement provoked by a remote external stimulus acting through a nerve center. **rolling m.,** the rolling of an animal on its long axis. **saccadic m.,** the quick movement of the eye in going from one fixation point to another. **scissors m.,** a movement of the pupillary reflex seen with a retinoscope, resembling the opening and shutting of scissors; it is indicative of irregular astigmatism. **segmentation m.,** one of the movements of the small intestine in digestion, consisting of small, irregular or rhythmic, circular contractions that segment a portion of the intestine into evenly spaced parts somewhat resembling a string of sausages; see also *pendular m.* **sleep m.,** a type of nastic movement in which leaves or plant parts change their position in the late afternoon or evening and return to their original position in the morning. Sleep movement is in no way related to animal sleep. **spontaneous m.,** one originated within the organism. **Swedish m.,** see under *gymnastics.* **synkinetic m's,** minor, unconscious movements that accompany major voluntary movements, such as the facial contortions in severe exertion. **vermicular m's,** the wormlike movements of the intestines in peristalsis.

moxa (mok′sah) [Japanese] a tuft of soft, combustible substance to be burned upon the skin, popularly used in the Orient as a cautery.

moxazocine (mok-sa′zo-sēn) chemical name: $[2R\text{-}(2\alpha,6\alpha,11R^*)]$-3-(cyclopropylmethyl)-1,2,3,4,5,6-hexahydro-11-methoxy-6-methyl-2,6-methano-3-benzazocin-8-ol; an analgesic and antitussive, $C_{18}H_{25}NO_2$.

moxibustion (mok″sĭ-bus′chun) cauterization by the burning of moxa upon the skin.

moxnidazole (moks-nid′ah-zōl) chemical name: 3-[[1-methyl-5-nitro-1H-imidazol-2-yl] methylene] amino]-5-(4-morpholinylmethyl)-2-oxazolidinone; an antiprotozoal, $C_{13}H_{18}N_6O_5$, effective against *Trichomonas.*

moyamoya (moi′ah-moi″ah) [Japanese] the arteriographic appearance of a filmy network of small vessels (resembling a puff of smoke) replacing the normal vascular pattern at the termination of the internal carotid artery; seen in patients with sudden cerebrovascular insufficiency.

Moynihan's cream, test (moin′yanz) [Berkeley George Andrew *Moynihan* (Lord Moynihan), British surgeon, 1865–1936] see under *cream* and *tests.*

6-MP 6-mercaptopurine.

mp. melting point.

M.P.D. maximum permissible dose; see under *dose.*

M.P.H. Master of Public Health.

M. Phys. A. Member of the Physiotherapists' Association (British).

M.P.U. Medical Practitioners Union (British).

mR milliroentgen.

μR microroentgen.

μr microroentgen.

M.R.A. Medical Record Administrator.

M.R.A.C.P. Member of Royal Australasian College of Physicians.

mrad millirad.

M.R.C. Medical Reserve Corps.

M.R.C.P. Member of the Royal College of Physicians.

M.R.C.P.E. Member of the Royal College of Physicians of Edinburgh.

M.R.C.P. (Glasg.) Member of the Royal College of Physicians and Surgeons of Glasgow *qua* Physician.

M.R.C.P.I. Member of the Royal College of Physicians of Ireland.

M.R.C.S. Member of the Royal College of Surgeons.

M.R.C.S.E. Member of the Royal College of Surgeons of Edinburgh.

M.R.C.S.I. Member of the Royal College of Surgeons of Ireland.

M.R.C.V.S. Member of the Royal College of Veterinary Surgeons.

M.R.D. minimum reacting dose.

MRF melanocyte-stimulating hormone releasing factor.

M.R.L. Medical Record Librarian; now called Medical Record Administrator.

mRNA messenger RNA; see *ribonucleic acid,* under *acid.*

MS multiple sclerosis.

M.S. Master of Surgery.

msec. millisecond.

μsec. microsecond.

MSH melanocyte-stimulating hormone (see under *hormone*); it occurs in two forms, α-MSH and β-MSH.

MSH-IF melanocyte-stimulating hormone inhibiting factor; see under *factor.*

M.S.L. midsternal line.

M.T. Medical Technologist; membrana tympani.

MTU methylthiouracil.

M.u. Mache unit.

mU. milliunit.

m.u. mouse unit.

μU. microunit.

mu (mu) the twelfth letter of the Greek alphabet, μ. In micrometry, a micron.

Muc. abbreviation for L. *mucila′go,* mucilage.

mucase (mu′kās) an enzyme that catalyzes the hydrolysis of mucin; a mucopolysaccharidase.

Much's granules, reaction (mooks) [Hans Christian R. *Much,* German physician, 1880–1932] see under *granule* and *reaction.*

Much-Holzmann reaction (mook-holts′man) [Hans *Much;* V. *Holzmann,* German physician] Much's reaction.

mucicarmine (mu″sĭ-kar′min) a specific stain for mucin consisting of carmine, aluminum chloride, and distilled water.

muciferous (mu-sif′er-us) [*mucus* + L. *ferre* to bear] secreting mucus.

mucification (mu″sĭ-fi-ka′shun) the mucus producing changes in the vaginal epithelium of laboratory animals during the progestational stage of the ovarian cycle.

muciform (mu′sĭ-form) [*mucus* + L. *forma* form] resembling mucus.

mucigen (mu′sĭ-jen) [*mucus* + Gr. *gennan* to produce] the substance from which mucin is derived.

mucigenous (mu-sij′ĕ-nus) producing mucus.

mucigogue (mu′sĭ-gog) [*mucus* + Gr. *agōgos* leading] 1. stimulating the secretion of mucus. 2. an agent that stimulates the secretion of mucus.

mucilage (mu′sĭ-lij) [L. *mucilago*] 1. an artificial viscid paste of gum or dextrin used in pharmacy as a vehicle or excipient, or in therapy as a demulcent. 2. a naturally formed viscid principle in a plant, consisting of a gum dissolved in the juices of the plant. **acacia m.,** a preparation of acacia and benzoic acid in purified water, used as a suspending agent for drugs. **tragacanth m.** [NF], a preparation of tragacanth, benzoic acid, and glycerin in distilled water, used as a protective.

mucilaginous (mu″sĭ-laj′ĭ-nus) of the nature of mucilage; slimy and adhesive.

mucilago (mu″sĭ-lah′go) [L.] mucilage. **m. aca′ciae,** acacia mucilage. **m. tragacan′thae,** tragacanth mucilage.

mucilloid (mu′sil-loid) a preparation of a mucilaginous substance. **psyllium hydophilic m.,** a powdered preparation of the mucilaginous portion of blond psyllium (*Plantago ovata*) seeds used in treatment of simple constipation resulting from lack of bulk.

mucin (mu′sin) a mucopolysaccharide or glycoprotein, the chief constituent of mucus. **gastric m.,** a substance derived from the lining of hog stomachs; formerly used for its protective and lubricating action in the treatment of peptic ulcer.

mucinase (mu′sĭ-nās) any enzyme which acts upon mucin.

mucinoblast (mu-sin′o-blast) [*mucin* + Gr. *blastos* germ] the progenitor of a mucous cell.

mucinogen (mu-sin′o-jen) [*mucin* + Gr. *gennan* to produce] a precursor of mucin.

mucinoid (mu′sĭ-noid) [*mucin* + Gr. *eidos* form] 1. resembling mucin. 2. mucoid, def. 2.

mucinolytic (mu″sĭ-no-lit′ik) [*mucin* + Gr. *lysis* dissolution] dissolving or splitting up mucin.

mucinosis (mu″sĭ-no′sis) a condition characterized by abnormal deposits of mucopolysaccharides (mucins) in the skin. The mucinoses have been classified as metabolic (myxedema, diffuse or pretibial; lichen myxedematosus; and gargoylism), secondary or catabolic (degeneration in a variety of neoplasms), and localized (follicular, papular, plaquelike, focal, and the myxoid [synovial] cyst. **follicular m.,** a disease of unknown cause, characterized clinically by plaques of folliculopapules and histologically by deposition of acid mucopolysaccharides in the sebaceous glands and outer root sheath of the pilosebaceous unit; alopecia (*alopecia mucinosa*) is usually evident if lesions occur among terminal hairs. Extensive and persistent lesions in patients over thirty years of age are associated with reticulosis in perhaps 20 per cent of cases. **papular m.,** lichen myxedematosus.

mucinous (mu′sĭ-nus) resembling or marked by the formation of mucin.

mucinuria (mu″sin-u′re-ah) [*mucin* + Gr. *ouron* urine + *-ia*] the occurrence of mucin in the urine; it may suggest vaginal contamination.

muciparous (mu-sip′ah-rus) [*mucus* + L. *parere* to produce] secreting mucus.

mucitis (mu-si′tis) inflammation of the mucous membrane.

muco- [L. *mucus*] a combining form denoting relationship to mucus.

mucoantibody (mu″ko-an′tĭ-bod-e) a local concentration of antibody (usually IgA) admixed with mucus at mucous surfaces.

mucocartilage (mu″ko-kar′tĭ-lij) a soft cartilage the cells of which are in a mucus-like matrix.

mucocele (mu′ko-sēl) [*mucus* + Gr. *kēlē* tumor] 1. dilatation of a cavity with accumulated mucous secretion. 2. a mucous polyp. **suppurating m.,** a mucocele whose contents are purulent.

mucoclasis (mu-kok′lah-sis) [*mucus* + Gr. *klasis* a breaking] surgical destruction of the mucous lining of any organ, as of the gallbladder mucosa with the thermo- or electrocautery.

mucocolitis (mu″ko-ko-li′tis) mucous colitis.

mucocolpos (mu″ko-kol′pos) [*mucus* + Gr. *kolpos* vagina] accumulation of mucus in the vaginal canal.

mucocutaneous (mu″ko-ku-ta′ne-us) [*mucus* + *cutaneous*] pertaining to or affecting the mucous membrane and the skin.

mucocyte (mu′ko-sīt) an oligodendroglial cell whose cytoplasm has undergone mucoid degeneration.

mucoderm (mu′ko-derm) lamina propria mucosae.

mucodermal (mu″ko-der′mal) pertaining to mucoderm.

mucoenteritis (mu″ko-en-ter-i′tis) mucous colitis.

mucoepidermoid (mu″ko-ep″ĭ-der′moid) composed of mucus-producing and epithelial cells; see under *carcinoma*.

mucofibrous (mu″ko-fi′brus) composed of mucus and fibrous tissue.

mucoflocculent (mu″ko-flok′u-lent) containing threads of mucus.

mucoglobulin (mu″ko-glob′u-lin) one of the class of glycoproteins.

mucoid (mu′koid) 1. mucinoid. 2. any one of a group of mucus-like conjugated proteins of animal origin. The mucoids differ from mucins in solubility. They are precipitated by acetic acid. They include colloid and ovomucoid. Called also *mucinoid*.

mucoitin sulfate (mu-ko′ĭ-tin) a sulfur-containing polysaccharide from gastric mucin and from the cornea of the eye.

mucolemma (mu″ko-lem′ah) mucin coat, a noncellular envelope secreted around the rabbit egg and its oolemma by the oviduct; formerly called *albumen layer*.

mucolipid (mu″ko-lip′id) any sphingolipid, such as ganglioside, containing sialic acid (*N*-acetylneuraminic acid).

mucolipidoses (mu″ko-lip″ĭ-do′sez) plural of *mucolipidosis*.

mucolipidosis (mu″ko-lip″ĭ-do′sis) any of a group of genetic disorders in which both mucopolysaccharides and lipids accumulate in tissues but without excess of mucopolysaccharides in the urine. **m. I,** a hereditary congenital disorder characterized by mild Hurler-like manifestations with moderate mental retardation, peculiar inclusions in the fibroblasts, and no excess mucopolysacchariduria. Called also *lipomucopolysaccharidosis*. **m. II,** a rapidly progressing disease of young children, characterized histologically by abnormal fibroblasts containing a large number of dark inclusions which fill the central part of the cytoplasm except for the juxtonuclear zone (I-cells), and clinically by severe growth impairment, minimal hepatomegaly, extreme mental and motor retardation, and clear corneas; inherited as an autosomal recessive trait, it is due to deficiency of multiple acid hydrolases. Called also *I-cell disease*. **m. III,** a disorder similar to but milder than mucolipidosis II and thought to be due to the same enzyme deficiency but to a lesser extent. Called also

pseudo-Hurler polydystrophy. **m. IV,** a form marked by early corneal clouding, psychomotor retardation, and the presence of lysosomal storage bodies; thought to be transmitted as an autosomal recessive trait.

mucolytic (mu″ko-lit′ik) destroying or dissolving mucus; an agent that so acts.

mucomembranous (mu″ko-mem′brah-nus) pertaining to or composed of mucous membrane.

Mucomyst (mu′ko-mist) trademark for a preparation of acetylcysteine.

mucoperichondrial (mu″ko-per″e-kon′dre-al) pertaining to the mucoperichondrium.

mucoperichondrium (mu″ko-per″e-kon′dre-um) perichondrium having a mucosal surface, as that of the nasal septum.

mucoperiosteal (mu″ko-per″e-os′te-al) consisting of mucous membrane and periosteum.

mucoperiosteum (mu″ko-per″e-os′te-um) periosteum having a mucous surface, as in parts of the auditory apparatus.

mucopolysaccharidase (mu″ko-pol″e-sak′ah-ri-dās) an enzyme that catalyzes the hydrolysis of mucopolysaccharides.

mucopolysaccharide (mu″ko-pol′e-sak′ah-rīd) a group of polysaccharides which contain hexosamine, which may or may not be combined with protein and which, dispersed in water, form many of the mucins. The major mucopolysaccharides include chondroitin and its sulfate forms (A, B, and C), heparin, and hyaluronic acid. Called also *glycosaminoglycan*.

mucopolysaccharidoses (mu″ko-pol″e-sak″ah-rĭ-do′sēz) plural of mucopolysaccharidosis.

mucopolysaccharidosis (mu″ko-pol″e-sak″ah-rĭ-do′sis) any of a group of closely related genetically determined disorders caused by a defect in mucopolysaccharide metabolism and characterized by skeletal changes, mental retardation, visceral involvement, and corneal clouding, with widespread tissue deposits and excessive urinary secretion of mucopolysaccharides. Hurler's syndrome is the prototype of this disorder. **m. I,** originally, Hurler's syndrome; it now encompasses any of the forms due to deficiency of α-L-iduronidase; see *m. I-H, m. I-H/S,* and *m. I-S*. **m. I-H,** Hurler's syndrome. **m. I-H/S,** a form intermediate between the Hurler and Scheie syndromes, with all the findings of Hurler's syndrome but in a milder and slowly progressive form; it is postulated to be due to heterozygosity for each of the two genes affecting α-L-iduronidase activity. Called also *Hurler-Scheie compound*. **m. I-S,** Scheie's syndrome. **m. II,** Hunter's syndrome. **m. III,** Sanfilippo's syndrome. **m. IV,** Morquio's syndrome. **m. V,** former name for Scheie's syndrome, now classified as m. I-S. **m. VI,** Maroteaux-Lamy syndrome. **m. VII,** a form resembling a mild form of Hurler's syndrome, but with pectus carinatum, short stature, moderate mental retardation, and striking granulocyte inclusion. It is due to deficiency of β-glucuronidase and is transmitted as an autosomal recessive trait.

mucopolysacchariduria (mu″ko-pol″e-sak″ah-rĭ-du′re-ah) an excess of mucopolysaccharides in the urine.

mucoprotein (mu″ko-pro′te-in) a compound present in all connective and supporting tissues, containing mucopolysaccharides as prosthetic groups; they are relatively resistant to denaturation.

mucopurulent (mu″ko-pu′roo-lent) containing both mucus and pus.

mucopus (mu′ko-pus) [*mucus* + *pus*] mucus which has the appearance of pus on account of the presence of leukocytes.

Mucor (mu′kor) [L.] a genus of fungi of the family Mucoraceae, order Mucorales, which form delicate, white tubular filaments and spherical, black sporangia. See *mucormycosis*. **M. corym′bifer,** a species of soil saprophytes frequently found growing on moldy bread and rotting potatoes, and on occasion isolated from otomycosis. **M. muce′do,** a species of common soil saprophytes causing rot of fruit, baked goods, and insects; it is sometimes isolated as a contaminant of the feet and skin, but has not been determined to be pathogenic in humans. **M. pusil′lus,** a species resembling *M. mucedo*, from moist bread. It is pathogenic for rabbits and is occasionally found in cases of otomycosis in man. **M. racemo′sus,** a mold from soil and diseased fruits; it has occasionally been isolated from otomycosis. **M. ramo′sus,** *Absidia ramosa*. **M. rhizopodifor′mis,** *Absidia corymbifera*.

Mucoraceae (mu″ko-ra′se-e) a family of phycomycetes of the order Mucorales, subclass Zygomycetes, in which the thallus is not segmented and ramified; it includes the genera *Absidia, Rhizopus, Mucor,* and *Thamnidium*.

mucoraceous (mu″ko-ra′shus) pertaining to fungi of the order Mucorales.

Mucorales (Mu″kor-a′lēz) an order of phycomycetous fungi of the subclass Zygomycetes made up of bread molds and related fungi, the majority of which are saprophytic; it includes the family Mucoraceae.

mucorin (mu′ko-rin) an albuminous substance prepared from mucoraceous fungi.

mucormycosis (mu″kor-mi-ko′sis) a mycosis due to fungi of the order Mucorales, including species of *Mucor, Absidia,* and especially *Rhizopus.* It usually occurs as a complication of a chronic debilitating disease, particularly uncontrolled diabetes, most often beginning in the upper respiratory tract or lungs, in which spores germinate and from which mycelial growths metastasize to other organs.

mucosa (mu-ko′sah) [L. "mucus"] a mucous membrane, or tunica mucosa.

mucosal (mu-ko′sal) pertaining to the mucous membrane.

mucosanguineous (mu″ko-sang-gwin′e-us) composed of mucus and blood.

mucosedative (mu″ko-sed′ah-tiv) soothing to the mucous surfaces.

mucoserous (mu″ko-se′rus) pertaining to or producing both mucus and serum.

mucosin (mu-ko′sin) a form of mucin peculiar to the more tenacious varieties of mucus, as that of the nasal and uterine cavities.

mucositis (mu″ko-si′tis) inflammation of a mucous membrane. **m. necrot′icans agranulocyt′ica,** necrotic inflammation of mucous membranes associated with agranulocytosis.

mucosocutaneous (mu-ko″so-ku-ta′ne-us) pertaining to a mucous membrane and the skin.

mucostatic (mu″ko-stat′ik) 1. arresting the secretion of mucus. 2. denoting the normal relaxed condition of the tissues of the mucosa of the jaws.

mucotome (mu′ko-tōm) a dermatome for removing mucous membrane for transplantation; see *Castroviejo electric dermatome,* under *dermatome.*

mucous (mu′kus) [L. *mucosus*] pertaining to or resembling mucus; also secreting mucus.

mucoviscidosis (mu″ko-vis″ĭ-do′sis) cystic fibrosis of the pancreas (q.v. under *fibrosis*); so called because of the abnormally viscous mucoid secretions observed in the disease.

mucro (mu′kro), pl. *mucro′nes* [L. "a sharp point"] the pointed end of a part or organ. **m. ba′seos cartilag′inis arytae-noi′deae,** processus vocales. **m. cor′dis,** the apex of the heart. **m. ster′ni,** processus xiphoideus.

mucronate (mu′kro-nāt) [L. *mucro* a sharp point] having a spinelike tip or end.

mucroniform (mu-kron′ĭ-form) spinelike.

Mucuna (mu-ku′nah) [Brazilian] a genus of leguminous plants. The pods of *M. pru′riens,* cowitch or cowage, bear easily detached hairs which may cause unbearable itching; the seeds contain L-dopa.

mucus (mu′kus) [L.] the free slime of the mucous membranes, composed of secretion of the glands, along with various inorganic salts, desquamated cells, and leukocytes.

muffle (muf′f'l) a part of a furnace, usually removable or replaceable, in which material may be placed for processing, without exposing it to the direct action of the fire.

muguet (moo-gwa′) [Fr.] thrush (1st def.).

Muirhead's treatment (mūr′hedz) [Archibald Laurence *Muirhead,* Omaha pharmacologist, 1863–1921] see under *treatment.*

mular (mu′lar) [L. *mulus* mule] pertaining to mules. The term has been applied to certain lesions of verruga peruana in man which resemble the characteristic lesions of this disease in mules.

mulberry (mul′ber-e) any tree of the genus *Morus.* From the juice of the edible fruit a syrup is made which is used as a drink in fevers. The leaves serve as food for the silkworm. See also under *molar.*

Mulder's angle (mul′derz) [Johannes *Mulder,* Dutch anatomist, 1769–1810] see under *angle.*

Mulder's test (mul′derz) [Gerardus Johann *Mulder,* Dutch chemist, 1802–1880] see under *tests.*

Mules' operation (mūlz) [Philip Henry *Mules,* English ophthalmologist, 1843–1905] see under *operation.*

muliebria (mu″le-eb′re-ah) [L.] the female genitalia.

muliebrity (mu″le-eb′rĭ-te) [L. *muliebritas*] 1. womanly quality; the sum of the characteristics typical of the female sex. 2. the assumption of female qualities by the male.

mull (mul) a variety of thin, soft muslin formerly used in surgery. **plaster m.,** a sheet of mull coated with gutta-percha.

Muller (mul′er), Hermann Joseph. American biologist, 1890–1967, noted for his research on genes; winner of the Nobel prize for physiology in 1946.

Müller (mil′er), Paul Herrmann. Swiss chemist, 1890–1965, noted for synthesis of D.D.T. and discovery of its insecticidal properties; winner of the Nobel prize for medicine in 1948.

Müller's capsule, duct (canal), maneuver (experiment), tubercle, etc. (mil′erz) [Johannes Peter *Müller,* German physiologist, 1801–1858; one of the most distinguished physiologists of Germany and the founder of scientific medicine in Germany] see *capsula glomeruli* and *ductus paramesonephricus,* and see under *maneuver* and *tubercle.*

Müller's fibers (cells, radial cells), muscle (mil′erz) [Heinrich *Müller,* German anatomist, 1820–1864] see under *fiber* and *muscle.*

Müller's fluid (liquid) (mil′erz) [Hermann Franz *Müller,* German histologist, 1866–1898] see under *fluid.*

Müller's sign [Friedrich von *Müller,* Munich physician, 1858–1941] see under *sign.*

Müller's test [Edward *Müller,* German physician, 1876–1928] see under *tests* (1) and (2).

Müller's test (reaction) [Rudolf *Müller,* Vienna dermatologist, 1877–1934] see under *tests* (3).

Müller-Haeckel law (mil′er hek″l) [Fritz *Müller,* German naturalist, 1821–1997; Ernst Heinrich *Haeckel,* German biologist, 1834–1919] biogenetic law; see under *law.*

Müller-Jochmann test (mil′er-yōk′man) [Edward *Müller;* George *Jochmann,* Berlin physician, 1874–1915] see under *tests.*

muller (mul′er) a kind of pestle, flat at the bottom, used for grinding drugs upon a slab of similar material.

müllerian (mil-e′re-an) named for Johannes Peter *Müller,* as müllerian duct.

müllerianoma (mil-e″re-ah-no′mah) a tumor of müllerian duct origin.

Müllerius (mil-ler′e-us) a genus of nematode lungworms. **M. capilla′ris,** a species of lungworms that is parasitic in sheep and goats.

multangular (mul-tang′gu-lar) having many angles or corners.

multi- [L. *multus* many, much] a combining form signifying many or much.

multiallelic (mul″te-ah-lel′ik) pertaining to or occupied by many different genes affecting the same or different hereditary characters.

multiarticular (mul″te-ar-tik′u-lar) pertaining to or affecting many joints.

multibacillary (mul″tĭ-bas′ĭ-la″re) pertaining to or made up of a number of bacilli.

multicapsular (mul″tĭ-kap′su-lar) having many capsules, as a lamellar (pacinian) corpuscle.

multicell (mul′tĭ-sel) any organ made up of many cells; any group of functionally active cells.

multicellular (mul″tĭ-sel′u-lar) [*multi-* + L. *cellula* cell] 1. composed of many cells. 2. containing many hollow spaces.

multicellularity (mul″tĭ-sel″u-lar′ĭ-te) the state of being composed of many cells; the state of being multicellular.

multicentric (mul″tĭ-sen′trik) [*multi-* + *center*] polycentric.

multicentricity (mul″tĭ-sen-tris′ĭ-te) polycentricity.

Multiceps (mul′tĭ-seps) a genus of tapeworms (family Taeniidae), the bladder worms of which are found in herbivorous animals and the adult forms in carnivorous animals. **M. mul′ticeps,** a species which in the adult stage is parasitic in dogs. Its larval stage (*Coenurus cerebralis*) usually develops in the central nervous system, but sometimes in other organs or tissues, of goats and sheep and occasionally in man, and is productive of gid in sheep. **M. seria′lis,** a species parasitic in dogs, its larval stage developing in rabbits, squirrels, and other rodents; the larvae have rarely been reported from man, generally developing, as in its other intermediate hosts, in the connective tissues.

multicontaminated (mul″tĭ-kon-tam′ĭ-nāt″ed) infected by several different species of microorganisms, or by several different contaminating agents.

multicuspidate (mul″tĭ-kus′pĭ-dāt) [*multi-* + L. *cuspis* point] having many cusps.

multicystic (mul″tĭ-sis′tik) polycystic.

multidentate (mul″tĭ-den′tāt) having many teeth or many indentations.

multifactorial (mul″tĭ-fak-to′re-al) 1. of or pertaining to, or arising through the action of many factors. 2. in genetics, arising as the result of the interaction of several genes and usually, to some extent, of nongenetic factors. Cf. *polygenic.*

multifamilial (mul″tĭ-fah-mil′e-al) affecting several successive generations of a family.

multifid (mul′tĭ-fid) cleft into many parts.

multifidus (mul-tif′ĭ-dus) [L., from *multus* many + *findere* to split] cleft into many parts, as the musculus multifidus.

multifocal (mul″tĭfo′kal) arising from or pertaining to many foci.

multiform (mul′tĭ-form) occurring in several forms; polymorphic.

multiganglionic (mul″tĭ-gang″gle-on′ik) pertaining to, affecting, or possessing many ganglia.

multigesta (mul″tĭ-jes′tah) multigravida.

multiglandular (mul″tĭ-glan′du-lar) pluriglandular.

multigravida (mul″tĭ-grav′ĭ-dah) [*multi-* + L. *gravida* pregnant] a woman who has been pregnant several times. Also written gravida II, III, etc., according to the number of pregnancies. **grand m.,** a woman who has had six or more previous pregnancies.

multihallucalism (mul″tĭ-hal′ŭ-kal-izm) [multi- + L. *hallux, hallucis,* great toe + -ism] a developmental anomaly characterized by the presence of more than one great toe on one foot.

multihallucism (mul″tĭ-hal′u-sizm) multihallucalism.

multi-infection (mul″tĭ-in-fek′shun) infection with several varieties of organisms.

multilobar (mul″tĭ-lo′bar) having numerous lobes.

multilobular (mul″tĭ-lob′u-lar) [multi- + L. *lobulus* lobule] having many lobules.

multilocular (mul″tĭ-lok′u-lar) [multi- + L. *loculus* cell] having many cells or compartments, as a multilocular cyst.

multimammae (mul″tĭ-mam′e) [multi- + L. *mamma* breast] the condition of having more than two breasts.

multinodular (mul″tĭ-nod′u-lar) composed of many nodules.

multinucleate (mul″tĭ-nu′kle-āt) [multi- + *nucleus*] having several nuclei; said of cells.

multipara (mul-tip′ah-rah) [multi- + L. *parere* to bring forth, produce] a woman who has had two or more pregnancies which resulted in viable fetuses, whether or not the offspring were alive at birth. Also written para II, III, IV, etc., according to the number of offspring. **grand m.,** a woman who has had six or more pregnancies which resulted in viable fetuses.

multiparity (mul″tĭ-par′ĭ-te) 1. the condition of being a multipara. 2. the production of several offspring in one gestation.

multiparous (mul-tip′ah-rus) 1. having had two or more pregnancies which resulted in viable fetuses. 2. producing several ova or offspring at one time.

multipartial (mul″tĭ-par′shal) made from cultures of several strains of the same microorganism rather than from one culture only; said of sera.

multiple (mul′tĭ-p'l) [L. *multiplex*] manifold; occurring in or affecting various parts of the body at once.

multiplicitas (mul″tĭ-plis′ĭ-tas) a multiplication; a developmental anomaly characterized by the presence of an abnormal multiplicity of organs, or of a specific organ. **m. cor′dis,** a developmental anomaly characterized by the presence of a number of separate hearts.

multipolar (mul″tĭ-po′lar) [multi- + L. *polus* pole] having more than two poles or processes.

multipollicalism (mul″tĭ-pol′ĭ-kal-izm) [multi- + L. *pollex, pollicis* thumb + -ism] a developmental anomaly characterized by the presence of more than one thumb on one hand.

multirooted (mul″tĭ-rōōt′ed) having many roots; said of molar teeth.

multisensitivity (mul″tĭ-sen″sĭ-tiv′ĭ-te) the condition of being sensitive (allergic) to more than one antigen (allergen).

multisynaptic (mul″te-sĭ-nap′tik) polysynaptic.

multiterminal (mul″tĭ-ter′mĭ-nal) having several sets of terminals so that several electrodes may be used.

multituberculate (mul″tĭ-tu-ber′ku-lāt) having many tubercles.

multivalent (mul″tĭ-va′lent) [multi- + L. *valere* to have value] 1. having the power of combining with three or more univalent atoms. 2. active against several strains of an organism.

mummification (mum″ĭ-fi-ka′shun) conversion into a state resembling that of a mummy, such as occurs in dry gangrene, or the shriveling and drying up of a dead fetus.

mummying (mum′e-ing) former term for a form of physical restraint in which the entire body is enclosed in a sheet or blanket, leaving only the head exposed; application of a wet-sheet pack.

mumps (mumps) a contagious paramyxovirus disease occurring mainly in children and conferring a resultant persisting immunity. It is acquired by aspiration, the heaviest inoculation of virus being in the salivary glands, the parotids more so than submandibular or sublingual. The incubation period is 18 to 22 days. Infection is symptomatic in approximately 75 per cent of cases. In these, parotitis occurs in 70 per cent, and meningitis in 10–15 per cent (with asymptomatic pleocytosis in half of these). Epididymo-orchitis develops in 20 per cent of postpubertal males, but subsequent sterility is rare. Other manifestations are less common and consist of pancreatitis, arthritis, myocarditis, oophoritis, thyroiditis, and mastitis. Fever and painful inflammation of the involved part are most pronounced during the first two days and subside slowly over the next four or five. More than one area may be involved simultaneously; occasionally the involvement is sequential, the entire disease lasting for two or three weeks. Meningoencephalitis with attendant lasting neurological injury is rare. Called also *epidemic parotitis.* **iodine m.,** swelling of the salivary and lacrimal glands as a toxic reaction to iodine therapy. **m. meningoencephalitis,** see under *meningoencephalitis.* **metastatic m.,** involvement of other glands or organs of the body occurring in association with mumps.

mumu (mu′mu) a condition characterized by swelling and edema of the spermatic cord, and sometimes swelling of the scrotum, epididymis, and testicle, and by the appearance of a hydrocele; probably an allergic manifestation developing after inoculation by filaria.

Münchausen's syndrome (men-chow′zenz) [named after Baron von *Münchhausen,* a reputed teller of exaggerated tales] see under *syndrome.*

Münchmeyer's disease (minch′mi-erz) [Ernst *Münchmeyer,* German physician, 1846–1880] see under *disease.*

Mundinus (mun-di′nus) [It. *Mondino* de Luzzi (?1275–1326) an Italian physician and anatomist—"the restorer of anatomy." His *Anothomia* (1316) was the first text devoted to human anatomy and, although not illustrated, it was greatly esteemed for some two hundred years.

munity (mu′nĭ-te) the state of being susceptible to infection.

Munk's disease (munks) [Fritz *Munk,* Berlin internist, born 1879] lipid nephrosis.

Munro's point (mun-rōz′) [John Cummings *Munro,* Boston surgeon, 1858–1910] see under *point.*

mural (mu′ral) [L. *muralis,* from *murus* wall] pertaining to or occurring in the wall of a cavity.

muramidase (mu-ram′ĭ-dās) lysozyme.

Murchison-Pel-Ebstein fever [Charles *Murchison,* British physician, 1830–1879; Pieter Klaases *Pel,* Dutch physician, 1852–1919; Wilhelm *Ebstein,* German physician, 1836–1912] Pel-Ebstein fever.

Murel (mu′rel) trademark for preparations of valethamate bromide.

Murex (mu′reks) a genus of mollusks. **M. purpu′rea,** a gastropodous mollusk of the Mediterranean from which murexine is obtained.

murexide (mu-rek′sĭd) [L. *murex* purple sea snail] ammonium purpurate, $C_8H_4O_6N_5 \cdot NH_4 \cdot H_2O$, a substance formed in Weidel's test for uric acid; a purple color is produced when uric acid is present. Formerly used as a dye. See also *Weidel's test* (1), under *tests.*

murexine (mu-rek′sin) [L. *murex, muricis* the purple fish or pointed rock + -ine, suffix for chemical compounds] chemical name: β-[imidazolyl-(4)]-acrylcholine. A neurotoxic substance derived from the median zone of the hypobranchial gland of gastropods of the genus *Murex* and related species; the substance is called *purpurine* when derived from snails of the genus *Purpura.*

muriate (mu′re-āt) [L. *muria* brine] an obsolete synonym of chloride.

muriatic (mu″re-at′ik) [L. *muriaticus; muria* brine] derived from common salt. See also under *acid.*

Murimyces (mu″rĭ-mi′sēz) a name once proposed for the pleuropneumonia-like organisms, now called *Mycoplasma.*

murine (mu′rin) [L. *mus, muris* mouse] pertaining to or affecting mice or rats.

murivirus (mu″rĭ-vi′rus) [from *m*ild *u*pper *r*espiratory *i*llness + *virus*] former name for rhinovirus.

murmur (mur′mur) [L.] an auscultatory sound, benign or pathologic, particularly a periodic sound of short duration of cardiac or vascular origin. **accidental m.,** a cardiac murmur due to some temporary and unimportant circumstance. **amphoric m.,** a respiratory murmur having a blowing musical character. **anemic m.,** a cardiac murmur heard in anemic patients. **aneurysmal m.,** a vascular murmur heard over an aneurysm. **aortic m.,** a sound generated by blood flowing through a diseased aorta or aortic valve. **apex m.,** one heard at the apex of the heart. **apical diastolic m's,** murmurs at the apex of the heart indicative of mitral stenosis and consisting essentially of low-frequency vibrations, which account for their rumble quality. **arterial m.,** a murmur (bruit) over an artery, sometimes aneurysmal and sometimes constricted. **attrition m.,** the sound produced by the friction of the pericardial surfaces in some cases of pericarditis. **Austin Flint m.,** a presystolic murmur at the apex in aortic regurgitation. **basal diastolic m's,** diastolic murmurs at the base of the heart, due to aortic or pulmonic insufficiency. **bellows m.,** to-and-fro sound. **blood m.,** one due to an abnormal, and commonly an anemic, condition of the blood. **brain m.,** a systolic murmur chiefly heard in the temporal region, and principally in cases of rickets. **bronchial m.,** one heard over the large bronchi resembling a laryngeal respiratory murmur. **cardiac m.,** a sound of finite length generated by blood flow through the heart. **cardiopulmonary m., cardiorespiratory m.,** a sound generated within lung tissue and related to movement of the heart. **Carey-Coombs m.,** a rumbling mid-diastolic prediastolic apical cardiac murmur occurring in the early stages of rheumatic fever and disappearing after the rheumatic attack abates. **continuous m.,** a humming cardiac murmur extending throughout systole into late diastole or to the end of diastole, and occurring in patent ductus arteriosus, arteriovenous fistulas, rupture of a syphilitic aortic aneurysm into the pulmonary artery, aorticopulmonary septal defect, bronchial artery anastomosis in pulmonary atresia, angioma of lung, and stenosis of a branch of the pulmonary artery. **cooing m.,** musical m. **crescendo m.,** a murmur marked by progressively increasing loudness, e.g., the late diastolic

A Table of Endocardial Murmurs

TIME OF OCCURRENCE	SITE OF GREATEST INTENSITY	DIRECTION OF TRANSMISSION	SEAT OF LESION	NATURE OF LESION
Systolic.	At cardiac apex.	Along left fifth and sixth ribs—in left axilla—in the back, at inferior angle of left scapula.	Mitral orifice.	Incompetency—Regurgitation.
Systolic.	At junction of right second costal cartilage with sternum.	To junction of right clavicle with sternum—in course of right carotid.	Aortic orifice.	Narrowing—Obstruction.
Systolic.	At ensiform cartilage.	Feebly transmitted.	Tricuspid orifice.	Incompetency—Regurgitation.
Systolic.	At left second intercostal space, close to sternum.	Feebly transmitted.	Pulmonary orifice.	Narrowing—Obstruction.
Diastolic.	At junction of right second costal cartilage with sternum.	To midsternum—in course of sternum.	Aortic orifice.	Incompetency—Regurgitation.
Diastolic.	At left second intercostal space, close to sternum.	In course of sternum.	Pulmonary orifice.	Incompetency—Regurgitation.
(Diastolic) presystolic.	Over body of heart.	To apex of heart.	Mitral orifice.	Narrowing—Obstruction.
(Diastolic) presystolic.	At ensiform cartilage.	Feebly transmitted.	Tricuspid orifice.	Narrowing—Obstruction.

murmur in mitral stenosis with sinus rhythm. **Cruveilhier-Baumgarten m.,** a venous murmur heard at the abdominal wall over veins connecting the portal and caval system. **deglutition m.,** one heard over the esophagus during the act of swallowing. **diamond-shaped m.,** the systolic murmur of aortic stenosis, named for its recorded shape on the phonocardiogram. **diastolic m.,** one occurring during diastole, i.e., after the second sound of the heart. Heard at the apex, it is a sign of mitral obstruction; at the base of the heart, it is due to aortic regurgitation; more rarely to pulmonary regurgitation. **direct m.** (*obs.*), the sound made by the forward flow of blood related to cardiac obstruction. **Duroziez's m.,** a double murmur over the femoral or other large peripheral artery, due to aortic insufficiency. **ejection m.,** systolic murmurs which occur predominantly in midsystole when ejection volume and velocity of blood flow are at their maximum; heard in aortic or pulmonary stenosis. **Flint's m.,** Austin Flint m. **friction m.,** see under *rub.* **functional m.,** a cardiac murmur generated within a structurally normal heart. **Gibson m.,** a long rumbling sound occupying most of systole and diastole, usually localized in the second left interspace near the sternum, and usually indicative of patent ductus arteriosus. **Graham Steell's m.,** one caused by pulmonary regurgitation in patients with pulmonary hypertension and mitral stenosis; it is a murmur heard in the third left intercostal space near the border of the sternum and thence propagated down the sternum. **Hamman's m.,** a crunching sound heard over the precordium synchronous with the heart beat; a sign of mediastinal emphysema, it is noted particularly in persons with pneumopericardium and is attributed to agitation of air bubbles by heart action. **heart m.,** cardiac m. **hemic m.,** blood m. **holosystolic m.,** pansystolic m. **hourglass m.,** a cardiac murmur characterized by two periods of maximum loudness joined by a period of decreased loudness. **humming-top m.,** venous hum. **incidental m.,** accidental m. **indirect m.** (*obs.*), the sound made by the backward flow of blood related to valvular regurgitation. **innocent m.,** functional m. **inorganic m.** (*obs.*), any cardiac murmur not due to a valvular or other lesion. **machinery m.,** Gibson m. **mitral m.,** cardiac murmur due to disease of the mitral valve. **muscle m.,** one heard over a muscle in a state of contraction. **musical m.,** a cardiac murmur, usually systolic, resulting when the responsible vibrations have a periodic harmonic pattern. **obstructive m.,** direct m. **organic m.,** one due to a structural change in the heart, in a vessel, or in the lung substance. **pansystolic m.,** a cardiac murmur that extends through systole; called also *holosystolic m.* **pericardial m.,** see *pericardial (friction) rub,* under *rub.* **pleuropericardial m.,** a pleural friction sound heard in the pericardial region and resembling a pericardial rub. **prediastolic m.,** one occurring just before and with the diastole. Heard at the apex, it is due to mitral obstruction; at the base of the heart, to aortic regurgitation; more rarely, to pulmonary regurgitation. **presystolic m.,** one occurring shortly before the onset of ventricular ejection, usually attributed to atrial contraction and the acceleration of blood flow through a narrowed atrial ventricular valve. **pulmonic m.,** one due to disease of the valves of the pulmonary artery. **regurgitant m.,** a murmur due to regurgitation of blood through a diseased valvular orifice. **Roger's m.,** bruit de Roger. **sea-gull m.,** a raucous murmur with musical qualities resembling the call of a sea gull, heard occasionally in aortic insufficiency, and attributed specifically to eversion or retroversion of the right anterior aortic cusp. **seesaw m.,** to-and-fro sound. **Steell's m.,** Graham Steell's m. **stenosal m.,** a sound produced in an artery by artificial pressure or by a stenosis. **Still's m.,** a functional cardiac murmur of childhood, occurring in midsystole and usually of maximal intensity at the lower left sternal border. **subclavicular m.,** a sound sometimes produced in the subclavian artery during systole, and due to a stenosis. **systolic m.,** one during systole; usually due to mitral or tricuspid regurgitation, or to aortic or pulmonary obstruction. **to-and-fro m.,** see under *sound.* **Traube's m.,** gallop rhythm. **tricuspid m.,** a murmur caused by disease of the tricuspid valves. **vascular m.,** a murmur heard over a blood vessel. **venous m.,** a murmur heard over a vein. **vesicular m.,** the normal breath sounds over the lungs.

Murphy (mur′fe), William Parry. American physician, born in 1892, co-winner with George Richards Minot and George Hoyt Whipple, of the Nobel prize for medicine and physiology in 1934, for their work on anemia.

Murphy button, etc. (mur′fe) [John Benjamin *Murphy*, Chicago surgeon, 1857–1916] see under *button, method, percussion, sign, tests,* and *treatment.*

Murri's disease (moor′ēz) [Augusto *Murri*, Italian clinician, 1841–1932] intermittent hemoglobinuria.

murrina (moo-re′nah) a form of trypanosomiasis among mules and horses in Panama, marked by fever, anemia, icterus, weakness, emaciation and edema, conjunctivitis, and posterior paralysis. It is caused by *Trypanosoma hippicum* (now considered to be identical with *T. evansi*), which is transmitted by flies of the genus *Glossina* and by vampire bats (*Desmodus rotundus*). Called also *derrengadera.*

Mus (mus) [L. "mouse"] a genus of mice. **M. alexandri′nus,** *Rattus rattus alexandrinus,* the Egyptian or roof rat. **M. decuma′nus,** *Rattus norvegicus,* the brown rat. **M. mus′-culus,** the common house mouse. **M. norve′gicus,** *Rattus norvegicus,* the brown rat. **M. rat′tus rat′tus,** the black rat.

Musca (mus′kah) [L. "fly"] a genus of flies of the family Muscidae which have their mouth parts adapted for suction only. **M. autumna′lis,** the face fly, a species commonly found in Europe, parts of Asia and Africa, and America. **M. domes′tica,** the common house fly. It may act as a mechanical carrier of the microorganisms of typhoid fever, cholera, dysentery, plague, anthrax, tetanus, trachoma, leprosy, and encephalitis, and

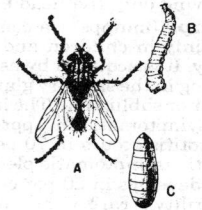

Musca domestica: A, fly; *B,* larva; *C,* pupa.

of pyogenic bacteria, cysts of some protozoa, and helminth ova. The larvae may cause myiasis. **M. domes′tica neb′ulo,** a subspecies of *M. domestica* found in India. **M. domes′tica vici′-na,** a subspecies of *M. domestica* common in Egypt and India. **M. lute′ola,** see *Auchmeromyia.* **M. sor′bens,** a species of Indonesia, Ethiopia, and Oriental areas, believed to transmit conjunctivitis, trachoma, and other infections. **M. vomito′-ria,** *Calliphora vomitoria.*

musca (mus′kah), pl. *mus′cae* [L.] a fly. **mus′cae his-pan′icae,** cantharides. **mus′cae volitan′tes** [L. "flitting flies"], specks seen floating before the eyes; see *floaters.*

muscacide (mus′kah-sīd) [L. *musca* fly + *caedere* to kill] 1. destructive to flies. 2. any agent that destroys flies.

muscae (mus′e) [L.] plural of *musca*.

muscardine (mus′kar-din) a disease of silkworms caused by *Beauvaria bassiana*.

muscarine (mus′kah-rin) [L. *muscarius* pertaining to flies] an active alkaloid, $C_9H_{20}O_2N$, obtained from the red variety of the mushroom *Amanita muscaria* (L.) Pers. (Agaricaceae). It produces a characteristic toxic syndrome in man when the fungus is ingested (see *mushroom poisoning*, under *poisoning*). Muscarine is used in pharmacologic and physiologic studies because it mimics the action of acetylcholine (see *muscarinic*).

muscarinic (mus″kah-rin′ik) denoting the acetylcholine-like (parasympathomimetic) effects of muscarine on postganglionic parasympathetic neural impulses, including decrease in heart rate and contractility, bronchoconstriction, dilatation of arterioles, increase in motility, tone, and secretion of stomach and intestine, and stimulation of salivary and lacrimal glands.

muscarinism (mus′kar-in-izm) poisoning by muscarine.

muscegenetic (mus″e-jĕ-net′ik) giving rise to muscae volitantes.

muscicide (mus′ĭ-sīd) muscacide.

Muscidae (mus′ĭ-de) a family of flies of the order Diptera. It includes the genera *Fannia, Haematobia, Glossina, Musca, Muscina,* and *Stomoxys.*

Muscina (mŭ-si′nah) the nonbiting stable flies, a genus of the family Muscidae which breeds in dung. It is closely related to the housefly and it also frequents dwellings.

muscle (mus′el) an organ which by contraction produces the movements of an animal organism. Called also *musculus* [NA]. Muscles are of two varieties: *striated,* or *striped,* including all the muscles in which contraction is voluntary and the heart muscle; *unstriated, nonstriated, smooth,* or *organic,* including all the involuntary muscles except the heart, such as the muscular layer of the intestines, bladder, blood vessels, etc. Striated muscles are covered with a thin layer of connective tissue (*epimysium*) from which septa (*perimysium*) pass, dividing the muscle into bundles of fibers, or *fasciculi*. Each fasciculus contains a number of parallel fibers separated by connective tissue septa (*endomysium*). Each fiber consists of sarcoplasm which is cross-striated or composed of alternate light and dark portions (whence the name *striated muscle*); each contains embedded in it the *myofibrils* and each is surrounded by *sarcolemma.* Smooth muscles are composed of elongated, spindle-shaped, nucleated cells arranged parallel to one another and to the long axis of the muscle, and these cells are often grouped into bundles of varying size. The muscles, bundles, and cells are enclosed in an indifferent connective tissue material much as is found in striated muscles. **abductor m. of great toe,** musculus abductor hallucis. **abductor m. of little finger,** musculus abductor digiti minimi manus. **abductor m. of little toe,** musculus abductor digiti minimi pedis. **abductor m. of thumb, long,** musculus abductor pollicis longus. **abductor m. of thumb, short,** musculus abductor pollicis brevis. **adductor m., great,** musculus adductor magnus. **adductor m., long,** musculus adductor longus. **adductor m., short,** musculus adductor brevis. **adductor m., smallest,** musculus adductor minimus. **adductor m. of great toe,** musculus adductor hallucis. **adductor m. of thumb,** musculus adductor pollicis. **Aeby's m.,** musculus depressor labii inferioris. **agonistic m.,** a muscle opposed in action by another muscle, called the antagonist. **Albinus' m.,** 1. musculus risorius. 2. musculus scalenus medius. **anconeus m.,** musculus anconeus. **anconeus m., lateral,** caput laterale musculi tricipitis brachii. **anconeus m., medial,** caput mediale musculi tricipitis brachii. **anconeus m., short,** caput laterale musculi tricipitis brachii. **antagonistic m.,** a muscle that counteracts the action of another muscle, called the agonist. **antigravity m's,** those muscles that by their tone resist the constant pull of gravity in the maintenance of normal posture. **m. of antitragus,** musculus antitragicus. **appendicular m's,** the muscles of a limb. **arrector m's of hair,** musculi arrectores pilorum. **articular m.,** a muscle that has one end attached to the capsule of a joint; called also *musculus articularis.* **articular m. of elbow,** musculus articularis cubiti. **articular m. of knee,** musculus articularis genus. **aryepiglottic m.,** musculus aryepiglotticus. **arytenoid m., oblique,** musculus arytenoideus obliquus. **arytenoid m., transverse,** musculus arytenoideus transversus. **m's of auditory ossicles,** musculi ossiculorum auditus. **auricular m., anterior,** musculus auricularis anterior. **auricular m., posterior,** musculus auricularis posterior. **auricular m., superior,** musculus auricularis superior. **Bell's m.,** the muscular strands between the ureteric orifices and the uvula vesicae, bounding the trigone of the urinary bladder. Called also *ureteric bridge.* **biceps m. of arm,** musculus biceps brachii. **biceps m. of thigh,** musculus biceps femoris. **bipennate m.,** musculus bipennatus. **Bowman's m.,** musculus ciliaris. **brachial m.,** musculus brachialis. **brachioradial m.,** musculus brachioradialis. **bronchoesophageal m.,** musculus bronchoesophageus. **Brücke's m.,** the longitudinal fibers of the ciliary muscle. **buccinator m.,** musculus buccinator. **buccopharyngeal m.,** pars buccopharyngea musculi constrictoris pharyngis superioris. **bulbocavernous m.,** musculus

bulbospongiosus. **canine m.,** musculus levator anguli oris. **cardiac m.,** the muscle of the heart, composed of striated muscle fibers. **Casser's m., casserian m.,** ligamentum mallei anterius. **ceratocricoid m.,** musculus ceratocricoideus. **ceratopharyngeal m.,** pars ceratopharyngea musculi constrictoris pharyngis medii. **Chassaignac's axillary m.,** an occasional muscle bundle extending from the lower edge of the latissimus dorsi across the hollow of the axilla to the brachial fascia or to the lower border of the pectoralis minor. **chondroglossus m.,** musculus chondroglossus. **chondropharyngeal m.,** pars chondropharyngea musculi constrictoris pharyngis medii. **ciliary m.,** musculus ciliaris. **coccygeal m's,** those connected with the coccyx, including the musculus coccygeus, musculus sacrococcygeus dorsalis, and musculus sacrococcygeus ventralis; called also *musculi coccygei* [NA]. **coccygeal m.,** musculus coccygeus. **compressor m. of naris,** pars transversa musculi nasalis. **congenerous m's,** muscles having a common action or function. **constrictor m. of pharynx, inferior,** musculus constrictor pharyngis inferior. **constrictor m. of pharynx, middle,** musculus constrictor pharyngis medius. **constrictor m. of pharynx, superior,** musculus constrictor pharyngis superior. **coracobrachial m.,** musculus coracobrachialis. **Crampton's m.,** the anterior portion of the ciliary muscle in birds. **cremaster m.,** musculus cremaster. **cricoarytenoid m., lateral,** musculus cricoarytenoideus lateralis. **cricoarytenoid m., posterior,** musculus cricoarytenoideus posterior. **cricopharyngeal m.,** pars cricopharyngea musculi constrictoris pharyngis inferioris. **cricothyroid m.,** musculus cricothyroideus. **cutaneous m.,** striated muscle that inserts into the skin; called also *musculus cutaneus.* **dartos m. of scrotum,** tunica dartos. **deltoid m.,** musculus deltoideus. **depressor m., superciliary,** musculus depressor supercilii. **depressor m. of angle of mouth,** musculus depressor anguli oris. **depressor m. of lower lip,** musculus depressor labii inferioris. **depressor m. of septum of nose,** musculus depressor septi nasi. **detrusor m.,** detrusor urinae. **diaphragmatic m.,** diaphragm. **digastric m.,** musculus digastricus. **dilator m. of nose,** pars alaris musculi nasalis. **dilator m. of pupil,** musculus dilator pupillae. **emergency m's,** muscles which ordinarily are not required in the performance of an act but which assist the prime movers when an act is performed with great force. **epicranial m.,** musculus epicranius. **epimeric m.,** a muscle derived from an epimere and innervated by a posterior ramus of a spinal nerve. **epitrochleoanconeus m.,** musculus epitrochleoanconaeus. **erector m. of penis,** musculus ischiocavernosus. **erector m. of spine,** musculus erector spinae. **eustachian m.,** musculus tensor tympani. **extensor m. of digits, common, extensor m. of fingers,** musculus extensor digitorum. **extensor m. of fifth digit, proper,** musculus extensor digiti minimi. **extensor m. of great toe, long,** musculus extensor hallucis longus. **extensor m. of great toe, short,** musculus extensor hallucis brevis. **extensor m. of index finger,** musculus extensor indicis. **extensor m. of little finger,** musculus extensor digiti minimi. **extensor m. of thumb, long,** musculus extensor pollicis longus. **extensor m. of thumb, short,** musculus extensor pollicis brevis. **extensor m. of toes, long,** musculus extensor digitorum longus. **extensor m. of toes, short,** musculus extensor digitorum brevis. **extraocular m's,** musculi bulbi. **extrinsic m.,** a muscle that does not originate in the same limb or part in which it is inserted. **m's of eye,** musculi bulbi. **fast m.,** white m. **m's of fauces,** musculi palati et faucium. **femoral m.,** musculus vastus intermedius. **fibular m., long,** musculus peroneus longus. **fibular m., short,** musculus peroneus brevis. **fibular m., third,** musculus peroneus tertius. **fixation m's, fixator m's,** accessory muscles that serve to steady a part. **fixator m. of base of stapes,** musculus fixator baseos stapedis. **flexor m., accessory,** musculus quadratus plantae. **flexor m. of fingers, deep,** musculus flexor digitorum profundus. **flexor m. of fingers, superficial,** musculus flexor digitorum superficialis. **flexor m. of great toe, long,** musculus flexor hallucis longus. **flexor m. of great toe, short,** musculus flexor hallucis brevis. **flexor m. of little finger, short,** musculus flexor digiti minimi brevis manus. **flexor m. of little toe, short,** musculus flexor digiti minimi brevis pedis. **flexor m. of thumb, long,** musculus flexor pollicis longus. **flexor m. of thumb, short,** musculus flexor pollicis brevis. **flexor m. of toes, long,** musculus flexor digitorum longus. **flexor m. of toes, short,** musculus flexor digitorum brevis. **Folius' m.,** ligamentum mallei laterale. **frontal m.,** venter frontalis musculi occipitofrontalis. **fusiform m.,** a spindle-shaped muscle; see *musculus fusiformis.* **gastrocnemius m.,** musculus gastrocnemius. **gastrocnemius m., lateral,** caput laterale musculi gastrocnemii. **gastrocnemius m., medial,** caput mediale musculi gastrocnemii. **Gavard's m.,** the oblique muscular elements of the stomach wall. **gemellus m., inferior,** musculus gemellus inferior. **gemellus m., superior,** musculus gemellus superior. **genioglossus m.,** musculus genioglossus. **geniohyoid m.,** musculus geniohyoideus. **glossopalatine m.,** musculus palatoglossus. **glossopharyngeal** m., pars glossopharyngea musculi constrictoris pharyngis superioris. **gluteal m., least,** musculus gluteus minimus. **gracilis m.,** musculus gracilis. **Guthrie's m.,** musculus sphincter urethrae. **hamstring m's,** the muscles of the back of the thigh, including the biceps femoris, the semitendinosus, and the semimembranosus. **Hilton's m.,** musculus aryepiglotticus. **Horner's m.,** pars lacrimalis musculi orbicularis oculi. **Houston's m.,** fibers of the bulbocavernosus muscle compressing the dorsal vein of the penis. **hyoglossal m., hyoglossus m.,** musculus hyoglossus. **m's of hyoid bone,** see *musculi infrahyoidei* and *musculi suprahyoidei.* **hypaxial m's,** musculus longus capitis, musculus longus colli, the vertebral portion of the diaphragm, and musculus sacrococcygeus anterior; called also *subvertebral m's.* **hypomeric m.,** a muscle derived from a hypomere and innervated by an anterior ramus of a spinal nerve. **iliac m.,** musculus iliacus. **iliococcygeal m.,** musculus iliococcygeus. **iliocostal m's,** see entries beginning *musculus iliocostalis.* **iliopsoas m.,** musculus iliopsoas. **incisive m's of inferior lip,** musculi incisivi labii inferioris. **incisive m's of lower lip,** musculi incisivi labii inferioris. **incisive m's of superior lip,** musculi incisivi labii superioris. **incisive m's of upper lip,** musculi incisivi labii superioris. **infrahyoid m's,** musculi infrahyoidei. **infraspinous m.,** musculus infraspinatus. **inspiratory m's,** the muscles that act in inspiration, such as the diaphragm, and the intercostal and pectoral muscles. **intercostal m's, external,** musculi intercostales externi. **intercostal m's, innermost,** musculi intercostales intimi. **intercostal m's, internal,** musculi intercostales interni. **interfoveolar m.,** ligamentum interfoveolare. **interosseous m's, palmar,** musculi interossei palmares. **interosseous m's, plantar,** musculi interossei plantares. **interosseous m's, volar,** musculi interossei palmares. **interosseous m's of foot, dorsal,** musculi interossei dorsales pedis. **interosseous m's of hand, dorsal,** musculi interossei dorsales manus. **interspinal m's,** musculi interspinales. **interspinal muscles of thorax,** musculi interspinales thoracis. **intertransverse m's,** musculi intertransversarii. **intertransverse m's, anterior,** musculi intertransversarii thoracis. **intertransverse m's of neck, anterior,** musculi intertransversarii anteriores cervicis. **intertransverse m's of neck, posterior,** musculi intertransversarii posteriores cervicis. **intertransverse m's of thorax,** musculi intertransversarii thoracis. **intraauricular m's,** the stapedius and tensor tympani muscles. **intraocular m's,** the intrinsic muscles of the eyeball. **intrinsic m.,** a muscle whose origin and insertion are both in the same limb or part. **involuntary m.,** a muscle that is not under the control of the will; such muscles are, for the most part, composed of nonstriated fibers. **iridic m's,** the muscles controlling the iris. **ischiocavernous m.,** musculus ischiocavernosus. **Jarjavay's m.,** a muscle arising from the ramus of the ischium and inserting in the constrictor muscle of the vagina, which acts to depress the urethra. **Jung's m.,** musculus pyramidalis auriculae. **Koyter's m.,** musculus corrugator supercilii. **Landström's m.,** minute muscle fibers in the fascia around and behind the eyeball, attached in front to the anterior orbital fascia and eyelids. **Langer's m.,** muscular fibers from the insertion of the pectoralis major muscle over the bicipital groove to the insertion of the latissimus dorsi. **latissimus dorsi m.,** musculus latissimus dorsi. **levator m. of angle of mouth,** musculus levator anguli oris. **levator ani m.,** musculus levator ani. **levator m. of prostate,** musculus levator prostatae. **levator m's of ribs,** musculi levatores costarum. **levator m's of ribs, long,** musculi levatores costarum longi. **levator m's of ribs, short,** musculi levatores costarum breves. **levator m. of scapula,** musculus levator scapulae. **levator m. of thyroid gland,** musculus levator glandulae thyroideae. **levator m. of upper eyelid,** musculus levator palpebrae superioris. **levator m. of upper lip,** musculus levator labii superioris. **levator m. of upper lip and ala of nose,** musculus levator labii superioris alaeque nasi. **levator muscle of velum palatini,** musculus levator velum palatini. **longissimus m.,** musculus longissimus. **longissimus m. of back,** musculus longissimus thoracis. **longissimus m. of head,** musculus longissimus capitis. **longissimus m. of neck,** musculus longissimus cervicis. **longissimus m. of thorax,** musculus longissimus thoracis. **longitudinal m. of tongue, inferior,** musculus longitudinalis inferior linguae. **longitudinal m. of tongue, superior,** musculus longitudinalis superior linguae. **lumbrical m's of foot,** musculi lumbricales pedis. **lumbrical m's of hand,** musculi lumbricales manus. **Luschka's m's,** the uterosacral ligaments, which contain muscular tissue. **masseter m.,** musculus masseter. **Merkel's m.,** musculus ceratocricoideus. **mesothenar m.,** musculus adductor pollicis. **Müller's m.,** 1. fibrae circulares musculi ciliaris. 2. musculus orbitalis. **multifidus m's,** musculi multifidi. **mylohyoid m.,** musculus mylohyoideus. **mylopharyngeal m.,** pars mylopharyngea musculi constrictoris pharyngis superioris. **nasal m.,** musculus nasalis. **m's of neck,** musculi colli. **nonstriated m.,** a type of muscle without transverse striations upon its constituent fibers; such muscles are almost always involuntary. Called also *smooth m.*

oblique m. of abdomen, external, musculus obliquus externus abdominis. **oblique m. of abdomen, internal,** musculus obliquus internus abdominis. **oblique m. of auricle,** musculus obliquus auriculae. **oblique m. of eyeball, inferior,** musculus obliquus inferior bulbi. **oblique m. of eyeball, superior,** musculus obliquus superior bulbi. **obturator m., external,** musculus obturatorius externus. **obturator m., internal,** musculus obturatorius internus. **occipital m.,** venter occipitalis musculi occipitofrontalis. **occipitofrontal m.,** musculus occipitofrontalis. **Ochsner's m.,** an inconstant muscular thickening of the duodenal muscle just distal to the opening of the common bile duct. **ocular m's,** musculi bulbi. **Oddi's m.,** musculus sphincter ductus choledochi, or the combination of this with musculus sphincter ampullae hepatopancreaticae when the ampulla is present. **omohyoid m.,** musculus omohyoideus. **opposing m. of little finger,** musculus opponens digiti minimi. **opposing m. of thumb,** musculus opponens pollicis. **orbicular m.,** a muscle that encircles a body opening, such as the eye or mouth; called also *musculus orbicularis* [NA]. **orbicular m. of eye,** musculus orbicularis oculi. **orbicular m. of mouth,** musculus orbicularis oris. **orbital m.,** musculus orbitalis. **organic m.,** visceral m. **m's of palate and fauces,** musculi palati et faucium. **palatoglossus m.,** musculus palatoglossus. **palatopharyngeal m.,** musculus palatopharyngeus. **palmar m., long,** musculus palmaris longus. **palmar m., short,** musculus palmaris brevis. **papillary m's,** musculi papillares. **papillary m. of left ventricle, anterior,** musculus papillaris anterior ventriculi sinistri. **papillary m. of left ventricle, posterior,** musculus papillaris posterior ventriculi sinistri. **papillary m. of right ventricle, anterior,** musculus papillaris anterior ventriculi dextri. **papillary m. of right ventricle, posterior,** musculus papillaris posterior ventriculi dextri. **papillary m's of right ventricle, septal,** musculi papillares septales ventriculi dextri. **pectinate m's,** musculi pectinati. **pectineal m.,** musculus pectineus. **pectoral m., greater,** musculus pectoralis major. **pectoral m., smaller,** musculus pectoralis minor. **penniform m.,** musculus unipennatus. **m's of perineum,** musculi perinei. **peroneal m., long,** musculus peroneus longus. **peroneal m., short,** musculus peroneus brevis. **peroneal m., third,** musculus peroneus tertius. **pharyngopalatine m.,** musculus palatopharyngeus. **Phillips' m.,** a muscular slip from the radial collateral ligament of the wrist and the styloid process of the radius to the phalanges. **piriform m.,** musculus piriformis. **plantar m.,** musculus plantaris. **platysma m.,** see *platysma.* **pleuroesophageal m.,** musculus pleuroesophageus. **popliteal m.,** musculus popliteus. **postaxial m.,** a muscle on the dorsal side of a limb. **preaxial m.,** a muscle on the ventral side of a limb. **procerus m.,** musculus procerus. **pronator m., quadrate,** musculus pronator quadratus. **pronator m., round,** musculus pronator teres. **psoas m., greater,** musculus psoas major. **psoas m., smaller,** musculus psoas minor. **pterygoid m., external,** musculus pterygoideus lateralis. **pterygoid m., internal,** musculus pterygoideus medialis. **pterygoid m., lateral,** musculus pterygoideus lateralis. **pterygoid m., medial,** musculus pterygoideus medialis. **pterygopharyngeal m.,** pars pterygopharyngea musculi constrictoris pharyngis superioris. **pubicoperitoneal m.,** ligamentum interfoveolare. **pubococcygeal m.,** musculus pubococcygeus. **puboprostatic m.,** musculus puboprostaticus. **puborectal m.,** musculus puborectalis. **pubovaginal m.,** musculus pubovaginalis. **pubovesical m.,** musculus pubovesicalis. **pyramidal m.,** musculus pyramidalis. **pyramidal m. of auricle,** musculus pyramidalis auriculae. **quadrate m. of lower lip,** musculus depressor labii inferioris. **quadrate m. of sole,** musculus quadratus plantae. **quadrate m. of thigh,** musculus quadratus femoris. **quadrate m. of upper lip,** musculus levator labii superioris. **quadriceps m. of thigh,** musculus quadriceps femoris. **rectococcygeus m.,** musculus rectococcygeus. **rectourethral m.,** musculus rectourethralis. **rectouterine m.,** musculus rectouterinus. **rectovesical m.,** musculus rectovesicalis. **red m.,** the darker-colored muscle tissue of some mammals, composed of small dark fibers rich in mitochondria, myoglobin, and sarcoplasm but with only faint cross-striping; red muscle is designed for slow but repetitive contraction for long periods of time. Called also *slow,* or *tonic, m.* Cf. *white m.* **Reisseisen's m's,** the smooth muscle fibers of the smallest bronchi. **rhomboid m., greater,** musculus rhomboideus major. **rhomboid m., lesser,** musculus rhomboideus minor. **ribbon m's,** musculi infrahyoidei. **rider's m's,** the adductor muscles of the thigh. **Riolan's m's,** 1. ciliary bundle of pars palpebralis musculi orbicularis oculi. 2. musculus cremaster. **risorius m.,** musculus risorius. **rotator m's,** musculi rotatores. **rotator m's, long,** musculi rotatores longi. **rotator m's, short,** musculi rotatores breves. **rotator m's of neck,** musculi rotatores cervicis. **rotator m's of thorax,** musculi rotatores thoracis. **Rouget's m.,** the circular portion of the ciliary muscle. **Ruysch's m.,** the muscular tissue of the fundus uteri. **sacrococcygeal m., anterior,** musculus sacrococcygeus ventralis. **sacrococcyg-**

Plate XXIX

muscle

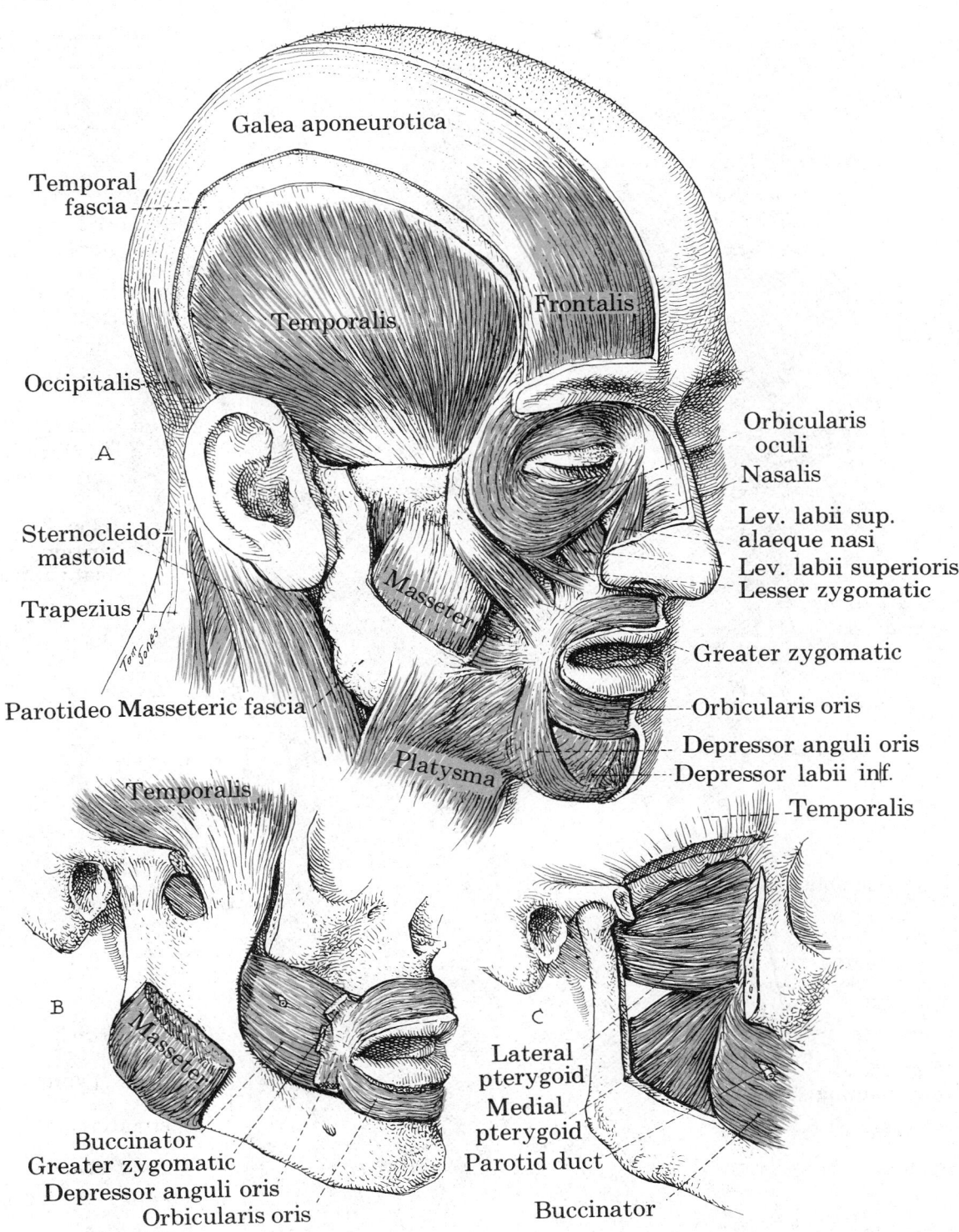

Galea aponeurotica

Temporal
fascia

Temporalis

Frontalis

Occipitalis

A

Orbicularis
oculi

Nasalis

Lev. labii sup.
alaeque nasi

Lev. labii superioris
Lesser zygomatic

Sternocleido-
mastoid

Masseter

Greater zygomatic

Trapezius

Orbicularis oris

Parotideo Masseteric fascia

Depressor anguli oris
Depressor labii inf.

Platysma

Temporalis

Temporalis

B

Masseter

Lateral
pterygoid

C

Medial
pterygoid

Parotid duct

Buccinator
Greater zygomatic
Depressor anguli oris
Orbicularis oris

Buccinator

MUSCLES OF THE HEAD AND FACE

A, muscles of face and scalp, showing insertion of platysma; B, buccinator and orbicularis oris;
C, pterygoid muscles. (Jones and Shepard.)

Plate XXX   muscle

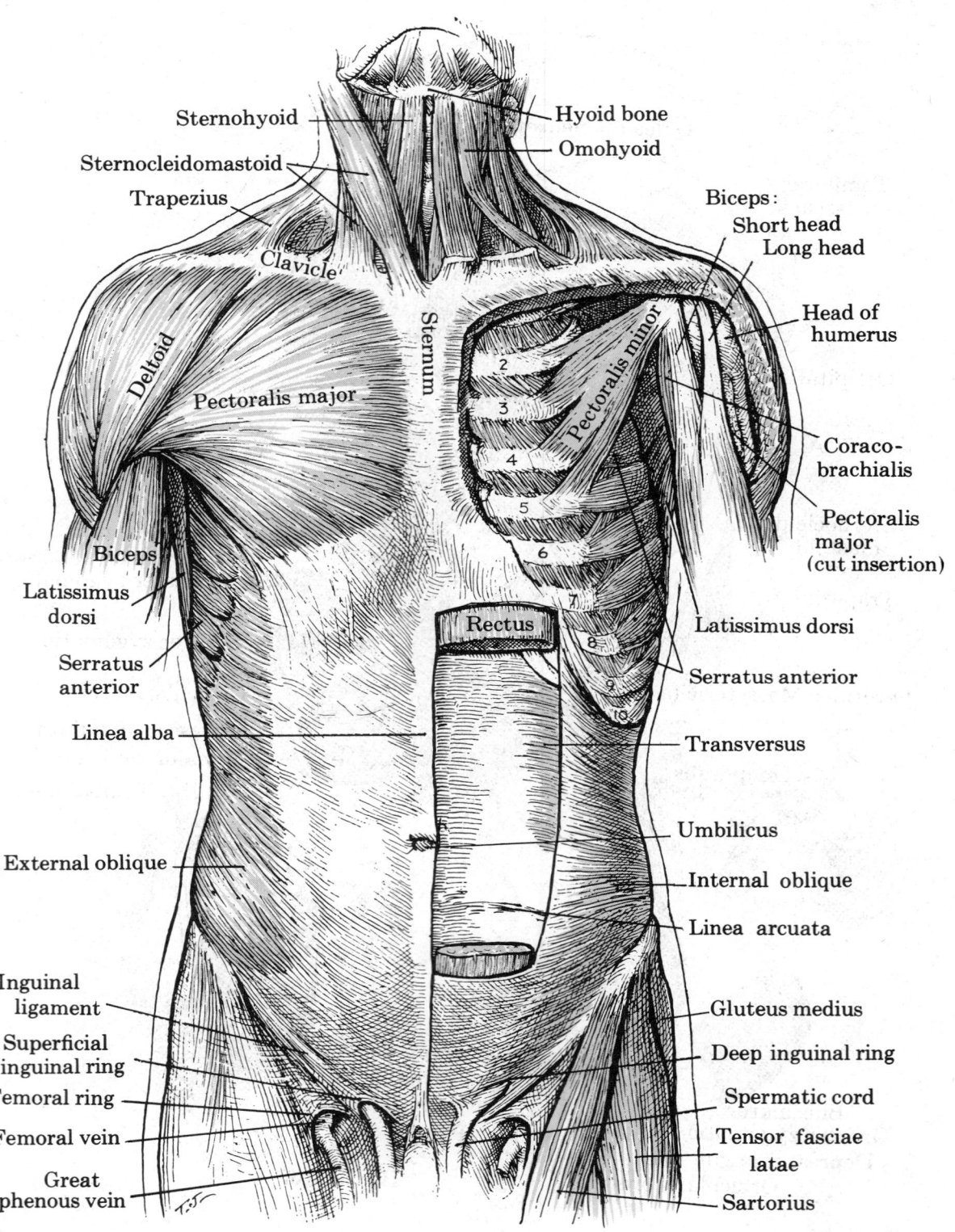

MUSCLES OF TRUNK, ANTERIOR VIEW

The left sternocleidomastoid, pectoralis major, external oblique, and a portion of the deltoid have been removed to show underlying muscles.
A portion of the rectus abdominis has been cut away to expose the posterior part of its sheath. (Jones and Shepard.)

Plate XXXI   muscle

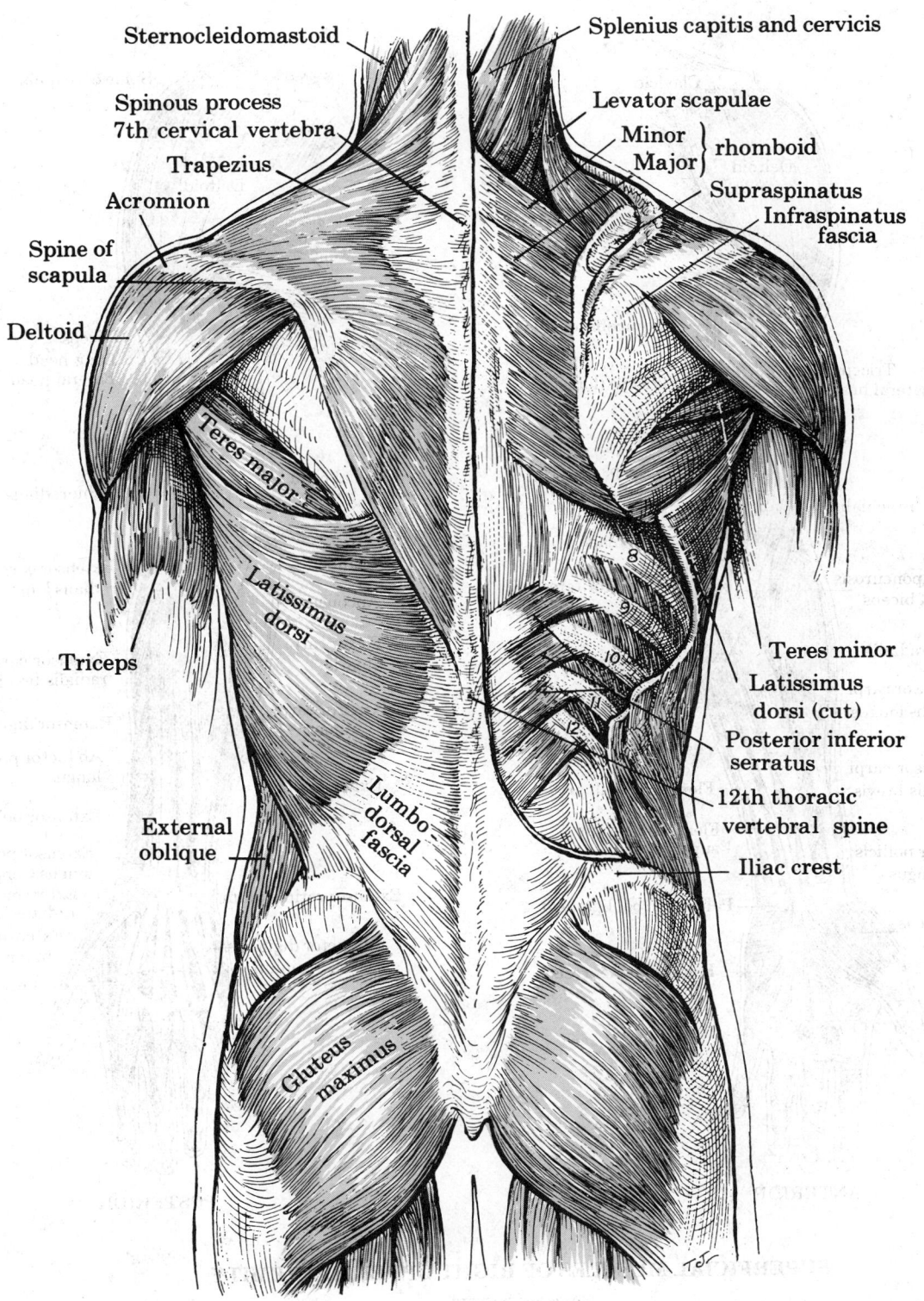

Sternocleidomastoid

Spinous process
7th cervical vertebra

Trapezius

Acromion

Spine of
scapula

Deltoid

Teres major

Latissimus
dorsi

Triceps

External
oblique

Lumbo-
dorsal
fascia

Gluteus
maximus

Splenius capitis and cervicis

Levator scapulae

Minor } rhomboid
Major }

Supraspinatus

Infraspinatus
fascia

8

9

10

12

Teres minor

Latissimus
dorsi (cut)

Posterior inferior
serratus

12th thoracic
vertebral spine

Iliac crest

MUSCLES OF TRUNK, POSTERIOR VIEW

The latissimus dorsi and trapezius on the right side have been cut away to expose the underlying muscles.
(Jones and Shepard.)

Plate XXXII

muscle

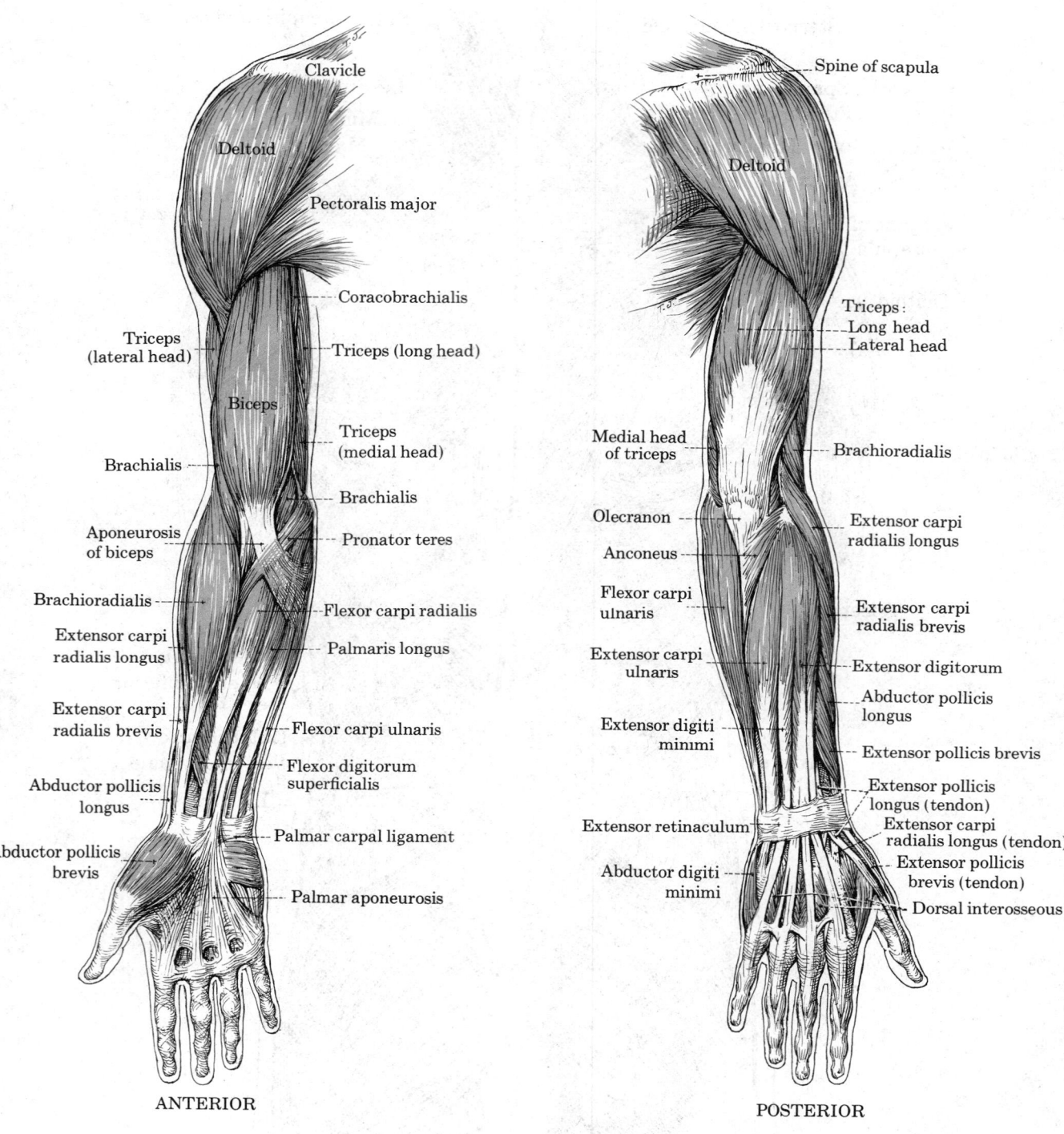

Clavicle

Deltoid

Pectoralis major

Coracobrachialis

Triceps (lateral head)

Triceps (long head)

Biceps

Triceps (medial head)

Brachialis

Brachialis

Aponeurosis of biceps

Pronator teres

Brachioradialis

Flexor carpi radialis

Extensor carpi radialis longus

Palmaris longus

Extensor carpi radialis brevis

Flexor carpi ulnaris

Abductor pollicis longus

Flexor digitorum superficialis

Abductor pollicis brevis

Palmar carpal ligament

Palmar aponeurosis

ANTERIOR

Spine of scapula

Deltoid

Triceps :
Long head
Lateral head

Medial head of triceps

Brachioradialis

Olecranon

Extensor carpi radialis longus

Anconeus

Flexor carpi ulnaris

Extensor carpi radialis brevis

Extensor carpi ulnaris

Extensor digitorum

Abductor pollicis longus

Extensor digiti minimi

Extensor pollicis brevis

Extensor retinaculum

Extensor pollicis longus (tendon)

Extensor carpi radialis longus (tendon)

Abductor digiti minimi

Extensor pollicis brevis (tendon)

Dorsal interosseous

POSTERIOR

SUPERFICIAL MUSCLES OF RIGHT UPPER EXTREMITY

(Jones and Shepard)

Plate XXXIII

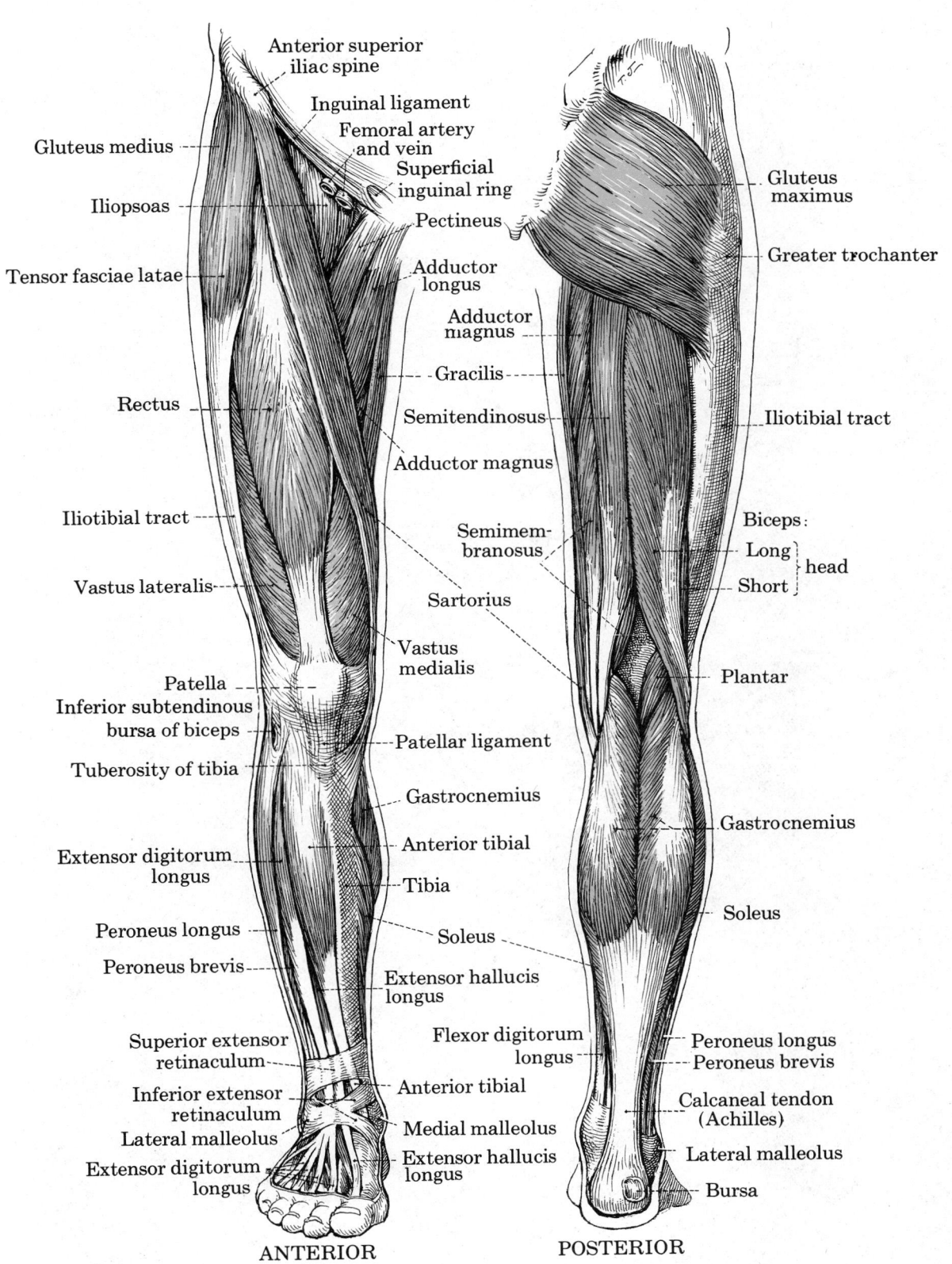

Anterior superior
iliac spine

Inguinal ligament

Femoral artery
and vein

Superficial
inguinal ring

Gluteus medius

Iliopsoas

Pectineus

Tensor fasciae latae

Adductor
longus

Adductor
magnus

Gracilis

Rectus

Semitendinosus

Adductor magnus

Iliotibial tract

Semimem-
branosus

Vastus lateralis

Sartorius

Vastus
medialis

Patella

Inferior subtendinous
bursa of biceps

Patellar ligament

Tuberosity of tibia

Gastrocnemius

Anterior tibial

Extensor digitorum
longus

Tibia

Peroneus longus

Soleus

Peroneus brevis

Extensor hallucis
longus

Superior extensor
retinaculum

Flexor digitorum
longus

Inferior extensor
retinaculum

Anterior tibial

Lateral malleolus

Medial malleolus

Extensor digitorum
longus

Extensor hallucis
longus

ANTERIOR

Gluteus
maximus

Greater trochanter

Iliotibial tract

Biceps

Long ⎱
      ⎰ head
Short ⎱

Plantar

Gastrocnemius

Soleus

Peroneus longus

Peroneus brevis

Calcaneal tendon
(Achilles)

Lateral malleolus

Bursa

POSTERIOR

SUPERFICIAL MUSCLES OF RIGHT LOWER EXTREMITY

(Jones and Shepard)

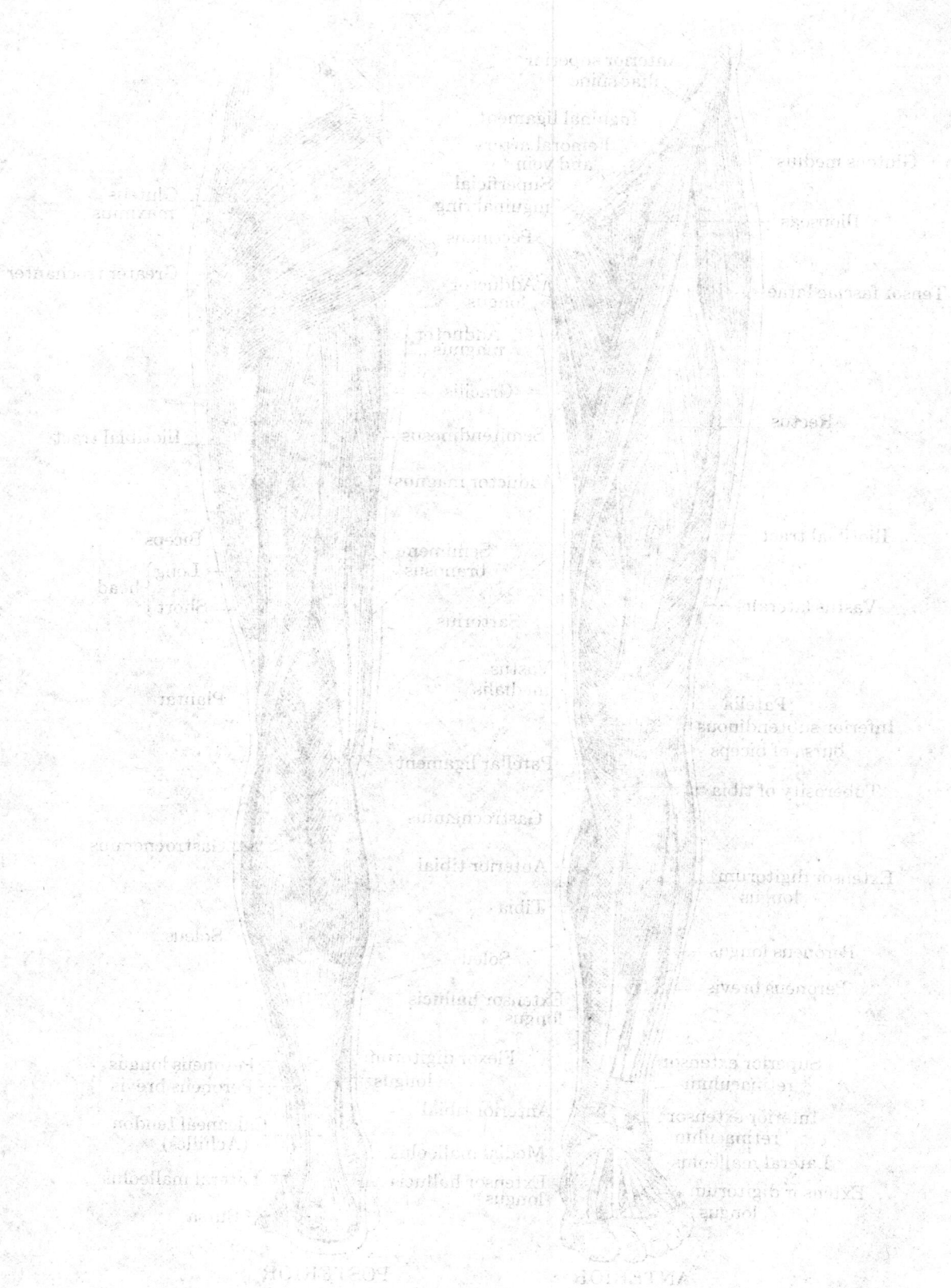

eal m., **dorsal,** musculus sacrococcygeus dorsalis. **sacrococcygeal m., posterior,** musculus sacrococcygeus dorsalis. **sacrococcygeal m., ventral,** musculus sacrococcygeus ventralis. **sacrospinal m.,** musculus erector spinae. **salpingopharyngeal m.,** musculus salpingopharyngeus. **Santorini's m.,** musculus risorius. **Santorini's m's, circular,** the nonstriated fibers that encircle the urethra beneath the sphincter urethrae. **sartorius m.,** musculus sartorius. **scalene m., anterior,** musculus scalenus anterior. **scalene m., middle,** musculus scalenus medius. **scalene m., posterior,** musculus scalenus posterior. **scalene m., smallest,** musculus scalenus minimus. **semimembranous m.,** musculus semimembranosus. **semispinal m.,** musculus semispinalis. **semispinal m. of head,** musculus semispinalis capitis. **semispinal m. of neck,** musculus semispinalis cervicis. **semispinal m. of thorax,** musculus semispinalis thoracis. **semitendinous m.,** musculus semitendinosus. **serratus m., anterior,** musculus serratus anterior. **serratus m., posterior, inferior,** musculus serratus posterior inferior. **serratus m., posterior, superior,** musculus serratus posterior superior. **skeletal m's,** striated muscles that are attached to bones and typically cross at least one joint; called also *musculi skeleti.* **slow m.,** red m. **smooth m.,** nonstriated, involuntary muscle. **soleus m.,** musculus soleus. **somatic m's,** musculi skeleti. **sphincter m.,** musculus sphincter. **sphincter m. of anus, external,** musculus sphincter ani externus. **sphincter m. of anus, internal,** musculus sphincter ani internus. **sphincter m. of bile duct,** musculus sphincter ductus choledochi. **sphincter m. of hepatopancreatic ampulla,** musculus sphincter ampullae hepatopancreaticae. **sphincter m. of membranous urethra,** musculus sphincter urethrae. **sphincter m. of pupil,** musculus sphincter pupillae. **sphincter m. of pylorus,** musculus sphincter pylori. **sphincter m. of urethra,** musculus sphincter urethrae. **sphincter m. of urinary bladder,** musculus sphincter vesicae urinariae. **spinal m.,** see *musculus spinalis.* **splenius m. of head,** musculus splenius capitis. **splenius m. of neck,** musculus splenius cervicis. **stapedius m.,** musculus stapedius. **sternal m.,** musculus sternalis. **sternocleidomastoid m.,** musculus sternocleidomastoideus. **sternohyoid m.,** musculus sternohyoideus. **sternomastoid m.,** musculus sternocleidomastoideus. **sternothyroid m.,** musculus sternothyroideus. **strap m's,** muscles of the neck, particularly those of the thyroid cartilage and hyoid bone. **striated m., striped m.,** any muscle whose fibers are divided by transverse bands into striations; such muscles are voluntary. See *muscle.* **styloglossus m.,** musculus styloglossus. **stylohyoid m.,** musculus stylohyoideus. **stylopharyngeus m.,** musculus stylopharyngeus. **subclavius m.,** musculus subclavius. **subcostal m's,** musculi subcostales. **subscapular m.,** musculus subscapularis. **subvertebral m's,** hypaxial m's. **supinator m.,** musculus supinator. **suprahyoid m's,** musculi suprahyoidei. **supraspinous m.,** musculus supraspinatus. **suspensory m. of duodenum,** musculus suspensorius duodeni. **synergic m's, synergistic m's,** muscles that assist one another in action. **tarsal m., inferior,** musculus tarsalis inferior. **tarsal m., superior,** musculus tarsalis superior. **temporal m.,** musculus temporalis. **temporoparietal m.,** musculus temporoparietalis. **tensor m. of fascia lata,** musculus tensor fasciae latae. **tensor m. of tympanic membrane, tensor m. of tympanum,** musculus tensor tympani. **tensor m. of velum palatini,** musculus tensor veli palatini. **teres major m.,** musculus teres major. **teres minor m.,** musculus teres minor. **thenar m's,** the abductor and flexor muscles of the thumb. **thyroarytenoid m.,** musculus thyroarytenoideus. **thyroepiglottic m.,** musculus thyroepiglotticus. **thyrohyoid m.,** musculus thyrohyoideus. **thyropharyngeal m.,** pars thyropharyngea musculi constrictoris pharyngis inferioris. **tibial m., anterior,** musculus tibialis anterior. **tibial m., posterior,** musculus tibialis posterior. **tonic m.,** red m. **tracheal m.,** musculus trachealis. **trachelomastoid m.,** musculus longissimus capitis. **m. of tragus,** musculus tragicus. **transverse m. of abdomen,** musculus transversus abdominis. **transverse m. of auricle,** musculus transversus auriculae. **transverse m. of chin,** musculus transversus menti. **transverse m. of nape,** musculus transversus nuchae. **transverse m. of perineum, deep,** musculus transversus perinei profundus. **transverse m. of perineum, superficial,** musculus transversus perinei superficialis. **transverse m. of thorax,** musculus transversus thoracis.

transverse m. of tongue, musculus transversus linguae. **transversospinal m.,** musculus transversospinalis. **trapezius m.,** musculus trapezius. **m. of Treitz,** musculus suspensorius duodeni. **triangular m.,** musculus depressor anguli oris. **triceps m. of arm,** musculus triceps brachii. **triceps m. of calf,** musculus triceps surae. **twitch m.,** white m. **unipennate m.,** musculus unipennatus. **unstriated m.,** nonstriated m. **m. of uvula,** musculus uvulae. **vertical m. of tongue,** musculus verticalis linguae. **vestigial m.,** a muscle that was once well developed but through evolution has become rudimentary. **visceral m.,** muscle fibers associated chiefly with the hollow viscera and largely of splanchnic mesodermal origin; except for the striated fibers in the wall of the heart, they are smooth-muscle fibers bound together by reticular fibers. **vocal m.,** musculus vocalis. **voluntary m.,** any muscle that normally is under the control of the will; such muscles are nearly always composed of striated fibers. **white m.,** the paler-colored muscle tissue of some mammals, composed of fibers with little sarcoplasm and prominent cross-striping and which are paler and of larger diameter than the fibers of red muscle. Called also *fast,* or *twitch, m. red m.* **Wilson's m.,** musculus sphincter urethrae. **yoked m's,** muscles that normally act simultaneously and equally, as in moving the eyes. **zygomatic m., greater,** musculus zygomaticus major. **zygomatic m., lesser,** musculus zygomaticus minor.

musculamine (mus″ku-lam′in) a base isolated from hydrolyzed calf's muscle; it is the same as spermine.

muscular (mus′ku-lar) [L. *muscularis*] 1. pertaining to or composing muscle. 2. having a well-developed musculature.

muscularis (mus″ku-la′ris) [L.] relating to muscles, specifically a muscular coat; see *tunica muscularis.*

muscularity (mus″ku-lar′ĭ-te) the condition or quality of being muscular.

muscularize (mus′ku-lar-īz) to change into muscle tissue.

musculation (mus″ku-la′shun) 1. the muscular system or apparatus. 2. the muscular activity or work.

musculature (mus′ku-lah-chur) the muscular apparatus of the body, or of any part of it.

musculi (mus′ku-li) [L.] plural of *musculus.*

musculoaponeurotic (mus″ku-lo-ap″o-nu-rot′ik) pertaining to a muscle and its aponeurosis.

musculocutaneous (mus″ku-lo-ku-ta′ne-us) pertaining to or supplying both muscles and skin.

musculodermic (mus″ku-lo-der′mik) musculocutaneous.

musculoelastic (mus″ku-lo-e-las′tik) composed of muscular and elastic tissue.

musculointestinal (mus″ku-lo-in-tes′tĭ-nal) pertaining to the muscles and the intestines.

musculomembranous (mus″ku-lo-mem′brah-nus) [L. *musculus* muscle + *membrana* membrane] both muscular and membranous.

Musculomyces (mus″ku-lo-mi′sēz) a name proposed for the pleuropneumonia-like bacteria found in mice.

musculophrenic (mus″ku-lo-fren′ik) [*muscular* + *phrenic*] pertaining to or supplying both the diaphragm and the adjoining muscles.

musculoprecipitin (mus″ku-lo-pre-sip′ĭ-tin) any one of a series of precipitins used in distinguishing various kinds of meat.

musculoskeletal (mus″ku-lo-skel′ĕ-tal) pertaining to or comprising the skeleton and the muscles, as musculoskeletal system.

musculospiral (mus″ku-lo-spi′ral) [L. *musculus* muscle + *spira* coil] pertaining to muscles and having a spiral direction, as the nervus radialis.

musculospiralis (mus″ku-lo-spi-ra′lis) nervus radialis.

musculotendinous (mus″ku-lo-ten′dĭ-nus) pertaining to or composed of muscle and tendon.

musculotonic (mus″ku-lo-ton′ik) pertaining to muscular contractility.

musculotropic (mus″ku-lo-trop′ik) having a special affinity for or exerting its principal effect upon muscular tissue.

musculus (mus′ku-lus), pl. *mus′culi* [L., dim. of *mus* mouse, because of a fancied resemblance to a mouse of a muscle moving under the skin] [NA] an organ which by its contraction and relaxation produces movements of certain organs or of the entire animal organism. See *muscle.* For names and description of specific muscles see *Table of Musculi.*

TABLE OF MUSCULI

Descriptions of muscles are given on NA terms, and include anglicized names of specific muscles.

mus′culi abdo′minis [NA], the muscles of the abdomen.
m. abduc′tor dig′iti min′imi ma′nus [NA], abductor muscle of little finger: *origin,* pisiform bone, flexor carpi ulnaris tendon;

insertion, medial surface of base of proximal phalanx of little finger; *innervation,* ulnar; *action,* abducts little finger.
m. abduc′tor dig′iti min′imi pe′dis [NA], abductor muscle

of little toe: *origin*, medial and lateral tubercles of calcaneus, plantar fascia; *insertion*, lateral surface of base of proximal phalanx of little toe; *innervation*, superficial branch of lateral plantar; *action*, abducts little toe.

m. abduc′tor dig′iti quin′ti ma′nus, m. abductor digiti minimi manus.

m. abduc′tor dig′iti quin′ti pe′dis, m. abductor digiti minimi pedis.

m. abduc′tor hal′lucis [NA], abductor muscle of great toe: *origin*, medial tubercle of calcaneus, plantar fascia; *insertion*, medial surface of base of proximal phalanx of great toe; *innervation*, medial plantar; *action*, abducts, flexes great toe.

m. abduc′tor pol′licis bre′vis [NA], short abductor muscle of thumb: *origin*, scaphoid, ridge of trapezium, transverse carpal ligament; *insertion*, lateral surface of base of proximal phalanx of thumb; *innervation*, median; *action*, abducts thumb.

m. abduc′tor pol′licis lon′gus [NA], long abductor muscle of thumb: *origin*, posterior surfaces of radius and ulna; *insertion*, radial side of base of first metacarpal bone; *innervation*, posterior interosseous; *action*, abducts, extends thumb.

m. adduc′tor bre′vis [NA], short adductor muscle: *origin*, outer surface of inferior ramus of pubis; *insertion*, upper part of linea aspera of femur; *innervation*, obturator; *action*, adducts, rotates, flexes thigh.

m. adduc′tor hal′lucis [NA], adductor muscle of great toe (2 heads): *origin*, CAPUT OBLIQUUM—bases of second, third, and fourth metatarsals, and sheath of peroneus longus, CAPUT TRANSVERSUM—capsules of metatarsophalangeal joints of three lateral toes; *insertion*, lateral side of base of proximal phalanx of great toe; *innervation*, lateral plantar; *action*, adducts great toe.

m. adduc′tor lon′gus [NA], long adductor muscle: *origin*, crest and symphysis of pubis; *insertion*, linea aspera of femur; *innervation*, obturator; *action*, adducts, rotates, flexes thigh.

m. adduc′tor mag′nus [NA], great adductor muscle (2 parts): *origin*, DEEP PART—inferior ramus of pubis, ramus of ischium, SUPERFICIAL PART—ischial tuberosity; *insertion*, DEEP PART—linea aspera of femur, SUPERFICIAL PART—adductor tubercle of femur; *innervation*, DEEP PART—obturator, SUPERFICIAL PART—sciatic; *action*, DEEP PART—adducts thigh, SUPERFICIAL PART—extends thigh.

m. adduc′tor min′imus, smallest adductor muscle: a name given the anterior portion of the adductor magnus muscle; *insertion*, ischium, body and ramus of pubis; *innervation*, obturator and sciatic; *action*, adducts thigh.

m. adduc′tor pol′licis [NA], adductor muscle of thumb (2 heads): *origin*, CAPUT OBLIQUUM—sheath of flexor carpi radialis, anterior carpal ligament, capitate bone, and bases of second and third metacarpals, CAPUT TRANSVERSUM—lower two-thirds of anterior surface of third metacarpal; *insertion*, medial surface of base of proximal phalanx of thumb; *innervation*, ulnar; *action*, adducts, opposes thumb.

m. anco′neus [NA], anconeus muscle: *origin*, back of lateral epicondyle of humerus; *insertion*, olecranon and posterior surface of ulna; *innervation*, radial; *action*, extends forearm.

m. antitrag′icus [NA], antitragus muscle: *origin*, outer part of antitragus; *insertion*, caudate process of helix and anthelix; *innervation*, temporal and posterior auricular.

mus′culi arrecto′res pilo′rum [NA], arrector muscles of hair: *origin*, papillary layer of skin; *insertion*, hair follicles; *innervation*, sympathetic; *action*, elevate hairs of skin.

m. articula′ris [NA], articular muscle: a muscle that is attached at one end to the synovial capsule of a joint.

m. articula′ris cu′biti [NA], articular muscle of elbow: a few fibers of the deep surface of the triceps brachii that insert into the posterior ligament and synovial membrane of the elbow joint.

m. articula′ris ge′nu, m. articularis genus.

m. articula′ris ge′nus [NA], articular muscle of knee: *origin*, distal fourth of anterior surface of shaft of femur; *insertion*, synovial membrane of knee joint; *innervation*, femoral; *action*, lifts capsule of knee joint.

m. aryepiglot′ticus [NA], aryepiglottic muscle: a name given to an inconstant fascicle of the oblique arytenoid muscle, originating from the apex of the arytenoid cartilage and inserting on the lateral margin of the epiglottis.

m. arytaenoi′deus obli′quus, m. arytenoideus obliquus.

m. arytaenoi′deus transver′sus, m. arytenoideus transversus.

m. arytenoi′deus obli′quus [NA], oblique arytenoid muscle: *origin*, dorsal aspect of muscular process of arytenoid cartilage; *insertion*, apex of opposite arytenoid cartilage; *innervation*, recurrent laryngeal; *action*, closes inlet of larynx.

m. arytenoi′deus transver′sus [NA], transverse arytenoid muscle: *origin*, dorsal aspect of muscular process of arytenoid cartilage; *insertion*, continuous with thyroarytenoid, apex of opposite cartilage; *innervation*, recurrent laryngeal; *action*, approximates arytenoid cartilages.

m. auricula′ris ante′rior [NA], anterior auricular muscle: *origin*, superficial temporal fascia; *insertion*, cartilage of ear; *innervation*, facial; *action*, draws the auricle forward.

m. auricula′ris poste′rior [NA], posterior auricular muscle: *origin*, mastoid process; *insertion*, cartilage of ear; *innervation*, facial; *action*, draws auricle backward.

m. auricula′ris supe′rior [NA], superior auricular muscle: *origin*, galea aponeurotica; *insertion*, cartilage of ear; *innervation*, facial; *action*, raises auricle.

m. bi′ceps bra′chii [NA], biceps muscle of arm (2 heads): *origin*, CAPUT LONGUM—upper border of glenoid cavity, CAPUT BREVE—apex of coracoid process; *insertion*, radial tuberosity and fascia of forearm; *innervation*, musculocutaneous; *action*, flexes forearm, supinates hand.

m. bi′ceps fem′oris [NA], biceps muscle of thigh (2 heads): *origin*, CAPUT LONGUM—ischial tuberosity, CAPUT BREVE—linea aspera of femur; *insertion*, head of fibula, lateral condyle of tibia; *innervation*, CAPUT LONGUM—tibial, CAPUT BREVE—peroneal, popliteal; *action*, flexes leg, extends thigh.

m. bipenna′tus [NA], bipennate muscle: a muscle in which the fibers approach the tendon of insertion from a wide area and are inserted through a large segment of its circumference.

m. brachia′lis [NA], brachial muscle: *origin*, anterior surface of humerus; *insertion*, coronoid process of ulna; *innervation*, radial, musculocutaneous; *action*, flexes forearm.

m. brachioradia′lis [NA], brachioradial muscle: *origin*, lateral supracondylar ridge of humerus; *insertion*, lower end of radius; *innervation*, radial; *action*, flexes forearm.

m. bronchoesopha′geus [NA], bronchoesophageal muscle: a name given muscular fasciculi arising from the wall of the left bronchus, reinforcing muscles of the esophagus.

m. bronchooesopha′geus, m. bronchoesophageus.

m. buccina′tor [NA], buccinator muscle: *origin*, buccinator ridge of mandible, alveolar process of maxilla, pterygomandibular ligament; *insertion*, orbicularis oris at angle of mouth; *innervation*, buccal branch of facial; *action*, compresses cheek and retracts angle of the mouth.

m. buccopharyn′geus, pars buccopharyngea musculi constrictoris pharyngis superioris.

mus′culi bul′bi [NA], extraocular muscles: the six voluntary muscles that move the eyeball, including the superior, inferior, middle, and lateral recti, and the superior and inferior oblique muscles.

m. bulbocaverno′sus, m. bulbospongiosus.

m. bulbospongio′sus [NA], bulbocavernous muscle: *origin*, central point of perineum, median raphe of bulb; *insertion*, fascia of penis (clitoris); *innervation*, pudendal; *action*, constricts bulbous urethra (urethra).

m. cani′nus, m. levator anguli oris.

mus′culi cap′itis [NA], the muscles of the head.

m. ceratocricoi′deus [NA], ceratocricoid muscle: a name given a muscular fasciculus arising from the cricoid cartilage and inserted on the inferior cornu of the thyroid cartilage.

m. ceratopharyn′geus, pars ceratopharyngea musculi constrictoris pharyngis medii.

m. chondroglos′sus [NA], chondroglossus muscle: *origin*, medial side and base of lesser cornu of hyoid bone; *insertion*, substance of tongue; *innervation*, hypoglossal; *action*, depresses, retracts tongue.

m. chondropharyn′geus, pars chondropharyngea musculi constrictoris pharyngis medii.

m. cilia′ris [NA], ciliary muscle: *origin*, LONGITUDINAL DIVISION (Brücke's muscles)—junction of cornea and sclera, CIRCULAR DIVISION (Müller's muscle)—sphincter of ciliary body; *insertion*, outer layers of choroid and ciliary processes; *innervation*, short ciliary; *action*, affects shape of lens in visual accommodation.

mus′culi coccyg′ei [NA], coccygeal muscles: the muscles acting upon the coccyx, including the coccygeal and the dorsal and ventral sacrococcygeal muscles.

m. coccyg′eus [NA], coccygeal muscle: *origin*, ischial spine; *insertion*, lateral border of lower part of sacrum, upper coccyx; *innervation*, third and fourth sacral; *action*, supports and raises coccyx.

mus′culi col′li [NA], the muscles of the neck, including the sternocleidomastoid and the longus colli, and the suprahyoid, infrahyoid, and scalene muscles.

m. compres′sor na′ris, pars transversa musculi nasalis.

m. constric′tor pharyn′gis infe′rior [NA], inferior constrictor muscle of pharynx: *origin*, under surfaces of cricoid and thyroid cartilages; *insertion*, median raphe of posterior wall of pharynx; *innervation*, glossopharyngeal, pharyngeal plexus, and external and recurrent laryngeal; *action*, constricts pharynx.

m. constric′tor pharyn′gis me′dius [NA], middle constrictor muscle of pharynx: *origin*, cornua of hyoid and stylohyoid ligament; *insertion*, median raphe of posterior wall of pharynx; *innervation*, pharyngeal plexus of vagus and glossopharyngeal; *action*, constricts pharynx.

m. constric′tor pharyn′gis supe′rior [NA], superior constrictor muscle of pharynx: *origin*, medial pterygoid plate, pterygomandibular raphe, mylohyoid ridge of mandible, and mucous membrane of floor of mouth; *insertion*, median raphe of posterior wall of pharynx; *innervation*, pharyngeal plexus of vagus; *action*, constricts pharynx.

m. coracobrachia′lis [NA], coracobrachial muscle: *origin*, coracoid process of scapula; *insertion*, medial surface of shaft of humerus; *innervation*, musculocutaneous; *action*, flexes, adducts arm.

m. corruga′tor supercil′ii [NA], *origin*, medial end of superciliary arch; *insertion*, skin of eyebrow; *innervation*, facial; *action*, draws eyebrow downward and medially.

m. cremas'ter [NA], cremaster muscle: *origin*, inferior margin of internal oblique muscle of abdomen; *insertion*, pubic tubercle; *innervation*, genital branch of genitofemoral; *action*, elevates testis.

m. cricoarytaenoi'deus latera'lis, m. cricoarytenoideus lateralis.

m. cricoarytaenoi'deus poste'rior, m. cricoarytenoideus posterior.

m. cricoarytenoi'deus latera'lis [NA], lateral cricoarytenoid muscle: *origin*, lateral surface of cricoid cartilage; *insertion*, muscular process of arytenoid cartilage; *innervation*, recurrent laryngeal; *action*, approximates vocal folds.

m. cricoarytenoi'deus poste'rior [NA], posterior cricoarytenoid muscle: *origin*, back of cricoid cartilage; *insertion*, muscular process of arytenoid cartilage; *innervation*, recurrent laryngeal; *action*, separates vocal folds.

m. cricopharyn'geus, pars cricopharyngea musculi constrictoris pharyngis inferioris.

m. cricothyreoi'deus, m. cricothyroideus.

m. cricothyroi'deus [NA], cricothyroid muscle: *origin*, front and side of cricoid cartilage; *insertion*, lamina of thyroid cartilage; *innervation*, superior laryngeal; *action*, tenses vocal folds.

m. cuta'neus [NA], cutaneous muscle: striated muscle that inserts into the skin.

m. deltoi'deus [NA], deltoid muscle: *origin*, clavicle, acromion, spine of scapula; *insertion*, deltoid tuberosity of humerus; *innervation*, axillary; *action*, abducts, flexes, extends arm.

m. depres'sor an'guli o'ris [NA], depressor muscle of angle of mouth: *origin*, lower border of mandible; *insertion*, angle of mouth; *innervation*, facial; *action*, pulls down angle of mouth.

m. depres'sor la'bii inferio'ris [NA], depressor muscle of lower lip: *origin*, anterior portion of lower border of mandible; *insertion*, orbicularis oris and skin of lower lip; *innervation*, facial; *action*, depresses lower lip.

m. depres'sor sep'ti na'si [NA], depressor muscle of nasal septum: *origin*, incisor fossa of maxilla; *insertion*, ala and septum of nose; *innervation*, facial; *action*, contracts nostril and depresses ala.

m. depres'sor supercil'ii [NA], superciliary depressor muscle: a name given a few fibers of the orbital part of the orbicularis oculi muscle that are inserted in the eyebrow, which they depress.

m. digas'tricus [NA], digastric muscle: *origin*, VENTER ANTERIOR—digastric fossa on deep surface of lower border of mandible near symphysis, VENTER POSTERIOR—mastoid notch of temporal bone; *insertion*, intermediate tendon on hyoid bone; *innervation*, VENTER ANTERIOR—mylohyoid, VENTER POSTERIOR—digastric branch of facial; *action*, elevates hyoid bone, lowers jaw.

m. dila'tor na'ris, pars alaris musculi nasalis.

m. dila'tor pupil'lae [NA], dilator muscle of pupil: a name given fibers extending radially from the sphincter pupillae to the ciliary margin; *innervation*, sympathetic; *action*, dilates iris.

mus'culi dor'si [NA], dorsal muscles: the muscles of the back.

m. epicra'nius [NA], epicranial muscle: a name given the muscular covering of the scalp, including the occipitofrontalis and temporoparietalis muscles, and the galea aponeurotica.

m. epitrochleoanconae'us, epitrochleoanconeus muscle: an occasional band of fibers originating at the back of the medial condyle of the humerus and inserting on the medial side of the olecranon process, innervated by a branch of the ulnar nerve.

m. erec'tor spi'nae [NA], erector muscle of spine: a name given the fibers of the more superficial of the deep muscles of the back, originating from the sacrum, spines of the lumbar and the eleventh and twelfth thoracic vertebrae, and the iliac crest, which split and insert as the iliocostalis, longissimus, and spinalis muscles (q.v.).

m. exten'sor car'pi radia'lis bre'vis [NA], short radial extensor muscle of wrist: *origin*, lateral epicondyle of humerus, *insertion*, base of third metacarpal bone; *innervation*, radial; *action*, extends and abducts wrist joint.

m. exten'sor car'pi radia'lis lon'gus [NA], long radial extensor muscle of wrist: *origin*, lateral supracondylar ridge of humerus; *insertion*, base of second metacarpal bone; *innervation*, radial; *action*, extends and abducts wrist joint.

m. exten'sor car'pi ulna'ris [NA], ulnar extensor muscle of wrist (2 heads): *origin*, CAPUT HUMERALE—lateral epicondyle of humerus, CAPUT ULNARE—dorsal border of ulna; *insertion*, base of fifth metacarpal bone; *innervation*, deep radial; *action*, extends and adducts wrist joint.

m. exten'sor dig'iti min'imi [NA], extensor muscle of little finger: *origin*, common extensor tendon; *insertion*, tendon of extensor digitorum to little finger; *innervation*, deep radial; *action*, extends little finger.

m. exten'sor dig'iti quin'ti pro'prius, m. extensor digiti minimi.

m. exten'sor digito'rum [NA], extensor muscle of fingers: *origin*, lateral epicondyle of humerus; *insertion*, common extensor tendon of each finger; *innervation*, deep radial; *action*, extends wrist joint and phalanges.

m. exten'sor digito'rum bre'vis [NA], short extensor muscle of toes: *origin*, dorsal surface of calcaneus; *insertion*, extensor tendons of first, second, third, fourth toes; *innervation*, deep peroneal; *action*, extends toes.

m. exten'sor digito'rum commu'nis, m. extensor digitorum.

m. exten'sor digito'rum lon'gus [NA], long extensor muscle of toes: *origin*, anterior surface of fibula, lateral condyle of tibia, interosseous membrane; *insertion*, common extensor tendon of four lateral toes: *innervation*, deep peroneal; *action*, extends toes.

m. exten'sor hal'lucis bre'vis [NA], short extensor muscle of great toe: a name given the portion of the extensor digitorum brevis muscle that goes to the great toe.

m. exten'sor hal'lucis lon'gus [NA], long extensor muscle of great toe: *origin*, front of fibula and interosseous membrane; *insertion*, dorsal surface of base of distal phalanx of great toe; *innervation*, deep peroneal; *action*, dorsiflexes ankle joint, extends great toe.

m. exten'sor in'dicis [NA], extensor muscle of index finger: *origin*, dorsal surface of body of ulna, interosseous membrane; *insertion*, common extensor tendon of index finger; *innervation*, deep radial; *action*, extends index finger.

m. exten'sor in'dicis pro'prius, m. extensor indicis.

m. exten'sor pol'licis bre'vis [NA], short extensor muscle of thumb: *origin*, dorsal surface of radius and interosseous membrane; *insertion*, dorsal surface of proximal phalanx of thumb; *innervation*, deep radial; *action*, extends thumb.

m. exten'sor pol'licis lon'gus [NA], long extensor muscle of thumb: *origin*, dorsal surface of ulna and interosseous membrane; *insertion*, dorsal surface of distal phalanx of thumb; *innervation*, deep radial; *action*, extends, abducts thumb.

mus'culi extremita'tis inferio'ris, musculi membri inferioris.

mus'culi extremita'tis superio'ris, musculi membri superioris.

m. fibula'ris bre'vis, NA alternative for *m. peroneus brevis*.

m. fibula'ris lon'gus, NA alternative for *m. peroneus longus*.

m. fibula'ris ter'tius, NA alternative for *m. peroneus tertius*.

m. fixa'tor ba'seos stape'dis, fixator muscle of base of stapes: fibers attaching to the base of the stapes.

m. flex'or accesso'rius, NA alternative for *m. quadratus plantae*.

m. flex'or car'pi radia'lis [NA], radial flexor muscle of wrist: *origin*, medial epicondyle of humerus; *insertion*, base of second metacarpal; *innervation*, median; *action*, flexes and abducts wrist joint.

m. flex'or car'pi ulna'ris [NA], ulnar flexor muscle of wrist (2 heads): *origin*, CAPUT HUMERALE—medial epicondyle of humerus, CAPUT ULNARE—olecranon, ulna, intermuscular septum; *insertion*, pisiform, hook of hamate, proximal end of fifth metacarpal; *innervation*, ulnar; *action*, flexes and adducts wrist joint.

m. flex'or dig'iti min'imi bre'vis ma'nus [NA], short flexor muscle of little finger: *origin*, hook of hamate bone, transverse carpal ligament; *insertion*, medial side of proximal phalanx of little finger; *innervation*, ulnar; *action*, flexes little finger.

m. flex'or dig'iti min'imi bre'vis pe'dis [NA], short flexor muscle of little toe: *origin*, base of fifth metatarsal, plantar fascia; *insertion*, lateral surface of base of proximal phalanx of little toe; *innervation*, lateral plantar; *action*, flexes little toe.

m. flex'or dig'iti quin'ti bre'vis ma'nus, m. flexor digiti minimi brevis manus.

m. flex'or dig'iti quin'ti bre'vis pe'dis, m. flexor digiti minimi brevis pedis.

m. flex'or digito'rum bre'vis [NA], short flexor muscle of toes: *origin*, medial tuberosity of calcaneus, plantar fascia; *insertion*, middle phalanges of four lateral toes; *innervation*, medial plantar; *action*, flexes toes.

m. flex'or digito'rum lon'gus [NA], long flexor muscle of toes: *origin*, posterior surface of shaft of tibia; *insertion*, distal phalanges of four lateral toes; *innervation*, posterior tibial; *action*, flexes toes and extends foot.

m. flex'or digito'rum profun'dus [NA], deep flexor muscle of fingers: *origin*, shaft of ulna, coronoid process; *insertion*, distal phalanges of fingers; *innervation*, ulnar and anterior interosseous; *action*, flexes distal phalanges.

m. flex'or digito'rum subli'mis, m. flexor digitorum superficialis.

m. flex'or digito'rum superficia'lis [NA], superficial flexor muscle of fingers (2 heads): *origin*, CAPUT HUMEROULNARE—medial epicondyle of humerus, coronoid process of ulna, CAPUT RADIALE—oblique line of radius, anterior border; *insertion*, middle phalanges of fingers; *innervation*, median; *action*, flexes middle phalanges.

m. flex'or hal'lucis bre'vis [NA], short flexor muscle of great toe: *origin*, under surface of cuboid, lateral cuneiform; *insertion*, base of proximal phalanx of great toe; *innervation*, lateral and medial plantar; *action*, flexes great toe.

m. flex'or hal'lucis lon'gus [NA], long flexor muscle of great toe: *origin*, posterior surface of fibula; *insertion*, base of distal phalanx of great toe; *innervation*, posterior tibial; *action*, flexes great toe.

m. flex'or pol'licis bre'vis [NA], short flexor muscle of thumb: *origin*, transverse carpal ligament, ridge of trapezium; *insertion*, base of proximal phalanx of thumb; *innervation*, median, ulnar; *action*, flexes and adducts thumb.

m. flex'or pol'licis lon'gus [NA], long flexor muscle of thumb: *origin*, anterior surface of radius and coronoid process of ulna; *insertion*, base of distal phalanx of thumb; *innervation*, anterior interosseous; *action*, flexes thumb.

m. fronta'lis, venter frontalis musculi occipitofrontalis.

m. fusifor'mis [NA], fusiform muscle: a spindle-shaped muscle in which the fibers are approximately parallel to the long axis of the muscle but converge upon a tendon at either end.

m. gastrocne'mius [NA], gastrocnemius muscle (2 heads): *origin*, CAPUT MEDIALE—popliteal surface of femur, upper part of medial condyle, and capsule of knee, CAPUT LATERALE—lateral condyle and capsule of knee; *insertion*, aponeurosis unites with tendon of soleus to form calcaneal tendon (Achilles tendon); *innervation*, tibial; *action*, plantar flexes ankle joint, flexes knee joint.

m. gemel'lus infe'rior [NA], inferior gemellus muscle: *origin*, tuberosity of ischium; *insertion*, greater trochanter of femur; *innervation*, sacral plexus; *action*, rotates thigh laterally.

m. gemel'lus supe'rior [NA], superior gemellus muscle: *origin*, spine of ischium; *insertion*, greater trochanter of femur; *innervation*, sacral plexus; *action*, rotates thigh laterally.

m. genioglos'sus [NA], genioglossus muscle: *origin*, mental spine of mandible; *insertion*, hyoid bone and under surface of tongue; *innervation*, hypoglossal; *action*, protrudes and depresses tongue.

m. geniohyoi'deus [NA], geniohyoid muscle: *origin*, mental spine of mandible; *insertion*, body of hyoid bone; *innervation*, a branch of first cervical nerve through hypoglossal; *action*, elevates, draws hyoid forward.

m. glossopalati'nus, m. palatoglossus.

m. glossopharyn'geus, pars glossopharyngea musculi constrictoris pharyngis superioris.

m. glu'teus max'imus [NA], greatest gluteal muscle: *origin*, lateral surface of ilium, dorsal surface of sacrum and coccyx, sacrotuberous ligament; *insertion*, iliotibial tract of fascia lata, gluteal tuberosity of femur; *innervation*, inferior gluteal; *action*, extends, abducts, and rotates thigh laterally.

m. glu'teus me'dius [NA], middle gluteal muscle: *origin*, lateral surface of ilium between anterior and posterior gluteal lines; *insertion*, greater trochanter of femur; *innervation*, superior gluteal; *action*, abducts thigh.

m. glu'teus min'imus [NA], least gluteal muscle: *origin*, lateral surface of ilium between anterior and inferior gluteal lines; *insertion*, greater trochanter of femur; *innervation*, superior gluteal; *action*, abducts, rotates thigh medially.

m. gra'cilis [NA], gracilis muscle: *origin*, inferior ramus of pubis; *insertion*, medial surface of shaft of tibia; *innervation*, obturator; *action*, adducts thigh, flexes knee joint.

m. hel'icis ma'jor [NA], *origin*, spine of helix; *insertion*, anterior border of helix; *innervation*, auriculotemporal and posterior auricular; *action*, tenses skin of auditory canal.

m. hel'icis mi'nor [NA], *origin*, anterior rim of helix; *insertion*, concha; *innervation*, temporal, posterior auricular.

m. hyoglos'sus [NA], hyoglossal muscle: *origin*, body and greater cornu of hyoid bone; *insertion*, side of tongue; *innervation*, hypoglossal; *action*, depresses and retracts tongue.

m. ili'acus [NA], iliac muscle: *origin*, iliac fossa and base of sacrum; *insertion*, lesser trochanter of femur; *innervation*, femoral; *action*, flexes thigh, trunk on limb.

m. iliococcyg'eus [NA], iliococcygeal muscle: a name given the posterior portion of the levator ani which originates as far forward as the obturator canal and inserts on the side of the coccyx and the anococcygeal body; *innervation*, third and fourth sacral; *action*, helps to support pelvic viscera and resist increases in intra-abdominal pressure.

m. iliocosta'lis [NA], iliocostal muscle: the lateral division of m. erector spinae, which includes the *m. iliocostalis cervicis, m. iliocostalis thoracis,* and *m. iliocostalis lumborum.*

m. iliocosta'lis cer'vicis [NA], iliocostal muscle of neck: *origin*, angles of third, fourth, fifth, and sixth ribs; *insertion*, transverse processes of fourth, fifth, and sixth cervical vertebrae; *innervation*, branches of cervical; *action*, extends cervical spine.

m. iliocosta'lis dor'si, m. iliocostalis thoracis.

m. iliocosta'lis lumbo'rum [NA], iliocostal muscle of loins: *origin*, iliac crest; *insertion*, angles of lower six or seven ribs; *innervation*, branches of thoracic and lumbar; *action*, extends lumbar spine.

m. iliocosta'lis thora'cis [NA], iliocostal muscle of thorax: *origin*, upper borders of angles of six lower ribs; *insertion*, angles of six upper ribs and transverse process of seventh cervical vertebra; *innervation*, branches of thoracic; *action*, keeps thoracic spine erect.

m. iliopso'as [NA], iliopsoas muscle: a compound muscle consisting of iliacus and psoas major.

mus'culi incisi'vi la'bii inferio'ris, incisive muscles of inferior lip: small bundles of muscle fibers, one arising from the incisive fossa of the mandible on each side and passing laterally to the angle of the mouth.

mus'culi incisi'vi la'bii superio'ris, incisive muscles of superior lip: small bundles of muscle fibers, one arising from the incisive fossa of the maxilla on each side and passing laterally to the angle of the mouth.

m. incisu'rae hel'icis [NA], an inconstant muscular slip continuing forward from the m. tragicus to bridge the incisure of the cartilaginous meatus.

m. incisu'rae hel'icis [Santori'ni], m. incisurae helicis.

mus'culi infrahyoi'dei [NA], infrahyoid muscles: the muscles that anchor the hyoid bone to the sternum, clavicle, and scapula, including the sternohyoid, omohyoid, sternothyroid, and thyrohyoid muscles.

m. infraspina'tus [NA], infraspinous muscle: *origin*, infraspinous fossa of scapula; *insertion*, greater tubercle of humerus; *innervation*, suprascapular; *action*, rotates humerus laterally.

mus'culi intercosta'les exter'ni [NA], external intercostal muscles (11 on each side): *origin*, inferior border of rib; *insertion*, superior border of rib below; *innervation*, intercostal; *action*, draw ribs together in respiration and expulsive movements.

mus'culi intercosta'les inter'ni [NA], internal intercostal muscles (11 on each side): *origin*, inferior border of rib and costal cartilage; *insertion*, superior border of rib and costal cartilage below; *innervation*, intercostal; *action*, draw ribs together in respiration and expulsive movements.

mus'culi intercosta'les in'timi [NA], innermost intercostal muscles: the layer of muscle fibers separated from the internal intercostal muscles by the intercostal nerves.

mus'culi interos'sei dorsa'les ma'nus [NA], dorsal interosseous muscles of hand (4): *origin*, by two heads from adjacent sides of metacarpal bones; *insertion*, extensor tendons of second, third, and fourth fingers; *innervation*, ulnar; *action*, abduct, flex proximal phalanges.

mus'culi interos'sei dorsa'les pe'dis [NA], dorsal interosseous muscles of foot (4): *origin*, surfaces of adjacent metatarsal bones; *insertion*, extensor tendons of second, third, and fourth toes; *innervation*, lateral plantar; *action*, abduct, flex toes.

mus'culi interos'sei palma'res [NA], palmar interosseous muscles (3): *origin*, sides of second, fourth, and fifth metacarpal bones; *insertion*, extensor tendons of second, fourth, and fifth fingers; *innervation*, ulnar; *action*, adduct, flex proximal phalanges.

mus'culi interos'sei planta'res [NA], plantar interosseous muscles (3): *origin*, medial surface of third, fourth, and fifth metatarsal bones; *insertion*, extensor tendons of third, fourth, and fifth toes; *innervation*, lateral plantar; *action*, adduct, flex toes.

mus'culi interos'sei vola'res, musculi interossei palmares.

mus'culi interspina'les [NA], interspinal muscles: short bands of muscle fibers between spinous processes of contiguous vertebrae, including the *musculi interspinales cervicis, musculi interspinales thoracis,* and *musculi interspinales lumborum.*

mus'culi interspina'les cer'vicis [NA], interspinal muscles of neck: paired bands of muscle fibers extending between spinous processes of contiguous cervical vertebrae, innervated by spinal nerves, and acting to extend the vertebral column.

mus'culi interspina'les lumbo'rum [NA], interspinal muscles of loins: paired bands of muscle fibers extending between spinous processes of contiguous lumbar vertebrae, innervated by spinal nerves, and acting to extend the vertebral column.

mus'culi interspina'les thora'cis [NA], interspinal muscles of thorax: paired bands of muscle fibers extending between spinous processes of contiguous thoracic vertebrae, innervated by spinal nerves, and acting to extend the vertebral column.

mus'culi intertransversa'rii [NA], intertransverse muscles: small muscles passing between the transverse processes of contiguous vertebrae, including the lateral and medial intertransverse muscles of the loins, the intertransverse muscles of the thorax, and the anterior and posterior intertransverse muscles of the neck.

mus'culi intertransversa'rii anterio'res, musculi intertransversarii thoracis.

mus'culi intertransversa'rii anterio'res cer'vicis [NA], anterior intertransverse muscles of neck: small muscles passing between the anterior tubercles of adjacent cervical vertebrae, innervated by spinal nerves, and acting to bend the vertebral column laterally.

mus'culi intertransversa'rii latera'les, musculi intertransversarii laterales lumborum.

mus'culi intertransversa'rii latera'les lumbo'rum [NA], small muscles passing between the transverse processes of adjacent lumbar vertebrae, innervated by spinal nerves, and acting to bend the vertebral column laterally.

mus'culi intertransversa'rii media'les musculi intertransversarii mediales lumborum.

mus'culi intertransversa'rii media'les lumbo'rum [NA], small muscles passing from the accessory process of one lumbar vertebra to the mamillary process of the contiguous lumbar vertebra, innervated by spinal nerves, and acting to bend the vertebral column laterally.

mus'culi intertransversa'rii posterio'res, musculi intertransversarii posteriores cervicis.

mus'culi intertransversa'rii posterio'res cer'vicis [NA], posterior intertransverse muscles of neck: small muscles, divided into medial and lateral parts, passing between the posterior tubercles of adjacent cervical vertebrae, innervated by spinal nerves, and acting to bend the vertebral column laterally.

mus'culi intertransversa'rii thora'cis [NA], intertransverse muscles of thorax: poorly developed muscle bundles extending between the anterior tubercles of adjacent thoracic vertebrae, innervated by spinal nerves, and acting to bend the vertebral column laterally.

m. ischiocaverno'sus [NA], ischiocavernous muscle: *origin*, ramus of ischium; *insertion*, crus penis (crus clitoridis); *innervation*, perineal; *action*, maintains erection of penis (clitoris).

mus′culi laryn′gis [NA], the intrinsic and extrinsic muscles of the larynx.

m. latis′simus dor′si [NA], *origin,* spines of thoracic and lumbar vertebrae, thoracolumbar fascia, iliac crest, lower ribs, inferior angle of scapula; *insertion,* crest of intertubercular sulcus of humerus; *innervation,* thoracodorsal; *action,* adducts, extends, and rotates humerus medially.

m. leva′tor an′guli o′ris [NA], levator muscle of angle of mouth: *origin,* canine fossa of maxilla; *insertion,* orbicularis oris and skin at angle of mouth; *innervation,* facial; *action,* raises angle of mouth.

m. leva′tor a′ni [NA], levator ani muscle: a name applied collectively to important muscular components of the pelvic diaphragm, including the pubococcygeus (levator prostatae and pubovaginalis), the puborectalis, and the iliococcygeus muscles.

mus′culi levato′res costa′rum [NA], levator muscles of ribs (12 on each side): originating from the transverse processes of the seventh cervical and first to eleventh thoracic vertebrae and inserting medial to the angle of a lower rib (see *musculi levatores costarum breves* and *musculi levatores costarum longi*); innervated by intercostal nerves and aiding in elevation of the ribs in respiration.

mus′culi levato′res costa′rum bre′ves [NA], short levator muscles of ribs: the levatores costarum muscles of each side that insert medial to the angle of the rib next below the vertebra of origin.

mus′culi levato′res costa′rum lon′gi [NA], long levator muscles of ribs: the lower levatores costarum muscles of each side, which have fascicles extending down to the second rib below the vertebra of origin.

m. leva′tor glan′dulae thyreoi′deae, m. levator glandulae thyroideae.

m. leva′tor glan′dulae thyroi′deae [NA], levator muscle of thyroid gland: an inconstant muscle originating on the isthmus or pyramid of the thyroid gland and inserting on the body of the hyoid bone.

m. leva′tor la′bii superio′ris [NA], levator muscle of upper lip: *origin,* lower orbital margin; *insertion,* muscle of upper lip; *innervation,* facial nerve; *action,* raises upper lip.

m. leva′tor la′bii superio′ris alae′que na′si [NA], levator muscle of upper lip and ala of nose: *origin,* nasal process of maxilla; *insertion,* cartilage of ala nasi and upper lip; *innervation,* infraorbital branch of facial; *action,* raises upper lip and dilates nostril.

m. leva′tor pal′pebrae superio′ris [NA], levator muscle of upper eyelid: *origin,* upper border of optic foramen; *insertion,* tarsal plate of upper eyelid; *innervation,* oculomotor; *action,* raises upper lid.

m. leva′tor prosta′tae [NA], levator muscle of prostate: a name applied to a part of the anterior portion of the pubococcygeus muscle, which is inserted in the prostate and the tendinous center of the perineum; innervated by sacral and pudendal nerves, it supports and compresses the prostate and is involved in control of micturition.

m. leva′tor scap′ulae [NA], levator muscle of scapula: *origin,* transverse processes of four upper cervical vertebrae; *insertion,* medial border of scapula; *innervation,* third and fourth cervical; *action,* raises scapula.

m. leva′tor ve′li palati′ni [NA], *origin,* apex of petrous portion of temporal bone and cartilaginous part of auditory tube; *insertion,* aponeurosis of soft palate; *innervation,* pharyngeal plexus of vagus; *action,* raises soft palate.

mus′culi lin′guae [NA], muscles of tongue: the extrinsic and intrinsic muscles that move the tongue.

m. longis′simus [NA], longissimus muscle: the largest element of the m. erector spinae, which includes the *m. longissimus capitis, m. longissimus cervicis,* and *m. longissimus thoracis.*

m. longis′simus cap′itis [NA], longissimus muscle of head: *origin,* transverse processes of four or five upper thoracic vertebrae, articular processes of three or four lower cervical vertebrae; *insertion,* mastoid process of temporal bone; *innervation,* branches of cervical; *action,* draws head backward, rotates head.

m. longis′simus cer′vicis [NA], longissimus muscle of neck: *origin,* transverse processes of four or five upper thoracic vertebrae; *insertion,* transverse processes of second to sixth cervical vertebrae; *innervation,* lower cervical and upper thoracic; *action,* extends cervical vertebrae.

m. longis′simus dor′si, m. longissimus thoracis.

m. longis′simus thora′cis [NA], longissimus muscle of thorax: *origin,* transverse and articular processes of lumbar vertebrae and thoracolumbar fascia; *insertion,* transverse processes of all thoracic vertebrae, nine or ten lower ribs; *innervation,* lumbar and thoracic; *action,* extends thoracic vertebrae.

m. longitudina′lis infe′rior lin′guae [NA], inferior longitudinal muscle of tongue: *origin,* under surface of tongue at base; *insertion,* tip of tongue; *innervation,* hypoglossal; *action,* changes shape of tongue in mastication and deglutition.

m. longitudina′lis supe′rior lin′guae [NA], superior longitudinal muscle of tongue: *origin,* submucosa and septum of tongue; *insertion,* margins of tongue; *innervation,* hypoglossal; *action,* changes shape of tongue in mastication and deglutition.

m. lon′gus cap′itis [NA], long muscle of head: *origin,* transverse processes of third to sixth cervical vertebrae; *insertion,* basal portion of occipital bone; *innervation,* branches from first, second, and third cervical; *action,* flexes head.

m. lon′gus col′li [NA], long muscle of neck: *origin,* SUPERIOR OBLIQUE PORTION—transverse processes of third to fifth cervical vertebrae, INFERIOR OBLIQUE PORTION—bodies of first to third thoracic vertebrae, VERTICAL PORTION—bodies of three upper thoracic and three lower cervical vertebrae; *insertion,* SUPERIOR OBLIQUE PORTION—tubercle of anterior arch of atlas, INFERIOR OBLIQUE PORTION—transverse processes of fifth and sixth cervical vertebrae, VERTICAL PORTION—bodies of second to fourth cervical vertebrae; *innervation,* anterior cervical; *action,* flexes and supports cervical vertebrae.

mus′culi lumbrica′les ma′nus [NA], lumbrical muscles of hand: *origin,* tendons of flexor digitorum profundus; *insertion,* extensor tendons of four lateral fingers; *innervation,* median and ulnar; *action,* flex metacarpophalangeal joint and extend middle and distal phalanges.

mus′culi lumbrica′les pe′dis [NA], lumbrical muscles of foot: *origin,* tendons of flexor digitorum longus; *insertion,* extensor tendons of four lateral toes; *innervation,* medial and lateral plantar; *action,* flex proximal phalanges.

m. masse′ter [NA], masseter muscle: *origin,* PARS SUPERFICIALIS—zygomatic process of maxilla and lower border of zygomatic arch, PARS PROFUNDA—lower border and medial surface of zygomatic arch; *insertion,* PARS SUPERFICIALIS—angle and ramus of mandible, PARS PROFUNDA—upper half of ramus and lateral surface of coronoid process of mandible; *innervation,* mandibular division of trigeminal; *action,* raises mandible, closes jaws.

mus′culi mem′bri inferio′ris [NA], the muscles acting on the thigh, leg, and foot.

mus′culi mem′bri superio′ris [NA], the muscles acting on the arm, forearm, and hand.

m. menta′lis [NA], *origin,* incisive fossa of mandible; *insertion,* skin of chin; *innervation,* facial; *action,* wrinkles skin of chin.

musculi multif′idi [NA], *origin,* sacrum, sacroiliac ligament, mamillary processes of lumbar, transverse processes of thoracic, and articular processes of cervical vertebrae; *insertion,* spines of contiguous vertebrae above; *innervation,* dorsal branches of spinal nerves; *action,* extends, rotates vertebral column.

m. mylohyoi′deus [NA], mylohyoid muscle: *origin,* mylohyoid line of mandible; *insertion,* body of hyoid bone and median raphe; *innervation,* mylohyoid branch of trigeminal; *action,* elevates hyoid bone, supports floor of mouth.

m. mylopharyn′geus, pars mylopharyngea musculi constrictoris pharyngis superioris.

m. nasa′lis [NA], nasal muscle: *origin,* maxilla; *insertion,* PARS ALARIS—ala of nose, PARS TRANSVERSA—by aponeurotic expansion with fellow of opposite side; *innervation,* facial; *action,* PARS ALARIS—aids in widening nostril, PARS TRANSVERSA—depresses cartilage of nose.

m. obli′quus auric′ulae [NA], oblique muscle of auricle: *origin,* cranial surface of concha; *insertion,* cranial surface of auricle above concha; *innervation,* posterior auricular and temporal.

m. obli′quus cap′itis infe′rior [NA], inferior oblique muscle of head: *origin,* spinous process of axis; *insertion,* transverse process of atlas; *innervation,* dorsal branches of spinal nerves; *action,* rotates atlas and head.

m. obli′quus cap′itis supe′rior [NA], superior oblique muscle of head: *origin,* transverse process of atlas; *insertion,* occipital bone; *innervation,* dorsal branches of spinal nerves; *action,* extends and moves head laterally.

m. obli′quus exter′nus abdom′inis [NA], external oblique muscle of abdomen; *origin,* lower eight ribs at costal cartilages; *insertion,* crest of ilium, linea alba through rectus sheath; *innervation,* lower intercostal; *action,* flexes and rotates vertebral column, compresses abdominal viscera.

m. obli′quus infe′rior bul′bi [NA], inferior oblique muscle of eyeball: *origin,* orbital plate of maxilla; *insertion,* sclera; *innervation,* oculomotor; *action,* rotates eyeball upward and outward.

m. obli′quus infe′rior oc′uli, m. obliquus inferior bulbi.

m. obli′quus inter′nus abdom′inis [NA], internal oblique muscle of abdomen: *origin,* inguinal ligament, iliac crest, lumbar aponeurosis; *insertion,* lower three or four costal cartilages, linea alba, conjoined tendon to pubis; *innervation,* lower intercostal; *action,* flexes and rotates vertebral column, compresses abdominal viscera.

m. obli′quus supe′rior bul′bi [NA], superior oblique muscle of eyeball: *origin,* lesser wing of sphenoid above optic foramen; *insertion,* sclera; *innervation,* trochlear; *action,* rotates eyeball downward and outward.

m. obli′quus supe′rior oc′uli, m. obliquus superior bulbi.

m. obtura′tor exter′nus, m. obturatorius externus.

m. obtura′tor inter′nus, m. obturatorius internus.

m. obturato′rius exter′nus [NA], external obturator muscle: *origin,* pubis, ischium, and superficial surface of obturator membrane; *insertion,* trochanteric fossa of femur; *innervation,* obturator; *action,* rotates thigh laterally.

m. obturato′rius inter′nus [NA], internal obturator muscle: *origin,* pelvic surface of hip bone, margin of obturator foramen, ramus of ischium, inferior ramus of pubis, internal surface of obturator membrane; *insertion,* greater trochanter of femur; *innervation,* first, second, and third sacral; *action,* rotates thigh laterally.

m. occipita′lis, venter occipitalis musculi occipitofrontalis.

m. occipitofronta′lis [NA], occipitofrontal muscle: *origin,* VENTER FRONTALIS—galea aponeurotica, VENTER OCCIPITALIS—highest nuchal line of occipital bone; *insertion,* VENTER FRONTALIS—skin of eyebrows and root of nose, VENTER OCCIPITALIS—galea aponeurotica; *innervation,* VENTER FRONTALIS—temporal branch of facial, VENTER OCCIPITALIS— posterior auricular branch of facial; *action,* VENTER FRONTALIS—raises eyebrows, VENTER OCCIPITALIS—draws scalp backward.

mus′culi oc′uli, musculi bulbi.

m. omohyoi′deus [NA], omohyoid muscle, comprising two bellies (superior and inferior) connected by a central tendon that is bound to the clavicle by a fibrous expansion of the cervical fascia; *origin,* superior border of scapula; *insertion,* lateral border of hyoid bone; *innervation,* upper cervical through ansa cervicalis; *action,* depresses hyoid bone.

m. oppo′nens dig′iti min′imi [NA], opposing muscle of little finger: *origin,* hook of hamate bone, transverse carpal ligament; *insertion,* medial aspect of fifth metacarpal; *innervation,* eighth cervical through ulnar; *action,* rotates, abducts fifth metacarpal.

m. oppo′nens dig′iti quin′ti ma′nus, m. opponens digiti minimi.

m. oppo′nens pol′licis [NA], opposing muscle of thumb: *origin,* ridge of trapezium, transverse carpal ligament; *insertion,* radial side of first metacarpal; *innervation,* sixth and seventh cervical through median; *action,* flexes and opposes thumb.

m. orbicula′ris [NA], orbicular muscle: a muscle that encircles a body opening, such as the eye or mouth.

m. orbicula′ris oc′uli [NA], orbicular muscle of eye; the oval sphincter muscle surrounding the eyelids, consisting of three parts: *origin,* PARS ORBITALIS—medial margin of orbit, including frontal process of maxilla, PARS PALPEBRALIS—medial canthus, medial palpebral ligament, PARS LACRIMALIS—posterior lacrimal crest; *insertion,* PARS ORBITALIS—near origin after encircling orbit, PARS PALPEBRALIS—lateral canthus, PARS LACRIMALIS—joins palpebral portion; *innervation,* facial; *action,* closes eyelids, wrinkles forehead, compresses lacrimal sac.

m. orbicula′ris o′ris [NA], orbicular muscle of mouth, comprising a *pars labialis,* fibers restricted to the lips, and a *pars marginalis,* fibers blending with those of adjacent muscles; *innervation,* facial; *action,* closes and protrudes lips.

m. orbita′lis [NA], orbital muscle: *origin,* orbital periosteum; *insertion,* fascia of inferior orbital fissure; *innervation,* sympathetic fibers; *action,* protrudes eye.

mus′culi ossiculo′rum audi′tus [NA], muscles of auditory ossicles: the two muscles of the middle ear, the tensor tympani and the stapedius.

mus′culi os′sis hyoi′dei, muscles of the hyoid bone; see *musculi infrahyoidei* and *musculi suprahyoidei.*

mus′culi pala′ti et fau′cium [NA], muscles of palate and fauces: the intrinsic and extrinsic muscles that act upon the soft palate and the adjacent pharyngeal wall.

m. palatoglos′sus [NA], palatoglossus muscle: *origin,* under surface of soft palate; *insertion,* side of tongue; *innervation,* pharyngeal plexus of vagus; *action,* elevates tongue, constricts fauces.

m. palatopharyn′geus [NA], palatopharyngeal muscle: *origin,* soft palate; *insertion,* aponeurosis of pharynx, dorsal border of thyroid cartilage; *innervation,* pharyngeal plexus of vagus; *action,* aids in deglutition.

m. palma′ris bre′vis [NA], short palmar muscle: *origin,* palmar aponeurosis; *insertion,* skin of medial border of hand; *innervation,* ulnar; *action,* tenses palm of hand.

m. palma′ris lon′gus [NA], long palmar muscle: *origin,* medial epicondyle of humerus; *insertion,* transverse carpal ligament, palmar aponeurosis; *innervation,* median; *action,* flexes wrist joint.

mus′culi papilla′res [NA], papillary muscles: conical muscular projections from the walls of the cardiac ventricles, attached to the cusps of the atrioventricular valves by the chordae tendineae. There is an anterior and a posterior papillary muscle in each ventricle, as well as a group of small papillary muscles on the septum in the right ventricle.

m. papilla′ris ante′rior ventric′uli dex′tri [NA], anterior papillary muscle of right ventricle: the papillary muscle arising from the sternocostal wall of the right ventricle.

m. papilla′ris ante′rior ventric′uli sinis′tri [NA], anterior papillary muscle of left ventricle: the papillary muscle arising from the anterior wall of the left ventricle.

m. papilla′ris poste′rior ventric′uli dex′tri [NA], posterior papillary muscle of right ventricle: the papillary muscle arising from the diaphragmatic wall of the right ventricle.

m. papilla′ris poste′rior ventric′uli sinis′tri [NA], posterior papillary muscle of left ventricle: the papillary muscle arising from the posterior wall of the left ventricle.

mus′culi papilla′res septa′les ventric′uli dex′tri [NA], septal papillary muscles of right ventricle: several small papillary muscles in the right ventricle of the heart, arising from the interventricular septum.

mus′culi pectina′ti [NA], pectinate muscles: small ridges of muscle fibers projecting from the inner walls of the auricles of the heart and extending in the right atrium from the auricle to the crista terminalis.

m. pectin′eus [NA], pectineal muscle: *origin,* iliopectineal line, spine of pubis; *insertion,* femur distal to lesser trochanter; *innervation,* obturator and femoral; *action,* flexes, adducts thigh.

m. pectora′lis ma′jor [NA], greater pectoral muscle: *origin,* clavicle, sternum, six upper ribs, aponeurosis of obliquus externus abdominis. These origins are reflected in the subdivision of the muscle into clavicular, sternocostal, and abdominal parts; *insertion,* crest of intertubercular groove of humerus; *innervation,* anterior thoracic; *action,* adducts, flexes, rotates arm medially.

m. pectora′lis mi′nor [NA], smaller pectoral muscle: *origin,* third, fourth, and fifth ribs; *insertion,* coracoid process of scapula; *innervation,* anterior thoracic; *action,* draws shoulder forward and downward.

mus′culi perine′i [NA], the muscles participating in formation of the perineum.

m. perone′us bre′vis [NA], short peroneal muscle: *origin,* lateral surface of fibula; *insertion,* base of fifth metatarsal bone; *innervation,* superficial peroneal; *action,* abducts, plantar flexes foot. Called also *m. fibularis brevis* [NA alternative] or *short fibular muscle.*

m. perone′us lon′gus [NA], long peroneal muscle: *origin,* lateral condyle of tibia, lateral surface of fibula; *insertion,* medial cuneiform, first metatarsal; *innervation,* superficial peroneal; *action,* abducts, everts, plantar flexes foot. Called also *m. fibularis longus* [NA alternative] or *long fibular muscle.*

m. perone′us ter′tius [NA], third peroneal muscle: *origin,* medial surface of fibula; *insertion,* fifth metatarsal; *innervation,* deep peroneal; *action,* everts, dorsiflexes foot. Called also *m. fibularis tertius* [NA alternative] or *third fibular muscle.*

m. pharyngopalati′nus, m. palatopharyngeus.

m. pirifor′mis [NA], piriform muscle: *origin,* ilium, second to fourth sacral vertebrae; *insertion,* upper border of greater trochanter; *innervation,* first and second sacral; *action,* rotates thigh laterally.

m. planta′ris [NA], plantar muscle: *origin,* lateral condyle of femur; *insertion,* posterior part of calcaneus; *innervation,* tibial; *action,* plantar flexes foot.

m. pleuroesopha′geus [NA], pleuroesophageal muscle: a bundle of smooth muscle usually connecting the esophagus with the left mediastinal pleura.

m. pleurooesopha′geus, m. pleuroesophageus.

m. poplite′us [NA], popliteal muscle: *origin,* lateral condyle of femur; *insertion,* posterior surface of tibia; *innervation,* fourth and fifth lumbar and first sacral; *action,* flexes leg, rotates leg medially.

m. proce′rus [NA], procerus muscle: *origin,* skin over nose; *insertion,* skin of forehead; *innervation,* facial; *action,* draws eyebrows down.

m. prona′tor quadra′tus [NA], *origin,* anterior surface and border of distal third or fourth of ulna; *insertion,* distal fourth of shaft of radius; *innervation,* anterior interosseous; *action,* pronates hand.

m. prona′tor te′res [NA], (2 heads): *origin,* CAPUT HUMERALE— medial epicondyle of humerus, CAPUT ULNARE— coronoid process of ulna; *insertion,* lateral surface of radius; *innervation,* median; *action,* pronates hand.

m. prostat′icus, substantia muscularis prostatae.

m. pso′as ma′jor [NA], greater psoas muscle: *origin,* lumbar vertebrae and fascia; *insertion,* lesser trochanter of femur; *innervation,* second and third lumbar; *action,* flexes trunk, flexes and rotates thigh medially.

m. pso′as mi′nor [NA], smaller psoas muscle: *origin,* last thoracic and first lumbar vertebrae; *insertion,* iliopectineal eminence; *innervation,* first lumbar; *action,* flexes trunk on pelvis.

m. pterygoi′deus exter′nus, m. pterygoideus lateralis.

m. pterygoi′deus inter′nus, m. pterygoideus medialis.

m. pterygoi′deus latera′lis [NA], lateral pterygoid muscle (2 heads): *origin,* UPPER HEAD—lateral surface of greater wing of sphenoid and infratemporal crest; LOWER HEAD—lateral surface of lateral pterygoid plate; *insertion,* neck of condyle of mandible, temporomandibular joint capsule; *innervation,* mandibular division of trigeminal; *action,* protrudes mandible, opens jaws, moves mandible from side to side.

m. pterygoi′deus media′lis [NA], medial pterygoid muscle: *origin,* lateral pterygoid plate, tuberosity of maxilla; *insertion,* medial surface of ramus and angle of mandible; *innervation,* mandibular division of trigeminal; *action,* closes jaws.

m. pterygopharyn′geus, pars pterygopharyngea musculi constrictoris pharyngis superioris.

m. pubococcyg′eus [NA], pubococcygeal muscle: a name applied to the anterior portion of the levator ani, originating in front of the obturator canal; *insertion,* anococcygeal ligament and side of coccyx; *innervation,* third and fourth sacral; *action,* helps support pelvic viscera and resist increases in intraabdominal pressure.

m. puboprostat′icus [NA], puboprostatic muscle: a name applied to smooth muscle fibers contained within the medial puboprostatic ligament, which pass from the prostate anteriorly to the pubis.

m. puborecta′lis [NA], puborectal muscle: a name applied to a portion of the levator ani having a more lateral origin from the pubic bone, and continuous posteriorly with the corresponding muscle of the opposite side; *innervation,* third and fourth sacral; *action,* helps support pelvic viscera and resist increases in intraabdominal pressure.

m. pubovagina′lis [NA], pubovaginal muscle: a name applied to a part of the anterior portion of the pubococcygeus muscle, which is inserted into the urethra and vagina; innervated by the sacral and pudendal nerves, it is involved in control of micturition.

m. pubovesica′lis [NA], pubovesical muscle: a name applied to smooth muscle fibers extending from the neck of the urinary bladder to the pubis.

m. pyramida′lis [NA], pyramidal muscle: *origin*, front of pubis, anterior pubic ligament; *insertion*, linea alba; *innervation*, last thoracic; *action*, tenses abdominal wall.

m. pyramida′lis auric′ulae [NA], pyramidal muscle of auricle: a prolongation of the fibers of the tragicus to the spina helicis.

m. quadra′tus fem′oris [NA], quadrate muscle of thigh: *origin*, upper part of lateral border of tuberosity of ischium; *insertion*, quadrate tubercle of femur; *innervation*, last lumbar and first sacral; *action*, adducts, rotates thigh laterally.

m. quadra′tus la′bii inferio′ris, m. depressor labii inferioris.

m. quadra′tus la′bii superio′ris, m. levator labii superioris.

m. quadra′tus lumbo′rum [NA], *origin*, crest of ilium, thoracolumbar fascia, lumbar vertebrae; *insertion*, twelfth rib, transverse processes of four upper lumbar vertebrae; *innervation*, first and second lumbar and twelfth thoracic; *action*, flexes lumbar vertebrae laterally.

m. quadra′tus plan′tae [NA], quadrate muscle of sole: *origin*, calcaneus and plantar fascia; *insertion*, tendons of flexor digitorum longus; *innervation*, lateral plantar; *action*, aids in flexing toes. Called also *m. flexor accessorius* [NA alternative] or *accessory flexor muscle*.

m. quad′riceps fem′oris [NA], quadriceps muscle of thigh: a name applied collectively to the rectus femoris, vastus intermedius, vastus lateralis, and vastus medialis, inserting by a common tendon that surrounds the patella and ends on the tuberosity of the tibia, and acting to extend the leg upon the thigh. See individual components.

m. rectococcyg′eus [NA], rectococcygeal muscle: smooth muscle fibers originating on the anterior surface of the second and third coccygeal vertebrae and inserting on the posterior surface of the rectum, innervated by autonomic nerves, and acting to retract and elevate the rectum.

m. rectourethra′lis [NA], rectourethral muscle: a band of smooth muscle fibers extending from the perineal flexure of the rectum to the membranous urethra in the male.

m. rectouteri′nus [NA], rectouterine muscle: a band of fibers running between the cervix of the uterus and the rectum, in the rectouterine fold.

m. rectovesica′lis [NA], rectovesical muscle: a band of fibers in the male, connecting the longitudinal musculature of the rectum with the external muscular coat of the bladder.

m. rec′tus abdom′inis [NA], *origin*, pubis; *insertion*, xiphoid process, cartilages of fifth, sixth, and seventh ribs; *innervation*, branches of lower thoracic; *action*, flexes lumbar vertebrae, supports abdomen.

m. rec′tus cap′itis ante′rior [NA], *origin*, lateral mass of atlas; *insertion*, basilar process of occipital bone; *innervation*, first and second cervical; *action*, flexes, supports head.

m. rec′tus cap′itis latera′lis [NA], *origin*, upper surface of transverse process of atlas; *insertion*, jugular process of occipital bone; *innervation*, first and second cervical; *action*, flexes, supports head.

m. rec′tus cap′itis poste′rior ma′jor [NA], *origin*, spinous process of axis; *insertion*, occipital bone; *innervation*, suboccipital and greater occipital; *action*, extends head.

m. rec′tus cap′itis poste′rior mi′nor [NA], *origin*, tubercle on dorsal arch of atlas; *insertion*, occipital bone; *innervation*, suboccipital and greater occipital; *action*, extends head.

m. rec′tus fem′oris [NA], *origin*, anterior inferior iliac spine, rim of acetabulum; *insertion*, patella, tubercle of tibia; *innervation*, femoral; *action*, extends leg, flexes thigh.

m. rec′tus infe′rior bul′bi [NA], *origin*, circumference of optic foramen; *insertion*, under side of sclera; *innervation*, oculomotor; *action*, adducts, rotates eyeball downward and medially.

m. rec′tus infe′rior oc′uli, m. rectus inferior bulbi.

m. rec′tus latera′lis bul′bi [NA], *origin*, lateral margin of optic foramen, margin of superior orbital fissure; *insertion*, lateral side of sclera; *innervation*, abducens; *action*, abducts eyeball.

m. rec′tus latera′lis oc′uli, m. rectus lateralis bulbi.

m. rec′tus media′lis bul′bi [NA], *origin*, circumference of optic foramen; *insertion*, medial side of sclera; *innervation*, oculomotor; *action*, adducts eyeball.

m. rec′tus media′lis oc′uli, m. rectus medialis bulbi.

m. rec′tus supe′rior bul′bi [NA], *origin*, upper border of optic foramen; *insertion*, upper aspect of sclera; *innervation*, oculomotor; *action*, adducts, rotates eyeball upward and medially.

m. rec′tus supe′rior oc′uli, m. rectus superior bulbi.

m. rhomboi′deus ma′jor [NA], greater rhomboid muscle: *origin*, spinous processes of second, third, fourth, and fifth thoracic vertebrae; *insertion*, medial margin of scapula; *innervation*, dorsal scapular; *action*, retracts, elevates scapula.

m. rhomboi′deus mi′nor [NA], lesser rhomboid muscle: *origin*, spinous processes of seventh cervical to first thoracic vertebrae, lower part of ligamentum nuchae; *insertion*, medial margin of scapula at root of the spine; *innervation*, dorsal scapular; *action*, adducts, elevates scapula.

m. riso′rius [NA], risorius muscle: *origin*, fascia over masseter; *insertion*, skin at angle of mouth; *innervation*, buccal branch of facial; *action*, draws angle of mouth laterally.

mus′culi rotato′res [NA], rotator muscles: a series of small muscles deep in the groove between the spinous and transverse processes of the vertebrae, including the *musculi rotatores cervicis, musculi rotatores thoracis,* and *musculi rotatores lumborum.*

mus′culi rotato′res bre′ves, short rotator muscles: a name given the musculi rotatores that insert on the lamina of the vertebra next above the vertebra of origin.

mus′culi rotato′res cer′vicis [NA], rotator muscles of neck: *origin*, transverse processes of cervical vertebrae; *insertion*, base of spinous process of suprajacent vertebrae; *innervation*, spinal nerves; *action*, extend vertebral column and rotate it toward the opposite side.

mus′culi rotato′res lon′gi, long rotator muscles: a name given the musculi rotatores that cross one or two segments of the vertebral column and insert into the spine of the vertebra next above.

mus′culi rotato′res lumbo′rum [NA], *origin*, transverse processes of lumbar vertebrae; *insertion*, base of spinous process of suprajacent vertebrae; *innervation*, spinal nerves; *action*, extend vertebral column and rotate it toward the opposite side.

mus′culi rotato′res thora′cis [NA], rotator muscles of thorax: *origin*, transverse processes of thoracic vertebrae; *insertion*, base of spinous process of suprajacent vertebrae; *innervation*, spinal nerves; *action*, extend vertebral column and rotate it toward the opposite side.

m. sacrococcyg′eus ante′rior, m. sacrococcygeus ventralis.

m. sacrococcyg′eus dorsa′lis [NA], dorsal sacrococcygeal muscle: a muscular slip passing from the dorsal aspect of the sacrum to the coccyx.

m. sacrococcyg′eus poste′rior, m. sacrococcygeus dorsalis.

m. sacrococcyg′eus ventra′lis [NA], ventral sacrococcygeal muscle: a musculotendinous slip passing from the lower sacral vertebrae to the coccyx.

m. sacrospina′lis, m. erector spinae.

m. salpingopharyn′geus [NA], salpingopharyngeal muscle: *origin*, auditory tube near its orifice; *insertion*, posterior part of palatopharyngeus; *innervation*, pharyngeal plexus of vagus; *action*, raises nasopharynx.

m. sarto′rius [NA], sartorius muscle: *origin*, anterior superior iliac spine; *insertion*, medial side of proximal end of tibia; *innervation*, femoral; *action*, flexes thigh and leg.

m. scale′nus ante′rior [NA], anterior scalene muscle: *origin*, transverse processes of third to sixth cervical vertebrae; *insertion*, tubercle of first rib; *innervation*, second to seventh cervical; *action*, raises first rib. Called also *m. scalenus anticus.*

m. scale′nus me′dius [NA], middle scalene muscle: *origin*, transverse processes of second to sixth cervical vertebrae; *insertion*, first rib; *innervation*, second to seventh cervical; *action*, raises first rib.

m. scale′nus min′imus [NA], smallest scalene muscle: a band occasionally found between the m. scalenus anterior and the m. scalenus medius.

m. scale′nus poste′rior [NA], posterior scalene muscle: *origin*, tubercles of fourth to sixth cervical vertebrae; *insertion*, second rib; *innervation*, second to seventh cervical; *action*, raises first and second ribs.

m. semimembrano′sus [NA], semimembranous muscle: *origin*, tuberosity of ischium; *insertion*, medial condyle of tibia; *innervation*, tibial; *action*, flexes leg, extends thigh.

m. semispina′lis [NA], a muscle composed of fibers extending obliquely from the transverse processes of the vertebrae to the spines, except for the semispinalis capitis; it includes the *m. semispinalis capitis, m. semispinalis cervicis,* and *m. semispinalis thoracis.*

m. semispina′lis cap′itis [NA], *origin*, transverse processes of five or six upper thoracic and four lower cervical vertebrae; *insertion*, occipital bone; *innervation*, suboccipital, greater occipital, and branches of cervical; *action*, extends head.

m. semispina′lis cer′vicis [NA], *origin*, transverse processes of five or six upper thoracic vertebrae; *insertion*, spinous processes of second to fifth cervical vertebrae; *innervation*, branches of cervical; *action*, extends, rotates vertebral column.

m. semispina′lis dor′si, m. semispinalis thoracis.

m. semispina′lis thora′cis [NA], *origin*, transverse processes of sixth to tenth thoracic vertebrae; *insertion*, spinous processes of two lower cervical and four upper thoracic vertebrae; *innervation*, spinal nerves; *action*, extends, rotates vertebral column.

m. semitendino′sus [NA], semitendinous muscle: *origin*, tuberosity of ischium; *insertion*, upper part of medial surface of tibia; *innervation*, tibial; *action*, flexes leg, extends thigh.

m. serra′tus ante′rior [NA], *origin*, eight or nine upper ribs; *insertion*, medial border of scapula; *innervation*, long thoracic; *action*, draws scapula forward; rotates scapula to raise shoulder in abduction of arm.

m. serra′tus poste′rior infe′rior [NA], *origin*, spines of two lower thoracic and two or three upper lumbar vertebrae; *insertion*, inferior border of four lower ribs; *innervation*, ninth to twelfth thoracic; *action*, lowers ribs in expiration.

m. serra′tus poste′rior supe′rior [NA], *origin*, ligamentum nuchae, spinous processes of upper thoracic vertebrae; *insertion*, second, third, fourth, and fifth ribs; *innervation*, upper four intercostal; *action*, raises ribs in inspiration.

mus′culi skel′eti [NA], skeletal muscles: striated muscles that are attached to bones and typically cross at least one joint.

m. so′leus [NA], soleus muscle: *origin*, fibula, popliteal fascia, tibia; *insertion*, calcaneus by tendo calcaneus; *innervation*, tibial; *action*, plantar flexes ankle joint.

m. sphinc′ter [NA], sphincter muscle: a ringlike muscle that closes a natural orifice; called also *sphincter*.

m. sphinc′ter ampul′lae hepatopancreat′icae [NA], muscle fibers investing the hepatopancreatic ampulla.

m. sphinc′ter a′ni exter′nus [NA], external sphincter muscle of anus: *origin*, tip of coccyx and surrounding fascia; *insertion*, tendinous center of perineum; *innervation*, inferior rectal and fourth sacral; *action*, closes anus.

m. sphinc′ter a′ni inter′nus [NA], internal sphincter muscle of anus: a thickening of the circular lamina of the tunica muscularis at the caudal end of the rectum.

m. sphinc′ter duc′tus chole′dochi [NA], an annular sheath of muscle that invests the bile duct within the wall of the duodenum.

m. sphinc′ter pupil′lae [NA], sphincter muscle of pupil: circular fibers of the iris, innervated by the oculomotor nerve (parasympathetic), and acting to contract the pupil.

m. sphinc′ter pylo′ri [NA], sphincter muscle of stomach: a thickening of the circular muscle of the stomach around its opening into the duodenum; called also *pyloric sphincter*.

m. sphinc′ter ure′thrae [NA], sphincter muscle of urethra: *origin*, ramus of pubis; *insertion*, median raphe behind and in front of urethra; *innervation*, pudendal; *action*, compresses urethra.

m. sphinc′ter ure′thrae membrana′ceae, m. sphincter urethrae.

m. sphinc′ter vesi′cae urina′riae, sphincter muscle of urinary bladder: a circular layer of fibers surrounding the internal urethral orifice, innervated by the vesical nerve, and acting to close the internal orifice of the urethra.

m. spina′lis [NA], the medial division of the erector spinae, including the *m. spinalis capitis, m. spinalis cervicis,* and *m. spinalis thoracis.*

m. spina′lis cap′itis [NA], *origin*, spines of upper thoracic and lower cervical vertebrae; *insertion*, occipital bone; *innervation*, spinal nerves; *action*, extends head.

m. spina′lis cer′vicis [NA], *origin*, spinous processes of fifth, sixth, and seventh cervical and two upper thoracic vertebrae; *insertion*, spinous processes of axis and sometimes of second to fourth cervical vertebrae; *innervation*, branches of cervical; *action*, extends vertebral column.

m. spina′lis dor′si, m. spinalis thoracis.

m. spina′lis thora′cis [NA], *origin*, spinous processes of two upper lumbar and two lower thoracic; *insertion*, spines of upper thoracic vertebrae; *innervation*, branches of spinal nerves; *action*, extends vertebral column.

m. sple′nius cap′itis [NA], *origin*, lower half of ligamentum nuchae, spines of seventh cervical and three upper thoracic vertebrae; *insertion*, occipital bone; *innervation*, middle and lower cervical; *action*, extends, rotates head.

m. sple′nius cer′vicis [NA], *origin*, spinous processes of third to sixth thoracic vertebrae; *insertion*, transverse processes of two or three upper cervical vertebrae; *innervation*, dorsal branches of lower cervical; *action*, extends, rotates head and neck.

m. stape′dius [NA], stapedius muscle: *origin*, interior of pyramid of tympanic cavity; *insertion*, posterior surface of neck of stapes; *innervation*, stapedial branch of facial; *action*, dampens stapedial movement.

m. sterna′lis [NA], sternal muscle: a band occasionally found parallel to the sternum on the sternocostal origin of the pectoralis major.

m. sternocleidomastoi′deus [NA], sternocleidomastoid muscle (2 heads): *origin*, sternum and clavicle; *insertion*, mastoid process and superior nuchal line of occipital bone; *innervation*, accessory nerve and cervical plexus; *action*, flexes vertebral column, rotates head.

m. sternohyoi′deus [NA], sternohyoid muscle: *origin*, manubrium sterni; *insertion*, body of hyoid bone; *innervation*, upper cervical; *action*, depresses hyoid bone and larynx.

m. sternothyreoi′deus, m. sternothyroideus.

m. sternothyroi′deus [NA], sternothyroid muscle: *origin*, manubrium sterni; *insertion*, thyroid cartilage; *innervation*, upper cervical; *action*, depresses thyroid cartilage.

m. styloglos′sus [NA], styloglossus muscle: *origin*, styloid process; *insertion*, margin of tongue; *innervation*, hypoglossal; *action*, raises and retracts tongue.

m. stylohyoi′deus [NA], stylohyoid muscle: *origin*, styloid process; *insertion*, body of hyoid bone; *innervation*, facial; *action*, draws hyoid and tongue upward.

m. stylopharyn′geus [NA], stylopharyngeal muscle: *origin*, styloid process; *insertion*, thyroid cartilage and pharyngeal constrictors; *innervation*, pharyngeal plexus, glossopharyngeal; *action*, raises and dilates pharynx.

m. subcla′vius [NA], subclavius muscle: *origin*, first rib and its cartilage; *insertion*, lower surface of clavicle; *innervation*, fifth and sixth cervical; *action*, depresses lateral end of clavicle.

mus′culi subcosta′les [NA], subcostal muscles: *origin*, inner surface of ribs: *insertion*, inner surface of first, second, third rib below; *innervation*, intercostal; *action*, raise ribs in inspiration.

m. subscapula′ris [NA], subscapular muscle: *origin*, subscapular fossa of scapula; *insertion*, lesser tubercle of humerus; *innervation*, subscapular; *action*, rotates humerus medially.

m. supina′tor [NA], supinator muscle: *origin*, lateral epicondyle of humerus, ulna, elbow joint fascia; *insertion*, radius; *innervation*, deep radial; *action*, supinates hand.

mus′culi suprahyoi′dei [NA], suprahyoid muscles: the muscles that attach the hyoid bone to the skull, including the digastric, stylohyoid, mylohyoid, and geniohyoid muscles.

m. supraspina′tus [NA], supraspinous muscle: *origin*, supraspinous fossa of scapula; *insertion*, greater tubercle of humerus; *innervation*, suprascapular; *action*, abducts humerus.

m. suspenso′rius duode′ni [NA], suspensory muscle of duodenum: a flat band of smooth muscle originating from the left crus of the diaphragm, and continuous with the muscular coat of the duodenum at its junction with the jejunum.

m. tarsa′lis infe′rior [NA], inferior tarsal muscle: *origin*, inferior rectus muscle; *insertion*, tarsal plate of lower eyelid; *innervation*, sympathetic; *action*, widens palpebral fissure.

m. tarsa′lis supe′rior [NA], superior tarsal muscle: *origin*, m. levator palpebrae superioris; *insertion*, tarsal plate of upper eyelid; *innervation*, sympathetic; *action*, widens palpebral fissure.

m. tempora′lis [NA], temporal muscle: *origin*, temporal fossa and fascia; *insertion*, coronoid process of mandible; *innervation*, mandibular division of trigeminal; *action*, closes jaws.

m. temporoparieta′lis [NA], temporoparietal muscle: *origin*, temporal fascia above ear; *insertion*, galea aponeurotica; *innervation*, temporal branches of facial; *action*, tightens scalp.

m. ten′sor fas′ciae la′tae [NA], tensor muscle of fascia lata: *origin*, iliac crest; *insertion*, iliotibial band of fascia lata; *innervation*, superior gluteal; *action*, flexes, rotates thigh medially.

m. ten′sor tym′pani [NA], tensor muscle of tympanic membrane: *origin*, cartilaginous portion of auditory tube; *insertion*, manubrium of malleus; *innervation*, mandibular division of trigeminal; *action*, tenses tympanic membrane.

m. ten′sor ve′li palati′ni [NA], *origin*, scaphoid fossa of sphenoid, wall of auditory tube; *insertion*, aponeurosis of soft palate, horizontal part of palatine bone; *innervation*, mandibular division of trigeminal; *action*, tenses soft palate, opens auditory tube.

m. te′res ma′jor [NA], teres major muscle: *origin*, inferior angle of scapula; *insertion*, crest of intertubercular sulcus of humerus; *innervation*, subscapular; *action*, adducts, extends, rotates arm medially.

m. te′res mi′nor [NA], teres minor muscle: *origin*, lateral margin of scapula; *insertion*, greater tuberosity of humerus; *innervation*, axillary; *action*, rotates arm laterally.

mus′culi thora′cis [NA], the muscles of the thorax.

m. thyreoarytaenoi′deus [exter′nus], m. thyroarytenoideus.

m. thyreoepiglot′ticus, m. thyroepiglotticus.

m. thyreohyoi′deus, m. thyrohyoideus.

m. thyreopharyn′geus, pars thyropharyngea musculi constrictoris pharyngis inferioris.

m. thyroarytenoi′deus [NA], thyroarytenoid muscle: *origin*, lamina of thyroid cartilage; *insertion*, muscular process of arytenoid cartilage; *innervation*, recurrent laryngeal; *action*, relaxes, shortens vocal folds.

m. thyroepiglot′ticus [NA], thyroepiglottic muscle: *origin*, lamina of thyroid cartilage; *insertion*, epiglottis; *innervation*, recurrent laryngeal; *action*, closes inlet to larynx.

m. thyrohyoi′deus [NA], thyrohyoid muscle: *origin*, thyroid cartilage; *insertion*, greater cornu of hyoid bone; *innervation*, upper cervical; *action*, raises and changes form of larynx.

m. tibia′lis ante′rior [NA], anterior tibial muscle: *origin*, tibia, interosseous membrane; *insertion*, medial cuneiform and first metatarsal; *innervation*, deep peroneal; *action*, dorsiflexes and inverts foot.

m. tibia′lis poste′rior [NA], posterior tibial muscle: *origin*, tibia, fibula, interosseous membrane; *insertion*, bases of metatarsals and tarsals, except talus; *innervation*, posterior tibial; *action*, plantar flexes and inverts foot.

m. trachea′lis [NA], tracheal muscle: a transverse layer of smooth fibers in the dorsal portion of the trachea; *insertion*, tracheal cartilages; *innervation*, autonomic fibers; *action*, lessens caliber of trachea.

m. trag′icus [NA], muscle of tragus: a short, flattened vertical band on the lateral surface of the tragus, innervated by the auriculotemporal and posterior auricular nerves.

m. transversospina′lis [NA], a general term including the semispinalis and multifidus muscles and the rotatores.

m. transver′sus abdom′inis [NA], transverse muscle of abdomen: *origin*, cartilages of six lower ribs, thoracolumbar fascia, iliac crest, inguinal ligament; *insertion*, linea alba through rectus sheath, conjoined tendon to pubis; *innervation*, lower intercostals, iliohypogastric, ilioinguinal; *action*, compresses abdominal viscera.

m. transver′sus auric′ulae [NA], transverse muscle of auricle: *origin*, cranial surface of auricle; *insertion*, circumference of auricle; *innervation*, great auricular and posterior auricular; *action*, retracts helix.

m. transver′sus lin′guae [NA], transverse muscle of tongue: *origin*, median septum of tongue; *insertion*, dorsum and margins of tongue; *innervation*, hypoglossal; *action*, changes shape of tongue in mastication and deglutition.

m. transver'sus men'ti [NA], transverse muscle of chin: superficial fibers of the depressor anguli oris which turn back and cross to the opposite side.

m. transver'sus nu'chae [NA], transverse muscle of nape: a small muscle often present, passing from the occipital protuberance to the posterior auricular muscle; it may be either superficial or deep to the trapezius.

m. transver'sus perine'i profun'dus [NA], deep transverse muscle of perineum: *origin*, inferior ramus of ischium; *insertion*, median raphe of perineum; *innervation*, pudendal; *action*, draws back central point of perineum.

m. transver'sus perine'i superficia'lis [NA], superficial transverse muscle of perineum: *origin*, tuberosity of ischium; *insertion*, central tendon of perineum; *innervation*, perineal branch of pudendal; *action*, tenses central point of perineum.

m. transver'sus thora'cis [NA], transverse muscle of thorax: *origin*, mediastinal surface of sternum and of xiphoid process; *insertion*, cartilages of second to sixth ribs; *innervation*, intercostal; *action*, narrows chest.

m. trape'zius [NA], trapezius muscle: *origin*, occipital bone, ligamentum nuchae, spinous processes of seventh cervical and all thoracic vertebrae; *insertion*, clavicle, acromion, spine of scapula; *innervation*, accessory nerve and cervical plexus; *action*, rotates scapula to raise shoulder in abduction of arm, draws scapula backward.

m. triangula'ris, m. depressor anguli oris.

m. tri'ceps bra'chii [NA], triceps muscle of arm (3 heads): *origin*, CAPUT LONGUM—infraglenoid tubercle of scapula, CAPUT LATERALE—posterior surface of humerus, lateral border of humerus, lateral intermuscular septum, CAPUT MEDIALE—posterior surface of humerus below radial groove, medial border of humerus, medial intermuscular septa; *insertion*, olecranon of ulna; *innervation*, radial; *action*, extends forearm, adducts and extends arm.

m. tri'ceps su'rae [NA], the gastrocnemius and soleus considered together.

m. unipenna'tus [NA], unipennate muscle: a muscle in which the fiber bundles approach the tendon of insertion from only one direction and are inserted through only a small segment of its circumference.

m. u'vulae [NA], muscle of uvula: *origin*, posterior nasal spine of palatine bone and aponeurosis of soft palate; *insertion*, uvula; *innervation*, pharyngeal plexus of vagus; *action*, raises uvula.

m. vas'tus interme'dius [NA], *origin*, anterior and lateral surfaces of femur; *insertion*, patella, common tendon of quadriceps femoris; *innervation*, femoral; *action*, extends leg.

m. vas'tus latera'lis [NA], *origin*, capsule of hip joint, lateral aspect of femur; *insertion*, patella, common tendon of quadriceps femoris; *innervation*, femoral; *action*, extends leg.

m. vas'tus media'lis [NA], *origin*, medial aspect of femur; *insertion*, patella, common tendon of quadriceps femoris; *innervation*, femoral; *action*, extends leg.

m. ventricula'ris, a name applied to fibers of the thyroarytenoid muscle running into the vestibular folds.

m. verti'calis lin'guae [NA], vertical muscle of tongue: *origin*, dorsal fascia of tongue; *insertion*, sides and base of tongue; *innervation*, hypoglossal; *action*, changes shape of tongue in mastication and deglutition.

m. vis'cerum, a term applied to muscle of a body organ.

m. voca'lis [NA], vocal muscle: *origin*, thyroid cartilage; *insertion*, vocal process of arytenoid cartilage; *innervation*, recurrent laryngeal; *action*, shortens vocal folds.

m. zygomat'icus, m. zygomaticus major.

m. zygomat'icus ma'jor [NA], greater zygomatic muscle: *origin*, zygomatic bone in front of temporal process; *insertion*, angle of mouth; *innervation*, facial; *action*, draws angle of mouth backward and upward.

m. zygomat'icus mi'nor [NA], lesser zygomatic muscle: *origin*, zygomatic bone near maxillary suture; *insertion*, orbicularis oris and levator labii superioris; *innervation*, facial; *action*, draws upper lip upward and laterally.

---

mushbite (mush'bīt) the making simultaneously of an impression of both upper and lower teeth and/or associated structures by having the subject bite on a mass of plastic material placed between the jaws; no longer a generally accepted prosthodontic procedure. See *wax bite*, under *bite*.

mushroom (mush'room) the fruiting body of any of a variety of basidiomycetous, fleshy fungi of the order Agaricales, especially one that is edible; poisonous species are popularly called *toadstools*. Called also *basidiocarp*. See also *agaric*.

musicogenic (mu″zĭ-ko-jen'ik) caused or produced by musical sounds.

musicotherapy (mu″zĭ-ko-ther'ah-pe) [Gr. *mousikē* music + *therapeia* treatment] the treatment of disease by music.

Musset's sign (mu-sāz') [Louis Charles Alfred de *Musset*, French poet, 1810–1857, who died of aortic insufficiency] see under *sign*.

mussitation (mus″ĭ-ta'shun) [L. *mussitare* to mutter] the moving of the lips with no utterance of articulate sounds.

Mussy see *Guéneau de Mussy*.

must (must) [L. *mustum*] the unfermented juice of grapes and other fruit.

mustard (mus'tard) [L. *sinapis*] 1. a plant of the genus *Brassica*. 2. the ripe seeds of *Brassica nigra* (L.) Koch (Cruciferae) (black mustard) and of *B. alba* (L.) Rabenh. (Cruciferae) (white mustard). When mustard seeds are crushed and moistened, volatile oils are liberated. These oils give mustard its counterirritant, stimulant, and emetic properties. **black m., brown m.,** *Brassica nigra* (L.) Koch, a source of mustard oil and allyl isothiocyanate, and used internally as an emetic and externally as a counterirritant. See *mustard plaster*, under *plaster*. **nitrogen m.,** mechlorethamine hydrochloride; see also *nitrogen m's*. **nitrogen m's,** a group of toxic, blistering alkylating agents (q.v.) homologous with dichlorodiethyl sulfide (mustard gas), some of which have been used as antineoplastics. The group includes nitrogen mustard itself (mechlorethamine hydrochloride), triethylenemelamine, cyclophosphamide, thiotepa, chlorambucil, and melphalan. **uracil m.** [USP], chemical name: 5-[bis(2-choroethyl) amino]-2,4(1*H*,3*H*)-pyrimidinedione. An analogue of nitrogen mustard, $C_8H_{11}Cl_2N_3O_2$, occurring as an off-white, crystalline powder, which acts as an alkylating agent on proliferating cells; used orally as an antineoplastic, especially for palliative treatment in chronic lymphocytic leukemia and malignant lymphomas. **white m., yellow m.,** *Brassica alba* (L.) Rabenh.; it is a source of mustard oil and acrynyl isothiocyanate, and used the same as black mustard (q.v.).

Mustargen (mus'tar-jen) trademark for a preparation of mechlorethamine hydrochloride.

mutacism (mu'tah-sizm) 1. the improper pronunciation of the sounds of mute letters. 2. mytacism.

mutafacient (mu″tah-fa'shent) mutagenic.

mutagen (mu'tah-jen) [*mutation* + *genesis*] a chemical or physical agent that induces genetic mutations.

mutagenesis (mu″tah-jen″ĕ-sis) [*mutation* + *genesis*] 1. the production of change. 2. the induction of genetic mutation.

mutagenic (mu″tah-jen'ik) 1. causing change. 2. inducing genetic mutation.

mutagenicity (mu″tah-jĕ-nis'ĭ-te) the property of being able to induce genetic mutation.

Mutamycin (mu″tah-mi'sin) trademark for a preparation of mitomycin.

mutant (mu'tant) [L. *mutare* to change] 1. an organism that has undergone genetic mutation. 2. produced by mutation.

mutarotase (mu″tah-ro'tās) aldose 1-epimerase.

mutarotation (mu″tah-ro-ta'shun) a special type of tautomerism involving either (*a*) the transformation of one optical isomer into another, or (*b*) the transformation of one structural isomer into another (both possessing asymmetric centers and optical activity). With each type the rotatory power of a freshly prepared solution of the compound will change, under a variety of conditions, until an equilibrium value is set up which (unlike in racemization) will not be zero.

mutase (mu'tās) [L. *mutare* to change + *-ase*] a group of enzymes (transferases) that catalyze the intramolecular shifting of a chemical group (acyl, phospho, amino, or other group) from one position to another. **aldehyde m.,** an enzyme that catalyzes the Cannizzaro reaction. **methylaspartate m.,** an enzyme that catalyzes the conversion of L-*threo*-3 methylaspartate to L-glutamate. **methylmalonyl-CoA m.,** an enzyme that catalyzes the conversion of methylmalonyl-CoA to succinyl-CoA.

mutation (mu-ta'shun) [L. *mutatio*, from *mutare* to change] 1. a change in form, quality, or some other characteristic. 2. in genetics, a permanent transmissible change in the genetic material, usually in a single gene; the change may be in the form of a loss (deletion), gain (translocation), or exchange (transduction) of genetic material. Also, an individual exhibiting such a change. Called also (in classical genetics) a *sport*. **genomic m.,** a mutation which alters the normal number of chromosomes of an individual; if the result is a whole multiple of the haploid set of the chromosomes, it is a ploidic mutation. **induced m.,** a genetic mutation caused by external factors which are experimentally or accidentally produced. **missense m.,** one that changes a codon so that it codes for a different amino acid. **natural m.,** a genetic mutation occurring without the intervention of any known external factors. **nonsense m.,** a mutation in which a codon for a particular amino acid is so changed that it no longer encodes any amino acid. **ploidic m.,** see *genomic m*. **point m.,** a mutation resulting from a change in a single base pair in the DNA molecule. **somatic m.,** a genetic mutation occurring in a somatic cell, providing the basis for a mosaic condition. **suppressor m.,** the correction of the effect of a mutation in one gene by a mutation in a different gene.

mutational (mu-ta′shun-al) pertaining to mutation.

mute (mūt) [L. *mutus*] 1. unable to speak. 2. one who cannot speak. **deaf m.,** see *deaf-mute.*

mutein (mu′te-in) [from *mut*ant-pro*tein*] a name suggested for a protein arising as a result of a mutation; it is analogous to the wild-type protein but does not necessarily have the same enzymological, immunological, or physicochemical properties.

mutilation (mu″tĭ-la′shun) [L. *mutilatio*] the act of depriving an individual of a limb, member, or other important part; deprival of an organ; castration.

Mutisia (mu-tiz′e-ah) a genus of plants. **M. viciaefo′lia,** a composite-flowered plant of South America, used there as a sedative and in various diseases of the heart, respiratory organs, and nervous system.

mutism (mu′tizm) [L. *mutus* unable to speak, inarticulate] inability or refusal to speak. **akinetic m.,** a state in which the individual makes no spontaneous movement or sound. **deaf m.,** inability to speak as a result of deafness and never having heard spoken words. **hysterical m.,** hysterical inability to utter words.

muton (mu′ton) [*mutation* + Gr. *on* neuter ending] in molecular genetics, the smallest element of DNA whose alteration can give rise to a mutant form of organism, possibly as small as one nucleotide base. Cf. *cistron* and *recon.*

mutualism (mu′tu-al-izm″) symbiosis in which both populations (or individuals) gain from the association and are unable to survive without it.

mutualist (mu′tu-al-ist) any organism or species associated with another in a relationship which is beneficial to both.

muzolimine (mu-zo′lĭ-mēn) chemical name: 5-amino-2-[1-(3,4-dichlorophenyl)ethyl]-2,4-dihydro-3*H*-pyrazol-3-one; a diuretic and antihypertensive, $C_{11}H_{11}Cl_2N_3O$.

M.V. abbreviation for L. *Med′icus Veterina′rius,* veterinary physician.

Mv chemical symbol for *mendelevium.*

mv. millivolt.

μv. microvolt.

μw. microwatt.

Mx Medex.

My. myopia.

my. mayer.

my- see *myo-.*

Myà's disease (me-āz′) [Giuseppe *Myà,* Italian physician, 1857–1911] see under *disease.*

myalgia (mi-al′je-ah) [*my-* + *algia*] pain in a muscle or muscles. **m. abdom′inis,** pain in the abdominal wall. **m. cap′itis,** pain in the scalp muscles; cephalalgia or headache. **m. cervica′lis,** torticollis. **epidemic m.,** epidemic pleurodynia. **lumbar m.,** lumbago.

Myambutol (mi-am′bu-tol) trademark for a preparation of ethambutol hydrochloride.

Myanesin (mi-an′ĕ-sin) trademark for a preparation of mephenesin.

myasis (mi-a′sis) myiasis.

myasthenia (mi″as-the′ne-ah) [*my-* + Gr. *astheneia* weakness] muscular debility; any constitutional anomaly of muscle. **angiosclerotic m.,** intermittent claudication. **m. gas′trica,** weakness and loss of tone in the muscular coats of the stomach; atony of the stomach. **m. gra′vis, m. gra′vis pseudoparalyt′ica,** a disorder of neuromuscular function thought to be due to the presence of antibodies to acetylcholine receptors at the neuromuscular junction; clinically there is fatigue and exhaustion of the muscular system with a tendency to fluctuate in severity and without sensory disturbance or atrophy. The disorder may be restricted to a muscle group or become generalized with severe weakness and, in some cases, ventilatory insufficiency. It may affect any muscle of the body, but especially those of the eye, face, lips, tongue, throat, and neck. **m. laryn′gis,** disability of the phonatory laryngeal muscles from overuse, debilitating conditions, or age. **neonatal m.,** a transient (a week to a month) myasthenia affecting offspring of myasthenic women, characteristically marked by difficulty in sucking and swallowing.

myasthenic (mi″as-then′ik) pertaining to or characterized by muscular weakness.

myatonia (mi″ah-to′ne-ah) [*my-* + *a* neg. + Gr. *tonos* tension] amyotonia. **m. congen′ita,** amyotonia congenita.

myatony (mi-at′o-ne) myatonia.

myatrophy (mi-at′ro-fe) [*my-* + *atrophy*] atrophy of a muscle; muscular atrophy.

myautonomy (mi″aw-ton′o-me) [*my-* + Gr. *autos* self + *nomos* law] a condition in which muscular contraction aroused by

stimulation is so long delayed that it appears to occur independently of the stimulation.

myc- see *myco-.*

mycelial (mi-se′le-al) pertaining to a mycelium.

mycelian (mi-se′le-an) mycelial.

mycelioid (mi-se′le-oid) having the radiate filamentous appearance of mold colonies.

mycelium (mi-se′le-um), pl. *myce′lia* [*myc-* + Gr. *hēlos* nail] the mass of threadlike processes (hyphae) constituting the fungal thallus.

mycete (mi′sēt) [Gr. *mykēs* fungus] a fungus, def. 1.

mycethemia (mi″se-the′me-ah) [*myceto-* + Gr. *haima* blood + *-ia*] the presence of fungi in the blood.

mycetism (mi′se-tizm) mycetismus.

mycetismus (mi″se-tiz′mus) poisoning caused by a fungus, as that resulting from ingestion of poisonous mushrooms. **m. cer′ebris,** a hallucinogenic intoxication following the ingestion of any of several species of mushrooms. **m. cholerifor′mis,** a serious and often fatal intoxication caused by ingestion of *Amanita phalloides, A. verna,* and probably other *Amanita* species which produce phalloidin; it is characterized by abdominal pain, vomiting, diarrhea, bloody stools, protein and casts in the urine, malaise, and cyanosis. **m. gastrointestina′lis,** a mild form of mycotoxicosis marked by nausea which may be followed by vomiting and diarrhea; it is caused by the ingestion of the orange jack-o-lantern mushroom (*Clitocybe illudens*) and many other species. **m. nervo′sus,** mushroom poisoning caused by ingestion of *Amanita patherina* and *A. muscaria,* which elaborate muscarine, a parasympathetic stimulant; it is marked by such symptoms as tearing, sweating, salivation, persistent peristalsis, retching and vomiting, contraction of the pupil and ciliary muscles, acute excitement, delirium, and coma. **m. sanguina′rius,** mushroom poisoning marked by hemoglobinuria, abdominal distress, and jaundice, caused by ingestion of *Helvella esculenta* and other *Helvella* species.

myceto- see *myco-.*

mycetogenic, mycetogenous (mi″se-to-jen′ik; mi″se-toj′e-nus) [*myceto-* + Gr. *gennan* to produce] caused by fungous growths.

mycetoma (mi″se-to′mah) [*myceto-* + *-oma*] 1. maduromycosis. 2. a tumor-like tangled mass of fungal mycelia. **white m.,** maduromycosis in which the granules are white, such as that caused by *Streptomyces madurae, Allescheria boydii,* or *Cephalosporium falciforme.*

Mycetozoa (mi-se″to-zo′ah) [*myceto-* + Gr. *zōon* animal] Mycetozoida.

Mycetozoida (mi″se-to-zoi′dah) a group of fungus-like microorganisms occurring as a mass of multinucleate protoplasm, frequently known as "slime molds" or "slime animals." Most forms are free-living and are found on the bark of trees, dead wood, and decaying vegetation, but some are intracellular parasites of plants. They have been classified by some as an order of amebae (Mycetozoa), by others as lower fungi (Myxomycetes).

mycid (mi′sid) dermatophytid.

Mycifradin (mi-sif′rah-din) trademark for preparations of neomycin sulfate.

myco-, myc-, mycet- [Gr. *mykēs* fungus] a combining form denoting relationship to fungus.

mycoagglutinin (mi″ko-ah-gloo′tĭ-nin) an agglutinin which has the power of agglutinating fungi.

mycobacteria (mi″ko-bak-te′re-ah) plural of *mycobacterium.*

Mycobacteriaceae (mi″ko-bak-te″re-a′se-e) a family of Schizomycetes, order Actinomycetales, made up of spherical to rod-shaped, gram-positive, aerobic, mesophilic cells showing no branching on ordinary media, found in soil and dairy products and occurring as parasites in man and other animals. It includes two genera, *Mycobacterium* and *Mycococcus.*

mycobacteriosis (mi″ko-bak-te″re-o′sis) any tuberculosis-like disease caused by mycobacteria other than *Mycobacterium tuberculosis;* these include Group I–IV mycobacteria. Called also *atypical tuberculosis.*

Mycobacterium (mi″ko-bak-te′re-um) a genus of microorganisms of the family Mycobacteriaceae, order Actinomycetales, occurring as gram-positive slender rods and distinguished by acid-fast staining. **M. a′vium,** the avian type of tubercle bacillus, commonly producing disease in chickens and swine, and only rarely infecting man; called also *M. tuberculosis* var. *avium.* **M. bal′nei,** the causative organism of swimming-pool granuloma; called also *M. marinum.* **M. bo′vis,** the bovine variety of tubercle bacillus, most commonly infecting cattle and acquired by man usually by infected milk, more commonly found in children and producing a hilar pulmonary infection, or a tracheobronchial lymphatic or mesenteric lymphatic infection with tendency to generalization. Called also *M. tuberculosis* var. *bovis.* **M. butyr′icum,** a saprophytic form found in milk and butter. **M. fortu′itum,** a species found naturally in soil but also associated with infection in man and other animals. **M. intracellula′ris,** a group III anonymous mycobacterium associated with chronic pulmonary infection in man. **M. kansas′ii,** a photochromogenic species which is the etiologic agent of a tuberculosis-like disease in man; see also *photochromogen*. **M. lep′rae,** a species found in enormous numbers in typical aggregates of parallel cells in nasal smears and other pathologic material from human leprosy; considered to be the etiologic agent of leprosy, although it has not been cultivated in vitro nor has the disease been reproduced experimentally. Called also *Hansen's bacillus*. **M. lep′rae bubalo′rum,** the causative agent of leprosy of water buffaloes. **M. lepraemu′rium,** the causative agent of murine leprosy (q.v. under *leprosy*). **M. lucifla′vum,** *M. kansasii.* **M. mari′num,** *M. balnei.* **M. micro′ti,** an organism infecting voles but not rabbits or fowls; nonpathogenic for man, and used for the preparation of experimental vaccines. **M. paratuberculo′sis,** the causative agent of Johne's disease, a chronic enteritis of cattle; nonpathogenic for man. Called also *Johne's bacillus.* **M. phle′i,** a saprophytic form found on grasses and in soil and water. **M. scrofula′ceum,** an anonymous scotochromogenic mycobacterium, apparently nonpathogenic. **M. smeg′matis,** a species found in human smegma, closely resembling *M. tuberculosis;* called also *smegma bacillus.* **M. tuberculo′sis,** the causative agent of tuberculosis, most commonly pulmonary, in mar; called also *M. tuberculosis* var. *hominis,* and *tubercle bacillus.* **M. tuberculo′sis** var. **a′vium,** see *M. avium.* **M. tuberculo′sis** var. **bo′vis,** see *M. bovis.* **M. tuberculo′sis** var. **hom′inis,** see *M. tuberculosis.* **M. tuberculo′sis** var. **mu′ris,** *M. microti.* **M. ul′cerans,** the causative agent of Buruli ulcer.

mycobacterium (mi″ko-bak-te′re-um), pl. *mycobacte′ria.* 1. an organism of the genus *Mycobacterium.* 2. a slender, acid-fast microorganism resembling the bacillus which causes tuberculosis. **anonymous mycobacteria, atypical mycobacteria,** acid-fast bacteria resembling the tubercle bacilli, found in pulmonary infections, usually of a chronic nature, in man, for which species names have not been established. They are divided into the chromogens and nonchromogens, the former including photochromogens (Group I), which produce yellow pigment in the presence of light, and scotochromogens (Group II), which produce orange pigment independent of light. The nonchromogens are subdivided into filamentous forms (Group III) and rapid growers (Group IV). **Group I–IV mycobacteria,** see *anonymous m.*

Mycocandida (mi″ko-kan′dĭ-dah) *Candida.*

mycocidin (mi″ko-si′din) an antibiotic substance extracted from a mold (Aspergillaceae); active in vivo against *Mycobacterium tuberculosis.*

Mycococcus (mi″ko-kok′us) a genus of microorganisms of the family Mycobacteriaceae, order Actinomycetales, made up of non-acid-fast, gram-positive, saprophytic rod-shaped microorganisms producing pigments and resembling actinomyces in mode of reproduction; found in soil and water.

Mycoderma (mi″ko-der′mah) [*myco-* + Gr. *derma* skin] a former genus of imperfect fungi of the order Moniliales, family Moniliaceae, most species of which are now included in the genus *Candida.* **M. ace′ti,** a name formerly given a combination of yeasts, which together with bacteria, such as *Acetobacter aceti,* grow on the surface of fermenting fluids and produce acetic acid from fermentation of alcohol. **M. dermati′tidis,** *Blastomyces dermatitidis.* **M. immi′te,** *Coccidioides immitis.*

mycoderma (mi″ko-der′mah) [Gr. *mykos* mucus + *derma* skin] mucous membrane (tunica mucosa [NA]).

mycodermatitis (mi″ko-der″mah-ti′tis) candidiasis.

mycodermomycosis (mi″ko-der″mo-mi-ko′sis) candidiasis.

mycoflora (mi″ko-flo′rah) the number and varieties of fungi present in or characteristic of a specific location.

mycohemia (mi″ko-he′me-ah) [*myco-* + Gr. *haima* blood + *-ia*] the presence of fungi in the blood.

mycologist (mi-kol′o-jist) a person specializing in mycology; a student of mycology.

mycology (mi-kol′o-je) [*myco-* + *-logy*] the science and study of fungi.

mycomyringitis (mi″ko-mir″in-ji′tis) [*myco-* + L. *myringa* membrana tympani + *-itis*] myringomycosis.

Myconostoc (mi″ko-nos′tok) a genus of microorganisms of the family Spirillaceae, suborder Pseudomonadineae, order Pseudomonadales, made up of curved cells occurring singly or in spiral or curved chains and in small gelatinous masses. The type species is *M. gregar′ium.*

mycopathology (mi″ko-pah-thol′o-je) the scientific study of the pathologic changes caused by fungi.

mycophage (mi′ko-fāj) [*myco-* + Gr. *phagein* to eat] a virus that infects fungi and may cause their lysis.

mycophagy (mi-kof′ah-je) ingestion of mushrooms and other fungi.

Mycoplana (mi″ko-pla′nah) a genus of microorganisms of the family Pseudomonadaceae, suborder Pseudomonadineae, order Pseudomonadales, occurring as branching cells in soil. It includes two species, *M. bulla′ta* and *M. dimor′pha.*

Mycoplasma (mi″ko-plaz′mah) [*myco-* + Gr. *plasma* anything formed or molded] a taxonomic name given a genus (family Mycoplasmataceae) of highly pleomorphic, gram-negative, aerobic

to facultatively anaerobic microorganisms differing from bacteria in that they lack a cell wall and are bounded by a triple-layered membrane. The smallest known free-living organisms, they include the pleuropneumonia-like organisms (PPLO) and are separated into species on the basis of source, glucose fermentation, and growth on agar media. **M. fermen′tans,** a species found in the genitourinary tract. **M. gallisep′ticum,** the causative agent of infectious arthritis in chickens and turkeys. **M. granula′rum,** a causative agent of swine arthritis. **m. hom′inis,** a species found in association with nongonococcal urethritis; it has been reported to cause mild pharyngitis in human volunteers. **M. hyoarthrino′sa,** a causative agent of swine arthritis distinct from *M. granularum* although their growth and morphological properties and the arthritis caused by them are similar. **M. hyorhi′nis,** a causative agent of swine arthritis; commonly a secondary invader in pneumonia in swine. **M. mycoi′des,** the type species of *Mycoplasma,* which is the etiologic agent of pleuropneumonia (def. 2); called also *Asterococcus mycoides* and *Bovimyces pleuropneumoniae.* **M. ora′le,** a species found in the upper respiratory tract; called also *M. pharyngis.* **M. pharyn′gis,** *M. orale.* **M. pneumo′niae,** an etiologic agent of primary atypical pneumonia; called also *Eaton agent.* **M. saliva′rium,** a species found in the upper respiratory tract.

mycoplasma (mi″ko-plaz′mah), pl. *mycopla′smas, mycoplas′mata.* Any member of the genus *Mycoplasma.* **T m.,** varieties isolated from the urogenital tract which form small colonies (T for *tiny*) and are otherwise poorly characterized.

mycoplasmal (mi″ko-plaz′mal) of, pertaining to, or caused by *Mycoplasma.*

Mycoplasmataceae (mi″ko-plaz″mah-ta′se-e) a family of the order Mycoplasmatales, which includes the genus *Mycoplasma.*

Mycoplasmatales (mi″ko-plaz″mah-ta′les) an order of bacteria, the members of which lack a true cell wall and are highly pleomorphic organisms reproducing, according to some investigators, by breaking of the filaments into coccoid elementary bodies. It includes a single family, Mycoplasmataceae. In some systems of classification, because of their unusual physical structure, the organisms in this order are considered different from bacteria and have been assigned to a separate class—the Mollicutes.

mycoplasmosis (mi″ko-plaz-mo′sis) infection with *Mycoplasma.*

mycoprecipitin (mi″ko-pre-sip′ĭ-tin) [*myco-* + *precipitin*] a precipitin which will precipitate extracts of yeast and fungi.

mycoproteination (mi″ko-pro″te-in-a′shun) inoculation with dead bacterial cells or fungi, or protein derived from them.

mycopus (mi′ko-pus) mucus containing pus.

mycorrhiza (mi″ko-ri′zah) [*myco-* + Gr. *rhiza* root] a growth occurring as a result of the symbiotic relationship between certain fungi and the roots of plants and trees; it is most frequently found in poor soil, and is associated with the absorption of minerals and nitrogenous material.

mycose (mi′kōs) [*myc-* + *-ose*] a sugar from ergot and also from trehala manna, $C_{12}H_{22}O_{11}$ + $2H_2O$; trehalose.

mycoside (mi′ko-sid) a type-specific glycolipid of mycobacterial origin.

mycosis (mi-ko′sis) [*myco-* + *-osis*] any disease caused by a fungus. **cutaneous m.,** dermatomycosis. **m. framboesioi′des** (*obs.*), yaws. **m. fungoi′des,** a rare, chronic, malignant, lymphoreticular neoplasm of the skin and, in the late stages, the lymph nodes and viscera, marked by the development of large, firm, reddish, painful tumors that ulcerate. The disease usually ends fatally after continuing a number of years. **m. fungoi′des d'emblée,** the tumor stage of mycosis fungoides unheralded by prodromal symptoms. **m. fungoi′des en plaques,** the infiltrative stage of mycosis fungoides. **Gilchrist's m.,** North American blastomycosis. **m. intestina′lis,** anthrax intestinalis. **m. leptoth′rica,** a benign conditon of the tonsil and pharynx produced by *Leptotrichia buccalis.* **Posada m.,** coccidioidomycosis. **splenic m.,** siderotic splenomegaly.

mycostasis (mi-kos′tah-sis) [*myco-* + Gr. *stasis* stoppage] prevention of the growth or multiplication of fungi.

mycostat (mi′ko-stat) an agent that inhibits the growth of fungi.

Mycostatin (mi″ko-stat′in) trademark for a preparation of nystatin.

mycosterol (mi-kos′ter-ol) zymosterol.

mycotic (mi-kot′ik) pertaining to a mycosis; caused by fungi.

mycoticopeptic (mi-kot″ĭ-ko-pep′tik) (*obs.*) both mycotic and peptic.

Mycotoruloides (mi″ko-tor″u-loi′dēz) *Candida.*

mycotoxicosis (mi″ko-tok″sĭ-ko′sis) 1. poisoning caused by a fungal or bacterial toxin. 2. poisoning resulting from ingestion of fungi, such as that caused by the fungus *Claviceps purpurea* (ergotism).

mycotoxin (mi″ko-tok′sin) a fungal toxin.

mycotoxinization (mi″ko-tok″sin-i-za′shun) inoculation with a fungal toxin.

mycteric (mik-ter′ik) [Gr. *myktēr* nostril] pertaining to the nasal cavities.

mycteroxerosis (mik″ter-o-ze-ro′sis) [Gr. *myktēr* nostril + *xēros* dry] dryness of the nostrils.

mydaleine (mi-da′le-in) [Gr. *mydaleos* damp, mouldy] a poisonous ptomaine from putrefied viscera. Poisoning by it is attended with salivation, dilatation of the pupils, rise of temperature followed by a fall, and arrest of the heart in diastole.

mydatoxine (mi″dah-tok′sin) [Gr. *mydan* to be damp + *toxin*] a deadly ptomaine, $C_6H_{13}NO_2$, from decaying flesh; also obtained from human intestines kept for a long time at a low temperature.

Mydriacyl (mǐ-dri′ah-sil) trademark for a preparation of tropicamide.

mydriasis (mǐ-dri′ah-sis) [Gr.] extreme or morbid dilatation of the pupil; dilatation of the pupil as the effect of a drug. **alternating m.,** varying inequality of the pupils, mydriasis occurring first on one side, then on the other; called also *bounding* or *springing m.* **bounding m.,** alternating mydriasis. **paralytic m.,** that caused by paralysis of the oculomotor nerve. **spasmodic m., spastic m.,** that due to spasm of the dilator of the iris or to overaction of the sympathetic. **spinal m.,** that due to lesion of the ciliospinal center of the spinal cord. **springing m.,** alternating m.

mydriatic (mid″re-at′ik) 1. dilating the pupil. 2. any drug that dilates the pupil.

myectomy (mi-ek′to-me) [*my-* + Gr. *ektomē* excision] excision of a portion of muscle.

myectopia (mi-ek-to′pe-ah) [Gr. *mys* muscle + *ektopos* displaced + *-ia*] displacement of a muscle.

myectopy (mi-ek′to-pe) myectopia.

myel- see *myelo-*.

myelacephalus (mi″el-ah-sel′ah-lus) [*myel-* + *a* neg. + Gr. *kephalē* head] the lowest grade of acephalous monster, being only slightly above a fetus amorphus.

myelalgia (mi″ĕ-lal′je-ah) [*myel-* + *-algia*] pain in the spinal cord.

myelanalosis (mi″el-an″ah-lo′sis) [*myel-* + Gr. *analiskein* to spend, waste + *-osis*] wasting of the spinal marrow; tabes dorsalis.

myelapoplexy (mi″el-ap′o-plek-se) [*myel-* + *apoplexy*] hematomyelia.

myelasthenia (mi″el-as-the′ne-ah) [*myel-* + *asthenia*] neurasthenia due to some cause which affects the spinal cord.

myelatelia (mi″el-ah-te′le-ah) [*myel-* + Gr. *ateleia* imperfection] imperfect development of the spinal cord.

myelatrophy (mi″el-at′ro-fe) [*myel-* + *atrophy*] atrophy of the spinal cord.

myelauxe (mi″el-awks′e) [*myel-* + Gr. *auxē* increase] morbid increase in size of the spinal cord.

myelemia (mi″ĕ-le′me-ah) [*myel-* + Gr. *haima* blood + *-ia*] myelocytosis.

myelencephalitis (mi″ĕ-len-sef″ah-li′tis) inflammation of the brain and spinal cord.

myelencephalon (mi″ĕ-len-sef′ah-lon) [*myel-* + Gr. *enkephalos* brain] 1. [NA] the posterior portion of the rhombencephalon, including the medulla oblongata and the lower part of the fourth ventricle; see Plate accompanying *brain.* 2. the posterior of the two brain vesicles formed by specialization of the rhombencephalon in the developing embryo.

myelencephalospinal (mi″ĕ-len-sef″ah-lo-spi′nal) pertaining to the myelencephalon and spinal cord.

myeleterosis (mi″ĕ-let″er-o′sis) [*myel-* + Gr. *heterōsis* alteration] morbid alteration of the spinal cord.

myelin (mi′ĕ-lin) [Gr. *myelos* marrow] 1. the substance of the cell membrane of Schwann's cells that coils to form the myelin sheath (see under *sheath*); it has a high proportion of lipid to protein and serves as an electrical insulator. Called also *white substance of Schwann.* 2. any one of a certain group of lipid substances found in various normal and pathologic tissues and differing from fats in being doubly refractive. 3. a monoaminomonophosphatide found in small quantities in the brain.

myelinated (mi′ĕ-lǐ-nāt″ed) having a myelin sheath.

myelination (mi″ĕ-lǐ-na′shun) myelinization.

myelinic (mi″ĕ-lin′ik) pertaining to or of the nature of myelin.

myelinization (mi″ĕ-li-ni-za′shun) the act of furnishing with or taking on myelin.

myelinoclasis (mi″ĕ-lin-ok′lah-sis) [*myelin* + Gr. *klasis* a breaking] destruction of myelin; demyelination. **acute perivascular m.,** postinfection encephalitis. **central pontine m.,** central pontine myelinolysis. **postinfection perivenous m.,** postinfection encephalomyelopathy.

myelinogenesis (mi″ĕ-lin″o-jen′ĕ-sis) myelinization.

myelinogenetic (mi″ĕ-lin″o-jĕ-net′ik) producing myelin; producing myelinization.

myelinogeny (mi″ĕ-lǐ-noj′ĕ-ne) [*myelin* + Gr. *gennan* to produce] the development of the myelin of nerve fibers; the myelinization of nerve fibers.

myelinolysin (mi″ĕ-lǐ-nol′ǐ-sin) [*myelin* + *lysin*] a lytic substance present in the serum of patients with multiple sclerosis which destroys myelin.

myelinolysis (mi″ĕ-lin-ol′ǐ-sis) destruction of myelin; demyelination. **central pontine m.,** a rare form of massive demyelination of the pons occurring in alcoholics; called also *central pontine myelinoclasis.*

myelinopathy (mi″ĕ-lǐ-nop′ah-the) any disease of the myelin; degeneration of the white matter of the brain.

myelinosis (mi″ĕ-lǐ-no′sis) a form of fatty necrosis in which myelin is formed.

myelinotoxic (mi″ĕ-lin-o-tok′sik) having a deleterious effect on myelin; causing demyelination.

myelinotoxicity (mi″ĕ-lin-o-tok-sis′ĭ-te) the property of being myelinotoxic.

myelitic (mi″ĕ-lit′ik) pertaining to myelitis.

myelitis (mi″ĕ-li′tis) [Gr. *myelos* marrow + *-itis*] 1. inflammation of the spinal cord (see *leukomyelitis, poliomyelitis*). The symptoms of myelitis vary with the location of the lesion, and include pain in the back, girdle sensation, hyperesthesia, formication, anesthesia, motor disturbances, paralysis, increase of the reflexes, paralysis of the sphincters, decubitus ulcers, and, in later stages, spasmodic contractions of the paralyzed limbs. In practice, the term is also used to denote noninflammatory lesions of the spinal cord; see *myelopathy.* 2. inflammation of the bone marrow; see *osteomyelitis.* **acute m.,** any inflammatory disease of the spinal cord. **apoplectiform m.,** see under *myelopathy.* **ascending m.,** see under *myelopathy.* **bulbar m.,** that which involves the medulla oblongata. **cavitary m.,** syringomyelitis. **central m.,** inflammation affecting chiefly the gray substance of the spinal cord. **chronic m.,** a slowly progressing inflammation of the spinal cord. **compression m.,** see under *myelopathy.* **concussion m.,** see under *myelopathy.* **cornual m.,** that which affects the horns of gray matter of the spinal cord. **descending m.,** see under *myelopathy.* **diffuse m.,** inflammation involving large and variously placed sections of the spinal cord. **disseminated m.,** a form with several distinct foci in the spinal cord. **focal m.,** see under *myelopathy.* **foudroyant m.,** central m. **funicular m.,** see under *myelopathy.* **hemorrhagic m.,** see under *myelopathy.* **interstitial m.,** sclerosing myelopathy. **neuro-optic m.,** neuromyelitis optica. **parenchymatous m.,** see under *myelopathy.* **periependymal m.,** myelitis surrounding the central canal of the spinal cord. **sclerosing m.,** see under *myelopathy.* **systemic m.,** see under *myelopathy.* **transverse m.,** see under *myelopathy.* **traumatic m.,** see under *myelopathy.* **m. vaccin′ia,** that which sometimes follows vaccination.

myelo-, myel- [Gr. *myelos* marrow] a combining form denoting relationship to marrow, often used in specific reference to the spinal cord.

myeloarchitecture (mi″ĕ-lo-ar′kǐ-tek″tūr) 1. the arrangement of nerve fibers in the cerebral and cerebellar cortices. 2. the organization of the nerve tracts in the spinal cord and brain stem.

myeloblast (mi′ĕ-lo-blast″) [*myelo-* + Gr. *blastos* germ] an immature cell found in the bone marrow and not normally in the peripheral blood; it is the most primitive precursor in the granulocytic series, which matures to develop into the promyelocyte and eventually the granular leukocyte. Myeloblasts have fine, evenly distributed chromatin, several nucleoli, and a nongranular basophilic cytoplasm. Called also *granuloblast.*

myeloblastemia (mi″ĕ-lo-blas-te′me-ah) [*myeloblast* + Gr. *haima* blood + *-ia*] presence of myeloblasts in the blood.

myeloblastoma (mi″ĕ-lo-blas-to′mah) [*myeloblast* + *-oma*] a focal malignant tumor, observed in acute myelogenous leukemia, composed of myeloblasts and lacking green coloration.

myeloblastomatosis (mi″ĕ-lo-blas″to-mah-to′sis) the presence of multiple myeloblastomas.

myeloblastosis (mi″ĕ-lo-blas-to′sis) the presence of an excess of myeloblasts in the blood.

myelocele (mi′ĕ-lo-sēl) [*myelo-* + Gr. *kēlē* hernia] protrusion of the substance of the spinal cord through a defect in the bony spinal canal.

myeloclast (mi′ĕ-lo-klast) [*myelo-* + Gr. *klan* to break] a cell which splits up myelin sheaths.

myelocoele (mi-el′o-sēl) [*myelo-* + Gr. *koilia* cavity] (*obs.*) the central canal of the spinal cord.

myelocone (mi′ĕ-lo-kōn) [*myelo-* + Gr. *konis* dust] a fatty matter from the brain.

myelocyst (mi′ĕ-lo-sist) [*myelo-* + *cyst*] a benign cyst developed from rudimentary medullary canals.

myelocystic (mi″ĕ-lo-sis′tik) both myeloid and cystic in structure.

myelocystocele (mi″ĕ-lo-sis′to-sēl) [*myelo-* + Gr. *kēlē* hernia] myelomeningocele.

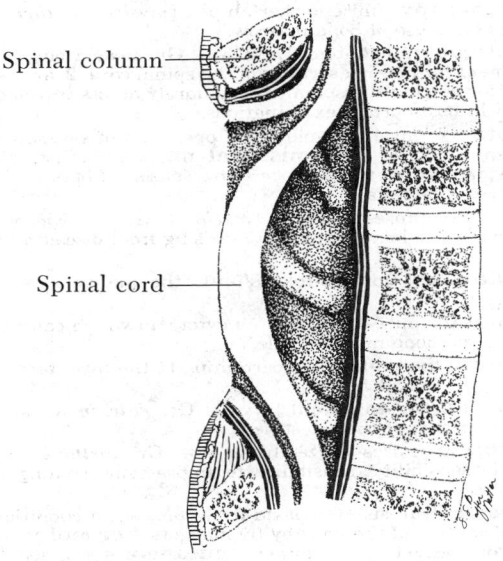

Spinal column

Spinal cord

Myelocele in cross-section (after Netter, from Ciba Collection).

myelocystomeningocele (mi″ĕ-lo-sis″to-mĕ-ning′go-sēl) myelomeningocele.

myelocyte (mi′ĕ-lo-sit) [myelo- + -cyte] 1. a precursor in the granulocytic series, being a cell intermediate in development between a promyelocyte and a metamyelocyte; in this stage, differentiation into specific cytoplasmic granules has begun. 2. any cell of the gray matter of the nervous system.

myelocythemia (mi″ĕ-lo-si-the′me-ah) [myelocyte + Gr. haima blood + -ia] excess of myelocytes in the blood.

myelocytic (mi″ĕ-lo-sit′ik) relating to or of the nature of myelocytes.

myelocytoma (mi″ĕ-lo-si-to′mah) chronic myelocytic leukemia; myeloma, def. 1.

myelocytomatosis (mi″ĕ-lo-si″to-mah-to′sis) 1. (obs.) a form of leukosis in which the myelocytes are chiefly involved. 2. a disease of fowl that is included in the avian leukosis complex, marked by the presence of tumors composed of myeloid cells. There may also be an increase of immature myeloid cells in the circulating blood.

myelocytosis (mi″ĕ-lo-si-to′sis) the presence of an excessive number of myelocytes in the blood; myelosis.

myelodysplasia (mi″ĕ-lo-dis-pla′se-ah) [myelo- + dys- + Gr. plassein to form] defective development of any part (especially the lower segments) of the spinal cord.

myeloencephalic (mi″ĕ-lo-en″sĕ-fal′ik) pertaining to the spinal cord and the brain.

myeloencephalitis (mi″ĕ-lo-en-sef″ah-li′tis) [myelo- + Gr. enkephalos brain + -itis] inflammation of the spinal cord and brain. **epidemic m.**, epidemic polioencephalitis.

myelofibrosis (mi″ĕ-lo-fi-bro′sis) replacement of the bone marrow by fibrous tissue, occurring in association with a myeloproliferative disorder or secondary to another, unrelated condition; called also myelosclerosis. See also myeloid metaplasia, under metaplasia. **osteosclerosis m.**, myelosclerosis, def. 2.

myelofugal (mi″ĕ-lof′u-gal) [myelo- + L. fugare to flee] moving away from the spinal cord.

myelogenesis (mi″ĕ-lo-jen′ĕ-sis) 1. the development of the nervous system, especially of the brain and spinal cord. 2. the deposition of myelin around the axon.

myelogenic (mi″ĕ-lo-jen′ik) myelogenous.

myelogenous (mi″ĕ-loj′ĕ-nus) [myelo- + Gr. gennan to produce] produced in the bone marrow.

myelogeny (mi″ĕ-loj′ĕ-ne) the maturation of the myelin sheaths of nerve fibers in the development of the central nervous system.

myelogone (mi′ĕ-lo-gōn″) a white blood cell of the myeloid series having a reticulate violaceous nucleus, well-stained nucleolus, and a deep blue rim of cytoplasm.

myelogonic (mi″ĕ-lo-go′nik) characterized by the presence of myelogones.

myelogonium (mi″ĕ-lo-go′ne-um) myelogone.

myelogram (mi′ĕ-lo-gram) 1. a roentgenogram of the spinal cord. 2. a graphic representation of the differential count of cells found in a stained preparation of bone marrow.

myelography (mi″ĕ-log′rah-fe) [myelo- + Gr. graphein to write] roentgenography of the spinal cord after injection of a contrast medium into the subarachnoid space. **oxygen m.**, myelography in which oxygen is used as the contrast medium.

myeloid (mi′ĕ-loid) [myelo- + Gr. eidos form] 1. pertaining to, derived from, or resembling bone marrow. 2. pertaining to the spinal cord. 3. having the appearance of myelocytes, but not derived from bone marrow.

myeloidin (mi″ĕ-loi′din) [myelin + Gr. eidos form] a substance resembling myelin, occurring in the pigmented cells of the retina.

myeloidosis (mi″ĕ-loi-do′sis) the development of myeloid tissue, especially hyperplastic development of such tissue.

myelokentric (mi″ĕ-lo-ken′trik) [myeloid + Gr. kentron stimulus] stimulating the formation of myeloid cells. Cf. lymphokentric.

myelolipoma (mi″ĕ-lo-li-po′mah) a rare benign tumor of the adrenal gland, several centimeters in diameter, composed in varying proportions of adipose tissue, lymphocytes, and primitive myeloid cell, probably a developmental abnormality.

myelolymphangioma (mi″ĕ-lo-lim-fan″je-o′mah) elephantiasis.

myelolysis (mi″ĕ-lol′ĭ-sis) [myelin + Gr. lysis dissolution] the dissolution of myelin.

myelolytic (mi″ĕ-lo-lit′ik) pertaining to, characterized by, or causing myelolysis.

myeloma (mi″ĕ-lo′mah) [myelo- + -oma] a tumor composed of cells of the type normally found in the bone marrow; see multiple m. **endothelial m.**, Ewing's tumor. **extramedullary m.**, a plasmacytoma (plasma cell tumor) occurring outside the bone marrow. **giant cell m.**, giant cell tumor of bone. **multiple m.**, a malignant neoplasm of plasma cells usually arising in the bone marrow and manifested by skeletal destruction, pathologic fractures, and bone pain, and by the presence of anomalous circulating immunoglobulins (paraproteins), Bence-Jones proteinuria, and anemia; it is the most common form of monoclonal gammopathy. Called also plasma cell m. See also plasmacytoma. **osteosclerotic m.**, multiple myeloma associated with osteosclerosis (rather than bone destruction) and often with peripheral neuropathy. **plasma cell m.**, multiple m. **plasma cell m., peripheral**, plasmacytoma.

myelomalacia (mi″ĕ-lo-mah-la′she-ah) [myelo- + Gr. malakia softening] morbid softening of the spinal cord.

myelomatoid (mi″ĕ-lo′mah-toid) resembling myeloma.

myelomatosis (mi″ĕ-lo-mah-to′sis) multiple myeloma.

myelomenia (mi″ĕ-lo-me′ne-ah) [myelo- + Gr. mēn month] menstrual hemorrhage into the spinal cord, associated with plaques of endometriosis in the spinal canal.

myelomeningitis (mi″ĕ-lo-men″in-ji′tis) [myelo- + meningitis] inflammation of the spinal cord and its membranes.

myelomeningocele (mi″ĕ-lo-mĕ-ning′go-sēl) [myelo- + meningocele] hernial protrusion of the cord and its meninges through a defect in the vertebral canal.

myelomere (mi′ĕ-lo-mēr) [myelo- + Gr. meros part] one of the segments of the developing brain and spinal cord.

myelomyces (mi″ĕ-lom′ĭ-sēz) [myelo- + Gr. mykēs fungus] medullary carcinoma.

myelon (mi′ĕ-lon) [Gr. myelos marrow] (obs.) the spinal cord (medulla spinalis [NA]).

myeloneuritis (mi″ĕ-lo-nu-ri′tis) inflammation of both spinal cord and peripheral nerves.

myelonic (mi″ĕ-lon′ik) pertaining to the myelon; myeloid.

myelo-opticoneuropathy (mi″ĕ-lo-op″tĭ-ko-nu-rop′ah-the) a disorder affecting the spinal cord and optic nerve. **subacute m.**, a clinical syndrome reported from Japan affecting the spinal cord, optic nerve, and peripheral nerves, preceded by diarrhea. Symptoms include paresthesia in both lower limbs, gait disturbances, visual disturbances, abnormalities of deep tendon reflexes, and psychic disorders. The hydroxyquinolones (especially clioquinol), taken for gastrointestinal disorders, have been implicated as an etiologic factor. Abbreviated SMON.

myelopathic (mi″ĕ-lo-path′ik) pertaining to or characterized by myelopathy.

myelopathy (mi″ĕ-lop′ah-the) [myelo- + Gr. pathos disease] 1. a general term denoting functional disturbances and/or pathological changes in the spinal cord; the term is often used to designate nonspecific lesions, in contrast to inflammatory lesions (myelitis). 2. pathological changes in the bone marrow. **apoplectiform m.**, myelopathy in which paralysis comes on suddenly. **ascending m.**, myelopathy that progresses cephalad along the spinal cord. **compression m.**, myelopathy due to pressure on the spinal cord, as from a tumor. **concussion m.**, myelopathy due to spinal concussion. **descending m.**, myelopathy that progresses caudad along the spinal cord. **focal m.**, myelopathy affecting a small area only, or several small areas. **funicular m.**, myelopathy involving the white matter of the spinal cord, especially the posterior funiculus; it is characteristic of pernicious anemia. **hemorrhagic m.**, myelopathy associated with hemorrhage. **interstitial m.**, sclerosing m. **parenchymatous m.**, myelopathy in which the proper nerve substance of the spinal cord is chiefly affected. **sclerosing m.**, myelopathy marked by hardening of the spinal cord and overgrowth of the glia; called also *interstitial m.* **spondylotic cervical m.,** myelopathy secondary to encroachment of cervical spondylosis upon a congenitally small cervical spinal canal. **systemic m.,** myelopathy which affects distinct tracts or systems in the spinal cord. **transverse m.,** myelopathy which extends across the spinal cord. **traumatic m.,** myelopathy which follows injury to the spinal cord.

myeloperoxidase (mi″ĕ-lo-per-ok′sĭ-das) a hemoprotein which has peroxidase activity, occurring in the primary granules of promyelocytes, myelocytes, and neutrophils, and which exhibits bactericidal, fungicidal, and viricidal properties.

myelopetal (mi″ĕ-lop′ĕ-tal) [*myelo-* + L. *petere* to seek for] moving toward the spinal cord.

myelophage (mi′ĕ-lo-fāj″) [*myelo-* + Gr. *phagein* to eat] a macrophage which digests or breaks down myelin.

myelophthisis (mi″ĕ-lof′thĭ-sis) [*myelo-* + Gr. *phthisis* wasting] 1. wasting of the spinal cord. 2. reduction of the cell-forming functions of the bone marrow; see *aleukia haemorrhagica.*

myeloplaque (mi-el′o-plak) myeloplax.

myeloplast (mi′ĕ-lo-plast″) [*myelo-* + Gr. *plastos* formed] any leukocyte of the bone marrow.

myeloplax (mi-el′o-plaks″) [*myelo-* + Gr. *plax* plate] any multinuclear giant cell of the bone marrow.

myeloplegia (mi″ĕ-lo-ple′je-ah) [*myelo-* + Gr. *plēgē* stroke] spinal paralysis.

myelopoiesis (mi″ĕ-lo-poi-e′sis) [*myelo-* + Gr. *poiein* to form] the formation of bone marrow or the cells that arise from it. **ectopic m., extramedullary m.,** the formation of myeloid tissue outside the bone marrow.

myelopore (mi′ĕ-lo-pōr) [*myelo-* + Gr. *poros* opening] a canal or opening in the spinal cord.

myeloproliferative (mi″ĕ-lo-pro-lif″er-a′tiv) pertaining to or characterized by medullary and extramedullary proliferation of bone marrow constituents; see *myeloproliferative syndrome.*

myeloradiculitis (mi″ĕ-lo-rah-dik″u-li′tis) [*myelo-* + L. *radiculus* rootlet + *-itis*] inflammation of the spinal cord and the posterior nerve roots.

myeloradiculodysplasia (mi″ĕ-lo-rah-dik″u-lo-dis-pla′ze-ah) developmental abnormality of the spinal cord and spinal nerve roots.

myeloradiculopathy (mi″ĕ-lo-rah-dik″u-lop′ah-the) disease of the spinal cord and spinal nerve roots.

myelorrhagia (mi″ĕ-lo-ra′je-ah) [*myelo-* + Gr. *rhēgnynai* to burst forth] hematomyelia.

myelosarcoma (mi″ĕ-lo-sar-ko′mah) a sarcomatous growth made up of myeloid tissue or bone marrow cells.

myelosarcomatosis (mi″ĕ-lo-sar-ko″mah-to′sis) myelomatosis.

myeloschisis (mi″ĕ-los′kĭ-sis) [*myelo-* + Gr. *schisis* cleft] a developmental anomaly characterized by a cleft spinal cord, owing to failure of the neural plate to form a complete tube or to rupture of the neural tube after closure.

myeloscintogram (mi″ĕ-lo-sin′to-gram) the graphic record of particles counted by a scintillation counter after injection into the subarachnoid space of a solution containing a radioactive isotope.

myelosclerosis (mi″ĕ-lo-skle-ro′sis) 1. sclerosis of the spinal cord. 2. a condition characterized by obliteration of the normal marrow cavity by the formation of small spicules of bone, the pathogenesis possibly being similar to that of myelofibrosis; called also *osteosclerosis myelofibrosis.* 3. myelofibrosis.

myelosis (mi″ĕ-lo′sis) 1. the proliferation of marrow tissue which produces the blood changes of myelocytic leukemia; myelocytosis. 2. the formation of a tumor of the spinal cord. **aleukemic m.,** agnogenic myeloid metaplasia; see also *pseudoleukemia.* **chronic nonleukemic m.,** agnogenic myeloid metaplasia. **erythremic m.,** a malignant blood dyscrasia regarded as one of the myeloproliferative disorders and characterized by progressive anemia, megaloblastic erythroid hyperplasia, myeloid dysplasia, hepatosplenomegaly, and hemorrhagic phenomena. Called also *Di Guglielmo's disease* or *syndrome.* Cf. *erythroleukemia.* **funicular m.,** myelosis marked by degenerative foci in the white substance of the spinal cord. **nonleukemic m.,** agnogenic myeloid metaplasia.

myelospasm (mi′ĕ-lo-spazm) [*myelo-* + *spasm*] (*obs.*) spasm due to disease of the spinal cord.

myelospongium (mi″ĕ-lo-spon′je-um) [*myelo-* + Gr. *spongos* sponge] the network from which the neuroglial tissue is developed: it pervades the embryonic neural tube, and is composed of the spongioblasts and their branching processes.

myelosuppressive (mi″ĕ-lo-sŭ-pres′iv) 1. inhibiting bone marrow activity, resulting in decreased production of blood cells and platelets. 2. an agent having such properties.

myelosyphilis (mi″ĕ-lo-sif′ĭ-lis) syphilis of the spinal cord.

myelosyphilosis (mi″ĕ-lo-sif″ĭ-lo′sis) any syphilitic affection of the spinal cord.

myelosyringosis (mi″ĕ-lo-sir″ing-go′sis) [*myelo-* + Gr. *syrinx* pipe] syringomyelia.

myelotherapy (mi″ĕ-lo-ther′ah-pe) [*myelo-* + *therapy*] the therapeutic use of bone marrow.

myelotome (mi-el′o-tōm) [*myelo-* + Gr. *tomē* a cut] 1. an instrument for making sections of the spinal cord. 2. an instrument used for cutting the spinal cord squarely across in removing the brain in postmortem examinations.

myelotomy (mi″ĕ-lot′o-me) the operation of severing tracts in the spinal cord. **commissural m.,** longitudinal division of the spinal cord, to sever crossing sensory fibers and produce localized analgesia.

myelotoxic (mi″ĕ-lo-tok′sik) [*myelo-* + Gr. *toxikon* poison] 1. destructive to bone marrow. 2. arising from diseased bone marrow.

myelotoxicity (mi″ĕ-lo-toks-is′ĭ-te) the quality of being myelotoxic.

myelotoxin (mi″ĕ-lo-tok′sin) a cytotoxin which causes destruction of the bone marrow cells.

myenteric (mi″en-ter′ik) pertaining to the myenteron; see also under *plexus* and *reflex.*

myenteron (mi-en′ter-on) [*my-* + Gr. *enteron* intestine] the muscular coat of the intestine.

myesthesia (mi″es-the′ze-ah) [*my-* + Gr. *aisthēsis* perception] muscle sensibility; sensibility to impressions coming from the muscles.

myiasis (mi′yah-sis) [Gr. *myia* fly + *-iasis*] a condition caused by infestation of the body by fly maggots. **creeping m.,** larva migrans caused by fly larvae. **cutaneous m.,** see *larva migrans.* **dermal m.,** see *larva migrans.* **m. dermato′sa,** infection of the skin with the larvae of flies. **intestinal m.,** the presence of living fly larvae in the intestines. **m. linea′ris,** larva migrans caused by fly larvae. **nasal m.,** myiasis produced by living fly larvae in the nasal passages. **traumatic m.,** maggot infestation of wounds or ulcers.

myiocephalon (mi″yo-sef′ah-lon) [Gr. *myia* fly + *kephalē* head] projection of the iris through a rent in the cornea.

myiocephalum (mi″yo-sef′ah-lum) myiocephalon.

myiodesopsia (mi″yo-des-op′se-ah) [Gr. *myiōdes* flylike + *opsis* vision + *-ia*] the appearance of muscae volitantes.

myiosis (mi-yo′sis) myiasis.

myitis (mi-i′tis) [*my-* + *-itis*] inflammation of a muscle; myositis.

myko- for words beginning thus, see those beginning *myco-.*

Mylaxen (mi-lak′sin) trademark for a preparation of hexafluorenium bromide.

Myleran (mil′er-an) trademark for a preparation of busulfan.

Mylicon (mi′lĭ-kon) trademark for preparations of simethicone.

myo-, my- [Gr. *mys* muscle] a combining form denoting relationship to muscle.

myoalbumin (mi″o-al-bu′min) an albumin constituting about one per cent of the protein of muscle.

myoarchitectonic (mi″o-ar″ke-tek-ton′ik) [*myo-* + *architectonic*] pertaining to the structure of muscle.

myoasthenia (mi″o-as-the′ne-ah) amyosthenia.

myoatrophy (mi″o-at′ro-fe) myatrophy.

myoblast (mi′o-blast) [*myo-* + Gr. *blastos* germ] an embryonic cell which becomes a cell of the muscle fiber.

myoblastic (mi″o-blas′tik) pertaining to a myoblast.

myoblastoma (mi″o-blas-to′mah) a benign circumscribed tumor-like lesion of soft tissue; see *granular cell tumor,* under *tumor.* **granular cell m.,** see under *tumor.*

myoblastomyoma (mi″o-blas″to-mi-o′mah) myoblastoma.

myobradia (mi″o-bra′de-ah) [*myo-* + Gr. *bradys* slow + *-ia*] a slow, sluggish reaction of muscle to electric stimulation.

myocardiac (mi″o-kar′de-ak) myocardial.

myocardial (mi″o-kar′de-al) pertaining to the muscular tissue of the heart; see also under *infarction.*

myocardiogram (mi″o-kar′de-o-gram) a tracing made by the myocardiograph.

myocardiograph (mi″o-kar′de-o-graf″) [*myo-* + Gr. *kardia* heart + *graphein* to record] an instrument for making a tracing of the movements of the heart muscles.

myocardiolysis (mi″o-kar″de-ol′ĭ-sis) local necrosis of the myocardial fibers due to arterial obstruction, in which the fibers are replaced by scar tissue and often, especially when complicated by thrombosis, leading to gross infarction.

myocardiopathy (mi″o-kar″de-op′ah-the) any noninflammatory disease of the muscular walls (myocardium) of the heart. **alcoholic m.,** a form attributed to ingestion of large amounts of alcohol over an extended period of time, characterized chiefly by enlargement of the heart and myocardial degenerative changes, particularly evident on electron microscopy. **chagasic m.,** myocardiopathy with saccular apical ventricular aneurysm associated with Chagas' disease.

myocardiorrhaphy (mi″o-kar″de-or′ah-fe) suture of wounds of the myocardium.

myocardiosis (mi″o-kar″de-o′sis) myocardosis.

myocarditic (mi″o-kar-dit′ik) pertaining to myocarditis.

myocarditis (mi″o-kar-di′tis) [*myo-* + Gr. *kardia* heart + *-itis*] inflammation of the myocardium; inflammation of the muscular walls of the heart. **acute bacterial m.,** acute myocarditis due to bacterial infection. **acute isolated m.,** acute interstitial myocarditis of unknown etiology, marked by sudden onset, absence of endocarditis or pericarditis, and frequently by a fatal outcome; called also *Fiedler's m.* and *idiopathic m.* **chronic m.,** chronic myocardial inflammatory disease; often used loosely to indicate any myocardial deficiency. **diphtheritic m.,** acute myocarditis leaving no permanent damage, occurring in diphtheria. **fibrous m.,** chronic interstitial m. **Fiedler's m.,** acute isolated m. **fragmentation m.,** fragmentation of the myocardium. **giant cell m.,** a granulomatous form of myocarditis in which large discrete foci form, each containing many lymphocytes and macrophages, and sometimes multinucleate giant cells not unlike those found in tuberculosis; called also *tuberculoid myocarditis.* **idiopathic m.,** acute isolated m. **interstitial m.,** myocarditis affecting chiefly the interstitial fibrous tissue. **parenchymatous m.,** myocarditis affecting chiefly the muscle substance itself. **rheumatic m.,** a common sequela of rheumatic fever characterized histologically by perivascular granulomata known as Aschoff bodies or nodules. **toxic m.,** myocarditis due to poisoning by drug or to toxins of infecting organisms reaching the heart through the blood stream, as in diphtheria. **tuberculoid m.,** giant cell m. **tuberculous m.,** tuberculosis of the myocardium.

myocardium (mi″o-kar′de-um) [*myo-* + Gr. *kardia* heart] [NA] the middle and thickest layer of the heart wall, composed of cardiac muscle.

myocardosis (mi″o-kar-do′sis) a general term for disorders of the myocardium which are not inflammatory, but which may result from hypertension, coronary sclerosis, and hyperthyroidism.

myocele (mi′o-sēl) [*myo-* + Gr. *kēlē* hernia] hernia of muscle; protrusion of a muscle through its ruptured sheath.

myocelialgia (mi″o-se′le-al′je-ah) [*myo-* + Gr. *koilia* belly + *-algia*] pain in the abdominal muscles.

myocelitis (mi″o-se-li′tis) [*myo-* + Gr. *koilia* belly + *-itis*] inflammation of the muscles of the abdomen.

myocellulitis (mi″o-sel″u-li′tis) myositis conjoined with cellulitis.

myoceptor (mi′o-sep″tor) [*myo-* + L. *capere* to take] end-plate.

myocerosis (mi″o-se-ro′sis) [*myo-* + Gr. *kēros* wax] waxy degeneration of muscle.

myochorditis (mi″o-kor-di′tis) [*myo-* + Gr. *chordē* cord + *-itis*] inflammation of the muscles of the vocal cords.

myochrome (mi′o-krōm) [*myo-* + Gr. *chrōma* color] any member of a group of muscle pigments; see *cytochrome* (def. 1) and *myohematin.*

Myochrysine (mi″o-kri′sin) trademark for a preparation of gold sodium thiomalate.

myocinesimeter (mi″o-sin″ĕ-sim′ĕ-ter) myokinesimeter.

myoclonia (mi″o-klo′ne-ah) any disorder characterized by myoclonus. **m. epilep′tica,** myoclonus epilepsy. **m. fibrilla′ris mul′tiplex,** myokymia. **fibrillary m.,** the twitching of the fibrils of a muscle; see *fibrillation,* def. 2. **pseudoglottic m.,** hiccup.

myoclonic (mi″o-klon′ik) relating to or marked by myoclonus.

myoclonus (mi-ok′lo-nus) [*myo-* + Gr. *klonos* turmoil] shock-like contractions of a portion of a muscle, an entire muscle, or a group of muscles, restricted to one area of the body or appearing synchronously or asynchronously in several areas. **m. mul′tiplex,** paramyoclonus multiplex. **palatal m.,** a condition characterized by a rapid rhythmic, up-and-down movement of one or both sides of the palate, often accompanied by ipsilateral synchronous clonic movements of muscles of the face, tongue, pharynx, and diaphragm. Called also *palatal nystagmus.*

myocoele (mi′o-sēl) [*myo-* + Gr. *koilia* cavity] the cavity within a myotome (def. 2).

myocolpitis (mi″o-kol-pi′tis) [*myo-* + Gr. *kolpos* vagina + *-itis*] inflammation of the muscular layers of the vaginal wall.

myocomma (mi″o-kom′ah) [*myo-* + Gr. *komma* cut] 1. a myotome or muscle segment, as in a fish. 2. the septum between two adjacent myotomes.

myocrismus (mi″o-kris′mus) [*myo-* + Gr. *krizein* to creak] a sound heard on auscultation over a contracting muscle.

myoctonine (mi-ok′to-nin) [*myo-* + Gr. *kteinein* to kill] a poisonous alkaloid, $C_{36}H_{42}N_2O_{10}$, from *Aconitum lycoctonum.*

myoculator (mi-ok′u-la″tor) [*myo-* + L. *oculus* eye] an ocular instrument, on the principle of the orthoptoscope, which allows fusion and movement laterally, vertically, and in rotation.

myocyte (mi′o-sīt) [*myo-* + *-cyte*] 1. a cell of the muscular tissue. 2. the innermost layer of myonemes in the ectoplasm of certain gregarine protozoons. **Anichkov's m.,** a myocyte found in Aschoff's bodies, having a serrated bar of chromatin in its nucleus; called also *cardiac histiocyte.*

myocytolysis (mi″o-si-tol′ĭ-sis) disintegration of muscle fibers. **focal m. of heart,** a miliary lesion characterized by loss of muscular syncytium, preservation of stroma, absence of inflammatory reaction, and eventual necrosis.

myocytoma (mi″o-si-to′mah) a tumor made up of myocytes or muscle cells.

myodegeneration (mi″o-de-jen″er-a′shun) [*myo-* + *degeneration*] degeneration of muscle.

myodemia (mi″o-de′me-ah) [*myo-* + Gr. *dēmos* fat] fatty degeneration of muscle.

myodesopsia (mi″o-des-op′se-ah) myiodesopsia.

myodiastasis (mi″o-di-as′tah-sis) [*myo-* + Gr. *diastasis* separation] separation of a muscle.

myodiopter (mi″o-di-op′ter) the force of ciliary muscle contraction necessary to raise the refraction of the emmetropic eye by 1 diopter from a state of rest.

myodynamic (mi″o-di-nam′ik) relating to muscular force.

myodynamics (mi″o-di-nam′iks) the physiology of muscular action.

myodynamometer (mi″o-di″nah-mom′ĕ-ter) [*myo-* + Gr. *dynamis* power + *metron* measure] a device for testing the power of the muscles.

myodynia (mi″o-din′e-ah) [*myo-* + Gr. *odynē* pain] pains in a muscle; myalgia. **hysterical m.,** muscular pain or tenderness, generally in the ovarian region, in hysteria.

myodystonia (mi″o-dis-to′ne-ah) [*myo-* + *dys-* + Gr. *tonos* tension + *-ia*] disorder of muscular tone.

myodystony (mi″o-dis′to-ne) myodystonia.

myodystrophia (mi″o-dis-tro′fe-ah) muscular dystrophy; myotonia atrophica. **m. feta′lis,** amyoplasia congenita.

myodystrophy (mi″o-dis′tro-fe) myodystrophia.

myoedema (mi″o-ĕ-de′mah) [*myo-* + Gr. *oidēma* swelling] 1. edema of a muscle. 2. mounding.

myoelastic (mi″o-e-las′tik) composed of elastic fibers associated with smooth muscle cells.

myoelectric, myoelectrical (mi″o-e-lek′trik; mi″o-e-lek′trĭkal) pertaining to the electric or electromotive properties of muscle.

myoendocarditis (mi″o-en″do-kar-di′tis) combined myocarditis and endocarditis.

myoepithelial (mi″o-ep″ĭ-the′le-al) pertaining to or composed of myoepithelium.

myoepithelioma (mi″o-ep″ĭ-the″le-o′mah) a tumor composed of outgrowths of myoepithelial cells from the acini or, occasionally, the ducts of a sweat gland; it is usually well delineated by a condensation of connective tissue around it.

myoepithelium (mi″o-ep″ĭ-the′le-um) [*myo-* + *epithelium*] tissue made up of contractile epithelial cells.

myofascitis (mi″o-fah-si′tis) [*myo-* + *fasciitis*] inflammation of a muscle and its fascia, particularly of the fascial insertion of muscle to bone.

myofibril (mi″o-fi′bril) a muscle fibril, one of the slender threads which can be rendered visible in a muscle fiber by maceration in certain acids. They run parallel with the long axis of the fiber, and are composed of numerous myofilaments (q.v.).

myofibrilla (mi″o-fi-bril′ah), pl. *myofibril′lae.* A myofibril.

myofibrillae (mi″o-fi-bril′e) plural of *myofibrilla.*

myofibrillar (mi″o-fi′bril-ar) relating to a myofibril.

myofibroblast (mi″o-fi′bro-blast) an atypical fibroblast combining the ultrastructural features of a fibroblast and a smooth muscle cell; it has a highly irregular nucleus, a large amount of rough endoplasmic reticulum, and a dense collection of myofilaments.

myofibroma (mi″o-fi-bro′mah) a tumor containing both muscular and fibrous elements; fibroid leiomyoma.

myofibrosis (mi″o-fi-bro′sis) [*myo-* + L. *fibra* fiber] replacement of muscle tissue by fibrous tissue. **m. cor′dis,** myofibrosis of the heart.

myofibrositis (mi″o-fi″bro-si′tis) inflammation of the perimysium; perimysiitis.

myofilament (mi″o-fil′ah-ment) [*myo-* + *filament*] any of the numerous ultramicroscopic threadlike structures occurring in bundles in the myofibrils of striated muscle fibers. The thick filaments are composed of myosin, the thin ones of actin; together they are responsible for the contractile properties of muscle.

myofunctional (mi″o-funk′shun-al) pertaining to muscular function: a term applied to various exercises prescribed to eliminate abnormal perioral muscle function associated with various types of malocclusion.

myogelosis (mi″o-jĕ-lo′sis) [*myo-* + L. *gelare* to freeze] an area of hardening in a muscle, especially in the gluteus muscle.

myogen (mi′o-jen) [*myo-* + Gr. *gennan* to produce] an albumin-like protein, constituting 10 per cent of the protein of muscle; it is spontaneously coagulable, passing first into soluble myogen fibrin, and then into myosin fibrin. Cf. *myosin.*

myogenesis (mi″o-jen′ĕ-sis) the development of muscle tissue, especially its embryonic development.

myogenetic (mi″o-jĕ-net′ik) pertaining to myogenesis.

myogenic (mi″o-jen′ik) giving rise to or forming muscle tissue.

myogenous (mi-oj′ĕ-nus) originating in muscle tissue.

myoglia (mi-og′le-ah) [*myo-* + Gr. *glia* glue] a fibrillar substance formed by muscle cells, and present only during early embryogenesis of muscle fibers; called also *border fibrils*.

myoglobin (mi″o-glo′bin) the oxygen-transporting pigment of muscle, a conjugated protein resembling a single subunit of hemoglobin, being composed of one globin polypeptide chain and one heme group (containing one iron atom); it combines with oxygen released by erythrocytes, stores it, and transports it to the mitochondria of muscle cells, where it generates energy by combustion of glucose to carbon dioxide and water.

myoglobinuria (mi″o-glo″bin-u′re-ah) the presence of myoglobin in the urine, as in deficiency of muscle phosphorylase, in crush injuries, and after vigorous and prolonged exercise in susceptible persons. **idiopathic m.,** Meyer-Betz disease. **spontaneous m.,** Meyer-Betz disease.

myoglobulin (mi″o-glob′u-lin) [*myo-* + *globulin*] a globulin found in muscle serum.

myoglobulinuria (mi″o-glob″u-lin-u′re-ah) the presence of myoglobulin in the urine.

myognathus (mi-og′nah-thus) [*myo-* + Gr. *gnathos* jaw] a monster with a supernumerary lower jaw attached to the normally placed lower jaw.

myogram (mi′o-gram) [*myo-* + Gr. *gramma* writing] the record or tracing made by a myograph.

myograph (mi′o-graf) [*myo-* + Gr. *graphein* to record] an apparatus for recording the effects of a muscular contraction.

myographic (mi″o-graf′ik) pertaining to a myograph or to myography.

myography (mi-og′rah-fe) [*myo-* + Gr. *graphein* to record] 1. the use of the myograph. 2. a description of the muscles. 3. roentgenography of muscle tissue after injection of an opaque medium.

myohematin (mi″o-hem′ah-tin) [*myo-* + *hematin*] MacMunn's name for the cytochrome of muscle tissue, an iron-containing catalyst of tissue oxidation; see *cytochrome*, def. 1.

myohemoglobin (mi″o-he″mo-glo′bin) myoglobin.

myohypertrophia (mi″o-hi″per-tro′fe-ah) muscular hypertrophy. **m. kymoparalyt′ica,** a muscular dystrophy, with paralysis, described by Oppenheim (1914).

myoid (mi′oid) [*myo-* + Gr. *eidos* form] 1. resembling or like a muscle. 2. a substance resembling muscle. **cone m.,** the contractile portion of the inner member of the visual cones. **rod m.,** the contractile portion of the inner member of the visual rods.

myoidem (mi-oi′dem) myoedema.

myoidema (mi″o-i-de′mah) myoedema.

myoideum (mi-oi′de-um) myoid tissue.

myoidism (mi-o-id′izm) [*myo-* + Gr. *idios* own] idiomuscular contraction.

myo-inositol (mi″o-in-o′sĭ-tol) inositol, def. 2.

myoischemia (mi″o-is-ke′me-ah) [*myo-* + *ischemia*] local deficiency of blood supply in muscle.

myokerosis (mi″o-ke-ro′sis) [*myo-* + Gr. *kēros* wax] myocerosis.

myokinase (mi″o-kin′ās) adenylate kinase.

myokinesimeter (mi″o-kin″ĕ-sim′ĕ-ter) [*myokinesis* + Gr. *metron* measure] an apparatus for measuring muscular contraction aroused by stimulation by an electric current.

myokinesis (mi″o-ki-ne′sis) [*myo-* + Gr. *kinēsis* motion] movement of muscles, especially displacement of muscle fibers in operation.

myokinetic (mi″o-ki-net′ik) 1. pertaining to or characterized by myokinesis. 2. pertaining to the motion or kinetic function of muscle, as contrasted with the myotonic or tonic function.

myokinin (mi″o-kin′in) a base, $C_{11}H_{28}N_2O_3$, found in muscle.

myokymia (mi″o-kim′e-ah) [*myo-* + Gr. *kyma* wave] a benign condition marked by brief spontaneous tetanic contractions of motor units or groups of muscle fibers, usually adjacent groups of fibers contracting alternately. Called also *myoclonia fibrillaris multiplex.*

myolemma (mi″o-lem′ah) [*myo-* + Gr. *lemma* sheath] the sarcolemma.

myolin (mi′o-lin) the supposed material of the muscular fibrils.

myolipoma (mi″o-li-po′mah) [*myo-* + Gr. *lipos* fat + *-oma*] myoma (leiomyoma) containing fatty or lipomatous elements; called also *benign mesenchymoma.*

myologia (mi″o-lo′je-ah) myology; in NA terminology, *myologia* encompasses the nomenclature relating to the muscles and to the bursae and synovial sheaths.

myology (mi-ol′o-je) [*myo-* + Gr. *logos* treatise] the scientific study of muscles, and the body of knowledge relating thereto.

myolysis (mi-ol′ĭ-sis) [*myo-* + Gr. *lysis* dissolution] disintegration or degeneration of muscle tissue. **m. cardiotox′ica,** degeneration of the heart muscle due to systemic intoxication, as in infectious diseases. **nodular m.,** a condition of the tongue characterized by the formation of a nodule composed of degenerated muscle tissue.

myoma (mi-o′mah), pl. *myomas* or *myo′mata* [*myo-* + *-oma*] a tumor made up of muscular elements. **ball m.,** one that is spherical. **m. levicellula′re** (obs.), leiomyoma. **myoblastic m.,** myoblastoma. **m. pre′vium,** leiomyoma uteri. **m. sarcomato′des,** leiomyosarcoma. **m. striocellula′re,** rhabdomyoma. **m. telangiecto′des,** vascular leiomyoma, a tumor consisting of a coil of blood vessels surrounded by a network of muscular fibers; angiomyoma.

myomagenesis (mi-o″mah-jen′ĕ-sis) the production or causation of myoma (leiomyoma).

myomalacia (mi″o-mah-la′she-ah) [*myo-* + Gr. *malakia* softening] morbid softening of a muscle.

myomata (mi-o′mah-tah) plural of *myoma.*

myomatectomy (mi″o-mah-tek′to-me) myomectomy, def. 1.

myomatosis (mi″o-mah-to′sis) the formation of multiple myomas (leiomyomas).

myomatous (mi-o′mah-tus) pertaining to or of the nature of a myoma (leiomyoma).

myomectomy (mi″o-mek′to-me) [*myoma* + Gr. *ektomē* excision] 1. surgical removal of a myoma (leiomyoma). 2. myectomy.

myomelanosis (mi″o-mel″ah-no′sis) [*myo-* + Gr. *melanōsis* blackening] melanosis, or black pigmentation of a portion of the muscular substance.

myomere (mi′o-mēr) [*myo-* + Gr. *meros* part] myotome, def. 2.

myometer (mi-om′ĕ-ter) [*myo-* + Gr. *metron* measure] an apparatus for measuring muscle contraction.

myometritis (mi″o-mĕ-tri′tis) [*myo-* + Gr. *mētra* womb + *-itis*] inflammation of the muscular substance, or myometrium, of the uterus.

myometrium (mi-o-me′tre-um) [*myo-* + Gr. *mētra* uterus] the smooth muscle coat of the uterus which forms the main mass of the organ. NA alternative term for tunica muscularis uteri.

myomohysterectomy (mi″o-mo-his″ter-ek′to-me) [*myoma* + Gr. *hystera* uterus + *ektomē* excision] surgical removal of a myomatous uterus.

myomotomy (mi″o-mot′o-me) incision into a myoma.

myon (mi′on) [Gr. *mys* muscle + *on* neuter ending] a muscular unit.

myonecrosis (mi″o-nĕ-kro′sis) necrosis or death of individual muscle fibers. **clostridial m.,** gas gangrene.

myoneme (mi′o-nēm) [*myo-* + Gr. *nēma* thread] one of the contractile fibrils in certain protozoa.

myonephropexy (mi″o-nef′ro-pek-se) [*myo-* + Gr. *nephros* kidney + *pēxis* fixation] the operation of fixing a movable kidney by suturing it to a strap of muscle tissue.

myoneural (mi″o-nu′ral) [*myo-* + Gr. *neuron* nerve] pertaining to both muscle and nerve; said of the nerve terminations in muscles.

myoneuralgia (mi″o-nu-ral′je-ah) [*myo-* + *-neuralgia*] muscular neuralgia.

myoneurasthenia (mi″o-nu″ras-the′ne-ah) [*myo-* + *neurasthenia*] weakness of the muscular system in neurasthenia.

myoneure (mi′o-nūr) [*myo-* + Gr. *neuron* nerve] a nerve cell which supplies a muscle.

myonosus (mi-on′o-sus) [*myo-* + Gr. *nosos* disease] myopathy.

myonymy (mi-on′ĭ-me) [*myo-* + Gr. *onoma* name] nomenclature of the muscles.

myopachynsis (mi″o-pah-kin′sis) [*myo-* + Gr. *pachynsis* thickening] hypertrophy of muscle.

myopalmus (mi″o-pal′mus) muscle twitching.

myoparalysis (mi″o-pah-ral′ĭ-sis) [*myo-* + *paralysis*] paralysis of a muscle.

myoparesis (mi″o-par′ĕ-sis) muscle weakness.

myopathia (mi″o-path′e-ah) myopathy. **m. cor′dis,** myocardosis. **m. infraspina′ta,** a condition marked by the sudden development of pain in the shoulder with tenderness in the infraspinatus muscle.

myopathic (mi″o-path′ik) of the nature of a myopathy.

myopathy (mi-op′ah-the) [*myo-* + Gr. *pathos* suffering] any disease of a muscle. **alcoholic m.,** myopathy affecting alcoholics, commonly characterized by acute myoglobinuria and sometimes by proximal limb weakness. **centronuclear m.,** myotubular m. **distal m.,** that affecting the distal muscles of the hands and feet first; see *late distal hereditary m.* **late distal hereditary m.,** a hereditary disorder, transmitted as an autosomal dominant trait, in which muscular dystrophy starts in the small muscles of the hands and feet and spreads proximally; the onset is usually after the age of 40. Called also *distal muscular dystrophy* and *Gowers type muscular dystrophy.* **myotubular m.,** myopathy characterized by myofibers resembling those of early fetal muscle, i.e., with the nucleus located centrally and surrounded by a halo of apparently empty space; called also *centronuclear m.* **nemaline m.,** a congenital myofibrillar abnormality in which small threadlike or rod-shaped bodies are scattered through the muscle fibers; it is marked by hypotonia and proximal muscle weakness; called also *rod m.* **ocular m.,** a slowly progressive muscular dystrophy marked by ptosis and progressive immobility of the eyes; usually beginning in adulthood, it is sometimes limited to the levator muscles of the eyes. **rod m.,** nemaline m.

myope (mi′ōp) [Gr. *myein* to shut + *ōps* eye] a nearsighted person; one affected with myopia.

myopericarditis (mi″o-per″ĭ-kar-di′tis) myocarditis combined with pericarditis.

myophage (mi′o-fāj) a phagocyte which destroys the contractile substance of muscle.

myophagism (mi-of′ah-jizm) [*myo-* + Gr. *phagein* to eat] the atrophy or wasting away of muscular tissue.

myophone (mi′o-fōn) [*myo-* + Gr. *phōnē* voice] a device which renders audible the sound of a muscular contraction.

myophosphorylase (mi″o-fos-fōr′ĭ-lās) the phosphorylase of muscle.

myopia (mi-o′pe-ah) [Gr. *myein* to shut + *ōps* eye + *-ia*] that error of refraction in which rays of light entering the eye parallel to the optic axis are brought to a focus in front of the retina, as a result of the eyeball being too long from front to back (*axial m.*) or of an increased strength in refractive power of the media of the eye (*index m.*). Called also *nearsightedness,* because the near point is less distant than it is in emmetropia with an equal amplitude of accommodation. **chromic m.,** defective color vision for objects at a distance. **curvature m.,** a form due to changes in the curvature of the refracting surfaces of the eye. **index m.,** a form due to abnormal refractivity of the mediums of the eye. **malignant m., pernicious m.,** progressive myopia, associated with grave disease of the choroid and leading to retinal detachment and blindness. **prodromal m.,** a condition marked by the return of the ability to do close work without eyeglasses; sometimes seen in incipient cataract. **progressive m.,** myopia that continues to increase in adult life.

myopic (mi-op′ik) pertaining to or affected with myopia; nearsighted.

myoplasm (mi′o-plazm) [*myo-* + Gr. *plasma* something formed] the contractile part of the muscle cell, or myofibril.

myoplastic (mi″o-plas′tik) [*myo-* + Gr. *plassein* to form] performed by the plastic use of muscle; said of operations.

myoplasty (mi′o-plas″te) plastic surgery on muscle; an operation in which portions of partly detached muscle are utilized, especially in the field of defects or deformities.

myopolar (mi″o-po′lar) [*myo-* + *polar*] applied to a muscle between the electrodes of a battery.

myoprotein (mi″o-pro′te-in) a protein obtained from muscle tissue.

myopsis (mi-op′sis) myiodesopsia.

myopsychic (mi″o-si′kik) pertaining to the muscles and the mind—denoting the memory images of muscular activity.

myopsychopathy (mi″o-si-kop′ah-the) [*myo-* + Gr. *psyche* soul + *pathos* disease] any neuromuscular affection associated with mental weakness or disorder.

myopsychosis (mi″o-si-ko′sis) myopsychopathy.

myoreceptor (mi″o-re-sep′tor) a proprioceptor occurring in skeletal muscle.

myorrhaphy (mi-or′ah-fe) [*myo-* + Gr. *rhaphē* suture] suturation of divided muscle; myosuture.

myorrhexis (mi″o-rek′sis) [*myo-* + Gr. *rhēxis* rupture] the rupture of a muscle.

myosalgia (mi″o-sal′je-ah) myalgia.

myosalpingitis (mi″o-sal″pin-ji′tis) [*myo-* + *salpingitis*] inflammation of the muscular tissue of the oviduct.

myosalpinx (mi″o-sal′pinks) the muscular tissue of the oviduct.

myosan (mi′o-san) a denatured and insoluble form of myosin.

myosarcoma (mi″o-sar-ko′mah) a malignant tumor derived from myogenic cells.

myoschwannoma (mi″o-shwan-no′mah) schwannoma.

myosclerosis (mi″o-skle-ro′sis) [*myo-* + Gr. *sklēros* hard] hardening or sclerosis of muscle tissue.

myoscope (mi′o-skōp) [*myo-* + Gr. *skopein* to examine] 1. an instrument for observing muscle contraction. 2. an ocular instrument, on the principle of the orthoptoscope, which allows fusion and movement laterally, vertically, and in rotation.

myoseism (mi′o-sīzm) [*myo-* + Gr. *seismos* shake] jerky, irregular muscular contractions.

myoseptum (mi″o-sep′tum) myocomma.

myoserum (mi″o-se′rum) the juice expressed from muscle.

myosin (mi′o-sin) a globin which is the most abundant protein (68 per cent) in muscle, occurring chiefly in the A band. It is soluble in salt solution, but on long standing it coagulates into an insoluble protein called *myosin fibrin.* Along with actin (q.v.), it is responsible for the contraction and relaxation of muscle. Myosin has enzymatic properties, acting as an ATP-ase. It is the main constituent of the thick filaments of muscle fibers. Cf. *myogen* and *actomyosin.* **vegetable m.,** a substance resembling myosin, from seeds of various plants.

myosinogen (mi″o-sin′o-jen) [*myosin* + Gr. *gennan* to produce] myogen.

myosinuria (mi″o-sin-u′re-ah) [*myosin* + Gr. *ouron* urine + *-ia*] the presence of myosin in the urine.

myosis (mi-o′sis) miosis.

myositic (mi″o-sit′ik) pertaining to myositis.

myositis (mi″o-si′tis) [Gr. *myos* of muscle + *-itis*] inflammation of a voluntary muscle. **acute disseminated m.,** primary multiple m. **acute progressive m.,** a rare disease in which the inflammation gradually involves the whole muscular system and ends in death by asphyxia and pneumonia. **epidemic m.,** epidemic pleurodynia. **m. fibro′sa,** a type in which there is a formation of connective tissue within the muscle substance. **m. a frigo′re,** muscular rheumatism resulting from cold or chilling. **infectious m., interstitial m.,** inflammation of the connective and septal elements of muscular tissue. **multiple m.,** polymyositis. **orbital m.,** see under *pseudotumor.* **m. ossif′icans,** myositis which is characterized by bony deposits or by ossification of muscles. **m. ossif′icans circumscrip′ta,** a form marked by the formation of a muscular osteoma, such as rider's bone. **m. ossif′icans progressi′va,** a progressive disease, beginning in early life, in which the muscles are gradually converted into bony tissue; called also *progressive ossifying m.* **m. ossif′icans traumat′ica,** myositis ossificans due to injury. **parenchymatous m.,** that which affects the essential substance of a muscle. **primary multiple m.,** an acute febrile disease characterized by edema and inflammation of the skin and muscles in various parts of the body; called also *acute disseminated m.* and *pseudotrichinosis.* **progressive ossifying m.,** myositis ossificans progressiva. **m. purulen′ta,** a suppurative and gangrenous type, due to a bacterial infection. **rheumatoid m.,** fibrositis. **m. sero′sa,** muscle inflammation characterized by a serous exudation. **suppurative m.,** inflammation of muscle resulting in muscular abscesses or in diffuse suppuration of muscles. **trichinous m.,** that which is caused by the presence of trichinae.

myospasia (mi″o-spa′ze-ah) clonic contraction of muscle; paramyoclonus.

myospasm (mi′o-spazm) [*myo-* + Gr. *spasmos* spasm] spasm of a muscle.

myospasmia (mi″o-spaz′me-ah) disease characterized by uncontrollable muscular spasm.

myosteoma (mi-os″te-o′mah) [*myo-* + Gr. *osteon* bone + *-oma*] osteogenic sarcoma of soft parts.

myosthenic (mi″os-then′ik) [*myo-* + Gr. *sthenos* strength] pertaining to strength of muscle.

myosthenometer (mi″o-sthen-om′ĕ-ter) [*myo-* + Gr. *sthenos* strength + *metron* measure] an instrument for measuring the power of muscle groups.

myostroma (mi″o-stro′mah) [*myo-* + *stroma*] the stroma or framework of muscle tissue.

myostromin (mi″o-stro′min) a protein occurring in muscle stroma.

myosuria (mi″o-su′re-ah) [*myo-* + Gr. *ouron* urine + *-ia*] myosin in the urine.

myosuture (mi″o-su′tūr) [*myo-* + L. *sutura* sewing] the suture of a muscle; myorrhaphy.

myosynizesis (mi″o-sin″i-ze′sis) [*myo-* + Gr. *synizēsis* a sinking down] adhesion of muscles.

myotactic (mi″o-tak′tik) [*myo-* + L. *tactus* touch] pertaining to the proprioceptive sense of muscles.

myotamponade (mi″o-tam′po-nād) extrapleural pneumonolysis in which the cavity is packed with a mass of attached muscle.

myotasis (mi-ot′ah-sis) [*myo-* + Gr. *tasis* stretching] stretching of muscle.

myotatic (mi″o-tat′ik) [*myo-* + Gr. *teinein* to stretch] performed or induced by stretching or extending a muscle.

myotenontoplasty (mi″o-ten-on′to-plas″te) tenomyoplasty.

myotenositis (mi″o-ten″o-si′tis) [*myo-* + Gr. *tenōn* tendon + *-itis*] inflammation of a muscle and its tendon.

myotenotomy (mi″o-ten-ot′o-me) [*myo-* + *tenotomy*] surgical division of the tendon of a muscle.

myothermic (mi″o-ther′mik) [*myo-* + Gr. *thermē* heat] pertaining to temperature changes in muscle produced by its activity.

myotic (mi-ot′ik) miotic (def. 2).

myotility (mi″o-til′ĭ-te) muscular contractility.

myotome (mi′o-tōm) [*myo-* + Gr. *tomē* a cut] 1. an instrument for performing myotomy. 2. the muscle plate or portion of a somite that develops into voluntary muscle; called also *myomere.* 3. a group of muscles innervated from a single spinal segment.

myotomic (mi″o-tom′ik) pertaining to or derived from a myotome.

myotomy (mi-ot′o-me) [*myo-* + Gr. *tomē* a cutting] the cutting or dissection of a muscle or of muscular tissue.

myotone (mi′o-tōn) myotonus.

myotonia (mi″o-to′ne-ah) [*myo-* + Gr. *tonos* tension] increased muscular irritability and contractility with decreased power of relaxation; tonic spasm of muscle. **m. acquis′ita,** tonic muscular spasm developed after injury or in consequence of disease; called also *Talma's disease.* **m. atroph′ica,** *myotonic dystrophy;* see under *dystrophy.* **m. congen′ita, m. heredita′ria,** congenital and hereditary disease characterized by tonic spasm and rigidity of certain muscles when an attempt is made to move them after a period of rest or when mechanically stimulated. The stiffness disappears as the muscles are used. It is transmitted as an autosomal dominant trait. Called also *paramyotonia congenita, Eulenburg's disease,* and *Thomsen's disease.* **m. dystroph′ica,** myotonic dystrophy. **m. neonato′rum,** tetanism.

myotonic (mi″o-ton′ik) 1. pertaining to or characterized by myotonia. 2. pertaining to the tonic function of muscle, as contrasted with the myokinetic or motion function.

myotonoid (mi-ot′o-noid) [*myo-* + Gr. *tonos* tension + *eidos* form] resembling myotonia; said of reactions in muscle which are marked by slow contraction or relaxation.

myotonometer (mi″o-to-nom′ĕ-ter) [*myotonia* + Gr. *metron* measure] an instrument for measuring muscular tonus.

myotonus (mi-ot′o-nus) tonic spasm of a muscle or of a group of muscles.

myotony (mi-ot′o-ne) myotonia.

myotrophic (mi′o-tro″fik) 1. increasing the weight of muscle. 2. pertaining to myotrophy.

myotrophy (mi-ot′ro-fe) [*myo-* + Gr. *trophē* nutrition] nutrition of muscle.

myotropic (mi″o-trop′ik) [*myo-* + Gr. *tropos* a turning] having an affinity for muscle, as myotropic organisms.

myotube (mi′o-tūb) myotubule.

myotubular (mi″o-tu′bu-lar) relating to a myotubule.

myotubule (mi″o-tu′būl) a developing muscle fiber with a centrally, rather than peripherally, located nucleus.

myovascular (mi″o-vas′ku-lar) [*myo-* + *vascular*] pertaining to a muscle and its blood vessels.

myrcene (mer′sēn) an essential oil from the oil of bay; it is an olefinic terpene, $C_{10}H_{16}$, used in perfumery and pharmaceuticals as an odorant.

myria- [Gr. *myrios* numberless] a combining form meaning a great number.

myriachit (mir-e′ah-chit) [Russian] Gilles de la Tourette's syndrome.

Myriangiales (mir″e-an″je-a′lēz) an order of ascomycetous fungi (subclass Loculoascomycetaceae), in which the asci are formed in locules scattered throughout the ascocarp (fruiting body). They are usually parasites of higher plants, although a few are insect parasites; the order includes the family Piedraiaceae.

myriapod (mir′e-ah-pod) a member of the Myriapoda; a centipede or millipede.

Myriapoda (mir″e-ap′o-dah) [*myria-* + Gr. *pous* foot] a superclass of arthropods, including the classes Chilopoda (centipedes) and Diplopoda (millipedes).

myrica (mir-i′kah) the dried bark of the root of *Myrica cerifera* L. (Myriaceae), bayberry or wax myrtle, formerly used internally as an emetic and astringent, and externally in the treatment of indolent ulcers.

myricin (mir′ĭ-sin) [L. *myrica* myrtle] 1. a crystallizable principle, $C_{30}H_{61}\cdot C_{16}H_{31}O_2$, from yellow wax (beeswax). 2. a medicinal concentration prepared from *Myrica cerifera,* or wax myrtle; used like myrica.

myricyl (mir′ĭ-sil) the radical, $C_{30}H_{61}$, occurring in beeswax and other waxes.

myringa (mĭ-ring′gah) [L.] the membrana tympani.

myringectomy (mir″in-jek′to-me) myringodectomy.

myringitis (mir″in-ji′tis) [*myringa* + *-itis*] inflammation of the membrana tympani. **m. bullo′sa, bullous m.,** a form of viral otitis media in which serous or hemorrhagic blebs appear on the membrana tympani and often on the adjacent wall of the auditory meatus.

myringo- [L. *myringa* drum membrane] a combining form denoting relationship to the membrana tympani.

myringodectomy (mĭ-ring″go-dek′to-me) [*myringo-* + Gr. *ektomē* excision] surgical removal of the membrana tympani.

myringodermatitis (mĭ-ring″go-der″mah-ti′tis) [*myringo-* + Gr. *derma* skin] inflammation of the outer layer of the membrana tympani, with the formation of blebs.

myringomycosis (mĭ-ring″go-mi-ko′sis) [*myringo-* + Gr. *mykēs* fungus] disease of the membrana tympani caused by a fungus;

otomycosis. **m. aspergilli′na,** infection of the membrana tympani by an aspergillus; see *otomycosis.*

myringoplasty (mĭ-ring′go-plas″te) [*myringo-* + Gr. *plassein* to form] surgical restoration of a perforated tympanic membrane by grafting. See also *tympanoplasty.*

myringorupture (mĭ-ring″go-rup′chur) rupture of the membrana tympani.

myringostapediopexy (mĭ-ring″go-stah-pe′de-o-pek″se) fixation of the pars tensa of the membrana tympani to the head of the stapes.

myringotome (mĭ-ring′go-tōm) a knife for use in operating upon the membrana tympani.

myringotomy (mir″in-got′o-me) [*myringo-* + Gr. *tomē* a cutting] surgical incision of the membrana tympani; tympanotomy.

myrinx (mi′rinks) membrana tympani.

myristate (mēr′is-tāt) tetradecanoate: the ionic form of myristic acid, a naturally occurring fatty acid. **isopropyl m.,** see under *isopropyl.*

Myristica (mĭ-ris′tĭ-kah) [L.; Gr. *myrizein* to anoint] a genus of trees of tropical countries. *M. fragrans* Houtt. (Myristicaceae), the nutmeg tree, is the source of myristica. *M. ocuba* is the source of ocuba wax.

myristica (mĭ-ris′tĭ-kah) nutmeg; the dried ripe seed of *Myristica fragrans* Houtt. (Myristicaceae) deprived of its seed coat and arillode and with or within a coating of lime. It is the source of nutmeg oil, which is used as a flavoring agent in pharmaceutical preparations. It has stimulating aromatic, carminative, and psychomimetic properties.

myristicene (mĭ-ris′tĭ-sēn) a fragrant eleopten, $C_{10}H_{14}$, from nutmeg (myristica) oil.

myristicol (mĭ-ris′tĭ-kol) a stearopten, or camphor, $C_{10}H_{16}O$, from nutmeg (myristica) oil.

myristin (mĭ-ris′tin) chemical name: glyceryl trimyristate, C_3-$H_5(C_{14}H_{27}O_2)_3$, found in spermaceti and many vegetable oils and fats, especially coconut oil and fixed nutmeg (myristica) oil.

myrmecia (mur-me′she-ah) [Gr. *myrmēx* ant + *-ia*] a wart resembling somewhat an anthill.

myronate (mi′ro-nāt) any salt of myronic acid (derivable from black mustard). **potassium m.,** sinigrin.

myrosin (mi′ro-sin) thioglucosidase.

myrosinase (mi-ro′sĭ-nās) thioglucosidase.

myrrh (mur) the oleo-gum-resin obtained from species of East Indian and African trees, e.g., *Commiphora abyssinica* (Berg) Eng. (Burseraceae); it has been used as a carminative and a topical oral stimulant.

myrrholin (mur′o-lin) a mixture of myrrh and fat in equal parts, used as a vehicle for the administration of creosote.

myrtenol (mur′tĕ-nol) a terpene alcohol, $(CH_3)_2C:C_6H_7\cdot CH_2OH$, from the volatile oil distilled from the leaves of *Myrtus communis* (Myrtaceae).

myrtiform (mur′tĭ-form) [L. *myrtiformis; myrtus* myrtle + *forma* shape] shaped like the leaf or berry of the myrtle.

Myrtus (mur′tus) [L.; Gr. *myrtos*] a genus of myrtaceous trees. **M. commu′nis,** L. (Myrtaceae), the Old World myrtle, a species affording leaves which are antiseptic and astringent.

Mysoline (mi′so-lēn) trademark for preparations of primidone.

mysophilia (mi″so-fil′e-ah) [Gr. *mysos* uncleanness of body or mind + Gr. *philein* to love] a form of paraphilia in which there is a lustful attitude toward excretions.

mysophobia (mi″so-fo′be-ah) [Gr. *mysos* uncleanness of body or mind + *phobia*] morbid dread of filth or contamination.

mysophobiac (mi″so-fo′be-ak) a person affected with mysophobia.

mysophobic (mi″so-fo′bik) pertaining to or characterized by mysophobia.

mystin (mis′tin) a milk preservative, consisting of formaldehyde and sodium nitrite.

mytacism (mi′tah-sizm) [Gr. *mytakismos*] too free use of *m* sounds in utterance.

Mytelase (mi′tĕ-lās) trademark for a preparation of ambenonium chloride.

mythomania (mith″o-ma′ne-ah) [Gr. *mythos* myth + *mania* madness] a morbid propensity to lie or to exaggerate.

mythophobia (mith″o-fo′be-ah) [Gr. *mythos* myth + *phobia*] morbid fear of myths or of stating an untruth.

mytilocongestin (mit″ĭ-lo-kon-jes′tin) [Gr. *mytilos* mussel + *congestion*] a toxic substance derived from mussels of the species *Mytilus edulis* which, when injected in laboratory animals, causes intense congestion of the splanchnic vessels, and hemorrhage.

mytilotoxin (mit″ĭ-lo-tok′sin) a neurotoxic substance from mussels of the genus *Mytilus;* see *gonyaulax poison,* under *poison.*

mytilotoxism (mit″ĭ-lo-tok′sizm) poisoning due to ingestion of mussels contaminated with mytilotoxin.

myx- see *myxo-.*

myxadenitis (miks″ad-ĕ-ni′tis) [*myxo-* + Gr. *adēn* gland + *-itis*] inflammation of a mucous gland. **m. labia'lis,** see *cheilitis glandularis.*

myxadenoma (miks″ad-ĕ-no′mah) [*myxo-* + *adenoma*] an epithelial tumor with the structure of a mucous gland; mucinous adenoma.

myxangitis (miks″an-ji′tis) [*myxo-* + Gr. *angeion* vessel + *-itis*] inflammation of the ducts of mucous glands.

myxangoitis (miks″an-go-i′tis) myxangitis.

myxasthenia (miks″as-the-ne′ah) [*myxo-* + Gr. *astheneia* weakness] deficiency in the secretion of mucus.

myxedema (mik″sĕ-de′mah) [*myxo-* + Gr. *oidēma* swelling] a condition characterized by a dry, waxy type of swelling, with abnormal deposits of mucin in the skin (mucinosis) and other tissues, and associated with hypothyroidism. The edema is of the nonpitting type, and the facial changes are strikingly distinctive, with swollen lips and a thickened nose. The term myxedema is sometimes used interchangeably with adult hypothyroidism. Cf. *lichen myxedematosus.* **circumscribed m.,** pretibial m. **congenital m.,** cretinism. **infantile m.,** myxedema beginning during infancy in association with hypothyroidism developing after birth; called also *Brissaud's infantilism.* **nodular m.,** pretibial m. **operative m.,** myxedema developing subsequent to surgical removal of the thyroid gland. **papular m.,** lichen myxedematosus. **pituitary m.,** myxedema associated with hypothyroidism occurring as a consequence of deficient secretion of thyrotropic hormone by the anterior pituitary gland. **pretibial m.,** localized myxedema associated with preceding hyperthyroidism and exophthalmos, occurring typically on the anterior (pretibial) surface of the legs, the mucin deposits appearing as both plaques and papules.

myxedematoid (mik″sĕ-dem′ah-toid) [*myxedema* + Gr. *eidos* form] resembling myxedema.

myxedematous (mik″sĕ-dem′ah-tus) pertaining to or characterized by myxedema.

myxidiocy (miks-id′e-o-se) myxidiotie.

myxidiotie (miks-id′e-o-te) myxedema accompanied by defective mental development.

myxiosis (mik″se-o′sis) a discharge of mucus.

myxo-, myx- [Gr. *myxa* mucus] combining form denoting relationship to mucus, or slime.

myxoadenoma (mik″so-ad″ĕ-no′mah) myxadenoma.

Myxobacterales (mik″so-bak-tĕ-ra′lēz) an order of class Schizomycetes, made up of unicellular rods which, in the vegetative state, occur in two characteristic shapes, the cylindrical cells having blunt rounded ends, or tapering toward the tips. The cells multiply by binary, transverse fission, and movement is a universal characteristic. The order includes five families, Archangiaceae, Cytophagaceae, Myxococcaceae, Polyangiaceae, and Sorangiaceae, all occurring as saprophytic soil microorganisms.

myxoblastoma (mik″se-o′blas-to′mah) myxoma.

Myxobolus (miks-ob′o-lus) a genus of sporozoan parasites of the order Myxosporidia, which infect fish. **M. cypri′ni,** a protozoan parasite causing carp-pox. **M. pfeif′feri,** a parasite of fish of the genus *Barbus.*

myxochondrofibrosarcoma (mik″so-kon″dro-fi″bro-sar-ko′mah) malignant mesenchymoma.

myxochondroma (mik″so-kon-dro′mah) chondroma with a stroma resembling primitive mesenchymal tissue.

myxochondrosarcoma (mik″so-kon″dro-sar-ko′mah) malignant mesenchymoma.

Myxococcaceae (mik″so-kok-ka′se-e) a family of Schizomycetes, order Myxobacterales, made up of saprophytic microorganisms found in soil and decaying organic matter, and including four genera, *Myxococcus, Chondrococcus, Angiococcus,* and *Sporocytophaga.*

Myxococcus (mik″so-kok′us) [*myxo-* + *coccus*] a genus of bacteria of the family Myxococcaceae, found in decaying organic matter.

myxocystitis (mik″so-sis-ti′tis) [*myxo-* + *cystitis*] inflammation of the mucosa of the bladder.

myxocystoma (mik″so-sis-to′mah) myxoma with cystic degeneration.

myxocyte (mik′so-sīt) [*myxo-* + *cyte*] one of the characteristic cells of mucous tissue.

myxoenchondroma (mik″so-en″kon-dro′mah) a chondroma in which some of the elements have undergone mucous degeneration.

myxoendothelioma (mik″so-en″do-the″le-o′mah) angioendothelioma with myxomatous degeneration.

myxofibroma (mik″so-fi-bro′mah) a fibroma containing myxomatous tissue.

myxofibrosarcoma (mik″so-fi″bro-sar-ko′mah) fibrosarcoma with myxomatous areas.

myxoglioma (mik″so-gli-o′mah) a glioma which has undergone myxomatous degeneration.

myxoglobulosis (mik″so-glob″u-lo′sis) [*myxo-* + *globule* + *-osis*] a cystic condition of the appendix marked by the presence in the cysts of globoid bodies of mucinous character.

myxoid (mik′soid) [*myxo-* + Gr. *eidos* form] resembling mucus.

myxoinoma (mik″so-in-o′mah) myxofibroma.

myxolipoma (mik″so-li-po′mah) lipoma with foci of myxomatous degeneration.

myxoma (mik-so′mah), pl. *myxomas* or *myxo′mata* [*myxo-* + *-oma*] a tumor composed of primitive connective tissue cells and stroma resembling mesenchyme. **atrial m.,** a benign gelatinous growth usually pedunculated and usually arising from the interatrial septum of the heart in the region of the fossa ovalis; symptoms may include effort dyspnea, loss of weight, fatigue, low-grade fever, polyneuritis, nausea, and palpitations, and sometimes sudden syncopal attacks related to obstruction. **cystic m.,** one that has undergone cystic degeneration. **enchondromatous m.,** one containing cartilage in the intercellular substance. **erectile m.,** an angioma with myxomatous areas. **m. fibro′sum,** myxofibroma. **infectious m.,** myxomatosis cuniculi. **lipomatous m.,** a lipoma with myxomatous degeneration. **odontogenic m.,** an uncommon tumor of the jaw, apparently arising from the mesenchymal portion of the tooth germ, and possibly produced by myxomatous degeneration of an odontogenic fibroma. **m. sarcomato′sum,** myxosarcoma. **vascular m.,** a myxoma containing many blood vessels.

myxomatosis (mik″so-mah-to′sis) 1. a condition marked by the development of multiple myxomas. 2. myxomatous degeneration. **m. cunic′uli, infectious m.,** an infectious, highly fatal, febrile disease of rabbits caused by a virus, and characterized by edematous swelling of the mucous membranes and the presence of myxoma-like tumors of the skin.

myxomatous (mik-so′mah-tus) of the nature of a myxoma.

Myxomycetes (mik″so-mi-se′tēz) [Gr. pl., from *myxo-* + *mykēs* fungus] a group of organisms considered to be closely related to the fungi, but classified by some as protozoa. See *Mycetozoida.*

myxomyoma (mik″so-mi-o′mah) a myoma with myxomatous degeneration.

myxoneurosis (mik″so-nu-ro′sis) [*myxo-* + *neurosis*] a neurosis characterized by deranged mucous secretion. **intestinal m., m. intestina′lis,** an intestinal neurosis marked by the passage of mucous shreds in the stools; mucous colitis.

myxopapilloma (mik″so-pap″ĭ-lo′mah) myxoma combined with papilloma.

myxopoiesis (mik″so-poi-e′sis) [*myxo-* + Gr. *poiēsis* a making, creation] the formation of mucus.

myxorrhea (mik″so-re′ah) [*myxo-* + Gr. *rhoia* flow] a flow of mucus; blennorrhea. **m. intestina′lis,** a flow of mucus from the bowel occurring in nervous individuals under mental strain.

myxosarcoma (mik″so-sar-ko′mah) a sarcoma containing myxomatous tissue.

myxosarcomatous (mik″so-sar-ko′mah-tus) relating to or affected with myxosarcoma.

Myxosporidia (mik″so-spo-rid′e-ah) [*myxo-* + *sporidia*] an order of endoparasitic ameboid sporozoa parasitic on lower vertebrates, including amphibians, reptiles, and especially fishes.

myxovirus (mik″so-vi′rus) a general name for a large group of viruses, including the viruses of influenza, parainfluenza, mumps, and Newcastle disease; the viruses are characterized by an RNA nucleocapsid in a loose membrane, and they typically agglutinate erythrocytes. Myxoviruses have been divided into paramyxoviruses and orthomyxoviruses.

myzesis (mi-ze′sis) [Gr. *myzan* to suck] sucking.

Myzomyia (mi″zo-mi′yah) [Gr. *myzan* to suck + *myia* fly] a subgenus of anopheline mosquitoes, several species of which act as the carriers of malarial parasites.

Myzorhynchus (mi″zo-ring′kus) [Gr. *myzan* to suck + *rhynchos* snout] a subgenus of anopheline mosquitoes, several species of which are the carriers of malarial parasites. *M. (Anopheles) barbiros′tris,* a species which transmits malaria and filariasis in the Orient. *M. palu′dis,* an African species. *M. pseudopic′tus,* a European species. *M. sinen′sis,* a Japanese species.

N

N 1. symbol for refractive index. 2. chemical symbol for *nitrogen*; this symbol is also used as a prefix to denote combination with the nitrogen atom of organic compounds. 3. symbol for *normal* (solution); the expressions 2N, N/2 or 0.5N, N/10 or 0.1N, N/50 or 0.02N, N/200 or 0.005N, N/1000 or 0.001N denote the strength of a solution in comparison with the normal, respectively double normal, half-normal, tenth-normal, fiftieth-normal, two-hundredth-normal, and thousandth-normal. 4. symbol for an antigenic determinant of erythrocytes; see *blood type*. 5. symbol for *newton*.

n symbol for index of refraction; chemical symbol for *normal*.

NA abbreviation for *Nomina Anatomica*, the official anatomical terminology approved by the Sixth International Congress of Anatomists at Paris in 1955, with later emendations.

N.A. numerical aperture.

Na chemical symbol for *sodium* (L. *natrium*).

nabidrox (nab'ĭ-droks) chemical name: (+)-3-(1,1-dimethylheptyl)-6aβ,7,8,9,10aα-hexahydro-6,6-dimethyl-6*H*-dibenzo[*b,d*]pyran-1,9-diol; an antihypertensive, $C_{24}H_{38}O_3$.

nabilone (nab'ĭ-lōn) chemical name: *trans*-(+)-3-(1,1-dimethylheptyl)-6,6a,7,8,10,10a-hexahydro-1-hydroxy-6,6-dimethyl-9*H*-dibenzo[*b,d*]pyran-9-one; a synthetic cannabinoid, $C_{24}H_{36}O_3$, which acts as a minor tranquilizer and antiemetic.

$Na_2B_4O_7 \cdot 1OH_2O$ borax.

Naboth's follicles (cysts, glands, ovules, vesicles) (na'bōths) [Martin *Naboth*, Leipzig anatomist, 1675–1721] see under *follicle*.

nabothian (nah-bo'the-an) described by or named in honor of Martin *Naboth*. See under *follicle*.

NaBr sodium bromide.

NaCl sodium chloride.

NaClO sodium hypochlorite.

NaClO₃ sodium chlorate.

Na₂CO₃ sodium carbonate.

Na₂C₂O₄ sodium oxalate.

nacreous (na'kre-us) [Fr. *nacre* mother of pearl] having a grayish-white, translucent color, with a pearl-like luster; said of bacterial colonies.

Nacton (nak'ton) trademark for a preparation of poldine methylsulfate.

NAD nicotinamide-adenine dinucleotide.

N.A.D. no appreciable disease.

NAD⁺ the oxidized form of NAD.

NADH the reduced form of NAD.

nadide (na'dīd) chemical name: adenosine 5'-(trihydrogen diphosphate)5'→5'-ester with 3-(aminocarbonyl)-1-β-D-ribofuranosylpyridinium, hydroxide inner salt; an alcohol and narcotic antagonist, $C_{21}H_{27}N_7O_{14}P_2$, it is the naturally occurring coenzyme nicotinamide-adenine dinucleotide.

nadolol (na-do'lol) chemical name: *cis*-5-[3-[(1,1-dimethylamino)amino]-2-hydroxypropoxy]-1,2,3,4-tetrahydro-2,3-naphthalenediol; an antiadrenergic (β-receptor), $C_{17}H_{27}NO_4$.

NADP nicotinamide-adenine dinucleotide phosphate.

NADP⁺ the oxidized form of NADP.

NADPH the reduced form of NADP.

Naegeli's law, leukemia (na'gĕ-lēz) [Otto *Naegeli*, Swiss hematologist, 1871–1937] see under *law*, and see *monocytic leukemia*, under *leukemia*.

Naegleria (na-gle'rĭ-ah) a genus of coprozoic amebae of the class Rhizopoda, which has both an ameboid and a flagellate stage in its life history; in the latter stage it possesses two flagella. Human infection may result in primary amebic meningoencephalitis. Called also *Dimastigamoeba* and *Wasielewskia*.

naepaine (ne'pān) chemical name: 2-*n*-pentylaminoethyl *p*-aminobenzoate. Dimorphic crystals, $C_{14}H_{22}N_2O_2$, with a bitter taste and soluble in water; its hydrochloride is a local anesthestic for ocular use.

NaF sodium fluoride.

nafcillin (naf-sil'in) chemical name: 6-(2-ethoxy-1-naphthamido)-3,3-dimethyl-7-oxo-4-thia-1-azabicyclo[3.2.0]heptane-2-carboxylate. A semisynthetic, acid- and penicillinase-resistant penicillin whose sodium salt [USP], $C_{21}H_{21}N_2NaO_5S$, a white to yellowish white powder, is used as an antibacterial in severe staphylococcal infections caused by penicillinase-positive organisms.

nafenopin (nah-fen'o-pin) chemical name: 2-methyl-2-[4-(1,2,3,4-tetrahydro-1-naphthalenyl)phenoxy]propanoic acid; an antihyperlipidemic, $C_{20}H_{22}O_3$.

Naffziger's operation, syndrome (naf'zig-erz) [Howard Chris-

tian *Naffziger*, American surgeon, 1884–1961] see under *operation*, and see *scalenus syndrome*, under *syndrome*.

nafomine malate (naf'o-mēn) chemical name: hydroxybutanedioic acid compound with *O*-[(2-methyl-1-naphthyl)methyl]hydroxylamine (1:1); a muscle relaxant, $C_{12}H_{13}NO \cdot C_4H_6O_5$.

nafoxidine hydrochloride (naf-oks'ĭ-dēn) chemical name: 1-[2-[4-(3,4-dihydro-6-methoxy-2-phenyl-1-naphthalenyl) phenoxy]ethyl]pyrrolidine hydrochloride; an antiestrogen, $C_{29}H_{31}NO_2 \cdot HCl$, which has been used in the treatment of breast cancer.

nafronyl oxalate (naf'fro-nil) chemical name: tetrahydro-α-(1-naphthalenylmethyl)-2-furanpropanoic acid 2-(diethylamino)-ethyl ester ethanedioate (1:1); a vasodilator, $C_{24}H_{33}NO_3 \cdot C_2H_2O_4$, which has been used in the treatment of peripheral and cerebral vascular disorders.

naftalofos (naf'tah-lo"fos) chemical name: 2-[(diethoxyphosphinyl)oxy]-1*H*-benz[*de*]isoquinoline-1,3(2*H*)-dione; a veterinary anthelmintic, $C_{16}H_{16}NO_6P$.

Naga sore (nah'gah) [*Naga*, a region in India] tropical ulcer, def. 1.

nagana (nah-gah'nah) a rapidly fatal trypanosomiasis of equines, dogs, pigs, goats, sheep, camels, and elephants, characterized by high fever, congestion of the mucous membranes, edema of the limbs, abdomen, and eyelids, anemia, icterus, and weakness. Widely distributed throughout Africa, it is caused by the parasite *Trypanosoma brucei*, which is transmitted by the bite of the tsetse fly, *Glossina morsitans*, and other species of *Glossina*. The term nagana also includes infections with *T. congolense* and *T. vivax*. Called also *tsetse-fly disease*.

naganol (nag'ah-nol) suramin sodium.

Nagel's test (nah'gelz) [Willibald A. *Nagel*, German physiologist, 1870–1911] see under *tests*.

Nägele's obliquity, pelvis, rule (na'gĕ-lēz) [Franz Karl *Nägele*, German obstetrician, 1777–1851] see under *obliquity*, *pelvis*, and *rule*.

Nägeli's maneuver (method, treatment) (na'gĕ-lēz) [Otto *Nägeli*, Swiss physician, 1843–1922] see under *maneuver*.

Nageotte bracelets, cell (nazh-yot') [Jean *Nageotte*, Paris histologist, 1866–1948] see under *bracelet* and *cell*.

Nagler effect (nahg'ler) [Joseph *Nagler*, Vienna radiologist] see under *effect*.

Nagler's reaction (test) (nag'lerz) [F. P. O. *Nagler*, British bacteriologist] see under *reaction*.

NaHCO₃ sodium bicarbonate.

NaH₂PO₄ monosodium acid phosphate (sodium biphosphate).

Na₂HPO₄ disodium acid phosphate (sodium phosphate).

nail (nāl) 1. [L. *unguis*; Gr. *onyx*] the horny cutaneous plate on the dorsal surface of the distal end of a finger or toe; see *unguis*. 2. a rod of metal, bone, or other material used for fixation of the

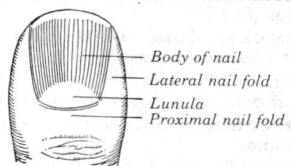

Body of nail
Lateral nail fold
Lunula
Proximal nail fold

Nail (Hill).

ends or the fragments of fractured bones. **double-edge n's,** malformed fingernails in which the normal transverse convexity is replaced by a flat plateau, with a deep slope on each side, occurring as a family trait. **eggshell n.,** a fingernail which has become thin and curved upward at its anterior edge. **fracture n.,** a steel nail used to fasten together the fragments of a broken bone. **hippocratic n.,** see *hippocratic fingers*, under *finger*. **ingrown n.,** aberrant growth of a toenail, with one or, less often, both lateral margins pushing deeply into the adjacent soft tissues. Called also *ingrowing toenail*, *onychocryptosis*, and *unguis incarnatus*. **Jewett n.,** a nail for internal fixation of a trochanteric fracture; the nail is fastened to a plate for fixing the head and neck of the bone to the shaft. **Küntscher n.,** a tubular metal nail for the intramedullary fixation of fractures. **Neufeld n.,** a device for internal fixation of intertrochanteric fracture of the femur, the **V** nail section being set at an angle of about 130 degrees to the plate portion. **parrot beak n.,** a curvature of the fingernail like that of a parrot's beak. **pitted n's,** nails with surface pits, usually under 1 mm. in diameter, most often seen in psoriasis, frequently in alopecia areata, and sometimes unexplained. **racket n.,** thumbnails that are much shorter than they are wide; rarely, other fingers may be affected. In the commonest form, the distal phalanges of affected digits are shortened as well. **reedy n.,** a fingernail marked by longitudinal furrows. **Smith-Petersen n.,** a flanged nail for fixing the head of the femur in fracture of the femoral neck. **spoon n.,** depression of the central portion of the fingernail, with raising of the edges at the sides. **turtle-back n.,** a fingernail which is greatly distorted, being more convex than normal. **watch-crystal n.,** a nail convex lengthwise as well as crosswise, and often as broad as it is long, seen in pulmonary osteoarthropathy and pachydermoperiostosis.

nailing (nāl′ing) the operation of fixing or fastening of a fractured bone with a nail. **intramedullary n., marrow n., medullary n.,** the fixation of a fractured long bone by insertion of a steel nail into the marrow cavity of the bone.

Nairobi eye, sheep disease (ni-ro′be) [*Nairobi*, the capital of Kenya, in East Africa] see under *disease* and *eye*.

naja (nah′jah) [Arabic] the cobra di capello, *Naja naja* (*N. tripudians*), a common cobra of India; also a homeopathic preparation of its venom. See *cobra*.

nalbuphine hydrochloride (nal′bu-fēn) chemical name: 17-(cyclobutylmethyl)-4,5α-epoxymorphinan-3,6α,14-triol hydrochloride; an analgesic and narcotic antagonist, $C_{21}H_{27}NO_4 \cdot HCl$.

Nalfon (nal′fon) trademark for a preparation of fenoprofen calcium.

nalidixate sodium (nal-ĭ-diks′āt) chemical name: 1-ethyl-1,4-dihydro-7-methyl-4-oxo-1,8-naphthyridine-3-carboxylate sodium salt monohydrate; an antibacterial, $C_{12}H_{11}N_2NaO_3H_2O$.

Nalline (nal′lēn) trademark for a preparation of nalorphine.

nalmexone hydrochloride (nal-meks′ōn) chemical name: 4,5α-epoxy-3,14-dihydroxy-17-(3-methyl-2-butenyl)morphinan-6-one hydrochloride; an antagonist and narcotic antagonist, $C_{21}H_{25}$-$NO_4 \cdot HCl$.

nalorphine (nal′or-fēn, nal-or′fēn) chemical name: 17-allyl-7,8-didehydro-4,5α-epoxymorphinan-3,6-α-diol. A drug structurally related to morphine, $C_{19}H_{21}NO_3$, which acts as an antagonist to morphine and related narcotics. Called also *allorphine* and *antorphine.* **n. hydrochloride** [USP], the hydrochloride salt of nalorphine, $C_{19}H_{21}NO_3 \cdot HCl$, occurring as a white or practically white, crystalline powder; used as a narcotic antagonist, chiefly to counteract respiratory depression due to narcotic overdosage, administered intravenously. It is also used to diagnose narcotic addiction; withdrawal symptoms occur following its subcutaneous administration to addicts.

naloxone hydrochloride (nal-oks′ōn) chemical name: 17-allyl-4,5α-epoxy-3,14-dihydroxymorphinan-6-one hydrochloride. A narcotic antagonist structurally related to oxymorphone, $C_{19}H_{21}$-NO_4HCl, occurring as a white to slightly off-white powder; used as an antidote to narcotic overdosage, and as an antagonist for pentazocine overdosage, administered parenterally.

naltrexone (nal-treks′ōn) chemical name: 17-(cyclopropylmethyl)-4,5α-epoxy-3,14-dihydroxymorphinan-6-one; a narcotic antagonist, $C_{20}H_{23}NO_4$.

nandrolone (nan′dro-lōn) chemical name: 17β-hydroxyestr-4-en-3-one. An anabolic steroid, $C_{18}H_{26}O_2$, differing from testosterone in not having a methyl group attached to carbon 10 of the steroid nucleus. Called also *norandrostenolone.* **n. cyclotate,** an ester of nandrolone, $C_{28}H_{38}O_3$. **n. decanoate** [USP], an ester of nandrolone, $C_{28}H_{44}O_3$, occurring as a fine, white to creamy white, crystalline powder, having the properties of other anabolic steroids and a long duration of action; used mainly as adjunctive therapy in senile and postmenopausal osteoporosis and in the treatment of severe growth retardation in children, administered intramuscularly. **n. phenpropionate** [USP], an ester of nandrolone, $C_{27}H_{34}O_3$, having a moderate duration of action and the appearance, properties, uses, and mode of administration of the decanoate ester.

nanism (na′nizm) [L. *nanus* dwarf] dwarfishness or marked undersize from whatever cause. **mulibrey n.,** a rare autosomal recessive disorder marked by dwarfism and constrictive pericarditis; called mulibrey to denote defects of *mu*scle, *li*ver, *br*ain, and *ey*es. Affected infants have a triangular face often with hypocephaloid skull, muscular hypotonia, squeaky voice, and yellowish dots and pigment dispersion in the ocular fundus. **Paltauf's n.,** nanism associated with lymphatism. **pituitary n.,** hypophyseal infantilism. **renal n.,** infantile renal osteodystrophy. **senile n.,** progeria. **symptomatic n.,** nanism with defective ossification, dentition, and sexual development.

Nannizzia (nah-niz′ĭ-ah) a genus of ascomycetous fungi (family Gymnoascaceae, order Eurotiales), in which the hyphae around the gymnothecium are verticillately branched and composed of cells with shallow constrictions; it contains the perfect (sexual) stages of *Microsporum.*

nano- (na′no) [Gr. *nanos*; L. *nanus* dwarf] a combining form designating small size; used in naming units of measurement to indicate one-billionth of the unit designated by the root with which it is combined (10^{-9}).

nanocephalia (nan″o-sĕ-fa′le-ah) nanocephaly.

nanocephalous (na″no-sef′ah-lus) [*nano-* + Gr. *kephalē* head] having a small head; pertaining to nanocephaly.

nanocephaly (na″no-sef′ah-le) abnormal smallness of the head.

nanocormia (na″no-kor′me-ah) [*nano-* + Gr. *kormos* trunk + *-ia*] a developmental anomaly characterized by abnormal smallness of the body, or trunk.

nanocurie (na″no-ku′re) a unit of radioactivity, being 10^{-9} curie, or the quantity of radioactive material in which the number of nuclear disintegrations is 3.7×10, or 37, per second; abbreviated nc. Called also *millimicrocurie.*

nanogram (na′no-gram) a unit of mass (weight) of the metric system, being one one-billionth (10^{-9}) gram; abbreviated ng. Called also *millimicrogram.*

nanoid (na′noid) [*nano-* + Gr. *eidos* form] dwarfish; resembling a dwarf.

nanoliter (na″no-le′ter) a unit of capacity equal to one-billionth (10^{-9}) of a liter; abbreviated nl. Called also *millimicroliter.*

nanomelia (na″no-me′le-ah) [*nano-* + Gr. *melos* limb + *-ia*] a developmental anomaly characterized by abnormal smallness of the limbs.

nanomelous (na-nom′ĕ-lus) pertaining to or characterized by nanomelia.

nanomelus (na-nom′ĕ-lus) an individual exhibiting nanomelia.

nanometer (na″no-me′ter) a unit of linear measure equal to one-billionth of a meter, 10^{-9} meter; abbreviated nm. Called also *millimicron.*

nanophthalmia (nan″of-thal′me-ah) nanophthalmos.

nanophthalmos (nan″of-thal′mus) [*nan(o)-* + Gr. *ophthalmos* eye] abnormal smallness in all dimensions of one or both eyes in the absence of other ocular defects; pure microphthalmos.

nanophthalmus (nan″of-thal′mus) 1. nanophthalmos. 2. a person affected with nanophthalmos.

Nanophyetus salmincola (na-no′fi-e-tus sal-min′ko-lah) *Troglotrema salmincola.*

nanoplankton (na″no-plank′ton) plankton of extremely minute size.

nanosecond (na″no-sek′ond) one-billionth (10^{-9}) of a second; abbreviated ns. or nsec.

nanosoma (na″no-so′mah) nanosomia.

nanosomia (na″no-so′me-ah) [*nano-* + Gr. *sōma* body + *-ia*] a dwarfish habit of body; nanism.

nanosomus (na-no-so′mus) [*nano-* + Gr. *sōma* body] a person of dwarfish stature and size; a dwarf.

nanounit (na″no-u′nit) one-billionth (10^{-9}) of a standard unit; abbreviated nU.

nanous (na′nus) dwarfish; stunted.

nanukayami (nah″nu-kah-yah′me) a leptospirosis marked by fever and jaundice, first reported in Japan and caused by *Leptospira hebdomidis;* the animal host is the field vole, *Microtus montebelli.* Called also *nanukayami disease* or *fever, akiyami, seven-day fever, autumn fever,* and *gikiyami.*

nanus (na′nus) [L.; Gr. *nanos*] a dwarf.

NaOH sodium hydroxide.

NAP see *angle of convexity.*

napelline (na-pel′in) [L. *napellus* aconite] an analgesic alkaloid, $C_{22}H_{33}O_3N$, from aconite.

napex (na′peks) the region of the scalp just below the occipital protuberance.

naphazoline hydrochloride (naf-az′o-lēn) [USP] chemical name: 4,5-dihydro-2-(1-naphthalenyl)-1*H*-imidazole monohydrochloride. An adrenergic, $C_{14}H_{14}N_2 \cdot HCl$, occurring as a white, crystalline powder; used as a vasoconstrictor, applied topically to the nasal or ocular mucous membranes.

naphtalin (naf′tah-lin) naphthalene.

naphtalinum, naphthalinum (naf″tah-li′num; naf″thah-li′num) [L.] naphthalene.

naphtha (naf′thah) [L., from Arabic] 1. petroleum benzin. 2. ligroin. **n. ace′ti, vinegar n.,** ethyl acetate. **wood n.,** methanol.

naphthalene (naf′thah-lēn) [L. *naphthalinum*] a silvery, crystalline hydrocarbon, $C_{10}H_8$, from coal tar oil. It is insoluble in cold water, but soluble in hot water, alcohol, ether, chloroform, and benzene. Formerly used as an antiseptic in diarrhea of typhoid fever.

naphthamine (naf′thah-min) methenamine.

naphthol (naf′thol) a crystalline, antiseptic substance, $C_{10}H_7$-OH, from coal tar, occuring in two forms, the α (alphanaphthol) and β (betanaphthol). **α-n., alpha-n.,** see *alphanaphthol.* **n. aristol,** betanaphthol diiodide. **β-n., beta-n.,** see *betanaphthol.*

naphtholate (naf′tho-lāt′) a naphthol compound in which a base takes the place of hydrogen in the hydroxyl.

naphtholism (naf′thol-izm) naphthol poisoning.

naphtholum (naf-tho′lum) [L.] naphthol.

naphthoresorcine (naf″tho-re-sor′sin) a principle in transparent crystals derived from naphthol and resorcinol.

naphthyl (naf′thil) the radical, $C_{10}H_7$. **n. alcohol,** naphthol.

M
N

n. benzoate, benzonaphthol.   **n. lactate,** lactol.   **n. phenol,** naphthol.

naphthylpararosaniline (naf″thil-par″ah-ro-san′ĭ-lin) a dye, isamine blue, which has been used experimentally in the treatment of malignant tumors.

naphtol (naf′tol) naphthol.

napiform (na′pĭ-form) [L. *napus* turnip + *forma* shape] having the shape or form of a turnip.

N.A.P.N.E.S. National Association for Practical Nurse Education and Services.

naprapath (nap′rah-path) a practitioner of naprapathy.

naprapathy (nah-prap′ah-the) [Bohemian *napravit* to correct + Gr. *pathos* disease] a system of therapy employing manipulation of connective tissue (ligaments, muscles, and joints) and dietary measures; said to facilitate the recuperative and regenerative processes of the body.

Naprosyn (nah-pro′sin) trademark for a preparation of naproxen.

naproxen (nah-proks′en) chemical name: (+)-6-methoxy-α-methyl-2-naphthaleneacetic acid; an anti-inflammatory, analgesic, and antipyretic, $C_{14}H_{14}O_3$. **n. sodium,** the sodium salt of naproxen, $C_{14}H_{13}NaO_3$, having the same actions as the base.

naproxol (nah-proks′ol) chemical name: (+)-6-methoxy-α-methyl-2-naphthaleneacetic acid. An anti-inflammatory, antipyretic, and analgesic, occurring as a white to off-white, crystalline powder; used in the treatment of rheumatoid arthritis, administered orally.

napsylate (nap′sĭ-lāt) USAN contraction for 2-naphthalenesulfonate.

Naqua (nak′wah) trademark for a preparation of trichlormethiazide.

naranol hydrochloride (nar′ah-nōl) chemical name: 8,-9,10,11,11a,12-hexahydro-8,10-dimethyl-7a*H*-naphtho[1′,2′:5,6]pyrano[3,2-c]pyridin-7a-ol; a tranquilizer, $C_{18}H_{21}NO_2 \cdot HCl$.

narasin (nar′ah-sin) chemical name: α-ethyl-6-[5-[2-(5-ethyltetrahydro-5-hydroxy-6-methyl-2*H*-pyran-2-yl)-15-hydroxy-2,10,12-trimethyl-1,6,8-trioxadispiro[4.1.5.3]pentadec-13-en-9-yl]-2-hydroxy-1,3-dimethyl-4-oxoheptyl] tetrahydro-3,5-dimethyl-2*H*-pyran-2-acetic acid; a veterinary coccidiostat and growth stimulant, $C_{43}H_{72}O_{11}$.

Narath's operation (nah′rats) [Albert *Narath*, Austrian surgeon, 1864–1924] see under *operation*.

Narcan (nar′kan) trademark for a preparation of naloxone hydrochloride.

narcism (nar′sizm) narcissism.

narcissine (nar-sis′in) a crystalline alkaloid, $C_{16}H_{17}NO_4$, having emetic properties, from the bulbs of many different plants, including the daffodil, *Narcissus pseudonarcissus* L. (Amaryllidaceae); identical with lycorine.

narcissism (nar′sĭ-sizm) [from *Narcissus*, a character in Greek mythology who fell in love with his own image reflected in water] self-love, which may or may not include genital excitation. In psychoanalysis, *primary n.* is the original energy embodied in the infantile ego; *secondary n.* denotes libidinous attachments withdrawn from others and directed back onto the self, as in schizophrenia.

narcissistic (nar″sĭ-sis′tik) pertaining to or characterized by narcissism.

narco- (nar′ko) [Gr. *narkē* numbness] a combining form denoting relationship to stupor or to a stuporous state.

narcoanalysis (nar″ko-ah-nal′ĭ-sis) a form of psychotherapy that utilizes the slow intravenous administration of barbiturates in order to release suppressed or repressed thoughts, i.e., to disinhibit communication of affect-laden and unacceptable ideas.

narcoanesthesia (nar″ko-an″es-the′ze-ah) [*narco-* + *anesthesia*] (*obs.*) anesthesia by the production of a stuporous condition by the hypodermic injection of scopolamine and morphine.

narcodiagnosis (nar″ko-di″ag-no′sis) narcoanalysis.

narcohypnia (nar″ko-hip′ne-ah) [*narco-* + Gr. *hypnos* sleep + *-ia*] numbness felt on waking from sleep.

narcohypnosis (nar″ko-hip-no′sis) hypnotic suggestions made while the patient is under the influence of a narcotic drug.

narcolepsy (nar′ko-lep″se) [*narco-* + Gr. *lēpsis* a taking hold, a seizure] a condition marked by an uncontrollable desire for sleep or by sudden attacks of sleep occurring at intervals; often associated with cataplexy. Called also *Gélineau's syndrome, paroxysmal sleep,* and *sleep epilepsy.*

narcoleptic (nar″ko-lep′tik) pertaining to, characterized by, or producing narcolepsy. By extension, sometimes used to denote an individual who exhibits narcolepsy.

narcoma (nar-ko′mah) a stuporous state produced by narcotics.

narcose (nar′kōs) stuporous; in a state of stupor.

narcosine (nar′ko-sēn) noscapine.

narcosis (nar-ko′sis) [Gr. *narkōsis* a benumbing] a nonspecific and reversible depression of function of the central nervous system marked by stupor or insensibility and produced by drugs.

basal n., basis n., narcosis marked by complete unconsciousness, amnesia, and analgesia; see *preanesthesia*. **insufflation n.,** insufflation anesthesia. **intravenous n.,** phlebonarcosis. **medullary n.,** narcosis produced by injection of a local anesthetic into the medullary subarachnoid space. **Nussbaum's n.,** general narcosis by the use of ether or chloroform after an injection of morphine. **rausch n.,** see *rausch*.

narcostimulant (nar″ko-stim′u-lant) having both narcotic and stimulant properties.

narcosynthesis (nar″ko-sin′thĕ-sis) narcoanalysis.

narcotic (nar-kot′ik) [Gr. *narkōtikos* benumbing, deadening] 1. pertaining to or producing narcosis. 2. an agent that produces insensibility or stupor.

narcotico-acrid (nar-kot″ĭ-ko-ak′rid) both narcotic and acrid.

narcotico-irritant (nar-kot″ĭ-ko-ir′ĭ-tant) both narcotic and irritant.

narcotile (nar′ko-tīl) ethyl chloride.

narcotine (nar′ko-tēn) noscapine.

narcotism (nar′ko-tizm) (*obs.*) 1. narcosis. 2. addiction to narcotics.

narcotize (nar′ko-tīz) to put under the influence of a narcotic.

narcous (nar′kus) narcose.

Nardil (nar′dil) trademark for a preparation of phenelzine sulfate.

nares (na′rēz) [L., pl. of *na′ris*, q.v.] [NA] the external orifices of the nose; called also *nostrils*. See *naris*.

naris (na′ris) pl. *na′res* [L.] one of the openings of the nasal cavity. **anterior n., external n.,** either of the external orifices of the nose (nares [NA]). **internal nares,** see *cavum nasi*. **posterior nares,** the openings between the nasal cavity and the nasopharynx (choanae [NA]).

Narone (nar′ōn) trademark for a preparation of dipyrone.

nasal (na′zal) [L. *nasalis*] pertaining to the nose.

nasalis (na-za′lis) [L.] relating to the nose.

nascent (nas′ent, na′sent) [L. *nascens*] 1. just born; just coming into existence. 2. just liberated from a chemical combination, and hence more reactive because uncombined.

N.A.S.E. National Association for the Study of Epilepsy.

nasioiniac (na″ze-o-in′e-ak) pertaining to the nasion and the inion.

nasion (na′ze-on) [L. *nasus* nose] 1. an anthropometric landmark, the point at which a horizontal line tangential to the highest points on the superior palpebral sulci is intersected by the midsagittal plane. Called also *nasal point*. 2. the depression at the root of the nose that indicates the position of the frontonasal suture.

nasitis (na-zi′tis) [L. *nasus* nose + *-itis*] inflammation of the nose.

Nasmyth's membrane (nas′miths) [Alexander *Nasmyth*, Scottish dental surgeon in London, died 1847] primary (enamel) cuticle.

NAS-NRC National Academy of Sciences–National Research Council.

Na₂SO₄ Na_2SO_4 sodium sulfate.

Na₂S₂O₃ $Na_2S_2O_3$ sodium thiosulfate.

naso- (na′zo) [L. *nasus* nose] a combining form denoting relationship to the nose.

nasoantral (na″zo-an′tral) pertaining to the nose and the maxillary antrum (sinus).

nasoantritis (na″zo-an-tri′tis) inflammation of the nose and antrum of Highmore.

nasoantrostomy (na″so-an-tros′to-me) surgical formation of a nasoantral window for drainage of an obstructed maxillary sinus.

nasobronchial (na″zo-brong′ke-al) pertaining to the nasal cavities and the bronchi.

nasociliary (na″zo-sil′e-a″re) pertaining to or affecting the eyes, brow, and root of the nose, as the nasociliary nerve.

nasofrontal (na″zo-frun′tal) pertaining to the nasal and frontal bones.

nasogastric (na″zo-gas′trik) pertaining to the nose and stomach, as in (nasogastric) aspiration of the stomach's contents.

nasograph (na′zo-graf) an instrument for measuring the nose.

nasolabial (na″zo-la′be-al) [*naso-* + L. *labium* lip] pertaining to the nose and lip.

nasolacrimal (na″zo-lak′rĭ-mal) pertaining to the nose and lacrimal apparatus.

nasomanometer (na″zo-mah-nom′ĕ-ter) a manometer for measuring intranasal pressure.

nasonnement (na″zon-maw′) [Fr.] a nasal quality of voice.

naso-oral (na″zo-o′ral) pertaining to or involving the nose and mouth.

nasopalatine (na″zo-pal′ah-tīn) [*naso-* + *palatine*] pertaining to the nose and palate.

nasopharyngeal (na″zo-fah-rin′je-al)   pertaining to the nasopharynx.

nasopharyngitis (na″zo-far″in-ji′tis)   inflammation of the nasopharynx.

nasopharyngolaryngoscope (na″zo-fah-ring″go-lah-ring′go-skōp)   a flexible fiberoptic endoscope for examining the nasopharynx and larynx.

nasopharyngoscope (na″zo-fah-rin′go-skōp)   a lighted, telescopic endoscope for use in examination of the nasopharynx and the pharyngeal end of the auditory tube.

nasopharynx (na″zo-far′inks) [naso- + pharynx]   the part of the pharynx which lies above the level of the soft palate (pars nasalis pharyngis [NA]).

nasorostral (na″zo-ros′tral)   pertaining to the rostrum of the nose.

nasoscope (na′zo-skōp) [naso- + Gr. skopein to examine]   an electrically lighted instrument for inspecting the nasal cavity.

nasoseptal (na″zo-sep′tal)   pertaining to the nasal septum.

nasoseptitis (na″zo-sep-ti′tis)   inflammation of the nasal septum.

nasosinusitis (na″zo-si″nu-si′tis)   inflammation of the accessory sinuses of the nose.

nasospinale (na″zo-spi-na′le)   the point at which a horizontal line tangential to the lower margins of the nasal aperture is intersected by the midsagittal plane.

nasoturbinal (na″zo-tur′bĭ-nal)   pertaining to the nose and turbinate bone.

nastic (nas′tik)   of or pertaining to a response of leaves or plant parts to external stimuli that is independent of the direction of origin of such stimuli; see under movement.

nasus (na′sus) [L.] [NA]   the nose: the specialized structure of the face that serves as an organ of the sense of smell and as part of the respiratory apparatus. **n. exter′nus** [NA] the external nose: the part of the nose that protrudes on the face; made up of an osteocartilaginous framework, covered externally by muscles and skin and lined internally by mucous membrane.

natal (na′tal)   1. [L. natus birth] pertaining to birth. 2. [L. nates buttocks] pertaining to the buttocks; pygal.

natality (na-tal′ĭ-te) [L. natalis pertaining to birth]   the birth rate in any community.

nataloin (na-tal′o-in)   an aloin or glycosidal bitter principle, $C_{25}H_{28}O_{11}$, derived from Natal aloes.

natamycin (nat″ah-mi′sin)   chemical name: pimaricin, a polyene antibiotic, $C_{33}H_{47}NO_{13}$, used in topical treatment of fungal keratitis, blepharitis, and conjunctivitis.

nates (na′tēz) [L., pl. of natis] [NA]   the prominences formed by the gluteal muscles on the lower part of the back; called also buttocks and clunes.

natimortality (na″te-mor-tal′ĭ-te) [L. natus birth + mortality]   the proportion of stillbirths to the general birth rate.

National Formulary   a book of standards for certain pharmaceuticals and preparations that are not included in the USP. It is revised every five years, and recognized as a book of official standards by the Pure Food and Drugs Act of 1906. Abbreviated NF.

natis (na′tis) [L. "rump"]   see nates.

native (na′tiv) [L. nativus]   normal to a location; unaltered from its natural state.

Natolone (nat′o-lōn)   trademark for a preparation of pregnenolone.

natremia (nah-tre′me-ah) [L. natrium sodium + Gr. haima blood + -ia]   hypernatremia.

natrium (na′tre-um), gen. na′trii [L.]   sodium.

natriuresis (na″tre-u-re′sis) [L. natrium sodium + Gr. ourēsis a making water]   the excretion of abnormal amounts of sodium in the urine.

natriuretic (na″tre-u-ret′ik)   1. pertaining to, characterized by, or promoting natriuresis. 2. an agent that promotes natriuresis.

natron (na′tron)   native sodium carbonate; also soda or sodium hydroxide.

natrum (na′trum)   sodium.

natruresis (nat″roo-re′sis)   natriuresis.

natruretic (nat″roo-ret′ik)   natriuretic.

natural (nat′u-ral) [L. naturalis, from natura nature]   neither artificial nor pathologic.

Naturetin (nat″u-re′tin)   trademark for preparations of bendroflumethiazide.

naturopath (na′tūr-o-path″)   a practitioner of naturopathy.

naturopathic (na″tūr-o-path′ik)   pertaining to naturopathy.

naturopathy (na″tūr-op′ah-the)   a drugless system of therapy, making use of physical forces such as air, light, water, heat, massage, etc.

Nauheim bath, treatment (now′hīm) [Bad-Nauheim, a town and watering place in Hessen, Germany]   see under bath, and see Schott's treatment, under treatment.

Naumanniella (naw-man″ne-el′lah)   a genus of microorganisms of the family Siderocapsaceae, suborder Pseudomonadineae, order Pseudomonadales, occurring as ellipsoidal or rod-shaped cells with rounded ends, found in iron-containing water. It includes five species, N. catena′ta, N. ellip′tica, N. mi′nor, N. neusto′nica, and N. pygmae′a.

Naunyn-Minkowski method (now′nin-min- kow′ske) [Bernard Naunyn; Oscar Minkowski, Lithuanian physician in Wiesbaden, 1858–1931]   see under method.

naupathia (naw-pa′the-ah, naw″pah-the′ah) [Gr. naus ship + pathos suffering + -ia]   (obs.) seasickness.

nausea (naw′se-ah) [L.; Gr. nausia seasickness]   an unpleasant sensation, vaguely referred to the epigastrium and abdomen, and often culminating in vomiting. **n. epidem′ica,** an epidemic disease, probably viral gastroenteritis, marked by nausea, vomiting, giddiness, and diarrhea. **n. gravida′rum,** the morning sickness of pregnancy. **n. mari′na, n. nava′lis,** seasickness.

nauseant (naw′se-ant)   1. inducing nausea. 2. an agent that causes nausea.

nauseate (naw′se-āt)   to affect with nausea.

nauseous (naw′shus, naw′se-us)   pertaining to or producing nausea.

Navane (nav′ān)   trademark for preparations of thiothixene.

navel (na′vel)   the umbilicus. **blue n.,** Cullen's sign. **enamel n.,** an indentation in the outer dental epithelium of a developing tooth, in the end of the enamel cord.

navicula (nah-vik′u-lah) [L.]   frenulum labiorum pudendi.

navicular (nah-vik′u-lar) [L. navicula boat]   boat-shaped, as the navicular bone.

navicularthritis (nah-vik″u-lar-thri′tis)   inflammation of the navicular joint of the horse's forefoot.

Nb   chemical symbol for niobium.

N.B.S.   National Bureau of Standards.

NBT   nitroblue tetrazolium; see under tests.

nc.   nanocurie.

N.C.A.   neurocirculatory asthenia.

NCI   National Cancer Institute.

N.C.M.H.   National Committee for Mental Hygiene.

N.C.N.   National Council of Nurses.

NCRP   National Committee on Radiation Protection and Measurements.

Nd   chemical symbol for neodymium.

n_D   symbol for refractive index.

N.D.A.   National Dental Association.

NDV   Newcastle disease virus.

Ne   chemical symbol for neon.

nealogy (ne-al′o-je) [Gr. nealēs young + -logy]   the study of the early infant stages of animals.

near-sight (nēr′sīt)   myopia.

nearsighted (nēr-sīt′ed)   myopic.

nearsightedness (nēr-sīt′ed-nes)   myopia.

nearthrosis (ne″ar-thro′sis) [Gr. neos new + arthron joint]   1. a false joint; pseudarthrosis. 2. an artificial joint constructed in the shaft of a bone by a surgical operation.

Nebcin (neb′sin)   trademark for a preparation of tobramycin sulfate.

nebenagglutinin (na″ben-ah-gloo′tĭ-nin) [Ger. neben near, beside + agglutinin]   partial agglutinin.

nebenkern (na″ben-kern) [Ger. neben near, beside + kern kernel, nucleus]   1. a name given to several structures of the cell, but especially to the paranucleus. 2. a large mitochondrial mass around the axial filament in the flagellum of the spermatozoon; it is formed by coalescence of smaller mitochondria during spermatogenesis.

nebramycin (neb″rah-mi′sin)   a complex of antibacterial antibiotic substances produced by Streptomyces tenebrarius, consisting of eight components, one of which, factor 6 (known as tobramycin), is used clinically.

Nebs (nebz)   trademark for preparations of acetaminophen.

nebula (neb′u-lah), pl. neb′ulae [L. "mist"]   1. a slight corneal opacity or scar that can be seen only by oblique illumination; it seldom interferes with vision. 2. cloudiness in urine. 3. an oily preparation for use in an atomizer.

nebularine (neb-u-lār′in)   chemical name: 9-β-D-ribofuranosyl-9H-purine. An antibiotic substance, $C_{10}H_{12}N_4O_4$, isolated from the juice of the fungus Clitocybe nebularis, which has tuberculostatic and antimitotic activity, and in high dilutions, preferentially inhibits growth of some cancer cells.

nebulization (neb″u-li-za′shun) [L. nebula mist]   1. conversion into a spray. 2. treatment by a spray.

nebulizer (neb′u-līz″er)   an atomizer; a device for throwing a spray.

Necator (ne-ka′tor) [L. "murderer"]   a genus of nematode parasites of the family Ancylostomidae. **N. america′nus,** the

American or New World hookworm, a nematode parasite resembling, but shorter and more slender than, *Ancylostoma duodenale*. It is characterized by its buccal cavity containing four plates, four pharyngeal lancets, and a dorsal conic tooth. Infection by this parasite produces hookworm disease. Called also *Ancylostoma americanum* and *Uncinaria americana*. See also *hookworm disease*, under *disease*.

necatoriasis (ne-ka″to-ri′ah-sis) the state of being infected with worms of the genus *Necator*. See *hookworm disease*, under *disease*.

necessity (ně-ses′ĭ-te) something necessary or indispensable. **pharmaceutic n., pharmaceutical n.,** a substance having slight or no value therapeutically, but used in the preparation of various pharmaceuticals, including preservatives, solvents, ointment bases, and flavoring, coloring, diluting, emulsifying, and suspending agents; called also *pharmaceutic* or *pharmaceutical aid*.

neck (nek) a constricted portion, such as the part connecting the head and trunk of the body (collum [NA]), or the constricted part of an organ, as of the uterus (cervix uteri), or other structure (e.g., collum dentis). **anatomical n. of humerus,** collum

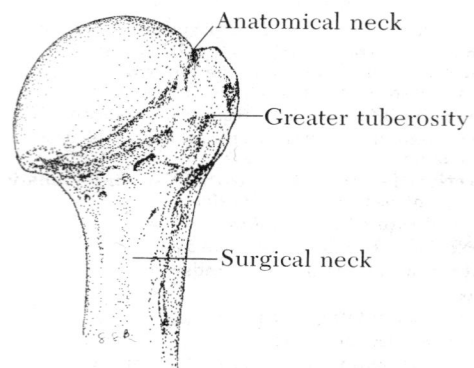

Anatomical neck

Greater tuberosity

Surgical neck

Head of humerus showing the anatomical and surgical necks.

anatomicum humeri. **n. of ankle bone,** collum tali. **big n.,** goiter. **bull n.,** massive swelling of the neck, as in malignant diphtheria. **n. of condyloid process of mandible,** collum mandibulae. **dental n.,** collum dentis. **Derbyshire n.,** goiter. **false n. of humerus,** collum chirurgicum humeri. **n. of femur,** collum femoris. **n. of gallbladder,** collum vesicae felleae. **n. of glans penis,** collum glandis penis. **n. of hair follicle,** collum folliculi pili. **n. of humerus,** collum anatomicum humeri. **lateral n. of vertebra,** pediculus arcus vertebrae. **Madelung's n.,** diffuse symmetrical lipomas of the neck. **n. of malleus,** collum mallei. **n. of mandible,** collum mandibulae. **Nithsdale n.,** goiter. **n. of pancreas,** a constricted portion marking the junction of the head and body of the pancreas. **n. of radius,** collum radii. **n. of rib,** collum costae. **n. of scapula,** collum scapulae. **n. of spermatozoon,** the portion of the tail of a spermatozoon beginning immediately behind the head and extending to the anterior centriole. See illustration under *spermatozoon*. **surgical n. of humerus,** collum chirurgicum humeri. **n. of talus,** collum tali. **n. of tooth,** the slightly constricted region of union of the crown and root or roots of a tooth; called also *collum dentis* [NA] and *cervix dentis*. **true n. of humerus,** collum anatomicum humeri. **turkey gobbler n.,** submental vertical skin folds. **n. of urinary bladder,** cervix vesicae. **uterine n., n. of uterus,** cervix uteri. **n. of vertebra, n. of vertebral arch,** pediculus arcus vertebrae. **webbed n.,** pterygium colli. **wry n.,** torticollis.

necklace (nek′las) an encircling band around the neck. **Casal's n.,** an area of erythema and pigmentation around the neck in pellagra; called also *Casal's collar*.

necrectomy (nek-rek′to-me) [*necro-* + Gr. *ektomē* excision] excision of necrotic tissue.

necrencephalus (nek″ren-sef′ah-lus) [*necro-* + Gr. *enkephalos* brain] softening of the brain.

necro- (nek′ro) [Gr. *nekros* dead] a combining form denoting relationship to death or to a dead body, cells, or tissue.

necrobacillosis (nek″ro-bas″ĭ-lo′sis) infection with Schmorl's bacillus, *Fusobacterium necrophorum*, which causes diphtheria with abscesses in cattle, gangrenous dermatitis in horses, areas of necrosis in hogs and cattle, and abscesses and areas of necrosis in rabbits. See also *calf diphtheria*, under *diphtheria*, and *Schmorl's disease*, under *disease*.

necrobiosis (nek″ro-bi-o′sis) [*necro-* + Gr. *biōsis* life] swelling, basophilia, and distortion of collagen bundles in the dermis, sometimes with obliteration of normal structure, but short of actual necrosis, characteristic especially of granuloma annulare

and necrobiosis lipoidica diabeticorum. Cf. *gangrene* and *necrosis*. **n. lipoi′dica,** n. lipoidica diabeticorum. **n. lipoi′dica diabetico′rum,** a dermatosis usually occurring in diabetics, characterized by necrobiosis of the elastic and connective tissue of the skin, with degenerating collagen occurring in irregular patches, especially in the upper dermis. The lesions are most commonly located on the mid or lower shins.

necrobiotic (nek″ro-bi-ot′ik) pertaining to or characterized by necrobiosis.

necrocytosis (nek″ro-si-to′sis) [*necro-* + Gr. *kytos* cell + *-osis*] death and decay of cells.

necrocytotoxin (nek″ro-si″to-tok′sin) a toxin that produces death of cells.

necrogenic (nek″ro-jen′ik) [*necro-* + Gr. *gennan* to produce] productive of necrosis or death.

necrogenous (ně-kroj′ě-nus) originating or arising from dead matter.

necrologic (nek″ro-loj′ik) pertaining to necrology.

necrologist (ně-krol′o-jist) an expert in necrology.

necrology (ně-krol′o-je, ne-krol′o-je) [*necro-* + *-logy*] the statistics or records of deaths.

necrolysis (ně-krol′ĭ-sis) [*necro-* + Gr. *lysis* dissolution] separation or exfoliation of tissue due to necrosis. **toxic epidermal n.,** an exfoliative skin disease in which erythema rapidly spreads over the entire body, followed by the formation of large flaccid bullae and later by skin that appears scalded and separates from the body in sheets, much as in a second degree burn. Staphylococci of phage group two (in infants) and a toxic reaction to various drugs (in adults) are the usual causes. Called *Lyell's syndrome* and *scalded skin syndrome*. Cf. *dermatitis exfoliativa neonatorum*.

necromania (nek″ro-ma′ne-ah) [*necro-* + Gr. *mania* madness] necrophilia.

necrometer (ně-krom′ě-ter) [*necro-* + Gr. *metron* measure] an instrument for measuring the organs of the dead body.

necromimesis (nek″ro-mi-me′sis) [*necro-* + Gr. *mimēsis* imitation] a delusion of being dead, or the feigning of death.

necronectomy (nek″ro-nek′to-me) [*necro-* + Gr. *ektomē* excision] the excision of necrotic tissue.

necrophagous (ně-krof′ah-gus) [*necro-* + Gr. *phagein* to eat] devouring or subsisting on dead bodies.

necrophilia (nek″ro-fil′e-ah) morbid attraction to corpses; sexual intercourse with a dead body.

necrophilic (nek″ro-fil′ik) 1. pertaining to or characterized by necrophilism. 2. showing preference for dead tissue, as necrophilic bacteria.

necrophilism (ně-krof′ĭ-lizm) [*necro-* + Gr. *philein* to love] necrophilia.

necrophilous (ně-krof′ĭ-lus) 1. showing preference for dead tissues; said of organisms. 2. pertaining to or characterized by necrophilia.

necrophily (ně-krof′ĭ-le) necrophilia.

necrophobia (nek″ro-fo′be-ah) [*necro-* + *phobia*] 1. morbid fear of death. 2. morbid dread of dead bodies.

necropneumonia (nek″ro-nu-mo′ne-ah) [*necro-* + Gr. *pneumōn* lung + *-ia*] gangrene of the lung.

necropsy (nek′rop-se) [Gr. *nekros* dead + *opsis* view] examination of a body after death; see *autopsy*.

necrosadism (nek″ro-sa′dism) [Gr. *nekros* dead + *sadism*] mutilation of a corpse for the purpose of exciting or gratifying sexual feelings.

necroscopy (ně-kros′ko-pe) [Gr. *nekros* dead + *skopein* to examine] necropsy.

necrose (nek′rōs) to become necrotic or to undergo necrosis.

necroses (ně-kro′sēz) [Gr.] plural of *necrosis*.

necrosin (nek′ro-sin) a substance liberated by injured cells, which produces the signs of inflammation, central necrosis, lymphatic blockade, injury to vascular endothelium, and swelling of collagen.

necrosis (ně-kro′sis), pl. *necro′ses* [Gr. *nekrōsis* deadness] the sum of the morphological changes indicative of cell death and caused by the progressive degradative action of enzymes; it may affect groups of cells or part of a structure or an organ. **arteriolar n.,** arteriolonecrosis. **aseptic n.,** increasing sclerosis and cystic changes in the head of the femur which sometimes follow traumatic dislocation of the hip. A similar condition sometimes develops in the head of the humerus after shoulder dislocation. **avascular n.,** that due to deficient blood supply. **bacillary n.,** necrobacillosis. **Balser's fatty n.,** gangrenous pancreatitis with omental bursitis and disseminated patches of necrosis of the fatty tissues; pancreatitis with fat necrosis. **caseous n.,** cheesy n. **central n.,** that which affects the central portion of a cell or of a bone or a lobule of the liver. **cerebrocortical n.,** a highly fatal condition due to abnormal utilization of thiamine or to anoxia, affecting calves and ewes and marked by circling movements, staggering gait, excitement, and convulsions. **cheesy n.,** necrosis in which the tissue is soft, dry and cheesy, thus resembling cottage cheese; it is seen mostly in tuberculosis and syphilis. Called also *caseous n.* **coagulation n.**, necrosis of a portion of some organ or tissue, with the formation of fibrous infarcts, in which a relatively small part seems to have been deprived of the afflux of blood by the plugging of its vessels with coagula. **colliquative n.**, necrosis in which the necrotic material becomes softened and liquefied. **cystic medial n.**, Erdheim's cystic medial n. **dry n.**, that in which the necrotic tissue becomes dry. **embolic n.**, coagulation necrosis of an infarct following embolism. **epiphyseal ischemic n.**, degeneration and eventual replacement of the osseous nucleus of an epiphysis, which collapses under pressure and causes distortion of the surrounding healthy tissue; attributed to interference with the blood supply of the epiphysis. It may affect the femur, tibia, tarsal navicular head, humerus, etc. Called also *osteochondrosis* (q.v.). **Erdheim's cystic medial n.**, changes in the medial layer of the aorta, consisting of degeneration and necrosis of elastic and muscle fibers, mucoid infiltration, and cyst formation, often resulting in dissecting aneurysm; called also *medionecrosis of aorta.* **exanthematous n.**, an acute necrotizing process involving the gingivae, jaw bones, and contiguous soft tissues, which primarily affects children; it resembles gangrenous stomatitis, except that there is slight odor, a tendency to be self-limited, low mortality rate, and normal leukocyte count. **fat n.**, a condition in which the neutral fats in the cells of adipose tissue are split into fatty acids and glycerol; it usually affects subcutaneous fat depots, particularly in the female breast, as a result of trauma, and forms a focal area felt on percussion as a firm circumscribed mass. Called also *steatonecrosis.* **focal n.**, the presence of small foci of necrosis often seen in the course of an infection. **gangrenous n.**, cell death caused by a combination of ischemia and superimposed bacterial infection, combining the features of coagulation and colliquative necrosis. **hyaline n.**, Zenker's degeneration. **ischemic n.**, coagulation n. **labial n. of rabbits**, a fatal necrobacillosis of rabbits that begins in the lower lip and extends down to the thorax. **liquefaction n.**, colliquative n. **massive hepatic n.**, acute yellow atrophy. **medial n.**, medionecrosis. **mercurial n.**, necrosis due to mercury poisoning. **moist n.**, that in which the dead tissue becomes wet and soft. **mummification n.**, dry gangrene. **Paget's quiet n.**, a process of local necrosis and sequestrum formation in the superficial layers of the shaft of a long bone with a minimal amount of suppuration around the sequestrum and without sinus formation. **peripheral n.**, necrosis of the peripheral portions of a liver lobule as in puerperal eclampsia. **phosphorus n.**, phosphonecrosis. **postpartum pituitary n.**, necrosis of the pituitary during the postpartum period, often associated with shock and excessive uterine bleeding during delivery, and leading to variable patterns of hypopituitarism; called also *Sheehan's syndrome.* **pressure n.**, necrosis due to insufficient local blood supply as in decubitus ulcers. **n. progre′diens**, progressive sloughing. **progressive emphysematous n.**, gas gangrene. **radiation n.**, a death of tissue caused by radiation. **radium n.**, necrosis of the jaw bone occurring in workers in radium plants. **n. of renal papillae, renal papillary n.**, an accompaniment of acute pyelonephritis, most often seen in diabetics, characterized by necrosis of the renal papillae of one or both kidneys, with sharp demarcation between necrotic and living tissue; called also *necrotizing papillitis* and *necrotizing renal papillitis.* **septic n.**, necrosis resulting from bacterial infection. **simple n.**, degeneration of the protoplasm and nucleus of the cells of a tissue without change in the appearance of the tissue. **subcutaneous fat n.**, adiponecrosis subcutanea neonatorum. **superficial n.**, that which affects only the outer layers of a bone. **syphilitic n.**, necrosis caused by syphilis. **total n.**, that which affects all parts of a bone. **n. ustilagin′ea**, dry gangrene from ergotism. **Zenker's n.**, see under *degeneration.*

necrospermia (nek″ro-sper′me-ah) [Gr. *nekros* dead + *sperm* + *-ia*] a condition in which the spermatozoa of the semen are dead or motionless.

necrospermic (nek″ro-sper′mik) pertaining to or characterized by necrospermia.

necrotic (ně-krot′ik) pertaining to or characterized by necrosis.

necrotizing (nek′ro-tīz″ing) causing necrosis.

necrotomy (ně-krot′o-me) [Gr. *nekros* + *tomē* a cutting] 1. dissection of a dead body. 2. the excision of a sequestrum. **osteoplastic n.**, removal of a sequestrum from a bone after first lifting a flap of the bone, which is replaced after the operation.

necrotoxin (nek″ro-tok′sin) a factor or substance, produced by certain staphylococci, which kills tissue cells.

necrozoospermia (nek″ro-zo″o-sper′me-ah) necrospermia.

Necturus (nek-tu′rus) a genus of salamanders having large external gills; employed in physiologic research.

needle (ne′d′l) [L. *acus*] 1. a sharp instrument for suturing or puncturing. 2. to puncture with a needle, as in discission of the lens for treatment of cataract. **Abrams′ n.**, a biopsy needle designed to reduce the danger of introducing air into tissues, as in pleural biopsy. **aneurysm n.**, one with a handle, used in ligating blood vessels. **aspirating n.**, a long hollow needle for removing fluid from a cavity. **Babcock′s n.**, a large hypodermic needle, provided with a stilet, for spinal puncture. **cata-**

ract n., one used in removing a cataract. **Cope′s n.**, a blunt-ended hooklike needle with a concealed cutting edge and snare, used in biopsy of the pleura, pericardium, peritoneum, and synovium. **Deschamps′ n.**, one with the eye near the point, and a long handle attached; used in ligating deep-seated arteries. **discission n.**, a special form of cataract needle. **Hagedorn′s n′s**, surgical needles which are flat from side to side, and have a straight cutting edge near the point and a large eye. **harelip n.**, a needle (or pin) introduced through edges of the wound in harelip operation, a figure-of-8 suture being applied over the needle. **hypodermic n.**, a short, slender, hollow needle used in injecting drugs beneath the skin. **knife n.**, a slender knife with a needle-like point, used in discission of a cataract and other ophthalmic operations, as in goniotomy and goniopuncture. **Kobak′s n.**, a needle used to inject anesthesia for vaginal delivery and cesarean section. **ligature n.**, a slender steel needle with a long handle and an eye in its curved end, used for passing a ligature underneath an artery. **Menghini n.**, a needle that does not require rotation to cut loose the tissue specimen in a biopsy of the liver. **Reverdin′s n.**, a surgical needle having an eye which can be opened and closed by means of a slide. **Silverman n.**, an instrument for taking tissue specimens, consisting of an outer cannula, an obturator, and an inner split needle with longitudinal grooves in which the tissue is retained when the needle and cannula are withdrawn. **stop n.**, a needle with a shoulder that prevents it from being inserted beyond a certain distance. **swaged n.**, one permanently attached to the suture material. **Vim-Silverman n.**, a needle used in liver biopsy.

Neef′s hammer (nāfs) [Christopher Ernst *Neef*, German physician, 1782–1849] see under *hammer.*

Neelsen (nēl′sen) see *Ziehl-Neelsen.*

neencephalon (ne″en-sef′ah-lon) [Gr. *neos* new + *enkephalos* brain] the cerebral cortex and its dependencies; the phylogenetically newer part of the brain.

NEFA nonesterified fatty acids.

nefluorophotometer (ně-floo″o-ro-fo-tom′ě-ter) fluoronephelometer.

nefopam hydrochloride (nef′o-pam) chemical name: 3,4,-5,6-tetrahydro-5-methyl-1-phenyl-1H-2,5-benzoxazocine hydrochloride; an analgesic and muscle relaxant, $C_{17}H_{19}NO \cdot HCl$.

Negatan (neg′ah-tan) trademark for a preparation of negatol.

negation (ne-ga′shun) refusal or denial; see *delusion of negation.*

negative (neg′ah-tiv) [L. *negativus*] 1. having a value of less than zero. 2. indicating a lack or absence, as chromatin negative or Wassermann negative. 3. characterized by resistance or opposition.

negativism (neg′ah-tiv-izm″) a morbid propensity to do the opposite of what most people would do under similar circumstances, or of what one is told to do or of what one's normal desires would suggest; e.g., it is not uncommon in catatonic schizophrenia for the patient to feel compelled to lower his arms if asked to raise them or to clench his fists if asked to open his hands.

negatol (neg′ah-tol) a colloidal product obtained by reacting meta-cresol sulfonic acid with formaldehyde; used as a parasiticide, germicide, and bacteriostatic, for topical application to the cervix.

negatoscope (neg′ah-to-skōp) an apparatus for showing radiographic negatives.

negatron (neg′ah-tron) the negative electron; see *positron* and *electron.*

NegGram (neg′gram) trademark for preparations of nalidixic acid.

Negri bodies (na′gre) [Adelchi *Negri*, Italian physician, 1876–1912] see under *body.*

Negro′s phenomenon (na′grōz) [Camillo *Negro*, Italian neurologist, 1861–1927] see *cogwheel phenomenon*, under *phenomenon.*

neighborwise (na′bor-wiz) descriptive of the plastic behavior of transplanted embryonic cells or tissue in a manner appropriate to its new and strange location. Cf. *selfwise.*

Neill-Mooser bodies, reaction [Mather Humphrey *Neill*, American physician, 1882–1930; H. *Mooser*, American physician] see under *body* and *reaction.*

Neisser′s diplococcus, syringe (ni′serz) [Albert Ludwig Siegmund *Neisser*, German physician, 1855–1916] see *Neisseria gonorrhoeae* and under *syringe.*

Neisser-Doering phenomenon (ni″ser-da′ring) [Ernst *Neisser*, German physician, born 1863; Hans *Doering*, German physician, born 1871] see under *phenomenon.*

Neisser-Wechsberg phenomenon, test (ni″ser-veks′berg) [Max *Neisser*, German physician, 1869–1938; Friedrich *Wechsberg*, German physician] see *complement fixation*, under *fixation*, and see under *tests.*

Neisseria (nīs-se′re-ah) [Albert Ludwig Siegmund *Neisser*] a genus of microorganisms of the family Neisseriaceae, order Eubacteriales; it includes the gonococcus, the several meningococcus types, pigmented forms occasionally associated with meningitis, and a number of saprophytic or parasitic but nonpathogenic species.

N. catarrha′lis, *Branhamella catarrhalis.* **N. gonor-rhoe′ae,** the specific etiologic agent of gonorrhea, occurring typically as pairs of flattened cells usually found intracellularly in heterophils in diagnostic smears of purulent material. **N. meningi′tidis,** a prominent cause of meningitis and the specific etiologic agent of epidemic cerebrospinal meningitis. It occurs as several serologic types, usually taken to be four, of which IIα or C, depending on the system of nomenclature used, is considered to be the most important pathogen. **N. muco′sus,** a species characterized by the production of a heavy mucoid growth resulting from its luxuriant capsule formation; it is found in the human rhinopharynx and is occasionally pathogenic for man. Called also *Diplococcus mucosus* and *Streptococcus mucosus.*

Neisseriaceae (nīs-se″re-a′se-e) a family of Schizomycetes, order Eubacteriales, made up of nonmotile gram-negative spherical cells occurring in pairs or masses; pigment may or may not be produced, and all known species are parasitic. There are two genera, *Neisseria,* the aerobic forms, and *Veillonella,* the obligate anaerobic forms.

neisserial (nīs-se′re-al) of, relating to, or caused by *Neisseria.*

neisseriology (ni-se″re-ol′o-je) former term for the branch of medicine which deals with gonorrhea and its treatment.

nekro- for words beginning thus, see those beginning *necro-.*

nekton (nek′ton) [Gr. *nēktos* swimming] collective term for marine organisms that swim actively, as contrasted with plankton.

Nélaton's catheter, etc. (na-lah-tawz′) [Auguste *Nélaton,* French surgeon, 1807–1873] see under *catheter, line, operation, probe,* and *sphincter.*

nelavane (nel′ah-van) African trypanosomiasis.

nem (nem) acronym for Nahrungs Einheit Milch [Ger. "nutritional unit milk"]. The unit of nutrition in Pirquet's system of feeding, equivalent to the nutritive value of 1 gm. of breast milk.

N.E.M.A. National Eclectic Medical Association.

Nema (ne′mah) trademark for a preparation of tetrachloroethylene.

nema (ne′mah) [Gr. *nēma* thread] a nematode.

nemathelminth (nem″ah-thel′minth) [*nemato-* + Gr. *helmins* worms] a worm of the phylum Nemathelminthes.

Nemathelminthes (nem″ah-thel-min′thēz) in some systems of classification, a phylum including the Acanthocephala and Nematoda.

nemathelminthiasis (nem″ah-thel′min-thi′ah-sis) infection by nematodes, or roundworms.

nematicide (ně-mat′ĭ-sīd) nematocide.

nematization (nem″ah-ti-za′shun) infection with nematodes, or roundworms.

nemato- (nem′ah-to) [Gr. *nēma* thread] a combining form denoting relationship to a nematode, or to a threadlike structure.

nematoblast (nem′ah-to-blast″) [Gr. *nēma* thread + *blastos* germ] spermatid.

Nematocerca (nem″ah-tos′er-ah) [Gr. *nēma* thread + *keras* horn] a suborder of Diptera characterized by having antennae of many segments and comprising the gnats, mosquitoes, midges, black flies, craneflies, gallflies, etc.

nematocide (nem′ah-to-sīd″) [*nemato-* + L. *caedere* to kill] 1. destructive to nematode worms. 2. an agent that destroys nematodes.

nematocyst (nem′ah-to-sist) a minute stinging structure, found in the cnidoblasts of jellyfish and other coelenterates, used for anchorage, for defense, and for the capture of prey.

Nematoda (nem″ah-to′dah) [Gr. *nēma* thread + *eidos* form] a class of tapered cylindrical helminths, the roundworms, of the phylum Aschelminthes, many species of which are parasites. They are characterized by longitudinally oriented muscles and by a triradiate esophagus. In some systems of classification, they are considered to be a separate phylum. Sometimes called *Nemathelminthes,* or a class under that phylum.

nematode (nem′ah-tōd) a roundworm; any individual belonging to the class Nematoda.

nematodiasis (nem″ah-to-di′ah-sis) infection by a nematode parasite. **nonpatent n.,** visceral larva migrans.

Nematodirus (nem″ah-to′di-rus) a genus of nematode parasites belonging to the family Trichostrongylidae, found in the duodenum of ruminants.

nematoid (nem′ah-toid) resembling a thread; pertaining to a nematode parasite.

nematologist (nem″ah-tol′o-jist) a specialist in nematology.

nematology (nem″ah-tol′o-je) the branch of zoology which deals with nematode worms.

Nematomorpha (nem″ah-to-mor′fah) [Gr. *nēma* thread + *morphē* form] a class of long, slender, cylindrical worms of the phylum Aschelminthes, commonly called "hairworms," "horse hairs," or "hair eels," which are parasitic as juveniles. In some systems of classification, they are considered to be a separate phylum. Called also *Gordiacea.*

nematosis (nem″ah-to′sis) the condition of being infected with nematodes, or roundworms.

nematospermia (nem″ah-to-sper′me-ah) [*nemato-* + Gr. *sperma* sperm] spermatozoa having elongated tails.

Nembutal (nem′bu-tal) trademark for preparations of sodium pentobarbital.

Nemertea (nem-er′te-ah) Rhynchocoela.

nemertean (nem-er-te′an) 1. pertaining to the Nemertea. 2. any individual of the Nemertea. See *Rhynchocoela.*

Nemertina (nem-er-ti′nah) Rhynchocoela.

nemic (nem′ik) pertaining to nematodes, or roundworms.

Nencki's test (nents′kēz) [Marcellus von *Nencki,* Polish physician, 1847–1901] see under *tests.*

neo- (ne′o) [Gr. *neos* new] a combining form meaning new or strange.

Neo-Antergan (ne″o-an′ter-gan) trademark for a preparation of pyrilamine maleate.

neoantigen (ne″o-an′tĭ-jen) an intranuclear antigen, e.g., a T antigen, present in tumor cells transformed by oncogenic papovaviruses or adenoviruses.

neoantimosan (ne″o-an-tim′o-san) stibophen.

neoarsphenamine (ne″o-ars-fen′ah-mēn) chemical name: [5-[(3-amino-4-hydroxyphenol)arseno]-2-hydroxyanilino]methanol sulfoxylate sodium. A modified soluble compound of arsphenamine, $C_{13}H_{13}As_2N_2NaO_4S$, formerly used as an antisyphilitic.

neoarthrosis (ne″o-ar-thro′sis) nearthrosis.

neobiogenesis (ne″o-bi″o-jen′ĕ-sis) [*neo-* + *biogenesis*] biopoiesis.

Neobiotic (ne″o-bi-ot′ik) trademark for a preparation of neomycin sulfate.

neoblastic (ne″o-blas′tik) [*neo-* + Gr. *blastos* germ] originating in or of the nature of new tissue.

Neo-Calglucon (ne″o-kal′gloo-kon) trademark for a preparation of calcium glubionate.

neocerebellum (ne″o-ser″ĕ-bel′um) [*neo-* + *cerebellum*] a term applied originally to the cerebellar hemispheres and later to those parts predominantly supplied by corticopontocerebellar fibers.

neocinchophen (ne″o-sin′ko-fen) chemical name: ethyl ester of 6-methylcinchopher. Yellow needles, $C_{19}H_{17}NO_2$, which have been used as an analgesic, antipyretic, and uricosuric.

neocinetic (ne″o-si-net′ik) neokinetic.

Neo-Cobefrin (ne″o-cob′ĕ-frin) trademark for a preparation of levonordefrin.

neocortex (ne″o-kor′teks) neopallium.

neocytosis (ne″o-si-to′sis) the presence of immature cell forms in the blood.

neodarwinism (ne″o-dar′win-izm) the concept that species evolve by natural selection only, thus ruling out the inheritance of acquired traits; see *darwinism.*

neodiathermy (ne″o-di′ah-ther″me) short wave diathermy.

Neo-Diloderm (ne″o-di′lo-derm) trademark for a preparation of dichlorisone containing neomycin sulfate.

neodymium (ne″o-dim′e-um) a rare element of atomic number, 60; atomic weight, 144.24; symbol, Nd.

neoencephalon (ne″o-en-sef′ah-lon) neencephalon.

neofetal (ne″o-fe′tal) pertaining to the transitional period between the embryonic and fetal stages of the developing human young.

neofetus (ne″o-fe′tus) the embryo at about the eighth week of intrauterine life.

neoformation (ne″o-for-ma′shun) a new growth or neoplasm.

neoformative (ne″o-for′mah-tiv) concerned in the formation of new tissue.

neogala (ne-og′ah-lah) [*neo-* + Gr. *gala* milk] the first milk developed after childbirth; see also *colostrum.*

neogenesis (ne″o-jen′ĕ-sis) [*neo-* + Gr. *genesis* production] a form of tissue regeneration that is slower than anagenesis.

neogenetic (ne″o-jĕ-net′ik) pertaining to neogenesis.

neogermitrine (ne″o-jer′mĭ-trēn) an alkaloid having antihypertensive properties, isolated from green hellebore (*Veratrum viride*).

neoglottic (ne″o-glot′ik) pertaining to a neoglottis.

neoglottis (ne″o-glot′is) a surgically constructed glottis created by suturing the pharyngeal musosa over the superior end of the transected trachea above the primary tracheostoma and making a permanent stoma in the mucosa; it is created to permit phonation after laryngectomy. Called also *pseudoglottis.*

neoglycogenesis (ne″o-gli″ko-jen′ĕ-sis) gluconeogenesis.

Neohetramine (ne″o-he′trah-min) trademark for a preparation of thonzylamine hydrochloride.

neo-hippocratism (ne″o-hip-pok′rah-tizm) a school of medicine which trends toward a humanistic view of disease focused on the individual patient and scientific observation by the physician, representing a return to the hippocratic theory and practice, with emphasis on observational and bedside medicine.

Neo-Hombreol (ne''o-hom'bre-ol) trademark for preparations of testosterone propionate.

neohymen (ne''o-hi'men) [*neo-* + Gr. *hymēn* membrane] a false membrane.

neokinetic (ne''o-ki-net'ik) [*neo-* + Gr. *kinētikos* pertaining to movement] a term applied to the nervous motor mechanism regulating voluntary muscular control. It is associated with the motor area of cerebral cortex, and receives its name because of the fact that it was developed more recently than the older paleokinetic system. Cf. *archeokinetic* and *paleokinetic.*

neolalia, neolalism (ne''o-lal'e-ah; ne''o-lal'izm) speech into which many neologisms are incorporated, as in schizophrenia.

neologism (ne-ol'o-jizm) [*neo-* + Gr. *logos* word] a newly coined word; in psychiatry, a new word whose meaning may be known only to the person using it and may be related to his conflicts.

Neoloid (ne'o-loid) trademark for a preparation of castor oil.

neomembrane (ne''o-mem'brān) a false membrane.

neomin (ne'o-min) neomycin.

neomorph (ne'o-morf) [*neo-* + Gr. *morphē* form] a part or organ recently acquired in the course of evolution.

neomorphism (ne''o-mor'fizm) the development of new form in the course of evolution.

neomycin (ne'o-mi''sin) a broad-spectrum antibacterial antibiotic produced by the growth of *Streptomyces fradiae*, effective against a wide range of gram-negative organisms, including *Escherichia coli, Aerobacter aerogenes, Proteus vulgaris, Salmonella* and *Shigella* species, *Pseudomonas aeruginosa*, and *Mycobacterium tuberculosis*, and most gram-positive bacteria. **n. palmitate**, the palmitate salt of neomycin; used topically as an antibacterial in the treatment of superficial skin infections, burns, wounds, and ulcers. **n. sulfate** [USP], the sulfate salt of neomycin, occurring as a white to slightly yellow powder or cryodessicated solid; used in the treatment of urinary tract, eye, skin, ear, and enteric infections due to susceptible bacteria and for preoperative disinfection, administered orally, intramuscularly, and topically.

neon (ne'on) [Gr. *neos* new] an inert gaseous element discovered in the air in 1898; symbol, Ne; atomic weight, 20.183; atomic number, 10.

neonatal (ne''o-na'tal) [*neo-* + L. *natus* born] pertaining to the first four weeks after birth.

neonate (ne'o-nāt) 1. newly born. 2. a new-born infant.

neonatologist (ne''o-na-tol'o-jist) a physician whose primary concern is in the specialty of neonatology.

neonatology (ne''o-na-tol'o-je) the art and science of diagnosis and treatment of disorders of the newborn infant.

neopallium (ne''o-pal'le-um) [*neo-* + L. *pallium* cloak] that portion of the pallium (cerebral cortex) showing stratification and organization characteristic of the most highly evolved type of cerebral tissue. It consists of six layers: layer I, the molecular or plexiform layer; layer II, the external granular layer; layer III, the pyramidal layer; layer IV, the internal granular layer; layer V, the ganglionic layer; layer VI, the multiform or polymorphic layer. Called also *homotypical cortex, isocortex, neocortex*, and *nonolfactory cortex.* Cf. *archipallium.*

neopathy (ne-op'ah-the) [*neo-* + Gr. *pathos* disease] (*obs.*) 1. a new disease. 2. a new condition or complication of disease in a patient.

neophrenia (ne''o-fre'ne-ah) [*neo-* + Gr. *phrēn* mind] Kahlbaum's term for mental disorder occurring in early youth; no longer in use.

neoplasia (ne''o-pla'ze-ah) the formation of a neoplasm, i.e., the progressive multiplication of cells under conditions that would not elicit, or would cause cessation of, multiplication of normal cells.

neoplasm (ne'o-plazm) [*neo-* + Gr. *plasma* formation] any new and abnormal growth; specifically a new growth of tissue in which the growth is uncontrolled and progressive (see neoplasia). Malignant neoplasms are distinguished from benign in that the former show a greater degree of anaplasia and have the properties of invasion and metastasis. Called also *tumor.* **histoid n.,** a neoplasm whose structure resembles that of the tissues in which it is situated. **organoid n.,** a neoplasm whose structure resembles that of some organ of the body.

neoplastic (ne''o-plas'tik) pertaining to or like a neoplasm; pertaining to neoplasia.

neoplastigenic (ne''o-plas''ti-jen'ik) tending to produce neoplasms.

Neopsylla (ne-op'sil-ah) a genus of fleas.

neoquassin (ne''o-kwas'in) a crystalline principle, $C_{24}H_{30}O_6$, from *Quassia amara* L. (Simarubaceae); it is a phenanthropyran derivative which forms quassin on oxidation.

Neorickettsia (ne''o-ri-ket'se-ah) a genus of the tribe Ehrlichieae, family Rickettsiaceae, order Rickettsiales. It includes a single species, *N. helmin'thoeca*, the etiologic agent of salmon poisoning (q.v.). It is found in the salmon fluke, *Troglotrema*

salmincola, a parasite of various fish, especially salmon and trout, and is transmitted by ingestion of raw infected fish.

Neoschoengastia (ne''o-shān-gas'te-ah) a genus of mites of the family Trombiculidae. **N. america'na,** a species of mites which infest chickens in the southern United States.

Neosporidia (ne''o-spo-rid'e-ah) [*neo-* + Gr. *sporos* seed] a former division of the Sporozoa, in which growth and sporulation proceed together and simultaneously.

neostibosan (ne''o-sti'bo-san) a pentavalent antimony compound, used as an antileishmanial. Called also *ethylstibamine.*

neostigmine (ne''o-stig'min) chemical name: 3-[[(dimethylamino)carbonyl]oxy]-*N,N,N*-trimethylbenzenaminium. A synthetic quaternary ammonium compound with anticholinesterase (cholinergic) activity. **n. bromide** [USP], the bromide salt of neostigmine, $C_{12}H_{19}BrN_2O_2$, occurring as a white, crystalline powder; used as a cholinergic in the symptomatic control of myasthenia gravis, and to produce miosis in certain forms of glaucoma, administered orally and applied to the conjunctiva. **n. methylsulfate,** [USP], the methylsulfate salt of neostigmine, $C_{13}H_{22}N_2O_6S$, occurring as a white crystalline powder; used as a cholinergic in the prevention and treatment of postoperative distention and urinary retention, as a screening test for pregnancy, in the treatment of delayed menstruation, in the symptomatic treatment of myasthenia gravis, as a diagnostic test for myasthenia gravis, and as an antidote for curare principles, administered intravenously and subcutaneously.

neostomy (ne-os'to-me) [*neo-* + Gr. *stoma* mouth] surgical creation of an artificial opening into an organ or between two organs.

neostriatum (ne''o-stri-a'tum) [*neo-* + *striatum*] the later developed portion of the corpus striatum represented by the caudate nucleus and the putamen; called also *striatum.* Cf. *paleostriatum.*

Neo-Synephrine (ne''o-sĭ-nef'rin) trademark for preparations of phenylephrine hydrochloride.

neoteny (ne-ot'ĕ-ne) [*neo-* + Gr. *teinein* to extend] the tendency to remain in the larval state, although gaining sexual maturity.

neothalamus (ne''o-thal'ah-mus) [Gr. *neos* new + *thalamus*] new thalamus; the phylogenetically new part of the thalamus, i.e., the part connected to the neocortex. Cf. *paleothalamus.*

Neothylline (ne''o-thil'lin) trademark for preparations of dyphylline.

Neotoma (ne-ot'o-mah) a genus of rodents of western North America, including the wood or pack rats. **N. lep'ida,** the desert wood rat, from which *Brucella neotome* has been isolated.

Neotrizine (ne''o-tri'zĕn) trademark for preparations of trisulfapyrinidenes.

neotype (ne'o-tīp) a strain of bacteria that replaces a type culture which no longer exists, and that agrees with the original description of the taxon and is accepted by international agreement.

nepenthic (ne-pen'thik) [Gr. *nēpenthēs* free from sorrow] pertaining to or inducing peace and forgetfulness.

Nepeta (nep'ĕ-tah) a genus of Eurasian mints that includes *Nepeta cataria*, L. (Labiatae), or catnip; see *cataria.*

nepetalactone (nep''ĕ-tah-lak'tōn) the chief constituent, $C_{10}H_{14}O_2$, of the aromatic volatile oil from the leaves and tops of catnip (*Nepeta cataria*), which is an attractant to cats.

nephelo- (nef'ĕ-lo) [Gr. *nephelē* cloud or mist] a combining form denoting relationship to cloudiness or mistiness.

nephelometer (nef''ĕ-lom'ĕ-ter) [*nephalo-* + Gr. *metron* measure] an instrument, similar in design to a visual colorimeter, which employs the Tyndall phenomenon for measurement of the concentration of substances in suspension. **photoelectric n.,** one in which photoelectric means of measurement is substituted for the human eye.

nephelometry (nef''ĕ-lom'ĕ-tre) [*nephelo-* + Gr. *metron* measure] measurement of the concentration of a suspension by means of a nephelometer.

nephelopia (nef''ĕ-lo'pe-ah) [*nephelo-* + Gr. *ōps* eye + *-ia*] defect of vision from cloudiness of the cornea.

nephelopsychosis (nef''ĕ-lo-si-ko'sis) [*nephelo-* + *psychosis*] an abnormal interest in clouds.

nephr- see *nephro-.*

nephradenoma (nef''rad-ĕ-no'mah) [*nephr-* + *adenoma*] adenoma of the kidney.

nephralgia (nĕ-fral'je-ah) [*nephr-* + *-algia*] pain in a kidney.

nephralgic (nĕ-fral'jik) pertaining to or characterized by nephralgia.

Nephramine (nef'rah-mēn) trademark for a crystalline solution of eight essential amino acids but no peptides; it is used as a component of total parenteral nutrition in renal failure.

nephrapostasis (nef''rah-pos'tah-sis) [*nephr-* + Gr. *apostasis* suppuration] abscess or suppurative inflammation of a kidney.

nephratonia (nef''rah-to'ne-ah) [*nephr-* + *a* neg. + Gr. *tonos* tension + *-ia*] atony of the kidney.

nephratony (nĕ-frat'o-ne) nephratonia.

nephrauxe (nef-rawk′se) [nephr- + Gr. auxē increase] nephromegaly.

nephrectasia (nef″rek-ta′ze-ah) [nephr- + Gr. ektasis distention + -ia] distention of the kidney; sacciform kidney.

nephrectasis (ně-frek′tah-sis) nephrectasia.

nephrectasy (ně-frek′tah-se) nephrectasia.

nephrectomize (ně-frek′to-mīz) to deprive of one or both kidneys by surgical removal.

nephrectomy (ně-frek′to-me) [nephr- + Gr. ektomē excision] excision of a kidney. **abdominal n., anterior n.,** nephrectomy through an incision in the abdominal wall. **lumbar n.,** nephrectomy through an incision in the loin. **paraperitoneal n.,** the surgical removal of a kidney by a cut through the side along the false rib. **posterior n.,** lumbar nephrectomy.

nephredema (nef″rě-de′mah) renal congestion; nephremia.

nephrelcosis (nef″rel-ko′sis) [nephr- + Gr. helkōsis ulceration] ulceration of the kidney.

nephremia (ně-fre′me-ah) [nephr- + Gr. haima blood + -ia] congestion of the kidney; nephredema.

nephric (nef′rik) pertaining to the kidney; renal.

nephridium (ně-frid′e-um) the excretory organ of the embryo; the embryonic tube whence the kidney is developed.

nephritic (ně-frit′ik) 1. pertaining to or affected with nephritis. 2. pertaining to the kidneys. 3. a drug or agent useful in kidney disease.

nephritides (ně-frit′ĭ-dēz) plural of nephritis, used as a collective term, to include all types of nephritis.

nephritis (ně-fri′tis), pl. nephrit′ides [Gr. nephros kidney + -itis] inflammation of the kidney; a focal or diffuse proliferative or destructive process which may involve the glomerulus, tubule, or interstitial renal tissue. See also glomerulonephritis. Cf. nephrosis. **acute n.,** nephritis in an acute and active stage with clinical manifestations usually including edema, weight gain, proteinuria, microhematuria, and cylindruria. When involvement is primarily glomerular, gross hematuria is common. **arteriosclerotic n.,** nephrosclerotic nephritis which may result primarily from the aging process, with hyaline changes of the large and small arterioles, or from hypertension, with hyaline and/or muscular changes of the small arterioles in the glomerular hilum. Renal damage occurs primarily through ischemic atrophy of the tubules with resultant focal or diffuse interstitial fibrosis. **azotemic n.,** nephritis which has resulted in anatomic and functional impairment leading to nitrogen retention. **bacterial n.,** nephritis caused by microorganisms. **Balkan n.,** a very slowly progressive interstitial nephritis occurring in several well-defined areas of Yugoslavia, Rumania, Bulgaria, and Greece; called also Balkan nephropathy. **capsular n.,** a form said to affect especially Bowman's capsules. **n. caseo′sa, caseous n.,** cheesy n. **cheesy n.,** a chronic suppurative form with caseous deposits. **chloro-azotemic n.,** nondematous renal failure with acidosis. **chronic n.,** active and slowly progressive parenchymal renal disease, usually with a predominantly glomerular lesion. **congenital n.,** nephritis existing at birth, as in congenital syphilis. **croupous n.,** acute n. **degenerative n.,** nephrosis. **n. doloro′sa,** nonspecific involvement of the kidney characterized by painful thickening of the renal capsule due to inflammation of indeterminate etiology, as in some forms of perinephritis. **dropsical n.,** nephrotic syndrome. **exudative n.,** nephritis with exudation of the blood serum. **fibrolipomatous n.,** perinephritis in which the perirenal fat has become enmeshed in fibrous tissue proliferation with scarring. **fibrous n.,** interstitial n. **glomerular n.,** that which principally affects the glomeruli; see glomerulonephritis. **glomerulocapsular n.,** a term sometimes used to describe glomerulopathy involving primarily the epithelial cells of Bowman's capsules. **n. gravida′rum,** nephritis or other glomerulopathies complicating pregnancy. **hemorrhagic n.,** glomerulopathy associated with gross hematuria. **hydremic n., hydropigenous n.,** nephrotic syndrome; glomerulopathy with hypoproteinemia, massive proteinuria, and edema. **indurative n.,** a condition marked by atrophy and gross scarring of the kidney due to glomerular, tubular, or interstitial renal disease. **interstitial n.,** primary or secondary disease of the renal interstitial tissue resulting from arterial, arteriolar, glomerular, or tubular disease which destroys individual nephrons, or from toxic involvement of interstitial cells and tubules due to systemic diseases such as gout, to drug exposure (as in phenacetin abuse), or to mercury poisoning. Clinically, it may be manifested primarily by loss of concentrating capacity, mineral wasting, proteinuria, and abnormal urine sediment. It may be seen in an acute form, particularly after specific bacterial infection, and may result in acute papillary necrosis. More commonly, the process is a chronic one with progressive renal atrophy and diminution of renal function. **interstitial n., acute,** nephritis in which the inflammatory changes are usually confined to the interstitial tissue. It almost always occurs as a secondary complication of a systemic infection, especially one due to beta-hemolytic streptococci, although it may possibly have an allergic etiology. The kidneys may be normal in size and appearance, or enlarged, soft, and pale or mottled red or gray. Other signs include a thickened cortex, focal or diffuse interstitial infiltration of leukocytes, and tubular degeneration. **Lancereaux's n.,** interstitial nephritis allegedly resulting from rheumatic disease. **lipomatous n.,** fatty replacement of renal nephrons associated with, but not causative of, a primary disease process; called also lipomatosis renis, lipoma diffusum renis. **lupus n.,** glomerulonephritis (diffuse, focal, or membranous) associated with systemic lupus erythematosus, marked by deposition of antigen-antibody complexes in the mesangium and basement membrane, by hematuria, and either by a fulminating course, with uremia and death in a few weeks, or by a chronic progressive course; hypertension is rare until late in the course of the disease. **Masugi n.,** experimental glomerulonephritis induced in one species, such as the rat, by the injection of antiglomerular basement membrane antibody raised in a heterologous host, such as a rabbit, immunized with rat glomerular basement membrane antigens. Glomerulonephritis develops within a few hours following the inoculation of a large dose of antiserum, whereas repeated smaller doses require several weeks to produce disease. **nephrotoxic n.,** nephritis produced in an animal by the injection of antikidney antibody, the antibody being taken from an animal of a different species that had previously received a preparation of glomerular basement membrane from an animal of the same species as the one to be inoculated. **parenchymatous n.,** renal parenchymal disease of specific or unknown etiology. **parenchymatous n., chronic,** chronic disease of the renal parenchyma of specific or nonspecific etiology, usually manifested as a diffuse glomerular, tubular, or interstitial fibrosis. **pneumococcus n.,** nephritis from infection with pneumococci, occurring usually as a complication of pneumonia or empyema. **potassium-losing n.,** persistent urinary potassium losses in the presence of hypokalemia. It may be seen in metabolic alkalosis, adrenocortical hormone excess, or in intrinsic renal disease (e.g., renal tubular acidosis or juxtaglomerular cell hyperplasia). Called also potassium-losing nephropathy. **n. of pregnancy,** n. gravidarum. **productive n.,** nephritis with the development of serous exudate and hypertrophy of the connective tissue stroma. **n. re′pens,** a condition in which the patient has advanced renal insufficiency and raised blood pressure but without an antecedent history of acute nephritis. **salt-losing n.,** intrinsic renal disease causing abnormal urinary sodium loss in persons ingesting normal amounts of sodium chloride; it usually affects the renal medulla (e.g., medullary cystic disease, polycystic kidney disease, pyelonephritis) and results in vomiting, dehydration, hypotension, and sudden death. Called also Thorn's syndrome. **saturnine n.,** a form due to chronic lead poisoning. **scarlatinal n.,** acute nephritis due to scarlet fever. **subacute n.,** parenchymatous n., chronic. **suppurative n.,** a form accompanied by abscess of the kidney. **suppurative n., acute,** a form due to septic infection, generally from operations on the genitourinary tract (then called surgical kidney), and marked by the development of multiple abscesses. **suppurative n., chronic,** is caused by infection with the tubercle bacillus; in this disease cavities are found in the kidney, filled with puslike, cheesy masses and tubercle bacilli. **syphilitic n.,** a form of nephritis occurring in tertiary syphilis. **tartrate n.,** acute nephritis produced by the subcutaneous injection of racemic tartaric acid. **transfusion n.,** a nephropathy following blood transfusion from a donor whose blood is incompatible with that of the recipient. **trench n.,** war n. **tubal n., tubular n.,** a variety that affects principally the tubules. **tuberculous n.,** see interstitial nephritis, chronic. **vascular n.,** nephrosclerosis. **war n.,** an acute diffuse glomerulonephritis affecting soldiers under war conditions.

nephritogenic (ně-frit″o-jen′ik) giving rise to inflammation of the kidney, or nephritis.

nephro-, nephr- [Gr. nephros kidney] combining form denoting relationship to the kidney.

nephroabdominal (nef″ro-ab-dom′ĭ-nal) pertaining to the kidney and the abdominal wall.

nephroangiosclerosis (nef″ro-an″je-o-skle-ro′sis) hypertension with renal lesions of arterial origin.

nephroblastoma (nef″ro-blas-to′mah) Wilms' tumor.

nephrocalcinosis (nef″ro-kal″si-no′sis) [nephro- + calcium + -osis] a condition characterized by precipitation of calcium phosphate in the tubules of the kidney, with resultant renal insufficiency.

nephrocapsectomy (nef″ro-kap-sek′to-me) [nephro- + L. capsula capsule + Gr. ektomē excision] excision of the renal capsule; decapsulation of the kidney.

nephrocardiac (nef″ro-kar′de-ak) pertaining to the kidney and the heart.

nephrocele (nef′ro-sēl) [nephro- + Gr. kēlē hernia] hernial protrusion of a kidney.

nephrocolic (nef″ro-kol′ik) [nephro- + colic] 1. pertaining to the kidney and the colon. 2. renal colic.

nephrocolopexy (nef″ro-ko′lo-pek″se) [nephro- + Gr. kolon colon + pēxis fixation] operative suspension of the kidney and colon by fixation to the nephrocolic ligament.

nephrocoloptosis (nef″ro-ko′lop-to′sis) [nephro- + Gr. kolon colon + *ptōsis* fall] downward displacement of the kidney and colon.

nephrocystanastomosis (nef″ro-sist″ah-nas″to-mo′sis) [*nephro*- + Gr. *kystis* bladder + *anastomōsis* an opening] the surgical formation of a communication between the kidney and the urinary bladder.

nephrocystitis (nef″ro-sis-ti′tis) [*nephro*- + Gr. *kystis* bladder + *-itis*] inflammation of the kidney and bladder.

nephrocystosis (nef″ro-sis-to′sis) [*nephro*- + *cyst* + *-osis*] development of cysts in the kidney.

nephroerysipelas (nef″ro-er″ĭ-sip′ĕ-las) erysipelas complicated with acute nephritis.

nephrogastric (nef″ro-gas′trik) pertaining to the kidney and the stomach; renogastric.

nephrogenic (nef″ro-jen′ik) [*nephro*- + Gr. *gennan* to produce] forming kidney tissue.

nephrogenous (nĕ-froj′ĕ-nus) originating or arising in the kidney.

nephrogram (nef′ro-gram) a roentgenogram of the kidney.

nephrography (nĕ-frog′rah-fe) [*nephro*- + Gr. *graphein* to write] roentgenography of the kidney.

nephrohemia (nef″ro-he′me-ah) [*nephro*- + Gr. *haima* blood + *-ia*] congestion of the kidney.

nephrohydrosis (nef″ro-hi-dro′sis) hydronephrosis.

nephrohypertrophy (nef″ro-hi-per′tro-fe) [*nephro*- + *hypertrophy*] hypertrophy of the kidney.

nephroid (nef′roid) [*nephro*- + Gr. *eidos* form] kidney-shaped, or resembling a kidney.

nephrolith (nef′ro-lith) [*nephro*- + Gr. *lithos* stone] a renal calculus; gravel in a kidney.

nephrolithiasis (nef″ro-lĭ-thi′ah-sis) a condition marked by the presence of renal calculi.

nephrolithotomy (nef″ro-lĭ-thot′o-me) [*nephrolith* + Gr. *tomē* a cutting] the removal of renal calculi by cutting through the body of the kidney.

nephrologist (nĕ-frol′o-jist) an expert in nephrology.

nephrology (nĕ-frol′o-je) [*nephro*- + *-logy*] scientific study of the kidney, its anatomy, physiology, and pathology.

nephrolysine (nĕ-frol′ĭ-sin) [*nephro*- + *lysine*] nephrotoxin.

nephrolysis (nĕ-frol′ĭ-sis) [*nephro*- + Gr. *lysis* dissolution] 1. solution of kidney substance. 2. the operation of separating the kidney from paranephric adhesions.

nephrolytic (nef″ro-lit′ik) pertaining to, characterized by, or producing nephrolysis.

nephroma (nĕ-fro′mah) [*nephr*- + *-oma*] a tumor of kidney tissue; a tumor of the kidney. **embryonal n.,** Wilms' tumor.

nephromalacia (nef″ro-mah-la′she-ah) [*nephro*- + Gr. *malakia* softness] softening of the kidney.

nephromegaly (nef″ro-meg′ah-le) [*nephro*- + Gr. *megas* great] enlargement of the kidney.

nephromere (nef′ro-mēr) [*nephro*- + Gr. *meros* part] nephrotome.

nephron (nef′ron) [Gr. *nephros* kidney + *on* neuter ending] the anatomical and functional unit of the kidney, consisting of the renal corpuscle, the proximal convoluted tubule, the descending and ascending limbs of Henle's loop, the distal convoluted tubule, and the collecting tubule. See illustration accompanying *kidney*. **lower n.,** the thick segment of the ascending limb of Henle's loop and the parts distal to it.

nephroncus (nef-rong′kus) [*nephr*- + Gr. *onkos* mass] nephroma.

nephronophthisis (nef″ron-of′thĭ-sis) [*nephron* + Gr. *phthisis* wasting] wasting disease of the kidney substance. **familial juvenile n.,** a progressive hereditary disease of the kidneys characterized clinically by anemia, polyuria, and renal loss of sodium, progressing to chronic renal failure; pathologically, there is tubular atrophy, interstitial fibrosis, glomerular sclerosis, and medullary cysts. Called also *medullary cystic disease.*

nephro-omentopexy (nef″ro-o-men′to-pek″se) the operation of grafting the omentum on to the decapsulated ischemic kidney; proposed for the relief of hypertension.

nephroparalysis (nef″ro-pah-ral′ĭ-sis) [*nephro*- + *paralysis*] paralysis of the kidney.

nephropathia (nef″ro-path′e-ah) nephropathy. **n. epidem′ica,** epidemic hemorrhagic fever.

nephropathic (nef″ro-path′ik) pertaining to, characterized by, or producing nephropathy.

nephropathy (nĕ-frop′ah-the) [*nephro*- + Gr. *pathos* disease] disease of the kidneys. **analgesic n.,** that due to renal damage associated with massive intake of analgesics containing phenacetin. **Balkan n.,** see under *nephritis.* **dropsical n.,** hypochloruric n. **gouty n.,** any of a group of kidney diseases associated with the abnormal production and excretion of uric acid. **hypazoturic n.,** kidney disease with retention of nitrogen. **hypochloruric n.,** kidney disease with sodium chloride retention. **IgA n.,** IgA glomerulonephritis. **membranous**

n., see under *glomerulonephritis.* **reflux r.,** childhood pyelonephritis in which the renal scarring results from vesicoureteric reflux, with radiological appearance of intrarenal reflux.

nephropexy (nef′ro-pek″se) [*nephro*- + Gr. *pēxis* fixation] the fixation or suspension of a floating kidney.

nephrophagiasis (nef″ro-fah-ji′ah-sis) [*nephro*- + Gr. *phagein* to eat] the devouring of the kidney by certain parasites.

nephrophthisis (nĕ-frof′thĭ-sis) [*nephro*- + Gr. *phthisis* wasting] 1. nephrotuberculosis. 2. nephronophthisis.

nephropoietic (nef″ro-poi-et′ik) [*nephro*- + Gr. *poiein* to make] forming kidney tissue.

nephropoietin (nef″ro-poi-e′tin) a substance thought to exist in the blood serum, in embryonic kidney, and in kidneys undergoing regeneration and to stimulate the formation of kidney tissue.

nephroptosia (nef″ro-to′se-ah) nephroptosis.

nephroptosis (nef″rop-to′sis) [*nephro*- + Gr. *ptōsis* falling] downward displacement of the kidney.

nephropyelitis (nef″ro-pi″ĕ-li′tis) [*nephro*- + *pyelitis*] pyelonephritis.

nephropyelography (nef″ro-pi″ĕ-log′rah-fe) radiography of the kidney and renal pelvis.

nephropyelolithotomy (nef″ro-pi″ĕ-lo-lĭ-thot′o-me) [*nephro*- + Gr. *pyelos* pelvis + *lithos* stone + *tomē* a cut] the operation of removing a calculus from the renal pelvis by an incision through the kidney substance.

nephropyeloplasty (nef″ro-pi′ĕ-lo-plas″te) [*nephro*- + Gr. *pyelos* pelvis + *plassein* to form] plastic operation on the pelvis of the kidney.

nephropyosis (nef″ro-pi-o′sis) [*nephro*- + Gr. *pyōsis* suppuration] suppuration of the kidney.

nephrorosein (nef″ro-ro′ze-in) a urinary pigment identified spectroscopically.

nephrorrhagia (nef″ro-ra′je-ah) [*nephro*- + Gr. *rhēgnynai* to burst forth] hemorrhage from the kidney.

nephrorrhaphy (nef-ror′ah-fe) [*nephro*- + Gr. *rhaphē* suture] the operation of suturing the kidney.

nephroscleria (nef′ro-skle′re-ah) nephrosclerosis.

nephrosclerosis (nef″ro-skle-ro′sis) [*nephro*- + Gr. *sklerōsis* hardening] sclerosis or hardening of the kidney; the condition of the kidney due to renovascular disease. **arteriolar n.,** nephrosclerosis involving chiefly the arterioles; it is frequently associated with hypertension, and characterized by insidious onset, cylindruria, edema, hypertrophy of the heart, degeneration of the renal tubules, and fibrotic thickening of the glomeruli (glomerulonephritis), resulting in renal insufficiency, congestive heart failure, and cerebral hemorrhage. Called also *intercapillary n.* and *glomerulosclerosis.* **benign n.,** arteriolar nephrosclerosis commonly occurring in patients sixty years of age or older, and frequently associated with benign hypertension and hyaline arteriolosclerosis; in younger persons, it may occur in diabetics with a predisposition to arteriosclerosis and in those who have hypertension resulting from an apparent underlying disease, such as pheochromocytoma. Called also *hyaline arteriolar n.* **hyaline arteriolar n.,** benign n. **hyperplastic arteriolar n.,** malignant n. **intercapillary n.,** arteriolar n. **malignant n.,** an uncommon form of arteriolar nephrosclerosis affecting all the vessels of the body, especially the small arteries and arterioles of the kidneys, and frequently associated with malignant hypertension and hyperplastic arteriolosclerosis. It may occur in the absence of previous history of hypertension, or may be superimposed on benign hypertension or primary renal disease, especially glomerulonephritis, benign nephrosclerosis, and pyelonephritis. Called also *hyperplastic arteriolar n.* and *Fahr-Volhard disease.* **senile n.,** nephrosclerosis which is just a part of the arteriosclerosis common in old age.

nephroscope (nef′ro-skōp) an instrument inserted into an incision in the renal pelvis for viewing the inside of the kidney, equipped with three channels for telescope, fiberoptic light input, and irrigation.

nephroscopy (nĕ-fros′ko-pe) visualization of the kidney by means of the nephroscope.

nephroses (nĕ-fro′sēz) plural of *nephrosis.*

nephrosis (nĕ-fro′sis), pl. *nephro′ses* [*nephr*- + *-osis*] any disease of the kidney, especially any disease of the kidneys characterized by purely degenerative lesions of the renal tubules—as opposed to nephritis—and marked by edema (noninflammatory), albuminuria, and decreased serum albumin (the nephrotic syndrome). **acute n.,** nephrosis marked by scanty urine but with little edema or albuminuria. **amyloid n.,** chronic nephrosis with amyloid degeneration of the median coat of the arteries and the glomerular capillaries; amyloid kidney. **cholemic n.,** renal disease associated with various types of hepatic or biliary dysfunction, especially those in which there is obstructive jaundice. **chronic n.,** renal disease characterized by chronic degeneration of the renal epithelium. **Epstein's n.,** a type of chronic tubular nephritis resulting from systemic metabolic disorder, occurring usually in young persons and in women, and frequently associated with hypothyroidism or other endocrine disturbance. **glycogen n.**, nephrosis associated with glycogen vacuolation within the proximal convoluted tubules and the loops of Henle. **hydropic n.**, vacuolar n. **hypokalemic n.**, vacuolar n. **infectious avian n.**, a sometimes fatal disease of chickens, usually four to nine weeks old, possibly caused by a variant of the infectious bronchitis virus; it is characterized by dehydration, swollen kidneys, and distention of the renal tubules and ureters with urates. In some outbreaks depression is observed, and in others mild respiratory symptoms. **larval n.**, a condition in which the renal lesions are slight and manifested clinically by albuminuria. **lipid n., lipoid n.**, nephrosis characterized by edema, albuminuria, and changes in the protein and lipids of the blood and the accumulation of globules of cholesterol esters in the tubular epithelium of the kidney. **lower nephron n.**, a condition of renal insufficiency leading to uremia, due to necrosis of the cells of the lower nephron, blocking the tubular lumens of this region. The condition is seen after severe injuries, especially crushing injury to muscles (*crush syndrome*). **necrotizing n.**, renal disease characterized by necrosis of tubular epithelium of the kidney. **osmotic n.**, vacuolar n. **toxic n.**, nephrosis caused by some toxic agent, most frequently and typically by bichloride of mercury. **vacuolar n.**, renal disease in which injury of the renal tubules is associated with vacuolization of the proximal convoluted tubules and sometimes of the loops of Henle and collecting tubules, presumed to be caused by disturbances in the normal osmotic relationships within the cells. These changes are seen in various clinical situations, as following the administration of hypertonic solutions, in diseases resulting in marked alterations in fluid balance, and in severe hypokalemia. Called also *hydropic n., hypokalemic n.,* and *osmotic n.*

nephrosonephritis (ně-fro″so-ně-fri′tis) [*nephrosis* + *nephritis*] renal disease with nephrotic and nephritic components. **hemorrhagic n., Korean hemorrhagic n.**, epidemic hemorrhagic fever.

nephrosonography (nef″ro-so-nog′rah-fe) ultrasonic scanning of the kidney.

nephrospasis (nef″ro-spas′is) [*nephro-* + Gr. *span* to draw] movable kidney in which the natural supports of the organ are so weakened that the organ hangs by its pedicle.

nephrosplenopexy (nef″ro-sple′no-pek″se) surgical fixation of the kidney and the spleen.

nephrostoma (ně-fros′to-mah) [*nephro-* + Gr. *stoma* mouth] one of the funnel-shaped and ciliated orifices of excretory tubules that open into the coelom in the embryo, best seen in lower vertebrates.

nephrostome (nef′ro-stōm) nephrostoma.

nephrostomy (ně-fros′to-me) [*nephro-* + Gr. *stomoun* to provide with an opening, or mouth] the creation of a permanent fistula leading directly into the pelvis of the kidney.

nephrotic (ně-frot′ik) pertaining to, resembling, or caused by nephrosis.

nephrotome (nef′ro-tōm) one of the segmented divisions of the mesoderm connecting the somite with the lateral plates of unsegmented mesoderm; it is the source of much of the urogenital system. Called also *intermediate cell mass* and *middle plate.*

nephrotomogram (nef″ro-to′mo-gram) the sectional radiograph of the kidney obtained by nephrotomography.

nephrotomography (nef″ro-to-mog′rah-fe) radiologic visualization of the kidney by tomography after intravenous introduction of contrast medium as a bolus or by infusion.

nephrotomy (ně-frot′o-me) [*nephro-* + Gr. *tomē* a cutting] a surgical incision into the kidney. **abdominal n.**, nephrotomy performed through an incision into the abdomen. **lumbar n.**, nephrotomy performed through an incision into the loin.

nephrotoxic (nef″ro-tok′sik) toxic or destructive to kidney cells.

nephrotoxicity (nef″ro-tok-sis′ĭ-te) the quality of being toxic or destructive to kidney cells.

nephrotoxin (nef″ro-tok′sin) [*nephro-* + Gr. *toxikon* poison] a toxin which has a specific destructive effect on kidney cells.

nephrotresis (nef″ro-tre′sis) [*nephro-* + Gr. *trēsis* boring] the operation of establishing a fistula into the kidney by stitching the edges of the kidney incision to the parietal muscles.

nephrotropic (nef″ro-trop′ik) having a special affinity for or exerting its principal effect upon kidney tissue.

nephrotuberculosis (nef″to-tu-ber″ku-lo′sis) [*nephro-* + *tuberculosis*] disease of the kidney due to *Mycobacterium tuberculosis.*

nephrotyphoid (nef″ro-ti′foid) typhoid fever complicated with acute nephritis.

nephrotyphus (nef″ro-ti′fus) [*nephro-* + *typhus*] typhus with nephritis and resultant hematuria.

nephroureterectomy (nef″ro-u″re-ter-ek′to-me) [*nephro-* + *ureterectomy*] excision of a kidney and a whole or part of the ureter.

nephroureterocystectomy (nef″ro-u-re″ter-o-sis-tek′to-me) [*nephro-* + Gr. *ourētēr* ureter + *kystis* bladder + *ektomē* excision] excision of the kidney, ureter, and a portion of the bladder wall.

nephrozymase (nef″ro-zi′mās) [*nephro-* + Gr. *zymē* leven] an enzyme, like diastase, found in the urine.

nephrozymosis (nef″ro-zi-mo′sis) zymotic or fermentative disease of the kidney.

nephrydrosis (nef″rĭ-dro′sis) [*nephro-* + Gr. *hydōr* water + *-osis*] hydronephrosis.

nephrydrotic (nef″rĭ-drot′ik) pertaining to nephrydrosis.

nepiology (nep″e-ol′o-je) [Gr. *nēpio* infant + *-logy*] (*obs.*) the department of pediatrics treating of young infants.

Neptazane (nep′tah-zān) trademark for a preparation of methazolamine.

neptunium (nep-tu′ne-um) [from planet Neptune] a radioactive element of atomic number 93 and atomic weight 237, occurring in certain earths and obtained by splitting the uranium atom with neutrons. It is unstable and changes into plutonium. Symbol Np.

nequinate (ně-kwin′āt) chemical name: 6-butyl-1,4-dihydro-4-oxo-7-(phenylmethoxy)-3-quinolinecarboxylic acid methyl ester; a coccidiostat for poultry, $C_{22}H_{23}NO_4$.

Nerium (ne′rĭ-um) a genus of evergreen apocynaceous shrubs of the Mediterranean region and Asia. *N. odorum* (*N. indicum*) is the sweet-scented oleander; *N. oleander* L. is the common oleander.

nerol (ne′rol) an essential oil, $(CH_3)_2C\!:\!CH\cdot CH_2\cdot CH_2\cdot C\text{-}(CH_3)\!:\!CH\cdot CH_2OH$, a constituent of orange flower oil.

neroli (ner′o-le) an essential oil distilled from orange blossoms; orange flower oil.

neropathy (ne-rop′ah-the) see *weltmerism.*

nerval (ner′val) (*obs.*) neural.

nerve (nerv) [L. *nervus;* Gr. *neuron*] a cordlike structure, visible to the naked eye, comprising a collection of nerve fibers which convey impulses between a part of the central nervous system and some other region of the body. Called also *nervus* [NA]. A nerve consists of a connective tissue sheath (epineurium) enclosing bundles (funiculi or fasciculi) of nerve fibers, each bundle being surrounded by its own sheath of connective tissue (perineurium), the inner surface of which is formed by a membrane of flattened mesothelial cells. Very small nerves may consist of only one funiculus derived from the parent nerve. Within each such bundle, the individual nerve fibers, which are microscopic in size, are surrounded by interstitial connective tissue (endoneurium). An individual nerve fiber (an axon with its covering sheath) consists of formed elements in a matrix of protoplasm (axoplasm), the entire structure being enclosed in a thin membrane (axolemma). Each nerve fiber is enclosed by a cellular sheath (neurilemma), from which it may or may not be separated by a lipid layer (myelin sheath) derived from neurilemmal cells. **abducent n.**, nervus abducens. **accelerator n's,** the cardiac sympathetic nerves, which, when stimulated, accelerate the action of the heart. **accessory n., accessory n., spinal,** nervus accessorius. **accessory n., vagal,** ramus internus nervi accessorii. **acoustic n.**, nervus vestibulocochlearis. **afferent n.**, any nerve that transmits impulses from the periphery toward the central nervous system; see *sensory n.* **alveolar n., inferior,** nervus alveolaris inferior. **alveolar n's, superior,** nervi alveolaris superior. **ampullar n., anterior,** nervus ampullaris anterior. **ampullar n., inferior,** nervus ampullaris posterior. **ampullar n., lateral,** nervus ampullaris lateralis. **ampullar n., posterior,** nervus ampullaris posterior. **ampullar n., superior,** nervus ampullaris anterior. **anabolic n.**, any nerve, such as the vagus, the stimulation of which serves to promote the anabolic processes. **Andersch's n.**, nervus tympanicus. **anococcygeal n's,** nervi anococcygei. **Arnold's n.**, ramus auricularis nervi vagi. **articular n.**, nervus articularis. **auditory n.**, nervus vestibulocochlearis. **auricular n's, anterior,** nervi auriculares anteriores. **auricular n., great,** nervus auricularis magnus. **auricular n., internal,** ramus posterior nervi auricularis magni. **auricular n., posterior,** nervus auricularis posterior. **auricular n. of vagus n.**, ramus auricularis nervi vagi. **auriculotemporal n.**, nervus auriculotemporalis. **autonomic n's,** nerves of the autonomic nervous system, see under *system.* **axillary n.**, nervus axillaris. **Bell's n.**, nervus thoracicus longus. **Bock's n.**, ramus pharyngeus ganglii pterygopalatini. **buccal n., buccinator n.**, nervus buccalis. **cardiac n., cervical, inferior,** nervus cardiacus cervicalis inferior. **cardiac n., cervical, middle,** nervus cardiacus cervicalis medius. **cardiac n., cervical, superior,** nervus cardiacus cervicalis superior. **cardiac n., inferior,** nervus cardiacus cervicalis inferior. **cardiac n., middle,** nervus cardiacus cervicalis medius. **cardiac n., superior,** nervus cardiacus cervicalis superior. **cardiac n's, supreme,** rami cardiaci cervicales superiores nervi vagi. **cardiac n's, thoracic,** nervi cardiaci thoracici. **caroticotympanic n's,** nervi caroticotympanici. **carotid n's, external,** nervi carotici externi. **carotid n., internal,** nervus caroticus internus. **cavernous n's of clitoris,** nervi cavernosi clitoridis. **cavernous n's of penis,** nervi cavernosi penis. **celiac n's,** rami celiaci nervi vagi. **centrifugal n.**, efferent n. **centripetal n.**, afferent n. **cerebral n's,** nervi craniales. **cervical n's,** the eight pairs

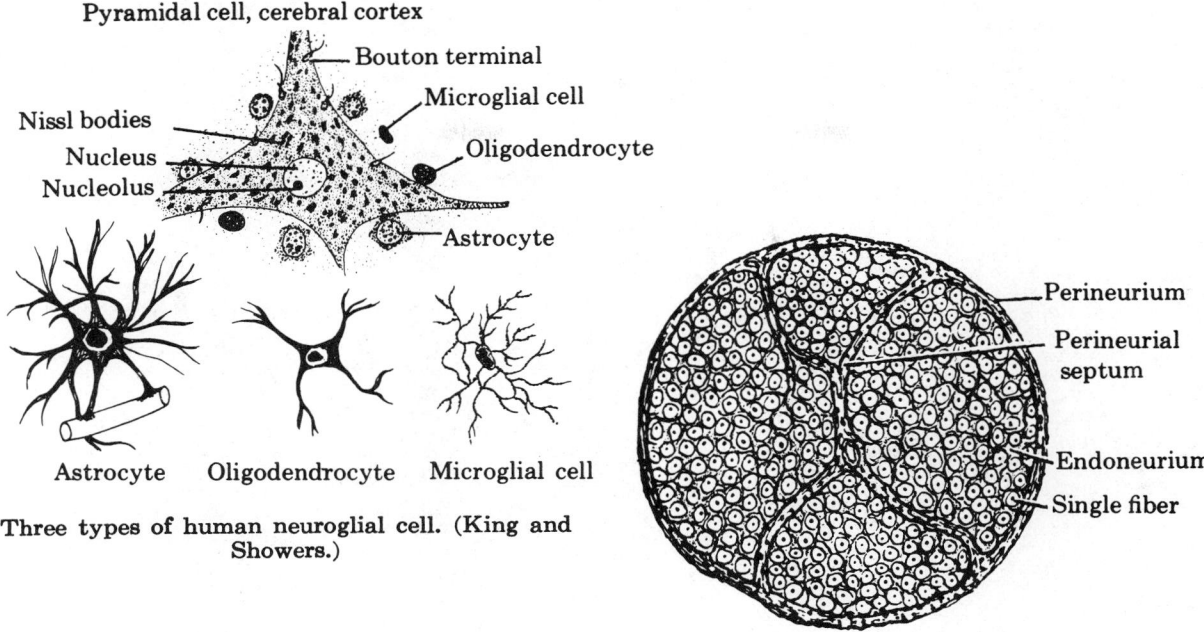

Plate XXXIV

Pyramidal cell, cerebral cortex

Bouton terminal

Microglial cell

Nissl bodies

Nucleus

Oligodendrocyte

Nucleolus

Astrocyte

Astrocyte   Oligodendrocyte   Microglial cell

Three types of human neuroglial cell. (King and Showers.)

Perineurium

Perineurial septum

Endoneurium

Single fiber

Transverse section of a nerve.

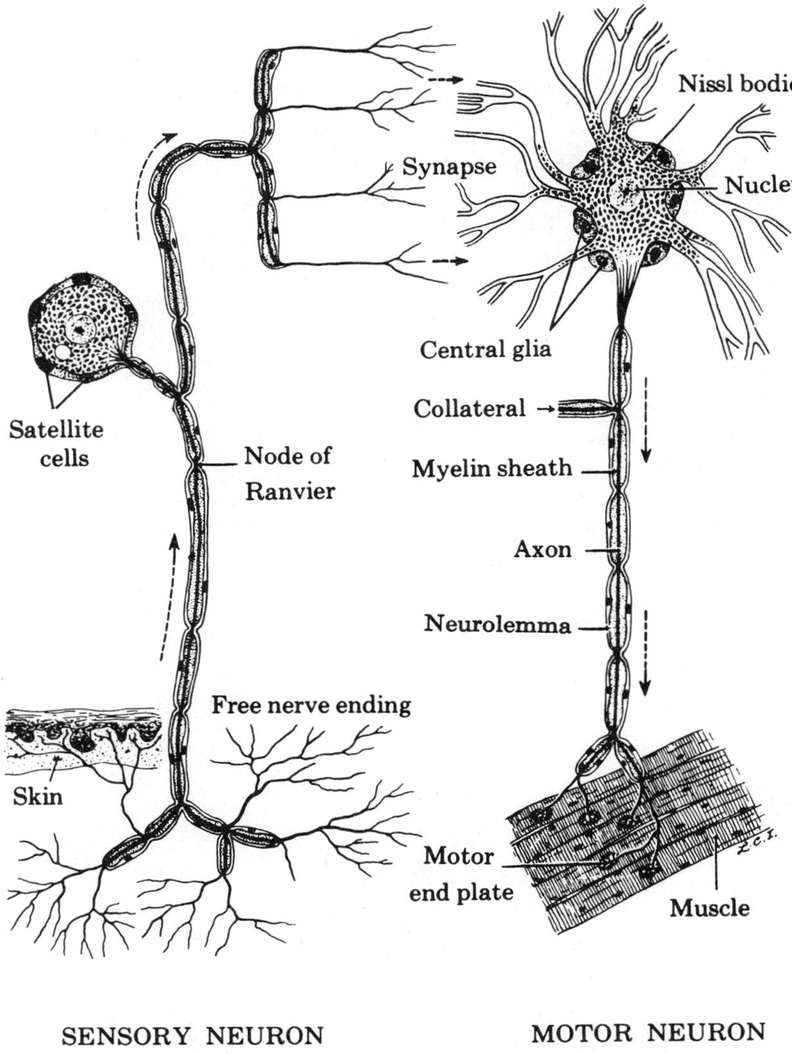

Nissl bodies

Synapse

Nucleus

Central glia

Collateral →

Myelin sheath

Axon

Neurolemma

Satellite cells

Node of Ranvier

Free nerve ending

Skin

Motor end plate

Muscle

Schmidt-Lantermann cleft

Node of Ranvier

Neurilemma

Nucleus of neurilemmal cell

Mitochondria

Axon (composed of fibrils)

Myelin (here dissolved, above blackened by fixation)

SENSORY NEURON   MOTOR NEURON

Diagrammatic representation of two types of neurons. (King and Showers.)

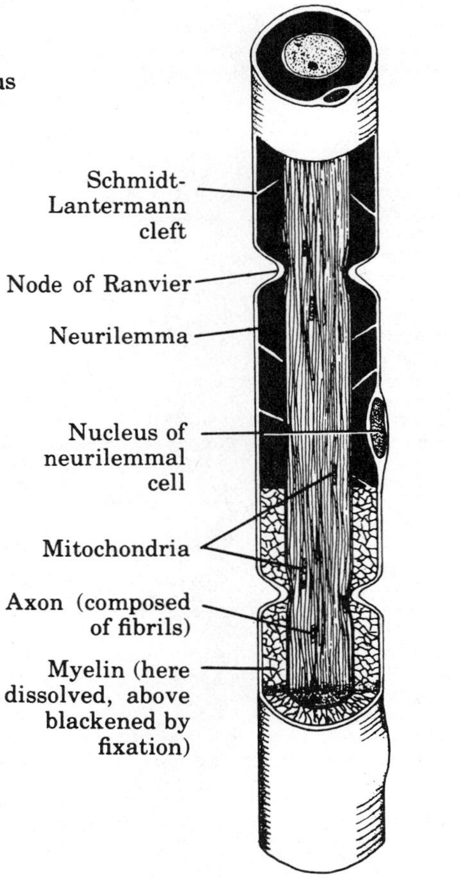

Longitudinal section of a nerve fiber (Leeson and Leeson).

DETAILS OF STRUCTURE OF COMPONENTS OF NERVE TISSUE

Plate XXXV

nerve

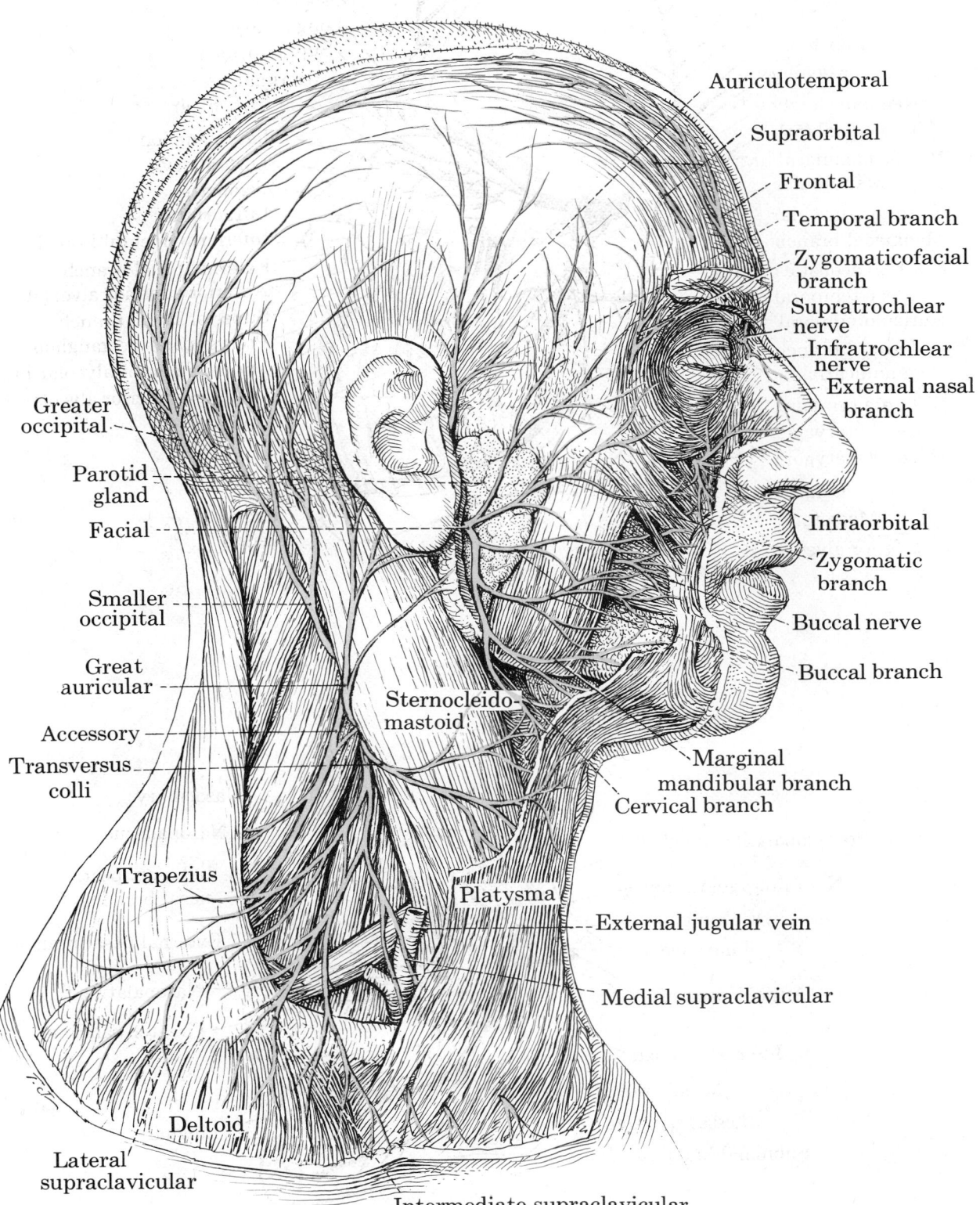

Auriculotemporal

Supraorbital

Frontal

Temporal branch

Zygomaticofacial branch

Supratrochlear nerve

Infratrochlear nerve

External nasal branch

Infraorbital

Zygomatic branch

Buccal nerve

Buccal branch

Marginal mandibular branch

Cervical branch

External jugular vein

Medial supraclavicular

Intermediate supraclavicular

Greater occipital

Parotid gland

Facial

Smaller occipital

Great auricular

Accessory

Transversus colli

Trapezius

Sternocleido-mastoid

Platysma

Deltoid

Lateral supraclavicular

SUPERFICIAL NERVES AND MUSCLES OF HEAD AND NECK

Portions of the parotid gland and platysma muscle are shown cut away. (Jones and Shepard.)

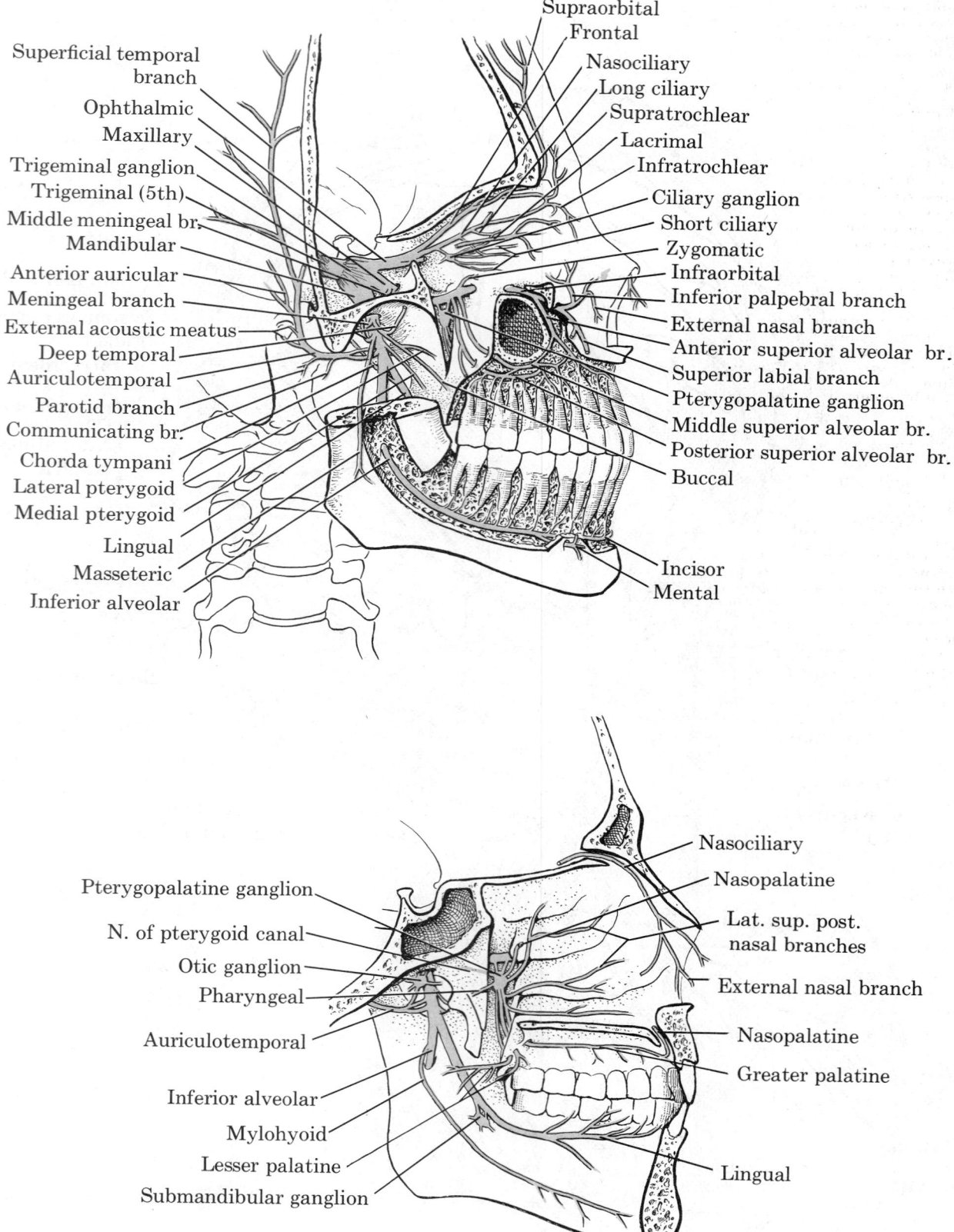

Superficial temporal branch
Ophthalmic
Maxillary
Trigeminal ganglion
Trigeminal (5th)
Middle meningeal br.
Mandibular
Anterior auricular
Meningeal branch
External acoustic meatus
Deep temporal
Auriculotemporal
Parotid branch
Communicating br.
Chorda tympani
Lateral pterygoid
Medial pterygoid
Lingual
Masseteric
Inferior alveolar

Supraorbital
Frontal
Nasociliary
Long ciliary
Supratrochlear
Lacrimal
Infratrochlear
Ciliary ganglion
Short ciliary
Zygomatic
Infraorbital
Inferior palpebral branch
External nasal branch
Anterior superior alveolar br.
Superior labial branch
Pterygopalatine ganglion
Middle superior alveolar br.
Posterior superior alveolar br.
Buccal
Incisor
Mental

Pterygopalatine ganglion
N. of pterygoid canal
Otic ganglion
Pharyngeal
Auriculotemporal
Inferior alveolar
Mylohyoid
Lesser palatine
Submandibular ganglion

Nasociliary
Nasopalatine
Lat. sup. post. nasal branches
External nasal branch
Nasopalatine
Greater palatine
Lingual

DEEP NERVES SHOWN IN RELATION TO BONES OF FACE

Plate XXXVII   nerve

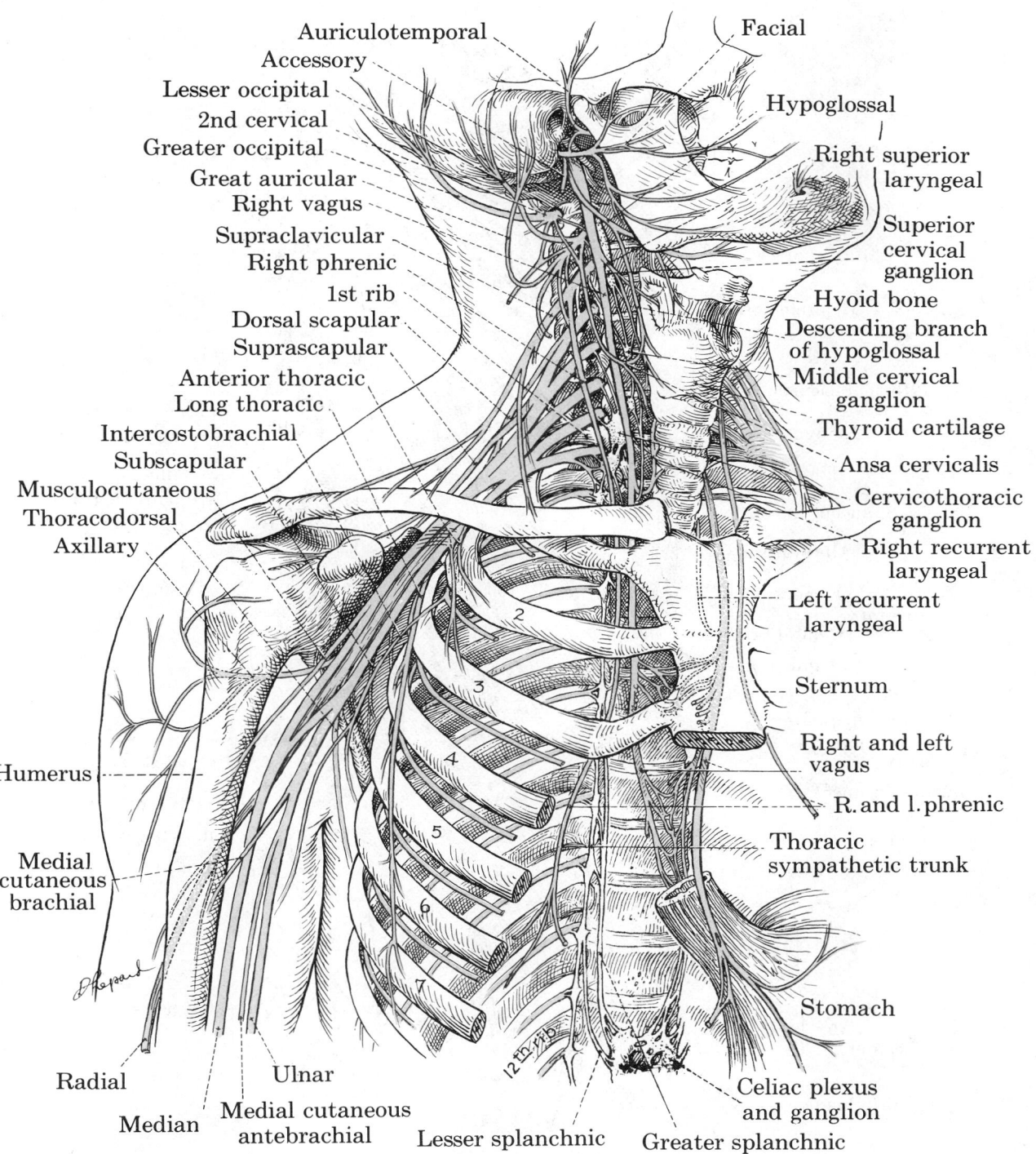

Auriculotemporal
Accessory
Lesser occipital
2nd cervical
Greater occipital
Great auricular
Right vagus
Supraclavicular
Right phrenic
1st rib
Dorsal scapular
Suprascapular
Anterior thoracic
Long thoracic
Intercostobrachial
Subscapular
Musculocutaneous
Thoracodorsal
Axillary
Humerus
Medial
cutaneous
brachial
Radial
Median
Medial cutaneous
antebrachial
Ulnar
Lesser splanchnic

Facial
Hypoglossal
Right superior
laryngeal
Superior
cervical
ganglion
Hyoid bone
Descending branch
of hypoglossal
Middle cervical
ganglion
Thyroid cartilage
Ansa cervicalis
Cervicothoracic
ganglion
Right recurrent
laryngeal
Left recurrent
laryngeal
Sternum
Right and left
vagus
R. and l. phrenic
Thoracic
sympathetic trunk
Stomach
Celiac plexus
and ganglion
Greater splanchnic

2
3
4
5
6
7
12 th rib

DEEP NERVES OF NECK, AXILLA, AND UPPER THORAX

The sympathetic nerves are uncolored. (Jones and Shepard.)

Plate XXXVIII

nerve

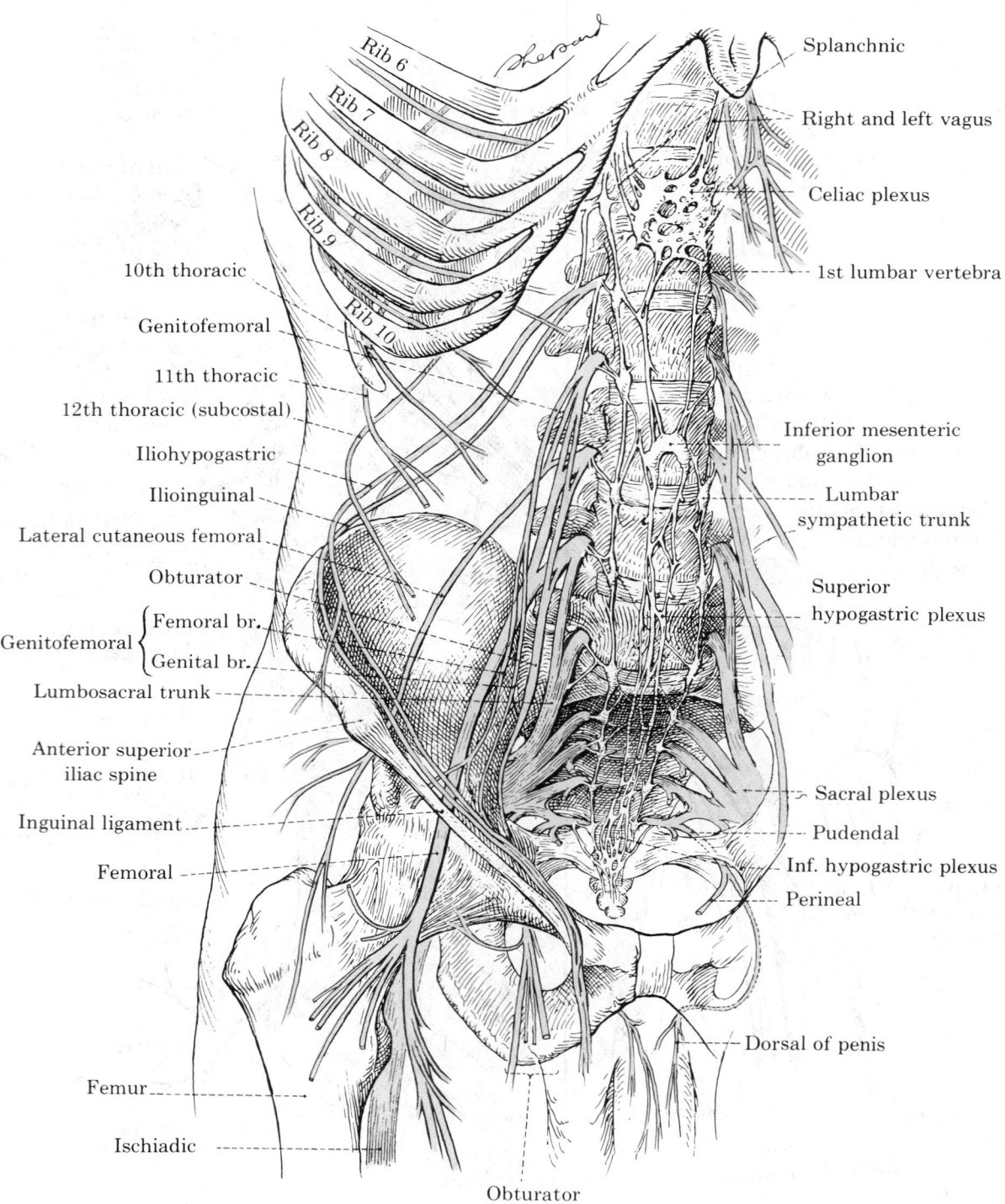

Rib 6

Shepard

Rib 7

Rib 8

Rib 9

10th thoracic

Genitofemoral

Rib 10

11th thoracic

12th thoracic (subcostal)

Iliohypogastric

Ilioinguinal

Lateral cutaneous femoral

Obturator

Genitofemoral { Femoral br.

Genital br.

Lumbosacral trunk

Anterior superior iliac spine

Inguinal ligament

Femoral

Femur

Ischiadic

Obturator

Splanchnic

Right and left vagus

Celiac plexus

1st lumbar vertebra

Inferior mesenteric ganglion

Lumbar sympathetic trunk

Superior hypogastric plexus

Sacral plexus

Pudendal

Inf. hypogastric plexus

Perineal

Dorsal of penis

DEEP NERVES OF LOWER TRUNK

The sympathetic nerves are uncolored. (Jones and Shepard.)

Plate XXXIX

nerve

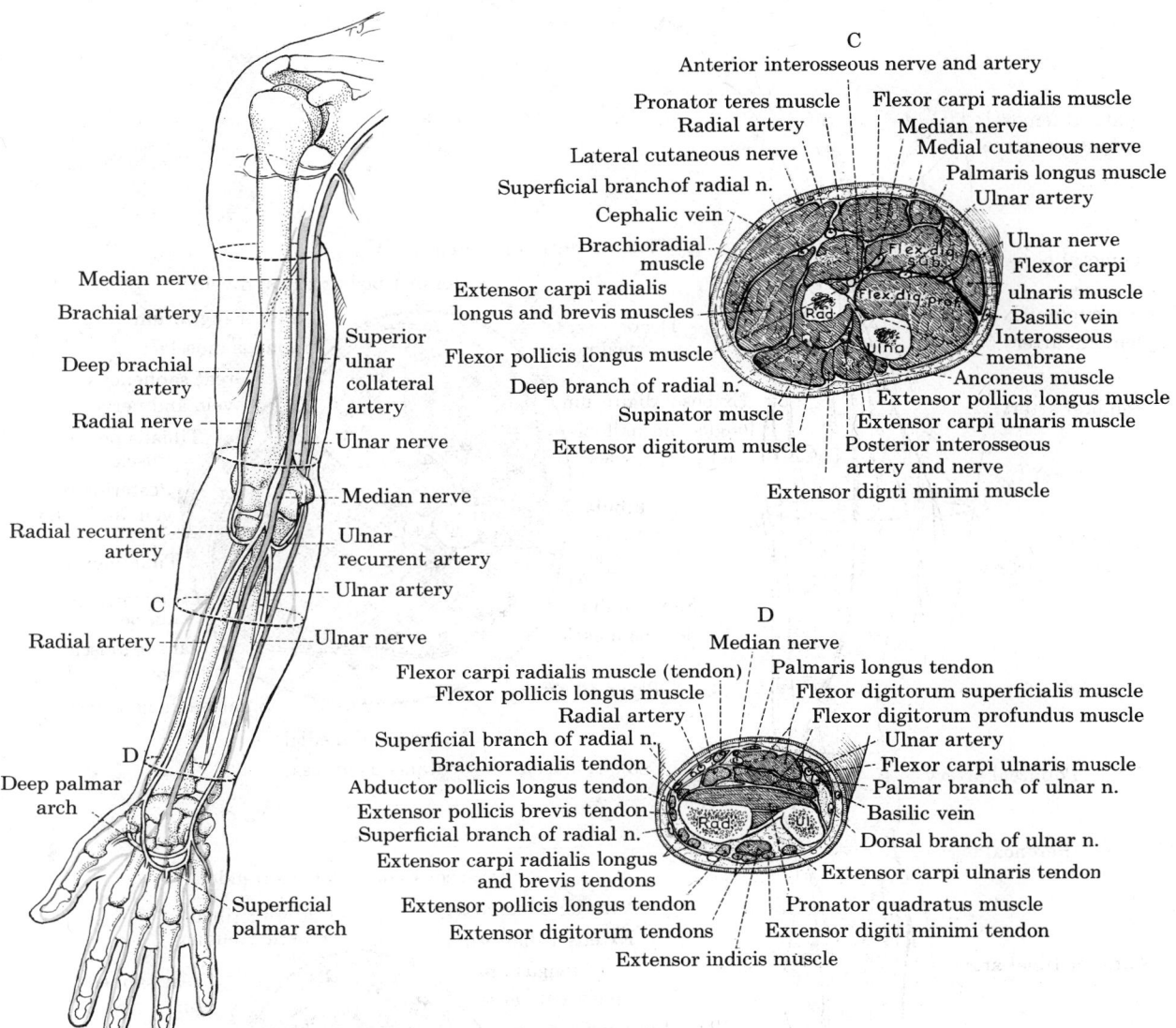

C

Anterior interosseous nerve and artery

Pronator teres muscle | Flexor carpi radialis muscle
Radial artery | Median nerve
Lateral cutaneous nerve | Medial cutaneous nerve
Superficial branch of radial n. | Palmaris longus muscle
Cephalic vein | Ulnar artery
Brachioradial muscle | Ulnar nerve
Extensor carpi radialis | Flexor carpi
longus and brevis muscles | ulnaris muscle
Flexor pollicis longus muscle | Basilic vein
Deep branch of radial n. | Interosseous membrane
Supinator muscle | Anconeus muscle
Extensor digitorum muscle | Extensor pollicis longus muscle
Extensor carpi ulnaris muscle
Posterior interosseous artery and nerve
Extensor digiti minimi muscle

Flex.dig. subl.
Flex.dig. prof.
Rad.
Ulna

D

Median nerve
Flexor carpi radialis muscle (tendon) | Palmaris longus tendon
Flexor pollicis longus muscle | Flexor digitorum superficialis muscle
Radial artery | Flexor digitorum profundus muscle
Superficial branch of radial n. | Ulnar artery
Brachioradialis tendon | Flexor carpi ulnaris muscle
Abductor pollicis longus tendon | Palmar branch of ulnar n.
Extensor pollicis brevis tendon | Basilic vein
Superficial branch of radial n. | Dorsal branch of ulnar n.
Extensor carpi radialis longus and brevis tendons | Extensor carpi ulnaris tendon
Extensor pollicis longus tendon | Pronator quadratus muscle
Extensor digitorum tendons | Extensor digiti minimi tendon
Extensor indicis muscle

Rad.
Ul.

Median nerve
Brachial artery
Deep brachial artery
Radial nerve
Radial recurrent artery
C
Radial artery

Superior ulnar collateral artery
Ulnar nerve
Median nerve
Ulnar recurrent artery
Ulnar artery
Ulnar nerve

D
Deep palmar arch
Superficial palmar arch

NERVES OF RIGHT UPPER EXTREMITY

Front view shows principal nerves and arteries (uncolored) in relation to the bones, *C* and *D* are cross sections made at levels indicated on drawing at left. (Jones and Shepard.)

Plate XL   nerve

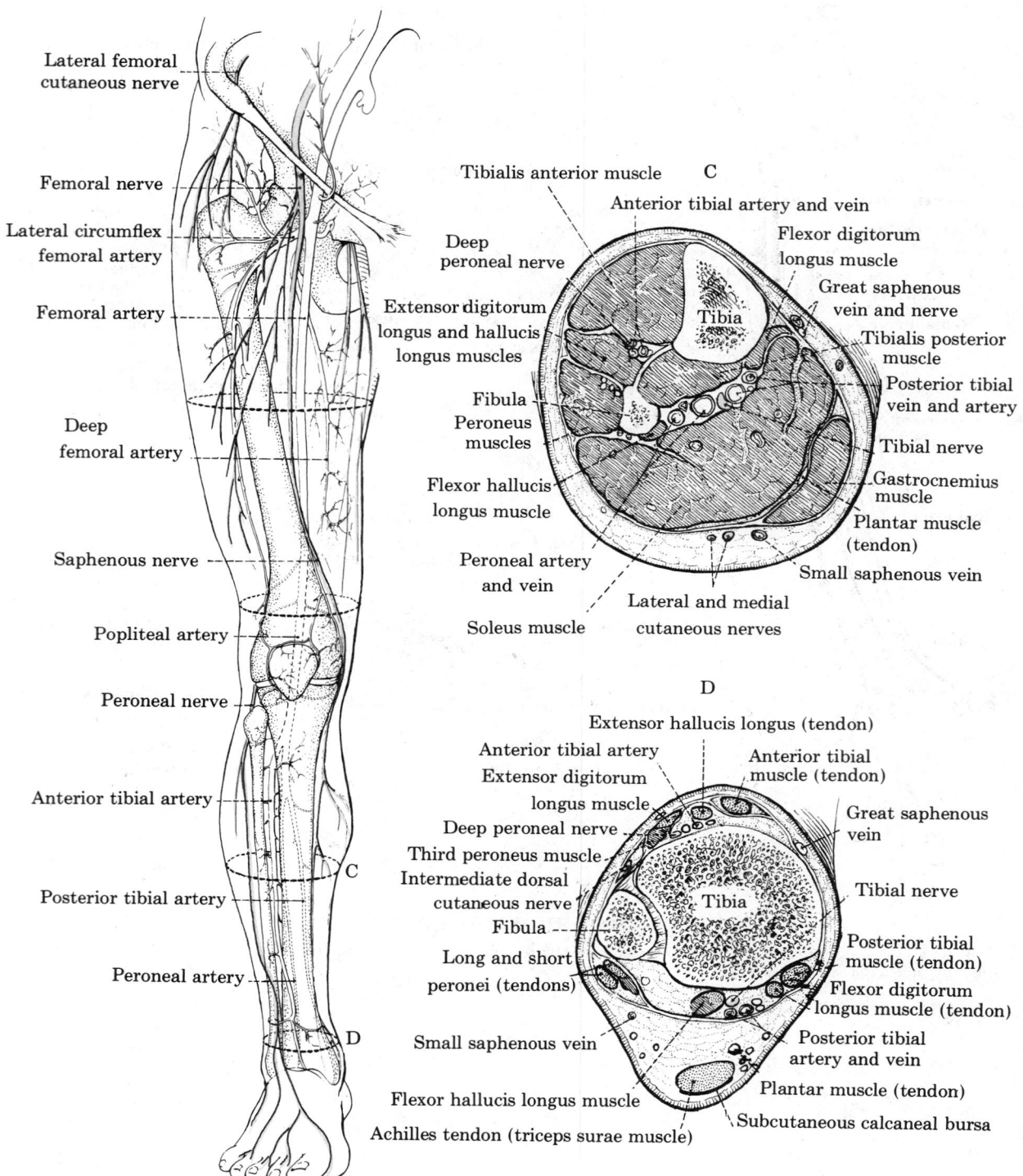

Lateral femoral
cutaneous nerve

Femoral nerve

Lateral circumflex
femoral artery

Femoral artery

Deep
femoral artery

Saphenous nerve

Popliteal artery

Peroneal nerve

Anterior tibial artery

Posterior tibial artery

Peroneal artery

Tibialis anterior muscle   C
Anterior tibial artery and vein

Deep
peroneal nerve

Extensor digitorum
longus and hallucis
longus muscles

Fibula
Peroneus
muscles

Flexor hallucis
longus muscle

Peroneal artery
and vein

Soleus muscle

Flexor digitorum
longus muscle

Great saphenous
vein and nerve

Tibia

Tibialis posterior
muscle

Posterior tibial
vein and artery

Tibial nerve

Gastrocnemius
muscle

Plantar muscle
(tendon)

Small saphenous vein

Lateral and medial
cutaneous nerves

D

Extensor hallucis longus (tendon)

Anterior tibial artery

Extensor digitorum
longus muscle

Deep peroneal nerve

Third peroneus muscle

Intermediate dorsal
cutaneous nerve

Fibula

Long and short
peronei (tendons)

Small saphenous vein

Flexor hallucis longus muscle

Achilles tendon (triceps surae muscle)

Anterior tibial
muscle (tendon)

Great saphenous
vein

Tibia

Tibial nerve

Posterior tibial
muscle (tendon)

Flexor digitorum
longus muscle (tendon)

Posterior tibial
artery and vein

Plantar muscle (tendon)

Subcutaneous calcaneal bursa

NERVES OF RIGHT LOWER EXTREMITY

Front view shows principal nerves and arteries (uncolored) in relation to the bones. *C* and *D* are cross sections made at levels indicated on
drawing at left. (Jones and Shepard.)

of nerves arising from the cervical segments of the spinal cord; see *nervi cervicales* [NA]. **cervical n., descending,** radix inferior ansae cervicalis. **cervical n., transverse,** nervus transversus colli. **chorda tympani n.,** see *chorda tympani.* **ciliary n's, long,** nervi ciliares longi. **ciliary n's, short,** nervi ciliares breves. **circumflex n.,** nervus axillaris. **clunial n's, inferior,** nervi clunium inferiores. **clunial n's, middle,** nervi clunium medii. **clunial n's, superior,** nervi clunium superiores. **coccygeal n.,** either of the thirty-first pair of spinal nerves, arising from the coccygeal segment of the spinal cord; called also *nervus coccygeus.* **cochlear n.,** pars cochlearis nervi vestibulocochlearis. **n. of Cotunnius,** nervus nasopalatinus. **cranial n's,** the twelve pairs of nerves connected with the brain; see *nervi craniales* [NA]. **cranial n., eighth,** nervus vestibulocochlearis. **cranial n., eleventh,** nervus accessorius. **cranial n., fifth,** nervus trigeminus. **cranial n's, first,** see *nervi olfactorii.* **cranial n., fourth,** nervus trochlearis. **cranial n., ninth,** nervus glossopharyngeus. **cranial n., second,** nervus opticus. **cranial n., seventh,** nervus facialis. **cranial n., sixth,** nervus abducens. **cranial n., tenth,** nervus vagus. **cranial n., third,** nervus oculomotorius. **cranial n., twelfth,** nervus hypoglossus. **crotaphitic n.,** nervus maxillaris. **cubital n.,** nervus ulnaris. **cutaneous n.,** nervus cutaneus. **cutaneous n. of abdomen, anterior,** ramus cutaneus anterior [pectoralis et abdominalis] nervorum intercostalium. **cutaneous n. of arm, lateral, inferior,** nervus cutaneus brachii lateralis inferior. **cutaneous n. of arm, lateral, superior,** nervus cutaneus brachii lateralis superior. **cutaneous n. of arm, medial,** nervus cutaneus brachii medialis. **cutaneous n. of arm, posterior,** nervus cutaneus brachii posterior. **cutaneous n. of calf, lateral,** nervus cutaneus surae lateralis. **cutaneous n. of calf, medial,** nervus cutaneus surae medialis. **cutaneous n. of foot, dorsal, intermediate,** nervus cutaneus dorsalis intermedius. **cutaneous n. of foot, dorsal, lateral,** nervus cutaneus dorsalis lateralis. **cutaneous n. of foot, dorsal, medial,** nervus cutaneus dorsalis medialis. **cutaneous n. of forearm, dorsal,** nervus cutaneus antebrachii posterior. **cutaneous n. of forearm, lateral,** nervus cutaneus antebrachii lateralis. **cutaneous n. of forearm, medial,** nervus cutaneus antebrachii medialis. **cutaneous n. of forearm, posterior,** nervus cutaneus antebrachii posterior. **cutaneous n. of thigh, lateral,** nervus cutaneus femoris lateralis. **cutaneous n. of thigh, posterior,** nervus cutaneus femoris posterior. **Cyon's n.,** a depressor nerve, the branch of the vagus nerve in the rabbit, stimulation of which results in lowering of the blood pressure. **dental n., inferior,** nervus alveolaris inferior. **depressor n.,** 1. a nerve that lessens the activity of an organ. 2. an inhibitory nerve whose stimulation depresses a motor center. **diaphragmatic n.,** nervus phrenicus. **digastric n.,** ramus digastricus nervi facialis. **digital n's, dorsal, radial,** nervi digitales dorsales nervi radialis. **digital n's, dorsal, ulnar,** nervi digitales dorsales nervi ulnaris. **digital n's of foot, dorsal,** nervi digitales dorsales pedis. **digital n's of lateral plantar nerve, plantar, common,** nervi digitales plantares communes nervi plantaris lateralis. **digital n's of lateral plantar nerve, plantar, proper,** nervi digitales plantares proprii nervi plantaris lateralis. **digital n's of lateral surface of great toe and of medial surface of second toe, dorsal,** nervi digitales dorsales hallucis lateralis et digiti secundi medialis. **digital n's of medial plantar nerve, plantar, common,** nervi digitales plantares communes nervi plantaris medialis. **digital n's of medial plantar nerve, plantar, proper,** nervi digitales plantares proprii nervi plantaris medialis. **digital n's of median nerve, palmar, common,** nervi digitales palmares communes nervi mediani. **digital n's of median nerve, palmar, proper,** nervi digitales palmares proprii nervi mediani. **digital n's of radial nerve, dorsal,** nervi digitales dorsales nervi radialis. **digital n's of ulnar nerve, dorsal,** nervi digitales dorsales nervi ulnaris. **digital n's of ulnar nerve, palmar, collateral,** nervi digitales palmares proprii nervi ulnaris. **digital n's of ulnar nerve, palmar, common,** nervi digitales palmares communes nervi ulnaris. **digital n's of ulnar nerve, palmar, proper,** nervi digitales palmares proprii nervi ulnaris. **dorsal n. of clitoris,** nervus dorsalis clitoridis. **dorsal n. of penis,** nervus dorsalis penis. **dorsal n. of scapula,** nervus dorsalis scapulae. **efferent n.,** any nerve that carries impulses from the central nervous system toward the periphery, as a motor nerve. **eighth n.,** nervus vestibulocochlearis. **eleventh n.,** nervus accessorius. **esodic n.,** afferent n. **ethmoidal n., anterior,** nervus ethmoidalis anterior. **ethmoidal n., posterior,** nervus ethmoidalis posterior. **exciter n.,** a nerve that transmits impulses resulting in an increase in functional activity. **excitoreflex n.,** a visceral nerve that produces reflex action. **exodic n.,** efferent n. **n. of external acoustic meatus,** nervus meatus acustici externi. **facial n.,** nervus facialis. **facial n., temporal,** see *rami temporales nervi facialis.* **femoral n.,** nervus femoralis. **fibular n., common,** nervus peroneus communis. **fibular n., deep,** nervus peroneus profundus. **fibular n., superficial,**

nervus peroneus superficialis. **fifth n.,** nervus trigeminus. **first n's,** see *nervi olfactorii.* **fourth n.,** nervus trochlearis. **frontal n.,** nervus frontalis. **furcal n.,** the fourth lumbar nerve, so called because its fibers pass to the lumbar and sacral plexuses. **fusimotor n's,** those with a special type of nerve ending that innervates intrafusal fibers of the muscle spindle. **gangliated n.,** any nerve of the sympathetic nervous system. **gastric n's,** truncus vagalis anterior and truncus vagalis posterior. **genitofemoral n.,** nervus genitofemoralis. **glossopharyngeal n.,** nervus glossopharyngeus. **gluteal n., inferior,** nervus gluteus inferior. **gluteal n's, inferior,** nervi clunium inferiores. **gluteal n's, middle,** nervi clunium medii. **gluteal n., superior,** nervus gluteus superior. **hemorrhoidal n's, inferior,** nervi rectales inferiores. **Hering's n.,** ramus sinus carotici nervi glossopharyngei. **hypogastric n.,** nervus hypogastricus [dexter et sinister]. **hypoglossal n.,** nervus hypoglossus. **iliohypogastric n.,** nervus iliohypogastricus. **ilioinguinal n.,** nervus ilioinguinalis. **infraoccipital n.,** nervus suboccipitalis. **infraorbital n.,** nervus infraorbitalis. **infratrochlear n.,** nervus infratrochlearis. **inhibitory n.,** a nerve that transmits impulses resulting in a decrease in functional activity. **intercostal n's,** rami ventrales nervorum thoracicorum. **intercostobrachial n's,** nervi intercostobrachiales. **intermediary n., intermediate n.,** nervus intermedius. **interosseous n. of forearm, anterior,** nervus interosseus antebrachii anterior. **interosseous n. of forearm, posterior,** nervus interosseus antebrachii posterior. **interosseous n. of leg,** nervus interosseus cruris. **ischiadic n.,** nervus ischiadicus. **Jacobson's n.,** nervus tympanicus. **jugular n.,** nervus jugularis. **labial n's, anterior,** nervi labiales anteriores. **labial n's, posterior,** nervi labiales posteriores. **lacrimal n.,** nervus lacrimalis. **n's of Lancisi,** stria longitudinalis lateralis corporis callosi and stria longitudinalis medialis corporis callosi. **Langley's n's,** pilomotor n's. **laryngeal n., inferior,** nervus laryngeus inferior. **laryngeal n., recurrent,** nervus laryngeus recurrens. **laryngeal n., superior,** nervus laryngeus superior. **laryngeal n., superior, internal,** ramus internus nervi laryngei superioris. **lingual n.,** nervus lingualis. **longitudinal n's of Lancisi,** stria longitudinalis lateralis corporis callosi and stria longitudinalis medialis corporis callosi. **lumbar n's,** the five pairs of nerves arising from the lumbar segments of the spinal cord; see *nervi lumbales.* **lumboinguinal n.,** ramus femoralis nervi genitofemoralis. **n. of Luschka,** 1. ramus meningeus nervorum spinalium. 2. nervus ethmoidalis posterior. **mandibular n.,** nervus mandibularis. **masseteric n.,** nervus massetericus. **maxillary n.,** nervus maxillaris. **median n.,** nervus medianus. **medullated n.,** myelinated n. **meningeal n.,** ramus meningeus nervi vagi. **mental n.,** nervus mentalis. **mixed n.,** a nerve composed of both sensory and motor fibers. **motor n.,** an efferent nerve that stimulates muscle contraction. **motor n. of tongue,** nervus hypoglossus. **musculocutaneous n.,** nervus musculocutaneus. **musculocutaneous n. of foot,** nervus peroneus superficialis. **musculocutaneous n. of leg,** nervus peroneus profundus. **musculospiral n.,** nervus radialis. **myelinated n.,** a nerve, especially a peripheral nerve, whose fibers (axons) are encased in a myelin sheath, which in turn is enclosed by a neurilemma. Called also *medullated n.* Cf. *unmyelinated n.* **mylohyoid n.,** nervus mylohyoideus. **nasociliary n.,** nervus nasociliaris. **nasopalatine n.,** nervus nasopalatinus. **ninth n.,** nervus glossopharyngeus. **nonmedullated n.,** unmyelinated n. **obturator n.,** nervus obturatorius. **occipital n., greater,** nervus occipitalis major. **occipital n., internal** (*obs.*), nervus occipitalis major. **occipital n., least,** nervus occipitalis tertius. **occipital n., lesser,** nervus occipitalis minor. **occipital n., third,** nervus occipitalis tertius. **oculomotor n.,** nervus oculomotorius. **olfactory n's,** nervi olfactorii. **ophthalmic n.,** nervus ophthalmicus. **optic n.,** nervus opticus. **pain n.,** a sensory nerve whose function is the conduction of stimuli which produce the sensation of pain. **palatine n., anterior,** nervus palatinus major. **palatine n., greater,** nervus palatinus major. **palatine n's, lesser,** nervi palatini minores. **palatine n., medial, palatine n., middle,** see *nervi palatini minores.* **palatine n., posterior,** see *nervi palatini minores.* **parasympathetic n.,** any of the nerves of the parasympathetic nervous system; see *parasympathetic system,* under *system.* **parotid n's,** rami parotidei nervi auriculotemporalis. **pectoral n., lateral,** nervus pectoralis lateralis. **pectoral n., medial,** nervus pectoralis medialis. **perineal n's,** nervi perineales. **peripheral n.,** any nerve outside the central nervous system (outside the brain and spinal cord). **peroneal n., accessory deep,** nervus peroneus profundus accessorius. **peroneal n., common,** nervus peroneus communis. **peroneal n., deep,** nervus peroneus profundus. **peroneal n., superficial,** nervus peroneus superficialis. **petrosal n., deep,** nervus petrosus profundus. **petrosal n., greater,** nervus petrosus major. **petrosal n., lesser,** nervus petrosus minor. **petrosal n., middle, superficial,** nervus petrosus minor. **phrenic n.,** nervus phrenicus. **phrenic n's, accessory,** nervi phrenici accessorii. **phrenicoabdominal n's,** rami phrenicoabdominales nervi phrenici. **pilomotor n's,** the nerves that supply the arrectores pilorum muscles. **plantar n., lateral,** nervus plantaris lateralis. **plantar n., medial,** nervus plantaris medialis. **pneumogastric n.,** nervus vagus. **popliteal n., external,** nervus peroneus communis. **popliteal n., internal,** nervus tibialis. **popliteal n., lateral,** nervus peroneus communis. **popliteal n., medial,** nervus tibialis. **presacral n.,** plexus hypogastricus superior. **pressor n.,** any afferent nerve whose irritation stimulates a vasomotor center and increases intravascular tension. **pterygoid n., external,** nervus pterygoideus lateralis. **pterygoid n., internal,** nervus pterygoideus medialis. **pterygoid n., lateral,** nervus pterygoideus lateralis. **pterygoid n., medial,** nervus pterygoideus medialis. **n. of pterygoid canal,** nervus canalis pterygoidei. **pterygopalatine n's,** nervi pterygopalatini. **pudendal n.,** nervus pudendus. **pudic n.,** nervus pudendus. **radial n.,** nervus radialis. **radial n., deep,** ramus profundus nervi radialis. **radial n., superficial,** ramus superficialis nervi radialis. **rectal n's, inferior,** nervi rectales inferiores. **recurrent n.,** nervus laryngeus recurrens. **recurrent n., ophthalmic,** ramus tentorii nervi ophthalmici. **saccular n.,** nervus saccularis. **sacral n's,** the five pairs of nerves arising from the sacral segments of the spinal cord; see *nervi sacrales.* **saphenous n.,** nervus saphenus. **Scarpa's n.,** nervus nasopalatinus. **sciatic n.,** nervus ischiadicus. **sciatic n., small,** nervus cutaneus femoris posterior. **scrotal n's, anterior,** nervi scrotales anteriores. **scrotal n's, posterior,** nervi scrotales posteriores. **second n.,** nervus opticus. **secretory n.,** any efferent nerve whose stimulation increases glandular activity. **sensory n.,** a peripheral nerve that conducts impulses from a sense organ to the spinal cord or brain. **seventh n.,** nervus facialis. **sinus n.,** ramus sinus carotici nervi glossopharyngei. **sinu-vertebral n.,** ramus meningeus nervorum spinalium. **sixth n.,** nervus abducens. **somatic n's,** the motor and sensory nerves that supply skeletal muscle and somatic tissues. **spermatic n., external,** ramus genitalis nervi genitofemoralis. **spinal n's,** the thirty-one pairs of nerves arising from the spinal cord; see *nervi spinales.* **splanchnic n's,** the nerves of the blood vessels and viscera, especially the visceral branches of the thoracic, lumbar, and pelvic parts of the sympathetic trunks. **splanchnic n., greater,** nervus splanchnicus major. **splanchnic n., inferior, splanchnic n., lesser,** nervus splanchnicus minor. **splanchnic n., lowest,** nervus splanchnicus imus. **splanchnic n's, lumbar,** nervi splanchnici lumbales. **splanchnic n's, pelvic,** nervi splanchnici pelvini. **splanchnic n's, sacral,** nervi splanchnici sacrales. **stapedial n., stapedius n.,** nervus stapedius. **stylohyoid n.,** ramus stylohyoideus nervi facialis. **stylopharyngeal n.,** ramus musculi stylopharyngei nervi glossopharyngei. **subclavian n.,** nervus subclavius. **subcostal n.,** nervus subcostalis. **suboccipital n.,** nervus suboccipitalis. **subscapular n's,** nervi subscapulares. **sudomotor n's,** the nerves that innervate the sweat glands. **supraclavicular n's,** nervi supraclaviculares. **supraclavicular n's, anterior,** nervi supraclaviculares mediales. **supraclavicular n's, intermediate,** nervi supraclaviculares intermedii. **supraclavicular n's, lateral,** nervi supraclaviculares laterales. **supraclavicular n's, medial,** nervi supraclaviculares mediales. **supraclavicular n's, middle,** nervi supraclaviculares intermedii. **supraclavicular n's, posterior,** nervi supraclaviculares laterales [posteriores]. **supraorbital n.,** nervus supraorbitalis. **suprascapular n.,** nervus suprascapularis. **supratrochlear n.,** nervus supratrochlearis. **sural n.,** nervus suralis. **sympathetic n.,** 1. truncus sympatheticus. 2. one of the nerves of the sympathetic nervous system; see *sympathetic system,* under *system.* **tem-**

poral n's, deep, nervi temporales profundi. **temporal n's, subcutaneous,** rami temporales superficiales nervi auriculotemporalis. **n. of tensor tympani,** nervus tensoris tympani. **n. of tensor veli palatini,** nervus tensoris veli palatini. **tenth n.,** nervus vagus. **terminal n's,** nervi terminales. **third n.,** nervus oculomotorius. **thoracic n's,** the twelve pairs of spinal nerves arising from the thoracic segments of the spinal cord; see *nervi thoracici.* **thoracic n., long,** nervus thoracicus longus. **thoracodorsal n.,** nervus thoracodorsalis. **tibial n.,** nervus tibialis. **Tiedemann's n.,** a name given a plexus of sympathetic nerve fibrils surrounding the central artery of the retina. **tonsillar n's,** rami tonsillares nervi glossopharyngei. **transverse n. of neck,** nervus transversus colli. **trigeminal n.,** nervus trigeminus. **trochlear n.,** nervus trochlearis. **trophic n.,** a nerve that aids in regulating nutrition. **twelfth n.,** nervus hypoglossus. **tympanic n.,** nervus tympanicus. **ulnar n.,** nervus ulnaris. **unmyelinated n.,** a nerve whose fibers (axons) are not encased in a myelin sheath, and which may or may not be enclosed by a neurilemma. Called also *nonmedullated n.* Cf. *myelinated n.* **utricular n.,** nervus utricularis. **utriculoampullar n.,** nervus utriculoampullaris. **vaginal n's,** nervi vaginales. **vagus n.,** nervus vagus. **vascular n.,** nervus vascularis. **vasoconstrictor n.,** a nerve whose stimulation causes contraction of the blood vessels. **vasodilator n.,** a nerve whose stimulation causes dilation of the blood vessels. **vasomotor n.,** any nerve concerned in controlling the caliber of vessels, whether as a vasodilator or a vasoconstrictor. **vasosensory n.,** any nerve supplying sensory fibers to the vessels. **vertebral n.,** nervus vertebralis. **vestibular n.,** pars vestibularis nervi octavi. **vestibulocochlear n.,** nervus vestibulocochlearis. **vidian n.,** nervus canalis pterygoidei. **vidian n., deep,** nervus petrosus profundus. **n. of Willis,** nervus accessorius. **Wrisberg's n.,** 1. nervus intermedius. 2. nervus cutaneus brachii medialis. **zygomatic n.,** nervus zygomaticus. **zygomaticofacial n.,** ramus zygomaticofacialis nervi zygomatici. **zygomaticotemporal n.,** ramus zygomaticotemporalis nervi zygomatici.

nervi (ner′vi) [L.] plural of *nervus.*

nervimotility (ner″vĭ-mo-til′ĭ-te) susceptibility to nervimotion.

nervimotion (ner″vĭ-mo′shun) motion effected through the agency of a nerve.

nervimotor (ner″vĭ-mo′tor) pertaining to a motor nerve.

nervimuscular (ner″vĭ-mus′ku-lar) pertaining to the nerve supply of muscles.

nervomuscular (ner″vo-mus′ku-lar) nervimuscular.

nervone (ner′vōn) a cerebroside, $C_{48}H_{91}O_8N$, isolated from nerve tissue.

nervosism (ner′vo-sizm) (*obs.*) 1. neurasthenia. 2. the theory that disease is dependent on variations in nerve force.

nervous (ner′vus) [L. *nervosus*] 1. pertaining to a nerve or to nerves. 2. unduly excitable.

nervous breakdown (ner′vus brāk′down) a nonspecific, popular name for any type of mental disorder that interferes with the affected individual's normal activities, and may include neurosis, depression, or psychosis.

nervousness (ner′vus-nes) morbid or undue excitability; a state of excessive irritability, with great mental and physical unrest.

nervous system see under *system.*

nervus (ner′vus), pl. *ner′vi* [L.] [NA] a nerve: a cordlike structure, visible to the naked eye, comprising a collection of nerve fibers which convey impulses between a part of the central nervous system and some other region of the body. See also *nerve.* For names and description of specific nerves, see *Table of Nervi.*

TABLE OF NERVI

Descriptions are given on NA terms, and include anglicized names of specific nerves.

n. abdu′cens [NA], abducens nerve (6th cranial): *origin,* a nucleus in the pons, beneath the floor of the fourth ventricle, emerging from the brain stem anteriorly between the pons and medulla oblongata; *distribution,* lateral rectus muscle of eye; *modality,* motor.

n. accesso′rius [NA], accessory nerve (11th cranial); *origin,* by cranial roots from the side of the medulla oblongata, and by spinal roots from the side of the spinal cord (from the upper three or more cervical segments); the roots unite and the nerve thus formed divides into an internal branch (cranial portion) and an external branch (spinal portion); *distribution,* the internal branch to the vagus and thereby to the palate, pharynx, larynx, and thoracic viscera; the external branch to the sternocleidomastoid and trapezius muscles; *modality,* parasympathetic and motor.

n. acus′ticus, n. vestibulocochlearis.

n. alveola′ris infe′rior [NA], inferior alveolar nerve: *origin,* mandibular nerve; *branches,* mylohyoid, inferior dental, mental, and inferior gingival nerves; *distribution—*see individual branches, in this table; *modality,* motor and general sensory.

ner′vi alveola′res superio′res [NA], superior alveolar nerves: a term denoting collectively the dental branches arising from the maxillary and infraorbital nerves. viz., *rami alveolares superiores anteriores nervi infraorbitalis, ramus alveolaris superior medius nervi infraorbitalis,* and *rami alveolares superiores posteriores nervi maxillaris.*

n. ampulla′ris ante′rior [NA], anterior ampullar nerve: the branch of the pars vestibularis nervi octavi that innervates the ampulla of the anterior semicircular duct, ending around the hair cells of the ampullary crest.

n. ampulla′ris infe′rior, n. ampullaris posterior.

n. ampulla′ris latera′lis [NA], lateral ampullar nerve: the branch of the pars vestibularis nervi octavi that innervates the ampulla of the lateral semicircular duct, ending around the hair cells of the ampullary crest.

n. ampulla′ris poste′rior [NA], posterior ampullar nerve: the branch of the pars vestibularis nervi octavi that innervates the ampulla of the posterior semicircular duct, ending around the hair cells of the ampullary crest.

n. ampulla′ris supe′rior, n. ampularis anterior.

ner′vi anococcyg′ei [NA], anococcygeal nerves: *origin,* coccygeal plexus; *distribution,* sacrococcygeal joint, coccyx, skin over the coccyx; *modality,* general sensory.

n. articula′ris [NA], articular nerve: a peripheral nerve that supplies a joint and its associated structures.

ner′vi auricula′res anterio′res [NA], anterior auricular nerves: *origin,* auriculotemporal nerve; *distribution,* skin of anterosuperior part of external ear; *modality,* general sensory.

n. auricula′ris mag′nus [NA], great auricular nerve: *origin,* cervical plexus—C2–C3; *branches,* anterior and posterior rami; *distribution,* skin over parotid gland and mastoid process, and both surfaces of auricle; see individual branches under *ramus; modality,* general sensory.

n. auricula′ris poste′rior [NA], posterior auricular nerve: *origin,* facial nerve; *branches,* occipital ramus; *distribution,* auricularis posterior and occipitofrontalis muscles and skin of external acoustic meatus; *modality,* motor and general sensory.

n. auriculotempora′lis [NA], auriculotemporal nerve: *origin,* by two roots from the mandibular nerve; *branches,* anterior auricular nerve, nerve of external acoustic meatus, parotid branches, branch to tympanic membrane, and branches communicating with facial nerve; its terminal branches are superficial temporal to the scalp; *distribution*—see individual branches, in this table and under *ramus; modality,* general sensory.

n. axilla′ris [NA], axillary nerve: *origin,* posterior cord of brachial plexus (C5–C6); *branches,* lateral superior brachial cutaneous nerve and muscular rami; *distribution,* deltoid and teres minor muscles, skin on back of arm; *modality,* motor and general sensory.

n. bucca′lis [NA], buccal nerve: *origin,* mandibular nerve; *distribution,* skin and mucous membrane of cheeks, gums, and perhaps first two molars and the premolars; *modality,* general sensory.

n. buccinato′rius, n. buccalis.

n. cana′lis pterygoi′dei [NA], nerve of pterygoid canal: *origin,* union of deep and greater petrosal nerves; *distribution,* pterygopalatine ganglion and branches; *modality,* parasympathetic and sympathetic. Called also *radix facialis* [NA alternative].

n. cardi′acus cervica′lis infe′rior [NA], inferior cervical cardiac nerve: *origin,* cervicothoracic ganglion; *distribution,* heart via cardiac plexus; *modality,* sympathetic (accelerator) and visceral afferent (chiefly pain).

n. cardi′acus cervica′lis me′dius [NA], middle cervical cardiac nerve: *origin,* middle cervical ganglion; *distribution,* heart; *modality,* sympathetic (accelerator) and visceral afferent (chiefly pain).

n. cardi′acus cervica′lis supe′rior [NA], superior cervical cardiac nerve: *origin,* superior cervical ganglion; *distribution,* heart; *modality,* sympathetic (accelerator).

n. cardi′acus infe′rior, n. cardiacus cervicalis inferior.

n. cardi′acus me′dius, n. cardiacus cervicalis medius.

n. cardi′acus supe′rior, n. cardiacus cervicalis superior.

ner′vi cardi′aci thora′cici [NA], thoracic cardiac nerves: *origin,* second through fourth or fifth thoracic ganglia of sympathetic trunk; *distribution,* heart; *modality,* sympathetic (accelerator) and visceral afferent (chiefly pain).

ner′vi caroticotympan′ici [NA], caroticotympanic nerves: *origin,* internal carotid plexus; *branches,* together with tympanic nerve, they form the tympanic plexus; *distribution,* tympanic region and parotid gland; *modality,* sympathetic.

n. caroticotympan′icus infe′rior, n. caroticotympan′icus supe′rior, see *nervi caroticotympanici.*

ner′vi carot′ici exter′ni [NA], external carotid nerves: *origin,* superior cervical ganglion; *distribution,* cranial blood vessels and glands via the external carotid plexus; *modality,* sympathetic.

n. carot′icus inter′nus [NA], internal carotid nerve: *origin,* superior cervical ganglion; *distribution,* cranial blood vessels and glands via internal carotid plexus; *modality,* sympathetic.

ner′vi caverno′si clitor′idis [NA], cavernous nerves of clitoris: *origin,* uterovaginal plexus; *distribution,* erectile tissue of clitoris; *modality,* parasympathetic, sympathetic, and visceral afferent.

n. caverno′sus clitor′idis ma′jor, ner′vi caverno′si clitor′idis mino′res, see *nervi cavernosi clitoridis.*

ner′vi caverno′si pe′nis [NA], cavernous nerves of penis: *origin,* prostatic plexus; *distribution,* erectile tissue of penis; *modality,* parasympathetic, sympathetic, and visceral afferent.

n. caverno′sus pe′nis ma′jor, ner′vi caverno′si pe′nis mino′res, see *nervi cavernosi penis.*

ner′vi cerebra′les, nervi craniales.

ner′vi cervica′les [NA], cervical nerves: the eight pairs of nerves that arise from the cervical segments of the spinal cord and, except for the last pair, leave the vertebral column above the correspondingly numbered vertebra. The ventral branches of the upper four, on either side, unite to form the cervical plexus, and those of the lower four, together with the ventral branch of the first thoracic nerve, form most of the brachial plexus.

ner′vi cilia′res bre′ves [NA], short ciliary nerves: *origin,* ciliary ganglion; *distribution,* smooth muscle and tunics of eye; *modality,* parasympathetic, sympathetic, and general sensory.

ner′vi cilia′res lon′gi [NA], long ciliary nerves: *origin,* nasociliary nerve, from ophthalmic nerve; *distribution,* dilator pupillae, uvea, cornea; *modality,* sympathetic and general sensory.

ner′vi clu′nium inferio′res [NA], inferior clunial nerves: *origin,* posterior femoral cutaneous nerve; *distribution,* skin of lower part of buttock; *modality,* general sensory.

ner′vi clu′nium me′dii [NA], middle clunial nerves: *origin,* plexus formed by lateral branches of dorsal rami of first four sacral nerves behind the sacrum and coccyx; *distribution,* ligaments of sacrum and skin over posterior part of buttock; *modality,* general sensory.

ner′vi clu′nium superio′res [NA], superior clunial nerves: *origin,* lateral branches of dorsal rami of upper lumbar nerves; *distribution,* skin of upper part of buttock; upper gluteal region; *modality,* general sensory.

n. coccyg′eus [NA], coccygeal nerve: one of the pair of nerves that arise from the coccygeal segment of the spinal cord.

n. coch′leae, pars cochlearis nervi vestibulocochlearis.

ner′vi crania′les [NA], cranial nerves: the twelve pairs of nerves that are connected with the brain, including the nervi olfactorii (I), and the opticus (II), oculomotorius (III), trochlearis (IV), trigeminus (V), abducens (VI), facialis (VII), vestibulocochlearis (VIII), glossopharyngeus (IX), vagus (X), accessorius (XI), and hypoglossus (XII). Called also *nervi cerebrales.*

n. cuta′neus [NA], cutaneous nerve: a peripheral nerve that supplies a region of the skin, many of them not being specifically named.

n. cuta′neus antebra′chii latera′lis [NA], lateral cutaneous nerve of forearm: *origin,* continuation of musculocutaneous nerve; *distribution,* skin over radial side of forearm and sometimes an area of skin of dorsum of hand; *modality,* general sensory.

n. cuta′neus antebra′chii media′lis [NA], medial cutaneous nerve of forearm: *origin,* medial cord of brachial plexus (C8, T1); *branches,* anterior and ulnar; *distribution,* skin of front, medial, and posteromedial aspects of forearm; *modality,* general sensory.

n. cuta′neus antebra′chii poste′rior [NA], posterior cutaneous nerve of forearm: *origin,* radial nerve; *distribution,* skin of dorsal aspect of forearm; *modality,* general sensory.

n. cuta′neus antibra′chii dorsa′lis, n. cutaneous antebrachii posterior.

n. cuta′neus bra′chii latera′lis infe′rior [NA], inferior lateral cutaneous nerve of arm: *origin,* radial nerve; *distribution,* skin of lateral surface of lower part of arm; *modality,* general sensory.

n. cuta′neus bra′chii latera′lis supe′rior [NA], superior lateral cutaneous nerve of arm: *origin,* axillary nerve; *distribution,* skin of back of arm; *modality,* general sensory.

n. cuta′neus bra′chii media′lis [NA], medial cutaneous nerve of arm: *origin,* medial cord of brachial plexus (T1); *distribution,* skin on medial and posterior aspects of arm; *modality,* general sensory.

n. cuta′neus bra′chii poste′rior [NA], posterior cutaneous nerve of arm: *origin,* radial nerve in the axilla; *distribution,* skin on back of arm; *modality,* general sensory.

n. cuta′neus col′li, n. transversus colli.

n. cuta′neus dorsa′lis interme′dius [NA], intermediate dorsal cutaneous nerve: *origin,* superficial peroneal nerve; *branches,* dorsal digital nerves of foot; *distribution,* skin of front of lower third of leg and dorsum of foot, and skin and joints of adjacent sides of third and fourth, and of fourth and fifth toes; *modality,* general sensory.

n. cuta′neus dorsa′lis latera′lis pe′dis [NA], lateral dorsal cutaneous nerve: *origin,* continuation of sural nerve; *distribution,* skin and joints of lateral side of foot and fifth toe; *modality,* general sensory.

n. cuta′neus dorsa′lis media′lis [NA], medial dorsal cutaneous nerve: *origin,* superficial peroneal nerve; *distribution,* skin and joints of medial side of foot and big toe, and adjacent sides of second and third toes; *modality,* general sensory.

n. cuta′neus fem′oris latera′lis [NA], lateral cutaneous nerve of thigh: *origin,* lumbar plexus—L2–L3; *distribution,* skin of lateral and front aspects of thigh; *modality,* general sensory.

n. cuta′neus fem′oris poste′rior [NA], posterior cutaneous nerve of thigh: *origin,* sacral plexus—S1–S3; *branches,* inferior clunial nerves and perineal rami; *distribution,* skin of buttock, external genitalia, and back of thigh and calf; *modality,* general sensory.

n. cuta′neus su′rae latera′lis [NA], lateral cutaneous nerve of calf: *origin,* common peroneal nerve; *distribution,* skin of lateral side of back of leg, rarely may continue as the sural nerve; *modality,* general sensory.

n. cuta′neus su′rae media′lis [NA], medial cutaneous nerve of calf: *origin,* tibial nerve; usually joins peroneal communicating branch of common peroneal nerve to form the sural nerve; *distribution,* may continue as the sural nerve; *modality,* general sensory.

ner′vi digita′les dorsa′les hal′lucis latera′lis et dig′iti secun′di media′lis [NA], dorsal digital nerves of lateral surface of great toe and of medial surface of second toe: *origin,* medial terminal division of deep peroneal nerve; *distribution,* skin and joints of adjacent sides of great and second toes; *modality*, general sensory.

ner'vi digita'les dorsa'les ner'vi radia'lis [NA], dorsal digital nerves of radial nerve: *origin*, superficial branch of radial nerve; *distribution*, skin and joints of back of thumb, index finger, and part of middle finger, as far distally as the distal phalanx; *modality*, general sensory.

ner'vi digita'les dorsa'les ner'vi ulna'ris [NA], dorsal digital nerves of ulnar nerve: *origin*, dorsal branch of ulnar nerve; *distribution*, skin and joints of medial side of little finger, dorsal aspects of adjacent sides of little and ring fingers and of ring and middle fingers; *modality*, general sensory.

ner'vi digita'les dorsa'les pe'dis [NA], dorsal digital nerves of foot: *origin*, intermediate dorsal cutaneous nerve; *distribution*, skin and joints of adjacent sides of third and fourth, and of fourth and fifth toes; *modality*, general sensory.

ner'vi digita'les palma'res commu'nes ner'vi media'ni [NA], common palmar digital nerves of median nerve: *number*, four; *origin*, lateral and medial divisions of median nerve; *branches*, proper palmar digital nerves; *distribution*, thumb, index, middle, and ring fingers, and first two lumbrical muscles—see individual branches, in this table; *modality*, motor and general sensory.

ner'vi digita'les palma'res commu'nes ner'vi ulna'ris [NA], common palmar digital nerves of ulnar nerve: *number*, two; *origin*, superficial branch of ulnar nerve; *branches*, proper palmar digital nerves; *distribution*, little and ring fingers—see individual branches, in this table; *modality*, general sensory.

ner'vi digita'les palma'res pro'prii ner'vi media'ni [NA], proper palmar digital nerves of median nerve: *origin*, common palmar digital nerves; *distribution*, first two lumbrical muscles, skin and joints of both sides and palmar aspect of thumb, index, and middle fingers, radial side of ring finger, and back of distal aspect of these digits; *modality*, general sensory and motor.

ner'vi digita'les palma'res pro'prii ner'vi ulna'ris [NA], proper palmar digital nerves of ulnar nerve: *origin*, the lateral of the two common palmar digital nerves from superficial branch of ulnar nerve; *distribution*, skin and joints of adjacent sides of fourth and fifth fingers; *modality*, general sensory.

ner'vi digita'les planta'res commu'nes ner'vi planta'ris latera'lis [NA], common plantar digital nerves of lateral plantar nerve: *number*, two; *origin*, superficial branch of lateral planter nerve; *branches*, the medial nerve gives rise to two proper plantar digital nerves; *distribution*, the lateral one to the musculus flexor digiti minimi brevis pedis and to skin and joints of lateral side of sole and little toe; the medial one to adjacent sides of fourth and fifth toes—see individual branches, in this table; *modality*, motor and general sensory.

ner'vi digita'les planta'res commu'nes ner'vi planta'ris media'lis [NA], common plantar digital nerves of medial plantar nerve: *number*, four; *origin*, medial plantar nerve; *branches*, muscular and proper plantar digital nerves; *distribution*, flexor hallucis brevis muscle and first lumbrical muscles, skin and joints of medial side of foot and big toe, and adjacent sides of first and second, second and third, and third and fourth toes—see individual branches, in this table; *modality*, motor and general sensory.

ner'vi digita'les planta'res pro'prii ner'vi planta'ris latera'lis [NA], proper plantar digital nerves of lateral plantar nerve: *origin*, common plantar digital nerves; *distribution*, flexor digiti minimi brevis muscle, and skin and joints of lateral side of sole and little toe, and adjacent sides of fourth and fifth toes; *modality*, motor and general sensory.

ner'vi digita'les planta'res pro'prii ner'vi planta'ris media'lis [NA], proper plantar digital nerves of medial plantar nerve: *origin*, common plantar digital nerves; *distribution*, skin and joints of medial side of first toe, and adjacent sides of first and second, second and third, and third and fourth toes; the nerves extend to the dorsum to supply nail beds and tips of toes; *modality*, general sensory.

ner'vi digita'les vola'res commu'nes ner'vi media'ni, nervi digitales palmares communes nervi mediani.

ner'vi digita'les vola'res commu'nes ner'vi ulna'ris, nervi digitales palmares communes nervi ulnaris.

ner'vi digita'les vola'res pro'prii ner'vi media'ni, nervi digitales palmares proprii nervi mediani.

ner'vi digita'les vola'res pro'prii ner'vi ulna'ris, nervi digitales palmares proprii nervi ulnaris.

n. dorsa'lis clitor'idis [NA], dorsal nerve of clitoris: *origin*, pudendal nerve; *distribution*, transversus perinei profundus and sphincter urethrae muscles, corpus cavernosum clitoridis, and skin, prepuce, and glans of clitoris; *modality*, general sensory and motor.

n. dorsa'lis pe'nis [NA], dorsal nerve of penis: *origin*, pudendal nerve; *distribution*, transversus perinei profundus and sphincter urethrae muscles, corpus cavernosum penis, and skin, prepuce, and glans of penis; *modality*, general sensory and motor.

n. dorsa'lis scap'ulae [NA], dorsal nerve of scapula: *origin*, brachial plexus—ventral ramus of C5; *distribution*, rhomboid muscles and occasionally the levator scapulae muscle; *modality*, motor.

ner'vi erigen'tes, NA alternative for *nervi splanchnici pelvini*.

n. ethmoida'lis ante'rior [NA], anterior ethmoidal nerve: *origin*, continuation of nasociliary nerve, from ophthalmic nerve; *branches*, internal, external, lateral, and medial rami; *distribution*,

mucosa of upper and anterior nasal septum, lateral wall of nasal cavity, skin of lower bridge and tip of nose; *modality*, general sensory.

n. ethmoida'lis poste'rior [NA], posterior ethmoidal nerve: *origin*, nasociliary nerve, from ophthalmic nerve; *distribution*, mucosa of posterior ethmoid cells and of sphenoidal sinus; *modality*, general sensory.

n. facia'lis [NA], facial nerve (7th cranial), consisting of two roots: a large motor root, which supplies the muscles of facial expression, and a smaller root, the nervus intermedius (q.v.). *Origin*, inferior border of pons, between olive and inferior cerebellar peduncle; *branches* (of motor root), stapedius and posterior auricular nerves, parotid plexus, digastric, temporal, zygomatic, buccal, lingual, marginal mandibular, and cervical rami, and a communicating ramus with the tympanic plexus; *distribution*—see individual branches, in this table and under *ramus; modality*, motor, parasympathetic, general sensory, special sensory.

n. femora'lis [NA], femoral nerve: *origin*, lumbar plexus—L2–L4; descending behind the inguinal ligament to the femoral triangle; *branches*, saphenous nerve, muscular and anterior cutaneous rami; *distribution*, the skin of the thigh and leg, the muscles of the front of the thigh, and the hip and knee joints—see individual branches, in this table and under *ramus; modality*, general sensory and motor.

n. fibula'ris commu'nis, NA alternative for *n. peroneus communis*.

n. fibula'ris profun'dus, NA alternative for *n. peroneus profundus*.

n. fibula'ris superficia'lis, NA alternative for *n. peroneus superficialis*.

n. fronta'lis [NA], frontal nerve: *origin*, ophthalmic division of trigeminal nerve; enters the orbit through the superior orbital fissure; *branches*, supraorbital and supratrochlear nerves; *distribution*, chiefly to the forehead and scalp—see individual branches, in this table; *modality*, general sensory.

n. genitofemora'lis [NA], genitofemoral nerve: *origin*, lumbar plexus—L1–L2; *branches*, genital and femoral rami; *distribution*—see individual branches, under *ramus; modality*, general sensory and motor.

n. glossopharyn'geus [NA], glossopharyngeal nerve (9th cranial): *origin*, several rootlets from lateral side of upper part of medulla oblongata, between the olive and the inferior cerebellar peduncle; *branches*, tympanic nerve, pharyngeal, stylopharyngeal, tonsillar, and lingual rami, ramus to the carotid sinus, and a ramus communicating with the auricular ramus of the vagus nerve; *distribution*, it has two enlargements (superior and inferior ganglia) and supplies the tongue, pharynx, and parotid gland—see individual branches, in this table and under *ramus; modality*, motor, parasympathetic, general, special, and visceral sensory.

n. glu'teus infe'rior [NA], inferior gluteal nerve: *origin*, sacral plexus—L5–S2; *distribution*, gluteus maximus muscle; *modality*, motor.

n. glu'teus supe'rior [NA], superior gluteal nerve: *origin*, sacral plexus—L4–S1; *distribution*, gluteus medius and minimus muscles, tensor fasciae latae, and hip joint; *modality*, motor and general sensory.

ner'vi haemorrhoida'les inferio'res, nervi rectales inferiores.

ner'vi haemorrhoida'les me'dii, former term for branches of the middle rectal plexus.

ner'vi haemorrhoida'les superio'res, former term for branches of the superior rectal plexus.

n. hypogas'tricus [dex'ter et sinis'ter] [NA], hypogastric nerve: a nerve trunk situated on either side (right and left), interconnecting the superior and inferior hypogastric plexuses.

n. hypoglos'sus [NA], hypoglossal nerve (12th cranial): *origin*, several rootlets in the anterolateral sulcus between the olive and the pyramid of the medulla oblongata; it passes through the hypoglossal canal to the tongue; *branches*, lingual rami; *distribution*, styloglossus, hypoglossus, and genioglossus muscles and intrinsic muscles of the tongue; *modality*, motor.

n. iliohypogas'tricus [NA], iliohypogastric nerve: *origin*, lumbar plexus—L1 (sometimes T12); *branches*, lateral and anterior cutaneous rami; *distribution*, the skin above the pubis and over the lateral side of the buttock, and occasionally the pyramidalis; *modality*, motor and general sensory.

n. ilioinguina'lis [NA], ilioinguinal nerve: *origin*, lumbar plexus—L1 (sometimes T12); accompanies the spermatic cord through the inguinal canal; *branches*, anterior scrotal or labial rami; *distribution*, skin of scrotum or labia majora, and adjacent part of thigh; *modality*, general sensory.

n. infraorbita'lis [NA], infraorbital nerve: *origin*, continuation of the maxillary nerve, entering the orbit through the inferior orbital fissure, and occupying in succession the infraorbital groove, canal, and foramen; *branches*, middle and anterior superior alveolar, inferior palpebral, internal and external nasal, and superior labial rami; *distribution*—see individual branches, under *ramus; modality*, general sensory.

n. infratrochlea'ris [NA], infratrochlear nerve: *origin*, nasociliary nerve from ophthalmic nerve; *branches*, palpebral rami; *distribution*, skin of root and upper bridge of nose and lower eyelid, conjunctiva, lacrimal duct; *modality*, general sensory.

ner'vi intercosta'les, NA alternative for rami ventrales nervorum thoracicorum.

ner'vi intercostobrachia'les [NA], intercostobrachial nerves: *origin*, second and third intercostal nerves; *distribution*, skin on back and medial aspect of arm; *modality*, general sensory.

n. interme'dius [NA], intermediate nerve: the smaller root of the facial nerve, lying between the main root and the vestibulocochlear nerve; it joins the main root at, or merges with the geniculate ganglion at the geniculum of the facial nerve; *branches*, chorda tympani and greater petrosal nerve; *distribution*, lacrimal, nasal, palatine, submandibular, and sublingual glands, and anterior two-thirds of tongue; *modality*, parasympathetic and special sensory.

n. interos'seus [antebra'chii] ante'rior [NA], anterior interosseous nerve of forearm: *origin*, median nerve; *distribution*, flexor pollicis longus, flexor digitorum profundus, and pronator quadratus muscles, wrist and intercarpal joints; *modality*, motor and general sensory.

n. interos'seus antebra'chii poste'rior [NA], posterior interosseous nerve of forearm: *origin*, continuation of deep branch of radial nerve; *distribution*, abductor pollicis longus, extensors of the thumb and second finger, and wrist and intercarpal joints; *modality*, motor and general sensory.

n. interos'seus [antebra'chii] dorsa'lis, n. interosseus antebrachii posterior.

n. interos'seus [antebra'chii] vola'ris, n. interosseus antebrachii anterior.

n. interos'seus cru'ris [NA], interosseous nerve of leg: *origin*, tibial nerve; *distribution*, interosseous membrane and tibiofibular syndesmosis; *modality*, general sensory.

n. ischiad'icus [NA], sciatic nerve, the largest nerve of the body: *origin*, sacral plexus—L4–S3; it leaves the pelvis through the greater sciatic foramen; *branches*, divides into the tibial and common peroneal nerves, usually in lower third of thigh; *distribution*—see individual branches, in this table; *modality*, general sensory and motor.

n. jugula'ris [NA], jugular nerve: a branch of the superior cervical ganglion which communicates with the vagus and glossopharyngeal nerves.

ner'vi labia'les anterio'res [NA], anterior labial nerves: *origin*, ilioinguinal nerve; *distribution*, skin of anterior labial region of labia majora, and adjacent part of thigh; *modality*, general sensory.

ner'vi labia'les posterio'res [NA], posterior labial nerves: *origin*, pudendal nerve; *distribution*, labium majus; *modality*, general sensory.

n. lacrima'lis [NA], lacrimal nerve: *origin*, ophthalmic division of trigeminal nerve, entering the orbit through the superior orbital fissure; *distribution*, lacrimal gland, conjunctiva, lateral commissure of eye, and skin of upper eyelid; *modality*, general sensory.

n. laryn'geus infe'rior [NA], inferior laryngeal nerve: *origin*, recurrent laryngeal nerve, especially the terminal portion of this nerve; *distribution*, intrinsic muscles of larynx, except cricothyroid; communicates with the internal laryngeal nerve; *modality*, motor.

n. laryn'geus recur'rens [NA], recurrent laryngeal nerve: *origin*, vagus nerve (chiefly the cranial part of the accessory nerve); *branches*, inferior laryngeal nerve, tracheal, esophageal, and inferior cardiac rami; *distribution*—see individual branches, in this table and under *ramus; modality*, parasympathetic, visceral afferent, and motor.

n. laryn'geus supe'rior [NA], superior laryngeal nerve: *origin*, inferior ganglion of vagus nerve; *branches*, external, internal, and communicating rami; *distribution*, inferior constrictor of pharynx, cricothyroid muscle, and mucous membrane of back of tongue and larynx—see individual branches, under *ramus; modality*, motor, general sensory, visceral afferent, and parasympathetic.

n. lingua'lis [NA], lingual nerve: *origin*, mandibular nerve, descending to the tongue, first medial to the mandible and then under cover of the mucous membrane of the mouth; *branches*, sublingual nerve, lingual ramus, ramus to the isthmus of the fauces, and rami communicating with the hypoglossal nerve and chorda tympani; *distribution*—see individual branches, in this table and under *ramus; modality*, general sensory.

ner'vi lumba'les [NA], lumbar nerves: the five pairs of nerves that arise from the lumbar segments of the spinal cord, each pair leaving the vertebral column below the correspondingly numbered vertebra. The ventral branches of these nerves participate in the formation of the lumbosacral plexus.

n. lumboinguina'lis, ramus femoralis nervi genitofemoralis.

n. mandibula'ris [NA], mandibular nerve, one of three terminal divisions of the trigeminal nerve, passing through the foramen ovale to the infratemporal fossa. *Origin*, trigeminal ganglion; *branches*, meningeal ramus, masseteric, deep temporal, lateral and medial pterygoid, buccal, auriculotemporal, lingual, and inferior alveolar nerves; *distribution*, extensive distribution to muscles of mastication, skin of face, mucous membrane of mouth, and teeth—see individual branches, in this table and under *ramus; modality*, general sensory and motor.

n. masseter'icus [NA], masseteric nerve: *origin*, mandibular division of trigeminal nerve; *distribution*, masseter muscle and temporomandibular joint; *modality*, motor and general sensory.

n. masticato'rius, former term for radix motoria nervi trigemini.

n. maxilla'ris [NA], maxillary nerve, one of the three terminal divisions of the trigeminal nerve, passing through the foramen rotundum, and entering the pterygopalatine fossa. *Origin*, trigeminal ganglion; *branches*, meningeal ramus, zygomatic nerve, posterior superior alveolar rami, infraorbital nerve, pterygopalatine nerves, and, indirectly, the branches of pterygopalatine ganglion; *distribution*, extensive distribution to skin of face and scalp, mucous membrane of maxillary sinus and nasal cavity, and teeth—see individual branches, in this table and under *ramus; modality*, general sensory.

n. mea'tus acus'tici exter'ni [NA], nerve of external acoustic meatus: *origin*, auriculotemporal nerve; *distribution*, skin lining external acoustic meatus, and tympanic membrane; *modality*, general sensory.

n. mea'tus audito'rii exter'ni, n. meatus acustici externi.

n. media'nus [NA], median nerve: *origin*, lateral and medial cords of brachial plexus—C6–T1; *branches*, anterior interosseous nerve of forearm, common palmar digital nerves, and muscular and palmar rami, and a communicating branch with the ulnar nerve; *distribution*, ultimately, skin on front of lateral part of hand, most of flexor muscles of front of forearm, most of short muscles of thumb, and elbow joint and many joints of hand—see individual branches, in this table and under *ramus; modality*, general sensory.

n. menin'geus [me'dius], ramus meningeus [medius] nervi maxillaris.

n. menta'lis [NA], mental nerve: *origin*, inferior alveolar nerve; *branches*, mental and inferior labial rami; *distribution*, skin of chin, and lower lip; *modality*, general sensory.

n. musculocuta'neus [NA], musculocutaneous nerve: *origin*, lateral cord of brachial plexus—C5–C7; *branches*, lateral cutaneous nerve of forearm, and muscular rami; *distribution*, coracobrachialis, biceps, brachialis muscles, the elbow joint, and skin of radial side of forearm; *modality*, general sensory and motor.

n. mylohyoi'deus [NA], mylohyoid nerve: *origin*, inferior alveolar nerve; *distribution*, mylohyoid muscle, anterior belly of digastric muscle; *modality*, motor.

n. nasocilia'ris [NA], nasociliary nerve: *origin*, ophthalmic division of trigeminal nerve; *branches*, long ciliary, posterior ethmoidal, anterior ethmoidal, and infratrochlear nerves, and a communicating branch to the ciliary ganglion; *distribution*—see individual branches, in this table; *modality*, general sensory.

n. nasopalati'nus [NA], nasopalatine nerve: *origin*, pterygopalatine ganglion; *distribution*, mucosa and glands of most of nasal septum and anterior part of hard palate; *modality*, parasympathetic and general sensory.

n. obturato'rius [NA], obturator nerve: *origin*, lumbar plexus—L3–L4; *branches*, anterior, posterior, and muscular rami; *distribution*, adductor muscles and gracilis muscle, skin of medial part of thigh, and hip and knee joints—see individual branches, under *ramus; modality*, general sensory and motor.

n. occipita'lis ma'jor [NA], greater occipital nerve: *origin*, medial branch of dorsal ramus of C2; *distribution*, semispinalis capitis muscle and skin of scalp as far forward as the vertex; *modality*, general sensory and motor.

n. occipita'lis mi'nor [NA], lesser occipital nerve: *origin*, superficial cervical plexus—C2–C3; *distribution*, ascends behind the auricle and supplies some of the skin on the side of the head and on the cranial surface of the auricle; *modality*, general sensory.

n. occipita'lis ter'tius [NA], third occipital nerve: *origin*, medial branch of dorsal ramus of C3; *distribution*, skin of upper part of back of neck and head; *modality*, general sensory.

n. octa'vus [L. "eighth nerve"], NA alternative for *n. vestibulocochlearis.*

n. oculomoto'rius [NA], oculomotor nerve (3rd cranial): *origin*, brain stem, emerging medial to cerebral peduncles and running forward in the cavernous sinus; *branches*, superior and inferior rami; *distribution*, entering the orbit through the superior orbital fissure, the branches supply the levator palpebrae superioris, all extrinsic eye muscles except the lateral rectus and superior oblique, and carry parasympathetic fibers for the ciliary muscle and sphincter pupillae; *modality*, motor and parasympathetic.

ner'vi olfacto'rii [NA], olfactory nerves (1st cranial): the nerves of smell, consisting of about 20 bundles which arise in the olfactory epithelium and pass through the cribriform plate of the ethmoid bone to the olfactory bulb.

n. ophthal'micus [NA], ophthalmic nerve, one of the three terminal divisions of the trigeminal nerve. *Origin*, trigeminal ganglion; *branches*, tentorial rami, frontal, lacrimal, and nasociliary nerves; *distribution*, eyeball and conjunctiva, lacrimal gland and sac, nasal mucosa and frontal sinus, external nose, upper eyelid, forehead, and scalp—see individual branches, in this table and under *ramus; modality*, general sensory.

n. op'ticus [NA], optic nerve (2nd cranial): the nerve of sight, consisting chiefly of axons and central processes of cells of the ganglionic layer of the retina, which leave the orbit through the optic canal, join the optic chiasm (the medial ones crossing over to opposite side), and continue as the optic tract.

ner'vi palati'ni, see *n. palatinus major* and *nervi palatini minores.*

n. palati'nus ante'rior, n. palatinus major.

n. palati'nus ma'jor [NA], greater palatine nerve: *origin*, pterygopalatine ganglion; *branches*, posterior inferior [lateral] nasal branches; *distribution*, emerges through the greater palatine foramen and supplies the palate; *modality*, parasympathetic, sympathetic, and general sensory.

n. palati'nus me'dius, see *nervi palatini minores*.

ner'vi palati'ni mino'res [NA], lesser palatine nerves: *origin*, pterygopalatine ganglion; *distribution*, emerge through the lesser palatine foramen and supply the soft palate and tonsil; *modality*, parasympathetic, sympathetic, and general sensory.

n. palati'nus poste'rior, see *nervi palatini minores*.

n. pectora'lis latera'lis [NA], lateral pectoral nerve: *origin*, lateral cord of brachial plexus or anterior divisions of upper and middle trunks (C5–C7); *distribution*, usually several nerves supplying the musculus pectoralis minor and acromioclavicular and shoulder joints; *modality*, motor and general sensory.

n. pectora'lis media'lis [NA], medial pectoral nerve: *origin*, medial cord or lower trunk of brachial plexus (C8, T1); *distribution*, usually several nerves supplying the musculus pectoralis major and pectoralis minor; *modality*, motor.

ner'vi perinea'les [NA], perineal nerves: *origin*, pudendal nerve in the pudendal canal; *branches*, muscular branches and posterior scrotal or labial nerves; *distribution*, muscular branches supply the bulbospongiosus, ischiocavernosus, superficial transversus perinei muscles and bulb of the penis and, in part, the sphincter ani externus and levator ani; the scrotal (labial) nerves supply the scrotum or labium majus; *modality*, general sensory and motor.

ner'vi perine'i, nervi perineales.

n. perone'us commu'nis [NA], common peroneal nerve: *origin*, sciatic nerve in lower part of thigh; *branches and distribution*, supplies short head of biceps femoris muscle (while still incorporated in sciatic nerve), gives off lateral sural cutaneous nerve and peroneal communicating branch as it descends in popliteal fossa, supplies knee and superior tibiofibular joints and tibialis anterior muscle, and divides into superficial and deep peroneal nerves; *modality*, general sensory and motor. Called also *n. fibularis communis* [NA alternative] or *common fibular nerve*.

n. perone'us profun'dus [NA], deep peroneal nerve: *origin*, a terminal branch of common peroneal nerve; *branches and distribution*, winds around the neck of the fibula and descends on the interosseous membrane to the front of the ankle; muscular branches are given off to the tibialis anterior, extensor hallucis longus, extensor digitorum longus, and peroneus tertius muscles, and a twig to the ankle joint; a lateral terminal division supplies the extensor digitorum brevis muscle and tarsal joints; the medial terminal division, or digital branch, divides into dorsal digital nerves for the skin and joints of the adjacent sides of the big and second toes; *modality*, general sensory and motor. Called also *n. fibularis profundus* [NA alternative] or *deep fibular nerve*.

n. perone'us profun'dus accesso'rius, the accessory deep peroneal nerve: the branch of the superficial peroneal nerve to the musculus peroneus brevis, often prolonged to the lateral malleolus and ending in twigs to the musculus extensor digitorum brevis and adjacent joints.

n. perone'us superficia'lis [NA], superficial peroneal nerve: *origin*, a terminal branch of common peroneal nerve; *branches and distribution*, descends in front of fibula, supplies peroneus longus and brevis muscles and, in the lower part of the leg, divides into the muscular rami, medial and intermediate dorsal cutaneous nerves— see also individual branches, in this table and under *ramus*; *modality*, general sensory and motor. Called also *n. fibularis superficialis* [NA alternative] or *superficial fibular nerve*.

n. petro'sus ma'jor [NA], greater petrosal nerve: *origin*, intermediate nerve via geniculate ganglion; *distribution*, running forward from the geniculate ganglion, it joins the deep petrosal nerve of the pterygoid canal, and reaches lacrimal, nasal, and palatine glands and nasopharynx, via pterygopalatine ganglion and its branches; *modality*, parasympathetic and general sensory.

n. petro'sus mi'nor [NA], lesser petrosal nerve: *origin*, tympanic plexus; *distribution*, parotid gland via otic ganglion and auriculotemporal nerve; *modality*, parasympathetic.

n. petro'sus profun'dus [NA], deep petrosal nerve: *origin*, internal carotid plexus; *distribution*, joins greater petrosal nerve to form nerve of pterygoid canal, and supplies lacrimal, nasal, and palatine glands via pterygopalatine ganglion and its branches; *modality*, sympathetic.

n. petro'sus superficia'lis ma'jor, n. petrosus major.

n. petro'sus superficia'lis mi'nor, n. petrosus minor.

n. phren'icus [NA], phrenic nerve: *origin*, cervical plexus —C4–C5; *branches*, pericardiac and phrenicoabdominal rami; *distribution*, pleura, pericardium, diaphragm, peritoneum, and sympathetic plexuses; *modality*, general sensory and motor.

ner'vi phren'ici accesso'rii [NA], accessory phrenic nerves: an inconstant contribution of the fifth cervical nerve to the phrenic nerve; when present, they run a separate course to the root of the neck or into the thorax before joining the phrenic nerve.

n. planta'ris latera'lis [NA], lateral plantar nerve: *origin*, the smaller of terminal branches of tibial nerve; *branches*, muscular, superficial, and deep rami; *distribution*, lying between first and second layers of muscles of sole, it supplies the quadratus plantae, abductor digiti minimi, flexor digiti minimi brevis, adductor hallucis, interossei, and second, third, and fourth lumbrical muscles, and gives off cutaneous and articular twigs to lateral side of sole and fourth and fifth toes—see individual branches, under *ramus*; *modality*, general sensory and motor.

n. planta'ris media'lis [NA], medial plantar nerve: *origin*, the larger of the terminal branches of tibial nerve; *branches*, common plantar digital nerves and muscular rami; *distribution*, abductor hallucis, flexor digitorum brevis, flexor hallucis brevis, and first lumbrical muscles, and cutaneous and articular twigs to the medial side of the sole, and to the first to fourth toes—see individual branches, in this table and under *ramus*; *modality*, general sensory and motor.

n. presacra'lis, NA alternative for *plexus hypogastricus superior*.

n. pterygoi'deus exter'nus, n. pterygoideus lateralis.

n. pterygoi'deus inter'nus, n. pterygoideus medialis.

n. pterygoi'deus latera'lis [NA], lateral pterygoid nerve: *origin*, mandibular nerve; *distribution*, lateral pterygoid muscle; *modality*, motor.

n. pterygoi'deus media'lis [NA], medial pterygoid nerve: *origin*, mandibular nerve; *distribution*, medial pterygoid, tensor tympani, and tensor veli palatini muscles; *modality*, motor.

ner'vi pterygopalati'ni [NA], pterygopalatine nerves: the two nerves which connect the maxillary nerve to the pterygopalatine ganglion; they are the sensory roots of the ganglion.

n. puden'dus [NA], pudendal nerve: *origin*, sacral plexus— S2–S4; *branches*, enters the pudendal canal, gives off the inferior rectal nerve, and then divides into the perineal nerve and dorsal nerve of the penis (clitoris); *distribution*, muscles, skin, and erectile tissue of perineum—see individual branches; *modality*, general sensory, motor, and parasympathetic. Called also *pudic nerve*.

n. radia'lis [NA], radial nerve: *origin*, posterior cord of brachial plexus—C6–C8, and sometimes C5 and T1; *branches*, posterior cutaneous and inferior lateral cutaneous nerves of arm, posterior cutaneous nerve of forearm, muscular, deep, and superficial rami; *distribution*, descending in the back of arm and forearm, it is ultimately distributed to skin on back of arm, forearm, and hand, extensor muscles on back of arm and forearm, and elbow joint and many joints of hand—see individual branches, in this table and under *ramus*; *modality*, general sensory and motor.

ner'vi recta'les inferio'res [NA], inferior rectal nerves: *origin*, pudendal nerve, or independently from sacral plexus; *distribution*, sphincter ani externus muscle, skin around anus, and lining of anal canal up to pectinate line; *modality*, general sensory and motor.

n. recur'rens, n. laryngeus recurrens.

n. saccula'ris [NA], saccular nerve: the branch of the pars vestibularis nervi octavi that innervates the macula of the saccule.

ner'vi sacra'les [NA], sacral nerves: the five pairs of nerves that arise from the sacral segments of the spinal cord; the ventral branches of the first four pairs participate in the formation of the sacral plexus.

n. saphe'nus [NA], saphenous nerve: *origin*, termination of femoral nerve, descending first with femoral vessels and then on medial side of leg and foot; *branches*, infrapatellar and medial crural cutaneous rami; *distribution*, knee joint, subsartorial and patellar plexuses, skin on medial side of leg and foot—see individual branches, under *ramus*; *modality*, general sensory.

ner'vi scrota'les anterio'res [NA], anterior scrotal nerves: *origin*, ilioinguinal nerve; *distribution*, skin of anterior scrotal region; *modality*, general sensory.

ner'vi scrota'les posterio'res [NA], posterior scrotal nerves: *origin*, perineal nerves; *distribution*, skin of scrotum; *modality*, general sensory.

n. spermat'icus exter'nus, ramus genitalis nervi genitofemoralis.

ner'vi sphenopalati'ni, nervi pterygopalatini.

ner'vi spina'les [NA], spinal nerves: the thirty-one pairs of nerves that arise from the spinal cord and pass out between the vertebrae, including the eight pairs of cervical, twelve of thoracic, five of lumbar, five of sacral, and one pair of coccygeal nerves.

n. spino'sus, former term for ramus meningeus nervi mandibularis.

n. splanch'nicus i'mus [NA], lowest splanchnic nerve: *origin*, last ganglion of sympathetic trunk or lesser splanchnic nerve; *distribution*, aorticorenal ganglion and adjacent plexus; *modality*, sympathetic and visceral afferent.

ner'vi splanch'nici lumba'les [NA], lumbar splanchnic nerves: *origin*, lumbar ganglia or sympathetic trunk; *distribution*, upper nerves join celiac and adjacent plexuses, middle ones go to intermesenteric and adjacent plexuses, and lower ones descend to superior hypogastric plexus; *modality*, preganglionic sympathetic and visceral afferent.

n. splanch'nicus ma'jor [NA], greater splanchnic nerve: *origin*, thoracic sympathetic trunk and fifth through tenth thoracic ganglia; *distribution*, descending through the diaphragm or its aortic opening, ends in celiac ganglia and plexuses, with a splanchnic ganglion commonly occurring near the diaphragm; *modality*, preganglionic sympathetic and visceral afferent.

n. splanch'nicus mi'nor [NA], lesser splanchnic nerve: *origin*, ninth and tenth thoracic ganglia of sympathetic trunk; *branches*, renal ramus; *distribution*, pierces the diaphragm, joins the aorticorenal ganglion and celiac plexus, and communicates with the renal and superior mesenteric plexuses; *modality*, preganglionic sympathetic and visceral afferent.

ner'vi splanch'nici pelvi'ni [NA], pelvic splanchnic nerves: *origin*, sacral plexus—S3–S4; *distribution*, leaving the sacral plexus, they enter the inferior hypogastric plexus and supply the pelvic organs; *modality*, preganglionic parasympathetic and visceral afferent. Called also *nervi erigentes* [NA alternative].

ner'vi splanch'nici sacra'les [NA], sacral splanchnic nerves: *origin*, sacral part of sympathetic trunk; *distribution*, pelvic organs and blood vessels via inferior hypogastric plexus; *modality*, preganglionic sympathetic and visceral afferent.

n. stape'dius [NA], stapedius nerve: *origin*, facial nerve; *distribution*, stapedius muscle; *modality*, motor.

n. subcla'vius [NA], subclavian nerve: *origin*, upper trunk of brachial plexus—C5; *distribution*, subclavius muscle and sternoclavicular joint; *modality*, motor and general sensory.

n. subcosta'lis [NA], subcostal nerve: *origin*, ventral ramus of twelfth thoracic nerve; *distribution*, skin of lower abdomen and lateral side of gluteal region, parts of transversus, oblique, and rectus muscles, and usually the pyramidalis muscle, and adjacent peritoneum; *modality*, general sensory and motor.

n. sublingua'lis [NA], sublingual nerve: *origin*, lingual nerve; *distribution*, sublingual gland and overlying mucous membrane; *modality*, parasympathetic and general sensory.

n. suboccipita'lis [NA], suboccipital nerve: *origin*, dorsal ramus of first cervical nerve; *distribution*, emerges above posterior arch of atlas and supplies muscles of suboccipital triangle and semispinalis capitis muscle; *modality*, motor.

n. subscapula'ris [NA], subscapular nerve: *origin*, posterior cord of brachial plexus—C5; *distribution*, usually two or more nerves, upper and lower, supplying subscapularis and teres major muscles; *modality*, motor.

ner'vi supraclavicula'res [NA], supraclavicular nerves: a term denoting collectively the common trunk, which is a branch of the cervical plexus (C3–C4) and which emerges under cover of the posterior border of the sternocleidomastoid muscle and divides into the nervi supraclaviculares intermedii, nervi supraclaviculares laterales, and nervi supraclaviculares mediales.

ner'vi supraclavicula'res anterio'res, nervi supraclaviculares mediales.

ner'vi supraclavicula'res interme'dii [NA], intermediate supraclavicular nerves: *origin*, cervical plexus—C3–C4; *distribution*, descends in the posterior triangle, crosses the clavicle, and supplies the skin over pectoral and deltoid region; *modality*, general sensory.

ner'vi supraclavicula'res latera'les [posterio'res] [NA], lateral supraclavicular nerves: *origin*, cervical plexus—C3–C4; *distribution*, descends in the posterior triangle, crosses the clavicle, and supplies the skin of superior and posterior parts of shoulder; *modality*, general sensory. Called also *nervi supraclaviculares posteriores* [NA alternative].

ner'vi supraclavicula'res media'les [NA], medial supraclavicular nerves: *origin*, cervical plexus—C3–C4; *distribution*, descends in posterior triangle, crosses the clavicle, and supplies the skin of medial infraclavicular region; *modality*, general sensory.

ner'vi supraclavicula'res me'dii, nervi supraclaviculares intermedii.

ner'vi supraclavicula'res posterio'res, NA alternative for *nervi supraclaviculares laterales*.

n. supraorbita'lis [NA], supraorbital nerve: *origin*, continuation of frontal nerve, from ophthalmic nerve; *branches*, lateral and medial rami; *distribution*, leaves orbit through supraorbital notch or foramen, and supplies the skin of upper eyelid, forehead, anterior scalp (to vertex), mucosa of frontal sinus; *modality*, general sensory.

n. suprascapula'ris [NA], suprascapular nerve: *origin*, brachial plexus—C5–C6; *distribution*, descends through suprascapular and spinoglenoid notches and supplies acromioclavicular and shoulder joints, and supraspinatus and infraspinatus muscles; *modality*, motor and general sensory.

n. supratrochlea'ris [NA], supratrochlear nerve: *origin*, frontal nerve, from ophthalmic nerve; *distribution*, leaves orbit at medial end of supraorbital margin and supplies the forehead and upper eyelid; *modality*, general sensory.

n. sura'lis [NA], sural nerve: *origin*, medial sural cutaneous nerve and peroneal communicating branch of common peroneal nerve; *branches*, lateral dorsal cutaneous nerve and lateral calcaneal rami; *distribution*, skin on back of leg, and skin and joints on lateral side of heel and foot—see individual branches, in this table and under *ramus; modality*, general sensory.

ner'vi tempora'les profun'di [NA], deep temporal nerves, usually two in number, anterior and posterior: *origin*, mandibular nerve; *distribution*, temporal muscles; *modality*, motor.

n. tempora'lis profun'dus ante'rior, the anterior of the two deep temporal nerves.

n. tempora'lis profun'dus poste'rior, the posterior of the two temporal nerves.

n. tenso'ris tym'pani [NA], nerve of tensor tympani: *origin*, mandibular nerve via nerve to medial pterygoid muscle and otic ganglion; *distribution*, tensor tympani muscle; *modality*, motor.

n. tenso'ris ve'li palati'ni [NA], nerve of tensor veli palatini: *origin*, mandibular nerve via nerve to medial pterygoid muscle and otic ganglion; *distribution*, tensor veli palatini muscle; *modality*, motor.

n. tento'rii, ramus tentorii nervi ophthalmici.

ner'vi termina'les [NA], terminal nerves: nerve filaments, collectively termed the nervus terminalis, found in the pia mater between the olfactory bulb and the crista galli, and passing through the cribriform plate to the nasal mucosa; ganglion cells occur along their course.

ner'vi thoraca'les, nervi thoracici.

ner'vi thoraca'les anterio'res, former term for the medial and lateral pectoral nerves.

ner'vi thoraca'les posterio'res, former term for dorsal scapular and long thoracic nerves collectively.

n. thoraca'lis lon'gus, n. thoracicus longus.

ner'vi thora'cici [NA], thoracic nerves: the twelve pairs of spinal nerves that arise from the thoracic segments of the spinal cord, each pair leaving the vertebral column below the correspondingly numbered vertebra. They innervate the body wall of the thorax and upper abdomen.

n. thora'cicus lon'gus [NA], long thoracic nerve: *origin*, brachial plexus—ventral rami of C5–C7; *distribution*, descends behind brachial plexus to serratus anterior muscle; *modality*, motor.

n. thoracodorsa'lis [NA], thoracodorsal nerve: *origin*, posterior cord of brachial plexus—C7–C8; *distribution*, latissimus dorsi muscle; *modality*, motor.

n. tibia'lis [NA], tibial nerve: *origin*, sciatic nerve in lower part of thigh; *branches*, interosseous nerve of leg, medial cutaneous nerve of calf, sural, and medial and lateral plantar nerves, and muscular and medial calcaneal rami; *distribution*, while still incorporated in the sciatic nerve, it supplies the semimembranosus and semitendinosus muscles, long head of biceps, and adductor magnus muscle; it supplies the knee joint as it descends in the popliteal fossa and, continuing into the leg, supplies the muscles and skin of the calf and sole of the foot, and the toes—see individual branches, in this table and under *ramus; modality*, general sensory and motor.

n. transver'sus col'li [NA], transverse nerve of neck: *origin*, cervical plexus—C2–C3; *branches*, superior and inferior rami; *distribution*, skin on side and front of neck; *modality*, general sensory.

n. trigem'inus [NA], trigeminal nerve (5th cranial), which emerges from the lateral surface of the pons as a motor and a sensory root, together with some intermediate fibers. The sensory root expands into the trigeminal ganglion, which contains the cells of origin of most of the sensory fibers, and from which the three divisions of the nerve arise. See *n. mandibularis, n. maxillaris,* and *n. ophthalmicus.* The trigeminal nerve is sensory in supplying the face, teeth, mouth, and nasal cavity, and motor in supplying the muscles of mastication.

n. trochlea'ris [NA], trochlear nerve (4th cranial): *origin*, the fibers of each trochlear nerve (one on either side) decussate across the median plane and emerge from the back of the brain stem below the corresponding inferior colliculus; *distribution*, runs forward in lateral wall of cavernous sinus, traverses the superior orbital fissure, and supplies superior oblique muscle of eyeball; *modality*, motor.

n. tympan'icus [NA], tympanic nerve: *origin*, inferior ganglion of glossopharyngeal nerve; *branches*, helps form tympanic plexus; *distribution*, mucous membrane of tympanic cavity, mastoid air cells, auditory tube, and, via lesser petrosal nerve and otic ganglion, the parotid gland; *modality*, general sensory and parasympathetic.

n. ulna'ris [NA], ulnar nerve: *origin*, medial and lateral cords of brachial plexus—C7–T1; *branches*, muscular, dorsal, palmar, superficial, and deep rami; *distribution*, ultimately to skin on front and back of medial part of hand, some flexor muscles on front of forearm, many short muscles of hand, elbow joint, many joints of hand—see individual branches, under *ramus; modality*, general sensory and motor.

n. utricula'ris [NA], utricular nerve: the branch of the pars vestibularis nervi octavi that innervates the macula of the utricle.

n. utriculoampulla'ris [NA], utriculoampullar nerve: a nerve that arises by peripheral division of the vestibular part of the eighth cranial nerve, and supplies the utricle and ampullae of the semicircular ducts.

ner'vi vagina'les [NA], vaginal nerves: *origin*, uterovaginal plexus; *distribution*, vagina; *modality*, sympathetic and parasympathetic.

n. va'gus [NA], vagus nerve (10th cranial): *origin*, by numerous rootlets from lateral side of medulla oblongata in the groove between the olive and the inferior cerebellar peduncle; *branches*, superior and recurrent laryngeal nerves, meningeal, auricular, pharyngeal, cardiac, bronchial, gastric, hepatic, celiac, and renal rami, pharyngeal, pulmonary, and esophageal plexuses, and anterior and posterior trunks; *distribution*, descending through the jugular foramen, it presents a superior and an inferior ganglion, and continues through the neck and thorax into the abdomen. It supplies sensory fibers to the ear, tongue, pharynx, and larynx, motor fibers to the pharynx, larynx, and esophagus, and parasympathetic and visceral afferent fibers to thoracic and abdominal viscera—see individual branches, in this table and under *ramus; modality*, parasympathetic, visceral afferent, motor, general sensory.

n. vascula'ris [NA], vascular nerve: a nerve branch that supplies the adventitia of a blood vessel.

n. vertebra'lis [NA], vertebral nerve: *origin*, cervicothoracic and vertebral ganglia; *distribution*, ascends with vertebral artery and gives fibers to spinal meninges, cervical nerves, and posterior cranial fossa; *modality*, sympathetic.

ner'vi vesica'les inferio'res plex'us puden'di, former term for a few small nerves to the bladder, thought to arise from the pudendal plexus (pudendal nerve).

ner'vi vesica'les inferio'res plex'us vesica'lis, former term for the nerves reaching the vesical plexus by way of the inferior vesical artery.

ner′vi vesica′les superio′res plex′us vesica′lis, former term for the nerves reaching the vesical plexus by way of the superior vesical artery.

n. vestib′uli, pars vestibularis nervi octavi.

n. vestibulocochlea′ris [NA], vestibulocochlear nerve (8th cranial), which emerges from the brain between the pons and the medulla oblongata, at the cerebellopontine angle and behind the facial nerve. It consists of two sets of fibers, the pars vestibularis

nervi octavi from the utricle, saccule, and semicircular ducts, and the pars cochlearis nervi octavi from the cochlea, and is connected with the brain by corresponding roots, the radix superior and the radix inferior nervi vestibulocochlearis. Called also *n. acusticus, n. octavus* [NA alternative], and *acoustic nerve.*

n. zygomat′icus [NA], zygomatic nerve: *origin,* maxillary nerve, entering the orbit through the inferior orbital fissure; *branches,* zygomaticofacial and zygomaticotemporal rami; *distribution,* communicates with the lacrimal nerve and supplies the skin of the temple and adjacent part of the face—see individual branches, under *ramus; modality,* general sensory.

Nesacaine (nes′ah-kān)   trademark for preparations of chloroprocaine hydrochloride.

nesidiectomy (ne-sid″e-ek′to-me) [Gr. *nēsidion* islet + *ektomē* excision]   excision of the islands of Langerhans of the pancreas.

nesidioblast (ne-sid′e-o-blast″) [Gr. *nēsidion* islet + *blastos* germ]   any one of the cells that build up the islet cells of the pancreas.

nesidioblastoma (ne-sid″e-o-blas-to′mah)   an islet-cell tumor of the pancreas.

nesidioblastosis (ne-sid″e-o-blas-to′sis)   diffuse proliferation of the islet cells of the pancreas.

Nessler's reagent (solution, test) (nes′lerz) [A. *Nessler,* German chemist, 1827–1905]   see under *reagent.*

nesslerization (nes″ler-i-za′shun)   treatment with Nessler's reagent.

nesslerize (nes′ler-īz)   to treat with Nessler's reagent.

nest (nest)   a small mass of cells foreign to the area in which it is found.   **birds′ n′s,** endocardial pockets.   **Brunn′s epithelial n′s,** solid or branched clusters of cells occurring in the healthy ureter.   **cancer n′s,** masses of concentrically arranged cells seen in cancerous growths.   **cell n.,** a mass of closely packed epithelial cells surrounded by a stroma of connective tissue.   **swallow′s n.,** nidus avis.

nesteostomy (nes″te-os′to-me) [*nestis* + Gr. *stomoun* to provide with an opening, or mouth]   creation of a permanent opening into the jejunum through the abdominal wall; also, the opening so established.

nestiatria (nes″te-a′tre-ah)   hunger cure.

nestitherapy (nes″tĭ-ther′ah-pe)   nestotherapy.

nestotherapy (nes″to-ther′ah-pe) [Gr. *nēstis* fasting + *therapy*]   hunger cure; the therapeutic use of fasting or of a restricted diet.

net (net)   a meshlike structure of interlocking fibers or strands; see also under *network.*   **achromatic n.,** the network within the cell which does not stain with dyes.   **chromidial n.,** a network of chromatin staining material in the cytoplasm of certain cells; it has the properties of active nuclear material.   **nerve n.,** a nonsynaptic protoplasmic network of nerve fibers; a form of free nerve fiber ending characteristic of connective tissue, consisting of a network of thin threads.   **Trolard′s n.,** plexus venosus canalis hypoglossi.

nethalide (neth′ah-līd)   pronethalol.

netilmicin sulfate (net″il-mi′sin)   chemical name: (2*S-cis*)-4-*O*-[3-amino-6-(aminomethyl)-3,4-dihydro-2*H*-pyran-2-yl]-2-deoxy-6-*O*-[3-deoxy-4-*C*-methyl-3-(methylamino)-β-*L*-arabinopyranosyl]-*N*′-ethyl-*d*-streptamine, sulfate (2:5) salt; an antibacterial, $(C_{21}H_{41}N_5O_7)_2 \cdot 5H_2SO_4$.

nettle (net′l)   any plant of the genus *Urtica,* having leaves covered with stinging hairs that secrete a poisonous and irritating fluid.

network (net′werk)   a meshlike structure of interlocking fibers or strands; see also under *net.*   **cell n.,** mitome.   **Chiari′s n.,** a network of fine fibers which sometimes extend across the interior of the right atrium of the heart from the thebesian and eustachian valves to the crista terminalis.   **Gerlach′s n.,** an apparent (but not real) interlacement of the dendritic processes of the ganglion cells of the spinal cord.   **n. of Gesvelst,** a reticular appearance sometimes seen on the myelin sheath of a neuron, perhaps artificial.   **neurofibrillar n.,** the network formed by the neurofibrils of a nerve cell.   **peritarsal n.,** a set of lymphatics in the eyelid.   **Purkinje′s n.,** a reticulation of immature muscle fibers in the subendocardial tissue of the ventricles of the heart.   **subpapillary n.,** rete subpapillare.   **venous n.,** rete venosum.

neu (nu)   neurilemma.

Neubauer's artery (noi′bow-erz) [Johann Ernst *Neubauer,* German anatomist, 1742–1777]   arteria thyroidea.

Neubauer-Fischer test (noi′bow-er-fish′er) [Otto *Neubauer,* Munich physician, born 1874]   see *glycyltryptophan test,* under *tests.*

Neuber's treatment, tubes (noi′berz) [Gustav Adolf *Neuber,* German surgeon, 1850–1932]   see under *treatment* and *tube.*

Neufeld nail (nu′feld) [Alonzo John *Neufeld,* American orthopedic surgeon, born 1906]   see under *nail.*

Neufeld's phenomenon, reaction (test) (noi′felts) [Fred *Neu-*

feld, German bacteriologist, 1861–1945]   see under *phenomenon* and *reaction.*

Neumann's cells, sheath (noi′manz) [Ernst *Neumann,* German pathologist, 1834–1918]   see under *cell,* and see *dental sheath,* under *sheath.*

Neumann's law [Franz Ernst *Neumann,* German physicist, 1798–1895]   see under *law.*

Neumann's method [Heinrich *Neumann,* otologist in Vienna, 1873–1939]   see under *method.*

neur-   see *neuro-.*

neurad (nu′rad)   toward a neural axis or aspect.

neuradynamia (nu″rah-di-na′me-ah) [*neur-* + *a* neg. + Gr. *dynamis* power]   neurasthenia.

neuragmia (nu-rag′me-ah) [*neur-* + Gr. *agmos* break]   the tearing of a nerve trunk.

neural (nu′ral) [L. *neuralis;* Gr. *neuron* nerve]   1. pertaining to a nerve or to the nerves.   2. situated in the region of the spinal axis, as the neural arch; cf. *hemal.*

neuralgia (nu-ral′je-ah) [*neur-* + *-algia*]   paroxysmal pain which extends along the course of one or more nerves. Many varieties of neuralgia are distinguished according to the part affected or to the cause, as brachial, facial, occipital, supraorbital, etc., or anemic, diabetic, gouty, malarial, syphilitic, etc.   **cardiac n.** (*obs.*), angina pectoris.   **cervicobrachial n.,** pain in the neck radiating to the arm, due to compression of nerve roots of the cervical spinal cord.   **cervico-occipital n.,** neuralgia in the upper cervical nerves, especially the posterior division of the second cervical nerve.   **cranial n.,** neuralgia along the course of a cranial nerve.   **n. facia′lis ve′ra,** geniculate n.   **Fothergill′s n.,** trigeminal n.   **geniculate n.,** Ramsay Hunt syndrome, def. 1.   **glossopharyngeal n.,** neuralgia affecting the petrosal and jugular ganglia of the glossopharyngeal nerve, marked by severe paroxysmal pain originating on the side of the throat and extending to the ear. Occasionally attacks are associated with cardiac slowing or arrest, and syncope.   **hallucinatory n.,** a mental impression of pain without any actual peripheral stimulus.   **Harris′ migrainous n.,** migrainous neuralgia.   **Hunt′s n.,** Ramsay Hunt syndrome, def. 1.   **idiopathic n.,** neuralgia of unknown etiology, unaccompanied by any structural change.   **intercostal n.,** neuralgia of the intercostal nerves.   **mammary n.,** neuralgic pain in the breast.   **mandibular joint n.,** vertex and occipital pain, otalgia, glossodynia, and pain about the nose and eyes, associated with disturbed function of the temporomandibular joint.   **migrainous n.,** a migraine variant characterized by attacks of unilateral excruciating pain over the eye and forehead, with temperature elevation, lacrimation, and rhinorrhea; attacks last 15 to 30 minutes and tend to occur in clusters. Because attacks identical to the spontaneous attacks may be induced in sufferers by subcutaneous injection of histamine diphosphate, it is also known as *histamine cephalalgia* or *headache.* Called also *cluster headache,* and *Horton′s headache* or *syndrome.*   **Morton′s n.,** see under *toe.*   **nasociliary n.,** pain in the eyes, brow, and root of the nose.   **otic n.,** geniculate n.   **peripheral n.,** pain along the course of a peripheral sensory nerve.   **postherpetic n.,** persistent burning pain and hyperesthesia along the distribution of a cutaneous nerve following an attack of herpes zoster; it may last for a few weeks or many months.   **red n.,** erythromelalgia.   **reminiscent n.,** a mental impression of neuralgic pain persisting after the actual pain has ceased.   **sciatic n.,** sciatica.   **Sluder′s n.,** neuralgia of the sphenopalatine ganglion, causing a burning and boring pain in the area of the superior maxilla and a radiation of the pain into the neck and shoulder. Called also *sphenopalatine n.*   **sphenopalatine n.,** Sluder′s n.   **stump n.,** neuralgia at the site of an amputation.   **supraorbital n.,** neuralgia of the supraorbital nerve.   **trifacial n.,** trigeminal n.   **trigeminal n.,** excruciating episodic pain in the area supplied by the trigeminal nerve, often precipitated by stimulation of well-defined trigger points. Called also *Fothergill′s n., trifocal n.,* and *tic douloureux.*   **vidian n.,** neuralgia affecting the vidian nerve (nervus canalis pterygoidei).   **visceral n.,** neurasthenic pain in the pelvic region.

neuralgic (nu-ral′jik)   pertaining to or of the nature of neuralgia.

neuralgiform (nu-ral′jĭ-form)   resembling neuralgia.

neuraminidase (nūr-ah-min′ĭ-dās)   an enzyme contained in the surface coat of myxoviruses that destroys the neuraminic acid of the cell surface during attachment, thereby preventing hemagglutination.

neuranagenesis (nu″ran-ah-jen′ĕ-sis) [*neur-* + Gr. *anagennan* to regenerate] regeneration or renewal of nerve tissue.

neurangiosis (nu″ran-je-o′sis) [*neur-* + Gr. *angeion* vessel] (*obs.*) a disorder of the nerves supplying blood vessels.

neurapophysis (nu″rah-pof′ĭ-sis) [*neur-* + *apophysis*] the structure forming either side of the neural arch; also the part supposedly homologous with this structure in a so-called cranial vertebra.

neurapraxia (nu″rah-prak′se-ah) [*neur-* + Gr. *apraxia* absence of action] failure of conduction in a nerve in the absence of structural changes, due to blunt injury, compression, or ischemia; return of function normally ensues. Called also *axonapraxia*. Cf. *axonotmesis* and *neurotmesis*.

neurarchy (nu′rar-ke) [*neur-* + Gr. *archē* rule] the control of the cerebrospinal system over the body.

neurarthropathy (nu″rar-throp′ah-the) neuroarthropathy.

neurasthenia (nu″ras-the′ne-ah) [*neur-* + Gr. *astheneia* debility] neurasthenic neurosis. **acoustic n.,** neurasthenia marked by hearing loss of varying degrees. **angioparalytic n., angiopathic n.,** a condition in neurasthenic patients in which there is a constant sense of the pulse beat. **cardiac n., cardiovascular n.,** neurocirculatory asthenia. **gastric n.,** a form characterized by functional stomach complications. **n. gra′vis,** a severe form of neurasthenia with great exhaustion on the slightest exertion. **grippal n.,** neurasthenia occurring as a sequel of influenza. **obsessive n.,** psychasthenia. **prostatic n.,** a neurasthenic condition due to prostatic hyperemia and hyperesthesia. **pulsating n.,** angioparalytic n. **sexual n.,** a variety associated with disorders of the sexual function. **traumatic n.,** neurasthenia following shock or injury.

neurastheniac (nu″ras-the′ne-ak) a person suffering from neurasthenic neurosis.

neurasthenic (nu″ras-then′ik) pertaining to or affected with neurasthenic neurosis.

neuratrophia (nu″rah-tro′fe-ah) [*neur-* + Gr. *atrophia* atrophy] impaired nutrition of the nervous system.

neuratrophic (nu″rah-trof′ik) 1. characterized by atrophy of the nerves. 2. a person affected with atrophy of the nerves.

neuratrophy (nu-rat′ro-fe) neuratrophia.

neuraxial (nu-rak′se-al) pertaining to the neuraxis.

neuraxis (nu-rak′sis) [*neur-* + *axis*] 1. an axon. 2. the central nervous system.

neuraxon (nu-rak′son) [*neur-* + Gr. *axōn* axis] an axon.

neure (nūr) neuron, def. 1.

neurectasia (nu″rek-ta′ze-ah) [*neur-* + Gr. *ektasis* stretching] neurotony.

neurectomy (nu-rek′to-me) [*neur-* + Gr. *ektomē* excision] the excision of a part of a nerve. **gastric n.,** surgical vagotomy. **opticociliary n.,** excision of the optic and ciliary nerves.

neurectopia (nu″rek-to′pe-ah) [*neur-* + Gr. *ektopos* out of place + *-ia*] displacement of a nerve or abnormal situation of a nerve.

neurectopy (nu-rek′to-pe) neurectopia.

neurenteric (nu″ren-ter′ik) [*neur-* + Gr. *enteron* intestine] pertaining to the neural tube and archenteron of the embryo, applied especially to the canal interconnecting them.

neurepithelial (nūr″ep-ĭ-the′le-al) neuroepithelial.

neurepithelium (nūr″ep-ĭ-the′le-um) neuroepithelium.

neurergic (nu-rer′jik) [*neur-* + Gr. *ergon* work] pertaining to or dependent on nerve action.

neurexeresis (nūr″ek-ser′ĕ-sis) [*neur-* + Gr. *exairein* to extract] operation of tearing out (avulsion) of a nerve.

neurhypnology (nūr″hip-nol′o-je) neurohypnology.

neuriatry (nu-ri′ah-tre) [*neur-* + Gr. *iatreia* medication] the treatment of nervous diseases.

neuridine (nu′rĭ-dēn) a base isolated from fresh human brain, identical with spermine.

neurilemma (nu″rĭ-lem′mah) [*neur-* + Gr. *lemma* rind, husk, a covering or wrapper] the thin membrane spirally enwrapping the myelin layers of certain, especially peripheral, myelinated nerve fibers or the axons of certain unmyelinated nerve fibers. Called also *neurolemma, Schwann's membrane, sheath of Schwann,* and *endoneural membrane.*

neurilemmal (nu″rĭ-lem′al) pertaining to a neurilemma.

neurilemmitis (nu″rĭ-lem-mi′tis) inflammation of the neurilemma.

neurilemmoma (nu″rĭ-lem-mo′mah) neurilemoma.

neurilemoma (nu″rĭ-lĕ-mo′mah) [*neur-* + Gr. *eilēma* a closely adhering sheath + *-oma*] a tumor of a peripheral nerve sheath (neurilemma). **acoustic n.,** acoustic neuroma.

neurility (nu-ril′ĭ-te) the sum of the attributes and functions of nerve tissue.

neurimotility (nu″rĭ-mo-til′ĭ-te) nervimotility.

neurimotor (nu″rĭ-mo′tor) nervimotor.

neurine (nu′rin) a poisonous ptomaine, vinyl trimethyl ammonium hydroxide, $CH_2{:}CHN(CH_3)_3OH$, found in decaying fish, fungi, and in the brain and in many other normal tissues.

neurinoma (nu″rĭ-no′mah) [*neur-* + Gr. *is* fiber + *-oma*] schwannoma. **acoustic n.,** acoustic neuroma.

neurite (nu′rīt) an axon.

neuritic (nu-rit′ik) pertaining to or affected with neuritis.

neuritis (nu-ri′tis) [*neur-* + *-itis*] inflammation of a nerve, a condition attended by pain and tenderness over the nerves, anesthesia and paresthesias, paralysis, wasting, and disappearance of the reflexes. In practice, the term is also used to denote noninflammatory lesions of the peripheral nervous system; see *neuropathy.* **adventitial n.,** that which affects the sheath of a nerve. **alcoholic n.,** see under *neuropathy.* **ascending n.,** see under *neuropathy.* **brachial n.,** neuralgic amyotrophy. **central n.,** parenchymatous n. **descending n.,** see under *neuropathy.* **dietetic n.,** beriberi. **disseminated n.,** polyneuritis. **endemic n.,** beriberi. **fallopian n.,** neuritis of the facial nerve in the fallopian canal. **Gombault's n.,** progressive hypertrophic interstitial neuropathy. **interstitial n.,** inflammation of the connective tissue of a nerve trunk. **interstitial hypertrophic n.,** progressive hypertrophic interstitial neuropathy. **intraocular n.,** neuritis of the retinal part of the optic nerve. **jake n.,** Jamaica ginger paralysis. **latent n.,** degeneration of the fibers of a nerve without corresponding clinical phenomena. **lead n.,** n. saturnina. **leprous n.,** a form associated with true leprosy. **malarial n.,** a form associated with malaria. **malarial multiple n.,** inflammation involving many nerves, and associated with malaria. **n. mi′grans, migrating n.,** neuritis affecting first one nerve and then another. **multiple n.,** polyneuritis. **n. mul′tiplex endem′ica,** beriberi. **n. nodo′sa,** a form characterized by the formation of nodes on the nerves. **optic n.,** inflammation of the optic nerve; it may affect the part of the nerve within the eyeball (*neuropapillitis*) or the portion behind the eyeball (*retrobulbar n.*). **orbital optic n.,** retrobulbar n. **parenchymatous n.,** neuritis affecting principally the axons and myelin of the peripheral nerves; called also *central n.* **periaxial n.,** segmental (demyelination) neuropathy. **peripheral n.,** inflammation of the nerve endings or of terminal nerves. **porphyric n.,** neuritis occurring as a manifestation of acute intermittent porphyria. **postfebrile n.,** that which mostly follows an attack of severe exanthematous disease. **postocular n.,** retrobulbar n. **pressure n.,** a form due to compression of the nerve. **n. puerpera′lis traumat′ica,** neuritis occurring in parturient women as a result of injury at childbirth. **radiation n.,** radioneuritis. **radicular n.,** neuritis involving the spinal roots of the nerves; radiculitis. **retrobulbar n.,** inflammation in that portion of the optic nerve which is posterior to the eyeball. **rheumatic n.,** a form associated with rheumatic symptoms. **n. saturni′na,** neuritis due to plumbism. **sciatic n.,** sciatica. **segmental n.,** segmental (demyelination) neuropathy. **senile n.,** a form occurring in aged persons, and affecting chiefly the nerves of the extremities. **serum n.,** see under *neuropathy.* **shoulder-girdle n.,** neuralgic amyotrophy. **syphilitic n.,** neuritis due to syphilis. **tabetic n.,** neuritis associated with tabes dorsalis. **toxic n.,** that which is due to some poison. **traumatic n.,** that which follows and is caused by an injury.

neuro-, neur- (nu′ro, nūr) [Gr. *neuron* nerve] combining form denoting relationship to a nerve or nerves, or to the nervous system.

neuroallergy (nu″ro-al′er-je) allergy in nervous tissue.

neuroamebiasis (nu″ro-am″e-bi′ah-sis) neuritis due to amebiasis.

neuroanastomosis (nu″ro-ah-nas″to-mo′sis) the operation of forming an anastomosis of nerves.

neuroanatomy (nu″ro-ah-nat′o-me) [*neuro-* + *anatomy*] that branch of neurology which is concerned with the anatomy of the nervous system.

neuroarthropathy (nu″ro-ar-throp′ah-the) [*neuro-* + Gr. *arthron* joint + *pathos* disease] any disease of joint structures associated with disease of the central or peripheral nervous system.

neuroastrocytoma (nu″ro-as″tro-si-to′mah) [*neuro-* + *astrocytoma*] a glioma composed mainly of astrocytes, closely resembling an astrocytoma and most commonly found in the floor of the third ventricle and the temporal lobes, although it may arise in almost any part of the central nervous system.

neurobehavioral (nu″ro-be-hāv′u-ral) relating to neurologic status as assessed by observation of behavior.

neurobiologist (nu″ro-bi-ol′o-jist) a specialist in neurobiology.

neurobiology (nu″ro-bi-ol′o-je) the biology of the nervous system.

neurobiotaxis (nu″ro-bi″o-tak′sis) [*neuro-* + *biotaxis*] the theory that nerve cell bodies have a tendency during development to migrate in the direction from which they habitually receive their stimuli.

neuroblast (nu′ro-blast) [*neuro-* + Gr. *blastos* germ] any embryonic cell which develops into a nerve cell or neuron; an immature nerve cell.

neuroblastoma (nu″ro-blas-to′mah) sarcoma of nervous system origin, composed chiefly of neuroblasts and affecting mostly infants and children up to 10 years of age. Most of such tumors arise in the autonomic nervous system (sympathicoblastoma) or in the adrenal medulla. When there is metastasis from the adrenal medulla to the cranium or to the liver, it is known as *Hutchinson's type* or *Pepper's syndrome*, respectively.

neurocanal (nu″ro-kah-nal′) [*neuro-* + *canal*] the vertebral canal (canalis vertebralis).

neurocardiac (nu″ro-kar′de-ak) [*neuro-* + Gr. *kardia* heart] pertaining to the nervous system and the heart.

neurocentral (nu″ro-sen′tral) pertaining to the centrum and the two lateral masses of a developing vertebra.

neurocentrum (nu″ro-sen′trum) one of the embryonic vertebral elements from which the spinous processes of the vertebrae develop.

neuroceptor (nu′ro-sep″tor) [*neuro-* + L. *capere* to take] one of the terminal elements of a dendrite which receives the stimulus from the neuromittor of the adjoining neuron; called also *ceptor*.

neuroceratin (nu″ro-ser′ah-tin) neurokeratin.

neurochemistry (nu″ro-kem′is-tre) that branch of neurology which is concerned with the chemistry of the nervous system.

neurochitin (nu″ro-ki′tin) [*neuro-* + Gr. *chitōn* frock, skin, membrane] the substance that forms the framework support of nerve fibers.

neurochondrite (nu″ro-kon′drīt) [*neuro-* + Gr. *chondros* cartilage] one of the embryonic cartilaginous elements which develop into the neural arch of a vertebra.

neurochorioretinitis (nu″ro-ko″re-o-ret″ĭ-ni′tis) [*neuro-* + *chorioretinitis*] inflammation of the optic nerve, choroid, and retina.

neurochoroiditis (nu″ro-ko″roi-di′tis) inflammation of the choroid coat and optic nerves.

neurocirculatory (nu″ro-cir′cu-lah-to″re) pertaining to the nervous and circulatory systems, as neurocirculatory asthenia.

neurocladism (nu-rok′lah-dizm) [*neuro-* + Gr. *klados* branch] the formation of new branches by the process of a neuron; especially the force by which, in regeneration of divided nerves, the newly formed axons of the proximal stump become attracted by the peripheral stump so as to form a bridge between the two ends. Called also *odogenesis*.

neuroclonic (nu″ro-klon′ik) [*neuro-* + Gr. *klonos* spasm] characterized by nervous spasms.

neurocommunications (nu″ro-kŏ-mu″nĭ-ka′shunz) the branch of neurology dealing with the transfer and integration of information within the nervous system.

neurocranial (nu″ro-kra′ne-al) pertaining to the neurocranium.

neurocranium (nu″ro-kra′ne-um) the portion of the cranium which encloses the brain.

neurocrine (nu′ro-krin) [*neuro-* + Gr. *krinein* to secrete] 1. denoting an endocrine influence on or by the nerves. 2. pertaining to neurosecretion.

neurocrinia (nu″ro-krin′e-ah) endocrine influence on the nerves.

neurocristopathy (nu″ro-kris-top′ah-the) [*neuro-* + L. *crista* crest + *-pathy*] any disease arising from maldevelopment of the neural crest.

neurocutaneous (nu″ro-ku-ta′ne-us) pertaining to the nerves and the skin; pertaining to the cutaneous nerves.

neurocyte (nu′ro-sīt) [*neuro-* + *-cyte*] a nerve cell of any kind; a neuron.

neurocytology (nu″ro-si-tol′o-je) that branch of neurology which is concerned with the cellular components of the nervous system.

neurocytolysin (nu″ro-si-tol′ĭ-sin) a constituent of the venom of certain snakes (rattler, coral, cobra), which lyses nerve cells.

neurocytoma (nu″ro-si-to′mah) a brain tumor consisting of undifferentiated cells of nervous origin, i.e., cells resembling medullary neural epithelium; called also *neuroepithelioma* and *medulloepithelioma*.

neurodealgia (nu-ro″de-al′je-ah) [Gr. *neurōdēs* retina + *-algia*] pain in the retina.

neurodeatrophia (nu-ro″de-ah-tro′fe-ah) [Gr. *neurōdēs* retina + *atrophia*] retinal atrophy.

neurodegenerative (nu″ro-de-jen′er-a-tiv) relating to or marked by nervous degeneration.

neurodendrite (nu″ro-den′drīt) [*neuro-* + Gr. *dendritēs* of a tree] dendrite.

neurodendron (nu″ro-den′dron) dendrite.

neuroderm (nu′ro-derm) the neural ectoderm; that portion of the ectoderm which develops into the neural tube.

neurodermatitis (nu″ro-der″mah-ti′tis) [*neuro-* + Gr. *derma* skin + *-itis*] a general term for a dermatosis presumed to be caused by itching due to emotional causes; it is also used to refer to n. circumscripta (*lichen simplex chronicus*) and sometimes n. disseminata (*atopic dermatitis*).

neurodiagnosis (nu″ro-di″ag-no′sis) [*neuro-* + *diagnosis*] the diagnosis of diseases of the nervous system.

neurodin (nu-ro′din) acetyl para-oxyphenylurethane, C_6H_4-$(OCOCH_3)NH\cdot COOC_2H_5$, used as an antineuralgic and antipyretic.

neurodynamic (nu″ro-di-nam′ik) [*neuro-* + Gr. *dynamis* force] relating to nervous energy.

neurodynia (nu″ro-din′e-ah) [*neuro-* + Gr. *odynē* pain] pain in a nerve or in nerves.

neuroectoderm (nu″ro-ek′to-derm) the portion of the ectoderm of the early embryo which gives rise to the central and peripheral nervous systems, including some glial cells.

neuroectodermal (nu″ro-ek″to-der′mal) pertaining or relating to the neuroectoderm.

neuroeffector (nu″ro-ef-fek′tor) of or relating to the junction between a neuron and the effector organ it innervates.

neuroelectricity (nu″ro-e″lek-tris′ĭ-te) the electrical signals, currents, or voltages generated by the nervous system.

neuroelectrotherapeutics (nu″ro-e-lek″tro-ther″ah-pu′tiks) the treatment of nervous diseases by electricity.

neuroencephalomyelopathy (nu″ro-en-sef″ah-lo-mi″ĕ-lop′-ah-the) [*neuro-* + Gr. *enkephalos* brain + *myelos* marrow + *pathos* disease] disease involving the brain, spinal cord, and nerves. **optic n.,** neuromyelitis optica.

neuroendocrine (nu″ro-en′do-krin) pertaining to neural and endocrine influence, and particularly to the interaction between the nervous and endocrine systems.

neuroendocrinology (nu″ro-en″do-kri-nol′o-je) the study of the interactions of the nervous system and endocrine system.

neuroenteric (nu″ro-en-ter′ik) neurenteric.

neuroepidermal (nu″ro-ep″ĭ-der′mal) [*neuro-* + *epidermis*] pertaining to or giving origin to the nervous and epidermal tissues.

neuroepithelial (nu″ro-ep″ĭ-the″le-al) pertaining to or composed of neuroepithelium.

neuroepithelioma (nu″ro-ep″ĭ-the″le-o′mah) neurocytoma.

neuroepithelium (nu″ro-ep″ĭ-the″le-um) [*neuro-* + *epithelium*] 1. simple columnar epithelium made up of cells specialized to serve as sensory cells for the reception of external stimuli, as the sensory cells of the cochlea, vestibule, nasal mucosa, and tongue. 2. the epithelium of the ectoderm, from which the central nervous system is developed. **n. of ampullary crest, n. cris′tae ampulla′ris** [NA], the specialized epithelium of the ampullary crest of the labyrinth, containing receptor cells from some of which sensory hairs project into the cupula. **n. of maculae, n. macula′rum** [NA], the specialized epithelium of the maculae of the labyrinth, containing receptor cells from some of which sensory hairs project into the statoconic membrane.

neurofibril (nu″ro-fi′bril) any of the delicate interlacing threads coursing through the cytoplasm of the body of a neuron and extending from one dendrite into another or into the axon; with the electron microscope, it can be seen to be formed by aggregations of neurofilaments and neurotubules.

neurofibrilla (nu″ro-fi-bril′ah), pl. *neurofibril′lae.* A neurofibril.

neurofibrillae (nu″ro-fi-bril′e) plural of *neurofibrilla.*

neurofibrillar (nu″ro-fi-bril′ar) pertaining to neurofibrils.

neurofibroma (nu″ro-fi-bro′mah) [*neuro-* + *fibroma*] a tumor of peripheral nerves caused by abnormal proliferation of Schwann cells.

neurofibromatosis (nu″ro-fi″bro-mah-to′sis) a familial condition characterized by developmental changes in the nervous system, muscles, bones and skin and marked superficially by the formation of multiple pedunculated soft tumors (neurofibromas) distributed over the entire body associated with areas of pigmentation. Called also *multiple neuroma, neuromatosis,* and *von Recklinghausen's disease.*

neurofilament (nu″ro-fil′ah-ment) one of the slender, fibrillar elements which, along with the neurotubules, forms a neurofibril; they seem to correspond to the microfilaments occurring in many cells outside the nervous system, and in addition to a cytoskeletal function, they may be involved in intracellular transport of metabolites.

neurofixation (nu″ro-fik-sa′shun) development of syphilis of the central nervous system after use of arsenical preparations for the treatment of the primary chancre or of the skin lesion of secondary syphilis.

neurogangliitis (nu″ro-gang″gle-i′tis) inflammation of a neuroganglion.

neuroganglion (nu″ro-gang′gle-on) a ganglion, or mass of nervous matter.

neurogastric (nu″ro-gas′trik) involving the nerves of the stomach.

neurogen (nu'ro-jen) 1. transmitter substance. 2. the chemical substance by means of which the primary organizer causes the development of the neural plate.

neurogenesis (nu″ro-jen'ĕ-sis) [*neuro-* + Gr. *genesis* production] the development of nervous tissue.

neurogenetic (nu″ro-jĕ-net'ik) pertaining to neurogenesis.

neurogenic (nu″ro-jen'ik) [*neuro-* + Gr. *gennan* to produce] 1. forming nervous tissue, or stimulating nervous energy. 2. originating in the nervous system.

neurogenous (nu-roj'ĕ-nus) arising in the nervous system; arising from some lesion of the nervous system.

neuroglia (nu-rog'le-ah) [*neuro-* + Gr. *glia* glue] the supporting structure of nervous tissue (Virchow, 1854). It consists of a fine web of tissue made up of modified ectodermal elements, in which are enclosed peculiar branched cells known as *neuroglial cells* or *glial cells*. The neuroglial cells are of three types: astrocytes and oligodendrocytes (collectively macroglia, which are of ectodermal origin, and microglia, said to be of mesodermal origin. Astrocytes and oligodendrocytes appear to play a role in myelin formation, transport of material to neurons, and maintenance of the ionic environment of neurons. Called also *bind web* and *glia*. **interfascicular n.,** oligodendroglia of white matter along the myelin sheaths. **peripheral n.,** the neurilemma, Schwann cells, and satellite cells of the peripheral nervous system.

neuroglial, neurogliar (nu-rog'le-al, nu-rog'le-ar) pertaining to the neuroglia.

neurogliocyte (nu-rog'le-o-sīt″) [*neuroglia* + *-cyte*] a cell of the neuroglia.

neurogliocytoma (nu-rog″le-o-si-to'mah) a tumor composed of neuroglial cells; a glioma.

neuroglioma (nu″ro-gli-o'mah) [*neuro-* + *glioma*] a tumor made up of neuroglial tissue. **n. gangliona're,** ganglioneuroma.

neurogliomatosis (nu″ro-gli″o-mah-to'sis) neurogliosis.

neurogliosis (nu-rog'le-o'sis) a condition marked by diffuse formation of neurogliomas. **n. gangliocellula'ris diffu'sa,** tuberous sclerosis.

neuroglycopenia (nu″ro-gli″ko-pe'ne-ah) [*neuro-* + Gr. *glykys* sweet + *penia* poverty] chronic hypoglycemia of a degree sufficient to impair brain function, resulting in personality changes and intellectual deterioration.

neurogram (nu'ro-gram) [*neuro-* + Gr. *gramma* mark] Prince's name for residua of past cerebral activities which make up the brain disposition and thus take part in the formation of personality.

neurography (nu-rog'rah-fe) [*neuro-* + Gr. *graphein* to write] a treatise on or description of the nerves.

neurohistology (nu″ro-his-tol'o-je) the histology of the nervous system.

neurohormonal (nu″ro-hor'mo-nal) both neural and hormonal.

neurohormone (nu'ro-hor″mōn) a hormone stimulating the neural mechanism.

neurohumor (nu″ro-hu'mor) a chemical substance formed in a neuron and able to activate or modify the function of a neighboring neuron, muscle, or gland.

neurohumoral (nu″ro-hu'mor-al) pertaining to the neurohumors.

neurohumoralism (nu″ro-hu'mor-al-izm) the theory that the action of the autonomic nerves on peripheral organs is produced through the medium of chemicals (neurohumors) which are liberated at the endings of activated nerves.

neurohypnologist (nu″ro-hip-nol'o-jist) an expert in neurohypnology.

neurohypnology (nu″ro-hip-nol'o-je) [*neuro-* + Gr. *hypnos* sleep + *-logy*] the sum of knowledge concerning hypnotic conditions.

neurohypophyseal (nu″ro-hi'po-fiz'e-al) pertaining to the neurohypophysis.

neurohypophysectomy (nu″ro-hi'po-fiz-ek'to-me) [*neuro-* + *hypophysectomy*] surgical removal of the neural lobe of the pituitary gland.

neurohypophysial (nu″ro-hi'po-fiz'e-al) neurohypophyseal.

neurohypophysis (nu″ro-hi-pof'ĭ-sis) [NA alternative] the posterior (neural) lobe of the pituitary gland as distinguished from the anterior lobe (adenohypophysis). See *pituitary gland,* under *gland.*

neuroid (nu'roid) [*neuro-* + Gr. *eidos* form] resembling a nerve.

neuroimmunologic (nu″ro-im″u-no-loj'ik) pertaining to neuroimmunology.

neuroimmunology (nu″ro-im″u-nol'o-je) that branch of science which deals with the interaction of the nervous and immune systems in health and disease, as in the effects of autonomic nervous activity on the immune response and the role of antibodies in myasthenia gravis.

neuroinduction (nu″ro-in-duk'shun) [*neuro-* + L. *inducere* to persuade] mental suggestion.

neuroinidia (nu″ro-ĭ-nid'e-ah) deficient nutrition of nerve cells.

neurokeratin (nu″ro-ker'ah-tin) [*neuro-* + Gr. *keras* horn] a variety of keratin said to form the supporting network of the myelin sheath of medullated nerve fibers.

neurokinet (nu″ro-kin'et) [*neuro-* + Gr. *kinein* to move] an apparatus for stimulating the nerve by percussion.

neurokyme (nu'ro-kīm) a nervous process in general.

neurolabyrinthitis (nu″ro-lab″ĭ-rin-thi'tis) inflammation of the nervous structures of the labyrinth.

neurolathyrism (nu″ro-lath'ĭ-rizm) lathyrism.

neurolemma (nu″ro-lem'ah) neurilemma.

neurolemmitis (nu″ro-lĕ-mi'tis) neurilemmitis.

neurolemmoma (nu″ro-lĕ-mo'mah) neurilemoma.

neuroleptanalgesia (nu″ro-lep″tan-al-je'ze-ah) [*neuro-* + Gr. *leptos* slender + *an* neg. + *algēsis* pain + *-ia*] a state of quiescence, altered awareness, and analgesia produced by the administration of a combination of a narcotic analgesic and a neuroleptic agent.

neuroleptanalgesic (nu″ro-lep″tan-al-je'zik) 1. pertaining to or producing neuroleptanalgesia. 2. an agent that produces neuroleptanalgesia.

neuroleptanesthesia (nu″ro-lep″tan-es-the'ze-ah) [*neuro-* + Gr. *leptos* slender + *an* neg. + *aisthēsis* sensation] a state of neuroleptanalgesia and unconsciousness, produced by the combined administration of a narcotic analgesic and a neuroleptic agent, together with the inhalation of nitrous oxide and oxygen.

neuroleptanesthetic (nu″ro-lep″tan-es-thet'ik) 1. pertaining to or producing neuroleptanesthesia. 2. an agent that produces neuroleptanesthesia.

neuroleptic (nu″ro-lep'tik) [*neuro-* + Gr. *lēpsis* a taking hold] 1. modifying psychotic behavior. 2. any drug that favorably modifies psychotic symptoms; the main categories of neuroleptics include the phenothiazines, butyrophenones, and thioxanthenes. Called also *antipsychotic* and *major tranquilizer.*

neurolipomatosis (nu″ro-lĭ-po″mah-to'sus) a condition characterized by the formation of subcutaneous multiple fat deposits, with pressure on the nerves resulting in tenderness, pain, and paresthesias. **n. doloro'sa,** adiposis dolorosa.

neurologia (nu″ro-lo'je-ah) neurology.

neurologic (nu-ro-loj'ik) pertaining to neurology or to the nervous system.

neurologist (nu-rol'o-jist) an expert in neurology or in the treatment of disorders of the nervous system.

neurology (nu-rol'o-je) [*neuro-* + *-logy*] that branch of medical science which deals with the nervous system, both normal and in disease. **clinical n.,** that specialty concerned with the diagnosis and treatment of disorders of the nervous system.

neurolues (nu″ro-loo'ēz) neurosyphilis.

neurolymph (nu'ro-limf) (*obs.*) the cerebrospinal fluid.

neurolymphomatosis (nu″ro-lim″fo-mah-to'sis) lymphoblastic infiltration of a nerve. **n. gallina'rum,** Marek's disease.

neurolysin (nu-rol'ĭ-sin) a cytolysin which has a specific destructive action upon nerve cells.

neurolysis (nu-rol'ĭ-sis) [*neuro-* + Gr. *lysis* dissolution] 1. release of a nerve sheath by cutting it longitudinally. 2. the operative breaking up of perineural adhesions. 3. the relief of tension upon a nerve obtained by stretching. 4. exhaustion of nervous energy. 5. destruction or dissolution of nerve tissue.

neurolytic (nu″ro-lit'ik) destructive of nerve substance.

neuroma (nu-ro'mah) [*neuro-* + *-oma*] a tumor or new growth largely made up of nerve cells and nerve fibers; a tumor growing from a nerve. **acoustic n.,** a progressively enlarging, benign tumor within the auditory canal arising from the eighth cranial (acoustic) nerve; the symptoms, which vary with the size and location of the tumor, may include hearing loss, headache, disturbances of balance and gait, facial numbness or pain, and tinnitus. It may be unilateral or bilateral. Called also *acoustic neurilemoma* or *neurinoma,* and *schwannoma.* **amputation n.,** traumatic neuroma occurring after amputation of an extremity or part. **amyelinic n.,** one containing only nonmedullated nerve fibers. **n. cu'tis,** neuroma seated in the skin. **cystic n.,** a false neuroma, or a neuroma which has become cystic. **false n.,** one which does not contain nerve elements. **fascicular n., medullated n.,** a neuroma made up of myelinated nerve fibers. **ganglionar n., ganglionated n., ganglionic n.,** one made up of nerve cells. **malignant n.,** sarcoma of a nerve structure, usually spindle celled. **multiple n.,** see *neuromatosis* and *neurofibromatosis.* **myelinic n.,** one that contains myelinated nerve fibers. **nevoid n.,** neuroma telangiectodes. **plexiform n.,** a neuroma made up of contorted nerve trunks; called also *Verneuil's n.* **n. telangiecto'des,** one which contains an excess of blood vessels; called also *nevoid n.* **traumatic n.,** an unorganized bulbous or nodular mass of nerve fibers and Schwann cells produced by hyperplasia of nerve fibers and their supporting tissues after accidental or purposeful sectioning of the nerve. **true n.,** a neuroma made up of nerve tissue. **Verneuil's n.,** plexiform n.

neuromalacia (nu″ro-mah-la'she-ah) [*neuro-* + Gr. *malakia* softening] morbid softening of the nerves.

neuromalakia (nu″ro-mah-la'ke-ah) neuromalacia.

neuromatosis (nu″ro-mah-to'sis) a disease condition characterized by the presence of many neuromas; see also *neurofibromatosis.*

neuromatous (nu-rom'ah-tus) affected with or of the nature of neuroma.

neuromechanism (nu″ro-mek'ah-nizm) the structure and arrangement of the nervous system in relation to function.

neuromeningeal (nu″ro-men-in'je-al) pertaining to or affecting nervous tissue and the meninges.

neuromere (nu'ro-mēr) [*neuro-* + Gr. *meros* part] 1. any of the series of transitory segmental elevations in the wall of the neural tube of the developing embryo; also commonly used to refer to such elevations in the wall of the mature rhombencephalon. 2. a part of the spinal cord to which a pair of dorsal roots and a pair of ventral roots are attached. Called also *neural segment.*

neuromimesis (nu″ro-mi-me'sis) [*neuro-* + *mimesis*] hysterical simulation of organic disease.

neuromimetic (nu″ro-mi-met'ik) 1. eliciting a response in effector organs that simulates that elicited by nervous impulses. 2. an agent that elicits such a response. 3. pertaining to neuromimesis.

neuromittor (nu″ro-mit'or) [*neuro-* + L. *mittere* to send] one of the terminal elements at the peripheral end of a neuron which transfers a stimulus to the neuroceptor of the adjoining neuron. Called also *mittor.*

neuromotor (nu″ro-mo'tor) involving both nerves and muscles; pertaining to nervous impulses to muscles.

neuromuscular (nu″ro-mus'ku-lar) pertaining to muscles and nerves.

neuromyal (nu″ro-mi'al) [*neuro-* + Gr. *mus* a muscle] neuromuscular.

neuromyasthenia (nu″ro-mi″as-the'ne-ah) [*neuro-* + *myasthenia*] muscular weakness associated with emotional lability. **epidemic n.,** benign myalgic encephalomyelitis.

neuromyelitis (nu″ro-mi″ĕ-li'tis) [*neuro-* + Gr. *myelos* marrow + *-itis*] inflammation of nervous and medullary substance; myelitis attended with neuritis. **n. op'tica,** combined demyelination of the optic nerve and the spinal cord; it is marked by diminution of vision and possibly blindness, flaccid paralysis of the extremities, and sensory and genitourinary disturbances. Called also *Devic's disease, optic neuroencephalomyelopathy,* and *neuro-optic myelitis.*

neuromyic (nu″ro-mi'ik) [*neuro-* + Gr. *mys* muscle] neuromuscular.

neuromyon (nu″ro-mi'on) [*neuro-* + Gr. *mys* muscle] (*obs.*) the neural elements in a muscle.

neuromyopathic (nu″ro-mi″o-path'ik) pertaining to or affecting the nervous system and muscle, including the heart.

neuromyositis (nu″ro-mi″o-si'tis) [*neuro-* + *myositis*] neuritis complicated with myositis.

neuron (nu'ron) [Gr. *neuron* nerve] 1. any of the conducting cells of the nervous system. A typical neuron consists of a cell body, containing the nucleus and the surrounding cytoplasm (perikaryon); several short radiating processes (dendrites); and one long process (the axon), which terminates in twiglike branches (telodendrons) and may have branches (collaterals) projecting along its course. The axon together with its covering or sheath forms the nerve fiber. See illustration accompanying *nerve.* Called also *nerve cell.* 2. (*obs.*) axon. 3. (*obs.*) the central nervous system. **afferent n.,** a neuron which conducts a nervous impulse from a receptor to a center. **bipolar n.,** a neuron having two processes, one projecting from each end of the cell body. **central n.,** a neuron which belongs entirely to the central nervous system. **connector n.,** one whose dendrites and axon both synapse with other neurons. **correlation n.,** a neuron which takes part in the function of correlating various stimuli into the appropriate response; see *correlation.* **efferent n.,** a neuron which conducts a nervous impulse from a center to an organ of response. **Golgi type I n's,** pyramidal neurons with very long axons, which leave the gray matter of the central nervous system, traverse the white matter, and terminate in the periphery; called also *Golgi cells.* **Golgi type II n's,** stellate neurons with short axons that do not pass out of the gray matter in which the cell body lies, and are especially numerous in the cerebral and cerebellar cortices and in the retina. Called also *Golgi cells* and *cells of van Gehuchten.* **intercalary n., internuncial n.,** interneuron. **long n.,** axon, def. 2. **motor n.,** any neuron possessing a motor function; an efferent neuron conveying motor impulses. See *motoneuron.* **multiform n.,** polymorphic n. **multipolar n.,** a neuron with several to many processes; such neurons vary in shape, depending on the arrangement of the processes, with pyramidal and stellate (star) shapes being common. Called also *polymorphic n.* **peripheral sensory n.,** a

neuron forming the first part of a peripheral reflex arc; situated outside the central nervous system, it has a peripheral branch which enters the central nervous system. Together with the interneurons and the peripheral motor neuron it forms a peripheral reflex arc. **polymorphic n.,** a neuron of irregular shape. **postganglionic n's,** neurons whose cell bodies are situated in the autonomic ganglia and whose purpose is to relay impulses beyond the ganglia. **preganglionic n's,** neurons whose cell bodies lie in the central nervous system and whose efferent fibers terminate in the autonomic ganglia. **premotor n.,** a neuron not connected directly with muscle, but serving as a connecting center to command excitation in one or more motor neurons. **projection n.,** one which serves for the transmission of nervous impulses, whether motor or sensory, between the cerebral cortex and the lower centers. **pseudounipolar n.,** a unipolar neuron which was originally bipolar but whose two processes fused during development to form a single process that bifurcates at a distance from the cell body. **pyramidal n.,** see under *cell.* **sensory n.,** any neuron possessing a sensory function; an afferent neuron conveying sensory impulses. See illustration accompanying *nerve.* **short n.,** a local process from a nerve cell or brain cell reaching only to a nearby gray mass. **unipolar n.,** a neuron with one process only; see also *pseudounipolar n.*

neuronagenesis (nu″rōn-ah-jen'ĕ-sis) [*neuron* + *a* neg. + Gr. *gennan* to produce] lack of development of neurons.

neuronal (nu'ro-nal) pertaining to a neuron or neurons.

neuronatrophy (nu″ron-at'ro-fe) Southard and Solomon's term for any nervous disease due to sclerosis of neurons.

neurone (nu'rōn) neuron.

neuronephric (nu″ro-nef'rik) pertaining to the nervous and renal systems.

neuronevus (nu″ro-ne'vus) a cellular or nevocytic nevus, especially a mature one with differentiation toward neural skin structures, such as Meissner corpuscles.

neuronic (nu-ron'ik) pertaining to or affecting a neuron.

neuronin (nu'ro-nin) the principal protein of the axon of a nerve.

neuronist (nu'ro-nist) (*obs.*) an adherent of the neuron theory.

neuronitis (nu″ro-ni'tis) a term applied by Foster Kennedy to a disorder of unknown origin involving the more proximal part of the peripheral nervous system, characterized by breakdown of nerve fibers, sometimes in association with inflammatory-cell reaction. Currently seldom used, it was in the past one of numerous synonyms used for *acute febrile polyneuritis.*

neuronophage (nu-ron'o-fāj) [*neuron* + Gr. *phagein* to eat] a phagocyte which destroys nerve cells.

neuronophagia (nu″ron-o-fa'je-ah) the destruction of nerve cells by phagocytic action.

neuronophagy (nu″ron-of'ah-je) neuronophagia.

neuronosis (nu″ro-no'sis) [*neuron* + Gr. *nosos* disease] any disease of nervous origin.

neuronotropic (nu-ron″o-trōp'ik) [*neuron* + Gr. *tropein* to turn] having a special affinity for neurons.

neuronymy (nu-ron'ĭ-me) [*neuron* + Gr. *onoma* name] the systematic naming of the parts of the nervous system.

neuro-ophthalmology (nu″ro-of″thal-mol'o-je) the field of specialization dealing with portions of the nervous system related to the eye.

neuro-otology (nu″ro-o-o-tol'o-je) that part of otology dealing especially with portions of the nervous system related to the ear.

neuropacemaker (nu″ro-pās'māk-er) an implant device that relieves pain due to nerve injury.

neuropapillitis (nu″ro-pap″ĭ-li'tis) optic neuritis.

neuroparalysis (nu″ro-pah-ral'ĭ-sis) paralysis due to disease of a nerve or nerves.

neuroparalytic (nu″ro-par″ah-lit'ik) pertaining to or characterized by neuroparalysis.

neuropath (nu'ro-path) a person with a tendency to neurosis.

neuropathic (nu″ro-path'ik) pertaining to or characterized by neuropathy.

neuropathogenesis (nu″ro-path″o-jen'ĕ-sis) development of disease of the nervous system.

neuropathogenicity (nu″ro-path″o-jĕ-nis'ĭ-te) the quality of producing or the ability to produce pathologic changes in nerve tissue.

neuropathology (nu″ro-pah-thol'o-je) the branch of medicine dealing with morphological and other aspects of disease of the nervous system.

neuropathy (nu-rop'ah-the) a general term denoting functional disturbances and/or pathological changes in the peripheral nervous system. The etiology may be known (e.g., *arsenical n., diabetic n., ischemic n., traumatic n.*), or unknown. *Encephalopathy* and *myelopathy* are corresponding terms relating to involvement of the brain and spinal cord, respectively. The term is also used to designate noninflammatory lesions in the peripheral nervous system, in contrast to inflammatory lesions (neuritis).

alcoholic n., neuropathy due to thiamine deficiency in chronic alcoholism; called *polyneuritis potatorum.* **ascending n.,** that which progresses from the feet upwards to affect the thigh, hip, trunk, etc. **descending n.,** that which starts proximately (shoulder, hip) and spreads distally toward the limb extremities (hands, feet). **diabetic n.,** a chronic, symmetrical sensory polyneuropathy affecting first the nerves of the lower limbs and often affecting autonomic nerves; pathologically, there is segmental demyelination of the peripheral nerves. An uncommon, acute form is marked by severe pain, weakness, and wasting of proximal and distal muscles, peripheral sensory impairment, and loss of tendon reflexes. With autonomic involvement there may be orthostatic hypotension, nocturnal diarrhea, retention of urine, impotence, and small diameter of the pupils with sluggish reaction to light. **entrapment n.,** any of a group of neuropathies, including the carpal tunnel syndrome, tarsal tunnel syndrome, and meralgia paresthetica, in which a peripheral nerve is injured by compression in its course through a fibrous or osseofibrous tunnel or at a point where it abruptly changes its course through deep fascia over a fibrous or muscular band. **hereditary sensory radicular n.,** a dominantly inherited disorder characterized by signs of radicular sensory loss in both the upper and lower extremities; shooting pains; chronic, indolent, trophic ulceration of the feet; and sometimes deafness. The pathologic findings are primary degeneration of the dorsal root ganglia together with evidence of degeneration of the olivary nuclei, optic nerves, and cerebellum. **periaxial n.,** segmental (demyelination) n. **progressive hypertrophic interstitial n.,** a condition characterized by hyperplasia of the interstitial connective tissue, causing thickening of peripheral nerve trunks and posterior roots, and by sclerosis of the posterior columns of the spinal cord. It is a slowly progressive familial disease beginning in early life, marked by atrophy of distal parts of the legs, and by diminution of tendon reflexes and of sensation. Called also *Dejerine-Sottas disease* or *atrophy,* and *interstitial hypertrophic neuritis.* **segmental (demyelination) n.,** neuropathy in which there is loss of myelin segments; called also *periaxial n.* **serum n.,** a neurologic disorder, usually involving the cervical nerves or brachial plexus, occurring two to eight days after the injection of foreign protein, as in immunization or serotherapy for tetanus, diphtheria, or scarlet fever, and characterized by local pain followed by sensory disturbances and paralysis. Called also *serum neuritis.*

neuropeptide (nu″ro-pep′tid) any of the molecules composed of short chains of amino acids (endorphins, enkephalins, vasopressin, etc.) found in brain tissue, often localized in axon terminals at synapses; they are classified as putative neurotransmitters, although some are also hormones.

neurophage (nu′ro-fāj) neuronophage.

neuropharmacological (nu″ro-fahr″mah-ko-loj′ĭ-k′l) pertaining to neuropharmacology.

neuropharmacology (nu″ro-fahr″mah-kol′o-je) that branch of pharmacology dealing especially with the action of drugs upon various parts and elements of the nervous system.

neurophilic (nu″ro-fil′ik) neurotropic.

neurophonia (nu″ro-fo′ne-ah) [*neuro-* + Gr. *phōnē* voice + *-ia*] a form of nervous disorder in which the patient utters peculiar cries, sometimes like those of certain animals.

neurophthalmology (nu″rof-thah-mol′o-je) neuro-ophthalmology.

neurophthisis (nu-rof′thĭ-sis) [*neuro-* + Gr. *phthisis* wasting] wasting of nerve tissue.

neurophysin (nu″ro-fi′sin) any of a group of soluble proteins (molecular weights 9500–10,500) secreted in the hypothalamus that serve as binding ("carrier") proteins for vasopressin and oxytocin and play a role in transport of these hormones in the neurohypophyseal tract and their storage in the posterior pituitary.

neurophysiology (nu″ro-fiz″e-ol′o-je) [*neuro-* + *physiology*] the physiology of the nervous system.

neuropil (nu′ro-pīl) [*neuro-* + Gr. *pilos* felt] a dense feltwork of interwoven cytoplasmic processes of nerve cells (dendrites and neurites) and of neuroglial cells in the central nervous system and in some parts of the peripheral nervous system.

neuropile (nu′ro-pīl) neuropil.

neuropilem (nu-ro-pi′lem) neuropil.

neuroplasm (nu′ro-plazm) [*neuro-* + Gr. *plasma* something formed] the undifferentiated basophilic protoplasm of a nerve cell.

neuroplasmic (nu″ro-plaz′mik) of or relating to neuroplasm.

neuroplasty (nu′ro-plas″te) [*neuro-* + Gr. *plassein* to form] plastic surgery of a nerve.

neuroplexus (nu″ro-plek′sus) a plexus of nerves.

neuropodia (nu″ro-po′de-ah) plural of *neuropodium.*

neuropodion (nu″ro-po′de-on) neuropodium.

neuropodium (nu″ro-po′de-um), pl. *neuropo′dia* [*neuro-* + Gr. *pous* foot] a bulbous termination of an axon in one type of synapse.

neuropore (nu′ro-pōr) [*neuro-* + Gr. *poros* pore] the open ante-

rior end (foramen anterius) or the open posterior end (foramen posterius) of the neural tube of the early embryo. These openings gradually close as the tube develops, the timing of each closure being so precise that they are used to define horizons XI and XII. **anterior n.,** the embryonic opening in the anterior portion of the forebrain, which closes at the 20-somite stage, marking the end of Streeter's horizon XI. **posterior n.,** the embryonic opening at the posterior end of the neural tube, which closes by about the 25-somite stage.

neuropotential (nu″ro-po-ten′shal) nerve energy; nerve potential.

neuroprobasia (nu″ro-pro-ba′se-ah) [*neuro-* + Gr. *pro* forward + *basis* walking] advance along the nerves; said of the action of certain viruses.

neuropsychiatrist (nu″ro-si-ki′ah-trist) a physician who specializes in neuropsychiatry.

neuropsychiatry (nu″ro-si-ki′ah-tre) the branch of medicine which includes both neurology and psychiatry.

neuropsychic (nu″ro-si′kik) [*neuro-* + Gr. *psyche* soul] pertaining to the nerve center concerned in mental processes.

neuropsychopathy (nu″ro-si-kop′ah-the) [*neuro-* + Gr. *psyche* soul + *pathos* disease] a disease condition of the nerves and mind.

neuropsychopharmacology (nu″ro-si″ko-fahr″mah-kol′o-je) the science of the effect of drugs in psychiatric disorders.

neuropsychosis (nu″ro-si-ko′sis) [*neuro-* + *psychosis*] (*obs.*) psychosis.

neuroradiology (nu″ro-ra″de-ol′o-je) radiology of the nervous system.

neurorecidive (nu″ro-res″ĭ-dēv′) neurorelapse.

neurorecurrence (nu″ro-re-kur′ens) neurorelapse.

neurorelapse (nu″ro-re-laps′) a peculiar outburst of neurosyphilis precipitated by insufficient treatment with arsphenamine, and characterized by various nervous symptoms; called also *neurorecidive* and *neurorecurrence.*

neuroretinitis (nu″ro-ret″ĭ-ni′tis) inflammation of the optic nerve and retina.

neuroretinopathy (nu″ro-ret″ĭ-nop′ah-the) [*neuro-* + *retina* + Gr. *pathos* disease] a disease of the optic disk and retina. **hypertensive n.,** swelling of the optic disk and formation of serous and fibrinous precipitates in the retina, occurring in severe hypertension.

neuroroentgenography (nu″ro-rent″gen-og′rah-fe) neuroradiology.

neurorrhaphy (nu-ror′ah-fe) [*neuro-* + Gr. *rhaphē* stitch] the suturing of a cut nerve.

Neurorrhyctes hydrophobiae (nu″ro-rik′tēz hi″dro-fo′be-e) Negri bodies.

neurosarcokleisis (nu″ro-sar″ko-kli′sis) [*neuro-* + Gr. *sarx* flesh + *kleisis* closure] an operation performed for neuralgia, done by relieving pressure on the affected nerve by partial resection of the bony canal through which it passes, and transplanting the nerve among soft tissues.

neurosarcoma (nu″ro-sar-ko′mah) a sarcoma with neuromatous elements.

neuroscience (nu″ro-si′ens) any of the branches of science dealing with the embryology, anatomy, physiology, biochemistry, pharmacology, etc., of the nervous system.

neuroscientist (nu″ro-si′en-tist) an expert in any of the branches of the neurosciences.

neurosclerosis (nu″ro-skle-ro′sis) [*neuro-* + Gr. *sklēros* hard] the hardening of the substance of a nerve or nerve center.

neurosecretion (nu″ro-se-kre′shun) [*neuro-* + *secretion*] 1. the secretory activities of nerve cells, as the secretion of releasing hormones, vasopressin, neurotransmitters, etc. 2. the product of such activities; a neurosecretory substance.

neurosecretory (nu″ro-se-kre′to-re) [*neuro-* + *secretory*] pertaining to neurosecretion.

neurosegmental (nu″ro-seg-men′tal) [*neuro-* + *segmental*] of or pertaining to a pair of spinal dorsal and ventral roots or to the area which they supply.

neurosensory (nu″ro-sen′so-re) pertaining to a sensory nerve.

neuroses (nu-ro′sēz) plural of *neurosis.*

neurosis (nu-ro′sis), pl. *neuro′ses* [*neur-* + *-osis*] an emotional disorder due to unresolved conflicts, anxiety being its chief characteristic. The anxiety may be expressed directly or indirectly, as by conversion, displacement, etc. In contrast to the psychoses, the neuroses do not involve gross distortions of external reality or disorganization of personality. Called also *psychoneurosis.* **accident n.,** a neurosis with hysterical symptoms caused by accident or injury. **anxiety n.,** neurosis characterized by morbid and unjustified dread, sometimes extending to panic and frequently associated with somatic symptoms; it occurs without apparent external cause. Called also *anxiety reaction.* **association n.** (*obs.*), a condition in which an abnormal mental experience tends to be reproduced, with all its original mental and physical phenomena, when an idea related to the original experience is brought into the mind. **cardiac n.,** neurocirculatory asthenia. **character n.,** a neurosis in which certain personality traits have become exaggerated or overdeveloped, but the behavior is socially acceptable and may not be easily recognized as symptomatic. **combat n.,** a neurosis resulting from battle experiences and conditions of military life; formerly called *combat fatigue.* **compensation n.,** the neurotic phenomena developing after an accident in persons who are insured or who believe that by being ill they may increase their chances of receiving compensation. **compulsion n.,** a neurosis marked by an imperative impulse toward some absurd act or speech. **conversion n.,** see under *reaction.* **craft n.,** occupation n. **depersonalization n.,** a syndrome characterized by a feeling of unreality and of estrangement from the self, one's body, or one's surroundings; it differs from the process of *depersonalization,* which may be part of another mental disorder or a manifestation of normal anxiety. Called also *depersonalization syndrome.* **depressive n.,** a neurosis characterized by an excessive reaction of depression due to an internal conflict or to an identifiable event. **expectation n.,** a neurotic condition in which the expectation of an occurrence induces mental tension, etc. **experimental n.,** a neurosis produced by deliberate exposure to biological or psychologic stress. **fatigue n.,** a neurosis due to nervous fatigue, as neurasthenia or psychasthenia. **fixation n.,** a neurosis based on fixation of the personality at a stage short of complete maturity, a psychoanalytic concept. **gastric n.,** a disorder of gastric digestion based on disturbance of the nervous system. **hypochondriacal n.,** a neurosis characterized by persistent preoccupation with the body and fear of presumed diseases of various organs. **hysterical n.,** a neurosis characterized by sudden involuntary psychogenic loss or disorder of function in response to emotional stress, occurring in two types: a *conversion type,* which is manifested by disorders of the special senses or the voluntary nervous system and produces such symptoms as blindness, deafness, anesthesia, paresthesia, paralysis, and impaired muscular coordination, and a *dissociative type,* which is manifested by alterations in the state of consciousness or in identity and produces such symptoms as amnesia, somnambulism, fugue, and multiple personality. **intestinal n.,** intestinal indigestion due to disturbance of innervation or of psychic control. **neurasthenic n.,** a neurosis characterized by chronic weakness, easy fatigability, and sometimes exhaustion; believed by some to be one of the psychophysiologic, or psychosomatic, disorders. Called also *neurasthenia, psychophysiologic asthenic reaction,* and *psychophysiologic nervous system reaction.* **obsessional n.,** a neurosis marked by obsessions which dominate the conduct of the patient. **obsessive-compulsive n.,** a neurosis marked by the persistent intrusion of unwanted and repetitive thoughts or urges, compelling the patient to perform rituals such as handwashing. **occupational n.,** a neurosis due to the patient's employment. **pension n.,** compensation n. **phobic n.,** a neurosis characterized by intense fear, usually leading to avoidance, of an object or situation that the individual consciously recognizes as harmless. **professional n.,** occupational n. **rectal n.,** a rectal disorder due to disturbance of innervation or of psychic control. **regression n.,** fixation n. **transference n.,** hysteria and compulsion neurosis. **traumatic n.,** one which results from an injury. **true n.,** in freudian theory, a neurosis resulting from present disruption of sexual activity; the true neuroses include neurasthenia and anxiety neurosis and are distinguished theoretically from the psychoneuroses, which are held to be derived from past (infancy and childhood) experiences. **vegetative n.,** acrodynia. **war n.,** a term referring to a number of conditions, chiefly hysterical conversion phenomena, seen in soldiers.

neuroskeletal (nu″ro-skel′ĕ-tal) pertaining to the nervous tissues and the skeletal muscular tissue.

neuroskeleton (nu″ro-skel′ĕ-ton) [*neuro-* + Gr. *skeleton* skeleton] endoskeleton.

neurosome (nu′ro-sōm) [*neuro-* + Gr. *sōma* body] 1. the body of a nerve cell. 2. any of a set of minute particles in the ground substance of the protoplasm of the neurons.

neurospasm (nu′ro-spazm) [*neuro-* + Gr. *spasmos* spasm] the nervous twitching of a muscle.

neurosplanchnic (nu″ro-splangk′nik) pertaining to the cerebrospinal and sympathetic nervous systems; neurovisceral.

neurospongioma (nu″ro-spon″je-o′mah) glioma.

neurospongium (nu″ro-spon′je-um) [*neuro-* + Gr. *spongos* sponge] 1. the fibrillar component of neurons. 2. a meshwork of nerve fibers, especially the inner reticular layer of the retina.

Neurospora (nu-ros′po-rah) a genus of ascomycetous fungi (family Sordariaceae, order Sphaeriales) comprising the bread molds, which are capable of converting tryptophan to nicotinic acid, and are extensively used in genetic and enzyme research.

neurostatus (nu″ro-sta′tus) the state or condition of neural symptoms in a case history.

neurosthenia (nu″ro-sthe′ne-ah) [*neuro-* + Gr. *sthenos* strength + *-ia*] great nervous power and excitement; cf. *neurasthenia.*

neurosurgeon (nu″ro-sur′jun) a physician who specializes in neurosurgery.

neurosurgery (nu″ro-sur′jer-e) surgery of the nervous system. **functional n.,** that designed (*a*) to restore normal conductivity in malfunctional nerve fibers or to improve blood flow in nerve tissue, or (*b*) to alleviate mental illness.

neurosuture (nu″ro-su′tūr) neurorrhaphy.

neurosyphilis (nu″ro-sif′ĭ-lis) syphilis of the central nervous system. **ectodermogenic n.,** neurosyphilis affecting the substance of the brain, cord, or nerves. **meningeal n.,** neurosyphilis affecting chiefly the meninges. **meningovascular n.,** neurosyphilis in which both the meninges and the vessels of the nervous system are involved. **mesodermogenic n.,** neurosyphilis affecting the meninges, blood vessels, and nerve sheaths. **paretic n.,** dementia paralytica. **tabetic n.,** tabes dorsalis.

neurotabes (nu″ro-ta′bēz) [*neuro-* + *tabes*] (*obs.*) pseudotabes.

neurotagma (nu″ro-tag′mah) [*neuro-* + Gr. *tagma* arrangement] a linear arrangement of the structural elements of a nerve cell.

neurotendinous (nu″ro-ten′dĭ-nus) pertaining to both nerve and tendon.

neurotensin (nu″ro-ten′sin) a tridecapeptide first isolated from the bovine hypothalamus that induces vasodilatation and hypotension; it is present in the brain tissue of man and is postulated to be a neurotransmitter.

neuroterminal (nu″ro-ter′mĭ-nal) an end organ of a peripheral nerve.

neurothele (nu″ro-the′le) [*neuro-* + Gr. *thele* nipple] a sensory papilla of the corium.

neurotherapeutics (nu″ro-ther″ah-pu′tiks) neurotherapy.

neurotherapy (nu″ro-ther′ah-pe) [*neuro-* + Gr. *therapeia* treatment] 1. the treatment of nervous disorders. 2. a term proposed for psychotherapy on the ground that the basis of such treatment is the employment of all sources of nervous activity.

neurotic (nu-rot′ik) 1. pertaining to or affected with a neurosis. 2. pertaining to the nerves. 3. a nervous person in whom emotions predominate over reason.

neurotica (nu-rot′ĭ-kah) functional nervous disorders.

neuroticism (nu-rot′ĭ-sizm) a state of perverted or excessive nervous action.

neurotigenic (nu-rot″ĭ-jen′ik) producing a neurosis.

neurotization (nu″rot-ĭ-za′shun) 1. the regeneration of a nerve after its division. 2. the operation of implanting a nerve into a paralyzed muscle.

neurotmesis (nu″rot-me′sis) [*neuro-* + Gr. *tmēsis* cutting apart] partial or complete severance of a nerve, with disruption of the axon and its myelin sheath and the connective tissue elements; regeneration does not occur. Cf. *axonotmesis* and *neurapraxia.*

neurotology (nu″ro-tol′o-je) neuro-otology.

neurotome (nu′ro-tōm) [*neuro-* + Gr. *tomē* a cut] 1. a needle-like knife for dissecting the nerves. 2. neuromere.

neurotomography (nu″ro-to-mog′rah-fe) tomography of the central nervous system.

neurotomy (nu-rot′o-me) [*neuro-* + Gr. *temnein* to cut] 1. the dissection or anatomy of the nerves. 2. the surgical cutting of a nerve. **retrogasserian n.,** see under *rhizotomy.*

neurotonia (nu″ro-to′ne-ah) instability of tonus of the vegetative nervous system.

neurotonic (nu″ro-ton′ik) [*neuro-* + *tonic*] having a tonic effect upon the nerves.

neurotonometer (nu″ro-to-nom′ĕ-ter) an apparatus for measuring minute differences in skin tonus.

neurotony (nu-rot′o-ne) [*neuro-* + Gr. *teinein* to stretch] the stretching of a nerve, chiefly to relieve pain; called also *nerve stretching.*

neurotoxia (nu″ro-tok′se-ah) a toxic condition of the nervous system; neurasthenia regarded as an autointoxication.

neurotoxic (nu″ro-tok′sik) poisonous or destructive to nerve tissue.

neurotoxicity (nu″ro-tok-sis′ĭ-te) the quality of exerting a destructive or poisonous effect upon nerve tissue.

neurotoxin (nu″ro-tok′sin) a substance that is poisonous or destructive to nerve tissue, especially an exotoxin which is characterized by a marked affinity for nerve tissue and which produces a fatty degeneration in the myelin sheath of peripheral nerves, in the white substance of the brain and spinal cord, and in certain other tissues, such as heart muscle.

neurotransducer (nu″ro-trans-du′ser) a neuron that synthesizes and releases hormones which serve as the functional link between the nervous system and the pituitary gland.

neurotransmitter (nu″ro-trans′mit-er) a substance (norepinephrine, acetylcholine, dopamine, etc.) that is released from the axon terminal of a presynaptic neuron on excitation, and that travels across the synaptic cleft to either excite or inhibit the target cell. Called also *transmitter substance.* **false n.,** an amine, e.g., octopamine, that can be stored in and released from presynaptic vesicles but that has little effect on postsynaptic receptors.

neurotrauma (nu″ro-traw′mah) [*neuro-* + *trauma*] mechanical injury of a nerve.

neurotrophasthenia (nu″ro-tro″fas-the′ne-ah) [*neuro-* + Gr. *trophē* nutrition + *astheneia* weakness] defective nutrition of the nervous system.

neurotrophic (nu″ro-trof′ik) pertaining to neurotrophy.

neurotrophy (nu-rot′ro-fe) [*neuro-* + Gr. *trophē* nutrition] the nutrition and maintenance of tissues as regulated by nervous influence.

neurotropic (nu″ro-trop′ik) having a selective affinity for nervous tissue, or exerting its principal effect on the nervous system; polioclastic; polioencephalotropic.

neurotropism (nu-rot′ro-pizm) [*neuro-* + Gr. *tropē* a turn, turning] 1. the quality of having a special affinity for nervous tissue. 2. the alleged tendency of regenerating nerve fibers to grow toward specific portions of the periphery.

neurotropy (nu-rot′ro-pe) neurotropism.

neurotrosis (nu″ro-tro′sis) [*neuro-* + Gr. *trōsis* wound] neurotrauma.

neurotubule (nu″ro-too′būl) [*neuro-* + *tubule*] any of the long, straight, parallel tubules within neurons, which along with the neurofilaments, form neurofibrils; they seem to correspond to the microtubules occurring in many cells outside the nervous system.

neurovaccine (nu″ro-vak′sin) vaccine virus prepared by growing the virus in the brain of a rabbit.

neurovaricosis (nu″ro-var″ĭ-ko′sis) [*neuro-* + *varicose* + *-osis*] a varicose state of the fibers of a nerve.

neurovariola (nu″ro-vah-ri′o-lah) neurovaccine.

neurovascular (nu″ro-vas′ku-lar) pertaining to both nervous and vascular elements; pertaining to the nerves that control the caliber of blood vessels.

neurovegetative (nu″ro-vej′ĕ-ta″tiv) pertaining to the vegetative (autonomic) nervous system.

neurovirulence (nu″ro-vir′u-lens) the competence of an infectious agent to produce pathologic effects on the nervous system.

neurovirulent (nu″ro-vir′u-lent) capable of producing pathologic effects on the nervous system.

neurovirus (nu″ro-vi′rus) a vaccine virus which has been modified by passing into nervous tissue.

neurovisceral (nu″ro-vis′er-al) neurosplanchnic.

neurula (nu′roo-lah) [*neuro-* + dim. *-ula*] the early embryo during the development of the neural tube from the neural plate, marking the first appearance of the nervous system; the next stage after the gastrula, and occurring 19 to 26 days after fertilization.

neurulation (nu″roo-la′shun) formation, in the early embryo, of the neural plate, followed by its closure with development of the neural tube.

neururgic (nu-rer′jik) [*neuro-* + Gr. *ergon* work] pertaining to nerve action.

neurypnology (nu″rip-nol′o-je) neurohypnology.

Neusser's granules (noi′serz) [Edmund von *Neusser*, Austrian physician, 1852–1912] see under *granule*.

neutral (nu′tral) [L. *neutralis; neuter,* neither] in chemistry, neither acid nor basic.

neutralism (nu′tral-izm) the absence of interaction between coexisting organisms of different species.

neutrality (nu-tral′ĭ-te) the state of being neutral.

neutralize (nu′tral-īz) to render neutral.

neutramycin (nu-trah-mi′sin) an antibacterial substance produced by *Streptomyces rimosus.*

Neutrapen (nu′trah-pen) trademark for a lyophilized preparation of penicillinase.

Neutra-Phos-K (nu″trah-fos′ka) trademark for a preparation of potassium phosphate.

neutretto (nu-tret′o) a particle similar in mass to a barytron but having no electrical charge.

neutrino (nu-tre′no) an elementary (subatomic) particle that has no electric charge and no rest mass, and that very rarely reacts with matter; it is a product of beta decay.

neutroclusion (nu″trŏ-kloo′zhun) malocclusion characterized by irregularities of individual teeth, but with normal mesiodistal or normal anteroposterior relation of the mandibular or the maxillary dental arch. Generally regarded as identical with class I in Angle's classification of malocclusion.

neutrocyte (nu′tro-sīt) a neutrophilic leukocyte; see *neutrophil,* def. 1.

neutrocytopenia (nu″tro-si″to-pe′ne-ah) neutropenia.

neutrocytosis (nu″tro-si-to′sis) neutrophilia.

neutroflavine (nu″tro-fla′vin) acriflavine.

neutron (nu′tron) an electrically neutral or uncharged particle of matter existing along with protons in the atoms of all elements except the mass 1 isotope of hydrogen. **epithermal n.,** a neutron having an energy level of a few hundredths electron volt to 100 electron volts. **fast n.,** a neutron having an energy level exceeding 10^5 electron volt. **intermediate n.,** a neutron having an energy level of 100 to 100,000 electron volts. **slow n.,** 1. thermal n. 2. any neutron having an energy level up to 100 electron volts. **thermal n.,** a neutron having an energy level of about 0.025 electron volt; called also *slow n.*

neutropenia (nu″tro-pe′ne-ah) [*neutrophil* + Gr. *penia* poverty] a decrease in the number of neutrophilic leukocytes in the blood; see *agranulocytosis.* **chronic benign n. of childhood,** a condition observed in children in which granulocytopenia and, often, recurrent infections may be present for a considerable time, with subsequent spontaneous remission. **chronic hypoplastic n.,** a syndrome of extreme chronicity, repeated infections of skin and oral cavity, moderate splenomegaly, and bone marrow markedly deficient in granulocyte precursors. **congenital n.,** a condition occurring in infants, characterized by absence of neutrophils from the peripheral blood; called also *congenital aleukia* and *congenital leukopenia.* **cyclic n.,** periodic n. **familial benign chronic n.,** a familial type of peripheral neutropenia, probably transmitted by an autosomal dominant gene. **hypersplenic n.,** primary splenic n. **idiopathic n., malignant n.,** agranulocytosis. **neonatal n., transitory,** a short-lived neutropenia, observed in the newborn, which may be of the isoimmune type. **periodic n.,** a chronic form of neutropenia characterized by its regular, periodic episodic recurrences, association with malaise, fever, stomatitis, and various types of infections. **peripheral n.,** decrease in the number of neutrophils in the circulating blood. **primary splenic n.,** a syndrome characterized by splenomegaly, profound leukopenia and neutropenia, susceptibility to infection, occasionally anemia and thrombocytopenia, and hypercellular bone marrow.

neutrophil (nu′tro-fil) [L. *neuter* neither + Gr. *philein* to love] 1. a granular leukocyte having a nucleus with three to five lobes connected by slender threads of chromatin, and cytoplasm containing fine inconspicuous granules; neutrophils have the properties of chemotaxis, adherence to immune complexes, and phagocytosis; called also *polymorphonuclear, polynuclear,* or *neutrophilic leukocytes.* Their counterparts in nonhuman mammals are heterophils. 2. any cell, structure, or histologic element readily stainable by neutral dyes. **filamented n.,** a neutrophil having two or more lobes connected by a filament of chromatin. **giant n.,** macropolycyte. **juvenile n.,** a metamyelocyte. **nonfilamented n.,** a neutrophil whose lobes are connected by thick strands of chromatin. **rod n., stab n.,** a neutrophil whose nucleus is not divided into segments.

neutrophilia (nu″tro-fil′e-ah) increase in the number of neutrophils in the blood; it is the most common form of leukocytosis and may result from many causes, among them acute infections, intoxications, hemorrhage, and rapidly growing malignant neoplasms.

neutrophilic (nu″tro-fil′ik) 1. stainable by neutral dyes. 2. neither anthropophilic nor zoophilous; said of certain mosquitoes.

neutropism (nu′tro-pizm) neutrotropism.

neutrotaxis (nu″tro-tak′sis) [*neutrophil* + Gr. *taxis* arrangement] the attractive or repellent influence exerted by neutrophilic leukocytes.

nevi (ne′vi) [L.] plural of *nevus.*

nevocarcinoma (ne″vo-kar″sĭ-no′mah) malignant melanoma.

nevocytic (ne-vo-sit′ik) pertaining to or composed of nevus cells.

nevoid (ne′void) resembling a nevus.

nevolipoma (ne″vo-lĭ-po′mah) a nevus containing a large amount of fibrofatty tissue.

nevoxanthoendothelioma (ne″vo-zan″tho-en″do-the″le-o′mah) juvenile xanthogranuloma.

Nevskia (nev′ske-ah) [*Neva,* a river in Russia] a genus of microorganisms of the family Caulobacteraceae, suborder Pseudomonadineae, order Pseudomonadales, occurring as stalked, rod-shaped cells, the long axis of the cell being at right angles to the axis of the stalk. The type species is *N. ramo′sa.*

nevus (ne′vus), pl. *ne′vi* [L. *naevus*] a circumscribed stable malformation of the skin and occasionally of the oral mucosa, which is not due to external causes and therefore presumed to be of hereditary origin. The excess (or deficiency) of tissue may involve epidermal, connective tissue, adnexal, nervous, or vascular elements. **amelanotic n.,** a nevocytic nevus which contains no pigment. **n. ane′micus,** a nevus characterized by the presence of circumscribed pale macules, which are often grouped; the condition seems to be a functional incapacity of the blood vessels to dilate. **n. arachnoi′deus, n. araneo′sus, n. araneus,** vascular spider. **bathing trunk n.,** a giant, hairy, darkly pigmented, usually congenital, nevocytic nevus affecting the lower portion of the body, or the area usually covered by bathing trunks. Its major importance is cosmetic, but it is also potentially a precursor of malignant melanoma. **Becker's n.,** a nevus composed of loosely clustered tan macules, usually occupying a single upper thoracic dermatome, most frequently appearing in late adolescence, and soon developing dark terminal hairs 2 or 3 cm. long; sometimes called *pigmented hairy epidermal nevus* or *nevus spilus tardus.* **blue n.,** a benign, slowly growing, light to dark blue nodular lesion, usually between 2 and 7 mm. in diameter, composed of closely grouped melanocytes and melanophages situated in the mid-dermis. Called also *Jadassohn-Tièche n.* and *dermal melanocytoma.* **blue rubber bleb n.,** a hereditary disorder, transmitted as an autosomal dominant trait, characterized by multiple bluish cutaneous hemangiomas with soft raised centers somewhat resembling nipples, frequently associated with hemangiomas scattered throughout the gastrointestinal tract. **cellular n.,** nevocytic nevus. **cellular blue n.,** a blue to blue-black nodule or tumor, usually present at birth in the region of the buttocks or sacrum, which differs from the blue nevus of Jadassohn-Tièche only in its larger size and its occasional, though infrequent, malignant transformation and metastasis. Called also *dermal melanocytoma.* **n. comedon′icus,** a rare epidermal nevus marked by one or more patches 2 to 5 cm. or more in diameter, in which there is a collection of large comedones or comedo-like lesions; these nevi usually occur unilaterally on the trunk in a linear manner and are frequently associated with ichthyosis hystrix. **compound n.,** a usually raised, flesh-colored to brown, nevocytic nevus, which may be papillomatous and may contain hairs; it is composed of both fully formed nevus-cell nests (theques) in the dermis and newly forming nevus cell nests in the epidermis, or of cells in transition from the lower epidermis down to the dermis (a process known as *abtropfung*). **connective tissue n.,** nevi occurring in the dermal connective tissue and characterized clinically by nodules, papules, or plaques, or by varying combinations of such lesions. Histological features include inconstant focal or diffuse thickening and abnormal staining of collagen fibers, and normal or diminished elastic fibers. Although attempts to differentiate distinct forms on the basis of clinical and histological features have resulted in terms such as juvenile elastoma, shagreen skin, nevus elasticus of Lewandowsky, and nodular connective tissue nevus, the evidence supporting distinct forms is inconclusive. Most connective tissue nevi apparently are isolated developmental anomalies and not of genetic origin. **connective tissue n., nodular,** a connective tissue nevus (q.v.) in which the lesions are smooth skin-colored or yellowish nodules, usually occurring between five and ten years of age, singly or in plaques, on the thighs, lower abdomen, and buttocks, and occasionally on the arms and legs. **n. elas′ticus,** 1. pseudoxanthoma elasticum. 2. connective tissue n. **n. elas′ticus of Lewandowsky,** a connective tissue nevus (q.v.) in which the lesions—patches of smooth ivory- or skin-colored papules—occur most frequently on the trunk, especially on the chest and back, usually with asymmetrical, and sometimes with zoniform or linear, distribution. Most lesions are present from birth or shortly thereafter and show no changes, although some may extend gradually for years. **epidermal nevi, epithelial nevi,** congenital skin tumors which do not contain melanocytes, ordinarily present at birth or appearing in early childhood, and showing some predilection for the flexor surfaces; they vary widely in appearance, size, and distribution, and are commonly hyperkeratotic. The term includes such lesions as nevus unius lateris, ichthyosis hystrix, nevus sebaceus, nevus comedonicus, and nevus syringocystadenomatosus papilliferus. **fatty n.,** n. lipomatosus. **n. flam′meus,** a diffuse, poorly defined area varying from pink to dark bluish red, involving otherwise normal

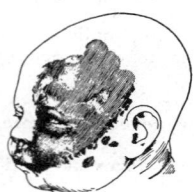

Nevus flammeus (Homans).

skin; called also *capillary hemangioma,* and *port-wine stain* or *mark.* **n. follicula′ris,** hair follicle n. **n. fuscoceru′leus acromiodeltoi′deus,** n. of Ito. **n. fuscoceru′leus ophthalmomaxilla′ris,** n. of Ota. **giant pigmented n.,** a very large, hairy, nevocytic nevus. **hair follicle n.,** a usually congenital nevus consisting of a nodule with a central crater from which hairs project; called also *n. follicularis.* **hairy n.,** a more or less pigmented nevus of variable size, with hairs growing from its surface. **halo n.,** a pigmented nevus, usually of the compound or intradermal type, surrounded by a concentric ring of depigmentation; called also *leukoderma centrifugum acquisitum,* and *Sutton's disease* or *nevus.* **hepatic n.,** hemorrhagic infarct of the liver. **intradermal n.,** a nevocytic nevus, clinically indistinguishable from a compound nevus, in which the nevus cells occur in nests (theques) in the upper part of the dermis, with no remaining evidence of the proliferative process (abtropfung) by which they originated. **n. of Ito,** a mongolian spot in the distribution of the posterior supraclavicular and lateral cutaneous brachial nerves, over the shoulder, usually on only one side; called also *n. fuscoceruleus acromiodeltoideus.* **Jadassohn-Tièche n.,** blue n. **junction n., junctional n.,** a brownish, smooth, hairless, flat or slightly elevated nevocytic nevus, varying in size from 1 to 8 mm. in diameter, which may occur anywhere on the body. Histologically, there are nests of nevus cells (theques) in the lower epidermis, which contain

melanin, and seem about to "fall off" into the dermis. **linear n.,** an epidermal nevus composed of a collection of papillary elevations, occurring in elongated streaks, and due to hypertrophy of epidermal and, to an extent, dermal elements. **n. lipomato′sus,** one containing much fibro-fatty tissue. **n. lipomato′sus cutane′us superficia′lis,** a nevus composed of masses of fat cells in the dermis, usually on the buttocks or thighs, manifested as yellowish papules, nodules, and plaques. **n. lymphangiecto′des, lymphatic n., n. lymphat′icus,** a skin growth containing lymph and blood elements intermediate in position between hemangioma and lymphangioma; hemolymphangioma. **melanocytic n.,** a usually pigmented nevus composed of melanocytes; it includes *n. spilus,* Becker's *n., n. of Ota, n. of Ito, blue n., cellular blue n., lentigo,* and *mongolian spot.* **nevocytic n.,** the common mole: a usually more or less hyperpigmented nevus, initially flat but soon becoming elevated, composed of nests of nevus cells (*theques*), possibly derived from Schwann cells or from melanocytes. Occasionally present at birth, they may arise at any age, but usually in adolescence or early adult life, and are divided, according to their stage of growth, into *junction nevi* (growing into the dermis from the epidermis), *compound nevi* (still growing, but largely static in the dermis), or *intradermal nevi* (no longer growing, but static in the dermis). Called also *cellular nevus* and *nevus-cell nevus.* **nevus-cell n.,** nevocytic nevus. **nonpigmented n.,** amelanotic n. **n. of Ota, Ota's n.,** a mongolian spot involving the conjunctiva and lids, as well as the adjacent facial skin, sclera, ocular muscles, and periosteum, usually on only one side. Rarely, malignant melanoma may occur, usually in the iris. Called also *n. fuscoceruleus ophthalmomaxillaris.* **pigmented n., n. pigmento′sus,** a nevus containing melanin; the term is usually restricted to nevocytic nevi, or moles, but may be applied to other pigmented nevi, e.g., nevus spilus and Becker's nevus. **pigmented hairy epidermal n.,** Becker's n. **pilose n., n. pilo′sus,** hairy n. **sebaceous n., sebaceous n. of Jadassohn,** an epidermal nevus of the scalp or less often the face, which frequently grows larger during puberty or early adult life, and may rarely give rise to a variety of new growths, including basal cell carcinoma. **n. seba′ceus,** sebaceous n. **spider n.,** vascular spider. **n. spi′lus,** a smooth-surfaced, tan to brown, macular, epidermal, melanocytic nevus, which is speckled with smaller, darker macules. **n. spi′lus tar′dus,** Becker's n. **spindle cell n.,** juvenile melanoma. **Spitz n.,** juvenile melanoma. **n. spongio′sus al′bus muco′sae,** white sponge n. **stellar n.,** vascular spider. **strawberry n.,** cavernous hemangioma. **Sutton's n.,** halo n. **n. syringocystadeno′sus papillif′erus,** an epidermal nevus usually involving the apocrine sweat glands, and with a predilection for the shoulders, axillae, genital and inguinal regions, and scalp; the lesions, occurring in groups, are rose-red papules of firm consistency, with vesicle-like inclusions filled with clear fluid. **n. un′ius lat′eris,** a verrucous epidermal nevus occurring as a linear band, patch, or streak, usually along the margin between two neurotomes, most often between L4 and 5 and S1, 2, and 3. **Unna's n.** (*obs.*), n. flammeus. **vascular n., n. vascula′ris, n. vasculo′sus,** a reddish swelling or patch on the skin due to hypertrophy of the skin capillaries; it includes nevus flammeus, blue rubber bleb nevus, vascular spider, and cavernous hemangioma. **verrucoid n., n. verruco′sus,** a pinkish, grayish, or brownish, raised nevus, with fine digitate excrescences on its surface. **white sponge n.,** a white spongy nevus of a mucous membrane, inherited as an autosomal dominant trait; called also *n. spongiosus albus mucosae.*

newborn (nu′born) 1. recently born. 2. a recently born infant.

Newcastle disease (nu′kas-el) [*Newcastle,* a seaport on the Tyne River in Northeast England] see under *disease.*

newton (nu′ton) [Sir Isaac *Newton,* English mathematician, physicist, and astronomer, 1643–1727] the SI unit of force which, when applied in a vacuum to a body having a mass of one kilogram, accelerates it at the rate of one meter per second. Symbol, N.

Newton's law, rings (nu′tonz) [Sir Isaac *Newton,* English mathematician, physicist, and astronomer, 1643–1727] see under *law* and *ring.*

nexeridine hydrochloride (nek-ser′ĭ-dēn) chemical name: 1-[2-(dimethylamino)-1-methylethyl]-2-phenylcyclohexanol acetate (ester) hydrochloride; an analgesic, $C_{19}H_{29}NO_2 \cdot HCl$.

nexin (neks′in) a substance which serves as a connecting link between the outer pairs of microtubules in cilia and flagella.

nexus (nek′sus), pl. *nex′us* [L. "bond"] 1. a bond, especially one between members of a series or group. 2. gap junction.

NF National Formulary.

N.F.L.P.N. National Federation for Licensed Practical Nurses.

ng. nanogram.

n'gana (na-gah′nah) nagana.

NGF nerve growth factor.

NH₃ ammonia.

NH₄Br ammonium bromide.

N.H.C. National Health Council.

NH₄Cl   ammonium chloride.

NH₄CNO   ammonium cyanate.

(NH₂)₂CO   urea.

(NH₄)₂CO₃   ammonium carbonate.

(NH₄)HS   ammonium hydrosulfide.

N.H.I.   National Health Insurance; National Heart Institute.

N.H.L.I.   National Heart and Lung Institute.

N.H.M.R.C.   National Health and Medical Research Council.

NH₄NO₃   ammonium nitrate.

NH₄O·CO·NH₂   ammonium carbamate.

N.H.S.   National Health Service (British).

(NH₄)₂·SO₂   ammonium sulfate.

NH₂-terminal (ter′min-al)   N-terminal.

Ni   chemical symbol for *nickel.*

niacin (ni′ah-sin)   chemical name: 3-pyridinecarboxylic acid. A water-soluble vitamin of the B complex, $C_6H_5NO_2$, occurring in various animal and plant tissues, especially liver, yeast, bran, peanuts, lean meats, poultry, and fish, and first prepared by the oxidation of nicotine. It is required by the body for the formation of the coenzymes nicotinamide-adenine dinucleotide (NAD) and nicotinamide-adenine dinucleotide phosphate (NADP), which are important in biochemical oxidations, and it also has a pellagra-curative property and a vasodilating action. The official preparation [USP], occurring as white crystals or crystalline powder, is administered orally and parenterally in the prophylaxis and treatment of pellagra, to improve the peripheral circulation, and to depress the blood cholesterol level. Called also *nicotinic acid.*

niacinamide (ni″ah-sin-am′īd)   chemical name: 3-pyridinecarboxamide. The amide of niacin, $C_6H_6N_2O$, which lacks the vasodilating action of the parent compound. The official preparation [USP], occurring as a white, crystalline powder, is administered in the prophylaxis and treatment of pellagra. Called also *nicotinamide.*

NIAID   National Institute of Allergy and Infectious Diseases.

nialamide (ni-al′ah-mīd)   chemical name: 4-pyridinecarboxylic acid 2-[3-oxo-3-[(phenylmethyl)amino]propyl]hydrazide. A monoamine oxidase inhibitor, $C_{16}H_{18}N_4O_2$, occurring as a white, crystalline powder; it has been used orally as an antidepressant.

NIAMD   National Institute of Arthritis and Metabolic Diseases.

Niamid (ni′ah-mid)   trademark for a preparation of nialamide.

nibroxane (ni-broks′ān)   chemical name: 5-bromo-2-methyl-5-nitro-1,3-dioxane; a topical antimicrobial, $C_5H_8BrNO_4$.

Nicalex (nik′ah-leks)   trademark for a preparation of aluminum nicotinate.

Nicander (nik-an′der) (3rd century B.C.)   a celebrated Greek physician and poet. Two of his works (on toxicology), the *Theriaca* and the *Alexipharmaca,* have survived. He is said to have been the first writer to describe the use of leeches in medicine.

niccolum (nik′o-lum), gen. *nic′coli* [L.]   nickel.

nicergoline (ni-ser′go-lēn)   chemical name: 10-methoxy-1,6-dimethylergoline-8β-methanol 5-bromo-3-pyridinecarboxylate (ester); a vasodilator, $C_{24}H_{26}BrN_3O_3$.

niche (nich)   a defect in an otherwise even surface, especially a depression or recess in the wall of a hollow organ, as seen in the roentgenogram, or such a depression in an organ visible to the naked eye.   **Barclay's n.,** a deformity of the cap in the roentgenogram in duodenal ulcer consisting of a small projection.   **ecologic n.,** the place of an organism within its community or ecosystem.   **enamel n.,** either of two depressions between the dental lamina and the developing tooth germ, one pointing distally (*distal enamel n.*) and the other mesially (*mesial enamel n.*).   **Haudek's n.,** see under *sign.*   **n. of round window,** fossula fenestrae cochleae.

NICHHD   National Institute of Child Health and Human Development.

Nichrome (nik′krōm)   trademark for an alloy of nickel and chromium, having a melting point between that of brass and that of iron, and being very durable because of its resistance to oxidation under heat; widely used for laboratory equipment.

nickel (nik′el) [L. *niccolum*]   a silver-white metallic element: symbol, Ni; specific gravity, 8.9; atomic number, 28; atomic weight, 58.71.   **n. carbonyl,** a volatile liquid, Ni(CO)₄, used in industry, which may produce serious pulmonary edema and dyspnea.

nicking (nik′ing)   localized constrictions in the retinal blood vessels seen in arterial hypertension.

Nicklès' test (ne-klēz′) [François Joseph J. *Nicklès,* a French chemist, 1821–1869]   see under *tests.*

niclosamide (ni-klo′sah-mīd)   chemical name: 5-chloro-N-(2-chloro-4-nitrophenyl)-2-hydroxybenzamide. An anthelmintic, $C_{13}H_8Cl_2N_2O_4$, occurring as a pale yellow, crystalline powder, effective against the tapeworms *Diphyllobothrium latum, Hymenolepsis nana, Taenia saginata,* and the adults of *T. solium;* administered orally.

Nicol prism (nik′ol) [William *Nicol,* Scottish physicist, 1768–1851]   see under *prism.*

Nicolas-Favre disease (ne-ko-lah fav′r) [Joseph *Nicolas,* born 1869; M. *Favre,* French physicians]   lymphogranuloma venereum.

Nicolle (ne-kol′)   see *Nicollella.*

Nicollella (nĭ-ko-lel′ah) [Charles Jules Henri *Nicolle,* French physician, 1866–1936, noted for his discovery of the role of body lice in the transmission of typhus fever; winner of the Nobel prize for medicine in 1928]   a genus of holotrichous ciliate protozoa found in the intestinal tract of the gundi (*Ctenodactylus gundi*), a northern African rodent.

Niconyl (ni′ko-nil)   trademark for a preparation of isoniazid.

Nicotiana (nik″o-she-a′nah) [Jean *Nicot* de Villemain, 1530–1600, who introduced tobacco chewing to Catherine de Medici]   a genus of solanaceous annual plants, native to tropical America, from which tobacco is derived, mainly from *N. tabacum* L. and its varieties.

nicotinamide (nik″o-tin′ah-mīd)   niacinamide.   **n.-adenine dinucleotide (NAD),** the dinucleotide of nicotinamide and of adenine, a coenzyme found widely in nature and involved in numerous enzymatic reactions, in which it serves as an electron carrier by being alternately oxidized (NAD⁺) and reduced (NADH). The products of hydrolysis are 1 molecule of adenine, 1 of nicotinamide, 2 of *d*-ribose, and 2 of phosphoric acid. Called also *codehydrogenase I, coenzyme I* (*CoI*), *dihydroenzyme I,* and formerly *diphosphopyridine nucleotide* (*DPN*).   **n.-adenine dinucleotide phosphate (NADP),** a coenzyme required for a limited number of reactions, and similar to nicotinamide-adenine dinucleotide, except for the inclusion of 3 phosphate units. It serves as an electron carrier linking catabolic reactions (in the reduced form, NADPH) to biosynthetic (anabolic) reactions, where it gives up an electron (oxidized form, NADP⁺). Called also *coenzyme II, codehydrogenase II* (*CoII*), *triphosphopyridine nucleotide* (*TPN*), and *Warburg's coenzyme.*

nicotinamidemia (nik″o-tin-am″ĭ-de′me-ah)   the presence of nicotinamide in the blood.

nicotine (nik′o-tēn, nik′o-tin) [L. *nicotiana* tobacco]   chemical name: β-pyridyl-α-N-methylpyrrolidine. A very poisonous colorless, soluble fluid alkaloid, $C_{10}H_{14}N_2$, with a pyridine-like odor and a burning taste, obtained from tobacco or produced synthetically. It is used as an agricultural insecticide and, in veterinary medicine, as an external parasiticide and is used in pharmacological and physiological studies for its neurological effects (see *nicotinic*).

nicotinic (nik″o-tin′ik)   denoting the effect of nicotine and other drugs in initially stimulating and subsequently, in high doses, inhibiting neural impulses at autonomic ganglia and the neuromuscular junction.

nicotinism (nik′o-tin-izm″)   poisoning by nicotine, characterized by stimulation and subsequent depression of the central and autonomic nervous systems, with death due to respiratory paralysis.

nicotinolytic (nik″o-tin-o-lit′ik) [*nicotine* + Gr. *lysis* dissolution]   destroying or suppressing the toxic action of nicotine.

β-nicotyrine (nik-o′ti-rin)   chemical name: 3-(1-methyl-2-pyrryl)pyridine. An alkaloid, $C_{10}H_{10}N_2$, from tobacco, which occurs as an oily liquid with a characteristic odor, and has insecticidal properties.

nicoumalone (ni-koo′mah-lōn)   acenocoumarin.

Nicozide (nik′o-zīd)   trademark for preparations of isoniazid.

nictation (nik-ta′shun)   nictitation.

nictitation (nik″tĭ-ta′shun) [L. *nictitare* to wink]   the act of winking.

nidal (ni′dal)   pertaining to a nidus.

nidation (ni-da′shun) [L. *nidus* nest]   implantation of the conceptus in the endometrium.

nidi (ni′di) [L.]   plural of *nidus.*

NIDR   National Institute of Dental Research.

nidus (ni′dus), pl. *ni′di* [L. "nest"]   1. the point of origin or focus of a morbid process. 2. nucleus, def. 2.   **n. a′vis,** a depression in the cerebellum between the posterior velum and the uvula, the location of the tonsil of the cerebellum.   **n. hirun′dinis,** n. avis.

Niemann's disease (splenomegaly) (ne′man) [Albert *Niemann,* German pediatrician, 1880–1921]   Niemann-Pick disease.

Niewenglowski's ray (nya-ven-glov′ske) [Gaston Henri *Niewenglowski,* French physicist]   see under *ray.*

nifedipine (ni-fed′ĭ-pēn)   chemical name: 1,4-dihydro-2,6-dimethyl-4-(2-nitrophenyl)pyridinedicarboxylic acid dimethyl ester. A coronary vasodilator, $C_{17}H_{18}N_2O_6$, used in the treatment of coronary insufficiency and angina of effort.

nifungin (ni-fun′jin)   an antifungal polypeptide derived from *Aspergillus giganteus.*

nifuradene (ni-fūr′ah-dēn)   chemical name: 1-[[(5-nitro-2-furanyl)methylene]amino]-2-imidazolidinone; an antibacterial, $C_8H_8N_4O_4$.

nifuraldezone (ni-fūr-al′de-zōn) chemical name: 5-nitro-2-fur-aldehyde semioxamazone; an antibacterial, $C_7H_6N_4$.

nifuratel (ni-fūr′ah-tel) chemical name: 5-[(methylthio)-methyl]-3-[[(5-nitro-2-furanyl)methylene]amino]-2-oxazolidinone; an antibacterial, antifungal, and antitrichomonal, $C_{10}H_{11}N_3O_5S$.

nifuratrone (ni-fūr′ah-trōn) chemical name: N-(2-hydroxy-ethyl)-α-(5-nitro-2-furyl)nitrone; an antibacterial, $C_7H_8N_2O_5$.

nifurdazil (ni-fūr′dah-zil) chemical name: 1-(2-hydroxyethyl)-3-[[(5-nitro-2-furanyl)methylene]amino]-2-imidazolidinone; an antibacterial, $C_{10}H_{12}N_4O_5$.

nifurimide (ni-fūr′ĭ-mīd) chemical name: (±)-4-methyl-1-[[(5-nitro-2-furanyl)methylene]amino]-2-imidazolidinone; an antibacterial, $C_9H_{18}N_4O_4$.

nifurmerone (ni-fūr′mer-ōn) chemical name: 2-chloro-1-(5-ni-tro-2-furanyl)ethanone; an antifungal agent, $C_6H_4ClNO_4$.

nifuroxime (ni′′fūr-ok′sēm) chemical name: 5-nitro-2-furancar-boxaldehyde oxime. A fungicide, $C_{13}H_8Cl_2N_2O_4$, occurring as a colorless to pale yellow, somewhat viscous liquid; used in combina-tion with furazolidone (an antibacterial and antiprotozoal agent) in the treatment of bacterial, candidal, and trichomonal vaginitis due to susceptible organisms, administered intravaginally.

nifurpirinol (ni′′fūr-pēr′ĭ-nōl) chemical name: 6-[2-(5-nitro-2-furanyl)ethenyl]-2-pyridinemethanol; an antibacterial, $C_{12}H_{10}N_2O_4$.

nifurquinazol (ni-fūr-kwin′ah-zōl) chemical name: 2,2′[[2-(5-nitro-2-furanyl)-4-quinazolinyl]imino]bisethanol; an antibacte-rial, $C_{16}H_{16}N_4O_5$.

nifursemizone (ni′′fūr-sem′ĭ-zōn) chemical name: 1-ethyl-2-[(2-nitro-2-furanyl)methylene]hydrazinecarboxamide. An antipro-tozoal, $C_8H_{10}N_4O_4$, effective against Histomonas; used in poultry.

nifursol (ni′fūr-sōl) chemical name: 2-hydroxy-3,5-dinitroben-zoic acid [(5-nitro-2-furanyl)methylene]hydrazide. An antiproto-zoal, $C_{12}H_7N_5O_9$, effective against Histomonas; used in poultry.

nightmare (nīt′mār) a terrifying dream; called also oneiro-dynia.

nightshade (nīt′shād) a plant of the genus Solanum. **deadly n.,** belladonna leaf.

NIGMS National Institute of General Medical Sciences.

nigra (ni′grah) [L. "black"] the substantia nigra.

nigral (ni′gral) pertaining to the substantia nigra.

nigricans (ni′grĭ-kans) [L.] blackish.

nigrities (ni-grish′e-ēz) [L.] blackness. **n. lin′guae,** black tongue.

nigrosin (ni′gro-sin) an aniline dye, $C_{36}H_{27}N_3$, having a special affinity for ganglion cells, used to stain tissues from the central nervous system for study under the microscope.

nigrostriatal (ni′′gro-stri-a′tal) projecting from the substantia nigra to the corpus striatum; said of a bundle of nerve fibers.

NIH National Institutes of Health.

nihilism (ni′hil-izm) [L. nihil nothing + -ism] a form of delu-sion in which, to the patient, everything no longer exists. **therapeutic n.,** skepticism regarding the therapeutic value of drugs.

nikethamide (nĭ-keth′ah-mīd) chemical name: N,N-diethyl-3-pyridinecarboxamide. A central and respiratory stimulant, $C_{10}H_{14}N_2O$, occurring as a colorless to pale yellow, somewhat viscous liquid; used to counteract respiratory and central nervous system depression and circulatory failure, administered intramuscularly and intravenously.

Nikiforoff's method (ne′′ke-for′ofs) [Mikhail Nikiforoff, Russian dermatologist, 1858–1915] see under method.

Nikolsky's sign (nĭ-kol′skēz) [Petr Vasilyevich Nikolsky, Russian dermatologist, 1858–1940] see under sign.

Nilevar (ni′lĕ-var) trademark for preparations of norethandro-lone.

nimazone (nim′ah-zōn) chemical name: 3-(4-chlorophenyl)-4-imino-2-oxo-1-imidazolideneacetonitrile; an anti-inflammatory, $C_{11}H_9ClN_4O$.

Nimeh's method (ne′mez) [William Nimeh, Lebanese gastroen-terologist, born 1891] see under method.

NIMH National Institute of Mental Health.

nimidane (nim′ĭ-dān) chemical name: 4-chloro-N-1,3-dithietan-2-ylidene-2-methylbenzeneamine; a veterinary acaricide, $C_9H_8ClNS_2$.

nimiety (nĭ-mi′ĕ-te) [L. nimis overmuch + -ety state or condition of] (obs.) repletion or excess, as that degree of repletion or ex-cess of water which, beyond satiety, elicits aversion to the ingestion of fluids.

NINDB National Institute of Neurological Diseases and Blind-ness.

Ninhydrin (nin-hi′drin) trademark for a preparation of trike-tohydrindene hydrate.

niobium (ni-o′be-um) [named for Niobe, of Greek mythology, who was turned into stone] the chemical element, atomic number, 41; atomic weight, 92.906; symbol, Nb. It was formerly called columbium.

Nionate (ni′o-nāt) trademark for a preparation of ferrous glu-conate.

NIOSH National Institute of Occupational Safety and Health.

niperyt (ni′per-it) pentaerythritol tetranitrate.

niphablepsia (nif′′ah-blep′se-ah) [Gr. nipha snow + ablepsia blindness] snow blindness.

niphotyphlosis (nif′′o-tif-lo′sis) [Gr. nipha snow + typhlōsis blindness] snow blindness.

nipple (nip′′l) the pigmented projection on the anterior surface of the mammary gland, surrounded by the areola; it gives outlet to milk from the breast. Called also papilla mammae [NA], mamilla, and thelium. Also, any similarly shaped structure.

Nippostrongylus (nip′′o-stron′jĭ-lus) a genus of hookworms of the family Trichostrongylidae. **N. mu′ris,** a species occurring in rats.

Nipride (nip′rid) trademark for a preparation of sodium nitro-prusside.

niridazole (nĭ-rid′ah-zōl) chemical name: 1-(5-nitro-2-thiazo-lyl)-2-imidazolidinone; an antischistosomal, $C_6H_6N_4O_3S$, occur-ring as a yellow, crystalline powder; it is also used in the treatment of intestinal and extraintestinal amebiasis and in dracunculiasis, administered orally.

nisbuterol mesylate (nis-bu′tĕ-rōl) chemical name: (±)-4-methoxy benzoic acid 2-(acetyloxy)-4-[2-[(1,1-dimethylethyl)-amino]-1-hydroxy ethyl]phenyl ester methanesulfonate (salt); a bronchodilator, $C_{22}H_{27}NO_6 \cdot CH_4O_3S$.

Nisentil (ni′sen-til) trademark for a preparation of alphapro-dine.

nisin (ni′sin) an antibiotic substance from cultures of lactic acid streptococci, said to be effective against gram-positive organisms, including Mycobacterium tuberculosis.

nisobamate (ni-so-bah′māt) chemical name: 2-(hydroxyme-thyl)-2,3-dimethylpentyl isopropylcarbamate carbamate(ester); a minor tranquilizer, sedative, and hypnotic, $C_{13}H_{26}N_2O_4$.

nisoxetine (nĭ-soks′ĕ-tēn) chemical name: (±)-γ-(2-methoxy-phenoxy)-N-methylbenzenepropanamine; an antidepressant, $C_{17}H_{21}NO_2$.

Nissl bodies (granules, substance), degeneration, method of staining (nis′′lz) [Franz Nissl, neurologist in Hei-delberg, 1860–1919] see under body, degeneration, and Table of Stains.

nisterime acetate (ni-stēr′ēm) chemical name: 17β-(acetyl-oxy)-2α-chloro-5α-androstan-3-one 3-[O-(4-nitrophenyl)oxime]; an androgen, $C_{27}H_{35}ClN_2O_5$.

nisus (ni′sus) [L.] an effort, strong tendency, or molimen.

nit (nit) the egg of a louse.

Nitabuch's layer (stria, zone) (ne′tah-books) [Raissa Nita-buch, German physician of 19th century] see under layer.

nitarsone (ni-tar′sōn) chemical name: (4-nitrophenyl) arsonic acid; an antiprotozoal, $C_6H_6AsNO_5$, effective against Histomonas; used in poultry.

nitavirus (ni′′tah-vi′rus) [nuclear inclusion type A] a name suggested, but not generally accepted, for herpesviruses that induce formation of single homogeneous eosinophilic inclusion bodies occupying most of the central area of the nucleus of the infected cells, and clearly separated from the marginated chroma-tin (A-type inclusions).

niter (ni′ter) nitre.

nithiamide (ni-thi′ah-mīd) chemical name: N-(5-nitro-2-thiazo-lyl)acetamide; a veterinary antibiotic, $C_5H_5N_3O_3S$.

niton (ni′ton) radon.

nitramine (ni-tram′in) a nitro derivative of an amine.

nitramisole hydrochloride (ni-tram′ĭ-sōl) chemical name: (±)-2,3,5,6-tetrahydro-6-(3-nitrophenyl)-imidazo[2,1-b]thiazole monohydrochloride; an anthelmintic, $C_{11}H_{11}N_3O_2S \cdot HCl$.

nitratase (ni′trah-tās) [nitrate + -ase] a bacterial enzyme cata-lyzing the reduction of nitrate to nitrite.

nitrate (ni′trāt) [L. nitratum] any salt of nitric acid. Organic ni-trates are used in the treatment of angina pectoris.

nitrazepam (ni-trah′zĕ-pam) chemical name: 1,3-dihydro-7-ni-tro-5-phenyl-2H-1,4-benzodiazepin-2-one. One of the benzodiaze-pine tranquilizers, $C_{15}H_{11}N_3O$, used as an anticonvulsant and hypnotic.

nitre (ni′ter) [L. nitrum; Gr. nitron] potassium nitrate, or saltpe-ter. **cubic n.,** sodium nitrate.

nitremia (ni-tre′me-ah) azotemia.

nitric (ni′trik) pertaining to or containing nitrogen, applied es-pecially to compounds containing nitrogen with a higher valence than that contained in the nitrous compounds.

nitridation (ni-trĭ-da′shun) combination with nitrogen to form a nitride.

nitride (ni′trīd) a binary compound of nitrogen with a metal.

nitrification (ni′′trĭ-fi-ka′shun) [nitric acid + L. facere to make] the bacterial oxidation of ammonia to nitrate and nitrite in the soil.

nitrifier (ni′trĭ-fi″er) a nitrifying microorganism.

nitrifying (ni′trĭ-fi″ing) oxidizing ammonia to nitrite and then to nitrate, the first step being carried out by *Nitrosomonas* and *Nitrosococcus* and the second by *Nitrobacter*.

nitrilase (ni′tril-ās) an enzyme which catalyzes the decomposition of nitriles.

nitrile (ni′tril) an organic compound containing trivalent nitrogen attached to one carbon atom, ·C::N.

nitrite (ni′trīt) any salt of nitrous acid. Organic nitrites are used in the treatment of angina pectoris.

nitritoid (ni′trĭ-toid) resembling a nitrite or the reaction caused by a nitrite.

nitrituria (ni″trĭ-tu′re-ah) [*nitrite* + Gr. *ouron* urine + -*ia*] the presence of nitrites in the urine.

nitro- (ni′tro) a prefix indicating presence of the group —NO_2.

nitro-amine (ni′tro-am′in) nitramine.

nitro-anisol (ni″tro-an′ĭ-sol) a nitro derivative of anisol, NO_2·· C_6H_4·O·CH_3.

Nitrobacter (ni″tro-bak′ter) [L. *nitrum* nitre + *bactrum* rod] a genus of microorganisms of the family Nitrobacteraceae, suborder Pseudomonadineae, order Pseudomonadales, occurring as rod-shaped cells which oxidize nitrites to nitrates. It includes two species, *N. ag′ilis* and *N. winograd′skyi*.

Nitrobacteraceae (ni″tro-bak″te-ra′se-e) a family of Schizomycetes (order Pseudomonadales, suborder Pseudomonadineae), occurring as rod-shaped, ellipsoidal, spherical or spirillar cells, deriving energy exclusively from oxidation of ammonia to nitrite, or of nitrite to nitrate; also known informally as the nitrifying bacteria. It includes seven genera, *Nitrobacter, Nitrocystis, Nitrosococcus, Nitrosocystis, Nitrosogloea, Nitrosomonas,* and *Nitrosospira.*

nitrobacteria (ni″tro-bak-te′re-ah) plural of *nitrobacterium.*

nitrobacterium (ni″tro-bak-te′re-um), pl. *nitrobacte′ria.* A microorganism that oxidizes ammonia to nitrites.

nitrobenzene (ni″tro-ben′zēn) a poisonous benzene derivative, $C_6H_5NO_2$, occurring as a colorless to pale yellow, oily liquid; used in the manufacture of aniline. Called also *nitrobenzol* and *oil of mirbane.*

nitrobenzol (ni″tro-ben′zol) nitrobenzene.

nitroblue tetrazolium (ni′tro-blu tet″rah-zo′le-um) a yellow water-soluble dye that on reduction is converted to a dark blue water-insoluble formazan; see also under *tests.*

nitrocellulose (ni″tro-sel′u-lōs) pyroxylin.

nitrocycline (ni-tro-si′klēn) chemical name: 4-(dimethylamino)-1,4,4a,5,5a,6,11,12a-octahydro-3,10,12,12a-tetrahydroxy-7-nitro-1,11-dioxo-2-naphthacenecarboxamide; an antibiotic, $C_{21}H_{21}N_3O_9$.

Nitrocystis (ni″tro-sis′tis) a genus of microorganisms of the family Nitrobacteraceae, suborder Pseudomonadineae, order Pseudomonadales, occurring as ellipsoidal or rod-shaped cells, which are embedded in slime to form zoogloea and which oxidize nitrites to nitrates. It includes two species, *N. micropuncta′ta* and *N. sarcinoi′des.*

nitrofuran (ni-tro-fu′ran) any of a group of antibacterials, including furazolidone, nitrofurazone, nitrofurantoin, and related compounds, which are effective against a wide range of bacteria.

nitrofurantoin (ni″tro-fu-ran′to-in) [USP] chemical name: 1-[[(5-nitro-2-furanyl)methyl]amino]-2,4-imidazolidinedione. A synthetic antibacterial, $C_8H_6N_4O_5$, occurring as lemon-yellow crystals or fine powder, effective against many gram-negative and gram-positive organisms, including *Escherichia coli, Staphylococcus pyogenes, Streptococcus pyogenes, Aerobacter aerogenes,* and *Paracolobactrum* species; used in the treatment of urinary tract infections due to susceptible bacteria, administered orally.

nitrofurazone (ni″tro-fu′rah-zōn) [USP] chemical name: 2-[(5-nitro-2-furanyl)methylene]hydrazinecarboxamide. An antibacterial $C_6H_6N_4O_4$, occurring as a lemon yellow, crystalline powder, effective against a wide variety of gram-negative and gram-positive organisms. It is used topically as a local anti-infective in many skin lesions, including wounds, burns, skin infections, and ulcers; to aid healing and prevent infection of skin grafts; and in the treatment of otitis media and externa, urethritis, and eye infections. It has also been used orally in the treatment of African trypanosomiasis.

nitrogen (ni′tro-jen) [Gr. *nitron* niter + *gennan* to produce] 1. a colorless, gaseous element found free in the air; symbol, N; specific gravity, 0.9713; atomic number, 7; atomic weight, 14.007. It constitutes part of the atmosphere, forming about four fifths of common air. Chemically, it is almost inert, but forms by combination nitric acid and ammonia. Nitrogen is important biologically, being a constituent of protein and nucleic acids and thus present in all living cells. It is a gas unfitted to support respiration; not a poison, but proving fatal if breathed alone, because of the want of oxygen. It is soluble in the blood and body fluids and when released as bubbles of gas by reduction of atmospheric pressure causes serious symptoms. See *decompression sickness,* under *sickness.* 2. [NF] N_2; nitrogen containing not less than 99 per cent, by volume, of N_2. It is used to replace air in pharmaceutical preparations. **amide n.,** that portion of the nitrogen in protein that exists in the form of acid amides. **n. dioxide,** a brownish, irritant gas, NO_2, generated by the decomposition of nitrogen tetroxide or the reaction of metals with concentrated nitric acid. **n. monoxide,** nitrous oxide. **n. mustards,** see under *mustard.* **nomadic n.,** free nitrogen from the air which enters into plant and animal growth. **nonprotein n.,** the nitrogenous constituents of the blood exclusive of the protein bodies. It consists of the nitrogen of urea, uric acid, creatine, creatinine, amino acids, polypeptides, and an undetermined part known as *rest nitrogen.* **n. pentoxide,** a crystalline compound, N_2O_5, or nitric anhydride, which combines with water to form nitric acid. **n. peroxide, n. tetroxide,** a poisonous volatile liquid, N_2O_4, decomposing at room temperature to nitrogen dioxide (q.v.). **rest n.,** see *nonprotein n.* **urea n.,** see under *urea.*

nitrogenase (ni′tro-jen-ās) as enzyme system of nitrogen-fixing bacteria and blue-green algae that catalyzes the reduction of molecular nitrogen (N_2) to ammonia (NH_3).

nitrogen-fixing (ni′tro-jen-fiks′ing) accomplishing nitrogen fixation (see under *fixation*); said of certain bacteria.

nitrogenization (ni″tro-jen-i-za′shun) the act of impregnating with nitrogen.

nitrogenous (ni-troj′ĕ-nus) containing nitrogen.

nitroglycerin (ni-tro-glis′er-in) chemical name: glyceryl trinitrate. A colorless to yellow liquid, $C_3H_5N_3O_9$, formed by the action of nitric and sulfuric acids on glycerine. It explodes on concussion, but is rendered safe when compounded in tablets with mannitol. The official preparation [USP] is used in medicine chiefly in the prophylaxis and treatment of angina pectoris, administered sublingually.

Nitroglyn (ni′tro-glin) trademark for a preparation of nitroglycerin.

Nitrol (ni′trol) trademark for preparations of nitroglycerin.

nitromannite (ni″tro-man′īt) mannitol hexanitrate.

nitromersol (ni″tro-mer′sol) [USP] chemical name: 5-methyl-2-nitro-7-oxa-8-mercurabicyclo[4.2.0]octa-1,3,5-triene. A mercurial compound, $C_7H_5HgNO_3$, occurring as brownish yellow to yellow granules or powder; used as a local anti-infective, applied topically to the skin and mucous membranes. It is also used to disinfect surgical and dental instruments.

nitrometer (ni-trom′-ĕ-ter) [*nitrogen* + Gr. *metron* measure] an apparatus for measuring the quantity of nitrogen given off in a reaction.

nitromethane (ni″tro-meth′ān) a nitrated form of methane, CH_3NO_2, which is a powerful explosive.

nitromifene citrate (ni-tro′mĭ-fēn) chemical name: 1-[2-[4-[1-(4-methoxyphenyl)-2-nitro-2-phenylethenyl]phenoxy]ethyl]pyrrolidene 2-hydroxy-1,2,3-propanetricarboxylate (1:1); an antiestrogen, $C_{27}H_{28}N_2O_4 \cdot C_6H_8O_7$.

nitron (ni′tron) the name suggested by Sir W. Ramsay and R. W. Gray for the molecular weight of a radium emanation.

nitronaphthalene (ni″tro-naf′thah-lēn) a substance, $C_{10}H_7$·· NO_2, whose vapors may cause vesication and opacity of the cornea.

nitronaphthalin (ni″tro-naf′thah-lin) nitronaphthalene.

nitrophenol (ni″tro-fe′nol) an indicator, para-nitrophenylic acid, $C_6H_4(NO_2)OH$, with a pH range of 5 to 7; being colorless at 5 and yellow at 7.

nitropropiol (ni″tro-pro′pe-ol) orthonitrophenylpropiolic acid, $NO_2 \cdot C_6H_4 \cdot C$:$C \cdot COOH$: used as a test for sugar.

nitroprotein (ni″tro-pro′te-in) a nitrated protein made by treating serum protein with nitric acid.

nitroprusside (ni″tro-prus′īd) a salt of nitroprussic acid; see also under *sodium.*

nitrosaccharose (ni″tro-sak′ah-rōs) nitrated sucrose, an explosive and vasodilator used like nitroglycerin.

nitrosalol (ni″tro-sal′ol) an ester, $C_6H_4(OH)CO_2 \cdot C_6H_4NO_2$, in a yellowish, crystalline powder.

nitrosamine (ni″trōs-ah′mēn) any of a group of *N*-nitroso derivatives of secondary amines, (R_2N—NO), formed by the combining of nitrates with amines; some nitrosamines show carcinogenic activity.

nitrosate (ni′tro-sāt) to convert into a nitroso compound.

nitrosation (ni″tro-sa′shun) conversion into a nitroso compound.

nitroscanate (ni″tro-skan′āt) chemical name: 1-isothiocyanato-4-(4-nitrophenoxy)benzene; a veterinary anthelmintic, $C_{13}H_8N_2O_3S$.

nitrose (ni′trōs) a term used to include nitric and nitrous acids.

nitrosification (ni-tro″sĭ-fi-ka′shun) the oxidation of ammonia into nitrites.

nitrosifying (ni-tro″sĭ-fi′ing) oxidizing ammonia into nitrites; said of certain nitrogen bacteria.

nitroso- (ni-tro′so) a prefix indicating presence of the group —N:O.

nitrosobacteria (ni-tro″so-bak-te′re-ah) plural of *nitrosobacterium*.

nitrosobacterium (ni-tro″so-bak-te′re-um), pl. *nitrosobacte′ria*. A microorganism that oxidizes nitrites to nitrates.

Nitrosococcus (ni″tro-so-kok′us) [L. *nitrosus* full of soda + Gr. *kokkos* berry] a genus of microorganisms of the family Nitrobacteraceae, suborder Pseudomonadineae, order Pseudomonadales, occurring as large spherical, nonmotile cells, which oxidize ammonia to nitrite. The type species is *N. nitro′sus*.

Nitrosocystis (ni-tro″so-sis′tis) a genus of microorganisms of the family Nitrobacteraceae, suborder Pseudomonadineae, order Pseudomonadales, occurring as ellipsoidal or elongated cells which unite in cystlike compact rounded aggregates, and oxidizing ammonia to nitrite. It includes two species, *N. coccoi′des* and *N. javanen′sis*.

Nitrosogloea (ni-tro″so-gle′ah) a genus of microorganisms of the family Nitrobacteraceae, suborder Pseudomonadineae, order Pseudomonadales, occurring as ellipsoidal or rod-shaped bacteria, embedded in slime to form zoogloea, and oxidizing ammonia to nitrite. It includes three species, *N. membrana′cea*, *N. merismoi′des*, and *N. schizobacteroi′des*.

nitroso-indol (ni-tro″so-in′dol) a compound which gives a red reaction when indol is treated with sulfuric acid and potassium nitrite.

Nitrosomonas (ni-tro″so-mo′nas) [L. *nitrosus* full of soda + Gr. *monas* unit] a genus of microorganisms of the family Nitrobacteraceae, suborder Pseudomonadineae, order Pseudomonadales, occurring as nonmotile ellipsoidal cells, which oxidize ammonia to nitrite more rapidly than other genera of the family. It includes two species, *N. europae′a* and *N. monocel′la*.

Nitrosospira (ni-tro″so-spi′rah) [L. *nitrosus* full of soda + *spira* coil] a genus of microorganisms of the family Nitrobacteraceae, suborder Pseudomonadineae, order Pseudomonadales, occurring as spiral-shaped cells which oxidize ammonia to nitrite very slowly. It includes two species, *N. antarc′tica* and *N. brien′sis*.

nitrososubstitution (ni-tro″so-sub″sti-tu′shun) the substitution of the radical nitroxyl for some other radical or atom in a compound.

nitrosourea (ni-tro″so-u-re′ah) any of a group of lipid-soluble proteins that function as alkylating agents, and which, because of their ability to penetrate the central nervous system, have been used as antineoplastics in the treatment of meningeal leukemia and brain tumors.

Nitrostat (ni′tro-stat) trademark for a preparation of nitroglycerin.

nitrosugars (ni″tro-shug′erz) a class of substances which have been used in the treatment of angina pectoris.

nitrosyl (ni′tro-sil) the univalent radical NO.

nitrous (ni′trus) pertaining to nitrogen in its lowest valency. **n. oxide**, a colorless gas, N_2O, having a sweetish taste and a pleasant odor and used as a general anesthetic or analgesic; called also *nitrogen monoxide*, *factitious air*, and *laughing gas*.

Nitrovas (ni′tro-vas) trademark for a preparation of nitroglycerin.

nitroxyl (ni-trok′sil) the radical NO_2.

nitryl (ni′tril) nitroxyl.

nivazol (ni′vah-zōl) chemical name: 2′(4-fluorophenyl)-2′*H*-pregna-2,4-dien-20-yno[3,2-*c*]pyrazol-17α-ol; a glucocorticoid, C_{28}-$H_{31}FN_2O$.

nivemycin (niv′ĕ-mi′sin) neomycin.

nivimedone sodium (nĭ-vi′mĕ-dōn) chemical name: 5,6-dimethyl-2-nitro-1*H*-indene-1,3(2*H*)-dione ion(1–)sodium monohydrate; an antiallergic agent, $C_{11}H_8NNaO_4 \cdot H_2O$.

NK. abbreviation for *Nomenklatur Kommission*, a committee of the Anatomical Society of Germany which has given supplementary names to the terminology of anatomy.

nl. nanoliter.

N.L.N. National League for Nursing.

Nm. abbreviation for L. *nux moscha′ta*, nutmeg.

nm. nanometer.

N.M.A. National Malaria Association; National Medical Association.

NMRI Naval Medical Research Institute, part of the National Naval Medical Center.

N.M.S.S. National Multiple Sclerosis Society.

N-Multistix (mul′tĭ-stiks) trademark for a reagent strip for testing urine specimens for protein, glucose, ketones, bilirubin, occult blood, urobilinogen, nitrite, and to indicate urinary pH.

nn. abbreviation for L. *nervi* (nerves).

N.N.D. *New and Nonofficial Drugs*, former annual publication of the American Medical Association containing descriptions of agents proposed for use in or on the human body in the prevention, diagnosis, or treatment of disease, which have been evaluated by the Council on Drugs of the A.M.A.

NO nitric oxide.

N_2O dinitrogen monoxide (nitrous oxide).

No chemical symbol for *nobelium*.

No. abbreviation of L. *nu′mero*, "to the number of."

Nobel prize (no-bel′) [Alfred Bernard *Nobel*, Swedish chemist and engineer, 1833–1896; the inventor of dynamite, under the terms of whose will the prizes were established] an award usually given annually for outstanding achievement in chemistry, physics, medicine and physiology, literature, and in the interest of world peace. First presented in 1901. An award for achievement in economics has since been added.

nobelium (no-be′le-um) [Alfred Bernard *Nobel*] the chemical element of atomic number 102, atomic weight 253, symbol No, obtained in 1958 by bombardment of ^{246}Cm with ^{12}C ions in a heavy ion linear accelerator.

Noble's position (no′b′lz) [Charles Percy *Noble*, American gynecologist, 1863–1935] see under *position*.

Nocard's bacillus [Edmond Isidore Étienne *Nocard*, French veterinarian, 1850–1903] *Salmonella typhimurium*.

Nocardia (no-kar′de-ah) [Edmond Isidore Étienne *Nocard*] a genus of actinomycetes of the family Actinomycetaceae, order Actinomycetales, separable into 40 or more species, of which a few are pathogenic and the remainder saprophytic forms. They are aerobic, fragment into bacillary or coccoid forms, and produce chains of spores by simple fragmentation of hyphal branches. Called also *Streptothrix*. **N. asteroi′des**, an acid-fast filamentous actinomycete producing pulmonary infection in man that simulates tuberculosis. The disease, considered to be an opportunistic infection, sometimes becomes systemic and may be fatal. See *nocardiosis*. **N. brasilien′sis**, an acid-fast species found in soil, which causes nocardiosis and maduromycosis in man. It is particularly prevalent in Mexico and South America, but has been reported worldwide. **N. ca′viae**, *N. otitidis-caviarum*. **N. farci′nica**, a species of acid-fast filamentous actinomycetes of uncertain classification, associated with a disease in cattle resembling tuberculosis; it is probably identical with *N. asteroides*. See *cattle farcy*, under *farcy*. **N. madu′rae**, *Actinomadura madurae*. **N. oti′tidis-cavia′rum**, a species isolated from an ear infection in guinea pigs and from soil in the United States and India; the species is related to *N. asteroides* and causes some cases of nocardiosis and maduromycosis.

nocardial (no-kar′de-al) pertaining to or caused by *Nocardia*.

nocardiasis (no″kar-di′ah-sis) nocardiosis.

nocardin (no-kar′din) an antibiotic substance from *Nocardia coeliaca*, active against tubercle bacilli.

nocardiosis (no-kar-de-o′sis) an acute or chronic suppurative infection, usually of the lungs but with a marked tendency to spread to any organ of the body, especially to the brain; abscess formation occurs in any organ, most commonly in the lungs, brain, or skin or subcutaneous tissue. Lung abscesses tend to cavitate with time. The causative agent in most instances is *Nocardia asteroides*, but *N. brasiliensis* and *N. caviae* cause occasional cases.

Nochtia (nok′te-ah) a genus of small nematode worms. **N. noch′ti**, a species of worms found in and apparently causing the production of tumors in the stomachs of Javanese monkeys.

noci- (no′se) [L. *nocere* to injure] a combining form denoting relation to injury or to a noxious or deleterious agent or influence.

nociassociation (no″se-ah-so″se-a′shun) the unconscious discharge of nervous energy under the stimulus of trauma, as in surgical shock.

nociceptive (no″se-sep′tiv) [*noci-* + L. *capere* to receive] receiving injury; said of a receptive neuron for painful sensations.

nociceptor (no″se-sep′tor) a receptor which is stimulated by injury; a receptor for pain. Cf. *beneceptor* and *ceptor* (def. 2).

nocifensor (no″se-fen′sor) [*noci-* + L. *fendere* to defend] Sir Thomas Lewis' name for a system of nerves in the skin and mucous membranes which are concerned with local defense against injury.

noci-influence (no″se-in′floo-ens) injurious or traumatic influence.

nociperception (no″se-per-sep′shun) the perception by the system of injurious (traumatic) stimuli.

nocodazole (no-ko′dah-zōl) chemical name: [5-(2-thienylcarbonyl)-1*H*-benzimidazolecarbamic acid methyl ester; an antineoplastic, $C_{14}H_{11}N_3O_3S$.

Noct. abbreviation for L. *noc′te*, at night.

noctalbuminuria (nok″tal-bu″mĭ-nu′re-ah) [L. *nox* night + *albuminuria*] the presence of excessive amounts of albumin in the urine secreted during the night.

noctambulation (nok″tam-bu-la′shun) [L. *noctambulatio*; *nox* night + *ambulare* to walk] somnambulism, def. 1.

noctambulic (nok″tam-bu′lik) pertaining to or marked by sleep walking (somnambulism).

Noctec (nok′tek) trademark for preparations of chloral hydrate.

noctiphobia (nok″te-fo′be-ah) [L. *nox* night + *phobia*] morbid dread of night and its darkness and silence.

Noct. maneq. abbreviation for L. *noc′te mane′que*, at night and in the morning.

nocturia (nok-tu′re-ah) [L. *nox* night + Gr. *ouron* urine + *-ia*] excessive urination at night.

nocturnal (nok-tur′nal) [L. *nocturnus*] pertaining to, occurring at, or active at night.

nocuity (nok-u′ĭ-te) (*obs.*) noxiousness.

nodal (no′dal) pertaining to a node, particularly the atrioventricular node.

node (nōd) [L. *nodus* knot] a small mass of tissue in the form of a swelling, knot, or protuberance, either normal or pathological. See also *nodule* and *nodus*. **Aschoff's n., n. of Aschoff and Tawara,** nodus atrioventricularis. **atrioventricular n.,** nodus atrioventricularis. **axillary n's, axillary lymph n's,** nodi lymphatici axillares; see under *nodus*. **Bouchard's n's,** cartilaginous and bony enlargements of the proximal interphalangeal joints of the fingers in degenerative joint disease. Such nodules in the terminal interphalangeal joints are called *Heberden's nodes*. **bronchopulmonary lymph n's,** nodi lymphatici bronchopulmonales. **buccal lymph n's,** nodi lymphatici buccales. **celiac lymph n's,** nodi lymphatici celiaci. **cervical lymph n's, deep,** nodi lymphatici cervicales profundae. **cervical lymph n's, superficial,** nodi lymphatici cervicales superficiales. **Cloquet's n., n. of Cloquet,** the highest of the deep inguinal lymph nodes; called also *Cloquet's gland*. **colic lymph n's, left,** nodi lymphatici colici sinistri. **colic lymph n's, middle,** nodi lymphatici colici medii. **colic lymph n's, right,** nodi lymphatici colici dextri. **cubital lymph n's,** nodi lymphatici cubitales. **Delphian n.,** a lymph node encased in the fascia in the midline, just anterior to the thyroid isthmus, so called because it is exposed first at surgery and, if diseased, is indicative of disease in the thyroid gland, but not of a specific disease process. **Dürck's n's,** granulomatous perivascular infiltrations in the cerebral cortex in trypanosomiasis. **epigastric lymph n's,** nodi lymphatici epigastrici. **Ewald's n.,** sentinel n. **Féréol's n's** (*obs.*), subcutaneous nodes sometimes occurring in acute rheumatism. **Flack's n.,** sinoatrial n. **gastric lymph n's, left,** nodi lymphatici gastrici sinistri. **gastric lymph n's, right,** nodi lymphatici gastrici dextri. **gastroepiploic lymph n's,** lymph nodes associated with the left and right gastroepiploic arteries. **gouty n.,** a nodule produced by gouty inflammation. **Haygarth's n's,** joint swellings in arthritis deformans. **Heberden's n's,** small hard nodules, formed usually at the distal interphalangeal articulations of the fingers, produced by calcific spurs of the articular cartilage and associated with interphalangeal osteoarthritis. Heredity is an important etiologic factor. Called also *Heberden's sign*. Cf. *Bouchard's n's*. **hemal n's,** nodes with a rich content of erythrocytes within sinuses, having an organization much like a lymph node but no lymphatic supply, found near large blood vessels along the ventral side of the vertebrae and near the spleen and kidneys in various mammals, especially ruminants; their functions are probably like those of the spleen. The presence of such nodes in man is doubtful. A special type of hemal node is found in the pig; see *hemolymph n's, def. 2*. Called also *hemal glands, hemolymph n's,* and *vascular glands.* **hemolymph n's,** 1. hemal n's. 2. special types of hemal nodes found in the pig, having characteristics midway between those of ordinary lymph nodes and typical hemal nodes, containing both blood and lymphatic vessels, the contents of both of which mix in the sinuses; called also *hemolymph glands.* **Hensen's n.,** primitive knot. **hepatic lymph n's,** nodi lymphatici hepatici. **ileocolic lymph n's,** nodi lymphatici ileocolici. **iliac lymph n's,** nodi lymphatici iliaci. **iliac lymph n's, common,** nodi lymphatici iliaci communes. **iliac lymph n's, external,** nodi lymphatici iliaci externi. **iliac lymph n's, internal,** nodi lymphatici iliaci interni. **inguinal lymph n's, deep,** nodi lymphatici inguinales profundi. **inguinal lymph n's, superficial,** nodi lymphatici inguinales superficiales. **intercostal lymph n's,** nodi lymphatici intercostales. **Keith's n., Keith-Flack n.,** sinoatrial n. **Koch's n.,** nodus atrioventricularis. **lumbar lymph n's,** nodi lymphatici lumbales. **lymph n.,** any of the accumulations of lymphoid tissue organized as definite lymphoid organs, varying from 1 to 25 mm. in diameter, situated along the course of lymphatic vessels (see illustration accompanying *lymph*), and consisting of an outer cortical and an inner medullary part. The lymph nodes are the main source of lymphocytes of the peripheral blood and, as part of the reticuloendothelial system, serve as a defense mechanism by removing noxious agents, such as bacteria and toxins, and probably play a role in antibody production. Called also *nodus lymphaticus* [NA]. **mandibular lymph n's,** nodi lymphatici mandibulares. **mediastinal lymph n's, anterior,** nodi lymphatici mediastinales anteriores. **mediastinal lymph n's, posterior,** nodi lymphatici mediastinales posteriores. **mesenteric lymph n's,** nodi lymphatici mesenterici. **mesenteric lymph n's, inferior,** nodi lymphatici mesenterici inferiores. **mesenteric lymph n's, superior,** nodi lymphatici mesenterici superiores. **Meynet's n's,** nodules in the capsules of joints and in tendons in rheumatic disorders, especially of children. **occipital lymph n's,** nodi lymphatici occipitales. **Osler's n's,** small, raised, swollen tender areas, about the size of a pea, characteristically bluish but sometimes pink or red, and sometimes having a blanched center, occurring most commonly in the pads of the fingers or toes, in the thenar or hypothenar eminences, or the soles of the feet; they are practically pathognomonic

of subacute bacterial endocarditis. **pancreaticosplenic lymph n's,** nodi lymphatici pancreaticolienales. **parasternal lymph n's,** nodi lymphatici parasternales. **paratracheal n.,** any of the minute lymph nodes situated alongside the recurrent nerves on the lateral aspect of the trachea and esophagus, which help drain the thyroid gland. **parotid lymph n's, superficial and deep,** nodi lymphatici parotidei superficiales et profundi. **Parrot's n.,** see *Parrot's sign* (def. 2), under *sign*. **phrenic lymph n's,** nodi lymphatici phrenici. **popliteal lymph n's,** nodi lymphatici poplitei. **prelaryngeal n.,** a lymph node deep in the neck that helps drain the thyroid gland. **pretracheal n.,** a lymph node deep in the neck that helps drain the thyroid gland. **primitive n.,** primitive knot. **pulmonary lymph n's,** nodi lymphatici pulmonales. **pyloric lymph n's,** nodi lymphatici pylorici. **n's of Ranvier,** constrictions occurring on myelinated nerve fibers at regular intervals of about 1 millimeter; at these sites the myelin sheath is absent and the axon is enclosed only by Schwann cell processes. **retroauricular lymph n's,** nodi lymphatici retroauriculares. **retropharyngeal lymph nodes,** nodi lymphatici retropharyngei. **Rosenmüller's n.,** 1. pars palpebralis glandulae lacrimalis. 2. [pl.] nodi lymphatici inguinales profundi. **Rotter's n's,** lymph nodes occasionally found between the pectoralis major and minor muscles which often contain metastases from mammary cancer. **sacral lymph n's,** nodi lymphatici sacrales. **Schmidt's n.,** the medullated interannular segment of a nerve fiber. **Schmorl's n.,** an irregular or hemispherical bone defect in the upper or lower margin of the body of the vertebra. **sentinel n., signal n.,** an enlarged supraclavicular node which is often the first sign of an abdominal tumor; called also *Virchow's n.* or *gland,* and *Troisier's n.* **singer's n.,** a small white nodule occurring on the vocal cord in chorditis tuberosa. Called also *vocal nodule.* **sinoatrial n., sinus n.,** a microscopic collection of atypical cardiac muscle fibers at the superior end of the sulcus terminalis, at the junction of the superior vena cava and right atrium. Called also *nodus sinuatrialis* [NA]. The cardiac rhythm normally takes its origin in this node which is, for that reason, also known as the pacemaker of the heart. **submandibular lymph n's,** nodi lymphatici submandibulares. **submental lymph n's,** nodi lymphatici submentales. **syphilitic n.,** a swelling on a bone due to syphilitic periostitis. **n. of Tawara,** nodus atrioventricularis. **teacher's n.,** singer's n. **tibial lymph n's, anterior,** nodi lymphatici tibialis anterior. **tracheal lymph n's,** nodi lymphatici tracheales. **tracheobronchial lymph n's, inferior,** nodi lymphatici tracheobronchiales inferiores. **tracheobronchial lymph n's, superior,** nodi lymphatici tracheobronchiales superiores. **triticeous n.,** cartilago triticea. **Troisier's n., Virchow's n.,** signal n. **vital n.,** an old name applied to the respiratory centers.

nodi (no′di) plural of *nodus.*

nodose (no′dōs) [L. *nodosus*] having nodes or projections.

nodosity (no-dos′ĭ-te) [L. *nodositas*] 1. the quality or condition of being nodose. 2. a node. **Haygarth's n's,** see under *node.*

nodular (nod′u-lar) 1. like a nodule or node. 2. marked with nodules.

nodulated (nod′u-lāt″ed) marked with nodules.

nodulation (nod″u-la′shun) the presence of nodules.

nodule (nod′ūl) [L. *nodulus* little knot] a small boss or node which is solid and can be detected by touch; see also *nodulus.* **accessory thymic n's,** noduli thymici accessorii. **aggregate n's,** folliculi lymphatici aggregati. **Albini's n's,** gray nodules of the size of small grains, sometimes seen on the free edges of the atrioventricular valves of infants; they are remains of fetal structures. Called also *Cruveilhier's n's.* **n's of aortic valve,** see *noduli valvularum semilunarium.* **apple jelly n's,** minute translucent nodules of a distinctive yellowish or reddish brown color, visible on diascopic examination of the lesions of lupus vulgaris. **n's of Arantius,** see *noduli valvularum semilunarium.* **Aschoff's n's,** Aschoff bodies. **Bianchi's n's,** nodules of aortic valve; see *noduli valvularum semilunarium.* **Bohn's n's,** small white or yellow nodules near the midline of the palate in the newborn, which disappear soon after birth; they are small retention cysts arising from mucus glands. **Bouchard's n's** (*obs.*), see under *node.* **Busacca n's,** an accumulation of epithelioid cells and lymphocytes occurring in chronic inflammation of the iris, usually on the anterior surface about the region of the ciliary zone. **cortical n's,** nodules of closely packed lymphocytes in the cortical portion of a lymph gland. **Cruveilhier's n's,** Albini's n's. **Dalen-Fuchs n's,** small hemispherical mounds principally composed of epithelioid cells and cells of the retinal epithelium, seen in sympathetic ophthalmia and certain other disorders. **Fraenkel's n's,** typhus nodules of the cutaneous blood vessels. **Gamna n's,** brown or yellow pigmented nodules seen in the spleen in certain cases of enlargement, such as Gamna's disease and sideerotic splenomegaly; called also *nodules tabac.* **Gandy-Gamna n's,** Gamna n's. **Guatamahri's n's** (*obs.*), nodules on the scalp and face in onchocerciasis. **Hoboken's n's,** dilatations of the outer surface of the umbilical arteries. **Jeanselme's n's,** gummata of tertiary syphilis and of nonvenereal treponemal diseases, located on joint capsules, bursae or tendon sheaths; called also *juxta-articular n's* and *Steiner's tumors*. **juxta-articular n's,** Jeanselme's n's. **n's of Kerckring,** nodules of aortic valve; see *noduli valvularum semilunarium.* **Koeppe n's,** white to gray nodules observed at the pupillary border in chronic inflammation of the iris, and consisting of accumulations of epithelioid cells and lymphocytes. **Koester's n.,** a tubercle composed of one giant cell enclosed by a double layer of cells. **Leishman's n's,** (*obs.*), pinkish nodules observed in cutaneous leishmaniasis. **lentiform n.,** processus lenticularis. **Lutz-Jeanselme n's,** Jeanselme's n's. **lymphatic n's,** a term applied to lymph nodes, as well as to one of the small collections of lymphoid tissue (folliculus lymphaticus [NA]) situated deep to epithelial surfaces, and also to temporary small (about 1 mm. in diameter), dense accumulations of lymphocytes located within the cortex of a lymph node and expressing the cytogenetic and defense functions of the tissue. **lymphatic n's, solitary, of large intestine,** folliculi lymphatici solitarii intestini crassi. **lymphatic n's, solitary, of small intestine,** folliculi lymphatici solitarii intestini tenuis. **lymphatic n's of stomach,** folliculi lymphatici gastrici. **milkers' n's,** hard circumscribed nodules on the hands of persons who milk cows suffering from cowpox. **Morgagni's n's,** nodules of aortic valve; see *noduli valvularum semilunarium.* **Paterson's n's,** molluscum bodies. **pearly n.,** one of the nodules of bovine tuberculosis. **primary n.,** a lymph nodule without a germinal center, or apart from a center. **n's of pulmonary trunk valves,** see *noduli valvularum semilunarium.* **pulp n.,** denticle, def. 2. **rheumatic n's,** small round or oval, mostly subcutaneous nodules made up chiefly of a mass of Aschoff bodies and seen in cases of rheumatic fever. **Schmorl's n.,** a nodule seen in roentgenograms of the spine, due to prolapse of a nucleus pulposus into an adjoining vertebra. **secondary n.,** germinal center. **siderotic n's,** focal fibrotic lesions characterized by the presence of crystals of iron on the degenerated elastic tissue fibers, seen in the spleen in Banti's disease. **singers' n.,** a small white node occurring on the vocal cord in chorditis tuberosa. **surfers' n's,** hyperplastic, fibrosing, rarely ulcerated granulomas 1 to 3 cm. in diameter, occurring over bony prominences of the feet and legs of surfers, occurring as a result of repeated trauma from kneeling on surfboards; called also *Malibu disease* and *surfers' knobs* or *knots*. **n's tabac,** Gamna n's. **teachers' n.,** a nodule of the vocal cords in chorditis tuberosa. **triticeous n.,** cartilago triticea. **typhoid n.,** a mass of macrophages and other necrotic cells observed in the liver in typhoid fever. **typhus n's,** minute nodules in the skin, formed by perivascular infiltration of mononuclear cells in typhus. **n. of vermis,** nodulus vermis. **vestigial n.,** tuberculum auriculae. **vocal n.,** singer's node. **warm n.,** a nodule in the thyroid gland which shows the same ^{131}I uptake as the rest of the gland; normally not carcinomatous.

noduli (nod′u-li) [L.] plural of *nodulus*.

nodulous (nod′u-lus) nodose.

nodulus (nod′u-lus), pl. *nod′uli* [L., dim. of *nodus*] a nodule or small knot; used in anatomical nomenclature as a general term to designate a comparatively minute collection of tissue. **nod′uli aggrega′ti proces′sus vermifor′mis,** folliculi lymphatici aggregati processus vermiformis. **n. cerebel′li,** n. vermis. **n. intercarot′icus,** glomus caroticum. **n. lymphat′icus,** folliculus lymphaticus. **nod′uli lymphat′ici aggrega′ti [Peyer′i],** folliculi lymphatici aggregati. **nod′uli lymphat′ici bronchia′les,** lymph nodules situated in the lining of the bronchi. **nod′uli lymphat′ici conjunctiva′les,** lymph nodules situated in the conjunctiva. **nod′uli lymphat′ici gas′trici,** folliculi lymphatici gastrici. **nod′uli lymphat′ici laryn′gei,** folliculi lymphatici laryngei. **nod′uli lymphat′ici liena′les [Malpig′hii],** folliculi lymphatici lienales. **nod′uli lymphat′ici rec′ti,** folliculi lymphatici recti. **nod′uli lymphat′ici solita′rii intesti′ni cras′si,** folliculi lymphatici solitarii intestini crassi. **nod′uli lymphat′ici solita′rii intesti′ni ten′uis,** folliculi lymphatici solitarii intestini tenuis. **nod′uli lymphat′ici tuba′rii tu′bae auditi′vae,** lymphatic follicles about the pharyngeal end and internally along the median wall of the auditory tube; called also *Gerlach's tonsil.* **nod′uli lymphat′ici vagina′les,** small collections of lymphatic tissue deep to the epithelial surface of the vagina. **nod′uli lymphat′ici vesica′les,** collections of lymphatic tissue in the lining of the urinary bladder. **nod′uli thy′mici accesso′rii** [NA], accessory thymic nodules: portions of thymus tissue that have been detached from the stalk and left behind in the caudal migration of the gland in embryonic development. **nod′uli valvula′rum aor′tae,** former NA term for nodules of aortic valve; see *noduli valvularum semilunarium.* **nod′uli valvula′rum semiluna′rium** [NA], small fibrous tubercles, one at the center of the free margin of each of the three cusps of the valve of the pulmonary trunk (called also *noduli valvularum semilunarium [ventriculi dextri]* and *nodules of pulmonary trunk valve*) and of the aortic valve (called also *noduli valvularum aortae* or *nodules of aortic valve*, and *nodules of Arantius*). **nod′uli valvula′rum semiluna′rium [Aran′tii],** nodules of aortic valve; see *noduli valvularum semilunarium.* **nod′uli valvula′rum semiluna′rium [ventric′uli dex′tri],** see *noduli val-*

nodus (no′dus), pl. no′di [L.] a node or knot; used in anatomical nomenclature as a general term to designate a small mass of tissue. **n. atrioventricula′ris** [NA], atrioventricular node: a microscopic collection of specialized cardiac muscle fibers (Purkinje's fibers), located beneath the endocardium of the right atrium, and continuous with atrial muscle fibers and with the atrioventricular bundle; it is similar to but somewhat smaller than the nodus sinuatrialis. Called also *Aschoff's, Koch's,* and *Tawara's node.* **n. cor′dis,** see *trigona fibrosa cordis.* **n. curso′rius,** a point in the corpus striatum of some animals, as the rabbit, stimulation of which causes the animal to rush forward. **n. lymphat′icus** [NA], one of the accumulations of lymphoid tissue interposed throughout the lymphatic system. See *lymph node,* under *node.* Called also *lymphoglandula* and *lymphonodus* [NA alternative]. **no′di lymphat′ici apica′les** [NA], see *nodi lymphatici axillares.* **no′di lymphat′ici axilla′res** [NA], axillary lymph nodes: the lymph nodes of the axilla, which receive lymph from the arm and the thoracic wall. They comprise five groups: the apical nodes (nodi lymphatici apicales), lying medial to the axillary vein; the central (nodi lymphatici centrales), near the base of the axilla; the lateral (node lymphatici laterales), behind the axillary vein; the pectoral (nodi lymphatici pectorales), along the lateral thoracic veins; and the subscapular (nodi lymphatici subscapulares), along the subscapular vein. Called also *lymphoglandulae axillares.* **no′di lymphat′ici bronchopulmona′les** [NA], bronchopulmonary lymph nodes: nodes embedded in and receiving lymph from the root of the lung. **no′di lymphat′ici bucca′les** [NA], buccal lymph nodes: a variable number of lymph nodes lying on a line between the angle of the mandible and the angle of the mouth; called also *lymphoglandulae faciales profundae.* **no′di lymphat′ici celi′aci** [NA], celiac lymph nodes: a few nodes along the celiac trunk, which receive lymph from the stomach, spleen, duodenum, liver, and pancreas; called also *lymphoglandulae coeliacae.* **no′di lymphat′ici centra′les** [NA], see *nodi lymphatici axillares.* **no′di lymphat′ici cervica′les profun′dae** [NA], deep cervical lymph nodes: the 15 to 30 nodes that lie along the course of the carotid artery and internal jugular vein, including the jugulodigastric, lingual, and jugulo-omohyoid nodes. They receive lymph from both superficial and deep structures. Called also *lymphoglandulae cervicales profundae superiores.* **no′di lymphat′ici cervica′les superficia′les** [NA], superficial cervical lymph nodes: nodes along the external jugular vein which receive lymph from the entire cervical skin surface; called also *lymphoglandulae cervicales superficiales.* **no′di lymphat′ici col′ici dex′tri** [NA], right colic lymph nodes: nodes accompanying the right colic vessels and receiving lymph from the adjacent region. **no′di lymphat′ici col′ici me′dii** [NA], middle colic lymph nodes: nodes accompanying the middle colic vessels and receiving lymph from the adjacent region. **no′di lymphat′ici col′ici sinis′tri** [NA], left colic lymph nodes: nodes situated along the left colic vessels and receiving lymph drained from the adjacent region. **no′di lymphat′ici cubita′les** [NA], cubital lymph nodes: a few lymph nodes situated in the deep part of the elbow. **no′di lymphat′ici epigas′trici** [NA], epigastric lymph nodes: lymph nodes along the deep epigastric vessels, receiving lymph from the lower abdominal wall; called also *lymphoglandulae epigastricae.* **no′di lymphat′ici gas′trici dex′tri** [NA], right gastric lymph nodes: a few nodes along the right gastric artery that receive lymph from the stomach, spleen, duodenum, liver, and pancreas: called also *lymphoglandulae gastricae inferiores.* **no′di lymphat′ici gas′trici sinis′tri** [NA], left gastric lymph nodes: a few nodes along the left gastric artery that receive lymph from the stomach, spleen, duodenum, liver, and pancreas; called also *lymphoglandulae gastricae superiores.* **no′di lymphat′ici gastroepiplo′ici dex′tri** [NA], lymph nodes associated with the right gastroepiploic artery. **no′di lymphat′ici gastroepiplo′ici sinis′tri** [NA], lymph nodes associated with the left gastroepiploic artery. **no′di lymphat′ici hepat′ici** [NA], hepatic lymph nodes: a few nodes along the common hepatic artery that receive lymph from the stomach, spleen, duodenum, liver, and pancreas; called also *lymphoglandulae hepaticae.* **no′di lymphat′ici ileocol′ici** [NA], ileocolic lymph nodes: nodes in the region of the ileocolic junction, draining adjacent structures. **no′di lymphat′ici ili′aci,** iliac lymph nodes: nodes located along the aorta and the common, internal, and external iliac arteries, receiving lymph from the pelvic viscera; called also *lymphoglandulae iliacae.* **no′di lymphat′ici ili′aci cummu′nes** [NA], common iliac lymph nodes: the four to six lymph nodes grouped at the sides and dorsal to the common iliac artery. **no′di lymphat′ici ili′aci exter′ni** [NA], external iliac lymph nodes: the eight to ten nodes along the external iliac vessels. **no′di lymphat′ici ili′aci inter′ni** [NA], internal iliac lymph nodes: nodes grouped around the origins of the branches of the internal iliac vessels, receiving lymph from the regions supplied by these various branches; called also *lymphoglandulae hypogastricae.* **no′di lymphat′ici inguina′les profun′di** [NA], deep inguinal lymph nodes: nodes deep to the fascia lata along the femoral vein, receiving lymph from adjacent areas; called also *lymphoglandulae subinguinales profundae*. **no′di lymphat′ici inguina′les superficia′les** [NA], superficial inguinal lymph nodes: nodes in the subcutaneous tissue inferior to the inguinal ligament; called also *lymphoglandulae subinguinales superficiales*. **no′di lymphat′ici intercosta′les** [NA], intercostal lymph nodes: lymph nodes in the back of the thorax, along the intercostal vessels; called also *lymphoglandulae intercostales*. **n. lymphat′icus jugulodigas′tricus** [NA], one of the deep cervical lymph nodes lying on the internal jugular vein at the level of the greater cornu of the hyoid bone. **n. lymphat′icus juguloomohyoi′- deus** [NA], one of the deep cervical lymph nodes lying on the internal jugular vein just above the tendon of the omohyoid muscle. **no′di lymphat′ici latera′les** [NA], see *nodi lymphatici axillares*. **no′di lymphat′ici lingua′les** [NA], deep cervical lymph nodes receiving afferent vessels from the tongue; called also *lymphoglandulae linguales*. **no′di lymphat′ici lumba′les** [NA], lumbar lymph nodes: a chain of nodes alongside the lower abdominal aorta, receiving most of the lymph from the abdominal structures; called also *lymphoglandulae lumbales*. **no′di lymphat′ici mandibula′res** [NA], mandibular lymph nodes: nodes near the angle of the mandible, into which lymph from some of the superficial tissues of the head and neck is drained. **no′di lymphat′ici mediastina′les anterio′res** [NA], anterior mediastinal lymph nodes: nodes along the great vessels of the superior mediastinum and on the anterior part of the diaphragm, receiving lymph from adjacent structures; called also *lymphoglandulae mediastinales anteriores*. **no′di lym- phat′ici mediastina′les posterio′res** [NA], posterior medi- astinal lymph nodes: 8 to 10 nodes along the thoracic aorta, receiving lymph from the mediastinal structures; called also *lymphoglandulae mediastinales posteriores*. **no′di lymphat′- ici mesenter′ici**, mesenteric lymph nodes: nodes that lie at the root of the mesentery, receiving lymph from the parts of the small intestine, cecum, appendix, and large intestine; called also *lympho- glandulae mesentericae*. **no′di lymphat′ici mesenter′ici inferio′res** [NA], inferior mesenteric lymph nodes: nodes situ- ated along the inferior mesenteric vessels and receiving lymph from the adjacent region. **no′di lymphat′ici mesenter′ici superio′res** [NA], superior mesenteric lymph nodes: nodes situ- ated along the superior mesenteric vessels, receiving lymph from the adjacent regions. **no′di lymphat′ici occipita′les** [NA], occipital lymph nodes: several small nodes near the occipital insertion of the semispinalis capitis muscle; called also *lympho- glandulae occipitales*. **no′di lymphat′ici pancreat- icoliena′les** [NA], pancreaticosplenic lymph nodes: a few nodes along the splenic artery that receive lymph from the stomach, spleen, duodenum, liver, and pancreas; called also *lymphoglandulae pancreaticolienales*. **no′di lymphat′ici parasterna′les** [NA], parasternal lymph nodes: nodes located along the course of the internal thoracic artery, which drain the mammary gland, abdominal wall, and diaphragm; called also *lymphoglandulae sternales*. **no′di lymphat′ici paroti′dei superficia′les et profun′di** [NA], superficial and deep pa- rotid lymph glands: a dozen or so nodes in the substance of the parotid gland, through which lymph drains from the adjacent area; called also *lymphoglandulae parotideae*. **no′di lym- phat′ici pectora′les** [NA], see *nodi lymphatici axillares*. **no′di lymphat′ici phren′ici** [NA], phrenic lymph nodes: sev- eral nodes on the thoracic surface of the diaphragm, receiving lymph from the intercostal spaces, pericardium, diaphragm, and liver. **no′di lymphat′ici poplite′i** [NA], popliteal lymph nodes: a few nodes deep to the fascia around the popliteal vessels, through which lymph drains from nearby areas; called also *lymphoglandulae poplitea*. **no′di lymphat′ici pulmo- na′les** [NA], pulmonary lymph nodes; nodes located along the larger bronchi within the lung substance, through which lymph from the lung drains; called also *lymphoglandulae pulmonales*. **no′di lymphat′ici pylo′rici** [NA], pyloric lymph nodes: nodes that lie in front of the head of the pancreas, receiving lymph from the pyloric part of the stomach, the adjacent part of the duodenum, and part of the inferior portion of the body of the stomach. **no′di lymphat′ici retroauricula′res** [NA], retroauricular lymph nodes: two small nodes on the insertion of the sternocleido- mastoid muscle; called also *lymphoglandulae auriculares posterio- res*. **no′di lymphat′ici retrophar′yn′gei** [NA], retrophar- yngeal lymph nodes: nodes deep in the neck behind the pharynx, receiving lymph from some of the deeper structures of the head and neck. **no′di lymphat′ici sacra′les** [NA], sacral lymph nodes: nodes located in the hollow of the sacrum, receiving lymph from the pelvic, perineal, and gluteal regions; called also *lymphoglandulae sacrales*. **no′di lymphat′ici subman- dibula′res** [NA], submandibular lymph nodes: the three to six nodes alongside the submandibular gland, through which lymph drains from the adjacent skin and mucous membrane; called also *lymphoglandulae submaxillares*. **no′di lymphat′ici sub- menta′les** [NA], submental lymph nodes: nodes under the chin into which the lymph from some of the superficial tissues of the head and neck is drained. **no′di lymphat′ici sub- scapula′res** [NA], see *nodi lymphatici axillares*. **no′di lym- phat′ici tibia′lis ante′rior** [NA], anterior tibial lymph nodes:

lymph nodes occasionally occurring along the anterior tibial vessels; called also *lymphoglandulae tibialis anterior*. **no′di lymphat′ici trachea′les** [NA], tracheal lymph nodes: nodes along each side of the trachea, receiving lymph from the trachea, esophagus, and tracheobronchial nodes; called also *lymphoglandu- lae tracheales*. **no′di lymphat′ici tracheobronchia′les inferio′res** [NA], inferior tracheobronchial lymph nodes: nodes in the angle of the bifurcation of the trachea, receiving lymph from adjacent structures. **no′di lymphat′ici tracheobron- chia′les superio′res** [NA], superior tracheobronchial lymph nodes: nodes between the trachea and the bronchus on either side, receiving lymph from the adjacent structures. **n. sinuatria′- lis** [NA], a microscopic collection of atypical cardiac muscle fibers (Purkinje's fibers) at the superior end of the sulcus terminalis, at the junction of the superior vena cava and the right atrium. See *sinoatrial node*, under *node*.

noematachograph (no-e″mah-tak′o-graf) [Gr. *noēma* thought + *tachys* swift + *graphein* to write] a device for registering the time required in a mental operation.

noematachometer (no-e″mah-tah-kom′ĕ-ter) [Gr. *noēma* thought + *tachys* swift + *metron* measure] a device for mea- suring the time required in a mental operation.

noematic (no″e-mat′ik) pertaining to thought or the operation of the mind.

noesis (no-e′sis) [Gr. *noēsis* thought] the operation of the intel- lect; cognition.

noetic (no-et′ik) pertaining to the intellect or to cognition.

noeud (nuh) [Fr.] knot, or node. **n. vital** (nuh ve-tal′) ["vital node"], an old term applied to the respiratory centers.

nogalamycin (no-gal-ah-mi′sin) an antineoplastic antibiotic produced by a variant of *Streptomyces nogalater*.

Noguchi's culture medium, leutin reaction, reagent, test (no-goo′chēz) [Hideyo *Noguchi*, Japanese pathologist in New York, 1876–1928] see *tissue culture medium*, under *culture me- dium*, and see under *reaction*, *reagent*, and *tests*.

Noguchia (no-goo′che-ah) [Hideyo *Noguchi*] a genus of micro- organisms of the family Brucellaceae, order Eubacteriales, made up of small, gram-negative rods, motile by means of peritrichous flagella, and found in the conjunctiva of man and animals having a follicular type of disease. **N. cuni′culi**, an organism that is said to be the cause of conjunctival folliculosis in rabbits. **N. granulo′sis**, an organism which at one time was thought to be the etiologic agent of trachoma. **N. si′miae**, an organism that is said to be the cause of conjunctival folliculosis in monkeys.

noli-me-tangere (no″li-me-tan′jer-e) [L. "touch me not"] a term believed to have been originally applied by the Romans to the ulcerative form of lupus, because of the unfortunate effects of certain types of treatment; frequently applied to different types of destructive lesions of the skin.

nolinium bromide (no-lin′e-um) chemical name: 2-[(3,4-di- chlorophenyl)amino]quinolizinium bromide; an antisecretory and antiulcerative, $C_{15}H_{11}BrCl_2N_2$.

Noludar (nol′u-dar) trademark for preparations of methypry- lon.

Nolvadex (nol′vah-deks) trademark for a preparation of tamoxifen.

noma (no′mah) [Gr. *nomai* eating sores] gangrene processes of the mouth (gangrenous stomatitis or cancrum oris) or genitalia (noma pudendi, noma vulvae, or phlegmonous vulvitis). In the mouth, it begins as a small gingival ulcer and results in gangre- nous necrosis of surrounding facial tissues. On the genitalia, it involves first one labium majus and then the other.

nomadic (no-mad′ik) wandering; unsettled; free.

nomenclature (no′men-kla″tūr, no-men′kla″tūr) [L. *nomen* name + *calare* to call] a classified system of names, as of anatomical structures, organisms, etc. See *Nomina Anatomica*. **binomial n.**, the Linnean system of designating plants and animals by two latinized words signifying the genus and species.

nomifensine maleate (no″mĭ-fen′sēn) chemical name: 1,2,3,4-tetrahydro-2-methyl-4-phenyl-8-isoquinolinamine (Z)-2- butenedioate (1:1). A central nervous system stimulant, $C_{16}H_{18}$- $N_2 \cdot C_4H_4O_4$, used as an antidepressant.

Nomina Anatomica (no′mĭ-nah an-ah-tom′ĭ-kah) [L. "anatomi- cal names"] the official body of anatomical nomenclature, ap- plied specifically to that revised by the International Anatomical Nomenclature Committee appointed by the Fifth International Congress of Anatomists held at Oxford in 1950, and approved by the Sixth, Seventh, and Eighth International Congresses of Anatomists held in Paris, 1955, New York, 1960, and Wiesbaden, 1965. Abbreviated NA.

nomo- (no′mo) [Gr. *nomos* law] a combining form denoting rela- tionship to usage or law.

nomogenesis (no″mo-jen′ĕ-sis) [*nomo-* + Gr. *genesis* generation] the theory of evolution according to which the course of evolution is fixed and predetermined by law, no place being left for chance.

nomogram (nom′o-gram) [*nomo-* + Gr. *gramma* mark] the graphic representation produced in nomography; a chart or diagram on which a number of variables are plotted, forming a computation chart for the solution of complex numerical formulae.

nomography (no-mog′rah-fe) [*nomo*- + Gr. *graphein* to write] a graphic method by which the relation between any number of variables may be represented graphically on a plane surface, such as a piece of paper.

nomotopic (no″mo-top′ik) [*nomo*- + Gr. *topos* place] occurring at a normal place; occurring normally.

nona (no′nah) a condition resembling lethargic encephalitis which appeared in epidemic form in southern Europe in 1889–1890.

nonacosane (non″ah-ko′sān) an aliphatic hydrocarbon, $C_{29}H_{60}$, extracted from plant waxes.

nonadherent (non″ad-he′rent) not adherent to or connected with adjacent structures.

nonan (no′nan) [L. *nonus* ninth] recurring every ninth day, or at intervals of eight days.

nonantigenic (non″an-tĭ-jen′ik) not eliciting an immune response (antibody formation or cell-mediated immunity); without antigenic effect, attributable to either the physical and chemical nature of the antigen or the genetically determined ability of the host to respond.

nonapeptide (non″ah-pep′tid) a peptide containing nine amino acids.

non compos mentis (non kom′pos men′tis) [L.] not of sound mind.

nonconductor (non″kon-duk′tor) any substance that does not readily transmit electricity, light, or heat.

nondepolarizer (non″de-po′lar-īz″er) a muscle relaxant that produces striate muscle paralysis by competitive interference with the transmission of nerve impulses from nerve ending to muscle receptor.

nondisjunction (non″dis-junk′shun) failure (*a*) of two homologous chromosomes to pass to separate cells during the first division of meiosis, or (*b*) of the two chromatids of a chromosome to pass to separate cells during mitosis or during the second meiotic division. As a result, one daughter cell has two chromosomes or two chromatids, and the other has none.

nonelectrolyte (non″e-lek′tro-lit) a substance which in solution is a nonconductor of electricity.

nonheme (non-hēm) not bound within a porphyrin ring; said of iron so contained within a protein.

nonhomogeneity (non-ho″mo-jĕ-ne′ĭ-te) the lack of homogeneity; the state of not being homogeneous.

nonigravida (no″ne-grav′ĭ-dah) [L. *nonus* ninth + *gravida* pregnant] a woman pregnant for the ninth time. Written gravida IX.

noninfectious (non″in-fek′shus) not infectious; not spread by contact, inhalation, etc.; not able to spread disease.

noninvolution (non″in-vo-lu′shun) failure of a part to return to normal size and condition after enlargement from functional activity, as noninvolution of the uterus after pregnancy.

nonipara (no-nip′ah-rah) [L. *nonus* ninth + *parere* to bring forth, produce] a woman who has had nine pregnancies which resulted in viable offspring. Written para IX.

nonmedullated (non-med′u-lāt″ed) unmyelinated.

nonmetal (non-met′al) any chemical element that is not a metal or a metalloid.

nonmyelinated (non-mi′ĕ-lĭ-nāt″ed) unmyelinated.

Nonne's syndrome, test (non′ez) [Max *Nonne*, Hamburg neurologist, 1861–1959] see *hereditary cerebellar ataxia*, and see *Ross-Jones test*, under *tests*.

Nonne-Apelt reaction (phase, test) (non′ĕ-ah′pelt) [Max *Nonne*; F. *Apelt*, German physician, 1877–1911] see under *reaction*.

Nonne-Milroy-Meige syndrome (non′e-mil′roy-mehzh′e) [Max *Nonne*; William Forsyth *Milroy*, American physician, 1855–1942; Henri *Meige*, French physician, 1866–1940] Milroy's disease.

non-neuronal (non″nu-ro′nal) pertaining to or composed of nonconducting cells of the nervous system, e.g., neuroglial cells.

non-nucleated (non-nu′kle-āt″ed) without a nucleus; cf. *anuclear*.

nonocclusion (non″ŏ-kloo′zhun) open bite malocclusion.

nonoliguric (non-ol″ĭ-gu′rik) not pertaining to, characterized by, or conducive to oliguria.

nononcogenic (non″on-ko-jen′ik) not giving rise to tumors or causing tumor formation.

nonopaque (non″o-pāk′) not opaque to the roentgen ray.

nonose (non′ōs) [L. *nonus* ninth] a carbohydrate containing nine atoms of carbon in the molecule.

nonoxynol (no-noks′ĭ-nōl) nonylphenoxypolyethoxyethanol. A group of compounds of the general composition $C_{15}H_{24}O(C_2H_4O)_n$, which are assigned numbers according to the approximate value of *n*: nonoxynol 4 is $C_{15}H_{24}O(C_2H_4O)_4$, or $C_{23}H_{40}O_5$; nonoxynol 9 is $C_{33}H_{60}O_{10}$; nonoxynol 15 is $C_{45}H_{84}O_{16}$; nonoxynol 30 is

$C_{75}H_{144}O_{31}$. Nonoxynol 4, 15, and 30 are nonionic surfactants, and nonoxynol 9 is used as a spermaticide. Nonoxynol 10 [NF], in which *n* varies from 6 to 16, is used as a pharmaceutical surfactant.

nonparous (non-par′us) nulliparous.

nonphotochromogen (non″fo-to-kro′mo-jen) a microorganism which is not conspicuously affected in color by exposure to light; specifically a member of Group III of the so-called "anonymous" or "unclassified" mycobacteria, e.g., Battey bacilli.

nonpolar (non-po′lar) not having poles; not exhibiting dipole characteristics.

nonradiable (non-ra′de-ah-b′l) impervious to rays, such as roentgen rays, cathode rays, etc.

non repetat. abbreviation for L. *non repeta′tur*, do not repeat.

nonrotation (non″ro-ta′shun) [*non*- + L. *rotare* to turn] failure of rotation of a part to the proper position. **n. of the intestine,** failure of rotation of the intestine during embryonic development, with the result that the small intestine lies on the right side of the abdomen and the large intestine on the left.

nonsecretor (non″se-kre′tor) an individual possessing A or B type blood whose saliva and other body secretions do not contain the particular (A or B) substance.

nonseptate (non-sep′tāt) without a septum or septa.

nonspecific (non-spĕ-sif′ik) 1. not due to any single known cause, as to a particular pathogen. 2. not directed against a particular agent, but rather having a general effect, as nonspecific therapy.

nontaster (non-tās′ter) an individual incapable of tasting a particular test substance, such as phenylthiocarbamide, used in certain genetic studies.

nonunion (non-ūn′yun) failure of the ends of a fractured bone to unite.

nonus (no′nus) [L. "ninth"] (*obs.*) the hypoglossal nerve (nervus hypoglossus [NA]); so called because formerly regarded as the ninth cranial nerve.

nonvalent (non-va′lent) [L. *non* not + *valere* to be able] having no chemical valency: not capable of entering into chemical composition; said of argon, helium, and the other inert gases.

nonviable (non-vi′ah-b′l) [L. *non* not + *viable*] not capable of living.

nonyl (no′nil) the monovalent radical C_9H_{19}.

noopsyche (no′o-si″ke) [Gr. *nous* mind + *psyche* soul] the intellectual processes of the mind.

Noorden treatment (noor′den) [Carl Harko von *Noorden*, German physician, 1858–1944] oatmeal treatment.

noothymopsychic (no″o-thi″mo-si′kik) pertaining to the intellectual and the affective processes of the mind.

nopalin G (no′pal-in) bluish eosin; see under *eosin*.

N.O.P.H.N. National Organization for Public Health Nursing.

nor- chemical prefix denoting (*a*) a compound (e.g., norleucine) of normal structure (having an unbranched chain of carbon atoms) that is isomeric with one (e.g., leucine) having a branched chain, or (*b*) a compound (e.g., norepinephrine) whose chain or ring contains one less methylene (CH_2) group than does that of its homologue (e.g., epinephrine).

noradrenalin (nor″ah-dren′ah-lin) norepinephrine.

noradrenergic (nor″ah-dren-er′jik) activated by or secreting norepinephrine.

noramidopyrine (nor-am″ĭ-do-pi′rēn) dipyrone.

norandrostenolone (nor-an″dro-sten′o-lōn) nandrolone.

Nordau's disease (nor′dowz) [Max Simon *Nordau*, German scientist, 1849–1923] degeneracy.

nordauism (nor-dow′izm) [named for M. S. *Nordau*] degeneracy.

nordefrin hydrochloride (nor-def′rin) chemical name: 4-(2-amino-1-hydroxypropyl)-1,2-benzenediol hydrochloride. An adrenergic agent isomeric with epinephrine, $C_9H_{13}NO_3$, having significant central stimulant action and almost no vasoconstrictor action; the levo-isomer, *levodefrin* (q.v.), is usually used when vasoconstriction is desired. Called also *homoarterenol hydrochloride*.

norepinephrine (nor″ep-ĭ-nef′rin) one of the naturally occurring catecholamines; a neurohormone released by the postganglionic adrenergic nerves, which is the principal neurotransmitter of adrenergic neurons, having predominately α-adrenergic but some β-adrenergic activity. It is also secreted by the adrenal medulla in response to splanchnic stimulation and is stored in the chromaffin granules, being released predominantly in response to hypotension. Norepinephrine is a powerful vasopressor and is used in the form of the bitartrate salt. Called also *arterenol* and *noradrenalin*. **n. bitartrate** [USP], the bitartrate salt of norepinephrine, $C_6H_{11}NO_3 \cdot C_4H_6O_6 \cdot H_2O$, occurring as a white or faintly gray, crystalline powder, having the vasoconstrictor actions of the parent compound; used to restore the blood pressure in certain cases of acute hypotension, and as an adjunct in the treatment of cardiac arrest and profound hypotension, administered by intravenous infusion. Called also *levarterenol bitartrate*.

norethandrolone (nor″eth-an′dro-lōn) [NF] chemical name: 17-hydroxy-19-nor-17α-pregn-4-en-3-one. A synthetic androgen, $C_{20}H_{30}O_2$, equal to testosterone in anabolic activity, but having less androgenic activity.

norethindrone (nor-eth′in-drōn) [USP] chemical name: 17β-hydroxy-19-nor-17α-pregn-4-en-20-yn-3-one. A progestin, $C_{20}H_{26}O_2$, occurring as a white to creamy white, crystalline powder, having some anabolic, estrogenic, and androgenic properties; used in the treatment of amenorrhea, abnormal uterine bleeding due to hormonal imbalance, and endometriosis, administered orally. Also used, alone or in combination with an estrogen component, as an oral contraceptive. **n. acetate** [NF], the acetate salt of norethindrone, $C_{22}H_{28}O_3$, having the same appearance, actions, uses, and route of administration as the base.

norethisterone (nor″eth-is′ter-ōn) norethindrone.

norethynodrel (nor″ĕ-thi′no-drel) [USP] chemical name: 17-hydroxy-19-nor-17α-pregn-5(10)-en-20-yn-3-one. A progestin, $C_{20}H_{26}O_2$, occurring as a white or nearly white, crystalline powder; used in combination with an estrogen component as an oral contraceptive, to control endometriosis, for the treatment of hypermenorrhea, to produce cyclic withdrawal bleeding, and to produce amenorrhea for medical or sociological reasons.

Norflex (nor′fleks) trademark for a preparation of orphenadrine citrate.

norflurane (nor-floor′ān) chemical name: 1,1,1,2-tetrafluoroethane; an inhalation anesthetic, $C_2H_2F_4$.

norgestimate (nor-jes′ti-māt) chemical name: (+)-17-(acetyloxy)-13-ethyl-18,19-dinor-17α-pregn-4-en-20-yn-3-one oxime; a progestin, $C_{23}H_{31}NO_3$.

norgestomet (nor-jes′to-met) chemical name: 17-(acetyloxy)-11β-methyl-19-norpregn-4-ene-3,20-dione; a progestin, $C_{23}H_{32}O_4$.

norgestrel (nor-jes′trel) [USP] chemical name: (+)13β-ethyl-17-hydroxy-18,19-dinor-17α-pregn-4-en-20-yn-3-one. A potent progestin, $C_{21}H_{28}O_2$, occurring as a white or nearly white, crystalline powder; used in combination with an estrogen component as an oral contraceptive.

norhyoscyamine (nor-hi″o-si′ah-mēn) chemical name: 1-tropic acid 3α-nortropanyl ester. An alkaloid, $C_{16}H_{21}NO_3$, from plants of the family Solanaceae, having properties like those of hyoscyamine. Called also *pseudohyoscyamine* and *solandrine*.

Norisodrine (nor-i′so-drin) trademark for preparations of isoproterenol.

norleucine (nor-lu′sin) chemical name: 2-aminohexanoic acid. A nonessential amino acid, $CH_3 \cdot (CH_2)_3 \cdot CH(NH_2) \cdot COOH$, extracted from the leucine fraction of the decomposition of the proteins of nervous tissue. It has been synthesized.

Norlutate (nor-lu′tāt) trademark for a preparation of norethindrone acetate.

Norlutin (nor-lu′tin) trademark for a preparation of norethindrone.

norm (norm) [L. *norma* rule] a fixed or ideal standard.

norma (nor′mah) [L.] an outline established to define the aspects of the cranium; also a norm or typical standard. **n. anterior,** norma frontalis. **n. basilaris,** the outline of the inferior aspect of the skull. **n. facialis,** norma frontalis. **n. frontalis,** the outline of the skull viewed from the front. **n. inferior,** norma basilaris. **n. lateralis,** the outline of the skull seen from either side. **n. occipitalis,** the outline of the skull seen from behind. **n. posterior,** norma occipitalis. **n. sagittalis,** the outline of a sagittal section through the skull. **n. superior,** norma verticalis. **n. temporalis,** norma lateralis. **n. ventralis,** the outline of the inferior aspect of the skull. **n. verticalis,** the outline of the skull viewed from above.

normal (nor′mal) [L. *norma* rule] 1. agreeing with the regular and established type. 2. in chemistry, (*a*) denoting a solution containing in each 1000 ml. 1 gram equivalent weight of the active substance; (*b*) denoting aliphatic hydrocarbons in which no carbon atom is combined with more than two other carbon atoms; (*c*) denoting salts formed from acids and bases in such a way that no acidic hydrogen of the acid remains nor any of the basic hydroxyl of the base. Abbreviated N, n. 3. in bacteriology, not immunized or otherwise bacteriologically treated.

normality (nor-mal′i-te) 1. the state of being normal. 2. the number of gram-equivalent weights of solute per liter of solution.

normalization (nor″mal-i-za′shun) the process of bringing or restoring to the normal standard.

normergic (norm-er′jik) [norm- + Gr. *ergon* work] reacting in a normal manner.

normetanephrine (nor-met″ah-nef′rin) α-(aminomethyl)-vanillyl alcohol (3-methylnorepinephrine): a metabolite of epinephrine excreted in the urine and found in certain tissues.

normo- (nor′mo) [L. *norma* rule] a combining form meaning conforming to the rule; normal or usual.

normoblast (nor′mo-blast) [normo- + Gr. *blastos* germ] a nucleated precursor cell in the erythrocyte series; four developmental stages are recognized: the pronormoblast and the basophilic, polychromatic, and orthochromatic normoblasts. **acidophilic**

n., orthochromatic n. **basophilic n.,** a nucleated immature erythrocyte. The cytoplasm in general is similar to that of the earlier pronormoblast but may be even more basophilic, and is usually regular in outline. The nucleus is still relatively large, but the chromatin strands are thicker and more deeply staining, giving a coarser appearance; the nucleoli have disappeared. Called also *prorubricyte, early normoblast,* and *early* or *basophilic erythroblast.* **early n.,** basophilic n. **eosinophilic n.,** orthochromatic n. **intermediate n.,** polychromatic n. **late n.,** orthochromatic n. **orthochromatic n.,** the final stage of the nucleated, immature erythrocyte, before nuclear loss. Typically the cytoplasm is described as acidophilic, but it still shows a faint polychromatic tint. The nucleus is small and initially may still have very coarse, clumped chromatin, as in its precursor, the polychromatic normoblast, but ultimately it becomes pyknotic, and appears as a deeply staining, blue-black, homogeneous structureless mass. The nucleus is often eccentric and is sometimes lobulated. Called also *late, acidophilic, oxyphilic,* or *eosinophilic normoblast; late, orthochromatic, acidophilic, oxyphilic,* or *eosinophilic erythroblast;* and *metarubricyte.* **oxyphilic n.,** orthochromatic n. **polychromatic n.,** a nucleated, immature erythrocyte in which the nucleus occupies a relatively smaller part of the cell than in its precursor, the basophilic normoblast. The cytoplasm is beginning to acquire hemoglobin and thus is no longer a purely blue color, but takes on an acidophilic tint, which becomes progressively more marked as the cell matures. The chromatin of the nucleus is arranged in coarse, deeply staining clumps. Called also *intermediate n., intermediate* or *polychromatic erythroblast,* and *rubricyte.*

normoblastic (nor″mo-blas′tik) relating to or having the character of a normoblast.

normoblastosis (nor″mo-blas-to′sis) excessive production of normoblasts by the bone marrow.

normocalcemia (nor″mo-kal-se′me-ah) a normal level of calcium in the blood.

normocalcemic (nor″mo-kal-se′mik) pertaining to or characterized by normocalcemia.

normocapnia (nor″mo-kap′ne-ah) a normal tension of carbon dioxide in the blood.

normocapnic (nor″mo-kap′nik) pertaining to or characterized by normocapnia.

normocholesterolemia (nor″mo-ko-les″ter-o-le′me-ah) a normal level of cholesterol in the blood.

normocholesterolemic (nor″mo-ko-les″ter-o-le′mik) pertaining to, characterized by, or tending to produce a normal level of cholesterol in the blood.

normochromasia (nor″mo-kro-ma′ze-ah) [normo- + Gr. *chrōma* color] 1. a normal staining reaction in a cell or tissue. 2. normal color of the red blood cells.

normochromia (nor″mo-kro′me-ah) normal color of the red blood cells.

normochromic (nor″mo-kro′mik) having a normal color; having a normal hemoglobin content.

normocrinic (nor″mo-krin′ik) pertaining to normal secretion or to normal endocrine action.

normocyte (nor′mo-sīt) [normo- + -cyte] an erythrocyte that is normal in size, shape, and color.

normocytic (nor″mo-sit′ik) relating to or having the character of a normocyte.

Normocytin (nor″mo-si′tin) trademark for preparations of concentrated crystalline vitamin B_{12}. See *cyanocobalamin.*

normocytosis (nor″mo-si-to′sis) a normal state of the blood in respect to the erythrocytes.

normoerythrocyte (nor″mo-ĕ-rith′ro-sīt) normocyte.

normoglycemia (nor″mo-gli-se′me-ah) the state of having the level of glucose in the blood within the normal range.

normoglycemic (nor″mo-gli-se′mik) pertaining to, characterized by, or conducive to normoglycemia.

normokalemia (nor″mo-kah-le′me-ah) a normal level of potassium in the blood.

normokalemic (nor″mo-kah-le′mik) pertaining to, characterized by, or conducive to normokalemia.

normolineal (nor″mo-lin′e-al) built on normal lines.

normomastic (nor″mo-mas′tik) see *Kafka's test,* under *tests.*

normo-orthocytosis (nor″mo-or″tho-si-to′sis) [normo- + Gr. *orthos* correct + -cyte + -osis] a condition of the blood leukocytes in which the total number is increased, but the proportion between the different varieties remains normal.

normosexual (nor″mo-seks′u-al) having normal sexuality.

normoskeocytosis (nor″mo-ske″o-si-to′sis) [normo- + Gr. *skaios* left + -cyte + -osis] a condition of the leukocytes of the blood in which the number is normal, but many immature forms (deviation to the left) are present.

normospermic (nor″mo-sper′mik) producing spermatozoa normal in number and motility.

normosthenuria (nor″mo-sthen-u′re-ah) [normo- + Gr. *sthenos* strength + *ouron* urine + -ia] 1. the secretion of urine of varying specific gravity within the normal range. 2. normally active urination.

normotension (nor″mo-ten′shun) normal tone, tension, or pressure.

normotensive (nor″mo-ten′siv) 1. characterized by normal tone, tension, or pressure, as by normal blood pressure. 2. a person with normal blood pressure.

normothermia (nor″mo-ther′me-ah) [normo- + Gr. thermē heat + -ia] a normal state of temperature, especially (a) normal body temperature (98.6° F.), or (b) that state of normal environmental temperature at which there is neither stimulation nor depression of the activity of the body cells (Herrmann).

normothermic (nor″mo-ther′mik) pertaining to or characterized by normal temperature; neither hyperthermic nor hypothermic.

normotonia (nor″mo-to′ne-ah) normal tone or tension.

normotonic (nor″mo-ton′ik) pertaining to or characterized by normotonia.

normotopia (nor″mo-to′pe-ah) [normo- + Gr. topos place + -ia] (obs.) normal location.

normotopic (nor″mo-top′ik) (obs.) normally located.

normotrophic (nor″mo-trof′ik) of normal development; exhibiting neither hypertrophy nor hypotrophy.

normouricemia (nor″mo-u″rĭ-se′me-ah) a normal value of uric acid in the blood.

normouricemic (nor″mo-u″rĭ-se′mik) pertaining to or characterized by normouricemia.

normouricuria (nor″mo-u″rĭ-ku′re-ah) a normal amount of uric acid in the urine.

normouricuric (nor″mo-u″rĭ-ku′rik) pertaining to or characterized by normouricuria.

normovolemia (nor″mo-vo-le′me-ah) [normo- + volume + Gr. haima blood + -ia] normal blood volume.

normovolemic (nor″mo-vo-le′mik) pertaining to or characterized by normovolemia; having a normal volume of circulating fluid (plasma) in the body.

Norodin (nor′o-din) trademark for a preparation of methamphetamine hydrochloride.

Norpace (nor′pās) trademark for a preparation of disopyramide phosphate.

Norpramin (nor′pram-in) trademark for a preparation of desipramine hydrochloride.

norpseudoephedrine (nor-su″do-ĕ-fed′rēn) a nervous system stimulant, $C_9H_{13}NO$, from the leaves of the shrub Catha edulis.

Norris' corpuscles (nor′is-ez) [Richard Norris, English physician, 1831–1916] see under corpuscle.

norsulfazole (nor-sul′fah-zōl) sulfathiazole.

Northrop (north′rup), John Howard. An American chemist (born 1891), co-winner, with J. B. Sumner and W. M. Stanley, of the Nobel prize in chemistry for 1946, for pioneering work in crystallizing protein.

nortriptyline hydrochloride (nor-trip′tĭ-lēn) [USP] chemical name: 3-(10,11-dihydro-5H-dibenzo[a,d]cyclohepten-5-ylidene)-N-methyl-1-propanamine hydrochloride. An antidepressant, $C_{19}H_{21}N·HCl$, occurring as a white to off-white powder; administered orally.

nortropinon (nor-tro′pĭ-non) a solid, fusible ketone, $C_6H_{11}NO$, derived from tropin.

nosazontology (nos-az″on-tol′o-je) nosetiology.

noscapine (nos′kah-pēn) chemical name: (S)-6,7-dimethoxy-3-(5,6,7,8-tetrahydro-4-methoxy-6-methyl-1,3-dioxolo[4,5-g]isoquinolin-5-yl)-1(3H)-isobenzofuranone. An alkaloid of opium, $C_{22}H_{23}-NO_7$, occurring as a white to nearly white, crystalline powder; used as an antitussive, administered orally. **n. hydrochloride,** the hydrochloride salt of noscapine, $C_{22}H_{23}NO_7·HCl$, having the same appearance, actions, uses, and route of administration as the base.

nose (nōz) [L. nasus; Gr. rhis] the specialized structure of the face that serves as an organ of the sense of smell and as part of the respiratory apparatus. The receptor cells for the sense of smell (olfactory cells) lie in the olfactory membrane, in the superior portion of each nostril. In its respiratory function, the nose serves to warm the inspired air as it passes along the surfaces of the septum and turbinate bones and to moisten and filter the air. Called also nasus [NA]. **brandy n.,** rosacea. **cleft n.,** a developmental anomaly resulting from incomplete union of the paired nasal primordia. **external n.,** nasus externus. **hammer n.,** rhinophyma. **potato n.,** rhinophyma. **saddle n., saddle-back n., swayback n.,** concavity of the contour of the bridge of the nose due to collapse of cartilaginous or bony support, or both; it was once most often due to congenital syphilis, but is now more commonly the result of congenital epidermal defect or of leprosy.

nosebrain (nōz′brān) (obs.) rhinencephalon, def. 1.

nosegay (nōz′ga) a name applied to an anatomical structure resembling a small bunch of flowers. **Riolan's n.,** the group of

muscles that take their origin from the styloid process of the temporal bone.

Nosema (no-se′mah) a genus of sporozoan parasites of the order Microsporidia. N. a′pis causes the nosema disease of bees. N. bomby′cis causes the disease pébrine in silkworms. **N. cunic′-uli,** the causative agent of spontaneous encephalomyelitis of the rabbit; it is found in intracellular cysts as well as free in the brain, kidney, and other organs.

nosema (no-se′mah), pl. nose′mas or nosem′ata [Gr. nosēma a sickness] (obs.) any illness or disease.

nosematosis (no-se″mah-to′sis) infection with Nosema.

nosencephalus (no″sen-sef′ah-lus) [noso- + Gr. enkephalos brain] a fetus with a defective cranium and brain.

nosepiece (nōz′pēs) the portion of a microscope nearest to the stage, which bears the objective or objectives, constructed so as to permit change of the objective without disturbing the focus of the instrument. **quick-change n.,** one bearing a single objective, which may be quickly attached to or removed from a microscope. **rotating n.,** one bearing more than one objective, designed to permit the one selected to be rotated into place, with its axis coincident with the optical axis of the microscope.

nosetiology (nos″e-te-ol′o-je) [noso- + Gr. aitia cause + -logy] the study of the causation of disease.

nosiheptide (no″sĭ-hep′tīd) a veterinary growth stimulant, $C_{51}-H_{43}N_{13}O_{12}S_6$.

noso- (nos′o) [Gr. nosos disease] a combining form denoting relationship to disease.

nosochthonography (nos″ok-tho-nog′rah-fe) [noso- + Gr. chthōn land + graphein to write] the geography of epidemic or other diseases; the study of the geographical distribution of diseases; nosogeography.

nosocomial (nos″o-ko′me-al) [Gr. nosokomeion from nosos disease + komeion to take care of] pertaining to or originating in a hospital, as nosocomial disease.

nosocomium (nos″o-ko′me-um) [Gr. nosokomeion, from nosos disease + komeion to take care of] (obs.) a hospital or an infirmary.

nosode (nos′ōd) any disease product used as a remedy.

nosogenesis (nos″o-jen′ĕ-sis) pathogenesis.

nosogenic (nos″o-jen′ik) pathogenic.

nosogeny (no-soj′ĕ-ne) [noso- + Gr. gennan to produce] pathogenesis.

nosogeography (nos″o-je-og′rah-fe) [noso- + Gr. gē earth + graphein to write] nosochthonography.

nosographer (no-sog′rah-fer) a writer of nosography.

nosography (no-sog′rah-fe) [noso- + Gr. graphein to write] a written account or description of diseases.

nosointoxication (nos″o-in-tok″sĭ-ka′shun) intoxication by the harmful products of disease.

nosologic (nos″o-loj′ik) pertaining to the classification of disease.

nosological (nos″o-loj′e-kal) pertaining to nosology.

nosology (no-sol′o-je) [noso- + -logy] the science of the classification of diseases.

nosomania (nos″o-ma′ne-ah) [noso- + Gr. mania madness] the incorrect belief of a patient that he has some special disease; hypochondriasis.

nosometry (no-som′ĕ-tre) [noso- + Gr. metron measure] the measurement of the morbidity rate.

nosomycosis (nos″o-mi-ko′sis) [noso- + Gr. mykēs fungus] a disease caused by a fungus.

nosonomy (no-son′o-me) [noso- + Gr. nomos law] the classification of diseases.

nosoparasite (nos″o-par′ah-sīt) [noso- + parasite] an organism found in conjunction with a disease which it is able to modify, but not to produce.

nosophilia (nos″o-fil′e-ah) [noso- + Gr. philein to love] a morbid desire to be sick.

nosophobe (nos′o-fōb) a person who has an abnormal fear of some particular disease, such as cancer, venereal disease, appendicitis, etc.

nosophobia (nos″o-fo′be-ah) [noso- + phobia] morbid dread of sickness or of any special disease.

nosophyte (nos′o-fīt) [noso- + Gr. phyton plant] a pathogenic plant microorganism.

nosopoietic (nos″o-poi-et′ik) [noso- + Gr. poiein to make] causing or producing disease.

Nosopsyllus (nos″o-sil′us) [noso- + Gr. psylla flea] a genus of fleas. **N. fascia′tus,** the common rat flea of North America and Europe; it is a vector of murine typhus and probably of plague. Formerly called Ceratophyllus fasciatus.

nosotaxy (nos′o-tak″se) [noso- + Gr. taxis arrangement] the classification of disease.

nosotherapy (nos″o-ther′ah-pe) the treatment of one disease by means of another, as in malaria therapy.

nosotoxic (nos″o-tok′sik) producing nosotoxicosis.

nosotoxicity (nos″o-tok-sis′ĭ-te) the quality of being nosotoxic.

nosotoxicosis (nos″o-tok″sĭ-ko′sis) [*noso-* + *toxicosis*] any disease due to or associated with poisoning.

nosotoxin (nos″o-tok′sin) [*noso-* + *toxin*] any toxin causing or associated with disease.

nosotrophy (no-sot′ro-fe) [*noso-* + Gr. *trophē* nourishment] the care and nursing of the sick.

nosotropic (no″so-trop′ik) [*noso-* + Gr. *tropos* a turning] directed against or opposed to a disease.

nostalgia (nos-tal′je-ah) [Gr. *nostein* to return home + *-algia*] homesickness; longing to return home or to one's native land.

nostology (nos-tol′o-je) [Gr. *nostein* to return home + *-logy*] (*obs.*) gerontology.

nostomania (nos″to-ma′ne-ah) [Gr. *nostein* to return home + *mania* madness] intense nostalgia.

nostril (nos′tril) one of the external orifices of the nose; called also *anterior* or *external naris*. See *nares*.

nostrum (nos′trum) [L.] a quack, patent, or secret remedy.

Nostyn (nos′tin) trademark for a preparation of ectylurea.

notalgia (no-tal′je-ah) [Gr. *nōton* back + *-algia*] pain in the back; dorsalgia.

notancephalia (no″tan-sĕ-fa′le-ah) [Gr. *nōton* + *an* neg. + *kephalē* head + *-ia*] congenital absence of the back of the skull.

notanencephalia (no″tan-en-sĕ-fa′le-ah) [Gr. *nōton* back + *an* neg. + *enkephalos* brain + *-ia*] absence of the cerebellum.

notatin (nō′tā-tĭn) glucose oxidase.

N.O.T.B. National Ophthalmic Treatment Board (British).

notch (noch) an indentation or depression, especially one on the edge of a bone or other organ. See also *incisura*. **acetabular n.,** incisura acetabuli. **aortic n.,** dicrotic n. **auricular n.,** incisura anterior auris. **cardiac n. of left lung,** incisura cardiaca pulmonis sinistri. **cardiac n. of stomach,** incisura cardiaca ventriculi. **cerebellar n., anterior,** incisura cerebelli anterior. **cerebellar n., posterior,** incisura cerebelli posterior. **clavicular n. of sternum,** incisura clavicularis sterni. **coracoid n.,** incisura scapulae. **costal n's of sternum,** incisurae costales sterni. **cotyloid n.,** incisura acetabuli. **dicrotic n.,** a small downward deflection in the arterial pulse or pressure contour immediately following the closure of the semilunar valves, sometimes used as a marker for the end of systole or the ejection period. **ethmoidal n. of frontal bone,** incisura ethmoidalis ossis frontalis. **fibular n.,** incisura fibularis tibiae. **frontal n.,** incisura frontalis. **n. of gallbladder,** fossa vesicae felleae. **gastric n.,** incisura angularis ventriculi. **interarytenoid n.,** incisura interarytenoidea laryngis. **interclavicular n.,** incisura jugularis sterni. **interclavicular n. of occipital bone,** incisura jugularis ossis occipitalis. **interclavicular n. of temporal bone,** incisura jugularis ossis temporalis. **intercondylar n. of femur,** fossa intercondylaris femoris. **interlobar n.,** incisura ligamenti teretis. **intertragic n.,** incisura intertragica. **intervertebral n.,** see *incisura vertebralis inferior* and *incisura vertebralis superior*. **ischiatic n., greater,** incisura ischiadica major. **ischiatic n., lesser,** incisura ischiadica minor. **jugular n. of occipital bone,** incisura jugularis ossis occipitalis. **jugular n. of sternum,** incisura jugularis sterni. **jugular n. of temporal bone,** incisura jugularis ossis temporalis. **lacrimal n. of maxilla,** incisura lacrimalis maxillae. **n. of ligamentum teres,** incisura ligamenti teretis. **mandibular n.,** incisura mandibulae. **marsupial n.,** incisura cerebelli posterior. **mastoid n.,** incisura mastoidea ossis temporalis. **nasal n. of maxilla,** incisura nasalis maxillae. **palatine n.,** fissura pterygoidea. **palatine n. of palatine bone,** incisura sphenopalatina ossis palatini. **pancreatic n.,** incisura pancreatis. **parietal n. of temporal bone,** incisura parietalis ossis temporalis. **parotid n.,** the notch between the ramus of the mandible and the mastoid process of the temporal bone. **popliteal n.,** fossa intercondylaris femoris. **preoccipital n.,** incisura preoccipitalis. **presternal n.,** incisura jugularis sterni. **pterygoid n.,** fissura pterygoidea. **radial n., radial n. of ulna,** incisura radialis ulnae. **rivinian n., n. of Rivinus,** incisura tympanica. **sacrosciatic n., greater,** incisura ischiadica major. **sacrosciatic n., lesser,** incisura ischiadica minor. **scapular n.,** incisura scapulae. **sciatic n., greater,** incisura ischiadica major. **sciatic n., lesser,** incisura ischiadica minor. **semilunar n. of mandible,** incisura mandibulae. **semilunar n. of scapula,** incisura scapulae. **Sibson's n.,** an inward bend of the left upward limit of precordial dullness in acute pericardial effusion. **sigmoid n.,** incisura mandibulae. **sphenopalatine n. of palatine bone,** incisura sphenopalatina ossis palatini. **sternal n.,** incisura jugularis sterni. **supraorbital n.,** 1. incisura supraorbitalis. 2. incisura frontalis. **suprascapular n.,** incisura scapulae. **suprasternal n.,** incisura jugularis sterni. **tentorial n.,** incisura tentorii cerebelli. **thyroid n., inferior,** incisura thyroidea inferior. **thyroid n., superior,** incisura thyroidea superior. **trigeminal n.,** a notch in the superior border of the petrosal portion of the temporal

bone, near the apex, for transmission of the trigeminal nerve. **trochlear n. of ulna,** incisura trochlearis ulnae. **tympanic n.,** incisura tympanica. **ulnar n., ulnar n. of radius,** incisura ulnaris radii. **umbilical n.,** incisura ligamenti teretis. **vertebral n., inferior,** incisura vertebralis superior. **vertebral n., superior,** incisura vertebralis superior.

Notechis (no-tek′is) a genus of extremely venomous snakes of Australia. *N. scuta′tus* is the tiger snake.

notencephalocele (no″ten-sĕ-fal′o-sēl″) [*noto-* + Gr. *enkephalos* brain + *kēlē* hernia] hernial protrusion of the brain from the back of the head.

notencephalus (no″ten-sef′ah-lus) [*noto-* + Gr. *enkephalos* brain] a monster affected with notencephalocele.

Nothnagel's bodies, syndrome, type (nōt′nah- gelz) [Carl Wilhelm Hermann *Nothnagel*, German physician, 1841–1905] see under *body, syndrome,* and *acroparathesia*.

notifiable (no′tĭ-fi″ah-b'l) denoting that which should be made known; said of diseases that are required to be made known to the board of health.

noto- [Gr. *nōton* back] a combining form denoting relationship to the back.

notochord (no′to-kord) [*noto-* + Gr. *chordē* cord] the rod-shaped body, composed of cells derived from the mesoblast, below the primitive groove of the embryo, defining the primitive axis of the body; it is the common factor of all species of the phylum Chordata. It is the center of development of the axial skeleton. Called also *chorda dorsalis*.

notochordoma (no″to-kor-do′mah) chordoma.

Notoedres (no″to-ed′rēz) a genus of mites. **N. ca′ti,** an itch mite which causes a very persistent and often fatal mange in cats; it also infests domestic rabbits, and may temporarily infest man.

notogenesis (no″to-jen′ĕ-sis) [*noto-* + Gr. *gennan* to produce] the development of the notochord.

notomelus (no-tom′ĕ-lus) [*noto-* + Gr. *melos* limb] a fetus with accessory limbs on the back.

notomyelitis (no″to-mi″ĕ-li′tis) [*noto-* + *myelitis*] (*obs.*) inflammation of the spinal cord.

not-self (not′self) a term introduced by Burnet and Fenner to denote antigenic constituents foreign to the organism (self), which are eliminated through humoral or cell-mediated immunity.

notum (no′tum) [Gr. *nōton* the back] 1. the dorsal part of the body. 2. the dorsal element of each segment of an arthropod.

noumenal (nu′me-nal) pertaining to the noumenon; pertaining to rational intuition independent of sensory perception.

noumenon (nu′me-non) [Gr. *nooumenon* a thing thought] an object of intuition by the understanding independent of sensory perception.

nousic (noo′sik) [Gr. *nous* mind] pertaining to or affecting cerebration or the intellectual powers.

Novaldin (no-val′din) trademark for preparations of dipyrone.

novobiocin (no″vo-bi′o-sin) chemical name: *N*-[7-[[3-*O*-(aminocarbonyl)-5,5-di-*C*-methyl-4-*O*-methyl-α-L-lyxopyranosyl]-oxy]-4-hydroxy-8-methyl-2-oxo-2*H*-1-benzopyran-3-yl]-4-hydroxy-3-(3-methyl-2-butenyl)benzamide. An antibiotic, $C_{13}H_{36}N_2O_{11}$, obtained from *Streptomyces niveus* and other *Streptomyces* species, effective chiefly against staphylococci and other gram-positive organisms. **n. calcium,** the calcium salt of novobiocin, $C_{62}H_{70}CaN_4O_{22} \cdot 2H_2O$, occurring as a white or nearly white, crystalline powder, having the same actions as the base; used in the treatment of infections in children due to susceptible bacteria resistant to other antibiotics, administered orally. **n. sodium,** the sodium salt of novobiocin, $C_{31}H_{35}N_2NaO_{11}$, having the same appearance, actions, uses, and mode of administration as the calcium salt; usually used in adults.

Novocain (no′vo-kān) trademark for preparations of procaine hydrochloride.

novoscope (no′vo-skōp) [L. *novus* new + *scope*] Fornai's instrument for auscultatory percussion.

Novrad (nov′rad) trademark for preparations of levopropoxyphene napsylate.

Novy's rat disease (no′vēz) [Frederick George *Novy*, American bacteriologist, 1864–1957] see under *disease*.

noxa (nok′sah), pl. *nox′ae* [L. "harm"] an injurious agent, act, or influence.

noxious (nok′shus) [L. *noxius*] hurtful; not wholesome; pernicious; damaging to tissue.

Np chemical symbol for *neptunium*.

NPN nonprotein nitrogen.

N.R.C. normal retinal correspondence.

NREM non-rapid eye movements (see under *sleep*).

ns. nanosecond.

N.S.A. Neurosurgical Society of America.

N.S.C.C. National Society for Crippled Children.

nsec. nanosecond.

N.S.N.A. National Student Nurse Association.

N.S.P.B. National Society for the Prevention of Blindness.

N.T.A. National Tuberculosis Association.

N-terminal (ter′min-al) the amino (NH₂) end of a polypeptide chain, conventionally written to the left; called also *NH₂-terminal*.

N.T.P. normal temperature and pressure.

nU. nanounit.

nubecula (nu-bek′u-lah) [L., dim. of *nubes* cloud] 1. a slight cloudiness of the cornea or of the urine; a nebula. 2. statoconia.

nubility (nu-bil′ĭ-te) [L. *nubilitas;* from *nubere* to marry] marriageableness; fitness to marry; said of the female.

nucha (nu′kah) [L.] [NA] the nape, or scruff, or back of the neck.

nuchal (nu′kal) pertaining to the nucha, or back of the neck.

nucin (nu′sin) [L. *nux, nucis,* nut] juglandic acid.

nucis (nu′sis) [L.] genitive of *nux.*

Nuck's canal, diverticulum, hydrocele (nuks) [Anton *Nuck,* Dutch anatomist, 1650–1692] see *processus vaginalis peritonei* and *hydrocele muliebris.*

nuclear (nu′kle-ar) pertaining to a nucleus.

nuclease (nu′kle-ās) an enzyme or a group of enzymes which split nucleic acid into mononucleotides and other products. They are present as digestive enzymes in the intestinal tract and as autolytic enzymes in many cells. Similar enzymes are found in bacterial cultures. Some are specific for RNA (ribonuclease) and others for DNA (deoxyribonuclease). **purine n.,** an enzyme that causes the hydrolysis of purine nucleotides so as to liberate the purine base; it has been found in the pancreas.

nucleated (nu′kle-āt″ed) [L. *nucleatus*] having a nucleus or nuclei.

nuclei (nu′kle-i) [L.] plural of *nucleus.*

nucleide (nu′kle-īd) any compound of nucleic acid with a metallic element.

nucleiform (nu′kle-ĭ-form) shaped like a nucleus.

nuclein (nu′kle-in) a decomposition product of nucleoprotein intermediate between native nucleoprotein and nucleic acid (F. Miescher, 1874). It is a colorless, amorphous compound, soluble in dilute alkalis, but insoluble in dilute acids. The nucleins consists of nucleic acid and bases which vary in the different nucleins.

nucleinase (nu′kle-in-ās) nuclease.

nucleocapsid (nu″kle-o-kap′sid) a unit of viral structure, consisting of a capsid (protein coat) with the enclosed nucleic acid; some viruses are naked nucleocapsids, while in others the nucleocapsids form part of a more complex structure.

nucleochylema (nu″kle-o-ki-le′mah) [*nucleus* + Gr. *chylos* juice] the ground substance of the nucleus of a cell as distinguished from that of the cytoplasm.

nucleochyme (nu′kle-o-kīm) [*nucleus* + Gr. *chymos* juice] karyolymph.

nucleocytoplasmic (nu″kle-o-si″to-plaz′mik) pertaining to the nucleus and the cytoplasm of cells.

nucleofugal (nu″kle-of′u-gal) [*nucleus* + L. *fugere* to flee] moving away from a nucleus.

nucleoglucoprotein (nu″kle-o-gloo″ko-pro′te-in) a combination of a nucleoprotein with a carbohydrate.

nucleohistone (nu″kle-o-his′tōn) a complex nucleoprotein made up of deoxyribonucleic acid (DNA) and a histone, the principal constituent of chromatin.

nucleohyaloplasm (nu″kle-o-hi-al′o-plazm) linin.

nucleoid (nu′kle-oid) 1. resembling a nucleus. 2. a nucleus-like body sometimes seen in the center of an erythrocyte. 3. the nuclear region of a bacterium, which contains the chromosomes but is not limited by a nuclear membrane. 4. the genetic material (nucleic acid) of a virus, situated in the center of the virion. **Ladovski's n.,** centrosome.

nucleokeratin (nu″kle-o-ker′ah-tin) a variety of keratin found in the nervous system.

nucleolar (nu-kle′o-lar) pertaining to a nucleolus.

nucleoli (nu-kle′o-li) plural of *nucleolus.*

nucleoliform (nu″kle-ol′ĭ-form) resembling a nucleolus.

nucleolin (nu-kle′o-lin) the substance composing the nucleolus of a cell.

nucleolinus (nu″kle-o-li′nus) a deeply staining granule in the nucleolus.

nucleoloid (nu′kle-o-loid) resembling a nucleolus.

nucleololus (nu″kle-ol′o-lus) a minute spot within the nucleolus.

nucleolonema (nu″kle-o″lo-ne′mah) [*nucleolus* + Gr. *nēma* thread] a network of strands formed by organization of a finely granular substance, perhaps containing ribonucleic acid, in the nucleolus of a cell.

nucleoloneme (nu″kle-o′lo-nēm) nucleolonema.

nucleolonucleus (nu″kle-o-lo-nu′kle-us) a nucleololus.

nucleolus (nu-kle′o-lus), pl. *nucle′oli* [L., dim. of *nucleus*] a rounded refractile body present in the nucleus of most cells, which is the site of synthesis of ribosomal RNA, becoming enlarged during periods of synthesis and atrophied during quiescent periods; it consists of a mixed granular (pars granulosa) and a fibrillar (pars fibrosa) portion. Multiple nucleoli occur in some cells. Called also *micronucleus* and *plasmosome.* **chromatin n., false n., nucleinic n.,** karyosome. **secondary n.,** a mass sometimes seen near a nucleolus, and looking like a separated portion of the latter.

nucleolymph (nu′kle-o-limf″) karyolymph.

nucleomicrosome (nu″kle-o-mi′kro-sōm) [*nucleus* + Gr. *mikros* small + *sōma* body] any of the minute segments of a chromatin fiber.

nucleon (nu′kle-on) 1. a particle of the atomic nucleus, a proton or a neutron. 2. phosphocarnic acid.

nucleonic (nu″kle-on′ik) pertaining to a nucleus.

nucleonics (nu″kle-on′iks) the study of atomic nuclei and their reactions; nuclear physics.

nucleopetal (nu″kle-op′e-tal) [*nucleus* + L. *petere* to seek] moving toward a nucleus.

Nucleophaga (nu″kle-of′ah-gah) [*nucleus* + Gr. *phagein* to eat] an organism that is parasitic in amebas, destroying the nucleus of the latter.

nucleophagocytosis (noo″kle-o-fag″o-si-to′sis) the engulfing of the nuclei of other cells by phagocytes; see *tart* n., under *cell.*

nucleophile (nu′kle-o-fil″) an electron donor in chemical reactions involving covalent catalysis in which the donated electrons bond other chemical groups (electrophiles).

nucleophilic (nu″kle-o-fil′ik) having an affinity for nuclei; being or serving as a nucleophile.

nucleophosphatase (nu″kle-o-fos′fah-tās) nucleotidase.

nucleoplasm (nu′kle-o-plazm″) [*nucleus* + *plasma*] the protoplasm composing the nucleus of a cell; karyoplasm. Cf. *cytoplasm.*

nucleoprotamine (nu″kle-o-pro-tam′in) a compound of protamine and nucleic acid found chiefly in fish sperm.

nucleoprotein (nu″kle-o-pro′te-in) a substance composed of a simple basic protein, usually a histone or protamine, combined with a nucleic acid. **deoxyribose n.,** a deoxyribonucleic acid–protein complex. **ribose n.,** a ribonucleic acid–protein complex.

nucleoreticulum (nu″kle-o-re-tik′u-lum) [*nucleus* + *reticulum*] any intranuclear network.

nucleosidase (nu″kle-o-si′dās) *N*-ribosyl-purine ribohydrolase: an enzyme that catalyzes the splitting of nucleosides. The nucleosidases are adenosin-hydrolase, guanosin-hydrolase, inosin-hydrolase, and xanthosin-hydrolase.

nucleoside (nu′kle-o-sīd″) one of the glycosidic compounds into which a nucleotide is split by the action of nucleotidase or by chemical means; it is a combination of a sugar (a pentose) with a purine or a pyrimidine base.

nucleosidediphosphatase (nu″kle-o-sīd-di-fos′fah-tās) nucleosidediphosphate phosphohydrolase: an enzyme occurring in the liver and kidney that catalyzes the hydrolysis of a nucleoside diphosphate to a nucleotide and an orthophosphate.

nucleosin (nu′kle-o-sin) thymin.

nucleosis (nu″kle-o′sis) nuclear proliferation; abnormal increase in the production of nuclei, such as occurs in the subsarcolemmal nuclei of muscle following injury.

nucleosome (nu′kle-o-sōm″) [*nucleus* + Gr. *sōma* body] any of the complexes of histone and DNA in eukaryotic cells, seen under the electron microscope as beadlike bodies on a string of DNA.

nucleospindle (nu″kle-o-spin′d'l) the spindle-shaped body in mitosis.

nucleotherapy (nu″kle-o-ther′ah-pe) [*nuclein* + *therapy*] the treatment of disease with nucleins.

nucleotidase (nu″kle-ot′ĭ-dās) ribonucleotide phosphohydrolase: an enzyme that splits nucleotides into nucleosides and phosphoric acid; called also *phosphonuclease* and *nucleophosphatase.*

nucleotide (nu′kle-o-tīd) one of the compounds into which nucleic acid is split by the action of nuclease; the nucleotides are composed of a base (purine or pyrimidine), a sugar (ribose or deoxyribose), and a phosphate group. See *mononucleotide.* **cyclic n's,** nucleotides in which the phosphate group forms a ring, as in AMP and GMP. **n. polymerase,** an enzyme that takes part in the polymerization of activated nucleoside triphosphate in DNA synthesis.

nucleotidyl (nu″kle-o-tīd′il) a nucleotide residue.

nucleotidyltransferase (nu″kle-o-tīd′il-trans′fer-ās) any enzyme that catalyzes the transfer of a nucleotidyl from nucleoside phosphates to polymer forms. **DNA n.,** an enzyme that catalyzes the formation of DNA from deoxyribonucleoside triphosphates, with single-stranded DNA serving as a template; called also *DNA polymerase.* **polyadenate n.,** an enzyme that catalyzes the transfer of a phosphate group from ATP to form pyrophosphate and an adenylate polymer. **polyribonucleotide n.,** polynucleotide phosphorylase. **RNA n.,** an enzyme that catalyzes the formation of RNA from the four ribonucleoside triphosphates (which contain the bases adenine, guanine, cytosine, and uracil), with single-stranded DNA serving as a template; called also *RNA polymerase*.

nucleotoxin (nu″kle-o-tok′sin) 1. a toxin from cell nuclei. 2. any toxin exerting a deleterious effect on cell nuclei.

nucleus (nu′kle-us), pl. *nu′clei* [L., dim. of *nux* nut] 1. a cell nucleus: a spheroid body within a cell, consisting of a number of characteristic organelles visible with the optical microscope, a thin nuclear membrane, a nucleolus or nucleoli, irregular granules of chromatin and linin, and a diffuse nucleoplasm. 2. [NA] a general term used to designate a group of nerve cells ordinarily located within the central nervous system and bearing a direct relationship to the fibers of a particular nerve. 3. in organic chemistry, the combination of atoms forming the central element or basic framework of the molecule of a specific compound or class of compounds. 4. see *atomic n.* **abducens n., n. of abducens nerve,** n. nervi abducentis. **n. accesso′rius** [NA], **accessory n.,** a collection of small cells located dorsal to the upper part of the somatic groups of the oculomotor nuclear complex, comprising the parasympathetic outflow via the ciliary ganglion to the ciliary muscle and sphincter pupillae of the eye; called also *Edinger-Westphal n.* and *n. autonomicus* [NA alternative]. **nuclei of acoustic nerve,** nuclei nervi vestibulocochlearis. **n. acus′ticus,** see *nuclei nervi vestibulocochlearis.* **n. acus′ticus, infe′rior et latera′lis,** see *nuclei cochleares, ventralis et dorsalis.* **n. acus′ticus supe′rior,** the superior vestibular nucleus; see *nuclei vestibulares.* **n. a′lae cine′reae,** n. dorsalis nervi vagi. **ambiguous n.,** n. ambiguus. **ambiguous n. of Quain,** n. nervi hypoglossi. **n. ambig′uus** [NA], ambiguous nucleus: the nucleus of origin of motor fibers of the vagus, glossopharyngeal, and accessory nerves that supply the striated muscles of the larynx and pharynx. It consists of an intermittent cell column in the middle of the lateral funiculus of the medulla oblongata, between the caudal end of the medulla and the level of exit of the glossopharyngeal nerve. **n. amyg′dalae, amygdaloid n.,** corpus amygdaloideum. **n. amygdalifor′mis of J. Stilling,** n. subthalamicus. **amygdaloid n.,** corpus amygdaloideum. **n. angula′ris, Bekhterev′i,** the superior vestibular nucleus; see *nuclei vestibulares.* **n. ante′rior thal′ami,** former NA term for nuclei anteriores thalami. **anterior nuclei of thalamus,** nuclei anteriores thalami. **nu′clei anterio′res thal′ami** [NA], anterior nuclei of thalamus: the three nuclei in the anterior part of the thalamus: the nucleus anteroventralis, nucleus anterodorsalis, and nucleus anteromedialis. Together, they receive connections from the mamillary body and fornix and project fibers to the cingulate body. Formerly called *n. anterior thalami.* **anterodorsal n., n. anterodorsa′lis** [NA], see *nuclei anteriores thalami.* **anteromedial n., n. anteromedia′lis** [NA], see *nuclei anteriores thalami.* **anteroventral n., n anteroventra′lis** [NA], see *nuclei anteriores thalami.* **nu′clei arcifor′mes,** nuclei arcuati. **nu′clei arcua′ti** [NA], arcuate nuclei of medulla oblongata: small, irregular areas of gray substance found on the ventromedial aspect of the pyramid of the medulla oblongata. **n. of atom, atomic n.,** the central core of an atom, constituting almost all of its mass but only a small part of its volume, and composed of protons and neutrons, the protons being positively charged and their number (atomic number) being fixed for all the atoms of each element and equal to the number of the orbiting electrons. The neutrons, which bear no charge, may vary in number, accounting for the isotopes of an element. **auditory nuclei,** see *nuclei cochleares, ventralis et dorsalis,* and *nuclei vestibularis.* **nuclei of auditory nerve,** nuclei nervi vestibulocochlearis. **n. of auditory nerve, accessory,** see *nuclei cochleares, ventralis et dorsalis.* **n. autonom′icus,** NA alternative for n. accessorius. **Balbiani′s n.,** yolk n. **basal n.,** 1. nucleus olivaris. 2. [pl.] the corpus striatum, amygdaloid body, and claustrum; see also *basal ganglia.* **n. basa′lis,** n. olivaris. **Béclard′s n.,** a vascular lentil-shaped center of ossification seen in the cartilage of the lower epiphysis of the femur during the latter part of fetal life. **Bekhterev′s n.,** the superior vestibular nucleus; see *nuclei vestibulares.* **Blumenau′s n.,** the lateral portion of the cuneate nucleus. **n. of Burdach′s column,** n. cuneatus. **n. cauda′lis centra′lis** [NA], central caudate nucleus: an unpaired collection of cells in the caudal third of the oculomotor nuclear complex, located in the median raphe somewhat dorsal to the lateral nuclei. **caudate n., n. cauda′tus** [NA], an elongated, arched gray mass closely related to the lateral ventricle throughout its entire extent and consisting of a head, body, and tail. The caudate nucleus and putamen form a functional unit (the neostriatum) of the corpus striatum. **cell n., cellular n.,** see *nucleus,* def. 1. **central n. of thalamus, n. centra′lis thal′ami,** a collection of cells lying close to the wall of the third ventricle, between the medial and the posterior ventral nuclei of the thalamus, medial to and partially embedded in the internal medullary lamina. **n. centromedia′nus thal′ami,** NA alternative for n. medialis centralis thalami. **n. cerebel′li,** n. dentatus. **n. of cerebellum, dentate,** n. dentatus. **n. of cerebellum, medullary,** corpus medullare cerebelli. **cervical n., cervical n., lateral,** n. lateralis cervicalis. **cho-**

lane n., a cyclopentanophenanthrene structure forming the basis of the specific compounds, found in the bile acids, the sterols, in toad poisons, in digitalis, strophanthus, ouabain, and other heart aglycones, in the sex hormones, and in some carcinogenic hydrocarbons. **n. cine′reum,** substantia grisea medullae spinalis. **Clarke′s n., n. of Clarke′s column,** n. thoracicus. **cleavage n.,** segmentation n. **cochlear n.,** see *nuclei cochleares, ventralis et doralis.* **cochlear n., ventral,** see *nuclei cochleares, ventralis et dorsalis.* **nu′clei cochlea′res, ventra′lis et dorsa′lis** [NA], the ventral and dorsal cochlear nuclei: the nuclei of termination of the sensory fibers of the pars cochlearis nervi vestibulocochlearis, which enter the brain through the inferior root of the nerve. The nuclei partly encircle the inferior cerebellar peduncle at the junction between the medulla oblongata and pons. The dorsal cochlear nucleus forms an eminence (the acoustic tubercle) on the most lateral part of the floor of the fourth ventricle. Called also *nuclei nervi cochlearis.* **nuclei of cochlear nerve,** nuclei cochlearis, ventralis et dorsalis. **n. collic′uli inferio′ris** [NA], nucleus of inferior colliculus: the large oval-shaped group of nerve cell bodies that makes up most of the substance of the inferior colliculus. **compact n.,** a cellular nucleus with an inconspicuous nuclear membrane and minute chromatin granules throughout its substance. **conjugation n.,** fertilization n. **n. cor′poris genicula′ti latera′lis** [NA], nucleus of lateral geniculate body: a nucleus within the lateral geniculate body, composed of a small ventral and a large dorsal part, the latter consisting of six concentrically arranged cell layers which receive crossed and uncrossed fibers of the optic tract and which are connected with the visual cortex. **n. cor′poris genicula′ti media′lis** [NA], nucleus of medial geniculate body: a nucleus within the medial geniculate body, composed of central and dorsal parts which receive ascending auditory fibers and project to the auditory cortex. **nu′clei cor′poris mamilla′ris** [NA], nuclei of mamillary body: three masses of cells within the mamillary body which comprise medial, intermediate, and lateral nuclei. The nuclei receive fibers from the basal olfactory areas and the fornix, and project to the thalamus and midbrain via mamillothalamic and mamillotegmental fasciculi. **nuclei cor′poris trapezoi′dei** [NA], the two nuclei of the trapezoid body in the pons: the dorsal (superior olive) and the ventral nuclei. **n. of corpus striatum, intraventricular,** n. caudatus. **nuclei of cranial nerves,** nuclei nervorum cranialium. **cuneate n.,** n. cuneatus. **cuneate n., accessory, cuneate n., lateral,** n. cuneatus accessorius. **n. cunea′tus** [NA], cuneate nucleus: a nucleus in the medulla oblongata at the rostral end of the fasciculus cuneatus, in which the fibers of this fasciculus synapse; the cells project to the thalamus via the medial lemniscus. Called also *n. funiculi cuneati.* **n. cunea′tus accesso′rius** [NA], accessory cuneate nucleus: a group of nerve cells lying lateral to the nucleus cuneatus that relay impulses from upper limb fibers in the fasciculus cuneatus to the cerebellum (rostral spinocerebellar tract) via external arcuate fibers and the inferior cerebellar peduncle; called also *lateral cuneate n.* **Darkshevich′s n.,** a small nucleus dorsal to the medial longitudinal fasciculus in the central gray matter at the rostral end of the cerebral aqueduct; it is believed to receive fibers from the fasciculus and from the superior colliculus. **daughter n.,** a new cell nucleus formed in mitosis by the diaster. **Deiters′ n.,** the lateral vestibular nucleus; see *nuclei vestibulares.* **dental n.,** pulpa dentis. **dentate n., n. denta′tus** [NA], the largest of the deep cerebellar nuclei lying in the white matter of the cerebellum just lateral to the emboliform nucleus, and receiving Purkinje cell fibers from the neocerebellum; its axons form most of the superior cerebellar peduncle and project chiefly to the contralateral red nucleus and thalamus. **diploid n.,** a cell nucleus containing the number of chromosomes typical of the somatic cells of the particular species. **dorsal n. of Clarke, n. dorsa′lis,** n. thoracicus. **dorsal lateral n.,** lateralis dorsalis. **n. dorsa′lis [Stillin′gi, Clark′ii],** n. thoracicus. **n. dorsa′lis cor′poris trapezoi′dei** [NA], dorsal nucleus of trapezoid body: a group of nerve cell bodies dorsolateral to the trapezoid body; it receives cochlear fibers and contributes to the formation of the trapezoid body and lateral lemniscus. Called also *n. olivaris superior* or *superior olivary n.* **n. dorsa′lis ner′vi glossopharyn′gei** [NA], dorsal nucleus of glossopharyngeal nerve: the rostral part of the column which forms the dorsal nucleus of the vagus nerve; it is believed to give some parasympathetic fibers to the glossopharyngeal nerve. **n. dorsa′lis ner′vi va′gi** [NA], dorsal nucleus of vagus nerve: the nucleus of origin of the parasympathetic fibers of the vagus nerve, situated just dorsal or dorsolateral to the nucleus intercalatus; called also *n. alae cinereae.* **dorsolateral n., n. dorsolatera′lis** [NA], dorsally placed cells in the lateral part of the oculomotor nuclear complex; they are very distinct from the ventrally placed cells in the middle third of the complex and have a somatic motor function. **dorsomedial n. of thalamus,** n. medialis thalami. **n. dorsomedia′lis hypothal′ami** [NA], dorsomedial nucleus of hypothalamus: the dorsal one of two main cell groups in the medial part of the tuberal region of the hypothalamus. **drumstick n.,** see *drumstick,* under D. **Duval′s n.,** a collection of multipolar ganglion cells situated ventrolaterally from the hypoglossal nucleus in the medulla oblongata. **Edinger's n.,** n. accessorius. **Edinger-Westphal n.,** n. accessorius. **emboliform n., n. embolifor'mis cerebel'li** [NA], a small mass that lies between the dentate nucleus and globose nucleus and contributes to the superior peduncles. **end nuclei,** terminal nuclei. **n. of facial nerve,** n. nervi facialis. **fastigial n., n. fasti'gii** [NA], the most medial of the deep cerebellar nuclei, near the midline in the roof of the fourth ventricle; it projects to the pons and medulla oblongata, chiefly to the vestibular nuclei. **fertilization n.,** the nucleus produced by fusion of the male and female pronuclei in the fertilized ovum; called also *conjugation n., zygote n.,* and *synkaryon.* **free n.,** a cell nucleus from which the other elements of the cell have disappeared. **n. funic'uli cunea'ti,** n. cuneatus. **n. funic'uli gra'cilis,** n. gracilis. **n. gelatino'sus,** n. pulposus disci intervertebralis. **germ n., germinal n.,** pronucleus. **gingival n.,** a part of the cerebellum in the third and fourth months of fetal life. **globose n., n. globo'sus cerebel'li** [NA], a deep cerebellar nucleus that lies between the emboliform nucleus and the fastigial nucleus and projects its fibers via the superior cerebellar peduncle. **n. of glossopharyngeal nerve, dorsal,** n. dorsalis nervi glossopharyngei. **n. of Goll's column,** n. gracilis. **gonad n.,** micronucleus, def. 1. **n. gra'cilis** [NA], a nucleus in the medulla oblongata at the rostral end of the fasciculus gracilis of the cord, in which the fibers of the fasciculus gracilis synapse; the cells project to the thalamus via the medial lemniscus. Called also *n. funiculi gracilis* and *Goll's tract.* **gray n.,** substantia grisea medullae spinalis. **nuclei of habenula, nu'clei haben'ulae** [NA], **habenular n.,** two nerve cell groups within the habenula which give rise to the fasciculus retroflexus. **haploid n.,** a cell nucleus containing half of the number of chromosomes typical of the somatic cells of a particular species. **hypoglossal n., n. of hypoglossal nerve,** n. nervi hypoglossi. **hypothalamic n., n. hypothalam'icus** (*obs.*), n. subthalamicus. **n. of hypothalamus, dorsomedial,** n. dorsomedialis hypothalami. **n. of hypothalamus, paraventricular,** n. paraventricularis hypothalami. **n. of hypothalamus, posterior,** n. posterior hypothalami. **n. of hypothalamus, supraoptic,** n. supraopticus hypothalami. **n. of hypothalamus, ventromedial,** n. ventromedialis hypothalami. **n. of inferior colliculus,** n. colliculi inferioris. **n. intercala'tus** [NA], a group of nerve cells between the dorsal nucleus of the vagus nerve and the nucleus of the hypoglossal nerve, forming part of the perihypoglossal nuclear complex; called also *Staderini's n.* **intermediolateral n., n. intermediolatera'lis,** a nucleus situated in the substantia intermedia lateralis of thoracic and upper lumbar levels of the spinal cord, which forms the lateral horn, and whose cells give rise to the preganglionic sympathetic outflow. **intermediomedial n., n. intermediomedia'lis,** a nucleus composed of scattered cells in the substantia intermedia centralis, medial to the nucleus intermediolateralis; it is most prominent in the cervical spinal cord and is thought to be propriospinal in its connections. **n. of internal geniculate body,** n. corporis geniculati medialis. **interpeduncular n., n. interpeduncula'ris** [NA], a nucleus situated between the cerebral peduncles immediately dorsal to the interpeduncular fossa, which receives the fasciculus retroflexus; called also *Ganser's ganglion.* **interstitial n., interstitial n. of Cajal, n. interstitia'lis** [NA], a nucleus at the rostral end of the medial longitudinal fasciculus in the mesencephalic tegmentum; its chief connections are reciprocal with vestibular nuclei and it also projects to the spinal cord. **intralaminar nuclei, nu'clei intralamina'res** [NA], the nuclei within the internal medullary lamina of the thalamus. **Kaiser's nuclei,** longitudinal motor nuclei in the cervical and lumbar enlargements of the cord, between the intermediolateral column and the median column. **Klein-Gumprecht nuclei** (*obs.*), unstainable nuclei seen in degenerating lymphocytes in leukemia. **Kölliker's n.,** substantia intermedia centralis. **large cell auditory n.,** the lateral vestibular nucleus; see *nuclei vestibulares.* **laryngeal n.,** the nucleus of origin (nucleus ambiguus) of the nerve fibers going to the larynx. **n. of lateral geniculate body,** n. corporis geniculati lateralis. **n. of lateral lemniscus,** n. lemnisci lateralis. **n. latera'lis cervica'lis,** lateral cervical nucleus: a small group of cells in the lateral funiculus of the first and second cervical segments of the spinal cord, comprising a relay station in a spinocervicothalamic path. **n. latera'lis dorsa'lis** [NA], dorsal lateral nucleus: one of the two dorsally placed nuclei in the lateral nuclei of the thalamus; its chief connections are with the cingulate gyrus. **n. latera'lis medul'lae oblonga'tae** [NA], a nucleus in the reticular substance of the medulla oblongata, dorsolateral to the olive; it relays spinal impulses to the cerebellum. Called also *lateral reticular n.* **nu'clei latera'les thal'ami** [NA], lateral nuclei of thalamus: a nuclear mass lying between the internal medullary lamina and the internal capsule, commonly divided into a larger ventral part and a smaller dorsal part. The ventral part comprises the n. ventralis anterolateralis, n. ventralis intermedius, n. ventralis posteromedialis, and n. ventralis posterolateralis; these nuclei (particularly the last two), together with the geniculate bodies, are concerned with relaying sensory impulses to specific areas of the

cerebral cortex. The dorsal part includes n. lateralis dorsalis, which has major connections with the cingulate gyrus, and n. posterior thalami, which has extensive connections with the cerebral cortex. **n. latera'lis thal'ami,** a term replaced by the plural form; see *n. laterales thalami.* **n. lemnis'ci latera'lis** [NA], nucleus of lateral lemniscus: several diffuse cell groups interposed in the course of the lateral lemniscus through the pons. **n. of lens,** n. lentis. **lenticular n., lentiform n.,** n. lentiformis. **n. lentifor'mis** [NA], lentiform nucleus: the part of the corpus striatum comprising the putamen and globus pallidus; it lies just lateral to the internal capsule. Called also *lenticular n.* **n. len'tis** [NA], nucleus of the lens: the harder internal part of the lens of the eye. **n. of Luys,** nucleus subthalamicus. **n. magnocellula'ris,** the lateral vestibular nucleus; see *nuclei vestibulares.* **nuclei of mamillary body,** nuclei corporis mamillaris. **n. of medial geniculate body,** n. corporis geniculati medialis. **n. media'lis centra'lis thal'ami** [NA], centromedian nucleus of thalamus: a prominent nucleus lying mostly within the internal medullary lamina of the thalamus, between the medial nucleus above and the ventral posteromedial nucleus below; it has complex connections with the corpus striatum and motor cortex. Called also *n. centromedianus thalami* [NA alternative] and *centrum medianum.* **n. media'lis thal'ami** [NA], medial nucleus of thalamus: a prominent nuclear mass lying between the internal medullary lamina and the periventricular gray matter. Composed of magnicellular and parvicellular parts, it has extensive intrathalamic, hypothalamic, subcortical, and cortical connections. Called also *dorsomedial n. of thalamus.* **n. of medulla oblongata, arcuate,** nuclei arcuati. **n. medulla'ris cerebel'li,** corpus medullare cerebelli. **n. of mesencephalic tract of trigeminal nerve,** n. tractus mesencephalicus nervi trigemini. **Monakow's n.,** the lateral part of the cuneate nucleus. **motion n.,** kinetoplast. **motor n.,** any collection of cells of the central nervous system giving origin to motor fibers of a nerve. **motor n. of trigeminal nerve, n. moto'rius ner'vi trigem'ini** [NA], the nucleus of origin of the motor fibers of the trigeminal nerve, located in the dorsolateral part of the pons, just medial to the main sensory nucleus and the entering sensory root. See also *n. sensorius principalis nervi trigemini.* **n. ner'vi abducen'tis** [NA], nucleus of abducens nerve: the nucleus of origin of the abducens nerve; it lies in the lower part of the pons and forms the lateral part of the facial colliculus in the floor of the fourth ventricle; fibers of the facial nerve form a complicated loop about the nucleus. **n. ner'vi accesso'rii** [NA], the nucleus of origin of the accessory nerve; situated in the medulla oblongata and upper five or six levels of the cervical spinal cord, it comprises the nucleus ambiguus (caudal part) and the spinal nucleus in the anterior horn. **nu'clei ner'vi acus'tici,** nuclei nervi vestibulocochlearis. **nu'clei nervo'rum cerebra'lium,** nuclei nervorum cranialium. **nu'clei ner'vi cochlea'ris,** nuclei cochleares, ventralis et dorsalis. **nu'clei nervo'rum crania'lium** [NA], nuclei of cranial nerves: groups of nerve cells in the central nervous system that give rise to, or transmit or receive impulses from, the motor and sensory components of the cranial nerves. **n. ner'vi facia'lis** [NA], nucleus of facial nerve: the nucleus of origin of the motor fibers of the facial nerve, which innervate the muscles of facial expression; the nucleus lies in the ventrolateral part of the lower pons, and its emerging fibers form a complicated loop about the nucleus of the abducent nerve. The term is also applied collectively to the motor nucleus, the superior salivatory nucleus, and the nucleus of the tractus solitarius. **n. ner'vi facia'lis of Arnold,** colliculus facialis. **n. ner'vi glossopharyn'gei** [NA], the nucleus of origin and termination of the glossopharyngeal nerve; located in the medulla oblongata, it comprises the inferior salivatory nucleus, the nucleus ambiguus (rostral part), and the nucleus of the tractus solitarius. **n. ner'vi hypoglos'si** [NA], nucleus of hypoglossal nerve: the nucleus of origin of the hypoglossal nerve, forming a column in the central gray matter of the medial eminence from below the level of the inferior olive to the upper part of the medulla oblongata. **n. ner'vi oculomoto'rii** [NA], nucleus of oculomotor nerve: the nucleus or origin of the fibers of the oculomotor nerve, situated in the tegmentum of the mesencephalon immediately ventral to the central gray matter, where its two cell groups form a complex between the medial longitudinal fasciculi; the complex comprises paired lateral somatic groups, an unpaired median somatic group, and paired dorsal autonomic (parasympathetic) groups. The somatic groups supply the levator palpebrae superioris and all the extrinsic eye muscles except the lateral rectus and superior oblique; the autonomic group supplies the ciliary muscle and sphincter pupillae. **nu'clei ner'vi trigem'ini** [NA], the nuclear complex of the trigeminal nerve, located chiefly in the pons and medulla oblongata, but also in the mesencephalon and upper cervical cord. See *n. motorius nervi trigemini, n. sensorius principalis nervi trigemini, n. tractus mesencephalicus nervi trigemini,* and *n. tractus spinalis nervi trigemini.* **n. ner'vi trochlea'ris** [NA], nucleus of trochlear nerve: the nucleus of origin of the motor fibers of the trochlear nerve; it lies in the central gray matter on the dorsal surface of the medial longitudinal fasciculus in the lower part of the mesencephalon. **n. ner'vi va'gi,** the nucleus of origin and termination of the vagus nerve; situated in the medulla oblongata, it comprises the nucleus dorsalis, the nucleus ambiguus, and the nucleus of the tractus solitarius. **nu′clei ner′vi vestibula′ris,** nuclei vestibulares. **nu′clei ner′vi vestibulocochlea′ris** [NA], vestibulocochlear nuclei: the nuclei of termination of the sensory fibers of the vestibular and cochlear divisions of the eighth cranial nerve, comprising the ventral and dorsal cochlear nuclei and the medial, lateral, superior, and inferior vestibular nuclei. Called also *nuclei nervi acustici.* **nutrition n.,** macronucleus. **n. of oculomotor nerve,** n. nervi oculomotorii. **n. oliva′ris** [NA], olivary nucleus: a folded band of gray substance enclosing a white core (hilus nuclei olivaris), and producing the elevation on the medulla oblongata known as the olive; it is a nuclear complex which receives heavy projections from the spinal cord, mesencephalon, and cerebral cortex, and projects fibers, via the opposite inferior cerebellar peduncle, partly to the vermis, but principally to the neocerebellum. Called also *n. olivaris inferior* or *inferior olivary n.* **n. oliva′ris accesso′rius dorsa′lis** [NA], dorsal accessory olivary nucleus: the band of cells that lies dorsal to the olivary nucleus and projects fibers to the opposite side of the cerebellum, especially to the vermis. **n. oliva′ris accesso′rius media′lis** [NA], medial accessory olivary nucleus: the band of gray substance that lies medial to the olivary nucleus and projects fibers to the opposite side of the cerebellum, especially to the vermis. **n. oliva′ris inferior,** n. olivaris. **n. oliva′ris supe′rior,** n. dorsalis corporis trapezoidei. **olivary n.,** 1. nucleus olivaris. 2. oliva. **olivary n., accessory, olivary n., dorsal accessory,** n. olivaris accessorius dorsalis. **olivary n., inferior,** n. olivaris. **olivary n., medial accessory,** n. olivaris accessorius medialis. **olivary n., superior,** n. dorsalis corporis trapezoidei. **n. of origin,** any collection of nerve cells giving origin to the fibers, or a part of the fibers, of a peripheral nerve. **nuclei of origin of cranial nerves, nu′clei ori′ginis nervo′rum cerebra′lium, nu′clei ori′-ginis nervo′rum crania′lium** [NA], groups of nerve cells in the central nervous system, the axons of which exit as the efferent fibers of various cranial nerves. **Pander's n.,** n. subthalamicus. **n. paraventricula′ris hypothal′ami** [NA], paraventricular nucleus of hypothalamus: a sharply defined band of cells in the wall of the third ventricle in the supraoptic part of the hypothalamus; many of its cells are neurosecretory in function (secreting oxytocin) and project to the neurohypophysis. **Perlia's n.,** a group of cells in the midline of the oculomotor nuclear complex, thought to be associated with ocular convergence. **phenanthrene n.,** cholane n. **polymorphic n.,** a cell nucleus that assumes an irregular form or splits up into more or less completely separated lobes, such as the nuclei in the polymorphonuclear leukocytes (neutrophils). **pontine nuclei, nu′clei pon′tis** [NA], groups of nerve cell bodies in the portion of the pyramidal tract within the pars ventralis of the pons upon which the fibers of the corticopontine tract synapse, and whose axons in turn cross to the opposite side and form the middle cerebellar peduncle, which projects fibers to the neocerebellum. **n. poste′rior hypothal′ami** [NA], posterior nucleus of hypothalamus: a group of nerve cell bodies in the posterior, mamillary part of the hypothalamus, above the nucleus of the mamillary body; the nucleus has major brain stem connections via periventricular fibers and the dorsal longitudinal fasciculus. **n. poste′rior thal′ami** [NA], the posterior nucleus of the thalamus, which receives fibers from the somatic, sensory, auditory, and visual projection areas of the cortex. Called also *pulvinar thalami* [NA alternative]. **pretectal n., n. pretecta′lis** [NA], several indistinct groups of cells in the pretectal area which receive impulses chiefly from the optic tract; they project to the nucleus accessorius of the oculomotor nerve and constitute the midbrain center for the pupillary light reflex. **n. pulpo′sus dis′ci interverte-bra′lis** [NA], pulpy n., a semifluid mass of fine white and elastic fibers that forms the central portion of an intervertebral disk; it has been regarded as the persistent remains of the embryonic notochord. **pyramidal n.,** n. olivaris accessorius medialis. **n. radi′cis descenden′tis ner′vi trigem′ini,** n. tractus mesencephalicus nervi trigemini. **red n.,** n. ruber. **reproductive n.,** micronucleus, def. 1. **reticular n., lateral,** n. lateralis medullae oblongatae. **n. reticula′ris tegmen′ti,** a nucleus in the tegmentum of the pons which receives fibers from the cerebral cortex and mesencephalon and which projects fibers to the neocerebellum via the middle cerebellar peduncle. **n. reticula′ris thal′ami** [NA], reticular nucleus of thalamus: a thin layer of cells on the lateral surface of the thalamus, within and lateral to the external medullary lamina. **Roller's n.,** 1. a sharply defined nucleus immediately anterior to the hypoglossal nucleus, forming part of the perihypoglossal nuclear complex; called also *sublingual n.* 2. cells near the hilus of the olivary nucleus. **n. of roof of cerebellum,** n. fastigii. **n. ru′ber** [NA], red nucleus: a distinctive oval nucleus (pink in fresh specimens because of relatively high vascularity) centrally placed in the upper mesencephalic reticular formation; it receives fibers from the deep cerebellar nuclei and cerebral cortex and projects fibers to the cerebellum, brain stem, spinal cord, and probably to the thalamus. **sacral n.,** the lumbosacral extension of the nucleus thoracicus. **n. salivato′rius**

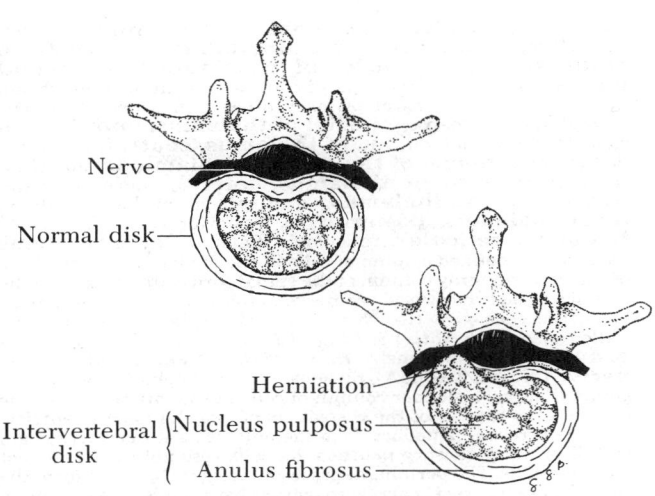

Nucleus pulposus in transverse section, showing normal intervertebral disk and herniation of the nucleus pulposus.

infe′rior [NA], inferior salivatory nucleus: the caudal part of the column of scattered cells in the dorsolateral part of the reticular formation in the lower pons and upper medulla oblongata, whose cells comprise the parasympathetic outflow of the glossopharyngeal nerve for the supply of the parotid gland. **n. salivato′rius supe′rior** [NA], superior salivatory nucleus: a column of scattered cells in the dorsolateral part of the reticular formation of the lower pons whose cells comprise the parasympathetic outflow of the facial nerve (via the nervus intermedius) for the supply of the lacrimal, nasal, palatine, submandibular, and sublingual glands; it is continuous with the nucleus salivatorius inferior. **salivatory n., inferior,** n. salivatorius inferior. **salivatory n., superior,** n. salivatorius superior. **n. of Sappey,** n. ruber. **Schwalbe's n.,** the medial vestibular nucleus; see *nuclei vestibulares.* **Schwann's n.,** the nucleus of a Schwann cell. **segmentation n.,** the fertilization nucleus after cleavage has begun. **n. senso′rius infe′rior ner′vi trigem′ini,** n. tractus spinalis nervi trigemini. **n. senso′rius principa′lis ner′vi trigem′ini** [NA], **n. senso′rius supe′rior ner′vi trigem′ini,** principal sensory nucleus of trigeminal nerve: the nucleus of termination of afferent fibers of the trigeminal nerve, carrying impulses for sensations of touch and pressure, located in the dorsolateral part of the middle of the pons, just lateral to the entering trigeminal root fibers. Called also *superior sensory n. of trigeminal nerve.* **sensory n.,** the nucleus of termination of the afferent (sensory) fibers of a peripheral nerve. **sensory n. of trigeminal nerve, lower,** n. tractus spinalis nervi trigemini. **sensory n. of trigeminal nerve, superior,** n. sensorius superior nervi trigemini. **Setchenow's (Sechenoff's) nuclei,** see under *center.* **shadow n.,** a cell nucleus that does not stain and appears as a faint shadow under the microscope. **Siemerling's n.,** one of the subdivisions of the oculomotor nuclear complex. **n. of solitary tract,** n. tractus solitarii. **somatic n.,** macronucleus. **sperm n.,** the male pronucleus. **spherical n.,** n. globosus. **spinal n. of accessory nerve,** n. spinalis nervi accessorii. **n. of spinal tract of trigeminal nerve,** n. tractus spinalis nervi trigemini. **n. spina′lis ner′vi acesso′rii** [NA], spinal nucleus of accessory nerve: the group of cells in the anterior horn of the upper five or six levels of the cervical spinal cord that form the spinal roots of the accessory nerve. **Spitzka's n.,** Perlia's n. **Staderini's n.,** n. intercalatus. **Stilling's n.,** 1. sacral n. 2. n. thoracicus. **Stilling's sacral n.,** sacral n. **striate n.,** a term loosely applied to the neostriatum, to a nucleus of the corpus striatum, or to the corpus striatum itself. **subependymal n.,** the dorsal cochlear nucleus. **sublingual n.,** Roller's n., def. 1. **subthalamic n., n. subthalam′icus** [NA], a biconvex mass of gray matter on the medial side of the junction of the internal capsule and the crus cerebri; its chief connections are with the globus pallidus. Called also *n. of Luys, corpus Luysi,* and *Luys' body.* **superior n.,** the superior vestibular nucleus; see *nuclei vestibulares.* **n. supraop′ticus hypothal′ami** [NA], supraoptic nucleus of hypothalamus: a sharply defined nucleus immediately above the lateral part of the optic chiasm; many of its cells are neurosecretory in function (secreting antidiuretic hormone) and project to the neurohypophysis; other cells are osmoreceptors which respond to increased osmotic pressure to signal the release of antidiuretic hormone by the neurohypophysis. **n. taeniaefor′mis,** corpus amygdaloideum. **n. tec′ti,** n. fastigii. **tegmental nuclei,** nuclei tegmenti mesencephalici. **nu′clei tegmen′ti mesencephal′ici** [NA], several nuclear masses of the reticular formations of the pons and midbrain, especially of the latter, where they are in close approximation to the superior cerebellar peduncles. **terminal nuclei, nu′clei terminia′les, nu′clei terminatio′nis nervo′rum crania′lium** [NA], nuclei of termination of cranial nerves, groups of nerve cells within the central nervous system upon which the axons of primary afferent neurons of various cranial nerves synapse. **nuclei of thalamus, anterior,** nuclei anteriores thalami. **n. of thalamus, central,** n. centralis thalami. **nuclei of thalamus, intralaminar,** nuclei intralaminares. **n. of thalamus, lateral,** nuclei laterales thalami. **n. of thalamus, medial,** n. medialis thalami. **n. of thalamus, posterior,** n. posterior thalami. **n. of thalamus, reticular,** reticularis thalami. **n. thorac′icus** [NA], a well-defined column of cells in the medial part of the base of the posterior gray column of the spinal cord, extending from the seventh or eighth cervical segments to the second or third lumbar level; the cells give rise to the posterior spinocerebellar tract. Called also *n. dorsalis* [*Stillingi, Clarkii*]. **n. of tongue, fibrous,** septum linguae. **n. trac′tus mesencephal′icus ner′vi trigem′ini** [NA], nucleus of mesencephalic tract of trigeminal nerve: a slender column of cells in the lateral part of the central gray matter of the rostral portion of the fourth ventricle and the cerebral aqueduct. It is the only central nervous system site of primary sensory neurons, its cells resembling dorsal root ganglion cells. The peripheral processes of its cells, which form the mesencephalic tract, carry proprioceptive impulses; the central processes have widespread cerebellar and brain stem connections, including the motor nucleus of the trigeminal nerve. Called also *n. descendentis nervi trigemini*. **n. trac′tus solita′rii** [NA], nucleus of solitary tract: the nucleus of termination of the visceral afferent fibers of the facial, glossopharyngeal, and vagus nerves, which enter the tractus solitarius. It surrounds the tractus solitarius and its caudal end joins with the caudal end of the corresponding nucleus of the opposite side. **n. trac′tus spina′lis ner′vi trigem′ini** [NA], nucleus of spinal tract of trigeminal nerve: a column of cells which lies along the medial aspect of the spinal tract, extending from the level of entry of the trigeminal nerve in the pons to the second cervical segment of the spinal cord, where it is continuous with the posterior gray column. The nucleus has several cytoarchitectonic subdivisions and the fibers of the spinal tract end in it. **n. of trapezoid body, dorsal,** n. dorsalis corporis trapezoidei. **triangular n.,** the medial vestibular nucleus; see *nuclei vestibulares.* **n. triangula′ris,** the medial vestibular nucleus; see *nuclei vestibulares.* **nuclei of trigeminal nerve,** see *n. motorius nervi trigemini, n. sensorius principalis nervi trigemini,* and *n. tractus spinalis nervi trigemini.* **n. of trochlear nerve,** n. nervi trochlearis. **trophic n.,** macronucleus. **tuberal nuclei, nu′clei tubera′les** [NA], **nu′clei tu′beris,** see *n. dorsomedialis hypothalami* and *n. ventromedialis hypothalami.* **vagoglossopharyngeal n.,** n. ambiguus. **n. of vagus nerve, dorsal,** n. dorsalis nervi vagi. **ventral n. of thalamus,** the nuclear group containing several ventral nuclei of the nuclei laterales thalami. **ventral n. of thalamus, anterior,** n. ventralis anterolateralis. **ventral n. of thalamus, intermediate,** n. ventralis intermedius. **ventral n. of thalamus, lateral,** n. ventralis intermedius. **ventral n. of thalamus, posterior,** see *n. ventralis thalami posterior.* **ventral n. of trapezoid body,** n. ventralis corporis trapezoidei. **n. ventra′lis anterolatera′lis** [NA], the anterolateral ventral nucleus of the thalamus, which receives fibers from the globus pallidus and sends other fibers back to the corpus striatum; called also *n. ventralis thalami anterior* or *anterior ventral n. of thalamus.* **n. ventra′lis cor′poris trapezoi′dei** [NA], ventral nucleus of trapezoid body: a group of nerve cells intermingled with the fibers of the trapezoid body, medial and ventral to the dorsal nucleus (superior olive); they contribute fibers to the lateral lemniscus. **n. ventra′lis interme′dius** [NA], the intermediate part of the ventral nucleus of the thalamus, which receives fibers from the superior cerebellar peduncle and sends fibers to the motor cortex and to the premotor cortex of the frontal lobe; called also *n. ventralis thalami intermedius* and *lateral ventral n. of thalamus.* **n. ventra′lis posterolatera′lis** [NA], the posterolateral part of the ventral nucleus of the thalamus, which is the terminus of the spinothalamic tract and medial lemniscus and projects to the postcentral gyrus. **n. ventra′lis posteromedia′lis** [NA], the posteromedial part of the posterior ventral nucleus of the thalamus, which receives the secondary trigeminal tract and sends axons to the somesthetic area of the postcentral gyrus for the face. **n. ventra′lis thal′ami,** the nuclear group containing the several ventral nuclei of the nuclei laterales thalami. **n. ventra′lis thal′ami ante′rior,** former NA term for n. ventralis anterolateralis. **n. ventra′lis thal′ami interme′dius,** former NA term for n. ventralis intermedius. **n. ventra′lis thal′ami poste′rior,** the posterior part of the ventral nucleus of the thalamus, which is the site of termination of the main ascending sensory pathways. It is divided into the n. ventralis posteromedialis and n. ventralis posterolateralis. **ventromedial n. of hypothalamus, n. ventromedia′lis hypothal′ami** [NA], the ventral one of two main groups of nerve cell bodies found in the middle, tuberal region of the hypothalamus; it appears to be involved in diverse functions, e.g., the control of food intake and of sexual behavior. **n. ventromedia′lis,**

ventrally placed cells in the lateral part of the oculomotor nuclear complex; they are very distinct from the dorsally placed cells in the middle third of the complex and have a somatic motor function. **vesicular n.,** a form of cell nucleus the membrane of which stains deeply, while the central part is rather pale. **vestibular nuclei, nu′clei vestibula′res** [NA], the four cellular masses in the floor of the fourth ventricle: the superior (n. acusticus, n. angularis, Bekhterevi's, or Bekhterev's n.), lateral (Deiter's n., n. magnocellularis, or large cell auditory n.), medial (Schwalbe's n., triangular n., or n. triangularis), and inferior vestibular nuclei, in which the short ascending and longer descending branches of the pars vestibularis nervi octavi terminate and in which cerebellar projections are received. The nuclei give rise to a widely dispersed special sensory system through projections to motor nuclei in the brain stem and cervical cord via the medial longitudinal fasciculi (from all the vestibular nuclei), to the cerebellum (chiefly from the inferior and medial nuclei), and to motor cells throughout the spinal cord (from the lateral nucleus). Additional connections of the nuclei provide for conscious perception of, and autonomic reactions to, labyrinthine stimulation. Called also *nuclei nervi vestibulares.* **vestibulocochlear nuclei,** nuclei nervi vestibulocochlearis. **Voit's n.,** a cerebellar nucleus accessory to the dentate nucleus. **Westphal's n.,** n. accessorius. **yolk n.,** a special area of the cytoplasm of an ovum in which the synthetic activities leading to the accumulation of food supplies in the oocyte are apparently initiated; called also *vitelline body, Balbiani's body,* and *Balbiani's n.* **zygote n.,** fertilization n.

nuclide (nu′klīd) a species of atom characterized by the charge, mass, number, and quantum state of its nucleus, and capable of existing for a measurable lifetime (generally greater than 10^{-10} sec.). Thus nuclear isomers are separate nuclides, but promptly decaying excited nuclear states and unstable intermediates in nuclear reactions are not so considered. **radioactive n.,** radionuclide.

nudophobia (nu″do-fo′be-ah) [L. *nudus* unclothed, bare + Gr. *phobos* fear + *-ia*] an abnormal aversion to being unclothed.

Nuel's space (ne-elz′) [Jean Pierre *Nuel,* Belgian oculist, 1847–1920] see under *space.*

nufenoxole (noo″fĕ-nok′sōl) chemical name: 2-[3-(5-methyl-1,-3,4-oxadiazol-2-yl)-3,3-diphenylpropyl]-2-azabicyclo[2.2.2]octane; an antiperistaltic, $C_{25}H_{29}N_3O$.

Nuhn's glands (noonz) [Anton *Nuhn,* German anatomist, 1814–1889] glandulae linguales anteriores.

nullipara (nuh-lip′ah-rah) [L. *nullus* none + *parere* to bring forth, produce] a woman who has never borne a viable child. Also written para 0.

nulliparity (nul″ĭ-par′ĭ-te) the condition or fact of being nulliparous.

nulliparous (nuh-lip′ah-rus) having never given birth to a viable infant.

nullisomatic (nul″ĭ-so-mat′ik) lacking one pair of chromosomes.

number (num′ber) a symbol, as a figure or word, expressive of a certain value or of a specified quantity determined by count. **acetyl n.,** the number of milligrams of KOH necessary to neutralize the acetic acid saponified from 1 gram of acetylated fat; it represents the extent to which hydroxyl groups are present. **acid n.,** the number of milligrams of potassium hydroxide necessary to neutralize the free fatty acids in 1 gram of fat; it represents a measure of the amount of free fatty acids in the fat. **atomic n.,** a number expressive of the number of protons in an atomic nucleus, or the positive charge of the nucleus in terms of the number of electrons outside the nucleus of a neutral atom. All atoms having the same atomic number exhibit the same chemical properties. **Avogadro's n.,** the number of particles, real or imaginary, of the type specified by the chemical formula of a certain substance in one mole of the substance; the value assigned to the number is 6.023×10^{23}. Called also *Avogadro's constant.* **Brinell hardness n.,** an expression of the hardness of a substance determined by use of the Brinell tester. **chromosome n.,** the number of chromosomes present in the somatic cells of an organism; the normal individual receives, at conception, one set of chromosomes (the haploid number, symbol n) from each of the gametes forming the zygote, thus acquiring the diploid number ($2n$). In humans, n equals 23. **dibucaine n.,** an expression of the percentage of inhibition of the enzyme cholinesterase in a serum sample by dibucaine; used to differentiate between normal and abnormal serum cholinesterase phenotypes. Normal or usual is about 80; intermediate is about 60; abnormal or atypical is about 20. Abbreviated DN. **Hehner n.,** the percentage of fatty acids not volatile with steam, obtainable from a fat. **Hittorf n.,** the fraction of the total current passing through an electrolysis cell that is carried by a given ion species; called also *transport n.* **Hounsfield n's,** a series of numbers used in computed tomography to represent the densities of various substances, structures, and growths. **Hübl n.,** iodine n. **hydrogen n.,** the amount of hydrogen that fats can take up; it represents the amount of unsaturated fatty acids present. **iodine n.,** the amount of iodine in grams which 100 grams of the fat can take up; it indicates the amount of unsaturated fatty acids present in the fat. **isotopic n.**, the number which added to twice the atomic number gives the atomic weight. **Knoop hardness n.**, an expression of the hardness (indentation) of a material determined by use of a special indenting tool. **Loschmidt's n.**, 1. Avogadro's number. 2. the number of molecules per unit volume of an ideal gas at 0° C. and normal pressure. **mass n.**, the whole number nearest to the atomic weight of an element or isotope. Symbol A. **polar n.**, the number of valences (positive or negative) possessed by an atom in any particular compound. **Polenske n.**, the number of milliliters of tenth normal KOH required to neutralize the insoluble, volatile fatty acids from 5 gm. of the fat. **Reichert-Meissl n.**, the number of milliliters of tenth normal KOH required to neutralize the soluble volatile fatty acids distilled from 5 gm. of fat after it has been saponified with KOH and then made acid with H_3PO_4 or H_2SO_4. **Reynold's n.**, the velocity of flow of a fluid multiplied by the diameter of the vessel and divided by the kinematic viscosity of the circulating fluid. **saponification n.**, the number of milligrams of potassium hydroxide required to neutralize the fatty acids in 1 gram of a fat or oil; it indicates the average size of the fatty acid molecules or the amount of the lower fatty acids present. **thiocyanogen n.**, the amount of thiocyanogen absorbed by a fat or oil. **transport n.**, Hittorf number. **turnover n.**, the number of molecules of substrate acted upon by one molecule of enzyme per minute. **wave n.**, in light waves, the reciprocal of the wavelength expressed as a fraction of a centimeter.

numbness (num′nes) a lack or diminution of sensation in a part.

nummular (num′u-lar) [L. *nummularis*] 1. coin-sized and coin-shaped. 2. made up of round, flat disks. 3. piled, like coins, in a rouleau.

Numorphan (nu-mor′fan) trademark for preparations of oxymorphone hydrochloride.

nunnation (nun-a′shun) [Heb. *nun* letter N] the too frequent use of *n* sounds, or the nasalizing of sounds or words.

Nupercainal (noo″per-kān′al) trademark for a preparation of dibucaine.

Nupercaine (nu′per-kān) trademark for preparations of dibucaine.

nuptiality (nup-shal′ĭ-te) [L. *nuptus* married] the proportion of marriages to the population.

N-Uristix (u′rĭ-stiks) trademark for a reagent strip designed for testing for nitrite, glucose, and protein in urine.

nurse (ners) 1. a person who is especially prepared in the scientific basis of nursing and who meets certain prescribed standards of education and clinical competence. 2. to provide services that are essential to or helpful in the promotion, maintenance, and restoration of health and well-being. 3. to breast-feed an infant. See also *nursing*. **charge n.**, one who is in charge of a patient care unit of a hospital or similar health agency; called also *head n.* **clinical n. specialist**, a registered nurse with a high degree of knowledge, skill, and competence in a specialized area of nursing. These skills are made directly available through the provision of nursing care to clients and are indirectly available through guidance and planning of care with other nursing personnel. Clinical nurse specialists hold a master's degree in nursing, preferably with an emphasis in clinical nursing. Called also *n. specialist*. **n. clinician**, a registered nurse, referred to as a *nurse clinician* or as a *nurse practitioner*, who has well-developed competencies in utilizing a broad range of cues. These cues are used for prescribing and implementing both direct and indirect nursing care and for articulating nursing therapies with other planned therapies. Nurse clinicians demonstrate expertise in nursing practice and ensure ongoing development of expertise through clinical experience and continuing education. Generally, minimal preparation for this role is the baccalaureate degree. **community n.**, the name given in Great Britain to a public health nurse, from the fact that such a nurse was placed in charge of each one of the districts into which the city or community was divided. See also *public health n.* **community health n.**, public health n. **district n.**, community n. **dry n.**, a woman who has charge of another's infant but does not breast-feed it. **general duty n.**, a registered nurse, usually one who has not undergone training beyond the basic nursing program, who sees to the general nursing care of patients in a hospital or other health agency. **graduate n.**, a graduate of a school of nursing; often used to designate one who has not been registered or licensed to practice. Called also *trained n.* **head n.**, charge n. **hospital n.**, one employed by a hospital. **licensed practical n.**, a graduate of a school of practical nursing whose qualifications have been examined by a state board of nursing and who has been legally authorized to practice as a licensed practical or vocational nurse (L.P.N. or L.V.N.), under the supervision of a physician or registered nurse. **licensed vocational n.**, see *licensed practical n.* **monthly n.**, a nurse who attends confinement cases. **occupational health n.**, an especially prepared registered nurse employed by an institution to apply nursing principles and procedures for the promotion, restoration, and maintenance of optimal health of its employees as compared to a nurse who performs normal nursing functions in an

occupational setting. **office n.**, a registered nurse employed by a physician in his office to perform or to assist him in the performance of certain procedures. **practical n.**, a person who has had practical experience in nursing care but who is not a graduate of any kind of nursing school; not to be confused with a licensed practical nurse. **n. practitioner**, see *n. clinician*. **private n., private duty n.**, one who attends an individual patient, usually on a fee-for-service basis, and who may specialize in a specific class of diseases; called also *special n.* **probationer n.**, a person who has entered a school of nursing and is under observation to determine her fitness for the nursing profession; applied principally to nursing students enrolled in hospital schools of nursing. **public health n.**, an especially prepared registered nurse employed in a community agency to safeguard the health of persons in the community, giving care to the sick in their homes, promoting health and well-being by teaching families how to keep well, and assisting in programs for the prevention of disease. Called also *community health n.* and *visiting n.* **Queen's n.**, in Great Britain, a district nurse who has been trained at or in accordance with the regulations of the Queen Victoria Jubilee Institute for Nurses. **registered n.**, a graduate nurse who has been legally authorized (registered) to practice after examination by a state board of nurse examiners or similar regulatory authority, and who is legally entitled to use the designation R.N. **school n.**, an especially prepared registered nurse employed in a school system or public health agency to assist in safeguarding the health of students and to teach health practices. **scrub n.**, one who directly assists the surgeon in the operating room. **special n.**, 1. a private nurse. 2. a nurse who specializes in a particular class of cases. **n. specialist**, clinical n. specialist. **student n.**, a person enrolled in a basic program of nursing education. **trained n.**, graduate n. **visiting n.**, see *public health n.* **wet n.**, a woman who breast-feeds the infant of another.

nurse-midwife (ners-mid′wīf) an individual educated in the two disciplines of nursing and midwifery, who possesses evidence of certification according to the requirements of the American College of Nurse-Midwives. Abbreviated C.N.M. (Certified Nurse-Midwife).

nurse-midwifery (ners-mid′wi-fer-e, ners-mid′wīf-ĕ-re) the independent management of care of essentially normal newborns and women, antepartally, intrapartally, postpartally, and/or gynecologically, occurring within a health care system which provides for medical consultation, collaborative management, or referral, and is in accord with the functions, standards, and qualifications as defined by the American College of Nurse-Midwives.

nursery (ner′sĕ-re) the department in a hospital where newborn infants are cared for. **day n., day care n.**, an institution devoted to the care of young children during the day.

nursing (ners′ing) the provision, at various levels of preparation, of services that are essential to or helpful in the promotion, maintenance, and restoration of health and well-being or in the prevention of illness, as of infants, of the sick and injured, or of others for any reason unable to provide such services for themselves. Sometimes designated according to the age of the patients being cared for (e.g., pediatric or geriatric nursing), or their particular health problems (e.g., gynecologic, medical, obstetrical, orthopedic, psychiatric, surgical, urological nursing, or the like), or the setting in which the services are provided (e.g., office, school, or occupational health nursing). See also *nurse.*

Nussbaum's bracelet, narcosis (noos′bowmz) [Johann Nepomuk *Nussbaum*, German surgeon, 1829– 1890] see under *bracelet* and *narcosis*.

Nussbaum's experiment (noos′bowmz) [Moritz *Nussbaum*, German histologist, 1850–1915] see under *experiment*.

nut (nut) [L. *nux;* Gr. *karyon*] a seed element, as of various trees, usually enclosed in a coating of variable hardness. **betel n.**, areca.

nutation (nu-ta′shun) [L. *nutatio*] the act of nodding, especially involuntary nodding.

nutatory (nu′tah-tor″e) [L. *nutare* to keep nodding, to sway] nodding, especially involuntarily.

nutgall (nut′gawl) [L. *galla*] an excrescence growing on oak trees, especially species of *Quercus* (e.g., *Q. infectoria* Oliv., Fagaceae), produced by insect eggs and larvae embedded in the plant tissues; it is a source of gallic and tannic acids, which are used in various pharmaceutics for their astringent properties. Called also *gall, Aleppo gall, Smyrna gall,* and *gallnut.*

nutmeg (nut′meg) myristica.

nutrient (nu′tre-ent) [L. *nutriens*] 1. nourishing; affording nutriment. 2. a nutritious substance; food, or a component of food. **essential n's**, those nutrients (proteins, minerals, carbohydrates, fat, vitamins) necessary for growth, normal functioning, and maintaining life; they must be supplied by food, since they cannot be synthesized by the body. **secondary n.**, a substance that stimulates the intestinal microflora to synthesize other nutrients.

nutrilite (nu′trĭ-līt) any organic substance which in minute amounts is important in the nutrition of a microorganism.

nutriment (nu′trĭ-ment) [L. *nutrimentum*] nourishment; nutritious material; food.

nutriology (nu‴tre-ol′o-je) the science of nutrition; the study of foods and their use in diet and therapy.

nutrition (nu-trish′un) [L. *nutritio*] 1. the sum of the processes involved in taking in nutriments and assimilating and utilizing them. 2. nutriment. **adequate n.**, see under *diet*. **heterotrophic n.**, that of organisms which, because they cannot synthesize their own food from inorganic substances, must live either by eating autotrophic organisms or dead or decaying organic matter. See also *holozoic n.*, *parasitic n.*, and *saprophytic n.* **holozoic n.**, heterotrophic nutrition in which organisms, including most animals, must obtain food as particles of some size which must be eaten and digested before it can be absorbed. **parasitic n.**, heterotrophic nutrition in which an organism lives on the body of another living organism and obtains its nourishment from it. **saprophytic n.**, heterotrophic nutrition in which organisms, such as many protozoa, as well as yeasts, molds, and most bacteria, absorb required nutrients through the cell membrane following extracellular digestion of nonliving organic material. **total parenteral n.**, parenteral hyperalimentation.

nutritional (nu-trish′un-al) relating to or affecting nutrition.

nutritionist (nu-trish′un-ist) a specialist in food and nutrition.

nutritious (nu-trish′us) [L. *nutritius*] affording nourishment.

nutritive (nu′trĭ-tiv) pertaining to nutrition.

nutriture (nu′trĭ-tūr‴) the status of the body in relation to nutrition, generally or in regard to a specific nutrient, such as protein.

nutrix (nu′triks) a wet nurse.

nutrose (nu′trōs) neutral casein sodium; a dry food preparation of milk for the use of invalids.

Nuttallia (nŭ-tal′e-ah) [George H. F. *Nutall*, biologist, Cambridge University, 1862–1937] *Babesia*. **N. e′qui**, *Babesia equi*. **N. gibso′ni**, *Babesia gibsoni*.

nux (nuks), gen. *nu′cis* [L.] nut. **n. moscha′ta**, myristica. **n. vom′ica**, the dried ripe seed of *Strychnos nux-vomica* L. (Loganiaceae), containing several alkaloids, principally strychnine and brucine. It has been used as a bitter tonic and central nervous system stimulant, and in veterinary medicine it is used as a bitter tonic and in the treatment of inappetence, atony of the rumen, and chronic indigestion.

nyacyne (ni′ah-sīn) neomycin.

nyad (ni′ad) the nymph form of certain arthropods.

nyctalgia (nik-tal′je-ah) [nycto- + -algia] pain that occurs in sleep only.

nyctalope (nik′tah-lōp) a person affected with nyctalopia.

nyctalopia (nik‴tah-lo′pe-ah) [Gr. *nyktalōps*] 1. night blindness (Galen); failure or imperfection of vision at night or in a dim light, with good vision only on bright days (Heberden, 1767). 2. in French (and incorrectly in English), day blindness (Hippocrates), or hemeralopia, a condition in which the patient sees better in an obscure light than in bright sunlight.

nyctaphonia (nik‴tah-fo′ne-ah) [nycto- + aphonia] loss of voice during the night.

nycterine (nik′ter-īn) [Gr. *nykterinos* by night] 1. occurring at night. 2. obscure.

nycterohemeral (nik‴ter-o-hem′er-al) nyctohemeral.

nycto- (nik′to) [Gr. *nyx* night] a combining form denoting relationship to night or to darkness.

nyctohemeral (nik‴to-hem′er-al) [nycto- + Gr. *hēmera* day] pertaining to both night and day.

nyctophilia (nik‴to-fil′e-ah) [nycto- + Gr. *philein* to love] abnormal preference for night over day.

nyctophobia (nik‴to-fo′be-ah) [nycto- + Gr. *phobein* to be affrighted by] morbid dread of darkness.

nyctophonia (nik‴to-fo′ne-ah) [nycto- + Gr. *phōnē* voice] loss of voice during the day but not at night.

Nyctotherus (nik-toth′er-us) [Gr. "one who hunts at night"] a genus of ciliate protozoa of the subclass Euciliatia, found as parasites of the large intestine of amphibians, fish, and invertebrates. *N. cordifor′mis* occurs in the rectums of frogs and tadpoles. *N. ova′lis*, occurs in the intestines of cockroaches.

nyctotyphlosis (nik‴to-tif-lo′sis) [nycto- + Gr. *typhlōsis* blindness] nyctalopia.

nycturia (nik-tu′re-ah) [nycto- + Gr. *ouron* urine + -ia] frequent urination during the night, especially the passage of more urine at night than during the day.

N.Y.D. not yet diagnosed.

Nydrazid (ni′dra-zid) trademark for preparations of isoniazid.

Nylander's test (reagent) (ni′lan-derz) [Emil Salomon *Nylander*, Swedish chemist, 1858–1936] see under *tests*.

nylestriol (ni-les′tre-ōl) chemical name: 3-(cyclopentyloxy)-19-nor-17α-pregna-1,3,5(10)-trien-20-yne-16,17-diol; an estrogen, $C_{25}H_{32}O_3$.

nylidrin hydrochloride (nil′ĭ-drin) [USP] chemical name: 4-hydroxy-α-[1-[(1-methyl-3-phenylpropyl)amino]ethyl] benzene-

methanol hydrochloride. A synthetic adrenergic, $C_{19}H_{25}NO_2 \cdot HCl$, occurring as a white, crystalline powder; used as a peripheral vasodilator, administered orally, intramuscularly, and subcutaneously.

nylon (ni′lon) a synthetic polymerized plastic which in fiber form is used as suture material.

nymph (nimf) [Gr. *nymphē* a bride] a stage in the life cycle of certain arthropods, as the ticks, between the larva and the adult. A nymph resembles the adult in appearance.

nympha (nim′fah), pl. *nym′phae* [L.; Gr. *nymphē*] labium minus pudendi. **n. of Krause**, clitoris.

nymphae (nim′fe) [L.] plural of *nympha*.

nymphectomy (nim-fek′to-me) [nympha + Gr. *ektomē* excision] excision of the nymphae.

nymphitis (nim-fi′tis) inflammation of the nymphae.

nympho- (nim′fo) [L. *nympha*: Gr. *nymphē*] a combining form denoting relationship to the nymphae, or labia minora.

nymphocaruncular (nim‴fo-kah-rung′ku-lar) pertaining to the labia minora and the caruncula hymenalis.

nymphohymeneal (nim‴fo-hi‴mĕ-ne′al) pertaining to the labia minora and the hymen.

nymphomania (nim‴fo-ma′ne-ah) [nympho- + Gr. *mania* madness] exaggerated sexual desire in a female. Cf. *satyriasis*.

nymphomaniac (nim‴fo-ma′ne-ak) 1. affected with nymphomania. 2. one who is affected with nymphomania.

nymphoncus (nim-fong′kus) [nympho- + Gr. *onkos* mass, bulk] swelling of the nymphae.

nymphotomy (nim-fot′o-me) [nympho- + Gr. *tomē* a cutting] surgical incision of the nymphae or clitoris.

Nyssorhynchus (nis‴o-ring′kus) [Gr. *nyssa* prick + *rhynchos* snout] a subgenus of anopheline mosquitoes, several species of which act as carriers of the malarial parasite in tropical America.

nystagmic (nis-tag′mik) pertaining to or characterized by nystagmus.

nystagmiform (nis-tag′mĭ-form) nystagmoid.

nystagmograph (nis-tag′mo-graf) [nystagmus + Gr. *graphein* to write] an instrument for recording the movements of the eyeball in nystagmus.

nystagmoid (nis-tag′moid) resembling nystagmus.

nystagmus (nis-tag′mus) [Gr. *nystagmos* drowsiness, from *nystazein* to nod] an involuntary rapid movement of the eyeball, which may be horizontal, vertical, rotatory, or mixed, i.e., of two varieties. **aural n.**, nystagmus due to disturbances in the labyrinth; the eye movements are rhythmic, with a fast and a slow component. **caloric n.**, that induced by irrigating the ears with warm or cold water or air; see *Bárány's symptom* (def. 2), under *symptom*. **Cheyne's n.**, **Cheyne-Stokes n.**, a peculiar rhythmical eye movement resembling Cheyne-Stokes respiration in its rhythm. **disjunctive n.**, nystagmus in which the eyes swing toward and away from each other. **dissociated n.**, nystagmus in which the movements in the two eyes are dissimilar. **end-position n.**, nystagmus occurring at extremes of gaze. **fixation n.**, nystagmus which appears only on gazing fixedly at an object. **gaze n.**, nystagmus made apparent by looking to the right or to the left. **head n.**, an oscillatory motion of the head of an animal which occurs when it is rotated. **jerk n., jerky n.**, nystagmus which consists of a slow movement in one direction, followed by a rapid return movement in the opposite direction; called also *resilient n.* and *rhythmical n.* **labyrinthine n.**, vestibular n. **latent n.**, nystagmus which occurs only when one eye is covered. **lateral n.**, nystagmus in which the movement of the eyes is from side to side. **miner's n.**, an occupational disease of coal miners consisting of abnormal eye movements associated with other signs and symptoms; it is considered by some to be related to poor lighting and by others as a functional disorder. **ocular n.**, nystagmus due to eye disease. **opticokinetic n., optokinetic n.**, the normal nystagmus occurring when looking at objects passing across the field of vision, as in viewing from a moving railroad car or automobile. **oscillating n.**, undulatory n. **palatal n.**, see under *myoclonus*. **paretic n.**, a false nystagmus occurring when there is a weakness of the ocular muscles. **pendular n.**, undulatory n. **positional n.**, that which occurs, or is altered in form or intensity, on assumption of certain positions of the head. **railroad n.**, optokinetic n. **resilient n.**, jerk n. **retraction n.**, **retracto′rius**, a spasmodic backward retraction of the eyeball occurring on attempted movement of the eye; it is a sign of disease of the midbrain. **rhythmical n.**, jerk n. **rotatory n.**, nystagmus in which the movement is about the visual axis. **see-saw n.**, that in which one eye moves up as the other moves down. **spontaneous n.**, that occurring without specific stimulation of the vestibular system. **undulatory n.**, one which consists of to-and-fro movements of equal velocity; called also *pendular n.*, *vibratory n.*, and *oscillating n.* **unilateral n.**, nystagmus manifest in only one eye. **vertical n.**, an up-and-down movement of the eyes. **vestibular n.**, nystagmus due to vestibular disturbance; eye movements are rhythmic, with a slow and a fast component. Called also *labyrinthine n.* **vibratory n.**, undulatory n. **visual n.**, nystagmus characterized by smooth pendulum-like movement. **voluntary n.,** rapid rhythmic eye movements which can be produced at will by some normal individuals.

nystagmus-myoclonus (nis-tag'mus-mi-ok'lo-nus) a rare congenital condition in which there is nystagmus together with abnormal involuntary movements of the extremities and trunk.

nystatin (nis'tah-tin) [USP] an antibiotic, $C_{46}H_{77}NO_{19}$, produced by the growth of *Streptomyces noursei*, occurring as a yellow

to tan powder, specifically effective against *Candida albicans;* used in the treatment of vaginal, intestinal, oral, or cutaneous candidal infections, administered orally and topically. Called also *fungicidin.*

nystaxis (nis-tak'sis) [Gr.] nystagmus.

Nysten's law (ne-stahz') [Pierre Hubert *Nysten*, French pediatrician, 1771–1818] see under *law.*

nyxis (nik'sis) [Gr. "pricking"] puncture, or paracentesis.

O

O chemical symbol for *oxygen.*

O symbol for the nonmotile strain of an organism and for its surface antigen. Cf. *H,* and see *O agglutinin.*

O. abbreviation for L. *oc'ulus,* eye; *octarius,* pint; and for *opening.*

o- chemical symbol for ortho-.

O₂ 1. symbol for the diatomic form of oxygen; molecular oxygen. 2. symbol for *both eyes.*

O₃ ozone.

oak (ōk) a cupuliferous tree of the genus *Quercus.* The bark of all species contains a large proportion of tannin. **poison o.,** the plants *Toxicodendron diversilobum* (T. and G.) Greene (true western poison oak) and *T. quercifolium* (Michx.) Greene (true eastern poison oak). The term is also used loosely to refer to *T. radicans* (L.) Kuntze (poison ivy). All contain toxic urishiol resin, whose major constituent is 3-*n*-pentadicylcatechol, a highly allergenic compound.

oakum (o'kum) prepared fiber from old ropes; formerly used in making surgical dressings.

oario- for words beginning thus, see those beginning *oophoro-* and *ovario-*.

oasis (o-a'sis), pl. *oa'ses* [Gr. "a fertile islet in a desert"] an island or spot of healthy tissue in a diseased area.

oath (ōth) a solemn declaration or affirmation. **o. of Hippocrates, hippocratic o.,** see under *Hippocrates.*

OB. obstetrics.

ob- [L. *ob* against] prefix signifying against, in front of, towards.

obcecation (ob''se-ka'shun) incomplete blindness.

obducent (ob-du'sent) [L. *obducere* to draw over, to cover] serving as a cover; covering.

obduction (ob-duk'shun) [L. *obductio*] a medicolegal autopsy.

O'Beirne's sphincter (o-birnz') [James *O'Beirne,* Irish surgeon, 1786–1862] see under *sphincter.*

obeliac (o-be'le-ak) pertaining to the obelion.

obeliad (o-be'le-ad) toward the obelion.

obelion (o-be'le-on) [Gr., *dim.* of *obelos* a spit] a point on the sagittal suture where it is crossed by a line which connects the parietal foramina.

Ober's operation, test (sign) (o'berz) [Frank Roberts *Ober,* Boston orthopedic surgeon, born 1881] see under *operation* and *tests.*

Obermayer's test (o'ber-mi''erz) [Friedrich *Obermayer,* physiologic chemist in Vienna, 1861–1925] see under *tests.*

Obermüller's test (o'ber-mil-erz) [Kuno *Obermüller,* German physician, born 1861] see under *tests.*

Oberst's method (o'bersts) [Maximilian *Oberst,* German surgeon, 1849–1925] see under *method.*

Obersteiner-Redlich area (zone) (o'ber-sti''ner-red'likh) [Heinrich *Obersteiner,* Austrian neurologist, 1847–1922; Emil *Redlich,* Austrian neurologist, 1866–1930] see under *area.*

obese (o-bēs') [L. *obesus*] excessively fat.

obesitas (o-be'sĭ-tas) [L.] obesity.

obesity (o-bēs'ĭ-te) [L. *obesitas*] an increase in body weight beyond the limitation of skeletal and physical requirement, as the result of an excessive accumulation of fat in the body. **adult-onset o.,** obesity beginning in adulthood and characterized by increase in size (hypertrophy) of adipose cell with no increase in number; called also *hypertrophic o.* **alimentary o.,** exogenous obesity. **endogenous o.,** obesity due to metabolic (endocrine) abnormalities. **exogenous o.,** obesity due to overeating. **hyperinsulinar o.,** obesity due to overactivity of insulin secretion, associated with hypoglycemia and increased appetite. **hyperinterrenal o.,** obesity associated with hyperfunction of the adrenal cortex. **hyperplasmic o.,** obesity due to increase in the body protoplasm, as distinguished from that due to accumulation of fat and water. **hyperplastic-hypertrophic o.,** lifelong o. **hypertrophic o.,** adult-onset o. **hypogonad o.,** obesity associated with hypofunction of the gonads. **hypoplasmic o.,** obesity due to increase of fat and water and marked by decrease of the body protoplasm. **hypo-**

thyroid o., obesity due to hypothyroidism. **lifelong o.,** obesity beginning in childhood and characterized by an increase both in number (hyperplasia) and in size (hypertrophy) of adipose cells; called also *hyperplastic-hypertrophic o.* **morbid o.,** the condition of weighing two or three, or more, times the ideal weight; so called because it is associated with many serious and life threatening disorders (diabetes mellitus, atherosclerosis, hypertension, pickwickian syndrome, etc.). **simple o.,** exogenous o.

obesogenous (o-bēs-oj'ĕ-nus) producing or causing obesity.

obex (o'beks) [L. "barrier"] [NA] the ependyma-lined junction of the teniae of the fourth ventricle of the brain at the inferior angle.

obfuscation (ob''fus-ka'shun) [L. *obfuscatio* a darkening] the act of rendering, or process of becoming, obscure; a darkening.

obidoxime chloride (ŏ-bĭ-doks'ēm) chemical name: 1,1'-(oxydimethylene)bis[4-formylpyridinium]dichloride, a cholinesterase reactivator, $C_{14}H_{16}Cl_2N_4O_3$, which has been used to counter organophosphorus poisoning.

objective (ob-jek'tiv) [L. *objectivus*] 1. perceptible to the external senses. 2. a result for whose achievement an effort is made. 3. the lens or system of lenses in a microscope (or telescope) that is nearest to the object under examination. **achromatic o.,** a microscope objective in which the chromatic aberration is corrected for light of two wavelengths and the spherical aberration is corrected for that of one wavelength. **apochromatic o.,** a microscope objective in which the chromatic aberration is corrected for light of three wavelengths and the spherical aberration is corrected for that of two. **dry o.,** a microscope objective designed to be used without a liquid between its tip and the cover glass over the specimen. **fluorite o.,** a microscope objective in which some of the lenses are made from fluorite instead of glass. **immersion o.,** a microscope objective designed to have its tip and the cover glass over the specimen connected by a liquid instead of by air. The liquid may be water (water immersion) or a specially prepared oil (oil immersion). **semiapochromatic o.,** a microscope objective in which the correction of chromatic and spherical aberrations is between those of the achromatic and apochromatic objectives.

obligate (ob'lĭ-gāt) [L. *obligatus*] not facultative; necessary; compulsory; pertaining to or characterized by the ability to survive only in a particular environment or to assume only a particular role, as an obligate anaerobe.

oblique (ŏ-blēk', ŏ-blīk') [L. *obliquus*] slanting; inclined; between a horizontal and a perpendicular direction.

obliquity (ob-lik'wĭ-te) the state of being oblique, or slanting. **Litzmann's o.,** inclination of the fetal head so that the posterior parietal bone presents to the parturient canal; called also *posterior asynclitism.* **Nägele's o.,** the position of the fetal head in which the anterior parietal bone presents to the parturient canal, the biparietal diameter being oblique in relation to the brim of the pelvis; called also *anterior asynclitism.* **o. of pelvis,** inclination of the pelvis.

obliquus (ob-li'kwus) [L.] oblique.

obliteration (ob-lit''er-a'shun) [L. *obliteratio*] complete removal, whether by disease, degeneration, surgical procedure, irradiation, etc. **cortical o.,** cortical achromia; a condition in which the cerebral cortex is marked by areas in which the ganglion cells have disappeared.

oblongata (ob''long-ga'tah, ob''long-gah'tah) a Latin adjective meaning oblong, sometimes used informally to refer to the medulla oblongata.

oblongatal (ob''long-ga'tal) pertaining to the medulla oblongata.

obnubilation (ob-nu''bĭ-la'shun) a clouded state of the mind.

O'Brien akinesia (o-bri'en) [Cecil Starling *O'Brien,* American ophthalmologist, born 1889] see under *akinesia.*

observerscope (ob-zer'ver-skōp) a form of endoscope with two ocular systems which permit two persons to inspect the same spot at the same time.

obsession (ob-sesh'un) [L. *obsessio*] preoccupation with an idea which morbidly dominates the mind, constantly suggesting irrational action.

obsessive (ob-ses′siv) pertaining to or characterized by obsession.

obsessive-compulsive (ob-ses″siv-kom-pul′siv) marked by compulsion to repetitively perform certain acts, or carry out certain rituals; see under *neurosis.*

obsolescence (ob′so-les′ens) [L. *obsolescere* to grow old] the cessation or the beginning of the cessation of any physiologic process.

obsolete (ob′so-lēt) [L. *obsoletus,* from *obsolere* to go out of use] indistinct; faded; gone out of use.

obstetric, obstetrical (ob-stet′rik; ob-stet′re-kal)[L. *obstetricius*] pertaining to obstetrics.

obstetrician (ob″stĕ-trish′un) [L. *obstetrix* midwife] one who practices obstetrics.

obstetrics (ob-stet′riks) [L. *obstetricia*] that branch of surgery which deals with the management of pregnancy, labor, and the puerperium.

obstipation (ob″stĭ-pa′shun) [L. *obstipatio*] intractable constipation.

obstruction (ob-struk′shun) [L. *obstructio*] 1. the act of blocking or clogging. 2. the state or condition of being clogged. **false colonic o.,** see *Ogilvie's syndrome,* under *syndrome.* **intestinal o.,** any hindrance to the passage of the intestinal contents. See also *ileus.*

obstruent (ob′stroo-ent) [L. *obstruens*] 1. causing obstruction or blocking. 2. any agent or agency that causes obstruction.

obtund (ob-tund′) [L. *obtundere*] to render dull or blunt; to render less acute.

obtundent (ob-tun′dent) [L. *obtundens*] 1. having the power to dull sensibility or to soothe pain. 2. a soothing or partially anesthetic medicine.

obturation (ob″tu-ra′shun) the act of closing or occluding; a form of intestinal obstruction.

obturator (ob′tu-ra″tor) [L.] a disk or plate, natural or artificial, which closes an opening, such as a prosthetic appliance used to close a congenital or acquired opening in the palate.

obtuse (ob-tūs′) [L. *obtusus*] 1. blunt; dull. 2. having a dull intellect.

obtusion (ob-tu′zhun) [L. *obtusio*] morbid bluntness or dullness of sensibility.

occipital (ok-sip′ĭ-tal) [L. *occipitalis*] pertaining to the occiput; located near the occipital bone, as the occipital lobe.

occipitalis (ok-sip″ĭ-ta′lis) [L.] the posterior part of the occipitofrontalis muscle.

occipitalization (ok-sip″ĭ-tal-i-za′shun) synostosis of the atlas with the occipital bone.

occipitoanterior (ok-sip″ĭ-to-an-te′re-or) having the occiput directed forward toward the pubis (designating the position of the fetus in relation to the maternal pelvis).

occipitoatloid (ok-sip″ĭ-to-at′loid) pertaining to the occipital bone and the atlas.

occipitoaxoid (ok-sip″ĭ-to-ak′soid) pertaining to the occipital bone and the axis.

occipitobasilar (ok-sip″ĭ-to-bas′ĭ-ler) pertaining to the occiput and the base of the skull.

occipitobregmatic (ok-sip″ĭ-to-breg-mat′ik) pertaining to the occiput and the bregma.

occipitocalcarine (ok-sip″ĭ-to-kal′kar-in) both occipital and calcarine.

occipitocervical (ok-sip″ĭ-to-ser′vĭ-kal) pertaining to the occiput and neck.

occipitofacial (ok-sip″ĭ-to-fa′shal) pertaining to the occiput and the face.

occipitofrontal (ok-sip″ĭ-to-fron′tal) pertaining to the occiput and the forehead.

occipitomastoid (ok-sip″ĭ-to-mas′toid) pertaining to the occipital bone and the mastoid process.

occipitomental (ok-sip″ĭ-to-men′tal) pertaining to the occiput and the chin.

occipitoparietal (ok-sip″ĭ-to-pah-ri′e-tal) pertaining to the occipital and parietal bones or lobes of the brain.

occipitoposterior (ok-sip″ĭ-to-pos-te′re-or) having the occiput directed toward the back, or turned toward the sacrum (designating the position of the fetus in relation to the maternal pelvis).

occipitotemporal (ok-sip″ĭ-to-tem′po-ral) pertaining to the occipital and the temporal bones.

occipitothalamic (ok-sip″ĭ-to-thah-lam′ik) pertaining to the occipital lobe and thalamus.

occiput (ok′sĭ-put) [L.] [NA] the back part of the head; called also *o. cra′nii* and *o. of cranium.*

occlude (ŏ-klood′) to fit close together; to close tight, as to bring the mandibular teeth into contact with the teeth in the maxilla; to obstruct or close off.

occluder (ŏ-klood′er) a form of dental articulator.

occlusal (ŏ-kloo′zal) pertaining to closure; applied to the masti-

cating surfaces of the premolar and molar teeth, or to the contacting surfaces of opposing occlusion rims, or designating a position toward the hypothetical plane passing between the mandibular and maxillary teeth when the jaws are brought into approximation.

occlusion (ŏ-kloo′zhun) [L. *occlusio*] 1. the act of closure or state of being closed; an obstruction or a closing off. 2. the trapping of a material, either liquid or gas, within cavities in a solid. 3. the relation of the maxillary and mandibular teeth when in functional contact during activity of the mandible. **abnormal o.,** malocclusion. **acentric o.,** a condition in which the habitual voluntary closure pattern of the mandible does not coincide with centric relation, producing primary premature tooth contacts in the centric path of closure. **afunctional o.,** malocclusion which prevents mastication. **anatomic o.,** occlusion in which all the teeth are present and occlude normally according to the anatomical standard. **anterior o.,** mesioclusion. **balanced o.,** that in which the occlusal contact of the teeth on the working side of the jaw is accompanied by the harmonious contact of the teeth of the opposite (balancing) side. The occlusion of artificial teeth may be *mechanically balanced,* as on an articulator, without reference to physiologic considerations, or *physiologically balanced,* functioning in harmony with the temporomandibular joint and the neuromuscular system. **buccal o.,** the position of a posterior tooth when it is outside (buccal to) the line of occlusion. **capsular o.,** surgical closure of the perinephric capsule for the relief of floating kidney. **central o.,** centric o. **centric o.,** occlusion of the teeth when the mandible is in centric relation to the maxilla, i.e., full occlusal surface contact of the upper and lower teeth in habitual occlusion, with the mandibular condyles in their most posterior, unstrained position on the posteroinferior third of the articular eminentia. It is a reference position from which all other horizontal positions are eccentric. **components of o.,** the various factors involved in occlusion, e.g., the temporomandibular joint, the associated neuromusculature, and the teeth, and in denture prosthetics, the denture-supporting structures. **coronary o.,** complete obstruction of an artery of the heart, usually from progressive atherosclerosis (sometimes complicated by thrombosis), rarely from embolism, arteritis, or dissecting aneurysm. **distal o.,** the position of a lower tooth when it is distal to its opposite number in the maxilla. **eccentric o.,** occlusion of the teeth when the lower jaw has moved from the centric position; see *centric o.* **edge-to-edge o.,** occlusion in which the anterior maxillary and mandibular teeth meet along their incisal edges when the mandible is in centric position. **end-to-end o.,** edge-to-edge o. **enteromesenteric o.,** obstruction of blood vessels in both the mesentery and the wall of the intestine. **functional o.,** such contact of the maxillary and mandibular teeth as will provide the highest efficiency in the centric position and during all excursive movements of the jaw that are essential to mastication, without producing trauma. **habitual o.,** the consistent relationship of the teeth in the maxilla to those of the mandible when the teeth in both jaws are brought into maximum contact, such relationship varying from individual to individual; the ideal habitual occlusion is centric occlusion, but it is seldom attained without corrective dental treatment. **hyperfunctional o.,** traumatic o. **ideal o.,** perfect interdigitation of the upper and lower teeth. **labial o.,** the position of an anterior tooth when it is outside (labial to) the line of occlusion. **lateral o.,** the occlusion of the teeth when the lower jaw is moved to the right or left of centric position. **lingual o.,** malocclusion in which the tooth is lingual to the line of the normal dental arch. **mesial o.,** the position of a lower tooth when it is mesial to its opposite number in the maxilla. **neutral o.,** normal o. **normal o.,** the contact of the upper and lower teeth in the centric relationship. **pathogenic o.,** an occlusal relationship that is capable of producing pathologic changes in the supporting tissues. **physiologic o.,** occlusion which is in harmony with the functioning of the temporomandibular joint and the neuromuscular system. **posterior o.,** distoclusion. **postnormal o.,** distal o. **prenormal o.,** mesial o. **protrusive o.,** anteroclusion. **o. of pupil,** closure of the opening in the iris of the eye by formation of an opaque membrane. **retrusive o.,** distoclusion. **spherical form of o.,** an arrangement of teeth that places their occlusal surfaces on the surface of an imaginary sphere, about 8 inches in diameter, with its center above the level of the teeth; see also *Monson curve,* under *curve.* **terminal o.,** the relationship of opposing occlusal surfaces that provides the maximum natural or planned contact and/or intercuspation. **traumatic o.,** occlusion in which the contact relation of the masticatory surfaces of the teeth is directly the result of trauma. **traumatogenic o.,** occlusion which, under biting pressure, produces injury to the periodontal tissues. **working o.,** the contact made between the teeth on the side toward which the mandible is moved.

occlusive (ŏ-kloo′siv) pertaining to or effecting occlusion.

occlusocervical (ŏ-kloo″so-ser′vĭ-kal) pertaining to the occlusal surface and the neck of a tooth.

occlusometer (ok″loo-som′ĕ-ter) gnathodynamometer.

occlusorehabilitation (ŏ-kloo″zo-re″hah-bil″ĭ-ta′shun) the employment of procedures designed to restore the dentition to an optimal functional relationship.

occult (ŏ-kult′) [L. *occultus*] obscure; concealed from observation; difficult to be understood.

occupancy (ok′ŭ-pan-se) the period of time during which a unit quantity of a substance, administered in a specified way, is present in, or occupies, a part of the body before it is excreted or broken down.

ocellus (o-sel′us) [L., dim. of *oculus* eye] 1. a small simple eye in insects and other invertebrates. 2. one of the elements of a compound eye of insects. 3. a roundish, eyelike patch of color.

ochlesis (ok-le′sis) [Gr. *ochlēsis* crowding] any disease due to overcrowding.

Ochoa (o-cho′ah), Severo. United States physician and biochemist, born 1905; co-winner, with Arthur Kornberg, of the Nobel prize in medicine and physiology for 1959, for work in the discovery of enzymes for producing nucleic acids artificially.

Ochrobium (o-kro′be-um) a genus of microorganisms of the family Siderocapsaceae, suborder Pseudomonadineae, order Pseudomonadales, occurring as ellipsoidal to rod-shaped cells partially surrounded by a marginal thickening heavily impregnated with iron, and contained in a delicate, transparent capsule. The type species is *O. tec′tum*.

ochrometer (o-krom′ĕ-ter) [Gr. *ōchros* paleness + *metron* measure] an instrument for measuring the capillary blood pressure by registering the force necessary to compress a finger by a rubber balloon until blanching of the skin occurs.

Ochromonadidae (ok″ro-mo-nad′ĭ-de) a family of free-swimming, colonial, flagellate protozoa of the order Chrysomonadina, class Phytomastigophora, including the genera *Uroglena* and *Uroglenopsis*.

Ochromyia (o″kro-mi′yah) Cordylobia.

ochronosis (o″kro-no′sis) [Gr. *ōchros* yellow + *nosos* disease] a peculiar discoloration of certain tissues of the body, caused by the deposit of alkapton bodies as the result of a metabolic disorder. **exogenous o.,** ochronosis allegedly resulting from exposure to some noxious substance in the internal environment, such as phenol, trinitrophenol, or benzene derivatives. **ocular o.,** a condition characterized by symmetrical, semilunar, or V-shaped accumulations of brown or gray pigment in the sclera, midway between the margin of the cornea and the inner or outer canthus. The eyelids and conjunctivae may also be affected.

ochronosus (o″kro-no′sus) ochronosis.

ochronotic (o″kro-not′ik) pertaining to, characterized by, or caused by ochronosis.

Ochsner's muscle, ring, treatment (oks′nerz) [Albert John *Ochsner*, surgeon in Chicago, 1858–1925] see under *muscle, ring,* and *treatment.*

Ocimum (os′ĭ-mum) a genus of herbs, including *O. basilicum* L. (Labiatae), or basil. They are a source of condiment and perfume oil.

ocrylate (ok′rĭ-lāt) chemical name: octyl 2-cyanoacrylate; a tissue adhesive, $C_{12}H_{19}NO_2$.

octa- (ok′tah) [Gr. *oktō,* L. *octo* eight] a combining form meaning eight.

octabenzone (ok-tah-ben′zōn) chemical name: 2-hydroxy-4-(octyloxy)benzophenone; an ultraviolet screen, $C_{21}H_{26}O_3$.

octacosane (ok″tah-ko′sān) an aliphatic hydrocarbon, $C_{28}H_{58}$, extracted from plant waxes.

octacosanol (ok″tah-ko-sa′nol) a solid white alcohol, $C_{28}H_{57}$-OH, from wheat oil and from the cuticular wax of apples.

octadecanoate (ok″tah-dek″ah-no′āt) systematic name for stearate, denoting that it has eighteen (*octa* eight + *deca* ten) carbon atoms in a straight chain.

octamethyl pyrophosphoramide (ok″tah-meth′il pir″o-fosfor′ah-mīd) chemical name: octamethyldiphosphoramide. A cholinesterase inhibitor, $C_8H_{24}N_4O_3P_2$, used as a systemic insecticide for plants. Called also *schradan.* Abbreviated OMPA.

octamylose (ok-tam′ĭ-lōs) a crystalline amylose, $(C_6H_{10}O_5)_8$.

octan (ok′tan) [L. *octo* eight] recurring every eighth day, or at intervals of seven days.

octane (ok′tān) an oily hydrocarbon, $CH_3(CH_2)_6CH_3$, occurring in petroleum.

octapeptide (ok″tah-pep′tid) a peptide which on hydrolysis yields eight amino acids.

octaploid (ok′tah-ploid) 1. pertaining to or characterized by octaploidy. 2. an individual or cell having eight sets of chromosomes.

octaploidy (ok′tah-ploi′de) the state of having eight sets of chromosomes (8n).

octarius (ok-ta′re-us) [L.; from *octo* eight] a pint; the eighth part of a gallon.

octavalent (ok″tah-va′lent) [L. *octo* eight + *valens* able] having a valency of eight.

octazamide (ok-ta′zah-mīd) chemical name: 5-benzoylhexahydro-1*H*-furo[3,4-*c*]pyrrole; an analgesic, $C_{13}H_{15}NO_2$.

octet (ok′tet) a group of eight identical or similar objects or entities, as the group of eight electrons (four pairs) in the outer, or valence, shell of an atom, which pairs may or may not be shared with another atom.

octicizer (ok″tĭ-si′zer) chemical name: 2-ethylhexyl diphenyl phosphate; a plasticizer, $C_{20}H_{27}O_4P$.

octigravida (ok″tĭ-grav′ĭ-dah) [L. *octo* eight + *gravida* pregnant] a woman pregnant for the eighth time; also written gravida VIII.

Octin (ok′tin) trademark for preparations of isometheptene.

octipara (ok-tip′ah-rah) [L. *octo* eight + *parere* to bring forth, produce] a woman who has had eight pregnancies which resulted in viable offspring; also written para VIII.

octodrine (ok′to-drēn) chemical name: 1,5-dimethylhexylamine; an adrenergic with vasoconstrictor and local anesthetic actions, $C_8H_{19}N$.

octofollin (ok′to-fol′in) benzestrol.

Octomitus (ok-tom′ĭ-tus) Hexamita. **O. hom′inis,** Trichomonas hominis.

Octomyces (ok″to-mi′sēz) a former genus of yeastlike fungi, now considered to be identical with Saccharomyces. **O. etien′nei,** yeastlike fungi of uncertain identity once isolated from a severe pleuropulmonary infection, probably as a contaminant.

octopamine (ok″to-pam′ēn) a sympathomimetic amine thought to result from inability of the diseased liver to metabolize tyrosine; it is called a false neurotransmitter, since it can be stored in presynaptic vesicles, replacing norepinephrine, but has little effect on postsynaptic receptors. It is used as the hydrochloride salt in treatment of hypotension.

octose (ok′tōs) [L. *octo* eight] a monosaccharide having the formula $C_8H_{16}O_8$.

octoxynol 9 (ok-toks′ĭ-nol) [NF] a clear, pale yellow, viscous liquid composed of an anhydrous mixture of mono[*p*-(1,1,3,3-tetramethylbutyl)phenyl]ethers of polyethylene glycols containing 5 to 15 oxyethylene groups in the polyoxyethylene chain, and having an average molecular weight of 647, corresponding to the formula $C_{34}H_{62}O_{11}$; used as a surfactant in pharmaceutical preparations. Called also *octylphenoxy polyethoxyethanol.*

octriptyline phosphate (ok-trip′tĭ-lēn) chemical name: 3-(1a, 10b-dihydrodibenzo[*a,e*]cyclopropa[*c*]cyclohepten-6(1*H*)-ylidene)-*N*-methyl-1-propanamine phosphate(1:1); an antidepressant, $C_{20}H_{21}N·H_3PO_4$.

octylphenoxy polyethoxyethanol (ok″til-fe″nok-se pol″eeth-ok″se-eth′ah-nol) octoxynol 9.

ocufilcon (ok″u-fil′kon) chemical name: 2-methyl-2-propenoic acid 2-hydroxyethyl ester polymer with 2-methyl-2-propenoic acid and 1,2-ethanediyl bis(2-methyl-2-propenoate); either of two hydrophilic contact lens materials, designated A or B, $(C_6H_{10}O_3)_x$-$(C_4H_6O_2)_y(C_{10}H_{14}O_4)_z$.

ocular (ok′u-lar) [L. *ocularis; oculus* eye] 1. of, pertaining to, or affecting the eye. 2. eyepiece.

oculentum (ok″u-len′tum), pl. *oculen′ta.* An eye ointment.

oculi (ok′u-li) [L.] plural of *oculus.*

oculist (ok′u-list) ophthalmologist.

oculistics (ok″u-lis′tiks) the treatment of diseases of the eye.

oculo- (ok′u-lo) [L. *oculus* eye] a combining form denoting relationship to the eye.

oculocephalogyric (ok″u-lo-sef″ah-lo-ji′rik) pertaining to the movements of the head in connection with vision.

oculocutaneous (ok″u-lo-ku-ta′ne-us) pertaining to or affecting both the eyes and the skin.

oculofacial (ok″u-lo-fa′she-al) pertaining to the eyes and the face.

oculogyration (ok″u-lo-ji-ra′shun) movement of the eye about the anteroposterior axis.

oculogyria (ok″u-lo-ji′re-ah) a condition characterized by oculogyration.

oculogyric (ok″u-lo-ji′rik) [*oculo-* + L. *gyrus* a turn] pertaining to, characterized by, or causing oculogyration; see also under *crisis.*

oculometroscope (ok″u-lo-met′ro-skōp) an instrument for performing retinoscopy in which the trial lenses are rotated before the eyes without effort on the part of the examiner.

oculomotor (ok″u-lo-mo′tor) [*oculo-* + L. *motor* mover] pertaining to or effecting movements of the eye.

oculomotorius (ok″u-lo-mo-to′re-us) [L.] nervum oculomotorius.

oculomycosis (ok″u-lo-mi-ko′sis) [*oculo-* + *mycosis*] any eye disease caused by a fungus.

oculonasal (ok″u-lo-na′zal) pertaining to the eye and the nose.

oculopathy (ok″u-lop′ah-the) [*oculo-* + Gr. *pathos* disease] any morbid condition of the eyes. **pituitarigenic o.,** abnormality of the eye caused by secretions of the pituitary gland.

oculoplastic (ok″u-lo-plas′tik) [*oculo-* + Gr. *plassein* to form, to mold] denoting plastic surgery of the eye, eyelids, ocular muscles, lacrimal apparatus, orbit.

oculopupillary (ok″u-lo-pu′pĭ-lār-e) pertaining to the pupil of the eye.

oculoreaction (ok″u-lo-re-ak′shun) the ophthalmic reaction; see under *reaction*.

oculospinal (ok″u-lo-spi′nal) pertaining to the eye and the spinal cord.

oculozygomatic (ok″u-lo-zi″go-mat′ik) pertaining to the eye and the zygoma.

oculus (ok′u-lus), pl. *oc′uli* [L.] [NA] the organ of vision; see *eye*.

O.D. abbreviation for *Doctor of Optometry*; L. *oc′ulus dex′ter*, right eye; and *outside diameter*; popular name for *drug overdose*.

od (od) [Gr. *hodos* pathway] (*obs.*) the influence supposedly exerted upon the nervous system by mesmerism.

O.D.A. abbreviation for L. *occipito-dextra anterior* (right occipito-anterior, a position of the fetus).

odaxesmus (o″dak-sez′mus) [Gr. *odaxēsmos* an itching] the biting of the tongue or cheek in an epileptic seizure.

odaxetic (o″dak-set′ik) [Gr. *odaxētikos*] causing a biting or itching sensation.

Oddi's muscle (sphincter) (od′ēz) [Ruggero *Oddi*, Italian physician of 19th century] see under *muscle*.

odditis (od-di′tis) inflammation of Oddi's muscle.

odogenesis (od″o-jen′ĕ-sis) [Gr. *hodos* pathway + *genesis* formation] neurocladism.

odon-eki (o″don-ek′e) [Japanese "icteric pestilence"] a disease resembling spirochetal jaundice.

odontalgia (o-don-tal′je-ah) [*odonto-* + *-algia*] pain in a tooth.

odontalgic (o-don-tal′jik) pertaining to or characterized by toothache.

odontectomy (o″don-tek′to-me) [*odonto-* + Gr. *ektomē* excision] excision of an erupted tooth, or of an unerupted or impacted tooth.

odontexesis (o″don-teks′e-sis) [*odonto-* + Gr. *xesis* scraping] (*obs.*) the removal of dental calculus and polishing of the teeth.

odontiatria (o-don″te-at′re-ah) [*odonto-* + Gr. *iatreia* treatment] dentistry.

odontiatrogenic (o-don″te-at′ro-jen′ik) [*odont* + Gr. *iatros* one who heals + *gennan* to produce] occurring as a result of treatment by a dentist.

odontic (o-don′tik) [Gr. *odous* tooth] pertaining to the teeth.

odonto- (o-don′to) [Gr. *odous* tooth] a combining form denoting relationship to a tooth or to the teeth.

odontoameloblastoma (o-don″to-am″ĕ-lo-blas-to′mah) ameloblastic odontoma.

odontoblast (o-don′to-blast) [*odonto-* + Gr. *blastos* germ] one of the columnar connective tissue cells which deposit dentin and form the outer surface of the dental pulp adjacent to the dentin.

odontoblastoma (o-don″to-blas-to′mah) a tumor made up of odontoblasts.

odontobothrion (o-don″to-both′re-on) [*odonto-* + Gr. *bothrion* a small trench] an alveolar crypt.

odontobothritis (o-don″to-both-ri′tis) inflammation of the alveolar process.

odontoclamis (o-don″to-kla′mis) [*odonto-* + Gr. *klamys* cloak] dental operculum.

odontoclast (o-don′to-klast) [*odonto-* + Gr. *klan* break] a multinucleated giant cell (osteoclast), found associated with absorption of the roots of a deciduous tooth.

odontogen (o-don′to-jen) [*odonto-* + Gr. *gennan* to produce] the substance which develops into the dentin of the tooth.

odontogenesis (o-don″to-jen′ĕ-sis) [*odonto-* + Gr. *genesis* production] the origin and histogenesis of the teeth. **o. imperfec′ta,** dentinogenesis imperfecta.

odontogenetic (o-don″to-jĕ-net′ik) pertaining to odontogenesis.

odontogenic (o-don″to-jen′ik) 1. forming teeth. 2. arising in tissues which give origin to the teeth.

odontogenous (o″don-toj′ĕ-nus) arising or originating in the teeth, or a dental condition.

odontogeny (o″don-toj′ĕ-ne) odontogenesis.

odontogram (o-don′to-gram) [*odonto-* + Gr. *gramma* mark] the tracing made by an odontograph.

odontograph (o-don′to-graf) [*odonto-* + Gr. *graphein* to write] an instrument for recording the unevenness of surface of tooth enamel.

odontography (o″don-tog′rah-fe) [*odonto-* + Gr. *graphein* to write] 1. a description of the teeth. 2. the use of the odontograph.

odontoiatria (o-don″to-i-at′re-ah) [*odonto-* + Gr. *iatreia* cure] dental therapeutics.

odontoid (o-don′toid) [*odonto-* + Gr. *eidos* form] toothlike; resembling a tooth.

odontolith (o-don′to-lith) [*odonto-* + Gr. *lithos* stone] dental calculus.

odontolithiasis (o-don″to-lĭ-thi′ah-sis) a condition marked by the presence of deposits of calcium on the teeth.

odontologist (o″don-tol′o-jist) a dentist.

odontology (o″don-tol′o-je) [*odonto-* + *-logy*] 1. the sum of knowledge regarding the teeth. 2. dentistry.

odontolysis (o-don-tol′ĭ-sis) [*odonto-* + Gr. *lysis* dissolution] the resorption of dental tissue.

odontoma (o-don-to′mah) [*odonto-* + Gr. *-ōma* tumor] any tumor of odontogenic origin; customarily used to designate a composite odontoma (q.v.); called also *coronodental cyst*. **o. adamanti′num,** ameloblastic o. **ameloblastic o.,** a rare neoplasm composed of enamel, dentin, and an odontogenic epithelium like that seen in ameloblastoma; called also *odontoameloblastoma*. **composite o.,** an odontogenic tumor in which both the epithelial and mesenchymal cells exhibit complete differentiation; this results in the formation, by functional ameloblasts and odontoblasts, of enamel and dentin which are usually laid down in an abnormal pattern because of failure of the odontogenic cells to reach a normal state of morphodifferentiation. **composite o., complex,** a composite odontoma in which the calcified dental tissues occur in an irregular mass, and there is no morphologic similarity to even rudimentary teeth. **composite o., compound,** a composite odontoma in which the enamel and dentin are laid down so that the structure bears a superficial anatomic resemblance to normal teeth. **coronal o., coronary o.,** odontoma associated with the crown of a tooth, or one formed at the time when the crown of the tooth was developing. **dilated o.,** dens in dente. **embryoplastic o.,** a soft odontoma formed in the period that precedes the formation of the dental tissues. **fibrous o.,** an odontoma containing fibrous elements. **mixed o.,** an odontogenic neoplasm containing different elements of the tooth structure. **radicular o.,** one associated with the root of a tooth, or one formed at the time when the root of the tooth was developing.

odontonomy (o″don-ton′o-me) [*odonto-* + Gr. *onoma* name] dental nomenclature.

odontopathic (o-don″to-path′ik) relating to disease of the teeth.

odontopathy (o″don-top′ah-the) [*odonto-* + Gr. *pathos* illness] any disease of the teeth.

odontoperiosteum (o-don″to-per″e-os′te-um) periodontium.

odontophobia (o-don″to-fo′be-ah) [*odonto-* + Gr. *phobein* to be affrighted by] a morbid fear associated with teeth, as that aroused by the sight of teeth, or abnormal dread of dental operations.

odontoplasty (o-don′to-plas″te) [*odonto-* + Gr. *plassein* to form] (*obs.*) orthodontics.

odontoprisis (o-don″to-pri′sis) [*odonto-* + Gr. *prisis* sawing] bruxism.

odontoradiograph (o-don″to-ra′de-o-graf) a roentgenogram of a tooth or of the teeth.

odontorthosis (o-don″tor-tho′sis) [*odonto-* + Gr. *orthōsis* a making straight] orthodontics.

odontoschism (o-don″to-skizm) [*odonto-* + Gr. *schisma* cleft] fissure of a tooth.

odontoscopy (o″don-tos′ko-pe) the taking of impressions of the teeth in order to make casts to be used as a means of personal identification.

odontoseisis (o-don″to-si′sis) [*odonto-* + Gr. *seisis* a shaking] looseness of the teeth.

odontosis (o″don-to′sis) [Gr. *odous* tooth] the formation or eruption of the teeth.

odontotechny (o-don′to-tek″ne) [*odonto-* + Gr. *technē* art] dentistry.

odontotheca (o-don″to-the′kah) [*odonto-* + Gr. *thēkē* case] the dental sac.

odontotomy (o″don-tot′o-me) [*odonto-* + Gr. *tomē* a cutting] the operation of cutting into a tooth, especially incision into an occlusal groove.

odontotripsis (o-don″to-trip′sis) [*odonto-* + Gr. *tripsis* rubbing] wearing away of the teeth.

odor (o′dor) [L.] a volatile emanation that is perceived by the sense of smell. **butcher shop o.,** a smell like that of a butcher shop given off by yellow fever patients. **minimal identifiable o.,** the lowest concentration of a substance in air, or in another medium, which still permits its identification by the sense of smell.

odorant (o′dor-ant) any substance capable of eliciting olfactory excitation, i.e., of stimulating the sense of smell.

odoratism (o″dor-a′tizm) osteolathyrism.

odoriferous (o″dor-if′er-us) [*odor* + L. *ferre* to bear] fragrant; emitting an odor.

odorimeter (o″dor-im′ĕ-ter) an instrument for performing odorimetry.

odorimetry (o″dor-im′ĕ-tre) the measurement of olfactory stimuli.

odoriphore (o-dor′ĭ-fōr) osmophore.

odorivector (o″dor-ĭ-vek′tor) a substance which gives off an odor.

odorography (o″dor-og′rah-fe) [odor + Gr. graphein to write] a description of odors.

O.D.P. abbreviation for L. occipito-dextra posterior (right occipitoposterior, a position of the fetus).

O.D.T. abbreviation for L. occipito-dextra transversa (right occipitotransverse, a position of the fetus).

O'Dwyer's tubes (o-dwi′erz) [Joseph P. O'Dwyer, American otolaryngologist, 1841–1898] intubation tube.

odynacusis (o″din-ah-ku′sis) [odyno- + Gr. akousis hearing] painful hearing.

-odynia (o-din′e-ah) [Gr. odynē pain] a word ending meaning pain.

odyno- (o-din′o) [Gr. odynē pain] a combining form meaning pain.

odynometer (o″din-om′ĕ-ter) [odyno- + Gr. metron measure] an instrument for measuring pain.

odynophagia (od″ĭ-no-fa′je-ah) [odyno- + Gr. phagein to eat] pain on deglutition.

odynphagia (o″din-fa′je-ah) odynophagia.

oe- for other words beginning thus, see also those beginning with e-.

Oeciacus (e-si′ah-kus) a genus of insects closely related to the bedbugs (Cimex), but distinguished by their hairy bodies covered by long silklike coats; they are found on birds and in their nests. O. hirudinis is found on barn swallows in Europe and sometimes invades homes and attacks man, causing a severe irritation; O. vicarius is found on swallows in North America.

oedipism (ed′ĭ-pizm) [see Oedipus complex] edipism.

Oedipus complex (ed′ĭ-pus) [Oedipus, a character in Greek tragedy who, raised by a foster parent, killed his actual father in a quarrel, and subsequently married his mother. Later, when he discovered the true relationship, he blinded himself (edipism)] see under complex.

Oehler's symptom (e′lerz) [Johannes Oehler, German physician, born 1879] see under symptom.

oenanthol (e-nan′thol) heptoic aldehyde, $CH_3(CH_2)_5CHO$; called also heptanal.

oersted (er′sted) [Hans Christian Oersted, Danish physicist, 1777–1851] the unit of magnetizing force, symbol H.

Oertel's treatment (er′telz) [Max Joseph Oertel, physician in Munich, 1835–1897] see under treatment.

oesophago- for words beginning thus, see those beginning esophago-.

oesophagostomiasis (e-sof″ah-go-sto-mi′ah-sis) infection with Oesophagostomum.

Œsophagostomum (e-sof″ah-gos′to-mum) [Œsophagus + Gr. stoma mouth] a genus of nematode worms of the family Strongylidae, parasitic in the intestines of various animals; the larvae often encyst in the intestinal wall, while the adults are mostly free in the lumen. **Œ. apios′tomum**, Œ. bifurcum. **Œ. bifur′cum**, a parasite that forms tumors in the large intestine of monkeys and occasionally of man in Africa and the Philippines. **Œ. brevicau′dum**, a species found in pigs. **Œ. brump′ti**, Œ. bifurcum. **Œ. columbia′num**, the nodular worm, infects sheep and goats in the southern United States; see nodular disease, under disease. **Œ. denta′tum**, a parasite of the pig. **Œ. infla′tum**, Œ. radiatum. **Œ. longicau′dum**, a parasite of pigs. **Œ. radia′tum**, a parasite of cattle. **Œ. stephanos′tomum**, a species, normally parasitic in gorillas; a single human case has been recorded from Brazil. **Œ. su′is**, Œ. brevicaudum.

oesophagus (e-sof′ah-gus) esophagus.

Oestreicher's reaction (est′ri-kerz) [A. Oestreicher] xanthydrol reaction.

oestriasis (es-tri′ah-sis) infestation with larvae of flies of the genus Oestrus.

Oestridae (es′trĭ-de) the family of the "bot," "heel," or "warble" flies. They are very hairy diptera with rudimentary mouth parts and with the antennae inserted into round pits. The family includes the following genera: Gasterophilus, Oestrus, Hypoderma, Dermatobia, Rhinoestrus, and Cuterebra.

oestrone (es′tron) estrone.

oestrous (es′trus) estrous.

oestrual (es′troo-al) estrual.

oestrum (es′trum) estrus.

oestrus (es′trus) estrus.

Oestrus (es′trus) [Gr. oistros gadfly] a genus of botflies of the family Oestridae, which may cause ophthalmomyiasis, called also Cephalomyia. **O. hom′inis**, O. ovis. **O. o′vis**, a species of botfly whose larvae infest nasal cavities and sinuses of sheep; they may cause ocular myiasis in man.

official (ŏ-fish′al) [L. officialis; officum duty] recognized by the current U. S. Pharmacopeia or National Formulary, and meeting the standards established by the respective authority.

officinal (ŏ-fis′ĭ-nal) [L. officinalis; officina shop] regularly kept for sale in the shops of druggists.

Ogata's method (o-gah′tahz) [M. Ogata, Japanese physician] see under method.

Ogen (o′jen) trademark for preparations of piperazine estrone sulfate; see under estrone.

ogive (o′jīv) a S-shaped curve; a term used in biometry.

ogo (o′go) gangosa.

Ogston's line, operation (og′stonz) [Sir Alexander Ogston, Scottish surgeon, 1844–1929] see under line and operation.

Ogston-Luc operation (og′ston-luk′) [Sir Alexander Ogston; Henry Luc, French laryngologist, 1855–1925] see under operation.

Oguchi's disease (o-goo′chēz) [Chuta Oguchi, Japanese ophthalmologist, born 1875] see under disease.

OH hydroxyl group; (with negative sign) hydroxide ion; a hydroxide.

Ohara's disease (o-hah′rahz) [Hachiro Ohara, Japanese physician, born 1882] see under disease.

ohm (ōm) [George S. Ohm, German physicist, 1787–1854] the SI unit of electrical resistance, being equivalent to that of a column of mercury one square millimeter in cross-section and one hundred and six contimeters long. Symbol Ω.

Ohm's law (ōmz) [George S. Ohm, German physicist, 1787–1854] see under law.

ohmammeter (ōm′am-me″ter) an ohmmeter and ammeter combined.

ohmmeter (ōm′me-ter) an instrument for measuring electric resistance in ohms.

ohne Hauch (o′nah-houkh) [Ger. "without breath"] see O, and also see H (def. 2).

-oid [Gr. eidos form, shape] a word termination signifying resemblance to the thing specified by the stem to which it is affixed, as ovoid.

Oidiomycetes (o-id″e-o-mi-se′tēz) former name for a group of fungi characterized by having mycelial threads and producing small spores by fragmentation.

oidiomycosis (o-id″e-o-mi-ko′sis) [oidium + Gr. mykēs fungus] infection with fungi of the genus Oidium.

oidiomycotic (o-id″e-o-mi-kot′ik) pertaining to oidiomycosis.

Oidium (o-id′e-um) [dim. of Gr. ōon egg] 1. a former name for a genus of fungi the species of which are now included in the genera Candida and Geotrichum. 2. the imperfect (sexual) stage of the powdery mildews (order Erysiphales), causing many plant diseases.

oikosite (oi′ko-sīt) ecosite.

oil (oil) [L. oleum] 1. an unctuous, combustible substance which is liquid, or easily liquefiable, on warming, and is soluble in ether but insoluble in water. Such substances, depending on their origin, are classified as animal, mineral, or vegetable oils. Depending on their behavior on heating, they are classified as volatile or fixed. 2. a fat that is liquid at room temperature. **allspice o.**, pimenta o. **almond o.** [NF], a preparation of the fixed oil obtained from the kernels of varieties of Prunus amygdalus; used as an emollient and perfume and as an ingredient of rose water ointment. Called also expressed or sweet almond o., and oleum amygdalae expressum. **almond o., bitter**, the volatile oil obtained from the dried ripe kernels of Prunus amygdalus var. amara Focke (Rosaceae) or from other kernels containing amygdalin; formerly used as a topical antipruritic; used also in perfumery and liqueurs. **almond o., expressed**, see almond o. **almond o., sweet**, see almond o. **anise o.** [NF], a volatile oil distilled from the dried, ripe fruit of Pimpinella anisum or of Illicium verum; used as a flavoring agent for drugs, and has been used as a carminative and expectorant. **apricot kernel o.**, persic o. **arachis o.**, peanut o. **argemone o.**, an oil from Argemona mexicana L. (Papaveraceae), the prickly poppy, which is toxic to humans; it is the cause of epidemic dropsy, and sometimes causes disturbances of the gastrointestinal tract and of vision. **bay o.**, myrcia o. **Benne o.**, sesame o. **bergamot o.**, a volatile oil obtained by expression from the rind of the fresh fruit of Citrus bergamia; used as a perfuming agent and insecticide. **betula o.**, methyl salicylate. **bhilawanol o.**, a fluid obtained from the nut of a tree, Semecarpus anacardium (ral tree, bella gutta tree), in India, used by native washermen for marking laundry, and the cause, through induction of eczematous contact sensitization, of dhobie itch. **birch o., sweet**, methyl salicylate. **birch tar o., rectified**, the pyroligneous oil obtained by the dry distillation of the bark and wood of Betula alba L. (Betulaceae) and other species of Betula, and rectified by steam distillation; used topically in the treatment of eczema and other dermatitides. **cade o.**, juniper tar. **o. of cajuput**, a volatile oil from the fresh leaves and twigs of Melaleuca leucadendron L. (Myrtaceae) and other species of Melaleuca; used as a stimulant, expectorant, counterirritant, and external parasiticide, and in veterinary medicine as a rubefacient and parasiticide in the treatment of ringworm. **camphorated o.**, camphor liniment. **caraway o.** [NF], a volatile oil distilled from the dried ripe fruit of *Carum carvi*, yielding at least 50 per cent by volume of carvone; used as a flavoring agent for drugs. Called also *oleum cari*. **cardamom o.** [NF], a volatile oil distilled from the seed of *Elettaria cardamomum* (cardamom seed), a perennial herb of the ginger family of tropical Asia; used as a flavoring agent in pharmaceutical preparations. Called also *oleum cardamomi*. **cassia o.,** cinnamon o. **castor o.** [USP], a fixed oil obtained from the seed of *Ricinus communis;* used as a cathartic and as a plasticizer for pharmaceutical preparations, and has been used as a bland emollient to the skin in certain dermatoses. **castor o., aromatic** [USP], a mixture of cinnamon, clove, and castor oils, with saccharin, vanillin, and alcohol, used as a cathartic. **cedar o.,** a volatile oil from cedar wood, used as a clearing agent in microscopical techniques; the thicker fraction is used as the immersion medium with oil-immersion objectives. **chaulmoogra o.,** a fixed oil expressed from the ripe seeds of *Taraktogenos kurzii, Hydnocarpus wightiana,* and *H. anthelmintica;* formerly used in the treatment of leprosy; ethyl esters of the fatty acids (ethyl chaulmoograte) obtained from this oil are now so used. **chenopodium o.,** a volatile oil obtained by steam distillation of fresh overground parts of the flowering and fruiting plant of *Chenopodium ambrosiodes,* L. (Chenopodiaceae); it contains 65 per cent of ascaridole, an active anthelmintic principle and was once used as an anthelmintic. **chloriodized o.,** an iodine monochloride addition product of vegetable oil; formerly used as a radiopaque medium in roentgenography of the uterus and uterine tubes, and of the bronchi. **cinnamon o.** [NF], a volatile oil distilled with steam from the leaves and twigs of *Cinnamomum cassia;* used as a flavoring agent for pharmaceuticals and as a carminative. **citronella o.,** a fragrant oil used as an insect repellent. **clove o.** [NF], a volatile oil distilled with steam from clover, the dried flowerbuds of *Eugenia caryophyllus;* used as a flavor in pharmaceutical preparations, and as a topical germicide and analgesic in dentistry. **coconut o.,** the fixed oil obtained by expression or extraction from the kernels of seeds of *Cocos nucifera;* used as an ointment base and edible oil and in soap, chocolate, and candle formulations. **cod liver o.** [USP], the partially destearinated fixed oil obtained from fresh livers of *Gadus morrhua* and other species of the family Gadidae; used as a source of vitamin A and vitamin D. In veterinary medicine, it is also used topically to promote wound-healing and in abscesses, burns, and dermatoses. **cod liver o., nondestearinated** [NF], the entire fixed oil obtained from fresh livers of *Gadus morrhua* and other species of the family Gadidae; used as a source of vitamins A and D. **o. of copaiba,** a volatile oil derived from copaiba, *Copaifera* spp. (Leguminosae), trees indigenous to central South America; it contains aromatic principles and was once used for chronic inflammations of mucous membranes. **coriander o.** [NF], a volatile oil distilled with steam from the dried ripe fruit of *Coriandrum sativum;* used as a flavoring agent. **corn o.** [NF], a refined fixed oil obtained from the embryo of *Zea mays;* used as a solvent and vehicle for various medicinal agents and as a vehicle for injections. It has also been promoted as a source of polyunsaturated fatty acids in special diets. **cottonseed o.** [NF], a refined fixed oil obtained from the seeds of cultivated plants of various varieties of *Gossypium hirsutum;* used as a solvent and vehicle for drugs. It has also been promoted as a source of polyunsaturated fatty acids in special diets. **croton o.,** the thick, fixed oil of the seeds of *Croton tiglium,* L. Euphorbiaceae, an Asiatic plant. A drastic purgative and counterirritant, unsafe for human use, it is used as standard irritant in pharmacological research. **o. of dill,** an oil distilled from the dried ripe fruits of *Anethum graveolens* L. (Umbelliferae); used as an aromatic carminative and as a source of carvone. **distilled o.,** volatile o. **drying o.,** a type of fixed oil which thickens and hardens on exposure to the air, especially when spread out in a thin layer, being converted to a solid by absorption and reaction with oxygen. **empyreumatic o.,** a volatile oil formed by the destructive distillation of organic material. **essential o.,** volatile o. **ethereal o.,** 1. a compound of ether with heavy oil of wine. 2. a volatile oil. **ethiodized o.** [USP], an iodine addition product of the ethyl ester of the fatty acids of poppyseed oil, containing 35.2 to 38.9 per cent of organically combined iodine; used as a radiopaque medium in hysterosalpingography and lymphography. **eucalyptus o.** [NF], a volatile oil distilled with steam from the fresh leaf of *Eucalyptus globulus* and other species of *Eucalyptus;* used as a flavor in pharmaceutical preparations, and as an expectorant and local antiseptic with mild anesthetic effect. Formerly used as a vermifuge. **expressed o., fatty o.,** fixed o. **fennel o.** [NF], a volatile oil distilled with steam from the dried ripe fruit of *Foeniculum vulgare;* used as a flavoring agent for pharmaceuticals and formerly as a carminative. **fixed o.,** an oil which does not evaporate on warming. Such oils, consisting of a mixture of fatty acids and their esters, are classified as solid (chiefly stearin), semisolid (chiefly palmitin), and liquid (chiefly olein). Fixed oils are also classified as *drying, semidrying,* and *nondrying,* depending on their tendency to solidify when exposed, in a thin film, to air. Called also *expressed o.* and *fatty o.* **flaxseed o.,** linseed o. **gaultheria o.,** methyl salicylate. **gingilli o.,** sesame o. **groundnut o.,** peanut o. **Haarlem o.,** juniper tar. **halibut liver o.,** a fixed oil obtained from fresh or suitably preserved livers of halibut species of the genus *Hippoglossus* Linné; used as a source of vitamins A and D. **heavy o.,** an oily product obtained by the action of sulfuric acid on alcohol. **hydnocarpus o.,** chaulmoogra o. **iodized o.,** an iodine addition product of vegetable oil; used as radiopaque medium in roentgenography of the uterus and uterine tubes. **juniper o.,** a volatile oil distilled with steam from the dried ripe fruit of *Juniperus communis;* used to preserve catgut sutures and has been used as a diuretic. **lavender o.** [NF], a volatile oil distilled with steam from the fresh flowering tops of *Lavandula officinalis;* used as a perfuming agent and flavor, and has been used as a carminative and aromatic. **lavender flowers o.,** lavender o. **lemon o.** [NF], the volatile oil obtained by expression from the fresh peel of the fruit of *Citrus limon;* used as a flavoring agent. **linseed o., raw linseed o.,** the fixed oil obtained from the dried ripe seed of *Linum usitatissimum* (L. Linaceae); used as an emollient in liniments, pastes, and medicinal soaps, and in veterinary medicine as a laxative. Called also *flaxseed o.* **o. of male fern,** an oleoresin from the root of the male fern, *Dryopteris filix-mas* (L.) Schott., Polypodiaceae; it contains about 24 per cent of crude filicin and is used as an anthelmintic. **mineral o.** [USP], a mixture of liquid hydrocarbons obtained from petroleum, with a specific gravity of 0.845–0.905; used as a cathartic and as a solvent and oleaginous vehicle in pharmaceutical preparations. Called also *heavy liquid petrolatum, liquid petrolatum, liquid paraffin, petrolatum liquidum,* and *white mineral o.* **mineral o., light** [USP], **mineral o., light white,** a mixture of liquid hydrocarbons obtained from petrolatum, with a specific gravity of 0.818–0.880; used as a vehicle for drugs and also as a laxative. Called also *light liquid paraffin* and *light liquid petrolatum.* **mineral o., white,** liquid petrolatum. **o. of mirbane,** nitrobenzene. **o. of mustard,** an oil derived from the seeds of species of *Brassica.* Volatile mustard oil is from the seeds of black mustard (see *allyl isothiocyanate*). Used internally as a condiment and emetic and externally as a counterirritant. **myrcia o.,** the volatile oil obtained by distilling the leaves of *Pimenta officinalis* Lindl. (Myrtaceae). It contains 55–65 per cent of eugenol and other related aromatic principles and is used in perfumes and such products as bay rum as an after-shave lotion and rub or liniment. Called also *bay o.* **myristica o.,** nutmeg o. **neroli o.,** orange flower o. **nutmeg o.,** [NF], the volatile oil distilled with steam from the dried kernels of the ripe seeds of *Myristica fragrans* Houtt. (Myristicaceae); used as a flavoring agent in pharmaceutical preparations. Called also *myristica o.* **olive o.** [NF], the fixed oil obtained from the ripe fruit of *Olea europaea;* used as a setting retardant for dental cements and as a topical emollient, and has been used as a laxative. Called also *sweet o.* **orange o.** [NF], the volatile oil obtained by expression from the fresh peel of the ripe fruit of *Citrus sinensis;* used as a flavoring agent in pharmaceuticals. Called also *sweet orange o.* **orange o., bitter,** a volatile oil obtained by expression from the fresh peel of the fruit of *Citrus aurantium* L. (Rutaceae); used as a flavoring agent. **orange o., sweet,** orange o. **orange flower o.** [NF], a volatile oil distilled from the fresh flowers of *Citrus aurantium;* used as a flavoring agent and perfume. Called also *neroli.* **o. of Palma Christi,** castor o. **peach kernel o.,** persic o. **peanut o.** [NF], the refined fixed oil obtained from the seed kernels of one or more of the cultivated varieties of *Arachis hypogaea;* used as a solvent and oleaginous vehicle for drugs, and as a laxative in veterinary medicine. **peppermint o.** [NF], the volatile oil distilled with steam from the fresh overground parts of the flowering plant of *Mentha piperita* L. (Labiate); used as a flavor in pharmaceutical preparations, and as a gastric stimulant and carminative. **persic o.** [NF], an oil expressed from the kernels of varieties of *Prunus armeniaca,* the apricot, or from *P. persica,* the peach; used as a vehicle for drugs. **pimenta o.,** the volatile oil distilled from the fruit of *Pimenta officinalis;* used as a flavoring agent for drugs. **pine o.,** the volatile oil obtained by steam distillation of the wood of *Pinus palustris* and of other species of *Pinus;* used as a deodorant and disinfectant. **pine needle o.** [NF], **pine needle o., dwarf,** the volatile oil distilled with steam from the fresh leaf of the dwarf pine, *Pinus mugo* and its variety *pumilio;* used as a perfume and flavoring agent. **ricinus o.,** castor o. **rose o.** [NF], the volatile oil distilled with steam from the fresh flowers of *Rosa gallica* L., *R. damascena* Mill., *R. alba* L., *R. centifolia,* and varieties of these species; used as a perfuming agent in pharmaceuticals. It has also been used as a flavoring agent in ointments and lozenges. Called also *attar of rose.* **rosemary o.,** the volatile oil distilled with steam from the fresh flowering tops of *Rosmarinus officinalis* L.; used as a flavoring or perfuming agent. **safflower o.,** an oily liquid extracted from the seeds of the safflower, *Carthamus tinctorius;* used as a dietary supplement in the management of hypercholesterolemia. **sandalwood o.,** santal o. **santal o.,** a pale yellow, somewhat viscid, oily liquid with characteristic odor and taste of sandalwood, distilled with steam from the dried heartwood of *Santalum album* L. (Santalaceae), or sandalwood; formerly used as a urinary antiseptic. **sassafras o.,** the volatile oil distilled with steam from the root of *Sassafras albidum;* used as a flavoring agent for liquid pharmaceutical preparations and to offset their disagreeable odor. It is also applied to insect bites and stings and has been used as a topical antiseptic, pediculicide, and carminative. It contains safrene and safrol. The oil is also the basis of the soda beverage known as root beer. **sesame o.** [NF], the refined fixed oil obtained from the seed of one or more cultivated varieties of *Sesamum indicum*; it is used as a solvent and oleaginous vehicle for drugs, and has been used internally as a laxative and externally as a skin softener. **spearmint o.** [NF], the volatile oil distilled with steam from the fresh overground parts of *Mentha spicata* (*M. viridis*) or *Mentha cardiaca*, yielding at least 55 per cent by volume of carvone; used as a flavoring agent and has been used as a carminative. **o. of spike**, a volatile oil obtained from a broad-leaved variety of lavender, *Lavandula latifolia*, growing wild in Europe; used in perfumery, and formerly in home remedies as an emmenagogue and abortive. **o. of spruce,** a volatile oil obtained from the hemlock tree, *Tsuga canadensis*, sometimes used in veterinary liniments. **sweet o.,** olive o. **tangan-tangan o.,** castor o. **tar o., rectified,** the volatile oil from pine tar rectified by steam distillation; used, in veterinary medicine, internally as a stimulant expectorant and externally as an antipruritic, antiseptic, and stimulant for diseases of the skin. Also widely used in disinfecting and deodorizing preparations. **teel o.,** sesame o. **theobroma o.,** cocoa butter. **thyme o.,** the volatile oil distilled from the flowering plant of *Thymus vulgaris*; used as a flavoring agent for drugs, and has been used as a rubefacient, expectorant, counterirritant, antiseptic, and carminative. **turpentine o.,** the volatile oil distilled from an oleoresin obtained from *Pinus palustris* Mill. (Pinaceae) and other species of *Pinus*. Its chief constituent is pinene, which is used in the synthetic production of camphor. It is used as a counterirritant and rubefacient. **turpentine o., rectified,** turpentine oil rectified by use of sodium hydroxide; used as an inhalation expectorant. **volatile o.,** an oil which evaporates readily. The volatile oils occur in aromatic plants, to which they give odor and other characteristics. Most volatile oils consist of a mixture of two or more terpenes or of a mixture of an eleopten with a stearopten. Called also *distilled o., essential o.,* and *ethereal o.* **wheat-germ o.,** oil derived from the germ of wheat kernels; it is rich in vitamin E. **wintergreen o.,** methyl salicylate. **wormseed o., American,** chenopodium o.

oinomania (oi″no-ma′ne-ah) alcholism.

ointment (oint′ment) [L. *unguentum*] a semisolid preparation for external application to the body, and usually containing a medicinal substance. Called also *unguent, unction,* and *salve.* **ammoniated mercury o.** [USP], a preparation of ammoniated mercury, liquid petrolatum, and white ointment, containing 4.5 to 5.5 per cent of HgNH₂Cl; used as a topical anti-infective. Called also *white precipitate o.* **anthralin o.** [USP], a preparation of anthralin in a petrolatum or other suitable base; used as a topical antipsoriatic. **bacitracin o.** [USP], a preparation of bacitracin or bacitracin zinc in an anhydrous ointment base, containing not less than 500 U.S.P. units per gram; used as an antibacterial, applied topically to the skin. **bacitracin ophthalmic o.** [USP], a preparation of bacitracin in an anhydrous ointment base, containing not less than 500 U.S.P. units per gram; used as an antibacterial, applied topically to the conjunctiva. **belladonna o.,** a preparation of pilular belladonna extract and diluted alcohol in yellow ointment; used locally as an analgesic. **benzocaine o.** [USP], a preparation of finely powdered benzocaine in white ointment, used as a local anesthetic; called also *ethyl aminobenzoate o.* **benzoic and salicylic acids o.** [USP], a preparation of benzoic acid and salicylic acid in a water-soluble base (polyethylene glycol ointment), formerly used topically as an antifungal agent. Called *Whitfield's o.* **betamethasone valerate o.** [USP], a preparation containing betamethasone valerate equivalent to 95 to 120 per cent of the labeled amount of betamethasone; used as an anti-inflammatory glucocorticoid. **blue o.,** mercurial o., mild. **boric acid o.,** a preparation of finely powdered boric acid and liquid petrolatum in white ointment, formerly used extensively for its emollient and protective action in superficial wounds, abrasions, and burns, and for ophthalmic application. **calamine o.,** a preparation containing calamine, yellow wax, anhydrous lanolin, and petrolatum; used as an astringent protective application. **calomel o.,** a preparation of calomel, hydrous wool fat, and white petrolatum, containing 28.5 to 31.5 per cent calomel; has been used to treat various infections and parasitic infestations of the skin. Called also *mild mercurous chloride o.* **candicidin o.** [USP], a semisolid preparation of candicidin in a suitable ointment base, containing 90 to 140 per cent of the labeled amount of candicidin; used as a local antifungal agent in the treatment of vaginal candidiasis, administered intravaginally. **carbolic acid o.,** phenol o. **chloramphenicol ophthalmic o.** [USP], an ointment containing between 90 and 130 per cent of the labeled amount of chloramphenicol; used as an antibacterial, applied topically to the conjunctiva. **chrysarobin o.,** a preparation of chrysarobin, chloroform, and white ointment; used topically in the treatment of psoriasis and other chronic skin diseases. **coal tar o.** [USP], a preparation of coal tar, polysorbate 80, and zinc oxide paste, used as a topical antieczematic and antipsoriatic. **Credé's o.,** one containing collargol, water, white wax, and benzoinated lard, used in septicemia, pyemia, boils, carbuncles, etc. **cyclomethycaine sulfate o.** [USP], a preparation containing

90 to 110 per cent of the labeled amount of cyclomethycaine sulfate in a suitable ointment base; used as a topical anesthetic. **dexamethasone sodium phosphate ophthalmic o.** [NF], an ointment containing 90 to 115 per cent of the labeled amount of dexamethasone sodium phosphate; used as an anti-inflammatory glucocorticoid applied to the conjunctiva. **dibucaine o.** [USP], a semisolid preparation of dibucaine in a suitable ointment base, containing 90 to 110 per cent of the labeled amount of dibucaine; used as a local anesthetic, especially for dry, encrusted lesions, applied topically to the skin and mucous membranes. **dimethisoquin hydrochloride o.** [USP], an ointment containing 90 to 110 per cent of the labeled amount of dimethisoquin hydrochloride; used as a local anesthetic, applied topically to the skin to relieve pain, itching, and burning. **diperodon o.** [USP], a preparation containing 90 to 110 per cent of the labeled amount of diperodon in a suitable ointment base; used as a local anesthetic, applied topically to the skin for abrasions, irritations, and pruritus or intrarectally for relief of discomfort associated with hemorrhoids. **erythromycin o.** [USP], a preparation containing 90 to 125 per cent of the labeled amount of erythromycin (the labeled amount being 10 mg. of erythromycin per gm. of ointment) in a suitable ointment base; used as a topical antibacterial in the treatment of superficial infections of the skin due to organisms susceptible to erythromycin. **erythromycin ophthalmic o.** [USP], a preparation containing 90 to 120 per cent of the labeled amount of erythromycin (the labeled amount being 5 mg. of erythromycin per gm. of ophthalmic ointment) in a suitable ointment base; used as a topical antibacterial in the treatment of superficial infections of the conjunctiva and/or cornea due to organisms susceptible to erythromycin. **ethyl aminobenzoate o.,** benzocaine o. **fluocinolone acetonide o.** [USP], an ointment containing 90 to 110 per cent of the labeled amount of fluocinolone acetonide; used as an anti-inflammatory in steroid-responsive dermatoses, applied topically. **flurandrenolide o.** [USP], an ointment containing 85 to 115 per cent of the labeled amount of flurandrenolide; used as a topical anti-inflammatory glucocorticoid in the treatment of steroid-responsive dermatoses. **gentamicin sulfate o.** [USP], a semisolid preparation of gentamicin sulfate in a suitable ointment base, containing 90 to 135 per cent of the labeled amount of gentamicin; used as a topical antibacterial. **gentamicin sulfate ophthalmic o.** [USP], a sterile preparation of gentamicin sulfate in a petroleum base, containing the equivalent of 90 to 135 per cent of the labeled amount of gentamicin; used as an antibacterial, applied topically to the conjunctiva. **hydrocortisone o.** [USP], a semisolid preparation of hydrocortisone in a suitable ointment base, containing 90 to 110 per cent of the labeled amount of hydrocortisone; used as an anti-inflammatory adrenocortical steroid. **hydrocortisone acetate o.** [USP], a preparation containing 1.00 to 1.25 per cent hydrocortisone acetate, equivalent to 0.9 to 1.1 per cent hydrocortisone, used as a topical adrenocortical steroid. **hydrocortisone acetate ophthalmic o.** [USP], a semisolid preparation of hydrocortisone acetate in a suitable ointment base, containing 90 to 110 per cent of the labeled amount of hydrocortisone acetate; used as an anti-inflammatory steroid applied to the conjunctiva. **hydrophilic o.** [USP], a water-in-oil emulsion consisting of methylparaben, propylparaben, sodium lauryl sulfate, propylene glycol, stearyl alcohol, white petrolatum, and purified water; used as an ointment base. **hydroquinone o.,** an ointment containing 94 to 106 per cent of the labeled amount of hydroquinone; used as a depigmenting agent. **ichthammol o.** [USP], a preparation of ichthammol in anhydrous lanolin and petrolatum, used in dermatolgic preparations. **idoxuridine ophthalmic o.** [USP], a semisolid preparation of idoxuridine in a petrolatum base, containing 0.45 to 0.55 per cent idoxuridine; used as an antiviral agent in the treatment of herpes simplex keratitis, applied to the conjunctiva. **iodochlorhydroxyquin o.** [USP], an ointment containing 90 to 110 per cent of the labeled amount of iodochlorhydroxyquin in a suitable ointment base; used as a local anti-infective in the treatment of a wide range of dermatoses, including all types of eczema, applied topically. **iodochlorhydroxyquin and hydrocortisone o.,** an ointment containing 90 to 110 per cent of the labeled amounts of iodochlorhydroxyquin and of hydrocortisone; used as a local anti-infective agent and glucocorticoid. **isoflurophate ophthalmic o.** [USP], an ointment containing 0.0225 to 0.0275 per cent of isoflurophate in a suitable anhydrous base; used as a cholinergic applied to the conjunctiva in the treatment of glaucoma. **lidocaine o.** [USP], a semisolid preparation of lidocaine in a suitable hydrophilic base, containing 95 to 105 per cent of the labeled amount of lidocaine; used as a topical anesthetic. **Löwenstein's o.,** an ointment prepared from a detoxicated unfiltered culture of diphtheria bacilli containing toxoid and killed bacteria; formerly used by inunction in attempted immunization against diphtheria. **mercurial o., diluted,** mercurial o., mild. **mercurial o., mild,** a preparation of mercury and mercury oleate, in solid bases, containing between 9 and 11 per cent mercury, used chiefly as a topical parasiticide. Called also *blue o.* **mercurial o., strong,** a preparation of mercury, mercury oleate, anhydrous lanolin, white wax, and white petrolatum, containing 47.5–52.5 per cent of mercury; used as a topical parasiticide. **mercuric oxide ophthalmic o., yellow,** a

mixture of finely powdered yellow mercuric oxide, liquid petrolatum, and white ointment, containing 0.9–1.1 per cent of mercuric oxide, used as a topical anti-infective in the treatment of blepharitis, conjunctivitis, and styes. **mercurous chloride o., mild** calomel o. **methylbenzethonium chloride o.** [USP], an ointment containing 0.1 per cent methylbenzethonium chloride; used as a local anti-infective, applied topically to the skin of the genitalia, rectum, thighs, and intertriginous areas in the treatment of ammonia dermatitis and in the treatment and prevention of dermatoses caused by contact with urine, feces, and perspiration. **monobenzone o.** [USP], an ointment containing 94 to 106 per cent of the labeled amount of monobenzene; used as a depigmenting agent. **neomycin sulfate o.** [USP], an ointment containing 3.5 mg. of neomycin base per gram, used as a topical antibacterial. **neomycin and polymyxin B sulfates, and bacitracin zinc o.** [USP], an ointment containing 90 per cent of the labeled amounts of neomycin sulfate, polymyxin B sulfate, and zinc bacitracin; used as a local anti-infective agent. **nitrofurazone o.** [USP], an ointment containing 95 to 105 per cent of the labeled amount of nitrofurazone in a suitable water-miscible base; used as a local anti-infective against a wide variety of gram-negative and gram-positive bacteria in the treatment of many skin lesions, especially second and third degree burns and to aid healing and prevent infection of skin grafts, applied topically. **nystatin o.** [USP], a semisolid preparation of nystatin in a suitable ointment base, containing in each gram, 90,000 to 130,000 units of nystatin activity, the labeled amount being 100,000 units per gram; used as a topical antifungal agent. **Pagenstecher's o.,** yellow mercuric oxide; see under *mercuric.* **penicillin o.,** a preparation of calcium penicillin, crystalline penicillin, or procaine penicillin in a suitable ointment base, with or without incorporation of a suitable anesthetic. **phenol o.,** a preparation of phenol, glycerin, and white ointment, containing 1.8–2.2 per cent of phenol; used as an antipruritic. Called also *carbolic acid o.* **pine tar o.,** a preparation of pine tar, yellow wax, and yellow ointment, used as a local antieczematic and rubefacient. **polyethylene glycol o.** [NF], a mixture of polyethylene glycol 4000 and polyethylene glycol 400, used as a water-soluble ointment base. **polymyxin B sulfate o.,** a semisolid preparation of polymyxin B sulfate in an anhydrous petrolatum base, containing 90 to 120 per cent of the labeled amount of polymyxin B, the labeled amount being 20,000 polymyxin B units per gram; used as a topical antibacterial agent. **resorcinol o., compound** [USP], a preparation of resorcinol, zinc oxide, bismuth subnitrate, juniper tar, yellow wax, petrolatum, anhydrous lanolin, and glycerin, used as a topical antifungal and keratolytic. **rose water o.** [USP], a preparation of spermaceti, white wax, almond oil, sodium borate, stronger rose water, purified water, and rose oil, used as an emollient and ointment base. **rose water o., petrolatum,** an ointment prepared with spermaceti, white wax, mineral oil, sodium borate, rose water, purified water, and rose oil. **scarlet red o.,** a preparation of scarlet red, olive oil, anhydrous lanolin, and petrolatum, applied locally as a protective agent. **simple o.,** white o. **sulfacetamide sodium ophthalmic o.** [USP], a sterile ointment containing 95 to 105 per cent of the labeled amount of sulfacetamide sodium; used as an antibacterial in sulfonamide-responsive eye infections, applied topically to the conjunctiva. **sulfisoxazole diolamine ophthalmic s.** [USP], a sterile ointment containing sulfisoxazole diolamine equivalent to 90 to 110 per cent of the labeled amount of sulfisoxazole; used as an antibacterial in the treatment of sulfonamide-responsive eye infections. **sulfur o.** [USP], a mixture of precipitated sulfur, mineral oil, and white ointment, used as a scabicide. **sutilains o.** [USP], a preparation of sutilains in a suitable ointment base; used as a proteolytic agent in wound débridement. **tar o., compound,** a preparation of rectified tar oil, benzoin tincture, zinc oxide, yellow wax, lard, and cottonseed oil, used locally as an antibacterial and irritant. **tetracaine o.** [USP], an ointment containing 5 per cent of tetracaine in a suitable ointment base; used as a local anesthetic, applied topically to the conjunctiva. **tetracaine ophthalmic o.** [USP], an ointment containing 0.45 to 0.55 per cent tetracaine in white petrolatum; used as a local anesthetic. **triamcinolone acetonide o.** [USP], a semisolid preparation of triamcinolone acetonide in a suitable ointment base, containing 90 to 115 per cent of the labeled amount of triamcinolone acetonide; used as a topical anti-inflammatory adrenocortical steroid. **triclobisonium chloride o.,** an ointment containing 90 to 110 per cent of the labeled amount of triclobisonium chloride; used as a topical anti-infective agent, primarily in gynecological infections. **undecylenic acid o., compound,** 1. [USP] a preparation of undecylenic acid, zinc undecylenate, and polyethylene glycol ointment, used as a topical antifungal. 2. a preparation of clove and cinnamon oils, salicylic acid, undecylenic acid, benzoic acid, and white petrolatum, used in podiatry. **Wertheim's o.** (*obs.*), a combination of ammoniated mercury, bismuth, and glycerin ointment, for application in chloasma. **white o.** [USP], an oleaginous ointment base prepared from white wax and white petrolatum. **Whitfield's o.,** benzoic and salicylic acid o. **yellow o.** [USP], a mixture of yellow wax and petrolatum, used as an ointment base for drugs. **zinc o.,** zinc oxide o. **zinc oxide o.** [USP], a

preparation of zinc oxide and mineral oil in white ointment, used topically as an astringent and protective.

Oken's body (corpus), canal (o'kenz) [Lorenz *Oken*, German physiologist, 1779–1851] see *mesonephros* and *ductus mesonephricus.*

O.L. abbreviation for L. *oc'ulus lae'vus,* left eye.

Ol. abbreviation for L. *o'leum,* oil.

-ol suffix indicating that the substance is an alcohol or a phenol, i.e., a hydroxyl derivative of a hydrocarbon.

O.L.A. abbreviation for L. *occipito-laeva anterior* (left occipito-anterior, a position of the fetus).

olaflur (o'lah-floor) chemical name: 2,2'-[[3-[(2-hydroxyethyl)octadecylamino]propyl]imino]bisethanol dihydrofluoride; a dental caries prophylactic, $C_{27}H_{58}N_2O_3 \cdot 2HF$.

olamine (ol'ah-mēn) USAN contraction for ethanolamine.

Olea (o'le-ah) a genus of small trees or shrubs having oily fruit, including the true wild olive (*O. oleaster*) and the common olive (*O. europaea* L.).

olea (o'le-ah) [L.] 1. olive. 2. plural of *oleum.*

oleaginous (o″le-aj'ĭ-nus) [L. *oleaginus*] oily; greasy; unctuous.

oleander (o″le-an'der) a poisonous evergreen apocynaceous shrub, *Nerium oleander,* whose roots, flowers, seeds, and bark contain a cardiac glycoside.

oleandomycin phosphate (o″le-an'do-mi″sin) a macrolide antibiotic, $C_{35}H_{61}NO_{12} \cdot H_3PO_4$, elaborated by the growth of *Streptomyces antibioticus,* resembling erythromycin in chemical structure, actions, and uses but having weaker antibacterial activity; it has been used chiefly in the treatment of infections due to staphylococci and other gram-positive bacteria resistant to other systemic antibiotics, administered parenterally.

oleandrin (o″le-an'drin) 1. a cardiac glycoside, $C_{30}H_{46}O_8$, from oleander, composed of digitalose and digitaligenin. 2. an alkaloid, $C_{32}H_{48}O_9$, from oleander which is a potent diuretic and has been used in cardiac insufficiency.

oleandrism (o″le-an'drizm) poisoning by oleander.

oleanol (o-le'ah-nol) a white solid alcohol, $C_{18}H_{35}OH$, from the liver oils of fish.

olease (o'le-ās) an enzyme from olive oil which produces rancidity and discoloration of the oil.

oleaster (o″le-as'ter) 1. the true wild olive, *Olea oleaster.* 2. any plant of the genus *Elaeagnus,* a large shrub or small tree native to Asia and southern Europe, but especially the Russian olive (*E. angustifolia*).

oleate (o'le-āt) 1. any salt of oleic acid. 2. [L. *oleatum*] a solution of a chemical substance or drug in oleic acid, used as an ointment.

olecranal (o-lek'rah-nal) pertaining to the olecranon.

olecranarthritis (o-lek″ran-ar-thri'tis) [*olecranon* + *arthritis*] inflammation of the elbow joint.

olecranarthrocace (o-lek″ran-ar-throk'ah-se) [*olecranon* + Gr. *arthron* joint + *kakē* badness] tuberculosis of the elbow joint.

olecranarthropathy (o-lek″ran-ar-throp'ah-the) [*olecranon* + Gr. *arthron* joint + *pathos* disease] disease of the elbow joint.

olecranoid (o-lek'rah-noid) resembling the olecranon.

olecranon (o-lek'rah-non) [Gr. *ōlekranon*] [NA] the proximal bony projection of the ulna at the elbow, its anterior surface forming part of the trochlear notch.

olefin (o'le-fin) [*oleo-* + L. *facere* to make] an unsaturated hydrocarbon; alkene.

olei (o'le-i) genitive of *oleum.*

olein (o'le-in) glycerotrioleate, $C_3H_5[CH_3(CH_2)_7CH:CH(CH_2)_7-CO \cdot O]_3$, found in various fixed oils and fats; it is a colorless, oily liquid, insoluble in water but freely soluble in ether and alcohol.

olenitis (o-len-i'tis) inflammation of the elbow joint.

oleo- (o'le-o) [L. *oleum* oil] a combining form denoting relationship to oil.

oleoarthrosis (o″le-o-ar-thro'sis) [*oleo-* + Gr. *arthron* joint + *-osis*] therapeutic injection of oil into a joint.

oleochrysotherapy (o″le-o-kris″o-ther'ah-pe) [*oleo-* + Gr. *chrysos* gold + *therapy*] therapeutic administration of gold salts in oily suspensions.

oleocreosote (o″le-o-kre'o-sōt) the oleic acid ester of creosote.

oleodipalmitin (o″le-o-di-pal'mĭ-tin) a fat found in soya bean oil, butter, cocoa fat, etc.

oleodistearin (o″le-o-di-ste'ah-rin) a fat found in the seeds of the Indian mango, *Mangifera indica.*

oleogranuloma (o″le-o-gran″u-lo'mah) paraffinoma.

oleoinfusion (o″le-o-in-fu'zhun) a preparation made by infusing a drug in oil.

oleoma (o″le-o'mah) [*oleo-* + *-oma*] paraffinoma.

oleomargarine (o″le-o-mar'jah-rin) margarine, def. 1.

oleometer (o″le-om'ĕ-ter) [*oleo-* + Gr. *metron* measure] an instrument for testing the purity of oil.

oleonucleoprotein (o″le-o-nu″kle-o-pro′te-in) the caseinogen and fat of milk regarded as forming one complex substance.

oleopalmitate (o″le-o-pal′mĭ-tāt) an oleate and a palmitate of the same base.

oleoperitoneography (o″le-o-per″ĭ-to-ne-og′rah-fe) roentgenography of the peritoneum following the injection of iodized oil.

oleoresin (o″le-o-rez′in) [L. *oleoresina*] 1. any natural combination of a resin and a volatile oil such as exudes from pines and other plants. 2. a compound prepared by exhausting a drug by percolation with a volatile solvent, such as acetone, alcohol, or ether, and evaporating the solvent. **aspidium o.,** a thick dark green liquid, an ether extract from aspidium, yielding not less than 24 per cent of crude filicin; used as an anthelmintic in the treatment of intestinal tapeworm infestation. **capsicum o.,** the extract from capsicum obtained by percolation, with either acetone or ether as the menstruum; used as an irritant and carminative.

oleoresina (o″le-o-re-zi′nah), pl. *oleoresi′nae* [L.] oleoresin.

oleosaccharum (o″le-o-sak′ah-rum) eleosaccharum.

oleostearate (o″le-o-ste′ar-āt) an oleate and a stearate of the same base.

oleosus (o″le-o′sus) [L.] oily; greasy.

oleotherapy (o″le-o-ther′ah-pe) [*oleo-* + *therapy*] treatment with oil, particularly treatment by the injection of oil.

oleothorax (o″le-o-tho′raks) [*oleo-* + *thorax*] intrapleural injection of oil in order to compress the lung in pulmonary tuberculosis.

oleotine (o″le-o′tĭn) a peptonized fat for use as a butter substitute.

oleovitamin (o″le-o-vi′tah-min) a preparation of fish liver oil or edible vegetable oil containing one or more fat-soluble vitamins or their derivatives. **o. A,** an oily preparation containing the natural or synthetic form of vitamin A. **o. A and D** [USP], an oily preparation containing vitamin A and natural or synthetic vitamin D; used as a dietary supplement. **o. D, synthetic,** a solution of calciferol or of activated 7-dehydrocholesterol in an edible vegetable oil, used as an antirachitic vitamin. **o. D₂,** calciferol. **o. D₃,** 7-dehydrocholesterol, activated.

oleum (o′le-um), gen. *o′lei,* pl. *o′lea* [L.] oil. **o. aethe′reum,** ethereal oil. **o. amyg′dalae ama′rae,** bitter almond oil. **o. amyg′dalae expres′sum,** almond oil. **o. ane′thi,** oil of dill. **o. arach′idis,** peanut oil. **o. auran′tii,** orange oil. **o. auran′tii ama′ri,** bitter orange oil. **o. auran′tii flo′ris,** orange flower oil. **o. bergamot′tae,** bergamot oil. **o. bet′ulae empyreumat′icum rectifica′tum,** rectified birch tar oil. **o. cardamo′mi,** cardamom oil. **o. ca′ri,** caraway oil. **o. caryophyl′li,** clove oil. **o. chaulmoo′grae,** chaulmoogra oil. **o. chenopo′dii,** chenopodium oil. **o. co′cois,** coconut oil. **o. eucalyp′ti,** eucalyptus oil. **o. gossyp′ii sem′inis,** cottonseed oil. **o. hippoglos′si,** halibut liver oil. **o. jec′oris asel′li,** cod liver oil. **o. junip′eri,** juniper oil. **o. junip′eri empyreumat′icum,** juniper tar. **o. li′ni,** linseed oil. **o. may′dis,** corn oil. **o. men′thae piperi′tae,** peppermint oil. **o. mor′rhuae,** cod liver oil. **o. myr′ciae,** myrcia oil. **o. pi′cis li′quidae rectifica′tum, o. pi′cis rectifica′tum,** rectified tar oil. **o. pi′ni,** pine oil. **o. pi′ni pumilio′nis,** dwarf pine needle oil. **o. ric′ini,** castor oil. **o. ric′ini aromat′icum,** aromatic castor oil. **o. rosmari′ni,** rosemary oil. **o. rus′ci,** rectified birch tar oil. **o. san′tali,** santal oil. **o. ses′ami,** sesame oil. **o. terebin′thinae,** turpentine oil. **o. terebin′thinae rectifica′tum,** rectified turpentine oil. **o. thy′mi,** thyme oil. **o. tig′lii,** croton oil.

olfact (ol′fakt) a unit of odor, the *minimum perceptible odor,* being the minimum concentration of a substance in solution which can be perceived by a large number of normal individuals, expressed in terms of grams per liter.

olfactie (ol-fak′te) a term applied by Zwaardemaker to a unit of the distance of withdrawal of the tube of his olfactometer at which an odorous substance was recognized, representing the exposed surface area of the odorous or solution-impregnated substance of which the cylinders were made.

olfaction (ol-fak′shun) [L. *olfacere* to smell] the act of smelling; the sense of smell.

olfactism (ol-fak′tizm) a sensation of smell produced by other than olfactory stimuli.

olfactology (ol″fak-tol′o-je) the science of the sense of smell.

olfactometer (ol″fak-tom′ĕ-ter) [L. *olfactus* smell + *metrum* measure] an apparatus for testing the sensitiveness of perception of odors.

olfactometry (ol″fak-tom′ĕ-tre) the study of the sense of smell.

olfactory (ol-fak′to-re) [L. *olfacere* to smell] pertaining to olfaction, or the sense of smell.

olfactus (ol-fak′tus) a unit of acuity of smell. See also under *organum.*

olfacty (ol-fak′te) olfactie.

oligakisuria (ol″ĭ-gak″ĭ-su′re-ah) [Gr. *oligakis* few times + *ouron* urine + *-ia*] a condition in which urination occurs at long intervals.

oligemia (ol″ĭ-ge′me-ah) [*oligo-* + Gr. *haima* blood + *-ia*] deficiency in the volume of the blood.

oligemic (ol″ĭ-ge′mik) pertaining to or characterized by oligemia.

oligergasia (ol″ig-er-ga′se-ah) an oligergastic disorder; a mental disorder based on intellectual inadequacy or feeblemindedness.

oligergastic (ol″ig-er-gas′tik) [*oligo-* + Gr. *ergon* work] Meyer's term for psychic disorders based on brain deficiency from lack of development.

oligo- (ol′ĭ-go) [Gr. *oligos* little] a combining form meaning few, little, or scanty.

oligoamnios (ol″ĭ-go-am′ne-os) [*oligo-* + *amnios*] oligohydramnios.

oligoblast (ol′ĭ-go-blast″) a primitive oligodendrocyte.

oligocardia (ol″ĭ-go-kar′de-ah) [*oligo-* + Gr. *kardia* heart] bradycardia.

oligocholia (ol″ĭ-go-ko′le-ah) [*oligo-* + Gr. *cholē* bile + *-ia*] (*obs.*) a lack or deficiency of the bile.

oligochromasia (ol″ĭ-go-kro-ma′se-ah) hypochromasia.

oligochromemia (ol″ĭ-go-kro-me′me-ah) [*oligo-* + Gr. *chrōma* color + *haima* blood + *-ia*] insufficiency of hemoglobin in the blood.

oligochylia (ol″ĭ-go-ki′le-ah) [*oligo-* + Gr. *chylos* chyle + *-ia*] (*obs.*) deficiency of chyle.

oligochymia (ol″ĭ-go-ki′me-ah) [*oligo-* + Gr. *chymos* juice + *-ia*] (*obs.*) deficiency of chyme.

oligocystic (ol″ĭ-go-sis′tik) [*oligo-* + Gr. *kystis* sac, bladder] containing only a few cysts.

oligocythemia (ol″ĭ-go-si-the′me-ah) [*oligo-* + *-cyte* + Gr. *haima* blood + *-ia*] reduction in the red cell mass of the blood; called also *oligocytosis.*

oligocythemic (ol″ĭ-go-si-them′ik) relating to or affected with oligocythemia.

oligocytosis (ol″ĭ-go-si-to′sis) oligocythemia.

oligodactyly (ol″ĭ-go-dak′tĭ-le) [*oligo-* + Gr. *daktylos* finger] a developmental anomaly characterized by a smaller than usual number of fingers or toes.

oligodendria (ol″ĭ-go-den′dre-ah) oligodendroglia.

oligodendroblastoma (ol″ĭ-go-den″dro-blas-to′mah) oligodendroglioma.

oligodendrocyte (ol″ĭ-go-den′dro-sīt) [*oligodendro*glia + *-cyte*] see *oligodendroglia.*

oligodendroglia (ol″ĭ-go-den-drog′le-ah) [*oligo-* + Gr. *dendron* dendron + *neuroglia*] 1. the non-neural cells of ectodermal origin forming part of the adventitial structure (neuroglia) of the central nervous system; projections of the surface membrane of each of these cells (oligodendrocytes) fan out and coil around the axon of many neurons to form myelin sheaths in the white matter. With microglia, they form the perineuronal satellites in the gray matter. 2. the tissue composed of such cells.

oligodendroglioma (ol″ĭ-go-den″dro-gli-o′mah) a neoplasm derived from and composed of oligodendrogliocytes in varying stages of differentiation; called also *oligodendroblastoma.*

oligodipsia (ol″ĭ-go-dip′se-ah) [*oligo-* + Gr. *dipsa* thirst + *-ia*] abnormally diminished thirst.

oligodontia (ol″ĭ-go-don′she-ah) [*oligo-* + Gr. *odous* tooth] presence of less than the normal number of teeth, some of them being congenitally absent.

oligodynamic (ol″ĭ-go-di-nam′ik) [*oligo-* + Gr. *dynamis* power] active in very minute quantities; said especially of heavy metal ions (Hg⁺⁺, Ag⁺).

oligoencephalon (ol″ĭ-go-en-sef′ah-lon) [*oligo-* + Gr. *enkephalos* brain] micrencephalon (def. 1).

oligogalactia (ol″ĭ-go-gah-lak′she-ah) [*oligo-* + Gr. *gala* milk + *-ia*] deficient secretion of milk.

oligogenic (ol″e-go-jen′ik) [*oligo-* + *gene*] produced by a few genes at most; used in reference to certain hereditary characters.

oligogenics (ol″ĭ-go-jen′iks) [*oligo-* + Gr. *gennan* to produce] limitation of the number of offspring; birth control.

oligoglia (ol″ĭ-go-gog′le-ah) oligodendroglia.

oligohemia (ol″ĭ-go-he′me-ah) oligemia.

oligohydramnios (ol″ĭ-go-hi-dram′ne-os) [*oligo-* + Gr. *hydōr* water + *amnion*] the presence of less than 300 ml. of amniotic fluid at term.

oligohydruria (ol″ĭ-go-hi-droo′re-ah) [*oligo-* + Gr. *hydōr* water + *ouron* urine + *-ia*] abnormally high concentration of the urine.

oligohypermenorrhea (ol″ĭ-go-hi″per-men″o-re′ah) infrequent menstruation with excessive menstrual flow.

oligohypomenorrhea (ol″ĭ-go-hi″po-men″o-re′ah) infrequent menstruation with diminished menstrual flow.

oligolecithal (ol″ĭ-go-les′ĭ-thal) [*oligo-* + Gr. *lekithos* yolk] possessing only a little yolk.

oligomeganephronia (ol″ĭ-go-meg″ah-nĕ-fro′ne-ah) [*oligo-* + Gr. *megas* great + *nephros* kidney] congenital renal hypoplasia in which there is a reduction in the number of lobes and of total number of nephrons, and hypertrophy of the nephrons.

oligomeganephronic (ol″ĭ-go-meg″ah-nef-ron′ik) 1. characterized by a reduced number of and hypertrophy of the nephrons. 2. pertaining to oligomeganephronia.

oligomenorrhea (ol″ĭ-go-men″o-re′ah) [*oligo-* + Gr. *mēn* month + *rhoia* flow] markedly diminished menstrual flow; relative amenorrhea.

oligometallic (ol″ĭ-go-mĕ-tal′ik) containing only small quantities of metals.

oligomorphic (ol″ĭ-go-mor′fik) [*oligo-* + Gr. *morphē* form] passing through only a few forms of growth; said of microorganisms.

oligonatality (ol″ĭ-go-na-tal′ĭ-te) [*oligo-* + L. *natus* birth] scanty birth rate.

oligonecrospermia (ol″ĭ-go-nek″ro-sper′me-ah) [*oligo-* + Gr. *nekros* dead + *sperma* sperm + *-ia*] a condition of the spermatic fluid in which there is diminution of the number of spermatozoa, some of which are dead.

oligonitrophilic (ol″ĭ-go-ni″tro-fil′ik) [*oligo-* + *nitrogen* + Gr. *philein* to love] absorbing nitrogen from the air and from media containing combined nitrogen; said of microorganisms.

oligonucleotide (ol″ĭ-go-nu′kle-o-tīd) [*oligo-* + *nucleotide*] a polymer made up of a few (2–10) nucleotides.

oligo-ovulation (ol″ĭ-go-ov″u-la′shun) maturation and discharge of fewer than the normal number of ova from the ovaries.

oligopeptide (ol″ĭ-go-pep′tīd) the structure formed by the linkage of a few amino acids.

oligophosphaturia (ol″ĭ-go-fos″fah-tu′re-ah) deficiency in the excretion of phosphates in the urine.

oligophrenia (ol″ĭ-go-fre′ne-ah) [*oligo-* + Gr. *phrēn* mind + *-ia*] defective mental development; mental deficiency. **moral o.,** see under *insanity*. **phenylpyruvic o., o. phenylpyru′vica,** mental deficiency associated with phenylketonuria. **polydystrophic o.,** Sanfilippo's syndrome.

oligophrenic (ol″ĭ-go-fren′ik) 1. pertaining to oligophrenia. 2. a person affected with oligophrenia.

oligoplastic (ol″ĭ-go-plas′tik) deficient tissue repair.

oligopnea (ol″ĭ-gop-ne′ah) [*oligo-* + Gr. *pnoia* breath] hypoventilation.

oligoposia (ol″ĭ-go-po′ze-ah) [*oligo-* + Gr. *posis* drinking + *-ia*] abnormally diminished ingestion of fluids.

oligoposy (ol″ĭ-gop′o-se) oligoposia.

oligoptyalism (ol″ĭ-go-ti′al-izm) [*oligo-* + Gr. *ptyalon* saliva + *-ism*] diminished secretion of saliva.

oligopyrene, oligopyrous (ol″ĭ-go-pi′rēn; ol″ĭ-go-pi′rus) [*oligo-* + Gr. *pyrēn* stone of fruit] deficient in nuclear or chromatin material.

oligosaccharide (ol″ĭ-go-sak′ah-rīd) a carbohydrate which on hydrolysis yields a small number (from two to four or as many as ten, according to various authorities) of monosaccharides. Cf. *polysaccharide.*

oligosialia (ol″ĭ-go-si-a′le-ah) [*oligo-* + Gr. *sialon* saliva + *-ia*] pathologically diminished secretion of saliva.

oligospermatism (ol″ĭ-go-sper′mah-tizm) oligospermia.

oligospermia (ol″ĭ-go-sper′me-ah) [*oligo-* + Gr. *sperma* seed + *-ia*] deficiency in the number of spermatozoa in the semen.

Oligosporidia (ol″ĭ-go-spo-rid′e-ah) former name for a suborder of sporozoan parasites of the order Coccidia.

oligosynaptic (ol″ĭ-go-sin-ap′tik) [*oligo-* + *synaptic*] involving a few synapses in series and therefore a sequence of only a few neurons; called also *paucisynaptic.* Cf. *polysynaptic.*

oligotrophia (ol″ĭ-go-tro′fe-ah) [*oligo-* + Gr. *trophē* nourishment + *-ia*] a state of poor (insufficient) nutrition.

oligotrophic (ol″ĭ-go-trof′ik) pertaining to, characterized by, or conducive to poor (insufficient) nutrition.

oligotrophy (ol″ĭ-got′ro-fe) oligotrophia.

oligozoospermatism (ol″ĭ-go-zo″o-sper′mah-tizm) oligospermia.

oligozoospermia (ol″ĭ-go-zo″o-sper′me-ah) oligospermia.

oliguresis (ol″ĭ-gu-re′sis) oliguria.

oliguria (ol″ĭ-gu′re-ah) [*oligo-* + Gr. *ouron* urine + *-ia*] secretion of a diminished amount of urine in relation to the fluid intake.

oliguric (ol″ĭ-gu′rik) pertaining to or characterized by oliguria.

olisthe (o-lis′the) olisthy.

olisthy (o-lis′the) [Gr. *olisthanein* to slip] a slipping, as the slipping of the bones of a joint from their normal relation in the joint.

oliva (o-li′vah), pl. *oli′vae* [L.] [NA] a rounded elevation, lateral to the upper part of each pyramid of the medulla oblongata. It is produced by an irregular mass of gray substance, the olivary nucleus, located just beneath its surface. Called also *olive, inferior olive,* and *olivary body* or *nucleus.* **o. cerebella′ris,** nucleus dentatus.

olivae (o-li′ve) [L.] plural of *oliva.*

olivary (ol′ĭ-ver″e) [L. *olivarius*] shaped like an olive, as the olivary nucleus.

olive (ol′iv) [L. *oliva*] 1. the tree *Olea europaea* L. (Oleaceae), and its fruit. The latter affords a fixed oil (*olive oil, sweet oil*), which consists chiefly of olein and palmitin, and is employed as a food, as a mild laxative, and as an application to wounds, bruises, etc. 2. a rounded elevation, lateral to the upper part of each pyramid of the medulla oblongata; see *oliva.* **inferior o.,** oliva. **spurge o.,** mezereum. **superior o.,** nucleus dorsalis corporis trapezoidei.

Oliver's sign (ol′ĭ-verz) [William Silver *Oliver,* English physician, 1836–1908] tracheal tugging.

Oliver's test (ol′ĭ-verz) [George *Oliver,* English physician, 1841–1915] see under *tests.*

olivifugal (ol″ĭ-vif′u-gal) [*olive* + L. *fugere* to flee] moving or conducting away from the oliva.

olivipetal (ol″ĭ-vip′e-tal) [*olive* + L. *petere* to seek] passing or conducting toward the oliva.

olivopontocerebellar (ol″ĭ-vo-pon″to-ser″ĕ-bel′ar) pertaining to the olivae, the middle peduncles, and the cortex of the cerebellum.

Ollier's disease, law, layer (ol″e-āz′) [Léopold Louis Xavier Edouard *Ollier,* French surgeon, 1830–1900] see *enchondromatosis,* and under *law* and *layer.*

Ollier-Thiersch graft (ol″e-a′tērsh′) [L.L.X.E. *Ollier;* Karl *Thiersch,* German surgeon, 1822–1895] see under *graft.*

Ol. oliv. abbreviation for L. *o′leum oli′vae,* olive oil.

olophonia (ol″lo-fo′ne-ah) [Gr. *oloos* destroyed, lost + *phōnē* voice + *-ia*] defective speech due to malformed vocal organs.

O.L.P. abbreviation for L. *occipito-laeva posterior* (left occipito-posterior, a position of the fetus).

Olpitrichum (ol-pĭ-trik′um) a genus of imperfect fungi of the order Moniliales, family Monidiaceae, which contains species of the former genera *Oidium* and *Acladium;* they are found in soil, and are sometimes isolated from infected wounds.

Olshausen's operation (ols′how-zenz) [Robert von *Olshausen,* obstetrician in Berlin, 1835–1915] see under *operation.*

Olshevsky tube (ol-shev′ske) [Dimitry E. *Olshevsky,* American physician, born 1900] see under *tube.*

O.L.T. abbreviation for L. *occipito-laeva transversa* (left occipito-transverse, a position of the fetus).

o.m. abbreviation for L. *om′ni ma′ne,* every morning.

-oma [Gr. *ōma,* perhaps adapted from *onkōma,* a swelling] a word termination meaning tumor or neoplasm, of the part indicated by the stem to which it is attached.

omacephalus (o″mah-sef′ah-lus) [Gr. *ōmos* shoulder + *a* neg. + *kephalē* head] a monster with deficient head and no upper extremities.

omagra (o-ma′grah) [Gr. *ōmos* shoulder + *agra* seizure] gout in the shoulder.

omalgia (o-mal′je-ah) [Gr. *ōmos* shoulder + *-algia*] pain in the shoulder.

omarthritis (o″mar-thri′tis) [Gr. *ōmos* shoulder + *arthron* joint + *-itis*] inflammation of the shoulder joint.

omasitis (o″mah-si′tis) inflammation of the omasum.

omasum (o-ma′sum) [L.] the third division of the stomach of ruminant animals; called also *manyplies* and *psalterium.*

Ombrédanne's operation (ahm-bra-danz′) [Louis *Ombrédanne,* Paris surgeon, 1871–1956] see under *operation.*

ombrophore (om′bro-fōr) [Gr. *ombros* rain + *phoros* bearer] an apparatus for applying a douche bath of water containing carbon dioxide.

omega (o-me′gah) the twenty-fourth, and final, letter of the Greek alphabet, Ω or ω. **o. melancho′licum,** a folding of the skin between the eyebrows like the Greek letter omega; a sign of melancholia. Called also *Schüle's sign.*

omeire (o-mi′re) a native drink of southwest Africa, made by permitting milk to ferment.

omenta (o-men′tah) [L.] plural of *omentum.*

omental (o-men′tal) pertaining to the omentum.

omentectomy (o″men-tek′to-me) [*omentum* + Gr. *ektomē* excision] excision of all or a portion of the omentum.

omentitis (o″men-ti′tis) inflammation of the omentum.

omentofixation (o-men″to-fik-sa′shun) omentopexy.

omentopexy (o-men′to-pek″se) [*omentum* + Gr. *pēxis* fixation] in general, an operation which fastens the omentum to some other tissue, and especially one which uses a part of the omentum as a circulatory bridge either to lessen congestion, as in the Talma operation for relief of the portal circulation, or to supply more vascular nutrition as to the heart in coronary disease.

omentoplasty (o-men′to-plas″te) [*omentum* + Gr. *plassein* to form] the use of omental grafts.

omentoportography (o-men″to-por-tog′rah-fe) roentgenography of the hepatic portal veins after injection of a contrast medium into the gastroepiploic vein in the base of the omentum.

omentorrhaphy (o″men-tor′ah-fe) [*omentum* + Gr. *rhaphē* suture] suture or repair of the omentum.

omentosplenopexy (o-men″to-sple′no-pek″se) combined omentopexy and splenopexy.

omentotomy (o″men-tot′o-me) [*omentum* + Gr. *temnein* to cut] incision of the omentum.

omentovolvulus (o-men″to-vol′vu-lus) volvulus of the omentum.

omentum (o-men′tum), pl. *omen′ta* [L. "fat skin"] a fold of peritoneum extending from the stomach to adjacent organs in the abdominal cavity; see *omentum majus* and *omentum minus.* **colic o., gastrocolic o.,** o. majus. **gastrohepatic o.,** o. minus. **gastrosplenic o.,** ligamentum gastrolienale. **greater o.,** o. majus. **lesser o.,** 1. ligamentum hepatogastricum. 2. omentum minus. **o. ma′jus** [NA], greater omentum: a prominent peritoneal fold suspended from the greater curvature of the stomach and passing inferiorly a variable distance in front of the intestines; it is attached to the anterior surface of the transverse colon. **o. mi′nus** [NA], lesser omentum: a peritoneal fold joining the lesser curvature of the stomach and the first part of the duodenum to the porta hepatis. **pancreaticosplenic o.,** a fold of peritoneum connecting the tail of the pancreas and the visceral surface of the spleen. **splenogastric o.,** ligamentum gastrolienale.

omentumectomy (o-men″tum-ek′to-me) [*omentum* + Gr. *ektomē* excision] omentectomy.

omitis (o-mi′tis) [*omo-* + *-itis*] inflammation of the shoulder.

ommatidium (om″ah-tid′e-um) [Gr. *omma* the eye] one of the elongated units of a compound eye of an arthropod.

ommochrome (om′o-krōm) [Gr. *omma* eye + *chrōma* color] a product of tryptophan metabolism which gives rise to pigments, particularly the eye pigments of certain animals; it is apparently not involved in the visual processes.

Omn. bih. abbreviation for L. *om′ni biho′ra,* every two hours

Omn. hor. abbreviation for L. *om′ni ho′ra,* every hour.

Omnipen (om′nĭ-pen) trademark for preparations of ampicillin.

omnipotence (om-nip′o-tens) the state of being all-powerful. **o. of thought,** the deluded belief of a patient that his thoughts and wishes are all powerful and will be fulfilled as soon as he expresses them.

omnivorous (om-niv′o-rus) [L. *omnis* all + *vorare* to eat] subsisting upon both plants and animals.

Omn. noct. abbreviation for L. *om′ni noc′te,* every night.

omo- (o′mo) [Gr. *ōmos* shoulder] a combining form denoting relationship to the shoulder.

omocephalus (o″mo-sef′ah-lus) [*omo-* + Gr. *kephalē* head] a fetus with no arms and an incomplete head.

omoclavicular (o″mo-klah-vik′u-lar) pertaining to the shoulder and the clavicle.

omodynia (o″mo-din′e-ah) [*omo-* + Gr. *odynē* pain] pain in the shoulder.

omohyoid (o″mo-hi′oid) pertaining to the shoulder and the hyoid bone.

omophagia (o″mo-fa′je-ah) [Gr. *ōmos* raw + *phagein* to eat] the eating of raw food.

omoplata (o″mo-plat′ah) [Gr. *ōmoplatē* the shoulder-blade] the scapula.

omosternum (o″mo-ster′num) the interarticular cartilage at the joint between the sternum and clavicle.

OMPA octamethyl pyrophosphoramide.

omphalectomy (om″fah-lek′to-me) [*omphalo-* + Gr. *ektomē* excision] excision of the umbilicus.

omphalelcosis (om″fal-el-ko′sis) [*omphalo-* + Gr. *helkōsis* ulceration] ulceration of the umbilicus.

omphalic (om-fal′ik) [Gr. *omphalikos*] pertaining to the umbilicus.

omphalitis (om″fah-li′tis) [*omphalo-* + *-itis*] inflammation of the umbilicus. **o. of birds,** infection of the yolk sac with bacteria normally found in the alimentary tract and on the skin of the hen, leading to death of the embryos and chicks, occurring up to ten days after hatching; called also *mushy chick disease.*

omphalo- (om′fah-lo) [Gr. *omphalos* the navel] a combining form denoting relationship to the umbilicus.

omphaloangiopagous (om″fah-lo-an″je-op′ah-gus) [*omphalo-* + Gr. *angeion* vessel + *pagos* thing fixed] allantoidoangiopagous.

omphaloangiopagus (om″fah-lo-an″je-op′ah-gus) allantoidoangiopagus.

omphalocele (om′fah-lo-sēl″) [*omphalo-* + Gr. *kēlē* hernia] protrusion, at birth, of part of the intestine through a large defect in the abdominal wall at the umbilicus, the protruding bowel being covered only by a thin transparent membrane composed of amnion and peritoneum.

omphalochorion (om″fah-lo-ko′re-on) the structure formed by fusion of the yolk sac with the chorion; a choriovitelline placenta.

omphalodidymus (om″fah-lo-did′ĭ-mus) [*omphalo-* + Gr. *didymos* twin] gastrodidymus.

omphalogenesis (om″fah-lo-jen′ĕ-sis) [*omphalo-* + Gr. *genesis* formation] development of the umbilicus or yolk sac in the embryo.

omphaloma (om″fah-lo′mah) [*omphalo-* + *-oma*] a tumor of the umbilicus.

omphalomesaraic (om″fah-lo-mes-ah-ra′ik) omphalomesenteric.

omphalomesenteric (om″fah-lo-mes″en-ter′ik) pertaining to the umbilicus and mesentery.

omphaloncus (om″fah-long′kus) [*omphalo-* + Gr. *onkos* mass, bulk] omphaloma.

omphalopagus (om″fah-lop′ah-gus) [*omphalo-* + Gr. *pagos* thing fixed] monomphalus.

omphalophlebitis (om″fah-lo-fle-bi′tis) [*omphalo-* + Gr. *phleps* vein + *-itis*] 1. inflammation of the umbilical veins. 2. a condition characterized by markedly suppurative lesions of the umbilicus in young animals, due to infection through the umbilicus; see *navel ill,* under *ill.*

omphalorrhagia (om″fah-lo-ra′je-ah) [*omphalo-* + Gr. *rhēgnynai* to burst forth] hemorrhage from the umbilicus.

omphalorrhea (om″fah-lo-re′ah) [*omphalo-* + Gr. *rhoia* flow] an effusion of lymph at the navel.

omphalorrhexis (om″fah-lo-rek′sis) [*omphalo-* + Gr. *rhēxis* rupture] rupture of the umbilicus.

omphalosite (om′fah-lo-sīt″) [*omphalo-* + Gr. *sitos* food] an underdeveloped member of allantoidoangiopagous twins, which is joined to the more developed member (autosite) by the vessels of the umbilical cord.

omphalotomy (om″fah-lot′o-me) [*omphalo-* + Gr. *tomē* a cutting] the cutting of the umbilical cord.

omphalus (om′fah-lus) [Gr. *omphalos*] the umbilicus.

Om. quar. hor. abbreviation for L. *om′ni quadran′te ho′ra,* every quarter of an hour.

omunono (om″u-no′no) yaws.

o.n. abbreviation for L. *om′ni noc′te,* every night.

onanism (o′nah-nizm) [*Onan,* son of Judah] 1. coitus interruptus. 2. masturbation.

onaye (o-nah′ye) an exceedingly virulent poison from the seeds of *Strophanthus hispidus.*

Onchocerca (ong″ko-ser′kah) [Gr. *onkos* tumor + *kerkos* tail] a genus of nematode parasites of the superfamily Filarioidea. The adults live and breed in subcutaneous fibroid nodules; the young (the microfilariae) are carried by the lymph and are found chiefly in the skin, subcutaneous connective tissues, and eyes. **O. caecu′tiens,** *O. volvulus.* **O. cervica′lis,** a species found in the cervical ligament of horses and mules. **O. gibso′ni,** a species that infects the subcutaneous tissues of cattle and zebra, producing nodular swellings on the flanks, knees, and shoulders. **O. volvulus,** the etiologic agent of onchocerciasis in man, found in tropical Africa and the Western Hemisphere, especially Guatemala, Mexico, and Venezuela. Transmitted by the bites of flies of the family Simuliidae, the parasites invade the skin, subcutaneous tissues, and other tissues, producing fibrous nodules. In the Western Hemisphere, subcutaneous lesions are usually seen on the head, most often the scalp, but in Africa they are primarily found on the trunk, axillae, and around the pelvis. Blindness occurs after ocular invasion (*Robles' disease, blinding filarial disease, river blindness*). Called also *mal morado* and *volvulosis.* See also *coast erysipelas,* under *erysipelas,* and *craw-craw.*

onchocerciasis (ong″ko-ser-ki′ah-sis) the state of being infected with worms of the genus *Onchocerca.* See individual species under *Onchocerca.*

onchocercosis (ong″ko-ser-ko′sis) onchocerciasis.

Onciolo (on-si′o-lah) a genus of acanthocephalous parasites. **O. ca′nis,** a species found in the intestines of dogs in Texas and Nebraska.

onco- (ong′ko) [Gr. *onkos* mass, bulk] a combining form denoting relationship to a tumor, swelling, or mass.

Oncocerca (ong″ko-ser′kah) *Onchocerca.*

oncocyte (on′ko-sit″) a large epithelial cell with an extremely acidophilic and granular cytoplasm, containing vast numbers of mitochondria; such cells undergo neoplastic transformation.

oncocytic (on″ko-sit′ik) composed of or containing oncocytes.

oncocytoma (ong″ko-si-to′ma) [*oncocyte* + *-oma*] Hürthle cell tumor; see under *tumor.*

oncodnavirus (on-kod′nah-vi″rus) [*onco-* + *DNA* + *virus*] any DNA virus that causes cancer.

oncofetal (on′ko-fe′tal) carcinoembryonic; see under *antigen.*

oncogene (ong′ko-jēn) hypothetical viral genetic material carrying the potential of cancer and passed from parent to offspring.

oncogenesis (ong″ko-jen′ĕ-sis) [*onco-* + Gr. *genesis* production, generation] the production or causation of tumors.

oncogenetic (ong″ko-jĕ-net′ik) pertaining to or characterized by oncogenesis.

oncogenic (ong″ko-jen′ik) giving rise to tumors or causing tumor formation; said especially of tumor- inducing viruses. Cf. *tumorigenic.*

oncogenicity (ong″ko-jĕ-nis′ĭ-te) the quality or property of being able to cause tumor formation.

oncogenous (ong-koj′ĕ-nus) arising in or originating from a tumor.

oncoides (ong-koi′dēz) [*onco-* + Gr. *eidos* form] turgid swelling; intumescence.

oncology (ong-kol′o-je) [*onco-* + *-logy*] the sum of knowledge concerning tumors; the study of tumors.

oncolysate (on-kol′ĭ-sāt) any agent that lyses or destroys tumor cells.

oncolysis (ong-kol′ĭ-sis) [*onco-* + Gr. *lysis* dissolution] the lysis or destruction of tumor cells.

oncolytic (ong″ko-lit′ik) pertaining to, characterized by, or causing oncolysis.

oncoma (ong-ko′mah) [Gr. *onkōma*] a swelling; tumor.

Oncomelania (ong″ko-mĕ-la′ne-ah) a genus of snails species of which transmit schistosomiasis japonica; formerly called *Katayama.*

oncometer (ong-kom′ĕ-ter) [*onco-* + Gr. *metron* measure] (*obs.*) an instrument for measuring variations in the size of various organs or parts of the body, as of the kidney or spleen.

oncornavirus (on-kor′nah-vi″rus) [*onco-* + *RNA* + *virus*] any RNA virus that causes cancer.

oncosis (ong-ko′sis) [*onco-* + *-osis*] a morbid condition characterized by the development of tumors.

oncosphere (ong′ko-sfēr) [Gr. *onkos* barb + *sphaira* sphere] the larva of the tapeworm contained within the external embryonic envelope and armed with six hooks; it may be found in the feces.

oncotherapy (ong″ko-ther′ah-pe) [*onco-* + *therapy*] the treatment of tumors.

oncothlipsis (ong″ko-thlip′sis) [*onco-* + Gr. *thlipsis* pressure] pressure caused by a tumor.

oncotic (ong-kot′ik) pertaining to, caused by, or marked by, swelling; see also under *pressure.*

oncotomy (ong-kot′o-me) [*onco-* + Gr. *temnein* to cut] the incision of a tumor or swelling.

oncotropic (ong″ko-trop′ik) [*onco-* + Gr. *tropos* a turning] having a special affinity or attraction for tumor cells.

Oncovin (on′ko-vin) trademark for a preparation of vincristine sulfate.

oncovirus (on′ko-vi″rus) [*onco-* + *virus*] any virus that causes cancer.

ondometer (on-dom′ĕ-ter) an apparatus for measuring the frequency of the oscillations in high frequency currents.

-one a suffix used in chemistry to indicate (*a*) quintivalent nitrogen, and (*b*) a compound having two hydrocarbon radicals attached to the carbonyl group; a ketone.

oneiric (o-ni′rik) pertaining to or characterized by dreaming.

oneirism (o-ni′rizm) a dreamlike waking hallucination; cerebral automatism, as in a dream prolonged into the waking state.

oneiro- (o-ni′ro) [Gr. *oneiros* dream] a combining form denoting relationship to a dream.

oneiroanalysis (o-ni″ro-ah-nal′ĭ-sis) the exploration of the conscious and unconscious personality through the interpretation of pharmacologically induced dreams.

oneirodynia (o-ni″ro-din′e-ah) [*oneiro-* + Gr. *odynē* pain] nightmare.

oneirogenic (o″ni-ro-jen′ik) producing a dreamlike state; capable of causing dreams.

oneirogmus (o″ni-rog′mus) [Gr. *oneirōgmos* an effusion during sleep] emission of semen accompanying dreams.

oneiroid (o′ni-roid) resembling a dream.

oneirology (o″ni-rol′o-je) [*oneiro-* + *-logy*] the science of dreams.

oneirophrenia (o-ni″ro-fre′ne-ah) [*oneiro-* + Gr. *phrēn* mind + *-ia*] Meduna's term for a form of schizophrenia characterized by disturbances of the sensorium (illusions, confusions, disorientation), amnesia, stupor, and hallucinations.

oneiroscopy (o″ni-ros′ko-pe) [Gr. *oneiroskopilkos* of the interpretation of dreams] analysis of dreams for the purpose of diagnosing the patient's mental state.

oniric (o-ni′rik) oneiric.

onirogenic (o″ni-ro-jen′ik) oneirogenic.

oniroid (o′ni-roid) oneiroid.

onium (o′ne-um) a term applied to a cation in which nitrogen has its maximum covalency, as in the ammonium ion $NH_4{}^+$. The compounds include betaines, cholines, and amine oxides.

onkinocele (on-kin′o-sēl) [Gr. *onkos* swelling + *is* fiber + *kēlē* hernia, tumor] a swollen condition of a tendon sheath.

onlay (on′la) a graft applied or laid on the surface of an organ or structure. **epithelial o.,** an epithelial graft, the edges of

which are not completely approximated to the edges of the wound, thus permitting new epithelium to grow out around the margin; see also under *inlay.*

onobaio (o″no-ba′yo) a powerful arrow poison from Obok, in Africa; it has a depressant action on the heart.

onomatology (on″o-mah-tol′o-je) [Gr. *onoma* name + *-logy*] the science of names and nomenclature.

onomatomania (on″o-mat″o-ma′ne-ah) [Gr. *onoma* name + *mania* madness] mental derangement with regard to words or names, marked by persistent dwelling on some particular word, by perplexed effort to recall some word, by attaching some special significance to certain words, or by showing disgust for certain words (Charcot and Magnan, 1885).

onomatophobia (on″o-mat″o-fo′be-ah) [Gr. *onoma* name + *phobia*] morbid dread of hearing a certain name or word.

onomatopoiesis (on″o-mat″o-poi-e′sis) [Gr. *onoma* name + *poiein* to make] the formation of meaningless words by the psychotic.

Ontjom the fermented product of peanut press cake, made by the natives of Java and Sumatra; occasionally this product causes poisoning of which one sign is jaundice.

ontogenesis (on″to-jen′ĕ-sis) ontogeny.

ontogenetic (on″to-jĕ-net′ik) ontogenic.

ontogenic (on″to-jen′ik) pertaining to ontogeny.

ontogeny (on-toj′ĕ-ne) [Gr. *ōn* existing + *gennan* to produce] the development of the individual organism. Cf. *phylogeny.*

onyalai, onyalia (o″ne-al′a-e; o″ne-a′le-ah) a nutritional disorder occurring among the blacks in various parts of Africa, and marked by the formation, on the palatal and buccal mucous membrane, of blebs containing semicoagulated blood and without signs of constitutional disorder. It is a form of thrombopenic purpura.

onych- (on′ik) see *onycho-.*

onychatrophia (o″nik-ah-tro′fe-ah)[*onych-* + a neg. + Gr. *trophē* nutrition + *-ia*] atrophy of a nail or of the nails.

onychatrophy (on″ik-at′ro-fe) onychatrophia.

onychauxis (on″ĭ-kawk′sis) [*onych-* + Gr. *auxein* to increase] overgrowth or, especially, thickening of the nails.

onychectomy (on″ĭ-kek′to-me) [*onych-* + Gr. *ektomē* excision] excision of a nail or nail bed, or of the claws of animals.

onychia (o-nik′e-ah) [*onych-* + *-ia*] inflammation of the matrix of the nail resulting in shedding of the nail; see *paronychia.*

onychitis (on″ĭ-ki′tis) [*onych-* + *-itis*] onychia.

onycho-, onych- (on′ĭ-ko, on′ik) [Gr. *onyx* nail] a combining form denoting relationship to the nails.

onychoclasis (on″ĭ-kok′lah-sis) [*onycho-* + Gr. *klasis* breaking] breaking of the nail.

onychocryptosis (on″ĭ-ko-krip-to′sis) [*onycho-* + Gr. *kryptein* to conceal] ingrown nail.

onychodystrophy (on″ĭ-ko-dis′tro-fe) [*onycho-* + *dystrophy*] malformation of a nail.

onychogenic (on″ĭ-ko-jen′ik) [*onycho-* + Gr. *gennan* to produce] producing or forming nail substance.

onychogram (o-nik′o-gram) a tracing made by the onychograph.

onychograph (o-nik′o-graf) [*onycho-* + Gr. *graphein* to write] an instrument for observing and recording the nail pulse and capillary circulation.

onychogryphosis (on″ĭ-ko-grĭ-fo′sis) [*onycho-* + Gr. *grypōsis* a crooking, hooking] a deformed overgrowth of the nails; hooked or incurved state of the nails.

onychogryposis (on″ĭ-ko-grĭ-po′sis) onychogryphosis.

onychoheterotopia (on″ĭ-ko-het″er-o-to′pǐ-ah) [*onycho-* + *heterotopia*] a condition in which the nails are abnormally situated.

onychoid (on′ĭ-koid) [*onycho-* + Gr. *eidos* form] resembling a fingernail.

onycholysis (on″ĭ-kol′ĭ-sis) [*onycho-* + Gr. *lysis* dissolution] loosening or separation of all or part of a nail from its nail bed; often a manifestation of psoriasis.

onychomadesis (on″ĭ-ko-mah-de′sis) [*onycho-* + Gr. *madēsis* loss of hair] complete shedding of the nails.

onychomalacia (on″ĭ-ko-mah-la′she-ah) [*onycho-* + Gr. *malakia* softness] softening of the fingernail.

onychomycosis (on″ĭ-ko-mi-ko′sis) [*onycho-* + Gr. *mykēs* fungus + *-osis*] a disease of the nails of the fingers and toes caused by *Epidermophyton floccosum,* by several species of *Trichophyton,* or by *Candida albicans.* The nails become opaque, white, thickened, friable, and brittle. Called also *tinea unguium* and *ringworm of the nails.*

onycho-osteodysplasia (on″ĭ-ko-os″te-o-dis-pla′ze-ah) nail-patella syndrome.

onychopathic (on″ĭ-ko-path′ik) pertaining to onychopathy or any disease of the nails.

onychopathology (on″ĭ-ko-pah-thol′o-je) [*onycho-* + *pathology*] the pathology of diseases of the nails.

onychopathy (on″ĭ-kop′ah-the) [onycho- + Gr. *pathos* disease] disease of the nails.

onychophagia (on″ĭ-ko-fa′je-ah) [onycho- + Gr. *phagein* to eat + -*ia*] the habit of biting the nails.

onychophagist (on″ĭ-kof′ah-jist) one who habitually bites the fingernails.

onychophagy (on″ĭ-kof′ah-je) [onycho- + Gr. *phagein* to eat] onychophagia.

onychophyma (on″ĭ-ko-fi′mah) [onycho- + Gr. *phyma* growth] (*obs.*) onychauxis.

onychoptosis (on″ĭ-kop-to′sis) [onycho- + Gr. *ptōsis* falling] onychomadesis.

onychorrhexis (on″ĭ-ko-rek′sis) spontaneous splitting or breaking of the nails.

onychoschizia (on″ĭ-ko-skiz′e-ah) [onycho- + Gr. *schizein* to divide + -*ia*] onycholysis.

onychosis (on″ĭ-ko′sis) [onycho- + -*osis*] disease or deformity of a nail or of the nails.

onychotillomania (on″ĭ-ko-til″o-ma′ne-ah) neurotic picking at the nails.

onychotomy (on″ĭ-kot′o-me) [onycho- + Gr. *tomē* a cutting] incision of a nail.

onym (on′im) [Gr. *onyma* name] a technical name or term; a combining form denoting relationship to a name or word.

onyx (on′iks) [Gr. "nail"] 1. a fingernail or toenail; see *unguis* [NA]. 2. a variety of hypopyon.

onyxis (o-nik′sis) ingrown nail.

oo- [Gr. *ōon* an egg] a combining form denoting relationship to an egg or ovum; see also words beginning *ovo-*.

ooblast (o′o-blast) [oo- + Gr. *blastos* germ] a primitive cell from which an ovum ultimately is developed.

oocenter (o″o-sen′ter) ovocenter.

oocephalus (o″o-sef′ah-lus) [oo- + Gr. *kephalē* head] an individual characterized by an egg-shaped head.

Oochoristica (o″o-ko-ris′tĭ-kah) a large genus of tapeworms, family Linstowiidae, which are parasitic in birds, reptiles, and mammals.

oocinesia (o″o-sĭ-ne′ze-ah) ookinesia.

oocinete (o″o-sin′ēt) ookinete.

oocyan (o″o-si′an) a blue-green pigment from the shells of birds' eggs; it is a dehydro bilirubin.

oocyanin (o″o-si′ah-nin) [oo- + Gr. *kyanos* blue] a bluish coloring matter from birds' eggs.

oocyesis (o″o-si-e′sis) [oo- + Gr. *kyēsis* pregnancy] ovarian pregnancy.

oocyst (o′o-sist) [oo- + Gr. *kystis* sac, bladder] the encysted or encapsulated ookinete in the wall of a mosquito's stomach; also, the analogous stage in the development of any sporozoon, as in Isospora.

oocytase (o″o-si′tās) an enzyme having a destructive effect on ovarian cells.

oocyte (o′o-sīt) [oo- + -*cyte*] a developing egg cell in one of two stages: The *primary* oocyte (one that has begun but not completed the first maturation division) is derived from an oogonium by differentiation near the time of birth. The *secondary* oocyte (one in the period between the first and second maturation division) is derived from a primary oocyte shortly before ovulation by a division that splits off the first polar body. Ovulation follows. If fertilized, the secondary oocyte divides into an ootid and the second polar body; otherwise it perishes.

oocytin (o″o-si′tin) a substance obtained from spermatozoa, leukocytes, and red blood cells which will cause the formation of fertilization membranes in ova.

oodeocele (o-o′de-o-sēl) [Gr. *ōoeidēs* egg-shaped + *kēlē* hernia] (*obs.*) obturator hernia.

oogamous (o-og′ah-mus) pertaining or relating to or produced by oogamy; heterogamous.

oogamy (o-og′ah-me) 1. the fertilization of a large nonmotile egg by a small, motile male gamete or sperm, as seen in certain algae. 2. the conjugation of two dissimilar gametes; heterogamy.

oogenesis (o″o-jen′ĕ-sis) [oo- + Gr. *genesis* production] the process of formation of the female gametes (ova).

oogenetic (o″o-jĕ-net′ik) pertaining to oogenesis.

oogenic (o″o-jen′ik) producing ova.

oogonium (o″o-go′ne-um), pl. *oogo′nia* [oo- + Gr. *gonē* generation] 1. an ovarian egg during fetal development; it is derived from primordial germ cell, multiplies rapidly, then becomes encapsulated in primordial follicle cells and, near time of birth, becomes a primary oocyte by entering into prophase of first maturation division. 2. in certain fungi and algae, the female gametangium containing one or more eggs (oospheres).

ookinesis (o″o-kĭ-ne′sis) [oo- + Gr. *kinēsis* motion] the mitotic movements of the egg during maturation and fertilization.

ookinete (o″o-kĭ-nēt′) the fertilized form of the malarial para-

site in the body of a mosquito; it is formed by fertilization of a macrogamete by a microgamete and develops into an oocyst.

oolemma (o″o-lem′ah) [oo- + Gr. *lemma* sheath] zona pellucida, def. 1.

Oomycetes (o″o-mi-se′tēz) [oo- + Gr. *mykēs* fungus] a subclass of phycomycetous fungi having sporangia of different kinds and cell walls made up of cellulose, in which reproduction takes place sexually by biflagellate spores; it includes the order Saprolegniales.

oophagia (o″o-fa′je-ah) oophagy.

oophagy (o-of′ah-je) [Gr. *ōophagein* to eat eggs] the eating of eggs; said of insects whose diet consists largely of eggs.

oophor- see *oophoro-*.

oophoralgia (o″of-or-al′je-ah) [oophor- + -*algia*] pain in an ovary.

oophorectomize (o″of-o-rek′to-mīz) to deprive of the ovaries by surgical removal.

oophorectomy (o″of-o-rek′to-me) [oophor- + Gr. *ektomē* excision] the removal of an ovary or ovaries; called also *ovariectomy*.

oophoritis (o″of-o-ri′tis) [oophor- + -*itis*] inflammation of an ovary. **o. parotid′ea,** oophoritis occurring in association with infection by the virus causing mumps.

oophoro-, oophor- (o-of′o-ro, o′o-fōr) [Gr. *ōophoros* bearing eggs] combining form denoting relationship to the ovary.

oophorocystectomy (o-of″o-ro-sis-tek′to-me) [oophoro- + *cyst* + Gr. *ektomē* excision] excision of an ovarian cyst.

oophorocystosis (o-of″o-ro-sis-to′sis) [oophoro- + *cyst* + -*osis*] the formation of ovarian cysts.

oophorogenous (o-of″o-roj′ĕ-nus) derived from the ovary.

oophorohysterectomy (o-of″o-ro-his″ter-ek′to-me) [oophoro- + Gr. *hystera* uterus + *ektomē* excision] surgical removal of the uterus and ovaries.

oophoroma (o-of″o-ro′mah) seldom used term for malignant tumor of the ovary. **o. follicula′re,** Brenner tumor.

oophoron (o-of′o-ron) [Gr. *ōon* egg + *pherein* to bear] an ovary (ovarium [NA]).

oophoropathy (o-of″o-rop′ah-the) [oophoro- + Gr. *pathos* disease] any disease of the ovaries.

oophoropexy (o-of′o-ro-pek″se) [oophoro- + Gr. *pēxis* fixation] ovariopexy.

oophoroplasty (o-of′o-ro-plas″te) plastic operation on the ovary.

oophorosalpingectomy (o-of″o-ro-sal″pin-jek′to-me) [oophoro- + Gr. *salpinx* tube + *ektomē* excision] salpingo-oophorectomy.

oophorosalpingitis (o-of″o-ro-sal″pin-ji′tis) salpingo-oophoritis.

oophorostomy (o-of″o-ros′to-me) [oophoro- + Gr. *stomoun* to provide with an opening, or mouth] the making of an opening into an ovarian cyst for drainage purposes.

oophorotomy (o-of″o-rot′o-me) [oophoro- + Gr. *tomē* a cutting] incision of the ovary.

oophorrhagia (o-of″o-ra′je-ah) [oophoro- + Gr. *rhēgnynai* to burst forth] severe hemorrhage from an ovary.

oophyte (o′o-fīt) [oo- + Gr. *phyton* plant] any member of the generation in the life history of mosses, ferns, etc., in which the sexual organs are produced.

ooplasm (o′o-plazm) the cytoplasm of the egg.

ooporphyrin (o″o-por′fir-in) protoporphyrin contained in egg shells.

oorhodein (o″o-ro′de-in) [oo- + Gr. *rhodon* rose] a red coloring matter from birds' eggs.

oosperm (o′o-sperm) [oo- + Gr. *sperma* seed] the recently fertilized ovum.

oosphere (o″o-sfēr) 1. an unfertilized female gamete of certain fungi. 2. the large, nonmotile, fertile gamete of certain algae and fungi.

Oospora (o-os′po-rah) [oo- + Gr. *sporos* seed] a genus of imperfect fungi of the family Moniliaceae, order Moniliales, which is associated with disease of citrus trees and potatoes. **O. catena′ta, O. frag′ilis,** species of uncertain classification which were once isolated from black tongue, probably as a contaminant. **O. lac′tis,** Geotrichum candidum. **O. tozeu′ri,** Madurella mycetomi.

oosporangium (o″o-spo-ran′je-um) the female element in the sexual formation of oospores.

oospore (o′o-spōr) [oo- + *spore*] 1. the final developmental stage after fusion of sexually differentiated gametes in certain fungi. 2. the thick-walled, resting zygote formed from a fertilized oosphere.

oosporosis (o″o-spo-ro′sis) (*obs.*) infection with an oospore; e.g., in chronic bronchitis.

ootheca (o″o-the′kah) [oo- + Gr. *thēkē* case] 1. an egg case, such as is found in some lower animals. 2. an ovary.

ootheco- [Gr. *ōon* egg + *thēkē* case] for words beginning thus, see those beginning *oophoro-* and *ovario-*.

ootherapy (o″o-ther′ah-pe) ovotherapy.

ootid (o′o-tid) a ripe ovum; one of four cells derived from the two consecutive divisions of the primary oocyte, and corresponding to the spermatids derived from division of the primary spermatocyte. In mammals, the second maturation division is not completed unless fertilization occurs, hence the ootid has male as well as female pronuclear (haploid) elements.

ootype (o′o-tīp) [oo- + Gr. typos impression] in some trematodes, a dilated portion of the uterus into which the oviduct opens and where the ovum is fertilized, provided with the yolk, and invested with a shell.

ooxanthine (o″o-zan′thin) [oo- + Gr. xanthos yellow] a yellow pigment found in egg shells.

oozooid (o″o-zo′oid) [oo- + Gr. zōo-eidēs like an animal] an individual developed from an ovum, that is, as a result of sexual reproduction. Cf. blastozooid.

opacification (o-pas″ĭ-fĭ-ka′shun) 1. the development of opacity, as of the cornea or lens. 2. the rendering opaque to radiation of a tissue or organ by introduction of a contrast medium.

opacity (o-pas′ĭ-te) [L. opacitas] 1. the condition of being opaque. 2. an opaque spot or area. See also cataract. **Caspar's ring o.,** a ring-shaped opacity of the cornea caused by contusion.

opalescent (o″pal-es′ent) showing a milky iridescence, like an opal.

opalescin (o″pal-es′in) an albuminoid derivable from milk; its solutions are opalescent.

opalgia (o-pal′je-ah) [Gr. ōps face + -algia] facial neuralgia.

Opalina (o″pah-li′nah) a genus of ciliate protozoa of the subclass Protociliata found as parasites in the colon of frogs and toads. **O. rana′rum,** a species found in the large intestine of the frog.

opaline (o′pah-lēn) [L. opalus opal] having the appearance of an opal.

opalisin (o-pal′ĭ-sin) an opalescent protein, obtainable from human milk.

opaque (o-pāk′) [L. opacus] impervious to light rays, or by extension to roentgen rays or other electromagnetic vibrations; neither transparent nor translucent.

OPD outpatient department.

opeidoscope (o-pi′do-skōp) [Gr. ops a voice + eidos form + skopein to examine] (obs.) an apparatus for studying the vibrations of the voice by means of light reflected from a mirror.

open (o′pen) 1. exposed to the air; not covered by unbroken skin. 2. interrupted (as a circuit) so that an electric current cannot pass. 3. not obstructed or closed.

opening (o′pen-ing) an aperture, orifice, or open space; see also ostium. **o. in adductor magnus muscle,** hiatus tendineus. **aortic o. in diaphragm,** hiatus aorticus. **o. of aqueduct of cochlea, external,** apertura externa canaliculi cochleae. **o. of bladder,** ostium urethrae internum. **cardiac o.,** ostium cardiacum. **cutaneous o. of male urethra,** ostium urethrae externum masculinae. **duodenal o. of stomach,** ostium pyloricum. **esophageal o. in diaphragm,** hiatus esophageus. **o. of Hunter's canal, inferior,** hiatus tendineus. **ileocecal o.,** ostium ileocecale. **o. to lesser sac of peritoneum,** foramen epiploicum. **o. for lesser superficial petrosal nerve,** apertura superior canaliculi tympanici. **nasal o. of facial skeleton,** apertura piriformis. **orbital o., o. of orbital cavity, anterior,** aditus orbitae. **ovarian o. of uterine tube,** ostium abdominale tubae uterinae. **o. of pelvis, inferior,** apertura pelvis inferior. **o. of pelvis, superior,** apertura pelvis superior. **pharyngeal o. of auditory tube,** ostium pharyngeum tubae auditivae. **piriform o.,** apertura piriformis. **o. of pulmonary trunk,** ostium trunci pulmonalis. **pyloric o.,** ostium pyloricum. **o. of sacral canal, inferior,** hiatus sacralis. **saphenous o.,** hiatus saphenus. **semilunar o. of ethmoid bone,** hiatus semilunaris. **o. for smaller superficial petrosal nerve,** apertura superior canaliculi tympanici. **o. of sphenoidal sinus,** apertura sinus sphenoidalis. **o. of stomach, anterior,** ostium pyloricum. **tendinous o.,** hiatus tendineus. **thoracic o., inferior, thoracic o., lower,** apertura thoracis inferior. **thoracic o., superior, thoracic o., upper,** apertura thoracis superior. **tympanic o. of auditory tube,** ostium tympanicum tubae auditivae. **o. for tympanic branch of glossopharyngeal nerve,** apertura inferior canaliculi tympanici. **o. of tympanic canal, superior,** apertura superior canaliculi tympanici. **uterine o. of uterine tube,** ostium uterinum tubae uterinae. **o. for vena cava,** foramen venae cavae. **o. of vermiform appendix,** ostium appendicis vermiformis. **vesicourethral o.,** ostium urethrae internum.

operable (op′er-ah-b′l) subject to being operated upon with a reasonable degree of safety; appropriate for surgical removal.

operant (op′ĕ-rant) in psychology, any response that is not elicited by specific external stimuli but that recurs at a given rate in a particular set of circumstances. See also conditioning.

operate (op′er-āt) 1. to perform an operation. 2. an individual

that has undergone a specific experimental surgical procedure, in contrast to the normal control.

operation (op″er-a′shun) [L. operatio] 1. any act performed with instruments or by the hands of a surgeon; a surgical procedure. 2. any effect produced by an agent employed in therapy. **Abbe's o.,** 1. a lateral intestinal anastomosis made with rings of catgut. 2. division of an esophageal stricture by string friction. 3. (obs.) intracranial resection of the second and third divisions of the fifth nerve for trigeminal neuralgia. **Abbé-Estlander o.,** the transfer of a full-thickness flap from one lip to fill a defect in the other lip, using an arterial pedicle to ensure survival of the graft. **Adams' o.,** 1. subcutaneous intracapsular division of the neck of the femur for ankylosis of the hip. 2. subcutaneous division of the palmar fascia at various points for Dupuytren's contracture. 3. excision of a wedge-shaped piece from the eyelid for relief of ectropion. 4. advancement of the round ligaments. 5. (obs.) operation of crushing the projecting portion of a deflected nasal septum with forceps and inserting a splint. **Adelmann's o.,** disarticulation of a finger with the attached head of the metacarpal bone. **Albee's o.,** 1. operation for ankylosis of the hip, consisting of cutting off the upper surface of the head of the femur and freshening a corresponding point on the acetabulum, and permitting the two freshened surfaces to rest in contact. 2. transplantation of a portion of the tibia into the split spinous processes of the vertebrae for tuberculous spondylitis. **Albee-Delbet o.,** an operation for fracture of the neck of the femur, done by drilling a hole through the trochanter and the neck and head of the femur and inserting a bone peg in this hole. **Albert's o.,** excision of the knee to secure ankylosis for the cure of flail joint. **Alexander's o.,** 1. [William Alexander] the shortening of the round ligaments of the uterus for displacement of that organ. 2. [William Alexander] (obs.) ligation of the vertebral arteries for the cure or relief of epilepsy. 3. [Samuel Alexander] prostatectomy by median suprapubic and median perineal incisions. **Alexander-Adams o.,** Alexander's o., def. 1. **Allarton's o.,** marian lithotomy. **Allingham's o.,** 1. [Herbert William Allingham] inguinal colotomy by an incision parallel with and one-half inch above Poupart's ligament. 2. [William Allingham] excision of the rectum by an incision into the ischiorectal fossae, about the rectum, and extending backward to the coccyx. **Alouette's o.,** see under amputation. **Ammon's o.,** 1. blepharoplasty by a flap from the cheek. 2. dacryocystotomy. 3. for epicanthus: resection of a spindle-shaped piece of skin over the bridge of the nose, undermining the flaps of the epicanthal fold and closing with sutures. **Amussat's o.,** a long transverse incision for exposure of the colon. **Anagnostakis' o.,** an operation for entropion; also an operation for trichiasis. **Anderson's o.,** longitudinal splitting of a tendon followed by sliding along of the cut surfaces to produce lengthening of the tendon. **Anel's o.,** dilatation of the lacrimal duct with a probe, followed by an astringent injection. **Annandale's o.,** 1. the removal of the condyles of the femur for genu valgum. 2. the fixation of displaced cartilages of the knee joint by stitches. **Arlt's o.,** any of several operations on the eye and the eyelid. **Arlt-Jaesche o.,** the transplantation of the ciliary bulbs from the edge of the lid for the correction of distichiasis. **Asch's o.** (obs.), an operation for the correction of deflection of the nasal septum, consisting of making a crucial incision over the deflection, taking up the segments, reducing the deflection, and inserting a tube to keep the segments in place. **Babcock's o.,** extirpation of the saphenous vein by inserting a long probe with an acorn tip and drawing out the vein by invagination; done for eradication of varicose veins. **Badal's o.** (obs.), laceration of the infratrochlear nerve for the pain of glaucoma. **Baldwin's o.,** formation of an artificial vagina by transplantation of a piece of the ileum between the bladder and the rectum. **Baldy's o., Baldy-Webster o.,** Webster's o. **Barkan's o.,** goniotomy. **Barker's o.,** 1. an excision of the hip joint by an anterior cut. 2. a special method of excising the astragalus by an incision extending from just above the external malleolus forward and inward to the dorsum of the foot. **Barraquer's o.,** phacoerysis. **Barsky's o.,** an operation for repair of a cleft hand with a missing central ray and a deep central V-shaped cleft, consisting in closing the cleft, bringing the ring and index fingers closer together, and correcting the associated syndactyly, if present. **Barton's o.,** an operation for ankylosis consisting of sawing through the bone and removing a V-shaped piece. **Barwell's o.,** a method of osteotomy for genu valgum by division of the upper end of the tibia below and the lower end of the tibia above their respective epiphyses. **Basset's o.,** a method of dissecting the inguinal glands in operation for cancer of the vulva. **Bassini's o.,** a method for the radical cure of inguinal hernia. **Bates' o.,** the division of a urethral stricture from within outward by means of a special form of urethrotome. **Battle's o.,** an operation for appendicitis in which the rectus muscle is temporarily retracted. **Baum's o.** (obs.), the stretching of the facial nerve by an incision below the ear. **Beatson's o.** (obs.), ovariotomy in cases of inoperable cancer of the breast, on the theory that lack of the internal secretion of the ovary will produce atrophy of the tumor. **Beck I o.,** an operation for supplying collateral circulation to the heart; the procedure includes abrasion of the epicardium and lining of the parietal pericardium, application of an irritant (0.2 gm. of powdered asbestos) to these surfaces, partial occlusion of the coronary sinus at its entrance to the right atrium, and grafting the parietal pericardium and mediastinal fat to the surface of the myocardium. **Beck II o.,** a two-stage operation for supplying collateral circulation to the heart: 1. a venous graft is placed between the aorta and coronary sinus to shunt the arterial blood. 2. two to three weeks later, the coronary sinus is partially occluded to raise the pressure therein and cause the arterialized blood entering from the aorta to flow back to the coronary vessels. **Beer's o.,** a flap method for cataract. **Belfield's o.,** vasotomy. **Bennett's o.,** operation for varicocele by partial excision of the pampiniform plexus, followed by suture of the divided ends of the plexus. **Bent's o.,** a form of shoulder excision with flap taken from the deltoid region. **Bergenhem's o.,** surgical implantation of the ureter into the rectum. **Berger's o.,** interscapulothoracic amputation. **Bergmann's o.,** incision of the tunica vaginalis, with removal of its parietal layer, performed for hydrocele. **Berke's o.,** an operation for ptosis of the upper eyelid, consisting of resection of the levator muscle through a skin incision, and excision of excess muscle. **Berke-Motais o.,** an operation for ptosis of the upper eyelid, consisting in suspension of the ptotic lid from the superior rectus muscle. **Bevan's o.,** an operation for undescended testicle, by which the testicle is brought down permanently into the scrotum. **Bier's o.,** see under *amputation.* **Biesenberger's o.,** reduction mammaplasty operation using transposition of the nipple, consisting in excision of the lateral portion of the mammary gland with rotation of the remaining glandular pedicle attached to the nipple, and formation of a skin brassiere. **Bigelow's o.,** litholapaxy or rapid lithotrity. **Billroth's o.,** 1. partial resection of the stomach with anastomosis of the severed end of the duodenum to the partially closed end of the resected stomach (Billroth I), or with anastomosis of the resected stomach to the jejunum through the transverse mesocolon (Billroth II). 2. pylorogastrectomy with anterior gastroenterostomy. 3. excision of the tongue by making a transverse incision below the symphysis of the jaw and joining it by two incisions, one on each side, parallel to the body of the mandible, with preliminary ligation of the lingual arteries. **Bissell's o.** (*obs.*), excision of a section of the round and the broad ligaments for uterine retroversion. **Blalock-Hanlen o.,** an operation to compensate for transposition of the great vessels, consisting in the creation of an interatrial septal defect. **Blalock-Taussig o.,** the anastomosis of the subclavian artery to the pulmonary artery in order to shunt some of the systemic circulation into the pulmonary circulation; performed in cases of congenital pulmonary stenosis. **Blaskovics o.,** for epicanthus: resection of a semilunar piece of skin from the canthal fold nearer to the side of the nose than the canthus, followed by closure with black silk sutures. **Boari's o.,** transplantation of the vasa deferentia so that they will empty into the urethra. **Bobroff's o.,** an osteoplastic operation for spina bifida. **Bogue's o.,** multiple ligation of the veins with catgut in varicocele. **Böhm's o.,** tenotomy of an ocular muscle for strabismus. **Bonzel's o.,** iridodialysis performed with a hook inserted through a corneal incision. **Bose's o.,** a method of performing tracheotomy. **Bottini's o.,** the operation of making a channel through the prostate with the galvanocautery for the cure of prostatic enlargement. **Bozeman's o.,** hysterocytocleisis. **Brailey's o.** (*obs.*), stretching of the supratrochlear nerve to relieve pain in glaucoma. **Brenner's o.,** a modification of Bassini's operation in which the abdominal muscles are sutured to the cremaster muscle. **Bricker's o.,** the surgical creation of an ileal conduit with a flat stoma for the collection of urine; the flat contour is achieved by suturing the ileal mucosa to the skin. **Brock's o.,** transventricular closed valvotomy. **Brophy's o.,** an operation for cleft palate. **Brunschwig's o.,** pancreatoduodenectomy performed in two stages. **Bryant's o.,** lumbar colotomy by an oblique incision between the lowest rib and the crest of the ilium. **Buck's o.,** cuneiform excision of the patella and the ends of tibia and fibula. **Burckhardt's o.** (*obs.*), incision into a retropharyngeal abscess from the outside of the neck. **(von) Burow's o.,** plastic operation for removal of tumors. **Buzzi's o.,** the creation of an artificial pupil by a needle passed through the cornea. **Caldwell-Luc o.,** the operation of opening into the maxillary sinus by way of an incision into the supradental fossa opposite the premolar teeth. **Calot's o.,** forcible reduction of kyphosis by stretching under narcosis. **Carnochan's o.** (*obs.*), removal of Meckel's ganglion and a considerable part of the fifth nerve for neuralgia; incision is made below the orbit, and the ganglion is reached by trephination through the maxillary antrum. **Carpue's o.,** the Indian method of rhinoplasty. **Carter's o.,** 1. formation of an artificial pupil by making a small opening in the cornea and doing an iridotomy. 2. [W. W. Carter] reconstruction of the bridge of the nose by transplanting a piece of bone from the rib. **Cassel's o.** (*obs.*), excision of exostoses of the ear through the external auditory meatus by means of a gouge. **Cecil's o.,** a three-stage operation for urethral stricture: 1. the entire strictured area is excised through an incision on the ventral surface of the penis. 2. a new urethral segment is constructed and buried in the scrotum. 3. the penis is separated from the scrotum; peri-

neal or suprapubic drainage of urine is continued until skin incisions are healed. **celsian o.,** 1. perineal lithotomy. 2. excision of epithelioma of the lip by a V-shaped incision. 3. circular amputation. **Cheever's o.** (*obs.*), complete tonsillectomy through the neck. **Chiene's o.,** 1. the removal of a wedge from the inner condyle of the femur for the cure of knock knee. 2. (*obs.*) exposure of the retropharyngeal space by lateral cervical incision along the posterior border of the sternocleidomastoid. **Chopart's o.,** 1. see under *amputation.* 2. a plastic operation on the lip. **Civiale's o.,** lithotrity. **Clark's o.,** a plastic operation for urethral fistula. **Coakley's o.,** (*obs.*), an operation for disease of the frontal sinus by incising through the cheek, removing the anterior wall, and curetting away the mucous membrane. **Cock's o.,** urethrotomy by a cut along the median line of the perineum. **Codivilla's o.,** an operation for pseudarthrosis by surrounding the pseudarthrosis with thin osteoperiosteal plates taken from the internal face of the tibia. **Colonna's o.,** 1. a reconstruction operation for intracapsular fracture of the femoral neck. 2. capsular arthroplasty of the hip. **Commando's o.,** an operation for management of oral cancer, consisting in resection of the primary lesion and the regional lymphatic nodes. **cosmetic o.,** one intended to remove or correct a deformity in an esthetically acceptable manner. **Cotte's o.,** removal of the presacral nerve. **Cotting's o.,** operation for ingrowing toe-nail, consisting in cutting off the side of the toe down to and including the ingrowing edge of the nail. **Crile and Matas's o.** (*obs.*), production of regional anesthesia by intraneural infiltration. **Critchett's o.,** excision of the anterior part of the eyeball. **Crosby-Cooney o.,** introduction of a flanged glass tube into the peritoneal cavity for drainage of fluid in ascites. **Cushing's o.,** 1. (*obs.*) exposure of the gasserian ganglion and three divisions of the fifth nerve by the direct infra-arterial route. 2. a method of performing ureterorrhaphy without support. **Dana's o.** (*obs.*), posterior rhizotomy. **Daniels' o.,** an exploratory operation for nonpalpable lymph nodes on the scalene muscles to determine the presence or absence of lymphoma, metastatic tumors, and sarcoidosis. **Davat's o.,** cure of varicocele by compressing the veins by acufilopressure. **Daviel's o.,** extraction of cataract through a corneal incision without cutting the iris. **Davies-Colley o.,** the removal of a wedge of bone from the outer side of the tarsus for the correction of talipes. **de Grandmont's o.,** an operation for ptosis of the lid. **Delorme's o.** (*obs.*), decortication of the heart in adhesive pericarditis; pericardiectomy. **Del Toro's o.,** destruction of the apex of a conical cornea by a white-hot knife. **Denonvilliers' o.,** plastic correction of a defective ala nasi by transferring a triangular flap from the adjacent side of the nose. **Dieffenbach's o.,** 1. amputation at the hip by a circular incision, with application of an elastic ligature, followed by removal of the ligature, securing of the vessels, and the making of an incision on the outer aspect from a point two inches above the great trochanter to the circular incision. 2. plastic closure of triangular defects by displacing a quadrangular flap toward one side of the triangle. **Dittel's o.,** the enucleation of the lateral lobes of an enlarged prostate through an external incision. **Doléris' o.,** an operation for retrodeviation of the uterus by shortening the round ligaments and fixing them on either side by an opening in the rectus muscle just above the spine of the ilium. **Doppler's o.,** bisection of, or injection of phenol into the tissues around, the sympathetic nerve leading to the gonads with the object of increasing hormone production and producing sexual rejuvenation; called also *sympathicodiaphtheresis.* **Doyen's o.,** eversion of the sac for the relief of hydrocele. **Duhamel o.,** the treatment of Hirschsprung's disease by a modification of the pull-through procedure and establishment of a longitudinal anastomosis between the proximal ganglionated segment of colon and the rectum, leaving the latter *in situ.* **Dührssen's o.,** vaginofixation of the uterus. **Duplay's o.,** a designation for several plastic operations upon the congenitally deformed penis (epispadias and hypospadias). **Dupuy-Dutemps o.,** blepharoplasty of the lower lid with tissue from the opposing lid. **Dupuytren's o.,** see under *amputation.* **Edebohls' o.,** decapsulation of the kidney for Bright's disease. **Elliot's o.,** a method of trephining the sclerocornea for the relief of increased tension in glaucoma. **Ely's o.,** skin grafting performed on the granulating surfaces in chronic suppurative otitis media. **Emmet's o.,** 1. a method of repairing a lacerated perineum. 2. trachelorrhaphy, or suture of the edges of a lacerated cervix uteri. 3. surgical creation of a vesicovaginal fistula to secure drainage of the bladder in cystitis. **equilibrating o.,** tenotomy of the direct antagonist of a paralyzed eye muscle. **Esser's o.,** epithelial inlay; see under *inlay.* **Estes' o.,** implantation of an ovary into a uterine cornu; performed for sterility when the tubes are absent. **Estlander's o.** (*obs.*), the resection of one or more ribs in empyema so as to allow the chest wall to collapse and close the abnormal cavity. **Eversbusch's o.,** an operation for the correction of ptosis. **exploratory o.,** surgical incision into an area of the body followed by inspection and palpation of organs and tissues to determine the cause of unexplained symptoms. **Fergusson's o.,** see under *incision.* **Finney's o.,** see under *pyloroplasty.* **Flajani's o.,** iridodialysis performed with a needle thrust through the cornea. **flap o.,** any operation involving the raising of a flap of tissue. In periodontics, an operation to secure greater access to granulation tissue and osseous defects, consisting in detachment of the gingivae, the alveolar mucosa, and/or a portion of the palatal mucosa. See also under *amputation*. **Förster's o.,** 1. (*obs.*) the operation of cutting intradurally the seventh, eighth, and ninth dorsal nerve roots on both sides in locomotor ataxia. 2. an operation to produce rapid artificial ripening of cataract (1884). **Förster-Penfield o.** (*obs.*), total excision of the scar tissue along with the epileptogenic cortical area in traumatic epilepsy. **Fothergill o.,** an operation for uterine prolapse by fixation of the cardinal ligaments. **Franco's o.,** suprapubic cystotomy. **Frank's o.,** a method of performing gastrostomy by shaping a valve out of a cone of the stomach, suturing it to the incision in the chest wall, and inserting a tube. **Franke's o.** (*obs.*), removal of the intercostal nerves for the visceral crises of tabes. **Frazier-Spiller o.,** division of the sensory root of the gasserian ganglion for relief of trigeminal neuralgia. **Fredet-Ramstedt o.,** the operation for congenital stenosis of the pylorus by longitudinally incising the thickened serosa and muscularis down to the mucosa; pyloromyotomy. **Freund's o.,** chondrotomy for congenital funnel breast. **Freyer's o.,** a method of performing suprapubic enucleation of the hypertrophied prostate. **Frommel's o.** (*obs.*), shortening of the uterosacral ligaments for retrodeviation of the uterus. **Frost-Lang o.,** insertion of a gold ball to take the place of an enucleated eyeball. **Fukala's o.,** removal of the lens of the eye for the treatment of marked myopia. **Fuller's o.,** incision of the seminal vesicles. **Gant's o.,** division of the shaft of the femur below the lesser trochanter for ankylosis of the hip joint. **Gaza's o.** (*obs.*), section or division of the rami communicantes; ramisection. **Gifford's o.,** 1. delimiting keratotomy. 2. destruction of the lacrimal sac by instilling trichloracetic acid into it. **Gigli's o.,** lateral section of the os pubis by means of Gigli's wire saw; done in difficult labor. **Gill's o.,** an operation for dropfoot or pes equinus done by inserting a wedge of bone in order to limit plantar flexion. **Gillespie's o.,** excision of the wrist by a lengthwise dorsal incision between the extensor communis and extensor medii digiti. **Gilliam's o.,** an operation for retroversion of the uterus by drawing a loop of each round ligament through the abdominal wall and fixing the loops to the abdominal fascia. **Gillie's o.,** a technique for reducing fractures of the zygoma and the zygomatic arch through an incision in the temporal region above the hairline. **Gillies' o.,** operation for correction of ectropion utilizing a split-skin graft known as an *epithelial outlay*. **Glenn's o.,** an operation for pulmonary atresia, consisting in anastomosis of the superior vena cava to the right pulmonary artery. **Gonin's o.,** treatment of retinal detachment by thermocautery of the fissure in the retina performed through an opening in the sclera. **Graber-Duvernay o.,** the operation of boring minute channels through the bone to the center of the head of the femur with the object of modifying the circulation within the bone in chronic arthritis. **Graefe's o.,** removal of the cataractous lens by a scleral cut, with laceration of the capsule and iridectomy. **Grant's o.,** excision of tumors of the lip by removing a square block of tissue containing the tumor, and then making oblique incisions extending down and out from each angle of the wound. The triangular flaps thus formed are drawn toward the center and sutured. **Gritti's o.,** see under *amputation*. **Grondahl-Finney o.,** esophagogastroplasty in which the orifice between the esophagus and stomach is enlarged. **Grossmann's o.,** treatment of retinal detachment by aspiration of the subretinal fluid and the slow injection of warm salt solution into the vitreous. **Gussenbauer's o.,** the cutting of an esophageal stricture through an opening above the stricture. **Guyon's o.,** see under *amputation*. **Hacker's o.,** an operation for balanitic hypospadias. **Hagner's o.,** drainage of gonorrheal epididymitis through an incision into the epididymis. **Hahn's o.,** Loreta's o. **Halpin's o.,** extirpation of the lacrimal gland by a curved incision through the middle of the eyebrow. **Halsted's o.,** 1. an operation for the radical cure of inguinal hernia. 2. radical mastectomy with removal of the supraclavicular nodes for cancer of the breast. **Hancock's o.,** see under *amputation*. **Hartmann's o.,** see under *procedure*. **Hartley-Krause o.** (*obs.*), excision of the gasserian ganglion and its roots to relieve facial neuralgia. **Haultain's o.,** a modification of the Huntington operation (q.v.) for replacement of a chronically inverted uterus, involving a posterior incision in the uterus through the cervical ring. **Haynes's o.** (*obs.*), the operation of draining the cisterna magna for acute suppurative meningitis. **Heath's o.,** division of the ascending rami of the lower jaw with a saw for ankylosis; performed within the mouth. **Heaton's o.,** an operation for inguinal hernia. **Heine's o.,** cyclodialysis in glaucoma. **Heineke's o.,** a multiple stage operation for resection of the colon to remove tumors. **Heineke-Mikulicz o.,** see under *pyloroplasty*. **Heisrath's o.,** excision of the tarsal folds for trachoma. **Heller's o.,** cardiomyotomy for relief of obstruction of the esophagogastric junction. **Herbert's o.,** displacement of a wedge-shaped flap of sclera in order to form a filtering cicatrix in glaucoma. **Hey's o.,** see under *amputation*. **Hibbs' o.,** an operation for Pott's disease by fracturing the spinous processes of the vertebrae and pressing the tip of each downward to rest in the denuded area caused by the

fracture of its elbow below. **Hochenegg's o.,** an operation for rectal cancer. **Hoffa's o., Hoffa-Lorenz o.,** Lorenz's o. **Holme's o.,** a method of excising the os calcis by an incision along its upper border and at the outer border of the foot to the calcaneocuboid joint, and another across the sole, the peroneal tendons being divided. **Holth's o.,** excision of the sclera by punch operation. **Horsley's o.** (*obs.*), excision of an area of motor cortex for relief of athetoid and convulsive movements of an upper extremity. **Hotchkiss' o.,** operation for epithelioma of the cheek, with resection of part of the mandible and maxilla and plastic restoration of the defect from the tongue and side of the neck. **Huggins' o.,** castration performed for cancer of the prostate. **Hunter's o.** (*obs.*), ligation of an artery in the proximal side of an aneurysm and at a distance from it. **Huntington's o.,** the replacement of a chronically inverted uterus through an opening made in the abdominal wall below the umbilicus, done by grasping the invaginated portion with vulsella placed on both sides of the rim; as the uterus is pulled up, additional vulsella are placed lower down and upward traction is applied. After the uterus is in place, it is packed through the vagina. **Indian o.,** see under *rhinoplasty*. **interposition o.,** Watkins' o. **interval o.,** an operation performed during the interval between two acute attacks of a disease, as in appendicitis. **Irving's sterilization o.,** a method of tubal ligation in which the uterine tubes are ligated and severed. **Italian o.,** see under *rhinoplasty*. **Jaboulay's o.,** interpelviabdominal amputation. **Jacobaeus o.,** the treatment of pleural adhesions by thoracoscopy and cauterization. **Jansen's o.,** operation for disease of the frontal sinus by removing the lower wall and a part of the anterior wall and curetting away the mucous membrane. **Jarvis's o.,** removal of the hypertrophied portion of the lower turbinated bone with a special wire snare écraseur. **Jelks's o.,** incision of the fibrous tissue around the rectum through incisions on each side of the anus; done for stricture of rectum. **Jonnesco's o.** (*obs.*), sympathectomy. **Kader's o., Kader-Senn o.,** gastrostomy by which the feeding tube is introduced through a valvelike flap which closes on withdrawal of the tube. **Kasai o.,** portoenterostomy. **Kazanjian's o.,** a technique of surgical extension of the buccal vestibular sulcus of edentulous ridges to increase their height and to improve denture retention. **Keegan's o.,** a modification of the Indian rhinoplasty for reconstructing the nose, the flap being taken mainly from one side of the forehead. **Kelly's o.,** 1. [Howard A. *Kelly*] an operation for correction of urinary incontinence (usually due to stress) in women, in which the site of the internal urethral sphincter is identified by means of a balloon catheter, and the connective tissue between the vagina and the urethra and the floor of the bladder are sutured to form a wide shelf of firm tissue to support the urethra and bladder. 2. [J. D. *Kelly*] arytenoidopexy. **Key's o.,** the lateral operation of lithotomy done with a straight staff. **Killian's o.,** excision of the anterior wall of the frontal sinus, removal of the diseased tissue, and formation of a permanent communication with the nose. **King's o.,** arytenoidopexy. **Kirmisson's o.,** transplantation of the Achilles tendon to the peroneus longus muscle in clubfoot. **Knapp's o.** (for cataract), the formation of a peripheral opening in the capsule behind the iris, without iridectomy. **Kocher's o.,** 1. a method of excising the ankle joint by a cut below the outer malleolus, division of the peroneal tendons, removal of the diseased tissues, and suture of the divided tendons. 2. a method of reducing a subcoracoid dislocation of the humerus. 3. excision of the tongue through an incision extending from the symphysis of the jaw to the hyoid bone and thence to the mastoid process. 4. a method of mobilizing the duodenum. 5. a method of pylorectomy. **Kocks's o.** (*obs.*), shortening of the base of the broad ligament by the vaginal route for uterine retroversion or prolapse. **Kolomnin's o.,** cauterization of the diseased tissues in hip joint disease by ignipuncture. **Kondoleon o.,** treatment of elephantiasis by the removal of strips of subcutaneous tissue. **König's o.,** operation for congenital dislocation of hip by reducing the dislocation and forming an edge on the upper border of the acetabulum by an osteoperiosteal flap from the ilium. **Körte-Ballance o.,** anastomosis of the facial and hypoglossal nerves. **Kortzeborn's o.,** an operation to relieve ape hand due to median nerve paralysis; the extensor tendons of the thumb are lengthened and the thumb is tied to the ulnar side of the hand by means of a strip of fascia. **Kraske's o.,** removal of the coccyx and part of the sacrum for access to a carcinoma of the rectum. **Krause's o.** (*obs.*), extradural excision of the gasserian ganglion for trigeminal neuralgia. **Krimer's o.,** uranoplasty in which mucoperiosteal flaps from each side of the palatal cleft are sutured together at the median line. **Krönlein's o.,** 1. (*obs.*) exposure of the third branch of the trigeminal nerve for facial neuralgia. 2. resection of the outer wall of the orbit for the removal of an orbital tumor without excising the eye. **Küstner's o.,** replacement of an inverted uterus through an incision made in the cervix and uterus along the posterior surface. **Lagrange's o.,** sclerectoiridectomy. **Landolt's o.,** the formation of a lower eyelid with a double pedicle or bridge flap of eyelid skin taken from the upper lid. **Lane's o.,** the operation of dividing the ileum near the cecum, closing the distal portion and anastomosing the proximal end with the upper part of the rectum or lower part of the sigmoid, thus eliminating the colon from the fecal current. **Lange's o.**, artificial tendon transplantation with strands of silk; see *silk implantation*, under *implantation*. **Lanz's o.**, an operation for elephantiasis of the leg in which the strips of fascia lata are inserted into an opening made in the femur. **Larrey's o.**, see under *amputation*. **Latzko's o.**, 1. see *cesarean section, Latzko's*, under *section*. 2. a method of repairing a vesicovaginal fistula by using mucosa denuded from the posterior wall of the vagina as a flap to cover the fistula. **Lauren's o.**, a plastic operation for closure of a cicatricial opening following mastoid operation. **Le Fort's o., Le Fort-Neugebauer o.**, the operation of uniting the anterior and posterior vaginal walls along the middle line for the repair of prolapse of the uterus. **Lempert's fenestration o.**, an operation for otosclerosis, consisting in drilling a small window into the lateral semicircular canal and then placing a flap of skin over the fistula; as long as the new passage remains patent, hearing is significantly improved. **Lisfranc's o.**, see under *amputation* (def. 3). **Liston's o.**, an operation for excision of the upper jaw. **Littre's o.**, a method of inguinal colostomy, proposed by Littre and reported in 1710. **Lizar's o.**, excision of the upper jaw by a curved incision extending from the angle of the mouth to the malar bone. **Longuet's o.**, extraserous transplantation of the testicle for varicocele and hydrocele. **Lorenz's o.**, an operation for congenital dislocation of the hip, consisting in reduction of the dislocation, and keeping the head of the femur fixed against the rudimentary acetabulum until a socket is formed. **Loreta's o.**, gastrotomy with distal dilatation of the pylorus. **Lowsley's o.**, an operation for repair of simple epispadias, consisting in closing the glandular cleft urethra, splitting the glans, and burying the repaired urethra deep in the soft tissue so that the orifice will be positioned at the normal site. **Luc's o.**, Caldwell-Luc o. **Ludloff's o.**, oblique osteotomy of the first metatarsal bone for the correction of hallux valgus. **Lund's o.**, removal of the astragalus for the correction of talipes. **McBurney's o.**, an operation for the radical cure of inguinal hernia: the sac is exposed, ligated, and cut off at the internal ring; the skin is turned in and stitched to the underlying tendinous and ligamentous structures. **Macewen's o.**, 1. supracondylar division of the femur for genu valgum. 2. an operation for the radical cure of hernia by closing the internal ring with a pad made of the hernial sac. **McGill's o.**, suprapubic transvesical prostatectomy. **Mackenrodt's o.**, vaginal fixation of the round ligaments for retrodisplacement of the uterus. **Madlener o.**, a method of sterilization in the female, in which the middle portion of the fallopian tube is crushed with a clamp, which is then replaced with a ligature of nonabsorbable material. **magnet o.**, removal of a fragment of steel or iron from the eyeball by means of a powerful magnet. **major o.**, a surgical procedure of major magnitude and risk. **Makka's o.**, an operation for ectopia of the bladder in which the cecum is utilized as a bladder and the appendix as a ureter. **Manchester o.**, Fothergill o. **Marian's o.**, a perineal median operation for stone in the bladder. **Marshall-Marchetti o.**, an operation for the correction of stress incontinence, the anterior portion of the urethra, vesical neck, and bladder being sutured to the posterior surface of the pubic bone. **Martin's o.**, an operation for radical cure of hydrocele. **mastoid o.**, mastoidotomy. **Matas' o.**, endoaneurysmorrhaphy. **Maydl's o.**, 1. colostomy in which the colon is drawn out through the wound and maintained in position by placing a glass rod beneath it until adhesions have formed. 2. insertion of the ureters into the rectum for exstrophy of the bladder. **Mayo's o.**, 1. excision of the pyloric end of the stomach, followed by closure of both duodenum and stomach and the construction of an independent posterior gastrojejunostomy. 2. for radical cure of umbilical hernia by excision of the hernial mass and overlapping the abdominal aponeuroses transversely. 3. subcutaneous removal of varicose veins with a long-handled stripper terminating in a small ring angled with the shaft of the instrument. **Meller's o.**, an operation for excision of the tear sac. **Mercier's o.**, prostatectomy. **mika o.**, the making of a permanent fistula in the bulbous urethra for the purpose of preventing or avoiding procreation. **Mikulicz's o.**, 1. removal of the sternocleidomastoid muscle for torticollis. 2. Heineke-Mikulicz pyloroplasty. 3. tarsectomy in which the heel, os calcis, and astragalus are removed, the articular surfaces of the tibia, fibula, cuboid, and scaphoid are excised, and the foot brought into line with the leg; called also *Wladimiroff's o.* 4. by anterior gastrotomy a dilating instrument is introduced into the esophagus, which is stretched up to 6 cm. 5. enterectomy in stages, including exteriorization of the section of intestine to be resected, usually the colon; resection of the exteriorized loop; elimination of the fecal fistula by crushing the spur between the two barrels of the anastomosis; and closure of the fecal fistula. **Miles' o.**, abdominoperineal resection for cancer of the lower sigmoid and rectum, which includes permanent colostomy, removal of the pelvic colon, mesocolon, and adjacent lymph nodes, and wide perineal excision of the rectum and anus. **Millin-Read o.**, an operation for the correction of stress incontinence employing the suprapubic approach. **Mingazzini-Förster o.** (*obs.*), Förster's o. **minor o.**, a surgical operation which is not serious in its magnitude or risk. **Moore's o.** (*obs.*), introduction of a coil of small wire into the sac of an aortic aneurysm to effect coagulation. **Moore-Corradi o.** (*obs.*), Moore's operation in which a strong galvanic current is passed through the wire. **Morestin's o.**, disarticulation of the knee with intracondyloid division of the femur. **Moschcowitz's o.**, an operation for the repair of a femoral hernia by the inguinal approach. **Motais's o.**, an operation for ptosis, consisting of transplanting the middle portion of the tendon of the superior rectus muscle of the eyeball into the upper lid. **Mules' o.**, evisceration of the eyeball, with insertion of an artificial vitreous. **Müller's o.**, 1. (*obs.*) a method of vaginal hysterectomy: the uterus is split into lateral halves, which are brought down in succession and removed. 2. (*obs.*) cesarean section in which the uterus is lifted out of the abdomen and then opened. 3. resection of the sclera for detachment of the retina. **Mustard's o.**, an intra-atrial operation to correct the hemodynamic fault in transposition of the great vessels. **Naffziger's o.**, excision of the superior and lateral walls of the orbit for exophthalmos. **Narath's o.**, fixing of the omentum to the subcutaneous tissue of the abdominal wall in order to establish collateral circulation in portal obstruction. **Nélaton's o.**, excision of the shoulder joint by a transverse incision. **Neuber's o.**, the operation of filling a cavity in bone with skin flaps taken from the sides of the wound. **Ober's o.**, cutting or division of a joint capsule. **Ogston's o.**, 1. removal of the inner condyle of the femur for knock knee. 2. excision of the wedge of the tarsus for the purpose of restoring the arch in flatfoot. **Ogston-Luc o.** (*obs.*), an operation for frontal sinus disease, the incision being made from the edge of the orbit, the sinus being opened on the outer side of the median line. **Olshausen's o.**, the operation of fixing or suturing the uterus to the abdominal wall for the cure of retroversion. **Ombrédanne's o.**, 1. an operation for hypospadias. 2. transscrotal orchiopexy. **open o.**, an operation in which the tissues and organs are exposed to view through a surgical incision. **Ord's o.**, an operation for breaking up fresh adhesions in joints. **Paci's o.**, a modification of Lorenz's bloodless operation for congenital dislocation of the hip. **Panas' o.**, the attachment of the upper eyelid to the occipitofrontalis muscle for ptosis. **Partsch's o.**, a technique for marsupialization of dental cyst. **Péan's o.**, 1. (*obs.*) vaginal hysterectomy bit by bit. 2. hip joint amputation in which the vessels are ligated as the operation goes on. **Petersen's o.**, a modification of high lithotomy. **Phelps' o.**, an open and direct incision through the sole and inner side of the foot, done for talipes. **Phemister o.**, use of an onlay graft of cancellous bone without internal fixation, for treatment of a stable but ununited fracture. **Physick's o.**, the removal of a circular piece of the iris by means of a cutting forceps to create an artificial pupil. **plastic o.**, one in which the shape of a part or the character of its covering is altered by transplantation of tissue, etc. **Politzer's o.** (*obs.*), 1. the creation of an artificial opening in the membrana tympani by incision and galvanocautery. 2. division of the anterior ligament of the malleus. **Pollock's o.**, amputation at the knee joint by a long anterior and short posterior flap, the patella being left. **Polya's o.**, anastomosis of the transected end of the stomach to the side of the jejunum following subtotal gastrectomy. **Pomeroy's o.**, a method of sterilization in the female, in which the fallopian tube is picked up about two inches from the uterine cornua, a chronic catgut ligature tied around the loop without crushing it, and the tied loop is then resected. **Poncet's o.**, 1. lengthening of the Achilles tendon for talipes equinus. 2. perineotomy. 3. perineal urethrostomy. **Potts-Smith-Gibson o.**, anastomosis between the aorta and the pulmonary artery in congenital pulmonary stenosis. **Power's o.**, removal of a corneal leukoma, followed by the insertion of a rabbit's cornea. **Puusepp's o.**, splitting of the central canal of the spinal cord for the treatment of syringomyelia. **Quaglino's o.**, sclerotomy done with a small knife and a spatula. **Quénu-Mayo o.**, excision of the rectum, together with the neighboring lymph glands, for cancer. **radical o.**, one involving extensive resection of tissue for the complete extirpation of disease. **Ramstedt's o.**, Fredet-Ramstedt o. **Rastelli's o.**, an operation to correct such cardiac anomalies as transposition of the great vessels (with pulmonary stenosis), truncus arteriosus, and pulmonary arterial atresia, in which an aortic allograft is used to carry blood from the right ventricle to the pulmonary artery. **Regnoli's o.**, excision of the tongue through a median opening below the lower jaw, reaching from the chin to the hyoid bone. **Reverdin's o.**, a method of taking an epidermic graft and transplanting it to a defect. **Ridell's o.**, excision of the anterior and inferior walls of the frontal sinus for chronic inflammation. **Rigaud's o.**, a plastic operation for urethral fistula: a square flap is taken from below the fistula, turned over it, and reinforced by flaps from each side. **Rose's o.**, gasserectomy. **Routier's o.**, a method of operating for Dupuytren's contracture. **Routte's o.**, venoperitoneostomy: the operation of suturing the saphenous vein so that it will open into the peritoneal cavity, so as to drain that cavity in cases of ascites with cirrhosis of the liver. **Roux-en-Y o.**, see under *anastomosis*. **Saemisch's o.**, transfixion of the cornea and of the base of the ulcer for the cure of hypopyon. **Sayre's o.**, the application of a plaster-of-Paris jacket in the treatment of spondylitis and Pott's disease.

Scanzoni's o., see under *maneuver.* **Scarpa's o.,** ligation of the femoral artery in Scarpa's triangle. **Schauta's o.,** extended vaginal hysterectomy for cancer of the cervix uteri. **Schauta-Wertheim o.,** Wertheim-Schauta o. **Schede's o.,** 1. resection of the thorax for chronic empyema. 2. an operation for varicose veins of the leg, done by a circular incision, rolling one cuff up and another down, so as to reach and remove the varices. 3. excision of the necrosed part of a bone, all dead bone and diseased tissue being scraped away, and the cavity permitted to fill with blood clot, the latter being kept moist and aseptic with a cover of gauze and rubber tissue, and eventually becoming organized. **Scheie's o.,** 1. scleral cauterization with peripheral iridectomy for treatment of glaucoma. 2. a technique for needling and aspiration of cataract. **Schlatter's o.,** total excision of the stomach for cancer. **Schmalz's o.,** the introduction of a thread into the lacrimal duct for the cure of stricture. **Schönbein's o.,** staphyloplasty in which a flap of mucous membrane from the posterior wall of the pharynx is stitched to the velum palati, shutting off the nose from the mouth. **Sédillot's o.,** 1. a method of staphylorrhaphy. 2. a flap operation for restoring the upper lip. **Semb's o.,** extrafascial apicolysis for pulmonary tuberculosis. **Senn's o.,** intestinal anastomosis by lateral approximation and the use of bone plates. **Serre's o.,** an operation for correction of skin contractures that distort the angle of the mouth, involving switching of a skin and subcutaneous tissue flap from one lip to another. **shelf o.,** a reconstructive arthroplasty. **shelving o.,** König's o. **Siebold's o.,** pubiotomy. **Sistrunk o.,** a surgical procedure for removal of thyroglossal cysts and sinuses. **Sluder's o.,** removal of the tonsil along with its capsule. **Smith's o.,** extraction of an immature cataract with an intact capsule. **Socin's o.,** enucleation of a goitrous or thyroidal tumor from the healthy part of the gland to avoid cachexia strumipriva. **Spinelli's o.,** the operation of splitting the anterior wall of the prolapsed inverted uterus, reversing the organ, and restoring it to the correct position. **Spivack's o.,** a method of cystostomy in which a tube, with a valve at its base, is formed from a flap on the anterior abdominal wall. **Ssabanejew-Frank o.,** Frank's o. **Stacke's o.,** the removal of the mastoid and the contents of the tympanum, so that the antrum, attic, tympanum, and meatus form a single cavity. **State o.,** the treatment of Hirschsprung's disease by end-to-end anastomosis of the colon from above the aganglionic segment to the upper part of the rectum. **Stein o.,** an operation for reconstruction of the lower lip with flaps taken from the upper lip. **Steinach's o.,** ligation of the vas deferens with resection of a portion of the vas; done with a view of rejuvenating the patient by causing atrophy of the spermatogenic apparatus and proliferation of the interstitial tissue of the testicle, thus increasing the patient's output of gonadal hormone. **Stokes's o.,** Gritti-Stokes amputation. **Sturmdorf's o.,** conical excision of the diseased endocervix. **subcutaneous o.,** operation on the subcutaneous tissues, as excision of a wen. **Swenson's o.,** an operation for Hirschsprung's disease, consisting in removal of the rectum and the aganglionic segment of the bowel, with preservation of the anal sphincters, by the pull-through surgical technique. **Syme's o.,** 1. see under *amputation.* 2. a method of external urethrotomy. **tagliacotian o.,** see under *rhinoplasty.* **Talma's o.,** the surgical production of artificial adhesions between the liver and spleen and the omentum and abdominal wall in cases of ascites due to cirrhosis of the liver. **Tanner's o.,** an operation for bleeding esophageal varices in which the left and short gastric veins are divided and the stomach is bisected and resutured just distal to the esophagus. **Tansini's o.,** 1. amputation of the breast with all the skin over it, the denuded area being covered by a flap from the back. 2. a method of removing a cyst of the liver. 3. a method of gastric resection. **Teale's o.,** see under *amputation.* **Textor's o.,** removal of thin, split-thickness skin grafts by means of a razor, skin-graft cutting knife, or a dermatome. **Thiersch's o.,** removal of skin grafts by means of a razor. **Torek o.,** 1. an operation for undescended testicle. 2. an operation for the excision of the thoracic part of the esophagus. **Torkildsen's o.,** ventriculocisternostomy. **Toti's o.,** dacryocystorhinostomy. **Trendelenburg' o.,** 1. excision of varicose veins. 2. ligation of the great saphenous vein for varicose veins. 3. synchondroseotomy. 4. pulmonary embolectomy for the treatment of postoperative embolism. **Treves' o.,** operation for Pott's disease by opening the abscess through the loin, irrigating and curetting the sac, and scraping away dead bone. **van Hook's o.,** ureteroureterostomy. **Verhoeff's o.,** posterior sclerotomy followed by electrolytic punctures, for detachment of the retina. **Vermale's o.,** amputation by double-flap transfixion. **Vidal's o.,** subcutaneous ligation of the veins for varicocele. **Vineberg's o.,** an operation to establish a collateral blood supply to the heart, in which an internal mammary artery is implanted in the myocardium, the artery being pulled into a myocardial tunnel after blunt dissection between the muscle bundles. **Volkmann's o.,** incision of the tunica vaginalis for hydrocele. **Voronoff's o.,** transplantation into man of the testes of an anthropoid ape, in the hope of rejuvenating the recipient. **Wagner's o.,** osteoplastic resection of the skull. **Water's o.,** a form of extraperitoneal cesarean section. **Watkins' o.,** an operation for prolapse and procidentia uteri in which the bladder is separated from the anterior wall of the uterus so that the uterus is left in a position to support the entire bladder. Called also *interposition o.* **Webster's o.,** for retrodisplacement of the uterus: the round ligaments are passed through the perforated broad ligaments and fixed to the back of the uterus. **Weir's o.,** appendicostomy. **Wertheim's o.,** radical hysterectomy; an operation for cancer of the cervix in which there is removed with the uterus as much of the parametrial tissue as possible and a wide margin of the vagina. **Wertheim-Schauta o.,** an operation for cystocele, consisting in the interposition of the uterus between the base of the bladder and the anterior vaginal wall. **Wheelhouse's o.,** a method of perineal section for impermeable stricture of the urethra by cutting the stricture on a fine staff passed through it. **Whipple's o.,** radical pancreatoduodenectomy. **White's o.,** castration for hypertrophy of the prostate. **Whitehead's o.,** 1. treatment of hemorrhoids by excision. 2. removal of the tongue with scissors, the operation being performed within the mouth. **Whitman's o.,** 1. an operation for arthroplasty of the hip joint. 2. a method of astragalectomy. **Winiwarter's o.,** cholecystoenterostomy. **Witzel's o.,** gastrostomy by drawing a cone of the stomach wall through an incision, and inserting a tube which is buried in the stomach wall and carried into the lumen; the stomach cone is replaced and the wound sutured. **Wladimiroff's o.,** Mikulicz's o., def. 3. **Wölfler's o.,** anterior gastrojejunostomy for pyloric obstruction. **Wützer's o.,** a process for the radical cure of inguinal hernia by invaginating the scrotum into the inguinal canal and fixing it in place with a suture. **Wyeth's o.,** amputation at the hip joint, hemorrhage being controlled by an elastic cord or tube fastened above large needles which transfix the tissues on each side of the articulation. **Yankauer's o.,** curettement of the bony end of the eustachian tube for the purpose of shutting off infection from the nasopharynx and thereby curing chronic suppuration of the middle ear. **Young's o.,** 1. partial prostatectomy by punch. 2. total excision of the seminal vesicles and partial excision of the ejaculatory ducts by a suprapubic T-shaped incision. **Ziegler's o.,** V-shaped iridectomy for forming an artificial pupil.

operative (op′er-ă-tiv) [L. *operativus*] 1. pertaining to an operation. 2. effective; not inert.

operator (op′er-a-tor) 1. one who performs an operation, or operates a mechanical device. 2. operator gene.

opercula (o-per′ku-lah) [L.] plural of *operculum.*

opercular (o-per′ku-lar) pertaining to an operculum.

operculectomy (o-per″ku-lek′to-me) the surgical removal of a mucosal flap partially or completely covering an unerupted tooth.

operculitis (o-per″ku-li′tis) pericoronitis.

operculum (o-per′ku-lum), pl. *oper′cula* [L.] 1. a lid or covering structure, such as the mucus plug obstructing the cervix of the gravid uterus in various animals. 2. the folds of the pallium covering the insula and forming part of the lips of the lateral sulcus; see *operculum frontale, o. frontoparietale,* and *o. temporale.* **cartilaginous o.,** discus articularis articulationis temporomandibularis. **dental o.,** the hood of gingival tissue overlying the crown of an erupting tooth. **frontal o., o. fronta′le** [NA], the part of the inferior frontal gyrus between the anterior and ascending branches of the lateral sulcus, covering over a part of the insula; called also *pars frontalis operculi.* **frontoparietal o., o. frontoparieta′le** [NA], the part of the inferior frontal gyrus behind the ascending branch of the lateral sulcus, together with the lower ends of the precentral and postcentral gyri, plus the anterior and lower part of the inferior parietal lobule, all covering over a part of the insula; called also *pars parietalis operculi.* **oper′cula in′sulae,** the folds of the pallium covering the insula; see *o. frontale, o. frontoparietale,* and *o. temporale.* **occipital o.,** a part of the occipital lobe of the brain demarcated by the sulcus lunatus, when the latter structure is present. **temporal o., o. tempora′le** [NA], the parts of the superior temporal gyrus and transverse temporal gyri that cover over a part of the insula; called also *pars temporalis operculi.* **trophoblastic o.,** the plug of trophoblast that helps close the gap in the endometrium made by the implanting blastocyst.

operon (op′er-on) [L. *opera* exertion + Gr. *on* neuter ending] in genetic theory, a segment of a chromosome comprising an operator gene and closely linked structural genes having related functions, the activity of the latter being controlled by the operator gene through its interaction with a regulator gene.

ophiasis (o-fi′ah-sis) [Gr.] a form of alopecia areata of long duration, involving the temporal and occipital margins of the scalp in a continuous band.

Ophidia (o-fid′e-ah) [Gr. *ophidion* serpent] a suborder of Reptilia which embraces the snakes.

ophidiasis (o″fĭ-di′ah-sis) ophidism.

ophidic (o-fid′ik) pertaining to, caused by, or derived from snakes.

ophidism (o′fĭ-dizm) poisoning by snake venom.

Ophiophagus hannah (o″fe-of′ah-gus han′ah) the king cobra of India; see *cobra.*

ophiotoxemia (o″fe-o-tok-se′me-ah) [Gr. *ophis* snake + *toxemia*] poisoning by snake venom.

ophtoxemia (o″fe-tok-se′me-ah) ophiotoxemia.

ophryitis (of″re-i′tis) [Gr. *ophrys* eyebrow + *-itis*] (*obs.*) dermatitis in the eyebrow region.

ophryon (of′re-on) [Gr. *ophrys* eyebrow + *on* neuter ending] the middle point of the transverse supraorbital line.

ophryosis (of″re-o′sis) [Gr. *ophrys* eyebrow] spasm of the eyebrow.

Ophthaine (of′thān) trademark for a preparation of proparacaine hydrochloride.

ophthalm- see *ophthalmo-*.

ophthalmagra (of″thal-mag′rah) [*ophthalm-* + Gr. *agra* seizure] sudden pain in the eye.

ophthalmalgia (of″thal-mal′je-ah) [*ophthalm-* + *-algia*] pain in the eye.

ophthalmatrophia (of″thal-mah-tro′fe-ah) [*ophthalm-* + Gr. *atrophia* atrophy] atrophy of the eye.

ophthalmectomy (of″thal-mek′to-me) [*ophthalm-* + Gr. *ektome* excision] the surgical removal of an eye; enucleation of the eyeball.

ophthalmencephalon (of″thal-men-sef′ah-lon) [*ophthalm-* + Gr. *enkephalos* brain] the retina, optic nerve, and visual apparatus of the brain.

ophthalmia (of-thal′me-ah) [Gr., from *ophthalmos* eye] severe inflammation of the eye or of the conjunctiva or deeper structures of the eye. **actinic ray o.**, electric o. **catarrhal o.**, a severe form of simple conjunctivitis. **caterpillar o.**, o. nodosa. **o. eczemato′sa**, phlyctenulosis. **Egyptian o.**, trachoma, def. 1. **electric o.**, conjunctivitis due to the effect of bright electric light, especially that of a welding arc. **flash o.**, electric o. **gonorrheal o.**, acute and severe purulent ophthalmia due to gonorrheal infection. **granular o.**, an acute and severe form of purulent conjunctivitis. **jequirity o.**, a form due to poisoning by jequirity, the poisonous seeds of *Abrus precatorius*. **metastatic o.**, choroiditis due to metastasis or to pyemia. **migratory o.**, sympathetic o. **mucous o.**, catarrhal o. **o. neonato′rum**, any hyperacute purulent conjunctivitis occurring during the first ten days of life, usually contracted during birth from infected vaginal discharge of the mother. Formerly it referred only to ocular gonorrheal infections. **neuroparalytic o.**, keratitis due to lesion of branches of the fifth nerve or of the gasserian ganglion. **o. nivia′lis**, snow blindness. **o. nodo′sa**, inflammation of the conjunctiva produced by caterpillar hairs, and marked by the formation of a round, gray swelling where each hair is embedded. **periodic o.**, a form of recurrent uveitis affecting horses. **phlyctenular o.**, see under *keratoconjunctivitis*. **purulent o.**, a form with a purulent discharge, commonly due to gonorrheal infection. **scrofulous o.**, keratoconjunctivitis associated with tuberculosis. **spring o.**, vernal conjunctivitis. **strumous o.**, phlyctenular keratoconjunctivitis. **sympathetic o.**, granulomatous inflammation of the uveal tract of the uninjured eye (the sympathizing eye) following some weeks after a wound involving the uveal tract of the other eye (the exciting eye). The end result is bilateral granulomatous inflammation of the entire uveal tract. Called also *sympathetic uveitis*. **transferred o.**, sympathetic o. **ultraviolet ray o.**, electric o. **varicose o.**, a variety associated with varicosity of the veins of the conjunctiva.

ophthalmiac (of-thal′me-ak) a person affected with ophthalmia.

ophthalmiatrics (of″thal-me-at′riks) [*ophthalm-* + Gr. *iatrike* surgery, medicine] the treatment of eye diseases.

ophthalmic (of-thal′mik) [Gr. *ophthalmikos*] pertaining to the eye.

ophthalmitic (of″thal-mit′ik) pertaining to ophthalmitis.

ophthalmitis (of″thal-mi′tis) [*ophthalm-* + *-itis*] inflammation of the eye.

ophthalmo-, ophthalm- [Gr. *ophthalmos* eye] a combining form denoting relationship to the eye.

ophthalmoblennorrhea (of-thal″mo-blen″o-re′ah) [*ophthalmo-* + Gr. *blenna* mucus + *rhoia* flow] gonorrheal or purulent ophthalmia.

ophthalmocele (of-thal′mo-sēl) [*ophthalmo-* + Gr. *kele* hernia, tumor] exophthalmos.

ophthalmocopia (of-thal″mo-ko′pe-ah) [*ophthalmo-* + Gr. *kopos* weariness] asthenopia, or eyestrain; fatigue of the eyes.

ophthalmodesmitis (of-thal″mo-dez-mi′tis) [*ophthalmo-* + Gr. *desmos* ligament + *-itis*] inflammation of the ocular tendons.

ophthalmodiaphanoscope (of-thal″mo-di-ah-fan′o-skōp) [*ophthalmo-* + *diaphanoscope*] an instrument for examining the back of the eye (retina) by transillumination through the buccal cavity.

ophthalmodiastimeter (of-thal″mo-di″as-tim′e-ter) [*ophthalmo-* + Gr. *diastema* interval + *metron* measure] an instrument for determining the proper distance at which to place lenses for the two eyes.

ophthalmodonesis (of-thal″mo-do-ne′sis) [*ophthalmo-* + Gr. *donesis* trembling] a trembling motion of the eyes.

ophthalmodynamometer (of-thal″mo-di″nah-mom′e-ter) 1. an instrument for measuring the retinal arterial pressure. 2. an instrument for determining the near point of convergence.

ophthalmodynamometry (of-thal″mo-di″nah-mom′e-tre) determination of the retinal arterial pressure.

ophthalmodynia (of-thal″mo-din′e-ah) [*ophthalmo-* + Gr. *odyne* pain] ophthalmalgia.

ophthalmoeikonometer (of-thal″mo-i″ko-nom′e-ter) an instrument used to determine both the refraction of the eye and the relative size and shape of the ocular images.

ophthalmograph (of-thal′mo-graf) [*ophthalmo-* + Gr. *graphein* to write] an instrument for photographing the movements of the eye during reading.

ophthalmography (of″thal-mog′rah-fe) [*ophthalmo-* + Gr. *graphein* to write] description of the eyes.

ophthalmogyric (of-thal″mo-ji′rik) [*ophthalmo-* + Gr. *gyros* circle] oculogyric.

ophthalmoleukoscope (of-thal″mo-lu′ko-skōp) [*ophthalmo-* + Gr. *leukos* white + *skopein* to examine] an apparatus for testing color perception by means of colors produced by polarized light.

ophthalmolith (of-thal′mo-lith) [*ophthalmo-* + Gr. *lithos* stone] a lacrimal calculus.

ophthalmologic (of″thal-mo-loj′ik) pertaining to ophthalmology.

ophthalmologist (of″thal-mol′o-jist) a physician who specializes in the diagnosis and medical and surgical treatment of diseases and defects of the eye and related structures.

ophthalmology (of″thal-mol′o-je) [*ophthalmo-* + *-logy*] that branch of medicine dealing with the eye, its anatomy, physiology, pathology, etc.

ophthalmomalacia (of-thal″mo-mah-la′she-ah) [*ophthalmo-* + Gr. *malakia* softness] abnormal softness of the eye.

ophthalmometer (of″thal-mom′e-ter) [*ophthalmo-* + Gr. *metron* measure] any instrument for measuring the eye, especially one for determining its refractive powers and defects by measuring the size of the images reflected from the cornea and lens. Called also *Javel's o.*

ophthalmometroscope (of-thal″mo-met′ro-skōp) an ophthalmoscope with an attachment for measuring the refraction of the eye.

ophthalmometry (of″thal-mom′e-tre) determination of the refractive powers and defects of the eye.

ophthalmomycosis (of-thal″mo-mi-ko′sis) [*ophthalmo-* + Gr. *mykes* fungus + *-osis*] any disease of the eye caused by a fungus.

ophthalmomyiasis (of-thal″mo-mi′yah-sis) [*ophthalmo-* + Gr. *myia* a fly + *-sis*] infection of the eye by the larvae of the fly *Oestrus ovis*.

ophthalmomyitis (of-thal″mo-mi-i′tis) [*ophthalmo-* + Gr. *mys* muscles + *-itis*] inflammation of the muscles that move the eyeball.

ophthalmomyositis (of-thal″mo-mi″o-si′tis) inflammation of the eye muscles.

ophthalmomyotomy (of-thal″mo-mi-ot′o-me) [*ophthalmo-* + *myotomy*] surgical division of the muscles of the eye.

ophthalmoneuritis (of-thal″mo-nu-ri′tis) inflammation of the ophthalmic nerve.

ophthalmoneuromyelitis (of-thal″mo-nu″ro-mi-e-li′tis) neuro-optic myelitis.

ophthalmopathy (of″thal-mop′ah-the) [*ophthalmo-* + Gr. *pathos* disease] any disease of the eye. **external o.**, any affection of the eyelids, cornea, conjunctiva, or eye muscles. **internal o.**, any affection of the deep or more essential parts of the eye.

ophthalmophacometer (of-thal″mo-fa-kom′e-ter) [*ophthalmo-* + Gr. *phakos* lens + *metron* measure] an ophthalometer used to determine the refractive power of the lens.

ophthalmophantom (of-thal″mo-fan′tom) 1. a model of the eye used in demonstration. 2. an apparatus for holding animals' eyes for operation.

ophthalmophlebotomy (of-thal″mo-flē-bot′o-me) [*ophthalmo-* + *phlebotomy*] phlebotomy to relieve congestion of the conjunctival veins.

ophthalmophthisis (of″thal-mof′thĭ-sis) [*ophthalmo-* + Gr. *phthisis* wasting] ophthalmomalacia.

ophthalmoplasty (of-thal″mo-plas″te) [*ophthalmo-* + Gr. *plassein* to mold] plastic surgery of the eye or of its appendages.

ophthalmoplegia (of-thal″mo-ple′je-ah) [*ophthalmo-* + Gr. *plege* stroke + *-ia*] paralysis of the eye muscles. **basal o.**, ophthalmoplegia due to a lesion at the base of the brain. **exophthalmic o.**, hyperophthalmopathic syndrome. **o. exter′na**, paralysis of the external ocular muscles. **fascicular o.**, ophthalmoplegia due to lesion in the pons varolii. **infectious o.**, encephalitis lethargica. **o. inter′na**, paralysis of the iris and ciliary apparatus. **internuclear o.,** that which is due to some lesion between the nuclei of the motor nerves of the eye; called also *internuclear paralysis.* **nuclear o.,** that which is due to some lesion of the nuclei of the motor nerves of the eye. **orbital o.,** ophthalmoplegia due to lesion in the orbit. **Parinaud's o.,** paralysis of conjugate upward movement of the eyes without paralysis of convergence, associated with lesions of the midbrain, such as a tumor of the pineal gland. Called also *Parinaud's syndrome.* **o. partia'lis,** paralysis of either one or two of the eye muscles. **o. progressi'va, progressive o.,** gradual paralysis affecting first one eye muscle and then another; called also *Graefe's disease.* **o. tota'lis,** that affecting both the extrinsic and intrinsic muscular apparatus of the eye.

ophthalmoplegic (of-thal″mo-ple′jik) pertaining to ophthalmoplegia.

ophthalmoptosis (of-thal″mop-to′sis) [*ophthalmo-* + Gr. *ptōsis* fall] exophthalmos.

ophthalmoreaction (of-thal″mo-re-ak′shun) see *ophthalmic reaction,* under *reaction.* **Calmette's o.,** ophthalmic reaction.

ophthalmorrhagia (of-thal″mo-ra′je-ah) [*ophthalmo-* + Gr. *rhēgnynai* to burst forth] hemorrhage from the eye.

ophthalmorrhea (of-thal″mo-re′ah) [*ophthalmo-* + Gr. *rhoia* flow] oozing of blood from the eye.

ophthalmorrhexis (of-thal″mo-rek′sis) [*ophthalmo-* + Gr. *rhēxis* rupture] rupture of the eyeball.

ophthalmoscope (of-thal′mo-skōp) [*ophthalmo-* + Gr. *skopein* to examine] an instrument containing a perforated mirror and lenses used to examine the interior of the eye. **binocular o.,** an instrument for stereoscopic examination of the eye. **direct o.,** one that produces an upright, or unreversed, image of approximately 15 times magnification. **ghost o.,** a form in which a portion of the reflected rays are deflected by a mirror. **indirect o.,** one that produces an inverted, or reversed, direct image of 2 to 5 times magnification, depending on the dioptic power to the examining lens.

ophthalmoscopy (of-thal-mos′ko-pe) the examination of that interior of the eye with the ophthalmoscope. **direct o.,** that performed with a direct ophthalmoscope. **indirect o.,** that performed with an indirect ophthalmoscope. **medical o.,** that performed for diagnostic purposes. **metric o.,** that performed for the measurement of refraction.

ophthalmostasis (of″thal-mos′tah-sis) [*ophthalmo-* + Gr. *stasis* standing] fixation of the eye with the ophthalmostat.

ophthalmostat (of-thal′mo-stat) [*ophthalmo-* + Gr. *histanai* to halt] an instrument for holding the eye steady during operation.

ophthalmostatometer (of-thal″mo-stah-tom′ĕ-ter) [*ophthalmo-* + Gr. *histanai* to halt + *metron* measure] an instrument for determining the degree of protrusion of the eyeball.

ophthalmosteresis (of-thal″mo-stĕ-re′sis) [*ophthalmo-* + Gr. *steresis* privation, loss] loss of an eye.

ophthalmosynchysis (of-thal″mo-sin′kĭ-sis) [*ophthalmo-* + Gr. *synchysis* a mixing] effusion into the eye.

ophthalmothermometer (of-thal″mo-ther-mom′ĕ-ter) [*ophthalmo-* + *thermometer*] an apparatus for recording the temperature of the eye.

ophthalmotomy (of″thal-mot′o-me) [*ophthalmo-* + Gr. *temnein* to cut] the operation of incising the eyeball.

ophthalmotonometer (of-thal″mo-to-nom′ĕ-ter) [*ophthalmo-* + Gr. *tonos* tension + *metron* measure] an instrument used in measuring the intraocular tension; a tonometer.

ophthalmotonometry (of-thal″mo-to-nom′ĕ-tre) the measurement of the intraocular tension; tonometry.

ophthalmotoxin (of-thal″mo-tok′sin) [*ophthalmo-* + *toxin*] 1. a toxin formed on injection of emulsion of the ciliary body. 2. a toxin acting on the eye.

ophthalmotrope (of-thal′mo-trōp) [*ophthalmo-* + Gr. *trepein* to turn] a mechanical eye that moves like a real eye, used for demonstrating the action of the ocular muscles.

ophthalmotropometer (of-thal″mo-tro-pom′ĕ-ter) [*ophthalmo-* + Gr. *tropos* a turning + *metron* measure] an instrument for measuring eye movements.

ophthalmovascular (of-thal″mo-vas′ku-lar) pertaining to the blood vessels of the eye.

ophthalmoxerosis (of-thal″mo-ze-ro′sis) xerophthalmia.

ophthalmoxyster (of-thal″moks-is′ter) [*ophthalmo-* + Gr. *xystēr* scraper] an instrument for scraping the conjunctiva.

Ophthetic (of-thet′ik) trademark for a preparation of proparacaine hydrochloride.

Ophthochlor (of′tho-klōr) trademark for a preparation of chloramphenicol.

opian (o′pe-an) noscapine.

opianine (o-pi′ah-nin) noscapine.

opiate (o′pe-at) a remedy containing or derived from opium; also any drug that induces sleep.

Opie paradox (o′pe) [Eugene Lindsay *Opie,* American pathologist, born 1873] see under *paradox.*

opilação (o″pil-ah-sah′o) [Port.] Chagas' disease.

opilation (o″pĭ-la′shun) Chagas' disease.

opioid (o′pe-oid) 1. any synthetic narcotic that has opiate-like activities but is not derived from opium. 2. denoting naturally occurring peptides, e.g., enkepalins, that exert opiate-like effects by interacting with opiate receptors of cell membranes.

opiomania (o″pe-o-ma′ne-ah) [*opium* + Gr. *mania* madness] a craving for opium.

opiomaniac (o″pe-o-ma′ne-ak) a person affected with opiomania.

opiophagism, opiophagy (o″pe-of′ah-jizm; o-pe-of′ah-je) [*opium* + Gr. *phagein* to eat] the habitual use or eating of opium.

opipramol hydrochloride (o-pip′rah-mōl) chemical name: 4-[3-(5*H*-dibenz[*b,f*]azepin-5-yl)propyl]-1-piperazineethanol dihydrochloride; a tricyclic antidepressant with mild tranquilizing properties, $C_{23}H_{29}N_3O \cdot 2HCl$.

Opisocrostis (o″pĭ-so-kros′tis) a genus of fleas. **O. bru′neri,** a squirrel flea said to be a vector of sylvatic plague.

opisthe (o-pis′the) [Gr. *opisthen* behind] the posterior daughter organism after transverse division of a protozoon; cf. *proter.*

opisthenar (o-pis′the-nar) [*opistho-* + Gr. *thenar* palm of the hand] the dorsum of the hand.

opisthencephalon (o-pis″then-sef′ah-lon) [*opistho-* + Gr. *enkephalos* brain] the cerebellum.

opisthiobasial (o-pis″the-o-ba′se-al) pertaining to or connecting the opisthion and basion.

opisthion (o-pis′the-on) [Gr. *opisthion* rear, posterior] the midpoint of the lower border of the foramen magnum.

opisthionasial (o-pis″the-o-na′ze-al) connecting the opisthion and nasion.

opistho- (o-pis′tho) [Gr. *opisthen* behind, at the back] a combining form meaning backward or denoting relationship to the back.

opisthogenia (o-pis″tho-je′ne-ah) defective development of the jaws following ankylosis of the jaw.

opisthognathism (o″pis-thog′nah-thizm) the condition of having receding jaws.

opisthoporeia (o-pis″tho-po-ri′ah) [*opistho-* + Gr. *poreia* walk] involuntary walking backward, as in parkinsonism; retropulsion.

opisthorchiasis (o-pis″thor-ki′ah-sis) infection of the biliary tract by the liver flukes *Opisthorchis felineus* and *O. viverrini.* In heavy infections, local injury to the distal bile capillaries and surrounding liver tissue develops; in severe infections, there may be cirrhosis of the liver with areas of necrosis and fatty degeneration.

Opisthorchis (o″pis-thor′kis) [*opistho-* + Gr. *orchis* testicle] a genus of trematodes or flukes characterized by having the testes near the posterior end of the body. **O. felin′eus,** the Siberian liver fluke found in the liver of cats, dogs, pigs, and man; infection (see *opisthorchiasis*) results from ingestion of infected fish (*Leuciscus rutilis, Idus melanotus,* and related species). **O. nover′ca,** *Amphimerus noverca.* **O. sinen′sis,** *Clonorchis sinensis.* **O. viverri′ni,** a species found in Thailand in the civet cat and sometimes in man (see *opisthorchiasis*).

opisthorchosis (o″pis-thor-ko′sis) infection with any species of *Opisthorchis.*

opisthotic (o″pis-thot′ik) [*opistho-* + Gr. *ous* ear] situated behind the ear.

opisthotonoid (o″pis-thot′o-noid) resembling opisthotonos.

opisthotonos (o″pis-thot′o-nos) [*opistho-* + Gr. *tonos* tension] a

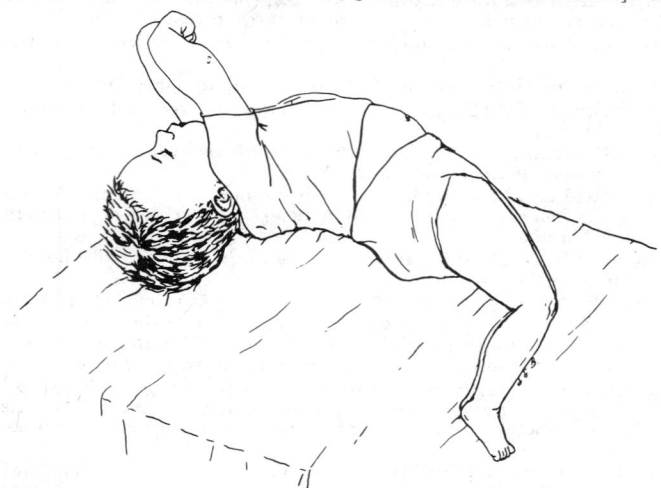

Opisthotonus

form of spasm in which the head and the heels are bent backward and the body bowed forward. **o. feta'lis,** an exaggerated deflection attitude of the fetus during labor, which may persist during the neonatal period, but which gradually changes to a more normal posture.

opisthotonus (o″pis-thot′o-nus) opisthotonos.

Opitz's disease (o′pitz) [Hans *Opitz*, German pediatrician, born 1888] see under *disease*.

opium (o′pe-um) [L.; Gr. *opion*] [*USP*] an air-dried milky exudate obtained by incising the unripe capsules of *Papaver somniferum* L. (Papaveraceae) or its variety, *album*, yielding not less than 9.5 per cent of anhydrous morphine. Called also *crude o.* and *gum o.* Various principles and derivatives of opium, including some 20 alkaloids, notably morphine, codeine, paperavine, and thebaine, are used for their narcotic and analgesic effects. Because it is highly addictive, the production of opium is restricted, and the cultivation of the plants from which it is obtained is prohibited by most nations under an international agreement. **crude o.,** see *opium*. **denarcotized o., o. deodora′tum, deodorized o.,** powdered opium freed from certain nauseating constituents by extraction with purified petroleum benzin. **granulated o., o. granula′tum,** opium reduced to a coarse powder. **gum o.,** see *opium*. **lettuce o.,** the bitter, inspissated juice of various species of lettuce, e.g., *Lactuca sativa* L. (Compositae), formerly used for mild hypnotic and sedative action. **powdered o.** [USP], **o. pulvera′tum,** opium dried at a temperature not exceeding 70° C., and reduced to a very fine powder, yielding not less than 10 per cent and not more than 10.5 per cent of anhydrous morphine. It may contain any of the diluents, except starch, permitted in powdered extracts. See *brown mixture*, under *mixture*, and see *paregoric*.

opobalsamum (o″po-bal′sah-mum) [Gr. *opos* juice + *balsamon* balsam] balsam of Gilead.

opocephalus (o″po-sef′ah-lus) [Gr. *ōps* face + *kephalē* head] a monster with the ears fused to the head, one orbit, no mouth, and no nose.

opodidymus (o″po-did′ĭ-mus) [Gr. *ōps* fact + *didymos* twin] a fetus with two fused heads and with the sense organs partially fused.

opodymus (o-pod′ĭ-mus) opodidymus.

opossum (o-pos′um) a marsupial animal, species of which (*Didelphis*) in South America are reservoirs of *Trypanosoma cruzi*.

opotherapy (o″po-ther′ah-pe) [Gr. *opos* juice + *therapeia* treatment] treatment by juices, especially treatment of disease by the administration of extract from animals' organs, as from endocrine organs.

Oppenheim's disease (syndrome), sign (reflex) (op′en-hīmz) [Hermann *Oppenheim*, neurologist in Berlin, 1858–1919] see *amyotonia congenita*, and see under *sign*.

oppilation (op″ĭ-la′shun) [L. *oppilatio*] (*obs.*) constipation.

oppilative (op′ĭ-la″tiv) (*obs.*) closing the pores; also constipating.

opponens (o-po′nenz) [L.] opposing; said of an opposing structure, as musculus opponens.

opportunistic (op″or-tu-nis′tik) 1. denoting a microorganism which does not ordinarily cause disease but which, under certain circumstances (e.g., impaired immune responses), becomes pathogenic. 2. denoting a disease or infection caused by such an organism.

oppositipolar (o-poz″ĭ-ti-po′lar) having two poles on opposite sides of a cell.

opsialgia (op″se-al′je-ah) [Gr. *ōps* face + *-algia*] geniculate neuralgia.

opsigenes (op-sij′ĕ-nēz) [Gr. *opsigenēs*] late born; a term sometimes applied to the third permanent molars (wisdom teeth).

opsin (op′sin) a protein of the retinal rods (scotopsin) and cones (photopsin) that combines with 11-*cis*-retinal to form visual pigments; see *retinal* (def. 2). The opsins are also named according to the color of pigment: iodopsin (violet), porphyropsin (red), rhodopsin (purple), etc.

opsinogen (op-sin′o-jen) a substance (antigen) with the power to induce the formation of opsonins in the body.

opsinogenous (op″sin-oj′ĕ-nus) able to form opsonins.

opsiometer (op″se-om′ĕ-ter) [Gr. *opsis* vision + *metron* measure] optometer.

opsiuria (op″se-u′re-ah) [Gr. *opse* late + *ouron* urine + *-ia*] the condition in which more urine is excreted during fasting than during digestion.

opsoclonia, opsoclonus (op″so-klo′ne-ah; op″so-klo′nus) a condition characterized by nonrhythmic horizontal and vertical oscillations of the eyes, observed in various disorders of the brain stem or cerebellum.

opsogen (op′so-jen) opsinogen.

opsomania (op″so-ma′ne-ah) [Gr. *opson* dainty + *mania* madness] a craving for some special food.

opsone (op′sōn) opsonin.

opsonic (op-son′ik) pertaining to opsonins.

opsoniferous (op″so-nif′er-us) bearing opsonin.

opsonification (op-son″ĭ-fi-ka′shun) opsonization.

opsonify (op-son′ĭ-fi) to subject to opsonization.

opsonin (op′so-nin) [Gr. *opsōnein* to buy victuals] 1. an antibody that renders bacteria and other cells susceptible to phagocytosis. 2. a nonantibody substance, which may be derived from the C3 component of complement, capable of rendering bacteria susceptible to phagocytosis. The basic proteins, protamine, globin, and lysozyme, have been shown to be opsonins. Two proteins, one a β-globulin and the other an α₁-globulin, are opsonic without the aid of complement and are not basic proteins. These are called P.P.F. (phagocytosis promoting factor). **immune o.,** an antibody that sensitizes a particulate antigen to phagocytosis, following combination with the homologous antigen in vivo or in vitro.

opsoninopathy (op-so″nin-op′ah-the) a condition marked by reduced levels of serum opsonins, leading to increased susceptibility to infection. **consumptive o.,** depletion of opsonins by consumption (i.e., by reacting with antigen) of specific antibody or complement components, or both, during infection. Fatal cases are usually associated with malnutrition.

opsonist (op′so-nist) one who is expert in opsonic technique.

opsonization (op″so-ni-za′shun) the rendering of bacteria and other cells subject to phagocytosis.

opsonize (op′so-nīz) to subject to opsonization.

opsonocytophagic (op″so-no-si″to-faj′ik) denoting the phagocytic activity of blood in the presence of serum opsonins and homologous leukocytes.

opsonogen (op-son′o-jen) opsinogen.

opsonology (op″so-nol′o-je) the study of opsonins and opsonic action.

opsonometry (op″so-nom′ĕ-tre) the measurement of the amount of opsonin present.

opsonophilia (op″so-no-fil′e-ah) [*opsonin* + Gr. *philein* to love] affinity for opsonins.

opsonophilic (op″so-no-fil′ik) having an affinity for opsonins.

opsonophoric (op″so-no-for′ik) bearing opsonin; the term applied to that group of an opsonin which acts on the bacterium or other cell to render it subject to phagocytosis.

opsonotherapy (op″so-no-ther′ah-pe) treatment by the use of bacterial vaccines to increase the opsonic action of the blood.

Optef (op′tef) trademark for a preparation of hydrocortisone.

optesthesia (op″tes-the′ze-ah) visual sensibility; ability to perceive visual stimuli.

optic (op′tik) [Gr. *optikos* of or for sight] of or pertaining to the eye.

optical (op′tĭ-kal) [L. *opticus*; Gr. *optikos*] pertaining to or subserving vision.

optician (op-tish′an) an expert in opticianry.

opticianry (op-tish′an-re) the science, craft, and art of optics as applied to the translation, filling, and adapting of ophthalmic prescriptions, products, and accessories.

opticist (op′tĭ-sist) an expert in the science of optics.

opticochiasmatic (op″tĭ-ko-ki″az-mat′ik) pertaining to the optic nerves and chiasma.

opticociliary (op″tĭ-ko-sil′e-a-re) pertaining to the optic and ciliary nerves.

opticocinerea (op″tĭ-ko-sĭ-ne′re-ah) [*optic* + *cinerea*] (*obs.*) the gray matter of the optic tract.

opticokinetic (op″tĭ-ko-ki-net′ik) pertaining to movement of the eyes.

opticonasion (op″tĭ-ko-na′se-on) the distance from the posterior edge of the optic foramen to the nasion.

opticopupillary (op″tĭ-ko-pu′pĭ-ler-e) pertaining to the optic nerve and the pupil.

optics (op′tiks) [Gr. *optikos* of or for sight] the science which treats of light and of vision. **fiber o.,** see *fiberoptics*.

optimal (op′tĭ-mal) the best; the most favorable.

optimeter (op-tim′ĕ-ter) optometer.

optimum (op′tĭ-mum) [L. "best"] 1. that condition of surroundings which is conducive to the most favorable activity or function. 2. Pirquet's term for the amount of food most desirable under given circumstances.

optist (op′tist) a person skilled in optometry.

opto- (op′to) [Gr. *optos* seen] a combining form meaning visible, or denoting relationship to vision or sight.

optoblast (op′to-blast) [*opto-* + Gr. *blastos* germ] one of the large ganglion cells of the retina.

optochiasmic (op″to-ki-az′mik) opticochiasmatic.

optogram (op′to-gram) [*opto-* + Gr. *gramma* mark] the retinal image formed by the bleaching of the visual purple under the influence of light.

optokinetic (op″to-ki-net′ik)   pertaining to movement of the eyes, as in nystagmus.

optomeninx (op″to-me′ningks) [opto- + Gr. *mēninx* membrane] the retina.

optometer (op-tom′ĕ-ter) [opto- + Gr. *metron* measure]   a device for measuring the power and range of vision.

optometrist (op-tom′ĕ-trist)   a person trained and licensed to examine and test the eyes and to treat visual defects by prescribing and adapting corrective lenses and other optical aids, and by establishing programs of visual training.

optometry (op-tom′ĕ-tre)   measurement of the powers of vision and the adaptation of prisms or lenses for the aid thereof, utilizing any means other than drugs. See *optometrist.*

optomyometer (op″to-mi-om′ĕ-ter) [opto- + Gr. *mys* muscle + *metron* measure]   a device used in measuring the power of the ocular muscles.

optophone (op′to-fōn) [opto- + Gr. *phōne* voice]   an instrument by means of which light and darkness are made discernible to the blind through their sense of hearing, the light waves being transformed into sound waves.

optotype (op′to-tīp) [opto- + *type*]   the test types used in testing vision.

Opuntia (o-pun′she-ah)   a genus of cacti. *O. vulgaris,* the prickly pear, is used as a remedy in homeopathic practice.

O.R.   operating room.

ora[1] (o′rah), pl. *o′rae* [L.]   an edge or margin.   **o. serra′ta ret′inae** [NA], the irregular anterior margin of the pars optica of the retina, lying internal and slightly posterior to the junction of the choroid and the ciliary body.

ora[2] (o′rah) [L.]   plural of *os,* mouth.

Orabilex (or″ah-bi′leks)   trademark for a preparation of bunamiodyl.

orad (o′rad) [L. *os, oris* mouth + *ad* toward]   toward the mouth.

orae (o′re) [L.]   plural of *ora,* edge.

Oragrafin (or″ah-graf′in)   trademark for a preparation of the calcium or the sodium salt of ipodate.

oral (o′ral) [L. *oralis*]   1. pertaining to the mouth, taken through or applied in the mouth, as an oral medication or an oral thermometer.   2. denoting that aspect of the teeth which faces the oral cavity or tongue.

orale (o-ra′le)   the point in the midline of the maxillary suture just lingual to the central incisors in the alveolar process.

orality (o-ral′ĭ-te)   a term embracing all of the aspects and components (sucking, mouthing, etc.) of the oral stage of psychosexual development.

oralogy (o-ral′o-je) [L. *oralis* pertaining to the mouth + -*logy*]   stomatology.

orange (or′anj) [L. *aurantium*]   1. the rutaceous tree, *Citrus aurantium* L., and its yellow, edible fruit (*aurantii fructus*). There are two varieties, *bitter orange* (*aurantii amara*) and *sweet orange* (*aurantii dulcis*). The peel of the two varieties is used in making various pharmaceutical preparations.   2. a color between red and yellow.   3. a dye or stain that produces an orange color.   **acridine o.,** see *acridine.*   **ethyl o.,** an indicator with a pH range of 2 to 4.   **o. G,** an acid azo dye used as a cytoplasmic stain, $C_6H_5 \cdot N{:}N \cdot C_{10}H_4(SO_2 \cdot ONa)_2 \cdot OH$.   **gold o.,** methyl o.   **o. III,** methyl o.   **methyl o.** [USP], an orange-yellow powder, the sodium salt of dimethylaminoazobenzene sulfonic acid, used as an indicator with a pH range of 3.2 to 4.4 and a color change from pink to yellow. Called also *gold o.* and *helianthin.*   **Poirrier's o.,** methyl o.   **victoria o.,** a salt of dinitrocresol used in histology as a stain.   **wool o.,** orange G.

orangeophil (or-an′je-o-fīl)   1. staining readily with orange dyes.   2. a cell or other histologic element that stains readily with orange dyes.   3. one of the acidophils, or alpha cells (*somatotropes*), of the adenohypophysis staining readily with orange G; called also *alpha acidophil.*

orangutan (o-rang′oo-tan″) [Malayan *orang* a human being + *utan* (*hutan*) wild]   one of the anthropoid apes, of the family Pongidae, frequently used for laboratory studies because it is susceptible to some of the same diseases as man.

Oranixon (or″ah-nik′son)   trademark for a preparation of mephenesin.

Ora-Testryl (o″rah-tes′tril)   trademark for a preparation of fluoxymesterone.

orb (orb) [L. *orbis* circle, disk]   a sphere; the eyeball.

Orbeli phenomenon (effect) (or-ba′le) [Leon Algarovich *Orbeli,* Russian physiologist, 1882–1958]   see under *phenomenon.*

orbicular (or-bik′u-lar) [L. *orbicularis*]   circular, or rounded.

orbiculare (or-bik″u-la′re) [L.]   processus lenticularis incudis.

orbiculi (or-bik′u-li)   plural of *orbiculus.*

orbiculus (or-bik′u-lus), pl. *orbic′uli* [L., dim. of *orbis* orb, circle] [NA], a general term denoting a structure shaped like a small circle, or disk.   **o. cilia′ris** [NA], the thin part of the ciliary body extending between its crown and the ora serrata retinae; called also *ciliary disk.*

orbit (or′bit)   the bony cavity that contains the eyeball; see *orbita* [NA].

orbita (or′bĭ-tah), pl. *or′bitae* [L. "mark of a wheel"] [NA]   the orbit: bony cavity that contains the eyeball and its associated muscles, vessels, and nerves; the ethmoidal, frontal, lacrimal, nasal, palatine, sphenoidal, and zygomatic bones, and the maxilla contribute to its formation.

orbitae (or′bĭ-te) [L.]   plural of *orbita.*

orbital (or′bĭ-tal) [L. *orbitalis*]   1. pertaining to the orbit.   2. a region in an atom that may contain either one or two opposite spin electrons; orbitals of various sizes and shapes may occur in a single atom. A set of orbitals is a housing arrangement for electrons.

orbitale (or′bĭ-ta′le)   an anthropometric landmark, the lowest point on the inferior margin of the orbit.

orbitalis (or′bĭ-ta′lis) [L.]   pertaining to the orbit.

orbitonasal (or″bĭ-to-na′zal)   pertaining to the orbit and the nose.

orbitonometer (or″bĭ-to-nom′ĕ-ter)   an instrument for measurement of the backward displacement of the eyeball produced by a given pressure exerted against its anterior aspect.

orbitonometry (or″bĭ-to-nom′ĕ-tre)   the measurement of the backward displacement of the eyeball under varying pressures.

orbitopagus (or″bĭ-top′ah-gus) [*orbit* + Gr. *pagos* thing fixed]   a twin monster composed of a small fetus attached to the orbit of the autosite.

orbitostat (or′bĭ-to-stat)   an instrument for measuring the axis of the orbit.

orbitotemporal (or″bĭ-to-tem′po-ral)   pertaining to the orbital and temporal regions.

orbitotomy (or″bĭ-tot′o-me) [*orbit* + Gr. *temnein* to cut]   the operation of incising or opening into the orbit through the orbital margin.

orbivirus (or′bĭ-vi″rus)   a group of RNA viruses, a subgroup of the diplornavirus.

orcein (or-se′in)   a brown coloring matter, $C_{28}H_{24}N_2O_7$, derived from orcin and soluble in alcohol; used as a specific stain for elastic tissue.

orchectomy (or-kek′to-me)   orchiectomy.

orchella (or-shel′ah)   a histologic stain composed of 5 ml. of acetic acid and 40 ml. each of alcohol and water, colored to a dark red with archil from which excess of ammonia has been driven off.

orchi-   see *orchio-.*

orchialgia (or″ke-al′je-ah) [orchi- + -*algia*]   pain in a testis.

orchic (or′kik)   orchidic.

orchichorea (or″ke-ko-re′ah) [orchi- + *chorea*]   a twitching or jerking movement of a testis.

orchidalgia (or″kĭ-dal′je-ah)   orchialgia.

orchidectomy (or″kĭ-dek′to-me)   orchiectomy.

orchidic (or-kid′ik)   pertaining to the testes.

orchiditis (or″kĭ-di′tis)   orchitis.

orchido- (or′kĭ-do) [Gr. *orchidion* dim. of *orchis*]   see *orchio-.*

orchidocelioplasty (or″kĭ-do-se′le-o-plas″te) [orchido- + Gr. *koilia* belly + *plassein* to form]   the operation of transplanting an undescended testis to the abdominal cavity.

orchidoepididymectomy (or″kĭ-do-ep″ĭ-did″ĭ-mek′to-me) [orchido- + *epididymis* + Gr. *ektome* excision]   the operation of excising the testis and epididymis.

orchidometer (or″kĭ-dom′ĕ-ter)   an instrument for measuring the testis.   **Prader o.,** a string of plastic models of testicular shape, marked according to their volume in cubic centimeters; used for measuring the size of the testes in genital development.

orchidoncus (or″kĭ-dong′kus) [orchido- + Gr. *onkos* tumor]   a tumor of a testis.

orchidopathy (or″kĭ-dop′ah-the)   orchiopathy.

orchidopexy (or′kĭ-do-pek″se)   orchiopexy.

orchidoplasty (or′kĭ-do-plas″te)   orchioplasty.

orchidoptosis (or″kĭ-dop-to′sis) [orchido- + Gr. *ptōsis*]   downward displacement of the testis, a condition due to varicocele or relaxation of the scrotum.

orchidorrhaphy (or″kĭ-dor′ah-fe)   orchiopexy.

orchidotherapy (or″kĭ-do-ther′ah-pe) [orchido- + Gr. *therapeia* treatment]   use of testicular extract in treating diseases.

orchidotomy (or″kĭ-dot′o-me)   orchiotomy.

orchiectomy (or″ke-ek′to-me) [orchio- + Gr. *ektome* excision]   excision of one or both testes.

orchiencephaloma (or″ke-en-sef″ah-lo′mah) [orchio- + *encephaloma*]   embryonal carcinoma.

orchiepididymitis (or″ke-ep″ĭ-did″ĭ-mi′tis) [orchio- + *epididymis* + -*itis*]   inflammation of a testis and an epididymis.

orchilytic (or″kĭ-lit′ik) [orchio- + Gr. *lytikos* dissolving]   destroying testicular tissue.

orchio-, orchi-, orchido- [Gr. *orchis* testis]   a combining form denoting relationship to the testes.

orchiocatabasis (or″ke-o-kah-tab′ah-sis) [*orchio-* + Gr. *katabasis* descent] the descent of the testes.

orchiocele (or′ke-o-sēl″) [*orchio-* + Gr. *kēlē* hernia] 1. hernial protrusion of a testis. 2. scrotal hernia. 3. tumor of a testis.

orchiococcus (or″ke-o-kok′us) [*orchio-* + Gr. *kokkos* berry] former term for diplococcus recovered from gonorrheal orchitis.

orchiodynia (or″ke-o-din′e-ah) orchialgia.

orchiomyeloma (or″ke-o-mi″ĕ-lo′mah) [*orchio-* + *myeloma*] plasmacytoma of the testis.

orchioncus (or″ke-ong′kus) [*orchio-* + Gr. *onkos* mass, tumor] tumor of the testis.

orchioneuralgia (or″ke-o-nu-ral′je-ah) [*orchio-* + *neuralgia*] orchialgia.

orchiopathy (or″ke-op′ah-the) [*orchio-* + Gr. *pathos* disease] any disease of the testis.

orchiopexy (or″ke-o-pek′se) [*orchio-* + G. *pēxis* fixation] surgical fixation in the scrotum of an undescended testis.

orchioplasty (or″ke-o-plas″te) [*orchio-* + Gr. *plassein* to form] plastic surgery of the testis.

orchiorrhaphy (or″ke-or′ah-fe) [*orchio-* + Gr. *rhaphē* suture] orchiopexy.

orchioscheocele (or″ke-os′ke-o-sēl″) [*orchio-* + Gr. *oscheon* scrotum + *kēlē* hernia] scrotal tumor with scrotal hernia.

orchioscirrhus (or″ke-o-skir′us) [*orchio-* + Gr. *skirrhos* hard] hardening of the testis.

orchiotomy (or″ke-ot′o-me) [*orchio* + Gr. *temnein* to cut] incision and drainage of a testis.

Orchis (or′kis) the typical genus of orchidaceous plants, so named because certain species bear root or rhizome systems that resemble testicles. Various species are medicinal.

orchis (or′kis) [Gr.] the testis.

orchitic (or-kit′ik) pertaining to, causing, or affected with orchitis.

orchitis (or-ki′tis) [*orchio-* + *-itis*] inflammation of a testis. The disease is marked by pain, swelling, and a feeling of weight. It may occur idiopathically, but is usually due to gonorrhea, syphilis, filarial disease, or tuberculosis. **metastatic o.,** an infection brought to the testis by the blood stream, as in mumps. **mumps o.,** o. parotidea. **o. parotid′ea,** orchitis occurring before, or as the only manifestation of, mumps. **spermatogenic granulomatous o.,** orchitis in which the normal structure of the testis has been replaced by gray-white granulomatous tissue without evident necrosis; it is thought to be in some way a reaction to spermatozoa. **traumatic o.,** orchitis following trauma, vas ligation, or surgical manipulation, without evidence of previous disease, believed to be due to an infectious process resulting from lowered resistance of the injured tissues to bacteria. **o. variolo′sa,** orchitis occurring in smallpox.

orchitolytic (or″kĭ-to-lit′ik) orchilytic.

orchotomy (or-kot′o-me) orchiotomy.

orcin (or′sin) orcinol.

orcinol (or′sĭ-nol) chemical name: 5-methylresorcinol. An antiseptic principle, $C_7H_8O_2 \cdot H_2O$, mainly derived from various lichens, used as a reagent in various tests; called also *orcin*.

Ord's operation [William Miller *Ord*, English surgeon, 1834–1902] see under *operation*.

order (or′der) [L. *ordo* a line, row, or series] a taxonomic category subordinate to a class and superior to a family; see *taxon*.

orderly (or′der-le) a male attendant in a hospital who does general work, attending especially to the preoperative preparation (shaving, catheterizing, etc.) of male patients.

ordinate (or′dĭ-nāt) one of the lines used as a base of reference in graphs; see *abscissa*.

ordure (or′dūr) excrement.

O.R.E.F. Orthopedic Research & Education Foundation.

oreoselinum (o″re-o-se-li′num) [L.] an umbelliferous plant of the Old World, *Peucedanum oreoselinum* (L.) Munch. (Umbelliferae); used in homeopathic practice as a diuretic.

Oretic (o-ret′ik) trademark for a preparation of hydrochlorothiazide.

Oreton (or′e-ton) trademark for preparations of testosterone propionate.

orexia (o-rek′se-ah) [Gr. *orexis*] appetite.

orexigenic (o-rek″sĭ-jen′ik) [Gr. *orexis* appetite + *gennan* to produce] increasing or stimulating the appetite.

oreximania (o-rek″sĭ-ma′ne-ah) [Gr. *orexis* appetite + *mania* madness] enormous increase in appetite and food intake due to fear of becoming thin.

orf 1. a contagious pustular dermatitis of sheep, caused by a virus and communicable to man. 2. sheep-pox.

Orfila museum (or″fĭ-lah′) a museum of anatomy at the Medical School of Paris, founded by Mathieu Joseph Bonaventure *Orfila* (1787–1853).

organ (or′gan) [L. *organum*: Gr. *organnon*] a somewhat independent part of the body that performs a special function or functions; see *organum* [NA]. **absorbent o.,** vascular granulation tissue interposed between the enamel epithelium of a growing permanent tooth and the dentin of the deciduous tooth that the former is replacing. **accessory o's of eye,** structures accessory to the eye, including the ocular muscles and fascia, and the eyebrows, eyelids, conjunctiva, and lacrimal apparatus (organa oculi accessoria [NA]). **acoustic o.,** organum spirale. **Bidder's o.,** an anterior portion, ovarian in character, of the gonad of male toads. **cell o.,** a structural part of a cell having some definite function in its life or reproduction, as a nucleus or a centrosome. **cement o.,** the embryonic tissue that develops into the cement layer of the tooth. **Chievitz's o.,** an embryonic outgrowth behind the parotid gland which may merge into the latter or may disappear. **o. of Corti,** organum spirale. **digestive o's,** those concerned with the ingestion, digestion, and assimilation of food (apparatus digestorius [NA]). **effector o.,** a muscle or gland that contracts or secretes, respectively, in direct response to nerve impulses. **enamel o.,** a process of epithelium forming a cap over a dental papilla and developing into the enamel. **end o.,** end-organ; see under *E*. **essential o. of thalamus,** some portion of the thalamus, possibly the medial nucleus, which functions as an integrating center in animals with little or no cerebral cortex and functioning in a more or less similar manner in higher forms. **genital o's,** the various internal and external organs that are concerned with reproduction (organa genitalia [NA]). **genital o's, external,** the pudendum and clitoris in the female (partes genitales femininae externae [NA]) and the scrotum and penis in the male (partes genitales masculinae externae [NA]). **genital o's, female,** the various organs in the female that are concerned with reproduction; see *organa genitalia feminina*. **genital o's, male,** the various organs in the male that are concerned with reproduction; see *organa genitalia masculina*. **o. of Giraldés,** paradidymis. **Golgi tendon o.,** a mechanoreceptor found in tendons of mammalian muscles; arranged in series with the muscle, it is sensitive to mechanical distortion induced by either passive stretch of the tendon or isometric contraction of the muscle and thus signals muscle tension, being the receptor responsible for the lengthening reaction, or clasp-knife reflex. Called also *tendon spindle*. **gustatory o.,** the organ concerned with the perception of taste; see *organum gustus* [NA]. **Jacobson's o.,** organum vomeronasale. **lateral line o's,** a system of sense organs arranged in longitudinal canals in the skin of fishes and amphibians which are sensitive to changes in pressure and current and to vibrations of low frequency and thus aid in localizing objects. **Marchand's o.,** see under *adrenal*. **o's of mastication,** the masticatory system; see under *system*. **Meyer's o.,** an area of circumvallate papillae on either side of the posterior part of the tongue. **olfactory o.,** the organ concerned with the perception of odors; see *organum olfactus* [NA]. **parapineal o.,** a median dorsal outgrowth of the pineal body in certain lower vertebrates, such as tailless amphibians, primitive fishes, and lizards, the principal cell type of which is an apparent photoreceptor. In some species, it may specialize to form an extracranial epiphyseal eye. Called also *parietal a.* **parenchymal o., parenchymatous o.,** organon parenchymatosum. **parietal a.,** parapineal o. **primitive fat o.,** brown adipose tissue. **reproductive o's,** those concerned with reproduction; see *organa genitalia* [NA], under *organum*. **reproductive o's, female,** organa genitalia feminina; see under *organum*. **reproductive o's, male,** organa genitalia masculina; see under *organum*. **o. of Rosenmüller,** epoophoron. **rudimentary o.,** 1. a primordium. 2. an imperfectly or incompletely developed organ. **o. of Ruffini,** brushes of Ruffini. **segmental o.,** the pronephros, mesonephros, and metanephros together. **sense o's, sensory o's,** organa sensuum. See under *organum*. **o. of shock, shock o.,** the organ which reacts in anaphylactic shock; those organs whose responses determine the nature and, to a large extent, the outcome of a given anaphylactic reaction. **o's of special sense,** organa sensuum; see under *organum*. **spiral o.,** organum spirale. **subcommissural o.,** a collection of columnar cells lining the roof of the caudal end of the third ventricle of the brain; thought to play a role in maintaining water and salt balance. **target o.,** the organ that is affected by a particular hormone. **terminal o.,** the organ situated at either end of a reflex neural arc. **urinary o's,** the organs that are concerned with the production and excretion of urine (organa uropoietica), including the kidneys, ureters, bladder, and urethra. **vestibulocochlear o's,** those structures outside the central nervous system which are concerned with vestibular and auditory function; see *organum vestibulocochleare* [NA]. **vestigial o.,** an undeveloped organ that, in the embryo or in some more or less remote ancestor, was well developed and functional. **o. of vision, visual o.,** organum visus. **vomeronasal o.,** organum vomeronasale. **Weber's o.,** utriculus prostaticus. **o's of Zuckerkandl,** corpora paraaortica.

organa (or′gah-nah) plural of *organum* [L.] and *organon* [Gr.].

organacidia (or″gan-ah-sid′e-ah) the presence of an organic acid, especially in the stomach.

organella (or″gan-el′ah), pl. *organel′lae* [L.] organelle.

organellae (or″gan-el′e) plural of *organella*.

organelle (or″gan-el′) [L. *organella*] 1. a specific particle of membrane-bound organized living substance present in practically all eukaryotic cells, including mitochondria, the Golgi complex, endoplasmic reticulum, lysosomes, ribosomes, centrioles, and the cell center, as well as the plastids of plant cells. 2. one of the minute organs of protozoa concerned with such functions as locomotion, metabolism, or the like.

organic (or-gan′ik) [L. *organicus*; Gr. *organikos*] 1. pertaining to an organ or the organs. 2. having an organized structure. 3. arising from an organism. 4. pertaining to substances derived from living organisms. 5. denoting chemical substances containing carbon. 6. pertaining to or cultivated by the use of animal or vegetable fertilizers, rather than synthetic chemicals.

organicism (or-gan′ĭ-sizm) 1. the theory that all symptoms are due to organic disease. 2. the theory that each of the various organs of the body has its own special constitution.

organicist (or-gan′ĭ-sist) one who believes that the symptoms of disease are due to organic changes.

Organidin (or-gan′ĭ-din) trademark for a preparation of iodinated glycerol.

organism (or′gah-nizm) any individual living thing, whether animal or plant. **consumer o's,** the organisms of an ecosystem, plants or animals, that eat other plants or animals. **Glover's o.,** a gram-positive microorganism isolated by Glover from various types of malignant tumor. **nitrifying o's,** those nitrogen bacteria which are capable of oxidizing nitrites to nitrates. **nitrosifying o's,** those nitrogen bacteria which are capable of oxidizing ammonia to nitrites. **pleuropneumonia-like o's,** a group of organisms of the genus *Mycoplasma*; abbreviated PPLO. See *pleuropneumonia-like*.

organization (or″gah-ni-za′shun) 1. the process of organizing or of becoming organized. 2. the replacement of blood clots by fibrous tissue. 3. an organized body, group, or structure.

organize (or′gah-nīz) to provide with an organic structure; to form into organs.

organizer (or′gah-nīz″er) a part of an embryo which so influences some other part as to bring about and direct its histological and morphological differentiation. Parts developing as a result of induction, and inducing in their turn are classified as organizers of the second grade, third grade, and so on. Cf. *activator*(def. 2) and *inductor*. **nucleolar o., nucleolus o.,** material responsible for organization of the nucleolus of a cell; it is thought to comprise slender strands of heterochromatin by which satellites are attached to the rest of the chromosome. **primary o.,** the dorsal lip region of the blastopore. **procentriole o.,** deuterosome. **secondary o.,** one of second grade, such as the optic cup, which exerts influence on the lens. **tertiary o.,** one of third grade, such as the tympanic ring, which exerts influence on the tympanic membrane.

organo- (or′gah-no) [Gr. *organon* organ] a combining form denoting relationship to an organ.

organochlorine (or″gah-no-klo′rēn) any compound of chlorine and organic elements, as an organochlorine pesticide, e.g., DDT.

organofaction (or″gah-no-fak′shun) the formation and development of an organ.

organoferric (or″gah-no-fer′ik) containing iron and some organic compound.

organogel (or-gan′o-jel) a gel in which an organic liquid takes the place of water.

organogen (or-gan′o-jen) any of the chemical elements—carbon, hydrogen, oxygen, nitrogen, sulfur, phosphorus, and chlorine—characteristic of organic substances.

organogenesis (or″gah-no-jen′ĕ-sis) [*organo-* + Gr. *genesis* generation] the origin and development of organs.

organogenetic (or″gah-no-jĕ-net′ik) pertaining to organogenesis.

organogenic (or″gah-no-jen′ik) originating in an organ.

organogeny (or″gah-noj′ĕ-ne) organogensis.

organography (or-gah-nog′rah-fe) [*organo-* + Gr. *graphein* to write] 1. the roentgenologic visualization of the organs of the body. 2. (*obs.*) a description of the organs of a living body.

organoid (or′gah-noid) [*organ* + Gr. *eidos* form] 1. resembling an organ. 2. a structure which resembles an organ. **cytoplasmic o's,** structures present in all cells which are probably able to divide and thus perpetuate themselves, in contrast to lifeless cell inclusions. Organoids include mitochondria, fibrils, Golgi apparatus, and centrosomes.

organoleptic (or″gah-no-lep′tik) [*organo-* + Gr. *lambanein* to seize] 1. making an impression on an organ of special sense. 2. capable of receiving a sense impression.

organology (or-gah-nol′o-je) [*organo-* + *-logy*] the sum of what is known regarding the organs of the body.

organoma (or-gah-no′mah) a tumor composed of organs or definite portions of an organ, or characterized by the presence in it of definite organs, as a dermoid cyst.

organomegaly (or″gah-no-meg′ah-le) [*organo-* + Gr. *megas* large] enlargement of the viscera; visceromegaly.

organomercurial (or″gah-no-mer-ku′re-al) any mercury-containing organic compound, e.g., the diuretic mercaptomerin.

organometallic (or-gah-no-mĕ-tal′ik) consisting of a metal in combination with an organic radical.

organon (or′gah-non), pl. *or′gana* [Gr.] a somewhat independent part of the body that performs a special function; see *organum*. **o. audi′tus,** organum vestibulocochleare. **or′gana genita′lia,** see under *organum*. **or′gana genita′lia mulie′bria,** see *organa genitalia feminina,* under *organum*. **or′gana genita′lia viril′ia,** see *organa genitalia masculina,* under *organum*. **o. gus′tus,** organum gustus. **or′gana oc′uli accesso′ria** see under *organum*. **o. olfac′tus,** organum olfactus. **o. parenchymato′sum,** a parenchymatous organ. **or′gana sen′suum,** see under *organum*. **o. spira′le [Cor′tii],** organum spirale. **or′gana uropoët′ica,** see *organa uropoietica,* under *organum*. **o. vi′sus,** organum visus. **o. vomeronasa′le [Jacobso′ni],** organum vomeronasale.

organonomy (or″gah-non′o-me) [*organo-* + Gr. *nomos* law] the laws of organic life and of living organisms.

organopathy (or″gah-nop′ah-the) [*organo-* + Gr. *pathos* disease] 1. organic disease. 2. organotherapy.

organopexia (or″gah-no-pek′se-ah) organopexy.

organopexy (or′gah-no-pek′se) [*organo-* + Gr. *pēxis* fixation] the surgical fixation of an organ, especially of the uterus.

organophilic (or″gah-no-fil′ik) [*organo-* + Gr. *philein* to love] organotropic.

organophilism (or-gah-nof′ĭ-lizm) organotropism.

organophosphate (or″gan-o-fos′fāt) phosphate esterified to organic compounds such as glucose or sorbitol; see *organophosphorus*.

organophosphorus (or″gah-no-fos′fŏ-rus) a compound containing phosphorus bound to an organic molecule; many organophosphorus compounds are powerful acetylcholinesterase inhibitors and are used as insecticides.

organoscopy (or-gah-nos′ko-pe) [*organo-* + Gr. *skopein* to examine] examination of the abdominal viscera by means of an endoscope inserted through an incision in the abdominal wall.

organotaxis (or″gah-no-tak′sis) [*organo-* + Gr. *taxis* arrangement] a tendency to selective migration to some particular organ.

organotherapy (or″gah-no-ther′ah-pe) [*organo-* + Gr. *therapeia* therapy] the treatment of disease by the administration of animal endocrine organs or their extracts; called also *Brown-Séquard's treatment*. See *opotherapy*. **heterologous o.,** organotherapy with substances that have no relation to the diseased organ of the patient. **homologous o.,** organotherapy by extractives of the organs of animals corresponding to the diseased organ of the patient.

organotrope (or-gan′o-trōp) an organotropic element or agent.

organotrophic (or″gah-no-trof′ik) 1. relating to the nutrition of organs of the body. 2. deriving energy from the oxidation of organic compounds; said of bacteria.

organotropic (or″gah-no-trop′ik) pertaining to or characterized by organotropism.

organotropism (or-gah-not′ro-pizm) [*organo-* + Gr. *tropē* a turning] the special affinity of chemical compounds or of pathogenic agents for particular tissues or organs of the body.

organotropy (or″gan-ot′ro-pe) organotropism.

organ-specific (or′gan-spĕ-sif′ik) restricted to, or having an effect only on, a particular organ, as an organ-specific antigen.

organule (or′gan-ūl) an end-organ of sensory receptors, such as a taste bud.

organum (or′gah-num), pl. *or′gana* [L.] [NA] an organ: a somewhat independent part of the body that is arranged according to a characteristic structural plan, and performs a special function or functions; it is composed of various tissues, one of which is primary in function. Called also *organon*. **or′gana genita′lia,** genital organs: the various internal and external organs that are concerned with reproduction; see Plate accompanying *system*. **or′gana genita′lia femini′na** [NA], female genital organs: the various organs in the female that are concerned with reproduction, including the ovary, uterine tube, uterus, vagina, labia, and clitoris. Called also *organa genitalia muliebria*. See Plate accompanying *system*. **or′gana genita′lia masculi′na** [NA], male genital organs: the various organs in the male that are concerned with reproduction, including the testis, epididymis, ductus deferens, seminal vesicle, ejaculatory duct, prostate, bulbourethral gland, and penis; called also *organa genitalia virilia*. See Plate accompanying *system*. **o. gus′tus** [NA], gustatory organ: the organ of taste, comprising the taste buds, most of which are found within the epithelial covering of the tongue. Called also *organon gustus*. **or′gana oc′uli accesso′ria** [NA], the accessory organs of the eye, including the ocular muscles and fascia, and the eyebrows, eyelids, conjunctiva, and lacrimal apparatus. Called also *adnexa oculi*. See Plate accompanying *eye*. **o. olfac′tus** [NA], olfactory organ: the specialized structures subserving the function of the sense of smell, including the olfactory region of the nasal mucosa containing the bipolar cells of origin of the olfactory nerves, together with the olfactory glands; called also *organon olfactus*. **or′gana sen′suum** [NA], sense organs: organs that receive stimuli which give rise to sensations, i.e., organs which translate certain forms of energy into nerve impulses that are perceived as special sensations; they are characterized by highly specialized neuroreceptors and relationships, and include the visual, vestibulocochlear, olfactory, and gustatory organs. Called also *organs of special sense*. **o. spira′le** [NA], spiral organ: the organ, resting on the basilar membrane in the cochlear duct, that contains the special sensory receptors for hearing; it consists of neuroepithelial hair cells and several types of supporting cells, including the inner and outer pillar cells, inner and outer phalangeal cells, border cells, and Hansen's cells. Called also *organon spirale* [*Cortii*] and *organ of Corti*. **or′gana uropoët′ica** [NA], **or′gana uropoiet′ica**, the organs concerned with the production and excretion of urine, including the kidneys, ureters, bladder, and urethra; called also *urinary organs*. See Plate accompanying *system*. **o. vestibulocochlea′re** [NA], vestibulocochlear organ: a collective term in official anatomical nomenclature applied to those structures outside the central nervous system that are concerned with balance and hearing, and comprising the internal, middle, and external ear. Called also *organon auditus*. See Plate accompanying *ear*. **o. vi′sus** [NA], organ of vision: a collective term in official anatomical nomenclature applied to those structures outside the central nervous system that are concerned with vision, comprising the eyeball and its fibrous, vascular, and internal tunics, and the accessory organs of the eye. Called also *organon visus*. See Plate accompanying *eye*. **o. vomeronasa′le** [NA], vomeronasal organ: a short rudimentary canal just above the vomeronasal cartilage, opening in the side of the nasal septum and passing from there blindly upward and backward; called also *organon vomeronasale* [*Jacobsoni*] and *Jacobson's organ*.

orgasm (or′gazm) [Gr. *orgasmos* swelling, or *organ* to swell, to be lustful] the apex and culmination of sexual excitement.

orgotein (or′go-tēn) any of a group of water-soluble congeners derived from red blood cells, liver, and other tissues, of molecular weight about 33,000 with compact conformation maintained by about 4 gram-atoms of divalent metal; produced from beef liver as a copper-zinc mixed chelate having superoxide dismutation activity. Orgotein has anti-inflammatory properties and has been used as an antirheumatic.

Oribasius (or″ĭ-ba′se-us) [325–403 A.D.] a famous physician and medical writer who became physician to the Emperor Julian. His *magnum opus* was an encyclopedia of medicine in seventy volumes, of which only some seventeen survive; these are invaluable for they contain extracts from the works of many important physicians of antiquity (e.g., Dioscorides, Galen, Antyllus).

orientation (o″re-en-ta′shun) [L. *oriens* arising] the determination of the east point; hence, the determination of one's position with respect to space and time.

orifice (or′ĭ-fis) [L. *orificium*] 1. the entrance or outlet of any cavity in the body. 2. any foramen, meatus, or opening. Called also *ostium* [NA] and *orificium*. **abdominal o. of uterine tube,** ostium abdominale tubae uterinae. **aortic o.,** the opening of the aorta in the left ventricle of the heart. **o. of aqueduct of vestibule, external,** apertura externa aqueductus vestibuli. **atrioventricular o., auriculoventricular o.,** see *ostium atrioventriculare dextrum* and *ostium atrioventriculare sinistrum*. **canal o.,** root canal o. **cardiac o.,** ostium cardiacum. **duodenal o. of stomach,** ostium pyloricum. **epiploic o.,** foramen epiploicum. **o. of female urethra, external,** ostium urethrae externum feminina. **hymenal o.,** ostium vaginae. **o. of male urethra, external,** ostium urethrae externum masculinae. **o. of maxillary sinus,** hiatus maxillaris. **mitral o.,** ostium atrioventriculare sinistrum. **pharyngeal o.,** ostium pharyngeum tubae auditivae. **pilosebaceous o's,** the openings of the hair follicles, giving egress to the secretion of the sebaceous glands whose ducts open into the follicles, and to the hairs. **pulmonary o.,** the opening of the pulmonary artery in the right ventricle of the heart. **o. of pulp canal,** foramen apicis dentis. **root canal o.,** an opening in the floor of the pulp chamber of a tooth, leading into a root canal. **o. of ureter,** ostium ureteris. **o. of urethra, internal,** ostium urethrae internum. **uterine o. of uterine tube,** ostium uterinum tubae uterinae. **o. of uterus, external,** ostium uteri. **vesicourethral o.,** ostium urethrae internum.

orificia (or″ĭ-fish′e-ah) plural of *orificium*.

orificial (or″ĭ-fish′al) pertaining to an orifice.

orificialist (or″ĭ-fish′al-ist) one who treats disease by dilating or otherwise operating upon the external orifices of the body.

orificium (or″ĭ-fish′e-um), pl. *orific′ia* [L.] an opening or orifice, especially the entrance or outlet of any cavity or tube. Called *ostium* [NA]. **o. exter′num isth′mi, o. exter′num u′teri,** ostium uteri. **o. hy′menis,** ostium vaginae. **o. inter′num isth′mi, o. inter′num u′teri,** the internal orifice of the cervix uteri, opening into the cavity of the uterus. **o. ure′teris,** ostium ureteris. **o. ure′thrae exter′num mulie′bris,** ostium urethrae externum feminina. **o. ure′thrae exter′num vir′ilis,** ostium urethrae externum masculinae.

o. ure′thrae inter′num, ostium urethrae internum. **o. vagi′nae,** ostium vaginae.

origin (or′ĭ-jin) [L. *origo* beginning] the source or beginning of anything, especially the more fixed end or attachment of a muscle (as distinguished from its insertion), or the site of emergence of a peripheral nerve from the central nervous system.

Orimune (or′ĭ-mūn) trademark for a preparation of live oral poliovirus vaccine.

Orinase (or′ĭ-nās) trademark for a preparation of tolbutamide.

orinotherapy (o-ri″no-ther′ah-pe) [Gr. *oreinos* pertaining to mountains + *therapeia* treatment] treatment by living in high, mountainous regions.

ormetoprim (or-met′o-prim) chemical name: 2,4-diamino-5-(6-methylveratryl)pyrimidine; an antibacterial, $C_{14}H_{18}N_4O_2$.

Orn ornithine.

ornidazole (or-nid′ah-zōl) chemical name: α-(chloromethyl)-2-methyl-5-nitro-1*H*-imidazole-1-ethanol; an anti-infective, $C_7H_{10}ClN_3O_3$.

ornithine (or′nĭ-thin) an amino acid, α,δ-diaminovalerianic acid, $NH_2(CH_2)_3 \cdot CH(NH_2) \cdot CO_2H$, it is produced in the urea cycle by the splitting off of urea from arginine and is itself converted into citrulline. On decomposition, it gives rise to putrescine.

Ornithodoros (or″nĭ-thod′o-ros) [Gr. *ornis, ornithos* bird + *doros* bag] a genus of argasid ticks, many species of which are the reservoirs and vectors of the spirochetes (*Borrelia*) of relapsing fevers. The chief vectors are: *O. as′perus* of Asia; *O. duge′si* of Mexico; *O. errat′icus* of Spain and North Africa; *O. gur′neyi* of Australia; *O. herm′si* of western United States; *O. mouba′ta,* the tampan or tampan tick of South Africa; *O. norman′di* of Tunisia; *O. par′keri* of western United States; *O. ru′dis* of Central and South America; *O. savign′yi* of Africa, Arabia, and India; *O. tala′je* of the tropics of North and South America; *O. tartakov′skyi* in Russia; *O. tholoza′ni* in Turkestan, Syria, and Palestine; *O. turica′ta* in Mexico, Texas, Arizona, Colorado, and California; *O. verrucosus* of North Caucasus. **O. coria′ceus,** the pajaroello, a venomous

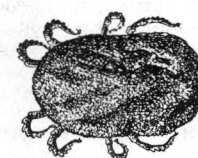

Ornithodoros moubata (after Chandler).

tick of California whose bite causes painful swellings; it is not known to transmit disease.

Ornithonyssus (or″nĭ-tho-nis′us) a genus of mites; formerly called *Liponyssus*. **O. baco′ti,** the rat mite or tropical rat mite; a species whose bite may cause a painful dermatitis (rat-mite dermatitis), and which experimentally transmits murine typhus; formerly called *Leiognathus bacoti* and *Liponyssus bacoti*. **O. bur′sa,** the tropical fowl mite, commonly found on chickens and wild birds or in their nests. **O. sylvia′rum,** the northern fowl mite, commonly a parasite of many domestic and wild fowl.

ornithosis (or″nĭ-tho′sis) [Gr. *ornis, ornithos* bird + *-osis*] a contagious disease of nonpsittacine birds caused by a strain of *Chlamydia psittaci* and marked by respiratory and systemic infection. In man and psittacine birds, it is known as *psittacosis*.

oro- (o′ro) 1. [L. *os, oris* mouth] a combining form denoting relationship to the mouth. 2. [Gr. *oros* the watery part of the blood (serum), or whey] see *orrho-*.

orodiagnosis (or″o-di″ag-no′sis) (*obs.*) serum diagnosis.

orogranulocyte (o″ro-gran′u-lo-sīt″) [*oro*-(1) + *granulocyte*] any of the polymorphonuclear leukocytes suspended in the mucus layer on the free surfaces of oral tissues.

orogranulocytic (o″ro-gran″u-lo-sit′ik) pertaining to orogranulocytes.

oro-immunity (o″ro-ĭ-mu′nĭ-te) [*oro*-(2) + *immunity*] passive immunity.

orokinase (o″ro-kin′ās) [*oro*-(1) + *kinase*] a kinase produced by the buccal glands of certain animals which converts inactive ptyalin into active ptyalin.

orolingual (o″ro-ling′gwal) [*oro*-(1) + L. *lingua* tongue] pertaining to the mouth and tongue.

oromaxillary (o″ro-mak′sĭ-ler″e) pertaining to the mouth and the maxillary region.

oromeningitis (or″o-men″in-ji′tis) orrhomeningitis.

oronasal (o″ro-na′zal) [*oro*-(1) + L. *nasus* nose] pertaining to the mouth and nose.

oropharynx (o″ro-far′inks) [*oro*-(1) + *pharynx*] that division of the pharynx which lies between the soft palate and the upper edge of the epiglottis (pars oralis pharyngis [NA]).

Oropsylla (o″ro-sil′ah) a genus of fleas. **O. idahoen′sis,** a rodent flea of the western United States, implicated in the transmission of sylvatic plague. **O. monta′na,** former name for *Diamanus montanus*. **O. silantiew′i,** a flea of the Manchuria marmot or tarbagan, capable of transmitting plague.

orosomucoid (or″ŏ-so-mu′koid) α_1-acid glycoprotein, a glycoprotein occurring in blood plasma.

orotherapy (o″ro-ther′ah-pe) [*oro*(2) + Gr. *therapeia* treatment] 1. whey cure; the treatment of disease by administering whey. 2. serotherapy.

oroticaciduria (o-rot″ik-as″ĭ-du′re-ah)   orotic aciduria; see under *aciduria*.

Oroya fever (o-ro′yah) [*Oroya*, a region in Peru]   see under *fever*.

orpanoxin (or″pah-nok′sin)   chemical name: 5-(4-chlorophenyl)-β-hydroxy-2-furanpropanoic acid; an anti-inflammatory, C_{13}-$H_{11}ClO_4$.

orphenadrine (or-fen′ah-drēn)   chemical name: *N,N*-dimethyl-2-(o-methyl-α-phenylbenzyl)oxyethylamine. The *ortho*-methyl analogue of diphenhydramine, $C_{18}H_{23}NO$; it possesses antihistaminic, antitremor, and antispasmodic activities. Called also *mephenamine*. **o. citrate** [USP], the citrate salt of orphenadrine, $C_{18}H_{23}NO·C_6H_8O_7$, occurring as a white, crystalline powder; used as a skeletal muscle relaxant in acute spasm of voluntary muscles, regardless of location, especially post-traumatic, discogenic, and tension spasms, administered orally, intramuscularly, and intravenously. **o. hydrochloride,** the hydrochloride salt of orphenadrine, $C_{18}H_{23}NO·HCl$, occurring as a white crystalline powder; used in the treatment of parkinsonism and drug-induced extrapyramidal reactions, administered orally.

Orr treatment (method, technic) [Hiram Winnett *Orr*, American orthopedic surgeon, 1877–1956]   see under *treatment*.

orrho- (or′o) [Gr. *orrhos* serum]   a combining form denoting relationship to serum.

orrhodiagnosis (or″o-di″ag-no′sis)   (*obs.*) serum diagnosis.

orrhoimmunity (or″o-ĭ-mu′nĭ-te) [*orrho-* + *immunity*]   passive immunity.

orrhology (or-ol′o-je) [*orrho-* + *-logy*]   the scientific study of serums; serology.

orrhomeningitis (or″o-men″in-ji′tis) [*orrho-* + *meningitis*]   inflammation of a serous membrane.

orrhoreaction (or″o-re-ak′shun) [*orrho-* + *reaction*]   seroreaction.

orrhorrhea (or-o-re′ah) [*orrho-* + Gr. *rhoia* flow]   (*obs.*) a watery or serous discharge.

orrhotherapeutic (or″o-ther″ah-pu′tik)   pertaining to or of the nature of orrhotherapy.

orrhotherapy (or″o-ther′ah-pe) [*orrho-* + *therapy*]   the therapeutic use of serums; serotherapy.

orris (or′is)   1. any of several species of herbs of the genus *Iris*, especially *I. florentina* L. (Iridaceae).   2. orris root: the peeled, dried, and powdered, fragrant root of *Iris florentina* and other species of *Iris;* used in dentifrices, toilet and dusting powders, perfumery, etc.

O.R.S.   Orthopedic Research Society.

Orsi-Grocco method (or″se-grok′o) [Francesco *Orsi*, 1828–1890; Pietro *Grocco*, 1857–1916, Italian physicians]   see under *method*.

orthergasia (or″ther-ga′ze-ah) [*ortho-* + Gr. *ergon* work]   a condition of normal mental functioning and adjustment; euergasia.

orthesis (or-the′sis), pl. *orthe′ses.*   Orthosis.

orthetic (or-thet′ik)   orthotic.

orthetics (or-thet′iks)   orthotics.

orthetist (or′thĕ-tist)   orthotist.

ortho- (or′tho) [Gr. *orthos* straight]   a combining form meaning straight, normal, correct, etc. In chemistry, this prefix indicates an isomer; also a cyclic derivative which has two substituents in adjacent positions.

ortho-acid (or″tho-as′id)   an acid containing as many hydroxyl groups as the valence of the acidulous element.

orthoarteriotony (or″tho-ar-te″re-ot′o-ne) [*ortho-* + Gr. *artēria* artery + *tonos* tension]   normal arterial pressure.

orthobiosis (or″tho-bi-o′sis) [*ortho-* + Gr. *biōsis* way of life]   proper living; living in accordance with all the laws of health.

orthocephalic (or″tho-sĕ-fal′ik) [Gr. *orthos* straight + *kephalē* head]   having a head with a vertical index of 70.1 to 75.

orthocephalous (or″tho-sef′ah-lus)   orthocephalic.

orthochorea (or″tho-ko-re′ah) [*ortho-* + *chorea*]   choreic movements in the erect posture.

orthochromatic (or″tho-kro-mat′ik)   1. normally colored or stained.   2. denoting a photographic emulsion sensitive to all colors except red.

orthochromia (or″tho-kro′me-ah) [*ortho-* + Gr. *chrōma* color + *-ia*]   normal hemoglobin content of the erythrocytes.

orthochromophil (or″tho-kro′mo-fil) [*ortho-* + Gr. *chrōma* color + *philein* to love]   staining normally with neutral stains.

orthocrasia (or″tho-kra′se-ah) [*ortho-* + Gr. *krasis* a mixing + *-ia*]   (*obs.*) a state in which the body reacts normally to ingested or injected drugs, proteins, etc.

orthocresol (or″tho-kre′sol)   one of the three isomeric forms of cresol.

orthocytosis (or″tho-si-to′sis) [*ortho-* + *-cyte* + *-osis*]   the presence of mature cells only in the blood.

orthodactylous (or″tho-dak′tĭ-lus) [*ortho-* + Gr. *daktylos* finger]   having straight digits.

orthodentin (or″tho-den′tin) [*ortho-* + *dentin*]   straight-tubed dentin, as seen in the teeth of mammals.

orthodeoxia (or″tho-de-ok′se-ah)   accentuation of arterial hypoxemia in the erect position, improved by assumption of a recumbent position.

orthodiagram (or″tho-di′ah-gram)   the print or record made by an orthodiagraph; the silhouette of an organ as traced in orthodiagraphy.

orthodiagraph (or″tho-di′ah-graf) [*ortho-* + Gr. *dia* through + *graphein* to write]   a radiographic apparatus for recording accurately the form and size of structures inside the body, doing away with the distortion of the ordinary roentgen-ray plate; called also *orthoskiagraph.*

orthodiagraphy (or″tho-di-ag′rah-fe)   the use of the orthodiagraph; called also *orthoskiagraphy.*

orthodiascope (or″tho-di′ah-skōp)   an instrument for orthodiascopy.

orthodiascopy (or″tho-di-as′ko-pe)   undistorted fluoroscopy, especially the direct tracing of the silhouette of an organ (e.g., the heart) as projected on a fluoroscopic screen.

orthodichlorobenzene (or″tho-di-klo″ro-ben′zēn)   an insecticide, $C_6H_4Cl_2$, used as a spray.

orthodigita (or″tho-dij′ĭ-tah) [*ortho-* + L. *digitus* finger or toe]   the art of correcting deformities of the toes and fingers.

orthodontia (or″tho-don′she-ah)   orthodontics.

orthodontic (or″tho-don′tik)   pertaining to the proper positioning and relationship of the teeth.

orthodontics (or″tho-don′tiks) [*ortho-* + Gr. *odous* tooth]   that branch of dentistry which deals with the development, prevention, and correction of irregularities of the teeth and malocclusion, and with associated facial abnormalities.   **corrective o.,** that phase of orthodontics which is concerned with the reduction or elimination of an existing malocclusion and its attendant sequelae.   **interceptive o.,** that phase of orthodontics which is concerned with elimination of a condition which might lead to the development of malocclusion.   **preventive o.,** that phase of orthodontics which is concerned with preservation of the integrity of what appears to be normal occlusion.

orthodontist (or″tho-don′tist)   a dentist who specializes in orthodontics.

orthodontology (or″tho-don-tol′o-je)   orthodontics.

orthodromic (or″tho-drom′ik) [Gr. *orthodromein* to run straight forward]   conducting impulses in the normal direction; said of nerve fibers. Cf. *antidromic.*

orthogenesis (or″tho-jen′ĕ-sis) [*ortho-* + *genesis*]   1. progressive evolution in a given direction, in contrast with variations in several directions.   2. the theory that the course of evolution is fixed and predetermined; monogenesis.

orthogenics (or″tho-jen′iks) [*ortho-* + Gr. *genikos* sexual]   eugenics.

orthoglycemic (or″tho-gli-se′mik) [*ortho-* + Gr. *glykys* sweet + *haima* blood]   having the normal amount of sugar in the blood.

Orthognatha (or-thog′nah-thah)   a suborder of spiders (order Araneae) of temperate and tropical areas of the world; Theraphosidae and Dipluridae are families of medical importance.

orthognathia (or″thog-nath′e-ah)   orthognathics.

orthognathic (or″thog-na′thik)   1. pertaining to orthognathics.   2. orthognathous.

orthognathics (or″thog-na′thiks)   the science dealing with the cause and treatment of malposition of the bones of the jaw.

orthognathous (or-thog′nah-thus) [*ortho-* + Gr. *gnathos* jaw]   having a gnathic index of less than 98.

orthograde (or′tho-grād) [*ortho-* + L. *gradi* to walk]   characterized by walking with the body upright; said of bipeds. Cf. *pronograde.*

orthomelic (or″tho-me′lik) [*ortho-* + Gr. *melos* limb]   correcting deformities of the limbs.

orthometer (or-thom′ĕ-ter) [*ortho-* + Gr. *metron* measure]   an instrument for finding the relative protrusion of the two eyeballs.

orthomolecular (or″tho-mo-lek′u-lar) [*ortho-* + *molecular*]   relating to or aimed at restoring the optimal concentrations and functions at the molecular level of the substances (e.g., vitamins) normally present in the body.

orthomorphia (or″tho-mor′fe-ah) [*ortho-* + Gr. *morphē* form]   the surgical and mechanical correction of deformities.

orthomyxovirus (or″tho-mik″so-vi′rus)   a subgroup of the myxoviruses that includes the viruses of human and animal influenza; cf. *paramyxovirus.*

orthoneutrophil (or″tho-nu′tro-fil)   orthochromophil.

orthopaedic (or″tho-pe′dik)   orthopedic.

orthopaedics (or″tho-pe′diks) orthopedics.

orthopantograph (or″tho-pan′to-graf″) panoramic radiograph.

Orthopantomograph (or″tho-pan′to-mo-graf) trademark for the equipment used in panoramic radiography.

orthopedic (or″tho-pe′dik) [*ortho-* + Gr. *pais* child] pertaining to the correction of deformities of the musculoskeletal system; pertaining to orthopedics.

orthopedics (or″tho-pe′diks) [*ortho-* + Gr. *pais* child] that branch of surgery which is specially concerned with the preservation and restoration of the function of the skeletal system, its articulations and associated structures. **dental o., dentofacial o.,** orthodontics; the correction of malformations of the face and jaws. **functional jaw o.,** utilization of muscle forces to effect changes in jaw position and tooth alignment by removable appliances, such as a function corrector or monobloc activator.

orthopedist (or″tho-pe′dist) an orthopedic surgeon.

orthopercussion (or″tho-per-kush′un) [*ortho-* + *percussion*] percussion in which the distal phalanx of the pleximeter finger is held perpendicularly to the chest wall.

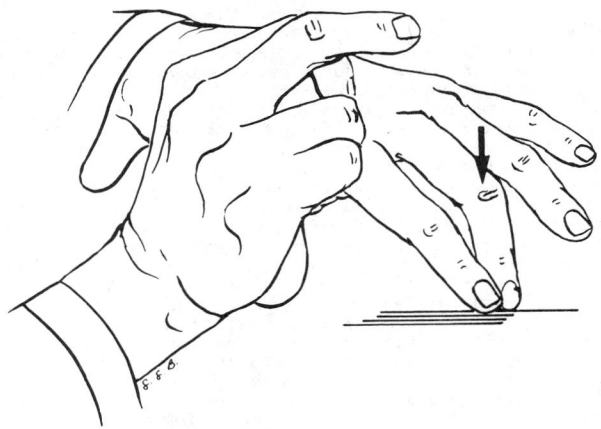

Orthopercussion.

orthophenanthrolene (or′tho-fe-nan′thro-lēn) a white powder, $C_{12}H_8N_2 \cdot H_2O$, used as an indicator.

orthophenolase (or″tho-fe′nol-ās) an enzyme in sweet potatoes which oxidizes catechol and orthocresol.

orthophony (or-thof′o-ne) [*ortho-* + Gr. *phōnē* voice] the direct and correct production of sound.

orthophoria (or″tho-fo′re-ah) [*ortho-* + Gr. *pherein* to bear + *-ia*] the normal or proper placement of organs, especially the condition in which visual axes remain parallel after the visual fusional stimuli have been partially or entirely eliminated. **asthenic o.,** general weakness of the eye muscles.

orthophoric (or″tho-for′ik) pertaining to or marked by orthophoria.

orthophosphate (or″tho-fos′fāt) a salt of orthophosphoric acid; a compound of the type M_3PO_4.

orthophrenia (or″tho-fre′ne-ah) [*ortho-* + Gr. *phrēn* mind + *-ia*] the condition of normal mental reactivity in social relations.

orthopia (or-tho′pe-ah) the prevention or correction of strabismus.

orthoplessimeter (or″tho-ple-sim′ĕ-ter) an instrument to take the place of the pleximeter finger in orthopercussion.

orthopnea (or″thop-ne′ah) [*ortho-* + Gr. *pnoia* breath] difficult breathing except in an upright position. Cf. *platypnea.* **two-pillow o.,** see under *position.*

orthopneic (or″thop-ne′ik) pertaining to or marked by orthopnea.

orthopod (or′tho-pod) orthopedist.

orthopraxis (or″tho-prak′sis) orthopraxy.

orthopraxy (or′tho-prak-se) [*ortho-* + Gr. *prassein* to make] the mechanical correction of deformities.

orthopsychiatry (or″tho-si-ki′ah-tre) [*ortho-* + *psychiatry*] that branch of psychiatry which deals with mental and emotional development, embracing child psychiatry and mental hygiene.

Orthoptera (or-thop′ter-ah) [*ortho-* + Gr. *pteron* wing] an order of biting insects which do not undergo metamorphosis; they include the grasshoppers, locusts, crickets, and cockroaches.

orthoptic (or-thop′tik) [*ortho-* + Gr. *optikos* of or for sight] correcting obliquity of one or both visual axes.

orthoptics (or-thop′tiks) a technique of eye exercises designed to correct the visual axes of eyes not properly coordinated for binocular vision.

orthoptist (or-thop′tist) an expert in orthoptics.

orthoptoscope (or-thop′to-skōp) [*ortho-* + Gr. *op-* to see + *skopein* to examine] an instrument for orthoptic or exercise treatment in anomalies of the ocular muscles.

orthorhombic (or″tho-rom′bik) having three unequal axes intersected at right angles.

orthoroentgenography (or″tho-rent″gen-og′rah-fe) orthodiagraphy.

orthorrhachic (or″tho-rak′ik) [*ortho-* + Gr. *rhachis* spine] having a vertebral column with practically no curvature in the lumbar region; cf. *koilorrhachic* and *kyrotorrhachic.*

orthoscope (or′tho-skōp) [*ortho-* + Gr. *skopein* to examine] an apparatus which neutralizes the corneal refraction by means of a layer of water; it is used in examining the eye.

orthoscopic (or″tho-skop′ik) affording a correct and undistorted view.

orthoscopy (or-thos′ko-pe) examination of the eye by means of the orthoscope.

orthosis (or-tho′sis), pl. ortho′ses [Gr. *orthōsis* making straight] an orthopedic appliance or apparatus used to support, align, prevent, or correct deformities or to improve the function of movable parts of the body.

orthoskiagraph (or″tho-ski′ah-graf) orthodiagraph.

orthoskiagraphy (or″tho-ski-ag′rah-fe) orthodiagraphy.

orthostatic (or″tho-stat′ik) [*ortho-* + Gr. *statikos* causing to stand] pertaining to or caused by standing erect.

orthostatism (or′tho-stat″izm) an erect standing position of the body.

orthostereoscope (or″tho-ste′re-o-skōp) an apparatus for stereoscopic radiography.

orthosympathetic (or″tho-sim″pah-thet′ik) a term applied to the sympathetic (thoracolumbar) division of the autonomic nervous system as contrasted with the parasympathetic (craniosacral) division.

orthotast (or′tho-tast) [*ortho-* + Gr. *tassein* to arrange] an apparatus for straightening curvatures of bones.

orthoterion (or″tho-te′re-on) [Gr. *orthōtēr* one who sets straight] a device for use in straightening crooked limbs.

orthotherapy (or″tho-ther′ah-pe) [*ortho-* + *therapy*] treatment of disorders by correction of posture.

orthotic (or-thot′ik) serving to protect or to restore or improve function; pertaining to the use or application of orthoses.

orthotics (or-thot′iks) the field of knowledge relating to orthoses and their use.

orthotist (or′tho-tist) [Gr. *orthōtēr* a restorer or preserver] a person skilled in orthotics and practicing its application in individual cases.

ortho-tolueno-azo-beta-naphthol (or″tho-tol″u-ēn′o-az″o-ba″tah-naf′thol) a poisonous dye used in processing citrus fruits.

orthotonos (or-thot′o-nos) [*ortho-* + Gr. *tonos* tension] tetanic fixation of the head, body, and limbs in a rigid straight line.

orthotonus (or-thot′o-nus) orthotonos.

orthotopic (or″tho-top′ik) [*ortho-* + Gr. *topos* place] occurring at the normal place or upon the proper part of the body; in tissue transplantation, said of a graft transferred to a position formerly occupied by tissue of the same kind.

orthotyphoid (or″tho-ti′foid) typhoid fever as distinguished from paratyphoid.

orthovoltage (or″tho-vol′tij) in x-ray therapy, voltage in the range of 140 to 400 kilovolts; cf. *supervoltage.*

Orthoxine (or-thok′sēn) trademark for preparations of methoxyphenamine.

orthropsia (or-throp′se-ah) [Gr. *orthros* the time just about daybreak + *opsis* vision] the ability of the human eye to see better during dawn or twilight than in bright sunlight.

orthuria (or-thu′re-ah) [*ortho-* + Gr. *ouron* urine + *-ia*] normal frequency of urination.

Oryza (o-ri′zah) [L.; Gr. *oryza* rice] a genus of cereal plants; *O. sativa* produces rice.

oryzenin (o-ri′zĕ-nin) [Gr. *oryza* rice] 1. an extractive from rice bran. 2. a glutelin from rice.

O.S. abbreviation for L. *oc′ulus sinis′ter,* left eye.

Os chemical symbol for *osmium.*

os¹ (os), gen. *o′ris,* pl. *o′ra* [L. "an opening, or mouth"] any orifice of the body; [NA] the mouth; the anterior or proximal opening of the digestive apparatus. See *mouth.* **o. exter′num u′teri,** ostium uteri. **o. of uterus, external,** ostium uteri.

os² (os), gen. *os′sis,* pl. *os′sa* [L.] bone; [NA] a general term which is qualified by the appropriate adjective to designate a specific type of bony structure or a specific segment of the skeleton. **o. acetab′uli,** acetabulum. **o. acromia′le,** a movable joint between the spine of the scapula and the epiphysis of the acromion. **o. acromia′le seconda′rium,** a round structure appearing in the roentgenogram just above the tuberosity of the humerus.

o. basila're, a term applied to the sphenoid and occipital bones. **o. bre've** [NA], short bone: any bone whose main dimensions are approximately equal. **o. cal'cis,** NA alternative of *calcaneus.* **o. capita'tum** [NA], capitate bone: the bone in the distal row of carpal bones lying between the trapezoid and hamate bones. **o. carpa'le dista'le pri'mum,** o. trapezium. **o. carpa'le dista'le quar'tum,** o. hamatum. **o. carpa'le dista'le secun'dum,** o. trapezoideum. **o. carpa'le dista'le ter'tium,** o. capitatum. **os'sa car'pi** [NA], carpal bones: the eight bones of the wrist (carpus), including the o. capitatum, o. hamatum, o. lunatum, o. pisiforme, o. scaphoideum, o. trapezium, o. trapezoideum, and o. triquetrum. **o. centra'le** [NA], central bone: an accessory bone sometimes found on the back of the carpus. **o. centra'le tar'si,** o. naviculare. **o. coc'cygis** [NA], coccygeal bone: the small bone caudad to the sacrum in man, formed by union of four (sometimes five or three) rudimentary vertebrae, and forming the caudal extremity of the vertebral column; called also *coccyx.* **o. coro'nae,** the small pastern bone of the horse. **o. costa'le** [NA], a rib bone. **o. cox'ae** [NA], the hip bone, which comprises the ilium, ischium, and pubis. **os'sa cra'nii** [NA], cranial bones: the bones of the cranium, or skull, including the occipital, sphenoidal, temporal, parietal, frontal, ethmoidal, lacrimal, and nasal bones, the concha nasalis, and vomer. **o. cuboi'deum** [NA], cuboid bone: a bone on the lateral side of the tarsus between the calcaneus and the fourth and fifth metatarsal bones. **o. cuneifor'me interme'dium** [NA], intermediate cuneiform bone: the intermediate and smallest of the three wedge-shaped tarsal bones located medial to the cuboid and between the navicular and the first three metatarsal bones; called also *o. cuneiforme secundum.* **o. cuneifor'me latera'le** [NA], lateral cuneiform bone: the most lateral of the three wedge-shaped tarsal bones located medial to the cuboid and between the navicular and the first three metatarsal bones; called also *o. cuneiforme tertium.* **o. cuneifor'me media'le** [NA], medial cuneiform bone: the medial and largest of the three wedge-shaped tarsal bones located medial to the cuboid and between the navicular and the first three metatarsal bones; called also *o. cuneiforme primum.* **o. cuneifor'me pri'mum,** o. cuneiforme mediale. **o. cuneifor'me secun'dum,** o. cuneiforme intermedium. **o. cuneifor'me ter'tium,** o. cuneiforme laterale. **os'sa digito'rum ma'nus** [NA], the 14 bones that compose the skeleton of the fingers; called also *phalanges digitorum manus* or *phalanges of fingers.* **os'sa digito'rum pe'dis** [NA], the 14 bones that compose the skeleton of the toes; called also *phalanges digitorum pedis* or *phalanges of toes.* **o. epitympan'icum,** a bone of very early fetal life which becomes the posterior portion of the squama that aids in forming the mastoid cells. **o. ethmoida'le** [NA], ethmoid bone: the cubical bone located between the orbits and consisting of the lamina cribrosa, the lamina perpendicularis, and the paired lateral masses. **os'sa extremita'tis inferio'ris,** ossa membri inferioris. **os'sa extremita'tis superio'ris,** ossa membri superioris. **os'sa fa'ciei** [NA], facial bones: the bones that constitute the facial part of the skull, including the maxilla, palatine bone, zygomatic bone, mandible, and hyoid bone. **o. fronta'le** [NA], frontal bone: a single bone that closes the front part of the cranial cavity and forms the skeleton of the forehead; it is developed from two halves, the line of separation sometimes persisting in adult life. **o. hama'tum** [NA], hamate bone: the medial bone in the distal row of carpal bones. **o. hyoi'deum** [NA], hyoid bone: a horseshoe-shaped bone situated at the base of the tongue, just above the thyroid cartilage. **o. il'ium** [NA], the ilium: the expansive superior portion of the hip bone (os coxae); it is a separate bone in early life. **o. in'cae,** o. interparietale. **o. incisi'vum** [NA], incisive bone: the portion of the maxilla that bears the incisor teeth. Developmentally it is the premaxilla, which in the human subsequently fuses with the maxilla proper to form the adult bone. In most other vertebrates it persists as an independent bone. **o. innomina'tum,** o. coxae. **o. intercuneifor'me,** an occasionally occurring bone situated between the medial and intermediate cuneiform bones. **o. interme'dium,** o. lunatum. **o. intermetatar'seum,** an occasionally occurring accessory bone situated between the proximal ends of the first and second metatarsal bones. **o. interparieta'le** [NA], interparietal bone: the part of the squama of the occipital bone that lies superior to the highest nuchal line when this portion remains separate throughout life. **o. is'chii** [NA], the ischium: the inferior dorsal portion of the hip bone (os coxae); it is a separate bone in early life. **o. lacrima'le** [NA], lacrimal bone: a thin scalelike bone at the anterior part of the medial wall of the orbit, articulating with the frontal and ethmoid bones and the maxilla and inferior nasal concha. **o. lon'gum** [NA], long bone: any bone whose length exceeds its breadth and thickness, as the bones of the limbs. **o. luna'tum** [NA], lunate bone: the bone in the proximal row of carpal bones lying between the scaphoid and triquetral bones. **o. mag'num,** o. capitatum. **o. mastoi'deum,** pars mastoidea ossis temporalis. **os'sa mem'bri inferio'ris** [NA], the bones of the lower limb; called also *ossa extremitatis inferioris.* **os'sa mem'bri superio'ris** [NA], the bones of the upper limb; called also *ossa extremitatis superioris.* **os'sa metacarpa'lia I–V** [NA], metacarpal bones: the five cylindric bones of the hand, articulat-

ing proximally with bones of the carpus and distally with the proximal phalanges of the fingers; numbered from that articulating with the proximal phalanx of the thumb to the most lateral one, articulating with the proximal phalanx of the little finger. *Os metacarpale III,* the middle metacarpal bone, is characterized by the presence of the styloid process at its base. **os'sa metatarsa'lia I–V** [NA], metatarsal bones: the five bones that extend from the tarsus to the phalanges of the toes, being numbered in the same sequence from the most medial to the most lateral. **o. multan'gulum ma'jus,** o. trapezium. **o. multan'gulum mi'nus,** o. trapezoideum. **o. nasa'le** [NA], nasal bone: either of the two small, oblong bones that together form the bridge of the nose. **o. navicula're** [NA], navicular bone: the ovoid-shaped tarsal bone that is situated between the talus and the three cuneiform bones; called also *o. naviculare pedis.* **o. navicula're ma'nus,** o. scaphoideum. **o. navicula're pe'dis,** o. naviculare. **o. navicula're ped'is retarda'tum,** see *Kohler's bone disease* (def. 1), under *disease.* **o. no'vum,** Orell's name for new bone produced following the subperiosteal implantation of os purum. **o. occipita'le** [NA], occipital bone: a single trapezoid-shaped bone situated at the posterior and inferior part of the cranium, articulating with the two parietal and two temporal bones, the sphenoid bone, and the atlas; it contains a large opening, the foramen magnum. **o. orbicula're,** 1. processus lenticularis incudis. 2. os pisiforme. **os in os,** a radiation-induced injury appearing on roentgenograms as a vertebra within a vertebra. **o. palati'num** [NA], palatine bone: the irregularly shaped bone forming the posterior part of the hard palate, the lateral wall of the nasal fossa between the medial pterygoid plate and the maxilla, and the posterior part of the floor of the orbit. **o. parieta'le** [NA], parietal bone: either of the two quadrilateral bones forming part of the superior and lateral surfaces of the skull, and joining each other in the midline at the sagittal suture. **o. pe'dis,** the coffin bone of the horse. **o. pe'nis,** baculum. **o. perone'um,** a sesamoid bone sometimes formed in the tendon of the peroneus longus muscle. **o. pisifor'me** [NA], pisiform bone: the medial bone of the proximal row of carpal bones. **o. pla'num,** 1. [NA], flat bone: any bone whose thickness is slight, sometimes consisting of only a thin layer of compact bone, or two layers with intervening spongy bone and marrow; usually bent or curved, rather than flat. 2. Lamina orbitalis ossis ethmoidalis. **o. pneumat'icum** [NA], pneumatic bone: a bone that contains air-filled cavities or sinuses. **o. pri'api,** baculum. **o. pu'bis** [NA], pubic bone: the anterior inferior part of the hip bone (os coxae) on either side, articulating with its fellow in the anterior midline at the pubic symphysis; it is a separate bone in early life; called also *pubis.* **o. pu'rum,** Orell's name for bone freed from connective tissue and fat, used for bone grafting; see also *os novum.* **o. radia'le,** o. scaphoideum. **o. sa'crum** [NA], the sacrum: the wedge-shaped bone formed usually by five fused vertebrae that are lodged dorsally between the two hip bones (ossa coxae). **o. scaphoi'deum** [NA], scaphoid bone: the most lateral bone of the proximal row of carpal bones; called also *o. naviculare manus.* **o. sedenta'rium,** tuber ischiadicum. **os'sa sesamoi'dea,** sesamoid bones: a type of short bone occurring mainly in the hands and feet, and found embedded in tendons and joint capsules. **os'sa sesamoi'dea ma'nus** [NA], the sesamoid bones of the hand. **os'sa sesamoi'dea pe'dis** [NA], the sesamoid bones of the foot. **o. sphenoida'le** [NA], sphenoid bone: a single irregular, wedge-shaped bone at the base of the skull, forming a part of the floor of the anterior, middle, and posterior cranial fossae. **o. subtibia'le,** an occasionally occurring bone found over the tip of the medial malleolus. **os'sa suprasterna'lia** [NA], suprasternal bones: ossicles occasionally occurring in the ligaments of the sternoclavicular articulation. **os'sa sutura'rum** [NA], sutural bones: small irregular bones in the sutures between the bones of the skull. **os'sa tarsa'lia,** ossa tarsi. **o. tarsa'le dista'le pri'mum,** o. cuneiforme mediale. **o. tarsa'le dista'le quar'tum,** o. cuboideum. **o. tarsa'le dista'le secun'dum,** o. cuneiforme intermedium. **o. tarsa'le dista'le ter'tium,** o. cuneiforme laterale. **os'sa tar'si** [NA], tarsal bones: the seven bones of the ankle (tarsus), including the calcaneus, o. cuboideum, ossa cuneiformia intermedium, laterale, and mediale, o. naviculare, and talus. **o. tar'si fibula're,** calcaneus. **o. tar'si tibia're,** talus, def. 1. **o. tempora'le** [NA], temporal bone: one of the two irregular bones forming part of the lateral surfaces and base of the skull, and containing the organs of hearing. **o. tibia'le exter'num,** a small anomalous bone situated in the angle between the navicular bone and the head of the talus. **o. trape'zium** [NA], trapezium bone: the most lateral bone of the distal row of carpal bones; called also *o. multangulum majus.* **o. trapezoi'deum** [NA], trapezoid bone: the bone in the distal row of carpal bones lying between the trapezium and capitate bones; called also *o. multangulum minus.* **o. trigo'num tar'si** [NA], triangular bone of tarsus: an external tubercle at the back of the talus, sometimes occurring as a separate bone. **o. trique'trum** [NA], triquetral bone: the bone in the proximal row of carpal bones lying between the lunate and pisiform bones; called also *triangular bone.* **o. un'guis,** o. lacrimale. **o. vesalia'num pe'dis,** vesalian bone: the proximal and external part of the tuberosity of the fifth metatarsal bone. **os′sa Wor′mi,** ossa suturarum. **o. zygomat′icum** [NA], zygomatic bone: the quadrangular bone of the cheek, articulating with the frontal bone, the maxilla, the zygomatic process of the temporal bone, and the great wing of the sphenoid bone.

O.S.A. Optical Society of America.

osamine (ōs′ah-mēn) a sugar with an amino group replacing one of the hydroxyl groups, e.g., glucosamine.

osazone (o′sa-zōn) any of a series of compounds obtained by heating a sugar with phenylhydrazine and acetic acid; see *glucosazone.*

Osbil (os′bil) trademark for a preparation of iobenzamic acid.

oscedo (os-se′do) [L.] the act of yawning.

oscheal (os′ke-al) [Gr. *oscheon* scrotum] pertaining to the scrotum.

oscheitis (os″ke-i′tis) [*oscheo-* + *-itis*] inflammation of the scrotum.

oschelephantiasis (osk″el-ĕ-fan-ti′ah-sis) elephantiasis of the scrotum.

oscheo- (os′ke-o) [Gr. *oscheon* scrotum] a combining form denoting relationship to the scrotum.

oscheocele (os′ke-o-sēl″) [*oscheo-* + Gr. *kēlē* hernia, tumor] 1. tumor or swelling of the scrotum. 2. (*obs.*) scrotal hernia.

oscheohydrocele (os″ke-o-hi′dro-sēl) [*oscheo-* + *hydrocele*] hydrocele in the sac of a scrotal hernia.

oscheolith (os′ke-o-lith) [*oscheo-* + Gr. *lithos* stone] a concretion in the sebaceous glands of the scrotum.

oscheoma (os″ke-o′mah) [*oscheo-* + *-oma*] a tumor of the scrotum.

oscheoncus (os″ke-ong′kus) [*oscheo-* + Gr. *onkos* mass, bulk] oscheoma.

oscheoplasty (os′ke-o-plas″te) [*oscheo-* + Gr. *plassein* to mold] plastic surgery of the scrotum.

oschitis (os-ki′tis) oscheitis.

Oscillaria (os″ĭ-la′re-ah) a genus of algae.

oscillation (os″ĭ-la′shun) [L. *oscillare* to swing] a backward and forward motion, like a pendulum; also vibration, fluctuation, or variation. **bradykinetic o.,** slow, recurring, choreiform movements seen in epidemic encephalitis.

oscillator (os′ĭ-la″tor) an apparatus for producing oscillations; an electric circuit designed to generate alternating current at a particular frequency.

oscillo- (os′ĭ-lo) [L. *oscillare* to swing] a combining form denoting relationship to oscillation.

oscillogram (o-sil′o-gram) the graphic record made by an oscillograph.

oscillograph (o-sil′o-graf) [*oscillo-* + Gr. *graphein* to write] an instrument for recording electric oscillations. Such an instrument, working on the plan of a string galvanometer, is used in recording the action of the heart.

oscillometer (os″ĭ-lom′ĕ-ter) an instrument for measuring oscillations of any kind, such as changes in the volume of the arteries accompanying the heart beat.

oscillometric (os″ĭ-lo-met′rik) pertaining to oscillometry or the oscillometer.

oscillometry (os″ĭ-lom′ĕ-tre) the use of the string galvanometer or similar apparatus.

oscillopsia (os″ĭ-lop′se-ah) [*oscillo-* + Gr. *opsis* vision + *-ia*] oscillating vision, a condition in which objects seem to move back and forth, to jerk, or to wiggle. It occurs in multiple sclerosis.

oscilloscope (ŏ-sil′o-skōp) [*oscillo-* + Gr. *skopein* to examine] an instrument that displays a visual representation of electrical variations on the fluorescent screen of a cathode-ray tube.

Oscillospira (os″sil-lo-spi′rah) a genus of Schizomycetes (order Caryophanales, family Oscillospiracae).

Oscillospiraceae (os″sil-lo-spi-ra′se-e) a family of Schizomycetes (order Caryophanales), made up of motile or nonmotile cells occurring in filaments of varying lengths each containing a central chromatin body, and found as nonpathogenic parasites in the intestinal tract of vertebrates. It includes a single genus, *Oscillospi′ra.*

oscine (os′in) a substance, $CH_3 \cdot N:C_6H_8:CH \cdot O$, obtained on the decomposition of scopolamine.

Oscinis pallipes (os′ĭ-nis pal′ĭ-pēz) *Hippelatus pallipes.*

oscitate (os′ĭ-tāt) to yawn.

oscitation (os″ĭ-ta′shun) [L. *oscitatio*] the act of yawning.

osculum (os′ku-lum), pl. *os′cula* [L.] a small aperture or minute opening.

-ose a suffix indicating that the substance is a carbohydrate.

Osgood-Haskins test (oz′good-haz′kinz) [Edwin Eugene *Osgood*, American physician, born 1899; Howard Davis *Haskins*, American physician, 1871–1933] see under *tests.*

Osgood-Schlatter disease (oz′good-shlat′er) [Robert Bayley *Osgood*, Boston orthopedist, born 1873; Carl *Schlatter*, surgeon in Zurich, 1864–1934] see under *disease.*

-osis a word termination denoting a process, especially a disease or morbid process, and sometimes conveying the meaning of abnormal increase. See also *-sis.*

Osler's disease, nodes, phenomenon, sign, triad (ōs′lerz) [Sir William *Osler*, Canadian-born physician, 1849–1919; successively professor of medicine in McGill University, the University of Pennsylvania, Johns Hopkins University, and the University of Oxford] see *hereditary hemorrhagic telangiectasia,* under *telangiectasia,* see *polycythemia vera,* and see under *node, phenomenon, sign,* and *triad.*

Osler-Vaquez disease (ōs′ler-vak-āz′) [Sir William *Osler;* Louis Henri *Vaquez,* French physician, 1860–1936] polycythemia vera.

Osler-Weber-Rendu disease (os′ler-web′er-ron-duh′) [Sir William *Osler;* Frederick Parkes *Weber,* British physician, 1863–1962; Henri Jules Louis Marie *Rendu,* French physician, 1844–1902] hereditary hemorrhagic telangiectasia.

Oslo meal (breakfast) [*Oslo,* Norway] see under *meal.*

osmate (oz′māt) a salt of osmic acid.

osmatic (oz-mat′ik) [Gr. *osmasthai* to smell] 1. pertaining to the sense of smell. 2. having a sense of smell; applied to a category of animals subdivided further into macrosmatic and microsmatic. Cf. *anosmatic.*

osmazome (oz′mah-zōm) [Gr. *osmē* odor + *zōmos* broth] a principle derivable from muscular fiber which gives the peculiar flavor and odor to roast meats and gravies.

osmesis (oz-me′sis) [Gr. *osmēsis* smelling] the act of smelling.

osmesthesia (oz″mes-the′ze-ah) [*osmo-* + Gr. *aisthēsis* perception] olfactory sensibility; ability to perceive and distinguish odors.

osmic (oz′mik) containing osmium.

osmicate (oz′mĭ-kāt) to stain or impregnate with osmic acid.

osmics (oz′miks) [Gr. *osmē* odor] the pure and applied science relating to the olfactory organs and the sense of smell, and to odoriferous organs and substances.

osmidrosis (oz″mĭ-dro′sis) [*osmo-*(1) + Gr. *hidrōs* sweat] bromhidrosis.

osmification (oz″mĭ-fĭ-ka′shun) treatment with osmium or osmic acid, as in histologic technic.

osmiophilic (oz″me-o-fil′ik) [*osmic* acid + Gr. *philein* to love] staining easily with osmium or osmic acid.

osmiophobic (oz″me-o-fo′bik) [*osmic* acid + *phobia*] resistant to staining with osmium or osmic acid.

Osmitrol (oz′mĭ-trōl) trademark for a preparation of mannitol.

osmium (oz′me-um) [Gr. *osmē* odor; so named because of the odor of the vapor, OsO_4, produced by oxidation of the element] 1. a very hard, gray, toxic, and nearly infusible metal; atomic number, 76; atomic weight, 190.2; symbol, Os. See *acid, osmic.* 2. a homeopathic trituration of metallic osmium. **o. tetroxide,** colorless or slightly yellow cyrstals or crystalline granules with a pungent odor, OsO_4, used as a fixative in preparing histologic specimens.

osmo- (oz′mo) 1. [Gr. *osmē* smell] a combining form denoting relationship to odors. 2. [Gr. *ōsmos* impulse] a combining form denoting relationship to an impulse, or to osmosis.

osmoceptor (oz′mo-sep′tor) osmoreceptor.

osmodysphoria (oz″mo-dis-fo′re-ah) [*osmo-*(1) + *dys-* + Gr. *pherein* to bear] (*obs.*) an intense and abnormal dislike of certain odors.

osmol (oz′mōl) the standard unit of osmotic pressure, being equal to the gram molecular weight divided by the number of particles or ions into which a substance dissociates in solution. Written also *osmole.* See also *milliosmol.*

osmolagnia (oz″mo-lag′ne-ah) [*osmo-*(1) + Gr. *lagneia* lust] (*obs.*) sexual excitation produced by odor.

osmolality (oz″mo-lal′ĭ-te) a property of a solution which depends on the concentration of the solute per unit of solvent.

osmolar (oz-mo′lar) pertaining to the concentration of osmotically active particles in solution.

osmolarity (oz″mo-lār′ĭ-te) the concentration of osmotically active particles in solution.

osmole (oz′mōl) osmol.

osmology (oz-mol′o-je) 1. [Gr. *osmē* smell + *-logy*] osphresiology. 2. [Gr. *ōsmos* impulse + *-logy*] that branch of physics that treats of osmosis.

osmometer (oz-mom′ĕ-ter) 1. [Gr. *ōsmos* impulse + *metron* measure] a device for measuring osmotic force. 2. [Gr. *osmē* smell + *metron* measure] an instrument for measuring the acuteness of the sense of smell. **freezing-point o.,** an osmometer using freezing-point depression measurement for analysis of osmotic pressure (number of particles, molecules, or ions) of solutions. **Hepp o.,** an osmometer in which very small quantities of material can be used and a direct reading of the osmotic pressure may be made. **membrane o.,** an osmometer in which diffusion through a semipermeable membrane indicates the osmotic pressure of macromolecules (number of molecules or ions) in a solution.

osmonosology (oz″mo-no-sol′o-je) [osmo-(1) + nosology] the study of disorders of the sense of smell.

osmophilic (oz″mo-fil′ik) [osmo-(2) + Gr. philein to love] having an affinity for solutions with a high osmotic pressure.

osmophore (oz′mo-fōr) [osmo-(1) + Gr. phoros bearing] the group of atoms in a molecule of a compound which is responsible for its characteristic odor.

osmoreceptor (oz″mo-re-cep′tor) 1. [osmo-(2)] any of a group of specialized neurons in the supraoptic nuclei of the hypothalamus that are stimulated by increased osmolality (chiefly, increased sodium concentration) of the extracellular fluid; their excitation promotes the release of antidiuretic hormone by the posterior pituitary. 2. [osmo-(1) +L. recipere to receive, accept] a specialized sensory nerve ending sensitive to stimulation giving rise to the sensation of odors.

osmoregulation (oz″mo-reg″u-la′shun) maintenance of osmolarity by a simple organism or body cell with respect to the surrounding medium.

osmoregulatory (oz″mo-reg′u-lah-to″re) pertaining to osmoregulation.

osmoscope (oz′mo-skōp) [osmo-(1) + Gr. skopein to examine] an apparatus for attachment to the nose for intensifying the sense of smell and enabling the user to make quantitative and qualitative analyses of odor.

osmose (os′mōs) to pass through a membrane by osmosis.

osmosis (oz-mo′sis, os-mo′sis) [Gr. ōsmos impulsion] the passage of pure solvent from a solution of lesser to one of greater solute concentration when the two solutions are separated by a membrane which selectively prevents the passage of solute molecules, but is permeable to the solvent.

osmosology (os″mo-sol′o-je) the science of osmosis.

osmostat (os′mo-stat″) the regulatory centers that control the osmolality of the extracellular fluid.

osmotaxis (os″mo-tak′sis) [osmo-(2) + Gr. taxis arrangement] the movement of cells as affected by the density of the liquid containing them.

osmotherapy (oz″mo-ther′ah-pe) [osmo-(2) + therapy] treatment by the intravenous injection of hypertonic solutions to produce dehydration.

osmotic (oz-mot′ik) pertaining to or of the nature of osmosis.

osmyl (oz′mil) an odor.

osone (o′sōn) a carbonyl sugar formed by heating an osazone with hydrochloric acid.

osphresio- (os-fre′ze-o) [Gr. osphrēsis smell] a combining form denoting relationship to odors.

osphresiolagnia (os-fre″ze-o-lag′ne-ah) [osphresio- + Gr. lagneia lust] (obs.) erotic stimulation produced by odors.

osphresiology (os″fre-ze-ol′o-je) [osphresio- + -logy] the sum of knowledge regarding odors and the sense of smell.

osphresiometer (os″fre-ze-om′ĕ-ter) [osphresio- + Gr. metron measure] an instrument for measuring the acuteness of the sense of smell.

osphresis (os-fre′sis) [Gr. osphrēsis smell] the sense of smell.

osphretic (os-fret′ik) pertaining to the sense of smell.

osphyarthrosis (os″fe-ar-thro′sis) inflammation of the hip joint.

osphyomyelitis (os″fe-o-mi″ĕ-li′tis) [Gr. osphys loin + myelitis] myelitis of the lumbar region of the spinal cord.

osphyotomy (os″fe-ot′o-me) [Gr. osphys loin + tomē a cutting] surgical incision through the loin.

ossa (os′ah) [L.] plural of os, bone. See os².

ossature (os′ah-tūr) the arrangement of bones in the body or in a part.

ossein (os′e-in) the collagen of bone.

osselet (os′ĕ-let) an exostosis on the inner aspect of a horse's knee or on the lateral aspect of the fetlock.

osseoalbumoid (os″ĕ-o-al′bu-moid) a protein derived from bone after hydration of the collagen.

osseoaponeurotic (os″e-o-ap″o-nu-rot′ik) pertaining to bone and the aponeurosis of a muscle.

osseocartilaginous (os″e-o-kar″tĭ-laj′ĭ-nus) pertaining to or composed of bone and cartilage.

osseofibrous (os″e-o-fi′brus) made up of fibrous tissue and bone.

osseomucin (os″e-o-mu′sin) the homogeneous ground substance which binds together the collagen and elastic fibrils of bony tissue.

osseomucoid (os″e-o-mu′koid) a mucin existing in bone.

osseosonometer (os″e-o-so-nom′ĕ-ter) an instrument used in osseosonometry.

osseosonometry (os″e-o-so-nom′ĕ-tre) [L. os, ossa bone + sonus sound + Gr. metron measure] the measurement of the conduction of sound through bone.

osseous (os′e-us) [L. osseus] of the nature or quality of bone; bony.

ossicle (os′sĭ-k'l) [L. ossiculum] a small bone. **Andernach's o's,** ossa suturarum. **auditory o's,** the malleus, incus, and stapes, of the middle ear; see ossicula auditus. **o's of Bertin,** see concha sphenoidalis. **epactal o's,** ossa suturarum. **episternal o's,** ossa suprasternalia. **intercalar o's,** ossa suturarum. **Kerckring's o.,** a small bone of early life which becomes the basilar process of the occipital bone. **Riolan's o's,** small bones occasionally seen in the suture between the mastoid portion of the temporal bone and the occipital bone. **sphenoturbinal o's,** see concha sphenoidalis. **wormian o's,** ossa suturarum.

ossicula (ŏ-sik′u-lah) [L.] plural of ossiculum.

ossiculectomy (os″ĭ-ku-lek′to-me) [ossiculum + Gr. ektomē excision] surgical removal of an ossicle, or of the ossicles, of the ear.

ossiculotomy (os″ĭ-ku-lot′o-me) [ossiculum + Gr. temnein to cut] surgical incision of the bonelets (ossicles) of the ear.

ossiculum (ŏ-sik′u-lum), pl. ossic′ula [L.] [NA] a general term for a small bone, or ossicle. **ossic′ula audi′tus** [NA], auditory ossicles: the malleus, incus, and stapes, the small bones of the middle ear, which transmit the vibrations from the tympanic membrane to the oval window.

ossidesmosis (os″ĭ-des-mo′sis) osteodesmosis.

ossiferous (ŏ-sif′er-us) [L. os bone + ferre to bear] producing bone.

ossific (ŏ-sif′ik) [L. os bone + facere to make] forming or becoming bone.

ossification (os″ĭ-fi-ka′shun) [L. ossificatio] the formation of bone or of a bony substance; the conversion of fibrous tissue or of cartilage into bone or a bony substance. **cartilaginous o.,** ossification that occurs in and replaces cartilage. **ectopic o.,** a pathological condition in which bone arises in tissues not in the osseous system and in connective tissues usually not manifesting osteogenic properties. **endochondral o.,** cartilaginous o. **intramembranous o.,** ossification that occurs in and replaces connective tissue, as occurs in the calvaria and in periosteal bone formation. **metaplastic o.,** the development of bony substance in normally soft structures. **perichondral o.,** that which occurs in a layered manner beneath the perichondrium or, later, the periosteum. **periosteal o.,** a type of intramembranous bone formation.

ossifluence (ŏ-sif′lu-ens) softening of bony tissue.

ossiform (os′ĭ-form) resembling bone.

ossifying (os′ĭ-fi″ing) changing or developing into bone.

ossiphone (os′ĭ-fōn) [L. os, ossa bone + Gr. phōnē voice] an apparatus for enabling deaf persons to hear by transmitting the sound from the instrument through the bony stucture of the body.

ostalgia (os-tal′je-ah) ostealgia.

ostarthritis (os″tar-thri′tis) osteoarthritis.

osteal (os′te-al) bony; osseous.

ostealbumoid (os″te-al′bu-moid) osseoalbumoid.

ostealgia (os″te-al′je-ah) [Gr. osteon bone + -algia] pain in a bone or in the bones.

osteameba (os″te-ah-me′bah) a bone cell.

osteanabrosis (os″te-an″ah-bro′sis) [osteo- + Gr. anabrōsis eating up] atrophy of bone.

osteanagenesis (os″te-an″ah-jen′ĕ-sis) osteoanagenesis.

osteanaphysis (os″te-ah-naf′ĭ-sis) [osteo- + Gr. anaphyein to reproduce] reproduction of bone.

ostearthritis (os″te-ar-thri′tis) osteoarthritis.

ostearthrotomy (os″te-ar-throt′o-me) [osteo- + Gr. arthron joint + temnein to cut] excision of an articular end of a bone.

ostectomy (os-tek′to-me) [osteo- + Gr. ektomē excision] the excision of a bone or a portion of a bone.

osteectomy (os″te-ek′to-me) ostectomy.

osteectopia (os″te-ek-to′pe-ah) [osteo- + Gr. ektopos out of place + -ia] displacement of a bone.

osteectopy (os″te-ek′to-pe) osteectopia.

ostein (os′te-in) ossein.

osteite (os′te-īt) an independent bony element or center of ossification.

osteitis (os″te-i′tis) [osteo- + -itis] inflammation of a bone, involving the haversian spaces, canals, and their branches, and generally the medullary cavity, and marked by enlargement of the bone, tenderness, and a dull, aching pain. See also osteomyelitis. **acute o.,** osteomyelitis, usually of septic origin. **o. albumino′sa,** osteitis with accumulation of a sticky, albuminous liquid. **alveolar o.,** dry socket; see under socket. **carious o.,** osteomyelitis. **o. carno′sa,** o. fungosa. **caseous o.,** tuberculous caries of bone. **central o.,** endosteitis. **chronic o.,** central caries or bone abscess; often due to tuberculosis, sometimes syphilitic. **chronic nonsuppurative o.,** sclerosing nonsuppurative osteomyelitis. **o. conden′sans,** condensing o. **o. conden′sans generalisa′ta,** osteopoikilosis. **o. conden′sans il′ii,** a condition marked by an area of dense sclerosis on the iliac side of the sacroiliac joint. **condensing o.,** osteitis with hard deposits of earthy salts in the affected bone; called also *formative o.* and *sclerosing o.* **cortical o.,** periostitis. **o. defor′mans,** a disease of bone marked by repeated episodes of increased bone resorption followed by excessive attempts at repair, resulting in weakened deformed bones of increased mass. There may be bowing of the long bones and deformation of flat bones; pain and pathological fractures are associated. When it affects the bones of the skull, deafness may result. Called also *Paget's disease.* **o. fibro′sa cys′tica, o. fibro′sa cys′tica generalisa′ta,** rarefying osteitis with fibrous degeneration and formation of cysts, and with the presence of fibrous nodules on the affected bones; it is due to marked osteoclastic activity secondary to hyperfunction of the parathyroid gland. Called also *Recklinghausen's* or *von Recklinghausen's disease of bone.* **o. fibro′sa dissemina′ta,** Albright's syndrome. **o. fibro′sa localisa′ta,** localized fibrous degeneration with weakening and deformity of a bone, as of the patella. **o. fibro′sa osteoplas′tica,** o. fibrosa cystica. **formative o.,** condensing o. **o. fragil′itans,** osteogenesis imperfecta. **o. fungo′sa,** chronic osteitis in which the haversian canals are dilated and filled with granulation tissue. **Garré's o.,** sclerosing nonsuppurative osteomyelitis. **o. granulo′sa,** o. fungosa. **gummatous o.,** a chronic form associated with syphilis. **localized alveolar o.,** dry socket; see under *socket.* **necrotic o.,** osteomyelitis. **o. ossif′icans,** condensing o. **parathyroid o.,** o. fibrosa cystica. **pedal o.,** inflammation of the pedal bone of the horse; called also *peditis.* **productive o.,** condensing o. **o. pu′bis,** 1. sclerosis of the pubic bones, in the region of the symphysis, usually observed as an incidental finding in roentgenography of the pelvis. 2. a symptom-producing inflammatory condition of the pubic bones in the region of the symphysis, which may be associated with surgical procedures on pelvic structures or with pregnancy, infection of the urinary tract, degenerative changes, rheumatic disease, or other conditions. **rarefying o.,** a bone disease in which the inorganic matter is lessened and the hard bone becomes cancelled. **sarcomatous o.,** former name for multiple myeloma. **sclerosing o.,** 1. sclerosing nonsuppurative osteomyelitis. 2. condensing osteitis. **secondary hyperplastic o.,** hypertrophic pulmonary osteoarthropathy. **o. tuberculo′sa cys′tica, o. tuberculo′sa mul′tiplex cystoi′des,** sarcoidosis. **vascular o.,** rarefying osteitis in which the spaces formed become occupied by blood vessels.

ostembryon (os-tem′bre-on) [*osteo-* + Gr. *embryon* fetus] ossification of a fetus.

ostempyesis (os″tem-pi-e′sis) [*osteo-* + Gr. *empyēsis* suppuration] suppuration within a bone.

Ostensin (os-ten′sin) trademark for a preparation of trimethidinium methosulfate.

osteo- (os′te-o) [Gr. *osteon* bone] a combining form denoting relationship to a bone or to the bones.

osteoacusis (os″te-o-ah-ku′sis) [*osteo-* + Gr. *akousis* hearing] bone conduction.

osteoanagenesis (os″te-o-an′ah-jen′ĕ-sis) [*osteo-* + Gr. *anagenesis*] regeneration of bone.

osteoanesthesia (os″te-o-an′es-the′ze-ah) the insensitiveness of bone.

osteoaneurysm (os″te-o-an′u-rizm) aneurysm in a bone.

osteoarthritis (os″te-o-ar-thri′tis) [*osteo-* + Gr. *arthron* joint + *-itis*] noninflammatory degenerative joint disease occurring chiefly in older persons, characterized by degeneration of the articular cartilage, hypertrophy of bone at the margins, and changes in the synovial membrane. It is accompanied by pain and stiffness, particularly after prolonged activity. Called also *degenerative arthritis, hypertrophic arthritis,* and *degenerative joint disease.* **o. defor′mans, endemic o.,** a condition endemic in portions of Russia, marked by thickening of the joints and softening of the articular ends of bones. **o. defor′mans endem′ica,** Kashin-Beck disease. **hyperplastic o.,** hypertrophic pulmonary osteoarthropathy. **interphalangeal o.,** a localized form of arthritis involving the finger joints, characterized by the formation of nodosities (Heberden's nodes) and degenerative changes with intermittent inflammatory episodes, and leading eventually to deformities and ankyloses.

osteoarthropathy (os″te-o-ar-throp′ah-the) [*osteo-* + *arthropathy*] any disease of the joints and bones. **familial o. of fingers,** Thiemann's disease. **hypertrophic pneumic o.,** hy-

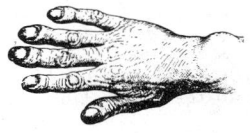

Osteoarthropathy (Homans).

pertrophic pulmonary o. **hypertrophic pulmonary o.,** symmetrical osteitis of the four limbs, chiefly localized to the phalanges and the terminal epiphyses of the long bones of the forearm and leg, sometimes extending to the proximal ends of the

limbs and the flat bones, and accompanied by a dorsal kyphosis and some affection of the joints. It is often secondary to chronic conditions of the lungs and heart. Called also *osteoarthropathie hypertrophiante pneumique* and *Marie-Bamberger disease.* **pulmonary o.,** hypertrophic pulmonary o. **secondary hypertrophic o.,** hypertrophic pulmonary o.

osteoarthrosis (os″te-o-ar-thro′sis) chronic arthritis of noninflammatory character.

osteoarthrotomy (os″te-o-ar-throt′o-me) osteoarthrotomy.

osteoarticular (os″te-o-ar-tik′u-lar) pertaining to or affecting bones and joints.

osteoblast (os′te-o-blast″) [*osteo-* + Gr. *blastos* germ] a cell which arises from a fibroblast and which, as it matures, is associated with the production of bone.

osteoblastic (os″te-o-blas′tik) pertaining to or composed of osteoblasts.

osteoblastoma (os″te-o-blas-to′mah) [*osteoblast* + *-oma*] a benign, painful, rather vascular tumor of bone characterized by the formation of osteoid tissue and primitive bone; called also *giant osteoid osteoma.*

osteocachectic (os″te-o-kah-kek′tik) pertaining to or characterized by osteocachexia.

osteocachexia (os″te-o-kah-kek′se-ah) cachexia due to chronic bone disease; also chronic disease of bone.

osteocamp (os′te-o-kamp) an instrument for bending the femur straight following osteotomy.

osteocampsia (os″te-o-kamp′se-ah) [*osteo-* + Gr. *kamptein* to bend] curvature or bending of a bone, as in rickets.

osteocampsis (os″te-o-kamp′sis) osteocampsia.

osteocartilaginous (os″te-o-kar″tĭ-laj′ĭ-nus) pertaining to or composed of bone and cartilage.

osteocele (os′te-o-sēl) [*osteo-* + Gr. *kēlē* tumor] 1. bony tumor of the testis or scrotum. 2. a hernia containing bone.

osteocementum (os″te-o-se-men′tum) the hard bonelike tissue of the secondary cementum, usually found at the apical third of a tooth root.

osteochondral (os″te-o-kon′dral) pertaining to bone and cartilage; pertaining to a bone and its articular cartilage.

osteochondritis (os″te-o-kon-dri′tis) [*osteo-* + Gr. *chondros* cartilage + *-itis*] inflammation of both bone and cartilage. **calcaneal o.,** Haglund's disease. **o. defor′mans juveni′lis,** osteochondrosis of the capitular epiphysis of the femur; see *osteochondrosis.* **o. defor′mans juveni′lis dor′si,** osteochondrosis of vertebrae; see *osteochondrosis.* **o. dis′secans,** osteochondritis resulting in the splitting of pieces of cartilage into the joint, particularly the knee joint or shoulder joint. **o. ischiopu′bica,** a condition observed in the roentgenogram, consisting of granular looking bodies at the junction of the ischium and os pubis in children. **o. necrot′icans,** a condition marked by necrosis and solution of continuity in the cartilage of the sesamoid bone of the great toe. **o. os′sis metacar′pi et metatar′si,** Thiemann's disease (q.v.) affecting both the fingers and toes.

osteochondrodysplasia (os″te-o-kon″dro-dis-pla′ze-ah) [*osteo-* + *chondro-* + *dys-* + Gr. *plassein* to form] any disorder of cartilage and bone growth.

osteochondrodystrophia (os″te-o-kon″dro-dis-tro′fe-ah) Morquio's syndrome. **o. defor′mans,** Morquio's syndrome.

osteochondrodystrophy (os″te-o-kon″dro-dys′tro-fe) Morquio's syndrome. **familial o.,** Morquio's syndrome.

osteochondrofibroma (os″te-o-kon″dro-fi-bro′mah) fibrosing osteochondroma.

osteochondrolysis (os″te-o-kon-drol′ĭ-sis) osteochondritis dissecans.

osteochondroma (os″te-o-kon-dro′mah) [*osteo-* + Gr. *chondros* cartilage + *-oma*] osteoma blended with chondroma, a benign tumor consisting of projecting adult bone capped by cartilage. Called also *chondrosteoma, enchondroma petrificum,* and *osteocartilaginous exostosis.* **fibrosing o.,** a tumor containing the elements of osteoma, chondroma, and fibroma.

osteochondromatosis (os″te-o-don″dro-mah-to′sis) a condition marked by the presence of multiple osteochondromas. **synovial o.,** a rare condition in which cartilage bodies are formed in the synovial membrane of the joints, tendon sheaths, or bursae, later undergoing secondary calcification and ossification; some of the bodies may become detached and remain as viable, growing structures in the synovial spaces.

osteochondromyxoma (os″te-o-kon″dro-mik-so′mah) osteochondroma blended with myxoma.

osteochondropathia (os″te-o-kon″dro-path′e-ah) osteochondropathy. **o. cretinoi′dea,** Läwen-Roth syndrome.

osteochondropathy (os″te-o-kon-drop′ah-the) [*osteo-* + Gr. *chondros* cartilage + *pathos* disease] any morbid condition affecting both bone and cartilage, or marked by abnormal enchondral ossification. **polyglucose (dextran) sulfate–induced o.,** an experimentally produced disorder of enchondral ossification characterized by a deficient formation of bone matrix in the metaphyses of long bones.

osteochondrophyte (os″te-o-kon′dro-fīt) [osteo- + Gr. chondros cartilage + phyton growth] osteochondroma.

osteochondrosarcoma (os″te-o-kon″dro-sar-ko′mah) sarcoma blended with osteoma and chondroma.

osteochondrosis (os″te-o-kon-dro′sis) a disease of the growth or ossification centers in children which begins as a degeneration or necrosis followed by regeneration or recalcification. Called also epiphyseal ischemic necrosis (q.v.). It may affect (1) the CALCANEUS (os calcis), a condition sometimes called apophysitis; (2) the CAPITULAR EPIPHYSIS (head) OF THE FEMUR, a condition known as Legg-Calvé-Perthes disease, Perthes disease, Waldenström's disease, coxa plana, and pseudocoxalgia; (3) the ILIUM; (4) the LUNATE (SEMILUNAR) BONE, known as Kienböck's disease; (5) HEAD OF THE SECOND METATARSAL BONE, known as Freiberg's infraction; (6) the NAVICULAR (TARSAL SCAPHOID), known as Köhler's tarsal scaphoiditis; (7) the TUBEROSITY OF THE TIBIA, called Osgood-Schlatter disease, Schlatter's disease; (8) the VERTEBRAE, called Scheuermann's disease or kyphosis, juvenile kyphosis, vertebral epiphysitis, and kyphosis dorsalis juvenilis. (9) the capitellum of the humerus, called Panner's disease. **o. defor′mans tib′iae**, aseptic necrosis of the medial condyle of the tibia, producing lateral bowing of the leg; called also Blount's disease, nonrachitic bowleg, and tibia vara.

osteochondrous (os″te-o-kon′drus) [osteo- + Gr. chondros cartilage] composed of bone and cartilage.

osteoclasia (os″te-o-kla′ze-ah) [osteo- + Gr. klasis a breaking + -ia] the absorption and destruction of bony tissue.

osteoclasis (os-te-ok′lah-sis) [osteo- + Gr. klasis a breaking] the surgical fracture or refracture of bones.

osteoclast (os′te-o-klast″) [osteo- + Gr. klan to break] 1. a large multinuclear cell associated with the absorption and removal of bone; osteoclasts become highly active in the presence of parathyroid hormone, causing increased bone resorption and release of bone salts (phosphorus and, especially, calcium) into the extracellular fluid. 2. an instrument for use in the surgical fracture or refracture of bones. **Collin's o.,** an osteoclast for fracturing a bone at any desired point. **Rizzoli's o.,** an osteoclast consisting of a rod on which are two sliding padded rings, and between these a padded plate that can be screwed down upon the part, thus fracturing the bone.

osteoclastic (os″te-o-klas′tik) pertaining to or of the nature of an osteoclast; destructive to bone.

osteoclastoma (os″te-o-klas-to′mah) giant cell tumor of bone.

osteoclasty (os″te-o-klas″te) osteoclasis.

osteocomma (os″te-o-kom′ah) [osteo- + Gr. komma fragment] any of the pieces or members of a series of bony structures, as a vertebra.

osteocope (os′te-o-kōp″) [osteo- + Gr. kopos pain] a severe pain in a bone or in the bones, generally a symptom of syphilitic bone disease.

osteocopic (os″te-o-kop′ik) pertaining to or characterized by osteocope.

osteocranium (os″te-o-kra′ne-um) [osteo- + Gr. kranion cranium] the fetal cranium during its stage of ossification.

osteocystoma (os″te-o-sis-to′mah) [osteo- + cystoma] a bone cyst.

osteocyte (os″te-o-sīt″) an osteoblast that has become embedded within the bone matrix, occupying a flat oval cavity (bone lacuna [q.v.]) and sending, through the canaliculi, slender cytoplasmic processes that make contact with processes of other osteocytes.

osteodentin (os″te-o-den′tin) [osteo- + dentin] dentin that resembles bone: seen in the teeth of certain fish and pathologically in other lower species, and in man, being produced by rapid formation of secondary dentin, with entrapment of cells.

osteodentinoma (os″te-o-den-tĭ-no′mah) an odontoma composed of bone and dentin.

osteodermia (os″te-o-der′me-ah) [osteo- + Gr. derma skin + -ia] osteoma cutis.

osteodesmosis (os″te-o-des-mo′sis) [osteo- + Gr. desmos tendon] 1. the formation of bone and tendon. 2. ossification of tendon.

osteodiastasis (os″te-o-di-as′tah-sis) [osteo- + Gr. diastasis separation] the separation of two adjacent bones.

osteodynia (os″te-o-din′e-ah) [osteo- + Gr. odynē pain] pain in a bone.

osteodysplasty (os″te-o-dis-plas′te) [osteo- + dys- + Gr. plassein to form] abnormal development of bone. **o. of Melnick and Needles,** a hereditary disorder, transmitted as an autosomal dominant trait, in which there are severe congenital bone abnormalities manifested by striking facies (exophthalmos, full cheeks, micrognathia, and malalignment of the teeth), flaring of the metaphyses of long bones, S-like curvature of the leg bones, irregular constrictions in the ribs, and sclerosis of the base of the skull.

osteodystrophia (os″te-o-dis-tro′fe-ah) osteodystrophy. **o. cys′tica,** osteitis fibrosa cystica. **o. fibro′sa,** osteitis fibrosa cystica.

osteodystrophy (os″te-o-dis′tro-fe) defective bone formation. **Albright's hereditary o.,** pseudo-pseudohypoparathyroidism. **renal o.,** a condition resulting from chronic disease of the kid-

neys with onset usually in childhood. It is characterized by impaired renal function, by elevated serum phosphorus and low or normal serum calcium levels, and by stimulation of parathyroid function. The resultant bone disease includes a variable admixture of osteitis fibrosa cystica, osteomalacia, osteoporosis, and sometimes osteosclerosis. If the onset is in childhood, renal dwarfism may result.

osteoectomy (os″te-o-ek′to-me) ostectomy.

osteoenchondroma (os″te-o-en″kon-dro′mah) osteochondroma.

osteoepiphysis (os″te-o-ĕ-pif′ĭ-sis) [osteo- + epiphysis] any bony epiphysis.

osteofibrochondrosarcoma (os″te-o-fi″bro-kon″dro-sar-ko′mah) malignant mesenchymoma.

osteofibroma (os″te-o-fi-bro′mah) [osteo- + fibroma] a tumor containing both osseous and fibrous elements.

osteofibromatosis (os″te-o-fi″bro-mah-to′sis) polyostotic form of fibrous dysplasia of bone. **cystic o.,** Jaffe-Lichtenstein disease.

osteofluorosis (os″te-o-floo″o-ro′sis) skeletal changes, usually consisting of osteomalacia and osteosclerosis, caused by the chronic intake of excessive quantities of fluorides. See also fluorosis, def. 2.

osteogen (os′te-o-jen″) [osteo- + Gr. gennan to produce] the substance composing the inner layer of the periosteum, from which bone is formed.

osteogenesis (os″te-o-jén′ĕ-sis) [osteo- + Gr. gennan to produce] formation of bone; the development of the bones. **o. imperfec′ta,** an inherited condition, usually transmitted as an autosomal dominant trait, in which the bones are abnormally brittle and subject to fractures. In o. imperfec′ta congen′ita the fractures occur in intrauterine life and the child is born with deformities. In o. imperfec′ta tar′da the fractures occur when the child begins to walk. The condition is usually attended by blue coloration of the sclera of the eyes (Lobstein's disease or syndrome) and sometimes also by otosclerotic deafness (Van der Hoeve's syndrome). Called also fragilitas ossium, brittle bones, osteopsathyrosis, and hypoplasia of the mesenchyme. **o. imperfec′ta cys′tica,** a disorder in which the marrow spaces contain myxomatous fibroid tissue, the x-ray showing cystic changes.

osteogenetic (os″te-o-jĕ-net′ik) forming bone; concerned in bone formation.

osteogenic (os″te-o-jen′ik) [osteo- + Gr. gennan to produce] derived from or composed of any tissue which is concerned in the growth or repair of bone.

osteogenous (os″te-oj′ĕ-nus) osteogenic.

osteogeny (os″te-oj′ĕ-ne) osteogenesis.

osteogram (os′te-o-gram) a semidiagram of the spine used as a record sheet for the charting of bone lesions.

osteography (os″te-og′rah-fe) [osteo- + Gr. graphein to write] a description of the bones.

osteohalisteresis (os″te-o-hah-lis″ter-e′sis) [osteo- + Gr. hals salt + sterein to deprive] loss or deficiency of the mineral elements of bones.

osteohemachromatosis (os″te-o-hem″ah-kro′mah-to′sis) [osteo- + Gr. haima blood + chrōma color + -osis] a disease of animals marked by discoloration of the bone by blood pigment.

osteohydatidosis (os″te-o-hi″dah-tid-o′sis) hydatid disease of bone.

osteoid (os′te-oid) [osteo- + Gr. eidos form] 1. resembling bone. 2. the organic matrix of bone; young bone which has not undergone calcification.

osteolathyrism (os″te-o-lath′ĭ-rizm) a skeletal disorder produced in laboratory animals by diets containing the sweet pea (Lathyrus odoratus) or its active principle, β-aminopropionitrile, or other aminonitriles. Characterized, in rats, by hernias, dissecting aortic aneurysms, lameness, of the hind legs, exostoses, and kyphoscoliosis and other skeletal deformities, apparently as the result of defective aging of collagen tissue.

osteolipochondroma (os″te-o-lĭ-po″kon-dro′mah) osteochondroma with fatty elements.

osteolipoma (os″te-o-lĭ-po′mah) lipoma with osseous metaplasia.

osteologia (os″te-o-lo′je-ah) osteology; in NA terminology it encompasses the nomenclature relating to the bones.

osteologist (os″te-ol′o-jist) a specialist in osteology.

osteology (os″te-ol′o-je) [osteo- + Gr. logos treatise] the scientific study of the bones; applied also to the body of knowledge relating to the bones.

osteolysis (os″te-ol′ĭ-sis) [osteo- + Gr. lysis dissolution] dissolution of bone; applied especially to the removal or loss of the calcium of bone.

osteolytic (os″te-o-lit′ik) relating to, characterized by, or promoting osteolysis.

osteoma (os″te-o′mah) [osteo- + -oma] a tumor composed of bone tissue; a hard tumor of bonelike structure developing on a bone (homoplastic o.) and sometimes on other structures (hetero-

plastic o.). **cavalryman's o.,** osteoma at the insertion of the adductor femoris longus muscle. **compact o.,** o. durum. **o. cu′tis,** a condition in which bone-containing nodules form on the skin; called also *osteodermia* and *osteosis cutis.* **o. du′rum, o. ebur′neum,** a tumor made up of hard bony tissue. **giant osteoid o.,** osteoblastoma. **o. medulla′re,** an osteoma containing marrow spaces. **osteoid o.,** a small, benign but painful, circumscribed tumor of spongy bone occurring especially in the bones of the extremities and vertebrae, most often in young persons. **o. sarcomato′sum,** osteogenic sarcoma. **o. spongio′sum,** osteoma containing cancellated bone.

osteomalacia (os″te-o-mah-la′she-ah) [*osteo-* + Gr. *malakia* softness] a condition marked by softening of the bones (due to impaired mineralization, with excess accumulation of osteoid), with pain, tenderness, muscular weakness, anorexia, and loss of weight, resulting from deficiency of vitamin D and calcium. **bovine o.,** aphosphorosis. **hepatic o.,** osteomalacia as a complication of cholestatic liver disease, which may lead to severe bone pain and multiple fractures. **infantile o., juvenile o.,** late rickets. **puerperal o.,** osteomalacia occurring as a consequence of exhaustion of skeletal stores of calcium and phosphorus by repeated pregnancies and lactation. **renal tubular o.,** osteomalacia occurring as a consequence of acidosis and hypercalciuria, resulting from inability to produce an acid urine or ammonia because of deficient activity of the renal tubules. **senile o.,** softening of bones in old age due to vitamin D deficiency.

osteomalacic (os″te-o-mah-la′sik) pertaining to or characterized by osteomalacia.

osteomalacosis (os″te-o-mal″ah-ko′sis) osteomalacia.

osteomatoid (os″te-o′mah-toid) resembling an osteoma.

osteomatosis (os″te-o-mah-to′sis) the formation of multiple osteomas.

osteomere (os′te-o-mēr″) [*osteo-* + Gr. *meros* part] one of a series of similar bony structures, such as the vertebrae.

osteometry (os″te-om′ĕ-tre) [*osteo-* + Gr. *metron* measure] the measurement of bones.

osteomiosis (os″te-o-mi-o′sis) [*osteo-* + Gr. *meiōsis* diminution] disintegration of bone.

osteomyelitic (os″te-o-mi″ĕ-lit′ik) marked by or characteristic of osteomyelitis.

osteomyelitis (os″te-o-mi″ĕ-li′tis) [*osteo-* + Gr. *myelos* marrow] inflammation of bone caused by a pyogenic organism. It may remain localized or may spread through the bone to involve the marrow, cortex, cancellous tissue, and periosteum. **conchiolin o.,** a condition seen in the workers in mother of pearl, probably due to the inhaled dust being deposited in the bone marrow. Cf. *coniosis.* **Garré's o.,** sclerosing nonsuppurative o. **malignant o.,** former name for multiple myeloma. **sclerosing nonsuppurative o.,** chronic idiopathic osteomyelitis involving the long bones, particularly the tibia and femur, and characterized by a diffuse inflammatory reaction, increased density and spindle-shaped sclerotic thickening of the cortex, and an absence of suppuration; called also *Garré's disease, osteitis,* or *osteomyelitis,* and *chronic nonsuppurative osteitis.* **typhoid o.,** osteomyelitis occurring as a concurrent or greatly delayed sequel of typhoid fever. **o. variolo′sa,** osteomyelitis due to, or occurring as a complication of, smallpox.

osteomyelodysplasia (os″te-o-mi″ĕ-lo-dis-pla′se-ah) [*osteo-* + Gr. *myelos* marrow + *dys-* + *plassein* to form] a condition characterized by thinning of the osseous tissue of bones and increase in size of the marrow cavities, attended with leukopenia and fever.

osteomyelography (os″te-o-mi″ĕ-log′rah-fe) roentgen visualization of bone marrow.

osteomyxochondroma (os″te-o-mik″so-kon-dro′mah) osteochondromyxoma.

osteon (os′te-on) [*osteo-* + Gr. *on* neuter ending] the basic unit of structure of compact bone, comprising a haversian canal and its concentrically arranged lamellae, of which there may be 4 to 20, each 3 to 7 microns thick, in a single (haversian) system; such units are directed mainly in the long axis of the bone.

osteone (os′te-ōn) osteon.

osteonecrosis (os″te-o-ne-kro′sis) [*osteo-* + Gr. *nekrōsis* death] death, or necrosis, of bone.

osteoneuralgia (os″te-o-nu-ral′je-ah) [*osteo-* + *neuralgia*] neuralgia of a bone.

osteonosus (os″te-on′o-sus) [*osteo-* + Gr. *nosos* disease] disease of bone.

osteo-odontoma (os″te-o-o″don-to′mah) ameloblastic odontoma.

osteopath (os′te-o-path) a practitioner of osteopathy.

osteopathia (os″te-o-path′e-ah) any disease of a bone; called also *osteopathy.* **o. conden′sans,** myelosclerosis, def. 2. **o. conden′sans dissemina′ta, o. conden′sans generalisa′ta,** osteopoikilosis. **o. hemorrha′gica infan′tum,** Moeller-Barlow disease. **o. hyperostot′ica congen′ita,** melorheostosis. **o. hyperostot′ica mul′tiplex infan′tilis,** diaphyseal dysplasia. **o. stria′ta,** an abnormality apparent only on roentgen examination, and occurring only in cancellous bone; it is characterized by multiple condensations beginning at the epiphyseal line and extending into the diaphysis.

osteopathic (os″te-o-path′ik) pertaining to osteopathy.

osteopathology (os″te-o-pah-thol′o-je) any disease of bone.

osteopathy (os″te-op′ah-the) [*osteo-* + Gr. *pathos* disease] 1. any disease of a bone. 2. a system of therapy founded by Andrew Taylor Still (1828–1917) and based on the theory that the body is capable of making its own remedies against disease and other toxic conditions when it is in normal structural relationship and has favorable environmental conditions and adequate nutrition. It utilizes generally accepted physical, medicinal, and surgical methods of diagnosis and therapy, while placing chief emphasis on the importance of normal body mechanics and manipulative methods of detecting and correcting faulty structure. **alimentary o.,** hunger o. **disseminated condensing o.,** osteopoikilosis. **hunger o.,** disturbances of the skeletal system observed in famine areas, characterized by a reduction in the amount of normally calcified bone, and attributed to dietary deficiencies and associated hormonal dysfunction. **myelogenic o.,** any bone disease due to the impaired relation between the medullary and osseous tissues.

osteopecilia (os″te-o-pĕ-sil′e-ah) [*osteo-* + Gr. *poikilia* spottedness] osteopoikilosis.

osteopedion (os″te-o-pe′de-on) [*osteo-* + Gr. *paidion* child] lithopedion.

osteopenia (os″te-o-pe′nĭ-ah) [*osteo-* + Gr. *penia* poverty] reduced bone mass due to a decrease in the rate of osteoid synthesis to a level insufficient to compensate normal bone lysis. The term is also used to refer to any decrease in bone mass below the normal.

osteopenic (os″te-o-pen′ik) pertaining to osteopenia.

osteoperiosteal (os″te-o-per″ĭ-os′te-al) pertaining to bone and its periosteum.

osteoperiostitis (os″te-o-per″ĭ-os-ti′tis) [*osteo-* + *periostitis*] inflammation of a bone and its periosteum. Called also *periosteitis.* **alveolodental o.,** periodontitis.

osteopetrosis (os″te-o-pe-tro′sis) [*osteo-* + Gr. *petra* stone + *-osis*] a rare hereditary disease characterized by abnormally dense bone, probably due to faulty bone resorption. The disorder occurs in two forms: a severe autosomal recessive form occurring in infancy or childhood, and a benign autosomal dominant form occurring in adolescence or adulthood. In the recessive form, the proliferation of bone obliterates the marrow cavity, causing anemia, and the nerve foramina of the skull, causing compression of cranial nerves, which may result in deafness and blindness. Fractures are common in both forms. Called also *Albers-Schönberg disease, ivory bones,* and *marble bones.* **o. gallina′rum,** see *avian leukosis,* under *leukosis.*

osteophage (os′te-o-fāj) [*osteo-* + Gr. *phagein* to eat] osteoclast, def. 2.

osteophagia (os″te-o-fa′je-ah) [*osteo-* + Gr. *phagein* to eat] the eating of bone due to a craving for phosphorus.

osteophlebitis (os″te-o-fle-bi′tis) [*osteo-* + Gr. *phleps* vein + *-itis*] inflammation of the veins of a bone.

osteophone (os′te-o-fōn″) [*osteo-* + Gr. *phōnē* voice] audiphone.

osteophony (os″te-of′o-ne) [*osteo-* + Gr. *phōnē* voice.] the conduction of sounds by bone; bone conduction.

osteophore (os′te-o-fōr) [*osteo-* + Gr. *pherein* to carry] a bone-crushing forceps.

osteophyma (os″te-o-fi′mah) [*osteo-* + Gr. *phyma* growth] a tumor or outgrowth of a bone.

osteophyte (os′te-o-fīt″) [*osteo-* + Gr. *phyton* plant] a bony excrescence or osseous outgrowth.

osteophytosis (os″te-o-fi-to′sis) a condition characterized by the formation of osteophytes.

osteoplaque (os′te-o-plak) a layer of bone.

osteoplast (os′te-o-plast) [*osteo-* + Gr. *plastos* formed] osteoblast.

osteoplastic (os″te-o-plas′tik) 1. osteogenic. 2. pertaining to osteoplasty.

osteoplastica (os″te-o-plas′tĭ-kah) osteitis fibrosa cystica.

osteoplasty (os′te-o-plas″te) [*osteo-* + Gr. *plassein* to form] plastic surgery of the bones.

osteopoikilosis (os″te-o-poi″kĭ-lo′sis) [*osteo-* + Gr. *poikilos* mottled] a hereditary condition characterized by the presence of multiple sclerotic foci in the ends of long bones and scattered stippling in round and flat bones, usually without symptoms and diagnosed fortuitously by x-ray examination. It is transmitted as an autosomal dominant trait.

osteopoikilotic (os″te-o-poi″kĭ-lot′ik) pertaining to or characterized by osteopoikilosis.

osteoporosis (os″te-o-po-ro′sis) [*osteo-* + Gr. *poros* passage + *-osis*] abnormal rarefaction of bone, seen most commonly in the elderly. Depending on the extent of demineralization of bone, it may be accompanied by pain, particularly of the lower back; deformities, such as loss of stature; and pathological fractures. It may be idiopathic or secondary to other diseases, such as thyrotoxicosis.

adipose o., osteoporosis in which the enlarged spaces in bone are filled with fat. **o. circumscrip′ta cra′nii,** demineralization of the bones of the skull, characteristic of the destructive or osteolytic phase of Paget's disease; called also *Schüller's disease.* **o. of disuse,** decrease in bone substance as a result of lack of re-formation of laminae in the absence of functional stress which ordinarily leads to their replacement in new stress lines. **post-traumatic o.,** loss of bone substance following an injury in which there is damage to a nerve, sometimes due to an increased blood supply caused by the neurogenic insult, or to disuse secondary to pain.

osteoporotic (os″te-o-po-rot′ik) pertaining to or characterized by osteoporosis.

osteopsathyrosis (os″te-op-sath″ĭ-ro′sis) [osteo- + Gr. *psathyros* friable] osteogenesis imperfecta.

osteoradionecrosis (os″te-o-ra″de-o-ne-kro′sis) necrosis of bone following irradiation.

osteorrhagia (os″te-o-ra′je-ah) [osteo- + Gr. *rhēgnynai* to burst out] hemorrhage from bone.

osteorrhaphy (os″te-or′ah-fe) [osteo- + Gr. *rhaphē* suture] the suturing or wiring of bones.

osteosarcoma (os″te-o-sar-ko′mah) [osteo- + *sarcoma*] osteogenic sarcoma. **telangiectatic o.,** an osteogenic sarcoma containing dilated capillaries.

osteosarcomatous (os″te-o-sar-ko′mah-tus) of the nature of osteosarcoma.

osteosclerosis (os″te-o-skle-ro′sis) [osteo- + Gr. *sklērōsis* hardening] the hardening or abnormal density of bone, as in eburnation and condensing osteitis. **o. congen′ita,** achondroplasia. **o. frag′ilis,** osteopetrosis. **o. frag′ilis generalisa′ta,** osteopoikilosis. **o. myelofibrosis,** myelosclerosis, def. 2.

osteosclerotic (os″te-o-skle-rot′ik) pertaining to or characterized by osteosclerosis.

osteoscope (os′te-o-skōp) [osteo- + Gr. *skopein* to examine] an instrument for testing a roentgen ray apparatus by examining a standard preparation of the bones of the forearm.

osteoseptum (os″te-o-sep′tum) [osteo- + *septum*] the bony part of the nasal septum.

osteosis (os″te-o′sis) the formation of bony tissue, especially the infiltration of connective tissue with bone. **o. cu′tis,** see under *osteoma.* **o. ebur′nisans monomel′ica,** melorheostosis. **parathyroid o.,** osteitis fibrosa cystica.

osteostixis (os″te-o-stik′sis) [osteo- + Gr. *stixis* puncture] surgical puncture of a bone.

osteosuture (os′te-o-su-tūr) [osteo- + L. *sutura* suture] osteorrhaphy.

osteosynovitis (os″te-o-sin′o-vi′tis) synovitis together with osteitis of the neighboring bones.

osteosynthesis (os″te-o-sin′thē-sis) [osteo- + Gr. *synthesis* a putting together] surgical fastening of the ends of a fractured bone by sutures, rings, plates, or other mechanical means.

osteotabes (os″te-o-ta′bēz) [osteo- + L. *tabes* wasting] a disease, chiefly of infants, in which the cells of the bone marrow are destroyed and the marrow disappears.

osteotelangiectasia (os″te-o-tě-lan″je-ek-ta′se-ah) [osteo- + *telangiectasia*] telangiectatic osteosarcoma.

osteothrombophlebitis (os″te-o-throm″bo-fle-bi′tis) inflammation extended through intact bone by a progressive thrombophlebitis of small venules, such as sometimes occurs in the mastoid bone.

osteothrombosis (os″te-o-throm-bo′sis) [osteo- + *thrombosis*] thrombosis of the veins of a bone.

osteotome (os′te-o-tōm″) [osteo- + Gr. *tomē* a cut] a chisel-like knife for cutting bone.

osteotomoclasia (os″te-o-to″mo-kla′se-ah) osteotomoclasis.

osteotomoclasis (os″te-o-to-mok′lah-sis) [osteo- + Gr. *tomos* section + *klasis* breaking] correction of curvature of bone by partial division with the osteotome, followed by forcible fracture.

osteotomy (os″te-ot′o-me) [osteo- + Gr. *temnein* to cut] the surgical cutting of a bone. **angulation o.,** in midhumeral amputation, the bending of a small terminal of the humerus at a right angle to the bone shaft so as to provide a projection that locks the prosthesis to the bone. **block o.,** osteotomy in which a section of bone is removed. **cuneiform o.,** the removal of a wedge of bone. **cup-and-ball o.,** osteotomy in which the distal fragment is pointed and the proximal fragment is recessed. **displacement o.,** surgical division of a bone and shifting of the divided ends to change the alignment of the bone or to alter weight-bearing stresses. **hinge o.,** curvilinear cutting of a bone. **innominate o.,** pelvic osteotomy to deepen the acetabulum in congenital dislocation of the hip. **linear o.,** the sawing or linear cutting of a bone. **Lorenz's o.,** osteotomy of the neck of the femur by a V-shaped cutting of the femur so as to prevent displacement of the shaft. **Macewen's o.,** see under *operation,* def. 1. **pelvic o.,** pubiotomy. **subtrochanteric o.,** Gant's operation. **transtrochanteric o.,** division of the femur through the lesser trochanter for deformity about the hip joint.

osteotribe, osteotrite (os′te-o-trīb″; os′te-o-trīt″) [osteo- + Gr. *tribein* to rub] an instrument for rasping carious bone.

osteotrophy (os″te-ot′ro-fe) [osteo- + Gr. *trophē* nutrition] nutrition of bone.

osteotylus (os″te-ot′ĭ-lus) [osteo- + Gr. *tylos* callus] the callus enclosing the end of a broken bone.

osteotympanic (os″te-o-tim-pan′ik) craniotympanic.

Ostertagia (os″ter-ta′je-ah) [Robert von *Ostertag,* German veterinarian, 1864–1940] a genus of attenuated nematode parasites belonging to the family Trichostrongylus, found mostly in cysts on the wall of the abomasum of cattle and other ruminants.

osthexia, osthexy (os-thek′se-ah; os′thek-se) [Gr. *osteon* bone + *hexis* condition] abnormal ossification.

ostia (os′te-ah) [L.] plural of *ostium.*

ostial (os′te-al) pertaining to an ostium.

ostiary (os′te-a-re) [L. *ostiarius* pertaining to a door] (*obs.*) pertaining to an orifice.

ostitis (os-ti′tis) osteitis.

ostium (os′te-um), pl. *os′tia* [L.] a door, or opening; used in anatomical nomenclature as a general term to designate an opening into a tubular organ, or between two distinct cavities within the body. Called also *orificium, orifice,* and *opening.* **o. abdomina′le tu′bae uteri′nae** [NA], abdominal orifice of uterine tube: the funnel-shaped opening by which the uterine tube communicates with the pelvic cavity. **o. aor′tae** [NA], the opening between the left ventricle and the aorta. **o. appen′dicis vermifor′mis** [NA], opening of vermiform appendix: the orifice between the vermiform appendix and the cecum. **o. arterio′sum cor′dis,** ostium atrioventriculare sinistrum. **o. atrioventricula′re dex′trum** [NA], the opening between the right atrium and the right ventricle of the heart, guarded by the right atrioventricular valve; called also *o. venosum cordis.* **o. atrioventricula′re sinis′trum** [NA], the opening between the left atrium and the left ventricle of the heart, guarded by the left atrioventricular valve; called also *o. arteriosum cordis* and *mitral orifice.* **o. cardi′acum** [NA], cardiac opening: the orifice between the esophagus and the cardiac part of the stomach. **coronary o.,** either of the two openings in the aortic sinus which mark the origin of the (left and right) coronary arteries. **o. ileoceca′le** [NA], **o. ileocaecocol′icum,** ileocecal opening: the orifice between the ileum and cecum. **o. inter′num u′teri,** o. uterinum tubae uterinae. **persistent o. pri′mum,** an endocardial cushion defect characterized by a cleft in the basal portion of the atrial septum, usually associated with cleft mitral valve. **o. pharyn′geum tu′bae auditi′vae** [NA], the pharyngeal opening of the auditory tube. **o. pri′mum,** an opening in the lowest aspect of the septum primum of the embryonic heart, posteriorly, in the neighborhood of the atrioventricular valve. **o. pylo′ricum** pyloric opening: the orifice between the stomach and the duodenum. **o. secun′dum,** an opening high in the septum primum of the embryonic heart, approximately where the foramen ovale will be later. **sinusoidal o.,** any of the openings of the veins of Vieussens in the chambers of the heart. **sphenoidal o.,** apertura sinus sphenoidalis. **o. trun′ci pulmona′lis** [NA], opening of pulmonary trunk: the opening between the right ventricle (from the conus arteriosus portion) and the pulmonary trunk. **o. tympan′icum tu′bae auditi′vae** [NA], tympanic opening of auditory tube: the opening of the auditory tube on the carotid wall of the tympanic cavity. **o. ure′teris** [NA], the opening of the ureter in the bladder; called also *orificium ureteris.* **o. ure′thrae exter′num femini′nae** [NA], external orifice of female urethra: the opening of the urethra into the vestibule; it is surrounded by a sphincter of striated muscle derived from the bulbocavernosus muscle. Called also *orificium urethrae externum muliebris.* **o. ure′thrae exter′num masculi′nae** [NA], external orifice of male urethra: the slitlike opening of the urethra on the tip of the glans penis; called also *orificium urethrae externum virilis.* **o. ure′thrae inter′num** [NA], internal orifice of urethra: the opening between the bladder and the urethra; called also *orificium urethrae internum.* **o. u′teri** [NA], the external opening of the cervix of the uterus into the vagina; called also *orificium externum uteri* and *external orifice of uterus.* **o. uteri′num tu′bae uteri′nae** [NA], uterine orifice of uterine tube: the point at which the cavity of the uterine tube becomes continuous with that of the uterus. **o. vagi′nae** [NA], the external orifice of the vagina, situated just posterior to the external urethral orifice; called also *orificium vaginae.* **o. ve′nae cav′ae inferio′ris** [NA], the opening of the inferior vena cava into the right atrium of the heart; it is accompanied by a valve which, in the adult, is usually rudimentary. **o. ve′nae cav′ae superio′ris** [NA], the opening of the superior vena cava into the right atrium of the heart; it is unaccompanied by a valve. **os′tia vena′rum pulmona′lium** [NA], the openings of the pulmonary veins (in the human, usually four) into the left atrium of the heart; they are unaccompanied by valves. **o. veno′sum cor′dis,** ostium atrioventriculare dextrum.

ostomate (os′to-māt) one who has undergone enterostomy or ureterostomy.

ostomy (os′to-me) a general term referring to any operation in which an artificial opening is formed between two hollow organs or between one or more such viscera and the abdominal wall for discharge of intestinal contents or of urine.

ostosis (os-to′sis) osteogenesis.

ostraceous (os-tra′shus) [Gr. *ostrakon* shell] shaped like or resembling an oyster shell.

ostracosis (os″trah-ko′sis) [Gr. *ostrakon,* shell] bony change which takes on the consistency of oyster shell.

ostreasterol (os″tre-as′ter-ol) a solid sterol, $C_{29}H_{48}O$, present in oysters.

ostreotoxismus (os″tre-o-tok-siz′mus) [Gr. *ostreon* oyster + *toxikon* poisoning] poisoning caused by the eating of contaminated oysters.

O.S.U.K. Ophthalmological Society of the United Kingdom.

Oswaldocruzia (oz-wal″do-kroo′ze-ah) [G. *Oswaldo Cruz,* Brazilian physician, 1872–1917] a genus of nematode parasites inhabiting the lungs and intestines of reptiles and batrachians.

OT 1. abbreviation for *old term* in anatomy. 2. old tuberculin.

ot- see *oto-.*

otagra (o-tag′rah) otalgia.

otalgia (o-tal′je-ah) [Gr. *ōtalgia*] pain in the ear; earache. **o. denta′lis,** reflex pain in the ear due to dental disease. **geniculate o.,** geniculate neuralgia. **o. intermit′tens,** otalgia of an intermittent type. **reflex o.,** otalgia dependent upon some lesion of the buccal cavity or nasopharynx. **secondary o.,** otalgia dependent on inflammation of the geniculate ganglion. **tabetic o.,** otalgia in tabes dorsalis due to degeneration of the nerve of Wrisberg.

otalgic (o-tal′jik) 1. pertaining to earache. 2. an earache remedy.

otaphone (o′tah-fōn) otophone.

OTC over the counter; applied to drugs not required by law to be sold on prescription only.

OTD organ tolerance dose; see under *dose.*

otic (o′tik) [Gr. *ōtikos*] pertaining to the ear; aural.

otiobiosis (o″te-o-bi-o′sis) otobiosis.

Otiobius (o″te-o′be-us) *Otobius.*

otitic (o-tit′ik) pertaining to otitis.

otitis (o-ti′tis) [*ot-* + *-itis*] inflammation of the ear, which may be marked by pain, fever, abnormalities of hearing, hearing loss, tinnitus, and vertigo. **aviation o.,** barotitis media. **o. croupo′sa,** that which is associated with the formation of a fibrinous membrane. **o. desquamati′va,** otitis externa or media in which there are overdevelopment and desquamation of the cutaneous or mucous epithelium. **o. diphtherit′ica,** o. crouposa. **o. exter′na,** inflammation of the external auditory canal. **o. exter′na circumscrip′ta,** that which affects a limited area or areas. **o. exter′na diffu′sa,** that which affects the greater part of the meatus. **o. exter′na furunculo′sa,** furuncular o. **furuncular o.,** the formation of furuncles in the external meatus. **o. inter′na,** inflammation of the internal ear; labyrinthitis. **o. labyrin′thica,** labyrinthitis. **o. mastoi′dea,** otitis which involves the mastoid spaces. **o. me′dia,** inflammation of the middle ear; tympanitis. **o. me′dia, adhesive,** otitis media resulting in the formation of adhesions between the tympanic membrane and the bony walls of the middle ear or the ossicles. **o. media, secretory,** a painless accumulation of serous or mucoid fluid in the middle ear, resulting from obstruction of the eustachian tube, and causing conduction hearing loss. **o. media, serous,** that marked by serous effusion into the middle ear. **o. me′dia catarrha′lis acu′ta,** an acute catarrhal form. **o. me′dia catarrha′lis chron′ica,** a chronic catarrhal form of several subvarieties. **o. me′dia purulen′ta acu′ta,** an acute suppurative form. **o. me′dia purulen′ta chron′ica,** otorrhea. **o. me′dia sclerot′ica,** dry catarrh of the middle ear. **o. me′dia sero′sa,** one marked by a serous exudation. **o. me′dia suppurati′va,** suppurative inflammation of the middle ear. **o. me′dia vasomotor′ica,** otitis media of vasomotor origin. **mucosis o., mucosus o.,** otitis media caused by *Streptococcus mucosus.* **o. mycot′ica,** that which is due to parasitic fungi. **parasitic o.,** otoacariasis. **o. sclerot′ica,** that which is marked by hardening of the ear structures.

oto-, ot- [Gr. *ous, ōtos* ear] a combining form denoting relationship to the ear.

otoacariasis (o″to-ak″ah-ri′ah-sis) [*oto-* + *acariasis*] infection of the ears of cats, dogs, and domestic rabbits with the mite *Otodectes;* called also *parasitic otitis.*

otoantritis (o″to-an-tri′tis) otitis involving the attic of the tympanum and the mastoid antrum.

otobiosis (o″to-bi-o′sis) infestation by *Otobius.*

Otobius (o-to′be-us) [*oto-* + Gr. *bios* manner of living] a genus of argasid ticks, the spinous ear ticks. The nymphs of *O. lagophilus* of rabbits and *O. megnini* of cattle and other domestic animals may attack the ears of man.

otoblennorrhea (o″to-blen″o-re′ah) [*oto-* + Gr. *blenna* mucus + *rhoia* flow] mucous discharge from the ear.

otocariasis (o″to-kah-ri′ah-sis) otoacariasis.

Otocentor (o″to-sen′tor) *Anocentor.* **O. ni′tens,** *Anocentor nitens.*

otocephalus (o″to-sef′ah-lus) [*oto-* + Gr. *kephalē* head] an individual exhibiting otocephaly.

otocephaly (o″to-sef′ah-le) [*oto-* + Gr. *kephalē* head] a congenital malformation characterized by lack of a lower jaw and by ears that are united below the face.

otocerebritis (o″to-ser″ĕ-bri′tis) [*oto-* + *cerebritis*] inflammation of the brain dependent upon disease of the middle ear.

otocleisis (o″to-kli′sis) [*oto-* + Gr. *kleisis* closure] closure of the auditory passages.

otoconia (o″to-ko′ne-ah) [*oto-* + Gr. *konis* dust] statoconia.

otoconite (o-tok′o-nīt) statoconium; see *statoconia.*

otoconium (o″to-ko′ne-um) [L.] singular of *otoconia.*

otocranial (o″to-kra′ne-al) pertaining to the otocranium.

otocranium (o″to-kra′ne-um) [*oto-* + Gr. *kranion* skull] 1. the chamber in the petrous bone that lodges the internal ear. 2. the auditory portion of the cranium; called also *petromastoid.*

otocyst (o′to-sist) [*oto-* + Gr. *kystis* sac, bladder] 1. the auditory vesicle of the embryo. 2. the auditory sac of some of the lower animals.

Otodectes (o″to-dek′tēz) [*oto-* + Gr. *dēktēs* a biter] a genus of mites; see *otoacariasis.*

otodynia (o″to-din′e-ah) [*oto-* + Gr. *odynē* pain] otalgia.

otoencephalitis (o″to-en-sef″ah-li′tis) [*oto-* + *encephalitis*] inflammation of the brain due to an extension from an inflamed middle ear.

otoganglion (o″to-gang′gle-on) [*oto-* + Gr. *ganglion* ganglion] the otic ganglion.

otogenic (o″to-jen′ik) otogenous.

otogenous (o-toj′ĕ-nus) [*oto-* + Gr. *gennan* to produce] originating within the ear.

otography (o-tog′rah-fe) [*oto-* + Gr. *graphein* to write] a description of the ear.

otohemineurasthenia (o″to-hem″e-nu″ras-the′ne-ah) [*oto-* + *hemi-* + *neurasthenia*] nervous defect of hearing in one ear.

otolaryngology (o″to-lar″in-gol′o-je) that branch of medicine concerned with medical and surgical treatment of the head and neck, including the ears, nose, and throat.

otolite (o′to-lit) otolith.

otolith (o′to-lith) [*oto-* + Gr. *lithos* stone] 1. see *statoconia.* 2. a calcareous mass in the inner ear of vertebrates or the otocyst of invertebrates.

otolithiasis (o″to-lĭ-thi′ah-sis) the presence of calculi in the ear.

otologic (o″to-loj′ik) pertaining to otology.

otologist (o-tol′o-jist) a physician who specializes in otology.

otology (o-tol′o-je) [*oto-* + *-logy*] that branch of medicine which deals with the medical treatment and surgery of the ear, and its anatomy, physiology, and pathology.

otomastoiditis (o″to-mas″toid-i′tis) mastoiditis combined with otitis.

Oto-Microscope (o″to-mi′kro-skōp) trademark for an operating microscope especially devised to improve visualization of the surgical field in operations on the ear, providing both magnification of the structures and illumination of the area.

otomucormycosis (o″to-mu″kor-mi-ko′sis) mucormycosis affecting the ear.

otomyasthenia (o″to-mi″as-the′ne-ah) [*oto-* + Gr. *mys* muscle + *astheneia* weakness] a debilitated state of the ear muscles, interfering with the normal attenuation and selection of sounds.

Otomyces (o″to-mi′sēz) [*oto-* + Gr. *mykēs* fungus] a former name for a genus of fungi which infest the ear; now considered the same as *Aspergillus.* **O. hage′ni, O. purpu′reus,** species of uncertain classification, which were once found in the human ear. *O. purpureus* is probably identical with *Aspergillus nidulans.*

otomycosis (o″to-mi-ko′sis) [*oto-* + Gr. *mykēs* fungus] fungal infection of the external auditory meatus, marked by pruritus and exudative inflammation; there may be secondary bacterial infection. **o. aspergilli′na,** any ear disease caused by the presence of an aspergillus; see *myringomycosis.*

otomyiasis (o″to-mi′yah-sis) infestation of the ear by larvae.

otoneuralgia (o″to-nu-ral′je-ah) [*oto-* + *neuralgia*] neuralgic pain in the ear.

otoneurasthenia (o″to-nu″ras-the′ne-ah) [*oto-* + *neurasthenia*] neurasthenia due to ear disease.

otoneurologic (o″to-nu″ro-loj′ik) pertaining to those portions of the nervous system relating to the ear.

otoneurology (o″to-nu-rol′o-je) that branch of otology dealing especially with those portions of the nervous system related to the ear.

otopathy (o-top′ah-the) [*oto-* + Gr. *pathos* disease] any disease of the ear.

otopharyngeal (o″to-fah-rin′je-al) pertaining to the ear and pharynx.

otophone (o′to-fōn) [oto- + Gr. *phōnē* sound] 1. an external appliance used to aid the hearing; a hearing aid. 2. a tube used in the auscultation of the ear.

otoplasty (o′to-plas″te) [oto- + Gr. *plassein* to form] plastic surgery of the ear; the surgical correction of ear deformities and defects.

otopolypus (o″to-pol′ĭ-pus) [oto- + *polypus*] a polyp of the ear.

otopyorrhea (o″to-pi″o-re′ah) [oto- + Gr. *pyon* pus + *rhein* to flow] a copious purulent discharge from the ear.

otopyosis (o″to-pi-o′sis) [oto- + Gr. *pyōsis* suppuration] a suppurative disease of the ear.

otor (o′tor) pertaining to the ear; aural.

otorhinolaryngology (o″to-ri″no-lar″in-gol′o-je) [oto- + Gr. *rhis* nose + *larynx* larynx + -*logy*] that branch of medicine concerned with medical and surgical treatment of the head and neck, including the ears, nose, and throat.

otorhinology (o″to-ri-nol′o-je) [oto- + Gr. *rhis* nose + -*logy*] that branch of medicine which treats of the nose and ear and their diseases.

otorrhagia (o″to-ra′je-ah) [oto- + Gr. *rhēgnynai* to burst forth] hemorrhage from the ear.

otorrhea (o″to-re′ah) [oto- + Gr. *rhoia* to flow] a discharge from the ear, especially a purulent one. **cerebrospinal fluid o.,** escape of cerebrospinal fluid through the external auditory meatus due to fracture of the temporal bone.

otosalpinx (o″to-sal′pinks) [oto- + Gr. *salpinx* trumpet] the auditory tube (tuba auditiva [NA]).

otosclerosis (o″to-skle-ro′sis) [oto- + Gr. *sklērōsis* hardening] a pathological condition of the bony labyrinth of the ear, in which there is formation of spongy bone (otospongiosis), especially in front of and posterior to the footplate of the stapes; it may cause bony ankylosis of the stapes, resulting in conductive hearing loss. Cochlear otosclerosis may also develop, resulting in sensorineural hearing loss.

otosclerotic (o″to-skle-rot′ik) characterized by otosclerosis.

otoscope (o′to-skōp) [oto- + Gr. *skopein* to examine] an instrument for inspecting or for auscultating the ear. **Brunton's o.,** an otoscope lighted by means of a funnel attached to the side. **Siegle's o.,** an otoscope which gives a view of the drum membrane when subjected to condensed or rarefied air. **Toynbee's o.,** a tube for insertion into the ear of the patient and of the observer for the purpose of auscultating the patient's ear during politzerization.

otoscopy (o-tos′ko-pe) examination of the ear by means of the otoscope.

otosis (o-to′sis) a false impression of sounds uttered by others.

otospongiosis (o″to-spon″je-o′sis) the formation of spongy bone in the bony labyrinth of the ear; see *otosclerosis*.

ototoxic (o″to-tok′sik) having a deleterious effect upon the eighth nerve, or upon the organs of hearing and balance.

ototoxicity (o″to-toks-is′ĭ-te) the quality of being poisonous to or of exerting a deleterious effect upon the eighth nerve or upon the organs of hearing and balance.

Otrivin (o′trĭ-vin) trademark for preparations of xylometazoline hydrochloride.

Ott's test (ots) [Isaac *Ott*, American physiologist, 1847–1916] see under *tests*.

Otto disease, pelvis (ot′o) [Adolph Wilhelm *Otto*, German surgeon, 1786–1845] see under *disease* and *pelvis*.

O.U. abbreviation for L. *oc′ulus uter′que*, each eye.

ouabain (wah-ba′in) [USP] chemical name: 3β-[(6-deoxy-α-L-mannopyranosyl)oxy]1β,5β,11α,19-pentahydroxycard-20(22)-enolide octahydrate. A cardiac glycoside, $C_{29}H_{44}O_{12} \cdot 8H_2O$, obtained principally from the seeds of *Strophanthus gratus* (Wall & Hock.) Baill. (Apocynaceae), occurring as white crystals or crystalline powder, and having the same actions as digitalis but producing digitalization more rapidly; used in the treatment of acute congestive heart failure, nodal paroxysmal tachycardia, and atrial flutter, administered intravenously. Called also *G-strophanthin* or *strophanthin-G*.

Oudin current, resonator (oo-da′) [Paul *Oudin*, French electrotherapist and roentgenologist, 1851–1923] see under *current* and *resonator*.

oulectomy (oo-lek′to-me) ulectomy.

oulitis (oo-li′tis) ulitis.

oulonitis (oo″lo-ni′tis) pulpitis.

oulorrhagia (oo″lo-ra′je-ah) ulorrhagia.

ounce (owns) [L. *uncia*] a measure of weight in both the avoirdupois and the apothecaries' system; abbreviation oz. The ounce *avoirdupois* is one sixteenth of a pound, or 437.5 grains (28.3495 gm.). The *apothecaries'* ounce is one twelfth of a pound, or 480 grains (31.103 gm.); symbol ℥. **fluid o.,** a unit of capacity (liquid measure) of the apothecaries' system, being 8 fluiddrams, or the equivalent of 29.57 ml. Abbreviated fl.oz.

outbreeding (owt′brēd-ing) the mating of totally unrelated individuals, which frequently results in the production of offspring that show more vigor, as measured in terms of growth, survival, and fertility, than the parents (heterosis); called also *crossbreeding*.

outlet (owt′let) a means by which something escapes. **pelvic o.,** the lower aperture of the pelvis (apertura pelvis inferior [NA]).

outpatient (owt′pa-shent) a patient who comes to the hospital, clinic, or dispensary for diagnosis and/or treatment but does not occupy a bed.

outpocketing (owt-pok′et-ing) evagination.

outpouching (owt′powch″ing) the obtrusion of a layer or part to form a pouch; evagination.

output (owt′poot) the yield, or the total of anything produced by any functional system of the body. **cardiac o.,** the effective volume of blood expelled by either ventricle of the heart per unit of time (usually volume per minute); it is equal to the stroke output multiplied by the number of beats per the time unit used in the computation. **energy o.,** the energy a body is able to manifest in work or activity. **stroke o.,** the amount of blood ejected by a ventricle at each beat of the heart. **urinary o.,** the amount of urine excreted by the kidneys.

ova (o′vah) [L.] plural of *ovum*.

oval (o′val) [L. *ovalis*] egg shaped; having the outline of the long section of an egg.

ovalbumin (o″val-bu′min) [L. *ovum* egg + *albumin*] an albumin obtainable from the whites of eggs.

ovalocytary (o″vah-lo-si′ter-e) elliptocytary.

ovalocyte (o′vah-lo-sīt″) elliptocyte.

ovalocytosis (o-val″o-si-to′sis) elliptocytosis.

ovarialgia (o-va″re-al′je-ah) oophoralgia.

ovarian (o-va′re-an) pertaining to an ovary or ovaries.

ovariectomy (o″va-re-ek′to-me) oophorectomy.

ovario- (o-va′re-o) [L. *ovarium* ovary] a combining form denoting relationship to the ovary.

ovariocele (o-va′re-o-sēl″) [ovario- + Gr. *kēlē* hernia] hernial protrusion of an ovary.

ovariocentesis (o-va″re-o-sen-te′sis) [ovario- + Gr. *kentēsis* puncture] surgical puncture of an ovary.

ovariocyesis (o-va″re-o-si-e′sis) [ovario- + Gr. *kyēsis* pregnancy] ovarian pregnancy.

ovariodysneuria (o-va″re-o-dis-nu′re-ah) [ovario- + *dys-* + Gr. *neuron* nerve + -*ia*] neuralgic pain in the ovary.

ovariogenic (o-va″re-o-jen′ik) arising in the ovary.

ovariohysterectomy (o-va″re-o-his″ter-ek′to-me) oophorohysterectomy.

ovariopathy (o-va″re-op′ah-the) [ovario- + Gr. *pathos* disease] ovarian disease.

ovariopexy (o-va″re-o-pek′se) [ovario- + Gr. *pēxis* fixation] the operation of elevating and fixing an ovary to the abdominal wall.

ovariorrhexis (o-va″re-o-rek′sis) [ovario- + Gr. *rhēxis* rupture] rupture of an ovary.

ovariosalpingectomy (o-va″re-o-sal″pin-jek′to-me) surgical removal of an ovary and oviduct.

ovariostomy (o-va″re-os′to-me) oophorostomy.

ovariotestis (o-va″re-o-tes′tis) ovotestis.

ovariotherapy (o-va″re-o-ther′ah-pe) ovotherapy.

ovariotomy (o-va″re-ot′o-me) [ovario- + Gr. *tomē* a cutting] surgical removal of an ovary, or removal of an ovarian tumor. **abdominal o.,** ovariotomy performed through the abdominal wall. **vaginal o.,** ovariotomy performed through the vagina.

ovariotubal (o-va″re-o-tu′bal) pertaining to the ovary and uterine tube.

ovaritis (o″vah-ri′tis) oophoritis.

ovarium (o-va′re-um) pl. *ova′ria* [L.] [NA] the ovary or female gonad: one of the two sexual glands in which the ova are formed. It is a flat oval body along the lateral wall of the pelvic cavity, attached to the posterior surface of the broad ligament. It consists of stroma and ovarian follicles in various stages of maturation, and is covered by a modified peritoneum. **o. masculi′num,** appendix testis.

ovarotherapy (o″vah-ro-ther′ah-pe) ovotherapy.

ovary (o′vah-re) the female gonad: one of the two sexual glands in which the ova are formed; see *ovarium*. **adenocystic o.,** an ovary containing numerous small serous cysts. **oyster o's,** hypertrophied, edematous ovaries usually seen in hydatidiform mole. **polycystic o.,** an ovary containing multiple, small follicular cysts filled with yellow or blood-stained, thin serous fluid; the condition may lead to the full-blown Stein-Leventhal syndrome.

ovaserum (o″vah-se′rum) an antiserum found on immunizing with egg albumin.

OVD occlusal vertical dimension; see *vertical dimension*, under *dimension*.

overbite (o′ver-bīt) that condition in which the incisal ridges of the maxillary anterior teeth extend below the incisal ridges of the mandibular anterior teeth when the jaws are in habitual occlusion. Cf. *overjet*. **horizontal o.,** see *overjet*. **vertical o.,** see *overbite*.

overclosure (o″ver-klo′sur) that condition in which the mandible raises too far before the teeth make contact, owing to the loss of occlusal vertical dimension. **reduced interarch distance o.,** an occlusal vertical dimension resulting in excessive interocclusal distance when the mandible is in rest position and in reduced interridge distance when the teeth are in contact.

overcompensation (o″ver-kom″pen-sa′shun) excessive compensation, especially an excessive drive for dominance to offset feelings of inferiority.

overcorrection (o″ver-ko-rek′shun) the use of too powerful lenses in correcting defect of vision.

overdenture (o″ver-den′chur) a complete denture supported both by soft tissue (mucosa) and by a few remaining natural teeth that have been altered, as by insertion of a long or short coping, to permit the denture to fit over them; called also *overlay denture*.

overdetermination (o″ver-de-ter″mǐ-na′shun) in psychoanalysis, the unconscious mechanism through which every mental symptom or every element of a dream is determined by more than one association: i.e., every element of the dream or symptom is the result of many factors.

overdose (o′ver-dōs″) 1. to administer an excessive dose. 2. an excessive dose.

overdosage (o″ver-do′sij) 1. the administration of an excessive dose. 2. the condition resulting from an excessive dose.

overdrive (o′ver-drīv) in cardiology, the process of increasing the heart rate to overcome ectopic heart rhythms; done by the use of drugs or electrical pacemakers.

overeruption (o″ver-e-rup′shun) supraclusion.

overextension (o″ver-eks-ten′shun) extension, as of a limb, beyond the normal limit.

overflow (o′ver-flo) the continuous escape of a fluid, as of the tears or the urine.

overgrafting (o″ver-graft′ing) the application of a second skin graft over a previously healed graft from which the epithelium has been removed, as a means of reinforcing split thickness grafts.

overgrowth (o′ver-grōth) excessive growth of a part, due either to increase in size of the constituent cells (hypertrophy) or to an increase in their number (hyperplasia).

overhang (o′ver-hang) the extension, over the margins of a tooth cavity, of an excessive amount of filling material.

overhydration (o″ver-hi-dra′shun) a state of excess fluids in the body.

overinflation (o″ver-in-fla′shun) excessive inflation or expansion, as of the lungs; hyperinflation. **nonobstructive pulmonary o.,** compensatory emphysema. **obstructive pulmonary o.,** localized obstructive emphysema.

overjet (o′ver-jet) that condition in which the incisal or buccal cusp ridges of the maxillary teeth extend labially or buccally to the incisal margins and ridges of the mandibular teeth when the jaws are in habitual occlusion. Cf. *overbite*.

overlap (o′ver-lap) anything that extends over and partially covers something else. **horizontal o.,** the projection of the upper anterior and/or posterior teeth beyond their antagonists in a horizontal direction. **vertical o.,** 1. the extension of the upper teeth over the lower teeth in a vertical direction when the opposing posterior teeth are in contact in centric occlusion. 2. the distance that teeth lap over their antagonists vertically. 3. the relationship of the maxillary incisors to the mandibular incisors when the incisal edges pass each other in centric occlusion.

overlay (o′ver-la) an increment; a later addition superimposed upon an already existing mass, state, or condition. **emotional o.,** psychogenic o. **psychogenic o.,** the emotionally determined increment to an existing symptom or disability which has been of an organic or of a physically traumatic origin.

overproductivity (o″ver-pro″duk-tiv′ĭ-te) mental activity characterized by volubility, psychomotor activity, flights of ideas, incoherence, destructiveness, noisiness, etc.

overreaching (o″ver-rēch′ing) an error of gait in the horse, in which the toe of the hind hoof strikes the heel of the forefoot.

overresponse (o″ver-re-spons′) abnormally intense response or reaction to a stimulus.

overriding (o″ver-rīd′ing) the slipping of either part of a fractured bone past the other.

overstain (o′ver-stān) to stain a tissue excessively, so that certain elements may be properly stained when the excess of stain is washed out.

overstrain (o′ver-strān) an abnormal degree of fatigue brought about by activity; it is intermediate between fatigue and actual exhaustion.

overstress (o′ver-stres) excessive activity resulting in overstrain.

overtoe (o′ver-to) hallux varus in which the great toe overlies its fellows.

overtone (o′ver-tōn) any whole number multiple of a fundamental tone. **psychic o.,** the consciousness of a fringe or halo of associated relations which surrounds every image presented to the mind.

overtransfusion (o″ver-trans-fu′shun) overloading of the circulation by excessive transfusion of blood or other fluid.

overventilation (o″ver-ven″tĭ-la′shun) hyperventilation.

overweight (o′ver-wāt) excessive increase in adipose tissue (obese overweight) or in muscle and skeletal tissue (muscular overweight).

ovi- see *ovo-*.

ovi (o′vi) [L.] genitive of *ovum*. **o. albu′min** [L.], the white of hens' eggs. **o. vitel′lus** [L.], the yolk of hens' eggs.

ovicide (o′vĭ-sīd) an agent destructive to the ova of certain organisms.

oviducal (o′vĭ-du-kal) pertaining to the oviducts.

oviduct (o′vĭ-dukt) [*ovi-* + L. *ductus* duct] 1. a passage through which ova leave the maternal organism or pass to an organ which communicates with the exterior of the body. 2. a uterine tube (tuba uterina [NA]).

oviductal (o″vĭ-duk′tal) pertaining to an oviduct.

oviferous (o-vif′er-us) [*ovi-* + L. *ferre* to bear] producing ova.

oviform (o′vĭ-form) [*ovi-* + L. *forma* shape] egg-shaped; ovoid.

ovigenesis (o″vĭ-jen′ĕ-sis) [*ovi-* + Gr. *gennan* to produce] oogenesis.

ovigenetic (o″vĭ-jĕ-net′ik) oogenetic.

ovigenic (o″vĭ-jen′ik) oogenic.

ovigenous (o-vij′ĕ-nus) oogenic.

ovigerm (o′vĭ-jerm) [*ovi-* + L. *germen* a bud] a cell which develops into an ovum.

ovigerous (o-vij′er-us) [*ovi-* + L. *gerere* to bear] producing or containing ova.

ovination (o″vĭ-na′shun) [L. *ovinus* of a sheep] inoculation with the virus of sheep-pox.

ovine (o′vīn) [L. *ovinus* of a sheep] pertaining to, characteristic of, or derived from sheep.

ovinia (o-vin′e-ah) [L. *ovis* sheep] sheep-pox.

oviparity (o″vĭ-par′ĭ-te) the quality of being oviparous.

oviparous (o-vip′ah-rus) [*ovi-* + L. *parere* to bring forth, produce] producing eggs from which the young are hatched outside the body of the maternal organism. Cf. *ovoviviparous* and *viviparous*.

oviposition (o″vĭ-po-zish′un) [*ovi-* + L. *ponere* to place] the act of laying or depositing eggs.

ovipositor (o″vĭ-pos′ĭ-tor) a specialized organ by means of which many female insects deposit their eggs in various plant structures or in the soil.

ovisac (o′vĭ-sak) [*ovi-* + L. *saccus* bag] a graafian follicle (folliculi ovarici vesiculosi [NA]).

ovist (o′vist) one who believes that the undeveloped embryo exists preformed in the ovum. Cf. *animalculist*.

ovium (o′ve-um) the mature ovum.

ovo-, ovi- [L. *ovum* egg] combining form denoting relationship to an egg, or to ova. See also words beginning *oo-*.

ovocenter (o′vo-sen″ter) oocenter.

ovocyte (o′vo-sīt) oocyte.

ovoflavin (o″vo-fla′vin) [L. *ovum* egg + *flavus* yellow] riboflavin derived from eggs.

ovogenesis (o″vo-jen′ĕ-sis) oogenesis.

ovoglobulin (o″vo-glob′u-lin) the globulin of white of egg.

ovogonium (o″vo-go′ne-um) oogonium.

ovoid (o′void) [*ovo-* + Gr. *eidos* form] egg-shaped.

ovolysin (o-vol′ĭ-sin) [*ovo-* + *lysin*] a lysin that acts on egg albumin.

ovolytic (o″vo-lit′ik) splitting up egg albumin.

ovomucin (o″vo-mu′sin) a glycoprotein from the white of egg.

ovomucoid (o″vo-mu′koid) [*ovo-* + *mucoid*] a mucus-like principle derivable from egg white.

ovoplasm (o′vo-plazm) [*ovo-* + Gr. *plasma* anything formed] the protoplasm of an unfertilized ovum.

ovoprecipitin (o″vo-pre-sip′ĭ-tin) a precipitin specific for the egg albumin.

ovoserum (o″vo-se′rum) the serum of an animal into which an egg albumin has been injected. This serum will precipitate the albumin from eggs of the same species as those from which the injection was made.

ovotestis (o″vo-tes′tis) a gonad containing both testicular and ovarian tissue.

ovotherapy (o″vo-ther′ah-pe) therapeutic use of ovarian extract, especially extract from the corpus luteum.

ovotransferrin (o″vo-trans-fer′in) an iron-binding protein in egg white having the same properties as transferrin.

ovoverdin (o″vo-ver′din) [*ovo-* + Fr. *verd* green] the green pigment of the chromoprotein of crawfish eggs.

ovovitellin (o″vo-vi-tel′in) vitellin.

ovoviparity (o″vo-viv″ĭ-par′ĭ-te) the quality of being ovoviviparous.

ovoviviparous (o″vo-vi-vip′ah-rus) [*ovo-* + L. *vivus* alive + *parere* to being forth, produce] bearing living young that hatch from large, yolk-filled eggs inside the body of the maternal organism, the embryo being nourished by food stored in the egg; said of lizards, etc. Cf. *oviparous* and *viviparous.*

Ovrette (ov-ret′) trademark for a preparation of norgestrel.

ovula (ov′u-lah) [L.] plural of *ovulum.*

ovular (o′vu-lar) pertaining to an ovule or an ovum.

ovulase (o′vu-lās) an enzyme once thought to be present in ova and to stimulate karyokinesis.

ovulation (o″vu-la′shun) the discharge of a secondary oocyte from a vesicular follicle of the ovary. **amenstrual o.,** that which occurs in the absence of menstrual bleeding. **anestrous o.,** that which occurs in animals unaccompanied by other events of estrus. **paracyclic o.,** supplementary o. **supplementary o.,** an extra ovulation in a particular estrous cycle; called also *paracyclic o.*

ovulatory (ov′u-lah-to″re) pertaining to ovulation.

ovule (o′vūl) [L. *ovulum*] 1. the ovum within the graafian follicle. 2. any small, egglike structure. 3. the megasporangium enclosed within one or more integuments which, after fertilization, becomes a plant seed. **graafian o's,** folliculi ovarici vesiculosi. **Naboth's o's,** Naboth's follicles. **primitive o., primordial o.,** a rudimentary ovum within the ovary.

ovulogenous (o″vu-loj′ĕ-nus) producing or developing from an ovule or ovum.

ovulum (ov′u-lum), pl. *ov′ula* [L. dim. of *ovum*] 1. ovum (def. 2). 2. any small, egglike structure. **ov′ula nabo′thi** ["Naboth's ovules"], Naboth's follicles.

ovum (o′vum), pl. *o′va,* gen. *o′vi* [L.] 1. the female reproductive cell which, after fertilization, develops into a new member of the same species (von Baer, 1827); an egg. 2. [NA] the human ovum: a round cell about 0.1 mm. in diameter, produced in the ovary, where there is deposited around it a noncellular covering (*oolemma; zona pellucida; zona radiata*). It consists of protoplasm which contains some yolk, enclosed by a thin cell wall (*vitelline membrane*). There is a large nucleus (*germinal vesicle*), within which is a nucleolus (*germinal spot*). By extension, the word is also used to designate any early stage of the conceptus, when the embryo itself constitutes a tiny and insignificant part of the whole. **alecithal o.,** one with only a small amount of yolk, or almost no

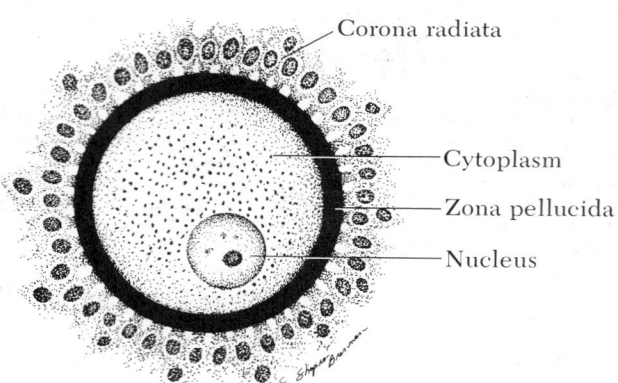

Human ovum.

yolk, as in the ova of mammals and many of the invertebrates; called also *oligolecithal o.* **blighted o.,** a fertilized ovum in which development has become arrested, and abnormality or degeneration is evident. **Bryce-Teacher o.,** a human ovum which was thought to be the youngest known ovum at the time of its study in 1908; now known to be a pathological specimen. **centrolecithal o.,** one in which the yolk is centrally located, and surrounded by a peripheral layer of cytoplasm, as the ova of arthropods. **cleidoic o.,** one which possesses within itself sufficient nutritive material for the production of a complete embryo and so needs to absorb nothing from its environment except oxygen, as a bird's egg. **ectolecithal o.,** one in which the yolk is situated peripherally. **Hertig-Rock ova,** 34 fertilized ova, ranging from 1 to 17 days of age, 21 of which were normal, and 13 abnormal to one degree or another; discovered between 1938 and 1953, they constitute the only series of such early human conceptuses in existence. **holoblastic o.,** one that undergoes total cleavage. **isolecithal o.,** one with yolk evenly distributed throughout the cytoplasm. **macrolecithal o.,** one with much yolk. **Mateer-Streeter o.,** a fertilized ovum about 18 days old, first described in 1920. **medialecithal o.,** one with a medium amount of yolk. **megalecithal o.,** macrolecithal o. **meroblastic o.,** one that undergoes partial cleavage. **mi-**

crolecithal o., miolecithal o. **Miller o.,** a fertilized ovum 10 or 11 days old, first described in 1913. **miolecithal o.,** one containing little yolk. **oligolecithal o.,** alecithal o. **permanent o.,** an ovum ready for fertilization. **Peters' o.,** a fertilized ovum about 13 or 14 days old, first described in 1899. **primitive o., primordial o.,** an egg cell very early in its development. **telolecithal o.,** one in which the yolk is increasingly concentrated toward one pole.

Owen's lines (o′enz) [Sir Richard *Owen,* English anatomist and paleontologist, 1804–1892] see under *line.*

oxacillin sodium, (oks″ah-sil′in) [USP] chemical name: [2*S*-(2α,5α,6β)]-3,3-dimethyl-6-[[(5-methyl-3-phenyl-4-isoxazolyl)carbonyl]amino]-7-oxo-4-thia-1-azabicyclo[3.2.0]heptane-2-carboxylic acid monosodium salt monohydrate. A semisynthetic penicillinase-resistant penicillin, $C_{19}H_{18}N_3NaO_5S \cdot H_2O$, occurring as a fine, white, crystalline powder; used primarily in the treatment of infections due to penicillinase-resistant staphylococci, administered orally, intramuscularly, or intravenously.

Oxaine (ok′sān) trademark for a preparation of oxethazaine.

oxalaldehyde (ok″sal-al′dĕ-hīd) glyoxal.

oxalate (ok′sah-lāt) a salt of oxalic acid. **ammonium o.,** odorless crystals or white granules, $(NH_4)_2C_2O_4$, formed by evaporation of the product obtained by the reaction of equivalent amounts of ammonia solution and oxalic acid. **balanced o.,** a mixture of ammonium and potassium oxalates in a 3:2 ratio, used as an anticoagulant in the collection of blood for laboratory examination. **calcium o.,** a salt of oxalic acid which, when formed in high concentrations in the urine, may lead to formation of urinary calculi. **potassium o.,** colorless, odorless crystals, $K_2C_2O_4 \cdot H_2O$, used extensively as a reagent. **sodium o.,** white, odorless, crystalline powder, $Na_2C_2O_4$, formerly used as an anticoagulant in collection of blood for laboratory examination.

oxalated (ok′sah-lāt″ed) treated with oxalate solution.

oxalation (ok″sah-la′shun) treatment with oxalate solution.

oxalemia (ok″sah-le′me-ah) [*oxalate* + Gr. *haima* blood + *-ia*] the presence of an excess of oxalates in the blood.

Oxalid (ok′sah-lid) trademark for a preparation of oxyphenbutazone.

oxalism (ok′sal-izm) poisoning by oxalic acid or an oxalate.

oxaloacetate (oks″ah-lo-as′ĕ-tāt) a salt of oxaloacetic acid; in biochemistry the term is often used interchangeably with oxaloacetic acid (see under *acid*).

oxalosis (ok″sah-lo′sis) generalized deposition of calcium oxalate in renal and extrarenal tissues, as may occur in primary hyperoxaluria.

oxaluria (ok″sah-lu′re-ah) hyperoxaluria.

oxalyl (ok′sah-lil) the divalent group, $(C:O)_2$, formed from oxalic acid by the loss of two hydroxyl groups.

oxalylurea (ok″sah-lil-u′re-ah) 1. oxaluric acid. 2. parabanic acid.

oxamide (ok-sam′id) the diamide of oxalic acid, $NH_2 \cdot CO \cdot CO \cdot NH_2$. It will give the biuret reaction.

oxamniquine (oks-am′nĭ-kwin) chemical name: 1,2,3,4-tetrahydro-2-[[(1-methylethyl)amino]methyl]-7-nitro-6-quinolinemethanol. An antischistosomal, $C_{14}H_{21}N_3O_3$, especially effective against *Schistosoma mansoni.*

oxanamide (ok-san′ah-mīd) chemical name: 2,3-epoxy-2-ethylhexanamide. Tasteless, odorless, white crystals, $C_8H_{15}NO_2$, used as a tranquilizer.

oxandrolone (ok-san′dro-lōn) [USP] chemical name: 17β-hydroxy-17-methyl-2-oxa-5α-androstan-3-one. An androgenic steroidal lactone, $C_{19}H_{30}O_3$, which promotes retention of nitrogen, potassium, and phosphorus, and is used to accelerate anabolism and/or to arrest excessive catabolism.

oxantel pamoate (oks′an-tel) chemical name: (*E*)-3-[2-(1,4,5,6-tetrahydro-1-methyl-2-pyrimidinyl)ethenyl]phenol 4,4′-methylenebis[3-hydroxy-2-naphthalenecarboxylate] (2:1) (salt); an anthelmintic effective against *Trichuris,* $(C_{13}H_{16}N_2O)_2 \cdot C_{23}H_{16}O_6$.

oxaprozin (ok″sah-pro′zin) chemical name: 4,5-diphenyl-2-oxazolepropanoic acid; an anti-inflammatory, $C_{18}H_{15}NO_3$.

oxarbazole (ok-sar′bah-zōl) chemical name: 9-benzoyl-2,3,4,9-tetrahydro-6-methoxy-1*H*-carbaxole-3-carboxylic acid; an antiasthmatic, $C_{21}H_{19}NO_4$.

oxatomide (ok-sa′to-mīd) chemical name: 1-[3-[4-(diphenylmethyl)-1-piperaxinyl]propyl]-1,3-dihydro-2*H*-benzimidazol-2-one; an antiallergic and antiasthmatic, $C_{27}H_{30}N_4O$.

oxazepam (oks-az′ĕ-pam) [USP] chemical name: 7-chloro-1,3-dihydro-3-hydroxy-5-phenyl-2*H*-1,4-benzodiazepin-2-one. One of the benzodiazepine tranquilizers, $C_{15}H_{11}ClN_2O_2$, occurring as a creamy white to pale yellow powder. It is used orally as a sedative in the treatment of anxiety, especially in the elderly, and may be used as an adjunct for acute withdrawal symptoms in chronic alcoholics.

oxethazaine (ok-seth′ah-zān) chemical name: 2,2′-(2-hydroxyethylimino)-bis-[*N*-α,α-dimethylphenethyl]-*N*-methylacetamide]. A topical anesthetic, $C_{28}H_{41}N_3O_3$, which has been administered orally to relieve gastric distress.

oxetorone fumarate (ok-set′o-rōn) chemical name: 3-benzofuro[3,2-*c*][1][benzoxepin-6(12*H*)-ylidene-*N,N*-dimethyl-1-propanamine(*E*)-2-butenedioate (1:1); an analgesic specific in migraine, $C_{21}H_{21}NO_2 \cdot C_4H_4O_4$.

oxfendazole (oks-fen′dah-zōl) chemical name: [5-(phenylsulfinyl)-1*H*-benzimidazol-2-yl]carbamic acid methyl ester; an anthelmintic, $C_{15}H_{13}N_3O_3S$.

oxgall (oks′gawl) see *ox bile extract,* under *extract.*

oxibendazole (ok″sĭ-ben′dah-zōl) chemical name: (5-propoxy-1*H*-benzimidazol-2-yl)carbamic acid methyl ester; a veterinary anthelmintic, $C_{12}H_{15}N_3O_3$.

oxidant (ok′sĭ-dant) the electron acceptor in an oxidation-reduction (redox) reaction.

oxidase (ok′sĭ-dās) any of a class of (metalloprotein) enzymes that catalyze the reduction of molecular oxygen independently of hydrogen peroxide. **amine o.,** monoamine o. **amino acid o.,** an enzyme that catalyzes the oxidative removal of alpha amino groups; it is a flavoprotein occurring in two forms: one reacting with L-amino acid, the other with D-amino acid. **ascorbate o., ascorbic acid o.,** L-ascorbate:oxygen oxidoreductase. An enzyme found in squash and other vegetables which catalyzes the oxidation of 2 L-ascorbic acid to dehydroascorbic acid. **diamine o.,** diamine:oxygen oxidoreductase (deaminating). An enzyme that catalyzes the change of diamines into the corresponding aldehydes, ammonia, and peroxide; it also oxidizes histamine. *p*-**diphenol o.,** *p*-diphenol oxygen oxidoreductase. An enzyme occurring in the latex of lac trees and in many vegetables; it oxidizes the latex to Japanese lacquer and many phenols to ortho- and para-quinones; called also *laccase.* **direct o.,** an oxidase that causes the direct transference of oxygen from the air. **dopa o.,** see *dopa-oxidase.* **glucose o.,** β-D-glucose:oxygen oxidoreductase. A toxic antibiotic flavoprotein from *Penicillium notatum* that catalyzes the oxidation of glucose to gluconic acid; called also *glucose aerodehydrogenase, notatin, penatin,* and *penicillin B.* **hypoxanthine o.,** xanthine o. **indirect o.,** an oxidase that acts only with a peroxide. **indophenol o.,** cytochrome o. **monamine o.,** monoamine:oxygen oxidoreductase (deaminating). A cuproprotein enzyme that catalyzes the oxidation of amines into the corresponding aldehydes, ammonia, and hydrogen peroxide; called also *amine o.* **monophenyl o.,** tyrosinase. **primary o.,** direct o. **tyramine o.,** tyrosinase. **xanthine o.,** xanthine:oxygen oxidoreductase. A flavoprotein enzyme that catalyzes the oxidation of various purine bases, including xanthine and hypoxanthine, as well as pterins and aldehydes. Called also *hypoxanthine o.*

oxidation (ok″sĭ-da′shun) the act of oxidizing or state of being oxidized. Chemically it consists in the increase of positive charges on an atom or the loss of negative charges. Most biological oxidations are accomplished by the removal of a pair of hydrogen atoms (dehydrogenation) from a molecule. Such oxidations must be accompanied by reduction of an acceptor molecule. *Univalent o.* indicates loss of one electron; *divalent o.,* the loss of two electrons. **beta o.** (β-oxidation), oxidation of a fatty acid at the beta carbon atom, the second carbon from the carboxyl group, with the result that the two end carbons are split off as acetic acid (acetylcoenzyme A) and with the formation of a fatty acid containing two less carbon atoms. **biological o.,** the enzymatic process by which food is metabolized, resulting in the release of energy. See also *oxidation.* **coupled o.,** the enzymatic oxidation of two donor molecules, with the incorporation of oxygen into one of the donors.

oxidation-reduction (ok″sĭ-da′shun-re-duk′shun) the chemical reaction whereby electrons are removed (oxidation) from atoms of the substance being oxidized and transferred to atoms being reduced (reduction). Called also *redox.*

oxide (ok′sīd) [L. *oxidum*] any compound of oxygen with an element or radical. **arsenous o.,** arsenic trioxide. **diethyl o.,** ether (def. 2).

oxidize (ok′sĭ-dīz) to combine or cause to combine with oxygen, or to lose electrons. See *oxidation.*

oxidopamine (oks″ĭ-do′pah-mēn) chemical name: 5-(2-aminoethyl-1,2,4-benzenetriol, $C_8H_{11}NO_3$; an ophthalmic adrenergic.

oxidoreductase (ok″sĭ-do-re-duk′tās) a class of enzymes that catalyze the reversible transfer of electrons from one substance to another (oxidation-reduction, or redox reaction). It includes dehydrogenases, reductases, oxidases, transhydrogenases, peroxidases, and oxygenases.

oxidosis (ok″sĭ-do′sis) acidosis.

oxifungin hydrochloride (ok″sĭ-fun′gin) chemical name: 1,2-dihydro-3-(phenoxymethyl)pyrido[3,4-*e*]-1,2,4-triazine monohydrochloride; an antifungal, $C_{13}H_{12}N_4O \cdot HCl$.

oxigram (ok′sĭ-gram) (*obs.*) oxyhemogram.

oxilorphan (ok′sil-or′fan) chemical name: 17-(cyclopropylmethyl)morphinan-3,14-diol; a narcotic antagonist, $C_{20}H_{27}NO_2$.

oxim, oxime (ok′sim) any of a series of compounds formed by the action of hydroxylamine upon an aldehyde or a ketone.

oximeter (ok-sim′ĕ-ter) a photoelectric device for determining the oxygen saturation of the blood. **ear o.,** an oximeter for attachment to the ear, by which oxygen saturation of the blood

flowing through the ear can be determined. **intracardiac o.,** an instrument for measuring the concentration of oxygen or dye in blood within the heart; see also *oxygen gas analyzer,* under *analyzer.* **whole blood o.,** an oximeter for determination of oxygen saturation of removed specimens of blood.

oximetry (ok-sim′ĕ-tre) determination of the oxygen saturation of arterial blood by means of bichromate photoelectric colorimetry.

oximinotransferase (ok-sim″ĭ-no-trans′fer-ās) an enzyme that catalyzes the transfer of oxime from pyruvateoxime to form pyruvate and acetoxime; called also *transoximinase.*

oxiperomide (ok″se-per′o-mīd) chemical name: 1,3-dihydro-1-[1-(2-phenoxyethyl)-4-piperidinyl]-2*H*-benzimidazol-2-one; a dopamine-receptor antagonist, $C_{20}H_{23}N_3O_2$, used as a tranquilizer.

oxiramide (ok-sēr′ah-mīd) chemical name: *cis*-(+)-*N*-[4-(2,6-dimethyl-1-piperidenyl)butyl]-α-phenoxybenzeneacetamide; a cardiac depressant, $C_{25}H_{34}N_2O_2$, with antiarrhythmic activity.

oxisuran (ok″se-sur′an) chemical name: (methylsulfinyl)methyl-2-pyridyl ketone; an antineoplastic, $C_8H_9NO_2S$.

oxogestone phenpropionate (ok″so-jes′tōn) chemical name: 20β-hydroxy-19-norpregn-4-en-3-one hydrocinnamate; a progestin, $C_{29}H_{38}O_3$.

oxonemia (ok″so-ne′me-ah) [L. *oxone* acetone + Gr. *haima* blood + -*ia*] (*obs.*) acetonemia.

oxonium (ok-so′ne-um) containing tetravalent basic oxygen.

oxonuria (ok″so-nu′re-ah) (*obs.*) acetonuria.

oxophenarsine hydrochloride (ok″so-phen-ar′sin) chemical name: 2-amino-arsenophenol hydrochloride. An arsenical, $C_6H_6AsNO_2 \cdot HCl$, with antispirochetal and antitrypanosomal properties; rarely used in the treatment of syphilis and trypanosomiasis, administered intravenously.

5-oxoproline (ok″so-pro′lēn) a ninhydrin-negative, acidic lactam of glutamic acid occurring at the N-terminus of several peptides and proteins. Called also *pyroglutamic acid* or *pyroglutamate.*

5-oxoprolinuria (ok″so-pro′lin-u′re-ah) an inborn error of metabolism marked by abnormally increased levels of 5-oxoproline in the urine, metabolic acidosis, and an increase in the rate of hemolysis; neurological symptoms may also occur. Called also *pyroglutamic aciduria.*

oxozone (ok′so-zōn) a hypothetical allotropic form of oxygen, O_4, supposed to be present in ozone.

oxpentifylline (oks″ĭ-pin-tif′ĭ-lēn) pentoxifylline.

oxprenolol hydrochloride (oks-pren′o-lōl) chemical name: 1-[(1-methylethyl)amino]-3-[2-(2-propenyloxy)-2-propanol hydrochloride; a beta-adrenergic blocking agent, $C_{15}H_{23}NO_3 \cdot HCl$, having the same actions as propanolol (q.v.)

Oxsoralen (ok-sor′ah-len) trademark for preparations of methoxsalen.

oxtriphylline (oks-trif′ĭ-lēn) [NF] chemical name: 2-hydroxy-*N,N,N*-trimethylethanaminium salt with 3,7-dihydro-1,3-dimethyl-1*H*-purine,2,6-dione. A compound of choline and theophylline, $C_{12}H_{21}N_5O_3$, occurring as a white crystalline powder, having the same actions as the parent compound; used chiefly as a bronchodilator, administered orally. Called also *choline theophyllinate* and *theophylline cholinate.*

oxy- [Gr. *oxys* keen] a combining form meaning (*a*) sharp, quick, or sour, or (*b*) denoting the presence of oxygen in a compound.

oxyachrestia (ok″se-ah-kres′te-ah) [*oxy-* + *a* neg. + Gr. *chrēsis* use] a condition of defective supply of glucose to the neurons, which is the cause of hypoglycemic coma.

oxyacoia (ok′se-ah-koi′ah) oxyecoia.

oxybenzene (ok″se-ben′zēn) phenol.

oxybenzone (ok″se-ben′zōn) [USP] chemical name: (2-hydroxy-4-methoxyphenyl)phenylmethanone. A sunscreening agent, $C_{14}H_{12}O_3$, occurring as a white to off-white powder; applied topically to the skin.

oxyblepsia (ok″se-blep′se-ah) [*oxy-* + Gr. *blepsis* vision + -*ia*] unusual acuity of vision.

oxybutynin chloride (ok″se-bu′tĭ-nin) chemical name: 4-(diethylamino)-2-butyl-α-phenylcyclohexaneglycolate. An anticholinergic, $C_{22}H_{31}NO_3 \cdot HCl$, which has a direct antispasmodic effect on smooth muscle; used in the treatment of uninhibited neurogenic bladder and reflex neurogenic bladder, administered orally.

oxybutyria (ok″se-bu-tir′e-ah) [*oxybutyric acid* + Gr. *ouron* urine + -*ia*] the presence of hydroxybutyric acid in urine.

oxybutyricacidemia (ok″se-bu-tir″ik-as″ĭ-de′me-ah) oxybutyria.

oxycalorimeter (ok″se-kal-o-rim′ĕ-ter) Benedict's apparatus for determining the caloric value of food by burning a sample in a combustion chamber and measuring the volume of oxygen consumed.

oxycanthine (ok-se-kan′thin) a white alkaloid, $C_{37}H_{40}O_6N_2$, from the root of *Berberis vulgaris,* the barberry; said to paralyze and irritate the brain and spinal cord.

Oxycel (ok′sĭ-sel) trademark for preparations of oxidized cellulose.

oxycephalia (ok″se-sĕ-fa′le-ah) oxycephaly.

oxycephalic (ok″se-sĕ-fal′ik) pertaining to or characterized by oxycephaly.

oxycephalous (ok″se-sef′ah-lus) oxycephalic.

oxycephaly (ok″se-sef′ah-le) [*oxy-* + Gr. *kephalē* head] a condition in which the top of the head is pointed or conical owing to premature closure of the coronal and lambdoid sutures. Called also *acrocephaly, hypsicephaly, turricephaly, steeple head* or *skull*, and *tower head* or *skull*.

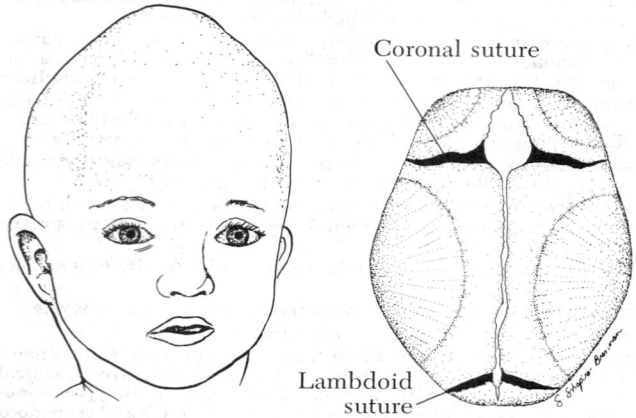

Coronal suture

Lambdoid suture

Oxycephaly, showing in black the sites of premature closure of cranial sutures.

oxychloride (ok″se-klo′rīd) an element or radical combined with oxygen and chlorine.

oxychlorosene (ok″se-klor′o-sēn) the hypochlorous acid complex of a mixture of the phenyl sulfonate derivatives of aliphatic hydrocarbons, $C_{20}H_{34}O_3S \cdot HOCl$, having actions similar to those of chlorine; used as a topical anti-infective. **o. sodium,** the sodium salt of oxychlorosene, used like the base.

oxycholine (ok″se-ko′lin) muscarine.

oxychromatic (ok″se-kro-mat′ik) [*oxy-* + Gr. *chrōma* color] staining with acid dyes; acidophilic.

oxychromatin (ok″se-kro′mah-tin) [*oxy-* + *chromatin*] that part of the chromatin that stains with acid aniline dyes; called also *lanthanin.*

oxycinesia (ok″se-si-ne′ze-ah) [*oxy-* + Gr. *kinēsis* movement + *-ia*] pain on motion.

oxycodone hydrochloride (ok″se-ko′dōn) chemical name: 4,5α-epoxy-14-hydroxy-3-methoxy-17-methylmorphinan-6-one. A morphine derivative, $C_{18}H_{21}NO \cdot HCl$, used as a narcotic analgesic.

oxycyanide (ox″se-si′ah-nīd) the oxide of any binary compound of cyanogen.

oxydase (ok′se-dās) oxidase.

oxydendron (ok″se-den′dron) [*oxy-* + Gr. *dendron* tree] a homeopathic remedy prepared from the leaves of *Oxydendrum arboreum,* an ericaceous tree of North America.

oxydesis (ok″se-de′sis) [*oxy-* + Gr. *desis* binding] (*obs.*) the acid-binding power especially of the blood. In the latter it represents the greatest amount of HCl (one hundredth normal) that can be added to oxalated blood without clumping the erythrocytes.

oxydetic (ok″se-det′ik) (*obs.*) pertaining to acid-binding power, especially of blood.

oxydoreductase (ok″sĕ-do-re-duk′tās) oxidoreductase.

oxyecoia (ok″se-e-koi′ah) [*oxy-* + Gr. *akoē* hearing + *-ia*] morbid acuteness of the sense of hearing.

oxyesthesia (ok″se-es-the′ze-ah) [*oxy-* + Gr. *aisthesis* perception + *-ia*] morbid or abnormal acuteness of the senses. Cf. *hyperesthesia.*

oxyetherotherapy (ok″se-e″ther-o-ther′ah-pe) [*oxy-* + *ether* + Gr. *therapeia* medical treatment] treatment by the inhalation of ether vapor which is carried along by a current of oxygen; formerly used in pulmonary infection and in whooping cough.

oxygen (ok′sĭ-jen) [Gr. *oxys* sour + *gennan* to produce] a gaseous element existing free in the air and in combination in most nonelementary solids, liquids, and gases; atomic number, 8; atomic weight, 15.999; symbol, O. Oxygen exists in three isotopes, with atomic weights of 16, 17 and 18 (heavy oxygen). Oxygen constitutes 20 per cent by weight of the atmospheric air; it is the essential agent in the respiration of plants and animals and, although noninflammable, is necessary to support combustion. It forms the characteristic constituent of ternary acids. It is administered by inhalation in some pulmonary and cardiac disorders. **excess o.,** the quantity of oxygen used over and above the resting requirements of the body. **heavy o.,** an isotope of oxygen of atomic weight 18. **high pressure o.,** hyperbaric o. **hyperbaric o.,** high-pressure oxygen, i.e., oxygen under greater than atmo-

spheric pressure. **molecular o.,** oxygen whose atoms are joined in pairs, as in the atmosphere; symbol O_2.

oxygenase (ok′sĭ-jĕ-nās″) any of the enzymes of the oxidoreductase class that catalyze the incorporation of both atoms of molecular oxygen into the substrate.

oxygenate (ok′sĭ-jĕ-nāt) to add oxygen to.

oxygenation (ok″sĭ-jĕ-na′shun) the act, process, or result of oxygenating.

oxygenator (ok″sĭ-jĕ-na′tor) a device which mechanically oxygenates venous blood extracorporeally. It is used in combination with one or more pumps for maintaining circulation during open heart surgery and for assisting the circulation in patients seriously ill with some cardiac and pulmonary disorders. **bubble o.,** a device in which pure oxygen is bubbled through an extracorporeal reservoir of blood, either directly or through a filter. **disk o.,** rotating disk o. **film o.,** a device, encased in a container of oxygen, which makes possible the production of a thin film of blood to facilitate the exchange of gases; see *rotating disk o.* and *screen o.* **membrane o.,** a device, usually consisting of a connected series of flat bags made of semipermeable material, such as cellophane, Teflon, or Silastic, encased in a container of oxygen. The exchange of gases between the blood in the bags and the oxygen in the container occurs across the membrane. **pump-o.,** see *pump-oxygenator.* **rotating disk o.,** a type of film oxygenator in which parallel disks in series rotate through an extracorporeal pool of venous blood in a container of oxygen; gaseous exchange occurs between the thin film of blood on the exposed surfaces of the disks and the oxygen in the container. **screen o.,** a type of film oxygenator in which the venous blood is passed over a series of screens in a container of oxygen, gaseous exchange taking place in the thin film of blood produced on the screens.

oxygenic (ok″sĭ-jen′ik) containing oxygen.

oxygeusia (ok″sĭ-gu′se-ah) [*oxy-* + Gr. *geusis* taste + *-ia*] unusual acuteness of the sense of taste.

oxyhematoporphyrin (ok″se-hem″ah-to-por′fĭ-rin) a pigment sometimes found in the urine, closely allied to hematoporphyrin.

oxyheme (ok′se-hēm) heme.

oxyhemochromogen (ok″se-he″mo-kro′mo-jen) heme.

oxyhemocyanine (ok″se-he″mo-si′ah-nin) hematocyanine charged with oxygen.

oxyhemoglobin (ok″se-he″mo-glo′bin) hemoglobin that contains bound O_2, a compound formed from hemoglobin on exposure to alveolar gas in the lungs, with formation of a covalent bond with oxygen and without change of the charge of the ferrous state.

oxyhemogram (ok″se-he′mo-gram) (*obs.*) a graphic record of the oxygen saturation of the blood as determined by use of the oxyhemograph.

oxyhemograph (ok″se-he′mo-graf) [*oxygen* + Gr. *haima* blood + *graphein* to write] (*obs.*) an apparatus for determining the oxygen content of the blood, by photoelectric registration of changes in the spectroscopic properties of hemoglobin.

oxyhydrocephalus (ok″se-hi″dro-sef′ah-lus) hydrocephalus in which the top of the head assumes a pointed shape.

oxyhyperglycemia (ok″se-hi″per-gli-se′me-ah) a condition in which there is slight glycosuria and an oral glucose tolerance curve which rises about 180–200 mg. per 100 ml. but returns to fasting values 2½ hours after ingestion of the glucose.

oxyiodide (ok″se-i′o-dīd) an element or radical combined with oxygen and iodine.

oxykrinin (ok-se-krin′in) secretin.

oxylalia (ok-se-la′le-ah) [*oxy-* + Gr. *lalein* to talk + *-ia*] swiftness of speech.

Oxylone (ok′sĭ-lōn) trademark for a preparation of fluorometholone.

oxyluciferin (ok-se-lu-sif′er-in) the product of the oxidation of luciferin catalyzed by luciferase.

oxymetazoline hydrochloride (ok″se-met-az′o-lēn) [USP] chemical name: 3-[(4,5-dihydro-1*H*-imidazol-2-yl)methyl]-6-(1,1-dimethylethyl)-2,4-dimethylphenol monohydrochloride. An adrenergic, $C_{16}H_{24}N_2O \cdot HCl$, occurring as a white to nearly white, crystalline powder; used topically as a vasoconstrictor to reduce swelling and congestion of the nasal mucosa.

oxymetholone (ok″se-meth′o-lōn) [NF] chemical name: 17β-hydroxy-2-(hydroxymethylene)-17α-methyl-5α-androstan-3-one. An anabolic-androgenic steroid, $C_{21}H_{32}O_3$, occurring as a white to creamy white, crystalline powder; administered orally.

oxymetry (ok-sim′ĕ-tre) oximetry.

oxymorphone hydrochloride (ok″se-mor′fōn) [USP] chemical name: 4,5α-epoxy-3,14-dihydroxy-17-methylmorphinan-6-one hydrochloride. A semisynthetic compound, $C_{12}H_{19}NO_4 \cdot HCl$, occurring as a white or slightly off-white, odorless powder; used as a narcotic analgesic.

oxymyoglobin (ok″se-mi″o-glo′bin) a compound formed from myoglobin on exposure to atmospheric conditions, with formation of a covalent bond with oxygen and without change of the charge of the ferrous state.

oxymyohematin (ok″se-mi″o-hem′ah-tin) oxidized myohematin from muscle.

oxynervon (ok″se-ner′von) a cerebroside isolated from the brain.

oxyneurine (ok″se-nu′rin) betaine.

oxynitrilase (ok″se-ni′tril-ās) an enzyme that splits mandelonitrite to benzaldehyde and HCN.

oxyntic (ok-sin′tik) [Gr. *oxynō* to make acid] secreting acid, as the parietal (oxyntic) cells.

oxyopia (ok″se-o′pe-ah) [*oxy-* + Gr. *ōpē* sight + *-ia*] acuteness of vision.

oxyopter (ok″se-op′ter) [*oxy-* + Gr. *ōps* vision] a unit of measurement of visual acuity, being the reciprocal value of the visual angle expressed in degrees. An oxyopter (1 degree) is equivalent to 60 Snellen units (60′) and corresponds to the counting of fingers at 1 meter (De Blaskovics).

oxyosis (ok″se-o′sis) [*oxy-* + *-osis*] acidosis.

oxyosmia (ok″se-os′me-ah) [*oxy-* + Gr. *osmē* odor + *-ia*] acuteness of the sense of smell.

oxyosphresia (ok″se-os-fre′ze-ah) [*oxy-* + Gr. *osphrēsis* smell + *-ia*] unusual acuteness of the sense of smell.

oxyparaplastin (ok″se-par″ah-plas′tin) the oxyphil part of paraplastin.

oxypathia (ok″se-pa′the-ah) acuteness of sensation. See *hyperesthesia.*

oxyperitoneum (ok″se-per″ĭ-to-ne′um) injection of oxygen into the peritoneal cavity.

oxypertine (ok″se-per′tēn) chemical name: 5,6-dimethoxy-2-methyl-3-[2-(4-phenyl-1-piperazinyl)ethyl]indole; an antidepressant, $C_{23}H_{29}N_3O_2$.

oxyphenbutazone (ok″se-fen-bu′tah-zōn) [USP] chemical name: 4-butyl-1-(4-hydroxyphenyl)-2-phenyl-3,5-pyrazolidinedione monohydrate. A derivative of phenylbutazone, $C_{19}H_{20}N_2O_3 \cdot H_2O$, having similar anti-inflammatory, analgesic, and antipyretic actions; administered orally in the treatment of arthritis, gout, and similar conditions.

oxyphencyclimine hydrochloride (ok″se-fen-si′klĭ-mēn) [USP] chemical name: α-cyclohexyl-α-hydroxybenzeneacetic acid (1,4,5,6-tetrahydro-1-methyl-2-pyrimidinyl)methyl ester monohydrochloride. An anticholinergic, $C_{20}H_{28}N_2O_3 \cdot HCl$, occurring as a white, crystalline powder, having antispasmodic, antisecretory, and antimotility activities; used especially in the treatment of peptic ulcer and spasm of the gastrointestinal tract, administered orally.

oxyphenisatin (ok″se-fĕ-ni′sah-tin) chemical name: 3,3-bis(4-hydroxyphenyl)-1,3-dihydro-2*H*-indol-2-one. A cathartic, $C_{20}H_{15}NO_3$, occurring as a white, crystalline powder; administered as an enema to cleanse the bowel before surgery or colon examination. **o. acetate,** the diacetyl derivative of oxyphenisatin, $C_{24}H_{19}NO_5$, occurring as a white, crystalline powder; used as a cathartic, administered orally.

oxyphenonium bromide (ok″se-fĕ-no′ne-um) chemical name: 2-[cyclohexylhydroxyphenylacetyl)oxy]-*N,N*-diethyl-*N*-methylethanaminium bromide. A quaternary ammonium anticholinergic, $C_{21}H_{34}BrNO_3$, occurring as a white, crystalline powder having antisecretory, antispasmodic, and antimotility activities; used in the treatment of peptic ulcer and other gastrointestinal disorders in which hypermotility and spasm are a feature, administered orally.

oxyphenylethylamine (ok″se-fen″il-eth″il-am′in) tyramine.

oxyphil (ok′se-fil) 1. Hürthle cell. 2. oxyphilic.

oxyphilic (ok″se-fil′ik) [*oxy-* + Gr. *philein* to love] stainable with an acid dye.

oxyphilous (oks-if′ĭ-lus) oxyphilic.

oxyphonia (ok″se-fo′ne-ah) [Gr. *oxyphōnia*] an abnormally sharp quality or pitch of the voice.

oxyphorase (ok′se-for′ās) an oxygen-carrying enzyme.

oxyplasm (ok′se-plazm) the oxyphil part of the cytoplasm.

oxypurinase (ok″se-pu′rĭ-nās) an enzyme that oxidizes oxypurines.

oxypurine (ok″se-pu′rin) a purine containing oxygen. The oxypurines include hypoxanthine or monoxypurine, xanthine or dioxypurine, and uric acid or trioxypurine.

oxypurinol (ok″se-pūr′ĭ-nol) chemical name: 1*H*-pyrazolo[3,4-*d*]pyrimidine-4,6-diol; the active metabolite of allopurinol, a xanthine oxidase inhibitor, $C_5H_4N_4O_2$.

oxyrenin (ok″se-re′nin) a term suggested for the hypertensive substance produced by the oxidation of renin.

oxyrhine (ok′se-rīn) [*oxy-* + Gr. *rhis* nose] having a sharp-pointed nose.

oxyrygmia (ok″se-rig′me-ah) [*oxy-* + Gr. *erygmos* eructation] (*obs.*) acid eructation.

oxysalt (ok′se-sawlt) any salt of an oxacid.

oxysantonin (ok″se-san′to-nin) a compound formed in the body from ingested santonin.

Oxyspirura (ok″se-spi-roo′rah) a genus of nematode parasites of the superfamily Spiruroidea. **O. manso′ni,** a species found beneath the nictitating membrane of chickens and other fowl in Asia, Africa, Australia, South America, Samoa, and in the United States in Florida, Texas, Louisiana, and Hawaii.

oxytalan (oks-it′ah-lan) a connective tissue fiber found typically in the periodontal membranes of man and certain other animals, including monkeys. It is stained with aldehyde fuchsin after appropriate oxidation. On electron microscopic examination, fibrillar and amorphous components are revealed.

oxytalanolysis (oks-it″ah-lan-ol′ĭ-sis) destruction of oxytalan fibers.

oxytetracycline (ok″se-tet″rah-si′klēn) [USP] chemical name: 4-(dimethyl-amino)-1,4,4α,5α,6,11,12a-octahydro-3,5,6,10,12a-hexahydroxy-6-methyl-1,11dioxa-2-naphthacenecarboxamide. A broad-spectrum antibiotic of the tetracycline group, produced by *Streptomyces rimosus,* $C_{22}H_{24}N_2O_9 \cdot 2H_2O$, occurring as a yellow crystalline powder, and used chiefly as an antibacterial, administered intramuscularly. **o. calcium** [USP], the calcium salt of oxytetracycline, $C_{44}H_{46}Ca_4O_{18}$, occurring as a yellow to light brown, crystalline powder; used as a antibacterial, administered orally. **o. hydrochloride** [USP], the monohydrochloride salt of oxytetracycline, $C_{22}H_{24}N_2O_9 \cdot HCl$, occurring as a yellow, crystalline powder; used as an antibacterial and antirickettsial, administered orally and by intravenous infusion.

oxytocia (ok-se-to′se-ah) [*oxy-* + Gr. *tokos* birth + *-ia*] rapid labor.

oxytocic (ok-se-to′sik) 1. pertaining to, characterized by, or promoting oxytocia. 2. an agent that hastens evacuation of the uterus by stimulating contractions of the myometrium.

oxytocin (ok″se-to′sin) 1. an octapeptide, one of two hormones formed by the neuronal cells of the hypothalamic nuclei and stored in the posterior lobe of the pituitary, the other being vasopressin. It has uterine-contracting and milk-ejection actions. 2. the same oxytocic principle obtained synthetically or from the posterior pituitary of domestic animals, prepared in accordance with USP standards; it is administered intramuscularly or by intravenous infusion to induce active labor, increase the force of contractions in labor, contract uterine muscle after delivery of the placenta, control postpartum hemorrhage, and stimulate milk ejection. Often used in veterinary medicine to stimulate the letdown of milk in cows and heifers affected with agalactia. **o. citrate,** the citrate salt of oxytocin, $C_{43}H_{66}N_{12}O_{12}S_2 \cdot C_6H_8O_7$, used to initiate or stimulate labor in selected patients, administered buccally.

oxytropism (oks-it′ro-pizm) [*oxygen* + Gr. *trepein* to turn] response of living cells to the stimulus of oxygen.

oxytuberculin (ok″se-tu-ber′ku-lin) a tuberculin from cultures of an extremely virulent bacillus, modified by oxidation.

oxyuria (ok″se-u′re-ah) oxyuriasis.

oxyuriasis (ok″se-u-ri′ah-sis) infection with *Enterobius vermicu′laris* (in humans) or with other oxyurids; enterobiasis.

oxyuricide (ok″se-u′rĭ-sīd) [*oxyuris* + L. *caedere* to kill] an agent that destroys oxyurids.

oxyurid (ok-se-u′rid) a pinworm, seatworm, or threadworm; any individual organism of the superfamily Oxyuroidea.

oxyurifuge (ok″se-u′rĭ-fūj) [*oxyuris* + L. *fugare* to put to flight] an agent that promotes the expulsion of oxyurids.

oxyuriosis (ok″se-u″re-o′sis) oxyuriasis.

Oxyuris (ok″se-u′ris) [Gr. *oxys* sharp + *oura* tail] a genus of intestinal nematode worms of the superfamily Oxyuroidea. **O. e′qui,** the largest known species of pinworm, found in the horse, mainly in the cecum, colon, and rectum. **O. incog′nita,** a name given to certain ova found in human stools; possibly identical with *Heterodera radicicola.* **O. vermicula′ris,** *Enterobius vermicularis.*

oxyuroid (ok-se-u′roid) oxyurid.

Oxyuroidea (ok″se-u″roi-de′ah) the oxyurids: a superfamily of small nematodes, the threadworms or pinworms, characterized by the presence of phasmids and a bulbous esophagus. They are usually found as parasites in the cecum and colon of vertebrates, but may also infect invertebrates, including insects. *Enterobius vermicularis* is the only oxyurid commonly infecting man. In some systems of classification, Oxyuroidea is considered to be an order.

oz. ounce.

ozena (o-ze′nah) [Gr. *ozaina* a fetid polypus in the nose] an atrophic rhinitis marked by a thick mucopurulent discharge, mucosal crusting, and fetor. **o. laryn′gis,** a condition of the larynx associated with a foul-smelling discharge usually related to atrophic rhinitis.

ozenous (o′zĕ-nus) pertaining to or of the nature of ozena.

ozolinone (o-zo′lĭ-nōn) chemical name: (*Z*)-[3-methyl-4-oxo-5-(1-piperidinyl)-2-thiazolidinylidene]acetic acid; a diuretic, $C_{11}H_{16}N_2O_3S$.

ozonator (o′zo-nāt″or) an instrument for generating ozone.

ozone (o′zōn) [Gr. *ozē* stench] a bluish explosive gas or blue liquid, which is an allotropic and more active form of oxygen, O₃: antiseptic and disinfectant. It is formed when oxygen is exposed to the silent discharge of electricity, and is both irritating and toxic in the pulmonary system. **o.-ether,** a mixture of ethylic ether, hydrogen peroxide, and alcohol, used as an antiseptic and for whooping cough and diabetes.

ozonide (o′zo-nīd) a compound of an olefin and ozone, the union taking place at the double bond.

ozonize (o′zo-nīz) to impregnate with ozone.

ozonizer (o′zo-nīz″er) (*obs.*) an apparatus for applying ozone to wounds, sinuses, etc.

ozonometer (o″zo-nom′ĕ-ter) [*ozone* + Gr. *metron* measure] an instrument for estimating the ozone in the air.

ozonophore (o-zo′no-fōr) [*ozone* + Gr. *phoros* bearing] 1. one of the granular elements of cell cytoplasm. 2. a red blood cell.

ozonoscope (o-zo′no-skōp) [*ozone* + Gr. *skopein* to examine] an instrument for studying ozone and its effects.

ozostomia (o″zo-sto′me-ah) [Gr. *ozē* stench + *stoma* mouth + *-ia*] foulness of the breath.

P

P chemical symbol for *phosphorus.*

P. abbreviation for *position, presbyopia,* L. *prox′imum* (near), L. *pugil′lus* (handful), *pulse, pupil,* and L. *pon′dere* (by weight).

P₁ symbol for *parental generation.*

P₂ pulmonic second sound.

³²P chemical symbol for the radioactive isotope of phosphorus of atomic mass 32; also written P³² and P 32.

p symbol for (1) the short arm of a chromosome or (2) the frequency of the more common allele of a pair.

p- chemical abbreviation for *para-.*

P.A. physician assistant.

Pa 1. chemical symbol for *protactinium.* 2. symbol for *pascal.*

Paas′ disease (pahz) [H. R. *Paas,* German physician] see under *disease.*

PAB, PABA para-aminobenzoic acid; see under *acid; see aminobenzoic acid,* under *acid.*

Pabanol (pab′ah-nol) trademark for a preparation of aminobenzoic acid.

pabular (pab′u-lar) pertaining to or of the nature of pabulum.

pabulin (pab′u-lin) the fatty and albuminous products of digestion which appear in the blood after eating.

pabulum (pab′u-lum) [L.] food or aliment.

Pacatal (pak′ah-tal) trademark for a preparation of mepazine.

pacchionian depressions, foramen, granulations (bodies, glands) (pak″e-o′ne-an) [Antonio *Pacchioni,* an Italian anatomist, 1665–1726] see *foveolae granulares, foramen diaphragmatis* [*sellae*], and *granulationes arachnoideales.*

pacemaker (pās′māk-er) an object or substance that influences the rate at which a certain phenomenon occurs; often used alone to indicate the natural cardiac pacemaker or an artificial cardiac pacemaker. In biochemistry, a substance whose rate of reaction sets the pace for a series of interrelated reactions. **artificial p.,** see *cardiac p., artificial.* **asynchronous p.,** an implanted cardiac pacemaker in which the induced ventricular rhythm is independent of the atrium; it is usually set at a fixed rate of ventricular stimulation. **cardiac p.,** the group of cells rhythmically initiating the heart beat, characterized physiologically by a slow loss of membrane potential during diastole. Usually the pacemaker site is the sinoatrial node. **cardiac p., artificial,** a device designed to stimulate, by electrical impulses, contraction of the heart muscle at a certain rate; used particularly in heart block or in absence of normal function of the sinoatrial node; it may be connected from the outside or implanted within the body. Popularly called *pacemaker.* **Chardack-Greatbatch p.,** an implanted asynchronous cardiac pacemaker, with the cardiac electrodes sewn into the myocardium. **cilium p.,** the biological regulator which controls the frequency of the beat of the cilia of cells by determining the rate of contraction and excitation. **demand p.,** an implanted cardiac pacemaker in which the generator stimulus is inhibited for a set interval (refractory period) by a signal derived from depolarization (normal or ectopic), thus minimizing the risk of pacemaker-induced ventricular fibrillation. **ectopic p.,** any biological cardiac pacemaker other than the sinus node. **external p.,** an artificial cardiac pacemaker located outside the body with output wires connected to circular chest electrodes, with a wire sewn directly into the heart, or with an electrode inserted through an intravenous catheter. **fixed-rate p.,** an implanted cardiac pacemaker in which the generator stimulates the heart at a predetermined rate, regardless of the heart's rhythm. **gastric p.,** a saddle-shaped area of the greater curvature of the stomach at the junction of its proximal and middle thirds, where originate electric potentials which regulate the frequency of gastric contractions. **p. of heart,** cardiac p. **implanted p.,** a cardiac pacemaker implanted into the subcutaneous tissue; called also *internal p.* **Nathan p.,** a synchronous pacemaker. **radio-frequency p.,** a cardiac pacemaker consisting of an antenna coil cemented to the skin and a subcutaneously implanted receiving coil with an electrode inserted into the ventricular myocardium. Pulses from a light-

weight radio transmitter carried by the patient are transmitted to the pacemaker. **synchronous p.,** an implanted cardiac pacemaker that synchronizes the electromechanical events in the atrium with those of the ventricle; the pacemaker stimulates the ventricle when triggered by the P wave from the atrium. **transvenous catheter p.,** an external cardiac pacemaker connected to the heart by an electrode inserted through a catheter. **wandering p.,** a condition in which the site of origin of the impulses controlling the heart rate shifts from the head of the sinoatrial node to a lower part of the node or to another part of the atrium.

pachismus (pah-kiz′mus) [Gr. *pachys* thick] thickening.

pachonychia (pak″o-nik′e-ah) pachyonychia.

pachy- [Gr. *pachys* thick, clotted] a combining form meaning thick.

pachyacria (pak″e-a′kre-ah) [*pachy-* + Gr. *akron* end + *-ia*] a condition characterized by enlargement of the soft parts of the extremities.

pachyblepharon (pak″e-blef′ah-ron) [*pachy-* + Gr. *blepharon* eyelid] a thickening of the eyelid, chiefly near the border.

pachyblepharosis (pak″e-blef″ah-ro′sis) pachyblepharon.

pachycephalia (pak″e-sĕ-fa′le-ah) pachycephaly.

pachycephalic (pak″e-sĕ-fal′ik) pertaining to or characterized by pachycephaly.

pachycephalous (pak″e-sef′ah-lus) pachycephalic.

pachycephaly (pak″e-sef′ah-le) [*pachy-* + Gr. *kephalē* head] abnormal thickness of the bones of the skull, as in acromegaly.

pachycheilia (pak″e-ki′le-ah) [*pachy-* + Gr. *cheilos* lip + *-ia*] thickening of the lips.

pachycholia (pak″e-ko′le-ah) [*pachy-* + Gr. *cholē* bile + *-ia*] (*obs.*) abnormal thickness of the bile.

pachychromatic (pak″e-kro-mat′ik) [*pachy-* + Gr. *chrōma* color] having thick chromatin threads.

pachychymia (pak″e-kim′e-ah) [*pachy-* + Gr. *chymos* juice + *-ia*] (*obs.*) undue thickness of the chyme.

pachycolpismus (pak″e-kol-piz′mus) [*pachy-* + Gr. *kolpos* vagina] pachyvaginitis.

pachydactylia (pak″e-dak-til′e-ah) pachydactyly.

pachydactyly (pak″e-dak′tĭ-le) [*pachy-* + Gr. *daktylos* finger] abnormal enlargement of the fingers and toes.

pachyderma (pak″e-der′mah) [*pachy-* + Gr. *derma* skin] abnormal thickening of the skin. **p. circumscrip′ta, p. laryn′gis,** localized warty epithelial thickenings on the larynx. **p. verruco′sa,** a condition characterized by papillomatous growths on the vocal cords. **p. vesi′cae,** a dry, thickened condition of the mucous membrane of the bladder.

pachydermatocele (pak″e-der-mat′o-sēl) [*pachy-* + Gr. *derma* skin + *kēlē* tumor] plexiform neuroma which attains large dimensions and produces a condition resembling elephantiasis; called also *elephantiasis neuromatosa.*

pachydermatous (pak″e-der′mah-tus) thick-skinned.

pachydermic (pak″e-der′mik) (*obs.*) characterized by abnormal thickness of the skin.

pachydermoperiostosis (pak″e-der″mo-per′e-os-to′sis) a condition characterized by thickening of the skin of the face and scalp, thickening of the bones of the distal parts of the limbs, and clubbing of the fingers and toes (acropachy). When it occurs secondary to severe pulmonary disease, it is probably synonymous with hypertrophic pulmonary osteoarthropathy (q.v.). Called also *Touraine-Salente-Golé syndrome.*

pachyglossia (pak″e-glos′e-ah) [*pachy-* + Gr. *glōssa* tongue + *-ia*] abnormal thickness of the tongue.

pachygnathous (pah-kig′nah-thus) [*pachy-* + Gr. *gnathos* jaw] having a large jaw.

pachygyria (pak″e-ji′re-ah) [*pachy-* + *gyrus* + *-ia*] macrogyria.

pachyhemia (pak″e-he′me-ah) pachyemia.

pachyleptomeningitis (pak″e-lep″to-men″in-ji′tis) [*pachy-* + Gr. *leptos* thin + *mēninx* membrane + *-itis*] inflammation of the dura and pia together.

pachymeninges (pak″e-me-nin′jēz) plural of *pachymeninx*.

pachymeningitis (pak″e-men″in-ji′tis) [*pachy-* + Gr. *mēninx* membrane + *-itis*] inflammation of the dura mater; the symptoms of the disease resemble those of meningitis. Cf. *leptomeningitis*. **cerebral p.,** inflammation of the dura of the brain. **circumscribed p.,** pachymeningitis limited to a definite area of the dura. **external p.,** inflammation of the outer layers of the dura. **hemorrhagic internal p.,** pachymeningitis associated with dural hematoma. **internal p.,** that which affects the inner layer of the dura. **p. intralamella′ris,** intradural abscess. **purulent p.,** abscess on the dura mater. **serous internal p.,** the so-called external hydrocephalus. **spinal p.,** inflammation of the dura of the spinal column. **syphilitic p.,** that which is caused by syphilis.

pachymeningopathy (pak″e-men″in-gop′ah-the) [*pachymeninx* + Gr. *pathos* disease] any noninflammatory disease of the dura mater.

pachymeninx (pak″e-me′ninks), pl. *pachymenin′ges* [*pachy-* + Gr. *mēninx* membrane] the dura mater.

pachymucosa (pak″e-mu-ko′sa) [*pachy-* + *mucosa*] abnormal thickening of the mucosa. **p. al′ba,** leukoplakia with thickening of the mucous membrane.

pachynema (pak″e-ne′mah) [*pachy-* + Gr. *nēma* thread] a postsynaptic stage of mitosis in which the chromatin is in the form of thick spireme threads.

pachynesis (pak″e-ne′sis) thickening and swelling of a chondriosome.

pachynsis (pah-kin′sis) [Gr.] a thickening, especially an abnormal thickening.

pachyntic (pah-kin′tik) pertaining to or characterized by abnormal thickening.

pachyonychia (pak″e-o-nik′e-ah) [*pachy-* + Gr. *onyx* nail + *-ia*] thickening of the nails. **p. congen′ita,** a rare, congenital, dominantly inherited disorder, characterized by excessive thickening of the nails that progresses to produce onychogryposis, hyperkeratosis of the palms, soles, knees, and elbows, leukoplakia of the oral mucous membranes, and, usually, hyperhidrosis of the hands and feet; widespread, tiny cutaneous horns may occur and bullae may develop on the palms and soles. Called also *Jadassohn-Lewandowsky syndrome.*

pachyostosis (pak″e-os-to′sis) [*pachy-* + Gr. *osteon* bone + *-osis*] a benign form of hypertrophy of the bones; found particularly in aquatic animals.

pachyotia (pak″e-o′she-ah) [*pachy-* + Gr. *ous* ear] (*obs.*) marked thickness of the auricles of the ears.

pachypelviperitonitis (pak″e-pel″ve-per″ĭ-to-ni′tis) [*pachy-* + *pelvis* + *peritonitis*] pelvic peritonitis with thickening of the affected parts.

pachyperiosteoderma (pak″e-per″e-os″te-o-der′mah) pachydermoperiostosis.

pachyperiostitis (pak″e-per″e-os-ti′tis) periostitis of long bones resulting in abnormal thickness of the bones.

pachyperitonitis (pak″e-per″ĭ-to-ni′tis) [*pachy-* + *peritonitis*] peritonitis with thickening of the affected membrane.

pachypleuritis (pak″e-ploo-ri′tis) [*pachy-* + *pleuritis*] fibrothorax.

pachypodous (pah-kip′o-dus) [*pachy-* + Gr. *pous* foot] having abnormally thick feet.

pachyrhizid (pak″ir-i′zid) a poisonous glycoside from *Pachyrhizus angulatus,* a plant of various tropical regions.

pachysalpingitis (pak″e-sal″pin-ji′tis) [*pachy-* + Gr. *salpinx* tube + *-itis*] chronic interstitial inflammation of the muscular coat of the oviduct, producing thickening; called also *mural salpingitis* and *parenchymatous salpingitis.*

pachysalpingo-ovaritis (pak″e-sal-ping″go-o″var-i′tis) chronic parenchymatous inflammation of the ovary and oviduct.

pachysomia (pak″e-so′me-ah) [*pachy-* + Gr. *sōma* body] abnormal thickening of parts of the body.

pachytene (pak′e-tēn) [Gr. *pachytēs* thickness] in meiosis (q.v.), the stage following synapsis (zygotene) in which the homologous chromosome threads (synaptonemal complex) shorten, thicken, and continue to intertwine, and each of the conjoined (bivalent) chromosomes separate into two sister chromatids, which are held together by a centromere, to form a tetrad. During this phase the chromatids break up and corresponding regions of the nonsister chromatids of the paired chromosomes are exchanged in a process known as crossing over. See also *diplotene, leptotene,* and *zygotene.*

pachyvaginalitis (pak″e-vaj″ĭ-nal-i′tis) [*pachy-* + *vaginalitis*] inflammatory thickening of the tunica vaginalis of the testis.

pachyvaginitis (pak″e-vaj″ĭ-ni′tis) [*pachy-* + *vaginitis*] chronic vaginitis with thickening of the vaginal walls. **cystic p.,** emphysematous vaginitis.

pacing (pās′ing) setting the pace, or regulation of the rate of.

cardiac p., regulation of the rate of contraction of the heart muscle by an artificial cardiac pacemaker.

Pacini's corpuscles (pah-che′nēz) [Filippo *Pacini,* Italian anatomist, 1812–1883] see under *corpuscle.*

pacinian corpuscles (pah-sin′e-an) [named for Filippo *Pacini*] see under *corpuscle.*

Paci's operation (pah′chēz) [Agostino *Paci,* Pisa surgeon] see under *operation.*

pack (pak) 1. treatment by wrapping a patient in blankets or sheets or a limb in towels, wet or dry and either hot or cold; also the blankets, sheets, or towels used for this purpose. 2. a tampon. **cold p.,** the wrapping of a patient in blankets, sheets, or towels dipped in cold water before application. **dry p.,** dry, hot blankets or towels for wrapping the body or an extremity. **full p.,** one which encloses the entire body. **half p.,** a pack applied from the axillae to below the knees. **hot p.,** the hot blankets or towels, wet or dry, for wrapping the body or an extremity. **ice p.,** a folded towel filled with crushed ice, often used in place of an icebag. **Mikulicz p.,** layers of mesh or gutta-percha sewn together at the edges, packed with strips of gauze, often placed in a denuded pelvic area to wall off the unperitonealized surfaces but also used for packing off abdominal viscera to improve operative exposure. **one sheet p.,** a wet pack consisting of only one large sheet. **partial p.,** a wet pack covering only a portion of the body. **periodontal p.,** a mixture which usually consists of a zinc oxide powder and eugenol liquid, applied to the gingiva around the teeth after surgical periodontal procedures, such as gingivectomy, to protect the tissues during the healing process. **salt p.,** a wet pack utilizing sheets or blankets wrung out after immersion in salt water. **three-quarters p.,** a wet pack extending upward from the toes as far as the axillae. **throat p.,** a moistened gauze pack used as a posterior pharyngeal seal around a non-cuffed endotracheal tube. **wet p., wet-sheet p.,** wet blankets or sheets, hot or cold, for wrapping an extremity or the entire body.

packer (pak′er) an instrument for introducing dressing into the uterus or vagina, or into another body cavity or wound.

packing (pak′ing) 1. the act of filling a wound or cavity with gauze, sponges, pads, or other material. 2. the material used for filling a cavity.

pad (pad) a cushion-like mass of soft material. **abdominal p.,** a pad for the absorption of discharges from abdominal wounds; also for packing off abdominal viscera to improve exposure during surgical procedures. **dinner p.,** a pad placed over the stomach before a plaster jacket is applied. The pad is then removed, leaving space under the jacket to take care of expansion of the stomach after eating. **fat p.,** 1. sucking pad. 2. a large pad of fat lying behind and below the patella, between the patellar ligament, the head of the tibia and the femoral condyles; called also *infrapatellar* and *retropatellar fat pad.* **gum p's,** edentulous segments of the maxilla and the mandible that correspond to the underlying primary teeth. **kidney p.,** a pad held in place by a belt or corset for the support of a movable kidney. **knuckle p's,** nodules about the size of a split pea on the dorsal surface of the interphangeal joints, consisting of new growths of fibrous tissue, with thickening of the dermis and epidermis, and frequently associated with camptodactyly and Dupuytren's contracture; they are probably of genetic origin. **Mikulicz's p.,** a pad composed of layers of folded gauze; used in surgical procedures. **occlusal p.,** a pad which covers the occlusal surface of a tooth. **Passavant's p.,** see under *bar.* **periarterial p.,** see *juxtaglomerular cells,* under *cell.* **retromolar p.,** a cushion-like mass of tissue situated at the distal termination of the mandibular residual ridge, immediately distal to the last mandibular molar in vivo. **sucking p., suctorial p.,** a lobulated mass of fat which occupies the space between the masseter and the external surface of the buccinator; it is well developed in infants. Called also *fatty ball of Bichat, fat pad, corpus adiposum buccae* [NA], and *adipose body of cheek.*

Padgett's dermatome (paj′ets) [Earl Calvin *Padgett,* American surgeon, 1893–1946] see under *dermatome.*

padimate A (pad′ĭ-māt) chemical name: 4-(dimethylamino)-benzoic acid pentyl ester; an ultraviolet screen, $C_{14}H_{21}NO_2$.

padimate O (pad′ĭ-mat) chemical name: 4-(dimethylamino)-benzoic acid 2-ethylhexyl ester; an ultraviolet screen, $C_{17}H_{27}NO_2$.

P. ae. abbreviation for L. *par′tes aequa′les,* equal parts.

pae- for words beginning thus, see also those beginning *pe-*.

Paecilomyces (pe-sil″o-mi′sēz) a genus of soil-inhabiting imperfect fungi of the family Moniliaceae, order Moniliales, morphologically resembling *Penicillium,* and often isolated as contaminants of skin and sputum. See *cladiosis.*

paed-, paedo-, etc. for words beginning thus, see those beginning *ped-, pedia-, pedio-, pedo-.*

Paederus (pe′der-us) a genus of blistering beetles of South America, Asia, and Africa, from which pederin has been isolated.

PAF platelet activating factor.

Pagenstecher's circle, ointment, linen, thread (pah′gen-stek″erz) [Alexander *Pagenstecher,* German ophthalmologist,

1828–1879] see under *circle, linen,* and *thread,* and see *yellow mercuric oxide,* under *mercuric.*

Paget's abscess, etc. (paj′ets) [Sir James *Paget,* English surgeon, 1814–1899] see under *abscess, cell, disease, necrosis,* and *tests.*

pagetic (pah-jet′ik) affected with or relating to Paget's disease (osteitis deformans).

pagetoid (paj′ĕ-toid) resembling Paget's disease; characteristic of Paget's disease.

Pagitane (paj′ĭ-tān) trademark for a preparation of cycrimine hydrochloride.

pagon (pag′on) [Gr. *pagos* frost] the plant and animal organisms occurring in ice.

pagophagia (pa″go-fa′je-ah) [Gr. *pagos* frost + *phagein* to eat] the ingestion of extraordinary amounts of ice, probably related to iron lack.

pagoplexia (pa″go-plek′se-ah) [Gr. *pagos* frost + *plēgē* stroke] frostbite.

-pagus [Gr. *pagos* that which is fixed or firmly set] a word termination denoting a monster composed of symmetrical twins conjoined at the site indicated by the stem to which it is affixed, as *craniopagus, pygopagus, thorocopagus.*

PAH, PAHA para-aminohippuric acid; see *aminohippuric acid,* under *acid.*

Pahvant Valley fever, plague (pah′vant) [*Pahvant,* a valley in Utah] tularemia.

pain (pān) [L. *poena, dolor;* Gr. *algos, odynē*] a more or less localized sensation of discomfort, distress, or agony, resulting from the stimulation of specialized nerve endings. It serves as a protective mechanism insofar as it induces the sufferer to remove or withdraw from the source. **bearing-down p.,** pain accompanying uterine contractions during the second stage of labor. **boring p.,** a sensation as of being pierced with a long, slender, twisting object; called also *terebrant p.* **Brodie's p.,** pain induced by folding the skin near a joint affected with neuralgia. **central p.,** pain due to a lesion in the central nervous system. **Charcot's p's,** rheumatism of a testicle. **dilating p's,** those of the first stage of labor. **expulsive p's,** those of the second stage of labor. **false p's,** ineffective pains which resemble labor pains, but which are not accompanied by effacement and dilatation of the cervix. **fulgurant p's,** lightning p's. **gas p's,** pains caused by distention of the stomach or intestines by accumulations of air or other gases, occurring as a result of ingestion of gas-forming foods. **girdle p.,** a painful sensation as of a cord about the waist. **growing p's,** recurrent quasirheumatic limb pains peculiar to early youth. **heterotopic p.,** referred pain. **homotopic p.,** pain that is felt at the point of injury. **hunger p.,** pain coming on at the time for feeling hunger for the next meal; it is a symptom of gastric disorder. **ideogenous p.,** pain caused by an erroneous idea; mentally produced pain. **imperative p.,** a persisting painful sensation felt in psychasthenia. **intermenstrual p.,** pain occurring during the period between the menses, usually about half way, accompanying extrusion of the ovum. **jumping p.,** a peculiar pain in joint diseases when the bone is laid bare by ulceration of the cartilage. **labor p's,** the rhythmic pains of increasing severity and frequency, caused by contractions of the uterus during childbirth. **lancinating p.,** a sharp, darting pain. **lightning p's,** the cutting and intense darting pains of tabes dorsalis; called also *fulgurant p's* and *shooting p's.* **middle p.,** intermenstrual pain. **mind p.,** psychalgia, def. 2. **osteocopic p.,** osteocope. **phantom limb p.,** pain felt as though arising in an absent (amputated) limb; see under *limb.* **postprandial p.,** abdominal pain occurring after eating a meal. **premonitory p's,** mild uterine contractions before the beginning of true labor. **referred p.,** pain felt in a part other than that in which the cause that produced it is situated. **rest p.,** a continuous burning pain of the distal portion of the lower limb, usually the forefoot, which begins or is aggravated after reclining and is relieved by sitting or standing; it is due to ischemia. **root p.,** pain caused by disease of the sensory nerve roots and felt in the cutaneous areas supplied by the affected roots. **shooting p's,** lightning p's. **soul p.,** psychalgia, def. 2. **spot p's,** pains which seem like patches on the integument. **starting p's,** pain and muscular spasm in the early stages of sleep. **terebrant p., terebrating p.,** boring p. **wandering p.,** a pain which repeatedly changes its location.

paint (pānt) 1. a liquid designed for application to the surface, as of the body or a tooth. 2. to apply a liquid to a specific area as a remedial or protective measure. **Castellani's p.,** carbol-fuchsin solution.

pair (pār) a combination of two related, similar, or identical entities or objects. **base p.,** either of the two pairs—guanine and cytosine, adenine and thymine—of purine-pyrimidine bases joined by hydrogen bonds that make up DNA. In RNA, uracil replaces thymine. **buffer p.,** a buffer system consisting of a weak acid and its conjugate base.

pairing (pār′ing) the act or process of joining into pairs. In transplantation immunology, the process of selecting a compatible donor and host, usually by typing or matching. **base p.,** the coalescing of purines and pyrimidines by forming hydrogen bonds;

see under *pair.* **somatic p.,** the close association of homologous pairs of polytene chromosomes, as in meiotic prophase; such chromosomes are considered to be in a permanent prophase.

pajaroello (pah-hah-ro-el′yo) *Ornithodoros coriaceus.*

Pajot's hook, law, maneuver, method (pahzh-ōz′) [Charles *Pajot,* French obstetrician, 1816–1896] see under the nouns.

pakurin (pak′u-rin) an arrow poison derived from the sap of a tree in Colombia; it has a digitalis-like action on the heart.

Pal's stain (pahlz) [Jacob *Pal,* Vienna clinician, 1863–1936] see *Table of Stains.*

Palade (pal-ād′), George Emil. American cytologist, born in Rumania in 1912; co-winner, with Albert Claude and Christian R. de Duve, of the Nobel prize in medicine or physiology for 1974, for his work on mitochondria, ribosomes, and microsomes.

palae- for words beginning thus, see those beginning *pale-.*

palata (pal-ah′tah) [L.] plural of palatum.

palatal (pal′ah-tal) pertaining to the palate; sometimes used to designate the lingual surface of a maxillary tooth.

palate (pal′at) the partition separating the nasal and oral cavities; see *palatum* [NA]. **artificial p.,** a prosthetic device used to close a cleft palate. **bony p., bony hard p.,** the osseous framework of the hard palate (palatum osseum [NA]). **cleft p.,** a palate having a congenital fissure in the median line, which may range from a simple cleft in the uvula to a cleft involving the uvula and hard palate; the latter cleft may extend anteriorly unilaterally or bilaterally (never in the midline) through the alveolar ridge. **falling p.,** 1. an abnormally elongated uvula. 2. a palate that has lost neuromuscular control. **gothic p.,** an unusually high and pointed hard palate. **hard p.,** the anterior, rigid portion of the palate; see *palatum durum* [NA]. **pendulous p.,** uvula. **premaxillary p.,** primary p. **primary p.,** that portion of the palate contributed by the median nasal process. **secondary p.,** the palate proper, formed by fusion of the lateral palatine processes. **smoker's p.,** a condition of the palate occurring in heavy smokers, particularly pipe smokers, characterized by a diffusely erythematous or whitened "cobblestone" surface with multiple inflamed orifices of mucous gland ducts. **soft p.,** the posterior, fleshy part of the palate; see *palatum molle* [NA].

palategraph (pal′at-graf) palatograph.

palatiform (pah-lat′ĭ-form) [L. *palatum* palate + *forma* form] resembling the palate.

palatine (pal′ah-tīn) [L. *palatinus*] pertaining to the palate.

palatitis (pal″ah-ti′tis) 1. inflammation of the palate. 2. lampas.

palato- [L. *palatum* palate] a combining form denoting relationship to the palate; sometimes used instead of linguo- in terms referring to the lingual surface of maxillary teeth.

palatoglossal (pal″ah-to-glos′al) pertaining to the palate and tongue.

palatognathous (pal″ah-tog′nah-thus) [*palato-* + Gr. *gnathos* jaw] having a congenitally cleft palate.

palatograph (pal′ah-to-graf) [*palato-* + Gr. *graphein* to write] an instrument to record the movements of the palate in speech.

palatography (pal″ah-tog′rah-fe) the making of graphic records of the movements of the palate in speech.

palatomaxillary (pal″ah-to-mak′sĭ-ler″e) pertaining to the palate and the maxilla.

palatomyograph (pal″ah-to-mi′o-graf) [*palato-* + Gr. *mys* muscle + *graphein* to write] an instrument used in registering palatal movements.

palatonasal (pal″ah-to-na′zal) [*palato-* + L. *nasus* nose] pertaining to the palate and nose.

palatopagus (pal″ah-top′ah-gus) [*palato-* + Gr. *pagos* that which is firmly set] symmetrical twins conjoined at the palate.

palatopharyngeal (pal″ah-to-fah-rin′je-al) pertaining to the palate and pharynx.

palatoplasty (pal′ah-to-plas″te) [*palato-* + Gr. *plassein* to form] plastic reconstruction of the palate, including cleft palate operations.

palatoplegia (pal″ah-to-ple′je-ah) [*palato-* + Gr. *plēgē* stroke] paralysis of the palate.

palatoproximal (pal″ah-to-prok′sĭ-mal) pertaining to the palatal (lingual) and proximal surface of a maxillary tooth.

palatorrhaphy (pal″ah-tor′ah-fe) surgical correction of a cleft palate, the cleft involving the soft palate and the soft tissues over the hard palate; cf. *staphylorrhaphy.*

palatosalpingeus (pal″ah-to-sal-pin′je-us) [*palato-* + Gr. *salpinx* tube] musculus tensor veli palatini.

palatoschisis (pal″ah-tos′kĭ-sis) [*palato-* + Gr. *schisis* cleft] cleft palate.

palatostaphylinus (pal″ah-to-staf″ĭ-li′nus) [*palato-* + Gr. *staphylē* uvula] a muscular slip going to the uvula.

palatouvularis (pal″ah-to-u″vu-la′ris) [*palato-* + L. *uvula* uvula] musculus uvulae.

palatum (pal-ah′tum), pl. *pala′ta* [L.] [NA] the palate: the partition separating the nasal and oral cavities, consisting anteriorly of a hard bony part and posteriorly of a soft fleshy part. **p. du′-rum** [NA], the hard palate: the anterior part of the palate, characterized by an osseous framework, covered superiorly by mucous membrane of the nasal cavity and, on its oral surface, by mucoperiosteum. **p. du′rum os′seum,** p. osseum. **p. fis′-sum,** cleft palate. **p. mol′le** [NA], the soft palate: the fleshy part of the roof of the mouth, extending from the posterior edge of the hard palate; from its free inferior border is a projection of variable length, the uvula. Called also *velum palatinum* [NA alternative]. **p. ogiva′le,** gothic palate. **p. os′seum** [NA], bony palate: the bony part of the anterior two-thirds of the roof of the mouth, formed by the palatine processes of the maxillae and the horizontal plates of the palatine bones. Called also *p. durum osseum* or *bony hard palate.*

paleencephalon (pa″le-en-sef′ah-lon) [*paleo-* + Gr. *enkephalos* brain] the (phylogenetically) old brain; all of the brain except the cerebral cortex and its dependencies.

paleo- [Gr. *palaios* old] a combining form meaning old.

paleocerebellar (pa″le-o-ser″ĕ-bel′ar) pertaining to or affecting the paleocerebellum.

paleocerebellum (pal″e-o-ser″ĕ-bel′um) [*paleo-* + *cerebellum*] a term applied originally to the phylogenetically older parts of the cerebellum, including the flocculonodular lobe; now applied specifically to those parts whose afferent inflow is predominantly supplied by spinocerebellar fibers, including in man the lingula, lobulus centralis, culmen, pyramis, and uvula of the vermis, and the tonsils of the hemispheres.

paleocinetic (pa″le-o-si-net′ik) paleokinetic.

paleocortex (pa″le-o-kor′teks) paleopallium.

paleoencephalon (pa″le-o-en-sef′ah-lon) paleencephalon.

paleogenesis (pa″le-o-jen′ĕ-sis) palingenesis, def. 2.

paleogenetic (pa″le-o-jĕ-net′ik) [*paleo-* + Gr. *gennan* to produce] originated in the past; not newly acquired. Said of traits, structures, etc., of species.

paleokinetic (pa″le-o-ki-net′ik) [*paleo-* + Gr. *kinētikos* pertaining to motion] old kinetic; a term applied to the nervous motor mechanism concerned in automatic associated movements. It is under the control of the corpus striatum and represents a primitive (that is, early developed) type of motor control. Cf. *archeokinetic* and *neokinetic.*

paleologic (pal″le-o-loj′ik) a type of abnormal reasoning in which, because two unlike things share a common property, the two are equated.

paleoneurology (pa″le-o-nu-rol′o-je) the study of the evidence of nervous systems of fossil animals.

paleontology (pa″le-on-tol′o-je) [*paleo-* + Gr. *ōn* existing + *-logy*] the sum of knowledge regarding the early forms of life upon the earth.

paleopallium (pa″le-o-pal′e-um) [*paleo-* + L. *pallium* mantle] that portion of the pallium (cerebral cortex) which, with the archipallium, develops in association with the olfactory system and which is phylogenetically older and less stratified than the neopallium. It is composed chiefly of the piriform cortex and parahippocampal gyrus. Called also *paleocortex.*

paleopathology (pa″le-o-pah-thol′o-je) [*paleo-* + *pathology*] the study of disease in bodies preserved from ancient times, such as mummies.

paleophrenia (pa″le-o-fre′ne-ah) [*paleo-* + Gr. *phrēn* mind + *-ia*] a term suggested as a substitute for schizophrenia on the basis that the disorder represents a regression to childhood level.

paleopsychology (pa″le-o-si-kol′o-je) [*paleo-* + *psychology*] the study of mental phenomena which are based on primitive or ancestral mentality.

paleosensation (pa″le-o-sen-sa′shun) [*paleo-* + *sensation*] the sensation of severe pain and marked variations of temperature, as compared with phylogenetically newer sensations such as those of light touch and moderate variations of temperature and the epicritic sensations.

paleostriatal (pa″le-o-stri-a′tal) pertaining to the paleostriatum.

paleostriatum (pa″le-o-stri-a′tum) [*paleo-* + *striatum*] the phylogenetically older part of the corpus striatum represented by the globus pallidus. Cf. *neostriatum.*

paleothalamus (pa″le-o-thal′ah-mus) [*paleo-* + *thalamus*] old thalamus; a term applied occasionally to the phylogenetically older part of the thalamus, i.e., the medial portion which lacks reciprocal connections with the neopallium.

pali-, palin- [Gr. *palin* backward, or again] a combining form meaning again, often denoting pathologic repetition.

palicinesia (pal″e-si-ne′se-ah) palikinesia.

palikinesia (pal″e-ki-ne′se-ah) [*pali-* + Gr. *kinēsis* movement] pathologic repetition of movements.

palilalia (pal″ĭ-la′le-ah) [*pali-* + Gr. *lalein* to babble] a condition characterized by the repetition of a phrase or word with increasing rapidity.

palin- see *pali-.*

palindromia (pal″in-dro′me-ah) [Gr. *palindromia* a running back] the recurrence of a disease.

palindromic (pal″in-dro′mik) returning; recurrent.

palinesthesia (pal″in-es-the′ze-ah) [palin- + Gr. *aisthēsis* sensation] the rapid termination of the anesthetic state and the restoration to consciousness of a person under general anesthesia: it may be induced by the injection of weak hydrochloric acid; now discontinued because it is ineffective and harmful.

palingenesis (pal″in-jen′ĕ-sis) [*palin-* + Gr. *genesis* birth] 1. the regeneration or restoration of a lost part. 2. the appearance of ancestral characters in successive generations. Cf. *cenogenesis.*

palingraphia (pal″in-gra′fe-ah) [*palin-* + Gr. *graphein* to write] pathologic repetition of letters, words, or parts of words in writing.

palinmnesis (pal″in-ne′sis) [*palin-* + Gr. *-mnēsis* memory] memory for past events or experiences.

palinopsia (pal″in-op′se-ah) [*palin-* + Gr. *opsis* vision + *ia*] visual perseveration; the continuance of a visual sensation after the stimulus is gone.

palinphrasia (pal″in-fra′ze-ah) [*palin-* + Gr. *phrasis* speech + *-ia*] pathologic repetition, in speaking, of words or phrases.

paliphrasia (pal″e-fra′ze-ah) palinphrasia.

palladium (pah-la′de-um) [L.] 1. a rare, hard, inert metal resembling platinum; symbol, Pd; specific gravity, 12.16; atomic number, 46; atomic weight, 106.4. It is comparatively light in weight and of a neutral color and is used for dentures and orthodontic appliances. 2. a homeopathic preparation of the same metal.

pallanesthesia (pal″an-es-the′ze-ah) [Gr. *pallein* to shake + *anesthesia*] loss of vibration senses; insensibility to the vibrations of a tuning fork.

pallesthesia (pal″es-the′ze-ah) [Gr. *pallein* to shake + *aisthēsis* perception] sensibility to vibrations; the peculiar vibrating sensation felt when a vibrating tuning-fork is placed against a subcutaneous bony prominence of the body. Called also *bone sensibility.*

pallesthetic (pal″es-thet′ik) pertaining to pallesthesia, or vibration sense.

pallhypesthesia (pal″hi-pes-the′ze-ah) [Gr. *pallein* to shake + *hypo* under + *aisthēsis* perception] diminished sensibility to vibrations.

pallial (pal′e-al) pertaining to the pallium.

palliate (pal′e-āt) to reduce the severity of; to relieve.

palliative (pal′e-a″tiv) [L. *palliatus* cloaked] 1. affording relief, but not cure. 2. an alleviating medicine.

pallidal (pal″ĭ-dal) pertaining to the globus pallidum.

pallidectomy (pal″ĭ-dek′to-me) surgical excision of the globus pallidus or extirpation of it by other means (chemopallidectomy).

pallidin (pal″ĭ-din) a suspension made from the lung of congenital syphilitics, rich in *Treponema pallidum;* used in cutaneous test for syphilis. See under *reaction.*

pallidoansection (pal″ĭ-do-an-sek′shun) surgical section of the globus pallidus and ansa lenticularis.

pallidoansotomy (pal″ĭ-do-an-sot′o-me) production of lesions in the globus pallidus and ansa lenticularis.

pallidofugal (pal″ĭ-dof′u-gal) [*pallidum* + L. *fugere* to flee] conducting impulses away from the globus pallidus.

pallidoidosis (pal″ĭ-doi-do′sis) rabbit syphilis.

pallidotomy (pal″ĭ-dot′o-me) [*pallidum* + Gr. *tomē* a cutting] a stereotaxic surgical technique for producing lesions in the globus pallidus for treatment of extrapyramidal disorders.

pallidum (pal′ĭ-dum) [L. "pale"] globus pallidus.

pallium (pal′e-um) [L. "cloak"] [NA] the cerebral cortex (q.v.) as viewed in its entirety, i.e., the mantle of gray matter covering both cerebral hemispheres. It is divided into the archipallium, paleopallium, and neopallium (some classifications include the paleopallium with the archipallium, and both are often loosely termed the rhinencephalon). Also, the cerebral cortex during its period of development.

pallor (pal′or) [L.] paleness; absence of the skin coloration.

palm (palm) [L. *palma*] 1. the hollow of the hand (palma manus [NA]). 2. any of various, chiefly tropical trees, the palm trees. **handball p.,** contusion of the palm of the hand occurring in handball players.

palma (pal′mah), pl. *pal′mae* [L.] 1. the palm. 2. the palm tree. **p. ma′nus** [NA], the palm, or flexor surface, of the hand. **pal′mae plica′tae,** the branching folds of the mucosa of the vagina.

palmae (pal′me) [L.] plural of *palma.*

palmanesthesia (pal″man-es-the′ze-ah) [Gr. *palmos* vibration + *anesthesia*] pallanesthesia.

palmar (pal′mar) [L. *palmaris; palma* palm] pertaining to the palm.

palmaris (pal-ma′ris) palmar; [NA] a general term designating relationship to the palm of the hand.

palmature (pal′mah-tūr) [L. *palma* palm] a webbed state of the fingers.

palmellin (pal-mel′in) a red pigment from the fresh-water alga *Palmella cruenta*.

palmesthesia (pal″mes-the′ze-ah) pallesthesia.

palmesthetic (pal″mes-thet′ik) pallesthetic.

palmital (pal′mĭ-tal) an aldehyde lipid, the aldehyde form of palmitate; see *plasmalogen*.

palmitate (pal′mĭ-tāt) hexadecanote: the ionic form of palmitic acid, the most abundant fatty acid in man.

palmitin (pal′mĭ-tin) a crystallizable and saponifiable fat, $C_3H_5(C_{16}H_{31}O_2)_3$, from various fats and oils; glycerol tripalmitate.

palmitone (pal′mĭ-tōn) a crystalline compound, $CH_3(CH_2)_{14}\cdot CO\cdot(CH_2)_{14}\cdot CH_3$, obtained when palmitic acid is distilled with lime.

palmus (pal′mus) [Gr. *palmos* a quivering motion] 1. palpitation. 2. saltatory spasm.

palp (palp) a sensory or feeding appendage, especially one of the jointed sensory appendages attached to the mouth of arthropods.

palpable (pal′pah-b′l) perceptible by touch.

palpate (pal′pāt) [L. *palpare* to touch] to examine by the hand; to feel.

palpation (pal-pa′shun) [L. *palpatio*] the act of feeling with the hand; the application of the fingers with light pressure to the surface of the body for the purpose of determining the consistence of the parts beneath in physical diagnosis. **bimanual p.**, examination with both hands. **light touch p.**, light palpation of the surface of the abdomen and thorax with the tip of a finger for the purpose of finding the outlines of the organs.

palpatometry (pal″pah-tom′ĕ-tre) [*palpation* + Gr. *metron* measure] measurement of the amount of pressure that can be borne without causing pain.

palpatopercussion (pal″pah-to-per-kush′un) palpation combined with percussion.

palpebra (pal′pĕ-brah), pl. *pal′pebrae* [L.] eyelid; either of the two movable folds that protect the anterior surface of the eyeball. **p. infe′rior** [NA], the lower eyelid: the lower of the two movable folds protecting the anterior surface of the eyeball. **p. supe′rior** [NA], the upper eyelid: the upper of the two movable folds protecting the anterior surface of the eyeball. **p. ter′tius,** nictitating membrane.

palpebrae (pal′pĕ-bre) [L.] plural of *palpebra*.

palpebral (pal′pĕ-bral) [L. *palpebralis*] pertaining to an eyelid.

palpebralis (pal″pĕ-bra′lis) [L.] pertaining to an eyelid.

palpebrate (pal′pĕ-brāt) [L. *palpebrare* to wink] 1. to wink. 2. having eyelids.

palpebration (pal″pĕ-bra′shun) [L. *palpebratio*] 1. the act of winking. 2. abnormally frequent winking.

palpebritis (pal″pĕ-bri′tis) blepharitis.

palpitation (pal″pĭ-ta′shun) [L. *palpitatio*] a subjective sensation of an unduly rapid or irregular heart beat.

palsy (pawl′ze) paralysis. **Bell's p.,** unilateral facial paralysis of sudden onset, due to lesion of the facial nerve and resulting in characteristic distortion of the face. **birth p.,** see under *paralysis*. **brachial p.,** see under *paralysis*. **bulbar p.,** see under *paralysis*. **cerebral p.,** a persisting qualitative motor disorder appearing before the age of three years, due to a nonprogressive damage to the brain. **crossed leg p.,** palsy of the peroneal nerve caused by sitting with one leg crossed over the other. **diver's p.,** decompression sickness. **Erb's p.,** see under *paralysis*. **facial p.,** Bell's p. **hammer p.,** a variety caused by hard work with the hammer. **ischemic p.,** see under *paralysis*. **Klumpke's p.,** see under *paralysis*. **Landry's p.,** acute febrile polyneuritis. **printer's p.,** a condition observed in printers due to chronic antimony poisoning, and marked by neuritis with paralysis, pain in the pubes, and papular eruption. **progressive supranuclear p.,** pseudobulbar paralysis. **pseudobulbar p.,** see under *paralysis*. **radial p.,** see under *paralysis*. **Saturday night p.,** musculospiral paralysis. **scriveners' p.,** writers' cramp. **shaking p.,** paralysis agitans. **spastic bulbar p.,** pseudobulbar paralysis. **tardy median p.,** carpal tunnel syndrome. **Todd's p.,** see under *paralysis*. **transverse p.,** crossed paralysis. **wasting p.,** spinal muscular atrophy.

Paltauf's dwarf, nanism (dwarfism) (pahl′towfs) [Arnold *Paltauf*, Austrian specialist in forensic medicine, 1860–1893] see *pituitary dwarf*, under *dwarf*, and see under *nanism*.

paludal (pal′u-dal) [L. *palus* marsh] pertaining to or arising from marshes.

paludism (pal′u-dizm) malaria.

Paludrine (pal′u-drin) trademark for a preparation of proguanil hydrochloride.

palustral (pah-lus′tral) [L. *paluster* marshy] 1. paludal; pertaining to marshes. 2. malarial.

2-PAM pralidoxime.

pamaquine (pam′ah-kwin) chemical name: 6-methoxy - 8 - (1-methyl-4-diethylamino)butylaminoquinoline. A toxic antimalarial compound, $C_{19}H_{29}N_3O_4$, derived from 8-aminoquinoline, which was discovered in Germany in 1924. It destroys the exoerythro-

cytic forms of human malarial parasites; now largely replaced by primaquine. Called also *Fourneau 694* or *710*. **p. naphthoate,** the methylene-bis-β-hydroxynaphthoate of pamaquine base, $C_{42}H_{45}N_3O_7$, occurring as a yellow to orange yellow powder; now largely replaced as an antimalarial by primaquine.

pamatolol sulfate (pam″ah-to′lŏl) chemical name: (±)-[2-[4-[2 - hydroxy - 3 - [(1-methylethyl)amino]propoxy]phenyl]ethyl] carbamic acid methyl ester sulfate (salt); an antiadrenergic (β-receptor), $(C_{16}H_{26}N_2O_4)_2\cdot H_2SO_4$.

Pamine (pam′ēn) trademark for preparations of methscopolamine bromide.

Pamisyl (pam′ĭ-sil) trademark for preparations of aminosalicylic acid.

pamoate (pam′oh-āt) USAN contraction for 4,4′-methylenebis-[3-hydroxy-2-naphthoate].

pampiniform (pam-pin′ĭ-form) [L. *pampinus* tendril + *forma* form] shaped like a tendril.

pampinocele (pam-pin′o-sēl) [L. *pampinus* tendril + Gr. *kēlē* tumor] varicocele.

pamplegia (pam-ple′je-ah) [Gr. *pan* all + *plēgē* stroke] total paralysis.

Pan (pan) the genus of primates containing the chimpanzee and gorilla.

pan- [Gr. *pan* all] prefix signifying all.

Panacea (pan″ah-se′ah) [Gr. *Panakeia*] one of two sisters, the other being Hygeia, who were the daughters of Æsculapius and, according to legend, assisted in the rites and fed the sacred snakes in the early Greek temples of healing.

panacea (pan″ah-se′ah) [Gr. *panakeia*] 1. a universal remedy. 2. an ancient name for a healing herb or its juice.

panagglutinable (pan″ah-gloo′tĭ-nah-b′l) agglutinable with every type of blood serum from the same species, e.g., red blood cells agglutinable with sera of all human blood groups.

panagglutination (pan″ah-gloo″tĭ-na′shun) agglutination (e.g., of red blood cells) by the serum of all blood groups of the same species.

panagglutinin (pan″ah-gloo′tĭ-nin) [*pan-* + *agglutinin*] an agglutinin which agglutinates the red blood cells of all blood groups in the same species.

panangiitis (pan″an-je-i′tis) [*pan-* + Gr. *angeion* vessel + *-itis*] inflammation involving all the coats of the vessel. **diffuse necrotizing p.,** panangiitis with extensive involvement of the blood vessels.

panaris (pan′ah-ris) paronychia. **analgesic p.,** Morvan's disease.

panaritium (pan″ah-rish′e-um) [L.] (*obs.*) paronychia. **p. anal′gicum,** Morvan's disease.

panarteritis (pan″ar-tĕ-ri′tis) diffuse arterial disease; periarteritis nodosa.

panarthritis (pan″ar-thri′tis) [*pan-* + Gr. *arthron* joint] inflammation of all the joints or of all the structures of a joint.

Panas' operation (pan-ahz′) [Photinos *Panas*, French ophthalmologist, 1832–1903] see under *operation*.

panasthenia (pan″as-the′ne-ah) [*pan-* + *a* neg. + Gr. *sthenos* strength] a term suggested as a substitute for neurasthenia.

panatrophy (pan-at′ro-fe) [*pan-* + *atrophy*] atrophy affecting several parts; general atrophy.

panautonomic (pan-aw″to-no-mik) pertaining to or affecting the entire autonomic (sympathetic and parasympathetic) nervous system.

panblastic (pan-blas′tik) [*pan-* + Gr. *blastos* germ] pertaining to each of the layers of the blastoderm.

pancarditis (pan″kar-di′tis) [*pan-* + Gr. *kardia* heart] diffuse inflammation of the heart, involving the pericardium, myocardium, and endocardium.

panchontee (pan-shon-te′) a gum from *Bassia elliptica*, a tree of India; it resembles gutta-percha.

panchrest (pan′krest) [Gr. *panchrēstos* useful for everything] a panacea, or remedy, for every disease.

panchromatic (pan″kro-mat′ik) [*pan-* + *chromatic*] sensitive to all colors; applied to photographic emulsions.

panchromia (pan-kro′me-ah) the condition of staining with various dyes.

Pancoast's suture (pan′kōsts) [Joseph *Pancoast*, American surgeon, 1805–1882] see under *suture*.

Pancoast's syndrome, tumor [Henry Khunrath *Pancoast*, Philadelphia radiologist, 1875–1939] see under *syndrome*, and see *pulmonary sulcus tumor*, under *tumor*.

pancolectomy (pan″ko-lek′to-me) excision of the entire colon with creation of an ileostomy.

pancrealgia (pan″kre-al′je-ah) pancreatalgia.

pancreas (pan′kre-as), pl. *pan′creata* [Gr. *pan* all + *kreas* flesh] a large, elongated, racemose gland situated transversely behind the stomach, between the spleen and the duodenum. Its right extremity, the *head*, is the larger, and directed downward; the left extremity, or *tail*, is transverse, and terminates close to the spleen.

The external secretion or juice of the pancreas, which passes into the duodenum through the pancreatic duct, contains a variety of digestive enzymes. An internal secretion, insulin, produced in the beta cells, is concerned with the regulation of carbohydrate metabolism. Glucagon, a glycogenolytic-hyperglycemic factor, is produced in the alpha cells. Both the alpha and beta cells, along with the delta cells, form aggregates known as islets of Langerhans, scattered throughout the pancreas. **aberrant p.,** an exclave of pancreatic tissue occurring most commonly as a firm yellow nodule in the stomach, duodenum, or jejunum, but encountered also in other sites. **p. accesso′rium** [NA], **accessory p.,** an inconstant separate part of the head of the pancreas, usually an unattached uncinate process. **annular p.,** a developmental anomaly in which the pancreas forms a ring entirely surrounding the duodenum. **Aselli's p.,** an assemblage of lymphatic glands at the root of the mesentery, especially in carnivora. **p. divi′sum,** a developmental anomaly in which the pancreas is present as two separate structures, each with its own duct. **dorsal p.,** an embryonic outpocketing from the entodermal lining of the gut on the dorsal wall cephalad to the level of the hepatic diverticulum, which forms much of the pancreas and its functional duct. **lesser p.,** the small, partially detached portion of the pancreas lying dorsad to its head (processus uncinatus pancreatis [NA]); called also *Willis' p.* and *Winslow's p.* **ventral p.,** an embryonic outpocketing from the entodermal lining of the gut on the ventral wall, in the caudal angle between the gut and the hepatic diverticulum, which forms part of the pancreas and the stem of its functional duct. **Willis' p., Winslow's p.,** lesser pancreas.

pancreata (pan-kre′ah-tah) [Gr.] plural of *pancreas*.

pancreatalgia (pan″kre-ah-tal′je-ah) [*pancreas* + *-algia*] pain in the pancreas.

pancreatectomy (pan″kre-ah-tek′to-me) [*pancreas* + Gr. *ektomē* excision] surgical removal of the pancreas.

pancreathelcosis (pan″kre-ath″el-ko′sis) [*pancreas* + Gr. *helkōsis* ulceration] (*obs.*) ulceration of the pancreas.

pancreatic (pan″kre-at′ik) [L. *pancreaticus*] pertaining to the pancreas.

pancreatico- a combining form denoting relationship to the pancreatic duct.

pancreaticoduodenal (pan″kre-at″ĭ-ko-du″o-de′nal) pertaining to the pancreas and duodenum.

pancreaticoduodenostomy (pan″kre-at″ĭ-ko-du″o-de-nos′to-me) surgical anastomosis of the pancreatic duct, or the divided end of the transected pancreas, with the duodenum.

pancreaticoenterostomy (pan″kre-at″ĭ-ko-en″ter-os′to-me) surgical anastomosis of the pancreatic duct, or the divided end of the transected pancreas, with the intestine.

pancreaticogastrostomy (pan″kre-at″ĭ-ko-gas-tros′to-me) surgical anastomosis of the pancreatic duct, or the divided end of the transected pancreas, with the stomach.

pancreaticojejunostomy (pan″kre-at″ĭ-ko-je″ju-nos′to-me) surgical anastomosis of the pancreatic duct, or the divided end of the transected pancreas, with the jejunum.

pancreaticosplenic (pan″kre-at″ĭ-ko-splen′ik) pertaining to the pancreas and spleen.

pancreatin (pan′kre-ah-tin) [USP] a substance obtained from the pancreas of the hog or the ox, which contains enzymes, chiefly amylase, protease, and lipase, and having the same action as do the enzymes of the pancreatic juice; used as a digestive aid in conditions of pancreatic insufficiency, and also to peptonize milk and other foods.

pancreatism (pan′kre-ah-tizm″) activity of the pancreas.

pancreatitis (pan″kre-ah-ti′tis) acute or chronic inflammation of the pancreas, which may be asymptomatic or symptomatic, and which is due to autodigestion of a pancreatic tissue by its own enzymes. It is caused most often by alcoholism or biliary tract disease; less commonly it may be associated with hyperlipemia, hyperparathyroidism, abdominal trauma (accidental or operative injury), vasculitis, or uremia. **acute p.,** a form characterized by sudden onset of abdominal pain, nausea, and vomiting. **acute hemorrhagic p.,** a condition due to autolysis of pancreatic tissue caused by the escape of enzymes into its substance, resulting in hemorrhage into the parenchyma and surrounding tissues. Blood staining of the lateral abdominal wall (Grey Turner's sign) or periumbilical area (Cullen's sign) may result. **calcereous p.,** pancreatitis accompanied by the formation of calculi; pancreatic calcification is usually associated with exocrine insufficiency and diabetes mellitus. **centrilobar p.,** pancreatitis located around the branches of the pancreatic duct. **chronic p.,** a form marked usually by chronic abdominal pain and by progressive fibrosis and loss of exocrine (steatorrhea) and endocrine (diabetes mellitus) function; recurrent attacks of acute pancreatitis (*chronic relapsing p.*) are often superimposed. **chronic relapsing p.,** see *chronic p.* **interstitial p.,** pancreatitis in which there is overgrowth of the inter- and intra-acinar connective tissue and frequently a corresponding atrophy of the glandular tissue. **perilobar p.,** fibrosis of the pancreas

surrounding collections of atrophic acini. **purulent p.,** purulent inflammation of the pancreas.

pancreato- a combining form denoting relationship to the pancreas.

pancreatoduodenectomy (pan″kre-ah-to-du″o-dĕ-nek′to-me) excision of the head of the pancreas along with the encircling loop of the duodenum.

pancreatoduodenostomy (pan″kre-ah-to-du″o-dĕ-nos′to-me) pancreaticoduodenostomy.

pancreatoenterostomy (pan″kre-ah-to-en″ter-os′to-me) pancreaticoenterostomy.

pancreatogenic (pan″kre-ah-to-jen′ik) pancreatogenous.

pancreatogenous (pan″kre-ah-toj′ĕ-nus) arising in or from the pancreas.

pancreatogram (pan″kre-at′o-gram) the x-ray film produced by pancreatography.

pancreatography (pan″kre-ah-tog′rah-fe) roentgenography of the pancreas performed during surgical exploration, a water-soluble contrast medium being injected into the pancreatic duct and the film being made while the abdomen is open. **endoscopic retrograde p.,** that in which the radiopaque medium is injected into the pancreatic duct at the ampulla of Vater via a cannula introduced through a fiberoptic endoscope.

pancreatoid (pan-kre′ah-toid) resembling the pancreas.

pancreatolipase (pan″kre-ah-to-lip′ās) pancreatic lipase.

pancreatolith (pan″kre-at′o-lith) [*pancreas* + Gr. *lithos* stone] a pancreatic calculus.

pancreatolithectomy (pan″kre-ah-to-lĭ-thek′to-me) [*pancreatolith* + Gr. *ektomē* excision] excision of a calculus from the pancreas.

pancreatolithiasis (pan″kre-ah-to-lĭ-thi′ah-sis) the presence of calculi in the ductal system or parenchyma of the pancreas.

pancreatolithotomy (pan″kre-ah-to-lĭ-thot′o-me) [*pancreatolith* + Gr. *tomē* a cutting] incision of the pancreas for the removal of a calculus.

pancreatolysis (pan″kre-ah-tol′ĭ-sis) pancreolysis.

pancreatolytic (pan″kre-ah-to-lit′ik) pancreolytic.

pancreatomy (pan-kre-at′o-me) pancreatotomy.

pancreatoncus (pan″kre-ah-ton′kus) [*pancreas* + Gr. *onkos* mass] a tumor of the pancreas.

pancreatopathy (pan″kre-ah-top′ah-the) [*pancreas* + Gr. *pathos* disease] any disease of the pancreas.

pancreatotomy (pan″kre-ah-tot′o-me) [*pancreas* + Gr. *tomē* a cutting] incision of the pancreas.

pancreatotropic (pan-kre″ah-to-trop′ik) [*pancreas* + Gr. *tropē* a turning] having an affinity for or an influence on the pancreas.

pancreatropic (pan″kre-ah-trop′ik) pancreatotropic.

pancrectomy (pan″kre-ek′to-me) pancreatectomy.

pancrelipase (pan″kre-li′pās) [USP] a standardized preparation of hog pancreas, containing enzymes, principally lipase, with amylase and protease, and having the same actions as those of the pancreatic juice; used as a digestive aid in conditions of pancreatic insufficiency.

pancreolithotomy (pan″kre-o-lĭ-thot′o-me) pancreatolithotomy.

pancreolysis (pan″kre-ol′ĭ-sis) [*pancreas* + Gr. *lysis* dissolution] destruction of pancreatic tissue by pancreatic enzymes.

pancreolytic (pan″kre-o-lit′ik) pertaining to or producing pancreolysis.

pancreopathy (pan″kre-op′ah-the) [*pancreas* + Gr. *pathos* disease] any disease of the pancreas.

pancreoprivic (pan″kre-o-priv′ik) lacking a pancreas.

pancreotherapy (pan″kre-o-ther′ah-pe) therapeutic use of pancreas tissue or of extracts of the pancreas containing digestive enzymes; pancreatic replacement therapy, used in pancreatic insufficiency with malabsorption.

pancreotropic (pan″kre-o-trop′ik) pancreatotropic.

pancreozymin (pan″kre-o-zi′min) a hormone of the duodenal mucosa which stimulates the external secretory activity of the pancreas, especially its production of amylase; identical with cholecystokinin (q.v.).

pancuronium bromide (pan″ku-ro′ne-um) chemical name: 1,1′-[(2β,3α,5α,16β,17β)-3,17-bis(acetyloxy)androstane-2,16-diyl]-bis[1-methyl]piperidinium dibromide. A nondepolarizing skeletal muscle relaxant, $C_{35}H_{60}Br_2N_2O_4$, with curariform action; used as an adjunct to anesthesia, and may be used to facilitate mechanical ventilation, administered intravenously.

pancystitis (pan″sis-ti′tis) cystitis involving the entire thickness of the wall of the urinary bladder, as occurs in interstitial cystitis.

pancytopenia (pan″si-to-pe′ne-ah) [*pan-* + *-cyte* + Gr. *penia* poverty] deficiency of all cell elements of the blood; aplastic anemia. **congenital p.,** Fanconi's syndrome, def. 1. **Fanconi's p.,** Fanconi's syndrome, def. 1.

pandemic (pan-dem′ik) [*pan-* + Gr. *dēmos* prople] 1. widely epidemic; distributed throughout a region or continent, or globally. 2. a widespread epidemic disease.

pandemicity (pan″dĕ-mis′ĭ-te) the state of being epidemic and widely spread.

Pander's islands, layer, nucleus (pan′derz) [Heinrich Christian *Pander*, German anatomist, 1794–1865] see under *island* and *layer*, and see *nucleus subthalamicus.*

pandiculation (pan″dik-u-la′shun) [L. *pandiculari* to stretch one's self] the act of stretching and yawning.

Pándy's test (reaction) (pan′dēz) [Kálmán *Pándy,* Hungarian neurologist, born 1868] see under *tests.*

panel (pan′el) a list of names, a number of individuals participating in a specific discussion or activity, especially a list of names of the medical men who are willing to care for insured persons for a stipulated yearly fee under the system of medical insurance carried on by insurance groups under the supervision of the government in Great Britain, or the list of the insured persons assigned as clients to a physician under the British National Health Insurance Act. **personality p.** (*obs.*), a list of the aspects of a person's constitution with reference to his predisposition to particular types of diseases.

panelectroscope (pan″e-lek′tro-skōp) an instrument for examining by electrical illumination the various organs of the body, as the stomach, rectum, urethra, etc.

panencephalitis (pan″en-sef″ah-li′tis) encephalitis, probably of viral origin, which produces intranuclear or intracytoplasmic inclusion bodies of type A (Cowdry's classification), which result in parenchymatous lesions affecting the gray and white matter of the brain simultaneously. **Pette-Döring p.,** a form of subacute encephalitis characterized by involvement of both the gray and white matter of the brain, and with a predilection for the basal ganglia. **subacute sclerosing p.,** a rare and devastating form of leukoencephalitis usually affecting children and adolescents. Insidious in onset, it characteristically produces progressive cerebral dysfunction over a course of several weeks or months and death within a year. Pathologically, in addition to the lesions of the white matter, there are demyelination and intranuclear inclusion bodies in nerve cells and oligodendroglia, suggesting a viral etiology. Called also *Dawson's encephalitis, subacute inclusion body encephalitis, subacute sclerosing leukoencephalopathy,* and *van Bogaert's encephalitis* or *sclerosing leukoencephalitis.*

panendography (pan″en-dog′rah-fe) the recording of events observed through a panendoscope.

panendoscope (pan-en′do-skōp) a cystoscope that permits wide-angle viewing of the urinary bladder. **oral p.,** an illuminated tubular device that permits visual observation and audiovisual recording of the larynx and vocal cords during production of speech sounds.

panendoscopy (pan″en-dos′ko-pe) observation by means of a panendoscope.

panepizootic (pan-ep″ĭ-zo-ot′ik) 1. attacking almost all the animals in a fairly large area; said of disease. 2. a widely diffused and rapidly spreading animal disease.

panesthesia (pan″es-the′ze-ah) [*pan-* + Gr. *aisthēsis* perception] the sum of the sensations experienced.

panesthetic (pan″es-thet′ik) relating to panesthesia.

Paneth's cells (pah′nāts) [Josef *Paneth,* German physician, 1857–1890] see under *cell.*

pang (pang) a sudden, piercing pain. **breast p.,** angina pectoris. **brow p.,** 1. supraorbital neuralgia. 2. hemicrania (def. 1).

pangamate (pan′gah-māt) any salt of pangamic acid.

pangen (pan′jen) [*pan-* + Gr. *gennan* to produce] one of the hypothetical units of idioplasm.

pangenesis (pan-jen′ĕ-sis) [*pan-* + *genesis*] the doctrine that in reproduction each cell of the parent body is represented by a particle; the hypothesis that all the units or cells of the body reside in the blood as gemmules, multiply by division, and throw off atoms which are transmitted to the offspring, accounting for the hereditary transmission of acquired mental habits and other phenomena of heredity; the theory implying that the whole organism, in the sense of every atom or unit, reproduces itself.

panglossia (pan-glos′e-ah) [Gr. *panglōssia*] abnormal or pathologic garrulity.

Pangonia (pan-go′ne-ah) a genus of flies, the zimbs of Ethiopia, which are exceedingly annoying to man and animals.

panhematopenia (pan-hem″ah-to-pe′ne-ah) [*pan-* + Gr. *haima* blood + *penia* poverty] pancytopenia. **primary splenic p.,** a form of hypersplenism of unknown etiology, marked by indiscriminate elimination of all circulating elements of the blood. Whether such an entity exists, as such, is moot, since the hypersplenism may be a manifestation of an underlying systemic disease.

Panheprin (pan-hep′rin) trademark for a preparation of heparin sodium.

panhydrometer (pan″hi-drom′ĕ-ter) [*pan-* + *hydrometer*] an instrument for ascertaining the specific gravity of any liquid.

panhyperemia (pan″hi-per-e′me-ah) [*pan-* + *hyperemia*] general plethora.

panhypogonadism (pan-hi″po-go′nad-izm) underdevelopment of all the genital tissues due to abnormally decreased functional activities of the gonads.

panhypopituitarism (pan-hi″po-pĭ-tu′ĭ-tar-izm) generalized hypopituitarism due to absence or damage to the pituitary gland, which, in its complete form, leads to absence of gonadal function and insufficiency of thyroid and adrenal function. Dwarfism, regression of secondary sex characteristics and loss of libido, weight loss, fatigability, bradycardia, hypotension, depression, and many other manifestations may occur. When cachexia is a prominent feature, it is called *hypophyseal* or *pituitary cachexia,* and *Simmonds' disease.* **prepubertal p.,** pituitary dwarfism.

panhysterectomy (pan″his-ter-ek′to-me) [*pan-* + Gr. *hystera* uterus + *ektomē* excision] complete extirpation of the uterus and cervix; total hysterectomy.

panhystero-oophorectomy (pan-his″ter-o-o″of-o-rek′to-me) excision of the body of the uterus, cervix, and ovary.

panhysterosalpingectomy (pan-his″ter-o-sal″pin-jek′to-me) excision of the body of the uterus, cervix, and uterine tube.

panhysterosalpingo-oophorectomy (pan-his″ter-o-sal″ping-go-o″of-o-rek′to-me) excision of the uterus, cervix, uterine tube, and ovary.

panic (pan′ik) extreme and unreasoning fear and anxiety. **acute homosexual p., homosexual p.,** an acute reaction due to unconscious conflicts involving homosexuality, marked by severe anxiety, excitement, great activity, sometimes accompanied by auditory hallucinations accusing the patient of homosexual practices or inclinations, and frequently assaultiveness. Called also *Kempf's disease.*

panimmunity (pan″ĭ-mu′nĭ-te) [*pan-* + *immunity*] immunity to several infections caused by bacteria and viruses.

panis (pa′nis) [L.] bread.

Panizza's plexus (pan-id′zaz) [Bartolomeo *Panizza,* Professor of anatomy at Pavia, 1785–1867] see under *plexus.*

panleukopenia (pan″lu-ko-pe′ne-ah) a viral disease of cats, characterized by leukopenia and marked by inactivity, refusal of food, diarrhea, and vomiting. Called also *infectious feline agranulocytosis, feline* or *cat enteritis, cat distemper,* and *cat plague.*

panmeristic (pan″mer-is′tik) [*pan-* + Gr. *meros* part] pertaining to the protoplasm of ova, made up of independent units or pangens.

panmixia (pan-mik′se-ah) [*pan-* + Gr. *mignynai* to mix] panmixis.

panmixis (pan-mik′sis) [*pan-* + Gr. *mignynai* to mix] random mating.

Panmycin (pan-mi′sin) trademark for preparations of tetracycline.

panmyeloid (pan-mi′ĕ-loid) pertaining to all the elements of the bone marrow.

panmyelopathia (pan″mi-ĕ-lo-path′e-ah) panmyelopathy.

panmyelopathy (pan″mi-ĕ-lop′ah-the) [*pan-* + Gr. *myelos* marrow + *pathos* disease] a pathologic condition of all the elements of the bone marrow. **constitutional infantile p.,** Fanconi's syndrome, def. 1.

panmyelophthisis (pan-mi″ĕ-lof′thĭ-sis) [*pan-* + Gr. *myelos* marrow + *phthisis* wasting] 1. aplastic anemia. 2. (*obs.*) aleukia hemorrhagica.

panneuritis (pan″nu-ri′tis) [*pan-* + Gr. *neuron* nerve + *-itis*] (*obs.*) multiple or general neuritis. **p. epidem′ica,** beriberi.

pannicualgia (pah-nik″u-lal′je-ah) adiposalgia.

panniculectomy (pah-nik″u-lek′to-me) surgical excision of the abdominal apron of superficial fat in the obese.

panniculitis (pah-nik″u-li′tis) inflammation of the panniculus adiposus. **LE p.,** a form of lupus erythematosus in which nontender firm nodules 1 to 4 cm. in diameter occur in the panniculus adiposus, usually beneath relatively normal-appearing skin. Infrequently, the lesions may ulcerate. Systemic involvement is common. See also *lupus erythematosus profundus.* **nodular nonsuppurative p., relapsing febrile nodular nonsuppurative p.,** a disease marked by fever and the formation of crops of tender nodules in the subcutaneous fatty tissues; called also *Weber-Christian p., disease,* or *syndrome.* **subacute nodular migratory p.,** a variety of nodular vasculitis, closely resembling erythema induratum, occurring on the legs of women; it is distinguished principally by its "migration," i.e., the coalescence and clearing of the lesions and the appearance of new lesions nearby. **Weber-Christian p.,** relapsing febrile nodular nonsuppurative p.

panniculus (pah-nik′u-lus), pl. *pannic′uli* [L., dim. of *pannus* cloth] a layer of membrane. **p. adipo′sus** [NA], the subcutaneous fat: a layer of fat underlying the corium, or dermis. Called also *pannus.* **p. carno′sus,** a thin muscular layer within the superficial fascia of animals with a hairy coat; in man it is represented mainly by the platysma myoides.

pannus (pan′us) [L. "a piece of cloth"] 1. superficial vascularization of the cornea with infiltration of granulation tissue. **2.** an inflammatory exudate overlying the lining layer of synovial cells on the inside of a joint, usually occurring in patients with rheumatoid arthritis or related articular rheumatism, and sometimes resulting in fibrous ankylosis of the joint. **3.** panniculus adiposus. **allergic p.,** pannus of the cornea as a result of allergy. **p. cara′teus,** pinta. **p. carno′sus, p. cras′sus,** pannus of the cornea characterized by extremely dense opacity. **degenerative p., p. degenerati′vus,** a connective-tissue growth between the epithelium of the cornea and Bowman's membrane. **glaucomatous p.,** degeneration and desquamation of corneal epithelium due to edema in avanced glaucoma. **inflammatory p.,** pannus which contains inflammatory cells and replaces Bowman's membrane. **phlyctenular p.,** pannus associated with phlyctenular keratitis, the vascularization running all the way around the periphery of the limbus and extending toward the center. **p. sic′cus,** pannus of the cornea associated with dryness of the cornea and conjunctiva. **p. ten′uis,** pannus of the cornea in which the opacity is very slight. **p. trachomato′sus,** pannus occurring secondarily to trachoma, the small fine branching vessels always appearing at the upper limbus and running down under the epithelium into the cornea.

panodic (pah-nod′ik) panthodic.

panophobia (pan″o-fo′be-ah) panphobia.

panophthalmia (pan″of-thal′me-ah) panophthalmitis.

panophthalmitis (pan″of-thal-mi′tis) [*pan-* + Gr. *ophthalmos* eye + *-itis*] inflammation of all the structures or tissues of the eye.

panoptic (pan-op′tik) [*pan-* + Gr. *optikos* of or for vision] rendering everything visible; said of a stain which differentiates all the tissues of a specimen. See *Giemsa's stain,* under *stain.*

panoptosis (pan″op-to′sis) [*pan-* + Gr. *ptōsis* falling] (*obs.*) general ptosis of the abdominal organs.

panosteitis (pan″os-te-i′tis) [*pan-* + Gr. *osteon* bone + *-itis*] inflammation of every part of a bone.

panostitis (pan″os-ti′tis) panosteitis.

panotitis (pan″o-ti′tis) [*pan-* + Gr. *ous* ear + *-itis*] an inflammation of all the parts or structures of the ear.

panphobia (pan-fo′be-ah) fear of everything; a vague morbid dread of some unknown evil.

panplegia (pan-ple′je-ah) pamplegia.

panproctocolectomy (pan-prok″to-ko-lek′to-me) excision of the entire rectum and colon, with creation of an ileal stoma for elimination of the feces.

Pansch's fissure (pansh′ez) [Adolf *Pansch,* German anatomist, 1841–1887] see under *fissure.*

pansclerosis (pan″skle-ro′sis) [*pan-* + Gr. *sklērōsis* hardening] complete induration of a part or organ.

panseptum (pan-sep′tum) the entire nasal septum, including bony and cartilaginous parts.

pansinuitis (pan″si-nu-i′tis) pansinusitis.

pansinusectomy (pan″si-nus-ek′to-me) excision of the diseased membrane of all of the paranasal sinuses on one side.

pansinusitis (pan″si-nu-si′tis) [*pan-* + *sinus* + *-itis*] inflammation involving all of the paranasal sinuses on one side.

panspermatism (pan-sper′mah-tizm) panspermia.

panspermia (pan-sper′me-ah) [*pan-* + Gr. *sperma* seed + *-ia*] **1.** the doctrine that disease germs and bacteria are everywhere present. **2.** biogenesis.

pansphygmograph (pan-sfig′mo-graf) [*pan-* + Gr. *sphygmos* pulse + *graphein* to record] a device for recording cardiac, pulse, and chest movements at the same time.

Panstrongylus (pan-stron′jĭ-lus) a genus of cone-nosed bugs of the family Reduviidae, species of which are vectors of *Trypanosoma.* **P. genicula′tus,** a vector of *Trypanosoma cruzi* in Panama and Brazil. **P. infes′tans,** *Triatoma infestans.* **P. megis′tus,** an important vector of *Trypanosoma cruzi* in Brazil. It frequently bites the face and so is called barbiero by the natives. Formerly called *Triatoma megista.*

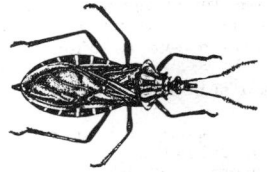

Panstrongylus megistus (female).

pant- see *panto-.*

pantachromatic (pan″tah-kro-mat′ik) [*pant-* + *achromatic*] entirely achromatic.

pantalgia (pan-tal′je-ah) [*pant-* + *-algis*] pain over the whole body.

pantamorphia (pan″tah-mor′fe-ah) [*pant-* + Gr. *amorphia* shapelessness] complete or general deformity.

pantamorphic (pan″tah-mor′fik) formless.

pantanencephaly (pan″tan-en-sef′ah-le) [*pant-* + *an* neg. + Gr. *enkephalos* brain] complete absence of the brain in a fetus.

pantankyloblepharon (pan-tang″kĭ-lo-blef′ah-ron) [*pant-* + Gr. *ankylē* noose + *blepharon* lid] general adhesion of the eyelids to the eyeball and to each other.

pantatrophia (pan″tah-tro′fe-ah) [*pant-* + Gr. *atrophia* atrophy] general or complete malnutrition.

pantatrophy (pan-tat′ro-fe) pantatrophia.

Panteric (pan-ter′ik) trademark for a preparation of pancreatin.

pantetheine (pan-tĕ-the′in) a naturally occurring amide of pantothenic acid and β-mercaptoethanolamine; it is an intermediate in the biosynthesis of CoA, a growth factor for *Lactobacillus bulgaricus,* and a cofactor in certain enzyme complexes (e.g., in fatty acid or polypeptide synthesis).

panthenol (pan′thĕ-nōl) chemical name: 2,4-dihydroxy-*N*-(3-hydroxypropyl)-3,3-dimethylbutanamide. The alcohol derivative of pantothenic acid, $C_9H_{19}NO_4$, which is converted in the body to pantothenic acid, a member of the B-complex vitamins. Called also *pantothenyl alcohol* and *pantothenol.* The term is sometimes used to refer to the $D^{(+)}$ form of panthenol; see *dexpanthenol.*

pantherapist (pan-ther′ah-pist) [*pan-* + Gr. *therapeia* treatment] a practitioner who is ready to draw his information from any and every source.

panthodic (pan-thod′ik) [*pan-* + Gr. *hodos* way] radiating in every direction; said of nerve impulses.

Pantholin (pan′tho-lin) trademark for a preparation of calcium pantothenate.

panting (pant′ing) swift and shallow breathing with a fast respiratory frequency and small tidal volume.

panto-, pant- [Gr. *pas, pantos* all] combining form meaning all, the whole.

pantochromism (pan″to-kro′mizm) [*panto-* + Gr. *chrōma* color] the phenomenon of existing in two or more differently colored forms, as a salt.

pantogamy (pan-tog′ah-me) [*panto-* + Gr. *gamos* marriage] promiscuous sexual intercourse.

pantograph (pan′to-graf) [*panto-* + Gr. *graphein* to write] an instrument for copying a plane figure to any desired scale.

pantomographic (pan-to″mo-graf′ik) pertaining to pantomography.

pantomography (pan″to-mog′rah-fe) a method of body-section roentgenography for visualization of curved surfaces at any depth.

pantomorphia (pan″to-mor′fe-ah) [*panto-* + Gr. *morphē* form + *-ia*] **1.** general or perfect symmetry. **2.** ability to assume various shapes, as an ameba.

pantomorphic (pan″to-mor′fik) able to assume any shape.

Pantopaque (pan-to-pāk′) trademark for a preparation of iophendylate.

pantophobia (pan″to-fo′be-ah) [*panto-* + *phobia*] panphobia.

pantophobic (pan″to-fo′bik) characterized by pantophobia.

pantoscopic (pan″to-skop′ik) [*panto-* + Gr. *skopein* to examine] adapted to view both near and distant objects; a term applied to bifocal lenses.

pantothen (pan′to-then) pantothenic acid.

pantothenate (pan-to′then-āt) a salt of pantothenic acid.

pantothenol (pan″to-the′nōl) **1.** panthenol. **2.** dexpanthenol.

pantotropic (pan″to-trop′ik) pantropic.

pantropic (pan-to-trop′ik) [*pan-* + Gr. *tropos* a turning] having an affinity for many tissues; capable of attacking derivatives of any of the three embryonic layers.

panturbinate (pan-ter′bĭ-nāt) the entire structure of a nasal concha, including bone and soft tissue.

Panum's casein (pah′nōōmz) [Peter Ludvig *Panum,* Danish physiologist, 1820–1885] serum globulin.

panus (pa′nus) [L. "swelling"] a lymphatic gland inflamed but not suppurating.

panuveitis (pan″u-ve-i′tis) inflammation of the entire uveal tract.

Panwarfin (pan-war′fin) trademark for a preparation of warfarin sodium.

panzerherz (pan′zer-herz) [Ger.] armored heart; see under *heart.*

panzootic (pan″zo-ot′ik) [*pan-* + Gr. *zōon* animal] occurring pandemically among animals.

pap (pap) any soft food, as bread soaked in milk.

Pap test (pap) Papanicolaou's test; see under *tests.*

papain (pah-pa′in, pah-pi′in) a crystalline proteolytic enzyme from the latex of the papaw, *Carica papaya* L. (Caricaceae), which catalyzes the hydrolysis of proteins and polypeptides to amino acids. It has a wide substrate specificity and is active in a broad pH range. Papain is the main constituent of meat tenderizers and is used in the brewing industry to chillproof beer. In medicine, it is used as a protein digestant and as a topical application for enzymatic débridement and promotion of normal healing of surface lesions.

Papanicolaou's stain, test (pap″ah-nik″o-la′ōōz) [George Nicolas *Papanicolaou*, Greek physician, anatomist, and cytologist in the United States, 1883–1962] see *Table of Stains*, and under *tests*.

Papaver (pah-pav′er) a genus of herbs of the family Papaveraceae, or poppies. *P. somnif′erum*, a pink to purplish-pink and purple species, and its variety *al′bum*, a silvery white species, are the source of opium. The unripe capsules when scarified yield a white latex which when dried is known as crude opium. It contains the opium alkaloids (morphine, codeine, etc.), which are used as narcotics and analgesics. The poppy seeds, devoid of the alkaloids, are used as a condiment on baked products. *P. orienta′lis* is the source of isothebaine.

papaverine hydrochloride (pah-pav′er-in) [USP] chemical name: 1-[(3,4-dimethoxyphenyl)methyl]-6,7-dimethoxyisoquinoline hydrochloride. The hydrochloride salt of an opium alkaloid, $C_{20}H_{21}NO_4 \cdot HCl$, which also may be synthesized, occurring as white crystals or as a white, crystalline powder; used as a smooth muscle relaxant, especially in the treatment of cerebral and peripheral ischemia associated with arterial spasm and myocardial ischemia complicated by arrhythmias, administered orally and intramuscularly.

papaw (pah-paw′) 1. a large herbaceous plant, the papaya, *Carica papaya* L. (Caricaceae) of Southern United States; also its fruit. The fruit contains papain, a proteolytic enzyme. 2. pawpaw; the tree *Asimina triloba* (L.) Duval (Annonaceae), which has edible fruit, although ingestion may cause severe skin irritation in sensitive persons.

papaya (pah-pa′yah) papaw, def. 1.

papayotin (pap″a-yo′tin) papain.

paper (pa′per) a substance manufactured in thin sheets, prepared from wood, rags, or other fibrous substance which has first been reduced to a pulp. **alkanin p.**, filter paper dipped in an alcoholic solution of alkanin; alkalis turn it blue, acids red. **amboceptor p.**, filter paper saturated with amboceptor serum; used in the Noguchi test for syphilis. **aniline acetate p.**, filter paper dipped into a mixture of aniline, water, and glacial acetic acid, and then dried. **antigen p.**, filter paper saturated with antigen solution; used in the Noguchi test for syphilis. **articulating p.**, carbon paper to be placed between the upper and lower teeth and bitten on, to record the contact relationships of the teeth. **asthma p.**, niter p. **azolitmin p.**, filter paper saturated with a solution of azolitmin; acids turn it from purple to bright red, alkalis turn it blue. **bibulous p.**, a paper which absorbs water readily. **biuret p.**, filter paper previously dipped in Gies' biuret reagent, dried, and cut into strips. **blue litmus p.**, see *litmus p*. **Congo red p.**, wet filter paper with a 0.2 per cent solution of Congo red in water, dry, and cut in strips. **filter p.**, a porous, unsized paper used as a filter. **lacmoid p.**, blotting paper impregnated with lacmoid; used in testing for alkalinity or acidity. **litmus p.**, bibulous paper impregnated with a solution of litmus, dried, and cut into strips. If slightly alkaline the paper is blue, and is used as a test for acids, which turn it red; if slightly acid it is red and alkalis turn it blue. **niter p.**, paper impregnated with potassium nitrate, ignited and used as a moxa or by inhalation in asthma; called also *saltpeter p*. **occluding p.**, articulating p. **potassium nitrate p.**, niter p. **red litmus p.**, see *litmus p*. **saltpeter p.**, niter p. **test p.**, paper that is impregnated with litmus or other indicator. **turmeric p.**, paper dyed yellow with turmeric; alkalis turn it brown.

papescent (pah-pes′ent) having the consistence of pap.

papilla (pah-pil′ah), pl. *papil′lae* [L.] a small nipple-shaped projection or elevation; [NA] a general term for such a structure. **acoustic p.**, organum spirale. **arcuate papillae of tongue**, papillae filiformes. **Bergmeister's p.**, a small mass of neuroglial cells in the center of the embryonic optic disk, surrounding the bulb of the hyaloid artery. Also, a congenital anomaly consisting of a glial veil attached to the anterior aspect of the optic disk, resulting from glial proliferation around the remnants of the posterior part of the hyaloid vessel system. **bile p.**, p. duodeni major. **calciform papillae, capitate papillae**, papillae vallatae. **circumvallate papillae**, papillae vallatae. **clavate papillae**, papillae fungiformes. **papil′lae con′icae** [NA], **conical papillae**, sparsely scattered large elevations on the tongue surface, often considered as a modified type of filiform papillae. **conical papillae of tongue, of Soemmering**, papillae filiformes. **conoid papillae of tongue**, papillae conicae. **papil′lae co′rii** [NA], **papillae of corium**, conical extensions of the collagen fibers, the capillary blood vessels, and sometimes the nerves of the corium into corresponding spaces among the downward- or inward-projecting rete ridges on the under surface of the epidermis. On the forehead and ear these are lacking; on the face, neck, and pubes the relations are reversed and "rete pegs" extend inward or downward into spaces among a network of dermal ridges. Called also *dermal papillae* and *skin papillae*. **corolliform papil-**

lae of tongue, papillae filiformes. **dental p., dentinal p.**, p. dentis. **p. den′tis** [NA], the small mass of condensed mesenchyme capped by each of the enamel organs. **dermal papillae**, papillae corii. **duodenal p., major**, p. duodeni major. **duodenal p., minor**, p. duodeni minor. **p. duode′ni ma′jor** [NA], major duodenal papilla: a small elevation at the site of the opening of the conjoined common bile duct and pancreatic duct into the lumen of the duodenum. Called also *p. duodeni* [*Santorini*]. See also *p. duodeni minor*. **p. duode′ni mi′nor** [NA], minor duodenal papilla: a small elevation at the site of the opening of the accessory pancreatic duct into the lumen of the duodenum. See also *p. duodeni major*. **p. duode′ni** [San-tori′ni], p. duodeni major. **filiform papillae, papil′lae filifor′mes** [NA], threadlike elevations that cover most of the tongue surface. **papil′lae folia′tae** [NA], **foliate papillae**, parallel mucosal folds on the margins of the tongue at the junction of its body and root. **fungiform papillae, papil′-lae fungifor′mes** [NA], knoblike projections on the tongue, scattered singly among the filiform papillae. **gingival p.**, septal gingiva; the triangular pad of gingiva filling the space between the proximal surfaces of two adjacent teeth; called also *interdental p*. **gustatory papillae**, papillae linguales. **hair p.**, p. pili. **p. incisi′va** [NA], **incisive p.**, a rounded projection at the anterior end of the raphe of the palate. **interdental p.**, gingival p. **interproximal p.**, the cone-shaped projection of the gingiva filling the interdental spaces between adjacent teeth up to the contact areas as viewed from the labial, buccal, or lingual aspect. **lacrimal p., p. lacrima′lis** [NA], a papilla in the conjunctiva near the medial angle of the eye. **papil′lae lacrima′les**, see *p. lacrimalis*. **lenticular papillae, papil′lae lenticula′res**, a series of papillae of the tongue resembling, but less elevated than, the fungiform papillae. **lingual papillae, papil′lae lingua′les** [NA], the filiform, fungiform, vallate, foliate, and conical papillae of the tongue. **major duodenal p.**, p. duodeni major. **p. mam′mae** [NA], **mammary p.**, nipple of the breast: the pigmented projection on the anterior surface of the mammary gland, surrounded by the areola. The lactiferous ducts open onto it. **medial papillae of tongue**, papillae fungiformes. **minor duodenal p.**, p. duodeni minor. **p. ner′vi op′tici**, discus nervi optici. **obtuse papillae of tongue**, papillae fungiformes. **optic p.**, discus nervi optici. **palatine p.**, p. incisiva. **parotid p.**, **paroti′dea** [NA], the small papilla marking the orifice of the parotid duct in the mucous membrane of the cheek. **p. pi′li** [NA], hair papilla: the fibrovascular mesodermal papilla enclosed within the hair bulb. **renal papillae, papil′lae rena′les** [NA], the blunted apices of the renal pyramids, which project into the renal sinus. **p. of Santorini**, p. duodeni major. **simple papillae of tongue**, papillae filiformes. **skin papillae**, papillae corii. **small papillae of tongue**, papillae filiformes. **p. spira′lis**, organum spirale. **sublingual p.**, caruncula sublingualis. **tactile papillae**, corpuscula tactus. **urethral p.**, a slight elevation in the vestibule of the vagina on which is situated the external orifice of the urethra. **papil′-lae valla′tae** [NA], **vallate papillae**, the largest papillae of the tongue, 8 to 12 in number, arranged in the form of a V in front of the sulcus terminalis of the tongue. **p. of Vater**, p. duodeni major. **villous papillae of tongue**, papillae filiformes.

papillae (pah-pil′e) [L.] plural of *papilla*.

papillary (pap′ĭ-ler″e) pertaining to or resembling a papilla, or nipple.

papillate (pap′ĭ-lāt) marked by nipple-like elevations.

papillectomy (pap″ĭ-lek′to-me) [*papilla* + Gr. *ektomē* excision] excision of a papilla, especially removal of one or more engorged papillae from a kidney for the cure of hematuria.

papilledema (pap″il-ĕ-de′mah) choked disk; edema of the optic disk (papilla), most commonly due to increased intracranial pressure, malignant hypertension, or thrombosis of the central retinal vein.

papilliferous (pap″ĭ-lif′er-us) [*papilla* + L. *ferre* to bear] bearing papillae.

papilliform (pah-pil′ĭ-form) [*papilla* + L. *forma* shape] shaped like a papilla.

papillitis (pap″ĭ-li′tis) [*papilla* + -*itis*] inflammation of the optic papilla (disk); see *optic neuritis*, under *neuritis*. **necrotizing p., necrotizing renal p.**, renal papillary necrosis.

papilloadenocystoma (pah-pil″o-ad″ĕ-no-sis-to′mah) papillary cystadenoma.

papillocarcinoma (pah-pil″o-kar″sĭ-no′mah) papillary carcinoma.

papilloma (pap″ĭ-lo′mah) [*papilla* + -*oma*] a branching or lobulated benign tumor derived from epithelium. **p. acumina′-tum** (*obs.*), condyloma acuminatum. **basal cell p.**, seborrheic keratosis. **cockscomb p.**, papilloma of the uterine cervix that occurs during pregnancy and regresses following delivery; it is a small, red lesion that projects above the surrounding mucosa and resembles a cockscomb. **cutaneous p.**, see under *tag*. **fibroepithelial p.**, a papilloma containing extensive fibrous tissue; fibropapilloma. **hirsutoid p's of penis**, pearly penile papules. **Hopmann's p.,** Hopmann's polyp. **intracanalicular p.,** a warty, nonmalignant growth within the substance of certain glands, especially of the breast. **intracystic p.,** a papilloma formed within a cystic adenoma. **rabbit p.,** a viral disease of rabbits marked by the formation of horny warts. These papillomas were the first mammalian tumors shown to be induced by a virus (by Shope in 1933) and the first to be transmitted by purified viral DNA. Called also *Shope p.* **rabbit oral p.,** a viral disease of wild rabbits, characterized by the appearance of nodules on the lower surface of the tongue. **Shope p.,** rabbit p. **villous p.,** a papilloma in which the papillary processes are slender and elongated, occurring usually in the urinary bladder or mammary gland, or as an outgrowth from the choroid plexus in a lateral ventricle of the brain.

papillomatosis (pap″ĭ-lo″mah-to′sis) the development of multiple papillomas. **confluent and reticulated p.,** a genetically determined, profuse papular eruption often occurring in the midline of the trunk and the elbow flexures, usually affecting girls at puberty or soon after. Initially, the lesions are discrete, but later become partially confluent warty papules 3 to 5 mm. in diameter; once established, the condition may remain unchanged for years. Called also *Gougerot-Carteaud syndrome.*

papillomatous (pap″ĭ-lo′mah-tus) of the nature of a papilloma.

papillomavirus (pap″ĭ-lo″mah-vi′rus) any of a subgroup of the papovaviruses causing papillomata in humans and in rabbits, cows, dogs, pigs, and various other animals. Cf. *polyomavirus.* **malignant p. of Degos,** malignant atrophic papulosis.

papilloretinitis (pah-pil″o-ret″ĭ-ni′tis) inflammation of the optic papilla extending to the retina.

papillosphincterotomy (pap″il-lo-sfingk″ter-ot′o-me) surgical division of the sphincter of the major duodenal papilla (Oddi's sphincter).

papillotome (pap′ĭ-lo-tōm″) a cutting instrument for incising the papilla of Vater.

papillotomy (pap″ĭ-lot′o-me) incision of a papilla, as of a duodenal papilla.

Papin's digester (pah-paz′) [Denis *Papin,* French physicist, 1647–1714] an apparatus for subjecting substances to the action of water at a heat greater than the boiling point.

papoid (pap′oid) a commercial preparation of papain.

papovavirus (pap″o-vah-vi′rus) [from *papilloma, polyoma,* and *vacuolating agent* + *virus*] any of a group of relatively small, morphologically similar, ether-resistant DNA viruses, many of which are oncogenic or potentially oncogenic; the group includes the papillomaviruses and polyomaviruses.

Pappenheim's stain (pahp′en-hīmz) [Artur *Pappenheim,* German physician, 1870–1916] see *Table of Stains.*

pappose (pap′pōs) having a downy surface.

pappus (pap′pus) [L.; Gr. *pappos*] 1. (*obs.*) the first downy growth of the beard. 2. the lanugo.

paprika (pap-re′kah) the fruit of *Capsicum annuum* and a condiment prepared from it; it is rich in vitamin C.

papular (pap′u-lar) [L. *papularis*] consisting of, characterized by, or pertaining to a papule.

papulation (pap″u-la′shun) the production of papules.

papule (pap′ūl) [L. *papula*] a small circumscribed, superficial, solid elevation of the skin. **dry p.,** the papule of chancre. **moist p., mucous p.,** condyloma acuminatum. **pearly penile p's,** numerous pearly white papules 1 to 2 mm. in diameter on the coronal edge of the glans penis; called also *hirsutoid papillomas of penis* and *papillomatosis coronae penis.* **prurigo p.,** the characteristic lesion of prurigo, a dome-shaped papule with a small vesicle on top; the vesicle is usually removed immediately by scratching so that a crusted or lichenified papule is most often seen. **split p's,** fissured papular syphilides sometimes seen at the corners of the mouth.

papuloerythematous (pap″u-lo-er″ĕ-them′ah-tus) marked by papules on an erythematous surface.

papuloid (pap′u-loid) resembling a papule; papular.

papulopustular (pap″u-lo-pus′tu-lar) characterized by the presence of papules and pustules.

papulosis (pap-u-lo′sis) a state marked by the presence of multiple papules. **lymphomatoid p.,** an eruption of hemorrhagic papules on the skin, the lesions constantly involuting as new ones are formed. Histologically, there are clusters of large mononuclear cells in the mid and upper dermis. **malignant p., malignant atrophic p.,** a progressive, often fatal, scarring, papular, atrophic, endovasculitis affecting the skin, gastrointestinal tract, and rarely the brain, eye, or kidney; usually occurring in young males, it is characterized clinically by the formation of umbilicated cutaneous papules leaving procelain-colored depressed scars, mostly on the trunk. Called also *Degos' syndrome* or *disease.*

papulosquamous (pap″u-lo-skwa′mus) both papular and scaly; used to denote a group of dermatoses so characterized, including psoriasis, pityriasis rosea, lichen planus, seborrheic dermatitis, and parapsoriasis.

papulovesicular (pap″u-lo-ve-sik′u-lar) characterized by the presence of papules and vesicles.

papyraceous (pap″ĭ-ra′shus) [L. *papyraceus*] like paper; chartaceous.

Paquelin's cautery (pah″kĕ-lanz′) [Claude André *Paquelin,* French physician, 1836–1905] see under *cautery.*

par (par) [L.] pair.

para (par′ah) [L. *parere* to bring forth, to bear] a woman who has produced viable young regardless of whether the child was living at birth. Used with Roman numerals to designate the number of pregnancies that have resulted in the birth of viable offspring, as *para 0* (none—nullipara), *para I* (one—primipara), *para II* (two—secundipara), *para III* (three—tripara), *para IV* (four—quadripara), etc. The number is not indicative of the number of offspring produced in event of a multiple birth. Cf. *gravida.*

para- [Gr. *para* beyond] a prefix meaning beside, beyond, accessory to, apart from, against, etc. In chemistry, the prefix indicates the substitution in a derivative of the benzene ring of two atoms linked to opposite carbon atoms in the ring. The abbreviation is *p-*.

para-actinomycosis (par″ah-ak″tĭ-no-mi-ko′sis) pseudoactinomycosis.

para-agglutinin (par″ah-ah-gloo′tĭ-nin) a partial agglutinin.

para-albuminemia (par″ah-al-bu″mĭ-ne′me-ah) bisalbuminemia.

para-aminobenzenesulfonamide sulfanilamide.

para-aminobenzoate (par″ah-am″ĭ-no-ben′zo-āt) a salt of para-aminobenzoic acid.

para-aminohippurate (par″ah-am″ĭ-no-hip′u-rāt) a salt of para-aminohippuric acid.

para-analgesia (par″ah-an″al-je′ze-ah) analgesia of the lower part of the body, including the lower limbs.

para-anesthesia (par″ah-an″es-the′ze-ah) anesthesia of the lower part of the body and of the legs.

para-appendicitis (par″ah-ah-pen″dĭ-si′tis) inflammation of tissues adjacent to the vermiform appendix.

parabion (par-ab′e-on) parabiont.

parabiont (par-ab′e-ont) [*para-* + Gr. *bioun* to live] one of two or more organisms living in a condition of parabiosis.

parabiosis (par″ah-bi-o′sis) [*para-* + Gr. *biōsis* living] 1. the union of two individuals, as of joined twins, or of experimental animals by surgical operation. 2. temporary suppression of conductivity and excitability in a nerve. **dialytic p.,** the circulation of the blood of two individuals through a dialyzer, separated by a membrane which permits the removal of harmful material from the recipient's blood and the contribution of essential factors from the donor's blood. **vascular p.,** the crossing of the circulation between two individuals by anastomosis of blood vessels.

parabiotic (par″ah-bi-ot′ik) pertaining to or characterized by parabiosis.

parablast (par′ah-blast) [*para-* + Gr. *blastos* germ] that part of the mesoblast from which the blood vessels, lymphatics, etc., are developed.

parablastic (par″ah-blas′tik) pertaining to the parablast.

parablepsia (par-ah-blep′se-ah) [*para-* + Gr. *blepsis* vision + *-ia*] false or perverted vision.

parabolus (pah-rab′o-lus) pl. *parab′oli* [Gr. *parabolos* venturesome] in medieval medicine, an agent of the church who sought out the indigent sick for care and treatment.

parabulia (par″ah-bu′le-ah) [*para-* + Gr. *boulē* will + *-ia*] perversion of the will, as when an individual intends to perform a particular action but halts and substitutes either an opposite action or an unrelated alternative.

paracarbinoxamine (par″ah-kar″bin-ok′sah-min) carbinoxamine.

paracardiac (par″ah-kar′de-ak) beside the heart.

paracarmine (par″ah-kar′min) a staining medium consisting of carminic acid, calcium chloride, and alcohol.

paracasein (par″ah-ka′se-in) the chemical product of the action of rennin on casein; see *casein.*

paracele (par′ah-sēl) paracoele.

paracellulose (par″ah-sel′u-lōs) a kind of cellulose found in the pith of plants.

paracelsian (par″ah-sel′se-an) pertaining to or named for Paracelsus.

Paracelsus (par-ah-sel′sus) [Philippus Aureolus Theophrastus Bombastus von Hohenheim] (1493–1541) a famous Swiss physician and alchemist; a controversial figure whose alchemical researches led to the introduction of such substances as lead, sulfur, iron, and arsenic into pharmaceutical chemistry. Although he was far ahead of his time in many of his observations (e.g., on metabolic and on occupational diseases), much of his thinking was made obscure by his mystic religiosity.

paracenesthesia (par″ah-se″nes-the′ze-ah) [*para-* + *cenesthesia*] any abnormality of the general sense of well being. Cf. *cenesthesiopathy.*

paracentesis (par″ah-sen-te′sis) [*para-* + Gr. *kentēsis* puncture] surgical puncture of a cavity for the aspiration of fluid. **abdominal p., p. abdom′inis,** paracentesis of the abdominal cavity. **aqueous p.,** puncture of the cornea, as in certain operations on the cornea; called also *keratocentesis* and *keratonyxis.* **p. bul′bi,** puncture of the eyeball. **p. cap′itis,** puncture of the cranium for the removal of effusion in hydrocephalus. **p. cor′dis,** puncture of the heart. **p. oc′uli,** p. bulbi. **p. pericar′dii,** puncture of the pericardial sac. **p. pulmo′nis,** puncture of the lung. **p. thora′cis,** thoracentesis. **p. tu′nicae vagina′lis,** puncture of the tunica vaginalis. **p. tym′pani,** incision of the tympanic membrane for drainage or irrigation. **p. vesi′cae,** puncture of the bladder wall.

paracentetic (par″ah-sen-tet′ik) pertaining to or accomplished by paracentesis.

paracentral (par″ah-sen′tral) near a center.

paracephalus (par″ah-sef′ah-lus) [*para-* + Gr. *kephalē* head] a fetus with a rudimentary or misshapen head, imperfect sense organs, and defective trunk or limbs.

paracerebellar (par″ah-ser″ĕ-bel′ar) pertaining to the lateral part of the cerebellum.

paracetaldehyde (par-as″et-al′de-hīd) paraldehyde.

paracetamol (par-as″et-am′ol) acetaminophen.

parachloralose (par″ah-klōr′al-ōs) a substance, $C_8H_{12}Cl_3O_6$, in iridescent plates, formed by a combination of dextrose and chloral.

parachloramine (par″ah-klōr′ah-men) meclizine.

parachlorophenol (par″ah-klo″ro-fe′nol) [USP] chemical name: 4-chlorophenol. An antibacterial, C_6H_5ClO, occurring as white to pink crystals, effective against most gram-negative organisms; used as a topical anti-infective. **camphorated p.** [USP], a preparation of 33 to 37 per cent parachlorophenol and 63 to 67 per cent camphor; used as a dental anti-infective, applied topically to the root canals and the periapical region.

paracholera (par″ah-kol′er-ah) a disease resembling Asiatic cholera, but caused by an organism other than the *Vibrio cholerae.*

paracholesterin (par″ah-ko-les′ter-in) a form of sterol occurring in vegetable tissue, probably related to sitosterol or phytosterol.

paracholia (par″ah-ko′le-ah) [*para-* + Gr. *cholē* bile + *-ia*] (*obs.*) disordered bile secretion.

parachordal (par″ah-kor′dal) [*para-* + Gr. *chordē* cord] situated beside the notochord; see *parachordal cartilages,* under *cartilage.*

Parachordodes (par″ah-kor-do′dēz) a genus of Gordiacea. A few cases of infection with this worm have been reported. *P. pustilo′sus,* from Italy. *P. tolosa′nus,* from France and from Italy. *P. viola′ceus,* from Italy, one specimen taken from the throat.

parachromatin (par″ah-kro′mah-tin) a chromatophil substance contained in the finer part of the nuclear substance, as in the nucleoplasm of the spindle in karyokinesis.

parachromatism (par″ah-kro′mah-tizm) [*para-* + Gr. *chrōma* color] color blindness; incorrect perception of colors.

parachromatopsia (par″ah-kro″mah-top′se-ah) [*para-* + Gr. *chrōma* color + *opsis* vision + *-ia*] color blindness.

paracinesia (par″ah-si-ne′se-ah) parakinesia.

paracinesis (par″ah-si-ne′sis) parakinesia.

paraclinical (par″ah-klin′ĭ-k′l) pertaining to abnormalities (e.g., morphological or biochemical) underlying clinical manifestations (e.g., chest pain or fever).

paracnemis, paracnemidion (par″ak-ne′mis; par″ak-ne-mi-d′e-on) [*para-* + Gr. *knēmē* shin] the fibula.

Paracoccidioides brasiliensis (par″ah-kok-sid′e-oi′dēz brah-sil″e-en′sis) an imperfect fungus of the family Moniliaceae, order Moniliales, which is the etiologic agent of paracoccidioidomycosis. The organisms proliferate multiple budding yeast cells in the tissues, and produce white aerial mycelia and single or double conidia in media at 25° C. or in soil. Called also *Blastomyces brasiliensis.*

paracoccidioidomycosis (par″ah-kok-sid′e-oi″do-mi-ko′sis) an often fatal infection caused by *Paracoccidioides brasiliensis.* The primary infection begins in the lungs and spreads to the mucocutaneous areas, particularly the buccal mucosa, and may extend to the adjacent skin, tonsils, gastrointestinal lymphatics, liver, and spleen. Called also *Almeida's* or *Lutz-Splendore-Almeida disease, Brazilian* or *South American blastomycosis,* and *paracoccidioidal granuloma.*

paracoele (par″ah-sēl) [*para-* + Gr. *koilos* hollow] (*obs.*) a lateral ventricle of the brain.

paracolitis (par″ah-ko-li′tis) inflammation of the outer coat of the colon.

Paracolobactrum (par″ah-ko′lo-bak′trum) a name once proposed for a genus of microorganisms of the tribe Escherichieae, family Enterobacteriaceae, order Eubacteriales, made up of short rods, characterized by a delayed (3 to 14 days) fermentation of lactose, and which are found in the intestinal tracts of animals, including man, and in surface waters, soil, and grains.

paracolpitis (par″ah-kol-pi′tis) [*para-* + Gr. *kolpos* vagina + *-itis*] inflammation of the tissues around the vagina.

paracolpium (par″ah-kol′pe-um) [*para-* + Gr. *kolpos* vagina] the connective and other tissues that surround the vagina.

paracone (par′ah-kōn) [*para-* + Gr. *kōnos* cone] the mesiobuccal cusp of any upper molar.

paraconid (par″ah-ko′nid) a lingual cusp of a lower molar in lower mammals.

paracousis (par″ah-koo′sis) paracusis.

paracoxalgia (par″ah-koks-sal′je-ah) a condition marked by pain simulating that of coxitis.

paracresol (par″ah-kre′sol) 1. one of the three isomeric forms or recognized varieties of cresol; see *cresol.* 2. a patented soluble and nearly odorless preparation of cresol: disinfectant.

paracrine (par′ah-krin) denoting the influence of the secretion of one kind of endocrine cell on that of another kind which is not the normal target cell.

paracrystals (par″ah-kris′tals) imperfect crystals, such as the "crystals" of tobacco mosaic virus which have only two dimensional symmetry instead of three dimensional.

paracusia (par-ah-ku′se-ah) paracusis. **p. a′cris,** intense and incessant acuity of hearing. **p. duplica′ta,** diplacusis. **p. lo′ci,** inability to locate correctly the origin of sounds. **p. willisia′na,** paracusis of Willis.

paracusis (par″ah-ku′sis) any perversion of the sense of hearing. **p. of Willis,** ability to hear best in a loud din (Thomas Willis, 1672).

paracyesis (par″ah-si-e′sis) [*para-* + Gr. *kyēsis* pregnancy] (*obs.*) ectopic pregnancy.

paracystic (par″ah-sis′tik) [*para-* + Gr. *kystis* bladder] situated near the bladder.

paracystitis (par″ah-sis-ti′tis) [*para-* + Gr. *kystis* bladder + *-itis*] inflammation of the tissues around the bladder.

paracystium (par″ah-sis′te-um) [*para-* + Gr. *kystis* bladder] the connective and other tissues around the bladder.

paracytic (par″ah-sit′ik) [*para-* + *-cyte*] denoting cell elements present in the blood or other part of the organism, but enthetic or not normal to it.

paradental (par″ah-den′tal) 1. having some connection with or relation to the science or practice of dentistry. 2. periodontal.

paradentitis (par″ah-den-ti′tis) periodontitis.

paradentium (par″ah-den′she-um) periodontium.

paradentosis (par″ah-den-to′sis) periodontosis.

paraderm (par′ah-derm) [*para-* + Gr. *derma* skin] the part of the vitellus of the ovum that furnishes cells which contribute to the body of the embryo.

paradidymal (par″ah-did′ĭ-mal) 1. pertaining to the paradidymis. 2. beside the testis.

paradidymis (par″ah-did′ĭ-mis) [*para-* + Gr. *didymos* testis] [NA] a body made up of a few convoluted tubules in the anterior part of the spermatic cord, considered to be a remnant of the mesonephros; called also *organ of Giraldés', parepididymis,* and *massa innominata.*

paradimethylaminobenzaldehyde (par″ah-di-meth″il-am″-ĭ-no-ben-zal′de-hīd) white or pale yellow crystals or crystalline powder, $(CH_3)_2NC_6H_4CHO$, used in the preparation of Ehrlich's aldehyde reagent and in the determination of urobilinogen and porphobilinogen.

Paradione (par″ah-di′ōn) trademark for preparations of paramethadione.

paradiphenylbiuret (par″ah-di-fen″il-bi′u-ret) a substance, $NH(CO \cdot NH \cdot C_6H_4OH)_2$, transformed into benzoic acid in the body.

paradipsia (par″ah-dip′se-ah) [*para-* + Gr. *dipsa* thirst + *-ia*] a perverted appetite for fluids, which are ingested without relation to bodily need.

paradox (par′ah-doks) [Gr. *paradoxos* incredible] a statement which seems to be, though it may not be, absurd or self-contradictory. **p. of Kretz,** while the injection of an accurately neutralized toxin-antitoxin mixture produces no adverse effects in a normal animal, the reverse is the case in an animal that has previously been actively immunized with toxin. **Opie p.,** necrotizing local anaphylaxis sometimes acts as a specific protective mechanism. **Weber's p.,** the elongation of a muscle which has been so stretched that it cannot contract.

paradoxical (par″ah-dok′se-kal) occurring at variance with the normal rule.

paradysentery (par″ah-dis′en-ter″e) a diarrhea resembling mild dysentery; see *Shigella flexneri.*

paraeccrisis (par″ah-ek′rĭ-sis) [*para-* + Gr. *ekkrisis* excretion] disordered secretion or excretion.

paraepilepsy (par″ah-ep′ĭ-lep-se) minor focal epilepsy.

paraequilibrium (par″ah-e″kwĭ-lib′re-um) vertigo due to disturbance of the vestibular apparatus of the ear.

paraesophageal (par″ah-ĕ-sof″ah-je′al) alongside, near, or about the esophagus.

parafalx (par″ah-falks′)   situated near the falx cerebri or falx cerebelli.

Par. aff.   abbreviation for L. *pars affec′ta,* the part affected.

paraffin (par′ah-fin) [L. *parum* little + *affinis* akin]   1. [NF] a purified mixture of solid hydrocarbons obtained from petroleum, occurring as an odorless, tasteless, colorless or white, more or less translucent mass; used as a stiffening agent in pharmaceutical preparations. 2. alkane. **chlorinated p.,** paraffin which has been reacted with chlorine to replace some of the hydrogen atoms with chlorine atoms. **hard p.,** paraffin which has a high melting point. **liquid p.,** mineral oil. **liquid p., light,** light mineral oil. **pliable p.,** a mixture of paraffin and other ingredients, used as a nonabsorbent protective dressing for burns and other wounds. **soft p., white,** white petrolatum. **soft p., yellow,** petrolatum.

paraffinoma (par″ah-fĭ-no′mah)   a chronic granuloma produced by prolonged continuous exposure to the irritation of paraffin.

Parafilaria multipapillosa (par″ah-fĭ-la′re-ah mul″te-pap″ĭ-lo′sah)   a parasitic worm causing dermatorrhagia parasitica.

Paraflex (par′ah-fleks)   trademark for a preparation of chlorzoxazone.

paraflocculus (par″ah-flok′u-lus)   accessory flocculus.

paraformaldehyde (par″ah-for-mal′de-hīd)   a white, crystalline polymer of formaldehyde.

Parafossarulus (par″ah-fos-sar′u-lus)   a genus of fresh-water snails. **P. manchou′ricus,** a species found throughout the Orient that is the foremost intermediate host of *Clonorchis sinensis* in Japan and the second most important in China, and also a carrier of *Opisthorchis felineus* and *Echinochasmus perfoliatus.*

parafunction (par′ah-funk″shun)   disordered or perverted function.

parafunctional (par″ah-funk′shun-al)   characterized by perverted or abnormal function.

paragammacism (par″ah-gam′ah-sizm) [*para-* + Gr. *gamma,* the Greek letter G]   the faulty utterance of *g, k,* and *ch* sounds.

paraganglia (par″ah-gang′gle-ah)   plural of *paraganglion.*

paraganglioma (par″ah-gang″gle-o′mah)   a tumor of the tissue composing the paraganglia. **medullary p.,** pheochromocytoma. **nonchromaffin p.,** chemodectoma.

paraganglion (par″ah-gang′gle-on), pl. *paragan′glia.* A collection of chromaffin cells, which are derived from neural ectoderm, occurring outside of the adrenal medulla, most commonly near the sympathetic ganglia and in relation to the aorta and its branches. Most, if not all, of the paraganglia secrete epinephrine (or norepinephrine). Called also *chromaffin* or *pheochrome bodies.*

paragelatose (par″ah-jel′ah-tōs)   a substance obtained by boiling gelatin.

paragenitalis (par″ah-jen″ĭ-ta′lis) [*para-* + L. *genitalis* genital]   1. in lower vertebrates, the urinary part of the mesonephros, caudal to the genital part. 2. in higher animals, the paradidymis or paraoophoron.

parageusia (par″ah-gu′se-ah) [*para-* + Gr. *geusis* taste + *-ia*]   1. perversion of the sense of taste. 2. a bad taste in the mouth.

parageusic (par″ah-gu′sik)   pertaining to or characterized by parageusia.

paragglutination (par″ah-gloo″tĭ-na′shun)   group agglutination.

paraglobulin (par″ah-glob′u-lin)   a globulin from blood serum, blood cells, lymph, and various connective tissues; called also *fibroplastin, fibrinoplastin,* and *serum globulin.*

paraglobulinuria (par″ah-glob″u-lĭ-nu′re-ah) [*paraglobulin* + Gr. *ouron* urine + *-ia*]   the discharge of paraglobulin in the urine.

paraglossia (par″ah-glos′e-ah) [*para-* + Gr. *glōssa* tongue + *-ia*]   inflammation of the oral tissues under the tongue.

paraglossitis (par″ah-glo-si′tis)   paraglossia.

paragnathus (par-ag′nah-thus) [*para-* + Gr. *gnathos* jaw]   1. a fetus with a supernumerary jaw. 2. a parasitic fetus attached laterally to the jaw of the autosite.

paragnosis (par″ag-no′sis) [*para-* + Gr. *gnōsis* knowledge]   diagnosis, after death, based on contemporaneous accounts of the diseases which affected historical characters.

paragonimiasis (par″ah-gon″ĭ-mi′ah-sis)   the state of being infected with flukes of the genus *Paragonimus.* See individual species.

paragonimosis (par″ah-gon″ĭ-mo′sis)   paragonimiasis.

Paragonimus (par″ah-gon′ĭ-mus) [*para-* + Gr. *gonimos* productive; having generative power]   a genus of trematode parasites; they have two invertebrate hosts, the first a snail (*Semisulcospira,* etc.) and the second a crab or crayfish (*Potamon, Eriocheir,* etc.). **P. africa′nus,** a species of the Congo and Cameroons that parasitizes man and carnivores. **P. heterotre′ma,** a species infecting man in Thailand and China. **P. kellicot′ti,** a species closely allied to *P. westermani,* found in cats, dogs, and hogs in the United States. **P. rin′geri,** *P. westermani.* **P. wester-**

man′i, the lung fluke, an oval or pear-shaped fluke of a pinkish or reddish brown color, found in cysts in the lungs and sometimes in the pleura, liver, abdominal cavity, and elsewhere. It causes the disease known as parasitic or oriental hemoptysis. It occurs especially in Asiatic countries, and infects lower animals as well as man; infection is acquired through ingestion of infected freshwater crabs or crayfish. Called also *Distoma westermani, D. ringeri,* and *D. pulmonale.*

Paragordius (par″ah-gor′de-us)   a genus of the class Nematomorpha. Human infection with *P. cintus, P. tricuspidatus,* and *P. varius* has been reported.

paragrammatism (par″ah-gram′ah-tizm)   impairment of speech, with confusion in the use and order of words and grammatical forms.

paragranuloma (par″ah-gran″u-lo′mah)   the most benign form of Hodgkin's disease, which is largely confined to the lymph nodes.

paragraphia (par″ah-gra′fe-ah) [*para-* + Gr. *graphein* to write + *-ia*]   a disorder in which the patient makes mistakes in spelling or writes one word in place of another.

parahemophilia (par″ah-he″mo-fil′e-ah)   a hemorrhagic tendency due to deficiency of coagulation Factor V; it varies greatly in intensity and is inherited as an autosomal recessive trait.

parahepatic (par″ah-he-pat′ik) [*para-* + Gr. *hēpar* liver]   beside the liver.

parahepatitis (par″ah-hep″ah-ti′tis)   perihepatitis.

paraheredity (par″ah-he-red′ĭ-te)   the alleged transmission of characters not from mother cell to daughter cell but through an external medium from affected cell to normal cell.

parahormone (par″ah-hor′mōn) [*para-* + *hormone*]   a substance, not a true hormone, which has a hormone-like action in controlling the functioning of some distant organ.

parahypnosis (par″ah-hip-no′sis) [*para-* + Gr. *hypnos* sleep]   abnormal or perverted sleep, as in hypnotism or somnambulism.

parahypophysis (par″ah-hi-pof′ĭ-sis)   an accessory pituitary body.

parakeratosis (par″ah-ker″ah-to′sis)   persistence of the nuclei of the keratinocytes into the stratum corneum (horny layer) of the skin. Parakeratosis is normal in the epithelium of true mucous membrane of the mouth and vagina. **p. ostra′cea,** p. scutularis. **p. scutula′ris,** an extremely rare disease of the legs and scalp marked by the formation of hard, cuplike or shieldlike crusts which envelop the hairs and send up incrustations around the hairs. **p. variega′ta,** 1. pityriasis lichenoides et varioliformis acuta. 2. poikiloderma atrophicans vasculare.

parakinesia (par″ah-ki-ne′se-ah) [*para-* + Gr. *kinēsis* motion + *-ia*]   perversion of motor function resulting in strange and unnatural movements. In ophthalmology, irregular action of an individual ocular muscle.

parakinetic (par″ah-ki-net′ik)   pertaining to or characterized by parakinesia.

Paral (pah-ral′)   trademark for preparations of paraldehyde.

paralalia (par″ah-la′le-ah) [*para-* + Gr. *lalia* speech]   any disturbance of the faculty of speech, especially the production of a vocal sound different from the one desired, or the substitution in speech of one letter for another. **p. litera′lis,** impairment of the power to utter the sounds of certain letters.

paralambdacism (par″ah-lam′dah-sizm) [*para-* + Gr. *lambdakismos*]   the faulty utterance of *l* sounds, or the substitution of other sounds for *l.*

paralbumin (par″al-bu′min) [*para-* + *albumin*]   an albumin or protein substance found in ovarian cysts.

paraldehyde (par-al′dĕ-hīd) [USP]   chemical name: 2,4,6-trimethyl-1,3,5-trioxane. A polymerization product of acetaldehyde, $C_6H_{12}O$, occurring as a colorless, transparent liquid and having rapid-acting sedative and hypnotic properties; used to control insomnia, excitement, agitation, delirium, and convulsions, administered rectally and intramuscularly and by intravenous infusion.

paraldehydism (par-al′de-hīd″izm)   a condition produced by excessive use of paraldehyde; paraldehyde poisoning.

paralepsy (par′ah-lep″se)   psycholepsy.

paralexia (par″ah-lek′se-ah) [*para-* + *alexia*]   impairment of the power of reading, marked by the transposition of words and syllables into meaningless combinations.

paralexic (par″ah-lek′sik)   pertaining to or affected with paralexia.

paralgesia (par″al-je′se-ah) [*para-* + Gr. *algesis* sense of pain + *-ia*]   any condition marked by abnormal and painful sensations; a painful paresthesia.

paralgesic (par″al-je′sik)   pertaining to or affected with paralgesia.

paralgia (par-al′je-ah)   paralgesia.

paralinin (par″ah-li′nin) [*para-* + *linin*]   karyolymph.

parallactic (par″ah-lak′tik)   pertaining to parallax.

parallagma (par″ah-lag′mah) [Gr.]   displacement of a bone or of the fragments of a broken bone.

parallax (par′ah-laks) [Gr. "in turn"] an apparent displacement of an object due to a change in the observer's position. **binocular p.**, the seeming difference in position of an object as seen separately by one eye and then by the other, the head remaining stationary. **crossed p.**, binocular parallax in which the object viewed seems to move away from the open eye. **direct p.**, binocular parallax in which the object viewed seems to move toward the open eye. **heteronymous p.**, crossed p. **homonymous p.**, direct p. **vertical p.**, binocular parallax in which the object seen seems to move vertically.

parallelism (par′ah-lel″izm) the doctrine that mental processes and brain processes run side by side and that they do not interact. Cf. *automatism*, def. 2.

parallelometer (par″ah-lel-om′ĕ-ter) [*parallel* + Gr. *metron* measure] an instrument used in artificial denture work to determine the exactness of the parallel relationship of lines and surfaces.

parallergia (par″ah-ler′je-ah) parallergy.

parallergic (par″ah-ler′jik) pertaining to or marked by parallergy.

parallergin (par-al′er-jin) an antigen which produces a parallergic reaction.

parallergy (par-al′er-je) a condition in which an allergic state, produced by specific sensitization, predisposes the body to react to other allergens with clinical manifestations that differ from the original reaction.

paralogia (par″ah-lo′je-ah) [*para-* + Gr. *logos* reason + *-ia*] a disordered state of the reason; impairment of the reasoning power marked by illogical or delusional speech. **thematic p.**, a perversion of the mind in which the patient dwells unduly upon one subject.

paralogism (pah-ral′o-jizm) the use of meaningless or illogical language by the psychotic.

paralogy (pah-ral′o-je) 1. paralogia. 2. anatomical similarity that has no phylogenetic or functional implication.

paralyses (pah-ral′ĭ-sēz) plural of *paralysis.*

paralysis (pah-ral′ĭ-sis), pl. *paral′yses* [*para-* + Gr. *lyein* to loosen] loss or impairment of motor function in a part due to lesion of the neural or muscular mechanism; also, by analogy, impairment of sensory function (sensory paralysis). In addition to the types named below, paralysis is further distinguished as *traumatic, syphilitic, toxic,* etc., according to its cause; or as *obturator, ulnar,* etc., according to the nerve, part, or muscle specially affected. For other varieties see also under *hemiplegia, palsy, paraplegia,* and *paresis.* **abducens p.**, paralysis of the external rectus muscle of the eye due to lesion of the abducens nerve, with internal strabismus and diplopia. **abducens-facial p., congenital,** Möbius' syndrome. **p. of accommodation,** paralysis of the ciliary muscles so as to prevent accommodation of the eye. **acoustic p.**, nerve deafness. **acute ascending spinal p.**, acute febrile polyneuritis. **acute atrophic p.**, see *poliomyelitis.* **acute bulbar p.**, bulbar paralysis usually caused by acute vascular lesions of the brain, most commonly hemorrhage or thrombosis; called also *acute bulbar polioencephalitis.* **acute infectious p.**, epidemic poliomyelitis. **acute wasting p.**, see *poliomyelitis.* **p. ag′itans,** a form of parkinsonism of unknown etiology usually occurring in late life, although a juvenile form has been described. It is a slowly progressive disease characterized by masklike facies, a characteristic tremor of resting muscles, a slowing of voluntary movements, a festinating gait, peculiar posture, and weakness of the muscles. There may be excessive sweating and feelings of heat. Pathologically, there is degeneration within the nuclear masses of the extrapyramidal system and a characteristic loss of melanin-containing cells from the substantia nigra and a corresponding reduction in dopamine levels in the corpus striatum. Called also *Parkinson's disease* and *shaking palsy.* **p. ag′itans, juvenile (of Hunt),** a condition developing in early life, usually familial but occasionally occurring sporadically, marked by increased muscle tonus with the characteristic attitude and facies of paralysis agitans, due to progressive degeneration of the globus pallidus; involvement of the substantia nigra and pyramidal tracts may occur. Called also *paleostriatal syndrome, pallidal atrophy, pallidal syndrome,* and *Ramsay Hunt syndrome.* **alcoholic p.**, paralysis caused by habitual drunkenness. **alternate p., alternating p.**, alternate hemiplegia. **ambiguo-accessorius p.**, Schmidt's syndrome. **ambiguo-accessorius-hypoglossal p.**, Jackson's syndrome. **ambiguohypoglossal p.**, Tapia's syndrome. **ambiguospinothalamic p.**, Avellis' syndrome. **anesthesia p.**, paralysis following anesthesia. **anterior spinal p.**, anterior poliomyelitis. **arsenical p.**, paralysis due to arsenical poisoning. **ascending p.**, spinal paralysis that progresses cephalad. **association p.**, bulbar p. **asthenic bulbar p.**, myasthenia gravis pseudoparalytica. **asthenobulbospinal p.**, myasthenia gravis. **atrophic spinal p.**, anterior poliomyelitis. **Avellis's p.**, see under *syndrome.* **Bell's p.**, see under *palsy.* **bilateral p.**, diplegia; paralysis on both sides. **birth p.**, paralysis due to injury received at birth. **brachial p.**, paralysis of an arm from lesion of the brachial plexus; see *Erb-Duchenne p.* and *Klumpke-Dejerine p.* **brachiofacial p.**,

paralysis affecting the face and an arm. **Brown-Séquard's p.**, 1. Brown-Séquard's syndrome. 2. a flaccid paralysis seen in disorders of the urinary tract. **bulbar p.**, paralysis due to changes in the motor centers of the medulla oblongata; a chronic, usually fatal disease, most commonly affecting persons over 50 years old but also occurring in the course of amyotrophic lateral sclerosis, syringobulbia, and multiple sclerosis. It is marked by progressive paralysis and atrophy of the muscles of the lips, tongue, mouth, pharynx, and larynx, and is due to degeneration of the nerve nuclei of the floor of the fourth ventricle. Called also *labioglossopharyngeal p., labioglossolaryngeal p.,* and *Duchenne's p.* **bulbospinal p.**, myasthenia gravis. **cage p.**, a complex nutritional deficiency sometimes seen in captive primates, which is said to resemble osteomalacia. **central p.**, any paralysis due to a lesion of the brain or spinal cord. **centrocapsular p.**, that which is due to lesions of the internal capsule. **cerebral p.**, any paralysis due to an intracranial lesion; see *cerebral palsy,* under *palsy.* **Chastek p.**, progressive ataxia and paralysis in silver foxes due to thiamine deficiency following the substitution of raw fish for meat in the diet. **circumflex p.**, paralysis of the circumflex nerve. **complete p.**, entire loss of motion, sensation, and function. **compression p.**, paralysis caused by pressure on a nerve, as by a crutch or during sleep. **congenital abducens-facial p.**, Möbius syndrome. **congenital oculofacial p.**, Möbius syndrome. **conjugate p.**, loss of ability to perform some of the parallel ocular movements. **cortical p.**, paralysis dependent upon a lesion of the brain cortex. **creeping p.**, tabes dorsalis. **crossed p., cruciate p.**, paralysis affecting one side of the face and the opposite side of the body. **crural p.**, that which chiefly affects the thigh or thighs. **crutch p.**, paralysis of one or both arms, due to pressure of the crutch in the axilla. **Cruveilhier's p.**, progressive muscular atrophy. **decubitus p.**, paralysis due to pressure on a nerve from lying for a long time in one position. **Dejerine-Klumpke p.**, Klumpke's p. **diaphragmatic p.**, unilateral paralysis of the diaphragm. **diphtheric p., diphtheritic p.**, a partial paralysis which often follows diphtheria, chiefly affecting the soft palate and throat muscles. **divers' p.**, paralysis occurring as a result of too rapid reduction of pressure on deep-sea divers. **Duchenne's p.**, 1. bulbar paralysis. 2. Erb-Duchenne paralysis. **Duchenne-Erb p.**, Erb-Duchenne p. **emotional p.**, paralysis with emotional excitement occurring in hysterical persons. **epidemic infantile p.**, epidemic poliomyelitis. **Erb's p.**, 1. Erb-Duchenne paralysis. 2. Erb's spastic paraplegia. 3. pseudohypertrophic muscular dystrophy. **Erb-Duchenne p.**, the upper-arm type of brachial paralysis; paralysis of the upper roots of brachial plexus due to destruction of the fifth and sixth cervical roots and characterized by absence of involvement of the small hand muscles. **essential p.**, see *poliomyelitis.* **facial p.**, weakening or paralysis of the facial nerve, as in Bell's palsy. **false p.**, pseudoparalysis. **familial periodic p.**, a rare dominantly inherited disorder, marked by recurring attacks of rapidly progressive flaccid paralysis, which may be associated with a fall in (*hypokalemic periodic p.*), a rise in (*hyperkalemic periodic p.*), or normal (*normokalemic periodic p.*) serum potassium levels. **Felton's p.**, a specific loss of immunologic reactivity to pneumococcal polysaccharides after exposure to large doses. **Féréol-Graux p.**, see under *palsy.* **flaccid p.**, paralysis with loss of tone of the muscles of the paralyzed part and absence of tendon reflexes. Cf. *spastic p.* **fowl p.**, Marek's disease. **functional p.**, a temporary paralysis which is apparently not caused by a nerve lesion. **p. of gaze,** paralysis due to pathological processes which implicate the supranuclear oculomotor centers or pathways, and result in either lateral or vertical gaze paralysis. **general p., general p. of the insane,** dementia paralytica. **ginger p.**, Jamaica ginger p. **glossolabial p., glossopharyngolabial p.**, bulbar p. **Gubler's p.**, alternate hemiplegia. **hereditary cerebrospinal p.**, (hemiplegia, diplegia, paraplegia, or tetraplegia), a hereditary condition which develops usually in early middle life, characterized by gradually developing paralyses which may be manifest in the upper or lower extremities, in the two extremities, or one side, or in all four extremities. **histrionic p.**, paralysis of certain muscles of the face, producing a facial expression of some emotion. **hyperkalemic periodic p.**, see *familial periodic p.* **hypoglossal p.**, paralysis due to a lesion of the hypoglossal nucleus or the hypoglossal nerve at any point. **hypokalemic periodic p.**, see *familial periodic p.* **hysterical p.**, apparent loss of power of movement in a part seen in hysteria, in the absence of a neurological cause. **immune p., immunological p.**, the absence of immune response to a specific antigen, usually induced with very large doses of antigen; see *immunological tolerance,* under *tolerance.* **incomplete p.**, partial paralysis or paresis. **Indian bow p.**, paralysis of the thyroarytenoid muscles. **infantile p.**, see *poliomyelitis.* **infantile, cerebral, ataxic p.**, a condition which is dependent upon faulty development of the frontal regions of the brain, is present at birth, affects all extremities, and is not definitely progressive; called also *diataxia infantilis cerebralis* and *cerebral diataxia.* **infantile cerebrocerebellar diplegic p.**, a condition developing in infants, affecting all extremities, and due to combined failure of development or destruction of the reciprocating portions of the cerebrum and the cerebellum. **infantile spastic p.**, cerebral palsy. **infantile spinal p.**, spinal paralytic poliomyelitis. **infectious bulbar p.**, pseudorabies. **internuclear p.**, see under *ophthalmoplegia*. **ischemic p.**, local paralysis due to an impairment of the circulation, as in certain cases of embolism or thrombosis; called also *Volkmann's ischemic paralysis*. **jake p.**, Jamaica ginger p. **Jamaica ginger p.**, paralysis of the extremities, especially the legs, following the use of Jamaica ginger as a beverage; called also *jake paralysis, jake neuritis, ginger paralysis, Jamaica ginger polyneuritis*. **juvenile p.**, general paralysis in young persons. **Klumpke's p.**, **Klumpke-Dejerine p.**, the lower-arm type of brachial paralysis; atrophic paralysis of the muscles of the arm and hand, from lesion of the eighth cervical and first dorsal nerves. It often occurs in infants delivered by breech extraction. **Kussmaul's p.**, **Kussmaul-Landry p.**, acute febrile polyneuritis. **labial p.**, **labioglossolaryngeal p.**, **labioglossopharyngeal p.**, bulbar p. **lambing p.**, pregnancy toxemia in ewes. **Landry's p.**, acute febrile polyneuritis. **laryngeal p.**, paralysis of one of the laryngeal muscles. **lead p.**, paralysis caused by lead poisoning, due to a peripheral neuritis, and marked by wristdrop. **lingual p.**, paralysis of the tongue. **Lissauer's p.**, an apoplectiform type of dementia paralytica. **local p.**, paralysis of one muscle or of a group of muscles. **masticatory p.**, paralysis of the muscles of mastication. **medullary tegmental p's**, paralyses due to lesions of the medullary tegmentum: they include alternate hemiplegia, Tapia's syndrome, syndrome of Babinski-Nageotte, and Cestan's syndrome. **Millard-Gubler p.**, see under *syndrome*. **mimetic p.**, paralysis of the facial muscles. **mixed p.**, combined motor and sensory paralysis. **motor p.**, paralysis of voluntary muscles. **musculospiral p.**, paralysis of the extensor muscles of the wrist and fingers, most often due to compression of the musculospiral (radial) nerve, and, depending upon the site of the nerve injury, sometimes accompanied by weakness of extension of the elbow; called also *radial p.* and *Saturday night palsy*. **myopathic p.**, paralysis due to disease of the muscle itself. **narcosis p.**, paralysis during anesthesia, caused by pressure, cold, curare, etc. **normokalemic periodic p.**, see *familial periodic p*. **p. notario'rum**, writers' cramp. **nuclear p.**, any paralysis due to a lesion in a nucleus of origin. **obstetric p.**, birth p. **ocular p.**, see *amaurosis, cycloplegia*, and *ophthalmoplegia*. **oculofacial p., congenital**, Möbius' syndrome. **oculomotor p.**, paralysis of the oculomotor nerve. **organic p.**, paralysis due to lesion of nerve tissue. **parotitic p.**, paralysis accompanying mumps. **parturient p.**, milk fever, def. 4. **periodic p.**, a recurrent paralysis; see also *familial periodic p*. **peripheral p.**, loss of power due to some lesion of the nervous mechanism between the nucleus of origin and the muscle. **peroneal p.**, crossed leg palsy. **phonetic p.**, paralysis of the muscles of speech. **postdiphtheric p.**, diphtheric paralysis. **posthemiplegic p.**, residual weakness after a stroke. **posticus p.**, paralysis of the posterior cricothyroid muscle. **Pott's p.**, see under *paraplegia*. **pressure p.**, paralysis, generally temporary, caused by pressure on a nerve trunk. **progressive bulbar p.**, see *bulbar p*. **pseudobulbar p.**, spastic weakness of the muscles innervated by the cranial nerves, i.e., the muscles of the face, pharynx, and tongue, due to bilateral lesions of the corticospinal tract; it is often accompanied by uncontrolled weeping or laughing. Called also *supranuclear p.* and *spastic bulbar palsy*. **pseudohypertrophic muscular p.**, see under *dystrophy*. **psychic p.**, hysterical p. **radial p.**, 1. musculospiral p. 2. a condition usually affecting horses, but also other domestic animals, in which paralysis of certain muscles of the elbow and knee occurs as a result of injury to the radial nerve. Called also *dropped elbow*. **Ramsay Hunt p.**, juvenile paralysis agitans. **range p.**, Marek's disease. **reflex p.**, one ascribable to peripheral irritation; in some cases secondary changes occur in the spinal cord, and the paralysis ceases to be truly reflex. **Remak's p.**, paralysis of the extensor muscles of the fingers and wrist; called also *Remak's type*. **rucksack p.**, a disorder of motor and sensory function of the upper extremities as a result of damage to the brachial plexus caused by the wearing of backpack. **Saturday night p.**, musculospiral p. **sensory p.**, loss of sensation resulting from a morbid process. **serum p.**, peripheral nerve paralysis following administration of serum. **spastic p.**, paralysis marked by spasticity of the muscles of the paralyzed part and increased tendon reflexes, due to upper motor neuron lesions. Cf. *flaccid p*. **spastic spinal p.**, lateral sclerosis of the spinal cord. **spinomuscular p.**, paralysis due to lesion of the gray matter of the spinal cord, or the nerves originating therefrom. **supranuclear p.**, pseudobulbar p. **tick p.**, a progressive ascending flaccid motor paralysis which follows the bite of certain ticks (*Dermacentor andersoni*) in children and in domestic animals in Oregon, British Columbia, and other parts of the world. A similar paralysis sometimes follows the bites of species of *Ixodes, Haemaphysalis*, and *Rhipicephalus*. **Todd's p.**, postepileptic hemiplegia or monoplegia lasting for a few minutes or hours, or occasionally for several days, after the epileptic attack. **trigeminal p.**, paralysis due to a lesion of the trigeminal (fifth) nerve, marked by sensory loss in the face and weakness of the muscles of mastication. **p. vacil'lans**, cho-

rea. **vasomotor p.**, cessation of vasomotor control. **Volkmann's ischemic p.**, ischemic p. **waking p.**, a form of hypnogogic helplessness that follows waking, especially in some cases of narcolepsy. **wasting p.**, spinal muscular atrophy. **Weber's p.**, see under *syndrome*. **Werdnig-Hoffmann p.**, a hereditary, progressive, infantile form of muscular atrophy, transmittted as an autosomal recessive trait, usually occurring in siblings rather than in successive generations, and resulting from degeneration of the anterior horn cells of the spinal cord. It is marked by early onset (usually at about six months of age, but sometimes in fetal life), hypotonia and wasting of the muscles, complete flaccid paralysis, and death, usually in early life. Called also *familial spinal muscular atrophy, Hoffmann-Werdnig syndrome*, and *progressive spinal muscular atrophy of infants*. Cf. *Kugelberg-Welander disease*. **writers' p.**, writers' cramp.

paralysor (par'ah-līz"or) paralyzer.

paralyssa (par"ah-lis'ah) rabies occurring in Central and South America caused by the bite of vampire bats.

paralytic (par"ah-lit'ik) [Gr. *paralytikos*] 1. affected with or pertaining to paralysis. 2. a person affected with paralysis.

paralytogenic (par"ah-lit"o-jen'ik) causing paralysis.

paralyzant (par'ah-līz"ant) 1. causing paralysis. 2. an agent that paralyzes.

paralyze (par'ah-līz) to put into a state of paralysis.

paralyzer (par'ah-līz"er) a substance which hinders or prevents a chemical reaction; an inhibitor.

paramagnetic (par"ah-mag-net'ik) characterized by or exhibiting paramagnetism.

paramagnetism (par"ah-mag'ne-tizm) [*para-* + Gr. *magnēs* magnet] the property of being attracted by a magnet, and of assuming a position parallel to that of a magnetic force, but not of becoming permanently magnetized.

paramania (par"ah-ma'ne-ah) [*para-* + *mania*] a form of parathymia in which one manifests joy by complaining.

paramastigote (par"ah-mas'tĭ-gōt) [*para-* + Gr. *mastix* lash] having an accessory flagellum by the side of a larger one.

paramastitis (par"ah-mas-ti'tis) [*para-* + Gr. *mastos* mamma + *-itis*] inflammation of the tissues around the mammary gland.

paramastoid (par"ah-mas'toid) near the mastoid process.

paramastoiditis (par"ah-mas"toid-i'tis) inflammation of the temporal bone in mastoiditis.

parameatal (par"ah-me-a'tal) situated near or around a meatus.

paramecia (par"ah-me'se-ah) plural of *paramecium*.

paramecin (par"ah-me'sin) an antibiotic compound secreted by a specially developed strain of paramecia; it is destructive to other strains of paramecia.

Paramecium (par"ah-me'she-um) [Gr. *paramēkēs* oblong] a genus of holotrichous ciliate protozoa (subclass Euciliatia) of elongated form. Certain strains have been employed in the protozoan test. See under *tests*. **P. co'li**, *Balantidium coli*.

paramecium (par"ah-me'she-um), pl. *parame'cia*. An organism belonging to the genus *Paramecium*.

paramedian (par"ah-me'de-an) [*para-* + L. *medianus* median] situated near the midline or midplane.

paramedical (par"ah-med'ĭ-kal) having some connection with or relation to the science or practice of medicine; adjunctive to the practice of medicine in the maintenance or restoration of health and normal functioning. Paramedical workers include physical, occupational, and speech therapists, medical social workers, pharmacists, technicians, and so on.

paramenia (par"ah-me'ne-ah) [*para-* + Gr. *mēniaia* menses] disordered or difficult menstruation.

parameningococcus (par"ah-me-ning"go-kok'us) a microorganism resembling the meningococcus, differing only in its serum reactions.

parameniscitis (par"ah-me-nĭ-si'tis) inflammation of the parameniscus.

parameniscus (par"ah-me-nis'kus) the structure or area around the menisci (semilunar fibrocartilages) of the knee.

paramesial (par"ah-me'se-al) [*para-* + Gr. *mesos* middle] paramedian.

parameter (pah-ram'ĕ-ter) [Gr. *parametrein* to measure one thing by another] 1. a variable whose measure is indicative of a quantity or function that cannot itself be precisely determined by direct methods; e.g., blood pressure and pulse rate are parameters of cardiovascular function, and the level of glucose in blood and urine is a parameter of carbohydrate metabolism. 2. a distinguishing feature that is subject to measurement, either directly or indirectly.

paramethadione (par"ah-meth"ah-di'ōn) [USP] chemical name: 5-ethyl-3,5-dimethyl-2,4-oxazolidinedione. An anticonvulsant, $C_7H_{11}NO_3$, occurring as a clear, colorless liquid, used especially in the treatment of petit mal epilepsy, administered orally.

paramethasone acetate (par"ah-meth'ah-sōn) [USP] chemical name: 21-(acetyloxy)-6α-fluoro-11β,17-dihydroxy-16α-methylpregna-1,4-diene-3,20-dione. A glucocorticoid, $C_{24}H_{31}FO_6$, occurring as a fluffy, white to creamy white, crystalline powder; used chiefly for its anti-inflammatory and antiallergic actions, administered orally.

parametrial (par″ah-me′tre-al) 1. pertaining to the parametrium. 2. parametric[1].

parametric[1] (par″ah-met′rik) [para- + Gr. *mētra* uterus] situated near the uterus; parametrial.

parametric[2] (par″ah-met′rik) [para- + *meter*] pertaining to or defined in terms of a parameter.

parametritic (par″ah-mĕ-trĭt′ik) pertaining to parametritis.

parametritis (par″ah-mĕ-tri′tis) inflammation of the parametrium. **posterior p.,** inflammation of the cellular tissue around the uterosacral ligaments.

parametrium (par″ah-me′tre-um) [para- + Gr. *mētra* uterus] [NA] the extension of the subserous coat of the supracervical portion of the uterus laterally between the layers of the broad ligament.

paramidoacetophenone (par-am″ĭ-do-as″ĕ-to-fe′nōn) NH_2-$C_6H_4·CO·CH_3$; used in Ehrlich's diazo reaction.

paramimia (par″ah-mim′e-ah) [para- + Gr. *mimēsis* imitation] a condition in which signs are misused in expressing thoughts; the use of wrong or improper gestures in speaking.

paramitome (par″ah-mi′tōm) [para- + Gr. *mitos* thread] hyaloplasm, def. 1.

paramnesia (par″am-ne′ze-ah) [para- + *amnesia*] 1. perversion of memory in which the person believes that he remembers events or circumstances which never happened; called also *retrospective falsification.* 2. a state in which words are remembered, but are used without a comprehension of their meaning.

Paramoeba (par″ah-me′ba) see *Craigia.*

paramolar (par″ah-mo′lar) a supernumerary tooth appearing adjacent to a molar tooth.

Paramonostomum parvum (par″ah-mo-nos′to-mum par′vum) a trematode infecting ducks and chickens in North America.

paramphistomiasis (par-am″fe-sto-mi′ah-sis) invasion of the body by trematode parasites of the order Paramphistomatoidea, particularly *Watsonius watsoni* and *Gastrodiscoides hominis.*

Paramphistomum (par″am-fis′to-mum) a genus of flukes. **P. cer′vi,** a species found in the rumen and reticulum of sheep, goats, cattle, and other ruminants. Formerly called *amphistoma conicum* and *Fasciola cervi.*

paramucin (par″ah-mu′sin) a colloid substance found in ovarian cysts, which differs from mucin and pseudomucin in the fact that it reduces Fehling's solution before boiling with acid.

paramusia (par″ah-mu′ze-ah) [para- + Gr. *mousa* music + -ia] perversion or partial loss of the power of correct musical expression.

paramutable (par″ah-mu′tah-b′l) the condition (of an allele) of being subject to paramutation.

paramutagenic (par″ah-mu″tah-jen′ik) denoting an allele that causes paramutation in another allele.

paramutation (par″ah-mu-ta′shun) a permanent transmissible change in an allele after passage through a heterozygote.

paramyelin (par″ah-mi′ĕ-lin) a mono-aminomonophosphatid from brain substance.

paramyloidosis (par-am″ĭ-loi-do′sis) accumulation of an atypical form of amyloid in tissues.

paramylum (pah-ram′ĭ-lum) a carbohydrate storage compound present in the euglenoids, chemically distinct from both starch and glycogen.

paramyoclonus (par″ah-mi-ok′lo-nus) [para- + Gr. *mys* muscle + *klonos* turmoil] a condition characterized by myoclonic contractions of various muscles. **p. mul′tiplex,** a condition occurring more often in males than in females, characterized by sudden shocklike contractions affecting first the proximal muscles of the arms and the shoulder girdle, with any muscles of the limbs and trunk being involved later, and finally involving the face and bulbar muscles.

paramyosin (par″ah-mi′o-sin) a muscle protein found in the catch muscle fibers of mollusks and annelids; it has a molecular weight of about 137,000 and shows pronounced symmetry; called also *tropomyosin A.*

paramyosinogen (par″ah-mi″o-sin′o-jen) a protein resembling myosinogen (myogen) derived from muscle plasma.

paramyotone (par″ah-mi′o-tōn) paramyotonus.

paramyotonia (par″ah-mi″o-to′ne-ah) [para- + Gr. *mys* muscle + *tonos* tension + -ia] a disease marked by tonic spasms due to disorder of muscular tonicity, especially a hereditary and congenital affection. **ataxia p.,** muscular spasm with slight ataxia on attempting to move. **p. congen′ita,** myotonia congenita. **symptomatic p.,** temporary stiffness on starting to walk, seen in paralysis agitans.

paramyotonus (par″ah-mi-ot′o-nus) a condition marked by tonic muscular spasm.

paramyxovirus (par″ah-mik″so-vi′rus) a subgroup of the myxoviruses, including the viruses of human and animal parainfluenza, mumps, and Newcastle disease; it may also include the viruses of measles, canine distemper, rinderpest, the rubella and pneumonia virus of mice, and the respiratory syncytial virus. Cf. *orthomyxovirus.*

paranalgesia (par″an-al-je′se-ah) analgesia of the lower extremities.

paranea (par″ah-ne′ah) paranoia.

paranephric (par″ah-nef′rik) 1. near the kidney. 2. pertaining to the adrenal gland.

paranephritis (par″ah-nĕ-fri′tis) [para- + Gr. *nephros* kidney + -itis] 1. inflammation of the paranephros. 2. inflammation of the connective tissue around and near the kidney. **lipomatous p.,** lipomatous nephritis.

paranephroma (par″ah-nĕ-fro′mah) a tumor of the adrenal gland.

paranephros (par″ah-nef′ros), pl. *paraneph′roi* [para- + Gr. *nephros* kidney] an adrenal gland.

paranesthesia (par″an-es-the′ze-ah) para-anesthesia.

paraneural (par″ah-nu′ral) [para- + Gr. *neuron* nerve] beside or alongside a nerve.

parangi (pah-ran′je) Ceylonese name for yaws.

para-nitrosulfathiazole (par″ah-ni″tro-sul″fah-thi′ah-zōl) chemical name: *p*-nitro-*N*-2-thiazolylbenzenesulfonamide. A sulfonamide, $C_9H_7N_3O_4S_2$, occurring as a yellow powder; used as an antibacterial in the treatment of nonspecific ulcerative colitis and of proctitis, administered by rectal injection.

paranoia (par″ah-noi′ah) [para- + Gr. *nous* mind + -ia] a chronic, slowly progressive mental disorder (personality disorder) characterized by the development of ambitions or suspicions into systematized delusions of persecution and grandeur which are built up in a logical form. The condition does not appear to interfere with the rest of the personality and thinking. Cf. *paranoid schizophrenia.* **acute hallucinatory p.,** paranoia in which hallucinations are combined with the delusions. **alcoholic p.,** a paranoic condition developing in chronic alcoholism. **p. hallucinato′ria,** acute hallucinatory paranoia. **heboid p.,** paranoid schizophrenia, or paranoia with schizoid features. **litigious p.,** paranoia characterized by a tendency to go to law for imaginary causes. **querulous p.,** paranoia marked by querulousness.

paranoiac (par″ah-noi′ak) an individual exhibiting paranoia.

paranoic (par″ah-no′ic) pertaining to or characterized by paranoia.

paranoid (par′ah-noid) resembling paranoia.

paranoidism (par″ah-noid′izm) a state resembling paranoia.

paranomia (par″ah-no′me-ah) [para- + Gr. *onoma* name + -ia] aphasia characterized by inability to name objects felt (*myotactic p.*) or seen (*visual p.*).

paranormal (par″ah-nor′mal) beyond the normal or natural; said of phenomena such as extrasensory perception.

paranosic (par″ah-no′sik) pertaining to paranosis.

paranosis (par″ah-no′sis) [para- + Gr. *nosos* disease] the primary advantage that is to be gained by illness. Cf. *epinosis.*

paranuclear (par″ah-nu′kle-ar) 1. beside a nucleus. 2. pertaining to a paranucleus.

paranucleolus (par″ah-nu-kle′o-lus) a small basophil body in the enclosing sac of the cell nucleus.

paranucleus (par″ah-nu′kle-us) [para- + *nucleus*] a body resembling the nucleus, sometimes seen in the cell cytoplasm near the nucleus.

paraomphalic (par″ah-om-fal′ik) [para- + Gr. *omphalos* navel] alongside the umbilicus.

paraoperative (par″ah-op′er-a″tiv) pertaining to the accessories essential to operative surgery, such as care of instruments and gloves, sterilization, etc.

paraoral (par″ah-o′ral) administered by some other route than by the mouth; said of medication.

paraosmia (par″ah-os′me-ah) parosmia.

parapancreatic (par″ah-pan″kre-at′ik) situated near the pancreas.

paraparesis (par″ah-par′ĕ-sis) [para- + Gr. *paresis* paralysis] a partial paralysis of the lower extremities.

parapedesis (par″ah-pĕ-de′sis) [para- + Gr. *pēdēsis* a leaping] passage of body substances into channels not normally conveying them, as of bile pigments into the blood capillaries.

paraperitoneal (par″ah-per″ĭ-to-ne′al) near the peritoneum.

parapestis (par″ah-pes′tis) ambulatory plague.

paraphasia (par″ah-fa′ze-ah) [para- + *aphasia*] partial aphasia in which the patient employs wrong words, or uses words in wrong and senseless combinations (*choreic p.*). **central p.,** partial aphasia due to brain lesion. **literal p.,** the replacement of one or more sounds in otherwise correct words. **verbal p.,** the substitution of one correct word or phrase for another, sometimes related in meaning and sometimes completely unrelated.

paraphasic (par″ah-fa′sik) characterized by paraphasia.

paraphasis (pah-raf′ah-sis) an evagination of the membranous roof of the telencephalon in front of the velum transversum in certain vertebrate brains.

paraphemia (par″ah-fe′me-ah) [*para-* + Gr. *phēmē* speech + *-ia*] aphasia marked by the employment of the wrong words.

paraphenylenediamine (par″ah-fen″il-ēn-di-am′in) a dye, $C_6H_4(NH_2)_2$, whose hydrochloride dyes the hair black, but may cause delayed contact-type hypersensitivity.

paraphia (par-a′fe-ah) [*para-* + Gr. *haphē* touch + *-ia*] a perversion of the sense of touch.

paraphilia (par″ah-fil′e-ah) [*para-* + Gr. *philein* to love + *-ia*] aberrant sexual activity; sexual deviation; expression of the sexual instinct in practices which are socially prohibited or unacceptable, or biologically undesirable.

paraphiliac (par″ah-fil′e-ak) 1. pertaining to paraphilia. 2. an individual exhibiting paraphilia; a sexual deviant.

paraphimosis (par″ah-fi-mo′sis) [*para-* + Gr. *phimoun* to muzzle + *-osis*] retraction of phimotic foreskin, causing a painful swelling of the glans that, if severe, may cause dry gangrene unless corrected. See also *phimosis*.

paraphobia (par″ah-fo′be-ah) [*para-* + Gr. *phobos* fear + *-ia*] a mild phobia.

paraphonia (par″ah-fo′ne-ah) [*para-* + Gr. *phōnē* voice + *-ia*] morbid alteration of the voice; partial aphonia. **p. pu′berum,** the change in the male voice at the time of puberty.

paraphora (par-af′o-rah) [*para-* + Gr. *pherein* to bear] a slight mental disorder.

paraphrasia (par″ah-fra′ze-ah) [*para-* + *aphrasia*] partial aphrasia; speech defect marked by disorderly arrangement of spoken words.

paraphrenia (par″ah-fre′ne-ah) [*para-* + Gr. *phrēn* mind + *-ia*] 1. Kraepelin's term for a small group of psychoses now classified as paranoid states, i.e., conditions classified between true paranoia and paranoid schizophrenia. 2. Freud's term for schizophrenia. 3. paraphrenitis. **p. confab′ulans,** paraphrenia distinguished by falsifications of memory. **p. expansi′va,** paraphrenia marked by delusions of grandeur, exalted mood, and mild excitement. **p. phantas′tica,** paraphrenia with somewhat unsystematized delusions. **p. systemat′ica,** paraphrenia with rigidly systematized delusions of persecution and no intellectual deterioration.

paraphrenic (par″ah-fre′nik) 1. pertaining to or characterized by paraphrenia. 2. an individual exhibiting paraphrenia.

paraphrenitis (par″ah-fre-ni′tis) [*para-* + Gr. *phrēn* diaphragm + *-itis*] inflammation of the diaphragm, or, more correctly, of the parts around it.

paraphronia (par″ah-fro′ne-ah) a condition of abnormal mentality marked by change in disposition and character.

paraphyseal (par″ah-fiz′e-al) pertaining to the paraphysis.

paraphysis (pah-raf′ĭ-sis) [Gr. "offshoot"] 1. a thin-walled derivative of the roof plate of the telencephalon, present only temporarily in the human embryo and fetus; called also *paraphyseal body.* 2. a sterile thread alongside the spore sac or sexual organs in the hymenial layer of some fungi, especially ascomycetes; also found in mosses and ferns.

parapineal (par″ah-pin′e-al) pertaining to the parapineal organ of certain lower vertebrates.

paraplasm (par′ah-plazm) [*para-* + Gr. *plasma* something formed] 1. hyaloplasm (def. 1). 2. an abnormal growth.

paraplasmic (par″ah-plaz′mik) pertaining to paraplasm.

paraplastic (par″ah-plas′tik) [*para-* + Gr. *plassein* to mold] exhibiting a perverted formative power; of the nature of a paraplasm.

paraplastin (par″ah-plas′tin) a substance resembling parachromatin in the cytoplasm and nucleus of a cell.

paraplectic (par″ah-plek′tik) [Gr. *paraplēktikos*] paraplegic.

paraplegia (par″ah-ple′je-ah) [*para-* + Gr. *plēgē* stroke + *-ia*] paralysis of the legs and lower part of the body. **alcoholic p.,** paraplegia due to chronic alcoholism, and probably dependent upon peripheral neuritis. **ataxic p.,** subacute combined degeneration of spinal cord; see under *degeneration.* **cerebral p.,** that which is due to a bilateral lesion. **Erb's spastic p., Erb's syphilitic spastic p.,** an uncommon form of meningovascular syphilis marked by progressive spasticity and weakness of the legs, paraplegia, muscular atrophy, paresthesia, increased knee and ankle reflexes, and incontinence. Called also *cerebrospinal syphilis, Erb's paralysis, Erb-Charcot disease,* and *syphilitic paraplegia.* **flaccid p.,** paraplegia with loss of muscle tone of the paralyzed part and absence of tendon reflexes. Cf. *spastic p.* See under *paralysis.* **peripheral p.,** that which is due to a lower motor neuron lesion. **Pott's p.,** that which is due to vertebral caries or spinal tuberculosis; called also *Pott's paralysis.* **reflex p.,** paralysis of the lower limbs due to peripheral irritation of the nerve centers. **senile p.,** a form marked by tonic spasm of the paralyzed muscles, with increased reflex irritability; it is usually caused by transverse lesions of the spinal cord or by anterolateral sclerosis. Called also *tetanoid p.* **spastic p.,** par-

aplegia marked by spasticity of the muscles of the paralyzed part and increased tendon reflexes, due to damage to the corticospinal tract. Cf. *flaccid p.* **spastic p., congenital,** spastic p., infantile. **spastic p., infantile,** spastic paralysis occurring in early childhood, due to injuries in birth, cerebral hemorrhage before birth, or abnormal development of the brain. **spastic p., primary,** a form of spastic paraplegia said to be due to primary degeneration in the pyramidal tracts. **p. supe′rior,** paralysis of both arms. **syphilitic p.,** Erb's spastic p. **toxic p.,** paraplegia due to poisons in the blood.

paraplegic (par″ah-plej′ik) pertaining to or of the nature of paraplegia; by extension, sometimes used to designate an individual affected with paraplegia.

paraplegiform (par″ah-plej′ĭ-form) resembling paraplegia.

parapleuritis (par″ah-plu-ri′tis) [*para-* + Gr. *pleura* side + *-itis*] inflammation in the wall of the chest.

paraplexus (par″ah-plek′sus) [*para-* + *plexus*] (*obs.*) the choroid plexus of the lateral ventricle.

parapneumonia (par″ah-nu-mo′ne-ah) a disease resembling pneumonia clinically.

parapophysis (par″ah-pof′ĭ-sis) [*para-* + *apophysis*] the lower transverse process of a vertebra (processus transversus vertebrarum [NA]), or its homologue.

parapoplexy (par-ap′o-plek″se) [*para-* + *apoplexy*] a condition resembling apoplexy.

parapraxia (par″ah-prak′se-ah) [*para-* + Gr. *praxis* doing + *-ia*] 1. irrational behavior. 2. inability to perform purposive movements properly, e.g., a slip of the tongue or misplacement of an article.

parapraxis (par″ah-prak′sis) parapraxia.

paraproctitis (par″ah-prok-ti′tis) [*paraproctium* + *-itis*] inflammation of the paraproctium; perirectal inflammation.

paraproctium (par″ah-prok′she-um) [*para-* + Gr. *prōktos* anus] the tissues that surround the rectum and the anus.

paraprofessional (par″ah-pro-fesh′un-al) 1. a person who is specially trained in a particular field or occupation to assist a professional, such as a physician or some other professional. 2. allied health professional. 3. pertaining to a paraprofessional.

paraprostatitis (par″ah-pros″tah-ti′tis) inflammation of the tissues near the prostate gland.

paraprotein (par″ah-pro′te-in) immunoglobulin produced by a clone of neoplastic plasma cells proliferating abnormally. Those derived from any individual patient are of a single immunoglobulin class, subclass, and (in humans) light chain (κ or γ) type. On electrophoresis of serum, they are normally demonstrable as a sharply localized band. Paraproteins include myeloma proteins, cryoglobulins, and the IgM of Waldenström's macroglobulinemia.

paraproteinemia (par″ah-pro″te-in-e′me-ah) presence in the blood of a paraprotein, such as a cryoglobulin or a macroglobulin, in amounts not normally observed.

parapsia (par-ap′se-ah) parapsis.

parapsis (par-ap′sis) [*para-* + Gr. *hapsis* touch] perversion of the sense of touch; paraphia.

parapsoriasis (par″ah-so-ri′ah-sis) a name applied by Brocq to a group of maculopapular scaly erythrodermas of slow development. They are marked by persistent red, scaling patches or papules devoid of subjective symptoms and resistant to treatment. There are three principal forms, the guttate, lichenoid, and patchy. **p. acu′ta, acute p.,** pityriasis lichenoides et varioliformis. **p. atro′phicans,** pityriasis lichenoides et varioliformis acuta. **p. gutta′ta, guttate p.,** p. lichenoides chronica. **p. lichenoi′des chron′ica,** a relatively benign, chronic, scaly, papular skin disorder occurring at any age and not much helped by any treatment. Called also *p. guttata, p. varioliformis chronica.* **p. en plaques,** a chronic eruption of slightly scaly erythematous patches on the trunk or extremities, with little or no itching; the risk of evolution into mycosis fungoides rises with itchiness and the amount of infiltration. Called also *xanthoerythrodermia perstans.* **p. variolifor′mis,** pityriasis lichenoides et varioliformis acuta. **p. variolifor′mis chron′ica,** p. lichenoides chronica.

parapsychology (par″ah-si-kol′o-je) [*para-* + *psychology*] a branch of psychology dealing with those psychical effects and experiences which appear to fall outside the scope of physical law, e.g., telepathy and clairvoyance.

parapyknomorphous (par″ah-pik″no-mor′fus) [*para-* + Gr. *pyknos* compact + *morphē* form] neither pyknomorphous nor apyknomorphous, but between the two; staining moderately well. Said of certain nerve cells.

parapyramidal (par″ah-pi-ram′ĭ-dal) beside or near a pyramid.

paraquat (par′a-kwat) a poisonous dipyridilium compound whose dichloride and dimethylsulfate salts are used as contact herbicides. Contact with concentrated solutions causes irritation of the skin, cracking and shedding of the nails, and delayed healing of cuts and wounds. After ingestion of large doses, renal and hepatic failure may develop, followed by pulmonary insufficiency.

paraqueduct (par-ak'we-dukt) (*obs.*) a lateral extension of the cerebral aqueduct.

pararabin (pah-rar'ah-bin) a carbohydrate residuum identified by Reichardt (1875) and obtained by depriving agar of its nitrogen (Bordet-Zung, 1914).

parareaction (par''ah-re-ak'shun) Meyer's term for paranoia and paranoid states.

pararectal (par''ah-rek'tal) beside the rectum.

parareducine (par''ah-re-du'sin) [*para-* + *reducin*] a leukomaine found in the urine.

parareflexia (par''ah-re-flek'se-ah) any disorder or derangement of the reflexes.

pararenal (par''ah-re'nal) beside the kidney.

pararhizoclasia (par''ah-ri''zo-kla'se-ah) [*para-* + Gr. *rhiza* root + *klasis* destruction + *-ia*] inflammatory destruction of the deep layers of the alveolar process and the periodontal membrane around the roots of a tooth. Cf. *perirhizoclasia*.

pararhotacism (par''ah-ro'tah-sizm) [*para-* + Gr. *rhō* the Greek letter *r*] imperfect pronunciation of the sound of the letter *r*.

pararosaniline (par''ah-ro-zan'ĭ-lin) a basic dye, triaminotriphenylmethane chloride; generally, the chief constituent of basic fuchsin. **p. pamoate,** chemical name: α-(p-aminophenyl)-α-(4-imino-2,5-cyclohexadien-1-ylidene)-p-toluidine-4',4'-methylenebis(3-hydroxy-2-naphthoate) (2:1) dihydrate; an antischistosomal, [(C$_{19}$H$_{18}$N$_3$)$_2$·C$_{23}$H$_{14}$O$_6$]·2H$_2$O.

pararrhythmia (par''ah-rith'me-ah) parasystole.

pararthria (par-ar'thre-ah) [*para-* + Gr. *arthron* articulation] disordered or imperfect utterance of speech.

Parasaccharomyces (par''ah-sak''ah-ro-mi'sēz) *Candida.*

parasacral (par''ah-sa'kral) situated near the sacrum.

Parasal (par'ah-sal) trademark for preparations of aminosalicylic acid.

parasalpingeal (par''ah-sal-pin'je-al) situated beside or in the wall of the fallopian or uterine tube.

parasalpingitis (par''ah-sal''pin-ji'tis) [*para-* + Gr. *salpinx* tube + *-itis*] inflammation of the tissues around a fallopian or uterine tube.

parascapular (par''ah-skap'u-lar) near the scapula.

Parascaris (par-as'kar-is) a genus of nematode worms of the family Ascarididae. **P. equo'rum,** a species found in horses.

parascarlatina (par''ah-skar''lah-ti'nah) Duke's disease.

parascarlet (par''ah-skar'let) Duke's disease.

parasecretion (par''ah-se-kre'shun) any disorder or derangement of secretion; also, hypersecretion.

parasellar (par''ah-sel'ar) near or around the sella turcica.

parasexual (par''ah-seks'u-al) accomplished by other than sexual means, as by genetic study of *in vitro* somatic cell hybrids rather than by pedigree studies.

parasexuality (par''ah-seks''u-al'ĭ-te) perverted sexuality.

parasigmatism (par''ah-sig'mah-tizm) [*para-* + Gr. *sigma* the Greek letter ς] imperfect pronunciation of *s* and *z* sounds.

parasinoidal (par''ah-si-noi'dal) [*para-* + *sinus*] situated along the course of a sinus.

parasite (par'ah-sīt) [Gr. *parasitos*] 1. a plant or animal which lives upon or within another living organism at whose expense it obtains some advantage. See *symbiosis.* 2. the smaller, less complete component of asymmetrical conjoined twins, which is attached to and dependent on the autosite. **accidental p.,** an organism parasitizing an animal other than the usual host, as *Dirofilaria* in man. **allantoic p.,** a twin embryonic parasite in which the weaker member takes its blood supply from the stronger through its umbilical circulation. **animal p.,** any parasite that is a member of the animal kingdom, including many protozoa, helminths, annelids, arthropods, etc. **celozoic p.,** a parasite which lives in a body cavity. **cytozoic p.,** a parasite which lives in body cells, as a plasmodium. **diheteroxenic p.,** a parasite which requires two intermediate hosts. **ectophytic p.,** a plant ectoparasite. **ectozoic p.,** an animal ectoparasite. **endophytic p.,** a plant endoparasite. **entozoic p.,** a parasite which lives in the lumen of the intestine. **eurytrophic p.,** an ectoparasite which can feed on various hosts. **facultative p.,** an organism which may be parasitic upon another but which is capable of independent existence. **hematozoic p.,** a parasite which lives in the blood. **incidental p.,** accidental p. **intermittent p.,** a parasite which lives in its host only at times, being free living during the interval; called also *occasional p.* **karyozoic p.,** a parasite which lives in cell nuclei. **malarial p.,** *Plasmodium.* **obligatory p.,** a parasite which cannot live apart from its host. **occasional p.,** intermittent p. **periodic p.,** a parasite that resides in its host for short periods. **permanent p.,** a parasite which lives in its host from early life until maturity or death. **plant p.,** any parasite of the vegetable kingdom. **specific p.,** one normal to its current host. **spurious p.,** an organism which is parasitic on hosts other than man, but which may pass through the human body without causing harm. **stenotrophic p.,** an ectoparasite which can feed on one host only. **temporary p.,** a para-

site which lives free of its host during part of its life cycle. **teratoid p.,** a fetal parasite which appears as a tumor-like mass. **vegetable p.,** any parasite of the vegetable kingdom, such as a fungus.

parasitemia (par''ah-si-te'me-ah) the presence of parasites (especially malarial parasites) in the blood.

parasitic (par''ah-sit'ik) [Gr. *parasitikos*] pertaining to, of the nature of, or caused by a parasite.

parasiticidal (par''ah-sit''ĭ-si'dal) destructive to parasites.

parasiticide (par''ah-sit''ĭ-sīd) [L. *parasitus* a parasite + *caedere* to kill] 1. destructive to parasites. 2. an agent that is destructive to parasites.

parasitifer (par''ah-sit''ĭ-fer) [*parasite* + L. *ferre* to bear] an organism which serves as the host of a parasite.

parasitism (par'ah-si''tizm) 1. symbiosis in which one population (or individual) adversely affects the other, but cannot live without it. 2. infection or infestation with parasites.

parasitization (par''ah-sit''i-za'shun) infection or infestation with a parasite.

parasitogenic (par''ah-si''to-jen'ik) [Gr. *parasitos* parasite + *gennan* to produce] caused by parasites.

parasitoid (par'ah-si''toid) resembling a parasite.

parasitologist (par''ah-si-tol'o-jist) an expert in parasitology.

parasitology (par''ah-si-tol'o-je) [Gr. *parasitos* parasite + *-logy*] the science or study of parasites and parasitism.

parasitosis (par''ah-si-to'sis) infection or infestation with parasites.

parasitotrope (par''ah-si'to-trōp) parasitotropic.

parasitotropic (par''ah-si''to-trop'ik) [*parasite* + Gr. *trepein* to turn] having special affinity for parasites.

parasitotropism (par''ah-si-tot'ro-pizm) parasitotropy.

parasitotropy (par''ah-si-tot'ro-pe) the affinity of a drug for infective parasites.

parasoma (par''ah-so'mah) paranucleus.

parasomnia (par''ah-som'ne-ah) a state in which there is no response to stimuli, verbal or mental, except that of a reflex nature.

paraspadias (par''ah-spa'de-as) [*para-* + Gr. *spadon* a rent] a developmental anomaly in which the urethra opens upon one side of the penis.

paraspasm (par'ah-spazm) [L. *paraspasmus;* Gr. *paraspasmos*] spasm of the corresponding muscles on both sides of the body.

paraspasmus (par'ah-spaz'mus) paraspasm. **p. facia'le,** a painless motor disturbance affecting both sides of the face.

paraspecific (par''ah-spě-sif'ik) having curative properties in addition to the specific one.

Paraspirillum (par''ah-spi-ril'um) a genus of microorganisms of the family Spirillaceae, suborder Pseudomonadineae, order Pseudomonadales, made up of spiral or S-shaped cells having a well-marked thickening at the middle and tapering toward the ends. The type species is *P. vejdov'skii.*

parasplenic (par''ah-sple'nik) beside the spleen.

parasternal (par''ah-ster'nal) [*para-* + Gr. *sternon* sternum] situated beside the sternum.

parasthenia (par''as-the'ne-ah) [*para-* + Gr. *sthenos* strength + *-ia*] a condition of organic tissue causing it to function at abnormal intervals.

parastruma (par''ah-stroo'mah) a goiter-like enlargement of a parathyroid gland or glands.

parasuicide (par''ah-soo'ĭ-sīd) an apparent attempt at suicide, as by self-poisoning or self-mutilation, in which death is not the desired outcome.

parasympathetic (par''ah-sim''pah-thet'ik) of or pertaining to that division of the autonomic nervous system made up of the ocular, bulbar, and sacral divisions; see under *system.*

parasympathicotonia (par''ah-sim-path''ě-ko-to'ne-ah) vagotonia.

parasympathin (par''ah-sim'pah-thin) a hypothetical product given off when a cranial autonomic nerve is stimulated, and having stimulating action on the parasympathetic nervous system.

parasympatholytic (par''ah-sim''pah-tho-lit'ik) [*parasympathetic* + Gr. *lytikos* dissolving] 1. producing effects resembling those of interruption of the parasympathetic nerve supply to a part. 2. an agent that opposes the effects of impulses conveyed by the parasympathetic nerves. Called also *anticholinergic.*

parasympathomimetic (par''ah-sim''pah-tho-mi-met'ik) [*parasympathetic* + Gr. *mimētikos* imitative] 1. producing effects resembling those of stimulation of the parasympathetic nerve supply to a part. 2. an agent that produces effects similar to those produced by stimulation of the parasympathetic nerves. Called also *cholinergic.*

parasynanche (par''ah-sin'an-ke) [Gr. *parasynanchē*] inflammation of a parotid gland or of the throat muscles.

parasynapsis (par''ah-sĭ-nap'sis) [*para-* + Gr. *synapsis* conjunction] the union of chromosomes side by side during meiosis. Cf. *telosynapsis*.

parasyndesis (par″ah-sin-de′sis) parasynapsis.

parasynovitis (par″ah-sin″o-vi′tis) [*para-* + *synovitis*] inflammation of the tissues about a synovial sac.

parasyphilis (par″ah-sif′ĭ-lis) a disease condition following and partly due to syphilis, but not itself syphilitic.

parasyphilitic (par″ah-sif′ĭ-lit′ik) pertaining to a sequel or result of syphilis, but not to syphilis itself.

parasyphilosis (par″ah-sif″ĭ-lo′sis) parasyphilis.

parasystole (par″ah-sis′to-le) [*para-* + Gr. *systolē* contraction] a cardiac irregularity attributed to the interaction of two foci that independently initiate cardiac impulses at different rates; as a rule, one of these foci is the sinoatrial node (the normal pacemaker), and the ectopic focus is usually in the ventricle. Each focus, and thus each rhythm, is protected from the influence of the other.

paratarsium (par″ah-tar′se-um) [*para-* + *tarsus*] the side of the tarsus of the foot.

paratenic (par″ah-ten′ik) denoting an intermediate host, sometimes called transfer host, of a parasite that is not essential to (neither hindering nor hastening) the completion of the parasite's life cycle.

paratenon (par″ah-ten′ōn) [*para-* + Gr. *tenōn* tendon] the fatty areolar tissue filling the interstices of the fascial compartment in which a tendon is situated.

paratereseomania (par″ah-ter-e″se-o-ma′ne-ah) [Gr. *paratērēsis* observation + *mania* madness] a mania for seeing new sights.

paratherapeutic (par″ah-ther″ah-pu′tik) (*obs.*) iatrogenic.

parathion (par″ah-thi′on) chemical name: diethyl-*p*-nitrophenyl thiophosphate. An agricultural insecticide, $C_{10}H_{14}NO_5PS$, highly toxic to humans and animals.

parathormone (par″ah-thor″mōn) parathyroid hormone.

parathymia (par″ah-thi′me-ah) [*para-* + Gr. *thymos* spirit] a perverted, contrary, or inappropriate mood.

parathyroid (par″ah-thi′roid) [*para-* + *thyroid*] 1. situated beside the thyroid gland. 2. one of the parathyroid glands; see under *gland*. 3. [USP] a sterile preparation of the water-soluble principle(s) of the parathyroid glands; administered parenterally as an antihypocalcemic, especially in the treatment of hypoparathyroidism with tetany.

parathyroidal (par″ah-thi-roi′dal) pertaining to the parathyroid glands.

parathyroidectomize (par″ah-thi″roid-ek′to-mīz) to deprive of the parathyroid glands by surgical removal.

parathyroidectomy (par″ah-thi″roi-dek′to-me) [*parathyroid* + Gr. *ektomē* excision] excision of a parathyroid gland.

parathyroidin (par″ah-thi-roi′din) an extract of the parathyroid glands. It increases absorption of calcium from the gut, increases resorption of calcium and phosphorus from bone, and increases reabsorption of calcium and excretion of phosphorus by the kidney.

parathyroidoma (par″ah-thi″roi-do′mah) parathyroid adenoma or carcinoma.

parathyropathy (par″ah-thi-rop′ah-the) any disease of the parathyroid glands.

parathyroprival (par″ah-thi″ro-pri′val) pertaining to or caused by absence of the parathyroid glands.

parathyroprivia (par″ah-thi-ro-pri′ve-ah) the condition resulting from the removal of the parathyroid glands.

parathyroprivic (par″ah-thi″ro-priv′ik) parathyroprival.

parathyroprivous (par″ah-thi-rop′rĭ-vus) parathyroprival.

parathyrotoxicosis (par″ah-thi″ro-tok″sĭ-ko′sis) an acute form of parathyroid intoxication; a morbid condition resulting from overactivity of the parathyroid glands.

parathyrotrophic (par″ah-thi-ro-trof′ik) parathyrotropic.

parathyrotropic (par″ah-thi-ro-trop′ik) having an affinity for the parathyroid glands.

paratoloid, paratoloidin (par″ah-to′loid; par″ah-to-loi′din) Koch's lymph, or tuberculin; see *tuberculin*.

paratonia (par″ah-to′ne-ah) [*para-* + Gr. *tonos* tension + *-ia*] a disorder of tone or tension.

paratope (par′ah-tōp) [*para* + Gr. *topos* a place] the site on the molecule of an antibody which attaches to an antigen; an antibody combining site. Cf. *epitope*.

paratose (par′ah-tōs) an unusual sugar found to be a polysaccharide somatic antigen of *Salmonella* species.

paratrachoma (par″ah-trah-ko′mah) [*para-* + Gr. *trachoma*] a conjunctivitis resembling trachoma, caused by the genital inclusion virus. See *inclusion blennorrhea*, under *blennorrhea*.

paratrimma (par″ah-trim′ah) [*para-* + Gr. *tribein* to rub] (*obs.*) 1. irritation; chafing. 2. intertrigo, especially between the buttocks.

paratripsis (par″ah-trip′sis) 1. (*obs.*) irritation or chafing. 2. suppression of tissue waste.

paratriptic (par″ah-trip′tik) 1. (*obs.*) pertaining to chafing. 2. pertaining to or preventing waste of body tissue. 3. an agent that prevents the waste of body tissue.

paratrophic (par″ah-trof′ik) [*para-* + Gr. *trophē* nutrition] requiring living material or complex protein matter for food. Cf. *metatrophic*.

paratrophy (par-at′ro-fe) [*para-* + Gr. *trophē* nutrition] dystrophy.

paratuberculosis (par″ah-tu-ber″ku-lo′sis) 1. a disease resembling tuberculosis but not due to *Mycobacterium tuberculosis*. 2. Johne's disease.

paratuberculous (par″ah-tu-ber″ku-lus) having an indirect relation to tuberculosis; due to conditions produced by tuberculosis; pertaining to paratuberculosis.

paratype (par′ah-tīp) any strain of bacteria, other than the holotype, that is specifically stated to be the one on which the original description of the taxon was based.

paratyphlitis (par″ah-tif-li′tis) [*para-* + Gr. *typhlos* blind + *-itis*] inflammation of the postperitoneal tissue of the cecum.

paratyphoid (par″ah-ti′foid) a term used originally for enteritis due to *Salmonella* species other than *S. typhosa*, and regarded as milder than typhoid. Properly used only as a generic term for infection due to *Salmonella* of all groups (principally B–E) except *S. typhosa*. Called also *Brion-Kayser disease, enteric fever, paratyphoid fever*, and *Schottmüller's disease*.

paratypic (par″ah-tip′ik) paratypical.

paratypical (par″ah-tip′ĭ-kal) differing from the type.

paraumbilical (par″ah-um-bil′ĭ-kal) alongside the umbilicus.

paraungual (par″ah-ung′gwal) [*para-* + L. *unguis* nail] near or beside a nail.

paraurethra (par″ah-u-re′thrah) an accessory urethral canal.

paraurethral (par″ah-u-re′thral) near the urethra.

paraurethritis (par″ah-u″re-thri′tis) inflammation of the tissues near the urethra.

parauterine (par″ah-u′ter-in) alongside the uterus.

paravaccinia (par″ah-vak-sin′e-ah) an eruption of red hemispherical tubercles which sometimes follows vaccination, but which is not vaccinial in nature.

paravaginal (par″ah-vaj′ĭ-nal) beside or alongside of the vagina.

paravaginitis (par″ah-vaj″ĭ-ni′tis) inflammation of the tissue about the vagina.

paravenous (par″ah-ve′nus) beside a vein.

paravertebral (par″ah-ver″tĕ-bral) beside the vertebral column.

paravitaminosis (par″ah-vi″tah-mĭ-no′sis) a vitamin deficiency disorder without specific lesions.

paraxial (par-ak′se-al) [*para-* + *axis*] situated alongside an axis.

paraxon (par-ak′son) [*para-* + *axon*] a collateral branch of an axon.

Parazoa (par-ah-zo′ah) a subdivision of Metazoa comprising the sponges, i.e., multicellular animals having incipient tissues, but no mouth or digestive tract or organ systems. Cf. *Eumetazoa*.

parazone (par′ah-zōn) one of the white bands alternating with the dark bands (diazones) in the layers of enamel prisms and seen in cross-section of a tooth.

parazoon (par″ah-zo′on) [*para-* + Gr. *zōon* animal] (*obs.*) an animal organism parasitic upon or within an animal; animal parasite.

parbendazole (par-ben′dah-zōl) chemical name: (5-butyl-1*H*-benzimidazol-2-yl)carbamic acid methyl ester; a veterinary anthelmintic with nematocidal action, $C_{13}H_{17}N_3O_2$.

parconazole hydrochloride (par-ko′nah-zōl) chemical name: *cis*-1-[[2-(2,4-dichlorophenyl)-4-[(2-propynyloxy)methyl]-1,-3-dioxolan-2-yl]methyl]-1*H*-imidazole monohydrochloride; an antifungal, $C_{17}H_{16}Cl_2N_2O_3 \cdot HCl$.

Paré (par-ā′), Ambroise (1510–1590). A French surgeon, the most celebrated surgeon of the Renaissance, who reformed the treatment of gunshot wounds by abolishing cauterization with boiling oil. He also practiced ligation of arteries after amputation, and re-introduced podalic version into obstetrics. His famous aphorism, *Je le pansay, et Dieu le guarit* ("I dressed him and God healed him"), first appeared in 1585, in the fourth edition of his collected works.

parectasia (par″ek-ta′se-ah) parectasis.

parectasis (par-ek′tah-sis) [*para-* + Gr. *ektasis* extension] excessive stretching or distention of a part or organ.

parectropia (par″ek-tro′pe-ah) [*para-* + Gr. *ek* out + *tropos* a turning] apraxia.

Paredrine (par′ah-drēn) trademark for preparations of hydroxyamphetamine hydrobromide.

paregoric (par″ě-gor′ik) [Gr. *parēgorikos* consoling] [USP] a preparation of powdered opium, anise oil, benzoic acid, camphor, diluted alcohol, and glycerin, each 100 ml. of which yields 35–45 mg. of anhydrous morphine; used as an antiperistaltic, especially in the treatment of diarrhea, administered orally. Formerly called *camphorated opium tincture.*

paregorism (par'ĕ-gor"izm) addiction to paregoric.

pareidolia (par"i-do'le-ah) [*para-* + Gr. *eidōlon* phantom + *-ia*] an illusion in which visual images are given a fantastic interpretation.

parelectronomic (par"e-lek"tro-nom'ik) giving no response to electromotive stimuli.

parelectronomy (par"e-lek-tron'o-me) [*para-* + *electric* + Gr. *nomos* law] a condition in which there is a decrease in strength of an electric current passed through a muscle.

pareleidin (par"el-e'i-din) the keratin of epidermal cells derived from eleidin of the stratum lucidum.

parencephalia (par"en-sĕ-fa'le-ah) [*para-* + Gr. *enkephalos* brain + *-ia*] congenital defect of the brain.

parencephalocele (par"en-sef'ah-lo-sēl) [*parencephalon* + Gr. *kēlē* hernia] hernial protrusion of the cerebellum.

parencephalon (par"en-sef'ah-lon) [*para-* + Gr. *enkephalos* brain] the cerebellum.

parencephalous (par"en-sef'ah-lus) [*para-* + Gr. *enkephalos* brain] having a congenital deformity of the brain.

parenchyma (pah-reng'kĭ-mah) [Gr. "anything poured in beside"] the essential elements of an organ; used in anatomical nomenclature as a general term to designate the functional elements of an organ, as distinguished from its framework, or stroma. **p. of lens,** substantia lentis. **p. tes'tis** [NA], **p. of testis,** the seminiferous tubules, which are located within the lobules of the testis.

parenchymal (pah-reng'kĭ-mal) pertaining to or of the nature of parenchyma.

parenchymatitis (par"eng-kim"ah-ti'tis) inflammation of a parenchyma.

parenchymatous (par"eng-kim'ah-tus) pertaining to or of the nature of parenchyma.

parenchymula (par"eng-kim'u-lah) the embryonic stage next succeeding that called the closed blastula.

Parendomyces (par"en-do-mi'sēz) a former genus of yeastlike fungi, species of which have now been included in the genus *Candida.*

Parenogen (pah-ren'o-jen) trademark for a preparation of fibrinogen (def. 2).

parental (pah-ren'tal) of, pertaining to, or derived from the parents.

parenteral (pah-ren'ter-al) [*para-* + Gr. *enteron* intestine] not through the alimentary canal but rather by injection through some other route, as subcutaneous, intramuscular, intraorbital, intracapsular, intraspinal, intrasternal, intravenous, etc.

parepicoele (par-ep'ĭ-sēl) (*obs.*) either of the lateral recesses of the fourth ventricle of the brain.

parepididymis (par"ep-ĭ-did'ĭ-mis) paradidymis.

parepigastric (par"ep-ĭ-gas'trik) near the epigastrium.

parergasia (par"er-ga'ze-ah) [*para-* + Gr. *ergasia* work] 1. Kraepelin's term for perverted functioning, such as closing the eyes instead of putting out the tongue. 2. Meyer's term for personality twist reactions such as schizophrenia.

parergastic (par"er-gas'tik) [*para-* + Gr. *ergon* work] Meyer's term for psychic disorders marked by twist reactions, i.e., incongruities, oddities, mannerisms, or fantastic or passivity projections (schizophrenia and paranoia).

paresis (pah-re'sis, par"ĕ-sis) [Gr. "relaxation"] slight or incomplete paralysis; often used alone to mean general paresis (dementia paralytica). **galloping p.,** an acutely and rapidly progressing paresis. **general p.,** dementia paralytica. **juvenile p.,** a form of general paresis occurring in children as a result of congenital syphilis. **stationary p.,** paresis which has become arrested.

Parest (par'est) trademark for a preparation of methaqualone hydrochloride.

paresthesia (par"es-the'ze-ah) [*para-* + Gr. *aisthēsis* perception] morbid or perverted sensation; an abnormal sensation, as burning, prickling, formication, etc. **Berger's p.,** paresthesia in young persons of one or both lower limbs, accompanied by weakness, but without objective symptoms. **Bernhardt's p.,** meralgia paresthetica. **visceral p.,** an abnormal sensation referred to some viscus; not a mere excess or defect of a normal visceral sensation.

paresthetic (par"es-thet'ik) pertaining to or marked by paresthesia.

paretic (pah-ret'ik) pertaining to or affected with paresis.

parfocal (par-fo'kal) [L. *par* equal + *focus* hearth] retaining correct focus on changing powers in microscopy.

pargyline hydrochloride (par'gĭ-lēn) [USP] chemical name: *N*-methyl-*N*-2-propynylbenzylamine hydrochloride. An antihypertensive, $C_{11}H_{13}N \cdot HCl$, occurring as a white or practically white crystalline powder; administered orally.

Parham band (pahr'am) [F. W. *Parham,* New Orleans surgeon, 1885–1927] see under *band.*

parhedonia (par"he-do'ne-ah) Freud's name for the abnormalities of sexuality, such as the obsessive desire to see, to exhibit, or to touch the sexual organs of oneself or another.

parhormone (par-hor'mōn) any metabolic substance of the body which influences the functions of other organs or tissues. For example, carbon dioxide.

parica (par"ĭ-kah') a narcotic snuff prepared from the leguminous seeds of *Piptadenia* (*Anadenanthera*) species, a tree of Brazil. The seeds contain dimethyltryptamine and related psychotomimetic indole alkaloids. Called also *cohoba.*

paricine (pah-ris'in) a quinoline alkaloid, $C_{16}H_{18}ON_2$, from the bark of *Cinchona succirubra* Parvon. (Rubiaceae), redbark cinchona.

paries (pa're-ez), pl. *pari'etes* [L.] a wall; [NA] a general term for the wall of an organ or body cavity. **p. ante'rior vagi'nae** [NA], the wall of the vagina that is intimately associated with the posterior wall of the bladder and urethra. **p. ante'rior ventric'uli** [NA], the wall of the stomach that is directed toward the ventral surface of the body. **p. carot'icus ca'vi tym'pani** [NA], the anterior wall of the tympanic cavity, related to the carotid canal in which is lodged the internal carotid artery. **p. exter'nus duc'tus cochlea'ris** [NA], the external wall of the cochlear duct, adjacent to the outer wall of the cochlea. **p. infe'rior or'bitae** [NA], the inferior wall of the orbit, formed by the orbital surfaces of the maxilla and the zygomatic and palatine bones; called also *floor of orbit.* **p. jugula'ris ca'vi tym'pani** [NA], the floor of the tympanic cavity, which is in intimate relation with the jugular fossa, which lodges the bulb of the internal jugular vein. **p. labyrin'thicus ca'vi tym'pani** [NA], the medial wall of the tympanic cavity. **p. latera'lis or'bitae** [NA], the lateral wall of the orbit, formed by the orbital surfaces of the great wing of the sphenoid bone, the zygomatic bone, and the zygomatic process of the frontal bone. **p. mastoi'deus ca'vi tym'pani** [NA], the posterior wall of the tympanic cavity, related to the mastoid portion of the temporal bone. **p. media'lis or'bitae** [NA], the medial wall of the orbit, formed by parts of the maxillary, lacrimal, ethmoid, and sphenoid bones. **p. membrana'ceus bron'chi** [NA], that part of the wall of the smaller bronchi where the cartilage is deficient. **p. membrana'ceus ca'vi tym'pani** [NA], the outer, or lateral, wall of the tympanic cavity, formed mainly by the tympanic membrane. **p. membrana'ceus tra'cheae** [NA], the posterior part of the wall of the trachea where the cartilaginous rings are deficient. **p. poste'rior vagi'nae** [NA], the wall of the vagina that is intimately associated with the anterior wall of the rectum. **p. poste'rior ventric'uli** [NA], the wall of the stomach that is directed toward the back of the body. **p. supe'rior or'bitae** [NA], the superior wall of the orbit, formed chiefly by the orbital plate of the frontal bone and by the orbital surface of the lesser wing of the sphenoid bone; called also *roof of orbit.* **p. tegmenta'lis ca'vi tym'pani** [NA], the roof of the tympanic cavity, related to part of the petrous portion of the temporal bone. **p. tympan'icus duc'tus cochlea'ris** [NA], tympanic wall of cochlear duct: the wall of the cochlear duct that separates it from the scala tympani, composed of the osseous spiral laminae and the basilar membrane. **p. vestibula'ris duc'tus cochlea'ris** [NA], vestibular wall of cochlear duct: the thin anterior wall of the cochlear duct, which separates it from the scala vestibuli; called also *membrana spiralis ductus cochlearis* [NA alternative] or *spiral membrane of cochlear duct.*

parietal (pah-ri'ĕ-tal) [L. *parietalis*] 1. of or pertaining to the walls of a cavity. 2. pertaining to or located near the parietal bone, as the parietal lobe.

parietes (pah-ri'ĕ-tēz) [L.] plural of *paries.*

parietitis (pah-ri"ĕ-ti'tis) inflammation of the wall of an organ.

parietofrontal (pah-ri"ĕ-to-fron'tal) pertaining to the parietal and frontal bones, gyri, or lobes.

parietography (pah-ri"ĕ-tog'rah-fe) roentgenographic visualization of the walls of an organ. **gastric p.,** roentgenographic visualization of the stomach wall by special technique, as a means of detecting early gastric neoplasm.

parieto-occipital (pah-ri"ĕ-to-ok-sip'ĭ-tal) pertaining to the parietal and occipital bones or lobes.

parietosphenoid (pah-ri"ĕ-to-sfe'noid) pertaining to the parietal and sphenoid bones.

parietosplanchnic (pah-ri"ĕ-to-splank'nik) parietovisceral.

parietosquamosal (pah-ri"ĕ-to-skwah-mo'sal) pertaining to the parietal bone and the squamous portion of the temporal bone.

parietotemporal (pah-ri"ĕ-to-tem'po-ral) pertaining to the parietal and temporal bones or lobes.

parietovisceral (pah-ri"ĕ-to-vis'er-al) both parietal and visceral; pertaining to the walls of a cavity and the viscera within it.

Parinaud's oculoglandular syndrome (conjunctivitis), ophthalmoplegia (pah-rĭ-nōz') [Henri *Parinaud,* French ophthalmologist, 1844–1905] see under *ophthalmoplegia* and *syndrome.*

pari passu (pa′re pas′u) [L., "at equal pace"] coincidentally with; to the same proportion or degree.

parity (par′ĭ-te) 1. [L. *parere* to bring forth, produce] para; the condition of a woman with respect to her having borne viable offspring. Cf. *gravidity.* 2. [L. *par* equal] equality; close correspondence or similarity.

Park's aneurysm (parks) [Henry *Park,* English surgeon, 1744–1831] see under *aneurysm.*

Parker's fluid (park′erz) [George Howard *Parker,* American zoologist, 1864–1955] see under *fluid.*

Parker's incision (park′erz) [William *Parker,* New York surgeon, 1800–1884] see under *incision.*

Parkinson's disease, facies (sign) (par′kin-sunz) [James *Parkinson,* English physician, 1755–1824] see *paralysis agitans,* and under *facies.* See also *parkinsonism.*

parkinsonian (par″kin-sun′e-an) pertaining to parkinsonism.

parkinsonism (par′kin-sun-izm″) a group of neurological disorders characterized by hypokinesia, tremor, and muscular rigidity. See *parkinsonian syndrome,* under *syndrome,* and see *paralysis agitans* (Parkinson's disease). **postencephalitic p.,** parkinsonian syndrome.

parlodion (par-lo′de-on) collodion in a shredded form, used as an embedding medium in microscopical technique.

Parnate (par′nāt) trademark for a preparation of tranylcypromine sulfate.

paroccipital (par″ok-sip′ĭ-tal) [*para-* + L. *occiput* occiput] near the occipital bone.

parodontal (par″o-don′tal) situated near or beside a tooth.

parodontid (par″o-don′tid) [*para-* + Gr. *odous* tooth] a tumor on the gingiva.

parodontitis (par″o-don-ti′tis) periodontitis.

parodontium (par″o-don′she-um) periodontium.

parodontopathy (par″o-don-top′ah-the) periodontopathy.

parodontosis (par″o-don-to′sis) periodontosis.

parolivary (par-ol′ĭ-var″e) [*para-* + *olivary*] situated near the olive or olivary nucleus.

paromomycin (par′o-mo-mi″sin) chemical name: *O*-2,6-diamino-2, 6-dideoxy-α-L-idopyranosyl-(1→3)-*O*-β-D-ribofuranosyl-(1→5)-*O*-[2-amino-2-deoxy-α-D-glucopyranosyl-(1→4)]-2-deoxystreptamine. An aminoglycoside antibiotic, $C_{23}H_{45}N_5O_{14}$, derived from *Streptomyces rimosus* var. *paromomycinus,* which is effective against a wide variety of gram-negative, gram-positive, and acid-fast bacteria. **p. sulfate** [USP], the sulfate salt of paromomycin, $C_{23}H_{45}N_5O_{14} \cdot xH_2SO_4$, occurring as a creamy white to yellow, amorphous powder; used orally as an antiamebic.

paromphalocele (par″om-fal′o-sēl) [*para-* + Gr. *omphalos* navel + *kēlē* hernia] hernia situated near the navel.

paroniria (par″o-ni′re-ah) [*para-* + Gr. *oneiros* dream + *-ia*] morbid dreaming.

paronychia (par″o-nik′e-ah) [*para-* + Gr. *onyx* nail + *-ia*] inflammation involving the folds of tissue surrounding the fingernail. Cf. *felon* and *eponychia,* and see *onychia.* **herpetic p.,** a herpesvirus infection marked by pyogenic and vesicular paronychia, occurring in hospital workers. **p. tendino′sa,** septic inflammation of the sheath of the tendon of a finger.

paronychial (par″o-nik′e-al) of or pertaining to paronychia; of or pertaining to the nail folds, as a paronychial wart.

paroophoric (par″o-o-fo′rik) pertaining to the paroophoron.

paroophoritis (par″o-of-o-ri′tis) 1. inflammation of the paroophoron. 2. inflammation of the tissues about the ovary.

paroophoron (par″o-of′o-ron) [*para-* + Gr. *ōon* egg + *pherein* to bear] [NA] an inconstantly present small group of coiled tubules between the layers of the mesosalpinx, being a remnant of the excretory part of the mesonephros.

parophthalmia (par″of-thal′me-ah) [*para-* + Gr. *ophthalmos* eye + *-ia*] inflammation of the connective tissue around the eye.

parophthalmoncus (par″of-thal-mong′kus) [*para-* + Gr. *opthalmos* eye + *onkos* mass] a tumor situated near the eye.

paropsis (par-op′sis) [*para-* + Gr. *opsis* vision] disorder of the sense of vision.

parorchidium (par″or-kid′e-um) [*para-* + Gr. *orchis* testicle] misplacement of a testis or testes.

parorchis (par-or′kis) the epididymis.

parorexia (par″o-rek′se-ah) [*para-* + Gr. *orexis* appetite] perversion of the appetite, with craving for special articles of diet or for articles that are not suitable for food.

parosmia (par-oz′me-ah) [*para-* + Gr. *osmē* smell] any disease or perversion of the sense of smell.

parosphresia (par″os-fre′ze-ah) [*para-* + Gr. *osphrēsis* smelling + *-ia*] disorder or perversion of the sense of smell.

parosphresis (par″os-fre′sis) parosphresia.

parosteal (par-os′te-al) pertaining to the outer surface of the periosteum.

parosteitis (par″os-te-i′tis) [*para-* + *osteitis*] inflammation of the tissues around a bone.

parosteosis (par″os-te-o′sis) [*para-* + Gr. *osteon* bone + *-osis*] ossification of the tissues outside of the periosteum.

parostitis (par″os-ti′tis) parosteitis.

parostosis (par″os-to′sis) parosteosis.

parotic (pah-rot′ik) [*para-* + Gr. *ous* ear] situated or occurring near the ear.

parotid (pah-rot′id) [*para-* + Gr. *ous* ear] situated or occurring near the ear, as the parotid gland.

parotidean (pah-rot″ĭ-de′an) pertaining to the parotid gland.

parotidectomy (pah-rot″ĭ-dek′to-me) [*parotid* + Gr. *ektomē* excision] excision of the parotid gland.

parotiditis (pah-rot″ĭ-di′tis) parotitis.

parotidoscirrhus (pah-rot″ĭ-do-skir′us) [*parotid* + Gr. *skirrhos* hardness] hardening of the parotid gland.

parotidosclerosis (pah-rot″ĭ-do-skle-ro′sis) hardening of the parotid gland.

parotin (par-o′tin) a proteinaceous factor extractable from human parotid gland, which supposedly has hormonal properties; in rabbits, it promotes mesenchymal growth and calcification of teeth, lowers serum calcium levels, and affects the leukocyte count.

parotitic (par″o-tit′ik) pertaining to parotitis.

parotitis (par″o-ti′tis) inflammation of the parotid gland caused by viruses, such as the mumps virus and coxsackievirus, and by bacteria, including *Staphylococcus aureus, Pneumococcus,* and *Streptococcus.* **celiac p.,** inflammation of the parotid gland after abdominal disease or injury. **epidemic p.,** mumps. **p. phlegmono′sa,** parotitis that goes on to suppuration. **postoperative p.,** an acute parotitis due to infection (usually with staphylococci) of the parotid gland following a surgical procedure; it is marked by rapid onset, frequently with severe pain and rapid swelling of the glands, and by trismus, low-grade fever, headache, malaise, and leukocytosis. It affects generally debilitated patients, usually middle-aged or older, suffering from dehydration, suppression of salivary secretion, vomiting, or mouth-breathing. **staphylococcal p.,** postoperative parotitis caused by staphylococci.

parous (pa′rus) [L. *parere* to bring forth, produce] having borne one or more viable offspring.

parovarian (par″o-va′re-an) 1. situated beside the ovary. 2. pertaining to the parovarium (epoophoron).

parovariotomy (par″o-va″re-ot′o-me) [*parovarium* + Gr. *tomē* a cutting] excision of a paroophoritic cyst.

parovaritis (par″o-vah-ri′tis) inflammation of the parovarium (epoophoron).

parovarium (par″o-va′re-um) [*para-* + L. *ovarium* ovary] epoophoron.

paroxia (pah-rok′se-ah) (*obs.*) pica.

paroxysm (par′ok-sizm) [Gr. *paroxysmos*] 1. a sudden recurrence or intensification of symptoms. 2. a spasm or seizure.

paroxysmal (par″ok-siz′mal) recurring in paroxysms.

Parpanit (par-pan′it) trademark for a preparation of caramiphen hydrochloride.

Parrot's atrophy of newborn, disease (pseudoparalysis), sign (node), ulcer (par-ōz′) [Jules Marie *Parrot,* French physician, 1839–1883] see *marasmus,* see *syphilitic pseudoparalysis,* under *pseudoparalysis,* and see under *sign* and *ulcer.*

Parry's disease (pār′ēz) [Caleb Hillier *Parry,* English physician, 1755–1822] Graves' disease.

pars (parz), pl. *par′tes* [L.] a division or part; [NA] a general term for a particular portion of a larger area, organ, or structure. **p. abdomina′lis esoph′agi** [NA], the part of the esophagus below the diaphragm, joining the stomach. **p. abdomina′lis et pelvi′na syste′matis autonom′ici** [NA], **p. abdomina′lis et pelvi′na syste′matis sympath′ici,** the portion of the autonomic nervous system contained within the abdomen and pelvis. Its parasympathetic components (vagus nerves) arise from the medulla oblongata and sacral spinal cord; its sympathetic components from the thoracic and upper lumbar cord. **p. abdomina′lis mus′culi pectora′lis majo′ris** [NA], the portion of the pectoralis major muscle originating from the aponeurosis of the obliquus externus abdominis. **p. abdomina′lis oesoph′agi,** p. abdominalis esophagi. **p. abdomina′lis ure′teris** [NA], that portion of the ureter extending from the kidney to the terminal line of the pelvis. **p. ala′ris mus′culi nasa′lis** [NA], dilator muscle of nose: the part of the nasal muscle that arises from the maxilla below the nose and inserts into the ala nasi. **p. alveola′ris mandib′ulae** [NA], the superior portion of the body of the mandible, which contains sockets for the teeth. **p. amor′pha,** the spherical, finely granular body surrounded by the nucleolonema of the nucleolus. **p. ana′lis rec′ti,** canalis analis. **p. ante′rior commissu′rae anterio′ris cer′ebri** [NA], the part of the anterior cerebral commissure that interconnects the two olfactory bulbs; it is rudimentary in man. **p. ante′rior fa′ciei diaphragmat′icae hep′atis** [NA], the portion of the diaphragmatic surface of the liver that is directed toward the ventral surface of the body. **p. ante′rior lob′uli quadrangula′ris,** the anterior portion of the quadrangular cerebellar lobule. **p. ante′rior rhinenceph′ali,** the anterior part of the rhinencephalon. **p. anula′ris vagi′nae fibro′sae digito′rum ma′nus** [NA], annular ligaments of fingers: a strong transverse band of fibrous tissue in the vagina fibrosa of the fingers, crossing the flexor tendons at the level of the upper half of the proximal phalanx. **p. anula′ris vagi′nae fibro′sae digito′rum pe′dis** [NA], annular ligaments of toes: a fibrous band in the toes resembling those of similar name in the fingers. **p. ascen′dens duode′ni** [NA], the terminal part of the duodenum, ending at the duodenojejunal flexure. **p. basila′ris fascic′uli pedunculomamilla′ris,** fibers in the basal or ventral part of the mamillary peduncle which connect the mamillary body and interpeduncular region. **p. basila′ris os′sis occipita′lis** [NA], a quadrilateral plate of the occipital bone that projects superiorly and anteriorly from the foramen magnum. **p. basila′ris pon′tis,** former NA term for *p. ventralis pontis.* **p. bucca′lis hypophys′eos,** Rathke's pouch. **p. buccopharyn′gea mus′culi constricto′ris pharyn′gis superio′ris** [NA], buccopharyngeal muscle: the part of the constrictor pharyngis superior muscle arising from the pterygomandibular raphe; called also *musculus buccopharyngeus.* **p. cae′ca oc′uli,** discus nervi optici. **p. cae′ca ret′inae,** the parts of the retina that are not sensitive to light, namely, the pars ciliaris retinae and pars iridica retinae. **p. calcaneocuboi′dea ligamen′ti bifurca′ti,** ligamentum calcaneocuboideum. **p. calcaneonavicula′ris ligamen′ti bifurca′ti,** ligamentum calcaneonaviculare. **p. cardi′aca ventric′uli** [NA], the part of the stomach immediately adjacent to and surrounding the gastric opening of the esophagus, distinguished only by the presence of the cardiac glands, and lacking acid (parietal) and pepsin (chief) cells. Called also *cardia.* **p. cartilagin′ea sep′ti na′si** [NA], cartilaginous part of nasal septum: the plate of cartilage forming the anterior part of the nasal septum; called also *septum cartilagineum nasi.* **p. cartilagin′ea tu′bae auditi′vae** [NA], the part of the auditory tube that is chiefly supported by the tubal cartilage; it extends from the pars ossea to the pharyngeal orifice of the auditory tube. **p. caverno′sa ure′threa vir′ilis,** p. spongiosa urethrae masculinae. **p. centra′lis ventric′uli latera′lis cer′ebri** [NA], the part of the lateral ventricle found within the parietal lobe of the cerebrum; it communicates with the anterior, posterior, and inferior horns. **p. cephal′ica et cervica′lis syste′matis autonom′ici** [NA], **p. cephal′ica et cervica′lis syste′matis sympath′ici,** the portion of the autonomic nervous system contained in the head and neck. Its sympathetic components arise from the upper thoracic cord, and are relayed by cervical sympathetic ganglia; its parasympathetic components arise from the brain stem via oculomotor, facial, glossopharyngeal, vagus, and accessory nerves, and are relayed by way of ciliary, pterygopalatine, otic, submandibular, and intrinsic ganglia. **p. ceratopharyn′gea mus′culi constricto′ris pharyn′gis me′dii** [NA], ceratopharyngeal muscle: the portion of the constrictor pharyngis medius muscle arising from the greater cornu of the hyoid bone; called also *musculus ceratopharyngeus.* **p. cervica′lis esoph′agi** [NA], the part of the esophagus that is located in the cervical region, related anteriorly to the trachea and the recurrent laryngeal nerves, posteriorly to the longus colli muscle and vertebral column, and laterally to the lobes of the thyroid gland and the common carotid arteries. **p. cervica′lis medul′lae spina′lis** [NA], that part of the spinal cord lodged within the cervical part of the vertebral canal and giving rise to the eight pairs of cervical spinal nerves. **p. cervica′lis oesoph′agi,** p. cervicalis esophagi. **p. cervica′lis syste′matis sympath′ici,** see *p. cephalica et cervicalis systematis autonomici.* **p. chondropharyn′gea mus′culi constricto′ris pharyn′gis me′dii** [NA], chondropharyngeal muscle: the portion of the constrictor pharyngis medius muscle arising from the lesser cornu of the hyoid bone; called also *musculus chondropharyngeus.* **p. cilia′ris ret′inae** [NA], the two layers of epithelium lining the basal lamina of the ciliary body. **p. clavicula′ris mus′culi pectora′lis majo′ris** [NA], the portion of the pectoralis major muscle originating from the clavicle. **p. cochlea′ris ner′vi octa′vi** [NA], the cochlear nerve: the part of the eighth cranial nerve concerned with hearing, consisting of fibers that arise from bipolar cells in the spiral ganglion and have their receptors in the spiral organ of the cochlea; called also *nervus cochleae.* **p. convolu′ta lob′uli cortica′lis re′nis** [NA], the part of the renal cortex surrounding the intracortical prolongations of the renal pyramids and composed of convoluted tubules. **par′tes corpo′ris huma′ni** [NA], the category in anatomical nomenclature embracing the names of the various parts of the human body, from head to foot. **p. costa′lis diaphrag′matis** [NA], the part of the respiratory diaphragm arising from the inner surfaces of the ribs and their cartilages. **p. cricopharyn′gea mus′culi constricto′ris pharyn′gis inferio′ris** [NA], cricopharyngeal muscle: the portion of the constrictor pharyngis inferior muscle arising from the cricoid cartilage; called also *musculus cricopharyngeus.* **p. crucifor′mis vagi′nae fibro′sae digito′rum ma′nus** [NA], cruciate ligaments of fingers: one of the diagonal bundles of the fascia of the fingers which cross each other on the dorsal

surface of each digit at the level of the distal end of the proximal phalanx; called also *ligamenta cruciata digitorum manus.* **p. crucifor′mis vagi′nae fibro′sae digito′rum pe′dis** [NA], cruciate ligaments of toes: one of the bundles of fascial fibers in the toes resembling those of similar name in the fingers; called also *ligamenta cruciata digitorum pedis.* **p. cupula′ris reces′sus epitympan′ici** [NA], cupular space: the part of the epitympanic recess above the head of the malleus. **p. descen′dens duode′ni** [NA], the part of the duodenum between the superior and inferior parts, into which the bile and pancreatic ducts open. **p. dex′tra faci′ei diaphragmat′icae hep′atis** [NA], the portion of the diaphragmatic surface of the liver that is directed toward the right side of the body. **p. dista′lis lo′bi anterio′ris hypophys′eos,** see *pituitary gland,* under *gland.* **p. dorsa′lis pon′tis** [NA], the tegmental part of the pons, which resembles the medulla oblongata in structure and is continuous with the tegmentum of the mesencephalon. **p. feta′lis placen′tae** [NA], fetal placenta: the nonmaternal part of the placenta, derived not from the fetus but from the trophoblast that envelops the fetus; from within outward, it consists of amnion, chorionic plate, and chorionic villi. Called also *placenta foetalis.* **p. fibro′sa,** the portion of the nucleolus containing chiefly filaments. **p. flac′cida membra′nae tym′pani** [NA], the small portion of the tympanic membrane, between the mallear folds. **p. fronta′lis cap′sulae inter′nae,** crus anterius capsulae internae. **p. fronta′lis coro′nae radia′tae,** the portion of the corona radiata contained within a frontal lobe of the brain. **p. fronta′lis oper′culi,** operculum frontale. **p. fronta′lis radiatio′nis corpo′ris callo′si,** the frontal part of the radiatio corporis callosi, composed of fibers sweeping forward from the genu into the frontal lobe. **p. functiona′lis,** stratum functionale. **par′tes genita′les exter′nae mulie′bres,** partes genitales femininae externae. **par′tes genita′les exter′nae vir′iles,** partes genitales masculinae externae. **par′tes genita′les femini′nae exter′nae** [NA], the external genitalia of the female, comprising the pudendum femininum, clitoris, and urethra femininum; called also *partes genitales externae muliebres.* **par′tes genita′les masculi′nae exter′nae** [NA], the external genitalia of the male, comprising the penis, scrotum, and urethra masculina; called also *partes genitales externae viriles.* **p. gla′bra,** a smooth zone or area, such as the outer smooth zone of the lip appearing early in its embryonic development. **p. glossopharyn′gea mus′culi constricto′ris pharyn′gis superio′ris** [NA], glossopharyngeal muscle: the part of the constrictor pharyngis superior muscle arising from the side of the root of the tongue. **p. granulo′sa,** the portion of the nucleolus containing chiefly granules. **p. gris′ea hypothal′ami,** the gray matter, i.e., nuclear masses, of the hypothalamus. **p. horizonta′lis duode′ni** [NA], that part of the duodenum situated between the descending and ascending parts, crossing from right to left ventral to the third lumbar vertebra; called also *p. inferior duodeni* [NA alternative] or *inferior part of duodenum.* **p. horizonta′lis os′sis palati′ni,** lamina horizontalis ossis palatini. **p. ili′aca lin′eae termina′lis,** linea arcuata ossis ilii. **p. infe′rior duode′ni,** NA alternative for p. horizontalis duodeni. **p. infe′rior fos′sae rhomboi′deae,** a space at the lower part of the floor of the fourth ventricle of the brain, between the restiform bodies. **p. infe′rior gy′ri fronta′lis me′dii,** the inferior portion of the middle frontal gyrus. **p. infe′rior par′tis vestibula′ris ner′vi octa′vi** [NA], the inferior of the branches into which the vestibular part of the eighth cranial nerve divides peripherally; it gives rise to the posterior ampullar and saccular nerves. **p. inflex′a,** the bar of a horse's hoof. **p. infraclavicula′ris plex′us brachia′lis** [NA], the part of the brachial plexus that lies in the axilla, below the level of the clavicle. In it arise the medial and lateral pectoral, musculocutaneous, medial brachial cutaneous, medial antebrachial cutaneous, median, ulnar, radial, subscapular, thoracodorsal, and axillary nerves. **p. infundibula′ris lo′bi anterio′ris hypophys′eos** [NA], see *pituitary gland,* under *gland.* **p. intercartilagin′ea ri′mae glot′tidis** [NA], the part of the rima glottidis between the arytenoid cartilages; called also *interarytenoid space.* **p. interme′dia fos′sae rhomboi′deae,** the middle part of the rhomboid fossa. **p. interme′dia lo′bi anterio′ris hypophys′eos** [NA], see *pituitary gland,* under *gland.* **p. intermembrana′cea ri′mae glot′tidis** [NA], the part of the rima glottidis between the vocal folds. **p. interstia′lis tu′bae uteri′nae,** pars uterina tubae uterinae. **p. irid′ica ret′inae** [NA], the two layers of pigmented epithelium lining the posterior part of the iris. **p. labia′lis mus′culi orbicula′ris o′ris** [NA], the part of the orbicular muscle of the mouth whose fibers are restricted to the lips. **p. lacrima′lis mus′culi orbicula′ris oc′uli** [NA], the part of the orbicularis oculi muscle that arises from the posterior lacrimal ridge of the lacrimal bone, to become continuous with the palpebral portion. **p. laryn′gea pharyn′gis** [NA], laryngopharynx: the portion of the pharynx that lies below the upper edge of the epiglottis and opens into the larynx and esophagus. **p. latera′lis ar′cus longitudina′lis pe′dis** [NA], that part of the longitudinal arch of the foot formed by the calcaneus, the cuboid bone, and the lateral two metatarsal bones.

p. latera′lis musculo′rum intertransversario′rum posterio′rum cer′vicis [NA], the lateral part of the posterior intertransverse muscles of the neck. **p. latera′lis os′sis occipita′lis** [NA], lateral part of occipital bone: one of the paired parts of the occipital bone which form the lateral boundaries of the foramen magnum, each being prominently characterized by the presence of one of the occipital condyles. **p. latera′lis os′sis sa′cri** [NA], the part or mass of the sacrum on either side lateral to the dorsal and pelvic sacral foramina; called also *lateral mass of sacrum.* **p. li′bera colum′nae for′nicis,** the postcommissural component of the columns of the fornix. **p. lumba′lis diaphrag′matis** [NA], the portion of the respiratory diaphragm that arises from the lumbar vertebrae, comprising the right and left diaphragmatic crura, the right crus arising from the upper three or four vertebrae, and the left from the upper two or three. **p. lumba′lis medul′lae spina′lis** [NA], that part of the spinal cord lodged within the lower thoracic part of the vertebral canal (in adults) and giving rise to the five pairs of lumbar spinal nerves. **p. mamilla′ris hypothal′ami,** the mamillary bodies. **p. margina′lis mus′culi orbicula′ris o′ris** [NA], the part of the orbicular muscle of the mouth whose fibers blend with those of adjacent muscles. **p. margina′lis sul′ci cin′guli,** the portion of the cingulate gyrus that turns off at a right angle and is directed toward the dorsal margin of the cerebral hemisphere. **p. mastoi′dea os′sis tempora′lis,** mastoid bone: the posterior portion of the petrous part of the temporal bone, bounded anteriorly by the external acoustic meatus and articulating superiorly with the parietal bone and posteriorly with the occipital bone. **p. media′lis ar′cus longitudina′lis pe′dis** [NA], that part of the longitudinal arch of the foot formed by the calcaneus, talus, and the navicular, cuneiform, and first three metatarsal bones. **p. media′lis musculo′rum intertransversario′rum posterio′rum cer′vicis** [NA], the medial part of the posterior intertransverse muscles of the neck. **p. mediastina′lis faci′ei media′lis pulmo′nis** [NA], the part of the medial surface of each lung that is adjacent to the mediastinum. **p. membrana′cea sep′ti atrio′rum,** p. membranacea septi interventricularis cordis. **p. membrana′cea sep′ti interventricula′ris cor′dis** [NA], the very small, completely membranous area of the interventricular septum of the heart; situated near the root of the aorta, it can be viewed between the opposed margins of the right and posterior semilunar valves of the aorta. Called also *septum membranaceum ventriculorum cordis.* **p. membrana′cea sep′ti na′si** [NA], membranous septum of nose: the anterior inferior part of the nasal septum, beneath the cartilaginous part; it is composed of skin and subcutaneous tissues. Called also *septum membranaceum nasi.* **p. membrana′cea ure′thrae masculi′nae** [NA], **p. membrana′cea ure′thrae viri′lis,** the portion of the male urethra between the pars prostatica and pars spongiosa, and traversing the urogenital diaphragm and the deep perineal space. **p. mo′bilis sep′ti na′si** [NA], mobile part of nasal septum: the part of the nasal septum at the apex of the nose, formed by skin, subcutaneous tissue, and the greater alar cartilages; called also *septum mobile nasi.* **p. muscula′ris sep′ti interventricula′ris cor′dis,** the thick muscular partition forming the greater part of the septum between the ventricles of the heart; called also *septum musculare ventriculorum cordis.* **p. mylopharyn′gea mus′culi constricto′ris pharyn′gis superio′ris** [NA], the part of the constrictor pharyngis superior muscle arising from the mylohyoid ridge of the mandible; called also *musculus mylopharyngeus.* **p. nasa′lis os′sis fronta′lis** [NA], the small, irregularly shaped process that projects downward from the medial part of the squama of the frontal bone to articulate with the nasal bones and the frontal processes of the maxillae. Called also *prefrontal bone* and *nasal process of frontal bone.* **p. nasa′lis pharyn′gis** [NA], nasopharynx: the part of the pharynx that lies above the level of the soft palate. **p. nervo′sa hypophys′eos,** see *pituitary gland,* under *gland.* **p. obli′qua mus′culi cricothyroi′dei** [NA], the fibers of the cricothyroid muscle that are inserted into the inferior horn, caudal margin, and inner surface of the thyroid cartilage. **p. occipita′lis cap′sulae inter′nae,** crus posterius capsulae internae. **p. occipita′lis coro′nae radia′tae,** the part of the corona radiata contained within the occipital lobe. **p. occipita′lis radiatio′nis corpo′ris callo′si,** the occipital part of the radiatio corporis callosi, composed of fibers from the splenium bending backward toward the occipital pole. **p. opercula′ris gy′ri fronta′lis inferio′ris,** former NA term for the part of the inferior frontal lobe adjacent to the parietal lobe and overhanging the insula. **p. op′tica hypothal′ami** (*obs.*), the optic chiasma and tracts. **p. op′tica ret′inae** [NA], the part of the retina that contains receptors sensitive to light, extending posteriorly from the ora serrata on the inner surface of the choroid and continuous at the optic disk with the optic nerve; it consists of an outer pigmented stratum and an inner, multilayered cerebral stratum. **p. ora′lis pharyn′gis** [NA], the division of the pharynx lying between the soft palate and the upper edge of the epiglottis; called also *oropharynx.* **p. orbita′lis glan′dulae lacrima′lis** [NA], the main part of the lacrimal gland, limited in front by the orbicularis muscle and the orbital septum; called also *glandulae lacrimalis superior.* **p.**

orbita′lis gy′ri fronta′lis inferio′ris, former NA term for the part of the inferior frontal gyrus rostral to the anterior branch of the lateral cerebral sulcus. **p. orbita′lis mus′culi orbicula′ris oc′uli** [NA], the part of the orbicularis oculi muscle that arises from the medial margin of the orbit and surrounds it and the palpebral part of the muscle, inserting near the site of origin. **p. orbita′lis os′sis fronta′lis** [NA], the horizontally placed part of the frontal bone that forms the greater part of the roof of the orbit and of the floor of the anterior cranial fossa; it is separated from its fellow of the other side by the ethmoid incisure. Called also *orbital plate of occipital bone.* **p. os′sea sep′ti na′si** [NA], the bony part of the nasal septum, composed posterosuperiorly of the perpendicular plate of the ethmoid bone and posteroinferiorly of the vomer. **p. os′sea tu′bae auditi′vae** [NA], the part of the auditory tube that lies within the temporal bone, extending from the tympanic orifice to the pars cartilaginea of the auditory tube. **p. palpebra′lis glan′dulae lacrima′lis** [NA], the part of the lacrimal gland that projects laterally into the upper eyelid; called also *glandula lacrimalis inferior,* and *Rosenmüller's gland* or *node.* **p. palpebra′lis mus′culi orbicula′ris oc′uli** [NA], palpebral part of orbicularis oculi muscle: the part of the orbicularis oculi muscle that is contained in the eyelids, originating from the medial palpebral ligament and inserting in the lateral canthus. **p. parasympath′ica syste′matis nervo′si autonom′ici** [NA], the craniosacral division of the autonomic nervous system, its preganglionic fibers traveling with cranial nerves III, VII, IX, X, and XI, and with the second to fourth sacral ventral roots; it innervates the heart, the smooth muscle and glands of the head and neck, and the thoracic, abdominal, and pelvic viscera. The ganglion cells with which these fibers synapse are in or near the organs innervated. Called also *parasympathetic nervous system.* **p. parieta′lis coro′nae radia′tae,** the part of the corona radiata contained in the parietal lobe. **p. parieta′lis oper′culi,** operculum frontoparietale. **p. parieta′lis radiatio′nis cor′poris callo′si,** the fibers of the radiatio corporis callosi passing into the parietal lobe. **p. pelvi′na syste′matis sympath′ici,** see *p. abdominalis et pelvina systematis autonomici.* **p. pelvi′na ure′teris** [NA], the portion of the ureter that extends from the terminal line of the pelvis to the urinary bladder. **p. perpendicula′ris os′sis palati′ni,** lamina perpendicularis ossis palatini. **p. petro′sa os′sis tempora′lis** [NA], petrous portion of temporal bone: a pyramid of dense bone located at the base of the cranium; one of the three parts of the temporal bone, it houses the organ of hearing. **p. pharyn′gea lo′bi anterio′ris hypophys′eos** [NA], the portion of the pituitary gland formed from Rathke's pouch. **p. pla′na cor′poris cilia′ris,** orbiculus ciliaris. **p. plica′ta cor′poris cilia′ris,** corona ciliaris. **p. poste′rior commissu′rae anterio′ris cer′ebri** [NA], the part of the anterior cerebral commissure that interconnects the middle and inferior temporal gyri, the parahippocampal gyri, and the amygdaloid bodies of the two sides. **p. poste′rior faci′ei diaphragmat′icae hep′atis** [NA], the portion of the diaphragmatic surface of the liver that is directed toward the dorsal surface of the body; called also *facies posterior hepatis.* **p. poste′rior lob′uli quadrangula′ris,** the posterior portion of the quadrangular cerebellar lobule. **p. poste′rior rhinenceph′ali,** the posterior portion of the rhinencephalon. **p. pri′ma radi′cis ner′vi facia′lis** (*obs.*), the ascending part of the root of the facial nerve. **p. profun′da glan′dulae parot′idis** [NA], that part of the parotid gland located deep to the facial nerve. **p. profun′da mus′culi masse′teris** [NA], the deep portion of the masseter muscle, the fibers of which arise from the medial surface of the zygomatic arch and the fascia over the temporal muscle, and are directed vertically downward. **p. profun′da mus′culi sphinc′teris a′ni exter′ni** [NA], the part of the sphincter ani externus muscle that surrounds the upper part of the anal canal. **p. prostat′ica ure′thrae masculi′nae** [NA], **p. prostat′ica ure′thrae viril′is,** the part of the male urethra that passes through the prostate. **p. pterygopharyn′gea mus′culi constricto′ris pharyn′gis superio′ris** [NA], pterygopharyngeal muscle: the part of the constrictor pharyngis superioris muscle arising from the caudal part and hamulus of the medial pterygoid plate; called also *musculus pterygopharyngeus.* **p. pu′bica lin′eae termina′lis,** the pubic part of the terminal line of the pelvis. **p. pylo′rica ventric′uli** [NA], the caudal one-third of the stomach, consisting of the pyloric antrum and canal, and distinguished by the presence of the pyloric glands and by the absence of parietal cells. **p. quadra′ta** [NA], the quadrilateral portion of the medial segment of the left hepatic lobe. **p. radia′ta lob′uli cortica′lis re′nis** [NA], any of the intracortical prolongations of the renal pyramids; called also *processus Ferreini lobuli corticalis renis* and *pyramid of Ferrein.* **p. rec′ta mus′culi cricothyroi′dei** [NA], the fibers of the cricothyroid muscle that are inserted into the caudal margin of the thyroid cartilage. **p. retrolentifor′mis cap′sulae inter′nae** [NA], that part of the internal capsule resting on the lateral surface of the thalamus behind the lentiform nucleus, and containing the posterior thalamic radiation. **p. sacra′lis lin′eae termina′lis,** the sacral part of the terminal line of the pelvis. **p. secun′da radi′cis ner′vi facia′lis** (*obs.*), the second portion of the root of the facial nerve. **p. spongio′sa ure′thrae masculi′nae** [NA], the portion of the male urethra found within the corpus spongiosum of the penis; called also *p. cavernosa urethrae virilis*. **p. squamo′sa os′sis tempora′lis** [NA], squamous part of temporal bone; the flat, scalelike, anterior and superior portion of the temporal bone; called also *squama temporalis*. **p. sterna′lis diaphrag′matis** [NA], the portion of the diaphragm that arises from the inner aspect of the xiphoid process of the sternum. **p. sternocosta′lis mus′culi pectora′lis majo′ris** [NA], the portion of the pectoralis major muscle that originates from the sternum and the ribs. **p. subcuta′nea mus′culi sphinc′teris a′ni exter′ni** [NA], the part of the sphincter ani externus muscle that surrounds the lowermost portion of the anal canal. **p. subfronta′lis sul′ci cin′guli,** the portion of the cingulate sulcus under the superior frontal gyrus. **p. sublentifor′mis cap′sulae inter′nae** [NA], the part of the internal capsule lying ventral to the back part of the lentiform nucleus, and containing the temporopontile, geniculocalcarine, and auditory radiation fibers. **p. superficia′lis glan′dulae parot′idis** [NA], that part of the parotid gland located superficial to the facial nerve. **p. superficia′lis mus′culi masse′teris** [NA], the superficial portion of the masseter muscle, the fibers of which arise from the anterior part of the zygomatic arch and are directed downward and backward. **p. superficia′lis mus′culi sphinc′teris a′ni exter′ni** [NA], the part of the sphincter ani externus muscle that lies just deep to the pars subcutanea, extending farther toward the rectum. **p. supe′rior duode′ni** [NA], the part of the duodenum adjacent to the pylorus, forming the superior flexure; called also *duodenal cap*. **p. supe′rior faci′ei diaphragmat′icae hep′atis** [NA], the portion of the diaphragmatic surface of the liver that is directed cranially. **p. supe′rior fos′sae rhomboi′deae,** the superior portion of the rhomboid fossa. **p. supe′rior gy′ri fronta′lis me′dii,** the superior portion of the middle frontal gyrus. **p. supe′rior par′tis vestibula′ris ner′vi octa′vi** [NA], the superior of the branches into which the vestibular part of the eighth cranial nerve divides peripherally; it gives rise to the utricular, anterior ampullar, and lateral ampullar nerves. **p. supraclavicula′ris plex′us brachia′lis** [NA], the part of the brachial plexus lying in the cervical region above the level of the clavicle, in which arise the dorsal scapular, long thoracic, and suprascapular nerves, and the nerve to the subclavius muscle. **p. sympath′ica syste′matis nervo′si autonom′ici** [NA], sympathetic nervous system: the portion of the autonomic nervous system that receives its fibers of connection with the central nervous system through the thoracolumbar outflow of visceral efferent fibers. These fibers (preganglionic) arise from cells in the thoracic and upper lumbar levels of the spinal cord, leave by way of ventral roots, and, by way of rami communicantes, enter sympathetic trunks, where some synapse with ganglion cells. The fibers (postganglionic) of these ganglion cells return to spinal nerves by way of rami communicantes to supply the blood vessels, smooth muscle, and glands of the trunk and limbs, or go as visceral branches to the blood vessels, smooth muscles, and glands of the head and neck, and the viscera of the thorax, abdomen, and pelvis. Some preganglionic fibers pass through the sympathetic trunks and synapse in the prevertebral ganglia; postganglionic fibers from those ganglia supply adjacent viscera. Called also *thoracicolumbar* or *thoracolumbar division*. **p. tec′ta colum′nae for′nicis,** the crura of the fornix. **p. tegmenta′lis fascic′uli pedunculomamilla′ris,** former term for a tegmental component of the mamillary peduncle. **p. tempora′lis coro′nae radia′tae,** the part of the corona radiata contained in the temporal lobe. **p. tempora′lis oper′culi,** operculum temporale. **p. tempora′lis radiatio′nis cor′poris callo′si,** the fibers of the radiatio corporis callosi passing into the temporal lobe. **p. ten′sa membra′nae tym′pani** [NA], the larger portion of the tympanic membrane. **p. thoraca′lis esoph′agi** [NA], the part of the esophagus located in the thoracic region, and related anteriorly to the trachea and pericardium and posteriorly to the vertebral column. **p. thoraca′lis medul′lae spina′lis,** p. thoracica medullae spinalis. **p. thoraca′lis oesoph′agi,** p. thoracalis esophagi. **p. thoraca′lis syste′matis autonom′ici** [NA], **p. thoraca′lis syste′matis sympath′ici,** the parts of the autonomic nervous system contained within the thorax; its sympathetic components are derived from the upper thoracic cord, and its parasympathetic components, from the vagus nerves. It also contains preganglionic sympathetic fibers which reach abdominal viscera by way of thoracic splanchnic nerves. **p. thora′cica medul′lae spina′lis** [NA], the part of the spinal cord contained in the upper three-fourths of the thoracic part of the vertebral canal (in the adult), and giving rise to the twelve pairs of thoracic spinal nerves. **p. thyropharyn′gea mus′culi constricto′ris pharyn′gis inferio′ris** [NA], thyropharyngeal muscle: the part of the constrictor pharyngis inferior muscle arising from the thyroid cartilage; called also *musculus thyreopharyngeus*. **p. tibiocalca′nea ligamen′ti media′lis** [NA], the middle portion of the superficial fibers of the medial ligament of the ankle joint; attached superiorly to the medial malleolus of the tibia and inferiorly into nearly the entire length of the sustentaculum tali

of the calcaneus. Called also *ligamentum calcaneotibiale* and *calcaneotibial ligament*. **p. tibionavicula′ris ligamen′ti media′lis** [NA], the anterior portion of the superficial fibers of the medial ligament of the ankle joint; attached superiorly to the anterior surface of the medial malleolus of the tibia and inferiorly to the navicular bone and the margin of the calcaneonavicular ligament. Called also *ligamentum tibionaviculare* and *tibionavicular ligament*. **p. tibiotala′ris ante′rior ligamen′ti media′lis** [NA], the deeper portion of the medial ligament of the ankle joint; attached superiorly to the medial malleolus of the tibia and inferiorly to the medial surface of the talus. Called also *ligamentum talotibiale anterius* and *anterior talotibial ligament*. **p. tibiotala′ris poste′rior ligamen′ti media′lis** [NA], the posterior portion of the superficial fibers of the medial ligament of the ankle joint; attached superiorly to the posterior part of the medial malleolus of the tibia and inferiorly to the medial surface of the talus. Called also *ligamentum talotibiale posterius* and *posterior talotibial ligament*. **p. transver′sa,** the transverse part of the left branch of the hepatic portal vein. **p. transver′sa mus′culi nasa′lis** [NA], the part of the nasal muscle that arises from the canine eminence of the maxilla and joins by common aponeurosis its fellow of the opposite side. **p. triangula′ris,** operculum frontale. **p. triangula′ris gy′ri fronta′lis inferio′ris** [NA], the wedge-shaped part of the inferior frontal lobe that lies between the anterior and ascending branches of the lateral sulcus of the cerebral hemisphere. **p. tubera′lis lo′bi anterio′ris hypophys′eos,** former NA term for pars infundibularis lobi anterioris hypophyseos; see *pituitary gland*, under *gland*. **p. tympan′ica os′sis tempora′lis** [NA], the part of the temporal bone that forms the anterior and inferior walls and part of the posterior wall of the external auditory meatus. **p. umbilica′lis** [NA], the part of the left branch of the hepatic portal vein that passes from the hilum of the liver to the umbilicus. **p. uteri′na placen′tae** [NA], uterine placenta: the maternally contributed part of the placenta, derived from the decidua basalis; called also *maternal placenta* and *placenta uterina*. **p. uteri′na tu′bae uteri′nae** [NA], the proximal part of the uterine tube, located within the wall of the uterus. **p. ventra′lis pon′tis** [NA], the part of the pons connecting the cerebrum, cerebellum, and medulla oblongata. It is a broad, transverse band that arches across the ventral surface of the rostral end of the rhombencephalon and on each side narrows to enter the cerebellum as the middle cerebellar peduncle. It comprises longitudinal fibers originating at the cerebral cortex, transverse fibers, and masses of gray matter, the pontine nuclei. Formerly called *p. basilaris pontis*. **p. verte-bra′lis faci′ei media′lis pulmo′nis** [NA], the part of the medial surface of each lung that is adjacent to the vertebral column. **p. vestibula′ris ner′vi octa′vi** [NA], vestibular nerve: the part of the eighth cranial nerve concerned with equilibration, consisting of fibers that arise from bipolar cells in the vestibular ganglion and divide peripherally into a superior and an inferior part, with receptors in the semicircular canals, utricle, and saccule. Called also *nervus vestibuli*. **p. villo′sa,** a villus-covered zone or area, such as the inner villus-covered zone of the lip appearing early in its embryonic development.

Parsidol (par′sĭ-dol) trademark for a preparation of ethopropazine hydrochloride.

Parsons′ disease (par′sunz) [James *Parsons*, English physician, 1705–1770] Graves′ disease.

pars planitis (pars pla-ni′tis) a granulomatous uveitis of the pars plana of the ciliary body.

part (part) [L. *pars* a portion, piece, share] a division or portion. For names of various other parts of various anatomical structures, see under *pars*. **broad p. of anterior annular ligament of leg,** retinaculum musculorum extensorum pedis superius. **colic p. of omentum,** omentum majus. **condylar p. of occipital bone,** pars lateralis ossis occipitalis. **exoccipital p. of occipital bone,** pars lateralis ossis occipitalis. **interstitial p. of uterine tube, intramural p. of uterine tube,** pars uterina tubae uterinae. **jugular p. of occipital bone,** pars lateralis ossis occipitalis. **lambdoidal (lower) p. of anterior annular ligament of leg,** retinaculum musculorum extensorum pedis inferius. **lateral p. of occipital bone,** pars lateralis ossis occipitalis. **mamillary p. of temporal bone,** pars mastoidea ossis temporalis. **occipital p. of occipital bone,** squama occipitalis. **parietal p. of pelvic fascia,** fascia diaphragmatis pelvis superior. **pectineal p. of inguinal ligament,** ligamentum lacunare. **presenting p.,** that portion of the fetus which is touched by the examining finger through the uterine cervix and, during labor, is bounded by the girdle of resistance. **squamous p. of occipital bone,** squama occipitalis. **squamous p. of temporal bone,** pars squamosa ossis temporalis. **sternocostal p. of diaphragm,** pars costalis diaphragmatis. **subphrenic p. of esophagus,** pars abdominalis esophagi. **superior p. of anterior annular ligament of leg,** retinaculum musculorum extensorum pedis superius. **tabular p. of occipital bone,** squama occipitalis. **tendinous p. of epicranius muscle,** galea aponeurotica. **third p. of quadriceps femoris muscle,** musculus adductor minimus. **transverse p. of anterior annular ligament of leg,** retinaculum musculorum extensorum pedis superius. **vaginal p. of cervix,** portio vaginalis cervicis. **vertebral p. of diaphragm,** pars lumbalis diaphragmatis. **visceral p. of pelvic fascia,** fascia pelvis visceralis.

Part. aeq. abbreviation for L. *par'tes aequa'les,* equal parts.

partal (par'tal) pertaining to parturition.

partes (par'tēz) [L.] plural of *pars.*

parthenocarpy (par"thĕ-no-kar'pe) the reproduction of fruit without fertilization; it may occur naturally or be artificially induced.

parthenogenesis (par"thĕ-no-jen'ĕ-sis) [Gr. *parthenos* virgin + *genesis* production] a modified form of sexual reproduction by the development of a gamete without fertilization, as occurs in some plants and invertebrates, especially arthropods, e.g., honey bees and wasps, and in certain lizards. It may occur as a natural phenomenon or be induced by chemical, thermal, or mechanical stimulation (*artificial p.*).

parthenophobia (par"thĕ-no-fo'be-ah) [Gr. *parthenos* virgin + *phobein* to be affrighted by] morbid dread of girls.

parthogenesis (par"tho-jen'ĕ-sis) parthenogenesis.

particle (par'tĕ-k'l) [L. *particula,* dim. of *partus* part] a tiny mass of material. **alpha p.,** a positively charged particle ejected from the nucleus of a radioactive atom, being a high-speed ionized atom of helium. A stream of these particles constitutes alpha rays. **attraction p.,** a small particle in the center of the centrosome. **beta p.,** an electron emitted from an atomic nucleus during beta decay. **C p.,** a noninfectious RNA virus that is postulated to be a normal inhabitant of all living cells and has been postulated as the single cause of all forms of cancer. **colloid p's,** in colloid chemistry the ultimate particles of a dispersed phase. In lyophilic colloids the particles are larger than a single molecule, being from 1 to 100 micromicrons in diameter, but not large enough to settle out by gravity; in a lyophobic colloid they may consist of one or more large organic molecules, as of starch or protein. **Dane p.,** a particle 42 nm. in diameter, containing hepatitis B antigen on its surface (HB_sAg and e antigen) and in its core (HB_cAg) and consisting of an outer lipoprotein coat surrounding a nucleocapsid which contains DNA. **disperse p's,** the dispersed phase of colloid system; the particles of colloid in a colloid system. **elementary p.,** any of the subatomic particles, including electrons, protons, neutrons, positrons, neutrinos, muons, etc. **elementary p's of mitochondria,** numerous minute, club-shaped granules with spherical heads attached to the inner membrane of a mitochondrion. **high-velocity p's,** nuclear particles, such as electrons, protons, and deuterons, given high speeds in an accelerator. **lens p's,** fine brown points of pigment on the anterior capsule of the lens, being the vestiges of the capsulopupillary membrane of the fetus. **ionizing p.,** one that directly produces ion pairs in its passage through matter. **nuclear p's,** Howell-Jolly bodies. **viral p.,** virion. **X-p.,** a hypothetical particle of matter, believed to arise from the collision of cosmic rays in the upper air. **Zimmermann's elementary p's,** blood platelets.

particulate (par-tik'u-lāt) composed of separate particles.

partigen (par'tĭ-jen) one of the hypothetical constituents of an antigen, which is considered as a mixture of partigens or partial antigens. See *hapten.*

partinium (par-tin'e-um) an alloy of aluminum and tungsten.

partition (par-tish'un) something that separates or divides into parts. **oropharyngeal p.,** a protective barrier between the oral cavity and the pharynx made of moistened gauze sponges, useful during general anesthesia when a nasal mask is used.

partricin (par-tri'sin) an antifungal and antiprotozoal produced by *Streptomyces aureofaciens,* consisting of a mixture in a constant ratio (about 1:1) of two polyene substances having very similar structures and biological properties. See also *mepartricin.*

parturient (par-tu're-ent) [L. *parturiens*] giving birth, or pertaining to childbirth; by extension, a woman in labor.

parturifacient (par"tu-re-fa'shent) [L. *parturire* to have the pains of labor + *facere* to cause] 1. inducing or facilitating childbirth. 2. an agent that induces or facilitates childbirth.

parturiometer (par"tu-re-om'ĕ-ter) [L. *parturitio* childbirth + *metrum* measure] a device used in measuring the expulsive power of the uterus.

parturition (par"tu-rish'un) [L. *parturitio*] the act or process of giving birth to a child; see *labor.*

partus (par'tus) [L.] (*obs.*) labor, or childbirth. **p. agrippi'nus** (*obs.*), breech delivery. **p. caesa'reus** (*obs.*), delivery by cesarean section. **p. immatu'rus** (*obs.*), premature labor. **p. matu'rus** (*obs.*), labor at full term. **p. precipita'tus** (*obs.*), precipitate labor. **p. prematu'rus** (*obs.*), premature labor. **p. seroti'nus** (*obs.*), postmature labor. **p. sic'cus** (*obs.*), dry labor.

Part. vic. abbreviation for L. *parti'tis vi'cibus,* in divided doses.

parulis (pah-roo'lis) [*para-* + Gr. *oulon* gum] a gumboil or subperiosteal abscess of the gum.

parumbilical (par"um-bil'ĭ-kal) alongside the navel.

paruria (par-u're-ah) [*para-* + Gr. *ouron* urine + *-ia*] any dis-

order of the urine or abnormal state of the urine or its discharge.

parvicellular (par"vĭ-sel'u-lar) [L. *parvus* small + *cellula* cell] composed of small cells.

Parvobacteriaceae (par"vo-bak-te"re-a'se-e) a name formerly given the family of schizomycetes later called Brucellaceae.

parvoline (par'vo-lin) an amber-colored liquid poison, $C_9H_{13}N$, from decaying fish or horse flesh.

parvovirus (par"vo-vi'rus) [L. *parvus* small + *virus*] a group of extremely small, morphologically similar, ether-resistant, DNA viruses; the group includes the osteolytic hamster viruses and adeno-associated viruses. Called also *picodnavirus.*

parvule (par'vūl) [L. *parvulus* very small] a very small pill, pellet, or granule.

Paryphostomum (par"e-fos'to-mum) a genus of flukes related to *Echinostoma.*

PAS para-aminosalicylic acid (see under *acid*); periodic acid-Schiff (see under *reaction*).

pascal (pas-kal', pas'kal) [after Blaise *Pascal*] the SI unit of pressure, which corresponds to a force of one newton per square meter; symbol, Pa.

Pascal's law (pas-kahlz') [Blaise *Pascal,* French scientist, 1623–1662] see under *law.*

Paschen's bodies, (corpuscles, granules) (pahs'kenz) [Enrique *Paschen,* Hamburg pathologist, 1860–1936] see under *body.*

Paschutin's degeneration (pas-ku'tinz) [Viktor Vasil'evich *Paschutin,* Russian pathologist, 1845–1901] see under *degeneration.*

paspalism (pas'pal-izm) poisoning due to the seeds of a grass, *Paspalum scrobiculatum,* of India.

passage (pas'ij) 1. a channel. 2. an evacuation of the bowels. 3. introduction of infectious material into an experimental animal or culture medium, followed by recovery of the infectious agent. 4. the act of moving from one place to another. 5. the introduction of a catheter, probe, sound, or bougie through a natural channel such as the urethra. **blind p.,** successive transfer of infection through experimental animals, chick embryo, or tissue culture, when overt lesions of disease are not apparent, at least in the earlier members of the series. **false p.,** an unnatural channel or meatus in a body structure, created by trauma or by disease. **serial p.,** the successive transfer of infection through a series of experimental animals by the inoculation of tissue, exudate, or other material containing the infectious agent.

Passavant's bar (cushion, pad, ridge) (pas'ah-vants) [Philip Gustav *Passavant,* German surgeon, 1815–1893] see under *bar.*

passenger (pas'en-jer) the fetus or any of the fetal membranes during labor.

Passiflora (pas"ĭ-flo'rah) [L. *passio* passion + *flos* flower] a genus of twining plants of the warmer parts of America; passion flower. Many species, e.g., *P. incarnata* L. (Passifloraceae), were formerly used medicinally for their sedative and anodyne properties.

passive (pas'iv) [L. *passivus*] neither spontaneous nor active; not produced by active efforts.

passivism (pas'ĭ-vizm) in psychiatry, sexual perversion with submission of the will to the partner.

passivity (pas-siv'ĭ-te) 1. in psychiatry, a state of dependency on others and of failure to take initiative or personal responsibility; the individual is more childlike than mature, as in the passive-dependent personality. Also, a state in which psychotic delusions of being influenced by others or by outside forces are experienced. 2. in dentistry, the condition of rest assumed by the teeth, surrounding tissue, and denture when a removable partial denture is in place but not under masticatory pressure.

Past. abbreviation for *Pasteurella.*

pasta (pas'tah), pl. *pas'tae* [L.] paste.

paste (pāst) [L. *pasta*] a semisolid preparation, generally for external use, of a fatty base, a viscous or mucilaginous base, or a mixture of starch and petrolatum. **aluminum p.,** a preparation of very finely powdered aluminum, liquid petrolatum, and zinc oxide ointment, used in dressing wounds, and applied topically to the skin around an intestinal stoma to prevent digestion. **arsenical p.,** a caustic paste containing arsenic. **bipp p.,** see *bipp.* **dextrinated p.,** a preparation of dextrin, glycerin, and distilled water, used as a vehicle. **Ihle's p.,** an ointment containing resorcin, starch, and zinc oxide in soft paraffin. **Lassar's p.,** zinc oxide and salicylic acid p. **Lassar's betanaphthol p.,** a paste containing betanaphthol, precipitated sulfur, soft soap, and petrolatum. **Lassar's plain zinc p.,** zinc oxide p. **Leunbach's p.,** a paste formerly used for injection into the uterus to induce abortion. **Morison's p.,** see under *method.* **Piffard's p.,** a paste made of copper sulfate, tartrated soda, and caustic soda, used in testing the urine for sugar. **triamcinolone acetonide dental p.** [USP], a preparation containing 90 to 115 per cent of the labeled amount of triamcinolone acetonide in a suitable emollient paste; used in the treatment of steroid-responsive oral inflammatory lesions and ulcerative lesions due to trauma, applied topically. **Vienna**

p., a caustic paste of potash and lime, applied for 10 to 15 minutes to the area to be cauterized. **zinc oxide p.** [USP], a preparation of zinc oxide and starch in white petrolatum, used topically as an astringent and protectant; called also *Lassar's plain zinc paste.* **zinc oxide and salicylic acid p.** [USP], **zinc oxide p. with salicylic acid,** a mixture of zinc oxide paste and salicylic acid, containing 23.5 to 25.5 per cent, by weight, of zinc oxide; used topically as an astringent and local protective. Called also *Lassar's p.* **zipp p.,** see *zipp.*

paster (pās'ter) the portion of a bifocal lens ground for near vision.

pastern (pas'tern) the portion of a horse's foot occupied by the first and second phalanges.

Pasteur's effect (reaction), method, solution (culture medium, fluid, liquid), theory (pas-terz') [Louis *Pasteur,* French chemist and bacteriologist, 1822–1895, who founded the science of microbiology and developed the technique of vaccination by attenuated virus, and whose discoveries embrace the entire field of microbial activity] see under *effect, method, solution,* and *theory.*

Pasteur-Chamberland filter (pas-ter'-shahm-ber-lah) [Louis *Pasteur;* Charles Edouard Chamberland, French bacteriologist, 1851–1908] see under *filter.*

Pasteurella (pas″tĕ-rel'ah) [Louis *Pasteur*] a genus of microorganisms of the family Brucellaceae, order Eubacteriales, made up of motile or nonmotile small, coccoid to rod-shaped, gram-negative cells occurring singly or in pairs, short chains, or groups. Many of the species in this genus have been reclassified as serotypes of *P. multocida.* **P. anapes'tifer,** an organism etiologically associated with septicemia in ducklings. **P. haemolyt'ica,** an etiologic agent of shipping fever in cattle and of mastitis in sheep. It is considered by some to be a separate species distinct from the *P. multocida* group. Called also *P. mastitis, P. haemolytica.* **P. multoci'da,** a species isolated from cattle, rabbits, fowl, sheep, and swine, which is the etiologic agent of the group of diseases known as the hemorrhagic septicemias. It is now considered that many species of *Pasteurella* are merely serotypes of *P. multocida.* Called also *P. septica.* **P. novi'cida,** *Francisella novicida.* **P. pes'tis,** *Yersinia pestis.* **P. pfaf'fii,** the etiologic agent of an epidemic septicemia in canaries, producing a necrotic enteritis. **P. pseudotuberculo'sis,** former name for *Yersinia pseudotuberculosis.* **P. sep'tica,** *P. multocida.* **P. septicae'miae,** an organism isolated from geese, and the cause of a fatal septicemia in young of the species. **P. tularen'sis** *Francisella tularensis.*

Pasteurelleae (pas″ter-el'e-e) a name formerly given a tribe of schizomycetes.

pasteurellosis (pas″ter-ĕ-lo'sis) infection by microorganisms of the genus *Pasteurella;* see individual species, under *Pasteurella.*

Pasteuria (pas-tu're-ah) a genus of microorganisms of the family Pasteuriaceae, order Hyphomicrobiales, made up of pear-shaped, nonmotile cells remaining attached in cauliflower-like masses, which are parasitic on fresh-water crustacea. The type species is *P. ramo'sa.*

Pasteuriaceae (pas-tu″re-a'se-e) a family of schizomycetes (order Hyphomicrobiales), made up of spherical or pear-shaped cells, sometimes growing on short stalks in a whorl-like arrangement. It includes two genera, *Blastocaulis* and *Pasteuria.*

pasteurization (pas″ter-i-za'shun) [Louis *Pasteur*] the process of heating milk or other liquids, e.g., urine, to a moderate temperature for a definite time, often to 60° C. for thirty minutes. This exposure kills most species of pathogenic bacteria and considerably delays other bacterial development.

pasteurizer (pas'ter-īz″er) an instrument used in effecting pasteurization.

Pastia's sign (lines) (pas'te-ahz) [C. *Pastia,* Rumanian physician] see under *sign.*

pastil (pas'til) pastille.

pastille (pas-tēl') [Fr.] 1. a troche in which the active ingredient is incorporated in a mass of sweetened gum, glycerin, and gelatin base. 2. an aromatic mass to be burnt as a fumigant. 3. a small disk of paper coated with platinocyanide of barium or other substance. The green color changes to brown when exposed to the roentgen ray. It was once used to estimate the amount of x-ray administered and also to test the intensity of ultraviolet radiation. **Sabouraud's p.,** a small disk of barium platinochloride with acetate of starch and collodion, used to indicate by change of color the strength of roentgen rays.

pasty (pās'te) like paste in consistency and color; puffy, pitting, or slightly edematous.

patch (pach) [L. *pittacium;* Gr. *pittakion*] an area differing from the rest of a surface, in either color or texture, or both, but not elevated above it; a macule more than 3 or 4 cm. in diameter. **Bitot's p's,** see under *spot.* **cottonwool p's,** see under *spot.* **gray p.,** the lesion of common ringworm (*Microsporum audouini*) of the scalp. **herald p.,** the initial lesion in pityriasis rosea, consisting of a solitary patch preceding the general eruption. **Hutchinson's p.,** a reddish or salmon-yellow patch of the cornea in syphilitic keratitis. **MacCallum's p.,** a sheet of granulation tissue in the deeper layers of the endocardium formed by extensive confluence of Aschoff nodules in the myocardium in rheumatic fever. **mucous p.,** a flat, rounded, grayish white erosion covered by a soggy membrane with an erythematous zone, occurring most often on the oral mucosa, and sometimes on the anogenital mucosa, in early active secondary syphilis. It contains vast numbers of treponemata and is therefore highly contagious. **Peyer's p's,** oval elevated areas of lymphoid tissue on the mucosa of the small intestine, composed of many lymphoid nodules closely packed together (folliculi lymphatici aggregati [NA]). **salmon p.,** a salmon-colored spot in the cornea in syphilis of that structure. **shagreen p.,** see under *skin.* **smokers' p.,** leukoplakia. **soldiers' p's,** milk spots, def. 1. **white p.,** a white opaque spot on the pericardium or on the capsule of the spleen, due to rubbing against a nodule of a rib in rachitis.

patchouli (pat-shoo'le) a labiate herb of India, *Pogostemon patchouli,* Pellet., used chiefly in perfumery and soaps.

patefaction (pat″ĕ-fak'shun) [L. *patefacere* to lay open] the act of laying open.

Patein's albumin (pat-anz') [*Patein,* French physician, died 1928] acetosoluble albumin.

patella (pah-tel'ah) [L., dim of *patera* a shallow dish] [NA] a triangular sesamoid bone, about 5 cm. in diameter, situated at the front of the knee in the tendon of insertion of the quadriceps extensor femoris muscle. Called also *knee cap.* **p. biparti'ta,** a patella that is divided into two parts. **p. cu'biti,** an anomalous sesamoid bone sometimes occurring over the extensor surface of the elbow joint. **floating p.,** a patella that is separated from the condyles by a large effusion in the knee. **p. parti'ta,** a patella that is divided into two or more parts. **slipping p.,** a patella that is easily movable and readily dislocated.

Patella's disease (pah-tel'ahz) [Vincenzo *Patella,* Italian physician, 1856–1928] see under *disease.*

patellapexy (pah-tel'ah-pek″se) [*patella* + Gr. *pēxis* fixation] the operation of suturing the patella to the lower end of the femur.

patellar (pah-tel'ar) [L. *patellarius*] of or pertaining to the patella.

patellectomy (pat″ĕ-lek'to-me) [*patella* + Gr. *ektomē* excision] excision or removal of the patella.

patelliform (pah-tel'ĭ-form) shaped like the patella.

patellofemoral (pah-tel'o-fem'o-ral) pertaining to the patella and the femur.

patellometer (pat″e-lom'ĕ-ter) [*patella* + Gr. *metron* measure] an instrument for measuring the patellar reflex.

patency (pa'ten-se) [L. *patens* open] the condition of being wide open.

patent (pa'tent) [L. *patens*] 1. open, unobstructed, or not closed. 2. apparent, evident.

Paterson's bodies, nodules [Robert *Paterson,* Scottish physician, 1814–1889] molluscum bodies.

Paterson's syndrome [Donald Rose *Paterson,* laryngologist in Cardiff (Wales), 1863–1939] Plummer-Vinson syndrome.

path (path) a particular course that is followed, or a route that is ordinarily traversed. In neurology, the set of nerve fibers along which a nervous impulse may move, whether esodic or exodic; particularly the intracranial or intraspinal portion of such a course. See also *pathway.* **condyle p.,** the course followed by the mandibular condyle in the temporomandibular joint during the various movements of the mandible. **copulation p.,** the course taken by the male and female pronuclei as they approach each other in a fertilized ovum. **generated occlusal p.,** a registration of the paths of movement of the occlusal surfaces of mandibular teeth on a plastic or abrasive surface attached to the maxillary arch. **incisor p.,** the course followed by the incisal edges of the lower anterior teeth in movement of the mandible from the position of normal occlusion to that of edge-to-edge contact with opposing incisors. **p. of insertion,** the direction in which a dental prosthesis is inserted in and removed from the mouth, seating and removing its attachments from the abutment teeth. **ionization p.,** the trail of ion pairs produced by ionizing radiation in its passage through matter; called also *ionization track.* **lateral condyle p.,** the path of the condyle in the glenoid fossa when a lateral mandibular movement is made. **milled-in p's,** 1. the contours carved by various mandibular movements into the occluding surface of an occlusion rim by teeth or studs placed in the opposing occlusion rim. The curves or contours may be carved into wax, modeling plastic, or plaster of Paris. 2. gliding movements of occlusion rims which are composed of materials, including abrasives. **occlusal p.,** the course followed by the occlusal surfaces of the lower teeth in movements of the mandible.

pathema (pah-the'mah), pl. *pathemas* or *pathem'ata* [Gr. *pathēma* disease] any disease state or morbid condition.

pathematology (path″ĕ-mah-tol'o-je) [*pathema* + -*logy*] (*obs.*) pathology, especially psychopathology.

pathergasia (path′er-ga″se-ah) [Gr. *pathos* disease + *ergasia* work] Meyer's term for mental malfunction, implying functional or structural damage and marked by abnormal behavior.

minor p's, minor somatic disorders and nervousness; minor psychoses or neuroses.

pathergia (pah-ther'je-ah)   pathergy.

pathergic (path'er-jik)   characterized by pathergy.

pathergization (path″er-ji-za'shun)   the process of becoming spontaneously or of being made pathergic.

pathergy (path'er-je) [Gr. *pathos* disease + *ergon* work]   1. a condition in which the application of a stimulus leaves the organism in a state in which it is unduly susceptible to subsequent stimuli of a different kind (Rössle). 2. the condition of being allergic to numerous antigens; polyvalent allergy.

pathetic (pah-thet'ik) [L. *patheticus;* Gr. *pathētikos*]   pertaining to the trochlear nerve.

pathfinder (path'find-er)   1. an instrument for locating strictures of the urethra. 2. a dental instrument for tracing the course of root canals. See *smooth broach,* under *broach.*

Pathilon   trademark for a preparation of tridihexethyl chloride.

patho- [Gr. *pathos* disease]   a combining form denoting relationship to disease.

pathoamine (path″o-am'in)   an amine causing disease, or formed as the product of a disease process; a ptomaine.

pathoanatomical (path″o-an″ah-tom'ĭ-kal)   pertaining to the anatomy of diseased tissues.

pathoanatomy (path″o-ah-nat'o-me)   pathologic anatomy.

pathobiology (path″o-bi-ol'o-je)   pathology.

pathobolism (pah-thob'o-lizm) [*patho-* + *metabolism*]   a condition of perverted metabolism of a disease nature.

Pathocil (path'o-sil)   trademark for a preparation of dicloxacillin sodium.

pathoclisis (path″o-klis'is)   a specific elemental sensitivity to specific toxins, or a specific affinity of certain toxins for certain systems of organs.

pathocrine (path'o-krin)   pertaining to pathocrinia.

pathocrinia (path″o-krin'e-ah) [*patho-* + endo*crine*]   disorder of endocrine function.

pathodontia (path″o-don'she-ah)   dental pathology.

pathoformic (path″o-for'mik) [*patho-* + L. *forma* form]   pertaining to the beginning of disease; said of symptoms at the beginning of mental disorder.

pathogen (path'o-jen) [*patho-* + Gr. *gennan* to produce]   any disease-producing microorganism.

pathogenesis (path″o-jen'ĕ-sis) [*patho-* + *genesis*]   the development of morbid conditions or of disease; more specifically the cellular events and reactions and other pathologic mechanisms occurring in the development of disease. **drug p.,** the production of symptoms of disease by the use of drugs.

pathogenesy (path″o-jen'ĕ-se)   pathogenesis.

pathogenetic (path″o-jĕ-net'ik)   pertaining to pathogenesis.

pathogenic (path-o-jen'ik)   giving origin to disease or to morbid symptoms.

pathogenicity (path″o-jĕ-nis'ĭ-te)   the quality of producing or the ability to produce pathologic changes or disease.

pathogeny (path-oj'ĕ-ne)   pathogenesis.

pathoglycemia (path″o-gli-se'me-ah) [*patho-* + Gr. *glykys* sweet + *haima* blood + *-ia*]   sugar in the blood (decreased carbohydrate tolerance) as a result of some disease.

pathognomonic (path″og-no-mon'ik) [*patho-* + Gr. *gnōmonikos* fit to give judgment]   specifically distinctive or characteristic of a disease or pathologic condition; a sign or symptom on which a diagnosis can be made.

pathognomy (path-og'no-me) [*patho-* + Gr. *gnōmē* a means of knowing]   the science of the signs and symptoms of disease.

pathognostic (path″og-nos'tik)   pathognomonic.

pathography (pah-thog'rah-fe) [*patho-* + Gr. *graphein* to write]   a history or description of disease.

pathoklisis (path″o-klis'is)   pathoclisis.

pathologic (path″o-loj'ik)   1. indicative of or caused by a morbid condition. 2. pertaining to pathology.

pathological (path″o-loj'ĭ-kal)   pertaining to pathology; pathologic.

pathologicoanatomic (path″o-loj″ĭ-ko-an-ah-tom'ik)   pertaining to pathologic anatomy.

pathologist (pah-thol'o-jist)   an expert in pathology. **speech p.,** a person skilled and certified in speech pathology.

pathology (pah-thol'o-je) [*patho-* + *-logy*]   1. that branch of medicine which treats of the essential nature of disease, especially of the structural and functional changes in tissues and organs of the body which cause or are caused by disease. 2. the structural and functional manifestations of disease. **cellular p.,** that which regards the cells as starting points of the phenomena of disease and that every cell descends from some preexisting cell (Virchow). **clinical p.,** pathology applied to the solution of clinical problems, especially the use of laboratory methods in clinical diagnosis. **comparative p.,** that which institutes comparisons between various diseases of the human body and

those of the lower animals. **dental p.,** the science which treats of disease of the teeth. Cf. *oral p.* **experimental p.,** the study of artificially induced disease processes. **functional p.,** the study of the changes of function due to morbid tissue changes. **general p.,** that which takes cognizance of pathologic conditions which may occur in various diseases and in different organs. **geographical p.,** pathology in its geographic and climatic relations. **humoral p.,** the opinion that disease is due to abnormal conditions of the fluids of the body. **internal p.,** medical p. **medical p.,** that which relates to morbid processes which are not accessible to operative intervention. Cf. *surgical p.* **mental p.,** psychopathology. **oral p.,** the science which treats of disease of the structures of the mouth, especially of the structural and functional changes which are caused by or which cause oral disease. **plant p.,** the pathology of diseases of plants. **solidistic p.,** that opinion which attributes disease to rarefaction or condensation of the solid tissues. **special p.,** the study of the pathology of particular diseases or organs. **speech p.,** a field of the health sciences dealing with the evaluation of speech, language, and voice disorders and the rehabilitation of patients with such disorders not amenable to medical or surgical treatment. **surgical p.,** the pathology of disease processes which are surgically accessible for diagnosis or treatment. **vegetable p.,** plant p.

patholysis (pah-thol'ĭ-sis) [*patho-* + Gr. *lysis* dissolution]   the dissolution of disease.

pathomaine (path'o-mān)   any of the pathogenic cadaveric alkaloids.

pathomania (path-o-ma'ne-ah) [*patho-* + Gr. *mania* madness]   moral insanity, i.e., mania without delirium.

pathometabolism (path″o-me-tab'o-lizm) [*patho-* + *metabolism*]   metabolism in disease.

pathometer (path-thom'ĕ-ter)   an apparatus for recording the incidence of disease in a given locality.

pathometry (path-thom'ĕ-tre) [*patho-* + Gr. *metrein* to measure]   (*obs.*) Sir Ronald Ross' term for the quantitative study of parasitic invasion and infection in individuals or groups of individuals.

pathomimesis (path″o-mi-me'sis) [*patho-* + Gr. *mimēsis* imitation]   malingering.

pathomimia (path″o-mim'e-ah)   malingering.

pathomimicry (path″o-mim'ĭ-kre)   malingering.

pathomorphism (path″o-mor'fizm)   perverted or abnormal morphology.

pathomorphology (path″o-mor-fol'o-je)   pathomorphism.

pathoneurosis (path″o-nu-ro'sis)   in psychoanalytic theory, a neurosis in which undue attention is given to a physical disorder; the libido is said to be inverted excessively in the diseased part.

pathonomia (path-o-no'me-ah) [*patho-* + Gr. *nomos* law]   the sum of knowledge regarding the laws of disease.

pathonomy (pah-thon'o-me)   pathonomia.

patho-occlusion (path″o-ŏ-kloo'zhun)   malocclusion.

pathophilia (path″o-fil'e-ah) [*patho-* + Gr. *philein* to love]   the condition in which a patient adapts himself and his mode of life to some chronic affection.

pathophoresis (path″o-fo-re'sis) [*patho-* + Gr. *phoros* bearing]   the transmission of disease.

pathophoric (path″o-for'ik)   pathophorous.

pathophorous (path-of'o-rus)   conveying or transmitting disease.

pathophysiology (path″o-fiz″e-ol'o-je)   the physiology of disordered function.

pathopoiesis (path″o-poi-e'sis) [*patho-* + Gr. *poiēsis* production]   1. the causation of disease. 2. the tendency of an individual to become diseased.

pathopsychology (path″o-si-kol'o-je) [*patho-* + *psychology*]   the psychology of mental disease.

pathopsychosis (path″o-si-ko'sis)   a psychosis arising from organic diseases, such as brain tumors, encephalitis, etc.

pathoradiography (path″o-ra″de-og'rah-fe)   pathoroentgenography.

pathoroentgenography (path″o-rent″gen-og'rah-fe)   the study of pathologic lesions by the roentgenogram.

pathosis (pah-tho'sis) [*patho-* + *-osis*]   a condition of disease; a morbid condition.

pathotropism (pah-thot'ro-pizm) [*patho-* + Gr. *tropos* a turning]   the tendency of drugs to pass to diseased areas.

pathway (path'wa)   a path or course, especially a course followed in the attainment of a specific end. In neurology, the nerve structures through which a sensory impression is conducted to the cerebral cortex (*afferent p.*) or through which an impulse passes from the brain to the skeletal musculature (*efferent p.*). See also *path.* Also used alone to indicate a sequence of reactions which convert one biological material to another (metabolic pathway). **alternative p.,** a pathway by which complement components C3 and C5 through C9 are activated without participation by C1, C2 and C4. Also known as the *properdin pathway,* it may be activated by human IgA, for example. **biosynthetic p.,** the sequence of enzymatic steps in the process by which a specific end-product is synthesized in a living organism; called also *anabolic p.* **Embden-Meyerhof p.** (of glucose metabolism), the series of enzymatic reactions in the anaerobic conversion of glucose to lactic acid, resulting in energy in the form of adenosine triphosphate (ATP). See Plate XLI. **Embden-Meyerhof-Parnas p.,** Embden-Meyerhof p. **final common p.,** the motor neurons by which nerve impulses from many central sources pass to a muscle or gland in the periphery. **internuncial p.,** a correlation tract connecting different centers or neurons within the central nervous system. **metabolic p.,** a series of enzymatic reactions that converts one biological material to another. **pentose phosphate p.,** a major branching of the Embden-Meyerhof pathway of carbohydrate metabolism: a pathway of hexose oxidation in which glucose-6-phosphate undergoes two successive oxidations by NADP, the final one being an oxidative decarboxylation to form a pentose phosphate. Called also *phosphogluconate p.*, *hexose monophosphate shunt*, and *pentose shunt.* **phosphogluconate p.,** pentose phosphate p. **reentrant p.,** a mechanism by which a premature or ectopic heart beat is coupled to the normal beat; see *reentry.*

-pathy (path′e) [Gr. *pathos* disease] a word termination denoting a morbid condition, or disease.

patient (pa′shent) [L. *patiens*] a person who is ill or who is undergoing treatment for disease.

Patrick's test (sign) (pat′riks) [Hugh Talbot *Patrick*, neurologist in Chicago, 1860–1938] see under *tests.*

patrilineal (pat″rĭ-lin′e-al) [L. *pater* father + *linea* line] descended through the male line.

patroclinous (pat″ro-kli′nus) [Gr. *patēr* father + *klinein* to incline] inheriting or inherited from the father; having characters inherited from the father. Cf. *matroclinous.*

patrogenesis (pat″ro-jen′ĕ-sis) [Gr. *patēr* father + *genesis*] androgenesis.

patten (pat′n) a metallic support to be worn under the sound foot in hip joint disease.

pattern (pat′ern) 1. a design to be followed or a device to be used in the construction or fabrication of something. 2. the particular design or arrangement of figures. 3. a characteristic set of traits or actions, as behavior patterns. **action p.,** the congenital or acquired manner in which certain stimuli produce certain actions in given individuals. **behavior p.,** the general grouping of behavior responses. **fixed action p.,** a sequence of stereotyped acts peculiar to a species, such as a courting dance. **muscle p.,** a number of muscles organized in a definite fashion and responding as a whole to a stimulus. **occlusal p.,** the form or design of the occluding surfaces of a tooth or teeth; these forms may be based upon natural or modified anatomic or nonanatomic concepts of teeth. **startle p.,** the various phenomena evidenced by an individual in reaction to a sudden, unexpected stimulus. **stimulus p.,** a group of stimuli resulting from a particular situation. **wax p.,** a form created in wax which, when invested and burned out, will produce a mold in which a positive reproduction of a structure can be cast; used in construction of dental inlays and crowns.

patulin (pat′u-lin) chemical name: 4-hydroxy-4*H*-furo-[3,2-*c*]pyran-2(6*H*)-one. A very toxic antibiotic substance, $C_7H_6O_4$, from cultures of various fungi, especially *Aspergillus* and *Penicillium;* used as an antimicrobial.

patulous (pat′u-lus) [L. *patulus*] spreading widely apart; open; distended.

paucibacillary (paw″se-bas′ĭ-ler-e) [L. *paucus* few] containing only a few bacilli.

paucine (paw′sin) a yellow, flaky alkaloid, $C_{27}H_{39}N_5O_5 \cdot 6\frac{1}{2}H_2O$, from the pauco nut, the fruit of *Pentaclethra macrophylla,* an African plant.

paucisynaptic (paw″sĕ-sin-ap′tik) [L. *paucus* few + *synaptic*] oligosynaptic.

Paul of Aegina (e-je′nah) (first half of 7th century) a celebrated Greek medical writer who practiced in Alexandria. Of his writings, only a seven-book compilation on medicine survives, the sixth book of which—on surgery—is of particular interest and importance.

Paul's test, treatment (pawlz) [Gustav *Paul,* Austrian physician, 1859–1935] see under *tests* and *treatment.*

Paul-Bunnell test (reaction) [John Rodman *Paul,* American physician, born 1893; Walls Willard *Bunnell,* American physician, born 1902] see under *tests.*

Paul-Mixter tube [Frank Thomas *Paul,* English surgeon, 1851–1941; Samuel Jason *Mixter,* Boston surgeon, 1855–1926] see under *tube.*

Paulus Aegineta (paw′lus ej″ĭ-ne′tah) see *Paul of Aegina.*

paunch (pawnch) rumen.

pause (pawz) an interruption, or rest. **compensatory p.,** the pause after a premature ventricular systole, related to blockage of one beat of the basic pacemaker.

pavementing (pāv′ment-ing) adhesion of leukocytes to the lining endothelium of the vessels of an injured part, which occurs when

the circulation slows down within the vessels in response to the inflammatory process.

Paveril (pav′er-il) trademark for preparations of dioxyline.

pavilion (pah-vil′yun) [L. *papilio* butterfly, tent] a dilated or flaring expansion at the end of a passage. **p. of the ear,** the auricle, def. 1. **p. of the oviduct,** the outer, or fimbriated, end of the fallopian or uterine tube. **p. of the pelvis,** the upper, flaring portion of the pelvis.

Pavlov's method, pouch, stomach (pahv′lovz) [Ivan Petrovich *Pavlov,* Russian physiologist, 1849– 1936; winner of the Nobel prize for medicine in 1904] see under *method, pouch,* and *stomach.*

pavor (pa′vor) [L.] terror. **p. diur′nus** [L. "day terrors"], attacks of fear in children occurring during the afternoon nap. **p. noctur′nus** [L. "night terrors"], a nightmare of children which causes them to cry out in fright and awake in panic.

Pavulon (pav′u-lon) trademark for a preparation of pancuronium bromide.

Pavy's disease (pa′vēz) [Frederick William *Pavy,* English physician, 1829–1911] cyclic proteinuria.

Pawlik's triangle (trigone) (pahv′liks) [Karel J. *Pawlik,* gynecologist in Prague, 1849–1914] see under *triangle.*

pawpaw (paw′paw) papaw, def. 2.

Payr's clamp, disease, method (pīrz) [Erwin *Payr,* German surgeon, 1871–1946] see under *clamp, disease,* and *method.*

pazoxide (pah-zok′sīd) chemical name: 6,7-dichloro-3-(3-cyclopenten-1-yl)-1,2,4-benzothiadiazine 1,1-dioxide; an antihypertensive, $C_{12}H_{10}Cl_2N_2O_2S.$

P.B. abbreviation for *Pharmacopoeia Britannica,* British Pharmacopoeia.

Pb chemical symbol for *lead* [L. *plumbum*].

Pb(C₂H₃O₂)₂ lead acetate.

$PbCO_3$ lead carbonate.

$PbCrO_4$ lead chromate.

PBE abbreviation for German *Perlsucht Bacillenemulsion,* a form of tuberculin prepared from a culture of bacilli of bovine tuberculosis.

PBI protein-bound iodine.

PbI_2 lead iodide.

$Pb(NO_3)_2$ lead nitrate.

PbO lead monoxide.

PbO_2 lead dioxide.

PbS lead sulfide.

$PbSO_4$ lead sulfate.

PBZ pyribenzamine.

PC phosphocreatine; sometimes used to designate phosphatidyl choline, or palmitoyl carnitine.

P.C. abbreviation for L. *pon′dus civi′le,* avoirdupois weight.

p.c. abbreviation for L. *post ci′bum,* after meals.

pc. picocurie.

PCA passive cutaneous anaphylaxis; see under *anaphylaxis.*

PCB polychlorinated biphenyl; see under *biphenyl.*

PcB abbreviation for *near point of convergence to the intercentral base line.*

P.Cc. periscopic concave.

PCG phonocardiogram.

P.C.M.O. Principal Colonial Medical Officer.

PCO_2 symbol for *carbon dioxide partial pressure* or *tension;* also written P_{CO_2}, pCO_2, and pCO_2.

Pcs. preconscious.

PCV packed cell volume; see under *volume.*

P.Cx. periscopic convex.

P.D. interpupillary distance.

Pd chemical symbol for *palladium.*

p.d. prism diopter; papilla diameter; pupillary distance.

peak (pēk) the top or upper limit of a graphic tracing or of any variable. **Bragg p. of proton beam,** the end of range of a beam of protons aimed from a cyclotron in nearly a straight line. **kilovolt p.,** the maximum amount of voltage that an x-ray machine is using; abbreviated kvp.

Péan's forceps, operation (pa-anz′) [Jules Émile *Péan,* French surgeon, 1830–1898] see under *operation.*

pearl (perl) 1. a small calcareous concretion from various species of mollusks, formerly regarded as having curative powers. 2. a small medicated granule, or a glass globule with a single dose of volatile medicine, as amyl nitrite. 3. a rounded mass of tough sputum as seen in the early stages of an attack of bronchial asthma. **Bohn's epithelial p's,** small retention cysts in the mouths of infants. **Elschnig's p's,** see under *body.* **enamel p.,** enameloma. **epidermic p's, epithelial p's,** rounded concentric masses of epithelial cells found in certain papillomas and epitheliomas; called also *pearly bodies.* **Epstein's p's,** small whitish-yellow masses on either side of the raphe of the hard palate of the newborn. **gouty p.,** a sodium

Plate XLI   pathway

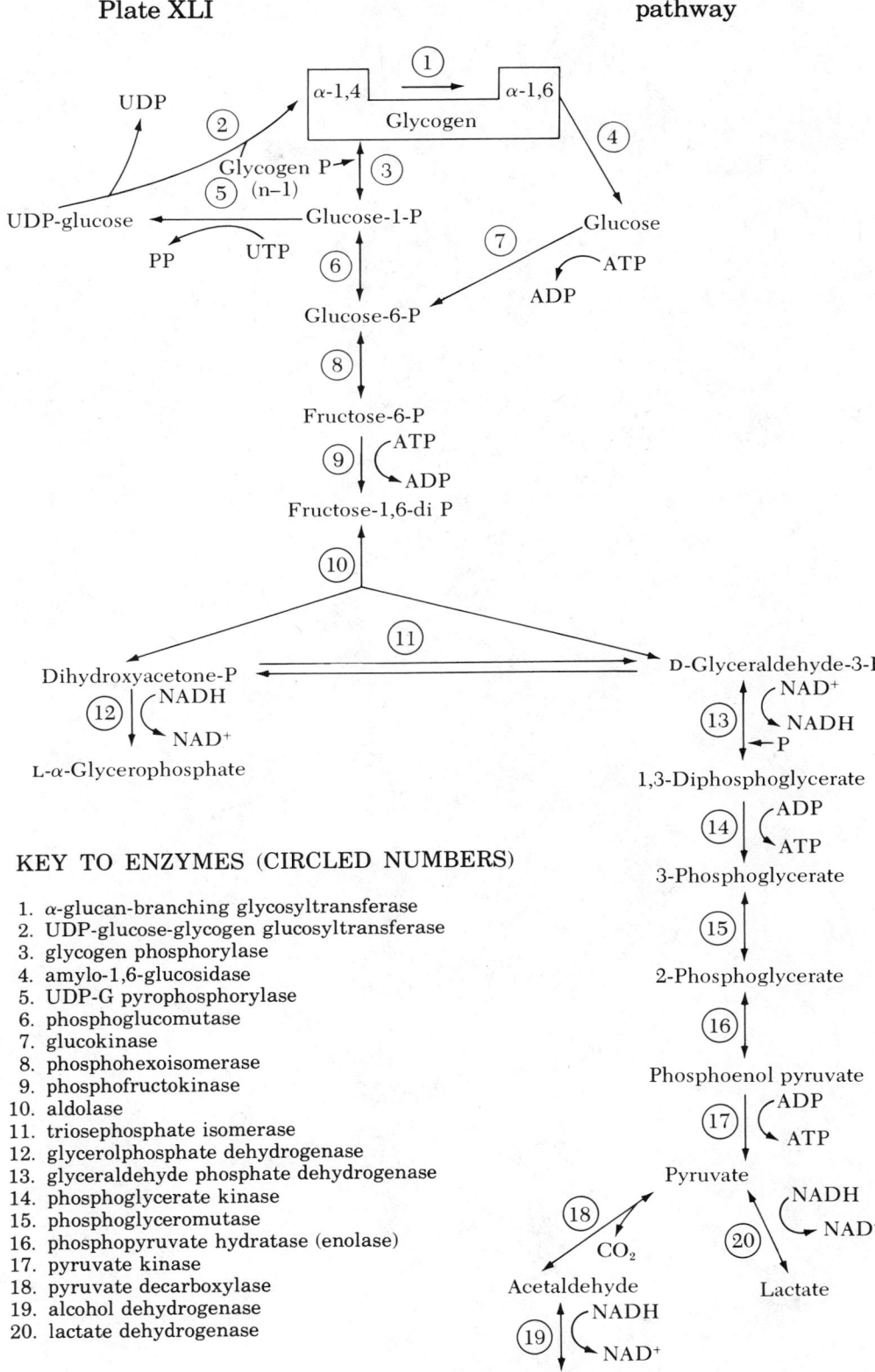

KEY TO ENZYMES (CIRCLED NUMBERS)

1. α-glucan-branching glycosyltransferase
2. UDP-glucose-glycogen glucosyltransferase
3. glycogen phosphorylase
4. amylo-1,6-glucosidase
5. UDP-G pyrophosphorylase
6. phosphoglucomutase
7. glucokinase
8. phosphohexoisomerase
9. phosphofructokinase
10. aldolase
11. triosephosphate isomerase
12. glycerolphosphate dehydrogenase
13. glyceraldehyde phosphate dehydrogenase
14. phosphoglycerate kinase
15. phosphoglyceromutase
16. phosphopyruvate hydratase (enolase)
17. pyruvate kinase
18. pyruvate decarboxylase
19. alcohol dehydrogenase
20. lactate dehydrogenase

EMBDEN-MEYERHOF PATHWAY OF GLUCOSE METABOLISM

(after Mazur and Harrow)

urate concretion on the cartilage of the ear in gouty persons. **Laennec's p's,** soft casts of the smaller bronchial tubes expectorated in bronchial asthma.

pearlash (perl'ash) impure potassium carbonate in crystals.

peat (pēt) carbonized vegetable matter found in bogs; used in peat baths and as a dry absorbent dressing.

peau (po) [Fr.] skin. **p. de chagrin** (po''duh shah-grin') [Fr.], shagreen skin. **p. d'orange** (po''do-rahnj') [Fr. "orange skin"], a dimpled condition of the skin, resembling that of an orange.

pebble (peb'l) a kind of rock crystal from which lenses are sometimes cut.

pébrine (pa-brēn') [Fr.] an infectious disease of silkworms caused by *Nosema bombycis*. Cf. *nosema disease*.

pecazine (pe'kah-zēn) mepazine.

peccant (pek'ant) [L. *peccans* sinning] unhealthy; causing illness or disease.

peccatiphobia (pek''kah-tĭ-fo'be-ah) [L. *peccata*, sins + *phobia*] morbid fear of sinning.

pechyagra (pek''e-a'grah) [Gr. *pēchys* forearm + *agra* seizure] gout of the elbow.

pecilo- for words beginning thus, see those beginning *poikilo-*.

Pecquet's cistern (reservoir), duct (pek-āz') [Jean *Pecquet*, French anatomist, 1622–1674] see *cisterna chyli* and *ductus thoracicus*.

pectase (pek'tās) pectinesterase.

pecten (pek'ten), pl. *pec'tines* [L.] 1. a comb; applied to certain anatomical structures because of a fancied resemblance to a comb. 2. a name given by Stroud, in 1895, to a narrow zone in the anal canal, bounded above by the pectinate line and possessing a comparatively dense connective tissue matrix with thick muscular and elastic components. 3. a triangular pleated membrane in the eye of birds, extending forward from the optic disk, which it covers, for a variable distance into the vitreous body. **p. os'sis pu'bis** [NA], the anterior border of the superior ramus of the pubis, beginning at the pubic tubercle and continuing to the iliopubic eminence; called also *pectineal line*.

pectenine (pek'tĕ-nin) a poisonous alkaloidal compound from a Mexican cactus, *Cereus pecten*.

pectenitis (pek''tĕ-ni'tis) inflammation of the pecten of the anus.

pectenosis (pek''tĕ-no'sis) stenosis of the anal canal caused by a rigid, inelastic ring of tissue of variable width and thickness, between the anal groove and anal crypts, producing pain on defecation, bleeding, and anal irritation.

pectenotomy (pek''tĕ-not'o-me) [*pecten* + Gr. *tomē* a cutting] surgical correction of pectenosis by incision of the ring of tissue causing it.

pectic (pek'tik) relating to pectin.

pectin (pek'tin) [Gr. *pēktos* congealed] a homosaccharidic polymer of sugar acids of fruit that forms gels with sugar at the proper pH. A purified form [USP] obtained from the acid extract of the inner portion of the rind of citrus fruits or from apple pomace is used as the protective component of various formulations employed in the treatment of diarrhea and as a suspending agent in pharmaceutical preparations. It is also used in the preparation of certain foods, such as jams and jellies.

pectinase (pek'tĭ-nās) polygalacturonase.

pectinate (pek'tĭ-nāt) [L. *pecten* comb] shaped like a comb.

pectineal (pek-tin'e-al) [L. *pecten*, comb, pubes] pertaining to the os pubis.

pectinesterase (pek''tin-es'ter-ās) pectin pectyl-hydrolase: an enzyme that catalyzes the hydrolysis of methyl ester groups of pectic substances, releasing the free acid.

pectiniform (pek-tin'ĭ-form) [L. *pecten* comb + *forma* form] comb-shaped.

pectization (pek''ti-za'shun) [Gr. *pēktikos* curdling] coagulation or gelatinization; a term used in colloidal chemistry.

pectolytic (pek''to-lit'ik) [*pectin* + Gr. *lytikos* dissolving] capable of effecting the digestion of pectin.

pectoral (pek'to-ral) [L. *pectoralis*] 1. of, or pertaining to, the breast or chest. 2. relieving disorders of the respiratory tract, as an expectorant.

pectoralgia (pek''to-ral'je-ah) [L. *pectus* breast + -*algia*] pain in the breast or pectoral muscles.

pectoralis (pek''to-ra'lis) [L.] pertaining to the breast or chest.

pectoriloquy (pek''to-ril'o-kwe) [L. *pectus* breast + *loqui* to speak] transmission of the sound of spoken words through the chest wall. **aphonic p.,** the sound of the whispered voice transmitted through a serous, but not through a purulent, exudate within the pleura. **whispered p., whispering p.,** the transmission of the sound of whispered words through the walls of the chest.

pectorophony (pek''to-rof'o-ne) [L. *pectus* breast + Gr. *phōnē* voice] exaggeration of the vocal resonance heard on auscultation.

pectose (pek'tōs) a principle in unripe fruits and plants from which pectin is derived.

pectous (pek'tus) pertaining to, composed of, or resembling pectin; having a firm, jelly-like consistence.

pectunculus (pek-tung'ku-lus) [L., dim of *pecten* comb] any one of the series of small longitudinal ridges on the aqueduct of Sylvius.

pectus (pek'tus) [L.] the breast: the chest or thorax. **p. carina'tum** [L. "keeled breast"], undue prominence of the sternum; called also *chicken* or *pigeon breast*. **p. excava'tum** [L. "hollowed breast"], undue depression of the sternum; called also *funnel breast* or *chest*. **p. gallina'tum,** p. carinatum. **p. recurva'tum,** p. excavatum.

pedal (ped'al) [L. *pedalis; pes* foot] pertaining to the foot or feet.

pedarthrocace (pe-dar-throk'ah-se) [Gr. *pais* child + *arthrocace*] caries of the joints in children.

pedatrophia (pe-dah-tro'fe-ah) [Gr. *pais* child + *atrophia*] 1. marasmus. 2. (*obs.*) tabes mesenterica.

pederast (ped'er-ast) one who practices pederasty.

pederasty (ped'er-as''te) [Gr. *pais* boy + *erastēs* lover] homosexual anal intercourse between men and boys, the latter as the passive partners.

pederin (ped'er-in) a crystalline toxin, $C_{25}H_{45}NO_9$, isolated from blister beetles of the genus *Paederus*.

pederosis (pe''der-o'sis) pedophilia.

pedes (pe'dēz) [L.] plural of *pes*.

pedia- [Gr. *pais, paidos* child] a combining form denoting relationship to a child. Cf. *pedo-*(1).

pediadontia (pe''de-ah-don'she-ah) pedodontics.

pediadontist (pe''de-ah-don'tist) pedodontist.

pediadontology (pe''de-ah-don-tol'o-je) pedodontics.

Pediaflor (pe'de-ah-floor) trademark for a preparation of sodium fluoride.

pedialgia (ped''e-al'je-ah) [L. *pes* foot + -*algia*] neuralgic pain in the foot.

Pediamycin (pe''de-ah-mi'sin) trademark for preparations of erythromycin ethylsuccinate.

pediatric (pe''de-at'rik) pertaining to pediatrics.

pediatrician (pe''de-ah-trish'un) a physician who specializes in pediatrics.

pediatrics (pe''de-at'riks) [*pedia-* + Gr. *iatrikē* surgery, medicine] that branch of medicine which treats of the child and its development and care and of the diseases of children and their treatment.

pediatrist (pe''de-at'rist) pediatrician.

pediatry (pe'de-at''re) pediatrics.

pedication (ped''ĭ-ka'shun) pederasty.

pedicel (ped'ĭ-sel) a footlike part, especially any of the secondary processes of a podocyte which interdigitate with those of other podocytes in a renal corpuscle.

pedicellate, pedicellated (pĕ-dis'ĭ-lāt; ped'ĭ-sel-āt''ed) pediculate; pedunculated.

pedicellation (ped''ĭ-sel-la'shun) the development or possession of a pedicle.

pedicle (ped'ĭ-k'l) a footlike, stemlike, or narrow basal part or structure, as the stalk by which a nonsessile tumor is attached to normal tissue, or the narrow strip of flap tissue through which it receives its blood supply. **cone p.,** the thick triangular or club-shaped ending of a retinal cone cell, which synapses with the bipolar and horizontal cells in the outer plexiform layer. **p. of vertebral arch,** pediculus arcus vertebrae.

pedicled (ped'ĭ-k'ld) having a pedicle.

pedicterus (pe-dik'ter-us) [*pedo-* + Gr. *ikteros* jaundice] (*obs.*) icterus neonatorum.

pedicular (pe-dik'u-lar) [L. *pedicularis*] pertaining to or caused by lice.

pediculate (pe-dik'u-lāt) [L. *pediculatus*] provided with a pedicle; pedunculated.

pediculation (pe-dik''u-la'shun) [L. *pediculatio*] 1. infestation with lice. 2. the formation of a pedicle.

pediculi (pe-dik'u-li) plural of *pediculus*.

pediculicide (pe-dik'u-lĭ-sīd) [*pediculus* + L. *caedere* to kill] 1. destroying lice. 2. an agent that destroys lice.

Pediculidae (ped''i-ku'li-de) a family of lice (order Anoplura) that includes the genera Pediculus and Phthirus, which feed on human blood.

Pediculoides (pe-dik''u-loi'dēz) former name for *Pyemotes*. **P. ventrico'sus,** *Pyemotes ventricosus*.

pediculosis (pe-dik''u-lo'sis) [*pediculus* + -*osis*] infestation with lice of the family Pediculidae, especially infestation with *Pediculus humanus*. **p. capillit'ii, p. cap'itis,** infestation of the hair of the head by lice. **p. cor'poris,** infestation of the body by lice. **p. inguina'lis,** phthiriasis inguinalis. **p. palpebra'rum,** infestation of the eyelashes by lice. **p. pu'bis,** phthiriasis inguinalis. **p. vestimen'ti, p. vestimento'rum,** infestation of the clothing by lice.

pediculous (pe-dik'u-lus) infested with lice.

Pediculus (pe-dik′u-lus) a genus of sucking lice of the family Pediculidae, order Anoplura, the sucking lice. **P. huma′nus,** a species that feeds on human blood, is a major vector of epidemic typhus, trench fever, and relapsing fever, and causes skin reactions, especially in sensitized persons. It includes two subspecies, *P. humanus capitis* and *P. humanus corporis.* **P. huma′nus cap′itis,** the head louse, found on the scalp hair. **P. huma′nus cor′poris,** the body or clothes louse, which lives on the clothing when feeding; it is not taking place; called also *P. humanus humanus, P. humanus vestimento′rum,* and *P. vestimenti.* **P. huma′nus huma′nus,** *P. humanus corporis.* **P. huma′nus vestimento′rum,** *P. humanus corporis.* **P. inguina′lis, P. pu′bis,** *Phthirus pubis.* **P. vestimen′ti,** *P. humanus corporis.*

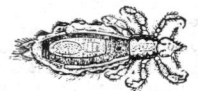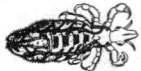

Pediculus humanus.

pediculus (pe-dik′u-lus), pl. *pedic′uli* [L.] 1. louse. 2. a footlike or stemlike part; called also *pedicle.* **p. ar′cus ver′tebrae** [NA], pedicle of vertebral arch: one of the paired parts of the vertebral arch that connect a lamina to the vertebral body; called also *radix arcus vertebrae.*

pedicure (ped′ĭ-kūr) [L. *pes* foot + *cura* care] 1. professional care and treatment of the feet. 2. a podiatrist.

pedigree (ped′ĭ-gre′) [L. *pedis* foot + *dē* of + *grūs* crane] a table, chart, diagram, or list of an individual's ancestors, used in human genetics in the analysis of mendelian inheritance.

pediluvium (ped″ĭ-lu′ve-um) [L. *pes* foot + *luere* to wash] a foot bath.

Pediococcus (pe″de-o-kok′us) in some systems of classification, a genus of microaerophilic, saprophytic, gram-positive, nonmotile cocci, usually occurring in pairs or tetrads, found most commonly in fermenting plant products; in other systems of classification, assigned to the family Streptococcaceae. **P. acidilacti′ci,** a species found in sauerkraut and fermenting mashes. **P. cerevi′siae,** a species found in spoiled beer and brewer's yeast. **P. pentosa′ceus,** a species occurring commonly in fermenting products, such as pickles, sauerkraut, etc. **P. halophi′lus,** a species found in anchovies and soy mash. **P. uri′nae-equi,** a species originally isolated from horse urine, which is often found in brewer's yeast.

pediodontia (pe″de-o-don′she-ah) pedodontics.

pedionalgia (pe″de-o-nal′je-ah) [Gr. *pedion* metatarsus + *-algia* pain] pain in the sole of the foot.

pediphalanx (ped″ĭ-fa′lanks) [L. *pes* foot + *phalanx*] a phalanx of a digit of the foot.

pedistibulum (ped″ĭ-stib′u-lum) [L.] the stapes.

peditis (pe-di′tis) [L. *pes* foot + *-itis*] pedal osteitis.

pedo- 1. [Gr. *pais, paidos* child] a combining form denoting relationship to a child. 2. [L. *pes, pedis* foot] a combining form denoting relationship to a foot.

pedodontia (pe″do-don′she-ah) pedodontics.

pedodontics (pe-do-don′tiks) [pedo(1) + Gr. *odous* tooth] the branch of dentistry concerned with the diagnosis and treatment of conditions of the teeth and mouth in children.

pedodontist (pe-do-don′tist) a dentist who specializes in pedodontics.

pedodynamometer (ped″o-di-nah-mom′ĕ-ter) [pedo(2) + *dynamometer*] an instrument for measuring the strength of a leg.

pedogamy (pe-dog′ah-me) [pedo(1) + Gr. *gamos* marriage] endogamy, def. 1.

pedogenesis (pe″do-jen′ĕ-sis) [pedo(1) + Gr. *genesis* reproduction] the production of offspring by young or larval forms.

pedograph (ped′o-graf) [pedo(2) + Gr. *graphein* to write] an imprint on paper of the weight-bearing surface of the foot, surrounded by a pencil-marked contour of the upper foot.

pedologist (pe-dol′o-gist) a specialist in pedology.

pedology (pe-dol′o-je) [pedo(1) + *-logy*] the systematical study of the life and development of children.

pedometer (pe-dom′ĕ-ter) [pedo- + Gr. *metron* measure] 1. an instrument for recording the number of steps taken in walking. 2. (*obs.*), an instrument for measuring infants.

pedomorphic (pe″do-mor′fik) pertaining to or characterized by pedomorphism.

pedomorphism (pe″do-mor′fizm) [pedo(1) + Gr. *morphē* form + *-ism*] the retention in the adult organism of highly progressive species of bodily characters which at an earlier stage of evolutionary history were actually only infantile.

pedopathy (pe-dop′ah-the) [pedo(2) + Gr. *pathos* disease] any disease of the foot.

pedophilia (pe″do-fil′e-ah) [pedo(1) + Gr. *philein* to love] abnormal fondness for children; sexual activity of adults with

children as the objects. Called also *p. erotica* and *pederosis.* **p. erot′ica,** pedophilia.

pedophilic (pe″do-fil′ik) 1. fond of children. 2. pertaining to or characterized by pedophilia.

pedophobia (pe″do-fo′be-ah) [pedo(1) + Gr. *phobein* to be affrighted by] fear or dread of children.

pedorthic (pĕ-dor′thik) pertaining to pedorthics.

pedorthics (pĕ-dor′thiks) [L. *pedis* foot + Gr. *orthōsis* making straight] the design, manufacture, fit, and modification of shoes and related foot appliances as prescribed for amelioration of painful and/or disabling conditions of the foot and limb.

pedorthist (pĕ-dor′thist) a person skilled in pedorthics and practicing its application in individual cases.

peduncle (pĕ-dung′k′l) a stemlike connecting part (called also *pedunculus* [NA]); the stalk by which a nonsessile tumor is attached to normal tissue. **cerebellar p., inferior,** pedunculus cerebellaris inferior. **cerebellar p., middle,** pedunculus cerebellaris medius. **cerebellar p., superior,** pedunculus cerebellaris superior. **cerebral p.,** pedunculus cerebri. **p. of flocculus,** pedunculus flocculi. **p. of hypophysis** (*obs.*), infundibulum hypothalami. **olfactory p.,** in comparative neuroanatomy, the olfactory stalk, especially the region of its attachment to the cerebral hemisphere. **pineal p., p. of pineal body,** habenula, def. 2. **p. of thalamus, inferior,** pedunculus thalami inferior.

peduncular (pĕ-dung′ku-lar) pertaining to a peduncle.

pedunculated (pĕ-dung′ku-lāt-ed) provided with a peduncle; opposed to sessile.

pedunculotomy (pĕ-dung″ku-lot′o-me) [L. *pedunculus* + Gr. *tomē* a cutting] incision of a cerebral peduncle, with division of both pyramidal and nonpyramidal fibers, for relief of the tremor of parkinsonism.

pedunculus (pĕ-dung′ku-lus) [L.] a stemlike part; [NA] a general term for collections of nerve fibers coursing between different areas in the central nervous system. Called also *peduncle.* **p. cerebella′ris infe′rior** [NA], inferior cerebellar peduncle: a large bundle of nerve fibers serving to connect the medulla oblongata and spinal cord with the cerebellum (especially the archicerebellum and paleocerebellum); it courses along the lateral border of the fourth ventricle and turns dorsally into the cerebellum. Called also *corpus restiforme* or *restiform body.* **p. cerebella′ris me′dius** [NA], middle cerebellar peduncle: a fiber tract originating in the contralateral pontine nuclei and entering the cerebellum, conveying impulses from the cerebral cortex to the neocerebellum; it is continuous with the pons at the line of attachment of the trigeminal nerve. Called also *brachium pontis.* **p. cerebella′ris supe′rior** [NA], superior cerebellar peduncle: a large fiber bundle arising chiefly in the dentate nucleus of each cerebellar hemisphere (neocerebellum) and ascending to decussate in the mesencephalon; its fibers end mostly in the red nucleus and thalamus. Spinocerebellar fibers to the paleocerebellum lie adjacent to each peduncle. Called also *brachium conjunctivum* [*cerebelli*]. **p. cer′ebri** [NA], cerebral peduncle: the ventral half of the mesencephalon; it is divisible into the tegmental, or dorsal, part and the crus cerebri, or ventral part, which are separated by the substantia nigra. Called also *caudex cerebri.* **p. cor′poris callo′si** (*obs.*), gyrus paraterminalis. **p. cor′poris pinea′lis,** habenula, def. 2. **p. floc′culi** [NA], peduncle of flocculus: the lateral expansion of the inferior medullary velum toward the flocculus. **p. thal′ami infe′rior** [NA], inferior peduncle of thalamus: a bundle of fibers forming one of the principal components of the ansa peduncularis; it curves around the medial margin of the internal capsule and turns dorsally into the thalamus.

peel (pēl) [L. *pilare* to deprive of hair] the outer rind of a fruit. **bitter orange p.** [NF], the dried rind of unripe but fully grown fruit of *Citrus aurantium* Linné, used as a pharmaceutical flavoring agent. **lemon p.,** the outer, yellow rind of the fresh ripe fruit of *Citrus limon,* used in preparing lemon oil and lemon tincture.

peenash (pe′nash) [India] rhinitis due to the presence of insect larvae in the nose.

PEEP positive end-expiratory pressure; see under *pressure.*

PEG pneumoencephalography.

peg (peg) a projecting structure. **rete p's,** the inward projections of the epidermis into the dermis at the dermoepidermal junction, as seen histologically in vertical sections.

Peganone (peg′ah-nōn) trademark for a preparation of ethotoin.

peglicol 5 oleate (pĕ-gli′kōl) a product obtained by alcoholysis of natural vegetable oils in the presence of polyethylene glycols of molecular weights between 200 and 400, consisting of a mixture of partially mixed esters of glycerin and these polyethylene glycols; the average number of ethylene glycol units is 5. It is used as an emulsifying agent in pharmaceutical preparations. Called also *polyoxyl 5 oleate.*

pegology (pe-gol′o-je) [Gr. *pēgē* fountain + *-logy*] the study of springs, particularly medicinal or mineral springs.

pegoterate (peg″o-ter′āt) a condensation polymer used as a suspending agent in pharmaceutical preparations.

pegoxol 7 stearate (peg-ok′sŏl) a mixture of mono- and distearic esters of ethylene glycol and of polyoxyethylene glycol, the latter having an average molecular weight of 450; the average number of ethylene glycol units is 7. It is used as an emulsifying agent in pharmaceutical preparations.

peinotherapy (pi″no-ther′ah-pe) [Gr. *peina* hunger + *therapeia* cure] hunger cure.

Pel's crises (pelz) [Pieter Klaases *Pel*, Dutch physician, 1852–1919] see under *crisis*.

Pel-Ebstein disease, fever (pyrexia, symptom) (pel-eb′stīn) [Pieter Klaases *Pel;* Wilhelm *Ebstein,* German physician, 1836–1912] see *Hodgkin's disease,* under *disease,* and see under *fever*

pelade (pel-ad′) [Fr.] alopecia areata.

pelage (pel′ij, pĕ-lahzh′) [Fr.] the hairy coat of mammals; the hairs of the body, limbs, and head collectively.

pelagic (pe-laj′ik) [Gr. *pelagios* living in the sea] pertaining to or inhabiting open, offshore waters, as in midocean.

pelagism (pel′ah-jism) seasickness.

Pelamis (pel′ah-mis) a genus of sea snakes. **P. bico′lor,** a poisonous sea snake of the Indian ocean.

Pelecypoda (pel″e-sip′o-dah) [Gr. *pelekys* hatchet + *podos* foot] the bivalves: a class of mollusks which are laterally compressed and have a pair of dorsally hinged lateral shells (valves) and a hatchet-shaped foot for digging; it includes the clams, oysters, and scallops. Called also *Bivalvia.*

Pelger's nuclear anomaly (pel′gerz) [Karel *Pelger,* Dutch physician, 1885–1931] see under *anomaly.*

Pelger-Huët nuclear anomaly (pel′ger-hyoo′et) [Karel *Pelger;* G. J. *Huët,* Dutch physician, born 1879] see under *anomaly.*

pelidisi (pel″ĭ-de′se) [term coined from L. *pondus decies linearis divisus sidentis* (altitudo) meaning weight ten line divided sitting height] the unit of Pirquet's index for determining the nutritive condition of children. It is obtained by dividing the cube root of ten times the weight (in grams) by the sitting height (in centimeters). A pelidisi of 94 or less indicates undernutrition; of 95–100, good nutrition, and of 101 or above, overnutrition.

peliosis (pe″le-o′sis) [Gr. *peliōsis* extravasation of blood] purpura. **p. hep′atis, p. of liver,** mottled blue liver, caused by blood-filled lacunae in the parenchyma.

Pelizaeus-Merzbacher disease (pa″le-zi′us- merz′bak-er) [Friedrich *Pelizaeus,* German physician, 1850–1917; Ludwig *Merzbacher,* German physician in Buenos Aires, born 1875] familial centrolobar sclerosis.

pellagra (pĕ-la′grah, pĕ-lag′rah) [It. *pelle* skin + *agra* rough] a clinical deficiency syndrome due to deficiency of niacin (or failure to convert tryptophan to niacin) and characterized by dermatitis, inflammation of mucous membranes, diarrhea, and psychic disturbances. The dermatitis occurs on the portions of the body exposed to light or trauma. Mental symptoms include depression, irritability, anxiety, confusion, disorientation, delusions, and hallucinations. **monkey p.,** a condition in caged monkeys manifested by loss of appetite, diarrhea, vomiting, emaciation, and finally death. **p. si′ne pella′gra,** pellagra in which the characteristic dermatitis is not present. **typhoid p.,** pellagra characterized by continued high temperature.

pellagragenic (pĕ-lag″rah-jen′ik) causing pellagra.

pellagral (pĕ-lag′ral) pertaining to or caused by pellagra.

pellagramin (pĕ-lag′rah-min) niacin.

pellagrazein (pel″ah-gra′ze-in) a poisonous ptomaine from damaged maize, formerly regarded as a probable cause of pellagra.

pellagrin (pĕ-la′grin, pĕ-lag′rin) a person affected with pellagra.

pellagrocein (pel″ah-gro′se-in) pellagrazein.

pellagroid (pĕ-lag′roid) a condition resembling pellagra.

pellagrologist (pel″ah-grol′o-jist) one who makes a special study of pellagra.

pellagrology (pel″ah-grol′o-je) the study of pellagra.

pellagrose (pĕ-lag′rōs) pellagrous.

pellagrosis (pel″ah-gro′sis) the dermal syndrome of pellagra characterized by skin pigmentation, erythema, and hyperkeratosis.

pellagrous (pĕ-lag′rus) affected with or of the nature of pellagra.

pellant (pel′ant) [L. *pellere* to drive] depurative.

pellate (pel′āt) to repel or tend to separate.

Pellegrini's disease (pel″a-gre′nēz) [Augusto *Pellegrini,* surgeon in Italy] see under *disease.*

Pellegrini-Stieda disease (pel″a-gre′ne-ste′dah) [A. *Pellegrini;* Alfred *Stieda,* German surgeon, born 1869–1945] see *Pellegrini's disease* under *disease.*

pellet (pel′et) a small pill or granule, such as a small rod- or ovoid-shaped, sterile mass composed of essentially pure steroid hormones, to be implanted under the skin to provide for their slow absorption, or a small pill made from sucrose and impregnated with a medicine, used in homeopathic practice.

pellicle (pel′ĭ-k'l) [L. *pellicula*] a thin skin or film, such as a thin film on the surface of a liquid. **brown p.,** a brownish gray to black film formed over a period of time on the surfaces of the teeth, resulting from the use of dentifrices that do not contain abrasives.

pellicular, pelliculous (pel-lik′u-lar; pel-lik′u-lus) characterized by a pellicle.

Pellizzi's syndrome (pel-le′zēz) [G. B. *Pellizzi,* Pisa physician] epiphyseal syndrome.

pellote (pa-yo′tah) peyote.

pellucid (pel-lu′sid) [L. *pellucidus,* from *per* through + *lucere* to shine] translucent.

pelo- (pe′lo) [Gr. *pelos* mud] a combining form denoting relationship to mud.

Pelodictyon (pe″lo-dik′te-on) [*pelo-* + Gr. *diktyon* net] a genus of microorganisms of the family Chlorobacteriaceae, suborder Rhodobacteriineae, order Pseudomonadales, occurring as ovoid to rod-shaped cells generally united into large colonies of characteristic shape. It includes three species, *P. aggrega′tum, P. clathrati-for′me,* and *P. paralle′lum.*

peloid (pe′loid) [*pelo-* + Gr. *eidos* form] mud used for therapeutic purposes, as in packs and baths.

pelology (pĕ-lol′o-je) [*pelo-* + *-logy*] the science of mud and similar substances.

Pelonema (pe″lo-ne′mah) [*pelo-* + Gr. *nēma* thread] a genus of microorganisms of the family Peloplocaceae, order Chlamydobacteriales, made up of long, straight, or spirally twisted, unbranched trichomes, enclosed in an extremely delicate sheath. It includes four species, *P. hyali′num, P. pseudovacuola′tum, P. ten′ue,* and *P. spira′le.*

pelopathy (pe-lop′ah-the) pelotherapy.

Peloploca (pĕ-lop′lo-kah) [*pelo-* + Gr. *plokē* anything twisted] a genus of microorganisms of the family Peloplocaceae, order Chlamydobacteriales, made up of colorless, filamentous, cylindrical cells containing false vacuoles which emit a reddish gleam of light. It includes two species, *P. taenia′ta* and *P. undula′ta.*

Peloplocaceae (pe″lo-plo-ka′se-e) a family of Schizomycetes, order Chlamydobacteriales, made up of long, unbranched filamentous cells usually enclosed in a delicate sheath. It includes two genera, *Pelone′ma* and *Pelo′plo′ca.*

pelosine (pe-lo′sin) bebeerine.

pelotherapy (pe″lo-ther′ah-pe) [*pelo-* + Gr. *therapeia* cure] the therapeutic use of earth or mud.

peltate (pel′tāt) [L. *pelta;* Gr. *peltē* shield] shield-shaped.

peltation (pel-ta′shun) the protective influence of inoculation with an antiserum or a vaccine.

pelves (pel′vēs) [L.] plural of *pelvis.*

pelvic (pel′vik) pertaining to the pelvis.

pelvicaliceal, pelvicalyceal (pel″ve-kal″ĭ-se-al) pertaining to the renal pelves and calices.

pelvicellulitis (pel″ve-sel′u-li′tis) pelvic cellulitis.

pelvicephalography (pel″ve-sef″ah-log′rah-fe) [*pelvis* + Gr. *kephalē* head + *graphein* to write] roentgenographic measurement of the fetal head and of the birth canal.

pelvicephalometry (pel″ve-sef″ah-lom′ĕ-tre) [*pelvis* + Gr. *kephalē* head + *metron* measure] measurement of the diameters of the head of the fetus in relation to those of the mother's pelvis.

pelvifemoral (pel″ve-fem′o-ral) pertaining to or affecting the pelvis and femur.

pelvifixation (pel″ve-fik-sa′shun) surgical fixation of a displaced or wandering pelvic organ.

pelvilithotomy (pel″ve-lĭ-thot′o-me) pyelolithotomy.

pelvimeter (pel-vim′ĕ-ter) [*pelvis* + Gr. *metron* measure] an instrument for measuring the diameters and capacity of the pelvis.

pelvimetry (pel-vim′ĕ-tre) the measurement of the dimensions and capacity of the pelvis. **combined p.,** pelvimetry in which measurements are made both within and outside the body. **digital p.,** pelvimetry performed with the hands. **external p.,** that in which the measurements are made outside the body. **instrumental p.,** measurement of the pelvis with the pelvimeter. **internal p.,** that in which the measurements are made within the vagina. **manual p.,** that which is performed with the hands.

pelviography (pel″ve-og′rah-fe) pelviroentgenography.

pelvioileoneocystostomy (pel″ve-o-il″e-o-ne′o-sis-tos′to-me) anastomosis of renal pelvis to an isolated segment of the ileum, which is then anastomosed to the urinary bladder.

pelviolithotomy (pel″ve-o-lĭ-thot′o-me) pyelolithotomy.

pelvioneostomy (pel″ve-o-ne-os′to-me) ureteroneopyelostomy.

pelvioperitonitis (pel″ve-o-per″ĭ-to-ni′tis) pelvic peritonitis.

pelvioplasty (pel′ve-o-plas″te) pyeloplasty.

pelvioradiography (pel″ve-o-ra″de-og′rah-fe) radiography of the organs of the pelvis; pelviroentgenography.

pelvioscopy (pel″ve-os′ko-pe) [*pelvis* + Gr. *skopein* to examine] 1. the inspection or visual examination of the pelvis or pelvic viscera. 2. pyeloscopy.

pelviostomy (pel″ve-os′to-me) pyelostomy.

pelviotomy (pel″ve-ot′o-me) [*pelvis* + Gr. *tomē* a cutting] 1. the cutting of the pelvic bones. 2. pyelotomy.

pelviperitonitis (pel″ve-per″ĭ-to-ni′tis) pelvic peritonitis.

pelviradiography (pel″ve-ra″de-og′rah-fe) pelviroentgenography.

pelvirectal (pel″ve-rek′tal) pertaining to the pelvis and the rectum.

pelviroentgenography (pel″ve-rent″gen-og′rah-fe) roentgenography of the organs of the pelvis.

pelvis (pel′vis), pl. *pel′ves* [L.; Gr. *pyelos* an oblong trough] [NA] the lower (caudal) portion of the trunk of the body, bounded anteriorly and laterally by the two hip bones and posteriorly by the sacrum and coccyx. The pelvis is divided by a plane passing through the terminal lines into the *false pelvis* (*p. major* [NA]) above and the *true pelvis* (*p. minor* [NA]) below. The upper boundary of the cavity of the pelvis is known as the *inlet, brim,* or *superior strait of the pelvis.* The true pelvis is limited below by the *inferior strait,* or *outlet,* bounded by the coccyx, the symphysis pubis, and the ischium of either side. The outlet of the pelvis is closed by the coccygeus and levator ani muscles and the perineal fascia, which form the *floor of the pelvis.* The inlet and outlet of the pelvis each have three important diameters—an anteroposterior (conjugate), an oblique, and a transverse, the relations of which determine types variously classified by different authors (see entries under *diameter*). The term pelvis is applied also to any basin-like structure, such as the renal pelvis (pelvis renalis [NA]). **android p.,** a pelvis characterized by a wedge-shaped inlet and narrowness of the anterior segment; used as a general designation of a female pelvis showing characters typical of the pelvis in the male. **anthropoid p.,** a female pelvis characterized by a long anteroposterior diameter of the inlet, which equals or exceeds the transverse diameter. **assimilation p.,** a pelvis in which the transverse processes of the last lumbar vertebra are fused with the sacrum (*high-assimilation p.*—including six vertebral segments), or the last sacral vertebra may fuse with the first coccygeal body (*low-assimilation p.*—including only four vertebral segments). **beaked p.,** one with the pelvic bones laterally compressed and their anterior junction pushed forward, as in osteomalacia. **bony p., p.** ossea. **brachypellic p.,** an oval type of pelvis, the transverse diameter of the inlet exceeding the anteroposterior diameter by 1 to 3 cm. **contracted p.,** a pelvis in which there is a diminution of 1.5 to 2 cm. in any important diameter; when all dimensions are proportionately diminished it is a *generally contracted pelvis* (*p. justo minor*). **cordate p., cordiform p.,** one that is somewhat heart shaped. **coxalgic p.,** one deformed in consequence of hip-joint disease. **dolichopellic p.,** an elongated pelvis, the anteroposterior diameter of the inlet being greater than the transverse diameter. **dwarf p.,** a small pelvis seen in several types of dwarfism. **extrarenal p.,** see under *renal p.* **false p., p.** major. **flat p.,** one in which the anteroposterior dimension is abnormally reduced. **frozen p.,** a condition, due to infection or carcinoma, in which the adnexa and uterus are fixed in the pelvis. **funnel-shaped p.,** a female pelvis with a normal inlet, but a greatly narrowed outlet. **giant p., p.** justo major. **greater p., p.** major. **gynecoid p.,** a pelvis having a rounded oval shape with a well rounded anterior and posterior segment; it represents the normal female pelvis. **high-assimilation p.,** see *assimilation p.* **infantile p.,** a generally contracted pelvis characterized by an oval shape, a high sacrum, and marked inclination of the walls. **p. jus′to ma′jor,** a pelvis that is unusually large, with all its dimensions equally increased. **p. jus′to mi′nor,** a pelvis that is unusually small, with all its dimensions equally reduced; see also *contracted p.* **juvenile p.,** infantile p. **kyphoscoliotic p.,** an irregularly contracted pelvis due to rachitic kyphoscoliosis. **kyphotic p.,** one characterized by increase of the conjugate diameter at the brim, with decrease of the transverse diameter at the outlet, due to close proximity of the ischial spines and tuberosities. **large p., p.** major. **lesser p., p.** minor. **lordotic p.,** one in which the vertebral column has an anterior curvature in the lumbar region. **low-assimilation p.,** see *assimilation p.* **p. ma′jor** [NA], the part of the pelvis superior to a plane passing through the ileopectineal lines. **mesatipellic p.,** a round type of pelvis, the transverse diameter of the inlet being equal to the anteroposterior diameter or being greater by 1 cm. or less. **p. mi′nor** [NA], the part of the pelvis inferior to a plane passing through the iliopectineal lines; see *pelvis.* **Nägele's p.,** one so distorted that the conjugate diameter takes an oblique direction. **p. na′na,** dwarf p. **oblique p.,** Nägele's p. **p. obtec′ta,** a kyphotic pelvis in which the vertebral column extends horizontally across the pelvic inlet. **p. os′sea** [NA], bony pelvis: the ring of bone forming the skeleton of the pelvis, supporting the vertebral column and resting upon the inferior members, and composed of the two hip bones anteriorly and laterally, and the sacrum and coccyx posteriorly. **osteomalacic p.,** deformity of the pelvis due to absorption by the bones of their calcium salts, as a result of which the bones

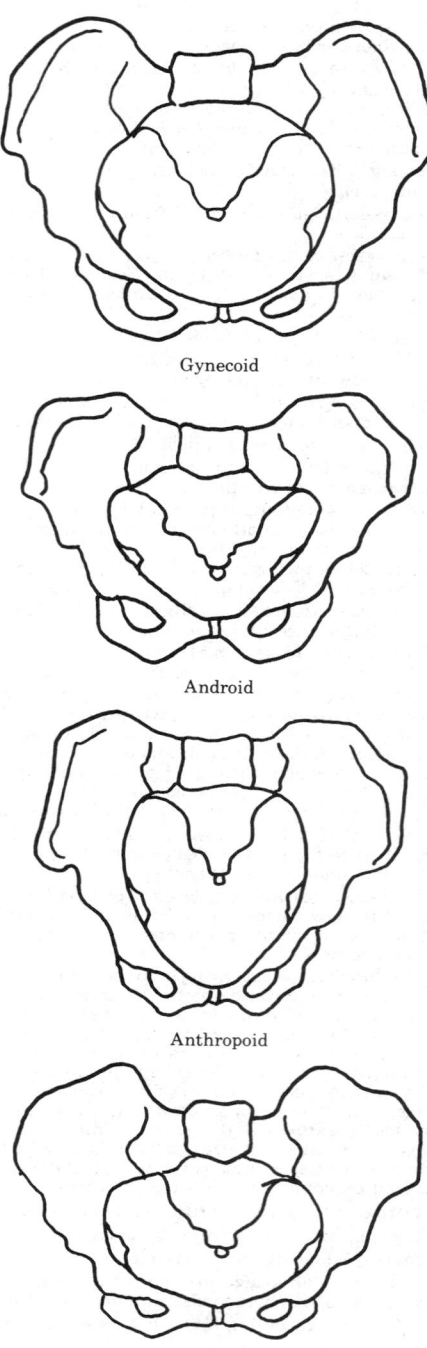

Gynecoid

Android

Anthropoid

Platypelloid

Various types of pelvic inlets (Greenhill and Friedman).

become soft and so flexible that they may be stretched or pushed together and cause narrowing of the pelvic inlet. **Otto p.,** a pelvis in which the acetabulum is depressed, permitting the head of the femur to protrude intrapelvically; see *arthrokatadysis.* **p. ova′lis,** fossula fenestrae vestibuli. **p. pla′na,** flat p. **platypellic p., platypelloid p.,** a pelvis characterized by flattening of the pelvic inlet, with a short anteroposterior and a wide transverse diameter. **Prague p.,** spondylolisthetic p. **pseudo-osteomalacic p.,** a deformed pelvis simulating one affected with osteomalacia, but resulting from other causes. **pseudospider p.,** a congenitally small, long, thin renal pelvis with calices that may simulate renal tumor urographically. **rachitic p.,** one distorted as a result of rickets. **renal p., p. rena′lis** [NA], the expansion from the upper end of the ureter into which the calices of the kidney open; ordinarily lodged within the renal sinus, under certain conditions, as in a long kidney or obstruction of the ureteropelvic junction, a large part of it may be outside the kidney (*extrarenal p.*). **Robert's p.,** a transversely contracted pelvis caused by osteoarthritis affecting both sacroiliac joints, the inlet becoming a narrow wedge. **Rokitansky's p.,** spondylolisthetic p. **p. rotun'da,** fossula fenestrae cochleae. **round p.,** one with an inlet of nearly circular outline. **scoliotic p.,** one deformed as a result of scoliosis. **simple flat p.,** one with a shortened anteroposterior diameter. **small p.,** p. minor. **spider p.,** a renal pelvis which in the pyelogram shows the calices as narrow, string-like extensions, resembling the legs of a spider. **p. spino'sa,** a rachitic pelvis with the crest of the pubis very sharp. **split p.,** one with a congenital separation at the symphysis pubis, often associated with exstrophy of the bladder. **spondylolisthetic p.,** one in which the last, or rarely the fourth or third, lumbar vertebra is dislocated in front of the sacrum, more or less occluding the pelvic brim. Called also *Prague p.* and *Rokitansky's p.* **p. spu'ria,** p. major. **triangular p.,** one with a triangular inlet. **true p.,** p. minor. **p. of ureter,** renal p.

pelvisacral (pel″ve-sa′kral) pertaining to the pelvis and the sacrum.

pelvisacrum (pel-ve-sa′krum) the pelvis and the sacrum together.

pelviscope (pel′ve-skōp) an apparatus for examining roentgenologically the contours of the pelvis.

pelvisection (pel″ve-sek′shun) [pelvis + L. sectio a cutting] a cutting of the pelvis bones, such as pubiotomy and symphysiotomy.

pelvisternum (pel″ve-ster′num) the cartilage of the symphysis pubis.

pelvitherm (pel′ve-therm) [pelvis + Gr. thermē heat] an apparatus for applying heat to the pelvic organs through the vagina.

pelvitomy (pel-vit′o-me) [pelvis + Gr. temnein to cut] the operation of cutting the pelvis at any point in order to facilitate delivery.

pelvitrochanterian (pel″ve-tro″kan-te″re-an) relating to the pelvis and the great trochanter of the femur.

pelviureteral (pel″ve-u-re′ter-al) relating to the renal pelvis and the ureter.

pelviureteroradiography (pel″ve-u-re″ter-o-ra″de-og′rah-fe) roentgenography of the ureter and renal pelvis.

pelvoscopy (pel-vos′ko-pe) [pelvis + Gr. skopein to examine] examination of a pelvis, particularly of the renal pelvis.

pelvospondylitis (pel″vo-spon″dĭ-li′tis) inflammation of the pelvic portion of the spine. **p. ossif'icans,** rheumatoid spondylitis.

pelyco- [Gr. pelyx pelvis] for words beginning thus, see those beginning pelvi- and pyelo-.

pemerid nitrate (pem′ĕ-rid) chemical name: 4-[3-(dimethylamino)propoxyl]-1,2,2,6,6-pentamethylpiperidine dinitrate; an antitussive, $C_{15}H_{32}N_2O \cdot 2HNO_3$.

pemoline (pem′o-lēn) chemical name: 2-imino-5-phenyl-4-oxazolidinone; a central nervous system stimulant, $C_9H_8N_2O_2$.

pemphigoid (pem′fĭ-goid) [Gr. pemphix blister + eidos form] 1. like or resembling pemphigus. 2. a name applied to a group of dermatological syndromes similar to but clearly distinguishable from those of the pemphigus group. Frequently used alone to designate bullous pemphigoid. **benign mucosal p.,** a chronic bullous disease of elderly persons, involving primarily the mucous membranes, particularly the conjunctiva and oral mucosa, with scarring; called also *cicatricial p.* and *ocular pemphigus.* **bullous p.,** a chronic generalized bullous eruption, occurring predominantly in elderly adults, and usually not fatal; the blisters are tense and there is separation at the dermoepidermal junction. IgE antibodies are found at the basement membrane. **cicatricial p.,** benign mucosal p. **localized chronic p.,** a form in which bulla formation is confined for many years to a circumscribed region, as of the face, scalp, limbs, etc., with scarring but without affecting the mucous membranes.

pemphigus (pem′fĭ-gus) [Gr. pemphix blister] a name applied to a distinctive group of diseases characterized by successive crops of bullae, the specific type usually being indicated by a modifying term. Frequently used alone to designate pemphigus vulgaris. **benign p.** (obs.), bullous pemphigoid. **benign familial p.,** a rare, hereditary, persistently recurring bullous and vesicular dermatitis most often involving the axillae, groin, and neck, but sometimes widespread. The lesions appear in crops and regress over several weeks or months. The disease is transmitted as an autosomal dominant trait. Called also *Hailey-Hailey disease.* **Brazilian p.,** fogo selvagem. **p. erythemato'sus,** chronic pemphigus in which the lesions, limited to the face and chest, resemble those of disseminated lupus erythematosus. Immunofluorescent studies suggest that, in some cases at least, pemphigus and lupus erythematosus may both be present. Called also *Senear-Usher syndrome.* **p. folia'ceus,** a chronic, generalized, vesicular and scaling skin eruption somewhat resembling dermatitis herpetiformis or, later in its course, exfoliative dermatitis. **p. neonato'rum,** impetigo bullosa. **ocular p.,** benign mucosal pemphigoid affecting the conjunctiva. **South American p.,** fogo selvagem. **p. veg'etans, benign,** dermatitis vegetans. **p. veg'etans (Hallopeau type),** dermatitis vegetans. **p. veg'etans (Neumann type),** a variant of pemphigus vulgaris in which the bullous lesions are replaced by verrucoid hypertrophic vegetative masses; called also *pyoderma*

verrucosum or *verrucous pyoderma.* Cf. *dermatitis vegetans.* **p. vulga'ris,** a rare relapsing disease manifested by suprabasal, intraepidermal bullae of the skin and mucous membranes; invariably fatal if untreated, but remission has been obtained by use of corticosteroid hormones and immunosuppressive drugs. **wildfire p.,** fogo selvagem.

pempidine tartrate (pem′pĭ-dēn) chemical name: 1,2,2,6,6-pentamethylpiperidine tartrate; a ganglion-blocking agent, $C_{10}H_{21}N$, occurring as a white, crystalline powder, which has been used as an antihypertensive.

penatin (pen′ah-tin) glucose oxidase.

Penbritin (pen-brit′in) trademark for preparations of ampicillin.

penbutolol sulfate (pen-bu′to-lōl) (S)-1-(2-cyclopentylphenoxy)-3-[(1,1-dimethylethyl)amino]-2-propanol sulfate (2:1) (salt); an antiadrenergic (β-receptor), $(C_{18}H_{29}NO_2)_2 \cdot H_2SO_4$.

Pende's sign (pen′dēz) [Nicola Pende, Italian physician, born 1880] André-Thomas sign.

pendular (pen′du-lar) having a pendulum-like movement.

pendulous (pen′joo-lus, pen′dŭ-lus) [L. pendere to hang] hanging; dependent.

penetrance (pen′ĕ-trans) [L. penetrare to enter into] the extent to which a substance is penetrated, or to which an object enters into a substance. In genetics, the frequency with which a heritable trait is manifested by individuals carrying the principal gene or genes conditioning it.

penetrating (pen′ĕ-trāt-ing) [L. penetrans] piercing; entering deeply.

penetration (pen″ĕ-tra′shun) [L. penetratio] 1. the act of piercing or entering deeply. 2. the focal depth of a lens, or its power of giving a clear definition at various depths.

penetrology (pen″ĕ-trol′o-je) the study of radiant energy.

penetrometer (pen″ĕ-trom′ĕ-ter) 1. an apparatus for measuring the penetrating power and intensity of the roentgen ray. The best known are those of Benoist, Walter, and Wehnelt. 2. an apparatus for registering the resistance of semisolid material to penetration.

penfluridol (pen-floor′ĭ-dōl) chemical name: 1-[4,4-bis(p-fluorophenyl)butyl]-4-(4-chloro-α,α,α-trifluoro-m-tolyl)-4-piperidinol; a tranquilizer, $C_{28}H_{27}ClF_5NO$.

-penia [Gr. penia poverty, need] a word termination indicating an abnormal reduction in number of the element denoted by the root to which it is affixed, as leukopenia.

penial (pe′ne-al) penile.

penicidin (pen″ĭ-si′din) patulin.

penicillamine (pen″ĭ-sil-ah-mēn) [USP] chemical name: 3-mercapto-D-valine. A degradation product of penicillin, $C_5H_{11}NO_2S$, occurring as a white or almost white, crystalline powder, which chelates certain heavy metals; used orally to reduce the blood copper level in the treatment of hepatolenticular degeneration and to promote excretion of cystine by forming a more soluble penicillamine-cystine disulfide. It has been used in the treatment of rheumatoid arthritis.

penicilli (pen″ĭ-sil′li) [L.] plural of penicillus.

penicilliary (pen″ĭ-sil′e-er′e) [L. penicillium, dim. of peniculus a brush] resembling a brush or broom.

penicillin (pen″ĭ-sil′in) any of a large group of natural or semisynthetic antibacterial antibiotics derived directly or indirectly from strains of fungi of the genus *Penicillium* and other soil-inhabiting fungi grown on special culture media, which exert a bacteriocidal as well as a bacteriostatic effect on susceptible bacteria by interfering with the final stages of the synthesis of peptidoglycan, a substance in the bacterial cell wall. The penicillins, despite their relatively low toxicity for the host, are active against many bacteria, especially gram-positive pathogens (streptococci, staphylococci, pneumococci); clostridia; some gram-negative forms (gonococci, meningococci); some spirochetes (*Treponema pallidum* and *T. pertenue*); and some fungi. Certain strains of some target species, e.g., staphylococci, secrete the enzyme penicillinase, which inactivates penicillin and confers resistance to the antibiotic. **aluminum p.,** the aluminum salt of penicillin prepared from extracts of cultures of *Penicillium notatum* or *P. chrysogenum.* **p. B,** glucose oxidase. **benzyl p. potassium,** potassium p. G. **benzyl p. sodium,** p. G. sodium. **clemizole p.,** the clemizole salt of penicillin G, $C_{16}H_{18}N_2O_4C_{19}H_{20}ClN_3$, the combination of which produces a respository form of penicillin G with antihistaminic properties. **dimethoxyphenyl p. sodium,** methicillin sodium. **p. G,** the most widely used form and the first of the penicillins developed for medicinal use. It is used in the form of the benzathine, potassium, procaine, and sodium salts, principally in the treatment of infections due to penicillin-susceptible gram-positive bacteria, gram-negative cocci, *Treponema pallidum*, and *Actinomyces israeli.* Called also *benzylpenicillin.* **p. G benzathine** [USP], a salt having a long-sustained action, $C_{16}H_{20}N_2 \cdot 2C_{16}H_{18}N_2O_4S \cdot 4H_2O$, obtained by combining penicillin G with N,N′-bis(phenylmethyl)-1,2-ethanediamine (2:1), occurring as a white, crystalline powder, and containing 57.9 to 71.6 per cent of penicillin G; administered orally and intramuscularly. **p. G potassium,** a salt $C_{16}H_{17}KN_2O_4S$, occurring as colorless or white crystals, or white, crystalline powder, and containing 80.8 to 94.3 per cent of penicillin G; administered orally and by intravenous injection or infusion. **p. G procaine** [USP], a salt having a long-sustained action, $C_{16}H_{18}N_2O_4\cdot S\cdot C_{13}H_{20}N_2H_2O$, obtained by combining penicillin G with procaine (1:1), occurring as white crystals or white, very fine, microcrystalline powder, and containing 51 to 59.6 per cent penicillin G; administered intramuscularly. **p. G sodium,** a salt, $C_{16}H_{17}N_2NaO_4S$, occurring as colorless or white crystals or as a white to slightly yellow, crystalline powder, containing not less than 85 per cent of penicillin G sodium; administered intramuscularly and intravenously. *Sterile penicillin G sodium* [USP] is suitable for parenteral use. **isoxazolyl p.,** a group of semisynthetic penicillins, including oxacillin, cloxacillin, and dicloxacillin, which combine resistance to penicillinase with acid stability and activity against gram-positive bacteria. **p. N,** adicillin. **p. O,** a penicillin produced biosynthetically by adding a precursor to the culture medium; penicillin O and its potassium and sodium salts have actions similar to those of penicillin G and are said to be hypoallergenic. **p. O chloroprocaine,** a salt of 2-chloroprocaine and penicillin O, having actions similar to penicillins G and O. **p. O potassium,** see *p. O.* **p. O sodium,** see *p. O.* **phenoxymethyl p.,** p. V. **potassium phenoxymethyl p.,** p. V potassium. **p. V** [USP], a semisynthetic oral penicillin prepared from cultures of the mold *Penicillium* in the presence of 2-phenoxyethanol with an autolysate of yeast as the source of nitrogen. It is a broad-spectrum antibiotic having pharmacologic and toxic properties similar to those of other penicillins, and is less potent than penicillin G. Called also *phenoxymethyl p.* **p. V benzathine** [USP], an oral penicillin, $(C_{16}H_{18}N_2O_5S)_2C_{16}H_{20}N_2$, occurring as practically white powder. **p. V hydrabamine** [USP], an oral penicillin, $(C_{16}H_{18}N_2O_5S)_2\cdot C_{42}H_{64}N_2$, occurring as a practically white powder. **p. V potassium** [USP], an oral penicillin, $C_{16}H_{17}KN_2O_5S$, occurring as a white crystalline powder.

penicillinase (pen″ĭ-sil′ĭ-nās)   penicillin amido-β-lactamhydrolase: an enzyme produced by certain bacteria which converts penicillin to an inactive product and thus increases resistance to the antibiotic. A purified preparation from cultures of a strain of *Bacillus cereus* is used in treatment of reactions to penicillin.

penicillin-fast (pen″ĭ-sĭl′in-fast)   resistant to the action of penicillin; said of certain strains of bacteria.

penicilliosis (pen″ĭ-sil″e-o′sis)   infection with *Penicillium*, usually a pulmonary infection.

Penicillium (pen″ĭ-sil′e-um) [L. *penicillum* brush, roll]   a genus of Fungi Imperfecti (family Moniliaceae, order Moniliales) that develop fruiting organs resembling a broom, or the bones of the hand and fingers. When identified, the perfect (sexual) stage is classified with the ascomycetous fungi in the family Eurotiaceae, order Eurotiales. See also *penicillin.* **P. chrysog′enum,** a

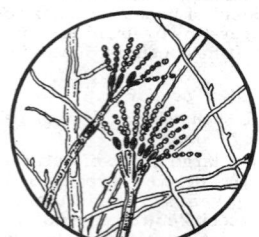

Penicillium (de Rivas).

species from which various penicillins are obtained. **P. ci-tri′num,** a species that produces the antibiotic citrinin. **P. crusta′ceum,** *P. glau′cum.* **P. glau′cum,** a species that is one of the sources green mold. **P. nota′tum,** a species that is one of the sources of various penicillins. **P. pat′ulum,** *P. uticale.* **P. utica′le,** one of the species that produces patulin; called also *P. patulum.*

penicilloyl-polylysine (pen″i-sil′oil-pol″ĕ-li′sēn)   an agent prepared from polylysine and a penicillenic acid; intradermal injection elicits a wheal and erythema response within 20 minutes in those sensitive to penicillin.

penicillus (pen″ĭ-sil′us), pl. *penicil′li* [L.]   a structure resembling a brush in appearance. **penicil′li arte′riae liena′lis** [NA], brushlike groups of arterial branches in the lobules of the spleen.

penile (pe′nīl)   pertaining to or affecting the penis.

penillamine (pen″il-am′in)   chemical name: 2-amino-3-mercapto-3-methylbutanoic acid or β,β-dimethylcysteine. An amine, $C_5H_{11}O_2NS$, derived from penillic acid by the removal of a molecule of carbon dioxide.

penilloaldehyde (pen″ĭ-lo-al′de-hīd)   an aldehyde derived from penicillin.

penis (pe′nis) [L.] [NA]   the male organ of copulation and of urinary excretion, comprising a root, body, and extremity, or glans penis. The root is attached to the descending portions of the pubic bone by the *crura,* the latter being the extremities of the corpora

cavernosa. The body consists of two parallel cylindrical bodies, the *corpora cavernosa,* and beneath them the *corpus spongiosum,* through which the urethra passes. The glans is covered with mucous membrane and ensheathed by the prepuce, or foreskin. The penis is homologous with the clitoris in the female. **clubbed p.,** a condition in which the penis is curved when erect. **concealed p.,** a rudimentary penis concealed beneath the skin of the scrotum, perineum, abdomen, or thigh. **double p.,** an anomaly resulting when the urethral groove completely divides the penile shaft during development of the embryo. **p. mulieb′ris** (*obs.*), clitoris. **p. palma′tus,** webbed p. **p. plas′tica,** Peyronie's disease. **webbed p.,** a penis that is enclosed by the skin of the scrotum; called also *p. palmatus.*

penischisis (pe-nis′kĭ-sis) [*penis* + Gr. *schisis* splitting]   a fissured state of the penis, as epispadias, hypospadias, or paraspadias.

penitis (pe-ni′tis)   inflammation of the penis.

Penjdeh sore, ulcer (penj′deh) [*Penjdeh,* a town of Turkestan]   cutaneous leishmaniasis.

Penn seroflocculation reaction [Harry Samuel *Penn,* Russian physician and zoologist in the United States, born 1891]   see under *reaction.*

pennate (pen′āt)   penniform.

penniform (pen′ĭ-form) [L. *penna* feather + *forma* form]   shaped like a feather; looking like a feather.

pennyroyal (pen″e-roi′al)   a popular name for various labiate plants, especially *Mentha pulegium* L. (*European p.*) and *M. canadensis* L. (American wild mint); the oil was formerly used as a diaphoretic, aromatic, and emmenagogue.

pennyweight (pen′e-wāt)   a unit of weight in the troy system, being 24 grains, or one twentieth of an ounce.

penology (pe-nol′o-je) [Gr. *poinē* penalty + *-logy*]   the science of punishment; that branch of criminology which deals with the treatment of criminals.

penoscrotal (pe″no-skro′tal)   relating to the penis and the scrotum.

penotherapy (pe″no-ther′ah-pe)   the medical examination and regulation of prostitutes in the control of venereal disease.

Penrose drain (pen′rōz) [Charles Bingham *Penrose,* Philadelphia gynecologist, 1862–1925]   see under *drain.*

pent-, penta- [Gr. *pente* five]   a combining form meaning five.

pentabasic (pen″tah-ba′sik)   having five replaceable atoms of hydrogen in the molecule.

pentachlorin (pen″tah-klo′rin)   chlorophenothane.

pentachromic (pen″tah-kro′mik) [*penta-* + Gr. *chrōma* color]   1. pertaining to or exhibiting five colors. 2. able to distinguish only five of the seven colors of the spectrum.

pentacyclic (pen″tah-sik′lik)   having a ring of five atoms in the molecule.

pentad (pen′tad)   1. any group of five. 2. a pentavalent element or radical.

pentadactyl (pen″tah-dak′til) [*penta-* + Gr. *daktylos* finger]   having five fingers or toes on the hand or foot.

pentaerythritol (pen″tah-ĕ-rith′rĭ-tol)   chemical name: 2,2-bis(hydroxymethyl)-1,3-propanediol. An alcohol, $(CH_2OH)_4C$, prepared by treating acetaldehyde with formaldehyde in an aqueous solution of calcium hydroxide; used in synthetic resins and in paints and varnishes. **p. chloral,** petrichloral. **p. tetranitrate,** the nitric acid ester of pentaerythritol, $C_5H_8N_4O_{12}$, having vasodilator action similar to nitroglycerin, occurring as a white, crystalline powder that may explode on percussion. Called also *niperyt, pentaerythrityl tetranitrate, penthrit, pentrinitrol,* and *PTEN. Diluted p. tetranitrate* [USP], a dry mixture of pentaerythritol tetranitrate with lactose, mannitol, or other inert excipients to render it nonexplosive is administered orally in the treatment of angina pectoris.

pentaerythrityl (pen″tah-ĕ-rith′rĭ-til)   pentaerythritol. **p. tetranitrate,** pentaerythritol tetranitrate.

pentagastrin (pen″tah-gas′trin)   a synthetic pentapeptide consisting of β-alanine and the C-terminal tetrapeptide of gastrin; used as a test of gastric secretory function.

pentalogy (pen-tal′o-je)   a combination of five elements or factors, as five concurrent defects or symptoms. **p. of Fallot,** the four defects included in the tetralogy of Fallot, occurring in association with patent foramen ovale or atrial septal defect.

pentamer (pen′tah-mer)   a polymer consisting of five monomers; a viral capsomer having five structural units.

pentamethazene (pen″tah-meth′ah-zēn)   azamethonium.

pentamethylenediamine (pen″tah-meth″il-ēn-di-am′in)   cadaverine.

pentamethylenetetrazol (pen-tah-meth″il-ēn-tet′rah-zol)   pentylenetetrazol.

pentamidine (pen-tam′ĭ-dēn)   chemical name: 4,4′-(pentamethylenedioxy)dibenzamidine; an anti-infective used as the isethionate salt and effective against *Pneumocystis carinii.*

pentane (pen′tān)   n-pentane; an aliphatic hydrocarbon of the methane series, C_5H_{12}, obtained by distillation of petroleum and occurring as a clear, colorless, flammable liquid. It produces anesthesia when inhaled, ingested, or injected.

pentapeptide (pen″tah-pep′tid) a polypeptide containing five amino acids.

pentapiperide methylsulfate (pen″tah-pi′per-īd) chemical name: 1,1,-dimethyl-4-[(3-methyl-1-oxo-2-phenylpentyl)oxy]piperidinium. A synthetic quaternary ammonium anticholinergic, $C_{20}H_{33}NO_6S$, used in the treatment of peptic ulcer and other disorders in which gastrointestinal hypermotility and hypersecretion are features, administered orally. Called also *pentapiperium methylsulfate.*

pentapiperium methylsulfate (pen-tah-pĭ-per′ĭ-um) pentapiperide methylsulfate.

pentaploid (pen′tah-ploid) 1. pertaining to or characterized by pentaploidy. 2. an individual or cell having five sets of chromosomes.

pentaploidy (pen′tah-ploi″de) the state of having five sets of chromosomes (5n).

pentapyrrolidinium bitartrate (pen″tah-pir-ro″lĭ-din′e-um) pentolinium tartrate.

pentasomy (pen″tah-so′me) [*penta-* + Gr. *sōma* body] the presence of three additional chromosomes of one type (e.g., 5 X chromosomes) in an otherwise diploid cell (2n + 3).

Pentastoma (pen-tas′to-mah) [*penta-* + Gr. *stoma* mouth] a genus of endoparasitic, wormlike arthropods of the class Porocephalidae. *P. denticulatum* (incorrectly assigned to this genus) is the larva of *Linguatulidae serrata.*

pentastomiasis (pen″tah-sto-mi′ah-sis) infection with pentastomids.

pentastomid (pen-tah-sto′mid) any individual of the class Pentastomida.

Pentastomida (pen″tah-sto′mid-ah) a class of Arthropoda, the tongue worms, consisting of degenerate wormlike parasites, without circulatory or respiratory systems. The adults, otherwise without appendages, possess two pairs of hooks near the mouth. The larvae bear two or three pairs of rudimentary legs. Adults live in the respiratory passages and head cavities of reptiles, birds, and mammals. Two genera, *Armillifer* and *Linguatula*, have been reported on several occasions from man as larval host. It includes the order Porocephalida.

pentatomic (pen″tah-tom′ik) [*penta-* + *atom*] 1. containing five atoms. 2. containing five replaceable hydrogen atoms.

Pentatrichomonas (pen″tah-trĭ-kom′o-nas) Trichomonas. **P. ar′din delte′ili,** *Trichomonas hominis.*

pentavaccine (pen″tah-vak′sēn) [*penta-* + *vaccine*] a vaccine comprised of five microorganisms, as one containing dead cultures of the bacteria of typhoid, paratyphoid A, paratyphoid B, cholera, and brucellosis.

pentavalent (pen″tah-va′lent, pen-tav′ah-lent) having a chemical valency of five; capable of combining with five atoms of hydrogen.

pentazocine (pen-taz′o-sēn) [USP] chemical name: 1,2,3,4,5,6-hexahydro-*cis*-6,11-dimethyl -3-(3-methyl-2-butenyl)-2,6-methano-3-benzazocin-8-ol. A synthetic analgesic, $C_{27}H_{27}NO$, occurring as a white or very pale tan-colored powder; used in the form of the hydrochloride and lactate salts. **p. hydrochloride** [USP], the hydrochloride salt of pentazocine, occurring as a white crystalline powder; administered orally. **p. lactate** [USP], the lactate salt of pentazocine, administered parenterally.

pentdyopent (pent-di′o-pent) [*penta* + Gr. *dyo* two + *pente* five = 525, referring to the spectroscopic line of the substance] a substance derived from blood pigment, occurring in the urine in certain diseases.

pentene (pen′tēn) amylene.

pentetate calcium trisodium (pen′tĕ-tāt) chemical name: [*N,N*-bis[2-[bis(carboxymethyl)amino]ethyl]glycinato(5−)]calcinate(3−)trisodium. The calcium trisodium salt of pentetic acid, $C_{14}H_{18}CaN_3Na_3O_{10}$, used as a chelating agent, especially in the treatment of plutonium poisoning. Called also *calcium trisodium pentetate.*

penthienate bromide (pen-thi′ĕ-nāt) chemical name: 2-[(cyclopentylhydroxy-2-thienylacetyl)oxy]-*N,N*-diethyl-*N*-methylethanaminium bromide. A quaternary ammonium anticholinergic, $C_{18}H_{30}BrNO_3S$, used orally, mainly in the treatment of gastric ulcer.

Penthrane (pen′thrān) trademark for a preparation of methoxyflurane.

penthrit (pen′thrit) pentaerythritol tetranitrate.

Pentids (pen′tidz) trademark for preparations of penicillin G potassium.

pentizidone sodium (pen-tiz′ĭ-dōn) chemical name: (*R*)-4-[(1-methyl-3-oxo-1-butenyl)amino]-3-isoxazolidinone monosodium salt hemihydrate; an antibacterial, $C_8H_{11}N_2NaO_3·\frac{1}{2}H_2O$.

pentobarbital (pen″to-bar′bĭ-tal) [USP] chemical name: 5-ethyl-5-(1-methylbutyl)-2,4,6(1*H*,3*H*,5*H*)-pyrimidinetrione. A short- to intermediate-acting barbiturate, $C_{11}H_{17}N_2O_3$, occurring as a white to practically white, fine powder, used as a sedative and

hypnotic, administered orally. Called also *pentobarbitone.* **p. sodium** [USP], the sodium salt of pentobarbital, a hypnotic used as a sedative, anticonvulsant, preanesthetic in surgery, an adjunct to anesthesia, and an amnesic in obstetrics.

pentobarbitone (pen″to-bar′bĭ-tōn) pentobarbital.

pentolinium tartrate (pen″to-lin′e-um) chemical name: 1,1′-(1,5-pentanediyl)bis[1-methylpyrrolidinium]. A ganglionic blocking agent, $C_{23}H_{42}N_2O_{12}$, occurring as a white or slightly cream-colored powder; used as an antihypertensive, administered orally, intramuscularly, and subcutaneously.

pentone (pen′tōn) valylene.

pentosan (pen′to-san) any member of a group of pentose polysaccharides having the composition $(C_5H_8O_4)_n$; found in various foods and plant juices. They yield pentose on hydrolysis. **methyl p.,** a pentosan which on hydrolysis yields methyl pentoses.

pentosazon (pen″to-sa′zon) a crystalline compound formed by treating a pentose with phenyl hydrazine, sometimes abnormally occurring in the urine.

pentose (pen′tōs) a monosaccharide containing five carbon atoms in a molecule.

pentosemia (pen″to-se′me-ah) the presence of pentose in the blood.

pentosidase (pen-tos′ĭ-dās) an enzyme that catalyzes the conversion of pentoses to some other form.

pentoside (pen′to-sid) a compound of a pentose with some other substance. Compounds of pentoses with purine and pyrimidine bases are found in the nucleic acids.

pentosuria (pen″to-su′re-ah) [*pentose* + Gr. *ouron* urine + *-ia*] a benign error of metabolism due to a defect in the activity of the enzyme L-xylulose dehydrogenase, which results in high levels of L-xylulose in the urine. It is transmitted as an autosomal recessive trait. Called also *L-xylulosuria.*

pentosuric (pen″to-su′rik) affected with pentosuria.

pentosyl (pen′to-sil) a radical of pentose.

pentosyltransferase (pen″to-sil-trans′fer-ās) an enzyme that catalyzes the transfer of a pentosyl group, as from uridine to orthophosphate to form uracil; called also *transpentosylase.*

Pentothal (pen′to-thol) trademark for preparations of thiopental.

pentoxide (pen-tok′sīd) an oxide containing five atoms of oxygen in a molecule.

pentoxifylline (pen-toks-i″fĭ-lin) chemical name: 2,2-bis[(nitrooxy)methyl]-1,3-propanediol mononitrate (ester); a coronary vasodilator, $C_5H_9N_3O_{10}$.

pentrinitrol (pen-tri-ni′trōl) pentaerythritol trinitrate.

Pentritol (pen′trĭ-tol) trademark for a preparation of pentaerythritol tetranitrate.

Pentryate (pen-tri′āt) trademark for preparations of pentaerythritol trinitrate.

pentylenetetrazol (pen″tĭ-lēn-tet′rah-zol) chemical name: 6,7,8,9-tetrahydro-5*H*-tetrazolo[1,5-*a*]azepine. A central nervous system stimulant, $C_8H_{10}N_4$, occurring as white crystals; used mainly to counteract the depressant action of overdoses of depressant drugs, administered orally, intravenously, and subcutaneously. Called also *pentamethylenetetrazol* and *leptazol.* See also *Metrazol shock therapy,* under *therapy.*

Pen-Vee (pen′ve) trademark for preparations of penicillin V.

Penzoldt's test, reagent (pen′zōldz) [Franz *Penzoldt,* physician in Erlangen, 1849–1927] see under *tests.*

Penzoldt-Fisher test (pen′zōld-fish′er) [Franz *Penzoldt;* Emil *Fisher,* German chemist, 1852–1919] see under *tests.*

peonin chloride (pe′o-nin) chemical name: 4′,7-dihydroxy-3,5-di-β-glucosido-3′-methoxyflavylium chloride. A deep purple dye, $C_{28}H_{33}ClO_{16}$, the coloring matter of deep purple peonies; called also *peonin.*

peotillomania (pe″o-til″o-ma′ne-ah) [Gr. *peos* penis + *tillein* to pull + *mania* madness] a ticlike movement consisting in constant pulling at the penis; called also *pseudomasturbation.*

peotomy (pe-ot′o-me) [Gr. *peos* penis + *temnein* to cut] surgical removal of the penis.

peplomer (pep′lo-mer) a subunit of the peplos, or envelope, of a virion.

peplos (pep′lohs) the lipoprotein envelope possessed by some types of virions, assembled in some cases from subunits called peplomers.

pepo (pe′po) [L. "pumpkin"] pumpkin seed; the dried ripe edible seeds of the pumpkin, *Cucurbita pepo* L. (Cucurbitaceae); used as an anthelmintic.

pepper (pep′er) [L. *piper*] black pepper; the dried unripe fruit of *Piper nigrum* L. (Piperaceae) and other plants of that genus. *White pepper* is the decorticated ripe fruit of black pepper, and is milder. Pepper contains piperine, an aromatic pungent volatile oil (5–9 per cent), minor alkaloids, fat, protein, and resins; used chiefly as a spice, but it also has diaphoretic, carminative, and gastric secretagogue properties. **cayenne p.,** capsicum.

Pepper's syndrome (type) (pep′erz) [William *Pepper*, Philadelphia physician, 1874–1947] see under *syndrome*.

peppermint (pep′er-mint) [USP] the dried leaves and flowering tops of *Mentha piperita* L. (Labiatae), having carminative, gastric stimulant, and counter-irritant properties; used as an oil, spirit, or water extract as a flavored vehicle for drugs.

pepsic (pep′sik) peptic.

pepsin (pep′sin) [L. *pepsinum*, from Gr. *pepsis* digestion] the proteolytic enzyme of gastric juice which catalyzes the hydrolysis of native or denatured proteins to form a mixture of polypeptides. It has an optimum pH of 1.5 to 2.0 and a specificity for peptide bonds involving aromatic amino acids (phenylalanine, tyrosine, tryptophan), although other bonds are also split. It is formed from pepsinogen in the presence of acid or, autocatalytically, in the presence of pepsin. It is freely soluble in water and has been obtained in pure crystalline form. Crude preparations from swine or beef stomach have been used as a digestive aid. **aromatic p.**, a mixture of 10 per cent of pepsin with tartaric acid, sodium chloride, and milk sugar. **Brücke's protein-free p.**, a purified pepsin that contains less nitrogen than crystalline pepsin and that hydrolyzes casein which has already been digested by crystalline pepsin. **ostrich p.**, a pepsin prepared in Argentina from the gizzard of the ostrich or rhea. **saccharated p.**, pepsin mixed with sugar of milk.

pepsinate (pep′sin-āt) to treat or charge with pepsin.

pepsinia (pep-sin′e-ah) the secretion of pepsin; it may be normal, excessive (hyperpepsinia), deficient (hypopepsinia), or totally absent (apepsinia).

pepsiniferous (pep″sin-if′er-us) [pepsin + L. *ferre* to bear] producing or secreting pepsin.

pepsinogen (pep-sin′o-jen) [pepsin + Gr. *gennan* to produce] a zymogen secreted by chief cells, mucous neck cells, and pyloric gland cells, which is converted into pepsin in the presence of gastric acid or of pepsin itself.

pepsinogenous (pep″sin-oj′ĕ-nus) producing pepsin.

pepsinum (pep-si′num) pepsin.

pepsinuria (pep″sĭ-nu′re-ah) the presence of pepsin in the urine; it may be associated with duodenal ulcer because of the increased volume of gastric secretion.

pepstatin (pep-stat′in) any of the pentapeptide pepsin inhibitors obtained from several species of *Streptomyces*, identified as pepstatin A, B, and C. The A component, $C_{34}H_{63}N_5O_9$, has been used in the treatment of gastric ulcer.

peptase (pep′tās) peptidase.

Peptavlon (pep-tav′lon) trademark for a preparation of pentagastrin.

peptic (pep′tik) [Gr. *peptikos*] pertaining to pepsin or to digestion; related to the action of gastric juices.

peptid (pep′tid) peptide.

peptidase (pep′tĭ-dās) any of a subclass of proteolytic enzymes that catalyze the hydrolysis of peptide linkages. **procollagen p.**, an enzyme that converts procollagen to collagen.

peptide (pep′tid) any member of a class of compounds of low molecular weight which yield two or more amino acids on hydrolysis. Formed by loss of water from the NH₂ and COOH groups of adjacent amino acids, they are known as di-, tri-, tetra-[etc.] peptides, depending on the number of amino acids in the molecule. Peptides form the constituent parts of proteins. **C p.**, the connecting peptide chain that is removed in the cleavage of proinsulin to form insulin. **vasoactive intestinal p. (VIP)**, a peptide hormone (approximately 3381 daltons, 28 amino acids) first isolated from the small intestine of the pig, which in addition to its vasoactive properties, stimulates intestinal secretion of water and electrolytes, inhibits gastric secretion, promotes glycogenesis, causes hyperglycemia, and stimulates production of pancreatic juice. Its physiologic role as a hormone is not yet known. Called also *vasoactive intestinal polypeptide*.

peptidergic (pep″tĭ-der′jĭk) of or pertaining to neurons like those that secrete peptide hormones which have a hypophyseotropic function.

peptidoglycan (pep″tĭ-do-gli′kan) a glycan (polysaccharide) attached to short cross-linked peptides; peptidoglycans are found in bacterial cell walls.

peptidolytic (pep″tĭ-do-lit′ik) [peptide + Gr. *lytikos* dissolving] capable of splitting peptide bonds.

peptinotoxin (pep″tĭ-no-tok′sin) a poisonous intestinal product of imperfect stomach digestion.

peptization (pep″ti-za′shun) increase in the degree of dispersion of a colloid solution; the liquefaction of a colloid gel to form a sol.

Peptococcus (pep″to-kok′us) a genus of gram-positive, anaerobic bacteria (cocci) of the family Micrococcaceae, order Eubacteriales, usually occurring singly, in pairs, or as irregular masses, which are chemo-organotrophic and capable of fermenting protein decomposition products. They have been found in the urogenital, respiratory, and intestinal tract in humans, but their pathogenicity is uncertain because they are often found in association with pathogens in such conditions as cystitis, pleurisy, and postpartum septicemia. **P. anaero′bius**, a microaerophilic or obligate anaerobe found in the appendix and the female genital tract, and in cystitis and draining sinus. Called also *Diplococcus magnus*. **P. constella′tus**, a microaerophilic or obligate anaerobe found in purulent pleurisy and in the tonsils, appendix, nose, throat, gums, and infrequently the skin and vagina. Called also *Diplococcus constellatus*.

peptogenic (pep″to-jen′ik) [Gr. *peptein* to digest + *gennan* to produce] 1. producing pepsin or peptones. 2. promoting digestion.

peptogenous (pep-toj′ĕ-nus) peptogenic.

peptolysis (pep-tol′ĭ-sis) [peptone + Gr. *lysis* dissolution] the splitting up of peptone.

peptolytic (pep″to-lit′ik) splitting up peptone.

peptone (pep′tōn) [Gr. *pepton* digesting] a derived protein, or a mixture of cleavage products produced by the partial hydrolysis of a native protein either by an acid or by an enzyme. Peptones are readily soluble in water, and are not precipitatable by heat, by alkalis, or by saturation with ammonium sulfate. **beef p.**, a peptone made from beef by treating it with extract of pancreas. **casein p.**, a light-brown powder, soluble in water; a nutrient for convalescents. **gelatin p.**, a peptone formed during the digestion of gelatin with pepsin. **glycerin-gelatin p.**, a bacteriologic culture medium. **Höchst's p.**, peptone obtained from silk, once used as a test for the presence of peptone-splitting enzymes, either by changes in optical activity or by the precipitation of tyrosine. **milk p.**, casein p. **venom p.**, a peptone from snake venom.

peptonic (pep-ton′ik) pertaining to or containing peptone.

peptonize (pep′to-nīz) to convert a protein into peptone by the action of an acid or enzyme.

peptonoid (pep′to-noid) a peptone-like substance.

peptonuria (pep″to-nu′re-ah) [peptone + Gr. *ouron* urine + -ia] the presence of peptones in the urine. **enterogenous p.**, that which is due to disease of the intestine. **hepatogenous p.**, that which is due to disease of the liver. **nephrogenic p.**, that which is due to disease of the kidney. **puerperal p.**, that which occurs during the puerperium. **pyogenic p.**, that which is associated with a suppurative process.

Peptostreptococcus (pep″to-strep″to-kok′us) a genus of microorganisms of the tribe Streptococceae, family Lactobacillaceae, order Eubacteriales, made up of obligate anaerobic streptococci occurring as parasitic inhabitants of the intestinal tract, and occasionally found in gangrenous and necrotic lesions probably as secondary invaders. It includes 13 species.

peptotoxin (pep″to-tok′sin) any toxin or poisonous base developed from a peptone; also a poisonous alkaloid or ptomaine occurring in certain peptones and putrefying proteins.

per- [L. *per* through] 1. a prefix meaning throughout, in space or time, or completely or extremely. 2. a prefix used in chemical terms to denote a large amount or to designate combination of an element in its highest valence.

peracephalus (per″ah-sef′ah-lus) [per- + *acephalus*] a monster with neither head nor arms, and with a defective thorax.

peracetate (per-as′ĕ-tāt) a salt or derivative of peracetic acid.

peracid (per-as′id) an acid containing more than the usual quantity of oxygen.

peracidity (per″ah-sid′ĭ-te) excessive acidity.

peracute (per″ah-kūt′) [L. *peracutus*] excessively acute or sharp.

Perandren (per-an′dren) trademark for a preparation of testosterone.

per anum (per a′num) [L.] through the anus.

perarticulation (per″ar-tik″u-la′shun) [per- + L. *articulatio* joint] diarthrosis.

peratodynia (per″at-o-din′e-ah) [Gr. *peran* to pierce + *odynē* pain] (*obs.*) cardialgia or heartburn.

Perazil (per′ah-zil) trademark for preparations of chlorcyclizine hydrochloride.

percentile (per-sen′tĭl, per-sen′til) 1. of, pertaining to, or used in percentage. 2. one of 100 equal parts of a series divided in order of their measurable magnitude.

percentual (per-sen′tu-al) pertaining to percentage; figured on the basis of 100.

percept (per′sept) the object perceived; the mental image of an object in space perceived by the senses.

perception (per-sep′shun) [L. *perceptio* a gathering together] the conscious mental registration of a sensory stimulus. **depth p.**, the proper recognition of depth or the relative distances to different objects in space, with ability to orient one's position in relation to them. **extrasensory p.**, knowledge of, or response to, an external thought or objective event not achieved as the result of stimulation of the sense organs. Abbreviated ESP. **facial p.**, see under *vision*. **stereognostic p.**, the recognition of objects by touch.

perceptive (per-sep′tiv) pertaining to perception.

perceptivity (per″sep-tiv′ĭ-te) ability to receive sense impressions.

perceptorium (per″sep-to′re-um) sensorium.

perchloride (per-klo′rīd) a chloride that contains more chlorine than the ordinary chloride; an organic compound in which all the hydrogen atoms are substituted by chlorine, as in perchloroethylene (tetrachloroethylene), C_2Cl_4.

perchlormethane (per″klōr-meth′ān) carbon tetrachloride.

perchlormethylformate (per″klor-meth″il-for′māt) diphosgene.

percine (per′sin) a protamine from the sperm of yellow perch, *Perca flavescens*.

percipient (per-sip′e-ent) 1. pertaining to perception. 2. an individual who perceives or is capable of perception.

percolate (per′ko-lāt) [L. *percolare*] 1. to strain; to submit to percolation. 2. to trickle slowly through a substance. 3. a liquid that has been submitted to percolation.

percolation (per″ko-la′shun) [L. *percolatio*] the extraction of the soluble parts of a drug by causing a liquid solvent to flow slowly through it.

percolator (per′ko-la″tor) a vessel used in percolating drugs.

percomorph (per′ko-morf) pertaining to Percomorphi, an order of fishes whose liver oil is rich in vitamins A and D.

per contiguum (per kon-tig′u-um) [L.] in contiguity: arranged in such a way that the edges touch.

per continuum (per kon-tin′u-um) [L.] in continuity: without separation or break.

Percorten (per-kor′ten) trademark for preparations of desoxycorticosterone.

percuss (per-kus′) [L. *percutere*] to subject to percussion.

percussible (per-kus′ĭ-b'l) discoverable on percussion.

percussion (per-kush′un) [L. *percussio*] 1. the act of striking a part with short, sharp blows as an aid in diagnosing the condition of the underlying parts by the sound obtained. 2. a method of massage; see *tapotement*. **auscultatory p.,** auscultation of the sound produced by percussion. **bimanual p.,** the usual manner of percussion in which the middle finger of the left hand is placed against the body wall and its nail is struck a quick blow with the end of the bent right middle finger. **coin p.,** see under *tests*. **comparative p.,** percussion of two or more areas in order to compare the sounds obtained. **deep p.,** percussion in which a firm blow is struck in order to obtain a note from a deep-seated tissue. **direct p.,** immediate percussion. **drop p., drop stroke p.,** instrumental percussion in which the plexor is allowed to fall by its own weight on to the pleximeter, the elements considered in the examination being the sound heard, the vibrations felt in the handle of the plexor, and the rebound of the plexor seen. Called also *Lerch's p.* **finger p.,** that in which the fingers of one hand are used as a plexor, and those of the other as a pleximeter. **fist p.,** percussion in which the fist is brought down with a moderate thump over the area to be tested. **Goldscheider's p.,** 1. threshold percussion. 2. orthopercussion. **immediate p.,** that in which no pleximeter is used. **instrumental p.,** that in which a plexor or hammer is used. **Kora′nyi's p.,** see under *auscultation*. **Krönig's p.,** auscul-

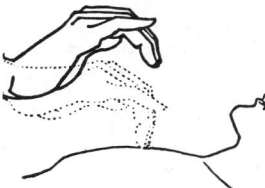

Immediate percussion (Külbs).

tatory percussion over the apexes of the lungs in the diagnosis of tuberculosis. **Lerch's p.,** drop p. **mediate p.,** that in which a pleximeter is employed. **Murphy's p.,** piano p. **palpatory p.,** a combination of palpation and percussion, affording tactile rather than auditory impressions. **paradoxical p.,** resonance of the chest combined with abundant rales as in acute edema of the lungs. **pencil p.,** Plesch's p. **piano p.,** percussion by striking the body by the four fingers one after the other, beginning with the little finger; called also *Murphy's p.* **Plesch's p.,** percussion within the intercostal spaces to avoid

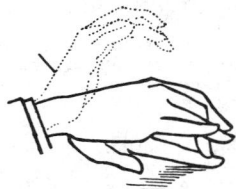

Strong percussion (Külbs).

setting the ribs into vibration, the pleximeter finger with the first interphalangeal joint flexed at a right angle. **pleximetric p.,**

mediate p. **respiratory p.,** percussion during respiration so as to bring out the difference in the percussion notes of inspiration and expiration. **slapping p.,** percussion made by a slapping blow: used in comparing the resonance. **strip p.,** percussion

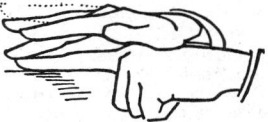

Weak percussion (Külbs).

which starts from above and progresses downward, thus covering a "strip" of the chest wall. **tangential p.,** percussion with the pleximeter placed vertically on the body, the strokes being applied to the pleximeter in a direction parallel with the surface of the skin. **threshold p.,** percussion performed by tapping lightly with the finger upon a glass rod pleximeter, one end of which, fitted with a rubber cap, rests upon an intercostal space, the rod being held at an angle to the surface of the thorax and parallel to the borders of the organ to be delimited. This method confines the percussion vibrations to a very restricted area. Called also *Goldscheider's p.* **topographic p.,** the demarcation and outlining of a dull area by percussion to determine the boundaries of organs or parts of organs.

percussopunctator (per-kus″o-punk′ta-tor) an instrument for performing multiple acupuncture.

percussor (per-kus′or) [L. "striker"] an instrument for use in performing percussion.

percutaneous (per″ku-ta′ne-us) [*per-* + L. *cutis*] performed through the skin, as injection of radiopaque material in radiological examination, or the removal of tissue for biopsy accomplished by a needle.

per cutem [L.] through the skin.

percuteur (per″koo-tūr′) [Fr.] an instrument for therapeutic or diagnostic percussion.

pereirine (per-e′ir-in) [Port. *pereira* brier] a white alkaloid, $C_{19}H_{24}N_2O$, from the bark of *Geissospermum vellosi* Allem. (Apocynaceae), a tree of tropical America; antiperiodic, antipyretic, and tonic.

perencephaly (per″en-sef′ah-le) [Gr. *pēra* pouch + *enkephalos* brain] porencephalia.

perennial (per-en′ĭ-al) [L. *perennis*, from *per* through + *annus* year] lasting through the year or for several years.

perethynol (per-eth′ĭ-nol) (*obs.*) a colloidal suspension prepared from fresh horse heart in chlorethylene and alcohol for Vernes' test for syphilis. See *Vernes' test* (def. 1), under *tests*.

Perez's sign (pa-rāths″) [Jorje *Perez*, Spanish physician, died 1920] see under *sign*.

perfectionism (per-fek′shun-izm) a personality trait characterized by the setting of impossible standards, leading to frustration and self-condemnation.

perfilcon A (per-fil′kon) chemical name: 2-methyl-2-propenoic acid 2-hydroxyethyl ester polymer with 1-ethenyl-2-pyrrolidinone and 2-methyl-2-propenoic acid; a hydrophilic contact lens material, $(C_6H_{10}O_3)_x(C_6H_9NO)_y(C_4H_6O_2)_z$.

perflation (per-fla′shun) [L. *perflatio*] the act of blowing air into a space in order to force out secretions or other substances.

perforans (per′fo-ranz) [L.] penetrating; a term applied to various muscles and nerves. **p. ma′nus,** musculus flexor digitorum profundus.

perforated (per′fo-rāt″ed) [L. *perforatus*] pierced with holes.

perforation (per″fo-ra′shun) [L. *perforare* to pierce through] 1. the act of boring or piercing through a part. 2. a hole made through a part or substance. **Bezold's p.,** perforation of the inner surface of the mastoid bone. **mechanical p.,** an artificial opening or hole made by boring, piercing, or cutting through a structure or surface, such as the root of a tooth. **pathologic p.,** an opening or hole produced in a tissue surface or structure by a pathologic process, as may occur in internal resorption of a tooth.

perforator (per′fo-ra″tor) an instrument for piercing the bones, and especially for perforating the fetal head.

perforatorium (per″fo-rah-to′re-um) acrosome.

perfrication (per″fri-ka′shun) [L. *perfricare* to rub] rubbing with an ointment or embrocation.

perfrigeration (per-frij″er-a′shun) [*per-* + L. *frigere* to be cold] frostbite.

perfusate (per-fu′zāt) a liquid that has been passed over or through the vessels of an organ or tissue.

perfuse (per-fūz′) to pour over or through.

perfusion (per-fu′zhun) 1. the act of pouring over or through, especially the passage of a fluid through the vessels of a specific organ. 2. a liquid poured over or through an organ or tissue.

perhexiline maleate (per-heks′ĭ-lēn) chemical name: 2-(2,2-dicylohexylethyl)piperidine (*Z*)-2-butenedioate. A coronary vasodilator, $C_{19}H_{35}N·C_4H_4O_4$; used in the prophylaxis of angina of effort and has been used to control certain cardiac arrhythmias.

peri- [Gr. *peri* around] a prefix meaning around.

periacinal (per″e-as′ĭ-nal) [peri- + L. *acinus* berry] situated around an acinus.

periacinous (per″e-as′ĭ-nus) around an acinus.

Periactin (per″e-ak′tin) trademark for preparations of cyproheptadine hydrochloride.

periadenitis (per″e-ad″ĕ-ni′tis) [peri- + Gr. *adēn* gland + -itis] inflammation of the tissues around a gland. **p. aph′thae,** p. mucosa necrotica recurrens. **p. muco′sa necrot′ica re-cur′rens,** a disease of the mouth, once considered a distinct entity, but now recognized as the more severe form of aphthous stomatitis (q.v.); it is marked by recurrent attacks of aphtha-like lesions that begin as small, firm nodules, which then enlarge, ulcerate, and heal by scar formation. After repeated attacks, numerous atrophied scars mark the oral mucosa. Called also *chronic intermittent recurrent aphthae, Mikulicz's aphthae, recurrent scarring aphthae, aphthae resistentiae, periadenitis aphthae,* and *Sutton's disease.*

periadventitial (per″e-ad″ven-tish′al) outside the adventitia.

perialienitis (per″e-āl″yen-i′tis) [peri- + L. *alienus* foreign + -itis] inflammation around a foreign body, as a biliary concretion.

periampullary (per″e-am′pu-lar″e) situated around an ampulla, as around the hepatopancreatic ampulla.

perianal (per″e-a′nal) [peri- + L. *anus* anus] located around the anus.

periangiitis (per″e-an″je-i′tis) [peri- + Gr. *angeion* vessel + -itis] inflammation of the tissue surrounding a blood or lymph vessel.

periangiocholitis (per″e-an″je-o-ko-li′tis) pericholangitis.

periangioma (per″e-an-je-o′mah) [peri- + Gr. *angeion* vessel + -oma] a tumor which surrounds a blood vessel.

perianth (per′e-anth) [peri- + Gr. *anthos* flower] the floral envelope, including the calyx and corolla.

periaortic (per″e-a-or′tik) around the aorta.

periaortitis (per″e-a″or-ti′tis) inflammation of the tissues around the aorta.

periapex (per″e-a′peks) the tissue which surrounds the root apex of a tooth (the periodontal ligament and alveolar bone).

periapical (per″e-ap′ĭ-kal) [peri- + L. *apex* tip] relating to tissues encompassing the apex of a tooth, including periodontal membrane and alveolar bone.

periappendicitis (per″e-ah-pen″dĭ-si′tis) [peri- + *appendix* + -itis] inflammation of the tissues around the vermiform appendix. **p. decidua′lis,** a condition in tubal pregnancy in which, on account of adhesions between the appendix and the fallopian tube, decidual cells are present in the peritoneum of the appendix.

periappendicular (per″e-ap″en-dik′u-lar) around the vermiform appendix.

periapt (per′e-apt) [Gr. *periapton* amulet] a substance worn in the belief that it wards off disease.

periaqueductal (per″e-ak″wĭ-duk′tal) around an aqueduct.

periarterial (per″e-ar-te′re-al) around an artery.

periarteritis (per″e-ar″tĕ-ri′tis) [peri- + Gr. *artēria* artery + -itis] inflammation of the external coats of an artery and of the tissues around the artery. **p. gummo′sa,** accumulation of gummas on the blood vessels in syphilis. **p. nodo′sa,** an inflammatory disease of the coats of the small and medium-sized arteries of the body, associated with a variety of systemic symptoms. Called also *polyarteritis* and *panarteritis.* **syphilitic p.,** periarteritis gummosa.

periarthric (per″e-ar′thrik) [peri- + Gr. *arthron* joint] around a joint.

periarthritis (per″e-ar-thri′tis) inflammation of the tissues around a joint. **p. of shoulder,** adhesive capsulitis.

periarticular (per″e-ar-tik′u-lar) [peri- + L. *articulus* joint] situated around a joint.

periatrial (per″e-a′tre-al) around the atrium of the heart.

periauricular (per″e-aw-rik′u-lar) 1. around the concha of the ear. 2. periatrial.

periaxial (per″e-ak′se-al) [peri- + Gr. *axōn* axis] situated around an axis.

periaxillary (per″e-ak′sĭ-ler″e) situated or occurring around the axilla.

periaxonal (per″e-ak′so-nal) [peri- + *axon*] occurring around an axon.

periblast (per′ĭ-blast) [peri- + Gr. *blastos* germ] the portion of the blastoderm of telolecithal eggs the cells of which lack complete cell membranes.

peribronchial (per″ĭ-brong′ke-al) situated around a bronchus.

peribronchiolar (per″ĭ-brong-ki′o-lar) situated around the bronchioles.

peribronchiolitis (per″ĭ-brong″ke-o-li′tis) inflammation of the tissues around the bronchioles.

peribronchitis (per″ĭ-brong-ki′tis) a form of bronchitis consisting of inflammation and thickening of the peribronchial tissue.

peribulbar (per″ĭ-bul′bar) surrounding the bulb of the eye.

peribursal (per″ĭ-ber′sal) surrounding a bursa.

pericaliceal (per″ĭ-kal′ĭ-se′al) situated near to or around a renal calix.

pericallosal (per″ĭ-kah-lo′sal) situated around the corpus callosum.

pericalyceal (per″ĭ-kal′ĭ-se′al) pericaliceal.

pericanalicular (per″ĭ-kan″ah-lik′u-lar) occurring around canaliculi.

pericapsular (per″ĭ-kap′su-lar) surrounding a capsule.

pericardectomy (per″ĭ-kar-dek′to-me) pericardiectomy.

pericardiac (per″ĭ-kar′de-ak) pericardial.

pericardial (per″ĭ-kar′de-al) pertaining to the pericardium.

pericardicentesis (per″ĭ-kar″de-sen-te′sis) pericardiocentesis.

pericardiectomy (per″ĭ-kar″de-ek′to-me) [*pericardium* + Gr. *ektomē* excision] excision of the pericardium.

pericardiocentesis (per″ĭ-kar″de-o-sen-te′sis) [*pericardium* + Gr. *kentēsis* puncture] surgical puncture of the pericardial cavity for the aspiration of fluid.

pericardiolysis (per″ĭ-kar″de-ol′ĭ-sis) [*pericardium* + Gr. *lysis* dissolution] the operation of freeing adhesions between the visceral and parietal pericardium.

pericardiomediastinitis (per″ĭ-kar″de-o-me″de-as-tĭ-ni′tis) pericarditis with mediastinitis; inflammation of the pericardium and mediastinum.

pericardiophrenic (per″ĭ-kar″de-o-fren′ik) pertaining to the pericardium and the diaphragm.

pericardiopleural (per″ĭ-kar″de-o-plu′ral) pertaining to the pericardium and the pleura.

pericardiorrhaphy (per″ĭ-kar″de-or′ah-fe) [*pericardium* + Gr. *rhaphē* suture] the operation of suturing a wound in the pericardium.

pericardiostomy (per″ĭ-kar″de-os′to-me) [*pericardium* + Gr. *stoma* mouth] the operation of making an opening into the pericardium usually for the drainage of effusions.

pericardiotomy (per″ĭ-kar″de-ot′o-me) [*pericardium* + Gr. *temnein* to cut] surgical incision of the pericardium.

pericarditic (per″ĭ-kar-dit′ik) pertaining to pericarditis.

pericarditis (per″ĭ-kar-di′tis) [*pericardium* + -itis] inflammation of the pericardium. **acute benign p.,** idiopathic p. **acute fibrinous p.,** inflammation of the pericardium marked by fibrinous exudate on the serous membrane. **adhesive p.,** a condition resulting from the presence of dense fibrous tissue between the parietal and visceral layers of the pericardium. There may be complete obliteration of the pericardial cavity, or there may be adhesions extending from the pericardium to the mediastinum (mediastinopericarditis), diaphragm, and chest wall (accretio cordis, accretio pericardii). **amebic p.,** pericarditis occurring as a result of rupture of an amebic abscess of the liver through the diaphragm. **bacterial p.,** pericarditis produced by bacterial infection. **p. calculo′sa,** pericarditis with a calcareous deposit in the pericardium. **carcinomatous p.,** that which is associated with malignant disease of the pericardium. **constrictive p.,** inflammation of the pericardium leading to thickening and sometimes to calcification with impaired diastolic filling, inflow stasis, or constrictive effect. **dry p.,** pericarditis unattended with effusion. **p. with effusion,** pericarditis associated with the collection of a serous or purulent exudate in the pericardial cavity. **p. epistenocardi′aca,** the symptom complex of stenocardia, fever, pericarditis, and myocardial insufficiency (Sternberg). **p. exter′na et inter′na,** inflammation of the outer and inner surfaces of the pericardium. **external p.,** that which chiefly affects the outer surface of the pericardium. **fibrinous p., fibrous p.,** chronic pericarditis characterized by the formation of fibrous tissue and probably adhesions. **hemorrhagic p.,** that in which there is a bloody exudate. **idiopathic p.,** an acute serofibrinous pericarditis of unknown cause; recurrent attacks are not unusual. Called also *acute benign p.* **localized p.,** a term usually denoting chronic pericarditis with thickened white or milky epicardial areas. **mediastinal p.,** inflammation of the exterior surface of the pericardium and the mediastinal tissue. **p. oblit′erans, obliterating p.,** an adhesive pericarditis which leads to the obliteration of the pericardial cavity. **purulent p.,** a form characterized by pus formation. **rheumatic p.,** the form associated with active rheumatic heart disease. **serofibrinous p.,** a variety attended with a serous fluid effusion with deposition of fibrin on the pericardial surfaces. **p. sic′ca,** acute fibrinous pericarditis without effusion. **suppurative p.,** purulent p. **tuberculous p.,** a variety caused by tuberculous disease. **uremic p.,** pericarditis occurring as a complication of uremia. **p. villo′sa,** cor villosum.

pericardium (per″ĭ-kar′de-um) [L.; peri- + Gr. *kardia* heart] [NA] the fibroserous sac that surrounds the heart and the roots of the great vessels, comprising an external layer of fibrous tissue (*pericardium fibrosum* [NA]) and an inner serous layer (*pericardium serosum* [NA]). The base of the pericardium is attached to the central tendon of the diaphragm. **adherent p.,** a pericardium that is abnormally connected with the heart by dense fibrous tissue, as in adhesive pericarditis. **bread-and-butter p.,** a pericardium having a thick fibrinous deposit on its surfaces. **calcified p.,** a pericardium containing deposits of lime salts. **cardiac p.,** visceral p. **p. fibro'sum** [NA], **fibrous p.,** the external layer of the pericardium, consisting of fibrous tissue. **parietal p.,** the parietal layer (lamina parietalis) of the serous pericardium, which is in contact with the fibrous pericardium. **p. sero'sum** [NA], **serous p.,** the inner serous portion of the pericardium consisting of two layers, the *lamina parietalis*, apposed to the fibrous pericardium, and another layer, the *lamina visceralis*, or epicardium, which is reflected onto the roots of the great vessels and the heart. The space between the two layers is the cavum pericardium. **shaggy p.,** a pericardium coated with a roughened layer of fibrinous exudate. **visceral p.,** the inner layer (lamina visceralis pericardii) of the serous pericardium, which is in contact with the heart and roots of the great vessels; called also *epicardium*.

pericardotomy (per″ĭ-kar-dot′o-me) pericardiotomy.

pericarp (per′ĭ-karp) [*peri-* + Gr. *karpos* fruit] the seed vessel or ripened ovary of a flower.

pericaryon (per″ĭ-kar′e-on) perikaryon.

pericecal (per″ĭ-se′kal) surrounding the cecum.

pericecitis (per″ĭ-sĕ-si′tis) inflammation of the tissues around the cecum.

pericellular (per″ĭ-sel′u-lar) [*peri-* + L. *cellula* cell] surrounding a cell.

pericemental (per″ĭ-se-men′tal) pertaining to the pericementum (periodontal ligament).

pericementitis (per″ĭ-se″men-ti′tis) [*pericementum* + *-itis*] periodontitis. **apical p.,** apical abscess. **chronic suppurative p.,** compound periodontitis.

pericementoclasia (per″ĭ-se-men″to-kla′ze-ah) [*pericementum* + Gr. *klasis* breaking] disintegration of the periodontal ligament (pericementum) and alveolar bone without loss of the overlying gingival tissue; it results in pocket formation. Cf. *compound periodontitis*.

pericementum (per″ĭ-se-men′tum) [*peri-* + L. *caementum* cement] the periodontal ligament.

pericentral (per″ĭ-sen′tral) surrounding a center.

pericentriolar (per″e-sen′tre-o′lar) situated around a centriole.

pericephalic (per″ĭ-sĕ-fal′ik) surrounding the head.

pericholangitis (per″ĭ-ko″lan-ji′tis) [*peri-* + Gr. *cholē* bile + *angeion* vessel + *-itis*] inflammation of the tissues that surround the bile ducts.

pericholecystitis (per″ĭ-ko″le-sis-ti′tis) inflammation of the tissues around the gallbladder. **gaseous p.,** emphysematous cholecystitis.

perichondrial (per″ĭ-kon′dre-al) pertaining to or composed of perichondrium.

perichondritis (per″ĭ-kon-dri′tis) inflammation of the perichondrium.

perichondrium (per″ĭ-kon′dre-um) [*peri-* + Gr. *chondros* cartilage] [NA] the layer of dense fibrous connective tissue which invests all cartilage except the articular cartilage of synovial joints.

perichondroma (per″ĭ-kon-dro′mah) a tumor arising from the perichondrium.

perichord (per′ĭ-kord) the investing sheath of the notochord.

perichordal (per″ĭ-kor′dal) [*peri-* + Gr. *chordē* cord] situated around the notochord.

perichorioidal (per″ĭ-ko″re-oi′dal) perichoroidal.

perichoroidal (per″ĭ-ko-roi′dal) surrounding the choroid coat.

perichrome (per′ĭ-krōm) [*peri-* + Gr. *chrōma* color] a nerve cell in which the Nissl bodies are arranged in rows beneath the cell membrane. Cf. *arkyochrome*, *gyrochrome*, and *stichochrome*.

periclasia (per″ĭ-kla′se-ah) periodontoclasia.

Periclor (pār′ĭ-klōr) trademark for a preparation of petrichloral.

pericolic (per″ĭ-ko′lik) around the colon, as pericolic membrane.

pericolitis (per″ĭ-ko-li′tis) [*peri-* + Gr. *kolon* colon + *-itis*] inflammation around the colon, especially of the peritoneal coat of the colon. **p. dex′tra,** pericolitis affecting the ascending colon. **membranous p.,** a morbid condition resulting from the presence of Jackson's membrane (q.v.). **p. sinis′tra,** inflammation of the surrounding connective tissue and peritoneum of the descending colon.

pericolonitis (per″ĭ-ko″lon-i′tis) pericolitis.

pericolpitis (per″ĭ-kol-pi′tis) [*peri-* + Gr. *kolpos* vagina + *-itis*] inflammation of the tissues around the vagina.

periconchal (per″ĭ-kong′kal) [*peri-* + Gr. *konchē* a shell-like cavity] situated around the concha.

periconchitis (per″ĭ-kong-ki′tis) [*peri-* + Gr. *konchē* a shell-like cavity + *-itis*] inflammation of the lining of the orbit.

pericorneal (per″ĭ-kor′ne-al) surrounding the cornea.

pericoronal (per″ĭ-kor′o-nal) around the crown of a tooth.

pericoronitis (per″ĭ-kor″o-ni′tis) [*peri-* + L. *corona* crown + *-itis*] inflammation of the gingiva surrounding the crown of a partially erupted tooth; called also *operculitis*.

pericoxitis (per″ĭ-kok-si′tis) inflammation of the tissues about the hip joint.

pericranial (per″ĭ-kra′ne-al) pertaining to the pericranium.

pericranitis (per″ĭ-kra-ni′tis) inflammation of the external periosteum of the skull.

pericranium (per″ĭ-kra′ne-um) [*peri-* + Gr. *kranion* cranium] [NA] the external periosteum of the skull.

pericycle (per″ĭ-si′k'l) [*peri-* + Gr. *kyklos* circle] a layer of parenchymal cells capable of being transformed into meristem to give rise to the root cambium and cork cambium and to branch roots.

pericystic (per″ĭ-sis′tik) situated about a cyst.

pericystitis (per″ĭ-sis-ti′tis) [*peri-* + Gr. *kystis* bladder + *-itis*] inflammation of the tissues around the bladder.

pericystium (per″ĭ-sis′te-um) the vascular envelope of certain cysts.

pericyte (per′ĭ-sit) [*peri-* + Gr. *kytos* cell] one of the peculiar elongated cells with the power of contraction, found wrapped about precapillary arterioles outside the basement membrane; called also *pericyte of Zimmermann* and *Rouget cell*.

pericytial (per″ĭ-si′shal) situated around a cell.

pericytoma (per″ĭ-si-to′mah) hemangiopericytoma.

peridectomy (per″ĭ-dek′to-me) peritectomy.

perideferentitis (per″ĭ-def″er-en-ti′tis) inflammation of the tissues surrounding the ductus deferens.

peridendritic (per″ĭ-den-drit′ik) surrounding the dendrites.

peridens (per″ĭ-dens) a supernumerary tooth appearing elsewhere than in the midline of the dental arch.

peridental (per″ĭ-den′tal) periodontal.

peridentium (per″ĭ-den′she-um) periodontium.

periderm (per′ĭ-derm) [*peri-* + Gr. *derma* skin] 1. the large-celled outer layer of the bilaminar fetal epidermis. In the human it is loosened by the hair which grows beneath it, and generally disappears before birth. Called also *epitrichium*. 2. the cuticle (eponychium and hyponychium), the only part of the periderm which persists after birth.

peridermal (per″ĭ-der′mal) pertaining to the periderm.

peridesmic (per″ĭ-dez′mik) around a ligament; pertaining to the peridesmium.

peridesmitis (per″ĭ-dez-mi′tis) inflammation of the peridesmium.

peridesmium (per″ĭ-dez′me-um) [*peri-* + Gr. *desmion* band] the areolar membrane which covers the ligaments.

perididymis (per″ĭ-did′ĭ-mis) [*peri-* + Gr. *didymos* testicle] the tunica vaginalis testis.

perididymitis (per″ĭ-did″ĭ-mi′tis) inflammation of the perididymis; called also *vaginitis testis*.

peridiverticulitis (per″ĭ-di″ver-tik″u-li′tis) inflammation of structures around a diverticulum of the intestine.

peridontoclasia (per″ĭ-don″to-kla′se-ah) periodontoclasia.

periductal (per″ĭ-duk′tal) surrounding a duct, particularly a duct of the mammary gland.

periductile (per″ĭ-duk′tīl) periductal.

periduodenitis (per″ĭ-du″o-dĕ-ni′tis) inflammation around the duodenum, a condition marked by a deformed duodenum surrounded and fixed by peritoneal adhesions.

peridural (per″ĭ-du′ral) around or external to the dura mater.

peridurogram (per″ĭ-du′ro-gram) the film obtained in peridurography.

peridurography (per″ĭ-du-rog′rah-fe) [*peri-* + *dura* + Gr. *graphein* to write] roentgenography of the spinal canal and interspaces after injection of a contrast medium in the peridural space.

periencephalitis (per″ĭ-en-sef′ah-li′tis) [*peri-* + Gr. *enkephalos* brain + *-itis*] inflammation of the surface of the brain; meningitis with cortical encephalitis.

periencephalography (per″e-en-sef″ah-log′rah-fe) roentgenography of the cerebral meninges.

periencephalomeningitis (per″e-en-sef″ah-lo-men″in-ji′tis) [*peri-* + Gr. *enkephalos* brain + *mēninx* membrane + *-itis*] chronic inflammation of the cerebral cortex and meninges; paresis or general paralysis of the insane.

perienteric (per″e-en-ter′ik) situated around the intestine.

perienteritis (per″e-en″ter-i′tis) [*peri-* + Gr. *enteron* intestine + *-itis*] inflammation of the peritoneal coat of the intestine; visceral peritonitis.

perienteron (per″e-en′ter-on) [*peri-* + Gr. *enteron* intestine] the primitive perivisceral cavity of the embryo.

periependymal (per″e-ep-en′dĭ-mal) situated around the ependyma.

periepithelioma (per″e-ep″ĭ-the-le-o′mah) adrenal cortical carcinoma.

periesophageal (per″e-ĕ-sof′ah-je-al) situated around the esophagus.

periesophagitis (per″e-ĕ-sof′ah-ji′tis) inflammation of the tissues around the esophagus.

perifascicular (per″e-fah-sik′u-lar) surrounding a fasciculus of nerve or muscle fibers.

perifistular (per″ĭ-fis′tu-lar) around a fistula.

perifocal (per″ĭ-fo′kal) around or surrounding a focus, such as a focus of infection.

perifollicular (per″ĭ-fŏ-lik′u-lar) surrounding a follicle.

perifolliculitis (per″ĭ-fŏ-lik″u-li′tis) inflammation around the hair follicles. **p. cap′itis absce′dens et suffo′diens,** a suppurating and cicatrizing disease of the scalp marked by numerous fluctuating abscesses, comedones, and scars. Called also *folliculitis abscedens et suffodiens* and *dissecting cellulitis of scalp.* **superficial pustular p.,** Bockhart's impetigo.

perigangliitis (per″ĭ-gang″gle-i′tis) inflammation of tissues around a ganglion.

periganglionic (per″ĭ-gang″gle-on′ik) situated around a ganglion.

perigastric (per″ĭ-gas′trik) situated around the stomach; pertaining to the peritoneal coat of the stomach.

perigastritis (per″ĭ-gas-tri′tis) [peri- + Gr. *gastēr* stomach + *-itis*] inflammation of the peritoneal coat of the stomach.

perigemmal (per″ĭ-jem′al) surrounding a taste bud or other bud.

periglandular (per″ĭ-glan′du-lar) surrounding a gland or glands.

periglandulitis (per″ĭ-glan″du-li′tis) inflammation of the tissues about a glandule or glandules.

periglial (per″ĭ-gli′al) surrounding the glial cells of the brain.

periglossitis (per″ĭ-glŏ-si′tis) inflammation of the tissues around the tongue.

periglottic (per″ĭ-glot′ik) situated around the tongue.

periglottis (per″ĭ-glot′is) [peri- + Gr. *glōtta* tongue] the mucous membrane of the tongue.

perihepatic (per″ĭ-he-pat′ik) [peri- + Gr. *hēpar* liver] situated or occurring around the liver.

perihepatitis (per″ĭ-hep″ah-ti′tis) [peri- + Gr. *hēpar* liver + *-itis*] inflammation of the peritoneal capsule of the liver and of the tissues around the liver. **p. chron′ica hyperplas′tica,** a disease in which the peritoneal covering of the liver becomes converted into a white mass resembling the icing of a cake; called also *frosted liver, icing liver, sugar-icing liver,* and *zuckergussleber.* **gonococcal p.,** perihepatitis due to extension of gonorrheal infection; see *Fitz-Hugh–Curtis syndrome,* under *syndrome.*

perihernial (per″ĭ-her′ne-al) situated or occurring around a hernia.

perihilar (per″e-hi′lar) around a hilus, e.g., around the pulmonary hilus.

peri-insular (per″e-in′su-lar) surrounding an island, particularly the insula.

peri-islet (per″e-i′let) situated around the islets of Langerhans.

perijejunitis (per″ĭ-je″ju-ni′tis) inflammation around the jejunum.

perikaryon (per″ĭ-kar′e-on) [peri- + Gr. *karyon* nucleus] the cell body as distinguished from the nucleus and the processes; applied particularly to neurons.

perikeratic (per″ĭ-ker-at′ik) surrounding the cornea.

perikymata (per″ĭ-ki′mah-tah) [pl., *peri-* + Gr. *kyma* wave] the numerous small transverse ridges on the exposed surface of the enamel of a permanent tooth.

perilabyrinth (per″ĭ-lab′ĭ-rinth) the tissue surrounding the labyrinth of the ear.

perilabyrinthitis (per″ĭ-lab″ĭ-rin-thi′tis) inflammation of the tissues around the labyrinth of the ear. It may lead to circumscribed labyrinthitis.

perilaryngeal (per″ĭ-lah-rin′je-al) situated around the larynx.

perilaryngitis (per″ĭ-lar″in-ji′tis) [peri- + Gr. *larynx* larynx + *-itis*] inflammation of the tissues around the larynx.

perilenticular (per″ĭ-len-tik′u-lar) surrounding the lens of the eye.

perilesional (per″ĭ-le′shun-al) located or occurring around a lesion.

periligamentous (per″ĭ-lig″ah-men′tus) situated around a ligament.

perilobar (per″ĭ-lo′bar) surrounding a lobe.

perilobulitis (per″ĭ-lob-u-li′tis) inflammation of the tissues surrounding the lobules of the lung.

perilymph (per′ĭ-limf) [peri- + L. *lympha* lymph] the fluid contained within the space separating the membranous from the osseous labyrinth of the ear; it is entirely separate from the endolymph. Called also *perilympha* [NA].

perilympha (per″ĭ-lim′fah) [NA] the perilymph.

perilymphadenitis (per″ĭ-lim″fad-ĕ-ni′tis) inflammation of the tissues around a lymph gland.

perilymphangeal (per″ĭ-lim-fan′je-al) located around a lymphatic vessel.

perilymphangitis (per″ĭ-lim″fan-ji′tis) inflammation of the tissues around a lymphatic vessel.

perilymphatic (per″ĭ-lim-fat′ik) 1. pertaining to the perilymph. 2. around a lymphatic vessel.

perimastitis (per″ĭ-mas-ti′tis) [peri- + Gr. *mastos* breast + *-itis*] inflammation of the connective tissue around the mammary gland.

perimedullary (per″ĭ-med′u-ler″e) surrounding a medulla, as the medulla oblongata or the marrow of a bone.

perimeningitis (per″ĭ-men″in-ji′tis) [peri- + Gr. *mēninx* membrane + *-itis*] pachymeningitis.

perimeter (pĕ-rim′ĕ-ter) [peri- + Gr. *metron* measure] 1. a line forming the boundary of a plane figure. 2. an apparatus for determining the extent of the peripheral visual field on a curved surface. **bed p.,** an apparatus for determining the limits of peripheral vision in a patient confined to bed. **dental p.,** an instrument for measuring the circumference of a tooth.

perimetric (per″ĭ-met′rik) 1. pertaining to a perimeter. 2. around the uterus. 3. pertaining to the perimetrium.

perimetritic (per″ĭ-me-trit′ik) pertaining to or characterized by perimetritis.

perimetritis (per″ĭ-mĕ-tri′tis) [peri- + Gr. *mētra* uterus + *-itis*] inflammation of the perimetrium.

perimetrium (per-ĭ-me′tre-um) [peri- + Gr. *mētra* uterus] the serous coat of the uterus; NA alternative for *tunica serosa uteri.*

perimetrosalpingitis (per″ĭ-met′ro-sal″pin-ji′tis) inflammation of the uterus and uterine tubes and of surrounding tissues. **encapsulating p.,** perimetrosalpingitis with formation of a membrane about the organs involved.

perimetry (pĕ-rim′ĕ-tre) [peri- + Gr. *metron* measure] determination of the extent of the peripheral visual field by use of a perimeter.

perimyelis (per″ĭ-mi′ĕ-lis) [peri- + Gr. *myelos* marrow] endosteum.

perimyelitis (per″ĭ-mi″ĕ-li′tis) 1. inflammation of the perimyelis (endosteum). 2. spinal meningitis.

perimyelography (per″ĭ-mi″ĕ-log′rah-fe) [peri- + Gr. *myelos* marrow + *graphein* to record] roentgen-ray examination after injecting iodized oil or other contrast fluid into the subarachnoid space of the spinal cord.

perimyocarditis (per″ĭ-mi″o-kar-di′tis) [peri + *myocarditis*] combined pericarditis and myocarditis.

perimyoendocarditis (per″ĭ-mi″o-en″do-kar-di′tis) pericarditis associated with myocarditis and endocarditis.

perimyositis (per″ĭ-mi″o-si′tis) inflammation of the connective tissue around muscles.

perimysia (per″ĭ-mis′e-ah) plural of perimysium.

perimysial (per″ĭ-mis′e-al) pertaining to the perimysium.

perimysiitis (per″ĭ-mis″e-i′tis) inflammation of the perimysium; myofibrositis.

perimysitis (per″ĭ-mis-i′tis) perimysiitis.

perimysium (per″ĭ-mis′e-um), pl. *perimys′ia* [peri- + Gr. *mys* muscle] [NA] the connective tissue demarcating a fascicle of skeletal muscle fibers; called also *internal p.,* or *p. internum.* **external p., p. exter′num,** epimysium. **internal p., p. inter′num,** perimysium.

perinatal (per″ĭ-na′tal) [peri- + L. *natus* born] pertaining to or occurring in the period shortly before and after birth; variously defined as beginning with completion of the twentieth to twenty-eighth week of gestation and ending 7 to 28 days after birth.

perinatologist (per″ĭ-na-tol′o-jist) a specialist in perinatology.

perinatology (per″ĭ-na-tol′o-je) [perinatal + *-logy*] the branch of medicine (obstetrics and pediatrics) dealing with the fetus and infant during the perinatal period.

perineal (per″ĭ-ne′al) pertaining to the perineum.

perineocele (per″ĭ-ne′o-sēl) [perineum + Gr. *kēlē* hernia] a hernia lying between the rectum and the prostate, or between the rectum and vagina; perineal hernia.

perineometer (per″ĭ-ne-om′ĕ-ter) an instrument for measuring the strength of contractions of the perivaginal muscles.

perineoplasty (per″ĭ-ne′o-plas″te) [perineum + Gr. *plassein* to shape] plastic surgery of the perineum.

perineorrhaphy (per″ĭ-ne-or′ah-fe) [perineum + Gr. *rhaphē* suture] suturation of the perineum, performed for the repair of a laceration.

perineoscrotal (per″ĭ-ne-o-skro′tal) pertaining to the perineum and scrotum.

perineosynthesis (per″ĭ-ne″o-sin′the-sis) [perineum + Gr. *syn-*

thesis a placing together] (*obs.*) surgical restoration of a completely lacerated perineum.

perineotomy (per″ĭ-ne-ot′o-me) [*perineum* + Gr. *temnein* to cut] surgical incision through the perineum.

perineovaginal (per″ĭ-ne″o-vaj′ĭ-nal) pertaining to or communicating with the perineum and vagina, as a perineovaginal fistula.

perineovaginorectal (per″ĭ-ne″o-vaj″ĭ-no-rek′tal) pertaining to the perineum, vagina, and rectum.

perineovulvar (per″ĭ-ne″o-vul′var) pertaining to the perineum and the vulva.

perinephrial (per″ĭ-nef′re-al) pertaining to the perinephrium.

perinephric (per″ĭ-nef′rik) around the kidney.

perinephritic (per″ĭ-ně-frit′ik) pertaining to or characterized by perinephritis.

perinephritis (per″ĭ-ně-fri′tis)[*peri-* + Gr. *nephros* kidney + *-itis*] inflammation of the perinephrium; it is marked by fever, local pain, and tenderness on pressure.

perinephrium (per″ĭ-nef′re-um) [*peri-* + Gr. *nephros* kidney] the peritoneal envelope and other tissues around the kidney.

perineum (per″ĭ-ne′um) [Gr. *perineos* the space between the anus and scrotum] 1. [NA] the pelvic floor and the associated structures occupying the pelvic outlet; it is bounded anteriorly by the pubic symphysis, laterally by the ischial tuberosities, and posteriorly by the coccyx. 2. the region between the thighs, bounded in the male by the scrotum and anus and in the female by the vulva and anus.

perineural (per″ĭ-nu′ral) surrounding a nerve or nerves.

perineurial (per″ĭ-nu′re-al) pertaining to the perineurium.

perineuritic (per″ĭ-nu-rit′ik) pertaining to or suffering from perineuritis.

perineuritis (per″ĭ-nu-ri′tis) inflammation of the perineurium.

perineurium (per″ĭ-nu′re-um) [*peri-* + Gr. *neuron* nerve] the connective tissue sheath surrounding each bundle of fibers (fasciculus) in a peripheral nerve.

perinuclear (per″ĭ-nu′kle-ar) situated or occurring around a nucleus.

periocular (per″e-ok′u-lar) situated or occurring around the eye.

period (pe′re-od) [*peri-* + Gr. *hodos* way] an interval or division of time; the time for the regular recurrence of a phenomenon. **absolute refractory p.,** the portion of the refractory period when a nerve or muscle fiber cannot respond to a stimulus, as contrasted with the relative refractory period. **child-bearing p.,** the duration of the reproductive ability in the human female, roughly from puberty to menopause. **ejection p.,** sphygmic p. **G₁ p.,** the period in the mitotic cycle from the end of the previous division to the start of DNA synthesis (S period). **G₂ p.,** the period of the mitotic cycle from the end of DNA synthesis (S period) to the beginning of mitosis. **gestational p.,** the duration of pregnancy, which in the human female averages about 266 days. **half-life p.,** see *half-life.* **incubation p.,** the interval of time required for development; the period of time between the moment of entrance of the infecting organism into the body and the first symptoms of the consequent disease, or between the moment of entrance into a vector and the time at which the vector is capable of transmitting the disease. Called also *incubative stage.* **isoelectric p.,** the moment in muscular contraction when the electrodes are so related to the contraction wave that no deflection of the galvanometer is produced. **p. of isometric contraction,** presphygmic p. **p. of isometric relaxation,** postsphygmic p. **isovolumic p.,** presphygmic p. **lag p.,** the time which elapses between the introduction of a microorganism into a nutrient medium and the initiation of exponential growth. **latency p.,** 1. see *latent p.* 2. in psychoanalytic theory, the period, usually between 5 years of age and adolescence, of relative quiescence in psychosexual development, with a cessation of interest in persons of the opposite sex and a tendency to associate mainly with persons of one's own sex. 3. see under *stage.* **latent p.,** a seemingly inactive period, as that between exposure of tissue to an injurious agent and the manifestation of response, or that between the instant of stimulation and the beginning of response. **M p.,** the period of active mitosis. **menstrual p., monthly p.,** the time of menstruation. **postsphygmic p.,** the short interval of ventricular diastole (0.08 second), immediately following the sphygmic period and lasting until the opening of the atrioventricular valves, during which the muscle fibers are relaxing and no blood is entering the ventricles; called also *period of isometric relaxation.* **prefunctional p.,** the time span during morphological and histological development before physiological activity begins. **presphygmic p.,** the first phase of ventricular systole, being the short period (0.04–0.06 second) immediately following closure of the atrioventricular valves and lasting until opening of the semilunar valves, during which the muscle fibers are contracting against the incompressible mass of fluid filling the ventricles; called also *period of isometric contraction* and *isovolumic p.* **quarantine p.,** the length of time, varying with the infection in question, which must elapse before a person exposed to contagion is regarded as incapable of

transmitting or acquiring the disease. **reaction p.,** 1. the stage of rallying from shock after trauma. 2. reaction time, the time that elapses between stimulation and the consequent reaction. **refractory p.,** the period of depolarization of the cell membrane after excitation, during which the nerve or muscle fiber cannot respond to a second stimulus. **relative refractory p.,** the brief period following the absolute refractory period, during which there is repolarization of the cell membrane to the extent that the fiber can respond to a strong stimulus, although the normal resting potential has not been reached. **S p.,** the period of DNA synthesis in the mitotic cycle. **safe p.,** the period of the menstrual cycle when conception is considered least likely to occur; it is approximately the ten days after menstruation begins, and the ten days preceding menstruation. **silent p.,** an interval in the course of a disease in which the symptoms become very mild or disappear for a time. **sphygmic p.,** the second phase of ventricular systole, being the period (0.21–0.30 second) intervening between the opening and closing of the semilunar valves, during which the blood is being discharged into the aortic and the pulmonary arteries; called also *ejection period.* **Wenckebach p.,** a form of partial heart block characterized by progressive lengthening of the P-R interval until ventricular response occurs; such a sequence is usually repetitive.

periodate (per-i′o-dāt) a salt of periodic acid.

periodic (pe″re-od′ik) [Gr. *periodikos*] recurring at regular intervals of time.

periodicity (pe″re-o-dis′ĭ-te) recurrence at regular intervals of time. **filarial p.,** the periodic increase of microfilariae in the peripheral blood: nocturnal periodicity occurs in *Wuchereria bancrofti* infection, in most endemic areas, and in *Brugia malayi* infection; diurnal periodicity occurs in *Loa loa* infection. **lunar p.,** recurrence synchronized with phases of the moon, as the reproductive phenomena in some lower animals. **malarial p.,** the more or less regular recurrence of paroxysms at intervals of one, two, or three days in malaria; see under *malaria.*

periodontal (per″e-o-don′tal) [*peri-* + Gr. *odous* tooth] situated or occurring around a tooth; pertaining to the periodontium.

periodontia (per″e-o-don′she-ah) 1. plural of *periodontium.* 2. periodontics.

periodontics (per″e-o-don′tiks) [*peri-* + Gr. *odous* tooth] that branch of dentistry dealing with the study and treatment of diseases of the periodontium.

periodontist (per″e-o-don′tist) a dentist who specializes in periodontics.

periodontitis (per″e-o-don-ti′tis) [*peri-* + Gr. *odous* tooth + *-itis*] inflammatory reaction of the tissues surrounding a tooth (periodontium), usually resulting from the extension of gingival inflammation (gingivitis) into the periodontium. **apical p.,** inflammatory reaction of the tissues surrounding the root of a tooth. **chronic apical p.,** see *apical granuloma,* under *granuloma.* **compound p.,** periodontitis in which the combination of local irritants and occlusal trauma produces an exacerbation of the clinical manifestations of simple periodontitis: there are more periodontal pockets formed, alveolar bone and cementum are resorbed, destruction of the periodontal ligament is combined with vascular, degenerative, and necrotic changes, and bone destruction is angular rather than horizontal; called also *chronic suppurative pericementitis, Riggs' disease,* and *pyorrhea alveolaris.* **simple p., p. sim′plex,** periodontitis due to a variety of local irritants, such as calculus, impaction of food, and rough edges of fillings, marked by chronic inflammation of the gingiva, formation of periodontal pockets usually with pus formation, horizontal bone resorption, destruction of the periodontal ligament, and loss of teeth.

periodontium (per″e-o-don′she-um), pl. *periodon′tia* [*peri-* + Gr. *odous* tooth] the tissues investing and supporting the teeth, including the cementum, periodontal ligament, alveolar bone, and gingiva. Anatomically [NA], the term is restricted to the connective tissue interposed between the teeth and their bony sockets, i.e., the periodontal ligament; called also *periosteum alveolare.*

periodontoclasia (per″e-o-don″to-kla′se-ah) [*peri-* + Gr. *odous* tooth + *klasis* breaking] a general term sometimes used for any degenerative and destructive disease of the periodontium.

periodontology (per″e-o-don-tol′o-je) [*peri-* + Gr. *odous* tooth + *-logy*] the scientific study of the periodontium and periodontal diseases.

periodontopathy (per″e-o-don-top′ah-the) a noninflammatory disorder of the periodontium.

periodontosis (per″e-o-don-to′sis) a degenerative, noninflammatory condition of the periodontium, originating in one or more of the periodontal structures and characterized by destruction of the tissues.

periomphalic (per″e-om-fal′ik) [*peri-* + Gr. *omphalos* navel] around the umbilicus.

perionychia (per″e-o-nik′e-ah) paronychia.

perionychium (per″e-o-nik′e-um) [*peri-* + Gr. *onyx* nail] the epidermis bordering a nail.

perionyx (per″e-o′niks) [*peri-* + Gr. *onyx* nail] a relic of the eponychium persisting as a band across the root of the nail, seen in the eighth month of fetal life.

perioophoritis (per″e-o-of″o-ri′tis) [*peri-* + Gr. *ōon* egg + *pherein* to bear + *-itis*] inflammation of the tissues around the ovary.

perioophorosalpingitis (per″e-o-of″o-ro-sal″pin-ji′tis) [*peri-* + Gr. *ōon* egg + *pherein* to bear + *salpinx* tube + *-itis*] inflammation of the tissues around the ovary and oviducts.

perioothecitis (per-e-o″o-the-si′tis) perioophoritis.

perioperative (per″e-op′er-ah-tiv) pertaining to the period extending from the time of hospitalization for surgery to the time of discharge.

periophthalmia (per″e-of-thal′me-ah) periophthalmitis.

periophthalmic (per″e-of-thal′mik) situated around the eye.

periophthalmitis (per″e-o-of″thal-mi′tis) inflammation of the tissues around the eye.

periople (per′e-o″p'l) [*peri-* + Gr. *hoplē* hoof] the layer of soft, light-colored horn covering the outer aspect of the hoof in ungulates.

perioptometry (per″e-op-tom′ĕ-tre) [*peri-* + Gr. *optos* visible + *metron* measure] the measurement of the peripheral acuity of vision or of the limits of the visual field.

perioral (per″e-o′ral) [*peri-* + L. *os* mouth] situated or occurring around the mouth.

periorbit (per″e-or′bit) periorbita.

periorbita (per″e-or′bi-tah) [*peri-* + L. *orbita* orbit] [NA] the periosteal covering of the bones forming the orbit, or eye socket.

periorbital (per″e-or′bĭ-tal) situated around the orbit, or eye socket.

periorbititis (per″e-or″bĭ-ti′tis) inflammation of the periorbita.

periorchitis (per″e-or-ki′tis) [*peri-* + Gr. *orchis* testis + *-itis*] inflammation of the tunica vaginalis testis. **p. adhaesi′va,** a variety in which the two layers of the tunica vaginalis are more or less adherent. **p. purulen′ta,** periorchitis which goes on to pus formation.

periorchium (per″e-or′ke-um) the parietal layer of the tunica vaginalis.

periost (per′e-ost) periosteum.

periosteal (per″e-os′te-al) pertaining to the periosteum.

periosteitis (per″e-os″te-i′tis) periostitis.

periosteodema (per″e-os″te-o-de′mah) periosteoedema.

periosteoedema (per″e-os″te-o-ĕ-de′mah) edema of the periosteum.

periosteoma (per″e-os-te-o′mah) a morbid bony growth surrounding a bone.

periosteomedullitis (per″e-os″te-o-med″u-li′tis) inflammation of the periosteum and bone marrow.

periosteomyelitis (per″e-os″te-o-mi″ĕ-li′tis) [*peri-* + Gr. *osteon* bone + *myelos* marrow + *-itis*] inflammation of the entire bone, including periosteum and marrow.

periosteophyte (per″e-os′te-o-fīt″) [*periosteum* + Gr. *phyton* growth] a bony outgrowth on the periosteum.

periosteorrhaphy (per″e-os″te-or′ah-fe) [*periosteum* + Gr. *rhaphē* suture] the suturing together of the margins of severed periosteum.

periosteosis (per″e-os″te-o′sis) periostosis.

periosteotome (per″e-os′te-o-tōm) an instrument for cutting the periosteum; also an instrument for separating the periosteum from the bone.

periosteotomy (per″e-os″te-ot′o-me) [*peri-* + Gr. *osteon* bone + *tomē* a cutting] surgical incision or slitting of the periosteum.

periosteous (per″e-os′te-us) pertaining to or of the nature of periosteum.

periosteum (per″e-os′te-um) [*peri-* + Gr. *osteon* bone] [NA] a specialized connective tissue covering all bones of the body, and possessing bone-forming potentialities; in adults, it consists of two layers that are not sharply defined, the external layer being a network of dense connective tissue containing blood vessels, and the deep layer composed of more loosely arranged collagenous bundles with spindle-shaped connective tissue cells and a network of thin elastic fibers. **alveolar p., p. alveola′re,** the periodontal ligament.

periostitis (per″e-os-ti′tis) inflammation of the periosteum. The condition is generally chronic, and is marked by tenderness and swelling of the bone and an aching pain. Acute periostitis is due to infection, is characterized by diffuse suppuration, severe pain, and constitutional symptoms, and usually results in necrosis. **p. albumino′sa, albuminous p.,** a form accompanied by the exudation of a clear, albuminous liquid into a flattened cavity beneath the periosteum; called also *serous abscess* and *periosteal ganglion.* **dental p.,** inflammation of the dental periosteum. **diffuse p.,** a noncircumscribed periostitis of the long bones. **hemorrhagic p.,** a form in which blood is extravasated beneath the periosteum. **p. hyperplas′tica,** hypertrophic pulmonary osteoarthropathy. **p. inter′na cra′nii,** inflammation of the endocranium; external pachymeningitis. **precocious p.,** syphilitic osteoperiostitis occurring as an early symptom.

periostoma (per″e-os-to′mah) periosteoma.

periostomedullitis (per″e-os″to-med″u-li′tis) periosteomedullitis.

periostosis (per″e-os-to′sis) the abnormal deposition of periosteal bone; the condition manifested by development of periosteomas. Called also *periosteosis.* **hyperplastic p.,** cortical infantile hyperostosis.

periostosteitis (per″e-os-tos″te-i′tis) osteoperiostitis.

periostotome (per″e-os′to-tōm) periosteotome.

periostotomy (per″e-os-tot′o-me) periosteotomy.

periotic (per″e-o′tik) [*peri-* + Gr. *ous* ear] 1. situated about the ear, especially the internal ear. 2. the petrous and mastoid portions of the temporal bone, at one stage a distinct bone.

periovaritis (per″e-o″vah-ri′tis) perioophoritis.

periovular (per″e-o′vu-lar) surrounding an ovum.

peripachymeningitis (per″ĭ-pak″e-men″in-ji′tis) [*peri-* + Gr. *pachys* thick + *mēninx* membrane + *-itis*] inflammation of the substance between the dura and the bony covering of the central nervous system.

peripancreatic (per″ĭ-pan″kre-at′ik) surrounding the pancreas.

peripancreatitis (per″ĭ-pan″kre-ah-ti′tis) [*peri-* + Gr. *pankreas* pancreas + *-itis*] inflammation of tissues around the pancreas.

peripapillary (per″ĭ-pap′ĭ-ler″e) located around the optic papilla.

peripartum (per″ĭ-par′tum) occurring during the last month of gestation or the first few months after delivery, with reference to the mother.

peripatellar (per″ĭ-pah-tel′ar) around the patella, or knee cap.

peripatetic (per″ĭ-pah-tet′ik) [Gr. *peripatētikos* given to walking about while teaching or disputing] walking about.

peripenial (per″ĭ-pe′ne-al) around the penis.

peripericarditis (per″ĭ-per″ĭ-kar-di′tis) inflammation around the pericardium producing adhesions of the pericardium to the pleura and chest wall.

periphacitis (per″ĭ-fah-si′tis) [*peri-* + Gr. *phakos* lens + *-itis*] inflammation surrounding the capsule of the lens of the eye.

periphakitis (per″ĭ-fah-ki′tis) periphacitis.

peripharyngeal (per″ĭ-fah-rin′je-al) situated around the pharynx.

peripherad (pĕ-rif′er-ad) toward the periphery.

peripheral (pĕ-rif′er-al) pertaining to or situated at or near the periphery; situated away from a center or central structure.

peripheraphose (pĕ-rif′er-ah-fōs) a subjective sensation of a dark spot in the line of vision, originating in the peripheral ocular mechanism.

peripheric (per″ĭ-fer′ik) peripheral.

peripherocentral (pĕ-rif′er-o-sen′tral) both peripheral and central.

peripheroceptor (pĕ-rif′er-o-sep′tor) any of the receptors at the peripheral ends of a sensory peripheral neuron which receive the stimulus.

peripheromittor (pĕ-rif″er-o-mit′or) a terminal mittor placed in connection with the ceptor of a muscle fiber or gland cell which transmits the impulse to the fiber or cell.

peripherophose (pĕ-rif′er-o-fōz) [*periphery* + *phose*] any phose or subjective sensation of light originating in the peripheral ocular mechanism.

periphery (pĕ-rif′er-e) [Gr. *periphereia,* from *peri* around + *pherein* to bear] the outward part or surface or structure; the portion of a system outside the central region.

periphlebitic (per″ĭ-flĕ-bit′ik) pertaining to periphlebitis.

periphlebitis (per″ĭ-flĕ-bi′tis) [*peri-* + Gr. *phleps* vein + *-itis*] inflammation of the tissues around a vein, or of the external coat of a vein. **sclerosing p.,** Mondor's disease.

periphoria (per″ĭ-fo′re-ah) [*peri-* + Gr. *phoros* bearing + *-ia*] cyclophoria.

periphrastic (per″ĭ-fras′tik) [Gr. *periphrastikos*] marked by the use of superfluous words and roundabout methods in expressing ideas; often seen in schizophrenic speech and writing.

periphrenitis (per″ĭ-fre-ni′tis) [*peri-* + Gr. *phrēn* diaphragm + *-itis*] inflammation of the diaphragm and structures around it.

Periplaneta (per″ĭ-plah-ne′tah) a genus of roaches. *P. america′na* is the American cockroach; *P. australa′siae* is the Australian cockroach.

periplasmic (per″ĭ-plas′mik) around the plasma membrane; between the plasma membrane and the cell wall of a bacterium.

peripleural (per″ĭ-ploo′ral) surrounding the pleura.

peripleuritis (per″ĭ-ploo-ri′tis) [*peri-* + *pleura* + *-itis*] inflammation of the tissues between the pleura and the chest wall.

periplocin (per″ĭ-plo′sin) a crystallizable glycoside, $C_{36}H_{56}O_{13}$, from a woody vine, *Periploca graeca* L. (Asclepiadaceae); it acts like digitalin as a heart tonic and slower of the pulse.

periplocymarin (per″ĭ-plo-si′mah-rin) a cardiac glycoside,

$C_{30}H_{46}O_8$, from the bark and wood of *Periploca graeca* L. (Asclepiadaceae).

periplogenin (per″ĭ-ploj′e-nin) chemical name: 3β,5,14-trihydroxy-5β-card-20(22)-enolide. An aglycone sterol derivative, $C_{23}H_{34}O_5$, from periplocin and periplocymarin.

peripneumonia (per″ĭ-nu-mo′ne-ah) [*peri-* + Gr. *pneumōn* lung + *-ia*] pneumonia; also pleuropneumonia. **p. no′tha,** a variety of acute bronchitis simulating pneumonia.

peripneumonitis (per″ĭ-nu″mo-ni′tis) peripneumonia.

peripolar (per″ĭ-po′lar) situated about a pole or poles.

peripolesis (per″ĭ-po-le′sis) [Gr. *peripolēsis* a going about] the clustering of lymphocytes around macrophages, a phenomenon occurring in tissue cultures of lymphoid tissue challenged by antigen. The immunological significance, if any, is unknown. Cf. *emperipolesis*.

periporitis (per″ĭ-por-i′tis) a staphylococcal infection complicating miliaria, with inflammation around the sweat pores, usually affecting infants; called also *periporitis staphylogenes*.

periportal (per″ĭ-por′tal) situated around the portal vein.

periproctic (per″ĭ-prok′tik) [*peri-* + Gr. *prōktos* anus] situated around the anus.

periproctitis (per″ĭ-prok-ti′tis) [*peri-* + Gr. *prōktos* anus + *-itis*] inflammation of the tissues surrounding the rectum and anus.

periprostatic (per″ĭ-pros-tat′ik) situated about the prostate.

periprostatitis (per″ĭ-pros″tah-ti′tis) inflammation of the tissues and structures around the prostate gland.

peripyema (per″ĭ-pi-e′mah) suppuration surrounding a part, as a tooth.

peripylephlebitis (per″ĭ-pi″le-flĕ-bi′tis) [*peri-* + Gr. *pylē* gate + *phleps* vein + *-itis*] inflammation of the tissue about the portal vein.

peripyloric (per″ĭ-pi-lor′ik) around the pylorus or the pyloric part of the stomach (see *pars pylorica ventriculi*).

periradicular (per″ĭ-rah-dik′u-lar) surrounding a root, especially the root of a tooth.

perirectal (per″ĭ-rek′tal) around the rectum.

perirectitis (per″ĭ-rek-ti′tis) periproctitis.

perirenal (per″ĭ-re′nal) [*peri-* + L. *ren* kidney] situated around a kidney.

perirhinal (per″ĭ-ri′nal) [*peri-* + Gr. *rhis* nose] situated about the nose.

perirhizoclasia (per″ĭ-ri″zo-kla′se-ah) [*peri-* + Gr. *rhiza* root + *klasis* destruction] inflammatory destruction of tissues immediately around the root of a tooth, i.e., the pericementum, cementum, and superficial layers of the alveolar process. Cf. *pararhizoclasia*.

perisalpingitis (per″ĭ-sal″pin-ji′tis) [*peri-* + Gr. *salpinx* tube + *-itis*] inflammation of the tissues and peritoneum around a uterine tube.

perisalpingo-ovaritis (per″ĭ-sal-ping″go-o″vah-ri′tis) inflammation involving the ovary and the tissues around the uterine tube.

perisalpinx (per″ĭ-sal′pinks) the peritoneal cover of the upper border of the uterine tube.

perisclerium (per″ĭ-skle′re-um) [*peri-* + Gr. *sklēros* hard] fibrous tissue surrounding ossifying cartilage.

periscopic (per″ĭ-skop′ik) [*peri-* + Gr. *skopein* to examine] affording a wide range of vision; said of microscopical and spectacle lenses.

perisigmoiditis (per″ĭ-sig″moi-di′tis) inflammation of the peritoneal covering of the sigmoid flexure.

perisinuitis (per″ĭ-si″nu-i′tis) perisinusitis.

perisinuous (per″ĭ-sin′u-us) situated around a sinus.

perisinusitis (per″ĭ-si″nŭ-si′tis) inflammation of the tissues around a sinus.

perispermatitis (per″ĭ-sper″mah-ti′tis) inflammation of the tissues about the spermatic cord. **p. sero′sa,** encysted hydrocele of the spermatic cord.

perisplanchnic (per″ĭ-splank′nik) [*peri-* + Gr. *splanchnon* viscus] around a viscus or the viscera.

perisplanchnitis (per″ĭ-splank-ni′tis) inflammation around the viscera; perivisceritis.

perisplenic (per″ĭ-splen′ik) occurring around the spleen.

perisplenitis (per″ĭ-splĕ-ni′tis) [*peri-* + Gr. *splēn* spleen + *-itis*] inflammation of the peritoneal coat of the spleen and of the structures around it. **p. cartilagin′ea,** inflammatory overgrowth of the capsule of the spleen, causing a thickening of cartilaginous hardness.

perispondylic (per″ĭ-spon-dil′ik) around a vertebra.

perispondylitis (per″ĭ-spon″dĭ-li′tis) [*peri-* + Gr. *spondylos* vertebra + *-itis*] inflammation of the parts around a vertebra. **Gibney's p.,** a painful condition of the spinal muscles.

Perisporiaceae (per″ĭ-spo″re-a′se-e) Moniliaceae.

Perissodactyla (pĕ-ris″so-dak′tĭ-lah) [Gr. *perissos* odd + *daktylos* finger] an order of ungulates having an odd number of toes, including the horse, tapir, and rhinoceros. Cf. *Artiodactyla*.

perissodactylous (pĕ-ris″so-dak′tĭ-lus) having an odd number of digits on a hand or foot.

peristalsis (per″ĭ-stal′sis) [*peri-* + Gr. *stalsis* contraction] the wormlike movement by which the alimentary canal or other tubular organs provided with both longitudinal and circular muscle fibers propel their contents. It consists of a wave of contraction passing along the tube for variable distances. **mass p.,** strong usually brief bursts of peristaltic movements, which propel intestinal contents through long stretches of the intestine or colon, often resulting in defecation. **retrograde p.,** reversed p. **reversed p.,** that which impels the contents of the intestine cephalad.

peristaltic (per″ĭ-stal′tik) of the nature of peristalsis.

peristaltin (per″ĭ-stal′tin) a glycoside, $C_{14}H_{18}O_8$, of cascara sagrada.

peristaphyline (per″ĭ-staf′ĭ-lin) [*peri-* + Gr. *staphylē* uvula] situated around the uvula.

peristasis (pĕ-ris′tah-sis) environment.

peristoma (pĕ-ris′to-mah) peristome.

peristomatous (per″ĭ-stom′ah-tus) around the mouth.

peristome (per′ĭ-stōm) [*peri-* + Gr. *stoma* mouth] a groove running from the cytostome in certain protozoa.

peristrumitis (per″ĭ-stroo-mi′tis) inflammation extending from an inflamed goiter to the surrounding structures.

peristrumous (per″ĭ-stroo′mus) around or near a goiter.

perisynovial (per″ĭ-sĭ-no′ve-al) around a synovial structure.

perisyringitis (per″ĭ-sir″in-ji′tis) inflammation of tissues around ducts of the sweat glands. **p. chron′ica na′si,** granulosis rubra nasi.

peritectomy (per″ĭ-tek′to-me) [*peri-* + Gr. *ektomē* excision] excision of a ring of conjunctiva behind the limbus, followed by cauterization of the trench thus made.

peritendineum (per″ĭ-ten-din′e-um) [NA] the connective tissue investing larger tendons and extending as septa between the fibers composing them.

peritendinitis (per″ĭ-ten″dĭ-ni′tis) tenosynovitis. **adhesive p.,** adhesive capsulitis. **p. calca′rea,** a painful condition marked by calcareous deposits in tendons and in peritendinous, capsular, and ligamentous tissues. **p. crep′itans,** tenosynovitis crepitans. **p. sero′sa,** ganglion, def. 2.

peritendinous (per″ĭ-ten′dĭ-nus) around a tendon.

peritenon (per″ĭ-te′non) [*peri-* + Gr. *tenōn* tendon] the connective tissue structures associated with a tendon.

peritenoneum (per″ĭ-ten″o-ne′um) the loose connective tissue covering the surface of tendons and ligaments and penetrating inside to separate the substance into bundles.

peritenonitis (per″ĭ-ten″o-ni′tis) tenosynovitis.

peritenontitis (per″ĭ-ten″on-ti′tis) tenosynovitis.

perithecium (per″ĭ-the′se-um) [*peri-* + Gr. *thēkē* case] the flask-shaped fruiting body, with a pore for the escape of spores, enclosing the asci and spores of certain ascomycetous fungi and molds. Cf. *apothecium, cleistothecium,* and *gymnothecium.*

perithelial (per″ĭ-the′le-al) pertaining to the perithelium.

perithelioma (per″ĭ-the″le-o′mah) hemangiopericytoma.

perithelium (per″ĭ-the′le-um) [*peri-* + Gr. *thēlē* nipple] the layer of connective tissue that surrounds the capillaries and smaller vessels. **Eberth's p.,** a partial layer of cells on the external surface of the capillaries.

perithoracic (per″ĭ-tho-ras′ik) surrounding the thorax.

perithyreoiditis (per″ĭ-thi″re-oid-i′tis) perithyroiditis.

perithyroiditis (per″ĭ-thi″roi-di′tis) inflammation of the capsule of the thyroid body.

peritomist (pĕ-rit′o-mist) one who performs peritomy (circumcision).

peritomize (pĕ-rit′o-mīz) to subject to peritomy.

peritomy (pĕ-rit′o-me) [*peri-* + Gr. *temnein* to cut] 1. surgical incision of the conjunctiva and subconjunctival tissue about the whole circumference of the cornea; usually done as part of enucleation and retinal detachment procedure. 2. circumcision.

peritoneal (per″ĭ-to-ne′al) pertaining to the peritoneum.

peritonealgia (per″ĭ-to″ne-al′je-ah) pain in the peritoneum.

peritonealize (per″ĭ-to-ne′al-īz) to cover with peritoneum.

peritoneocentesis (per″ĭ-to″ne-o-sen-te′sis) [*peritoneum* + Gr. *kentēsis* puncture] puncture of the peritoneal cavity with a needle for the purpose of obtaining fluid.

peritoneoclysis (per″ĭ-to″ne-o-kli′sis) injection of water or other fluids into the peritoneal cavity.

peritoneography (per″ĭ-to-ne-og′rah-fe) roentgenography of the peritoneum.

peritoneomuscular (per″ĭ-to-ne″o-mus′ku-lar) pertaining to or composed of peritoneum and muscle.

peritoneopathy (per″ĭ-to-ne-op′ah-the) [*peritoneum* + Gr. *pathos* disease] any disease of the peritoneum.

peritoneopericardial (per″ĭ-to-ne″o-per″ĭ-kar′de-al) pertaining to the peritoneum and pericardium.

peritoneopexy (per″ĭ-to′ne-o-pek″se) [*peritoneum* + Gr. *pēxis* fixation] fixation of the uterus by the vaginal route.

peritoneoplasty (per″ĭ-to′ne-o-plas″te) [*peritoneum* + Gr. *plassein* to form] the operation of covering denuded areas of abdominal viscera or of the abdominal cavity with peritoneum; peritonization.

peritoneoscope (per″ĭ-to′ne-o-skōp″) an instrument for performing peritoneoscopy.

peritoneoscopy (per″ĭ-to′ne-os′ko-pe) [*peritoneum* + Gr. *skopein* to examine] examination of the peritoneal cavity by an instrument inserted through the abdominal wall.

peritoneotome (per″ĭ-to′ne-o-tōm) an area of the peritoneum supplied with afferent nerve fibers by a single posterior root.

peritoneotomy (per″ĭ-to′ne-ot′o-me) [*peritoneum* + Gr. *tomē* a cutting] incision into the peritoneal cavity.

peritoneovenous (per″ĭ-to-ne″o-ve′nus) communicating with the peritoneal cavity and the venous system; see under *shunt*.

peritoneum (per″ĭ-to-ne′um) [L.; Gr. *peritonaion,* from *per* around + *teinein* to stretch] [NA] the serous membrane lining the abdominopelvic walls (*parietal p.*) and investing the viscera (*visceral p.*). A strong, colorless membrane with a smooth surface, it forms a closed sac in the male and is continuous with the mucous membrane of the uterine tubes in the female. **abdominal p.,**

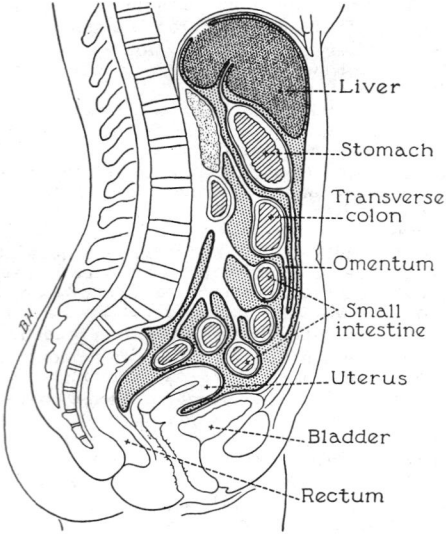

Course of the peritoneum (heavy black line) in a median sagittal section of a female.

Labels in figure: Liver, Stomach, Transverse colon, Omentum, Small intestine, Uterus, Bladder, Rectum

p. parietale. **p. of cranium** (*obs.*), pericranium. **intestinal p.,** p. viscerale. **parietal p., p. parieta′le** [NA], the peritoneum that lines the abdominal and pelvic walls and the undersurface of the diaphragm. **visceral p., p. viscera′le** [NA], a continuation of the parietal peritoneum reflected at various places over the viscera, forming a complete covering for the stomach, spleen, liver, ascending portion of the duodenum, jejunum, ileum, transverse colon, sigmoid flexure, upper end of rectum, uterus, and ovaries; it also partially covers the descending and transverse portions of the duodenum, the cecum, ascending and descending colon, the middle part of the rectum, the posterior wall of the bladder, and the upper portion of the vagina. The peritoneum serves to hold the viscera in position by its folds, some of which form the *mesenteries,* connecting portions of the intestine with the posterior abdominal wall; other folds, the *omenta,* are attached to the stomach; and still others form the *ligaments* of the liver, spleen, stomach, kidneys, bladder, and uterus. The potential space between the visceral and the parietal peritoneum is the peritoneal cavity, which consists of the *pelvic peritoneal cavity* below and the *general peritoneal cavity* above. The general peritoneal cavity communicates by the epiploic foramen with the cavity of the greater omentum, which is also known as the *lesser peritoneal cavity.*

peritonism (per′ĭ-to-nizm) a condition of shock simulating peritonitis, but without inflammation of the peritoneum.

peritonitis (per″ĭ-to-ni′tis) inflammation of the peritoneum; a condition marked by exudations in the peritoneum of serum, fibrin, cells, and pus. It is attended by abdominal pain and tenderness, constipation, vomiting, and moderate fever. **adhesive p.,** that which is characterized by adhesions between adjacent serous surfaces. **benign paroxysmal p.,** familial Mediterranean fever. **bile p., biliary p.,** choleperitoneum. **chemical p.,** peritonitis due to chemical irritation. **p.**

chron′ica fibro′sa encap′sulans, a chronic peritonitis marked by the formation on the intestine of a white coating of fibrous tissue undergoing hyaline degeneration; called also *iced intestine* and *zuckergussdarm.* **circumscribed p.,** that which is limited to a portion of the peritoneum. **p. defor′-mans,** chronic peritonitis producing shortening of the mesentery so that the intestines are drawn up in loops toward the spine. **diaphragmatic p.,** that which affects the peritoneal surface of the diaphragm. **diffuse p.,** that which is not limited to a portion of the peritoneum. **p. encap′sulans, encysted p.,** that in which a collection of pus or serum is enclosed by adhesions; peritoneal abscess. **fibrocaseous p.,** tubercular peritonitis with fibrous and caseous degeneration. **gas p.,** peritonitis with the accumulation of gas within the peritoneum. **general p.,** inflammation of the greater part of the peritoneum. **hemorrhagic p.,** that which is attended with hemorrhagic effusion. **localized p.,** circumscribed p. **meconium p.,** peritonitis resulting from perforation of the bowel into the peritoneal cavity *in utero* or shortly after birth, resulting in escape of meconium into the peritoneal cavity; it occurs most often as a complication of meconium ileus in fibrocystic disease of the pancreas. **pelvic p.,** perimetritis; peritonitis situated in the pelvis. **perforative p.,** that which is due to a perforation in the digestive tract. **periodic p.,** familial Mediterranean fever. **puerperal p.,** that which occurs following childbirth. **purulent p.,** peritonitis with the formation of pus. **septic p.,** that which is due to a pyogenic microorganism. **serous p.,** that which is attended by a copious liquid exudation. **silent p.,** asymptomatic peritonitis. **terminal p.,** primary peritonitis in the late stages of a wasting disease. **traumatic p.,** simple acute peritonitis due to trauma. **tuberculous p.,** peritonitis caused by the tubercle bacillus.

peritonization (per″ĭ-to-ni-za′shun) the operation of covering a denuded surface of an abdominal organ or the abdominal wall with peritoneum; peritoneoplasty.

peritonize (per′ĭ-to-nīz) to cover with peritoneum.

peritonsillar (per″ĭ-ton′sĭ-lar) situated around a tonsil.

peritonsillitis (per″ĭ-ton″sĭ-li′tis) inflammation of the peritonsillar tissues.

peritracheal (per″ĭ-tra′ke-al) situated around the trachea.

Peritrate (per′ĭ-trāt) trademark for preparations of pentaerythritol tetranitrate.

peritrichal, peritrichic (pe-rit′rĭ-kal; per″e-trik′ik) peritrichous.

Peritrichida (per″ĭ-trik′ĭ-dah) an order of primarily free-living protozoa of the subphylum Ciliophora, class Euciliatia, in which cilia form a spiral around the cystostome; it includes the genera *Trichodina* and *Vorticella.*

peritrichous (pĕ-rit′rĭ-kus) [*peri-* + Gr. *thrix* hair] 1. having flagella over the entire surface; said of a bacterial cell; see *flagellum.* 2. having cilia around the cytostome only; said of Ciliophora.

peritrochanteric (per″ĭ-tro″kan-ter′ik) situated about a trochanter.

perituberculosis (per″ĭ-tu-ber″ku-lo′sis) paratuberculosis.

perityphlic (per″ĭ-tif′lik) [*peri-* + Gr. *typhlon* cecum] around the cecum; pericecal.

perityphlitis (per″ĭ-tif-li′tis) [*peri-* + Gr. *typhlon* cecum + *-itis*] inflammation of the peritoneum surrounding the cecum; appendicitis. **p. actinomycot′ica,** actinomycosis whose principal seat is pericecal.

periumbilical (per″e-um-bil′ĭ-kal) situated around the umbilicus.

periungual (per″e-ung′gwal) around the nail.

periureteral (per″ĭ-u-re′ter-al) around the ureter.

periureteric (per″e-u″re-ter′ik) about the ureter.

periureteritis (per″e-u″re-tĕ-ri′tis) [*peri-* + Gr. *ourētēr* ureter + *-itis*] inflammation of the tissues around a ureter.

periurethral (per″e-u-re′thral) occurring around the urethra.

periurethritis (per″e-u″re-thri′tis) [*peri-* + Gr. *ourēthra* urethra + *-itis*] inflammation of the tissues around the urethra; spongiitis.

periuterine (per″e-u′ter-ĭn) around the uterus.

periuvular (per″e-u′vu-lar) around the uvula.

perivaginal (per″ĭ-vaj′ĭ-nal) around the vagina.

perivaginitis (per″ĭ-vaj″ĭ-ni′tis) pericolpitis.

perivascular (per″ĭ-vas′ku-lar) situated around a vessel.

perivascularity (per″ĭ-vas′ku-lar′ĭ-te) an infiltrate of cellular elements of mesodermal origin (polymorphonuclear leukocytes, lymphocytes, etc.) in the perivascular spaces, as in those of the cerebral parenchyma.

perivasculitis (per″ĭ-vas″ku-li′tis) inflammation of a perivascular sheath and of the tissues surrounding it.

perivenous (per″ĭ-ve′nus) around a vein.

periventricular (per″ĭ-ven-trik′u-lar) around a ventricle; see also under *system.*

perivertebral (per″ĭ-ver′tĕ-bral) around a vertebra.

perivesical (per″ĭ-ves′ĭ-kal) [peri- + L. vesica bladder] occurring around the bladder.

perivesicular (per″ĭ-vĕ-sik′u-lar) around a seminal vesicle.

perivesiculitis (per″ĭ-vĕ-sik″u-li′tis) inflammation of tissue around the seminal vesicle.

perivisceral (per″ĭ-vis′er-al) occurring around a viscus or the viscera.

perivisceritis (per″ĭ-vis″er-i′tis) inflammation around a viscus or around the viscera.

perivitelline (per″ĭ-vi-tel′īn) situated around a vitellus or yolk.

perixenitis (per″ĭ-zĕ-ni′tis) [peri- + Gr. xenos strange + -itis] inflammation occurring around a foreign body in a tissue or organ.

perkeratosis (per″ker-ah-to′sis) hyperkeratosis, def. 3.

perkinism, perkinsism (per′kin-izm; per′kin-sizm) [Elisha Perkins, of Norwich, Connecticut, 1741–1799] an obsolete form of metallotherapy, embracing the therapeutic use of metallic appliances, such as Perkins' tractors.

perlapine (per′lah-pēn) chemical name: 6-(4-methyl-1-piperazinyl)morphanthridine; a hypnotic, $C_{19}H_{21}N_3$.

perlèche (per-lesh′) [Fr.] superficial erosions and fissuring of the commissures of the lips, the causes and contributing factors of which include candidiasis, streptococcal or staphylococcal infection, overclosure of an edentulous mouth, ariboflavinosis, and excess salivation with drooling at the corners of the lips. Called also *angular cheilitis, angular cheilosis,* and *angular stomatitis.*

Perlia's nucleus (per′le-ahz) [Richard Perlia, German ophthalmologist] see under *nucleus.*

Perls' anemia bodies, test (stain) (perlz) [Max Perls, German pathologist, 1843–1881] see under *body* and *tests.*

perlsucht (perl′sookt) [Ger.] tuberculosis of the mesentery and peritoneum in cattle.

permanganate (per-man′gah-nāt) any salt of permanganic acid.

permeability (per″me-ah-bil′ĭ-te) the property or state of being permeable; see also *osmosis.*

permeable (per′me-ah-b'l) [L. per through + meare to pass] not impassable; pervious; permitting passage of a substance.

permease (per′me-ās) a collective term for genetically controlled, stereospecific membrane transport systems, e.g., a membrane-bound carrier protein (M protein) of bacteria involved in the transport of β-galactosides across the cell membrane. In *Escherichia coli,* called *M protein.*

permeate (per′me-āt″) 1. to penetrate or pass through, as through a filter. 2. the constituents of a solution or suspension that pass through a filter.

permeation (per″me-a′shun) the act of spreading through or penetrating a substance, tissue, or organ, as by a disease process, such as cancer.

Permitil (per′mĭ-til) trademark for a preparation of fluphenazine hydrochloride.

perna (per′nah) a chlorinated naphthalin, which may cause a serious acne in persons handling it.

pernasal (per-na′sal) [L. per through + nasus nose] performed through the nose.

perneiras (pār-na′ras) Brazilian name for beriberi.

perniciosiform (per-nish″e-o′sĭ-form) seemingly pernicious; a term applied to a condition which is apparently, but not actually, pernicious or malignant.

pernicious (per-nish′us) [L. perniciosus] tending to a fatal issue.

pernio (per′ne-o), pl. *pernio′nes* [L.] chilblain.

perniosis (per″ne-o′sis) (obs.) a general term for skin affections caused by cold; the presence of chilblains on various portions of the body.

pero- (pe′ro) [Gr. pēros maimed] a combining form meaning maimed or deformed.

perobrachius (pe″ro-bra′ke-us) [pero- + Gr. brachiōn arm] a fetus with deformed arms.

perocephalus (pe″ro-sef′ah-lus) [pero- + Gr. kephalē head] a fetus with a deformed head.

perochirus (pe″ro-ki′rus) [pero- + Gr. cheir hand] a fetus with malformed hands.

perocormus (pe″ro-kor′mus) [pero- + Gr. kormos trunk] perosomus.

perodactylus (pe″ro-dak′tĭ-lus) [pero- + Gr. daktylos finger] a fetus with deformity of fingers or toes, or both, especially absence of one or more digits.

peromelia (per″o-me′le-ah) congenital deformity of the limbs.

peromelus (pe-rom′ĕ-lus) [pero- + Gr. melos limb] a fetus with malformed limbs.

peronarthrosis (per″o-nar-thro′sis) [Gr. peronē anything pointed for piercing or pinning + arthron joint] an articulation in which the surfaces are convex in one direction and concave in the other.

perone (per-o′ne) the fibula.

peroneal (per″o-ne′al) pertaining to the fibula or to the outer side of the leg; fibular.

peroneotibial (per″o-ne″o-tib′e-al) pertaining to the fibula and tibia.

peronia (pe-ro′ne-ah) [Gr. pēros maimed] a developmental malformation or mutilation.

Per. op. emet. abbreviation for L. *perac′ta operatio′ne emet′ici,* when the action of the emetic is over.

peropus (pe′ro-pus) [pero- + Gr. pous foot] a fetus with malformed legs and feet.

peroral (per-o′ral) [L. per through + os, oris the mouth] performed through or administered through the mouth.

per os (per os) [L.] by mouth.

perosis (pĕ-ro′sis) a disease of chicks marked by bone deformities and associated with deficiency of certain dietary factors, such as choline and manganese.

perosomus (pe″ro-so′mus) [pero- + Gr. sōma body] a fetus with greatly deformed body or trunk.

perosplanchnia (pe″ro-splank′ne-ah) [pero- + Gr. splanchnon viscus + -ia] a developmental anomaly characterized by malformation of the viscera.

perosseous (per-os′e-us) [L. per through + os bone] transmitted through bone.

perotic (pĕ-rot′ik) pertaining to or characterized by perosis.

peroxidase (pĕ-rok′sĭ-dās) any of a group of iron-porphyrin enzymes which catalyze the oxidation of some organic substrates in the presence of hydrogen peroxide. They occur widely in plants (e.g., horseradish); in animals there is weak peroxidase activity in the kidney, and leukocytes contain verdoperoxidase, which may explain the peroxidative activity of pus. Substrates which have been reported, in addition to peroxides, include phenols, reduced glutathione, ferrocytochrome C, and NADH.

peroxide (pĕ-rok′sīd) that oxide of any element which contains more oxygen than any other. More correctly applied to compounds having such linkage as —O—O—; for instance, hydrogen peroxide, H—O—O—H.

peroxisome (pĕ-roks′ĭ-sōm) 1. any of the microbodies present in vertebrate animal cells, especially liver and kidney cells, which are rich in the enzymes peroxidase, catalase, D-amino acid oxidase, and, to a lesser extent, urate oxidase; their functions are not fully understood, but they participate in metabolic oxidations involving hydrogen peroxide, purine metabolism, and gluconeogenesis. Similar structures (*glyoxysomes*), containing the enzymes of the glyoxylate cycle, are found in certain plants and microorganisms. 2. microbody.

peroxydase (pĕ-rok′sĭ-dās) peroxidase.

peroxydol (pĕ-rok′sĭ-dol) sodium perborate.

perphenazine (per-fen′ah-zēn) [USP] chemical name: 4-[3-(2-chloro-10H-phenothiazin-10-yl)propyl]-1-piperazineethanol. A major tranquilizer, $C_{21}H_{26}ClN_3OS$, occurring as a white to creamy white powder; used orally and intramuscularly as an antipsychotic agent, and also used as an antiemetic.

per primam (per pri′mam) [L.] see *per primam intentionem.*

per primam intentionem (per pri′mam in-ten″she-o′nem) [L.] by first intention; see under *healing.*

per rectum (per rek′tum) [L.] by way of the rectum.

Perrin-Ferraton disease (per′an-fer′ah-ton′) [Maurice Perrin, Paris surgeon, 1826–1889; Louis Ferraton, French surgeon, born 1860] snapping hip.

Perroncito's apparatus (spirals) (per″on-se′tōz) [Aldo Perroncito, Italian histologist, 1882–1929] see under *apparatus.*

persalt (per′sawlt) a salt of a peracid; a salt the acid radical of which has a higher valence than the protosalt.

per saltum (per sal′tum) [L.] by a leap or bound; denoting a sudden evolutionary development without intermediate stages.

Persantine (per-san′tēn) trademark for preparations of dipyridamole.

per secundam (per se-kun′dam) [L.] see *per secundam intentionem.*

per secundam intentionem (per se-kun′dam in-ten″she-o′nem) [L.] by second intention; see under *healing.*

perseveration (per-sev″er-a′shun) persistent repetition of the same verbal or motor response to varied stimuli; continuance of an activity after cessation of the causative stimulus. **clonic p.,** a condition in which a movement is repeated. **tonic p.,** a condition in which a position is maintained.

persona (per-so′nah) [L. "mask"] Jung's term for the personality "mask" or facade presented by a person to the outside world, as opposed to the *anima* (def. 3).

personalistics (per″sun-al-is′tiks) the study of personality.

personality (per″sŭ-nal′ĭ-te) that which constitutes, distinguishes, and characterizes a person as an entity over a period of time; the total reaction of a person to his environment. **affective p.,** cyclothymic p. **alternating p.,** see *multiple p.* **anankastic p.,** obsessive-compulsive p. **antisocial p.,** a personality disorder marked by a basic lack of socialization, behavior resulting in repeated conflict with society, and an incapacity to be loyal to individuals, groups, or social codes; it is associated with low tolerance to frustration, impulsiveness, selfishness, inability to feel guilty and to learn from experience and punishment, callousness, and a tendency to blame others for inappropriate behavior or to offer rationalizations for it, and by irresponsibility. Those who exhibit this type of personality have been called psychopaths and sociopaths. Called also *psychopathic p.* and *sociopathic p.* **asthenic p.,** a personality disorder characterized by easy fatigability, low energy level, lack of enthusiasm, marked incapacity for enjoyment, and oversensitivity to physical and emotional stress. **compulsive p.,** see *obsessive-compulsive p.* **cycloid p.,** cyclothymic p. **cyclothymic p.,** a personality characterized by alternating moods of elation and sadness, with mood swings out of proportion to apparent stimuli, and by a predisposition to the development of manic-depressive or affective psychoses. Called also *affective p., cycloid p.,* and *cyclothymia.* **double p., dual p.,** see *multiple p.* **dyssocial p.,** a personality disorder in which the individual is not antisocial, but disregards social codes and may come in conflict with them, is predatory, follows more or less criminal activities, and may be loyal to his own socially deviant group; narcotics dealers, racketeers, prostitutes, and dishonest gamblers are those who may exhibit this type of personality. **explosive p.,** a personality disorder characterized by gross outbursts of rage or of verbal or physical agressiveness, which are strikingly different from the patient's usual behavior, and for which he may be regretful or repentant. **hysterical p.,** a personality characterized by shifting emotional feelings, susceptibility to suggestion, impulsiveness, attention-seeking, and self-absorption. **inadequate p.,** a personality disorder characterized by ineffectual responses to emotional, social, intellectual, and physical demands; while the affected individual seems neither physically nor mentally deficient, he does manifest inadaptability, ineptness, poor judgment, social inability, and lack of physical and emotional stamina. **multiple p.,** a dissociative reaction in which an individual adopts two or more separate and distinct personalities, in none of which is he aware of his experiences in the other. **obsessive p.,** see *obsessive-compulsive p.* **obsessive-compulsive p.,** a personality disorder characterized by excessive concern with conformity and adherence to rigid standards of conscience, typically manifested by overinhibition, overconscientiousness, overdutifulness, indecisiveness, perfectionism, and inability to relax easily. This disorder may lead to an obsessive-compulsive neurosis (q.v.). Called also *anankastic p.* **paranoid p.,** a personality disorder characterized by hypersensitivity, rigidity, unwarranted suspicion, envy, jealousy, excessive self-importance and a tendency to blame others and ascribe evil motives to them. **passive-aggressive p.,** a personality characterized by aggression exhibited in passive ways, as by pouting, stubbornness, procrastination, and passive obstructionism. **passive-dependent p.,** a personality characterized by lack of self-confidence, indecisiveness, and emotional dependency. **psychopathic p.,** antisocial p. **schizoid p.,** a personality disorder marked by timidness, self-consciousness, introversion, feelings of isolation and loneliness, and failure to form close interpersonal relationships; the individual is frequently ambitious, meticulous, and a perfectionist. **seclusive p., shut-in p.,** schizoid p. **sociopathic p.,** antisocial p. **split p.,** a popular and erroneous name for schizophrenia.

perspiratio (per″spĭ-ra′she-o) [L.] perspiration. **p. insensib′ilis,** insensible perspiration.

perspiration (per″spĭ-ra′shun) [L. *perspira′re* to breathe through] 1. sweating; the functional secretion of sweat. 2. sweat. **insensible p.,** those evaporative losses of water from the moist surfaces of the body (such as the skin and respiratory tree) not due to the secretory activity of glands. **sensible p.,** perspiration due to secretory activity of sweat glands.

persuasion (per-swa′zhun) in psychiatry, a therapeutic approach based on direct suggestion and guidance intended to influence favorably attitudes, behavior, and goals.

persulfate (per-sul′fāt) a salt of persulfuric acid.

persulfide (per-sul′fīd) a sulfide which contains more sulfur than the ordinary sulfide.

per tertiam (per ter′she-am) [L.] see *per tertiam intentionem.*

Perthes' disease, incision, test (per′tēz) [Georg Clemens *Perthes,* German surgeon, 1869–1927] see under *osteochondrosis* and *incision,* and see *tourniquet test,* under *tests.*

Pertik's diverticulum (per′tiks) [Otto *Pertik,* Hungarian physician, 1852–1913] see under *diverticulum.*

Pertofrane (per′to-frān) trademark for a preparation of desipramine hydrochloride.

per tubam (per tu′bam) [L.] through a tube.

pertubation (per″tu-ba′shun) perflation or insufflation of the uterine tubes to render them patent.

pertussis (per-tus′is) [L. *per* intensive + *tussis* cough] whooping cough.

pertussoid (per-tus′oid) [*pertussis* + Gr. *eidos* form] 1. resem-

bling whooping cough; 2. an influenzal cough resembling that of whooping cough.

per vaginam (per vah-ji′nam) through the vagina.

perversion (per-ver′shun) [L. *per* through + *versio* a turning] a turning aside from the normal course; a morbid alteration of function which may occur in emotional, intellectual, or volitional fields. In psychiatry, sexual deviation. **sexual p.,** paraphilia.

pervert (per′vert) a perverted person, especially a person who indulges in unnatural sexual acts (*sexual p.,* or *paraphiliac*).

per vias naturales (per vi′as nat″u-ra′lēz) [L.] by the natural ways.

pervigilium (per″vĭ-jil′e-um) [L.] sleeplessness.

pervious (per′ve-us) [L. *pervius*] permeable.

pes (pes), pl. *pe′des,* gen. *pe′dis* [L.] [NA] the foot: the terminal organ of the leg, or lower limb. Used also as a general term to designate a footlike part. **p. abduc′tus,** a deformed foot in which the anterior part is displaced so that it lies laterally to the vertical axis of the leg. **p. adduc′tus,** a deformed foot in which the anterior part is displaced so that it lies medially to the vertical axis of the leg. **p. anseri′nus** [L. "goose's foot"], 1. plexus parotideus nervi facialis. 2. the combined insertion of the tendinous expansions of the sartorius, gracilis, and semitendinosus muscles. **p. ca′vus,** exaggerated height of the longitudinal arch of the foot, present from birth or appearing later because of contractures or disturbed balance of the muscles. **p. cer′ebri,** crus cerebri. **congenital convex p. val′gus,** rocker-bottom foot (def. 1). **p. corvi′nus** [L. "crow's foot"] (*obs.*), a set of wrinkles radiating from the lateral canthus of the eye. **p. equinovalgus,** talipes equinovalgus. **equinovarus p.,** talipes equinovarus. **p. febric′itans,** elephantiasis. **p. gi′gas,** macropodia. **p. hippocam′pi** [NA], a formation of two or three elevations on the rostral end of the ventricular surface of the hippocampus; called also *digitationes hippocampi.* **p. hippocam′pi ma′jor,** hippocampus. **p. hippocam′pi mi′nor,** calcar avis. **p. pedun′culi,** crus cerebri. **p. planoval′gus, p. pla′nus,** flatfoot, a deformed foot in which the position of the bones relative to each other has been altered, with lowering of the longitudinal arch. **p. prona′tus,** a deformed foot in which the outer border of the anterior part is higher than the inner border. **p. supina′tus,** a deformed foot in which the inner border of the anterior part is higher than the outer border. **p. val′gus,** flatfoot. **p. varus,** talipes varus.

pessary (pes′ah-re) [L. *pessarium*] 1. an instrument placed in the vagina to support the uterus or rectum or as a contraceptive device. 2. a medicated vaginal suppository. **cup p.,** a pessary

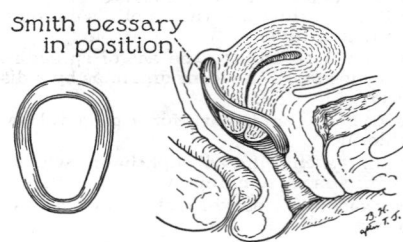

Smith pessary (Curtis).

the top of which has a cuplike shape to fit the os uteri. **diaphragm p.,** a diaphragm for insertion into the vagina as an occlusive contraceptive. **doughnut p.,** an inflated soft rubber pessary shaped like a doughnut. **Gehrung p.** (*obs.*), a pessary for cystocele, being a Hodge pessary bent on itself so as to form a double horseshoe, one lever being a little shorter than the other. **Gellhorn p.** (*obs.*), a single stem pessary for use in uterine prolapse. **Hodge's p.,** a pessary for retrodeviations of the uterus. **lever p.,** a pessary which acts on the principle of the lever. **Menge's p.,** a ring pessary with a fixed crossbar holding a detachable stem. **ring p.,** a round or ring-shaped pessary. **Smith's p.,** a pessary for use in retrodisplacement of the uterus. **stem p.,** a pessary with a stem for introduction into the canal of the cervix uteri.

pessimism (pes′ĭ-mizm) [L. *pes′simus* worst] a morbid disposition to put the worst construction upon everything. **therapeutic p.,** a tendency to undervalue the curative properties of drugs.

pessimum (pes′ĭ-mum) a weakened muscular contraction following a strong initial reaction after the stimulation of the neuromuscular system with high-frequency electric current.

pest (pest) plague. **avian p.,** Newcastle disease. **chicken p., fowl p.,** fowl plague.

pesticemia (pes″tĭ-se′me-ah) [L. *pestis* plague + Gr. *haima* blood + *-ia*] 1. the presence of plague germs (*Yersinia pestis*) in the blood. 2. septicemic plague.

pesticide (pes′tĭ-sīd) a poison used to destroy pests of any sort; the term includes fungicides, herbicides, insecticides, rodenticides, etc.

pestiferous (pes-tif′er-us) [L. *pestiferus; pestis* plague + *ferre* to bear] causing or propagating a pestilence.

pestilence (pes′tĭ-lens) [L. *pestilentia*] any virulent contagious or infectious epidemic disease; also an epidemic of such a disease.

pestilential (pes″tĭ-len′shal) of the nature of a pestilence; producing an epidemic disease.

pestis (pes′tis) [L.] plague. **p. am′bulans,** ambulatory plague. **p. bubon′ica,** bubonic plague. **p. equo′rum,** African horse sickness. **p. ful′minans, p. ma′jor,** the severe form of bubonic plague. **p. mi′nor,** ambulatory plague. **p. sid′erans,** septicemic plague. **p. variolo′sa,** smallpox.

pestle (pes″l) [L. *pestillum*] an implement for pounding drugs in a mortar.

pestology (pes-tol′o-je) the branch of science concerned with pests.

-petal [L. *petere* to seek] a word termination meaning directed or moving toward, the point of reference being indicated by the word stem to which it is affixed, as centripetal (toward a center), corticipetal (toward the cortex), etc.

petalo- (pet′ah-lo) [Gr. *petalon* leaf] a combining form denoting relationship to a leaf.

petalobacteria (pet″ah-lo-bak-te′re-ah) [petalo- + *bacteria*] bacteria which become so aggregated as to form thin pellicles.

petechia (pe-te′ke-ah), pl. *pete′chiae* [L.] a pinpoint, nonraised, perfectly round, purplish red spot caused by intradermal or submucous hemorrhage. Cf. *ecchymosis.*

petechiae (pe-te′ke-e) plural of *petechia.*

petechial (pe-te′ke-al) characterized by or of the nature of petechiae.

Peter of Abano (1250–c. 1316) physician, philosopher, astrologer; an outstanding professor in the University of Padua whose opinions caused him to be tried for heresy during the Inquisition. His works include the *Conciliator differentiarum* (an attempt to reconcile Arabian and Greek medicine) and *De venenis* (a book on poisons). He was also known as Pietro d'Abano and Petrus Apponus.

Peterman test (pe′ter-man) [Mynie Gustav *Peterman,* American physician, born 1896] see under *tests.*

Peters' ovum (pa′terz) [Hubert *Peters,* Budapest gynecologist, 1859–1934] see under *ovum.*

Petersen's bag (pa′ter-senz) [C. F. *Petersen,* surgeon in Kiel, 1845–1908] see under *bag.*

pethidine hydrochloride (peth′ĭ-din hi″dro-klo′rīd) meperidine hydrochloride.

petiolate, petiolated (pet′e-o-lāt; pet′e-o-lāt″ed) having a stalk or petiole.

petiole (pet′e-ōl) a stem, stalk, or pedicle. **epiglottic p.,** petiolus epiglottidis.

petioled (pet′e-ōld) petiolate.

petiolus (pĕ-ti′o-lus) [L., dim. of *pes* foot] a stem, stalk, or pedicle. **p. epiglot′tidis** [NA], epiglottic petiole: the pointed lower end of the epiglottic cartilage, which is attached to the back of the thyroid cartilage.

Petit's canal, sinus (ptēz) [François Pourfour du *Petit,* French anatomist and surgeon, 1664–1741] see *spatia zonularia* and *sinus aortae.*

Petit's hernia, ligament, triangle (ptēz) [Jean Louis *Petit,* French surgeon, 1674–1750] see under *hernia,* see *uterosacral ligament,* under *ligament,* and see *trigonum lumbale.*

Petit's law (ptēz) [Alexis Therese *Petit,* French physicist, 1791–1820] see *Dulong and Petit's law,* under *law.*

petit mal (pĕ-te′ mahl′) [Fr. "little illness"] see under *epilepsy.*

Petrén's diet (treatment) (pa-trenz′) [Karl Anders *Petrén,* Swedish physician, 1869–1927] see under *diet.*

Pétrequin's ligament (pātr-kanz′) [Joseph Pierre Eléonor *Pétrequin,* Lyons surgeon, 1809–1876] see under *ligament.*

Petri dish, plate, test (reaction) (pa′tre) [Julius Richard *Petri,* German bacteriologist, 1852–1921] see under *dish, plate,* and *tests.*

petrichloral (pet″rĭ-klo′ral) chemical name: pentaerythritol chloral. A derivative, $C_{13}H_{16}Cl_{12}O_8$, of chloral with pharmacological properties similar to those of chloral hydrate; used as a hypnotic and sedative.

petrifaction (pet″rĭ-fak′shun) [L. *petra* stone + *facere* to make] conversion into a stonelike substance.

pétrissage (pa″trĭ-sahzh′) [Fr.] foulage.

petroccipital (pet″rok-sip′ĭ-tal) petro-occipital.

petrolate (pet′ro-lāt) petrolatum.

petrolatoma (pet″ro-lah-to′mah) a tumor developing consequent to injection of liquid petrolatum; a discontinued procedure.

petrolatum (pet″ro-la′tum) [L.] [USP] a purified mixture of semisolid hydrocarbons obtained from petroleum; used as an ointment base. It is also used as a protective dressing and soothing application to the skin. Called also *mineral jelly, petroleum jelly, yellow soft paraffin,* and *petrolate.* **p. al′bum,** white p. **hydrophilic p.** [USP], a mixture of cholesterol, stearyl alcohol, and white wax, in white petrolatum; used as an absorbent ointment base and topical protectant. **liquid p.,** mineral oil; see under *oil.* **liquid p., heavy,** mineral oil; see under *oil.* **liquid p., light,** light mineral oil; see under *oil.* **p. liq′uidum,** mineral oil; see under *oil.* **p. liq′uidum le′ve,** light mineral oil; see under *oil.* **white p.** [USP], a wholly or nearly decolorized, purified mixture of semisolid hydrocarbons obtained from petroleum; used as an oleaginous ointment base and topical protectant.

petroleum (pĕ-tro′le-um) [L. *petra* stone + *oleum* oil] a thick natural oil obtained from beneath the earth. It consists of a mixture of various hydrocarbons of the paraffin and olefin series. It has been used as an expectorant, diaphoretic, and vermifuge; also in skin diseases, etc.

petrolization (pet″rol-i-za′shun) the spreading of petroleum on water for the purpose of destroying mosquito larvae therein.

petromastoid (pet″ro-mas′toid) 1. pertaining to the petrous portion of the temporal bone and its mastoid process. 2. otocranium (def. 2).

petro-occipital (pet″ro-ok-sip′ĭ-tal) pertaining to the petrous portion of the temporal bone and to the occipital bone.

petropharyngeus (pet″ro-fah-rin′je-us) an occasional muscle arising from the lower surface of the petrous portion of the temporal bone and inserted into the pharynx.

petrosal (pĕ-tro′sal) pertaining to the petrous portion of the temporal bone.

petrosalpingostaphylinus (pet″ro-sal-ping″go-staf″ĭ-li′nus) [Gr. *petra* stone + *salpinx* tube + *staphylē* uvula] musculus levator veli palatini.

petrosectomy (pet″ro-sek′to-me) [*petrous* + Gr. *ektomē* excision] excision of the cells of the apex of the petrous portion of the temporal bone.

petrositis (pet″ro-si′tis) inflammation of the petrous portion of the temporal bone.

petrosomastoid (pĕ-tro″so-mas′toid) petromastoid.

petrosphenoid (pet″ro-sfe′noid) pertaining to the sphenoid bone and the petrous portion of the temporal bone.

petrosphere (pet′ro-sfēr) the solid structure of the earth as distinguished from the atmosphere and the aquasphere.

petrosquamosal (pet″ro-skwah-mo′sal) pertaining to the petrous and squamous portions of temporal bone.

petrosquamous (pet″ro-skwa′mus) petrosquamosal.

petrostaphylinus (pet″ro-staf″ĭ-li′nus) musculus levator veli palatini.

petrous (pet′rus) [L. *petrosus*] resembling a rock; hard; stony.

petrousitis (pet″rus-i′tis) petrositis.

Petruschky's litmus whey, spinalgia (pĕ-trush′kēz) [Johannes *Petruschky,* German bacteriologist, born 1863] see *litmus whey,* under *whey,* and see under *spinalgia.*

Pettenkofer's test, theory (pet′en-kof″erz) [Max Josef von *Pettenkofer,* chemist in Munich, 1818–1901] see under *tests* and *theory.*

pettymorrel (pet″e-mor′rel) *Aralia.*

Petzetaki's test (reaction) (pet″za-tah′kēz) see under *tests.*

Peucetia (pu-se′te-ah) a genus of spiders. **P. vir′idans,** a lynx spider that is capable of producing painful burns of the eye by squirting a corrosive spray.

pexia (pek′se-ah) pexis.

pexic (pek′sik) [Gr. *pēxis* fixation] having the power of fixing substances; said of tissues.

pexin (pek′sin) [Gr. *pēxis* fixation] rennet.

pexinogen (pek-sin′o-jen) [*pexin* + Gr. *gennan* to produce] prerennin.

pexis (pek′sis) [Gr. *pēxis*] 1. the fixation of matter by a tissue. 2. surgical fixation, usually by suturing.

-pexy [Gr. *pēxis* a fixing, putting together] a word termination meaning fixation.

Peyer's patches (glands, insulae, plaques) (pi′erz) [Johann Conrad *Peyer,* Swiss anatomist, 1653–1712] folliculi lymphatici aggregati.

peyote (pa-o′te) 1. any of several Mexican cacti of the genus *Lophophora,* especially *L. williamsii* or mescal. 2. a stimulant drug from mescal buttons, the flowering heads of *L. williamsii,* used by North American Indians in ceremonies and feasts to produce a state of intoxification marked by feelings of ecstasy. The active euphoric principle is the major alkaloid, mescaline. Called also *peyotl.*

peyotl (pa-o′t'l) peyote.

Peyronie's disease (pa-ron-ēz′) [François de la *Peyronie,* French surgeon, 1678–1747] see under *disease.*

Peyrot's thorax (pa-roz′) [Jean Joseph *Peyrot,* surgeon in Paris, 1843–1917] see under *thorax.*

Pfannenstiel's incision (pfan′en-stēlz) [Hermann Johann *Pfannenstiel,* gynecologist in Breslau, 1862–1909] see under *incision.*

Pfeiffer's bacillus, law, phenomenon (reaction) (pfi′erz)

[Richard Friedrich Johann *Pfeiffer*, bacteriologist in Breslau, 1858–1945] see *Hemophilus influenzae*, and see under *law* and *phenomenon*.

Pfeiffer's disease, glandular fever (pfi′ferz) [Emil *Pfeiffer*, German physician, 1846–1921]   infectious mononucleosis.

Pfeifferella (pfi″fer-el′ah) [Richard F. J. *Pfeiffer*]   a genus name formerly given certain bacteria now included in the family Brucellaceae.   **P. anapes′tifer,** *Pasteurella anapestifer.*   **P. mal′lei,** *Pseudomonas mallei.*

Pflüger's cords, law, tubes (pfle′gerz) [Edward Friedrich Wilhelm *Pflüger*, physiologist in Bonn, 1829–1910]   see under *law*, and see *ovarian* and *salivary tubes*, under *tube*.

pfropfhebephrenia (pfropf″he-bĕ-fre′ne-ah) [Ger. *Pfropf* a plug or graft]   hebephrenic schizophrenia associated with mental retardation (Kraepelin).

pfropfschizophrenia (pfropf″skiz-o-fre′ne-ah)   schizophrenia associated with mental retardation (Kraepelin).

Pfuhl's sign (pfoolz) [Adam *Pfuhl*, German physician, 1842–1905]   see under *sign*.

PG   abbreviation for prostaglandin.

P.G.   abbreviation of *Pharmacopoeia Germanica*, German pharmacopeia.

pg.   picogram.

P.G.A.   pteroylglutamic acid (folic acid).

PGH   pituitary growth hormone.

Ph   chemical symbol for *phenyl*.

Ph.   Pharmacopeia.

pH   the symbol relating the hydrogen ion (H$^+$) concentration or activity of a solution to that of a given standard solution. Numerically the pH is approximately equal to the negative logarithm of H$^+$ concentration expressed in molarity. pH 7 is neutral; above it alkalinity increases and below it acidity increases.

phacitis (fah-si′tis)   phakitis.

phaco- (fak′o) [Gr. *phakos* a lentil, or lentil-shaped object]   a combining form denoting relationship to a lens, as the crystalline lens; see also words beginning *phako-*.

phacoanaphylaxis (fak″o-an″ah-fi-lak′sis) [*phaco-* + *anaphylaxis*]   hypersensitivity to the protein of the crystalline lens of the eye, induced by escape of material from the lens capsule.

phacocele (fak′o-sēl) [*phaco-* + Gr. *kēlē* hernia]   the dislocation of the eye lens from its proper place; hernia of the eye lens.

phacocyst (fak′o-sist) [*phaco-* + Gr. *kystis* sac, bladder]   the capsule of the lens (capsula lentis [NA]).

phacocystectomy (fak″o-sis-tek′to-me) [*phacocyst* + Gr. *ektomē* excision]   excision of a portion of the capsule of the lens for cataract.

phacocystitis (fak″o-sis-ti′tis) [*phacocyst* + *-itis*]   inflammation about the capsule of the crystalline lens.

phacoemulsification (fak″o-e-mul″si-fi-ka′shun)   a method of cataract extraction in which the lens is fragmented by ultrasonic vibrations and simultaneously irrigated and aspirated.

phacoerysis (fak″o-er-e′sis) [*phaco-* + Gr. *eryein* to drag away]   removal of the lens in cataract by means of suction with an instrument known as an erysiphake; called also *Barraquer's method* or *operation*.

phacoglaucoma (fak″o-glaw-ko′mah) [*phaco-* + *glaucoma*]   the structural changes in the lens produced by glaucoma.

phacohymenitis (fak″o-hi″men-i′tis) [*phaco-* + Gr. *hymēn* membrane + *-itis*]   inflammation about the capsule of the crystalline lens.

phacoid (fak′oid) [*phaco-* + Gr. *eidos* form]   shaped like a lens or a lentil.

phacoiditis (fak″oi-di′tis)   phakitis.

phacoidoscope (fah-koi′do-skōp) [*phaco-* + Gr. *eidos* form + *skopein* to examine]   phacoscope.

phacolysin (fah-kol′ĭ-sin)   an albumin from the lens of the eye; used in the treatment of early cataract.

phacolysis (fah-kol′ĭ-sis) [*phaco-* + Gr. *lysis* dissolution]   discission of the crystalline lens, followed by extraction.

phacolytic (fak″o-lit′ik)   pertaining to or causing dissolution of the crystalline lens.

phacoma (fah-ko′mah)   phakoma.

phacomalacia (fak″o-mah-la′she-ah) [*phaco-* + Gr. *malakia* softness]   softening of the lens; a soft cataract.

phacomatosis (fak″o-mah-to′sis)   phakomatosis.

phacometachoresis (fak″o-met″ah-ko-re′sis) [*phaco-* + Gr. *metachōrēsis* displacement]   displacement of the eye lens.

phacometecesis (fak″o-met″ĕ-se′sis) [*phaco-* + Gr. *metoikēsis* migration]   phacometachoresis.

phacometer (fah-kom′ĕ-ter) [*phaco-* + Gr. *metron* measure]   an instrument of measuring the refractive power of lenses.

phacopalingenesis (fak″o-pal″in-jen′ĕ-sis) [*phaco-* + Gr. *palin* again + *genesis* production]   re-formation of the crystalline lens.

phacoplanesis (fak″o-plah-ne′sis) [*phaco-* + Gr. *planēsis* wandering]   abnormal mobility of the eye lens.

phacosclerosis (fak″o-skle-ro′sis) [*phaco-* + Gr. *sklērōsis* hardening]   hardening of the eye lens; a hard cataract.

phacoscope (fak′o-skōp) [*phaco-* + Gr. *skopein* to examine]   an instrument for viewing accommodative changes of the eye lens.

phacoscopy (fah-kos′ko-pe)   the examination of the eye with a phacoscope.

phacoscotasmus (fak″o-sko-taz′mus) [*phaco-* + Gr. *skotasmos* a clouding]   the clouding of the lens of the eye.

phacotherapy (fak″o-ther′ah-pe) [*phaco-* + Gr. *therapeia* treatment]   heliotherapy.

phacotoxic (fak″o-tok′sik)   exerting a deleterious effect upon the crystalline lens.

phacozymase (fak″o-zi′mās)   an enzyme derived from an aqueous extract of the crystalline lens.

Phaenicia (fen-ĭ-she′ah)   a genus of greenbottle flies of the family Calliphoridae that are metallic green or blue.   **P. cupri′na,** a sheep maggot fly of worldwide distribution; its larvae cause various forms of myiasis in humans. Called also *Lucilia cuprina.*   **P. serica′ta,** a sheep maggot fly of the British Isles which lays its eggs in wounds of sheep and soiled wool; its larvae have been introduced into infected wounds to facilitate healing. Called also *Lucilia sericata*. See also *maggot*.

phaeo-   for terms beginning thus, see also terms beginning *pheo-*.

phaeohyphomycosis (fe″o-hi″fo-mi-ko′sis)   any opportunistic infection caused by dematiacious fungi.

phage (fāj)   bacteriophage.

phagedena (faj″ĕ-de′nah) [Gr. *phagedaina; phagein* to eat]   (*obs.*) rapidly spreading and sloughing ulceration.

phagelysis (fāj′li-sis) [*phage* + Gr. *lysis* dissolution]   the destruction or solution of phage; the destructive or solvent action of phage.

-phagia, -phagy [Gr. *phagein* to eat]   a word termination denoting a perversion of appetite (pica), such as geophagia, or relationship to eating or swallowing, e.g., aerophagy.

phago- (fag′o) [Gr. *phagein* to eat]   a combining form denoting relationship to eating or consumption by ingestion or engulfing.

phagocaryosis (fag″o-kar″e-o′sis)   phagokaryosis.

phagocytable (fag′o-sīt″ah-b′l)   capable of being subject to phagocytosis.

phagocyte (fag′o-sīt) [*phago-* + *-cyte*]   any cell that ingests microorganisms or other cells and foreign particles. In many cases but not always the ingested material is digested within the phagocyte. Fixed phagocytes (fixed macrophages) are potentially phagocytic, and free phagocytes (free macrophages, polymorphonuclear leukocytes) are intensely phagocytic.   **alveolar p's,** rounded granular phagocytic cells within the alveoli of the lungs, which ingest inhaled material; called also *alveolar macrophages* and *dust cells.*   **endothelial p.,** endotheliocyte.   **globuliferous p.,** one which takes up the blood corpuscles.   **maloniferous p.,** one which takes up the blood pigment.   **mobile p.,** a free phagocyte.   **mononuclear p.,** see under *system.*   **sessile p.,** a fixed phagocyte.

phagocytic (fag″o-sit′ik)   pertaining to or produced by phagocytes.

phagocytin (fag″o-si′tin)   a bactericidal heat-stable protein contained in neutrophilic leukocytes.

phagocytize (fag′o-sīt″īz)   to exert a phagocytic action on.

phagocytoblast (fag″o-si′to-blast) [*phagocyte* + Gr. *blastos* germ]   a cell which gives rise to phagocytes.

phagocytolysis (fag″o-si-tol′ĭ-sis) [*phagocyte* + Gr. *lysis* dissolution]   solution or destruction of phagocytes.

phagocytolytic (fag″o-si″to-lit′ik)   pertaining to phagocytolysis.

phagocytose (fag″o-si′tōs)   to envelop and perhaps destroy bacteria and other foreign bodies.

phagocytosis (fag″o-si-to′sis)   the engulfing of microorganisms, other cells, and foreign particles by phagocytes.   **induced p.,** phagocytosis aided by subjecting bacteria to the action of opsonins in the blood.   **spontaneous p.,** phagocytosis of bacteria taking place in an indifferent medium, or phagocytosis of nonantigenic particles.   **surface p.,** phagocytosis of cellular antigens adsorbed on a rough surface, but not of the free-floating antigens; it occurs in the absence of opsonin.

phagocytotic (fag″o-si-tot′ik)   pertaining to or characterized by phagocytosis.

phagodynamometer (fag″o-di″nah-mom′ĕ-ter) [*phago-* + Gr. *dynamis* force + *metron* measure]   an apparatus for measuring the force exerted in chewing food.

phagokaryosis (fag″o-kar″e-o′sis) [*phago-* + Gr. *karyon* nucleus + *-osis*]   the alleged phagocytic action of the cell nucleus.

phagological (fag″o-loj′ĕ-kal)   pertaining to phage.

phagology (fah-gol′o-je) [*phago-* + *-logy*]   the subject of eating or feeding.

phagolysis (fah-gol′ĭ-sis) phagocytolysis.

phagolysosome (fag″o-li′so-sōm) the digestive vacuole formed when the membranes of pre-existent lysosomes within the cytoplasm merge with the phagosome; the lysosomes then discharge their hydrolytic enzymes, resulting in digestion of the phagocytized material.

phagolytic (fag″o-lit′ik) phagocytolytic.

phagomania (fag″o-ma′ne-ah) [*phago-* + Gr. *mania* madness] an insatiable craving for food, or an obsessive preoccupation with the subject of eating.

phagophobia (fag″o-fo′be-ah) [*phago-* + Gr. *phobein* to be affrighted by] morbid fear of eating.

phagosome (fag′o-sōm) [*phago* + Gr. *soma* body] the membrane-bounded vesicle in a phagocyte formed by invagination of the cell membrane and the phagocytized material; see also *phagolysosome*.

phagotherapy (fag″o-ther′ah-pe) [*phago-* + Gr. *therapeia* treatment] (*obs.*) treatment by feeding so as to strengthen the body's response to infection.

phagotrophy (fah-got′ro-fe) [*phago-* + Gr. *trophē* nutrition] the uptake of fluid or particulate matter by ciliary movement of the matter into a cytostome, with invagination of the matter by the cell membrane to form a food vacuole, a process of food intake occurring in ciliate protozoa.

phagotype (fag′o-tīp) phage type; see under *type*.

phakitis (fa-ki′tis) [Gr. *phakos* lens + *-itis*] inflammation of the crystalline lens.

phako- [Gr. *phakos* a lentil, or lentil-shaped object; a spot on the body, a freckle] for words beginning thus, see also those beginning *phaco-*.

phakoma (fah-ko′mah) [*phaco-* + *-oma*] 1. an occasional small, grayish white tumor seen microscopically in the retina in tuberous sclerosis. 2. a patch of myelinated nerve fibers seen very infrequently in the retina in neurofibromatosis.

phakomatosis (fak″o-mah-to′sis), pl. *phakomato′ses* [Gr. *phakos* mother spot] an ophthalmologic term for any of four hereditary syndromes (neurofibromatosis, tuberous sclerosis, encephalotrigeminal angiomatosis, and cerebroretinal angiomatosis) characterized by disseminated hamartomas of the eye, skin, and brain.

phalacrosis (fal″ah-kro′sis) [Gr. *phalakrōsis* baldness] alopecia.

phalangeal (fah-lan′je-al) pertaining to a phalanx.

phalangectomy (fal″an-jek′to-me) excision of a phalanx of a finger or toe.

phalanges (fah-lan′jēz) plural of *phalanx*.

phalangette (fal″an-jet′) the distal phalanx of a digit. **drop p.**, dropping of the distal phalanx of a finger and loss of power to extend it when the hand is prone.

phalangitis (fal″an-ji′tis) inflammation of one or more phalanges.

phalangization (fal″an-ji-za′shun) surgical separation of the terminal portion of fused digits, without complete extirpation of the connecting web.

phalangophalangeal (fah-lan″go-fah-lan′je-al) pertaining to two adjoining phalanges of a finger or toe.

phalangosis (fal″an-go′sis) a condition in which the eyelashes grow in rows.

phalanx (fa′lanks), pl. *phalan′ges* [Gr. "a line or array of soldiers"] 1. [NA] a general term for any bone of a finger or toe. 2. any one of a set of plates (made up of supporting cells, q.v.) disposed in rows which makes up the reticular membrane of the organ of Corti. **Deiters' phalanges**, modified cuticular plates forming the ends of sustentacular epithelial cells of the reticular membrane of the organ of Corti. **phalan′ges digito′rum ma′nus**, the fourteen bones composing the skeleton of the fingers (ossa digitorum manus [NA]). **phalan′ges digito′rum pe′dis**, the fourteen bones composing the skeleton of the toes (ossa digitorum pedis [NA]). **phalanges of fingers**, ossa digitorum manus. **p. dista′lis digito′rum ma′nus** [NA], distal phalanx of fingers: any one of the five terminal bones of the fingers, articulating, except in the thumb, with the distal phalanx; called also *p. tertia digitorum manus*. **p. dista′lis digito′rum pe′dis** [NA], distal phalanx of toes: any one of the five terminal bones of the toes, articulating, except in the great toe, with the phalanx media; called also *p. tertia digitorum pedis*. **p. me′dia digito′rum ma′nus** [NA], middle phalanx of fingers: any one of the four bones of the fingers (excluding the thumb) situated between the proximal and distal phalanges; called also *p. secunda digitorum manus*. **p. me′dia digito′rum pe′dis** [NA], middle phalanx of toes: any one of the four bones of the toes (excluding the great toe) situated between the proximal and distal phalanges; called also *p. secunda digitorum pedis*. **p. pri′ma digito′rum ma′nus**, p. proximalis digitorum manus. **p. pri′ma digito′rum pe′dis**, p. proximalis digitorum pedis. **p. proxima′lis digito′rum ma′nus** [NA], proximal phalanx of fingers: any one of the five bones of the fingers that articulate with the metacarpal bones and, except in the thumb, with the phalanx media; called also *p. prima digitorum manus*. **p. proxima′lis digito′rum pe′dis** [NA], proximal phalanx of

toes: any one of the five bones of the toes that articulate with the metatarsal bones and, except in the great toe, with the phalanx media; called also *p. prima digitorum pedis*. **p. secun′da digito′rum ma′nus**, p. media digitorum manus. **p. secun′da digito′rum pe′dis**, p. media digitorum pedis. **p. ter′tia digito′rum ma′nus**, p. distalis digitorum manus. **p. ter′tia digito′rum pe′dis**, p. distalis digitorum pedis. **phalanges of toes**, ossa digitorum pedis. **ungual p. of fingers**, p. distalis digitorum manus. **ungual p. of toes**, p. distalis digitorum pedis.

Phallales (fah-la′lēz) an order of basidiomycetes of the Gasteromycetes, characterized by the presence of a fetid mucinous substance around the basidiospores that are exposed by an internal stalk which grows and breaks out of the basidiocarp.

phallalgia (fal-al′je-ah) [*phallus* + *-algia*] pain in the penis.

phallanastrophe (fal″an-as′tro-fe) [*phallus* + Gr. *anastrophē* a turning upward] upward distortion of the penis.

phallaneurysm (fal-an′u-rizm) [*phallus* + Gr. *aneurysma* aneurysm] aneurysm of the penis.

phallectomy (fal-ek′to-me) [*phallos* + Gr. *ektomē* excision] amputation of the penis.

phallic (fal′ik) [Gr. *phallikos*] pertaining to the phallus, or penis.

phalliform (fal′ĭ-form) [*phallus* + L. *forma* form] shaped like the phallus or penis.

phallin (fal′in) a poisonous hemolytic glycoside from *Amanita phalloides*.

phallitis (fal-i′tis) [*phallus* + *-itis*] inflammation of the penis; penitis.

phallo- [Gr. *phallos* penis] combining form denoting relationship to the penis.

phallocampsis (fal″o-kamp′sis) [*phallo-* + Gr. *kampsis* bending] curvature of the penis when erect.

phallocrypsis (fal″o-krip′sis) [*phallo-* + Gr. *krypsis* hiding] retraction of the penis.

phallodynia (fal″o-din′e-ah) [*phallo-* + Gr. *odynē* pain] pain in the penis.

phalloid (fal′oid) [*phallo-* + Gr. *eidos* form] resembling a penis.

phalloidin, phalloidine (fah-loid′in) a heat-stable, bicyclic hexapeptide poison from the mushroom *Amanita phalloides*, which causes asthenia, vomiting, diarrhea, convulsions, and death.

phalloncus (fal-ong′kus) [*phallo-* + Gr. *onkos* mass] a morbid swelling or tumor of the penis.

phalloplasty (fal′o-plas″te) [*phallo-* + Gr. *plassein* to shape] plastic surgery of the penis.

phallorrhagia (fal″o-ra′je-ah) [*phallo-* + Gr. *rhēgnynai* to burst forth] hemorrhage from the penis.

phallorrhea (fal″o-re′ah) [*phallo-* + Gr. *rhoia* flow] (*obs.*) gonorrhea in the male.

phallotomy (fal-ot′o-me) [*phallo-* + Gr. *tomē* a cutting] incision of the penis.

Phallus (fal′us) a genus of basidiomycetous fungi of the order Phallales, series Gasteromycetes, including the stinkhorns.

phallus (fal′us) [Gr. *phallos*] 1. the rudiment of embryonic or fetal tissue that develops into the penis or clitoris. 2. the penis or clitoris. 3. the penis or a representation of the penis.

phanero- (fan′er-o) [Gr. *phaneros* visible] a combining form meaning visible or apparent.

phanerogam (fan′er-o-gam) [*phanero-* + Gr. *gamos* marriage] a true seed-bearing plant.

phanerogenetic (fan″er-o-jĕ-net′ik) phanerogenic.

phanerogenic (fan″er-o-jen′ik) [*phanero-* + Gr. *gennan* to produce] having a known cause. Cf. *cryptogenic*.

phaneroplasm (fan′er-o-plazm) [Gr. *phaneros* visible + *plasm*] membranous organelles and nonmembranous inclusions in the cytoplasm; cf. *cytosol*.

phaneroscope (fan′er-o-skōp) [Gr. *phaneros* visible + *skopein* to examine] (*obs.*) an instrument for illuminating the skin and rendering it translucent for examination.

phanerosis (fan″er-o′sis) [Gr. *phanerōsis*] the act of becoming visible; the setting free of a substance which has previously been undemonstrable owing to its being held in combination. **fat p.**, conversion in the tissues of invisible fatty substances into fat which can be stained and seen.

phanerosterol (fan″er-os′ter-ol) a sterol of one of the higher plants.

Phanodorn (fan′o-dorn) trademark for a preparation of cyclobarbital.

phantasia (fan-ta′ze-ah) fantasy.

phantasm (fan′tazm) [Gr. *phantasma* appearance] an impression or image not evoked by actual stimuli; called also *phantom*.

phantasmatology (fan″taz-mah-tol′o-je) [*phantasm* + *-logy*] the sum of what is known regarding apparitions and phantasms.

phantasmatomoria (fan-taz″mah-to-mo′re-ah) [*phantasm* +

Gr. *mōria* folly] childishness or dementia with absurd delusions.

phantasmology (fan″taz-mol′o-je) phantasmatology.

phantasy (fan″tah-se) [Gr. *phantasia* imagination; the power by which an object is made apparent to the mind] fantasy.

phantom (fan′tom) [Gr. *phantasma* an appearance] 1. an impression or image not evoked by actual stimuli. 2. a model of the body or of a specific part thereof. 3. in radiology, a device that simulates the conditions encountered when radiation or radioactive material is deposited *in vivo* and permits a quantitative estimation of its effects.

phanurane (fan′u-rān) canrenone.

phao- for words beginning thus, see those beginning *pheo-*.

phar., pharm. pharmacy; pharmaceutical; pharmacopeia.

Phar. B. abbreviation for L. *Pharmaciae Baccalaureus*, Bachelor of Pharmacy.

Phar. C. Pharmaceutical Chemist.

pharcidous (fahr′sĭ-dus) [Gr. *pharkis* wrinkled] wrinkled.

Phar. D. abbreviation for L. *Pharmaciae Doctor*, Doctor of Pharmacy.

Phar. G. Graduate in Pharmacy.

Phar. M. abbreviation for L. *Pharmaciae Magister*, Master of Pharmacy.

pharmacal (fahr′mah-kal) pertaining to pharmacy.

pharmaceutic (fahr-mah-su′tik) [Gr. *pharmakeutikos*] pertaining to pharmacy or to drugs.

pharmaceutical (fahr″mah-su′tĭ-kal) 1. pertaining to pharmacy or to drugs. 2. a medicinal drug.

pharmaceutics (fahr″mah-su′tiks) 1. pharmacy (def. 1). 2. pharmaceutical preparations.

pharmaceutist (fahr″mah-su′tist) a pharmacist.

pharmacist (fahr′mah-sist) one who is licensed to prepare and sell or dispence drugs and compounds, and to make up prescriptions; an apothecary, druggist, or (British) chemist.

pharmaco- (fahr′mah-ko) [Gr. *pharmakon* medicine] a combining form denoting relationship to a drug or medicine.

pharmacochemistry (fahr″mah-ko-kem′is-tre) pharmaceutical chemistry.

pharmacodiagnosis (fahr″mah-ko-di″ag-no′sis) [*pharmaco-* + *diagnosis*] the employment of drugs in the diagnosis of disease.

pharmacodynamic (fahr″mah-ko-di-nam′ik) [*pharmaco-* + Gr. *dynamis* power] pertaining to pharmacodynamics.

pharmacodynamics (fahr″mah-ko-di-nam′iks) [*pharmaco-* + Gr. *dynamis* power] the study of the biochemical and physiological effects of drugs and the mechanisms of their actions, including the correlation of actions and effects of drugs with their chemical structure; also, such effects on the actions of a particular drug or drugs.

pharmacoendocrinology (fahr″mah-ko-en″do-kri-nol′o-je) the study of the influence of drugs on the activity of the endocrine glands.

pharmacogenetics (fahr″mah-ko-jĕ-net′iks) the scientific study of the relationship between genetic factors and the nature of responses to drugs.

pharmacognostics (fahr″mah-kog-nos′tiks) pharmacognosy.

pharmacognosy (fahr″mah-kog′no-se) [*pharmaco-* + Gr. *gnōsis* knowledge] that branch of pharmacology which deals with the biological, biochemical, and economic features of natural drugs and their constituents.

pharmacography (fahr″mah-kog′rah-fe) [*pharmaco-* + Gr. *graphein* to write] an account or written description of drugs.

pharmacokinetics (fahr″mah-ko-ki-net′iks) the action of drugs in the body over a period of time, including the processes of absorption, distribution, localization in tissues, biotransformation, and excretion.

pharmacologic (fahr″mah-ko-loj′ik) pertaining to pharmacology or to the properties and reactions of drugs.

pharmacologist (fahr″mah-kol′o-jist) one who makes a study of the actions of drugs.

pharmacology (fahr″mah-kol′o-je) [*pharmaco-* + *-logy*] the science that deals with the origin, nature, chemistry, effects, and uses of drugs; it includes pharmacognosy, pharmocokinetics, pharmacodynamics, pharmacotherapeutics, and toxicology.

pharmacomania (fahr″mah-ko-ma′ne-ah) [*pharmaco-* + Gr. *mania* madness] uncontrollable desire to take or to administer medicines.

pharmacometrics (fahr″mah-ko-met′riks) [*pharmaco-* + Gr. *metron* measure] the comparative evaluation of drug activity, distinguished from bioassay in that substances with different chemical constitutions are compared.

pharmacon (fahr′mah-kon) [Gr. *pharmakon*] a drug.

pharmaco-oryctology (fahr″mah-ko-or″ik-tol′o-je) [*pharmaco-* + Gr. *oryktos* excavated + *-logy*] the study of mineral drugs.

pharmacopedia, pharmacopedics (fahr″mah-ko-pe′de-ah; fahr″mah-ko-pe′diks) [*pharmaco-* + Gr. *paideia* instruction]

the science which deals with the properties and preparations of drugs.

pharmacopeia (fahr″mah-ko-pe′ah) [*pharmaco-* + Gr. *poiein* to make] an authoritative treatise on drugs and their preparations; a book containing a list of products used in medicine, with descriptions, chemical tests for determining identity and purity, and formulas for certain mixtures of these substances. It also generally contains a statement of average dosage. The first United States pharmacopeia was published on December 15, 1820, printed in both Latin and English, and its 272 pages included 217 drugs which were considered worthy of recognition. See *U.S.P.*

pharmacopeial (fahr″mah-ko-pe′al) pertaining to or recognized by the pharmacopeia.

pharmacophilia (fahr″mah-ko-fil′e-ah) [*pharmaco-* + Gr. *philein* to love] morbid fondness for drugs; see *drug addiction*, under *addiction*.

pharmacophobia (fahr″mah-ko-fo′be-ah) [*pharmaco-* + Gr. *phobein* to be affrighted by] morbid dread of drugs or medicines.

pharmacophore (fahr′mah-ko-fōr″) [*pharmaco-* + Gr. *phoros* bearing] the group of atoms in a drug molecule which is responsible for the action of the compound.

pharmacopoeia (fahr″mah-ko-pe′ah) pharmacopeia.

pharmacopsychosis (fahr″mah-ko-si-ko′sis) [*pharmaco-* + *psychosis*] Southard's term for any one of the group of mental diseases due to alcohol, drugs, or poisons.

pharmacoradiography (fahr″mah-ko-ra″de-og′rah-fe) pharmacoroentgenography.

pharmacoroentgenography (fahr″mah-ko-rent″gen-og′rah-fe) roentgenographic examination of a body organ under the influence of a drug which best facilitates such examination.

pharmacotherapeutics (fahr″mah-ko-ther″ah-pu′tiks) [*pharmaco-* + *therapeutics*] study of the uses of drugs in the treatment of disease.

pharmacotherapy (fahr″mah-ko-ther′ah-pe) [*pharmaco-* + Gr. *therapeia* treatment] the treatment of disease by medicines.

pharmacy (fahr′mah-se) [Gr. *pharmakon* medicine] 1. the branch of the health sciences dealing with the preparation, dispensing, and proper utilization of drugs. 2. a place where drugs are compounded or dispensed. **chemical p.**, pharmaceutical chemistry. **galenic p.**, the pharmacy of vegetable medicines.

Pharm.D. abbreviation for Doctor of Pharmacy.

pharyngalgia (far″in-gal′je-ah) [*pharyngo-* + *-algia*] pain in the pharynx.

pharyngeal (fah-rin′je-al) [L. *pharyngeus*] pertaining to the pharynx.

pharyngectasia (far″in-jek-ta′se-ah) pharyngocele.

pharyngectomy (far″in-jek′to-me) [*pharyngo-* + Gr. *ektomē* excision] surgical removal of a part of the pharynx.

pharyngemphraxis (far″in-jem-frak′sis) [*pharyngo-* + Gr. *emphraxis* stoppage] obstruction of the pharynx.

pharyngeus (far-in-je′us) [L.] pharyngeal.

pharyngism (far′in-jism) pharyngismus.

pharyngismus (far″in-jiz′mus) muscular spasm of the pharynx.

pharyngitic (far″in-jit′ik) affected with or of the nature of pharyngitis.

pharyngitid (fah-rin′ji-tid) a cutaneous eruption occurring in pharyngitis.

pharyngitis (far″in-ji′tis) [*pharyngo-* + *-itis*] inflammation of the pharynx. **acute p.**, inflammation with pain in the throat, especially on swallowing, dryness, followed by moisture of the pharynx, congestion of the mucous membrane, and fever; called also *catarrhal p.* **atrophic p.**, a chronic pharyngitis which leads to wasting of the submucous tissue accompanied by dryness and thickened secretions. **catarrhal p.**, acute p. **chronic p.**, that which results from repeated acute attacks or is due to tuberculosis or syphilis; it is attended with excessive secretion, and in the severe ulcerated varieties by pain and dysphagia. **croupous p.**, membranous p. **diphtheric p.**, diphtheria of the pharynx. **follicular p.**, sore throat with enlargement of the pharyngeal glands. **gangrenous p.**, a form characterized by gangrenous patches. **glandular p.**, follicular p. **granular p.**, a chronic variety in which the mucous membrane becomes granular. **p. herpet′ica**, membranous or aphthous sore throat; a form of acute pharyngitis characterized by the formation of vesicles, which give place to excoriations. **hypertrophic p.**, a chronic form which leads to thickening of the submucous tissues. **p. kerato′sa**, pharyngomycosis. **membranous p.**, pharyngitis with a fibrous exudate leading to the formation of a false membrane. **phlegmonous p.**, acute parenchymatous tonsillitis attended with the formation of abscesses. **p. sic′ca**, an atrophic pharyngitis in which the throat becomes dry. **p. ulcero′sa**, the formation of ulcers covered by a yellow, membrane-like deposit in the pharynx, with fever, pain, and prostration.

pharyngo- (fah-ring′go) [Gr. *pharynx* pharynx] a combining form denoting relationship to the pharynx.

pharyngocele (fah-ring′go-sēl) [*pharyngo-* + Gr. *kēlē* hernia] hernial protrusion of a part of the pharynx; a hernial pouch or other cystic deformity of the pharynx.

pharyngoceratosis (fah-ring″go-ser′ah-to′sis) pharyngokeratosis.

pharyngoconjunctivitis (fah-ring″go-kon-junk″tĭ-vi′tis) inflammation involving the pharynx and conjunctiva, the result of a viral infection.

pharyngodynia (fah-ring″go-din′e-ah) [*pharyngo-* + Gr. *odynē* pain] pain in the pharynx.

pharyngoepiglottic (fah-ring″go-ep″ĭ-glot′ik) pertaining to the pharynx and epiglottis.

pharyngoepiglottidean (fah-ring″go-ep″ĭ-glŏ-tid′e-an) pharyngoepiglottic.

pharyngoesophageal (fah-ring″go-e-sof′ah-je′al) pertaining to the pharynx and esophagus.

pharyngoglossal (fah-ring″go-glos′al) pertaining to the pharynx and the tongue.

pharyngoglossus (fah-ring″go-glos′us) the muscular fibers from the superior constrictor of the pharynx to the tongue.

pharyngokeratosis (fah-ring″go-ker′ah-to′sis) keratosis of the pharynx.

pharyngolaryngeal (fah-ring″go-lah-rin′je-al) pertaining to the pharynx and the larynx.

pharyngolaryngitis (fah-ring″go-lar″in-ji′tis) [*pharyngo-* + Gr. *larynx* larynx + *-itis*] inflammation of the pharynx and the larynx.

pharyngolith (fah-ring′go-lith) [*pharyngo-* + Gr. *lithos* stone] a concretion in the walls of the pharynx.

pharyngology (far″ing-gol′o-je) [*pharyngo-* + *-logy*] the sum of what is known regarding the pharynx.

pharyngolysis (far″ing-gol′ĭ-sis) [*pharyngo-* + Gr. *lysis* dissolution] paralysis of the pharynx.

pharyngomaxillary (fah-ring″go-mak′sĭ-ler″e) pertaining to the pharynx and the maxillae.

pharyngomycosis (fah-ring″go-mi-ko′sis) [*pharyngo-* + Gr. *mykēs* fungus + *-osis*] any fungal disease of the pharynx.

pharyngonasal (fah-ring″go-na′sal) pertaining to the pharynx and the nose.

pharyngo-oral (fah-ring″go-o′ral) pertaining to the pharynx and the mouth.

pharyngopalatine (fah-ring″go-pal′ah-tīn) pertaining to the pharynx and the palate.

pharyngoparalysis (fah-ring″go-pah-ral′ĭ-sis) [*pharyngo-* + *paralysis*] paralysis of the pharyngeal muscles.

pharyngopathy (far″ing-gop′ah-the) [*pharyngo-* + Gr. *pathos* disease] disease of the pharynx.

pharyngoperistole (fah-ring″go-pĕ-ris′to-le) [*pharyngo-* + Gr. *peristolē* contracture] narrowing of the pharynx.

pharyngoplasty (fah-ring′go-plas″te) [*pharyngo-* + Gr. *plassein* to form] plastic operation on the pharynx. **Hynes p.,** a technique of pharyngoplasty accomplished by muscle transposition.

pharyngoplegia (far″ing-go-ple′je-ah) [*pharyngo-* + Gr. *plēgē* stroke] paralysis of the muscles of the pharynx.

pharyngorhinitis (fah-ring″go-ri-ni′tis) inflammation of the nasopharynx.

pharyngorhinoscopy (fah-ring″go-ri-nos′ko-pe) examination of the nasopharynx and posterior nares with rhinoscope.

pharyngorrhagia (far″ing-go-ra′je-ah) [*pharyngo-* + Gr. *rhēgnynai* to break forth] hemorrhage from the pharynx.

pharyngorrhea (far″ing-go-re′ah) [*pharyngo-* + Gr. *rhoia* flow] a discharge of mucus from the pharynx.

pharyngosalpingitis (fah-ring″go-sal″pin-je′tis) inflammation of the pharynx and the eustachian tube.

pharyngoscleroma (fah-ring″go-skle-ro′mah) scleroma of the pharynx.

pharyngoscope (fah-ring′go-skōp) [*pharyngo-* + Gr. *skopein* to examine] an instrument for inspecting the pharynx.

pharyngoscopy (far″ing-gos′ko-pe) direct visual examination of the pharynx.

pharyngospasm (fah-ring′go-spazm) [*pharyngo-* + Gr. *spasmos* spasm] spasm of the pharyngeal muscles.

pharyngostenosis (fah-ring″go-ste-no′sis) [*pharyngo-* + Gr. *stenōsis* narrowing] narrowing of the lumen of the pharynx.

pharyngostoma (fah″ring-gos′to-mah) [*pharyngo* + Gr. *stoma* mouth] the opening formed by pharyngostomy.

pharyngostomy (fah″ring-gos′to-me) [*pharyngo* + Gr. *stomoun* to provide with an opening, or mouth] the surgical creation of an artificial opening into the pharynx.

pharyngotherapy (fah-ring″go-ther′ah-pe) [*pharyngo-* + *therapy*] the treatment of pharyngeal disorders, and especially the irrigation of the nasopharynx in infectious diseases.

pharyngotome (fah-ring′go-tōm) a cutting instrument used in pharyngeal surgery.

pharyngotomy (far″ing-got′o-me) [*pharyngo-* + Gr. *tomē* a cutting] surgical incision of the pharynx. **external p.,** pharyngotomy done from the outside. **internal p.,** that which is performed from within the pharynx. **lateral p.,** the opening of the pharynx from one side. **subhyoid p.,** section of the pharynx through the thyrohyoid membrane.

pharyngotonsillitis (fah-ring″go-ton″sĭ-li′tis) inflammation of the pharynx and the tonsil.

pharyngotyphoid (fah-ring″go-ti′foid) enteric fever with angina and sore patches on the tonsils.

pharyngoxerosis (fah-ring″go-ze-ro′sis) [*pharyngo-* + Gr. *xērōsis* dryness] dryness of the pharynx.

pharynx (far′inks) [Gr. "the throat"] [NA] the musculomembranous passage between the mouth and posterior nares and the larynx and esophagus. The part above the level of the soft palate is the *nasopharynx,* which communicates with the auditory tube. The lower portion consists of two sections—the *oropharynx,* which lies between the soft palate and the upper edge of the epiglottis, and the *hypopharynx,* which lies below the upper edge of the epiglottis and opens into the larynx and esophagus.

phase (fāz) [Gr. *phasis* an appearance] 1. the view that a thing presents to the eye. 2. any one of the varying aspects or stages through which a disease or process may pass. 3. in physical chemistry, any physically or chemically distinct, homogenous, and mechanically separable part of a system, e.g., the ice and steam phases of water. **alpha p.,** the estrous stage of the ovarian cycle. **anal p.,** see under *stage.* **apophylactic p.,** negative p. **beta p.,** the progestational stage of the ovarian cycle. **cholesteric p.,** a liquid crystal phase that exhibits molecular orientation and arrangement both within and between equispaced planes. **continuous p.,** a phase that is physically continuous; the continuous portion of a colloid system (see *dispersion medium*). **p. of decline,** the stage in the growth of a bacterial culture in which the number of live organisms gradually decreases. **disperse p.,** the internal or discontinuous portion of a colloid system; it is analogous to the solute in a solution. Called also *internal p.* Cf. *dispersion medium.* **erythrocytic p.,** that phase in the life cycle of a malarial plasmodium in which the parasites multiply in the red blood cells. **estrin p.,** proliferative stage. **external p.,** dispersion medium. **genital p.,** see under *stage.* **hematic p.,** a liquid crystal phase that exhibits molecular orientation without periodicity. **inductive p.,** the time that elapses between the administration of antigen and the development of a detectable immune response. **internal p.,** disperse p. **lag p.,** lag, def. 2. **logarithmic p.,** the stage in the growth of a bacterial culture at which, if the logarithms of their members are plotted against the time, a straight upward line will be formed. **meiotic p.,** that stage in meiosis in which the reduction of the chromosomes occurs; called also *reduction p.* **motofacient p.,** see *motofacient.* **negative p.,** the initial lowering of the antibody content of blood following the injection of corresponding antigen. **nonmotofacient p.,** see *motofacient.* **Nonne-Apelt p.,** see under *reaction.* **oral p.,** see under *stage.* **phallic p.,** see under *stage.* **positive p.,** the rise above unity in the opsonic index which follows the negative phase. **postmeiotic p.,** the stage following the reduction of the chromosomes in meiosis. **premeiotic p., prereduction p.,** the stage in meiosis which precedes the reduction of the chromosomes. **reduction p.,** meiotic p. **resting p.,** former term for interphase. **smectic p.,** a liquid crystal phase that exhibits molecular orientation and arrangement in equispaced planes, but no periodicity within the planes. **stationary p.,** the stage in the growth of a bacterial culture at which multiplication of organisms gradually decreases, the number of bacteria remaining practically constant. **synaptic p.,** synapsis.

phaseolin (fa-se′o-lin) a globulin, $C_{20}H_{18}O_4$, from the kidneybean, *Phaseolus vulgaris,* which has antifungal properties.

phaseolunatin (fa″se-o-lu′nah-tin) linamarin.

phasin, phasein (fa′sin) any of a group of nitrogenous substances found in seeds, bark, and other plant tissues, which agglutinate red blood corpuscles.

phasmid (faz′mid) 1. one of a pair of caudal chemoreceptors occurring in certain nematodes. The class Nematoda is sometimes divided into two subclasses, Phasmidia and Aphasmidia, on the basis of the presence or absence of these organs. 2. a nematode belonging to the Phasmidia. Cf. *aphasmid.*

Phasmidia (faz-mid′e-ah) a subclass of Nematoda comprising those organisms possessing phasmids. The following superfamilies are of medical or veterinary importance: Rhabditoidea, Strongyloidea, Oxyuroidea, Ascarioidea, Spiruroidea, Filarioidea, and Dracunculoidea.

phatnoma (fat-no′mah), pl. *phatnomas* or *phatno′mata* [Gr. *phatnōma*] a tooth socket.

phatnorrhagia (fat″no-ra′je-ah) hemorrhage from a tooth socket, or dental alveolus.

Ph.B. British Pharmacopoeia.

Ph.D. Doctor of Philosophy.

Phe phenylalanine.

phellandrene (fĕ-lan′drēn) chemical name: 5-isopropyl-2-methyl-1,3-cyclohexadiene. A liquid hydrocarbon, $C_{10}H_{16}$, occurring in fennel oil, elemi oil, the oil of water hemlock, and the Australian eucalyptus.

Phelps' operation (felps) [Abel Mix *Phelps*, surgeon in New York, 1851–1902] see under *operation*.

Phe-Mer-Nite (fe′mer-nīt) trademark for preparations of phenylmercuric nitrate.

Phemerol (fe′mer-ol) trademark for preparations of benzethonium.

phemfilcon A (fem-fil′kon) chemical name: 2-methyl-2-propenoic acid 2-hydroxyethyl ester polymer with 2-ethoxyethyl 2-methyl-2-propenoate; a hydrophilic contact lens material, $(C_6H_{10}O_3)_x(C_8H_{14}O_3)_y$.

phemitone (fem′ĭ-tōn) mephobarbital.

phen- see *pheno-*.

phenacaine hydrochloride (fen′ah-kān) [USP] chemical name: N,N′-bis(4-ethoxphenyl)ethanimidamide monohydrochloride monohydrate. A local anesthetic, $C_{18}H_{22}N_2O_2 \cdot HCl$, occurring as small, white crystals; applied topically to the conjunctiva.

phenacemide (fĕ-nas′ĕ-mīd) [USP] chemical name: N-(aminocarbonyl)-benzeneacetamide. An oral anticonvulsant, $C_9H_{10}N_2O_2$, occurring as a white to almost white, fine crystalline powder; used in the treatment of psychomotor, grand mal, and petit mal epilepsy, and in the management of mixed seizures.

phenacetin (fĕ-nas′ĕ-tin) [USP] chemical name: N-(4-ethoxyphenyl)acetamide. An analgestic and antipyretic, $C_{10}H_{13}NO_2$, occurring as white, glistening crystals or fine, white, crystalline powder; administered orally. Called also *acetophenetidin* and *acetphenetidin*.

phenacetolin (fen″ah-set′o-lin) a red powder, $C_{16}H_{12}O_2$, used as an indicator: it has a pH range of 5 to 6, being yellow at 5 and red at 6.

phenacetylurea (fen″ah-set′ah-mīd) phenacemide.

phenaglycodol (fen″ah-gli′ko-dol) chemical name: 2-(4-chlorophenyl)-3-methyl-2,3-butanediol. A tranquilizer, $C_{11}H_{15}ClO_2$, occurring as a white, crystalline powder; administered orally.

phenakistoscope (fe″nah-kis′to-skōp) [Gr. *phenakistēs* deceiver + *skopein* to examine] a device consisting of a revolving disk with figures near the center that appear to be in motion when viewed through slots at the periphery of the disk by means of a mirror.

phenanthrene (fe-nan′thrēn) a colorless, crystalline hydrocarbon, $(C_6H_4 \cdot CH)_2$.

phenanthrolene (fe-nan′thro-lēn) orthophenanthrolene.

phenate (fe′nāt) phenolate.

phenazocine hydrobromide (fĕ-naz′o-sēn) chemical name: 1,2,3,4,5,6-hexahydro-8-hydroxy-6, 11-dimethyl-3-phenethyl-2,6-methano-3-benzazocine-8-ol hydrobromide. A synthetic narcotic analgesic, $C_{22}H_{27}NO \cdot HBr$, occurring as a white or nearly white, crystalline powder; administered intramuscularly and intravenously.

phenazone (fen′ah-zōn) antipyrine.

phenazopyridine hydrochloride (fen″ah-zo-pēr′ĭ-dēn) [USP] chemical name: 3-(phenylazo)-2,6-pyridinediamine monohydrochloride. A urinary analgesic, $C_{11}H_{11}N_5 \cdot HCl$, occurring as a light or dark red to dark violet, crystalline powder; used orally in cystitis, urethritis, pyelonephritis, and prostatitis. Formerly used as a urinary antiseptic.

phenbutazone sodium glycerate (fen-bu′tah-zōn) chemical name: 4-butyl-3-hydroxy-1,2-diphenyl-3-pyrazolin-5-one sodium salt compound with glycerol (1:1); an anti-inflammatory, $C_{19}H_{19}N_2NaO_2 \cdot C_3H_8O_3$.

phencyclidine hydrochloride (fen-si′klĭ-dēn) chemical name: 1-(1-phenylcyclohexyl)piperidine hydrochloride; a potent analgesic and anesthetic, $C_{17}H_{25}N \cdot HCl$, used in veterinary medicine. Abuse of this drug may lead to serious psychological disturbances. Abbreviated PCP.

phene (fēn) the characters assigned to certain genes or a configuration of genes, which may or may not be expressed in the phenotype.

phenelzine sulfate (fen′el-zēn) [USP] chemical name: (2-phenylethyl)hydrazine sulfate. A monoamine oxidase inhibitor, $C_8H_{12}N_2 \cdot H_2SO_4$, occurring as a white to yellowish white powder; used as an antidepressant, administered orally.

Phenergan (fen′er-gan) trademark for preparations of promethazine hydrochloride.

phenethicillin (fĕ-neth″ĭ-sil′in) chemical name: 3,3-dimethyl-7-oxo-6-[(1-oxo-2-phenoxypropyl)amino]-4-thia-1-azabicyclo[3.2.0]-heptane-2-carboxylic acid. A semisynthetic acid-resistant penicillin, $C_{17}H_{20}N_2O_5S$, which is a methyl analogue of penicillin V. **p. potassium** [USP], the monopotassium salt of phenethicillin, $C_{17}H_{19}KN_2O_5S$, occurring as a white to almost white, fine crystalline powder; used as an antibacterial, especially in certain infections due to susceptible organisms, such streptococcal infections of the upper respiratory tract, pneumococcal infections of the

respiratory tract, staphylococcal infections of skin and soft tissues, and fusospiroketosis. It is administered orally.

phenethylbiguanide (fen-eth″il-bi′gwan-īd) phenformin.

phenetidin (fe-net′ĭ-din) the ethyl ester of para-aminophenol, $NH_2 \cdot C_6H_4 \cdot OC_2H_5$; used in preparing acetophenetidin. It often appears in the urine after the administration of acetophenetidin.

phenetidinuria (fe-net″ĭ-dĭ-nu′re-ah) the presence of phenetidin in the urine.

phenetole (fen′ĕ-tol) ethyl phenyl ether, an oily liquid, $C_6H_5 \cdot O \cdot C_2H_5$.

phenformin hydrochloride (fen-for′min) chemical name: N-(2-phenylethyl)imidodicarbonimidic diamide monohydrochloride; an oral hypoglycemic agent, $C_{10}H_{15}N_5 \cdot HCl$, no longer available in the United States.

phengophobia (fen″go-fo′be-ah) [Gr. *phengos* light + *phobein* to be affrighted by] photophobia.

phenidin (fen′ĭ-din) (*obs.*) phenacetin.

phenin (fe′nin) (*obs.*) phenacetin.

phenindamine tartrate (fĕ-nin′dah-mēn) chemical name: 2,3,4,9-tetrahydro-2-methyl-9-phenyl-1H-indene[2,1-c]pyridine. An antihistaminic, $C_{19}H_{19}N \cdot C_4H_6O_6$, occurring as a creamy white powder; administered orally.

phenindione (fen″in-di′ōn) [USP] chemical name: 2-phenyl-1H-indene-1,3,(2H)-dione. One of the indanedione anticoagulants, $C_{15}H_{10}O_2$, occurring as creamy white to pale yellow crystals or as a crystalline powder and having a rapid onset and short duration of action; administered orally.

pheniramine maleate (fen-ir′ah-mēn) chemical name: N,N-dimethyl-γ-phenyl-2-pyridinepropanamine. An antihistaminic, $C_{16}H_{20}N_2 \cdot C_4H_4O_4$, occurring as a white crystalline powder; administered orally. Called also *prophenpyridamine maleate*.

phenmetrazine hydrochloride (fen-met′rah-zēn) [USP] chemical name: 3-methyl-2-phenyl morpholine hydrochloride. A central nervous system stimulant, $C_{11}H_{15}NO \cdot HCl$, occurring as a white to off-white crystalline powder, used as an anorexic. Abuse of this drug may lead to habituation; see *amphetamine*.

pheno-, phen- [Gr. *phainein* to show] 1. a combining form indicating a showing or displaying. 2. a combining form indicating derived from or related to benzene, or containing phenyl.

phenobarbital (fe″no-bar′bĭ-tal) [USP] chemical name: 5-ethyl-5-phenyl-2,4,6(1H,3H,5H)pyrimidinetrione. A long-acting barbiturate, $C_{12}H_{12}N_2O_3$, occurring as white, glistening, small crystals, or white, crystalline powder; used as a sedative, hypnotic, and anticonvulsant, administered orally. Called also *phenobarbitone* and *phenylethylbarbituric acid*. **p. sodium** [USP], the monosodium salt of phenobarbital, $C_{12}H_{11}N_2NaO_3$, occurring as flaky crystals, or white, crystalline granules, or white powder, having the actions and uses of the base; administered orally, rectally, intravenously, intramuscularly, and subcutaneously.

phenobarbitone (fe″no-bar′bĭ-tōn) phenobarbital.

phenocopy (fe′no-kop″e) [Gr. *phainein* to show + *copy*] 1. an environmentally induced phenotype mimicking one usually produced by a specific genotype. 2. an individual exhibiting such a phenotype. 3. the simulated trait in a phenocopy. Cf. *genocopy*.

phenodeviant (fe″no-de′ve-ant) an individual whose phenotype differs significantly from that of the typical phenotype in the population.

phenogenetics (fe″no-jĕ-net′iks) the science which attempts to explain the chain of causality between genotype and phenotype.

phenol (fe′nol) 1. [USP] an extremely poisonous, colorless to light pink, crystalline compound, $C_6H_5 \cdot OH$, obtained by the distillation of coal tar, and converted, by the addition of 10 per cent water, into a clear liquid with a peculiar odor and a burning taste. Used as an antimicrobial agent. Called also *carbolic acid, hydroxybenzene, oxybenzene, phenic acid, phenylic acid,* and *phenylic alcohol*. See also under *poisoning*. 2. a generic term for any organic compound containing one or more hydroxyl groups attached to an aromatic or carbon ring. **p. liquefac′tum, liquefied p.** [USP], an aqueous solution of phenol containing not less than 89 per cent by weight of phenol; used as a topical antipruritic. Called also *phenylic alcohol*. **p. red,** phenolsulfonphthalein. **p. salicylate,** phenyl salicylate.

phenolase (fe′no-lās) a copper-containing enzyme which catalyzes the oxidation of mono-phenols and dihydroxybenzenes to quinones; it occurs in potatoes and mushrooms.

phenolate (fe′no-lāt) 1. to treat with phenol for purposes of sterilization. 2. a salt formed by union of a base with phenol, in which a monovalent metal, such as sodium or potassium, replaces the hydrogen of the hydroxyl group.

phenolated (fe′no-lāt″ed) charged with phenol.

Phenolax (fe′no-laks) trademark for a preparation of phenolphthalein.

phenolemia (fe″no-le′me-ah) the presence of phenols in the blood.

phenolic (fe-nol′ik) pertaining to or derived from phenol.

phenolization (fe′nol-i-za′shun) treatment by subjection to the action of phenol.

phenologist (fe-nol′o-jist) an expert or specialist in phenology.

phenology (fe-nol′o-je) [Gr. *phainesthai* to appear + *-logy*] a study of the effects of climate upon the life and health of living organisms.

phenolphthalein (fe″nol-thal′e-in) [USP] chemical name: 3,3-bis-(4-hydroxyphenyl)-1(3*H*)-isobenzofuranone. A cathartic, $C_{20}H_{14}O_4$, occurring as a white or faintly white, crystalline powder; administered orally.

phenolsulfonphthalein (fe″nol-sul″fŏn-thal′e-in) [USP] chemical name: 4,4′-(3*H*-2,1-benzoxathiol-3-ylidene)bis(*S, S*-dioxide)phenol. A bright to dark red, crystalline powder, $C_{19}H_{14}O_5S$, administered by intramuscular or intravenous injection as a test of renal function. Called also *phenol red*. Abbreviated PSP.

phenoltetrachlorophthalein (fe″nol-tet″rah-klōr′o-thal′e-in) a coal tar derivative, used intravenously in tests of liver function.

phenoltetraiodophthalein (fe″nol-tet″rah-i″o-do-thal′e-in) phentetiothalein.

phenoluria (fe″nol-u′re-ah) the presence of phenols in the urine.

phenom (fe′nom) in some systems of classification, a group or "cluster" of strains of phenotypically related organisms. Called also *phenon*. See also *numerical taxonomy*, under *taxonomy*.

phenomenology (fe-nom″e-nol′o-je) the study of phenomena; especially that part of a science, as of psychopathology, which treats of the recognition, classification, and description of the phenomena observed in that science.

phenomenon (fĕ-nom′ĕ-non), pl. *phenom′ena* [Gr. *phainomenon* thing seen] any sign or objective symptom; any observable occurrence or fact. **abstinence p.,** withdrawal symptoms; see under *symptom*. **anaphylactoid p.,** pseudoanaphylaxis. **Anderson's p.,** clumps of red blood cells in the stools of amebic dysentery; seen on microscopic examination. **aqueous-influx p.,** entrance into conjunctival or subconjunctival vessels of clear fluid (aqueous humor), deriving from an aqueous vein during compression of its recipient vessel. Formerly called *glass-rod phenomenon*, because of resemblance of the aqueous-filled vessel to a glass rod. Cf. *blood-influx p.* **arm p.,** Pool's p., def. 2. **p. of Arthus,** see *Arthus reaction*, under *reaction*. **Ascher's glass-rod p.,** aqueous-influx p. **Aschner's p.,** slowing of the pulse following pressure on the eyeball; it is indicative of cardiac vagus irritability. See *oculocardiac reflex*, under *reflex*. **Ashman's p.,** aberrant ventricular activation resulting in a short cardiac cycle following a normal or long cycle; it is associated with supraventricular premature beats and with atrial fibrillation. **Aubert's p.,** by an optic illusion, when the head is turned toward one side a vertical line appears to incline toward the other side. **Auer's p.,** inflammation or necrosis in the ear of a rabbit that is rubbed with Merck's xylol shortly after the rabbit receives its second intraperitoneal injection of horse serum—the rabbit having previously been sensitized. **Austin Flint p.,** Flint murmur; see under *murmur*. **autokinetic visible light p.,** the apparent spontaneous movement of a pin-point source of light as seen by certain susceptible persons when they gaze steadily at it in a completely blacked-out room. **Babinski's p.,** dorsiflexion of the large toe and spreading of the other toes instead of plantar flexion of all the toes when the sole is stimulated; it is a sign of damage to the corticospinal tract. **Becker's p.,** increased pulsation of the retinal arteries in Graves' disease. **Bell's p.,** an outward and upward rolling of the eyeball on the attempt to close the eye; it occurs on the affected side in peripheral facial paralysis (Bell's palsy). **Berry-Dedrick p.,** the transformation of fibroma viruses into myxoma viruses. **blanching p.,** Schultz-Charlton reaction. **blood-influx p.,** filling of conjunctival or subconjunctival vessels with blood during compression of the recipient vessel of an aqueous vein. This and the aqueous-influx phenomenon, depending on minute pressure differences between blood and aqueous humor, differ in glaucomatous eyes and those with normal intraocular pressure. **Bordet's p.,** see *serum test*, under *tests*. **Bordet-Gengou p.,** fixation of the complement. **borrowing-lending hemodynamic p.,** the phenomenon of the shifting of blood from one part of the body to another, as from the skin to the internal organs, according to physiologic need; hematometakinesis. **brake p.,** the tendency of a muscle to maintain itself in its normal resting position; called also *Rieger's p.* **break-off p.,** a state of disconnectedness or unreality experienced by high-altitude pilots. Its symptomatic sensations are apparently indescribable in understandable physical terms, but the condition could be the result of a loss of all the physical sense perceptions. **Chase-Sulzberger p.,** Sulzberger-Chase p. **cheek p.,** in meningitis if pressure is exerted on both cheeks just under the zygomas there is reflex upward jerking of both arms with simultaneous bending of both elbows. **Christensen's p.,** when the mandible is protruded, a separation occurs, in the region of the molars, between the surfaces which are in contact in centric occlusion, the degree of separation depending on the downward pitch of the condyle paths. **cogwheel p.,** when a hypertonic muscle is passively stretched it resists, and this resistance sometimes takes the form of an irregular jerkiness; called also *Negro's p.* **Collie p.,** when pure neon is enclosed in a glass tube with a globule of mercury and shaken it glows with a bright,

orange-red color, and when the globule rolls it appears to be followed by a flame. **Cushing's p.,** a rise in systemic blood pressure as a result of an increase in intracranial pressure. **Dale p.,** see under *reaction*. **Danysz's p.,** decrease of the neutralizing influence of an antitoxin when a toxin is added to it in divided portions instead of all at once. **Debre's p.,** absence of measles rash at the site of injection of convalescent measles serum which has not prevented the appearance of the eruption. **Dejerine-Lichtheim p.,** Lichtheim sign. **dental p.,** thermal and tactile sensations in the gums with toothache, produced by repeated faradic stimulation of hyperesthetic lines on the body (Calligaris). **Denys-Leclef p.,** phagocytosis taking place in a test tube on mixing therein leukocytes, bacteria, and immune serum specific for the bacteria. **d'Herelle's p.,** Twort-d'Herelle p. **diaphragm p., diaphragmatic p.,** the movement of the diaphragm as seen through the walls of the body; called also *phrenic phenomenon* and *phrenic wave*. **doll's head p.,** an abnormal extraocular muscle manifestation of many ophthalmologic syndromes and conditions: the eyes depress as the head is bent backward. **Donath p.,** blood from a person with paroxysmal hemoglobinuria if cooled to 5° C. outside the body and then warmed to body temperature undergoes hemolysis. See also *Donath-Landsteiner test*, under *tests*. **Doppler p.,** see under *effect*. **Duckworth's p.,** arrest of breathing before stoppage of the heart's action in certain fatal brain conditions. **Du Noüy p.,** the addition of sodium oleate to blood serum reduces the surface tension of the serum for a short time only. **Erb's p.,** Erb's sign, def. 1. **Erben's p.,** temporary slowness of the pulse on stooping or sitting down; said to characterize certain cases of neurasthenia. **face p., facia′lis p.,** Chvostek's sign. **fall-and-rise p.,** the drop in the number of bacteria that occurs at the beginning of drug treatment and the gradual rise that follows, even while treatment continues. **fern p.,** see *ferning*. **Fick's p.,** a fogging of vision, with the appearance of halos around light, occurring in individuals wearing contact lenses. **finger p.** (in hemiplegia), 1. extension of all the fingers or of the thumb and index finger, on pressure against the pisiform bone; called also *Gordon's sign*. 2. Souques' p. **fixation p.,** fixation of the complement. **flicker p.,** see under *flicker*. **Friedreich's p.,** the tympanic note of skodaic resonance in pleuritis with effusion varies in pitch during inspiration and expiration, being raised on inspiration. **Galassi's pupillary p.,** Westphal-Piltz p. **Gärtner's p.,** the degree of fulness of the veins of the arm as it is raised to varying heights indicates the degree of pressure in the right atrium. **Gengou p.,** fixation of the complement. **Gerhardt's p.,** see under *sign*. **glass-rod p.,** aqueous-influx p. **glass-rod p., negative,** blood-influx p. **Goldblatt p.,** ischemic tubular atrophy, a characteristic of renovascular hypertension. **Grasset's p., Grasset-Gaussel p.,** inability of a patient to raise both legs at the same time, though he can raise either alone; seen in incomplete organic hemiplegia. **Gunn's p.,** see under *syndrome*. **Gunn's pupillary p.,** swinging flashlight sign. **halisteresis p.,** selective withdrawal of bone salt from already calcified tissue. **Hamburger p.,** chloride shift. **Hammerschlag's p.,** abnormal fatigability toward continuous sounds of gradually decreasing intensity. **Hata p.,** increase in severity of an infectious disease when a small dose of a chemotherapeutical remedy is given. **Hecht p.,** Rumpel-Leede p. **Hektoen p.,** when antigens are introduced into the animal body in allergic states, there may exist an increased range of new antibody production which may include production of antibodies concerned in previous infections and immunizations. **d'Herelle's p.,** Twort-d'Herelle p. **Hering's p.,** a faint murmur heard with the stethoscope over the lower end of the sternum for a short time after death. **Hertwig-Magendie p.,** skew deviation. **hip-flexion p.,** in paraplegia, when the patient attempts to rise from a lying position, he flexes the hip of the paralyzed side. **Hochsinger's p.,** pressure on the inner side of the biceps muscle produces closure of the fist in tetany. **Hoffmann's p.,** increased excitability to electrical stimulation in the sensory nerves; the ulnar nerve is usually tested. **Holmes' p., Holmes-Stewart p.,** rebound p. **Houssay p.,** hypoglycemia and marked increase in sensitiveness to insulin produced by hypophysectomy in depancreatized experimental animals. **Huebener-Thomsen-Friedenreich p.,** the *in vivo* or *in vitro* polyagglutinability of red cells by all normal human sera as a result of activation by a bacterial enzyme of a latent "T" receptor common to all erythrocytes. Called also *Thomsen p.* **Hunt's paradoxical p.,** in dystonia musculorum deformans, if the examiner attempts forcible plantar flexion of the foot that is in dorsal spasm there is produced increase of the dorsal spasm, but if the patient is ordered to extend the foot he will perform plantar flexion. **interference p.,** 1. the interference of one drug with the therapeutic activity of another drug; especially a sort of drug-fastness toward full therapeutic doeses of one drug conferred on a parasite by subtherapeutic doses of another drug. 2. the interference with the replication or virulence of a virus by the simultaneous infection with another that may or may not be related; called also *preemptive immunity*. **jaw-winking p.,** Gunn's syndrome. **Kienböck's p.,** paradoxical diaphragm contraction: the hemidiaphragm on one side rises on inspiration and falls on expiration.

Koch's p., if a guinea pig which has been previously infected with tuberculosis organisms is reinjected intracutaneously, the skin over the injected area undergoes necrosis and a superficial ulcer develops. The ulcer heals quickly and infection of regional lymph nodes is retarded. The phenomenon demonstrates development of ability to localize tubercle bacilli. **Koebner's p.,** the appearance of isomorphic lesions at the site of an injury in psoriasis, verruca plana, lichen nitidus, or lichen planus; called also *isomorphic effect.* **Kohnstamm's p.,** after-movement. **Kühne's muscular p.,** Porret's p. **LE p.,** the process by which the LE cell is formed. **Leede-Rumpel p.,** Rumpel-Leede p. **Le Grand-Geblewics p.,** a flickering source of colored light (40–50 per second) when observed indirectly is perceived as a constant white light. **Leichtenstern's p.,** see under *sign.* **Lewis' p.,** hydrophagocytosis. **Liesegang's p.,** the peculiar periodic formation of a precipitate in concentric banded rings, waves, or spirals, when two electrolytes diffuse into and meet in a colloid gel. **Litten's diaphragm p.,** a movable horizontal depression of the lower part of the sides of the thorax, seen in respiration. **Lucio's p.,** a reaction occurring in diffuse lepromatous leprosy, most frequently in Mexico and Central America, marked by the eruption of crops of small red skin lesions with an area of central necrosis; the eschar may be shed, revealing ulceration, with eventual scar formation. **Lust's p.,** abduction with dorsal flexion of the foot on tapping the external popliteal nerve just below the head of the fibula; indicative of spasmophilia. **Marcus Gunn pupillary p.,** swinging flashlight sign. **Meirowsky p.,** darkening of existing melanin, perhaps by oxidation, beginning within seconds and complete within minutes to a few hours after exposure to long-wave ultraviolet radiation. See also *tan* (def. 2). **Metchnikoff's p.,** in Pfeiffer's phenomenon, if the animals are given an intraperitoneal injection of bouillon or other material, twelve hours before the test, lytic phenomena are replaced by phagocytosis. **Mills-Reincke p.,** the mortality from all diseases decreases as a result of water purification. **Moreschi p.,** fixation of the complement. **muscle p.,** the tendency of striated muscle to contract in hard lumps upon tapping. **Narsaroff's p.,** the difference in rectal temperature before and after a cold bath gradually decreases as cold baths are repeated. **Negro's p.,** cogwheel p. **Neisser-Doering p.,** suppression of the normal hemolytic action of human serum due to the presence of some antihemolytic substance; sometimes seen in renal cirrhosis and arteriosclerosis. **Neisser-Wechsberg p.,** complement deviation. **Neufeld's p.,** the dissolution of pneumococci in a solution of bile salts. **Orbeli p.,** when the response of a nerve-muscle preparation is diminishing because of fatigue, stimulation of the sympathetic nerve increases the height of the contractions. **orbicularis p.,** Westphal-Piltz p. **paradoxical diaphragm p.,** one hemidiaphragm moves upward on inspiration and downward on expiration, opposite to the movements on the contralateral side; seen in phrenic nerve paralysis and eventration. **paradoxical p. of dystonia,** Hunt's paradoxical p. **paradoxical pupil p.,** Westphal-Piltz p. **paragglutination p.,** a form of nonspecific agglutination of erythrocytes caused by certain blood sera. It disappears at 37° C. and is often due to bacterial contamination of the serum. **peroneal-nerve p.,** Lust's p. **Pfeiffer's p.,** cholera vibrios, introduced into the peritoneal cavity of a guinea pig that has been immunized against cholera, lose their motility and disintegrate. The disintegration can be followed under the microscope by removing a portion of the peritoneal contents from time to time. The same result is observed if a bacteriolytic serum (against cholera) is introduced along with the bacteria into the peritoneal cavity of a normal guinea pig. **phi p.,** the perception of the sequential flashing of a stationary row of lights as a moving light. **phrenic p.,** diaphragm p. **Piltz-Westphal p.,** Westphal-Piltz p. **Pool's p.,** 1. Schlesinger's sign. 2. contraction of the muscles of the arm following the raising of the arm above the head with the forearm extended, so as to cause stretching of the brachial plexus; seen in postoperative tetany. **Porret's p.,** the passage of a continuous current through a living muscle fiber causes an undulation proceeding from the positive toward the negative pole. **prezone p.,** prozone p. **prozone p.,** see *prozone.* **psi p.** [*psyche*], an experience or effect produced without physical agency or intermediation. **Purkinje's p.,** the phenomenon that fields of equal brightness but different color become unequally bright if the intensity of the illumination is decreased. **Queckenstedt's p.,** see under *sign.* **radial p.,** the involuntary dorsal flexion of the wrist which occurs on palmar flexion of the fingers. **rash-extinction p.,** Schultz-Charlton reaction. **Raynaud's p.,** intermittent bilateral attacks of ischemia of the fingers or toes and sometimes of the ears or nose, marked by severe pallor, and often accompanied by paresthesia and pain; it is brought on characteristically by cold or emotional stimuli and relieved by heat, and is due to an underlying disease or anatomical abnormality. When the condition is idiopathic or primary it is termed *Raynaud's disease.* **rebound p.,** a manifestation of loss of coordination between groups of antagonistic muscles of the extremities in cerebellar dysfunction. It may be demonstrated by having the patient extend both arms horizontally, the examiner then tapping both outstretched arms sharply. The normal arm returns to position

promptly, whereas the affected arm overshoots the original position and may oscillate several times before achieving it. Or, the patient rests his elbow on a table and tries to flex his arm against the resistance of the examiner. When the resistance is suddenly withdrawn, the affected arm rebounds to the patient's chest, whereas the normal arm flexes only slightly, the flexion being arrested by contraction of antagonistic muscles (the triceps). **reclotting p.,** thixotropy. **release p.,** the unhampered activity of a lower center when a higher inhibiting control is removed. **Rieger's p.,** brake p. **Ritter-Rollet p.,** flexion of the foot upon a gentle electric stimulation, and its extension upon energetic stimulation. **Rumpel-Leede p.,** the appearance of minute subcutaneous hemorrhages below the area at which a rubber bandage is applied not too tightly for ten minutes upon the upper arm; characteristic of scarlet fever and hemorrhagic diathesis. **Rust's p.,** in caries or cancer of the upper cervical vertebrae, the patient supports his head with his hands when rising from or assuming a lying position; see also under *syndrome.* **satellite p.,** the more luxuriant development of a colony of microorganisms when in the neighborhood of a foreign colony, as shown by *Hemophilus influenzae* when contaminated by *Staphylococcus pyogenes* var. *aureus.* **Schellong-Strisower p.,** fall of systolic blood pressure on assuming an erect posture from the lying down position. **Schlesinger's p.,** see under *sign.* **Schramm's p.,** visibility with the cystoscope of a whole or part of the posterior urethra; seen in spinal cord disease. **Schüller's p.,** in hemiplegia due to organic lesion, the patient walks sideward more easily to the affected side than to the healthy side. **Schültz-Charlton p.,** see under *reaction.* **second set p.,** the accelerated and intensified rejection by the recipient of a second graft of tissue from the same donor as a consequence of the primary immune response (i.e., antibody production and cell-mediated immunity) induced by the first graft. **Sherrington p.,** the response of the hind limb musculature on stimulation of a motor nerve which has previously been degenerated. **shot-silk p.,** see under *retina.* **Shwartzman p.,** a severe hemorrhagic reaction with necrosis, observed in rabbits which are first injected with 0.25 ml. of typhoid or certain other culture filtrates into the skin of the abdomen and which then twenty-four (eighteen to thirty-two) hours later are injected intravenously with 0.01 ml. of the same filtrate. The site of the later injection turns blue at the center and red at the periphery, the skin is glossy, smooth, and edematous, the blood vessels below the surface are ruptured and the numerous leukocytes are dead. **Simonsen p.,** a type of graft-versus-host (GVH) reaction with an immunological basis. The injection of 10- to 11-day-old chick embryos with adult spleen cells, whole blood, or leukocyte concentrates is almost invariably fatal before hatching. Injections of these cells shortly before or after hatching are likewise fatal for many of the hosts. In all cases the principal symptoms are splenomegaly and a severe hemolytic anemia accompanied by lesions in the liver, bone marrow, and other tissues (Simonsen, 1957). **Sinkler's p.,** in an extremity with spastic paralysis, sharp flexion of the toe may be followed by flexion of the knee and hip. **Soret p.,** see under *effect.* **Souques' p.,** a phenomenon seen in incomplete hemiplegia, consisting of involuntary extension and separation of the fingers when the arm is raised; called also *finger p.* **springlike p.,** André-Thomas sign. **staircase p.,** treppe. **Staub-Traugott p.,** after a glucose load is administered, subsequent loads, given after a short interval, are disposed of at an accelerated rate. **Straus' p.,** see under *reaction.* **Strümpell p.,** dorsiflexion and supination of the foot on flexing the extended leg against resistance offered by the examiner. **Sulzberger-Chase p.,** immunological unresponsiveness to chemical synthesizing agents (haptens) normally capable of inducing delayed-type hypersensitivity; induced by oral administration of the hapten, it results in decreased reactivity to that hapten when it is administered as an antigen, as when conjugated to its protein carrier. **Theobald Smith's p.,** guinea pigs which have been used for standardizing diphtheria antitoxin and have thus been injected with a small dose of blood serum become highly susceptible to the serum and may die very promptly if given a rather large second dose of the same serum a few weeks later. See *anaphylaxis.* **Thomsen p.,** Huebener-Thomsen-Friedenreich p. **toe p.,** Babinski's reflex. **tongue p.,** a slight blow upon the tongue produces a contraction with the appearance of deep depressions; seen in tetany. Called also *Schultze's sign* and *tongue test.* **Trousseau's p.,** spasmodic contractions of muscles provoked by pressure upon the nerves which go to them; seen in tetany. **Twort-d'Herelle p.,** the phenomenon of transmissible bacterial lysis; bacteriophagia. When to a broth culture of typhoid or dysentery bacilli there is added a drop of filtered broth emulsion of the stool from a convalescent typhoid or dysentery patient, complete lysis of the bacterial culture will occur in a few hours. If a drop of this lysed culture is added to another culture of the bacilli, lysis will take place exactly as in the first. A drop of this culture will then dissolve a third culture, and so on through hundreds of transfers. d'Herelle attributes this phenomenon to the action of an ultramicroscopic parasite of bacteria which he named the *bacteriophage.* See *bacterial virus,* under *virus.* **Tyndall p.,** the rendering visible of a transverse beam of light through its being broken up by solid particles suspended in a liquid or gas.

Wedensky's p., on applying a series of rapidly repeated stimuli to a nerve, the muscle contracts quickly in response to the first stimulus and then fails to respond further; but if the stimuli are applied to the nerve at a slower rate, the muscle responds to all of them. **Wenckebach p.,** the generation of impulses by the sinus node of the heart at a constant rate while the P-R interval grows progressively longer during several beats until an atrial complex is not followed by a ventricular complex. **Westphal's p.,** 1. Westphal-Piltz phenomenon. 2. Westphal's sign. **Westphal-Piltz p.,** contraction of the pupil, followed by dilatation, after vigorous closing of the lids; caused by tension of the orbicularis muscle. **Wever-Bray p.,** cochlear microphonics. **Williams' p.,** the tympanic note of skodaic resonance in pleuritis with effusion varies in pitch with the opening and closing of the patient's mouth. **zone p.,** in precipitation reactions, three zones may appear in the supernatant: a zone of antibody excess, in which uncombined antibody is present; a zone of equivalence, in which both antigen and antibody are completely precipitated and no uncombined antigen or antibody is present; and a zone of antigen excess, in which all antibody has combined with antigen and additional uncombined antigen is present (in this zone, precipitation is partly or completely inhibited because, in the presence of excess antigen, soluble antigen-antibody complexes form).

phenon (fe′non) phenom.

phenopropazine (fe″no-pro′pah-zēn) ethopropazine hydrochloride.

phenothiazine (fe″no-thi′ah-zēn) 1. a greenish, tasteless compound, $C_{12}H_9NS$, prepared by fusing diphenylamine with sulfur; used as a veterinary anthelmintic. Called also *dibenzothiazine, thiodiphenylamine.* 2. any of a group of psychotherapeutic agents (e.g., chlorpromazine) resembling phenothiazine in molecular structure, i.e., all sharing a three-ring structure in which two benzene rings are joined by a sulfur and nitrogen atom. They are potent adrenergic blocking agents, their pharmacologic actions including central nervous system depression, prolongation and potentiation of the effects of narcotic and hypnotic drugs, hypotensive activity, and antispasmodic, antihistaminic, and antiemetic activity.

phenotype (fe′no-tīp) [Gr. *phainein* to show + *typos* type] 1. the entire physical, biochemical, and physiological makeup of an individual as determined both genetically and environmentally, as opposed to genotype. Also, any one or any group of such traits. 2. an individual or group of individuals exhibiting a certain phenotype. **Bombay p.,** a rare phenotype produced by the interaction of genes of the ABO blood group and a rare recessive gene at a different locus, resulting in a complete lack of H antigen. Cells of individuals possessing the Bombay phenotype lack A, B, and H antigen, and their serum contains anti-A, anti-B and anti-H antigen.

phenotypic (fe″no-tip′ik) pertaining to or expressive of the phenotype.

Phenoxene (fĕ-nok′sēn) trademark for a preparation of chlorphenoxamine hydrochloride.

phenoxide (fen-ok′sīd) phenolate.

phenoxy- a prefix indicating the presence of the group OC_6H_5, composed of phenyl and an atom of oxygen.

phenoxybenzamine hydrochloride (fĕ-nok″se-ben′zah-mēn) [USP] chemical name: N-(2-chloroethyl)-N-(1-methyl-2-phenoxyethyl)benzenemethanamine hydrochloride. A potent α-adrenergic blocking agent, $C_{18}H_{22}ClNO \cdot HCl$, occurring as a white, crystalline powder; used as an antihypertensive, administered orally.

phenozygous (fe″no-zi′gus) [Gr. *phainein* to show + *zygon* yoke] having the cranium much narrower than the face, so that the zygomatic arches are seen when the skull is viewed from above. Cf. *cryptozygous.*

phenprocoumon (fen-pro′koo-mon) [USP] chemical name: 4-hydroxy-3-(1-phenylpropyl)-2H-1-benzopyran. One of the synthetic coumarin anticoagulants, $C_{13}H_{16}O_3$, occurring as a fine, white, crystalline powder, having a more rapid onset and longer-acting effects than dicumarol and having a marked cumulative effect; administered orally.

phenpromethamine hydrochloride (fen″pro-meth′ah-mēn) phenylpropylmethylamine hydrochloride.

phenpropionate (fen-pro′pe-o-nāt″) USAN contraction for 3-phenylpropionate.

phensuximide (fen-suk′sĭ-mīd) [USP] chemical name: 1-methyl-3-phenyl-2,5-pyrrolidinedione. An anticonvulsant, $C_{11}H_{11}NO_2$, occurring as a white to off-white, crystalline powder; used mainly in the treatment of petit mal epilepsy, administered orally.

phentermine (fen′ter-mēn) chemical name: α,α,-dimethylbenzeneethanamine. An adrenergic isomeric with amphetamine, $C_{10}H_{15}N$, occurring as a colorless, oily liquid; used as an anorexic, administered orally as a complex with an ion-exchange resin to produce a sustained action. **p. hydrochloride,** the water-soluble hydrochloride salt of phentermine, $C_{10}H_{15}N \cdot HCl$, occurring as a white, crystalline powder; used as an anorexic, administered orally.

phentolamine (fen-tol′ah-mēn) chemical name: 3-[[(4,5-dihydro-1H-imidazol-2-yl)methyl](4-methylphenyl)amino]phenol. An antiadrenergic, $C_{17}H_{19}N_3O$, which blocks the hypertensive action of epinephrine and norepinephrine and most smooth muscle responses involving alpha-adrenergic cell receptors. **p. hydrochloride** [USP], the monohydrochloride salt of phentolamine, $C_{17}H_{19}N_3O \cdot HCl$, occurring as a white to off-white, crystalline powder, having the same antiadrenergic actions as the base; used mainly in the treatment of peripheral vascular diseases and to prevent and control hypertension due to pheochromocytoma, administered orally. **p. mesylate** [USP], the methanesulfonate salt of phentolamine, $C_{17}H_{19}N_3O \cdot CH_4O_3S$, occurring as a white, crystalline powder, having the same antiadrenergic actions as the base; used mainly in the diagnosis of pheochromocytoma and in the prevention and treatment of cutaneous necrosis and sloughing when extravasation of norepinephrine occurs after intravenous administration, administered intramuscularly and intravenously.

Phenurone (fen′u-rōn) trademark for a preparation of phenacemide.

phenyl (fen′il, fe′nil) the univalent radical, C_6H_5. Symbol Ph. **p. aminosalicylate,** chemical name: 4-amino-2-hydroxybenzoic acid phenyl ester; a tuberculostatic antibacterial, $C_{13}H_{11}NO_3$. **p. carbinol,** benzyl alcohol. **p. hydrate, p. hydroxide,** phenol. **p. mercury acetate** phenylmercuric acetate. **p. mercury nitrate,** phenylmercuric nitrate. **p. salicylate,** a compound occurring in fine white crystals, or as a white crystalline powder, $C_{13}H_{10}O_3$; formerly used as an analgesic, antipyretic, intestinal antiseptic, enteric coating for tablets, and in preparations used in the prevention of sunburn. In veterinary medicine, it is sometimes used internally as an antipyretic and externally as an antiseptic. Called also *salol.*

phenylalaninase (fen″il-al′ah-nin-ās) phenylalanine hydroxylase.

phenylalanine (fen″il-al′ah-nīn) a naturally occurring amino acid, $C_6H_5 \cdot CH_2CH(NH_2)COOH$, discovered in 1879 by Schulze; essential for optimal growth in infants and for nitrogen equilibrium in human adults.

phenylbutazone (fen″il-bu′tah-zōn) [USP] chemical name: 4-butyl-1,2-diphenyl-3,5-pyrazolidinedione. A congener of aminopyrine and antipyrine, $C_{19}H_{20}N_2O_2$, occurring as a white to off-white, crystalline powder, having analgesic, antipyretic, anti-inflammatory, and mild uricosuric properties; used especially in the treatment of gout, rheumatoid arthritis, ankylosing spondylitis, and other rheumatoid conditions, administered orally. Called also *diphebuzol.*

phenylcarbinol (fen″il-kar′bĭ-nol) benzyl alcohol.

phenyldimethylpyrazolon (fen″il-di-meth″il-pi-ra′zo-lon) antipyrine.

phenylene (fe′nĭ-lēn) a divalent radical, $=C_6H_4$.

phenylephrine hydrochloride (fen″il-ef′rin) [USP] chemical name: (S)-3-hydroxy-α-[(methylamino)methyl]benzenemethanol hydrochloride. An adrenergic with strong alpha-receptor stimulant activity, $C_9H_{13}NO_2 \cdot HCl$, occurring as white or nearly white crystals; used as vasoconstrictor to decongest nasal and laryngeal mucous membranes, to produce mydriasis without cycloplegia, to maintain blood pressure during spinal and inhalation anesthesia, to treat vascular failure in drug-induced shock, shocklike states, and hypotension, to prolong spinal anesthesia, and to treat supraventricular tachycardia. It is applied topically or administered by intramuscular or intravenous injection or infusion.

phenylhydrazine (fen″il-hi′drah-zin) an oily liquid principle, $C_6H_5NH \cdot NH_2$, used as a reagent for sugars, ketones, and aldehydes. Its hydrochloride is also used as a reagent, and has been used as an oral hemolytic in the treatment of polycythemia vera. See also *Kowarsky's test* (def. 1) and *von Jaksch's test* (def. 2), under tests.

phenylic (fe-nil′ik) pertaining to phenyl.

phenylindanedione (fen″il-in-dān′de-ōn) phenindione.

phenylketonuria (fen″il-ke″to-nu′re-ah) an inborn error of metabolism attributable to a deficiency of or a defect in phenylalanine hydroxylase, the enzyme that catalyzes the conversion of phenylalanine to tyrosine. The lack permits the accumulation of phenylalanine and its metabolic products in the body fluids. It results in mental retardation (phenylpyruvic oligophrenia), neurologic manifestations (including hyperkinesia, epilepsy, and microcephaly), light pigmentation, eczema, and a mousy odor, unless treated by administration of a diet low in phenylalanine. The disorder is transmitted as an autosomal recessive trait. Abbreviated PKU. Two variants of classic phenylketonuria have been recognized: a mild variant, in which the patient tolerates higher levels of phenylalanine in the diet, and a transient variant, in which tolerance increases during infancy and early childhood.

phenylmercuric (fen″il-mer-ku′rik) denoting a compound containing the radical $C_6H_5Hg—$, forming various antiseptic, antibacterial, and fungicidal salts. **p. acetate,** chemical name: (aceto-O)phenylmercury. 1. a crystalline salt, $C_8H_8HgO_2$. 2. [NF] a compound with properties similar to those of phenylmercuric nitrate, occurring as a white to creamy white, crystalline powder or as small white prisms or leaflets; used as a bacteriostatic preservative in pharmaceutical preparation, and in solution as a vaginal douche for adjunctive therapy in trichomonal, candidal, bacterial, and mixed infections and nonspecific leukorrhea. It is also widely used as a herbicide, especially for crabgrass. Called also *phenyl mercury acetate*. **p. nitrate,** chemical name: (nitrato-*O*)phenylmercury. 1. the normal salt, $C_6H_5HgNO_3$, which is converted to the basic compound (see def. 2) in aqueous solution or in moist air. 2. [NF] *basic p. nitrate:* an antibacterial and antifungal compound of phenylmercuric nitrate and its hydroxide, containing 87 to 87.9 per cent of $C_6H_5Hg^+$(phenylmercuric ion), and 62.75 to 63.50 per cent Hg (mercury), occurring as a white, crystalline powder; used as a bacteriostatic preservative in pharmaceuticals, and as an antiseptic for various topical uses. Called also *phenyl mercury nitrate*.

phenylmethanol (fen″il-meth′ah-nol) benzyl alcohol.

phenylpropanolamine hydrochloride (fen″il-pro′pah-nol′-ah-mēn hi″dro-klo′rĭd) [USP] chemical name: (±)(*R**,*S**)-α-(1-aminoethyl)benzenemethanol hydrochloride. An adrenergic structurally and pharmacologically related to amphetamine and ephedrine, $C_9H_{13}NO\cdot HCl$, occurring as a white, crystalline powder; used as a vasoconstrictor to decongest mucous membranes, applied topically, and to produce bronchodilation in the symptomatic control of allergic manifestations, administered orally. It has also been used as a central nervous system stimulant and as an anorexic.

phenylpropylmethylamine hydrochloride (fen″il-pro″pil-meth″il-am′ēn) chemical name: *N,β*-dimethylphenethylamine hydrochloride. An adrenergic with chiefly alpha-receptor activity, $C_{10}H_{15}N\cdot HCl$, used mainly as a vasoconstrictor to decongest mucous membranes, applied topically by inhalation. Called also *phenpromethamine hydrochloride*.

phenylpyruvicaciduria (fen″il-pi-ru″vik-as″ĭ-du′re-ah) phenylketonuria.

phenylthiocarbamide (fen″il-thi″o-kar-bam′id) phenylthiourea.

phenylthiourea (fen″il-thi″o-u-re′ah) a compound, C_6H_5-$NHCSNH_2$, used in genetic research in dry crystal form or in 5 per cent solution. The ability to taste it is inherited as a dominant trait, the compound being intensely bitter to approximately 70 per cent of the population, and nearly tasteless to the rest. Called also *phenylthiocarbamide* or *PTC*.

phenyltoloxamine citrate (fen″il-tol-ok′sah-mēn) chemical name: *N,N*-dimethyl-2-[2-(phenylmethyl)phenoxy]ethanamine citrate. An isomer of diphenhydramine, $C_{17}H_{21}NO$, used as an antihistaminic, mainly to decongest the nasal mucosa, administered orally.

phenyramidol hydrochloride (fen″ĭ-ram′ĭ-dol) chemical name: α-[(2-pyridylamino)methyl]benzyl alcohol hydrochloride. A compound, $C_{13}H_{14}N_2O\cdot HCl$, used as an analgesic and skeletal muscle relaxant.

phenytoin (fen′ĭ-to-in) [USP] chemical name: 5,5-diphenyl-2,4-imidazolidinedione. An anticonvulsant and cardiac depressant, $C_{15}H_{12}N_2O_2$, occurring as a white powder; used in the treatment of all forms of epilepsy except petit mal and as an antiarrhythmic, administered orally. Called also *diphenylhydantoin*. **p. sodium** [USP], the monosodium salt of phenytoin, $C_{15}H_{22}N_2NaO_2$, having the same appearance, actions, and uses as the base; administered orally and intravenously.

pheo- [Gr. *phaios* dun, dusky] a combining form denoting relationship to brown, dun, or dusky.

pheochrome (fe′o-krōm) [Gr. *phaios* dusky + *chrōma* color] staining dark with chromium salts; said of certain embryonic cells; chromaffin.

pheochromoblast (fe″o-kro′mo-blast) any of the embryonic structures which develop into pheochrome (chromaffin) cells.

pheochromoblastoma (fe″o-kro″mo-blas-to′mah) pheochromocytoma.

pheochromocyte (fe″o-kro′mo-sīt) [*pheochrome* + Gr. *kytos* hollow vessel] a chromaffin cell.

pheochromocytoma (fe-o-kro″mo-si-to′mah) [*pheochromocyte* + *-oma*] a well encapsulated, lobular, vascular tumor of chromaffin tissue of the adrenal medulla or sympathetic paraganglia. The cardinal symptom, reflecting the increased secretion of epinephrine and norepinephrine, is hypertension, which may be persistent or intermittent. During severe attacks, there may be headache, palpitation, apprehension, tremor, pallor or flushing of the face, nausea and vomiting, pain in the chest and abdomen, and paresthesias of the extremities.

pheophytin (fe″o-fi′tin) [Gr. *phaios* dusky + *phyton* plant] a brown pigment derived from chlorophyll by removal of magnesium.

pheresis (fĕ-re′sis) [Gr. *aphairesis* removal] any procedure in which blood is withdrawn from a donor, a portion (plasma, leukocytes, etc.) is separated and retained, and the remainder is retransfused into the donor. It includes plasmapheresis, leukapheresis, etc. More properly called *apheresis*.

pheromone (fer′o-mōn) a substance secreted to the outside of the body by an individual and perceived (as by smell) by a second individual of the same species, releasing a specific reaction of behavior in the percipient. **alarm p.,** a mucus secreted by the earthworm on noxious stimulation, which is aversive to other members of the species.

phetharbital (feth-ar′bĭ-tal) chemical name: 5,5-diethyl-1-phenylbarbituric acid. A nonhypnotic barbiturate, $C_{14}H_{16}N_2O_3$, which has been used as an anticonvulsant and in the treatment of unconjugated hyperbilirubinemia.

Ph.G. Graduate in Pharmacy; Pharmacopoeia germanica (German pharmacopeia).

phial (fi′al) a vial or small bottle.

phialide (fi′ah-līd) [Gr. *phialis*, dim. of *phialē* a broad flat vessel] 1. a flask-shaped projection from the mycelium of certain fungi that gives rise to endogenous basipetally produced spores. 2. the end cell of a phialophore.

Phialophora (fi″ah-lof′o-rah) a genus of imperfect fungi of the family Dematiaceae, order Moniliales. *P. verrucosa* is a cause of chromomycosis, a chronic subcutaneous fungous infection, and *P. jeanselmi* is an etiologic agent of maduromycosis.

phialophore (fi′ah-lo-fōr) the branch of the mycelium which bears at its tip the phialospores of certain fungi.

phialospore (fi′ah-lo-spōr) a spore which is borne at the end of a phialide or a phialophore.

philagrypnia (fi″lah-grip′ne-ah) [Gr. *philein* to love + *agrypnia* sleeplessness] the ability to live with far less than the amount of sleep normally required by most people.

-philia (fil′e-ah) [Gr. *philein* to regard with affection, to love] a word termination designating notable or abnormal fondness or attraction for the subject indicated by the stem to which it is affixed.

philiater (fĭ-li′ah-ter) [Gr. *philos* fond + *iatreia* healing] a person interested in medical science, particularly a medical student.

Philinos (fĭ-li′nos) **of Cos** (c. 250 B.C.) a Greek physician who was a pupil of Herophilus, and is believed to have been one of the founders of the Empiric school of medicine.

Philip's glands (fil′ips) [Sir Robert William *Philip*, Scottish physician, 1857–1939] see under *gland*.

Philippe-Gombault tract (fe-lēp′-gom-bo′) [Claudius *Philippe*, French pathologist, 1866–1903; François Alexis Albert *Gombault*, French neurologist, 1844– 1904] Gombault-Philippe triangle.

phillyrin (fil′ĭ-rin) a crystalline substance, $C_{27}H_{34}O_{11}$, from the leaves and bark of various species of *Phillyrea*, a genus of evergreen shrubs, e.g., *P. latifolia* L. (Oleaceae), which has antimalarial properties.

philothion (fi″lo-thi′on) [Gr. *philein* to love + *theion* sulfur] glutathione.

philter (fil′ter) a substance or object alleged to provoke love or carnal appetite.

philtrum (fil′trum) [Gr. *philtron* love potion] 1. [NA] the vertical groove in the median portion of the upper lip, a part of the prolabium. 2. a philter.

Philumenus (fil″u-me′nus) [2nd century A.D.] a Greek physician of the Eclectic school whose works are quoted by Oribasius and Aëtius.

phimosiectomy (fi-mo″se-ek′to-me) [*phimosis* + Gr. *ektomē* excision] circumcision for phimosis.

phimosis (fi-mo′sis) [Gr. *phimōsis* a muzzling or closure] constriction of the preputial orifice so that the prepuce cannot be retracted back over the glans. **labial p., oral p.,** atresia of the mouth. **p. vagina′lis,** atresia of the vagina.

phimotic (fi-mot′ik) pertaining to phimosis.

pHisoHex (fi′so-heks) trademark for an emulsion containing hexachlorophene.

phleb- see *phlebo-*.

phlebalgia (flĕ-bal′je-ah) [*phleb-* + *-algia*] pain due to varices within or on the surface of a nerve.

phlebanesthesia (fleb″an-es-the′ze-ah) phlebonarcosis.

phlebangioma (fleb″an-je-o′mah) [*phleb-* + *angioma*] a venous aneurysm.

phlebarteriectasia (fleb″ar-te″re-ek-ta′ze-ah) [*phleb-* + Gr. *artēria* artery + *ektasis* extension] general dilatation of veins and arteries.

phlebasthenia (fleb″as-the′ne-ah) [*phleb-* + *a* neg. + Gr. *sthenos* strength + *-ia*] impairment of the vitality of the walls of blood vessels.

phlebectasia (fleb″ek-ta′ze-ah) [*phleb-* + Gr. *ektasis* dilatation + *-ia*] a varicosity; a dilatation of a vein. **p. laryn′gis,** permanent dilatation of the veins of the larynx, especially those of the vocal cords.

phlebectasis (fle-bek′tah-sis) phlebectasia.

phlebectomy (fle-bek′to-me) [*phleb-* + Gr. *ektomē* excision] excision of a vein, or of a part of a vein.

phlebectopia (fleb″ek-to′pe-ah) [*phleb-* + Gr. *ektopos* out of place + *-ia*] displacement of a vein.

phlebectopy (fle-bek′to-pe) phlebectopia.

phlebemphraxis (fleb″em-frak′sis) [*phleb-* + Gr. *emphraxis* stoppage] the stoppage of a vein by a plug or clot.

phlebexairesis (fleb″ek-si′rĕ-sis) [*phleb-* + Gr. *exairesis* a taking out] surgical removal of a vein.

phlebismus (fle-biz′mus) obstruction and consequent turgescence of veins.

phlebitic (flĕ-bit′ik) pertaining to phlebitis.

phlebitis (flĕ-bi′tis) [*phleb-* + *-itis*] inflammation of a vein. The condition is marked by infiltration of the coats of the vein and the formation of a thrombus. The disease is attended by edema, stiffness, and pain in the affected part, and in the septic variety by pyemic symptoms. **adhesive p.,** phlebitis which tends to the obliteration of the vein; called also *plastic p.* and *proliferative p.* **anemic p.,** a form associated with anemia or chlorosis. **blue p.,** phlegmasia cerulea dolens. **chlorotic p.,** anemic p. **gouty p.,** a variety associated with the gouty diathesis, often recurrent, and sometimes occlusive; a causal relation to gout is in question. **p. mi′grans, migrating p.,** recurrent phlebitis in peripheral veins. **obliterating p., obstructive p.,** phlebitis that permanently closes the lumen of a vein. **plastic p.,** adhesive p. **productive p.,** phlebosclerosis. **proliferative p.,** adhesive p. **puerperal p.,** septic inflammation of uterine or other veins following childbirth. **septic p.,** that which is related to a septic process, as in erysipelas, peritonitis, or endometritis. In it the thrombus breaks down and septic emboli are carried to distant parts of the body. Called also *suppurative p.* **sinus p.,** inflammation of a cerebral sinus. **suppurative p.,** septic p.

phlebo-, phleb- [Gr. *phleps, phlebos* vein] a combining form denoting relationship to a vein or veins. See also words beginning *veno-.*

phleboclysis (flĕ-bok′lĭ-sis) [*phlebo-* + Gr. *klysis* injection] injection of fluid into a vein. **drip p., slow p.,** phleboclysis in which the solution is instilled slowly, drop by drop.

phlebofibrosis (fleb″o-fi-bro′sis) fibrosis of the veins, as in phlebosclerosis.

phlebogenous (flĕ-boj′ĕ-nus) originating in a vein.

phlebogram (fleb′o-gram) [*phlebo-* + Gr. *gramma* a writing] 1. roentgenogram of a vein filled with contrast medium. 2. a tracing of the venous pulse made with a phlebograph or sphygmograph.

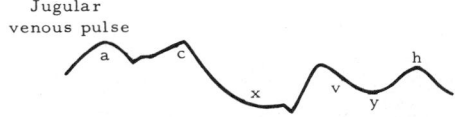

Jugular venous pulse

Phlebogram: *a,* a positive wave due to contraction of the right atrium; *c,* a venous wave due to contraction of the right ventricle, with downward movement of the tricuspid valve; *x,* a small negative wave due to atrial relaxation; *v,* the early diastolic wave, a positive wave occurring during ventricular contraction and reflecting the filling of the right atrium (also [not shown] the exaggerated positive wave related to reflux of blood through an incompetent atrioventricular valve); *y,* a negative wave due to emptying of the right atrium; *h,* an occasional, late filling wave.

phlebograph (fleb′o-graf) [*phlebo-* + Gr. *graphein* to write] an instrument for recording the venous pulse.

phlebography (flĕ-bog′rah-fe) [*phlebo-* + Gr. *graphein* to write] 1. roentgenography of a vein or veins by use of contrast medium. 2. the graphic recording of the venous pulse. 3. a description of the veins.

phleboid (fleb′oid) [*phlebo-* + Gr. *eidos* form] resembling a vein, or composed of veins.

phlebolith (fleb′o-lith) [*phlebo-* + Gr. *lithos* stone] a calculus or concretion in a vein; a vein stone.

phlebolithiasis (fleb″o-lĭ-thi′ah-sis) [*phlebo-* + *lithiasis*] a condition characterized by the development of vein stones.

phlebology (flĕ-bol′o-je) [*phlebo-* + *-logy*] the study of the veins and their diseases.

phlebomanometer (fleb″o-mah-nom′ĕ-ter) [*phlebo-* + *manometer*] an instrument for the direct measurement of venous blood pressure (Burch and Winsor).

phlebometritis (fleb″o-mĕ-tri′tis) [*phlebo-* + Gr. *metra* uterus + *-itis*] inflammation of the veins of the uterus.

phlebonarcosis (fleb″o-nar-ko′sis) narcosis produced by intravenous injections.

phlebopexy (fleb′o-pek″se) [*phlebo-* + Gr. *pēxis* fixation] extraserous transplantation of the testicle, with preservation of the reticulum of veins; done for varicocele.

phlebophlebostomy (fleb″o-fle-bos′to-me) [*phlebo-* + Gr. *phleps* vein + *stomoun* to provide with an opening, or mouth] operative anastomosis of vein to vein.

phlebophthalmotomy (fleb″of-thal-mot′o-me) [*phlebo-* + Gr. *ophthalmos* eye + *tomē* a cutting] ophthalmophlebotomy.

phlebopiezometry (fleb″o-pi″ĕ-zom′ĕ-tre) [*phlebo-* + Gr. *piesis*

pressure + *metron* measure] measurement of the venous pressure.

phleboplasty (fleb′o-plas″te) [*phlebo-* + Gr. *plassein* to form] plastic operation for the repair of a vein.

phleborrhagia (fleb″o-ra′je-ah) [*phlebo-* + Gr. *rhēgnynai* to burst forth] copious hemorrhage from a vein; venous hemorrhage.

phleborrhaphy (flĕ-bor′ah-fe) [*phlebo-* + Gr. *rhaphē* suture] the suturing of a vein.

phleborrhexis (fleb″o-rek′sis) [*phlebo-* + Gr. *rhēxis* rupture] rupture of a vein.

phlebosclerosis (fleb″o-skle-ro′sis) [*phlebo-* + Gr. *sklērōsis* hardening] fibrous thickening of the wall of the veins.

phlebosis (flĕ-bo′sis) abnormal noninflammatory changes in the veins.

phlebostasia (fleb″os-ta′ze-ah) phlebostasis.

phlebostasis (flĕ-bos′tah-sis) [*phlebo-* + Gr. *stasis* stoppage] 1. retardation of the flow of blood in the veins. 2. temporary sequestration of a portion of the blood from the general circulation by application of tourniquets on an extremity.

phlebostenosis (fleb″o-stĕ-no′sis) [*phlebo-* + Gr. *stenōsis* narrowing] stenosis or constriction of a vein.

phlebothrombosis (fleb″o-throm-bo′sis) [*phlebo-* + *thrombosis*] presence of a clot in a vein, unassociated with inflammation of the wall of the vein. Cf. *thrombophlebitis.*

phlebotome (fleb′o-tōm) a knife or lancet for use in phlebotomy.

phlebotomist (fle-bot′o-mist) one who practices phlebotomy.

phlebotomize (fle-bot′o-mīz) to bleed; to take blood from by phlebotomy.

Phlebotomus (flĕ-bot′o-mus) [*phlebo-* + Gr. *tomos* a cutting] a genus of biting flies of the family Psychodidae, containing some 60 species, the females of which suck blood. **P. argen′tipes,** the species which transmits kala-azar in India. **P. chinen′sis,** the species which transmits kala-azar in China. **P. interme′dius,** a species suspected of being a transmitter of leishmaniasis in South America. **P. macedon′icum,** a species found in Italy. **P. marti′ni,** the principal vector of kala-azar in East Africa. **P. nogu′chi,** a species found in Peru which may transmit *Bartonella bacilliformis,* the etiologic agent of *Carrión's disease;* called also *Lutzomyia noguchii.* **P. orienta′lis,** the vector of kala-azar in the Sudan. **P. papatas′ii,** the sandfly, a dipterous insect of India and the Mediterranean countries, which conveys by its bite an infection known as *phlebotomus fever.* **P. pernicio′sus,** the principal vector of kala-azar in the Medi-

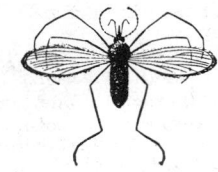

Phlebotomus papatasii.

terranean. **P. sergen′ti,** a vector of *Leishmania tropica,* the etiologic agent of cutaneous leishmaniasis. **P. verruca′rum,** a fly abounding in Peru; it is a vector of *Bartonella bacilliformis,* the etiologic agent of Carrión's disease (bartonellosis). **P. vexa′tor,** a species found in the United States which is not a disease vector.

phlebotomy (flĕ-bot′o-me) [*phlebo-* + Gr. *tomē* a cutting] incision of a vein, as for the letting of blood; venesection. **bloodless p.,** phlebostasis, def. 2.

phlegm (flem) [Gr. *phlegma*] 1. one of the four humors of the body, according to the obsolete humoral pathology. 2. morbid or viscid mucus secreted in abnormally large amount; applied especially to such mucus discharged through the mouth.

phlegmasia (fleg-ma′ze-ah) [Gr. "heat, inflammation"] inflammation or fever. **p. al′ba do′lens,** phlebitis of the femoral vein, occasionally following parturition or an acute febrile illness; it is characterized by swelling of the leg, usually without redness. Called also *leukophlegmasia* and *white leg.* **p. al′ba do′lens puerpera′rum,** postpartum iliofemoral thrombophlebitis. **cellulitic p.,** swelling and inflammation of the leg after childbirth from infection of the connective tissue. **p. ceru′lea do′lens,** an acute fulminating form of deep venous thrombosis, with reactive arterial spasm and pronounced edema of the extremity and severe cyanosis, purpuric areas, and petechiae; called also *blue phlebitis.* **p. malabar′ica,** elephantiasis. **thrombotic p.,** phlegmasia alba dolens.

phlegmatic (fleg-mat′ik) [Gr. *phlegmatikos*] characterized by an excess of the supposed humor called phlegm; hence, heavy, dull, and apathetic.

phlegmon (fleg′mon) [Gr. *phlegmonē*] diffuse inflammation of the soft or connective tissue due to infection; see *cellulitis.* **Holz p.,** a chronic cellulitis of the floor of the mouth and neck. **periurethral p.,** an extensive fulminating phlegmon originating in and about the urethra and usually accompanied by massive gangrene of the genital and perigenital tissues; called also *periurethral cellulitis.*

phlegmona (fleg'mo-nah) phlegmon. **p. diffu'sa,** phlegmonous cellulitis.

phlegmonosis (fleg"mo-no'sis) phelgmasia.

phlegmonous (fleg'mon-us) pertaining to or attended by phlegmon; see under *cellulitis.*

phlobaphene (flo'bah-fēn) [Gr. *phloios* bark + *baphē* dye] one of a series of compounds resembling resins and differing from the latter only in that they dissolve in dilute ammonia water. They are derived from tannin by boiling with acids and are characterized by their brown color.

phloem (flo'em) [Gr. *phloios* bark] a form of vascular tissue in plants which conducts synthesized nutrients, such as glucose, both up and down the stem or root, characterized by the presence of sieve tubes. Cf. *xylem.*

phlogistic (flo-jis'tik) [Gr. *phlogistos*] inflammatory.

phlogisticozymoid (flo-jis"tĭ-ko-zi'moid) a hypothetical substance supposed to supply the necessary feeding ground for inflammatory processes.

phlogiston (flo-jis'ton) [Gr. *phlogistos* burnt] the supposed principle of fire and combustion; a term proposed in 1697 by Stahl, who supposed that combustible substances were compounds of phlogiston and that combustion is due to the removal or liberation of phlogiston leaving the other structures of the substance behind.

phlogo- [Gr. *phlox, phlogos* flame] a combining form denoting relation to inflammation.

phlogocyte (flo'go-sīt) [*phlogo-* + *-cyte*] a cell characteristic of tissue in an inflamed state; a plasma cell.

phlogocytosis (flo"go-si-to'sis) presence of phlogocytes (plasma cells) in the blood.

phlogogen (flo'go-jen) a body that has the power of causing inflammation.

phlogogenic (flo"go-jen'ik) [*phlogo-* + Gr. *gennan* to produce] causing inflammation.

phlogogenous (flo-goj'ĕ-nus) phlogogenic.

phlogotherapy (flog"o-ther'ah-pe) [*phlogo-* + Gr. *therapeia* treatment] nonspecific therapy; see under *therapy.*

phlogotic (flo-got'ik) inflammatory.

phlorhizin (flo-ri'zin) [Gr. *phloios* bark + *rhiza* root] a bitter glycoside, $C_{21}H_{24}O_{10} + 2H_2O$, from the root bark of apple, cherry, plum, and pear trees; it causes glycosuria by blocking the tubular reabsorption of glucose.

phlorhizinize (flo-ri'zi-nīz) to bring under the influence of phlorhizin.

phloridzin (flo-rid'zin) phlorhizin.

phloridzinize (flo-rid'zi-nīz) phlorhizinize.

phlorizin (flo-ri'zin) phlorhizin.

phloroglucin (flo"ro-gloo'sin) [*phlorhizin* + Gr. *glykys* sweet] chemical name: 1,3,5-trihydroxybenzene. The aglycone of many glycosides, $C_6H_6O_3$, obtained from the bark of apple and other trees, and used as a reagent for pentoses, pentosans, glycuronates, hydrochloric acid in gastric juice, etc. It is an excellent decalcifier of bone specimens. See under *tests,* and see *Günzburg's test,* under *tests.*

phloroglucinol (flo"ro-gloo'sĭ-nol) phloroglucin.

phlorol (flo'rol) an oily liquid, $C_6H_5(OC_2H_5)$, derived from creosote; see *phenetole.*

phlorose (flor'ōs) a sugar formed when phlorhizin is boiled with dilute acids; glucose.

phlorrhizin (flo-ri'zin) phlorhizin.

phloryl (flo'ril) a principle obtainable from creosote.

phloxine (flok'sin) a brick-red acid dye said to have a destructive action on cancer cells.

P.H.L.S. Public Health Laboratory Service (British).

phlycten (flik'ten) phlyctena.

phlyctena (flik-te'nah), pl. *phlycte'nae* [Gr. *phlyktaina*] 1. a blister made by a burn. 2. a small vesicle containing lymph seen on the conjunctiva in certain conditions.

phlyctenar (flik'tĕ-nar) pertaining to or marked by phlyctenae.

phlyctenoid (flik'tĕ-noid) [*phlyctena* + Gr. *eidos* form] resembling a phlyctena.

phlyctenosis (flik"tĕ-no'sis) [Gr. *phlyktainōsis*] (*obs.*) any phlyctenular disease or lesion.

phlyctenotherapy (flik"tĕ-no-ther'ah-pe) [*phlyctenule* + Gr. *therapeia* treatment] treatment by the subcutaneous injection of the serum from blisters raised on the patient's own body by applying cantharides.

phlyctenula (flik-ten'u-lah), pl. *phlycten'ulae* [L.] phlyctenule.

phlyctenular (flik-ten'u-lar) associated with the formation of phlyctenules or vesicles, or of prominences that look like vesicles.

phlyctenule (flik'ten-ūl) [L. *phlyctaenulaly;* Gr. *phlyktaina* blis-

---

ter] a small vesicle, or an ulcerated nodule of the cornea or of the conjunctiva.

phlyctenulosis (flik"ten-u-lo'sis) the condition marked by the formation of phlyctenules, as phlyctenular keratoconjunctivitis, conjunctivitis, or ophthalmia. **allergic p.,** phlyctenulosis due to allergy. **tuberculous p.,** phlyctenulosis due to tuberculous allergy.

phobia (fo'be-ah) [Gr. *phobos* fear (*phobein* to be affrighted by) + *-ia*] any persistent abnormal dread or fear. Used as a word termination designating abnormal or morbid fear of or aversion to the subject indicated by the stem to which it is affixed.

phobic (fo'bik) of the nature of or pertaining to phobia or morbid fear.

phobophobia (fo-bo-fo'be-ah) [Gr. *phobos* fear + *phobein* to be affrighted by] a condition in psychasthenia marked by fear of one's own fears.

Phocas' disease (fo-kahz') [B. G. Phocas, French physician] see under *disease.*

phocomelia (fo"ko-me'le-ah) [Gr. *phōkē* seal + *melos* limb + *-ia*] a developmental anomaly characterized by absence of the proximal portion of a limb or limbs, the hands or feet being attached to the trunk of the body by a single small, irregularly shaped bone. Cf. *amelia.*

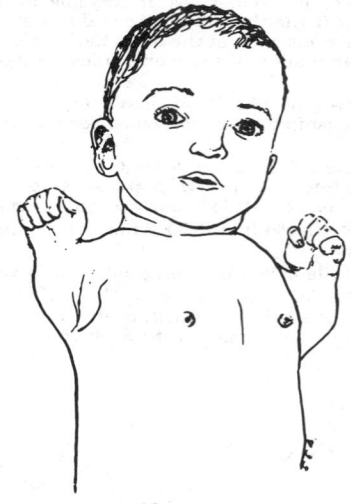

Phocomelia of arms.

phocomelus (fo-kom'ĕ-lus) [Gr. *phōkē* seal + *melos* limb] an individual exhibiting phocomelia.

phon (fōn) [Gr. *phōnē* voice] a unit of the subjective loudness of a sound.

phon- see *phono-.*

phonacoscope (fo-nak'o-skōp) the apparatus used in phonacoscopy.

phonacoscopy (fo"nah-kos'ko-pe) [*phon-* + Gr. *skopein* to examine] combined auscultation and percussion by means of a bell-shaped resonating chamber containing a percussion hammer, which is held on the anterior thoracic wall while the examiner listens at the back of the thorax.

phonal (fo'nal) pertaining to the voice.

phonarteriogram (fōn"ar-te'/re-o-gram") a tracing or graphic record of arterial sounds obtained in phonarteriography.

phonarteriographic (fōn"ar-te"re-o-graf'ik) pertaining to phonarteriography or to a phonarteriogram.

phonarteriography (fōn"ar-te"re-og'rah-fe) the recording of arterial sounds by means of a phonocardiograph.

phonasthenia (fo"nas-the'ne-ah) [*phon-* + *asthenia*] weakness of the voice; difficult phonation from fatigue.

phonation (fo-na'shun) the utterance of vocal sounds. **subenergetic p.,** hypophonia. **superenergetic p.,** hyperphonia.

phonatory (fo'nah-to"re) subserving or pertaining to phonation.

phonautograph (fōn-aw'to-graf) [*phon-* + Gr. *autos* self + *graphein* to write] an apparatus which registers the vibrations of the air caused by the voice.

phoneme (fo'nēm) [Gr. *phōnēma* a sound made, a thing spoken] 1. a speech sound that is the basic unit of spoken language. 2. (*obs.*) a hallucination of hearing voices.

phonendoscope (fōn-en'do-skōp) [*phon-* + Gr. *endon* within + *skopein* to examine] a stethoscopic device that intensifies auscultatory sounds.

phonendoskiascope (fōn-en″do-ski′ah-skōp) a phonendoscope combined with a fluorescent screen for observing the heart movements at the same time as the heart sounds are heard.

phonetic (fo-net′ik) [Gr. *phonētikos*] pertaining to the voice or to articulate sounds.

phonetics (fo-net′iks) the science of vocal sounds; phonology.

phoniatrician (fo″ne-ah-trish′an) a person who specializes in treating voice and speech defects.

phoniatrics (fo″ne-at′riks) [phon- + Gr. *iatrikē* surgery, medicine] the treatment of voice and speech defects.

phonic (fon′ik, fo′nik) pertaining to the voice.

phonism (fo′nizm) a form of synesthesia in which a sensation of hearing is produced by the effect of something seen, felt, tasted, smelled, or thought of.

phono-, phon- [Gr. *phōnē* voice] a combining form denoting relationship to sound, often specifically to the sound of the voice.

phonoangiography (fo″no-an″je-og′rah-fe) the recording and analysis of arterial bruits to estimate the extent of arterial stenosis.

phonoauscultation (fo″no-aws″kul-ta′shun) auscultation in which a tuning-fork is placed over the organ to be examined and its vibrations are listened to through a stethoscope placed over the same organ.

phonocardiogram (fo″no-kar′de-o-gram) [phono- + Gr. *kardia* heart + *gramma* a writing] the graphic record produced by phonocardiography.

phonocardiograph (fo″no-kar′de-o-graf) the instrument used in phonocardiography. **fetal p.,** an instrument which provides continuous, instantaneous recording of beat-to-beat changes in fetal heart rate.

phonocardiographic (fo″no-kar″de-o-graf′ik) pertaining to phonocardiography or to a phonocardiogram.

phonocardiography (fo″no-kar″de-og′rah-fe) the graphic representation of heart sounds and murmurs; by extension, the term also includes pulse tracings (carotid, apex, and jugular pulse). **intracardiac p.,** the graphic registration of sounds produced by action of the heart by means of a phonocatheter passed into one of the heart chambers.

phonocatheter (fo″no-kath′ĕ-ter) a device similar in appearance to a conventional catheter, with a microphone at the tip.

phonocatheterization (fo″no-kath″ĕ-ter-i-za′shun) the use of a phonocatheter for the detection of sounds produced by the circulatory system. **intracardiac p.,** the passage of a phonocatheter into a chamber of the heart, for the detection of sounds as an aid in diagnosis of cardiac defects.

phonoelectrocardioscope (fo″no-e-lek″tro-kar″de-o-skōp) an instrument incorporating a double beam cathode ray oscilloscope with a fluorescent screen of long afterglow, which permits the simultaneous direct visual recording of two phenomena such as the phonocardiogram and the electrocardiogram, the phonocardiogram and the sphygmogram, or the electrocardiogram and the sphygmogram.

phonogram (fo′no-gram) [phono- + Gr. *gramma* mark] a graphic record of a sound, as of a heart sound.

phonology (fo-nol′o-je) [phono- + -logy] the science which treats of vocal sounds; phonetics.

phonomania (fon″o-ma′ne-ah) [Gr. *phonē* murder + *mania* madness] psychosis marked by a tendency to commit murder.

phonomyoclonus (fo″no-mi-ok′lo-nus) myoclonus in which a sound is heard on auscultation of an affected muscle, indicating fibrillar contractions.

phonomyogram (fo″no-mi′o-gram) [phono- + Gr. *mys* muscle + *gramma* mark] a tracing of the sound produced by muscle action.

phonomyography (fo″no-mi-og′rah-fe) the recording of muscle sounds by an oscillograph to which the sounds are transmitted by a microphone placed over the muscle.

phonophobia (fo″no-fo′be-ah) [phono- + Gr. *phobein* to be affrighted by] morbid dread of sounds or of speaking aloud.

phonopsia (fo-nop′se-ah) [phono- + Gr. *opsis* vision + -ia] a subjective sensation of seeing colors, caused by the hearing of sounds.

phonorenogram (fo″no-re′no-gram) a graphic representation by means of a paper recording of pulsations of the renal artery obtained by use of a phonocatheter passed through a ureter into the pelvis of the kidney.

phonoscope (fo′no-skōp) [phono- + Gr. *skopein* to examine] 1. an apparatus for recording photographically the movements of a diaphragm set up by the sounds of the heart. 2. an instrument for auscultatory percussion.

phonoscopy (fo-nos′ko-pe) 1. the delimiting of solid and hollow organs (liver, heart, lungs, etc.) by listening with a stethoscope while percussion is made in the vicinity. 2. the use of the phonoscope.

phonoselectoscope (fo″no-se-lek′to-skōp) [phono- + *select* + Gr. *skopein* to examine] an instrument for auscultation by means of which the lower (normal) range of the pulmonary sounds are eliminated, thus emphasizing the higher-pitched pathologic elements.

phonostethograph (fo″no-steth′o-graf) an instrument by which the chest sounds are amplified, filtered, and recorded.

Phorandendron flavescens (for″ah-den′dron fla-ves′enz) American mistletoe; see *mistletoe*.

-phore (fōr) [Gr. *phoros* bearing] a word termination signifying a carrier of the element designated by the stem to which it is affixed, as a melanophore.

-phoresis (fo-re′sis) [Gr. *phorēsis* a being borne] a word termination indicating transmission, as electrophoresis, immunophoresis, etc.

phoria (fo′re-ah) [Gr. *pherein* to bear] any tendency to deviation of the eyes from the normal when fusional stimuli are absent or fusion is otherwise prevented; a latent or usually unmanifested tropia. Heterophoria. See *cyclophoria, esophoria, exophoria, hyperphoria,* and *hypophoria.*

phoriascope (fo′re-ah-skōp) a prism-refracting instrument for use in orthoptic training.

Phormia (for′me-ah) the blackbottle flies, a genus of blue, black, or green flies of the family Calliphoridae. **P. regi′na,** a blowfly which causes a cutaneous myiasis of sheep in the United States and Canada. The larvae have been introduced into infected wounds to facilitate healing. Called also *Lucilia regina.* See also *maggot.*

phoroblast (fo′ro-blast) [Gr. *phoros* carrying + *blastos* germ] fibroblast.

phorocyte (fo′ro-sīt) a connective tissue cell.

phorocytosis (fo″ro-si-to′sis) proliferation of connective tissue cells.

phorologist (fo-rol′o-jist) one skilled in tracing the sources of endemic and epidemic diseases.

phorology (fo-rol′o-je) [Gr. *phoros* carrying + -logy] the study of disease carriers.

phorometer (fo-rom′ĕ-ter) [Gr. *pherein* to bear + *metron* measure] an instrument for ascertaining the degree and kind of heterophoria.

phorometry (fo-rom′ĕ-tre) use of the phorometer.

phorone (fo′rōn) chemical name: 2,6-dimethyl-2,5-heptadien-4-one. A yellowish, oily, unsaturated ketone, $C_9H_{14}O$, obtained from acetone, camphoric acid, etc.

phoroplast (fo′ro-plast) [Gr. *phoros* carrying + *plastos* formed] connective tissue.

Phoroptor (fo-rop′tor) trademark for a phorometer fitted with a battery of cylindrical lenses.

phoroscope (fo′ro-skōp) a fixed trial frame for eye testing, with a head rest which may be fastened to the table or the wall.

phorotone (fo′ro-tōn) [Gr. *phora* motion, movement + *tonos* tension] an instrument for exercising the muscles of the eye.

phorozoon (fo″ro-zo′on) [Gr. *phoros* fruitful + *zōon* animal] the asexual stage in the life history of an organism.

phose (fōz) [Gr. *phōs* light] any subjective sensation, as of light or color; see *aphose, centraphose, centrophose, chromophose, peripheraphose, peripherophose,* etc.

phosgene (fos′jēn) a suffocating and highly poisonous war gas, carbonyl chloride, $COCl_2$; called also *CG.*

phosgenic (fos-jen′ik) [Gr. *phōs* light + *gennan* to produce] producing light.

phosis (fo′sis) the production of a phose.

phosphagen (fos′fah-jen) a group of compounds, including phosphocreatine and phosphoarginine, which occur in tissue and which yield inorganic phosphate with release of energy on cleavage. They are therefore classed as high-energy phosphate compounds.

phosphagenic (fos″fah-jen′ik) producing or forming phosphate.

phosphaminase (fos-fam′ĭ-nās) an enzyme that catalyzes the hydrolysis of amino phosphoric compounds into amines and phosphoric acid.

phosphatase (fos′fah-tās″) [phosphate + -ase] an enzyme that hydrolyzes monophosphoric esters, with liberation of inorganic phosphate, found in practically all tissues, body fluids, and cells, including erythrocytes and leukocytes. **acid p.,** a phosphatase active in an acid medium; such enzymes are found in mammalian erythrocytes and yeast (optimal activity at pH 6), prostatic tissue, epithelium, spleen, kidney, blood plasma, liver, and pancreas, and in rice bran (optimal activity at pH 5) and Taka-diastase (optimal activity at pH 3–4). **alkaline p.,** a phosphatase active in an alkaline medium; such enzymes are found in blood plasma or serum, bone, kidney, mammary gland, spleen, lung, leukocytes, adrenal cortex, and seminiferous tubules (optimal activity at about pH 9.3). **serum p.,** the phosphatase of the blood serum.

phosphate (fos′fāt) [L. *phosphas*] any salt or ester of phosphoric acid. Phosphates are distributed throughout the body. Inorganic phosphates occur chiefly in the skeleton in association with calcium, where they play a role in the mineralization of bone, and in body fluids, where they play a role in the regulation of acid-base balance. Organic phosphates are incorporated in such macromolecules as sugar phosphates, phospholipids, phosphoproteins, and nucleic acids. **acid p.,** any phosphate in which only one or two of the three replaceable hydrogen atoms are taken up or replaced. **alkaline p.,** a phosphate of an alkaline metal, as sodium or potassium. **ammoniomagnesium p.,** a double salt of ammonium and magnesium with orthophosphoric acid, $Mg(NH_4)PO_4 \cdot 6H_2O$; closely allied to and often associated with triple phosphate. **arginine p.,** phosphoarginine. **calcium p.,** a compound containing calcium and the phosphate radical (PO_4). **carbamyl p.,** an important intermediate compound in the formation of pyrimidine and citrulline, the latter being a step in urea formation. **creatine p.,** phosphocreatine. **earthy p.,** a phosphate of any one of the alkaline earth metals. **ferric p.,** a yellowish white powder, $FePO_4 \cdot 4H_2O$, insoluble in water or acetic acid, used as a feed and food supplement, especially to enrich bread, and as a fertilizer. **ferric p., soluble,** ferric phosphate rendered soluble by the presence of sodium citrate; used as a hematinic. **guanidine p.,** phosphoguanidine. **magnesium p., dibasic,** a salt, $MgHPO_4 \cdot 3H_2O$, occurring as a white, crystalline powder; it has been used as a mild saline laxative. **magnesium p., tribasic,** a powdered, white salt, $Mg_3(PO_4)_2 \cdot 5H_2O$, used as a gastric antacid; called also *trimagnesium p.* **normal p.,** any phosphate in which all the replaceable hydrogen atoms in phosphoric acid are replaced. **polyestradiol p.,** a polymeric ester of phosphoric acid and estradiol, used as a palliative in prostatic carcinoma. **stellar p.,** calcium phosphate occurring in star-shaped masses of crystals in urinary sediment. **trimagnesium p.,** magnesium p., tribasic. **triorthocresyl p.,** a poisonous compound, $(CH_3C_6H_4 \cdot O)PO$, contained in Jamaica ginger, ingestion of which causes paralysis. **triose p.,** phosphotriose. **triple p.,** a calcium, ammonium, and magnesium phosphate, sometimes found in the urine.

phosphated (fos'fāt-ed) containing phosphates.

phosphatemia (fos"fah-te'me-ah) [*phosphate* + Gr. *haima* blood + -*ia*] an excess of phosphates in the blood.

phosphatic (fos-fat'ik) pertaining to or containing phosphates.

phosphatidate (fos"fah-tid-āt') a phospholipid from which choline, ethanolamine, or serine has been split off.

phosphatide (fos'fah-tīd) phospholipid.

phosphatidosis (fos"fah-tǐ-do'sis), pl. *phosphatido'ses* [*phosphatide* + -*osis*] lipidosis in which the fatty accumulations are phosphatides.

phosphatidylcholine (fos-fat"ǐ-dil-ko'lēn) lecithin.

phosphatidylethanolamine (fos-fat"ǐ-dil-eth"ah-nol-am'ēn) one of the prothromboplastic phosphatides contained in blood platelets.

phosphatidylinositide (fos-fat"ǐ-dil-in-o'sǐ-tīd) any of a group of compounds containing residues of inositol and phosphatide, occurring in a variety of tissues and especially concentrated in the brain. Called also *phosphoinositide.*

phosphatidylinositol (fos-fat"ǐ-dil-in-o'sǐ-tol) a phosphatidic acid combined with inositol.

phosphatidylserine (fos-fat"ǐ-dil-se'rin) one of the prothromboplastic phosphatides contained in blood platelets.

phosphatoptosis (fos"fah-top-to'sis) [*phosphate* + Gr. *ptōsis* fall] the spontaneous precipitation of phosphates from the urine; phosphaturia.

phosphaturia (fos"fah-tu're-ah) [*phosphate* + Gr. *ouron* urine + -*ia*] 1. a high percentage of phosphates in any given specimen of urine. 2. ready precipitation of the earthy phosphates from the urine; phosphatoptosis.

phosphene (fos'fēn) [Gr. *phōs* light + *phainein* to show] an objective visual sensation that appears with the eyes closed and in the absence of visual light. **accommodation p.,** the streak of light surrounding the visual field seen in the dark after accommodation.

phosphide (fos'fīd) any binary compound of phosphorus and another element or radical.

phosphine (fos'fēn) 1. hydrogen phosphide, PH_3; a toxic malodorous gas and radical. 2. a coal tar dye extremely destructive to infusorial life; it is used as a stain. Called also *Philadelphia yellow.*

phosphite (fos'fīt) any salt of phosphorous acid.

phosphoamidase (fos"fo-am'ǐ-dās) an enzyme (a lyase) that catalyzes the conversion of phosphocreatine to creatine and orthophosphate.

phosphoarginine (fos"fo-ar'jǐ-nin) an arginine phosphoric acid compound homologous with phosphocreatine but found in invertebrate muscles.

phosphocozymase (fos"fo-ko-zi'mās) nicotinamide-adenine dinucleotide phosphate (NADP); see under *dinucleotide.*

phosphocreatine (fos"fo-kre'ah-tin) a creatine–phosphoric acid compound, $(OH)_2PO \cdot NH \cdot C(:NH) \cdot N(CH_3) \cdot CH_2 \cdot COOH$, occurring in muscle metabolism, being broken down into creatine and inorganic phosphorus. It is an important storage form of high-energy phosphate, the energy source in muscle contraction.

The phosphate group is transferred to ADP on muscle contraction to yield creatine and ATP. Called also *creatine phosphate.*

phosphodiesterase (fos"fo-di-es'ter-ās) an enzyme that hydrolyzes —O—P—O— bonds in RNA and DNA.

phosphoesterase (fos"fo-es'ter-ās) phosphatase.

phosphofructaldolase (fos"fo-frukt-al'do-lās) an enzyme that catalyzes the cleavage of fructose-1,6-diphosphate into two isomeric triose phosphates: the aldose (D-glyceraldehyde-3-phosphate) and the ketose (dihydroxyacetone phosphate); it is elevated in the serum of patients with viral hepatitis, decreasing in activity as the disease subsides and becoming normal when recovery takes place.

phosphofructokinase (fos"fo-fruk"to-ki'nās) an enzyme produced by spermatozoa, allowing the spermatocyte to utilize fructose as an energy source; it catalyzes the conversion of ATP and fructose-6-phosphate to ADP and fructose-1,6-diphosphate. Formerly called *phosphohexokinase.*

phosphoglobulin (fos"fo-glob'u-lin) a phosphoprotein with globulin as the protein moiety.

phosphoglucokinase (fos"fo-gloo"ko-ki'nās) an enzyme (a transferase) that catalyzes the conversion of ATP and glucose-1-phosphate to ADP and glucose-1,6-phosphate.

phosphoglucomutase (fos"fo-gloo"ko-mu'tās) an enzyme of the phosphotransferase group that catalyzes the change of glucose-1-phosphate into glucose-6-phosphate. Found in plants and animals.

phosphoglucoprotein (fos"fo-gloo"ko-pro'te-in) a phosphorus-containing glucoprotein.

3-phosphoglyceraldehyde (fos"fo-glis"er-al'de-hīd) a triose phosphate, $CH2 \cdot O \cdot PO(OH)_2 \cdot CHOH \cdot CHO$, which results from the splitting of fructose-1,6-diphosphate in muscle metabolism.

phosphoglycerate (fos"fo-glis'er-āt) a salt of phosphoglyceric acid; it is an intermediate in the metabolic formation of pyruvate, its phosphate group being transferred from the 3-carbon of the glycerate to the 2-carbon.

phosphoglyceride (fos"fo-glis'er-īd) a class of phospholipids, including lecithin and cephalin, consisting of a glycerol backbone, two fatty acid chains, and a phosphorylated alcohol, the common alcohol moieties being choline, ethanolamine, serine, and inositol. Phosphatidic acid is the parent compound. The phosphoglycerides are a major component of cell membranes.

phosphoglyceromutase (fos"fo-glis"er-o-mu'tās) an enzyme of the phosphotransferase group that catalyzes the change of 3-phosphoglyceric acid into 2-phosphoglyceric acid.

phosphoguanidine (fos"fo-gwan'ǐ-dēn) a guanidine phosphoric acid compound which on hydrolysis yields low-energy phosphate linkages.

phosphohexoisomerase (fos"fo-hek"so-i-som'er-ās) glucosephosphate isomerase.

phosphohexokinase (fos"fo-hek"so-ki'nās) phosphofructokinase.

phosphoinositide (fos"fo-in-o'sǐ-tīd) phosphatidylinositide.

phosphoketolase (fos"fo-ke'to-lās) an enzyme (a lyase) that catalyzes the conversion of xylulose-5-phosphate and orthophosphate to acetylphosphate, glyceraldehyde-3-phosphate, and water.

phosphokinase (fos"fo-ki'-nās) kinase.

phospholecithinase (fos"fo-les'ǐ-thin-ās) any of a group of enzymes that split phosphoric acid from lecithin and some other phospholipids; usually designated as phospholipase A, B, C, D, etc., according to bond specificity.

Phospholine (fos'fo-lēn) trademark for a preparation of echothiophate iodide.

phospholipase (fos"fo-lip'ās) any of four enzymes that catalyze the splitting of a phospholipid: *Phospholipase A* occurs in the pancreas, liver, kidney, heart, muscle, and adrenals, and in cobra venom, and hydrolyzes the conversion of lecithin and cephalin to lysolecithin and lysocephalin. *Phospholipase B* has the same occurrence as A and hydrolyzes the splitting of a fatty acid from lysolecithin and lysocephalin. *Phospholipase C* occurs in the pancreas, intestinal mucosa, kidney, liver, and brain, and hydrolyzes the splitting of glycerylphosphorylcholine into a diglyceride and choline phosphate. *Phospholipase D* occurs in the toxin of *Clostridium welchii,* and hydrolyzes the splitting of phosphatidylcholine into choline and phosphatidate. Called also *lecithinase.*

phospholipid (fos"fo-lip'id) any lipid that contains phosphorus, including those with a glycerol backbone (phosphoglycerides and plasmalogens) or a backbone of sphingosine or related substance (sphingomyelins). Phospholipids are the major form of lipid in all cell membranes.

phospholipidemia (fos"fo-lip"ǐ-de'me-ah) the presence of phospholipid in the blood.

phospholipin (fos"fo-lip'in) phospholipid.

phosphomonoesterase (fos"fo-mon"o-es'ter-ās) a phosphatase that catalyzes the hydrolysis of simple esters held by P—O bonds.

phosphomutase (fos"fo-mu'tās) an enzyme of the isomerase class that catalyzes the intermolecular transfer of phosphoryl groups. **phosphoglycerate p.,** an enzyme that catalyzes the conversion of 2- to 3-phospho-D-glycerate.

phosphonate (fos′fo-nāt) a carbon-phosphate compound. Such compounds may be related to inorganic pyrophosphates in structure but possess stable P—C—P bonds instead of P—O—P bonds; they are stable to both enzymatic and chemical hydrolysis.

phosphonecrosis (fos″fo-ne-kro′sis) necrosis of the jaw bone due to exposure to phosphorus; called also *phossy jaw.*

phosphonium (fos-fo′ne-um) the univalent radical, PH₄, forming compounds analogous to those of ammonium.

phosphonuclease (fos″fo-nu′kle-ās) nucleotidase.

phosphopenia (fos″fo-pe′ne-ah) [*phosphorus* + Gr. *penia* poverty] deficiency of phosphorus in the body.

phosphoprotein (fos″fo-pro′te-in) a conjugated protein, such as the vitelline of egg yolk and casein of milk, in which phosphoric acid is esterified with a hydroxy amino acid, especially with serine.

phosphoptomaine (fos″fo-to′mān) any of a class of toxic compounds found in the blood in phosphorus poisoning.

phosphorated (fos′fo-rāt″ed) charged or combined with phosphorus.

phosphorescence (fos″fo-res′ens) the emission of light without appreciable heat; it is characterized by the emission of absorbed light after a delay and at a considerably longer wavelength than that of the absorbed light. Cf. *fluorescence.*

phosphorescent (fos″fo-res′ent) pertaining to or exhibiting phosphorescence.

phosphoretted (fos′fo-ret″ed) phosphorated.

phosphoribokinase (fos″fo-ri″bo-ki′nās) an enzyme (a transferase) that catalyzes the conversion of ATP and ribose-5-phosphate to ADP and ribose-1,5-diphosphate.

phosphoribosylamine (fos″fo-ri″bo-sil′ah-mēn) an intermediate product in the synthesis of purines formed from phosphoribosylpyrophosphate and glutamine; excessive production is often a factor in primary gout.

phosphoribosylpyrophosphate (fos″fo-ri″bo-sil- pi″ro-fos′fāt) an intermediate in the formation of purines and of purine and pyrimidine nucleotides; abbreviated as PRPP.

phosphoribulokinase (fos″fo-ri″bu-lo-ki′nās) an enzyme (a transferase) that catalyzes the conversion of ATP and D-ribulose 5-phosphate to ADP and D-ribulose 1,5-diphosphate.

phosphorism (fos′fo-rizm) chronic phosphorus poisoning; see under *poisoning.*

phosphorized (fos′fo-rīzd) containing phosphorus.

phosphorolysis (fos″fo-rol′ĭ-sis) cleavage of a chemical bond with simultaneous addition of the elements of phosphoric acid to the residues, as in the splitting of the glycosidic bonds of glycogen catalyzed by the enzyme phosphorylase in carbohydrate metabolism. The reaction is analogous to hydrolysis.

phosphoroscope (fos′fōr-o-skōp) an instrument for measuring phosphorescence.

phosphorous (fos′fo-rus) pertaining to or containing phosphorus.

phosphorpenia (fos″fōr-pe′ne-ah) phosphopenia.

phosphoruria (fos″fōr-u′re-ah) [*phosphorus* + Gr. *ouron* urine + *-ia*] the presence of free phosphorus in the urine.

phosphorus (fos′fŏ-rus) [Gr. *phōs* light + *phorein* to carry] a nonmetallic, allotropic element: poisonous and highly inflammable; symbol, P; atomic number, 15; atomic weight, 30.974. It occurs in three forms—*white* (yellow), *red,* and *black.* It is obtainable from bones, urine, and especially minerals, such as apatite. Ordinary white phosphorus is the kind once used in medicine, and is very inflammable and exceedingly poisonous. Phosphorus is an essential element in the diet; it is a major component of the mineral phase of bone and is abundant in all tissues, being involved in some form in almost all metabolic processes. Free phosphorus causes a fatty degeneration of the liver and other viscera, and the inhalation of its vapor often leads to necrosis of the lower jaw. Therapeutically, it was once used in rickets, osteomalacia, nervous and cerebral diseases, scrofula, and tuberculosis, as a genital stimulant in sexual exhaustion, and as a tonic in conditions of exhaustion. **amorphous p.,** red p. **black p.,** black lustrous crystals, resembling coal, insoluble in organic solvents, produced by heating white phosphorus under very high pressure. **labeled p.,** radioactive p. **ordinary p.,** white p. **radioactive p.,** ³²P, radiophosphorus. **red p.,** a dark red amorphous powder, which is infusible and insoluble in carbon disulfide, and is not poisonous; called also *amorphous p.* **white p.,** a usually white, sometimes yellow, waxy solid, which is soluble in carbon disulfide, and very inflammable and exceedingly poisonous; it is the form that was once used in medicine in the treatment of various disorders. Called also *ordinary p.* **yellow p.,** white p.

phosphoryl (fos′fōr-il) the trivalent chemical radical ≡P:O.

phosphorylase (fos-fōr′ĭ-lās) an enzyme which, in the presence of inorganic phosphate, is able to catalyze reversibly the phosphorolytic cleavage of the α-1.4-linkage of glycogen to yield glucose-1-phosphate; it occurs in plants and animals. In animals,

it may exist in an inactive form, phosphorylase "b," which when phosphorylated, using ATP in the presence of kinase, becomes active, phosphorylase "a." **polynucleotide p.,** an enzyme that catalyzes the phosphorylation of RNA, freeing a nucleoside diphosphate; called also *polyribonucleotide nucleotidyltransferase.*

phosphorylation (fos″fōr-ĭ-la′shun) the metabolic process of introducing a phosphate group into an organic molecule. **oxidative p.,** the formation of high-energy phosphate bonds by phosphorylation of ADP to ATP, in which electrons are transferred from the substrate to oxygen in a series of steps: from substrate in succession to NAD, ubiquinone, cytochrome C, and oxygen; it occurs in the mitochondria.

phosphorylysis (fos″fo-ril′ĭ-sis) phosphorolysis.

phosphosugar (fos″fo-shug′ar) a sugar combined with a phosphate; a pentose or hexose phosphate.

phosphotransacetylase (fos″fo-trans″ah-set′ĭ-lās) phosphate acetyltransferase.

phosphotransferase (fos″fo-trans′fer-ās) any of a subclass of enzymes that catalyze the transfer of a phosphate group; see *kinase* (def. 1).

phosphotriose (fos″fo-tri′ōs) a compound consisting of a 3-carbon sugar combined with a phosphate radical. Two such compounds are formed from hexosediphosphate: 3-phosphoglyceraldehyde and 1-phosphodihydroxyacetone. Called also *triose phosphate.*

phosphotungstate (fos″fo-tung′stāt) a salt of phosphotungstic acid.

phosphovitellin (fos″fo-vi-tel′in) phosvitin.

phosphuresis (fos″fu-re′sis) the urinary excretion of phosphorus (phosphates).

phosphuret (fos′fu-ret) phosphide.

phosphuretic (fos″fu-ret′ik) pertaining to, characterized by, or promoting the urinary excretion of phosphorus (phosphates).

phosphuretted (fos″fu-ret″ed) phosphorated.

phosphuria (fos-fu′re-ah) phosphaturia.

phosvitin (fos-vi′tin) a phosphoprotein isolated from vitellin in egg yolk; called also *phosphovitellin.*

phot (fōt) phote.

phot- see *photo-.*

photalgia (fo-tal′je-ah) [*phot-* + *-algia*] pain, as in the eye, caused by light.

photallochromy (fo-tal′o-kro″me) [*phot-* + Gr. *allos* different + *chrōma* color] allotropic change with color alteration due to light, as the change of yellow into red phosphorus.

photaugiaphobia (fo-taw″je-ah-fo′be-ah) [Gr. *phōtaugeia* glare + *phobein* to be affrighted by] abnormal intolerance of a glare of light.

phote (fōt) [Gr. *phōs* light] the C.G.S. unit of illumination, being one lumen per square centimeter.

photechy (fo′tek-e) [*phot-* + Gr. *ēchō* echo] the power shown by certain substances of becoming radioactive after having been exposed to radiation.

photerythrous (fo″te-rith′rus) [*phot-* + Gr. *erythros* red] sensitive to the red rays of the spectrum; said of a form of color blindness in which green is not clearly recognized.

photesthesis (fo″tes-the′sis) [*phot-* + Gr. *aisthēsis* perception] sensitiveness to light.

photic (fo′tik) pertaining to light.

photism (fo′tizm) a visual image; a sensation of color associated with a sensation of hearing, taste, smell, or touch.

photo-, phot- [Gr. *phōs, phōtos* light] combining form denoting relationship to light.

photoactinic (fo″to-ak-tin′ik) giving off both luminous and actinic rays.

photoactive (fo″to-ak′tiv) reacting chemically to sunlight or ultraviolet radiation.

photoallergic (fo″to-al-ler′jik) pertaining to or characterized by heightened delayed contact–type sensitivity to light.

photoallergy (fo″to-al′er-je) an allergic type of sensitivity to light.

Photobacterium (fo″to-bak-te′re-um) a genus of microorganisms of the family Pseudomonadaceae, suborder Pseudomonadineae, order Pseudomonadales, occurring usually as coccoid or rod-shaped cells, producing luminescent substances, and found on dead fish and other salt-water animals, and in sea water. It includes four species, *P. fisch′eri, P. har′veyi, P. phospho′reum,* and *P. pieranto′nii.*

photobacterium (fo″to-bak-te′re-um) 1. a bacterium producing luminescent substances. 2. an individual organism of the genus *Photobacterium.*

photobiologic, photobiological (fo″to-bi″o-loj′ik; fo″to-bi″o-loj′ĭ-kal) pertaining to photobiology or to the effect of light on living organisms.

photobiology (fo″to-bi-ol′o-je) [*photo-* + *biology*] that department of biology which deals with the effect of light on living organisms, including the study of photosynthesis.

photobiotic (fo″to-bi-ot′ik) [*photo-* + Gr. *bios* life]　living or thriving only in the light; said of certain organisms such as green plants.

photocatalysis (fo″to-kah-tal′ĭ-sis)　the promotion or stimulation of a reaction by light.

photocatalyst (fo″to-kat′ah-list)　a substance by means of which sunlight is utilized, as chlorophyll in the photosynthesis of carbohydrates by green plants.

photocatalytic (fo″to-kat′ah-lit′ik)　promoted or stimulated by light; pertaining to, characterized by, or causing photocatalysis.

photocatalyzer (fo″to-kat′ah-līz′er)　photocatalyst.

photoceptor (fo′to-sep′tor)　photoreceptor.

photochemical (fo″to-kem′e-kal)　pertaining to the chemical properties of light; chemically reactive in the presence of light or other radiation.

photochemistry (fo″to-kem′is-tre) [*photo-* + *chemistry*]　the branch of chemistry which deals with the chemical properties or effects of light rays or other radiation.

photochemotherapy (fo″to-ke″mo-ther′ah-pe)　treatment by means of drugs (e.g., methoxsalen) that react to ultraviolet radiation or sunlight.

photochromogen (fo″to-kro′mo-jen) [*photo-* + Gr. *chrōma* color + *gennan* to produce]　a microorganism whose pigmentation develops as a result of exposure to light, specifically *Mycobacterium kansasii* (pathogenic for man), which is yellow-orange if grown in the light, and almost colorless if grown in the dark.

photochromogenic (fo″to-kro′mo-jen′ik)　pertaining to or characterized by photochromogenicity.

photochromogenicity (fo″to-kro′mo-je-nis′ĭ-te)　the property of microorganisms of forming pigment consequent to light exposure; induction occurs within a few minutes in the shorter wavelengths of visible light, pigmentation then occurring within 24 hours if conditions permit continued growth.

photocinetic (fo″to-si-net′ik)　(*obs.*) photokinetic.

photocoagulation (fo″to-ko-ag″u-la′shun)　condensation of protein material by the controlled use of an intense beam of light (e.g., xenon arc light or argon laser); used especially in treatment of retinal detachment and destruction of abnormal retinal vessels, or of intraocular tumor masses.

photoconvulsive (fo″to-kon-vul′siv)　photoparoxysmal.

photocutaneous (fo″to-ku-ta′ne-us)　relating to skin manifestations in the production of which light is an important factor.

photodermatitis (fo″to-der″mah-ti′tis)　an abnormal state of the skin in which light is an important causative factor.

photodermatosis (fo″to-der″mah-to′sis)　a morbid condition produced in the skin by exposure to light.

photodromy (fo-tod′ro-me) [*photo-* + Gr. *dromos* running]　the phenomenon of moving toward (*positive p.*) or away from (*negative p.*) light; as in the case of particles in suspension.

photodynamic (fo″to-di-nam′ik) [*photo-* + Gr. *dynamis* power]　powerful in the light; said of the action exerted by fluorescent substances in the light.

photodynamics (fo″to-di-nam′iks)　the science of the activating effects of light.

photodynesis (fo″to-di-ne′sis)　the initiation of cytoplasmic streaming (cyclosis) in plant cells by visible light.

photodynia (fo″to-din′e-ah) [*photo-* + Gr. *odynē* pain]　photalgia.

photodysphoria (fo″to-dis-fo′re-ah) [*photo-* + Gr. *dysphoria* distress]　intolerance of light; photophobia.

photoelectric (fo″to-e-lek′trik)　pertaining to the electric effects of light or other radiation.

photoelectron (fo″to-e-lek′tron)　an electron emitted from a metallic surface when the latter is illuminated with light, especially with light of short wavelength.

photoelement (fo″to-el′e-ment)　a galvanic element which is decomposed under the influence of light and produces photoelectricity.

photoerythema (fo″to-er″ĭ-the′mah)　erythema due to exposure to light.

photoesthetic (fo″to-es-thet′ik) [*photo-* + Gr. *aisthēsis* perception]　pertaining to or having the sensation of light.

photofluorogram (fo″to-floo-or′o-gram)　the film produced in photofluorography.

photofluorography (fo″to-floo″or-og′rah-fe)　the photographic recording of fluoroscopic images on small films, using a fast lens; a procedure used in mass roentgenography of the chest. Called also *fluororoentgenography,* and sometimes *abreuography,* in honor of Manoel de Abreu, Brazilian physician, who discovered the technique.

photofluoroscope (fo″to-floo-or′o-skōp)　a form of fluoroscope used in making either observations or photographs by means of roentgen rays.

photogastroscope (fo″to-gas′tro-skōp) [*photo-* + Gr. *gastēr* stomach + *skopein* to examine]　an apparatus for photographing the interior of the stomach.

photogene (fo′to-jēn)　after-image.

photogenic (fo′to-jen′ik)　1. produced by light, as photogenic epilepsy. 2. producing or emitting light; phosphorescent.

photogram (fo′to-gram) [*photo-* + Gr. *gramma* mark]　the photographic record of a physiologic experiment.

photography (fo-tog′rah-fe)　the process of making images on a sensitized material by exposure to light or other radiant energy. **Kirlian p.,** the taking of photographs of ordinarily invisible emanations (an aura or halo) from living organisms, plant and animal, that change in color and size. The object under study, a leaf, fingertip, etc., is placed on a piece of photographic paper or negative film on a metal plate in which a generator induces an electromagnetic field in a dark enclosure.

photohalide (fo″to-hal′īd)　any halogen salt that is sensitive to light.

photohematachometer (fo″to-hem″ah-tah-kom′ĕ-ter) [*photo-* + Gr. *haima* blood + *tachys* swift + *metron* measure]　a device for making a photographic record of the speed of the blood current.

photohenric (fo″to-hen′rik) [*photo-* + *henry*]　denoting a change in inductive capacity due to the action of light.

photohmic (fo-to′mik)　denoting a change in electric resistance produced by light.

photoinactivation (fo″to-in-ak″tĭ-va′shun)　inactivation, as of complement, by light.

photokinetic (fo″to-ki-net′ik) [*photo-* + Gr. *kinētikos* pertaining to motion]　moving in response to the stimulus of light.

photokymograph (fo″to-ki′mo-graf)　a camera with a moving film for recording movements as of the string in a string galvanometer; called also *recording camera.*

photolethal (fo″to-le′thal)　pertaining to the lethal or destructive action of light.

photology (fo-tol′o-je) [*photo-* + *-logy*]　the branch of physics which treats of light.

photoluminescence (fo″to-lu″mĭ-nes′ens)　the quality of being luminescent after being exposed to light.

photolysis (fo-tol′ĭ-sis)　1. chemical decomposition by the action of light. 2. lysis or solution of cells under the influence of light.

photolyte (fo′to-līt) [*photo-* + Gr. *lyein* to dissolve]　any substance decomposable by the action of light.

photolytic (fo′to-lit′ik)　decomposed by light or radiant energy.

photoma (fo-to′mah)　a flash of light sparks or color with no objective basis.

photomagnetism (fo″to-mag′nĕ-tizm)　magnetism induced by the action of light.

photometer (fo-tom′ĕ-ter) [*photo-* + Gr. *metron* measure]　a device for measuring the intensity of light. **flame p.,** an instrument for analyzing the light emitted by a substance in a flame; commonly used for determination of sodium, potassium, lithium, and calcium in biological materials. **flicker p.,** an instrument in which the frequency of a flickering light can be controlled, for use in performing the flicker test; called also *flicker meter.* **Förster's p.,** phototometer.

photomethemoglobin (fo″to-met-he″mo-glo′bin)　a compound formed by the action of light on methemoglobin.

photometry (fo-tom′ĕ-tre) [*photo-* + Gr. *metron* measure]　the measurement of light. **flicker p.,** see *flicker test,* under *tests.*

photomicrograph (fo″to-mi′kro-graf) [*photo-* + Gr. *mikros* small + *graphein* to record]　the photograph of a minute object as seen under the light microscope, produced by ordinary photographic methods. Cf. *microphotograph.*

photomicrography (fo″to-mi-krog′rah-fe)　the production of photomicrographs.

photomicroscope (fo″to-mi′kro-skōp)　a microscope and camera combined for making photomicrographs.

photomicroscopy (fo″to-mi-kros′ko-pe)　photography of enlarged pictures of minute objects with the photomicroscope.

photomorphogenesis (fo″to-mor″fo-jen′ĕ-sis)　the regulation of form by light, as in the induction of flowering in plants by a minimal period of daylight.

photomyoclonic (fo″to-mi″o-klon′ik)　photomyogenic.

photomyogenic (fo″to-mi″o-jen′ik)　photomyoclonic; denoting an electroencephalographic response to photic stimulation (brief flashes of light) marked by myoclonus of the facial muscles.

photon (fo′ton)　a particle (quantum) of radiant energy.

photoncia (fo-ton′se-ah) [*photo-* + Gr. *onkos* mass]　swelling due to the action of light.

photone (fo′tōn)　a visualization or hallucination of light.

photo-onycholysis (fo″to-o″nĭk-ol′ĭ-sis)　onycholysis resulting from exposure to sunlight or ultraviolet rays, as after treatment with the tetracyclines or methoxypsoralen.

photo-ophthalmia (fo″to-of-thal′me-ah) [*photo-* + *ophthalmia*]　ophthalmia caused by intense light, such as electric light, rays of welding arc, or reflection from snow (ophthalmia nivialis). **flash p.,** ophthalmia produced by exposure to a welding arc.

photoparoxysmal (fo″to-par″oks-is′mal)　photoconvulsive; denoting an abnormal electroencephalographic response to photic stimulation (brief flashes of light), marked by diffuse paroxysmal discharge recorded as spike-wave complexes; the response may be accompanied by minor seizures.

photopathy (fo-top'ah-the) [*photo-* + Gr. *pathos* affection] a pathologic effect produced by light.

photoperceptive (fo"to-per-sep'tiv) [*photo-* + *perceptive*] able to perceive light.

photoperiod (fo"to-pēr'e-od) the period of time per day that an organism is exposed to daylight or to artificial light.

photoperiodic (fo"to-pēr'e-od'ik) pertaining to the photoperiod or to photoperiodism.

photoperiodicity (fo"to-pe"re-o-dis'ĭ-te) the regularly recurring changes in the relation of light and darkness in various areas of the world, noted in the annual passage of the earth about the sun; applied also to rhythm of certain biological phenomena as determined by those changes.

photoperiodism (fo"to-pe're-od-izm) the physiologic and behavioral reactions brought about in organisms by changes in the duration of daylight and darkness in a 24-hour period. Called also *photoperiodicity*.

photopharmacology (fo"to-far"mah-kol'o-je) [*photo-* + *pharmacology*] the study of the effects of light and other radiations on drugs and on their pharmacological action.

photophilic (fo"to-fil'ik) [*photo-* + Gr. *philein* to love] thriving in light; said of organisms.

photophobia (fo"to-fo'be-ah) [*photo-* + Gr. *phobein* to be affrighted by] abnormal visual intolerance of light.

photophobic (fo"to-fo'bik) pertaining to or characterized by photophobia.

photophosphorylation (fo"to-fos"for-ĭ-la'shun) the formation of ATP occurring in chloroplasts during photosynthesis; it is analogous to oxidative phosphorylation. **cyclic p.,** that in which ATP formation is coupled with liberation of the energy arising from a cyclic flow of electrons from the ferredoxin-reducing system back to the chlorophyll.

photophthalmia (fo"tof-thal'me-ah) photo-ophthalmia.

photopia (fo-to'pe-ah) [*photo-* + Gr. *ōpē* sight + *-ia*] day vision; see also *light adaptation*.

photopic (fo-top'ik) pertaining to vision in the light; said of the eye which has become light-adapted.

photoproduct (fo'to-prod"ukt) a substance synthesized in the body by the action of light.

photoprotection (fo"to-pro-tek'shun) the protection of some cells by exposure to light in the near ultraviolet light range prior to exposure to light in the far ultraviolet range.

photopsia (fo-top'se-ah) [*photo-* + Gr. *opsis* vision + *-ia*] an appearance as of sparks or flashes due to retinal irritation.

photopsin (fo-top'sin) the protein moiety of the cones of the retina that combines with retinal to form photochemical pigments.

photopsy (fo-top'se) photopsia.

photoptarmosis (fo"to-tar-mo'sis) [*photo-* + Gr. *ptarmos* sneezing + *-osis*] sneezing caused by the influence of light.

photoptometer (fo"top-tom'ĕ-ter) [*photo-* + Gr. *optos* seen + *metron* measure] a device for testing the acuity of vision by determining the smallest amount of light that will render an object just visible.

photoptometry (fo"top-tom'ĕ-tre) measurement of light perception.

photoradiometer (fo"to-ra"de-om'ĕ-ter) an apparatus for measuring the quantity of roentgen rays penetrating any given surface.

photoreaction (fo"to-re-ak'shun) a chemical reaction produced by the influence of light; a photochemical reaction.

photoreactivation (fo"to-re-ak"tĭ-va'shun) the reversal of the biological effects of ultraviolet radiation on cells by subsequent exposure to visible light; called also *photoreversal*.

photoreception (fo"to-re-sep'shun) [Gr. *phōs* light + L. *receptio*, from *recipere* to receive] the process of detecting radiant energy, usually of wavelengths between 3900 and 7700 Å, being the range of visible light.

photoreceptive (fo"to-re-sep'tiv) sensitive to stimulation by light.

photoreceptor (fo"to-re-sep'tor) [*photo-* + *receptor*] a nerve end-organ or receptor sensitive to light.

photorespiration (fo"to-res"pĭ-ra'shun) a process carried out by certain plants, occurring as a result of oxidation of glycolic acid (a product of photosynthesis released by chloroplasts) by glycolic acid oxidase, an enzyme present in the glyoxosomes, ultimately causing an increased output of carbon dioxide.

photoretinitis (fo"to-ret"ĭ-ni'tis) inflammation of the retina due to exposure to intense light, which may result in transient central scotoma.

photoreversal (fo"to-re-ver'sal) photoreactivation.

photoscan (fo'to-skan) a two-dimensional representation (map) of the gamma rays emitted by a radioisotope, revealing its varying concentration in a body tissue, differing only from a scintiscan in

that the printout mechanism is a light source exposing a photographic film.

photoscanner (fo"to-skan'ner) the system of equipment used in the making of a photoscan.

photoscope (fo'to-skōp) [*photo-* + Gr. *skopein* to examine] a kind of fluoroscope.

photoscopy (fo-tos'ko-pe) [*photo-* + Gr. *skopein* to examine] skiascopy.

photosensitive (fo"to-sen'sĭ-tiv) exhibiting an abnormally heightened reactivity to sunlight.

photosensitivity (fo"to-sen"sĭ-tiv'ĭ-te) abnormal reactivity of the skin to sunlight.

photosensitization (fo"to-sen"sĭ-ti-za'shun) the development of abnormally heightened reactivity of the skin to sunlight. **contactant p.,** cutaneous sensitization produced by exposure to a contactant sensitizer followed by exposure to light, resulting in photocontact dermatitis.

photosensitize (fo"to-sen'sĭ-tīz) [*photo-* + *sensitize*] to sensitize a substance or an organism, cell, or tissue to the influence of light.

photostable (fo'to-sta'b'l) unchanged by the influence of light.

photostethoscope (fo"to-steth'o-skōp) a lamp which transforms sounds amplified by a microphone into pulsations of light; used for recording the heartbeats of the fetus.

photosynthesis (fo"to-sin'thĕ-sis) [*photo-* + Gr. *synthesis* putting together] a chemical combination caused by the action of light; specifically the formation of carbohydrates (with release of molecular oxygen) from carbon dioxide and water in the chlorophyll tissue of plants and blue-green algae under the influence of light. In bacteria, photosynthesis employs hydrogen sulfide, molecular hydrogen, and other reduced compounds in place of water, so that molecular oxygen is not released. See also *light reaction* and *dark reaction*, under *reaction*. Cf. *chemosynthesis*.

phototaxis (fo"to-tak'sis) [*photo-* + Gr. *taxis* arrangement] the movement of cells and microorganisms under the influence of light, which may be toward (*positive p.*) or away (*negative p.*) from the source of light stimulus; called also *heliotaxis*.

phototherapy (fo"to-ther'ah-pe) [*photo-* + *therapy*] the treatment of disease, e.g. bilirubinemia, by exposure to light, especially by variously concentrated light rays.

photothermal (fo"to-ther'mal) pertaining to the heat produced by radiant energy.

photothermy (fo"to-ther"me) [*photo-* + Gr. *thermē* heat] the heat effects produced by radiant energy.

phototimer (fo"to-tīm'er) a timer used in photography and radiography to give a desired interval for exposure.

phototonus (fo-tot'o-nus) [*photo-* + Gr. *tonos* tension] an irritable state of protoplasm due to the influence of light.

phototoxic (fo"to-tok'sik) pertaining to or characterized by heightening of the sunburn response to ultraviolet light, without any allergic effect (immune response) being involved; see under *dermatitis*.

phototoxicity (fo"tō-tok-sis'ĭ-te) the quality of being phototoxic.

phototrophic (fo"to-trof'ik) [*photo-* + Gr. *trophē* nourishment] capable of deriving energy from light, as in certain green plants and bacteria.

phototropic (fo"to-trop'ik) exhibiting phototropism.

phototropism (fo-tot'ro-pizm) [*photo-* + Gr. *tropos* a turning] 1. the tendency of an organism to turn or move toward (*positive p.*) or away from (*negative p.*) light. 2. change of color produced in a substance by the action of light.

phototurbidometric (fo"to-tur-bid"o-met'rik) pertaining to the determination of the turbidity of a solution by optic methods; used in study of the activity of various enzymes.

photoxylin (fo-tok'sĭ-lin) [*photo-* + Gr. *xylon* wood] a nitrocellulose from wood pulp used in preparing a collodion-like film; employed in microscopy and minor surgery.

photronreflectometer (fo"tron-re"flek-tom'ĕ-ter) an apparatus for measuring turbidity.

photuria (fo-tu're-ah) [*photo-* + Gr. *ouron* urine + *-ia*] the excretion of urine having a luminous appearance.

Phoxinus laevis (fok'sĭ-nus le'vis) a minnow used to demonstrate the presence of chromatophore-stimulating hormone. When an extract of posterior pituitary is injected into the minnow, a red coloration appears at the point of attachment of the thoracic, abdominal, and anal fins.

Phragmidiothrix (frag-mid'e-o-thriks") a genus of microorganisms of the family Crenotrichaceae, order Chlamydobacteriales, made up of small disk-shaped cells occurring in attached trichomes which are articulated and unbranched, and are enclosed in extremely delicate, colorless sheaths with no deposits of iron or magnesium compounds. The type species is *P. multisepta'ta*.

phragmoplast (frag'mo-plast) [Gr. *phragmos* inclosure + *plastos* formed] the barrel-shaped spindle formed in the equatorial plane during mitosis of plant cells; it precedes the formation of the cell plate.

phren (fren) [Gr. *phrēn*] 1. the diaphragm. 2. the mind, as seat of the intellect, or the heart, as seat of the passions.

phren- (fren) [Gr. *phrēn* diaphragm, mind] a combining form denoting relationship to the diaphragm or to the mind.

phrenalgia (fre-nal′je-ah) [*phren-* + *-algia*] 1. pain in the diaphragm. 2. psychalgia.

phrenectomy (fre-nek′to-me) the removal of all or a part of the diaphragm.

phrenemphraxis (fren″em-frak′sis) [*phrenic* nerve + Gr. *emphraxis* stoppage] the operation of crushing the phrenic nerve; phrenicotripsy.

phrenetic (frĕ-net′ik) 1. maniacal. 2. a maniac.

phrenic (fren′ik) [L. *phrenicus*; Gr. *phrēn* mind; diaphragm] 1. pertaining to the diaphragm; diaphragmatic. 2. pertaining to the mind.

phrenicectomized (fren″ĭ-sek′to-mīzd) having the phrenic nerve excised or resected.

phrenicectomy (fren″ĭ-sek′to-me) [*phrenic* nerve + Gr. *ektomē* excision] resection of the phrenic nerve; phreniconeurectomy.

phreniclasia, phreniclasis (fren″ĭ-kla′ze-ah; fren″ĭ-kla′sis) [*phrenic* nerve + Gr. *klasis* crushing] crushing of the phrenic nerve with a clamp.

phrenicoexairesis (fren″ĭ-ko-ek-si′re-sis) phrenicoexeresis.

phrenicoexeresis (fren″ĭ-ko-ek-ser′ĕ-sis) [*phrenic* nerve + Gr. *exairesis* a taking out] avulsion of the phrenic nerve.

phreniconeurectomy (fren″ĭ-ko-nu-rek′to-me) [*phrenic* + Gr. *neuron* nerve + *ektomē* excision] excision of a whole or a portion of the phrenic nerve; phrenicectomy.

phrenicotomy (fren″ĭ-kot′o-me) [*phrenic* nerve + Gr. *tomē* a cutting] surgical division of the phrenic nerve and its accessory for the purpose of causing one-sided paralysis of the diaphragm, which then becomes pushed up by the viscera so as to compress a diseased lung.

phrenicotripsy (fren″ĭ-ko-trip′se) [*phrenic* nerve + Gr. *tripsis* a crushing] crushing of the phrenic nerve; phrenemphraxis.

phrenitis (frĕ-ni′tis) [*phren-* + *-itis*] 1. delirium or frenzy. 2. inflammation of the diaphragm; diaphragmitis.

phrenocardia (fren″o-kar′de-ah) [*phren-* + Gr. *kardia* heart] neurocirculatory asthenia.

phrenocolic (fren″o-kol′ik) pertaining to or connecting the diaphragm and colon.

phrenocolopexy (fren″o-ko′lo-pek-se) [*phren-* + Gr. *kolon* colon + *pēxis* fixation] operative fixation of the colon to the diaphragm.

phrenodynia (fren″o-din′e-ah) [*phren-* + Gr. *odynē* pain] pain in the diaphragm.

phrenogastric (fren″o-gas′trik) pertaining to the diaphragm and the stomach.

phrenoglottic (fren″o-glot′ik) pertaining to the diaphragm and the glottis.

phrenograph (fren′o-graf) [*phren-* + Gr. *graphein* to write] an apparatus for recording the movements of the diaphragm.

phrenohepatic (fren″o-hĕ-pat′ik) [*phren-* + Gr. *hēpar* liver] pertaining to the diaphragm and the liver.

phrenologist (frĕ-nol′o-jist) a person who practices phrenology.

phrenology (frĕ-nol′o-je) [*phren-* + *-logy*] the study of the mind and character from the shape of the skull.

phrenopathy (frĕ-nop′ah-the) [*phren-* + Gr. *pathos* disease] (*obs.*) any mental disease or disorder.

phrenopericarditis (fren″o-per″ĭ-kar-di′tis) [*phren-* + *pericarditis*] a condition in which the apex of the heart is attached to the diaphragm by adhesions.

phrenoplegia (fren″o-ple′je-ah) [*phren-* + Gr. *plēgē* stroke] 1. a sudden attack of mental disorder. 2. loss or paralysis of the mental faculties. 3. paralysis of the diaphragm.

phrenoptosis (fren″op-to′sis) [*phren-* + Gr. *ptōsis* falling] downward displacement of the diaphragm.

phrenosin (fren′o-sin) a cerebroside, probably $C_{48}H_{93}O_9N$, obtained from brain substance; it yields on hydrolysis galactose, sphingosine, and cerebronic acid.

phrenospasm (fren′o-spazm) [*phren-* + *spasm*] spasm of the diaphragm.

phrenosplenic (fren″o-splen′ik) pertaining to or connecting the diaphragm and the spleen.

phrenosterol (fren″o-ste′rol) a sterol from brain substance.

phrenotropic (fren″o-trop′ik) [*phreno-* + Gr. *tropē* a turn, turning] exerting its principal effect upon the mind.

phrictopathic (frik″to-path′ik) [Gr. *phriktos* producing a shudder + *pathos* disease] causing a shudder; a term applied to a peculiar sensation caused by irritating a hysterical anesthetic area during recovery.

phronema (fro-ne′mah) [Gr. *phronēma* mind] that portion of the cortex of the brain which is occupied by thought centers or association centers.

phrynin (fri′nin) a poisonous substance obtainable from the skin and secretions of various toads; its properties resemble those of digitalin.

phrynoderma (frin″o-der′mah) [Gr. *phrynē* toad + *derma* skin] a papular dry skin eruption (follicular hyperkeratosis), frequently accompanied by mild neuritic and eye symptoms, seen in East Indian laborers fed on a diet of maize meal; probably due to deficiency of vitamin A or of essential fatty acids. Called also toadskin.

phrynolysin (fri-nol′ĭ-sin) [Gr. *phrynē* toad + *lysis* dissolution] the lysin or toxin from the venom of the fire toad (*Bombinator igneus*).

phthalate (thal′āt) a salt of phthalic acid.

phthalein (thal′e-in) any one of a series of coloring matters formed by the condensation of phthalic anhydride with the phenols; some of them have a purgative action. See *phenolphthalein*. **alpha-naphthol p.,** an indicator used in the determination of hydrogen ion concentration; it has a pH range of 9.3–10.5. **orthocresol p.,** an indicator used in the determination of hydrogen ion concentration; it has a pH range of 8.2–9.8.

phthaleinometer (thal″e-in-om′ĕ-ter) an instrument for use in performing phenolsulfonphthalein tests.

phthalin (thal′in) any one of a series of colorless compounds formed by reduction of phthalein.

phthalylsulfacetamide (thal″il-sul″fah-set′ah-mīd) [USP] chemical name: 2-[[[4-(acetylamino)sulfonyl]phenyl]amino]carbonyl]benzoic acid. A sulfonamide, $C_{16}H_{14}N_2O_6S$, occurring as white or creamy white crystals or a crystalline powder; used as an intestinal antibacterial, administered orally. Called also phthalylsulfonazole.

phthalylsulfathiazole (thal″il-sul″fah-thi′ah-zōl) [NF] chemical name: 2-[[[4-[(2-thiazolylamino)sulfonyl]phenyl]amino]carbonyl]benzoic acid. A sulfonamide, $C_{17}H_{13}N_3O_5S_2$, occurring as a white or faintly yellowish white, crystalline powder; used as an intestinal antibacterial, administered orally.

phthalylsulfonazole (thal″il-sul-fon′ah-zōl) phthalylsulfacetamide.

phthinoid (thi′noid) resembling phthisis; consumptive; tuberculous.

phthiocerol (thi″o-se′rol) an alcohol, $C_{35}H_{72}O_3$, isolated from the wax of human tubercle bacilli.

phthiocol (thi′o-kol) chemical name: 2-hydroxy-3-methyl-1,4-naphthoquinone. An antibiotic substance produced by *Mycobacterium tuberculosis* and having some vitamin K activity.

phthiriasis (thir-i′ah-sis) [Gr. *phtheiriasis*, from *phtheir* louse] infestation with crab or pubic lice; see *pediculosis*. **p. inguina′lis, pubic p.,** infestation with lice of the species *Phthirus pubis;* it is usually limited to the pubic hairs but may occur on other areas, as the eyelashes.

Phthirus (thir′us) [Gr. *phtheir* louse] a genus of sucking lice of the family Pediculidae, order Anoplura, which feed on human blood. **P. pu′bis,** the pubic or crab louse, which infests the hair of the pubic region and which is sometimes found in other hairy areas of the body, such as the eyebrows, eyelashes, and axillae.

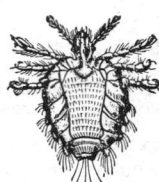
Phthirus pubis.

phthisic (tiz′ik) [Gr. *phthisikos*] 1. affected with phthisis (tuberculosis). 2. a former name for asthma.

phthisical (tiz′ĕ-kal) affected with phthisis, or of the nature of phthisis (tuberculosis).

phthisicky (tiz′e-ke) asthmatic.

phthisiogenesis (tiz″e-o-jen′ĕ-sis) the development of phthisis (tuberculosis).

phthisiogenetic (tiz″e-o-jĕ-net′ik) causing or pertaining to the causation of phthisis (tuberculosis).

phthisiogenic (tiz″e-o-jen′ik) phthisiogenetic.

phthisiologist (tiz″e-ol′o-jist) former name for a physician who specializes in pulmonary tuberculosis.

phthisiology (tiz″e-ol′o-je) [*phthisis* + *-logy*] the sum of knowledge relating to tuberculosis.

phthisiotherapeutical (tiz″e-o-ther″ah-pu′tĕ-kal) of or relating to the treatment of phthisis (tuberculosis).

phthisiotherapeutics (tiz″e-o-ther″ah-pu′tiks) phthisiotherapy.

phthisiotherapeutist, phthisiotherapist (tiz″e-o-ther″ah-pu′tist, tiz″e-o-ther″ah-pist) (*obs.*) one who makes a specialty of the treatment of phthisis (tuberculosis).

phthisiotherapy (tiz″e-o-ther′ah-pe) [*phthisis* + *therapy*] the treatment of phthisis.

phthisis (ti′sis) [Gr. *phthisis*, from *phthien* to decay] 1. a wasting away of the body or a part of the body. 2. tuberculosis especially of the lungs. **abdominal p.**, tuberculosis of the intestines and mesenteric glands. **aneurysmal p.**, the clinical symptoms of chest pain and cough, at first dry and later productive, sometimes with hemoptysis, produced by aneurysm of the ascending aorta and the aortic arch. **bacillary p.**, that due to *Mycobacterium tuberculosis*. **black p.**, pneumoconiosis of coal workers. **p. bul′bi**, shrinkage and wasting of the eyeball. **colliers′ p.**, pneumoconiosis of coal workers. **p. cor′neae**, the shriveling and disappearance of the cornea after suppurative keratitis. **diabetic p.**, caseous tuberculous bronchopneumonia in diabetic patients. **dorsal p.**, tuberculosis of the spine. **essential p.** (of the eye), ophthalmomalacia. **fibroid p.**, chronic tuberculosis in which fibrous tissue is developed in the lung; fibrotuberculosis. **flax dressers′ p.**, a form of pneumoconiosis occurring in flax dressers. **glandular p.**, tuberculous lymphadenitis. **grinders′ p.**, a combination of tuberculosis and pneumoconiosis occurring among grinders. **hepatic p.**, tuberculosis of the liver. **laryngeal p.**, tuberculosis of the larynx. **Mediterranean p.**, brucellosis. **miner's p.**, pneumoconiosis of coal workers. **p. nodo′sa**, acute miliary tuberculosis. **nonbacillary p.**, presumptive tuberculosis without demonstration of *Mycobacterium tuberculosis*. **ocular p.**, ophthalmomalacia. **p. pancreat′ica**, a wasted condition associated with disease of the pancreas. **potters′ p.**, a combination of tuberculosis and silicosis of the lungs in potters. **pulmonary p.**, tuberculosis of the lung. **p. rena′lis**, tuberculosis of the kidney. **stone cutters′ p.**, tuberculosis and pneumoconiosis of stone cutters. **p. ventric′uli** (*obs.*), atrophy of the mucous membrane of the stomach and alimentary canal.

phyco- [Gr. *phykos* seaweed] a combining form denoting relationship to seaweed or algae.

phycobilin (fi″ko-bil′in) any of a group of protein-linked pigments including phycoerythrin (red pigment) and phycocyanin (blue pigment), which are found in the red and the blue-green algae.

phycochrome (fi′ko-krōm) [*phyco-* + Gr. *chrōma* color] 1. a blue-green pigment from various fresh-water algae of the simplest type. 2. any of the algae that contain both chlorophyll and a blue pigment; the blue-green algae.

phycochromoprotein (fi″ko-kro′mo-pro′te-in) a colored, conjugated protein, with respiratory function, found in various seaweeds.

phycocyanin (fi″ko-si′an-in) a blue chromoprotein found in blue-green algae.

phycocyanogen (fi″ko-si-an′o-jen) a blue pigment derived from blue-green algae.

phycoerythrin (fi″ko-er′ĭ-thrin) a red chromoprotein found in red algae.

phycologist (fi-kol′o-jist) a specialist in phycology; called also *algologist*.

phycology (fi-kol′o-je) [*phyco-* + *-logy*] the scientific study of algae; algology.

Phycomycetae (fi″ko-mi-se′te) Phycomycetes.

Phycomycetes (fi″ko-mi-se′tēz) [*phyco-* + Gr. *mykēs* fungus] a group of fungi comprising the common water, leaf, and bread molds, and including the classes Chytridiomycetes, Oomycetes, and Zygomycetes. In some classifications, considered to be a class of the Eumycetes, with the subordinate categories as subclasses.

phycomycetosis (fi″ko-mi-sĕ-to′sis) infection with fungi of the group Phycomycetes; see *phycomycosis*. **subcutaneous p.**, subcutaneous phycomycosis.

phycomycetous (fi″ko-mi-se′tus) of or pertaining to fungi of the group Phycomycetes.

phycomycosis (fi″ko-mi-ko′sis) any of a group of acute mycoses caused by fungi of the group Phycomycetes, including species of *Absidia, Mucor, Rhizopus, Hyphomyces, Basidiobolus, Entomophthora*, and *Mortierella*; it may involve the sinuses, orbital tissue, central nervous system, lungs, gastrointestinal tract, skin, and subcutaneous tissue. Except in the subcutaneous form, it is characterized by inflammation and vascular thrombosis of the blood vessels of the organ involved. Most infections occur in diabetics; other predisposing factors include primary debilitating disease and therapy with antimetabolites, steroids, or antibiotics. **cerebral p.**, a form affecting the brain, due to extension of rhinophycomycosis through the ophthalmic and carotid arteries, resulting in orbital involvement, infarction of the brain, and meningitis; it usually develops in acidotic diabetics. **p. entomoph′thorae**, rhinophycomycosis. **subcutaneous p.**, a chronic infection caused by *Basidiobolus haptosporus*, in which gradually enlarging nodules (eosinophilic granulomas) form in the subcutaneous tissues of the arms, chest, and trunk. Multiple purulent ulcers may develop. It occurs in Indonesia, central Africa, and India, affecting chiefly children and adolescents. Unlike the other phycomycoses, it is unassociated with any apparent predisposing factors.

phygogalactic (fi″go-gah-lak′tik) [Gr. *pheugein* to avoid + *gala* milk] checking the secretion of milk; galactophygous.

phyla (fi′lah) plural of *phylum*.

phylacagogic (fi-lak″ah-goj′ik) [Gr. *phylakē* a guarding + *agōgos* leading] inducing the formation of phylaxins or protective antibodies.

phylactic (fi-lak′tik) [Gr. *phylaktikos* preservative] serving to protect; pertaining to or producing phylaxis.

phylactotransfusion (fi-lak′to-trans-fu′zhun) immunotransfusion.

phylaxiology (fi-lak″se-ol′o-je) [Gr. *phylaxis* a guarding + *-logy*] the study and practice of phylaxis or protection against infection.

phylaxis (fi-lak′sis) [Gr. "a guarding"] protection against infection; the bodily defense against infection.

phyletic (fi-let′ik) pertaining to a phylum, or to phylogeny.

Phyllanthus (fil-lan′thus) a genus of plants. **P. eng′leri**, a plant of northern Rhodesia known as suicide plant; when the bark or root is smoked it causes death.

phyllidea (fil-id′e-ah) bothridium.

phyllo- [Gr. *phyllon* leaf] a combining form denoting relationship to leaves.

phyllochlorin (fil″o-klo′rin) a compound of chlorophyll and protein.

phyllode (fil′ode) [Gr. *phyllon* leaf + *eidos* form] resembling a leaf; a term applied to tumors which on section show a lobulated, leaflike appearance.

phylloerythrin (fil″o-er′ĭ-thrin) a derivative of chlorophyll formed in the intestinal canal of ruminant animals and found also in their bile.

phyllolith (fil′o-lith) a small concretion 100 to 200 μ in diameter formed of concentric strata, occurring in cavities in renal tuberculosis.

phylloporphyrin (fil″o-por′fĭ-rin) a compound, $C_{32}H_{34}N_4O_2$, from chlorophyll, very similar to hematoporphyrin.

phyllopyrrole (fil″o-pir′ol) trimethylethylpyrrole, $(CH_3)_3C_4$-$(NH)C_2H_5$, from bile pigments.

phylloquinone (fil″o-kwin′ōn) phytonadione.

phylloxanthine (fil″o-san′thin) a compound formed together with phyllocyanic acid by treating chlorophyll with hydrochloric acid.

phylobiology (fi″lo-bi-ol′o-je) [Gr. *phylon* tribe + *biology*] the application of scientific methods in the field of human behavior.

phylogenesis (fi″lo-jen′ĕ-sis) phylogeny.

phylogenetic (fi″lo-jĕ-net′ik) phylogenic.

phylogenic (fi-lo-jen′ik) pertaining to phylogeny.

phylogeny (fi-loj′ĕ-ne) [Gr. *phylon* tribe + *genesis* generation] the complete developmental history of a race or group of animals. Cf. *ontogeny*.

phylum (fi′lum), pl. **phy′la** [L.; Gr. *phylon* race] a primary or main division of the animal or of the vegetable kingdom, grouping organisms which are assumed to have a common ancestry.

phyma (fi′mah), pl. **phy′mata** [Gr. "a growth"] any skin tumor or cutaneous tubercle, especially a circumscribed swelling on the skin, larger than a tubercle, and produced by exudation into the subcutaneous tissue or the corium.

phymata (fi′mah-tah) [Gr.] plural of *phyma*.

phymatology (fi″mah-tol′o-je) [Gr. *phyma* a growth + *-logy*] the study of tumors, now called oncology.

phymatorhusin (fi″mah-to-roo′sin) [Gr. *phyma* a growth + *rhysis* flow] a dark pigment from hair and melanotic tumors; it is a form of melanin.

phymatorrhysin (fi″mah-to-ris′in) phymatorhusin.

Physalia (fi-sa′le-ah) a genus of hydrozoans, the Portuguese man-of-war, characterized by a large, purple air sac that allows them to float on the surface of the water, and from which many long tentacles of stinging polyps hang. The tentacles are equipped with nematocysts that are able to penetrate the skin of man, causing intense pain; paralysis sometimes results from numerous stings.

physalides (fi-sal′ĭ-dēz) plural of *physalis*.

physaliferous (fis″ah-lif′er-us) [*physalis* + L. *ferre* to bear] physaliphorous.

physaliform (fi-sal′ĭ-form) [*physalis* + L. *forma* shape] resembling bubbles.

physaliphore (fi-sal′ĭ-fōr) [*physalis* + Gr. *phorein* to carry] a globular cavity in certain brood cells of cancers; more correctly, the cell itself which contains such a cavity.

physaliphorous (fis″ah-lif′o-rus) [*physalis* + Gr. *phoros* bearing] containing bubbles or vacuoles.

physalis (fis′ah-lis), pl. **physal′ides** [Gr. *physallis* bubble] 1. a large brood cell from a cancer. 2. a spherical cavity found in certain cells, such as the large brood cells of cancers or the giant cells of sarcoma.

physallization (fis″al-i-za′shun) [Gr. *physallis* bubble] the formation of a permanent froth when a liquid is shaken together with a gas.

Physaloptera (fis"ah-lop'ter-ah) [Gr. *physallis* bubble + *pteron* wing] a genus of nematode worms of the family Spiruroidea, found in the stomach and intestine of man and other vertebrates. **P. caucas'ica,** a species occurring in the Caucasus and in Africa. **P. mor'dens,** *P. caucasica.* **P. ra'ra,** a species found in the stomach of dogs. **P. trunca'ta,** a species found in the proventriculus of chickens and pheasants.

physalopteriasis (fis"ah-lop-ter-i'ah-sis) infection with *Physaloptera.*

physeal (fiz'e-al) pertaining to growth, or to the segment of tubular bone which is concerned mainly with growth (the physis).

physiatrician (fiz"e-ah-trish'an) physiatrist.

physiatrics (fiz"e-at'riks) [*physio-* + Gr. *iatrike* surgery, medicine] that branch of medicine which deals with the diagnosis, treatment, and prevention of disease with the aid of physical agents, such as light, heat, cold, water, and electricity, or with mechanical apparatus; physical medicine.

physiatrist (fiz"e-at'rist) a physician who specializes in physiatrics.

physiatry (fiz'e-at"re) physiatrics.

physic (fiz'ik) [Gr. *physikos* natural] 1. the art of medicine and of therapeutics. 2. a medicine, especially a cathartic.

physical (fiz'e-kal) [Gr. *physikos*] pertaining to the body, to material things, or to physics.

physician (fi-zish'un) 1. an authorized practitioner of medicine, as one graduated from a college of medicine or osteopathy and licensed by the appropriate board. See also *doctor.* 2. one who practices medicine as distinct from surgery. **p. assistant,** one who has been trained in an accredited program and certified by an appropriate board to perform certain of a physician's duties, including history taking, physical examination, diagnostic tests, treatment, certain minor surgical procedures, etc., all under the responsible supervision of a licensed physician. Abbreviated P.A. See also *Medex.* **attending p.,** a physician who attends a hospital at stated times to visit the patients and give directions as to their treatment. **emergency p.,** a specialist in emergency medicine. **family p.,** a medical specialist who plans and provides the comprehensive primary health care of all members of a family, regardless of age or sex, on a continuing basis. **resident p.,** a graduate and licensed physician resident in a hospital.

Physick's operation, pouches (fiz'iks) [Philip Syng *Physick,* American surgeon, 1768–1837] see under *operation* and *pouch.*

physicochemical (fiz"i-ko-kem'i-kal) pertaining to physics and chemistry.

physicogenic (fiz"i-ko-jen'ik) due to physical causes; of physical origin, as opposed to *psychogenic.*

physicotherapeutics, physicotherapy (fiz"i-ko-ther"ah-pu'-tiks; fiz"i-ko-ther'ah-pe) physical therapy.

physics (fiz'iks) [Gr. *physis* nature] the science of the laws and phenomena of nature, but especially of the forces and general properties of matter and energy.

physio- (fiz'e-o) [Gr. *physis* nature] a combining form denoting relationship to nature, as in *physionomy,* or to physiology, as in *physiochemistry,* or denoting physical, as in *physiotherapy.*

physiochemical (fiz"e-o-kem'i-kal) pertaining to physiologic chemistry, or clinical chemistry.

physiochemistry (fiz"e-o-kem'is-tre) physiologic chemistry, or clinical chemistry.

physiocracy (fiz"e-ok'rah-se) [*physio-* + Gr. *kratein* to rule] the passive tendency in therapeutics which permits nature to take its course with little interference by man. Cf. *anthropocracy.*

physiogenesis (fiz"e-o-jen'e-sis) embryology.

physiognomy (fiz"e-og'no-me) [*physio-* + Gr. *gnomon* a judge] 1. the determination of mental or moral character and qualities by the face. 2. the countenance, or face. 3. the facial expression and appearance as a means of diagnosis.

physiognosis (fiz"e-og-no'sis) [*physio-* + Gr. *gnosis* knowledge] diagnosis by means of the facial expression or appearance.

physiologic (fiz"e-o-loj'ik) normal; not pathologic; characteristic of or conforming to the normal functioning or state of the body or a tissue or organ; physiological.

physiological (fiz"e-o-loj'i-kal) pertaining to physiology; physiologic.

physiologicoanatomical (fiz"e-o-loj"e-ko-an"ah-tom'e-kal) pertaining to physiology and anatomy.

physiologist (fiz"e-ol'o-jist) a specialist in the study of physiology.

physiology (fiz"e-ol'o-je) [*physio-* + -*logy*] 1. the science which treats of the functions of the living organism and its parts, and of the physical and chemical factors and processes involved. 2. the basic processes underlying the functioning of a species or class of organism, or any of its parts or processes. **animal p.,** the physiology of animals. **comparative p.,** a study of organ functions in various types of animals, vertebrate and invertebrate, in an effort to find fundamental relations in the physiology of

members of the entire animal kingdom. **dental p.,** the study of the function and functional form of the teeth and supporting tissues. **general p.,** the science of the general laws of life and functional activity. **hominal p.,** human physiology. **morbid p., pathologic p.,** the study of disordered function or of function in diseased tissues. **special p.,** the physiology of particular organs. **vegetable p.,** the physiology of plants.

physiolysis (fiz"e-ol'i-sis) [*physio-* + Gr. *lysis* dissolution] natural dissolution and disintegration of tissue.

physiomedical (fiz"e-o-med'i-kal) of or relating to physiomedicalism.

physiomedicalism (fiz"e-o-med'i-kal-izm) [*physio-* + *medicalism*] a system of medical treatment in which only plant remedies are used, excluding those which are poisonous.

physiometry (fiz"e-om'e-tre) [*physio-* + Gr. *metron* measure] measurement of the physiologic functions of the body by serologic and physiologic methods.

physioneurosis (fiz"e-o-nu-ro'sis) true neurosis.

physionomy (fiz"e-on'o-me) [*physio-* + Gr. *nomos* law] the science of the laws of nature.

physiopathic (fiz"e-o-path'ik) [*physio-* + Gr. *pathos* disease] Babinski's term for the nonpsychopathic functional nervous disorders.

physiopathologic (fiz"e-o-path"o-loj'ik) pertaining to both the physiologic and pathologic conditions.

physiopathology (fiz"e-o-pah-thol'o-je) [*physio-* + *pathology*] the science of functions in disease, or as modified by disease.

physiophyly (fiz"e-of'i-le) [*physio-* + Gr. *phylon* tribe] the evolution of bodily functions.

physiotherapeutist (fiz"e-o-ther"ah-pu'tist) physical therapist.

physiotherapist (fiz"e-o-ther'ah-pist) physical therapist.

physiotherapy (fiz"e-o-ther'a-pe) [*physio-* + Gr. *therapeia* cure] physical therapy.

physique (fi-zek') bodily structure, organization, and development.

physis (fi'sis) [Gr. *phyein* to generate] the segment of tubular bone which is concerned mainly with growth in length of the bone. It consists of four zones: zone of resting cartilage, zone of proliferating cartilage, zone of hypertrophy, and zone of calcification.

physo- (fi'so) [Gr. *physa* air] a combining form denoting relationship to air or gas.

physocele (fi'so-sel) [*physo-* + Gr. *kele* tumor] 1. a tumor filled with gas. 2. a hernial sac filled with gas.

Physocephalus (fi"so-sef'ah-lus) a genus of nematode worms of the superfamily Spiruroidea. **P. sexala'tus,** a species found in the stomach of pigs.

physocephaly (fi"so-sef'ah-le) [*physo-* + Gr. *kephale* head] emphysematous swelling of the head.

physohematometra (fi"so-hem"ah-to-me'trah) [*physo-* + Gr. *haima* blood + *metra* uterus] the presence of gas and blood within the uterus.

physohydrometra (fi"so-hi"dro-me'trah) [*physo-* + Gr. *hydor* water + *metra* uterus] the presence of gas and fluid within the uterus.

physometra (fi"so-me'trah) [*physo-* + Gr. *metra* uterus] air or gas in the uterine cavity.

Physopsis (fi-sop'sis) a subgenus of snails (genus *Bulinus*), several species of which are the intermediate hosts of *Schistosoma haematobium* and other animal schistosomes.

physopyosalpinx (fi"so-pi"o-sal'pinks) [*physo-* + Gr. *pyon* pus + *salpinx* tube] presence of pus and gas in the uterine tube.

Physostigma (fi"so-stig'mah) [*physo-* + Gr. *stigma* stigma] a genus of tropical leguminous plants. The poisonous seed of *P. venenosum* Balf., Calabar bean, a climbing plant of Africa, contains the alkaloid, physostigmine.

physostigmine (fi"so-stig'men) [USP] chemical name: (3a-*cis*)-1,2,3,3a,8,8a-hexahydro-1,3a,8-trimethylpyrrolo[2,3-*b*]indol-5-ol methylcarbamate (ester). An alkaloid, $C_{15}H_{21}N_3O_2$, occurring as a white odorless crystalline powder, usually obtained from the dried ripe seed (Calabar bean) of *Physostigma venenosum* Balf. (Leguminosae); it is a cholinergic that functions as an anticholinesterase. Called also *eserine.* **p. salicylate** [USP], the salicylate salt of physostigmine, $C_{15}H_{21}N_3O_2C_7H_6O_3$, occurring as white, shining crystals or white powder; used mainly as an ophthalmic cholinergic to produce miosis and to decrease intraocular pressure in the treatment of glaucoma, applied to the conjunctiva. It is also administered intramuscularly and intravenously to reverse the toxic effects upon the central nervous system due to drugs capable of causing anticholinergic poisoning. **p. sulfate** [USP], the sulfate salt of physostigmine, $(C_{15}H_{21}N_3O_2)_2 \cdot H_2SO_4$, occurring as a white, microcrystalline powder; used mainly as an ophthalmic cholinergic to decrease intraocular pressure in the treatment of glaucoma, applied topically to the conjunctiva.

physostigminism (fi"so-stig'min-izm) poisoning by physostigmine.

phytagglutinin (fi″tah-gloo′tĭ-nin) a phytotoxin which has the power of agglutinating red blood corpuscles.

phytalbumin (fi″tal-bu′min) [*phyto-* + *albumin*] vegetable albumin.

phytalbumose (fi-tal′bu-mōs) [*phyto-* + *albumose*] an albumose of vegetable origin.

phytase (fi′tās) an enzyme (a hydrolase) of plants that catalyzes the hydrolysis of phytic acid to inositol and phosphoric acid.

phytate persodium (fi′tāt) chemical name: *myo*-inositol hexakis(dihydrogen phosphate) dodecasodium salt; a pharmaceutic aid, $C_6H_6Na_{12}O_{24}P_6$.

phytin (fi′tin) the calcium-magnesium salt of phytic acid; a form of inositol found in plants, it is used as a dietary supplement.

phyto- (fi′to) [Gr. *phyton* plant] a combining form denoting relationship to a plant or plants.

phytoalexin (fi″to-ah-lek′sin) any of a group of compounds formed in plants in response to elicitors released by plant pathogens; they inhibit or destroy the pathogen.

phytoanaphylactogen (fi″to-an″ah-fi-lak′to-jen) [*phyto-* + *anaphylactogen*] an antigen of plant origin that is capable of inducing anaphylaxis; called also *phytosensitinogen*.

phytobezoar (fi″to-be′zōr) [*phyto-* + *bezoar*] a gastric concretion composed of vegetable matter such as skins, seeds, and the fibers of fruit and vegetables.

phytochemistry (fi″to-kem′is-tre) [*phyto-* + *chemistry*] the study of plant chemistry, including the chemical processes that take place in plants, the nature of plant chemicals, and the various applications of such chemicals to science and industry.

phytochinin (fi″to-kin′in) a substance isolated from the leaves of certain grasses, said to have an effect on carbohydrate metabolism resembling that of insulin.

phytocholesterol (fi″to-ko-les′ter-ol) phytosterol.

phytochrome (fi″to-krōm) [*phyto-* + Gr. *chrōma* color] a bluish conjugated protein occurring in plants, whose response to relative periods of light and darkness regulates photoperiodism (e.g., the flowering cycle); it occurs in two forms, one responding to the red end of the spectrum, the other to far red.

phytodemic (fi″to-dem′ik) [*phyto-* + *epidemic*] an epidemic attack of any disease of plants.

phytodetritus (fi″to-de-tri′tus) detritus produced by the disintegration and decomposition of vegetable organisms. Cf. *zoodetritus*.

phytogenesis (fi″to-jen′ĕ-sis) [*phyto-* + Gr. *genesis* generation] the origin and development of plants.

phytogenetic, phytogenic (fi″to-jĕ-net′ik; fi″to-jen′ik) phytogenous.

phytogenous (fi-toj′ĕ-nus) [*phyto-* + Gr. *gennan* to produce] derived from a plant, or caused by a vegetable growth.

phytohemagglutinin (fi″to-hem″ah-gloo′tĭ-nin) a hemagglutinin of plant origin.

phytohormone (fi″to-hor′mōn) [*phyto-* + *hormone*] plant hormone; any of the hormones produced naturally in plants and which are active in minute amounts in controlling growth and other functions at a site remote from the place of production. There are three principal types: auxins, cytokinins, and gibberellins.

phytoid (fi′toid) [*phyto-* + Gr. *eidos* form] resembling a plant.

phytol (fi′tol) chemical name: 3,7,11,15-tetramethylhexadecen-2-ol-1. An unsaturated aliphatic alcohol, $CH_3[CH(CH_3)\text{-}(CH_2)_3]_3C(CH_3):CH\cdot CH_2OH$, which is related to xanthophyll, to the carotenoids, and to vitamin A, and exists in chlorophyll as an ester; used in the preparation of vitamin E and phytonadione.

Phytomastigophora (fi″to-mas″tĭ-gof′o-rah) a class of small, plantlike, flagellate protozoa of the subphylum Mastigophora that closely resemble algae. Most are free-living, but some are parasitic, and most have chromatophores containing chlorophyll and secrete a cellulose covering which varies in thickness. It includes the orders Chrysomonadina, Dinoflagellata, Euglenoidina, and Phytomonadina.

phytomelin (fi″to-mel′in) rutin.

phytomenadione (fi″to-men″ah-di′ōn) phytonadione.

phytomitogen (fi″to-mi′to-jen) a substance of plant origin that induces mitosis in human cells.

Phytomonadina (fi″to-mon-ah-di′nah) an order of protozoa of the class Phytomastigophora, subphylum Mastigophora, comprising plantlike flagellates. In former classifications, it was included, along with the order Protomonadina, in the group Monadina.

Phytomonas (fi-tom′o-nas) 1. a genus of flagellate parasitic protozoa of the family Trypanosomatidae, order Protomastigida, morphologically similar to the genus *Leptomonas;* the organisms are found in hemipterous insects and latex plants, being transmitted from plant to plant by the insect vector. 2. formerly, a genus of bacteria producing pathogenic necroses in plants, whose members are now included in the genera *Pseudomonas* and *Xanthomonas.*

phytonadione (fi″to-nah-di′ōn) 1. chemical name: [*R*-[*R**,*R**-(*E*)]]-2-methyl-3-(3,7,-11,15-tetramethyl-2-hexadecenyl)-1,4-naph-

thalenedione. A fat-soluble vitamin of the K group, $C_{31}H_{46}O_2$, found in green plants or prepared synthetically and having prothrombinogenic properties. 2. [USP] a clear, yellow to amber, very viscous liquid containing 97 to 103 per cent phytonadione; used as a prothrombinogenic agent in the treatment of hypoprothrombinemia due to various causes, administered orally and parenterally. Called also *phylloquinone* and *vitamin K₁*.

phytone (fi′tōn) a peptone made from plant protein.

phytonosis (fi-ton′o-sis) [*phyto-* + Gr. *nosos* disease] any morbid condition due to a plant.

phytoparasite (fi″to-par′ah-sīt) [*phyto-* + *parasite*] any parasitic vegetable organism or species.

phytopathogenic (fi″to-path′o-jen′ik) producing disease in plants.

phytopathology (fi″to-pah-thol′o-je) [*phyto-* + *pathology*] 1. the study of plant diseases and their control. 2. the pathology of morbid conditions caused by schizomycetes and other vegetable parasites.

phytopathy (fi-top′ah-the) [*phyto-* + Gr. *pathos* disease] any disease of plants.

phytophagous (fi-tof′ah-gus) [*phyto-* + Gr. *phagein* to eat] eating vegetable food.

phytopharmacology (fi″to-fahr″mah-kol′o-je) [*phyto-* + *pharmacology*] the study of the effect of drugs on plant growth.

phytophotodermatitis (fi″to-fo″to-der″mah-ti′tis) phototoxic dermatitis induced by exposure to certain plants (meadow grass, lime, fig, bergamot, etc.) and then to sunlight.

phytoplankton (fi″to-plank′ton) [*phyto-* + Gr. *planktos* wandering] the minute plant (vegetable) organisms which, with those of the animal kingdom, make up the plankton of natural waters.

phytoplasm (fi′to-plazm) [*phyto-* + Gr. *plasma* thing formed] vegetable protoplasm.

phytoprecipitin (fi″to-pre-sip′ĭ-tin) a precipitin produced by immunization with protein substances of plant origin.

phytosensitinogen (fi″to-sen″sĭ-tin′o-jen) [*phyto-* + *sensitinogen*] phytoanaphylactogen.

phytosis (fi-to′sis) [*phyto-* + *-osis*] any disease caused by a phytoparasite.

phytosterin (fi-tos′ter-in) [*phyto-* + Gr. *stear* fat] phytosterol.

phytosterol (fi″to-ste′rol) a plant sterol.

phytosterolin (fi″to-ste′rol-in) a glucosidic union of a sterol and glucose.

phytotherapy (fi″to-ther′ah-pe) [*phyto-* + Gr. *therapeia* treatment] treatment by use of plants.

phytotoxic (fi″to-tok′sik) 1. pertaining to a phytotoxin, or plant poison. 2. inhibiting the growth of plants.

phytotoxin (fi″to-tok′sin) an exotoxin produced by certain species of higher plants, notably *Abrus precatorius* (abrin), *Ricinus communis* (ricin), *Croton tiglium* (crotin), and *Robinia pseudacacia* (robin). Phytotoxins are resistant to proteolytic digestion, and are effective when taken by mouth. In the broadest sense a phytotoxin is any toxic substance of plant origin.

phytotrichobezoar (fi″to-tri″ko-be′zōr) [*phyto-* + Gr. *thrix* hair + *bezoar*] a bezoar composed of both plant fibers and hair.

phytotron (fi′to-tron) a laboratory in which virtually any climatic condition can be simulated for plant growth studies.

phytovitellin (fi″to-vi-tel′in) vitellin of vegetable origin.

phytoxylin (fi-tok′sĭ-lin) [*phyto-* + Gr. *xylon* wood] a substance resembling pyroxylin; used in preparing celloidin sections.

P.I. protamine insulin.

pI the pH of a solution containing a solute at its isoelectric point.

pia (pi′ah) [L.] 1. tender; soft. 2. pia mater. **p. ma′ter,** see *pia mater*, below.

pia-arachnitis (pi″ah-ar″ak-ni′tis) inflammation of the pia-arachnoid; leptomeningitis.

pia-arachnoid (pi″ah-ah-rak′noid) [*pia* + *arachnoid*] the pia mater and the arachnoid considered together as one functional unit; the leptomeninges.

pia-glia (pi″ah-gli′ah) a membrane formed by the fusion of the pia mater and the marginal glia, and constituting one of the layers of the pia-arachnoid.

pial (pi′al) pertaining to the pia mater.

pia mater (pi′ah ma′ter) [L. "tender mother"] the innermost of the three membranes (meninges) covering the brain and spinal cord, investing them closely and extending into the depths of the fissures and sulci; it consists of reticular, elastic, and collagenous fibers. **p. m. enceph′ali** [NA], the pia mater covering the brain, very thin over the cerebral cortex, and thicker over the brain stem; the blood vessels for the brain ramify within it and, as they enter the brain, are accompanied for a short distance by a pial sheath. **p. m. spina′lis** [NA], the pia mater covering the spinal cord and consisting of collagenous fibers, which also form the denticulate ligament, and reticular fibers, which closely invest the cord, form the various septa, and form an investment for the rootlets.

piamatral (pi″ah-ma′tral) pial.

pian (pe-ahn′) [Fr.] yaws. **p. bois,** a form of cutaneous leishmaniasis of the New World, caused by *Leishmania brasiliensis guyanensis,* transmitted by the sandfly *Lutzomyia anduzei,* occurring in the forests of the Guyanas and into Brazil and Venezuela, and characterized by multiple, widespread, deep skin ulcers with occasional involvement of the oronasal mucosa. Called also *forest yaws.* **hemorrhagic p.,** verruga peruana.

piarachnitis (pi″ar-ak-ni′tis) pia-arachnitis.

piarachnoid (pi″ar-ak′noid) pia-arachnoid.

piarhemia (pi″ar-he′me-ah) [Gr. *piar* fat + *haima* blood + *-ia*] the presence of fat in the blood; lipemia.

piastrinemia (pi-as″trĭ-ne′me-ah) [It. *piastre* coin + Gr. *haima* blood + *-ia*] thrombocythemia.

piblokto (pĭ-blok′to) [Eskimo] a psychic disturbance seen chiefly among Eskimo women, marked by attacks of hysteria and running naked through the snow, sometimes with suicidal or homicidal tendencies.

pica (pi′kah) [L.] a craving for unnatural articles of food; a depraved appetite, as seen in hysteria, pregnancy, and in malnourished children.

piceous (pi′se-us) [L. *piceis*] of the nature of or resembling pitch.

Pick's cell, disease (piks) [Ludwig *Pick,* Berlin physician, born 1868] see under *cell,* and *Niemann-Pick disease,* under *disease.*

Pick's convolution atrophy, disease (piks) [Arnold *Pick,* Prague psychiatrist, 1851–1924] see *lobar atrophy,* under *atrophy.*

Pick's disease, syndrome [Friedel *Pick,* Prague physician, 1867–1926] see under *disease* (def. 2), and under *syndrome.*

pickling (pik′ling) the process of cleansing metallic surfaces of the product of oxidation and other impurities by immersion in acid.

Pickrell's solution, spray (method) (pik′rel) [Kenneth LeRoy *Pickrell,* American physician, born 1910] see under *solution* and *spray.*

pickwickian syndrome (pik-wik′e-an) [from the description of the fat boy in Dickens' *Pickwick Papers*] see under *syndrome.*

pico- [Sp. *pico* small amount; It. *piccolo* small] a combining form used in naming units of measurement to indicate one-trillionth of the unit designated by the root with which it is combined (10^{-12}).

picocurie (pi″ko-ku′re) a unit of radioactivity, being 10^{-12} curie, or that quantity of radioactive material in which the number of nuclear disintegrations is 3.7×10^{-2}, or 0.037, per second. Abbreviated pc. Called also *micromicrocurie.*

picodnavirus (pi-kod″nah-vi′rus) [*pico-* + *d*eoxyribo*n*ucleic *a*cid + *virus*] parvovirus.

picogram (pi′ko-gram) a unit of mass (weight) of the metric system, being 10^{-12} gram. Abbreviated pg. Called also *microgamma* and *micromicrogram.*

picopicogram (pi″ko-pi′ko-gram) a unit of mass (weight) of the metric system, being 10^{-12} picogram, or 10^{-24} gram. Abbreviated ppg.

picornavirus (pi-kor″nah-vi′rus) [*pico-* + *ribo*nucleic *acid* + *virus*] a name applied to one of the extremely small ether-resistant RNA viruses, the group comprising the enteroviruses and the rhinoviruses.

picounit (pi″ko-u′nit) one trillionth part of a unit (10^{-12}).

picrate (pik′rāt) any salt of picric acid; a carbozoate.

picro- (pik′ro) [Gr. *pikros* bitter] a combining form meaning bitter.

picrocarmine (pik″ro-kar′min) a stain prepared from picric acid and carmine and used in microscopy. It consists of a mixture of carmine, ammonia, and distilled water, to which is added an aqueous solution of picric acid.

picrogeusia (pik″ro-gu′se-ah) [*picro-* + Gr. *geusis* taste + *-ia*] a pathologic bitter taste.

picrol (pik′rol) chemical name: potassium diiodoresorcin monosulfonate. A colorless and odorless, bitter, antiseptic powder, $(OH)_2 \cdot C_6HI_2 \cdot SO_2OK$, which contains about 53 per cent iodine; used as a substitute for iodoform and corrosive sublimate.

picronigrosin (pik″ro-ni-gro′sin) a solution of picric acid and nigrosin in alcohol, used as a stain.

picropodophyllin (pik″ro-pod″o-fil′in) chemical name: picropodophyllinic acid lactone. A crystalline principle, $C_{22}H_{22}O_8$, from *Podophyllum peltatum* L. (Berberidaceae): medicinally active. It is obtainable from podophyllotoxin also, and is an isomer of it.

Picrorrhiza (pik″ro-ri′zah) [*picro-* + Gr. *rhiza* root] a genus of herbs; the rhizome of *P. kurroa* Royle (Scrophulariaceae) is tonic and antiperiodic.

picrosaccharometer (pi″kro-sak″ah-rom′ĕ-ter) an instrument used in estimating diabetic sugar.

picrosclerotine (pik″ro-skle′ro-tin) a poisonous alkaloid occurring in ergot of rye.

picrotoxin (pik″ro-tok′sin) [NF] an active principle, $C_{30}H_{34}O_{13}$, obtained from the seed (cocculus indicus) of *Anamirta cocculus* L. Wight & Arn. (Menispermaceae), and occurring as flexible, shining, prismatic crystals or as a microcrystalline powder; it stimulates all portions of the central nervous system by blocking presynaptic inhibition of neural impulses and has been used as a central and respiratory stimulant in the treatment of poisoning by central nervous system depressant drugs, especially the barbiturates, administered intravenously. Called also *cocculin.*

picrotoxinism (pik″ro-tok′sĭ-nizm) poisoning by picrotoxin.

pictograph (pik′to-graf) a chart of silhouette pictures used for testing acuteness of vision of children.

piebald (pi′bawld) exhibiting piebaldism.

piebaldism (pi-bawld′izm) 1. a condition in which the skin is partly brown and partly white, as in partial albinism and vitiligo. 2. partial albinism.

piece (pēs) a part or portion. **chief p.,** principal p. **connecting p.,** 1. middle p. 2. the neck of a spermatozoon. **end p.,** 1. end-piece; see under E. 2. the terminal portion of the tail, or flagellum, of a spermatozoon; called also *terminal filament.* See illustration under *spermatozoon.* **middle p.,** the portion of the tail of a spermatozoon limited by the anterior centriole and by the annulus; called also *connecting p.* See also illustration under *spermatozoon.* **principal p.,** the main portion of the tail of a spermatozoon, beginning at the annulus and gradually tapering toward the end piece; called also *chief p.* See illustration under *spermatozoon.* **secretory p.,** a glycopeptide component of secretory (exocrine) IgA. Called also *secretory component.* See also *immunoglobulin.*

piedra (pe-a′drah) [Sp.] a fungal disease of the hair in which the shafts bear either white or black hard gritty nodular masses of fungi. **black p.,** a fungal disease that affects the hairs of the scalp in man and other primates, occurs mainly in tropical regions, and is caused by *Piedraia hortai.* **white p.,** piedra that affects the beard is caused by *Trichosporon cutaneum,* and occurs chiefly in temperate regions.

Piedraia (pi″ĕ-dri′ah) a genus of ascomycetous fungi of the family *Piedraiaceae,* one species of which, *P. hortae,* is parasitic on hair, forming small black adherent nodules; see *black piedra,* under *piedra.*

Piedraiaceae (pi″ĕ-dri-a′se-e) a family of ascomycetous fungi of the order Myriangiales, subclass Loculoascomycetidae, which includes the genus *Piedraia.*

pier (pēr) a natural tooth or root which helps support a partial denture elsewhere than at its termination; called also *intermediate abutment.*

Pierre Robin (pe-yair′ro-ba′) [*Pierre Robin,* French dentist, 1867–1950] see under *syndrome.*

Piersol's point (pēr′solz) [George Arthur *Piersol,* Philadelphia anatomist, 1856–1924] see under *point.*

piesesthesia (pi-e″zes-the′ze-ah) [Gr. *piesis* pressure + *aisthēsis* perception] pressure sensibility; the sense by which pressure stimuli are felt.

piesimeter (pi″e-sim′ĕ-ter) [Gr. *piesis* pressure + *metron* measure] an instrument for testing the sensitiveness of the skin to pressure. **Hales' p.,** a glass tube inserted into an artery for the purpose of ascertaining the blood pressure by the height to which the blood rises in the tube.

-piesis (pi-e′sis) [Gr. *piesis* a pressing or squeezing] a word termination meaning pressure, as in otopiesis.

piezallochromy (pi″e-zal′o-kro-me) [Gr. *piesis* pressure + *allochromy*] change of color of a substance caused by crushing.

piezesthesia (pi″e-zes-the′ze-ah) piesesthesia.

piezocardiogram (pi-e″zo-kar′de-o-gram″) a graphic tracing of the changes in pressure caused by pulsation of the heart, often recorded through the esophagus.

piezochemistry (pi-e″zo-kem″is-tre) [Gr. *piesis* pressure + *chemistry*] that branch of chemistry which deals with the effect of pressure on chemical phenomena.

piezometer (pi″e-zom′ĕ-ter) [Gr. *piezein* to press + *metron* measure] 1. piesimeter. 2. orbitonometer.

PIF proliferation-inhibiting factor; see under *factor.*

pifarnine (pĭ-far′nēn) chemical name: 1-(1,3-benzodioxol-5-ylmethyl)-4-(3,7,11-trimethyl-2,6,10-dodecatrienyl) piperazine; a gastric antiulcerative, $C_{27}H_{40}N_2O_2$.

pigment (pig′ment) [L. *pigmentum* paint] 1. any normal or abnormal coloring matter of the body. 2. a paintlike medicinal preparation to be applied to the skin. **autochthonous p.,** endogenous p. **bile p.,** any one of the coloring matters of the bile; they are bilirubin, biliverdin, bilifuscin, biliprasin, choleprasin, bilihumin, and bilicyanin. **blood p.,** any of the pigments derived from hemoglobin; they are heme, hematoidin, hemosiderin, hematoporphyrin, methemoglobin, and hemofuscin. **ceroid p.,** a coarsely globular, yellow, waxlike pigment found in the cirrhotic livers of rats kept on a low protein, low fat diet. **endogenous p.,** a pigment produced by the body's own metabolism. **exogenous p., extraneous p.,** a pigment which enters the body from without. **hematogenous p.,** any pigment derived from the blood or from the blood pigment. **hepatoge-**

nous p., bile pigment formed by disintegration of hemoglobin in the liver. **Lake's p.,** a mixture of lactic acid, formaldehyde solution, phenol, and water, suggested for relief of pain in laryngeal tuberculosis. **lipochrome p.,** lipochrome. **malarial p.,** a pigment formed by the malarial parasite from the pigment of the blood and deposited largely in the spleen and liver. **melanotic p.,** melanin. **metabolic p.,** any pigment produced by the metabolic actions of cells. **respiratory p's,** substances, such as hemoglobin, myoglobin, or the cytochromes, which take part in the oxidation processes of the animal body. **wear and tear p's,** lipochromes.

pigmentary (pig′men-ta″re) pertaining to or of the nature of a pigment.

pigmentation (pig″men-ta′shun) 1. the deposition of coloring matter; the coloration or discoloration of a part by a pigment. 2. coloration, especially abnormally increased coloration, by melanin. **carotinoid p.,** skin pigmentation by carotin and its congeners, usually a result of excessive ingestion of deep green or yellow fruits and vegetables. **exogenous p., extraneous p.,** pigmentation caused by coloring matter introduced from outside of the body. **hematogenous p.,** pigmentation produced by the accumulation of hemoglobin derivatives such as hematoidin or hemosiderin. **malarial p.,** a pigmentation due to the accumulation, especially in the spleen and liver, of the dark-brown pigment liberated by those red blood cells which are destroyed by malarial parasites. **vagabonds' p.** (obs.), see under disease.

pigmented (pig′ment-ed) colored by deposit of pigment.

pigmentogenesis (pig″men-to-jen′ĕ-sis) [pigment + genesis] the production of pigment.

pigmentogenic (pig″men-to-jen′ik) inducing the formation or deposit of pigment.

pigmentolysin (pig″men-tol′ĭ-sin) a lysin causing destruction of pigment.

pigmentolysis (pig″men-tol′ĭ-sis) [pigment + Gr. lysis dissolution] destruction of pigment.

pigmentophage (pig-men′to-fāj) [pigment + Gr. phagein to eat] any pigment-devouring cell, especially such a cell of the hair; called also chromophage.

pigmentophore (pig-men′to-for) a cell that transports pigment.

pigmentum (pig-men′tum) [L.] pigment.

Pignet's formula, (index, standard) (pēn-yāz′) [Maurice Charles-Joseph Pignet, French physician, born 1871] see under formula.

piitis (pi-i′tis) inflammation of the pia mater.

pikromycin (pik-ro-mi′sin) proactinomycin A.

Pil. abbreviation of L. pilula, pill, or pil′ulae, pills.

Pila (pi′lah) a genus of freshwater snails. **P. con′ica,** the second intermediate host of Echinostoma ilocanum in the Philippines.

pila (pi′lah), pl. pi′lae [L.] a pillar or pillar-like structure, such as a trabecula of spongy bone.

pilae (pi′le) [L.] plural of pila.

pilar, pilary (pi′lar, pil′a-re) [L. pilaris] pertaining to the hair.

pilaster (pi-las′ter) a ridge or fluting. **p. of Broca,** linea aspera femoris.

Pilcher bag (pil′cher) [Lewis Stephen Pilcher, Brooklyn surgeon, 1845–1934] see under bag.

pile (pīl) 1. [L. pila pillar] an aggregation of similar elements for generating electricity. In nucleonics, a chain-reacting fission device for producing slow neutrons and for the preparation of radioactive isotopes. 2. [L. pila a ball] a hemorrhoid. **esophageal p.,** a varix in the esophagus. **muscular p.,** layers of muscular tissue so arranged as to generate an electric current. **prostatic p.,** enlarged prostate attended by hemorrhage. **sentinel p.,** a hemorrhoid-like thickening of the mucous membrane at the lower end of a fissure of the anus. **thermoelectric p.,** a set of slender metallic bars which, on exposure to heat, generates a current of electricity that moves an index and is made to register delicate changes of temperature. **voltaic p.,** a battery for current electricity made up of a series of metallic disks.

piles (pīlz) hemorrhoids.

pileus (pi′le-us) [L. "a close fitting felt cap"] the membrane which sometimes covers a child's head at birth; caul.

pili (pi′li) [L.] plural of pilus.

pilial (pi′le-al) pertaining to a pilus or pili.

piliate (pi′le-at) having pili; said of bacteria.

Pilidae (pil′ĭ-de) a family of fresh-water snails (order Mesogastropoda) that includes the species Pila conica, the second intermediate host of Echinostoma ilocanum.

piliform (pi′lĭ-form) shaped like or resembling hair.

pilimictio (pi″lĭ-mik′she-o) pilimiction.

pilimiction (pi″lĭ-mik′shun) [L. pilus hair + mictio micturition] passing of urine containing hair or hairlike threads of mucus.

pilin (pi′lin) the protein that composes bacterial pili.

pill (pil) [L. pilula] a small globular or oval medicated mass to be swallowed. Pills contain, in addition to the active drug, a diluent (or filler) and an excipient to give the mass adhesiveness, firmness, and plasticity, so that the pill can be worked by hand or machine to the desired pillular form. Cf. tablet. **A.B.S. p.,** a laxative pill, containing aloin, extract of belladonna, and strychnine. **blue p.,** mercury mass. **chalybeate p's,** ferrous carbonate p's. **compound cathartic p.,** a pill of colocynth, calomel, jalap, and gamboge. **enteric p.,** one coated with a substance, such as salol, which will not dissolve in the stomach. **ferrous carbonate p's,** pills containing ferrous sulfate, potassium carbonate, sucrose, tragacanth, althea, glycerin, water; used as a hematinic. **ferruginous p's,** ferrous carbonate p's. **Fothergill's p.** (obs.), a pill of calomel, squill, and digitalis. **Guy's p.,** a pill composed of digitalis, squill, extract of hyoscyamus, and mercury mass. **hexylresorcinol p's** [NF], a pill consisting of hexylresorcinol covered with a rupture-resistant coating that disintegrates in the digestive tract; used as an anthelmintic against intestinal nematodes and trematodes. **radio p.,** telemetering capsule.

pillar (pil′ar) [L. pila] a supporting column, usually occurring in pairs. **p. of Corti's organ,** see pillar cells, under cell. **p's of diaphragm,** see pars lumbalis diaphragmatis. **p. of fauces, anterior,** arcus palatoglossus. **p. of fauces, posterior,** arcus palatopharyngeus. **p. of fornix, anterior,** columna fornicis. **p. of fornix, posterior,** crus fornicis. **p's of soft palate,** see arcus palatoglossus and arcus palatopharyngeus. **Uskow's p's,** two folds of the embryo attached to the dorsolateral portion of the body wall; from these pillars and the septum transversum the diaphragm is formed.

pillet (pil′et) a little pill, or pellet.

pillion (pil-yon′) a temporary replacement for an amputated leg.

pilo- (pi′lo) [L. pilus hair] a combining form denoting relationship to hair, resembling or composed of hair.

pilobezoar (pi″lo-be′zor) trichobezoar.

pilocarpine (pi″lo-kar′pin) chemical name: (3S-cis)-3-ethyldihydro-4-[(1-methyl-1H-imidazol-5-yl)methyl]-2(3H)-furanone. An alkaloid, $C_{11}H_{16}N_2O_2$, obtained from the leaves of Pilocarpus jaborandi or P. microphyllus, which has cholinergic activity. **p. hydrochloride** [USP], the monohydrochloride salt of pilocarpine, $C_{11}H_{16}N_2O_2 \cdot HCl$, occurring as colorless, translucent crystals; used mainly as an ophthalmic cholinergic to produce miosis and to decrease intraocular pressure in the treatment of glaucoma, applied topically to the conjunctiva. **p. nitrate** [USP], the nitrate salt of pilocarpine, $C_{11}H_{16}N_2O_2 \cdot HNO_3$, occurring as shining, white crystals, having the same actions and uses as the hydrochloride salt.

Pilocarpus (pi″lo-kar′pus) [Gr. pilos wool or hair wrought into felt + Gr. karpos fruit] a genus of rutaceous shrubs of tropical America; the leaves of P. jaborandi and P. microphyllus yield pilocarpine.

pilocystic (pi″lo-sis′tik) [pilo- + cystic] hollow, or cystlike, and containing hairs; said of certain dermoid tumors.

pilocytic (pi″lo-si′tik) composed of fiber-shaped cells.

piloerection (pi″lo-e-rek′shun) [pilo- + erection] erection of the hair.

pilojection (pi″lo-jek′shun) [pilo + L. jacere to throw] the introduction of one or more hairs into the sac of an aneurysm by means of a pneumatic gun, to furnish the nucleus for a blood clot inside the sac; used in the treatment of intracranial saccular aneurysms.

pilology (pi-lol′o-je) [pilo- + -logy] the study of the hair.

pilomatricoma (pi″lo-mah-trik-o′mah) a benign, sharply circumscribed, calcifying epithelial neoplasm derived from hair matrix cells, manifested as a firm intracutaneous spheroid mass from one to several centimeters in diameter, usually on the face, neck, and arms. Called also calcified epithelioma and calcifying epithelioma of Malherbe.

pilomatrixoma (pi″lo-ma-trik-so′mah) pilomatricoma.

pilomotor (pi″lo-mo′tor) [pilo- + L. motor mover] pertaining to the arrector muscles the contraction of which produces cutis anserina (goose flesh) and the erection of the hairs.

pilonidal (pi″lo-ni′dal) [pilo- + L. nidus nest] having hairs for a nidus; see under cyst and sinus.

pilose (pi′lōs) [L. pilosus] hairy; covered with hair.

pilosebaceous (pi″lo-sĕ-ba′shus) pertaining to the hair follicles and sebaceous glands.

Piltz's reflex, sign (pilts′ez) [Jan Piltz, Polish neurologist, 1870–1930] see attention reflex of pupil, under reflex, and Westphal-Piltz phenomenon, under phenomenon.

Piltz-Westphal phenomenon (pilts-vest′fahl) [Jan Piltz; A. K. O. Westphal, German neurologist, 1863–1941] see Westphal-Piltz phenomenon, under phenomenon.

pilula (pil′u-lah), pl. pil′ulae [L.] pill.

pilular (pil′u-lar) resembling or pertaining to a pill.

pilule (pil′ūl) [L. pilula] a small pill, or pellet.

pilus (pi′lus), pl. pi′li [L.] 1. [NA] any of the filamentous appendages of the skin, consisting of modified epidermal tissue; see hair.

2. [pl.] in microbiology, the minute filamentous appendages of certain bacteria; they are considerably smaller and less rigid than flagella and are associated with antigenic properties of the cell surface; called also *fimbria.* **p. annula′tus** (pl. *pi′li annula′ti*), a condition in which the individual hairs appear to be marked by alternating bands of white as a result of some barrier in the hair which prevents passage of light and causes the rays to be reflected back, giving the appearance of white bands. **p. cunicula′tus** (pl. *pi′li cunicula′ti*), burrowing hair. **p. incarna′tus** (pl. *pi′li incarna′ti*), ingrown hair. **p. incarna′tus recur′vus** (pl. *pi′li incarna′ti recur′vi*), ingrown hair that has repenetrated the skin after growing from the hair follicle. **pi′li multigem′ini,** multiple hairs growing from the same follicle, as a result of deep division of its base, producing, in effect, a cluster of separate papillae. **p. tor′tus** (pl. *pi′li tor′ti*), twisted hair.

Pima (pim′ah) trademark for a preparation of potassium iodide.

pimelitis (pim″ĕ-li′tis) [*pimelo- + -itis*] inflammation of the adipose tissue.

pimelo- (pim′ĕ-lo) [Gr. *pimelē* fat] a combining form denoting relationship to fat.

pimeloma (pim″ĕ-lo′mah) [*pimelo- + -oma*] a fatty tumor; lipoma.

pimelopterygium (pim″ĕ-lo-ter-ij′e-um) [*pimelo- +* Gr. *pterygion* wing] a fatty outgrowth upon the conjunctiva.

pimelorthopnea (pim″el-or″thop-ne′ah) [*pimelo- + orthopnea*] difficulty in breathing while lying down, due to excessive fatness.

pimelosis (pim″ĕ-lo′sis) [*pimelo- + -osis*] 1. conversion into fat. 2. fatness, or obesity.

pimeluria (pim″el-u′re-ah) [*pimelo- +* Gr. *ouron* urine *+ -ia*] the presence of fat in the urine.

Pimenta (pĭ-men′tah) [Sp. "allspice"] a genus of myrtaceous trees and shrubs of warm regions. The dried fruit of *P. officinalis* Lindl. (*Eugenia pimenta,* DC.), furnishes pimenta and pimenta oil.

pimenta (pĭ-men′tah) the dried, nearly ripe fruit of *Pimenta officinalis* Lindl. (Myrtaceae), once used as an aromatic, stimulant, and carminative; called also *allspice.*

piminodine esylate (pĭ-min′o-dēn) chemical name: 4-phenyl-1-[3-(phenylamino)propyl]-4-piperidinecarboxylic acid ethyl ester monoethanesulfonate. A synthetic narcotic analgesic, $C_{23}H_{30}N_2O_2 \cdot C_2H_6O_3S$, occurring as a colorless, crystalline solid; administered orally, intramuscularly, and subcutaneously.

pimozide (pim′o-zīd) chemical name: 1-[1-[4,4-bis(4-fluorophenyl)butyl]-4-piperidinyl]-1,3-dihydro-2*H*-benzimidazol-2-one; a tranquilizer that has been used in the treatment of schizophrenia, $C_{28}H_{29}F_2N_3O$.

Pimpinella (pim″pĭ-nel′ah) [L.] a genus of umbelliferous plants. The roots of *P. saxifraga* L., Burnet saxifrage, are tonic, diuretic, emmenagogue, and carminative, and are the source of pimpinellin. *P. anisum* L. yields anise and anise oil.

pimpinellin (pim″pĭ-nel′in) a bitter, crystallizable principle, $C_{13}H_{10}O_5$, seen in colorless needles, from the root of *Pimpinella saxifraga* L. (Umbelliferae).

pimple (pim′p'l) a papule or pustule, usually of the face, neck, or upper trunk, most often due to acne vulgaris.

pin (pin) 1. a long slender metal rod for the fixation of the ends of fractured bones. 2. in dentistry, a peg or dowel by means of which an artificial crown is fixed to the root of a tooth or by which supplemental retention is provided to any dental restoration. **Steinmann's p.,** a metal rod for the internal fixation of fractures; see *nail extension,* under *extension.*

pinacyanole (pin″ah-si′ah-nōl) an aniline dye, $C_{25}H_{25}N_2I$, used as a tissue stain, and for sensitizing photographic plates for red.

Pinard's maneuver (pe-nahrz′) [Adolphe *Pinard,* French obstetrician, 1844–1934] see under *maneuver.*

pince-ciseaux (pans″se-zo′) [Fr. "forceps-scissors"] a cutting forceps used in iridotomy.

pincement (pans-maw′) [Fr.] the pinching of the flesh in massage.

pincers (pin′serz) 1. forceps (def. 1). 2. the median deciduous incisor teeth in the horse.

pindolol (pin′do-lōl) chemical name: 1-(1*H*-indol-4-yloxy)-3-[(1-methylethyl)amino]-2-propanol; a beta-adrenergic blocking agent, $C_{14}H_{20}N_2O_2$, having the same actions as propranolol (q.v.).

pine (pīn) [L. *pinus*] the name of many coniferous trees, chiefly of the genus *Pinus.* The pines afford turpentine, volatile oils, rosin, pitch, tar, etc. **white p.,** the dried inner bark of *Pinus strobus* L. (Pinaceae), the Easter white pine; used as an ingredient in compound white pine syrup.

pineal (pin′e-al) [L. *pinealis; pinea* pine cone] 1. pertaining to the pineal body. 2. shaped like a pine cone.

pinealectomy (pin″e-al-ek′to-me) [*pineal* body + Gr. *ektomē* excision] excision of the pineal body.

pinealism (pin′e-al-izm″) the condition due to derangement of the secretion of the pineal body.

pinealoblastoma (pin″e-ah-lo-blas-to′mah) pinealoma in

which the pineal cells are not well differentiated. Called also *pineoblastoma.*

pinealocyte (pin′e-ah-lo-sīt″) the principal cell of the pineal body, being an epithelioid cell with pale-staining cytoplasm, prominent nucleoli, and large nuclei that are often irregularly infolded or lobulated; cords of these cells make up the body of the pineal body. Called also *chief cell* and *pineal cell.* See also *interstitial cells,* under *cell.*

pinealocytoma (pin″e-ah-lo-si-to′mah) pinealoma.

pinealoma (pin″e-ah-lo′mah) a rare tumor of the pineal body composed of neoplastic nests of large epithelial cells; symptoms include hydrocephalus, conjugate paralysis of upward gaze, disturbances of gait, and precocious puberty, the last due to the suppression of pineal secretion of melatonin. Called also *pinealocytoma.* **ectopic p.,** pinealoma arising from pineal rests in the midline area, resulting in diabetes insipidus, compression of the optic chiasm, and hypopituitarism.

pinealopathy (pin″e-ah-lop′ah-the) any disease of the pineal gland.

Pinel's system (pe-nelz′) [Philippe *Pinel,* psychologist in Paris, 1745–1826] see under *system.*

pinene (pi′nēn) a terpene, $C_{10}H_{16}$, found in turpentine and many essential oils; used as a solvent and in the manufacture of camphor. Called also *firpene.* **p. hydrochloride,** bornyl chloride.

pineoblastoma (pin″e-o-blas-to′mah) pinealoblastoma.

pineocytoma (pin″e-o-si-to′mah) pinealoma.

pinguecula (ping-gwek′u-lah) [L. *pinguis* fat] a yellowish spot of proliferation on the bulbar conjunctiva near the sclerocorneal junction, usually on the nasal side; seen in elderly people.

pinguicula (pin-gwik′u-lah) pinguecula.

piniform (pin′ĭ-form) [L. *pinea* pine cone + *forma* form] conical or cone shaped.

pinkeye (pink′i) acute contagious conjunctivitis.

Pinkus' disease (pin′koos) [Felix *Pinkus,* German dermatologist, born 1868] lichen nitidus.

pinna (pin′nah) [L. "wing"] the projecting part of the ear lying outside of the head (auricula [NA]).

pinnaglobin (pin″ah-glo′bin) a brown respiratory pigment found in the wedge-shaped mollusk *Pinna squamosa,* which contains manganese instead of iron.

pinnal (pin′al) pertaining to the pinna.

pinocarveol (pi″no-kar′ve-ol) a terpene alcohol, $(CH_3)_2C:C_6H_7\text{-}$ $(OH):CH_2$, from *Eucalyptus globulus;* called also *isocarveol.*

pinocyte (pi″no-, pi′no-sīt) a cell that exhibits pinocytosis.

pinocytic (pin″o-sit′ik) pertaining to a pinocyte or to pinocytosis.

pinocytosis (pi″no-, pin″-o-si-to′sis) [Gr. *pinein* to drink + *kytos* cell + -*osis*] the imbibition of liquids by cells, especially the mechanism by which cells ingest extracellular fluid and its contents; it involves the formation of minute incuppings or invaginations (caveolae) by the cell membrane, which close and pinch off to form free, fluid-filled vesicles (*pinosomes*) in the cytoplasm. It is thought to be a method of active transport across the cell membrane.

pinocytotic (pi″no-, pin″no-si-tot′ik) pertaining to or characterized by pinocytosis.

pinosome (pi″no-, pin′o-sōm) [Gr. *pinein* to drink + *sōma* body] any of the small fluid-filled vesicles found in the cytoplasm during pinocytosis, formed by invaginations of the cell membrane (caveolae) which pinch off and become free. Called also *pinocytotic vesicle.*

Pinoyella (pi″no-yel′ah) *Trichophyton.* **P. sim′ii,** *Trichophyton simii.*

Pins' sign [Emil *Pins,* Vienna physician, 1845–1913] Ewart's sign.

pint (pīnt) a measure of capacity (liquid measure), being 16 fluidounces, or the equivalent of 473.17 milliliters; symbol O (L. *octarius*), or abbreviated pt. The imperial pint is equal to 20 fluidounces.

pinta (pēn′tah) [Sp. "painted"] a form of treponematosis, being a chronic dyschromic dermatosis endemic in certain parts of tropical America and characterized by the presence on the skin of spots, which may be white, coffee colored, blue, red, or violet. It is caused by *Treponema carateum* (the Wassermann, reaction is usually positive), and is believed to be transmitted usually by direct person-to-person contact. Results of penicillin therapy are excellent. Called also *mal del pinto, carate, azul, tina, lota,* or *empeines.*

pintado (pēn-tah′do) a person affected with pinta.

pintid (pin′tid) one of the flat erythematous skin lesions constituting the spreading eruption occurring in the second stage of pinta.

pinto (pēn′to) pinta.

pinus (pi′nus) [L.] the pineal body.

pinworm (pin′werm) any oxyurid, especially *Enterobius vermicularis.*

pio- [Gr. *piōn* fat] a combining form denoting relationship to fat. See also words beginning *lipo-*.

pioepithelium (pi″o-ep″ĭ-the′le-um) [*pio-* + *epithelium*] epithelium in which fatty matter is deposited.

pion (pi′on) a nuclear particle with mass intermediate between an electron and a proton.

pionemia (pi″o-ne′me-ah) [Gr. *pion* fat + *haima* blood + *-ia*] the presence of fat or oil in the blood; lipemia.

Piophila (pi-of′ĭ-lah) a genus of flies. **P. ca′sei**, the fly whose larvae are the "cheese skippers" and a common cause of intestinal myiasis.

piorthopnea (pi″or-thop-ne′ah) [*pio-* + Gr. *orthos* upright + *pnoia* breath] dyspnea when lying down, due to obesity.

pioscope (pi′o-skōp) [*pio-* + Gr. *skopein* to examine] an instrument for estimating the fat content of milk by comparing its color with the six shades painted on the instrument.

Piotrowski's sign (pe″o-trov′skēz) [Alexander *Piotrowski*, neurologist in Berlin, born in 1878] see under *sign*.

pipamazine (pi-pam′ah-zēn) chemical name: 1-[3-(2-chlorophenothiazin-10-yl)propyl]-isonipecotamide. A crystal substance, $C_{21}H_{24}ClN_3OS$; used as an antiemetic.

pipamperone (pi-pam′pě-rōn) chemical name: 1′-[4-(4-fluorophenyl)-4-oxobutyl]-[1,4′-biperidine]-4′-carboxamide; a tranquilizer that has been used in the treatment of schizophrenia, $C_{21}H_{30}FN_3O_2$.

Pipanol (pip′ah-nol) trademark for a preparation of trihexyphenidyl hydrochloride.

pipazethate hydrochloride (pi-paz′ě-thāt) chemical name: 10H-pyrido[3,2-b][1,4]benzothiadiazine-10-carboxylic acid 2-(2-piperidinoethoxy)ethyl ester hydrochloride. A non-narcotic antitussive, $C_{21}H_{25}N_3O_3S\cdot HCl$, occurring as a white, crystalline powder; administered orally.

pipenzolate bromide (pi-pen′zo-lāt) chemical name: 1-ethyl-3-[(hydroxydiphenylacetyl)oxy]-1-methylpiperidinium bromide. A synthetic quaternary nitrogen anticholinergic, $C_{22}H_{28}BrNO_3$, occurring as a white, crystalline powder; used mainly for adjunctive therapy in the treatment of peptic ulcer, administered orally.

Piper (pi′per) [L. "pepper"] a genus of plants producing betel, cubeb, matico, and pepper.

piperacetazine (pip″er-ah-set′ah-zēn) [USP] chemical name: 1-[10-[3-[4-(2-hydroxyethyl)-1-piperidinyl]propyl]-10H-phenothiazin-2-yl]ethanone. An antipsychotic, $C_{24}H_{30}N_2O_2S$, occurring as a yellow, granular powder; used in the treatment of various forms of schizophrenia in adults, administered orally.

piperacillin sodium (pi-per′ah-sil″in) chemical name: [2S-[2α,5α,6β(S^*)]]-6-[[[[(4-ethyl-2,3-dioxo-1-piperazinyl)carbonyl]amino]phenylacetyl]amino]-3,3-dimethyl-7-oxo-4-thia-1-azabicyclo[3.2.0]heptane-2-carboxylic acid monosodium salt; an antibacterial, $C_{23}H_{26}N_5NaO_7S$.

piperazine (pi-per′ah-zēn) [USP] a compound, $C_4H_{10}N_2$, prepared by the action of alcoholic ammonia on ethylene chloride, or by other methods, occurring as white to slightly off-white lumps or flakes. Its salts are used orally as anthelmintics. See also *diethyl diamine*, *dispermine*, and *p. hexahydrate*. **p. citrate** [USP], the citrate salt of piperazine, $(C_4H_{10}N_2)_3\cdot 2C_6H_8O_7\cdot xH_2O$, occurring as a white, crystalline powder; used in the treatment of intestinal roundworm and pinworm infections, administered orally. **p. edetate calcium**, a compound, $C_{14}H_{24}CaN_4O_8\cdot 2H_2O$, prepared by the reaction of edetate with calcium carbonate and piperazine; used like the citrate salt. **p. estrone sulfate**, see under *estrone*. **p. phosphate** [USP], the phosphate salt of piperazine, $C_4H_{10}N_2\cdot H_3PO_4\cdot H_2O$, occurring as a white, crystalline powder; used in the treatment of intestinal roundworm and trematode infections. **p. tartrate**, the tartrate salt of piperazine, $C_8H_{16}N_2O_6$; used like the citrate salt.

piperidione (pi″per-ĭ-di′ōn) dihyprylone.

piperidolate hydrochloride (pi″per-id′o-lāt) [USP] chemical name: α-phenylbenzeneacetic acid 1-ethyl-3-piperidinyl ester hydrochloride. A synthetic tertiary anticholinergic, $C_{21}H_{25}NO_2\cdot HCl$, occurring as a white or cream-colored powder, having the ability to reduce motility of smooth muscle, especially that of the gastrointestinal tract; used as an antispasmodic in functional gastrointestinal disorders, administered orally.

piperine (pi′per-in) [L. *piperinum*] chemical name: 1-piperoylpiperidine. A crystallizable, slightly soluble alkaloid, $C_5H_{10}N\cdot CO\cdot(CH)_3CH\cdot C_6H_3\cdot O_2\cdot CH_2$, from *Piper nigrum* (black pepper), used as an insecticide.

piperism (pi′per-izm) [L. *piper* pepper] poisoning by pepper.

piperocaine hydrochloride (pi′per-o-kān″) chemical name: 2-methyl-1-piperidinepropanol benzoate hydrochloride. A local anesthetic, $C_{16}H_{23}NO_2\cdot HCl$, occurring as small, white crystals or white, crystalline powder; used for topical, infiltration, regional, spinal, and caudal anesthesia.

piperoxan hydrochloride (pi″per-oks′an) chemical name: 2-(1-piperidylmethyl)-1,4-benzodioxan hydrochloride. An alpha-adrenergic blocking agent, $C_{14}H_{19}NO_2$, formerly used in diagnostic tests for pheochromocytoma. Also used to counteract the effects of

epinephrine release before and during surgery for removal of pheochromocytoma.

pipet (pi-pet′) pipette.

pipette (pi-pet′) [Fr.] 1. a glass or transparent plastic tube used in measuring or transferring small quantities of liquid or gas. 2. to dispense fluid or gas by means of a pipette.

pipitzahoac (pi-pit″zah-ho-ak′) [Mex.] the root and rhizome of the Mexican plant *Trixis pipitzahuac* Shaffner (*Perezia adnata* Gr., Compositae); used as a cathartic.

Pipizan (pi′pĭ-zan) trademark for a preparation of piperazine.

pipobroman (pi″po-bro′man) [USP] chemical name: 1,4-bis(3-bromo-1-oxopropyl)piperazine. An antineoplastic alkylating agent, $C_{10}H_{16}Br_2N_2O_2$, occurring as a white to practically white, crystalline powder; used primarily in the treatment of polycythemia vera, and has been found to be useful in the treatment of chronic granulocytic leukemia, administered orally.

piposulfan (pĭ-po-sul′fan) chemical name: 1,4-dihydracryloylpiperazine dimethanesulfonate (ester); an antineoplastic, $C_{12}H_{22}N_2O_8S_2$.

pipotiazine palmitate (pip″o-ti′ah-zēn) chemical name: 2-[1-[3-[2-(dimethylamino)sulfonyl]-10H-phenothiazine-10-yl]propyl]-4-piperidinyl]ethyl ester hexanoic acid; a tranquilizer, $C_{40}H_{63}N_3O_4S_2$.

pipoxolan hydrochloride (pĭ-poks′o-lan) chemical name: 5,5-diphenyl-2-(2-piperidinoethyl)-1,3-dioxolan-4-one hydrochloride; a muscle relaxant, $C_{22}H_{25}NO_3\cdot HCl$.

pipradrol hydrochloride (pi′prah-drol) chemical name: α,α-diphenyl-2-piperidinemethanol hydrochloride. A central nervous system stimulant, $C_{18}H_{21}NO\cdot HCl$, occurring as small, white crystals or crystalline powder; used mainly as an antidepressant, administered orally.

piprozolin (pĭ-pro-zo′lin) chemical name: ethyl 3-ethyl-4-oxo-5-piperidino-$\Delta^{2,\alpha}$-thiazolidineacetate; a choleretic, $C_{14}H_{22}N_2O_3S$.

Piptal (pip′tal) trademark for preparations of pipenzolate methylbromide.

Piptocephalus (pip″to-sef″ah-lus) a genus of molds, some species of which cause alimentary toxic aleukia.

piqueur (pe-ker′) a fetishist who stabs his victims in the buttocks or breast.

piquizil hydrochloride (pik′wĭ-zil) chemical name: isobutyl 4-(6,7-dimethoxy-4-quinazolinyl)-1-piperazinecarboxylate monohydrochloride; a bronchodilator, $C_{19}H_{26}N_4O_4\cdot HCl$.

piqûre (pe-koor′) [Fr.] puncture, especially Bernard's (diabetic) puncture.

Piracaps (pi′rah-kaps) trademark for a preparation of tetracycline hydrochloride.

pirandamine hydrochloride (pēr-an′dah-mēn) chemical name: 1,3,4,9-tetrahydro-N,N,1-trimethylindeno[2,1-c]pyran-1-ethanamine hydrochloride; a tricyclic antidepressant, $C_{17}H_{23}NO\cdot HCl$.

pirbenicillin sodium (pēr-ben″ĭ-sil″in) chemical name: [2S-[2α,5α,6β(S^*)]]-6-[[[[(imino-4-pyridinylmethyl)amino]acetyl]amino]phenylacetyl]amino]-3,3-dimethyl-7-oxo-4-thia-1-azabicyclo[3.2.0]heptane-2-carboxylic acid monosodium salt; an antibacterial, $C_{24}H_{25}N_6NaO_5S$.

pirbuterol hydrochloride (pēr-bu′ter-ōl) chemical name: α^6-[[(1,1-dimethylethyl)amino]methyl]-3-hydroxy-2,6-pyridinedimethanol dihydrochloride; a bronchodilator, $C_{12}H_{20}N_2O_3\cdot 2HCl$.

Pirenella (pi″rě-nel′ah) a genus of snails. **P. con′ica**, the host of the intestinal fluke, *Heterophyes heterophyes*, in Egypt.

pirfenidone (pēr-fen′ĭ-don) chemical name: 5-methyl-1-phenyl-2(1H)-pyridinone; an anti-inflammatory and antipyretic, $C_{12}H_{11}NO$.

piriform (pir′ĭ-form) [L. *pirum* a pear + *forma* shape] pearshaped.

Pirogoff's amputation, angle (pir″o-gofs′) [Nikolai Ivanovich *Pirogoff*, Russian surgeon, 1810–1881] see under *amputation*, and see *venous angle*, under *angle*.

pirolate (pēr′o-lāt) chemical name: 1,4-dihydro-7,8-dimethoxy-4-oxopyrimido[4,5-b]quinoline-2-carboxylic acid ethyl ester; an antiasthmatic, $C_{16}H_{15}N_3O_5$.

pirolazamide (pēr″o-la′zah-mīd) chemical name: hexahydro-α,α-diphenylpyrrolo[1,2-a]pyrazine-2(1H)-butanamide; a cardiac depressant with antiarrhythmic action, $C_{23}H_{29}N_3O$.

Piroplasma (pi″ro-plaz′mah) [L. *pirum* pear + Gr. *plasma* something formed] a name formerly given to a genus of protozoan parasites found in the red blood cells of animals. Now called *Babesia*. See also *Nuttalia* and *Theileria*.

piroplasmosis (pi″ro-plaz-mo′sis) infection with *Piroplasma* (*Babesia*); babesiasis. **bovine p.**, see *Texas fever*, under *fever*. **canine p.**, an infectious jaundice of dogs caused by *Babesia canis*; called also *biliary fever of dogs* and *malignant jaundice of dogs*. **equine p.**, biliary fever of horses.

piroxicam (pēr-ok′sĭ-kam) chemical name: 4-hydroxy-2-methyl-N-2-pyridinyl-2H-1,2-benzothiazine-3-carboxamide; an anti-inflammatory, $C_{15}H_{13}N_3O_4S$.

pirprofen (pēr-pro′fen) chemical name: 3-chloro-4-(2,5-dihydro-1H-pyrrol-1-yl)-α-methylbenzeneacetic acid; an anti-inflammatory, $C_{13}H_{14}ClNO_2$.

Pirquet's reaction (cutireaction, test) (per-kāz′) [Clemens Freiherr von *Pirquet*, Austrian pediatrician, 1874–1929] see *cutaneous reaction*, under *reaction*.

pis (pe) [Fr.] urination. **p. en deux temps** installment emptying of the bladder, as in diverticulum or vesical hernia.

piscicide (pis′ĭ-sīd) any substance poisonous to fish.

Piscidia (pĭ-sid′e-ah) [L. *piscis* fish + *caedere* to kill] a genus of leguminous trees; the bark of *P. piscipula* (L.) Sarg. (*P. erythrina* L.), Jamaica dogwood, is a mild anodyne.

piscidin (pĭ-si′din) a neutral principle from *Piscidia piscipula* (L.) Sarg., an anodyne and antispasmodic.

pisiform (pi′sĭ-form) [L. *pisum* pea + *forma* shape] resembling a pea in shape and size.

pisiformis (pi″sĭ-for′mis) [L.] pisiform.

Piskacek's sign (pis′kach-eks) [Ludwig *Piskacek*, Hungarian obstetrician, 1854–1933] see under *sign*.

pistil (pis′til) [L. *pistillus* a pestle] gynecium.

pit (pit) 1. a hollow fovea or indentation. 2. a pockmark. 3. to indent, or to become and remain for a few minutes indented, by pressure. **anal p.**, the proctodeum. **arm p.**, the axillary fossa. **auditory p.**, a distinct depression appearing in each auditory placode, marking the beginning of the embryonic development of the internal ear. Called also *otic p.* **basilar p.**, a pit in the crown of an incisor tooth above its neck. **chrome p's**, deep ulcers in the skin caused by contact with chromium. **costal p.**, fovea costalis inferior. **ear p.**, a slight depression anterior to the helix and superior to the tragus, sometimes leading to a congenital preauricular cyst or fistula. **gastric p's**, foveolae gastricae. **Gaul's p's**, depressions in the corneal epithelium seen in neuroparalytic keratitis. **Herbert's p's**, a characteristic defect left after the healing of a limbal follicle in trachoma. **lens p.**, a pitlike depression in the ectoderm of the fetal head where the lens is developed. **nasal p.**, olfactory p. **oblong p. of arytenoid cartilage**, fovea oblonga cartilaginis arytenoideae. **olfactory p.**, the primordium of a nasal cavity. **otic p.**, auditory p. **postanal p.**, foveola coccygea. **primitive p.**, a depression at the cranial end of the primitive groove; it may open into a neurenteric canal. **pterygoid p.**, see under *fovea*. **p. of the stomach**, the epigastrium or fossa epigastrica. **triangular p. of arytenoid cartilage**, fovea triangularis cartilaginis arytenoideae.

pita (pe′tah) tinea imbricata.

pitch (pich) [L. *pix*] 1. a dark, lustrous, more or less viscous residue from the distillation of tar and other substances. 2. natural asphalt of various kinds. 3. the quality of sound dependent principally on its frequency. **black p.**, an inflammable substance obtainable from the tar of various species of pine. **Burgundy p.**, an aromatic, oily resin from *Abies* (or *Picea*) *excelsa*, the Norway spruce of Europe, much used in plasters. **Canada p.**, a resin from *Tsuga canadensis*, the hemlock tree, useful in plasters, etc. **liquid p.**, ordinary wood tar. **mineral p.**, bitumen. **naval p.**, black p.

pitchblende (pich′blend) a black mineral containing uranium oxide; from it are obtained radium, polonium, and uranium.

pith (pith) 1. to pierce the spinal cord or brain; see *pithing*. 2. the soft tissue found in plant stems that often disappears so that the stem becomes hollow. 3. the central core of colorless parenchymatous cells in stems and some roots.

pithecoid (pith′e-koid) [Gr. *pithēkos* ape + *eidos* form] apelike.

pithiatic (pith″e-at′ik) curable by persuasion; said of hysterical symptoms.

pithiatism (pith-i′ah-tizm) [Gr. *peithein* to persuade + *iatos* curable] 1. a condition which is caused by suggestion and which renders the patient subject to persuasion. 2. the cure of nervous and mental disorders by persuasion.

pithiatric (pith″e-at′rik) pertaining to persuasion as a means of treatment; capable of being cured by persuasion and suggestion.

pithiatry (pith-i′ah-tre) medical treatment by persuasion or suggestion.

pithing (pith′ing) destruction of the brain and spinal cord by thrusting a blunt needle into the spinal canal and cranium; done on animals to destroy sensibility preparatory to experimenting on their living tissues.

pithode (pi′thōd) [Gr. *pithos* wine cask + *eidos* form] the nuclear barrel figure in mitosis.

Pithomyces (pith″o-mi′sez) a genus of molds of the class Deuteromycetes. *P. charta′rum* causes facial eczema of ruminants.

Pitocin (pĭ-to′sin) trademark for preparations of oxytocin.

Pitres' sections, sign (pe-tres′) [Jean Albert *Pitres*, physician in Bordeaux, 1848–1927] see under *section* and *sign*.

Pitressin (pĭ-tres′in) trademark for vasopressin injection.

pitting (pit′ting) 1. the formation, usually by scarring, of a small depression. 2. the removal from erythrocytes, by the spleen, of certain structures, such as iron granules, without

destruction of the cells. 3. remaining indented for a few minutes after removal of firm finger-pressure, distinguishing fluid edema from myxedema.

pituicyte (pĭ-tu′ĭ-sīt) [*pituitary* + *-cyte*] any of the dominant and distinctive fusiform cells of the neurohypophysis, which are intermingled with nerve fibers and are regarded as specialized neuroglial cells. According to their morphological appearance on staining with silver, four subtypes are distinguished: adeno-, fibro-, reticulo-, and micropituicytes.

pituita (pĭ-tu′ĭ-tah) [L.] a glutinous mucus.

pituitarigenic (pĭ-tu″ĭ-tār″ĭ-jen′ik) [*pituitary* + *gennan* to produce] produced by secretions of the pituitary gland.

pituitarism (pĭ-tu″ĭ-tar-izm″) disorder of pituitary function; see *hyperpituitarism* and *hypopituitarism*.

pituitarium (pĭ-tu″ĭ-ta′re-um) [L.] pituitary. **p. ante′rius**, anterior pituitary. **p. poste′rius**, posterior pituitary. **p. to′tum**, whole pituitary.

pituitary (pĭ-tu′ĭ-tār″e) 1. pertaining to the pituitary gland. 2. the pituitary gland; see under *gland*. 3. a preparation of some part of the pituitary gland of animals, used therapeutically. Because of the abundant supply, the pituitary glands of healthy domesticated animals used as food for human consumption constitute the source. **anterior p.**, the anterior lobe of the pituitary gland. Also a preparation of the dried, partially defatted, powdered anterior lobe of the pituitary gland of hogs, sheep, or cattle. **pharyngeal p.**, pharyngeal hypophysis. **posterior p.**, 1. the posterior lobe of the pituitary gland; the neurohypophysis. 2. a powder prepared from the dried posterior pituitary lobe of those domestic animals used for food by man, having the pharmacological actions of its hormones, *oxytocin* and *vasopressin*; used mainly as an antidiuretic in the treatment of diabetes insipidus, administered subcutaneously or by nasal inhalation or topical application to the nasal mucosa. It may be used to stimulate smooth muscle tissue, especially to produce vasoconstriction in the presence of hemorrhage. **whole p.**, a preparation of the dried, partially defatted, powdered whole pituitary gland of domesticated animals.

pituitectomy (pĭ-tu″ĭ-tek′to-me) excision of the pituitary gland.

pituitous (pĭ-tu′ĭ-tus) [L. *pituitosus*] pertaining to mucus or characterized by its secretion.

Pituitrin (pĭ-tu′ĭ-trin) trademark for posterior pituitary injection.

pituitrism (pĭ-tu′ĭ-trizm) disorder of pituitary function.

pityriasis (pit″ĭ-ri′ah-sis) [Gr. *pityron* bran + *-iasis*] a name originally applied to a group of skin diseases characterized by the formation of fine, branny scales, but now used only with a modifier. **p. al′ba**, an extremely common skin disorder occurring on the face and neck in children and adolescents, which consists of one or many unevenly round or oval, hypopigmented, sometimes slightly reddened, finely scaling macules 1 to 4 cm. in diameter. If untreated, it usually persists for a year or several years, and often recurs. Called also *impetigo sicca, impetigo pityroides*, and *erythema streptogenes*. **p. amianta′cea**, tinea amiantacea. **p. capitis**, dandruff, def. 2. **p. furfura′cea**, dandruff, def. 2. **Gibert's p.** (*obs.*), p. rosea. **Hebra's p.** (*obs.*), dermatitis exfoliativa. **p. lichenoi′des**, a variety of parapsoriasis. **p. lichenoi′des et variolifor′mis acu′ta**, a disease characterized by the sudden appearance of a polymorphous skin eruption composed of macules, papules, and occasional vesicles, with hemorrhage, which may run an acute, subacute, or chronic course; called also *parapsoriasis lichenoides et varioliformis* and *parakeratosis variegata*. **p. lin′guae**, geographic tongue. **p. macula′ta**, p. alba. **p. pila′ris** (*obs.*), keratosis pilaris. **p. ro′sea**, a dermatosis characterized by scaling pink oval macules arranged with the long axes parallel to the lines of cleavage of the skin. **p. rotun′da**, a chronic dermatosis, usually affecting adults, manifested as perfectly circular patches of dry, ichthyosiform scaliness, 20 to 60 mm. in diameter, mostly on the buttocks, thighs, back, or upper arms. **p. ru′bra pila′ris**, a rare chronic inflammatory disease of the skin, characterized by the presence of pink scaling macules and fine acuminate, horny, follicular papules, and appearing in children or adults. It begins usually with severe seborrhea of the scalp and seborrheic dermatitis of the face, and is associated with striking keratoderma of palms and soles; it is thought by some to be a follicular variant of psoriasis. **p. sic′ca**, dandruff, def. 2. **p. sim′plex**, p. alba. **p. steatoi′des**, seborrheic dermatitis. **p. versic′olor**, tinea versicolor.

pityroid (pit′ĭ-roid) [Gr. *pityron* bran + *eidos* form] furfuraceous; branny.

Pityrosporon (pit″ĭ-ros′po-ron) a genus of imperfect fungi of the family Cryptococcaceae, which are yeastlike and produce no mycelium; called also *Malassezia*. **P. orbic′ulare**, a species which is a customary resident of normal skin, but is capable of causing disease (tinea versicolor) in susceptible hosts; called also *Malassezia furfur, M. macfadyani, M. tropica*, and *Microsporum furfur*. **P. ova′le**, a lipid-dependent species which is abundant in sebaceous areas, such as the skin of the face and scalp, but is not known to be pathogenic.

Pityrosporum (pit″ĭ-ros′po-rum) *Pityrosporon.*

pivalate (piv′ah-lāt) USAN contraction for trimethylacetate.

pivampicillin hydrochloride (piv-am″pĭ-sil′in) chemical name: 6-[(aminophenylacetyl)amino]-3,3-dimethyl-7-oxo-4-thia-1-azabicyclo[3.2.0]heptane-2-carboxylic acid (2,2-dimethyl-1-oxo-propoxy)methyl ester. A derivative of ampicillin, $C_{22}H_{29}N_3O_6S$, having the same broad spectrum of antibacterial activity and uses as ampicillin. Available as *p. hydrochloride, p. pamoate,* and *p. probenate.*

pivot (piv′ut) a dowel, or post; in dentistry the point of rotation for a removable partial denture. **occlusal p.,** an elevation contrived on the occlusal surface, usually in the molar region, designed to act as a fulcrum and to induce sagittal mandibular rotation.

pix (piks), gen. *pi′cis* [L.] pitch or tar.

pizotyline (pĭ-zo′tĭ-lēn) chemical name: 4-(9,10-dihydro-4*H*-benzo[4,5]cyclohepta[1,2-*b*]thien-4-ylidene)-1-methylpiperidine; an anabolic, antidepressant, and serotonin inhibitor (specific in migraine), $C_{19}H_{21}NS$.

PK psychokinesis.

pK the negative logarithm of the ionization constant (K) of an acid; the buffering power of a buffer system is greatest when its pK equals the pH.

PKU phenylketonuria.

P.L. light perception.

placebo (plah-se′bo) [L. "I will please"] an inactive substance or preparation given to satisfy the patient's symbolic need for drug therapy, and used in controlled studies to determine the efficacy of medicinal substances. Also, a procedure with no intrinsic therapeutic value, performed for such purposes. **active p., impure p.,** a substance having pharmacologic properties that are not relevant to the condition being treated.

placement (plās′ment) position or arrangement, as of the teeth. **lingual p.,** displacement of a tooth toward the tongue.

placenta (plah-sen′tah), pl. *placentas* or *placen′tae* [L. "a flat cake"] an organ characteristic of true mammals during pregnancy, joining mother and offspring, providing endocrine secretion and selective exchange of soluble, but not particulate, blood-borne substances through an apposition of uterine and trophoblastic vascularized parts. According to species, the area of vascular apposition may be diffuse, cotyledonary, zonary, or discoid; the nature of apposition may be labyrinthine or villous; the intimacy of apposition may vary according to what layers are lost of those originally interposed between maternal and fetal blood (maternal endothelium, uterine connective tissue, uterine epithelium, chorion, extraembryonic mesoderm, and endothelium of villous capillary). The chorion may be joined by and receive blood vessels from either the yolk sac or the allantois, and the uterine lining may be largely shed with the chorion at birth (deciduate) or may separate from the chorion and remain (nondeciduate). The human placenta is discoid, villous, hemochorial, chorioallantoic, and deciduate. After birth, it weighs about 600 gm. and is about 16 cm. in diameter and 2 cm. thick, the maternal blood in the intervillous space (which leaks out at birth) into which the chorionic villi dip. The villi are grouped into adjoining cotyledons making about 20 velvety bumps on the side of the placenta facing outward to the uterus; the inner side of the placenta facing the fetus is smooth, being covered with amnion, a thin avascular layer that continues past the edges of the placenta to line the entire hollow sphere of chorion except where it is reflected to cover the umbilical cord, which joins fetus and placenta. The cord usually joins the placenta near the center but may insert at the edge, on the nonplacental chorion, or on an accessory placenta. **accessory p.,** a placenta separate from the main placenta. **p. accre′ta,** abnormal adherence of part or all of the placenta to the uterine wall, with partial or complete absence of the decidua basalis, especially of the spongiosum layer. **adherent p.,** one which adheres closely to the uterine wall. **annular p.,** one which extends around the interior of the uterus like a ring or belt. **battledore p.,** one with marginal insertion of the cord. **bidiscoidal p.,** one consisting of two separate discoidal masses, as in the macaques. **bilobate p., bilobed p.,** a placenta consisting of two lobes. **p. biparti′ta, bipartite p.,** bilobate p. **chorioallantoic p.,** one in which the allantois joins the chorion or provides its major blood supply. **choriovitelline p.,** one in which the yolk sac becomes an intermediary in the fetal-maternal relationship. **p. circumval-la′ta, circumvallate p.,** a placenta in which a dense peripheral ring is raised from the surface and the attached membranes are doubled back over the edge of the placenta. **cirsoid p., p. cirsoi′des,** a placenta the vessels of which appear to be varicose. **deciduate p., deciduous p.,** a placenta or type of placentation in which the decidua or maternal parts of the placenta separate from the uterus and are cast off together with the fetal (or more precisely, trophoblastic) parts. **p. diffu′sa,** a placenta in which placental tissue is distributed over the chorionic membrane, as in swine. **p. dimidia′ta, dimidiate p.,** bilobate p. **discoid p., p. discoi′dea,** a disk-shaped placenta. **Duncan p.,** one that is expelled with the chorionic surface outward; cf. *Schultze's p.* **duplex p.,** bilobate p. **endotheliochorial**

p., one in which syncytial trophoblast embeds maternal vessels bared to their endothelial lining. **epitheliochorial p.,** one in which the uterine epithelial lining is not eroded but merely lies in apposition to the chorion. **p. fenestra′ta,** one which has spots where placental tissue is lacking. **fetal p., p. foeta′lis,** pars fetalis placentae. **fundal p.,** one which is attached to the fundus of the uterus in the normal manner. **furcate p.,** lobed p. **hemochorial p.,** one in which maternal blood comes in direct contact with the chorion. **hemoendothelial p.,** one in which maternal blood comes in contact with the endothelium of chorionic vessels. **horseshoe p.,** a crescentic form of placenta sometimes occurring in twin pregnancy. **incarcerated p.,** retained p. **p. incre′ta,** placenta accreta with penetration of the myometrium. **labyrinthine p.,** one in which maternal blood courses in channeled trophoblast. **lobed p.,** one that is more or less subdivided into lobes. **p. margina′lis, p. margina′ta,** a placenta surrounded by an unusual margin of elevated infarcted tissue. **maternal p.,** the maternally contributed part of the placenta, derived from the decidua basalis; called also *pars uterina placentae* [NA]. **p. membrana′cea,** a placenta which is abnormally thin and spread out over a large area of the uterine wall. **multilobate p., multilobed p., p. multiparti′ta,** a placenta consisting of more than three lobes. **p. nappifor′mis, p. circumvallata. nondeciduate p., nondeciduous p.,** one in which the maternal component remains in the uterus instead of being cast off together with the trophoblastic derivatives. **panduriform p., p. panduri-for′mis,** a placenta composed of two halves side by side, resembling a violin in shape. **p. percre′ta,** placenta accreta with invasion of the myometrium all the way to its peritoneal covering, sometimes resulting in rupture of the uterus. **p. pre′via,** a placenta which develops in the lower uterine segment, in the zone of dilatation, so that it covers or adjoins the internal os; painless hemorrhage in the last trimester, particularly during the eighth month, is the most common symptom. **p. pre′via centra′lis,** placenta previa in which the placenta entirely covers the internal os; called also *complete, total,* or *central placenta previa.* **p. pre′via margina′lis,** placenta previa in which the placenta is just palpable at the margin of the os; called also *lateral* or *marginal placenta previa.* **p. pre′via partia′lis,** placenta previa in which the internal os is partially covered; called also *incomplete* or *partial placenta previa.* **p. reflex′a,** one in which the margin is thickened, appearing to turn back on itself. **p. renifor′mis,** a kidney-shaped placenta. **retained p.,** one which is either adherent or incarcerated by irregular uterine contractions, and which in consequence fails to be expelled after childbirth. **Schultze's p.,** a placenta which is expelled with the gestation sac inside out, the amnion providing a smooth, glistening surface. Cf. *Duncan p.* **p. spu′ria,** an accessory portion having no blood vessel attachment to the main placenta. **p. succenturia′ta, succenturiate p.,** an accessory portion attached to the main placenta by an artery and vein. **syndes-mochorial p.,** one in which the lining epithelium of the uterus is the only maternal tissue eroded. **p. tri′loba, trilobate p.,** a placenta having three lobes. **p. triparti′ta, tripartite p.,** trilobate p. **p. trip′lex,** trilobate p. **p. uteri′na, uterine p.,** maternal p. **velamentous p.,** one in which the umbilical cord is attached on the adjoining membranes. **villous p.,** one characterized by the presence of villi which are outgrowths of the chorion. **yolk-sac p.,** choriovitelline p. **zonary p., zonular p.,** 1. annular placenta. 2. a belt-shaped placenta, as occurs in carnivores.

placental (plah-sen′tal) pertaining to the placenta.

Placentalia (pla″sen-ta′le-ah) a division of mammals whose embryos are nourished through a placenta; it includes all mammals except marsupials and monotremes.

placentation (plas″en-ta′shun) the process of placenta formation and the result, especially with respect to taxonomically relevant aspects of structure. See *placenta.*

placentin (plah-sen′tin) a defatted desiccation product of beef placenta.

placentitis (plas″en-ti′tis) inflammation of the placenta.

placentogenesis (plah-sen″to-jen′ĕ-sis) [*placenta* + *genesis*] the origin and development of the placenta.

placentogram (plah-sen′to-gram) a film taken in placentography.

placentography (plas″en-tog′rah-fe) radiological visualization of the placenta after the injection of a contrast medium. **indirect p.,** roentgenographic measurement of the space between the placenta and the presenting head of the fetus, for the recognition of placenta previa.

placentoid (plah-sen′toid) resembling the placenta.

placentologist (plas″en-tol′o-jist) a specialist in placentology.

placentology (plas″en-tol′o-je) the scientific study of the development, structure, and functioning of the placenta. **comparative p.,** the scientific study of the development, structure, and functioning of the placenta in different species of animals.

placentolysin (plas″en-tol′ĭ-sin) [*placenta* + Gr. *lysis* dissolution] a lysin formed in the serum of an animal into which have been injected placenta cells from another animal. It is destructive to the placenta of animals of the species from which the cells were originally taken.

placentoma (plas″en-to′mah) a neoplasm derived from a portion of the placenta retained after an abortion.

placentopathy (plas″en-top′ah-the) any placental disease.

Placido's disk (plah-si′dōz) [A. *Placido*, Portuguese ophthalmologist] see under *disk*.

Placidyl (plas′ĭ-dil) trademark for a preparation of ethchlorvynol.

placode (plak′ōd) [Gr. *plax* plate + *eidos* form] a platelike structure, especially a thickened plate of ectoderm in the early embryo, from which a sense organ develops. **auditory p.,** a thickened epidermal plate located midway alongside the hindbrain in the early embryo, from which the internal ear ultimately develops. Called also *otic p.* and *auditory saucer.* **dorsolateral p's,** a series of placodes giving rise to the acoustic and lateral line organs. **epibranchial p's,** a series of placodes located dorsal to the branchial grooves that contribute to adjacent cerebral ganglia. **lens p.,** a thickened area of ectoderm directly overlying the optic vesicle in the early embryo, from which the lens develops. **olfactory p.,** an oval area of thickened ectoderm on either ventrolateral surface of the head of the early embryo, constituting the first indication of the olfactory organ. **otic p.,** auditory p.

placoderm (plak′o-derm) [Gr. *plakos* a tablet or flat plate + *derma* skin] any of the primitive jawed fishes of the class Placodermi.

Placodermi (plak′o-der″mi) a class of primitive jawed fishes of the Paleozoic era, having a bony head shield movably articulated with a thoracic shield; known only from fossils, and believed to be ancestral to both bony and cartilaginous fishes.

placoid (plak′oid) platelike or plaquelike.

plagiocephalic (pla″je-o-se-fal′ik) characterized by plagiocephaly.

plagiocephalism (pla″je-o-sef′ah-lism) plagiocephaly.

plagiocephaly (pla″je-o-sef′ah-le) [Gr. *plagios* oblique + *kephalē* head] an unsymmetrical and twisted condition of the head, resulting from irregular closure of the cranial sutures.

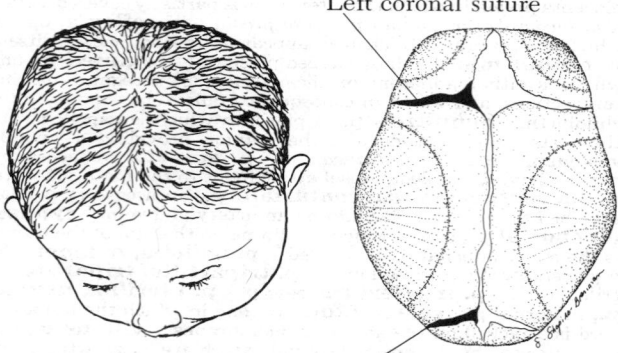

Left coronal suture

Left lambdoid suture

Plagiocephaly showing the sites of premature closure of cranial sutures.

plague (plāg) [L. *plaga, pestis*; Gr. *plēgē* stroke] an acute febrile, infectious disease with a high fatality rate, caused by *Yersinia pestis*; it begins with fever and chills, quickly followed by prostration, and frequently attended with delirium, headache, vomiting, and diarrhea. It is primarily a disease of rats and other rodents and is transmitted to man from infected rodents by the bite of fleas of several genera, or communicated from patient to patient. Called also *pest* and *oriental plague*. See also *bubonic plague, pneumonic plague*, and *septicemic plague*. **ambulatory p.,** a mild form of bubonic plague, with little or no toxemia. **avian p.,** fowl p. **black p.,** hemorrhagic p. **Brunswick bird p.,** fowl p. **bubonic p., p. bubon′ica,** plague which is marked by swelling of the lymph nodes, forming buboes in the femoral, inguinal, axillary and cervical regions. The severe form, with septicemia producing petechial hemorrhages, is known as *black death, pestis fulminans,* and *pestis major.* **canine p.,** black tongue of dogs; it is caused by niacin deficiency. **cat p.,** panleukopenia. **cattle p.,** a viral disease of cattle, which sometimes affects sheep and goats, marked by fever and croupous, ulcerative diphtheritic lesions of the intestinal tract; called also *rinderpest.* **cellulocutaneous p.,** plague marked by inflammation and necrosis of the skin and subcutaneous tissues and often associated with involvement of the lymph nodes. **defervescing p.,** a form which ends by a crisis. **equine p.,** African horse sickness. **fowl p.,** a viral disease of domestic fowls caused by a highly pathogenic strain of the avian influenza virus; called also *fowl pest.* **glandular p.,** bubonic p. **hemorrhagic p.,** a severe form of bubonic plague with hemorrhages into the mucous membrane and the skin. **larval p.,** ambulatory p. **lung p.,** pleuropneumonia, def. 2. **Pahvant**

Valley p., tularemia. **pneumonic p.,** that in which there is extensive involvement of the lungs, and the sputum is loaded with the causative organisms. **premonitory p.,** a mild form that sometimes foreruns the typical endemic variety. **rodent p.,** that affecting rodents. **septicemic p.,** that in which there is massive bacteremia, resulting in death before the appearance of buboes or of pulmonic manifestations. **siderating p.,** septicemic p. **Stuttgart dog p.,** Stuttgart disease. **swine p.,** hemorrhagic septicemia of swine. **sylvatic p.,** plague of the woods, as for example, the plague widely spread and still spreading among the ground squirrels and other wild rodents of the western U.S.A. **Vanin p.,** parangi. **white p.,** tuberculosis.

plakins (pla′kinz) substances similar to leukins that can be extracted from blood platelets.

plana (pla′nah) plural of *planum.*

planarian (plah-nar′ĭ-an) any of the free-living flatworms of the class Turbellaria, which are used extensively in biologic studies of regeneration.

planchet (plan′chet) a metal disk on which radioactive samples are deposited.

Planck's constant, theory (planks) [Max Karl Ernst Ludwig *Planck*, German physicist, 1858–1947] see under *constant,* and see *quantum theory,* under *theory.*

plane (plān) [L. *planus*] 1. a flat surface determined by the position of three points in space. 2. a specified level, as the plane of anesthesia. 3. to rub away or abrade; see *planing.* 4. a superficial incision in the wall of a cavity or between tissue layers, especially in plastic surgery, made so that the precise point of entry into the cavity or between the layers can be determined. **Addison's p's,** a series of planes used as landmarks in the topography of the thorax and abdomen. **Aeby's p.,** one passing through the nasion and basion, perpendicular to the median plane of the cranium. **auricular p. of sacral bone,** facies auricularis ossis sacri. **auriculoinfraorbital p.,** Frankfort horizontal p. **axial p.,** one parallel with the long axis of a structure. **axiobuccolingual p.,** one parallel with the long axis of a posterior tooth and passing through its buccal and lingual surfaces. **axiolabiolingual p.,** one parallel with the long axis of an anterior tooth and passing through its labial and lingual surfaces. **axiomesiodistal p.,** one parallel with the long axis of a tooth and passing through its mesial and distal surfaces. **Baer's p.,** one passing through the upper border of the zygomatic arches. **base p.,** an imaginary plane upon which is estimated the retention of an artificial denture. **bite p.,** occlusal p. **Blumenbach's p.,** a plane determined by the base of a skull from which the lower jaw has been removed. **Bolton-nasion p.,** nasion-postcondylare p. **Broadbent-Bolton p.,** nasion-postcondylare p. **Broca's p.,** visual p. **buccolingual p.,**

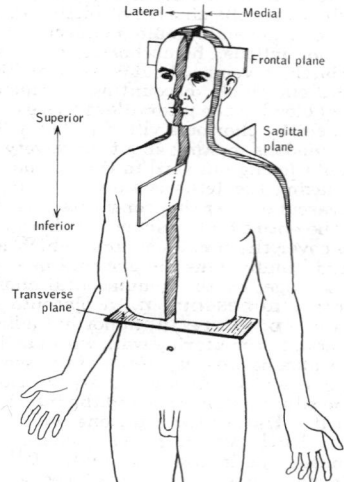

Planes of the body (Davenport). Anterior view, in the anatomical position, with standard planes of reference shown by cleavages.

one passing through the buccal and lingual surfaces of a posterior tooth. **coronal p.,** frontal p. **cove p.,** the ST-T segment of the electrocardiogram in which an inverted T wave is preceded by an isoelectric plateau. **cusp p.,** the small imaginary plane in which buccal cusp tips and lingual cusp tips are located on posterior teeth. **datum p.,** a given plan from which craniometric measurements are made. **Daubenton's p.,** one passing through the opisthion and the lower edges of the orbits. **eye-ear p.,** Frankfort horizontal p. **facial p's,** various planes determined by certain landmarks of the face, such as the Frankfort horizontal plane, and the orbital plane. **Frankfort horizontal p.,** a horizontal plane represented in profile by a line between the lowest point on the margin of the orbit and the highest point on the margin of the auditory meatus. **frontal p.**, any plane passing longitudinally through the body from side to side, at right angles to the median plane, and dividing the body into front and back parts. So called because such a plane roughly parallels the frontal suture of the skull. Called also *coronal p.* because one of these planes passes through the coronal suture. **guide p.**, 1. any plane that guides movement. 2. an orthodontic appliance used to correct crossbite of anterior teeth. **Hensen's p.**, one passing through the center of a series of sarcous elements of a muscle fibril. **Hodge's p's**, a series of planes running parallel with the pelvic inlet, the first parallel being in the inlet, the second parallel touching the arch of the pubis and striking the lower part of the second sacral vertebra, the third cutting the spines of the ischia, and the fourth passing through the tip of the coccyx. **horizontal p.**, any plane passing through a body, at right angles to both the median and the frontal plane, and dividing the body into upper and lower parts; in dentistry, a plane passing through a tooth at right angles to its long axis. Called also *transverse p.* **interparietal p. of oc-**

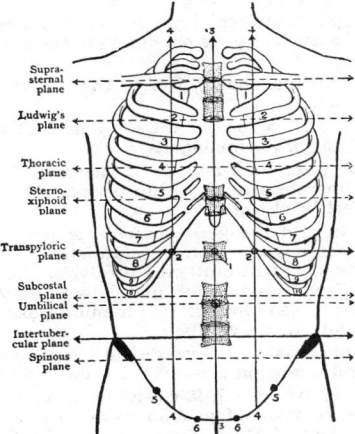

Planes of the trunk (Rawling).

cipital bone, planum occipitale. **intertubercular p.**, a horizontal plane transecting the trunk at the level of the tubercle of the iliac crest. **labiolingual p.**, one passing through the labial and lingual surfaces of an anterior tooth. **Listing's p.**, a transverse vertical plane perpendicular to the anteroposterior axis of the eye, and containing the center of motion of the eyes; in it lie the transverse and vertical axes of ocular rotation. **Ludwig's p.**, a horizontal plane transecting the trunk at about the level of the joint between the fourth and fifth thoracic vertebrae. **mean foundation p.**, the mean of the various irregularities in form and inclination of the basal seat (denture-supporting tissues). The ideal condition for denture stability exists when the mean foundation plane is most nearly at right angles to the direction of force. **Meckel's p.**, one passing through the auricular and alveolar points. **median p.**, the imaginary plane passing longitudinally through the middle of the body from front to back and dividing it into right and left halves. **median-raphe p.**, the median plane of the head. **mesiodistal p.**, one passing through the mesial and distal surfaces of a tooth. **midpelvic p.**, pelvic p., narrow. **midsagittal p.**, median p. **Morton's p.**, one passing through the most projecting points of the parietal and occipital protuberances. **nasion-postcondylare p.**, one passing at right angles to the median plane, and determined in profile by a line connecting the nasion and postcondylare. **nuchal p.**, planum nuchale. **occipital p.**, planum occipitale. **occlusal p., p. of occlusion,** the hypothetical horizontal plane formed by the contacting surfaces of the upper and lower teeth when the jaws are closed. **orbital p.**, 1. planum orbitale. 2. visual plane. **orbital p. of frontal bone,** pars orbitalis ossis frontalis. **parasagittal p.**, sagittal p. **pelvic p.**, one determined by certain landmarks of the hip bone. **pelvic p., narrow,** an ovoid plane passing through the apex of the pubic arch, the spines of the ischia, and the end of the sacrum. **pelvic p., wide,** an irregularly ovoid plane passing from the middle of the pubis to the junction of the second and third sacral vertebrae, at about the center of the excavation of the pelvis. **pelvic p. of outlet,** a plane passing through the arch of the pubis, the rami of the pubis, the ischial tuberosities, and the tip of the coccyx; see *apertura pelvis inferior.* **popliteal p. of femur,** facies poplitea femoris. **principal p.**, in radiology, the plane which contains the central ray of a radiation beam. **p's of reference,** planes which are referred to as a guide to the location of specific anatomical sites, or of other planes. **p. of regard,** one passing through the center of rotation and the point of fixation in the eye. **sagittal p.**, any vertical plane that passes through the body parallel to the median plane (or to the

sagittal suture) and divides the body into left and right portions. **semicircular p. of frontal bone,** facies temporalis ossis frontalis. **semicircular p. of parietal bone,** planum temporale. **semicircular p. of squama temporalis,** facies temporalis partis squamosae. **spinous p.**, a horizontal plane transecting the trunk at the level of the anterior superior iliac spine. **sternal p.**, planum sternale. **sternoxiphoid p.**, a horizontal plane transecting the trunk at about the level of the xiphisternal joint. **subcostal p.**, a horizontal plane transecting the trunk at the level of the lower margin of the tenth rib. **suprasternal p.**, a horizontal plane transecting the trunk at the level of the jugular notch. **temporal p.**, planum temporale. **thoracic p.**, a horizontal plane transecting the trunk at about the level of the fourth intercostal space. **tooth p.**, any hypothetical plane passing through a tooth. **transpyloric p.**, a horizontal plane transecting the trunk at about the level of the eighth intercostal space. **transverse p.**, a horizontal plane of the body dividing the body into upper and lower portions, or a plane at right angles to the longitudinal axis of a structure. **umbilical p.**, a horizontal plane transecting the trunk at the level of the umbilicus. **vertical p.**, any plane of the body perpendicular to a horizontal plane and dividing the body into left and right, or front and back portions, as the sagittal and frontal planes. **visual p.**, one passing through the visual axes of the two eyes; called also *Broca's p.* and *orbital p.*

planigram (pla'nĭ-gram) a roentgenogram of a structure at a selected level, made by body section roentgenography.

planigraphy (plah-nig'rah-fe) body section roentgenography; see under *roentgenography.*

planimeter (pla-nim'ĕ-ter) [L. *planus* plane + Gr. *metron* measure] an instrument used in measuring the area of surfaces.

planing (pla'ning) the plastic surgery procedure of abrading disfigured skin to promote reepithelialization with minimal scarring. It may be done by means of sandpaper, emery paper, low- or high-speed wire brushes, etc. (surgical planing; dermabrasion), or by application of caustic substances such as phenol or trichloracetic acid (chemical planing; chemabrasion).

planithorax (plan″ĭ-tho'raks) a diagram of the front and back of the chest.

plankton (plank'ton) [Gr. *planktos* wandering] a collective name for the minute free-floating organisms, vegetable and animal, which live in practically all natural waters.

planocellular (pla″no-sel'u-lar) made up of flat cells.

Planococcus (plan″o-kok'us) in some systems of classification, a genus of bacteria of the family Micrococcaceae, found in sea water, and made up of spherical, gram-positive cells, occurring singly, in pairs, in threes, or in tetrads.

planoconcave (pla″no-kon'kāv) flat on one side and concave on the other; see under *lens.*

planoconvex (pla″no-kon'veks) flat on one side and convex on the other; see under *lens.*

planocyte (pla'no-sīt) [Gr. *planē* wandering + -*cyte*] a wandering cell.

planogram (pla'no-gram) planigram.

planography (plah-nog'rah-fe) planigraphy.

planorbid (plah-nor'bid) 1. a snail of the family Planorbidae. 2. pertaining to snails of the family Planorbidae.

Planorbidae (plah-nor'bĭ-de) [L. *planus* flat + *orbis* ring + *idae*] a large family of pulmonate fresh-water snails (suborder Basommatophora, order Pulmonata), many species of which are intermediate hosts of pathogenic trematodes; it includes the genera *Biomphalaria, Planorbis* (the type genus), and *Bulinus.*

Planorbis (plan-or'bis) a genus of snails. Several species act as intermediate hosts for *Schistosoma mansoni* and others for *Fasciolopsis buski* and echinostomes.

planotopokinesia (pla″no-top″o-ki-ne'ze-ah) [Gr. *planē* wandering + *topos* place + *kinēsis* movement] disturbance of the power of orientation in space.

planta pedis (plan'tah pe'dis) [L.] [NA] the undersurface (sole) of the foot. Called also *regio plantaris pedis.*

plantaginis semen (plan-taj'ĭ-nis se'men) [L.] the seed of *Plantago psyllium* L., Plantaginaceae.

Plantago (plan-ta'go) a genus of herbs (family Plantaginaceae), including three species, *P. in'dica* L., *P. ova'ta* Forskal (blond psyllium), and *P. psyllium* L. (Spanish psyllium), whose seeds (plantago, or psyllium seeds) are used as a cathartic. A preparation of the separated mucilaginous outer layers of the seeds of *P. ovata* is used in the preparation of psyllium hydrophilic mucilloid (q.v.).

plantalgia (plan-tal'je-ah) [L. *planta* sole + -*algia*] a painful condition of the sole of the foot.

plantar (plan'tar) pertaining to the sole of the foot.

plantaris (plan-tah'ris) [L.] plantar; [NA] a term designating relationship to the sole of the foot.

plantation (plan-ta'shun) [L. *plantare* to plant] the insertion or application of tissue, such as a tooth, or of other material, in or on the human body. It includes *implantation,* the insertion of similar or other material within the body tissues, as of an artificial or natural tooth into a new socket, or of a therapeutic agent or device;

replantation, return of body tissue to its original site, as reinsertion of a tooth into the socket from which it was dislodged; and *transplantation,* the insertion or application of tissue derived from another individual, or from a different site in the same individual.

plantigrade (plan'tĭ-grād) [L. *planta* sole + *gradi* to walk] characterized by walking on the full sole of the foot, applied to animals whose entire sole touches the ground, such as the bear and man.

planula (plan'u-lah) a larval coelenterate. **invaginate p.,** the gastrula.

planum (pla'num), pl. *pla'na* [L.] a flat surface, determined by the position of three points in space. Called also *plane.* Used in anatomical nomenclature to designate a more or less flat surface of a bone or other structure. **p. nucha'le,** nuchal plane: the outer surface of the occipital bone between the foramen magnum and the superior nuchal line. **p. occipita'le,** occipital plane: the outer surface of the occipital bone above the superior nuchal line. **p. orbita'le,** orbital plane: a plane passing through the two orbital points and perpendicular to the Frankfort horizontal plane. **p. poplite'um fem'oris,** facies poplitea femoris. **p. semiluna'tum,** the rounded end of a crista in a semicircular canal. **p. sterna'le,** sternal plane: the anterior surface of the sternum. **p. tempora'le,** temporal plane: the depressed area on the side of the skull below the inferior temporal line.

planuria (pla-nu're-ah) [Gr. *planasthai* to wander + *ouron* urine + *-ia*] the discharge of urine from an abnormal site.

plaque (plak) [Fr.] any patch or flat area. **argyrophile p's,** amorphous argyrophilic masses, 40 to 80 microns in diameter, between the neurons of the brain in old people, particularly in the frontal cortex and the hippocampus. **attachment p's,** small regions of increased density along the sarcolemma of skeletal muscles to which myofilaments seem to attach; cf. *dense bodies,* under *body.* **bacterial p.,** dental p. **bacteriophage p.,** a cleared area in a bacterial culture, produced by bacteriophage that has been applied to it. **dental p.,** a mass adhering to the enamel surface of a tooth, composed of a mixed colony of bacteria in an intercellular matrix of bacterial and salivary polymers and remnants of epithelial cells and leukocytes. It may serve as a cause of caries, dental calculi, and periodontal disease. **fibromyelinic p's,** areas of overgrowth of medullated fibers and sheaths in areas of incomplete arteriosclerotic necrosis in the cerebral cortex. **Hollenhorst p's,** atheromatous emboli containing cholesterol crystals in the retinal arterioles, a warning sign of impending serious cardiovascular disease such as stroke, myocardial infarction, aortic aneurysm, or occlusion of the retinal arterioles. **Lichtheim p's,** areas of degeneration in the cerebral white matter that are seen in pernicious anemia. **mucous p., p. muqueuse',** condyloma latum. **opaline p.,** the gray plaque of secondary syphilis. **Peyer's p's,** Peyer's patches (folliculi lymphatici aggregati). **Randall's p's,** small calcium concretions within the tip of the renal papillae; they may project through the surface and serve as foci for the deposition of urinary calculi. **Redlich-Fisher miliary p's,** thickened, dark colored areas in the neuroglia reticulum of the brain, seen in cases of senile psychoses. **senile p's,** areas of incomplete necrosis in the senile cerebral cortex. **talc p's,** opaque material visible roentgenographically on pleural surfaces in talc miners and processors.

Plaquenil (pla'kwĕ-nil) trademark for a preparation of hydroxychloroquine sulfate.

plasm (plazm) plasma; formative substance. **germ p.** (*obs.*), Weismann's term for the reproductive and hereditary substance of individuals which is passed on from the germ cell in which an individual originates in direct continuity to the germ cells of succeeding generations. By it new individuals are produced and hereditary characters are transmitted. Cf. *somatoplasm.*

plasma (plaz'mah) [Gr. "anything formed or molded"] 1. the fluid portion of the blood in which the particulate components are suspended. *Plasma* is to be distinguished from *serum,* which is the cell-free portion of the blood from which the fibrinogen has been separated in the process of clotting. See *blood plasma,* under *blood.* 2. the lymph deprived of its corpuscles or cells. 3. a glycerite of starch used in preparing ointments. 4. cytoplasm or protoplasm. **antihemophilic human p.,** normal human plasma that has been processed promptly to preserve the antihemophilic properties of the original blood; used for temporary correction of bleeding tendency in hemophilia. **blood p.,** see under *B.* **citrated p.,** blood plasma treated with sodium citrate, which prevents clotting. **muscle p.,** a liquid expressible from muscular tissue; it clots spontaneously. **normal human p.,** sterile plasma obtained by pooling approximately equal amounts of the liquid portion of citrated whole blood from eight or more adult humans, used as a blood volume replenisher. **oxalate p.,** blood plasma to which 1 per cent of ammonium oxalate has been added, to prevent clotting. **peptone p.,** albumose p. **pooled p.,** a mixture of plasma from several donors. **salt p.,** blood plasma to which a neutral salt has been added to prevent clotting. **seminal p.,** the fluid portion of the semen, in which the spermatozoa are suspended. **true p.,** blood plasma drawn direct from the blood without any change in its gas content.

plasmablast (plaz'mah-blast) [*plasma* + Gr. *blastos* germ] the earliest precursor in the plasmacytic series, which matures to form the proplasmacyte and ultimately the mature plasma cell; it may itself be a derivative of the lymphoblast.

plasmacyte (plaz'mah-sīt) [*plasma* + *-cyte*] plasma cell.

plasmacytic (plaz"mah-sit'ik) pertaining to, characterized by, or of the nature of a plasma cell. See also under *series.*

plasmacytoma (plaz"mah-si-to'mah) [*plasmacyte* + *-oma*] any focal neoplasm of plasma cells, including those of multiple myeloma. Isolated plasma cell tumors may occur outside the bone marrow (extramedullary plasmacytomas), affecting such tissues as the nasal, oral, and pharyngeal mucosa and visceral organs. Called also *peripheral plasma cell myeloma* and *plasma cell tumor.* **extramedullary p.,** see *plasmacytoma.* **multiple p. of bone,** multiple myeloma. **peripheral p.,** see *plasmacytoma.*

plasmacytosis (plaz"mah-si-to'sis) the presence of excess plasma cells in the blood.

plasmagel (plas'mah-jel) a relatively rigid peripheral layer of cytoplasm which is devoid of granules.

plasmagene (plaz'mah-jēn) [*cytoplasm* + *gene*] a self-reproducing copy of a nuclear gene persisting in the cytoplasm of a cell. Cf. *chromogene.*

plasmahaut (plaz'mah-howt) [Ger.] the superficial layer of the protoplasm of a cell.

plasmal (plas'mal) a long-chain fatty acid aldehyde produced during hydrolysis of plasmalogens.

plasmalemma (plaz"mah-lem'ah) [*plasma* + Gr. *lemma* husk] 1. the plasma membrane. 2. a thin peripheral layer of the ectoplasm in a fertilized egg.

plasmalogen (plaz-mal'o-jen) a term applied to a member of a group of phospholipids, present in platelets, that liberate higher fatty aldehydes (e.g., palmital) on hydrolysis, and may be related to the specialized function of platelets in blood coagulation. Plasmalogens are also found in cell membranes of muscle and of the myelin sheath of nerve fibers.

Plasmanate (plaz'mah-nāt) trademark for a commercial preparation of human plasma protein fraction.

plasmapheresis (plaz"mah-fĕ-re'sis) [*plasma* + Gr. *aphairesis* removal] the removal of plasma from withdrawn blood, with retransfusion of the formed elements into the donor; generally, type-specific fresh frozen plasma or albumin is used to replace the withdrawn plasma. The procedure may be done for purposes of collecting plasma components or for therapeutic purposes.

plasmarrhexis (plaz"mah-rek'sis) [*plasma* + Gr. *rhēxis* rupture] dissolution of the cytoplasm.

plasmatherapy (plaz"mah-ther'ah-pe) the therapeutic use of blood plasma.

plasmatic (plaz-mat'ik) pertaining to or of the nature of the plasma.

plasmatogamy (plaz"mah-tog'ah-me) [*plasma* + Gr. *gamos* marriage] union of cells in which the nucleus of each cell is preserved.

plasmatorrhexis (plaz"mah-to-rek'sis) [*plasma* + Gr. *rhēxis* rupture] the bursting of a cell due to the pressure exerted from within.

plasmatosis (plaz"mah-to'sis) the liquefaction of the substance of a cell.

plasmic (plaz'mik) 1. plasmatic. 2. rich in protoplasm.

plasmid (plaz'mid) [*plasm* + *-id*] any extrachromosomal self-replicating element of a cell. In bacteria, plasmids are circular DNA molecules that reproduce themselves and are thus conserved, apart from the chromosome, through successive cell divisions; they include the F factor and R factor. Plasmids that may also become integrated into the chromosome are sometimes called *episomes.* **R p.,** see *R factor,* under *factor.*

plasmin (plaz'min) the active portion of the fibrinolytic or clot-lysing system, a proteolytic enzyme with a high specificity for fibrin, with the particular ability to dissolve formed fibrin clots but also having a similar effect on other plasma proteins and clotting factors and proteins in general. Called also *fibrinolysin.*

plasminogen (plaz-min'o-jen) the inactive precursor of plasmin to which it is converted by the proteolytic action of urokinase; called also *profibrinolysin.*

plasmo- (plaz'mo) [Gr. *plasma* anything formed] a combining form denoting relationship to plasma, or to the substance of a cell.

plasmocyte (plaz'mo-sīt) [*plasmo-* + *-cyte*] plasma cell.

plasmocytoma (plas"mo-si-to'mah) plasmacytoma.

plasmodesm, plasmodesma (plas'mo-dezm; plaz"mo dez'mah) singular of *plasmodesmata.*

plasmodesmata (plas"mo-dez'mah-tah), sing. *plas'modesm* or *plasmodes'ma* [*plasmo-* + Gr. *desmos* a band or bond] cytoplasmic bridges found in some plant cells, which pass between the pores in the plasma membranes of adjacent cells and serve to establish continuity between cells.

plasmodia (plaz-mo'de-ah) plural of *plasmodium.*

plasmodial (plaz-mo'de-al) pertaining to plasmodia.

plasmodiblast (plaz-mo'dĭ-blast) syncytiotrophoblast.

plasmodicidal (plaz"mo-dĭ-si'dal) [*plasmodia* + L. *caedere* to kill] destructive to plasmodia.

plasmodicide (plaz-mo'dĭ-sīd) an agent that is destructive to plasmodia.

Plasmodiidae (plaz"mo-di'ĭ-de) a family of protozoa of the order Haemosporidia, subphylum Sporozoa, containing the genus *Plasmodium*.

Plasmodiophora brassicae (plaz"mo-di-of'o-rah bras'ĭ-ke) a mycetozoan organism which causes a disease of cabbages and other cruciferous plants, called *finger and toe disease, stump root,* or *root-hernia.*

plasmoditrophoblast (plaz-mo"di-trof'o-blast) syncytiotrophoblast.

Plasmodium (plaz-mo'de-um) a genus of sporozoa of the family Plasmodiidae, order Haemosporidia, parasitic in the red blood cells of lizards, birds, and mammals; the malarial parasite. The organism is transmitted to the bloodstream of man by the bite of anopheline mosquitoes, in whose saliva the sporozoites are concentrated. From the blood stream, the sporozoites migrate directly to the liver (exoerythrocytic stage), where they develop and multiply within the parenchymal cells as merozoites, which then burst the liver cells and invade erythrocytes. Erythrocytic schizogeny then occurs, with merozoites escaping infected erythrocytes and invading others. Some of the merozoites develop into gametocytes, which are ingested by mosquitoes, beginning the sexual stage, which ends with the development of sporozoites. **P. brasilia'num,** a species found in monkeys in South America that is much like *P. malariae,* some authorities considering it to be identical. **P. ca'nis,** a species found in dogs in India. **P. capistra'ni, P. catheme'rium,** forms which cause malaria in birds. **P. cynomol'gi,** a species causing malaria in monkeys of the genus *Macacus;* it is similar to *P. vivax,* some authorities considering it to be identical. **P. danilews'kyi,** a species named in honor of Danilewsky, who first described intracorpuscular parasites from birds. This parasite was used by Ross to trace the development of *Plasmodium* in the mosquito, but its exact identification is uncertain. **P. du'rae,** a species pathogenic for turkeys. **P. e'qui,** a species found in the horse. **P. falcip'arum,** the species which causes falciparum malaria in man; it is characterized by thin "signet-ring" forms of trophozoites and the "crescent" form of the gametes. **P. gallina'ceum,** one of the numerous plasmodia of avian malaria. **P. in'ui,** a species pathogenic for monkeys (*Macacus*). **P. knowle'si,** a species causing malaria in monkeys. **P. ko'chi,** a species pathogenic for chimpanzees and monkeys. **P. lophu'rae,** a species recovered from a Borneo fireback pheasant, *Lophura igniti igniti* (Shaw and Nodd), and pathogenic for the domestic fowl. **P. mala'riae,** the species which causes quartan malaria in man. It is characterized by bandlike trophozoites and schizonts with six to twelve merozoites usually arranged in a rosette-like configuration. **P. ova'le,** a species found in the Congo and adjacent regions, causing ovale malaria, and characterized by oval or fimbriated infected red blood cells. **P. pithe'ci,** a species found in the orangutan and chimpanzees; it resembles *P. vivax* except that man is not susceptible. **P. relic'tum,** a form causing malaria in birds. **P. relic'tum** var. **matuti'num,** an organism isolated from the robin, which is morphologically similar to *P. relictum* but biologically very different. It possesses strict quotidian periodicity and a high degree of synchronism of segmentation, rupture of the infected red cells occurring daily about 9 A.M. **P. richeno'wi,** a species found in anthropoid apes. **P. schwet'zi,** a species found in chimpanzees. **P. ten'ue,** *P. falciparum.* **P. vas'sali,** a species found in the squirrel. **P. vi'vax,** the species causing vivax malaria, characterized by the ameboid activity and irregular form of its trophozoites, and by Schüffner's dots in parasitized red blood cells. **P. vi'vax minu'ta,** *P. ovale.*

plasmodium (plaz-mo'de-um), pl. *plasmo'dia* [*plasmo-* + Gr. *eidos* form] 1. a parasite of the genus *Plasmodium.* 2. a multinucleate continuous mass of protoplasm. **exoerythrocytic p.,** a malarial parasite outside a red blood corpuscle.

Plasmodroma (plaz"mo-dro'mah) in some classifications, a subphylum of the Protozoa, including the organisms that do not have cilia, but possess flagella or pseudopodia and one or more similar nuclei, i.e., the Mastigophora, Sporozoa, and Sarcodina. Cf. *Ciliophora.*

plasmogamy (plaz-mog'ah-me) [*plasmo-* + Gr. *gamos* marriage] cytoplasmic fusion of cells.

plasmogen (plaz'mo-jen) [*plasmo-* + Gr. *gennan* to produce] the essential part of protoplasm; bioplasm, def. 2.

plasmoid (plas'moid) an abnormal protein cellular element; see also under *humor.*

plasmology (plaz-mol'o-je) [*plasmo-* + *-logy*] the study of the most minute particles or ultimate corpuscles of living matter.

plasmolysis (plaz-mol'ĭ-sis) [*plasmo-* + Gr. *lysis* dissolution] contraction or shrinking of the protoplasm of a plant cell due to the loss of water from osmotic action.

plasmolytic (plaz"mo-lit'ik) tending toward, pertaining to, or characterized by plasmolysis.

plasmolyzability (plaz"mo-līz"ah-bil'ĭ-te) the power of undergoing plasmolysis.

plasmolyzable (plaz"mo-līz"ah-b'l) capable of undergoing plasmolysis.

plasmolyze (plaz'mo-līz) to subject to plasmolysis.

plasmoma (plaz-mo'mah) a tumor made up of plasma cells; plasmacytoma.

plasmon (plaz'mon) the hereditary factors of the egg cytoplasm. Cf. *genome.*

plasmoptysis (plaz-mop'tĭ-sis) [*plasmo-* + Gr. *ptyein* to spit] escape of protoplasm from a cell through a ruptured cell wall.

plasmorrhexis (plaz"mo-rek'sis) [*plasmo-* + Gr. *rhēxis* splitting] plasmatorrhexis.

plasmoschisis (plaz-mos'kĭ-sis) [*plasmo-* + Gr. *schisis* fission] the splitting of protoplasm into fragments.

plasmosin (plaz'mo-sin) a protein constituent of cytoplasm.

plasmosome (plaz'mo-sōm) [*plasmo-* + Gr. *sōma* body] 1. the true nucleolus of a cell. 2. [pl.] mitochondria.

plasmotomy (plaz-mot'o-me) [*plasmo-* + Gr. *temnein* to cut] reproduction by the separation from the mother cell of smaller masses of protoplasm, each containing several nuclei.

plasmotrophoblast (plaz"mo-trof'o-blast) syncytiotrophoblast.

plasmotropic (plaz"mo-trop'ik) pertaining to or causing plasmotropism.

plasmotropism (plaz-mot'ro-pizm) [Gr. *plasma* plasm + *tropos* a turning] solution or destruction of erythrocytes in the liver, spleen, or marrow, as contrasted with their destruction in the circulation.

plasome (plaz'ōm) [Gr. *plassein* to form] the hypothetical unit of living protoplasm; see *micelle.*

plasson (plas'on) [Gr. *plassōn* forming] the protoplasm of a cytode, or non-nucleated cell.

-plast [Gr. *plastos* formed] a word termination denoting any primitive living cell.

plastein (plas'te-in) the protein synthesized by pepsin from the peptic digestion products of protein.

plaster (plas'ter) [L. *emplastrum*] 1. a gypseum material which hardens when mixed with water, used for immobilizing or making impressions of body parts, as *dental plaster,* or *plaster of Paris.* 2. a pastelike mixture which can be spread over the skin and which is adhesive at body temperature. Plasters may be protectant, counterirritant, etc. **adhesive p.,** see under *tape.* **adhesive p., sterile,** see under *tape.* **belladonna p.,** a plaster containing 30 per cent of extract of belladonna leaves and an adhesive; useful as an anodyne application in neuralgic and rheumatic pains. **p. of cantharidin,** a mixture of cantharidin and other ingredients, formerly applied to the skin as a blistering agent. **capsicum p.,** an active counterirritant which may be used in place of liquid liniments for sprains, rheumatism, and other inflammations. **dental p.,** a gypsum preparation used for the making of impressions of structures of the mouth. **diachylon p.,** lead p. **lead p.,** a plaster containing lead oxide, olive oil, lard, and water, triturated and boiled, formerly used for applying to minor wounds and bruises and also in the preparation of other plasters. Called also *diachylon p.* **mercurial p.,** a plaster containing mercury, oleate of mercury, hydrous wool fat, and lead. **mustard p.,** a uniform mixture of powdered black mustard and a solution of suitable adhesive, spread on an appropriate backing material; used as a local irritant. **opium p.,** a plaster containing extract of opium, water, and an adhesive; used as an anodyne application. **p. of Paris,** calcium sulfate dihydrate, with about three fourths of the water of crystallization driven off, and reduced to a fine powder; the addition of water produces a porous mass that has been used extensively in making casts and bandages to support or immobilize body parts, and in dentistry for taking dental impressions. **resin p., rosin p.,** a plaster containing rosin, lead, and yellow wax. **salicylic acid p.** [USP], a uniform mixture of salicylic acid in a suitable base, spread on paper, cotton cloth, or other suitable backing material, containing between 90 and 110 per cent of the labeled amount of salicylic acid; used as a topical keratolytic. **soap p.,** a discutient plaster made of dried soap and lead, sometimes applied to tumors when a dressing is required.

plastic (plas'tik) [L. *plasticus;* Gr. *plastikos*] 1. tending to build up tissues or to restore a lost part. 2. conformable; capable of being molded. 3. a substance produced by chemical condensation or by polymerization. 4. material that can be molded.

plasticity (plas-tis'ĭ-te) 1. the quality of being plastic or conformable. 2. the ability of early embryonic cells to alter in conformity with the immediate environment.

plasticizer (plas'tĭ-si"zer) any of a group of agents added to other organic or synthetic substances to make them soft and flexible.

plastics (plas'tiks) 1. plastic materials used in surgery or dentistry. 2. plastic surgery.

plastid (plas'tid) [Gr. *plastos* formed] 1. any elementary constructive unit, as a cell. 2. any of the specialized organelles of plant cells that contain pigments (e.g., chlorophyll and carotenoids) or that synthesize and accumulate reserve substances (e.g., starch); they include chloroplasts and amyloplasts.

plastidogenetic (plas-tid″o-jĕ-net′ik)   producing plastids or cells.

plastin (plas′tin)   1. linin.   2. spongioplasm (def. 1).

plastiosome (plas′te-o-sōm)   [pl.] mitochondria.

plastochondria (plas″to-kon′dre-ah)   granular mitochondria.

plastocont (plas′to-kont)   chondriocont.

plastodynamia (plas″to-di-na′me-ah)   [Gr. *plastos* formed + *dynamis* power]   power or ability to develop.

plastogamy (plas-tog′ah-me)   [Gr. *plastos* formed matter + *gamos* marriage]   conjugation in protozoa in which the protoplasm of two or more individuals undergoes amalgamation, the nuclei remaining separate. See *karyogamy* and *plasmatogamy.*

plastogel (plas′to-jel)   a gel possessing great plasticity.

plastokont (plas′to-kont)   chondriocont.

plastomere (plas′to-mēr)   cytomere.

plastoquinone (plas″to-kwin′ōn)   a quinone occurring in chloroplasts, involved in the transport of electrons during photosynthesis.

plastosome (plas′to-sōm)   [Gr. *plastos* formed + *sōma* body]   one of the stainable granules or threads of the cytoplasm; [pl.] mitochondria.

plastron (plas′tron)   [Fr. "breast-plate"]   the sternum and costal cartilages.

-plasty (plas′te)   [Gr. *plassein* to form, mold, shape]   a word termination meaning the shaping or the surgical formation of.

plate (plāt)   [Gr. *platē*]   1. a flat structure or layer, such as a thin layer of bone; see also *lamina, layer,* etc.   2. a dental plate. Sometimes, by extension, incorrectly used to designate a complete denture.   3. to apply a culture medium to a glass plate.   4. to cultivate bacteria on such plates.   **alar p.,** lamina alaris. **anal p.,** cloacal membrane.   **auditory p.,** the bony roof of the auditory meatus.   **axial p.,** the primitive streak of the embryo.   **basal p.,**   1. lamina basalis.   2. the fused parachordal cartilages, precursors of the occipital bone.   3. the portion of the decidua basalis that becomes an integral part of the placenta. **base p.,** see *baseplate.*   **bite p.,** see *biteplate.*   **blood p′s,** blood platelets.   **bone p.,** a metal bar with perforations for the insertion of screws, used to immobilize fractured segments. **cardiogenic p.,** an area of splanchnic mesoderm, at first cephalad and later in the pharyngeal region of the embryo, from which the heart arises.   **cell p.,** a thickening midway of the mitotic spindle in plants that forms a dividing septum between the future daughter cells.   **chorionic p.,** the inner part of the fetal placenta that gives rise to chorionic villi.   **clinoid p.,** the portion of the sphenoid bone behind the sella turcica.   **collecting p.,** the electronegative element of a galvanic battery, where the hydrogen and other decomposition products collect.   **cortical p.,** the dense outer superficial portion of the alveolar process. **cough p.,** a plate of culture medium on which a patient with a respiratory infection, especially pertussis, coughs.   **p. of cranial bone, inner,** lamina interna ossis cranii.   **p. of cranial bone, outer,** lamina externa ossis cranii.   **cribriform p.,** fascia cribrosa.   **cribriform p. of ethmoid bone,** lamina cribrosa ossis ethmoidalis.   **cuticular p.,** terminal web. **cutis p.,** dermatome, def. 3.   **deck p.,** roof p.   **dental p.,** a plate of acrylic resin, metal, or other material, which is fitted to the shape of the mouth and serves for the support of artificial teeth.   **dermomyotome p.,** the portion of the embryonic somite remaining after migration of the sclerotomic tissue.   **die p.,** a plate of metal containing dies for forming the cusps in shell crowns.   **dorsal p.,** roof p.   **dorsolateral p.,** lamina alaris. **Eggers' p.,** bone plate used for maintaining apposition of bone segments.   **end p.,** see *end-plate.*   **epiphyseal p.,** the thin plate of cartilage between the epiphysis and the newly forming tissue (metaphysis) of a growing long bone.   **equatorial p.,** the platelike collection of chromosomes at the equator of the spindle in karyokinesis.   **ethmovomerine p.,** the central part of the ethmoid bone in the fetus.   **floor p.,** the unpaired ventral longitudinal zone of the neural tube, forming the floor of that tube; called also *ventral plate* and *bodenplatte.*   **foot p.,** see *footplate.*   **frontal p.,** a fetal plate of cartilage between the sides of the ethmoid cartilage and the sphenoid bone.   **frontonasal p.,** a fetal plate from which the external nose is developed. **gray p.** (*obs.*), lamina terminalis hypothalami.   **growth p.,** the area between the epiphysis and diaphysis of long bones, within which growth in length occurs.   **horizontal p. of palatine bone,** lamina horizontalis ossis palatini.   **Kühne's terminal p′s,** the motor end-plates of nerves in the muscle spindles. **Lane p′s,** steel plates with holes for screws, used in fixing the fragments of a fractured bone.   **lateral mesoblastic p.,** the thickened portion of either side of the mesoblast.   **lingual p.,** a major partial denture connector formed as a lingual bar extended to cover the cingula of the lower anterior teeth. **medullary p.,** neural p.   **mesial p.,** nephrotome.   **metaphase p.,** equatorial p.   **middle p.,** nephrotome.   **Moe p.,** a stainless steel plate for internal fixation of intertrochanteric

fractures of the femur.   **motor p.,** end-plate.   **muscle p.,** myotome, def. 2.   **nail p.,**   1. stratum corneum unguis.   2. stratum germinativum unguis.   **nephrotome p.,** nephrotome.   **neural p.,** the thickened plate of ectoderm in the embryo from which the neural tube develops.   **notochordal p.,** head process.   **oral p.,** fascia pharyngobasilaris.   **orbital p. of ethmoid bone,** lamina orbitalis ossis ethmoidalis.   **orbital p. of frontal bone,** pars orbitalis ossis frontalis.   **palate p.,** that part of the palatine bone which forms a lateral half of the roof of the mouth.   **paper p.,** lamina orbitalis ossis ethmoidalis.   **parachordal p.,** basal p., def. 2.   **parietal p.,** a thin lamina of the ethmoid bone that forms part of the nasal septum. **perpendicular p. of ethmoid bone,** lamina perpendicularis ossis ethmoidalis.   **perpendicular p. of palatine bone,** lamina perpendicularis ossis palatini.   **Petri p.,** a Petri dish containing a nutrient medium ready for inoculation with the microorganism to be cultured.   **pharyngeal p.,** pharyngeal membrane.   **polar p′s, pole p′s,** platelike bodies at the end of the spindle in certain forms of mitosis.   **pour p.,** a bacterial culture poured into a Petri dish from a test tube in which the medium has been inoculated.   **prechordal p., prochordal p.,** thickened entoderm, cephalad of the notochord, that combines with ectoderm to become the pharyngeal membrane.   **pterygoid p., external,** lamina lateralis processus pterygoidei. **pterygoid p., internal,** lamina medialis processus pterygoidei. **pterygoid p., lateral,** lamina lateralis processus pterygoidei. **pterygoid p., medial,** lamina medialis processus pterygoidei. **quadrigeminal p.,** lamina tecti mesencephali.   **retaining p.,** an appliance used in orthodontics.   **reticular p.,** a form of nerve ending in the ciliary body consisting of very fine reticulations of granular nerve fiber.   **roof p.,** the unpaired dorsal longitudinal zone of the neural tube, forming the roof of that tube; called also *deck plate, dorsal plate,* and *deckplatte.*   **segmental p.,** a plate of mesoblast on either side of the notochord at the posterior end of the embryo, from which the mesoblastic segments are formed.   **Sherman p.,** a chrome-cobalt alloy or stainless steel bone plate which can be affixed to a fracture site with screws. **sole p.,** a mass of protoplasm in which motor nerve endings are embedded.   **spiral p.,** lamina spiralis ossea.   **spring p.,** a dental prosthesis held in place by the elasticity of the base material which abuts against natural teeth.   **Strasburger's cell p.,** midbody, def. 1.   **streak p.,** a plate of solid culture medium in which the infectious material is inoculated in streaks across the surface.   **subgerminal p.,** a sheet of protoplasm forming the floor of the segmentation cavity of the ovum.   **tarsal p′s,** see *tarsus superior palpebrae* and *tarsus inferior palpebrae.*   **terminal p.,** lamina terminalis hypothalami.   **trial p.,** see *baseplate.*   **tympanic p.,** a bony plate which forms the floor and sides of the meatus acusticus internus.   **urethral p.,** an entodermal plate that gives rise to the terminal portion of the cavernous urethra.   **vascular foot p.,** sucker foot.   **ventral p.,** floor p.   **ventrolateral p.,** lamina basalis.   **vertical p. of palatine bone,** lamina perpendicularis ossis palatini.   **wing p.,** lamina alaris.

plateau (plah-to′)   an elevated and level area.   **tibial p.,** either of the bony surfaces of the tibia, internal and external, closest to the condyles of the femur.   **ventricular p.,** a nearly level part of the intraventricular curve of blood pressure corresponding to the mid-ejection period of the ventricle.

platelet (plāt′let)   a disk-shaped structure, 2 to 4μ in diameter, found in the blood of all mammals and chiefly known for its role in blood coagulation; platelets, which are formed in the megakaryocyte and released from its cytoplasm in clusters, lack a nucleus and DNA but contain active enzymes and mitochondria. See also under *factor,* and see *thrombocytic series,* under *series.* Called also *blood platelet* and *thrombocyte.*   **blood p.,** platelet.

plateletpheresis (plāt″let-fĕ-re′sis)   [platelet + Gr. (*a*)*phairesis* removal]   thrombocytapheresis.

platinectomy (plat″ĭ-nek′to-me)   [Fr. *platine* (for footplate of stapes) + Gr. *ektomē* excision]   excision of the footplate in surgical mobilization of the stapes, in treatment of hearing loss.

plating (plāt′ing)   1. the act of applying bacterial culture mediums to glass plates; the cultivation of bacteria on plates.   2. the application of plates to fractured bones for the purpose of holding the fragments in place.

platinic (plah-tin′ik)   containing platinum in its higher valency.

platinode (plat′ĭ-nōd)   [platinum + Gr. *hodos* way]   the collecting plate of an electric battery.

platinosis (plat″ĭ-no′sis)   [platinum + -osis]   a morbid condition resulting from exposure to soluble platinum salts, with involvement of the upper respiratory tract and allergic manifestations of the skin.

platinous (plat′ĭ-nus)   containing platinum in its lower valency.

platinum (plat′ĭ-num)   [L.]   a heavy, soft, whitish metal, resembling tin: symbol, Pt; atomic number, 78; atomic weight, 195.09; specific gravity, 21.37. It also occurs as a black powder (*p. black*) and a spongy substance (*spongy p.*). Metallic platinum is insoluble except in nitrohydrochloric acid, and is fusible only at very high temperatures; it is therefore used in the manufacture of chemical apparatus. Platinum black and spongy platinum have a strong affinity for oxygen, and act as powerful oxidizing and catalytic agents. **p. chloride,** platinic tetrachloride, a poisonous substance, $PtCl_4 \cdot 5H_2O$, used as a chemical reagent and formerly in syphilis. **p. diamminodichloride,** cisplatin.

platy- (plat'e) [Gr. *platys* broad] a combining form meaning broad or flat.

platybasia (plat″e-ba-se-ah) [*platy-* + Gr. *basis* base (of the skull) + *-ia*] basilar impression; see under *impression*.

platycelous (plat″e-se'lus) [*platy-* + Gr. *koilos* hollow] having vertebrae flat in front, or cephalad, and concave caudad.

platycephalic (plat″e-se-fal'ik) [*platy-* + Gr. *kephale* head] wide headed; having a breadth-height index of less than 70.

platycephalous (plat″e-sef'ah-lus) platycephalic.

platycephaly (plat″e-sef'ah-le) the state of being platycephalic.

platycnemia (plat″ik-ne'me-ah) compression of the tibia from side to side.

platycnemic (plat″ik-ne'mik) [*platy-* + Gr. *kneme* leg] having the tibia compressed from side to side.

platycoria (plat″e-ko're-ah) [*platy-* + Gr. *kore* pupil] a dilated condition of the pupil.

platycrania (plat″e-kra'ne-ah) [*platy-* + Gr. *kranion* skull + *-ia*] artificial flattening of the skull.

platycyte (plat'e-sīt) [*platy-* + *-cyte*] a variety of epithelioid cell found in tubercle nodules, intermediate between a leukocyte and a giant cell.

platyglossal (plat″e-glos'al) [*platy-* + Gr. *glossa* tongue] having a broad, flat tongue.

platyhelminth (plat″e-hel'minth) one of the Platyhelminthes.

Platyhelminthes (plat″e-hel-min'thez) [*platy-* + Gr. *helmins* worm] a phylum of acoelomate, dorsoventrally flattened, bilaterally symmetrical animals, commonly known as flatworms, and including the classes Turbellaria, Trematoda, and Cestoidea.

platyhieric (plat″e-hi-er'ik) [*platy-* + Gr. *hieron* sacrum] having a wide sacrum; having a sacral index exceeding 100.

platyknemia (plat″ik-ne'me-ah) platycnemia.

platymeria (plat″e-me're-ah) the condition of being platymeric.

platymeric (plat″e-me'rik) [*platy-* + Gr. *meros* thigh] having a femur that is excessively compressed from before backwards.

platymorphic (plat″e-mor'fik) [*platy-* + Gr. *morphe* form] having a shallow or presbyopic eye.

platymyarial, platymyarian (plat″e-mi-a're-al; plat″e-mi-a're-an) [*platy-* + Gr. *mys* muscle] having all muscle cells lying next to the subcuticula, their sarcoplasm being uncovered on three sides next to the body cavity; said of the muscle arrangement in certain nematodes.

platymyoid (plat″e-mi'oid) [*platy-* + Gr. *mys* muscle + *eidos* form] having the contractile stratum arranged in an even lamina; said of certain muscle cells.

platyonychia (plat″e-o-nik'e-ah) [*platy-* + Gr. *onyx* nail + *-ia*] (*obs.*) abnormal flatness and broadness of the nails.

platyopia (plat″e-o'pe-ah) [*platy-* + Gr. *ops* face + *-ia*] broadness across the face.

platyopic (plat″e-op'ik) marked by platyopia; having a broad face.

platypellic (plat″e-pel'ik) [*platy-* + Gr. *pella* bowl] having a wide pelvis, i.e., a pelvis index below 90.

platypelloid (plat″e-pel'oid) platypellic.

platyphylline (plat″e-fil'in) an alkaloid, $C_{18}H_{27}O_5N$, from *Senecio platyphyllus* D.C. (Compositae) and other species of *Senecio*.

platypnea (plah-tip'ne-ah) [*platy-* + Gr. *pnoia* breath] dyspnea induced by assumption of the upright position and relieved by assumption of a recumbent position; the opposite of orthopnea.

platypodia (plat″e-po'de-ah) [*platy-* + Gr. *pous* foot + *-ia*] abnormal flatness of the foot; flatfoot.

Platyrrhina (plat″ĭ-ri'nah) [*platy-* + Gr. *rhis* nose] a superfamily of the order Primates (suborder Anthropoidea), characterized by a broad nasal septum and often a prehensile tail, and including the New World monkeys.

platyrrhine (plat'e-rīn) [*platy-* + Gr. *rhis* nose] having a broad nose; having a nasal index exceeding 53.

platysma (plah-tiz'mah) [Gr.] [NA] a platelike muscle that originates from the fascia of the cervical region and inserts in the mandible and the skin around the mouth. It is innervated by the cervical branch of the facial nerve, and acts to wrinkle the skin of the neck and to depress the jaw.

platysmal (plah-tiz'mal) pertaining to the platysma.

platyspondylia (plat″e-spon-dil'e-ah) platyspondylisis.

platyspondylisis (plat″e-spon-dil'ĭ-sis) [*platy-* + Gr. *spondylos* vertebra] congenital flattening of the vertebral bodies.

platystaphyline (plat″e-staf'ĭ-lin) [*platy-* + Gr. *staphyle* palate] having a broad, flat palate.

platystencephalia (plat″e-sten″se-fa'le-ah) platystencephaly.

platystencephalic (plat″e-sten-se-fal'ik) exhibiting or pertaining to platystencephaly.

platystencephalism (plat″e-sten-sef'ah-lizm) platystencephaly.

platystencephaly (plat″e-sten-sef'ah-le) [Gr. *platystatos* widest + *enkephalos* brain + *-ia*] a form of dolichocephalism in which the occiput is very wide and pentagonal, the jaws prognathic; observed among South Africans.

platytrope (plat'e-trōp) [*platy-* + Gr. *trepein* to turn] either of two symmetrical parts on opposite sides of the body; a lateral homologue.

plauracin (plaw'rah-sin) an antibiotic complex produced by *Actinoplanes auranticolor*, the structure of the components of which are not fully confirmed; a veterinary growth stimulant.

Plaut's angina, ulcer (plowts) [Hugo Carl *Plaut*, German physician, 1858–1928] see *necrotizing ulcerative gingivostomatitis*, under *gingivostomatitis*, and *necrotizing ulcerative gingivitis*, under *gingivitis*.

Playfair's treatment (pla'fārz) [William Smoult *Playfair*, British physician, 1836–1903] see under *treatment*.

Plectomycetes (plek″to-mi-se'tēz) a series of ascomycetous fungi of the subclass Euascomycetidae that includes the order Eurotiales; their fruiting body is a cleistothecium or a gymnothecium.

plectron (plek'tron) [Gr. *plektron* anything to strike with] the hammer form assumed by certain bacilli during sporulation.

plectrum (plek'trum) [L. from Gr. *plektron* anything to strike with] 1. the uvula. 2. the malleus. 3. the styloid process of the temporal bone.

pledge (plej) a solemn statement of intention. **Nightingale p.,** a statement of principles for the nursing profession, formulated by a committee in 1893 and subscribed to by student nurses at the time of the capping ceremonies.

pledget (plej'et) a small compress or tuft, as of wool or lint.

plegaphonia (pleg″ah-fo'ne-ah) [Gr. *plege* stroke + *aphonia*] auscultation of the chest during percussion over the larynx or trachea in cases in which the patient cannot or is not allowed to speak. The vibrations produced by the percussion take the place of those of the vocal cords.

-plegia (ple'je-ah) [Gr. *plege* a blow, stroke] a word termination meaning paralysis, or a stroke.

pleiades (pli'ah-dēz) [in Greek mythology, seven daughters of Atlas who were placed by Zeus among the stars and form part of the constellation Taurus] a mass of enlarged lymph nodes.

pleiochloruria (pli″o-klo-roo're-ah) an excess of chlorides in the urine.

pleiochromia (pli″o-kro'me-ah) [Gr. *pleion* more + *chroma* color + *-ia*] (*obs.*) increased coloration, especially increased secretion of bile pigments.

pleionexia (pli″o-nek'se-ah) pleonexia.

pleiotropia (pli″o-tro'pe-ah) pleiotropy.

pleiotropic (pli″o-trop'ik) pertaining to or characterized by pleiotropy; producing many effects in the phenotype.

pleiotropism (pli-ot'ro-pizm) pleiotropy.

pleiotropy (pli-ot'ro-pe) [Gr. *pleion* more + *trope* a turning] the quality of a gene to manifest itself in a multiplicity of ways, i.e., to produce many effects in the phenotype.

pleiston (pli'ston) [Gr. *pleistos* most, very many] a group of very similar strains of bacteria.

plektron (plek'tron) [Gr.] plectron.

pleniloquence (ple-nil'o-kwens) [L. *plenus* full + *loqui* to talk] (*obs.*) abnormal talkativeness.

pleo- (ple'o) [Gr. *pleon* more] a combining form meaning more.

pleocaryocyte (ple'o-kar'e-o-sīt) pleokaryocyte.

pleochroic (ple″o-kro'ik) [*pleo-* + Gr. *chroia* color] pleochromatic.

pleochroism (ple-ok'ro-izm) the condition of being pleochromatic.

pleochromatic (ple″o-kro-mat'ik) [*pleo-* + Gr. *chroma* color] exhibiting pleochromatism.

pleochromatism (ple″o-kro'mah-tizm) [*pleo-* + Gr. *chroma* color] the property possessed by some crystals of transmitting one color in one position and the complementary color in a position at right angles to the first.

pleocytosis (ple″o-si-to'sis) presence of a greater than normal number of cells in the cerebrospinal fluid.

pleokaryocyte (ple″o-kar'e-o-sīt) a large nucleated cell found in cachectic disease such as cancer and tuberculosis.

pleomastia (ple″o-mas'te-ah) [*pleo-* + Gr. *mastos* breast + *-ia*] polymastia.

pleomastic (ple″o-mas'tik) polymastic.

pleomazia (ple″o-ma'ze-ah) [*pleo-* + Gr. *mazos* breast + *-ia*] polymastia.

pleomorphic (ple″o-mor'fik) [*pleo-* + Gr. *morphe* form] occurring in various distinct forms; exhibiting pleomorphism.

pleomorphism (ple″o-mor′fism) the assumption of various distinct forms by a single organism or species; also the property of crystallizing in two or more forms.

pleomorphous (ple″o-mor′fus) pleomorphic.

pleonasm (ple′o-nazm) [Gr. *pleonasmos* exaggeration] an excess in the number of parts.

pleonectic (ple″o-nek′tik) [Gr. *pleonexia* greediness] (*obs.*) taking up more than the average amount of oxygen; said of blood which has a higher than normal O₂ content at a given Po₂. Cf. *mesectic* and *mionektic*.

pleonexia (ple″o-nek′se-ah) [Gr. "greediness"] 1. the condition of being pleonectic. 2. morbid desire for acquisition; morbid greediness.

pleonexy (ple″o-nek′se) pleonexia.

pleonosteosis (ple″on-os″te-o′sis) [*pleo-* + Gr. *osteon* bone + *-osis*] abnormally increased ossification; premature and excessive ossification. **Léri's p.,** a hereditary syndrome resulting from premature ossification of epiphyses of the long bones, with broadening and deformity of the digits, flexion contractures of the fingers, broadening and stiffness of the toes and joints, shortening of stature, limitation of movement, and mongolian facies. Inherited as an autosomal dominant trait, the deformities become apparent during the first few years of life.

pleonotia (ple″o-no′she-ah) [*pleo-* + Gr. *ous* ear] a developmental anomaly characterized by the presence of a supernumerary ear located on the neck.

pleoptics (ple-op′tiks) [*pleo-* + Gr. *optikos* of or for sight] a technique of eye exercises designed to develop fuller vision of an amblyopic eye and assure proper binocular cooperation.

plerocercoid (ple″ro-ser′koid) [Gr. *plēroun* to complete + *kerkos* tail + *eidos* form] the wormlike completed larval stage of certain cestode tapeworms, found in the tissues of vertebrates and invertebrates.

plerosis (ple-ro′sis) the restoration of lost tissue, as after illness.

Plesch's percussion, test (plesh′ez) [Johann *Plesch*, German physician in England, born 1878] see under *percussion* and *tests*.

plesiomorphism (ple″se-o-mor′fizm) [Gr. *plesios* near + *morphē* form] similarity in form.

plesiomorphous (ple″se-o-mor′fus) pertaining to or characterized by plesiomorphism.

plessesthesia (ples″es-the′ze-ah) [Gr. *plēssein* to strike + *aisthēsis* perception] palpatory percussion; percussion with one hand against a palpating finger of the other hand.

plessigraph (ples′i-graf) [Gr. *plessein* to strike + *graphein* to write] a form of pleximeter designed to enable the user to mark out the limits of an area.

plessimeter (ples-sim′ĕ-ter) pleximeter.

plessimetric (ples″i-met′rik) pleximetric.

plessor (ples′or) plexor.

plethora (pleth′o-rah) [L.; Gr. *plēthōrē* fullness, satiety] a general term denoting a red florid complexion, or specifically, an excessive amount of blood. **p. hydrae′mica,** increase in amount of blood due to increase in the watery element alone.

plethoric (ple-thor′ik) pertaining to or characterized by plethora.

plethysmogram (ple-thiz′mo-gram) a tracing made by the plethysmograph.

plethysmograph (ple-thiz′mo-graf) [Gr. *plēthysmos* increase + *graphein* to write] an instrument for determining and registering variations in the volume of an organ, part, or limb and in the amount of blood present or passing through it; also used for recording variations in the size of parts and in the blood supply. **body p.,** a device for measuring change in body volume, used especially in measuring pulmonary ventilation. **digital p., finger p. finger p.,** one that registers the change in volume taking place in a single finger. **Franck's p.,** one consisting of an upright glass jar into which the hand and wrist are inserted. **jerkin p.,** a double-layered garment resembling a jerkin, filled with air at slightly positive pressure, used to monitor changes in pressure produced by movements of the chest wall in respiration. **Mosso's p.,** one consisting of a glass tube filled with warm water into which the hand and forearm are placed. The changes in water level, caused by the changes in volume of the limb, are graphically recorded.

plethysmography (pleth″iz-mog′rah-fe) the recording of the changes in the size of a part as modified by the circulation of the blood in it.

pleur- see *pleuro-*.

pleura (ploor′ah), pl. *pleur′ae* [Gr. "rib," "side"] [NA] the serous membrane investing the lungs and lining the thoracic cavity, completely enclosing a potential space known as the pleural cavity. There are two pleurae, right and left, entirely distinct from each other. The pleura is moistened with a serous secretion which facilitates the movements of the lungs in the chest. **cervical p.,** cupula pleurae. **costal p., p. costa′lis** [NA], the part of

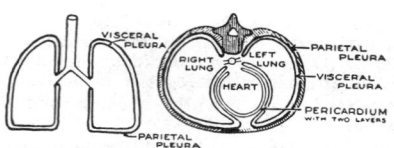

Pleura; for purposes of illustration, the pleural cavity is shown as an actual space. (Williams.)

the parietal pleura lining the rib cage. **diaphragmatic p., p. diaphragmat′ica** [NA], the part of the parietal pleura covering the diaphragm. **mediastinal p., p. mediastina′lis** [NA], a continuation of each pleura, medially, over the lateral face of the mediastinum and the structures within it. **parietal p., p. parieta′lis** [NA], the portion of the pleura lining the walls of the thoracic cavity. **pericardiac p., p. pericardi′aca,** the portion of the mediastinal pleura covering the pericardium and firmly attached to it. **p. pulmona′lis** [NA], **pulmonary p.,** the portion of the pleura investing the lungs and lining their fissures, completely separating the different lobes. **visceral p.,** p. pulmonalis.

pleuracentesis (ploor″ah-sen-te′sis) thoracentesis.

pleuracotomy (ploor″ah-kot′o-me) [*pleura* + Gr. *tomē* a cutting] incision into the pleural cavity.

pleurae (ploor′e) [L.] plural of *pleura.*

pleural (ploor′al) pertaining to the pleura.

pleuralgia (ploor-al′je-ah) [*pleur-* + *-algia*] pain in the pleura, or in the side.

pleuralgic (ploor-al′jik) pertaining to or affected with pleuralgia.

pleuramnion (ploor-am′ne-on) an amnion that develops by a process of folding of the somatopleure, a characteristic of many mammals but not man.

pleurapophysis (ploor″ah-pof′ĭ-sis) [*pleur-* + *apophysis*] a rib, or its homologue; a rib considered as part of a vertebra.

pleurectomy (ploor-ek′to-me) [*pleur-* + Gr. *ektomē* excision] excision of a portion of the pleura.

pleurisy (ploor′ĭ-se) [Gr. *pleuritis*] inflammation of the pleura, with exudation into its cavity and upon its surface. It may occur as either an acute or a chronic process. In acute pleurisy the pleura becomes reddened, then covered with an exudate of lymph, fibrin, and cellular elements (the *dry* stage); the disease may progress to the second stage, in which a copious exudation of serum occurs (stage of *liquid effusion*). The inflamed surfaces of the pleura tend to become united by adhesions, which are usually permanent. The symptoms are a stitch in the side, a chill, followed by fever and a dry cough. As effusion occurs there is an onset of dyspnea and a diminution of pain. The patient lies on the affected side. **acute p.,** a form marked by sharp, stabbing pain, fever, friction fremitus, and to-and-fro friction sounds, or by rapid development of pleural effusion. **adhesive p.,** that in which exudate forms dense adhesions between the visceral and parietal pleurae, which partially or totally obliterate the pleural space. **blocked p.,** pleurisy in which the exudate is imprisoned in a pocket so that it cannot be aspirated; loculated pleural effusion. **cholesterol p.,** accumulation of cholesterol-containing fluid in the pleural cavity. **chronic p.,** a dry serofibrinous or purulent form, which is long continued. **chyliform p., chyloid p.,** a form in which the effused fluid has a milky appearance. **chylous p.,** pleurisy in which the effusion consists of a turbid milky fluid, with sometimes a high percentage of fat; chylothorax. **circumscribed p.,** pleurisy in which the inflammation is limited to a portion of the pleura. **costal p.,** inflammation of the parietal pleura. **diaphragmatic p.,** parietal inflammation limited to parts near the diaphragm. **diffuse p.,** pleurisy in which the inflammation involves the entire surface of the pleura. **double p.,** inflammation involving the pleurae of both lungs. **dry p.,** a variety with comparatively dry fibrinous exudate, usually chronic. **encysted p.,** a form with adhesions which circumscribe the effused material; loculated pleural effusion. **epidemic p.,** epidemic pleurodynia. **exudative p.,** pleurisy with effusion. **fibrinous p.,** pleurisy characterized by deposition of large amounts of fibrin in the pleural space. **hemorrhagic p.,** a variety in which there is a bloody exudate. **ichorous p.,** empyema with a thin, offensive pus. **indurative p.,** pleurisy marked by thickening and hardening of the pleura. **interlobular p.,** a variety enclosed between the lobes of the lung. **latent p.,** a form attended with but little pain or inconvenience. **mediastinal p.,** a variety that affects the pleural folds about the mediastinum. **metapneumonic p.,** pleurisy following pneumonia; pneumococcal empyema. **plastic p.,** a form characterized by the deposition of a soft, semisolid exudate in a layer; fibrothorax. **primary p.,** a form not consequent upon pneumonia or any other observed disease. **proliferating p.,** plastic p. **pulmonary p.,** inflammation of the pleura which covers the lungs. **pulsating p.,** a form in which the heart's action conveys a perceptible throbbing to the effused fluid. **purulent p.,** thoracic empyema. **sacculated p.,** pleurisy characterized by an adhesion pocket filled with fluid. **secondary p.,** any pleurisy consequent upon an attack of some other disease. **serofibrinous p.,** one with a watery exudate and deposition of fibrin. **serous p.,** a form characterized by free exudation of fluid. **single p.,** pleurisy involving only one pleural space. **suppurative p.,** thoracic empyema. **typhoid p.,** pleurisy with symptoms of severe prostration. **visceral p.,** pleurisy involving the visceral pleural layer. **wet p., p. with effusion,** pleurisy marked by serous exudation.

pleuritic (ploo-rit′ik) pertaining to or of the nature of pleurisy.

pleuritis (ploo-ri′tis) pleurisy.

pleuritogenous (ploor″ĭ-toj′ĕ-nus) causing pleurisy.

pleuro-, pleur- [Gr. *pleura* rib, side] combining form denoting relationship to the pleura, to the side, or to a rib.

pleurobronchitis (ploor″o-brong-ki′tis) pleurisy and bronchitis combined.

pleurocele (ploor′o-sēl) [*pleuro-* + Gr. *kēlē* hernia] hernia of lung tissue or of pleura.

pleurocentesis (ploor″o-sen-te′sis) [*pleuro-* + *kentēsis* puncture] thoracentesis.

pleurocentrum (ploor″o-sen′trum) [*pleuro-* + Gr. *kentron* center] the lateral element of the vertebral column.

Pleuroceridae (ploor″o-ser′ĭ-de) a family of snails (order Mesogastropoda) that includes the medically important genera *Hua, Semisulcospira,* and *Goniobasis.*

pleurocholecystitis (ploor″o-ko″le-sis-ti′tis) [*pleuro-* + *cholecystitis*] inflammation of the pleura and the gallbladder.

pleuroclysis (ploo-rok′lĭ-sis) [*pleuro-* + Gr. *klysis* washing] injection of fluid into the pleural cavity; the flushing out of a pleural cavity.

pleurocutaneous (ploor″o-ku-ta′ne-us) pertaining to the pleura and the skin.

pleurodesis (ploo-rod′ĕ-sis) [*pleuro-* + Gr. *desis* binding] the production of adhesions between the parietal and the visceral pleura.

pleurodont (ploor′o-dont) [*pleur-* + Gr. *odous* tooth] having teeth attached by one side on the inner surface of the jaw elements, as in certain lizards.

pleurodynia (ploor″o-din′e-ah) [*pleuro-* + Gr. *odynē* pain] paroxysmal pain in the intercostal muscles due to muscular rheumatism (fibrositis) or irritation of pleural surfaces. **epidemic p.,** an epidemic disease caused by coxsackievirus B and marked by a sudden attack of violent pain in the chest or epigastrium, fever of brief duration, and a tendency to recrudescence on the third day; called also *devil's grip, epidemic myalgia, epidemic myositis,* and *Bornholm disease.*

pleurogenic (ploor″o-jen′ik) pleurogenous.

pleurogenous (ploor-oj′ĕ-nus) [*pleuro-* + Gr. *gennan* to produce] originating in the pleura.

pleurography (ploo-rog′rah-fe) [*pleuro-* + Gr. *graphein* to write] roentgenographic examination of the pleural cavity.

pleurohepatitis (ploor″o-hep″ah-ti′tis) [*pleuro-* + Gr. *hēpar* liver + *-itis*] hepatitis with inflammation of a portion of the pleura near the liver.

pleurolith (ploor′o-lith) [*pleuro-* + Gr. *lithos* stone] a concretion found in the pleura; calcified pleural plaque.

pleurolysis (ploo-rol′ĭ-sis) [*pleuro-* + Gr. *lysis* dissolution] surgical separation of the pleura from its attachments.

pleuromelus (ploor″o-me′lus) [*pleuro-* + Gr. *melos* limb] an individual with a supernumerary limb arising laterally from the thorax.

Pleuromonas (ploor″o-mo′nas) a genus of flagellate, somewhat ameboid protozoa of the family Bodonidae, order Protomastigida.

pleuroparietopexy (ploor″o-pah-ri′ĕ-to-pek″se) [*pleuro-* + *parietal* + Gr. *pēxis* fixation] the operation of fixing the visceral pleura to the parietal pleura, thus binding the lung to the chest wall.

pleuropericardial (ploor″o-per-ĭ-kar′de-al) pertaining to both the pleura and the pericardium.

pleuropericarditis (ploor″o-per″ĭ-kar-di′tis) inflammation involving both the pleura and the pericardium.

pleuroperitoneal (ploor″o-per″ĭ-to-ne′al) pertaining to both the pleura and the peritoneum, or communicating with both the pleural and the peritoneal cavity, as a pleuroperitoneal fistula.

pleuropneumonia (ploor″o-nu-mo′ne-ah) 1. pleurisy complicated with pneumonia. 2. a contagious or infectious pneumonia of cattle, combined with pleurisy, caused by *Mycoplasma mycoides;* called also *pleuropneumonia contagiosa bovum* and *lung plague.*

pleuropneumonia-like (ploor″o-nu-mo′nyah-līk) a term applied to a group of filtrable microorganisms similar to *Mycoplasma mycoides,* the causative agent of pleuropneumonia in cattle. Such organisms have been isolated from sheep and goats (contagious agalactia), dogs, rats and mice, and also in humans. They are also known as *PPLO.* See also *Mycoplasma.*

pleuropneumonolysis (ploor″o-nu″mo-nol′ĭ-sis) [*pleuro-* + Gr. *pneumōn* lung + *lysis* destruction] division of adhesions between the lung and the parietal pleura to permit the lung to collapse.

pleuropulmonary (ploor″o-pul′mo-ner″e) pertaining to the pleura and lungs.

pleurorrhea (ploor″o-re′ah) [*pleuro-* + Gr. *rhoia* flow] a pleural or pleuritic effusion.

pleuroscopy (ploor-os′ko-pe) [*pleuro-* + Gr. *skopein* to examine] examination of the pleural cavity through an endoscope by way of a small incision in the chest wall.

pleurosoma (ploor″o-so′mah) pleurosomus.

pleurosomus (ploor″o-so′mus) [*pleuro-* + Gr. *sōma* body] a fetus with protrusion of the intestine and imperfect development of the arm of one side.

pleurothotonos (ploor″o-thot′o-nos) [Gr. *pleurothen* from the side + *tonos* tension] tetanic bending of the body to one side.

pleurothotonus (ploor″o-thot′o-nus) pleurothotonos.

pleurotin (ploor-o′tin) a toxic antibiotic substance, $C_{20}H_{22}O_5$, obtained from the mushroom *Pleurotus griseus;* it shows activity against staphylococcus (of boils) and tubercle bacillus.

pleurotome (ploor′o-tōm) an area of the lung supplied with afferent nerve fibers by a single posterior spinal root.

pleurotomy (ploor-ot′o-me) [*pleuro-* + Gr. *tomē* a cutting] surgical incision of the pleura.

pleurotyphoid (ploor″o-ti′foid) acute pleurisy followed by and complicated with typhoid fever.

pleurovisceral (ploor″o-vis′er-al) pertaining to the pleura and the viscera.

plexal (plek′sal) pertaining to a plexus.

plexalgia (plek-sal′je-ah) [Gr. *plēxis* stroke + *-algia*] a condition seen in troops after long exposure; it is marked by pains in various parts of the body, fatigue, excitability, and insomnia.

plexectomy (plek-sek′to-me) [*plexus* + Gr. *ektomē* excision] surgical excision of a plexus.

plexiform (plek′sĭ-form) [L. *plexus* plait + *forma* form] resembling a plexus or network.

pleximeter (plek-sim′ĕ-ter) [Gr. *plēxis* stroke + *metron* measure] 1. a plate to be struck in mediate percussion. 2. a diascope; a glass plate used to show the condition of the skin under pressure.

pleximetric (plek″sĭ-met′rik) pertaining to or performed by a pleximeter.

pleximetry (plek-sim′ĕ-tre) the use of the pleximeter.

plexitis (plek-si′tis) inflammation of a nerve plexus.

plexogenic (plek′so-jen″ik) giving rise to a plexus or plexiform structure.

plexometer (plek-som′ĕ-ter) pleximeter.

plexopathy (pleks-op′ah-the) any disorder of a plexus, especially of nerves. **lumbar p.,** neuropathy of the lumbar plexus.

plexor (plek′sor) a hammer used in performing percussion.

plexus (plek′sus), pl. *plexus* or *plexuses* [L. "braid"] a network or tangle; [NA] a general term for a network of lymphatic vessels, nerves, or veins. **annular p.,** a plexus of nerve fibers encircling the corneal margin. **anserine p., p. anseri′nus, p. parotideus nervi facialis. aortic p., abdominal,** p. aorticus abdominalis. **aortic p., thoracic,** p. aorticus thoracicus. **p. aor′ticus,** a network of lymphatic vessels about the aorta. **p. aor′ticus abdomina′lis** [NA], abdominal aortic plexus: an unpaired plexus composed of interconnecting bundles of fibers that arise from the celiac and superior mesenteric plexuses and descend along the aorta. Receiving branches from the lumbar splanchnic nerves, it becomes the superior hypogastric plexus below the bifurcation of the aorta. Branches of the plexus are distributed along the adjacent branches of the aorta. **p. aor′ticus thoraca′lis, p. aor′ticus thora′cicus** [NA], thoracic aortic plexus: a plexus around the thoracic aorta formed by filaments from the sympathetic trunks and vagus nerves, and from which fine twigs accompany branches of the aorta. It is continuous below with the celiac plexus and the plexus of the abdominal aorta. **areolar p.,** p. venosus areolaris. **p. arte′riae cer′ebri anterio′ris,** a thin plexus of sympathetic nerve fibers accompanying the anterior cerebral artery. **p. arte′riae cer′ebri me′diae,** a thin plexus of sympathetic nerve fibers accompanying the middle cerebral artery. **p. arte′riae chorioi′deae,** delicate nerve plexuses accompanying the choroid arteries. **p. arte′riae ovar′icae,** p. ovaricus. **Auerbach's p.,** p. myentericus. **p. auricula′ris poste′rior,** a sympathetic nerve plexus on the posterior auricular artery. **autonomic p's, p. autonom′ici** [NA], extensive networks of nerve fibers and cell bodies associated with the autonomic nervous system; found particularly in the thorax, abdomen, and pelvis, and containing sympathetic, parasympathetic, and visceral afferent fibers. Called also *p. sympathici.* **p. axilla′ris, axillary p.,** a plexus of lymph vessels and nodes in the axilla. **basilar p., p. basila′ris** [NA], a venous plexus of the dura mater situated over the basilar part of the occipital bone and the posterior portion of the body of the sphenoid, extending from the cavernous sinus to the foramen magnum, and communicating with other dural sinuses. **biliary p.,** a network of bile ducts said to be sometimes observable in the liver. **brachial p., p. brachia′lis** [NA], a plexus originating from the ventral branches of the last four cervical spinal nerves and most of the ventral branch of the first thoracic spinal nerves. Situated partly in the neck and partly in the axilla, it is composed successively of ventral branches and trunks (supraclavicular part) which are related to the subclavian artery and which give off the dorsal scapular, long thoracic, subclavius, and suprascapular nerves. The infraclavicular part consists of divisions which lie approximately behind the clavicle and cords and branches in the axilla in relation to the axillary artery. Its branches are medial and lateral pectoral, medial brachial cutaneous, medial antebrachial cutaneous, median, ulnar radial, subscapular, thoracodorsal, and axillary nerves. **cardiac p.,** p. cardiacus. **cardiac p., anterior,** superficial cardiac p. cardiacus. **cardiac p., deep,** the larger part of the cardiac plexus, situated between the aortic arch and the tracheal bifurcation. **cardiac p., great,** deep cardiac p. **cardiac p., superficial,** the part of the cardiac plexus that lies beneath the aortic arch to the right of the ligamentum arteriosum. **p. cardi'acus** [NA], cardiac plexus: the plexus around the base of the heart, chiefly in the epicardium. It is formed by cardiac branches from the vagus nerves and the sympathetic trunks and ganglia, contains visceral afferent fibers, and shows subdivisions related to the arch of the aorta, right and left atria, and right and left coronary arteries. The cardiac plexus is continuous with the right and left pulmonary plexuses. **p. cardi'acus profun'dus,** the deep cardiac plexus. **p. cardi'acus superficia'lis,** the superficial cardiac plexus. **p. carot'icus commun'nis** [NA], common carotid plexus: a nerve plexus on the common carotid artery, formed by branches of the internal and external carotid plexuses and the cervical sympathetic ganglia. **p. carot'icus exter'nus** [NA], external carotid plexus: a nerve plexus located around the external carotid artery, formed by the external carotid nerves from the superior cervical ganglion, and supplying sympathetic fibers which accompany the branches of the external carotid artery. **p. carot'icus inter'nus** [NA], internal carotid plexus: a nerve plexus on the internal carotid artery, formed by the internal carotid nerve, which supplies sympathetic fibers to the branches of the internal carotid artery, to the tympanic plexus, to the nerves in the cavernous sinus, and, directly or indirectly, to the cranial parasympathetic ganglia through which they pass. Called also *carotid p.* **carotid p.,** caroticus internus. **carotid p., common,** p. caroticus communis. **carotid p., external,** p. caroticus externus. **carotid p., internal,** p. caroticus internus. **p. caverno'sus,** cavernous plexus: a plexus of sympathetic nerve fibers related to the cavernous sinus of the dura mater. **p. caverno'sus clitor'idis,** cavernous plexus of clitoris: a plexus of nerve fibers at the root of the clitoris, derived from the vesical plexus and supplying the corpora cavernosa clitoridis. **p. caverno'si concha'rum** [NA], cavernous plexuses of conchae: numerous venous plexuses in the thick mucous membrane of the nasal conchae. **p. caverno'sus pe'nis,** cavernous plexus of penis: a plexus of nerve fibers at the root of the penis, derived from the vesical plexus and supplying the corpora cavernosa penis. **cavernous p.,** p. cavernosus. **cavernous p. of clitoris,** p. cavernosus clitoridis. **cavernous p's of conchae,** p. cavernosi concharum. **cavernous p. of penis,** p. cavernosus penis. **celiac p.,** 1. plexus celiacus. 2. plexus coeliacus (def. 2). **p. celi'acus** [NA], celiac plexus: that portion of the prevertebral plexus which lies on the front and sides of the aorta at the origins of the celiac trunk and superior mesenteric and renal arteries. It contains the paired celiac ganglia, the superior mesenteric ganglion (or ganglia), and small unnamed ganglionic masses. Branches of the plexus extend along all of the adjacent arteries; called also *solar plexus.* **cervical p.,** p. cervicalis. **cervical p., posterior,** a plexus in the posterior cervical region, formed by dorsal rami of the first three or four cervical spinal nerves. **p. cervica'lis** [NA], cervical plexus: a nerve plexus formed by the ventral branches of the upper four cervical nerves; arranged as an irregular series of loops, it gives off superficial branches (lesser occipital, greater auricular, transverse cervical, and supraclavicular nerves), and deep branches (phrenic, accessory phrenic, ansa cervicalis, and muscular nerves). **p. cervicobrachia'lis,** the cervical and brachial plexuses together. **p. chorioi'deus ventric'uli latera'lis,** p. choroideus ventriculi lateralis. **p. chorioi'deus ventric'uli quar'ti,** p. choroideus ventriculi quarti. **p. chorioi'deus ventric'uli ter'tii,** p. choroideus ventriculi tertii. **choroid p.,** infoldings of blood vessels of the pia mater covered by a thin coat of ependymal cells that form tufted projections into the third, fourth, and lateral ventricles of the brain; they secrete the cerebrospinal fluid. See *p. choroideus ventriculi lateralis, p. choroideus ventriculi quarti,* and *p. choroideus ventriculi tertii.* **choroid p., inferior,** choroid p. of fourth ventricle, p. choroideus ventriculi quarti. **choroid p. of lateral ventricle,** p. choroideus ventriculi lateralis. **choroid p. of third ventricle,** p. choroideus ventriculi tertii. **p. choroi'deus ventric'uli latera'lis** [NA], choroid plexus of lateral ventricle: vascular, fringelike folds of the pia mater in the floor of the pars centralis and the roof of the inferior horn of the lateral ventricle, concerned with production of the cerebrospinal fluid. **p. choroi'deus ventric'uli quar'ti** [NA], choroid plexus of fourth ventricle: vascular fringelike folds of the pia mater in the roof of the posterior part of the fourth ventricle and extending into and through the lateral

recesses, concerned with production of the cerebrospinal fluid. **p. choroi'deus ventric'uli ter'tii** [NA], choroid plexus of third ventricle: vascular, fringelike folds of the pia mater in the roof of the third ventricle, concerned with production of the cerebrospinal fluid. **coccygeal p., p. coccyg'eus** [NA], a small plexus formed by the ventral branches of the coccygeal and the fifth sacral nerve, and a communication from the fourth sacral nerve, and giving off the anococcygeal nerves. **p. coeli'acus,** 1. plexus celiacus. 2. a plexus made up of lymphatic vessels and the superior mesenteric lymph nodes and the celiac lymph nodes behind the stomach, duodenum, and pancreas. Called also *celiac p.* **colic p., left,** the part of the inferior mesenteric plexus that accompanies the left colic artery. **colic p., middle,** the part of the superior mesenteric plexus that accompanies the middle colic artery. **colic p., right,** the part of the superior mesenteric plexus that accompanies the right colic artery. **p. corona'rius cor'dis ante'rior,** anterior coronary plexus of heart: a plexus of sympathetic nerve fibers anterior to the heart and related chiefly to the branches of the left coronary artery. **p. corona'rius cor'dis poste'rior,** posterior coronary plexus of heart: a plexus of sympathetic nerve fibers posterior to the heart and related chiefly to the branches of the right coronary artery. **coronary p's, gastric,** p. gastrici. **coronary p. of heart, anterior,** p. coronarius cordis anterior. **coronary p. of heart, posterior,** p. coronarius cordis posterior. **coronary p's of stomach, superior,** p. gastrici. **crural p.,** p. femoralis. **Cruveilhier's p.,** 1. posterior cervical plexus. 2. a form of angioma made up of a knot of varicose veins. **cystic p.,** a nerve plexus near the gallbladder, related to the cystic artery. **deferential p., p. deferentia'lis** [NA], the subdivision of the inferior hypogastric plexus that supplies nerve fibers to the ductus deferens. **dental p., inferior,** p. dentalis inferior. **dental p., superior,** p. dentalis superior. **p. denta'lis infe'rior** [NA], inferior dental plexus: a plexus of nerve fibers from the inferior alveolar nerve, situated around the roots of the lower teeth. **p. denta'lis supe'rior** [NA], superior dental plexus: a plexus of fibers from the superior alveolar nerves, situated around the roots of the upper teeth. **diaphragmatic p.,** p. phrenicus. **enteric p., p. enter'icus** [NA], a plexus of autonomic nerve fibers within the wall of the digestive tube, and made up of the submucosal, myenteric, and subserosal plexuses; it contains visceral afferent fibers, sympathetic postganglionic fibers, parasympathetic preganglionic and postganglionic fibers, and parasympathetic postganglionic cell bodies. **epigastric p.,** p. celiacus. **esophageal p., p. esopha'geus** [NA], a plexus surrounding the esophagus, formed by branches of the left and right vagi and sympathetic trunks, and containing also visceral afferent fibers from the esophagus; it is sometimes subdivided into anterior and posterior parts. **Exner's p.,** superficial tangential fibers in the molecular layer of the cerebral cortex; called also *molecular p.* **facial p., p. of facial artery,** a nerve plexus along the facial artery. **femoral p., p. femora'lis** [NA], a plexus accompanying the femoral artery, derived chiefly from the aortic plexus by way of the common and external iliac plexuses. **fundamental p.,** deep stroma p. **p. ganglio'sus cilia'ris,** a network of nerve fibers about the ciliary body. **gastric p's, p. gas'trici** [NA], subdivisions of the celiac portion of the prevertebral plexuses, accompanying the gastric arteries and branches and supplying nerve fibers to the stomach. **p. gas'tricus ante'rior,** see *rami gastrici anteriores nervi vagi.* **p. gas'tricus infe'rior,** a plexus of nerve fibers on the greater curvature of the stomach. **p. gas'tricus poste'rior,** see *rami gastrici posteriores nervi vagi.* **p. gas'tricus supe'rior,** a plexus of nerve fibers on the lesser curvature of the stomach. **gastroepiploic p., left,** a nerve plexus near the greater curvature of the stomach. **p. haemorrhoida'lis,** p. venosus rectalis. **p. haemorrhoida'lis me'dius,** see *p. rectales medii.* **p. haemorrhoida'lis supe'rior,** p. rectalis superior. **Heller's p.,** an arterial network in the submucosa of the intestine. **hemorrhoidal p.,** p. venosus rectalis. **hemorrhoidal p., middle,** see *p. rectales medii.* **hemorrhoidal p., superior,** p. rectalis superior. **hepatic p., p. hepat'icus** [NA], a subdivision of the celiac plexus accompanying the hepatic artery to the liver. **Hovius' p.,** a venous plexus in the ciliary region connected with the sinus venosus sclerae. **hypogastric p.,** the hypogastric portion of the prevertebral plexuses; see *p. hypogastricus inferior* and *p. hypogastricus superior.* **hypogastric p., inferior,** p. hypogastricus inferior. **hypogastric p., superior,** p. hypogastricus superior. **p. hypogas'tricus,** 1. see *p. hypogastricus inferior* and *hypogastricus superior.* 2. a plexus of lymphatic vessels in the hypogastric region. **p. hypogas'tricus infe'rior** [NA], inferior hypogastric plexus: the plexus formed on each side at the front of the lower part of the sacrum by the junction of the hypogastric and pelvic splanchnic nerves; branches are given off to the pelvic organs. Called also *p. pelvinus* [NA alternative] or *pelvic p.* **p. hypogas'tricus supe'rior** [NA], superior hypogastric plexus: the downward continuation of the aortic plexus; it lies in front of the upper part of the sacrum, just below the bifurcation of the aorta, receives fibers from the lower lumbar splanchnic nerves, and divides into the right and left hypogastric nerves. Called also *nervus presacralis* [NA alternative] or *presacral* *nerve.* **ileocolic p.,** the part of the superior mesenteric plexus that accompanies the ileocolic artery. **iliac p's, p. ili'aci** [NA], plexuses derived chiefly from the aortic plexus and accompanying the common iliac arteries. **p. ili'acus exter'nus,** a lymphatic plexus situated about the external iliac vessels. **infraorbital p.,** a nerve plexus situated deep to the levator labii superioris muscle, formed by superior labial branches of the infraorbital nerve and branches of the facial nerve. **inguinal p., p. inguina'lis,** a lymphatic plexus situated near the end of the long saphenous vein and along the femoral artery and vein in the iliopectineal fossa. **intercavernous p.,** a network of venous channels connecting the two cavernous sinuses across both the roof and the floor of the pituitary fossa. **intermesenteric p.,** p. intermesentericus. **intermesenteric p., lumboaortic p.,** p. aorticus abdominalis. **p. intermesenter'icus** [NA], intermesenteric plexus: the part of the aortic plexus that is located between the origins of the superior and inferior mesenteric arteries. **internal carotid venous p.,** p. venosus caroticus internus. **interradial p.,** Baillarger's lines. **intestinal p., submucous,** p. submucosus. **intramural p.,** a plexus of autonomous intrinsic nerve cells and fibers which are confined entirely to the intestinal and bladder walls, and which take part in or regulate local reflexes and activity. **intrascleral p.,** a network of vessels in the sclera, receiving junctional branches from the sinus venosus sclerae. **ischiadic p.,** p. sacralis. Jacobson's p., p. tympanicus. **jugular p., p. jugula'ris,** a plexus of lymphatic vessels along the internal jugular vein. **laryngeal p.,** a nerve plexus on the outer surface of the inferior constrictor of the pharynx; it is an offshoot of the pharyngeal plexus and is made up of fibers from the sympathetic and external laryngeal nerves. **lateral p.,** p. choroideus ventriculi lateralis. **Leber's p.,** Hovius' p. **lienal p., p. liena'lis** [NA], a subdivision of the celiac plexus, which accompanies the splenic artery; called also *splenic p.* **lingual p., p. lingua'lis,** a nerve plexus accompanying the lingual artery. **p. lumba'lis,** 1. [NA] lumbar plexus: a plexus formed by the ventral branches of the second to fifth lumbar nerves in the psoas major muscle (the branches of the first lumbar nerve often are included). The lower division of the fourth lumbar nerve joins the fifth, and the lumbosacral trunk thus formed becomes part of the sacral plexus. The branches of the first lumbar nerve are the ilioinguinal and iliohypogastric nerves; branches of the plexus proper are the genitofemoral, lateral femoral cutaneous, obturator, and femoral nerves. 2. a lymphatic plexus in the lumbar region. **lumbar p.,** p. lumbalis. **lumbosacral p., p. lumbosacra'lis** [NA], a term applied to the lumbar and sacral nerve plexuses together, because of their continuous nature. **lymphatic p., p. lymphat'icus** [NA], an interconnecting network of lymph vessels. **p. mamma'rius,** a plexus of lymph vessels along the internal mammary artery. **p. mamma'rius inter'nus,** a plexus accompanying the internal thoracic artery and its branches. **p. maxilla'ris exter'nus,** p. of facial artery. **p. maxilla'ris inter'nus,** a nerve plexus accompanying the internal maxillary artery. **maxillary p.,** see *p. maxillaris externus* and *p. maxillaris internus.* **Meissner's p.,** p. submucosus. **p. menin'geus,** a nerve plexus accompanying the middle meningeal artery. **mesenteric p., inferior,** p. mesentericus inferior. **mesenteric p., superior,** p. mesentericus superior. **p. mesenter'icus infe'rior** [NA], inferior mesenteric plexus: a subdivision of the aortic plexus accompanying the inferior mesenteric artery. **p. mesenter'icus supe'rior** [NA], superior mesenteric plexus: a subdivision of the celiac plexus accompanying the superior mesenteric artery. **molecular p.,** Exner's p. **myenteric p., p. myenter'icus** [NA], that part of the enteric plexus within the tunica muscularis. **nasopalatine p.,** a nerve plexus near the incisor foramen. **nerve p.,** a plexus made up of intermingled nerve fibers. **p. nervo'rum spina'lium** [NA], plexus of spinal nerves: a plexus formed by the intermingling of the fibers of two or more spinal nerves, such as the brachial or lumbosacral plexus. **nervous p.,** a plexus made up of intermingled nerve fibers. **occipital p., p. occipita'lis,** a nerve plexus accompanying the occipital artery. **p. oesophage'us ante'rior,** see *p. esophageus.* **p. oesopha'gus poste'rior,** see *p. esophageus.* **ophthalmic p., p. ophthal'micus,** a nerve plexus accompanying the ophthalmic artery. **ovarian p., p. ova'ricus** [NA], a subdivision of the aortic plexus, accompanying the ovarian arteries; called also *p. arteriae ovaricae.* **pampiniform p., p. pampinifor'mis** [NA], 1. in the male, a plexus of veins from the testicle and the epididymis, constituting part of the spermatic cord. 2. in the female, a plexus of ovarian veins in the broad ligament. **pancreatic p., p. pancreat'icus** [NA], subdivision of the celiac plexus, accompanying pancreatic arteries. **Panizza's p's,** two plexuses of the lymph vessels in the lateral fossae of the frenum of the prepuce. **parotid p. of facial nerve, p. paroti'deus ner'vi facia'lis** [NA], a plexus formed by anastomosis of the terminal branches of the temporal, zygomatic, buccal, marginal mandibular, and cervical rami of the facial nerve, arising in the parotid gland. **patellar p.,** a plexus of nerve fibers in front of the knee, formed by communications between branches of the saphenous nerves and the femoral cutaneous nerves. **pelvic p.,** p. hypogastricus inferior. **p. pelvi'nus,** NA alterna-

tive for *p. hypogastricus inferior.* **periarterial p., p. periarteria'lis** [NA], a network of autonomic and sensory nerve fibers in the adventitia of an artery, some of which are following the course of the artery to reach and innervate other structures and some of which innervate the artery itself. **pericorneal p.,** anastomosing branches of the anterior conjunctival arteries, arranged in a superficial conjunctival and a deep episcleral layer about the cornea. **pharyngeal p., p. pharyngeus. pharyngeal p. of vagus nerve,** p. pharyngeus nervi vagi. **p. pharyn'geus** [NA], pharyngeal plexus: a venous plexus posterolateral to the pharynx, formed by the pharyngeal veins, communicating with the pterygoid venous plexus, and draining into the internal jugular vein. **p. pharyn'geus ascen'dens,** a nerve plexus accompanying the ascending pharyngeal artery. **p. pharyn'geus ner'vi va'gi** [NA], pharyngeal plexus of vagus nerve: a plexus formed chiefly by fibers from branches of the vagus nerves, but also containing fibers from the glossopharyngeal nerves and sympathetic trunks, and supplying motor, general sensory, and sympathetic innervation to the muscles and mucosa of the pharynx and soft palate, except for the tensor veli palatini muscle. **phrenic p., p. phren'icus,** a nerve plexus accompanying the inferior phrenic artery to the diaphragm and suprarenal glands. **popliteal p., p. poplite'us,** a plexus of nerve fibers accompanying the popliteal artery. **presacral p.,** p. venosus sacralis. **prevertebral p's,** autonomic nerve plexuses situated in the thorax, abdomen, and pelvis, anterior to the vertebral column; they consist of visceral afferent fibers, preganglionic parasympathetic fibers, preganglionic and postganglionic sympathetic fibers, and ganglia containing sympathetic ganglion cells, and they give rise to postganglionic fibers. The major plexuses are cardiac, pulmonary, esophageal, celiac, mesenteric, and hypogastric. All are closely related to the aorta; those in the abdomen and pelvis supply adjacent viscera by subdivisions which accompany the branches of the aorta and which are named usually after these branches, but sometimes according to the organ supplied. **primary p.,** a network of capillaries that arise from superior hypophyseal arteries, extend into the median eminence of the hypothalamus, then return to the surface, where they are collected into veins that supply the sinusoids of the adenohypophysis. **prostatic p.,** 1. plexus prostaticus. 2. plexus venosus prostaticus. **prostaticovesical p.,** the plexus venosus vesicalis in the male. **p. prostat'icus** [NA], prostatic plexus: a subdivision of the inferior hypogastric plexus that supplies nerve fibers to the prostate and adjacent organs. **pterygoid p., p. pterygoi'deus** [NA], a network of veins corresponding to the second and third parts of the maxillary artery; situated on the lateral surface of the medial pterygoid muscle and on both surfaces of the lateral pterygoid muscle, and draining into the facial vein. **pudendal p.,** plexus venosus prostaticus. **p. pudenda'lis,** p. venosus prostaticus. **p. pulmona'lis** [NA], pulmonary plexus: a nerve plexus formed by several strong trunks of the vagus nerve which are joined at the root of the lung by branches from the sympathetic trunk and cardiac plexus. The plexus is often described as having anterior and posterior parts; filaments from each accompany the blood vessels and bronchi into the lungs. **p. pulmona'lis ante'rior,** anterior pulmonary plexus: the smaller portion of the pulmonary plexus, in front of the root of the lung and interconnected with the posterior plexus; see *p. pulmonalis.* **p. pulmona'lis poste'rior,** posterior pulmonary plexus: the larger portion of the pulmonary plexus behind the root of the lung and interconnected with the anterior plexus; see *p. pulmonalis.* **pulmonary p.,** p. pulmonalis. **pulmonary p., anterior,** p. pulmonalis anterior. **pulmonary p., posterior,** p. pulmonalis posterior. **pyloric p.,** a nerve plexus that supplies the region of the pylorus. **p. of Raschkow,** a delicate plexus of nerve fibers beneath the odontoblasts in the dental papilla during the formation of dentin. **rectal p's, inferior,** p. rectales inferiores. **rectal p's, middle,** p. rectales medii. **rectal p., superior,** p. rectalis superior. **p. recta'les inferio'res** [NA], inferior rectal plexuses: a plexus accompanying the inferior rectal artery, derived chiefly from the inferior rectal nerve. **p. recta'les me'dii** [NA], subdivisions of the inferior hypogastric plexus, in proximity with and supplying nerve fibers to the rectum; called also *p. haemorrhoidalis medius.* **p. recta'lis supe'rior** [NA], superior rectal plexus: a plexus accompanying the superior rectal artery to the rectum, derived from the inferior mesenteric and hypogastric plexuses. Called also *p. haemorrhoidalis superior.* **Remak's p.,** former name for p. submucosus. **renal p., p. rena'lis** [NA], a subdivision of the celiac plexus, accompanying the renal artery. **sacral p.,** 1. plexus sacralis. 2. plexus venosus sacralis. **sacral p., anterior,** p. venosus sacralis. **sacral lymphatic p.,** p. sacralis medius. **p. sacra'lis** [NA], sacral plexus: a plexus arising from the ventral branches of the last two lumbar nerves (which form the lumbosacral trunk) and the first four sacral nerves. The plexus, which lies in front of the piriformis, has twelve named branches; five supply pelvic structures (the nerves to the piriformis, to levator ani and coccygeus, and to sphincter ani muscles, the pelvic splanchnic nerves and the pudendal nerve); seven help to supply the buttock and lower limb (superior and inferior gluteal, posterior femoral cutaneous, perforating cutaneous, and sciatic nerves, and nerves to the quadratus femoris and obturator internus muscles). **p. sacra′lis ante′rior,** p. venosus sacralis. **p. sacra′lis me′dius,** a fine network of lymphatic vessels in the hollow of the sacrum. **Santorini′s p.,** 1. plexus prostaticus. 2. plexus venosus prostaticus. **Sappey′s subareolar p.,** a lymphatic plexus situated beneath the areola of the nipple. **solar p.,** p. celiacus. **spermatic p.,** 1. plexus testicularis. 2. plexus pampiniformis (def. 1). **p. spermat′icus,** p. testicularis. **sphenoid p.** (*obs.*), the upper portion of the internal carotid plexus. **p. of spinal nerves,** p. nervorum spinalium. **splenic p.,** p. lienalis. **Stenson′s p.,** the venous network around the parotid duct. **stroma p.,** a network formed by ramifications of nerve fibrils within the substantia propria of the cornea. **stroma p., deep,** the more deeply seated portion of the stroma plexus. **subbasal p.,** the superficial stroma plexus. **subclavian p., p. subcla′vius** [NA], a sympathetic nerve plexus on the subclavian artery, arising from the cervicothoracic ganglion, contributing fibers to the phrenic nerve and to the branches of the subclavian artery, and continuing to the axillary artery. **submucosal p., p. submuco′sus** [NA], **submucous p.,** the part of the enteric plexus that is situated in the submucosa. **subsartorial p.,** a nerve plexus deep to the sartorius muscle, formed by communications between branches of the medial femoral cutaneous nerve and the saphenous and obturator nerves. **subserosal p., p. subsero′sus** [NA], the part of the enteric plexus situated deep to the serosal surface of the tunica serosa. **subtrapezius p.,** a term occasionally applied to a small plexus situated deep to the trapezius muscle, formed by communications between branches of the accessory nerve and cervical nerves. **supraradial p.,** Bechterew′s layer. **suprarenal p., p. suprarena′lis** [NA], a subdivision of the celiac plexus, in proximity with and supplying nerve fibers to a suprarenal (adrenal) gland. **p. sympath′ici,** p. autonomici. **p. tempora′lis superficia′lis,** a plexus of nerve fibers accompanying the superficial temporal artery. **testicular p., p. testicula′ris** [NA], a subdivision of the aortic plexus accompanying the testicular arteries; called also *p. spermaticus.* **p. thyreoi′deus im′par,** p. thyroideus impar. **p. thyreoi′deus infe′rior,** inferior thyroid plexus: a nerve plexus accompanying the inferior thyroid artery to the larynx, pharynx, and thyroid region. **p. thyreoi′deus supe′rior,** superior thyroid plexus: a nerve plexus accompanying the superior thyroid artery to the larynx, pharynx, and thyroid region. **thyroid p., inferior,** p. thyreoideus inferior. **thyroid p., superior,** p. thyreoideus superior. **thyroid p., unpaired,** p. thyroideus impar. **p. thyroi′deus im′par** [NA], unpaired thyroid plexus: a venous plexus investing the surface of the thyroid gland. **tonsillar p.,** a plexus around the tonsil, formed by communications between the middle and posterior palatine nerves and the tonsillar branches of the glossopharyngeal nerve; fibers are supplied to the tonsil, soft palate, and region of the fauces. **Trolard′s p.,** p. venosus canalis hypoglossi. **tympanic p., p. tympan′icus** [NA], **p. tympan′icus** [Jacobso′ni], a nerve plexus on the promontory of the middle ear, formed by the tympanic and caroticotympanic nerves. It gives off the lesser petrosal nerve and a branch of the greater petrosal nerve and sends sensory fibers to the mucous membrane of the tympanic cavity, the auditory tube, and the mastoid air cells. **ureteric p., p. ureter′icus** [NA], a plexus supplying the ureter and derived from the renal and hypogastric plexuses. **uterine p.,** 1. the part of the uterovaginal plexus that supplies nerve fibers to the cervix and lower part of the uterus. 2. plexus venosus uterinus. **uterovaginal p., p. uterovagina′lis,** 1. [NA] the subdivision of the inferior hypogastric plexus that supplies nerve fibers to the uterus, ovary, vagina, urethra, and erectile tissue of the vestibule. 2. see *p. venosus uterinus* and *p. venosus vaginalis.* **vaginal p.,** 1. the part of the uterovaginal plexus that supplies nerve fibers to the walls of the vagina. 2. plexus venosus vaginalis. **vascular p.,** p. vasculosus. **vascular p., coccygeal,** glomus coccygeum. **p. vasculo′sus** [NA], vascular plexus: a network of intercommunicating blood vessels. **p. veno′sus** [NA], venous plexus: a network of interconnecting veins. **p. veno′sus areola′ris** [NA], areolar venous plexus: a venous plexus in the areola around the nipple, formed by branches of the internal thoracic veins and draining into the lateral thoracic vein. Called also *p. venosus mamillae.* **p. veno′sus cana′lis hypoglos′si** [NA], venous plexus of hypoglossal canal: a venous plexus surrounding the hypoglossal nerve in its canal, and connecting the occipital sinus with the vertebral vein and with the longitudinal vertebral venous sinuses. Called also *rete canalis hypoglossi.* **p. veno′sus carot′icus inter′nus** [NA], internal carotid venous plexus: a venous plexus around the petrosal portion of the internal carotid artery, through which the cavernous sinus communicates with the internal jugular vein. **p. veno′sus foram′inis ova′lis** [NA], venous plexus of foramen ovale: a venous plexus that connects the cavernous sinus through the foramen ovale with the pterygoid plexus and the pharyngeal plexus; called also *rete foraminis ovalis.* **p. veno′sus mamil′lae,** p. venosus areolaris. **p. veno′sus prostat′icus,** prostatic venous plexus: a venous plexus around the prostate gland, receiving the deep dorsal vein of the penis and draining through the vesical plexus and the prostatic

veins; called also *p. pudendalis.* **p. veno′sus recta′lis** [NA], rectal venous plexus: a venous plexus that surrounds the lower part of the rectum and drains into the rectal veins; called also *p. haemorrhoidalis.* **p. veno′sus sacra′lis** [NA], sacral venous plexus: the plexus on the pelvic surface of the sacrum that receives the sacral intervertebral veins, anastomoses with neighboring lumbar and pelvic veins, and drains into the middle and lateral sacral veins; called also *p. sacralis anterior.* **p. veno′sus suboccipita′lis** [NA], suboccipital venous plexus: that part of the external vertebral plexus which lies on and in the suboccipital triangle, receives the occipital veins of the scalp, and drains into the vertebral vein. **p. veno′sus uteri′nus** [NA], uterine venous plexus: the venous plexus around the uterus, draining into the internal iliac veins by way of the uterine veins. **p. veno′sus vagina′lis** [NA], vaginal venous plexus: a venous plexus in the walls of the vagina, which drains into the internal iliac veins by way of the internal pudendal veins. **p. veno′si vertebra′les anterio′res,** plexuses of veins on the anterior aspect of the vertebral column; see *p. venosi vertebrales externi* [*anterior et posterior*]. **p. veno′si vertebra′les exter′ni,** plexuses of veins ramifying external to the bodies of the vertebrae; see *p. venosi vertebrales externi* [*anterior et posterior*]. **p. veno′si vertebra′les exter′ni** [**ante′rior et poste′rior**] [NA], external vertebral plexuses [anterior and posterior]: venous plexuses situated on the anterior aspect of the bodies of the vertebra and on the posterior aspect of the vertebral arches, spines, and transverse processes. **p. veno′si vertebra′les inter′ni,** plexuses of venous plexuses ramifying external to the dura mater, within the vertebral canal; see *p. venosi vertebrale interni* [*anterior et posterior*]. **p. veno′si vertebra′les inter′ni** [**ante′rior et poste′rior**] [NA], internal vertebral plexuses [anterior and posterior]: networks of venous sinuses communicating freely within the vertebral foramina and ramifying externally to the dura mater, anterior and posterior to the spinal cord. **p. veno′si vertebra′les posterio′res,** plexuses of veins on the posterior aspect of the vertebral column; see *p. venosi vertebrales externi* [*anterior et posterior*]. **p. veno′sus vesica′lis** [NA], vesical venous plexus: a venous plexus surrounding the upper part of the urethra and the neck of the bladder, communicating with the vaginal plexus in the female and with the prostatic plexus in the male. **venous p.,** a network of interconnecting veins (p. venosus [NA]). **venous p., areolar,** p. venosus areolaris. **venous p., hemorrhoidal,** p. venosus rectalis. **venous p., prostatic,** p. venosus prostaticus. **venous p., rectal,** p. venosus rectalis. **venous p., sacral,** p. venosus sacralis. **venous p., suboccipital,** p. venosus suboccipitalis. **venous p., uterine,** p. venosus uterinus. **venous p., vaginal,** p. venosus vaginalis. **venous p., vesical,** p. venosus vesicalis. **venous p. of foot, dorsal,** rete venosum dorsale pedis. **venous p. of foramen ovale,** p. venosus foraminis ovalis. **venous p. of hand, dorsal,** rete venosum dorsale manus. **venous p. of hypoglossal canal,** p. venosus canalis hypoglossi. **vertebral p.,** a plexus of veins related to the vertebral column; see terms beginning *p. venosi vertebrales.* **vertebral p′s, internal,** see *p. venosi vertebrales interni* [*anterior et posterior*]. **vertebral p′s, external,** see *p. venosi vertebrales externi* [*anterior et posterior*]. **p. vertebra′lis** [NA], vertebral plexus: a nerve plexus accompanying the vertebral artery, formed by fibers from the vertebral and cervicothoracic ganglia and carrying sympathetic fibers to the posterior cranial fossa via cranial nerves. **vesical p.,** 1. plexus vesicale. 2. plexus venosus vesicalis. **p. vesica′le** [NA], vesical plexus: the subdivision of the inferior hypogastric plexus that supplies sympathetic nerve fibers to the urinary bladder and parts of the ureter, ductus deferens, and seminal vesicle; called also *p. vesicalis.* **p. vesica′lis,** 1. plexus venosus vesicalis. 2. plexus vesicale. **vesicoprostatic p.,** the plexus venosus vesicalis in the male. **vidian p.,** nervus canalis pterygoidei.

-plexy (plek′se) [Gr. *plēxis* a stroke] word termination meaning a stroke, or seizure.

plica (pli′kah), pl. *pli′cae* [L.] a fold; [NA] a general term for a ridge or fold, as of peritoneum or other membrane. **pli′cae adipo′sae pleu′rae,** folds of fat in the pleura. **pli′cae ala′res** [NA], alar folds: a pair of folds of the synovial membrane of the knee joint; attached to the medial and lateral margins of the articular surface of the patella, they pass posteriorly, converge, and become continuous with the infrapatellar synovial fold. **pli′cae ampulla′res tu′bae uteri′nae,** the folds of the mucous coat lining the ampulla of the uterine tube. **p. aryepiglot′tica** [NA], aryepiglottic fold: a fold of mucous membrane extending on each side between the lateral border of the epiglottis and the summit of the arytenoid cartilage. **p. axilla′ris ante′rior** [NA], the fold of skin forming the anterior boundary of the axilla. **p. axilla′ris poste′rior** [NA], the fold of skin forming the posterior boundary of the axilla. **p. caeca′lis,** see *plicae cecales.* **pli′cae ceca′les** [NA], cecal folds: peritoneal folds on either side of the retrocecal recess, which may connect the cecum to the abdominal wall. **p. ceca′lis vascula′ris** [NA], vascular cecal fold: the fold of peritoneum that covers the anterior cecal vessels, forming the superior ileocecal recess. **p. chor′dae tym′pani** [NA], a fold in the mucous membrane of the tympanic cavity overlying the chorda tympani nerve. **pli′cae**

cilia′res [NA], ciliary folds: low ridges in the furrows between the ciliary processes. **pli′cae circula′res** [NA], **pli′cae circula′res** [Kerk′ringi], **pli′cae conniven′tes,** circular folds: the permanent transverse folds of the luminal surface of the small intestine, involving both the mucosa and submucosa. **p. cor′dae utero-inguina′lis,** ligamentum teres uteri. **p. duodena′lis infe′rior** [NA], inferior duodenal fold: a thin fold of peritoneum that bounds the inferior duodenal recess; called also *p. duodenomesocolica* [NA alternative] or *duodenomesocolic fold.* **p. duodena′lis supe′rior** [NA], superior duodenal fold: a fold of peritoneum covering the inferior mesenteric vein and the ascending branch of the left colic artery; called also *p. duodenojunalis* [NA alternative] or *duodenojejunal fold.* **p. duodenojejuna′lis,** NA alternative for p. duodenalis superior. **p. duodenomesocol′ica,** NA alternative for p. duodenalis inferior. **p. epigas′trica,** p. umbilicalis lateralis, def. 1. **p. epigas′trica peritonae′i,** p. umbilicalis lateralis, def. 2. **epiglottic p.,** a fold of mucous membrane between the tongue and the epiglottis. **p. fimbria′ta** [NA], fimbriated fold: the lobulated fold running backward and outward from the anterior extremity of the frenulum of the tongue. **pli′cae gas′tricae** [NA], gastric folds: the series of folds in the mucous membrane of the stomach; they are oriented chiefly longitudinally and partially disappear when the stomach is distended. **p. gastropancreat′ica,** see *plicae gastropancreaticae.* **pli′cae gastropancreat′icae** [NA], gastropancreatic folds: two folds of peritoneum, one covering the left gastric artery, the other the common hepatic artery, between the pancreas and the lesser curvature of the stomach. **p. glossoepiglot′tica latera′lis,** either of two folds of mucous membrane extending, one on either side, between the base of the tongue and the epiglottis. **p. glossoepiglot′tica media′na,** a single fold of mucous membrane between the two lateral glossoepiglottic folds, connecting the base of the tongue and the epiglottis. **p. hypogas′trica,** p. umbilicalis medialis. **p. ileocaeca′lis, p. ileoceca′lis** [NA], ileocecal fold: a fold of peritoneum at the left border of the cecum, extending from the ileum above to the appendix below. **p. incu′dis** [NA], incudal fold: a variable fold in the tunica mucosa of the tympanic cavity, passing from the roof of the cavity to the body and short crus of the incus. **p. interdigita′lis,** the free border of the web connecting the bases of adjoining digits. **p. interureter′ica,** interureteric fold: a fold of mucous membrane extending across the bladder between the two ureteric orifices; called also *p. ureterica.* **pli′cae i′ridis** [NA], iridial folds: the numerous minute folds on the posterior surface of the iris. **pli′cae isth′micae tu′bae uteri′nae,** a fold of peritoneum at the junction of uterine tube and uterus. **p. lacrima′lis** [NA], **p. lacrima′lis** [Has′neri], lacrimal fold: a fold of mucous membrane at the lower opening of the nasolacrimal duct. **p. longitudina′lis duode′ni** [NA], longitudinal fold of duodenum: a mucosal ridge running longitudinally on the inner surface of the medial wall of the descending part of the duodenum. **p. luna′ta,** p. semilunaris conjunctivae. **p. mallea′ris ante′rior membra′nae tym′pani** [NA], anterior mallear fold of tympanic membrane: the line in the tympanic membrane that extends anteriorly from the mallear prominence and demarks the pars tensa from the pars flaccida; called also *p. malleolaris anterior membranae tympani.* **p. mallea′ris ante′rior tu′nicae muco′sae ca′vi tym′pani** [NA], anterior mallear fold of mucous coat of tympanic cavity: a fold in the tunica mucosa of the tympanic cavity, reflected from the tympanic membrane over the anterior process and ligament of the malleus and part of the chorda tympani nerve; called also *p. malleolaris anterior tunicae mucosae tympanicae.* **p. mallea′ris poste′rior membra′nae tym′pani** [NA], posterior mallear fold of tympanic membrane: the line in the tympanic membrane that extends posteriorly from the mallear prominence and demarks the pars tensa from the pars flaccida; called also *p. malleolaris posterior membranae tympanicae.* **p. mallea′ris poste′rior tu′nicae muco′sae ca′vi tym′pani** [NA], posterior mallear fold of mucous coat of tympanic cavity: a fold of the tunica mucosa of the tympanic cavity, extending from the manubrium of the malleus to the posterior wall of the cavity; called also *p. malleolaris posterior tunicae mucosae cavi tympani.* **p. malleola′ris ante′rior membra′nae tym′pani,** p. mallearis anterior membranae tympani. **p. malleola′ris ante′rior tu′nicae muco′sae tympan′icae,** p. mallearis anterior tunicae mucosae cavi tympani. **p. malleola′ris poste′rior membra′nae tym′pani,** p. mallearis posterior membranae tympani. **p. malleola′ris poste′rior tu′nicae muco′sae tympan′icae,** p. mallearis posterior tunicae mucosae cavi tympani. **p. membra′nae tym′pani exter′na ante′rior,** p. mallearis anterior membranae tympani. **p. membra′nae tym′pani exter′na poste′rior,** p. mallearis posterior membranae tympani. **p. muco′sa,** a mucous fold; a fold of mucous membrane. **p. ner′vi laryn′gei,** a fold of mucous membrane in the larynx, overlying the laryngeal nerve. **pli′cae palatinae transver′sae** [NA], transverse palatine folds: four to six transverse ridges on the anterior part of the hard palate. **pli′cae palma′tae** [NA], palmate folds: a system of folds on the anterior and posterior walls of the cervical canal of the uterus, consisting of a median longitudinal ridge and shorter elevations

extending laterally and upward. **p. palpebronasa′lis** [NA], palpebronasal fold: a vertical fold of skin on either side of the nose, covering the medial canthus of the eye; called also *epicanthus.* **p. paraduodena′lis** [NA], paraduodenal fold: an occasionally found peritoneal fold containing a branch of the left colic artery. **p. pubovesica′lis,** a fold of peritoneum between the pubis and bladder. **p. rec′ti,** see *plicae transversales recti.* **p. rectouteri′na** [NA], **p. rectouteri′na** [Doug′lasi], rectouterine fold: a crescentic fold of peritoneum extending from the rectum to the base of the broad ligament on either side, forming the rectouterine pouch. **p. salpingopalati′na** [NA], salpingopalatine fold: the mucosal fold passing caudally from the auditory tube to the lateral pharyngeal wall. **p. salpingopharyn′gea** [NA], salpingopharyngeal fold: a mucosal fold passing caudally from the posterior lip of the pharyngeal orifice of the auditory tube to the lateral pharyngeal wall. **p. semiluna′ris** [NA], semilunar fold: a curved fold interconnecting the palatoglossal and palatopharyngeal arches and forming the upper boundary of the supratonsillar fossa. **pli′cae semiluna′res co′li** [NA], semilunar folds of colon: crescentic folds in the wall of the large intestine, projecting into the lumen between the haustra. **p. semiluna′ris conjuncti′vae** [NA], semilunar fold of conjunctiva: a fold of mucous membrane at the medial angle of the eye. **p. sero′sa,** serosal fold; a fold of serous membrane. **p. sigmoi′dea co′li,** see *plicae semilunares coli.* **p. spira′lis** [NA], spiral fold: a spirally arranged elevation in the mucosa of the first part of the cystic duct; called also *valvula spiralis* [*Heisteri*]. **p. stape′dis** [NA], stapedial fold: a mucosal fold that passes from the posterior wall of the tympanic cavity along the tympanic membrane and surrounds the stapes. **p. sublingua′lis** [NA], sublingual fold: the elevation on the floor of the mouth under the tongue, covering part of the sublingual gland and containing its excretory ducts. **p. synovia′lis** [NA], synovial fold: an extension of the synovial membrane from its free inner surface into the joint cavity. **p. synovia′lis infrapatella′ris** [NA], **p. synovia′lis patella′ris,** infrapatellar synovial fold: a large process of synovial membrane, containing some fat, which projects into the knee joint; attached to the infrapatellar adipose body, it passes posteriorly and superiorly to the intercondylar fossa of the femur. **pli′cae transversa′les rec′ti** [NA], transverse folds of rectum: permanent transverse folds in the rectum, usually three in number (two on the left and one on the right), involving the tunica mucosa and tela submucosa, and the circular layer of the tunica muscularis. Called also *Houston's valves.* **p. triangula′ris** [NA], triangular fold: a fold of mucous membrane extending backward from the palatoglossal arch and covering the anteroinferior part of the palatine tonsil. **pli′cae tuba′riae tu′bae uteri′nae** [NA], tubal folds of uterine tube: the folds of the mucous lining of the uterine tube, which are high and complex in the ampulla. **pli′cae tu′nicae muco′sae ves′icae fel′leae** [NA], the folds in the mucosa of the gallbladder that bound the polygonal spaces, giving the interior a honeycombed appearance. **p. umbilica′lis latera′lis,** 1. [NA] lateral umbilical fold: a laterally placed indistinct line on either side of the inferior part of the anterior abdominal wall, overlying the inferior epigastric vessels; called also *p. epigastrica* or *epigastric fold.* 2. [NA] the fold of peritoneum covering the inferior epigastric vessels; called also *plica epigastrica peritonaei.* 3. plica umbilicalis medialis. **p. umbilica′lis me′dia,** p. umbilicalis mediana. **p. umbilica′lis media′lis** [NA], medial umbilical fold: the fold of peritoneum that covers the obliterated umbilical artery; called also *p. umbilicalis lateralis.* **p. umbilica′lis media′na** [NA], median umbilical fold: the fold of peritoneum that covers the median umbilical ligament; called also *p. umbilicalis media.* **p. ura′chi,** umbilicalis mediana. **p. ureter′ica,** p. interureterica. **pli′cae vagi′nae,** rugae vaginales. **p. ve′nae ca′vae sinis′trae** [NA], a fold of visceral pericardium enclosing the remnant of the embryonic left anterior cardinal vein; called also *ligamentum venae cavae sinistrae.* **p. ventricula′ris,** p. vestibularis. **p. vesica′lis transver′sa** [NA], transverse vesical fold: a transverse fold of the peritoneum extending from the bladder onto the pelvic wall when the bladder is empty. **p. vestibula′ris** [NA], vestibular fold: a fold of mucous membrane in the larynx, separating the ventricle from the vestibule; called also *false vocal cord.* **pli′cae villo′sae ventric′uli** [NA], villous folds of stomach: a fine network of furrows, marking off areas of the stomach. **p. voca′lis** [NA], a fold of mucous membrane in the larynx, forming the inferior boundary of the ventricle, the vocalis muscle being situated deep to it; called also *true vocal cord* and *vocal fold.*

plicadentin (pli″kah-den′tin) [*plica* + *dentin*] a modification of the dentin in which the fibers diverge in many lines from the central pulp cavity of the tooth, as in the teeth of reptiles and certain fish.

plicae (pli′se) plural of *plica.*

plicate (pli′kāt) [L. *plicatus*] plaited or folded.

plication (pli-ka′shun) the taking of tucks in any structure to shorten it, or in the walls of a hollow viscus; a folding.

plicidentin (pli″sĭ-den′tin) plicadentin.

plicotomy (pli-kot′o-me) [*plica* + Gr. *tomē* a cutting] surgical division of the posterior fold of the tympanic membrane.

pliers (pli′erz)   small tong-jawed pincers for bending metals or holding small objects; various forms are much used in dentistry.

Plimmer's bodies, salt (plim′erz) [Henry George *Plimmer*, English zoologist, 1857–1918] see under *body*, and see *antimony sodium tartrate*.

plint (plint)   plinth.

plinth (plinth)   a padded table for a patient to sit or lie on while performing therapeutic exercises.

-ploid [Gr. *-ploos* a fold, as in *diploos*, + *eidos* form]   a word termination denoting (in adjectives) the condition in regard to degree of multiplication of chromosome sets in the karyotype, or (in nouns) an individual or cell having chromosome sets of the particular degree of multiplication in the karyotype indicated by the root to which it is added, as aneuploid, polyploid, etc.

ploidy (ploi′de) [Gr. *-ploos* a fold, as in *diploos* + *eidos* form]   the status of the chromosome set in the karyotype; used also as a word termination denoting the condition in regard to the degree of multiplication of chromosome sets, as aneuploidy, diploidy, haploidy, etc.

plombage (plom-bahzh′) [Fr., "sealing, stopping"]   the surgical filling of an empty space in the body with inert material, as the filling of part of the chest with methyl methacrylate balls as a substitute for injection of air in artificial pneumothorax.

plotolysin (plo′′to-li′sin)   the hemotoxic fraction of plototoxin.

plotospasmin (plo′′to-spaz′min)   the neurotoxic fraction of plototoxin.

plototoxin (plo′′to-tok′sin)   a toxic substance derived from the catfish, *Plotosus lineatus*, said to be composed of a hemotoxic fraction (plotolysin) and a neurotoxic fraction (plotospasmin).

PLT   abbreviation for *psittacosis-lymphogranuloma venereum-trachoma* (group of organisms); see *Chlamydia*.

plug (plug)   a lumpy mass, which closes or obstructs an opening. **copulation p.**, vaginal p. **Corner's p.**, a piece of omentum inserted into a duodenal perforation as a temporary measure in cases which cannot be operated on at the time. **Dittrich's p's**, yellowish or gray caseous masses, of varying size, consisting of granular debris, fat globules, fatty acid crystals, and bacteria frequently found in the sputum, or expectorated alone, in cases of putrid bronchitis or bronchiectasis. **Ecker's p.**, a plug of cells in the primitive mouth of the gastrula. **epithelial p.**, a mass of ectodermal cells that temporarily closes the external naris of the fetus. **Imlach's fat p.**, a mass of fatty tissue sometimes found at the mesial angle of the external inguinal ring. **mucous p.**, a plug formed by secretions of the mucous glands of the cervix uteri and closing the cervical canal during pregnancy. **Traube's p's**, Dittrich's p's. **vaginal p.**, a plug consisting of a mass of coagulated sperm and mucus which forms in the vagina of animals after coitus; called also *copulation p.* **yolk p.**, the mass of yolk cells protruding from the blastopore of amphibians at the end of gastrulation.

Plugge's test (plug′ēz) [Pieter Cornelis *Plugge*, Dutch biochemist, 1847–1897] see under *tests*.

plugger (plug′er)   a dental instrument used for packing, condensing, and compacting filling material into a tooth cavity. **amalgam p.**, an instrument for condensing amalgam in a tooth cavity. **automatic p.**, one which operates by means of a spring, by attachment to a dental engine, or by a pneumatic or electronic device. **back-action p.**, one having a bent shank so that the direction of the force applied is toward the operator. **electromagnetic p.**, one activated by an electromagnet. **foil p.**, one for condensing foil in a tooth cavity. **foot p.**, one having a long, angled, foot-shaped nib. **gold p.**, an instrument for condensing gold in a tooth cavity. **reverse p.**, back-action p.

plumbage (ploom-bahzh′)   plombage.

plumbagin (plum-ba′jin)   chemical name: 5-hydroxy 2-methyl 1,4-naphthoquinone, $CH_3 \cdot C_{10}H_4(:O)_2 \cdot OH$. A yellow, needle-like irritant substance, obtained from various species of plants of the genus *Plumbago*, e.g., *P. europa* L., which has been used as an abortifacient.

plumbago (plum-ba′go)   see *graphite*.

plumbi (plum′bi) [L.]   genitive of *plumbum*, lead. **p. ace′tas,** lead acetate. **p. chlo′ridum,** lead chloride. **p. monox′-idum,** lead monoxide. **p. ni′tras,** lead nitrate. **p. ox′-idum,** lead monoxide.

plumbic (plum′bik) [L. *plumbicus* leaden]   pertaining to or containing lead.

plumbism (plum′bizm)   lead poisoning; see under *poisoning*.

plumbotherapy (plum′′bo-ther′ah-pe) [L. *plumbum* lead + *therapy*]   the therapeutic use of lead, especially its salts.

plumbum (plum′bum), gen. *plum′bi* [L.]   lead[1].

plumericin (ploo′′mer-i′sin)   a principle, $C_{15}H_{14}O_6$, isolated from the roots of *Plumeria multiflora* Muell.-Arg., Apocynaceae, which shows *in vitro* activity against fungi and bacteria, including *Mycobacterium tuberculosis*.

Plummer's disease, sign (plum′erz) [Henry Stanley *Plummer*, American physician, 1874–1937] see under *disease* and *sign*.

Plummer-Vinson syndrome (plum′er-vin′son) [Henry Stanley *Plummer*; Porter Paisley *Vinson*, American surgeon, born 1890] see under *syndrome*.

plumose (plu′mōs) [L. *plumosus*, Fr. *pluma* feather]   feathery; resembling a feather.

plumula (plum′u-lah)   a set of delicate cross-furrows occasionally found on the upper wall of the aqueduct of Sylvius.

pluri- [L. *plus* more]   combining form meaning several or more.

pluriceptor (ploor′′i-sep′tor) [*pluri-* + L. *capere* to take]   a receptor which has more than two complementophil groups.

pluridyscrinia (ploor′′i-dis-krin′e-ah) [*pluri-* + *dyscrinia*]   coincident disorder of several endocrine organs.

pluriglandular (ploor′′i-glan′du-lar) [*pluri-* + L. *glandula*]   pertaining to, derived from, or affecting several glands.

plurigravida (ploor′′i-grav′i-dah) [*pluri-* + L. *gravida* pregnant]   multigravida.

plurilocular (ploor′′i-lok′u-lar)   multilocular.

plurimenorrhea (ploor′′i-men′′o-re′ah)   increased frequency of menstrual periods.

plurinatality (ploor′′i-na-tal′i-te)   large birth rate.

plurinuclear (ploor′′i-nu′kle-ar) [*pluri-* + *nucleus*]   multinucleate.

pluriorificial (ploor′′e-or′′i-fish′al) [*pluri-* + L. *orificium* orifice]   pertaining to or affecting several orifices of the body.

pluripara (ploo-rip′ah-rah) [*pluri-* + L. *parere* to bear]   multipara.

pluriparity (ploor′′i-par′i-te)   multiparity.

pluripolar (ploor′′i-po′lar)   multipolar.

pluripotent (ploo-rip′o-tent)   pluripotential.

pluripotential (ploor′′i-po-ten′shal)   pertaining to or characterized by pluripotentiality.

pluripotentiality (ploor′′i-po-ten′′she-al′i-te) [*pluri-* + L. *potentia* power]   possession of the power of developing (as embryonic cells) or acting in any one of several possible ways, or of affecting more than one organ or tissue.

pluriresistant (ploor′′i-re-zis′tant)   resistant to several drugs.

pluritissular (ploor′′i-tis′u-lar)   composed of several tissues.

plurivisceral (ploor′′i-vis′er-al) [L. *pluri-* + *visceralis*, from *viscus* a body organ]   pertaining to or affecting several viscera, or organs.

plutonium (ploo-to′ne-um) [named from the planet *Pluto*]   a heavy, metallic, radioactive element of atomic number 94, atomic weight 242, obtained by the addition of neutrons to uranium, thereby changing it into neptunium and then into plutonium. Symbol Pu.

Pm   chemical symbol for *promethium*.

PMA   an expression of the prevalence of gingivitis in large groups of persons, *P* representing the papillary portion of the gingiva, *M* the marginal portion, and *A* the attached portion.

P.M.B.   polymorphonuclear basophil leukocytes; see *granular leukocytes*, under *leukocyte*.

P.M.E.   polymorphonuclear eosinophil leukocytes; see *granular leukocytes*, under *leukocyte*.

P.M.I.   point of maximal impulse; see under *point*.

P.M.N.   polymorphonuclear neutrophil leukocytes; see *granular leukocytes*, under *leukocyte*.

PMSG   pregnant mare serum gonadotropin.

P.N.   percussion note.

-pnea (ne′ah) [Gr. *pnoia* breath]   a word termination denoting relationship to breathing, as in orthopnea.

pneo- [Gr. *pnein* to breathe]   combining form denoting relationship to the breath or to breathing. For words beginning thus, see also those beginning *spiro-* (2).

pneogaster (ne′o-gas′′ter) [*pneo-* + Gr. *gaster* the belly]   the respiratory tract of the embryo.

pneogram (ne′o-gram)   spirogram.

pneograph (ne′o-graf) [*pneo-* + Gr. *graphein* to write]   spirograph.

pneometer (ne-om′ĕ-ter) [*pneo-* + Gr. *metron* measure]   spirometer.

pneoscope (ne′o-skōp) [*pneo-* + Gr. *skopein* to examine]   a device for determining movements of the chest wall in respiration.

pneuma-   see *pneumato-*.

pneumal (nu′mal)   pertaining to the lungs.

pneumarthrogram (nu-mar′thro-gram) [*pneumo-* + Gr. *arthron* joint + *gamma* that which is written]   a roentgenogram of a joint after it has been injected with air.

pneumarthrography (nu′′mar-throg′rah-fe)   roentgenography of a joint after it has been injected with air or gas as a contrast medium; called also *pneumoarthrography*.

pneumarthrosis (nu′′mar-thro′sis) [*pneumo-* + Gr. *arthron* joint + *-osis*]   1. the presence of gas or air in a joint. 2. the inflation of a joint with air or gas for the purpose of aiding roentgenographical examination.

pneumascope (nu′mah-skōp) spiroscope.

pneumathemia (nu″mah-the′me-ah) [*pneumo-* + Gr. *haima* blood + *-ia*] the presence of air or gas in the blood vessels; air embolism.

pneumatic (nu-mat′ik) [L. *pneumaticus;* Gr. *pneumatikos*] of or pertaining to air or respiration.

pneumatics (nu-mat′iks) the science which deals with the physical properties of gases.

pneumatinuria (nu″mah-tĭ-nu′re-ah) pneumaturia.

pneumatism (nu′mah-tizm) the doctrine of the Pneumatist school or sect of ancient medicine.

Pneumatist (nu′mah-tist) 1. a school or sect of ancient medicine, founded by Athenaeus of Attalia, and based on the action and constitution of the *pneuma,* or vital air, which passed from the lungs into the heart and arteries and was then disseminated throughout the body. Among other members of this school were Agathinus of Sparta, Archigenes of Apamea, Aretaeus of Cappadocia, and Antyllus. 2. a believer in or practitioner of the Pneumatist theory of medicine.

pneumatization (nu″mah-ti-za′shun) the formation of pneumatic cells or cavities in tissue, especially such formation in the temporal bone.

pneumatized (nu′mah-tīzd) filled with air; containing pneumatic cells.

pneumato-, pneuma- [Gr. *pneuma, pneumatos* air] combining form denoting relationship to air or gas, or to respiration.

pneumatocardia (nu″mah-to-kar′de-ah) [*pneumato-* + Gr. *kardia* heart] the presence of air in the heart.

pneumatocele (nu-mat′o-sēl) [*pneumato-* + Gr. *kēlē* hernia] 1. hernial protrusion of lung tissue, as through a congenital fissure of the chest. 2. a usually benign, thin-walled, air-containing cyst of the lung, as in staphylococcal pneumonia. 3. a tumor or sac containing gas, especially a gaseous swelling of the scrotum. **p. cra′nii, extracranial p.,** gaseous tumors beneath the scalp after a fracture of the skull that communicates with the paranasal sinuses. **intracranial p.,** pneumocephalus.

pneumatocephalus (nu″mah-to-sef′ah-lus) pneumocephalus.

pneumatodyspnea (nu″mah-to-disp′ne-ah) [*pneumato-* + *dyspnea*] difficulty in breathing due to emphysema.

pneumatogram (nu-mat′o-gram) spirogram.

pneumatograph (nu-mat′o-graf) spirograph.

pneumatometer (nu″mah-tom′e-ter) [*pneumato-* + Gr. *metron* measure] a form of spirometer, or instrument for measuring the air inspired and expired.

pneumatometry (nu″mah-tom′ĕ-tre) the measurement of the air inspired and expired; spirometry.

pneumatophore (nu-mat′o-fōr) [*pneumato-* + Gr. *phoros* bearing] an apparatus consisting of a bag with a tube and mouthpiece, which may be attached to the body; the bag contains oxygen, to be breathed by the wearer in rescue work in mines, etc.

pneumatorrhachis (nu″mah-tor′ah-kis) [*pneumato-* + Gr. *rhachis* spine] the presence of gas in the vertebral canal.

pneumatoscope (nu-mat′o-skōp) [*pneumato-* + Gr. *skopein* to examine] an instrument devised by Gabritschewsky for auscultating the percussion of the thorax from the mouth.

pneumatosis (nu″mah-to′sis) [Gr. *pneumatōsis*] the presence of air or gas in an abnormal situation in the body. **p. cystoi′des intestina′lis, p. cystoi′des intestino′rum,** a condition characterized by the presence of thin-walled, gas-containing cysts in the wall of the intestines; the lesions may be subserosal or submucosal. **intestinal p., p. intestina′lis,** p. cystoides intestinalis. **p. pulmo′num,** pulmonary emphysema.

pneumatotherapy (nu″mah-to-ther′ah-pe) [*pneumato-* + *therapy*] the treatment of disease by rarefied or condensed air. **cerebral p.,** injection of pure oxygen into the subarachnoid space; once used in treatment of psychoses.

pneumaturia (nu″mah-tu′re-ah) [*pneumato-* + Gr. *ouron* urine + *-ia*] passage of urine charged with air or gas.

pneumatype (nu′mah-tīp) [*pneuma-* + Gr. *typos* type] a breath picture; a deposition of moisture upon a glass surface or a shiny metal plate from the exhaled air; used in the diagnosis of nasal obstructions.

pneumectomy (nu-mek′to-me) [Gr. *pneumōn* lung + *ektomē* excision] pneumonectomy.

pneumencephalography (nūm″en-sef″ah-log′rah-fe) pneumoencephalography.

pneumo-, pneumono- [Gr. *pneumōn* lung] a combining form denoting relationship to the lungs. *Pneumo-* is also used as a combining form to denote relationship to air or to the breath.

pneumoalveolography (nu″mo-al″ve-o-log′rah-fe) roentgenography of the alveoli of the lungs.

pneumoamnios (nu″mo-am′ne-os) the presence of gas in the amniotic fluid.

pneumoangiogram (nu″mo-an′je-o-gram″) a composite of radiographs obtained by pneumoencephalography and cerebral angiography.

pneumoangiography (nu″mo-an″je-og′rah-fe) roentgenography of the blood vessels of the lungs.

pneumoarthrography (nu″mo-ar-throg′rah-fe) pneumarthrography.

pneumobacillus (nu″mo-bah-sil′us) [*pneumo-* + *bacillus*] *Klebsiella pneumoniae.* **Friedländer′s p.,** *Klebsiella pneumoniae.*

pneumobulbar (nu″mo-bul′bar) pertaining to the lungs and to the respiration center in the medulla oblongata.

pneumobulbous (nu″mo-bul′bus) pneumobulbar.

pneumocardial (nu″mo-kar′de-al) pertaining to the lungs and the heart.

pneumocardiograph (nu″mo-kar′de-o-graf) the instrument used in pneumocardiography.

pneumocardiography (nu″mo-kar′de-og′rah-fe) the recording of variations in heart function through sensors that monitor respiratory changes, e.g., changes in thoracic dimensions, in pressure changes in the bronchi, or in temperature differences between inspired and expired air.

pneumocele (nu′mo-sēl) [*pneumo-* + Gr. *kēlē* tumor] pneumatocele.

pneumocentesis (nu″mo-sen-te′sis) [*pneumo-* + Gr. *kentēsis* puncture] pneumonocentesis.

pneumocephalon (nu″mo-sef′ah-lon) pneumocephalus. **p. artificia′le,** treatment by insufflation of air into the cranial cavity.

pneumocephalus (nu″mo-sef′ah-lus) [Gr. *pneuma* air + *kephalē* head] the presence of air in the intracranial cavity; intracranial pneumatocele.

pneumocholecystitis (nu″mo-ko″le-sis-ti′tis) emphysematous cholecystitis.

pneumochysis (nu-mok′ĭ-sis) pulmonary edema, or serous infiltration of the lung.

pneumococcal (nu″mo-kok′al) pertaining to or caused by pneumococci.

pneumococcemia (nu″mo-kok-se′me-ah) the presence of pneumococci in the blood.

pneumococci (nu″mo-kok′si) plural of *pneumococcus.*

pneumococcic (nu″mo-kok′sik) pertaining to or caused by pneumococci.

pneumococcidal (nu″mo-kok-si′dal) destroying pneumococci.

pneumococcolysis (nu″mo-kok-kol′ĭ-sis) [*pneumococcus* + Gr. *lysis* dissolution] solubilization of pneumococci.

pneumococcosis (nu″mo-kok-ko′sis) infection with pneumococci.

pneumococcosuria (nu″mo-kok″o-su′re-ah) the presence in the urine of pneumococci or of pneumococcus polysaccharide.

pneumococcus (nu″mo-kok′us), pl. *pneumococ′ci* [*pneumo-* + Gr. *kokkos* berry] an individual organism of the species *Diplococcus pneumoniae.*

pneumocolon (nu″mo-ko′lon) [*pneumo-* + *colon*] the presence of air in the colon, often introduced as an aid to diagnosis.

pneumoconiosis (nu″mo-ko″ne-o′sis) [*pneumo-* + Gr. *konis* dust] a condition characterized by permanent deposition of substantial amounts of particulate matter in the lungs, usually of occupational or environmental origin, and by the tissue reaction to its presence. It may range from relatively harmless forms of anthracosis or siderosis to the destructive fibrosis of silicosis. See *aluminosis, anthracosis, asbestosis, siderosis, silicosis,* etc. **bauxite p.,** rapidly progressive pneumoconiosis leading to extreme pulmonary emphysema, frequently accompanied by pneumothorax, caused by inhalation of bauxite fumes containing fine particles of alumina and silica. Called also *bauxite workers′ disease* and *Shaver′s disease.* **p. of coal workers,** a form caused by deposition of large amounts of coal dust in the lungs, and typically characterized by centrilobular emphysema; called also *coalminer′s* or *miner′s lung, black phthisis,* and *miner′s phthisis.* Cf. *anthracosis.* **collagenous p.,** that in which permanent scarring results, due to fibrogenic dust, such as asbestos or silica, or to altered tissue response to nonfibrogenic dust. **noncollagenous p.,** that in which the stromal reaction is minimal, consisting chiefly of reticulin fibers. **rheumatoid p.,** Caplan′s syndrome. **p. siderot′ica,** siderosis, def. 1. **talc p.,** pneumoconiosis produced by the inhalation of talc; symptoms include shortness of breath, cough, fatigue, weakness, and weight loss. Prolonged exposure to large quantities of talc may result in pulmonary fibrosis.

pneumocrania (nu″mo-kra′ne-ah) pneumocephalus.

pneumocranium (nu″mo-kra′ne-um) pneumocephalus.

pneumocystic (nu″mo-sis′tik) relating to or caused by *Pneumocystis.*

Pneumocystis (nu″mo-sis′tis) a genus of organisms of uncertain status, but considered to be protozoa, probably sporozoa. **P. cari′nii,** the causative agent of a highly contagious, epidemic, interstitial plasma cell pneumonia, particularly of infants; see under *pneumonia.*

pneumocystography (nu″mo-sis-tog′rah-fe) cystography following the injection of air into the bladder.

pneumocystosis (nu″mo-sis-to′sis) interstitial plasma cell pneumonia.

pneumocystotomography (nu″mo-sis″to-to-mog′rah-fe) body section roentgenography after inflation of the bladder with air.

pneumocyte (nu-mo-sīt′) pneumonocyte.

pneumoderma (nu″mo-der′mah) [pneumo- + Gr. derma skin] subcutaneous emphysema.

pneumodograph (nu-mod′o-graf) [pneumo- + Gr. hodos way + graphein to write] an apparatus for registering the degree of respiratory nasal efficiency.

pneumodynamics (nu″mo-di-nam′iks) [pneumo- + Gr. dynamis force] the dynamics of the respiratory process; the study of the forces exerted in the act of breathing.

pneumoempyema (nu″mo-em″pi-e′mah) empyema marked by the presence of gas; pyopneumothorax.

pneumoencephalitis (nu″mo-en-sef″ah-li′tis) Newcastle disease.

pneumoencephalogram (nu″mo-en-sef′ah-lo-gram) the roentgenogram obtained by pneumoencephalography.

pneumoencephalography (nu″mo-en-sef″ah-log′rah-fe) radiographic visualization of the fluid-containing structures of the brain after cerebrospinal fluid is intermittently withdrawn by lumbar puncture and replaced by air, oxygen, or helium.

pneumoencephalomyelogram (nu″mo-en-sef″ah-lo-mi-el′o-gram) the roentgenogram obtained by pneumoencephalomyelography.

pneumoencephalomyelography (nu″mo-en-sef″ah-lo-mi″e-log′rah-fe) radiographic visualization of the brain and spinal cord after cerebrospinal fluid is removed by lumbar puncture and replaced by gas.

pneumoencephalos (nu″mo-en-sef′ah-los) [pneumo- + Gr. enkephalos brain] the presence of air or gas in the intracranial cavity.

pneumoenteritis (nu″mo-en″ter-i′tis) [pneumo- + Gr. enteron intestine + -itis] inflammation of the lung and intestine. **p. of calves,** white scours in calves.

pneumoerysipelas (nu″mo-er″ĭ-sip′e-las) (obs.) erysipelas complicated with pneumonia.

pneumofasciogram (nu″mo-fas′e-o-gram) a roentgenogram of tissue after injection of air into the fascial spaces.

pneumogalactocele (nu″mo-gah-lak′to-sēl) [pneumo- + Gr. gala milk + kēlē tumor] a tumor containing gas and milk.

pneumogastric (nu″mo-gas′trik) [pneumo- + Gr. gastēr stomach] pertaining to the lungs and stomach.

pneumogastrography (nu″mo-gas-trog′rah-fe) [pneumo- + gastrography] roentgenography of the stomach after the injection of air.

pneumogastroscopy (nu″mo-gas-tros′ko-pe) endoscopic examination of the stomach after injection of air.

pneumogram (nu′mo-gram) 1. the tracing or graphic record of respiratory movements. 2. a roentgenogram made after the injection of air into the part.

pneumograph (nu′mo-graf) [pneumo- + Gr. graphein to write] an instrument for registering the respiratory movements.

pneumography (nu-mog′rah-fe) [pneumo- + Gr. graphein to write] 1. an anatomical description of the lungs. 2. graphic recording of the respiratory movements. 3. roentgenography of a part after injection of a gas. **cerebral p.,** roentgenography of the brain by pneumoencephalography or ventriculography. **retroperitoneal p.,** roentgenography of the abdominal organs after retroperitoneal injection of air or oxygen.

pneumogynogram (nu″mo-gi′no-gram) a roentgenogram of the female reproductive organs after injection of air into the uterus.

pneumohemia (nu″mo-he′me-ah) [pneumo- + Gr. haima blood + -ia] the presence of air or gas in the blood vessels; air embolism.

pneumohemopericardium (nu″mo-he″mo-per″ĭ-kar′de-um) [pneumo- + Gr. haima blood + pericardium] the presence of air or gas and blood in the pericardial cavity.

pneumohemothorax (nu″mo-he″mo-tho′raks) [pneumo- + Gr. haima blood + thōrax chest] the presence of air or gas and blood in the pleural cavity.

pneumohydrometra (nu″mo-hi″dro-me′trah) [pneumo- + Gr. hydōr water + mētra uterus] a collection of gas and fluid in the uterine cavity.

pneumohydropericardium (nu″mo-hi″dro-per″ĭ-kar′de-um) [pneumo- + Gr. hydōr water + pericardium] the presence of air or gas and fluid in the pericardial cavity.

pneumohydrothorax (nu″mo-hi″dro-tho′raks) [pneumo- + Gr. hydōr water + thōrax chest] a collection of air or gas and fluid in the pleural cavity.

pneumokidney (nu″mo-kid″ne) [pneumo- + kidney] the presence of gas in the kidney pelvis.

pneumokoniosis (nu″mo-ko″ne-o′sis) pneumoconiosis.

pneumolith (nu′mo-lith) [pneumo- + Gr. lithos stone] a pulmonary calculus or concretion.

pneumolithiasis (nu″mo-lĭ-thi′ah-sis) the presence of concretions in the lungs.

pneumology (nu-mol′o-je) [pneumo- + -logy] the study of disease of the air passages.

pneumolysis (nu-mol′ĭ-sis) pneumonolysis.

pneumomalacia (nu″mo-mah-la′she-ah) [pneumo- + Gr. malakia softness] morbid softening of lung tissue.

pneumomassage (nu″mo-mah-sahzh′) [pneumo- + massage] air massage of the tympanum by the alternate compression and rarefaction of the air in the external auditory canal.

pneumomediastinogram (nu″mo-me″de-as-ti′no-gram) the film produced by pneumomediastinography.

pneumomediastinography (nu″mo-me″de-as″tĭ-nog′rah-fe) roentgenography of the mediastinum after injection of nitrous oxide or oxygen through a needle introduced back of the trachea or behind the manubrium.

pneumomediastinum (nu″mo-me″de-as-ti′num) [pneumo- + mediastinum] the presence of air or gas in the mediastinum, which may interfere with respiration and circulation and may lead to pneumopericardium, pneumothorax, or pneumoperitoneum. It is due to leakage of air from the tracheobronchial tree, usually as a result of trauma; sometimes the air is deliberately introduced as an aid to examination and diagnosis. Called also mediastinal emphysema.

pneumomelanosis (nu″mo-mel″ah-no′sis) [pneumo- + melanosis] the blackening of the lung tissue by inhaled coal dust; see anthracosis.

pneumometer (nu-mom′ĕ-ter) pneumatometer.

pneumomycosis (nu″mo-mi-ko′sis) [pneumo- + mycosis] any fungal disease of the lungs.

pneumomyelography (nu″mo-mi″ĕ-log′rah-fe) [pneumo- + Gr. myelos marrow + graphein to write] roentgen-ray examination after withdrawal of cerebrospinal fluid and injection of air or gas into the spinal canal.

pneumonectasia (nu″mon-ek-ta′ze-ah) pneumonectasis.

pneumonectasis (nu″mo-nek′tah-sis) [pneumo- + Gr. ektasis extension] emphysema of the lungs; overdistention of lung tissue.

pneumonectomy (nu″mo-nek′to-me) [pneumono- + Gr. ektomē excision] the excision of lung tissue, especially of an entire lung. **total p.,** surgical excision of an entire lung.

pneumonedema (nu″mo-ne-de′mah) [pneumo- + edema] edema of the lungs.

pneumonemia (nu″mo-ne′me-ah) [pneumo- + Gr. haima blood + -ia] congestion of the lungs.

pneumonere (nu′mo-nēr) one of the end-buds which cap the primitive bronchi.

pneumonia (nu-mo′ne-ah) [Gr. pneumōnia] inflammation of the lungs with consolidation. **abortive p.,** a form with a short and favorable course. **acute p.,** severe pneumonia of rapid onset. **p. al′ba,** a fatal desquamative pneumonia of the newborn resulting from congenital syphilis and characterized by white fatty degeneration of the lungs, which appear pale, and virtually airless. Called also white p. and white lung. **alcoholic p.,** pneumonia associated with alcoholism. **amebic p.,** pneumonia resulting from so-called amebic abscesses in the lung caused by Entamoeba histolytica. **anthrax p.,** pulmonary anthrax. **apex p., apical p.,** lobar pneumonia limited to the apex of the lung. **p. apostemato′sa,** suppurative p. **aspiration p.,** pneumonia due to the entrance of foreign matter, such as food particles, into the respiratory passages (bronchi). **atypical p.,** primary atypical p. **bacterial p.,** pneumonia caused by bacteria, chief among which are Streptococcus pneumoniae, S. hemolytica, Staphylococcus aureus, and Klebsiella pneumoniae. **bilious p.,** lobar pneumonia attended with jaundice. **bronchial p.,** bronchopneumonia. **brooder p.,** a pneumonic disease (aspergillosis) of chicks acquired from moldy grain or straw. **Buhl's desquamative p.,** cheesy p. **caseous p.,** cheesy p. **cat p.,** a lung disease of cats probably due to the agent (Chlamydia) of psittacosis. **catarrhal p.,** bronchopneumonia. **central p.,** lobar pneumonia beginning in the hilum of a lobe of the lung. **cerebral p.,** pneumonia associated with neurologic symptoms and disturbances of consciousness. **cheesy p.,** pneumonia, usually tuberculous, in which necrotic lung tissue is of semisolid consistency and the cut surface looks like cheese. **chronic p.,** a long-continuing form. **cold agglutinin p.,** primary atypical p. **congenital aspiration p.,** see respiratory distress syndrome, under syndrome. **contagious p. of horses,** a condition that may follow equine influenza, characterized by high fever, pneumonia, and necrosis of the lungs. **contusion p.,** pneumonia following an injury. **core p.,** central p. **Corrigan's p.,** Kaufman's p. **croupous p.,** lobar p. **deglutition p.,** aspiration pneumonia due to the entrance of food into the lungs, usually associated with dysphagia. **der-**

mal p., a condition produced by injection of virulent pneumococci into the skin of rabbits. **desquamative p.,** chronic pneumonia with hardening of the fibrous exudate and proliferation of the interstitial tissue and epithelium of the lung; called also *parenchymatous p.* **desquamative interstitial p.,** chronic pneumonia of unknown etiology, with desquamation of large alveolar cells and thickening of the walls of distal air passages; it is characterized by dyspnea and often by a nonproductive and harsh cough. **p. dis′secans,** pneumonia interlobularis purulenta. **double p.,** that which affects both lungs. **Eaton agent p.,** mycoplasmal p. **embolic p.,** pneumonia due to embolism of a blood vessel or vessels of the lungs. **ephemeral p.,** that in which the signs of pneumonia disappear after a short period. **ether p.,** pneumonia occurring after anesthesia by ether. **fibrinous p.,** pneumonia characterized by abundant exudation of fibrin into the air passages. **fibrous p.,** a form characterized by an increase in scar tissue during the healing process. **fibrous p., chronic,** interstitial pulmonary fibrosis. **Friedländer's p., Friedländer's bacillus p.,** an acute specific infectious disease characterized by massive mucoid inflammatory exudates in the lung, and caused by *Klebsiella pneumoniae.* **gangrenous p.,** gangrene of the lung. **giant cell p.,** a rare, usually fatal form of interstitial pneumonia caused by the measles virus, affecting children with disease of the reticuloendothelial system (such as leukemia), and marked by the presence of multinucleate giant-cell inclusion bodies; called also *Hecht's p.* **Hecht's p.,** giant cell p. **hypostatic p.,** pneumonia due to dorsal decubitus in weak or aged persons. **indurative p.,** pneumonia associated with dense fibrous scar tissue. **infective p. of goats,** a fatal disease of goats in South Africa. **influenzal p., influenza virus p.,** a severe, usually fatal disease caused by influenza virus and characterized by abrupt onset, high fever, prostration, sore throat, aching pains, and profound dyspnea and anxiety, and by massive pulmonary hemorrhagic edema and consolidation. It may be complicated by bacterial pneumonia, in which case the symptoms of that disease (shaking chills, pleuritic pain, etc.) are superimposed on the primary influenza virus pneumonia. **inhalation p.,** 1. aspiration pneumonia. 2. bronchopneumonia due to the inhalation of irritating vapors. **p. interlobula′ris purulen′ta,** pneumonia in which the lobules are separated from one another. **interstitial p.,** a chronic form of pneumonia with increase of the interstitial tissue and decrease of the proper lung tissue, with induration; called also *chronic fibrous p.* **interstitial plasma cell p.,** a pulmonary disease of infants and debilitated persons, including those receiving cytotoxic drugs, immunosuppressive drugs, cortisone, etc., in which cellular detritus containing plasma cells appears in the lung tissue; it is caused by *Pneumocystis carinii.* Called also *pneumocystis pneumonia.* **intrauterine p.,** pneumonia contracted by the fetus *in utero;* it may result in the death of the fetus or the birth of an infant with fully developed pneumonia. **Kaufman's p.,** acute interstitial pneumonia, a rare fatal form of pneumonia in young infants. **lipid p., lipoid p.,** a pneumonia-like reaction of the lung tissue to the aspiration of oils; called also *oil-aspiration p.* and *pneumonolipoidosis.* **lobar p.,** an acute febrile disease produced by the *Streptococcus pneumoniae,* and marked by inflammation of one or more lobes of the lung, together with consolidation. It is attended with chill, followed by sudden elevation of temperature, dyspnea, rapid breathing, pain in the side, and cough, with blood-stained expectoration. The symptoms abate after a week. It usually begins in the lower lobe, the lung being at first intensely congested (*stage of congestion* or *engorgement*), and afterward becoming red and solid from accumulation of exudate and blood cells in the alveoli (*red hepatization*), and later gray (*gray hepatization*), from degeneration of the exudates, which are finally absorbed. Called also *croupous p., fibrinous p.,* and *lung fever.* **lobular p.,** bronchopneumonia. **Löffler's p.,** Löffler's syndrome. **Louisiana p.,** a form of pneumonia encountered in Louisiana, caused by a strain of *Chlamydia psittaci.* **p. malleo′sa,** pneumonia caused by or associated with glanders. **massive p.,** lobar pneumonia with extensive solidification of the air cells, or even an entire lung. **metastatic p.,** suppurative pneumonia due to bloodborne infection in bacteremia. **migratory p.,** pneumonia gradually involving one lobe of the lung after another. **mycoplasmal p.,** the most common form of primary atypical pneumonia (q.v.), caused by *Mycoplasma pneumoniae* and occurring most frequently in young adults; called also *Eaton agent p.* **obstructive p.,** that due to obstruction of the air passages, as by bronchogenic carcinoma. **oil-aspiration p.,** lipid p. **parenchymatous p.,** desquamative p. **plague p.,** pneumonic plague. **plasma cell p.,** interstitial plasma cell p. **pleuritic p.,** pleuropneumonia. **pleurogenetic p., pleurogenic p.,** that which is secondary to pleural disease. **pneumococcal p.,** lobar p. **pneumocystis p., Pneumocystis carinii p.,** interstitial plasma cell p. **primary atypical p.,** a general term applied to an acute infectious pulmonary disease caused by *Mycoplasma pneumoniae,* species of *Rickettsia* and *Chlamydia,* and various viruses, including adenoviruses and parainfluenza virus; it is marked by extensive but tenuous pulmonary infiltration and by fever, malaise, myalgia, sore throat, and a cough which at first is nonproductive but becomes productive and paroxysmal. Called also *atypical p.,* atypical bronchopneu-

monia, acute interstitial pneumonitis, cold agglutinin p., and *viral p.* **purulent p.,** a form characterized by the expectoration of copious pus. **rheumatic p.,** a rare, usually fatal complication of acute rheumatic fever characterized by extensive pulmonary consolidation and rapidly progressive functional deterioration and by alveolar exudate (with the presence of Masson bodies), interstitial infiltrates, and necrotizing arteritis. **Riesman's p.,** a peculiar form of chronic bronchopneumonia. **secondary p.,** inflammation of the lungs coming on as a complication of some systemic disorder. **septic p.,** pneumonia invasive virulent infectious agents. **staphylococcal p.,** pneumonia caused by infection with *Staphylococcus,* many strains of which are antibiotic-resistant; it has a strong tendency to extend beyond the original site of infection. **streptococcal p.,** pneumonia caused by infection with *S. pyogenes,* usually occurring as a complication of influenza. **superficial p.,** a form which affects only the parts near the pleura. **suppurative p.,** pneumonia with formation of abscesses in the lungs. **terminal p.,** pneumonia developing during some other disease and hastening a fatal termination. **toxemic p.,** infection of the system with pneumococci without marked lung involvement. **transplantation p.,** an unusual pneumonia affecting the recipients of transplanted kidneys, possibly as a result of altered immunologic response in the lung. **traumatic p.,** inflammation of the lung following physical injury to the thorax. **tuberculous p.,** the simplest form of pulmonary tuberculosis, often the earliest reaction to infection. **tularemic p.,** pneumonia caused by *Pasteurella tularensis;* see *tularemia.* **typhoid p.,** a form of pneumonia with typhoid symptoms. **unresolved p.,** pneumonia in which the lung signs fail to clear up within the usual period. **vagus p.,** pneumonia associated with injury of the pneumogastric nerve. **varicella p.,** pneumonia developing two to six days after the appearance of varicella (chickenpox) eruption and apparently due to the same virus. Symptoms may be severe, with violent cough, hemoptysis, and severe chest pains. Radiologically, there are numerous nodular densities, which may coalesce, at the base of each lung and, often, enlarged lymph nodes in the hilar region. Small nodular calcifications may persist. **viral p.,** pneumonia caused by a virus, as by adenoviruses, influenza virus, parainfluenza virus, and varicella virus; see also *influenza virus p.* and *primary atypical p.* **wandering p.,** migratory p. **white p.,** p. alba. **woolsorter's p.,** pulmonary anthrax.

pneumonic (nu-mon′ik) [Gr. *pneumonikos*] pertaining to the lung or to pneumonia; see also under *plague.*

pneumonitis (nu″mo-ni′tis) [Gr. *pneumōn* lung + *-itis*] inflammation of the lungs. **acute interstitial p.,** primary atypical pneumonia. **aspiration p.,** aspiration pneumonia. **chemical p.,** pneumonitis caused by the inhalation of chemical irritants; the extent of the injury reflects the concentration of the irritants and the duration of exposure. **cholesterol p.,** pneumonitis characterized by chronic inflammatory changes and deposition of excessive amounts of cholesterol in the lungs. It is often lobar or segmental in distribution and may resemble primary or metastatic tumor. **feline p.,** a fatal pneumonitis with conjunctivitis in cats, caused by a strain of *Chlamydia psittaci.* **granulomatous p.,** inflammation of the lung which may result from inhalation of organic dusts by persons who have become sensitized to antigens in the dusts. The term is sometimes used to designate farmer's lung. **hypersensitivity p.,** allergic alveolitis. **malarial p.,** pneumonitis caused by *Plasmodium falciparum,* characterized by cough with bloody sputum and coarse rales; in severe cases thromboses may result from the agglutination of parasitized erythrocytes in small blood vessels of the lung. **mouse p.,** a bronchopneumonia of laboratory mice caused by a strain of *Chlamydia trachomatis.* **pneumocystis p.,** interstitial plasma cell pneumonia. **uremic p.,** pneumonitis associated with uremia; a butterfly or bat-wing configuration of opacities as seen on the chest roentgenogram is indicative of pulmonary edema.

pneumono- see *pneumo-.*

pneumonocele (nu-mon′o-sēl) pneumatocele.

pneumonocentesis (nu-mo″no-sen-te′sis) [*pneumono-* + Gr. *kentesis* puncture] surgical puncturing of a lung for aspiration.

pneumonocirrhosis (nu-mo″no-sĭ-ro′sis) [Gr. *pneumōn* lung + *cirrhosis*] cirrhosis, or hardening, of a lung; pulmonary fibrosis.

pneumonococcus (nu″mo-no-kok′us) pneumococcus.

pneumonoconiosis (nu-mo″no-ko-ne-o′sis) pneumoconiosis.

pneumonocyte (nu-mon′o-sīt) a collective term for the alveolar epithelial cells types I and II alveolar cells) and alveolar phagocytes of the lungs. **granular p.,** type II alveolar cell. **membranous p.,** type I alveolar cell.

pneumonoenteritis (nu-mo″no-en″ter-i′tis) pneumoenteritis.

pneumonoerysipelas (nu-mo″no-er″ĭ-sip′ĕ-las) pneumoerysipelas.

pneumonograph (nu-mon′o-graf) a roentgenogram of the lungs.

pneumonography (nu″mo-nog′rah-fe) [*pneumono-* + Gr. *graphein* to write] roentgenography of the lungs.

pneumonokoniosis (nu-mo″no-ko′ne-o′sis) pneumoconiosis.

pneumonolipoidosis (nu-mo″no-lip″oi-do′sis) [*pneumono-* + Gr. *lipos* fat + *-osis*] see *lipoid pneumonia*, under *pneumonia*.

pneumonolysis (nu″mo-nol′ĭ-sis) [*pneumono-* + Gr. *lysis* dissolution] division of the tissues attaching the lung to the wall of the chest cavity, to permit collapse of the lung. **extraperiosteal p.,** that in which the division is between the inner surface of the ribs and the periosteum, which, with the intercostal muscle bundles, remains attached to the parietal pleura. **extrapleural p.,** that in which the separation is between the parietal pleura and the chest wall. **intrapleural p.,** that in which the separation is between the pulmonary and the parietal pleura.

pneumonomelanosis (nu-mo″no-mel″ah-no′sis) [*pneumono-* + Gr. *melas* black + *-osis*] melanosis of the lung tissue.

pneumonometer (nu″mo-nom′ĕ-ter) [*pneumono-* + Gr. *metron* measure] a form of spirometer.

pneumonomoniliasis (nu-mo″no-mo″nĭ-li′ah-sis) moniliasis (candidiasis) of the lungs.

pneumonomycosis (nu″mo-no-mi-ko′sis) pneumomycosis.

pneumonopaludism (nu-mo″no-pal′u-dizm) pneumopaludism.

pneumonopathy (nu″mo-nop′ah-the) [*pneumono-* + Gr. *pathos* disease] any disease of the lung. **eosinophilic p.,** Löffler's syndrome, or other conditions associated with eosinophilic infiltration of the lung parenchyma.

pneumonopexy (nu-mo′no-pek″se) [*pneumono-* + Gr. *pēxis* fixation] surgical fixation of the lung to the thoracic wall.

pneumonophthisis (nu″mon-of-thi′sis) pulmonary tuberculosis.

pneumonopleuritis (nu-mo″no-ploo-ri′tis) pneumopleuritis.

pneumonoresection (nu-mo″no-re-sek′shun) surgical resection of a portion of the lung.

pneumonorrhagia (nu-mo″no-ra′je-ah) pneumorrhagia.

pneumonorrhaphy (nu″mo-nor′ah-fe) [*pneumono-* + Gr. *rhaphē* suture] suture of the lung.

pneumonosis (nu″mo-no′sis) [*pneumo-* + Gr. *nosos* disease] any lung disease.

pneumonotherapy (nu-mo″no-ther′ah-pe) treatment of disease of the lung.

pneumonotomy (nu″mo-not′o-me) [*pneumono-* + Gr. *tomē* a cutting] surgical incision of the lung.

Pneumonyssoides (nu″mo-nis-oi′dēz) a genus of mites. *P. cani′num* is found in the sinuses and nasal passages of dogs.

Pneumonyssus (nu″mo-nis′us) a genus of mites. *P. simicola* is found in the lungs of monkeys.

pneumopaludism (nu″mo-pal′u-dizm) [*pneumo-* + L. *palus* swamp] disease of the lungs of malarial origin.

pneumopathy (nu-mop′ah-the) pneumonopathy.

pneumopericardium (nu″mo-per″ĭ-kar′de-um) [*pneumo-* + *pericardium*] the presence of air or gas in the cavity of the pericardium.

pneumoperitoneal (nu″mo-per″ĭ-to-ne′al) pertaining to or characterized by pneumoperitoneum.

pneumoperitoneum (nu″mo-per″ĭ-to-ne′um) [*pneumo-* + *peritoneum*] the presence of gas or air in the peritoneal cavity; it may occur spontaneously, as in subphrenic abscess, or be deliberately introduced as an aid to radiologic examination and diagnosis (*diagnostic p.*).

pneumoperitonitis (nu″mo-per″ĭ-to-ni′tis) [*pneumo-* + *peritonitis*] peritonitis with the accumulation of air or gas in the peritoneal cavity.

pneumopexy (nu′mo-pek″se) pneumonopexy.

pneumophagia (nu″mo-fa′je-ah) [*pneumo-* + Gr. *phagein* to eat + *-ia*] aerophagia.

pneumophonia (nu″mo-fo′ne-ah) a form of dysphonia characterized by a breathy voice.

pneumopleuritis (nu″mo-ploo-ri′tis) inflammation of the lungs and pleura.

pneumopleuroparietopexy (nu″mo-ploor″o-pah-ri′ĕ-to-pek″se) [*pneumo-* + *pleura* + *parieto-* + Gr. *pēxis* fixation] the operation of suturing the lung with its parietal pleura to the margin of a thoracic wound.

pneumoprecordium (nu″mo-pre-kor′de-um) the presence of air in the precordial space.

pneumopreperitoneum (nu″mo-pre-per″ĭ-to-ne′um) the presence of air or gas in the preperitoneal space; it may occur spontaneously or be deliberately introduced as an aid to radiologic examination and diagnosis.

pneumopyelography (nu″mo-pi″ĕ-log′rah-fe) [*pneumo-* + Gr. *pyelos* pelvis + *graphein* to write] pyelography in which oxygen or air, instead of an opaque solution, is injected into the renal pelvis.

pneumopyopericardium (nu″mo-pi″o-per″ĭ-kar′de-um) [*pneumo-* + Gr. *pyon* pus + *pericardium*] the presence of air or gas and pus in the pericardium.

pneumopyothorax (nu″mo-pi″o-tho′raks) [*pneumo-* + Gr. *pyon* pus + *thōrax* thorax] the presence of air and pus in the pleural cavity, usually due to empyema and bronchopleural fistula.

pneumorachicentesis (nu″mo-ra″ke-sen-te′sis) [*pneumo-* + Gr. *rhachis* spine + *kentēsis* puncture] the introduction of air or gas into the spinal canal as a contrast medium for roentgen examination.

pneumorachis (nu″mo-ra′kis) [*pneumo-* + Gr. *rhachis* spine] 1. the presence of a gaseous collection in the spinal cord. 2. the injection of gas into the spinal canal for the facilitation of roentgenological examination.

pneumoradiography (nu″mo-ra″de-og′rah-fe) [*pneumo-* + *radiography*] radiography of a part following the injection of air or oxygen, as in pneumoperitoneum.

pneumoresection (nu″mo-re-sek′shun) pneumonoresection.

pneumoretroperitoneum (nu″mo-re″tro-per″ĭ-to-ne′um) the presence of air or gas in the retroperitoneal space.

pneumoroentgenogram (nu″mo-rent-gen′o-gram) a roentgenogram of a part after the injection of air or gas into it.

pneumoroentgenography (nu″mo-rent″gen-og′rah-fe) roentgenography of a part into which air or gas has been injected.

pneumorrhagia (nu″mo-ra′je-ah) [*pneumo-* + Gr. *rhēgnynai* to burst forth] hemorrhage from the lungs; severe hemoptysis.

pneumosepticemia (nu″mo-sep″tĭ-se′me-ah) pneumonia of an extreme and fatal form associated with septicemia.

pneumoserosa (nu″mo-se-ro′sah) injection of air into a joint cavity for roentgenoscopy.

pneumoserothorax (nu″mo-se″ro-tho′raks) [*pneumo-* + *serum* + Gr. *thōrax* thorax] the presence of gas and serum in the thoracic cavity.

pneumosilicosis (nu″mo-sil″ĭ-ko′sis) the deposition of silica-bearing particles of foreign matter in the lungs; silicosis.

pneumotachograph (nu″mo-tak′o-graf) pneumotachygraph.

pneumotachometer (nu″mo-tak-om′ĕ-ter) a transducer used in measuring expired air flow.

pneumotachygraph (nu″mo-tak′e-graf) [*pneumo-* + Gr. *tachys* swift + *graphein* to write] an instrument for recording the velocity of the respired air.

pneumotaxic (nu″mo-tak′sik) [*pneumo-* + Gr. *taxis* arrangement] relating to the regulation of the rate of respiration; see under *center*.

pneumotherapy (nu″mo-ther′ah-pe) 1. pneumatotherapy. 2. the treatment of diseases of the lungs.

pneumothermomassage (nu″mo-ther″mo-mah-sahzh′) [*pneumo-* + Gr. *thermē* heat + *massage*] the application to the body of hot condensed air that has been medicated.

pneumothorax (nu″mo-tho′raks) [*pneumo-* + Gr. *thōrax* thorax] an accumulation of air or gas in the pleural space, which may occur spontaneously or as a result of trauma or a pathological process, or be introduced deliberately. See *artificial p.* and *diagnostic p.* **artificial p.,** pneumothorax induced intentionally by artificial means, employed for the purpose of allowing the lung to collapse in the treatment of pulmonary tuberculosis. Called also *induced p.* and *therapeutic p.* Cf. *collapse therapy*, under *therapy*. **clicking p.,** pneumothorax in which the patient is conscious of a clicking sound synchronous with the heart beat. Cf. *precardial knock*, under *knock*. **closed p.,** pneumothorax in which pulmonary air leaks into the pleural cavity through a wound in a lung. **diagnostic p.,** temporary artificial pneumothorax employed for the purpose of clearly demonstrating the parietal or visceral pleura on chest films in order to detect and localize tumors of the pleura. **extrapleural p.,** production of collapse of the lung by formation of an air pocket by stripping the pleural layers from the inner surface of the ribs and intercostal muscle sheaths. **induced p.,** artificial p. **open p.,** pneumothorax in which the pleural cavity is exposed to the atmosphere through an open wound in the chest wall. **pressure p.,** tension p. **spontaneous p.,** pneumothorax without known cause. **tension p.,** closed pneumothorax in which the tissues surrounding the opening into the pleural cavity act as valves, allowing air to enter but not to escape. The resultant positive pressure in the cavity displaces the mediastinum to the opposite side, with consequent embarrassment of respiration. Called also *pressure p.* **therapeutic p.,** artificial p. **valvular p.,** pneumothorax in which an aperture in the pleura has a valvelike action.

pneumotomography (nu″mo-to-mog′rah-fe) body section radiography after injection of air or other gas into the region or organ being visualized roentgenographically.

pneumotomy (nu-mot′o-me) pneumonotomy.

pneumotropic (nu″mo-trop′ik) 1. having a selective affinity for pulmonary tissue; exerting its principal effect upon the lungs. 2. having a selective affinity for pneumococci.

pneumotropism (nu-mot′ro-pizm) the predilection of an agent or organism for lung tissue.

pneumotympanum (nu″mo-tim′pah-num) air in the middle ear.

pneumotyphoid (nu″mo-ti′foid) typhoid with localization of the lesions in the lungs.

pneumotyphus (nu″mo-ti′fus) pneumonia concurrent with typhoid fever.

pneumouria (nu″mo-u′re-ah) pneumaturia.

Pneumovax (nu′mo-vaks″) trademark for a pneumococcal vaccine containing the capsular polysaccharides (antigens) of 14 types of pneumococci.

pneumoventricle (nu″mo-ven′trĭ-k'l) pneumoventriculi.

pneumoventriculi (nu″mo-ven-trik′u-li) [pneumo- + L. ventriculus ventricle] presence of air in the cerebral ventricles.

pneumoventriculography (nu″mo-ven-trik″u-log′rah-fe) roentgenography of the cerebral ventricles after the injection of air or gas; see ventriculography.

pneusis (nu′sis) [Gr. pneusis a blowing] respiration.

P.O. abbreviation for L. per os, by mouth, orally.

Po chemical symbol for polonium.

PO₂ symbol for oxygen partial pressure (tension); also written P$_{O_2}$, pO_2, and pO₂.

Pocill. abbreviation for L. pocil′lum, a small cup.

pock (pok) a pustule, especially one of the lesions of smallpox.

pocket (pok′et) a saclike space or cavity, such as an abnormal extension of a gingival sulcus (periodontal pocket). **absolute p.**, a dental condition in which the deepening of the gingival sulcus entails migration of the epithelial attachment along the root and destruction of the periodontal ligament. It may be either gingival or infrabony. **complex p.**, a spiral type of periodontal pocket involving more than one surface of the tooth, but communicating with the gingival margin only along the surface at which it originates. **compound p.**, a periodontal pocket involving more than one tooth surface, and communicating with the gum margin along each of the involved surfaces. **endocardial p's**, sclerotic thickenings of the mural endocardium, occurring most often on the left ventricular septum below an insufficient aortic valve; called also regurgitant p's and birds' nests. **gingival p.**, a periodontal pocket in which the bottom is coronal to the level of the underlying alveolar bone. **infrabony p.**, a periodontal pocket in which the bottom is attached to the tooth in an area apical to the level of the adjacent alveolar bone. **intra-alveolar p.**, infrabony p. **intrabony p.**, infrabony p. **periodontal p.**, a gingival sulcus pathologically deepened by periodontal disease. **Rathke's p.**, see under pouch. **regurgitant p's**, endocardial p's. **relative p.**, a dental condition in which the deepening of the gingival sulcus results primarily from an increase in bulk of the gingiva, without apical migration of the epithelial attachment or appreciable destruction of the underlying tissues. **Seessel's p.**, see under pouch. **simple p.**, a periodontal pocket involving only one tooth surface. **subcrestal p.**, infrabony p. **supracrestal p.**, **supragingival p.**, gingival p. **p's of Zahn**, shallow pockets with miniature leaflets, resembling cusps of the semilunar valve, produced in the endocardium of the left ventricle by the regurgitant aortic stream in the presence of insufficiency of the aortic valve.

pockmark (pok′mark) a depressed scar left by a pustule, especially one left by a lesion of smallpox.

Pocul. abbreviation for L. poc′ulum, cup.

poculum (pok′u-lum) [L.] cup. **p. Diog′enis** ["Diogenes' cup"], the concave palm of the hand.

pod- see podo-.

podagra (po-dag′rah) [pod- + Gr. agra seizure] gouty pain in the great toe.

podagral (pod′ah-gral) pertaining to or characterized by podagra.

podagric (po-dag′rik) podagral.

podagrous (pod′ah-grus) podagral.

podalgia (po-dal′je-ah) [pod- + -algia] pain in the foot, as from gout or rheumatism.

podalic (po-dal′ik) [Gr. pous foot] accomplished by means of the feet; see under version.

Podalirius (po″dah-lir′e-us) the younger of two brothers, the older being Machaon, who were the sons of Æsculapius and, according to legend, the chief medical officers attached to the Greek forces during the Trojan war.

Podangium (po-dan′je-um) a genus of Schizomycetes of the order Myxobacterales, family Polyangiaceae.

podarthritis (pod″ar-thri′tis) [pod- + arthritis] inflammation of the joints of the feet.

podedema (pod″e-de′mah) edema of the feet.

podencephalus (pod″en-sef′ah-lus) [pod- + Gr. enkephalos brain] a fetus whose brain, without a cranium, hangs by a pedicle.

podia (po′de-ah) [L.] plural of podium.

podiatrist (po-di′ah-trist) a specialist in podiatry; formerly called chiropodist.

podiatry (po-di′ah-tre) [Gr. pous foot + iatreia healing] the specialized field that deals with the study and care of the foot,

including its anatomy, pathology, medical and surgical treatment, etc. Formerly called chiropody.

podium (po′de-um), pl. po′dia [L.] a footlike projection; a sucker foot; see under foot.

podo-, pod- [Gr. pous, podos foot] a combining form denoting relationship to the foot.

podocyte (pod′o-sīt) [podo- + Gr. kytos hollow vessel] a modified epithelial cell of the visceral layer (capsular epithelium) of the renal glomerulus, having a small perikaryon and a number of primary and secondary footlike radiating processes (pedicels) which interdigitate with those of other podocytes and which embrace the basal lamina of glomerular capillaries.

pododerm (pod′o-derm) [podo- + L. derma skin] that portion of the skin which is continued downward within the horn capsule of the hoof of an animal.

pododynamometer (pod″o-di″nah-mom′ĕ-ter) a device for determining the strength of the leg muscles.

pododynia (pod″o-din′e-ah) [podo- + Gr. odynē pain] neuralgic pain of the heel and sole; burning pain without redness in the sole of the foot.

podogram (pod′o-gram) [podo- + Gr. gramma mark] a print of, or an outline tracing of, the sole of the foot.

podograph (pod′o-graf) [podo- + Gr. graphein to write] the instrument used in the making of a podogram.

podology (po-dol′o-je) [podo- + -logy] podiatry.

podophyllin (pod″o-fil′in) see podophyllum resin, under resin.

podophyllotoxin (pod″o-fil′o-tok′sin) a highly toxic compound, $C_{22}H_{22}O_8$, the main active component of podophyllum; it has cathartic and antineoplastic properties.

podophyllous (po-dof′ĭ-lus) [podo- + Gr. phyllon leaf] designating the tissues which constitute the sensitive wall of the hoofs of animals.

Podophyllum (pod″o-fil′um) [podo- + Gr. phyllon leaf] a genus of perennial North American herbs, including P. peltatum L. (Berberidaceae), which is the source of podophyllum resin.

podophyllum (pod″o-fil′um) [USP] the dried rhizome and roots of Podophyllum peltatum L. (Berberidaceae), yielding not less than 5 per cent of resin (see under resin); its main active component is podophyllotoxin. Called also Indian apple, mandrake, mandrake root, May apple, and vegetable calomel.

podopompholyx (po″do-pom′fo-liks) [podo + Gr. pompholyx a bubble] pompholyx of the soles.

podotrochilitis (pod″o-tro-kĭ-li′tis) [podo- + Gr. trochilea pulley + -itis] inflammation of the navicular bone of the horse's foot.

poe- for words beginning thus, see those beginning pe.

poecil- for words beginning thus, see those beginning poikil-.

Poecilia (pe-sil′e-ah) a genus of minnows; called also Girardinus. **P. reticula′ta**, a species used, especially in tropical America, to control mosquitoes; they eat the larvae of Anopheles. Called also Girardinus poeciloides.

Poehl's test (pelz) [Alexander Vasilyevich von Poehl, Russian chemist, 1850–1908] see under tests.

pogoniasis (po″go-ni′ah-sis) [Gr. pōgōn beard + -iasis] 1. excessive growth of the beard. 2. the growth of a beard upon a woman.

pogonion (po-go′ne-on) [Gr., dim. of pōgōn beard] the most anterior point of the chin in the sagittal plane.

pOH an infrequently used symbol used in expressing the approximate concentration of hydroxide ions in a solution.

poi (poi) a Hawaiian food made from the root of the taro plant, Colocasia esculenta (L.) Schott., Araceae. It is used as a cereal substitute for allergic infants.

-poiesis (poi-e′sis) [Gr. poiein to make] a word termination meaning formation, as in hematopoiesis.

poietin (poi-e′tin) any of the hormones involved in regulation of the numbers of various cell types in the peripheral blood.

poikilergasia (poi″kil-er-ga′se-ah) [poikilo- + Gr. ergasia work] Meyer's term for psychopathic constitution.

poikilo- [Gr. poikilos spotted, mottled; varied] a combining form meaning varied or irregular.

poikiloblast (poi′kĭ-lo-blast″) [poikilo- + Gr. blastos germ] an abnormally shaped erythroblast.

poikilocarynosis (poi″kĭ-lo-kar″ĭ-no′sis) [poikilo- + Gr. karyon nucleus + -osis] Darier's term for the formation of various types and arrangements of cells which occurs in Bowen's disease.

poikilocyte (poi′kĭ-lo-sīt″) [poikilo- + -cyte] an erythrocyte showing abnormal variation in shape.

poikilocythemia (poi″kĭ-lo-si-the′me-ah) poikilocytosis.

poikilocytosis (poi″kĭ-lo-si-to′sis) [poikilocyte + -osis] presence in the blood of erythrocytes showing abnormal variation in shape.

poikilodentosis (poi″kĭ-lo-den-to′sis) [poikilo- + L. dens tooth + -osis] a mottled condition of the teeth.

poikiloderma (poi″kĭ-lo-der′mah) a condition characterized by pigmentation and atrophic changes in the skin, giving it a mottled appearance. **p. atroph′icans vascula′re** (Jacobi), a rare, slowly progressive atrophic skin disorder, usually of early adult life, which resembles radiodermatitis, with telangiectasia, atrophy, and variegated or mottled pigmentation of the skin. **p. of Civatte,** reddish-brown reticular pigmentation of the face, neck, and upper chest, occurring symmetrically, the result of exposure to sunlight perhaps aided by chemicals in cosmetics. **p. congenita′le,** Rothmund-Thomson syndrome.

poikilodermatomyositis (poi″ki-lo-der″mah-to-mi″o-si′tis) dermatomyositis with poikiloderma-like skin changes.

poikilonymy (poi″ki-lon′i-me) [poikilo- + Gr. *onoma* name] the mingling of names or terms from different systems of nomenclature.

poikiloploid (poi′ki-lo-ploid″) 1. pertaining to or characterized by poikiloploidy. 2. an individual having different cells with varying numbers of chromosomes.

poikiloploidy (poi′ki-lo-ploi″de) the state of having varying numbers of chromosomes in different cells.

poikilosmosis (poi″kil-oz-mo′sis) the processes by which a cell or tissue adjusts the osmolarity of its fluid to that of its immediate environment.

poikilosmotic (poi″kil-oz-mot′ik) pertaining to poikilosmosis.

poikilostasis (poi″ki-lo-sta′sis) [poikilo- + Gr. *stasis* standing] the maintenance of stability in the body state (internal environment) by behavioral activities involving movement and selection by the whole organism.

poikilotherm (poi-kil′o-therm″) an animal that exhibits poikilothermy; a so-called cold-blooded animal or ectotherm.

poikilothermal (poi″ki-lo-ther′mal) poikilothermic.

poikilothermic (poi″ki-lo-ther′mik) pertaining to or characterized by poikilothermy.

poikilothermism (poi″ki-lo-ther′mizm) poikilothermy.

poikilothermy (poi″ki-lo-ther′me) [poikilo- + Gr. *thermē* heat] 1. the exhibition of body temperature which varies with the environmental temperature. 2. the ability of organisms to adapt themselves to variations in the temperature of their environment.

poikilothrombocyte (poi-kil″o-throm′bo-sīt) [poikilo- + *thrombocyte*] a blood platelet of abnormal shape.

poikilothymia (poi″ki-lo-thi′me-ah) [poikilo- + Gr. *thymos* spirit] a mental condition characterized by abnormal variations of mood.

poin (poin) an uncharacterized antibiotic material produced by the fungus *Fusarium sporotrichiella* var. *paoe* Bilai, and cultured from cases involving septic tonsillitis. It is active against staphylococci and streptococci *in vitro*.

point (point) [L. *punctum*] 1. a small area or spot; the sharp end of an object. 2. to approach the surface, like the pus of an abscess, at a definite spot or place. **p. A,** a roentgenographic, cephalometric landmark, determined on the lateral head film; it is the most retruded part of the curved bony outline from the anterior nasal spine to the crest of the maxillary alveolar process. Called also *subspinale*. **p. of an abscess,** the place at which the pus comes nearest to the surface. **absorbent p.,** a cone of variable width and taper, most commonly composed of paper or a paper product, used in drying or maintaining a liquid disinfectant in the root canal of a tooth. **Addison's p.,** the midpoint of the epigastric region. **alveolar p.,** prosthion. **apophysiary p.,** 1. subnasal point. 2. see *Trousseau's apophysiary points*. **p. Ar,** a cephalometric landmark, the point of intersection of the dorsal contours of the process articularis mandibulae and os temporale; called also *articulare*. **p. of Arrhigi,** an electrode site in electrocardiography, 2 to 3 cm. to the left of the seventh thoracic vertebra. **auricular p.,** the center of the opening of the external auditory meatus; called also *Broca's point*. **p. B,** a roentgenographic, cephalometric landmark, determined on the lateral head film; it is the most posterior midline point in the concavity between the infradentale and pogonion. Called also *supramentale*. **p. Ba,** a cephalometric landmark, the most inferior point on the anterior margin of the foramen magnum in the midsagittal plane; called also *basion*. **Barker's p.,** a point 1¼ inches above and 1¼ inches behind the middle external auditory meatus, the proper spot to apply the trephine in abscess of the temporosphenoid lobe. **p. Bo,** Bolton p. **Boas' p.,** a tender area to the left of the twelfth thoracic vertebra in patients with gastric ulcer. **boiling p.,** the temperature at which a liquid will boil (at sea level water boils at 100° C., or 212° F.); specifically, the temperature at which the equilibrium vapor pressure of a liquid phase equals the atmospheric pressure. **boiling p., normal,** the temperature at which a liquid boils at one standard atmosphere pressure. **Bolton p.,** the upper part of the notch in the shadow cast by the occipital bone in the x-ray of the lateral aspect of the skull. **Brewer's p.,** the point of the costovertebral angle, tenderness over which points to kidney infection. **Broadbent's registration p.,** a cephalometric landmark, being the midpoint on a perpendicular line from the center of the sella turcica to the nasion-postcondylare plane. **Broca's p.,** auricular p. **Cannon's p.,** see under *ring*. **cardinal p's,** 1. principal points; points on the optic axis which include the nodal points, the principal foci, and the optic center; may include conjugate focal points of object and image. 2. four points within

the pelvic inlet—the two sacroiliac articulations and the two iliopectineal eminences. **Chauffard's p.,** a point of tenderness in gallbladder disease, situated under the right clavicle. **cold rigor p.,** that point of low temperature at which the activity of a cell ceases. **conjugate p.,** conjugate focus. **contact p.,** see under *area*. **convenience p.,** a groove or depression cut in the wall of a tooth cavity in such a way as to retain the first piece of the gold placed for its filling. **p. of convergence,** the point nearest to the patient to which both eyes can converge on an object moved toward them. **corresponding p's,** points upon the two retinae whose impressions unite to produce a single perception. Cf. *disparate p's*. **Cova's p.,** a point at the apex of the costolumbar angle which is tender on pressure in cases of pyelitis of pregnancy. **craniometric p.,** any one of a numerous set of points of reference assumed for use in craniometry. **critical p.,** the temperature at or above which a gas cannot be liquefied by pressure alone. **deaf p.,** one of certain points near the ear where a vibrating tuning-fork cannot be heard. **de Mussy's p.,** a point, exceedingly painful on pressure on the line of the left border of the sternum, at the level of the end of the tenth rib; it is a symptom of diaphragmatic pleurisy. **Desjardins' p.,** a point on the abdomen 5 to 7 cm. from the umbilicus, on a line joining it to the right axilla; it lies over the head of the pancreas. **dew p.,** the temperature of the atmosphere at which the moisture begins to be deposited as dew. **p. of direction,** see *position*, def. 2. **disparate p's,** points on the retina which are not paired exactly. Cf. *corresponding p's*. **p. of dispersion,** in optics, the virtual focus. **p. of divergence,** the conjugate focus from which the light proceeds. **dorsal p.,** in hepatic colic, a point, tender on pressure, situated between the spinous processes of the vertebrae at the border of the right scapula at the level of the fourth and fifth intercostal spaces at a distance of about 2 or 3 cm. from the middle line. Called also *Pauly's p.* **p's douloureux** (pwă doo-loo-ruh′) [Fr.], Valleix's p's. **p. of election,** that point at which any particular surgical operation is done by preference. **Erb's p.,** a point two or three centimeters above the clavicle and beyond the posterior border of the sternomastoid, at the level of the transverse process of the sixth cervical vertebra; stimulation here contracts various arm muscles. **eye p.,** 1. the bright circle seen at the crossing point or nearest the approximation of the rays above the microscopical ocular. 2. See under *spot*. **far p.,** the remotest point at which an object is clearly seen when the eye is at rest. **fixation p.,** the point or object on which the vision is fixed. **focal p.,** see *focus* (def. 1), and *cardinal p.* (def. 1). **freezing p.,** the temperature at which a liquid begins to freeze; that of pure water is 0° C., or 32° F. **fusion p.,** melting point. **glenoid p.,** the center of the glenoid cavity of the scapula. **Guéneau de Mussy's p.,** see *de Mussy's p.* **gutta-percha p.,** a fine, plastic, radiopaque cone made from gutta-percha and various compounding ingredients, used as a root canal filling material. **Hallé's p.,** a point on the surface of the abdomen corresponding to the point where the ureter crosses the pelvic brim. It is the point of intersection between a horizontal line connecting the anterior superior iliac spines and a vertical line projected upward from the pubic spine. **Hartmann's p., Hartmann's critical p.,** p. of Sudeck. **hinge-axis p.,** a reference point on the skin corresponding with the terminal hinge axis of the mandible. **hysteroepileptogenous p., hysterogenic p.,** a point on which, if pressure be made, a hysteric or hysteroepileptic attack may be produced. **ice p.,** the temperature of equilibrium between ice and air-saturated water under one atmosphere pressure. **identical p's,** corresponding p's. **p. of incidence,** see *refraction*, def. 2. **isobestic p.,** the wavelength at which two interconvertible substances (e.g., oxyhemoglobin and reduced hemoglobin) have the same absorptivity. **isoelectric p.,** the pH of a solution at which a charged molecule does not migrate in an electric field. **isoionic p.,** the pH of a solution at which a specific ion (usually a protein) contains as many negative charges as positive charges. **jugal p.,** the point of the angle formed by the masseteric and maxillary edges of the malar bone (os zygomaticum). **jugomaxillary p.,** the point at the anteroinferior angle of the malar bone (os zygomaticum). **Keen's p.,** a point for puncture of the lateral ventricles; 3 cm. above and 3 cm. behind the external auditory meatus. **Kienböck-Adamson p's,** points and lines to be marked on the scalp to indicate the areas for the application of x-ray therapy in order to produce temporary epilation for the treatment of tinea capitis. **Kocher's p.,** a point for puncture of the lateral ventricles; 2.5 cm. from the midline, 3.5 cm. in front of the bregma. **Krafft p.,** the temperature above which conjugated bile salts form polymolecular aggregates (micelles) of about 3 to 10 nm. in diameter. **lacrimal p.,** the punctum lacrimale; any of the outlets of the lacrimal canaliculi. **Lanz's p.,** a point which indicates the position of the vermiform appendix; it is situated on a line connecting the two anterior superior iliac spines one third of the distance from the right spine. **leak p.,** renal threshold for glucose; see under *threshold*. **McBurney's p.,** a point of special tenderness in acute appendicitis, situated about one-half to 2 inches from the right anterior superior iliac spine on a line between this spine and the umbilicus. It corresponds with the normal position of the base of the appendix. **McEwen's p.,** a point above the inner canthus of the eye which is tender in acute frontal sinusitis. **Mackenzie's p.,** a point of tenderness in gallbladder disease in the upper segment of the rectus muscle. **malar p.,** a point on the external tubercle of the malar bone (os zygomaticum). **marginal p's,** *Anaplasma marginale.* **p. of maximal impulse,** the point on the chest where the impulse of the left ventricle is felt most strongly, normally in the fifth costal interspace inside the left mamillary line; abbreviated P.M.I. **maximum occipital p.,** the point in the occipital bone situated furthest from the glabella. **median mandibular p.,** a point on the anteroposterior center of the mandibular ridge in the median sagittal plane. **Méglin's p.,** a point where the greater palatine nerve emerges from the great palatine foramen. **melting p.,** the minimum temperature at which a solid begins to liquify. **mental p.,** pogonion. **metopic p.,** glabella. **motor p.,** 1. the point at which a motor nerve enters a muscle. 2. any point on the skin over a muscle at which the application of galvanic stimulation will cause contraction of a corresponding muscle. **Munro's p.,** a point midway between the umbilicus and the left anterior iliac spine, usually selected as the point for performing abdominal puncture. **Mussy's p.,** see *de Mussy's p.* **nasal p.,** nasion. **near p.,** the nearest point at which the eye can distinctly perceive an object; the nearest point of clear vision. **near p., absolute,** the near point for either eye alone with accommodation relaxed. **near p., relative,** the near point for both eyes with the employment of accommodation. **nodal p's,** one of two points on the axis of an optical system so situated that a ray falling on one will produce a parallel ray emerging through the other. **occipital p.,** 1. the posterior point on the occipital bone. 2. (*obs.*) the pointed posterior end of the occipital lobe of the brain (occipital pole). **ossification p.,** a center of ossification in bone. **painful p.,** Valleix's p's. **paper p.,** absorbent p. **Pauly's p's,** dorsal p. **phrenic-pressure p.,** a point along the phrenic nerve between the sternocleidomastoid and the scalenus anticus on the right side; pressure on the point suggests gallbladder disease. **Piersol's p.,** a point indicating the location of the vesical orifice. **pour p.,** the temperature at which a liquid just begins to flow. **preauricular p.,** a point on the posterior root of the zygomatic arch just in front of the auricular point. **pressure p.,** 1. a point of extreme sensibility to pressure. 2. one of various locations on the body at which digital pressure may be applied for the control of hemorrhage. **pressure-arresting p.,** a point at which pressure arrests spasm. **pressure-exciting p.,** a point at which pressure produces spasm. **principal p's,** cardinal p's, def. 1. **R p.,** a cephalometric landmark determined by the midpoint of a line perpendicular to the Bolton-nasion plane from the sella turcica. **Ramond's p.,** a point of tenderness in gallbladder disease between the heads of the sternocleidomastoid muscle. **reflection p.,** the point from which a ray of light is reflected. **refraction p.,** the point at which a ray of light is refracted. **p. of regard,** the point at which the eye is directly looking. **retromandibular tender p.,** a point behind the superior extremity of the inferior maxilla below the lobule of the ear and in front of the mastoid process. Pressure on this point elicits extreme pain in meningitis. **Robson's p.,** the point of greatest tenderness in gallbladder inflammation, situated opposite the junction of the middle and lower third of a line drawn from the right nipple to the umbilicus. **silver p.,** a solid-core root canal filling material composed of silver; its diameter and taper usually correspond to the variations in diameter and taper of the root canal instruments. **spinal p.,** subnasal p. **stereoidentical p's,** points in space outside of the region within which fusion of double images occurs. **subnasal p.,** the central point of the root of the anterior nasal spine. **subtemporal p.,** the point where the sphenotemporal suture and infratemporal crest intersect. **Sudeck's critical p., p. of Sudeck,** the portion of the rectum between the last sigmoid artery and the bifurcation of the superior hemorrhoidal artery; the former belief that ligation of the latter below this point would lead to gangrene of the rectum has not been borne out by clinical experience. Called also *Hartmann's p.* **supra-auricular p.,** a point at the root of the zygomatic process of the temporal bone, directly above the auricular point. **supraclavicular p.,** a point above the clavicle and outside of the sternomastoid where the application of a stimulus causes contraction of the biceps brachii, deltoideus, brachialis, and brachioradialis muscles. **supranasal p.,** ophryon. **supraorbital p.,** 1. the ophryon. 2. in neuralgia, a tender spot just above the supraorbital notch. **sylvian p.,** a point on the surface of the skull from 29 to 32 mm. behind the external angular process of the frontal bone. **thermal death p.,** the degree of heat required to kill a given microorganism in a stated length of time. **trigger p.,** a particular spot on the body on which pressure or other stimulus will give rise to specific sensations or symptoms. **triple p.,** the temperature and pressure at which three different phases of a substance are in equilibrium. The *triple point of water* (ice, liquid, vapor) is 273.15°K. **Trousseau's apophysiary p's,** points sensitive to pressure along the dorsal and lumbar vertebrae in certain cases of neuralgia. **vaccine p.,** a piece of bone or quill, one end of which is coated with vaccine lymph. **Valleix's p's,** tender points on the course of certain nerves in neuralgia. **vital p.,** a

point in the medulla oblongata, at the respiratory center, puncture of which causes immediate death. **Vogt's p., Vogt-Hueter p.,** a point of the intersection of a horizontal line, two finger-breadths above the zygoma, with a vertical line a thumb-breadth behind the ascending sphenofrontal process; here trephination may be performed in traumatic meningeal hemorrhage. **Voillemier's p.,** a point on the linea alba 6.5 cm. below the line which joins the anterior superior iliac spinous processes; here the bladder may be punctured in obese or edematous patients. **p. Z,** a point formed by a line perpendicular to the nasion-menton line through the anterior nasal spine. **Ziemssen's motor p's,** the places of entrance of motor nerves into muscles; they are points of election in the therapeutical application of electricity to muscles.

pointer (point′er) a contusion at a bony eminence. **hip p.,** contusion of the bone of the iliac crest or avulsion of muscle attachments of the iliac crest.

pointillage (pwahn″te-yahzh′) [Fr.] massage with the points of the fingers.

Poirier's glands, line (pwah-re-āz′) [Paul *Poirier,* surgeon in Paris, 1853–1907] see under *gland* and *line.*

poise (poiz; Fr. pwahz) [J. M. *Poiseuille*] the unit of viscosity of a liquid, being number of grams per centimeter per second. The commonly used unit is the *centipoise,* or one one-hundredth of a poise.

Poiseuille's law, space (pwah-zuh′yez) [Jean Leonard Marie *Poiseuille,* physiologist in Paris, 1799–1869] see under *law* and *space.*

poison (poi′zn) [L. *potio* draft; *toxicum;* Gr. *toxikon*] any substance which, when ingested, inhaled or absorbed, or when applied to, injected into, or developed within the body, in relatively small amounts, by its chemical action may cause damage to structure or disturbance of function. See also *toxin.* **acrid p.,** one which produces irritation or inflammation, as the mineral acids, oxalic acid, the caustic alkalis, antimony, arsenic, the salts of copper, some of the compounds of lead, silver nitrate, the salts of zinc, iodine, cantharides, phosphorus, etc. **acronarcotic p., acrosedative p.,** poisons which produce sometimes irritation, sometimes narcotism (or sedation), or both together. They are chiefly derived from the vegetable kingdom. Stramonium and belladonna are examples of the acronarcotic and aconite is an example of the acrosedative poisons. **arrow p.,** a preparation of plant alkaloids used on their arrows by members of certain primitive tribes. **catalyst p.,** a substance firmly bound to the active areas on the surface of a catalyst, which prevents the adsorption of the reactants for the desired chemical reaction. **clam p.,** gonyaulax p. **corrosive p.,** any poison which acts by directly destroying tissue. **fatigue p.,** fatigue toxin. **fugu p.,** tetrodotoxin. **gonyaulax p.,** the neurotoxic principle produced by members of the genus *Gonyaulax* and related dinoflagellates; ingestion of shellfish that feed on these organisms causes a severe neurologic reaction which may end in paralysis and death. Called also *clam p., mussel p., paralytic shellfish p., mytilotoxin,* and *saxitoxin.* **hemotropic p.,** a poison which has a special affinity for erythrocytes. **irritant p.,** acrid p. **microbial p.,** a toxic substance produced by a microorganism. **mitotic p.,** a toxic principle that interferes with cell division. **muscle p.,** one that interferes with normal action or functioning of muscle. **mussel p.,** gonyaulax p. **narcotic p's,** poisons causing stupor or delirium, as opium, hyoscyamus, etc. **paralytic shellfish p.,** gonyaulax p. **puffer p.,** tetrodotoxin. **sedative p's,** those which directly depress the vital centers, as hydrocyanic acid, potassium cyanide, hydrogen sulfide, and other of the poisonous gases. **toot p.,** a poison from *Coriaria sarmentosa,* a plant of New Zealand. **vascular p.,** a poison which acts by affecting the blood vessels. **whelk p.,** a toxic substance which is localized in the salivary gland of whelks, members of the phylum Mollusca, class Gastropoda; its principal ingredient is tetramethylammonium hydroxide. See also under *poisoning.*

poison ivy (poi′zn i′ve) *Rhus.*

poison oak (poi′zn ōk) *Rhus.*

poison sumac (poi′zn soo′mak) *Rhus.*

poisoning (poi′zuh-ning) the morbid condition produced by a poison; see also *intoxication.* **akee p.,** Jamaica vomiting sickness. **antimony p.,** poisoning due to ingestion of antimony compounds, rarely to industrial exposure; the symptoms are similar to those of acute arsenic poisoning, with vomiting a prominent symptom. **argemone oil p.,** see *argemone oil,* under *oil.* **arsenic p.,** poisoning due to systemic exposure to inorganic pentavalent arsenic. *Acute arsenic poisoning,* which may result in shock and death, is marked by erythematous skin eruptions, vomiting, diarrhea, abdominal pain, muscular cramps, and swelling of the eyelids, feet, and hands. *Chronic arsenic poisoning,* due to the ingestion of small amounts over a long period of time, is marked by pigmentation of the skin accompanied by scaling, hyperkeratosis of the palms and soles, transverse white lines on the fingernails (Mees' lines), headache, peripheral neuropathy, and confusion. Called also *arsenicalism* and *arsenism.* **blood p.,** septicemia. **bongkrek p.,** see under *intoxication.* **broom p.,** poisoning caused by eating *Cytisus scoparius,* or broom, a leguminous shrub which contains both sparteine and cytisine. **callistin shellfish p.,** poisoning caused by ingestion of gastropods of the genus *Callista*, believed to be due to a choline present in large quantities in the ovaries of the shellfish; called also *esowasure-gai p.* **carbon disulfide p.,** a condition occurring in workers in rubber and viscose products caused by carbon disulfide and marked by weakness, sleeplessness, visual impairment, gastric ulcer, and paralysis. **carbon monoxide p.,** poisoning due to the inhalation of carbon monoxide and the resulting change of oxyhemoglobin to carboxyhemoglobin, which may result in damage to the central nervous system and death. **cheese p.,** tyrotoxicosis. **corncockle p.,** githagism. **dural p.,** poisoning in aircraft workers caused by the magnesium in the aluminum-magnesium alloy (Duralumin) used in airplanes. **elasmobranch p.,** a form of ichthyosarcotoxism produced by the ingestion of certain toxic sharks and skates. **ergot p.,** ergotism. **esowasure-gai p.,** Japanese name for callistin shellfish. **fish p.,** ichthyosarcotoxism. **fluoride p., chronic, fluorine p., chronic,** fluorosis, def. 2. **food p.,** a group of acute illnesses caused by the ingestion of contaminated food, characterized by vomiting, diarrhea, enteritis, and prostration. It may result from allergy; toxemia from foods, such as those inherently poisonous or those accidentally contaminated by poisons; foods containing poisons formed by bacteria, such as *Clostridium botulinum* (botulism), *C. perfringens* (clostridial food poisoning), and *Staphylococcus aureus* (staphylococcal food poisoning); and foodborne infections, including infection by species of *Salmonella* (salmonellal food poisoning). **food p., clostridial,** 1. food poisoning caused by *Clostridium botulinum.* See *allantiasis* and *botulism.* 2. food poisoning caused by *Clostridium perfringens;* meat, particularly poultry, is usually the vehicle of infection. **food p., salmonellal,** food poisoning caused by the ingestion of foods containing large numbers of *Salmonella typhimurium, S. enteritidis, S. paratyphi B,* or *S. choleraesuis;* the foods involved are usually meat and other protein foods, but almost any kind may carry the organisms. It is characterized by abrupt onset, 8 to 48 hours after ingestion of the infected food, with fever, chills, nausea, vomiting, diarrhea, headache, and abdominal pain and tenderness; the attack usually lasts 2 to 5 days. **food p., staphylococcal,** food poisoning caused by the ingestion of foods containing enterotoxin, usually produced by *Staphylococcus aureus* in such foods as cream-filled pastries, custards, and cottage cheese, but also in meat. It is characterized by sudden onset, headache, salivation, nausea, vomiting, diarrhea, abdominal cramps, and sweating; the attack usually lasts from 5 to 6 hours. **forage p.,** a disease of domestic animals, especially of horses, resulting from ingestion of moldy or fermented food, or from an encephalomyelitic infection; certain forms occurring in Australia are caused by *Clostridium botulinum.* **fugu p.,** tetrodotoxism. **gossypol p.,** poisoning from eating cottonseed cake. **gymnothorax p.,** a form of ichthyosarcotoxism produced by ingestion of certain moray eels of the genus *Gymnothorax.* **heavy metal p.,** poisoning with any of the heavy metals, particularly arsenic, lead, mercury, antimony, cadmium, or thallium. **larkspur p.,** poisoning from the fresh leaves and roots of larkspur, which contain aconite. Ingestion may result in instantaneous death, probably from paralysis of the heart. **lead p.,** poisoning due to the absorption or ingestion of lead or one of its salts. The symptoms include loss of appetite, weight loss, colic, constipation, insomnia, headache, dizziness, irritability, moderate hypertension, albuminuria, anemia, a blue line at the edge of the gums (lead line), encephalopathy (especially in children), and peripheral neuropathy leading to paralysis. Called also *plumbism.* **loco p.,** locoism. **manganese p.,** a condition usually caused by inhalation of manganese dust; symptoms include mental disorders accompanying a syndrome resembling paralysis agitans, and inflammation throughout the respiratory system. **meat p.,** acute, often severe gastroenteritis, caused by salmonella, clostridium, staphylococcus, streptococcus, or some similar organism. **mercury p.,** acute or chronic disease caused by mercury and its salts. The *acute* form, due to ingestion, is marked by severe abdominalgia, metallic taste in the mouth, vomiting, bloody diarrhea with watery stools, oliguria or anuria (usually at onset), and corrosion and ulceration of the entire digestive tract. The *chronic* form, due to absorption by the skin and mucous membranes, inhalation of vapors, or ingestion of mercury salts, is marked by stomatitis, metallic taste in the mouth, a blue line along the border of the gum, sore hypertrophied gums that bleed easily, loosening of the teeth, erethism, excessive secretion of saliva, tremors, and incoordination. Called also *mercurialism* and *hydrargyrism.* **milk p.,** trembles. **molybdenum p.,** poisoning due to ingestion of large amounts of molybdenum, characterized by weakness and diarrhea; no cases of molybdenum poisoning in man have been reported. **mushroom p.,** poisoning resulting from ingestion of poisonous mushrooms, including *Amanita verna, A. phalloides, A. muscaria,* and *A. pantherina.* The clinical course usually begins with nausea, vomiting, abdominal pain, and diarrhea, followed by a period (up to 48 hours) of improvement, and then culminating in signs and symptoms of severe hepatic, renal, and central nervous system damage. Called also *mycetismus.* **mussel p.,** see *gonyaulax poison,* under *poison.* **naphthol p.,** the toxic condition brought on by the ex-

cessive or continued use of naphthol, characterized by anemia, jaundice, convulsions, and coma. **nitroaniline p.,** poisoning by nitroaniline, a dye used in paints, paint removers, printing inks, cloth marking inks, and solvents; intense methemoglobinemia is produced. **nutmeg p.,** severe toxic symptoms produced by as little as 1 teaspoonful of powdered nutmeg; narcosis with periods of delirium and excitability may occur within 1 to 6 hours. **O_2 p.,** see under *toxicity.* **paraldehyde p.,** paraldehydism. **parathyroid p.,** the sudden increase in the extent of metastatic calcification of organs, particularly the kidneys, when a high calcium diet is given a hyperparathyroid patient. **phenol p.,** poisoning due to ingestion or absorption through the skin of phenol; the symptoms include colic, weakness, collapse, and local irritation and corrosion. Called also *carbolism.* **phosphorus p.,** a condition resulting from ingestion or inhalation of phosphorus, manifested by toothache and mandibular necrosis (phossy jaw), anorexia, weakness, and anemia. **pitch p.,** a usually fatal disorder of pigs that eat clay pigeons or lick the tarred walls and floors of pigpens, marked by inappetence, depression, weakness, jaundice, anemia. **puffer p.,** tetrodotoxism. **salmon p.,** a hemorrhagic enteritis, particularly affecting canines but which may also affect man and other animals. It is acquired by the ingestion of raw fish, especially salmon and trout, parasitized by the fluke *Troglotrema salmincola,* which serves as a vector of the etiologic agent, *Neorickettsia helminthoeca.* **salt p.,** poisoning of animals, especially pigs and birds, due to ingestion of too much salt in the absence of available water, marked by excessive thirst, diarrhea, and vomiting, often culminating in death. **saturnine p.,** lead p. **sausage p.,** see *allantiasis* and *botulism.* **scombroid p.,** a form of ichthyosarcotoxism caused by the ingestion of a toxic histamine-like substance produced by the action of bacteria on histidine, a normal component of fish flesh. Scombroid fish (tuna, bonito, mackeral, etc.) are particularly susceptible to bacterial decomposition, and when inadequately preserved contaminated fish are eaten the symptoms of the illness, including epigastric pain, nausea, vomiting, headache, dysphagia, thirst, urticaria, and pruritus, develop and usually last for less than 24 hours. **selenium p.,** a form of poisoning of livestock of the North Central Great Plains region of the United States due to the feeding on plants which have absorbed selenium from the soil and characterized by cirrhosis of the liver, anemia, loss of hair, erosions of long bones, emaciation. **shellfish p.,** see *gonyaulax poison,* under *poison.* **tempeh p.,** bongkrek intoxication. **tetrachlorethane p.,** a form of poisoning in munition workers caused by inhalation of fumes of tetrachlorethane, and marked by toxic jaundice, headache, anorexia, and gastrointestinal disturbance. **tetraodon p.,** tetrodotoxism. **thallium p.,** poisoning, particularly of children, due to ingestion of thallium compounds, marked by alopecia, by a variety of neurologic and psychic symptoms, including ataxia, restlessness, delirium, hallucinations, delusions, semicoma, blindness, and by liver and kidney damage. **T.N.T. p.,** trinitrotoluene p. **tobacco p.,** tabacosis. **trinitrotoluene p.,** a form of poisoning in munition workers, characterized by dermatitis, gastritis with abdominal pain, vomiting, constipation, flatulence, and blood changes. Abbreviated *T.N.T. p.* **whelk p.,** a form of intoxication characterized by intense headache, dizziness, nausea, and vomiting resulting from the ingestion of whelks, members of the phylum Mollusca, class Gastropoda. See also under *poison.* **zinc p.,** poisoning due to inhalation or ingestion of zinc; the symptoms include colic, diarrhea, vomiting, and fever.

poisonous (poi′son-us) pertaining to, due to, or of the nature of a poison; toxic; venomous.

poitrinaire (pwah″tre-nār′) [Fr.] a patient with a chronic disease of the chest.

pokeroot (pōk′root) pokeweed.

pokeweed (pōk′wēd) a tall perennial herb, *Phytolacca americana,* of North America; its root has emetic and purgative properties and has been used as an antirheumatic. Mitogen from pokeweed induce lymphocyte transformation and stimulate erythropoiesis. Called also *pokeroot.*

polacrilin (pol-ah-kril′in) methacrylic acid ester with divinylbenzene; a synthetic ion-exchange resin, supplied in the hydrogen or free acid form; a pharmaceutic aid. **p. potassium,** a synthetic ion exchange resin, prepared through polymerization of methacrylic acid and divinylbenzene, and then further neutralized with potassium hydroxide to form the potassium salt of methacrylic acid and divinylbenzene. It is supplied as a pharmaceutical-grade ion-exchange resin in a particle size of 100- to 500-mesh; a tablet disintegrant.

polar (po′lar) [L. *polaris, polus;* Gr. *polos*] 1. of or pertaining to a pole; see also under *compound.* 2. being at opposite ends of a spectrum of manifestations, as polar forms of leprosy.

Polaramine (po-lar′ah-mēn) trademark for preparations of dexchlorpheniramine maleate.

polarimeter (po″lah-rim′ĕ-ter) [*polar* + Gr. *metron* measure] a device for measuring the rotation of plane polarized light; a polariscope.

polarimetry (po″lah-rim′ĕ-tre) measurement of the rotation of plane polarized light by a liquid or solid.

polariscope (po-lar'ĭ-skōp) [*polar* + Gr. *skopein* to examine] an instrument for the measurement of polarized light.

polariscopic (po″lar-ĭ-skop'ik) pertaining to the polariscope or to polariscopy.

polariscopy (po″lar-is'ko-pe) the science of polarized light and the use of the polariscope.

polaristrobometer (po-lar″is-tro-bom'ĕ-ter) a form of polarimeter used for delicate analyses.

polarity (po-lar'ĭ-te) 1. the fact or condition of having poles. 2. the exhibition of opposite effects at the two extremities. 3. the presence of an axial gradient and exhibition by a nerve of both anelectrotonus and catelectrotonus. 4. the orientation of intracellular structures to the tissue as a whole. **dynamic p.,** the specialization of a nerve cell with reference to the flow of impulses.

polarization (po″lar-i-za'shun) 1. the production of that condition in light by virtue of which its vibrations take place all in one plane or else in circles and ellipses. 2. the accumulation of bubbles of hydrogen gas on the negative plate of a galvanic battery, so that the generation of electricity is impeded. **circular p.,** that polarization which causes vibration in circles. **elliptical p.,** that which causes the vibration in ellipses. **plane p.,** the production of polarization such that the light vibrations are all in one plane. **rotatory p.,** circular or elliptical polarization, as distinguished from plane polarization.

polarize (po'lar-īz) 1. to embue with polarity. 2. to put into a state of polarization.

polarizer (po'lah-rīz″er) an appliance for polarizing light.

polarogram (po-lar'o-gram) the curve of current versus voltage obtained in polarography.

polarographic (po″lah-ro-graf'ik) pertaining to polarography.

polarography (po″lar-og'rah-fe) an electrochemical technique for identifying and estimating the concentration of reducible elements by means of the dual measurement of the current flowing through an electrochemical cell (which contains the test solution) and the electrical potential between the two electrodes as the potential is increased at a constant rate by an external voltage source. As the voltage reaches the standard electrode potential of the test substance, there is a sharp increase in current flow. The indicator electrode is usually a dropping mercury electrode.

Polaroid (po'lar-oid) trademark for a sheet (film) polarizer utilizing oriented crystals used as a substitute for Nicol prisms and for reducing glare through lenses and windshields.

poldine methylsulfate (pol'dēn) [USP] chemical name: 2-[[(hydroxydiphenylacetyl)oxy]methyl]-1,1-dimethylpyrrolidinium methyl sulfate. A synthetic quaternary nitrogen anticholinergic, $C_{22}H_{29}NO_7S$, occurring as a creamy white, crystalline powder; used as an adjunct in the treatment of peptic ulcer and gastrointestinal disorders associated with hyperacidity, hypermotility, and spasm, administered orally.

pole (pōl) [L. *polus*; Gr. *polos*] 1. either extremity of an axis, as of the fetal ellipse, or of an organ of the body; called also *polus* or *extremitas.* 2. either one of two points which have opposite physical qualities (electric or other). **animal p.,** the site of an ovum to which the nucleus is approximated, and from which the polar bodies pinch off. Also, in nonmammalian species, the pole of an egg less heavily laden with yolk than the vegetal pole and therefore exhibiting faster cell division. **anterior p. of eyeball,** polus anterior bulbi oculi. **anterior p. of lens,** polus anterior lentis. **antigerminal p.,** vegetal p. **cephalic p.,** the end of the fetal ellipse at which the head of the fetus is situated. **frontal p. of hemisphere of cerebrum,** polus frontalis hemispherii cerebri. **germinal p.,** animal p. **inferior p. of kidney,** extremitas inferior renis. **inferior p. of testis,** extremitas inferior testis. **negative p.,** cathode. **nutritive p.,** vegetal p. **occipital p. of hemisphere of cerebrum,** polus occipitalis hemispherii cerebri. **pelvic p.,** the end of the fetal ellipse at which the breech of the fetus is situated. **positive p.,** anode. **posterior p. of eyeball,** polus posterior bulbi oculi. **posterior p. of lens,** polus posterior lentis. **temporal p. of hemisphere of cerebrum,** polus temporalis hemispherii cerebri. **twin p.,** that part of a spiral-fibered nerve cell from which both the straight and spiral fibers spring. **upper p. of kidney,** extremitas superior renis. **upper p. of testis,** extremitas superior testis. **vegetal p., vegetative p., vitelline p.,** that pole of an ovum at which the greater amount of food yolk is deposited. Cf. *animal p.*

poli (po'li) plural of *polus.*

policapram (pol'ĕ-ka'pram) chemical name: poly[imino(1-oxo-1,6-hexanediyl)]; a linear polymer of ε-aminocaproic lactam, $(C_6H_{11}NO)_n$, as microcrystals of colloid dimensions; used as a tablet binder for pharmaceutical preparations.

policeman (po-lēs'man) a glass rod with a piece of rubber tubing on one end, used as a stirring rod and transfer tool in chemical analysis.

policlinic (pol'e-klin'ik) [Gr. *polis* city + *klinē* bed] a city hospital, infirmary, or clinic. Cf. *polyclinic.*

poliencephalitis (pol'e-en-sef″ah-li'tis) polioencephalitis.

poliencephalomyelitis (pol'e-en-sef″ah-lo-mi″ĕ-li'tis) polioencephalomyelitis.

polio (po'le-o) poliomyelitis.

polio- (po'le-o) [Gr. *polios* gray] a combining form denoting relationship to the gray matter of the nervous system.

poliocidal (po'le-o-si'dal) neutralizing the poliomyelitis virus.

polioclastic (po'le-o-klas'tik) [*polio-* + Gr. *klastos* breaking] destroying the gray matter of the nervous system; a term applied to the viruses of poliomyelitis, epidemic encephalitis, and rabies; neurotropic.

poliodystrophia (po'le-o-dis-tro'fe-ah) poliodystrophy. **p. cer'ebri,** a rare disease of young children, characterized by neuron degeneration of the cerebral cortex and elsewhere, accompanied by progressive mental deterioration, motor disturbances, and early death; called also *Alper's disease.*

poliodystrophy (po'le-o-dis'tro-fe) [*polio-* + *dystrophy*] atrophy of the cerebral gray matter.

polioencephalitis (po″le-o-en-sef″ah-li'tis) [*polio-* + *encephalitis*] 1. inflammatory disease of the gray substance of the brain. 2. cerebral poliomyelitis. **p. acu'ta hemorrha'gica,** Wernicke's encephalopathy. **p. acu'ta infan'tum,** an acute variety seen in children under six years of age, and marked by fever, vomiting, and convulsions; it is usually followed by permanent paralysis of the limbs which were affected with convulsions. **acute bulbar p.,** acute bulbar paralysis. **p. hemorrha'gica supe'rior,** Wernicke's encephalopathy. **inferior p.,** bulbar paralysis. **posterior p.,** inflammation of the gray matter of the posterior part of the fourth ventricle. **superior hemorrhagic p.,** Wernicke's encephalopathy.

polioencephalomeningomyelitis (po″le-o-en-sef″ah-lo-mĕ-nin″go-mi″ĕ-li'tis) inflammation of the gray matter of the brain and spinal cord and of the meninges covering it.

polioencephalomyelitis (po″le-o-en-sef″ah-lo-mi″ĕ-li'tis) inflammatory disease of the gray matter of the brain and spinal cord.

polioencephalopathy (po″le-o-en-sef″ah-lop'ah-the) [*polio-* + Gr. *enkephalos* brain + *pathos* disease] disease of the gray matter of the brain.

polioencephalotropic (po″le-o-en-sef″ah-lo-trop'ik) having a special affinity for the gray substance of the brain; neurotropic.

poliomyelencephalitis (po″le-o-mi″el-en-sef″ah-li'tis) [*polio-* + Gr. *myelos* marrow + *enkephalos* brain + *-itis*] poliomyelitis combined with polioencephalitis.

poliomyeliticidal (po″le-o-mi″ĕ-li'tĭ-si″dal) having the power of destroying poliomyelitis virus.

poliomyelitis (po″le-o-mi″ĕ-li'tis) [*polio-* + Gr. *myelos* marrow + *-itis*] an acute viral disease, occurring sporadically and in epidemics, and characterized clinically by fever, sore throat, headache, and vomiting, often with stiffness of the neck and back. In the *minor illness* these may be the only symptoms. The *major illness,* which may or may not be preceded by the minor illness, is characterized by involvement of the central nervous system, stiff neck, pleocytosis in the spinal fluid, and perhaps paralysis. There may be subsequent atrophy of groups of muscles, ending in contraction and permanent deformity. The major illness is called *acute anterior p., infantile paralysis,* and *Heine-Medin disease.* The disease is now largely controlled by vaccines. See also *poliovirus* and *spinal paralytic p.* **acute anterior p.,** see *poliomyelitis.* **acute lateral p.,** spinal paralytic p. **anterior p.,** inflammation of the anterior horns of the gray substance of the spinal cord. **ascending p.,** a paralytic affection which is first manifested in the legs and rapidly ascends cephalad. **bulbar p.,** a serious form of poliomyelitis in which the medulla oblongata is affected, and in which there may be dysfunction of the swallowing mechanism, and respiratory and circulatory distress. **cerebral p.,** poliomyelitis in which the areas most likely to be involved are the brain stem and the motor cortex; called also *polioencephalomyelitis.* **endemic p.,** poliomyelitis occurring sporadically or in a small number of cases, particularly during periods of warm weather, in most countries throughout the world. **epidemic p.,** poliomyelitis occurring in epidemic form. **mouse p., murine p.,** Theiler's disease. **porcine p.,** infectious porcine encephalomyelitis. **postinoculation p.,** acute poliomyelitis appearing within three weeks after some type of inoculation. **post-tonsillectomy p.,** acute poliomyelitis appearing within a short time after tonsillectomy. **postvaccinal p.,** acute poliomyelitis appearing within three weeks after some type of vaccination. **spinal paralytic p.,** the classic form of acute anterior poliomyelitis, in which the appearance of flaccid paralysis, usually of one or more limbs, makes the diagnosis quite definite.

poliomyeloencephalitis (po″le-o-mi″ĕ-lo-en-sef″ah-li'tis) [*polio-* + Gr. *myelos* marrow + *enkephalos* brain + *-itis*] polioencephalomyelitis.

poliomyelopathy (po″le-o-mi″ĕ-lop'ah-the) [*polio-* + Gr. *myelos* marrow + *pathos* disease] any disease primarily affecting the gray matter of the spinal cord.

polioneuromere (po″le-o-nu'ro-mēr) [*polio-* + Gr. *neuron* nerve + *meros* part] one of the primitive segments of the gray matter of the spinal cord.

polioplasm (pol'e-o-plazm″) [*polio-* + Gr. *plasma* something formed] the internal, granular protoplasm proper of a cell.

poliosis (pol″e-o'sis) premature grayness of the hair. **p. cir-**

cumscrip'ta, grayness of the hair in a circumscribed area of the scalp.

poliothrix (pol'e-o-thriks) [polio- + Gr. *thrix* hair] poliosis.

poliovirus (po''le-o-vi'rus) the etiologic agent of poliomyelitis, separable, on the basis of specificity of neutralizing antibody, into three serotypes, designated types 1, 2, and 3. Over the years, type 1 has been responsible for about 85 per cent of all paralytic poliomyelitis and for most epidemics, and type 3 for about 10 per cent of paralytic poliomyelitis and for occasional epidemics. Type 2 has been responsible for about 5 per cent of paralytic poliomyelitis. Epidemics caused by poliovirus are now largely controlled by vaccines. **p. mu'ris,** Theiler's virus.

polipropene (pol''ĕ-pro'pēn) chemical name: 1-propene homopolymer; a tablet excipient for pharmaceutical preparations, $(C_3H_6)_n$.

polishing (pol'ish-ing) 1. the creation of a smooth and glossy finish on a surface, as of a denture. 2. [Pl.] material obtained by abrasion of a solid, such as that (*rice polishings* or *perpolitiones oryzae,* a rich source of vitamin B) produced by the milling of rice.

polisography (pol''ĕ-sog'rah-fe) [Gr. *polys* many + *isos* same + *graphein* to write] roentgenography in which several exposures are made in the same film.

Politzer's bag, etc. (pol'it-zerz) [Adam *Politzer,* Hungarian otologist, 1835–1920] see under *bag, cone, operation, speculum, test,* and *treatment.*

politzerization (pol''it-zer-i-za'shun) [Adam *Politzer*] inflation of the middle ear by means of a Politzer bag. **negative p.,** displacement of secretion from a cavity through negative pressure produced by means of a Politzer bag.

polkissen (pōl-kis'en) [Ger. "pole cushion"] juxtaglomerular cells.

poll (pōl) the back part of the head, especially that of an animal.

pollakidipsia (pol''ah-kĭ-dip'se-ah) [Gr. *pollakis* often + *dipsa* thirst + -*ia*] a condition characterized by abnormally frequent occurrence of the sensation of thirst.

pollakisuria (pol''ah-kĭ-su're-ah) pollakiuria.

pollakiuria (pol''ah-ke-u're-ah) [Gr. *pollakis* often + *ouron* urine + -*ia*] unduly frequent passage of the urine.

pollantin (pol-lan'tin) an antitoxin derived from the blood serum of horses previously inoculated with extracts of the pollen of certain plants; once used in the treatment of hay fever.

polled (pōld) having no horns; said of cattle that have been bred for this inherited trait.

pollen (pol'en) the mass of microspores (male fertilizing elements) of flowering plants. Many pollens, especially the airborne pollens, are allergens; i.e., they produce proteinaceous antigens capable of sensitizing susceptible persons and producing allergic symptoms.

pollenarium (pol''ĕ-na're-um) a building or room for the collection and storing of pollens.

pollenogenic (pol''ĕ-no-jen'ik) [*pollen* + Gr. *gennan* to produce] caused by the pollen of plants.

pollenosis (pol''ĕ-no'sis) pollinosis.

pollex (pol'eks), pl. *pol'lices* [L.] [NA] the first digit of the hand, or thumb. **p. exten'sus,** backward deviation of the thumb. **p. flex'us,** permanent flexion of the thumb. **p. val'gus,** deviation of the thumb toward the ulnar side. **p. va'rus,** deviation of the thumb toward the radial side.

pollicization (pol''is-i-za'shun) [L. *pollex* thumb] the replacement or rehabilitation of a thumb, especially surgical construction of a thumb from a portion of the index finger.

pollination (pol''ĭ-na'shun) the transfer of pollen from anther to stigma of a flowering plant.

pollinium (pol''ĭ-ne'um) an aggregation of pollen grains held together by a mucilaginous fluid and transported as a whole during pollination.

pollinosis (pol''ĭ-no'sis) the allergic reaction in the body to the airborne pollen of plants, resulting in the seasonal type of hay fever or rose cold. See *seasonal hay fever,* under *fever.*

pollodic (pol-lo'dik) [Gr. *polloi* many + *hodos* way] panthodic.

pollution (pŏ-lu'shun) [L. *pollutio*] 1. the act of defiling or making impure. 2. the discharge of semen without coition. **diurnal p., p. nim'iae,** spermatorrhea.

polocyte (po'lo-sīt) [Gr. *polos* pole + -*cyte*] see *polar bodies,* under *body.*

polonium (po-lo'ne-um) [L. *Polonia* Poland] a rare metal resembling bismuth, discovered in 1898 in pitchblende; atomic number, 84; atomic weight, 210; symbol, Po. It is radioactive, but less so than radium.

poloxalene (pol-oks'ah-lēn) a liquid poloxamer, having a molecular weight of approximately 3000; used as a surfactant in pharmaceutical preparations and in the prevention of bloat in ruminants.

poloxalkol (pol-ok'sal-kol) poloxamer 188.

poloxamer (pol-oks'ah-mer) any of a series of nonionic surfactants of the polyoxypropylene-polyoxyethylene copolymer type,

having the general formula $HO(C_2H_4O)_a(C_3H_6O)_b(C_2H_4O)_cH$, where $a = c$; the molecular weights of the members of the series vary from about 1000 to more than 16000. The term is used in conjunction with a numerical suffix for individual unique identification of products that may be used as a food, drug, or cosmetic. Poloxamers may be surfactants, emulsifiers, or stabilizers. **p. 182L,** a liquid poloxamer, having an average molecular weight of 2450; used as a food additive and pharmaceutic aid. **p. 188,** a waxy poloxamer, having an average molecular weight of 8350; used as a cathartic, administered orally. Called also *poloxalkol.* **p. 331,** a liquid poloxamer, having an average molecular weight of 3800; used as a food additive.

polster (pōl'ster) a small bulge, as on a vessel wall. **Sanderson p's,** collections of small follicles scattered throughout the thyroid gland, so arranged that each produces a characteristic bulge.

poltophagy (pol-tof'ah-je) [Gr. *poltos* porridge + *phagein* to eat] thorough chewing of the food so that it becomes reduced to a porridge-like mass.

polus (po'lus), pl. *po'li* [L.] a pole: either extremity of an axis; [NA] a general term for the extremity of an organ. **p. ante'rior bul'bi oc'uli** [NA], anterior pole of eyeball: the center of the anterior curvature of the eyeball. **p. ante'rior len'tis** [NA], anterior pole of lens: the central point of the anterior surface of the lens. **p. fronta'lis hemisphe'rii cer'ebri** [NA], frontal pole of hemisphere of cerebrum: the most prominent part of the anterior end of each hemisphere of the brain. **p. occipita'lis hemisphe'rii cer'ebri** [NA], occipital pole of hemisphere of cerebrum: the most posterior prominence of the occipital lobe of the cerebral hemisphere. **p. poste'rior bul'bi oc'uli** [NA], posterior pole of eyeball: the center of the posterior curvature of the eyeball. **p. poste'rior len'tis** [NA], posterior pole of lens: the central point of the posterior surface of the lens. **p. tempora'lis hemisphe'rii cer'ebri** [NA], temporal pole of hemisphere of cerebrum: the prominent anterior end of the temporal lobe of the brain.

poly (pol'e) colloquial name for a polymorphonulear leukocyte; see *neutrophil,* def. 1.

poly- [Gr. *polys* many] a combining form meaning many or much.

Polya's operation (pōl'yahz) [Jenö (Eugene) *Polya,* Budapest surgeon, 1876–1944] see under *operation.*

polyacid (pol'e-as'id) capable of neutralizing several molecules of an acid radical; said of a base or basic radical.

polyacrylamide (pol'e-ah-kril'ah-mīd) a polymer of acrylamide.

polyadenia (pol''e-ah-de'ne-ah) [*poly-* + Gr. *adēn* gland + -*ia*] pseudoleukemia.

polyadenitis (pol''e-ad''ĕ-ni'tis) [*poly-* + Gr. *adēn* gland + -*itis*] inflammation of several or many glands. **malignant p.,** bubonic plague.

polyadenoma (pol''e-ad''ĕ-no'mah) adenoma of many glands.

polyadenomatosis (pol''e-ad''ĕ-no-mah-to'sis) multiple adenomas in a part.

polyadenopathy (pol''e-ad''ĕ-nop'ah-the) any disease affecting several glands at once.

polyadenosis (pol''e-ad''ĕ-no'sis) disorder of several glands, particularly of several endocrine glands.

polyadenous (pol''e-ad'ĕ-nus) [*poly-* + Gr. *adēn* gland] having or affecting many glands.

polyagglutinability (pol''e-ah-gloo''tĭ-nah-bil'ĭ-te) the susceptibility to agglutination by a number of agents not necessarily corresponding to the antigenic structure of the agglutinogen.

polyalcoholism (pol''e-al'ko-hol-izm) intoxication or poisoning by a mixture of different alcohols.

polyalgesia (pol''e-al-je'se-ah) [*poly-* + Gr. *algēsis* sense of pain + -*ia*] a condition in which a single pin-prick feels as if several had been made.

polyamine (pol''e-am'in) any compound, e.g., spermine and spermidine, containing two or more amine groups.

polyandry (pol''e-an'dre) [*poly-* + Gr. *anēr* man] 1. the concurrent marriage of a woman to more than one man, as practiced by certain peoples. 2. union of two or more male pronuclei with a female pronucleus, resulting in polyploidy of the zygote. Cf. *polygyny.*

Polyangiaceae (pol''e-an''je-a'se-e) a family of schizomycetes, order Myxobacterales, made up of saprophytic microorganisms found in soil and decaying organic matter, and including four genera, *Chondromy'ces, Podan'gium, Polyan'gium,* and *Synan'gium.*

polyangiitis (pol''e-an''je-i'tis) inflammation involving multiple blood or lymph vessels.

Polyangium (pol''e-an'je-um) a genus of Schizomycetes of the order Myxobacterales, family Polyangiaceae.

polyarteritis (pol''e-ar''tĕ-ri'tis) [*poly-* + Gr. *artēria* artery + -*itis*] a condition marked by multiple sites of inflammatory and destructive lesions in the arterial system; see *periarteritis nodosa.*

polyarthric (pol″e-ar′thrik) [poly- + Gr. arthron joint] pertaining to or affecting many joints.

polyarthritis (pol″e-ar-thri′tis) [poly- + Gr. arthron joint + -itis] an inflammation of several joints together. **benign p.,** polyarthritis that is usually mild, but may be severe, though without permanent joint changes; attacks usually occur in winter and last only a few months. **chronic secondary p.,** Jaccoud's syndrome. **chronic villous p.,** chronic inflammation of the synovial membrane of several joints. **p. des′truens,** rheumatoid arthritis. **p. nodo′sa,** periarteritis nodosa. **peripheral p.,** that in which the knees and ankles tend to be involved more commonly than the small joints of the hands or feet; asymmetric involvement is common and the number of joints affected tends to be limited. **p. rheumat′ica acu′ta,** rheumatic fever. **tuberculous p.,** pulmonary hypertrophic osteoarthropathy. **vertebral p.,** disease of the intervertebral substance without caries of the bodies of the vertebrae.

polyarticular (pol″e-ar-tik′u-lar) [poly- + L. articulus joint] affecting many joints.

polyatomic (pol″e-ah-tom′ik) [poly- + Gr. atomon atom] composed of several atoms.

polyauxotroph (pol″e-awk′so-trōf) [poly- + Gr. auxein to increase + trophē nourishment] an organism, especially a mutant, which requires multiple growth factors.

polyauxotrophic (pol″e-awk″so-trōf′ik) requiring multiple growth factors; used especially with reference to a single mutation that causes a multiple requirement.

polyavitaminosis (pol″e-a-vi″tah-min-o′sis) [poly- + avitaminosis] a deficiency disease in which more than one vitamin is lacking in the diet.

polyaxon (pol″e-ak′son) [poly- + Gr. axōn axis] a nerve cell from the horizontal dendrites of which four or more axons or branches are given off.

polyaxonic (pol″e-ak-son′ik) having several axons.

polyazin (pol″e-az′in) an organic chemical compound whose molecules contain atoms two or more of which are nitrogen.

polybasic (pol″e-ba′sik) [poly- + Gr. basis base] 1. denoting any acid which has several hydrogen atoms replaceable by a base. 2. denoting any salt of a polybasic acid formed by replacing some or all of its hydrogen atoms by a base.

polyblast (pol′e-blast) [poly- + Gr. blastos germ] Maximow's name for the mononuclear exudate cells in inflamed tissues. According to him they arise from the wandering cells of the tissues and from hypertrophied nongranular leukocytes which have left the blood stream. As now used, the term is synonymous with macrophage.

polyblennia (pol″e-blen′e-ah) [poly- + Gr. blenna mucus + -ia] the secretion of an excessive quantity of mucus.

Polybrene (pol′e-brēn) trademark for a preparation of hexadimethrine bromide.

polybutilate (pol″e-bu′tĭ-lāt) chemical name: poly[oxy-1,4-butanediyloxy(1,6-dioxo-1,6-hexanediyl)]; a surgical suture coating, $(C_{10}H_{16}O_4)_n$.

polycarbophil (pol″e-kar′bo-fil) [USP] a pharmacologically inert, polyacrylic acid cross-linked with divinyl glycol, occurring as white to creamy white granules; used as a gastrointestinal absorbent in the treatment of diarrhea.

polycellular (pol″e-sel′u-lar) multicellular.

polycentric (pol″e-sen′trik) having many centers.

polycentricity (pol″e-sen-tris″ĭ-te) the state or quality of being polycentric.

polyceptor (pol″e-sep′tor) [poly- + ceptor] in early immunological theory, an amboceptor capable of binding a number of different complements.

polycheiria (pol″e-ki′re-ah) [poly- + Gr. cheir hand + -ia] the condition of having more than two hands.

polychemotherapy (pol″e-ke″mo-ther′ah-pe) treatment by the simultaneous administration of several chemotherapeutic agents.

polychloruria (pol″e-klo-roo′re-ah) an increased excretion of chlorine in the urine.

polycholia (pol″e-ko′le-ah) [poly- + Gr. cholē bile + -ia] excessive flow or secretion of bile.

polychondritis (pol″e-kon-dri′tis) inflammation involving many cartilages of the body. **chronic atrophic p., p. chron′ica atro′phicans,** relapsing p. **relapsing p.,** an acquired disease of unknown etiology, having a chronic course and a tendency to recurrence, and marked by inflammatory and degenerative lesions of various cartilaginous structures, including those of the joints, ears, nose, trachea, and bronchi, resulting in such deformities as floppy ear and saddle nose; if the tracheal or bronchial wall collapses, respiratory obstruction may occur. The aorta and the sclera and cornea are also affected. Called also chronic atrophic p., p. chronica atrophicans, and polychondropathia.

polychondropathia (pol″e-kon″dro-path′e-ah) relapsing polychondritis.

polychondropathy (pol″e-kon-drop′ah-the) relapsing polychondritis.

polychrest (pol′e-krest) [poly- + Gr. chrēstos useful] 1. useful in many conditions. 2. a remedy useful in many diseases.

polychromasia (pol″e-kro-ma′ze-ah) 1. variation in the hemoglobin content of the erythrocytes of the blood. 2. polychromatophilia.

polychromate (pol″e-kro′māt) a person who can distinguish many colors.

polychromatia (pol″e-kro-ma′she-ah) polychromatophilia.

polychromatic (pol″e-kro-mat′ik) [poly- + Gr. chrōma color] exhibiting many colors. Cf. monochromatic.

polychromatocyte (pol″e-kro-mat′o-sīt) a cell that is stainable with various stains or colors.

polychromatocytosis (pol″e-kro″mah-to-si-to′sis) polychromatophilia.

polychromatophil (pol″e-kro-mat′o-fil) [poly- + Gr. chrōma color + philein to love] a cell or other element that is stainable with various stains or colors.

polychromatophilia (pol″e-kro″mah-to-fil′e-ah) 1. the quality of being stainable with various stains or tints; affinity for all sorts of stains. 2. a condition in which the erythrocytes, on staining, show various shades of blue combined with tinges of pink.

polychromatophilic (pol″e-kro″mah-to-fil′ik) pertaining to or characterized by polychromatophilia.

polychromatosis (pol″e-kro″mah-to′sis) an excess of abnormally staining erythrocytes in the blood; see polychromatophilia, def. 2.

polychromemia (pol″e-kro-me′me-ah) [poly- + Gr. chrōma color + haima blood + -ia] increase in the coloring matter of the blood.

polychromic (pol″e-kro′mik) pertaining to or exhibiting many colors.

polychromophil (pol″e-kro′mo-fil) polychromatophil.

polychromophilia (pol″e-kro-mo-fil′e-ah) polychromatophilia.

polychylia (pol″e-ki′le-ah) [poly- + Gr. chylos chyle + -ia] excessive production of chyle.

Polycillin (pol″e-sil′in) trademark for preparations of ampicillin.

polyclinic (pol″e-klin′ik) [poly- + Gr. klinē bed] a hospital and school where diseases and injuries of all kinds are studied and treated clinically.

polyclonal (pol″e-klōn′al) derived from different cells; of or pertaining to several clones.

polyclonia (pol″e-klo′ne-ah) [poly- + Gr. klonos clonus + -ia] a disease marked by many clonic spasms, resembling tic and chorea, but distinct from either.

polycopria (pol″e-kop′re-ah) [poly- + Gr. kopros filth + -ia] (obs.) excessive formation of feces.

polycoria (pol″e-ko′re-ah) 1. [poly- + Gr. korē pupil + -ia] the existence of more than one pupil in an eye. 2. [poly- + Gr. koros surfeit + -ia] the deposit of reserve material in an organ or tissue so as to produce enlargement. **p. spu′ria,** a condition in which the iris contains several openings or holes. **p. ve′ra,** the existence in the eye of several pupils, each with its own sphincter.

polycrotic (pol″e-krot′ik) [poly- + Gr. krotos beat] having several secondary waves to each pulse beat.

polycrotism (pol-ik′ro-tizm) the fact or quality of being polycrotic.

polycyclic (pol″e-si′klik) [poly- + Gr. kyklos ring] containing more than one ring or cycle (frequency).

Polycycline (pol″e-si′klēn) trademark for preparations of tetracycline.

polycyesis (pol″e-si-e′sis) [poly- + Gr. kyēsis pregnancy] multiple pregnancy.

polycystic (pol″e-sis′tik) [poly- + Gr. kystis cyst] containing or made up of many cysts.

polycystoma (pol″e-sis-to′mah) a condition in which a part, especially the breast, is riddled with cysts.

polycyte (pol′e-sīt) [poly- + Gr. kytos cell] a hypersegmented polymorphonuclear leukocyte of normal size. Cf. macropolycyte.

polycythemia (pol″e-si-the′me-ah) [poly- + Gr. kytos cell + haima blood + -ia] an increase in the total red cell mass of the blood; see absolute p. and relative p. **absolute p.,** an increase in red cell mass caused by a sustained overactivity of the erythroid component of the bone marrow, which may occur as a compensatory physiologic response to tissue hypoxia (see secondary p.), or as the principal manifestation of polycythemia vera. Cf. relative p. **appropriate p.,** see secondary p. **benign p.,** stress p. **compensatory p.,** see secondary p. **p. hyperton′ica,** stress p. **inappropriate p.,** see secondary p. **myelopathic p., primary p.,** p. vera. **relative p.,** a decrease in plasma volume without change in red blood cell mass so that the erythrocytes become more concentrated (elevated hematocrit); it may occur as an acute transient condition due to marked loss of body fluid or lowered fluid intake or a combination of both, or it may be a chronic condition associated with a low normal plasma volume and a high normal red cell mass or with other factors (see stress *p.*). Cf. *absolute p.* **p. ru'bra, p. ru'bra ve'ra,** p. vera. **secondary p.,** any absolute increase in the total red cell mass other than polycythemia vera, occurring as a physiologic response to tissue hypoxia. It may be compensatory and *appropriate*, adjusting for general tissue hypoxia, such as that occurring in association with pulmonary disease, alveolar hypoventilation, cardiovascular disease, and prolonged exposure to high altitude or occurring as a result of defective hemoglobin or drugs. Or it may be *inappropriate*, reflecting excessive erythropoietin production due to renal or extrarenal disorders. Called also *erythrocytosis*. **splenomegalic p.,** p. vera. **spurious p.,** 1. relative p. 2. stress p. **stress p.,** chronic relative polycythemia (q.v.) usually affecting white, middle-aged, mildly obese males who are active, anxiety-prone, and hypertensive, occurring without the characteristic symptoms associated with polycythemia vera, i.e., without leukocytosis, splenomegaly, and thrombocytosis. Called also *benign p., Gaisböck's disease* or *syndrome,* and *stress erythrocytosis.* **p. ve'ra,** a myeloproliferative disorder of unknown etiology, characterized by abnormal proliferation of all hematopoietic bone marrow elements and an absolute increase in red cell mass and total blood volume, associated frequently with splenomegaly, leukocytosis, and thrombocythemia. Hematopoiesis is also reactive in extramedullary sites (liver and spleen). In time, myelofibrosis occurs. Called also *erythremia, erythrocythemia, p. ruba, splenomegalic p., myelopathic p., erythrocytosis megalosplenica, Osler's disease, Vaquez's disease,* and *Vasquez-Osler disease.* Cf. *secondary p.*

polydactylia (pol″e-dak-til'e-ah) polydactyly.

polydactylism (pol-e-dak'til-izm) polydactyly.

polydactyly (pol″e-dak'tĭ-le) [*poly-* + Gr. *daktylos* finger + *-ia*] a developmental anomaly characterized by the presence of supernumerary digits (fingers or toes) on the hands or feet.

polydentia (pol″e-den'she-ah) polyodontia.

polydipsia (pol″e-dip'se-ah) [*poly-* + Gr. *dipsa* thirst + *-ia*] excessive thirst persisting for long periods of time, as in diabetes mellitus.

polydispersoid (pol″e-dis-per'soid) a colloid in which the disperse phase consists of particles having different degrees of dispersion.

polydyscrinia (pol″e-dis-krin'e-ah) pluridyscrinia.

polydysplasia (pol″e-dis-pla'ze-ah) [*poly-* + *dysplasia*] faulty development in several types of tissue or several organs or systems. **hereditary ectodermal p.,** congenital ectodermal defect; see under *defect*.

polydysspondylism (pol″e-dis-spon'dĭ-lizm) malformation of several vertebrae, associated with dwarfed stature, low intelligence, and malformation of the sella turcica.

polydystrophic (pol″e-dis-tro'fik) pertaining to or exhibiting polydystrophy.

polydystrophy (pol″e-dis'tro-fe) dystrophy of several tissues or structures, as may occur in congenital anomalies. **pseudo-Hurler p.,** mucolipidosis III.

polyelectrolyte (pol″e-e-lek'tro-līt) an ion containing more than two charges.

polyembryony (pol″e-em-bri'o-ne) [*poly-* + *embryo*] the production of two or more embryos from the same ovum or seed.

polyendocrine (pol″e-en'do-krīn) pertaining to or affecting several endocrine glands; see under *adenomatosis*.

polyendocrinoma (pol″e-en″do-kri-no'mah) polyendocrine adenomatosis.

polyene (pol-e'ēn) a chemical compound in which there are several conjugated double bonds.

polyerg (pol'e-erg) [*poly-* + Gr. *ergon* work] a monogenic antiserum which reacts with heterologous antigens.

polyergic (pol″e-er'jik) able to act in several different ways.

polyesthesia (pol″e-es-the'ze-ah) [*poly-* + Gr. *aisthēsis* perception + *-ia*] a condition in which a single object seems to be felt in several different places.

polyesthetic (pol″e-es-thet'ik) pertaining to or affecting several senses or sensations.

polyestradiol phosphate (pol″e-es″trah-di'ol, pol″e-es-tra'-de-ol) a polymer of estradiol phosphate having estrogenic activity similar to that of estradiol; used in the palliative therapy of prostatic carcinoma, administered intramuscularly.

polyestrous (pol″e-es'trus) completing two or more estrus cycles in each sexual season.

polyethadene (pol-e-eth'ah-dēn) chemical name: 1,2:3,4-di-epoxybutane polymer with ethylenimine; an antacid, $(C_4H_6O_2)_m \cdot (C_2H_5N)_n$.

polyethylene (pol″e-eth'ĭ-lēn) polymerized ethylene, $(CH_2—CH_2)_n$, a synthetic plastic material, forms of which have been used in reparative surgery.

polyethylene glycol (pol″e-eth'ĭ-lēn gli'kol) [NF] a generic name for mixtures of condensation polymers of ethylene oxide and water, represented by the general formula $H(OCH_2CH_2)_n OH$, in which *n* is greater than or equal to 4. The term is used in combination with a numeric suffix which indicates the approximate average molecular weight. Those with average molecular weights between 200 and 700 are liquid and those above 1000 are waxlike solids: *p. glycol 3000* (*n* varies from 5 to 5.75) is used as a solvent and dispensing agent in pharmaceutical preparations; *p. glycol 400* (*n* varies from 8.2 to 9.1), *p. glycol 600* (*n* varies from 12.5 to 13.9), and *p. glycol 1500* (*n* varies from 29 to 36) are used as ointment and suppository bases; *p. glycol 1540* (*n* varies from 28 to 36) is used as a vehicle in pharmaceutical preparations; *p. glycol 4000* (*n* varies from 68 to 84) and *p. glycol 6000* (*n* varies from 158 to 204) are used as ointment and suppository bases and as tablet excipients. Called also *macrogal.*

polyferose (pol-ĭ-fer'ōs) a chelate complex of iron and a polymerized derivative of sucrose; a hematinic.

polyfolliculinic (pol″e-fo-lik″u-lin'ik) marked by extensive secretion of folliculin (estrone).

Polygala (po-lig'ah-lah) [*poly-* + Gr. *gala* milk] a genus of plants (milkworts) of many species. *P. senega* L. (Polygalaceae), or seneca snakeroot, is found in North America. See *senega*.

polygalactia (pol″e-gah-lak'she-ah) [*poly-* + Gr. *gala* milk] excessive secretion of milk.

polygalacturonase (pol″e-gah-lak-tu″ro-nās) poly-α-1,4-galacturonide glycanohydrolase: an enzyme present in most plants that catalyzes the hydrolysis of pectin to sugars and galacturonic acid; called also *pectinase*.

polygalin (po-lig'ah-lin) senegenin.

polygamy (po-lig'ah-me) [*poly-* + Gr. *gamos* marriage] the concurrent marriage of a woman or man to more than one mate, as opposed to monogamy. See also *polyandry* and *polygyny*.

polyganglionic (pol″e-gang″gle-on'ik) [*poly-* + Gr. *ganglion* ganglion] 1. having or pertaining to several or many ganglia. 2. affecting several lymphatic glands.

polygen (pol'ĕ-jen) 1. an element which is able to combine in two or more proportions. 2. a complex antigen comprised of two or more kinds of antigenic specificities (antigenic determinants) each of which stimulates the production of specific antibodies following inoculation of the complex antigen into the animal body.

polygene (pol'ĕ-jēn) a group of nonallelic genes (multiple factors or cumulative genes) that interact to influence the same character in the same way so that the effect is cumulative.

polygenic (pol″ĕ-jēn'ik) [*poly-* + *gene*] pertaining to or determined by the action of several different genes. Cf. *multifactorial*.

polyglactin 910 (pol″e-glak'tin) chemical name: 2-hydroxy-propanoic acid polymer with hydroxyacetic acid; an absorbable surgical suture material, $(C_2H_2O_2)_m (C_3H_4O_2)_n$.

polyglandular (pol″e-glan'du-lar) pertaining to or affecting several different glands.

polygnathus (po-lig'nah-thus) [*poly-* + Gr. *gnathos* jaw] a monster in which a parasitic twin is attached to the jaw of the autosite.

Polygonatum (pol″e-go-na'tum) [*poly-* + Gr. *gony* knee] a genus of liliaceous plants. *P. biflorum* (Walt.) Ell., or Solomon's seal, is a perennial herb of eastern North America, tonic, vulnerary, diuretic, emetic, and purgative; in a considerable dose it is a cardiac poison. The starchy rootstock was once used as a food by certain Indians.

polygram (pol'ĕ-gram) a tracing made by a polygraph.

polygraph (pol'ĕ-graf) [*poly-* + Gr. *graphein* to write] an instrument for simultaneously recording various physiological responses as represented by mechanical or electrical impulses, such as respiratory movements, pulse wave, blood pressure, and the psychogalvanic reflex. Such phenomena reflect emotional reactions which are of use in detecting deception. Popularly known as *lie detector.*

polygyny (po-lij'ĭ-ne) [*poly-* + Gr. *gynē* woman] 1. the concurrent marriage of a man to more than one woman, as practiced by certain peoples. 2. union of two or more female pronuclei with a male pronucleus, resulting in polyploidy of the zygote. Cf. *polyandry.*

polygyria (pol″e-ji're-ah) [*poly-* + Gr. *gyros* gyrus + *-ia*] a condition in which there is more than the normal number of convolutions in the brain.

polyhedral (pol″e-he'dral) [*poly-* + Gr. *hedra* seat, base] having many faces or sides.

polyhexose (pol″e-hek'sōs) polysaccharide formed by the enzymatic condensation of hexose sugars.

polyhidrosis (pol″e-hid-ro'sis) [*poly-* + Gr. *hidrōs* sweat + *-osis*] hyperhidrosis.

polyhybrid (pol″e-hi'brid) a hybrid whose parents differ from each other in more than three characters.

polyhydramnios (pol″e-hi-dram'ne-os) [*poly-* + Gr. *hydōr* water + *amnion* amnion] hydramnios.

polyhydric (pol″e-hi'drik) containing more than two hydroxyl groups.

polyhydruria (pol″e-hi-droo′re-ah) [*poly-* + Gr. *hydōr* water + *ouron* urine + *-ia*] abnormal dilution of the urine.

polyhypermenorrhea (pol″e-hi″per-men″o-re′ah) [*poly-* + Gr. *hyper* over + *menorrhea*] frequent menstruation with abnormally profuse discharge.

polyhypomenorrhea (pol″e-hi″po-men″o-re′ah) [*poly-* + Gr. *hypo* under + *menorrhea*] frequent menstruation with deficient amount of discharge.

polyidrosis (pol″e-id-ro′sis) hyperhidrosis.

polyinfection (pol″e-in-fek′shun) [*poly-* + *infection*] infection with more than one organism.

polyionic (pol″e-i-on′ik) containing several different ions (e.g., potassium, sodium, etc.), as a polyionic solution.

polykaryocyte (pol″e-kar′e-o-sīt) [*poly-* + Gr. *karyon* nucleus + *-cyte*] a giant cell containing several nuclei.

Polykol (pol′ĕ-kol) trademark for preparations of poloxalkol.

polylecithal (pol″e-les′ĭ-thal) [*poly-* + Gr. *lekithos* yolk] macrolecithal.

polyleptic (pol″e-lep′tik) [*poly-* + Gr. *lambanein* to seize] having many remissions and exacerbations.

polylysine (pol″e-li′sin) a polypeptide composed of lysine molecules in peptide linkage; used with penicillenic acid in the detection of penicillin sensitivity; see *penicilloyl-polylysine*.

polymacon (pol″e-ma′kon) chemical name: 2-methyl-2-propenoic acid 1,2-ethanediyl ester polymer with 2-hydroxyethyl 2-methyl-2-propenoate; a hydrophilic contact lens material, $(C_6H_{10}O_3)_n$.

polymastia (pol″e-mas′te-ah) [*poly-* + Gr. *mastos* breast] the presence of more than one pair of mammae, or breasts.

Polymastigida (pol″e-mas″tĭ-gi′dah) an order of protozoa of the class Zoomastigophora, subphylum Mastigophora, consisting of small organisms possessing three to eight or more flagella and usually one or two nuclei, although some are multinucleate; they are found in the digestive tract of various arthropods and vertebrates. It includes the genera *Callimastix, Enteromonas, Eutrichomastix, Copromastix, Chilomastix, Hexamita, Giardia,* and *Trichomonas.*

polymastigote (pol″e-mas′tĭ-gōt) [*poly-* + Gr. *mastix* lash] 1. having several flagella. 2. any member of the Polymastigida.

polymazia (pol″e-ma′ze-ah) polymastia.

polymelia (pol″e-me′le-ah) [*poly-* + Gr. *melos* limb + *-ia*] a developmental anomaly characterized by the presence of supernumerary limbs.

polymelus (po-lim′ĕ-lus) an individual exhibiting polymelia.

polymenia (pol″e-me′ne-ah) polymenorrhea.

polymenorrhea (pol″e-men″o-re′ah) [*poly-* + *menorrhea*] abnormally frequent menstruation.

polymer (pol′ĭ-mer) [*poly-* + Gr. *meros* part] a compound, usually of high molecular weight, formed by the linear combination of simpler repeating molecules, or monomers. In immunology, immunoglobulins that form aggregates of more than one four-chain monomeric unit structure. For example, IgM and IgA both contain J chains which are associated with polymerization of the molecules. **addition p.,** a compound formed by the repeated combination of smaller molecules (monomers) without the formation of any other products (e.g., polyethylene). **condensation p.,** a compound formed by the repeated reaction of smaller molecules, involving at the same time the elimination of water or other simple compound (e.g., nylon).

polymerase (pol-im′er-ās) any enzyme that catalyzes polymerization. **DNA p.,** DNA nucleotidyltransferase. **RNA p.,** RNA nucleotidyltransferase. **RNA-dependent DNA p.,** an enzyme found in the white cells of leukemia patients, but not in normal patients.

polymeria (pol″ĭ-me′re-ah) [*poly-* + Gr. *meros* part + *-ia*] a developmental anomaly characterized by the presence of supernumerary parts or organs of the body.

polymeric (pol″ĭ-mer′ik) exhibiting the characteristics of a polymer.

polymerid (po-lim′er-id) a polymer.

polymerism (po-lim′ĕ-rizm, pol″ĭ-mĕ-rizm) the phenomenon, or process, which results in the formation of a polymer.

polymerization (pol″ĭ-mer″ĭ-za′shun) the act or process of forming a compound (polymer), usually of high molecular weight, by the combination of simpler molecules.

polymerize (pol′ĭ-mer-īz) to subject to or to undergo polymerization.

polymetacarpia (pol″e-met″ah-kar′pe-ah) [*poly-* + *metacarpus* + *-ia*] presence of more than the normal number of metacarpal bones.

polymetatarsia (pol″e-met″ah-tar′se-ah) [*poly-* + *metatarsus* + *-ia*] presence of more than the normal number of metatarsal bones.

polymicrobial (pol″e-mi-kro′be-al) [*poly-* + *microbe*] characterized by the presence of several species of microorganisms.

polymicrobic (pol″e-mi-kro′bik) polymicrobial.

polymicrogyria (pol″e-mi″kro-ji′re-ah) [*poly-* + Gr. *mikros* small + *gyros* convolution + *-ia*] a malformation of the brain characterized by development of numerous small convolutions (microgyri).

polymicrolipomatosis (pol″e-mi″kro-lip″o-mah-to′sis) [*poly-* + Gr. *mikros* small + *lipomatosis*] lipomatosis marked by the presence in the subcutaneous tissues of numerous small lipomas.

polymicrotome (pol″e-mi′kro-tōm) [*poly-* + *microtome*] a microtome which cuts several sections at once.

Polymnia (po-lim′ne-ah) [Gr.; one of the nine Muses] a genus of composite-flowered plants. *P. uvedalia* L., leafcup or bearsfoot, is anthelmintic, alterative, antispasmodic, and laxative.

polymorph (pol′e-morf) colloquial term for a polymorphonuclear leukocyte; see *neutrophil,* def. 2.

polymorphic (pol″e-mor′fik) [*poly-* + Gr. *morphē* form] occurring in several or many forms; appearing in different forms at different stages of development.

polymorphism (pol″e-mor′fizm) [*poly-* + Gr. *morphē* form] the quality or character of occurring in several different forms. **balanced p.,** an equilibrium mixture of homozygotes and heterozygotes maintained by separate and opposing forces of natural selection. **genetic p.,** the occurrence together in the same population of two or more genetically determined phenotypes in such proportions that the rarest of them cannot be maintained merely by recurrent mutation.

polymorphocellular (pol″e-mor″fo-sel′u-lar) [*poly-* + Gr. *morphē* form + L. *cellula* cell] having cells of many forms.

polymorphocyte (pol″e-mor′fo-sīt) a cell with a polymorphic nucleus.

polymorphonuclear (pol″e-mor″fo-nu′kle-ar) [*poly-* + Gr. *morphē* form + *nucleus*] 1. having a nucleus deeply lobed or so divided that it appears to be multiple. 2. a polymorphonuclear leukocyte; see *neutrophil,* def. 1. **filament p.,** one whose nuclear segments are joined by the filaments. **nonfilament p.,** one whose nuclear segments are joined by wide bands.

polymorphous (pol″e-mor′fus) polymorphic. **p. perverse,** a term applied to infantile sexual impulses which have not become repressed into normal mature sexuality, but appear as sexual perversions or the bases of neuroses.

Polymox (pol′ĕ-moks) trademark for preparations of amoxicillin.

polymyalgia (pol″e-mi-al′je-ah) myalgia affecting several muscles. **p. arterit′ica,** p. rheumatica. **p. rheumat′ica,** a syndrome in the elderly characterized by proximal joint and muscle pain, high erythrocyte sedimentation rate, and a self-limiting course; it is frequently associated with temporal arteritis.

polymyarian (pol″e-mi-a′re-an) [*poly-* + Gr. *mys* muscle] having many muscle cells in each quadrant of a cross section, the cells being coelomyarian in type; said of the muscle arrangement in certain nematodes.

polymyoclonus (pol″e-mi-ok′lo-nus) [*poly-* + Gr. *mys* muscle + *klonos* clonus] 1. a fine or minute muscular tremor. 2. polyclonia.

polymyopathy (pol″e-mi-op′ah-the) disease affecting several muscles simultaneously.

polymyositis (pol″e-mi″o-si′tis) [*poly-* + Gr. *mys* muscle + *-itis*] inflammation of several or many muscles at once, along with degenerative and regenerative changes marked by muscle weakness out of proportion to the loss of muscle bulk. When developing in adults, it is often associated with cancer. When accompanied by skin lesions, it is known as *dermatomyositis.* **p. hemorrha′gica,** inflammation of muscles associated with edema, dermatitis, and the presence of hemorrhages into and between the muscles. **trichinous p.,** trichinosis.

polymyxin (pol″e-mik′sin) the generic name for five polypeptide antibiotics (designated A, B, C, D, and E) derived from strains of the soil bacterium *Bacillus polymyxa,* having specific activity against gram-negative bacteria, including *Pseudomonas aeruginosa, Proteus vulgaris, Escherichia coli, Hemophilus influenzae, Aerobacter aerogenes,* and *Klebsiella pneumoniae.* The least toxic members of the group are polymyxins B, usually used in the form of the sulfate salt, and E (see *colistin*). **p. B sulfate** [USP], the sulfate salt of the least toxic member of the polymyxin group, occurring as a buff-colored powder; used in the treatment of various systemic, urinary tract, ophthalmic, otic, and cutaneous infections due to susceptible gram-negative bacteria, especially *Pseudomonas aeruginosa,* administered orally, parenterally, and topically.

polynesic (pol″e-ne′sik) [*poly-* + Gr. *nēsos* island] multiple and insular; occurring in many foci.

polyneural (pol″e-nu′ral) [*poly-* + Gr. *neuron* nerve] pertaining to or supplied by several nerves.

polyneuralgia (pol″e-nu-ral′je-ah) neuralgia of several nerves.

polyneuric (pol″e-nu′rik) polyneural.

polyneuritic (pol″e-nu-rit′ik) pertaining to or affected with polyneuritis.

polyneuritis (pol″e-nu-ri′tis) [*poly-* + Gr. *neuron* nerve + *-itis*] inflammation of many nerves at once; multiple, or disseminated, neuritis. **acute febrile p., acute idiopathic p., acute infective p., acute postinfectious p.,** rapidly progressive ascending motor neuron paralysis of unknown etiology, frequently following an enteric or respiratory infection. An autoimmune mechanism following viral infection has been postulated. It begins with paresthesias of the feet, followed by flaccid paralysis and weakness of the legs, ascending to the arms, trunk, and face, and is attended by slight fever, bulbar palsy, absent or lessened tendon reflexes, and an increase in the protein of the cerebrospinal fluid without corresponding increase in cells. Called also *Barré-Guillain syndrome, Guillain-Barré polyneuritis* or *syndrome, acute ascending spinal paralysis, acute postinfectious polyneuropathy, neuronitis,* and *postinfectious p.* **anemic p.,** polyneuritis seen in subacute combined degeneration of the spinal cord which occurs in pernicious anemia. **p. cerebra′lis menierifor′mis,** symptoms of cochlear, vestibular, facial, and trigeminal nerve irritation occurring in the early period of syphilis; called also *Frankl-Hochwart's disease.* **endemic p., p. endem′ica,** beriberi. **p. gallina′rum,** a form of polyneuritis seen in fowls fed a thiamine-deficient diet. **Guillain-Barré p.,** acute febrile p. **Jamaica ginger p.,** see under *paralysis.* **postinfectious p.,** acute febrile p. **p. potato′rum,** alcoholic neuropathy. **uveoparotitic p.,** uveoparotid fever.

polyneuromyositis (pol″-nu″ro-mi″o-si′tis) inflammation of the muscles and peripheral nerves, with loss of reflexes, sensory loss, and paresthesias.

polyneuropathy (pol″e-nu-rop′ah-the) [*poly-* + Gr. *neuron* nerve + *pathos* disease] a disease which involves several nerves. **acute postinfectious p.,** acute febrile polyneuritis. **erythredema p.,** acrodynia.

polyneuroradiculitis (pol″e-nu″ro-rah-dik″u-li′tis) [*poly-* + Gr. *neuron* nerve + L. *radix* root + *-itis*] inflammation of the spinal ganglia, the nerve roots, and the peripheral nerves.

polynuclear (pol″e-nu′kle-ar) 1. pertaining to or having several nuclei. 2. polymorphonuclear.

polynucleate (pol″e-nu′kle-āt) having many nuclei.

polynucleated (pol″e-nu′kle-āt″ed) polynuclear.

polynucleolar (pol″e-nu-kle′o-lar) having several nucleoli.

polynucleotidase (pol″e-nu″kle-o′ti-dās) an enzyme or a group of enzymes that catalyze the depolymerization of nucleic acids of high molecular weight to form mononucleotides; found in pancreatic fluid and elsewhere.

polynucleotide (pol″e-nu′kle-o-tīd) any polymer of mononucleotides; nucleic acid.

polyodontia (pol″e-o-don′she-ah) [*poly-* + Gr. *odous* tooth] the presence of supernumerary teeth.

polyoma (pol″e-o′mah) a tumor caused by an oncogenic virus of broad host range, originally isolated from parotid gland tumors of mice inoculated with Gross leukemia virus.

polyomavirus (pol″e-o-mah-vi′rus) any of a subgroup of the papovaviruses causing neoplastic disease in mice and hamsters; the subgroup includes the K virus and vacuolating virus. Also written *polyoma virus.* Cf. *papillomavirus.*

polyonychia (pol″e-o-nik′e-ah) [*poly-* + Gr. *onyx* nail + *-ia*] the occurrence of supernumerary nails.

polyopia (pol″e-o′pe-ah) [*poly-* + Gr. *opsis* vision + *-ia*] the condition in which one object appears as two or more objects. **binocular p.,** diplopia. **p. monophthal′mica,** a condition in which an object looked at by one eye appears double.

polyopsia (pol″e-op′se-ah) polyopia.

polyopy (pol′e-o″pe) polyopia.

polyorchidism (pol″e-or′kĭ-dizm) a developmental anomaly characterized by the presence of more than two testes.

polyorchis (pol″e-or′kis) [*poly-* + Gr. *orchis* testis] a person with more than two testes.

polyorchism (pol″e-or′kizm) polyorchidism.

polyorrhomeningitis (pol″e-or″o-men″in-ji′tis) (*obs.*) polyserositis.

polyorrhymenitis (pol″e-or″hi-mĕ-ni′tis) [*poly-* + Gr. *orrhos* serum + *hymēn* membrane + *-itis*] (*obs.*) polyserositis.

polyostotic (pol″e-os-tot′ik) [*poly-* + L. *os* bone] pertaining to or affecting many bones.

polyotia (pol″e-o′she-ah) [*poly-* + Gr. *ous* ear] the condition of having more than two ears.

polyovular (pol″e-o′vu-lar) pertaining to or produced from more than one ovum, as polyovular twins.

polyovulatory (pol″e-ov′u-lah-to″re) ordinarily discharging several ova in one ovarian cycle.

polyoxyethylene 50 stearate (pol″e-oks″e-eth′ah-lēn) [NF] a mixture of the mono- and distearate esters of mixed polyoxyethylene diols and the corresponding free diols, the average polymer length being equivalent to about 50 oxyethylene units, occurring as a soft, cream-colored, waxy solid; used as a surfactant and emulsifying agent in pharmaceutical preparations. Called also *polyoxyl 50 stearate.*

polyoxyl (pol″e-oks′il) any of various mixtures of the mono- and distearate esters of mixed polyoxyethylene diols and the corresponding free diols. The term is used in combination with an identifying number which indicates the average polymer length in oxyethylene units: *p. 8 stearate* and *p. 40 stearate* [USP], in which the average polymer lengths in oxyethylene units are equivalent to about 8 and 40, respectively, are used as surfactants in pharmaceutical preparations. **p. 5 oleate,** peglicol 5 oleate. **p. 10 oleyl ether,** see under *ether.* **p. 20 celostearyl ether,** see under *ether.* **p. 50 stearate,** polyoxyethylene 50 stearate.

polyp (pol′ip) [Gr. *polypous* a morbid excrescence] a morbid excrescence, or protruding growth, from mucous membrane; classically applied to a growth on the mucous membrane of the nose, the term is now applied to such protrusions from any mucous membrane. **adenomatous p.,** a benign polypoid adenoma. **cardiac p.,** a ball thrombus or tumor attached by a pedicle to the inside of the heart. **cervical p.,** a common, relatively innocuous tumor of the uterine cervix, usually of the endocervical canal, composed of a loose fibromyxomatous stroma containing mucus-secreting endocervical glands; they vary widely in size and may produce irregular vaginal bleeding. **choanal p's,** nasal polyps that project posteriorly into the nasopharynx. **endometrial p's,** small, sessile, benign projecting masses on the endometrium, composed of an edematous stroma containing cystically dilated glands. **fibrinous p.,** an intrauterine polyp made up of fibrin from retained blood; it may grow from portions of an ovum or from a thrombus at the placental site. **gelatinous p.,** myxoma. **gum p.,** a small pedunculated growth on the gingiva. **Hopmann's p.,** a mass produced by papillary hypertrophy of the nasal mucosa, having something of the appearance of a papilloma. **hydatid p.,** polypus cysticus. **juvenile p's,** small, benign hemispheric hamartomas of the large intestine occurring sporadically in children; histologically, there is an abundant loose fibrovascular stroma containing widely spaced glands; called also *retention p.* **p's of larynx,** smooth, rounded, sessile or pedunculated swellings, occurring on the true vocal cords; caused by edema in the lamina propria of the mucous membrane. **lymphoid p's,** rare, benign tumors of the colon composed of aggregates of lymphoid tissue, usually covered by a fairly regular colonic mucosa. **nasal p's,** focal accumulations of edema fluid in the mucosa of the nose, with hyperplasia of the associated submucosal connective tissue. **retention p's,** juvenile p's.

polypapilloma tropicum (pol″e-pap″ĭ-lo′mah trop′ĭ-kum) yaws.

polyparasitism (pol″e-par′ah-si-tizm) infection or infestation by more than one variety of parasite.

polyparesis (pol″e-pah-re′sis) [*poly-* + Gr. *paresis* slackening] dementia paralytica.

polypathia (pol″e-path′e-ah) [*poly-* + Gr. *pathos* disease + *-ia*] the presence of several diseases at once.

polypectomy (pol″ĭ-pek′to-me) [*polyp* + Gr. *ektomē* excision] surgical removal of a polyp.

polypeptidase (pol″e-pep′tĭ-dās) an enzyme that catalyzes the hydrolysis of polypeptides.

polypeptide (pol″e-pep′tīd) [*poly-* + *peptide*] a peptide which on hydrolysis yields more than two amino acids; called tripeptides, tetrapeptides, etc., according to the number of amino acids contained. See *peptide.* **adrenocorticotropic p.,** a hydroxylate of adrenocorticotropic hormone; abbreviated ACTP. **vasoactive intestinal p.,** see under *peptide.*

polypeptidemia (pol″e-pep″tĭ-de′me-ah) [*polypeptide* + Gr. *haima* blood + *-ia*] the presence of polypeptides in the blood.

polypeptidorrhachia (pol″e-pep″tĭ-do-ra′ke-ah) [*polypeptide* + Gr. *rhachis* spine + *-ia*] the presence of polypeptides in the spinal fluid.

polyperiostitis (pol″e-per″e-os-ti′tis) inflammation of the periosteum of several bones. **p. hyperesthet′ica,** a chronic disease of the periosteum attended by extreme hyperesthesia of the skin and soft parts.

polyphagia (pol″e-fa′je-ah) [*poly-* + Gr. *phagein* to eat] 1. excessive or voracious eating. Cf. *bulimia.* 2. omnivorousness; craving for all kinds of food.

polyphalangia (pol″e-fah-lan′je-ah) side-by-side duplication of one or more of the phalanges of a digit.

polyphalangism (pol″e-fah-lan′jizm) polyphalangia.

polypharmaceutic (pol″e-fahr″mah-su′tik) pertaining to several drugs, especially to the administration of several drugs together.

polypharmacy (pol″e-fahr″mah-se) [*poly-* + Gr. *pharmakon* drug] 1. the administration of many drugs together. 2. the administration of excessive medication.

polyphase (pol′e-fāz) [*poly-* + *phase*] having several phases; containing colloids of several types.

polyphasic (pol″e-fa′zik) having or existing in many phases; having unlike particles in the disperse phase.

polyphenic (pol″e-fen′ik) see *pleiotropism.*

polyphenoloxidase (pol″e-fe″nol-ok″sĭ-dās) a copper-containing oxidizing enzyme which oxidizes phenols and their amino compounds (but not tyrosine) to quinones; occurring, for example, in potatoes and mushrooms.

polyphobia (pol″e-fo′be-ah) [*poly-* + Gr. *phobein* to be affrighted by] morbid dread or fear of many things.

polyphrasia (pol″e-fra′ze-ah) [*poly-* + Gr. *phrasis* speech] morbid volubility or loquacity. Cf. *verbigeration.*

polyphyletic (pol″e-fi-let′ik) [*poly-* + Gr. *phylē* tribe] arising or descending from more than one cell type.

polyphyletism (pol″e-fi′lĕ-tizm) polyphyletic theory; see under *theory.*

polyphyletist (pol″e-fi′lĕ-tist) an adherent of the polyphyletic theory, as in blood origin.

polyphyodont (pol″e-fi′o-dont) [*poly-* + Gr. *phyein* to produce + *odous* tooth] developing several sets of teeth successively throughout life.

polypi (pol′ĭ-pi) [L.] plural of *polypus.*

polypiform (po-lip′ĭ-form) resembling a polyp; polypoid.

polypionia (pol″e-pi-o′ne-ah) [*poly-* + Gr. *piōn* fat + *-ia*] obesity.

polyplastic (pol″e-plas′tik) [*poly-* + Gr. *plastos* molded] 1. containing many structural or constituent elements. 2. undergoing many changes of form.

Polyplax (pol′e-plaks) a sucking louse of rats and mice. *P. miacan′thus,* a form found infrequently on rats; *P. serra′tus,* a louse of rabbits which transmits tularemia; and *P. spinulo′sa,* the common louse of rats, which transmits murine typhus.

polyplegia (pol″e-ple′je-ah) [*poly-* + Gr. *plēgē* stroke + *-ia*] simultaneous paralysis of several muscles.

polypleurodiaphragmotomy (pol″e-ploo″ro-di″ah-fram-ot′o-me) [*poly-* + Gr. *pleura* rib + *diaphragm* + *tomē* a cutting] the operation of resecting several ribs and cutting through the diaphragm for access to the convex aspect of the liver.

polyploid (pol′e-ploid) [*poly-* + ha*ploid*] 1. having more than two full sets of homologous chromosomes. There may be three (triploid), four (tetraploid), five (pentaploid), six (hexaploid), seven (heptaploid), eight (octaploid), etc. 2. an individual or cell having more than two full sets of homologous chromosomes. Polyploid organisms, especially plants, are larger than normal and have larger cells. Affected animals are often abnormal in appearance and usually infertile. Cf. *aneuploid.*

polyploidy (pol′e-ploi″de) the state of having more than two full sets of homologous chromosomes (see *polyploid*).

polypnea (pol″ip-ne′ah) [*poly-* + Gr. *pnoia* respiration] a condition in which the rate of respiration is increased; hyperpnea.

polypodia (pol″e-po′de-ah) [*poly-* + Gr. *pous* foot] the presence of supernumerary feet.

polypoid (pol′e-poid) [*polyp* + Gr. *eidos* form] resembling a polyp.

polypoidosis (pol″e-poi-do′sis) a condition of multiple polypoid adenomas or carcinomas; diffuse adenomatosis.

polyporin (pol-ip′o-rin) a mixture of antibiotic substances from species of *Polyporus,* which is active against some bacteria.

polyporous (pol-ip′o-rus) having many pores.

Polyporus (pol-ip′o-rus) [*poly-* + Gr. *poros* pore] basidiomycetous fungi of the order Polyporales, series Hymenomycetes, containing many species, some of which are important pathogens of trees. *P. officinalis* (larch agaric, purging agaric, white agaric) is the source of agaric acid. See also *agaric.*

polyposia (pol″e-po′ze-ah) [*poly-* + Gr. *posis* + *-ia*] ingestion of abnormally increased amounts of fluids for long periods of time. Cf. *hyperposia.*

polyposis (pol″e-po′sis) the development of multiple polyps on a part. **p. co′li,** familial p. **familial p.,** multiple adenomatous polyps with high malignant potential, lining the mucous membrane of the intestine, particularly the colon, beginning at about puberty. It occurs in several autosomal dominant forms: In Gardner's syndrome, colonic polyposis is associated with epidermoid cysts, fibromas, osteomas of the skull, supernumerary teeth, and less commonly ampullary tumors. In Peutz-Jeghers syndrome, mucocutaneous pigmentation (particularly of the lips) is associated with hamartomas of the intestine, particularly the small bowel. In Canada-Cronkhite syndrome, familial polyposis is associated with ectodermal abnormalities. In Turcot syndrome, colonic polyposis is associated with gliomas of the central nervous system. Called also *p. coli, familial intestinal p.,* and *multiple familial p.* **familial intestinal p.,** familial p. **p. gas′trica,** the presence of multiple polyps on the gastric mucosa, usually associated with atrophic gastritis. **p. intestina′lis,** a condition in which polyps occur in the intestine and rectum. **multiple familial p.,** familial p. **p. ventric′uli,** p. gastrica.

polypotome (po-lip′o-tōm) a cutting instrument for removing polyps.

polypotrite (po-lip′o-trīt) [*polyp* + L. *terere* to crush] an instrument for crushing polyps.

polypous (pol′e-pus) of the nature of a polyp; polyp-like.

polypragmasy (pol″e-prag′mah-se) [*poly-* + Gr. *pragma* a doing] polypharmacy.

polyptychial (pol″e-ti′ke-al) [*poly-* + Gr. *ptychē* fold] arranged in several layers; said of glands whose cells are arranged on the basement membrane in several layers. Cf. *monoptychial.*

polypus (pol′ĭ-pus), pl. *pol′ypi* [L.; Gr. *polypous*] a polyp. **p. angiomato′des,** a polyp rich in blood vessels. **p. cys′ticus,** a polyp in which the fibrous network is coarse, thus stimulating or actually producing cysts. **p. hydatido′sus,** p. cysticus. **p. telangiecto′des,** a polyp which contains many dilated blood vessels.

polyradiculitis (pol″e-rah-dik″u-li′tis) [*poly-* + L. *radix* root + *-itis*] inflammation of the nerve roots.

polyradiculoneuritis (pol″e-rah-dik″u-lo-nu-ri′tis) [*poly-* + L. *radix* root + Gr. *neuron* nerve + *-itis*] acute febrile polyneuritis which involves the peripheral nerves, the spinal nerve roots, and the spinal cord.

polyradiculoneuropathy (pol″e-rah-dik″u-lo-nu- rop′ah-the) Guillain-Barré syndrome.

polyribosome (pol″e-ri′bo-sōm) a complex made up of ribosomal subunits assembled among themselves by the filaments of messenger RNA containing the genetic information; they play a role in the synthesis of peptides. Called also *ergosome* and *polysome.*

polyrrhea (pol″ĕ-re′ah) [*poly-* + Gr. *rhoia* flow] a copious fluid discharge.

polysaccharide (pol″e-sak′ah-rīd) a carbohydrate which on hydrolysis yields a large number (variously defined as five or more to eleven or more) of monosaccharides. Cf. *oligosaccharide.* **bacterial p's,** polysaccharides found in bacteria and especially in bacterial capsules. **capsular p.,** specific capsular substance. **gastric p.,** the mucopolysaccharide found in gastric mucus. **immune p's,** polysaccharides which can function as specific antigens, such as capsular substances. **pneumococcus p.,** a polysaccharide derived from the capsule of a pneumococcus. Over 70 types, each of specific sequence, are known; Type III consists of alternating amounts of glucose and glucuronic acid. **specific p's,** soluble polysaccharides obtained from various microorganisms which in high dilution precipitate specifically the antisera to the corresponding organisms.

polysaccharose (pol″e-sak′ah-rōs) polysaccharide.

polysarcia (pol″e-sar′se-ah) [*poly-* + Gr. *sarx* flesh] corpulence or obesity.

polysarcous (pol″e-sar′kus) corpulent; obese; affected with polysarcia.

polyscelia (pol″e-se′le-ah) [*poly-* + Gr. *skelos* leg + *-ia*] a developmental anomaly characterized by the presence of more than two legs.

polyscelus (pŏ-lis′ĕ-lus) [*poly-* + Gr. *skelos* leg] an individual exhibiting polyscelia.

polyscope (pol′e-skōp) [*poly-* + Gr. *skopein* to examine] diaphanoscope.

polysensitivity (pol″e-sen″sĭ-tiv′ĭ-te) sensitivity to a number of different stimuli.

polysensory (pol″e-sen′so-re) capable of responding to more than one kind of sensory input; said of certain neurons of the cerebral cortex and subcortical regions.

polyserositis (pol″e-se-ro-si′tis) general inflammation of serous membranes with serous effusion; see also Concato's disease. **familial recurrent p.,** familial Mediterranean fever. **periodic p.,** familial Mediterranean fever. **recurrent p.,** familial Mediterranean fever.

polysialia (pol″e-si-a′le-ah) [*poly-* + Gr. *sialon* saliva + *-ia*] ptyalism.

polysinuitis (pol″e-sin″u-i′tis) polysinusitis.

polysinusectomy (pol″e-si″nŭ-sek′to-me) excision of the diseased membrane of several of the paranasal sinuses.

polysinusitis (pol″e-si-nŭ-si′tis) [*poly-* + *sinusitis*] inflammation of several sinuses at once.

polysomatic (pol″e-so-mat′ik) characterized by or pertaining to polysomaty.

polysomaty (pol″e-so′mah-te) [*poly-* + chromo*some*] the state of having reduplicated chromatin in the nucleus. The term is applied both to the condition of increase in chromosome number resulting from a previous endomitotic cycle (endopolyploidy, def. 3) and to increase in the amount of chromatin per chromosome (polyteny).

polysome (pol′e-sōm) polyribosome.

polysomia (pol″e-so′me-ah) [*poly-* + Gr. *sōma* body + *-ia*] a doubling or tripling of the body of a fetus.

polysomic (pol″e-so′mik) 1. pertaining to or exhibiting polysomy. 2. an individual exhibiting polysomy.

polysomus (pol″e-so′mus) [*poly-* + Gr. *sōma* body] a monster exhibiting polysomia.

polysomy (pol″e-so′me) [*poly-* + chromo*some*] an excess of a particular chromosome, resulting from meiotic chromosomal nondisjunction. The chromosome may be duplicated three (trisomy), four (tetrasomy), or more times.

polysorbate (pol''e-sor'bāt) a generic name for esters of sorbitol and its anhydrides condensed with polymers of ethylene oxide, used as surfactant agents: *p. 20*, $C_{58}H_{114}O_{26}$, is polyoxyethylene 20 sorbitan monolaurate; *p. 40*, $C_{62}H_{122}O_{26}$, is polyoxyethylene 20 sorbitan monopalmitate; *p. 60*, $C_{64}H_{126}O_{26}$, is polyethylene 20 sorbitan monostearate; *p. 65*, $C_{100}H_{194}O_{28}$, is polyethylene 20 sorbitan tristearate; *p. 80*, $C_{64}H_{124}O_{26}$, is polyethylene 20 sorbitan monooleate; *p. 85*, $C_{100}H_{188}O_{26}$, is polyethylene 20 sorbitan trioleate. *Polysorbates 20, 40, 60, and 80* are official in NF.

polyspermia (pol''e-sper'me-ah) [*poly-* + Gr. *sperma* seed + *-ia*] 1. excessive secretion of semen. 2. polyspermy.

polyspermism (pol''e-sper'mizm) polyspermia.

polyspermy (pol''e-sper'me) fertilization of an ovum by more than one spermatozoon. **pathological p.,** entrance of more than one spermatozoon in an ovum when entrance of only one is the rule; usually development is abnormal and the embryo is not viable. **physiological p.,** entrance of more than one spermatozoon in an ovum, occurring normally in certain species, but with only one spermatozoon participating fully in the development of the embryo.

polystichia (pol''e-stik'e-ah) [*poly-* + Gr. *stichos* row + *-ia*] the presence of two or more rows of eyelashes upon a lid.

polystyrene (pol''e-sti'rēn) the resin produced by polymerization of styrol, a clear resin of the thermoplastic type, used to a limited extent in the construction of denture bases.

polysuspensoid (pol''e-sus-pen'soid) a suspensoid in which the particles are of different degrees of dispersion.

polysynaptic (pol''e-sĭ-nap'tik) involving many synapses in series and therefore a sequence of many neurons; called also *multisynaptic.* Cf. *oligosynaptic.*

polysyndactyly (pol''e-sin-dak'til-e) a hereditary association of polydactyly and syndactyly of varying degrees of both the hand and foot.

polysynovitis (pol''e-sin''o-vi'tis) [*poly-* + *synovitis*] general inflammation of the synovial membranes.

polysyphilide (pol''e-sif'ĭ-līd) characterized by many syphilitic lesions.

polytef (pol'ĕ-tef) a polymer of tetrafluoroethylene, used as a surgical implant material for many prostheses, such as artificial vessels and orbital floor implants and for many applications in skeletal augmentation and skeletal fixation. Also used in industry for many purposes, e.g., as an antistick coating for cooking utensils. Called also *polytetrafluoroethylene* (PTFE). See also *polymer fume fever,* under *fever.*

polytendinitis (pol''e-ten''dĭ-ni'tis) inflammation affecting several tendons.

polytendinobursitis (pol''e-ten''dĭ-no-bur-si'tis) associated bursitis and tendinitis in several parts of the body.

polytene (pol'e-tēn) [*poly-* + Gr. *tainia* (L. *taenia*) band] composed of or containing many strands of chromatin (chromonemata).

polytenosynovitis (pol''e-ten''o-sin''o-vi'tis) inflammation of several or many tendon sheaths at the same time.

polyteny (pol''ĕ-te'ne) reduplication of chromonemata in the chromosome without separation into distinct daughter chromosomes. See also *polysomaty.*

polytetrafluoroethylene (pol''e-tet''rah-floo''o-ro-eth'ĭ-lēn) polytef.

polythelia (pol''e-the'le-ah) [*poly-* + Gr. *thēlē* nipple + *-ia*] the condition of having more than one pair of nipples.

polythelism (pol''e-the'lizm) polythelia.

polythene (pol'e-thēn) polyethylene.

polythetic (pol''e-thet'ik) [*poly-* + Gr. *thetikos* fit for placing] denoting a taxonomic group classified on the basis of several characters, as opposed to a monothetic group.

polythiazide (pol''e-thi'ah-zīd) [USP] chemical name: 6-chloro-3,4-dihydro-2-methyl-3-[[2,2,2-trifluoroethyl)-thio]-methyl]-2*H*-1,2,4-benzothiadiazine-7-sulfonamide 1,1-dioxide. An orally effective diuretic and antihypertensive, $C_{11}H_{13}ClF_3N_3O_4S_3$, occurring as a white crystalline powder.

polytocous (po-lit'o-kus) [*poly-* + Gr. *tokos* birth] giving birth to several offspring at one time.

polytomogram (pol''e-tom'o-gram) the record produced by polytomography.

polytomographic (pol''e-to''mo-graf'ik) pertaining to polytomography.

polytomography (pol''e-to-mog'rah-fe) tomography of tissue at several predetermined planes.

polytrichia (pol''e-trik'e-ah) [*poly-* + Gr. *thrix* hair] hypertrichosis.

polytrichosis (pol''e-tri-ko'sis) hypertrichosis.

Polytrichum (po-lit'rĭ-kum) [*poly-* + Gr. *thrix* hair] a genus of mosses, *P. juniperi'num* Willd. haircap, or juniper moss, is diuretic.

polytrophia (pol''e-tro'fe-ah) [*poly-* + Gr. *trophē* nourishment] excessive nutrition.

polytrophic (pol''e-trof'ik) pertaining to or characterized by polytrophia.

polytrophy (po-lit'ro-fe) polytrophia.

polytropic (pol''e-trop'ik) [*poly-* + Gr. *tropē* a turning] affecting many kinds of bacteria or many varieties of tissue. Cf. *monotropic.*

polytropous (po-lit'ro-pus) polytropic.

polyunguia (pol''e-ung'gwe-ah) polyonychia.

polyunsaturated (pol''e-un-sach'ĕ-ra-ted) denoting a fatty acid, e.g., linoleic acid, having more than one double bond in its hydrocarbon chain.

polyuria (pol''e-u're-ah) [*poly-* + Gr. *ouron* urine + *-ia*] the passage of a large volume of urine in a given period, a characteristic of diabetes.

polyvalent (pol''e-va'lent; po-liv'ah-lent) having more than one valency.

polyvinyl (pol''e-vi'nil) a polymerization product of a monomeric vinyl compound, as vinyl chloride.

polyvinylacetate (pol''e-vi'nil-as'ĕ-tāt) a light- and heat-stable resin formed by the polymerization of vinyl acetate.

polyvinylbenzene (pol''e-vi'nil-ben'zēn) polystyrene.

polyvinylchloride (pol''e-vi'nil-klor'īd) a substance formed by the polymerization of vinyl chloride; a tasteless, odorless, clear hard resin, which changes color on exposure to ultraviolet light or heat.

polyvinylpyrrolidone (pol''e-vi''nil-pir-rol'ĭ-dōn) povidone.

pomade (po-mād') pomatum.

Pomatiopsis (po-mat''e-op'sis) a genus of amphibious fresh-water snails of the United States; *P. cincinnatien'sis* and *P. lapida'ria* have been shown to be hosts of *Paragonimus kellicotti.*

pomatum (po-ma'tum) [L., from *pomum* apple] a medicated ointment for the hair.

pomegranate (pum-gran'et) [L. *pomum granatum* grained apple] the punicaceous tree, *Punica granatum* L. (Punicaceae), and its fruit. The root and the dried bark of the stem were formerly used as teniacides. Called also *granatum.*

pompholyhemia (pom''fo-le-he'me-ah) [*pompholyx* + Gr. *haima* blood + *-ia*] the presence of bubbles of gas in the blood, as in decompression sickness.

pompholyx (pom'fo-liks) [Gr. "bubble"] a skin eruption on the sides of the fingers or toes or on the palms or soles, consisting of discrete round intraepidermal vesicles 1 or 2 mm. in diameter, accompanied by intense itching, and typically manifesting itself in repeated self-limited attacks lasting one or two weeks.

pomum (po'mum) [L.] apple. **p. ada'mi** ["Adam's apple"], the prominence in the neck produced by the thyroid cartilage; prominentia laryngea.

ponceau B (pon so') Biebrich scarlet; see under *scarlet.* **p. 3 B,** scarlet red; see under *red.*

Poncet's disease, operation, rheumatism (pahw-sāz') [Antonin *Poncet,* French surgeon, 1849– 1913] see under *disease, operation,* and *rheumatism.*

Pond. abbreviation for L. *pon'dere,* by weight.

ponderable (pon'der-ah-b'l) [L. *ponderabilis; pondus* weight] having weight.

ponderal (pon'der-al) [L. *pondus,* weight] pertaining to weight.

Pondimin (pon'dĭ-men) trademark for a preparation of fenfluramine hydrochloride.

pondostatural (pon''do-stat'u-ral) pertaining to weight and stature.

ponesiatrics (po-ne''ze-ah'triks) [Gr. *ponēsis* toil, exertion + *iatrike* surgery, medicine] a system of therapy in which misdirected neurophysiologic reactions are made perceptible (as by the oscilloscope, electromyograph, etc.) and used as a guide in recognizing and correcting such undesirable responses (dysponesis). Called also *effort training.*

Ponfick's shadow (pon'fiks) [Clemens Emil *Ponfick,* German pathologist, 1844–1913] phantom corpuscle; see under *corpuscle.*

Pongidae (pon'jĭ-de) a family of primates, including the anthropoid apes, which together with the family Hominidae (man), comprise the superfamily Hominoidea.

pono- [Gr. *ponos* toil, suffering, pain] a combining form denoting relationship to hard work or to pain.

ponograph (po'no-graf) [*pono-* + Gr. *graphein* to write] an instrument for estimating and recording sensitiveness to pain.

ponopalmosis (po''no-pal-mo'sis) [*pono-* + Gr. *palmos* palpitation] (*obs.*) palpitation on effort; Sir Clifford Albutt's term for soldier's heart or neurocirculatory asthenia.

pons (ponz), pl. *pon'tes,* gen. *pon'tis* [L. "bridge"] 1. any slip of tissue connecting two parts of an organ; called also *bridge.* 2. [NA] that part of the central nervous system lying between the medulla oblongata and the mesencephalon, ventral to the cerebellum, and consisting of a pars dorsalis and a pars ventralis; called also *bridge of Varolius, p. cerebelli, p. varolii,* and *commissura cerebelli.* See Plate accompanying *brain.* See also *brain stem,* under B. **p. cerebel′li,** pons [NA]. **p. hep′atis,** an occasional projection of fibers partially bridging the longitudinal fissure of the liver. **p. tari′ni,** substantia perforata posterior. **p. varo′lii,** pons [NA].

pons-oblongata (ponz″ob-lon-ga′tah) the pons and medulla oblongata considered together.

Ponstel (pon′stel) trademark for a preparation of mefenamic acid.

pontes (pon′tēz) plural of *pons.*

pontibrachium (pon″te-bra′ke-um) pedunculus cerebellaris medius.

pontic (pon′tik) [L. *pons, pontis* bridge] the portion of a bridge which substitutes for an absent tooth, both esthetically and functionally; it usually, but not necessarily, occupies the space formerly filled by a natural tooth.

ponticular (pon-tik′u-lar) pertaining to the ponticulus (propons).

ponticulus (pon-tik′u-lus), pl. *pontic′uli* [L., dim. of *pons* bridge] propons. **p. auric′ulae,** a point on the eminence of the concha where the posterior auricular muscle is attached. **p. promonto′rii,** a ridge on the median wall of the tympanic cavity connecting the promontory with the pyramid.

pontil (pon′til) pontile; pontine.

pontile (pon′tīl, pon′tēl) pertaining to the pons; pontine.

pontine (pon′tīn, pon′tēn) pertaining to the pons; pontile.

pontobulbar (pon″to-bul′bar) pertaining to, affecting, or regulated by the pons and the region of the medulla oblongata situated dorsad to it.

pontobulbia (pon″to-bul′be-ah) a condition in which cavities exist in the pons and medulla oblongata; syringobulbia.

Pontocaine (pon′to-kān) trademark for preparations of tetracaine.

pontocerebellar (pon″to-ser″ĕ-bel′ar) pertaining to the pons and the cerebellum.

pontomedullary (pon″to-med′u-lār″e) pertaining to the pons and the medulla oblongata.

pontomesencephalic (pon″to-mes″en-sĕ-fal′ik) pertaining to or involving the pons and the mesencephalon.

pontoon (pon-tōōn′) [Fr. *ponton;* L. *ponto* boat] a loop or knuckle of the small intestine.

pontopeduncular (pon″to-pĕ-dung′ku-lar) pertaining to, affecting, or communicating with the pons and cerebral peduncles.

pool (pōōl) 1. a common reservoir on which to draw. 2. to mix plasma from several donors. 3. an accumulation, as of blood in any part of the body due to retardation of the venous circulation. **gene p.,** the totality of the genes possessed by all of the members of a population. **metabolic p.,** the entire mass of labile and reactive substances in the body, to which and from which innumerable substances continuously pass; also used in a restricted sense to mean the extracellular pool or the potassium pool.

Pool's phenomenon (pōōlz) [Eugene Hillhouse *Pool,* New York surgeon, 1874–1949] 1. see under *phenomenon.* 2. Schlesinger's sign.

Pool-Schlesinger sign (pōōl-shla′zing-er) [E. H. *Pool;* Hermann *Schlesinger,* Austrian physician, 1868–1934] Schlesinger's sign.

popin (pop′in) a glycoside of unknown origin which is used in Barbados for amebic dysentery.

poples (pop′lez) [L. "ham"] [NA] the posterior surface of the knee.

popliteal (pop-lit′e-al; pop″lĭ-te′al) [L. *poples* ham] pertaining to the posterior surface of the knee; see also under *ligament.*

poppy (pop′e) any member of the poppy or Papaveraceae family. See *Papaver.*

population (pop″u-la′shun) [L. *populatio*] 1. the individuals collectively constituting a certain category or inhabiting a specified geographic area. 2. a contiguously distributed grouping of a single community that is characterized by both genetic and cultural continuity through several generations.

POR problem oriented record.

poradenia (pōr″ah-de′ne-ah) poradenitis.

poradenitis (pōr″ad-ĕ-ni′tis) [Gr. *poros* pore + *adēn* gland + *-itis*] a disease of the iliac lymph nodes characterized by the formation of small abscesses. **p. nos′tras, subacute inguinal p., p. vene′rea,** lymphogranuloma venereum.

poradenolymphitis (por-ad″ĕ-no-lim-fi′tis) lymphogranuloma venereum.

poral (pōr′al) pertaining to or having pores.

porcelain (por′sĕ-lin) a fused mixture of kaolin, felspar, quartz, and other substances, used in the making of artificial teeth, jacket crowns, facings, and veneers.

porcelaneous (por″sĕ-la′ne-us) pertaining to or resembling porcelain.

porcine (por′sīn) [L. *porcus* a pig, hog] pertaining to, characteristic of, or derived from swine.

pore (pōr) [L. *porus;* Gr. *poros*] a small opening; called also *porus* [NA]. **acoustic p., osseous, external,** porus acusticus externus osseus. **acoustic p., osseous, internal,** porus acusticus internus osseus. **alveolar p's,** openings between adjacent pulmonary alveoli that permit passage of air from one to another; called also *pores of Kohn.* **biliary p.,** ductus choledochus. **birth p.,** metraterm. **cranionasal p.** (*obs.*), foramen cecum ossis frontalis. **Galen's p.,** canalis inguinalis. **gustatory p.,** porus gustatorius. **interalveolar p's, p's of Kohn,** alveolar p's. **nuclear p's,** small octagonal openings in the nuclear envelope at sites where the two nuclear membranes are in contact, which together with the annuli form the pore complex. See also Plate XI. **slit p's,** small slitlike spaces between the pedicels of the podocytes of the renal glomerulus; called also *filtration slits.* **sweat p., p. of sweat duct,** porus sudoriferus. **taste p.,** porus gustatorius.

porencephalia (po″ren-sĕ-fa′le-ah) [Gr. *poros* pore + *enkephalos* brain + *-ia*] 1. the presence of cysts or cavities in the brain cortex communicating to a "pore" with the arachnoid space (Heschl, 1850). 2. the presence of cavities in the brain developed in fetal life or early infancy, whether or not they communicate with the arachnoid space; the cavities are usually the residues of destructive lesions (*encephaloclastic p.*), but sometimes are the result of maldevelopment (*schizencephalic p., schizencephaly*).

porencephalic (po″ren-sĕ-fal′ik) pertaining to or characterized by porencephalia.

porencephalitis (po″ren-sef″ah-li′tis) porencephalia associated with an inflammatory process, such as polioencephalitis.

porencephalous (po″ren-sef′ah-lus) porencephalic.

porencephaly (po″ren-sef′ah-le) porencephalia.

porfiromycin (por″fi-ro-mi′sin) chemical name: 6-amino-8-[[(aminocarbonyl)oxy]methyl]-1,1a,2,8,8a,8b-hexahydro-8a-methoxy-1,5-dimethylazirino[2′,3′:3,4]pyrrolo[1,2-*a*]indole-4,7-dione. An antineoplastic antibiotic with antitumor activity, $C_{16}H_{20}N_4O_5$, derived from *Streptomyces ardus;* it is the methyl derivative of mitomycin C.

Porges-Hermann-Perutz reaction (por′ges-her′man-pa′root) [Otto *Porges,* Vienna bacteriologist, born 1879; Otto *Hermann,* Vienna physician; Alfred *Perutz,* Austrian dermatologist, born 1885] Perutz reaction.

Porges-Meier test (reaction) [Otto *Porges;* Georg *Meier,* German serologist, born 1875] see under *tests.*

Porges-Salomon test [Otto *Porges;* Hugo *Salomon,* German physician in Buenos Aires, 1872–1954] see under *tests.*

pori (po′ri) [L.] plural of *porus.*

Porifera (po-rif′ĕ-rah) [L. *porus* pore + *ferre* to bear] the phylum of sponges; the body is perforated with many pores to admit water, from which food is strained.

poriomania (po″re-o-ma′ne-ah) [Gr. *poreia* walking + *mania* madness] an impulsive tendency to wander away from home; ambulatory automatism.

porion (po′re-on) [Gr. *poros* pore + *-on* neuter ending] 1. a cephalometric landmark, being the midpoint on the upper edge of the porus acusticus externus, situated about 5 mm. above the superior margin of the cutaneous external auditory meatus. 2. in roentgenographic cephalometrics, the top of the radiopaque ear rod, inserted in the external auditory meatus.

porocele (po′ro-sēl) [Gr. *pōros* callus + *kēlē* hernia] scrotal hernia with thickening and hardening of the coverings of the testes.

porocephaliasis (po″ro-sef″ah-li′ah-sis) infection with parasites of the order Porocephalida.

Porocephalida (por″o-sĕ-fal′ĭ-dah) an order of the class Pentastomida, wormlike degenerate arthropods, including the families Porocephalidae and Linguatulidae.

Porocephalidae (por″o-sĕ-fal′ĭ-de) a family of the order Porocephalida, class Pentastomida, having cylindrical bodies. Adults are found in the lungs of reptiles, and the larvae are found in various vertebrates, including man. It includes the genera *Armillifer, Porocephalus,* and *Pentastoma.*

porocephalosis (po″ro-sef″ah-lo′sis) porocephaliasis.

Porocephalus (po″ro-sef′ah-lus) [Gr. *poros* pore + *kephalē* head] a genus of wormlike arthropods of the order Porocephalida, family Porocephalidae. The species which parasitize man, formerly classified in this genus, are now assigned to other genera. **P. armilla′tus,** Armillifer armillatus. **P. constric′tus,** Armillifer armillatus. **P. denticula′tus,** Pentastoma denticulatum (the larva of *Linguatula serrata*).

porofocon (por″o-fo′kon) chemical name: cellulose acetate dibutanoate; either of two hydrophobic contact lens materials, designated A or B, $(C_{32}H_{48}O_{16})_n$.

porokeratosis (po″ro-ker″ah-to′sis) [Gr. *poros* pore + *keratosis*] a rare, chronic, hereditary disease of the skin, usually of the hands and feet, although it may be found on any part of the body. It is characterized by hypertrophy of the stratum corneum about the ducts of the sweat glands, followed by centrifugally spreading, indurated patches surrounded by an elevated keratotic border. It is transmitted as an autosomal dominant trait. Called also *p. excentrica* and *p. of Mibelli.* **disseminated superficial ac-**

tinic p., a form occurring on sun-exposed areas of the skin in persons 30 to 40 years of age; the lesions may enlarge to as much as 5 cm. in diameter. **p. excen′trica,** porokeratosis. **p. of Mibelli,** porokeratosis. **p. palma′ris et planta′ris dissemina′ta,** a distinctive form of porokeratosis inherited as an autosomal dominant trait, in which hundreds of gyrate and annular porokeratotic plaques occur on the soles or palms or both, and later elsewhere.

porokeratotic (po″ro-ker″ah-tot′ik) pertaining to or affected with porokeratosis.

poroma (po-ro′mah) [Gr. *pōrōma* callus] a general term for a neoplasm arising in or from the eccrine pore. **eccrine p.,** a benign tumor arising from the intraepidermal portion of the eccrine sweat duct, often on the palm or sole.

poropathy (po-rop′ah-the) an alleged system of healing in which medicines are supposed to reach the diseased organs through the pores of the skin.

poroplastic (po″ro-plas′tik) both porous and plastic.

porosis (po-ro′sis) 1. [Gr. *pōrōsis* callosity] the formation of the callus in the repair of a fractured bone. 2. [Gr. *pōros* pore] cavity formation. **cerebral p.,** a condition in which there are cavities in the brain substance; porencephalia.

porosity (po-ros′ĭ-te) 1. the condition of being porous. 2. a pore.

porotic (po-rot′ik) pertaining to or characterized by porosis favoring the growth of connective tissue.

porotomy (po-rot′o-me) [Gr. *poros* pore + *tomē* a cutting] meatotomy.

porous (po′rus) penetrated by pores and open spaces.

porphin (por′fin) the fundamental ring structure of four linked pyrrole nuclei around which porphyrins, hemin, the cytochromes, and chlorophyll are built.

porphobilin (por″fo-bi′lin) a dark brown nonporphyrin pigment of unknown chemical structure.

porphobilinogen (por″fo-bi-lin′o-jen) the parent compound of the porphyrins, itself formed by condensation of two molecules of 5-aminolevulinic acid; four molecules of porphobilinogen combine to make uroporphyrin and by a series of decarboxylations and oxidations, the other porphyrins, and finally heme. Not in evidence under normal circumstances, it characteristically appears in the urine in acute intermittent porphyria.

porphobilinogenuria (por″fo-bi-lin″o-jen-u′re-ah) the excretion of urine containing porphobilinogen.

porphyran (por′fĭ-ran) a combination of a porphyrin with a metal; a metalloporphyrin.

porphyria (por-fē′re-ah, por-fi′re-ah) [Gr. *porphyra* purple] any of a group of disturbances of porphyrin metabolism, characterized by marked increase in formation and excretion of porphyrins or their precursors. **acute p.,** acute intermittent p. **acute intermittent p.,** hereditary hepatic porphyria manifested by recurrent attacks of abdominal pain, gastrointestinal dysfunction, and neurologic disturbances and by excessive amounts of aminolevulinic acid and porphobilinogen in the urine; it is due to an abnormality of pyrrole metabolism transmitted as an autosomal dominant trait. Called also *acute p., p. hepatica, Swedish genetic p.,* and *pyrroloporphyria.* **congenital erythropoietic p.,** hereditary porphyria in which the excessive porphyrin formation occurs in bone marrow normoblasts; it is characterized by cutaneous photosensitivity, leading to mutilating skin lesions, by hemolytic anemia and splenomegaly, and by excessive urinary excretion of uroporphyrin. Erythrodontia and hypertrichosis are invariably present. It is transmitted as an autosomal recessive trait. Called also *congenital photosensitive p., Günther's disease,* and *erythropoietic uroporphyria.* **congenital photosensitive p.,** congenital erythropoietic p. **p. cuta′nea tar′da hereditar′ia,** hepatic porphyria resembling variegate porphyria except that abdominal and neurologic symptoms are absent or mild; called also *protocoproporphyria hereditaria.* **p. cuta′nea tar′da symptomat′ica,** a sporadic form of porphyria characterized by chronic skin lesions ranging from slight skin fragility to severe chronic scarring, by hepatomegaly, and by excessive urinary excretion of uroporphyrin and coproporphyrin; it is usually associated with chronic alcoholism. Called also *urocoproporphyria.* **cutaneous p.,** that characterized by skin manifestations; see *p. cutanea tarda hereditaria* and *symptomatica.* **erythropoietic p., p. erythropoiet′ica,** porphyria in which excessive formation of porphyrin or its precursors occurs in bone marrow normoblasts; it includes congenital erythropoietic porphyria and erythropoietic protoporphyria. **hepatic p.,** porphyria in which the excess formation of porphyrin or its precursors is found in the liver; it includes acute intermittent porphyria, variegate porphyria, and hereditary coproporphyria. **p. hepat′ica,** acute intermittent p. **mixed p.,** variegate p. **South African genetic p.,** variegate p. **Swedish genetic p.,** acute intermittent p. **p. variega′ta, variegate p.,** hereditary hepatic porphyria characterized by chronic cutaneous manifestations, notably extreme mechanical fragility of the skin, particularly areas exposed to sunlight, and by episodes of abdominal pain and neuropathy. There is typically an excess of coproporphyrin and protoporphyrin in the bile and feces. It is transmitted as an autosomal dominant trait. Called also *mixed p.* and *South African genetic p.* See also *p. cutanea tarda hereditaria.*

porphyrin (por′fĭ-rin) any one of a group of iron-free or magnesium-free cyclic tetrapyrrole derivatives which occur universally in protoplasm. They form the basis of the respiratory pigments of animals and plants. The porphyrins are protoporphyrin, mesoporphyrin, hematoporphyrin, deuteroporphyrin, etioporphyrin, coproporphyrin, uroporphyrin, rhodoporphyrin, pyrroporphyrin, pyrroetioporphyrin, and chlorophyll.

porphyrinemia (por″fĭ-rin-e′me-ah) the presence of porphyrin in the blood.

porphyrinogen (por″fĭ-rin′o-jen) a reduced, colorless nonfluorescing compound, fully hydrogenated and readily giving rise to the corresponding porphyrin by oxidation.

porphyrinopathy (por″fir-in-op′ah-the) any disorder of porphyrin metabolism.

porphyrinuria (por″fĭ-rĭ-nu′re-ah) [*porphyrin* + Gr. *ouron* urine + *-ia*] the presence in the urine of porphyrin (coproporphyrin or uroporphyrin) in excess of the normal amount.

porphyrism (por′fĭ-rizm) porphyria.

porphyrismus (por″fĭ-ris′mus) the triggering action attributed to psychic and emotional disturbances in attacks of acute intermittent porphyria.

porphyrization (por″fĭ-ri-za′shun) pulverization; reduction to a powder: so called because it was performed on a porphyry tablet.

porphyropsin (por″fĭ-rop′sin) a purple pigment in the retinal rods of certain fresh-water fishes.

porphyroxine (por″fĭ-rok′sin) an opium alkaloid, $C_{19}H_{23}O_4N$.

porphyruria (por″fir-u′re-ah) porphyrinuria.

porphyryl (por′fĭ-ril) a name for hemin from which iron has been removed.

Porro's cesarean section (por′ōz) [Edoardo *Porro,* obstetrician in Milan, 1842–1902] see *ceaseran section,* under *section.*

porta (por′tah), pl. *por′tae* [L.] an entrance or portal; used in anatomical nomenclature to designate an opening, especially the site of entrance to an organ of the blood vessels and other structures supplying or draining it. **p. hep′atis** [NA], hepatic portal: the transverse fissure on the visceral surface of the liver where the portal vein and hepatic artery enter the liver and the hepatic ducts leave. **p. labyrin′thi,** fenestra cochleae. **p. lie′nis,** hilus lienis. **p. of lung,** hilus pulmonis. **p. omen′ti, p. of omentum,** foramen epiploicum. **p. pulmo′nis,** hilus pulmonis. **p. re′nis,** hilus renalis. **p. of spleen,** hilus lienis.

portacaval (por″tah-ka′val) pertaining to or connecting the portal vein and the vena cava.

portacid (port-as′id) a dropper for the local application of an acid.

portal (por′tal) 1. an entrance or gateway; called also *porta.* 2. pertaining to a porta, or entrance, especially to the porta hepatis. **p. of entry,** the pathway by which bacteria or other pathogenic agents gain entry to the body. **hepatic p.,** porta hepatis. **intestinal p., anterior,** the region of opening of the embryonic foregut into the yolk sac or unclosed midgut. **intestinal p., posterior,** the region of opening of the embryonic hindgut into the yolk sac or unclosed midgut. **velopharyngeal p.,** the opening between the velum palatinum (soft palate) and the pharynx, which must be susceptible to closure by muscular action to permit normal speech and deglutition.

portcaustic (port-kaws′tik) [Fr. *porte-caustique*] a handle for holding a caustic substance.

porte-acid (port-as′id) portacid.

porte-aiguille (port″a-gēl′) [Fr.] a surgeon's needle holder.

porte-caustique (port″ko-stēk′) portcaustic.

porte-ligature (port-lig′ah-tūr) portligature.

porte-meche (port-mesh′) [Fr.] a probe or director with a fork at one end for introducing a drain into a wound or fistula.

porte-noeud (port-ned′) [Fr, "knot-carrier"] an instrument for applying a ligature to the pedicle of a tumor.

porte-polisher (pōrt-pol′ish-er) a hand instrument constructed to hold a wooden point, to be used in a dental engine for applying polishing paste to and burnishing teeth.

Porter (por′ter), Rodney. British biochemist, co-winner, with Gerald Maurice Edelman, of the Nobel prize for physiology and medicine in 1972, for his work on the chemical structure of antibodies.

Porter's sign (por′terz) [William Henry *Porter,* Dublin physician, 1790–1861] tracheal tugging; see under *tugging.*

Porter's test (por′terz) [William Henry *Porter,* New York physician, 1853–1933] see under *tests.*

Porteus maze test (por′te-us) [David Stanley *Porteus,* Hawaii psychologist, born 1883] see under *tests.*

portio (por′she-o), pl. *portio′nes* [L.] a part, or division; [NA] general term for a particular portion of an organ or structure. **p. du′ra pa′ris sep′timi,** nervus facialis (formerly considered as forming one nerve with the portio mollis paris septimi). **p.**

interme′dia ner′vi acus′tici, nervus intermedius. **p. ma′jor ner′vi trigem′ini,** radix sensoria nervi trigemini. **p. mi′nor ner′vi trigem′ini,** radix motoria nervi trigemini. **p. mol′lis pa′ris sep′timi,** nervus vestibulocochlearis (formerly considered as forming one nerve with the portio dura paris septimi). **p. supravagina′lis cer′vicis** [NA], the part of the cervix uteri that does not protrude into the vagina. **p. vagina′lis cer′vicis** [NA], the part of the cervix uteri that protrudes into the vagina.

portiones (por″she-o′nēz) [L.] plural of *portio.*

portligature (port-lig″ah-tūr) an instrument for applying a ligature in a deep wound.

portoenterostomy (por″to-en″ter-os′to-me) surgical anastomosis of the jejunum to a decapsulated area of liver in the porta hepatis region, and to the duodenum; done to establish a conduit from the intrahepatic bile ducts to the intestine in biliary atresia. Called also *hepatic p.*

portogram (por′to-gram) a roentgenogram of the portal vein.

portography (por-tog′rah-fe) roentgenography of the portal vein after injection of opaque material. **portal p.,** portography after injection of opaque material into the superior mesenteric vein or one of its branches after laparotomy has been performed. **splenic p.,** portography after percutaneous injection into the substance of the spleen, usually through the ninth intercostal space in the midaxillary line, of opaque material, which passes immediately into the splenic vein, and then into the portal vein, permitting visualization of those two vessels.

portosystemic (por″to-sis-tem′ik) connecting the portal and systemic venous circulation.

portovenogram (por″to-ve′no-gram) portogram.

portovenography (por″to-ve-nog′rah-fe) portography.

porus (po′rus) pl. *po′ri* [L.; Gr. *poros* passage] a pore; a small opening; [NA] a general term for certain openings in the body. **p. acus′ticus exter′nus** [NA], the outer end of the external acoustic meatus. **p. acus′ticus exter′nus os′seus** [NA], external osseous acoustic pore: the outer end of the bony external acoustic meatus in the tympanic portion of the temporal bone. **p. acus′ticus inter′nus** [NA], the opening of the internal acoustic meatus. **p. acus′ticus inter′nus os′seus** [NA], internal osseous acoustic pore: the opening into the internal acoustic meatus, found on the posteromedial portion of the internal surface of the petrous part of the temporal bone. **p. gale′ni,** canalis inguinalis. **p. gustato′rius** [NA], gustatory pore: the small opening of a taste bud onto the surface of the tongue. **p. op′ticus,** the opening in the sclera for passage of the optic nerve. **p. sudorif′erus** [NA], sweat pore: the opening of the duct of the sweat gland on the surface of the skin; called also *pore of sweat duct.*

Posada's mycosis (po-sah′dahz) [Alejandro *Posada,* Argentine pathologist, 1870–1902] coccidioidomycosis.

Posada-Wernicke disease (po-sah′dah-ver′nĭ-ke) [Alejandro *Posada;* Robert *Wernicke,* Argentine pathologist of 19th century] coccidioidomycosis.

posed (pōsd) placed; in dentistry, a term applied to the position of a tooth. **normally p., regularly p.,** in normal position. Cf. *malposed.*

-posia [Gr. *posis* drinking + *-ia*] a word termination denoting relationship to drinking, or to intake of fluids.

position (po-zish′un) [L. *positio*] 1. a bodily posture or attitude assumed by the patient to achieve comfort in certain conditions, or the particular disposition of the body and extremities to facilitate the performance of certain diagnostic or therapeutic procedures. 2. in obstetrics, the situation of the fetus in the pelvis, determined and described by the relation of a given arbitrary point (point of direction or reference point) in the presenting part to a given arbitrary point in the coronal plane of the maternal pelvis. For the various possible positions see the table (from Greenhill and Friedman's Obstetrics). Cf. *presentation.* **Albert's p.,** a semirecumbent position of the patient for roentgenography as a means of determining the diameters of the superior strait of the pelvis. **anatomical p.,** the position of the human body, standing erect, with the palms of the hands turned forward; used as the position of reference in description of site or direction of various structures or parts as established in official anatomical nomenclature. **batrachian p.,** a lying position of infants in which the lower limbs are flexed, abducted, and resting on the bed on their outer aspects, somewhat resembling the legs of a frog. Called also *froglike p.* **Bonner's p.,** flexion, abduction, and outward rotation of the thigh in coxitis. **Bozeman's p.,** one in which the patient is strapped to supports in the knee-elbow position. **Brickner p.,** a position for treating shoulder disability, secured by tying the patient's wrist to the head of the bed with his arm supported on a pillow and raising the head of the bed; thus traction with abduction and external rotation is obtained. **Caldwell p.,** a roentgenographic position with the forehead and nose against the x-ray plate, giving a posteroanterior projection for demonstration of frontal sinuses and the anterior ethmoidal cells. **Casselberry's p.,** a prone position employed after intubation so that the patient may swallow without danger of fluid entering the tube. **centric p.,** see under *relation.*

POSITIONS OF THE FETUS IN VARIOUS PRESENTATIONS

CEPHALIC PRESENTATION

1. Vertex—occiput, the point of direction

Left occipito-anterior	L.O.A.
Left occipitotransverse	L.O.T.
Right occipitoposterior	R.O.P.
Right occipitotransverse	R.O.T.
Right occipito-anterior	R.O.A.
Left occipitoposterior	L.O.P.

2. Face—chin, the point of direction

Right mentoposterior	R.M.P.
Left mento-anterior	L.M.A.
Right mentotransverse	R.M.T.
Right mento-anterior	R.M.A.
Left mentotransverse	L.M.T.
Left mentoposterior	L.M.P.

3. Brow—the point of direction

Right frontoposterior	R.F.P.
Left fronto-anterior	L.F.A.
Right frontotransverse	R.F.T.
Right fronto-anterior	R.F.A.
Left frontotransverse	L.F.T.
Left frontoposterior	L.F.P.

BREECH OR PELVIC PRESENTATION

1. Complete Breech—sacrum, the point of direction (feet crossed and thighs flexed on abdomen)

Left sacro-anterior	L.S.A.
Left sacrotransverse	L.S.T.
Right sacroposterior	R.S.P.
Right sacro-anterior	R.S.A.
Right sacrotransverse	R.S.T.
Left sacroposterior	L.S.P.

2. Incomplete breech—sacrum, the point of direction. Same designations as above, adding the qualifications footling, knee, etc.

TRANSVERSE LIE OR SHOULDER PRESENTATION

Shoulder—scapula, the point of direction

Left scapulo-anterior	L.Sc.A.	Back anterior positions
Right scapulo-anterior	R.Sc.A.	
Right scapuloposterior	R.Sc.P.	Back posterior positions
Left scapuloposterior	L.Sc.P.	

coiled p., the attitude of a patient on his side with hips and knees flexed and thighs drawn up to the body. **decubitus p.,** the position of an individual lying on a horizontal surface, designated, according to the portion of the body resting on the surface, *dorsal decubitus* (lying on the back), *left lateral decubitus* (on the left side), *right lateral decubitus* (on the right side), or *ventral decubitus* (on the abdomen). **Depage's p.,** a prone position with the pelvis raised to form the apex of an inverted V, while the trunk and lower limbs form the branches of the V. **dorsal p.,** the posture of a person lying on his back; called also *supine p.* **dorsal elevated p.,** position of the patient lying on the back, with shoulders and head elevated. **dorsal inertia p.,** the position of a patient on his back and tending to slide toward the foot of the bed; observed in conditions of great inertia. **dorsal recumbent p.,** position of patient on back, with lower limbs flexed and rotated outward; used in vaginal examination, application of obstetrical forceps, etc. **dorsal rigid p.,** position on the back with hips and knees flexed and thighs drawn up to the body. **dorsosacral p.,** lithotomy p. **Duncan's p.,** the position of the placenta with its margin presenting at the os for delivery. **eccentric p.,** see under *relation.* **Edebohls' p.,** a dorsal position, the knees and thighs drawn up, legs flexed on the thighs, and thighs flexed on the belly, the hips raised, and the thighs abducted; called also *Simon's p.* **Elliot's p.,** position of a patient on the operating table with lower chest elevated by placing a support under the lower costal margin; used in operations on the gallbladder. **emprosthotonos p.,** emprosthotonos. **English p.,** the patient on the left side, the right thigh and knee drawn up; called also *lateral recumbent p.* and *obstetrical p.* **Fowler's p.,** the position in which the head of the patient's bed is raised 18 or 20 inches above the level; the knees are also elevated. **froglike p.,** batrachian p. **frontal anterior p.,** frontoanterior p. **frontal posterior p.,** frontoposterior p. **frontal transverse p.,** frontotransverse p. **frontoanterior p.,** a position of the fetus in cephalic presentation in labor, with its brow directed toward the right (R.F.A) or left (L.F.A.) anterior quadrant of the maternal pelvis. **frontoposterior p.,** a position of the fetus in cephalic presentation in labor, with its brow directed toward the right (R.F.P.) or left (L.F.P.) posterior quadrant of the maternal pelvis. **frontotransverse p.,** a position of the fetus in cephalic presentation in labor, with its brow directed toward the right (R.F.T) or left (L.F.T.) iliac fossa of the maternal pelvis. **Fuchs p.,** a roentgenographic position which gives an oblique view of the zygomatic arch projected free of superimposed structures. **genucubital p.,** knee-elbow p. **genufacial p.,** the position of the patient resting on his knees and face. **genupectoral p.,** knee-chest p. **hinge p.,** the position of the condyle in the temporomandibular joint from which an opening by hinge movement is possible beyond the amplitude of rest position. **hinge p., condylar,** 1. hinge p. 2. the maxillomandibular relation from which a consciously stimulated, true, hinge movement can be executed. **hinge p., mandibular,** the most posterior mandibular position from which a consciously stimulated hinge movement can be executed. **hinge p., terminal,** the mandibular hinge position from which further opening of the mandible would produce translatory rather than hinge movement; the most retruded hinge position. **horizontal p.,** the position assumed by a person lying on his back with limbs extended. **jackknife p.,** position of patient on his back, with the shoulders elevated, legs flexed on thighs, and thighs at right angles to the abdomen; used in passing the urethral sound. **Jones' p.,** acute flexion of the forearm for the treatment of fracture of the internal condyle of the humerus. **knee-chest p.,** the position of a patient on his knees with the chest resting on the table. See illustration. **knee-elbow p.,** the position of a patient resting on knees and elbows with the chest elevated from the table. **kneeling-squatting p.,** squatting position with the knees flexed acutely and pressed against the abdomen while the body is held erect; often effective in digital palpation of high rectal lesions. **Kraske's p.,** a prone position with the buttocks raised on a kidney elevator. **lateral recumbent p.,** English p. **lithotomy p.,** the patient in dorsal decubitus with hips and knees flexed and the thighs abducted and externally rotated; called also *dorsosacral p.* **Mayer p.,** a roentgenographic position that gives a unilateral superoinferior view of the temporomandibular joint, external auditory canal, and mastoid and petrous processes; helpful in demonstrating fractures and malformations of the temporomandibular joint and in the study of bony atresia of the external auditory canal. **mentoanterior p.,** a position of the fetus in cephalic presentation in labor, with its chin directed toward the right (R.M.A.) or left (L.M.A.) anterior quadrant of the maternal pelvis. **mentoposterior p.,** a position of the fetus in cephalic presentation in labor, with its chin directed toward the right (R.M.P.) or left (L.M.P.) posterior quadrant of the maternal pelvis. **mentotransverse p.,** a position of the fetus in cephalic presentation in labor, with its chin directed toward the right (R.M.T.) or left (L.M.T.) iliac fossa of the maternal pelvis. **mentum anterior p.,** mentoanterior p. **mentum posterior p.,** mentoposterior p. **mentum transverse p.,** mentotransverse p. **Noble's p.,** position of the patient standing up, leaning forward and supporting the upper body on the arms; used in examining the kidney. **obstetrical p.,** English p. **occipitoanterior p.,** a position of the fetus in cephalic presentation in labor, with its occiput directed toward the right (R.O.A.) or left (L.O.A.) anterior quadrant of the maternal pelvis. **occipitoposterior p.,** a position of the fetus in cephalic presentation in labor, with its occiput directed toward the right (R.O.P.) or left (L.O.P.) posterior quadrant of the maternal pelvis. **occipitosacral p.,** a position of the fetus in cephalic presentation in labor, with the occiput presenting directly behind, or rotated squarely into the hollow of the sacrum. **occipitotransverse p.,** a position of the fetus in cephalic presentation in labor, with its occiput directed toward the right (R.O.T.) or left (L.O.T.) iliac fossa of the maternal pelvis. **occiput anterior p.,** occipitoanterior p. **occiput posterior p.,** occipitoposterior p. **occiput sacral p.,** occipitosacral p. **occiput transverse p.,** occipitotransverse p. **occlusal p.,** the relationship of the mandible and maxillae when the jaw is closed and the teeth are in contact. **opisthotonos p.,** opisthotonos. **orthopnea p., orthopneic p.,** the patient assumes an upright or a semivertical position by using two or more pillows to support his head and chest from the recumbent position, or he sits upright in a chair. Used when the patient has difficulty in breathing except in the upright position (orthopnea). **orthotonos p.,** orthotonos. **physiologic rest p.,** rest p. **posterior border p.,** the most posterior position of the mandible at any specific vertical relation to the maxillae. **prone p.,** patient lying face down. **rest p.,** the position passively assumed by the mandible when its musculature is relaxed, in the upright standing or sitting position, with eyes focused to distance. **Robson's p.,** the patient lying on his back with a sand-bag placed beneath the eleventh and twelfth ribs; used in surgery on the biliary tract. **Rose's p.,** one intended to prevent aspiration or swallowing of blood, as from an injured lip: the patient on his back with head hanging over the end of the table in full extension so as to enable the patient to bleed over the margins of the inverted upper incisors. **sacroanterior p.,** a position of the fetus in breech presentation in labor, with its sacrum directed toward the right (R.S.A.) or left (L.S.A.) anterior quadrant of the maternal pelvis. **sacroposterior p.,** a position of the fetus in breech presentation in labor, with its sacrum directed toward the right (R.S.P.) or left (L.S.P.) posterior quadrant of the maternal pelvis. **sacrotransverse p.,** a position of the fetus in breech presentation in labor, with its sacrum directed toward the right (R.S.T.) or left (L.S.T.) iliac fossa of the maternal pelvis. **sacrum anterior p.,** sacroanterior p. **sacrum posterior p.,** sacroposterior p. **sacrum transverse p.,** sacrotransverse p. **scapula anterior p.,** scapuloanterior p. **scapula posterior p.,** scapuloposterior p. **scapuloanterior p.,** a position of the fetus in transverse lie in labor, with its head to the right (R.Sc.A.) or left (L.Sc.A.) of the maternal pelvis, and its back anterior. **scapuloposterior p.,** a position of the fetus in transverse lie in labor, with its head to the right (R.Sc.P.) or left (L.Sc.P.) of the maternal

pelvis, and its back posterior. **scorbutic p.,** a pseudoparalytic position characteristic of advanced infantile scurvy, in which the infant lies quietly with the legs flexed at the knees and the hips flexed and externally rotated. **semiaxial p.,** Titterington p. **semiprone p.,** Sims' p. **semireclining p.,** a partly reclining position seen in heart disease, asthma, and pleural effusion. **Simon's p.,** Edebohls' p. **Sims' p.,** the patient on the left side with the chest, the right knee, and thigh drawn up, the left arm along the back; for vaginal examination. Called also *semiprone p.* **Stern's p.,** the patient supine with the head lowered over the end of the table, the murmur of tricuspid insufficiency being heard more distinctly. **submentovertex p.,** a roentgenographic position opposite of the verticosubmental position. **supine p.,** dorsal p. **Titterington p.,** a roentgenographic position used to demonstrate fractures of the zygomatic arches, lateral walls of the maxilla, orbital floors, and orbital margins. Called also *semiaxial p.* **trans p.,** trans configuration. **Trendelenburg's p.,** one in which the patient is supine on the table or bed, the head of which is tilted downward 30 to 40 degrees, and the table or bed angulated beneath the knees. See illustration. **tripod p.,** 1. a position assumed by the patient with abdominal weakness or meningeal irritation while sitting in bed, in which he supports himself with his hands in a plane posterior to his pelvis. 2. a sitting position assumed by the patient with respiratory insufficiency, in which his hands are placed anterior to the frontal plane. See also *tripoding.* **Valentine's p.,** the patient supine and the hips flexed by means of a double inclined plane; used in irrigating the urethra. **verticosubmental p.,** a roentgenographic position that gives an axial projection of the mandible, including the coronoid and condyloid processes of the rami, the base of the skull and its foramina, the petrous pyramids, the sphenoidal, posterior ethmoid, and maxillary sinuses, and the nasal septum. **Waters p.,** a roentgenographic position that gives a posteroanterior view of the maxillary sinus, maxilla, orbits, and zygomatic arches; helpful in demonstrating fractures of nasal bones and nasal processes of the maxilla. **Waters p., reverse,** a mento-occipital roentgenographic position used to demonstrate the facial bones when the patient cannot be placed in a prone position; helpful in demonstrating fractures of the orbits, maxillary sinuses, zygomatic bones, and zygomatic arches.

positioner (po-zish′un-er) a resilient elastoplastic removable appliance fitted over the occlusal surfaces of the teeth to obtain limited tooth movement and stabilization, usually at the end of orthodontic treatment. **tooth p.,** see *positioner.*

positive (poz′ĭ-tiv) [L. *positivus*] having a value greater than zero; indicating existence or presence of a condition, organism, etc., as chromatin positive or Wassermann positive; characterized by affirmation or cooperation.

positrocephalogram (poz″ĭ-tro-sef′ah-lo-gram″) [*positron* + Gr. *kephalos* head + *gramma* a mark] a record produced by the emission of positrons by isotopes of arsenic administered to facilitate localization of brain tumors.

positron (poz′ĭ-tron) the positive electron, a particle having the mass of the electron but with a positive electric charge; a free positive electron.

Posner's test (reaction) (pōs′nerz) [Carl *Posner*, Berlin urologist, 1854–1929] see under *tests.*

posologic (po″so-loj′ik) pertaining to doses.

posology (po-sol′o-je) [Gr. *posos* how much + *-logy*] the science of dosage, or a system of dosage.

Possum (pos′um) [*Patient-Operated Selector Mechanism*] trademark for a machine designed for the disabled by which, when breathed into in the correct manner, the individual can operate the telephone, ring bells, turn on the television, switch off a light, type a letter, or perform any of a number of other functions by no movement other than that involved in respiration.

post (pōst) dowel.

post- (pōst) [L. *post* after] a prefix signifying after or behind.

postabortal (pōst-ah-bor′tal) occurring after abortion.

postaccessual (pōst-ak-sesh′u-al) occurring after a paroxysm.

postacetabular (pōst″as-ĕ-tab′u-lar) behind the acetabulum.

postacidotic (pōst″as-ĭ-dot′ik) occurring after the cessation of acidosis.

postadolescence (pōst″ad-o-les′ens) the period following adolescence.

postadolescent (pōst″ad-o-les′ent) 1. pertaining to or occurring in the period following adolescence. 2. a young adult.

postalbumin (pōst″al-bu′min) a serum protein which has an electrophoretic mobility between albumin and alpha-globulin at pH 8.6.

postanal (pōst-a′nal) situated behind the anus.

postanesthetic (pōst″an-es-thet′ik) after anesthesia.

postapoplectic (pōst″ap-o-plek′tik) occurring after an attack of apoplexy.

postaurale (pōst″aw-ra′le) an anthropometric landmark, the most posterior point on the helix of the ear.

postauricular (pōst″aw-rik′u-lar) located or performed behind the auricle of the ear.

Plate XLII

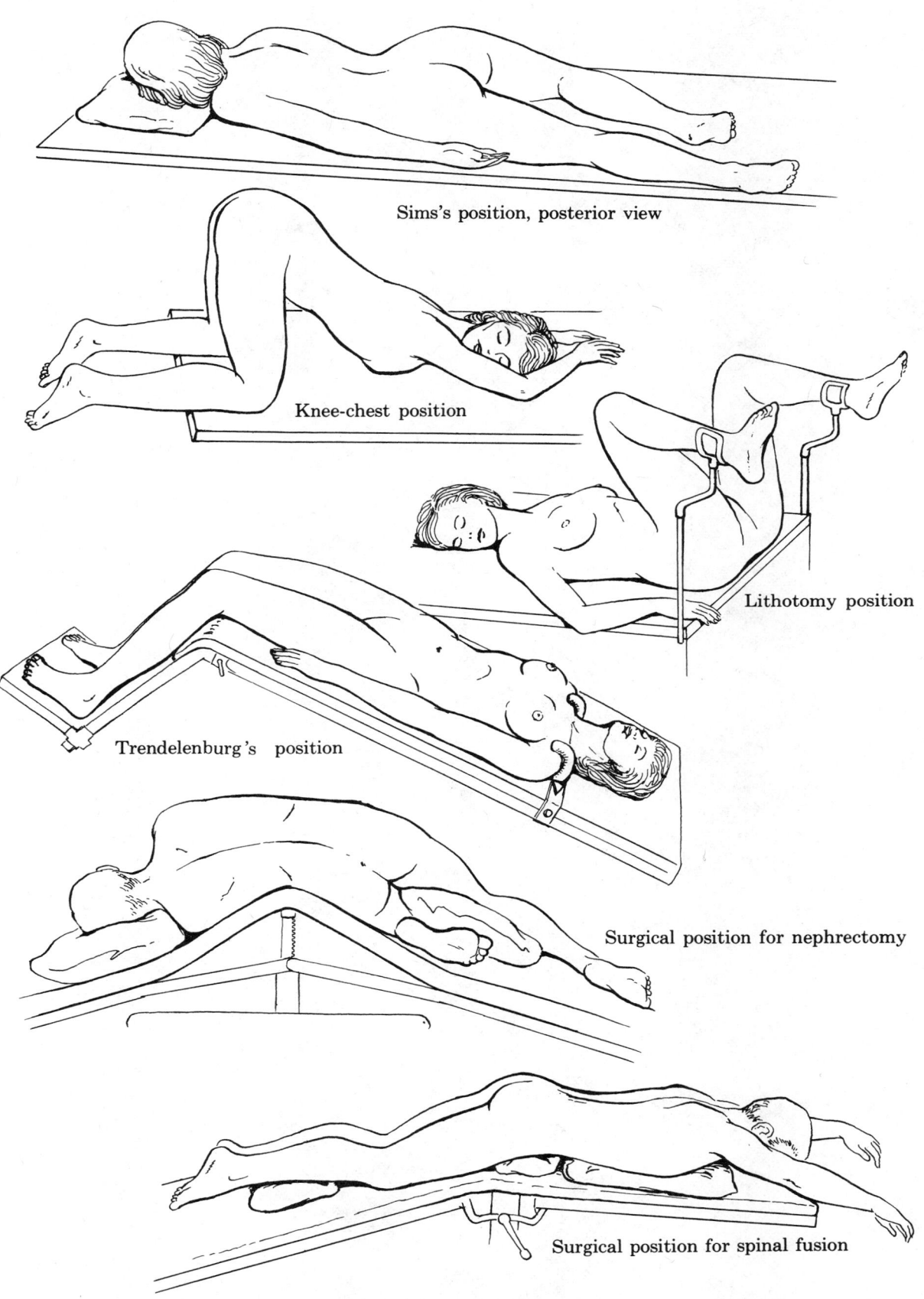

Sims's position, posterior view

Knee-chest position

Lithotomy position

Trendelenburg's position

Surgical position for nephrectomy

Surgical position for spinal fusion

VARIOUS POSITIONS USED IN EXAMINATION OR TREATMENT

postaxial (pōst-ak′se-al) situated behind an axis. In anatomical usage, postaxial refers to the medial (ulnar) aspect of the upper limb, and the lateral (fibular) aspect of the lower limb.

postbrachial (pōst-bra′ke-al) on the posterior part of the upper arm.

postbrachium (pōst-bra′ke-um) brachium colliculi inferioris.

postbuccal (pōst-buk′al) behind the buccal region.

postbulbar (pōst-bul′bar) situated behind or distal to a bulb as behind the medulla oblongata, or distal to the pileus ventriculi (duodenal bulb).

postcapillary (pōst-kap′ĭ-lar′e) a venous capillary.

postcardiotomy (pōst-kar′de-ot′o-me) occurring after or as a consequence of incision (open surgery) of the heart.

postcava (pōst-ka′vah) the vena cava inferior.

postcaval (pōst-ka′val) pertaining to the postcava.

postcecal (pōst-se′kal) retrocecal.

postcentral (pōst-sen′tral) situated or occurring behind a center, as the postcentral gyrus.

postcentralis (pōst″sen-tra′lis) the postcentral fissure.

postcesarean (pōst″se-za′re-an) following cesarean operation.

postcibal (pōst-si′bal) [post- + L. cibum food] occurring after ingestion of food; postprandial.

post cibum (pōst si′bum) [L.] after meals (after food).

postcisterna (pōst″sis-ter′nah) cisterna cerebellomedullaris.

postclavicular (pōst″klah-vik′u-lar) [post- + clavicle] situated or occurring behind the clavicle.

postclimacteric (pōst″kli-mak′ter-ik, pōst″kli-mak- ter′ik) 1. occurring after the climacteric. 2. postmenopausal.

postcoital (post-ko′ĭ-tal) pertaining to the time after coitus.

post coitum (pōst ko-i′tum) after coitus.

postcondylar (pōst-kon′dĭ-lar) behind a condyle.

postcondylare (pōst″kon-dĭ-lah′re) the highest point of the curvature behind the occipital condyle.

postconnubial (pōst″kŏ-nu′be-al) [post- + L. connubium marriage] occurring after marriage.

postconvulsive (pōst″kon-vul′siv) occurring after a convulsion.

postcordial (pōst-kor′de-al) back of the heart.

postcornu (pōst-kor′nu) cornu posterius ventriculi lateralis.

postcranial (pōst-kra′ne-al) situated posterior or inferior to the cranium, or skull.

postcubital (pōst-ku′bĭ-tal) on the dorsal side of the forearm.

postcyclodialysis (pōst-si″klo-di-al′ĭ-sis) occurring after or as a consequence of cyclodialysis.

postdevelopmental (pōst″de-vel″op-men′tal) occurring after the period of development.

postdiastolic (pōst″di-as-tol′ik) occurring after or following the diastole.

postdicrotic (pōst″di-krot′ik) occurring after the dicrotic elevation of the sphygmogram.

postdigestive (pōst″di-ges′tiv) after digestion.

postdiphtheric (pōst″dif-ther′ik) postdiphtheritic.

postdiphtheritic (pōst″dif-ther-it′ik) occurring after or as a consequence of diphtheria, as postdiphtheritic myocarditis.

postdormital (pōst-dor′mĭ-tal) pertaining to or occurring during the postdormitum.

postdormitum (pōst-dor′mĭ-tum) the period of increasing consciousness interposed between sound sleep and wakening.

postecdysis (pōst-ek′dĭ-sis) [post- + Gr. ekdysis a way out] the concluding phase of ecdysis in certain crustaceans and arthropods, during which the endocuticle is secreted and calcification of the skeleton occurs.

postembryonic (pōst″em-bre-on′ik) [post- + Gr. embryon embryo] occurring after the embryonic stage.

postencephalitic (pōst″en-sef″ah-lit′ik) occurring after or as a consequence of encephalitis.

postepileptic (pōst″ep-ĭ-lep′tik) occurring after or as a consequence of an epileptic attack.

posteriad (pos-te′re-ad) toward the posterior surface of the body.

posterior (pos-tēr′e-or) [L. "behind"; neut. posterius] situated in back of, or in the back part of, or affecting the back part of a structure; [NA] a term used in reference to the back or dorsal surface of the body. In lower animals, it refers to the caudal end of the body.

postero- (pos′ter-o) [L. posterus behind] a combining form denoting relationship to the posterior part.

posteroanterior (pos″ter-o-an-tēr′e-or) from back to front, or from the posterior (dorsal) to the anterior (ventral) surface. In roentgenology, denoting direction of the beam from the x-ray source to the beam exit surface.

posteroclusion (pos″ter-o-kloo′zhun) distoclusion.

posteroexternal (pos″ter-o-ek-ster′nal) situated on the outer side of a posterior aspect.

posteroinferior (pos″ter-o-in-fēr′e-or) posterior and inferior.

posterointernal (pos″ter-o-in-ter′nal) situated within and toward the back.

posterolateral (pos″ter-o-lat′er-al) situated behind and to one side.

posteromedial (pos″ter-o-me′de-al) situated toward the middle of the back.

posteromedian (pos″ter-o-me′de-an) situated on the midline of the back.

posteroparietal (pos″ter-o-pah-ri′ĕ-tal) situated at the back part of the parietal bone.

posterosuperior (pos″ter-o-soo-pēr′e-or) situated behind and above.

posterotemporal (pos″ter-o-tem′po-ral) situated at the back part of the temporal bone.

posterula (pos-ter′u-lah) [L.] the space between the nasal conchae and the posterior nares.

postesophageal (pōst-ĕ-sof″ah-je′al) retroesophageal.

postethmoid (pōst-eth′moid) behind the ethmoid bone.

postexed (pōs-tekst′) bent backward.

postexion (pōs-teks′yun) posterior flexion.

postfebrile (pōst-feb′ril) occurring after or as the result of a fever.

postganglionic (pōst″gang-gle-on′ik) situated posterior or distal to a ganglion; said especially of autonomic nerve fibers so located.

postglenoid (pōst-gle′noid) situated behind the glenoid fossa.

postglomerular (pōst″glo-mer′u-lar) located or occurring distal to a glomerulus of the kidney.

postgrippal (pōst-grip′al) occurring after grippe or influenza.

posthemiplegic (pōst″hem-ĭ-ple′jik) occurring after or as a consequence of hemiplegia.

posthemorrhage (pōst-hem′o-rāj) secondary hemorrhage.

posthemorrhagic (pōst-hem″o-raj′ik) occurring after hemorrhage.

posthepatic (pōst″he-pat′ik) situated behind the liver.

posthepatitic (pōst″hep-ah-tit′ik) occurring after or as a consequence of hepatitis.

postherpetic (pōst″her-pet′ik) occurring after or as a consequence of herpes zoster; postzoster.

posthetomy (pos-thet′o-me) [Gr. posthē foreskin + tomē a cutting] circumcision.

posthioplasty (pos′the-o-plas″te) [Gr. posthē foreskin + plastos formed] plastic surgery of the prepuce.

posthitis (pos-thi′tis) [Gr. posthē foreskin + -itis] inflammation of the prepuce.

postholith (pos′tho-lith) [Gr. posthē foreskin + lithos stone] a preputial concretion or calculus.

posthumous (pos′tu-mus) [L. postumus coming after] occurring after death; born after the father's death.

posthyoid (pōst-hi′oid) situated or occurring behind the hyoid bone.

posthypnotic (pōst″hip-not′ik) succeeding the hypnotic state.

posthypoglycemic (pōst-hi″po-gli-se′mik) occurring after or as a consequence of hypoglycemia.

posthypophysis (pōst″hi-pof′ĭ-sis) the posterior part of the hypophysis, or pituitary gland.

posthypoxic (pōst″hĭ-pok′sik) occurring after or as a consequence of hypoxia.

postictal (pōst-ik′tal) following a stroke or seizure, such as an acute epileptic attack.

posticus (pos-ti′kus) [L.] posterior.

postinfluenzal (pōst″in-flu-en′zal) occurring after influenza.

postischial (pōst-is′ke-al) situated behind the ischium.

postligation (pōst″li-ga′shun) following ligation of a blood vessel.

postmalarial (pōst″mah-la′re-al) occurring after malaria.

postmastectomy (pōst″mas-tek′to-me) following mastectomy.

postmastoid (pōst-mas′toid) situated behind the mastoid process of the temporal bone.

postmature (pōst″ma-tūr′) overly developed, as a postmature infant.

postmaturity (pōst″mah-tu′rĭ-te) overdevelopment; the condition of a postmature infant.

postmaximal (pōst-mak′sĭ-mal) after a maximum.

postmeatal (pōst″me-a′tal) behind a meatus, or passage.

postmediastinal (pōst″me-de-as″tĭ-nal) behind the mediastinum; pertaining to the posterior mediastinum.

postmediastinum (pōst″me-de-as-ti′num) mediastinum posterius.

postmeiotic (pōst″mi-ot′ik) [post- + Gr. *meioun* to decrease] occurring after or pertaining to the time following meiosis.

postmenopausal (pōst″men-o-paw′zal) occurring after the menopause.

postmenstrua (pōst-men′stroo-ah) the period immediately following cessation of menstrual flow.

postmesenteric (pōst″mes-en-ter′ik) behind or in the posterior part of the mesentery; retromesenteric.

postminimus (pōst-min′ĭ-mus), pl. *postmin′imi* [post- + L. *minimus* small] digitus postminimus.

postmiotic (pōst″mi-ot′ik) postmeiotic.

postmitotic (pōst″mi-tot′ik) 1. pertaining to the time following or occurring after mitosis in normally dividing cells. 2. pertaining to cells that stop dividing after reaching maturity, as cells of the mammalian heart or central nervous system.

postmortal (pōst-mor′tal) occurring after death.

post mortem (pōst mor′tem) [L.] after death.

postmortem (pōst-mor′tem) occurring or performed after death; pertaining to the period after death.

postnares (pōst-na′rēs) the posterior naris.

postnarial (pōst-na′re-al) pertaining to the posterior nares.

postnasal (pōst-na′zal) [post- + L. *nasus* nose] situated or occurring behind the nose.

postnatal (pōst-na′tal) occurring after birth, with reference to the newborn. Cf. *postpartum.*

postnecrotic (pōst″ne-krot′ik) after death of a part.

postneuritic (pōst″nu-rit′ik) occurring after neuritis.

postocular (pōst-ok′u-lar) [post- + L. *oculus* eye] situated or occurring behind the eye.

postoperative (pōst-op′er-a″tiv) occurring after a surgical operation.

postoral (pōst-o′ral) [post- + L. *os* mouth] behind the mouth.

postorbital (pōst-or′bĭ-tal) behind the orbit.

postpalatine (pōst-pal′ah-tin) behind the palate, or behind the palatine bone.

postpaludal (pōst-pal′u-dal) postmalarial.

postparalytic (pōst″par-ah-lit′ik) following an attack of paralysis.

post partum (pōst par′tum) [L.] after childbirth, or after delivery.

postpartum (pōst-par′tum) occurring after childbirth, or after delivery, with reference to the mother. Cf. *postnatal.*

postpharyngeal (pōst-fah-rin′je-al) situated or occurring behind the pharynx.

postpituitary (pōst-pĭ-tu′ĭ-ta-re) pertaining to the posterior lobe of the pituitary body.

postpneumonic (pōst″nu-mon′ik) following pneumonia.

postponent (pōst-po′nent) [post- + L. *ponere* to place] having a more or less delayed recurrence.

postprandial (pōst-pran′de-al) occurring after dinner, or after a meal; postcibal.

postpuberal (pōst-pu′ber-al) postpubertal.

postpubertal (pōst-pu′ber-tal) occurring in or pertaining to the period following puberty.

postpuberty (pōst-pu′ber-te) the period following puberty.

postpubescence (pōst″pu-bes′ens) postpuberty.

postpubescent (pōst″pu-bes′ent) postpubertal.

postpyknotic (pōst″pik-not′ik) occurring after the stage of pyknosis.

postradiation (pōst″ra-de-a′shun) following exposure to a source of radiation.

postrolandic (pōst″ro-lan′dik) situated behind the fissure of Rolando (sulcus centralis).

postsacral (pōst-sa′kral) behind or below the sacrum.

postscapular (pōst-skap′u-lar) behind the scapula.

postscarlatinal (pōst″skar-lah-ti′nal) occurring after or as a consequence of scarlatina.

Post sing. sed. liq. abbreviation for L. *post sin′gulas se′des liq′uidas,* after every loose stool.

postsphenoid (pōst-sfe′noid) the basisphenoid, pterygoid, and alisphenoid bones together; separate bones in infancy, they usually become united with the sphenoid.

postsphygmic (pōst-sfig′mik) occurring after the pulse wave; see under *period.*

postsplenectomy (pōst″sple-nek′to-me) occurring after splenectomy.

postsplenic (pōst-splen′ik) behind the spleen.

poststenotic (pōst″stĕ-not′ik) located or occurring distal to or beyond a stenosed segment.

poststertorous (pōst-ster′tor-us) occurring after stertor has begun in anesthesia.

postsylvian (pōst-sil′ve-an) behind the sylvian fissure (sulcus lateralis).

postsynaptic (pōst″sĭ-nap′tik) situated distal to a synapse, or occurring after the synapse is crossed.

post-tarsal (pōst-tar′sal) behind the tarsus.

post-tibial (pōst-tib′e-al) behind the tibia.

post-traumatic (pōst″traw-mat′ik) occurring as a result of or after injury.

post-tussis (pōst-tus′is) [L.] after coughing.

post-typhoid (pōst-ti′foid) occurring after typhoid.

postulate (pos′tu-lāt) [L. *postulatum* demanded] anything assumed or taken for granted. **Ehrlich's p.,** see *Ehrlich's side-chain theory,* under *theory.* **Koch's p's,** a statement of the kind of experimental evidence required to establish the etiologic relationship of a given microorganism to a given disease. The conditions included are (1) the microorganism must be observed in every case of the disease; (2) it must be isolated and grown in pure culture; (3) the pure culture must, when inoculated into a susceptible animal, reproduce the disease; and (4) the microorganism must be observed in, and recovered from, the experimentally diseased animal.

postural (pos′chur-al) pertaining to posture or position.

posture (pos′chur) [L. *postura*] the attitude of the body. **Drosin's p's,** three postures for eliciting tenderness in appendicitis.

postuterine (pōst-u′ter-in) situated behind the uterus.

postvaccinal (pōst-vak′sĭ-nal) occurring after or as a consequence of vaccination for smallpox.

postvaccinial (pōst″vak-sin′e-al) occurring after or as a consequence of vaccinia.

postvital (pōst-vi′tal) see *postvital staining,* under *staining.*

postzoster (pōst-zos′ter) occurring after or as a consequence of herpes zoster; postherpetic.

postzygotic (pōst″zi-got′ik) occurring after the completion of fertilization and formation of the zygote.

potable (po′tah-b'l) [L. *potabilis*] fit to drink; drinkable.

Potain's apparatus, sign (po-tānz′) [Pierre Carl Edouard *Potain,* French physician, 1825–1901] see under *apparatus* and *sign.*

Potamon (pot′ah-mon) a genus of fresh-water crabs; *P. dentricularis, P. dehaani,* and *P. rathbuni* are hosts of the metacercariae of *Paragonimus westermani* in the Orient.

potash (pot′ash) impure potassium carbonate. **caustic p.,** potassium hydroxide. **sulfurated p.** [USP], a mixture of potassium polysulfides and potassium thiosulfate, containing 12.8 per cent of sulfur in combination as sulfide; used as a source of sulfide in pharmaceutic preparations. See *white lotion,* under *lotion.* In veterinary medicine, it is used as a bath for mange. Called also *hepar sulfuris, liver of sulfur,* and *potassa sulfurata.*

potassa (po-tas′ah) [L.] potassium hydroxide. **p. caus′tica,** potassium hydroxide. **p. sulfura′ta,** sulfurated potash.

potassemia (pot″ah-se′me-ah) [potassa + Gr. *haima* blood + *-ia*] the presence of an abnormally large amount of potassium in the blood; hyperkalemia.

potassic (po-tas′ik) containing potash.

potassiomercuric (po-tas″e-o-mer-ku′rik) (obs.) containing potassium and mercury in its divalent form. **p. iodide,** potassium mercuric iodide.

potassium (po-tas′e-um) [L.] a metallic element of the alkali group, many of whose salts are used in medicine. It is a soft, silver-white metal, melting at 58° F.; atomic number, 19; atomic weight, 39.102; specific gravity, 0.87; symbol, K (L. *kalium*). Potassium is the chief cation of muscle and most other cells (intracellular fluid); see also *sodium-potassium pump,* under *pump.* **p. acetate** [USP], $CH_3 \cdot COOK$, occurring as colorless, monoclinic crystals or white, crystalline powder; used as an electrolyte replenisher and as a urinary and systemic alkalizer, administered by intravenous infusion and orally. Formerly used as a diuretic and expectorant. Called also *diuretic salt* and *sal diureticum.* **p. alum,** see *alum.* **p. antimonyltartrate,** antimony potassium tartrate; see under *antimony.* **p. arsenite,** a compound formed by the interaction of arsenic trioxide and potassium hydroxide. **p. aspartate and magnesium aspartate,** a mixture of $C_4H_6KNO_4 \cdot \frac{1}{2}H_2O$ and $C_8H_{12}MgN_2O_8 \cdot 4H_2O$; used as a nutrient. **p. bicarbonate** [USP], $KHCO_3$, occurring as colorless, transparent, monoclinic prisms or as a white, granular powder; used as a pharmaceutic necessity in the preparation of Randall's solution, and may be used as an electrolyte replenisher, antacid, and urinary alkalizer. **p. bichromate,** an orange-red, crystalline salt, formerly used as an external astringent, antiseptic, and caustic; in veterinary medicine, it is used as a caustic in the treatment of superficial growths. Called also *p. dichromate.* **p. bismuth tartrate,** bismuth potassium tartrate; see under *bismuth.* **p. bitartrate,** a mild cathartic, $C_4H_5KO_6$, occurring as opaque crystals or a white crystalline powder; administered orally. It is sometimes used in veterinary medicine as a laxative for small animals and as a diuretic for large animals. Called also *cream of tartar.* **p. bromide,** a sedative, KBr, occurring as white, cubical crystals or granular powder; used occasionally for grand mal seizures. See also *bromide.* **p. carbonate,** K_2CO_3, occurring as a white, crystalline or granular powder; formerly used as a systemic alkalizer and diuretic, but now used chiefly in pharmaceutical and chemical manufacturing procedures. **p. chlorate,** an explosive compound, $KClO_3$, occurring as colorless crystals or as white granules or powder, formerly used as an antiseptic for the skin and mucous membranes and in the treatment of hyperthyroidism and thyrotoxicosis. It is sometimes used in veterinary medicine in solution to treat stomatitis and vaginitis. **p. chloride** [USP], KCl, occurring as colorless, elongated, prismatic, or cubical crystals, or white, granular powder; used as an electrolyte replenisher, administered orally or by intravenous infusion. **p. citrate** [USP], $C_6H_5K_3O_7/H_2O$, occurring as transparent crystals or as a white, granular powder; used as a systemic alkalizer, and as an electrolyte replenisher, diuretic, and expectorant, usually administered orally. It is sometimes used in veterinary medicine as a nonirritating diuretic. **p. cyanide,** an extremely poisonous compound, KCN, occurring as a white granular powder or as fused pieces; formerly used in solution to remove silver nitrate stains from the conjunctiva. **p. dichromate,** p. bichromate. **p. dihydrogen phosphate,** p. phosphate, monobasic. **p. ferricyanide,** deep-red crystals, $K_3Fe(CN)_6$, used in a delicate test for ferrous salts. **p. glucaldrate,** chemical name: potassium diaqua[gluconato(2–)]dihydroxyaluminate(1–); an antacid, $C_6H_{16}AlKO_{11}$. **p. gluconate** [USP], chemical name: D-gluconic acid monopotassium salt. A salt, $C_6H_{11}KO_7$, occurring as a white to yellowish white, crystalline powder or as granules; used as an electrolyte replenisher in the prophylaxis and treatment of hypokalemia, administered orally. **p. glycerophosphate,** a colorless to slightly yellow viscous substance, $K_2C_3H_5(OH)_2PO_4$, formerly used as a tonic. **p. guaiacolsulfonate,** $C_7H_7KO_5S$, occurring as white crystals or crystalline powder; used as an expectorant. **p. hydroxide** [NF], KOH, white or nearly white, fused masses or small pellets, or flakes, or sticks, or other forms; used as an alkalizer in pharmaceutical preparations. Called also *caustic potash, potassa,* and *potassa caustica.* **p. hypophosphite,** a white, crystalline salt, KH_2PO_2, formerly used in the treatment of tuberculosis. **p. iodate,** a compound, KIO_3, occurring as white crystals or crystalline powder, formerly used as a topical antiseptic in the treatment of infections of the mucous membranes. It is added to animal feed as a source of iodine. **p. iodide** [USP], KI, occurring as crystals that are colorless and transparent or somewhat opaque and white, or as a white, granular powder; used as an expectorant, as a source of iodine in thyrotoxic crisis and in the preparation of thyrotoxic patients for thyroidectomy, and as an antifungal in the treatment of lymphocutaneous sporotrichosis; administered orally. **p. mercuric iodide,** a complex, K_2Hg-I_4, containing about 25.5 per cent of mercury; used as a germicide, and as an ingredient of various reagents. **p. metaphosphate** [NF], KPO_3, a white powder used as a buffering agent in pharmaceutical preparations. **p. nitrate,** KNO_3, occurring as a white granular or crystalline powder or as colorless transparent prisms; formerly used as an oral diuretic. **p. penicillin G,** penicillin G potassium. **p. perchlorate,** $KClO_4$, occurring as colorless crystals or white, crystalline powder; a thyroid inhibitor, it has been used in the treatment of thyrotoxicosis. **p. permanganate** [USP], the potassium salt of permanganic acid, $KMnO_4$, occurring as dark purple crystals, having bactericidal, fungicidal, astringent, and oxidizing properties; used in solution as a topical anti-infective. Because of its oxidizing activity, it is also used in solutions as a gastric lavage for certain poisons. **p. phenoxymethyl penicillin,** penicillin V potassium. **p. phosphate,** K_2HPO_4, occurring as colorless or white, granules or powder; has been used as a cathartic. Called also *dipotassium phosphate.* **p. phosphate, dibasic,** p. phosphate. **p. phosphate, monobasic** [NF], KH_2PO_4, occurring as colorless crystals or as a white, granular or crystalline powder; used as a buffering agent in pharmaceutical preparations. Called also *p. dihydrogen phosphate.* **radioactive p.,** radiopotassium. **p. silicate,** soluble glass, $K_2Si_2O_3$, sometimes used like plaster of Paris in making rigid dressings. **p. sodium tartrate** [USP], $C_4H_4KNaO_6 \cdot 4H_2O$, occurring as colorless crystals or as a white crystalline powder; used as a cathartic. Called also *Preston's salt, Rochelle salt,* and *Seignette's salt.* **p. sorbate** [NF], chemical name: 2,4-hexadienoic acid potassium salt. A mold and yeast inhibitor, $C_6H_7O_2$, occurring as white crystals or as a powder; used as a preservative in pharmaceutical preparations. **p. sulfate,** K_2SO_4, occurring as colorless or white crystals or as a white powder or granules, which has an extremely irritant action on the stomach and intestines; has been used as a cathartic. **p. sulfite,** $K_2SO_3 + 2H_2O$, occurring as white crystals or crystalline powder; formerly used as a cathartic and diuretic. **p. sulfocyanate,** p. thiocyanate. **p. tartrate,** $K_2C_4H_4O_6 + \frac{1}{2}H_2O$; occurring as white crystals or granular powder; has been used as a cathartic. **p. tellurate,** K_2TeO, occurring in white crystals; formerly used in tuberculosis. **p. thiocyanate,** KSCN, occurring as colorless, transparent, prismatic crystals; used as a reagent, and formerly as an antihypertensive agent. Called also *p. sulfocyanate.*

Potassium Triplex (po-tas′e-um tri′pleks) trademark for Randall's solution.

potency (po′ten-se) [L. *potentia* power] power; especially (1) the

ability of the male to perform sexual intercourse; (2) the power of a medicinal agent to produce the desired effects; (3) the ability of an embryonic part to develop and complete its destiny. **prospective p.,** the total developmental possibilities of which an embryonic part is capable. **reactive p.,** see *competence.*

potentia (po-ten′she-ah) [L.] power.

potential (po-ten′shal) [L. *potentia* power] 1. existing and ready for action, but not yet active. 2. electric tension or pressure, as measured by the capacity of producing electric effects in bodies of a different state of electrization. When bodies of different potentials are brought into communication, a current is set up between them; if they are of the same potential, no current passes between them. **action p.,** the electrical activity developed in a muscle or nerve cell during activity. It may be elicited by electrical, chemical, or mechanical stimulation, by temperature change, and so on. **after-p.,** the period following termination of the spike potential; it has a negative and positive phase. **after-p., negative,** the period following termination of the spike potential during which there is a lag in the return of the potential of an excitable cell membrane to resting potential. **after-p., positive,** the period following termination of the negative after-potential, during which the potential of an excitable cell membrane is more negative than the resting potential. It is paradoxically called *positive* because it was first detected outside the cell, where the polarity is reversed. **bioelectric p.,** the varying electric potential which accompanies all biochemical processes, as those manifested in the electrocardiogram and the electroencephalogram. **caries-producing p.,** decalcification p. **cochlear p.,** see under *microphonics.* **decalcification p.,** the amount of acid produced by oral bacteria from a unit amount of foodstuff, multiplied by the number of such units adhering to the teeth after ingestion of the particular food. **demarcation p.,** the difference in electrical potential between the intact longitudinal surface and the injured end of a muscle or nerve. **evoked cortical p's,** the various discrete electrical charges in the cerebral cortex which can be produced by stimulation of sense organs or of some point along the ascending pathways to the cerebral cortex. **excitatory postsynaptic p.,** a transient decrease in membrane polarization induced in a postsynaptic neuron when subjected to a volley of impulses over an excitatory afferent pathway; summation of such potentials may cause discharge by the neuron. Abbreviated EPSP. **generator p.,** the depolarization produced in neural receptors in response to specific kinds of physical stimuli; called also *receptor p.* **inhibitory postsynaptic p.,** a transient hyperpolarization of membrane potential induced in a postsynaptic neuron when subjected to a volley of impulses over an inhibitory afferent pathway, resulting in a diminished responsiveness of the neuron. Abbreviated IPSP. **membrane p.,** the electric potential which exists on the two sides of a membrane or across the wall of a cell. **morphogenetic p.,** the degree of strength or ability of an embryonic part to develop into a specific structure. **negative summating p.,** a decrease in voltage difference between the cochlear duct and the vestibule caused by moderate to strong stimulation; it is maintained as long as sound stimulation persists. **pacemaker p.,** the slow diastolic depolarization of cell membranes in the sinoatrial node. **receptor p.,** generator p. **resting p.,** the potential difference across the membrane of a normal cell at rest, i.e., the difference in potential between the outside and inside of a cell at rest; cf. *action potential.* **spike p.,** the initial very large change in potential of an excitable cell membrane during excitation.

potentialization, potentiation (po-ten″she-al-i-za′shun, po-ten″she-a′shun) the synergistic action of two drugs, being greater than the sum of the effects of each used alone.

potentiator (po-ten′she-a-tor) an agent that enhances another agent so that the combined effect is greater than the sum of the effects of each one alone.

potentiometer (po-ten″she-om′ĕ-ter) an instrument for the accurate measuring of voltage.

potification (po″tĭ-fĭ-ka′shun) the process of making water fit to drink. Applied to sea water, it is the process of removing sufficient salts to render the remaining fluid safe for drinking.

potion (po′shun) [L. *po′tio* draft] a draft; a large dose of liquid medicine. **Rivière's p.,** an effervescing drink produced by combining a solution of citric acid with one of sodium or potassium bicarbonate.

potocytosis (po″to-si-to′sis) [Gr. *potos* drinking + *kytos* cell + *-osis*] the hypothetical action of cells passing fluids through themselves from one place to another.

potomania (po″to-ma′ne-ah) [Gr. *potos* drinking + *mania* madness] 1. an abnormal desire to drink. 2. delirium tremens.

Pott's aneurysm, disease, etc. (pots) [Sir Percivall *Pott,* English surgeon, 1714–1788] see *aneurysmal varix,* under *varix;* see *tuberculosis of spine;* and see under *abscess, curvature, fracture,* and *paraplegia.*

Pottenger's sign (pot′en-jerz) [Francis Morison *Pottenger,* American physician, born 1869] see under *sign.*

Potter treatment (pot′er) [Caryl Ashley *Potter,* American physician, 1886–1933] see under *treatment.*

Potter version (pot′er) [Irving W. *Potter*, American obstetrician, 1868–1956] see under *version*.

Potts-Smith-Gibson operation [Willis John *Potts*, Chicago surgeon, born 1895; Sidney *Smith*, Chicago surgeon, born 1912; Stanley *Gibson*, Chicago pediatrician, born 1883] see under *operation*.

potus (po′tus) [L. "drink"] a potion. **p. imperia′lis,** imperial drink, a solution of ½ oz. of cream of tartar in 3 pts. of water, sweetened, and flavored with lemon peel.

pouch (powch) a pocket-like space or sac, as of the peritoneum. **abdominovesical p.,** the pouch formed by reflection of the peritoneum from the anterior abdominal wall to the distended bladder. **anterior p. of Tröltsch,** recessus membranae tympani anterior. **branchial p.,** pharyngeal p. **Broca's p.,** a pear-shaped sac in the labium majus, its extremity directed downward and backward, and its smaller one upward, forward, and outward toward the opening of the inguinal canal; composed of elastic fibers, and containing connective tissue and fat. **craniobuccal p., craniopharyngeal p.,** Rathke's p. **p. of Douglas,** excavatio rectouterina. **enterocoelic p.,** a diverticulum of the enteron of the embryo. **guttural p's,** large mucous sacs in the horse, which are ventral diverticula of the eustachian tube, situated between the base of the cranium and the atlas dorsally and the pharynx ventrally. **Hartmann's p.,** an abnormal sacculation of the neck of the gallbladder. **Heidenhain p.,** a small pocket of the stomach which has been surgically separated from the body of the stomach, and thus vagally denervated, and which drains to the exterior; used in the experimental study of gastric physiology. Cf. *Pavlov p.* **ileocecal p.,** a peritoneal pouch at the ileocecal junction. **laryngeal p.,** sacculus laryngis. **Morison's p.,** a pouch of peritoneum below the liver and to the right of the right kidney and extending downward to the transverse mesocolon. **neurobuccal p.,** Rathke's p. **obturator p.,** paravesical p. **paracystic p.,** the lateral part of the excavatio vesicouterina. **pararectal p.,** the lateral part of the excavatio rectouterina. **paravesical p.,** the lateral part of the uteroabdominal pouch, beside the bladder and in which the obturator canal opens; called also *obturator p.* **Pavlov p.,** a pocket of stomach which has been surgically separated from the body of the stomach by a mucosal septum, but which retains vagal innervation and muscular connection, and which drains to the exterior; used in the experimental study of gastric physiology. Cf. *Heidenhain p.* **pharyngeal p.,** a lateral diverticulum of the pharynx that meets a corresponding groove in the ectoderm, forming a closing plate that may rupture and complete the gill slit condition observed in lower vertebrates. **Physick's p's,** inflamed sacculations between the rectal valves, with mucous discharge. **posterior p. of Tröltsch,** recessus membranae tympani posterior. **Prussak's p.,** recessus membranae tympani superior. **Rathke's p.,** a diverticulum from the embryonic buccal cavity, from which the anterior lobe of the pituitary gland is developed. The lumen of Rathke's pouch persists in adults as small colloid-filled cysts and clefts at the juncture of the pars distalis and the neurohypophysis. Called also *craniobuccal p.* and *neurobuccal p.* **rectouterine p., rectovaginal p.,** excavatio rectouterina. **rectovesical p.,** excavatio rectovesicalis. **Seessel's p.,** a transient outpouching of the embryonic pharynx rostrad of the pharyngeal membrane and caudal to Rathke's pouch. **uteroabdominal p.,** the compartment of the pelvic cavity anterior to the uterus and broad ligaments. **uterovesical p., vesicouterine p.,** excavatio vesicouterina. **visceral p.,** pharyngeal p. **Willis' p.,** omentum minus. **Zenker's p.,** pulsion diverticulum.

poudrage (poo-drahzh′) [Fr.] the application of powder to a surface, as between the visceral and parietal layers of the pericardium or pleura, to promote their fusion. **pleural p.,** the application of an irritating powder on the surfaces of the pleura to promote adhesion.

poultice (pōl′tis) [L. *puls* pap; Gr. *kataplasma*] a soft, moist, mass about the consistency of cooked cereal, spread between layers of muslin, linen, gauze, or towels and applied hot to a given area in order to create moist local heat or counterirritation. **mustard p.,** see under *plaster*.

pound (pownd) [L. *pondus* weight; *libra* pound] a unit of mass (weight) of both the avoirdupois and the apothecaries' system. The avoirdupois pound contains 16 ounces, or 7000 grains, and is the equivalent of 453.592 gm. The apothecaries' pound contains 12 ounces, or 5760 grains, and is the equivalent of 373.242 gm. Abbreviated lb.

Poupart's ligament, line (poo-parts′) [François *Poupart*, French anatomist, 1661–1708] see *ligamentum inguinale*, and see under *line*.

Povan (po′van) trademark for a preparation of pyrvinium pamoate.

poverty (pov′er-te) the absence or scarcity of requisite substance or elements. **emotional p.,** diminution in the normal emotional qualities of the mind, such as love, sympathy, honor, etc. **p. of movement,** the relative immobility and stationariness of position seen in subjects with parkinsonism; akinesia.

povidone (po′vĭ-dōn) [USP] chemical name: 1-ethenyl-2-pyrrol-

idinone homopolymer. A synthetic polymer occurring as a white to creamy white, odorless powder, principally consisting of linear 1-vinyl-2-pyrrolidone groups, produced as a series of products having mean molecular weights ranging from about 10,000 to about 700,000; used as a dispersing and suspending agent, and has been used as a tablet binder, coating agent, and viscosity-increasing agent in pharmaceutical preparations. Formerly called *polyvinylpyrrolidone* (PVP). See also *povidone-iodine*.

povidone-iodine (po′vĭ-dōn i′o-dīn) [USP], a complex produced by reacting iodine with the polymer povidone, which slowly releases iodine; it occurs as a yellowish brown, amorphous powder and is used as a topical anti-infective. Abbreviated PVP-I.

powder (pow′der) [L. *pulvis*] a substance made up of an aggregation of small particles, as that obtained by the grinding or trituration of a solid drug. **aromatic p.,** powder of cinnamon, ginger, cardamon seed, and myristica. **bleaching p.,** calx chlorinata. **p. of chalk, aromatic,** a preparation of chalk, cinnamon, myristica, clove, cardamom, and sucrose; formerly used as an antacid, stimulant, and astringent. **p. of chalk, aromatic, with opium,** aromatic powder of chalk containing 2.5 per cent of powdered opium. **chalk p., compound,** a powder containing prepared chalk, finely powdered acacia, and sucrose; it is an antacid used in treatment of diarrhea. **chiniofon p.,** chiniofon. **Dalmatian insect p.,** pyrethrum flowers; see under *flower*. **Dover's p.,** ipecac and opium p. **dusting p.,** a fine powder used as a substitute for talc. **dusting p., absorbable,** an absorbable powder prepared by processing cornstarch, with not more than 2 per cent of magnesium oxide; used for dusting surgeons' rubber gloves and other purposes for which talc is used in the hospital. **effervescent p's, compound,** Seidlitz p's. **furazolidone and nifuroxime p.,** a preparation containing 0.09 to 0.11 per cent furazolidone and 0.45 to 0.55 per cent nifuroxime in a suitable, slightly acidified powder base; used in the treatment of candidal, trichomonal, and bacterial vaginitis, administered intravaginally. **glycyrrhiza p., compound,** senna p., compound. **Goa p.,** a bitter, brownish yellow to umber brown powder deposited in irregular interspaces of the wood of *Andira araroba* Aguiar. (Leguminosae), a large leguminous tree common in Brazil. It is the source of chrysarobin. **impalpable p.,** a powder so fine that its particles cannot be felt as distinct bodies. **iodochlorhydroxyquin p., compound** [USP], a preparation of iodochlorhydroxyquin, boric acid, lactic acid, zinc stearate, and lactose; used as a local anti-infective in the treatment of vaginitis due to *Trichomonas vaginalis, Candida albicans, Trichophyton,* or mixed bacteria, administered by intravaginal sufflation. **ipecac and opium p.,** a pale brown powder prepared by triturating 100 gm. of finely powdered ipecac, 100 gm. of powdered opium, and 800 gm. of coarsely powdered lactose to a very fine, uniform powder; formerly widely used as a sedative and diaphoretic. **p. of jalap, compound,** a mixture of jalap and potassium bitartrate, formerly used in treatment of dropsy. **licorice p., compound, p. of liquorice, compound,** senna p., compound. **methylbenzethonium chloride p.** [USP], a preparation containing 85 to 115 per cent of the labeled amount of methylbenzethonium chloride in a suitable fine powder base, free from grittiness; used topically as a local anti-infective, applied to the skin of the genitalia, rectum, thighs, and intertriginous area in the treatment of ammonia dermatitis and in the treatment and prevention of dermatoses caused by contact with urine, feces, and perspiration. **nystatin topical p.** [USP], a preparation containing 90 to 130 per cent of the labeled amount of nystatin; used as an antifungal. **Persian insect p.,** pyrethrum flowers; see under *flower*. **p. of rhubarb, compound,** a preparation of rhubarb, ginger, and magnesium oxide; formerly used as a laxative antacid. **Seidlitz p's,** a combination of sodium bicarbonate, potassium sodium tartrate, and tartaric acid, used as a cathartic; called also *compound effervescent p's.* See also under *tests*. **senna p., compound,** a weak or dusky yellow powder prepared from fennel oil, finely powdered sucrose, powdered senna, powdered glycyrrhiza, and washed sulfur; used as a laxative. **Sippy p. No. 1,** sodium bicarbonate and calcium carbonate p. **Sippy p. No. 2,** sodium bicarbonate and magnesium oxide p. **sodium bicarbonate and calcium carbonate p.,** a mixture of precipitated calcium carbonate and sodium bicarbonate: antacid; widely used in treatment of peptic ulcer in combination with sodium bicarbonate and magnesium oxide powder. **sodium bicarbonate and magnesium oxide p.,** a mixture of magnesium oxide and sodium carbonate; used as an antacid and laxative. **tolnaftate p.** [USP], a preparation containing 90 to 110 per cent of the labeled amount of tolnaftate; used topically as an antifungal. **triacetin p.,** a preparation containing 90 to 110 per cent of the labeled amount of triacetin in a suitable powder base; used as an antifungal in superficial skin infections, applied topically. **zinc sulfate p., compound,** a preparation of salicylic acid, zinc sulfate, phenol, eucalyptol, menthol, thymol, and boric acid; used as an antiseptic.

power (pow′er) [L. *posse* to have power] 1. capability; potency; the ability to act. 2. a measure of magnification, as of a microscope. **candle p.,** the numerical expression, in international candles, of the luminous intensity of a light source. **carbon dioxide-combining p., CO₂-combining p.,** ability of the blood plasma to combine with carbon dioxide; often, but probably inappropriately, referred to as the alkali reserve. **defining p.,** the ability of a lens to make an object clearly visible. **resolving p.,** the ability of the eye or of a lens to make separately visible small objects that are close together, thus revealing the structure of an object; see also *resolution*.

pox (poks) 1. any eruptive or pustular disease, especially one caused by a virus; see specific entries: *chickenpox, cowpox, horsepox, rabbitpox,* etc. 2. former name for syphilis. **Kaffir p.,** variola minor.

poxvirus (poks-vi′rus) any of a group of relatively large, morphologically similar, and immunologically related DNA viruses, including the viruses of vaccinia (cowpox), variola (smallpox), and those producing pox diseases in lower animals.

P.P. abbreviation for L. *punc′tum prox′imum,* near point of accommodation.

P.P.D. purified protein derivative (of tuberculin); see under *tuberculin*.

ppg. picopicogram.

PPLO pleuropneumonia-like organisms; see *pleuropneumonia-like,* and *Mycoplasma*.

ppm. parts per million.

Ppt. precipitate; prepared.

PR prosthion.

P.R. abbreviation for L. *punc′tum remo′tum,* far point of accommodation.

Pr chemical symbol for *praseodymium*.

Pr. presbyopia; prism.

practice (prak′tis) [Gr. *praktikē*] the utilization of one's knowledge in a particular profession, the practice of medicine being the exercise of one's knowledge in the practical recognition and treatment of disease. **contract p.,** the treatment of the members of a specified group for a lump sum, or at so much per member. **family p.,** the medical specialty concerned with the planning and provision of the comprehensive primary health care of all members of a family, regardless of age or sex, on a continuing basis. **general p.,** the provision of comprehensive medical care as a continuing responsibility regardless of age of the patient or of the condition that may temporarily require the services of a specialist. **group p.,** see under *medicine*. **panel p.,** see under *panel*.

practitioner (prak-tish′un-er) one who has complied with the requirements of and who is engaged in the practice of medicine. **nurse p.,** see *nurse clinician,* under *nurse*.

practolol (prak′to-lōl) chemical name: *N*-[4-[2-hydroxy-3-[(1-methylethyl)amino]propoxy]phenyl]acetamide; a beta-adrenergic blocking agent, $C_{14}H_{22}N_2O_3$, having the same actions as propranolol (q.v.). Its use has been found to be associated with an allergic reaction of the eyes, skin, mucous membranes, and ears.

prae- for words beginning thus, see also those beginning *pre-*.

praecox (pre′koks) [L.] beforetime; early; see *dementia praecox*.

praeputium (pre-pu′she-um) [L.] preputium. **p. clitor′idis,** preputium clitoridis. **p. pe′nis,** preputium penis.

praevia, praevius (pre′ve-a, pre′ve-us) [L.] going before, leading the way; see under *placenta*.

pragmatagnosia (prag″mat-ag-no′ze-ah) [Gr. *pragma* object + *agnōsia* absence of recognition] inability to recognize formerly known objects.

pragmatamnesia (prag″mat-am-ne′ze-ah) [Gr. *pragma* object + *amnesia* forgetfulness] loss of power of remembering the appearance of objects.

pragmatic (prag-mat′ik) pertaining to pragmatism; dealing with practical aspects.

pragmatism (prag′mah-tizm) the doctrine that the whole meaning of a conception lies in its practical consequences.

pralidoxime (pral″ĭ-doks′ēm) chemical name: 2-[(hydroxyimino)methyl]-1-methylpyridinium. A cholinesterase reactivator, $C_7H_9N_2O^+$, capable of acting as an antagonist to certain anticholinesterases. Called also *2-PAM*. **p. chloride** [USP], the chloride salt of pralidoxime, $C_7H_9ClN_2O$, occurring as a white to pale-yellow, crystalline powder; used as an antidote in the treatment of poisoning due to organophosphates having anticholinesterase activity and to counteract the effects of overdosage by anticholinesterases used in the treatment of myasthenia gravis, administered orally and by intravenous infusion. **p. iodide,** the iodide salt of pralidoxime, $C_7H_9IN_2O$, having the actions and uses of the chloride salt. **p. mesylate,** the methanesulfonate salt of pralidoxime, $C_8H_{12}N_2O_4S$, having the actions and uses of the chloride salt.

pramoxine hydrochloride (pram-ok′sēn) [USP] chemical name: 4-[3-(4-butoxyphenoxy)propyl]morpholine hydrochloride. A local anesthetic, $C_{17}H_{27}NO_3 \cdot HCl$, occurring as a white to nearly white, crystalline powder; applied topically.

prandial (pran′de-al) [L. *prandium* breakfast] pertaining to a meal, especially dinner.

pranolium chloride (pra-no′le-um) chemical name: 2-hydroxy-*N,N*-dimethyl-*N*-(1-methylethyl)-3-(1-naphthalenyloxy)-1-

propanaminium chloride; a cardiac depressant with antiarrhythmic actions, $C_{18}H_{26}ClNO_2$.

Prantal (pran′tal) trademark for preparations of diphemanil methylsulfate.

praseodymium (pra″ze-o-dim′e-um, pra″se-o-dim′e-um) a rare earth element; atomic number, 59; atomic weight, 140.907; symbol, Pr.

P. rat. aetat. abbreviation for L. *pro ratio′ne aeta′tis,* in proportion to age.

pratique (prah-tek′) [Fr.] a certificate which releases an incoming vessel from quarantine. It is given by the quarantine officer to the master, and when presented to the collector of the port admits the boat to entry.

Pratt's sign (symptom), test (prats) [Joseph Hersey *Pratt,* American physician, 1872–1956] see under *sign* and *tests*.

Prausnitz-Küstner reaction (test) (prows′nits- kist′ner) [Carl Willy *Prausnitz,* German hygienist, born 1876; Heinz *Küstner,* German gynecologist, born 1897] see under *reaction*.

Praxagoras (prak-sag′o-ras) **of Cos** (c. 340 B.C.) a Greek physician who succeeded Diocles as leader of the Dogmatists. He was apparently the first Greek physician to recognize the difference between arteries and veins, and to comment on the pulse.

praxiology (prak″se-ol′o-je) [Gr. *praxis* action + *-logy*] the study of conduct, rather than of thought or consciousness.

praxis (prak′sis) [Gr. "action"] the doing or performance of action; Edinger's term for the execution of pallial impulses. Cf. *gnosis*.

prazepam (prah′zĕ-pam) chemical name: 7-chloro-1-(cyclopropylmethyl)-1,3-dihydro-5-phenyl-2*H*-1,4-benzodiazepin-2-one. A benzodiazepine derivative, $C_{19}H_{17}ClN_2O$, used as a muscle relaxant and a tranquilizer in the treatment of conditions in which anxiety is a prominent feature, administered orally.

praziquantel (pra″zĭ-kwon′tel) chemical name: 2-(cyclohexylcarbonyl)-1,2,3,6,7,11b-hexahydro-4*H*-pyrazino[2,1-*a*]isoquinolin-4-one; a veterinary anthelmintic, $C_{19}H_{24}N_2O_2$.

prazosin hydrochloride (prah′zo-sin) chemical name: 1-(4-amino-6,7-dimethoxy-2-quinazolinyl)-4-(2-furanylcarbonyl)piperazine monohydrochloride. A quinazoline derivative with vasodilator properties, $C_{19}H_{21}N_5O_4 \cdot HCl$; used as an oral antihypertensive.

pre- [L. *prae* before] prefix signifying before.

preadult (pre″ah-dult′) prior to adult life.

preagonal (pre-ag′o-nal) preceding the death agony.

preagonic (pre″ah-gon′ik) preagonal.

prealbuminuric (pre″al-bu″mĭ-nu′rik) occurring before albuminuria sets in.

preanal (pre-a′nal) in front of the anus.

preanesthesia (pre″an-es-the′ze-ah) preliminary anesthesia; light anesthesia or narcosis induced by medication as a preliminary to administration of a general anesthetic.

preanesthetic (pre″an-es-thet′ik) 1. pertaining to or inducing preanesthesia. 2. an agent that induces preanesthesia.

preantiseptic (pre″an-tĭ-sep′tik) pertaining to the time before the discovery of antisepsis.

preaortic (pre″a-or′tik) in front of the aorta.

preaseptic (pre″a-sep′tik) pertaining to the time before aseptic surgery was practiced.

preataxic (pre″ah-tak′sik) occurring before or preceding ataxia.

preaurale (pre″aw-ra′le) a cephalometric landmark, the point at which a straight line from the postaurale, perpendicular to the long axis of the auricle, meets the base of the auricle.

preauricular (pre″aw-rik′u-lar) situated in front of the auricle of the ear.

preaxial (pre-ak′se-al) situated or occurring before an axis; in anatomical usage, preaxial refers to the lateral (radial) aspect of the upper limb, and the medial (tibal) aspect of the lower limb.

prebacillary (pre-bas′ĭ-ler″e) occurring before the entrance of bacilli into the system, or before they become discoverable.

prebacteriological (pre″bak-te″re-o-log′ĭ-kal) before the development of bacteriology.

prebase (pre′bās) that part of the dorsum of the tongue lying in front of the base.

prebetalipoprotein (pre″ba″tah-lip″o-pro′te-in) very low-density lipoprotein; see under *lipoprotein*.

prebetalipoproteinemia (pre″ba″tah-lip″o-pro′te-in-e′me-ah) hyperprebetalipoproteinemia.

prebiotic (pre″bi-ot′ik) denoting the period before the existence of life on earth.

prebladder (pre-blad′er) an extensive cavity formed in front of the orifice of the bladder within the capsule of the prostate.

prebrachium (pre-bra′ke-um) brachium colliculi superioris.

precancer (pre′kan-ser) a condition which tends eventually to become malignant.

precancerosis (pre″kan-ser-o′sis) a precancerous condition; a condition of early cancer.

precancerous (pre-kan′ser-us) pertaining to a pathologic process that tends to become malignant.

precapillary (pre-kap′ĭ-ler″e) a vessel lacking complete coats, intermediate between an arteriole and a true capillary, and containing scattered smooth muscle cells in its wall; these vessels usually have sphincter areas, which control blood flow into capillaries. Called also *metarteriole*.

precarcinomatous (pre″kar-sĭ-nom′ah-tus) preceding the development of carcinoma.

precardiac (pre-kar′de-ak) situated ventrad from the heart.

precardium (pre-kar′de-um) [*pre-* + Gr. *kardia* heart] precordium.

precartilage (pre-kar′tĭ-lij) embryonic cartilaginous tissue.

precava (pre-ka′vah) the vena cava superior.

precentral (pre-sen′tral) situated in front of a center, as the precentral gyrus.

prechordal (pre-kor′dal) situated in front of the notochord.

precipitable (pre-sip′ĭ-tah-b′l) capable of being precipitated.

precipitant (pre-sip′ĭ-tant) a substance which causes a chemical or mechanical precipitation.

precipitate (pre-sip′ĭ-tāt) [L. *praecipitare* to cast down] 1. to cause a substance in solution to settle down in solid particles. 2. [L. *praecipitatum*] a deposit made or substance thrown down by precipitation. 3. occurring with undue rapidity, as precipitate labor. 4. in immunology, the product of interaction between soluble macromolecular antigen and the homologous antibody (e.g., the antigen-antibody complex formed as a consequence of the reaction of pneumococcus capsular polysaccharide in solution with specific antiserum). **keratic p's,** see under *keratitis punctata*. **sweet p.,** calomel (mild mercurous chloride). **white p.,** ammoniated mercury.

precipitation (pre-sip″ĭ-ta′shun) [L. *praecipitatio*] the act or process of precipitating. **group p.,** precipitation by a precipitin in a specific antiserum of an antigen common to a group of closely related microorganisms.

precipitin (pre-sip′ĭ-tin) an antibody to soluble antigen that specifically aggregates the macromolecular antigen in vivo or in vitro to give a visible precipitate. **heat p.,** coctoprecipitin.

precipitinogen (pre-sip″ĭ-tin′o-jen) the soluble antigen which stimulates the formation of precipitins and is capable of reacting with them in vitro and in vivo.

precipitinoid (pre-sip′ĭ-tin-oid) (*obs.*) a precipitin in which the zymophore group has been changed or lost so that it cannot cause precipitation, although it still retains its affinity for the antigen.

precipitinophoric (pre-sip″ĭ-tin-o-for′ik) (*obs.*) denoting the active precipitating element or group in a precipitin.

precipitogen (pre-sip′ĭ-to-jen) precipitinogen.

precipitogenoid (pre-sip″ĭ-toj′e-noid) (*obs.*) a precipitogen which has lost its power of causing precipitation.

precipitoid (pre-sip′ĭ-toid) precipitinoid.

precipitophore (pre-sip′ĭ-to-fōr″) (*obs.*) the group in a precipitin which causes the actual precipitation.

precipitum (pre-sip′ĭ-tum) (*obs.*) the precipitate resulting from the action of a precipitin.

precirrhosis (pre″sir-ro′sis) the early stages of cirrhosis of the liver.

preclavicular (pre″klah-vik′u-lar) in front of the clavicle.

preclinical (pre-klin′ĭ-kal) before a disease becomes clinically recognizable.

preclival (pre-kli′val) in front of the clivus of the cerebellum.

precocious (pre-ko′shus) developed more than is usual at a given age.

precocity (pre-kos′ĭ-te) unusually early development of mental or physical traits.

precognition (pre″kog-nish′un) [*pre-* + *cognition*] the extrasensory perception of a future event.

precoid (pre′koid) resembling dementia praecox.

precollagenous (pre″kŏ-laj′ĕ-nus) [*pre-* + *collagen*] denoting an incomplete stage in the formation of collagen.

precoma (pre-ko′mah) the neuropsychiatric state preceding coma, as in hepatic encephalopathy.

preconscious (pre-kon′shus) in freudian terminology, all the mental processes that are "out of mind" at the time, but can be recalled with little or no effort.

preconvulsant (pre″kon-vul′sant) preceding the occurrence of convulsions.

preconvulsive (pre″kon-vul′siv) occurring before the convulsive stage.

precordia (pre-kor′de-ah) [L. *praecordia*] precordium.

precordial (pre-kor′de-al) pertaining to the precordium.

precordialgia (pre″kor-de-al′je-ah) [*precordia* + *-algia*] pain in the precordium.

precordium (pre-kor′de-um) the region over the heart and lower part of the thorax.

precornu (pre-kor′nu) cornu anterius ventriculi lateralis.

precostal (pre-kos′tal) in front of the ribs.

precritical (pre-krit′ĭ-kal) previous to the occurrence of the crisis.

precuneal (pre-ku′ne-al) situated in front of the cuneus.

precuneate (pre-ku′ne-āt) pertaining to the precuneus.

precuneus (pre-ku′ne-us) [*pre-* + L. *cuneus* wedge] [NA] a small, square-shaped convolution on the medial surface of the parietal lobe of the cerebrum, bounded posteriorly by the medial part of the parietooccipital sulcus and anteriorly by the paracentral lobule.

precursor (pre′kur-sor) [L. *praecursor* a forerunner] something that precedes. In biological processes, a substance from which another, usually more active or mature substance is formed. In clinical medicine, a sign or symptom that heralds another.

predation (pre-da′shun) the derivation by an organism of elements essential for its existence from organisms of other species which it consumes and destroys.

predator (pred′ah-tor) [L. *praedator* a plunderer, pillager] an organism that derives elements essential for its existence from organisms of other species, which it consumes and destroys.

predentin (pre-den′tin) the soft fibrillar substance composing the primitive dentin and forming the inner layer of the circumpulpar dentin; called also *dentinoid*.

prediabetes (pre-di″ah-be′tēz) a state of latent impairment of carbohydrate metabolism, in which the criteria for diabetes mellitus are not all satisfied; sometimes controllable by diet alone.

prediastole (pre″di-as′to-le) the interval immediately preceding diastole in the cardiac cycle.

prediastolic (pre″di-ah-stol′ik) 1. pertaining to the beginning of the diastole. 2. occurring just before the diastole.

predicrotic (pre″di-krot′ik) occurring before the dicrotic wave of the sphygmogram.

predigestion (pre″di-jes′chun) the partial artificial digestion of food before its ingestion.

predisposing (pre″dis-pōz′ing) conferring a tendency to disease.

predisposition (pre″dis-po-zish′un) [*pre-* + L. *disponere* to dispose] a latent susceptibility to disease which may be activated under certain conditions, as by stress.

prediverticular (pre-di″ver-tik′u-lar) denoting a condition of thickening of the muscular wall of the colon and increased intraluminal pressure but without herniation of the mucosa, i.e., without evidence of diverticulosis.

prednisolone (pred-nis′o-lōn) [USP] chemical name: 11β17α-21-trihydroxypregna-1,4-diene-3,20-dione. A synthetic glucocorticoid derived from cortisol, $C_{21}H_{28}O_5$, occurring as a white to practically white, crystalline powder; administered orally in the treatment of various conditions responsive to the anti-inflammatory action of glucocorticoids, including rheumatoid arthritis and other collagen diseases, allergic conditions, neoplastic and gastrointestinal disease, and blood dyscrasias. **p. acetate** [USP], the 21-acetate ester of prednisolone, $C_{23}H_{30}O_4$, occurring as a white to practically white, crystalline powder, having actions and uses similar to those of the base; administered by intra-articular or intramuscular injection. **p. butylacetate,** p. tebutate. **p. sodium phosphate** [USP], the sodium phosphate ester salt of prednisolone, $C_{21}H_{27}Na_2O_8P$, occurring as white or slightly yellow, friable granules or powder, having actions and uses similar to those of the base; administered by intravenous or intramuscular injection when rapid effect is needed, or applied topically to the conjunctiva. **p. sodium succinate for injection** [NF], sterile prednisolone sodium succinate prepared from prednisolone succinate with the aid of sodium carbonate, containing between 90 and 110 per cent of prednisolone; used as a glucocorticoid. **p. succinate** [USP], the succinate ester of prednisolone, $C_{25}H_{32}O_8$, occurring as a fine, creamy white powder with friable lumps, which on solubilization with sodium carbonate produces *prednisolone sodium succinate*, a form administered by intravenous or intramuscular injection when rapid effect is needed. **p. tebutate** [USP], an ester of prednisolone, $C_{27}H_{38}O_6$, occurring as a white to slightly yellow, free-flowing powder that may have some soft lumps; used as a pharmaceutic necessity for the sterile suspension dosage form intended for intra-articular, intrabursal, and soft-tissue injection. Called also *p. butylacetate*.

prednisone (pred′nĭ-sōn) [USP] chemical name: 17α,21-dihydroxypregna-1,4-diene-3,11,20-trione. A synthetic glucocorticoid derived from cortisone, $C_{21}H_{26}O_5$, but having reduced mineralocorticoid activity; it occurs as a white to practically white, crystalline powder and is used orally in the treatment of various conditions responsive to the anti-inflammatory action of glucocorticoids. Called also *deltacortisone*.

predormital (pre-dor′mĭ-tal) pertaining to or occurring in the predormitum.

predormitium (pre″dor-mish′e-um) predormitum.

predormitum (pre-dor′mĭ-tum) the period of waning consciousness interposed between the waking state and sound slumber.

preeclampsia (pre″e-klamp′se-ah) a toxemia of late pregnancy characterized by hypertension, edema, and proteinuria; when convulsions and coma are associated, it is called *eclampsia*.

preelacin (pre-el′ah-sin) a precursor of elacin in the circulating blood.

preenzyme (pre′en-zīm″) zymogen.

preepiglottic (pre″ep-ĭ-glot′ik) situated or occurring in front of the epiglottis.

preeruptive (pre″e-rup′tiv) preceding an eruption.

preexcitation (pre-ek″si-ta′shun) 1. premature excitation of a portion of the ventricle occurring in Wolff-Parkinson-White syndrome. It is caused by cardiac impulses transmitted along an accessory pathway not subject to the physiologic delay of the artioventricular node, and is characterized electrocardiographically by a short P-R interval and a wide QRS interval. 2. Wolff-Parkinson-White syndrome. **ventricular p.,** Wolff-Parkinson-White syndrome.

preflagellate (pre-flaj′ĕ-lāt) preceding the flagellate state; said of protozoa.

preformation (pre″for-ma′shun) the theory of early physiologists that the fully formed animal or plant exists in a minute form in the germ cell. Opposed to the theory of *epigenesis*. See *animalculist* and *ovist*.

preformationist (pre″for-ma′shun-ist) a believer in the theory of preformation.

prefrontal (pre-fron′tal) 1. situated in the anterior part of the frontal lobe or region. 2. the central part of the ethmoid bone.

prefunctional (pre-funk′shun-al) denoting the period in embryological development during which the organ rudiments are formed but are incapable of performing their specific functions.

preganglionic (pre″gang-gle-on′ik) situated anterior or proximal to a ganglion; said especially of autonomic nerve fibers so located.

pregenital (pre-jen′ĭ-tal) pertaining to the early infantile stage of sexual life before the genitals have become the dominant zone.

Pregl's test (pra′g′lz) [Fritz *Pregl*, Austrian chemist, 1869–1930] see under *tests*.

preglomerular (pre″glo-mer′u-lar) located or occurring proximal to a glomerulus of the kidney.

pregnancy (preg′nan-se) [L. *praegnans* with child] the condition of having a developing embryo or fetus in the body, after union of an ovum and spermatozoon. In women duration of pregnancy is about 266 days. Pregnancy is marked by cessation of the menses; nausea on arising in the morning (morning sickness); enlargement of the breasts and pigmentation of the nipples; progressive enlargement of the abdomen. The absolute signs of pregnancy are fetal movements, sounds of the fetal heart, and demonstration of the fetus by x-ray or ultrasound. **abdomi-**

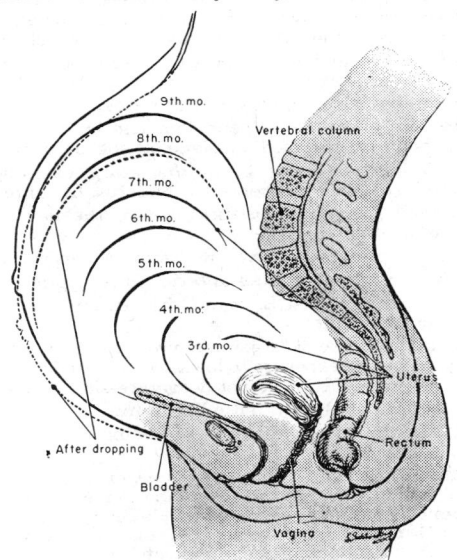

Pregnancy—Uterine levels.

nal p., ectopic pregnancy with development of the fetus in the abdominal cavity. **ampullar p.,** ectopic pregnancy in which the ovum has been arrested in the ampulla of the oviduct. **angular p.,** pregnancy in which the fertilized ovum becomes implanted in the angle or cornu of the uterus. **bigeminal p.,** twin p. **broad ligament p.,** ectopic pregnancy with development of the fertilized ovum in the broad ligament. **cervical**

p., ectopic pregnancy with the development of the ovum within the cervical canal. **combined p.,** simultaneous existence of intrauterine and ectopic pregnancy. **compound p.,** superimposition of an intrauterine pregnancy on a previously existing ectopic pregnancy, generally a lithopedion. **cornual p.,** pregnancy in one of the horns of a bicornate uterus. **ectopic p.,** development of the fertilized ovum outside of the uterine cavity; called also *extrauterine p.* **exochorial p.,** graviditas exocho-

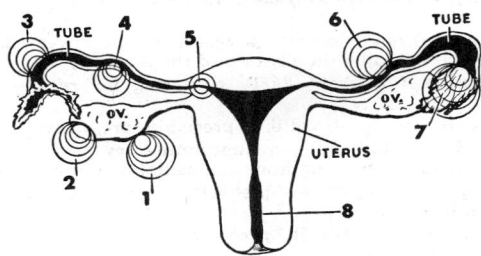

Diagram showing locations of ectopic (extrauterine) pregnancy: (1) primary abdominal; (2) ovarian; (3) ampullar, (4) tubal—rupture into broad ligament; (5) interstitial; (6) tubal—rupture into peritoneal cavity; (7) tubo-ovarian; (8) cervical (Greenhill).

rialis. **extrauterine p.,** ectopic p. **fallopian p.,** tubal p. **false p.,** absence of the menses and presence of other signs of pregnancy, without occurrence of conception and development of an embryo. It may be due to psychogenic factors, to a tumor or mole, or to endocrine disorders. Called also *pseudocyesis, pseudopregnancy,* and *spurious p.* **gemellary p.,** twin p. **heterotopic p.,** combined p. **hydatid p.,** that which is accompanied with the formation of a hydatid mole. **hysteric p.,** false pregnancy due to psychogenic factors. **incomplete p.,** pregnancy which is interrupted prematurely: abortion (up to the 16th week); immature delivery (16th to 28th week); premature delivery (28th to 36th week). **interstitial p.,** ectopic pregnancy with gestation in that part of the oviduct which is within the wall of the uterus. **intraligamentary p., intraligamentous p.,** ectopic pregnancy within the broad ligament. **intramural p.,** interstitial p. **intraperitoneal p.,** ectopic pregnancy within the peritoneal cavity. **membranous p.,** pregnancy in which the fetus has broken through its membranous envelope and lies in contact with the uterine walls. **mesenteric p.,** tuboligamentary p. **molar p.,** conversion of the ovum into a mole. **multiple p.,** pregnancy resulting in the birth of more than one infant; it may be *monovular* (resulting from the fertilization of a single ovum) or *polyovular* (resulting from the fertilization of more than one ovum). When more than two fetuses co-exist, they may come from one ovum or be the result of combined monovular and polyovular twinning. **mural p.,** interstitial p. **nervous p.,** false pregnancy due to psychogenic factors. **ovarian p.,** ectopic pregnancy occurring within an ovary. **ovario-abdominal p.,** ectopic pregnancy which begins ovarian, but afterward becomes abdominal. **oviductal p.,** tubal p. **parietal p.,** interstitial p. **phantom p.,** false pregnancy due to psychogenic factors. **plural p.,** pregnancy with more than one fetus. **prolonged p.,** pregnancy continuing beyond the normal duration, usually beyond 294 days after the beginning of the last menses. **pseudointraligamentary p.,** an ectopic pregnancy in which a sac has been formed in such a way as to simulate an intraligamentary pregnancy. **sarcofetal p.,** pregnancy with both a fetus and a mole. **sarcohysteric p.,** false pregnancy due to a mole. **spurious p.,** false p. **stump p.,** pregnancy at the stump remaining after a supracervical hysterectomy. **tubal p.,** ectopic pregnancy within an oviduct. **tuboabdominal p.,** ectopic pregnancy occurring partly in the fimbriated end of the oviduct and partly in the abdominal cavity. **tuboligamentary p.,** ectopic pregnancy partly in the tube and partly in the broad ligament. **tubo-ovarian p.,** ectopic pregnancy occurring partly in the ovary and partly in the oviduct. **tubouterine p.,** ectopic pregnancy partly within the uterus and partly in an oviduct. **twin p.,** gestation with development of two fetuses. **uteroabdominal p.,** pregnancy with one fetus in the uterus and another in the abdominal cavity. **utero-ovarian p.,** pregnancy with one fetus in the uterus and another in the ovary. **uterotubal p.,** tubouterine pregnancy.

pregnane (preg′nān) a crystalline saturated steroid hydrocarbon, $C_{21}H_{36}$. 5β-Pregnane is the form from which several hormones, including progesterone, are derived. 5α-Pregnane, or allopregnane, is the form excreted in the urine.

pregnanediol (preg″nān-di′ol) a crystalline, biologically inactive dihydroxy derivative of pregnane, formed by reduction of progesterone and found especially in urine of women during pregnancy or the secretory phase of the menstrual cycle.

pregnanetriol (preg″nān-tri′ol) a metabolite of 17-hydroxyprogesterone, normally occurring in small amounts in body fluids and urine, but greatly increased in disorders of the adrenal cortex in which 21-hydroxylation of the steroid nucleus is impaired.

pregnant (preg′nant) [L. *praegnans*] with child; gravid.

pregnene (preg′nēn) a crystalline unsaturated steroid with one double bond and three methyl groups, $C_{21}H_{34}$; $\triangle^4$-pregnene forms the nucleus of the corpus luteum principle, progesterone.

pregneninolone (preg″nēn-in′o-lōn) ethisterone.

pregnenolone succinate (preg-nēn′o-lōn) chemical name: (3β-carboxy-1-oxopropoxy)-pregn-5-en-20-one. A glucocorticoid, $C_{25}H_{36}O_5$, which has been used in the treatment of rheumatoid arthritis.

pregonium (pre-go′ne-um) a recess on the lower edge of the body of the mandible in advance of the angle.

pregranular (pre-gran′u-lar) occurring before the granular stage.

pregravidic (pre″grah-vid′ik) preceding pregnancy.

prehallux (pre-hal′uks) a supernumerary bone of the foot sometimes found growing from the medial border of the scaphoid.

prehemiplegic (pre″hem-ĭ-ple′jik) forerunning an attack of hemiplegia.

prehensile (pre-hen′sil) [L. *prehendere* to lay hold of] adapted for grasping or seizing.

prehension (pre-hen′shun) [L. *prehensio*] the act of seizing or grasping.

prehepaticus (pre″he-pat′ĭ-kus) [*pre-* + Gr. *hēpar* liver] a mass of vascular and connective tissue in the embryo which develops into the interstitial tissue of the liver.

prehormone (pre-hor′mōn) a precursor of a hormone.

prehyoid (pre-hi′oid) in front of the hyoid bone.

prehypophyseal (pre″hi-po-fiz′e-al) pertaining to or derived from the anterior lobe of the pituitary gland (lobus anterior hypophyseos [NA]).

prehypophysial (pre″hi-po-fiz′e-al) prehypophyseal.

prehypophysis (pre″hi-pof′ĭ-sis) the anterior lobe of the pituitary gland.

preictal (pre-ik′tal) [*pre-* + L. *ictus* stroke] occurring before a stroke or an attack, as before an acute epileptic attack.

preicteric (pre-ik-ter′ik) denoting the phase of hepatic disease before jaundice (icterus) appears.

preimmunization (pre-im″u-ni-za′shun) artificial immunization produced in very young infants, as by the BCG vaccine.

preinduction (pre″in-duk′shun) an environmental influence on the germ cells of an individual which does not produce a modification until the third generation of his descendants, i.e., in the grandchildren.

preinvasive (pre″in-va′siv) not yet invading other tissues; see *carcinoma in situ.*

preiotation (pre″i-o-ta′shun) [*pre-* + Gr. *iōta*, the Greek letter ι] the conversion of the initial sound of *i* into *y.*

Preiser's disease (pri′zerz) [Georg Karl Felix *Preiser*, orthopedic surgeon, Hamburg, Germany, 1879–1913] see under *disease.*

Preisz-Nocard bacillus (prīs-no-kard′) [Hugo von *Preisz*, Budapest bacteriologist, 1860–1940; E. I. E. *Nocard*] *Corynebacterium pseudotuberculosis.*

prelacrimal (pre-lak′rĭ-mal) in front of the lacrimal sac.

prelacteal (pre-lak′te-al) preceding the establishment of milk flow; a term applied to the feeding of a newborn baby with carbohydrate-electrolyte solutions to reduce initial weight loss until breast feeding is fully established.

prelaryngeal (pre″lah-rin′je-al) in front of the larynx.

preleukemia (pre-lu-ke′me-ah) a stage of varying duration preceding the development of overt acute myelogenous monocytic or stem-cell leukemia, characterized by bone marrow dysfunction as manifested by anemia, neutropenia, thrombocytopenia, or a combination of these. Splenomegaly, hepatomegaly, or lymphadenopathy may not appear until the onset, often explosive, of the overt leukemia itself.

preleukemic (pre-lu-ke′mik) pertaining to or affected with preleukemia.

prelimbic (pre-lim′bik) situated before a limbus; specifically, anterior to the limbus fossae ovalis.

prelipoid (pre-li′poid) 1. preceding or before the lipoid state. 2. a preliminary stage of lipoid substance.

prelocalization (pre″lo-kal-i-za′shun) the localization in the egg or blastomere of materials which will develop into a particular tissue or organ.

prelocomotion (pre″lo-ko-mo′shun) the movements of a child made with the intention of moving from place to place before motor coordination is sufficently developed to enable it to walk.

prelum (pre′lum) [L.] press.

premalignant (pre″mah-lig′nant) precancerous.

premaniacal (pre″ma-ni′ah-kal) preceding an attack of mania.

Premarin (prem′ah-rin) trademark for preparations of conjugated estrogens.

premature (pre-mah-tūr′) [L. *praematurus* early ripe] 1. occurring before the proper time. 2. a premature infant; see under *infant.*

prematurity (pre″mah-tu′rĭ-te) underdevelopment; the condition of a premature infant.

premaxilla (pre″mak-sil′ah) a separate element derived from the median nasal processes in the embryo, which later fuses with the maxilla; see also *os incisivum.*

premaxillary (pre-mak′sĭ-ler″e) 1. situated in front of the maxilla proper. 2. os incisivum. 3. pertaining to the premaxilla or to the os incisivum.

premedical (pre-med′ĭ-kal) preceding and preparing for the regular medical course of study, as premedical education.

premedicant (pre-med′ĭ-kant) a drug used for premedication.

premedication (pre″med-ĭ-ka′shun) preliminary medication, particularly internal medication to produce narcosis prior to inhalation anesthesia.

premeiotic (pre″mi-ot′ik) [*pre-* + Gr. *meioun* to decrease] occurring before or pertaining to the time preceding meiosis.

premenarchal (pre″mĕ-nar′kal) pertaining to the period before menstruation is established; occurring prior to the menarche.

premenarche (pre″mĕ-nar′ke) the period before menstruation is established; preceding the menarche.

premenarcheal (pre″mĕ-nar′ke-al) premenarchal.

premenstrua (pre-men′stroo-ah) plural of *premenstruum.*

premenstrual (pre-men′stroo-al) occurring before menstruation.

premenstruum (pre-men′stroo-um), pl. *premenstrua* [L.] the period immediately preceding occurrence of the menstrual flow.

premitotic (pre″mi-tot′ik) occurring before or pertaining to the time preceding mitosis.

premolar (pre-mo′lar) [*pre-* + L. *molaris* molar] 1. one of the eight permanent teeth (two on either side of each jaw) anterior to the molars and posterior to the canine teeth; in zoology, those teeth which succeed the deciduous molars regardless of the number to be succeeded. See under *tooth.* 2. situated in front of the molar teeth.

premonitory (pre-mon′ĭ-to-re) [L. *praemonitorius*] serving as a warning.

premonocyte (pre-mon′o-sīt) promonocyte.

premorbid (pre-mor′bid) occurring before the development of disease.

premortal (pre-mor′tal) occurring just before death.

premunition (pre″mu-nish′un) relative immunity; infection immunity; a state of resistance to infection which is established after an acute infection has become chronic and which lasts as long as the infecting organisms remain in the body.

premunitive (pre-mu′nĭ-tiv) pertaining to or produced by preventive vaccination.

premyeloblast (pre-mi′ĕ-lo-blast″) an early form of a myeloblast.

premyelocyte (pre-mi′ĕ-lo-sīt″) promyelocyte.

prenarcosis (pre″nar-ko′sis) narcosis induced as a preliminary to full general anesthesia or previous to local anesthesia.

prenarcotic (pre″nar-kot′ik) previous to the occurrence of narcosis.

prenares (pre-na′rēz) the nostrils or nares.

prenasale (pre″na-sa′le) a cephalometric landmark, the most projecting point, in the median plane, at the tip of the nose.

prenatal (pre-na′tal) [*pre-* + L. *natalis* natal] existing or occurring before birth, with reference to the fetus. Cf. *antepartal.*

preneoplastic (pre″ne-o-plas′tik) before the development or existence of a tumor.

preoperative (pre-op′er-a″tiv) preceding an operation.

preoptic (pre-op′tik) situated anterior to the optic chiasma.

preoral (pre-o′ral) [*pre-* + L. *os* mouth] situated in front of the mouth, or cranial to it.

preoxygenation (pre-ok″sĭ-jen-a′shun) the prolonged breathing of oxygen before exposure to low atmospheric pressure at high altitudes, as prophylaxis against decompression sickness.

prepalatal (pre-pal′ah-tal) situated in front of the palate.

preparalytic (pre″par-ah-lit′ik) preceding the appearance of paralysis.

preparation (prep′ah-ra′shun) [L. *praeparatio*] 1. the act or process of making ready. 2. a medicine made ready for use. 3. an anatomic or pathologic specimen made ready and preserved for study. **allergenic protein p's,** extracts of various substances such as pollens, foods, dusts, etc., that are used for the diagnosis, prophylaxis, and desensitization in allergic cases. **biomechanical p.,** the procedures involved in exposing, enlarging, cleansing, and shaping the pulp chamber and root canal of a tooth by mechanical means. **cavity p.,** the removal of carious tissue and the shaping of the cavity in a tooth preliminary to insertion of filling material. **corrosion p.,** an anatomical preparation made by injecting the parts to be retained and eating away the rest of the tissues with some corrosive substance. **Ehrlich-Hata p.,** arsphenamine. **Hata p.,** arsphenamine. **heart-lung p.,** an animal in which only the heart and lungs are kept alive, the blood from the aorta being diverted into an external system of tubes, simulating the systemic circulation, and back via a reservoir to the right atrium; used in studies of heart function. **impression p.**, a preparation of bacteria on a slide for examination, made by lightly touching a coverglass to a colony.

preparative (pre-par'ah-tiv) amboceptor, i.e., antibody.

preparator (prep'ah-ra''tor) amboceptor, i.e., antibody.

prepartal (pre-par'tal) [pre- + L. *partus* labor] occurring before, or just previous to, labor.

prepatellar (pre''pah-tel'ar) situated in front of the patella.

prepatent (pre-pa'tent) before becoming apparent or manifest; in malariology the term is applied to the period elapsing between infection and appearance of parasites in blood.

preperception (pre''per-sep'shun) in psychology, anticipation of a perception.

preperforative (pre-per'fo-ra''tiv) before the occurrence of perforation.

preperitoneal (pre''per-ĭ-to-ne'al) situated between the parietal peritoneum and the abdominal wall, or occurring in front of the peritoneum.

prephthisis (pre-thi'sis) pretuberculosis.

preplacental (pre''plah-sen'tal) previous to the formation of the placenta.

preponderance (pre-pon'der-ans) [pre- + L. *pondere* to weigh] the condition of having greater weight, force, or influence. **ventricular p.**, disproportionate hypertrophy between the ventricles of the heart; diagnosed by the electrocardiograph.

prepotency (pre-po'ten-se) [L. *praepotentia*] power superior to that of the other parent in transmitting inheritable characters to the offspring.

prepotent (pre-po'tent) [L. *praepotens*] having superior force; having greater power than the other parent in transmitting inheritable characters to the offspring.

prepotential (pre''po-ten'shal) the slow diastolic depolarization of the cell membranes of the cardiac pacemaker.

preprandial (pre-pran'de-al) before meals.

preproinsulin (pre''pro-in'su-lin) the precursor of proinsulin, containing an additional polypeptide sequence at the N-terminal.

preprophage (pre-pro'fāj) [pre- + *prophage*] a postulated stage in the life cycle of a temperate bacteriophage, occurring after infection of a bacterium and before establishment of the prophage.

preproprotein (pre''pro-pro'te-in) any precursor (e.g., preproinsulin) of a proprotein.

preprosthetic (pre''pros-thet'ik) performed or occurring before insertion of a prosthesis.

prepuberal (pre-pu'ber-al) prepubertal.

prepubertal (pre-pu'ber-tal) occurring before puberty; pertaining to the period of accelerated growth preceding gonadal maturity.

prepuberty (pre-pu'ber-te) the period preceding puberty.

prepubescence (pre''pu-bes'ens) prepuberty.

prepubescent (pre''pu-bes'ent) prepubertal.

prepuce (pre'pūs) a covering fold of skin; often used alone to designate the preputium penis. **p. of clitoris,** preputium clitoridis. **p. of penis,** preputium penis. **redundant p.,** a condition in which there is excessive growth of the foreskin, so that it cannot be drawn back over the glans.

preputial (pre-pu'shal) pertaining to the prepuce.

preputiotomy (pre-pu''she-ot'o-me) [*preputium* + Gr. *tomē* a cutting] incision of the preputium penis on the dorsum or side of the penis, to relieve the constriction in phimosis.

preputium (pre-pu'she-um) a covering fold of skin, as the preputium penis. **p. clitor'idis** [NA], a fold formed by the union of the labia minora anterior with the clitoris; called also *prepuce of clitoris.* **p. pe'nis** [NA], the fold of skin covering the glans penis; called also *prepuce of penis* and *foreskin.*

prepyloric (pre''pi-lor'ik) in front of or just proximal to the pylorus or the pyloric part of the stomach (see *pars pylorica ventriculi*).

prerectal (pre-rek'tal) situated in front of or just proximal to the rectum.

prerenal (pre-re'nal) in front of the kidney.

prerennin (pre-ren'in) the zymogen existing in the gastric glands, which, after secretion, is converted into rennin; called also *prorennin* and *renninogen.*

prereproductive (pre''re-pro-duk'tiv) pertaining to childhood, or the stage preceding puberty.

preretinal (pre-ret'ĭ-nal) in front of the retina.

presacral (pre-sa'kral) situated in front of the sacrum.

Presamine (pres'ah-mēn) trademark for a preparation of imipramine hydrochloride.

presby- (pres'be) [Gr. *presbys* old] a combining form meaning old or denoting relationship to old age.

presbyacusia (pres''be-ah-ku'se-ah) presbycusis.

presbyatrics (pres-be-at'riks) [*presby-* + Gr. *iatrikē* surgery, medicine] geriatrics.

presbycardia (pres''bĭ-kar'de-ah) impaired cardiac function attributed to the aging process, occurring in association with recognizable changes of senescence in the body and in the absence of convincing evidence of other forms of heart disease.

presbycusis (pres''bĕ-ku'sis) [*presby-* + Gr. *akousis* hearing] a progressive, bilaterally symmetrical perceptive hearing loss occurring with age.

presbyesophagus (pres''be-ĕ-sof'ah-gus) a condition characterized by alteration in motor function of the esophagus as a result of degenerative changes occurring with advancing age.

presbyope (pres'be-ōp) [*presby-* + Gr. *ōps* eye] one who is presbyopic.

presbyophrenia (pres''be-o-fre'ne-ah) [*presby-* + Gr. *phrēn* mind + *-ia*] a mental condition often seen in old age, consisting of defective memory, loss of sense of location, and confabulation; called also *Wernicke's syndrome.*

presbyopia (pres''be-o'pe-ah) [*presby-* + Gr. *ōps* eye + *-ia*] hyperopia and impairment of vision due to advancing years or to old age; it is dependent on diminution of the power of accommodation from loss of elasticity of the crystalline lens, causing the near point of distinct vision to be removed farther from the eye.

presbyopic (pres''be-op'ik) pertaining to presbyopia.

presbytia (pres-bish'e-ah) presbyopia.

presbytism (pres'bĭ-tizm) presbyopia.

prescapula (pre-skap'u-lah) the suprascapular portion of the scapula.

prescapular (pre-skap'u-lar) 1. in front of the scapula. 2. pertaining to the prescapula.

presclerotic (pre''skle-rot'ik) occurring before sclerosis takes place.

prescribe (pre-skrīb') [L. *praescribere* to write before] to designate in writing a remedy for administration.

prescription (pre-skrip'shun) [L. *praescriptio*] a written direction for the preparation and administration of a remedy. A prescription consists of the heading or *superscription*—that is, the symbol ℞ or the word Recipe, meaning "take"; the *inscription*, which contains the names and quantities of the ingredients; the *subscription*, or directions for compounding; and the *signature*, usually introduced by the sign S. for *sig'na*, "mark," which gives the directions for the patient which are to be marked on the receptacle. **shotgun p.,** an irrational presciption that contains a number of ingredients given with the idea that one or more of them may be effective.

presecretin (pre''se-kre'tin) prosecretion.

presegmenter (pre''seg-men'ter) a full-grown malarial parasite in the stage in which the pigment is accumulated into masses just previous to segmentation.

presenile (pre-se'nīl) pertaining to a condition resembling senility, but occurring in early or middle life.

presenility (pre''sĕ-nil'ĭ-te) premature old age.

presenium (pre-se'ne-um) the period immediately preceding old age.

present (pre-zent') [L. *praesentare* to show] to appear or to show, as to appear first at the os uteri (said of various parts of the fetus), or to appear for examination, treatment, etc. (said of a patient).

presentation (pre''zen-ta'shun) [L. *praesentatio*] in obstetrics: (*a*) the relationship of the long axis of the fetus to that of the mother (called also *lie*); (*b*) the presenting part, i.e., that portion of the fetus which is touched by the examining finger through the cervix, or during labor, is bounded by the girdle of resistance. Cf. *position.* **antigen p.,** the hypothesis that macrophages not only ingest and process antigen, refining and complexing it with SRNA, but also present it in concentrated form at their surfaces to lymphocytes, thus inducing an immune response by the lymphocytes. **breech p.,** presentation of the buttocks or feet of the fetus in labor; see also *longitudinal p.* **breech p., complete,** presentation of the buttocks of the fetus in labor, with the feet alongside of the buttocks, the fetus being in the same attitude as in vertex presentation, but with polarity reversed. **breech p., double,** complete breech p. **breech p., frank,** presentation of the buttocks of the fetus in labor, with the legs extended against the trunk and the feet lying against the face. **breech p., incomplete,** presentation of the buttocks of the fetus in labor, with one or both feet or one or both knees of the fetus prolapsed into the maternal vagina. **breech p., single,** frank breech p. **brow p.,** presentation of the fetal brow in labor. **cephalic p.,** presentation of any part of the fetal head in labor, including occiput, brow, or face; see also *longitudinal p.* **compound p.,** prolapse of an extremity of the fetus (an arm or leg, or both), alongside the head, or of one or both arms alongside a presenting breech, at the beginning of labor. **face p.,** the presentation of the face of the fetus in labor. **footling p.,** presentation of the fetus in labor with one (single footling) or both feet (double footling) prolapsed into the maternal vagina. **funis p.,** presentation of the umbilical cord in labor. **longitudinal p.,** the

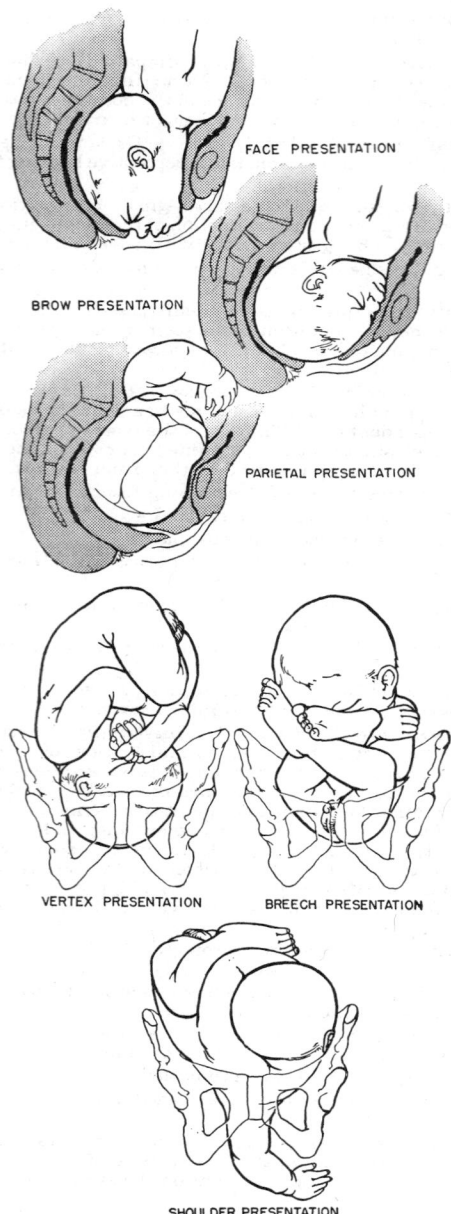

FACE PRESENTATION

BROW PRESENTATION

PARIETAL PRESENTATION

VERTEX PRESENTATION   BREECH PRESENTATION

SHOULDER PRESENTATION

situation of the fetus in labor in which the long axis of the fetal body lies parallel to that of the mother. Normally, the head presents first, but sometimes the breech is the first to appear. **oblique p.,** the situation of the fetus in labor in which the long axis of the fetal body lies obliquely to that of the mother; the shoulder presents first. **parietal p.,** presentation of the parietal portion of the fetal head in labor. **pelvic p.,** breech p. **placental p.,** placenta previa. **polar p.,** longitudinal p. **shoulder p.,** presentation of the fetal shoulder in labor; see also *oblique p.* and *transverse lie,* under *lie.* **torso p.,** transverse lie. **transverse p.,** see under *lie.* **trunk p.,** transverse lie. **vertex p.,** the presentation of the vertex of the fetal head in labor.

preservative (pre-zer′vah-tiv) "a substance or preparation added to a product for the purpose of destroying or inhibiting the multiplication of microorganisms" (Council on Pharmacy and Chemistry).

presomite (pre-so′mīt) [*pre-* + *somite*] referring to embryos before the appearance of somites; in the human, before Horizon IX or 19 days postfertilization.

prespermatid (pre-sper′mah-tid) a secondary spermatocyte.

presphenoid (pre-sfe′noid) the anterior portion of the body of the sphenoid bone.

presphygmic (pre-sfig′mik) occurring before the pulse wave; see under *period.*

prespinal (pre-spi′nal) situated in front of the spine.

prespondylolisthesis (pre-spon″dĭ-lo-lis-the′sis) a congenital defect in the last lumbar vertebra consisting of a bilateral defect in the neural arches at the pedicles.

pressometer (pres-som′ĕ-ter) manometer. **Jarcho p.,** an instrument especially designed for measuring pressure during injection of radiopaque material into the uterus in hysterosalpingography.

pressor (pres′or) tending to increase blood pressure, as a pressor substance.

pressoreceptive (pres″o-re-sep′tiv) sensitive to stimuli due to vasomotor activity, such as blood pressure.

pressoreceptor (pres″o-re-sep′tor) a receptor or nerve ending sensitive to stimuli of vasomotor activity.

pressosensitive (pres″o-sen′sĭ-tiv) pressoreceptive.

pressure (presh′ur) [L. *pressura*] stress or strain, whether by compression, pull, thrust, or shear. **after p.,** a sense of pressure which lasts for a short period after removal of the actual pressure. **arterial p.,** the pressure of the blood within the arteries. **atmospheric p.,** the pressure exerted by the atmosphere; it is about 15 pounds to the square inch at the level of the sea. **back p.,** the pressure caused by the damming back of the blood in a heart chamber and its tributaries, due to an obstructive heart valve or failing myocardium. **biting p.,** occlusal p. **blood p.,** the pressure of the blood on the walls of the arteries, dependent on the energy of the heart action, the elasticity of the walls of the arteries, and the volume and viscosity of the blood. The maximum pressure occurs near the end of the stroke output of the left ventricle of the heart and is termed *maximum* or *systolic* pressure. The minimum pressure occurs late in ventricular diastole and is termed *minimum* or *diastolic* pressure. *Mean blood pressure* is the average of the blood pressure levels. *Basic blood pressure* is the pressure during quiet rest or basal conditions. See also *hypertension* and *hypotension.* **brain p.,** the capillary venous pressure in the brain. **capillary p.,** the blood pressure in the capillaries. **central venous p. (CVP),** the venous pressure as measured at the right atrium, done by means of a catheter introduced through the median cubital vein to the superior vena cava, the distal end of the catheter being attached to a manometer. **cerebrospinal p.,** the pressure or tension of the cerebrospinal fluid, normally 100–150 mm. as measured by the manometer. **diastolic p.,** see *blood p.* **Donders' p.,** increase of manometric pressure with the instrument placed on the trachea on opening the chest of a dead body; due to collapse of the lung. **endocardial p.,** pressure of blood within the heart. **hydrostatic p.,** the pressure at any level on water at rest due to the weight of the water above it. **intra-abdominal p.,** the pressure between the viscera within the abdominal cavity. **intracranial p.,** the pressure in the space between the skull and the brain, i.e., the pressure of the subarachnoidal fluid. **intraocular p.,** the pressure of the fluids of the eye against the tunics. It is produced by continual renewal of the fluids within the interior of the eye, and is altered in certain pathological conditions (e.g., glaucoma). It may be roughly estimated by palpation of the eye or measured, directly or indirectly, with specially devised instruments, the tonometers. **intrathecal p.,** pressure within a sheath, particularly the pressure of the cerebrospinal fluid within the subarachnoid membrane. **intraventricular p.,** the pressure within one ventricle of the heart. **mean circulatory filling p.,** a measure of the average (arterial and venous) pressure necessary to cause filling of the circulation with blood; it varies with blood volume and is directly proportional to the rate of venous return and thus to cardiac output. **negative p.,** a pressure less than that of the atmosphere. **occlusal p.,** pressure exerted on the occlusal surfaces of the teeth when the jaws are brought into apposition. **oncotic p.,** the osmotic pressure due to the presence of colloids in a solution; in the case of plasma–interstitial fluid interaction, it is the force that tends to counterbalance the capillary blood pressure. **osmotic p.,** the potential pressure of a solution directly related to its solute osmolar concentration; it is the maximum pressure developed by osmosis in a solution separated from another by a semipermeable membrane, i.e., the pressure that will just prevent osmosis between two such solutions. **osmotic p., effective,** that part of the total osmotic pressure of a solution which governs the tendency of its solvent to pass through a semipermeable bounding membrane or across another boundary. **partial p.,** the pressure exerted by each of the components of a gas mixture. **perfusion p.,** the difference between the arterial and venous pressures at the brain level. **positive p.,** pressure greater than that of the atmosphere. **positive end-expiratory p. (PEEP),** a method of mechanical ventilation in which pressure is maintained to increase the volume of gas remaining in the lungs at the end of expiration, thus reducing the shunting of blood through the lungs and improving gas exchange; done in acute respiratory failure to allow reduction of inspired O_2 concentrations. **pulse p.,** the difference between the systolic and diastolic pressures. **selection p.,** an effect produced by a given gene that determines the frequency of a given allele; it may be advantageous for survival (*positive selection pressure*) or disadvantageous (*negative selection pressure*). **solution p.,** the force which tends to bring into solution the molecules of a solid contained in the solvent. **systolic p.,** see *blood p.* **venous p.,** the blood pressure in a vein, usually utilized to reflect filling pressure to the ventricle. **wedge p.,** intravascular pressure as measured by a catheter introduced into the pulmonary artery; it permits indirect measurement of the mean left atrial pressure.

presternum (pre-ster′num) manubrium sterni.

presubiculum (pre″su-bik′u-lum) a modified six-layered cortex situated between the subiculum and the main part of the parahippocampal gyrus.

presumptive (pre-zump′tiv) referring to the expected fate of an embryonic part on the basis of established fate mapping.

presuppurative (pre-sup′u-ra″tiv) occurring before suppuration.

presylvian (pre-sil′ve-an) pertaining to the anterior or ascending branch of the sylvian fissure (sulcus lateralis).

presymptom (pre-simp′tom) an indication which is a forerunner of the actual symptoms of a condition.

presymptomatic (pre″simp-to-mat′ik) existing before the appearance of symptoms.

presynaptic (pre″sĭ-nap′tik) situated proximal to a synapse, or occurring before the synapse is crossed.

presystole (pre-sis′to-le) an interval of time just preceding the systole.

presystolic (pre″sis-tol′ik) [*pre-* + *systole*] 1. pertaining to the beginning of the systole. 2. occurring just before the systole.

pretarsal (pre-tar′sal) situated in front of the tarsus.

pretectal (pre-tek′tal) located anterior to the tectum mesencephali.

prethcamide (preth′kah-mīd) a respiratory stimulant composed of equal parts by weight of cropropamide and crotethamide.

prethyroideal, prethyroidean (pre″thi-roi′de-al; pre″thi-roi-de′an) situated in front of the thyroid gland or thyroid cartilage.

pretibial (pre-tib′e-al) situated in front of the tibia.

pretracheal (pre-tra′ke-al) situated in front of the trachea.

pretragal (pre-tra′gal) situated in front of the tragus.

pretuberculosis (pre″tu-ber″ku-lo′sis) tuberculosis in an incipient and occult stage before any symptoms of the disease have appeared.

pretuberculous (pre″tu-ber′ku-lus) preceding the development of tuberculosis.

pretympanic (pre″tim-pan′ik) situated in front of the tympanum.

preurethritis (pre″u-re-thri′tis) inflammation of the vestibule of the vagina around the urethral orifice.

prevalence (prev′ah-lens) the total number of cases of a disease in existence at a certain time in a designated area. Cf. *incidence.*

preventive (pre-ven′tiv) serving to avert the occurrence of.

preventorium (pre″ven-to′re-um) an institution where persons are confined for the purpose of checking the systemic spread of disease, usually for prophylaxis of children who have been exposed to tuberculosis.

preventriculus (pre″ven-trik′u-lus) the cardiac opening of the stomach (ostium cardiacum [NA]).

prevertebral (pre-ver′tĕ-bral) situated in front of a vertebra.

prevesical (pre-ves′ĭ-kal) [*pre-* + L. *vesica* bladder] situated in front of the bladder.

previable (pre-vi′ah-b′l) not yet viable; said of a fetus incapable of extrauterine existence.

previtamin (pre-vi′tah-min) a precursor of a vitamin. **p. H,** carotene.

Prévost's law, sign (pra-vōz′) [Jean Louis *Prévost,* Swiss physician, 1838–1927] see under *law* and *sign.*

Preyer's reflex, test (pri-erz′) [Thierry Wilhelm *Preyer,* German physiologic chemist and physiologist, 1841–1897] see under *reflex* and *tests.*

prezone (pre′zōn) prozone.

prezygapophysis (pre″zi-gah-pof′ĭ-sis) processus articularis superior vertebrarum.

prezygotic (pre-zi-got′ik) occurring before the completion of fertilization.

prezymogen (pre-zi′mo-jen) a substance existing in the cell which becomes converted into zymogen or pre-enzyme.

PRF prolactin releasing factor.

priapism (pri′ah-pizm) [L. *priapismus;* Gr. *priapismos*] persistent abnormal erection of the penis, usually without sexual desire, and accompanied by pain and tenderness. It is seen in diseases and injuries of the spinal cord, and may be caused by vesical calculus and certain injuries to the penis. **secondary p.,** priapism caused by obstruction to the outflow of blood through the dorsal vein at the root of the penis.

priapitis (pri″ah-pi′tis) inflammation of the penis.

priapus (pri-ā′-pus) the penis.

Price-Jones curve (method) [Cecil *Price-Jones,* English physician, 1863–1943] see under *curve.*

Priessnitz compress (bandage) (prēs′nitz) [Vincenz *Priessnitz,* a Silesian farmer, 1799–1852] see under *compress.*

Priestley's mass (prēst′lēz) [Joseph *Priestley,* English naturalist, the discoverer of oxygen, 1733–1804] see under *mass.*

prilocaine hydrochloride (pril′o-kān) [USP] chemical name: *N*-(2-methyphenyl)-2-(propylamino)propanamide monohydrochloride. A local anesthetic, $C_{13}H_{20}N_2O \cdot HCl$, occurring as a white, crystalline powder; used to produce peripheral nerve block, epidural or caudal block, and infiltration and regional anesthesia.

primaquine phosphate (prim′ah-kwin) [USP] chemical name: *N*⁴-(6-methoxy-8-quinolinyl)-1,4-pentanediamine phosphate (1:2). An antimalarial, $C_{15}H_{21}N_3O \cdot 2H_3PO_4$, occurring as an orange-red crystalline powder, especially effective against exoerythrocytic forms of *Plasmodium vivax* and *P. falciparum;* used especially in the treatment of relapsing vivax malaria, administered orally, sometimes in conjunction with other antimalarials.

primary (pri′mer-e; pri′mah-re) [L. *primarius* principal; *primus* first] first in order or in time of development; principal.

primate (pri′māt) an individual belonging to the order Primates.

Primates (pri-ma′tez) [L. *primus* first] the highest order of mammals, including man, apes, monkeys, and lemurs.

primed (prīmd) immunologically activated by initial exposure to antigen; said of cells of the immune system.

prime mover (prīm′ mov′er) a muscle that acts directly to bring about a desired movement.

primer (prīm′er) a substance which prepares for or facilitates the action of another. **cavity p.,** a material which is used to increase the ability of resin material to adapt or adhere to the cavity wall.

primeverose (pri-mev′er-ōs) a disaccharide, 6-(β-D-xylosido)-D-glucose, $C_{11}H_{20}O_{10}$, from the cowslip, *Primula veris* L.

primidone (prim′ĭ-dōn) [USP] chemical name: 5-ethyldihydro-5-phenyl-4,6(1*H*,5*H*)-pyrimidinedione. An anticonvulsant, $C_{12}H_{14}N_2O_2$, occurring as a white, crystalline powder; used in the treatment of grand mal, focal, and psychomotor epileptic seizures, administered orally. Called also *desoxyphenobarbital.*

primigravid (pri″mĭ-grav′id) pregnant for the first time.

primigravida (pri″mĭ-grav′ĭ-dah) [L. *prima* first + *gravida* pregnant] a woman pregnant for the first time; also written gravida I.

primipara (pri-mip′ah-rah), pl. *primip′arae* [L. *prima* first + *parere* to bring forth, produce] a woman who has had one pregnancy which resulted in a viable child, regardless of whether the child was living at birth, and regardless of whether it was a single or multiple birth. Also written para I or *I-para.*

primiparity (pri″mĭ-par′ĭ-te) the condition or fact of being a primipara.

primiparous (pri-mip′ah-rus) bearing or having borne but one child.

primite (pri′mīt) the anterior of a pair of gregarines undergoing syzygy.

primitiae (pri-mish′e-e) [L. pl., "first things"] that part of the amniotic fluid discharged before the fetus is extruded.

primitive (prim′ĭ-tiv) [L. *primitivus*] first in point of time; existing in a simple or early form; showing little evolution.

primordial (pri-mor′de-al) [L. *primordialis*] original or primitive; of the simplest and most undeveloped character.

primordium (pri-mor′de-um), pl. *primor′dia* [L. "the beginning"] the earliest discernible indication during embryonic development of an organ or part; called also *anlage* or *rudiment.*

primverose (prim′ver-ōs) a disaccharide occurring in zein.

Prinadol (prin′ah-dol) trademark for a preparation of phenazocine.

princeps (prin′seps) [L.] principal; chief.

Principen (prin′sĭ-pen) trademark for preparations of ampicillin.

principle (prin′sĭ-p′l) [L. *principium*] 1. a chemical component. 2. a substance on which certain of the properties of a drug depend. 3. a law of conduct. **active p.,** any constituent of a drug which helps to confer upon it a medicinal property. **antianemia p.,** the constituent in liver (vitamin B₁₂) and certain other tissues that produces the hematopoietic effect in pernicious anemia. **Doppler p.,** see under *effect.* **Fick p.,** a restatement of the law of conservation of mass used in making indirect measurements, e.g., of cardiac output: the amount of blood traversing the pulmonary capillaries per unit of time is a measure of cardiac output and, because gas diffusion across the pulmonary alveolar walls depends on pulmonary blood flow, the cardiac output (liters per min.) equals O_2 absorption (cc. per minute) divided by the arterial O_2 minus the mixed venous O_2 (cc. per liter). **follicle-stimulating p.,** prolan A. **hematinic p.,** antianemia p. **immediate p.,** any one of the more or less complex substances of definite chemical constitution into which a heterogeneous substance can be readily resolved. **Le Chatelier p.,** if a biological system is subjected to stress, it will act in such a way as to reduce the stress. **luteinizing p.,** prolan B. **organic p.,** immediate p. **pleasure p.,** in freudian terminology, the automatic instinct or tendency to avoid pain and secure pleasure. **prothrombin converting p.,** in theoretical hematology, a principle in the plasma that converts prothrombin to thrombin. **proximate p.,** immediate p. **reality p.,** in freudian terminology, the mental activity which develops to control the pleasure principle under the pressure of necessity or the demands of reality. **ultimate p.,** a chemical element.

Pringle's disease (pring'g'lz) [John James *Pringle*, British dermatologist, 1855–1922] adenoma sebaceum.

Prinos verticellatus (pri'nos ver''tĭ-sil-la'tus) [Gr. *prinos* oak] *Ilex verticellata.*

Priscoline (pris'ko-lēn) trademark for preparations of tolazoline.

prism (prizm) [Gr. *prisma*] a solid with a triangular or polygonal cross section. A triangular prism splits up a ray of light into its constituent colors, and turns or deflects light rays toward its base. Prisms are used to correct deviations of the eyes, since they alter the apparent situation of objects. **adamantine p's, enamel p's,** prismata adamantina; see under *prisma.* **Maddox p.,** two prisms with their bases together; used in testing for torsion of the eyeball. **Nicol p.,** two slabs of Iceland spar cemented together and deflecting a ray of light in such a way that it is split in two, one part (the ordinary ray) being totally reflected and the other (polarized ray) passing through. **Risley's p.,** a prism which rotates in a metal frame marked with a scale; used in testing ocular muscles for imbalance.

prisma (priz'mah), pl. *pris'mata* [Gr.] prism. **pris'mata adaman'tina** [NA], adamantine or enamel prisms: the microscopic prisms or columns, arranged perpendicular to the surface, that make up the enamel of the teeth.

prismata (priz'mah-tah) plural of *prisma.*

prismatic (priz-mat'ik) shaped like a prism; produced by a prism.

prismoid (priz'moid) resembling a prism.

prismoptometer (priz''mop-tom'ĕ-ter) [*prism* + *optometer*] an instrument for testing the eye by means of a revolving prism.

prismosphere (priz''mo-sfēr) [*prism* + *sphere*] a prism combined with a globular lens.

prisoptometer (priz''op-tom'ĕ-ter) prismoptometer.

Privine (pri'vēn) trademark for preparations of naphazoline.

p.r.n. abbreviation for L. *pro re na'ta,* according as circumstances may require.

Pro proline.

pro- [L., Gr. *pro* before] 1. a prefix signifying before or in front of. 2. a prefix denoting a precursor, as of an enzyme or hormone.

proaccelerin (pro''ak-sel'er-in) Factor V; see *coagulation factors,* under *factor.*

pro-actinium (pro''ak-tin'e-um) protactinium.

Proactinomyces (pro''ak-tĭ-no-mi'sēz) *Nocardia.*

proactinomycin (pro-ak''tĭ-no-mi'sin) a group of antibiotic substances, designated A, B, and C, from cultures of *Nocardia gardneri,* which acts against gram-positive bacteria.

proactivator (pro-ak'tĭ-va''tor) the inactive precursor form of an activator, or a factor that requires a chemical change, usually by an enzyme, to become an activator, e.g., a substance present in plasma (*plasminogen proactivator*), which is absorbed onto fibrin during clotting and which, when activated, will convert plasminogen to plasmin.

proadifen hydrochloride (pro-ad'ĭ-fen) chemical name: 2-(diethylamino)ethyl-2,2-diphenylvalerate hydrochloride; a nonspecific synergist.

proagglutinoid (pro''ah-gloo'tĭ-noid) (*obs.*) an agglutinoid that has a stronger affinity for the agglutinogen than has the agglutinin.

proal (pro'al) characterized by forward movement.

proamnion (pro-am'ne-on) that part of the embryonal area at the front and side of the head which remains without mesoderm for some time.

proatlas (pro-at'las) a rudimentary vertebra which in some animals lies in front of the atlas; sometimes seen as an anomaly in man.

proazamine (pro-az'ah-mēn) promethazine.

probacteriophage (pro''bak-te're-o-fāj'') prophage.

proband (pro'band) [Ger.; from L. *probare* to prove] propositus.

probang (pro'bang) a flexible rod with a ball, tuft, or sponge at one end; used in applying medications to or removing matter from the esophagus or larynx. **ball p.,** a probang with a ball or bulb at the end. **bristle p., horse hair p.,** one with an expansible tuft of bristles or horse hairs at the end. **sponge p.,** one which is tufted with sponge at the end.

Pro-Banthine (pro-ban-thīn') trademark for preparations of propantheline bromide.

probarbital (pro-bar'bĭ-tal) chemical name 5-ethyl-5-(1-methylethyl)-2,4,6(1H,3H,5H)-pyrimidinetrione. A barbiturate of intermediate duration, $C_9H_{14}N_2O_3$, used as a sedative in the form of its calcium and sodium salts.

probe (prōb) [L. *proba; probare* to test] a slender, flexible instrument designed for introduction into a wound, cavity, or sinus tract for purposes of exploration. **Amussat's p.,** a probe used in lithotrity. **Anel's p.,** a delicate probe for the lacrimal puncta and canals. **blood flow p.,** an implanted cuff that fits around a surgically exposed artery or vein to detect blood flow. **blunt p.,** a probe with a blunt end. **Bowman's p.,** one of a set of probes for use on the nasal ducts. **Brackett's p's,** delicate and flexible probes of silver wire for exploring dental fistulas. **bullet p.,** one used for detecting the presence or determining the location of a bullet. **drum p.,** a probe with an attachment which emits a sound when it comes in contact with a foreign body. **electric p.,** one which on contact with a foreign body completes an electric circuit, thereby producing a sound. **eyed p.,** one with a slit near one end through which a ligature or tape may be drawn. **fiberoptic p.,** a flexible probe made up of a bundle of fine glass fibers optically aligned to transmit an image. **Girdner's p.,** an electric probe. **lacrimal p.,** one designed for use on the lacrimal passages. **Lente's p.,** a silver probe having a bulb coated with silver nitrate. **Lilienthal's p.,** an apparatus designed to explore for bullets. It consists of a probe composed of two or four pieces of metal attached to two insulated copper wires which run to a mouth piece consisting of two plates, one of copper and one of zinc. These plates are applied to the side of the tongue and the probe inserted in the wound. If the probe touches a bullet, a distinct metallic taste is perceived. **Lucae's p.,** a probe in a hollow handle, operated by a spring to apply massage in treating catarrhal otitis media. **meerschaum p.,** a probe with a meerschaum tip, which on contact with a lead bullet becomes darkened. **Nélaton's p.,** a bullet probe with an unglazed porcelain head. **pocket p.,** a dental instrument having a tapered, rodlike blade with a blunt, rounded tip and graduated in millimeters, used to measure the depth and determine the outline of a periodontal pocket. **scissors p.,** a long, delicate pair of scissors that can be used as a probe. **telephonic p.,** electric p. **uterine p.,** a probe for uterine exploration. **vertebrated p.,** a flexible probe made up of joined links. **wire p.,** a steel wire probe.

probenecid (pro-ben'ĕ-sid) [USP] chemical name: 4-[(dipropylamino)sulfonyl]benzoic acid. An oral uricosuric, $C_{13}H_{19}$-NO_4S, occurring as a white or nearly white, fine, crystalline powder; used in the treatment of hyperuricemia associated with gout and gouty arthritis and as an adjuvant to increase plasma levels of certain drugs, especially the penicillins.

probit (pro'bit) the normal deviate of the gaussian curve plus 5, the addition being made to avoid the use of negative numbers in the calculation of a 50 per cent end-point by the probit method. See also under *method.*

proboscis (pro-bos'is) [*pro-* + Gr. *boskein* to feed, graze] any tubular process or structure of the head or snout of an animal, usually used in feeding.

probucol (pro'bu-kōl) chemical name: 4,4'-[(1-methylethylidene)bis(thio)]bis[2,6-bis(1,1-dimethylethyl)phenol]. An anticholesteremic, $C_{31}H_{48}O_2S_2$, used especially as an adjunct to diet for the reduction of elevated serum cholesterol in primary cholesterolemia, administered orally.

procainamide· hydrochloride (pro-kān'ah-mīd) [USP] chemical name: 4-amino-N-(2-diethylaminoethyl)benzamide. A cardiac depressant, $C_{13}H_{21}N_3O·HCl$, occurring as a white to tan, crystalline powder; used in the treatment of cardiac arrhythmias, administered orally and intramuscularly, and by intravenous infusion. Called also *procaine amide hydrochloride.*

procaine (pro'kān) chemical name: 4-aminobenzoic acid 2-(diethylamino)ethyl ester; a local anesthetic, $C_{13}H_{20}N_2O_2$. **p. amide hydrochloride,** procainamide hydrochloride. **p. hydrochloride** [USP], the monohydrochloride salt of procaine, C_{13}-$H_{20}N_2O_2·HCl$, occurring as small white crystals or white crystalline powder; used to produce infiltration, epidural, and peripheral nerve block, and spinal anesthesia. **p. penicillin G,** see under *penicillin.*

procallus (pro-kal'us) the granulation tissue formed about the site of fracture of a bone, which develops into callus.

procarbazine hydrochloride (pro-kar'bah-zēn) [USP] chemical name: N-(1-methylethyl-4-[(2-methylhydrazino)methyl]benzamide monohydrochloride. An antineoplastic, $C_{12}H_{19}N_3$-$O·HCl$, occurring as a white to pale yellow, crystalline powder; used in the treatment of Hodgkin's disease, administered orally.

procarboxypeptidase (pro''kar-bok''se-pep'tĭ-dās) the inactive precursor of carboxypeptidase, which is converted to the active enzyme by the action of trypsin.

procarcinogen (pro''kar-sin'o-jen) a chemical substance that becomes carcinogenic only after it is altered by metabolic processes.

procaryosis (pro''kar-e-o'sis) prokaryosis.

Procaryotae (pro-kar″e-o′te) [pro- + Gr. *karyon* nucleus] in some systems of classification, a kingdom comprising all prokaryotic organisms, and separated into two divisions: the Cyanophyceae (blue-green algae, blue-green bacteria, or Cyanobacteria) and the Bacteria. Sometimes, prokaryotes without a true cell wall are considered to be unrelated to the Bacteria and have been placed in a separate class—the Mollicutes. Written also *Prokaryotae*. Cf. *Eucaryotae*.

procaryote (pro-kar′e-ōt) prokaryote.

procaryotic (pro″kar-e-ot′ik) prokaryotic.

procatarctic (pro″kah-tark′tik) predisposing: said of a cause of disease.

procatarxis (pro″kah-tark′sis) [Gr. *prokatarxis* a first beginning] 1. a predisposing cause. 2. predisposition. 3. the production of a disease partially as a result of predisposition.

procedure (pro-se′jur) [L. *procedere*, from *pro* forward + *cedere* move] a series of steps by which a desired result is accomplished. **Anderson p.,** reconstruction of the hypopharynx and cervical esophagus by the use of bilateral rectangular flaps. **Blair-Brown p.,** repair of a cleft lip by the use of a lateral flap one-half the length of the lip. **Bucknall's p.,** reconstruction of the urethra using skin flaps taken from the ventral surface of the penis and scrotum. **Denis Browne's p.,** a two stage operation for repair of hypospadias: the first stage consists of correction of the chordee and a meatotomy; the second stage is a urethroplasty. **Glenn p.,** anastomosis of the superior vena cava to the pulmonary artery for the treatment of tricuspid atresia. **Gomori-Takamatsu p.,** a method for localizing the alkaline phosphatase enzyme: a tissue secretion is incubated in a buffered solution containing the substrate, glycerophosphate, and calcium ions; hydrolysis of the substrate releases phosphoric acid, and it combines with calcium and precipitates as calcium phosphate. This colorless precipitate is converted to brown cobalt sulfide, which is readily visualized with the microscope. **Hartmann's p.,** resection of a diseased portion of the colon, with the proximal end of the colon brought out as a colostomy and the distal stump or rectum being closed by suture. Bowel continuity can later be restored. Called also *Hartmann's colostomy* or *operation*. **Heller p.,** pyloromyotomy or other drainage procedure combined with the surgery on the esopohagogastric junction. **Hunt-Transley p.,** a suspension procedure for ptosis of the upper eyelid; a vertical strip of lid skin with its lower end attached to the lid margin is raised, and a transverse ellipse of skin between the lid margin and eyebrow is excised. The distal portion of the skin strip is then denuded of epithelium and the strip is tunneled under the eyebrow area. The excess portion of the skin strip is excised and the wound is closed. **lip-switch p.,** a procedure which makes a tightly contracted repaired cleft lip more pliable and esthetically pleasing: a full thickness triangular flap of tissue from the lower lip with a pedicle containing the inferior labial artery is elevated and transferred by rotation to the upper lip. **push-back p.,** a surgical maneuver designed to reposition the soft palate posteriorly and reestablish velopharyngeal competence. **Rochet's p.,** reconstruction of the urethra using a tubed pedicle flap taken from the scrotum. **Swenson's p.,** a procedure for the treatment of obstinate constipation in newborn infants in which the aganglionic segment of colon is resected near the anus, with end-to-end anastomosis of the normally innervated upper colon to the stump of the rectum just inside the anus. **V-Y p.,** a method of repairing a skin defect in which a V-shaped incision is made next to the defect, creating a flap; the flap is transferred to the defect and closed; and the secondary defect thus created is closed with a Y-shaped suture.

procelous (pro-se′lus) [pro- + Gr. *koilos* hollow] concave on the anterior surface; applied to the vertebral centra of certain animals.

procentriole (pro-sen′tre-ol) the immediate precursor of centrioles and ciliary basal bodies; it is developed in proximity to either a preexisting centriole or a deuterosome.

procephalic (pro″sĕ-fal′ik) [pro- + Gr. *kephalē* head] pertaining to the anterior part of the head.

procercoid (pro-ser′koid) one of the larval stages of fish tapeworms.

procerus (pro-se′rus) [L.] long; slender.

process (pros′es; pro′ses) [L. *processus*] 1. a prominence or projection, as of bone; for names of specific anatomical structures, see official Latinized terms under *processus*. 2. a series of operations, events, or steps leading to the achievement of a specific result; used also as a verb to designate subjection to such a series designed to produce desired changes in the original material, or achieve other result. **A.B.C. p.,** see under *method*. **accessory p. of sacrum, spurious,** crista sacralis lateralis. **acromial p. of sacrum, spurious,** crista sacralis lateralis. **acromial p.,** acromion. **acute p. of helix,** spina helicis. **alar p. of sacrum,** crista sacralis lateralis. **aliform p. of sphenoid bone,** ala minor ossis sphenoidalis. **alveolar p.,** that portion of bone in either the maxilla or the mandible which surrounds and supports the teeth. In the maxilla, it is called *processus alveolaris maxillae* (q.v.); in the mandible, *pars alveolaris mandibulae.* **anconeal p. of ulna,** olecranon. **angular p. of frontal bone, external,** processus

zygomaticus ossis frontalis. **articular p. of axis, anterior,** facies articularis anterior axis. **articular p. of coccyx, false,** cornu coccygeum. **articular p. of sacrum, spurious,** crista sacralis intermedia. **ascending p's of vertebrae,** see *processus articularis superior vertebrarum*. **axis-cylinder p.,** axon. **basilar p.,** pars basilaris ossis occipitalis. **Beccari p.,** a method of garbage disposal involving bacterial fermentation in closed cells. **p. of Blumenbach,** processus uncinatus ossis ethmoidalis. **capitular p.,** the articular process on a vertebra for the head of a rib. **p. of cartilage of nasal septum, posterior,** processus posterior sphenoidalis. **caudate p.,** processus caudatus hepatis. **ciliary p's,** processus ciliares. **Civinini's p. of external pterygoid plate,** processus pterygospinosus. **clinoid p.,** any of three processes of the sphenoid bone; see *processus clinoideus anterior, medius,* and *posterior*. **condyloid p. of vertebrae, inferior,** processus articularis inferior vertebrarum. **condyloid p. of vertebrae, superior,** processus articularis superior vertebrarum. **conoid p.,** tuberculum conoideum. **coracoid p.,** processus coracoideus scapulae. **coronoid p.,** see entries beginning *processus coronoideus*. **cubital p. of humerus,** see *trochlea humeri* and *capitulum humeri*. **Deiters' p.,** axon, def. 2. **dendritic p.,** the branched process of a nerve cell; a dendrite. **dental p.,** processus alveolaris maxillae. **dentoid p. of axis,** dens axis. **descending p's of vertebrae,** see *processus articularis inferior vertebrarum*. **ensiform p. of sphenoid bone,** ala minor ossis sphenoidalis. **ensiform p. of sternum,** processus xiphoideus. **epiphyseal p.,** epiphysis. **ethmoidal p. of Macalister,** crista sphenoidalis. **falciform p. of cerebellum,** falx cerebelli. **falciform p. of cerebrum,** falx cerebri. **falciform p. of fascia lata,** margo falciformis hiatus saphenus. **falciform p. of fascia pelvis,** arcus tendineus fasciae pelvis. **falciform p. of rectus abdominis muscle,** falx inguinalis. **floccular p.,** flocculus, def. 2. **folian p., p. of Folius,** processus anterior mallei. **foot p.,** pedicel. **frontal p., external,** spina nasalis ossis frontalis. **frontonasal p.,** an expansive facial process in the embryo, which develops into the forehead and bridge of the nose. **funicular p.,** the portion of the tunica vaginalis surrounding the spermatic cord. **Gottstein's basal p.,** any attenuated basal process connecting the basilar membrane with an outer hair cell of the organ of Corti. **greater p. of ethmoid bone, hamate p. of ethmoid bone,** processus uncinatus ossis ethmoidalis. **hamular p. of lacrimal bone,** hamulus lacrimalis. **hamular p. of sphenoid bone,** hamulus pterygoideus. **hamular p. of unciform bone,** hamulus ossis hamati. **head p.,** an axial strand of cells in the embryo extending forward from the primitive knot; called also *notochordal plate*. **inframalleolar p. of calcaneus,** trochlea peronealis calcanei. **infundibular p.,** see *pituitary gland,* under *gland.* **Ingrassias' p.,** ala minor ossis sphenoidalis. **intercondylar p. of tibia,** eminentia intercondylaris. **internal p. of humerus,** processus supracondylaris humeri. **jugular p. of occipital bone, lateral,** processus paramastoideus ossis occipitalis. **jugular p. of occipital bone, middle,** processus intrajugularis ossis occipitalis. **jugular p. of occipital bone, posterior, of Krause,** processus paramastoideus ossis occipitalis. **lacrimal p.,** a process of the inferior nasal concha that articulates with the lacrimal bone. **lateral p. of calcaneus,** sustentaculum tali. **MacLachlan's p.,** see under *method.* **malar p.,** processus zygomaticus maxillae. **mamillary p's of sacrum, oblique,** see *crista sacralis intermedia.* **mamillary p. of temporal bone,** processus mastoideus ossis temporalis. **mandibular p.,** the ventral process formed by bifurcation of the first branchial arch (mandibular arch) in the embryo, which unites ventrally with its fellow to form the lower jaw. **marginal p. of malar bone,** tuberculum marginale ossis zygomatici. **mastoid p.,** processus mastoideus ossis temporalis. **maxillary p.,** the dorsal process formed by bifurcation of the first branchial arch in the embryo, which joins with the ipsilateral median nasal process in the formation of the upper jaw. **mental p.,** protuberantia mentalis. **nasal p., lateral,** the lateral one of the two limbs of the horseshoe-shaped elevation bounding a nasal pit in the embryo, which participates in formation of the side and wing of the nose. **nasal p., median,** the central one of the two limbs of the horseshoe-shaped elevation bounding a nasal pit in the embryo, which participates with the ipsilateral maxillary process in forming half of the upper jaw. **nasal p. of frontal bone,** pars nasalis ossis frontalis. **nasal p. of inferior turbinate bone,** processus lacrimalis conchae nasalis inferioris. **oblique p. of vertebrae, inferior,** processus articularis inferior vertebrarum. **oblique p. of vertebrae, superior,** processus articularis superior vertebrarum. **occipital p. of occipital bone,** pars basilaris ossis occipitalis. **odontoid p. of axis,** dens axis. **olecranon p. of ulna,** olecranon. **olivary p.** (*obs.*), tuberculum sellae turcicae. **palatine p., lateral,** a shelflike projection developing from each maxillary process region of the upper jaw in the embryo, later fusing with each other and with the nasal septum to form the palate. **palatine p., median,** a shelflike projection developing from each median nasal process in the embryo, which participates with its fellow in forming the premaxillary portion of the upper jaw. **palpebral p.,** pars palpebralis glandulae lacrimalis. **paracondyloid p. of occipital bone, paroccipital p. of occipital bone,** processus paramastoideus ossis occipitalis. **petrosal p., anterior,** lingula sphenoidalis. **petrosal p., middle,** processus clinoideus medius. **petrosal p., posterior superior,** processus clinoideus posterior. **pterygoid p.,** processus pyerygoideus ossis sphenoidalis. **Rau's p., ravian p.,** processus anterior mallei. **restiform p. of Henle,** pedunculus cerebellaris inferior. **small p. of Soemmering,** tuberculum marginale ossis zygomatici. **spinous p.,** a slender, more or less sharp-pointed projection; see *spina.* **spinous p. of sacrum, spurious,** crista sacralis mediana. **spinous p. of tibia,** 1. eminentia intercondylaris. 2. tuberculum intercondylare mediale. **spinous p. of vertebrae,** processus spinosus vertebrarum. **Stieda's p.,** processus posterior tali. **styloid p. of fibula,** apex capitis fibulae. **sucker p.,** see under *foot.* **synovial p.,** plica synovialis. **temporal p. of mandible,** processus coronoideus mandibulae. **Todd's p.,** see *fibrae intercrurales.* **Tomes' p.,** a cytoplasmic process of the ameloblasts, or enamel-forming cells, around which calcification of enamel occurs. **transverse p. of sacrum,** crista sacralis lateralis. **transverse p. of vertebrae, accessory,** processus accessorius vertebrarum lumbalium. **trochlear p. of calcaneus,** trochlea peronealis calcanei. **uncifuorm p. of scapula,** processus coracoideus scapulae. **uncinate p. of ethmoid bone,** processus uncinatus ossis ethmoidalis. **uncinate p. of lacrimal bone,** hamulus lacrimalis. **uncinate p. of pancreas,** processus uncinatus pancreatis. **uncinate p. of unciform bone,** hamulus ossis hamati. **uncinate p's of vertebra,** hook-shaped processes on the lateral borders of the superior surface of the bodies of vertebrae C3 to T1; they are frequent sites of formation of spurs (osteophytes), leading to spondylosis uncovertebralis. **ungual p. of third phalanx of foot,** tuberositas phalangis distalis pedis. **vermiform p.,** appendix vermiformis. **vermiform p. of cerebellum,** vermis cerebelli. **xiphoid p.,** the pointed process of cartilage, supported by a core of bone, connected with the lower end of the body of the sternum; called also *processus xiphoideus* and *xiphisternum.* **xiphoid p. of sphenoid bone,** ala minor ossis sphenoidalis. **zygomatico-orbital p. of maxilla,** processus zygomaticus maxillae.

processus (pro-ses′us), pl. *processus* [L.] a process: a prominence or projection; [NA] a general term for such a mass projecting from a larger structure. **p. accesso′rii spur′ii,** crista sacralis lateralis. **p. accesso′rius vertebra′rum lumba′lium** [NA], accessory process of lumbar vertebrae: a small nodule that projects backward from the posterior surface of the transverse process of a lumbar vertebra. It is situated lateral to and below the mamillary process and varies in size. **p. ala′ris os′sis ethmoida′lis,** ala cristae galli. **p. alveola′ris maxil′lae** [NA], alveolar process of maxilla: the thick parabolically curved ridge that projects downward and forms the free lower border of the maxilla; it is in front of and lateral to the palatine process and it bears the teeth. Called also *dental process.* **p. ante′rior mal′lei** [NA], **p. ante′rior mal′lei [Fo′lii],** anterior process of malleus: a slender process that arises from the anterior aspect of the neck of the malleus, passes anteriorly and inferiorly to the petrotympanic fissure, and is attached to the petrous portion of the temporal bone by ligamentous fibers. **p. articula′res inferio′res vertebra′rum,** see *p. articularis inferior vertebrarum.* **p. articula′ris infe′rior vertebra′rum** [NA], inferior articular process of vertebrae: a process on either side of the vertebrae, springing from the inferior surface of the arch near the junction of the lamina and pedicle; it bears a surface that faces anteriorly and inferiorly, articulating with the superior articular process of the vertebra below. Called also *zygapophysis* [NA alternative]. **p. articula′ris supe′rior os′sis sa′cri** [NA], superior articular process of sacrum: either of two processes projecting backward and medialward from the first sacral vertebra at the junctions between the body and the alae; they articulate with the inferior articular processes of the fifth lumbar vertebra. **p. articula′res superio′res vertebra′rum,** see *p. articularis superior vertebrarum.* **p. articula′ris supe′rior vertebra′rum** [NA], superior articular process of vertebrae: a process on either side of the vertebrae, springing from the superior surface of the arch near the junction of the lamina and pedicle; it bears a surface that faces posteriorly and superiorly, articulating with the inferior articular process of the vertebra above. **p. bre′vis incu′dis,** ligamentum incudis superius. **p. bre′vis mal′lei,** p. lateralis mallei. **p. cauda′tus hep′atis** [NA], caudate process: the right of the two processes seen on the caudate lobe of the liver. **p. cilia′res** [NA], ciliary processes: about 70 meridionally arranged ridges or folds projecting from the crown of the ciliary body; they secrete the aqueous humor into the posterior chamber of the eye. **p. clinoi′deus ante′rior** [NA], anterior clinoid process: the bony process found on the medial extremity of the posterior border of the small wing of the sphenoid bone. **p. clinoi′deus me′dius** [NA], middle clinoid process: either of two small inconstant eminences on the internal surface of the sphenoid bone, one on either side of the anterior part of the hypophyseal fossa.

p. clinoi′deus poste′rior [NA], posterior clinoid process: either of two tubercles found on the superior angle of either side of the dorsum sellae of the sphenoid bone, and giving attachment to the tentorium of the cerebellum. **p. cochlearifor′mis** [NA], cochleariform process: a small hollow cone of bone at the end of the semicanalis tubae auditivae, just anterior to the vestibular window, with an opening through which the tendon of the tensor tympani passes. **p. condyla′ris mandib′ulae** [NA], **p. condyloi′deus mandib′ulae,** condylar process of mandible: the posterior process on the ramus of the mandible that articulates with the mandibular fossa of the temporal bone. **p. coracoi′deus scap′ulae** [NA], coracoid process of scapula: a strong curved process that arises from the upper part of the neck of the scapula and overhangs the shoulder joint. **p. coronoi′deus mandib′ulae** [NA], coronoid process of mandible: the anterior part of the upper end of the ramus of the mandible, to which the temporal muscle is attached. **p. coronoi′deus ul′nae** [NA], coronoid process of ulna: a wide eminence at the proximal end of the ulna, forming the anterior and inferior part of the trochlear incisure. **p. costa′rius ver′tebrae** [NA], costal process of vertebra: in a cervical vertebra, the part of the transverse process anterior to the transverse foramen. **p. e cerebel′lo ad medul′lam,** pedunculus cerebellaris inferior. **p. e cerebel′lo ad pon′tem,** pedunculus cerebellaris medius. **p. e cerebel′lo ad tes′tes,** pedunculus cerebellaris superior. **p. ethmoida′lis con′chae nasa′lis inferio′ris** [NA], ethmoidal process of inferior nasal concha: a bony projection above and behind the maxillary process of the inferior nasal concha. **p. falcifor′mis ligamen′ti sacrotubero′si** [NA], falciform process of sacrotuberal ligament: a prolongation of the sacrotuberal ligament, continuing forward along the inner border of the ramus of the ischium from the point of attachment of the ligament on the tuber of the ischium. **p. Ferrei′ni lob′uli cortica′lis re′nis,** pars radiata lobuli corticalis renis. **p. fronta′lis maxil′lae** [NA], frontal process of maxilla: a large, strong, irregular process of bone that projects upward from the body of the maxilla, its medial surface forming part of the lateral wall of the nasal cavity. **p. fronta′lis os′sis zygomat′ici** [NA], **p. frontosphenoida′lis os′sis zygomat′ici,** frontal process of zygomatic bone: the strong, upward projecting triangular process of the zygomatic bone lying behind the malar surface and between the orbital and temporal surfaces; it unites above with the zygomatic process of the frontal bone and behind with the great wing of the sphenoid bone. **p. gra′cilis,** p. anterior mallei. **p. of Ingrassias,** ala minor ossis sphenoidalis. **p. intrajugula′ris os′sis occipita′lis** [NA], intrajugular process of occipital bone: a small process that subdivides the jugular notch of the occipital bone into a lateral and a medial part. **p. intrajugula′ris os′sis tempora′lis** [NA], intrajugular process of temporal bone: a small ridge on the petrous part of the temporal bone that separates the jugular notch into a medial and a lateral part, corresponding to similar parts of the jugular notch of the facing occipital bone. **p. jugula′ris os′sis occipita′lis** [NA], jugular process of occipital bone: either of two processes on the occipital bone that project laterally from the occipital condyles and form the posterior boundary of the jugular foramen. **p. lacrima′lis con′chae nasa′lis inferio′ris** [NA], lacrimal process of inferior nasal concha: a process of the inferior nasal concha that articulates with the lacrimal bone. **p. latera′lis mal′lei** [NA], lateral process of malleus: a small tapered process that projects laterally from the base of the manubrium mallei and produces the mallear prominence. **p. latera′lis ta′li** [NA], lateral process of talus: a large low process on the lateral surface of the talus, articulating with the lateral malleolus. **p. latera′lis tu′beris calca′nei** [NA], lateral process of tuberosity of calcaneus: a rough process projecting downward from the lower lateral portion of the tuber calcanei. **p. lenticula′ris incu′dis** [NA], lenticular process of incus: a small process on the medial side of the tip of the long limb of the incus, which articulates with the head of the stapes. **p. mamilla′ris vertebra′rum** [NA], mamillary process of vertebrae: a tubercle on each superior articular process of the lumbar vertebrae. **p. margina′lis os′sis zygomat′ici,** tuberculum marginale ossis zygomatici. **p. mastoi′deus os′sis tempora′lis** [NA], mastoid process of temporal bone: a conical process projecting forward and downward from the external surface of the petrous part of the temporal bone just posterior to the external acoustic meatus. **p. maxilla′ris con′chae nasa′lis inferio′ris** [NA], maxillary process of inferior nasal concha: a bony process descending from the ethmoid process of the inferior nasal concha. **p. media′lis tu′beris calca′nei** [NA], medial process of tuberosity of calcaneus: a rough process projecting downward from the lower medial portion of the tuber calcanei. **p. muscula′ris cartilag′inis arytenoi′deae** [NA], muscular process of arytenoid cartilage: the lateral and posterior lower angular projection of the arytenoid cartilage to which the cricoarytenoid muscles are attached. **p. orbita′lis os′sis palati′ni** [NA], orbital process of palatine bone: a pyramidal process on the uppermost part of the palatine bone, one surface of it forming the posterior angle of the floor of the orbit. **p. palati′nus maxil′lae** [NA], palatine process of maxilla: a horizontally arched plate of bone that helps to form the lower part of the maxilla and with its fellow of

the opposite side the anterior two-thirds of the hard palate.
p. papilla′ris hep′atis [NA], papillary process of liver: the left of the two processes seen on the caudate lobe of the liver. **p. paramastoi′deus os′sis occipita′lis** [NA], paramastoid process of occipital bone: a process that in man is represented by a tubercle on the under surface of the jugular process. **p. poste′rior sphenoida′lis** [NA], posterior process of cartilage of nasal septum: a narrow flat strip of cartilage that extends backward and upward along the groove on the upper margin of the vomer and below the perpendicular plate of the ethmoid bone, from the septal cartilage nearly to the sphenoid bone. Called also *p. sphenoidalis septi cartilaginei.* **p. poste′rior ta′li** [NA], posterior process of talus: a backward projection from the posterior portion of the talus, divided into two unequal parts by the sulcus tendinis musculi flexoris hallucis longi tali. **p. pterygoi′deus os′sis sphenoida′lis** [NA], pterygoid process of sphenoid bone: either of two processes on the sphenoid bone descending from the points of junction of the great wings and body of the bone, and each consisting of a lateral and a medial plate. **p. pterygospino′sus** [NA], **p. pterygospino′sus [Civini′ni]**, pterygospinous process: a small spine on the posterior edge of the lateral pterygoid plate of the sphenoid bone, giving attachment to the pterygospinous ligament. **p. pyramida′lis os′sis palati′ni** [NA], pyramidal process of palatine bone: a strong process projecting downward, backward, and laterally from the lateral part of the posterior margin of the palatine bone and helping to form the pterygoid fossa. **p. retromandibula′ris glan′dulae parot′idis,** an irregularly wedge-shaped portion of the parotid gland passing medially behind the ramus of the mandible almost to the wall of the pharynx. **p. sphenoida′lis os′sis palati′ni** [NA], sphenoid process of palatine bone: an irregular mass of bone that projects upward and medially from the posterior portion of the superior margin of the perpendicular portion of the palatine bone, and articulates with the body of the sphenoid bone and with the ala vomeris. **p. sphenoida′lis sep′ti cartilagin′ei,** processus posterior sphenoidalis. **p. spino′sus vertebra′rum** [NA], spinous process of vertebrae: a part of the vertebrae projecting backward from the arch, giving attachment to muscles of the back. **p. styloi′deus fib′ulae,** apex capitis fibulae. **p. styloi′deus os′sis metacarpa′lis III** [NA], styloid process of third metacarpal bone: a prominent process projecting proximally from the base of the third metacarpal bone. **p. styloi′deus os′sis tempora′lis** [NA], styloid process of temporal bone: a long spine projecting downward from the inferior surface of the temporal bone just anterior to the stylomastoid foramen, giving attachment to three muscles and two ligaments. **p. styloi′deus ra′dii** [NA], styloid process of radius: a blunt projection from the lateral surface of the distal end of the radius. **p. styloi′deus ul′nae** [NA], styloid process of ulna: the medial, non-articular process on the distal extremity of the ulna. **p. supracondyla′ris hu′meri** [NA], **p. supracondyloi′deus hu′meri,** supracondylar process of humerus: a small inconstant process just proximal to the medial epicondyle of the humerus. **p. tempora′lis os′sis zygomat′ici** [NA], temporal process of zygomatic bone: the posterior blunt process of the zygomatic bone that articulates with the zygomatic process of the temporal bone. **p. transver′sus vertebra′rum** [NA], transverse process of vertebrae: a process on either side of the vertebrae, projecting laterally from the junction between the lamina and the pedicle. **p. trochlea′ris calca′nei,** trochlea peronealis calcanei. **p. uncina′tus os′sis ethmoida′lis** [NA], uncinate process of ethmoid bone: a curved plate of bone that extends inferiorly and posteriorly from the anterior part of the ethmoid labyrinth. **p. uncina′tus pancrea′tis** [NA], uncinate process of pancreas: the left and caudal part of the head of the pancreas, which hooks around behind the pancreatic vessels; called also *Winslow's pancreas.* **p. vagina′lis os′sis sphenoida′lis** [NA], vaginal process of sphenoid bone: a small plate on the inferior surface of the body of the sphenoid bone on either side, running medially from the medial pterygoid plate to articulate with the ala of the vomer and with the sphenoid process of the palatine bone. **p. vagina′lis peritone′i** [NA], a diverticulum of the peritoneal membrane extending into the inguinal canal, accompanying the round ligament in the female, or the testis in its descent into the scrotum in the male (*processus vaginalis testis*); usually completely obliterated in the female. Called also *canal of Nuck* or *Nuck's diverticulum.* **p. vermifor′mis,** appendix vermiformis. **p. voca′lis** [NA], vocal process: the process of the arytenoid cartilage to which the vocal ligament is attached. **p. xiphoi′deus** [NA], xiphoid process: the pointed process of cartilage, supported by a core of bone, connected with the lower end of the body of the sternum. **p. zygomat′icus maxil′lae** [NA], zygomatic process of maxilla: the rough triangular eminence that articulates with the zygomatic bone and marks the separation of the facies anterior, infratemporalis, and orbitalis. **p. zygomat′icus os′sis fronta′lis** [NA], zygomatic process of frontal bone: a thick, strong process of the frontal bone, situated at the lateral end of the supraorbital margin and articulating with the zygomatic bone, and from which the temporal line starts. **p. zygomat′icus os′sis tempora′lis** [NA], zygomatic process of temporal bone: a long, strong process arising from the lower portion of the squamous part of the temporal bone, passing forward from just

above the entrance of the external acoustic meatus to join the zygomatic bone and thus forming the zygomatic arch.

procheilon (pro-ki′lon) [*pro-* + Gr. *cheilon* lip + *-on* neuter ending] the central prominence of the upper border between the skin and the mucous membrane of the upper lip, marking the distal termination of the philtrum (tuberculum labii superioris [NA]).

prochlorpemazine (pro″klōr-pem′ah-zēn) prochlorperazine.

prochlorperazine (pro″klōr-per′ah-zēn) [USP] chemical name: 2-chloro-10-[3-(4-methyl-1-piperazinyl)propyl]-10*H*-phenothiazine. A phenothiazine derivative, $C_{20}H_{24}ClN_3S$, occurring as a clear, pale yellow, viscous liquid; used chiefly as an antiemetic, administered rectally. Called also *prochlorpemazine.* **p. edisylate** [USP], the ethanedisulfonate salt of prochlorperazine, occurring as a white to very light yellow, crystalline powder; used as an antiemetic and tranquilizer, administered orally, intramuscularly, and intravenously. **p. maleate** [USP], the maleate salt of prochlorperazine, occurring as a white or pale yellow, crystalline powder; used as an antiemetic and tranquilizer, administered orally.

prochondral (pro-kon′dral) occurring previous to the formation of cartilage.

prochordal (pro-kor′dal) in front of the notochord.

prochorion (pro-ko′re-on) [Gr. *pro-* before + *chorion* skin] an old term for the noncellular covering of the dog egg; it has tufts that are casts of uterine glands producing secretion, but were once mistakenly thought to resemble chorionic villi and to be their predecessors.

Prochownick's diet, method (pro-kov′niks) [Ludwig *Prochownick,* German obstetrician, 1851–1923] see under *diet* and *method.*

prochromatin (pro-kro′mah-tin) the substance composing the true nucleoli; paranuclein.

prochromosome (pro-kro′mo-sōm) a chromosome-like body occurring in resting nuclei.

prochymosin (pro-ki′mo-sin) renninogen.

procidentia (pro″si-den′she-ah) [L.] a prolapse, or falling down, especially prolapse of the uterus to such a degree that the cervix protrudes from the vaginal outlet. See also *prolapse.*

procinonide (pro-sin′o-nīd) chemical name: 6α,9-difluoro-11β-hydroxy-16α,17-[(1-methylethylidene)bis(oxy)]-21-(1-oxopropoxy)pregna-1,4-diene-3,20-dione; an adrenocortical steroid, $C_{27}H_{34}F_2O_7$.

procoagulant (pro″ko-ag′u-lant) 1. tending to favor the occurrence of coagulation. 2. a precursor of a natural substance necessary to coagulation of the blood.

procoelia (pro-se′le-ah) [*pro-* + Gr. *koilia* hollow] (*obs.*) ventriculus lateralis cerebri.

procollagen (pro-kol′ah-jen) the precursor molecule of collagen, synthesized in the fibroblast, osteoblast, etc., and cleaved to form collagen extracellularly.

procollagenase (pro″ko-laj′ĕ-nās) the inactive precursor of collagenase.

proconceptive (pro″kon-sep′tiv) 1. aiding or favoring conception. 2. an agent that facilitates or promotes conception.

proconvertin (pro″kon-ver′tin) Factor VII; see *coagulation factors,* under *factor.*

procreation (pro″kre-a′shun) [L. *procreatio*] the entire process of bringing a new individual into the world.

procreative (pro′kre-a″tiv) concerned in procreation; able to beget.

proct- see *procto-.*

proctalgia (prok-tal′je-ah) [*proct-* + *-algia*] neuralgia of the lower rectum. **p. fu′gax,** episodic severe pain in the rectum, often awakening the individual at night; it is attributed to spasm of the levator ani and coccygeal muscles.

proctatresia (prok″tah-tre′ze-ah) [*proct-* + *a* neg. + Gr. *trēsis* perforation] imperforation of the anus.

proctectasia (prok″tek-ta′ze-ah) [*proct-* + Gr. *ektasis* dilatation + *-ia*] dilatation of the rectum or of the anus.

proctectomy (prok-tek′to-me) [*proct-* + Gr. *ektomē* excision] surgical removal of the rectum.

proctencleisis (prok″ten-kli′sis) [*proct-* + Gr. *enkleiein* to shut in] constriction, or stenosis, of the lower rectum; a rectal stricture.

procteurynter (prok″tu-rin″ter) [*proct-* + Gr. *eurynein* to widen] a baglike device used in dilating the rectum.

procteurysis (prok-tu′rĭ-sis) dilatation of the rectum by means of a procteurynter.

proctitis (prok-ti′tis) [*proct-* + *-itis*] inflammation of the rectum. **epidemic gangrenous p.,** a disease of the northern part of South America and the Fiji and other islands of the South Pacific, marked by rapidly spreading ulceration of the anus and lower bowel, with bloody discharges, fever, and great prostration. **factitial p.,** radiation p. **radiation p.,** proctitis resulting from radiation therapy, as of the cervix or uterus, marked by tenesmus, pain, rectal bleeding, and diarrhea and by telangiectasis, it may progress to ulceration. Called also *factitial p.*

procto-, proct- [Gr. *prōktos* anus, hence the hinder parts] combining form designating relationship to the rectum.

proctocele (prok'to-sēl) [*procto-* + Gr. *kēlē* hernia] rectocele.

proctoclysis (prok-tok'lĭ-sis) [*procto-* + Gr. *klysis* a drenching] the slow introduction of large quantities of liquid into the rectum; called also *Murphy drip*. See *Murphy's method* (2d def.), under *method*.

proctococcypexy (prok"to-kok'sĭ-pek"se) [*procto-* + Gr. *kokkyx* coccyx + *pēxis* fixation] fixation of the rectum to the coccyx by sutures.

proctocolectomy (prok"to-ko-lek'to-me) surgical removal of the rectum and colon.

proctocolitis (prok"to-ko-li'tis) coloproctitis.

proctocolonoscopy (prok"to-ko"lon-os'ko-pe) the inspection of the interior of the rectum and lower portion of the colon.

proctocolpoplasty (prok"to-kol'po-plas"te) [*procto-* + Gr. *kolpos* vagina + *plassein* to form] operative closure of a rectovaginal fistula.

proctocystoplasty (prok"to-sis'to-plas"te) [*procto-* + Gr. *kystis* bladder + *plassein* to form] a plastic operation on the rectum and bladder; operative closure of a rectovesical fistula.

proctocystotomy (prok"to-sis-tot'o-me) [*procto-* + Gr. *kystis* bladder + *tomē* a cutting] the rectovesical operation for stone in the bladder.

proctodaeum (prok"to-de'um) proctodeum.

proctodeum (prok"to-de'um) [*proct-* + Gr. *hodaios* pertaining to a way] an invagination of the ectoderm of the embryo at the point where later the anus is formed; called also *anal pit*.

proctodone (prok'to-dōn) a hormone said to be secreted by cells of the anterior intestine of insects and to terminate diapause.

proctodynia (prok"to-din'e-ah) [*proct-* + Gr. *odynē* pain] pain in or about the anus.

Proctofoam-HC (prok'to-fōm) trademark for an aerosol foam containing 1 per cent hydrocortisone acetate and 1 per cent pramoxine hydrochloride; used to relieve anorectal inflammation, pain, swelling, and pruritus.

proctogenic (prok"to-jen'ik) [*procto-* + Gr. *gennan* to produce] derived from the anus or rectum.

proctologic (prok"to-loj'ik) pertaining to proctology.

proctologist (prok-tol'o-jist) a physician who specializes in proctology.

proctology (prok-tol'o-je) [*procto-* + *-logy*] the branch of medicine concerned with disorders of the rectum and anus.

proctoparalysis (prok"to-pah-ral'ĭ-sis) [*procto-* + *paralysis*] paralysis of the muscles of the anus and rectum.

proctoperineoplasty (prok"to-per"ĭ-ne'o-plas"te) plastic repair of the anus and perineum.

proctoperineorrhaphy (prok"to-per"ĭ-ne-or'ah-fe) proctoperineoplasty.

proctopexy (prok'to-pek"se) [*procto-* + Gr. *pexis* fixation] fixation of the rectum to some adjacent tissue or organ by suture.

proctoplasty (prok'to-plas"te) [*procto-* + Gr. *plassein* to form] plastic surgery of the rectum.

proctoplegia (prok"to-ple'je-ah) [*procto-* + Gr. *plēgē* stroke] proctoparalysis.

proctopolypus (prok"to-pol'ĭ-pus) [*procto-* + *polypus*] polyp of the rectum.

proctoptoma (prok"top-to'mah) (*obs.*) proctoptosis.

proctoptosis (prok"top-to'sis) [*procto-* + Gr. *ptōsis* fall] prolapse of the anus.

proctorrhagia (prok"to-ra'je-ah) bleeding from the rectum.

proctorrhaphy (prok-tor'ah-fe) [*procto-* + Gr. *rhaphē* seam] surgical repair of the rectum.

proctorrhea (prok"to-re'ah) [*procto-* + Gr. *rhoia* flow] a mucous discharge from the anus.

proctoscope (prok'to-skōp) [*procto-* + Gr. *skopein* to examine] a speculum or tubular instrument with appropriate illumination for inspecting the rectum. **Tuttle's p.,** a rectal speculum with an electric light at its extremity and an arrangement for inflating the rectal ampulla.

proctoscopy (prok-tos'ko-pe) [*procto-* + Gr. *skopein* to examine] inspection of the rectum with a proctoscope.

proctosigmoid (prok"to-sig'moid) the rectum and sigmoid colon.

proctosigmoidectomy (prok"to-sig"moi-dek'to-me) [*procto-* + *sigmoid* + Gr. *ektomē* excision] excision of the anus, rectum, and sigmoid flexure.

proctosigmoiditis (prok"to-sig"moi-di'tis) inflammation of the rectum and sigmoid.

proctosigmoidopexy (prok"to-sig-moid'o-pek"se) the surgical fixation of the rectum and sigmoid colon.

proctosigmoidoscope (prok"to-sig-moid'o-skōp) an instrument for illuminating and viewing the rectum and sigmoid colon.

proctosigmoidoscopy (prok"to-sig"moi-dos'ko-pe) examination of the rectum and sigmoid with the sigmoidoscope.

proctospasm (prok'to-spazm) [*procto-* + *spasm*] spasm of the rectum.

proctostasis (prok-tos'tah-sis) [*procto-* + Gr. *stasis* stoppage] constipation due to anesthesia of the rectum to the stimulus of defecation.

proctostenosis (prok"to-stĕ-no'sis) [*procto-* + Gr. *stenōsis* narrowing] stricture of the rectum.

proctostomy (prok-tos'to-me) [*procto-* + Gr. *stomoun* to provide with an opening, or mouth] surgical creation of a permanent artificial opening from the body surface into the rectum.

proctotome (prok'to-tōm) a knife for proctotomy.

proctotomy (prok-tot'o-me) [*procto-* + Gr. *tomē* a cutting] incision into the rectum, as for relief of rectal stricture. **external p.,** that done on or near the sphincter. **internal p.,** transabdominal incision of the rectum from within above the sphincter.

proctotoreusis (prok"to-to-roo'sis) [*procto-* + Gr. *toreusis* boring] the construction of an artificial anus.

proctotresia (prok-to-tre'se-ah) proctotoreusis.

proctovalvotomy (prok"to-val-vot'o-me) incision of the rectal valves.

procumbent (pro-kum'bent) lying on the face; prone.

procursive (pro-kur'siv) [L. *procursivus*] characterized by a tendency to run forward.

procurvation (pro"kur-va'shun) [L. *procurvare* to bend forward] a bending forward, as of the body.

procuticle (pro-ku'tĭ-k'l) [*pro-* + L. *cuticula*] the layer of the exoskeleton of certain crustaceans and arthropods beneath the epicuticle, which contains chitin as the principal constituent; it is composed of an endocuticle and an exocuticle.

procyclidine hydrochloride (pro-si'klĭ-dēn) [USP] chemical name: 1-cyclohexyl-1-phenyl-3-pyrrolidino hydrochloride. A synthetic anticholinergic, $C_{19}H_{29}NO\cdot HCl$, occurring as a white crystalline powder; used as a skeletal muscle relaxant in the treatment of parkinsonism, administered orally.

prodigiosin (pro-dij"e-o'sin) chemical name: 2,2'-[3- methoxy-4'-amyl-5'-methyl-5- (2"-pyrryl)] dipyrrylmethene. An antibiotic dye from *Serratia marcescens*, $C_{20}H_{25}N_3O$, formerly used as an antifungal agent.

prodroma (pro-dro'mah), pl. *prodro'mata* [Gr. *prodromē* a running forward] prodrome.

prodromal (pro-dro'mal) premonitory; indicating the onset of a disease or morbid state.

prodromata (pro-dro'mah-tah) [Gr.] plural of *prodroma*.

prodrome (pro'drōm) [L. *prodromus;* Gr. *prodromos* forerunning] a premonitory symptom or precursor; a symptom indicating the onset of a disease.

prodromic (pro-dro'mik) prodromal.

pro-drug (pro'drug) [L. *pro-* before + *drug*] a compound that, on administration, must undergo chemical conversion by metabolic processes before becoming an active pharmacological agent; a precursor of a drug.

product (prod'ukt) something produced. **cleavage p.,** a substance formed by the splitting of a compound molecule into simpler molecules. **contact activation p.,** a product of the interaction of blood coagulation Factors XII and XI, which functions to activate Factor IX during the formation of intrinsic thromboplastin. **decay p.,** a nuclide, which may be stable or radioactive, resulting from the radioactive disintegration of a radionuclide, being formed either directly or as the result of successive transformations in a radioactive series. Called also *daughter*. **end p.,** the final product in a chain of metabolic reactions. **fibrinolytic split p's,** fragments of fibrinogen or fibrin degraded by plasmin. **fission p.,** an isotope, usually radioactive, of an element in the middle of the periodic table, produced by fission of a heavy element, such as uranium, under bombardment by high energy particles. **gene p., primary,** the specific protein or polypeptide molecules, frequently enzymes, which depend on the presence of a gene. **spallation p's,** the many different chemical elements produced in small quantities in nuclear fission. **substitution p.,** a chemical product obtained by substituting for one element in a molecule an atom or a radical of some other substance. **Vaughan's split p's,** a protein which has been split up into a poisonous and a nonpoisonous part by treatment with a solution of 2 per cent sodium hydroxide in ethanol; the toxic fraction is soluble in the menstruum, the latter is not. The former is called the "poison"; the latter, the "residue." Cf. *petit serum*.

productive (pro-duk'tiv) producing or forming; said especially of an inflammation that produces new tissue or of a cough that brings forth sputum or mucus.

proecdysis (pro-ek'dĭ-sis) [*pro-* + Gr. *ekdysis* a way out] the period of preparation for the process of ecdysis, during which the new cuticle is laid down and the old one ultimately detached from it.

proelastase (pro"e-las'tās) the inactive precursor of elastase, formed in the pancreas.

proemial (pro-e'me-al) [L. *prooemium* a prelude] introductory;

serving as an introduction or indication; prodromal; potentially dangerous.

proencephalon (pro″en-sef′ah-lon) prosencephalon.

proencephalus (pro″en-sef′ah-lus) [*pro-* + Gr. *enkephalos* brain] a fetus with a part of the brain protruding from a frontal fissure.

proenzyme (pro-en′zīm) an inactive precursor that is converted to the active enzyme by the action of acid, another enzyme, or by other means. Called also *pre-enzyme* and *zymogen.*

proerythroblast (pro″ĕ-rith′ro-blast) pronormoblast.

proerythrocyte (pro″ĕ-rith′ro-sīt) a precursor of an erythrocyte; the term is without standing in any scheme of morphological development.

proesterase (pro-es′ter-ās) the inactive precursor of an esterase.

proestrogen (pro-es′tro-jen) a substance which is without estrogenic activity but which is metabolized in the body to active estrogen.

proestrum (pro-es′trum) proestrus.

proestrus (pro-es′trus) [*pro-* + L. *oestrus*] the period of heightened follicular activity preceding estrus in female mammals.

Proetz position, treatment (prets) [Arthur Walter *Proetz,* American otolaryngologist, born 1888] see under *position* and *treatment.*

profadol hydrochloride (pro′fah-dōl) chemical name: 3-(1-methyl-3-propyl-3-pyrrolidinyl)phenol hydrochloride; a narcotic analgesic, $C_{14}H_{21}NO \cdot HCl$.

profenamine (pro-fen′ah-mēn) ethopropazine.

proferment (pro-fer′ment) proenzyme; zymogen.

professional (pro-fesh′un-al) 1. pertaining to one's profession or occupation. 2. one who is a specialist in a particular field or occupation. **allied health p.,** a person with special training and licensed when necessary, who works under the supervision of a health professional with responsibilities bearing on patient care. Called also *paraprofessional.*

Professional Standards Review Organization See *PSRO.*

Profeta's immunity, law (pro-fa′tahz) [Giuseppe *Profeta,* Italian dermatologist, 1840–1910] see under *immunity* and *law.*

profibrinolysin (pro″fi-bri-no-li′sin) the inactive precursor of fibrinolysin; plasminogen.

Profichet's syndrome (disease) (pro″fe-shāz′) [Georges Charles *Profichet,* French physician, born 1873] see under *syndrome.*

profile (pro′fīl) a simple outline of the shape or form of an object, such as the head or face, viewed from the side. By extension, a graph representing quantitatively a set of characteristics subjected to tests.

proflavine (pro-fla′vin) chemical name: 3,6-diaminoacridine. An acriflavine derivative, $C_{13}H_{11}N_3$, which is a disinfectant bacteriostatic against many gram-positive bacteria. It has been used in the form of the dihydrochloride and hemisulfate salts as a topical antiseptic, and was formerly used as a urinary antiseptic. Called also *diamino-acridine.*

profluvium (pro-floo′ve-um) [L.] a flowing forth. **p. sem′-inis,** a flowing from the vagina of the semen deposited during coitus.

profondometer (pro″fon-dom′ĕ-ter) an apparatus for locating a foreign body by the fluoroscope by obtaining three lines of sight which intersect at the foreign body.

profundaplasty (pro-fun′dah-plas″te) reconstruction of the occluded or stenosed deep femoral artery (profunda femoris artery).

profundoplasty (pro-fun′do-plas″te) profundaplasty.

profundus (pro-fun′dus) [L.] deep; [NA] a term denoting a structure situated deeper than another from the surface of the body.

progamous (prog′ah-mus) [*pro-* + Gr. *gamos* marriage] previous to fertilization of the ovum.

progaster (pro′gas-ter) [*pro-* + Gr. *gastēr* stomach] the archenteron.

progastrin (pro-gas′trin) an inactive precursor of gastrin.

progenia (pro-je′ne-ah) [*pro-* + L. *gena* chin] prognathism.

progenital (pro-jen′ĭ-tal) on the external surface of the genitals.

progenitor (pro-jen′ĭ-tor) [L.] a parent or ancestor.

progeny (proj′ĕ-ne) [L. *progignere* to bring forth] offspring, or descendants.

progeria (pro-je′re-ah) [*pro-* + Gr. *gēras* old age + *-ia*] premature old age; a form of infantilism marked by small stature, absence of facial and pubic hair, wrinkled skin, gray hair, and the facial appearance, attitude, and manner of old age. Cf. *infantilism* and *hypophyseal infantilism.*

progestagen (pro-jes′tah-jen) progestogen.

progestational (pro″jes-ta′shun-al) 1. a term applied to that phase of the menstrual cycle, just before menstruation, when the corpus luteum is active and the endometrium secreting. 2. de-

noting a class of pharmaceutical preparations that have effects similar to those of progesterone; used in such disorders as dysfunctional uterine bleeding and recurrent abortion. See also under *agent.*

progesteroid (pro-jes′tĕ-roid) a progesterone-like compound; sometimes used to include progesterone and all other compounds having progestational effects.

progesterone (pro-jes′tĕ-ron) chemical name: pregn-4-ene-3,20-dione. The principal progestational hormone of the body, $C_{21}H_{30}O_2$, liberated by the corpus luteum, adrenal cortex, and placenta, whose function it is to prepare the uterus for the reception and development of the fertilized ovum by transformation of the endometrium from the proliferative to the secretory stage. Also [USP], the same principle isolated from pregnant sows or prepared synthetically, occurring as a white or creamy white, crystalline powder, and containing, calculated on the dry basis, between 98 and 102 per cent of progesterone; used, usually in the form of synthetic derivatives, as a progestin in the treatment of functional uterine bleeding, abnormalities of the menstrual cycle, and threatened abortion, administered orally and intramuscularly. Called also *luteohormone* and *progestational hormone.*

progestin (pro-jes′tin) the name originally given (Corner and Allen, 1930) to the crude hormone of the corpora lutea. It has since been isolated in pure form and is now known as *progesterone.* The name progestin is used for certain synthetic or natural progestational agents. See *progestational agents,* under *agent.*

progestogen (pro-jes′to-jen) a term applied to any substance possessing progestational activity.

progestomimetic (pro-jes″to-mi-met′ik) having physiologic activity similar to that of progesterone.

proglossis (pro-glos′is) [Gr. *proglōssis*] the tip of the tongue.

proglottid (pro-glot′id) [*pro-* + *glottis*] one of the segments making up the body of a tapeworm. See *strobilia.*

proglottis (pro-glot′is), pl. *proglot′tides.* Proglottid.

proglumide (pro-gloo′mīd) chemical name: (+)-4-benzamido-*N,N*-dipropylglutaramic acid; an anticholinergic, $C_{18}H_{26}N_2O_4$.

prognathic (prog-na′thik) prognathous.

prognathism (prog′nah-thizm) the condition of being prognathous; marked protrusion of the jaw.

prognathometer (prog″nah-thom′ĕ-ter) [*prognathous* + Gr. *metron* measure] an instrument for measuring the form and degree of prognathism.

prognathous (prog′nah-thus, prog-na′thus) [*pro-* + Gr. *gnathos* jaw] having projecting jaws, having a gnathic index above 103, the teeth being in mesioclusion.

prognose (prog-nōs′) to forecast the course and outcome of a disease.

prognosis (prog-no′sis) [Gr. *prognōsis* foreknowledge] a forecast as to the probable outcome of an attack of disease; the prospect as to recovery from a disease as indicated by the nature and symptoms of the case. **dental p.,** an evaluation of the results to be achieved from any dental treatment.

prognostic (prog-nos′tik) 1. affording an indication as to prognosis. 2. a symptom or sign on which a prognosis may be based.

prognosticate (prog-nos′tĭ-kāt) to forecast the probable outcome of an attack of disease.

prognostician (prog″nos-tish′an) one who is skilled in prognosis.

progoitrin (pro-goi′trin) an inactive compound found in the seeds of most plants belonging to the genus Brassica, which liberates goitrin through specific enzymatic hydrolysis.

progonoma (pro″go-no′mah) [Gr. *pro* before + *gonos* sperm + *-oma*] a tumor due to misplacement of tissue as the result of fetal atavism to a stage which does not occur in the life history of the species, but which does occur in ancestral forms of the species. **melanotic p.,** melanotic neuroectodermal tumor.

progranulocyte (pro-gran′u-lo-sīt″) promyelocyte.

progravid (pro-grav′id) [*pro-* + L. *gravidus* pregnant] denoting the phase of the endometrium, under the influence of the corpus luteum, during which it is prepared for pregnancy.

progression (pro-gresh′un) the act of moving or walking forward; the process of spreading or becoming more severe. **backward p.,** walking backward; an act seen in certain nervous diseases. **cross-legged p.,** a walk in which the toes are turned in and the foot is placed in front of its fellow. **metadromic p.,** one of the sequelae of epidemic encephalitis, consisting in the fact that a person who is barely able to walk may have no difficulty in running.

progressive (pro-gres′iv) advancing; going forward; going from bad to worse; increasing in scope or severity.

proguanil hydrochloride (pro-gwan′il) chemical name: *N*-(4-chlorophenyl)-*N*′-(1-methylethyl)imidodicarbonimidic diamide hydrochloride. An antimalarial, $C_{11}H_{17}Cl_2N_5$, occurring as a white, crystalline powder; used in the prophylaxis and treatment of malaria, administered orally. Seldom used in the United States because of the development of resistance by the malarial parasite to proguanil. Called also *chloroguanide hydrochloride.*

Progynon (pro-jin'on) trademark for preparations of estradiol.

prohormone (pro-hor'mōn) a precursor of a hormone, for example, proinsulin, being of larger molecular size than the active hormone.

proinsulin (pro-in'su-lin) a precursor of insulin, with a molecular weight of 8,000 to 10,000; it has minimal hormonal activity and is converted to insulin by removal of the connecting C chain, leaving the two (A and B)-chains, active insulin molecule.

pro-invasin (pro''in-va'sin) a precursor of invasin (hyaluronidase).

projection (pro-jek'shun) [pro- + L. *jacere* to throw] 1. a throwing forward, especially the act of referring impressions made on the sense organs to their improper source, so as to locate correctly the objects producing them. 2. the connection between the cerebral cortex and other parts of the nervous system or organs of special sense. 3. the act of extending or jutting out, or a part that juts out. 4. a mental mechanism by which a repressed complex is disguised by being regarded as belonging to the external world or to someone else. **eccentric p.,** see *referred sensation,* under *sensation.* **erroneous p.,** a misjudging of the position of an object, due to weakness or palsy of the eye muscles.

prokaryon (pro-kar'e-on) [pro- + Gr. *karyon* nucleus] 1. nuclear material that is scattered in the cytoplasm of the cell, rather than bounded by a membrane; found in some unicellular organisms, such as bacteria. 2. prokaryote.

prokaryosis (pro''kar-e-o'sis) [pro- + Gr. *karyon* + *-osis*] the state of not having a true nucleus, the nuclear membrane being absent and the nuclear material being either scattered in the cytoplasm of the cell or collected in a nucleoid region; a characteristic of bacteria and the blue-green algae. Cf. *eukaryosis.*

Prokaryotae (pro-kar''e-o'te) [pro- + Gr. *karyon* nucleus] Procaryotae.

prokaryote (pro-kar'e-ōt) [pro- + Gr. *karyon* nucleus] an organism (e.g., a bacterium or a blue-green alga), which does not have a true nucleus, the nuclear membrane being absent and the nuclear structures being collected in a nuclear region, or nucleoid, and the chromosomes lying naked (not combined with protein) in the cytoplasm of the cell. Most prokaryotes (except mycoplasmas) have a true cell wall, and all reproduce by cell division. See also *Procaryotae.* Cf. *eukaryote.*

prokaryotic (pro''kar-e-ot'ik) pertaining to a prokaryon or to a prokaryote or to prokaryosis.

Proketazine (pro-ke'tah-zēn) trademark for preparations of carphenazine maleate.

prolabium (pro-la'be-um) [pro- + L. *labium* lip] the prominent central part of the upper lip, in its full thickness, which overlies the premaxilla.

prolactin (pro-lak'tin) [pro- + L. *lac* milk] one of the hormones of the anterior pituitary gland that stimulates and sustains lactation in postpartum mammals, the mammary glands having been prepared by other hormones, including estrogens, progesterone, growth hormone, and corticosteroids; it also stimulates the formation of milk in the crop sac of certain birds, as in pigeons and doves, and shows luteotropic activity in certain mammals. Called also *lactogen* and *lactogenic hormone.*

prolactinoma (pro-lak''tǐ-no'mah) a pituitary tumor, usually a microadenoma of the mammotropic cells, which secretes prolactin; a mammotropic tumor.

prolamin (pro-lam'in, pro'lah-min) any one of a group of proteins found in cereals. They are soluble in alcohol (70–80 per cent), but insoluble in water and absolute alcohol. They are also called *alcohol-soluble proteins.*

prolan (pro'lan) Zondek's term for the gonadotropic principle of human pregnancy urine, responsible for the biologic pregnancy tests. Originally, the response of rodents to pregnancy urine was ascribed to two hormones, *prolan A,* follicle-stimulating, and *prolan B,* luteinizing. It is now known that the gonadotropic principle in human pregnancy is a single entity and differs from the gonadotropic substance of the anterior pituitary. The term prolan has fallen into disuse but is of historic value. See *chorionic gonadotropin.*

prolapse (pro-laps') [L. *prolapsus; pro* before + *labi* to fall] 1. the falling down, or sinking, of a part or viscus; procidentia. 2. to undergo such displacement. **anal p., p. of anus,** protrusion of modified anal skin through the anal orifice. **p. of the cord,** premature expulsion of the umbilical cord in labor before the fetus is delivered. **frank p.,** prolapse of the uterus in which the vagina is inverted and hangs from the vulva. **p. of the iris,** protrusion of the iris through a wound in the cornea. **Morgagni's p.,** chronic inflammatory hyperplasia of the mucosa and submucosa of the sacculus laryngis. **rectal p., p. of rectum,** protrusion of the rectal mucous membrane through the anus in varying degree, classified as *incomplete* or *partial* with no displacement of anal sphincter muscle, *complete with displacement* of anal sphincter muscle, *complete with no displacement* of anal muscles but usually with herniation of bowel, and *internal complete (concealed)* with intussusception of the rectosigmoid and upper portion of the rectum into the lower rectum. **p. of**

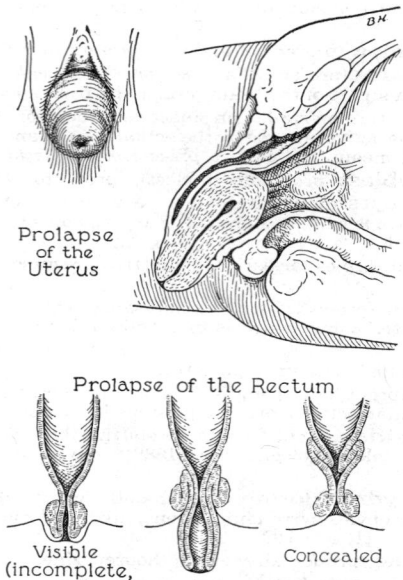

Prolapse
of the
Uterus

Prolapse of the Rectum

Visible   Complete   Concealed
(incomplete,
anal)   (Buie)

uterus, downward displacement of the uterus so that the cervix is within the vaginal orifice (*first-degree p.*), the cervix is outside the orifice (*second-degree p.*), or the entire uterus is outside the orifice (*third-degree p.*).

prolapsus (pro-lap'sus) [L.] prolapse. **p. a'ni,** prolapse of the anus. **p. rec'ti,** prolapse of the rectum. **p. u'teri,** prolapse of the uterus.

prolepsis (pro-lep'sis) the return of a paroxysm before the expected time.

proleptic (pro-lep'tik) occurring prior to the usual time; said of a periodic disease whose paroxysms return at successively shorter intervals.

proleukocyte (pro-lu'ko-sīt) a precursor of a leukocyte; the term is without standing in any current scheme of morphological development.

prolidase (pro'lǐ-dās) an enzyme which catalyzes the hydrolysis of an imide bond between an α-carboxyl group and proline or hydroxyproline; it may occur in intestines.

proliferate (pro-lif'er-āt) to grow by the reproduction of similar cells.

proliferation (pro-lif''ě-ra'shun) [L. *proles* offspring + *ferre* to bear] the reproduction or multiplication of similar forms, especially of cells and morbid cysts. **fibroplastic p.,** an overgrowth of collagenous connective tissue involving many organs of the body, as occurs in systemic lupus erythematosus, scleroderma, and other collagen diseases.

proliferative (pro-lif'er-a-tiv) characterized by proliferation.

proliferous (pro-lif'er-us) proliferative.

prolific (pro-lif'ik) [L. *prolificus*] fruitful; productive.

proligerous (pro-lij'er-us) [L. *proles* offspring + *gerere* to bear] producing offspring.

prolinase (pro'lǐ-nās) an enzyme which catalyzes the hydrolysis of dipeptides containing proline or hydroxyproline as N-terminal groups; occurs in the kidney and intestines. Called also *iminadipeptidase.*

proline (pro'lin) an amino acid, 2-pyrrolidine-carboxylic acid, discovered by Fischer in 1901; it is a major constituent of collagen (see *tropocollagen*).

prolinemia (pro''lǐ-ne'me-ah) hyperprolinemia.

prolintane hydrochloride (pro-lin'tān) chemical name: 1-(α-propylphenethyl)pyrrolidine hydrochloride; an antidepressant, $C_{15}H_{23}N \cdot HCl$.

Prolixin (pro-lik'sin) trademark for preparations of fluphenazine hydrochloride.

Proloid (pro'loid) trademark for a preparation of thyroglobulin (def. 2).

Proluton (pro-lu'ton) trademark for preparations of progesterone.

prolymphocyte (pro-lim'fo-sīt) a developmental form of the lymphocytic series intermediate between the lymphoblast and lymphocyte.

promanide (pro'man-id) glucosulfone sodium.

promastigote (pro-mas'tǐ-gōt) [pro- + Gr. *mastix* whip] the morphologic stage in the development of certain protozoa of the family Trypanosomatidae, characterized by a free anterior flagellum and resembling the typical adult form of *Leptomonas*. Called also *leptomonad stage* or *form*. Cf. *amastigote*, *epimastigote*, and *trypomastigote*.

promazine hydrochloride (pro′mah-zēn) [USP] chemical name: *N,N*-dimethyl-10*H*-phenothiazine-10-propanamine monohydrochloride. A phenothiazine derivative, $C_{17}H_{20}N_2S \cdot HCl$, occurring as a white to slightly yellow, crystalline powder; used as an antipsychotic agent, as an antiemetic, and as an analgesic- and anesthetic-potentiating agent, administered orally, intramuscularly, and intravenously.

promegakaryocyte (pro″meg-ah-kar′e-o-sīt″) a precursor in the thrombocytic series, being a cell intermediate between the megakaryoblast and the megakaryocyte.

promegaloblast (pro-meg′ah-lo-blast″) the earliest developmental form in the abnormal red cell maturation sequence occurring in vitamin B_{12} and folic acid deficiencies; it corresponds to the pronormoblast, but differs from it by its larger size, abundant basophilic cytoplasm, and reticulated, unclumped nuclear chromatin. Several nucleoli are usually present.

prometaphase (pro-met′ah-fāz) the phase of mitosis which generally begins with the disintegration of the nuclear membrane. When this has occurred a more fluid zone is noted in the center of the cell in which the chromosomes move freely and in apparent disorder, making their way toward the equator.

promethazine hydrochloride (pro-meth′ah-zēn) [USP] chemical name: *N,N,α*-trimethyl-10*H*-phenothiazine-10-ethanamine. A phenothiazine derivative, $C_{17}H_{20}N_2S \cdot HCl$, occurring as a white to faint yellow, crystalline powder, having marked antihistaminic activity as well as sedative and antiemetic actions; used to provide bedtime, surgical, and obstetrical sedation, to potentiate the action of central depressants, and to manage nausea and vomiting associated with surgery, pregnancy, and motion sickness, administered orally, intramuscularly, and intravenously.

promethestrol dipropionate (pro-meth′es-trol) chemical name: 4,4′-(1,2-diethyl-1,2-ethanediyl)bis[2-methylphenol]dipropanoate. An orally effective, synthetic, nonsteroid estrogenic agent, $C_{26}H_{34}O_4$, occurring as a white, crystalline powder, having actions and uses similar to those of diethylstilbestrol (q.v.). Called also *methestrol dipropionate*.

promethium (pro-me′the-um) the radioactive metallic chemical element of atomic number 61, atomic weight 147, and symbol Pm. Formerly called *florentium* and *illinium*.

promine (pro′mēn) a substance widely distributed in animal cells, characterized by its ability to promote cell division and growth. Cf. *retine*.

prominence (prom′ĭ-nens) a protrusion or projection; for names of specific anatomical structures see under *prominentia*. **Ammon's scleral p.,** a prominence on the globe of the eye of the fetus. **tubal p.,** torus tubarius.

prominentia (prom″ĭ-nen′she-ah), pl. *prominen′tiae* [L.] a prominence, protrusion, or projection; [NA] a general term for a small protrusion on another structure or part. **p. cana′lis facia′lis** [NA], prominence of facial canal: an elongated elevation on the medial wall of the tympanic cavity, just inferior to the prominence of the lateral semicircular canal and superior and posterior to the vestibular window. **p. cana′lis semicircula′ris latera′lis** [NA], prominence of lateral semicircular canal: a large rounded prominence on the upper portion of the medial wall of the tympanic cavity, between the vestibular window and the mastoid antrum. **p. laryn′gea** [NA], laryngeal prominence: a subcutaneous prominence on the front of the neck produced by the thyroid cartilage of the larynx; called also *Adam's apple*. **p. mallea′ris membra′nae tym′pani** [NA], **p. malleola′ris membra′nae tym′pani,** mallear prominence of tympanic membrane: a small projection at the upper extremity of the stria mallearis, formed by the lateral process of the malleus. **p. spira′lis** [NA], a prominence on the external wall of the cochlear duct, separating the stria vascularis from the external spiral sulcus. **p. styloi′dea** [NA], styloid prominence: an irregular nodule on the posterior portion of the floor of the tympanic cavity, corresponding to the base of the styloid process.

prominentiae (prom″ĭ-nen′she-e) plural of *prominentia*.

promitosis (pro″mi-to′sis) a simple form of cell division seen in tumor cells, in which the nucleolus or karyosome divides as in mitosis, the rest of the division simulating amitosis.

promonocyte (pro-mon′o-sīt) a precursor in the monocytic series, being a cell intermediate in development between the monoblast and monocyte.

promontorium (prom″on-to′re-um), pl. *promonto′ria* [L.] promontory, a projecting eminence or process; [NA] a general term for such a structure. **p. faci′ei,** nasus externus. **p. os′sis sa′cri** [NA], promontory of sacrum: the prominent anterior border of the pelvic surface of the body of the first sacral vertebra. **p. tym′pani** [NA], promontory of tympanic cavity: the prominence on the medial wall of the tympanic cavity, formed by the first turn of the cochlea.

promontory (prom′on-to″re) a projecting eminence or process;

for names of specific anatomical structures see under *promontorium*.

promoter (pro-mo′ter) a substance in a catalyst which increases the rate of activity of the latter. Cf. *protector*.

promoxolane (pro-mok′so-lān) chemical name: 2,2-diisopropyl-1,3-dioxolane-4-methanol. A liquid, $C_{10}H_{20}O_3$, used as a skeletal muscle relaxant and tranquilizer.

promyelocyte (pro-mi′ĕ-lo-sīt″) a precursor in the granulocytic series, being a cell intermediate in development between a myeloblast and myelocyte, and containing a few, as yet undifferentiated, cytoplasmic granules.

pronate (pro′nāt) to assume or place in a prone position.

pronation (pro-na′shun) [L. *pronatio*] the act of assuming the prone position, or the state of being prone. Applied to the hand, the act of turning the palm backward (posteriorly) or downward, performed by medial rotation of the forearm. Applied to the foot, a combination of eversion and abduction movements taking place in the tarsal and metatarsal joints and resulting in lowering of the medial margin of the foot, hence of the longitudinal arch. Cf. *supination*.

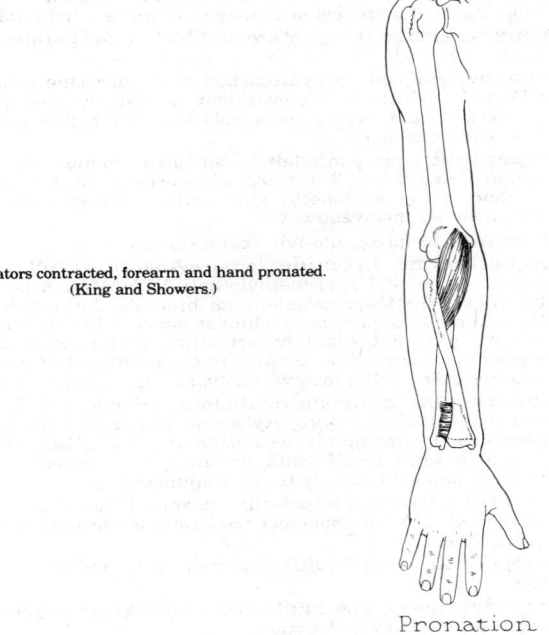

Pronators contracted, forearm and hand pronated. (King and Showers.)

Pronation

pronatoflexor (pro-na″to-flek′sor) both pronator and flexor.

pronator (pro-na′tor) [L.] a muscle that serves to pronate.

prone (prōn) [L. *pronus* inclined forward] lying face downward; see also *pronation*.

pronephron (pro-nef′ron) pronephros.

pronephros (pro-nef′ros), pl. *pronephroi* [*pro-* + Gr. *nephros* kidney] the primordial kidney; an excretory structure or its rudiments developing in the embryo before the mesonephros. Its duct is later used by the mesonephros, which arises caudal to it.

Pronestyl (pro-nes′til) trademark for preparations of procainamide hydrochloride.

pronetalol (pro-net′ah-lōl) pronethalol.

pronethalol (pro-neth′ah-lōl) chemical name: α-[(isopropylamino)methyl]-2-naphthalenemethanol; a beta-adrenergic blocking agent, $C_{15}H_{19}NO$, having the same actions as propranolol (q.v.). Called also *nethalide* and *pronetalol*.

prong (prong) a conical projection, such as a conical root of a tooth.

pronograde (pro′no-grād) [L. *pronus* bent downward + *gradi* to walk] characterized by walking with the body approximately horizontal; applied to quadrupeds. Cf. *orthograde*.

pronometer (pro-nom′ĕ-ter) an instrument for measuring the amount of pronation or supination of the forearm.

pronormoblast (pro-nor′mo-blast) the earliest of the immature forms recognizable as a normal precursor of the mature erythrocyte. It is round, with a relatively large nucleus which occupies most of the cell and is surrounded by a small amount of cytoplasm. The cytoplasm is of clear deep blue color, often staining slightly unevenly, and showing a pale perinuclear halo. The nucleus is round, and consists of a network of fairly uniformly distributed chromatin strands, giving a finely reticular appearance; it is reddish purple in color and contains several nucleoli. Called also *rubriblast* and *proerythroblast*. See also *normoblast*.

Prontosil (pron′to-sil) trademark for the hydrochloride salt of *p*-[(2,4-diaminophenyl)azo]benzenesulfonamide(sulfamidochrysoidine), $C_{12}H_{13}N_5O_2S \cdot HCl$, occurring as orange-red crystals. The forerunner of the sulfonamide drugs, it was first prepared in 1932, and is no longer used therapeutically. Called also *P. flavum* and *P. rubrum*.

pronucleus (pro-nu′kle-us) the precursor of a nucleus. **female p.,** the haploid nucleus of the fully mature ovum which loses its nuclear envelope and liberates its chromosomes to meet in synapsis with those similarly derived from the male pronucleus. **male p.,** the nuclear material of the head of a spermatozoon, after it has penetrated the ovum and acquired a pronuclear membrane.

pro-otic (pro-ot′ik) [*pro-* + Gr. *ous* ear] anterior to the ear.

Propadrine (pro′pah-drēn) trademark for preparations of phenylpropanolamine hydrochloride.

propagation (prop″ah-ga′shun) reproduction.

propagative (prop′ah-ga″tiv) pertaining to or concerned in propagation.

propagule (prop′ah-gūl) in ecology, the minimum number of individuals of a species necessary to colonize a habitable island.

propancreatitis (pro-pan″kre-ah-ti′tis) (obs.) purulent pancreatitis.

propane (pro′pān) a hydrocarbon of the methane series, $CH_3 \cdot CH_2 \cdot CH_3$, which is a constituent of natural gas and crude petroleum, and occurs as a colorless flammable gas with a characteristic odor.

propanidid (pro-pan′ĭ-did) chemical name: 4-[2-(diethylamino)-2-oxoethoxy]-3-methoxybenzeneacetic acid propyl ester. A short-acting anesthetic, $C_{18}H_{27}NO_5$, derived from eugenol; administered intravenously.

propanolide (pro-pan′o-līd) betapropiolactone.

propantheline bromide (pro-pan′thĕ-lēn) [USP] chemical name: *N*-methyl-*N*-(1-methylethyl)-*N*-[2-[(9*H*-xanthen-9-ylcarbonyl)oxy]ethyl]-2-propanaminium bromide. An anticholinergic, $C_{23}H_{30}BrNO_3$, occurring as white or nearly white crystals, which inhibits gastrointestinal hypermotility and hyperacidity; used especially as adjunctive therapy in the treatment of peptic ulcer, administered orally, intravenously, and intramuscularly.

proparacaine hydrochloride (pro-par′ah-kān) [USP] chemical name: 3-amino-4-propoxybenzoic acid 2-(diethylamino)ethyl ester monohydrochloride. An anesthetic, $C_{16}H_{26}N_2O_3 \cdot HCl$, occurring as a white to off-white, or faintly buff-colored, crystalline powder; applied topically to the conjunctiva.

propatyl nitrate (pro′pah-til) chemical name: 2-ethyl-2-(hydroxymethyl)-1,3-propanediol trinitrate; a coronary vasodilator, $C_6H_{11}N_3O_9$.

propedeutic (pro″pĕ-du′tik) pertaining to preliminary instruction.

propedeutics (pro″pĕ-du′tiks) [Gr. *propaideia* preparatory teaching] preliminary instruction.

propene (pro′pēn) propylene.

propenyl (pro-pe′nil) a three-carbon radical with one double bond between two of the carbons, $CH_3CH{=}CH{-}$.

propepsin (pro-pep′sin) pepsinogen.

propeptone (pro-pep′tōn) hemialbumose.

propeptonuria (pro″pep-to-nu′re-ah) hemialbumosuria.

properdin (pro′per-din) a relatively heat-labile, normal serum protein (a euglobulin) that, in the presence of complement component C3 and magnesium ions, acts nonspecifically against gram-negative bacteria and viruses and plays a role in lysis of erythrocytes. It migrates as a β-globulin, and although not an antibody, may act in conjunction with complement-fixing antibody.

properitoneal (pro″per-ĭ-to-ne′al) situated between the parietal peritoneum and the abdominal wall; preperitoneal.

prophage (pro′fāj) [*pro-* + *phage*] the latent stage of a phage in a lysogenic bacterium, in which the viral genome becomes inserted into a specific portion of the host chromosome and is duplicated each cell generation.

prophase (pro′fāz) the first stage in cell reduplication. In mitosis, the stage during which the chromosomes become visible (because of supercoiling of DNA), the cell nucleus starts to lose its identity, and the centrioles begin to migrate. In meiosis, the prophase of the first division consists of five stages: leptotene, zygotene, pachytene, diplotene, and diakinesis. In the second meiotic division, prophase resembles that in mitotic division. See *meiosis* and *mitosis*.

prophenpyridamine (pro″fen-pi-rid′ah-mēn) pheniramine.

prophylactic (pro″fi-lak′tik) [Gr. *prophylaktikos*] 1. tending to ward off disease; pertaining to prophylaxis. 2. an agent that tends to ward off disease.

prophylaxis (pro″fi-lak′sis) [Gr. *prophylassein* to keep guard before] the prevention of disease; preventive treatment. **causal p.,** removal of the cause of a disease. **chemical p.,** the use of chemicals in preventing the transmission of disease, especially venereal disease. **collective p.,** the protection of the community from infection. **dental p.,** the use of appropriate procedures and/or techniques to prevent dental and oral disease and malformations. **drug p.,** the use of drugs in the prevention of infection. **gametocidal p.,** the use of drugs, such as primaquine, to destroy the gametocytes of malaria. **individual p.,** the prevention of infection in an individual. **mechanical p.,** prevention of the transmission of venereal disease by mechanical means (e.g., a condom). **oral p.,** dental p. **serum p.,** prevention of disease by the use of immune serums.

propicillin (pro″pĭ-sil′in) levopropylcillin potassium.

propiodal (pro-pi′o-dal) chemical name: 2-hydroxytrimethylene-bis-(trimethylammonium) iodide. A white crystalline powder, $C_9H_{24}I_2N_2O$, formerly used as a source of iodine.

propiolactone (pro″pe-o-lak′tōn) chemical name: 2-oxetanone. A disinfectant, $C_3H_4O_2$, effective against gram-positive, gram-negative, and acid-fast bacteria, fungi, and viruses. It is also used to prepare inactivated vaccines, because it destroys the nucleic acid core of viruses but does not damage the capsid. Called also *beta-propiolactone*.

propiomazine hydrochloride (pro″pe-o-ma′zēn) [USP] chemical name: 1-[10-[2-(dimethylamino)propyl]-10*H*-phenothiazin-2-yl]-1-propanone monohydrochloride. A phenothiazine derivative, $C_{20}H_{24}N_2OS \cdot HCl$, occurring as a yellow powder; used to provide bedtime, perisurgical, and obstetrical sedation and as an antiemetic during labor, administered intramuscularly and intravenously.

propionate (pro′pe-o-nāt) any salt of propionic acid.

Propionibacteriaceae (pro″pe-on″e-bak-te″re-a′se-e) a family of Schizomycetes, order Eubacteriales, occurring as nonmotile, irregularly shaped rods. It includes three genera, *Butyribacterium*, *Propionibacterium*, and *Zymobacterium*.

Propionibacterium (pro″pe-on″e-bak-te′re-um) [*pro-* + Gr. *piōn* fat + *baktērion* little rod] a genus of microorganisms of the family Propionibacteriaceae, order Eubacteriales, made up of non–spore-forming, anaerobic, gram-positive bacilli found as saprophytes in dairy products.

propionicacidemia (pro″pĭ-on″ik-ah″sĭ-de′me-ah) propionic acidemia.

propionitrile (pro″pe-o-ni′tril) ethyl cyanide.

propionyl (pro′pe-o-nil) the acyl radical of propionic acid.

propiram fumarate (pro′pĭ-ram) chemical name: *N*-(1-methyl-2-piperidinoethyl)-*N*-2-pyridylpropionamide; an analgesic, $C_{16}H_{25}N_3O \cdot C_4H_4O_4$.

proplasmacyte (pro-plaz′mah-sīt) a precursor in the plasmacytic series, being a cell intermediate in development between the plasmablast and the plasma cell.

proplasmin (pro-plaz′min) plasminogen.

proplastid (pro-plas′tid) any of the cytoplasmic bodies resembling mitrochondria or chloroplasts, from which plastids are formed.

proplex, proplexus (pro′pleks, pro-plek′sus) (obs.) the choroid plexus of the lateral ventricle of the brain.

propons (pro′pons) [L. *pro* before + *pons* bridge] the delicate plates of white substance which pass transversely across the anterior end of the pyramid and just below the pons; called also *ponticulus*.

propositi (pro-poz′ĭ-ti) [L.] plural of *propositus*.

propositus (pro-poz′ĭ-tus), pl. *propos′iti* [L. *proponere* to put on view] the original person presenting with, or likely to be subject to, a mental or physical disorder and whose case serves as the stimulus for a hereditary or genetic study; called also *proband*. Cf. *index case*, under *case*.

propoxycaine hydrochloride (pro-pok′se-kān) [USP] chemical name: 4-amino-2-propoxybenzoic acid 2-(diethylamino)ethyl ester monohydrochloride. A local anesthetic, $C_{16}H_{26}N_2O_3 \cdot HCl$, occurring as a white, crystalline solid; used for infiltration and block anethesia.

propoxyphene (pro-pok′se-fēn) chemical name: (*S*)-α-[2-(dimethylamino)-1-methylethyl]-α-phenylbenzeneethanol propanoate. An analgesic, $C_{22}H_{29}NO_2$, structurally related to methadone. Called also *dextropropoxyphene*. See also *levopropoxyphene napsylate*. **p. hydrochloride** [USP], the hydrochloride salt of propoxyphene, $C_{22}H_{29}NO_2 \cdot HCl$, occurring as a white, crystalline powder; used as an analgesic to provide relief in mild to moderate pain, administered orally. **p. napsylate,** [USP], the napsylate salt of propoxyphene, $C_{22}H_{29}NO_2 \cdot C_{10}H_8O_3S \cdot H_2O$, occurring as a white powder, used the same as the hydrochloride salt.

propranolol (pro-pran′o-lōl) chemical name: 1-[(1-methylethyl)amino]-3-(1-naphthalenyloxy)-2-propanol. A beta-adrenergic blocking agent, $C_{16}H_{21}NO_2$, which decreases cardiac rate and output, reduces blood pressure, and is effective in the prophylaxis of migraine. **p. hydrochloride,** [USP], the hydrochloride salt of propranolol, $C_{16}H_{21}NO_2 \cdot HCl$, occurring as a white to off-white, crystalline powder. It is used as an antiarrhythmic, and also as an antihypertensive, in the management of hypertrophic aortic stenosis, and in conjunction with an alpha-adrenergic blocking agent in the symptomatic treatment of inoperable pheochromocytoma. It is also effective in the prophylaxis of migraine. Administered orally or intravenously.

proprietary (pro-pri′ĕ-ta-re)   a proprietary medicine; "any chemical, drug, or similar preparation used in the treatment of diseases, if such article is protected against free competition as to name, product, composition, or process of manufacture by secrecy, patent, trademark, or copyright, or by any other means."

proprioception (pro″pre-o-sep′shun)   perception mediated by proprioceptors or proprioceptive tissues.

proprioceptive (pro″pre-o-sep′tiv)   receiving stimuli within the tissues of the body, as within muscles and tendons. See *proprioceptor.*

proprioceptor (pro″pre-o-sep′tor)   sensory nerve terminals which give information concerning movements and position of the body; they occur chiefly in the muscles, tendons, and the labyrinth. See *exteroceptor, interoceptor,* and *receptor,* def. 3.

propriodentium (pro″pre-o-den′she-um)   the tissues of a tooth.

propriospinal (pro″pre-o-spi′nal)   pertaining wholly to the spinal cord; said of ascending and descending nerve fibers that interconnect segments of the spinal cord.

proprotein (pro-pro′te-in)   any precursor (e.g., proinsulin) of a protein.

proptometer (pro-tom′ĕ-ter) [Gr. *proptōsis* a fall forward + *metron* measure]   an instrument for measuring protrusion, especially a scale for measuring the degree of exophthalmos; exophthalmometer.

proptosis (prop-to′sis) [Gr. *proptōsis* a fall forward]   a forward displacement or bulging, especially of the eye; see *exophthalmos.*

propulsion (pro-pul′shun) [*pro-* + L. *pellere* to thrust]   1. tendency to fall forward in walking.   2. festination.

propyl (pro′pil)   the univalent chemical radical, C_3H_7 or $CH_3 \cdot CH_2 \cdot CH_2$.   **p. gallate** [NF], chemical name: 3,4,5-trihydroxybenzoic acid propyl ester. An antioxidant, $C_{10}H_{12}O_5$, occurring as a white, crystalline powder having a very slight characteristic odor; used in pharmaceutical preparations.

propylene (pro′pĭ-lēn)   chemical name: propene. A gaseous hydrocarbon, $CH_3 \cdot CH:CH_2$, of the olefin series, which has anesthetic properties.   **p. glycol** [USP], chemical name: 1,2-propanediol. A clear, colorless, viscous liquid, $C_3H_8O_2$, used as a humectant and solvent in pharmaceutical preparations.

propylhexedrine (pro″pil-hek′sĕ-drēn) [USP]   chemical name: *N,α*-dimethyl-2-cyclohexylethylamine. An adrenergic compound, $C_{10}H_{21}N$, occurring as a clear, colorless liquid; used as a vasoconstrictor to decongest nasal mucosa, administered by inhalation.

propyliodone (pro″pil-i′o-dōn) [USP]   chemical name: 3,5-diiodo-4-oxo-1(4*H*)-pyridineacetic acid propyl ester. A radiopaque medium, $C_{10}H_{11}I_2NO_3$, occurring as a white to almost white, crystalline powder; used in bronchography, administered intratracheally.

propylparaben (pro″pil-par′ah-ben) [NF]   chemical name: 4-hydroxybenzoic acid propyl ester. An antifungal agent, $C_{10}H_{12}O_3$, occurring as small colorless crystals or white powder; used as a preservative in pharmaceutical preparations.

propylthiouracil (pro″pil-thi″o-u′rah-sil) [USP]   chemical name: 2,3-dihydro-6-propyl-2-thioxo-4(1*H*)-pyrimidinone. A thyroid inhibitor, $C_7H_{10}N_2OS$, occurring as a white, powdery, crystalline substance; used in the treatment of hyperthyroidism, particularly to prepare patients for thyroid surgery and to maintain those who are poor surgical risks, administered orally.

proquazone (pro′kwah-zōn)   chemical name: 1-isopropyl-7-methyl-4-phenyl-2(1*H*)-quinazolinone; an anti-inflammatory, $C_{18}H_{18}N_2O$.

pro re nata (pro re na′tah) [L.]   according to circumstances. Abbreviated p.r.n.

prorennin (pro-ren′in)   prerennin.

prorenoate potassium (pro-ren′o-āt)   chemical name: potassium 6,7-dihydro-17-hydroxy-3-oxo-3′*H*-cyclopropa[6,7]-17α-pregna-4,6-diene-21-carboxylate; an aldosterone antagonist, $C_{23}H_{31}KO_4$.

proroxan hydrochloride (pro-rok′san)   chemical name: 1-(2,3-dihydro-1,4-benzodioxin-6-yl)-3-(3-phenyl-1-pyrrolidinyl)-1-propanone hydrochloride; an anti-adrenergic (α-receptor), $C_{21}H_{23}NO_3 \cdot HCl$.

prorrhaphy (pro′rah-fe) [*pro-* + Gr. *rhaphē* suture]   advancement.

prorsad (pror′sad) [L. *prorsum* forward]   in a forward direction.

prorubricyte (pro-roo′bri-sīt)   basophilic normoblast.

proscillaridin (pro-sil-ar′ĭ-din)   chemical name: 3β-[(6-deoxy-α-L-mannopyranosyl)-14-hydroxybufa-4,20,22-trienolide. A cardiac glycoside, $C_{30}H_{42}O_8$, which yields rhamnose on hydrolysis; used as a cardiotonic.

prosecretin (pro″se-kre′tin)   the supposed precursor of secretin,

thought to be contained in epithelial cells and to be converted into secretin on hydrolysis with acids.

prosection (pro-sek′shun)   a carefully programmed dissection for demonstration of anatomic structure.

prosector (pro-sek′tor) [L.]   one who dissects anatomical subjects for demonstration.

prosencephalon (pros″en-sef′ah-lon) [Gr. *prosō* before + *enkephalos* brain]   1. [NA] the part of the brain developed from the anterior of the three primary vesicles of the embryonic neural tube; it comprises the diencephalon and telencephalon.   2. the most anterior of the three primary brain vesicles in the embryo, later dividing into the telencephalon and the diencephalon. Called also *forebrain.*

prosimian (pro″sim′ĭ-an) [*pro-* + L. *simia* an ape]   a primitive living primate or an early ancestral primate.

proso- [Gr. *prosō* forward]   a prefix meaning forward, or anterior.

prosocele (pros′o-sēl)   prosocoele.

prosocoele (pros′o-sēl) [*proso-* + Gr. *koilia* a hollow]   the foremost cavity of the brain; the ventricular cavity of the prosencephalon.

prosodemic (pros″o-dem′ik) [*proso-* + Gr. *dēmos* people]   passing from one person to another instead of reaching a large number at once, through some means such as water supply; said of a disease progressing in that way.

prosody (pros′o-de) [Gr. *prosodos* a solemn procession]   the variation in stress, pitch, and rhythm of speech by which different shades of meaning are conveyed.

prosogaster (pros′o-gas″ter) [*proso-* + Gr. *gastēr* stomach]   foregut.

prosopagnosia (pros″o-pag-no′se-ah) [*prosopo-* + *a* neg. + Gr. *gnōsis* perception + *-ia*]   a variety of visual agnosia characterized by inability to recognize the faces of other people, or even one's own face in a mirror; it is due to damage to the underside of both occipital lobes, extending to the inner surface of the temporal lobes.

prosopalgia (pros″o-pal′je-ah) [*prosopo-* + *-algia*]   trigeminal neuralgia.

prosopalgic (pros″o-pal′jik)   pertaining to or affected with prosopalgia (trigeminal neuralgia).

prosopantritis (pros″o-pan-tri′tis) [*prosopo-* + Gr. *antron* cavity + *-itis*]   inflammation of the frontal sinuses.

prosopectasia (pros″o-pek-ta′ze-ah) [*prosopo-* + Gr. *ektasis* expansion + *-ia*]   oversize of the face.

prosoplasia (pros″o-pla′se-ah) [*proso-* + Gr. *plassein* to form]   1. abnormal differentiation of tissue.   2. development into a higher level of organization or of function.

prosopo- (pros′o-po) [Gr. *prosōpon* face]   a combining form denoting relationship to the face.

prosopoanoschisis (pros″o-po-ah-nos′kĭ-sis) [*prosopo-* + Gr. *ana* up + *schisis* cleft]   oblique facial cleft.

prosopodiplegia (pros″o-po-di-ple′je-ah) [*prosopo-* + Gr. *dis* (di-) twice + *plēgē* stroke]   paralysis of the face and one lower extremity.

prosopodysmorphia (pros″o-po-dis-mor′fe-ah) [*prosopo-* + *dys-* + Gr. *morphē* form + *-ia*]   facial hemiatrophy.

prosoponeuralgia (pros″o-po-nu-ral′je-ah)   pain in the nerves of the face.

prosopopagus (pros″o-pop′ah-gus) [*prosopo-* + Gr. *pagus* thing fixed]   unequal conjoined twins in which the parasite is attached to the face elsewhere than at the jaw.

prosopoplegia (pros″o-po-ple′je-ah) [*prosopo-* + Gr. *plēgē* stroke]   facial paralysis.

prosopoplegic (pros″o-po-ple′jik)   pertaining to or affected with prosopoplegia (facial paralysis).

prosoposchisis (pros″o-pos′kĭ-sis) [*prosopo-* + Gr. *schisis* cleft]   congenital fissure of the face.

prosopospasm (pros′o-po-spazm) [*prosopo-* + *spasm*]   spasm of the muscles of the face.

prosoposternodymus (pros″o-po-ster″no-di′mus) [*prosopo-* + Gr. *sternon* sternum + *didymos* twin]   a double monster joined face to face and sternum to sternum.

prosopothoracopagus (pros″o-po-tho″rah-kop′ah-gus) [*prosopo-* + Gr. *thōrax* chest + *pagos* thing fixed]   conjoined symmetrical twins united in the frontal plane, the fusion extending from the oral region through the thorax.

prostacyclin (pros″tah-si′klin)   an intermediate in the metabolic pathway of arachidonic acid, formed from prostaglandin endoperoxides in the walls of arteries and veins; an unstable substance, it is a potent vasodilator and a potent inhibitor of platelet aggregation.

prostaglandin (pros″tah-glan′din)   a group of naturally occurring, chemically related, long-chain hydroxy fatty acids that stimulate contractility of the uterine and other smooth muscle and have the ability to lower blood pressure, regulate acid secretion of the stomach, regulate body temperature and platelet aggregation, and to control inflammation and vascular permeability; they also affect the action of certain hormones. First found in semen, prostaglandins have since been found in menstrual fluid and various tissues of many species, and have been synthesized chemically. There are six types, A, B, C, D, E, and F, the degree of saturation of the side chain of each being designated by subscripts 1, 2, and 3. The types of prostaglandin are abbreviated PGE_2, PGF_2, and so on. Prostaglandin E_2 is also known as *dinoprostone*; $PGF_{2\alpha}$ as *dinoprost*. **p. E_1,** alprostadil. **p. E_2,** dinoprostone. **p. $F_{2\alpha}$,** dinoprost. **p. $F_{2\alpha}$ tromethamine,** dinoprost tromethamine.

prostalene (pros'tah-lēn) chemical name: $(\pm)$-methyl 7-[(1R^*, 2R^*,3R^*,5S^*)-3,5-dihydroxy-2-[(E)-3-hydroxy-3-methyl-1-octenyl]cyclopentyl]-4,5-heptadienoate; a prostaglandin, $C_{22}H_{36}O_5$.

Prostaphlin (pro-staf'lin) trademark for preparations of oxacillin sodium.

prostata (pros'tah-tah) [NA] a gland in the male which surrounds the neck of the bladder and part of the urethra; see *prostate*.

prostatalgia (pros"tah-tal'je-ah) [*prostate* + *-algia*] pain in the prostate.

prostatauxe (pros"tah-tawk'se) [*prostate* + Gr. *auxē* increase] enlargement of the prostate.

prostate (pros'tāt) [Gr. *prostates* one who stands before, from *pro* before + *histanai* to stand] a gland in the male which surrounds the neck of the bladder and the urethra. Called also *prostata* [NA]. It consists of a median lobe and two lateral lobes, and is made up partly of glandular matter, the ducts from which

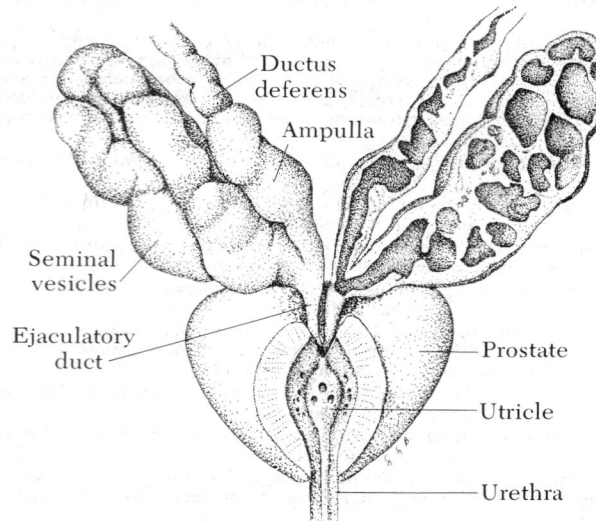

Prostate and seminal vesicles.

empty into the prostatic portion of the urethra, and partly of muscular fibers which encircle the urethra. The prostate contributes to the seminal fluid a secretion containing acid phosphatase, citric acid, and proteolytic enzymes which account for the liquefaction of the coagulated semen.

prostatectomy (pros"tah-tek'to-me) [*prostate* + *ektomē* excision] surgical removal of the prostate or of a part of it. **perineal p.,** removal of the prostate through an incision in the perineum. **retropubic prevesical p.,** removal of the prostate through a suprapubic incision but without entering the urinary bladder. **suprapubic transvesical p.,** removal of the prostate through an incision above the pubis and through the urinary bladder. **transurethral p.,** see under *resection*.

prostatelcosis (pros"tat-el-ko'sis) [*prostate* + Gr. *helkōsis* ulceration] ulceration of the prostate.

prostateria (pros"tah-te're-ah) prostatism.

prostatic (pros-tat'ik) pertaining to the prostate.

prostaticovesical (pros-tat"ĭ-ko-ves'ĭ-kal) pertaining to the prostate and the bladder.

prostaticovesiculectomy (pros-tat"ĭ-ko-ve-sik"u-lek'to-me) excision of the prostate and seminal vesicles.

prostatism (pros'tah-tizm) a symptom complex resulting from compression or obstruction of the urethra, due most commonly to hyperplasia of the prostate; symptoms include diminution in the caliber and force of the urinary stream, hesitancy in initiating voiding, inability to terminate micturition abruptly (with postvoiding dribbling), a sensation of incomplete bladder emptying, and, occasionally, urinary retention. **vesical p.,** a condition of retention of the urine resembling that of prostatic disease, but existing in the absence of any affection of the prostate.

prostatisme (pros'tah-tizm) prostatism. **p. sans prostate,** the symptoms of prostatic obstruction without enlargement of the prostate.

prostatitic (pros"tah-ti'tik) pertaining to prostatitis.

prostatitis (pros"tah-ti'tis) inflammation of the prostate. **allergic p., eosinophilic p.,** a condition seen in patients with certain allergies, characterized by diffuse infiltration of the prostate by eosinophils, with the development of small foci of fibrinoid necrosis. **nonspecific granulomatous p.,** prostatitis characterized histologically by focal or diffuse infiltration of the tissues by peculiar, large, pale macrophages.

prostatocystitis (pros-ta"to-sis-ti'tis) [*prostate* + Gr. *kystis* bladder + *-itis*] inflammation of the neck of the bladder (prostatic urethra) and the bladder cavity.

prostatocystotomy (pros-ta"to-sis-tot'o-me) [*prostate* + Gr. *kystis* bladder + *tomē* a cutting] surgical incision of the bladder and prostate.

prostatodynia (pros"tah-to-din'e-ah) [*prostate* + Gr. *odynē* pain] pain in the prostate.

prostatography (pros"tah-tog'rah-fe) roentgenography of the prostate.

prostatolith (pros-tat'o-lith) a prostatic calculus.

prostatolithotomy (pros-tat"o-lĭ-thot'o-me) incision of the prostate for the removal of calculus.

prostatomegaly (pros"tah-to-meg'ah-le) [*prostate* + Gr. *megalē* great] hypertrophy of the prostate.

prostatometer (pros"tah-tom'ĕ-ter) [*prostate* + Gr. *metron* measure] an instrument for measuring the prostate.

prostatomy (pros-tat'o-me) prostatotomy.

prostatomyomectomy (pros-ta"to-mi"o-mek'to-me) [*prostate* + *myomectomy*] the surgical removal of a prostatic myoma.

prostatorrhea (pros"tah-to-re'ah) [*prostate* + Gr. *rhoia* flow] a catarrhal discharge from the prostate.

prostatotomy (pros"tah-tot'o-me) [*prostate* + Gr. *tomē* a cutting] surgical incision of the prostate.

prostatotoxin (pros"tah-to-tok'sin) a toxin formed on injection of an extract of the prostate; it is destructive to prostatic cells.

prostatovesiculectomy (pros"tah-to-ve-sik"u-lek'to-me) excision of the prostate and seminal vesicles.

prostatovesiculitis (pros"tah-to-ve-sik"u-li'tis) inflammation of the prostate and seminal vesicles.

prostaxia (pro-stak'se-ah) a stabilized condition of protein dispersion in the body.

prosternation (pro"ster-na'shun) camptocormia.

prostheses (pros-the'sēz) [Gr.] plural of *prosthesis*.

prosthesis (pros-the'sis), pl. *prosthe'ses* [Gr. "a putting to"] an artificial substitute for a missing body part, such as an arm or leg, eye or tooth, used for functional or cosmetic reasons, or both. **Cape Town p.,** an aortic valve replacement developed at the University of Cape Town, inserted in conjuction with a cardiopulmonary bypass. **cleft palate p.,** an appliance used to restore integrity of the roof of the mouth in patients with cleft palate. **Cutter SCDK p.,** a double-cage modification of the Starr-Edwards prosthesis, with the additional cage extending into the proximal chamber or upstream of the orifice; designed to achieve optimal flow conditions by permitting the use of a larger orifice or a smaller ball. **dental p.,** a replacement for one or more of the teeth or other oral structure, ranging from a single tooth to a complete denture. **Magovern-Cromie p.,** a modified Starr-Edwards prosthesis equipped with multiple curved recessed pins which are ejected into the adjacent tissue for fixation, thus eliminating the need for suturing. **maxillofacial p.,** a replacement for parts of the upper jaw or of the face missing because of disease or injury. **ocular p.,** 1. an artificial substitute for the eyeball. 2. eyeglasses. **Sauerbruch's p.,** an artificial limb with which the tissues of the stump are used to secure motion. **Starr-Edwards p.,** a caged-ball cardiac valve prosthesis consisting of a retaining cage made of silicone-coated nonferrous metal containing a Silastic ball for occluding the orifice and preventing the reflux of blood. **Vanghetti's p.,** an artificial limb similar to Sauerbruch's prosthesis, designed to be moved by muscles of the stump.

prosthetic (pros-thet'ik) serving as a substitute; pertaining to the use or application of prostheses.

prosthetics (pros-thet'iks) the field of knowledge relating to prostheses, their design, use, etc. **dental p.,** prosthodontics. **facial p.,** prosthetics concerned only with the replacement of parts of the face.

prosthetist (pros'thĕ-tist) [Gr. *prosthetes* one who adds] a person skilled in prosthetics and practicing its application in individual cases.

prosthion (pros'the-on) [Gr. *prosthios* the foremost + *-on* neuter ending] 1. the lowest anterior point on the gum between the maxillary central incisors. 2. the point of the alveolar process that projects most anteriorly in the midline. Called also *alveolar point*.

prosthodontia (pros"tho-don'she-ah) prosthodontics.

prosthodontics (pros″tho-don′tiks) [*prosthesis* + Gr. *odous* tooth] that branch of dentistry concerned with the construction of artificial appliances designed to restore and maintain oral function by replacing missing teeth and sometimes other oral structures or parts of the face.

prosthodontist (pros″tho-don′tist) a dentist who specializes in prosthodontics.

Prosthogonimus (pros″tho-gon′ĭ-mus) a genus of trematode parasites. **P. macror′chis,** a species parasitizing chickens, turkeys, pheasants, and other birds.

prosthokeratoplasty (pros″tho-ker′ah-to-plas″te) surgical replacement of corneal tissue (as in cataract) by an inert transparent prosthesis.

Prostigmin (pro-stig′min) trademark for preparations of neostigmine.

Prostin E2 (pros′tin) trademark for preparations of dinoprostone.

Prostin F2 Alpha (pros′tin) trademark for preparations of dinoprost tromethamine.

prostration (pros-tra′shun) [L. *prostratio*] extreme exhaustion or powerlessness. **heat p.,** heat exhaustion. **nervous p.,** neurasthenia.

prot- see *proto-*.

protactinium (pro″tak-tin′e-um) a radioactive metallic chemical element occurring along with radium in pitchblende, carnotite and other minerals; atomic weight, 231; atomic number, 91; symbol Pa.

protagon (pro′tah-gon) [*prot-* + Gr. *agein* to lead] a crystalline mass, $C_{108}H_{360}N_5PO_{35}$, which separates from an alcoholic extract of brain substance on cooling.

protal (pro′tal) congenital; first; dating from the beginning.

Protalba (pro-tal′bah) trademark for preparations of protoveratrine A.

protalbumose (pro-tal′bu-mōs) a primary proteose.

protaminase (pro-tam′ĭ-nās) carboxypeptidase B.

protamine (pro′tah-min) [*prot-* + *amine*] any of a class of basic proteins of low molecular weight, occurring in combination with nucleic acids in the sperm of salmon and certain other fish and having the property of neutralizing heparin. **p. sulfate** [USP], a purified mixture of simple protein principles obtained from the sperm or testes of suitable species of fish; it has the property of neutralizing heparin, and is used as an antidote to overdosage with heparin, administered intravenously.

Protaminobacter (pro″tah-mĭ′no-bak″ter) a genus of microorganisms of the family Pseudomonadaceae, suborder Pseudomonadineae, order Pseudomonadales, occurring as motile or nonmotile, frequently pigmented cells in soil or water. It includes two species, *P. albofla′vus* and *P. ru′ber.*

protan (pro′tan) an individual exhibiting protanomalopia or protanopia, marked by derangement or loss of the red-green sensory mechanism, with a noticeable shift or shortening of the spectrum and luminancy loss in the long-wave (red) end. Cf. *deutan.*

protandrous (pro-tan′drus) exhibiting protandry.

protandry (prōt-an′dre) [Gr. *prōtos* first + *aner, andros* man] hermaphroditism in which the male gonad matures before the female gonad; cf. *protogyny.*

protanomalopia (pro″tah-nom″ah-lo′pe-ah) [*prot-* + Gr. *anōmalos* irregular + *ōpē* sight + *-ia*] a problematic variant of normal color vision, in which none of the constituents for complete chromatic perception are lacking, but a greater than usual proportion of lithium red light to thallium green is required to match a fixed sodium yellow. Sometimes called "red weakness," and viewed as a transitional stage to complete loss of color vision. Cf. the correlative terms *deuteranomalopia* and *tritanomalopia.*

protanomalopsia (pro″tah-nom″ah-lop′se-ah) protanomalopia.

protanomalous (pro″tah-nom′ah-lus) pertaining to or characterized by protanomalopia.

protanomaly (pro″tah-nom′ah-le) protanomalopia.

protanope (pro′tah-nōp) an individual exhibiting protanopia; a color deviant.

protanopia (pro″tah-no′pe-ah) [*prot-* + *an-* neg. + Gr. *ōpē* sight + *-ia*] defective color vision of the dichromatic type, characterized by retention of the sensory mechanism for two hues only (blue and yellow) of the normal 4-primary quota, and lacking that for red and green and their derivatives, with loss of luminance and shift of brightness and hue curves toward the short-wave end of the spectrum, as in twilight vision. Coined by von Kries (1897) to replace "red blindness." Cf. the correlative terms *deuteranopia, tritanopia,* and *tetartanopia* (def. 2), in which the color vision deficiency is in the second, third, and fourth primary, respectively.

protanopic (pro″tah-nop′ik) pertaining to or characterized by protanopia.

protanopsia (pro″tah-nop′se-ah) protanopia.

Protea (pro′te-ah) [L.] a genus of trees of many species from various wet and warm regions; some are medicinal, e.g.,

P. mellifera L., Proteaceae, the sugar protea, is made into a syrup used for coughs and pulmonary affections.

protean (pro′te-an) [Gr. *Prōteus* a many-formed deity] 1. assuming different shapes; changeable in form. 2. an insoluble derivative of protein, being the first product of the action of water, dilute acids, or enzymes.

proteantigen (pro″te-an′tĭ-jen) a protein antigen.

protease (pro′te-ās) a general term for a proteolytic enzyme. See *peptidase.* **fig-tree p.,** ficin.

protectant (pro-tek′tant) protective.

protectin (pro-tek′tin) thin paper coated on one side with an adhesive caoutchouc plaster; used in surgery.

protective (pro-tek′tiv) [L. *protegere* to cover over] 1. affording defense or immunity. 2. an agent that affords defense against a deleterious influence, such as a substance applied to the skin (*skin p.*) to avoid the effects of the sun's rays (*solar p.*) or other noxious influences; called also *screen.*

protector (pro-tek′tor) a substance in a catalyst which prolongs the rate of activity in the latter. Cf. *promotor.* **LATS p.,** an antibody in hyperthyroid patients with the capacity to block LATS (long acting thyroid stimulator) from combining with thyroid microsomes.

Proteeae (pro-te′e-e) a taxonomic tribe of the family Enterobacteriaceae, order Eubacteriales, made up of straight, motile, gram-negative rods, which are found primarily in fecal matter and other putrefying material. It includes a single genus, *Proteus.*

proteid (pro′te-id) protein.

proteidic (pro″te-id′ik) pertaining to a protein or proteins.

proteidin (pro″te-ĭ-din) an obsolete term for a bacteriolytic substance derived from certain microorganisms, and used at one time for protective inoculation against certain diseases. **pyocyanase p.,** a bacteriolytic substance derived from *Pseudomonas aeruginosa,* and used at one time for protective inoculation against diphtheria.

proteidogenous (pro″te-ĭ-doj′ĕ-nus) giving rise to or producing proteins.

protein (pro′te-in) [Gr. *prōtos* first] any of a group of complex organic compounds which contain carbon, hydrogen, oxygen, nitrogen, and usually sulfur, the characteristic element being nitrogen, and which are widely distributed in plants and animals. Proteins, the principal constituents of the protoplasm of all cells, are of high molecular weight and consist essentially of combinations of α-amino acids in peptide linkages. Twenty different amino acids are commonly found in proteins, and each protein has a unique, genetically defined amino-acid sequence which determines its specific shape and function. They serve as enzymes, structural elements, hormones, immunoglobulins, etc., and are involved in oxygen transport, muscle contraction, electron transport, and other activities throughout the body, and in photosynthesis. They may be classified as: 1. *Simple* or *globular proteins,* including most of the proteins in the body, are generally soluble in water or salt solution and yield only α-amino acids on complete hydrolysis. Based mainly on their chemical properties, this class includes albumins, globulins, histones, and protamines. 2. *Fibrous* or *fibrillar proteins,* the principal structural proteins of the body, are generally insoluble. The major types of this class are collagens, elastins, keratins, and actin and myosin. 3. *Conjugated* or *compound proteins* are those in which the protein molecule is united with a nonprotein molecule or molecules (the prosthetic group) otherwise than as a salt. They include nucleoproteins, mucoproteins, lipoproteins, chromoproteins, phosphoproteins, and metalloproteins. **alcohol-soluble p.,** prolamin. **allosteric p.,** any protein whose biological properties are changed by binding specific small molecules at sites other than the active site. **bacterial p.,** a protein formed by bacterial activity. **bacterial cellular p.,** a protein that forms part of the substance of a bacterium. **Bence Jones p.,** a low–molecular weight, thermosensitive urinary protein, which is found almost exclusively in multiple myeloma and constitutes the light-chain component of myeloma globulin. Its outstanding characteristic is its unique property of coagulating on heating at 45°–55° C. and of redissolving partially or wholly on boiling. **carrier p.,** a protein which, when coupled to hapten *in vivo* or *in vitro,* renders the hapten capable of eliciting an immune response. See *hapten.* **coagulated p.,** an insoluble form which certain proteins assume when denatured at their isoelectric point by heat, alcohol, ultraviolet rays, or other agents. **complete p.,** a protein composed of amino acids in appropriate proportion to each other so that they all can be properly used by the body, and therefore more valuable for nutrition than is the partial protein (q.v.). **compound p., conjugated p.,** see *protein.* **constitutive p's,** proteins produced in fixed amounts, regardless of the organism's need for them. **cord p's,** the proteins of blood from the umbilical cord. **C-reactive p.,** a globulin that forms a precipitate with the somatic C-polysaccharide of the pneumococcus *in vitro;* its demonstration in the serum is a sensitive indicator of inflammation of infectious or noninfectious origin. Abbreviated *CRP.* **defensive p.,** any protein formed within the body and serving as a protection against disease; any alexin, phylaxin, or sozin. Called also *Buchner body.* **denatured p.,** see *protein* denaturation, *under* denaturation. **derived p.,** derivatives of the protein molecule formed by hydrolytic changes, including proteans, metaproteins, coagulated proteins, proteoses, peptones, and peptides. **fibrillar p.,** see *protein.* **floating p.,** a protein which does not constitute part of the tissues, but simply circulates in the body and is then excreted. **globular p.,** see *protein.* **Hektoen, Kretschmer, and Welker p.,** a protein found in urine which resembles Bence Jones protein in solubility, but differs in its crystalline form, in its behavior toward heat, and in its precipitin reactions. **p. hydrolysate,** an artificial digest of protein derived by acid, enzymatic, or other hydrolysis of casein, lactalbumin, fibrin, or other suitable proteins that supply the approximate nutritive equivalent of the source protein in the form of its constituent amino acids; used intravenously as a fluid and nutrient replenisher. **immune p's,** immunoglobulins. **incomplete p.,** partial p. **insoluble p.,** a substance left behind after the other proteins have been extracted from a cell. **iodized p.,** a protein treated with iodine. **M p.,** see *permease.* **maintenance p.,** the smallest amount of protein upon which the normal conditions of the body can be maintained. **myeloma p.,** a homogeneous monoclonal immunoglobulin produced by a plasmacytoma, or partial immunoglobulin molecules, such as Bence Jones protein, produced by plasma cells that have undergone neoplastic transformation. **native p.,** unchanged animal or vegetable protein, especially as it occurs in foods. **partial p.,** a protein having a ratio of amino acids different from that of the average body protein, and therefore less valuable for nutrition than is the complete protein (q.v.). Called also *incomplete p.* **plasma p's,** all proteins present in the blood, including albumin, fibrinogen, and globulin. In addition to their other functions, all serve to provide colloid osmotic pressure, which prevents plasma loss from the capillaries. **plasma p. fraction,** see under *fraction.* **prophylactic measles p.,** an immune substance for prophylaxis against measles; an immunoglobulin fraction of serum that contains antibodies active against the measles virus. It may be a convalescent serum, and was formerly a placental extract. **protective p.,** defensive p. **pyocyanic p.** (*obs.*), a substance prepared by treating the *Pseudomonas aeruginosa* with potassium hydroxide; used in suppuration. **pyogenic p.** (*obs.*), the protein portion of a bacterium which is the suppuration-producing element of the bacterium. **racemized p.,** protein so changed by chemical or other agents, usually dilute alkali, that its optical activity is lowered and it becomes more resistant to enzymatic hydrolysis. Acid hydrolysis of a racemized protein shows inactivation (racemization) of several of its constituent amino acids. **serum p's,** proteins in the serum component of blood, including immunoglobulins, albumin, complement, clotting factors, and enzymes. **silver p., mild,** see under *silver.* **silver p., strong,** see under *silver.* **simple p.,** see *protein.* **split p.,** see *Vaughan's split product,* under *product.* **synthetic p.,** highly complex polypeptides made in the laboratory; they show most of the characteristics of native protein. **whole p.,** protein which has not been split.

proteinaceous (pro″te-in-a′shus) pertaining to or of the nature of a protein.

proteinase (pro′te-in-ās″) any enzyme that catalyzes the splitting of interior peptide bonds in a protein; an endopeptidase. **clothes-moth p.,** an enzyme found in the intestine of the clothes moth, *Tineola biselliella,* which will digest wool keratin at pH 9.3 after the keratin has been reduced. **serine p.,** any of a series of proteolytic enzymes that contain serine, histidine, and aspartic acid at their active site; they include enzymes active in digestion (e.g., trypsin), blood coagulation, immune reactions, and fertilization of the ovum. So called, because serine was the first amino acid found at the active site.

proteinemia (pro″te-in-e′me-ah) an excess of protein in the blood.

proteinic (pro″te-in′ik) pertaining to protein.

proteinochrome (pro″te-in′o-krōm) [*protein* + Gr. *chrōma* color] any one of a series of coloring matters formed by the action of bromine or chlorine on tryptophan.

proteinochromogen (pro″te-in-o-kro′mo-jen) former name for tryptophan; so called because it gave a red color with bromine.

proteinogen (pro″te-in′o-jen) Northrop's name for the hypothetical mother substance of all proteins.

proteinogenous (pro″te-in-oj′ĕ-nus) formed by or from a protein.

proteinogram (pro″te-in′o-gram) a graphic representation of the proteins present in the blood serum.

proteinology (pro″te-in-ol′o-je) [*protein* + -*logy*] the scientific study of proteins or of the protein status of the body.

proteinosis (pro″te-in-o′sis) the accumulation of excess protein in the tissues. **lipid p., lipoid p.,** a hereditary disturbance of lipid metabolism marked by yellowish deposits of a hyalin lipid-carbohydrate mixture on the inner surface of the lips, under the tongue, on the oropharynx and larynx, and in many other sites. There may be nodular masses on the face and extremities. Hoarseness due to laryngeal nodules is a common early symptom. A light-sensitive form is now thought to be a variety of erythropoietic protoporphyria. Called also *hyalinosis cutis et mucosae,* *lipoidosis cutis et mucosae,* and *Urbach Wiethe disease.* **pulmonary alveolar p.,** a chronic lung disease characterized by dyspnea, productive cough, chest pain, weakness, weight loss, and hemoptysis, and by the filling of the distal alveoli with a bland, eosinophilic, probably endogenous, proteinaceous material that prevents ventilation of affected areas. **tissue p.,** see *amyloidosis.*

proteinotherapy (pro-te″in-o-ther′ah-pe) treatment of disease by the parenteral injection of foreign protein.

proteinphobia (pro″te-in-fo′be-ah) [*protein* + Gr. *phobein* to be affrighted by + -*ia*] morbid aversion to protein foods.

proteinpolysaccharide (pro″te-in-pol″e-sak′ah-rīd) proteoglycan.

proteinuria (pro″te-in-u′re-ah) [*protein* + Gr. *ouron* urine + -*ia*] the presence of an excess of serum proteins in the urine; called also *albuminuria.* **accidental p.,** adventitious p. **p. of adolescence,** cyclic p. **adventitious p.,** that which is not due to a kidney disease; called also *accidental* or *false p.* **athletic p.,** functional proteinuria occuring in athletes; effort p. **Bence Jones p.,** the presence in the urine of Bence Jones protein. **cardiac p.,** proteinuria caused by cardiac disease. **colliquative p.,** proteinuria which is at first mild, but increases suddenly and markedly during convalescence; it is seen in several systemic and renal diseases. **cyclic p.,** a term once used to denote the appearance at stated times each day of a small amount of protein in the urine; it is observed principally in young persons (p. of adolescence). Called also *recurrent p.* and *Pavy's disease.* **dietetic p., digestive p.,** that produced by the use of certain foods. **effort p.,** functional proteinuria occurring as a result of vigorous and prolonged exercise of the lower limbs; called also *athletic p.* **emulsion p.,** proteinuria in which the turbidity does not disappear on filtration, heating, or adding acid; seen in puerperal eclampsia. **enterogenic p.,** that due to intestinal decomposition. **essential p.,** a form of functional proteinuria which is not associated with or followed by renal disease; it includes effort and orthostatic proteinuria. **false p.,** adventitious p. **febrile p.,** proteinuria due to fever. **functional p.,** any proteinuria which is not truly pathologic, such as the transient proteinurias of pregnancy or of adolescence; also known variously as *intermittent, paroxysmal, physiologic,* and *transient p.* **globular p.,** proteinuria due to renal excretion of red blood cells and dependent on blood in the urine. **gouty p.,** functional proteinuria, with excessive secretion of uric acid. **hematogenous p., hemic p.,** a variety due to abnormal condition of the blood, as in some intoxications. **intermittent p.,** functional p. **intrinsic p.,** true p. **light-chain p.,** increased urinary excretion of light-chain fragments of immunoglobulins, as in Fanconi syndrome. **lordotic p.,** postural proteinuria due to lordotic deformity of the spine. **mixed p.,** true proteinuria occurring concurrently with adventitious proteinuria. **nephrogenous p.,** that caused by renal disease; called also *renal p.* **neurotic p.,** a variety dependent on nervous diseases. **orthostatic p., orthotic p.,** a form of functional proteinuria, usually seen between the ages of ten and twenty, which occurs on standing erect and disappears on lying down. **palpatory p.,** temporary proteinuria produced by bimanual palpation of the kidneys. **paroxysmal p.,** functional p. **physiologic p.,** functional p. **postrenal p.,** proteinuria which has arisen at some point beyond the uriniferous tubule, such as the renal pelvis, ureter, bladder, prostate, or urethra. **postural p.,** proteinuria related to body position, as orthostatic and lordotic proteinuria. **p. praetuberculo′sa,** that occurring in the incipient stage of pulmonary tuberculosis. **prerenal p.,** proteinuria due primarily to a disease other than one of the kidney, such as heart disease, liver disease, fever, hyperthyroidism. **pseudo-p.,** adventitious p. **pyogenic p.,** that due to the absorption of pus cells or exudates, as in pneumonia, septic processes, etc. **recurrent p.,** cyclic p. **regulatory p.,** proteinuria or the transitory elimination of protein after excessive physical exercise, etc. **renal p.,** nephrogenous p. **residual p.,** persistence of protein in the urine after an attack of acute nephritis. **serous p.,** true p. **transient p.,** functional p. **true p.,** that which is characterized by the discharge with the urine of some of the protein elements of the blood; called also *intrinsic p.* and *serous p.*

proteinuric (pro″te-in-u′rik) pertaining to or marked by proteinuria.

proteoclastic (pro″te-o-klas′tik) [*protein* + Gr. *klasis* breakage] splitting up proteins or the protein molecule.

proteoglycan (pro″te-o-gli′kan) any of a group of glycoproteins present in connective tissue and formed of subunits of disaccharides linked together and joined to a protein core; the proteoglycans, which include the mucopolysaccharides with their protein moiety, serve as a binding or cementing material. Called also *proteinpolysaccharide.*

Proteoglypha (pro″te-og′li-fah) Proteroglypha.

proteohormone (pro″te-o-hor′mōn) a hormone that is a peptide or a protein and so is destroyed in the intestinal tract.

proteolipid (pro″te-o-lip′id) a combination of a peptide or protein with a lipid, having the solubility characteristics of lipids. Cf. *lipoprotein.*

proteolipin (pro″te-o-lip′in) proteolipid.

proteolysin (pro″te-ol′ĭ-sin) a specific substance causing proteolysis.

proteolysis (pro″te-ol′ĭ-sis) [*protein* + Gr. *lysis* dissolution] the splitting of proteins by hydrolysis of the peptide bonds with formation of smaller polypeptides; the process may be catalyzed by proteolytic enzymes, by acids, or by bases.

proteolytic (pro″te-o-lit′ik) 1. pertaining to, characterized by, or promoting proteolysis. 2. an enzyme that promotes proteolysis.

proteometabolic (pro″te-o-met″ah-bol′ik) pertaining to proteometabolism.

proteometabolism (pro″te-o-mě-tab′o-lism) the metabolism of protein.

Proteomyces (pro″te-o-mi′sēz) Trichosporon.

proteopectic (pro″te-o-pek′tik) proteopexic.

proteopepsis (pro″te-o-pep′sis) [*protein* + Gr. *pepsis* digestion] the digestion of protein.

proteopeptic (pro″te-o-pep′tik) digesting protein; pertaining to the digestion of protein.

proteopexic (pro″te-o-pek′sik) fixing protein within the organism.

proteopexy (pro′te-o-pek″se) [*protein* + Gr. *pēxis* fixation] the fixation of proteins within the organism.

proteophilic (pro″te-o-fil′ik) growing best in a protein-rich medium; said of certain bacteria.

proteose (pro′te-ōs) [*protein* + *-ose*] a secondary protein derivative or a mixture of split products formed by a hydrolytic cleavage of the protein molecule more complete than that which occurs with the primary protein derivatives, but not so complete as that which forms amino-acids. The *primary* proteoses are precipitated by half saturation with ammonium sulfate, the *secondary,* by full saturation.

Proteosoma (pro″te-o-so′mah) [*proteus* + Gr. *sōma* body] a former name for a genus of parasitic protozoa infecting birds and reptiles.

proteosotherapy (pro″te-o-so-ther′ah-pe) treatment of disease by the subcutaneous or intravenous injection of foreign proteose.

proteosuria (pro″te-o-su′re-ah) [*proteose* + Gr. *ouron* urine + *-ia*] the presence of proteose in the urine.

proteotherapy (pro″te-o-ther′ah-pe) proteinotherapy.

proteotoxin (pro″te-o-tok′sin) a toxic protein (e.g., anaphylatoxin) formed as a consequence of the interaction between a bacterial protein and the host's serum; endotoxin.

proter (pro′ter) [Gr. *proteros* front] the anterior daughter organism after transverse division of a protozoon; cf. *opisthe.*

Proteroglypha (pro″ter-o-glif′ah) a group of venomous snakes that have small stationary fangs which are grooved rather than hollow and so must be held in the wound if the poison is to reach the deeper tissues. Examples are the Indian cobra and the Sonoran coral snake. Called also *Ankyloproglypha* and *Proteoglypha.*

Proteromonas (pro″ter-o-mo′nahz) a genus of elongate, piriform, biflagellate protozoa of the family Bodonidae, order Protomastigida, found as parasites in the gut of various species of lizards. Called also *Prowazekella.*

proteuria (pro″te-u′re-ah) [*protein* + Gr. *ouron* urine + *-ia*] proteinuria.

proteuric (pro″te-u′rik) proteinuric.

Proteus (pro′te-us) [Gr. *Prōteus* a many-formed deity] a genus of microorganisms of the tribe Proteeae, family Enterobacteriaceae, order Eubacteriales, made up of gram-negative, generally active, motile, rod-shaped bacteria of limited pathogenicity, usually found in fecal and other putrefying material. **P. hydroph′ilus,** a bacillus closely related to the *Proteus* group and found to be the etiological agent of red leg of frogs, ulcer disease of brook trout, and red sore of pike. **P. incon′stans,** a species isolated from patients with gastroenteritis, and also found in urinary tract infections; more than 150 different serotypes have been recognized. **P. melanovog′enes,** the cause of black rot. **P. mirab′ilis,** a species which is usually saprophytic and occasionally found as a human pathogen. **P. morga′ni,** an organism found in the intestinal tract and associated with summer diarrhea of infants. **P. rettge′ri,** a causative agent of diarrheal diseases of birds; also isolated from patients with sporadic and epidemic gastroenteritis. **P. vulga′ris,** the type species of Proteus, occurring, often as a secondary invader, in a variety of localized suppurative pathologic processes, and being a common cause of cystitis. It occurs as several serotypes; the X strains agglutinate in antiserum to certain of the rickettsia, X-19 strains in antisera to the typhus group, and X-K in antisera to the tsutsugamushi group, in the Weil-Felix reaction used for diagnostic purposes. See Plate accompanying *bacterium.*

prothallus (prō-thăl′us) the independent, free living gametophyte generation of ferns and related lower vascular plants.

prothesis (proth′e-sis) [Gr. "a placing in public"] prosthesis.

prothetic (pro-thet′ik) prosthetic.

prothipendyl hydrochloride (pro-thi′pen-dil) chemical name: *N,N*-dimethyl-10*H*-pyrido[3,2-*b*][1,4]benzothiazine-10-propanamine hydrochloride monohydrate; an antihistaminic and sedative, $C_{16}H_{19}N_3S \cdot HCl \cdot H_2O$.

prothrombin (pro-throm′bin) [*pro-* + Gr. *thrombos* clot + *-in* chemical suffix] Factor II; see *coagulation factors,* under *factor.*

prothrombinase (pro-throm′bin-āse) thromboplastin. **extrinsic p.,** extrinsic thromboplastin. **intrinsic p.,** intrinsic thromboplastin.

prothrombinogenic (pro-throm″bĭ-no-jen′ik) promoting the production of prothrombin (Factor II).

prothrombinopenia (pro-throm″bĭ-no-pe′ne-ah) hypoprothrombinemia.

prothyl (pro′thil) protyl.

protide (pro′tīd) protein.

protidemia (pro″tĭ-de′me-ah) proteinemia.

protinium (pro-tin′e-um) protium.

protiodide (pro-ti′o-did) that one of the series of iodides of the same base which contains the smallest amount of iodine.

protirelin (pro-ti′re-lin) thyrotropin releasing hormone.

protist (pro′tist) any member of the kingdom Protista; a single-celled organism. **eukaryotic p.,** protists having a true nucleus bounded by a nuclear membrane, and which exhibits mitosis, including protozoa, fungi, slime molds, and algae other than blue-green algae. Called also *higher p's.* **higher p's,** eukaryotic p's. **lower p's,** prokaryotic p's. **prokaryotic p.,** protists having no true nucleus, the nuclear material being a naked ring in the cytoplasm of the cell, and which reproduce primarily by fission, including bacteria and blue-green algae. Called also *lower p's.*

Protista (pro-tis′tah) [Gr. *prōtista* the very first, from *prōtos* first] in some systems of classification, a kingdom comprising bacteria, algae, slime molds, fungi, and protozoa. It includes all the single-celled organisms, some of which are plantlike, some are animal-like, while others are distinctly different from either plants or animals. In other classifications the bacteria and blue-green algae are excluded (see *Monera* and *Procaryotae*).

protistologist (pro″tis-tol′o-jist) a microbiologist.

protistology (pro″tis-tol′o-je) [*Protista* + *-logy*] microbiology.

protium (pro′te-um) the mass one isotope of hydrogen, symbol ^1H; ordinary, or light, hydrogen. See *hydrogen.* Cf. *deuterium* and *tritium.*

proto-, prot- [Gr. *prōtos* first] a combining form meaning first.

proto-actinium (pro″to-ak-tin′e-um) protactinium.

protoalbumose (pro″to-al′bu-mōs) a primary proteose.

protoanemonin (pro″to-ah-nem′o-nin) chemical name: 5-methylene-2-oxodihydrofuran. An antibiotic substance, $C_5H_4O_2$, from the flowering herb, *Anemone pulsatilla,* active against certain gram-positive and gram-negative bacteria. Its mechanism of action is not well understood.

Protobacterieae (pro″to-bak″te-ri′e-e) a tribe of the family Nitrobacteriaceae that obtain their life energy by the oxidation of simple inorganic compounds of carbon or hydrogen.

protobe (pro′tōb) protobios.

protobiology (pro″to-bi-ol′o-je) [*proto-* + Gr. *bios* life + *-logy*] the science which deals with the forms of life more minute than bacteria, such as viruses.

protobios (pro″to-bi′os) [*proto-* + Gr. *bios* life] a name proposed by d'Herelle for the bacteriophage (protobios bacteriophagus).

protoblast (pro′to-blast) [*proto-* + Gr. *blastos* germ] 1. a cell with no cell wall; an embryonic cell. 2. the nucleus of an ovum. 3. a blastomere from which a particular organ or part develops.

protoblastic (pro″to-blas′tik) pertaining to a protoblast.

protobrochal (pro″to-bro′kal) [*proto-* + Gr. *brochos* mesh] denoting the first stage in the development of an ovary.

Protocalliphora (pro″to-kah-lif′o-rah) a genus of flies whose larvae feed on nesting birds.

protocaryon (pro″to-kar′e-on) [*proto-* + Gr. *karyon* nucleus] a cell nucleus formed of a single karyosome in a network of linin.

protochloride (pro″to-klo′rid) that one of a series of chlorides of the same element which contains the least amount of chlorine.

protochlorophyll (pro″to-klo′ro-fil) a substance in plant tissue which is changed by the action of light into chlorophyll.

protochondral (pro″to-kon′dral) pertaining to the protochondrium or to centers of condrification.

protochondrium (pro″to-kon′dre-um) [*proto-* + Gr. *chondros* cartilage] the basophil substance developed from precartilage which constitutes the intermediate stage in cartilage formation.

protociliate (pro″to-sil′e-āt) any member of the subclass Protociliatia.

Protociliatia (pro″to-sil-e-a′she-ah) a subclass of parasitic protozoa of the class Ciliata, subphylum Ciliophora, found in the colon of reptiles, amphibians, and fish, and characterized by two or more nuclei of the same type, cilia of equal length, and absence of a cytostome. It includes the genus *Opalina.*

protocol (pro'to-kol) the original notes made on a necropsy, an experiment, or on a case of disease.

protocone (pro'to-kōn) [*proto-* + Gr. *kōnos* cone] the primary inner, central, or lingual cusp in the evolutionary development of the upper molar teeth of placental mammals.

protoconid (pro''to-ko'nid) the labial cusp of a primitive lower molar; the primitive cusps become greatly modified in many higher mammals and have completely disappeared in some.

protocooperation (pro''to-co-op''er-a'shun) 1. symbiosis in which both populations (or individuals) gain from the association but are able to survive without it. 2. the tendency of animals to cluster in groups and thereby to mutually facilitate the survival of individual organisms.

protocoproporphyria (pro''to-kop''ro-por-fir'e-ah) porphyria with an excess of protophyrin and coproporphyrin in the bile and feces; see *porphyria cutanea tarda hereditaria.*

protodiastolic (pro''to-di''ah-stol'ik) pertaining to early diastole, i.e., immediately following the second heart sound.

protoduodenum (pro''to-du-o-de'num) the first or proximal portion of the duodenum, extending from the pylorus to the duodenal papilla, and developed embryonically from the foregut.

protoelastose (pro''to-e-las'tōs) hemielastin.

protofibril (pro''to-fi'bril) the first elongated unit appearing in the process of formation of any type of fiber.

protogaster (pro''to-gas''ter) [*proto-* + Gr. *gastēr* stomach] archenteron.

protoglobulose (pro''to-glob'u-lōs) a primary product formed in the digestion of globulin.

protogonocyte (pro''to-go'no-sīt) [*proto-* + *gonocyte*] one of the two cells resulting from division of the impregnated ovum and, in certain lower forms, constituting the primordial germ cell from which all gametes derive.

protogonoplasm (pro''to-go'no-plazm) [*proto-* + Gr. *gōnē* seed + *plasma* anything formed or molded] (*obs.*) idiochromidia.

protogynous (pro-toj'ĭ-nus) exhibiting protogyny.

protogyny (pro-toj'ĭ-ne) [*proto-* + Gr. *gyne* woman] hermaphroditism in which the female gonad matures before the male gonad. Cf. *protandry.*

protoheme (pro''to-hēm) the prosthetic group of cytochrome *b*, consisting of protoporphyrin and iron.

protohemin (pro''to-hem'in) hemin.

protohydrogen (pro''to-hi'dro-jen) protium.

protoiodide (pro''to-i'o-dīd) protiodide.

protokylol hydrochloride (pro''to-ki'lol) chemical name: 4-[2-[[2-(1,3-benzodioxol-5-yl)-1-methylethyl]amino]-1-hydroxyethyl]-1,2-benzenediol hydrochloride. An adrenergic, C_{18} $H_{21}NO_5$, occurring as a white crystalline powder; used as a bronchodilator for the treatment of bronchospasm associated with bronchial asthma, pulmonary emphysema, bronchitis, and bronchiectasis, administered orally.

Protomastigida (pro''to-mas-tij'ĭ-dah) an order of generally small protozoa of the class Zoomastigophora, subphylum Mastigophora, characterized by the presence of one or two flagella and a plastic rather than ameboid body. Many are free-living, but some are parasites in plants, invertebrates, and vertebrates, including man. It includes the families Trypanosmatidae, Cryptobiidae, and Bodonidae.

protomedicus (pro''to-med'ĭ-kus) [*proto-* + L. *medicus* physician] a medieval term for physician-in-chief.

protomerite (pro''to-me'rīt) [*proto-* + Gr. *meros* part] the anterior portion of certain gregarine protozoa. Cf. *deutomerite.*

protometer (pro-tom'ĕ-ter) [L. *pro-* + Gr. *metron* measure] an instrument for measuring the forward protrusion of the eyeball.

Protominobacter (pro-tom'ĭ-no-bak''ter) a genus of bacteria containing several species found in soil and water.

Protomonadina (pro''to-mon-ah-di'nah) an order of protozoa of the class Zoomastigophora, subphylum Mastigophora, comprising heterogeneous primitive animal flagellates. In former classifications, it was included, along with the order Phytomonadina, in the group Monadina. It includes the families Monodidae and Protomonadina.

proton (pro'ton) [Gr. *prōtos* first + *-on* neuter ending] 1. (*obs.*) the primitive rudiment of a part; a primordium or anlage. 2. an elementary particle of positive charge which forms the nucleus of the ordinary hydrogen atom of mass 1; protons, along with the neutrons, form the nucleus of atoms of all other elements. The proton is the unit of positive electricity, being equivalent to the electron in charge and approximately to the hydrogen ion in mass.

protonephridium (pro''to-nef-rid'e-um) an osmoregulatory tubule of some invertebrates; its inner end contains a flame cell or bulb.

protonephron (pro''to-nef'ron) pronephros.

protonephros (pro''to-nef'ros) pronephros.

protoneuron (pro''to-nu'ron) [*proto-* + Gr. *neuron* nerve] 1. the first neuron in a peripheral reflex arc. 2. a unit of the nerve net of low metazoa that lacks polarization.

protonic (pro-ton'ik) (*obs.*) primordial.

protonitrate (pro''to-ni'trāt) that one of several nitrates of the same base which contains the least amount of nitric acid.

Protopam (pro'to-pam) trademark for preparations of pralidoxime.

protopathic (pro''to-path'ik) [*proto-* + Gr. *pathos* disease] primary; idiopathic. See *protopathic sensibility,* under *sensibility.*

protopecten (pro''to-pek'ten) pectose.

protophyllin (pro''to-fil'in) chlorophyll hydride, a colorless substance which is changed into chlorophyll by the action of air or carbon dioxide.

Protophyta (pro''to-fi'tah) [*proto-* + Gr. *phyton* plant] the lowest division of the vegetable kingdom, made up of unicellular organisms and including the algae, bacteria, and viruses.

protophyte (pro''to-fīt) [*proto-* + Gr. *phyton* plant] a unicellular plant or vegetable organism; an individual of the division Protophyta.

protophytology (pro''to-fi-tol'o-je) the scientific study of the simplest forms of plants (protophytes).

protopine (pro''to-pin) 1. an alkaloid, $C_{20}H_{19}NO_5$, from *Eschscholtzia californica,* the California poppy, and many other plants; it is an anodyne and hypnotic. 2. a poisonous alkaloid from various species of perennial herbs of the genus *Dicentra.*

protoplasia (pro-to-pla'se-ah) primary formation of tissue.

protoplasm (pro'to-plazm) [*proto-* + Gr. *plasma* plasm] the viscid, translucent, polyphasic colloid with water as the continuous phase that makes up the essential material of all plant and animal cells. It is composed mainly of nucleic acids, proteins, lipids, carbohydrates, and inorganic salts. The protoplasm surrounding the nucleus is known as the *cytoplasm* and that composing the nucleus is the *nucleoplasm.* **functional p.,** kinoplasm. **granular p.,** protoplasm having granular inclusions, including those in the planeroplasm. **superior p.,** endoplasmic reticulum. **totipotential p.,** protoplasm which has the power of performing all the functions of the cell.

protoplasmatic (pro''to-plaz-mat'ik) protoplasmic.

protoplasmic (pro''to-plaz'mik) pertaining to or consisting of protoplasm.

protoplast (pro'to-plast) [*proto-* + Gr. *plastos* formed] 1. the type or model of some organic being. 2. a cell (Hanstein, 1880). 3. a bacterial or plant cell deprived of its rigid wall, but with its plasma membrane still intact; the cell is dependent for its integrity on an isotonic or hypertonic medium. Cf. *spheroplast.*

protoporphyria (pro''to-por-fir'e-ah) porphyria characterized by intense pruritus, erythema, and edema after short exposure of the skin to sunlight and by excessive protoporphyrin in erythrocytes, plasma, and feces; the skin lesions usually fade without scarring or pigmentation, but a chronic weatherbeaten appearance is characteristic. Called also *erythrohepatic p.* or *erythropoietic p.*

protoporphyrin (pro''to-por'fĭ-rin) the porphyrin, $C_{34}H_{34}N_4$-O_4, whose iron complex, united with protein, occurs as hemoglobin, myoglobin, catalase, and certain respiratory pigments. Two of its four pyrrole groups have both a methyl and a propionate side chain; the other two have both a methyl and a vinyl side chain.

protoporphyrinuria (pro''to-por''fĭ-rin-u're-ah) [*protoporphyrin* + Gr. *ouron* urine + *-ia*] the presence of protoporphyrin in the urine.

protoproteose (pro''to-pro'te-ōs) a primary proteose.

protopsis (pro-top'sis) protrusion of the eye; exophthalmos.

protosalt (pro'to-sawlt) that one of a series of salts of the same base which contains the smallest amount of the substance combining with the base.

protospasm (pro'to-spazm) [*proto-* + Gr. *spasmos* spasm] a spasm which begins in a limited area and extends to other parts; the earlier and minor spasm of jacksonian epilepsy.

Protospirura (pro''to-spi-roo'rah) a genus of nematode parasites. **P. grac'ilis,** a species found in cats.

protostoma (pro''to-sto'mah) blastopore.

protostome (pro'to-stōm) [*proto-* + Gr. *stoma* mouth] an individual of the Protostomia.

Protostomia (pro''to-sto'me-ah) a series of the Eucoelomata, including the mollusks, annelids, and arthropods, in all of which the mouth arises from the blastopore.

Protostrongylus (pro''to-stron'jĭ-lus) a genus of lung worms. **P. rufes'cens,** a species that infects sheep, goats, deer, and domestic rabbits.

protosulfate (pro''to-sul'fāt) that one of several sulfates of the same base which contains the smallest proportion of sulfate ion.

protosyphilis (pro''to-sif'ĭ-lis) primary syphilis.

Prototheria (pro''to-the'rĭ-ah) [*proto-* + Gr. *thērion* beast, animal] in some systems of classification, a subclass of the Mammalia, including the order Monotremata, the egg-laying mammals.

prototoxin (pro''to-tok'sin) [*proto-* + *toxin*] (*obs.*) that portion or constituent of a toxin which has the greatest combining capacity for the antitoxin; see *deuterotoxin, hemotoxin, heterotoxin, tritotoxin.*

prototoxoid (pro″to-tok′soid) protoxoid.

prototroph (pro′to-trōf) [*proto-* + Gr. *trophē* nourishment] a prototrophic organism.

prototrophic (pro″to-trof′ik) having the same growth factor requirements as the ancestral or prototype strain; said of microbial mutants.

prototropy (pro-tot′ro-pe) [*proton* + Gr. *trope* a turning] the more usual type of tautomerism, which is the result of a mobile hydrogen ion. For example, acetoacetic ester, $CH_3CCH_2COOC_2$-

$$H_5 \rightleftharpoons CH_3C=CHCOOC_2H_5.$$ Cf. *anionotropy.*

prototype (pro′to-tīp) [*proto-* + Gr. *typos* type] the original type or form after which other types or forms are developed.

protoveratrine (pro″to-ver′ah-trēn) an ester alkaloid obtained from the liliaceous plants *Veratrum album* L. and *V. viride* Aiton, occurring in two forms, designated A and B, both of which possess antihypertensive properties. Protoveratrine A is said to be more active than the B form; the two are usually administered in combination.

protovertebra (pro′to-ver′te-brah) 1. somite. 2. the caudal half of a somite that forms most of a vertebra.

protoxeoid (pro-tok′se-oid) protoxoid.

protoxide (pro-tok′sid) that one of a series of oxides of the same metal which contains the smallest amount of oxygen.

protoxoid (pro-tok′soid) any toxoid which has a greater affinity for the antitoxin than has the toxin; see *toxoid.*

Protozoa (pro″to-zo′ah) a phylum comprising the simplest organisms of the animal kingdom, consisting of unicellular organisms that range in size from submicroscopic to macroscopic; most are free-living, but some lead commensalistic, mutualistic, or parasitic existences. Protozoa are usually divided into four subphyla: Sarcodina (amebae), having pseudopodia during most of the life cycle; Mastigophora (flagellates), having one or more flagella during most of the life cycle; Ciliophora (ciliates and suctorians), having cilia during some stage of development; and Sporozoa, having no locomotor organs in the adult stages and reproducing by sporulation. Cf. *Metazoa.*

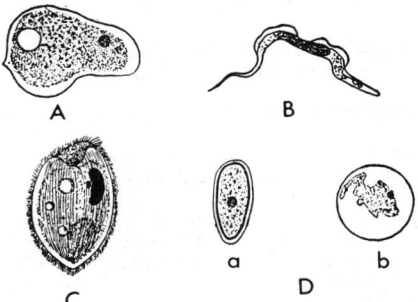

Subphyla of Protozoa: *A,* Sarcodina, represented by *Entamoeba histolytica* of amebic dysentery. *B,* Mastigophora, represented by *Trypanosoma gambiense* of African sleeping sickness. *C,* Ciliophora, represented by *Balantidium coli,* causative organism of a certain oriental dysentery (redrawn after Leuckart). *D,* Sporozoa, represented by (*a*) *Eimeria stiedae* from liver of rabbit, (*b*) *Plasmodium vivax,* of malaria, shown in a red blood cell (all greatly enlarged). (Herms.)

protozoa (pro″to-zo′ah) plural of *protozoon.*

protozoacide (pro″to-zo′ah-sīd) destructive to protozoa; an agent destructive to protozoa.

protozoagglutinin (pro″to-zo″ah-gloo′ti-nin) an agglutinin formed in the blood in protozoan infections which has the power of agglutinating the infecting protozoa.

protozoal (pro″to-zo′al) pertaining to or caused by protozoa.

protozoan (pro″to-zo′an) 1. of or pertaining to Protozoa. 2. an organism belonging to the Protozoa.

protozoiasis (pro″to-zo-i′ah-sis) any disease caused by protozoa.

protozoology (pro″to-zo-ol′o-je) the study of protozoa. **clinical p.,** the study of protozoan parasites causing diseases in man and other animals.

protozoon (pro″to-zo′on), pl. *protozoa* [*proto-* + Gr. *zōon* animal] a primitive animal organism consisting of a single cell; any individual organism belonging to the Protozoa.

protozoophage (pro″to-zo′o-fāj) [*protozoa* + Gr. *phagein* to eat] a cell which has a phagocytic action on protozoa.

protozoosis (pro″to-zo-o′sis) protozoiasis.

protozootherapy (pro″to-zo″o-ther′ah-pe) the treatment of diseases caused by protozoa, particularly the chemotherapy of such diseases.

protraction (pro-trak′shun) [L. *protrahere* to drag forth from a place] a facial anomaly in which a cephalometric landmark or facial structure stands farther forward than usual. **mandibular p.,** a facial anomaly in which the gnathion is anterior to the orbital plane. **maxillary p.,** a facial anomaly in which the subnasion is anterior to the orbital plane.

protractor (pro-trak′tor) [*pro-* + L. *trahere* to draw] an instrument for extracting bits of bone, bullets, or other foreign material from wounds.

protransglutaminase (pro-tranz″gloo-tam″in-ās) the inactive precursor of transglutaminase; called also *coagulation Factor XIII.*

protriptyline hydrochloride (pro-trip′ti-lēn) [USP] chemical name: *N*-methyl-5*H*-dibenzo [*a,d*] cycloheptene-5-propylamine hydrochloride; a tricyclic antidepressant, $C_{19}H_{21}N \cdot HCl$, occurring as a white to yellowish powder; administered orally.

protrusio (pro-troo′ze-o) [L.] the state of being thrust forward; projection. **p. acetab′uli,** arthrokatadysis.

protrusion (pro-troo′zhun) [L. *protrusi* to push forward] the state of being thrust forward or laterally, as in masticatory movements of the mandible. **bimaxillary p.,** the projection of both the maxilla and the mandible beyond normal limits in relation to the cranial base. **bimaxillary dentoalveolar p.,** the positioning of the entire dentition forward with respect to the facial profile. **intrapelvic p.,** arthrokatadysis.

protrypsin (pro-trip′sin) a substance convertible into trypsin.

protuberance (pro-tu′ber-ans) [*pro-* + L. *tuber* bulge] a projecting part, or prominence; an apophysis, process, or swelling. For names of specific anatomical structures not included here, see under *protuberantia.* **p. of chin,** protuberantia mentalis. **laryngeal p.,** prominentia laryngea. **occipital p., transverse,** torus occipitalis. **palatine p.,** torus palatinus. **tubal p.,** torus tubarius.

protuberantia (pro-tu″ber-an′she-ah) [L.] protuberance: a projecting part, or prominence. **p. menta′lis** [NA], mental protuberance: a more or less distinct and triangular prominence on the anterior surface of the body of the mandible, on or near the median line. **p. occipita′lis exter′na** [NA], external occipital protuberance: a prominence at the center of the outer surface of the squama of the occipital bone which gives attachment to the ligamentum nuchae. **p. occipita′lis inter′na** [NA], internal occipital protuberance: the projection of bone at the midpoint of the cruciform eminence, on the internal surface of the squama of the occipital bone, sometimes presenting as a ridge (*crista occipitalis interna* [NA]).

protyl, protyle (pro′til) [*proto-* + Gr. *hyle* matter] a theoretical substance from which all the chemical elements were formerly supposed to be derived.

proud (prowd) characterized by exuberant granulation tissue.

Provell (pro-vel′) trademark for a preparation of protoveratrines A and B.

Provera (pro-ver′ah) trademark for preparations of medroxyprogesterone acetate.

provertebra (pro-ver′te-brah) protovertebra.

provirus (pro-vi′rus) the genome of an animal virus integrated (by crossing over) into the chromosome of the host cell, and thus replicated in all of its daughter cells.

provisional (pro-vizh′un-al) formed or performed for temporary purposes; temporary.

provitamin (pro-vi′tah-min) a precursor of a vitamin; a substance from which the animal organism can form vitamin. Provitamin A is carotene. Ergosterol has been spoken of as provitamin D.

provocative (pro-vok′ah-tiv) stimulating the appearance of a sign, reflex, reaction, or therapeutic effect.

Prowazek's bodies (pro-vaht′seks) [Stanislas Joseph Matthias von *Prowazek,* zoologist in Hamburg, 1875–1915] see under *body.*

Prowazek-Greeff bodies (pro-vaht′sek-grāf) [S. J. M. von *Prowazek;* Carl Richard *Greeff,* German ophthalmologist, 1862–1938] trachoma bodies.

Prowazekella (pro-vaht″ze-kel′ah) *Proteromonas.*

Prowazekia (pro″vaht-zek′e-ah) *Bodo.*

proxazole (prok′sa-zōl) chemical name: *N,N*-diethyl-3-(1-phenylpropyl)-1,2,4-oxadiazole-5-ethanamine; a smooth muscle relaxant, analgesic, and anti-inflammatory, $C_{17}H_{25}N_3O$. **p. citrate,** the citrate salt of proxazole having the same actions as the base.

proxemics (prok-se′miks) the study of the effects of spatial distance between persons interacting with each other, and of their orientation toward each other.

proximad (prok′si-mad) toward the proximal end or in a proximal direction.

proximal (prok′si-mal) [L. *proximus* next] nearest; closer to any point of reference: opposed to *distal.*

proximalis (prok″si-ma′lis) proximal; [NA] a term denoting proximity to the point of origin or attachment of an organ or part.

proximate (prok′sĭ-māt) [L. *proximatus* drawn near] immediate or nearest.

proximoataxia (prok″sĭ-mo-ah-tak′se-ah) ataxia affecting the proximal part of an extremity, as the arm, forearm, thigh, or leg.

proximobuccal (prok″sĭ-mo-buk′al) pertaining to the proximal and buccal surfaces of a posterior tooth.

proximoceptor (prok″sĭ-mo-sep′tor) contiguous receptor.

proximolabial (prok″sĭ-mo-la′be-al) pertaining to the proximal and labial surfaces of an anterior tooth.

proximolingual (prok″sĭ-mo-ling′gwal) pertaining to the proximal and lingual surfaces of a tooth.

prozonal (pro′zo-nal) 1. situated before a sclerozone. 2. pertaining to a prozone.

prozone (pro′zōn) [*pro-* + *zone*] the phenomenon exhibited by some sera, which give effective agglutination reactions when diluted several hundred- or thousandfold but do not visibly react with the antigen particles when undiluted or only slightly diluted. The phenomenon is not due simply to antibody excess, but often involves a special class of antibodies, blocking or incomplete antibodies, which react with the corresponding particulate antigen in an anomalous manner. The bound antibody not only fails to elicit agglutination, but actively inhibits it. Called also *prezone*, *prozone phenomenon*, and *agglutinoid reaction*.

prozymogen (pro-zi′mo-jen) a precursor of a pre-enzyme, or zymogen.

PRPP phosphoribosylpyrophosphate.

prual (proo′al) a very violent poison from the root of the tropical flowering vine, *Coptosapelta flavescens;* used as a dart poison.

pruinate (proo′ĭ-nāt) [L. *pruina* hoarfrost] having the appearance of being covered with hoarfrost.

Prulet (pru′let) trademark for a preparation of oxyphenisatin acetate.

Prunella (proo-nel′ah) a genus of labiatę plants. *P. vulgaris* L. (heal-all or self-heal) is astringent and tonic.

prunin (proo′nin) a concentration prepared from the wild black cherry, *Prunus serotina* Ehrh. (Rosaceae), formerly used in thoracic and nervous diseases.

Prunus (proo′nus) [L. "plum-tree"] a genus of rosaceous trees and shrubs, including the plums, cherries, sloes, apricots, and peaches. **P. america′na**, Marsh., American wild plum or river plum. **P. amyg′dalus** Batsch., almond. **P. arMenia′ca**, apricot. **P. commu′nis** L., almond. **P. domes′tica** L., garden plum. **P. laurocer′asus** L., cherry laurel. **P. per′sica**, peach. **P. serot′ina** Ehrh., a large American cherry tree with dark bark and thick oval leaves; called also *wild cherry*. **P. spino′sa** L., a species of plum, the sloe, or blackthorn sloe. **P. virginia′na** L., the choke cherry of North America; its bark has sedative, pectoral, and astringent qualities and its fruit is highly astringent.

pruriginous (proo-rij″ĭ-nus) of the nature of or tending to cause prurigo.

prurigo (proo-ri′go) [L. "the itch"] a name applied to several itchy skin eruptions of unknown cause, in which the characteristic lesion (prurigo papule) is dome-shaped with a small transient vesicle on top, followed by crusting or lichenification; specific types are usually indicated by a modifying term. **p. ag′ria**, a severe prurigo persisting into adulthood, characterized chiefly by hard excoriated prurigo papules and lichenification, with sparse urticarial elements. **Besnier's p.**, a form of dermatitis which is known to pediatricians as infantile eczema (q.v.) when it occurs in infants and young children and to dermatologists as atopic dermatitis (q.v.) when it occurs in infants, adolescents, and adults. **p. chron′ica multifor′mis**, papular urticaria. **p. estiva′lis** (*obs.*), a papular type of polymorphous light eruption. **p. of Hebra**, p. mitis. **melanotic p.**, a form associated with primary biliary cirrhosis in women, characterized by reticulated hyperpigmentation and intense itching. **p. mi′tis**, a mild form of prurigo thought by some to be a mild papular variant of atopic dermatitis or of papular urticaria. **p. nodula′ris**, a type of neurodermatitis, with discrete, firm, rough-surfaced, dark brownish-gray, intensely itchy nodules up to 1 or 2 cm. broad; it mostly occurs on the extensor surfaces of the extremities, and chiefly affects middle-aged women. **p. sim′plex**, papular urticaria. **summer p.**, p. estivalis.

pruritic (proo-rit′ik) pertaining to or characterized by pruritus.

pruritogenic (proo″rĭ-to-jen′ik) capable of causing or tending to cause pruritus.

pruritus (proo-ri′tus) [L. from *prurire* to itch] itching; also, the name of various conditions characterized by itching, the specific site or type being indicated by a modifying term. **p. a′ni**, intense chronic itching in the anal region. **essential p.**, pruritus occurring idiopathically, without other discoverable abnormality. **p. hiema′lis**, winter itch. **p. scro′ti**, intense itching in the scrotal area. **senile p.**, **p. seni′lis**, an itching in the aged, possibly due to dryness of the skin occurring as a result of decreased sweat and sebum secretion, or bathing too frequently, or both. **symptomatic p.**, itching associated with and symptomatic of some other abnormality or disease, such as jaundice.

uremic p., generalized itching associated with chronic renal failure and not attributable to other internal or skin disease. **p. vul′vae**, intense itching of the external genitals of the female, as in kraurosis vulvae.

Prussak's fibers, pouch, space (proo′sahks) [Alexander *Prussak*, Russian otologist, 1839–1897] see under *fiber*, and see *recessus membranae tympani superior*.

prussiate (prus′e-āt) cyanide.

p.s. abbreviation for *per second*.

psalis (sa′lis) [Gr. "arch"] the fornix of the cerebrum (fornix cerebri [NA]).

psalterial (sal-te′re-al) pertaining to the psalterium.

psalterium (sal-te′re-um) [L.; Gr. *psaltērion* harp] 1. commissura fornicis. 2. the omasum.

Psalydolytta (sal″ĭ-do-lit′tah) a genus of blister beetles. *P. fusca* and *P. substrigata* of Africa produce a severe vesicular dermatitis.

psammo- (sam′o) [Gr. *psammos* sand] a combining form denoting relation to sand or to sandlike material.

psammocarcinoma (sam″o-kar″sĭ-no′mah) [*psammo-* + *carcinoma*] carcinoma containing calcareous matter.

psammoma (sam-o′mah) [*psammo-* + *-oma*] a tumor, especially a meningioma, that contains psammoma bodies; formerly sometimes called *Virchow's psammoma*.

psammosarcoma (sam″o-sar-ko′mah) [*psammo-* + *sarcoma*] a sarcoma containing a sandy deposit.

psammotherapy (sam″o-ther′ah-pe) [*psammo-* + Gr. *therapeia* treatment] ammotherapy.

psammous (sam′us) sandy.

psauoscopy (saw-os′ko-pe) [Gr. *psauein* to touch + *skopein* to examine] a method of physical examination by passing the ball of the index finger back and forth lightly over the margin of an abnormal area. Over the pathological area the finger seems to encounter greater resistance and the skin seems more tense and less supple.

pselaphesia (sel-ah-fe′ze-ah) [Gr. *psēlaphēsis* touching] the tactile sense.

psellism (sel′izm) [Gr. *psellisma* stammer] stammering or stuttering; see *stuttering*.

pseud- see *pseudo-*.

pseudacousis (soo″dah-koo′sis) [*pseud-* + Gr. *akousis* hearing] pseudacousma.

pseudacousma (soo″dah-kōōz′mah) [*pseud-* + Gr. *akousma* thing heard] a subjective sensation as if sounds were altered in pitch and quality.

pseudactinomycosis (soo-dak″tĭ-no-mi-ko′sis) pseudoactinomycosis.

pseudagraphia (soo″dah-gra′fe-ah) pseudoagraphia.

pseudalbuminuria (soo″dal-bu″mĭ-nu′re-ah) adventitious proteinuria.

Pseudamphistomum (sood″am-fis′to-mum) [*pseud-* + *amphi-* + Gr. *stoma* mouth] a genus of flukes; called also *Metorchis* and *Pseudoamphistomum*. **P. trunca′tum**, a species found in the bile ducts of cats, dogs, seals, and deer, and occasionally in man in Europe and India.

pseudangina (soo″dan-ji′nah) pseudoangina.

pseudankylosis (soo″dang-kĭ-lo′sis) pseudoankylosis.

pseudaphia (soo-da′fe-ah) [*pseud-* + Gr. *haphē* touch + *-ia*] defect in the power of perceiving touch.

pseudarrhenia (soo″dah-re′ne-ah) female pseudohermaphroditism.

pseudarthritis (soo″dar-thri′tis) [*pseud-* + *arthritis*] a hysterical affection of the joints.

pseudarthrosis (soo″dar-thro′sis) [*pseud-* + Gr. *arthrōsis* joint] a pathologic entity characterized by deossification of a weight-bearing long bone, followed by bending and pathologic fracture, with inability to form normal callus leading to existence of the "false joint" that gives the condition its name.

Pseudechis (soo-dek′is) [*pseud-* + Gr. *echis* viper] a genus of venomous elapid snakes of Australia, including *P. porphyria′cus*, the blacksnake. See table accompanying *snake*.

pseudencephalus (soo″den-sef′ah-lus) [*pseud-* + Gr. *enkephalos* brain] a monster with a vascular tumor in place of the brain.

pseudesthesia (soo″des-the′ze-ah) [*pseud-* + Gr. *aisthēsis* perception] any imaginary sensation; a sensation which is felt without any external stimulus, or a sensation which does not correspond to the stimulus that causes it.

pseudinoma (soo″dĭ-no′mah) [*pseud-* + *-oma*] phantom tumor.

pseudo-, pseud- [Gr. *pseudēs* false] combining form signifying false or spurious.

pseudoacanthosis (soo″do-ak″an-tho′sis) [*pseudo-* + *acanthosis*] a condition clinically resembling acanthosis. **p. ni′gricans**, a benign form of acanthosis nigricans associated with obesity; the obesity is sometimes associated with endocrine disturbance.

pseudoacephalus (soo″do-a-sef′ah-lus) [*pseudo-* + *acephalus*] a placental parasitic twin, apparently headless, but with a rudimentary cranium contained in the autosite.

pseudoactinomycosis (soo″do-ak″tĭ-no-mi-ko′-sis) [*pseudo-* + *actinomycosis*] a variety of chronic pulmonary disease resembling actinomycosis, usually nocardiosis.

pseudoagglutination (soo″do-ah-gloo″tĭ-na′shun) pseudohemagglutination.

pseudoagraphia (soo″do-ah-graf′e-ah) a condition in which the patient can copy writing, but cannot write except in a meaningless and illegible manner.

pseudoalbuminuria (soo″do-al″bu-mĭ-nu′re-ah) adventitious proteinuria.

pseudoalleles (soo″do-ah-lēlz′) [*pseudo-* + *allele*] 1. genes which are seemingly allelic, but which can eventually be shown to have distinct but closely linked loci. 2. allelic genes which form heterozygotes resembling the wild type rather than either mutant type.

pseudoallelic (soo″do-ah-lel′ik) pertaining to pseudoalleles; seemingly allelic but located at different sites on homologous chromosomes.

pseudoallelism (soo″do-al′lĕ-lizm) the possession of pseudoalleles.

pseudoalveolar (soo″do-al-ve′o-lar) simulating an alveolar structure.

Pseudoamphistomum (soo″do-am-fĭs′to-mum) *Pseudamphistomum.*

pseudoanaphylactic (soo″do-an″ah-fi-lak′tik) pertaining to pseudoanaphylaxis.

pseudoanaphylaxis (soo″do-an″ah-fi-lak′sis) [*pseudo-* + *anaphylaxis*] a reaction the symptoms of which resemble those of the anaphylactic reaction, produced by the injection of serum which has been acted upon by agar, kaolin, starch, and other substances, and also by the injection of other nonspecific proteins.

pseudoanemia (soo″do-ah-ne′me-ah) [*pseudo-* + *anemia*] marked pallor with no clinical or hematological evidence of anemia. **p. angiospas′tica,** a form due to vasoconstriction.

pseudoaneurysm (soo″do-an′u-rizm) dilatation and tortuosity of a vessel, giving the appearance of an aneurysm.

pseudoangina (soo″do-an-ji′nah) [*pseudo-* + *angina*] false angina; a syndrome occurring in nervous individuals, marked by precordial pain, fatigue, and lassitude, without evidence of organic disease of the heart. See *angina pectoris vasomotoria.*

pseudoankylosis (soo″do-ang″kĭ-lo′sis) a false ankylosis.

pseudoanodontia (soo″do-an″o-don′she-ah) the condition in which teeth develop but do not erupt.

pseudoantagonist (soo″do-an-tag′o-nist) a muscle which by flexing a joint enhances the effect of another muscle crossing that joint to act on a more distant one.

pseudoapoplexy (soo″do-ap′o-plek″se) [*pseudo-* + *apoplexy*] a condition resembling apoplexy, but without cerebral hemorrhage.

pseudoappendicitis (soo″do-ah-pen″dĭ-si′tis) a condition with symptoms simulating appendicitis, sometimes hysterical and sometimes of syphilitic origin, but without affection of the appendix. **p. zooparasit′ica,** a condition in which parasites are present in the vermiform appendix.

pseudoarthrosis (soo″do-ar-thro′sis) pseudarthrosis.

pseudoasthma (soo″do-as′mah) paroxysmal dyspnea.

pseudoathetosis (soo″do-ath″e-to′sis) movements of the fingers elicited when the patient closes his eyes and extends his arms, associated with impairment of joint position sense.

pseudoatrophoderma colli (soo″do-at″ro-fo-der′mah kol′le) a skin disease characterized by papillomatous, depigmented, glossy lesions on the sides of the neck; the depigmented areas resemble vitiligo. It probably differs from confluent reticulated papillomatosis chiefly in its location.

pseudobacillus (soo″do-bah-sil′us) an exceedingly small, rodlike poikilocyte, resembling a microorganism.

pseudobacterium (soo″do-bak-te′re-um) [*pseudo-* + Gr. *baktērion* stick] a cell that resembles a bacterium.

pseudobasedow (soo″do-bas′e-dow) basedow.

pseudobronchiectasis (soo″do-brong″ke-ek′tah-sis) a condition in which a bronchiectasis-like pattern appears in the bronchogram of partially atelectatic pulmonary segments when the larger bronchi have become shortened and broadened in outline; these reversible changes do not indicate destruction of the bronchial walls.

pseudobulbar (soo″do-bul′bar) apparently, but not really, due to a bulbar lesion.

pseudocartilage (soo″do-kar′tĭ-lij) chondroid tissue.

pseudocartilaginous (soo″do-kar″tĭ-laj′ĭ-nus) composed of a substance resembling cartilage.

pseudocast (soo″do-kast) a false cast: a form of urinary sediment resembling true casts, but being an accidental formation, taking the shape of casts by adherence to mucus threads, cotton fibers, etc.

pseudocele (soo′do-sēl) the cavum septi pellucidi.

pseudocephalocele (soo″do-sef′ah-lo-sēl) a hernia of the brain not congenital, but due to disease or injury of the skull.

pseudochancre (soo″do-shang′ker) an indurated lesion resembling or simulating chancre. **p. re′dux,** a gummatous recurrence at the site of a primary syphilitic lesion.

pseudocholecystitis (soo″do-ko″le-sis-ti′tis) a syndrome resembling cholecystitis but occurring as an allergic response to eating certain foods.

pseudocholesteatoma (soo″do-ko″les-te-ah-to′mah) a mass of cornified epithelial cells resembling cholesteatoma in the tympanic cavity in chronic middle ear inflammation.

pseudocholinesterase (soo″do-ko″lin-es′ter-ās) cholinesterase.

pseudochorea (soo″do-ko-re′ah) [*pseudo-* + *chorea*] a condition of complete general incoordination with symptoms like those of chorea.

pseudochromesthesia (soo″do-kro″mes-the′ze-ah) [*pseudo-* + Gr. *chrōma* color + *aisthēsis* perception + *-ia*] a false sensation of color.

pseudochromidrosis (soo″do-kro″mid-ro′sis) [*pseudo-* + *chromidrosis*] sweating with the presence on the skin of pigment due to the action of bacteria.

pseudochromosome (soo″do-kro′mo-sōm) rodlike Golgi bodies of the spermatocytes.

pseudochylous (soo″do-ki′lus) resembling chyle, but containing no fat.

pseudocirrhosis (soo″do-sĭ-ro′sis) [*pseudo-* + *cirrhosis*] a clinical condition suggestive of, but not due to, cirrhosis; it is often due to pericarditis (*pericardial p.*). See also *Pick's disease,* def. 2. **pericardial p. of the liver, pericarditic p.,** Pick's disease, def. 2.

pseudoclaudication (soo″do-claw″dĭ-ka′shun) intermittent claudication due to compression of the cauda equina.

pseudoclonus (soo″do-klo′nus) a short-lived clonic response.

pseudocoarctation (soo″do-ko″ark-ta′shun) a substandard term used to refer to a condition roentgenologically resembling coarctation, but without compromise of the lumen of the affected structure; a "kinked aorta," possibly an aortic arch anomaly. **p. of the aorta,** an uncommon congenital anomaly of the arch of the aorta that simulates roentgenologically coarctation but does not produce occlusion of the vessel.

pseudocoele (soo′do-sēl) [*pseudo-* + Gr. *koilia* hollow] the cavum septi pellucidi.

pseudocoelom (soo″do-se′lom) in zoology, a body cavity between the mesoderm and endoderm; a persistent blastocoele.

pseudocoelomate (soo″do-sēl′o-māt) 1. having a pseudocoelom. 2. an animal having a pseudocoelom, as the aschelminths.

pseudocolloid (soo″do-kol′oid) a mucoid substance sometimes found in ovarian cysts. **p. of lips,** Fordyce's spots.

pseudocoloboma (soo″do-kol″o-bo′mah) a line or scar on the iris giving the appearance of a coloboma.

pseudocolony (soo″do-kol′o-ne) a small aggregation of crystalline or other materials which sometimes appears on the surface of sterile serum agar or other culture plates, especially after long incubation or drying.

pseudocopulation (soo″do-kop′u-la′shun) bodily association of male and female associated with liberation of gametes in proximity of space and time but without sexual union.

pseudo-corpus luteum (soo″do-kor″pus loo′te-um) a maturing graafian follicle which does not rupture but retains its ovum and then becomes luteinized.

pseudocowpox (soo″do-kow′poks) milker's nodules; see under *nodule.*

pseudocoxalgia (soo″do-kok-sal′je-ah) osteochondrosis of the capitular epiphysis of the femur; see under *osteochondrosis.*

pseudocrisis (soo-dok′rĭ-sis) [*pseudo-* + Gr. *krisis* crisis] a false crisis; a sudden but temporary abatement of febrile symptoms.

pseudocroup (soo″do-kroōp′) 1. laryngismus stridulus. 2. thymic asthma.

pseudocyanin (soo″do-si′ah-nin) pseudoisocyanin.

pseudocyesis (soo″do-si-e′sis) [*pseudo-* + Gr. *kyēsis* pregnancy] false pregnancy.

pseudocylindroid (soo″do-sĭ-lin′droid) a shred of mucin in the urine resembling a cylindroid; sometimes of spermatic origin.

pseudocyst (soo′do-sist) [*pseudo-* + *cyst*] an abnormal or dilated space resembling a cyst but not lined by epithelium as is a true cyst. **pancreatic p.,** an encapsulated collection of pancreatic juice and cellular debris that has escaped from the pancreas, the wall being formed by inflammatory fibrosis of serosal surfaces of adjacent organs; pseudocysts most commonly occur in the lesser sac of the peritoneum.

pseudodementia (soo″do-de-men′she-ah) an extreme condition of general apathy simulating dementia, but with no actual defect of intelligence. **hysterical p.,** a condition marked by failure of memory, with seeming inability to answer simple questions, and by a psychotic-like state accompanied by bizarre behavior and episodes of excitement or stupor.

pseudodextrocardia (soo″do-deks″tro-kar′de-ah) a condition in which the heart is displaced to the right, but the ventricles are not inverted nor are the great vessels transposed.

pseudodiabetes (soo″do-di″ah-be′tēz) subclinical diabetes.

pseudodiastolic (soo″do-di″ah-stol′ik) apparently but not truly diastolic.

pseudodiphtheria (soo″do-dif-the′re-ah) the presence of a false membrane not due to *Corynbacterium diphtheriae.*

pseudodominant (soo″do-dom′ĭ-nant) giving the appearance of being dominant; said of a recessive genetic trait appearing in the offspring of a homozygous and a heterozygous parent, the trait being manifested only in the homozygous parent and offspring.

pseudodysentery (soo″do-dis′en-ter″e) a condition marked by the symptoms of dysentery, but due to some local irritation and not to the organisms of dysentery.

pseudoedema (soo″do-ĕ-de′mah) a puffy state resembling edema.

pseudoembryonic (soo″do-em″bre-on′ik) apparently, but not truly, embryonic.

pseudoemphysema (soo″do-em″fĭ-ze′mah) a condition resembling emphysema, but due to temporary blocking of the bronchial tubes.

pseudoencephalomalacia (soo″do-en-sef″ah-lo-mah-la′she-ah) a highly fatal disease of cattle, sheep, and pigs, marked by edema of the brain, with muzzle twitching, opisthotonos, blindness, and inability to stand.

pseudoendometritis (soo″do-en″do-mĕ-tri′tis) a condition simulating endometritis, in which there are changes in the blood vessels, hyperplasia of the stroma and glands, and atrophy.

pseudoeosinophil (soo″do-e″o-sin′o-fil) neutrophilic leukocytes with granules showing a predilection for acid dyes.

pseudoephedrine (soo″do-ĕ-fed′rin) chemical name: [S-(R*,-R*)]-α-[1-(methylamino)ethyl]benzenemethanol. One of the stereoisomers of ephedrine, $C_{10}H_{15}NO$, having less pressor action and central stimulant effects than ephedrine. **p. hydrochloride** [USP], the hydrochloride salt of pseudoephedrine, $C_{10}H_{15}NO \cdot HCl$, occurring as fine, white to off-white crystals or as a powder; used as a nasal decongestant, and as a bronchodilator, administered orally.

pseudoepiphysis (soo″do-e-pif′ĭ-sis) an accessory bone at the distal and the proximal end of the second metacarpal bone.

pseudoesthesia (soo″do-es-the′ze-ah) pseudesthesia.

pseudoexfoliation (soo″do-eks″fo-le-a′shun) a condition resembling exfoliation but actually resulting from deposition, as from the deposition of small grayish particles on the capsule of the crystalline lens.

pseudoexophoria (soo″do-ek″so-fo′re-ah) an outward tendency of the visual axis excited by diminishing the activity of the accommodative centers.

pseudoexophthalmos (soo″do-eks″of-thal′mos) any condition, other than exophthalmos, that gives a prominent appearance to the eyes, e.g., marked lid retraction, shallow orbits, congenital macroophthalmos, and high myopia.

pseudoextrophy (soo″do-ek′stro-fe) a developmental anomaly marked by the characteristic musculoskeletal defects of exstrophy of the bladder but with no major defect of the urinary tract.

pseudofarcy (soo″do-far′se) lymphangitis epizootica.

pseudofluctuation (soo″do-fluk′tu-a′shun) a tremor resembling fluctuation, such as is sometimes seen on tapping lipomas.

pseudofollicutitis (soo″do-fo-lik″u-li′tis) a chronic disorder occurring chiefly in the beard of Negroes, most often in the submandibular region of the neck, the characteristic lesions of which are erythematous papules, less commonly pustules, containing buried hairs whose tips can easily be freed up; in contrast to sycosis barbae (q.v.), which is most frequently seen in bearded men, this disorder affects exclusively those who shave.

pseudofracture (soo″do-frak′tūr) a condition seen in the roentgenogram of a bone as a thickening of the periosteum and formation of new bone over what looks like an incomplete fracture.

pseudofructose (soo″do-fruk′tōs) a form of fructose, differing from it in the carbon atom configuration.

pseudoganglion (soo″do-gang′gle-on) a thickening of a nerve simulating a ganglion. **Bochdalek's p.,** plexus dentalis superior. **Cloquet's p.,** see under *ganglion.* **Valentin's p.,** intumescentia tympanica.

pseudogestation (soo″do-jes-ta′shun) false pregnancy.

pseudogeusesthesia (soo″do-gūs″es-the′ze-ah) [*pseudo-* + Gr. *geusis* taste + *aisthēsis* perception + *-ia*] a false sensation of taste associated with a sensation of another modality.

pseudogeusia (soo″do-gu′ze-ah) [*pseudo-* + Gr. *geusis* taste + *-ia*] a sensation of taste inappropriate to the exciting stimulus or occurring in the absence of a stimulus.

pseudoglanders (soo″do-glan′derz) lymphangitis ulcerosa pseudofarcinosa.

pseudoglioma (soo″do-gli-o′mah) a condition resembling glioma, a membrane being produced back of the lens because of failure of the posterior vascular sheath of the lens to atrophy, or because of its replacement by connective tissue.

pseudoglobulin (soo″do-glob′u-lin) one of a class of globulins characterized by being soluble in water in the absence of neutral salts and thus not a true globulin (euglobulin); see also under *globulin.*

pseudoglottic (soo″do-glot′ik) pertaining to the pseudoglottis.

pseudoglottis (soo″do-glot′is) 1. the aperture between the false vocal cords. 2. neoglottis.

pseudoglucosazone (soo″do-gloo″ko-sa′zōn) a crystalline substance sometimes developed in normal urine in testing for sugar.

pseudogonorrhea (soo″do-gon″o-re′ah) gonococcal urethritis.

pseudogout (soo″do-gowt) an apparently hereditary, arthritic condition marked by attacks of goutlike symptoms, usually affecting a single joint (particularly the knee) and associated with chondrocalcinosis.

pseudographia (soo″do-graf′e-ah) [*pseudo-* + Gr. *graphein* to write + *-ia*] the production of meaningless written symbols.

pseudogynecomastia (soo″do-jin″ĕ-ko-mas′te-ah) an excess of adipose tissue in the male breast with no increase in glandular tissue.

pseudohallucination (soo″do-hah-loo″sĭ-na′shun) a hallucination brought about by the exercise of memory and imagination; the individual experiencing it realizes that it is morbid rather than real.

pseudohaustration (soo″do-haw-stra′shun) a false appearance of normal sacculation of the wall of the colon, the roentgenographic appearance being produced by edematous islands of mucosa regularly placed between deep areas of ulceration in the muscle layers.

pseudohelminth (soo″do-hel′minth) [*pseudo-* + Gr. *helmins* worm] a structure or object that resembles an endoparasitic worm.

pseudohemagglutination (soo″do-hem″ah-gloo″tĭ-na′shun) a clumping of erythrocytes due to rouleau formation.

pseudohematuria (soo″do-he″mah-tu′re-a) the presence in the urine of pigments that impart to it a pink or red color, but with no detectable hemoglobin or blood cells.

pseudohemophilia (soo″do-he″mo-fil′e-ah) von Willebrand's disease.

pseudohemoptysis (soo″do-he-mop′tĭ-sis) spitting of blood which comes from some source other than the lungs or bronchial tubes.

pseudohereditary (soo″do-hĕ-red′ĭ-tār″e) occurring in successive generations because of imposition of the same environmental factors and not because of genetic transmission.

pseudohermaphrodism (soo″do-her-maf′ro-dizm) pseudohermaphroditism.

pseudohermaphrodite (soo″do-her-maf′ro-dīt) an individual who has gonadal tissue of one sex and shows one or more contradictions of the morphological criteria of sex. See also *intersex* and *hermaphrodite.* **female p.,** a genetic and gonadal female, with partial masculinization; called also *female intersex.* **male p.,** a genetic and gonadal male with incomplete masculinization; called also *male intersex.*

pseudohermaphroditism (soo″do-her-maf′ro-dīt-izm″) a condition in which the gonads are of one sex but one or more contradictions exist in the morphologic criteria of sex. See also *intersexuality* and *hermaphroditism.* **female p.,** a form in which the affected individual is a genetic and gonadal female with partial masculinization. **male p.,** a form in which the affected individual is a genetic and gonadal male with incomplete masculinization.

pseudohernia (soo″do-her′ne-ah) an inflamed sac or gland simulating strangulated hernia.

pseudoheterotopia (soo″do-het″er-o-to′pe-ah) displacement of gray or white matter of the brain or cord, produced by unskillful manipulation in the autopsy.

pseudohydrocephalus (soo″do-hi″dro-sef′ah-lus) abnormally large appearance of a normal-sized head, due to smallness of the face and body, as in Russell's syndrome.

pseudohydronephrosis (soo″do-hi″dro-ne-fro′sis) a paranephritic cyst.

pseudohyoscyamine (soo″do-hi″o-si′ah-min) norhyoscyamine.

pseudohyperkalemia (soo″do-hi″per-kal-e′me-ah) spurious elevation of serum levels of potassium, as by release of potassium from platelets in thrombocytosis or from leukocytes in chronic myelogenous leukemia.

pseudohypertrichosis (soo″do-hi″per-trĭ-ko′sis) persistence after birth of the fine hair present during fetal life, owing to inability of the skin to throw it off.

pseudohypertrophic (soo″do-hi″per-trof′ik) characterized by apparent, but not real, hypertrophy.

pseudohypertrophy (soo″do-hi-per′tro-fe) false hypertrophy;

increase of size without true hypertrophy. **muscular p.,** an increase in the size of a muscle which is not due to enlargement of muscle fibers but to infiltration of the muscle with other tissue.

pseudohypoaldosteronism (soo″do-hi″po-al-dos′ter-ōn-izm) a hereditary disorder of infancy characterized by severe salt loss by the kidneys despite elevated secretion and urinary excretion of aldosterone; it is thought to be due to unresponsiveness of the distal renal tubule to aldosterone. Affected infants outgrow the need for dietary salt supplements in early childhood. The term is also applied to the endocrine abnormality associated with sodium-losing nephropathy, usually due to chronic pyelonephritis, in adults.

pseudohypoparathyroidism (soo″do-hi″po-par″ah-thi′roi-dizm) a hereditary condition clinically resembling hypoparathyroidism, but caused by failure of response to rather than deficiency of parathyroid hormone. It is characterized by hypocalcemia and hyperphosphatemia, and is commonly associated with short stature, obesity, short metacarpals, and ectopic calcification.

pseudohypophosphatasia (soo″do-hi″po-fos″fah-ta′ze-ah) a condition resembling hypophosphatasia, characterized by osteopathy of the skull and long bones, muscular hypotonia, hypercalcemia, and phosphoethanolaminuria. It is distinguished by normal alkaline phosphatase activity.

pseudohypothyroidism (soo″do-hi″po-thi′roi-dizm) the inability to utilize thyroxine in tissue cells, despite normal thyroid function, leading to development of the symptoms and certain stigmata of hypothyroidism.

pseudoicterus (soo″do-ik′ter-us) pseudojaundice.

pseudoinfarction (soo″do-in-fark′shun) the simulation in the electrocardiographic pattern of myocardial infarction, due to other cardiopathies.

pseudoion (soo″do-i′on) one of the electrically charged particles of a colloidal solution.

pseudoisochromatic (soo″do-i″so-kro-mat′ik) seemingly of the same color throughout: applied to solutions for testing color blindness, containing two pigments which will be distinguished by the normal eye, but not by the color blind. Cf. *anisochromatic.*

pseudoisocyanin (soo″do-i″so-si′ah-nin) an orange metachromatic dye, *N,N¹*-diethyl pseudoisocyanin, used for the selective demonstration of insulin in pancreatic islet beta cells.

pseudojaundice (soo″do-jawn′dis) skin discoloration caused by blood changes and not due to liver disease, as in carotinemia.

pseudokeratin (soo″do-ker′ah-tin) false keratin, found in the skin and the nervous system.

pseudolamellar (soo″do-lah-mel′ar) resembling lamellae.

pseudoleukemia (soo″do-lu-ke′me-ah) an obsolete term for a group of conditions resembling one another in showing enlargement of the lymph glands and in characteristics which resemble the conditions present in leukemia, but without leukemic blood findings. The term included aleukemic lymphadenosis, aleukemic myelosis, Hodgkin's disease, Kundrat's lymphosarcoma, multiple myeloma, and tuberculosis and syphilis of the lymph glands. See *lymphogranulomatosis,* and *agnogenic myeloid metaplasia,* under *metaplasia.* **p. cu′tis,** pseudoleukemia with the development of skin lesions. **p. gastrointestina′lis,** a condition characterized by extensive lymphocytic infiltration of the gastrointestinal tract, without the typical clinical picture of leukemia. **p. lymphat′ica,** nonsplenic leukemia, a state associated with Hodgkin's disease and also with lymphomatous tumors of the kidneys and intestines in children. **myelogenous p.,** former term for multiple myeloma.

pseudoleukocythemia (soo″do-lu″ko-si-the′me-ah) pseudoleukemia.

pseudolipoma (soo″do-lĭ-po′mah) localized edema of neuropathic origin simulating lipoma; it occurs in hysteria and certain lesions of the nervous system. Called also *neuropathic edema.*

pseudolithiasis (soo″do-lĭ-thi′ah-sis) a condition with symptoms of spasm resembling biliary colic.

pseudologia (soo″do-lo′je-ah) [*pseudo-* + Gr. *logos* word + *-ia*] the writing of anonymous letters to people of prominence, to one's self, etc. **p. fantas′tica,** a tendency to tell extravagant and fantastic falsehoods centered about one's self.

pseudoluxation (soo″do-luk-sa′shun) partial dislocation of a bone.

Pseudolynchia (soo″do-linch′e-a) a genus of parasitic flies of the family Hippoboscidae. **P. canarien′sis, P. mau′rah,** a species of pigeon flies that are vectors of *Haemoproteus columbae;* called also *Lynchia maura.*

pseudomalignancy (soo″do-mah-lig′nan-se) a lesion, especially of skin, histologically malignant but clinically benign, as in keratoacanthoma, juvenile melanoma, dermatofibroma, etc.

pseudomamma (soo″do-mam′ah) a structure resembling a nipple, or even a complete breast, sometimes found on ovarian dermoids.

pseudomania (soo″do-ma′ne-ah) [*pseudo-* + Gr. *mania* madness] 1. false or pretended mental disorder. 2. pathologic lying.

pseudomasturbation (soo″do-mas″tur-ba′shun) peotillomania.

pseudomegacolon (soo″do-meg′ah-ko″lon) dilatation of the colon in adults. Cf. *megacolon.*

pseudomelanosis (soo″do-mel″ah-no′sis) a staining of the tissue after death with pigments from the blood.

pseudomelia (soo″do-me′le-ah) [*pseudo-* + Gr. *melos* limb + *-ia*] phantom limb. **p. paraesthet′ica,** the perception of various morbid or perverted sensations as occurring in an absent or paralyzed limb.

pseudomembrane (soo″do-mem′brān) false membrane; see under *membrane.*

pseudomembranous (soo″do-mem′brah-nus) marked by or pertaining to a *pseudomembrane.*

pseudomeningitis (soo″do-men″in-ji′tis) pial inflammation with symptoms resembling meningitis.

pseudomenstruation (soo″do-men″stroo-a′shun) uterine discharge unattended with endometrial changes of menstruation, usually occurring in newborn babies.

pseudomethemoglobin (soo″do-met-he″mo-glo′bin) methemalbumin.

pseudomicrocephalus (soo″do-mi″kro-sef′ah-lus) an individual with a small brain due to the atrophy of one hemisphere, probably acquired secondarily.

pseudomilium (soo″do-mil′e-um) see *colloid milium,* under *milium.*

Pseudomonadaceae (soo″do-mo″nah-da′se-e) a family of microorganisms (order Pseudomonadales, suborder Pseudomonadineae), occurring as elongate straight rods or coccoid cells in soil and fresh or salt water. It includes 12 genera, *Acetobacter, Aeromonas, Alginomonas, Azotomonas, Halobacterium, Mycoplana, Photobacterium, Protaminobacter, Pseudomonas, Xanthomonas, Zoogloea,* and *Zymomonas.*

Pseudomonadales (soo″do-mo″nah-da′lēz) an order of class Schizomycetes, made up of straight, curved, or spiral, rigid, rod-shaped, gram-negative microorganisms, rarely occurring in pairs or chains, and including two suborders, Pseudomonadineae and Rhodobacteriineae.

Pseudomonadineae (soo″do-mo″nah-di′ne-e) a suborder of Schizomycetes (order Pseudomonadales), made up of cells of various shapes and sizes, containing unique pigments, soluble in water or organic solvents. It includes seven families, Caulobacteraceae, Methanomonadaceae, Nitrobacteraceae, Pseudomonadaceae, Siderocapsaceae, Spirillaceae, and Thiobacteriaceae.

Pseudomonas (soo″do-mo′nas) a genus of microorganisms of the family Pseudomonadaceae, suborder Pseudomonadineae, order Pseudomonadales, occurring usually as monotrichous, lophotrichous, or nonmotile straight rods. Some of the 149 described species are pathogenic for plants or for warm- and cold-blooded vertebrates. **P. aerugino′sa,** the type species of the genus, and the only one pathogenic for man, made up of microorganisms which produce the blue-green pigment, pyocyanin, which gives the color to "blue pus" observed in certain suppurative infections. It is the causative agent of a variety of human diseases, including some cases of endocarditis, pneumonia, and meningitis, and sometimes causes a type of otitis known as *hot weather ear.* Formerly called *P. pyocyanea, Bacillus pyocyaneus,* and *Bacterium aeruginosa.* **P. eisenber′gii,** a species of nonpathogenic fluorescent microorganisms found in water, which do not liquefy gelatin. **P. fluores′cens,** a species of nonpathogenic fluorescent microorganisms found in feces, sewage, soil, and water, and which liquefy gelatin. **P. mal′lei,** the etiologic agent of glanders. **P. nonliquefa′ciens,** *P. eisenbergii.* **P. pseudomal′lei,** the causative agent of melioidosis, a glanders-like infection observed in rodents and occasionally in man. **P. pyocya′nea,** *P. aeruginosa.* **P. reptiliv′ora,** a species which is pathogenic for lizards. **P. sep′tica,** a species which causes a disease of caterpillars. **P. syncya′nea,** a species isolated from blue milk, which produces the blue pigment responsible for its color.

Pseudomonilia (soo″do-mo-nil′e-ah) *Candida.*

pseudomorphine (soo″do-mor′fin) a compound, $C_{34}H_{36}N_2O_6 \cdot 3H_2O$, occurring in opium and prepared by the oxidation of morphine; called also *dehydromorphine.*

pseudomotor (soo″do-mo′tor) producing movements which are not normal.

pseudomucin (soo″do-mu′sin) a substance resembling mucin found in ovarian cysts.

pseudomucinous (soo″do-mu′sĭ-nus) pertaining to pseudomucin.

pseudomyiasis (soo″do-mi-i′ah-sis) the presence of fly maggots in the digestive tract due to ingestion; if present in large numbers, they may cause diarrhea and other symptoms.

pseudomyopia (soo″do-mi-o′pe-ah) defective vision, not myopia, which causes the patient to hold objects nearer than normal to the eyes, thus simulating myopia.

pseudomyxoma (soo″do-mik-so′mah) a colloid growth developed upon the peritoneum, often secondary to an ovarian dermoid cyst. **p. peritone′i,** the presence in the peritoneal cavity of mucoid matter from a ruptured ovarian cyst or a ruptured mucocele of the appendix; called also *hydrops spurius.*

pseudonarcotic (soo″do-nar-kot′ik) sedative and apparently, but not directly, narcotic.

pseudonarcotism (soo″do-nar′ko-tizm) a hysterical condition simulating narcosis.

pseudoneoplasm (soo″do-ne′o-plazm) [*pseudo-* + *neoplasm*] 1. a temporary formation resembling a tumor. 2. a phantom tumor.

pseudoneuritis (soo″do-nu-ri′tis) a hyperemic condition of the optic papilla, occurring as a congenital anomaly.

pseudoneuroma (soo″do-nu-ro′mah) [*pseudo-* + *neuroma*] a tumor on a nerve simulating a neuroma; false neuroma.

pseudoneuronophagia (soo″do-nu-ro″no-fa′je-ah) a false appearance of phagocytosis of nerve cells.

pseudonit (soo′do-nit) [*pseudo:* + *nit*] hair cast, def. 2.

pseudonucleolus (soo″do-nu-kle′o-lus) [*pseudo-* + *nucleolus*] karyosome.

pseudonystagmus (soo″do-nis-tag′mus) large rhythmic jerking movements of the eye occurring in association with other diseases.

pseudo-obstruction (soo″do-ob-struk′shun) a condition simulating obstruction. **intestinal p.,** a condition characterized by constipation, colicky pain, and vomiting, but without evidence of organic obstruction apparent at laparotomy.

pseudo-ochronosis (soo″do-o-kro′no-sis) a condition resembling ochronosis, but not caused by a disorder of metabolism.

pseudo-optogram (soo″do-op′to-gram) an optogram in which the rods strip off from the illuminated spot and only the cones remain.

pseudo-osteomalacia (soo″do-os″te-o-mah-la′she-ah) rachitic contraction of the pelvis.

pseudo-ovum (soo″do-o′vum) a large prominent cell, resembling an ovum, seen in granuloma-cell tumor.

pseudopannus (soo″do-pan′nus) a disorder of the cornea resembling pannus, as sometimes occurs in molluscum contagiosum.

pseudopapilla (soo″do-pah-pil′ah) a false papilla formed by the presence of deeply depressed lines or grooves on the gingival papillae or the marginal gingivae but without the separation of the tissue seen with cleft formation.

pseudopapilledema (soo″do-pap″ĭ-lĕ-de′mah) anomalous elevation of the optic disk.

pseudoparalysis (soo″do-pah-ral′ĭ-sis) false paralysis: apparent loss of muscular power, without true paralysis, marked by defective coordination of movements or by repression of movement on account of pain. **p. ag′itans,** paralysis agitans. **arthritic general p.,** a condition resembling general paralysis, dependent on intracranial atheroma in arthritic persons; called also *Klippel's disease.* **congenital atonic p.,** amyotonia congenita. **Parrot's p., syphilitic p.,** pseudoparalysis of one or more of the extremities in infants caused by syphilitic osteochondritis of an epiphysis.

pseudoparaphrasia (soo″do-par″ah-fra′ze-ah) complete general incoherence in which the patient calls everything by a wrong name.

pseudoparaplegia (soo″do-par″ah-ple′je-ah) spurious paralysis of the lower limbs, as in malingering or hysteria.

pseudoparasite (soo″do-par′ah-sīt) any object resembling or mistaken for a parasite.

pseudoparesis (soo″do-pah-re′sis) a hysterical or other nonorganic condition simulating paresis.

pseudopelade (soo″do-pe′lād) patchy alopecia of the scalp roughly simulating, and rarely accompanying, alopecia areata; it may be due to various diseases of the follicles, some of which are associated with scarring and some are not.

pseudopellagra (soo″do-pĕ-lag′rah) a condition in alcoholics once thought to be similar but not known to be identical to pellagra.

pseudopeptone (soo″do-pep′tōn) ovomucoid.

pseudopericardial (soo″do-per″ĭ-kar′de-al) seemingly, but not actually, arising from the pericardium.

pseudoperitonitis (soo″do-per″ĭ-to-ni′tis) peritonism.

pseudophakia (soo″do-fa′ke-ah) a condition in which the degenerated crystalline lens is replaced by mesodermal tissue. **p. adipo′sa,** a condition in which the crystalline lens is replaced by a mass of fatty tissue. **p. fibro′sa,** replacement of the crystalline lens by a mass of connective tissue that represents hyperplasia of both the anterior and posterior vascular sheaths of the lens.

pseudophotesthesia (soo″do-fo″tes-the′ze-ah) the perception of light on receipt of a stimulus other than light.

pseudophthisis (soo-dof′thi-sis) a wasting disease not of the nature of tuberculosis.

Pseudophyllidea (soo″do-fĭ-lid′e-ah) an order of cestodes in which the scolex typically has two opposing sucking organs. It includes the family Diphyllobothriidae.

pseudophyllidean (soo″do-fil-lid′e-an) pertaining to or caused by tapeworms of the order Pseudophyllidea.

pseudoplasm (soo′do-plazm) a new growth which disappears spontaneously.

pseudoplegia (soo″do-ple′je-ah) [*pseudo-* + Gr. *plēgē* stroke + *-ia*] hysterical paralysis or pseudoparalysis.

pseudopneumonia (soo″do-nu-mo′ne-ah) a condition marked by the symptoms of pneumonia, but without any lesions in the lungs.

pseudopod (soo′do-pod) pseudopodium.

pseudopodia (soo″do-po′de-ah) plural of *pseudopodium.*

pseudopodiospore (soo″do-po′de-o-spōr) [*pseudopodium* + *spore*] amebula, def. 2.

pseudopodium (soo″do-po′de-um), pl. *pseudopo′dia* [*pseudo-* + Gr. *pous* foot] a temporary protrusion of the cytoplasm of an ameba, serving for purposes of locomotion or to engulf food. There are four types: axopodium, filopodium, lobopodium, and rhizopodium.

pseudopoliomyelitis (soo″do-po″le-o-mi″ĕ-li′tis) a poliomyelitis-like disease caused by an enterovirus other than poliovirus.

pseudopolycythemia (soo″do-pol″e-si-the′me-ah) 1. stress polycythemia. 2. relative polycythemia.

pseudopolymelia (soo″do-pol″e-mi-e′le-ah) an illusory sensation which may be referred to many extreme portions of the body, including the nose, nipples, and glans penis, as well as the hands and feet. **p. paraesthet′ica,** the perception of various morbid or perverted sensations, referred to various extreme portions of the body.

pseudopolyp (soo″do-pol′ip) a hypertrophied tab of mucous membrane resembling a polyp, but caused by ulceration surrounding and sometimes undermining a portion of intact mucosa; frequently observed in chronic inflammatory diseases, such as ulcerative colitis.

pseudopolyposis (soo″do-pol″ĭ-po′sis) the occurrence of numbers of pseudopolyps in the colon and rectum, as the result of long-standing inflammation.

pseudopregnancy (soo″do-preg′nan-se) 1. false pregnancy. 2. the premenstrual stage of the endometrium; so called because it resembles the endometrium just before implantation of the blastocyst.

pseudoprognathism (soo″do-prog′nah-thizm) a deformity which gives the appearance of a true anteroposterior jaw malrelationship, but which primarily affects the teeth, rather than basal bone.

pseudoproteinuria (soo″do-pro″te-in-u′re-ah) adventitious proteinuria.

pseudopseudohypoparathyroidism (soo″do-soo″do-hi″po-par″ah-thi′roid-izm) an incomplete form of pseudohypoparathyroidism characterized by the same constitutional features but by normal levels of calcium and phosphorus in the serum.

pseudopsia (soo-dop′se-ah) [*pseudo-* + Gr. *opsis* vision + *-ia*] false or perverted vision.

pseudopterygium (soo″do-ter-ij′e-um) a conjunctival scar attached to the cornea, superficially resembling a true pterygium, but usually not firmly adherent to the underlying tissue.

pseudoptosis (soo″do-to′sis) [*pseudo-* + Gr. *ptōsis* fall] decrease in the size of the palpebral aperture.

pseudoptyalism (soo″do-ti′al-izm) accumulation and drooling of saliva due to dysphagia.

pseudorabies (soo″do-ra′be-ēz) a highly contagious disease affecting the central nervous system of swine, cattle, dogs, cats, rats, and other animals; in swine the infection usually runs a milder course than in other species. Caused by a herpesvirus, it is characterized by sudden onset, severe pruritus, late paralysis, convulsions, and death within three to four days after onset. Called also *Aujeszky's disease, mad itch,* and *infectious bulbar paralysis.* **bovine p.,** pseudorabies of cattle.

pseudoreaction (soo″do-re-ak′shun) a false or deceptive reaction; a skin reaction in intradermal tests which is not due to the specific protein used in the test but to the protein of the medium employed in producing the toxin.

pseudoreduction (soo″do-re-duk′shun) the apparent halving of the chromosome number by synapsis.

pseudoreminiscence (soo″do-rem″ĭ-nis′ens) confabulation.

pseudoretinitis pigmentosa (soo″do-ret″in-i′tis pig″men-to′sah) pigmentary degeneration of the retina mimicking retinitis pigmentosa, but arising from intrauterine viral infections, vascular lesions, and other causes.

pseudorheumatism (soo″do-roo′mah-tizm) a condition resembling rheumatic fever, due to some nonrheumatic disease, as gonorrhea.

pseudorickets (soo″do-rik′ets) renal osteodystrophy.

pseudoscarlatina (soo″do-skar″lah-ti′nah) a febrile condition with an eruption like that of scarlet fever, but due to septic poisoning.

pseudosclerema (soo″do-skle-re′mah) adiponecrosis subcutanea neonatorum.

pseudosclerosis (soo″do-skle-ro′sis) [*pseudo-* + Gr. *sklērōsis* hardening] a condition with the symptoms but without the lesions of multiple sclerosis. **spastic p., p. spas′tica,** Creutzfeldt-Jakob syndrome. **Strümpell-Westphal p.,** hepatolenticular degeneration. **Westphal-Strümpell p.,** hepatolenticular degeneration.

pseudoscrotum (soo″do-skro′tum) a solid partition with a median raphe, resembling the scrotum in the male, obliterating the opening into the vagina in female pseudohermaphrodites.

pseudosmia (soo-doz′me-ah) [*pseudo-* + Gr. *osmē* odor + *-ia*] a delusion as to smell.

pseudosolution (soo″do-so-lu′shun) solutions which do not act according to the usual physical laws of solutions; the term is sometimes applied to colloidal solutions.

pseudostoma (soo-dos′to-mah) [*pseudo-* + Gr. *stoma* mouth] an apparent communication between silver-stained endothelial cells.

pseudostrabismus (soo″do-strah-bis′mus) apparent strabismus due to an overhanging epicanthus which narrows the visible width of the sclera medial to the iris.

pseudostrophanthin (soo″do-stro-fan′thin) a poisonous glycoside, $C_{40}H_{60}O_{16} \cdot H_2O$, from the African shrub *Strophanthus hispidus* DC. (Apocynaceae).

pseudostructure (soo″do-struk′chur) reticular substance.

pseudotabes (soo″do-ta′bēz) [*pseudo-* + L. *tabes* wasting] (*obs.*) any neuropathy with symptoms like those of tabes dorsalis but not due to syphilis, which may be associated with various conditions such as diabetes, alcoholism, and arsenic poisoning. Called also *Leyden's ataxia* and *neurotabes*. **p. mesenter′ica,** hysterical pseudotabes, chiefly of young women. **p. peripher′ica** (*obs.*), an acute syphilitic disease involving the nerve roots and the meninges and simulating tabes. **pupillotonic p.,** Adie's syndrome.

pseudotetanus (soo″do-tet′ah-nus) persistent muscular contractions resembling tetanus but not associated with the presence of *Clostridium tetani.*

pseudothrill (soo″do-thril) a condition that simulates a true thrill.

pseudotoxin (soo″do-tok′sin) a poisonous extract from belladonna leaves.

pseudotrachoma (soo″do-trah-ko′mah) a disease of the eye and lids resembling trachoma.

pseudotrismus (soo″do-tris′mus) a motor disorder of the mouth with symptoms similar to those of trismus.

pseudotropine (soo-dot′ro-pin) a dark-brown, syrupy, liquid base, a decomposition product of tropine.

pseudotruncus arteriosus (soo″do-trunk′us ar-te″re-o′sus) the most severe form of tetralogy of Fallot.

pseudotubercle (soo″do-tu′ber-k'l) a tubercle resembling that of tuberculosis, but not due to the tubercle bacillus.

pseudotuberculoma (soo″do-tu-ber″ku-lo′mah) a tumor resembling in structure a tuberculoma. **p. silicot′icum,** a pseudotuberculoma due to the presence in the tissue of silica.

pseudotuberculosis (soo″do-tu-ber″ku-lo′sis) a fatal disease of rodents, especially guinea pigs and rabbits, caused by *Yersinia* (*Pasteurella*) *pseudotuberculosis,* marked by caseous swellings and nodules (pseudotubercles) in various organs. Rarely, *Corynebacterium pseudotuberculosis* causes the disease in sheep, goats, and other domestic animals. **p. hom′inis streptoth′rica,** a disease of man closely resembling tuberculosis, but due to a streptothrix.

pseudotumor (soo″do-tu′mor) phantom tumor. **p. cer′ebri,** a condition caused by cerebral edema, marked by raised intracranial pressure with headache, nausea, vomiting, and papilledema without neurological signs except occasional sixth-nerve palsy. Called also benign *intracranial hypertension* and *meningeal hydrops.* **orbital p.,** a distinctive, chronic inflammatory reaction in the orbital tissues of the eye, of unknown etiology, that may closely resemble a neoplasm and often becomes bilateral. Symptoms include exophthalmos and congestion of the lids with edema. When limitation of ocular motility also occurs, it is sometimes called *orbital myositis.*

pseudotympanites, pseudotympany (soo″do-tim″pah-ni′tēz, soo″do-tim′pah-ne) (*obs.*) false tympanites, as in accordion abdomen.

pseudotyphus (soo″do-ti′fus) a disease of Sumatra resembling scrub typhus (tsutsugamushi disease).

pseudouremia (soo″do-u-re′me-ah) uremia-like symptoms occurring in acute glomerulonephritis and in hypertensive vascular disease (hypertensive encephalopathy).

pseudouridine (soo″do-ūr′ĭ-dēn) 5-ribosyluracil, a constituent of transfer-RNA differing from uridine in having the linkage between the 5-carbon of uracil and the 1-carbon of ribose.

pseudovacuole (soo″do-vak′u-ōl) a round space within certain red blood corpuscles containing an animal microorganism.

pseudovalve (soo′do-valv) a peculiar formation on the parietal

endocardium of the left ventricle, seen especially in insufficiency of the aortic valves.

pseudoventricle (soo″do-ven′tre-k'l) cavum septi pellucidi.

pseudovermicule, pseudovermiculus (soo″do-ver′mĭ-kūl, soo″do-ver-mik′u-lus) ookinete.

pseudovoice (soo″do-vois) the vocal sounds produced under proper training by a person who has lost his larynx.

pseudovomiting (soo″do-vom′it-ing) regurgitation of matter from the stomach.

pseudoxanthine (soo″do-zan′thin) 1. a compound, $C_4H_5N_5O$, from muscle tissue or nucleic acids. 2. a compound, $C_5H_4N_4O_2$, from uric acid.

pseudoxanthoma elasticum (soo″do-zan-tho′mah e-las′tĭ-kum) a rare skin disease marked by small yellowish macules and papules, individual or confluent, or massed into plaques, and exaggeration of the normal creases and folds of the skin. The histologic features are masses of swollen and calcified elastic fibers with degeneration of the collagen fibers in the lower and middle layers of the dermis and in the gastrointestinal tract and heart.

pseudozooglea (soo″do-zo″o-gle′ah) a clump of bacteria not disintegrating readily in water, arising from imperfect separation or more or less fusion of the components, but not having the degree of compactness and gelatinization seen in zooglea.

p.s.i. pounds per square inch.

psilocin (si′lo-sin) a hallucinogenic substance closely related to psilocybin.

psilocybin (si″lo-si′bin) chemical name: 3-[2-(dimethylamino)-ethyl]indol-4-ol dehydrogen phosphate ester. A hallucinogenic crystalline compound, $C_{13}H_{18(20)}O_3N_2P_2$, possessing indole characteristics, isolated from the mushroom *Psilocybe mexicana* Heim.

psilosis (si-lo′sis) [Gr. *psilōsis* a stripping bare] (*obs.*) sprue (def. 1). **p. pigmento′sa,** pellagra.

psittacine (sit′ah-sīn) [Gr. *psittakos* parrot] of or relating to an order of birds including the parrot and related birds (parakeets, macaws, etc.)

psittacosis (sit-ah-ko′sis) [Gr. *psittakos* parrot + *-osis*] a disease caused by a strain of *Chlamydia psittaci,* first observed in parrots but later discovered to exist in other birds and domestic fowl (see *ornithosis*). In psittacine birds, it is characterized by respiratory and systemic infection. When transmitted to man, it usually takes the form of a pneumonia accompanied by fever, cough, and often by splenomegaly. Other clinical forms include hepatitis, myocarditis, delirium, and coma. The pulmonary form may be transmitted by contact with pigeons, parakeets, budgerigars, ducks, turkeys, pheasant, and probably chickens.

psoas (so′as) see *Table of Musculi.*

psodymus (sod′ĭ-mus) [Gr. *psoa* muscle of the loin + *didymos* twin] a monster with two heads and bodies, but single at and below the loins.

psoitis (so-i′tis) [Gr. *psoa* muscle of the loin + *-itis*] inflammation of a psoas muscle or of its sheath.

psomophagia (so″mo-fa′je-ah) [Gr. *psōmos* morsel + *phagein* to eat] bolting of food; swallowing of food without thorough chewing.

psomophagy (so-mof′ah-je) psomophagia.

psoralen (sor′ah-len) any of the constituents of certain plants (*Ammi majus, Psoralea corylifolia,* etc.) collectively known as "psoralens"; exposure to substances containing psoralens, such as certain perfumes and drugs (including methoxsalen and trioxsalen) and then to sunlight may produce phototoxic dermatitis (q.v.).

psorenteritis (so″ren-ter-i′tis) [*psora* + *enteritis*] a condition of the intestinal mucosa thought to be peculiar to cholera, marked by loss of villi and a granular debris in the surface mucous sheath.

psoriasiform (so″re-as′ĭ-form) resembling psoriasis.

psoriasis (so-ri′ah-sis) [Gr. *psōriasis*] a chronic, hereditary, recurrent, papulosquamous dermatosis, the distinctive lesion of which is a vivid red macule, papule, or plaque covered almost to its edge by silvery lamellated scales. It usually involves the scalp and extensor surfaces of the limbs, especially the elbows, knees, and shins. **p. annula′ris, p. annula′ta,** psoriasis with lesions occurring in ring-shaped patches; called also *p. circinata.* **p. arthropath′ica,** psoriasis associated with arthritis, probably of the rheumatoid type. **p. bucca′lis,** a rare form of psoriasis affecting the oral mucosa. **p. circina′ta,** p. annularis. **p. discoi′dea,** psoriasis occurring in solid persistent patches. **p. figura′ta,** psoriasis in which the lesions coalesce to form marked patterns. **flexural p.,** inverse p. (def. 1). **p. follicula′ris,** psoriasis with small scaly lesions located at the openings of sebaceous and sweat glands. **p. gutta′ta, guttate p.,** psoriasis in which the lesions are small (about the size of drops of water) and distinct. This form may begin suddenly after sunburn or an acute infection, such as streptococcal sore throat, and has a better prognosis than other forms. **p. gyra′ta,** psoriasis in which the lesions have coalesced to form a serpentine pattern. **inverse p.,** 1. psoriasis primarily involving the skin folds and flexures, including those of the nails, with little or no scaling, and sometimes with the formation of pustules; called also *flexural p.* 2. **p. palmaris et plantaris. p. invetera′ta,** a form with confluent lesions and with thickening and hardening of the skin. **p. lin′guae,** a rare form of psoriasis affecting the mucosa of the tongue. **p. ostra′cea,** psoriasis in which the lesions form thick, tough patches covered with scales, giving them a resemblance to the outside of an oyster shell. **p. palma′ris et planta′ris,** psoriasis of the palms and soles; called also *volar p.* **pustular p.,** psoriasis characterized by small pustules which may occur diffusely or in clusters on the palms and soles, or which may occur suddenly as an acute, generalized, febrile, pustular eruption (*von Zumbusch's type*), with persistent relapses and sometimes serious systemic involvement. **p. rupioi′des,** psoriasis with rupia-like crusts. **p. universa′lis,** psoriasis in which the lesions occur over the entire body. **volar p.,** p. palmaris et plantaris. **von Zumbusch's p.,** see *pustular p.*

psoriatic (so″re-at′ik) 1. pertaining to, affected with, or of the nature of, psoriasis. 2. a person affected with psoriasis.

Psorophora (so-rof′o-rah) a genus of large, annoying mosquitoes, the larvae of which prey on the larvae of other kinds of mosquitoes. Some species, particularly *P. ferox* and *P. lutzii,* act as carrier hosts of the eggs of *Dermatobia hominis.*

psorophthalmia (so″rof-thal′me-ah) [Gr. *psōrophthalmia*] a form of ulcerative marginal blepharitis.

Psoroptes (so-rop′tēz) a genus of mites. **P. bo′vis,** *P. ovis.* **P. cunic′uli,** a common external parasite of rabbits, leading to secondary infections that may extend to the inner ear and involve the central nervous system. **P. e′qui,** a species causing skin lesions (psoroptic mange) in horses, especially in areas covered with long hair. **P. o′vis,** a species which causes the most common type of mange in sheep (sheep scab), cattle (bovine scabies), and horses, with intense itching and sometimes general symptoms.

psorosperm (so′ro-sperm) [Gr. *psōros,* rough, scabby + *sperma* seed] (*obs.*) any parasitic sporozoon, especially of the order Myxosporidia.

P.S.P. phenolsulfonphthalein.

PSRO Professional Standards Review Organization: an organization of physicians and in some cases allied health professionals in a designated area, state, or community established to monitor health care services paid for through Medicare, Medicaid, and Maternal and Child Health programs to assure that services provided are medically necessary, meet professional standards, and are provided in the most economic medically appropriate health care agency or institution. The requirement for the establishment of PSRO's was added to the Social Security Amendments of 1972 (Public Law 92-603).

psych- see *psycho-.*

psychalgalia (si″kal-ga′le-ah) psychalgia.

psychalgia (si-kal′je-ah) a pain of mental or hysterical origin, such as neurasthenic headache, clavus hystericus, etc; pain attending or resulting from a mental effort.

psychalgic (si-kal′jik) pertaining to or characterized by psychalgia.

psychanalysis (si-kah-nal′ĭ-sis) psychoanalysis.

psychanopsia (si-kah-nop′se-ah) [psych- + *an* neg. + Gr. *opsis* vision + *-ia*] psychic blindness.

psychasthene (si′kas-thēn) (*obs.*) a person afflicted with psychasthenia.

psychasthenia (si″kas-the′ne-ah) (*obs.*) a functional neurosis marked by stages of pathologic fear or anxiety, obsessions, fixed ideas, tics, feelings of inadequacy, self-accusation, and peculiar feelings of strangeness, unreality, and depersonalization.

psychasthenic (si″kas-then′ik) (*obs.*) marked by, or characteristic of psychasthenia.

psychataxia (si″kah-tak′se-ah) a disordered mental condition marked by inability to fix the attention, agitation, etc.

psyche (si′ke) [Gr. *psyche* the organ of thought and judgment] the human faculty for thought, judgment, and emotion; the mental life, including both conscious and unconscious processes.

psychedelic (si″kĕ-del′ik) [psyche + Gr. *dēlos* manifest, evident] pertaining to or characterized by visual hallucinations, intensified perception, and, sometimes, behavior similar to that seen in psychosis. By extension, a drug that produces such effects.

psychergograph (si-ker′go-graf) [psyche + Gr. *ergon* work + *graphein* to write] an instrument for recording serial responses to a series of stimuli.

psychiatric (si″ke-at′rik) pertaining to or within the purview of psychiatry.

psychiatrics (si″ke-at′riks) psychiatry.

psychiatrist (si-ki′ah-trist) a physician who specializes in psychiatry.

psychiatry (si-ki′ah-tre) [psyche + Gr. *iatreia* healing] that branch of medicine which deals with the study, treatment, and prevention of mental illness. **biological p.,** that which emphasizes physical, chemical, and neurological causes and treatment approaches. **community p.,** a broad term referring to the mobilization of community resources to provide and deliver a coordinated program of mental health directed at diagnosis, treatment, rehabilitation, aftercare, early case-finding, and promoting mental health and preventing psychosocial disorders. The term is sometimes used synonymously with preventive psychiatry and with social psychiatry. **cross-cultural p.,** the comparative study of mental illness and mental health among different societies, nations, and cultures; called also *transcultural p.* **cultural p.,** the branch of social psychiatry concerned with the mentally ill in relation to their cultural environment. **descriptive p.,** psychiatry based upon the observation and study of external factors which can be readily seen, felt, or heard, as differentiated from dynamic psychiatry. **dynamic p.,** the study of emotional processes, their origins, and the mental mechanisms underlying them. **existential p.,** that based on the existential philosophy of Kierkegaard, Heidegger, Jaspers, etc. **forensic p.,** psychiatry which deals with the legal aspects of mental disorders. **industrial p.,** occupational p. **occupational p.,** that concerned with the diagnosis and prevention of mental illness in industry, with the return of the psychiatric patient to work, and with psychiatric aspects of absenteeism, accident proneness, personnel policies, occupational fatigue, vocational adjustment, retirement, and related phenomena. Called also *industrial p.* **organic p.,** 1. that dealing with the psychological aspects of organic brain disease. 2. biological p. **orthomolecular p.,** the study of mental disease on the basis of the molecular environment of the brain, especially as compared to the concentrations of substances normally present in the body. **preventive p.,** a broad term referring to the amelioration, control, and limitation of psychiatric disability. It is often categorized as *primary*—measures to prevent a disorder; *secondary*—therapeutic measures to limit a disorder; and *tertiary*—measures and intervention to reduce impairment or disability following a disorder. The term is sometimes used synonymously with community psychiatry and social psychiatry. **social p.,** that concerned with the cultural, ecologic, and sociologic facts that engender, precipitate, intensify, prolong, or otherwise complicate maladaptive patterns of behavior and their treatment. The term is sometimes used synonymously with community psychiatry and preventive psychiatry. **transcultural p.,** cross-cultural p.

psychic (si′kik) [Gr. *psychikos*] pertaining to the psyche or to the mind; mental.

psychics (si′kiks) psychology.

psychism (si′kizm) the theory that there is a fluid diffused through all living beings, animating all alike.

psycho-, psych- [Gr. *psyche* the organ of thought and reason] a combining form denoting relationship to the psyche, or to the mind.

psychoactive (si″ko-ak′tiv) affecting the mind or behavior, as psychoactive drugs.

psychoalgalia (si″ko-al-ga′le-ah) psychalgia.

psychoanaleptic (si″ko-an″ah-lep′tik) [psycho- + Gr. *analēpsis* a taking up] exerting a stimulating effect upon the mind.

psychoanalysis (si″ko-ah-nal′ĭ-sis) the method of eliciting from patients an idea of their past emotional experiences and the facts of their mental life, in order to discover the mechanism by which a pathologic mental state has been produced, and to furnish hints for psychotherapeutic procedures; the method employs free association, recall and interpretation of dreams, and interpretation of transference and resistance phenomena. Also, a system of theoretical psychology. **existential p.,** that based on the existential philosophy of Kierkegaard, Heidegger, Jaspers, etc.

psychoanalyst (si″ko-an′ah-list) a practitioner of psychoanalysis.

psychoanalytic (si″ko-an″ah-lit′ik) pertaining to psychoanalysis.

psychoauditory (si″ko-aw′dĭ-to″re) pertaining to the consciousness and intelligent perception of sound.

psychobacillosis (si″ko-bas″ĭ-lo′sis) (*obs.*) inoculation of bacteria for the treatment of schizophrenia.

psychobiological (si″ko-bi″o-loj′e-kal) pertaining to the interactions between mind and body in the formation and continuation of the personality.

psychobiology (si″ko-bi-ol′o-je) that branch of biology which considers the interactions between body and mind in the formation and functioning of personality; the scientific study of the personality function.

psychocatharsis (si″ko-kah-thar′sis) [psycho- + Gr. *katharsis* purging] see *abreaction* and *catharsis,* def. 2.

psychocentric (si″ko-sen′trik) [psycho- + Gr. *kentrikos* of or from a center] denoting or relating to the concept that control of the personality centers in the mind, the subjective system of the individual, as distinguished from the physical organs of the nervous system. Cf. *cerebrocentric.*

psychochemistry (si″ko-kem′is-tre) the application of chemistry to the study of psychology and behavior.

psychochrome (si″ko-krōm) [psycho- + Gr. *chrōma* color] a subjective mental association between any bodily sensation and some particular color.

psychochromesthesia (si″ko-krōm″es-the′ze-ah) [*psycho-* + Gr. *chrōma* color + *aisthēsis* perception + *-ia*] the condition in which auditory or other nonvisual stimuli produce sensations or associated sensations of color.

psychocortical (si″ko-kor′te-kal) pertaining to the mind and to the cortex of the brain as the site of mental functions.

psychocutaneous (si″ko-ku-ta′ne-us) pertaining to the relations between mental or emotional factors and skin disorders.

psychodelic (si″ko-del′ik) psychedelic.

psychodiagnosis (si″ko-di″ag-no′sis) the use of psychological testing in the diagnosis of disease.

psychodiagnostics (si″ko-di″ag-nos′tiks) psychodiagnosis.

Psychodidae (si-ko′dĭ-de) a family of flies, the owl flies or sandflies, of the order Diptera, characterized by small size, long legs, and abundant hair on both wings and body. It includes the genus *Phlebotomus*.

psychodometer (si″ko-dom′e-ter) an instrument for measuring the time factor in mental activity.

psychodometry (si″ko-dom′e-tre) [*psycho-* + Gr. *hodos* way + *metron* measure] the measurement of the rate of mental action.

psychodrama (si″ko-dram′ah) the psychiatric group-therapy technique of having patients dramatize their individual conflicting situations of daily life.

psychodynamics (si″ko-di-nam′iks) [*psycho-* + Gr. *dynamis* power] the science of mental processes.

psychodysleptic (si″ko-dis-lep′tik) [*psycho-* + Gr. *dys-* bad + *lēpsis* a taking hold] inducing a dreamlike or delusional state of mind.

psychogalvanometer (si″ko-gal″vah-nom′e-ter) a galvanometer for recording the electrical agitations produced by emotional stresses.

psychogenesis (si″ko-jen′e-sis) 1. mental development. 2. production of a symptom or illness by psychic, as opposed to organic, factors.

psychogenic (si″ko-jen′ik) of intrapsychic origin; having an emotional or psychologic origin (in reference to a symptom), as opposed to a physicogenic, or organic, basis.

psychogenous (si-koj′e-nus) psychogenic.

psychogeriatrics (si″ko-jer″e-at′riks) management of the psychologic and psychiatric problems of the aged.

psychogogic (si″ko-goj′ik) increasing intrapsychic tensions and acting as a stimulant.

psychogram (si′ko-gram) [*psycho-* + Gr. *gramma* a writing] 1. psychograph. 2. a visual sensation associated with a mental idea as of a certain number which appears visualized when it is thought of.

psychograph (si′ko-graf) [*psycho-* + Gr. *graphein* to write] 1. a chart for recording graphically the personality traits of an individual. 2. a written description of the mental functioning of an individual.

psychokinesia (si″ko-ki-ne′ze-ah) [*psycho-* + Gr. *kinēsis* motion + *-ia*] explosive cerebral action due to defective inhibition.

psychokinesis (si″ko-ki-ne′sis) [*psycho-* + Gr. *kinēsis* motion] 1. the direct influence of volitional action on a physical object, or the influence of mind on matter without the intermediation of physical force. 2. psychokinesia.

psychokym (si′ko-kim) a psychic process conceived physiologically; that something which flows through the central nervous system and which is at the basis of psychic processes.

psycholagny (si′ko-lag′ne) [*psycho-* + Gr. *lagneia* lust] the experiencing of sexual enjoyment from imagining or thinking of sexual acts.

psycholepsy (si′ko-lep′se) [*psycho-* + Gr. *lēpsis* a taking hold, a seizure] a condition characterized by sudden changes of mood.

psycholeptic (si″ko-lep′tik) [*psycho-* + Gr. *lēptikos* assimilative] Delay's term for drugs which affect the mental state (psyche). Cf. *neuroleptic*.

psycholinguistics (si″ko-ling-gwis′tiks) the study of factors affecting activities involved in communicating and comprehending verbal information.

psychologic, psychological (si″ko-loj′ik; si″ko-loj′e-kal) pertaining to psychology.

psychologist (si-kol′o-jist) a qualified specialist in psychology.

psychology (si-kol′o-je) [*psycho-* + *-logy*] that branch of science which deals with the mind and mental processes, especially in relation to human and animal behavior. **abnormal p.,** the study of derangements or deviations of mental functions. **analytic p., analytical p.,** psychology by introspective methods, founded by Carl Gustav Jung, as opposed to experimental psychology. **animal p.,** the study of the mental activity of animals. **behavioristic p.,** see *behaviorism*. **child p.,** the study of the development of the mind of the child. **clinical p.,** the use of psychologic knowledge and techniques in the treatment of persons with emotional difficulties. **cognitive p.,** that branch of psychology which deals with the human mind as it receives and interprets impressions from the external world. **community**

p., a broad term referring to the organization of community resources around multiple levels of professionals, paraprofessionals, and nonprofessionals for the prevention of mental disorders. **comparative p.,** the study of the mental action of animals. **constitutional p.,** the relation of the psychology of the individual to the morphology and physiology of his body. **criminal p.,** the study of the mentality, the motivation, and the social behavior of criminals. **depth p.,** the psychology of the unconscious; psychoanalysis. **dynamic p.,** psychology which stresses the element of energy in mental processes. **experimental p.,** the study of the mind and mental operations by the employment of experimental methods. **genetic p.,** that branch of psychology which deals with the development of mind in the individual and with its evolution in the race. **gestalt p.,** see *gestaltism*. **hormic p.,** a psychology which asserts that active striving toward a goal is a fundamental category of psychology (McDougall). **individual p.,** the system of Alfred Adler in psychiatric theory, research, and therapy, stressing the concepts of organ inferiority, the inferiority complex, and overcompensation. **physiologic p., physiological p.,** the branch of psychology that studies the relationship between physiologic processes and behavior. **social p.,** psychology which treats of the social aspects of mental life.

psychomathematics (si″ko-math″e-mat′iks) mathematics applied to the study of psychology.

psychometer (si-kom′e-ter) an instrument used in psychometry.

psychometrician (si″ko-mĕ-trish′an) a person skilled in psychometry.

psychometrics (si″ko-met′riks) ·psychometry.

psychometry (si-kom′e-tre) [*psycho-* + Gr. *metron* measure] 1. measurement of the duration and force of mental processes. 2. the measurement of intelligence.

psychomotor (si″ko-mo′tor) pertaining to motor effects of cerebral or psychic activity.

psychoneural (si″ko-nu′ral) relating to the totality of neural events initiated by a sensory input and leading to storage, to discrimation, or to an output of any kind.

psychoneuroses (si″ko-nu-ro′sēz) [Gr.] plural of *psychoneurosis*.

psychoneurosis (si″ko-nu-ro′sis), pl. *psychoneuroses* [*psycho-* + Gr. *neuron* nerve + *-osis*] an emotional disorder due to unresolved conflicts, anxiety being its chief characteristic. The anxiety may be expressed directly or indirectly, as by conversion, displacement, etc. In contrast to the psychoses, the psychoneuroses do not involve gross distortions of external reality or disorganization of personality. Called also *neurosis*. **defense p.,** a psychosis or neurosis whose symptoms are due to the attempt to repress a painful idea. The idea is excluded from the mind, but remains in subconsciousness, where it acts as a cause of disturbance. The term includes hysteria as well as various neuroses and psychoses.

psychonomy (si″kon-o′me) [*psycho-* + Gr. *nomos* law] the science of the laws of mental activity.

psychopath (si′ko-path) a person who has an antisocial (psychopathic) personality (q.v.); see *antisocial personality*, under *personality*. **sexual p.,** an individual whose sexual behavior is manifestly antisocial and criminal.

psychopathia (si″ko-pa′the-ah) psychopathy. **p. sexua′lis,** mental disease marked by perversion of the sexual feelings.

psychopathic (si″ko-path′ik) 1. pertaining to a person with an antisocial (psychopathic) personality (q.v.); antisocial. 2. (*obs.*) pertaining to mental disease.

psychopathology (si″ko-pah-thol′o-je) [*psycho-* + *pathology*] the pathology of mental disorders; the branch of medicine which deals with the causes and nature of mental disease.

psychopathy (si-kop′ah-the) [*psycho-* + Gr. *pathos* disease] a disorder of the psyche, whether or not associated with subnormal intelligence.

psychopharmacology (si″ko-fahr″mah-kol′o-je) 1. the study of the action of drugs on psychological functions and mental states. 2. the use of drugs to modify psychological functions and mental states.

psychophylaxis (si″ko-fi-lak′sis) prophylaxis in mental disease; mental hygiene.

psychophysical (si″ko-fiz′e-kal) pertaining to the mind and its relation to physical manifestations.

psychophysics (si″ko-fiz′iks) [*psycho-* + Gr. *physikos* natural] the science dealing with the quantitative relationships between the characteristics or patterns of physical stimuli and the resultant sensations.

psychophysiologic (si″ko-fiz″e-o-loj′ik) [*psycho-* + *physiology*] pertaining to psychophysiology; having bodily symptoms of a psychogenic origin. Called also *psychosomatic*. See also under *disorder*.

psychophysiology (si″ko-fiz″e-ol′o-je) the science that deals with the relationship between psychologic and physiologic processes.

psychoplasm (si′ko-plazm) protyl.

psychoplegia (si″ko-ple′je-ah) [psycho- + Gr. *plēgē* stroke + -ia] a sudden attack of dementia.

psychoplegic (si″ko-ple′jik) an agent that lessens cerebral activity or excitability.

psychopneumatology (si″ko-nu″mah-tol′o-je) [psycho- + Gr. *pneuma* breath + -logy] the study of the interactions of mind, body, and soul.

psychoprophylactic (si″ko-pro″fĭ-lak′tik) pertaining to psychoprophylaxis.

psychoprophylaxis (si″ko-pro″fĭ-lak′sis) a technique of psychophysical training aimed at the suppression of all painful sensation associated with normal childbirth.

psychoreaction (si″ko-re-ak′shun) Much's reaction.

psychorrhexis (si″ko-rek′sis) [phycho- + Gr. *rhēxis* rupture] a malignant form of anxiety neurosis, marked by perplexity and anguish; it is sometimes produced by shock and occasionally terminates in hyperpyrexia and death.

psychosedation (si″ko-sĕ-da′shun) a procedure whereby the patient is rendered free from fear and apprehension through the administration of a psychosedative agent.

psychosedative (si″ko-sed′ah-tiv) an agent that allays apprehension by its action on subcortical centers, while producing minimal motor and sensory impairment because of its limited effect on the cerebral cortex.

psychosensorial (si″ko-sen-so′re-al) psychosensory.

psychosensory (si″ko-sen′so-re) pertaining to the conscious perception of sensory impulses to the mind and to sensation.

psychoses (si-ko′sēz) [Gr.] plural of *psychosis*.

psychosexual (si″ko-seks′u-al) pertaining to the psychic or emotional aspects of sex.

psychosin (si-ko′sin) a galactoside, $C_{23}H_{45}N_7O$, resulting from the decomposition of phrenosin. On hydrolysis it yields galactose and sphingosine.

psychosis (si-ko′sis), pl. *psycho′ses* [psych- + -osis] 1. a general term for any major mental disorder of organic and/or emotional origin characterized by derangement of the personality and loss of contact with reality, often with delusions, hallucinations, or illusions. Cf. *neurosis*. 2. formerly, a generic name for any mental disorder. **affective p.,** major affective disorder. **alcoholic p.,** mental disorder in which excessive use of alcohol is the chief etiologic factor, such as delirium tremens and Korsakoff's psychosis. **bipolar p.,** see *manic-depressive p*. **Cheyne-Stokes p.,** a condition resembling cardiac asthma, with intense motor agitation, sometimes seen along with the onset of Cheyne-Stokes respiration in chronic heart disease. **circular p.,** see *manic-depressive p*. **depressed p.,** see *manic-depressive p*. **drug p.,** a toxic psychosis due to the ingestion of drugs. **epileptic p.,** psychosis occurring in a person suffering from epilepsy. **exhaustion p.,** mental disorder due to some exhausting or depressing occurrence, as an operation. **famine p.,** a mental condition resulting from malnutrition among destitute civilians under conditions of oppression. **febrile p.,** febrile delirium. **functional p.,** a psychosis in which organic disease or dysfunction does not play a part. **gestational p.,** a psychosis developing during pregnancy. **hysterical p.,** an acute situational reaction occurring in individuals with hysterical personalties, usually manifested by the sudden onset of hallucinations, delusions, bizarre behavior, and volatile affect; the term includes certain culture-specific syndromes such as amok, koro, and latah. **infection exhaustion p.,** exhaustion delirium. **involutional p.,** see under *melancholia*. **Korsakoff's p.,** alcoholic psychosis, believed to be a chronic form of Wernicke's encephalopathy (q.v.). It is accompanied by disturbance of orientation, susceptibility to external stimulation and suggestion, amnesia, hallucinations, and especially by confabulation. The signs of polyneuritis (wristdrop, etc.) are usually present. Called also *polyneuritic psychosis, cerebropathia psychica toxaemica,* and *chronic alcoholic delirium*. **manic p.,** see *manic-depressive p*. **manic-depressive p.,** a major affective disorder characterized by severe mood swings and a tendency to remission and recurrence. It is seen in a *manic type,* consisting of manic episodes characterized by excessive elation, irritability, talkativeness, flight of ideas, and psychomotor overactivity; in a *depressed* or *unipolar type,* consisting of depressive episodes characterized by severely depressed mood and by mental and motor retardation that may progress to stupor; and in a *circular* or *bipolar type,* consisting of at least one depressive episode and a manic episode. Called also *manic-depressive illness* or *reaction*. **organic p.,** organic brain syndrome; see under *syndrome*. **paranoiac p., paranoid p.,** paranoia. **periodic p.,** a condition in which intermittent periods of depression or hypomania recur regularly in a seemingly mentally healthy or nearly healthy individual. **polyneuritic p., p. polyneurit′ica,** Korsakoff's p. **postpartum p.,** a psychotic episode, usually schizophrenic in nature, occurring during the postpartum period, which may be precipitated by organic and/or toxic factors; called also *puerperal p*. **prison p.,** any psychosis for which prison environment has been a precipitating factor. **puerperal p.,** postpartum p. **purpose p.,** a psychotic state motivated by a clear-cut wish, such as a wish to appear insane and therefore irresponsible. **schizo-**

affective p., a psychotic state characterized by mixed schizophrenic and manic-depressive symptoms. **senile p.,** mental deterioration in old age associated with organic brain changes and characterized by numerous symptoms, including impaired memory of recent events, confabulation, irritability, self-interest, decreased capacity for abstract thought, and sometimes symptoms of paranoia, especially delusions of persecution. **situational p.,** a transitory mental disorder caused by an unbearable situation over which the patient has no control. **symbiotic p., symbiotic infantile p.,** a condition seen in two- to four-year-old children having an abnormal relationship to the mothering figure, characterized by intense separation anxiety, severe regression, giving up of useful speech, and autism. **toxic p.,** a psychosis due to the ingestion of toxic agents (e.g., alcohol, opium) into the body, or to presence of toxins within the body. **unipolar p.,** see manic-depressive p.

psychosocial (si″ko-so′shal) pertaining to or involving both psychic and social aspects.

psychosolytic (si-ko″so-lit′ik) [psychosis + Gr. *lytikos* dissolving] tending to relieve or abolish psychotic symptoms.

psychosomatic (si″ko-so-mat′ik) [psycho- + Gr. *sōma* body] pertaining to the mind-body relationship; having bodily symptoms of psychic, emotional, or mental origin; called also *psychophysiologic*. See also under *disorder*.

psychosomaticist (si″ko-so-mat′ah-sist) one who practices psychosomatic medicine.

psychosomimetic (si-ko″so-mi-met′ik) psychotomimetic.

psychostimulant (si″ko-stim′u-lant) 1. producing a transient increase in psychomotor activity. 2. a drug that produces such effects.

psychosurgery (si″ko-ser′jer-e) brain surgery performed for the relief of mental and psychic symptoms.

psychotechnics (si″ko-tek′niks) [psycho- + Gr. *technē* art] the employment of psychological methods in studying sociological and other problems.

psychotherapeutics (si″ko-ther″ah-pu′tiks) psychotherapy.

psychotherapy (si-ko-ther′ah-pe) [psycho- + Gr. *therapeia* treatment] treatment designed to produce a response by mental rather than by physical effects, including the use of suggestion, persuasion, re-education, reassurance, and support, as well as the techniques of hypnosis, abreaction, and psychoanalysis which are employed in the so-called deep psychotherapy. **group p.,** see under *therapy*. **supportive p.,** a technique aimed at reinforcing a patient's defenses and helping suppress disturbing psychological material, while avoiding the probing of emotional conflicts; used when symptoms are insufficient to warrant intensive psychotherapy.

psychotic (si-kot′ik) 1. pertaining to, characterized by, or caused by psychosis. 2. a person exhibiting psychosis.

psychotogenic (si-kot″o-jen′ik) producing a state of psychosis.

psychotomimetic (si-kot″o-mi-met′ik) [psychosis + Gr. *mimētikos* imitative] pertaining to, characterized by, or producing manifestations resembling those of a psychosis, e.g., visual hallucinations, distortion of perception, and schizophrenia-like behavior. By extension, applied to a drug that produces these effects.

psychotonic (si″ko-ton′ik) [psycho- + Gr. *tonos* tone] exerting an elevating or stimulating effect upon the mind.

psychotropic (si″ko-trop′pik) [psycho- + Gr. *tropē* a turning] exerting an effect upon the mind; capable of modifying mental activity; usually applied to drugs that affect the mental state.

psychro- (si′kro) [Gr. *psychros* cold] a combining form denoting relationship to cold.

psychroalgia (si″kro-al′je-ah) a painful feeling of cold.

psychroesthesia (si″kro-es-the′ze-ah) [psychro- + Gr. *aisthēsis* perception + -ia] a state in which a part of the body, though warm, seems cold.

psychrolusia (si″kro-loo′se-ah) [psychro- + Gr. *louein* to wash] bathing in cold water.

psychrometer (si-krom′ĕ-ter) [psychro- + Gr. *metron* measure] an apparatus for measuring atmospheric moisture by the difference in reading of two thermometers, one with a dry bulb and one with a wet bulb. **sling p.,** an instrument in which the thermometers are swung through the air to facilitate evaporation from the wet bulb.

psychrophile (si′kro-fīl) an organism which grows best at low temperatures.

psychrophilic (si″kro-fil′ik) [psychro- + Gr. *philein* to love] fond of cold; said of bacteria that grow in the cold, often growing best between 15° and 20° C. See also *mesophilic* and *thermophilic*.

psychrophore (si′kro-fōr) [psychro- + Gr. *pherein* to bear] a double catheter for applying cold to the urethra.

psychrotherapy (si″kro-ther′ah-pe) [psychro- + Gr. *therapeia* treatment] the treatment of disease by the application of cold.

psyllium (sil′e-um) a plant of the genus *Plantago*. Blond p. is *P. ovata* Forskal; Spanish p. is *P. psyllium* L. See also *plantago (psyllium)* seed, under *seed*.

Pt chemical symbol for *platinum*.

PTA plasma thromboplastin antecedent (blood coagulation Factor XI).

PTAP a purified diphtheria toxoid precipitated by aluminum phosphate.

ptarmic (tar′mik) [Gr. *ptarmikos* making to sneeze] relating to or producing spasmodic sneezing.

ptarmus (tar′mus) [Gr. *ptarmos*] spasmodic sneezing.

PTC plasma thromboplastin component (blood coagulation Factor IX); phenylthiocarbamide.

PTEN pentaerythritol tetranitrate.

pteridine (ter′ĭ-dēn) a bicyclic nitrogenous base characteristic of the pterins and folic acids.

Pteridophyta (ter″ĭ-dof′ĭ-tah) [Gr. *pteris* fern + *phyton* plant] a division of the plant kingdom including the ferns.

pteridophyte (ter′ĭ-do-fīt″) one of the Pteridophyta.

pterin (ter′in) [Gr. *pteron* wing] any compound containing pteridine; the pterins are derivatives of 2-amino-4-hydroxypteridine and are constituents of folic acids. They were first identified in the wings of butterflies. See also *aminopterin, leucopterin, uropterin,* and *xanthopterin.*

pterion (te′re-on) [Gr. *pteron* wing] a point at the junction of the frontal, parietal, temporal, and great wing of the sphenoid bone; about 3 cm. behind the external angular process of the orbit.

pternalgia (ter-nal′je-ah) [Gr. *pterna* heel + *algos* pain + *-ia*] pain in the heel.

pteroylglutamate (ter″o-il-gloo′tah-mate) a salt of pteroylglutamic (folic) acid. See *folic acid,* under *acid.*

pterygium (tĕ-rij′e-um) [Gr. *pterygion* wing] a winglike structure, applied especially to an abnormal triangular fold of membrane, in the interpalpebral fissure, extending from the conjunctiva to the cornea, being immovably united to the cornea at its apex, firmly attached to the sclera throughout its middle portion, and merged with the conjunctiva at its base. **p. col′li,** a thick

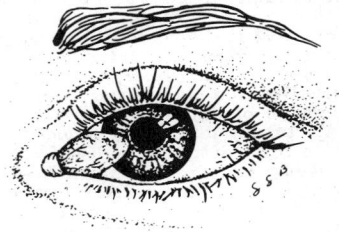

Pterygium.

fold of skin on the lateral aspect of the neck, extending from the mastoid region to the acromion, producing congenital webbed neck. **congenital p.,** epitarsus.

pterygoid (ter′ĭ-goid) [Gr. *pterygōdēs* like a wing] shaped like a wing.

pterygomandibular (ter″ĭ-go-man-dib′u-lar) pertaining to the pterygoid process and the mandible.

pterygomaxillary (ter″ĭ-go-mak′sĭ-ler″e) pertaining to a pterygoid process and the upper jaw.

pterygopalatine (ter″ĭ-go-pal′ah-tin) pertaining to a pterygoid process and to the palate bone.

PTFE abbreviation for polytetrafluroethylene; see *polytef.*

ptilosis (ti-lo′sis) [Gr. *ptilōsis*] 1. a falling out or loss of the eyelashes. 2. a form of pneumoconiosis caused by inhaling the dust from ostrich feathers.

ptisan (tiz′an) [L. *ptisana;* Gr. *ptisanē*] (*obs.*) sweetened barley water, or other similar preparation; a decoction or medicinal tea.

P.T.O. abbreviation for Ger. *Perlsucht Tuberculin Original;* see *Klemperer's tuberculin,* under *tuberculin.*

ptomaine (to′mān, to-mān′) [Gr. *ptōma* carcass] any one of a nonspecific and vague class of toxic bases, usually considered to be formed by the action of bacterial metabolism. Some are formed by the decarboxylation of amino acids. The ptomaines include cadaverine, muscarine, neurine, ptomatropine, putrescine, and many other compounds. Called also *animal alkaloid, putrefactive alkaloid,* and *cadaveric alkaloid.*

ptomainemia (to″mān-e′me-ah) [*ptomaine* + Gr. *haima* blood + *-ia*] the presence of ptomaines in the blood.

ptomainotoxism (to″mān-o-tok′sizm) poisoning by a ptomaine.

ptomatine (to′mah-tin) ptomaine.

ptomatopsia (to″mah-top′se-ah) [Gr. *ptōma* corpse + *opsis* vision + *-ia*] necropsy.

ptomatopsy (to″mah-top′se) necropsy.

ptomatropine (to-mat′ro-pin) [*ptomaine* + *atropine*] a poison from putrid sausages and the viscera of corpses of those dead from typhoid fever; it has effects somewhat like those of atropine.

ptosed (tōst) affected with ptosis; prolapsed.

ptosis (to′sis) [Gr. *ptōsis* fall] 1. prolapse of an organ or part. 2. drooping of the upper eyelid from paralysis of the third nerve or from sympathetic innervation. **abdominal p.** (*obs.*), splanchnoptosis. **p. adipo′sa, false p.,** an apparent ptosis caused by a fold of skin and fat hanging down below the border of the eyelid. **Horner's p.,** moderate ptosis of an eye, with retraction of the eyeball, miosis, and flushing of the affected side of the face, due to lesions of the cervical sympathetic. **p. lipomato′sis,** ptosis produced by lipoma of the eyelid. **morning p.,** waking ptosis. **p. sympath′ica,** ptosis associated with miosis, vasomotor facial paralysis, and diseases of the cervical sympathetic system. **visceral p.** (*obs.*), splanchnoptosis. **waking p.,** temporary paralysis of the upper lid on awakening from sleep.

-ptosis (to′sis) [Gr. *ptōsis* fall] a word termination indicating downward displacement.

ptotic (tot′ik) pertaining to or affected with ptosis.

P.T.R. abbreviation for Ger. *Perlsucht Tuberculin Rest;* see under *tuberculin.*

PTT partial thromboplastin time; see under *test.*

ptyal-, ptyalo- [Gr. *ptyalon* spittle] a combining form denoting relationship to the saliva. See also words beginning *sial-* and *sialo-*.

ptyalagogue (ti-al′ah-gog) [*ptyalo-* + Gr. *agōgos* leading] sialagogue.

ptyalectasis (ti″ah-lek′tah-sis) [*ptyalo-* + Gr. *ektasis* distention] 1. operative dilatation of a salivary duct. 2. dilatation of one of the ducts of the salivary glands.

ptyalin (ti′ah-lin) [Gr. *ptyalon* spittle] α-amylase occurring in saliva.

ptyalinogen (ti″ah-lin′o-jen) [*ptyalin* + Gr. *gennan* to produce] pre-α-amylase, a hypothetical proenzyme in the salivary glands.

ptyalism (ti′ah-lizm) [Gr. *ptyalismos*] excessive secretion of saliva, as seen in chronic mercury poisoning; called also *salivation* and *polysialia.*

ptyalith (ti′ah-lith) [*ptyalo-* + Gr. *lithos* stone] (*obs.*) a salivary calculus.

ptyalize (ti′ah-līz) to increase or stimulate the secretion of saliva.

ptyalocele (ti-al′o-sēl) [*ptyalo-* + Gr. *kēlē* tumor] a cystic tumor containing saliva. **sublingual p.,** ranula.

ptyalogenic (ti″ah-lo-jen′ik) [*ptyalo-* + Gr. *gennan* to produce] formed from or by the action of saliva.

ptyalography (ti″ah-log′rah-fe) [*ptyalo-* + Gr. *graphein* to write] sialography.

ptyalolith (ti′ah-lo-lith) (*obs.*) a salivary calculus.

ptyalolithiasis (ti″ah-lo-lĭ-thi′ah-sis) the presence of salivary calculi.

ptyalolithotomy (ti″ah-lo-lĭ-thot′o-me) sialolithotomy.

ptyaloreaction (ti″ah-lo-re-ak′shun) a reaction occurring in the saliva.

ptyalorrhea (ti″ah-lo-re′ah) [*ptyalo-* + Gr. *rhoia* flow] ptyalism.

ptyalose (ti′ah-lōs) maltose produced by the action of ptyalin on starch.

ptyocrinous (ti-ok′rĭ-nus) [Gr. *ptyon* a winnowing shovel, or fan + *krinein* to separate] elaborating secretion in the form of granules which are eventually extruded; said of unicellular glands, as globlet cells, which secrete in this way. Cf. *diacrinous.*

Pu chemical symbol for *plutonium.*

pubarche (pu-bar′ke) the beginning of growth of the pubic hair.

puberal (pu′ber-al) [L. *puber* of marriageable age] pubertal.

puberphonia (pu″ber-fo′ne-ah) a failure of adolescent voice change, usually of psychogenic origin.

pubertal (pu′ber-tal) pertaining to or characteristic of puberty.

pubertas (pu-ber′tas) [L.] puberty. **p. prae′cox,** precocious puberty.

puberty (pu′ber-te) [L. *pubertas*] the period during which the secondary sex characteristics begin to develop and the capability of sexual reproduction is attained. **precocious p.,** unusually early sexual maturity, either idiopathic or pathological and either isosexual or with development of sex characters of the opposite sex; called also *pubertas praecox.*

pubes (pu′bēz) [L., pl. of *pubis*] 1. [NA] the hairs growing over the pubic region. 2. regio pubica.

pubescence (pu-bes′ens) the state of being pubescent.

pubescent (pu-bes′ent) [L. *pubescens* becoming hairy] 1. arriving at the age of puberty. 2. covered with down or lanugo.

pubic (pu′bik) pertaining to or lying near the pubes.

pubioplasty (pu″be-o-plas″te) a plastic operation on the pubes.

pubiotomy (pu″be-ot′o-me) [*pubis* + Gr. *tomē* a cutting] surgical separation of the pubic bone lateral to the median line.

pubis (pu′bis), pl. *pu′bes* [L.] the os pubis.

pubisure (pu′bĭ-sūr) pubes.

pubococcygeal (pu″bo-kok-sij′e-al) pertaining to the pubis and coccyx or to the musculus pubococcygeus.

pubofemoral (pu″bo-fem′o-ral) pertaining to the os pubis and femur.

puboprostatic (pu″bo-pros-tat′ik) pertaining to the os pubis and prostate gland.

puborectal (pu″bo-rek′tal) pertaining to the pubis and rectum or to the musculus puborectalis.

pubotibial (pu″bo-tib′e-al) pertaining to the pubes and tibia.

pubovesical (pu″bo-ves′ĭ-kal) pertaining to the pubes and bladder.

pudenda (pu-den′dah) [L.] plural of *pudendum*.

pudendal (pu-den′dal) pertaining to the pudenda.

pudendum (pu-den′dum), pl. *puden′da* [L., from *pudere* to be ashamed.] the external genitalia of humans, especially of the female; see *p. femininum*. **female p.,** p. femininum. **p. femini′num** [NA], female pudendum: that portion of the female genitalia comprising the mons pubis, labia majora, labia minora, vestibule of the vagina, bulb of the vestibule, greater and lesser vestibular glands, and vaginal orifice. Commonly used to denote the entire external female genitalia (partes genitales femininae externae). Called also *p. muliebre* and *vulva*. **p. mulie′bre,** p. femininum.

pudic (pu′dik) [L. *pudicus*] pertaining to the pudenda.

puericulture (pu′er-ĭ-kul″tūr) [L. *puer* child + *cultura* culture] the art of rearing and training children.

puericulturist (pu″er-ĭ-kul′tūr-ist) a specialist in the training of children.

puerile (pu′er-il) [L. *puerilis*; *puer* child] pertaining to childhood or to children; childish.

puerpera (pu-er′per-ah) [L. *puer* child + *parere* to bring forth, to bear] a woman who has just given birth to an infant.

puerperal (pu-er′per-al) [L. *puerperalis*] pertaining to the puerperium.

puerperalism (pu-er′per-al-izm) a disease condition incident to childbirth.

puerperant (pu-er′per-ant) 1. giving birth. 2. a puerpera.

puerperium (pu″er-pe′re-um) [L.] the period or state of confinement after labor.

puff (puf) 1. a short, blowing, auscultation sound. 2. in genetics, any of the regions of the giant chromosomes of certain flies at which disorganized arrangement and most of RNA synthesis occurs. **chromosome p's,** active loci of RNA and DNA synthesis in the giant salivary gland chromosomes of insects. **veiled p.,** a faint, muffled pulmonary murmur.

puffing (puf′ing) enlargement in giant polytene chromosomes of fly larval organs; these chromosome puffs are repositories of RNA and DNA synthesis.

pugil, pugillus (pu′jil, pu-jil′us) [L. *pugillus*] a handful.

pukateine (pu-kat′e-in) chemical name: 1,2-methylenedioxy-11-hydroxyaporphine. A crystalline alkaloid, $C_{18}H_{17}NO_3$, from the bark of *Laurelia novaezelandiae* A. Cunn., Lauraceae.

pulegone (pu′le-gōn) chemical name: *p*-menth-4(8)-en-3-one. A volatile oil, a menthene, $(CH_3)_2C:C_6H_7(O)\cdot CH_3$, from pennyroyal oil.

Pulex (pu′leks) [L. "flea"] a genus of fleas which are parasitic on man, dogs, cats, and badgers. **P. cheo′pis,** *Xenopsylla cheopis*. **P. duge′si,** *P. irritans*. **P. ir′ritans,** the common flea or human flea, which is parasitic on the skin of man, its bite producing itching. **P. pen′etrans,** *Tunga penetrans;* see *chigoe*. **P. serrat′iceps,** *Ctenocephalides canis*.

pulex (pu′leks), pl. *pu′lices* [L.] an organism of the genus *Pulex;* a flea.

Pulheems (pul′hēmz) a system of medical classification for recording the physical and mental status of recruits in the British armed services, representing: P, physical capacity; U, upper limbs; L, lower limbs; H, hearing (acuity); EE, eyesight (visual acuity); M, mental capacity; S, stability (emotional).

pulicicide (pu-lis′ĭ-sīd) [L. *pulex* flea + *caedere* to kill] an agent destructive to fleas.

Pulicidae (pu-lis′ĭ-de) a family of the Siphonaptera which includes most of the fleas. Four genera are important to man: *Ctenocephalides, Hoplopsyllus, Pulex,* and *Xenopsylla*.

pull (pul) 1. to strain a muscle. 2. the injury sustained in a muscle strain.

pullorin (pul′o-rīn) a preparation containing the soluble antigens of *Salmonella pullorum*.

Pullularia (pul″u-la′re-ah) *Aureobasidium*. **p. pul′lulans,** *Aureobasidium pullulans*.

pullulate (pul′u-lāt) to germinate.

pullulation (pul″u-la′shun) [L. *pullulare* to sprout] the act or process of budding, as in yeast, or of sprouting; germination.

pulmo (pul′mo), gen. *pulmo′nis,* pl. *pulmo′nes* [L.] [NA] the organ of respiration; see *lung*.

pulmo- [L. *pulmo* lung] a combining form denoting relationship to the lungs; see also words beginning *pulmono-*.

pulmoaortic (pul″mo-a-or′tik) pertaining to the lungs and the aorta.

pulmogram (pul′mo-gram) a roentgenogram of the lungs.

pulmolith (pul′mo-lith) [*pulmo-* + Gr. *lithos* stone] a lung calculus.

pulmometer (pul-mom′ĕ-ter) [*pulmo-* + L. *metrum* measure] a form of spirometer for measuring the capacity of the lungs for air.

pulmometry (pul-mom′ĕ-tre) the measurement of the lung capacity.

pulmonal (pul′mo-nal) pulmonary.

pulmonary (pul′mo-ner″e) [L. *pulmonarius*] pertaining to the lungs.

pulmonectomy (pul″mo-nek′to-me) pneumonectomy.

pulmonic (pul-mon′ik) 1. pertaining to the lungs; pulmonary. 2. pertaining to the pulmonary artery.

pulmonitis (pul″mo-ni′tis) inflammation of the lungs; pneumonia.

pulmono- [L. *pulmo, pulmonis* lung] a combining form denoting relationship to the lungs; see also words beginning *pulmo-*.

pulmonohepatic (pul″mo-no-hĕ-pat′ik) pertaining to or communicating with the lungs and the liver; hepatopulmonary.

pulmonologist (pul″mo-nol′o-jist) an individual skilled in pulmonology.

pulmonology (pul″mo-nol′o-je) the science concerned with the anatomy, physiology, and pathology of the lungs.

pulmonoperitoneal (pul″mo-no-per″ĭ-to-ne′al) pertaining to or communicating with the lungs and the peritoneum.

pulmotor (pul′mo-tor) [*pulmo-* + L. *motor* mover] an apparatus for producing artificial respiration by forcing oxygen into the lungs, and, when they are distended, sucking out the air.

pulp (pulp) [L. *pulpa* flesh] any soft, juicy animal or vegetable tissue, such as that contained within the spleen or the pulp chamber of a tooth (see *dental pulp*). **coronal p.,** the part of the dental pulp contained in the crown portion of the pulp cavity. **dead p.,** necrotic p. **dental p.,** the richly vascularized and innervated connective tissue contained in the pulp cavity of a tooth, constituting the formative, nutritive, and sensory organ of the dentin; called also *pulpa dentis* [NA]. **devitalized p.,** necrotic p. **digital p.,** the mass of tissue forming the soft cushion on the palmar or plantar surface of the distal phalanx of a finger or toe. **enamel p.,** stellate reticulum. **exposed p.,** dental pulp which, through trauma or disease, has become exposed to the external environment. **mummified p.,** dental pulp which has undergone caseation necrosis. **necrotic p.,** dental pulp which has been deprived of its blood and nerve supply and is no longer composed of living tissue, as evidenced by its insensitivity to stimulation by electricity, heat, cold, or trauma. **nonvital p.,** necrotic p. **putrescent p.,** a necrotic pulp which has been invaded by putrefactive microorganisms and is characterized by a particularly foul odor. **radicular p.,** the part of the dental pulp contained in the root canal of a tooth. **red p., splenic p.,** the dark, reddish brown substance which fills up the interspaces of the sinuses of the spleen; called also *pulpa lienis* [NA]. **tooth p.,** dental p. **vertebral p.,** the soft central portion of an intervertebral disk. **vital p.,** a dental pulp which is characterized by vascularity and sensation. **white p.,** sheaths of lymphatic tissue surrounding the arteries of the spleen. **wood p.,** a purified cellulose prepared from finely shredded wood and used in the manufacture of paper; sometimes used also as an absorbent dressing.

pulpa (pul′pah), pl. *pul′pae* [L. "flesh"] pulp. **p. corona′le** [NA], the portion of the dental pulp in the crown portion of the pulp cavity. **p. den′tis** [NA], dental pulp: the richly vascularized and innervated connective tissue contained in the pulp cavity of a tooth. **p. lie′nis** [NA], the dark, reddish-brown substance that fills up the interspaces of the sinuses of the spleen; called also *red pulp* and *pulp of spleen*. **p. radicula′ris** [NA], the portion of the dental pulp in the root canal of a tooth.

pulpal (pul′pal) pertaining to the pulp.

pulpalgia (pul-pal′je-ah) pain in the pulp of a tooth.

pulpation (pul-pa′shun) pulpefaction.

pulpectomy (pul-pek′to-me) [*pulp* + Gr. *ektomē* excision] extirpation of the pulp from the pulp chamber and root canals of a tooth.

pulpefaction (pul″pĕ-fak′shun) [*pulp* + L. *facere* to make] conversion into pulp.

pulpiform (pul′pĭ-form) resembling pulp.

pulpitides (pul-pit′ĭ-dēz) [Gr.] plural of *pulpitis;* applied to all types of pulp inflammation collectively.

pulpitis (pul-pi′tis), pl. *pulpit′ides*. Inflammation of the dental pulp. **anachoretic p.,** pulpitis caused by bacteria attracted to the pulp because of local irritation; see also *anachoresis*. **closed p.,** pulpitis in which the dental pulp is not exposed to the oral environment. **hyperplastic p.,** pulpitis characterized by exuberant proliferation of chronically inflamed dental pulp. **open p.,** pulpitis in which the dental pulp is obviously exposed to the oral environment through a carious lesion.

pulpless (pulp′les) without pulp; having the pulp removed.

pulpoaxial (pul″po-ak′se-al) pertaining to or formed by the pulpal and axial walls of a tooth cavity.

pulpobuccoaxial (pul″po-buk″o-ak′se-al) pertaining to or formed by the pulpal, buccal, and axial walls of a tooth cavity.

pulpodistal (pul″po-dis′tal) pertaining to or formed by the pulpal and distal walls of a tooth cavity.

pulpodontia (pul″po-don′she-ah) pulpodontics.

pulpodontics (pul″po-don′tiks) that branch of dentistry dealing with the dental pulp.

pulpolabial (pul″po-la′be-al) pertaining to or formed by the pulpal and labial walls of a tooth cavity.

pulpolingual (pul″po-ling′gwal) pertaining to or formed by the pulpal and lingual walls of a tooth cavity.

pulpolinguoaxial (pul″po-ling″gwo-ak′se-al) pertaining to or formed by the pulpal, lingual, and axial walls of a tooth cavity.

pulpomesial (pul″po-me′ze-al) pertaining to or formed by the pulpal and mesial walls of a tooth cavity.

pulpotomy (pul-pot′o-me) [*pulp* + Gr. *tomē* a cutting] surgical excision of the coronal portion of a vital pulp.

pulpy (pul′pe) soft or pulpaceous.

pulque (pul′ke) a fermented drink made in Mexico and Central America from the juice of *Agave;* it is the source of mescal (def. 2).

pulsate (pul′sāt) to beat rhythmically, as the heart.

pulsatile (pul′sah-tīl) characterized by a rhythmical pulsation.

pulsatilla (pul″sah-til′ah) the dried herb of the ranunculaceous flowering plants *Anemone pulsatilla* L., *A. pratensis* L., or *A. patens* L. Formerly used in a variety of conditions, such as dysmenorrhea, epididymitis, and orchitis, its use has been largely abandoned.

pulsation (pul-sa′shun) [L. *pulsatio*] a throb or rhythmical beat, as of the heart. **expansile p.,** a pulsation which is seen or felt to become larger and wider with each impact of the pulse; it reflects an increase in volume of a mass, usually an aneurysm. **suprasternal p.,** arterial pulsation in the region of the suprasternal notch, due to dilatation and/or elongation of the aortic arch or to aneurysm.

pulsator (pul′sa-tor) an apparatus for maintaining respiration. **Bragg-Paul p.,** a pulsator consisting of an air bag placed around the patient's chest and abdomen and rhythmically inflated and deflated by an electric pump.

pulse (puls) [L. *pulsus* stroke] 1. the rhythmic expansion of an artery which may be felt with the finger. The *pulse rate* or number of pulsations of an artery per minute normally varies from 50 to 100. See also *beat.* 2. a brief surge, as of current or voltage. **abdominal p.,** the pulse over the abdominal aorta. **abrupt p.,** a pulse which strikes the finger rapidly; a quick or rapidly rising pulse. **allorhythmic p.,** a pulse marked by irregularities in rhythm. **alternating p.,** pulsus alternans. **anacrotic p.,** one in which the ascending limb of the tracing shows a transient drop in amplitude, or a notch. **anadicrotic p.,** one in which the ascending limb of the tracing shows two small additional waves or notches. **anatricrotic p.,** one in which the ascending limb of the tracing shows three small additional waves or notches. **atrial liver p.,** a presystolic pulse corresponding to the atrial venous pulse, sometimes occurring in tricuspid stenosis. **atrial venous p., atriovenous p.,** a cervical venous pulse having an accentuated "a" wave during atrial systole, owing to increased force of contraction of the right atrium; a characteristic of tricuspid stenosis. **biferious p., bisferious p.,** pulsus bisferiens. **bigeminal p.,** a pulse in which two beats follow each other in rapid succession, each group of two being separated from the following by a longer interval, usually related to regularly occurring ventricular premature beats. **cannon ball p.,** Corrigan's p. **capillary p.,** Quincke's p. **carotid p.,** the pulse in the carotid artery, tracings of which are used in timing the phases of the cardiac cycle. **catadicrotic p.,** one in which the descending limb of the tracing shows two small additional waves or notches. **catatricrotic p.,** one in which the descending limb of the tracing shows three small additional waves or notches. **centripetal venous p.,** a venous pulse caused by a systolic volume expansion passed from the arteries through the capillaries and venules into the larger veins. **collapsing p.,** Corrigan's p. **Corrigan's p.,** a jerky pulse with a full expansion, followed by a sudden collapse, occurring in aortic regurgitation; called also *water-hammer p.* See also *Corrigan's sign* (def. 2), under *sign.* **coupled p.,** bigeminal p. **dicrotic p.,** a pulse characterized by two peaks, the second peak occurring in diastole and being an exaggeration of the dicrotic wave. **dropped-beat p.,** intermittent p. **elastic p.,** a full pulse which gives an elastic feeling to the finger. **entoptic p.,** the subjective sensation of seeing in the dark a flash of light at each heart beat. **epigastric p.,** abdominal p. **equal p.,** one in which all of the beats are of the same strength. **febrile p.,** a pulse characteristic of fever, often described as full and bounding. **filiform p.,** thready p. **formicant p.,** a small, nearly imperceptible pulse. **frequent p.,** one which is faster in rate than normal. **full p.,** an easily felt pulse; one with a large amplitude of expansion of the vessel palpated. **fu-**

nic p., the arterial tide in the umbilical cord. **hard p.,** one which is characterized by very high tension. **hepatic p.,** the pulsations of the liver. **high-tension p.,** one characterized by a gradual impulse, long duration, slow subsidence, and a firm, cordy state of the artery between the beats. **infrequent p.,** one which is slower in rate than normal. **intermittent p.,** one in which various beats are dropped. **irregular p.,** one in which the beats occur at irregular intervals. **jerky p.,** one in which the artery is suddenly and markedly distended. **jugular p.,** a pulsation seen or felt over the jugular vein. **Kussmaul's p.,** paradoxical p. **labile p.,** a pulse which is normal when the patient is resting, but which is increased by sitting, standing, or exercise. **low-tension p.,** a pulse with sudden onset, short duration, and quick decline, and which is easily obliterated by pressure. **Monneret's p.,** a full, slow, and soft pulse said to be characteristic of jaundice. **monocrotic p.,** one in which the tracing shows only one expansion in one beat of the artery. **nail p.,** the pulsation of blood under the nails; sometimes demonstrated by the onychograph. **paradoxical p.,** a pulse that markedly decreases in size during inspiration, as that which often occurs in constrictive pericarditis. **pistol-shot p.,** a form in which the arteries are subject to sudden distention and collapse. **plateau p.,** a pulse which is slowly rising and sustained. **polycrotic p.,** one in which the tracing shows secondary pulse waves. **quadrigeminal p.,** one with a pause after every fourth beat. **quick p.,** 1. one which strikes the finger smartly and leaves it quickly; called also *short p.* 2. one with a faster rate than normal. **Quincke's p.,** alternate blanching and flushing of the skin that may be elicited in several ways, e.g., by observing the nail bed or skin at the root of the nail while pressing on the end of the nail. Caused by pulsation of subpapillary arteriolar and venous plexuses, it is sometimes seen in aortic insufficiency and other disorders, but may occur in normal persons under certain conditions. It was originally thought to be due to pulsation of the capillaries, hence the name *capillary pulse.* Called also *Quincke's sign.* **radial p.,** that felt over the radial artery. **respiratory p.,** a pulsation observed even in health in the superficial cervical veins after rapid exercise. **retrosternal p.,** a venous pulse perceptible just above the suprasternal notch. **Riegel's p.,** a pulse which is diminished in size during expiration. **running p.,** a pulse with small irregular excursions. **sharp p.,** jerky p. **short p.,** quick p., def. 1. **slow p.,** one with less than the usual number of pulsations per minute. **soft p.,** a pulse of low tension. **strong p.,** a forcible pulse; a pulse of high amplitude. **tense p.,** a pulse that is hard and full, but without wide excursions. **thready p.,** one that is very fine and scarcely perceptible. **trembling p., tremulous p.** (obs.), running p. **tricrotic p.,** one in which the tracing shows three marked expansions in one beat of the artery. **trigeminal p.,** one with a pause after every third beat. **trip-hammer p.,** Corrigan's p. **undulating p.,** a pulse giving the sensation of successive waves. **unequal p.,** a pulse in which some of the beats are strong and others weak. **vagus p.,** a slow pulse. **venous p.,** the pulsation which occurs in a vein, usually observed at the right jugular vein just above the sternoclavicular junction. **vermicular p.,** a small rapid pulse giving to the finger a sensation of wormlike movement. **vibrating p.,** jerky p. **water-hammer p.,** Corrigan's p. **wiry p.,** a small, tense pulse.

pulsimeter (pul-sim′ĕ-ter) [*pulse* + L. *metrum* measure] (obs.) an apparatus for measuring the force of the pulse.

pulsion (pul′shun) a pushing forward, or outward or to either side.

pulsus (pul′sus), pl. *pul′sus* [L.] pulse. **p. abdomina′lis,** abdominal pulse. **p. aequa′lis,** equal pulse. **p. alter′nans,** alternating pulse: a pulse in which there is regular alternation of weak and strong beats without changes in cycle length. **p. bifer′iens, p. bisfer′iens,** a pulse characterized by two strong systolic peaks separated by a midsystolic dip, most commonly occurring in pure aortic regurgitation and aortic regurgitation with stenosis. **p. bigem′inus,** bigeminal pulse. **p. ce′ler,** quick pulse. **p. cor′dis** (obs.), the pulse felt over the apex of the heart. **p. dele′tus** (obs.), absence of pulse, seen in aortic aneurysm. **p. dif′ferens,** inequality of the pulse observable at corresponding sites on either side of the body. **p. du′plex** (obs.), dicrotic pulse. **p. du′rus** (obs.), hard pulse. **p. filifor′mis,** thready pulse. **p. for′micans,** formicant pulse. **p. for′tis,** a strong pulse. **p. fre′quens,** frequent pulse. **p. irregula′ris perpet′uus,** a pulse which is wholly irregular. **p. mag′nus,** a large, full pulse. **p. mag′nus et ce′ler,** a large, full, and rapid pulse. **p. mol′lis,** soft pulse. **p. monoc′rotus,** monocrotic pulse. **p. oppres′sus,** a pulse which appears to be pushing its way through a contracted artery. **p. paradox′us,** paradoxical pulse. **p. par′vus,** a small pulse. **p. par′vus et tar′dus,** a small hard pulse which rises and falls slowly. **p. ple′nus,** full pulse. **p. pseudointermit′tens** (obs.), a pulse showing an occasional intermittence, owing to a feeble contraction of the ventricle. **p. ra′rus** (obs.), a slow pulse due to prolongation of the heart's pause. **p. tar′dus,** an abnormally slow pulse due to a prolongation of the systole or diastole. **p. trigem′inus,** trigeminal pulse. **p. undulo′sus,** undulating pulse. **p. vac′uus,** an extremely weak pulse. **p. veno'sus,** venous pulse. **p. vi'brans** (obs.), jerky pulse.

pultaceous (pul-ta'shus) [L. *pultaceus*] like a pulp or poultice.

pulv. abbreviation for L. *pulvis* powder.

pulverization (pul″ver-i-za'shun) [L. *pulvis* powder] the reduction of any substance to powder.

pulverulent (pul-ver'u-lent) [L. *pulverulentus*] powdery; dust-like.

pulvinar (pul-vi'nar) [L. "a cushioned seat"] [NA] the prominent medial portion of the posterior end of the thalamus, which is cushion-like and partly overhangs the superior colliculus; it receives fibers from other thalamic nuclei and gives off widespread cortical projections. **p. thal'ami,** NA alternative for nucleus posterior thalami.

pulvinate (pul'vĭ-nāt) [L. *pulvinus* cushion] shaped like a cushion.

pulvis (pul'vis) [L.] powder.

pumex (pu'meks) [L. "foam"] pumice.

pumice (pum'is) [USP] a substance of volcanic origin, consisting chiefly of complex silicates of aluminum, potassium, and sodium, occurring as a very light, hard, rough, porous, grayish powder; used in dentistry as an abrasive or polishing agent, the effect achieved depending on the particle size.

pump (pump) 1. an apparatus for drawing or forcing fluids or gases. 2. to draw or force fluids or gases. **air p.,** a pump for exhausting or forcing in air. **Alvegniat's p.,** a mercurial air pump used in measuring the free gaseous constituents of the blood. **blood p.,** a machine used to propel blood through the tubing of extracorporeal circulation devices, especially designed to achieve this without causing damage to the blood constituents, particularly the erythrocytes. **breast p.,** a manual or electric pump for abstracting milk from the breast. **calcium p.,** the mechanism of active transport of calcium (Ca^{++}) across a membrane, as of the sarcoplasmic reticulum of muscle cells, against a concentration gradient; the mechanism is driven by hydrolysis of ATP by the membrane-bound enzyme ATPase. **cardiac balloon p.,** a device for augmenting blood flow to the heart while relieving the cardiac work load. **infusion p.,** a device for injecting a measured amount of fluid during a specific interval of time. **infusion-withdrawal p.,** a pump for the simultaneous injection and withdrawal of fluid at the same rate. **Lindbergh p.,** a perfusion apparatus by means of which an organ removed from the body may be kept alive indefinitely. **Na$^+$-K$^+$ p.,** sodium p. **peristaltic p.,** a pump that moves liquid through tubing by alternate contractions and relaxations on the tubing. **sodium p., sodium-potassium p.,** the mechanism of active transport, involving membrane-bound ATPase, by which sodium (Na$^+$) is extruded from a cell and potassium (K$^+$) is brought in, so as to maintain the low concentration of Na$^+$ and the high concentration of K$^+$ within the cell with respect to the surrounding medium, the high concentration of K$^+$ being necessary for vital processes such as protein biosynthesis, certain enzymes activities, and maintenance of the membrane potential of excitable cells. Called also Na$^+$-K$^+$ p. **stomach p.,** a pump for removing the contents from the stomach.

pumpkin (pump'kin) the edible fruit of the plant *Cucurbita pepo* L. (Curcurbitaceae), whose dried, ripe seeds were once used as an anthelmintic.

pump-oxygenator (pump'-ok″sĭ-jĕ-na'tor) an apparatus, usually extracorporeal, comprising an arterial pump and blood oxygenator plus filters and traps, for saturating blood with oxygen; used to relieve the heart and lungs during heart surgery.

puna (poo'nah) mountain sickness.

punch (punch) 1. an instrument for indenting, perforating, or excising a disk or segment of tissue or material. 2. an instrument for extracting the root of a tooth. **Caulk p.,** a cautery punch for the removal of median bar prostatic enlargements. **kidney p., Murphy's kidney p.,** see *Murphy's test,* under *tests.* **pin p.,** an instrument for piercing the metal plate to receive the pins for fastening artificial teeth. **plate p.,** a tool for cutting out parts of an artificial dental plate.

punchdrunk (punch'drunk) a traumatic encephalopathy of prizefighters resulting from cumulative cerebral concussions; it is characterized by the general slowing of mental functions, occasional bouts of confusion, and scattered memory loss.

punched-out (puncht'owt) having the appearance of substance or tissue having been removed with a punch.

puncta (punk'tah) [L.] plural of *punctum.*

punctate (punk'tāt) [L. *punctum* point] resembling or marked with points or dots.

punctiform (punk'tĭ-form) [L. *punctum* point + *forma* shape] like a point; located in a point. In bacteriology, said of very minute colonies.

punctio (punk'she-o) [L.] the act of puncturing, pricking or dotting.

punctograph (punk'to-graf) [L. *punctum* point + Gr. *graphein* to write] an instrument for the roentgenographic localization of foreign bodies in the tissues.

punctum (punk'tum), pl. *punc'ta* [L.] an extremely small spot, or point; used in anatomical nomenclature as a general term to designate an extremely small area, or point of projection. **p. cae'cum,** blind spot; see under *spot.* **punc'ta doloro'sa,** Valleix's points. **p. lacrima'le** [NA], lacrimal point: the opening on the lacrimal papilla of an eyelid, near the medial angle of the eye, into which tears from the lacrimal lake drain to enter the lacrimal canaliculi. **punc'ta lacrima'lia,** see *punctum lacrimale.* **p. lu'teum,** macula retinae. **p. nasa'le infe'rius,** the rhinion. **p. ossificatio'nis,** ossification center. **p. prox'imum,** near point. **p. remo'tum,** far point. **punc'ta vasculo'sa,** minute red spots marking the cut surface of the white substance of the brain, produced by blood from divided vessels.

punctumeter (punk-tum'ĕ-ter) [L. *punctum* point + *metrum* measure] an instrument for measuring the range of accommodation.

punctura (punk-tu'rah) [L.] puncture. **p. explorato'ria,** exploratory puncture.

puncturatio (punk″tu-ra'she-o) [L.] the act of puncturing.

puncture (punk'tūr) [L. *punctura*] 1. the act of piercing or penetrating with a pointed object or instrument. 2. a wound so made. **Bernard's p.,** in experimental medicine, puncture on a definite point of the floor of the fourth ventricle causing glycosuria; called also *diabetic p.* **cisternal p.,** puncture of the cisterna cerebellomedullaris through the occipitoatlantoid ligament for the purpose of withdrawing cerebrospinal fluid. **Corning's p.,** lumbar p. **cranial p.,** cisternal p. **diabetic p.,** Bernard's p. **epigastric p.,** pericardiocentesis in which the trocar is passed just below the xiphoid cartilage in the middle line, directed obliquely from below upward, passing 2 cm. along the posterior surface of the sternum. It is then directed somewhat obliquely backward, passing into the gap in the sternal insertion of the diaphragm, entering the pericardium at its base. Called also *Marfan's method* and *Marfan's epigastric p.* **exploratory p.,** puncture of a cavity or tumor and removal of some portion of the contents for examination. **heat p.,** elevation of the temperature of the animal body produced by puncturing the base of the brain. **intracisternal p.,** cisternal p. **Kronecker's p.,** in experimental medicine, puncture of the inhibitory nerve center of the heart by means of a long fine needle. **lumbar p.,** the tapping of the subarachnoid space in the lumbar region, usually between the third and fourth lumbar vertebrae. **Marfan's epigastric p.,** epigastric p. **Quincke's p., spinal p.,** lumbar p. **splenic p.,** puncture of the spleen to obtain a specimen of splenic tissue for examination. **sternal p.,** removal of bone marrow from the manubrium of the sternum through an appropriate needle. **suboccipital p.,** cisternal p. **thecal p.,** puncture of the spinal membranes. **transethmoidal p.,** a technique for obtaining postmortem biopsy specimens of the brain, using a tracer inserted through the nostril. **ventricular p.,** puncture of a cerebral ventricle for the purpose of withdrawing fluid.

pungent (pun'jent) [L. *pungens* pricking] sharp or biting; somewhat acrid.

punizin (pu'nĭ-zin) a purple dye formed by the action of light and air on a colorless chromogen found in the secretions of the snails *Murex trunculus* and *Purpura lapillus.*

Puntius (pun'te-us) a genus of fresh-water fish. **P. javan'icus,** a species placed in fresh-water ponds in certain areas of the world, because it eliminates the weeds necessary for the propagation of mosquitoes.

P.U.O. *py*rexia of *u*nknown *o*rigin.

pupa (pu'pah) [L. "a doll"] the second stage in the development of an insect, between the larva and the imago.

pupal (pu'pal) pertaining to a pupa.

pupil (pu'pil) [L. *pupilla* girl] the opening at the center of the iris of the eye, through which light enters the eye; see *iris.* Called also *pupilla* [NA]. **Adie's p.,** tonic p. **Argyll Robertson p.,** one which is miotic and which responds to accommodation effort, but not to light. **artificial p.,** one made by iridectomy. **Behr's p.,** contralateral dilatation of the pupil in lesions of the optic tract. **bounding p.,** a pupil which shows alternating dilatation and contraction. **Bumke's p.,** dilatation of the pupil following a psychic stimulus; it is said not to occur in schizophrenia. **cat's-eye p.,** one with a narrow vertical aperture. **cornpicker's p's,** dilated pupils resulting from exposure to dust from Jimsonweed (which contains stramonium) in the cornfield. **fixed p.,** a pupil which does not react either to light or on convergence, or in accommodation. **Horner's p.,** a pupil that is smaller both in light and in darkness than the normal pupil, due to a lesion of the peripheral sympathetic innervation of the eye. **Hutchinson's p.,** a condition of the pupils in which one is dilated and the other not. **keyhole p.,** a pupil with a coloboma or a sector iridectomy on one side of the margin. **pinhole p.,** one which is extremely contracted. **skew p's,** a condition in which one of the ocular axes deviates upward and the other downward. **stiff p.,** Argyll Robertson p. **tonic p.,** a usually unilateral condition of the eye in which the affected pupil is larger than the other, responds to accommodation and convergence in a slow, delayed fashion, and reacts to light only after prolonged exposure to dark or light. Called also *Adie's pupil* and *papillotonia*. See also *Adie's syndrome*, under *syndrome*.

pupilla (pu-pil′ah) [L. "girl"], pl. *pupil′lae* [NA] the pupil: the opening at the center of the iris of the eye, through which light enters the eye; see *iris*.

pupillary (pu′pĭ-ler-e) pertaining to the pupil.

pupillatonia (pu″pil-ah-to′ne-ah) tonic pupil.

Pupillidae (pu-pil′ĭ-de) a family of small to minute terrestrial gastropods (suborder Stylommatophora, order Pulmonata) that are commonly found in moist wooded regions in North America; the genus *Chondrina* serves as a host of *Dicrocoelium dentriticum*.

pupillo- (pu′pĭ-lo) [L. *pupilla* pupil] a combining form denoting relationship to the pupil.

pupillograph (pu-pil′o-graf) an instrument that detects responses of the pupil of the eye.

pupillometer (pu″pĭ-lom′ĕ-ter) [*pupillo-* + L. *metrum* measure] an instrument for measuring the width or diameter of the pupil.

pupillometry (pu″pil-lom′ĕ-tre) measurement of the diameter or width of the pupil of the eye.

pupillomotor (pu″pĭ-lo-mo′tor) pertaining to the movement of the pupil.

pupilloplegia (pu″pĭ-lo-ple′je-ah) [*pupillo-* + Gr. *plēgē* stroke] tonic pupil.

pupilloscope (pu-pil′o-skōp) von Hess's instrument for measuring reactions of the pupil.

pupilloscopy (pu″pĭ-los′ko-pe) [*pupillo-* + Gr. *skopein* to examine] retinoscopy.

pupillostatometer (pu-pil″o-stah-tom′ĕ-ter) [*pupillo-* + Gr. *statos* placed + *metron* measure] an instrument for measuring the distance between the pupils.

pupillotonia (pu″pĭ-lo-to′ne-ah) tonic pupil.

Purdy's method, test (per′dēz) [Charles Wesley *Purdy*, American physician, 1846–1901] see under *method* and *tests*.

pure (pūr) [L. *purus*] free from mixture with or contamination by other materials; a reagent is *chemically pure* when it contains no other chemicals that might interfere with its action.

purgación (poor″gah-se-on′) [Sp.] a Peruvian term for gonorrhea.

purgation (pur-ga′shun) [L. *purgatio*] catharsis; purging effected by a cathartic medicine.

purgative (pur′gah-tiv) [L. *purgativus*] 1. cathartic (def. 1); causing evacuation of the bowels. 2. a cathartic, particularly one that stimulates peristaltic action.

purge (purj) [L. *purgare* to cleanse, to purify] 1. to relieve of fecal matter. 2. a purgative remedy or dose.

puric (pu′rik) 1. pertaining to pus. 2. pertaining to purine.

puriform (pu′rĭ-form) [L. *pus* pus + *forma* form] resembling pus; the term is applied to the contents of cold abscesses which resemble pus.

purinase (pu′rĭ-nās) an enzyme that catalyzes purine conversions.

purine (pu′rin) [L. *purum* pure + *urine*] a colorless crystalline heterocyclic compound, $C_5H_4N_4$, which is not found free in nature, but is variously substituted to produce a group of compounds known as *purines* or *purine bases* (purine bodies), of which uric acid is a metabolic end product. The purine bases include adenine and guanine, which are constituents of nucleic acids, and hyoxanthine and xanthine. **amino p.**, aminopurine. **methyl p's**, alkaloids formed from purines by substituting methyl groups, usually in positions 1, 3, 7. The principal ones are caffeine, theobromine, and theophylline.

purinemia (pu″rĭ-ne′me-ah) [*purine* + Gr. *haima* blood + *-ia*] the presence of purine bases in the blood.

purinemic (pu″rĭ-ne′mik) pertaining to or characterized by purinemia.

Purinethol (pu′rēn-thol) trademark for a preparation of mercaptopurine.

purinolytic (pu″rin-o-lit′ik) [*purine* + Gr. *lytikos* loosing] splitting up purines.

purinometer (pu″rin-om′ĕ-ter) [*purine* + Gr. *metron* measure] an apparatus for estimating the quantity of purine bodies in the urine.

Purkinje's cells, fibers, etc. (pur-kin′jēz) [Johannes Evangelista von *Purkinje*, Bohemian anatomist, physiologist, and microscopist, 1787–1869] see under *cell, fiber, image, layer, network, phenomenon, shift,* and *vesicle.*

Purkinje-Sanson mirror images (pur-kin′je-sah-sōz′) [J. E. *Purkinje*; Louis Joseph *Sanson*, French physician, 1790–1841] Purkinje's images; see under *image.*

Purmann's method (poor′manz) [Matthaeus Gottfried *Purmann*, German surgeon, 1648–1711] see under *method.*

Purodigin (pu′ro-di′jin) trademark for a preparation of crystalline digitoxin.

purohepatitis (pu″ro-hep″ah-ti′tis) [*pus* + *hepatitis*] hepatic abscess.

puromucous (pu″ro-mu′kus) consisting of or containing pus and mucus; mucopurulent.

puromycin (pūr″o-mi′sin) chemical name: (S)-3′-[(2-amino-3-(4-methoxyphenyl)-1-oxopropyl]amino-3′-deoxy-N,N-dimethyladenosine. An antibiotic produced by *Streptomyces alboniger*, $C_{22}H_{29}N_7O_5$, which has the ability to inhibit protein synthesis and so has been used experimentally as an antineoplastic. It also has trypanosomicidal and amebicidal activity, and was formerly used in the treatment of African trypanosomiasis and amebic dysentery. **p. hydrochloride,** the dihydrochloride salt of puromycin, $C_{22}H_{29}N_7O_5 \cdot 2HCl$, having the same actions as the base.

puron (pu′ron) a compound $C_5H_8N_4O_2$, obtained by electrolysis of uric acid.

purple (pur′p'l) 1. a color, between blue and red. 2. a substance of this color used as a dye or indicator. **bromcresol p.,** an indicator, dibromorthocresol sulfonphthalein, used in the determination of hydrogen ion concentration; it has a pH range of 5.2 to 6.8, being yellow at 5.2 and purple at 6.8. **royal p.,** tyrian purple. **Stewart's p.,** 1 grain of iodine in 1 oz. of petrolatum. **tyrian p.,** a dye of the ancients which was obtained from the snails *Murex trunculus* and *Purpura lapillus.* **visual p.,** rhodopsin.

Purpura (pur′pu-rah) a genus of marine snails, some species of which furnish a purple dye. See *purpurine.*

purpura (pur′pu-rah) [L. "purple"] a group of disorders characterized by purplish or brownish red discoloration, easily visible through the epidermis, caused by hemorrhage into the tissues. Small punctate hemorrhages are called *petechiae;* large hemorrhages are called *ecchymoses* (bruises; black and blue marks). **p. abdomina′lis,** Henoch's p. **allergic p., anaphylactoid p.,** Schönlein-Henoch p. **p. annula′ris telangiecto′des,** a rare purpuric eruption, commonly beginning on the lower extremities and becoming generalized, the original punctate erythematous lesions coalescing to form an annular or serpiginous pattern; involution is gradual, sometimes followed by atrophy and loss of hair in the area. Called also *Majocchi's purpura* or *disease.* **brain p.,** cerebral toxic pericapillary hemorrhage. **p. bullo′sa,** pemphigus hemorrhagicus. **fibrinolytic p., p. fibrinolyt′ica,** purpura secondary to and accompanied by increased fibrinolytic activity of the blood; called also *p. thrombolytica.* **p. ful′minans,** a form of nonthrombocytopenic purpura, observed mainly in children, usually following an infectious disease such as scarlet fever, and characterized by fever, shock, anemia, and sudden and rapidly spreading symmetrical skin hemorrhages of the lower extremities, often associated with extensive intravascular thromboses and gangrene. **p. hemorrha′gica,** thrombocytopenic p., idiopathic. **Henoch's p.,** a variety of Schönlein-Henoch purpura characterized by acute visceral symptoms such as vomiting, diarrhea, abdominal distention, hematuria, and renal colic, and without articular symptoms. Called also *p. nervosa.* **Henoch-Schönlein p.,** Schönlein-Henoch p. **p. hyperglobuline′mica,** originally used to designate prolonged, repetitive episodes of purpura associated with an increase in gamma globulins; no longer considered a specific entity inasmuch as the clinical and laboratory findings are observed in a variety of hematologic conditions. **idiopathic p.,** see *thrombocytopenic p., idiopathic.* **Landouzy's p.,** a term originally used to designate a form of purpura with grave systemic manifestations. **Majocchi's p.,** p. annularis telangiectodes. **malignant p.,** epidemic cerebrospinal meningitis. **p. nervo′sa,** Henoch's p. **p. of newborn,** a form of thrombocytopenia observed soon after birth, presumed in certain instances to be due to the passage of anti-platelet factor(s) across the placenta. **nonthrombocytopenic p.,** purpura without any decrease in the platelet count of the blood. **p. pigmento′sa chron′ica,** chronic purpuric dermatosis with hemosiderosis. **psychogenic p.,** a condition clinically identical with autoerythrocyte sensitization syndrome, but without erythrocyte sensitivity. **p. rheumat′ica,** Schönlein's p. **Schönlein's p.,** Schönlein-Henoch purpura with articular symptoms and without gastrointestinal symptoms. **Schönlein-Henoch p.,** a form of nonthrombocytopenic purpura probably due to a vasculitis of unknown cause, most commonly observed in children and associated with a variety of clinical symptoms including urticaria and erythema, arthropathy and arthritis, gastrointestinal symptoms, and renal involvement. Called also *allergic p., anaphylactoid p.,* and *Schönlein-Henoch disease.* **p. seni′lis,** dark purplish red ecchymoses occurring on the forearms and back of the hands in the elderly. **p. sim′plex,** a general designation for nonthrombocytopenic purpura unaccompanied by defined vascular or intravascular abnormalities. **p. sim′plex, pigmented familial,** a form of nonthrombocytopenic purpura occurring in certain families; an autosomal dominant gene seems to be responsible. **steroid p.,** bizarre-shaped broad hemorrhages beneath the skin of the back of the forearms, hands, or shins caused by attrition of dermal and vascular connective tissue due to long-term treatment with adrenocortical steroid hormones. Identical with purpura senilis in appearance. **thrombocytolytic p.,** fibrinolytic p. **thrombocytopenic p's,** any form of purpura in which the platelet count is decreased; it may be either primary (idiopathic) or secondary. **thrombocytopenic p., idiopathic,** thrombocytopenic purpura unassociated with any definable systemic disease but often accompanied by the presence of a serum antiplatelet factor, now characterized as an IgG immunoglobulin. **thrombocytopenic p., secondary,** thrombocytopenic purpura occurring as a consequence of a primary hematologic disease such as leukemia, or an underlying systemic nonhematologic entity. **thrombocytopenic p., thrombotic,** a disease of undefined cause, characterized by thrombocytopenia, hemolytic anemia, bizarre neurological manifestations, azotemia, fever, and thromboses in terminal arterioles and capillaries; called also *microangiopathic hemolytic anemia* and *Moschcowitz's disease.* **p. thrombolyt′ica,** fibrinolytic p. **thrombopenic p.,** thrombocytopenic p. **p. variolo′sa** (*obs.*), hemorrhagic smallpox.

purpurate (pur′pu-rāt) a salt of purpuric acid.

purpureaglycoside (pur-pu″re-ah-gli′ko-sīd) a cardiac glycoside, $C_{47}H_{74}O_{18}$, from the leaves of *Digitalis purpurea* L. (Schrophulariaceae). **p. C.,** see *deslanoside.*

purpuric (pur-pu′rik) of the nature of, pertaining to, or affected with purpura.

purpuriferous (pur″pu-rif′er-us) [L. *purpura* purple + *ferre* to bear] producing a purple pigment.

purpurin (pur′pu-rin) 1. a glycoside from madder root that has been used as a nuclear stain. It is 1,2,4-trihydroxyanthraquinone, $C_6H_4(CO)_2C_6H(OH)_3$. 2. uroerythrin. 3. purpurine.

purpurine (pur′pu-rēn) 1. a neurotoxic substance derived from the median zone of the hypobranchial or purple gland of gastropods of the genus *Purpura*, thought to be an ester or a mixture of esters of choline; the substance is called *murexine* when derived from snails of the genus *Murex.* 2. purpurin.

purpurinuria (pur″pu-rin-u′re-ah) the presence of uroerythrin in the urine.

purpuriparous (pur″pu-rip′ah-rus) [L. *purpura* purple + *parere* to produce] purpuriferous.

purpurogenous (pur″pu-roj′ĕ-nus) [L. *purpura* purple + Gr. *gennan* to produce] producing visual purple (rhodopsin).

purr (pur) a low vibratory murmur, or purring sound.

purring (pur′ing) having a tremulous quality, like the purr of a cat.

purshianin (pur-shi′ah-nin) a brown, oily liquid glycoside mixture from *Rhamnus purshiana* D.C. (Rhamnaceae), having laxative action.

Purtscher's disease (angiopathic retinopathy) (poor′cherz) [Otmar *Purtscher*, Swiss ophthalmologist, 1852–1927] see under *disease.*

puru (poo′roo) the native name in the Malay States for yaws.

purulence (pu′roo-lens) [L. *purulentia*] the condition or fact of being purulent.

purulency (pu′roo-len″se) purulence.

purulent (pu′roo-lent) [L. *purulentus*] consisting of or containing pus; associated with the formation of or caused by pus.

puruloid (pu′roo-loid) resembling pus; puriform.

pus (pus), pl. *pu′ra*, gen. *pu′ris* [L.] a liquid inflammation product made up of cells (leukocytes) and a thin fluid called liquor puris. **anchovy sauce p.,** the brownish pus seen in amebic abscess of the liver. **blue p.,** pus with a bluish tint, seen in certain suppurative infections, the color occurring as a result of the presence of an antibiotic pigment (pyocyanin) produced by *Pseudomonas aeruginosa.* **p. bo′num et laudab′ile,** laudable pus. **burrowing p.,** pus which is not walled off but may extend between fascial planes for considerable distances. **cheesy p.,** thick, nearly solid pus. **curdy p.,** pus mixed with cheesy flakes. **green p.,** pus having a greenish tint. **ichorous p.,** a thin, acrid pus, often having an ill smell, secreted by unhealthy surfaces. **laudable p., p. laudan′dum,** a term once applied to a creamy yellow, inodorous pus, secreted by a healthy granulating surface, and regarded as indicative of less danger than other varieties. **sanious p.,** bloody pus, often ichorous and ill smelling.

Pusey's emulsion (pu′sēz) [William Allen *Pusey*, American dermatologist, 1865–1940] see under *emulsion.*

pustula (pus′tu-lah), pl. *pus′tulae* [L.] pustule.

pustular (pus′tu-lar) pertaining to or of the nature of a pustule; consisting of pustules.

pustulation (pus″tu-la′shun) the formation of pustules.

pustule (pus′tūl) [L. *pustula*] a visible collection of pus within or beneath the epidermis, often in a hair follicle or sweat pore. **multilocular p.,** a pustule with several compartments, indicating origin from a spongiotic vesicle within the epidermis rather than from infection arising in a follicle or sweat pore, or beneath the epidermis. **primary p.,** one formed without any previous lesion. **secondary p.,** one which is preceded by a vesicle or papule. **simple p.,** unilocular p. **spongiform p. of Kogoj,** a multilocular microabscess formed in the epidermis by spongiosis, followed by infiltration with large numbers of polymorphonuclear leukocytes, as in acrodermatitis continua and impetigo herpetiformis. **unilocular p.,** one consisting of a single cavity filled with pus, suggesting origin within a follicle or sweat

pore or from beneath the epidermis, rather than within it; called also *simple p.*

pustulosis (pus″tu-lo′sis) a condition marked by an outbreak of pustules. **p. vaccinifor′mis acu′ta, p. variolifor′mis acu′ta,** Kaposi's varicelliform eruption; see under *eruption.*

putamen (pu-ta′men) [L. "shell"] [NA] the larger and more lateral part of the lentiform nucleus, separated from the globus pallidus by the lateral medullary lamina.

Putnam type (put′nam) [James Jackson *Putnam*, Boston neurologist, 1846–1918] subacute combined degeneration of the spinal cord; see under *degeneration.*

Putnam-Dana syndrome (put′nam-da′nah) [J. J. *Putnam*; Charles Loomis *Dana*, neurologist in New York, 1852–1935] subacute combined degeneration of spinal cord (see under *degeneration*).

putrefaction (pu″trĕ-fak′shun) [L. *putrefactio*] enzymic decomposition, especially of proteins, with the production of foul-smelling compounds, such as hydrogen sulfide, ammonia, and mercaptans. Cf. *fermentation.*

putrefactive (pu″trĕ-fak′tiv) pertaining to or of the nature of putrefaction.

putrefy (pu′trĕ-fi) to decompose, with the production of foul-smelling compounds; a term applied especially to the decomposition of proteins and organic matter.

putrescence (pu-tres′ens) partial or complete rottenness.

putrescent (pu-tres′ent) [L. *putrescens* decaying] rotting; undergoing putrefaction.

putrescine (pu-tres′in) chemical name: tetra-methylene-diamine. A polyamine, $NH_2(CH_2)_4NH_2$, first found in decaying animal tissues but now known to occur in almost all tissues and in cultures of certain bacteria. It is formed by decarboxylation of ornithine and is itself a precursor of spermidine.

putrid (pu′trid) [L. *putridus*] characterized by putrefaction; rotten or corrupt.

putrilage (pu′trĭ-lij) [L. *putrilago*] putrescent or putrid matter.

putromaine (pu-tro′mān) any poison produced by the decomposition of food within the living body.

putty (put′e) a pliable, sticky material. **Horsley's p.,** see under *wax.*

Puusepp's operation, reflex (poos′eps) [Lyudvig Martinovich *Puusepp*, Estonian neurosurgeon, 1875– 1942] see under *operation* and *reflex.*

PVP polyvinylpyrrolidone.

PVP-I povidone-iodine.

Px. pneumothorax.

pyarthrosis (pi″ar-thro′sis) [Gr. *pyon* pus + *arthron* joint + -*osis*] suppuration within a joint cavity; acute suppurative arthritis.

Pycnanthemum (pik-nan′the-mum) [Gr. *pyknos* dense + *anthemon* bloom] a genus of American mints, called *mountain basil* and *mountain mint*, aromatic and carminative; resembling pennyroyal and spearmint in taste and smell.

pycno- for words thus beginning, see those beginning *pykno-*.

pyecchysis (pi-ek′kĭ-sis) [Gr. *pyon* pus + *ek* out + *chein* to pour] the effusion of purulent matter.

pyel- see *pyelo-*.

pyelectasia (pi″ĕ-lek-ta′ze-ah) pyelectasis.

pyelectasis (pi″ĕ-lek′tah-sis) [*pyel-* + Gr. *ektasis* distention] dilatation of the renal pelvis.

pyelic (pi-el′ik) pertaining to the pelvis of the kidney.

pyelitic (pi″ĕ-lit′ik) pertaining to or affected with pyelitis.

pyelitis (pi″ĕ-li′tis) [*pyel-* + -*itis*] inflammation of the pelvis of the kidney. It is attended by pain and tenderness in the loins, irritability of the bladder, remittent fever, bloody or purulent urine, diarrhea, vomiting, and a peculiar pain on flexion of the thigh. See also *pyelonephritis.* **calculous p.,** that which is caused by calculi. **p. cys′tica,** pyelitis with the formation of multiple submucosal cysts. **defloration p.,** pyelitis in women after the first sexual intercourse, as a result of infection following rupture of the hymen. **encrusted p.,** pyelitis with ulcers which are encrusted with urinary salts. **p. glandula′ris,** pyelitis with conversion of transitional mucosal into cylindrical epithelium, with formation of glandular acini. **p. granulo′sa,** pyelitis marked by the presence of exuberant granulations. **p. gravida′rum,** inflammation of the kidney and ureter occurring in pregnancy. **hematogenous p.,** pyelitis in which the infection comes from the blood. **hemorrhagic p.,** that which is attended with hemorrhage. **suppurative p.,** a form with development of pus which causes abscess of the kidney, or pyonephrosis. **urogenous p.,** pyelitis in which the infection comes from the urine.

pyelo-, pyel- [Gr. *pyelos* pelvis] combining form denoting relationship to the pelvis of the kidney.

pyelocaliectasis (pi″ĕ-lo-kal″e-ek′tah-sis) [*pyelo-* + *calix* + *ektasis* distention] dilatation of the kidney pelvis and calices.

pyelocystanastomosis (pi″ĕ-lo-sist″ah-nas″to-mo′sis) pyelocystostomosis.

pyelocystitis (pi″ĕ-lo-sis-ti′tis) [*pyelo-* + Gr. *kystis* bladder + *-itis*] inflammation of the renal pelvis and of the bladder.

pyelocystostomosis (pi″ĕ-lo-sis″to-sto-mo′sis) [*pyelo-* + Gr. *kystis* bladder + ana*stomosis*] the surgical formation of a communication between the renal pelvis and the bladder.

pyelofluoroscopy (pi″ĕ-lo-floo″o-ros′ko-pe) examination of the renal pelvis by means of the fluoroscope.

pyelogram (pi′ĕ-lo-gram″) [*pyelo-* + Gr. *gramma* mark] a roentgenogram of the kidney and ureter, especially showing the pelvis of the kidney. **dragon p.,** bizarre forms in the pyelogram seen in polycystic kidney.

pyelograph (pi′ĕ-lo-graf) pyelogram.

pyelography (pi″ĕ-log′rah-fe) [*pyelo-* + Gr. *graphein* to draw] roentgenography of the renal pelvis and ureter after the structures have been filled with a contrast solution. **air p.,** pneumopyelography. **antegrade p.,** that in which the contrast medium is introduced by percutaneous needle puncture into the renal pelvis. **ascending p.,** retrograde p. **p. by elimination,** intravenous p. **excretion p.,** intravenous p. **intravenous p.,** pyelography in which an intravenous injection is made of a contrast medium which passes quickly into the urine. **lateral p.,** pyelography in which the patient lies in lateral position with his questionable side next to the film. **respiration p.,** pyelography with a diphasic film showing the kidney under several phases of the respiratory cycle. **retrograde p.,** pyelography in which the contrast fluid is injected into the renal pelvis through the ureter. **wash-out p.,** that in which the roentgenogram is taken after the kidneys have been filled with a contrast solution and then "washed-out" by water diuresis; this procedure increases the contrast between a normal and a malfunctioning kidney.

pyeloileocutaneous (pi″ĕ-lo-il″e-o-ku-ta′ne-us) pertaining to the kidney pelvis, ileum, and skin; see under *anastomosis*.

pyelointerstitial (pi″ĕ-lo-in″ter-stish′al) pertaining to the interstitial tissue of the renal pelvis.

pyelolithotomy (pi″ĕ-lo-lĭ-thot′o-me) [*pyelo-* + Gr. *lithos* stone + *tomē* a cutting] the operation of excising a renal calculus from the pelvis of the kidney.

pyelometry (pi″ĕ-lom′e-tre) [*pyelo-* + Gr. *metron* measure] the measurement by tracings of the waves of contraction and relaxation of the renal pelvis, recorded by changes of pressure through a ureteral catheter.

pyelonephritis (pi″ĕ-lo-nĕ-fri′tis) [*pyelo-* + Gr. *nephros* kidney + *-itis*] inflammation of the kidney and its pelvis, beginning in the interstitium and rapidly extending to involve the tubules, glomeruli, and blood vessels; due to bacterial infection. **acute p.,** pyelonephritis of sudden onset characterized by fever, shaking chills, pain in the costovertebral region or flanks, and symptoms of bladder inflammation; it is a self-limited bacterial disease caused most often by gram-negative enteric bacilli. **chronic p.,** pyelonephritis attributed to cicatricial effects of a previous infection or to recurring or progressive infection. Typically, it is of insidious onset, manifested by symptoms of chronic renal insufficiency, with fatigue, headache, loss of appetite, weight loss, excessive thirst, and polyuria. **p. of pregnancy,** a renal infection during pregnancy characterized by dilatation of the renal pelvis and the ureters; some degree of ureteric obstruction may be caused by the gravid uterus.

pyelonephrosis (pi″ĕ-lo-nĕ-fro′sis) [*pyelo-* + Gr. *nephros* kidney + *-osis*] any disease of the kidney and its pelvis.

pyelopathy (pi″ĕ-lop′ah-the) [*pyelo-* + Gr. *pathos* disease] any disease of the renal pelvis.

pyelophlebitis (pi″ĕ-lo-fle-bi′tis) [*pyelo-* + Gr. *phleps* vein + *-itis*] inflammation of the veins of the renal pelvis.

pyeloplasty (pi′ĕ-lo-plas″te) [*pyelo-* + Gr. *plassein* to form] a plastic operation on the pelvis of the kidney.

pyeloplication (pi″ĕ-lo-pli-ka′shun) [*pyelo-* + L. *plica* fold] reduction in size of a dilated renal pelvis by infolding its walls by Lembert sutures.

pyeloscopy (pi″ĕ-los′ko-pe) [*pyelo-* + Gr. *skopein* to examine] observation of the kidney pelvis under the fluoroscope after intravenous or retrograde injection of a contrast medium.

pyelostomy (pi″ĕ-los′to-me) [*pyelo-* + Gr. *stomoun* to provide with an opening, or mouth] the operation of forming an opening into the renal pelvis for the purpose of temporarily diverting the urine from the ureter.

pyelotomy (pi″ĕ-lot′o-me) [*pyelo-* + Gr. *tomē* a cutting] incision of the pelvis of the kidney.

pyeloureterectasis (pi″ĕ-lo-u-re″ter-ek′tah-sis) dilatation of a renal pelvis and a ureter.

pyeloureterography (pi″ĕ-lo-u-re″ter-og′rah-fe) pyelography.

pyeloureterolysis (pi″ĕ-lo-u-re″ter-ol′ĭ-sis) [*pyelo-* + *ureter* + Gr. *lysis* dissolution] the surgical freeing of fibrous bands or adhesions near the junction of the kidney pelvis and ureter.

pyeloureteroplasty (pi″ĕ-lo-u-re′ter-o-plas″te) plastic operation on the renal pelvis and ureter.

pyelovenous (pi″ĕ-lo-ve′nus) pertaining to the kidney pelvis and renal veins.

pyemesis (pi-em′ĕ-sis) [Gr. *pyon* pus + *emesis* vomiting] vomiting of purulent matter.

pyemia (pi-e′me-ah) [Gr. *pyon* pus + *haima* blood + *-ia*] a general septicemia in which secondary foci of suppuration occur and multiple abscesses are formed. The condition is marked by fever, chills, sweating, jaundice, and abscess in various parts of the body. Called also *metastatic infection*. **arterial p.,** a form due to the dissemination of septic emboli from the heart. **cryptogenic p.,** that in which the source of infection is in an unidentified tissue. **otogenous p.,** that which originates from inflammation in the ear. **portal p.,** suppurative pylephlebitis; see *pylephlebitis*.

pyemic (pi-e′mik) pertaining to or marked by pyemia.

Pyemotes (pi-ĕ-mo′tez) a genus of parasitic mites; formerly called *Pediculoides*. **P. ventrico′sus,** a predaceous mite which attacks the larvae of a number of insects. Found in the straw of various cereals, it produces a vesiculopapular dermatitis (grain itch) in man. Formerly known as *Pediculoides ventricosus* and *Acarus tritici*.

pyencephalus (pi″en-sef′ah-lus) [Gr. *pyon* pus + *enkephalos* brain] abscess of the brain.

pyesis (pi-e′sis) suppuration.

pygal (pi′gal) [Gr. *pygē* rump] pertaining to the buttocks; natal.

pygalgia (pi-gal′je-ah) [*pygo-* + *-algia*] pain in the buttocks.

pygist (pi′jist) [Gr. *pygē* rump] a pederast.

pygmalionism (pig-ma′le-on-izm) [*Pygmalion*, a Greek sculptor who fell in love with a statue he had carved] the falling in love with an object made by one's self.

pygmy (pig′me) [Gr. *pygmaios* dwarfish] a small individual; a dwarf.

pygo- [Gr. *pygē* rump] a combining form denoting relationship to the buttocks.

pygoamorphus (pi″go-ah-mor′fus) asymmetrical conjoined twins, in which the parasite, or teratoma, is an amorphous mass attached to the sacral region of the autosite.

pygodidymus (pi″go-did′ĭ-mus) [*pygo-* + Gr. *didymos* twin] a fetus with double hips and pelvis.

pygomelus (pi-gom′ĕ-lus) [*pygo-* + Gr. *melos* limb] a fetus with a supernumerary limb or limbs attached to or near the buttock.

pygopagus (pi-gop′ah-gus) [*pygo-* + Gr. *pagos* thing fixed] a double monster consisting of two nearly complete individuals joined at the sacrum, so the two components are back to back. **p. parasit′icus,** an asymmetrical double monster in which the parasitic component is attached to the sacral region of the autosite.

pygopagy (pi-gop′ah-je) the condition of being a pygopagus.

pyic (pi′ik) of or pertaining to pus.

pyin (pi′in) [Gr. *pyon* pus] an albuminoid mucus-like substance found in pus, and separated from it by adding sodium chloride and filtering.

pyknic (pik′nik) [Gr. *pyknos* thick] having a short, thick, stocky build. Cf. *macrosplanchnic* and *microsplanchnic*.

pykno- [Gr. *pyknos* thick, frequent] a combining form meaning thick, compact, or frequent.

pyknocyte (pik″no-sīt) a distorted and contracted, occasionally spiculed erythrocyte normally occurring in small numbers in the full-term infant, but in greater numbers in hemolytic disorders.

pyknocytoma (pik″no-si-to′mah) oxyphilic granular cell adenoma.

pyknocytosis (pik″no-si-to′sis) conspicuous increases in the numbers of pyknocytes.

pyknodysostosis (pik″no-dis″os-to′sis) a symptom complex inherited as an autosomal recessive trait, consisting of dwarfism, osteopetrosis, partial agenesis of the terminal digits of the hands and feet, cranial anomalies, frontal and occipital bossing, and hypoplasia of the angle of the mandible.

pyknoepilepsy (pik″no-ep′ĭ-lep″se) [*pykno-* + Gr. *epilēpsia* seizure] petit mal epilepsy.

pyknolepsy (pik″no-lep′se) [*pykno-* + Gr. *lepsis* seizure] petit mal epilepsy.

pyknometer (pik-nom′ĕ-ter) [*pykno-* + Gr. *metron* measure] an instrument for determining the specific gravity of fluids.

pyknometry (pik-nom′ĕ-tre) measurement by the pyknometer.

pyknomorphic (pik″no-mor′fik) pyknomorphous.

pyknomorphous (pik″no-mor′fus) [*pykno-* + Gr. *morphē* form] having the stainable elements compactly arranged; a term applied to certain nerve cells.

pyknophrasia (pik″no-fra′ze-ah) [*pykno-* + Gr. *phrasis* speech + *-ia*] thickness of speech.

pyknoplasson (pik″no-plas′on) [*pykno-* + *plasson*] the plasson in its unexpanded form. Cf. *chasmatoplasson*.

pyknosis (pik-no′sis) [Gr. *pyknōsis* condensation] a thickening, especially degeneration of a cell in which the nucleus shrinks in size and the chromatin condenses to a solid, structureless mass or masses.

pyknotic (pik-not′ik) [Gr. *pyknōtikos*] 1. serving to close the pores. 2. pertaining to pyknosis.

pyle- [Gr. *pylē* gate] a combining form denoting relationship to the portal vein.

pylephlebectasis (pi″le-fle-bek′tah-sis) [*pyle-* + Gr. *phleps* vein + *ektasis* dilatation] dilatation of the portal vein.

pylephlebitis (pi″le-fle-bi′tis) [*pyle-* + Gr. *phleps* vein + *-itis*] inflammation of the portal vein; it usually results from intestinal disease. Suppurative pylephlebitis, or portal pyemia, is marked by symptoms of pyemia. **adhesive p.,** inflammation of the portal vein producing thrombosis; pylethrombophlebitis.

pylethrombophlebitis (pi″le-throm″bo-fle-bi′tis) [*pyle-* + Gr. *thrombos* clot of blood + *phleps* vein + *-itis*] thrombosis and inflammation of the portal vein.

pylethrombosis (pi″le-throm-bo′sis) thrombosis of the portal vein, as in adhesive pylephlebitis.

pylic (pi′lik) [Gr. *pylē* gate] pertaining to the portal vein.

pylometer (pi-lom′ĕ-ter) [Gr. *pylē* gate + *metron* measure] an instrument for measuring obstruction at the ureteral opening of the bladder.

pylon (pi′lon) a temporary artificial leg.

pyloralgia (pi″lo-ral′je-ah) [*pylorus* + Gr. *algos* pain + *-ia*] pain in the region of the pylorus.

pylorectomy (pi″lo-rek′to-me) [*pylorus* + Gr. *ektomē* excision] excision of the pylorus.

pyloric (pi-lor′ik) pertaining to the pylorus or to the pyloric part of the stomach (pars pylorica ventriculi).

pyloristenosis (pi-lor″e-stĕ-no′sis) [*pylorus* + Gr. *stenōsis* narrowing] stenosis, or narrowing, of the caliber of the pylorus; pyloric stenosis.

pyloritis (pi″lo-ri′tis) inflammation of the pylorus.

pyloro- (pi-lo′ro) [Gr. *pylōros*, from *pylē* gate + *ouros* guard] a combining form denoting relationship to the pylorus.

pylorodiosis (pi-lo″ro-di-o′sis) [*pyloro-* + Gr. *diōsis* pushing asunder] the operation of dilating a stricture of the pylorus with the finger, which is inserted either directly through a gastrotomy incision (*Loreta's method*) or indirectly by invaginating the anterior gastric wall (*Hahn's method*).

pyloroduodenitis (pi-lo″ro-du″o-de-ni′tis) inflammation of the pyloric and duodenal mucosa.

pylorogastrectomy (pi-lo″ro-gas-trek′to-me) excision of the pylorus and adjacent portion of the stomach.

pyloromyotomy (pi-lo″ro-mi-ot′o-me) incision of the longitudinal and circular muscles of the pylorus; Fredet-Ramstedt's operation.

pyloroplasty (pi-lo′ro-plas″te) [*pyloro-* + Gr. *plassein* to form] a plastic operation to relieve pyloric obstruction or to accelerate gastric emptying. **double p.,** posterior pyloromyotomy combined with the Heineke-Mikulicz pyloroplasty. **Finney p.,** enlargement of the pyloric canal by means of a longitudinal incision through the pylorus and adjacent walls of the stomach and duodenum and the establishment of an inverted U-shaped anastomosis between the stomach and duodenum. **Heineke-Mikulicz p.,** enlargement of a pyloric stricture by incising the pylorus longitudinally and suturing the incision transversely.

pyloroptosis (pi″lo-ro-to′sis) [*pyloro-* + Gr. *ptōsis* falling] (*obs.*) displacement of the pyloric end of the stomach.

pyloroscopy (pi″lo-ros′ko-pe) [*pyloro-* + Gr. *skopein* to examine] inspection of the pylorus with an endoscope.

pylorospasm (pi-lo′ro-spazm) [*pyloro-* + Gr. *spasmos* spasm] spasm of the pylorus or of the pyloric portion of the stomach. **congenital p.,** spasm of the pylorus in infants due to prenatal conditions. **reflex p.,** pylorospasm due to extragastric conditions.

pylorostenosis (pi-lo″ro-stĕ-no′sis) pyloristenosis.

pylorostomy (pi″lo-ros′to-me) [*pyloro-* + Gr. *stomoun* to provide with an opening, or mouth] surgical formation of an opening through the abdominal wall into the stomach near the pylorus.

pylorotomy (pi″lo-rot′o-me) [*pyloro-* + Gr. *tomē* a cutting] surgical incision of the pylorus.

pylorus (pi-lo′rus) [Gr. *pyloros*, from *pylē* gate + *ouros* guard] [NA] the distal aperture of the stomach surrounded by a strong band of circular muscle, and through which the stomach contents are emptied into the duodenum. It is variously used to mean pyloric part of the stomach, pyloric antrum, pyloric canal, pyloric opening, and pyloric sphincter.

pyo- [Gr. *pyon* pus] a combining form denoting relationship to pus.

pyoarthrosis (pi″o-ar-thro′sis) pyarthrosis.

pyoblennorrhea (pi″o-blen″o-re′ah) suppurative blennorrhea.

pyocalix (pi″o-ka′liks) the presence of pus in a calix of the renal pelvis.

pyocele (pi′o-sēl) [*pyo-* + Gr. *kēlē* hernia] distention of a cavity or tube with pus due to retention; as an accumulation of pus in the scrotum.

pyocelia (pi″o-se′le-ah) [*pyo-* + Gr. *koilia* cavity] pus in the abdominal cavity.

pyocephalus (pi″o-sef′ah-lus) [*pyo-* + Gr. *kephalē* head] the presence of purulent fluid in the cerebral ventricles.

pyochezia (pi″o-ke′ze-ah) [*pyo-* + Gr. *chezein* to defecate + *-ia*] presence of pus in the stools.

pyococcic (pi″o-kok′sik) pertaining to or produced by pus-forming cocci.

pyococcus (pi″o-kok′us) any pus-forming coccus.

pyocolpocele (pi″o-kol′po-sēl) [*pyo-* + Gr. *kolpos* vagina + *kēlē* tumor] a tumor of the vagina containing pus.

pyocolpos (pi″o-kol′pos) [*pyo-* + Gr. *kolpos* vagina] a collection of pus within the vagina.

pyoculture (pi′o-kul″tūr) [*pyo-* + *culture*] the comparison of a bacteriologic culture of pus with uncultured pus from the same lesion, as an indication of the resistance of the patient to the infection.

pyocyanase (pi″o-si′ah-nās) an antibacterial material from cultures of *Pseudomonas aeruginosa* (*pyocyanea*), which is bactericidal for many bacteria and lytic for some (*Vibro comma*). It is composed of three fractions, one of which is the blue pigment, pyocyanin.

pyocyanic (pi″o-si-an′ik) pertaining to blue pus, or to *Pseudomonas aeruginosa* (*P. pyocyanea*).

pyocyanin (pi″o-si′ah-nin) [*pyo-* + Gr. *kyanos* blue + *-in*, a chemical suffix] a blue-green antibiotic pigment produced by *Pseudomonas aeruginosa*; it gives the color to blue pus.

pyocyanogenic (pi″o-si″ah-no-jen′ik) producing pyocyanin.

pyocyanosis (pi″o-si″ah-no′sis) any disease due to infection with *Pseudomonas aeruginosa* (*P. pyocyanea*).

pyocyst (pi′o-sist) [*pyo-* + *cyst*] a cyst containing pus.

pyocystis (pi″o-sis′tis) pus in the urinary bladder.

pyoderma (pi″o-der′mah) [*pyo-* + Gr. *derma* skin] any purulent skin disease. **chancriform p., p. chancrifor′me faci′ei,** an ulcerated nodular solitary lesion of the face resembling a chancre. **p. facia′le,** a condition characterized by formation of a few or many abscesses and cysts on the face, with intense erythema, and sinus tracts linking the deep-seated lesions. Untreated, the lesions persist for months, and leave severe scars. **p. gangreno′sum,** a rapidly evolving cutaneous ulcer or ulcers, characterized by marked undermining of the border; once regarded as a complication peculiar to ulcerative colitis, it also occurs with other wasting diseases. **p. veg′etans,** dermatitis vegetans. **p. verruco′sum, verrucous p.,** dermatitis vegetans.

pyodermatitis (pi″o-der″mah-ti′tis) (*obs.*) pyoderma. **p. veg′etans,** dermatitis vegetans.

pyodermatosis (pi″o-der″mah-to′sis) (*obs.*) pyoderma.

pyodermia (pi″o-der′me-ah) pyoderma.

pyodermitis (pi″o-der-mi′tis) (*obs.*) pyoderma. **p. veg′etans,** dermatitis vegetans.

pyofecia (pi″o-fe′se-ah) pus in the feces.

pyogenesis (pi″o-jen′ĕ-sis) [*pyo-* + Gr. *genesis* production] the formation of pus; pyopoiesis.

pyogenic (pi″o-jen′ik) producing pus; pyopoietic.

pyogenin (pi-oj′e-nin) a compound, $C_{63}H_{128}N_2O_{19}$, derived from the body of pus cells.

pyogenous (pi-oj′ĕ-nus) caused by pus.

pyohemia (pi″o-he′me-ah) pyemia.

pyohemothorax (pi″o-he″mo-tho′raks) [*pyo-* + Gr. *haima* blood + *thōrax* chest] a collection of pus and blood in the pleural space.

pyohydronephrosis (pi″o-hi″dro-nĕ-fro′sis) the accumulation of pus and urine in the kidney.

pyoid (pi′oid) [*pyo-* + Gr. *eidos* form] 1. resembling pus. 2. a puslike substance from raw or granulating surfaces, but free from bacteria and nontoxic.

pyolabyrinthitis (pi″o-lab″ĭ-rin-thi′tis) inflammation of the labyrinth of the ear, with suppuration.

pyometra (pi″o-me′trah) [*pyo-* + Gr. *mētra* womb] an accumulation of pus within the uterus.

pyometritis (pi″o-mĕ-tri′tis) purulent inflammation of the uterus.

pyometrium (pi″o-me′tre-um) pyometra.

pyomyositis (pi″o-mi″o-si′tis) myositis purulenta. **tropical p.,** a disease of West Africa characterized by fever and the development of suppurating tumors in the muscles; it is probably caused by *Staphylococcus albus* and *S. aureus*. Called also *bung pagga*.

pyonephritis (pi″o-nĕ-fri′tis) purulent inflammation of the kidney.

pyonephrolithiasis (pi″o-nef″ro-lĭ-thi′ah-sis) [*pyo-* + Gr. *nephros* kidney + *lithos* stone + *-iasis*] the presence of stones and pus in the kidney.

pyonephrosis (pi″o-nĕ-fro′sis) [*pyo-* + Gr. *nephros* kidney + *-osis*] suppurative destruction of the parenchyma of the kidney, with total or almost complete loss of renal function.

pyonephrotic (pi″o-ně-frot′ik) pertaining to or characterized by pyonephrosis.

pyonychia (pi″o-nik′e-ah) [*pyo-* + Gr. *onyx* nail + *-ia*] paronychia.

pyo-ovarium (pi″o-o-va′re-um) abscess of an ovary.

Pyopen (pi′o-pen) trademark for a preparation of carbenicillin disodium.

pyopericarditis (pi″o-per″ĭ-kar-di′tis) purulent inflammation of the pericardium.

pyopericardium (pi″o-per″ĭ-kar′de-um) the presence of pus in the pericardial cavity.

pyoperitoneum (pi″o-per″ĭ-to-ne′um) [*pyo-* + *peritoneum*] pus in the peritoneal cavity.

pyoperitonitis (pi″o-per″ĭ-to-ni′tis) purulent inflammation of the peritoneum.

pyophagia (pi″o-fa′je-ah) [*pyo-* + Gr. *phagein* to eat] the swallowing of pus.

pyophthalmia (pi″of-thal′me-ah) a suppurative condition of the eye.

pyophthalmitis (pi″of-thal-mi′tis) purulent inflammation of the eye.

pyophylactic (pi″o-fi-lak′tik) [*pyo-* + Gr. *phylaktikos* guarding] serving as a defense against purulent infection.

pyophysometra (pi″o-fi″so-me′trah) [*pyo-* + Gr. *physa* air + *mētra* uterus] a collection of pus and gas in the uterus.

pyoplania (pi″o-pla′ne-ah) [*pyo-* + Gr. *planē* wandering] wandering of pus from one part to another.

pyopneumocholecystitis (pi″o-nu″mo-ko″le-sis-ti′tis) [*pyo-* + Gr. *pneuma* air + *cholecyst* + *-itis*] distention of the gallbladder with pus and gas.

pyopneumocyst (pi″o-nu′mo-sist) [*pyo-* + Gr. *pneuma* air + *cyst*] a cyst containing pus and gas.

pyopneumohepatitis (pi″o-nu″mo-hep″ah-ti′tis) abscess of the liver with pus and gas in the abscess cavity.

pyopneumopericardium (pi″o-nu″mo-per″ĭ-kar′de-um) [*pyo-* + Gr. *pneuma* air + *pericardium*] the presence of pus and gas in the pericardial cavity.

pyopneumoperitoneum (pi″o-nu″mo-per″ĭ-to-ne′um) the presence of pus and gas in the peritoneal cavity.

pyopneumoperitonitis (pi″o-nu″mo-per″ĭ-to-ni′tis) [*pyo-* + Gr. *pneuma* air + *peritonitis*] peritonitis with the presence of pus and gas in the peritoneal cavity.

pyopneumothorax (pi″o-nu″mo-tho′raks) [*pyo-* + Gr. *pneuma* air + *thōrax* chest] a collection of pus and air or gas in the pleural cavity.

pyopoiesis (pi″o-poi-e′sis) [*pyo-* + Gr. *poiein* to make] the formation of pus; pyogenesis.

pyopoietic (pi″o-poi-et′ik) producing pus; pyogenic.

pyoptysis (pi-op′tĭ-sis) [*pyo-* + Gr. *ptysis* spitting] spitting of purulent matter.

pyopyelectasis (pi″o-pi″ĕ-lek′tah-sis) [*pyo-* + Gr. *pyelos* pelvis + *ektasis* dilatation] dilatation of the renal pelvis with purulent fluid.

pyorrhea (pi″o-re′ah) [*pyo-* + Gr. *rhoia* flow] a discharge of pus. **p. alveola′ris**, compound periodontitis. **paradental p.**, pyorrhea in which the pockets are deep and the discharge of pus persists in spite of the removal of all local irritation. **Schmutz p.**, paradental p. with a pocket formation around the tooth with pus, caused by unhygienic local conditions.

pyorrheal (pi″o-re′al) pertaining to or characterized by pyorrhea.

pyorubin (pi″o-roo′bin) a bright-red, water-soluble, nonfluorescent pigment produced by *Pseudomonas aeruginosa*.

pyosalpingitis (pi″o-sal″pin-ji′tis) [*pyo-* + Gr. *salpinx* tube + *-itis*] purulent salpingitis.

pyosalpingo-oophoritis (pi″o-sal-ping″go-o″of-o-ri′tis) inflammation of the ovary and oviduct, with the formation and accumulation of pus.

pyosalpingo-oothecitis (pi″o-sal-ping″go-o″o-the-si′tis) pyosalpingo-oophoritis.

pyosalpinx (pi″o-sal′pinks) [*pyo-* + Gr. *salpinx* tube] a collection of pus in an oviduct.

pyosapremia (pi″o-sap-re′me-ah) [*pyo-* + Gr. *sapros* rotten + *haima* blood + *-ia*] infection of the blood with purulent matter.

pyosclerosis (pi″o-skle-ro′sis) an inflammatory, purulent sclerosis.

pyosepticemia (pi″o-sep″tĭ-se′me-ah) pyemia combined with septicemia.

pyosin (pi′o-sin) a compound, $C_{57}H_{110}N_2O_{15}$, derived from the plasma of pus cells.

pyosis (pi-o′sis) (*obs.*) suppuration.

pyospermia (pi″o-sper′me-ah) [*pyo-* + Gr. *sperma* seed + *-ia*] presence of pus in the semen.

pyostatic (pi″o-stat′ik) [*pyo-* + Gr. *statikos* halting] 1. arresting suppuration. 2. an agent that arrests the formation of pus.

pyostomatitis (pi″o-sto″mah-ti′tis) inflammation of the mouth with suppuration. **p. veg′etans**, inflammation of the mouth beginning with minute flat miliary abscesses of uniform size, tending to conglomerate and spreading to involve the whole mouth, the mucosa becoming proliferative, soft, red, folded, and verrucose; it is sometimes associated with ulcerative colitis.

pyotherapy (pi″o-ther′ah-pe) [*pyo-* + Gr. *therapeia* treatment] treatment with pus.

pyothorax (pi″o-tho′raks) [*pyo-* + Gr. *thōrax* chest] thoracic empyema.

pyotoxinemia (pi″o-tok″sĭ-ne′me-ah) [*pyo-* + *toxin* + Gr. *haima* blood + *-ia*] presence in the blood of the toxins of pus-forming organisms.

pyoumbilicus (pi″o-um-bil′ĭ-kus) infection of the umbilicus.

pyourachus (pi″o-u′rah-kus) the presence of pus in the urachus.

pyoureter (pi″o-u-re′ter) [*pyo-* + *ureter*] an accumulation of pus in a ureter.

pyovesiculosis (pi″o-vě-sik″u-lo′sis) an accumulation of pus in the seminal vesicles.

pyoxanthine (pi″o-zan′thin) a brownish red pigment derivable by oxidation from pyocyanin.

pyoxanthose (pi″o-zan′thōs) [*pyo-* + Gr. *xanthos* yellow] a yellow pigment produced by the oxidation of pyocyanin in blue pus when exposed to air.

pyrabrom (pēr′ah-brom) chemical name: 8-bromotheophylline compound with 2-[[2-dimethylamino) ethyl] (*p*-methoxyenzyl) amino]pyridine (1:1); an antihistaminic, $C_{24}H_{30}BrN_7O_3$.

pyracin (pi′rah-sin) a derivative of pyridoxine.

Pyralis (pēr′ah-lis) a genus of small, widely distributed moths. **P. farina′lis**, the grain-infesting meal moth that serves as an intermediate host of helminthic parasites, such as *Hymenolepis*.

pyramid (pēr′ah-mid) [Gr. *pyramis*] a pointed or cone-shaped structure or part; called also *pyramis* [NA]. The term is often used alone to indicate the pyramis medullae oblongatae. **p. of cerebellum**, pyramis vermis. **p. of Ferrein**, pars radiata lobuli corticalis renis. **p's of kidney**, pyramides renales; see under *pyramis*. **Lalouette's p.**, lobus pyramidalis glandulae thyroideae. **p. of light**, a triangular reflection seen upon the membrana tympani. **Malacarne's p.**, the posterior end of the pyramid of the vermis. **p's of Malpighi**, pyramides renales; see under *pyramis*. **p. of medulla oblongata**, pyramis medullae oblongatae. **p. of medulla oblongata, anterior** (*obs.*), pyramis medullae oblongatae. **p. of medulla oblongata, posterior** (*obs.*), fasciculus gracilis medullae oblongatae. **olfactory p.** (*obs.*), trigonum olfactorium. **petrous p.**, pars petrosa ossis temporalis. **renal p's**, pyramides renales; see under *pyramis*. **p. of temporal bone**, pars petrosa ossis temporalis. **p. of temporal bone, of Arnold**, pars mastoidea ossis temporalis. **p. of thyroid**, lobus pyramidalis glandulae thyroideae. **p. of tympanum**, eminentia pyramidalis. **p. of vermis**, pyramis vermis. **p. of vestibule**, pyramis vestibuli. **Wistar's p's**, see *concha sphenoidalis*.

pyramidal (pĭ-ram′ĭ-dal) [L. *pyramidalis*] shaped like a pyramid; see also under *tract*.

pyramidale (pi-ram″ĭ-da′le) os triquetrum.

pyramidalis (pi-ram″ĭ-da′lis) [L.] pyramidal.

pyramides (pi-ram′ĭ-dēz) [Gr.] plural of *pyramis*.

Pyramidon (pi-ram′ĭ-don) trademark for a preparation of aminopyrine.

pyramidotomy (pēr″am-ĭ-dot′o-me) section of the pyramidal tract.

pyramis (pēr′ah-mis), pl. *pyram′ides* [Gr.] pyramid; [NA] a general term for a part or structure resembling a pyramid. **p. cerebel′li**, p. vermis. **pyram′ides Malpig′hii**, pyramides renales. **p. medul′lae oblonga′tae** [NA], pyramid of medulla oblongata: either of two rounded masses, one on either side of the anterior median fissure of the medulla oblongata, composed of motor fibers (pyramidal tract) from the cerebral cortex to the spinal cord and medulla oblongata. **p. os′sis tempora′lis**, pars petrosa ossis temporalis. **pyram′ides rena′les** [NA], **pyram′ides rena′les [Malpig′hii]**, renal pyramids: the conical masses that make up the medullary substance of the kidney; they contain the loops of Henle, the collecting ducts, and the arteriolae rectae renis. **p. ver′mis** [NA], pyramid of vermis: the part of the vermis of the cerebellum between the tuber vermis and the uvula. **p. vestib′uli** [NA], pyramid of vestibule: the triangular-shaped anterior end of the vestibular crest.

pyran (pi′ran) 1. a cyclic compound, C_5H_6O, in which the ring consists of 5 carbon atoms and 1 oxygen atom. 2. (*obs.*) an antineuralgic and antirheumatic preparation of benzoic acid, salicylic acid, and thymol.

pyranisamine maleate (pi″rah-nis′ah-mēn) pyrilamine maleate.

pyranose (pi′rah-nōs) a hexose in which the oxygen ring bridges carbon atoms 1 and 5 in the aldoses or carbon atoms 2 and 6 in the ketoses.

pyrantel (pĭ-ran′tel) chemical name: (E)-1,4,5,6-tetrahydro-1-methyl-2-[2-(2-thienyl)vinyl]pyrimidine. An anthelmintic, $C_{11}H_{14}$-N_2S, effective against pinworms (Enterobius vermicularis) and roundworms (Ascaris lumbricoides). **p. pamoate** [USP], the pamoate salt of pyrantel, $C_{11}H_{14}N_2S \cdot C_{23}H_{16}O_6$, occurring as a yellow to tan solid; used in the treatment of ascariasis and enterobiasis, administered orally. **p. tartrate**, the tartrate salt of pyrantel, $C_{11}H_{14}N_2S \cdot C_4H_6O_6$, occurring as a white to greenish-yellow, crystalline powder, having the same actions as the pamoate salt.

pyranyl (pi′ran-il) the radical C_5H_5O, of which pyran is the hydride.

pyrathiazine hydrochloride (per″rah-thi′ah-zēn) chemical name: 10-[2-(1-pyrrolidinyl)ethyl]-phenothiazine hydrochloride, $C_{18}H_{20}N_2S_4HCl$; used as an antihistaminic.

pyrazinamide (pi″rah-zin′ah-mīd) [USP] chemical name: pyrazinecarboxamide. An antibacterial derived from nicotinic acid, $C_5H_5N_3O$, occurring as a white to practically white, crystalline powder; used as a tuberculostatic, administered orally.

pyrazine (pi′rah-zēn) a volatile compound, $C_4H_4N_2$, with the odor of heliotrope.

pyrazofurin (per″ah-zo-fūr′in) chemical name: 4-hydroxy-3-β-D-ribofuranosyl-1H-pyrazole-5-carboxamide; an antineoplastic, $C_9H_{13}N_3O_6$.

pyrectic (pi-rek′tik) [Gr. pyrektikos feverish] 1. pertaining to or of the nature of fever. 2. an agent that induces fever.

pyrene (pi′ren) a polycyclic hydrocarbon, $C_{16}H_{10}$.

pyrenoid (pi′rĕ-noid) [Gr. pyrēn fruit stone + eidos form] one of the refringent bodies seen in the chromatophores of certain protozoa; it is active in carbohydrate metabolism.

pyrenolysis (pi″rĕ-nol′ĭ-sis) [Gr. pyrēn fruit stone + lysis solution] the breaking down of the nucleolus of a cell.

Pyrenomycetes (pi-re″no-mi-se′tēz) a series of ascomycetous fungi of subclass Euascomycetidae, including the orders Clavicipitales and Erysiphales; their fruiting body is a perithecium.

pyretherapy (pi″rĕ-ther′ah-pe) [Gr. pyr fever + therapy] pyretotherapy.

pyrethron (pi′rĕ-thron) a neutral ester from pyrethrum.

pyrethrum (pi-re′thrum) [Gr. pyrethron] see under flower.

pyretic (pi-ret′ik) [Gr. pyretos fever] pertaining to or of the nature of fever.

pyreticosis (pi-ret″ĭ-ko′sis) any febrile affection.

pyreto- [Gr. pyretos fever] a combining form denoting relationship to fever.

pyretogen (pi-ret′o-jen) a substance which excites fever.

pyretogenesis (pi″rĕ-to-jen′ĕ-sis) [pyreto- + Gr. genesis production] the origin and causation of fever.

pyretogenetic (pi″rĕ-to-jĕ-net′ik) pertaining to pyretogenesis.

pyretogenic (pi″rĕ-to-jen′ik) producing fever.

pyretogenous (pi″rĕ-toj′ĕ-nus) 1. caused by high body temperature. 2. pyrogenic.

pyretography (pi″rĕ-tog′rah-fe) [pyreto- + Gr. graphein to write] a description of fever.

pyretology (pi″rĕ-tol′o-je) [pyreto- + -logy] the sum of what is known regarding fevers; the science of fevers.

pyretolysis (pi″rĕ-tol′ĭ-sis) [pyreto- + Gr. lysis dissolution] 1. reduction of fever. 2. lysis which is hastened by fever.

pyretotherapy (pi″rĕ-to-ther′ah-pe) [pyreto- + Gr. therapeia treatment] 1. treatment of a disease by raising the patient's temperature, especially by means of injecting fever-producing vaccines. 2. the treatment of fever.

pyretotyphosis (pi″rĕ-to-ti-fo′sis) [pyreto- + Gr. typhōsis delirium] the delirium of fever.

pyrexia (pi-rek′se-ah), pl. pyrex′iae [Gr. pyressein to be feverish] a fever, or a febrile condition; abnormal elevation of the body temperature. **Pel-Ebstein p.,** see under fever.

pyrexial (pi-rek′se-al) pertaining to or characterized by pyrexia.

pyrexiogenic (pi-rek″se-o-jen′ik) pyrogenic.

pyrexy (pi′rek-se) pyrexia.

Pyribenzamine (per″ĭ-ben′zah-mēn) trademark for preparations of tripelennamine.

pyridine (per′ĭ-dēn) 1. a colorless, liquid, basic coal tar derivative, C_5H_5N, derived also from tobacco and various organic matters. 2. any one of a large group of substances homologous with normal pyridine.

Pyridium (pĭ-rid′e-um) trademark for preparations of phenazopyridine hydrochloride.

pyridostigmine bromide (per″ĭ-do-stig′mēn) [USP] chemical name: 3-[[(dimethylamino)carbonyl]oxy]-1-methyl pyridinium bromide. A cholinergic, $C_9H_{13}BrN_2O_2$, occurring as a white or almost white, crystalline powder; used in the treatment of

myasthenia gravis and as an antidote for nondipolarizing muscle relaxants, such as curariform drugs, administered orally and parenterally.

pyridoxal (per″ĭ-dok′sal) chemical name: 2-methyl-3-hydroxy-4-formyl-5-hydroxymethylpyridine. One of the forms of vitamin B_6; see Table of Vitamins, under vitamin. **p. phosphate,** a major coenzyme involved in amino acid metabolism.

pyridoxamine (per″ĭ-doks′ah-mēn) one of the three active forms of vitamin B_6.

pyridoxine (per″ĭ-dok′sēn) chemical name: 5-hydroxy-6-methyl-3,4-pyridinedimethanol. One of the forms of vitamin B_6; see Table of Vitamins, under vitamin. **p. hydrochloride** [USP], the hydrochloride salt of pyridoxine, $C_8H_{11}NO_3 \cdot HCl$, occurring as colorless or white crystals or white crystalline powder; used in the prophylaxis and treatment of vitamin B_6 deficiency. It has also been used in neuromuscular and neurological diseases, in dermatoses, and in the management of nausea and vomiting of pregnancy and irradiation sickness. **p. phosphate,** a coenzyme involved in many amino acid reactions.

pyriform (per′ĭ-form) piriform.

pyrilamine maleate (per-il′ah-mēn) [USP] chemical name: N-[(4-methoxyphenyl)methyl]-N′,N′-dimethyl-N-2-pyridinyl-1,2-ethane diamine (Z)-2-butenedioate (1:1). An antihistaminic, C_{17}-$H_{23}N_3O \cdot C_4H_4O_4$, occurring as a white, crystalline powder; administered orally. Called also mepyramine maleate and pyranisamine maleate.

pyrimethamine (per″ĭ-meth′ah-mēn) [USP] chemical name: 5-(4-chlorophenyl)-6-ethyl-2,4-pyrimidinediamine. A folic acid antagonist, $C_{12}H_{13}ClN_4$, occurring as a white crystalline powder; used as an antimalarial, especially for suppressive prophylaxis, and also used concomitantly with a sulfonamide in the treatment of toxoplasmosis, administered orally.

pyrimidine (pi-rim′ĭ-dēn) an organic compound, a metadiazine, $C_4H_4N_2$, which is the fundamental form of the pyrimidine bases. These are mostly oxy or amino derivatives, for example, 2,4-dioxypyrimidine is uracil, 2-oxy-4-aminopyrimidine is cytosine, and 2,4-dioxy-5-methylpyrimidine is thymine. Some of these are constituents of nucleic acid (uracil, thymine, and cytosine). It is also the parent substance of the barbiturates.

pyrinoline (per-in′o-lēn) chemical name: 3-(di-2-pyridylmethylene)-α,α-di-2-pyridyl-1,4-cyclopentadiene-1-methanol; an antiarrhythmic cardiac depressant, $C_{27}H_{20}N_4O$.

pyrithiamine (per″ĭ-thi′ah-min) a synthetic compound, CH_3--$C_4N_2H(NH_2) \cdot CH_2 \cdot C_5NH_3(CH_3) \cdot CH_2 \cdot CH_2OH$, which by metabolic competition can cause symptoms of thiamine deficiency.

pyro- (pi′ro) [Gr. pyr fire] a combining form meaning fire or heat, or, in chemistry, produced by heating.

pyroborate (pi-ro-bo′rāt) any salt of pyroboric acid.

pyrocatechin (pi″ro-kat′ĕ-kin) [pyro- + catechu] pyrocatechol.

pyrocatechol (pi″ro-kat′ĕ-kol) chemical name: 1,2-benzenediol. A compound, $C_6H_4(OH)_2$, comprising the aromatic portion in the synthesis of endogenous catecholamines; it is obtained by distilling catechu, etc., or produced synthetically, and has been used as a topical antiseptic and as a reagent. Called also catechol and pyrocatechin.

pyrodextrin (pi″ro-deks′trin) a brown substance produced by the action of heat upon starch.

pyrogallol (pi″ro-gal′ol) chemical name: 1,2,3-trihydroxybenzene. A poisonous acid, $C_6H_6O_3$, derived from gallic acid, and used externally as an antimicrobial and irritant; it is also used as a reagent. Called also pyrogallic acid.

pyrogen (pi′ro-jen) [pyro- + Gr. gennan to produce] a fever-producing substance. **bacterial p.,** a fever-producing agent of bacterial origin; endotoxin. **distilled water p.,** filtrable thermostable products of bacterial activity that accumulate in distilled water and tend to cause a severe chill when the water is injected.

pyrogenetic (pi″ro-jĕ-net′ik) pyrogenic.

pyrogenic (pi″ro-jen′ik) [pyro- + Gr. gennan to produce] inducing fever.

pyrogenous (pi-roj′ĕ-nus) pyretogenous.

pyroglobulin (pi″ro-glob′u-lin) [pyro- + globulin] a blood globulin which precipitates from serum on heating (56°C.).

pyroglobulinemia (pi″ro-glob″u-li-ne′me-ah) presence in the blood of an abnormal protein constituent which is precipitated by heat; observed in myeloma and lymphosarcoma and sometimes in patients for whom no diagnosis can be established.

pyroglutamate (pi″ro-gloo′tah-māt) 5-oxoproline.

pyrolagnia (pi″ro-lag′ne-ah) [pyro- + Gr. lagneia lust] sexual gratification from witnessing or making fires.

pyroligneous (pi″ro-lig′ne-us) [pyro- + L. lignum wood] pertaining to the destructive distillation of wood.

pyrolusite (pi″ro-lu′sīt) native manganese dioxide, a black powder used in dry-cell batteries.

pyrolysis (pi-rol′ĭ-sis) [pyro- + Gr. lysis dissolution] decomposition of organic substances under the influence of a rise in temperature.

pyromania (pi″ro-ma′ne-ah) [*pyro-* + Gr. *mania* madness] obsessive preoccupation with fires; compulsion to set fires; incendiarism. **erotic p.,** pyrolagnia.

pyrometer (pi-rom′ĕ-ter) [*pyro-* + Gr. *metron* measure] an instrument for measuring the intensity of heat, especially for temperatures which cannot be measured with a mercury thermometer.

pyrone (pi′rōn) a principle, $CO(CH)_4O$, found in opium, from which several other constituents are derived by substitution.

Pyronil (pi′ro-nil) trademark for a preparation of pyrrobutamine.

pyronin (pi′ro-nin) a dye used in histology; the pyronines are methylated diamine xanthines. **p. B,** a basic dye, the tetraethylpyronine chloride, $(C_2H_5)_2N \cdot C_6H_3(O)CH \cdot C_6H_3 \cdot N(C_3H_5)_2Cl$. **p. G,** a basic dye, the tetramethylpyronine chloride, $(CH_3)_2N \cdot C_6H_3(O)CH \cdot C_6H_3N(CH_3)_2Cl$.

pyroninophilia (pi″ro-nin″o-fil′e-ah) [*pyronine* + Gr. *philein* to love] increased affinity for pyronine, sometimes observed in plasma and reticuloendothelial cells.

pyronyxis (pi″ro-nik′sis) [*pyro-* + Gr. *nyxis* a pricking] ignipuncture.

pyrophobia (pi″ro-fo′be-ah) [*pyro-* + Gr. *phobein* to be affrighted by] abnormal dread of fire.

pyrophosphatase (pi″ro-fos′fah-tās) any enzyme that catalyzes the hydrolysis of central pyrophosphate linkages. **inorganic p.,** pyrophosphate phosphohydrolase: an enzyme occurring in many tissues that catalyzes the hydrolysis of pyrophosphate to two orthophosphates. **nucleotide p.,** dinucleotide nucleotidohydrolase: an enzyme occurring in the liver and kidney that catalyzes the hydrolysis of a dinucleotide to two mononucleotides.

pyrophosphate (pi″ro-fos′fāt) any salt of pyrophosphoric acid. **stannous p.,** chemical name: diphosphoric acid ditin (2+) salt; a diagnostic aid (bone imaging), $Sn_2P_2O_7$.

pyrophosphokinase (pi″ro-fos″fo-ki′nās) an enzyme (a transferase) that catalyzes the transfer of a pyrophosphate from ATP to a substrate.

pyrophosphotransferase (pi″ro-fos″fo-trans′fer-ās) an enzyme that catalyzes the transfer of a pyrophosphate, as from ATP to thiamine to form AMP and thiamine pyrophosphate.

Pyroplasma (pi″ro-plaz′mah) *Babesia.*

pyropuncture (pi′ro-punk″tūr) [*pyro-* + *puncture*] ignipuncture.

pyroscope (pi′ro-skōp) [*pyro-* + Gr. *skopein* to examine] an instrument for measuring the intensity of heat radiations.

pyrosis (pi-ro′sis) [Gr. *pyrōsis* burning] heartburn.

Pyrosoma (pi″ro-so′mah) [*pyro-* + Gr. *sōma* body] *Babesia.*

pyrotic (pi-rot′ik) [Gr. *pyrōtikos*] caustic; burning.

pyrotoxin (pi″ro-tok′sin) [*pyro-* + Gr. *toxikon* poison] 1. a toxin developed during a fever. 2. a toxic principle obtained from many bacteria; even if ordinarily nonpathogenic, when injected it causes fever and wasting.

pyrovalerone hydrochloride (pēr-o-val′er-ōn) chemical name: 4′-methyl-2-(1-pyrrolidinyl)valerophenone hydrochloride; a central nervous systemic stimulant, $C_{16}H_{23}NO \cdot HCl$.

pyroxamine maleate (pēr-oks′ah-mēn) chemical name: 3-[(*p*-chloro-α-phenylbenzyl)oxy]-1-methylpyrrolidine maleate (1:1); an antihistaminic, $C_{18}H_{20}ClNO \cdot C_4H_4O_4$.

pyroxylin (pi-rok′sĭ-lin) [Gr. *pyr* fire + *xylon* wood] [USP] a product of the action of a mixture of nitric and sulfuric acids on cotton, consisting chiefly of cellulose tetranitrate; a necessary ingredient of collodion. Called also *colloxylin, dinitiocellulose, nitrocellulose,* and *guncotton.*

pyrrobutamine phosphate (pēr″ro-bu′tah-mēn) [USP] chemical name: 1-[4-(4-chlorophenyl)-3-phenyl-2-butenyl]pyrrolidine phosphate (1:2). A long-acting antihistaminic, $C_{20}H_{22}Cl \cdot N \cdot 2H_3PO_4$, occurring as a white, or almost white, crystalline powder; administered orally.

pyrrocaine (pēr′o-kān) chemical name: *N*-(2,6-dimethylphenyl)-1-pyrrolidineacetamide; a local anesthetic, $C_{14}H_{20}N_2O$. **p. hydrochloride,** the monohydrochloride salt of pyrrocaine, occurring as a white, crystalline powder; used as a local anesthetic in dentistry to produce infiltration and nerve block anesthesia.

pyrroetioporphyrin (pēr″o-e″te-o-por′fĭ-rin) a porphyrin, $C_{30}H_{34}N_4$.

pyrrole (pēr′ol) a liquid, basic, cyclic substance, $(CH)_4NH$, obtained in the destructive distillation of various animal substances. Four pyrrole groups (tetrapyrrole) are formed into a ring in the biosynthesis of the porphyrins.

pyrrolidine (pĭ-rol′ĭ-din) a simple base, tetramethylene imine, $(CH_2)_4NH$, which may be obtained from tobacco or prepared from pyrrole.

pyrrolin (pir′o-lin) an oily liquid, C_4H_6NH, formed by the action of acetic acid and zinc dust on pyrrole.

pyrrolnitrin (pēr-ōl-ni′trin) chemical name: 3-chloro-4-(3-chloro-2-nitrophenyl)-1*H*-pyrrole; an antifungal antibiotic isolated from *Pseudomonas pyrrocinia,* $C_{10}H_6Cl_2N_2O_2$, effective against *Trichophyton* species.

pyrroloporphyria (pir″o-lo-por-fir′e-ah) acute intermittent porphyria.

pyrroporphyrin (pir″o-por′fĭ-rin) a porphyrin, $C_{31}H_{34}O_2N_4$, derived from chlorophyll.

pyruvate (pi′roo-vāt) a salt, ester, or dissociated form of py-

$$ruvic acid, CH_3C—C—O^-.$$

In biochemistry, the term is used interchangeably with pyruvic acid, even though pyruvate tehnically refers to the negatively charged ion. Pyruvate is the end product of glycolysis, and it in turn may be converted to lactate or acetyl CoA or to ethanol (as in yeasts).

pyruvemia (pi″roo-ve′me-ah) a condition characterized by an increased amount of pyruvic acid in the blood.

pyrvinium pamoate (pir-vin′e-um) [USP] chemical name: 6-(dimethylamino)-2-[2-(2,5-dimethyl-1-phenyl-1*H*-pyrrol-3-yl)ethenyl]-1-methylquinolinium salt with 4,4′-methylenebis[3-hydroxy-2-naphthalenecarboxylic acid] (2:1). An anthelmintic, $C_{75}H_{70}N_6O_6$, occurring as a bright orange or orange-red to almost black, crystalline powder; used in the treatment of enterobiasis, administered orally.

Pythagoras (pĭ-thag′o-ras) **of Samos** (5th century B.C.) the famous Greek philosopher whose interest in mathematics is reflected in his concept of "critical days" in disease which, in Greek medicine of antiquity, was believed to enter a critical phase on certain days of the illness. Similar number lore (e.g., 4 humors, 4 elements, 4 qualities) is also found later in other concepts of disease and medicine (e.g., galenism).

pythogenesis (pi″tho-jen′ĕ-sis) [Gr. *pythein* to rot + *genesis* production] 1. the origination of a process of decay or decomposition. 2. generation from filth.

pythogenic (pi″tho-jen′ik) [Gr. *pythein* to rot + *gennan* to produce] causing decay or decomposition.

pythogenous (pi-thoj′ĕ-nus) caused by putrefaction or filth.

pyuria (pi-u′re-ah) [Gr. *pyon* pus + *ouron* urine + *-ia*] the presence of pus in the urine. **miliary p.,** the presence in the urine of miliary bodies consisting of pus cells, blood cells, and epithelium.

PZI protamine zinc insulin; see under *insulin.*

Q

Q. electric quantity.

Q₁₀ symbol for *temperature coefficient;* see under *coefficient.*

q symbol for (1) the long arm of a chromosome or (2) the frequency of the rarer allele of a pair.

qcepo (ksa′po) the tubercle type of cutaneous leishmaniasis.

q.d. abbreviation for L. *qua′que di′e,* every day.

Q fever (Q for *query)* see under *fever.*

q.h. abbreviation for L. *qua′que ho′ra,* every hour.

q.i.d. abbreviation for L. *qua′ter in di′e,* four times a day.

q.l. abbreviation for L. *quan′tum li′bet,* as much as desired.

Q.N.S. abbreviation for *Queen's Nursing Sister* (of Queen's Institute of District Nursing).

q.n.s. quantity not sufficient.

Q.P. abbreviation for *quanti-Pirquet reaction;* see under *reaction.*

q.p. abbreviation for L. *quan′tum pla′ceat,* as much as desired.

q.q.h. abbreviation for L. *qua′que quar′ta ho′ra,* every four hours.

Qq.hor. abbreviation for L. *qua′que ho′ra,* every hour.

q.s. abbreviation for L. *quan′tum sa′tis,* sufficient quantity.

q-sort (ku′sort) a technique of personality assessment in which the subject (or an observer) indicates the degree to which a standardized set of descriptive statements applies to the subject.

q.suff. abbreviation for L. *quan′tum suf′ficit,* as much as suffices.

Quaalude (kwa′lood) trademark for a preparation of methaqualone.

quack (kwak) one who fraudulently misrepresents his ability and experience in the diagnosis and treatment of disease or the effects to be achieved by the treatment he offers.

quackery (kwak′er-e) the fraudulent misrepresentation of one's ability and experience in the diagnosis and treatment of disease or of the effects to be achieved by the treatment offered.

quacksalver (kwak-sal′ver) one claiming special merit for treatment with his medications and salves.

Quadramoid (quad′rah-moid) trademark for an oral suspension of trisulfapyrimidines.

quadrangle (kwod′rang-g'l) 1. a figure having four angles, or sides. 2. Black's term for a dental instrument having four angulations in the shank connecting the handle, or shaft, with the working portion of the instrument, known as the blade, or nib.

quadrangular (kwod-rang′gu-lar) [L. *quadri* four + *angulus* angle] having four angles.

quadrant (kwod′rant) [L. *quadrans* quarter] 1. one quarter of a circle; that portion of the circumference of a circle that subtends an angle of 90 degrees. 2. any one of four corresponding parts or quarters, as of the abdominal surface or of the eardrum.

quadrantal (kwod-ran′tal) resembling or affecting a quadrant.

quadrantanopia (kwod″rant-ah-no′pe-ah) [L. *quadrans* a fourth part + Gr. *an-* neg. + *ōpē* vision + *-ia*] defective vision or blindness in one fourth of the visual field, bounded by a vertical and a horizontal radius. Called also *tetartanopia.*

quadrantanopsia (kwod″ran-tah-nop′se-ah) quadrantanopia.

quadrat (kwod′rat) [L. *quadratus* squared] a rectangular, usually square, sample plot used in ecological studies, especially a plot containing 1 square meter. A sample plot of larger area is often called a *major quadrat.*

quadrate (kwod′rāt) [L. *quadratus* squared] square or squared; four sided.

quadratipronator (kwod-ra″te-pro-na′tor) musculus pronator quadratus.

quadratus (kwod-ra′tus) [L.] squared; four sided.

quadri- (kwod″ri) [L. *quattuor* four; in combination, *quadri-*] a prefix signifying four, or fourfold.

quadribasic (kwod″ri-ba′sik) having four replaceable atoms of hydrogen.

quadriceps (kwod′ri-seps) [*quadri-* + L. *caput* head] four headed; possessing four heads. See *Table of Musculi.*

quadricepsplasty (kwod″ri-seps′plas-te) plastic repair of a ruptured quadriceps femoris muscle.

quadriceptor (kwod″ri-sep′tor) [*quadri-* + L. *ceptor*] an intermediary body having four combining groups.

quadricuspid (kwod″ri-kus′pid) [*quadri-* + L. *cuspis* point] 1. having four cusps; said of a tooth, or of a semilunar (aortic or pulmonary) valve with four cusps. 2. a tooth with four cusps.

quadridigitate (kwod″ri-dij′i-tāt) tetradactylous.

quadrigemina (kwod″ri-jem′i-nah) [L.] plural of *quadrigeminum.*

quadrigeminal (kwod″ri-jem′i-nal) [L. *quadrigeminus*] fourfold, or in four parts; forming a group of four.

quadrigeminum (kwod″ri-jem′i-num), pl. *quadrigem′ina* [L.] fourfold.

quadrigeminus (kwod″ri-jem′i-nus) [L.] quadrigeminal.

quadrilateral (kwod″ri-lat′er-al) [*quadri-* + L. *latus* side] 1. having four sides. 2. a four-sided figure, or postulate. **Celsus' q.,** "Notae vero inflammationis sunt quatuor, rubor et tumor, cum calore et dolore." (The four cardinal symptoms of inflammation, redness, swelling, heat, and pain.)

quadrilocular (kwod″ri-lok′u-lar) [*quadri-* + L. *loculus* a small space] having four cells, cavities, or chambers.

quadripara (kwod-rip′ah-rah) [*quadri-* + L. *parere* to bring forth, produce] a woman who has had four pregnancies which resulted in viable offspring; also written *para IV.*

quadripartite (kwod″ri-par′tīt) having four parts or divisions.

quadriplegia (kwod″ri-ple′je-ah) paralysis of all four limbs; tetraplegia.

quadripolar (kwod″ri-po′lar) having four poles, as a cell.

quadrisect (kwod′ri-sekt) [*quadri-* + L. *secare* to cut] to cut into four parts.

quadrisection (kwod″ri-sek′shun) [*quadri-* + L. *sectio* cut] division into four parts.

quadritubercular (kwod″ri-tu-ber′ku-lar) having four tubercles or cusps.

quadrivalent (kwod″ri-va′lent, kwod-riv′ah-lent) [*quadri-* + L. *valere* to be worth] having a chemical valence or combining power of four.

quadruped (kwod′roo-ped) [*quadri-* + L. *pes* foot] 1. four footed. 2. an animal having four feet.

quadrupl. abbreviation for L. *quadruplica′to,* four times as much.

quadruplet (kwod′rup-let) [L. *quadrupulus* fourfold] one of four offspring produced in one gestation period.

Quain's degeneration, fatty heart (kwānz) [Sir Richard *Quain,* British physician, 1816–1898] see under *degeneration* and *heart.*

quale (kwa′le) the quality of a thing; especially the quality of a sensation or other conscious process.

qualifying (kwol′i-fi′ing) in psychology, signifying a form of facial deceit in which an individual adds another facial expression to one that has just been shown, e.g., a smile may be shown after an angry expression as a sign that the individual is not as angry as he may seem.

qualimeter (kwah-lim′ĕ-ter) [L. *qualis* of what sort + *metrum* measure] penetrometer, def. 1.

qualitative, qualitive (kwol′i-ta″tiv) [L. *qualitativus*] pertaining to quality.

quality (kwol′i-te) in radiology, the ability of a particular form or type of ionizing radiation to penetrate matter.

quanta (kwon′tah) [L.] plural of *quantum.*

quantasome (kwon′tah-sōm) [L. *quantum* + Gr. *sōma* body] one of the uniform oblate spheroids of about 100 by 200 Å, which are present within the chloroplasts and are postulated to be the units of photosynthesis, each consisting of 250 molecules of chlorophyll, the minimum amount found necessary for photosynthesis.

quantatrope (kwon′tah-trōp) [L. *quantum* + Gr. *tropos* a turning] the site of the quantasome that is directly involved in the transfer of electrons.

quantimeter (kwon-tim′ĕ-ter) [L. *quantus* how much + *metrum* measure] an apparatus for measuring the quantity of roentgen rays generated by a tube.

quantitative (kwon′ti-ta-tiv) [L. *quantitativus*] denoting or expressible as quantity; relating to the proportionate quantities or to the amount of the constituents of a compound.

quantity (kwon′ti-te) 1. a characteristic, as of energy or mass, susceptible of precise physical measurement. 2. a measurable amount. **scalar q.,** a quantity that is expressed only in terms of magnitude. **vector q.,** a quantity that is expressed in terms of magnitude and direction.

quantum (kwon′tum), pl. *quan′ta* [L. "as much as"] a unit of energy under the quantum theory. It is hν, in which h is Planck's constant, 6.55×10^{-27}, and ν is the frequency of vibration with which the energy is associated. See *quantum theory,* under *theory.* **q. of light,** a quantity of light (radiant energy) equivalent to the frequency of the light times 6.55×10^{-27} erg. sec.

quantum libet (kwon′tum li′bet) [L.] as much as desired.

quantum satis (kwon′tum sat′is) a sufficient quantity.

quantum sufficit (kwon′tum suf′fi-sit) [L.] as much as suffices.

quarantine (kwor′an-tēn) [Ital. *quarantina*] 1. a period (usually of forty days' duration) of detention of ships or persons coming

1104

from infected or suspected ports. **2.** the place where persons are detained for inspection. **3.** to detain or isolate on account of suspected contagion. **4.** restrictions placed on the entrance to and exit from the place or premises where a case of communicable disease exists.

quart (kwort) [L. *quartus* fourth] the fourth part of a gallon (946 ml.).

quartan (kwor′tan) [L. *quartanus*, pertaining to the fourth] recurring every 72 hours (fourth day, counting the day of the previous paroxysm). See *malaria*. **double q.**, a fever in which the paroxysms occur on each of two successive days followed by an afebrile day, and continuing in this pattern. **triple q.**, a fever in which the paroxysms occur every day i.e., quotidian, because of infection with three different groups of quartan parasites.

quarter (kwor′ter) the part of a horse's hoof lying between the heel and the toe. **false q.**, a cleft in the quarter of a horse's hoof from the top to the bottom.

quartile (kwor′tīl) [L. *quartus* one fourth] the middle term of each half of a series of variables.

quartipara (kwor-tip′ah-rah) quadripara.

quartisect (kwor′tĭ-sekt) [L. *quartus* fourth + *secare* to cut] to cut into four parts.

quartisternal (kwor″tĭ-ster′nal) [L. *quartus* fourth + *sternum* sternum] pertaining to the fourth sternebra, or the bony segment of the sternum opposite the fourth intercostal space.

quartz (kwarts) a crystalline form of silicon dioxide (silica), Si-O₂; called also *rock crystal*.

Quarzan (kwahr′zan) trademark for a preparation of clidinium bromide.

quasi- [L. *quasi* as if, as though] a prefix signifying almost, seemingly, or resembling.

quasidominance (kwa″zi-dom′ĭ-nans, kwah″zĭ-dom′ĭ-nans) [*quasi-* + *dominance*] the direct transmission, generation to generation, of a recessive trait in populations in which the gene is frequent or inbreeding is intense, produced by mating of a recessive homozygote and a heterozygote, the proportion of affected offspring thus resembling that in dominant inheritance.

quasidominant (kwa″zi-dom′ĭ-nant, kwah-zĭ-dom′ĭ-nant) pertaining to or exhibiting quasidominance.

quassation (kwŏ-sa′shun) [L. *quassatio*] the crushing of drugs, or their reduction to small pieces.

Quassia (kwosh′e-ah) [after *Quassi*, a Negro who used it as a remedy] a genus of simaroubaceous tropical trees, the wood of which was first used in the 18th century in the treatment of fevers.

quassia (kwash′e-ah) [after *Quassi*, black slave of Surinam who used it in the treatment of malignant fevers in the 18th century] the dried, intensely bitter heart-wood of the simaroubaceous trees *Picrasma excelsa* (Sw.) Planch. (Jamaica quassia), or *Quassia amara* L. (Surinam quassia); it has been used as an enema for seatworms.

quassin (kwash′in) the major bitter principle, C₂₂H₃₀O₆, of quassia.

Quat., quat. abbreviation for L. *quat′tuor*, four.

quater in die (kwah′ter in de′a) [L.] four times a day.

quaternary (kwah′ter-ner″e, kwah-ter′nah-re) [L. *quaternarius*, from *quattuor* four] **1.** fourth in order. **2.** containing four elements or groups.

Quatrefages′ angle (katr′fazh-ez) [Jean Louis Armand de *Quatrefages* de Bréau, French naturalist, 1810–1892] parietal angle.

quazepam (kwah′zĕ-pam) chemical name: 7-chloro-5-(2-fluorophenyl)-1,3-dihydro-1-(2,2,2-trifluoroethyl)-2*H*-1,4-benzodiazepine-2-thione; a sedative and hypnotic, C₁₇H₁₁ClF₄N₂S.

quazodine (kwa′zo-dēn) chemical name: 4-ethyl-6,7-dimethoxyquinazoline; a cardiotonic and bronchodilator, C₁₂H₁₄N₂O₂.

quebrachitol (ka-brah′chĭ-tol) chemical name: 1-methyl-inositol. A sugar from quebracho bark, which has been suggested as a sugar substitute in diabetes.

Queckenstedt's sign (phenomenon, test) (kwek′en-stets″) [Hans Heinrich Georg *Queckenstedt*, German physician, 1876–1918] see under *sign*.

Quelicin (kwel′ĭ-sin) trademark for a preparation of succinylcholine.

quenching (kwench′ing) to put out, extinguish, or suppress; to cool (as hot metal) by immersing in water. In liquid scintillation counting, any process taking place within the sample container which results in a decrease in number or intensity of the light flashes produced, thus lowering the amount of energy recorded. **fluorescence q.**, a technique for measuring the primary interaction of antigen and antibody by determination of the amount of light absorbed by bound antigen from fluorescent-labeled antibody exposed to ultraviolet light.

Quénu-Mayo operation (ka′nuh-ma′o) [Eduard André Victor Alfred *Quénu*, French surgeon, 1852–1933; William James *Mayo*, American surgeon, 1861–1939] see under *operation*.

Quénu-Muret sign (ka′nu-mŭ-rě′) [E.A.V.A. *Quénu*; Paul Louis *Muret*, French surgeon, born 1878] see under *sign*.

quenuthoracoplasty (kwe″nu-tho′rah-ko-plas″te) [E.A.V.A. *Quénu*] division of the ribs to promote retraction of the chest wall in empyema.

quercetin (kwer′sĕ-tin) chemical name: 3,3′,4′,5,7-pentahydroxyflavone. The aglycon of rutin and other glycosides, which has been used to reduce abnormal capillary fragility; called also *meletin* and *sophoretin*. **q.-3-rutinoside,** rutin.

Quercus (kwer′kus) [L.] a genus of trees including the oaks, certain species of which (e.g., *Q. infectoria* Oliv., Fagaceae) harbor nutgalls, a source of gallic and tannic acids, which are used in various pharmaceuticals for their astringent properties.

Quervain's disease (kār′vanz) [Fritz de *Quervain*, Swiss surgeon, 1868–1940] see under *disease*.

Questran (kwes′tran) trademark for a preparation of cholestyramine resin.

Quetelet's rule (ket″ĕ-lāz′) [Lambert Adolphe Jacques *Quetelet*, Belgian mathematician, 1796–1874] see under *rule*.

Queyrat's erythroplasia (ka-rahz′) [Auguste *Queyrat*, French dermatologist, born 1872] see under *erythroplasia*.

quick (kwik) **1.** rapid. **2.** alive. **3.** pregnant and able to feel the fetal movements.

Quick test (kwik) [Armand James *Quick*, Milwaukee physician, born 1894] see under *tests*.

quicklime (kwik′līm) calcium oxide.

quickening (kwik′en-ing) the first recognizable movements of the fetus, appearing usually from the sixteenth to the eighteenth week of pregnancy.

quidding (kwid′ing) a condition in horses in which food is taken into the mouth, repeatedly chewed, and then expelled; it may be caused by injuries to the mouth, disorders of the teeth or gums, paralysis of the muscles of mastication, or some other condition causing inability to swallow. Called also *cudding*.

Quide (kwīd) trademark for a preparation of piperacetazine.

quigila (kwij′ĭ-lah) Brazilian name for ainhum.

quillaia (kwil-la′yah) the dried inner part of the bark of *Quillaja saponaria* Molina (Rosaceae); formerly used in medicine for its local irritant action. Its chief constituent is quillaic acid, and it is used in the manufacture of saponin, in shampoo formulations for its foaming qualities, and as a detergent in the film industry. Called also *soap bark, soap tree bark,* and *quillay bark*.

Quillaja (kwil-la′yah) [Chilian *quillai*] a genus of rosaceous trees. *Q. sapona′ria* Molina, a species native to South America, which was first described in 1782. See also *quillaia*.

quinacrine hydrochloride (kwin′ah-krin) [USP] chemical name: *N*⁴-(6-chloro-2-methoxy-9-acridinyl)-*N*¹,*N*¹-diethyl-1,4-pentanediamine dihydrochloride dihydrate. An antimalarial, antiprotozoal, and anthelmintic, C₂₃H₃₀ClN₃·2HCl·2H₂O, occurring as a bright yellow, crystalline powder; used especially for suppressive therapy of malaria and in the treatment of giardiasis and tapeworm infestations, administered orally. Called also *chinacrin hydrochloride* and *mepacrine hydrochloride*.

quinalbarbitone (kwin″al-bar′bĭ-tōn) secobarbital.

Quincke's disease, edema, meningitis, pulse (sign), puncture, (kwink′ez) [Heinrich Irenaeus *Quincke*, physician in Kiel, 1842–1922] see *angioneurotic edema*, under *edema*, see *lumbar puncture*, under *puncture*, and see under *meningitis* and *pulse*.

quinestrol (kwin-es′trōl) chemical name: 3-(cyclopentyloxy)-19-nor-17α-pregna-1,3,5(10)-trien-20-yn-17-ol; an estrogen, C₂₅H₃₂O₂.

quinethazone (kwin-eth′ah-zōn) [USP] chemical name: 7-chloro-2-ethyl-1,2,3,4-tetrahydro-4-oxo-6-quinazolinesulfonamide. An orally effective diuretic, C₁₀H₁₂ClN₃O₃S, occurring as a white to yellowish white, crystalline powder; used in the treatment of edema associated with various conditions and of hypertension.

quinfamide (kwin′fah-mīd) chemical name: 1-(dichloroacetyl)-1,2,3,4-tetrahydro-6-quinolinyl ester 2-furancarboxylic acid; an antiamebic, C₁₆H₁₃Cl₂NO₄.

quingestanol acetate (kwin-jes′tah-nōl) chemical name: 3-(cyclopentyloxy)-19-nor-17α-pregna-3,5-dien-20-yn-17-ol acetate; a progestin, C₂₇H₃₆O₃.

quingestrone (kwin-jes′trōn) chemical name: 3-(cyclopentyloxy)pregna-3,5-dien-20-one; a progestin, C₂₆H₃₈O₂.

Quinidex (kwin′ĭ-deks) trademark for a preparation of quinidine sulfate.

quinidine (kwin′ĭ-din) chemical name: 6-methoxycinchonan-9-ol. The dextrorotatory isomer of quinine, C₂₀H₂₄N₂O₂, obtained from various species of *Cinchona* and their hybrids, and from *Remijia pedunculata*, or prepared from quinine. It has cardiac depressant activity, and is as potent an antimalarial as quinine but is rarely used for the latter effect except in those having an idiosyncrasy to quinine. **q. gluconate** [USP], the gluconate salt of quinidine, occurring as an odorless, white powder with a very bitter taste; administered intramuscularly or intravenously for the treatment of cardiac arrhythmias. **q. polygalacturonate,** a salt of quinidine, (C₂₀H₂₄N₂O₂·C₆H₁₀O₇·H₂O)ₓ, having actions and uses the same as the other salts of quinidine; administered orally. **q. sulfate** [USP], the sulfate salt of quinidine, occurring as fine, needle-like crystals or as a fine, white powder, which is odorless, has a bitter taste, and darkens on exposure to light; administered orally for the treatment of cardiac arrhythmias.

quinine (kwin′in, kwin-ēn′, kwi′nīn) [L. *quinina*] an alkaloid of cinchona, $C_{20}H_{24}N_2O_2 \cdot 3H_2O$, occurring as a white microcrystalline powder, which suppresses the asexual erythrocytic forms of all malarial parasites and has a slight effect on the gametocytes of *Plasmodium vivax* and *P. malariae* but none on those of *P. falciparum*. Once widely used to prevent and control malaria, it has been largely replaced by less toxic and more effective synthetic antimalarials, and is now used chiefly (usually in the form of one of its soluble salts) in the treatment of falciparum malaria resistant to other antimalarials. Quinine also has analgesic antipyretic, mild oxytocic, cardiac depressant, and sclerosing properties, and it decreases the excitability of the motor endplate. **q. and urea hydrochloride,** a double salt of quinine and urea hydrochloride, $C_{20}H_{24}N_2O_2 \cdot HCl \cdot CH_4N_2O \cdot HCl \cdot 5H_2O$, occurring as colorless translucent prisms, white granules, or white powder. It has been used to produce sclerosing, thrombosis, and obliteration of internal hemorrhoids and varicose veins, and as a local anesthetic. **q. bismuth iodide,** a compound of quinine and bismuth iodide formerly used in the treatment of syphilis. **q. bisulfate,** a colorless, crystalline cinchona salt, $C_{20}H_{24}O_2N_2 \cdot H_2SO_4 + 7H_2O$. It is much more soluble than the ordinary sulfate, and was formerly used in solution in the treatment of various ophthalmic disorders. **q. dihydrochloride,** the dihydrochloride salt of quinine, $C_{20}H_{24}N_2O_2 \cdot 2HCl$, occurring as a white powder, having the same actions and uses as the base; administered intravenously. **q. ethylcarbonate,** a white crystalline compound, $C_2H_5 \cdot O \cdot CO \cdot O \cdot C_{20}H_{23}N_2O$, formed by the action of ethyl chlorocarbonate on quinine; it has been used like quinine sulfate. **q. hydrobromide,** a salt, $C_{20}H_{24}N_2O_2 \cdot HBr + H_2O$, formerly used in the treatment of hyperthyroidism and pneumococcal pneumonia. **q. hydrochloride,** a white salt, $C_{20}H_{24}O_2N_2 \cdot HCl + 2H_2O$, resembling the sulfate in taste and uses. **q. salicylate,** a salt, $C_{20}H_{24}N_2O_2 \cdot C_7H_6O_3 + H_2O$, in slender white needles, formerly used as an antipyretic and antirheumatic. **q. sulfate** [USP], the dihydrate sulfate salt of quinine, $(C_{20}H_{24}N_2O_2) \cdot H_2SO_4 \cdot 2H_2O$, occurring as white, fine needle-like crystals, having the same actions and uses as the base, and also used to prevent noctural cramps in the legs and feet; administered orally. **q. tannate,** a yellowish powder, containing 33 per cent anhydrous quinine, formerly used in whooping cough and diarrhea.

quininism (kwin′ĭ-nizm) cinchonism.

quinoid (kwin′oid) containing the chromatophoric group:

$$=C\left\langle\begin{array}{c}C{=}C\\C\quad C\end{array}\right\rangle C=$$

quinoline (kwin′o-lēn) a tertiary amine or alkaloid, C_6H_4-$(CH)_3N$, a yellowish, aromatic liquid derivable from quinine, coal tar, and various other sources, which has antiseptic, antipyretic, and antiperiodic properties.

quinometry (kwĭ-nom′ĕ-tre) the standardization of the alkaloids of quinine.

quinone (kwi-nōn′, kwin′ōn) 1. a substance, $CO(CH \cdot CH)_2CO$, in golden-yellow crystals, obtained by oxidizing quinic acid. 2. any benzene derivative in which two hydrogen atoms are replaced by two oxygen atoms.

Quinora (kwin′o-rah) trademark for a preparation of quinidine sulfate.

quinovin (kwin-o′vin) a bitter glycosidal mixture from cinchona.

quinovose (kwin′o-vōs) isorhodeose; 6-deoxy-D-glucose.

quinoxin (kwin-ok′sin) nitrosophenol, $C_6H_4(NO)OH$, a pale yellow, crystalline substance prepared from phenol by the action of nitrous acid.

Quinq. abbreviation for L. *quin′que,* five.

Quinquaud's sign (kang-kōz′) [Charles Eugène *Quinquaud,* French physician, 1843–1894] see under *sign.*

quinquecuspid (kwin″kwe-kus′pid) [L. *quinque* five + *cuspis* point] 1. having five cusps. 2. a tooth with five cusps.

quinquetubercular (kwin″kwe-tu-ber′ku-lar) having five tubercles or cusps.

quinquevalent (kwing″kwĕ-va′lent, kwin-kwev′ah-lent) [L. *quinque* five + *valens* able] 1. having five different valencies. 2. pentavalent.

quinquina (kin-ke′nah) cinchona.

quinsy (kwin′ze) [L. *cynanche* sore throat] peritonsillar abscess. **lingual q.,** suppurative inflammation of the lingual tonsil.

Quint. abbreviation for L. *quin′tus,* fifth.

quintan (kwin′tan) [L. *quintanus* of the fifth] recurring every fifth day, as a fever.

quintessence (kwin-tes′ens) [L. *quintus* fifth + *essentia* essence] the highly concentrated extract of any substance.

quintipara (kwin-tip′ah-rah) [L. *quintus* fifth + *parere* to bring forth, produce] a woman who has had five pregnancies which resulted in viable offspring; also written para V.

quintisternal (kwin″tĭ-ster′nal) [L. *quintus* fifth + *sternum*] denoting the fifth bony portion of the sternum, or the part above the xiphoid process and adjacent to the fifth intercostal space.

quintuplet (kwin′tup-let) [L. *quintuplex* five-fold] one of five offspring produced in one gestation period.

quittor (kwit′or) a fistulous sore on the quarters or the coronet of a horse's foot. **simple q.,** local inflammation resulting in a slough, with formation of pus immediately above the hoof. **skin q.,** a very painful ulcer of the skin above the hoof. **subhorny q.,** inflammation beginning at the coronary band and extending beneath the hoof and producing pus formation in the sensitive tissue. **tendinous q.,** a condition in which the inflammation has extended into the tendons of the leg and the ligaments of the joint.

quoad vitam (kwo′ad vi′tam) [L.] so far as life is concerned.

Quotane (kwo′tān) trademark for preparations of dimethisoquin hydrochloride.

Quotid. abbreviation for L. *quotid′ie,* daily.

quotidian (kwo-tid′e-an) [L. *quotidianus* daily] 1. recurring every day; amphemerous. 2. a form of intermittent malaria with daily recurrent paroxysms.

quotient (kwo′shent) a number obtained as the result of division. **achievement q.,** a percentage statement of the extent to which a child has progressed in learning in proportion to his ability. Abbreviated A.Q. **albumin q.,** the amount of albumin in the blood plasma divided by the amount of albumin present in the blood. **Ayala's q.,** a quotient in examination of the cerebrospinal pressure, obtained by dividing the pressure after removal of 10 ml. of cerebrospinal fluid by that registered before such removal, and multiplying by 10. Normal values are 5.5 to 6.5 A result under 5 indicates a small reservoir, as in subarachnoid block; over 7 means a large reservoir, as may be encountered in serous meningitis or hydrocephalus. **caloric q.,** the quotient obtained by dividing the heat evolved (expressed in calories) by the oxygen consumed (expressed in milligrams) in a metabolic process. **D q.,** the ratio of glucose to nitrogen in the urine. **growth q.,** that portion of the entire food energy which is utilized for the purpose of growth. **intelligence q.,** the measure of intelligence obtained by dividing the patient's mental age, as ascertained by the Binet-Simon scale, by his chronological age and multiplying the result by 100. Abbreviated I.Q. **protein q.,** the number obtained by dividing the quantity of globulin of the blood plasma by the quantity of albumin. **rachidian q.,** Ayala's q. **respiratory q.,** the ratio of the volume of carbon dioxide given off by the body tissues to the volume of oxygen absorbed by them; usually equal to the corresponding volumes given off and taken up by the lungs. Abbreviated R.Q. **spinal q.,** Ayala's q.

q.v. abbreviation for L. *quan′tum vis,* as much as you please, and for *quod vi′de,* which see.

R

R symbol for *roentgen;* chemical symbol for an *organic radical.*

R. abbreviation for *Rankine* (scale), *Réaumur* (scale), *remotum* (far), *respiration, Rickettsia, right,* and *Behnken's unit;* also for *rough* colony (see under *colony*).

℞ symbol for L. *rec'ipe,* take. See *prescription.*

r symbol for *ring chromosome;* former symbol for *roentgen,* officially replaced by capital R.

Ra chemical symbol for *radium.*

Raabe's test (rah'bez) [Gustav *Raabe,* German physician, born 1875] see under *tests.*

rabbetting (rab'et-ing) impaction of the denticulated broken surfaces of a fractured bone.

rabbia (rab'be-ah) rabies.

rabbitpox (rab'it-poks) an acute eruptive disease of laboratory rabbits, caused by a virus closely related to the vaccinia virus.

rabelaisin (rab″ĕ-la'ĭ-sin) a poisonous glycoside from *Rabelaisia philippinensis,* a plant of the Philippine Islands: a heart stimulant.

rabic (ra'bik) pertaining to rabies.

rabicidal (ra″be-si'dal) destructive to the rabies virus.

rabid (rab'id) [L. *rabidus*] affected with rabies.

rabies (ra'bēz, ra'be-ēz) [L. *rabere* to rage] an acute infectious disease of the central nervous system usually fatal in mammal species ranging from bats to cattle. It is caused by an RNA virus (rhabdoviridae). Human infection results from the bite of a rabid animal, such as a bat, wolf, dog, cat, mongoose, or other mammal. The incubation period in man is from one to three months, being shorter following bites near the brain than after those farther away. The earliest symptoms are numbness and tingling around the site of infection; soon afterwards generalized hyperexcitability occurs, followed by fever, by paralysis of the muscles of deglutition and glottal spasm at first provoked by the drinking of fluids or by the sight of fluids, and by maniacal behavior. Convulsions, tetany, and respiratory paralysis are the inevitable terminal event. The diagnosis can be confirmed during life by viral isolation (from saliva, cerebrospinal fluid, urine) or by demonstration of neutralizing antibody, and after death by the appearance of cytoplasmic inclusion bodies (Negri bodies) in degenerated neurons. Called also *hydrophobia* and *lyssa.* See also under *vaccine.* **dumb r.,** rabies in which paralysis is an early, predominant symptom, the animal showing no signs of viciousness or tendency to bite. **furious r.,** a form in which there is very pronounced excitement. **paralytic r.,** rabies in which paralysis is a marked symptom —usually an ascending spinal paralysis.

rabiform (ra'bĭ-form) resembling rabies.

race (rās) 1. an ethnic stock, or division of mankind; in a narrower sense, a national or tribal stock; in a still narrower sense, a genealogic line of descent; a class of persons of a common lineage. In genetics, races are considered as populations having different distributions of gene frequencies. 2. a class or breed of animals; a group of individuals having certain characteristics in common, owing to a common inheritance; a subspecies.

racemase (ra'se-mās) an enzyme that catalyzes the racemization of an optically active substance, such as lactic acid. **alanine r.,** an enzyme that catalyzes the conversion of L-alanine to D-alanine. **glutamate r.,** an enzyme that catalyzes the conversion of L-glutamate to D-glutamate. **lactate r.,** an enzyme that catalyzes the conversion of L-lactate to D-lactate. **lysine r.,** an enzyme that catalyzes the conversion of L-lysine to D-lysine. **mandelate r.,** an enzyme that catalyzes the conversion of L-mandelate to D-mandelate. **methionine r.,** an enzyme that catalyzes the conversion of L-methionine to D-methionine. **methylmalonyl-CoA r.,** an enzyme that catalyzes the conversion of D-methylmalonyl-CoA to L-methylmalonyl-CoA. **proline r.,** an enzyme that catalyzes the conversion of L-proline to D-proline. **threonine r.,** an enzyme that catalyzes the conversion of L-threonine to D-threonine.

racemate (ra'se-māt) an equimolecular mixture of two enantiomorphic isomers, being optically inactive in solution because of the presence of the same number of dextro- and levo-rotatory molecules. In the solid state it may have the properties of a loosely bound molecular compound. Called also *racemic form, racemic mixture,* or *racemic modification.*

raceme (ra-sēm') [L. *racemus* a bunch of grapes] 1. a form of inflorescence in which the individual flowers are borne on stalks which spring from a long central stem. 2. racemate.

racemethionine (rās″ĕ-mĕ-thi'o-nēn) [USP] chemical name: DL-methionine. A compound, $C_5H_{11}NO_2S$, occurring as white, crystalline platelets or powder. It is used as a dietary supplement with lipotropic action.

racemic (ra-se'mik) made up of two enantiomorphic isomers and therefore optically inactive.

racemization (ra″sĕ-mi-za'shun) the transformation of one half of the molecules of an optically active compound into molecules which possess exactly the opposite (mirror-image) configuration, with complete loss of rotatory power because of the statistical balance between equal numbers of dextro- and levorotatory molecules. Cf. *mutarotation.*

racemose (ras'e-mōs) [L. *racemosus*] resembling a bunch of grapes on its stalk.

racephedrine hydrochloride (ra-sef'ĕ-drin) chemical name: *dl*-α-[1-(methylamino)ethyl]benzyl alcohol hydrochloride. The racemic form of ephedrine hydrochloride, $C_{10}H_{15}NO \cdot HCl$, occurring as fine, white crystals or as a powder and used as a sympathomimetic.

racephenicol (rās-ĕ-fen'ĭ-kōl) chemical name: (±)-*threo*-2,2-dichloro-*N*-[β-hydroxy-α-(hydroxymethyl)-*p*-(methylsulfonyl)-phenethyl]acetamide; an antibacterial, $C_{12}H_{15}Cl_2NO_5S$.

rachi- see *rachio-.*

rachial (ra'ke-al) rachidial.

rachialbuminimeter (ra″ke-al-bu″mĭ-nim'ĕ-ter) an apparatus for measuring the albumin in a specimen of the cerebrospinal fluid.

rachialbuminimetry (ra″ke-al-bu″mĭ-nim'ĕ-tre) the measurement of the amount of albumin in the cerebrospinal fluid.

rachialgia (ra″ke-al'je-ah) [*rachi-* + Gr. *algos* pain + *-ia*] pain in the vertebral column.

rachianalgesia (ra″ke-an″al-je'ze-ah) rachianesthesia.

rachianesthesia (ra″ke-an″es-the'ze-ah) spinal anesthesia; anesthesia produced by the injection of the anesthetic into the spinal canal.

rachicentesis (ra″ke-sen-te'sis) [*rachi-* + Gr. *kentēsis* puncture] lumbar puncture.

rachidial (ra-kid'e-al) pertaining to the spine.

rachidian (ra-kid'e-an) pertaining to the spine.

rachigraph (ra'ke-graf) [*rachi-* + Gr. *graphein* to write] an instrument for recording the outlines of the spine and back.

rachilysis (ra-kil'ĭ-sis) [*rachi-* + Gr. *lysis* dissolution] mechanical treatment of a curved vertebral column by combined traction and pressure.

rachio-, rachi- (ra'ke-o, ra'ke) [Gr. *rhachis* spine] combining form denoting relation to the spine.

rachiocampsis (ra″ke-o-kamp'sis) [*rachio-* + Gr. *kampsis* curve] curvature of the spinal column.

rachiocentesis (ra″ke-o-sen-te'sis) [*rachio-* + Gr. *kentēsis* puncture] lumbar puncture.

rachiochysis (ra″ke-ok'ĭ-sis) [*rachio-* + Gr. *chysis* a pouring] the effusion of a fluid within the vertebral canal.

rachiocyphosis (ra″ke-o-si-fo'sis) kyphosis.

rachiodynia (ra″ke-o-din'e-ah) [*rachio-* + Gr. *odynē* pain + *-ia*] pain in the spinal column.

rachiokyphosis (ra″ke-o-ki-fo'sis) kyphosis.

rachiometer (ra″ke-om'ĕ-ter) [*rachio-* + Gr. *metron* measure] an instrument for measuring curvatures of the vertebral column.

rachiomyelitis (ra″ke-o-mi″ĕ-li'tis) [*rachio-* + Gr. *myelos* marrow + *-itis*] inflammation of the spinal cord.

rachiopagus (ra″ke-op'ah-gus) [*rachio-* + Gr. *pagos* thing fixed] symmetrical conjoined twins united back to back in the sagittal plane, fusion being limited to the upper trunk and cervical region.

rachiopathy (ra″ke-op'ah-the) [*rachio-* + Gr. *pathos* disease] any disease of the spine.

rachioscoliosis (ra″ke-o-sko″le-o'sis) lateral curvature of the spine.

rachiotome (ra'ke-o-tōm) an instrument for cutting the vertebrae.

rachiotomy (ra″ke-ot'o-me) [*rachio-* + Gr. *tomē* a cutting] incision of a vertebra, or of the vertebral column.

rachipagus (ra-kip'ah-gus) [*rachi-* + Gr. *pagos* thing fixed] a double monster joined at the vertebral column.

rachiresistance (ra″ke-re-zis'tans) a condition in which the injection of a spinal anesthetic produces little or no effect.

rachiresistant (ra″ke-re-zis'tant) abnormally insensitive to spinal anesthetics.

rachis (ra'kis) [Gr. *rhachis* spine] the vertebral column.

rachisagra (ra″kis-ag'rah) [*rachis* + Gr. *agra* seizure] pain or gout in the spine.

rachischisis (ra-kis'kĭ-sis) [*rachi-* + Gr. *schisis* cleft] congenital fissure of the spinal column. See illustration on following page. **r. partia'lis,** fissure of the spinal column of limited extent; merorachischisis. **r. poste'rior,** spina bifida. **r. tota'lis,** holorachischisis.

rachisensibility (ra″ke-sen″sĭ-bil'ĭ-te) the condition of being abnormally sensitive to spinal anesthetics.

1107

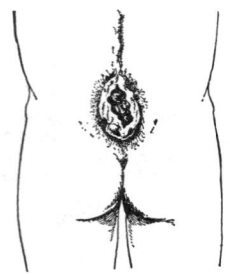

Rachischisis (Babcock).

rachisensible (ra″ke-sen′sĭ-b'l)   abnormally sensitive to spinal anesthetics.

rachitic (ra-kit′ik)   pertaining to or affected with rickets.

rachitis (ra-ki′tis) [Gr. *rachitis*]   1. rickets. 2. inflammatory disease of the vertebral column.   **r. feta′lis annula′ris**, the formation before birth of annular thickenings on the long bones. **r. feta′lis micromel′ica**, deficient longitudinal growth of the bones of the fetus.   **r. tar′da**, late rickets.

rachitism (rak′ĭ-tizm)   a tendency to rickets.

rachitogenic (rah-kit″o-jen′ik)   causing rickets.

rachitome (rak′ĭ-tōm)   a cutting instrument used in opening the spinal canal.

rachitomy (rah-kit′o-me) [*rachi-* + Gr. *tomē* a cutting]   the surgical or anatomical opening of the vertebral canal.

racial (ra′shal)   pertaining to a particular race.

rad [acronym for r*adiation* a*bsorbed* d*ose*]   a unit of measurement of the absorbed dose of ionizing radiation; it corresponds to an energy transfer of 100 ergs per gram of any absorbing material (including tissues). The biological effect of 1 rad varies with the kind of radiation the tissue is exposed to. Cf. *gray* (def. 3.).

rad.   abbreviation for L. *ra′dix*, root.

radarkymography (ra″dar-ki-mog′rah-fe)   the recording on a television monitor, by means of a radar tracking instrument, of cardiac motion displayed on a fluoroscope.

radectomy (ra-dek′to-me) [L. *radix* root + Gr. *ektomē* excision]   excision of a portion of the root of a tooth.

Rademacher's system (rah′dĕ-mah″kerz) [Johann Gottfried *Rademacher*, German physician, 1772–1850]   the belief that there should be a specific remedy for every disease.

radiability (ra″de-ah-bil′ĭ-te)   the property of being readily penetrated by the roentgen or other ray.

radiable (ra′de-ah-b'l)   capable of being examined by the roentgen ray.

radiad (ra′de-ad)   toward the radius or radial side.

radial (ra′de-al) [L. *radialis*]   1. pertaining to the radius of the forearm or to the radial (lateral) aspect of the arm as opposed to the ulnar (medial) aspect; pertaining to a radius. 2. radiating; spreading outward from a common center.

radialis (ra″de-a′lis) [L.]   radial; [NA] a term designating relationship to the radius.

radian (ra′de-an)   in ophthalmometry, an arc whose length equals the radius of its curvature. It is an arc of 57.295 degrees.

radiant (ra′de-ant) [L. *radians*]   1. diverging from a common center. 2. any radioactive substance.

radiate (ra′de-āt) [L. *radiare, radiatus*]   1. to diverge or spread from a common point. 2. arranged in a radiating manner.

radiathermy (ra-di″ah-ther′me)   short wave diathermy.

radiatio (ra-de-a′she-o), pl. *radiatio′nes* [L.]   a radiation or radiating structure; used in anatomical nomenclature to designate a collection of nerve fibers connecting different portions of the brain. **r. acus′tica** [NA], acoustic radiation: a fiber tract arising in the medial geniculate nucleus and passing laterally in the sublenticular portion of the internal capsule to terminate in the transverse temporal gyri of the temporal lobe; the radiation provides reciprocal connections and forms part of the inferior thalamic peduncle.   **r. cor′poris callo′si** [NA], radiation of corpus callosum: the fibers of the corpus callosum radiating to all parts of the neopallium.   **r. cor′poris stria′ti**, the extension of fibers from the thalamus and hypothalamus to the corpus striatum. **r. occipitothalam′ica** [Gratiole′ti], **r. optica**.   **r. op′tica** [NA], optic radiation: a fiber tract which begins at the lateral geniculate body, passes laterally through the pars retrolentiformis of the internal capsule, and finally projects posteriorly to end in the striate area on the medial surface of the occipital lobe, on either side of the calcarine sulcus; the radiation provides reciprocal connections and forms part of the posterior thalamic peduncle. Called also *geniculocalcarine tract*, *r. occipitothalamica* [*Gratioleti*], and *radiation of Gratiolet*.   **r. pyramida′lis**, pyramidal radiation: the projection of fibers from the cerebral cortex to the pyramidal tract.

radiation (ra-de-a′shun) [L. *radiatio*]   1. divergence from a common center. 2. a structure made up of divergent elements, as

one of the fiber tracts in the brain; for official names of specific structures, see under *radiatio*. 3. electromagnetic waves, such as those of light, or particulate rays, such as alpha, beta, and gamma rays, given off from some source.   **acoustic r.**, radiatio acustica.   **adaptive r.**, evolution from a generalized, primitive species to diverse, specialized species, each adapted to a distinct mode of life.   **alpha r.**, α-r., see under *ray*. **auditory r.**, radiatio acustica.   **background r.**, radiation arising from radioactive material other than that directly under consideration or study. Background radiation due to cosmic rays and natural radioactivity in the environment is always present; additional background radiation may be due to the presence of other radioactive material in the vicinity, or radioactive components of building materials, etc.   **beta r.**, β-r., see under *ray*. **Cerenkov r.**, energy produced when swiftly travelling electrons pass through a liquid with a speed greater than the speed of light in that liquid.   **r. of corpus callosum**, radiatio corporis callosi.   **corpuscular r's**, radiations other than x-ray and γ-rays, such as alpha-, beta-, proton-, neutron-, positron-, and deuteron-rays.   **electromagnetic r.**, see under *wave*. **gamma r.**, γ-r., see under *ray*.   **r. of Gratiolet**, radiatio optica.   **heterogeneous r.**, radiation consisting of a beam of particles of various energies, or having different frequencies, or containing different types of particles; see also *white r*.   **homogeneous r.**, radiation consisting of an extremely narrow band of frequencies or a beam of monoenergetic particles of a single type; see also *characteristic r*. and *monochromatic r*.   **Huldshinsky's r.**, a course of three months' treatment with ultraviolet rays from the quartz-mercury vapor lamp.   **interstitial r.**, energy emitted by radium or radon inserted directly into the tissue.   **ionizing r.**, high-energy radiation (x-rays and gamma rays) which interacts to produce ion pairs in matter.   **irritative r.**, radiation with ultraviolet rays to the point of erythema. **mitogenetic r., mitogenic r.**, specific energy allegedly given off by a cell undergoing mitosis.   **monochromatic r.**, see under *ray*.   **monoenergetic r.**, radiation of a given type, as of alpha, beta, or gamma rays, in which all particles or photons originate with and have the same energy.   **occipitothalamic r., optic r.**, radiatio optica.   **photochemical r.**, that part of the radiant spectrum which produces chemical changes.   **pyramidal r.**, radiatio pyramidalis.   **Rollier's r.**, exposure of the tuberculous patient to gradually increasing doses of the ultraviolet rays of the sun.   **tegmental r.**, fibers radiating laterally from the red nucleus.   **thalamic r.**, fibers which reciprocally connect the thalamus and cerebral cortex by way of the internal capsule; usually grouped into four subradiations (peduncles): anterior or frontal, superior or centroparietal, posterior or occipital, and inferior or temporal.   **thalamotemporal r.**, radiatio acustica.   **white r.**, a spectral distribution of x-rays ranging from very low energy photons to those produced by the peak kilovoltage applied across an x-ray tube; analogous to the continuous optical spectrum obtained from white light.

radiationes (ra-de-a″she-o′nēz) [L.]   plural of *radiatio*.

radical (rad′ĭ-kal) [L. *radicalis*]   1. directed to the cause; directed to the root or source of a morbid process, as radical surgery. 2. a group of atoms which enters into and goes out of chemical combination without change, and which forms one of the fundamental constituents of a molecule.   **acid r.**, 1. the electronegative element which combines with hydrogen to form an acid. 2. all of the acid except the hydroxyl group.   **alcohol r.**, all of the alcohol molecule except the hydrogen atom of the –OH group; an alkoxy radical.   **color r.**, chromophore.   **free r.**, a radical, extremely reactive and having a very short half-life (10^{-5} seconds or less in an aqueous solution), which carries an unpaired electron.

radices (rad′ĭ-sēz) [L.]   plural of *radix*.

radiciform (ra-dis′ĭ-form) [L. *radix* root + *forma* shape]   shaped like a root; shaped like the root of a tooth.

radicle (rad′ĭ-k'l) [L. *radicula*]   1. any one of the smallest branches of a vessel or nerve. 2. the embryonic, or primary, root that grows out of the hypocotyl of seed plants.

radicotomy (rad″ĭ-kot′o-me)   rhizotomy.

radicula (rah-dik′u-lah) [L.]   radicle, def. 1.

radiculalgia (rah-dik″u-lal′je-ah)   pain due to disease of the spinal nerve roots.

radicular (rah-dik′u-lar)   of or pertaining to a radical or root.

radiculectomy (rah-dik″u-lek′to-me) [L. *radicula* radicle + Gr. *ektomē* excision]   excision of a rootlet, especially resection of spinal nerve roots.

radiculitis (rah-dik″u-li′tis) [L. *radicula* radicle + *-itis*]   inflammation of the root of a spinal nerve, especially of that portion of the root which lies between the spinal cord and the intervertebral canal.

radiculoganglionitis (rah-dik″u-lo-gang″gle-o-ni′tis)   inflammation of the posterior spinal nerve roots and their ganglions.

radiculomedullary (rah-dik″u-lo-med′u-ler″e)   pertaining to or affecting the nerve roots and the spinal cord.

radiculomeningomyelitis (rah-dik″u-lo-mĕ-ning″go-mi′ĕ-li′tis)   inflammation of the nerve roots, the meninges, and the spinal cord.

radiculomyelopathy (rah-dik″u-lo-mi″ĕ-lop′ah-the) disease of the nerve roots and spinal canal.

radiculoneuritis (rah-dik″u-lo-nu-ri′tis) acute febrile polyneuritis.

radiculoneuropathy (rah-dik″u-lo-nu-rop′ah-the) disease of the nerve roots and nerve.

radiculopathy (rah-dik″u-lop′ah-the) disease of the nerve roots. **spondylotic caudal r.,** compression of the cauda equina due to encroachment upon a congenitally small spinal canal by spondylosis, resulting in pseudoclaudication or more profound neural disorders of the lower limbs.

radiectomy (ra″de-ek′to-me) [L. *radix* root + Gr. *ektomē* excision] excision of the root of a tooth.

radiferous (ra-dif′er-us) containing radium.

radii (ra′de-i) [L.] plural of *radius*.

radio- (ra′de-o) [L. *radius* ray] a combining form denoting relationship to a ray or radiation; sometimes used with specific reference to the emission of radiant energy, to radium, or to the radius (bone of the forearm). It is also affixed to the name of a chemical element to designate a radioactive isotope of that particular element, as radiocarbon, radioiodine, etc.

radioactinium (ra″de-o-ak-tin′e-um) a substance formed by the disintegration of actinium.

radioaction (ra″de-o-ak′shun) radioactivity.

radioactive (ra″de-o-ak′tiv) having the property of radioactivity.

radioactivity (ra″de-o-ak-tiv′ĭ-te) the quality of emitting or the emission of corpuscular or electromagnetic radiations consequent to nuclear disintegration, a natural property of all chemical elements of atomic number above 83, and possible of induction in all other known elements. **artificial r., induced r.,** radioactivity produced by bombarding an element with high velocity particles, as the radioactivity of synthetic nuclides.

radioactor (ra″de-o-ak′tor) an apparatus used for collecting and purifying radium emanation.

radioallergosorbent (ra″de-o-al″er-go-sor′bent) denoting a radioimmunoassay technique for the measurement of specific IgE antibody to a variety of allergens; see under *tests*.

radioanaphylaxis (ra″de-o-an″ah-fi-lak′sis) anaphylactic sensitization to the roentgen ray or other form of radiant energy.

radioautogram (ra″de-o-aw′to-gram) autoradiograph.

radioautograph (ra″de-o-aw′to-graf) autoradiograph.

radioautography (ra″de-o-aw-tog′rah-fe) autoradiography.

radiobe (ra′de-ōb) [*radio-* + Gr. *bios* life] one of the peculiar microscopical condensations of sterilized bouillon produced by radium, discovered by J. B. Burke, which, by their appearance and the way in which they divide, have suggested the similar phenomena of bacteria.

radiobicipital (ra″de-o-bi-sip′ĭ-tal) pertaining to the radius and the biceps muscle of the arm.

radiobiological (ra″de-o-bi″o-loj′ĭ-kal) pertaining to radiobiology: concerning cellular and tissue response to irradiation.

radiobiologist (ra″de-o-bi-ol′o-jist) one who devotes his studies to radiobiology.

radiobiology (ra″de-o-bi-ol′o-je) that branch of science which is concerned with the effect of light and of ultraviolet and ionizing radiations upon living tissue or organisms.

radiocalcium (ra″de-o-kal′se-um) a radioactive isotope of calcium. ^{45}Ca, with a half-life of 180 days, is used as a tracer in the study of calcium metabolism.

radiocarbon (ra″de-o-kar′bon) a radioactive isotope of carbon such as ^{14}C, with a half-life of over 5000 years.

radiocarcinogenesis (ra″de-o-kar″sĭ-no-jen′ĕ-sis) cancer formation caused by exposure to radiation.

radiocardiogram (ra″de-o-kar′de-o-gram) the graphic record obtained by radiocardiography.

radiocardiography (ra″de-o-kar′de-og′rah-fe) 1. the graphic recording of the variation with time of the concentration, in a selected chamber of the heart, of a radioactive isotope, usually injected intravenously. 2. radioelectrocardiography.

radiocarpal (ra″de-o-kar′pal) pertaining to the radius and carpus.

radiocarpus (ra″de-o-kar′pus) musculus flexor carpi radialis.

radiochemistry (ra″de-o-kem′is-tre) the branch of chemistry which treats of radioactive materials.

radiochemy (ra″de-o-kem′e) the effects produced by radioactive rays.

radiochroism (ra″de-o-kro′izm) [*radio-* + Gr. *chroa* color] the capacity of a substance to absorb certain radioactive and roentgen rays.

radiocinematograph (ra″de-o-sin″ĕ-mat′o-graf) an apparatus combining the moving picture camera and the roentgen ray machine, making possible moving pictures of the internal organs.

radiocolloids (ra″de-o-kol′oids) radioisotopes in pure form in solution, which tend to behave more like colloids than solutes.

radiocurable (ra″de-o-kūr′ah-b'l) curable by radiation therapy.

radiocystitis (ra″de-o-sis-ti′tis) acute or chronic inflammatory tissue changes in the urinary bladder caused by ionizing irradiation.

radiode (ra′de-ōd) an instrument for the therapeutic application of a radioactive source.

radiodense (ra′de-o-dens″) radiopaque.

radiodensity (ra′de-o-den′sĭ-te) the property of being relatively resistant to the passage of radiant energy; the property of being radiopaque.

radiodermatitis (ra″de-o-der-mah-ti′tis) a cutaneous inflammatory reaction occurring as a result of exposure to biologically effective levels of ionizing radiation.

radiodiagnosis (ra″de-o-di″ag-no′sis) diagnosis by means of roentgen rays and roentgenograms.

radiodiagnostics (ra″de-o-di″ag-nos′tiks) the art of roentgen-ray diagnosis.

radiodiaphane (ra″de-o-di′ah-fān) an instrument for performing transillumination by means of radium.

radiodigital (ra″de-o-dig′ĭ-tal) pertaining to the radius and to the fingers.

radiodontics (ra″de-o-don′tiks) dental radiology.

radiodontist (ra″de-o-don′tist) a dentist who specializes in dental radiology.

radioecology (ra″de-o-e-kol′o-je) the science dealing with the effects of radiation on species of plants and animals in natural communities or ecosystems.

radioelectrocardiogram (ra″de-o-e-lek″tro-kar′de-o-gram) the graphic recording obtained by radioelectrocardiography.

radioelectrocardiograph (ra″de-o-e-lek″tro-kar′de-o-graf″) a battery-operated device by means of which cardiographic signals from electrodes attached at desired body sites are transmitted to a recorder close to or at a distance from the subject.

radioelectrocardiography (ra″de-o-e-lek″tro-kar′de-og′rah-fe) electrocardiography in which impulses are beamed by radio from the subject to a receiver close to or at a distance from the subject.

radioelement (ra″de-o-el′ĕ-ment) any chemical element having radioactive properties.

radioencephalogram (ra″de-o-en-sef′ah-lo-gram″) a curve showing the passage of an injected tracer through the cerebral blood vessels as revealed by an external scintillation counter.

radioencephalography (ra″de-o-en-sef″ah-log′rah-fe) the recording of changes in the electric potential of the brain without direct attachment between the recording apparatus and the subject, the impulses being beamed by radio waves from the subject to the receiver.

radioepidermitis (ra″de-o-ep″ĭ-der-mi′tis) radiodermatitis.

radioepithelitis (ra″de-o-ep″ĭ-the-li′tis) radiodermatitis.

radiogen (ra′de-o-jen) any radioactive substance.

radiogenesis (ra″de-o-jen′ĕ-sis) the production of rays or radioactivity; actinogenesis.

radiogenic (ra″de-o-jen′ik) [*radio-* + Gr. *gennan* to produce] produced by irradiation.

radiogold (ra′de-o-gold) a radioactive isotope of gold, viz., ^{195}Au, ^{198}Au, or ^{199}Au. The isotope ^{198}Au is the most commonly used in solid form or in colloidal solution. It has a half-life of 2.7 days and emits gamma (0.411 MeV) as well as beta radiation (E max = 0.96 MeV). The gamma rays contribute from 6 to 10 per cent of the total dose. It is used both as a diagnostic scintiscanning agent and as a therapeutic cancericidal agent.

radiogram (ra′de-o-gram″) radiograph.

radiograph (ra′de-o-graf″) a film produced by radiography. **cephalometric r.,** cephalograph. **panoramic r.,** a type of extraoral body-section radiograph on which an entire maxilla or both maxillae are depicted on a single film. Called also *Orthopantograph*.

radiographic (ra″de-o-graf′ik) pertaining to or produced by radiography.

radiography (ra″de-og′rah-fe) [*radio-* + Gr. *graphein* to write] the making of film records (radiographs) of internal structures of the body by passage of x-rays or gamma rays through the body to act on specially sensitized film. See also *roentgenography*. **neutron r.,** that in which a narrow beam of neutrons from a nuclear reactor is passed through tissues, especially useful in visualizing bony tissue. **urine r.,** a technique for measuring the quantity of organic iodide excreted by the kidneys, by comparison of the roentgenographic density of a specimen of urine voided at completion of intravenous urography with that of a calibrated scale.

radiohumeral (ra″de-o-hu′mer-al) pertaining to the radius and humerus.

radioimmunity (ra″de-o-ĭ-mu′nĭ-te) a condition of decreased sensitivity to radiation sometimes produced by repeated irradiation.

radioimmunoassay (ra″de-o-im″u-no-as′a) an immunological technique for the measurement of minute quantities of antigen or antibody, hormones, certain drugs, and other substances. The substance under test (e.g., a hormone) is mixed with diluted antiserum (antihormone antibody) in the presence of radioactively labeled antigen (hormone). The concentration of the test substance will then be inversely proportional to amount of labeled antigen bound to the specific antibody and directly related to the amount of free labeled antigen.

radioimmunodiffusion (ra″de-o-im″u-no-dif-fu′zhun) immunodiffusion conducted with radioisotope-labeled antibodies or antigens.

radioimmunoelectrophoresis (ra″de-o-im″u-no-e-lek″tro-fo-re′sis) electrophoresis in which any layer of precipitates is identified by adding the corresponding radioactive-labeled antigen or antibody and subjecting it to autoradiography.

radioimmunoprecipitation (ra″de-o-im″u-no-pre-sip″-ĭ-ta′-shun) immunoprecipitation conducted with radioisotope-labeled antibody or antigen.

radioimmunosorbent (ra″de-o-im″u-no-sor′bent) denoting a radioimmunoassay technique for measuring IgE in samples of serum; see under *tests*.

radioiodine (ra″de-o-i′o-dīn) a radioactive isotope of iodine; of the nine isotopes, ^{131}I and ^{125}I are the most commonly used in the diagnosis and treatment of both benign and malignant disease of the thyroid gland and in the scintiscanning of such organs as the lung, liver, kidney, etc. ^{131}I has a half-life of 8.04 days and emits both beta and gamma rays. ^{125}I has a half-life of 60 days and emits only gamma radiation.

radioiron (ra″de-o-i′ern) a radioactive isotope of iron. ^{55}Fe has a half-life of about 4 years, ^{59}Fe, a half-life of 47 days. A mixture of these has been used in study of the blood.

radioisotope (ra″de-o-i′so-tōp) an isotope which is radioactive, i.e., one having an unstable nucleus, which gives it the property of decay by one or more of several processes. It may be produced from the stable isotope of the element by irradiation in a cyclotron or nuclear reactor. Radioisotopes have important diagnostic and therapeutic uses in clinical medicine and research. **carrier-free r.**, see *carrier-free*.

radiokymography (ra″de-o-ki-mog′rah-fe) roentgenkymography.

radiolead (ra″de-o-led′) a radioactive isotope of lead.

radiolesion (ra″de-o-le′zhun) a lesion caused by exposure to radiation.

radioligand (ra″de-o-li′gand, rad″de-o-lig′and) a radioactive-labeled substance, e.g., an antigen, used in the quantitative measurement of an unlabeled substance by its binding reaction to a specific antibody or other receptor site.

radiologic, radiological (ra″de-o-loj′ik; ra″de-o-loj′e-kal) pertaining to radiology.

radiologist (ra″de-ol′o-jist) a specialist in the use of radiant energy (x-rays, etc.) in the diagnosis and treatment of disease.

radiology (ra″de-ol′o-je) the science of radiant energy and radiant substances, especially that branch of the health sciences which deals with the use of radiant energy in the diagnosis and treatment of disease.

radiolucency (ra″de-o-lu′sen-se) the property of being radiolucent.

radiolucent (ra-de-o-lu′sent) [*radio-* + L. *lucere* to shine] permitting the passage of radiant energy, such as x-rays, yet offering some resistance to it, the representative areas appearing dark on the exposed film.

radiolus (ra-de′o-lus) [L., dim. of *radius* ray] a probe, staff, or sound.

radiometallography (ra″de-o-met″ah-log′rah-fe) the radiography of metals.

radiometer (ra″de-om′ĕ-ter) 1. an instrument for estimating roentgen-ray quantity. 2. an instrument in which radiant heat and light may be directly converted into mechanical energy. 3. an instrument for measuring radiant energy. **pastille r.,** an apparatus consisting of a color index by means of which the color changes in the pastilles, before and after radiation, may be estimated. **photographic r.,** a radiometer that uses strips of photographic paper which, after exposure and development, are compared with a half-tone color index.

radiomicrometer (ra″de-o-mi-krom′ĕ-ter) [*radio-* + Gr. *mikros* small + *metron* measure] an instrument for detecting minute changes of radiant energy.

radiomimetic (ra″de-o-mi-met′ik) [*radio-* + Gr. *mimētikos* imitative] exerting effects similar to those of ionizing radiation.

radiomuscular (ra″de-o-mus′ku-lar) going from the radial artery or nerve to the muscles.

radiomutation (ra″de-o-mu-ta′shun) change in the character of cells caused by exposure to radiation.

radion (ra′de-on) one of the radiant particles thrown off by a radioactive substance.

radionecrosis (ra″de-o-ne-kro′sis) destruction of tissue caused by radiant energy.

radioneuritis (ra″de-o-nu-ri′tis) a form of neuritis resulting from exposure to roentgen rays or other radiant energy.

radionitrogen (ra″de-o-ni′tro-jen) a radioactive substance produced by bombarding boron with alpha rays.

radionuclide (ra″de-o-nu′klīd) a radioactive nuclide; one that disintegrates with the emission of corpuscular or electromagnetic radiations.

radio-opacity (ra″de-o-o-pas′ĭ-te) radiopacity.

radiopacity (ra″de-o-pas′ĭ-te) the property of being radiopaque.

radiopaque (ra″de-o-pāk′) [*radio-* + L. *opacus* dark, obscure] not permitting the passage of radiant energy, such as x-rays, the representative areas appearing light or white on the exposed film.

radioparency (ra″de-o-par′en-se) the property of being radioparent.

radioparent (ra″de-o-par′ent) permitting the passage of roentgen rays.

radiopathology (ra″de-o-pah-thol′o-je) pathology having to do with the effects of radiation on tissues.

radiopelvimetry (ra″de-o-pel-vim′ĕ-tre) measurement of the pelvis by roentgen-ray examination.

radiopharmaceutical (ra″de-o-fahr″mah-su′tĭ-kal) a radioactive pharmaceutical or chemical (e.g., radioactive iodine, cobalt, etc.) used for diagnostic or therapeutic purposes.

radiopharmacy (ra″de-o-fahr′mah-se) the preparation of radioactive pharmaceuticals and radionuclides.

radiophobia (ra″de-o-fo′be-ah) morbid anxiety about the damaging effects of x-rays and radium.

radiophosphorus (ra″de-o-fos′fo-rus) either of two radioactive isotopes of phosphorus, ^{32}P and ^{33}P. The former, a pure beta emitter, has a half-life of 14.3 days and is used in solution or colloidal form as a diagnostic and therapeutic agent.

radiophotography (ra″de-o-fo-tog′rah-fe) photography of the fluorescent image produced by an x-ray beam.

radiophylaxis (ra″de-o-fi-lak′sis) the modifying effect of a small dose of radiation on the reaction to a large subsequent radiation.

radiophysics (ra″de-o-fiz′iks) the physics of radiology.

radioplastic (ra″de-o-plas′tik) a term used to designate a method of making a plaster image of an organ, such as the heart, from roentgenoscopic measurements.

radiopotassium (ra″de-o-po-tas′e-um) a radioactive isotope of potassium, ^{42}K, with a half-life of 12.4 hours, is used in tracer studies of potassium interchange in the body.

radiopotentiation (ra″de-o-po-ten″-she-a′shun) the action of a drug in enhancing the effect of irradiation.

radiopraxis (ra″de-o-prak′sis) [*radio-* + Gr. *praxis* practice] use of rays of light, electricity, etc., in treatment of disease.

radiopulmonography (ra″de-o-pul″mo-nog′rah-fe) a rapid method for estimation of ventilation of localized lung areas, based on measurement of variation in intensity of low-voltage x-rays passed through the lungs during breathing.

radioreaction (ra″de-o-re-ak′shun) a bodily reaction, especially a skin reaction, to radiation.

radioreceptor (ra″de-o-re-sep′tor) a receptor for the stimuli which are excited by radiant energy, such as light or heat.

radioresistance (ra″de-o-re-zis′tans) resistance, as of tissue or cells to irradiation.

radioresistant (ra″de-o-re-zis′tant) resisting the effects of radiation.

radioresponsive (ra″de-o-re-spon′siv) reacting favorably to radiation.

radiosclerometer (ra″de-o-skle-rom′ĕ-ter) penetrometer, def. 1.

radioscope (ra′de-o-skōp) [*radio-* + Gr. *skopein* to examine] an instrument for detecting or studying roentgen rays or other forms of radioactivity.

radioscopy (ra″de-os′ko-pe) [*radio-* + Gr. *skopein* to examine] fluoroscopy.

radiosensibility (ra″de-o-sen″sĭ-bil′ĭ-te) radiosensitivity.

radiosensitive (ra″de-o-sen′sĭ-tiv) sensitive to radiant energy, as roentgen ray or other radiations; said of skin, tumor tissue, etc.

radiosensitiveness (ra″de-o-sen′sĭ-tiv-nes) radiosensitivity.

radiosensitivity (ra″de-o-sen″sĭ-tiv′ĭ-te) sensitivity, as of the skin or other tissue, to radiant energy, such as roentgen-ray or other radiations.

radiosodium (ra″de-o-so′de-um) a radioactive isotope of sodium, ^{24}Na and ^{22}Na are used in the study of blood flow, water balance, and peripheral vascular diseases.

radiostereoscopy (ra″de-o-ster″e-os′ko-pe) [*radio-* + Gr. *stereos* solid + *skopein* to examine] the inspection of the interior organs by means of the roentgen rays.

radiostrontium (ra″de-o-stron′she-um) a radioactive isotope of strontium, of which there are four: ^{85}Sr, ^{87}Sr, ^{89}Sr, and ^{90}Sr. The half-lives are, respectively 65 days, 2.8 hours, 51 days, and 28 years. Their importance in clinical scintiscanning and nuclear fallout is primarily due to their affinity for bone.

radiosulfur (ra″de-o-sul′fur) a radioactive isotope of sulfur.

radiotelemetry (ra″de-o-tel-em′ĕ-tre) the determination of measurement of various factors, the specific data being transmitted by radio waves from the object of measurement to the recording apparatus.

radiotellurium (ra″de-o-tel-lu′re-um) any radioactive isotope of the element tellurium.

radiothanatology (ra″de-o-than″ah-tol′o-je) [radio- + Gr. thanatos death + logos treatise] the study of the effect of radiant energy on dead tissue.

radiotherapeutics (ra″de-o-ther″ah-pu′tiks) 1. the body of knowledge comprising the available information regarding the therapeutic use of ionizing radiation. 2. radiotherapy.

radiotherapist (ra″de-o-ther′ah-pist) a specialist in radiotherapy.

radiotherapy (ra″de-o-ther′ah-pe) [radio- + Gr. therapeia cure] the treatment of disease by ionizing radiation. **interstitial r.,** that administered with the radioactive element contained in devices (e.g., needles or wire) inserted directly into the tissues. **intracavitary r.,** that in which the radioactive element is introduced into a natural body cavity.

radiothermy (ra″de-o-ther′me) [radio- + Gr. thermē heat] 1. therapeutic use of radiant heat or of heat emanating from radioactive substances. 2. short wave diathermy.

radiothorium (ra″de-o-tho′re-um) a radioactive isotope of thorium.

radiotomy (ra″de-ot′o-me) [radio- + Gr. tomē a cutting] see body section roentgenography, under roentgenography.

radiotoxemia (ra″de-o-tok-se′me-ah) toxemia produced by radiation or a radioactive substance.

radiotracer (ra″de-o-tra′ser) a radioactive tracer.

radiotransparency (ra″de-o-trans-par′en-se) the quality of being pervious to roentgen rays or other forms of radiation.

radiotransparent (ra″de-o-trans-par′ent) permitting the passage of roentgen rays or of other forms of radiation.

radiotropic (ra″de-o-trop′ik) influenced by radiation.

radiotropism (ra″de-ot′ro-pizm) a tropism with regard to radiation.

radioulnar (ra″de-o-ul′nar) pertaining to the radius and ulna.

radium (ra′de-um) [so called from its radiant quality] a rare radioactive element in the uranium decay series. It has an atomic weight of 226, an atomic number of 88, and a half-life of 1622 years. It is found mainly in pitchblende and undergoes spontaneous disintegration with formation of a gas called radon (half-life = 3.85 days). In this process it emits alpha particles. Radon (alpha emitter) on deposit in solid form disintegrates into a series of decay products: radium A (half-life = 3 minutes), radium B (half-life = 26.7 minutes), and radium C (half-life = 19.5 minutes). The beta particles and gamma radiations used in clinical therapy originate from radium B and C. With radium in a sealed container and the same number of atoms of each decay product disintegrating per second, radium and its decay products are in equilibrium. In this state, the formation of beta particles and gamma rays reaches its maximum. In clinical gamma-ray therapy, shielding off of the beta particles can be accomplished by a metallic container, e.g., of gold or platinum. A glass wall container permits irradiation with beta particles as well as gamma rays.

radius (ra′de-us), pl. ra′dii [L. "spoke" (of a wheel)] 1. a line radiating from a center, or the circular limit defined by a fixed distance from an established point or center. 2. [NA] the bone on the outer or thumb side of the forearm, articulating proximally with the humerus and ulna and distally with the ulna and carpus; see Plate accompanying skeleton. **r. cur′vus,** Madelung's deformity. **r. fix′us,** a straight line from the hormion to the inion. **radii of lens, ra′dii len′tis** [NA], imaginary lines extending from the midpoint of the axis of the lens of the eye to the capsule of the lens. **Van der Waals r.,** the distance at which there is a balance between Van der Waals attractive and repulsive forces in the formation of chemical bonds.

radix (ra′diks), pl. rad′ices [L.] the lowermost part, or a structure by which something is firmly attached; [NA] a general term for the lowermost part, or a part by which a structure is anchored, as the portion of a hair, nail, or tooth that is buried in the tissues, or the part of a nerve adjacent to the center to which it is connected. Called also root. **r. ante′rior,** r. ventralis. **r. ar′cus ver′tebrae,** pediculus arcus vertebralis. **r. bre′vis gan′glii cilia′ris,** r. oculomotoria ganglii ciliaris. **r. clin′ica** [NA], clinical root: that portion of a tooth below the clinical crown, being attached to the gingiva or alveolus. **r. cochlea′ris ner′vi acus′tici,** r. inferior nervi vestibulocochlearis. **rad′ices crania′les ner′vi accesso′rii** [NA], the cranial roots of the accessory nerve. Originating from the nucleus ambiguus and emerging from the side of the medulla oblongata below the roots of the vagus nerve, they unite with the spinal portion in the

jugular foramen. Their constituent fibers then form the internal branch, which joins the vagus nerve and is distributed to the soft palate, constrictors of the pharynx, and the larynx. **r. den′tis** [NA], root of tooth: the portion of a tooth which is covered by cementum, proximal to the neck of the tooth and ordinarily embedded in the dental alveolus; called also anatomical root. **r. descen′dens [mesencephalica] ner′vi trigem′ini,** tractus mesencephalicus nervi trigemini. **r. dorsa′lis** [NA], dorsal root (of spinal nerves): the posterior, or sensory division of each spinal nerve, attached centrally to the spinal cord and joining peripherally with the ventral, or motor, root to form the nerve

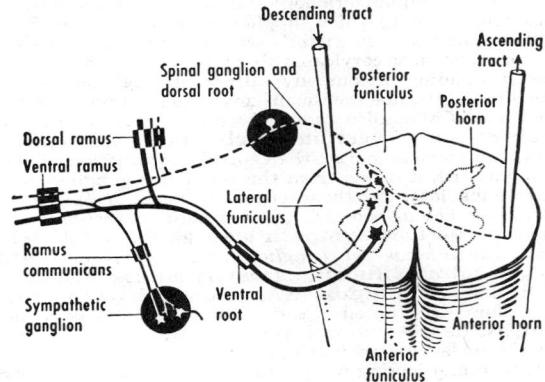

Diagram of a horizontal section of the spinal cord, with dorsal and ventral roots and a spinal nerve (Gardner, Gray, and O'Rahilley).

before it emerges through the intervertebral foramen: each dorsal root bears a spinal ganglion and conveys sensory fibers to the spinal cord. Called also r. posterior. **r. facia′lis,** NA alternative for nervus canalis pterygoidei. **r. infe′rior an′sae cervica′lis** [NA], inferior foot of ansa cervicalis: a strand of filaments connecting the ansa cervicalis with branches of the second and third cervical nerves. **r. infe′rior ner′vi vestibuloco-chlea′ris** [NA], inferior root of vestibulocochlear nerve: the central continuation of the pars cochlearis nervi octavi from the spiral ganglion, passing dorsal to the inferior cerebellar peduncle to enter the brain; called also r. cochlearis nervi acustici. **r. latera′lis ner′vi media′ni** [NA], lateral root of median nerve: the fibers contributed to the median nerve by the lateral cord of the brachial plexus. **r. latera′lis trac′tus op′tici** [NA], lateral root of optic tract: fibers from the optic tract that enter the lateral geniculate body. **r. lin′guae** [NA], root of tongue: the portion of the tongue posterior to the sulcus terminalis, being attached below to the hyoid bone, and directed backward as well as upward. **r. lon′ga gan′glii cilia′ris,** ramus communicans nervi nasociliaris cum ganglione ciliari. **r. media′lis ner′vi media′ni** [NA], medial root of median nerve: the fibers contributed to the median nerve by the medial cord of the brachial plexus. **r. media′lis trac′tus op′tici** [NA], medial root of optic tract: fibers from the optic tract that enter the superior colliculus and the pretectal region. **r. mesencephal′ica ner′vi trigem′ini,** tractus mesencephalicus nervi trigemini. **r. mesente′rii** [NA], root of mesentery: the line of attachment of the mesentery to the posterior abdominal wall, extending from the duodenojejunal flexure at the left of the second lumbar vertebra diagonally downward to the upper border of the right sacroiliac articulation. **rad′ices mol′les gan′glii cilia′re,** see ramus sympathicus ad ganglion ciliare. **r. moto′ria ner′vi trigem′ini** [NA], motor root of trigeminal nerve: the smaller of the two roots by which the trigeminal nerve is attached to the side of the pons; it contains proprioceptive as well as motor fibers, and continues deep to the trigeminal ganglion to join the mandibular nerve. Called also portio minor nervi trigemini. **r. na′si** [NA], root of nose: the upper portion of the nose, which is attached to the frontal bone. **r. ner′vi facia′lis,** the root of the facial nerve, consisting of fibers passing from the nucleus of the facial nerve to the facial colliculus, and from there to the ventral surface of the lower portion of the pons. **r. oculomo-to′ria gan′glii cilia′ris** [NA], oculomotor root of cilary ganglion: a short collection of fibers passing from the inferior branch of the oculomotor nerve to the posterior inferior portion of the ciliary ganglion; it contains preganglionic parasympathetic fibers for the sphincter pupillae and ciliary muscle. Called also r. brevis ganglii ciliaris. **rad′ices parieta′les ve′nae ca′vae infe′rio′ris,** vessels draining blood from the abdominal wall into the inferior vena cava, including the venae lumbales and vena phrenica inferior. **r. pe′nis** [NA], root of penis: the proximal, attached portion of the penis, consisting of the diverging crura of the corpora cavernosa and the bulb. **r. pi′li** [NA], root of hair: the proximal portion of a hair embedded in the hair follicle. **r. poste′rior,** r. dorsalis. **r. pulmo′nis** [NA], root of lung: the attachment of either lung, comprising the structures entering and emerging at the hilus. **r. senso′ria ner′vi trigem′ini**

[NA], sensory root of trigeminal nerve: the larger of the two roots by which the trigeminal nerve is attached to the side of the pons. It contains sensory fibers and expands into a large flat ganglion (the trigeminal ganglion) which gives rise to the ophthalmic, maxillary, and mandibular nerves. Called also *portio major nervi trigemini*. **rad′ices spina′les ner′vi accesso′rii** [NA], the spinal roots of the accessory nerve. Originating from the gray matter of the spinal cord and emerging from the side of the cord as far down as a level between the third and seventh cervical nerves, they form a trunk that ascends in the vertebral canal, passes through the foramen magnum, and unites with the cranial portion in the jugular foramen. The constituent fibers then form the external branch, which supplies the sternocleidomastoid and trapezius muscles. **r. supe′rior an′sae cervica′lis** [NA], superior root of ansa cervicalis: fibers of the first or second cervical nerve, descending in company with the hypoglossal nerve, connecting it and the ansa cervicalis and helping supply the infrahyoid muscles. Called also *ramus descendens nervi hypoglossi*. **r. supe′rior ner′vi vestibulocochlea′ris** [NA], superior root of vestibulocochlear nerve: the central continuation of the pars vestibularis nervi octavi from the vestibular ganglion, entering the brain just lateral to the intermediate nerve and in front of the inferior cerebellar peduncle. Called also *r. vestibularis nervi acustici*. **rad′ices sympath′icae gan′glii cilia′ris**, see *ramus sympathicus ad ganglion ciliare*. **r. sympath′ica gan′glii submaxilla′ris**, ramus sympathicus ad ganglion submandibulare. **r. un′guis** [NA], root of nail: the proximal portion of the nail, situated in the sulcus of the matrix of the nail. **r. ventra′lis** [NA], ventral root (of spinal nerves): the anterior, or motor, division of each spinal nerve, attached centrally to the spinal cord and joining peripherally with the dorsal, or sensory, root to form the nerve before it emerges through the intervertebral foramen. It conveys motor fibers to skeletal muscle and contains preganglionic autonomic fibers at thoracolumbar and sacral levels. Called also *r. anterior*. **r. vestibula′ris ner′vi acus′tici**, r. superior nervi vestibulocochlearis. **rad′ices viscera′les ve′nae ca′vae inferio′ris**, vessels draining blood from the viscera of the abdominal and pelvic cavities to the inferior vena cava, including the venae hepaticae, renales, and suprarenales, the vena spermatica, testicularis, and ovaricus, and the plexus pampiniformis.

radon (ra′don) a heavy, colorless, gaseous, radioactive element, symbol Rn, atomic weight 222, atomic number 86, obtained by the breaking up of radium, and used in radiotherapy. Called also *radium emanation (RE)*. Cf. *radium*. ²¹⁹Rn is a radioactive isotope of the actinium radioactive series. ²²⁰Rn is a radioactive isotope of the thorium radioactive series.

raffinase (raf′ĭ-nās) an enzyme which catalyzes the hydrolytic cleavage of raffinose.

raffinose (raf′ĭ-nōs) melitose.

rafoxanide (rah-foks′ah-nīd) chemical name: 3′-chloro-4′-(p - chlorophenoxy)-3,5-diiodosalicylanilide; an anthelmintic, $C_{19}H_{11}Cl_2I_2NO_3$.

rage (rāj) a state of violent anger. **sham r.**, an outburst of behavior in a decorticated animal, resembling that manifested in fear and anger; a similar phenomenon may be observed in man in cases of insulin hypoglycemia or carbon monoxide poisoning.

ragocyte (rag′o-sīt) a cell found in the joints in rheumatoid arthritis. Such cells are produced when polymorphonuclear leukocytes ingest aggregated IgG, rheumatoid factor, fibrin, and complement.

raigan (ra′ĭ-gan) a native Chinese name for dried mushrooms, *Omphalia lapidescens*; anthelmintic.

Raillietina (ri″le-ĕ-ti′nah) a genus of tapeworms of the family Davaineidae, many species of which infect birds, domestic fowl, and mammals. *R. madagascarien′sis* (*Taenia madagascariensis*, Madagascar tapeworm), *R. asiat′ica*, *R. formosa′na*, *R. demararien′sis* (*Taenia demarariensis*), and *R. loechesal′avezi* have been reported from man.

raillietiniasis (ri″le-ĕ-ti-ni′ah-sis) infection with a parasite of the genus *Raillietina*.

Rainey′s corpuscles, tubes, tubules (ra′nēz) [George *Rainey*, English anatomist, 1801–1884] sarcosporidian cysts; see under *cyst*.

rale (rahl) [Fr. *râle* rattle] an abnormal respiratory sound heard in auscultation, and indicating some pathologic condition. Rales are distinguished as *dry* or *moist*, according to the absence or presence of fluid in the air passages, and are classified according to their site of origin as *bronchial, cavernous, laryngeal, pleural, tracheal,* and *vesicular, (crepitant)*. **amphoric r.**, a coarse, musical, and tinkling rale caused by the splashing of fluid in a cavity connected with a bronchus. **atelectatic r.**, a nonpathologic rale which is dissipated by deep breathing or coughing. Such rales are frequently heard in those who breathe feebly and superficially, when on deep inspiration the moist walls of the unexpanded alveoli are suddenly forced apart by the entering air; after a few deep inspirations such rales become lost. These rales are best observed at the margins or borders of the lung and are sometimes known as *marginal* or *border rales*. **border r.**, atelectatic r. **bronchial r.**, a rale produced in a bronchus.

bubbling r., a moist rale, finer than a subcrepitant rale, heard in bronchitis, in the resolving stage of croupous pneumonia, and over small cavities. **cavernous r.**, a hollow and metallic rale caused by the alternate expansion and contraction of a pulmonary cavity during respiration. **cellophane r.**, a dry crackling chest sound, as heard in interstitial pulmonary fibrosis. **clicking r.**, a small, sticky sound heard in inspiration, and caused by the passage of air through secretions in the smaller bronchi. **collapse r.**, a fine crepitant rale heard over collapsed lung tissue; also at the base of the healthy lung of a bedridden patient, due to incomplete expansion of the air vesicles. **consonating r.**, a clear, ringing sound produced in bronchial tubes that are surrounded by consolidation tissues. **crackling r.**, subcrepitant r. **crepitant r.**, a very fine rale, resembling the sound produced by rubbing a lock of hair between the fingers or by particles of salt thrown on fire; heard at the end of inspiration. **dry r.**, a rale produced by the presence of viscid secretion in the bronchial tubes or by spastic contraction of the walls of the tubes; it has a whistling, musical, or squeaking quality. Dry rales are heard in asthma and bronchitis. **extrathoracic r.**, a rale produced in the larynx or trachea. **gurgling r.**, a very coarse rale resembling the bursting of large bubbles; in pulmonary edema, heard over large cavities that contain fluid, and in the trachea in the "death rattle." **guttural r.**, a rale produced in the throat. **r. in′dux**, a crepitant rale heard in the stage of beginning consolidation in pneumonia. **laryngeal r.**, a rale produced in the larynx. **marginal r.**, atelectatic r. **metallic r.**, consonating r. **moist r.**, a rale produced by the presence of liquid in the bronchial tubes. **mucous r., r. mu-queux**, a modified subcrepitant rale resembling the sound produced by blowing through a pipe into soapy water; it is caused by the bursting of viscid bubbles in the bronchial tubes. **pleural r.**, a pleural friction sound. **r. redux, r. de retour**, an unequal crackling sound produced by air passing through fluid in a bronchial tube; heard in the resolution stage of pneumonia. **sibilant r.**, a hissing sound resembling that produced by suddenly separating two oiled surfaces. It is produced by the presence of a viscid secretion in the bronchial tubes or by thickening of the walls of the tubes; heard in asthma and bronchitis. **sonorous r.**, a fine, moist sound resembling the cooing of a dove, produced by the passage of air through mucus in the capillary bronchial tubes; heard in capillary bronchitis and asthma. **subcrepitant r.**, a fine, moist rale heard in conditions that are associated with liquid in the smaller tubes; called also *crackling r.* **tracheal r.**, a rale produced in the trachea. **vesicular r.**, crepitant r. **whistling r.**, sibilant r.

Ralfe′s test (ralfs) [Charles Henry *Ralfe*, English physician, 1842–1896] see under *tests*.

ramal (ra′mal) pertaining to a ramus; branching.

Raman effect (ram′an) [Sir Chandrasekhara Venkata *Raman*, Indian physicist, born 1888; winner of the Nobel prize for physics in 1930] see under *effect*.

ramaninjana (ram″an-in-jah′nah) a form of palmus, or jumping disease, prevailing in Madagascar.

R.A.M.C. Royal Army Medical Corps.

ramex (ra′meks) [L.] 1. (*obs*.) a hernia. 2. varicocele.

rami (ra′mi) [L.] plural of *ramus*.

Ramibacterium (ra″me-bak-te′re-um) [L. *ramus* branch + *bacterium*] a genus of microorganisms of the tribe Lactobacilleae, family Lactobacillaceae, order Eubacteriales, made up of nonsporulating, anaerobic, gram-positive bacilli found in the intestinal tract and occasionally associated with purulent infections. **R. ramo′sum**, *Bacteroides ramosus*.

ramicotomy (ram″ĭ-kot′o-me) [*ramus* + Gr. *tomē* a cutting] ramisection.

ramification (ram″ĭ-fĭ-ka′shun) [*ramus* + L. *facere* to make] 1. distribution in branches. 2. a branch or set of branches. 3. the manner of branching.

ramify (ram′ĭ-fi) [*ramus* + L. *facere* to make] 1. to branch; to diverge in various directions. 2. to traverse in branches.

ramisection (ram″ĭ-sek′shun) [*ramus* + L. *sectio* a cutting] the operation of cutting the appropriate rami communicantes of the sympathetic nervous system (*sympathetic ramisection*).

ramisectomy (ram″ĭ-sek′to-me) ramisection.

ramitis (ram-i′tis) [*ramus* + -*itis* inflammation] inflammation of a ramus.

Rammstedt (rahm′stet) see *Ramstedt*.

ramollissement (rah″mol-ēs-maw′) [Fr.] softening.

Ramon′s flocculation, flocculation test [Gaston *Ramon*, French bacteriologist 1886–1963] see under *tests*.

Ramón y Cajal (rah-mōn e ka-hal′) [Santiago *Ramón y Cajal*, Spanish histologist, 1852–1934] see *Cajal*.

Ramond′s sign (ram-onz′) [Louis *Ramond*, French internist, 1879–1952] see under *sign*.

ramose (ra′mos) [L. *ramus* branch] branching; having many branches.

rampart (ram′part) a board, encircling embankment. **maxillary r.**, a ridge or mound of epithelial cells that is seen in that portion of the jaw of the embryo which is to become the alveolar border.

Ramsay Hunt disease, syndrome (ram′se hunt) [James *Ramsay Hunt,* American neurologist, 1872–1937] see *dyssynergia cerebellaris progressiva;* see *juvenile paralysis agitans (of Hunt),* under *paralysis;* and see under *syndrome,* def. 1.

Ramsden's eyepiece (ramz′denz) [Jesse *Ramsden,* English instrument maker and optician, 1735–1800] see under *eyepiece.*

Ramstedt operation (rahm′stet) [Wilhelm Conrad *Ramstedt,* surgeon in Münster, born 1867] Fredet-Ramstedt operation.

ramulus (ram′u-lus), pl. *ram′uli* [L., dim. of *ramus*] a small branch or terminal division.

ramus (ra′mus), pl. *ra′mi* [L.] a branch; [NA] a general term for a smaller structure given off by a larger one, or into which the larger structure, such as a blood vessel or nerve, divides. **r. acetabula′ris arte′riae circumflex′ae fem′oris media′lis** [NA], acetabular branch of medial circumflex femoral artery: a branch of the medial circumflex artery of the thigh, distributed to the head of the femur and to the acetabulum (hip joint); called also *r. acetabuli arteriae circumflexae femoris medialis.* **r. acetabula′ris arte′riae obturato′riae** [NA], acetabular branch of obturator artery: it is distributed to the hip joint; called also *arteria acetabuli.* **r. acetab′uli arte′riae circumflex′ae fem′oris media′lis,** r. acetabularis arteriae circumflexae femoris medialis. **r. acromia′lis arte′riae suprascapula′ris** [NA], acromial branch of suprascapular artery: it is distributed to the acromion process; called also *r. acromialis arteriae transversae scapulae.* **r. acromia′lis arte′riae thoracoacromia′lis** [NA], acromial branch of thoracoacromial artery: it is distributed to the deltoid muscle and acromion process. **r. acromia′lis arte′riae transver′sae scap′ulae,** r. acromialis arteriae suprascapularis. **ra′mi ad pon′tem arte′riae basila′ris** [NA], pontine branches of basilar artery: they are distributed to the pons and adjacent parts of the brain. **ra′mi alveola′res superio′res anterio′res ner′vi infraorbita′lis** [NA], anterior superior alveolar branches of infraorbital nerve: branches from the infraorbital nerve that innervate the incisor and canine teeth of the upper jaw, help form the superior dental plexus, and give terminal twigs to the floor of the nose; modality, general sensory. **r. alveola′ris supe′rius me′dius ner′vi infraorbita′lis** [NA], middle superior alveolar branch of infraorbital nerve: a branch from the infraorbital nerve that innervates the premolar teeth of the upper jaw by way of the superior dental plexus; modality, general sensory. **ra′mi alveola′res superio′res posterio′res ner′vi maxilla′ris** [NA], posterior superior alveolar branches of maxillary nerve: they innervate the maxillary sinus, cheek, gums, and molar and premolar teeth of the upper jaw; they form part of the superior dental plexus; modality, general sensory. **r. anastomot′icus,** a structure connecting one nerve to another; see terms beginning *r. communicans.* **r. anastomot′icus arte′riae menin′geae me′diae cum arte′ria lacrima′li** [NA], a branch of the middle meningeal artery that is distributed to the orbit and anastomoses with the recurrent meningeal branch of the lacrimal artery. **r. anastomot′icus gan′glii o′tici cum chor′da tym′pani,** r. communicans ganglii otici cum chorda tympani. **r. anastomot′icus gan′glii o′tici cum ner′vo auriculotempora′li,** r. communicans ganglii otici cum nervo auriculotemporali. **r. anastomot′icus gan′glii o′tici cum ner′vo spino′so,** r. communicans ganglii otici cum ramo meningeo nervi mandibularis. **ra′mi anastomot′ici ner′vi auriculotempora′lis cum ner′vo facia′li,** rami communicantes nervi auriculotemporalis cum nervo faciali. **r. anastomot′icus ner′vi facia′lis cum ner′vo glossopharyn′geo,** r. communicans nervi facialis cum nervo glossopharyngeo. **r. anastomot′icus ner′vi facia′lis cum plex′u tympan′ico,** r. communicans nervi facialis cum plexu tympanico. **r. anastomot′icus ner′vi glossopharyn′gei cum ra′mo auricula′ri ner′vi va′gi,** r. communicans nervi glossopharyngei cum ramo auriculari nervi vagi. **r. anastomot′icus ner′vi lacrima′lis cum ner′vo zygomat′ico,** r. communicans nervi lacrimalis cum nervo zygomatico. **ra′mi anastomot′ici ner′vi lingua′lis cum ner′vo hypoglos′so,** rami communicantes nervi lingualis cum nervo hypoglosso. **r. anastomot′icus ner′vi media′ni cum ner′vo ulna′ri,** r. communicans nervi mediani cum nervo ulnari. **r. anastomot′icus ner′vi va′gi cum ner′vo glossopharyn′geo,** r. communicans nervi vagi cum nervo glossopharyngeo. **r. anastomot′icus peronae′us ner′viperonae′i commu′nis,** r. communicans peroneus nervi peronei communis. **r. anastomot′icus ulna′ris ner′vi radia′lis,** r. communicans ulnaris nervi radialis. **ra′mi anterio′res arteria′rum intercosta′lium,** anterior branches of intercostal arteries. **r. ante′rior arte′riae obturato′riae** [NA], anterior branch of obturator artery: it passes forward around the medial margin of the obturator foramen, on the obturator membrane, and is distributed to the obturator and adductor muscles. **r. ante′rior arte′riae recurren′tis ulna′ris** [NA], anterior branch of ulnar recurrent artery: it helps supply the pronator teres and brachialis muscles and runs to the front of the medial epicondyle, supplying the elbow joint and

adjacent structures. **r. ante′rior arte′riae rena′lis** [NA], the anterior branch of the renal artery, supplying the anterior, superior, and inferior segments of the kidney. **r. ante′rior arte′riae thyroi′deae superio′ris** [NA], anterior branch of superior thyroid artery: it helps supply the upper part of the gland, anastomosing with its fellow of the opposite side along the upper border of the isthmus. **r. ante′rior ascen′dens fissu′rae cer′ebri latera′lis [Syl′vii],** r. ascendens sulci lateralis cerebri. **r. ante′rior duc′tus hepat′ici dex′tri** [NA], the anterior branch of the right hepatic duct. **r. ante′rior horizonta′lis fissu′rae cer′ebri latera′lis [Syl′vii],** r. anterior sulci lateralis cerebri. **r. ante′rior ner′vi auricula′ris mag′ni** [NA], anterior branch of great auricular nerve; it is distributed to the skin of the face over the parotid gland; modality, general sensory. **ra′mi anterio′res nervo′rum cervica′lium,** rami ventrales nervorum cervicalium. **r. ante′rior ner′vi coccyg′ei,** r. ventralis nervi coccygei. **r. ante′rior ner′vi cuta′nei antebrach′ii media′lis** [NA], anterior branch of medial cutaneous nerve of forearm; it innervates the skin of the front and medial aspect of the forearm; modality, general sensory; called also *r. volaris nervi cutanei antibrachii medialis.* **r. ante′rior ner′vi laryn′gei inferio′ris,** anterior branch of inferior laryngeal nerve. **ra′mi anterio′res nervo′rum lumba′lium,** rami ventrales nervorum lumbalium. **r. ante′rior ner′vi obturato′rii** [NA], anterior branch of obturator nerve; it supplies the gracilis and the adductor longus and brevis muscles and the pectineus, and occasionally gives off a branch to the skin of the medial side of the thigh and leg; modality, motor and general sensory. **ra′mi anterio′res nervo′rum sacra′lium,** rami ventrales nervorum sacralium. **r. ante′rior nervo′rum spina′lium,** r. ventralis nervorum spinalium. **ra′mi anterio′res nervo′rum thoraca′lium,** rami ventrales nervorum thoracicorum. **r. ante′rior ramo′rum cutaneo′rum latera′lium [pectora′lium et abdomina′lium] arterio′rum intercosta′lium,** the anterior branch of the lateral cutaneous branches of the intercostal arteries. **r. ante′rior ramo′rum cutaneo′rum latera′lium [pectora′lium et abdomina′lium] nervo′rum intercosta′lium,** the anterior branch of the lateral cutaneous branches of the intercostal nerve. **r. ante′rior sul′ci latera′lis cer′ebri** [NA], anterior branch of lateral cerebral sulcus; it runs forward a short distance into the inferior frontal gyrus; called also *r. anterior horizontalis fissurae cerebri lateralis [Sylvii].* **ra′mi arterio′si interlobula′res hep′atis,** arteriae interlobulares hepatis. **ra′mi articula′res arte′riae ge′nu supre′mae, ra′mi articula′res arte′riae ge′nus descenden′tis** [NA], articular branches of descending genicular artery; they pass downward in the vastus medialis muscle and help supply the knee joint. **r. ascen′dens arte′riae circumflex′ae fem′oris latera′lis** [NA], ascending branch of lateral circumflex femoral artery: it runs upward along the trochanteric line of the femur and between the gluteus medius and minimus muscles, and anastomoses with branches of the superior gluteal artery. It helps supply the upper thigh muscles. **r. ascen′dens arte′riae circumflex′ae fem′oris media′lis** [NA], ascending branch of medial circumflex femoral artery: it ascends in front of the quadratus femoris muscle to the trochanteric fossa, and there anastomoses with gluteal arteries. **r. ascen′dens arte′riae circumflex′ae il′ium profun′dae** [NA], ascending branch of deep circumflex iliac artery: a branch leaving the deep circumflex iliac artery near the anterior superior iliac spine, rising between and distributing to the transversus abdominis and internal oblique muscles. **r. ascen′dens arte′riae transver′sae col′li,** r. superficialis arteriae transversae colli. **r. ascen′dens sul′ci latera′lis cer′ebri** [NA], ascending branch of lateral cerebral sulcus: it runs superiorly a short distance into the inferior frontal gyrus; called also *r. anterior ascendens fissurae cerebri lateralis [Sylvii].* **ra′mi auricula′res anterio′res arte′riae tempora′lis superficia′lis** [NA], anterior auricular branches of superficial temporal artery: they supply the lateral aspect of the pinna and the external acoustic meatus. **r. auricula′ris arte′riae auricula′ris posterio′ris** [NA], auricular branch of posterior auricular artery: a branch supplying the pinna and adjacent skin. **r. auricula′ris arte′riae occipita′lis** [NA], auricular branch of occipital artery: an inconstant branch of the occipital artery that helps supply the medial aspect of the pinna. **r. auricula′ris ner′vi va′gi** [NA], auricular branch of vagus nerve: a branch arising from the superior ganglion of the vagus, innervating the cranial surface of the auricle, the floor of the external acoustic meatus, and the adjacent part of the tympanic membrane; modality, general sensory. **ra′mi bronchia′les anterio′res ner′vi va′gi,** see *rami bronchiales nervi vagi.* **ra′mi bronchia′les aor′tae thora′cicae** [NA], bronchial branches of thoracic aorta: branches arising from the thoracic aorta to supply the bronchi and lower trachea, and passing along the posterior sides of the bronchi to ramify along the respiratory bronchioles; distributed also to adjacent lymph nodes, pulmonary vessels, and pericardium, and to part of the esophagus. Called also *arteriae bronchiales* or *bronchial arteries.* **ra′mi bronchia′les arte′riae mamma′riae inter′nae,** rami bronchiales arteriae thoracicae internae. **ra′mi bronchia′les ar-**

te′riae thora′cicae inter′nae [NA], bronchial branches of internal thoracic artery: small, variable branches of the internal thoracic artery, with distribution to the bronchi and trachea; called also *rami bronchiales arteriae mammariae internae.* **ra′mi bronchia′les bron′chi,** a name applied to the first, extrapulmonary divisions of the main bronchi, the eparterial and hyparterial bronchial rami. **r. bronchia′lis eparteria′lis,** a name given to the superior lobar bronchus on the right, which arises above the level of the pulmonary artery; called also *eparterial bronchus.* **r. bronchia′les hyparteria′les,** a name given to the middle and inferior lobar bronchi on the right and the lobar bronchi on the left, all of which arise below the level of the pulmonary artery; called also *hyparterial bronchi.* **ra′mi bronchia′les ner′vi va′gi** [NA], branches of the vagus that supply the bronchi and the pulmonary vessels, both directly and by way of the anterior and posterior parts of the pulmonary plexus; modality, parasympathetic and visceral afferent. **ra′mi bronchia′les posterio′res ner′vi va′gi,** see *rami bronchiales nervi vagi.* **ra′mi bronchia′les pulmo′nis,** a name given to intrapulmonary bronchial divisions smaller than the main bronchi and larger than the bronchioles; in NA, they are classified as lobar and segmental bronchi, and branches (rami) of the latter. **ra′mi bronchia′les segmento′rum** [NA], intrasegmental bronchial branches: smaller branches arising from the segmental bronchi. **ra′mi bucca′les ner′vi facia′lis** [NA], buccal branches of facial nerve: they innervate the zygomatic, levator labii superioris, buccinator, and orbicularis oris muscles; modality, motor and general sensory. **ra′mi calca′nei latera′les arte′riae peronae′ae,** rami calcanei ramorum malleolarium lateralium arteriae peroneae. **ra′mi calca′nei latera′les ner′vi sura′lis** [NA], lateral calcaneal branches of sural nerve: they innervate the skin on the back of the leg and the lateral side of the foot and heel; modality, general sensory. **ra′mi calca′nei media′les arte′riae peronae′ae,** rami calcanei ramorum malleolarium medialium arteriae tibialis posterioris. **ra′mi calca′nei media′les ner′vi tibia′lis** [NA], medial calcaneal branches of tibial nerve: branches supplying the medial side of the heel and of the posterior part of the sole; modality, general sensory. **ra′mi calca′nei ramo′rum malleola′rium latera′lium arte′riae perone′ae** [NA], calcaneal branches of lateral malleolar branches of peroneal artery: branches arising from the lateral malleolar branches of the peroneal artery and distributed to the lateral aspect and back of the heel; called also *rami calcanei laterales arteriae peronaeae.* **ra′mi calca′nei ramo′rum malleola′rium media′lium arte′riae tibia′lis posterio′ris** [NA], calcaneal branches of medial malleolar branches of posterior tibial artery: branches that arise from the medial malleolar branches of the posterior tibial artery and are distributed to the medial aspect and back of the heel; called also *rami calcanei mediales arteriae peronaeae.* **ra′mi capsula′res arte′riae re′nis** [NA], capsular branches of renal artery: they supply the renal capsule. **ra′mi cardi′aci cervica′les inferio′res ner′vi va′gi** [NA], inferior cardiac branches of the vagus nerve: branches (sometimes called cervicothoracic) arising from the vagi and from the recurrent laryngeal nerves at the thoracic inlet, and joining cervicothoracic sympathetic cardiac nerves, the combined nerves passing to the cardiac plexus; modality, parasympathetic and visceral afferent. Called also *inferior cardiac branches of recurrent laryngeal nerve.* **ra′mi cardi′aci cervica′les superio′res ner′vi va′gi** [NA], superior cervical cardiac branches of vagus nerve: variable branches arising from the vagus in the cervical region and usually joining the cervical sympathetic cardiac nerves. The conjoined nerves then descend in front of, or behind, the arch of the aorta to the cardiac plexus; modality, parasympathetic and visceral afferent. **ra′mi cardi′aci infe′rio′res ner′vi recurren′tis,** r. cardiaci cervicales inferiores nervi vagi. **ra′mi cardi′aci thora′cici ner′vi va′gi** [NA], thoracic cardiac branches of the vagus nerve: branches which arise in the thorax from the right and left vagus and left recurrent laryngeal nerves. They go directly to the posterior walls of the atria, to the coronary plexuses, and to the anterior pulmonary plexuses. **ra′mi caroticotympan′ici arte′riae carot′idis inter′nae** [NA], caroticotympanic branches of internal carotid artery: branches that supply the tympanic cavity. **r. car′peus dorsa′lis arte′riae radia′lis** [NA], dorsal carpal branch of radial artery: it runs medially deep to the extensor tendons, and helps form the dorsal carpal rete. **r. car′peus dorsa′lis arte′riae ulna′ris** [NA], dorsal carpal branch of ulnar artery: a variable branch of the ulnar artery that runs laterally deep to the tendons of the ulnar muscles of the wrist, helping to form the dorsal carpal rete. **r. car′peus palma′ris arte′riae radia′lis** [NA], palmar carpal branch of radial artery: a branch that passes medially behind the flexor tendons on the palmar aspect of the wrist and forms a network with a corresponding branch of the ulnar artery; called also *r. carpeus volaris arteriae radialis.* **r. car′peus palma′ris arte′riae ulna′ris** [NA], palmar carpal branch of ulnar artery: a branch that passes laterally behind the flexor tendons on the palmar aspect of the wrist and forms a network with a corresponding branch of the radial artery; called also *r. carpeus volaris arteriae ulnaris.* **r. car′peus vola′ris arte′riae radia′lis,** r. car-

peus palmaris arteriae radialis. **r. car′peus vola′ris arte′riae ulna′ris,** r. carpeus palmaris arteriae ulnaris. **ra′mi cauda′ti** [NA], the caudate branches of the transverse part of the left branch of the portal vein. **ra′mi celi′aci ner′vi va′gi** [NA], celiac branches of vagus nerve: branches that arise from both the anterior and posterior vagal trunks and join the celiac plexus; modality, parasympathetic and visceral afferent; called also *rami coeliaci plexus gastrici posterioris* and *celiac nerves.* **ra′mi centra′les arte′riae cer′ebri anterio′ris** [NA], central branches of anterior cerebral artery: they ascend into the base of the brain in front of the optic chiasma and are distributed to the hypothalamus, caudate nucleus, and internal capsule. **ra′mi centra′les arte′riae cer′ebri me′diae** [NA], central branches of medial cerebral artery: central branches that pass through the anterior perforated substance, comprising chiefly the rami striati. **ra′mi centra′les arte′riae cer′ebri posterio′ris** [NA], central branches of posterior cerebral artery: they supply the thalamic area and, by way of the choroid branches, the choroid plexuses of the third and lateral ventricles. **r. choroi′deus arte′riae cer′ebri posterio′ris** [NA], choroid branch of posterior cerebral artery: it supplies the choroid plexuses of the third and lateral ventricles. **ra′mi choroi′dei posterio′res arte′riae cer′ebri posterio′ris** [NA], a name applied to the posterior choroidal branches of the posterior cerebral artery when it supplies more than one branch to the choroid plexus. **r. circumflex′us arte′riae corona′riae sinis′trae** [NA], circumflex branch of left coronary artery: it curves around to the back of the left ventricle in the coronary sulcus, supplying the left ventricle and left atrium. **r. circumflex′us fib′ulae arte′riae tibia′lis posterio′ris** [NA], fibular circumflex branch of posterior tibial artery: it winds laterally around the neck of the fibula, helping supply the soleus muscle and contributing to the anastomosis around the knee joint; called also *r. fibularis arteriae tibialis posterioris.* **r. clavicula′ris arte′riae thoracoacromia′lis** [NA], clavicular branch of thoracoacromial artery: a vessel that passes medially to supply the subclavius muscle. **r. coch′leae arte′riae auditi′vae inter′nae,** r. cochleae arteriae labyrinthi. **r. cochlea′ris arte′riae labyrin′thi,** cochlear branch of labyrinthine artery: it supplies the cochlea. **ra′mi coeli′aci plex′us gas′trici posterio′ris,** rami celiaci nervi vagi. **r. collatera′lis arteria′rum intercosta′lium posterio′rum [III–XI]** [NA], collateral branch of posterior intercostal arteries [III–XI]: a branch helping supply the thoracic wall, arising from the posterior intercostal arteries near the angle of the rib and running forward in the lower part of the corresponding intercostal space. **r. col′li ner′vi facia′lis** [NA], cervical branch of facial nerve: it lies deep to and innervates the platysma muscle; modality, motor. **r. commu′nicans,** 1. [NA] a communicating branch between two nerves. 2. a branch connecting two arteries. **r. commu′nicans arte′riae perone′ae** [NA], communicating branch of peroneal artery: a communicating branch between the peroneal and the posterior tibial arteries, distributed to the interosseous membrane and supramalleolar region. **r. commu′nicans gan′glii cilia′ris cum ner′vo nasocilia′ri** [NA], communicating branch of ciliary ganglion with nasociliary nerve: a branch or branches carrying sensory fibers from the cornea, iris, ciliary body, and choroid, and passing through the ciliary ganglion to the nasociliary nerve. Called also *sensory root of ciliary ganglion.* **r. commu′nicans gan′glii o′tici cum chor′da tym′pani** [NA], communicating branch of otic ganglion with chorda tympani: a small branch that interconnects the otic ganglion and the chorda tympani; called also *r. anastomoticus ganglii otici cum chorda tympani.* **r. commu′nicans gan′glii o′tici cum ner′vo auriculotempora′li** [NA], communicating branch of otic ganglion with auriculotemporal nerve: a branch carrying postganglionic parasympathetic fibers from the otic ganglion to the auriculotemporal nerve for distribution to the parotid gland; called also *r. anastomoticus ganglii otici cum nervo auriculotemporali.* **r. commu′nicans gan′glii o′tici cum ra′mo menin′geo ner′vi mandibula′ris** [NA], communicating branch of otic ganglion with meningeal branch of mandibular nerve: a branch that carries autonomic fibers destined for the meninges from the otic ganglion to the meningeal branch of the mandibular nerve; called also *r. anastomoticus ganglii otici cum ramo meningeo nervi mandibularis.* **ra′mi communican′tes gan′glii submandibula′ris cum ner′vo lingua′li** [NA], **ra′mi communican′tes gan′glii submaxilla′ris cum ner′vo lingua′li,** communicating branches of submandibular ganglion with lingual nerve: branches which interconnect the lingual nerve and the submandibular ganglion, and by which the ganglion is suspended from the nerve; they carry preganglionic fibers that derive from the chorda tympani and synapse in the submandibular ganglion, and postganglionic fibers. Called also *motor root(s) of submandibular ganglion.* **ra′mi communican′tes ner′vi auriculotempora′lis cum ner′vo facia′li** [NA], communicating branches of auriculotemporal nerve with facial nerve: branches containing sensory fibers from the auriculotemporal nerve that join the facial nerve within the parotid gland, to be distributed with branches of the latter; called also *rami anastomotici nervi auriculotemporalis cum nervo faciali.* **r. commu′nicans ner′vi facia′-**

lis cum ner′vo glossopharyn′geo [NA], communicating branch of facial nerve with glossopharyngeal nerve: a branch that interconnects the glossopharyngeal nerve and the facial nerve after emergence of the latter from the stylomastoid foramen; called also *r. anastomoticus nervi facialis cum nervo glossopharyngeo.* **r. commu′nicans ner′vi facia′lis cum plex′u tympan′ico** [NA], communicating branch of facial nerve with tympanic plexus: a branch that interconnects the facial nerve and the tympanic plexus of the glossopharyngeal nerve; called also *r. anastomoticus nervi facialis cum plexu tympanico.* **r. commu′nicans ner′vi glossopharyn′gei cum ra′mo auricula′ri ner′vi va′gi** [NA], communicating branch of glossopharyngeal nerve with auricular branch of vagus nerve: a small branch connecting the glossopharyngeal nerve with the auricular branch of the vagus nerve; called also *r. anastomoticus nervi glossopharyngei cum ramo auriculari nervi vagi.* **r. commu′nicans ner′vi lacrima′lis cum ner′vo zygomat′ico** [NA], communicating branch of lacrimal nerve with zygomatic nerve: a branch that carries parasympathetic postganglionic fibers originating in the pterygopalatine ganglion and destined for the lacrimal gland; called also *r. anastomoticus nervi lacrimalis cum nervo zygomatico.* **r. commu′nicans ner′vi laryn′gei inferio′ris cum ra′mo laryn′geo inter′no** [NA], communicating branch of inferior laryngeal nerve with internal laryngeal branch: a small branch interconnecting the inferior laryngeal nerve with the internal branch of the superior laryngeal nerve, behind or in the posterior cricoarytenoid muscle. **r. commu′nicans ner′vi laryn′gei recurren′tis cum ra′mo laryn′geo inter′no,** r. communicans nervi laryngei inferioris cum ramo laryngeo interno. **r. commu′nicans ner′vi laryn′gei superio′ris cum ner′vo laryn′geo inferio′re** [NA], communicating branch of superior laryngeal nerve with inferior laryngeal nerve: a small branch interconnecting the internal branch of the superior laryngeal nerve with the inferior laryngeal nerve, behind or in the posterior cricoarytenoid muscle; called also *r. anastomoticus nervi laryngei superioris cum nervo laryngeo inferiore.* **r. commu′nicans ner′vi lingua′lis cum chor′da tym′pani** [NA], communicating branch of lingual nerve with chorda tympani: the chorda tympani as it joins the lingual nerve in the infratemporal fossa medial to the lateral pterygoid muscle; modality, parasympathetic and special sensory. **ra′mi communican′tes ner′vi lingua′lis cum ner′vo hypoglos′so** [NA], communicating branches of lingual nerve with hypoglossal nerve: plexiform terminal branches interconnecting the lingual and hypoglossal nerves just in front of the hyoglossus muscle; called also *rami anastomotici nervi lingualis cum nervo hypoglosso.* **r. commu′nicans ner′vi media′ni cum ner′vo ulna′ri** [NA], communicating branch of median nerve with ulnar nerve: a small branch across the flexor digitorum profundus muscle, connecting the median with the ulnar nerve; called also *r. anastomoticus nervi mediani cum nervo ulnari.* **r. commu′nicans ner′vi nasocilia′ris cum ganglio′ne cilia′ri** [NA], communicating branch of nasociliary nerve with ciliary ganglion: a branch or branches carrying sensory fibers from the cornea, iris, ciliary body, and choroid, and passing through the ciliary ganglion to the nasociliary nerve; called also *radix longa ganglii ciliaris.* **ra′mi communican′tes ner′vo′rum spina′lium** [NA], communicating branches of spinal nerves: branches connecting spinal nerves with sympathetic ganglia, each spinal nerve receiving a gray communicating ramus, and the thoracic and upper lumbar spinal nerves having in addition a white communicating ramus. **r. commu′nicans ner′vi va′gi cum ner′vo glossopharyn′geo** [NA], communicating branch of vagus nerve with glossopharyngeal nerve: a small branch connecting the auricular branch of the vagus nerve with the glossopharyngeal nerve; called also *r. anastomoticus nervi vagi cum nervo glossopharyngeo.* **r. commu′nicans perone′us ner′vi perone′i commu′nis** [NA], peroneal communicating branch of common peroneal nerve: a small branch arising from the common peroneal nerve either with the lateral sural cutaneous nerve or separately; distally it joins the medial sural cutaneous to form the sural nerve; called also *r. anastomoticus peronaeus nervi peronaei communis.* **r. commu′nicans ulna′ris ner′vi radia′lis** [NA], ulnar communicating branch of radial nerve: a small branch in the hand that interconnects the most medial dorsal digital nerve from the superficial branch of the radial nerve with the adjacent most lateral dorsal digital nerve from the dorsal branch of the ulnar nerve; called also *r. anastomoticus ulnaris nervi radialis.* **ra′mi cortica′les arte′riae cer′ebri anterio′ris** [NA], cortical branches of anterior cerebral artery: orbital, frontal, and parietal branches of the anterior cerebral artery that supply the cortex of the frontal and parietal lobes. **ra′mi cortica′les arte′riae cer′ebri me′diae** [NA], cortical branches of middle cerebral artery: orbital, frontal, temporal, and parietal branches from the middle cerebral artery, distributed to the cortex over the insula and the lateral surface of the hemisphere. **ra′mi cortica′les arte′riae cer′ebri posterio′ris** [NA], cortical branches of posterior cerebral artery: temporal, occipital, and parieto-occipital branches from the posterior cerebral artery, distributed to the cortex of the inferior and medial surfaces of the temporal and occipital lobes. **r. costa′lis latera′lis arte′riae mamma′riae inter′nae,**

r. costalis lateralis arteriae thoracicae internae. **r. costa′lis latera′lis arte′riae thora′cicae inter′nae** [NA], lateral costal branch of internal thoracic artery: an occasional branch passing inferolaterally behind the ribs, supplying ribs and costal cartilages, and anastomosing with the posterior intercostal arteries. **r. cricothyroi′deus arte′riae thyroi′deae superio′ris** [NA], cricothyroid branch of superior thyroid artery: a vessel running medially over the cricothyroid muscle, toward the cricothyroid ligament, and anastomosing with its fellow of the opposite side. **ra′mi cuta′nei anterio′res ner′vi femora′lis** [NA], anterior cutaneous branches of femoral nerve: they innervate the skin on the front and medial aspect of the thigh and patella and contribute to the subsartorial and patellar plexuses; modality, general sensory. **r. cuta′neus ante′rior ner′vi iliohypogas′trici** [NA], anterior cutaneous branch of iliohypogastric nerve: it runs forward between the internal and external oblique muscles and innervates the skin over the pubis; modality, general sensory. **r. cuta′neus ante′rior [pectora′lis et abdomina′lis] nervo′rum intercosta′lium** [NA], a branch arising from the intercostal nerves and helping innervate the skin in the anteromedial thoracic and abdominal regions, with medial mammary branches given off in the breast region; modality, general sensory. **ra′mi cuta′nei anterio′res [pectora′les et abdomina′les] ramo′rum anterio′rum arteria′rum intercosta′lium,** anterior cutaneous branches (thoracic and abdominal) of the anterior branches of the intercostal arteries. **ra′mi cuta′nei arte′riae mamma′riae inter′nae,** cutaneous branches of the internal mammary artery. **ra′mi cuta′nei cru′ris media′les ner′vi saphe′ni** [NA], medial crural cutaneous branches of saphenous nerve: branches distributed by the saphenous nerve to the skin of the medial aspect of the leg; modality, general sensory. **r. cuta′neus latera′lis arteria′rum intercosta′lium posterio′rum [III–XI]** [NA], lateral cutaneous branch of posterior intercostal arteries [III–XI]: a branch arising from the posterior intercostal arteries, supplying the anterolateral thoracic wall. The branches of the third through fifth give off small mammary branches. Called also (pl.) *rami cutanei laterales [pectorales et abdominales] ramorum anteriorum arteriarum intercostalium.* **r. cuta′neus latera′lis ner′vi iliohypogas′trici** [NA], lateral cutaneous branch of iliohypogastric nerve: it is distributed to the skin over the side of the buttock; modality, general sensory. **r. cuta′neus latera′lis [pectora′lis et abdomina′lis] nervo′rum intercosta′lium** [NA], lateral cutaneous branch (thoracic and abdominal) of intercostal nerves: a branch arising from the intercostal nerves, and dividing further into anterior and posterior branches to innervate the skin of the lateral and posterior body wall; modality, general sensory. The branches of the fourth through sixth intercostal nerves give off lateral mammary branches. **ra′mi cuta′nei latera′les [pectora′les et abdomina′les] ramo′rum anterio′rum arteria′rum intercosta′lium,** see *r. cutaneus lateralis arteriarum intercostalium posteriorum [III–XI].* **r. cuta′neus latera′lis ra′mi dorsa′lis arteria′rum intercosta′lium posterio′rum [III–XI]** [NA], lateral cutaneous branch of dorsal branch of posterior intercostal arteries [III–XI]: it supplies the posterolateral aspect of the thorax. The branches of the third through fifth arteries give off small mammary branches. Called also *r. cutaneus lateralis ramorum posteriorum arteriarum intercostalium.* **r. cuta′neus latera′lis ramo′rum dorsa′lium nervo′rum thoracico′rum** [NA], lateral cutaneous branch of dorsal branches of thoracic nerves: the lateral of the two terminal divisions of the dorsal branch of each thoracic nerve; each supplies first the corresponding levator costae muscle, then the longissimus thoracis and iliocostalis thoracis muscles; the lower ones pierce the latissimus dorsi and supply the skin of the back. Called also *r. cutaneus lateralis ramorum posteriorum nervorum thoracalium.* **r. cuta′neus latera′lis ramo′rum posterio′rum arteria′rum intercosta′lium,** r. cutaneus lateralis ramorum dorsalium arteriarum intercostalium posteriorum [III–XI]. **r. cuta′neus latera′lis ramo′rum posterio′rum nervo′rum thoraca′lium,** r. cutaneus lateralis ramorum dorsalium nervorum thoracicorum. **r. cuta′neus media′lis ra′mi dorsa′lis arteria′rum intercosta′lium posterio′rum [III–XI]** [NA], medial cutaneous branch of dorsal branch of posterior intercostal arteries [III–XI]: it supplies the skin adjacent to the vertebral column; called also *r. cutaneus medialis ramorum posteriorum arteriarum intercostalium.* **r. cuta′neus media′lis ramo′rum dorsa′lium nervo′rum thoracico′rum** [NA], medial cutaneous branch of dorsal branches of thoracic nerves: the medial of the two terminal divisions of the dorsal branch of a thoracic nerve; those of the upper nerves supplying the skin of the back, and those of the lower ones chiefly supplying the erector spinae muscle. Both groups supply adjacent periosteum, ligaments, and joints. Called also *r. cutaneus medialis ramorum posteriorum nervorum thoracalium.* **r. cuta′neus media′lis ramo′rum posterio′rum arteria′rum intercosta′lium,** r. cutaneus medialis rami dorsalis arteriarum intercostalium posteriorum [III–XI]. **r. cuta′neus media′lis ramo′rum posterio′rum nervo′rum thoraca′lium,** r. cutaneus medialis ramorum dorsalium nervorum thoracicorum. **r. cuta′neus ner′vi obturato′rii**

[NA], cutaneous branch of obturator nerve: a variable branch arising from the anterior branch of the obturator nerve, forming part of the subsartorial plexus, and supplying the skin of the medial aspect of the thigh and leg; modality, general sensory. **r. cuta′neus palma′ris ner′vi ulna′ris,** r. palmaris nervi ulnaris. **r. deltoi′deus arte′riae profun′dae bra′chii** [NA], deltoid branch of deep brachial artery: it is distributed to the brachialis and deltoid muscles and anastomoses with the posterior circumflex humeral artery; called also *deltoid artery.* **r. deltoi′deus arte′riae thoracoacromia′lis** [NA], deltoid branch of thoracoacromial artery: a branch of the thoracoacromial artery descending with the cephalic vein and helping to supply the deltoid and pectoralis major muscles. **ra′mi denta′les arte′riae alveola′ris inferio′ris** [NA], dental branches of inferior alveolar artery: branches arising from the inferior alveolar artery in the mandibular canal and supplying the inferior teeth. **ra′mi denta′les arteria′rum alveola′rium superio′rum anterio′rum** [NA], dental branches of anterior superior alveolar arteries: they supply the incisor and canine teeth. **ra′mi denta′les arte′riae alveola′ris superio′ris posterio′ris** [NA], dental branches of posterior superior alveolar artery: they supply the molar and premolar teeth. **ra′mi denta′les inferio′res plex′us denta′lis inferio′ris** [NA], inferior dental branches of inferior dental plexus: they supply the lower teeth; modality, general sensory. **ra′mi denta′les superio′res plex′us denta′lis superio′ris** [NA], superior dental branches of superior dental plexus: they innervate the teeth of the upper jaw; modality, general sensory. **r. descen′dens ante′rior arte′riae corona′riae [cor′dis] sinis′trae,** r. interventricularis anterior arteriae coronariae sinistrae. **r. descen′dens arte′riae circumflex′ae fem′oris latera′lis** [NA], descending branch of lateral circumflex femoral artery: a branch passing from the lateral circumflex artery (sometimes directly from the deep femoral) to the knee, and supplying the thigh muscles. **r. descen′dens arte′riae occipita′lis** [NA], descending branch of occipital artery: a branch that arises from the occipital artery on the obliquus capitis superior muscle and divides into superficial and deep branches, supplying the trapezius and deep neck muscles. **r. descen′dens arte′riae transver′sae col′li,** r. profundus arteriae transversae colli. **r. descen′dens ner′vi hypoglos′si,** radix superior ansae cervicalis. **r. descen′dens poste′rior arte′riae corona′riae [cor′dis] dex′trae,** r. interventricularis posterior arteriae coronariae dextrae. **r. dex′ter arte′riae hepat′icae pro′priae** [NA], right branch of proper hepatic artery: the right of the two branches into which the proper hepatic artery normally divides; it supplies the right lobe of the liver and a branch, the cystic artery, to the gallbladder. **r. dex′ter arte′riae pulmona′lis,** arteria pulmonalis dextra. **r. dex′ter ve′nae por′tae** [NA], the right branch of the portal vein, distributed to the right lobe of the liver. **r. digas′tricus ner′vi facia′lis** [NA], digastric branch of facial nerve: a branch that innervates the posterior belly of the digastric muscle; modality, motor; called also *digastric nerve.* **r. dorsa′lis arteria′rum intercosta′lium posterio′rum [III–XI]** [NA], dorsal branch of posterior intercostal arteries: a branch arising from a posterior intercostal artery, passing backward with the dorsal branch of the corresponding intercostal nerve to supply the posterior thoracic wall; it has a spinal branch and a medial and a lateral cutaneous branch. Called also (pl.) *rami posteriores arteriarum intercostalium.* **ra′mi dorsa′les arte′riae intercosta′lis supre′mae** [NA], dorsal branches of highest intercostal artery: the dorsal branches arising from the first two posterior intercostal arteries, which stem from the highest intercostal artery. Their distribution is similar to that of the other posterior intercostals; see *ramus dorsalis arteriarum intercostalium posteriorum.* **r. dorsa′lis arteria′rum lumba′lium** [NA], dorsal branch of lumbar arteries: the larger of the two branches into which each lumbar artery (four or five) divides; it supplies lumbar back muscles and gives off a spinal branch. **r. dorsa′lis arte′riae subcosta′lis** [NA], dorsal branch of subcostal artery: a branch supplying back muscles, its distribution being similar to that of the dorsal branches of the lower posterior intercostal arteries. **ra′mi dorsa′les lin′guae arte′riae lingua′lis** [NA], dorsal lingual branches of lingual artery: branches of the lingual artery arising beneath the hyoglossus muscle and supplying the tonsil and the back of the tongue. **r. dorsa′lis ma′nus ner′vi ulna′ris,** r. dorsalis nervi ulnaris. **ra′mi dorsa′les nervo′rum cervica′lium** [NA], the dorsal branches of the eight cervical spinal nerves; called also *rami posteriores nervorum cervicalium.* **r. dorsa′lis ner′vi coccyg′ei** [NA], dorsal branch of coccygeal nerve: the dorsal branch of the last spinal nerve, which helps innervate the skin over the coccyx; called also *r. posterior nervi coccygei.* **ra′mi dorsa′les nervo′rum lumba′lium** [NA], the dorsal branches of the five lumbar spinal nerves; called also *rami posteriores nervorum lumbalium.* **ra′mi dorsa′les nervo′rum sacra′lium** [NA], the dorsal branches of the five sacral spinal nerves, which emerge from the sacrum through the dorsal sacral foramina; called also *rami posteriores nervorum sacralium.* **r. dorsa′lis nervo′rum spina′lium** [NA], dorsal branch of spinal nerves: the smaller of the two chief branches into which each spinal nerve divides almost

as soon as it emerges from the intervertebral foramen. The dorsal branches supply the skin, muscles, joints, and bone of the dorsal part of the neck and trunk. Commonly each branch divides into a medial and a lateral portion. Called also *r. posterior nervorum spinalium.* **ra′mi dorsa′les nervo′rum thoracico′rum** [NA], the dorsal branches of the twelve thoracic spinal nerves; called also *rami posteriores nervorum thoracalium.* **r. dorsa′lis ner′vi ulna′ris** [NA], dorsal branch of ulnar nerve: a large cutaneous branch that arises from the ulnar nerve and passes down the distal portion of the forearm to the medial side of the back of the hand, where it divides usually into three, sometimes four, dorsal digital nerves; modality, general sensory. Called also *r. dorsalis manus nervi ulnaris.* **r. dorsa′lis vena′rum intercosta′lium,** r. dorsalis venarum intercostalium posteriorum [IV–XI]. **r. dorsa′lis vena′rum intercosta′lium posterio′rum [IV–XI]** [NA], the dorsal branch of the posterior intercostal veins, corresponding to the dorsal branch of the posterior intercostal arteries. **ra′mi duodena′les arte′riae pancreaticoduodena′lis superio′ris** [NA], duodenal branches of superior pancreaticoduodenal artery: vessels supplying the duodenum. **ra′mi epiplo′ici arte′riae gastroepiplo′icae dex′trae** [NA], epiploic branches of right gastroepiploic artery: vessels that supply the greater omentum. **ra′mi esopha′gei aor′tae thora′cicae** [NA], esophageal branches of thoracic aorta: branches, usually two, that arise from the front of the aorta to supply the esophagus; called also *arteriae oesophageae* or *esophageal arteries.* **ra′mi esopha′gei arte′riae gas′tricae sinis′trae** [NA], esophageal branches of left gastric artery: vessels that supply the esophagus. **ra′mi esopha′gei arte′riae thyroi′deae inferio′ris** [NA], esophageal branches of inferior thyroid artery: vessels supplying the esophagus. **ra′mi esopha′gei ner′vi laryn′gei recurren′tis** [NA], esophageal branches of recurrent laryngeal nerve: branches of the recurrent laryngeal nerve that help innervate the esophagus; modality, visceral afferent and general sensory. **r. exter′nus ner′vi accesso′rii** [NA], external branch of accessory nerve: the branch of the eleventh cranial nerve that originates from the spinal roots of the nerve; it supplies the sternomastoid and trapezius muscles. **r. exter′nus ner′vi laryn′gei superio′ris** [NA], external branch of superior laryngeal nerve: the smaller of the two branches into which the superior laryngeal nerve divides, descending under cover of the sternothyroid muscle and innervating the cricothyroid and the inferior constrictor of the pharynx; modality, motor. **r. femora′lis ner′vi genitofemora′lis** [NA], femoral branch of genitofemoral nerve: a branch arising by division of the genitofemoral nerve above the inguinal ligament; entering the femoral sheath, it turns forward and supplies the skin of the femoral triangle; modality, general sensory. Called also *nervus lumboinguinalis.* **r. fibula′ris arte′riae tibia′lis posterio′ris,** r. circumflexus fibulae arteriae tibialis posterioris. **ra′mi fronta′les arte′riae cer′ebri anterio′ris** [NA], frontal branches of anterior cerebral artery: branches of the anterior cerebral artery that supply the cortex of the frontal lobe on the median and superior surfaces and the superior part of the lateral surface. **ra′mi fronta′les arte′riae cer′ebri me′diae** [NA], frontal branches of middle cerebral artery: branches of the middle cerebral artery that supply the cortex of the frontal lobe on the lateral surface. **r. fronta′lis arte′riae menin′geae me′diae** [NA], frontal branch of middle meningeal artery: a branch lodged in grooves on the sphenoid and parietal bones, and supplying the dura mater of the front of the brain. A part of it is sometimes enclosed in a bony canal. **r. fronta′lis arte′riae tempora′lis superficia′lis** [NA], frontal branch of superficial temporal artery: a tortuous terminal branch that supplies the forehead and frontal scalp. **r. fronta′lis ner′vi fronta′lis,** the frontal branch of the frontal nerve. **ra′mi gas′trici anterio′res ner′vi va′gi** [NA], anterior gastric branches of vagus nerve: branches arising from the anterior trunk of the vagus near the cardiac end of the stomach, innervating the anterior aspect of the lesser curvature and the anterior surface of the stomach almost to the pylorus; modality, parasympathetic and visceral afferent. Called also *plexus gastricus anterior.* **ra′mi gas′trici ner′vi va′gi,** see *rami gastrici anteriores nervi vagi* and *rami gastrici posteriores nervi vagi.* **ra′mi gas′trici posterio′res ner′vi va′gi** [NA], posterior gastric branches of vagus nerve: branches arising from the posterior vagal trunk near the cardiac end of the stomach, and innervating the cardiac orifice and fundus, the posterior aspect of the lesser curvature, and the posterior surface of the stomach to the pyloric antrum; modality, parasympathetic and visceral afferent. Called also *plexus gastricus posterior.* **r. genita′lis ner′vi genitofemora′lis** [NA], genital branch of genitofemoral nerve: a branch arising from the genitofemoral nerve above the inguinal ligament; entering the inguinal canal through the deep ring, it supplies the cremaster and continues to the skin of the scrotum or of the labium majus, and that of the adjacent area of the thigh; modality, general sensory and motor. Called also *nervus supermaticus externus.* **ra′mi gingiva′les inferio′res plex′us denta′lis inferio′ris** [NA], inferior gingival branches of inferior dental plexus: branches originating from the inferior dental plexus and innervating the gingivae of the lower jaw; modality, general sensory. **ra′mi gingiva′les su-**

perio′res plex′us denta′lis superio′ris [NA], superior gingival branches of superior dental plexus: branches arising from the superior dental plexus and innervating the gingivae of the upper jaw; modality, general sensory. **ra′mi glandula′res arte′riae facia′lis** [NA], **ra′mi glandula′res arte′riae maxilla′ris exter′nae,** glandular branches of facial artery: branches given off to the submandibular gland by the facial artery as it passes over the lateral surface of the gland. **ra′mi glandula′res arte′riae thyreoi′deae inferio′ris,** glandular branches of the inferior thyroid artery. **ra′mi glandula′res arte′riae thyreoi′deae superio′ris,** glandular branches of the superior thyroid artery. **ra′mi glandula′res gan′glii submandibula′ris** [NA], glandular branches of submandibular ganglion: short branches running from the submandibular ganglion to innervate the submandibular gland, bearing postganglionic parasympathetic (secretory) fibers from this ganglion and sympathetic fibers that are postganglionic from the superior cervical ganglion. Called also *rami submaxillares ganglii submaxillaris* and *submaxillary nerves.* **ra′mi hepat′ici ner′vi va′gi** [NA], hepatic branches of vagus nerve: branches (sometimes only one) arising from the anterior vagal trunk, contributing to the hepatic plexus, and helping innervate the liver, gallbladder, pancreas, pylorus, and duodenum; modality, parasympathetic and visceral afferent. **r. hyoi′deus arte′riae lingua′lis,** r. suprahyoideus arteriae lingualis. **r. hyoi′deus arte′riae thyreoi′deae superio′ris,** r. infrahyoideus arteriae thyroideae superioris. **r. ili′acus arte′riae iliolumba′lis** [NA], iliac branch of iliolumbar artery: one of the two branches into which the iliolumbar artery divides in the iliac fossa; it supplies the iliacus muscle and sends a large nutrient branch to the ilium. **r. infe′rior arte′riae glu′teae superio′ris** [NA], inferior branch of superior gluteal artery: the lower division of the deep branch of the superior gluteal artery, accompanied by the superior gluteal artery, accompanied by the superior gluteal nerve and helping supply the gluteus medius, gluteus minimus, and tensor fasciae latae muscles and the hip joint and ilium. **ra′mi inferio′res ner′vi cuta′nei col′li,** rami inferiores nervi transversi colli. **r. infe′rior ner′vi oculomoto′rii** [NA], inferior branch of oculomotor nerve: the branch of the oculomotor nerve that innervates the medial and inferior rectus and inferior oblique muscles of the eyeball and, via the motor root of the ciliary ganglion and then the short ciliary nerves, supplies the sphincter pupillae and ciliary muscles; modality, motor and parasympathetic. **ra′mi inferio′res ner′vi transver′si col′li** [NA], inferior branches of transverse nerve of neck: the more inferior of the branches that arise from the transverse cervical nerve near the anterior border of the sternocleidomastoid muscle, innervating skin and subcutaneous tissue in the anterior cervical region; modality, general sensory. Called also *rami inferiores nervi cutanei colli.* **r. infe′rior os′sis is′chii,** r. ossis ischii. **r. infe′rior os′sis pu′bis** [NA], **inferior r. of pubis,** the short flattened bar of bone that projects from the body of the pubic bone in a posteroinferolateral direction to meet the ramus of the ischium. **r. infrahyoi′deus arte′riae thyroi′deae superio′ris** [NA], infrahyoid branch of superior thyroid artery: a vessel running along the inferior border of the hyoid bone, supplying the infrahyoid region, and anastomosing with its fellow of the opposite side; called also *r. hyoideus arteriae thyreoideae superioris.* **r. infrapatella′ris ner′vi saphe′ni** [NA], infrapatellar branch of saphenous nerve: a branch running inferolaterally from the saphenous nerve to the patellar plexus; modality, general sensory. **ra′mi inguina′les arte′riae femora′lis** [NA], inguinal branches of femoral artery: branches arising from the external pudendal arteries and supplying the inguinal region. **ra′mi intercosta′les anterio′res arte′riae thora′cicae inter′nae** [NA], **ra′mi intercosta′les arte′riae mamma′riae inter′nae,** anterior intercostal branches of internal thoracic artery: twelve branches, two in each of the upper six intercostal spaces, that supply the intercostal spaces and the pectoralis major muscle. Within each space both branches run laterally, the upper anastomosing with the posterior intercostal artery, the lower with the collateral branch of that artery. **r. interfunicula′ris** (*obs.*), a branch connecting the two trunks of the sympathetic nervous system. **ra′mi intergangliona′res** [NA], interganglionic branches: the branches that interconnect the ganglia of the sympathetic trunk. **r. inter′nus ner′vi accesso′rii** [NA], internal branch of accessory nerve: the branch that continues from the cranial roots of the nerve, carrying motor fibers that are distributed by branches of the vagus to the soft palate, pharyngeal constrictors, and larynx. **r. inter′nus ner′vi laryn′gei superio′ris** [NA], internal branch of superior laryngeal nerve: the larger of the two branches of the superior laryngeal nerve, which innervates the mucosa of the epiglottis, base of the tongue, and larynx; modality, general sensory. **r. interventricula′ris ante′rior arte′riae corona′riae sinis′trae** [NA], anterior interventricular branch of left coronary artery: the branch of the left coronary artery that runs to the apex of the heart in the anterior interventricular sulcus, supplying the ventricles and most of the interventricular septum; called also *r. descendens anterior arteriae coronariae* [*cordis*] *sinistrae.* **r. interventricula′ris poste′rior arte′riae corona′riae dex′trae**

[NA], posterior interventricular branch of right coronary artery: a branch running toward the apex of the heart in the posterior interventricular sulcus, supplying the diaphragmatic surface of the ventricles and part of the interventricular septum. Called also *r. descendens posterior arteriae coronariae* [*cordis*] *dextrae.* **r. of ischium,** r. ossis ischii. **ra′mi isth′mi fau′cium ner′vi lingua′lis** [NA], branches from the lingual nerve to the isthmus of the fauces; modality, general sensory. **r. of jaw,** r. mandibulae. **ra′mi labia′les anterio′res arte′riae femora′lis** [NA], anterior labial branches of femoral artery: branches that arise from the external pudendal arteries and supply the labium majus; called also *arteriae labiales anteriores vulvae.* **ra′mi labia′les inferio′res ner′vi menta′lis** [NA], inferior labial branches of mental nerve: branches of the mental nerve that innervate the lower lip; modality, general sensory. **ra′mi labia′les posterio′res arte′riae puden′dae inter′nae** [NA], posterior labial branches of internal pudendal artery: two branches arising from the internal pudendal artery in the anterior part of the ischiorectal fossa, helping to supply the ischiocavernosus and bulbospongiosus muscles, and supplying the labium majus and labium minus. Called also *arteriae labiales posteriores vulvae.* **ra′mi labia′les superio′res ner′vi infraorbita′lis** [NA], superior labial branches of infraorbital nerve: branches of the infraorbital nerve that are distributed to mucous membrane of the mouth and skin of the upper lip; modality, general sensory. **ra′mi laryngopharyn′gei gan′glii cervica′lis superio′ris** [NA], laryngopharyngeal branches of superior cervical ganglion: branches from the superior cervical ganglion to the larynx and walls of the pharynx; modality, sympathetic. **r. latera′lis duc′tus hepat′ici sinis′tri** [NA], the lateral branch of the left hepatic duct. **r. latera′lis ner′vi supraorbita′lis** [NA], lateral branch of supraorbital nerve: a branch of the supraorbital nerve that supplies the frontal sinus, upper eyelid, and skin and subcutaneous tissue of the forehead and scalp laterally as far as the temporal region; modality, general sensory. **r. latera′lis ramo′rum dorsa′lium nervo′rum cervica′lium** [NA], lateral branch of dorsal branches of cervical nerves: the lateral branch that arises from the dorsal branch of each of the eight cervical nerves, supplying adjacent muscles; called also *r. lateralis ramorum posteriorum nervorum cervicalium.* **r. latera′lis ramo′rum dorsa′lium nervo′rum lumba′lium** [NA], lateral branch of dorsal branches of lumbar nerves: the branch that runs inferolaterally from the dorsal branch of each lumbar nerve, innervating adjacent muscle; the upper of these branches terminally constitute the superior cluneal nerves, supplying skin of the buttock. Called also *r. lateralis ramorum posteriorum nervorum lumbalium.* **r. latera′lis ramo′rum dorsa′lium nervo′rum sacra′lium** [NA], lateral branch of dorsal branches of sacral nerves: the lateral branch that arises from the dorsal branch of each of the three upper sacral nerves; called also *r. lateralis ramorum posteriorum nervorum sacralium.* **r. latera′lis ramo′rum posterio′rum nervo′rum cervica′lium,** r. lateralis ramorum dorsalium nervorum cervicalium. **r. latera′lis ramo′rum posterio′rum nervo′rum lumba′lium,** r. lateralis ramorum dorsalium nervorum lumbalium. **r. latera′lis ramo′rum posterio′rum nervo′rum sacra′lium,** r. lateralis ramorum dorsalium nervorum sacralium. **ra′mi liena′les arte′riae liena′lis** [NA], splenic branches of splenic artery: the terminal branches of the splenic artery, which follow the trabeculae. **ra′mi liena′les plex′us coeli′aci,** splenic branches of celiac plexus. **r. lingua′lis ner′vi facia′lis** [NA], lingual branch of facial nerve: an inconstant branch of the facial nerve sometimes arising together with the stylohyoid branch, and helping to supply the styloglossal and glossopalatine muscles; modality, motor. **ra′mi lingua′les ner′vi glossopharyn′gei** [NA], lingual branches of glossopharyngeal nerve: branches of the glossopharyngeal nerve that innervate the posterior third of the tongue; modality, general and special sensory. **ra′mi lingua′les ner′vi hypoglos′si** [NA], lingual branches of hypoglossal nerve: branches of the hypoglossal nerve that innervate the intrinsic and extrinsic muscles of the tongue; modality, motor. **ra′mi lingua′les ner′vi lingua′lis** [NA], lingual branches of lingual nerve: branches that innervate the anterior two-thirds of the tongue, adjacent areas of the mouth, and the gums; modality, general and special sensory. **r. lumba′lis arte′riae iliolumba′lis** [NA], lumbar branch of iliolumbar artery: a branch that arises from the iliolumbar artery in the iliac fossa and ascends to supply the psoas and quadratus lumborum muscles, sending a spinal branch through the intervertebral foramen just above the sacrum. **ra′mi malleola′res latera′les arte′riae perone′ae** [NA], lateral malleolar branches of peroneal artery: vessels supplying the lateral aspect of the ankle and giving off calcaneal branches to the lateral aspect and back of the heel; called also *arteria malleolaris posterior lateralis.* **ra′mi malleola′res media′les arte′riae tibia′les posterioris** [NA], medial malleolar branches of posterior tibial artery: vessels supplying the area of the medial malleolus and giving off calcaneal branches to the medial aspect and back of the heel; called also *arteria malleolaris posterior medialis.* **ra′mi mamma′rii arte′riae mamma′riae inter′nae,** rami mammarii arteriae thoracicae internae. **ra′mi mamma′rii arte′riae thora′ciae inter′nae** [NA], mammary branches of internal thoracic artery: branches arising from the second, third, and fourth perforating branches of the internal thoracic artery and helping to supply the mammary gland. **ra′mi mamma′rii exter′ni arte′riae thoraca′- lis latera′lis**, rami mammarii laterales arteriae thoracicae lateralis. **ra′mi mamma′rii latera′les arte′riae thora′cicae latera′lis** [NA], lateral mammary branches of lateral thoracic artery: they supply the mammary gland. **r. mamma′rii latera′les ramo′rum anterio′rum arteria′rum intercosta′lium**, lateral mammary branches of anterior branches of intercostal arteries. **ra′mi mamma′rii latera′les ramo′rum cutaneo′rum latera′lium nervo′rum intercosta′lium** [NA], lateral mammary branches of lateral cutaneous branches of intercostal nerves: branches given to the lateral part of the mammary gland by lateral cutaneous branches of intercostal nerves; modality, general sensory. **r. mamma′rii media′les arteria′rum intercosta′lium**, medial mammary branches of the intercostal arteries. **ra′mi mamma′rii media′les ramo′rum cutaneo′rum anterio′rum nervo′rum intercosta′lium** [NA], medial mammary branches of anterior cutaneous branches of intercostal nerves: branches given to the medial part of the mammary gland by anterior cutaneous branches of intercostal nerves; modality, general sensory. **ra′mi mamma′rii ra′mi cuta′nei latera′lis arteria′rum intercosta′lium posterio′rum** [NA], mammary branches of lateral cutaneous branch of posterior intercostal arteries: branches arising from the lateral cutaneous branches of the third through fifth posterior intercostal arteries and supplying the mammary region. **r. of mandible, r. mandib′ulae** [NA], a quadrilateral process projecting superiorly from the posterior part of either side of the mandible. **r. margina′lis mandib′ulae ner′vi facia′lis** [NA], marginal mandibular branch of facial nerve: a branch of the facial nerve that runs forward from the front of the parotid gland along the border of the mandible, deep to the platysma and depressor anguli oris muscles, supplying the latter and the risorius, depressor labii inferioris, and mentalis muscles; modality, motor. **ra′mi mastoi′dei arte′riae auricula′ris posterio′ris** [NA], mastoid branches of posterior auricular artery: they supply the mastoid cells. **r. mastoi′deus arte′riae occipita′lis** [NA], mastoid branch of occipital artery: it enters the cranial cavity through the mastoid foramen and supplies the dura mater, diploe, and mastoid cells. **r. media′lis duc′tus hepat′ici sinis′- tri** [NA], the medial branch of the left hepatic duct. **r. media′lis ner′vi supraorbita′lis** [NA], medial branch of supraorbital nerve: it supplies the frontal sinus, upper eyelid, and skin and subcutaneous tissue of the forehead and scalp as far back as the parietal bone; modality, general sensory. **r. media′lis ramo′rum dorsa′lium nervo′rum cervica′lium** [NA], medial branch of dorsal branches of cervical nerves: the medial branch arising from the dorsal branch of each of the eight cervical nerves, supplying muscle, periosteum, ligaments, and joints; also, except for those of the first, and generally the sixth, seventh, and eighth cervical nerves, having an eventual cutaneous distribution. Called also *r. medialis ramorum posteriorum nervorum cervicalium.* **r. media′lis ramo′rum dorsa′lium nervo′rum lumba′lium** [NA], medial branch of dorsal branches of lumbar nerves: the medial branch that arises from the dorsal branch of each lumbar nerve, mainly innervating deep muscle, but also helping supply ligaments, periosteum, and joints; called also *r. medialis ramorum posteriorum nervorum lumbalium.* **r. media′lis ramo′rum dorsa′lium nervo′rum sacra′lium** [NA], medial branch of dorsal branches of sacral nerves: the medial branch that arises from the dorsal branch of each of the upper three sacral nerves; called also *r. medialis ramorum posteriorum nervorum sacralium.* **r. media′lis ramo′rum posterio′rum nervo′rum cervica′lium**, r. medialis ramorum dorsalium nervorum cervicalium. **r. media′lis ramo′rum posterio′rum nervo′rum lumba′lium**, r. medialis ramorum dorsalium nervorum lumbalium. **r. media′lis ramo′rum posterio′rum nervo′rum sacra′lium**, r. medialis ramorum dorsalium nervorum sacralium. **ra′mi mediastina′les aor′tae thoraca′lis, ra′mi mediastina′les aor′tae thora′cicae** [NA], mediastinal branches of thoracic aorta: small vessels supplying connective tissue and lymph nodes in the posterior mediastinum. **ra′mi mediastina′les arte′riae thora′cicae inter′nae** [NA], mediastinal branches of internal thoracic artery: they supply areolar tissue, pericardium, lymph nodes, and the thymus in the anterior and superior mediastina; called also *arteriae mediastinales anteriores.* **r. membra′nae tym′pani ner′vi auriculotempora′lis** [NA], branch to tympanic membrane of auriculotemporal nerve: a branch given to the tympanic membrane by the nerve of the external acoustic meatus, a branch of the auriculotemporal nerve; modality, general sensory. **r. menin′geus accesso′rius arte′riae menin′geae me′diae** [NA], accessory meningeal branch of middle meningeal artery: a branch arising from the middle meningeal artery, or directly from the maxillary artery, and entering the middle cranial fossa through the foramen ovale to supply the trigeminal ganglion, walls of the cavernous sinus, and neighboring dura mater. **r. menin′geus arte′riae oc-**

cipita′lis [NA], meningeal branch of occipital artery: one or more variable branches of the occipital artery that enter the posterior fossa and supply the dura mater. **r. menin′geus arte′riae vertebra′lis** [NA], meningeal branch of vertebral artery: a branch arising from the vertebral artery in the foramen magnum, and ramifying in the posterior cranial fossa to supply the dura mater, including the falx cerebelli, and bone. **r. menin′geus [me′dius] ner′vi maxilla′ris** [NA], middle meningeal branch of maxillary nerve: a branch arising from the maxillary nerve in the middle cranial fossa, accompanying the middle meningeal artery, and supplying the dura mater; modality, general sensory. Called also *nervus meningeus [medius].* **r. menin′geus ner′vi mandibula′ris** [NA], meningeal branch of mandibular nerve: a branch that arises from the trunk of the mandibular nerve, re-enters the cranium through the foramen spinosum, accompanies the middle meningeal artery to supply the dura mater, and also helps innervate the mucous membrane of the mastoid air cells. Called also *nervus spinosus.* **r. menin′geus nervo′rum spina′lium** [NA], meningeal branch of spinal nerves: the small branch of each spinal nerve that re-enters the intervertebral foramen to supply the dura mater, vertebral column, and associated ligaments. **r. menin′geus ner′vi va′gi** [NA], meningeal branch of vagus nerve: a branch that arises in the jugular foramen from the superior ganglion of the vagus nerve, innervating dura mater of the posterior cranial fossa. **ra′mi menta′les ner′vi menta′lis** [NA], mental branches of mental nerve: they innervate the skin of the chin; modality, general sensory. **ra′mi muscula′res** [NA], muscular branches: any branches of a peripheral nerve or vessel that supply muscle, many not being more specifically named. **ra′mi muscula′res ner′vi axilla′ris** [NA], muscular branches of axillary nerve: they innervate the deltoid and teres minor muscles; modality, motor. **ra′mi muscula′res ner′vi femora′lis** [NA], muscular branches of femoral nerve: they innervate the anterior thigh muscles; modality, motor. **ra′mi muscula′res ner′vi fibula′ris profun′di**, NA alternative for *rami musculares nervi peronei profundi.* **ra′mi muscula′res ner′vi fibula′ris superficia′lis**, NA alternative for *rami musculares nervi peronei superficialis.* **ra′mi muscula′res ner′vi iliohypogas′trici**, muscular branches of iliohypogastric nerve; modality, probably sensory except for an occasional motor twig to the pyramidalis. **ra′mi muscula′res ner′vi ilioinguina′lis**, muscular branches of ilioinguinal nerve, probably sensory in nature. **ra′mi muscula′res nervo′rum intercosta′lium**, muscular branches of the intercostal nerves. **ra′mi muscula′res ner′vi ischiad′ici**, muscular branches of the sciatic nerve. **ra′mi muscula′res ner′vi media′ni** [NA], muscular branches of median nerve: they innervate most of the flexor muscles on the front of the forearm and most of the short muscles of the thumb; modality, motor. **ra′mi muscula′res ner′vi musculocuta′nei** [NA], muscular branches of musculocutaneous nerve: they innervate the coracobrachialis, biceps, and brachialis muscles; modality, motor and general sensory. **ra′mi muscula′res ner′vi obturato′rii** [NA], muscular branches of obturator nerve: branches arising from the anterior and posterior rami of the obturator nerve and innervating the obturator externus, gracilis, and adductor muscles, and sometimes the pectineus; modality, motor. **ra′mi muscula′res ner′vi peronae′i commu′nis**, muscular branches of the common peroneal nerve. **ra′mi muscula′res ner′vi perone′i profun′di** [NA], muscular branches of deep peroneal nerve: they innervate the tibialis anterior, extensor hallucis longus, extensor digitorum longus, and peroneus tertius muscles; modality, motor. **ra′mi muscula′res ner′vi perone′i superficia′lis** [NA], muscular branches of superficial peroneal nerve: they innervate the peroneus longus and peroneus brevis muscles; modality, motor; called also *rami musculares nervi fibularis superficialis* [NA alternative]. **ra′mi muscula′res ner′vi radia′lis** [NA], muscular branches of radial nerve: they innervate the triceps, anconeus, brachioradialis, and extensor carpi radialis muscles; a branch to the brachialis muscle is probably sensory; modality, motor and sensory. **ra′mi muscula′res ner′vi tibia′lis** [NA], muscular branches of tibial nerve: they supply muscles of the back of the leg; modality, motor. **ra′mi muscula′res ner′vi ulna′ris** [NA], muscular branches of ulnar nerve: they innervate the flexor carpi ulnaris muscle and the ulnar half of flexor digitorum profundus; modality, motor. **ra′mi muscula′res plex′us lumba′lis**, muscular branches of the lumbar plexus. **r. mus′culi stylopharyn′gei ner′vi glossopharyn′gei** [NA], stylopharyngeal branch of glossopharyngeal nerve: it supplies the stylopharyngeal muscle; modality, motor; called also *r. stylopharyngeus nervi glossopharyngei.* **r. mylohyoi′deus arte′riae alveola′ris inferio′ris** [NA], mylohyoid branch of inferior alveolar nerve: it descends with the mylohyoid nerve in the mylohyoid sulcus to supply the floor of the mouth. **ra′mi nasa′les anterio′res ner′vi ethmoida′lis anterio′ris**, rami nasales nervi ethmoidalis anterioris. **r. nasa′lis exter′nus ner′vi ethmoida′lis anterio′ris** [NA], external nasal branch of anterior ethmoidal nerve: essentially a continuation, or terminal branch, of the anterior ethmoidal nerve, it innervates the skin of the dorsal part of the nose; modality, general sensory. **ra′mi nasa′les exter′ni**

ner′vi infraorbita′lis [NA], external nasal branches of infraorbital nerve: they innervate the skin of the side of the nose; modality, general sensory. **ra′mi nasa′les inter′ni ner′vi ethmoida′lis anterio′ris** [NA], internal nasal branches of anterior ethmoidal nerve: through medial and lateral branches, they innervate the nasal septum and the mucous membrane of the lateral wall of the nasal cavity; modality, general sensory. **ra′mi nasa′les inter′ni ner′vi infraorbita′lis** [NA], internal nasal branches of infraorbital nerve: they innervate the mobile septum of the nose; modality, general sensory. **ra′mi nasa′les latera′les ner′vi ethmoida′lis anterio′ris** [NA], lateral nasal branches of anterior ethmoidal nerve: branches arising from the internal nasal branches of the anterior ethmoidal nerve and innervating the mucosa of the lateral wall of the nasal cavity; modality, general sensory. **ra′mi nasa′les media′les ner′vi ethmoida′lis anterio′ris** [NA], medial nasal branches of anterior ethmoidal nerve: branches arising from the internal nasal branches of the anterior ethmoidal nerve and supplying the nasal septum; modality, general sensory. **ra′mi nasa′les ner′vi ethmoida′lis anterio′ris** [NA], nasal branches of anterior ethmoidal nerve: the internal and external nasal branches of the anterior ethmoidal nerve, and their subdivisions; called also *rami nasales anteriores nervi ethmoidalis anterioris*. **ra′mi nasa′les posterio′res inferio′res [latera′les] gan′glii ptergopalati′ ni** [NA], **ra′mi nasa′les posterio′res inferio′res [latera′les] gan′glii sphenopalati′ni,** [lateral] inferior posterior nasal branches of pterygopalatine ganglion: they are usually branches of the greater palatine nerve and they supply the middle and inferior nasal meatuses and inferior concha; modality, general sensory. **ra′mi nasa′les posterio′res superio′res [latera′les] gan′glii pterygopalati′ni** [NA], **ra′mi nasa′les posterio′res superio′res [latera′les] gan′glii sphenopalati′ni,** [lateral] superior posterior nasal branches of pterygopalatine ganglion: they supply the superior and middle nasal conchae and the posterior ethmoidal sinuses; modality, general sensory. **ra′mi nasa′les posterio′res superio′res media′les gan′glii pterygopalati′ni** [NA], **ra′mi nasa′les posterio′res superio′res media′les gan′glii sphenopalati′ni,** medial superior posterior nasal branches of pterygopalatine ganglion: they are usually branches of the nasopalatine nerve, and they supply the nasal septum; modality, general sensory. **r. obturato′rius arte′riae epigas′tricae inferio′ris** [NA], obturator branch of inferior epigastric artery: a vessel connecting the pubic branches of the inferior epigastric and the obturator arteries. The obturator artery is sometimes replaced by an accessory obturator that arises from the inferior epigastric artery by way of this communication. **r. occipita′lis arte′riae auricula′ris posterio′ris** [NA], occipital branch of posterior auricular artery: it is distributed to the epicranius muscle. **ra′mi occipita′les arte′riae cer′ebri posterio′ris** [NA], occipital branches of posterior cerebral artery: they supply the cortex of the occipital lobe. **ra′mi occipita′les arte′riae occipita′lis** [NA], occipital branches of occipital artery: a medial and a lateral branch of the occipital artery, distributed to the scalp and, through the meningeal branch, to the dura mater. **r. occipita′lis ner′vi auricula′ris posterio′ris** [NA], occipital branch of posterior auricular nerve: a branch supplying the occipital belly of the occipitofrontalis muscle; modality, motor. **ra′mi oesopha′gei arte′riae gas′tricae sinis′trae,** rami esophagei arteriae gastricae sinistrae. **ra′mi oesopha′gei arte′riae thyreoi′deae inferio′ris,** rami esophagei arteriae thyroideae inferioris. **ra′mi oesopha′gei ner′vi recurren′tis,** rami esophagei nervi laryngei recurrentis. **ra′mi oesopha′gei ner′vi va′gi,** esophageal branches of vagus nerve. **ra′mi orbita′les arte′riae cer′ebri anterio′ris** [NA], orbital branches of anterior cerebral artery: branches from the anterior cerebral artery to the cortex of the medial part of the orbital surface of the frontal lobe. **ra′mi orbita′les arte′riae cer′ebri me′diae** [NA], orbital branches of middle cerebral artery: they pass to the cortex of the lateral part of the orbital surface of the frontal lobe. **ra′mi orbita′les gan′glii pterygopalati′ni** [NA], **ra′mi orbita′les gan′glii sphenopalati′ni,** orbital branches of pterygopalatine ganglion: branches passing from the pterygopalatine ganglion through the inferior orbital fissure to supply orbital periosteum and the ethmoidal and sphenoidal sinuses; modality, general sensory and parasympathetic. **r. os′sis is′chii** [NA], ramus of ischium: the flattened bar of bone that projects from the inferior end of the body of the ischium in an anterosuperomedial direction to meet the inferior ramus of the pubis. It forms part of the border of the obturator foramen. Called also *r. inferior ossis ischii*. **r. os′sis pu′bis,** see *r. inferior ossis pubis* and *r. superior ossis pubis*. **r. ova′ricus arte′riae uteri′nae** [NA], **r. ova′rii arte′riae uteri′nae,** ovarian branch of uterine artery: the terminal branch of the uterine artery, which supplies the ovary and anastomoses with the ovarian artery. **r. palma′ris ner′vi media′ni** [NA], palmar branch of median nerve: a branch arising from the median nerve in the lower part of the forearm and supplying the skin of the outer part of the palm; modality, general sensory. **r. palma′ris ner′vi ulna′ris** [NA], palmar branch of ulnar nerve: it arises from the ulnar nerve in the lower part of

the forearm, supplying the cutaneous structures of the medial part of the palm; modality, general sensory. Called also *r. volaris manus nervi ulnaris.* **r. palma′ris profun′dus arte′riae ulna′ris** [NA], deep palmar branch of ulnar artery: it accompanies the deep palmar branch of the ulnar nerve and joins the radial artery to form the deep palmar arch; called also *r. volaris profundus arteriae ulnaris.* **r. palma′ris superficia′lis arte′riae radia′lis** [NA], superficial palmar branch of radial artery: a branch arising from the radial artery in the lower part of the forearm and supplying the thenar eminence; called also *r. volaris superficialis arteriae radialis.* **ra′mi palpebra′les inferio′res ner′vi infraorbita′lis** [NA], inferior palpebral branches of infraorbital nerve: they supply the skin and conjunctiva of the lower eyelid; modality, general sensory. **r. palpebra′lis infe′rior ner′vi infratrochlea′ris,** see *rami palpebrales nervi infratrochlearis.* **ra′mi palpebra′les ner′vi infratrochlea′ris** [NA], palpebral branches of infratrochlear nerve: they help supply the eyelids; modality, general sensory. **r. palpebra′lis supe′rior ner′vi infratrochlea′ris,** see *rami palpebrales nervi infratrochlearis.* **ra′mi pancreat′ici arte′riae liena′lis** [NA], pancreatic branches of splenic artery: branches that supply the pancreas, arising from the splenic artery during its tortuous course along the superior border of the body of the pancreas. **ra′mi pancreat′ici arte′riae pancreaticoduodena′lis superio′ris** [NA], pancreatic branches of superior pancreaticoduodenal artery: vessels that help supply the pancreas from its anterior and inferior surfaces. **ra′mi parieta′les aor′tae abdomina′lis,** parietal branches of the abdominal aorta. **ra′mi parieta′les aor′tae thoraca′lis,** parietal branches of the thoracic aorta. **ra′mi parieta′les arte′riae cer′ebri anterio′ris** [NA], parietal branches of anterior cerebral artery: they supply the cortex of the parietal lobe except on the lower part of the lateral surface. **ra′mi parieta′les arte′riae cer′ebri me′diae** [NA], parietal branches of middle cerebral artery: they supply the cortex of the lower lateral surface of the parietal lobe. **ra′mi parieta′les arte′riae hypogas′tricae,** parietal branches of the hypogastric artery. **r. parieta′lis arte′riae menin′geae me′diae** [NA], parietal branch of middle meningeal artery: a vessel that arises in the middle cranial fossa, grooves the temporal and parietal bones, and supplies the posterior dura mater. **r. parieta′lis arte′riae tempora′lis superficia′lis** [NA], parietal branch of superficial temporal artery: the posterior terminal branch of the superficial temporal artery, supplying the scalp in the parietal region. **r. parietooccipita′lis arte′riae cer′ebri posterio′ris** [NA], parietooccipital branch of posterior cerebral artery: a vessel that supplies the cortex of the medial surface of the hemisphere up to the area of the parietooccipital sulcus. **ra′mi paroti′dei arte′riae tempora′lis superficia′lis** [NA], parotid branches of superficial temporal artery: vessels supplying the parotid gland and the temporomandibular joint. **ra′mi paroti′dei ner′vi auriculotempora′lis** [NA], parotid branches of auriculotemporal nerve: branches that bear postganglionic fibers from the otic ganglion to the parotid gland; modality, parasympathetic. **ra′mi paroti′dei ve′nae facia′lis** [NA], parotid branches of facial vein: small veins from the substance of the parotid gland which follow the parotid duct and open into the facial vein; called also *venae parotideae anteriores.* **ra′mi pectora′les arte′riae thoracoacromia′lis** [NA], pectoral branches of thoracoacromial artery: they descend between the pectoralis major and minor muscles, supplying these muscles and the mammary gland. **ra′mi perforan′tes arte′riae mamma′riae inter′nae,** rami perforantes arteriae thoracicae internae. **ra′mi perforan′tes arteria′rum metacarpea′rum palma′rium** [NA], **ra′mi perforan′tes arteria′rum metacarpea′rum vola′rium,** perforating branches of palmar metacarpal arteries: vessels connecting the palmar metacarpal arteries and deep palmar arch with the dorsal metacarpal arteries, between the bases of the metacarpal bones and in the interosseous spaces. **ra′mi perforan′tes arteria′rum metatarsea′rum planta′rium** [NA], perforating branches of plantar metatarsal arteries: vessels connecting the plantar metatarsal arteries with the dorsal metatarsal arteries through the interosseous spaces. **r. per′forans arte′riae perone′ae** [NA], perforating branch of peroneal artery: a branch passing forward from the peroneal artery where the interosseous membrane and the tibiofibular syndesmosis are continuous, and descending to supply the syndesmosis and the ankle joint. **ra′mi perforan′tes arte′riae thora′cicae inter′nae** [NA], perforating branches of internal thoracic artery: six branches, one in each of the upper six intercostal spaces, supplying the pectoralis major muscle and adjacent skin; the second, third, and fourth branches give off mammary branches. Called also *rami perforantes arteriae mammariae internae.* **ra′mi pericardi′aci aor′tae thoraca′lis,** rami pericardiaci aortae thoracicae. **ra′mi pericardi′aci aor′tae thora′cicae** [NA], pericardiac branches of thoracic aorta: small branches from the aorta distributed to the surface of the pericardium. **r. pericardi′acus ner′vi phren′ici** [NA], pericardiac branch of phrenic nerve: a branch arising from the phrenic or accessory phrenic nerve and supplying the pericardium; modality, general sensory. **ra′mi perinea′les ner′vi cuta′nei fem′oris posterio′ris**

[NA], perineal branches of posterior femoral cutaneous nerve: branches arising from the posterior femoral cutaneous nerve at the lower margin of the gluteus maximus muscle and innervating the skin of the external genitalia; modality, general sensory. **r. petro′sus arte′riae menin′geae me′diae** [NA], **r. petro′sus superficia′lis arte′riae menin′geae me′diae**, petrosal branch of middle meningeal artery: a branch that arises in the region of the petrous part of the temporal bone, entering the hiatus for the greater petrosal nerve and anastomosing with the stylomastoid artery. **ra′mi pharyn′gei arte′riae pharyn′geae ascenden′tis** [NA], pharyngeal branches of ascending pharyngeal artery: irregular vessels supplying the pharynx. **ra′mi pharyn′gei arte′riae thyroi′deae inferio′ris** [NA], pharyngeal branches of inferior thyroid artery: vessels that supply the pharynx. **r. pharyn′geus gan′glii pterygopalati′ni** [NA], a nerve branch running from the posterior part of the pterygopalatine ganglion, through the pharyngeal canal with the pharyngeal branch of the maxillary artery, to the mucous membrane of the nasal part of the pharynx posterior to the auditory tube; called also *pharyngeal branch of pterygopalatine ganglion*. **ra′mi pharyn′gei ner′vi glossopharyn′gei** [NA], pharyngeal branches of glossopharyngeal nerve: they innervate the mucous membrane of the oropharynx; modality, general sensory. **ra′mi pharyn′gei ner′vi va′gi** [NA], pharyngeal branches of vagus nerve: they innervate pharyngeal muscles and mucosa; modality, motor and general sensory. **ra′mi phrenicoabdomina′les ner′vi phren′ici** [NA], phrenicoabdominal branches of phrenic nerve: branches of the phrenic or accessory phrenic nerve that supply the diaphragm and contribute to the celiac plexus; modality, general sensory and motor. **r. planta′ris profun′dus arte′riae dorsa′lis pe′dis** [NA], deep plantar branch of dorsalis pedis artery: the main terminal branch of the dorsalis pedis artery, which passes through the first intermetatarsal space to the sole to form the plantar arch. **ra′mi posterio′res arteria′rum intercosta′lium**, see *r. dorsalis arteriarum intercostalium posteriorum [III–XI]*. **r. poste′rior arte′riae obturato′riae** [NA], posterior branch of obturator artery: it passes backward around the lateral margin of the obturator foramen, on the obturator membrane, supplying muscles around the ischial tuberosity and giving off an acetabular branch. **r. poste′rior arte′riae recurren′tis ulna′ris** [NA], posterior branch of ulnar recurrent artery: it runs to the back of the medial epicondyle, supplying the elbow joint and neighboring muscles. **r. poste′rior arte′riae rena′lis** [NA], the posterior branch of the renal artery, supplying the posterior segment of the kidney. **r. poste′rior arte′riae thyroi′deae superio′ris** [NA], posterior branch of superior thyroid artery: a vessel supplying the posterior part of the thyroid gland. **r. poste′rior duc′tus hepat′ici dex′tri** [NA], the posterior branch of the right hepatic duct. **r. poste′rior fissu′rae cer′ebri latera′lis** [Syl′vii], r. posterior sulci lateralis cerebri. **r. poste′rior ner′vi auricula′ris mag′ni** [NA], posterior branch of great auricular nerve: a branch, formed by division of the great auricular nerve, that innervates the skin over the mastoid process and the back of the external ear; modality, general sensory. **ra′mi posterio′res nervo′rum cervica′lium**, rami dorsales nervorum cervicalium. **r. poste′rior ner′vi coccyg′ei**, r. dorsalis nervi coccygei. **r. poste′rior ner′vi laryn′gei inferio′ris**, posterior branch of inferior laryngeal nerve. **ra′mi posterio′res nervo′rum lumba′lium**, rami dorsales nervorum lumbalium. **r. poste′rior ner′vi obturato′rii** [NA], posterior branch of obturator nerve: a branch that descends to innervate the knee joint, giving muscular branches to the obturator externus, adductor magnus, and sometimes the adductor brevis muscle; modality, general sensory and motor. **ra′mi posterio′res nervo′rum sacra′lium**, rami dorsales nervorum sacralium. **r. poste′rior nervo′rum spina′lium**, r. dorsalis nervorum spinalium. **ra′mi posterio′res nervo′rum thoraca′lium**, rami dorsales nervorum thoracicorum. **r. poste′rior ramo′rum cutaneo′rum latera′lium [abdomina′lium et pectora′lium] arteria′rum intercosta′lium**, posterior branch of (abdominal and thoracic) lateral cutaneous branches of intercostal arteries. **r. poste′rior ramo′rum cutaneo′rum latera′lium [abdomina′lium et pectora′lium] nervo′rum intercosta′lium**, posterior branch of (abdominal and thoracic) lateral cutaneous branches of intercostal nerves. **r. poste′rior sul′ci latera′lis cer′ebri** [NA], posterior branch of lateral cerebral sulcus: the part of the lateral cerebral sulcus that runs obliquely posteriorly between the temporal and the parietal lobes; called also *r. posterior fissurae cerebri lateralis* [Sylvii]. **r. profun′dus arte′riae cervica′lis ascenden′tis**, deep branch of ascending cervical artery. **r. profun′dus arte′riae circumflex′ae fem′oris media′lis** [NA], deep branch of medial circumflex femoral artery: a branch ascending toward the trochanteric fossa, and anastomosing with gluteal branches. **r. profun′dus arte′riae glu′teae superio′ris** [NA], deep branch of superior gluteal artery: a branch passing forward between the gluteus medius and minimus muscles, and dividing into superior and inferior branches. **r. profun′dus arte′riae planta′ris media′lis** [NA], deep branch of medial plantar artery: it supplies the anteromedial aspect of the sole,

anastomosing with the medial three plantar metatarsal arteries. **r. profun′dus arte′riae transver′sae col′li** [NA], deep branch of transverse cervical artery: it descends to supply medial and deep back muscles; sometimes replaced by an artery stemming directly from the subclavian artery (arteria scapularis descendens). Called also *arteria scapularis descendens* [*dorsalis*] [NA alternative] and *r. descendens arteriae transversae colli*. **r. profun′dus ner′vi planta′ris latera′lis** [NA], deep branch of lateral plantar nerve: it accompanies the lateral plantar artery on its medial side and the plantar arch, innervating the interossei, the second, third, and fourth lumbrical, and the adductor hallucis muscles, and some articulations; modality, general sensory. **r. profun′dus ner′vi radia′lis** [NA], deep branch of radial nerve: a branch arising from the radial nerve and winding laterally around the radius to the back of the forearm, supplying the supinator, extensor digitorum, extensor digiti minimi, and extensor carpi ulnaris muscles, and often the extensor carpi radialis brevis muscle. Its continuation, the posterior interosseous nerve, supplies distal forearm muscles and the carpal and intercarpal joints; modality, motor. **r. profun′dus ner′vi ulna′ris** [NA], deep branch of ulnar nerve: the deep branch that is accompanied by the deep palmar branch of the ulnar artery, rounds the hook of the hamate bone, and follows the deep palmar arch beneath the flexor tendons, supplying the wrist joint, the interossei, third and fourth lumbrical, and adductor pollicis muscles, and usually the deep head of the flexor pollicis brevis muscle; modality, general sensory and motor. **ra′mi pterygoi′dei arte′riae maxilla′ris** [NA], **ra′mi pterygoi′dei arte′riae maxilla′ris inter′nae**, pterygoid branches of maxillary artery: they supply the pterygoid muscles. **r. pu′bicus arte′riae epigas′tricae inferio′ris** [NA], pubic branch of inferior epigastric artery: it arises from the inferior epigastric artery near the deep inguinal ring and descends on the back of the pubis, anastomosing through an obturator branch with the pubic branch of the obturator artery. **r. pu′bicus arte′riae obturato′riae** [NA], pubic branch of obturator artery: it ascends on the pelvic surface of the ilium, anastomosing with its fellow of the other side and with the pubic branch of the inferior epigastric artery. **r. of pubis**, see *r. inferior ossis pubis* and *r. superior ossis pubis*. **r. of pubis, ascending**, r. superior ossis pubis. **r. of pubis, descending**, r. inferior ossis pubis. **ra′mi pulmona′les plex′us cardi′aci**, rami pulmonales systematis autonomici. **ra′mi pulmona′les systema′tis autonom′ici** [NA], pulmonary branches of autonomic system: branches from the sympathetic trunks and cardiac plexus, which, via the pulmonary plexuses, accompany the blood vessels and bronchi into the lungs; modality, sympathetic and visceral afferent. **r. rena′lis ner′vi splanch′nici mino′ris** [NA], renal branch of lesser splanchnic nerve: a branch from the lesser splanchnic nerve to the aorticorenal ganglion; modality, sympathetic preganglionic fibers and visceral afferent. **ra′mi rena′les ner′vi va′gi** [NA], **ra′mi rena′les plex′us coeli′aci**, renal branches of vagus nerve: branches passing from the vagal trunks via the celiac plexus to the kidney; modality, parasympathetic and visceral afferent. **r. saphe′nus arte′riae ge′nus descen′dens** [NA], saphenous branch of descending genicular artery: a vessel that accompanies the saphenous nerve between the sartorius and gracilis muscles on the medial side of the knee, supplying the skin and anastomosing with the medial inferior genicular artery. **r. saphe′nus arte′riae ge′nu supre′mae**, r. saphenus arteriae genus descendens. **ra′mi scrota′les anterio′res arte′riae femora′lis** [NA], anterior scrotal branches of femoral artery: branches arising from the external pudendal arteries and supplying the anterior scrotal region in the male; called also *arteriae scrotales anteriores*. **ra′mi scrota′les posterio′res arte′riae puden′dae inter′nae** [NA], posterior scrotal branches of internal pudendal artery: two branches arising from the internal pudendal artery in the anterior part of the ischiorectal fossa, helping to supply the ischiocavernosus and bulbospongiosus muscles, and distributed to the scrotum; called also *arteriae scrotales posteriores*. **r. sinis′ter arte′riae hepat′icae pro′priae** [NA], left branch of proper hepatic artery: it supplies the left lobe of the liver. **r. sinis′ter arte′riae pulmona′lis**, arteria pulmonalis sinistra. **r. sinis′ter ve′nae por′tae** [NA], the left branch of the portal vein, distributed to the left lobe of the liver. **r. si′nus carot′ici ner′vi glossopharyn′gei** [NA], branch of glossopharyngeal nerve to carotid sinus: a branch that supplies the pressoreceptors and chemoreceptors of the carotid sinus and carotid body with visceral afferent fibers. **ra′mi spina′les arte′riae cervica′lis ascenden′tis** [NA], spinal branches of ascending cerivcal artery: they help supply the vertebral canal. **r. spina′lis arte′riae iliolumba′lis**, r. spinalis rami lumbalis arteriae iliolumbalis. **ra′mi spina′les arte′riae intercosta′lis supre′mae** [NA], spinal branches of highest intercostal artery: vessels arising from the dorsal branches of the first two posterior intercostal arteries, entering intervertebral foramina with the corresponding two spinal nerves to help supply the contents of the vertebral canal. **r. spina′lis arteria′rum lumba′lium** [NA], spinal branch of lumbar arteries: a branch arising from the dorsal branch of the lumbar arteries and entering an intervertebral foramen with the spinal nerve to help supply the contents of the vertebral canal. **ra′mi spina′les arteria′rum sacra′lium latera′lium** [NA], spinal branches of lateral sacral arteries: vessels arising from the two lateral sacral arteries and entering the pelvic sacral foramina to help supply the contents of the vertebral canal. **r. spina′lis arte′riae subcosta′lis** [NA], spinal branch of subcostal artery: a spinal branch corresponding to those arising from the dorsal branches of the posterior intercostal arteries; it enters the vertebral canal to help supply the contents of the canal. **ra′mi spina′les arte′riae vertebra′lis** [NA], spinal branches of vertebral artery: vessels supplying the contents of the cervical part of the vertebral canal. **r. spina′lis ra′mi dorsa′lis arteria′rum intercosta′lium posterio′rum [III–XI]** [NA], **r. spina′lis ramo′rum posterio′rum arteria′rum intercosta′lium**, spinal branch of dorsal branch of posterior intercostal arteries [III–XI]: one of the two branches into which the dorsal branch of a posterior intercostal artery divides, passing through the intervertebral foramen with the corresponding spinal nerve to help supply the contents of the vertebral canal. **r. spina′lis ra′mi lumba′lis arte′riae iliolumba′lis** [NA], spinal branch of lumbar branch of iliolumbar artery; it passes through the intervertebral foramen between the fifth lumbar vertebra and the sacrum to help supply the contents of the vertebral canal. **r. spina′lis vena′rum intercosta′lium**, r. spinalium venarum intercostalium posteriorum [IV–XI]. **r. spina′lis vena′rum intercosta′lium posterio′rum [IV–XI]** [NA], spinal branch of posterior intercostal veins: a vessel, the vena comitans of the arterial spinal branch, that emerges from the vertebral canal and contributes to the dorsal branch of each posterior intercostal vein. **r. stape′dius arte′riae stylomastoi′deae** [NA], stapedial branch of stylomastoid artery: a variable branch supplying the stapedius muscle and tendon. **ra′mi sterna′les arte′riae mamma′riae inter′nae**, rami sternales arteriae thoracicae internae. **ra′mi sterna′les arte′riae thora′cicae inter′nae** [NA], sternal branches of internal thoracic artery: they supply the sternum and the transversus thoracis muscle. **ra′mi sternocleidomastoi′dei arte′riae occipita′lis** [NA], sternocleidomastoid branches of occipital artery: branches of the occipital artery, usually an upper and a lower, that supply the sternocleidomastoid and adjacent muscles. **r. sternocleidomastoi′deus arte′riae thyroi′deae superio′ris** [NA], sternocleidomastoid branch of superior thyroid artery: a branch that arises from the superior thyroid artery, but sometimes directly from the external carotid artery, passing across the carotid sheath to supply the middle portion of the sternocleidomastoid muscle. **ra′mi stria′ti arte′riae cer′ebri me′diae** [NA], striate branches of middle cerebral artery: central branches that supply the basal ganglia, thalamus, and internal capsule. **r. stylohyoi′deus ner′vi facia′lis** [NA], stylohyoid branch of facial nerve: a branch that arises from the facial nerve just below the base of the skull to innervate the stylohyoid muscle; modality, motor. **r. stylopharyn′geus ner′vi glossopharyn′gei**, r. musculi stylopharyngei nervi glossopharyngei. **ra′mi submaxilla′res gan′glii submaxilla′ris**, rami glandulares ganglii submandibularis. **ra′mi subscapula′res arte′riae axilla′ris** [NA], subscapular branches of axillary artery: they supply the subscapularis muscle. **r. superficia′lis arte′riae circumflex′ae fem′oris media′lis**, the superficial branch of the medial circumflex femoral artery. **r. superficia′lis arte′riae glu′teae superio′ris** [NA], superficial branch of superior gluteal artery: it ramifies to supply the gluteus maximus muscle. **r. superficia′lis arte′riae planta′ris media′lis** [NA], superficial branch of medial plantar artery: it supplies the medial side of the great toe. **r. superficia′lis arte′riae transver′sae col′li** [NA], superficial branch of transverse cervical artery: a branch that arises from the transverse cervical artery at the anterior border of the levator scapulae muscle, supplying the levator scapulae, trapezius, and splenius muscles. When there is no deep branch, the superficial branch is the continuation of the transverse cervical called the superficial cervical artery. Called also *arteria cervicalis superficialis* [NA alternative] and *r. ascendens arteriae transversae colli*. **r. superficia′lis ner′vi planta′ris latera′lis** [NA], superficial branch of lateral plantar nerve: a branch that arises from the lateral plantar nerve at the lateral border of the quadratus plantae muscle and passes forward, dividing into a lateral part that innervates skin of the lateral side of the sole and little toe, joints of the toe, and the flexor digiti minimi brevis muscle, and a medial part, a common plantar digital nerve, that gives two proper plantar digital nerves to the adjacent sides of the fourth and fifth toes; modality, general sensory. **r. superficia′lis ner′vi radia′lis** [NA], superficial branch of radial nerve: the continuation of the radial nerve that accompanies the radial artery in the forearm, winds dorsalward, supplies the lateral side of the back of the hand, and divides into dorsal digital nerves that supply the skin of the dorsal surface and adjacent surfaces of the thumb, index, and middle fingers, and sometimes the radial side of the ring finger; modality, general sensory. **r. superficia′lis ner′vi ulna′ris** [NA], superficial branch of ulnar nerve: the branch of the ulnar nerve in the hand that supplies the palmaris brevis muscle and divides into a proper palmar digital nerve for

the medial side of the little finger, a common palmar digital nerve giving off two proper nerves to supply adjacent sides of the little and fourth fingers, and sometimes palmar digital nerves also for the adjacent sides of the third and fourth fingers; modality, general sensory and motor. **r. supe′rior arte′riae glu′teae superio′ris** [NA], superior branch of superior gluteal artery: the upper division of the deep branch of the superior gluteal artery, extending as far as the anterior superior iliac spine and helping supply the gluteus medius, gluteus minimus, and tensor fasciae latae muscles. **ra′mi superio′res ner′vi cuta′nei col′li**, rami superiores nervi transversi colli. **r. supe′rior ner′vi oculomoto′rii** [NA], superior branch of oculomotor nerve: the upper and smaller of the two branches of the oculomotor nerve, which supplies the superior rectus muscle and, terminally, the levator palpebrae superioris; modality, motor. **ra′mi superio′res ner′vi transver′si col′li** [NA], superior branches of transverse cervical nerve: the upper of the branches that arise from the transverse cervical nerve near the anterior border of the sternocleidomastoid muscle, innervating skin and subcutaneous tissue in the anterior cervical region; modality, general sensory. Called also *rami superiores nervi cutanei colli*. **r. supe′rior os′sis is′chii**, a name formerly given to what is now considered the lower part of the body of the ischium (corpus ossis ischii). **r. supe′rior os′sis pu′bis** [NA], **superior r. of pubis**, the bar of bone projecting from the body of the pubic bone in a posterosuperolateral direction to the iliopubic eminence, and forming part of the acetabulum. **r. suprahyoi′deus arte′riae lingua′lis** [NA], suprahyoid branch of lingual artery: it passes along the upper border of the hyoid bone, supplying suprahyoid muscles and anastomosing with its fellow of the other side; called also *r. hyoideus arteriae lingualis*. **ra′mi suprarena′les superio′res arte′riae phren′icae inferio′ris**, see *arteria suprarenalis superior*. **r. sympath′icus ad gan′glion cilia′re** [NA], sympathetic branch to ciliary ganglion: a branch bearing sympathetic fibers, postganglionic from the superior cervical ganglion and derived from the internal carotid plexus, to the ciliary ganglion, for distribution by the short ciliary nerves to the dilator pupillae, orbitalis, and tarsal muscles, and blood vessels of the eyeball. Called also *radices sympathicae ganglii ciliaris*. **r. sympath′icus ad gan′glion submandibula′re** [NA], sympathetic branch to submandibular ganglion: a branch bearing sympathetic fibers, postganglionic from the superior cervical ganglion and derived from a plexus on the facial artery, to the submandibular ganglion, for distribution to the submandibular gland. Called also *radix sympathica ganglii submaxillaris*. **ra′mi tempora′les arte′riae cer′ebri me′diae** [NA], temporal branches of middle cerebral artery: vessels that supply the cortex of the lateral surface of the temporal lobe, and the temporal pole. **ra′mi tempora′les arte′riae cer′ebri posterio′ris** [NA], temporal branches of posterior cerebral artery: vessels that supply the cortex of the inferior and medial surfaces of the temporal lobe. **ra′mi tempora′les ner′vi facia′lis** [NA], temporal branches of facial nerve: terminal branches of the facial nerve that innervate the anterior and superior auricular muscles, the frontal belly of the occipitofrontal muscle, and the orbicularis oculi and corrugator muscles; modality, motor. **ra′mi tempora′les superficia′les ner′vi auriculotempora′lis** [NA], superficial temporal branches of auriculotemporal nerve: branches to the skin of the scalp in the temporal region; modality, general sensory. **r. tento′rii ner′vi ophthal′mici** [NA], tentorial branch of ophthalmic nerve: a branch that arises from the ophthalmic nerve close to its origin from the trigeminal ganglion, turning back to innervate the dura mater of the tentorium cerebelli and falx cerebri; modality, general sensory. Called also *nervus tentorii*. **ra′mi thy′mici arte′riae thora′cicae inter′nae** [NA], thymic branches of internal thoracic artery: branches distributed to the thymus gland in the anterior mediastinum; called also *arteriae thymicae*. **r. thyreohyoi′deus ner′vi hypoglos′si**, r. thyrohyoideus ansae cervicalis. **r. thyrohyoi′deus an′sae cervica′lis** [NA], thyrohyoid branch of ansa cervicalis: a branch from the superior root of the ansa cervicalis, innervating the thyrohyoid muscle; modality, motor. **r. tonsilla′ris arte′riae facia′lis** [NA], **r. tonsilla′ris arte′riae maxilla′ris exter′ni**, tonsillar branch of facial artery: a vessel ascending from the facial artery on the pharynx to supply the tonsil and the root of the tongue. **ra′mi tonsilla′res ner′vi glossopharyn′gei** [NA], tonsillar branches of glossopharyngeal nerve: they supply the mucosa over the palatine tonsil and the adjacent portion of the soft palate; modality, general sensory. **ra′mi trachea′les arte′riae thyroi′deae inferio′ris** [NA], tracheal branches of inferior thyroid artery: vessels supplying the trachea. **ra′mi trachea′les ner′vi laryn′gei recurren′tis** [NA], **ra′mi trachea′les ner′vi recurren′tis**, tracheal branches of recurrent laryngeal nerve: they are distributed to the tracheal mucosa; modality, general sensory. **r. transver′sus arte′riae circumflex′ae fem′oris latera′lis** [NA], transverse branch of lateral circumflex femoral artery: a branch that pierces the vastus lateralis muscle, turning around the femur to anastomose with the transverse branch of the medial circumflex femoral artery and with other arteries, deep to the gluteus maximus muscle. **r. transver′sus arte′riae circumflex′ae fem′oris media′-**

lis [NA], transverse branch of medial circumflex femoral artery: it passes between the quadratus femoris and adductor magnus muscles, supplying them, and then turning around the femur to anastomose with the transverse branch of the lateral circumflex femoral artery and with other arteries, deep to the gluteus maximus muscle. **r. tu′bae plex′us tympan′ici [Jacobso′ni]**, r. tubarius plexus tympanici. **r. tuba′rius arte′riae uteri′nae** [NA], tubal branch of uterine artery: it supplies the uterine tube and the round ligament. **r. tuba′rius plex′us tympan′ici** [NA], tubal branch of tympanic plexus: a branch given to the auditory tube from the tympanic plexus; modality, general sensory. Called also *r. tubae plexus tympanici [Jacobsoni]*. **r. ulna′ris ner′vi cuta′nei antebra′chii media′lis** [NA], ulnar branch of medial antebrachial cutaneous nerve: a branch that innervates the skin of the posteromedial and medial aspects of the forearm; modality, general sensory. **ra′mi ureter′ici arte′riae duc′tus deferen′tis** [NA], ureteral branches of artery of ductus deferens: they supply the lower portion of the ureter. **ra′mi ureter′ici arte′riae ova′ricae** [NA], ureteral branches of ovarian artery: they are distributed to the ureter. **ra′mi ureter′ici arte′riae rena′lis** [NA], ureteral branches of renal artery: they supply the upper portion of the ureter. **ra′mi ureter′ici arte′riae testicula′ris** [NA], ureteral branches of testicular artery: they are distributed to the ureter. **ra′mi ventra′les nervo′rum cervica′lium** [NA], ventral branches of cervical nerves: the upper four form the cervical plexus, and the lower four form most of the brachial plexus; called also *rami anteriores nervorum cervicalium*. **r. ventra′lis ner′vi coccyg′ei** [NA], ventral branch of coccygeal nerve: the ventral branch of the last spinal nerve, which emerges from the sacral hiatus and helps form the coccygeal plexus; called also *r. anterior nervi coccygei*. **ra′mi ventra′les nervo′rum lumba′lium** [NA], ventral branches of lumbar nerves: the ventral branches of the five lumbar sacral nerves. The upper four branches form the lumbar plexus, and the fifth and a part of the fourth participate in formation of the sacral plexus. Called also *rami anteriores nervorum lumbalium*. **ra′mi ventra′les nervo′rum sacra′lium** [NA], ventral branches of sacral nerves: the ventral branches of the five sacral spinal nerves. The upper four branches emerge from the sacrum through the anterior sacral foramina and help form the sacral plexus; the fifth emerges through the sacral hiatus and, with a communication from the fourth, participates in formation of the coccygeal plexus. Called also *rami anteriores nervorum sacralium*. **r. ventra′lis nervo′rum spina′lium** [NA], ventral branch of spinal nerves: the larger, usually, of the two branches into which each spinal nerve divides almost as soon as it emerges from the intervertebral foramen; the ventral branches supply the ventral and lateral parts of the trunk and all parts of the limbs. Called also *r. anterior nervorum spinalium*. **ra′mi ventra′les nervo′rum thoracico′rum** [NA], ventral branches of thoracic nerves: the ventral branches of the first eleven thoracic spinal nerves situated between the ribs, the first three of which give branches to the brachial plexus as well as to the thoracic wall, the fourth, fifth, and sixth supply only the thoracic wall, and the seventh to eleventh are thoracoabdominal in distribution. Called also *intercostal nerves, nervi intercostales* [NA alternative], and *r. anteriores nervorum thoracalium*. The anterior primary division of the twelfth thoracic nerve is subcostal rather than intercostal in position, differing in course and relationships from the other ventral branches, and is known as the subcostal nerve (*nervus subcostalis* [NA]). **ra′mi vestibula′res arte′riae audi′ti′vae inter′nae**, rami vestibulares arteriae labyrinthi. **ra′mi vestibula′res arte′riae labyrin′thi** [NA], vestibular branches of labyrinthine artery: vessels supplying the vestibule of the ear. **ra′mi viscera′les aor′tae abdomina′lis**, visceral branches of the abdominal aorta. **ra′mi viscera′les aor′tae thoraca′lis**, visceral branches of the thoracic aorta. **ra′mi viscera′les arte′riae hypogas′tricae**, visceral branches of the hypogastric artery. **r. vola′ris ma′nus ner′vi ulna′ris**, r. palmaris nervi ulnaris. **r. vola′ris ner′vi cuta′nei antibrach′ii media′lis**, r. anterior nervi cutanei antebrachii medialis. **r. vola′ris profun′dus arte′riae ulna′ris**, r. palmaris profundus arteriae ulnaris. **r. vola′ris superficia′lis arte′riae radia′lis**, r. palmaris superficialis arteriae radialis. **ra′mi zygomat′ici ner′vi facia′lis** [NA], zygomatic branches of facial nerve: branches that cross the zygomatic bone and innervate the orbicularis oculi muscle; modality, motor. **r. zygomaticofacia′lis ner′vi zygomat′ici** [NA], zygomaticofacial branch of zygomatic nerve: a branch that passes from the lateral wall of the orbit, piercing the zygomatic bone to supply overlying skin; modality, general sensory. **r. zygomaticotempora′lis ner′vi zygomat′ici** [NA], zygomaticotemporal branch of zygomatic nerve: a branch that passes from the lateral wall of the orbit, piercing the zygomatic bone to innervate the skin of the anterior temporal region; modality, general sensory.

rancid (ran′sid) [L. *rancidus*] having a musty, rank taste or smell; applied to fats that have undergone decomposition, with the liberation of fatty acids.

rancidify (ran-sid′ĭ-fi) to decompose, with the liberation of fatty acids; a term applied especially to the decomposition of fats.

rancidity (ran-sid′ĭ-te) the quality of being rancid.

Randolph's test (ran′dolfs) [Nathaniel Archer *Randolph*, American physician, 1858–1887] see under tests.

range (rānj) 1. the difference between the upper and lower limits of a variable or of a series of values. 2. the portion of the earth in which a given species is found. **r. of accommodation**, the alteration in the refractive state of the eye produced by accommodation. It is the difference in diopters between the refraction by the eye adjusted for its far point and that when adjusted for its near point. Called also *amplitude of accommodation*. **r. of audibility**, see under *limit*. **r. of motion**, the range, measured in degrees of a circle, through which a joint can be extended and flexed.

ranimycin (ran-i-mi′sin) an antibacterial antibiotic derived from a variant of *Streptomyces lincolnensis*.

ranine (ra′nīn) [L. *raninus; rana* frog] pertaining to (*a*) a frog; (*b*) a ranula, or to the lower surface of the tongue; (*c*) the sublingual vein.

Ranke's angle (rahn′kēz) [Hans Rudolph *Ranke*, Dutch anatomist, 1849–1887] see under *angle*.

Ranke's complex, formula, stages (rahn′kēz) [Karl Ernst *Ranke*, Munich internist, 1870–1926] see *primary complex*, under *complex*, and see under *formula* and *stage*.

ranula (ran′u-lah) [L., dim. of *rana* frog] a cystic tumor beneath the tongue, due to obstruction and dilatation of the sublingual or submaxillary duct or of a mucous gland. **pancreatic r.**, a retention cyst of the pancreatic duct.

ranular (ran′u-lar) pertaining to or of the nature of ranula.

Ranunculus (rah-nung′ku-lus) a genus of plants, the crowfoots and buttercups, certain species of which are poisonous; see also *risus sardonicus*.

Ranvier's crosses, etc. (rahn-ve-āz′) [Louis Antoine *Ranvier*, French pathologist, 1835–1922] see under *cross, disk, membrane, node,* and *segment*.

Raoult's law (rah-ōlz′) [François Marie *Raoult*, French physicist, 1830–1901] see under *law*.

raphania (rah-fa′ne-ah) [L. *raphanus*; Gr. *rhaphanos* radish] a chronic poisoning ascribed to the seeds of wild radish.

raphe (ra′fe) [Gr. *rhaphē* a seam; [NA] a general term for the line of union of the halves of various symmetrical parts. **abdominal r.**, linea alba. **amniotic r.**, the line of junction of the amniotic folds in the amnion of those vertebrates in which it is formed by folding. **r. anococcyg′ea, anococcygeal r.**, ligamentum anococcygeum. **r. cor′poris callo′si**, see *stria longitudinalis medialis corpus callosi* and *stria longitudinalis lateralis corporis callosi*. **longitudinal r. of tongue**, sulcus medianus linguae. **median r. of neck, posterior**, ligamentum nuchae. **r. of medulla oblongata, r. medul′lae oblonga′tae** [NA], the line of union of the two halves of the medulla oblongata. **r. pala′ti** [NA], **palatine r.**, a narrow whitish streak in the midline of the palate, extending from the incisive papilla to the tip of the uvula; it may present as a ridge in front and as a groove posteriorly. **palpebral r., lateral, r. palpebra′lis latera′lis** [NA], a thin horizontal band of connective tissue extending from the external angle of the rima palpebralis to the lateral margin of the orbit. **r. pe′nis** [NA], a narrow dark streak or ridge continuous posteriorly with the raphe scroti and extending forward for a variable distance along the midline on the under side of the penis; in the newborn it may extend to the tip of the glans. **r. perine′i** [NA], **r. of perineum**, a ridge along the median line of the perineum, continuous anteriorly with the raphe scroti and ending posteriorly at the anus. **r. pharyn′gis** [NA], **r. of pharynx**, a more or less distinct band of connective tissue extending downward from the base of the skull along the posterior wall of the pharynx in the median plane, and giving attachment to the constrictor muscles of the pharynx. **r. of pons, r. pon′tis** [NA], the line of union of the right and left halves of the pons. **pterygomandibular r., r. pterygomandibula′ris** [NA], a tendinous line between the buccinator and the constrictor pharyngis superior muscles, from which the middle portions of both muscles originate. **r. scro′ti** [NA], **r. of scrotum**, a ridge along the surface of the scrotum in the median line, dividing it into nearly equal lateral parts.

rapport (rah-por′) [Fr.] a relation of harmony and accord between two persons, as between patient and physician.

raptus (rap′tus) [L.] a sudden, violent attack. **r. haemorrha′gicus**, a sudden massive hemorrhage. **r. mani′acus**, a sudden, violent maniacal attack. **r. melanchol′icus**, an attack of frenzy or agitation occurring in melancholia. **r. nervo′rum**, a sudden, violent attack of nervousness.

rarefaction (rār″ĕ-fak′shun) [L. *rarefactio*] the condition of being or becoming less dense; diminution in density and weight, but not in volume.

Ras. abbreviation for L. *rasu′rae*, scrapings or filings.

rash (rash) a temporary eruption on the skin, as in urticaria; a drug eruption or viral exanthem. **brown-tail r.**, see under *dermatitis*. **butterfly r.**, see *butterfly* (def. 4). **cable r.**, chloracne. **caterpillar r.**, a local eruption attributed to poisoning by the hairs of caterpillars. **crystal r.** (*obs.*), miliaria crystallina. **diaper r.**, a cutaneous reaction in an infant, localized to the areas ordinarily covered by, and in contact with, the diaper, and sparing the folds of skin. It is due to various primary irritants, such as ammonia in decomposed urine, with histopathological changes varying with the causative factor; improperly processed diapers and other contact factors may also be responsible for such irritation. **drug r.**, drug eruption. **heat r.**, miliaria rubra. **hydatid r.**, an urticarial eruption which sometimes follows tapping or rupture of a hydatid cyst. **lily r.**, dermatitis affecting those who pick daffodils and narcissi in early spring. **mulberry r.** (*obs.*), a peculiar eruption of typhus, looking like that of measles. **nettle r.** (*obs.*), urticaria. **nickel r.**, a rash sometimes occurring in refiners of nickel. **rose r.**, roseola. **wandering r.**, geographic tongue.

rasion (ra′zhun) [L. *rasio*] the grating of drugs with a file.

Rasmussen's aneurysm (ras′mus-ens) [Fritz Waldemar *Rasmussen*, Danish physician, 1834–1877] see under *aneurysm.*

raspatory (ras′pah-to-re) [L. *raspatorium*] a file or rasp for surgical use; a xyster.

RAST radioallergosorbent test; see under *tests.*

rasura (rah-su′rah) [L.] scrapings or filings.

rat (rat) a small, aggressive, and omnivorous rodent of the genus *Rattus* and related genera of the family Muridae, commonly found about human habitations. Rats not only cause great economic loss, but are vectors of human disease; they harbor at least eleven different species of intestinal parasites that may be transmitted to man, such as tapeworms, roundworms, and trichinae; they are the reservoirs for the infective agents of plague, typhus, Weil's disease, and rat-bite fever. Albino mutants of *R. norvegicus* are used as laboratory animals. **albino r.**, white r. **black r.**, *Rattus rattus*, the European black rat and the one most commonly responsible for transmitting plague to man by means of its flea (*Xenopsylla cheopis*). **brown r.**, *Rattus norvegicus;* also called the barn rat, gray rat, Norway rat, sewer rat, and wharf rat. It is larger than the black rat, has a brownish gray color, and short ears and tail. **Egyptian r.**, *Rattus rattus alexandrinus,* a black rat originally found in North Africa, but now distributed worldwide. **Holtzman r.**, a strain of albino rat descended originally from S–D strain which originated from Wistar Institute sometime before 1929. **Long-Evans r.**, a strain of rat, developed at the University of Rochester, characterized by a brownish to black color of the head and shoulders. **roof r.**, Egyptian r. **Sprague-Dawley r.**, a strain of albino rat developed by the Sprague-Dawley Animal Company, which is widely used in experimental work because of its calmness and ease of handling. **white r.**, an albino form of *Rattus rattus* or of *R. norvegicus* which is much used as a laboratory animal. **Wistar r.**, a strain of albino rat developed at the Wistar Institute but which has spread so widely to other institutions that there is probably marked dilution of the strain. **wood r.**, a rat of the genus *Neotoma;* they are hosts of fleas and ticks. Called also *pack rat, trade rat, mountain rat,* and *brush rat.*

rate (rāt) an expression of the speed or frequency with which a certain event or circumstance occurs in relation to a certain period of time, a specific population, or some other fixed standard. **attack r.**, the rate at which new cases of a specific disease occur; see *incidence.* **basal metabolic r.**, an expression of the rate at which oxygen is utilized by the body cells, or the calculated equivalent heat production by the body, in a fasting subject at complete rest. Abbreviated B.M.R. See also *basal metabolism,* under *metabolism.* **birth r.**, an expression of the number of births occurring during one year. The *crude birth rate* is the ratio of births to the total population; the *refined birth rate* is the ratio of births to the female population; the *true birth rate* is the ratio of births to the female population of child-bearing age, that is, between the ages of 15 and 45. **case r.**, morbidity r. **case fatality r.**, the number of deaths caused by a specific disease, expressed as a percentage of or otherwise related to the total number of cases of the disease. **circulation r.**, an expression of the amount of blood pumped per minute by the heart through the body. **death r.**, the ratio of the total number of deaths in a specified area to the population, generally figured in terms of number of deaths per 1,000, 10,000, or 100,000 of population. The *crude death rate* is the ratio of the number of deaths within a given time (as one year) to the number of people alive at the middle of the period. The *specific death rate* is the proportion of deaths per annum in an age group or other specified group of the population per 1,000 of the mean annual number of people in that group. Called also *mortality r.* See also *mortality* (def. 2). **dose r.**, the amount of any agent administered per unit of time. **erythrocyte sedimentation r.**, an expression of the extent of settling of erythrocytes, per unit time, in a column of fresh citrated or otherwise treated blood. **fatality r.**, the number of deaths caused by a specific circumstance or disease, expressed as the absolute or relative number of deaths among the individuals encountering the circumstance or having the disease. **five-year survival r.**, an expression of the number of survivors with no trace of disease five years after each has been diagnosed or treated for the same disease. **glomerular filtration r.**, an expression of the quantity of glomerular filtrate formed each minute in all nephrons of both kidneys, calculated by measuring the clearance of a specific substance, e.g., inulin or creatinine. **growth r.**, an expression of the increase in size of an organic object per unit time, calculations usually being made as to both the absolute and the relative increment. **heart r.**, the number of contractions of the ventricles of the heart per unit of time (usually a minute). It usually corresponds to the pulse rate, but occasionally some of the contractions of the left ventricle fail to produce peripheral pulse waves, so that the rate of the pulse at the wrist is less than that of the heart. **lethality r.**, fatality r. **mendelian r.**, an expression of the numerical relations of the occurrence of distinctly contrasted mendelian characters in succeeding generations of hybrid offspring. **morbidity r.**, the number of cases of a given disease occurring during a specified period per 1,000, 10,000, or 100,000 of population. **mortality r.**, death r. **oocyst r.**, the percentage of wild female mosquitoes found to contain oocysts in the midgut. **output exposure r.**, in radiology, the exposure to radiation at a specified point per unit of time, usually expressed in roentgens per minute. **parasite r.**, the percentage of persons, in a particular age group or area, in whom parasites, especially malarial parasites, can be found. **pulse r.**, the rate of pulsation noted in a peripheral artery per minute, normally from 50 to 100. **respiration r.**, an expression of the number of movements of the chest, indicative of inspiration and expiration, occurring per minute. **sedimentation r.**, the rate at which a sediment is deposited in a given volume of solution, especially when subjected to the action of a centrifuge; see also *erythrocyte sedimentation r.* **sickness r.**, morbidity r. **sporozoite r.**, the percentage of wild female mosquitoes found to contain sporozoites in the glands. **stillbirth r.**, an expression of the relation of the number of stillbirths to the total number of births.

Rathke's pouch, etc. (rahth′kez) [Martin Heinrich *Rathke,* German anatomist, 1793–1860] see under *column, cyst, fold, pouch, trabecula,* and *tumor.*

raticide (rat′i-sīd) an agent destructive to rats.

ratio (ra′she-o) [L.] an expression of the quantity of one substance or entity in relation to that of another; the relationship between two quantities expressed as the quotient of one divided by the other. **A-G r., albumin-globulin r.,** the ratio of albumin to globulin in the blood serum, plasma, or the urine in various types of renal disease. **arm r.,** a figure expressing the relation of the length of the longer arm of a mitotic chromosome to that of the shorter arm. **birth-death r.,** vital index. **body-weight r.,** body weight in grams divided by stature in centimeters. **cardiothoracic r.,** the ratio of the transverse diameter of the heart to the internal diameter of the chest at its widest point just above the level of the dome of the diaphragm, a rough guide to cardiac enlargement, being normally less than 0.5. **cell color r.,** the result obtained by dividing the percentage of red cells by the percentage of hemoglobin. **concentration r.,** the ratio of the average concentration of a solid in the urine to its concentration in the blood. **curative r.,** therapeutic r. **D-N r., dextrose-nitrogen r.,** the ratio between the dextrose and the nitrogen of the urine. **expiratory exchange r.,** the ratio of carbon dioxide output to oxygen uptake in respiration. **G-N r., glucose-nitrogen r.,** D-N r. **grid r.,** in radiology, the ratio of the height of the lead strips to the width of the interspacing of a grid. **hand r.,** the ratio of the length of the hand to its width. **holdaway r.,** a means of expressing the relationship of the pogonion and the lower incisor to the nasion-basion plane; used in cephalometrics as a diagnostic aid. **karyoplasmic r.,** nucleocytoplasmic r. **ketogenic-antiketogenic r.,** the proportion between substances that form glucose in the body and those that form fatty acids. **lecithin-sphingomyelin r. (L/S r.),** the ratio of lecithin to sphingomyelin concentration in the amniotic fluid, used to predict the degree of pulmonary maturity of the fetus and thus the risk of respiratory difficulties. **nucleocytoplasmic r., nucleoplasmic r.,** the ratio of nuclear to cytoplasmic volume. **nutritive r.,** the ratio between the digestible protein and the digestible fats and carbohydrates in a ration in stock feeding. **respiratory exchange r.,** expiratory exchange r. **sex r.,** an expression of the number of males in a population to the number of females, usually stated as the number of males per 100 females. **therapeutic r.,** the fraction of the minimal lethal dose of a drug that is therapeutically effective; called also *curative r.* **urea excretion r.,** the ratio of the number of milligrams of urea in the urine excreted in one hour to the number of milligrams of urea in 100 ml. of blood; the normal ratio is 50.

ration (ra′shun) [L. *ratio* proportion] a fixed allowance of food or drink per day or other unit of time. **basal r.,** a ration giving the required energy, but lacking in one or more vitamins.

rational (rash′un-al) [L. *rationalis* reasonable] based upon reason; characterized by possession of one's reason.

rationale (rash″un-al′) [L.] a rational exposition of principles; the logical basis of a procedure.

rationalization (rash″un-al-i-za′shun) an unconscious defense mechanism by which one justifies attitudes and behavior that would otherwise be intolerable.

rat-tails (rat′tālz) a swollen condition of the hair papillae over the flexor tendons of a horse's legs, due to filth and bacteria.

rattlesnake (rat′'l-snāk) any of the New World pit vipers of the genera *Crotalus* and *Sistrurus*, having a series of cornified interlocking segments at the tip of the tail; when disturbed they vibrate the tail to produce the characteristic rattling or buzzing sound. See table accompanying *snake*.

Rattus (rat′us) a genus of small rodents, the rats (see *rat*). **R. norve′gicus,** the brown rat. **R. rat′tus,** the black rat. **R. rat′tus alexandri′nus,** the Egyptian, or roof, rat.

Rau's apophysis, process (row) [Johann J. *Rau* (Ravius), Dutch anatomist, 1658–1719] processus anterior mallei.

Rauber's layer (row′berz) [August Antinous Rauber, German anatomist, 1841–1917] see under *layer*.

Rauchfuss' sling, triangle (rowsh′foos) [Karl Andreyevich *Rauchfuss*, pediatrician in Leningrad, 1835–1915] see under *sling*, and see *Grocco's sign* (def. 1), under *sign*.

rausch (rowsh) [Ger. "intoxication"] light general anesthesia with ether only to the point where, if questioned sharply, the patient will not reply; called also *etherrausch*.

rauschbrand (rowsh′brahnt) [Ger.] blackleg.

Rau-Sed (row′sed) trademark for a preparation of reserpine.

Rauserpa (raw-ser′pah) trademark for a preparation of rauwolfia serpentina.

Rauwiloid (row′wĭ-loid) trademark for preparations of alseroxylon.

Rauwolfia (raw-wul′fe-ah) a genus of apocyanaceous tropical trees and shrubs, including over 100 species, and providing numerous alkaloids, including reserpine, of medical interest. Many species have been used in South America, Africa, and Asia, as a source of several medicines. **R. serpenti′na,** (L.) Benth. ex Kurz, a small shrub native to India and the Orient, containing many alkaloids, of which reserpine and rescinnamine are the most important therapeutically; the root is used as the whole root or as isolated alkaloids as a hypotensive, tranquilizer, and sedative.

rauwolfia (raw-wol′fe-ah) any member of the genus *Rauwolfia;* the dried root or an extract of the dried root of *Rauwolfia.* **r. serpenti′na** [USP], the dried root of *Rauwolfia serpentina,* sometimes with fragments of rhizome and aerial stem bases attached, containing not less than 0.15 per cent of reserpine-rescinnamine group alkaloids, calculated as reserpine; used as an antihypertensive. It is also used as a sedative and tranquilizer. **r. serpenti′na, powdered** [USP], rauwolfia serpentina reduced to a very fine powder adjusted, if necessary, to contain between 0.15 and 0.20 per cent of reserpine-rescinnamine group alkaloids.

RAV Rous associated virus.

Ravius (ra′ve-us) see *Rau*.

ray (ra) [L. *radius* spoke] a line emanating from a center, as (*a*) a more or less distinct portion of radiant energy (light or heat), proceeding in a specific direction (used in the plural as a general term for any form of radiant energy, whether vibratory or particulate), or (*b*) one of the individual elements at the distal end of the limb of an early embryo, foretelling development of the metacarpal or metatarsal bones and the phalanges of the digits. **actinic r.,** a light ray which produces chemical changes. In general, light rays become more actinic as one passes from the red through the spectrum to the violet and even into the ultraviolet. **alpha r's, α-r's,** high-speed helium nuclei which have been ejected from radioactive substances. Owing to their high velocity (one tenth that of light) their kinetic energy is so great that a single alpha particle produces a microscopic flash of light when it hits a spinthariscope; when it hits another atom (as of nitrogen) it may cause it to disintegrate. **anode r's,** positive r's. **antirachitic r's,** ultraviolet rays between 2700 and 3020 A.U. **astral r.,** one of the rays of an aster. Called also *polar r.* **bactericidal r's,** rays that are destructive to bacteria, i.e., those from 1850 to 2600 A.U. **Becquerel r's,** former name for rays emitted from uranium and other radioactive substances, and now known as alpha, beta, and gamma rays. **beta r's, β-r's,** electrons ejected from radioactive substances with velocities which may be as high as 0.98 of the velocity of light. **Blondlot r's,** n r's. **border r's, borderline r's,** grenz r's. **Bucky's r's,** grenz r's. **caloric r.,** radiant energy which is converted into heat when applied to the body. **canal r's,** positive rays in a vacuum tube; so called from having been first obtained by allowing the discharge from the anode to pass through a perforated (canalized) cathode. **cathode r's,** negative particles of electricity streaming out in a vacuum tube at right angles to the surface of the cathode and away from it irrespective of the position of the anode. They move in a straight line unless deflected by a magnet. By striking on solids they generate roentgen rays. See also *electron stream*. **central r.,** the straight line passing through the center of the radiation source and the center of the final beam-limiting diaphragm. **characteristic r.,** whan a metallic surface is exposed to roentgen rays a secondary radiation, called its characteristic ray, is emitted which is nearly homogeneous as to wavelength and is approximately proportional to the reciprocal of the square of the atomic weight of the metal. **chemical r.,**

actinic r. **convergent r.,** a ray which is approaching a focus; it may be produced by passage through a convex lens or by reflection from a concave mirror. **cosmic r's,** a form of very penetrating radiations which apparently move through interplanetary space in every direction; called also *Millikan rays* and *ultra x-rays*. **delta r's, δ-r's,** secondary beta rays produced in a gas by the passage of alpha particles. **digital r.,** a digit of the hand or foot and the corresponding portion of the metacarpus or metatarsus, considered as a continuous structural unit. **direct r.,** primary r. **direction r.,** the path of a ray of light from the point of fixation to the retina. **divergent r's,** rays coming from a source nearer than infinity. **Dorno's r's,** the active biological ultraviolet rays, i.e., those below 2890 A.U. **dynamic r's,** rays that are active physically or therapeutically. **erythema-producing r's,** rays that cause erythema, 2050 to 3100 A.U. **Finsen r's,** see under *light*. **gamma r's, γ-r's,** electromagnetic radiation of short wavelengths emitted by the nucleus of an atom during a nuclear reaction. They consist of high energy photons, have no mass and no electric charge, and travel with the speed of light and are usually associated with beta rays. **glass r's,** the rays formed in a roentgen-ray tube by the cathode rays striking the glass wall of the tube, so called to distinguish them from the roentgen rays originating at the anticathode. **Goldstein's r's,** rays formed when roentgen rays pass through some transparent medium; called also *s r's*. **grenz r's,** very soft roentgen rays having electromagnetic vibrations of wavelength about 2 A.U., lying between the roentgen rays and ultraviolet rays. **H r's,** a stream of hydrogen nuclei. **hard r's,** roentgen rays of short wavelength and great penetrative power. **heat r's,** see *radiant heat*, under *heat*. **hertzian r's,** see under *wave*. **incident r.,** see reflection, def. 2., and refraction, def. 2. **indirect r's,** rays formed at the surface of the glass of the cathode ray tube. **infrared r's,** radiations just beyond the red end of the spectrum; their wavelengths range between 0.75 and 1000 μm; see *infrared*. **infra-roentgen r's,** grenz r's. **intermediate r's,** wavelengths between the ultraviolet and the roentgen rays. **Lenard r's,** cathode rays after they have passed outside the discharge tube. **luminous r's,** the visible rays of the spectrum. **Lyman r's,** electromagnetic vibrations of wavelength between 600 and 12,300 A.U. **medullary r.,** any cortical extension of a bundle of tubules from a malpighian pyramid of the kidney. **Millikan r's,** cosmic r's. **minin r's,** rays generated by passing incandescent light through dark-blue glass. **monochromatic r's,** rays characterized by a definite wavelength, as secondary rays. **n r's,** an alleged form of radiation, the identity of which is not well established. Called also *Blondlot r's*. A variety of n rays (called *n′ rays*) differ from n rays in diminishing the luminosity of light and of faintly luminous surfaces. **necrobiotic r's,** short ultraviolet rays which kill living cells. **Niewenglowski's r's,** luminous rays given out by substances which have been exposed to the sun. **paracathodic r's,** rays formed by the impaction of cathode rays against a body (the anticathode) in their path. **parallel r's,** rays which come from a source at an infinite distance; divergent rays may be made parallel by means of a convex lens or a concave mirror. **pigment-producing r's,** rays that cause pigmentation, with a wavelength of 2500–3000 A.U. **polar r.,** astral r. **positive r's,** streams of positively charged atoms traveling at high speed from the anode of a partially evacuated tube under the influence of an applied voltage. **primary r.,** a ray given off directly from a radioactive substance. **reflected r.,** see *reflection*, def. 3. **refracted r.,** see *refraction*, def. 2. **roentgen r's,** electromagnetic vibrations of short wavelengths (from 5 A.U. down) or corresponding quanta (wave mechanics) that are produced when electrons moving at high velocity impinge on various substances, especially the heavy metals. They are commonly generated by passing a current of high voltage (from 10,000 volts up) through a Coolidge tube (see under *tube*). They are able to penetrate most substances to some extent, some much more readily than others, and to affect a photographic plate. These qualities make it possible to use them in taking roentgenograms of various parts of the body, thus revealing the

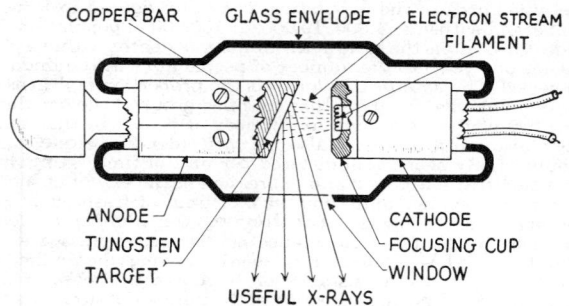

Standard stationary anode x-ray tube; diagram in longitudinal section. (Meschan.)

presence and position of fractures or foreign bodies or of radiopaque substances that have been purposely introduced. They can also cause certain substances to fluoresce and this makes fluoroscopy possible, by which the size, shape and movements of various organs such as the heart, stomach and intestines can be observed. By reason of the high energy of their quanta, they strongly ionize tissue through which they pass by means of the photoelectrons, both primary and secondary, which they liberate. Because of this effect they are used in treating various pathological conditions. Called also *x-rays*. **s r's**, Goldstein's r's. **Sagnac r's**, secondary beta rays formed when gamma rays are reflected from a metal surface. **scattered r's**, roentgen rays which, during their passage through a substance, have been deviated in direction and modified by an increase in wavelength. **Schumann's**, rays of wavelengths between 1850 and 1220 A.U. **secondary r.**, rays emitted by the matter on which a beam of roentgen ray impinges. **soft r's**, roentgen rays of long wavelength and little penetrative power. **titanium r.**, the radiation produced between metallic electrodes which consist of a tungsten alloy containing titanium. **transition r's**, grenz r's. **ultraviolet r's**, those invisible rays of the spectrum which are beyond the violet rays; their wavelengths range between 4 and 400 nm.; see *ultraviolet*. **ultra x-r.**, Millikan r's. **vital r's**, ultraviolet rays, between 2900 and 3200 A.U., which are the rays that act on the body therapeutically. **W r's**, intermediate r's. **x-r's**, the name given by Röntgen to roentgen rays.

Raymond's apoplexy (ra-mawz′) [Fulgence *Raymond*, French neurologist, 1844–1910] see under *apoplexy*.

Raymond-Cestan (ra-maw′-ses-tan′) [F. *Raymond*; Etienne Jacques Marie Raymond *Cestan*, French surgeon, 1867–1912] see under *syndrome*.

Raynaud's disease (gangrene), phenomenon (ra-nōz′) [Maurice *Raynaud*, French physician, 1834–1881] see under *disease* and *phenomenon*.

Rb chemical symbol for *rubidium*.

R.B.C. red blood cell; red blood [cell] count (see *blood count*, under *count*).

RBE relative biological effectiveness; see under *effectiveness*.

R.C.M. Royal College of Midwives.

R.C.N. Royal College of Nursing.

R.C.O.G. Royal College of Obstetricians and Gynaecologists.

R.C.P. Royal College of Physicians.

R.C.S. Royal College of Surgeons.

R.C.V.S. Royal College of Veterinary Surgeons.

R.D. reaction of degeneration; see under *reaction*.

rd. abbreviation for *rutherford*.

RDE receptor-destroying enzyme.

R.E. radium emanation (see *radon*); right eye.

Re chemical symbol for *rhenium*.

re- [L.] a prefix signifying *back, again, contrary*, etc.

reablement (re-a′b′l-ment) rehabilitation.

reabsorb (re″ab-sorb′) to absorb again; to undergo or to subject to reabsorption (q.v.); to resorb.

reabsorption (re″ab-sorp′shun) 1. the act or process of absorbing again, as the selective absorption by the kidneys of substances (glucose, proteins, sodium, etc.) already secreted into the renal tubules, and their return to the circulating blood. 2. resorption.

react (re-akt′) 1. to respond to a stimulus. 2. to enter into chemical action.

reactance (re-ak′tans) the weakening of an alternating electric current caused by passage through a coil of wire.

reactant (re-ak′tant) an original substance entering into a chemical reaction.

reaction (re-ak′shun) [*re-* + L. *agere* to act] 1. opposite action, or counteraction; the response to stimulation. 2. the phenomena caused by the action of chemical agents; a chemical process in which one substance is transformed into another substance or substances. For specially named reactions not defined here, see under *tests*. 3. in psychology, the mental and/or emotional state that develops in any particular situation. **Abderhalden's r.**, a serum reaction based upon the obsolete hypothesis that when a foreign protein gets into the blood the body reacts by elaborating a ferment which causes disintegration of the protein. Such a ferment, called a *protective ferment* (*defensive ferment, protective enzyme, abwehrfermente*), is specific for the particular protein which caused its formation. This reaction was first applied to the diagnosis of pregnancy on the principle that in the blood of pregnant women there is present a proteolytic ferment which will cause cleavage of placental albumin and placental peptone. The same principle has been applied to the diagnosis of cancer because the blood of cancer patients contains a ferment which digests coagulated cancer protein. Similarly, in schizophrenia, the brain becomes degenerated and furnishes to the blood substances which excite the formation of a ferment capable of decomposing proteins of human brain. This is the *Abderhalden-Fauser* or the *Fauser reaction*. The same principle has also been applied to the diagnosis of syphilis, tuberculosis, and the acute infections. **Abderhal-**

den-Fauser r., see under *Abderhalden's r.* **Abelin's r.**, a reaction for ascertaining the presence of arsphenamine in the urine. **accelerated r.**, a reaction or response which occurs in a shorter time than is usual. **acetic acid r.**, Rivalta's r. **acetonitrile r.**, Hunt's r. **acid r.**, 1. a surplus of hydrogen ions in a solution or a pH below 7. 2. any test by which an acid reaction is recognized, such as the reddening of blue litmus. **Acree-Rosenheim r.**, see under *tests*. **acrosome r.**, a sequence of structural changes that occur in spermatozoa when in the vicinity of an ovum in the oviduct, and that are believed to facilitate entry of a spermatozoon into the ovum: the outer membrane of the acrosome fuses at multiple points with the overlying plasma membrane of the sperm head, creating openings through which the enzymes of the acrosome are liberated. **acute situational r.**, a transient disorder, occurring in an individual without underlying mental disorder, in response to overwhelming environmental stress. **Adamkiewicz's r.**, see under *tests*. **adjustment r.**, one elicited by a change in situation or environment, sometimes evidenced as a transient personality disorder. **agglutinoid r.**, see *prozone*. **alarm r.**, the total of all nonspecific phenomena elicited by sudden exposure to stimuli which affect large portions of the body and to which the organism is not adapted quantitatively or qualitatively. One of the most striking manifestations of this reaction is the rapid involution of the lymphoid tissues due to the action of hormones. Abbreviated AR. **alkaline r.**, 1. the presence in a solution of more hydroxyl ions than hydrogen ions, i.e., a pH greater than 7. 2. any test by which an alkaline reaction is recognized, such as the bluing of red litmus. **allergic r.**, a local or general reaction characterized by altered reactivity of the animal body to an antigenic substance. **allograft r.**, the rejection of an allogeneic graft by a normal host; called also *homograft r.* **alpha-naphthol r.**, Molisch's test, defs. 2 and 3. **anamnestic r.**, see under *response*. **anaphylactic r.**, the reaction which occurs in anaphylactic shock; see *anaphylaxis*. **anaphylactoid r.**, pseudoanaphylaxis. **anatoxin r.**, an intradermic reaction in which anatoxin (toxoid) is used. **anergastic r.**, a psychosis due to a brain lesion and manifested by impairment of memory and judgment and by fits, palsy, and coma. **antalgic r.**, a bodily reaction or response having the purpose of avoiding pain. **antigen r. of Debré and Paraf**, a complement fixation reaction for the diagnosis of urinary tuberculosis, using for antigen the patient's urine, for antibody a known tuberculosis serum. **antigen-antibody r.**, the specific combination of antigen with homologous antibody resulting in the reversible formation of antigen-antibody complexes that differ in solubility according to the antigen-antibody ratio. The binding of a ligand by an antibody molecule may be considered a competitive partitioning of ligand between the active site and aqueous medium, with the complex being stabilized by the interaction of both polar and apolar forces. The relative stability of antigen-antibody complexes is dependent upon the ability of the ligand to interact with the apolar active site rather than with the polar aqueous medium. Antigen-antibody reactions may result in precipitation, agglutination, complement-dependent reactions, neutralization, or cytotropic effects. **antiglobulin r.**, the agglutination of particles (usually erythrocytes) that have been (1) sensitized by the adsorption of soluble antigen, (2) treated with antibody to that antigen, and (3) treated with antiserum to the serum globulin of the animal species that produced the antibody. **antitryptic r.**, the reaction produced by the blood upon mixtures of trypsin and casein solutions. Such reaction is modified by various disease conditions, such as cancer and tuberculosis, and by pregnancy. **anxiety r.**, see under *neurosis*. **Arakawa's r.**, see under *reagent*. **Arias-Stella r.**, changes in the cells of the endometrial epithelium consisting chiefly of bizarre-shaped hyperchromatic enlarged nuclei associated with a loss of cellular polarity; cytoplasmic vacuolization is occasionally present. The changes are thought to be associated with the presence of chorionic tissue in an intrauterine or extrauterine site, and are seen in some cases of ectopic pregnancy. **arsphenamine r.**, Abelin's r. **Arthus r.**, the development of an inflammatory lesion, classically an ulcer, marked by edema, hemorrhage, and necrosis, that occurs within hours after interdermal injection of an antigen to which the animal already has precipitating antibody. It is generally considered an immediate hypersensitivity, or is classed as a type III reaction. Antigen-antibody complexes formed in the presence of complement adhere to the vascular epithelium and are encircled by fibrin, blood platelets, and polymorphonuclear neutrophils. Plugging of the vessels is followed by exudation into surrounding tissues of fluid laden with the neutrophils. *Arthus-type reaction* refers to numerous hypersensitivity states in which antigen-antibody complexes initiate the lesion, including serum sickness, glomerulonephritis, and farmer's lung. Called also *Arthus phenomenon*. **Ascoli's r.**, miostagmin r. **associative r.**, a reaction in which the response is withheld until the idea presented has suggested an associated idea. **axon r., axonal r.**, the series of changes in the ganglion cell (central chromatolysis with displacement of the nucleus) following the severing of its axon. **Bachman r.**, see under *tests*. **bacteriolytic r.**, the reaction which brings about specific bacteriolysis. **Bareggi's r.**, the formation in a test tube of an unretracted clot, with but little serum, from the blood of typhoid fever; if the blood is from a patient with tuberculosis, the clot retracts with the separation of much serum. **Bekhterev's r.,** in cases of tetany the minimum of electric current needed to arouse muscular contraction needs to be diminished at every interruption or change of density in order to prevent tetanic contraction. **Bence Jones r.,** the precipitation of protein by heat followed by its redissolving on boiling and being precipitated again on cooling. **Besredka's r.,** a complement deviation reaction for tuberculosis. **biphasic r.,** a reaction made up of two parts, as flexion followed by extension. Cf. *uniphasic r.* **Bittorf's r.,** in renal colic the pain produced by squeezing the testicle or pressing the ovary radiates to the kidney. **biuret r.,** see under *tests.* **Blackman r.,** the fundamental thermochemical dark reaction in which carbon dioxide fixation takes place during photosynthesis. **blanching r.,** Schultz-Charlton r. **Boltz's r.,** see under *tests.* **Bordet and Gengou r.,** complement fixation. **Braun-Husler r.,** see under *tests.* **Brieger's cachexia r.,** cachexia r. **Brodie r.,** the extremely sensitive reaction of cats to foreign proteins. Intravenous doses of egg white or blood serum that have no appreciable effect on guinea pigs or rabbits produce marked fall of blood pressure in anesthetized cats. **Brown's r.,** see under *tests,* def. 1. **Bruck's nitric acid r.** (*for syphilis*), the precipitate formed when nitric acid is added to syphilitic serum is less soluble in an excess of dilute nitric acid than the precipitate from normal serum. **Buscaino r.,** see under *tests.* **cachexia r.,** increase in the antitryptic power of the blood serum seen in malignant disease and other diseases characterized by cachexia. **cadaveric r.,** total loss of electrical response in the affected muscles in familial periodic paralysis. **Calmette's r.,** ophthalmic r. **Cammidge's r.,** pancreatic r. **cancer r.,** see specific reactions, including *antitryptic r., cachexia r., Freund's r., Klein's r., miostagmin r., Penn seroflocculation r., Stammler's r.* See also *cancer test,* under *tests.* **Cannizzaro's r.,** the reaction which aldehydes may undergo in alkali or when brought in contact with animal tissue; one molecule of the aldehyde is reduced to the corresponding alcohol and another molecule is simultaneously oxidized to the corresponding acid. Cf. *aldehyde mutase.* **capsular r.,** the reaction of the capsular substance of bacteria with a homologous antibody. **carbamino r.,** alpha-amino acids unite with CO_2 in the presence of alkalis or alkaline earths to form salts of carbamino-carboxylic acids. This reaction is used in studying the course of protein digestion. See *formol titration,* under *method.* **Casoni's r.,** see *Casoni's intradermal test,* under *tests.* **chain r.,** a nuclear (neutron) reaction which once started will proceed and multiply of its own accord by emitting particles that propagate the reaction in adjacent nuclei. **Chantemesse's r.,** the ophthalmic reaction for typhoid fever; see *ophthalmic r.* **Chediak's r.,** see under *tests.* **Chopra antimony r.,** dilute the patient's serum with ten volumes of physiological salt solution and add an equal volume of 4 per cent antimony solution. A flocculent precipitate denotes a positive reaction, which may occur in sera of patients with kala-azar or with splenomegaly due to other causes. **chromaffin r.,** see *chromaffin.* **citochol r.,** see *Sachs-Witebsky test,* under *tests.* **coagulation r., coagulo r.,** a test for syphilis based on the fact that syphilitic sera inhibit the coagulation of the blood by interference with thrombin production more than do normal sera; called also *Hirschfeld-Klinger r.* **cockade r.,** see *Römer's test,* under *tests.* **colloidal gold r.,** see under *tests.* **complement fixation r.,** see under *fixation.* **compluetic r.,** Wassermann r. **conglobation r.,** see *Müller's test* (def. 3), under *tests.* **conglutination r.,** a characteristic agglutination reaction obtained by a mixture of conglutinin, cells (e.g., bacteria or red cells), fresh complement, and a cell-specific immune serum from which the agglutinins have been removed by absorption. See *conglutinin.* **conjunctival r.,** ophthalmic r. **consensual r.,** 1. crossed reflex. 2. a reaction that takes place independently of the will. See *consensual.* **conversion r.,** the conversion type of hysterical neurosis; see under *neurosis.* **coupled r.,** a series of linked reactions. **Cronin Lowe r.,** see under *tests.* **cross r.,** the interaction of an antibody with antigen that did not specifically stimulate its synthesis; it may be weaker than the reaction of an antibody with its homologous antigen; the interaction of an antigen with an antibody formed against a different antigen with which the first antigen shares identical or closely related antigenic determinants. **cutaneous r.,** 1. cutireaction. 2. a reaction produced by applying to an abrasion or by injecting into the skin a solution of a protein or a pollen to which the patient is sensitive. **cutituberculin r.,** Moro's r. **Dale r.,** an *in vitro* test for anaphylactic sensitization in the guinea pig: a small amount of the antigen added to a tissue bath in which is immersed the excised uterine horn (smooth muscle) of an anaphylactically sensitized guinea pig, causes contraction of the sensitized uterine muscle. Called also *Schultz-Dale reaction.* Schultz employed intestinal muscle; Dale used uterine muscle from virgin guinea pigs. **D'Amato's r.,** see under *tests.* **dark r.,** in photosynthesis, the series of reactions by which fixation of carbon dioxide into carbohydrate is accomplished; these reactions are driven by the products of the light reaction and do not require the presence of light. **Deehan's typhoid r.,** a cutaneous test for typhoid fe-

ver. **defense r.,** 1. a mental reaction which shuts out from consciousness ideas that are not acceptable to the ego. 2. conduct that tends to conceal some aspects of one's life from others. **r. of degeneration,** the reaction to electric stimulation of muscles whose nerves have degenerated. It consists of a loss of response to a faradic stimulus in a muscle, and to galvanic and faradic stimulus in a nerve. Galvanic irritability of the muscle is increased. Abbreviated Ea. R. (Ger. *Entartungs-Reaktion*) and R.D. **r. of degeneration, franklinic,** a form of reaction elicited by static electricity and similar to the reaction produced by the faradic current. **delayed r.,** a reaction, such as an allergic reaction, occurring hours to days after exposure to an inducer; called also *delayed response.* **delayed-blanch r.,** an unusual, paradoxical reaction to the intradermal injection of acetylcholine or methacholine, associated with atopic disease; characteristically, instead of the usual erythematous wheal and flare, a delayed blanch occurs within the flare 3 to 5 minutes after the injection and persists for 15 to 30 minutes. **depot r.,** a red reaction of the skin around the point of entrance of the needle in the subcutaneous tuberculin test. **depressive r.,** any neurotic depressive reaction in which insight is impaired to a lesser degree than in psychotic depression; see also *depression* (def. 3). **dermotuberculin r.,** Pirquet's r. **desmoid r.,** (for gastric secretion and motility): a bag of rubber tissue containing methylene blue and iodoform, and tied with a string of soft catgut, is administered to the patient: normal gastric juice will digest the string and liberate the stain, which will appear in the urine after five or six hours. **desmoplastic r.,** see *desmoplastic.* **Detre's r.** (*obs.*), differential cutireaction. **diazo r.,** Ehrlich's diazo r. **Dick r.,** see under *tests.* **digitonin r.,** the formation of a precipitate on treating a sterol, such as cholesterol or ergosterol, with digitonin; employed to define cholesterol esters which do not precipitate in total serum cholesterol determinations. **displacement r.,** a chemical reaction in which a reactant displaces a functional group from a substrate and becomes bound in the position formerly occupied by the leaving group; see also *displacement.* **dissociative r.,** the dissociative type of hysterical neurosis; see under *neurosis.* **Dochez and Avery's r.,** see *precipitin r.,* def. 1. **Dold's r.,** see under *tests.* **dopa r.,** the reaction by which dopa is changed into melanin under the influence of dopa-oxidase. **dysergastic r.,** a disorder characterized by disorientation, hallucinations, daydreams and fears, due to impaired cerebral circulation and to the resulting reduced nutrition of the brain. **E-E r.,** Foshay's r. **egg yellow r.,** a yellow foam appearing in Ehrlich's diazo reaction before the addition of ammonia; believed to indicate acute pneumonia. **Ehrlich's diazo r.,** a reaction of a pure pink or red color resulting from the action of diazotized sulfanilic acid and ammonia upon certain aromatic substances, e.g., urobilinogen, found in the urine in some conditions. This reaction has diagnostic value in hepatic disease, typhoid fever, and measles and prognostic value in tuberculosis. **electric r.,** a reaction, such as muscular contraction, caused by the application of electricity to the body. **epiphanin r.,** on the introduction of Weichardt's reagent into a solution of sera and antigen, the solution is rendered more alkaline (positive reaction); the reaction was used especially in the serodiagnosis of syphilis. **erythematous-edematous r.,** Foshay's r. **erythrocyte sedimentation r.,** see under *rate.* **erythrophore r.,** a red coloration appearing in certain male fishes after the injection of gonadal hormone. **r. of exhaustion,** reaction to electric stimulation seen in conditions of exhaustion. In it the reaction normally produced by a certain current can be reproduced only by an increase in the current. **Fahraeus r.,** erythrocyte sedimentation rate. **fatigue r.,** rise of temperature on muscular effort. **Fauser r.,** see under *Abderhalden's r.* **Felix-Weil r.,** Weil-Felix r. **Fernandez r.,** a reaction analogous to the tuberculin reaction, occurring three to four days after intradermal injection of lepromin; see also *lepromin test,* under *tests.* Cf. *Mitsuda r.* **Feulgen's r.,** see under *tests.* **fixation r.,** complement fixation. **flocculation r.,** see *Sachs-Georgi test,* under *tests.* **Florence's r.,** see under *tests.* **focal r.,** the reaction that occurs at or about the site of an infection or the point of an injection. It may be induced by the injection of a specific agent, such as tuberculin, mallein, or a bacterial vaccine, or by the use of nonspecific agents. **Fornet's r.,** a reaction for syphilis: the serum of the patient is treated with serum taken from a paretic; if syphilis is present, a flocculent ring will appear at the line of contact of the two serums. **Foshay's r.,** a spreading redness about a slightly elevated central edema developing at the site of the intradermal injection of an antiserum specific for the infection from which the patient is suffering; called also *erythematous-edematous r.* and *E-E reaction.* **Freund's r., Freund-Kaminer r.,** the serum of noncancerous persons destroys cancer cells, while that of cancer patients has no lytic effect. **fright r.,** involuntary contraction of extraocular and facial muscles of animals during states of fright and anger. **fuchsinophil r.,** certain substances when stained with fuchsin retain the stain on being treated with picric acid alcohol. **Gangi's r.,** a test of a liquid to determine whether it is a transudate or exudate, utilizing hydrochloric acid. **Gerhardt's r.,** see under *tests.* **Ghilarducci's r.,** contraction of the muscles of a limb when the active electrode is placed on a part somewhat removed from them. **Gmelin's r.,** see under *tests.* **Goetsch's skin r.,** a test for hyperthyroidism based on local reaction to hypodermic injection of epinephrine. **gold r.,** colloidal gold test. **graft-vs.-host r.,** the immunological reaction of a graft rich in immunologically competent cells against the genetically nonidentical tissues of the recipient. The graft is not rejected because of the recipient's immunological immaturity (as in the newborn) or its genetic make-up (as in F_1 hybrid disease), or because it has been treated with whole-body irradiation or immunosuppression. Tissues especially rich in immunologically competent cells capable of inducing a graft-vs.-host reaction include the spleen, lymph nodes, thoracic duct lymph, and to a lesser degree the bone marrow and peripheral blood. Clinical symptoms include skin rash, diarrhea, and evidence of hepatic dysfunction. Called also *graft-versus-host disease.* See also *runt disease.* **Grignard's r.,** see under *reagent.* **gross stress r.,** an acute emotional reaction incident to severe environmental stress, e.g., in military operations or civilian disasters; called also *stress r.* **group r.,** see *group agglutination,* under *agglutination.* **Gruber's r., Gruber-Widal r.,** Widal's test. **Gubler's r.,** the formation of a brown color on gradually adding nitrosonitric acid to urine; seen in urobilin jaundice. **Gunning's r.,** see under *tests.* **Hanganatziu-Deicher r.,** following the parenteral administration of heterogenic serum, human blood serum agglutinates certain heterogenic erythrocytes, particularly those of sheep, horses, hares, and guinea-pigs. **Hecht-Weinberg-Gradwohl modification of the Wassermann r.** (*obs.*), the natural antisheep amboceptor and the natural hemolytic complement found in the patient's fresh serum are utilized instead of the antisheep-rabbit amboceptor and guinea-pig complement of the regular test. **hemagglutination-inhibition r.,** the inhibition by antibodies of viral agglutination of red cells. **hemiopic pupillary r.,** reaction in certain cases of hemianopia in which the stimulus of light thrown upon one side of the retina causes the iris to contract, while light thrown on the other side arouses no response. Called also *Wernicke's r.* **hemoclastic r.,** laking of blood due to hemolysis; see *hemoclastic crisis,* under *crisis.* **Henle's r.,** the medullary cells of the adrenals stain dark brown on treatment with chromium salts. **Henry's melanin r.,** see under *tests.* **Herxheimer's r.,** Jarisch-Herxheimer r. **heterophil antibody r.,** a reaction produced by antibody against a heterophil antigen, as in the Paul-Bunnell test. **Hill r.,** the primary reaction of photosynthesis in which light is absorbed and used by chlorophyll. **Hirschfeld-Klinger r.,** coagulation r. **homograft r.,** allograft r. **Hunt's r.,** the acetonitrile resistance of white mice is increased by treatment of the mice with blood from a patient with hyperthyroidism; called also *acetonitrile reaction.* **hunting r.,** periods of vasoconstriction alternating with periods of vasodilatation in a finger or other part exposed to temperatures below 15° C. **hypersensitivity r.,** see *hypersensitivity.* **Ide r.,** see under *tests.* **r. of identity,** if the antigens in two solutions are identical, a continuous line of precipitation will be formed between them and a solution of homologous antibody when the three solutions are placed in separate wells forming a triangle on a gel diffusion plate (as in the Ouchterlony test). If the line of precipitation is continuous but has a spurlike projection (*r. of partial identity*), the antigens are not identical but share antigenic determinants. If two intersecting lines are formed (*r. of nonidentity*), the antigens are unrelated. **immediate r.,** a reaction, such as an allergic reaction, occurring seconds to minutes after exposure to an inducer; called also *immediate response.* **immune r.,** 1. specifically altered reactivity of the animal body following exposure to antigen, manifested as antibody production, cell-mediated immunity, or immunological tolerance; called also *immune response.* 2. the formation of a papule and areola without the development of a vesicle following smallpox vaccination; indicative of a high degree of immunity. **indophenol r.,** see under *tests.* **intracutaneous r.,** a reaction following an injection into the substance of the skin; such a reaction may have diagnostic value as in the Schick test, Dick test, tuberculin test, etc. **intracuti r.,** see *Frei test,* under *tests.* **intradermal r.,** intracutaneous r. **involutional psycotic r.,** involutional melancholia. **Israelson's r.,** see under *tests.* **Ito-Reenstierna r.,** see under *tests.* **Jaffé r.,** creatinine when treated with picric acid in strongly alkaline solution gives an intense red color. **Jarisch-Herxheimer r.,** transiently increased discomfort in skin lesions and temperature elevation occurring within two hours after the start of antibiotic treatment of secondary syphilis and of relapsing fever (*Borrelia recurrentis*); it occurs in many but not all who receive antibiotic therapy. **johnin r.,** a skin reaction like the tuberculin reaction, produced by filtrates of cultures of *Mycobacterium paratuberculosis* (johnin); used in the diagnosis of Johne's disease. **Jolly's r.,** failure of response to faradic stimulation in a muscle, the power of voluntary contraction as well as the response to galvanic stimulation being retained. **Jones-Mote r.,** a mild skin reaction of the delayed hypersensitivity type occurring after challenge with protein antigens. **Kafka's r.,** see under *tests.* **Kahn's albumin A r.,** see under *tests,* def. 2. **Keller-Killian r.** (*for 2-desoxy sugars*): dissolve the sugar in glacial acetic acid that contains some ferric chloride, underlay it with concentrated sulfuric acid and the

upper layer will take on a deep blue color. **K. H. r.,** a combined complement fixation and hemagglutination reaction used in the diagnosis of glanders. **Klein r.,** a modification of Freund's reaction for cancer, using for carcinolysis a cell suspension from an adenocarcinoma of the mouse. **Koch's r.,** see *tuberculin test,* under *tests.* **Koler r.,** Adamkiewicz's test. **Konsuloff's r.,** see under *tests.* **Kottmann's r.,** see under *tests.* **Landau's r.,** see under *tests.* **Lange's r.,** 1. colloidal gold test. 2. see under *tests.* **lengthening r.,** the elongation of the extensor muscles which permits flexion of a limb; called also *clasp-knife reflex.* **lentochol r.,** see *Sachs-Georgi test,* under *tests.* **lepra r.,** a recurring episode in the course of lepromatous leprosy, characterized by fever, malaise, neuralgia, aggravation and extension of existing lesions, and appearance of new ones, and often by erythema multiforme, sometimes by erythema bullosum or exudativum, but most often by erythema nodosum leprosum, with tender intradermal and subcutaneous red nodules 1 to 3 cm. in diameter scattered over the extremities and, to a lesser extent, the trunk. **lepromin r.,** see under *tests.* **leukemic r., leukemoid r.,** a peripheral blood picture resembling that of leukemia or indistinguishable from it on the basis of morphologic appearance alone. **Lewis' r.,** the urticaria produced by histamine; see *histamine test,* def. 2, under *tests.* **Lieben's r.,** see under *tests.* **Liebermann-Burchardt r.,** a green color is produced when concentrated sulfuric acid in acetic anhydride is added to a mixture of chloroform solution of cholesterol. **light r.,** in photosynthesis, the photochemical process in which a series of reactions driven by light energy results in the generation of ATP and reduced coenzymes (NADH or NADPH); these substances then drive the dark reaction. **Lignières' r.,** see under *tests.* **lignin r.,** a color reaction given by wood cellulose, consisting of a yellow color with aniline salts and a red color with a solution of phloroglucinol in concentrated hydrochloric acid. **local r.,** a reaction similar to a focal reaction occurring at the point of injection. **Loeb's decidual r.,** the presence of a glass bead or other irritant causes the formation of a small deciduoma in the uterine mucosa when corpora lutea are developing normally. **Loewi's r.,** see under *tests.* **Lohmann r.,** an easily reversible reaction occurring in muscle, in which the high-energy phosphate bond of ATP is transferred to creatine, forming creatine phosphate; the reaction is catalyzed by creatine kinase. **luetin r.,** Noguchi's luetin r. **Machado r., Machado-Guerreiro r.,** see under *tests.* **Malmejde r.,** see under *tests.* **manic-depressive r.,** see under *psychosis.* **Manoiloff's (Manoilov's) r.,** 1. a blood reaction once used in comparing the blood of the parents and of their alleged child for the determination of the paternity of the child. 2. an obsolete test for pregnancy: the serum of a pregnant woman decolorizes to yellow the blue mixture prepared by mixing serum with 2 per cent aqueous solution of theobromine sodium salicylate colored with Nile blue; called also *Manoiloff's test.* **Mantoux r.,** see under *tests.* **Marañón's r.,** see under *sign.* **Marchi's r.,** failure of the myelin sheath of a nerve to become discolored when treated with osmic acid. **Mátéfy's r.,** see under *tests.* **Meinicke r.,** see under *tests.* **Millon's r.,** see under *tests.* **miostagmin r., miostagminic r.,** an obsolete blood serum test to confirm the diagnosis of malignant tumors, syphilis, typhoid, etc., based on the fact that when the antibodies of a disease and its corresponding antigens are brought together, there is a lowering of the surface tension of the mixture. **Mitsuda r.,** a reaction marked by the development of a papulonodular lesion at the site of intradermal injection of lepromin, occurring three to four weeks after injection; it indicates cellular immunity (rather than infection with) *Mycobacterium leprae.* See also *lepromin test,* under *tests.* Cf. *Fernandez r.* **mixed cell agglutination r.,** the mixed clumping of different cell types owing to the reaction of antibody with different antigenic determinants on the cells. **mixed leukocyte r., mixed lymphocyte r.,** the appearance of blast cells in a culture of leukocytes from two individuals; histocompatibility varies inversely with the number of blast cells. **Moeller's r.,** see *rhinoreaction.* **Molisch's r.,** see under *tests.* **Moloney r.,** the intradermal injection of diluted diphtheria toxoid as a control in the Schick test. **Montenegro r.,** see under *tests.* **Morelli's r.,** see under *tests.* **Moritz r.,** Rivalta's r. **Moro's r.,** an eruption of pale or red papules on a cutaneous area after application of an ointment of 5 ml. of old tuberculin and 5 gm. of anhydrous lanolin; other percutaneous tests, e.g., the Vollmer patch test, have replaced Moro's test. **mouse tail r.,** stiffening of the tail in rats and mice following the adminstration of a small dose of morphine. **Much's r., Much-Holzmann r.,** inhibition of the hemolytic action of cobra venom on the red blood cells, reported to occur in schizophrenia and manic-depressive psychosis but not confirmed by subsequent research; called also *psychoreaction.* **Müller's r.,** see *Müller's test,* def. 3, under *tests.* **myasthenic r.,** progressively diminished response of a muscle to repeated electric stimuli. **myotonic r.,** failure of muscle to relax immediately upon cessation of voluntary or electrically induced contraction. **Nadi r.,** the production of a blue color when alphanaphthol and dimethyl paraphenylenediamine are injected into animals; see *indophenol test.* **Nagler's r.,** the production of turbidity in human blood serum by the addition of the toxin of *Clostridium perfringens* indicates the presence of that organism. The development of opalescence is due to the toxin's lecithinase action. Antiserum specifically inhibits the reaction. **near-point r.,** constriction of the pupil when the gaze is fixed on a near point. **Neill-Mooser r.,** a reaction in laboratory animals produced by inoculation with rickettsiae of murine typhus. The inflammatory exudate of the scrotal swelling contains large mononuclear cells filled with rickettsiae. **Neisser's r.,** a general reaction sometimes following an initial dose of arsphenamine, characterized by transitory increase of headache in cerebral syphilis and of the lightning pains in tabes. **Neufeld's r.,** when pneumococci and other capsulated microorganisms are mixed with specific immune serum there occurs in addition to agglutination a swelling (quellung) of the capsules of the organisms, owing to the binding of antibody with the capsular polysaccharide; called also *capsular swelling* and *quellung r.* **neurotonic r.,** muscular contraction persisting after the stimulus which produced it has ceased. **neutral r.,** the presence of an equal number of H^+ and OH^- ions in a solution, i.e., a pH of 7.0. **ninhydrin r.,** see *triketohydrindene hydrate test,* under *tests.* **nitritoid r.,** see under *crisis.* **Noguchi's r.** 1. a modification of the Wassermann reaction. Noguchi modifies as follows: (*a*) He prepares the antigen by extracting a lipoid substance from the liver and heart of dogs and cows. (*b*) Instead of using sheep's corpuscles in the hemolytic series, he employs human corpuscles, owing to the fact that a certain percentage of human sera tested produced hemolysis of the sheep's corpuscles. (*c*) In his test, therefore, he obtains the hemolytic amboceptor by immunizing rabbits with washed normal human corpuscles. (*d*) Another important improvement in the technique is the preservation of the specific antigen and the hemolytic amboceptor, which rapidly lose their strength in solution, in a dried form by soaking measured strips of filter paper (0.5 mm. square) with each. 2. a reaction seen in general paralysis and tabes. To 1 ml. of the cerebrospinal fluid is added 0.5 ml. of a solution of 10 per cent butyric acid in normal salt solution. This is heated, and then there is added 0.1 ml. of a 4 per cent sodium hydroxide solution. This is again heated. In about three hours the tube is examined. In tabes and general paralysis a characteristic flocculent precipitate forms, which gradually settles so that after twenty-four hours there is a bulky precipitate at the bottom of the tube, the supernatant fluid being clear. The test indicates an increased amount of globulin in the cerebrospinal fluid. **Noguchi's luetin r.** (1909), a papular response 6 to 24 hours after intradermal injection of killed *Treponema pallidum,* occurring in tertiary but not in primary or secondary syphilis; the procedure is no longer used. See *luetin.* **r. of nonidentity,** see *r. of identity.* **Nonne-Apelt r.,** 2 ml. of cerebrospinal fluid is mixed with an equal quantity of a neutral saturated solution of ammonium sulfate and compared after three minutes with another tube containing spinal fluid only; if there is no difference or only a faint opalescence the reaction is said to be *negative.* If there is an opalescence or turbidity the reaction is said to be *positive phase 1,* which indicates an excess of globulin in the fluid and points to nervous disorder. A normal fluid treated with heat and acetic acid only becomes turbid and is called *positive phase 2.* **nucleal r.,** upon the addition of fuchsin-sulfonic acid to any solution containing aldehydes, a bluish-red color is produced. **obsessive-compulsive r.,** a neurotic reaction pattern marked by the intrusion of insistent, repetitive, and unwanted thoughts, or the compulsion to repetitively perform certain acts or carry out certain rituals. **Oestreicher's r.,** xanthydrol r. **ophthalmic r.,** local reaction of the conjunctiva following instillation into the eye of toxins of typhoid fever and tuberculosis. The reaction is much more severe in persons affected with these diseases than in the healthy or those affected with some other disease. Called also *Calmette's ophthalmoreaction.* See also *Calmette's tuberculin,* under *tuberculin.* **orbicularis r.,** Westphal-Piltz phenomenon. **oxidase r.,** the formation of dark-blue granulations in myeloid cells when treated with alphanaphthol and dimethyl paraphenylenediamine. See *indophenol test,* under *tests.* **Pagano's r.,** an obsolete tuberculin reaction following application of the tuberculin to the urinary meatus. **pain r.,** dilatation of the pupil on a feeling of pain. **pallidin r.,** a red papular response in a syphilitic patient on intradermal injection of an extract prepared from the lung of an infant with syphilitic pneumonia. The reaction is said to be negative in the uninfected. The test is of historical interest only. **pancreatic r.** (*for ascertaining the presence of pancreatitis or malignant disease of the pancreas*): two specimens of urine, one of which is treated with mercuric chloride, are boiled with hydrochloric acid for ten minutes, and after the excess of acid has been neutralized with lead carbonate, are examined by the phenylhydrazine test. A difference in the amount of deposit yielded by the two specimens indicates the presence of pancreatic disease. Called also *Cammidge's r.* **Pándy's r.,** see under *tests.* **parallergic r.,** see *parallergy.* **paraserum r.,** agglutination of strains of typhoid and dysentery bacilli with those of paratyphoid, *Escherichia coli,* mutable cholera, and other infections. **Parish's r.,** an allergic reaction which follows the making of a Schick test; the symptoms appear within a few hours and may be quite severe. **passive cutaneous anaphylaxis r.,** passive cutaneous anaphylaxis. **Pasteur's r.,** see under *effect.* **paternity r.,** Manoiloff's r., def 1. See also *paternity test,* under *tests.*

Paul-Bunnell r., see under *tests.* **PCA r.,** passive cutaneous anaphylaxis. **Penn seroflocculation r.** (*for cancer*): plasma separated from a small amount of the patient's blood is mixed with a lipoid fraction derived from the liver of a patient who died of cancer. Resulting turbidity constitutes a negative reaction. **percutaneous r.,** Moro's r. **periodic acid–Schiff r.,** a tissue section is exposed to periodic acid, which oxidizes hydroxyl groups on adjacent carbon atoms or adjacent hydroxyl groups and amino groups to aldehydes, and then is stained with Schiff's reagent, which forms an additional product with aldehydes to produce a red or magenta reaction product; used to test for glycogen, epithelial mucins, neutral polysaccharides, and glycoproteins; called also *PAS r.* **peroxidase r.,** the appearance of deep-blue granules in leukocytes of marrow origin when stained with Goodpasture's stain, distinguishing them from cells of lymphatic origin. **Petri r.,** see under *tests.* **Petzetaki's r.,** see under *tests.* **Pfeiffer's r.,** see under *phenomenon.* **phobic r.,** a neurosis in which the principal feature is the presence of a specific irrational fear that is out of proportion to apparent stimuli; see also *phobia.* **photochemical r.,** photoreaction. **Piazza's r.,** see under *tests.* **Pinkerton-Moorer r.,** swelling and redness of guinea pig scrotum on intraperitoneal injection of *Rickettsia prowazeki;* formerly used to distinguish between murine and epidemic typhus. **Pirquet's r.,** appearance of a papule with a red areola 24–48 hours after introduction of two small drops of old tuberculin by slight scarification; a positive test indicates previous infection but does not distinguish clinical disease. Called also *dermotuberculin r., Pirquet's test, scarification test,* and *von Pirquet's cutireaction* or *test.* **P-K r.,** Prausnitz-Küstner r. **Porges-Meier r.,** see under *tests.* **Porter-Silber r.,** the reaction of the dihydroxyacetone side chains of 17-hydroxycorticosteroids with phenylhydrazine in acid, which produces a yellow color in the steroids; a sensitive index of adrenocortical function. **Posner's r.,** see under *tests.* **postpartum r.,** any emotional disturbance occurring after childbirth. **Prausnitz-Küstner r.,** a skin reaction for the detection and assay of human reagin (IgE). The intradermal inoculation of a nonatopic individual with serum containing reaginic antibody results in fixation of the reaginic antibody to the epidermal mast cells and diffusion of the other immunoglobulins away from the site of injection. Injection of specific antigen into the site of reagin attachment 48 hours later results in the immediate appearance of a wheal-and-flare response that can be graded in intensity. The danger of transferring serum hepatitis has precluded the use of this test clinically. The test was also used to determine a doner's sensitivity to various antigens. **precipitin r.,** 1. (*for pneumococcus infection of types I, II, III*): equal volumes of clear urine are mixed with antipneumococcus sera of types I, II, and III, and incubated for an hour. A cloudy to heavy flocculent precipitate indicates a positive reaction. Called also *Dochez and Avery's r.* 2. the specific precipitation of a soluble divalent ligand (i.e., antigen) in liquid or in gel by its specific antibody in the presence of electrolytes. **prozone r.,** see *prozone.* **psychogalvanic r.,** variations in the electric current passed through the body when the subject undergoes emotional disturbance of any kind. **psychophysiologic asthenic r.,** psychologic nervous system r., neurasthenic neurosis. **psychotic depressive r.,** severe nonrecurrent depression of psychotic intensity, sometimes characterized by loss of contact with reality and, frequently, by psychomotor retardation, feelings of guilt, impaired thinking ability, and suicidal attempts. **puncture r.,** swelling and redness at the point where tuberculin is injected subcutaneously; diagnostic of tuberculosis. **quanti-Pirquet r.,** the Pirquet reaction applied with a view to the amount or activity of the tuberculous infection; dilutions of 1 in 10 and 1 in 100 of old tuberculin rather than undiluted tuberculin are applied to the scarified cuticle. Abbreviated Q.P. **quellung r.** [Ger. "swelling"], Neufeld's r. **recurrent r.,** revivescence, def. 2. **reflex-like r.,** a reaction to physical agents, consisting of urticaria with systemic symptoms such as asthma, dermatoses, etc. **reverse passive Arthus r.,** the reaction produced when precipitating antibody is inoculated into a skin site in an experimental animal followed in 30 minutes to 2 hours by the intravenous inoculation of the homologous antigen. Thus the usual anatomical locations of precipitating antibody and antigen in an Arthus reaction are reversed. **reversible r.,** a chemical reaction which occurs in either direction, depending on conditions; a reaction in which the products react to re-form the reactants. **Rivalta's r.,** a reaction for distinguishing fluids of transudation and exudation, utilizing acetic acid. **Roger's r.,** the existence of albumin in the sputum, indicating tuberculosis. **Römer's r.,** see under *tests.* **Rosenbach's r.,** the formation of a deep-red color when concentrated nitric acid containing a small amount of nitrous acid is gradually added to boiling urine, indicative of an increase in the putrefactive processes of the intestine. **Rubino's r.** (*for leprosy*), the inactivated blood serum of leprous individuals when added to a suspension of washed and formalinized sheep erythrocytes causes the latter to agglutinate and to sediment rapidly. The test is correct in about 70 per cent of the cases. **Rumpf's traumatic r.,** see *Rumpf's sign* (def. 1), under *sign.* **Russo r.,** a reaction of the urine of typhoid patients on adding 4 drops of a solution of methylene blue to 15 ml. of urine. In the first stage of typhoid the urine becomes light green; at the height of the disease, an emerald color; and during the decline a bluish color. **Sachs-Georgi r.**, see under *tests*. **Sachs-Witebsky r.**, see under *tests*. **Sahli's r.**, desmoid r. **Schardinger's r.**, a reaction of oxidation or reduction made possible by a simulatneous and compensating reaction of reduction or oxidation. Cf. *Cannizzaro's reaction*. This reaction is used to distinguish between fresh milk and milk which has been heated. The milk is treated with aldehyde and methylene blue or indigo blue; if the milk is fresh the dye is reduced to a colorless compound. **Schick r.**, see under *tests*. **Schönbein's r.**, iodine is set free when potassium iodide and iron sulfate are added to a solution of hydrogen peroxide. **Schultz-Charlton r.**, when scarlet fever antitoxin or scarlet fever convalescent serum is injected into an area of the skin showing a bright red rash, a blanching of the skin at the site of the injection occurs. Serum from scarlet fever patients does not produce this reaction. **Schultz-Dale r.**, see *Dale r.* **second-set r.**, see under *phenomenon*. **sedimentation r.**, erythrocyte sedimentation rate. **Seifert's r.**, epiphanin r. **Selivanoff's r., Seliwanow's r.**, see under *tests*. **seroanaphylactic r.**, an anaphylactic reaction produced by the use of blood serum. **seroenzyme r.**, Abderhalden's r. **serum r.**, seroreaction. **shortening r.**, the shortening that succeeds the lengthening reaction when a limb is brought back into the extended position. **Shwartzman r.**, see under *phenomenon*. **sigma r.**, a flocculation reaction for the diagnosis of syphilis, being a modification of the Sachs-Georgi reaction in which a series of tests are made to determine which one of the tests produces flocculation. **skin r.**, cutaneous r. See also *cutireaction*. **small-drop r.**, miostagmin r. **Smith's r.**, anaphylaxis produced by the injection of a relatively large second dose of foreign blood serum (e.g., horse antitoxin) into a guinea pig sensitized by an earlier injection of a small dose of the same serum; see also *Theobald Smith phenomenon*, under *phenomenon*. **Stammler's r.**, cancer serum when added to a tumor extract clears up the opalescence normal to the extract: normal sera fail to act in this manner. **startle r.**, the various psychophysiological phenomena, including involuntary motor and autonomic reactions, evidenced by an individual in reaction to a sudden, unexpected stimulus, as a loud noise. **stemming r.**, resistance in the leg of a standing animal to forward displacement. **Straus' r.**, when material containing virulent glanders bacilli is inoculated into the peritoneal cavity of male guinea-pigs, scrotal lesions develop. **stress r.**, 1. gross stress r. 2. alarm r. **syphilis r.**, see specific reactions, including *Bruck's nitric acid r., coagulation r., D'Amato's r., epiphanin r., false positive r., Fornet's r., Hecht-Weinberg-Gradwohl modification of Wassermann r., Jarisch-Herxheimer r., miostagmin r., Noguchi's r., Noguchi's luetin r., pallidin r., Targowla r., Wassermann r., Wasserman r., provocative*. See also *syphilis test*, under *tests*. **Szent-Györgyi r.**, a deep violet color develops when a 1 per cent solution of ascorbic acid is mixed with a solution of ferrous sulfate; this color disappears on reduction with sodium hyposulfite. **Tanret's r.**, see under *tests*. **Targowla r.**, a reaction for the presence of syphilis based on the fact that a mixture of normal cerebrospinal fluid with elixir paregoric produces a colloidal suspension, whereas if the spinal fluid is syphilitic a precipitate is formed. **tendon r.**, see under *reflex*. **thyroid function r.**, see specific reactions, including *Goetsch's skin r.* and *Hunt's r.* See also *thyroid function test*, under *tests*. **toxin-antitoxin r.**, see *immunoreaction*. **Trambusti's r.**, tuberculin is injected into the skin by a needle inserted parallel to the cutaneous surface; any reddening within the site of the injection is positive. Called also *endodermoreaction*. **trigger r.**, see under *action*. **tryptophan r.**, see under *tests*. **tuberculin r.**, see under *tests*. **tuberculosis r.**, see specific reactions including *antigen r. of Debré and Paraf, antitryptic r., Besredka's r., depot r., Ehrlich's diazo r., Lignières' r., Malmejde r., Moro's r., Pagano's r., Pirquet's r., puncture r., quanti-Pirquet r., Trambusti's r.* See also *tuberculosis test*, under *tests*. **Turnbull's blue r.**, blue-black coloration produced when tissue containing chemically active iron is treated with potassium ferrocyanide and hydrochloric acid. **typhoid fever r.**, see specific reaction, including *Bareggi's r., Chantemesse's r., D'Amato's r., Deehan's typhoid r., Ehrlich's diazo r., miostagmin r., Russo's r.* See also *typhoid fever test*, under *tests*. **uniphasic r.**, a reaction consisting of flexion only. Cf. *biphasic r.* **vaccination r.**, the local and systemic reaction to vaccination. **vestibular pupillary r.**, dilatation of the pupils arising from stimulation of the external auditory canal. **Voges-Proskauer r.**, see under *tests*. **von Pirquet's r.**, Pirquet's r. **Wassermann r.**, a test for syphilis based on the fixation of complement. **Wassermann r., provocative**, a Wassermann reaction preceded by administration of arsphenamine. This procedure may result in a positive reaction in a patient who had previously given negative results. **Weichbrodt's r.**, three parts of a 1 per cent solution of sublimate solution are added to seven parts of cerebrospinal fluid; cloudiness of the mixture indicates pathologic changes in the fluid, especially syphilis. **Weil-Felix r.**, the diagnostic agglutination of Proteus X bacteria by the blood sera of typhus fever cases due, apparently, to the presence of a common antigen. **Weinberg's r.**, see under

tests. **Wernicke's r.**, hemiopic pupillary r. **wheal-flare r.**, a cutaneous sensitivity reaction to skin injury or administration of antigen, due to production of histamine and characterized by edematous elevation and erythematous flare; see also *triple response*, under *response*. **white-graft r.**, an immune reaction to a tissue graft, e.g., a skin graft, as a result of which the grafted tissue does not become vascularized and is rapidly rejected. **Widal's r.**, see under *tests*. **Wolff-Calmette r.**, ophthalmic r. **Wolff-Eisner r.**, ophthalmic r. **xanthoproteic r.**, see *Mulder's test*, under *tests*. **xanthydrol r.**, when tissue from a uremic patient is fixed in a solution of xanthydrol in glacial acetic acid, a large deposit of xanthydrol occurs in the tissue. **zed r.**, a reaction which appears in infants in cases of starvation after the starvation is relieved; it consists of a slight gain in weight, elevation of temperature, and the appearance of watery stools containing a large number of cells.

reaction-formation (re-ak′shun for-ma′shun) a psychic mechanism by which a person unconsciously assumes an attitude which is the reverse of, and a substitute for, a repressed antisocial impulse.

reactivate (re-ak′tĭ-vāt) to make active again; especially the restoring of the activity to immune serum that has had its activity destroyed.

reactivation (re-ak″tĭ-va′shun) the restoration of activity to something that has been inactivated. **r. of serum**, restoration of immunological activity to serum by adding fresh complement.

reactivity (re″ak-tiv′ĭ-te) the process or property of reacting.

reactor (re-ak′tor) a person or thing that reacts. **nuclear r.**, a device in which the chain reaction of neutron-induced nuclear fission is sustained in a self-supporting reaction at a controlled rate.

Reactrol (re-ak′trol) trademark for a preparation of clemizole hydrochloride.

Read's formula (rēdz) [Jay Marion *Read*, American physician, born 1889] see under *formula*.

reading (rēd′ing) understanding of written or printed symbols representing words. **lip r., speech r.**, the understanding of speech through observation of the movement of the lips of the speaker.

reagent (re-a′jent) [*re-* + L. *agere* to act] 1. a substance employed to produce a chemical reaction so as to detect, measure, produce, etc., other substances. 2. the subject of a psychological experiment, especially one who reacts to a stimulus. **acid molybdate r.**, Folin's acid molybdate r. **Acree-Rosenheim r.**, solution of formaldehyde, 1 part; water, 5000 parts. **Almén's r.**, to 5 grains of tannic acid in 240 ml. of 50 per cent alcohol add 10 ml. of 25 per cent acetic acid. **amino-acid r.**, a 0.5 per cent solution of the sodium salt of beta-naphthaquinone sulfonate acid freshly prepared. **Anstie's r.**, potassium dichromate 3.33 gm., concentrated sulfuric acid 250 ml., water to make 500 ml. **Arakawa's r.**, a complicated mixture containing guaiac resin and benzidine for use in testing for peroxidase in milk. If the peroxidase content of breast milk is adequate, the presence of maternal beriberi is excluded. **arsenic-sulfuric acid r.**, Rosenthaler's r. **Barfoed's r.**, see under *tests*. **Benedict-Hopkins-Cole r.**, 250 ml. of a saturated solution of oxalic acid is added slowly to 10 gm. of powdered magnesium kept cool. Filter, acidify with acetic acid, and make up to 1 liter. **benzidine r.**, saturate 2 ml. of glacial acetic acid with benzidine and add 1 ml. of 3 per cent hydrogen peroxide. **Bertrand's r.**, *A.* copper solution: Copper sulfate, 40 gm., to 1 liter of water. *B.* alkaline solution: Rochelle salt, 200 gm., sodium hydroxide, 150 gm., to 1 liter of water. *C.* iron solution: ferric sulfate, 50 gm., sulfuric acid, 200 gm., to 1 liter of water. *D.* permanganate solution: potassium permanganate, 5 gm., to 1 liter of water. By heating the alkaline copper solution (made from solutions *A* and *B*) with dextrose, cuprous oxide is formed. This is treated with the ferric sulfate solution, and the ferrous sulfate so formed is titrated with the solution of potassium permanganate. **Bial's r.**, orcinol 1.5 gm., fuming hydrochloric acid 500 gm., ferric chloride (10 per cent) 20–30 drops. **biuret r.**, see *Gies' biuret test*, under *tests*. **Black's r.**, 5 gm. of ferric chloride and 0.4 gm. of ferrous chloride dissolved in 100 ml. of water. **Blum's r.**, see under *tests*. **Bogg's r.**, dissolve 25 gm. of phosphotungstic acid in 125 ml. of water. Dilute 25 ml. of concentrated HCl to 100 ml. Mix the two solutions. **Bohme's r.**, two reagents for use in testing for indol. **Bonchardat's r.**, a general alkaloidal reagent, consisting of 1 per cent of iodine dissolved in a 1 per cent solution of potassium iodide. **Bruecke's r.**, 50 gm. of KI, 120 gm. of HgI₂, water up to 1000 ml.: a modification of Meyer's reagent. **Cramer's 2.5 r.**, 0.4 gm. of mercuric oxide and 6 gm. of potassium iodide dissolved in 100 ml. of water with the reagent so adjusted that 10 ml. will be neutralized to the phenolphthalein end point by 2.5 ml. of N/10 acid. **Cross and Bevan's r.**, two parts of concentrated hydrochloric acid and 1 part of zinc chloride by weight; used for dissolving cellulose. **Denigès' r.**, the reagent used in Denigès' test (def. 2). **diazo r.**, a reagent consisting of two solutions which are mixed just prior to the test in the proportion of 25 ml. of solution *A* to 0.75 ml. of *B.* Solution *A:* sulfanilic acid, 1 gm.; distilled water, 1000 ml.

Solution *B*: sodium nitrite, 0.5 gm.: distilled water, 100 ml. **dinitrosalicylic acid r.,** Sumner's r. **Edlefsen's r.,** an alkaline permanganate solution for testing for sugar in the urine. **Ehrlich's aldehyde r.,** 4 gm. of paradimethylaminobenzaldehyde in a mixture of 80 ml. of concentrated hydrochloric acid and 380 ml. of ethyl alcohol. **Ehrlich's diazo r.,** Solution *A*: dissolve 5 gm. of sodium nitrite in 1 liter of distilled water. Solution *B*: dissolve 5 gm. of sulfanilic acid and 50 ml. of HCl in 1 liter of distilled water. For use mix 1 part of *A* with 50 to 100 parts of *B*. **Erdmann's r.,** a reagent for testing for alkaloids, consisting of nitric and sulfuric acids. **Esbach's r.,** a mixture of a 1 per cent aqueous solution of picric acid and a 2 per cent solution of citric acid; used in quantitative estimation of albumin in urine. **Exton's r.,** dissolve 200 gm. of Na$_2$SO$_4 \cdot$10H$_2$O in 800 ml. of water. Cool and add 50 gm. sulfosalicylic acid and 25 ml. of a 0.4 per cent solution of bromphenol blue. Make up to 1 liter. **Folin's r.,** boil 100 gm. of sodium tungstate and 80 ml. of 85 per cent orthophosphoric acid in 750 ml. of water for two hours. Cool and dilute 1 liter. **Folin's acid molybdate r.,** dissolve 150 gm. of sodium molybdate in 300 ml. of water. Filter and add 2 to 3 drops of bromine and shake. Later add 225 ml. of 85 per cent phosphoric acid and 150 ml. of 25 per cent sulfuric acid. Aerate off the bromine, add 75 ml. of 90 per cent acetic acid, and dilute to 1 liter. **Folin's alkaline copper tartrate r.,** dissolve 12 gm. of sodium tartrate (or 15 gm. of Rochelle salt), 7 gm. of anhydrous sodium carbonate, and 20 gm. of sodium bicarbonate in 600 ml. of water. Dissolve 5 gm. of copper sulfate in 200 ml. of water. Mix the solutions and dilute to 1 liter. **Folin's sugar r.,** solution *A*: dissolve 5 gm. copper sulfate in 100 ml. of hot water, cool, and add 60 to 70 ml. of glycerin. Solution *B*: dissolve 125 gm. of anhydrous potassium carbonate in 400 ml. of water. Mix 1 part of solution *A* and 2 parts of solution *B* just before using. **Folin-McEllroy r.,** dissolve 100 gm. of sodium pyrophosphate, 30 gm. of disodium phosphate, and 50 gm. of dry sodium carbonate in 1 liter of water. Dissolve 13 gm. of copper sulfate in 200 ml. of water and pour into the first solution. **formalin-sulfuric acid r.,** see *Marquis' test,* under *tests.* **Fröhde's r.,** see under *tests.* **Frohn's r.,** see under *tests.* **general r.,** a reagent that indicates the general class of bodies to which a substance belongs. **Gies' biuret r.,** see under *tests.* **Grignard's r.,** any of several compounds of magnesium with an organic radical and a halogen; these reagents undergo reactions with many substances producing important products. **Hager's r.,** a reagent for detecting sugar in the urine, consisting of iron ferrocyanide and potassium hydroxide. **Hahn oxine r.,** a 5 per cent solution of hydroxyquinoline in alcohol. **Haines' r.,** copper sulfate, 2 parts; potassium hydroxide, 7.5 parts; glycerin, 15 parts; distilled water, 150 parts. **Ilosvay's r.,** a reagent used as a test for nitrites. It is prepared by treating a mixture of 0.5 gm. of sulfanilic acid and 150 ml. of dilute acetic acid with 0.1 gm. of naphthylamine, and then with 20 ml. of boiling water. The sediment produced by this reaction is dissolved in 150 ml. of dilute acetic acid. The suspected substance is heated with this reagent to 80° C., when a red color is formed if nitrites are present. **Izar's r.,** equal parts of linoleic acid and ricinoleic acid. **Lloyd's r.,** a specially fine preparation of fuller's earth obtained by elutriation; used to absorb alkaloids from solutions. **Mandelin's r.** (*for alkaloids*), 1 part of ammonium vanadate in 200 parts of cold concentrated sulfuric acid. **Marme's r.,** a solution of cadmium iodide and potassium iodide for the precipitation of alkaloids. **Marquis' r.,** see under *tests.* **Mayer's r.,** see under *tests.* **Mecke's r.,** 1 part of selenious acid in 200 parts of concentrated sulfuric acid. **Meyer's r.,** phenolphthalein, 0.032 part; decinormal sodium hydroxide, 21 parts; enough water to make 100 parts; used in testing for blood, which even in minute quantities gives the solution a purple color. **Millon's r.,** see under *tests.* **Mörner's r.,** a solution of 1 volume of formalin, 45 volumes of distilled water, 55 volumes of concentrated sulfuric acid; used as a test for tyrosine. See under *tests.* **Nadi r.,** a mixture of alphanaphthol and dimethyl paraphenylenediamine, which combine to form indophenol blue from cytochrome C under the influence of cytochrome oxidase. See *indophenol test,* under *tests.* **Nakayama r.,** ferric chloride, 0.4 gm., concentrated hydrochloric acid, 1 ml., 95 per cent alcohol, 99 ml. **Nessler's r.,** an aqueous solution of 5 per cent of potassium iodide, 2.5 per cent of mercuric chloride, and 16 per cent of potassium hydroxide; used as a test for ammonia. **Ninhydrin r.,** trademark for a preparation of triketohydrindene hydrate (q.v.). **Noguchi's r.,** butyric acid 10 parts, 0.9 per cent sodium chloride 90 parts. **Nylander's r.,** see under *tests.* **Obermayer's r.,** a solution of 2 gm. of ferric chloride in 1 liter of hydrochloric acid. **Penzoldt's r.,** see under *tests.* **Porges-Meier r.,** see under *tests.* **Rosenthaler's r.** (*for alkaloids*), 1 part of potassium arsenate in 100 parts of concentrated sulfuric acid. **Sahli's r.,** mix equal parts of a 48 per cent solution of potassium iodide and an 8 per cent solution of potassium iodate. **Schaer's r.** (*for alkaloids*), one volume of 30 per cent pure hydrogen peroxide in 10 volumes of concentrated sulfuric acid. Use while fresh. **Scheibler's r.,** a reagent made by boiling sodium tungstate with half as much phosphoric acid and water, precipitating with barium chloride, dissolving in hot dilute hydrochloric acid, treating with sulfuric acid, and evaporating. **Schiff's r.,** a reagent for testing for the presence of aldehydes, prepared by dissolving 0.25 gm. of fuchsin in 1 liter of water and decolorizing by passing sulfur dioxide into it. In the presence of aldehyde the blue color is restored. **Schweitzer's r.,** a solution of cupric hydroxide, Cu(OH)$_2$, in ammonia water; used as a solvent for cellulose. Called also *cuprammonia.* **Scott-Wilson r.,** (1) mercuric cyanide, 5 gm., (2) sodium hydroxide, 90 gm., (3) silver nitrate, 1.45 gm. Dissolve each separately in water and cool. Add (2) to (1), then add (3) with constant stirring. **selenious-sulfuric acid r.,** Mecke's r. **Soldaini's r.,** see under *tests.* **Sörensen's r.,** an acetate buffer solution for combining with Pardy's test for albumin: 188 gm. of sodium acetate and 56.5 gm. of glacial acetic acid brought up to 1 liter with distilled water. **Spiegler's r.,** see under *tests.* **splenic r.,** any drug or stimulus which causes the spleen to contract. **Stokes' r.** (*for oxyhemoglobin*), a solution containing 2 per cent of ferrous sulfate and 3 per cent of tartaric or citric acid; for use, add ammonium hydroxide to a small portion until the precipitate redissolves, thus forming ammonium ferrotartrate. **Sumner's r.,** to 10 gm. crystallized phenol add 22 ml. of 10 per cent NaOH and dilute to 100 ml. To 6.9 gm. of sodium bisulfite add 69 ml. of the alkaline phenol solution. To this add a solution containing 300 ml. of 4.5 per cent NaOH, 255 gm. NaKC$_4$H$_4$O$_6 \cdot$4H$_2$O, and 880 ml. of 1 per cent dinitrosalicylic acid; used for the estimation of sugar in normal and diabetic urine. **Takata's r.,** the reagent (a mixture of mercuric chloride solution and basic fuchsin solution) used in Takata-Ara test. **Tanret's r.** (*for albumin in urine, etc.*): mercuric chloride, 1.35 gm.; potassium iodide, 3.32 gm.; acetic acid, 20 ml.; distilled water, to make 80 ml.; it gives a white precipitate with albumin. **Triboulet's r.,** bichloride of mercury, 3.5 gm., acetic acid, 1 ml., water, 100 ml. **Tsuchiya r.,** an acid alcoholic solution of phosphotungstic acid for detecting small amounts of protein in the urine. **Uffelmann's r.,** see under *tests.* **vanadic-sulfuric acid r.,** Mandelin's r. **Weichardt's r.,** a system composed of sulfuric acid, and barium hydroxide, together with catalytic agents; it was added to the solution of serum and antigen in the epiphanin reaction. **Wolff's r.,** phosphotungstic acid, 0.3 gm.; concentrated hydrochloric acid, 1 ml.; absolute alcohol, 20 ml.; distilled water, 200 ml.

reagin (re′ah-jin) 1. antibody of a specialized immunoglobulin class (IgE) which attaches to tissue cells of the same species from which it is derived, and which interacts with its antigen to induce the release of histamine and other vasoactive amines. A form of cytotropic antibody, it is present in the serum of naturally hypersensitive individuals and can confer specific immediate hypersensitivity in nonreactive individuals. Called also *Prausnitz-Küstner* (*P-K*) *antibody* and *reaginic antibody.* 2. a complement-fixing antibody interacting with cardiolipin in the Wassermann reaction. **atopic r.,** the reagin of humans.

reaginic (re′ah-jin-ik) pertaining to reagin.

realgar (re″al-gar′) [Arabic *rahj al-ghar* powder of the mine] arsenic disulfide, As$_2$S$_2$: a pigment.

reamer (re′mer) an instrument used in dentistry for enlarging root canals.

reamputation (re″am-pu-ta′shun) the repeated performance of an amputation.

reattachment (re″ah-tach′ment) 1. the recementing of a dental crown or other prosthesis. 2. the reattachment to the alveolus of a tooth that has been loosened or replanted.

Réaumur's scale, thermometer (ra″o-merz′) [René Antoine Ferschault *Réaumur,* French natural philosopher, 1683–1757] see under *scale* and *thermometer.*

rebase (re-bās′) to replace the base material of a denture without changing the occlusal relations of the teeth.

rebound (re′bownd) a reversed response on the withdrawal of a stimulus; see also under *phenomenon* and *tenderness.* **REM r.,** the phenomenon in which a subject deprived of REM (rapid eye movement) sleep for a prolonged period will, on being permitted to sleep undisturbed, compensate by having about 60 per cent more REM sleep than he normally would.

recalcification (re-kal″sĭ-fi-ka′shun) the restoration of calcium salts to the bodily tissues.

recall 1. (rĕ-kol′) to remember or recollect. 2. (rĕ-kol′, re′kol) the process of bringing a memory into consciousness.

recapitulation (re″kah-pit′u-la′shun) see under *theory.*

receiver (re-sēv′er) 1. a vessel for collecting a gas or a distillate. 2. the portion of an apparatus by which electric energy is converted into signals which may be seen or heard.

receptaculum (re″sep-tak′u-lum), pl. *receptac′ula* [L.] a receptacle or container; that which serves for receiving or containing something. **r. chy′li,** cisterna chyli. **r. gan′glii petro′si,** fossula petrosa. **r. Pecquet′i,** cisterna chyli.

receptolysin (re″sep-tol′ĭ-sin) a substance that splits up or hydrolyzes receptors or receptor materials.

receptor (re-sep′tor) 1. a specific molecule on the surface or within the cytoplasm of a cell that recognizes and binds with other specific molecules, as the chemical group on the surface of an immunocompetent cell that binds with antigen, or the cell molecules that bind with hormone or neurotransmitter molecules and react with other molecules that respond in a specific way.

2. a term first used by Ehrlich to describe a hypothetical group in a cell, which has the power of combining with and thus anchoring a haptophore group of a toxin or other substance. Receptors may remain attached to cells or may be cast off into the blood serum. In either case, they retain their combining power and so function as antibodies. See *Ehrlich's side-chain theory,* under *theory.* 3. a sensory nerve terminal which responds to stimuli of various kinds; see *exteroceptive, interoceptive,* and *proprioceptive.* **adrenergic r's,** postulated sites on effector organs innervated by postganglionic adrenergic fibers of the sympathetic nervous system, classified as α-adrenergic and β-adrenergic receptors according to their reaction to norepinephrine and epinephrine, respectively, and to certain blocking and stimulating agents. Called also *adrenoceptor* and *adrenoreceptor.* **α-adrenergic r's,** adrenergic receptors that respond to norepinephrine and to such blocking agents as phenoxybenzamine and phentolamine. **β-adrenergic r.,** adrenergic receptors that respond to epinephrine and to such blocking agents as propanolol; they are of two types: β₁ (lipolysis and cardiostimulation) and β₂ (bronchodilation and vasodilation). **cholinergic r.,** receptor sites on effector organs innervated by cholinergic nerve fibers and which respond to the acetylcholine secreted by these fibers. **complement r.,** a cell-surface receptor structure capable of binding activated complement components. For example, component C3b is bound to neutrophils, B-lymphocytes, and macrophages. **contact r.,** a sense organ which responds to stimuli from objects in contact with the body. **contiguous r.,** a receptor which must be in direct contact with the stimulant, such as touch and taste receptors. **distance r.,** a sense organ which responds to stimuli from objects remote from the body, as a receptor for the stimuli of hearing, vision, or smell. **dominant r.,** an unknown physiologic configuration located at the site of action of a drug which by combining with the drug enables it to exert its physiologic action. **r. of the first order,** in Ehrlich's side-chain theory, a receptor which possesses a haptophore group only, and therefore serves only as a connecting link between the toxin and the tissues; this order of receptors includes only the antitoxins. **gustatory r.,** a receptor for the sense of taste; a taste bud. **H₁,H₂ r's,** see *histamine.* **pressure r.,** a receptor for stimuli of pressure or touch; a touch corpuscle. **r. of the second order,** in Ehrlich's side-chain theory, a receptor which possesses both a haptophore group for anchoring or holding the foreign toxin, and a zymophore group for its digestion; this group includes the agglutinins, the precipitins, and the opsonins. **secondary r's,** unknown substances, other than the dominant receptor, located at points other than the site of action which combine with a drug and so lessen its combination with the dominant receptor and its physiologic activity. **sessile r.,** in Ehrlich's side-chain theory, a receptor which cannot be given off to form an antibody. **r. of the third order,** in Ehrlich's side-chain theory, a receptor which possesses two combining groups only, a haptophore group for combining with the foreign toxin, and a complementophile group which combines with the complement that carries the zymotoxic element; this group includes the lysins. **visual r.,** the layer of rods and cones of the retina. **volume r's,** postulated receptors which respond to increased plasma extracellular fluid volume and stimulate corrective measures.

recess (re′ses) a small empty space, hollow, or cavity; called also *recessus.* **accessory r. of elbow,** recessus sacciformis articulationis cubiti. **acetabular r.,** fossa acetabuli. **Arlt's r.,** a small sinus occasionally present in the lower part of the lacrimal sac. **chiasmatic r.,** recessus opticus. **cochlear r. of vestibule,** recessus cochlearis vestibuli. **conarial r.,** recessus pinealis. **costodiaphragmatic r. of pleura,** recessus costodiaphragmaticus pleurae. **costomediastinal r. of pleura,** recessus costomediastinalis pleurae. **duodenal r., inferior,** recessus duodenalis inferior. **duodenal r., superior,** duodenojejunal r., recessus duodenalis superior. **elliptical r. of vestibule,** recessus ellipticus vestibuli. **epitympanic r.,** recessus epitympanicus. **r. of fourth ventricle, lateral,** recessus lateralis ventriculi quarti. **hepatorenal r.,** recessus hepatorenalis. **Hyrtl's r.,** recessus epitympanicus. **ileocecal r., inferior,** recessus ileocecalis inferior. **ileocecal r., superior,** recessus ileocecalis superior. **infundibular r.,** recessus infundibuli. **infundibuliform r.,** recessus pharyngeus. **r. of infundibulum,** recessus infundibuli. **intersigmoidal r.,** recessus intersigmoideus. **laryngopharyngeal r.,** recessus piriformis. **r. of lesser omental cavity,** recessus lienalis. **r. of nasopharynx, lateral,** recessus pharyngeus. **omental r., inferior,** recessus inferior omentalis. **omental r., superior,** recessus superior omentalis. **optic r.,** recessus opticus. **paracolic r's,** sulci paracolici. **paraduodenal r.,** recessus paraduodenalis. **r. of pelvic mesocolon,** recessus intersigmoideus. **pharyngeal r., middle,** bursa pharyngea. **pharyngeal r.,** recessus pharyngeus. **phrenicohepatic r's,** see *recessus subhepatici, recessus subphrenici,* and *recessus hepatorenalis.* **pineal r.,** recessus pinealis. **piriform r.,** recessus piriformis. **pleural r's,** recessus pleurales. **Reichert's r.,** recessus cochlearis vestibuli. **retroannular r.,** a deep groove formed by the cell membrane immediately behind the annulus of spermatozoa of some species. **retrocecal r.,** recessus retrocecalis.

retroduodenal r., recessus retroduodenalis. **r. of Rosenmüller,** recessus pharyngeus. **sacciform r. of articulation of elbow,** recessus sacciformis articulationis cubiti. **sacciform r. of distal radioulnar articulation,** recessus sacciformis articulationis radioulnaris distalis. **sphenoethmoidal r.,** recessus sphenoethmoidalis. **sphenoethmoidal r., bony,** recessus sphenoethmoidalis osseus. **spherical r. of vestibule,** r. sphericus vestibuli. **splenic r.,** recessus lienalis. **subhepatic r's,** recessus subhepatici. **subphrenic r's,** recessus subphrenici. **subpopliteal r.,** recessus subpopliteus. **suprapineal r.,** recessus suprapinealis. **supratonsillar r.,** fossa supratonsillaris. **Tarini's r.,** recessus anterior fossae interpeduncularis [Tarini]. **triangular r.,** recessus triangularis. **r's of Tröltsch,** see *recessus membranae tympani anterior* and *recessus membranae tympani posterior.* **r. of tympanic membrane, anterior,** recessus membranae tympani anterior. **r. of tympanic membrane, posterior,** recessus membranae tympani posterior. **r. of tympanic membrane, superior,** recessus membranae tympani superior. **utricular r.,** utriculus, def. 2. **r. of vestibule,** recessus sphericus vestibuli.

recession (re-sesh′un) [L. *recedere* to draw back or away] the act of drawing away or back. In dentistry, the retraction of the gingival margin and underlying tissue away from the neck of a tooth, resulting in exposure of the cementum. **angle r.,** recession of the angle of the anterior chamber of the eye; see also under *glaucoma.* **clitoral r.,** surgical displacement of the clitoris by suturing the corpus back to the ramus; done to reduce its apparent size in clitoral hypertrophy. **r. of ocular muscle,** surgical displacement of the insertion of an ocular muscle posteriorly; done to weaken the stronger muscle in strabismus.

recessive (re-ses′iv) 1. tending to recede; not exerting a ruling or controlling influence; in genetics, incapable of expression unless (the responsible allele is) carried by both members of a pair of homologous chromosomes. 2. a recessive allele or trait.

recessus (re-ses′sus), pl. *reces′sus* [L.] a recess; a small empty space, hollow, or cavity; [NA] a general term for such potential spaces. **r. ante′rior fos′sae interpeduncula′ris [Tari′ni],** the portion of the interpeduncular fossa that passes under the corpora mamillaria; called also *Tarini's recess* and *Tarin's space.* **r. chi′asmatis,** r. opticus. **r. cochlea′ris vestib′uli** [NA], cochlear recess of vestibule: a small depressed area on the medial wall of the vestibule of the ear, situated just below the posterior end of the crista vestibuli, and perforated with foramina through which nerve fibers pass to the posterior portion of the ductus cochlearis. Called also *Reichert's recess.* **r. costodiaphragmat′icus pleu′rae** [NA], costodiaphragmatic recess of pleura: the pleural recess situated at the junction of the costal and diaphragmatic pleurae; called also *sinus phrenicocostalis.* **r. costomediastina′lis pleu′rae** [NA], costomediastinal recess of pleura: a wedge-shaped space, not completely filled with lung tissue, along the line at which the costal pleura meets the mediastinal pleura in front; called also *sinus costomediastinalis pleurae.* **r. duodena′lis infe′rior** [NA], inferior duodenal recess: a pocket in the peritoneum on the left side of the ascending portion of the duodenum, bounded by the inferior duodenal fold. **r. duodena′lis supe′rior** [NA], **r. duodenojejuna′lis,** superior duodenal recess: a peritoneal pocket behind the superior duodenal fold. **r. ellip′ticus vestib′uli** [NA], elliptical recess of the vestibule: an oval depressed area in the roof and medial wall of the vestibule of the inner ear, situated above and behind the crista and pierced by 25 to 30 small foramina through which nerves come from the internal acoustic meatus to the utricle, which occupies the depression. **r. epitympan′icus** [NA], epitympanic recess: the upper portion of the tympanic cavity, extending above the level of the tympanic membrane and containing the greater part of the incus and the upper half of the malleus. **r. hepatorena′lis** [NA], hepatorenal recess: a peritoneal pouch between the liver and the kidney. **r. ileoceca′lis infe′rior** [NA], inferior ileocecal recess: a peritoneal pocket situated behind the ileocecal fold, above the vermiform appendix, below the ileum, and medial to the cecum. **r. ileoceca′lis supe′rior** [NA], superior ileocecal recess: a peritoneal pocket situated behind and below the vascular cecal fold, above the ileum and medial to the lower end of the ascending colon. **r. infe′rior omenta′lis** [NA], inferior omental recess: the lower portion of the omental bursa, including its extension down into the great omentum. It is bounded in front by the posterior wall of the stomach, and behind by the pancreas, the transverse colon and its mesocolon, the left suprarenal gland, and part of the left kidney. **r. infundib′uli** [NA], recess of infundibulum: a funnel-shaped depression in the anterior part of the floor of the third ventricle of the brain, within the infundibulum of the hypophysis. **r. intersigmoi′deus** [NA], intersigmoidal recess: a shallow peritoneal pocket running downward and to the left at the base of the sigmoid mesocolon. **r. latera′lis fos′sae rhomboi′dei,** r. lateralis ventriculi quarti. **r. latera′lis ventric′uli quar′ti** [NA], lateral recess of fourth ventricle: a narrow, curved prolongation of the cavity of the fourth ventricle of the brain, extending laterally onto the dorsal surface of the inferior cerebellar peduncle; it contains a lateral prolongation of the choroid plexus and provides for the passage of cerebrospinal fluid into the subarachnoid space. **r. liena′lis** [NA], splenic recess: an extension of the omental bursa to the left behind the gastrolienal ligament almost to the spleen. **r. membra′nae tym′pani ante′rior** [NA], anterior recess of tympanic membrane: a pocket in the tympanic membrane formed by the tunica mucosa between the anterior mallear fold and the anterior superior part of the pars tensa of the membrane, ending blindly above. **r. membra′nae tym′pani poste′rior** [NA], posterior recess of tympanic membrane: a pocket in the tympanic membrane formed by the tunica mucosa between the posterior mallear fold and the posterior superior part of the pars tensa of the membrane, ending blindly above. **r. membra′nae tym′pani supe′rior** [NA], superior recess of tympanic membrane: a recess in the tympanic membrane formed by the tunica mucosa between the neck of the malleus and the pars flaccida of the membrane, and ending blindly below. Called also *Prussak's pouch* or *space*. **r. op′ticus** [NA], optic recess: a depression in the floor of the third ventricle of the brain, between the chiasma behind and the lamina terminalis in front. **r. paracol′ici,** sulci paracolici. **r. paraduodena′lis** [NA], paraduodenal recess: a pocket occasionally found in the peritoneum behind a fold containing a branch of the left colic artery. **r. pharyn′geus** [NA], **r. pharyn′geus [Rosenmül′leri],** pharyngeal recess: a wide, slitlike lateral extension in the wall of the nasopharynx, cranial and dorsal to the pharyngeal orifice of the auditory tube; called also *Rosenmüller's cavity, fossa,* or *cavity.* **r. phrenicohepat′ici,** see *r. subhepatici, r. subphrenici,* and *r. hepatorenalis.* **r. pinea′lis** [NA], pineal recess: an extension of the third ventricle into the stalk of the pineal body. **r. pirifor′mis** [NA], piriform recess: a pear-shaped fossa in the wall of the laryngeal pharynx lateral to the arytenoid cartilage and medial to the lamina of the thyroid cartilage. **r. pleura′les** [NA], pleural recesses: the spaces where the different portions of the pleura join at an angle and which are never completely filled by lung tissue; called also *sinus pleurae.* **r. pneumatoenter′icus,** either of the paired embryonic excavations alongside the dorsal mesogastricum, the right one sometimes persisting as the infracardiac bursa. **r. poste′rior fos′sae interpeduncula′ris [Tari′ni],** the portion of the interpeduncular fossa that slightly undermines the anterior margin of the pons. **r. pro utric′ulo,** r. ellipticus vestibuli. **r. retroceca′lis** [NA], retrocecal recess: a peritoneal pocket extending upward behind the cecum and sometimes behind the colon. **r. retroduodena′lis** [NA], retroduodenal recess: an occasional peritoneal pocket extending behind the horizontal and ascending parts of the duodenum. **r. saccifor′mis articulatio′nis cu′biti,** sacciform recess of articulation of elbow: the distal bulging of the articular capsule of the elbow joint, situated between the incisura radialis ulnae and the circumferentia articularis radii. **r. saccifor′mis articulatio′nis radioulna′ris dista′lis** [NA], sacciform recess of distal radioulnar articulation: a bulging of the synovial membrane of the articular capsule of the distal radioulnar joint, which extends proximally between the radius and ulna beyond the point of their articular surfaces. **r. sphenoethmoida′lis** [NA], sphenoethmoidal recess: the most superior and posterior part of the nasal cavity, above the superior nasal concha, into which the sphenoidal sinus opens. **r. sphenoethmoida′lis os′seus** [NA], bony sphenoethmoidal recess: a small region in the skull, posterosuperior to the superior nasal concha and just anterior to the body of the sphenoid bone; the sphenoid sinus opens into it. **r. spher′icus vestib′uli** [NA], spherical recess of vestibule: a circular depressed area in the anteroinferior portion of the medial wall of the vestibule of the inner ear. It is pierced by 12 to 15 small foramina through which nerves come from the internal acoustic meatus to the saccule, which occupies the depression. **r. splenia′lis,** r. lienalis. **r. subhepat′ici** [NA], subhepatic recesses: peritoneal pockets located beneath the liver. **r. subphren′ici** [NA], subphrenic recesses: peritoneal pockets located beneath the diaphragm. **r. subpoplite′us** [NA], subpopliteal recess: a prolongation of the synovial tendon sheath of the popliteus muscle outside the knee joint into the popliteal space; called also *bursa musculi poplitei.* **r. supe′rior omenta′lis** [NA], superior omental recess: a rather long, narrow peritoneal pocket leading from the vestibule upward toward the liver, between the inferior vena cava on the right, the esophagus on the left, the gastrohepatic ligament in front, and the diaphragm behind. **r. suprapinea′lis** [NA], suprapineal recess: the posterior extension of the third ventricle of the brain above and around the pineal body. **r. triangula′ris,** triangular recess: a small triangular recess on the anterior wall of the third ventricle of the brain, its base below on the anterior commissure and its sides formed by the converging columns of the fornix.

recidivation (re-sid″ĭ-va′shun) recidivism.

recidivism (re-sid′ĭ-vizm) 1. the repetition of an offense, or crime. 2. the relapse or recurrence of a disease.

recidivist (re-sid′ĭ-vist) [Fr. *récidiviste,* from L. *recidere* to fall back] one who tends to relapse, especially a person who tends to return to criminal habits after treatment or punishment.

recipe (res′ĭ-pe) 1. [L.] take; used at the head of a physician's prescription, and usually indicated by the symbol ℞. See *prescrip-*

tion. 2. a formula for the preparation of a specific combination of ingredients.

recipient (re-sip′e-ent) one who receives, as blood in transfusion, or a tissue or organ graft. **universal r.,** a person thought to be able to receive blood of any "type" without agglutination of the donor cells.

recipiomotor (re-sip″e-o-mo′tor) [L. *recipere* to receive + *motor* mover] pertaining to the reception of motor impressions.

reciprocation (re-sip″ro-ka′shun) [L. *reciprocare* to move backward and forward] the complementary interaction of two distinct entities. Applied in dentistry to the means by which one part of a prosthesis or orthodontic appliance is made to counter the effect created by another part, as in a properly designed partial denture clasp.

Recklinghausen's canals, disease, disease of bone (rek′ling-how″zenz) [Friedrich Daniel von *Recklinghausen,* German pathologist, 1833–1910] see under *canal,* and see *neurofibromatosis* and *osteitis fibrosa cystica.*

reclination (rek″lĭ-na′shun) [L. *reclinatio*] (*obs.*) couching.

Reclus' disease (ra-klez′) [Paul *Reclus,* French surgeon, 1847–1914] see under *disease.*

recognin (re-kog′nin) any of a group of protein fragments produced from cancer cells that are capable of recognizing specific cells; they include astrocytin and malignin.

recognition (rek″og-nish′un) 1. the act of recognizing or state of being recognized. 2. in immunology, a term used to describe the functional changes occurring in immunologically competent cells on contact with antigen, involving recognition of antigen and resulting in combination of antigen with a receptor on the cell surface; called also *antigen r.*

recombinant (re-kom′bĭ-nant) 1. the new cell or individual that results from genetic recombination. 2. pertaining or relating to such cells or individuals. See also under *DNA.* **r. DNA,** see under *DNA.*

recombination (re″kom-bĭ-na′shun) the reunion, in the same or a different arrangement, of formerly united elements which have become separated. In genetics, the formation of new combinations of genes as a result of crossing over between homologous chromosomes. **bacterial r.,** the Mendelian segregation of marker characters, usually nutritional requirements, in mixed cultures of variant strains of bacteria derived from a common parent strain; studied most extensively with a strain of coliform bacillus designated K-12.

recompression (re″kom-presh′un) the restoration of pressure, especially the return to conditions of normal pressure after exposure to greatly diminished atmospheric pressure.

recon (re′kon) [*rec*ombination + Gr. *on* neuter ending] the smallest unit of genetic material capable of recombination, presumably a series of three nucleotide bases (a triplet). Cf. *cistron* and *muton.*

reconstitution (re″kon-stĭ-tu′shun) 1. a type of regeneration in which a new organ forms by the rearrangement of tissues rather than from new formation at an injured surface. 2. The restoration to original form of a substance previously altered for preservation and storage, as the restoration to a liquid state of blood serum or plasma that has been dried and stored.

reconstruction (re″kon-struk′shun) to reassemble or re-form from constituent parts. **image r. from projections,** radiography in which two- or three-dimensional images of an object are reconstructed from a set of mathematical projections, as in transverse axial tomography.

recontour (re-kon′toor) to give new shape or contour to. In dentistry, to change the contour of a crown or a complete or partial denture.

record (rek′ord) a permanent or long-lasting account of something (as on film, in writing, etc.); in dentistry, a registration. **face-bow r.,** a registration by means of a face-bow of the position of the hinge axis and/or the condyles; used to orient the maxillary cast to the opening and closing axis of the articulator. **functional chew-in r.,** a record of the natural chewing movements of the mandible made on an occlusion rim by teeth or scribing studs. **interocclusal r.,** a record of the positional relation of the teeth or jaws to each other, made on occlusal surfaces of occlusion rims or teeth in a plastic material which hardens, such as plaster of Paris, wax, or zinc oxide and eugenol paste. **interocclusal r., centric,** a record of the centric jaw position (relation). **interocclusal r., eccentric,** a record of a jaw relation other than the centric relation. **interocclusal r., lateral,** a record of a lateral eccentric jaw position. **interocclusal r., protrusive,** a record of a protruded eccentric jaw position. **jaw relation r.,** a registration of any positional relationship of the mandible in reference to the maxillae; these records may be of any of the many vertical, horizontal, or orientation relations. **maxillomandibular r.,** a record of the relation of the mandible to the maxillae. **occluding centric relation r.,** a registration of centric relation made at the established occlusal vertical dimension. **problem-oriented r. (POR),** an approach to patient care record keeping that focuses on those specific health problems of the patient that require immediate attention and on the structuring of a cooperative health care plan designed to cope with the identified problems. The components basic to the POR are: *the data base*, which provides information obtained from the variety of sources required for each patient regardless of diagnosis or presenting problems; *the problem list*, which contains those major problems currently needing attention and serves as the basis of a plan of care; *the plan*, which specifies what is to be done with regard to each problem; *the progress notes*, which document the observations, assessments, nursing care plans, physician's orders, etc., of all health care personnel directly involved in the care of the patient. See also *SOAP*. **profile r.**, a registration or record of the profile of a patient. **protrusive r.**, a registration of a forward position of the mandible with reference to the maxillae. **terminal jaw relation r.**, a record of the relationship of the mandible to the maxilla made at the vertical relation of occlusion and at the centric position.

recrement (rek′rĕ-ment) [L. *recrementum*] the saliva or other material which, after secretion, is reabsorbed into the blood.

recrementitious (rek″rĕ-men-tish′us) of the nature of a recrement.

recrudescence (re″kroo-des′ens) [L. *recrudescere* to become sore again] the recurrence of symptoms after a temporary abatement. See *relapse*. The chief distinction between a recrudescence and a relapse is the time interval, a recrudescence occurring after some days or weeks, a relapse after some weeks or months.

recrudescent (re″kroo-des′ent) [L. *recrudescens*] breaking out afresh.

recruitment (re-kroot′ment) 1. the gradual increase to a maximum in a reflex when a stimulus of unaltered intensity is prolonged. 2. in audiology, an abnormally rapid increase in the loudness of a sound caused by a slight increase in its intensity.

Rect. abbreviation for L. *rectifica′tus*, rectified.

rectal (rek′tal) pertaining to the rectum.

rectalgia (rek-tal′je-ah) [*rectum* + *-algia*] proctalgia.

rectectomy (rek-tek′to-me) [*rectum* + Gr. *ektomē* excision] proctectomy.

rectification (rek″tĭ-fi-ka′shun) [L. *rectificatio*] 1. the act of making straight, pure, or correct. 2. redistillation of a liquid to purify it. 3. conversion of alternating current to direct current. **spontaneous r.**, a transverse lie which rectifies itself before labor begins.

rectified (rek′tĭ-fīd) refined; made straight; converted to direct current (DC).

rectifier (rek′tĭ-fi″er) a device for obtaining a direct (unidirectional) current from an alternating current. **thermionic r.**, a rectifier consisting of an electric valve in which the electrons are supplied by a heated electrode.

rectischiac (rek-tis′ke-ak) pertaining to the rectum and the ischium.

rectitis (rek-ti′tis) proctitis. **epidemic gangrenous r.**, see under *proctitis*.

recto- [L. *rectum*] a combining form designating relationship to the rectum. See also words beginning *procto-*.

rectoabdominal (rek″to-ab-dom′ĭ-nal) pertaining to the rectum and abdomen.

rectocele (rek′to-sēl) [*recto-* + Gr. *kēlē* hernia] hernial protrusion of part of the rectum into the vagina; called also *proctocele*.

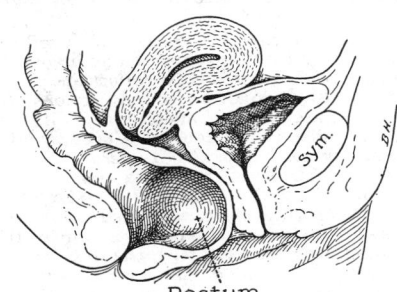

Rectocele.

rectoclysis (rek-tok′lĭ-sis) proctoclysis.

rectococcygeal (rek″to-kok-sij′e-al) pertaining to the rectum and the coccyx.

rectococcypexy (rek″to-kok′sĭ-pek-se) proctococcypexy.

rectocolitis (rek″to-ko-li′tis) coloproctitis.

rectocutaneous (rek″to-ku-ta′ne-us) pertaining to the rectum and the skin.

rectocystotomy (rek″to-sis-tot′o-me) proctocystotomy.

rectolabial (rek″to-la′be-al) pertaining to or communicating with the rectum and a labium majus, as a rectolabial fistula.

rectoperineorrhaphy (rek″to-per″ĭ-ne-or′ah-fe) proctoperineorrhaphy.

rectopexy (rek′to-pek″se) proctopexy.

rectoplasty (rek′to-plas″te) proctoplasty.

rectoromanoscope (rek″to-ro-man′o-skōp) an endoscope for examining the rectum and sigmoid.

rectoromanoscopy (rek″to-ro″mah-nos′ko-pe) [*rectum* + L. *romanum* sigmoid + Gr. *skopein* to examine] inspection of the rectum and sigmoid through an endoscope.

rectorrhaphy (rek-tor′ah-fe) [*rectum* + Gr. *rhaphē* suture] proctorrhaphy.

rectoscope (rek′to-skōp) proctoscope.

rectoscopy (rek-tos′ko-pe) proctoscopy.

rectosigmoid (rek″to-sig′moid) the lower portion of the sigmoid and upper portion of the rectum.

rectosigmoidectomy (rek″to-sig″moi-dek′to-me) excision of the rectum and sigmoid.

rectostenosis (rek″to-stĕ-no′sis) stenosis, or stricture, of the rectum.

rectostomy (rek-tos′to-me) [*rectum* + Gr. *stomoun* to provide with a mouth, or opening] surgical formation of a permanent opening into the rectum for the relief of stricture.

rectotome (rek′to-tōm) prototome.

rectotomy (rek-tot′o-me) proctotomy.

rectourethral (rek″to-u-re′thral) pertaining to or communicating with the rectum and urethra, as a rectourethral fistula.

rectouterine (rek″to-u′ter-in) pertaining to the rectum and uterus.

rectovaginal (rek″to-vaj′ĭ-nal) pertaining to or communicating with the rectum and vagina, as a rectovaginal fistula.

rectovesical (rek″to-ves′ĭ-kal) pertaining to or communicating with the rectum and urinary bladder, as a rectovesical fistula.

rectovestibular (rek″to-ves-tib′u-lar) pertaining to or communicating with the rectum and the vestibule of the vagina, as a rectovestibular fistula.

rectovulvar (rek″to-vul′var) pertaining to or communicating with the rectum and vulva, as a rectovulvar fistula.

Rectules (rek′tūlz) trademark for a preparation of chloral hydrate.

rectum (rek′tum) [L. "straight"] [NA] the distal portion of the large intestine, beginning anterior to the third sacral vertebra as a continuation of the sigmoid and ending at the anal canal; called also *intestinum rectum*.

rectus (rek′tus) [L.] straight; [NA] a general term denoting a straight structure, as a muscle (see entries beginning *musculus rectus*).

recumbent (re-kum′bent) lying down.

recuperation (re-ku″per-a′shun) [L. *recuperatio*] the recovery of health and strength.

recurrence (re-kur′ens) [L. *re-* again + *currere* to run] the return of symptoms after a remission.

recurrent (re-kur′ent) [L. *recurrens* returning] 1. running back, or toward the source. 2. returning after intermissions.

recurvation (re″kur-va′shun) [L. *recurvatio*] a backward bending or curvature.

red (red) [L. *rubrum*] 1. one of the primary colors produced by the longest waves of the visible spectrum. 2. a red dye or stain. **alizarin r.**, the sodium salt of alizarin monosulfonate. **alizarin r. S, alizarin water-soluble r.**, sodium alizarinsulfonate. **aniline r.**, basic fuchsin. **bordeaux r.**, cerasine. **bromphenol r.**, an indicator, dibromphenol-sulfonphthalein, (CH₂Br₂OH)₂C·C₆H₄·SO₂·ONa. **carmine r.**, a stain, C₁₁H₁₂O₇, derived from carmine. **cerasine r.**, sudan III. **cholera r.**, see *cholera red test*, under *tests*. **Congo r.**, chemical name: 3,3′-[4,4′-biphenylylene-bis(azo)]bis[4-amino-1-naphthalenesulfonic acid] disodium salt. An odorless dark red or reddish brown powder, C₃₂H₂₂N₆Na₂O₆S₂, which decomposes on exposure to acid fumes. It is used as a diagnostic aid in amyloidosis, and has been used as an antihemolytic and detoxicant. See also under *tests*. **cotton r.**, Congo r. **cotton r. 4 B**, benzopurpurine 4 B. **cresol r.**, an indicator, ortho-cresol-sulfonphthalein, (CH₃·C₆H₃·OH)₂C·C₆H₄·SO₂·ONa, used in the determination of the hydrogen ion concentration. It has a pH range of 7.2 to 8.8, being yellow at 7.2 and red at 8.8. **dianil r. 4 C, dianin r. 4 B**, benzopurpurine 4 B. **direct r.**, Congo r. **direct r. 4 B**, benzopurpurine 4 B. **fast r.**, amaranth. **fast r. B** or **P**, cerasine. **indigo r., indoxyl r.**, a coloring matter produced by heating an aqueous solution of indoxyl to 130° C. **magdala r.**, a basic dye used for staining connective tissue. It is a mixture of monoamino- and diamino-naphthosafranins. The diamino compound is NH₂C₁₀H₅·N₂Cl(C₁₀H₇)·C₁₀H₅·NH₂. **methyl r.**, a dye, para-dimethyl-amino-azo-benzene-ortho-carboxylic acid, (CH₃)₂N·C₆H₄·-N:N·C₆H₄·COOH, used as an indicator in the determination of hydrogen ion concentration and has a pH range of 4.4 to 6, being red at 4.4, and yellow at 6. **naphthaline r.**, magdala r. **naphthol r.**, amaranth. **neutral r.**, a dye, amino-dimethyl-amino-toluphenazonium chloride, (CH₃)₂N·C₆H₃·N₂C₆H₂(CH₃)·-NH₂HCl. As an indicator it has a pH range of 6.8 to 8, being red at 6.8 and yellow at 8. **oil r.**, sudan III. **oil r. IV**, scarlet r.

orange r., the red oxide of lead, Pb_3O_4, used as a pigment. **phenol r.,** phenolsulfonphthalein. **provisional r.,** a colored lipin obtained from rhodopsin. **scarlet r.,** chemical name: ortho-tolylazo-ortho-tolylazo-beta-naphthol. A fat-soluble azo dye, $C_{24}H_{20}N_4O$, which has some power to stimulate the proliferation of cells, and has been used to enhance wound healing. Called also *oil r. IV, ponceau 3B, rubrum scarlatinum, scarlet R, scharlach R,* and *Sudan IV.* **scarlet r. sulfonate,** the sodium salt of azo-benzene-disulfonic acid azobeta-naphthol; used for the same purpose as scarlet red. **senitol r.,** a dye, $C_2H_5 \cdot NC_9H_6(CH)_3 \cdot - C_9H_6N(I) \cdot C_2H_5$, with a highly selective germicidal action on staphylococci; it is also used to sensitize photographic plates to red rays of light. **sudan r.,** magdala r. **toluylene r.,** the base, the hydrochloride of which is neutral red. **tony r.,** sudan III. **trypan r.,** an acid azo dye used as a vital stain and which possesses some trypanocidal activity. **vital r.,** chemical name: 3-amino-4-[[4′-[(2-amino-6-sulfo-1-naphthyl)azo]-3,3′-dimethyl-4-biphenylyl]azo]-2,7-naphthalene disulfonic acid trisodium salt. A dye, which is introduced directly into the circulation by venipuncture for the purpose of estimating the volume of the blood in the body by determining the concentration of the dye in the blood plasma. **wool r.,** amaranth.

redecussate (re″de-kus′āt) to form a secondary decussation.

redfoot (red′foot) a fatal condition of unknown etiology affecting newborn lambs, in which the sensitive lamina of the feet become exposed owing to detachment of the overlying horn.

redia (re′de-ah), pl. *re′diae* [named after F. *Redi,* Italian naturalist, 1626–1698] a larval stage of certain trematode parasites, which develops in the body of a snail host and gives rise to daughter rediae, or to the cercariae.

rediae (re′de-e) plural of *redia.*

redifferentiation (re″dif-er-en″she-a′shun) the return of a dedifferentiated tissue or part to its original or another more or less similar condition.

Redig. in pulv. abbreviation for L. *rediga′tur in pul′verem,* let it be reduced to powder.

Red. in pulv. abbreviation for L. *reduc′tus in pul′verem,* reduced to powder.

redintegration (red-in″tĕ-gra′shun) [L. *redintegratio*] 1. the restoration or repair of a lost or damaged part. 2. that type of psychic process in which a part of a complex stimulus provokes the complete reaction that was previously made to the complex stimulus as a whole (Hollingworth).

redislocation (re″dis-lo-ka′shun) dislocation recurring after reduction.

Redisol (red′ĭ-sol) trademark for a preparation of crystalline vitamin B_{12}; see *cyanocobalamin.*

Redlich-Obersteiner (red′likh o″ber-sti′ner) see *Obersteiner-Redlich.*

redox (red′oks) oxidation-reduction.

redressement (rĕ-dres-maw′) [Fr.] 1. a second or repeated dressing. 2. correction of a deformity. **r. forcé,** forcible correction of a deformity, especially a procedure for the immediate correction of knock knee.

red tide (red tīd) see *Gonyaulax.*

reduce (re-dūs′) [re- + L. *ducere* to lead] 1. to restore to the normal place or relation of parts, as to *reduce* a fracture. 2. in chemistry, to submit to reduction. 3. to decrease in weight.

reduced (re-dūst′) 1. returned to the proper place or position, as a *reduced* fracture. 2. restored to a metallic form, as, *reduced* iron. 3. altered by a chemical change involving a gain of electrons.

reducible (re-du′sĭ-b′l) permitting of reduction; capable of being reduced.

reductant (re-duk′tant) the electron donor in an oxidation-reduction (redox) reaction.

reductase (re-duk′tās) any enzyme that has a reducing action on chemical compounds; a hydrogenase. **5α-r.,** an enzyme that catalyzes the irreversible reduction of testosterone to dihydrotestosterone. **acetaldehyde r.,** an enzyme that catalyzes the reduction of acetaldehyde to alcohol. It consists of a protein and a prosthetic group, nicotinamide adenine dinucleotide (NAD). **acetoacetyl-CoA r.,** an enzyme that catalyzes the conversion of D-3-hydroxyacyl CoA and NADP to 3-oxo-acyl-CoA and reduced NADP. **cytochrome r.,** a flavoprotein enzyme that catalyzes the simultaneous reduction of cytochrome C and the oxidation of reduced nicotinamide adenine dinucleotide (NADH). **quinone r.,** an enzyme that catalyzes the transfer of hydrogen from reduced pyridine nucleotides to suitable quinones—mostly 1,4-naphthoquinones or benzoquinones.

reduction (re-duk′shun) [L. *reductio*] 1. the correction of a fracture, luxation, or hernia. 2. in chemistry, the addition of hydrogen to a substance, or more generally, the gain of electrons. **r. of chromosomes,** the passing of the members of a chromosome pair to the daughter cells during meiosis, each daughter cell receiving half the diploid number. **closed r.,** the manipulative reduction of a fracture without incision. **r. en masse,** reduction of a strangulated hernia included within its sac, so that the

strangulation is not relieved. **open r.,** reduction of a fracture after incision into the fracture site. **tuberosity r.,** the surgical excision of excessive fibrous or bony tissue in the area of the maxillary tuberosity prior to the construction of prosthetic appliances. **weight r.,** the lessening of one's body weight by a specific regimen which is especially designed for that purpose.

reductone (re-duk′tōn) glucic acid.

redundant (re-dun′dant) more than necessary; superfluous.

reduplication (re″du-plĭ-ka′shun) [L. *reduplicatio*] 1. a doubling back. 2. the recurrence of paroxysms of a double type. 3. a doubling of parts, connected at some point, the extra part being usually a mirror image of the other.

reduviid (re-du′vĭ-id) belonging to the family Reduviidae.

Reduviidae (re″du-vi′ĭ-de) a family of winged hemipterous insects of the suborder Heteroptera, called cone-nose bugs or kissing bugs; they are also known as assassin bugs because they prey on other insects. They attack man and other mammals; some species transmit Chagas' disease. It includes the genera *Eratyrus, Eutriatoma, Panstrongylus, Reduvius* (type genus), *Rhodnius,* and *Triatoma.*

Reduvius (re-du′ve-us) a genus of hemipterous blood-sucking insects. **R. perso′natus,** a species whose bite may cause nausea, generalized urticaria, or other allergic symptoms.

redwater (red′wah-ter) 1. Texas fever. 2. bacillary hemoglobinuria.

Reed's cells (rēdz) [Dorothy *Reed,* American pathologist] Sternberg-Reed cells.

re-education (re″ed-u-ka′shun) the training of a disabled or mentally disordered person in the endeavor to restore his lost competence.

reef (rēf) an infolding or tuck of tissue, as a tuck made in plication.

reentry (re-en′tre) in cardiology, a postulated mechanism by which a premature heart beat can be coupled to the normal beat: the normal sinus impulse activates the heart except for an area of diminished responsiveness; by the time this abnormal area is activated, the remainder of the heart has recovered, and the impulse "reenters" the normal zone from the abnormal area, eliciting a premature contraction.

Rees's test (rēs′ez) [George Owen *Rees,* English physician, 1813–1889] see under *tests.*

refect (re-fekt′) to induce refection.

refection (re-fek′shun) [L. *reficere* to restore] recovery; repair: applied specifically to the ability of the flora of the cecum of rats to synthesize vitamins of the B group from deficient diets and supply them to the host animal.

refectious (re-fek′shus) capable of causing, or pertaining to, refection.

refine (re-fīn′) to purify or free from foreign matter.

reflected (re-flekt′ed) turned or bent back; mirrored.

reflection (re-flek′shun) [L. *reflexio*] 1. a turning or bending back; a bending back upon its course. 2. an image produced by reflection. 3. in physics, the turning back of a ray of light, sound, or heat when it strikes against a surface that it does not penetrate. The ray before reflection is known as the *incident ray;* after reflection, it is the *reflected ray.*

reflector (re-flek′tor) a device for reflecting light or sound. **dental r.,** a mouth mirror.

reflex (re′fleks) [L. *reflexus*] 1. reflected. 2. a reflected action or movement; the sum total of any particular involuntary activity. See *reflex arc* and *reflex action.* 3. a reflection or a reflected image of an object. **abdominal r's,** contractions of the abdominal muscles on scratching the abdominal wall. **abdomino-cardiac r.,** any reflex in the heart produced by stimulating the abdominal sympathetic nerves. Cf. *Livierato's sign* and *Prevel's sign,* under *sign.* **Abrams' r.,** reflex contraction of the lung following stimulation of the chest wall. **Abrams' heart r.,** contraction of the myocardium, with reduction in the area of cardiac dullness, which results when the skin of the precordial region is irritated. It is observed with the fluoroscope. **accommodation r.,** the coordinated changes that occur when the eye adapts itself for near vision; they are constriction of the pupil, convergence of the eyes, and increased convexity of the lens. **Achilles tendon r.,** triceps surae jerk. **acoustic r.,** contraction of the stapedius muscle in response to intense sound. Called also *stapedial r.* **acquired r.,** conditioned response. **adductor r.,** on tapping the tendon of the adductor magnus with the thigh in abduction, contraction of the adductors results. **adductor r. of foot,** Hirschberg's sign. **allied r's,** reflexes in which two afferent stimuli use the same common pathway or produce effects on two synergistic muscles. **anal r.,** contraction of the anal sphincter on irritation of the skin of the anus. **ankle r.,** triceps surae jerk. **antagonistic r's,** reflex movements occurring not in the muscle which has been stretched but in its antagonist. **anticus r.,** Piotrowski's sign. **Aschner's r.,** oculocardiac r. **atriopressor r.,** rise in arterial blood pressure (vasoconstriction) attributed to a change of pressure in the right atrium and great veins. **attention r. of pupil,** alteration of size in the pupil when the attention is suddenly fixed; called also *Piltz's r.* **attitudinal r's,** those reflexes having to do with the position of the body. **audito-oculogyric r.,** a turning of both eyes in the direction of a sudden sound. **auditory r.,** any reflex caused by stimulation of the auditory nerve, especially momentary closure of both eyes produced by a sudden sound. **aural r.,** any reflex connected with the auditory apparatus. **auricle r.,** involuntary movement of the ear produced by auditory stimuli. **auriculocervical nerve r.,** Snellen's r. **auriculopalpebral r.,** Kehrer's r. **autonomic r.,** a response of smooth muscle, glands, and conducting tissue of the heart, which alters the functional state of the innervated organ. **axon r.,** a reflex resulting from a stimulus applied to one branch of a nerve which sets up an impulse that moves centrally to the point of division of the nerve where it is reflected down the other branch to the effector organ. **Babinski's r.** (1896), dorsiflexion of the big toe on stimulating the sole of the foot; it occurs in lesions of the pyramidal tract, and indicates organic, as distinguished from hysteric, hemiplegia. Called also *Babinski's sign* or *toe sign.* **Babkin r.,** pressure by the examiner's thumbs on the palms of both hands of the infant results in opening of the infant's mouth; it is elicited in many newborn infants, normal and abnormal, except when lethargic or comatose. **Bainbridge r.,** rise in pressure in, or increased distention of, the large somatic veins or the right atrium, with acceleration of the heart beat. **Barkman's r.,** contraction of the rectus abdominis muscle on the same side after stimulation of the skin just below one of the nipples. **basal joint r.,** finger-thumb r. **behavior r.,** conditioned response. **Bekhterev's r.,** 1. *deep:* passive flexion of the toes and foot in a plantar direction is followed by flexion in a dorsal direction and by flexive movements of the knee and hip. 2. *hypogastric:* contraction of the muscles of the lower abdomen on stroking the skin of the inner surface of the thigh. 3. *pupil:* dilatation of the pupil on exposure to light; sometimes seen in tabes and general paralysis. 4. tickling of the mucosa of the nasal cavity with a feather or piece of paper produces contraction of the facial muscles on the same side of the face; called also *nasal r.* **Bekhterev-Mendel r.,** Mendel-Bekhterev r. **biceps r.,** contractions of the biceps muscle of the arm when its tendon is tapped; this reflex is normal but when greatly increased it indicates the same disease as increased knee jerk. **bladder r.,** any of the reflexes of the bladder necessary for effortless evacuation of urine and subconscious maintenance of continence: vesical contraction following distention of the bladder, vesical contraction evoked by urethral flow, vesical contraction evoked by proximal urethral distention, relaxation of the urethra resulting from running liquid in the urethra, distention of the bladder resulting in relaxation of the external sphincter, relaxation of the proximal urethral smooth muscle by distention of the bladder, and vesical contraction related to running liquid through the urethra. **blink r.,** corneal r. **Brain's r.,** an extension of the hemiplegic flexed arm when the patient assumes the quadrupedal position; called also *quadrupedal extensor reflex.* **bregmocardiac r.,** pressure upon the bregmatic fontanel slows the action of the heart. **Brissaud's r.,** contraction of the tensor muscle of fascia lata on tickling the sole. **Brudzinski's r.,** see under *sign.* **bulbocavernous r.,** a tap on the dorsum of the penis causes retraction of the bulbocavernous portion. **bulbomimic r.,** in coma from apoplexy, pressure on the eyeball causes contraction of the facial muscles on the side opposite to the lesion; in coma from toxic causes the reflex occurs on both sides. Called also *facial r.* and *Mondonesi's r.* **carotid sinus r.,** pressure on, or in, the carotid artery at the level of its bifurcation causing reflex slowing of the heart rate; this reflex originates in the wall of the sinus of the internal carotid artery. See *carotid sinus syndrome,* under *syndrome.* **cerebral cortex r.,** Haab's r. **Chaddock r.,** stimulation below the external malleolus produces extension of the great toe; it occurs in lesions of the pyramidal tract. **chain r.,** a series of reflexes, each serving as a stimulus to the next one, representing a complete activity. **chin r.,** stroking of the chin causes closing of the mouth. **chocked r.,** in skiascopy, absence of movement of the retinal illumination on reaching the point of reversal. **ciliary r.,** the movement of the pupil in accommodation. **ciliospinal r.,** painful stimulation of the skin of the neck dilates the pupil. **clasp-knife r.,** lengthening reaction. **cochleo-orbicular r., cochleopalpebral r.,** contraction of the orbicularis palpebrarum muscle when a sharp, sudden noise is made close to the ear; does not occur in total deafness from labyrinthine disease. **cochleopupillary r.,** a reaction of the iris (contraction of the pupil followed by dilatation) to a loud sound. **cochleostapedial r.,** the reflex contraction of the stapedius muscle from noises. **concealed r.,** one elicited by a stimulus but concealed by a more dominant reflex elicited by the same stimulus. **conditional r.,** conditioned response. **conditioned r.,** see under *response.* **conjunctival r.,** closure of the eyelid when the conjunctiva is touched. **consensual r.,** crossed r. **consensual light r.,** stimulation of one eye by light produces a reflex response in the opposite pupil. **convergency r.,** convergence of the visual axes with fixation on a near point. **convulsive r.,** one in which several muscles contract convulsively without coordination. **coordinated r.,** one in which several muscles react so as to produce an orderly and

useful movement. **corneal r.,** irritation of the cornea results in reflex closure of the lids; called also *blink r., eyelid closure r.,* and *lid r.* **corneomandibular r., corneopterygoid r.,** movement of the lower jaw toward the side opposite the eye whose cornea is lightly touched, the mouth being open. **corneomental r.,** unilateral wrinkling of the muscles of the chin when pressure is applied to the cornea. **coronary r.,** the reflex that controls the caliber of the coronary blood vessels. **cough r.,** the sequence of events initiated by the sensitivity of the lining of the airways of the lung and mediated by the medulla as a consequence of impulses transmitted by the vagus nerve, resulting in coughing, i.e., the clearing of the passageways of foreign matter. **cranial r.,** any reflex whose paths are connected directly with the brain. **cremasteric r.,** stimulation of the skin on the front and inner side of the thigh retracts the testis on the same side. The presence of this reflex indicates integrity of the first lumbar nerve segment of the spinal cord or its root; absence indicates damage of the first lumbar nerve segment or its root or lesion of the corticospinal tract. Cf. *Geigel's r.* **crossed r.,** stimulation of one side of the body often causes also a corresponding response on the other side, especially in the eye. **cuboidodigital r.,** Mendel-Bekhterev r. **cutaneous pupillary r.,** dilatation of the pupil on pinching the skin of the cheek or neck. **dartos r.,** the patient stands with his feet wide apart and the examiner suddenly applies cold to the perineum; the dartos muscle undergoes vermicular contraction. **dazzle r.,** a reflex by which a strong light shining on the eyes causes an immediate closing of the eyelids which lasts as long as the stimulus. **deep r.,** one elicited by a sharp tap on the appropriate tendon or muscle to induce brief stretch of the muscle, followed by contraction. Called also *tendon r.* **defecation r., rectal r.,** contraction and extension motions in a paralyzed limb produced by plantar flexion of the toes. **delayed r.,** a reflex which occurs some time after the stimulus provoking it has been received. **depressor r.,** a reflex to stimulation resulting in decreased activity of the motor center. **digital r.,** see *Hoffmann's sign,* def. 2, under *sign.* **direct r.,** a contraction on the same side as that of the stimulation. **direct light r.,** when a ray of light is thrown upon the retina through the pupil there is immediate contraction of the sphincter iridis, reducing the size of the pupillary aperture. **diving r.,** a reflex involving cardiovascular and metabolic adaptations to conserve oxygen occurring in animals during diving into water; observed in reptiles, birds, and mammals, including man. **doll's eye r.,** when the premature infant's head is rotated laterally, the eyes are pulled synergistically in the opposite direction, then return to the middle of the palpebral fissure. **dorsal r.,** contraction of the back muscles in response to stimulation of the skin along the erector spinae. **dorsocuboidal r.,** Mendel-Bekhterev r. **elbow r.,** triceps r. **embrace r.,** Moro's r. **emergency light r.,** excessive stimulation of the retina by light produces contraction of the pupils, closure of the eyelids, and lowering of the eyebrows. **enterogastric r.,** inhibition of gastric motility when irritants enter the duodenum. **epigastric r.,** contraction of the abdominal muscles caused by stimulating the skin of the epigastrium or over the fifth and sixth intercostal spaces near the axilla. **Erben's r.,** slowing down of the pulse upon bending head and trunk strongly forward; said to indicate vagal excitability. **erector spinae r.,** contraction of the erector spinae muscle on irritation of the skin along its border. **Escherich's r.,** see under *sign.* **esophagosalivary r.,** Roger's r. **ether r.,** the sudden and increased flow of duodenal secretion following the introduction of ether and certain other substances into the duodenum. **external auditory meatus r.,** Kisch's r. **eyeball compression r., eyeball-heart r.,** oculocardiac r. **eyelid closure r.,** 1. corneal r. 2. conjunctival r. **facial r.,** bulbomimic r. **faucial r.,** reflex vomiting caused by irritation of the fauces. **femoral r.,** Remak's r. **finger-thumb r.,** passive flexion of the metacarpophalangeal joint of one of the fingers causes flexion of the basal joint and extension of the terminal joint of the thumb. **flexion r. of leg,** tapping of the tendons of the semimembranosus and semitendinosus muscles causes flexion of the leg. **flexor r., paradoxical,** dorsiflexion of the great toe or of all the toes when the deep muscles of the calf are pressed upon. **fontanel r.,** Grünfelder's r. **foveolar r.,** the ophthalmoscopic reflex in the form of a dot caused by the foveola. **front-tap r.,** a tap on the skin muscles of the extended leg contracts the gastrocnemius. **fusion r.,** the reflex which tends to merge the images on the two retinas into a single impression. **gag r.,** pharyngeal r. **gastrocolic r.,** an increase in intestinal and colonic peristaltic activity following entrance of food into the empty stomach. **gastroileal r.,** an increase in ileal motility and opening of the ileocecal valve when food enters the empty stomach. **gastropancreatic r.,** an increase in pancreatic secretion induced by distention of the corpus of the stomach; it is mediated by the vagus nerve. **Gault's cochleopalpebral r.,** cochleopalpebral r. **Geigel's r.,** a reflex in the female corresponding to the cremasteric reflex in the male; i.e., on stroking of the inner anterior aspect of the upper thigh there is a contraction of the muscular fibers at the upper edge of Poupart's ligament. **genital r.,** any reflex irritability due to disorder of the genital organs. **Gifford's r., Gifford-Galassi r.,** contraction of the pupil when an effort is made to close the lids, which are held apart. **gluteal r.,** a stroke over the skin of the buttock contracts the glutei muscles. **Gordon's r.,** flexor r., paradoxical. **grasp r., grasping r.,** a reflex consisting of a grasping motion of the fingers or of the toes in response to stimulation. **Grünfelder's r.,** dorsal flexion of the great toe with a fan-wise spreading of the other toes elicited by continued pressure at the corner of the posterior lateral fontanel; occurs in the presence of disease of the middle ear in children up to the age of five years. **gustolacrimal r.,** an anomalous reflex by which food taken into the mouth tends to stimulate the secretion not only of saliva but also of tears. **H-r.,** a monosynaptic reflex elicited by stimulating a nerve, particularly the tibial nerve, with an electric shock. **Haab's r.,** bilateral pupillary contraction when the patient sits in a darkened room, and without accommodation or convergence directs his attention to a bright object already within the field of vision. Called also *cerebral cortex r.* **heart r.,** Abrams' heart r. **heel-tap r.,** a reflex occurring in disease of the pyramidal tract and consisting of fanning and plantar flexion of the toes produced by tapping the patient's heel. **hepatojugular r.,** see under *reflux.* **Hering-Breuer r.,** the nervous mechanism which tends to limit the respiratory excursions. Stimuli from the sensory endings in the lungs and perhaps in other parts passing up the vagi tend to limit both inspiration and expiration in ordinary breathing. **Hirschberg's r.,** tickling of the sole at the base of the great toe causes adduction of the foot. **Hoffmann's r.,** see under *sign,* def. 2. **Hughes's r.,** see *virile r.,* def. 2. **hypochondrial r.,** sudden inspiration caused by quick pressure beneath the lower border of the ribs. **ileogastric r.,** inhibition of gastric motility by distension of the ileum. **inborn r.,** unconditioned r. **indirect r.,** crossed r. **infraspinatus r.,** obtained by tapping a certain spot over the shoulder blade, on a line bisecting the angle formed by the spine of the bone and its inner border; outward rotation of the arm occurs, with simultaneous straightening of the elbow. **inguinal r.,** Geigel's r. **interscapular r.,** a stimulus applied between the scapulae contracts the scapular muscles; called also *scapular r.* **intestinointestinal r.,** when a part of the intestine becomes overdistended or its mucosa becomes excessively irritated, activity in other parts of the intestine is inhibited as long as the distention persists. **inverted radial r.,** a flexion of the fingers without movement of the forearm, produced by tapping the lower end of the radius; it indicates disease of the fifth cervical segment of the spinal cord associated with damage of the pyramidal tract below that level. **iris contraction r.,** pupillary r. **ischemic r.,** the elevation of arterial pressure in response to cerebral ischemia. **jaw r., jaw jerk r.,** closure of the mouth caused by a downward blow on the lower jaw while it hangs passively open. It is seen only rarely in health, but is very noticeable in lesions of the corticospinal tract. **Joffroy's r.,** twitching of the gluteal muscles on pressure against the nates in spastic paralysis. **Juster r.,** extension of the fingers instead of flexion on stimulation of the palm. **juvenile r.,** a glistening white reflection from the smooth surface of the retina in young people. **Kehrer's r., Kisch's r.,** closure of the eye as a result of tactile or thermal stimulation of the deepest part of the external auditory meatus and tympanum. **knee jerk r.,** quadriceps jerk. **Kocher's r.,** contraction of the abdominal muscle on compression of the testicle. **lacrimal r.,** secretion of tears elicited by touching the conjunctiva over the cornea. **Landau r.,** when an infant is held in the prone position, the entire body forms a convex upward arc; gentle pressure on the head or gravity flexes the neck and hip, reversing the arc. **laryngeal r.,** irritation of the fauces and larynx causing cough. **laughter r.,** laughter brought on by tickling. **let-down r.,** the ejection or release of milk from the alveoli of the breast into the ducts, caused by a combination of neurogenic and hormonal reflexes involving the hormone oxytocin and, to a lesser extent, vasopressin; called also *milk ejection* and *milk let-down r.* **lid r.,** corneal r. **Liddell and Sherrington r.,** stretch r. **light r.,** 1. a luminous image reflected from the membrana tympani. 2. a circular spot of light seen reflected from the retina with the retinoscopic mirror. 3. contraction of the pupil when light falls on the eye. **lip r.,** a reflex movement of the lips of sleeping babies which occurs on tapping near the angle of the mouth. **Livierato's r.,** Abrams' heart r. **Lovén r.,** general vasodilatation of an organ when its afferent nerve is stimulated; this secures a maximal supply of blood to the organ, together with a general rise of blood pressure. **lumbar r.,** dorsal r. **Lust's r.,** abduction of the foot with dorsal flexion on percussion of the common peroneal nerve. **McCarthy's r.,** contraction of the orbicularis oculi muscle on tapping the supraorbital nerve. **McCormac's r.,** percussing the patellar tendon produces adduction of the opposite leg. **McDowall r.,** a decrease in systemic blood pressure following vagotomy, due to abolishment of the afferent impulses from the atria, which normally induce vasoconstriction. **Magnus and de Kleijn neck r's,** extension of both ipsilateral limbs, or one, or part of a limb, and increase of tonus on the side to which the chin is turned when the head is rotated to the side, and flexion with loss of tonus on the side to which occiput points. Essentially it is a sign of *decerebrate rigidity.* **mandibular r.,** jaw r. **Marinesco-**

Radovici r., palm-chin r. **mass r.,** a reflex exhibited by the entire area controlled by the portion of the spinal cord which has been injured. **Mayer's r.,** opposition and adduction of the thumb combined with flexion at the metacarpophalangeal joint and extension at the interphalangeal joint, on downward pressure of the index finger. **Mendel's r., Mendel's dorsal r. of foot,** Mendel-Bekhterev r. **Mendel-Bekhterev r.,** percussion of the dorsum of the foot normally causes dorsal flexion of the second to fifth toes; in certain organic nervous conditions it causes plantar flexion of the toes. Called also *cuboidodigital r., dorsocuboidal r., Mendel-Beckterew r.,* and *tarsophalangeal r.* **milk ejection r., milk let-down r.,** let-down r. **Mondonesi's r.,** bulbomimic r. **Morley's peritoneocutaneous r.,** when any of the cerebrospinal nerve endings in the peritoneum or subperitoneal tissues are irritated, pain will be referred to the corresponding segmental skin area. **Moro's r., Moro embrace r.,** flexion of an infant's thighs and knees, fanning and then clenching of the fingers, with the arms first thrown outward then brought together in an embrace attitude, produced by a sudden stimulus, such as striking the table on either side of the child. It is seen normally in infants up to 3 to 4 months of age. Called also *embrace r.* and *startle r.* **motor r.,** a reflex brought about by stimulation upon the periphery of the motor mechanism. **muscular r.,** a reflex movement due to the stretching of a muscle. **myenteric r.,** contraction of the intestine above and relaxation below a portion of the intestine that is irritated or distended. **myopic r.,** Weiss's r. **myotatic r.,** stretch r. **nasal r.,** 1. irritation of the schneiderian membrane provokes sneezing. 2. see *Bekhterev's r.,* def. 4. **nasolabial r.,** sudden retroversion of the head, stretching of the back, retroversion of the arms at the shoulder, extension and pronation of the forearms, and extension and adduction of the legs, elicited by a slight vertical sweeping motion touching the tip of the nose; it frequently occurs in healthy infants, and disappears around the fifth month of age. **nasomental r.,** contraction of the mentalis muscle on tapping the side of the nose with a percussion hammer. **neck righting r.,** rotation of the trunk in the direction in which the head of the supine infant is turned; this reflex is absent or decreased in infants with spasticity. **nociceptive r's,** reflexes initiated by painful stimuli. **nostril r.,** reduction of the size of the opening of the naris, said to occur on the affected side in pulmonary disease. **obliquus r.,** stimulation of the skin below Poupart's ligament contracts a part of the external oblique muscle. **oculocardiac r.,** a slowing of the rhythm of the heart following compression of the eyes or pressure on the carotid sinus. A slowing of from 5 to 13 beats per minute is normal; one of from 13 to 50 or more is exaggerated; one of from 1 to 5 is diminished. If ocular compression produces acceleration of the heart, the reflex is called *inverted.* See also *Aschner's phenomenon,* under *phenomenon.* **oculocephalogyric r.,** the reflex by which the movements of the eye, the head, and the body are directed in the interest of visual attention. **oculopharyngeal r.,** rapid deglutition together with spontaneous closing of the eyes. **oculopupillary r.,** trigeminus r. **oculosensory cell r.,** trigeminus r. **oculovagal r.,** pressure on the eyeball induces atrioventricular beats or rhythm. **Oppenheim's r.,** see under *sign.* **opticofacial winking r.,** closure of the lids when an object is brought suddenly into the field of vision. **orbicular oculi r.,** normal contraction of the orbicularis oculi muscle, with resultant closing of the eye, on percussion at the outer aspect of the supraorbital ridge, over the glabella, or around the margin of the orbit. **orbicularis r.,** Westphal's pupillary r. **orthocardiac r.,** see *Livierato's test,* 2d def. **palatal r., palatine r.,** stimulation of the palate causing swallowing. **palm-chin r.,** twitching of the chin produced by stimulating (scratching) the palm. **palmomental r.,** palm-chin r. **paraserum r.,** group agglutination; paragglutination. **patellar r.,** quadriceps jerk. **patelloadductor r.,** crossed adduction of the thigh produced by tapping the quadriceps tendon as in the patellar reflex. **pathologic r.,** one which is not normal, but is the result of a pathologic condition, and may serve as a sign of disease. **pectoral r.,** the subject's arm is placed half way between adduction and abduction and the examiner's finger in the muscle tendon near the humerus: a sharp blow of the finger elicits adduction and slight internal rotation. **penile r., penis r.,** bulbocavernous r. **perception r.,** a reflex movement occurring when a perception is formed in consciousness. **perianal r.,** anal r. **peritoneointestinal r.,** inhibition of motility of the stomach and intestine resulting from retroperitoneal irritation or hemorrhage. **pharyngeal r.,** contraction of the constrictor muscle of the pharynx elicited by touching the back of the pharynx; called also *gag r.* **phasic r.,** an active and coordinated movement occurring as a response to stimulation. **Philippson's r.,** excitation of the knee extensor in one leg induced by inhibition in the knee extensor of the other leg. **pilomotor r.,** the production of goose flesh on stroking the skin; trichography. **Piltz's r.,** attention r. of pupil. **placing r.,** flexion followed by extension of the leg when the infant is held erect and the dorsum of the foot is drawn along the under edge of a table top; it is obtainable in the normal infant up to the age of six weeks. **plantar r.,** irritation of the sole contracts the toes. **platysmal r.,** the act of nipping the platysma contracts the pupil.

postural r., a reflex which consists of some assumption of posture. **prepotential r's,** instincts. **pressor r.,** a reflex to stimulation resulting in increased activity of a motor center. **Preyer's r.,** involuntary movements of the ears produced by auditory stimulation. **proprioceptive r.,** a reflex that is initiated by stimuli arising from some function of the reflex mechanism itself. **psychic r.,** a reflex aroused by a stored-up impression of memory, such as the secretion of saliva at the sight or thought of good tasting food. **psychocardiac r.,** increase in the pulse rate on recalling an individual emotional experience. **psychogalvanic r.,** decreased electric resistance of the body as a result of mental or emotional agitation. **pulmonocoronary r.,** reflex vasoconstriction of the coronary arteries, mediated by the vagus nerves. **pupillary r.,** 1. contraction of the pupil on exposure of the retina to light. 2. any reflex involving the iris, resulting in change in the size of the pupil, occurring in response to various stimuli, e.g., change in illumination or point of fixation, sudden loud noise, emotional stimulation. **pupillary r., paradoxic,** stimulation of the retina by light dilates the pupil. **Puusepp's r.,** abduction of the little toe on stimulating the posterior external part of the sole of the foot; indicative of lesion of the extrapyramidal and pyramidal tracts. **quadriceps r.,** contraction of the quadriceps and extension of the leg when the quadriceps tendon is tapped between the patella and the tibial tubercle. **quadrupedal extensor r.,** Brain's r. **radial r.,** flexion of the forearm, following tapping on the lower end of the radius; when the fingers flex as well, it indicates hyperreflexia. **rectal r.,** the process by which the accumulation of feces in the rectum excites defecation; called also *defecation r.* **red r.,** a luminous red appearance seen upon the retina. **regional r.,** segmental r. **Remak's r.,** plantar flexion of the first three toes and sometimes of the foot, with extension of the knee on stroking of the upper anterior surface of the thigh. **renointestinal r.,** inhibition of motility of the intestine resulting from renal irritation. **renorenal r.,** a reflex pain or anuria in a sound kidney in cases in which the other kidney is diseased. **resistance r.,** Babinski r. **retrobulbar pupillary r.,** slight dilatation of the pupil which contracts under light stimulation, and then dilates while the light stimulation is still present. **Riddoch's mass r.,** in severe injury of the spinal cord, stimulation below the level of the lesion produces flexion reflexes of the lower extremity, evacuation of the bowels and bladder, and sweating of the skin below the level of the lesion. **righting r.,** the ability to assume optimal position when there has been a departure from it. **Roger's r.,** salivation on irritation of the esophagus. **rooting r.,** a reflex in the newborn in which stimulation of the side of the cheek or the upper or lower lip causes the infant to turn his mouth and face to the stimulus. **Rossolimo's r.,** on tapping the plantar surface of the toes, plantar flexion of the toes occurs when there are lesions of the pyramidal tract. **Ruggeri's r.,** acceleration of the pulse following strong convergence of the eyeballs toward something very close to the eyes; it indicates sympathetic excitability. **Saenger's r.,** see under *sign*. **scapular r.,** interscapular r. **scapulohumeral r.,** adduction with outward rotation of the humerus produced by percussing along the inner edge of the scapula. **Schäffer's r.,** flexion of the foot and toes on pinching the Achilles tendon at its middle third; seen in organic hemiplegia. **scrotal r.,** a slow, vermicular contraction of the dartos muscle obtained by stroking the perineum or by applying a cold object to it. **segmental r.,** a reflex controlled by a single segment or region of the spinal cord. **senile r.,** a gray reflection from the pupil of aged people due to hardening of the lens. **sexual r.,** the reflex of erection and ejaculation produced by stimulation of the genitals. **shot-silk r.,** see *shot-silk retina*, under *retina*. **simple r.,** a reflex involving a single muscle. **skin r.,** a reflex which occurs on stimulation of the skin. **skin pupillary r.,** dilatation of the pupil produced by irritation of the skin of the neck. **Snellen's r.,** unilateral congestion of the ear upon stimulation of the distal end of the divided auriculocervical nerve. **sole r.,** plantar r. **Somagyi's r.,** widening of the pupils on deep inspiration and their contraction on expiration; said to indicate irritable weakness or instability of the cardiac vagus. **somatointestinal r.,** inhibition of intestinal motility when the skin over the abdomen is stimulated. **spinal r.,** any reflex whose arc is connected with a center in the spinal cord. **stapedial r.,** acoustic r. **startle r.,** Moro's r. **static r.,** the reflex pose and righting of the body. **statotomic r's,** attitudinal r's. **stepping r.,** 1. movements of progression elicited when the infant is held upright and inclined forward with the soles of the feet touching a flat surface; it is obtainable in the normal infant up to the age of six weeks. 2. extension of the hind leg of a dog on pressing the plantar surface of the foot. **Stookey r.,** with the leg semiflexed at the knee, the tendons of the semimembranosus and the semitendinosus muscles are tapped: flexion of the leg results. **stretch r.,** reflex contraction of a muscle in response to passive longitudinal stretching; called also *Liddell and Sherrington r.* and *myotatic reflex*. **Strümpell's r.,** leg movement with adduction of the foot produced by stroking the thigh or abdomen. **sucking r.,** sucking movements of the mouth elicited by the touching of an object to an infant's lips. **superficial r.,** any withdrawal reflex elicited by noxious or tactile stimulation of the skin, cornea, or mucous membrane, including the corneal reflex, pharyngeal reflex, cremasteric reflex, etc. **supinator longus r.,** tapping on the lower end of the radius produces flexion of the forearm. **supraorbital r.,** McCarthy's r. **suprapatellar r.,** with the leg extended the index finger of the examiner is crooked above the patella and is struck; the result is a kick-back of the patella. **suprapubic r.,** stroking the abdomen above Poupart's ligament causes deviation of the linea alba toward the side that is stroked. **supraumbilical r.,** epigastric reflex. **swallowing r.,** palatal r. **tapetal light r.,** the glowing of eyes in the dark, just as do the eyes of carnivorous animals. **tarsophalangeal r.,** Mendel-Bekhterev r. **tendon r.,** involuntary contraction of a muscle after brief stretching caused by percussion of its tendon; tendon reflexes include the biceps reflex, triceps reflex, quadriceps reflex, etc. Called also *deep r., tendon jerk* or *reaction*. **threat r.,** sudden closure of the eyes at a sign of danger. **Throckmorton's r.,** a variation of the Babinski reflex elicited by percussion of the metatarsophalangeal region in the dorsum of the foot. **tibioadductor r.,** tapping of the tibia on the inner side of the leg results either in homolateral adduction of the leg or crossed adduction from side to side. **toe r.,** strong flexion of the great toe flexes all the muscles of the lower extremity; it is seen in pathologic states in which there is hyperreflexia. **tonic r.,** the passing of an appreciable period of time after the occurrence of a reflex before relaxation; a reflex which maintains the reflex contractions that are the basis of posture and attitude. **tonic neck r.,** a reflex in the newborn consisting of extension of the arm and sometimes of the leg on the side to which the head is forcibly turned, with flexion of the contralateral limbs. **trained r.,** conditioned response. **triceps r.,** contraction of the belly of the triceps muscle and slight extension of the arm when the tendon of the muscle is tapped directly, with the arm flexed and fully supported and relaxed. **triceps surae r.,** plantar flexion of the foot elicited by a tap on the Achilles tendon preferably while the patient kneels on a bed or chair, the feet hanging free over the edge; ankle jerk. **trigeminus r.,** stimulation of the cornea or of the eyelid results in dilatation of the ipsilateral and the contralateral pupil; called also *oculopupillary r.* and *oculosensory cell r.* **ulnar r.,** tapping of the styloid process of the ulna results in pronation of the hand. **unconditioned r.,** see under *response*. **urinary r's,** bladder r. **vaccinoid r.,** a slight cutaneous reaction to vaccination in a person partially immune to smallpox. **vagus r.,** abnormal sensitiveness to pressure over the course of the vagus nerve. **vascular r.,** constriction of an artery produced by peripheral irritation. **vasopressor r's,** rise in pressure from reflex vasoconstriction. **vertebra prominens r.,** pressure upon the last cervical vertebra of an animal reduces the tone of all four limbs. **vesical r.,** desire to urinate produced by moderate distention of the bladder. **vesicointestinal r.,** inhibition of intestinal motility due to irritation of the bladder. **vestibular r's,** the reflexes for maintaining the position of the eyes and body in relation to changes in orientation of the head; the neural pathways are complex, traveling from the vestibular nerve to the vestibular nuclei and thence to the involved muscles of the eye and body. **vestibulo-ocular r.,** nystagmus or deviation of the eyes in response to stimulation of the vestibular system by angular acceleration or deceleration or by irrigation of the ears with warm or cool water or air (caloric test). **virile r.,** 1. bulbocavernous reflex. 2. a reflex in the flaccid penis elicited by pulling upward the foreskin or glans penis, when a sudden downward jerk results. Called also *Hughes's r.* **visceral r.,** that in which the stimulus is set up by some state of an internal organ. **viscerocardiac r.,** reflex alteration in cardiac rhythm or contractility caused by visceral excitation. **visceromotor r.,** contraction of abdominal muscles (abdominal rigidity) over a diseased viscus. **viscerosensory r.,** a region of sensitiveness to pressure on some part of the body due to disease of some internal organ. **viscerotrophic r.,** degeneration of any peripheral tissue as a result of chronic inflammation of any of the viscera. **von Mering r.,** relaxation of overlying abdominal muscles following ingestion of food. **water-silk r.,** see *shot-silk retina*, under *retina*. **Weiss's r.,** a curved reflection seen with the ophthalmoscope on the fundus of the eye to the nasal side of the disk; believed to be indicative of myopia. **Westphal's pupillary r., Westphal-Piltz r.,** contraction of the pupil associated with closure or attempted closure of the eye. **zygomatic r.,** lateral motion of the lower jaw to the percussed side on percussion over the zygoma.

reflexogenic (re-flek″so-jen′ik) [*reflex* + Gr. *gennan* to produce] producing or increasing reflex action.

reflexogenous (re″fleks-oj′ĕ-nus) reflexogenic.

reflexograph (re-flek′so-graf) [*reflex* + Gr. *graphein* to write] an instrument for graphically recording a reflex.

reflexology (re″flek-sol′o-je) the science or study of reflexes.

reflexometer (re″flek-som′ĕ-ter) [*reflex* + L. *metrum* measure] an instrument for measuring the force necessary to produce myotatic contraction.

reflexophil (re-flek′so-fil) [*reflex* + Gr. *philein* to love] characterized by activity of reflexes.

reflexotherapy (re-flek″so-ther′ah-pe) treatment by irritation of any area of the body distant from the lesion.

reflux (re′fluks) [*re-* + L. *fluxus* flow] a backward or return flow. **esophageal r., gastroesophageal r.,** reflux of the stomach contents into the esophagus. **hepatojugular r.,** distention of the jugular vein induced by pressure over the liver; it suggests insufficiency of the right heart; formerly called *hepatojugular reflex*. **intrarenal r.,** reflux of urine into the renal parenchymal tissue. **urethrovesiculo-differential r.,** the passage of a liquid, sperm, or injected substance from the posterior urethra into the genital system. **vesicoureteral r., vesicoureteric r.,** the passage of urine from the bladder back into a ureter; called also *vesicoureteral regurgitation*.

refract (re-frakt′) [L. *refringere* to break apart] 1. to cause to deviate. 2. to ascertain errors of ocular refraction.

refracta dosi (re-frak′tah do′si) [L.] in repeated and divided doses.

refractile (re-frak′til) capable of refracting.

refraction (re-frak′shun) 1. the act or process of refracting; specifically the determination of the refractive errors of the eye and their correction by glasses. 2. the deviation of light in passing obliquely from one medium to another of different density. The deviation occurs at the surface of junction of the two mediums, which is known as the refracting surface. The ray before refraction is called the *incident ray;* after refraction it is the *refracted ray.* The point of junction of the incident and the refracted ray is known as the *point of incidence.* The angle between the incident ray and a line perpendicular to the refracting surface at the point of incidence is known as the *angle of incidence;* that between the refracted ray and this perpendicular is called the *angle of refraction.* The sine of the angle of incidence divided by the sine of the angle of refraction gives the *relative index of refraction.* **double r.,** that in which the incident ray is divided into two refracted rays, so as to produce a double image. Double refraction is produced by Iceland spar. See *Nicol prism,* under *prism.* **dynamic r.,** the normal accommodation of the eye which is being continually exerted without conscious effort. **ocular r.,** the refraction of light produced by the mediums of the normal eye and resulting in the focusing of images upon the retina. **static r.,** the refraction of the eye when its accommodation is paralyzed.

refractionist (re-frak′shun-ist) one skilled in determining the refracting power of the eyes and correcting refractive defects.

refractive (re-frak′tiv) pertaining to or subserving a process of refraction; having the power to refract.

refractivity (re″frak-tiv′ĭ-te) the quality of being refractive; the power or ability to refract.

refractometer (re″frak-tom′ĕ-ter) [*refraction* + Gr. *metron* measure] 1. an instrument for measuring the refractive power of the eye. 2. an instrument for determining the indexes of refraction of various substances, particularly for determining the strength of lenses of spectacles.

refractometry (re″frak-tom′ĕ-tre) the measurement of refractive power with the refractometer.

refractor (re-frakt′or) a device for retinoscopic examination of the eye to determine its refractive power.

refractory (re-frak′to-re) [L. *refractorius*] not readily yielding to treatment.

refracture (re-frak′chur) the operation of breaking over again a bone which has been fractured and has united with a deformity; called also *anaclasis*.

refrangibility (re-fran″jĭ-bil′ĭ-te) susceptibility of being refracted; the quality of being refrangible.

refrangible (re-fran′jĭ-b'l) susceptible of being refracted.

refresh (re-fresh′) to freshen; to denude a wound of epithelium to enhance tissue repair.

refrigerant (re-frij′er-ant) [L. *refrigerans*] 1. relieving fever and thirst. 2. a cooling remedy. The refrigerants consist of cooling, acidulous drinks and evaporating lotions. Called also *algefacient*.

refrigeration (re-frij″er-a′shun) [L. *refrigeratio*] the therapeutic application of or exposure to low temperatures.

refringent (re-frin′jent) [L. *refringens*] refractive.

Refsum's disease (syndrome) (ref′soomz) [Sigvald *Refsum,* Norwegian physician] see under *disease*.

refusion (re-fu′shun) [L. *refusio*] the temporary removal and subsequent return of blood to the circulation.

R.E.G. radioencephalogram.

regainer (re-gān′er) a spacing appliance used to restore space in the dental arches.

regel (ra′gel) [Ger.] menstruation. **klei′ne r.** ["small menstruation"], a slight bloody discharge from the uterus at the time of ovulation.

regeneration (re-jen″er-a′shun) [*re-* + L. *generare* to produce, bring to life] the natural renewal of a structure, as of a lost tissue or part. **epimorphic r.,** epimorphosis. **morphallactic r.,** morphallaxis.

regimen (rej′ĭ-men) [L. "guidance"] a strictly regulated scheme of diet, exercise, or other activity designed to achieve certain ends.

regio (re′je-o), pl. *regio′nes* [L. "a space enclosed by lines"] a region: a plane area with more or less definite boundaries; [NA] a general term for certain areas on the surface of the body within certain defined boundaries. **r. abdomina′lis latera′lis,** r. lateralis abdominis [dextra et sinistra]. **regio′nes abdo′minis** [NA], the various anatomical regions of the abdomen, including [NA] the hypochondriac, epigastric, lateral, umbilical, inguinal, and pubic regions. See illustration under *abdomen.* **r. acromia′lis,** the region of the shoulder overlying the acromion. **r. ana′lis** [NA], anal region: the portion of the perineal region surrounding the anus. **r. antebra′chii ante′rior** [NA], anterior antebrachial region: the anterior, or palmar, region of the forearm; called also *regio antibrachii volaris.* **r. antebra′chii poste′rior** [NA], **r. antibra′chii dorsa′lis,** posterior antebrachial region: the posterior, or dorsal, region of the forearm. **r. antibra′chii radia′lis,** radial antebrachial region: the radial aspect of the forearm. **r. antibra′chii ul na′ris,** ulnar antebrachial region: the ulnar aspect of the forearm. **r. antibra′chii vola′ris,** r. antebrachii anterior. **r. auricula′ris,** auricular region: the region of the head on either side, about the ear. **r. axilla′ris** [NA], axillary region: the region of the chest about the axilla. **r. bra′chii ante′rior** [NA], anterior brachial region: the anterior region of the arm. **r. bra′chii latera′lis,** the lateral aspect of the arm. **r. bra′chii media′lis,** the medial aspect of the arm. **r. bra′chii poste′rior** [NA], posterior brachial region: the posterior region of the arm. **r. bucca′lis** [NA], buccal region: the region of the cheek. **r. calca′nea** [NA], calcaneal region: the region about the heel. **regio′nes cap′itis** [NA], the various anatomical regions of the head, including the frontal, parietal, occipital, temporal, and inframtemporal regions. **r. clavicula′ris,** clavicular region: the region of the front of the chest, overlying the clavicle. **regio′nes col′li** [NA], the various anatomical regions of the neck, including the anterior, sternocleidomastoid, lateral, and posterior regions. **r. col′li ante′rior** [NA], the anteromedial region of the neck. **r. col′li latera′lis** [NA], posterior region of neck: the region of the neck lateral to the regio sternocleidomastoidea; called also *trigonum colli laterale.* **r. col′li poste′rior** [NA], the posterior region of the neck, between the regio occipitalis above and the regions of the back below. **regio′nes cor′poris** [NA], **regio′nes cor′poris huma′ni,** regions of the body: the various anatomical areas, or subdivisions, demarcated on the surface of the human body for purpose of topographical description. **r. costa′lis latera′lis,** the lateral region of the thorax, or chest, overlying the ribs. **r. cox′ae,** the region of the hip. **r. cru′ris ante′rior** [NA], anterior crural region: the anterior region of the leg. **r. cru′ris latera′lis,** the lateral aspect of the leg. **r. cru′ris media′lis,** the medial aspect of the leg. **r. cru′ris poste′rior** [NA], posterior crural region: the posterior region of the leg. **r. cu′biti ante′rior** [NA], anterior cubital region: the anterior region about the elbow. **r. cu′biti latera′lis,** the lateral aspect of the elbow. **r. cu′biti media′lis,** the medial aspect of the elbow. **r. cu′biti poste′rior** [NA], posterior cubital region: the posterior or dorsal region about the elbow. **r. deltoi′dea** [NA], deltoid region: the region overlying the deltoid muscle. **regio′nes digita′les ma′nus,** the regions of the fingers. **regio′nes digita′les pe′dis,** the regions of the toes. **regio′nes dorsa′les digito′rum ma′nus,** the dorsal aspect of the several fingers. **regio′nes dorsa′les digito′rum pe′dis,** the dorsal aspect of the several toes. **r. dorsa′lis ma′nus,** dorsum manus. **r. dorsa′lis pe′dis,** dorsum pedis. **regio′nes dor′si** [NA], the various anatomical regions of the back, including the vertebral, sacral, scapular, infrascapular, and lumbar regions. **r. epigas′trica** [NA], epigastric region: the upper middle region of the abdomen, located within the sternal angle; called also *antecardium* and *epigastrium.* **regio′nes extremita′tis inferio′ris,** regiones membri inferioris. **regio′nes extremita′tis superio′ris,** regiones membri superioris. **regio′nes faci′ei** [NA], the various anatomical regions of the face. **r. fem′oris ante′rior** [NA], the anterior region of the thigh. **r. fem′oris latera′lis,** the lateral aspect of the thigh. **r. fem′oris media′lis,** the medial aspect of the thigh. **r. fem′oris poste′rior** [NA], the posterior region of the thigh. **r. fronta′lis** [NA], frontal region: the region of the head overlying the frontal bone; the forehead. **r. ge′nu ante′rior,** r. genus anterior. **r. ge′nu poste′rior,** r. genus posterior. **r. ge′nus ante′rior** [NA], the anterior region about the knee; called also *r. genu anterior.* **r. ge′nus poste′rior** [NA], the posterior region about the knee; called also *r. genu posterior.* **r. glu′tea** [NA], gluteal region: the region overlying the gluteal muscles. **r. hyoi′dea,** hyoid region: the part of the anterior region of the neck about the hyoid bone. **r. hypochondri′aca [dex′tra et sinis′tra]** [NA], hypochondriac region (right and left): the upper lateral region of the abdomen, about the costal cartilages, on either side of the epigastric region. **r. hypogas′trica,** r. pubica. **r. infraclavicula′ris** [NA], infraclavicular region: the region of the chest just below the clavicle. **r. inframamma′lis,** inframammary region: the region of the front of the chest situated below either mamma and above the lower border of the twelfth rib. **r. infraorbita′lis** [NA], infraorbital region: the region beneath the eye, adjacent to the regio nasalis. **r. infrascapula'ris** [NA], infrascapular region: the region of the back below the scapula and lateral to the lower thoracic vertebrae. **r. infratempora'lis** [NA], infratemporal region: the region of the head on either side, about the infratemporal fossa. **r. inguina'lis [dex'tra et sinis'tra]** [NA], inguinal region (right and left): the region of the abdomen on either side, lateral to the pubic region and about the inguinal canal. Called also *iliac region*. **r. interscapula'ris**, interscapular region: the region of the back between the scapulae. **r. labia'lis infe'rior**, inferior labial region: the region of the face about the lower lip. **r. labia'lis supe'rior**, superior labial region: the region of the face about the upper lip. **r. laryn'gea**, laryngeal region: the part of the anterior region of the neck overlying the larynx. **r. latera'lis abdo'minis [dex'tra et sinis'tra]**, [NA], lateral abdominal region (right and left): the region of the abdomen on either side of the umbilical region; called also *regio abdominalis lateralis*, *external abdominal region*, and *lumbar region*. **r. lumba'lis** [NA], lumbar region: the region of the back lying lateral to the lumbar vertebrae. **r. malleola'ris latera'lis**, the region overlying the lateral malleolus. **r. malleola'ris media'lis**, the region overlying the medial malleolus. **r. mamma'lis** [NA], mammary region: the region of the front of the chest, about the mammary gland. **r. mastoi'dea**, mastoid region: the region of the head on either side, about the mastoid process of the temporal bone. **r. media'na dor'si**, r. vertebralis. **regio'nes mem'bri inferio'ris** [NA], the various anatomical regions of the lower limb; called also *regiones extremitatis inferioris*. **regio'nes mem'bri superio'ris** [NA], the various anatomical regions of the upper limb; called also *regiones extremitatis superioris*. **r. menta'lis** [NA], mental region: the region of the chin. **r. nasa'lis** [NA], nasal region: the region of the face about the nose. **r. nu'chae**, nuchal region: the part of the posterior region of the neck adjoining the regio lateralis colli. **r. occipita'lis** [NA], occipital region: the region of the head overlying the occipital bone. **r. olec'rani**, olecranal region: the region of the elbow overlying the olecranon. **r. olfacto'ria** [NA], olfactory region: the upper part of the nasal cavity, the mucosa of which contains most of the receptors of the sense of smell. **r. ora'lis** [NA], oral region: the region of the face about the mouth. **r. orbita'lis** [NA], orbital region: the region of the face about the eye; called also *ocular region*. **r. palpebra'lis infe'rior**, inferior palpebral region: the region of the lower eyelid. **r. palpebra'lis supe'rior**, superior palpebral region: the region of the upper eyelid. **r. parieta'lis** [NA], parietal region: the region of the head on either side, about the parietal bone. **r. parotideomasseter'ica** [NA], parotideomasseteric region: the region of the face on either side, about the parotid gland and masseter muscle. **r. patella'ris**, the region of the knee overlying the patella. **regio'nes pecto'ris** [NA], pectoral regions: the various regions of the chest, including the infraclavicular, mammary, and axillary regions. **r. pecto'ris ante'rior**, the anterior aspect of the thorax, or chest. **r. pecto'ris latera'lis**, the lateral aspect of the thorax, or chest. **r. perinea'lis** [NA], perineal region: the region overlying the pelvic outlet, including the anal and urogenital regions. **regio'nes planta'res digito'rum pe'dis**, the plantar aspect of the several toes. **r. planta'ris pe'dis**, planta pedis. **r. pu'bica** [NA], pubic region: the middle portion of the most inferior region of the abdomen, located below the umbilical region and between the inguinal regions. Called also *r. hypogastrica*, *hypogastric region*, and *hypogastrium*. **r. puden-da'lis**, the region of the external genital organs (scrotum or vulva). **r. respirato'ria** [NA], respiratory region: the part of the nasal cavity below the olfactory region. **r. retromalleola'ris latera'lis**, the region back of the lateral malleolus. **r. retromalleola'ris media'lis**, the region back of the medial malleolus. **r. sacra'lis** [NA], sacral region: the region of the back overlying the sacrum. **r. scapula'ris** [NA], scapular region: the region of the back overlying the scapula. **r. sterna'lis**, the region of the front of the chest overlying the sternum. **r. sternocleidomastoi'dea** [NA], sternocleidomastoid region: the region of the neck overlying the sternocleidomastoid muscle. **r. subhyoi'dea**, subhyoid region: the part of the anterior region of the neck below the hyoid bone. **r. submaxilla'ris**, trigonum submandibulare. **r. submenta'lis**, submental region: the part of the anterior region of the neck beneath the chin. **r. supraorbita'lis**, supraorbital region: the region of the head immediately above the orbit. **r. suprascapula'ris**, suprascapular region: the region of the back above the scapula. **r. suprasterna'lis**, suprasternal region: the part of the anterior region of the neck above the sternum. **r. sura'lis**, the posterior aspect of the leg, overlying the calf. **r. tempora'lis** [NA], temporal region: the region of the head on either side, about the temporal bone. **r. thyreoi'dea**, thyroid region: the part of the anterior region of the neck about the thyroid gland. **r. trochanter'ica**, the portion of the lateral region of the thigh overlying the greater trochanter. **r. umbilica'lis** [NA], umbilical region: the region of the abdomen about the umbilicus. **regio'nes unguicula'res digito'rum ma'nus**, the region of the several fingers about the nails. **regio'nes unguicula'res digito'rum pe'dis**, the region of the several toes

about the nails. **r. urogenita'lis** [NA], urogenital region: the portion of the perineal region surrounding the urogenital organs. **r. vertebra'lis** [NA], vertebral region: the middle region of the back, overlying the vertebral column; called also *r. mediana dorsi*. **regio'nes vola'res digito'rum ma'nus**, volar region of fingers: the palmar aspect of the several fingers. **r. vola'ris ma'nus**, palma manus. **r. zygomati'ca** [NA], zygomatic region: the region of the face on either side, about the zygomatic bone.

region (re'jun) a plane area with more or less definite boundaries; see also *regio*. **abdominal r's**, the various anatomical regions of the abdomen; see *regiones abdominis* [NA], and illustration under *abdomen*. **abdominal r., external**, **abdominal r., lateral**, see *regio lateralis abdominis* [dextra et sinistra]. **r. of accommodation**, the space including all points to which the eye can be adjusted by accommodation. **anal r.**, regio analis. **antebrachial r., anterior**, regio antebrachii anterior. **antebrachial r., posterior**, regio antebrachii posterior. **antebrachial r., radial**, regio antibrachii radialis. **antebrachial r., ulnar**, regio antibrachii ulnaris. **antebrachial r., volar**, regio antebrachii anterior. **anterior r. of neck**, regio colli anterior. **auricular r.**, regio auricularis. **axillary r.**, regio axillaris. **basilar r.**, the base of the skull. **brachial r., anterior**, regio brachii anterior. **Broca's r.**, see under *convolution*. **buccal r.**, regio buccalis. **calcaneal r.**, regio calcanea. **ciliary r.**, the part of the eye occupied by the ciliary body and its adjuncts. **clavicular r.**, regio clavicularis. **crural r., anterior**, regio cruris anterior. **crural r., posterior**, regio cruris posterior. **cubital r., anterior**, regio cubiti anterior. **cubital r., posterior**, regio cubiti posterior. **deltoid r.**, regio deltoidea. **dorsal r's of fingers**, regiones dorsales digitorum manus. **dorsal r's of toes**, regiones dorsales digitorum pedis. **dorsal lip r.**, the mesodermal tissue around the dorsal lip of the blastopore; it is the organizer which by induction initiates and controls the early development of the embryo. **encephalic r.**, lamina alaris. **epigastric r.**, regio epigastrica. **extrapolar r.**, that region of the body which lies outside the influence of the poles in electrotherapy. **facial r's**, the areas into which the face is divided, including the *buccal* (side of oral cavity), *infraorbital* (below the eye), *mental* (chin), *nasal* (nose), *oral* (lips), *orbital* (eye), *parotideomasseter* (angle of the jaw), and *zygomatic* (cheek bone); called also *regiones faciei* [NA]. **frontal r.**, regio frontalis. **genitourinary r.**, regio urogenitalis. **gluteal r.**, regio glutea. **homology r's**, looped structures, comprising approximately 100 amino acid residues and fastened by disulfide bonds, that show similarities in primary structure from one region to another. They represent the building blocks or units of immunoglobulin molecules. **hyoid r.**, regio hyoidea. **hypochondriac r.**, see *regio hypochondriaca* [dextra et sinistra]. **hypogastric r.**, regio pubica. **I r.**, that part of the major histocompatibility complex where immune response genes are present. **iliac r.**, regio inguinalis. **infraclavicular r.**, regio infraclavicularis. **inframammary r.**, regio inframammalis. **infraorbital r.**, regio infraorbitalis. **infrascapular r.**, regio infrascapularis. **infratemporal r.**, regio infratemporalis. **inguinal r.**, see *regio inguinalis* [dextra et sinistra]. **interscapular r.**, regio interscapularis. **labial r., inferior**, regio labialis inferior. **labial r., superior**, regio labialis superior. **laryngeal r.**, regio laryngea. **lumbar r.**, 1. regio lumbalis. 2. regio lateralis abdominis. **mammary r.**, regio mammalis. **mastoid r.**, regio mastoidea. **mental r.**, regio mentalis. **motor r.**, the ascending frontal and parietal convolutions of the cerebrum; called also *rolandic r.* **mylohyoid r.**, the region on the lingual surface of the mandible to which the mylohyoid muscle is attached. **r. of nape**, regio nuchae. **nasal r.**, regio nasalis. **nuchal r.**, regio nuchae. **occipital r.**, regio occipitalis. **ocular r.**, regio orbitalis. **olecranal r.**, regio olecrani. **olfactory r.**, regio olfactoria. **opticostriate r.**, the basal ganglia and the capsule. **oral r.**, regio oralis. **orbital r.**, regio orbitalis. **palpebral r., inferior**, regio palpebralis inferior. **palpebral r., superior**, regio palpebralis superior. **parietal r.**, regio parietalis. **parietotemporal r.**, sensory r. **parotideomasseteric r.**, regio parotideomasseterica. **pectoral r's**, the areas into which the anterior surface of the chest is divided; see *regiones pectoris* [NA]. **perineal r.**, regio perinealis. **plantar r's of toes**, regiones plantares digitorum pedis. **posterior r. of neck**, regio colli posterior. **precordial r.**, a part of the anterior surface of the body covering the heart and the pit of the stomach. **prefrontal r.**, the part of the frontal lobe of the cerebrum in front of the precentral fissures. **presumptive r.**, an area of the blastula which has been proved under normal conditions to develop into a specific organ or type of tissue. **pterygomaxillary r.**, the region of the face about the zygoma and the prominences of the lower jaw. **pubic r.**, regio pubica. **respiratory r.**, regio respiratoria. **rolandic r.**, motor r. **sacral r.**, regio sacralis. **scapular r.**, regio scapularis. **sensory r.**, a part of the cerebral cortex located in part behind the central sulcus; called also *parietotemporal r.* **sternocleidomastoid r.**, regio sternocleidomastoidea. **subauricular r.**, fossa retromandibularis. **subhyoid r.**, regio subhyoidea. **submaxillary r.**, trigonum submandibulare.

submental r., regio submentalis. **supraclavicular r.,** the region above the clavicle. **supraorbital r.,** regio supraorbitalis. **suprasternal r.,** regio suprasternalis. **temporal r.,** regio temporalis. **thyroid r.,** regio thyreoidea. **trabecular r.,** the region of the embryonic skull from which the sphenoid bone is developed. **umbilical r.,** regio umbilicalis. **urogenital r.,** regio urogenitalis. **vertebral r.,** regio vertebralis. **vestibular r.,** the lowest and the movable portion of the nose; it is lined with stratified squamous cell epithelium and possesses hairs and sebaceous glands. **volar r's of fingers,** regiones volares digitorum manus. **volar r. of hand,** palma manus. **zygomatic r.,** regio zygomatica.

regional (re'jun-al) pertaining to, limited to, or affecting a certain region or regions.

regiones (re"je-o'nēz) [L.] plural of *regio*.

registrant (rej'is-trant) a nurse who is listed on the books of a registry as available for duty.

registrar (rej'is-trar) 1. an official keeper of records. 2. in British hospitals, a resident specialist who acts as assistant to the chief or attending specialist.

registration (rej"is-tra'shun) the act of recording. In dentistry, the making of a record of the jaw relations present, or of those desired, in order to transfer them to an articulator to facilitate proper construction of a dental prosthesis. **maxillomandibular r.,** see under *record*.

registry (rej'is-tre) 1. an office where a nurse may have his or her name listed as being available for duty. 2. a central agency for the collection of pathologic material and related clinical, laboratory, x-ray, and other data in a specified field of pathology, so organized that the data can be properly processed and made available for study.

Regitine (rej'ĭ-tēn) trademark for a preparation of phentolamine.

regression (re-gresh'un) [L. *regressio* a return] 1. a return to a former or earlier state. 2. a subsidence of symptoms or of a disease process. 3. in biology, the tendency in successive generations toward the mean; see *Galton's law of regression,* under *law.* 4. the turning backward of the libido to an early fixation at infantile levels because of inability to function in terms of reality. **atavistic r.,** a process by which the mind ceases to function at a logical critical level and reverts to a biologically more primitive mode of functioning.

regressive (re-gres'iv) going back; subsiding; characterized by regression.

regular (reg'u-lar) [L. *regularis; regula* rule] normal or conforming to rule; occurring at proper or fixed intervals.

regulation (reg"u-la'shun) [L. *regula* rule] 1. the act of adjusting or state of being adjusted to a certain standard. 2. in biology, the adaptation of form or behavior of an organism to changed conditions. 3. the power of a pregastrula stage to form a whole embryo from a part. **menstrual r.,** removal of the uterine contents, without dilatation, by application of a vacuum through a cannula introduced into the uterus.

Reg. umb. abbreviation for L. *re'gio umbili'ci,* umbilical region.

regurgitant (re-gur'jĭ-tant) [*re-* + L. *gurgitare* to flood] flowing back or in the opposite direction from normal.

regurgitation (re-gur"jĭ-ta'shun) [*re-* + L. *gurgitare* to flood] a backward flowing, as the casting up of undigested food, or the backward flowing of blood into the heart, or between the chambers of the heart when a valve is incompetent. **aortic r.,** the backflow of blood from the aorta into the left ventricle, owing to imperfect functioning (insufficiency or incompetence) of the aortic semilunar valve. **mitral r.,** the backflow of blood from the left ventricle into the left atrium, owing to inadequate functioning (insufficiency) of the mitral valve. **pulmonic r.,** the backflow of blood from the pulmonary artery into the right ventricle, owing to inadequate functioning (insufficiency) of the pulmonic semilunar valve. **tricuspid r.,** the backflow of blood from the right ventricle into the right atrium, owing to imperfect functioning (insufficiency) of the tricuspid valve. **valvular r.,** regurgitation of the blood through the orifices of the heart valves owing to imperfect closing (insufficiency or incompetence) of the valves; named, according to the valve affected, *aortic, mitral, pulmonic,* or *tricuspid r.* **vesicoureteral r.,** see under *reflux.*

rehabilitation (re"hah-bil'ĭ-ta'shun) 1. the restoration of normal form and function after injury or illness. 2. the restoration of an ill or injured patient to self-sufficiency or to gainful employment at his highest attainable skill in the shortest possible time.

rehabilitee (re"hah-bil'ĭ-te") the subject of rehabilitation.

rehalation (re"hah-la'shun) [*re-* + L. *halare* to breathe] rebreathing.

Rehfuss' test (method), tube (ra'fus) [Martin Emil *Rehfuss,* American physician, 1887–1964] see under *tests* and *tube.*

rehydration (re"hi-dra'shun) the restoration of water or of fluid content to a body or to substance which has become dehydrated.

Reichel's cloacal duct (ri'kelz) [Friedrich Paul *Reichel,* German obstetrician, born 1858] see under *duct.*

Reichert's canal, etc. [Karl Bogislaus *Reichert,* German anatomist, 1811–1883] see under *canal, cartilage, membrane, recess, scar,* and *substance.*

Reichmann's disease (syndrome) (rīk'manz) [Nikolas *Reichmann,* Warsaw physician, 1851–1918] gastrosuccorrhea.

Reichstein (rīk'stīn), Tadeus. Polish chemist in Switzerland, born 1897; co-winner, with E. C. Kendall and P. S. Hench, of the Nobel prize for medicine and physiology in 1950.

Reid's base line (rēdz) [Robert William *Reid,* Scottish anatomist, 1851–1939] see *base line,* under *line.*

Reid Hunt's reaction, test [*Reid Hunt,* American pharmacologist, 1870–1948] see *Hunt's reaction,* under *reaction.*

Reil's ansa, etc. (rīlz) [Johann Christian *Reil,* German anatomist, 1759–1813] see under *ansa, insula, ribbon, sulcus,* and *trigone.*

reimplantation (re"im-plan-ta'shun) replacement of tissue or a structure, such as a tooth, in the site from which it was previously lost or removed.

reinfection (re"in-fek'shun) a second infection by the same pathogenic agent, or a second infection of an organ such as the kidney by a different pathogenic agent.

reinforcement (re"in-fors'ment) the increasing of force or strength. In behavioral science, the presentation of a stimulus so as to modify a response; the stimulus may take the form of a reward or a punishment. **r. of reflex,** the increasing of a reflex response by causing the patient to perform some mental or physical concentration while the reflex is being elicited.

reinforcer (re"in-fors'er) anything that produces reinforcement; a reinforcing stimulus.

reinfusate (re'in-fu"sāt) fluid for reinfusion into the body, usually after being subjected to a treatment process.

reinfusion (re"in-fu'zhun) infusion of body fluid that has previously been withdrawn from the same individual, e.g., reinfusion of ascitic fluid after ultrafiltration.

reinnervation (re"in-er-va'shun) the operation of grafting a live nerve to restore the function of a paralyzed muscle.

reinoculation (re"in-ok"u-la'shun) an inoculation that follows a previous one with the same virus.

reintegration (re"in-te-gra'shun) 1. biological integration after a state of disruption. 2. the resumption of normal mental and physical activity after disappearance of the catatonic state or other psychic disturbance.

reintubation (re"in-tu-ba'shun) intubation performed a second time.

reinversion (re"in-ver'zhun) restoration to its normal place of an inverted organ, especially restoration of an inverted uterus.

reinvocation (re"in-vo-ka'shun) reactivation.

Reisseisen's muscles (rīs'ī-senz) [Franz Daniel *Reisseisen,* German anatomist, 1773–1828] see under *muscle.*

Reissner's fiber, membrane (rīs'nerz) [Ernst *Reissner,* German anatomist, 1824–1878] see under *fiber,* and see *paries vestibularis ductus cochlearis.*

Reiter's syndrome (ri'terz) [Hans *Reiter,* German hygienist, born 1881] see under *syndrome.*

reiterature (re-it"er-a-tu're) [L.] repeat or renew, as a prescription.

rejection (re-jek'shun) an immune reaction against grafted tissue. In *hyperacute rejection,* there is an immediate response against the graft because of the presence of preformed antibody, resulting in fibrin deposition, platelet aggregation, neutrophilic infiltration, and eventual graft failure. In *acute rejection,* the response occurs after the sixth day and then proceeds rapidly. It is characterized by loss of function of the transplanted organ and by pain and swelling, with leukocytosis and thrombocytopenia. In *chronic rejection,* there is gradual progressive loss of function of the transplanted organ with less severe symptoms than in the acute form. **second-set r.,** see under *phenomenon.*

rejuvenescence (re-ju"vě-nes'ens) [*re-* + L. *juvenescere* to become young] a renewal of youth or of strength and vigor.

relapse (re-laps') [L. *relapsus*] the return of a disease after its apparent cessation. Cf. *recrudescence.* **intercurrent r.,** a relapse occurring before the temperature has reached a normal level. **mucocutaneous r.,** the reappearance of infectious lesions of the mucous membranes and skin after the disappearance of the initial secondary lesions of syphilis. **rebound r.,** return of some of the symptoms of a disease on cessation of treatment, applied especially to the relapse of patients with rheumatoid arthritis on withdrawal of cortisone or ACTH (Hench).

relation (re-la'shun) [L. *relatio* a carrying back] the condition or state of one object or entity when considered in connection with another. **acentric r.,** eccentric jaw r. **buccolingual r.,** the position of a tooth or space in the dental arch in relation to the tongue and the cheek. **centric jaw r.,** the most retruded position of the mandible in respect to the maxilla when the condyles are in the most posterior unstrained position in the glenoid fossae from which lateral movement can be made at any given degree of jaw separation. **dynamic r's,** those existing between two objects or entities when one or both of them are moving or constantly changing. **eccentric jaw r.,** any relation of the mandible to the maxillae other than the centric relation; called also *acentric r.* and *eccentric position.* **eccentric jaw r., acquired,** an eccentric relation of the mandible to the maxilla that is assumed in order to bring the teeth into centric occlusion. **jaw r.,** any relation of the mandible to the maxilla, variously designated as centric, eccentric, median, occlusal, protrusive, and the like. **lateral r.,** the relation of the mandible to the maxilla when the lower jaw is in a position to either side of centric relation. **maxillomandibular r.,** jaw r. **median jaw r.,** any relation of the jaws when the mandible is not moved to either side. **median retruded jaw r.,** centric jaw r. **object r's,** the emotional bonds existing between an individual and another person, as contrasted with his interest in, and love for, himself; usually described in terms of his capacity for loving and reacting appropriately to others. **occlusal jaw r.,** the relation of the mandibular teeth to the maxillary teeth when the jaws are in contact; designated, depending on the relative position of the mandibular teeth, as lateral, protrusive, or retrusive. **posterior border jaw r.,** the most posterior relation of the mandible to the maxilla at any specific vertical relation. **protrusive jaw r.,** that resulting from protrusion of the mandible. **rest jaw r.,** that maintained when the patient is resting comfortably in the upright position, the rest position. **ridge r.,** the relation in space of the mandibular ridge to the maxillary ridge. **static r's,** those existing between two objects or entities when neither one of them is moving or changing in any way. **unstrained jaw r.,** that maintained when a state of balanced tonus exists among all the muscles involved, being achieved without undue or unnatural force and causing no distortion of the tissues of the temporomandibular joints.

relaxant (re-lak′sant) [L. *relaxare* to loosen] 1. lessening or reducing tension. 2. an agent that lessens tension. **muscle r.,** an agent that specifically aids in reducing muscle tension, as those acting at the polysynaptic neurons of motor nerves (e.g., meprobamate) or at the myoneural junction (curare and related compounds).

relaxation (re″lak-sa′shun) 1. a lessening of tension. 2. a mitigation of pain. **isometric r.,** relaxation of a muscle without shortening.

relaxin (re-lak′sin) a water-soluble protein-like principle secreted by the corpus luteum during pregnancy; it produces relaxation of the pubic symphysis and dilation of the uterine cervix in certain animal species. A pharmaceutical preparation, extracted from the ovaries of pregnant sows, has been used in treatment of dysmenorrhea and premature labor, and to facilitate labor at term.

relief (re-lēf′) [L. *relevatio*] the mitigation or removal of pain or distress.

relieve (re-lēv′) [L. *relevare* to lighten] to mitigate or remove pain or distress.

reline (re-līn′) to resurface the tissue side of a denture with new base material in order to achieve a more accurate fit.

reluxation (re″luk-sa′shun) redislocation.

REM rapid eye movements (see under *sleep*).

rem (rem) [roentgen-equivalent–*man*] the quantity of any ionizing radiation which has the same biological effectiveness as 1 rad of x-rays; 1 rem = 1 rad × RBE (relative biological effectiveness).

Remak's band, fibers, ganglion, plexus, etc. (ra′maks) [Robert *Remak,* German neurologist, 1815–1865] see *axon;* see *gray fibers,* under *fiber;* see under *ganglion;* and see *plexus submucosus.*

Remak's paralysis (type), reflex, symptom (sign) (ra′maks) [Ernst Julius *Remak,* German neurologist, 1848–1911] see under *paralysis, reflex,* and *symptom.*

remedial (re-me′de-al) [L. *remedialis*] curative, acting as a remedy.

remedy (rem′ĕ-de) [L. *remedium*] anything that cures, palliates, or prevents disease. **concordant r's,** a homeopathic term for remedies of similar action, but of dissimilar origin. **Ehrlich-Hata r.,** arsphenamine. **inimic r's,** a homeopathic term for remedies whose actions are antagonistic. **tissue r's,** the twelve remedies which, according to the biochemical school of homeopathy, form the mineral bases of the body.

Remijia (re-mij′e-ah) a genus of rubiaceous shrubs. *R. pedunculata* Flueck. furnishes cuprea bark, a source of hydroxycinchonidine.

remineralization (re-min″er-al-i-za′shun) the restoration of mineral elements, as to the human body.

remission (re-mish′un) [L. *remissio*] a diminution or abatement of the symptoms of a disease; also the period during which such diminution occurs.

remittence (re-mit′ens) temporary abatement, without actual cessation, of symptoms.

remittent (re-mit′ent) [L. *remittere* to send back] having periods of abatement and of exacerbation.

remnant (rem′nant) something remaining; a residue; a vestige. **acroblastic r.,** the peripheral part of the acroblast which recedes into the protoplasm of the spermatid and later disintegrates.

remotivation (re-mo″tĭ-va′shun) in psychiatry, a group therapy technique administered by the nursing staff in a mental hospital, which is used to stimulate the communication skills and an interest in the environment of long-term, withdrawn patients.

ren (ren), pl. *re′nes,* gen. *re′nis* [L.] [NA] either of the two organs (i.e., the kidneys) in the lumbar region that excrete the urine; see *kidney.* **r. mo′bilis,** hypermobile kidney. **r. ungulifor′-mis,** horseshoe kidney.

renacidin (re-nas′ĭ-din) hemiacidrin.

renal (re′nal) [L. *renalis*] pertaining to the kidney; nephric.

Renaut's bodies (ren-ōz′) [Joseph Louis *Renaut,* French physician, 1844–1917] see under *body.*

renculi (ren′ku-li) [L.] plural of *renculus.*

renculus (ren′ku-lus), pl. *ren′culi* [L.] reniculus.

Rendu's tremor (ron-duz′) [Henri Jules Louis Marie *Rendu,* French physician, 1844–1902] see under *tremor.*

Rendu-Osler-Weber disease, syndrome (ron-duh′-ōs′ler-web′er) [H. J. L. M. *Rendu;* Sir William *Osler,* Canadian-born physician, 1849–1919; Frederick Parkes *Weber,* British physician, 1863–1962] hereditary hemorrhagic telangiectasia.

renes (re′nēz) 1. [L.] plural of *ren.* 2. (*obs.*) a therapeutic extract of the kidneys of pigs or sheep.

Renese (ren′ēz) trademark for preparations of polythiazide.

renicapsule (ren′ĭ-kap″sūl) [*ren* + L. *capsula* capsule] an adrenal gland.

reniculi (rĕ-nik′u-li) [L.] plural of *reniculus.*

reniculus (rĕ-nik′u-lus), pl. *renic′uli* [L.] one of the lobules composing the kidney, and consisting of a pyramid and its enclosing cortical substance.

reniform (ren′ĭ-form) [*ren* + L. *forma* form] shaped like a kidney.

renin (re′nin) a proteolytic enzyme synthesized, stored, and secreted by the juxtaglomerular cells of the kidney; it plays a role in regulation of blood pressure by catalyzing the conversion of angiotensinogen to angiotensin I. Its secretion is induced by lowered renal arterial pressure. **big r.,** a relatively inactive protein with a higher molecular weight than normal renin, which is activated after exposure to low pH or to proteolytic enzymes.

reninism (re′nin-izm) a condition marked by overproduction of renin. **primary r.,** a syndrome of hypertension, hypokalemia, hyperaldosteronism, and elevated plasma renin activity, due to proliferation of juxtaglomerular cells.

renipelvic (ren″ĭ-pel′vik) pertaining to the pelvis of the kidney.

reniportal (ren″ĭ-pōr′tal) [*ren* + L. *porta* gate] pertaining to the portal system of the kidneys.

renipuncture (ren″ĭ-punk′tūr) [*ren* + L. *punctura* puncture] surgical incision or puncture of the capsule of the kidney: done for relief of albuminuric pain.

rennet (ren′et) an extract of calf's stomach which contains rennin and is used for curdling the milk in cheese making.

rennin (ren′in) the milk-curdling enzyme, an endopeptidase that converts casein to paracasein, found in the gastric juice of human infants (before pepsin formation) and abundantly in that of the calf and other ruminants. A preparation from the stomach of the calf is used to coagulate milk protein to facilitate its digestion. Called also *chymosin.*

renninogen (rĕ-nin′o-jen) prerennin.

renocortical (re″no-kor′tĭ-kal) pertaining to the cortex of a kidney.

renocutaneous (re″no-ku-ta′ne-us) pertaining to the kidneys and skin.

renocystogram (re″no-sis′to-gram) renogram.

renogastric (re″no-gas′trik) pertaining to the kidney and stomach; nephrogastric.

Renografin (re″no-graf′in) trademark for a solution of diatrizoate meglumine and diatrizoate sodium for injection.

renogram (re′no-gram) a graphic record of kidney function produced by externally monitoring the level of radioactivity in the bladder as a radiopharmaceutical agent enters it from the kidney via the ureters; called also *renocystogram.*

renography (re-nog′rah-fe) [*ren* + Gr. *graphein* to write] radiography of the kidney.

renointestinal (re″no-in-tes′tĭ-nal) pertaining to the kidney and intestine.

renopathy (ne-nop′ah-the) [*ren* + Gr. *pathos* disease] nephropathy.

renoprival (re″no-pri′val) pertaining to, characterized by, or resulting from deprivation of kidney function.

Renoquid (re′no-kwid) trademark for a preparation of sulfacytine.

renotrophic (re″no-trof′ik) having the ability to increase kidney size.

renotropic (re″no-trop′ik) having a special affinity for kidney tissue.

renule (ren′ūl) an area of the kidney supplied by a branch of the renal artery, usually consisting of three or four medullary pyramids and their corresponding cortical substance.

renunculus (re-nung′ku-lus) reniculus.

reovirus (re″o-vi′rus) [*respiratory* and *enteric origin* + *virus*] a group of ether-resistant RNA viruses, formerly classified as a subgroup of the echoviruses. Reoviruses are separable into three serotypes, and have been isolated from healthy children, children with febrile and afebrile upper respiratory disease, children with diarrhea, and many animals.

reoxidation (re-ok″si-da′shun) the act of taking up oxygen again, as the hemoglobin of the blood.

reoxygenation (re-ok″si-jen-a′shun) in radiobiology, the phenomenon in which hypoxic (and thus radioresistant) tumor cells become more exposed to oxygen (and thus more radiosensitive) by coming into closer proximity to capillaries after death and loss of other tumor cells due to previous irradiation.

Rep. abbreviation for L. *repeta′tur*, let it be repeated.

rep (rep) [*r*oentgen *e*quivalent *p*hysical] an unofficial unit of amount of radiation of any kind which yields an amount of energy transferred to the tissue equal to that transferred by 1 roentgen of hard x- or γ-radiation (200 kv. or greater). This amount of energy turns out to be about 93 ergs per gram of water or soft tissue.

repair (re-pār′) the physical or mechanical restoration of damaged or diseased tissues by the growth of healthy new cells or by surgical apposition.

repatency (re-pa′ten-se) [*re-* + L. *patens* open] reestablishment of the opening in a part or vessel which has been closed.

repellent (re-pel′ent) [L. *repellere* to drive back] 1. able to repel or drive off; also an agent so acting, as *insect repellent*. 2. (*obs.*) capable of dispersing a swelling; also an agent or remedy which causes a swelling to disappear.

repeller (re-pel′er) an instrument used in labor of animals to push back the fetus until the head and limbs can be properly placed for normal delivery.

repercolation (re″per-ko-la′shun) [L. *re-* again + *percolare* to filter] a second or repeated percolation with the same materials.

repercussion (re″per-kush′un) [L. *repercussio* rebound] 1. the driving in of an eruption or the scattering of a swelling. 2. ballottement.

repercussive (re″per-kus′iv) 1. causing or pertaining to repercussion. 2. an agent causing repercussion; a repellent.

repetatur (re″pe-ta′tūr) [L.] let it be renewed.

replant (re-plant′) to restore a structure to its original site, as to reinsert a tooth into the alveolar socket from which it has been displaced.

replantation (re″plan-ta′shun) the restoration of an organ or other structure to its original site. In dentistry, the reinsertion of a tooth into the alveolus from which it was removed or otherwise lost.

replenisher (re-plen′ish-er) an agent that restores what has been lost, used up, or is lacking.

repletion (re-ple′shun) [L. *repletio*] the condition of being full.

replication (rep″li-ka′shun) 1. a turning back of a part so as to form a duplication. 2. repetition of an experiment to ensure accuracy. 3. the process of duplicating or reproducing, as the replication of an exact copy of a polynucleotide strand of DNA or RNA. **conservative r.,** replication of DNA in which the original molecule remains intact and a completely new molecule is formed. **dispersive r.,** nonconservative r. **nonconservative r.,** replication of DNA in which parental nucleotide bases are distributed in both strands of each daughter molecule; called *dispersive r.* **semiconservative r.,** replication of DNA in which the strands separate longitudinally and each strand serves as a template for its new mate, so that each daughter molecule has one new and one parental strand.

replicon (rep′li-kon) an autonomously replicating aggregate of DNA in a bacterium (e.g., chromosome, plasmid).

Repoise (re-pōz′) trademark for preparations of butaperazine.

repolarization (re-po″lar-ĭ-za′shun) the reestablishment of polarity, especially the return of cell membrane potential to resting potential after depolarization.

reposition (re″po-zish′un) [L. *repositio*] replacement in the normal position.

repositioning (re″po-zish′un-ing) the replacing of a structure or part to its normal site. **jaw r.,** the changing of any relative position of the mandible to the maxilla, usually by altering the occlusion of the natural or artificial teeth. **muscle r.,** surgical replacement of a muscle attachment into a more acceptable functional position.

repositor (re-poz′ĭ-tor) an instrument used in returning displaced organs to the normal position. **Aveling's r.,** an apparatus for exerting continuous pressure on the fundus of the inverted uterus in order to secure replacement.

repository (re-poz′ĭ-to-re) a place where something is stored; used in pharmacology to refer to the injection, usually intramuscularly, of a long-acting drug, which is slowly absorbed and is therefore prolonged in its action.

repression (re-presh′un) the act of restraining, inhibiting, or suppressing. In psychiatry, the thrusting back from consciousness into the unconscious sphere of ideas or perceptions of a disagreeable nature. In genetic theory, inhibition of gene transcription by a repressor; called also *gene r.* Cf. *derepression*, def. 2. **coordinate r.,** parallel diminution of the concentrations of the several enzymes of a metabolic pathway, resulting from increases in the level of repressor. **endproduct r.,** enzyme r. **enzyme r.,** interference, usually by the endproduct of a pathway, with synthesis of the enzymes of that pathway. **gene r.,** see *repression*. **reactive r.,** a psychosis resulting from repression.

repressor (re-pres′or) [L. "a restrainer"] that which restrains or inhibits. In genetic theory, a substance produced by a regulator gene which acts through the cytoplasm to prevent initiation by the operator gene of protein synthesis by the operon.

reproduction (re″pro-duk′shun) [L. *re-* again + *productio* production] 1. the production of offspring by organized bodies. 2. the creation of a similar object or situation; duplication; replication. **asexual r.,** reproduction without the fusion of sexual cells, as by fission or budding. **bisexual r.,** see *sexual r.* **cytogenic r.,** reproduction in which the new individual proceeds from a single germ cell or zygote. **sexual r.,** reproduction by the fusion of a female sexual cell with a male sexual cell (*bisexual r., amphigony, gamogenesis, syngamy*) or by the development of an unfertilized egg (*unisexual r., parthenogenesis*). **somatic r.,** reproduction in which the new individual proceeds from a multicellular fragment produced by fission or budding. **unisexual r.,** see *sexual r.*

reproductive (re″pro-duk′tiv) subserving or pertaining to the production of offspring.

repromicin (rep″ro-mi′cin) chemical name: 12,13-deepoxy-12,13-didehydro-4′-deoxycirramycin A$_1$; an antibiotic, $C_{31}H_{51}NO_8$.

reproterol hydrochloride (re″pro-ter′ōl) chemical name: 7-[3-[[2-(3,5-dihydroxyphenyl)-2-hydroxy ethyl]amino]propyl]-3,7-dihydro-1,3-dimethyl-1*H*-purine-2,6-dione monohydrochloride; a bronchodilator, $C_{18}H_{23}N_5O_5 \cdot HCl$.

reptilase (rep′til-ās) an enzyme from Russell's viper venom used in determining blood clotting time.

reptile (rep′til) any member of the class Reptilia.

Reptilia (rep-til′e-ah) a class of aquatic or terrestrial, cold-blooded vertebrates, including snakes, lizards, turtles, alligators, and crocodiles, as well as the extinct dinosaurs, which have bodies covered with horny scales or plates and breathe by means of lungs; most lay eggs outside of the body.

repullulation (re-pul″u-la′shun) [L. *re-* back + *pullulare* to sprout out] renewed growth by sprouting.

repulsion (re-pul′shun) [L. *re-* back + *pellere* to drive] the act of driving apart or away; a force which tends to drive two bodies apart. It is the opposite of attraction. In genetics, occurrence on opposite chromosomes in a double heterozygote of the two mutant alleles of interest. Cf. *coupling.*

RES reticuloendothelial system.

rescinnamine (re-sin′ah-min) [NF] an alkaloid, the 3,4,5-trimethoxycinnamic acid ester of methyl reserpate, obtained from *Rauwolfia serpentina* and other species of *Rauwolfia.* It occurs as a white or pale buff to cream colored crystalline powder, $C_{35}H_{42}N_2O_9$; used as an antihypertensive and also as a tranquilizer.

resect (re-sekt′) to remove part of an organ or tissue.

resectable (re-sek′tah-b'l) capable of being resected; lending itself to resection.

resection (re-sek′shun) [L. *resectio*] excision of a portion of an organ or other structure. **gastric r.,** partial gastrectomy; see *gastrectomy.* **root r.,** apicoectomy. **Schede's r.,** see under *operation* (def. 1). **submucous r.,** excision of a portion of a deviated nasal septum after first laying back a flap of mucous membrane, which is replaced, or repositioned, after the operation. **transurethral r.,** resection of the prostate by means of an instrument passed through the urethra. **wedge r.,** removal of a triangular wedge of tissue, as from the ovary in an operation designed to stimulate ovarian function in patients with Stein-Leventhal syndrome.

resectoscope (re-sek′to-skōp) an instrument with a wide-angle telescope and an electrically activated wire loop for transurethral removal or biopsy of lesions of the bladder, prostate, or urethra.

resectoscopy (re″sek-tos′ko-pe) resection or biopsy of lesions by means of the resectoscope.

resene (res′ēn) any one of a class of resin derivatives.

reserpine (res′er-pēn, rĕ-ser′pin) [USP] chemical name: 3,4,5-trimethoxybenzoyl methyl reserpate. An alkaloid, $C_{33}H_{40}N_2O_9$, isolated from the root of *Rauwolfia serpentina* and other species of *Rauwolfia,* and occurring as a white or pale buff to slightly yellowish crystalline powder; used as an antihypertensive, and also as a sedative, administered orally and intramuscularly.

Reserpoid (res′er-poid) trademark for a preparation of reserpine.

reserve (re-zerv′) 1. to hold back for future use. 2. a supply, beyond that ordinarily used, which may be utilized in an emergency. **alkali r., alkaline r.,** the amount of conjugate base components of the blood buffers; since bicarbonate is the most important of these conjugate bases, the term blood bicarbonate is often preferred to alkali reserve. **cardiac r.,** the potential ability of the heart to perform a wide range of work beyond that required under basal conditions, depending on changing demands of various physiological or pathological states.

reservoir (rez′er-vwar) a place or cavity for storage; for anatomical structures serving as a storage space for fluids, see *cisterna* [NA]. Also, an alternate host or passive carrier of a pathogenic organism. **chromatin r.,** karyosome. **r. of infection,** the nonclinical source of infection, such as the alternate host or the passive carrier of a pathogenic organism. **Pecquet's r.,** cisterna chyli. **r. of virus,** the alternate host or the passive carrier of a virus, from which the virus is transmitted to a person who shows clinical signs of infection.

reshaping (re-shāp′ing) a restoration or change of shape, as of a crown, bridge, or denture.

resident (rez′ĭ-dent) a graduate and licensed physician receiving training in a specialty in a hospital.

residua (re-zid′u-ah) [L.] plural of *residuum*.

residual (re-zid′u-al) [L. *residuus*] remaining or left behind.

residue (rez′ĭ-du) [L. *residuum*, from *re*- back + *sidere* to sit] 1. a remainder; that which remains after the removal of other substances. In biochemistry, the portion of a molecule that remains after it has lost some of its components, as an amino acid residue, which loses a water molecule when it is joined to another amino acid. 2. see *Vaughn's split products*, under *product*. **day r.,** an occurrence or experience from the preceding day which may induce a dream at night.

residuum (re-zid′u-um), pl. *resid′ua* [L.] a residue or remainder. **gastric r.,** the contents of the stomach during the interdigestive period, as in the morning before eating. **sporal r.,** residual body.

resilience (re-zil′e-ens) [L. *resilire* to leap back] elasticity; the property of returning to the former shape, size, or state after distortion.

resiliency (re-zil′yen-se) the property of being resilient; resilience. In orthodontics, usually applied to the amount of energy absorbed by a wire when it is stressed, not to exceed its proportional limit. This is energy absorbed owing to elastic deformation.

resilient (re-zil′e-ent) [L. *resiliens*] elastic; returning to its former shape or size after distortion.

resilin (rĕ-zil′in) an elastic protein present in the wing-hinge of dragonflies, locusts, and fleas, which stores and releases energy with extremely high efficiency.

resin (rez′in) [L. *resina*] 1. a solid or semisolid, amorphous, organic substance, of vegetable origin or produced synthetically. True resins are insoluble in water, but are readily dissolved in alcohol, ether, and volatile oils. 2. rosin. **acrylic r′s,** a class of thermoplastic resins, ethylene derivatives containing a vinyl group, produced by polymerization of acrylic or methacrylic acid or their derivatives; used in the fabrication of medical prostheses and dental restorations and appliances. **activated r.,** self-curing r. **anion-exchange r.,** see *ion-exchange r.* **auto-polymer r.,** self-curing r. **azure A carbacrylic r.,** azuresin. **carbacrylamine r′s,** a mixture of 87.5 per cent of cation exchangers, carbacrylic resin, and potassium carbacrylic resin, with 12.5 per cent of the anion exchanger, polyaminemethylene resin; used to increase fecal excretion of sodium in the treatment of edema. **cation-exchange r.,** see *ion-exchange r.* **cholestyramine r.** [USP], a strongly basic anion exchange resin in the chloride form, consisting of styrene-divinylbenzene copolymer with quaternary ammonium functional groups, having an affinity for bile acids, which it binds into an insoluble complex that is excreted in the feces, resulting in elimination of bile acids from the enterohepatic circulation and in increased oxidation of cholesterol to bile acids; administered orally for the relief of pruritus associated with cholestasis occurring in partial biliary obstruction and as adjunctive therapy to diet in the management of patients with elevated cholesterol due to primary type II hyperlipoproteinemia (patients with pure hypercholesterolemia). **cold-curing r.,** self-curing r. **composite r.,** an acrylic resin to which a filler substance, e.g., glass beads and rods or quartz, has been added to produce a material whose properties are better than or radically different from those of its components; used in dental restorations. **copolymer r.,** one that is produced by the concurrent and joint polymerization of two or more different monomers or polymers. **direct filling r.,** a synthetic resin used for direct filling of dental cavities. **heat-curing r.,** one that requires the use of heat to effect its polymerization. **ion exchange r.,** a high molecular weight, insoluble polymer of simple organic compounds with the ability to exchange its attached ions for other ions in the surrounding solution. They are classified as (*a*) cation or anion exchange resins, depending on

which ions the resin exchanges, and (*b*) carboxylic, sulfonic, etc., depending on the nature of the active groups. *Cation exchange resins* are used to restrict intestinal sodium absorption in edematous states; *anion exchange resins* are used as antacids in the treatment of ulcers. **podophyllum r.** [USP], a powdered mixture of resins removed from podophyllum by percolation with alcohol and subsequent precipitation upon addition of acidified water; used as a topical caustic in the treatment of certain papillomas as a 25 per cent dispersion in compound benzoin tincture, or as a solution is alcohol. Formerly used as a cathartic. Called also *podophyllin*. **polyamine-methylene r.,** a polyethylene polyamine methylene substituted resin of diphenylol dimethylmethane and formaldehyde in basic form; because of its exchange-resin action it has been used as a gastric antacid. **quick-cure r.,** self-curing r. **self-curing r.,** any resin which can be polymerized by the addition of an activator and a catalyst without the use of external heat. **styrene r.,** polystyrene. **synthetic r.,** an amorphous, organic, semisolid or solid material produced from simpler compounds by polymerization or condensation. **vinyl r.,** a thermoplastic resin, an ethylene derivative containing the vinyl radical, $CH_2{:}CH{-}$.

resina (re-zi′nah) [L.] resin.

Resinat (rez′ĭ-nat) trademark for preparations of polyaminemethylene resin.

resinoid (rez′ĭ-noid) 1. resembling a resin. 2. a substance resembling a resin. 3. a dry therapeutic precipitate prepared from a vegetable tincture.

resinotannol (rez″ĭ-no-tan′ol) any resin alcohol which gives a tannin reaction.

resinous (rez′ĭ-nus) [L. *resinosus*] of the nature of a resin.

resistance (re-zis′tans) [L. *resistentia*] 1. opposition, or counteracting force, as the opposition by a conductor to the passage of an electric current or the opposition to air flow produced by the air passages. 2. in psychoanalysis, opposition to the coming into consciousness of repressed material. 3. the natural ability of a normal organism to remain unaffected by noxious agents in its environment, such as poisons, toxins, irritants, and pathogenic microorganisms. Resistance is for the most part a genetic endowment of an entire species with respect to a particular agent. If the resistance is absolute, all members of the species are insusceptible to a specific agent. If the resistance is relative, racial and individual differences become manifest within the species, one race or member being more resistant than another. See also *immunity.* **acid alcohol r.,** the power of a bacterium to resist the action of acid and alcohol. **drug r.,** the ability of a microorganism to withstand the effects of a drug that are lethal to most members of its species. Primary drug resistance refers to initial infection by a resistant organism; secondary drug resistance to resistance that develops during the course of therapy. **essential r.,** the resistance within the cells of a battery to a galvanic current. **external r., extraordinary r.,** the resistance in the part of a circuit outside the battery cells. **hemolytic r.,** erythrocyte fragility. **inductive r.,** see *reactance.* **internal r.,** essential r. **peripheral r.,** the resistance to the passage of the blood through the small blood vessels, especially the arterioles. **vital r.,** the natural resistance of an individual to the untoward effects of infections, diseases in general, fatigue, overwork, etc.

resite (res′ĭt) an insoluble, infusible compound formed by further reaction of resole under heat.

resole (res′ōl) a condensation polymer of an alcohol formed by interaction of phenol and formaldehyde, which is of relatively low molecular weight, thermoplastic, and alcohol soluble.

resolution (rez″o-lu′shun) [L. *resolutum*, from *resolvere* to unbind] 1. the subsidence of a pathologic state, as the subsidence of an inflammation, or the softening and disappearance of a swelling. 2. the perception as separate of two adjacent objects or points. In microscopy, it is the minimal distance at which two adjacent objects can be distinguished as separate. The resolving power of an instrument depends on the wavelength of the radiation used and the numerical aperture of the system; it is expressed in microns distance or lines per millimeter.

resolve (re-zolv′) [L. *resolvere*] 1. to restore to the normal state after some pathologic process. 2. to separate a thing into its component parts.

resolvent (re-zol′vent) [L. *resolvens* dissolving] 1. promoting resolution or the dissipation of a pathologic growth. 2. an agent that promotes resolution.

resonance (rez′o-nans) [L. *resonantia*] 1. the prolongation and intensification of sound produced by the transmission of its vibrations to a cavity, especially a sound elicited by percussion. Decrease of resonance is called *dullness*; absence of resonance, *flatness*. 2. a vocal sound as heard in auscultation. 3. mesomerism. **amphoric r.,** a sound resembling that produced by blowing over the mouth of an empty bottle. **bandbox r.,** the extremely resonant sound elicited by percussion in cases of emphysema of the lungs. **bell-metal r.,** a peculiar sound heard in pneumothorax when a coin placed on the chest wall is struck by another coin. **cough r.,** a peculiar auscultatory sound elicited by coughing. **cracked-pot r.,** a peculiar sound elicited by percussion over a pulmonary cavity that communicates with a bronchus. **electron spin r.**, in spectrometry, a measure of electron spin as an indication of the extent of activity of free radicals in an organic reaction. **hydatid r.**, a peculiar sound heard in the combined auscultation and percussion of a hydatid cyst. **nuclear magnetic r.**, a measure of the magnetic moment of atomic nuclei to determine the nature of covalent bonds in an organic reaction. **osteal r.**, the sound elicited by percussion over a bony structure. **shoulder-strap r.**, pulmonary resonance in the apex of the lung above the clavicle. **skodaic r.**, increased percussion resonance at the upper part of the chest, with flatness below it. **tympanic r.**, the drumlike reverberation of a cavity full of air. **tympanitic r.**, the peculiar sound elicited by percussing a tympanitic abdomen. **vesicular r.**, the normal pulmonary resonance. **vesiculotympanic r.**, a resonance partly vesicular and partly tympanic. **vocal r.**, the sound of ordinary speech as heard through the chest wall. **whispering r.**, the auscultatory sound of whispered words heard through the chest wall. **wooden r.**, vesiculotympanic r.

resonant (rez′o-nant)   giving a vibrant sound on percussion.

resonator (rez′o-na″ter)   an instrument used to intensify sounds. In electricity, an electrical circuit in which oscillations of a certain frequency are set up by oscillations of the same frequency in another circuit. **Oudin r.**, a coil of wire of adjustable number of turns which is designed to be connected to a source of high-frequency current, such as a spark gap and induction coil, for the purpose of applying an effluve to a patient.

resorb (re-sorb′, re-zorb′)   to take up or absorb again; to undergo resorption.

resorcin (rĕ-zor′sin)   resorcinol.

resorcinism (rĕ-zor′sĭ-nizm)   chronic poisoning by resorcinol, resulting in methemoglobinemia, paralysis, and damage to the capillaries, kidneys, heart, and nervous system.

resorcinol (rĕ-zor′sĭ-nol) [USP]   chemical name: 1,3-benzenediol. A bactericidal, fungicidal, keratolytic, exfoliative, and antipruritic agent, $C_6H_6O_2$, occurring as white, or nearly white, needle-shaped crystals or powder; used especially as a topical keratolytic in the treatment of acne and other dermatoses, such as seborrheic dermatitis. Called also *resorcin*. **r. monoacetate** [USP], a viscous, pale yellow or amber liquid with a faint odor and a burning taste; applied topically to the scalp as a keratolytic and antiseborrheic.

resorcinolphthalein (re-zor″si-nol-thal′e-in)   fluorescein.

resorcinum (re″zor-si′num)   resorcinol.

resorption (re-sorp′shun) [L. *resorbere* to swallow again]   the loss of substance through physiologic or pathologic means, such as loss of dentin and cementum of a tooth, or of the alveolar process of the mandible or maxilla. **bone r.**, a type of bone loss (resorption) due to osteoclastic activity. **idiopathic r.**, resorption of calcified tissues without apparent cause. **internal r. of teeth**, an unusual form of tooth resorption beginning centrally in a tooth, and apparently initiated by inflammatory hyperplasia of the pulp. **root r.**, a type of resorption in which cementum and/or dentin is lost from the roots, usually the apical portion, of teeth. Depending on the site of origin, the condition may be qualified as internal or external root resorption. **tubular r.**, resorption by renal tubular cells of elements of the fluid filtered at the glomerulus.

respirable (rĕ-spir′ah-b′l)   suitable for respiration, or able to be respired.

respiration (res″pĭ-ra′shun) [L. *respiratio*]   1. the exchange of oxygen and carbon dioxide between the atmosphere and the cells of the body. The process includes ventilation (inspiration and expiration), the diffusion of oxygen from pulmonary alveoli to the blood and of carbon dioxide from the blood to the alveoli, and the transport of oxygen to and carbon dioxide from the body cells. 2. the exergonic metabolic processes in living cells by which molecular oxygen is taken in, organic substances are oxidized, free energy is released, and carbon dioxide, water, and other oxidized products are given off by the cell; called also *cell r.* **abdominal r.**, respiration maintained by contribution of the diaphragm and respiratory muscles. Cf. *thoracic r.* **absent r.**, that in which the respiratory sounds are suppressed. **accelerated r.**, respiration at a faster than normal frequency. **aerobic r.**, the oxidative transformation of certain substrates into secretory products, the released energy being used in the process of assimilation. **amphoric r.**, that which is characterized by amphoric resonance, or a quality like that of the sound produced by blowing over the mouth of an empty jar. It is heard over tuberculous or bronchiectatic cavities, in pneumothorax, in compression of lung from effusion. **anaerobic r.**, a form of respiration in which energy is released from chemical reactions in which free oxygen takes no part. **artificial r.**, that which is maintained by artificial means. Among the various methods of artificial respiration are the following: *Buist's method* is employed in asphyxiation of the newborn, and consists of holding the infant alternately on the stomach and back. *Eve's method:* ". . . the victim is laid face downward on a stretcher and is well wrapped with blankets. His wrists and ankles are lashed to the handles. Then he is hoisted on

a trestle or sling and rocking is begun. The first tilt should be head down and steep (50 degrees) and should produce full expiration by the weight of the abdominal contents pressing on the diaphragm. It will also force aortic blood through the coronaries and empty the stomach and lungs of water. Then full inspiration is produced by tilting the foot end down to 50 degrees. The rocking is done a dozen times a minute through an angle of 45 degrees each way." (J.A.M.A.) *Method of Marshall Hall:* Put the body prone, gently press on the back, then removing the back pressure, turn the body on its side and press a little more, repeating this formula sixteen times every minute. It is known as the method of *prone* or *postural respiration*, or "ready method." *Howard method:* Place the body supine, with a cushion under the back, so that the head is lower than the abdomen; the arms are held over the head, forcible pressure is made with both hands inward and upward, over the lower ribs, about sixteen times per minute. *Mouth-to-mouth method:* The rescuer applies his mouth directly to the mouth of the patient and regularly inflates the patient's lungs with his own expired air. *Schafer's method:* Patient prone with forehead on one of his arms: straddle across patient with knees on either side of his hips, and press with both hands firmly upon the back over the lower ribs; then raise your body slowly, at the same time relaxing the pressure with your hands. Repeat this forward and backward movement about every five seconds. *Silvester's method:* Patient supine. The arms are pulled firmly over the head to raise the ribs, and kept there until air ceases to enter the chest. The arms are brought down to the chest, and are pressed against it for a second or so after air ceases to escape. This formula is repeated sixteen times per minute. See also *respirator.* **asthmoid r.**, respiration in which expiration is accompanied by a wheezing sound like that of bronchial asthma. **Austin Flint r.**, cavernous r. **Biot's r.**, breathing characterized by irregular periods of apnea alternating with periods in which four or five breaths of identical depth are taken; seen in patients with increased intracranial pressure. **Bouchut's r.**, respiration in which the inspiratory phase is shorter than the expiratory phase; seen in children with bronchopneumonia. **bronchial r.**, tubular r. **bronchocavernous r.**, that which is intermediate in character between bronchial and cavernous; it is heard over a lung cavity with solidified lung tissue adjacent to it. **bronchovesicular r.**, a variety intermediate between the bronchial and vesicular forms. **cavernous r.**, a respiration marked by a peculiar prolonged hollow resonance, usually due to a cavity in the lung; it is heard in the same conditions as amphoric respiration. **cell r.**, respiration, def. 2. **cerebral r.**, Corrigan's r. **Cheyne-Stokes r.**, breathing characterized by rhythmic waxing and waning of the depth of respiration, with regularly recurring periods of apnea; seen especially in coma resulting from affection of the nervous centers. **cogwheel r.**, a form with a peculiar jerky inspiration; breathing in which the expiratory and inspiratory sounds are not continuous, but are split into two or more separate sounds. Called also *interrupted r.* **collateral r.**, the entrance of air into alveoli through pulmonary alveolar pores and other pathways so that a lobule may remain aerated even though its bronchiole is obstructed. **controlled diaphragmatic r.**, the intentional use of abdominal respiration for the purpose of limiting the motion of the apices of the lung. **Corrigan's r.**, a shallow and frequent blowing respiration in a low fever. **costal r.**, that which is performed mainly by the rib muscles. **diaphragmatic r.**, that which is mainly performed by the diaphragm. **divided r.**, respiration marked by a pause between the inspiratory and expiratory sounds. **electrophrenic r.**, artificial respiration induced by electric stimulation of the phrenic nerve. Abbreviated EPR. **external r.**, the exchange of gases between the lungs and the blood. **fetal r.**, gaseous interchange through the placenta. **forced r.**, deliberate hyperventilation. **granular r.**, a vesicular respiration, giving a sound as if the air were passing through a tube with an uneven surface. **harsh r.**, bronchovesicular r. **indefinite r.**, a respiratory sound so feeble or so confused that it is difficult to assign to it a definite character. **internal r.**, the exchange of gases between the body cells and the blood; called also *tissue r.* **interrupted r.**, cogwheel r. **jerky r.**, cogwheel r. **Kussmaul's r.**, **Kussmaul Kien r.**, air hunger; see under *hunger.* **labored r.**, that which is performed with difficulty. **meningitic r.**, short and rapid breathing interrupted by pauses of ten to thirty seconds; occurring in healthy persons during sleep it has no important significance, but in meningitis it is regarded as an unfavorable sign. **metamorphosing r.**, bronchocavernous r. **nervous r.**, Corrigan's r. **paradoxical r.**, respiration in which a lung, or a portion thereof, is deflated during inspiration and inflated during expiration. **periodic r.**, Cheyne-Stokes r. **puerile r.**, that in which the breathing sounds are more intense than those of normal adult respiration and resemble those of childhood. **rude r.**, bronchovesicular r. **Seitz's metamorphosing r.**, a variety of bronchial respiration consisting of an inspiratory murmur, beginning as a tubular bronchial sound and ending as either a cavernous or an amphoric tone. **slow r.**, that in which there are less than twelve respirations in each minute. **stertorous r.**, that which is accompanied by abnormal snoring sounds. **supplementary r.**, puerile r. **suppressed r.**, respiration without any appreciable sound, as may occur in

Plate XLIII
respiration

Place one hand under the patient's chin and the other on top of his head. Lift up on the chin and push down on the top of the head to tilt the head backwards.

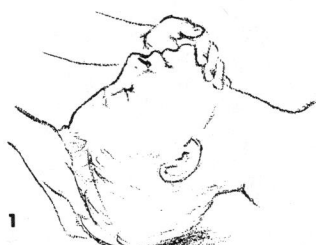

1

Put the thumb of the hand under the jaw into the patient's mouth; grasp the jaw and pull it forward.

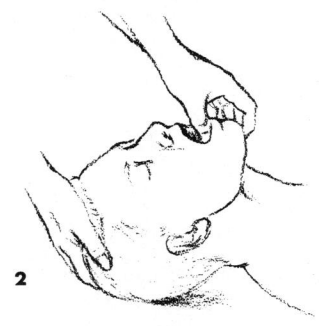

2

While holding the jaw forward pinch the nostrils closed with the other hand to prevent leakage of air through the nose.

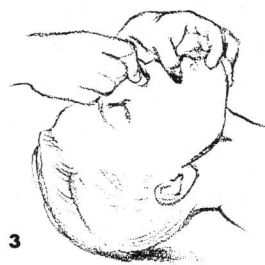

3

Take a deep breath; place your mouth tightly over the patient's and blow forcefully into his lungs.

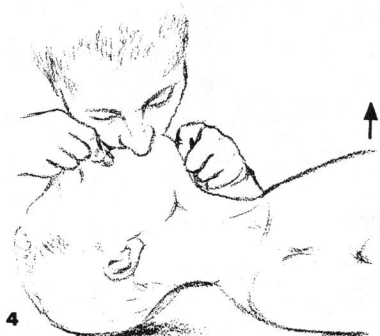

4

Blowing into the lungs causes the chest to expand. When the chest has expanded adequately remove your mouth from the patient's so that he can exhale.

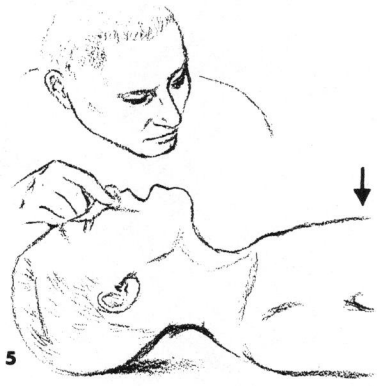

5

Repeat this sequence of maneuvers every 3 to 4 seconds until other means of ventilation are available.

If you cannot open his mouth blow through his nose. In infants cover both mouth and nose with your mouth. Blow gently into a child's mouth, and in infants use only small puffs from your cheeks.

The patient is placed in a supine position on a rigid support so that there is no give under the patient as pressure is applied. The individual applying the pressure stands or kneels at right angles to the patient. He places the heel of one hand with the heel of the other on top of it on the sternum, just cephalad to the xiphoid process.

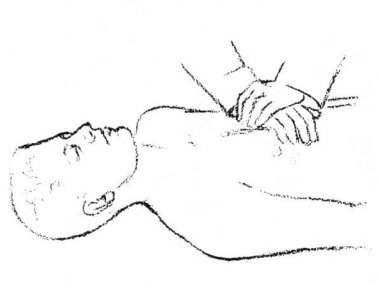

Firm pressure is applied vertically downward about 60 times a minute. At the end of each pressure stroke the hands are relaxed to permit full expansion of the chest. The position of the operator should be such that he can use his body weight while applying the pressure. Sufficient pressure should be exerted to move the sternum 3 or 4 cm. toward the vertebral column.

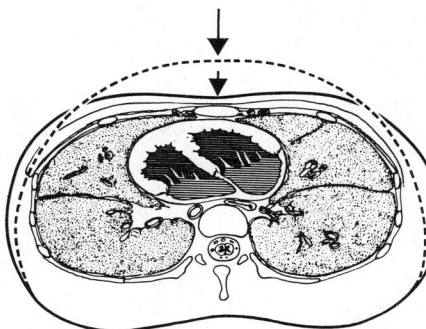

Children up to 10 years of age require the force of only one hand.

Only moderate pressure by the finger tips on the middle third of the sternum should be used on infants.

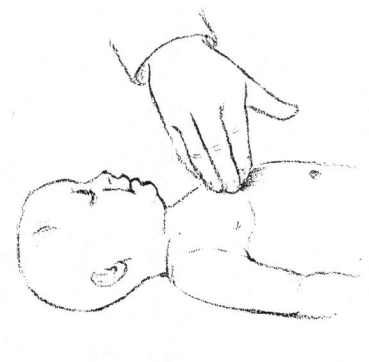

° Kouwenhoven, W. B., Jude, J. R., and Knickerbocker, G. G.: Closed Chest Cardiac Massage. J.A.M.A. 173:1064, 1960.

TECHNIQUE OF RESUSCITATION BY CLOSED CHEST CARDIAC MASSAGE

(Kouwenhoven, Jude, and Knickerbocker, J.A.M.A. 173:1064, 1960.)

extensive consolidation of the lung, or pleuritic effusion. **thoracic r.,** respiration performed by the intercostal and other thoracic muscles. Cf. *abdominal r.* **tissue r.,** internal r. **transitional r.,** bronchovesicular r. **tubular r.,** that which has high-pitched sounds, not unlike those made by blowing through a tube; it is heard in consolidation of lung, compression of lung, and sometimes over lung infiltrated with tumor. **vesiculocavernous r.,** cavernous respiration with a vesicular quality; it indicates a cavity surrounded by healthy lung tissue. **vicarious r.,** increased action in one lung when that of the other lung is diminished. **wavy r.,** cogwheel r.

respirator (res′pĭ-ra″tor) an apparatus to qualify the air that is breathed through it, or a device for giving artificial respiration or to assist in pulmonary ventilation. **cabinet r.,** one which encloses the entire body. **cuirass r.,** an apparatus which is applied only to the chest, either completely surrounding the trunk or applied only to the front of the chest and abdomen. **Drinker r.,** an apparatus for producing artificial respiration over long periods of time, consisting of a metal tank, enclosing the body of the patient, with his head outside, and within which artificial respiration is maintained by alternating negative and positive pressure. Popularly called *iron lung.* **Engström r.,** a volume-controlled respirator used after open-heart surgery as short-term prophylaxis to avoid hypoxia and respiratory acidosis and to prevent excessive fatigue caused by the increased work of breathing in the early postoperative period.

respiratory (re-spi′rah-to″re) [re- + L. *spirare* to breathe] pertaining to respiration.

respiratory system see under *system.*

respirometer (res″pĭ-rom′ĕ-ter) an instrument for determining the character of the respiratory movements.

response (re-spons′) [L. *respondere* to answer, reply] an action or movement due to the application of a stimulus. **anamnestic r.,** in immunology, the rapid reappearance of antibody in the blood following the administration of an antigen to which the subject had previously developed a primary immune response; called also *memory r., recall r., booster r., second set r.,* and *secondary immune r.* **autoimmune r.,** the immune response in which antibodies or immune lymphoid cells are produced against the body's own tissues. **booster r.,** anamnestic r. **conditioned r.,** one that does not occur naturally in the animal but that may be developed by regular association of some physiological function with an unrelated outside event, such as ringing of a bell or flashing of a light. Soon the physiological function starts whenever the outside event occurs (Pavlov, 1911). Called also *conditioned reflex.* **delayed r.,** see under *reaction.* **galvanic skin r.,** the alteration in electrical resistance of the skin associated with sympathetic nerve discharge. **immediate r.,** see under *reaction.* **immune r.,** specifically altered reactivity of the animal body following exposure to antigen, manifested as antibody production, cell-mediated immunity, or immunological tolerance; called also *immune reaction.* **memory r.,** anamnestic r. **primary immune r.,** the immune response to initial stimulation by an antigen; it is characterized by a latent period before the synthesis of specific antibody is begun. **recall r.,** anamnestic r. **recall titer r.,** an increase in specific agglutinins stimulated by a booster injection, as of tetanus toxoid; similar to the nonspecific anamnestic reaction. **reticulocyte r.,** increase in the formation of reticulocytes in response to a bone marrow stimulus, such as that provided by administration of a hematinic agent. **secondary immune r.,** anamnestic r. **second set r.,** anamnestic r. **triple r. (of Lewis),** a physiologic reaction of the skin to stroking with a blunt instrument: first a red line develops at the site of stroking, owing to the release of histamine or a histamine-like substance, then a flare develops around the red line, and lastly a wheal is formed as a result of local edema. **unconditioned r.,** an unlearned response, i.e., one that occurs naturally; called also *unconditioned reflex.* Cf. *conditioned r.*

rest (rest) 1. repose after exertion. 2. a fragment of embryonic tissue that has been retained within the adult organism; called also *embryonic, epithelial,* and *fetal r.* 3. in dentistry, a metallic extension from a removable partial denture which contacts a tooth or dental restoration and aids in supporting the prosthesis. **aberrant r.,** choristoma. **adrenal r.,** accessory adrenal tissue, sometimes found in the ovary or testis. **bed r.,** confinement of a patient to bed. **carbon r.,** the amount of carbon in the deproteinized blood. **embryonic r., epithelial r., fetal r.,** see *rest,* def. 2. **incisal r.,** a metallic extension from a removable partial denture which engages on the incisal surface of an anterior tooth to aid in supporting the prosthesis. **lingual r.,** a metallic extension from a removable partial denture onto the lingual surface of an anterior tooth to aid in supporting or acting as an indirect retainer for the prosthesis. **Malassez's r.,** an epithelial remnant of Hertwig's sheath in the periodontal membrane, which sometimes develops into a dental cyst. **occlusal r.,** a metallic extension from a removable partial denture which engages on the occlusal surface of a tooth to aid in supporting the prosthesis. **precision r.,** a partial denture rest that consists of closely interlocking parts. **recessed r.,** a rigid extension of a partial denture which contacts a definite seat prepared in the

surface of a tooth. **suprarenal r.,** adrenal r. **surface r.,** a rigid extension of a partial denture which contacts the unaltered extracoronal surface of a tooth. **Walthard's cell r's,** see under *islet.*

restbite (rest′bīt) the relation of the teeth when the jaw is at rest.

restenosis (re″stĕ-no′sis) recurrent stenosis, especially of a valve of the heart, after surgical correction of the primary condition. **false r.,** stenosis recurring after failure to divide either commissure of the cardiac valve beyond the area of incision of the papillary muscles. **true r.,** restenosis occurring after complete opening of one or both of the commissures of the cardiac valve involved.

restibrachium (res″tĭ-bra′ke-um), pl. *restibra′chia* [L. *restis* rope + *brachium* arm] (obs.) pedunculus cerebellaris inferior.

restiform (res′tĭ-form) [L. *restis* rope + *forma* form] shaped like a rope.

restis (res′tis), pl. *res′tes* [L. "rope"] (obs.) pedunculus cerebellaris inferior.

restitutio (res″tĭ-tu′she-o) [L.] restitution. **r. in′tegrum,** complete return to health.

restitution (res″tĭ-tu′shun) [L. *restitutio*] 1. an active process of restoration. 2. the spontaneous realignment of the fetal head with the fetal body, after delivery of the head.

restoration (res″to-ra′shun) 1. reconstruction to effect return to a previous state, as of health. 2. the partial or complete reconstruction of a body part, or the device used as its replacement. In dentistry, the act of restoring a tooth to its original condition by the filling of a cavity and replacement of lost parts, or the material used in such a procedure. **buccal r.,** the replacement, usually with silver alloy, gold, or plastic, of the buccal portion of a posterior tooth lost through caries or injury. **prosthetic r.,** the replacement of a lost or absent body part with an artificial structure, or the device or material used for such replacement, such as, in dentistry, an inlay, crown, bridge, or partial or complete denture, or other appliance to replace tissues missing from the mouth.

restorative (re-stōr′ah-tiv) (obs.) 1. promoting a return to health or to consciousness. 2. a remedy that aids in restoring health, vigor, or consciousness; called also *anastatic.*

restraint (re-strānt′) the forcible confinement of a violently psychotic or irrational person. **chemical r.,** the quieting of a violently psychotic or irrational person by means of narcotics.

resublimed (re″sub-līmd′) subjected to repeated processes of sublimation.

resultant (re-zul′tant) any of the products of a chemical reaction.

resupination (re″su-pĭ-na′shun) [L. *resupinare* to turn on the back] 1. the act of turning upon the back or dorsum. 2. the position of one lying upon the back.

resuscitation (re-sus″ĭ-ta′shun) [L. *resuscitare* to revive] the restoration to life or consciousness of one apparently dead; it includes such measures as artificial respiration and cardiac massage. **cardiopulmonary r. (CPR),** the reestablishing of heart and lung action as indicated for cardiac arrest or apparent sudden death resulting from electric shock, drowning, respiratory arrest, and other causes. The two major components of CPR are artificial ventilation and closed chest cardiac massage; see illustration accompanying *respiration.* **r. of the heart,** restoration of spontaneous cardiac contractions. See illustration accompanying *respiration.*

resuscitator (re-sus′ĭ-ta″tor) an apparatus for initiating respiration in cases of asphyxia. **cardiopulmonary r.,** an apparatus that simultaneously assists the patient's breathing and applies external cardiac massage.

resuture (re-soo′tūr) secondary suture.

retainer (re-tān′er) an appliance or device for retaining anything in position. In dentistry, an appliance which aids in maintaining in the proper position a tooth whose malposition has been corrected, or which helps keep a fixed or removable partial denture in place. **continuous bar r.,** Kennedy bar. **direct r.,** a clasp or attachment applied to an abutment tooth, by which a removable partial denture is maintained in position; called also *clasp.* **Hawley r.,** a removable palatal wire and acrylic appliance used as a stabilizing appliance or, with modifications, to move teeth. It usually incorporates a labial wire and an acrylic palate. **indirect r.,** a removable partial denture component which aids the action of a direct retainer by functioning through lever action on the opposite side of the fulcrum line. **matrix r.,** a mechanical device designed to engage the ends of a matrix band or strip and to tighten the matrix around the tooth.

retamine (ret′ah-min) an alkaloid, $C_{15}H_{26}N_2O$, from the young branches and bark of *Genista sphaerocarpa.*

retardate (re-tar′dāt) a mentally retarded individual.

retardation (re″tar-da′shun) [L. *retardare* to slow down, impede] delay; hindrance; delayed development. **mental r.,** subnormal general intellectual development, originating during the developmental period, and associated with impairment of either learning and social adjustment or maturation, or both. The disorder is classified according to intelligence quotient as follows: *borderline,* 68–83; *mild,* 52–67; *moderate,* 36–51; *severe,* 20–35; and *profound,* less than 20. Formerly called *feeblemindedness* and *mental deficiency.* **psychomotor r.,** underactivity of both mind and body, as seen in depressive disorders. **r. of thought,** delay in thinking in which either the process of thought is set in motion slowly (*initial r.*), or the thought or action once having started is performed slowly (*executive r.*).

retching (rech′ing) a strong involuntary effort to vomit.

rete (re′te), pl. *re′tia* [L. "net"] a net or meshwork; used in anatomical nomenclature as a general term to designate a network, especially of arteries or veins. **acromial r., r. acromia′le** [NA], a network formed by ramification of the acromial branch of the thoracoacromial artery on the acromion process. **r. arterio′sum** [NA], an anastomotic network formed by arteries just before they become arterioles or capillaries. **articular r.,** a network of anastomosing blood vessels in or around a joint. **articular cubital r., articular r. of elbow,** r. articulare cubiti. **articular r. of knee,** r. articulare genus. **r. articula′re cu′biti** [NA], articular rete of elbow: an arterial network formed on the posterior aspect of the elbow by the posterior ulnar recurrent, inferior and superior ulnar collateral, and interosseous recurrent arteries. **r. articula′re ge′nu,** r. articulare genus. **r. articula′re ge′nus** [NA], articular rete of knee: an extensive arterial rete on the capsule of the knee joint, supplying branches to the contiguous bones and joints. It is formed by the genicular arteries, the termination of the deep femoral artery, the descending branch of the lateral circumflex artery, and the tibial recurrent artery. **calcaneal r., r. calca′nei, r. calca′neum** [NA], an arterial rete on the posterior and lower surfaces of the calcaneus, receiving branches from the calcaneal branches of the peroneal artery and the lateral malleolar branches of the peroneal artery. **r. cana′lis hypoglos′si,** plexus venosus canalis hypoglossi. **carpal r., dorsal,** r. carpi dorsale. **r. car′pi dorsa′le** [NA], dorsal carpal rete: an arterial rete formed by the dorsal radial carpal and dorsal ulnar carpal arteries and giving off the second, third, and fourth dorsal metacarpal arteries to the dorsum of the hand and the second, third, and fourth fingers. **r. cuta′neum,** the network of arteries at the boundary between the corium and the tela subcutanea. **dorsal venous r. of foot,** r. venosum dorsale pedis. **dorsal venous r. of hand,** r. venosum dorsale manus. **r. dorsa′le pe′dis,** an arterial rete on the dorsum of the foot. **epidermal r.,** stratum germinativum epidermidis [Malpighii]. **r. foram′inis ova′lis,** plexus venosus foraminis ovalis. **r. of Haller, r. Halle′ri,** r. testis. **malleolar r., lateral,** r. malleolare laterale. **malleolar r., medial,** r. malleolare mediale. **r. malleola′re latera′le** [NA], lateral malleolar rete: a small arterial rete on the lateral malleolus, formed by the lateral anterior malleolar artery, the perforating branch of the peroneal artery, and the lateral tarsal artery. **r. malleola′re media′le** [NA], medial malleolar rete: a small arterial rete on the medial malleolus, formed by the medial anterior malleolar artery and branches from the posterior tibial artery. **r. Malpig′hi,** stratum germinativum epidermidis (Malpighii). **r. mira′bile,** 1. [NA], a vascular network formed by division of an artery or a vein into a large number of smaller vessels that subsequently reunite into a single vessel; in the human this occurs only in the arterioles that supply the glomeruli of the kidney. 2. arterial anastomosis of the brain occurring between the external and internal carotid arteries as a result of longstanding thrombosis of the internal carotid arteries. **r. na′si,** a venous plexus in the inferior nasal concha. **r. olec′rani,** r. articulare cubiti. **r. ova′rii,** a homologue of the rete testis, developed in the early female fetus, but vestigial in the adult. **r. of patella, r. patel′lae** [NA], a network of arterial branches surrounding the patella, and derived from the various arteries of the knee. **plantar r., plantar venous r.,** r. venosum plantare. **r. subpapilla′re,** the network of arteries at the boundary between the papillary and reticular layers of the corium. **r. test′is** [NA], **r. test′is [Halle′ri],** a network of channels, formed by the straight seminiferous tubules, traversing the mediastinum testis and draining into the efferent ductules; called also *rete of Haller.* **r. vasculo′sum,** a network of anastomosing blood vessels. **r. veno′sum** [NA], venous network: an anastomotic network of small veins. **r. veno′sum dorsa′le ma′nus** [NA], dorsal venous rete of hand: a venous network on the back of the hand, formed by the dorsal metacarpal veins. **r. veno′sum dor′sale pe′dis** [NA], dorsal venous rete of foot: a superficial network of anastomosing veins on the dorsum of the foot proximal to the transverse venous arch, draining into the great and the small saphenous veins. **r. veno′sum planta′re** [NA], plantar venous rete: a thick venous rete in the subcutaneous tissue of the sole of the foot. **re′tia veno′sa vertebra′rum,** networks of veins inside the vertebral canal.

retention (re-ten′shun) [L. *retentio,* from *retentare* to hold firmly back] the process of keeping in position, as (*a*) the persistent keeping within the body of matters normally excreted, or (*b*) in dentistry, the maintaining of a dental prosthesis in proper position in the mouth, against all forces that might tend to dislodge it. **direct r.,** maintenance of the position of a removable partial denture in the mouth by means of direct retainers. **indirect r.,** retention in the mouth of a removable partial denture by means of indirect retainers. **surgical r.,** retention in the mouth of a dental prosthesis by means of attachments embedded in the oral tissues. **r. of urine,** accumulation of urine within the bladder because of inability to urinate.

retethelioma (re″te-the-le-o′mah) malignant lymphoma.

retia (re′te-ah) [L.] plural of *rete.*

retial (re′te-al) pertaining to or of the nature of a rete.

reticula (rĕ-tik′u-lah) [L.] plural of *reticulum.*

reticular (rĕ-tik′u-lar) [L. *reticularis*] pertaining to or resembling a net.

reticulated (rĕ-tik′u-lāt″ed) reticular.

reticulation (rĕ-tik″u-la′shun) [L. *reticulum* a net] in radiology, a network of wrinkles or corrugations in the emulsion of an x-ray film resulting from sharp temperature differences between processing solutions. **dust r.,** an early stage of pneumoconiosis, seen especially in coal miners, which may go on to an anthracosilicosis.

reticulin (rĕ-tik′u-lin) a scleroprotein from the connective fibers of reticular tissue. **r. M,** an internal secretion produced by the reticuloendothelial system.

reticulitis (rĕ-tik″u-li′tis) inflammation of the reticulum of a ruminant animal.

reticulocyte (rĕ-tik′u-lo-sīt″) a young red blood cell showing a basophilic reticulum under vital staining.

reticulocytogenic (rĕ-tik″u-lo-si″to-jen′ik) causing the formation of reticulocytes.

reticulocytopenia (rĕ-tik″u-lo-si″to-pe′ne-ah) [*reticulocyte* + Gr. *penia* poverty] a decrease in the number of reticulocytes of the blood.

reticulocytosis (rĕ-tik″u-lo-si-to′sis) an increase in the number of reticulocytes in the peripheral blood.

reticuloendothelial (rĕ-tik″u-lo-en″do-the′le-al) pertaining to tissues having both reticular and endothelial attributes; see under *system.*

reticuloendothelioma (rĕ-tik″u-lo-en″do-the-le-o′mah) malignant lymphoma.

reticuloendotheliosis (rĕ-tik″u-lo-en″do-the-le-o′sis) hyperplasia of reticuloendothelial tissue. **leukemic r.,** leukemia marked by splenomegaly and by an abundance of large, mononuclear abnormal cells with numerous, irregular cytoplasmic projections that give them a flagellated or hairy appearance in the bone marrow, spleen, liver, and peripheral blood; called also *hairy-cell leukemia.* See also *hairy cell,* under *cell.* **systemic aleukemic r.,** Letterer-Siwe disease.

reticuloendothelium (rĕ-tik″u-lo-en″do-the′le-um) the tissue of the reticuloendothelial system.

reticulohistiocytary (re-tik″u-lo-his″te-o-si′ter-e) pertaining to or composed of histiocytes of the reticuloendothelial system.

reticulohistiocytoma (re-tik″u-lo-his″te-o-si-to′mah) a granulomatous aggregation of lipid-laden histiocytes and multinucleated giant cells; it may be solitary with no systemic involvement (*reticulohistiocytic granuloma*), or multiple with systemic involvement (*multicentric reticulohistiocytosis*).

reticulohistiocytosis (re-tik″u-lo-his″te-o-si-to′sis) the formation of multiple reticulohistiocytomas. **multicentric r.,** a rare systemic disease, usually affecting women, manifested by polyarthritis of the hands and large joints, frequently leading to crippling absorption of the phalanges, and the development of reticulohistiocytomas of the skin and mucous membranes. The course varies—there may be involution, it may remain stationary, or it may progress, terminating in death. Called also *lipid* or *lipoid dermatoarthritis.* Cf. *reticulohistiocytic granuloma.*

reticuloid (rĕ-tik′u-loid) 1. resembling reticulosis. 2. a condition resembling reticulosis. **actinic r.,** dermatosis aggravated by exposure to light, usually affecting the elderly, characterized by a chronic eczematous eruption predominantly on the exposed skin of the face, hands, and forearms, and extending to contiguous unexposed areas. Often there are episodes of almost universal erythroderma. In severe cases, edematous plaques produce gross furrowing and distortion of features. The eruption clears slowly on avoidance of light.

reticuloma (rĕ-tik″u-lo′mah) histiocytic malignant lymphoma.

reticulopenia (rĕ-tik″u-lo-pe′ne-ah) reticulocytopenia.

reticuloperithelium (rĕ-tik″u-lo-per″ĭ-the′le-um) retoperithelium.

reticulopituicyte (rĕ-tik″u-lo-pĭ-tu′ĭ-sīt) see *pituicyte.*

reticulopod (rĕ-tik″u-lo-pod) rhizopodium.

reticulopodium (rĕ-tik″u-lo-po′de-um) rhizopodium.

reticulosarcoma (rĕ-tik″u-lo-sar-ko′mah) malignant lymphoma, undifferentiated or histiocytic.

reticulosis (rĕ-tik″u-lo′sis) an abnormal increase in cells derived from or related to reticuloendothelial cells. **familial hemophagocytic r.,** familial histiocytic r. **familial histiocytic r.,** a fatal hereditary disorder transmitted as an autosomal recessive trait, characterized by anemia, granulocytopenia, thrombocytopenia, phagocytosis of blood cells, diffuse proliferation of histiocytes of various organs, and enlargement of the liver, spleen, and lymph nodes; called also *familial hemophagocytic r.* and *histiocytic medullary r.* **histiocytic medullary r.,** familial histiocytic r. **lipomelanic r.,** dermatopathic lymphadenopathy. **malignant mast cell r.,** a very rare, occasionally fatal form of systemic mastocytosis in which there is massive mast cell infiltration of various organs, resulting in impairment of their function. **midline malignant r.,** lethal midline granuloma thought to be due to lymphoma.

reticulothelium (rĕ-tik″u-lo-the′le-um) the retothelium. **agranular r.,** see *endoplasmic r.*

reticulum (rĕ-tik′u-lum), pl. *retic′ula* [L., dim. of *rete* net] 1. a network, especially a protoplasmic network in cells, as the flattened double membrane sheets of the endoplasmic reticulum. 2. reticular tissue. 3. the second division of the stomach of a ruminant animal. **Chiari's r.,** Chiari's network. **Ebner's r.,** a network of cells in the seminiferous tubules. **endoplasmic r.,** an ultramicroscopic organelle of nearly all cells of higher plants and animals, consisting of a more or less continuous system of membrane-bound cavities that ramify throughout the cytoplasm of a cell. Two forms have been distinguished: *granular reticulum* (chromidial substance, ergastoplasm), which bears large numbers of ribosomes on the outer surface of its membrane and is basophilic, and *agranular reticulum,* which contains no ribosomes and has no distinctive staining properties. Called also *superior protoplasm.* **granular r.,** see *endoplasmic r.* **retic′ula lie′nis,** trabeculae lienis. **sarcoplasmic r.,** a special form of agranular reticulum found in the sarcoplasm of striated muscle and comprising a system of smooth-surfaced tubules forming a plexus around each myofibril. **stellate r.,** the soft, middle part of the enamel organ of a developing tooth, the cells being separated by an increase in the gelatinous intercellular substance which forces the cells apart without breaking the intercellular connections, giving them a stellate appearance and providing protection later for the enamel-forming cells.

retiform (re′tĭ-form, ret′ĭ-form) [L. *rete* net + *forma* form] resembling a network.

retina (ret′ĭ-nah) [L.] [NA] the innermost of the three tunics of the eyeball, surrounding the vitreous body and continuous posteriorly with the optic nerve. It is divided into the *pars optica,* which rests upon the choroid, the *pars ciliaris,* which rests upon the ciliary body, and the *pars iridica,* which rests upon the posterior surface of the iris. Grossly, the retina is composed of an outer, pigmented layer (stratum pigmenti) and an inner, transparent layer, the optic part of which is the cerebral stratum (stratum cerebrale). The latter consists of nine layers, named from within outward, as follows (see illustration): (1) the membrana limitans interna; (2) the nerve fiber layer; (3) the layer of ganglion cells; (4) the inner molecular, or plexiform, layer; (5) the inner nuclear layer; (6) the outer molecular, or plexiform, layer; (7) the outer nuclear layer; (8) the membrana limitans externa; (9) the layer of rods and cones (called also *Jacob's membrane* and *bacillary layer*). The pigmentary layer overlying the optic portion is continued forward over the inner surface of the ciliary body, constituting the *pars ciliaris retinae.* The various layers are connected transversely by fibers of connective tissue (*fibers of Müller*). The layer of rods and cones forms the percipient element of the retina (i.e., the element that responds to visual stimuli by a photochemical reaction), and is connected with the nerve fiber layer by nerve fibers which join to form the optic nerve. In the center of the posterior part of the retina is the *macula lutea,* the most sensitive portion of the retina; and in the center of the macula lutea is a depression, the *fovea centralis,* from which the rods are absent.

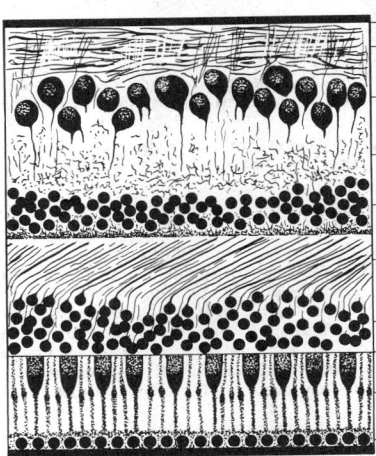

- Internal limiting membrane
- Nerve fiber layer
- Ganglion cell layer
- Inner molecular layer
- Inner nuclear layer
- Outer molecular layer
- Outer nuclear layer
- Outer limiting membrane
- Layer of rods and cones
- Pigment layer

Schematic representation of the layers of the adult human retina.

About 0.25 cm. inside the fovea is the point of entrance of the optic nerve and its central artery (*central artery of the retina*). At this point the retina is incomplete and forms the *blind spot.* **coarctate r.,** a funnel-shaped condition of the retina caused by a fluid exudation between the retina and the choroid. **lower r.,** the lower half of the retina. **nasal r.,** the nasal half of the retina. **physiological r.,** the part of the retina that contains receptors sensitive to light (pars optica retinae [NA]). **shot-silk r.,** an opalescent effect, as of changeable silk, sometimes seen in the retinas of young persons. **temporal r.,** the outer half of the retina. **tigroid r.,** the "striped" retina seen in a blond fundus in which the choroidal vessels can be seen, or in certain tapetoretinal degenerations. **upper r.,** the upper half of the retina. **watered-silk r.,** shot-silk retina.

Retin-A (ret′in) trademark for a preparation of tretinoin.

retinaculum (ret′ĭ-nak′u-lum), pl. *retinac′ula* [L. "a rope, cable"] 1. a structure which retains an organ or tissue in place; [NA] a general term for such a structure. 2. an instrument or device for retracting tissues during surgery. See *tenaculum.* **r. of arcuate ligament,** r. ligamenti arcuati. **r. cap′sulae articula′ris cox′ae,** one of the longitudinal folds of the cervical portion of the articular capsule of the hip. **caudal r., r. cauda′le** [NA], a fibrous band that extends from the tip of the coccyx to the adjacent skin and thus forms the foveola coccygea; called also *ligamentum caudale integumenti communis.* **r. cos′tae ul′timae,** ligamentum lumbocostale. **retinac′ula cu′tis** [NA], bands of connective tissue attaching the corium to the subcutaneous tissue. **extensor r. of foot, inferior,** r. musculorum extensorum pedis inferioris. **extensor r. of foot, superior,** r. musculorum extensorum pedis superius. **extensor r. of hand,** r. extensorum manus. **r. extenso′rum ma′nus** [NA], extensor retinaculum of hand: the distal part of the antebrachial fascia, overlying the extensor tendons; called also *ligamentum carpi dorsale.* **flexor r. of foot,** r. musculorum flexorum pedis. **flexor r. of hand,** r. flexorum manus. **r. flexo′rum ma′nus** [NA], flexor retinaculum of hand: a heavy fibrous band continuous with the distal part of the antebrachial fascia, completing the carpal canal through which pass the tendons of the flexor muscles of the hand and fingers; called also *ligamentum carpi transversum.* **r. ligamen′ti arcua′ti,** retinaculum of arcuate ligament: a band of converging fibers passing from the convex lower margin of the arcuate popliteal ligament to the head of the fibula. **r. musculo′rum extenso′rum pe′dis infe′rius** [NA], inferior extensor of foot: a thickened band of the fascia cruris passing from each malleolus across the front of the ankle joint, there crossing the other and passing onto the dorsum of the foot; called also *ligamentum cruciatum cruris.* **r. musculo′rum extenso′rum pe′dis supe′rius** [NA], superior extensor retinaculum of foot: the thickened lower portion of the fascia on the front of the leg, attached to the tibia on one side and the fibula on the other, and serving to hold in place the extensor tendons that pass beneath it; called also *ligamentum transversum cruris.* **r. musculo′rum fibula′rium infe′rius,** NA alternative for *r. musculorum peroneorum inferius.* **r. musculo′rum fibula′rium supe′rius,** NA alternative for *r. musculorum peroneorum superius.* **r. musculo′rum flexo′rum pe′dis** [NA], a strong band of fascia that extends from the medial malleolus down onto the calcaneus. It holds in place the tendons of the tibialis posterior, flexor digitorum, and flexor hallucis muscles as they pass to the sole of the foot, and gives protection to the posterior tibial vessels and tibial nerve. Called also *ligamentum laciniatum* and *flexor r. of foot.* **r. musculo′rum peronaeo′rum infe′rius,** r. musculorum peroneorum inferius. **r. musculo′rum peronaeo′rum supe′rius,** r. musculorum peroneorum superius. **r. musculo′rum peroneo′rum infe′rius** [NA], a fibrous band that arches over the tendons of the peroneal muscles and holds them in position on the lateral side of the calcaneus; called also *inferior peroneal r.* **r. musculo′rum peroneo′rum supe′rius** [NA], a fibrous band that arches over the peroneal tendons and helps to hold them in place below and behind the lateral malleolus; it extends from the malleolus downward and backward to the calcaneus. Called also *superior peroneal r.* **r. patel′lae latera′le** [NA], lateral patellar retinaculum: a fibrous membrane from the tendon of the vastus lateralis muscle, attached to the lateral margin of the patella and then along the side of the patellar ligament, and inserted into the tibia as far distal as the fibular collateral ligament; it also blends with the iliotibial tract of the fascia lata. Called also *lateral patellar ligament.* **r. patel′lae media′le** [NA], medial patellar retinaculum: a fibrous membrane from the tendon of the vastus medialis muscle, attached to the medial margin of the patella and then along the side of the patellar ligament, and inserted into the tibia as far distal as the tibial collateral ligament. **patellar r., lateral,** r. patellae laterale. **patellar r., medial,** r. patellae mediale. **peroneal r., inferior,** r. musculorum peroneorum inferius. **peroneal r., superior,** r. musculorum peroneorum superius. **r. ten′dinum,** a tendinous restraining structure, such as an annular ligament. **r. ten′dinum musculo′rum extenso′rum,** r. extensorum manus. **r. ten′dinum musculo′rum extenso′rum infe′rius,** r. musculorum extensorum pedis inferius. **r. ten′dinum musculo′rum extenso′rum supe′rius,** r.

musculorum extensorum pedis superius. **r. ten′dinum mus-culo′rum flexo′rum,** r. flexorum manus. **retinac′ula un′guis** [NA], structures homologous to the retinacula cutis, attaching the nail to underlying tissue. **Weitbrecht′s r.,** retinacular fibers attached to the neck of the femur.

retinal (ret′ĭ-nal) 1. pertaining to the retina. 2. the aldehyde of retinol, derived by the oxidative enzymatic splitting of absorbed dietary carotene, and having vitamin A activity. In the retina, retinal combines with opsins to form visual pigments. One isomer, 11-*cis* retinal combines with opsin in the rods (scotopsin) to form rhodopsin, or visual purple. Another, all-*trans* retinal (*trans*-r.; visual yellow; xanthopsin), results from the bleaching of rhodopsin by light, in which the 11-*cis* form is converted to the all-*trans* form. Retinal also combines with opsins in the cones (photopsins) to form the three pigments responsible for color vision. Called also *retinal₁* and *retinene₁*.

retinal₁ (ret′ĭ-nal) retinal.

retinal₂ (ret′ĭ-nal) dehydroretinal.

retinascope (ret′ĭ-nah-skōp) retinoscope.

retine (ret′ēn) a substance stated to be widely distributed in animal cells, which is characterized by its ability to retard cell division and growth. Cf. *promine.*

retinene (ret′ĭ-nēn) the aldehyde of vitamin A, occurring in two forms: *retinene₁* is the aldehyde of retinol (see *retinal*, def. 2), and *retinene₂* is the aldehyde of dehydroretinol.

retinitis (ret″ĭ-ni′tis) inflammation of the retina; used in the older ophthalmological literature to denote impairment of sight, perversion of vision, edema, and exudation into the retina, and occasionally by hemorrhages into the retina. **actinic r.,** retinitis due to exposure to actinic light rays. **r. albuminu′rica,** that which is associated with kidney disease. **apoplectic r.,** that which is characterized by extravasations of blood within the retina. **central angiospastic r., r. centra′lis sero′sa,** central serous retinopathy. **r. circina′ta, circinate r.,** circinate retinopathy. **Coats′ r.,** exudative retinopathy. **diabetic r.,** see under *retinopathy.* **r. discifor′mans,** a degenerative disease of the retina marked by an elevated grayish white mass in the macular region of both eyes; called also *central disk-shaped retinopathy.* **exudative r.,** exudative retinopathy. **r. gravida′rum,** gravidic r. **gravidic r.,** inflammation of the retina occurring along with the albuminuria of pregnancy. **r. haemorrha′gica,** retinitis marked by profuse retinal hemorrhage. **hypertensive r.,** retinitis occurring in the course of arterial hypertension. **Jacobson′s r.,** syphilitic r. **Jensen′s r.,** retinochoroiditis juxtapapillaris. **leukemic r.,** a variety seen in leukemia, and marked by hemorrhage and paleness of the retina; called also *splenic r.* **metastatic r.,** retinitis caused by the location of septic emboli in the retinal vessels. **r. nephrit′ica,** retinal changes associated with nephritis; called also *renal r.* **r. pigmento′sa,** a group of diseases, frequently hereditary, marked by progressive loss of retinal response (as elicited by the electroretinogram), retinal atrophy, attenuation of the retinal vessels, and clumping of the pigment, with contraction of the field of vision. It may be transmitted as a dominant, recessive, or X-linked trait and is sometimes associated with other genetic defects. **r. prolif′erans, proliferating r.,** a condition sometimes resulting from intraocular hemorrhage, with neovascularization and the formation of fibrous tissue bands extending into the vitreous from the surface of the retina; retinal detachment is sometimes a sequel. **r. puncta′ta albes′-cens,** a variety characterized by the presence of minute white spots in the fundus. **punctate r.,** a form marked by the presence of a number of white or yellowish spots scattered over the fundus. **renal r.,** r. nephritica. **serous r.,** simple inflammation of the superficial layers of the retina. **solar r.,** retinitis due to excessive exposure to sunlight. **splenic r.,** leukemic r. **r. stella′ta,** a star-shaped figure in the macular area of the retina seen in various conditions. **striate r.,** a form marked by the presence of gray or yellowish streaks just back of the retinal vessels. **suppurative r.,** retinitis due to pyemic infection. **syphilitic r., r. syphilit′ica,** retinitis complicating syphilitic iritis. **uremic r.,** retinitis occurring in uremia.

retinoblastoma (ret″ĭ-no-blas-to′mah) a tumor arising from retinal germ cells.

retinochoroid (ret″ĭ-no-ko′roid) pertaining to the retina and the choroid.

retinochoroiditis (ret″ĭ-no-ko-roi-di′tis) inflammation of the retina and choroid. **r. juxtapapilla′ris,** a condition seen in young healthy subjects marked by a small inflammatory area on the fundus close to the papilla; called also *Jensen′s retinitis* or *retinochoroiditis.*

retinodialysis (ret″ĭ-no-di-al′ĭ-sis) [*retina* + Gr. *dialysis* separation] disinsertion of the retina; detachment of the retina at its peripheral insertion.

retinograph (ret′ĭ-no-graf) a photograph of the retina.

retinography (ret″ĭ-nog′rah-fe) photography of the retina.

retinoid (ret′ĭ-noid) 1. resembling the retina. 2. any derivative of retinal, whether naturally occurring or synthetic. 3. [Gr. *rhētinē* resin + *eidos* form] resembling a resin.

retinol (ret′ĭ-nol) vitamin A₁, the form of vitamin A found in mammals; it is a 20-carbon alcohol, $C_{20}H_{30}O$, that is reversibly dehydrogenated by enzymatic action into its aldehyde, retinal (q.v.). Called also *retinol₁.*

retinol₁ (ret′ĭ-nol) retinol.

retinol₂ (ret′ĭ-nol) dehydroretinol.

retinomalacia (ret″ĭ-no-mah-la′she-ah) [*retina* + Gr. *malakos* soft + *-ia*] softening of the retina.

retinopapillitis (ret″ĭ-no-pap″ĭ-li′tis) inflammation of the retina and the optic papilla.

retinopathy (ret″ĭ-nop′ah-the) [*retina* + Gr. *pathos* disease] any noninflammatory disease of the retina. **central disk-shaped r.,** retinitis disciformans. **central serous r.,** a usually self-limiting condition marked by acute localized detachment of the neural retina or retinal pigment epithelium in the region of the macula, with hypermetropia; called also *central angiospastic retinitis* and *retinitis centralis serosa.* **circinate r.,** a condition marked by a circle of white spots enclosing the macular area, leading to complete foveal blindness; called also *retinitis circinata* or *circinate retinitis.* **diabetic r.,** retinopathy associated with diabetes mellitus, which may be of the background type, progressively characterized by microaneurysms, intraretinal punctate hemorrhages, yellow, waxy exudates, cotton-wool patches, and macular edema, or of the proliferative type, characterized by neovascularization of the retina and optic disk, which may project into the vitreous, proliferation of fibrous tissue, vitreous hemorrhage, and retinal detachment. Called also *diabetic retinitis.* **exudative r.,** a condition marked by masses of white or yellowish exudate in the posterior part of the fundus oculi, with deposit of cholesterin and blood debris from retinal hemorrhage, and leading to destruction of the macula and blindness. Called also *exudative retinitis,* and *Coats′ disease* or *retinitis.* **hypertensive r.,** that associated with essential or malignant hypertension; changes may include irregular narrowing of the retinal arterioles, hemorrhages in the nerve fiber layers and the outer plexiform layer, exudates and cotton-wool patches, arteriosclerotic changes, and, in malignant hypertension, papilledema. **leukemic r.,** a condition occurring in leukemia, with paleness of the fundus resulting from infiltration of the retina and choroid with leukocytes, and swelling of the disk with blurring of its margin. **pigmentary r.,** see *retinitis pigmentosa.* **proliferative r.,** the proliferative type of diabetic retinopathy (q.v.). **Purtscher′s angiopathic r.,** Purtscher′s disease.

retinoschisis (ret″ĭ-nos′kĭ-sis) [*retina* + Gr. *schisis* division] splitting of the retina: in the *juvenile form* the splitting occurs in the nerve fiber layer, and in the *adult form* in the external plexiform layer. The disorder is usually more benign and slowly progressive than retinal detachment.

retinoscope (ret′ĭ-no-skōp″) an instrument for performing retinoscopy.

retinoscopy (ret″ĭ-nos′ko-pe) [*retina* + Gr. *skopein* to examine] an objective method for investigating, diagnosing, and evaluating refractive errors of the eye, by projection of a beam of light into the eye and observation of the movement of the illuminated area on the retina surface and of the refraction by the eye of the emergent rays. Called also *pupilloscopy, skiascopy, skiametry,* and *shadow test.*

retinosis (ret″ĭ-no′sis) a general term for degenerative, noninflammatory conditions of the retina.

retinotopic (ret″ĭ-no-top′ik) relating to the organization of the visual pathways and visual area of the brain.

retinotoxic (ret″ĭ-no-tok′sik) exerting a toxic or deleterious effect upon the retina.

retisolution (ret″ĭ-so-lu′shun) [L. *rete* net + *solution*] dissolution of the Golgi apparatus.

retispersion (ret″ĭ-sper′shun) [L. *rete* net + *spargere* to throw about] migration of the Golgi apparatus from its normal position to the periphery of the cell.

retoperithelium (re″to-per″ĭ-the′le-um) [L. *rete* net + Gr. *peri* around + *thēlē* papilla] the layer of cells covering a reticular framework.

retort (re-tort′) [L. *retorta* bent back] a long-necked globular vessel formerly used in distillation.

Retortamonas (re″tor-tam′o-nas) [L. *retortus* bent back + Gr. *monas* unit] a genus of biflagellate protozoa of the family Bodonidae, order Protomastigida, usually having a piriform or fusiform body tapered at the posterior end; they are parasites in the intestines of various animals. *R. blattae* is found in the intestine of cockroaches, *R. caviae* in the cecum of guinea pigs, *R. intestinalis* in the human intestine, *R. ovis* in the intestine of sheep, and *R. cuniculi* in the cecum of rabbits. Called also *Embadomonas.*

retothel (re′to-thel) reticuloendothelial.

retothelial (re″to-the′le-al) pertaining to the retothelium; containing reticulum cells.

retothelium (re″to-the′le-um) [L. *rete* net + Gr. *thēlē* papilla] the layer of cells covering a reticular tissue.

retractile (re-trak′til) [L. *retractilis*] susceptible of being drawn back.

retraction (re-trak′shun) [L. *retractio*, from *re-* back + *trahere* to draw] the act of drawing back; the condition of being drawn back. **clot r.,** the drawing away of a blood clot from the wall of a vessel; it is a function of blood platelets. **gingival r.,** the apical advancement of the line of attachment of the gingiva on a tooth surface. **mandibular r.,** the condition of the mandible when the gnathion lies posterior to the orbital plane.

retractor (re-trak′tor) 1. an instrument for maintaining operative exposure by separating the edges of a wound and holding back underlying organs and tissues; many shapes, sizes, and styles are available. 2. any retractile muscle. **Emmet's r.,** a self-retaining vaginal speculum. **Moorehead's r.,** a retractor used in dentistry.

retrad (re′trad) [L. *retro* backward] toward a posterior or dorsal part.

retrieval (re-tre′val) in psychology, the process of obtaining memory information from wherever it has been stored.

retro- (ret′ro, re′tro) [L. *retro* backward] a prefix signifying backward, or located behind.

retroaction (ret″ro-ak′shun) action in a reversed direction; reaction.

retroauricular (ret″ro-aw-rik′u-lar) behind the auricle.

retrobronchial (ret″ro-brong′ke-al) behind the bronchi.

retrobuccal (ret″ro-buk′al) pertaining to the back part of the mouth.

retrobulbar (ret″ro-bul′bar) [*retro-* + L. *bulbus* bulb] 1. behind the pons. 2. behind the eyeball.

retrocalcaneobursitis (ret″ro-kal-ka″ne-o-bur-si′tis) achillobursitis.

retrocardiac (ret″ro-kar′de-ak) behind the heart.

retrocatheterism (ret″ro-kath′ĕ-ter-izm) the passing of a catheter through a suprapubic opening downward through the urethra to the external meatus.

retrocecal (ret″ro-se′kal) behind the cecum.

retrocervical (ret″ro-ser′ve-kal) behind the cervix uteri.

retrocession (ret″ro-sesh′un) [L. *retrocessio*] a going backward; backward displacement; specifically a dropping backward of the entire uterus.

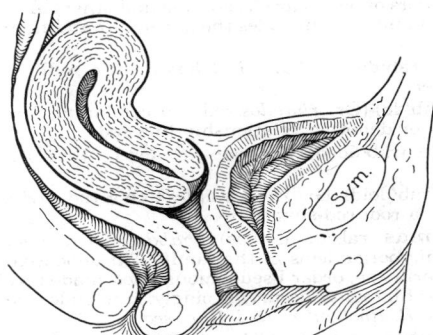

Retrocession of uterus.

retroclavicular (ret″ro-klah-vik′u-lar) behind the clavicle.

retroclusion (ret″ro-kloo′zhun) [*retro-* + L. *claudere* to close] closure of a bleeding artery by means of a pin passed over, behind, and under the vessel.

retrocochlear (ret″ro-kok′le-ar) 1. behind the cochlea. 2. denoting the eighth cranial nerve and cerebellopontine angle as opposed to the cochlea.

retrocolic (ret″ro-kol′ik) behind the colon.

retrocollic (ret″ro-kol′ik) pertaining to the back of the neck; nuchal.

retrocollis (ret″ro-kol′is) [*retro-* + L. *collum* neck] spasmodic wryneck in which the head is drawn directly backward.

retrocrural (re″tro-kru′ral) situated at the back of the leg, or crus.

retrocursive (re″tro-kur′siv) [*retro-* + L. *curro* to run] marked by stepping backward.

retrodeviation (re″tro-de″ve-a′shun) a general term inclusive of retroversion, retroflexion, retroposition, etc.

retrodisplacement (re″tro-dis-plās′ment) backward or posterior displacement.

retroesophageal (re″tro-ĕ-sof″ah-je′al) posterior to the esophagus.

retrofilling (ret″ro-fil′ing) a method of filling the root canal of a tooth from the apex of a root which has been surgically exposed.

retroflexed (ret′ro-flekst) [*retro-* + L. *flexus* bent] bent backward; in a state of retroflexion.

retroflexion (ret″ro-flek′shun) [L. *retroflexio*] the bending of an organ so that its top is turned backward; specifically, the bending backward of the body of the uterus toward the cervix, resulting in a sharp angle at the point of bending.

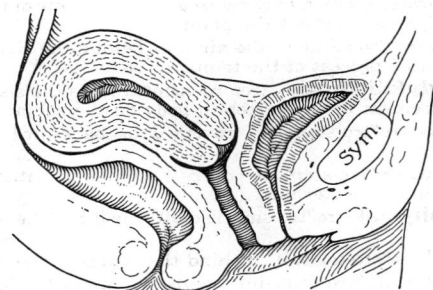

Retroflexion of uterus.

retrogasserian (ret″ro-gas-se′re-an) pertaining to the sensory (posterior) root of the trigeminal (gasserian) ganglion.

retrognathia (ret″ro-nath′e-ah) [*retro-* + Gr. *gnathos* jaw + *-ia*] position of the jaws back of the frontal plane of the forehead.

retrognathic (ret″ro-nath′ik) pertaining to or characterized by retrognathia.

retrognathism (ret″ro-nath′ism) retrognathia.

retrograde (ret′ro-grād) [*retro-* + L. *gradi* to step] going backward; retracing a former course; catabolic.

retrography (re-trog′rah-fe) [*retro-* + Gr. *graphein* to write] mirror writing.

retrogression (ret″ro-gresh′un) [*retro-* + L. *gressus* course] degeneration; deterioration; regression; return to an earlier, less complex condition.

retroinfection (re″tro-in-fek′shun) infection of the mother by the fetus.

retroinsular (ret″ro-in′su-lar) [*retro-* + L. *insula* island] situated or occurring behind the insula.

retroiridian (re″tro-i-rid′e-an) behind the iris.

retrojection (ret″ro-jek′shun) [*retro-* + L. *jacere* to throw] irrigation of a cavity by injection of fluid.

retrolabyrinthine (re″tro-lab″ĭ-rin′thēn) behind the labyrinth of the ear.

retrolental (re″tro-len′tal) behind the lens of the eye.

retrolenticular (re″tro-len-tik′u-lar) [*retro-* + *lenticular*] retrolental.

retrolingual (ret″ro-ling′gwal) behind the tongue.

retromammary (ret″ro-mamm′ar-e) behind the mammary gland.

retromandibular (re″tro-man-dib′u-lar) behind the mandible of the lower jaw.

retromastoid (re″tro-mas′toid) behind the mastoid process.

retromesenteric (ret″ro-mes″en-ter′ik) behind the mesentery.

retromorphosis (re″tro-mor-fo′sis) [*retro-* + Gr. *morphē* form] retrograde metamorphosis.

retronasal (ret″ro-na′zal) [*retro-* + L. *nasus* nose] behind the nose.

retro-ocular (ret″ro-ok′u-lar) [*retro-* + L. *oculus* eye] behind the eye.

retroparotid (re″tro-pah-rot′id) behind the parotid gland.

retropatellar (ret″ro-pah-tel′ar) situated behind the patella.

retroperitoneal (re″tro-per″ĭ-to-ne′al) behind the peritoneum.

retroperitoneum (re″tro-per″ĭ-to-ne′um) the retroperitoneal space.

retroperitonitis (re″tro-per″ĭ-to-ni′tis) inflammation in the retroperitoneal space.

retropharyngeal (re″tro-fah-rin′je-al) [*retro-* + *pharyngeal*] situated or occurring behind the pharynx.

retropharyngitis (re″tro-far″in-ji′tis) inflammation of the posterior part of the pharynx.

retropharynx (re″tro-far′inks) the posterior part of the pharynx.

retroplacental (re″tro-plah-sen′tal) behind the placenta.

retroplasia (ret″ro-pla′se-ah) [*retro-* + Gr. *plasis* formation + *-ia*] retrograde metaplasia; degeneration of a tissue or cell into a more primitive type.

retropleural (re″tro-ploor′al) behind the pleura; posterior to the pleural cavity.

retroposed (re″tro-pōzd) [*retro-* + L. *positus* placed] displaced backward or posteriorly.

retroposition (re″tro-po-zish′un) backward displacement.

retropulsion (re″tro-pul′shun) [*retro-* + L. *pellere* to drive] 1. a driving back, as of the fetal head in labor. 2. a tendency to walk backward, as in some cases of tabes dorsalis; opisthoporeia. 3. an abnormal gait in which the body is bent backward.

retrorectal (re″tro-rek′tal) behind the rectum.

retrorsine (ret′ror-sin) a poisonous alkaloid, $C_{18}H_{25}O_6N$, from *Senecio retrorsus*, which may cause a fatal cirrhosis of the liver in horses and cattle that eat the plant.

retrosinus (ret″ro-si′nus) the air cells behind the sigmoid sinus in the mastoid process of the temporal bone.

retrospondylolisthesis (ret″ro-spon″dĭ-lo-lis-the′sis) posterior displacement of one vertebral body on the subjacent body.

retrostalsis (re″tro-stal′sis) reversed or backward peristaltic action.

retrosternal (re″tro-ster′nal) [*retro-* + *sternum*] situated or occurring behind the sternum.

retrosymphysial (re″tro-sim-fiz′e-al) behind the symphysis pubis.

retrotarsal (re″tro-tar′sal) behind the tarsus of the eye.

retrouterine (re″tro-u′ter-in) [*retro-* + *uterus*] behind the uterus.

retrovaccination (re″tro-vak″sĭ-na′shun) the inoculation of a heifer with vaccine virus from a human subject, also vaccination with virus obtained from a cow which has been previously thus inoculated.

retroversioflexion (re″tro-ver″se-o-flek′shun) retroversion combined with retroflexion.

retroversion (ret″ro-ver′zhun) [L. *retroversio;* retro back + versio turning] the tipping of an entire organ backward. **r. of uterus,** the turning backward of the entire uterus in relation to the pelvic axis.

retroverted (ret″ro-vert′ed) in a condition of retroversion.

retrovesical (ret″ro-ves′ĭ-kal) behind the urinary bladder.

retrovirus (re″tro-vi′rus, ret″ro-vi′rus) a large group of RNA viruses that includes the leukoviruses and lentiviruses.

retrusion (re-troo′zhun) [L. *re-* back + *trudere* to shove] 1. the state of being located posterior to the normal position, as malposition of a tooth posteriorly in the line of occlusion. 2. the backward movement or position of the mandible.

Retzius' fibers, space (cavity), veins (ret′ze-us) [Anders Adolf *Retzius*, Swedish anatomist, 1796–1860] see under *fiber* and *vein*, and see *spatium retropubicum*.

Retzius' foramen, lines (striae, stripes) (ret′ze-us) [Magnus Gustav *Retzius*, Swedish anatomist, 1842–1919] see *apertura lateralis ventriculi*, and see *incremental lines*, under *line*.

reunient (re-ūn′yent) [L. *re-* again + *unire* to unite] effecting the union of divided tissues or organs.

Reuss's color charts (tables) (rois′ez) [August Ritter von *Reuss*, Vienna ophthalmologist, 1841–1924] see under *chart*.

revaccination (re″vak-sĭ-na′shun) a second vaccination.

revascularization (re-vas′ku-lar-i-za′shun) the restoration of an adequate blood supply to a part by means of a blood vessel graft, as in aortocoronary bypass.

revellent (re-vel′ent) [L. *re-* back + *vellere* to draw] causing revulsion; revulsive.

Reverdin's graft (method, operation) needle (ra-ver-danz′) [Jacques Louis *Reverdin*, surgeon at Geneva, 1842–1929] see *epidermic graft*, under *graft*, and see under *needle*.

reversal (re-ver′sal) a turning or change in the opposite direction. **r. of gradient,** a changing of direction of the fecal stream due to an area of irritation causing local spasticity of the intestine with higher tonus than that of the proximal area.

reversible (re-ver′sĭ-b'l) capable of going through a series of changes in either direction, forward or backward, as a reversible chemical reaction.

reversion (re-ver′zhun) [L. *re* back + *versio* turning] 1. a returning to a previous condition; regression. 2. in genetics, inheritance from some remote ancestor of a character which has not been manifest for several generations. Cf. *atavism.* **antigenic r.,** a change in the antigenic structure of adult cells to that of immature cells; such reversion may follow neoplastic change. **Mantoux r.,** a term suggested to designate the change from the tuberculin-positive to the tuberculin-negative state, occasionally observed with the passage of time in subjects immunized with B.C.G. vaccine. Mantoux reversion, the opposite of Mantoux conversion, may be an indication for revaccination with B.C.G. vaccine.

Revilliod's sign (ra-ve-yōz′) [Jean Léonard Adolphe *Revilliod*, Swiss physician, 1835–1918] see under *sign*.

revivescence (re″vi-ves′ens) [L. *revivescere* to revive] 1. the renewal of vital activities. 2. the reappearance of a local (cutaneous) reaction on the subcutaneous administration of tuberculin to a patient who has previously had a diagnostic (cutaneous) tuberculin test. Called also *recurrent reaction*.

revivification (re-viv″ĭ-fĭ-ka′shun) [L. *re-* again + *vivus* alive + *facere* to make] 1. restoration to life or consciousness. 2. refreshing of diseased surfaces to promote their union.

revolute (rev′o-lūt) turned back or curled back.

revulsant (re-vul′sant) [L. *revulsans*] revulsive.

révulseur (ra″vul-ser′) [Fr.] (*obs.*) an instrument with many fine needle points used in the performance of baunscheidtism.

revulsion (re-vul′shun) [L. *revulsio;* from re- back + *vellere* to draw] the act of drawing blood from one part to another, as in counterirritation; the diminution of morbid action in any part of the body by irritation in another.

revulsive (re-vul′siv) [L. *re-* back + *vellere* to draw] 1. effecting revulsion. 2. an agent causing revulsion; a counterirritant.

Reynals see *Duran-Reynals*.

Reynold's test (ren′oldz) [James Emerson *Reynold*, Scottish physician, 1844–1920] see under *tests*.

Rezipas (rez′ĭ-pas) trademark for a preparation of para-aminosalicylic acid.

RF rheumatoid factor.

Rf symbol for *rutherfordium*.

R.F.A. right fronto-anterior (position of the fetus).

R.F.P. right frontoposterior (position of the fetus).

R.F.P.S.(Glasgow) Royal Faculty of Physicians and Surgeons of Glasgow.

R.F.T. right frontotransverse (position of the fetus).

R.G.N. Registered General Nurse (Scotland).

Rh 1. chemical symbol for *rhodium*. 2. symbol for *rhesus factor* (see under *factor*).

Rh$_{null}$ symbol for a rare blood type in which all Rh factors are lacking; see also under *syndrome*.

Rhabdiasoidea (rab″dĭ-ah-soi′de-ah) in some classifications, a superfamily of phasmids, including the genus *Strongyloides*.

rhabditic (rab-dit′ik) pertaining or belonging to *Rhabditis*, or to the Rhabditoidea.

rhabditiform (rab-dit′ĭ-form) rhabdoid.

Rhabditis (rab-di′tis) [Gr. *rhabdos* rod] a genus of minute phasmid nematodes of the superfamily Rhabditoidea, living mostly in damp earth, and as an accidental parasite in man. *R. hominis* and *R. intestinalis* have been found in the stools. *R. niellyi* is found in the skin. *R. pellio* (*R. genitalis, Leptodera pellio*) is sometimes found in the genitourinary organs.

rhabditoid (rab′dĭ-toid) rhabdoid.

Rhabditoidea (rab″dĭ-toi′de-ah) a superfamily of phasmids, some members of which are free-living and others are parasites of plants and animals; it includes the genera *Rhabditis* and *Strongyloides*.

rhabdium (rab′de-um) [Gr. *rhabdion* a little rod] a voluntary muscle fiber.

rhabdo- (rab′do) [Gr. *rhabdos* rod] a combining form meaning rod-shaped or denoting relationship to a rod.

rhabdocyte (rab′do-sīt) [*rhabdo-* + *-cyte*] (*obs.*) metamyelocyte.

rhabdoid (rab′doid) [Gr. *rhabdo-eides* like a rod, striped looking] resembling a rod; rod-shaped.

Rhabdomonas (rab″do-mo′nas) [*rhabdo-* + Gr. *monas* unit] a genus of microorganisms of the family Thiorhodaceae, suborder Rhodobacteriineae, order Pseudomonadales, made up of irregular long rods or filaments, occurring singly. It includes three species, *R. gra'cilis, R. linsbau'eri,* and *R. ro'sea.*

rhabdomyoblastoma (rab″do-mi″o-blas-to′mah) [*rhabdo-* + Gr. *mys* muscle + *blastos* germ + *-oma*] rhabdomyosarcoma.

rhabdomyochondroma (rab″do-mi″o-kon-dro′mah) benign mesenchymoma.

rhabdomyolysis (rab″do-mi-ol′ĭ-sis) [*rhabdo-* + Gr. *mys* muscle + *lysis* dissolution] disintegration or dissolution of muscle, associated with excretion of myoglobin in the urine. **exertional r.,** that due to intense, prolonged physical exertion, with symptoms often resembling those elicited by exercise in persons with occlusive arterial disease.

rhabdomyoma (rab″do-mi-o′mah) a benign tumor derived from striated muscle; called also *myoma striocellulare*.

rhabdomyomyxoma (rab″do-mi″o-mik-so′mah) benign mesenchymoma.

rhabdomyosarcoma (rab″do-mi″o-sar-ko′mah) a highly malignant tumor of striated muscle derived from primitive mesenchymal cells and exhibiting differentiation along rhabdomyoblastic lines, including but not limited to the presence of cells with recognizable cross striations. It occurs in three forms: the *pleomorphic* form affects predominantly the extremities of adults; the *alveolar* form, occurring mainly in adolescents and young adults, affects muscles of the extremities, trunk, orbital region, etc.; the *embryonal* form, occurring predominantly in infants and children, affects the head and neck, the lower genitourinary tract, pelvis, and extremities.

Rhabdonema (rab″do-ne′mah) *Rhabditis*.

rhabdosarcoma (rab″do-sar-ko′mah) rhabdomyosarcoma.

rhabdovirus (rab″do-vi′rus) [*rhabdo-* + *virus*] any of a group of morphologically similar, bullet-shaped or bacilliform RNA viruses, including the viruses of vesicular stomatitis and rabies.

rhachi- for words beginning thus, see those beginning *rachi-*.

rhacoma (ra-ko′mah) [Gr. *rhakōma* rags] a pendulous scrotum.

rhaebocrania (re″bo-kra′ne-ah) [Gr. *rhaibos* crooked + *kranion* skull + -*ia*] torticollis, or wryneck.

rhaeboscelia (re″bo-se′le-ah) [Gr. *rhaibos* crooked + *skelos* leg + -*ia*] genu varum (bowleg), or genu valgum (knock knee).

rhaebosis (re-bo′sis) [Gr. *rhaibos* crooked + -*osis*] crookedness of the legs or of any normally straight part.

rhagades (rag′ah-dēz) [pl. of Gr. *rhagas* rent] fissures, cracks, or fine linear scars in the skin, especially such lesions around the mouth or other regions subjected to frequent movement.

rhagadiform (ra-gad′ĭ-form) [Gr. *rhagas* rent + L. *forma* shape] resembling rhagades.

-rhage [Gr. *rhēgnynai* to burst forth] word termination meaning a breaking or bursting forth, a profuse flow, as hemorrhage.

rhagiocrine (raj′e-o-krīn) [Gr. *rhax* grape + *krinein* to separate] denoting colloid vacuoles in the cytoplasm of gland cells that represent a stage in the development of secretory granules.

rhagionid (raj″e-on′id) a fly of the family Rhagionidae.

Rhagionidae (raj″e-on′ĭ-de) a family of biting flies, the snipe flies, of the order Diptera; the genera, *Spaniopsis*, *Suragina*, and *Symphoromyia*, contain species that are vicious biters.

rhamninose (ram′nĭ-nōs) a trisaccharide which occurs in the glycosides rutin and xanthorhamnin.

rhamnose (ram′nōs) 6-deoxy-L-mannose, $C_6H_{12}O_5$.

rhamnoside (ram′no-sīd) a glycoside which on hydrolysis yields rhamnose.

Rhamnus (ram′nus) [L.; Gr. *rhamnos* a kind of prickly shrub] a genus of rhamnaceous trees and shrubs, often with a purgative bark and fruit. Among them are *R. cathar′tica* L., or buckthorn, *R. purshia′na* D.C. (the source of cascara sagrada), and *R. fran′gula* L. *R. califor′nica* L., California buckthorn or coffee tree, has been used in rheumatism. *R. cro′ceus* Nutt. is a species of buckthorn with edible red fruit, the excessive use of which tinges the skin red.

rhaphania (rah-fa′ne-ah) raphania.

rhaphe (ra′fe) [Gr. *rhaphē*] raphe.

-rhaphy [Gr. *rhaphē* a seam] a word termination meaning joining in a seam, or suture of the part designated by the stem to which it is affixed, as blepharorrhaphy.

rhatany (rat′ah-ne) [Port. *ratanhia*] Krameria. **Brazilian r.,** *Krameria argentea*. **Peruvian r.,** *Krameria triandra*.

Rhazes (ra′zes) (c. 860 to c. 932 A.D.) a famous Arabian physician (although born in Persia), who was distinguished for his many writings, his treatise on smallpox and measles being particularly outstanding.

rhe (re) [Gr. *rheos* current] the unit of fluidity, being the reciprocal of the unit of velocity or centipoise.

-rhea [Gr. *rhein* to flow, run, gush] a word termination meaning flow.

rhegma (reg′mah) [Gr. *rhēgma* rent] a rupture, rent, or fracture.

rhegmatogenous (reg″mah-toj′ĕ-nus) [*rhegma* + Gr *gennan* to produce] arising from a rhegma, as rhegmatogenous detachment of the retina.

Rhein's picks (rīnz) [M. L. *Rhein*, American dentist, 1860–1928] instruments for opening and enlarging root canals at the apex.

rhenium (re′ne-um) a chemical element, atomic number 75, atomic weight 186.2, symbol Re.

rheo- (re′o) [Gr. *rheos* current] a combining form denoting relationship to an electric current, or to a flow, as of fluids.

rheobase (re′o-bās) [*rheo-* + Gr. *basis* step] the minimal electric current necessary to produce stimulation (L. Lapicque, 1909).

rheobasic (re″o-ba′sik) pertaining to a rheobase.

rheocord (re′o-kord) [*rheo-* + Gr. *chordē* chord] rheostat.

rheology (re-ol′o-je) the science of the deformation and flow of matter, such as the flow of blood through the heart and blood vessels.

Rheomacrodex (re″o-mak′ro-deks) trademark for a preparation of dextran 40.

rheometer (re-om′ĕ-ter) [*rheo-* + Gr. *metron* measure] galvanometer.

rheonome (re′o-nōm) [*rheo-* + Gr. *nemein* to distribute] an apparatus for determining the effect of irritation on a nerve.

rheophore (re′o-fōr) [*rheo-* + Gr. *phoros* carrying] an electrode.

rheoscope (re′o-skōp) [*rheo-* + Gr. *skopein* to examine] an instrument for detecting the presence of an electric current.

rheostat (re′o-stat) [*rheo-* + Gr. *histanai* to place] an appliance for regulating the resistance and thus controlling the amount of current entering an electric circuit.

rheostosis (re″os-to′sis) [*rheo-* + *ostosis*] a condition of hyperostosis marked by the presence of streaks in the bones; see also *melorheostosis*.

rheotachygraphy (re″o-tah-kig′rah-fe) [*rheo-* + Gr. *tachys* swift

+ *graphein* to write] the photographic record of the curve of variation in experiments upon the electromotive action of muscles.

rheotaxis (re″o-tak′sis) [*rheo-* + Gr. *taxis* arrangement] the orientation of an organism in a stream of liquid, with its long axis parallel with the direction of fluid flow. **negative r.,** rheotaxis with movement of the organism in the same direction as that of the liquid. **positive r.,** rheotaxis with movement of the organism in the opposite direction to that of the liquid.

rheotome (re′o-tōm) [*rheo-* + Gr. *tomē* a cutting] a device in a faradic battery for interrupting the current with an adjustable speed control.

rheotrope (re′o-trōp) [*rheo-* + Gr. *rheos* current + *trepein* to turn] an instrument for reversing an electric current.

rheotropism (re-ot′ro-pizm) rheotaxis.

rhestocythemia (res″to-si-the′me-ah) [Gr. *rhaiein* to break, ruin + -*cyte* + *haima* blood + -*ia*] (*obs.*) the occurrence of broken-down erythrocytes in the blood.

Rheum (re′um) a genus of cathartic polygonaceous plants; see *rhubarb*.

rheum, rheuma (rōōm, roo′mah) [Gr. *rheuma* flux] any watery or catarrhal discharge. **epidemic r.,** influenza.

rheumapyra (roo″mah-pi′rah) [Gr. *rheuma* flux + *pyr* fire] acute rheumatism; rheumatic fever.

rheumarthritis (roo″mar-thri′tis) rheumatoid arthritis.

rheumatalgia (roo″mah-tal′je-ah) chronic rheumatic pain.

rheumatic (roo-mat′ik) [Gr. *rheumatikos*] pertaining to or affected with rheumatism.

rheumaticosis (roo-mat″ĭ-ko′sis) a term suggested to express the general condition seen in the rheumatism of childhood.

rheumatid (roo′mah-tid) any skin lesion or eruption etiologically associated with rheumatism.

rheumatism (roo′mah-tizm) [L. *rheumatismus*; Gr. *rheumatismos*] any of a variety of disorders marked by inflammation, degeneration, or metabolic derangement of the connective tissue structures of the body, especially the joints and related structures, including muscles, bursae, tendons and fibrous tissue. It is attended by pain, stiffness, or limitation of motion of these parts. Rheumatism confined to the joints is classified as arthritis. **apoplectic r.,** rheumatism associated with brain hemorrhage. **articular r., acute,** rheumatic fever. **articular r., chronic,** see *rheumatoid arthritis*, under *arthritis*, and *osteoarthritis*. **Besnier's r.,** chronic arthrosynovitis. **cerebral r.,** acute rheumatic fever marked by chorea, delirium, convulsions, and coma. **desert r.,** the primary stage of coccidioidomycosis. **gonorrheal r.,** acute articular rheumatism associated with gonorrheal urethritis, and frequently producing ankylosis of the joints. **r. of the heart,** involvement of the heart by the rheumatic fever process. **Heberden's r.,** rheumatism of the finger joint, marked by the formation of nodosities. **inflammatory r.,** rheumatic fever. **lumbar r.,** lumbago. **MacLeod's capsular r.,** a rheumatoid arthritis with effusion into the synovial capsules, bursae, and sheaths. **muscular r.,** fibrositis. **nodose r.,** 1. articular rheumatism with the formation of nodules in the region of the joints. 2. rheumatoid arthritis. **osseous r.,** rheumatoid arthritis. **palindromic r.,** a condition in which there are repeated episodes of arthritis and periarthritis without fever and without producing irreversible changes in the joints. **Poncet's r.,** tuberculous rheumatism. **subacute r.,** a mild but protracted form of rheumatism. **tuberculous r.,** see under *arthritis*. **visceral r.,** that which involves a viscus, more commonly the heart or pericardium.

rheumatismal (roo″mah-tiz′mal) pertaining to or of the nature of rheumatism.

rheumatogenic (roo″mah-to-jen′ik) [*rheumatism* + Gr. *gennan* to produce] producing or causing rheumatism.

rheumatoid (roo′mah-toid) [Gr. *rheuma* flux + *eidos* form] resembling rheumatism.

rheumatologist (roo″mah-tol′o-jist) a specialist in rheumatic conditions.

rheumatology (roo″mah-tol′o-je) the branch of medicine dealing with rheumatic disorders, their causes, pathology, diagnosis, treatment, etc.

rheumatopyra (roo″mah-to-pi′rah) rheumapyra.

rheumatosis (roo″mah-to′sis) any disorder attributed to rheumatic origin.

rheumic (roo′mik) pertaining to a rheum or flux.

rhexis (rek′sis) [Gr. *rhēxis* a breaking forth, bursting] the rupture of an organ or vessel.

Rh factor see under *factor*.

rhigosis (rĭ-go′sis) [Gr. *rhigōsis* a shivering] the cold sense; the perception of cold.

rhigotic (rĭ-got′ik) pertaining to rhigosis.

rhin- see *rhino-*.

rhinal (ri′nal) [Gr. *rhis* nose] pertaining to the nose.

rhinalgia (ri-nal′je-ah) [*rhin-* + -*algia*] pain in the nose.

rhinallergosis (rīn″al-er-go′sis) [rhin- + allergy + -osis] allergic rhinitis.

rhinedema (ri″nĕ-de′mah) [rhin- + edema] edema of the nose.

rhinencephalia (ri″nen-sĕ-fa′le-ah) rhinocephaly.

rhinencephalon (ri″nen-sef′ah-lon) [rhin- + Gr. enkephalos brain] 1. a term generally applied to certain parts of the brain previously thought to be concerned entirely with olfactory mechanisms, including the olfactory nerves, bulbs, tracts, and subsequent connections (all olfactory in function) and the limbic system (not primarily olfactory in function); it is homologous with the olfactory portions of the brain in lower animals. Called also olfactory brain and smell brain. 2. one of the portions of the telencephalon in the embryo.

rhinencephalus (ri″nen-sef′ah-lus) rhinocephalus.

rhinenchysis (ri-nen′kĭ-sis) [rhin- + enchein to pour in] injection of a medicinal fluid into the nose.

rhinesthesia (ri″nes-the′ze-ah) [rhin- + Gr. aisthēsis perception] the sense of smell.

rhineurynter (rīn″u-rin′ter) [rhin- + Gr. eurynein to widen] a dilatable rubber bag for distending a nostril.

rhinion (rin′e-on) [Gr., dim. of rhis] the lower end of the suture between the nasal bones.

rhinism (ri′nizm) a nasal quality of voice.

rhinitis (ri-ni′tis) [rhin- + -itis] inflammation of the mucous membrane of the nose. **acute catarrhal r.,** coryza, or cold in the head; an acute congestion of the mucous membrane of the nose, marked by dryness, followed by increased mucous secretion from the membrane, impeded respiration through the nose, and some pain. **allergic r., anaphylactic r.,** a general term used to denote any allergic reaction of the nasal mucosa; it may occur perennially (nonseasonal allergic rhinitis) or seasonally (hay fever). **atopic r.,** nonseasonal allergic r. **atrophic r.,** a chronic form marked by wasting of the mucous membrane and the glands. **atrophic r. of swine,** a disease of very young swine that may result in marked displacement or atrophy of the turbinate bones in severe cases, due to severe persistent inflammation of the nasal mucosa; the primary inflammatory reaction may be caused by a variety of agents, including a virus (see inclusion-body r.). **r. caseo′sa,** rhinitis with a caseous, gelatinous, and fetid discharge. **chronic catarrhal r.,** a form characterized by hypertrophy and later by atrophy of the mucous and submucous tissues. **croupous r.,** fibrinous r. **dyscrinic r.,** rhinitis associated with and dependent on endocrine imbalance. **fibrinous r.,** a form characterized by the development of a false membrane; called also croupous r. **gangrenous r.,** a gangrene-like inflammation of the nasal mucosa. **hypertrophic r.,** a form in which the mucous membrane thickens and swells. **inclusion-body r.,** atrophic rhinitis of swine due to a viral infection, frequently marked by atrophy of the turbinate bones and distortion of the snout, sneezing, stunting of growth, and, histologically, by the presence of inclusion bodies in scrapings of the nasal mucous membranes. **membranous r.,** chronic rhinitis with the formation of a membranous exudate. **nonseasonal allergic r.,** allergic rhinitis that may occur continuously or intermittently all year round; it is caused by an allergen to which the individual is more or less always exposed, such as house dust, danders, and food, and is characterized by sudden attacks of sneezing, swelling of the nasal mucosa with a profuse watery discharge, itching of the eyes, and lacrimation. Called also atopic or perennial r. Cf. hay fever. **perennial r.,** nonseasonal allergic r. **pseudomembranous r.,** a form in which the inflamed region is covered with an opaque exudation. **purulent r.,** chronic rhinitis with the formation of pus. **scrofulous r.,** tuberculous rhinitis. **r. sic′ca,** a variety of atrophic rhinitis in which the secretion is entirely absent. **syphilitic r.,** a variety caused by syphilis, and marked by ulceration, caries of the nasal bone, and a fetid discharge. **tuberculous r.,** a variety due to tuberculosis, and attended with ulceration, caries of the nasal bone, and ozena. **vasomotor r.,** 1. a form of nonallergic rhinitis in which transient changes in vascular tone and permeability, with the same symptoms as in allergic rhinitis, are brought on by such stimuli as mild chilling, fatigue, anger, and anxiety. 2. any condition of allergic or nonallergic rhinitis, as opposed to infectious rhinitis.

rhino-, rhin- (ri′no, rīn, rin) [Gr. rhis nose] a combining form denoting relationship to the nose, or a noselike structure.

rhinoanemometer (ri″no-an″ĕ-mom′ĕ-ter) [rhino- + anemometer] an apparatus for measuring the air passing through the nose during respiration.

rhinoantritis (ri″no-an-tri′tis) [rhino- + antrum + -itis] inflammation of the nasal cavity and the antrum of Highmore.

rhinobyon (ri-no′be-on) [rhino- + Gr. byein to plug] a nasal tampon.

rhinocanthectomy (ri″no-kan-thek′to-me) rhinommectomy.

rhinocele (ri′no-sēl) rhinocoele.

Rhinocephalus annulatus (ri″no-sef′ah-lus an″u-la′tus) Boophilus annulatus.

rhinocephalus (ri″no-sef′ah-lus) a fetus exhibiting rhinocephaly.

rhinocephaly (ri″no-sef′ah-le) [rhino- + Gr. kephalē head + -ia] a developmental anomaly characterized by the presence of a proboscis-like nose above eyes partially or completely fused into one.

rhinocheiloplasty (ri″no-ki′lo-plas″te) [rhino- + Gr. cheilos lip + plassein to form] plastic surgery of the nose and lip.

rhinocleisis (ri″no-kli′sis) [rhino- + Gr. kleisis closure] obstruction of the nasal passages.

rhinocoele (ri′no-sēl) [rhino- + Gr. koilia hollow] the ventricle of the olfactory lobe of the brain.

rhinodacryolith (ri″no-dak′re-o-lith″) [rhino- + Gr. dakryon tear + lithos stone] a lacrimal concretion in the nasal duct.

rhinodynia (ri″no-din′e-ah) [rhino- + Gr. odynē pain + -ia] pain in the nose.

rhinoentomophthoromycosis (ri″no-en″to-mof″tho-ro-mi-ko′sis) rhinophycomycosis.

Rhinoestrus (rīn-es′trus) a genus of flies of the family Oestridae whose larvae occur in the nasal passages of horses in Europe, Asia and Africa; they may deposit larvae in the human eye.

rhinogenous (ri-noj′ĕ-nus) [rhino- + Gr. gennan to produce] arising in the nose.

rhinokyphosis (ri″no-ki-fo′sis) [rhino- + Gr. kyphos hump] the presence of an abnormal hump in the ridge of the nose.

rhinolalia (ri″no-la′le-ah) [rhino- + Gr. lalia speech] a nasal quality of voice due to some disease or defect of the nasal passages. **r. aper′ta,** that which is caused by undue patency of the posterior nares. **r. clau′sa,** that which is due to undue closure of the nasal passages. **open r.,** r. aperta.

rhinolaryngitis (ri″no-lar″in-ji′tis) inflammation of the mucous membrane of the nose and larynx.

rhinolaryngology (ri″no-lar″in-gol′o-je) [rhino- + Gr. larynx larynx + -logy] the sum of knowledge concerning the nose and larynx and their diseases.

rhinolith (ri′no-lith) [rhino- + Gr. lithos stone] a nasal stone or concretion.

rhinolithiasis (ri″no-lĭ-thi′ah-sis) a condition associated with the formation of rhinoliths.

rhinologist (ri-nol′o-jist) a specialist in rhinology.

rhinology (ri-nol′o-je) [rhino- + -logy] the sum of knowledge regarding the nose and its diseases.

rhinomanometer (ri″no-mah-nom′ĕ-ter) [rhino- + manometer] a manometer used in rhinomanometry.

rhinomanometry (ri″no-mah-nom′ĕ-tre) measurement of the airflow and pressure within the nose during respiration; nasal resistance or obstruction can be calculated from the data obtained.

rhinometer (ri-nom′ĕ-ter) [rhino- + Gr. metron measure] an instrument for measuring the nose or its cavities.

rhinommectomy (ri″nom-mek′to-me) [rhin- + Gr. omma eye + ektomē excision] excision of the inner canthus of the eye.

rhinomycosis (ri″no-mi-ko′sis) fungal infection of the nasal mucosa.

rhinonecrosis (ri″no-nĕ-kro′sis) necrosis of the nasal bones.

rhinonemmeter (ri″no-nem′ĕ-ter) a device for measuring nasal air flow rates.

rhinoneurosis (ri″no-nu-ro′sis) a neurosis or functional disease of the nose.

rhinopathia (ri″no-path′e-ah) rhinopathy. **r. vasomoto′ria,** vasomotor rhinitis.

rhinopathy (ri-nop′ah-the) [rhino- + Gr. pathos disease] any disease of the nose.

rhinopharyngeal (ri″no-fah-rin′je-al) nasopharyngeal.

rhinopharyngitis (ri″no-far″in-ji′tis) inflammation of the nasopharynx. **r. mu′tilans,** gangosa.

rhinopharyngocele (ri″no-fah-ring′go-sēl) a tumor, usually an aerocele, of the nasopharynx.

rhinopharyngolith (ri″no-fah-ring′go-lith) [rhino- + Gr. pharynx pharynx + lithos stone] calculus of the nasal pharynx.

rhinopharynx (ri″no-far′inks) nasopharynx (pars nasalis pharyngis [NA]).

rhinophonia (ri″no-fo′ne-ah) [rhino- + Gr. phōnē voice] a nasal twang or quality of voice.

rhinophore (ri′no-fōr) [rhino- + Gr. phoros bearing] a nasal cannula to facilitate breathing.

rhinophycomycosis (ri″no-fi″ko-mi-ko′sis) a fungal infection caused by Entomophthora coronata, marked by development of large polyps in the subcutaneous tissues of the nose and paranasal sinuses; orbital involvement with unilateral blindness may follow. It usually leads to cerebral involvement. Called also phycomycosis entomophthorae and rhinoentomophthoromycosis.

rhinophyma (re″no-fi′mah) [rhino- + Gr. phyma growth] a form of rosacea characterized by redness, sebaceous hyperplasia, and nodular swelling and congestion of the skin of the nose.

rhinoplastic (ri″no-plas′tik) pertaining to rhinoplasty.

rhinoplasty (ri′no-plas″te) [rhino- + Gr. plassein to form] a plastic surgical operation on the nose, either reconstructive,

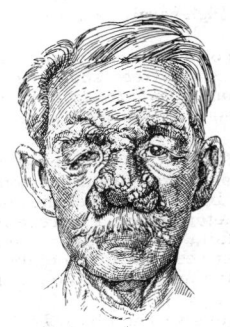

Rhinophyma (Homans).

restorative, or cosmetic. **Carpue's r.,** Indian r. **English r.,** that in which a nose is formed out of flaps from the cheeks. **Indian r.,** the reconstruction of a nose by a flap of skin taken from the forehead, with its pedicle at the root of the nose; called also *Carpue's operation*. **Italian r.,** tagliacotian r. **tagliacotian r.,** the reconstruction of a nose by a flap of skin taken from the arm, the flap remaining attached to the arm until union has taken place; called also *Italian* or *tagliacotian operation*.

rhinopneumonitis (ri″no-nu″mo-ni′tis) [*rhino-* + Gr. *pneumōn* lung + *-itis*] inflammation of the nasal and pulmonary mucous membranes. **equine viral r.,** a highly contagious disease of horses caused by a herpesvirus, which is marked by a mild respiratory infection in young animals and abortion in young mares exposed to the infection for the first time; in the latter instance, it is called *equine virus abortion*.

rhinopolypus (ri″no-pol′ĭ-pus) a nasal polyp.

rhinoptia (ri-nop′she-ah) esotropia.

rhinoreaction (ri″no-re-ak′shun) the nasal tuberculin reaction; an exudation appearing on the nasal mucous membrane after the application thereto of a solution of tuberculin in patients affected with tuberculosis. Called also *Moeller's reaction*.

rhinorrhagia (ri″no-ra′je-ah) [*rhino-* + Gr. *rhēgnynai* to burst forth] nosebleed; epistaxis.

rhinorrhaphy (ri-nor′ah-fe) [*rhino-* + Gr. *rhaphē* suture] an operation for epicanthus performed by excising a fold of skin from the nose and closing the opening with sutures.

rhinorrhea (ri″no-re′ah) [*rhino-* + Gr. *rhoia* flow] the free discharge of a thin nasal mucus. **cerebrospinal r.,** discharge of cerebrospinal fluid through the nose.

rhinosalpingitis (ri″no-sal-pin-ji′tis) [*rhino-* + Gr. *salpinx* tube + *-itis*] inflammation of the nasal mucosa and the eustachian tube.

rhinoscleroma (ri″no-skle-ro′mah) [*rhino-* + Gr. *sklērōma* a hard swelling] a granulomatous disease involving the nose and nasopharynx. The growth forms hard patches or nodules, which tend to increase in size and are painful on pressure. The disease occurs in Egypt, Eastern Europe, and Central and South America and is ascribed to the presence of the *Klebsiella rhinoscleromatis*.

rhinoscope (ri′no-skōp) [*rhino-* + Gr. *skopein* to examine] a speculum for use in nasal examinations.

rhinoscopic (ri″no-skop′ik) pertaining to rhinoscopy.

rhinoscopy (ri-nos′ko-pe) the examination of the nasal passages, either through the anterior nares (*anterior r.*) or through the nasopharynx (*posterior r.*). **median r.,** examination of the nasal cavity and the openings of the ethmoid cells, etc., by means of a long nasal speculum.

rhinosporidiosis (ri″no-spo-rid″e-o′sis) a fungal disease caused by *Rhinosporidium seeberi*, which is endemic in India and Ceylon and sporadic in other parts of the world; the fungus reproduces in tissue by endospores in a spherule similar to that seen in coccidioidomycosis. It affects man and other animals, and is characterized by the development of large pedunculated polyps on the mucosa of the nose, eyes, ears, and sometimes on the penis or vagina.

Rhinosporidium seeberi (ri″no-spo-rid′e-um se′ber-i) the fungus which causes rhinosporidiosis.

rhinostegnosis (ri″no-steg-no′sis) [*rhino-* + Gr. *stegnōsis* obstruction] obstruction of a nasal passage.

rhinostenosis (ri″no-stĕ-no′sis) narrowing of a nasal passage.

rhinotomy (ri-not′o-me) [*rhino-* + Gr. *tomē* a cutting] incision into the nose.

rhinotracheitis (ri″no-tra″ke-i′tis) [*rhino-* + L. *trachea* + *-itis*] inflammation of the nasal mucous membranes and trachea. **feline r., feline viral r.,** an acute, febrile, herpesvirus infection of the upper respiratory tract and conjunctivae affecting young kittens; it is marked by a mucopurulent discharge from the eyes and nose, photophobia, coughing, and sneezing. **infectious r., infectious bovine r.,** an acute, infectious, febrile disease of cattle, caused by a herpesvirus and marked by inflammation and ulceration of the upper respiratory tract, which may be followed

by pneumonia, coughing, profuse discharge from the eyes and nose, excessive salivation, anorexia, and, in pregnant cows, abortion.

rhinovaccination (ri″no-vak″sĭ-na′shun) the application of vaccine or other immunizing material to the mucous membrane of the nose.

rhinoviral (ri″no-vi′ral) pertaining to or caused by rhinoviruses.

rhinovirus (ri″no-vi′rus) any of a subgroup of the picornaviruses considered to be etiologically associated with the common cold and certain other upper respiratory ailments; over 90 antigenically distinct strains are known to cause the common cold. Called also *coryzavirus*.

rhiotin (ri′o-tin) a biotin vitamin which is active for *Rhizobium* but not for yeast, is avidin-combinable, and stable to acid or neutral autoclaving.

Rhipicentor (ri″pĭ-sen′tor) [Gr. *rhipis* fan + *kentein* to prick or stab] a genus of ticks. The bite of *R. bicor′nis* (*Ixodes bicornis*), a Mexican tick that infests the cougar, may cause a high fever in the human adult and may kill a child.

Rhipicephalus (ri″pĭ-sef′ah-lus) [Gr. *rhipis* fan + *kephalē* head] a genus of cattle ticks, species of which are the agents in transmitting *Babesia* of cattle fever, and other diseases. **R. appendicula′tus,** the brown tick; it transmits *Theileria parva*, the cause of East Coast fever in African cattle. **R. bur′sa,** a species that transmits *Babesia ovis*, which causes icterohematuria and carceag of sheep. **R. capen′sis,** an African species found on cattle and horses, which may transmit *Theileria parva*, the cause of East Coast fever. **R. decolora′tus,** a species regarded as the transmitter of *Borrelia theileri*, the cause of tickborne relapsing fever, of *Rickettsia conorii*, causing tickborne typhus, and of bovine anaplasmosis in some parts of Africa. **R. evert′si,** an African species found on horses and cattle; it may transmit *Theileria parva* and *Rickettsia conorii*. **R. sanguin′eus,** the brown dog tick, a species found on many domestic animals; it transmits *Rickettsia rickettsii*, the cause of Rocky Mountain spotted fever, *R. conorii*, the cause of tickborne typhus and Boutonneuse fever in man, and *Babesia canis*, the cause of malignant jaundice in dogs. **R. si′mus,** the black pitted tick, a species which transmits *Theileria parva*, the cause of East Coast fever.

rhitid- for words beginning thus, see those beginning *rhytid-*.

rhizagra (ri-zag′rah) [*rhizo-* + Gr. *agra* seizure] an ancient forceps which was used for extracting roots of teeth.

rhizanesthesia (ri-zan″es-the′ze-ah) anesthesia produced by injecting a local anesthetic into the spinal arachnoid space.

rhizo- (ri′zo) [Gr. *rhiza* root] a combining form denoting relationship to a root.

Rhizobiaceae (ri-zo″be-a′se-e) a family of Schizomycetes (order Eubacteriales), made up of rod-shaped, sparsely flagellated cells without endospores; it includes three genera, *Agrobacterium*, *Chromobacterium*, and *Rhizobium*.

Rhizobium (ri-zo′be-um) a genus of microorganisms of the family Rhizobiaceae, order Eubacteriales, made up of gram-negative, rod-shaped, symbiotic nitrogen-fixing bacteria, producing nodules on the roots of leguminous plants and fixing free nitrogen in this symbiosis. It includes six species, *R. japo′nicum*, *R. leguminosa′rum*, *R. lupi′ni*, *R. melilo′ti*, *R. phase′oli*, and *R. trifo′lii*.

rhizoblast (ri′zo-blast) a delicate fibril connecting the basal granule and nucleus of a protozoon.

rhizodontropy (ri″zo-don′tro-pe) [*rhizo-* + Gr. *odous* tooth + *tropos* a turn] the fixation of an artificial crown upon the natural root of a tooth.

rhizodontrypy (ri″zo-don′trĭ-pe) perforation of the root of a tooth for the escape of morbid matter.

Rhizoglyphus (ri-zog′lĭ-fus) a genus of mites. **R. parasit′icus,** the coolie-itch mite, which lives on the ground in India and is reported to cause sore feet in the tea plantation workers.

rhizoid (ri′zoid) [*rhizo-* + Gr. *eidos* form] rootlike; resembling a root.

rhizoidal (ri-zoi′dal) rhizoid.

rhizolysis (ri-zol′ĭ-sis) interruption of spinal nerve roots by coagulation with radiofrequency waves.

Rhizomastigida (ri″zo-mas-tij′ĭ-dah) an order of protozoa of the class Zoomastigophora, subphylum Mastigophora, embracing organisms having both flagella and pseudopodia; it includes the genus *Histomonas*.

rhizome (ri′zōm) [Gr. *rhizōma* root stem] the subterraneous root stock of a plant.

rhizomelic (ri-zo-mel′ik) [*rhizo-* + Gr. *melos* limb] pertaining to or involving the hip joint and shoulder joint.

rhizomeningomyelitis (ri″zo-mĕ-nin″go-mi″ĕ-li′tis) radiculomeningomyelitis.

rhizoneure (ri′zo-nūr) [*rhizo-* + Gr. *neuron* nerve] a nerve cell which forms a nerve root.

rhizoplast (ri′zo-plast) [*rhizo-* + Gr. *plastos* formed] a fibril that connects the blepharoplast to the nucleus in some flagellate protozoa; called also *zygoplast*.

Rhizopoda (ri-zop′o-dah) [*rhizo-* + Gr. *pous* foot] 1. a class of protozoa of the subphylum Sarcodina, having lobopodia, filopodia, or rhizopodia, and including the orders Amoebida and Mycetozoida. 2. Sarcodina.

rhizopodium (ri″zo-po′dĭ-um), pl. *rhizopo′dia* [*rhizo-* + Gr. *pous* foot] a filamentous pseudopodium, finer than a filopodium, characterized by branching and anastomosis of the branches; cf. *axopodium, filopodium,* and *lobopodium*.

Rhizopus (ri-zo′pus) a genus of fungi of the family Mucoraceae, order Mucorales; see *mucormycosis. R. arrhizus* and *R. oryzae* have been isolated from uncontrolled acidotic diabetics demonstrating cerebral infections, and *R. rhizopodoformis* has been isolated from cutaneous lesions of diabetics and severely burned patients.

rhizotomist (ri-zot′o-mist) in Greek medicine, a vagrant gatherer of medicinal herbs and simples.

rhizotomy (ri-zot′o-me) [*rhizo-* + Gr. *tomē* a cutting] interruption of the roots of spinal nerves within the spinal canal. **anterior r.,** division of the anterior or motor spinal nerve roots; done for relief of essential hypertension. **posterior r.,** division of the posterior or sensory spinal nerve roots; done for relief of intractable pain. **retrogasserian r.,** transection of the sensory root fibers of the trigeminal nerve for the permanent relief of trigeminal neuralgia; called also *retrogasserian neurotomy*.

rhodamine (ro-dah′min) [Gr. *rhodon* rose + *amine*] a red fluorescent dye.

rhodanate (ro′dah-nāt) a salt of thiocyanic acid.

rhodanine (ro-dah′nin) chemical name: 2-thioxo-4-thiazolidinone. An acid, $C_3H_3NOS_2$, used in the synthesis of phenylalanine. Called also *rhodanic acid*.

rhodium (ro′de-um) [Gr. *rhodon* rose] a hard and rare metal of the platinum group; atomic number, 45; atomic weight, 102.905; symbol, Rh.

Rhodnius prolixus (rod′ne-us pro-lik′sus) a reduviid bug from South America capable of transmitting *Trypanosoma cruzi,* the etiologic agent of Chagas' disease.

rhodo- (ro′do) [Gr. *rhodon* rose] a combining form meaning red.

Rhodobacteriineae (ro″do-bak″ter-e-i′ne-e) a suborder of Schizomycetes (order Pseudomonadales), made up of spherical or rod-, vibrio-, or spiral-shaped cells containing bacteriochlorophyll or other green pigments resembling chorophyll, and usually one or more carotenoid pigments. It includes three families, *Athiorhodaceae, Chlorobacteriaceae,* and *Thiorhodaceae*.

rhodogenesis (ro″do-jen′ĕ-sis) [*rhodo-* + Gr. *genesis* production] the restoration of the purple tint to rhodopsin after it has become bleached by the action of light.

Rhodomicrobium (ro″do-mi-kro′be-um) a genus of microorganisms of the family Hyphomicrobiaceae, order Hyphomicrobiales, made up of ovoid cells connected by filaments, growing in colonies which are salmon pink to orange red. The type species is *R. vanniel′ii*.

rhodophane (ro′do-fān) [*rhodo-* + Gr. *phainein* to show] a red pigment, or chromophane, from the retinal cones of birds and fishes.

rhodophylactic (ro″do-fi-lak′tik) tending to preserve or restore the retinal purple; pertaining to rhodophylaxis.

rhodophylaxis (ro″do-fi-lak′sis) [*rhodo-* + Gr. *phylaxis* defense] the supposed property of the retinal epithelium of protecting and increasing the power of the retinal purple to regain its color after bleaching.

rhodoporphyrin (ro″do-por′fĭ-rin) a porphyrin, $C_{32}H_{34}O_4N_4$, derived from chlorophyll.

Rhodopseudomonas (ro″do-su″do-mo′nas) a genus of microorganisms of the family Athiorhodaceae, suborder Rhodobacteriineae, order Pseudomonadales, occurring as motile, spherical or rod-shaped cells. It includes four species, *R. capsula′ta, R. gelatino′sa, R. palus′tris,* and *R. spheroi′des*.

rhodopsin (ro-dop′sin) [*rhodo-* + Gr. *opsis* vision] visual purple: a photosensitive purple-red chromoprotein in the retinal rods which is bleached to visual yellow (all-*trans* retinal) by light, thereby producing stimulation of the retinal sensory endings. It is a conjugated protein, the prosthetic group of which is 11-*cis* retinal.

Rhodospirillum (ro″do-spi-ril′lum) a genus of microorganisms of the family Athiorhodaceae, suborder Rhodobacteriineae, order Pseudomonadales, occurring as motile, spiral-shaped cells. It includes four species, *R. ful′vum, R. molischia′num, R. photome′tricum,* and *R. ru′brum*.

Rhodothece (ro″do-the′se) a genus of microorganisms of the family Thiorhodaceae, suborder Rhodobacteriineae, order Pseudomonadales, occurring as single spherical cells, each with a wide capsule. The type species is *R. pen′dens*.

Rhodotorula (ro″do-tor′u-lah) a genus of imperfect yeasts. **R. glu′tinis,** a nonpathogenic species from air, potatoes, and the skin in seborrhea; its cells are cylindrical, oval, or spherical and it forms a rosy pigment. Called also *Saccharomyces glutinis*.

R. ru′bra, a skin contaminant which rarely causes opportunistic infections in man.

rhodotoxin (ro″do-tok′sin) a poisonous compound from the flowers and leaves of various shrubs and trees, such as *Rhododendron;* it is also found in honey from *Rhododendron* flowers.

RhoGAM (ro′gam) trademark for a preparation of Rho (D) immune globulin.

rhombencephalon (rom″ben-sef′ah-lon) [Gr. *rhombos* rhomb + *enkephalos* brain] 1. [NA] the part of the brain developed from the posterior of the three primary brain vesicles of the embryonic neural tube; it comprises the metencephalon (cerebellum and pons) and myelencephalon (medulla oblongata). 2. the most caudal of the three primary brain vesicles in the embryo, later dividing into the metencephalon and myelencephalon. Called also *hindbrain*.

rhombocoele (rom′bo-sēl) [Gr. *rhombos* rhomb + *koilia* cavity] the terminal distention of the canal of the spinal cord.

rhomboid (rom′boid) [Gr. *rhombos* rhomb + *eidos* form] having a shape similar to a rectangle that has been skewed to one side so that the angles are oblique. **Michaelis's r.,** a diamond-shaped area over the posterior aspect of the pelvis formed by the dimples of the posterior-superior spines of the ilia, the lines formed by the gluteal muscles, and the groove at the end of the spine.

rhombomere (rom′bo-mēr) neuromere, def. 1.

rhonchal, rhonchial (rong′kal, rong′ke-al) pertaining to, or of the nature of, a ronchus.

rhonchus (rong′kus), pl. *rhon′chi* [L.; Gr. *rhonchos* a snoring sound] a rattling in the throat; also a dry, coarse rale in the bronchial tubes, due to a partial obstruction. See *rale*.

Rhopalopsyllus cavicola (ro″pah-lo-sil′us kah-vik′o-lah) the South American cavy flea, which transmits *Pasteurella pestis*.

rhotanium (ro-ta′ne-um) a gold-palladium alloy said to possess the same physical qualities as platinum.

rhubarb (roo′barb) the dried rhizome and root of *Rheum officinale* Baill., used in fluidextract or aromatic tincture as a cathartic. The common garden rhubarb, *R. rhaponticum* L., is edible and devoid of cathartic principles.

Rhuphos (roo′fos) see *Rufus of Ephesus*.

Rhus (rus) [L., gen. *rhois*] a genus of anacardiaceous vines and shrubs, many of them poisonous. Some species contain a highly allergenic oleoresin mixture known as *urushiol;* contact with these species produces a severe dermatitis in sensitive persons (see *rhus dermatitis,* under *dermatitis*). The most important toxic species are *R. radicans* L. (poison ivy), *R. diversiloba* L. (poison oak or western poison oak), and *R. vernix* L. (poison sumac). Extracts of the leaves and twigs of these plants (poison ivy extract, poison oak extract) have been used in the prophylaxis and treatment of dermatitis associated with these species. Called also *Toxicodendron*.

Rhynchocoela (rin-ko-sēl′ah) [Gr. *rhynchos* snout, bill, beak + *-coele*] the ribbon worms, a phylum of slender, flat, soft, often brightly colored, acoelmate worms which have unsegmented bodies and an eversible proboscis that lies in a special cavity in front of the mouth; most species are marine inhabitants. Called also *Nemertea* and *Nemertina*.

rhynchocoelan (rin-ko-sēl′an) a ribbon worm; any individual of the Rhynchocoela; called also *nemertean*.

rhyostomaturia (ri″o-sto″mah-tu′re-ah) [Gr. *rhein* to flow + *stoma* mouth + *ouron* urine + *-ia*] the excretion of urinary elements by the salivary glands.

rhyparia (ri-pa′re-ah) [Gr. "filth"] materia alba.

rhythm (rith′m) [L. *rhythmus;* Gr. *rhythmos*] a measured movement; the recurrence of an action or function at regular intervals. **alpha r.,** a uniform rhythm of waves in the normal electroencephalogram, showing an average frequency of 10 per second; called also *Berger r.* See under *wave*. **atrioventricular r.,** nodal r. **Berger r.,** alpha r. **beta r.,** a rhythm in the electroencephalogram consisting of waves smaller than those of the alpha rhythm, having an average frequency of 25 per second; see under *wave*. **biological r.,** the established regularity with which certain phenomena recur in living organisms. **cantering r.,** gallop r. **circadian r.,** the regular recurrence in cycles of approximately 24 hours from one stated point to another, as certain biological activities which occur at that interval, regardless of constant darkness or other conditions of illumination. **circus r.,** circus movement or contraction; a movement travelling in circular fashion around a ring of muscle. **coupled r.,** heart beats occurring in pairs, the second beat of the pair usually being a ventricular premature beat; see also *bigeminal pulse* and *bigeminy*. **delta r.,** see under *wave*. **ectopic r.,** a heart rhythm initiated by a focus outside the sinoatrial node. **escape r.,** a heart rhythm initiated by lower centers when the sinoatrial node fails to initiate impulses, its rhythmicity is depressed, or its impulses are completely blocked. **fetal r.,** embryocardia. **gallop r.,** an auscultatory finding of three (*triple r.*) or four heart sounds, the extra sound(s) by convention being in diastole and related than to atrial contraction (*fourth sound, presystolic gallop*), to early rapid filling of a ventricle with an altered ventricular compliance (*protodiastolic gallop*), or to concurrence of atrial contraction and ventricular early rapid filling (*summation gallop*). **gallop r., systolic,** systolic gallop. **gamma r.,** a rhythm of waves in the electroencephalogram having a frequency of 50 per second. **idioventricular r.,** a cardiac rhythm wherein the ventricle follows an intrinsic pacemaker different from that of the atrium; see *atrioventricular dissociation,* under *dissociation.* **infradian r.,** the regular recurrence in cycles of more than 24 hours from one stated point to another, as certain biological activities which occur at such intervals, regardless of conditions of illumination. **isochronal r.,** see *cilium* (def. 3). **metachronal r.,** see *cilium* (def. 3). **nodal r.,** heart rhythm initiated in the specialized junctional tissue, i.e., the atrioventricular node and the main (His) bundle. Called also *nodal arrhythmia.* **nyctohemeral r.,** a day and night rhythm. **pendulum r.,** alternation in the rhythm of the heart sounds in which the diastolic sound is equal in time, character, and loudness to the systolic sound, the beat of the heart resembling the tick of a watch. **reciprocal r.,** a heart rhythm produced with the occurrence of many reciprocal beats. **sinus r.,** normal heart rhythm originating in the sinoatrial node. **theta r.,** see under *wave.* **triple r.,** the cadence produced when three heart sounds recur in successive cardiac cycles; see also *gallop r.* **ultradian r.,** the regular recurrence in cycles of less than 24 hours from one stated point to another, as certain biological activities which occur at such intervals, regardless of conditions of illumination. **ventricular r.,** the ventricular contractions which occur in cases of complete heart block.

rhythmeur (rith-mer′) a device for making rhythmic interruptions of the current in an x-ray machine.

rhythmical (rith′me-kal) characterized by rhythm.

rhythmicity (rith-mis′ĭ-te) in cardiology, the ability to beat, or the state of beating, rhythmically without external stimuli.

rhythmophone (rith′mo-fōn) [Gr. *rhythmos* rhythm + *phōnē* voice] (*obs.*) an instrument for magnifying the sounds of the heart beat.

rhythmotherapy (rith″mo-ther′ah-pe) [Gr. *rhythmos* rhythm + *therapeia* treatment] the use of rhythm in treating disease, as the beating of time in treating stammering.

rhytidectomy (rit″ĭ-dek′to-me) [Gr. *rhytis* wrinkle + *ektomē* excision] excision of skin for the elimination of wrinkles.

rhytidoplasty (rit′ĭ-do-plas″te) plastic surgery for the elimination of wrinkles from the skin.

rhytidosis (rit″ĭ-do′sis) [Gr. *rhytidōsis; rhytis* wrinkle] a wrinkling of the cornea.

rib (rib) any one of the paired elastic arches of bone, twelve on either side, that extend from the thoracic vertebrae toward the median line on the ventral aspect of the trunk, forming the major part of the thoracic skeleton. The upper seven (true ribs) are connected ventrally with the sternum. The lower five (false ribs) are not. Collectively called *costae* [NA]. **abdominal r's, asternal r's,** false r's. **bicipital r.,** an anomalous rib resulting from fusion of the anterior part of the seventh cervical vertebra with the first thoracic rib. **cervical r.,** a supernumerary rib arising from a cervical vertebra. **false r's,** the lower five ribs on either side, which are not directly attached to the sternum; called also *costae spuriae* [NA]. **floating r's,** the lower two ribs on either side, which ordinarily have no ventral attachment. **slipping r.,** a rib whose attaching cartilage is repeatedly dislocated. **spurious r's,** false r's. **sternal r's,** true r's. **Stiller's r.,** an abnormally movable tenth rib. **true r's,** the upper seven ribs on either side, which are connected to the sides of the sternum by their costal cartilages; called also *costae verae* [NA]. **vertebral r's,** floating r's. **vertebrocostal r's,** the upper three false ribs of either side, articulating with the vertebrae and connected by cartilage to the costal cartilage of the ipsilateral seventh rib. **vertebrosternal r's,** true r's. **Zahn's r's,** see under *line.*

ribaminol (ri-bah′mĭ-nōl) chemical name: ribonucleic acid compound with 2-(diethylamino)ethanol; a memory adjuvant.

ribavirin (ri″bah-vi′rin) chemical name: 1β-D-ribofuranosyl-1*H*-1,2,4-triazole-3-carboxamide; an antiviral, $C_8H_{12}N_4O_5$.

Ribbert's theory (rib′erts) [Moritz Wilhelm Hugo *Ribbert,* German pathologist, 1855–1920] see under *theory.*

ribbon (rib′un) a band-like structure. **r. of Reil,** the rostral part of the lemniscus medialis. **synaptic r.,** 1. a dense lamella surrounded by a halo of synaptic vesicles, found at a right angle to the apex of the synaptic ridge in the outer plexiform layer of the retina. 2. a similar structure found in varying numbers in the cytoplasm of the hair cells of the ear.

Ribes's ganglion (rēbz) [François *Ribes,* French surgeon, 1800–1864] see under *ganglion.*

ribitol (ri′bĭ-tol) an alcohol corresponding to the sugar ribose; it is a constituent of a class of teichoic acids.

ribodesose (ri-bo′des-ōs) D-2-deoxyribose.

riboflavin (ri″bo-fla′vin) the heat-stable factor of the vitamin B complex, 6,7-dimethyl-9-[1′-D-ribityl]-isoalloxazin, $C_{17}H_{20}N_4O_6$; called also *lactoflavin* and *vitamin B₂.* A water-soluble vitamin, it serves as a component of two coenzymes or prosthetic groups (FAD and FMN) of flavoproteins, which function as hydrogen

carriers in oxidation-reduction processes. It occurs in milk, muscle, liver, kidney, eggs, grass, malt, leafy young vegetables, and various algae, and is an essential nutrient for man, the requirement being related to body size, metabolic rate, and growth rate. Deficiency of the vitamin is known as *ariboflavinosis* (q.v.). A standardized preparation [USP], occurring as a yellow to orange-yellow, crystalline powder, containing 98 to 102 per cent of riboflavin, calculated on the dried basis, is used in the treatment and prophylaxis of riboflavin deficiency, administered orally and parenterally. **r. kinase,** an enzyme (a phosphotransferase) that catalyzes the conversion of free riboflavin and ATP to flavin mononucleotide (FMN) and ADP. **r. phosphate,** flavin mononucleotide.

ribonuclease (ri″bo-nu″kle-ās) an enzyme of the transferase class which catalyzes the depolymerization of ribonucleic acid.

ribonucleoprotein (ri″bo-nu″kle-o-pro′te-in) a substance composed of both protein and ribonucleic acid.

ribonucleoside (ri″bo-nu′kle-o-sīd) a nucleoside in which the purine or pyrimidine base is combined with ribose.

ribonucleotide (ri″bo-nu′kle-o-tīd) a nucleotide in which the purine or pyrimidine base is combined with ribose.

riboprine (ri′bo-prēn) chemical name: *N*-(3-methyl-2-butenyl)-adenosine; an antineoplastic, $C_{43}H_{58}N_2O_{13}$.

ribopyranose (ri″bo-pi′rah-nōs) ribose in cyclic hemiacetal form.

ribose (ri′bōs) an aldopentose, $CH_2OH(CHOH)_3CHO$, found in ribonucleic acid (RNA) and in adenosine triphosphate (ATP).

ribosome (ri′bo-sōm) any of the intracellular ribonucleoprotein particles concerned with protein synthesis; they consist of reversibly dissociable units and are found either bound to membranes or free in the cytoplasm. They may occur singly or in clusters (polysomes). Ribosomes within cell organelles and in prokaryotic cells generally are smaller than the cytoplasmic ribosomes of eukaryotic cells. Ribosomes of glandular cells have been called *ergastoplasm,* and those of nerve cells *Nissl bodies.*

ribosyl (ri′bo-sil) a glycosyl radical, $C_5H_9O_4$, formed from ribose.

5-ribosyluridine (ri″bo-sil-u′rĭ-dēn) pseudouridine.

ribothymidine (ri″bo-thi′mĭ-dēn) the ribosyl analogue of thymidine, a rare base found in small amounts in transfer-RNA.

ribulose (ri′bu-lōs) the 2-ketose isomer of ribose.

R.I.C. Royal Institute of Chemistry.

rice (rīs) the cereal plant, *Oryza sativa;* also its seed or grain. The grain consists mainly of starch, and is used as a food and as a dusting powder. **r. polishings,** fine yellowish powder from the pericarp and germ of rice; used in vitamin B deficiency. **white r.,** rice from which the outer brown coats have been removed; a diet composed too exclusively of white rice is apt to produce beriberi.

Richards (rich′ardz), Dickinson W. United States physician, born 1895; co-winner, with Werner T. O. Forssmann and André F. Cournand, of the Nobel prize for medicine and physiology in 1956, for developing new techniques to measure more precisely lung and heart function.

Richardson's sign (rich′ard-sunz) [Sir Benjamin Ward *Richardson,* London physician, 1828–1896] see under *sign.*

Richet (re-shā′), Charles Robert. French physiologist, 1850–1935, noted for his discovery of anaphylaxis; winner of the Nobel prize for medicine and physiology in 1913.

Richet's aneurysm (re-shāz′) [Didier Dominique Alfred *Richet,* French surgeon, 1816–1891] a fusiform aneurysm.

Richter's hernia (rik′terz) [August Gottlieb *Richter,* surgeon in Göttingen, 1742–1812] see under *hernia.*

Richter-Monro line (rik′ter mon-ro′) see *Monro-Richter,* and under *line.*

ricin (ri′sin) a poisonous substance (phytotoxin) found in the seeds of the castor oil plant (*Ricinus communis*).

ricinism (ri′sĭ-nizm) intoxication caused by inhalation or ingestion of a poisonous principle of castor bean, producing superficial inflammation of the respiratory mucosa with hemorrhages into the lungs, or edema of the gastrointestinal tract with hemorrhages.

Ricinus (ris′ĭ-nus) [L.] the name of a genus of euphorbiaceous plants. The seeds of *R. commu′nis,* or castor oil plant, are highly poisonous but afford castor oil. The leaves of the castor oil plant are galactagogic.

rickets (rik′ets) [thought to be a corruption of Gr. *rhachitis* a spinal complaint] a condition caused by deficiency of vitamin D, especially in infancy and childhood, with disturbance of normal ossification. The disease is marked by bending and distortion of the bones under muscular action, by the formation of nodular enlargements on the ends and sides of the bones, by delayed closure of the fontanels, pain in the muscles, and sweating of the head. Vitamin D and sunlight with an adequate diet are curative, provided that the parathyroid glands are functioning properly. **acute r.,** infantile scurvy. **adult r.,** osteomalacia. **beryllium r.,** a form of rickets produced by adding beryllium to an otherwise normal diet. **fat r.,** a form in which the infant is plump and seems well nourished. **fetal r.,** achondroplasia. **glissonian r.,** rickets as described by Glisson. **hemorrhagic r.,** infantile scurvy. **hepatic r.,** a rickets-like condition with cirrhosis of the liver. **late r.,** rickets occurring in older children. **lean r.,** rickets with wasting and progressive emaciation. **pseudodeficiency r.,** vitamin D–resistant r. **refractory r.,** vitamin D–resistant r. **renal r.,** a condition characterized by rachitic changes in the skeleton and resulting from dysfunction of the kidneys; see *renal osteodystrophy,* under *osteodystrophy.* **scurvy r.,** rachitic changes in the skeleton associated with infantile scurvy. **tardy r.,** late r. **vitamin D–refractory r.,** vitamin D–resistant r. **vitamin D–resistant r.,** a condition almost indistinguishable from ordinary rickets clinically but resistant to unusually large doses of vitamin D; it is often familial but may occur sporadically. In *hypophosphatemic vitamin D–resistant rickets,* hypophosphatemia is the main characteristic, while in *hypocalcemic vitamin D–resistant rickets,* the serum concentration of phosphate is within normal limits or nearly so, and the concentration of calcium is abnormally low. Called also *pseudodeficiency r.* and *vitamin D–refractory r.*

rickettsemia (rik″et-se′me-ah) the presence of rickettsiae in the blood.

Rickettsia (rĭ-ket′se-ah) [Howard Taylor *Ricketts,* American pathologist, 1871–1910] a genus of the tribe Rickettsieae, family Rickettsiaceae, order Rickettsiales, made up of small rod-shaped to coccoid, often pleomorphic microorganisms occurring intracytoplasmically or free in the lumen of the gut in lice, fleas, ticks, and mites, by which they are transmitted to man and other animals. The various species are separated into a typhus group, a spotted fever group, a tsutsugamushi group, and a miscellaneous group. **R. akamu′shi,** *R. tsutsugamushi.* **R. ak′ari,** the etiologic agent of rickettsialpox, transmitted by the mite *Allodermanyssus sanguineus* from the reservoir of infection in house mice. **R. austra′lis,** the etiologic agent of North Queensland tick typhus, possibly transmitted by Ixodes ticks. **R. burnet′ii,** *Coxiella burnetii.* **R. ca′nis,** the etiologic agent of canine rickettsiosis in Africa, the Mediterranean region, and India. **R. cono′rii,** the etiologic agent of boutonneuse fever (Marseilles fever, Mediterranean fever), and possibly also Indian tick typhus, Kenya typhus, and South African tick-bite fever; transmitted by *Rhipicephalus* and *Haemaphysalis* ticks. **R. diapor′ica,** *Coxiella burneti.* **R. moo′seri,** *R. typhi.* **R. murico′la,** *R. typhi.* **R. nippon′ica, R. orienta′lis,** *R. tsutsugamushi.* **R. pedic′uli,** *R. quintana.* **R. prowaze′kii,** the etiologic agent of epidemic typhus and the latent infection Brill's disease, which are transmitted from man to man via *Pediculus humanus* var. *corporis.* **R. quinta′na,** the probable etiologic agent of trench fever, observed in World Wars I and II, and transmitted by the human body louse. **R. rickett′sii,** the etiologic agent of Rocky Mountain spotted fever, transmitted by *Dermacentor, Rhipicephalus, Haemaphysalis, Amblyomma* and *Ixodes* ticks. **R. sennet′sui,** a species isolated in Japan, associated with a disease having all the characteristics of infectious mononucleosis. **R. siber′ica,** or **R. siber′icus,** a species closely related to *R. conorii;* it is the causative agent of Siberian tick typhus. Called also *Dermacentroxenus sibericus.* **R. tsutsugamu′shi,** the etiologic agent of scrub typhus, transmitted by larval mites of the genus *Trombicula,* including *T. akamushi* and *T. deliensis,* from rodent reservoirs of infection; called *Dermacentroxenus orientalis, R. akamushi, R. nipponica,* and *R. orientalis.* **R. ty′phi,** the etiologic agent of fleaborne murine typhus. **R. wolhyn′ica,** *R. quintana.*

rickettsia (rĭ-ket′se-ah), pl. *rickett′siae.* An individual organism of the family Rickettsiaceae.

Rickettsiaceae (rĭ-ket″se-a′se-e) a family of the order Rickettsiales, made up of small rod-shaped, ellipsoidal, coccoid, or diplococcus-shaped, often pleomorphic microorganisms often occurring intracellularly in arthropods, by which they are transmitted to man and other animals, causing disease. It includes three tribes, Ehrlichieae, Rickettsieae, and Wolbachieae.

rickettsiae (rik-et′se-e) plural of *rickettsia.*

rickettsial (rĭ-ket′se-al) caused by rickettsiae.

Rickettsiales (rĭ-ket″se-a′lēz) a taxonomic order made up of small, rod-shaped or coccoid, often pleomorphic microorganisms occurring as elementary bodies that typically multiply only inside the cells of the host. Found as parasites in both vertebrates and invertebrates, which may serve as vectors, they may be pathogenic for both man and other animals. The order includes three families, Anaplasmataceae, Bartonellaceae, and Rickettsiaceae.

rickettsialpox (rĭ-ket′se-al-poks″) a febrile disease marked by a vesiculopapular eruption, resembling chickenpox clinically and caused by *Rickettsia akari,* transmitted from mice to men by the mite *Allodermanyssus sanguineus.* Recognized first in New York, the condition is also called *Kew Gardens spotted fever.*

rickettsicidal (rĭ-ket″sĭ-si′dal) destructive to rickettsiae.

Rickettsieae (rik″et-si′e-e) a tribe of the family Rickettsiaceae, order Rickettsiales, made up of small pleomorphic forms, mostly intracellular organisms occurring as parasites in arthropods and causing disease in vertebrate hosts. It includes three genera, *Coxiella, Rickettsia,* and *Cowdria.*

Rickettsiella (rĭ-ket″se-el′ah) [*rickettsia* + *-ella* diminutive ending] a genus of tribe Wolbachieae, family Rickettsiaceae, order Rickettsiales, made up of minute intracellular rickettsia-like organisms, parasitic on the Japanese beetle (*Popillia japonica*) and nonpathogenic for mammals. The type species is *R. popil′liae.*

rickettsiosis (rĭ-ket″se-o′sis) infection with rickettsiae. **canine r.,** an often fatal febrile disease of dogs in Africa, the Mediterranean area, and India, caused by *Rickettsia canis,* which is transmitted by the brown dog tick (*Rhipicephalus sanguineus*). It is characterized by high fever, mucopurulent discharge from the nose and eyes, gastritis, thirst, anorexia, emaciation, fetid breath, enlargement of lymph and spleen, erythematous pustules on the axilla and groin, hysteria, convulsions, meningoencephalitis, and paralysis; dogs that recover may become carriers.

rickettsiostatic (rĭ-ket″se-o-stat′ik) inhibiting the growth and activity of rickettsiae.

Ricolesia (ri″ko-le′ze-ah) [*Rickettsia* + J. D. W. A. *Coles*] a genus (incertae sedis) of coccoid microorganisms, occurring as four species, *R. bo′vis, R. ca′prae, R. conjuncti′vae,* and *R. lestoquar′dii,* producing a keratoconjunctivitis in cattle, goats, fowl, and swine, respectively.

Ricord's treatment (re-korz′) [Philippe *Ricord,* French physician, 1800–1889] see under *treatment.*

rictal (rik′tal) pertaining to a fissure.

rictus (rik′tus) [L.] 1. a fissure or cleft. 2. a gaping, as of the mouth.

Riddoch's reflex (rid′oks) [George *Riddoch,* British neurologist, 1888–1947] see under *reflex.*

Rideal-Walker coefficient (rid′e-al-waw′ker) [Samuel *Rideal,* English chemist, 1863–1929; J. F. Ainslie *Walker,* English chemist] phenol coefficient.

ridge (rij) a projection or projecting structure; see also *crest* and *crista.* **alveolar r., residual,** the bony ridge remaining after disappearance of the alveoli from the alveolar process following removal or loss of the teeth. **basal r.,** cingulum. **bicipital r., anterior,** crista tuberculi minoris. **bicipital r., external,** crista tuberculi majoris. **bicipital r., internal,** crista tuberculi minoris. **bicipital r., outer, bicipital r., posterior,** crista tuberculi majoris. **buccocervical r.,** a ridge on the buccal surface just above the cementoenamel junction of posterior teeth. **buccogingival r.,** buccocervical r. **bulbar r's,** spiral endocardial thickenings in the bulbus cordis that fuse and form the bulbar septum, separating the bulbus cordis into aortic and pulmonary trunks. **center of r.,** the buccolingual midline of the residual alveolar ridge. **cerebral r's of cranial bones,** juga cerebralia ossium cranii. **crest of r.,** the highest continuous surface of the residual alveolar ridge, but not necessarily the center of the ridge. **deltoid r.,** tuberositas deltoidea humeri. **dental r.,** any linear elevation on the crown of a tooth named according to the surface on which it is located, such as buccal or lingual, or in recognition of some other characteristic. **dermal r's,** cristae cutis. **epicondylic r., lateral,** supracondylar r., lateral. **epicondylic r., medial,** supracondylar r., medial. **epipericardial r.,** a ventral ridge separating the ventral ends of the branchial arches in the embryo from the pericardial swelling. **gastrocnemial r.,** a ridge on the posterior surface of the femur, giving attachment to the gastrocnemius muscle. **genital r.,** the more medial portion of the urogenital ridge, which gives rise to the gonad. **germ r.,** genital r. **gluteal r. of femur,** tuberositas glutea femoris. **healing r.,** an indurated ridge that normally forms deep to the skin along the length of a healing wound and extends about 1 cm. on each side of the wound. **r. of humerus,** tuberositas deltoidea humeri. **incisal r.,** that portion of the crown of an anterior tooth which makes up the actual incisal portion. **interarticular r. of head of rib,** crista capitis costae. **interosseous r. of fibula,** margo interosseus fibulae. **interosseous r. of radius,** margo interosseus radii. **interosseous r. of tibia,** margo interosseus tibiae. **interosseous r. of ulna,** margo interosseus ulnae. **intertrochanteric r.,** crista intertrochanterica. **interureteric r.,** a smooth ridge extending across the bladder from one ureteral opening to the other, produced by a transverse bundle of muscle fibers; called also *plica interureterica* [NA], and *plica ureterica.* **linguocervical r.,** cingulum. **linguogingival r.,** linguocervical r. **longitudinal r. of hard palate,** raphe palati. **Mall's r.,** pulmonary r. **mammary r.,** milk line. **r. of mandibular neck,** a blunt, smooth ridge passing obliquely downward and forward from the mandibular condyle on the medial surface of the mandibular neck and ramus, serving as their buttress. **marginal r's,** rounded borders of the enamel which form the mesial and distal margins of the occlusal surfaces of posterior teeth and the lingual surfaces of anterior teeth. **mesonephric r.,** the more lateral portion of the urogenital ridge, which gives rise to the mesonephros. **middle r. of femur,** linea pectinea femoris. **milk r.,** see under *line.* **mylohyoid r.,** linea mylohyoidea mandibulae. **r. of neck of rib,** crista colli costae. **r. of nose,** agger nasi. **oblique r.,** 1. a variable linear elevation obliquely crossing the occlusal surface of a maxillary molar tooth, formed by union of two triangular ridges. 2. tuberositas masseterica. **oblique r's of scapula,** lineae musculares scapulae. **palatine r's,**

transverse, plicae palatinae transversae. **Passavant's r.,** see under *bar*. **pectoral r.,** crista tuberculi majoris. **pharyngeal r.,** Passavant's bar. **pterygoid r.,** crista infratemporalis. **pulmonary r.,** a ridge along the common cardinal vein in the embryo, which develops into the pleuropericardial membrane. **radial r. of wrist,** eminentia carpi radialis. **residual r.,** alveolar r., residual. **rough r. of femur,** linea aspera femoris. **semicircular r. of parietal bone, inferior,** linea temporalis inferior ossis parietalis. **semicircular r. of parietal bone, superior,** linea temporalis superior ossis parietalis. **sublingual r.,** frenulum linguae. **superciliary r.,** arcus superciliaris. **supinator r.,** crista musculi supinatoris. **supplemental r.,** an abnormal ridge on the surface of a tooth. **supracondylar r., lateral,** a prominent, curved ridge on the lateral surface of the humerus, giving attachment in front to the brachioradialis and extensor carpi radialis longus muscles. **supracondylar r., medial,** a prominent, curved ridge on the medial surface of the humerus, giving attachment to the brachialis muscle in front and to the medial head of the triceps behind. **supraorbital r.,** arcus superciliaris. **suprarenal r.,** a caudal projection of the dorsal portion of the pleuroperitoneal membrane of the embryo, in which the adrenal cortex develops. **synaptic r.,** a wedge-shaped projection in the retina of a cone pedicle or of a rod spherule, on either side of which lie the horizontal cells whose dendrites are inserted into the ridge. **taste r's,** papillae foliatae. **tentorial r.,** a ridge on the inner surface of the cranium just above the groove for the transverse sinus, to which the tentorium is attached. **transverse r.,** a linear elevation extending transversely across the occlusal surface of a posterior tooth, formed by union of two triangular ridges. **transverse r's of sacrum,** lineae transversae ossis sacri. **transverse r's of vaginal wall,** rugae vaginales. **trapezoid r.,** linea trapezoidea. **triangular r.,** a linear elevation descending from the tip of a cusp toward the central part of the occlusal surface of a posterior tooth. **tubercular r. of sacrum,** crista sacralis mediana. **ulnar r. of wrist,** eminentia carpi ulnaris. **urethral r.,** carina urethralis vaginae. **urogenital r.,** a longitudinal ridge or fold in the embryo, lateral to the root of the mesentery, which later subdivides longitudinally into the mesonephric and the genital ridge. **wolffian r.,** mesonephric r.

ridgel (rid′jel) ridgling.

ridging (rij′ing) in plastic surgery, a visible line or ridge at the margin of an area that has been surgically planed; occasionally encountered when beveling at the junction of treated and untreated areas has not been performed.

ridgling (rij′ling) an animal, especially a horse, with one or both testes undescended.

Ridley's sinus (rid′lēz) [Humphrey *Ridley*, English anatomist, 1653–1708] sinus circularis.

Riedel's lobe, struma (disease, thyroiditis) (re′delz) [Bernhard Moritz Carl Ludwig *Riedel*, surgeon in Jena, 1846–1916] see under *lobe* and *struma*.

Rieder's cell, cell leukemia, lymphocyte (re′derz) [Hermann *Rieder*, German roentgenologist, 1858–1932] see under *cell*, *leukemia*, and *lymphocyte*.

Riegel's pulse (re′-gelz) [Franz *Riegel*, German physician, 1843–1904] see under *pulse*.

Riegler's test (reg′lerz) [Emanuel *Riegler*, German chemist, 1854–1929] see under *tests*.

Riehl's melanosis (rēlz) [Gustav *Riehl*, Vienna dermatologist, 1855–1943] see under *melanosis*.

Riesman's pneumonia, sign (rēs′manz) [David *Riesman*, American physician, 1867–1940] see under *pneumonia* and *sign*.

Rieux's hernia (re-uhz′) [*Léon Rieux*, French surgeon] retrocecal hernia.

R.I.F. right iliac fossa.

Rifadin (rif′ah-din) trademark for a preparation of rifampin.

rifamide (rif′ah-mīd) chemical name: 4-*O*-[2-(diethylamino)-2-oxoethyl]rifamycin. A semisynthetic antibacterial antibiotic, $C_{43}H_{58}N_2O_{13}$, derived from rifamycin B, having the actions of the other rifamycins; it has been used in the treatment of respiratory infections due to gram-positive cocci and in biliary tract infections due to gram-negative and gram-positive organisms. See also *rifamycin*.

rifampicin (rif′am-pĭ-sin) the international nonproprietary name for rifampin.

rifampin (rif′am-pin) [USP] chemical name: 3-[[(4-methyl-1-piperazinyl)imino]methyl]rifamycin. A semisynthetic derivative of rifamycin SV, $C_{43}H_{58}N_4O_{12}$, occurring as a red-brown, crystalline powder, having the antibacterial actions of rifamycin (q.v.) group of antibiotics; administered orally. Called also *rifampicin*.

rifamycin (rif″ah-mi′sin) any of a family of antibiotics biosynthesized by a strain of *Streptomyces mediterranei*, effective against a broad spectrum of bacteria, including gram-positive cocci, some gram-negative bacilli and *Mycobacterium tuberculosis* and certain other mycobacteria. The five components are designated A, B, C, D, and E; rifamycins O, S, and SV are derivatives of the B component, and AG and X are derivatives of the O component. In the United States the rifamycins are used only for the initial treatment and re-treatment of pulmonary tuberculosis and for treatment of asymptomatic nasopharyngeal carriers of *Neisseria meningitidis;* they have been used in other countries to treat various infectious diseases due to susceptible organisms, such as leprosy, gonorrhea, and biliary tract and respiratory infections. Formerly called *rifomycin*.

rifomycin (rif″o-mi′sin) former name for rifamycin.

Riga-Fede disease [Antonio *Riga*, Francesco *Fede*, Italian physicians of the nineteenth century] see under *disease*.

right-handed (rīt-han′ded) using the right hand preferentially, or more skillfully than the left, in voluntary motor acts. See also *laterality*.

rigidity (rĭ-jid′ĭ-te) [L. *rigiditas; rigidus* stiff] stiffness or inflexibility, chiefly that which is abnormal or morbid; rigor. **anatomical r.,** rigidity of the cervix uteri in labor so that it dilates to only a limited extent, beyond which uterine contractions are of no avail. **cadaveric r.,** rigor mortis. **clasp-knife r.,** increased resistance of the extensors (induced by passive flexion of a joint), which suddenly gives way on exertion of further pressure. **cogwheel r.,** rigidity of a muscle which gives way in a series of little jerks when the muscle is passively stretched. **decerebrate r.,** the posture produced in an experimental animal by decerebration (q.v.), marked by rigid extension of the legs. It occurs in man as a result of lesions of the upper part of the brain stem and is manifested as follows: the patient lies in rigid extension with his arms internally rotated at the shoulder, extended at the elbow, and pronated, his fingers flexed at the interphalangeal joints and extended at the metacarpophalangeal joints, and his legs extended at the hips and knees, with the ankles and toes flexed. **hemiplegic r.,** rigidity of the paralyzed limbs in hemiplegia. **lead-pipe r.,** the diffuse muscular rigidity seen in parkinsonism. **muscle r., muscular r.,** tetanus, def. 2. **mydriatic r.,** Westphal's pupillary reflex. **pathologic r.,** rigidity of the cervix uteri in labor from some disease. **postmortem r.,** rigor mortis. **spasmodic r.,** rigidity of the cervix uteri due to spasmodic contraction.

rigor (rig′or, ri′gor) [L.] 1. a chill. 2. rigidity. **acid r.,** coagulation of the protein of muscle produced by acids. **calcium r.,** systolic cardiac arrest caused by an excess of calcium. **heat r.,** rigidity of muscles induced by heat. **r. mor′tis,** the stiffening of a dead body, accompanying the depletion of adenosine triphosphate in the muscle fibers. **r. nervo′rum,** tetanus, def. 2. **r. tre′mens,** parkinsonism. **water r.,** a condition of rigor in a muscle caused by immersing it in water.

rim (rim) a border, or edge. **bite r.,** occlusion r. **occlusion r.,** a border constructed on temporary or permanent denture bases for the purpose of recording the maxillomandibular relation and for positioning the teeth. **record r.,** occlusion r.

rima (ri′mah), pl. *ri′mae* [L.] a cleft or crack; [NA] a general term for such an opening. **r. a′ni, r. clu′nium,** crena ani. **r. cornea′lis,** corneal fissure. **ri′mae cu′tis,** sulci cutis. **r. glot′tidis** [NA], the elongated opening between the true vocal cords and between the arytenoid cartilages; called also *fissure of glottis*. **r. glot′tidis cartilagin′ea,** pars intercartilaginea rimae glottidis. **r. glot′tidis membrana′cea,** pars intermembranacea rimae glottidis. **intercartilaginea r.,** pars intercartilaginea rimae glottidis. **intermembranous r.,** pars intermembranacea rimae glottidis. **r. o′ris** [NA], the longitudinal opening of the mouth, between the lips; called also *oral fissure*. **r. palpebra′rum** [NA], the longitudinal opening between the eyelids; called also *palpebral fissure*. **r. puden′di** [NA], the cleft between the labia majora in which the urethra and vagina open; called also *pudendal fissure*. **r. respirato′ria,** pars intercartilaginea rimae glottidis. **r. vestib′uli** [NA], the space between the right and left vestibular folds of the larynx; called also *fissure of vestibule*. **r. voca′lis,** pars intermembranacea rimae glottidis. **r. vul′vae,** r. pudendi.

Rimactane (rim-ak′tān) trademark for a preparation of rifampin.

rimae (ri′me) [L.] plural of *rima*.

rimal (ri′mal) pertaining to a rima.

rimantadine hydrochloride (ri-man′tah-dēn) chemical name: α-methyl-1-adamantanemethylamine. An antiviral agent, $C_{12}H_{21}N \cdot HCl$, which has been used in the prophylaxis of influenza type A.

Rimifon (rim′ĭ-fon) trademark for a preparation of isoniazid.

rimiterol hydrobromide (rim″ĭ-ter′ōl) chemical name: (*R**,*S**)-α-(3,4-dihydroxyphenyl)-2-piperidinemethanol hydrobromide. An adrenergic, $C_{12}H_{17}NO_3 \cdot HBr$, used as a bronchodilator.

rimose (rim′ōs) [L. *rima* crack] marked by cracks and fissures.

rimula (rim′u-lah), pl. *rim′ulae* [L.] a minute fissure, especially of the spinal cord or brain.

rinderpest (rind′er-pest) [Ger. *Rinder* cattle + *pest* plague] cattle plague.

Rindfleisch's cells, folds (rint″flish-ez) [Georg Eduard *Rindfleisch*, German physician, 1836–1908] see *eosinophil*, and under *fold*.

ring (ring) [L. *annulus, circulus, orbiculus*] 1. any annular or circular organ or area; for names of specific anatomical structures, see under *anulus.* 2. in chemistry, a collection of atoms united in a continuous or closed chain. **abdominal r., deep,** anulus inguinalis profundus. **abdominal r., external,** anulus inguinalis superficialis. **abdominal r., internal,** anulus inguinalis profundus. **abdominal r., superficial,** anulus inguinalis superficialis. **Albl's r.,** a ring-shaped shadow observed in a roentgenogram of the skull, caused by an aneurysm of a cerebral artery. **amnion r.,** the attached margin of the amnion about the umbilicus of the fetus. **annular r's,** round or oval opacities surrounding a translucent area in the roentgenogram, indicative of cavitation of the lung in tuberculosis; called also *pleural rings.* **atrial r.,** the ring surrounding the opening between the atrium and ventricle of the primitive vertebrate heart; represented in the mammalian heart by the atrioventricular node. **Balbiani's r's,** a series of loops of the chromonemata of polytene chromosomes, similar in nature to chromosome puffs and in appearance to lampbrush chromosomes. **Bandl's r.,** pathologic retraction r.; see *retraction r.* **benzene r.,** the closed hexagon of carbon atoms in benzene (C_6H_6), from which the different benzene compounds are derived by replacement of the hydrogen atoms. **Bickel's r.,** Waldeyer's tonsillar ring. **Braun's r.,** pathologic retraction r.; see *retraction r.* **Cabot's r's,** see *Cabot's ring bodies,* under *body.* **Cannon's r.,** in the roentgenogram after a barium meal, a narrow area or focal contraction at the mid-third of the transverse colon, representing the junction of the primitive midgut and hindgut and marking an area of overlap between the superior and inferior nerve plexuses. **carbocyclic r.,** a chemical ring which includes only carbon atoms. **casting r.,** refractory flask. **ciliary r.,** orbiculus ciliaris. **ciliary r. of iris,** anulus iridis major. **closing r. of Winkler-Waldeyer,** a slight thickening at the edge of the placenta, due to piling up of fetal and maternal tissues. **conjunctival r.,** anulus conjunctivae. **constriction r.,** a contracted area of the uterus, allegedly possible at any level, occurring where the resistance of the uterine contents is slight, as over a depression in the contour of the fetal body, or below the presenting part. Cf. *retraction r.* **contact r.,** the wound inflicted at the site of entrance of a bullet on the surface of the body. **contraction r.,** see *constriction r.* and *retraction r.* **coronary r.,** see under *band.* **crural r.,** anulus femoralis. **Döllinger's r.,** Schwalbe's r. **femoral r.,** anulus femoralis. **fibrocartilaginous r. of tympanic membrane,** anulus fibrocartilagineus membranae tympani. **fibrous r., interpubic,** discus interpubicus. **fibrous r's of heart,** anuli fibrosi cordis. **fibrous r. of intervertebral disk,** anulus fibrosus disci intervertebralis. **Fleischer keratoconus r.,** an incomplete annular pigmented line at the base of the cone in keratoconus. **Fleischer-Strümpell r.,** Kayser-Fleischer r. **furan r.,** a ring containing four atoms of carbon and one of oxygen. **germ r.,** the proliferating marginal zone of the early blastoderm that is about to become the lips of the blastopore. **glaucomatous r.,** a light yellowish ring around the optic disk in glaucoma, indicating atrophy of the choroid. **Gräfenberg's r.,** a flexible ring of silver wire inserted into the uterus to prevent conception. **greater r. of iris,** anulus iridis major. **heterocyclic r.,** a chemical ring which includes atoms of different elements. **homocyclic r.,** a chemical ring in which all the members are atoms of the same element. **infancy r.,** a line of arrested calcification sometimes seen near the incisal edges of anterior permanent teeth; it forms at approximately one year of age. **inguinal r., deep,** anulus inguinalis profundus. **inguinal r., external,** anulus inguinalis superficialis. **inguinal r., internal,** anulus inguinalis profundus. **inguinal r., superficial,** anulus inguinalis superficialis. **isocyclic r.,** homocyclic r. **Kayser-Fleischer r.,** a gray-green to red-gold pigmented ring at the outer margin of the cornea, seen in progressive lenticular degeneration and pseudosclerosis; called also *Fleischer-Strümpell r.* **lesser r. of iris,** anulus iridis minor. **Liesegang r's,** see under *phenomenon.* **Löwe's r.,** a ring in the visual field caused by the macula lutea. **Lower's r's,** anuli fibrosi cordis. **lymphoid r.,** Waldeyer's tonsillar ring. **Maxwell's r.,** a ring resembling Löwe's, but smaller and fainter. **neonatal r.,** a line of demarcation in the enamel and dentin of a deciduous tooth, indicating the transition from prenatal to postnatal calcification. **Newton's r's,** colored rings seen on the surface of thin, transparent membranes, as soap-bubbles, due to light wave interference. **Ochsner's r.,** a circular mucosal thickening at the opening of the pancreatic duct into the common bile duct. **periosteal bone r.,** see under *collar.* **pleural r's,** annular r's. **pyran r.,** a ring containing five atoms of carbon and one of oxygen. **retraction r.,** a ringlike thickening and indentation occurring in normal labor at the junction of the isthmus and corpus uteri, delineating the upper contracting portion and the lower dilating portion (*physiologic retraction r.*), or a persistent retraction ring in abnormal or prolonged labor that obstructs expulsion of the fetus (*pathologic retraction r.*). Cf. *constriction r.* **Schatzki's r.,** a web or ring in the lower esophagus in some patients with dysphagia; revealed radiographically after barium swallow. **Schwalbe's r.,** **Schwalbe's anterior border r.,** a circular ridge composed of collagenous fibers surrounding the outer margin of Descemet's membrane (lamina limitans posterior corneae). Called also *Schwalbe's line* and *Döllinger's r.* **signet r.,** the stage in the erythrocytic cycle of a malarial plasmodium consisting of a thin ring of protoplasm with a nucleus at one side; called also *ring stage.* **Soemmering's r.,** a doughnut-shaped opacity behind the pupil, occurring after cataract surgery or secondary to trauma as a result of contact between the anterior capsule and the posterior capsule, which traps varying amounts of lens substance peripherally; called also *Soemmering's ring cataract.* **tendinous r., common,** anulus tendineus communis. **tracheal r's,** cartilagines tracheales. **tympanic r.,** anulus tympanicus. **umbilical r.,** anulus umbilicalis. **vascular r.,** a developmental anomaly of the aortic arches wherein the trachea and esophagus are encircled by vascular structures, many variations being possible. **r. of Vieussens,** limbus fossae ovalis. **Vossius' lenticular r.,** a ring of pigment on the crystalline lens caused by pressure of the pupillary margin against the lens following a contusion injury. **Waldeyer's tonsillar r.,** the circular series of lymphoid tissue formed by the lingual, pharyngeal, and faucial tonsils. **Zinn's r.,** anulus tendineus communis.

ring-bone (ring'bōn) exostosis involving the first or second phalanx of the horse, resulting in lameness if the articular surfaces are affected. **low r.,** buttress foot.

Ringer's injection, irrigation (mixture, solution) (ring'-erz) [Sydney *Ringer,* English physiologist, 1835–1910] see under *injection* and *irrigation.*

ringschwiele (ring'shve-lĕ) [Ger. *ring* ring + *schwiele* callosity, wheal] a large pigmented plaque at the ora serrata, caused by a laminated proliferation of the retinal pigment epithelium, occurring as a result of long-standing retinal detachment or other injury to the eye.

ringworm (ring'wurm) a popular name for a group of fungal diseases of the skin of man and domestic animals, marked by the formation of ring-shaped pigmented patches covered with vesicles or scales, and caused by dermatophytes. See also *tinea.* Among domestic animals, *Trichophyton* is the most common cause in cattle; it also causes fur-slipping in chinchillas. *Microsporum* is the usual cause in dogs and cats. **r. of the beard,** tinea barbae. **black-dot r.,** tinea capitis caused by *Trichophyton violaceum* or *T. tonsurans,* with a distinctive appearance resulting from the breaking of the hairs at the scalp surface. **r. of the body,** tinea corporis. **r. of feet,** tinea pedis. **r. of groin,** tinea cruris. **r. of the nails,** onychomycosis. **r. of the scalp,** tinea capitis. **Tokelau r.,** tinea imbricata.

Rinne's test (rin'nēz) [Heinrich Adolf *Rinne,* German otologist, 1819–1868] see under *tests.*

Riolan's anastomosis, arch, etc. (re"o-lanz') [Jean *Riolan,* French physician and physiologist, 1580–1657] see under *anastomosis, arch, bone, muscle, nosegay,* and *ossicle.*

riomitsin (ri"o-mit'sin) oxytetracycline.

Riopan (ri'o-pan) trademark for preparations of magaldrate.

Ripault's sign (re-pōz') [Louis Henry Antoine *Ripault,* French physician, 1807–1856] see under *sign.*

ripazepam (rĭ-pah'zĕ-pam) chemical name: 1-ethyl-4,6-dihydro-3-methyl-8-phenypyrazolo[4,3-*e*][1,4]diazepin-5(1*H*)-one; a minor tranquilizer, $C_{15}H_{16}N_4O$.

R.I.P.H. Royal Institute of Public Health.

R.I.P.H.H. Royal Institute of Public Health and Hygiene.

Risley's prism (riz'lēz) [Samuel Doty *Risley,* American ophthalmologist, 1845–1920] see under *prism.*

risocaine (rīz'o-kān) chemical name: 4-aminobenzoic acid propyl ester; a local anesthetic and antipruritic, $C_{10}H_{13}NO_2$.

RIST radioimmunosorbent test; see under *tests.*

Ristella melaninogenica (ris-tel'ah mel"ah-nin-o-jen'ĭ-kah) *Bacteroides melaninogenicus.*

ristocetin (ris"to-se'tin) an antibiotic substance produced by the fermentation of *Nocardia lurida;* formerly used in treatment of severe staphylococcal infections resistant to other antibiotics.

risus (ri'sus) [L.] laughter. **r. cani'nus,** r. sardonicus. **r. sardon'icus,** a grinning expression produced by spasm of the facial muscles; so called from a plant of Sardinia, probably one of the genus *Ranunculus,* or crowfoot, which was believed to produce it.

Ritalin (rit'ah-lin) trademark for preparations of methylphenidate hydrochloride.

Ritgen maneuver (method) (rit'gen) [Ferdinand August Marie Franz von *Ritgen,* German gynecologist, 1787–1867] see under *maneuver.*

ritodrine (rit'o-drēn) chemical name: (*R*,S**)-4-hydroxy-α-[1-[[2-(4-hydroxyphenyl)ethyl]amino]ethyl]benzene methanol. A beta$_2$-adrenergic agent, $C_{17}H_{21}O_3$, used as a smooth muscle (uterine muscle) relaxant to delay uncomplicated premature labor.

Ritter's disease (rit'erz) [Gottfried *Ritter* von Rittershain, German physician, 1820–1883] dermatitis exfoliativa neonatorum.

Ritter's law, tetanus (rit'erz) [Johann Wilhelm *Ritter,* German physicist, 1776–1810] see under *law* and *tetanus.*

Ritter-Rollet phenomenon (sign) (rit′er-ro-la′) [J. W. *Ritter*] see under *phenomenon.*

Ritter-Valli law [J. W. *Ritter;* Eusebio *Valli,* Italian physician, 1755–1816] see under *law.*

ritual (rich′u-al) in psychiatry, a series of repetitive acts performed compulsively to relieve anxiety, as in obsessive-compulsive neurosis.

rivalry (ri′val-re) a state of competition or antagonism. **binocular r., retinal r.,** the apparent alternate displacement of two figures when viewed together, there being no fusion into a continuous picture of the images of the two eyes. **sibling r.,** competition between siblings for the love, affection, and attention of one or both parents for other recognition or gain.

Rivalta's reaction (test) (re-val′tahz) [Fabio *Rivalta,* pathologist in Bologna, born 1863] see under *reaction.*

Riva-Rocci sphygmomanometer (re″vah-ro′che) [Scipione *Riva-Rocci,* Italian physician, 1863–1937] see under *sphygmomanometer.*

Riverius' draft (re-ve′re-us) Rivière's potion.

Rivière's potion (re″ve-ārz′) [Lazare *Rivière,* French physician, 1589–1655] see under *potion.*

Riviere's sign (riv-ērz′) [Clive *Riviere,* British physician, 1873–1929] see under *sign.*

Rivinus's ducts (canals), gland, incisure (foramen, notch, segment) (re-ve′nus) [Augustus Quirinus *Rivinus,* anatomist and botanist in Leipzig, 1652–1723] see *ductus sublinguales minores, glandula sublinguales,* and *incisura tympanica* [*Rivini*].

rivus (ri′vus), pl. *ri′vi* [L.] a brook, or little stream. **r. lacrima′lis** [NA], the pathway by which the tears reach the lacrimal lake from the excretory ductules of the lacrimal gland.

riziform (riz′ĭ-form) resembling grains of rice.

RKY roentgenkymography.

RLF retrolental fibroplasia.

R.L.L. right lower lobe (of lungs).

R.M.A. right mentoanterior (position of the fetus).

R.M.L. right middle lobe (of lungs).

R.M.N. Registered Mental Nurse (England and Wales).

R.M.O. Regional Medical Officer (British).

R.M.P. right mentoposterior (position of the fetus).

R.M.T. right mentotransverse (position of the fetus).

R.N. Registered Nurse.

Rn chemical symbol for *radon.*

RNA (ar′en-a) ribonucleic acid (see under *acid*). **messenger RNA, ribosomal RNA, soluble RNA, transfer RNA,** see definitions on *ribonucleic acid,* under *acid.*

RNase ribonuclease.

R.N.M.S. Registered Nurse for the Mentally Sub-Normal.

R.O.A. right occipitoanterior (position of the fetus).

roach (rōch) see *Blatta.*

roaring (rōr′ing) a condition in the horse marked by a rough sound on inspiration and sometimes on expiration, due to some obstruction in the respiratory tract or to paralysis of the vocal cords.

Robalate (ro′bah-lāt) trademark for preparations of dihydroxyaluminum aminoacetate.

Robaxin (ro-bak′sin) trademark for preparations of methocarbamol.

Robbins (rob′binz), Frederick C. American pediatrician, born 1916; co-winner, with John F. Enders and Thomas H. Weller, of the Nobel prize in medicine and physiology for 1954, for the discovery that poliomyelitis viruses multiply in human tissue.

robenidine hydrochloride (ro-ben′ĭ-dēn) chemical name: 1,3-bis[(*p*-chlorobenzylidene)amino]guanidine monohydrochloride; a coccidiostat for poultry, $C_{15}H_{13}Cl_2N_5 \cdot HCl$.

Robert's ligament (ro-bārz′) [Cesar Alphonse *Robert,* French surgeon, 1801–1862] see under *ligament.*

Robert's pelvis (ro′bārts) [Heinrich Ludwig Ferdinand *Robert,* German gynecologist, 1814–1874] see under *pelvis.*

Roberts test (rob′erts) [Sir William *Roberts,* English physician, 1830–1899] see under *tests.*

Robertson's pupil (rob′ert-sunz) see *Argyll Robertson,* and under *pupil.*

Robertson's sign (rob′ert-sunz) [William Egbert *Robertson,* American physician, 1869–1956] see under *sign.*

robin (ro′bin) a poisonous substance (phytotoxin) found in the bark of the North American locust tree (*Robinia pseudacacia*).

Robin's syndrome (ro-bāz′) [Pierre *Robin,* French pediatrician, 1867–1950] Pierre Robin syndrome.

Robinson's circle (rob′in-sunz) [Frederick Byron *Robinson,* American anatomist, 1857–1910] see under *circle.*

Robinul (ro′bĭ-nul) trademark for preparations of glycopyrrolate.

Robison ester, ester degeneration (ro′bĭ-sun) [Robert Robi-

son, British chemist, 1884–1941] see under *ester,* and *degeneration.*

Robitussin (ro″bĭ-tus′in) trademark for preparations of guaifenesin.

roborant (rob′o-rant) [L. *roborans* strengthening] conferring strength; strengthening.

Robson's point, position (rōb′sonz) [Sir Arthur William Mayo *Robson,* London surgeon, 1853–1933] see under *point* and *position.*

Rochalimaea (ro″kah-li-me′ah) a genus of the tribe Rickettsieae, family Rickettsiaceae, order Rickettsiales, resembling the genus *Rickettsia,* but usually found extracellularly in the arthropod host. **R. quinta′na,** the etiologic agent of trench fever, transmitted by the body louse *Pediculus humanus;* formerly called *Rickettsia quintana.*

rod (rod) a straight, slim mass of substance; specifically, one of the rodlike bodies of the retina. See *retinal r's.* **Corti's r's,** *pillar cells;* see under *cell.* **enamel r's,** the approximately parallel rods or prisms forming the enamel of teeth. They are enclosed in a sheath of organic matter (the enamel rod sheath, or prism sheath) and are embedded in the interprismatic or cement substance. **germinal r.,** a sporozoite. **r's of Heidenhain,** the rodlike cells of the renal tubules. **König's r's,** a series of steel bars each of which gives a note of certain pitch when struck. **Maddox r's,** a set of parallel cylindrical glass rods used in testing for heterophoria. **Meckel's r.,** Meckel's cartilage. **muscle r.,** myofibril. **olfactory r.,** the slender apical portion of an olfactory bipolar neuron, a modified dendrite, extending as a cylindrical process from the nucleus to surface of the epithelium. **Reichmann's r.,** a short ivory rod with circular grooves and intervening projections, used in auscultatory percussion of the stomach. **retinal r's,** highly specialized cylindrical segments of the visual cells containing rhodopsin; together with the retinal cones they form the light-sensitive elements of the retina; called also *rod cells.*

rodenticide (ro-den′tĭ-sīd) 1. destructive to rodents. 2. any agent for destroying rodents.

rodentine (ro-den′tin) pertaining to a rodent.

rodocaine (ro′do-kān) chemical name: *trans*-(2-chloro-6-methylphenyl)octahydropyrindine-1-propanamide; a local anesthetic, $C_{18}H_{25}ClN_2O$.

roentgen (rent′gen) [for Wilhelm Conrad *Röntgen,* German physicist, 1845–1923, who discovered roentgen rays in 1895; winner of the Nobel prize in physics for 1901] the international unit of x- or γ-radiation. It is the quantity of x- or γ-radiation such that the associated corpuscular emission per 0.001293 gm. of air produces in air ions carrying 1 electrostatic unit of electrical charge of either sign. Abbreviated R.

roentgenkymograph (rent′gen-ki′mo-graf) the apparatus used in roentgenkymography.

roentgenkymography (rent″gen-ki-mog′rah-fe) a technique of graphically recording the movements of an organ or structure on a single x-ray film; abbreviated RKY.

roentgenocardiogram (rent″gen-o-kar′de-o-gram) a polygraphic tracing of cardiac pulsation made by the roentgen rays.

roentgenocinematography (rent″gen-o-sin″ĕ-mah-tog′rah-fe) moving picture roentgenography.

roentgenogram (rent-gen′o-gram″) a film produced by roentgenography. **cephalometric r.,** a roentgenogram of the full lateral view of the head, for the purposes of making cranial measurements; called also *cephalogram.* **lateral oblique jaw r.,** a roentgenogram of the mandible that unilaterally reveals the mandible from symphysis to condyle. **lateral ramus r.,** a roentgenogram of the mandibular ramus and condyle. **lateral skull r.,** a roentgenogram of the sinuses and lateral aspects of the skeletal structures of the cranium. **maxillary sinus r.,** a roentgenogram of the maxillary sinuses and the zygomas that permits direct comparison of the two sides; called also *Water's view r.* **submental vertex r.,** a roentgenogram that permits visualization of the lateral movements of the condyle, lateral displacement of the condyle and/or the coronoid process, and the contour of the zygomatic arches. **Towne projection r.,** a roentgenogram of the mandibular condyles and the midfacial skeleton. **Water's view r.,** maxillary sinus r.

roentgenograph (rent′gen-o-graf″) roentgenogram.

roentgenographic (rent″gen-o-graf′ik) pertaining to or produced by roentgenography.

roentgenography (rent″gen-og′rah-fe) [*roentgen* + Gr. *graphein* to write] the making of a record (roentgenogram) of internal structures of the body by passage of x-rays through the body to act on specially sensitized film. See also *radiography.* **body section r.,** a special technique to show in detail images of structures lying in a predetermined plane of tissue, while blurring or eliminating detail in images of structures in other planes. See *tomography.* Called also *analytical roentgenography* and *sectional roentgenography.* Various mechanisms and methods for such roentgenography have been given various names, such as *laminagraphy, laminography, planigraphy, radiotomy, stratigraphy,* and *vertigraphy.* **double contrast r.,** mucosal relief roentgenography. **mass r.,** examination by x-rays of the general population or of large groups of the population. **miniature r.,** the taking of miniature x-ray photographs. **miniature r., mass,** the use of miniature x-ray film in mass roentgenography. **mucosal relief r.,** a technique for revealing any abnormality of the intestinal mucosa, involving injection and evacuation of a barium enema, followed by inflation of the intestine with air under light pressure. The light coating of barium on the walls of the inflated intestine in the roentgenogram reveals clearly even small abnormalities. **selective r.,** roentgenography of certain segments of the population, chosen on some specific basis such as symptoms, or some other basis. **serial r.,** the taking of several exposures of a selected area at arbitrary intervals. **spot-film r.,** the making of localized instantaneous roentgenographic exposures during the course of a fluoroscopic examination.

roentgenokymograph (rent″gen-o-ki′mo-graf) roentgenkymograph.

roentgenologist (rent″gĕ-nol′o-jist) a physician who specializes in diagnosis and treatment by the roentgen rays; radiologist.

roentgenology (rent″gĕ-nol′o-je) [*roentgen rays* + *-logy*] the branch of radiology which deals with the diagnostic and therapeutic use of roentgen rays.

roentgenolucent (rent″gen-o-lu′sent) allowing roentgen rays to pass through; radiolucent.

roentgenometer (rent″gĕ-nom′ĕ-ter) an instrument for measuring the intensity of roentgen rays.

roentgenometry (rent″gĕ-nom′ĕ-tre) 1. measurement of the intensity of x-rays. 2. the direct measurement of structures shown in the roentgenogram with or without the necessity of correcting for magnification.

roentgenopaque (rent″gen-o-pāk′) radiopaque.

roentgenoparent (rent″gen-o-par′ent) radioparent.

roentgenoscope (rent-gen′o-skōp) a fluoroscope; an apparatus for examining the body by means of the fluorescent screen excited by the roentgen rays.

roentgenoscopy (rent″gĕ-nos′ko-pe) [*roentgen rays* + Gr. *skopein* to examine] examination by means of roentgen rays; fluoroscopy.

roentgenotherapy (rent″gen-o-ther′ah-pe) [*roentgen rays* + Gr. *therapeia* treatment] therapeutic use of roentgen rays.

roeteln (ret′eln) [Ger.] rubella.

Roger's disease, reaction, symptom (ro-zhāz′) [Henri Louis *Roger*, French physician, 1809–1891] see under *disease, reaction,* and *symptom*.

Roger-Josué test (ro-zha′ zho-zu-a′) [H. L. *Roger*; Otto *Josué*, French physician, 1869–1923] see *blister test,* under *tests*.

Rogers' sphygmomanometer (roj′erz) [Oscar H. *Rogers*, American physician, born 1857] see under *sphygmomanometer*.

Röhl's marginal corpuscles (rālz) [Wilhelm *Röhl*, German physician, 1881–1929] see under *corpuscle*.

roka (ro′kah) a tree of Arabia and Africa, *Trichilia emetica* Vahl.; it affords various remedial products.

Rokitansky's disease, diverticulum, pelvis (ro″kĭ-tan′skēz) [Karl Freiherr von *Rokitansky*, pathologist in Vienna, 1804–1878] see *acute yellow atrophy,* under *atrophy,* see *spondylolisthetic pelvis,* under *pelvis,* and see under *diverticulum*.

rolandic (ro-lan′dik) described by or named in honor of Luigi *Rolando*.

Rolando (ro-lan′do), Luigi. An Italian anatomist (1773–1831), known for his studies on the brain and spinal cord, who had a number of anatomical structures named in his honor. See under *angle, area, cell, column, fasciculus, fiber, fissure, funiculus, line, point, substance, tubercle,* and *zone*.

rolandometer (ro″lan-dom′ĕ-ter) an instrument for determining the positions of the various fissures of the surface of the brain.

role (rōl) the behavior pattern that an individual presents to others. **gender r.,** the image projected by a person that identifies him or her as being boy or girl, man or woman. It is the public expression of gender identity. Cf. *gender identity,* under *identity.*

roletamide (ro-let′ah-mīd) chemical name: 3′,4′,5′-trimethoxy-3-(3-pyrrolin-1-yl)acrylophenone; a hypnotic, $C_{16}H_{19}NO_4$.

rolitetracycline (ro″le-tet″rah-si′klēn) [USP] chemical name: 4-(dimethylamino)-1,4,4a,5,5a,6,11,12a-octahydro-3,6,10,12,12a-pentahydroxy-6-methyl-1,11,dioxo-*N*-(1-pyrrolidinylmethyl)-2-naphthacenecarboxamide. A semisynthetic broad-spectrum antibiotic of the tetracycline group, $C_{27}H_{33}N_3O_8$, occurring as a light yellow crystalline powder having an amine-like odor; used as an antibacterial administered intravenously or intramuscularly. **r. nitrate,** a salt of rolitetracycline, having the same actions and uses as the base.

roll (rōl) a cylindrical structure. **cotton r.,** a small cylinder of cotton, for use in dentistry. **iliac r.,** a mass shaped like a sausage, located in the left iliac fossa and produced by a collection of feces or by induration of the walls of the sigmoid flexure; called also *sigmoid sausage.* **jelly r.,** see under *hypothesis.* **scleral r.,** the posterior lip of the internal scleral furrow to which the ciliary body is attached.

roller (rōl′er) a small cylinder of rolled cotton, linen, or flannel for surgical use. **massage r.,** a proprietary apparatus for use in electric massage.

Roller's nucleus (rol′erz) [Christian Friedrich Wilhelm *Roller,* German neurologist, 1802–1878] see under *nucleus.*

Rolleston's rule (rol′es-tonz) [Sir Humphrey Davy *Rolleston,* London physician, 1862–1944] see under *rule.*

Rollet's chancre (ro-lāz′) [Joseph Pierre Martin *Rollet,* French surgeon and syphilographer, 1824–1894] mixed chancre.

Rollet's stroma (rol′ets) [Alexander *Rollet,* Austrian physiologist, 1834–1903] see under *stroma.*

Rollier's radiation, treatment (rol-yāz′) [Auguste *Rollier,* Swiss physician, 1874–1954] see under *radiation* and *treatment.*

Romaña's sign (ro-mahn′yahz) [Cecilio *Romaña,* Brazilian physician] see under *sign.*

romanopexy (ro-man′o-pek″se) [L. *romanum* the sigmoid + Gr. *pēxis* fixation] sigmoidopexy.

romanoscope (ro-man′o-skōp) sigmoidoscope.

Romanovsky's (Romanowsky's) stain (method) (ro″man-of′skēz) [Dimitri Leonidovich *Romanovsky,* Russian physician, 1861–1921] see *Table of Stains.*

Romberg's disease (trophoneurosis), sign, spasm, station (rom′bergz) [Moritz Heinrich *Romberg,* physician in Berlin, 1795–1873] see *facial hemiatrophy,* under *hemiatrophy,* and see under *sign, spasm,* and *station.*

rombergism (rom′berg-izm) the tendency of a patient to fall when he closes his eyes while standing still with his feet close together (Romberg's sign), due to loss of joint position sensation, as in tabes dorsalis.

Römer's test (reaction) (re′merz) [Paul Heinrich *Römer,* hygienist in Greifswald, (c)1876–1916] see under *tests.*

Romilar (ro′mil-ar) trademark for preparations of dextromethorphan hydrobromide.

Rommelaere's sign (rom″el-a-erz′) [Guillaume *Rommelaere,* Belgian physician, 1836–1916] see under *sign.*

Rondomycin (ron″do-mi′sin) trademark for a preparation of methacycline hydrochloride.

rongeur (raw-zhur′) [Fr. "gnawing, biting"] an instrument for cutting tissue, particularly bone.

Roniacol (ro-ni′ah-kol) trademark for preparations of nicotinyl alcohol.

ronidazole (ro-nid′ah-zōl) chemical name: 1-methyl-5-nitro-1*H*-imidazole-2-methanol carbamate (ester); a veterinary antiprotozoal, $C_6H_8N_4O_4$.

Rönne's nasal step (ren′ēz) see under *step.*

ronnel (ron′el) chemical name: phosphorothioic acid, *O,O*-dimethyl *O*-(2,4,5-trichlorophenyl) ester; a cholinesterase inhibitor, $C_8H_8Cl_3O_3PS$, used as an insecticide, effective against flies, roaches, screw worms, and cattle grub.

röntgenography (rent″gen-og′rah-fe) roentgenography.

roof (roof) a covering structure. **r. of orbit,** paries superior orbitae. **r. of skull,** calvaria. **r. of tympanum,** tegmen tympani, def. 1.

room (rōōm) a place in a building enclosed and set apart for occupancy or for performance of certain procedures. **anechoic r.,** an echo-free room used for acoustical testing. **delivery r.,** a hospital room to which an obstetrical patient is taken for delivery. **intensive therapy r.,** intensive care unit. **labor r.,** predelivery room. **operating r.,** a room in a hospital equipped and used for surgical operations. **postdelivery r.,** a recovery room for the care of obstetrical patients immediately after delivery. **predelivery r.,** a hospital room where an obstetrical patient remains during the first stage of labor, i.e., from the time the pains begin until she is ready for delivery; called also *labor r.* **recovery r.,** a hospital unit adjoining operating or delivery rooms, with special equipment and personnel for the care of postoperative or postpartum patients until they may safely be returned to general nursing care in their own rooms or wards.

rooming-in (rōōm′ing-in) the practice of keeping a newly born infant in a crib near the mother's bed, instead of in a nursery, during the hospital stay.

root (root) the lowermost part, or a structure by which something is firmly attached. For official names of various anatomical structures, see under *radix.* **anatomical r.,** the portion of a tooth that is covered by cementum; see *radix dentis* [NA]. **r. of ansa cervicalis, inferior,** radix inferior ansae cervicalis. **r. of ansa cervicalis, superior,** radix superior ansae cervicalis. **r. of arch of vertebra,** pediculus arcus vertebrae. **belladonna r.,** the dried root of *Atropa belladonna,* which contains various anticholinergic alkaloids; called also *deadly nightshade root.* See *belladonna.* **bitter r.,** gentian. **clinical r.,** radix clinica. **r. of clitoris,** crus clitoridis. **cochlear r. of acoustic nerve,** radix inferior nervi vestibulocochlearis. **cranial r's of accessory nerve,** radices craniales nervi accessorii. **dandelion r.,** taraxacum. **deadly nightshade r.,** belladonna r. **facial r.,** radix nervi facialis. **r. of hair,** radix pili. **insane r.,** hyoscyamus. **intermediate r. of olfactory trigone,** stria intermedia trigoni olfactorii. **licorice r.,** glycyrrhiza. **lingual r.,** that root of a posterior tooth, especially a maxillary molar, which is situated nearest the tongue. **long r. of ciliary ganglion,** ramus communicans nervi nasociliaris cum ganglione ciliari. **r. of lung,** radix pulmonis. **mandrake r.,** podophyllum. **r. of median nerve, lateral,** radix lateralis nervi mediani. **r. of median nerve, medial,** radix medialis nervi mediani. **r. of mesentery,** radix mesenterii. **motor r. of ciliary ganglion,** radix oculomotoria ganglii ciliaris. **motor r. of spinal nerves,** radix ventralis. **motor r's of submandibular ganglion,** rami communicantes ganglii submandibularis cum nervo linguali. **motor r. of trigeminal nerve,** radix motoria nervi trigemini. **r. of nail,** radix unguis. **nerve r's,** the series of paired bundles of nerve fibers which emerge at each side of the spinal cord, termed dorsal or posterior (see *radix dorsalis*), or ventral or anterior (see *radix ventralis*) according to their position. There are 31 pairs (8 cervical, 12 thoracic, 5 lumbar, 5 sacral, and 1 coccygeal), each corresponding dorsal and ventral root joining to form a spinal nerve. Called also *spinal r's.* Certain cranial nerves, e.g., the trigeminal, also have nerve roots. **r. of nose,** radix nasi. **oculomotor r. of ciliary ganglion,** radix oculomotoria ganglii ciliaris. **olfactory r., internal,** stria medialis trigoni olfactorii. **r. of optic tract, lateral,** radix lateralis tractus optici. **r. of optic tract, medial,** radix medialis tractus optici. **orizaba jalap r.,** ipomea. **orris r.,** orris. **palatine r.,** that root of a maxillary molar tooth which is situated nearest the palate; lingual root. **r. of penis,** radix penis. **physiological r.,** the portion of a tooth proximal to the gingival crevice, or embedded in the dental alveolus. **puccoon r., red r.,** sanguinaria. **retained r.,** a tooth root, or part of a root, remaining in the soft tissue or in bone following trauma, extensive tooth decay, or incomplete extraction. **sensory r. of ciliary ganglion,** ramus communicans ganglii ciliaris cum nervo nasociliaris. **sensory r. of spinal nerves,** radix dorsalis. **sensory r. of trigeminal nerve,** radix sensoria nervi trigemini. **short r. of ciliary ganglion,** radix oculomotoria ganglii ciliaris. **spinal r's,** nerve r's. **spinal r's of accessory nerve,** radices spinales nervi accessorii. **r. of spinal nerves, anterior,** radix ventralis. **r. of spinal nerves, dorsal, r. of spinal nerves, posterior,** radix dorsalis. **r. of spinal nerves, ventral,** radix ventralis. **sweet r.,** glycyrrhiza. **r. of tongue,** radix linguae. **r. of tooth,** radix dentis. **vestibular r. of acoustic nerve,** radix superior nervi vestibulocochlearis. **vestibular r. of auditory nerve,** radix superior nervi vestibulocochlearis. **r. of vestibulocochlear nerve, inferior,** radix inferior nervi vestibulocochlearis. **r. of vestibulocochlear nerve, superior,** radix superior nervi vestibulocochlearis.

R.O.P. right occipitoposterior (position of the fetus).

ropizine (ro′pĭ-zēn) chemical name: 4-(diphenylmethyl)-*N*-[(6-methyl-2-pyridinyl)methylene]-1-piperazinamine; an anticonvulsant, $C_{24}H_{26}N_4$.

Rorschach test (ror′shahk) [Hermann *Rorschach,* Swiss psychiatrist, 1884–1922] see under *tests.*

rosacea (ro-za′she-ah) a chronic disease affecting the skin of the nose, forehead, and cheeks, marked by flushing, followed by red coloration due to dilatation of the capillaries, with the appearance of papules and acne-like pustules. Called *acne rosacea.* Long-standing rosacea is associated with rhinophyma.

rosamicin (ro″zah-mi′sin) a macrolide antibiotic, $C_{31}H_{51}NO_9$, derived from *Micromonospora rosaria,* having a broad spectrum of antibacterial activity against gram-positive bacteria and some activity against gram-negative bacteria; the butyrate, propionate, sodium phosphate, and stearate salts have antibacterial activity similar to that of the base.

rosaniline (ro-zan′ĭ-lin) a basic dye derived from triphenylmethane, $C_{20}H_{21}N_3O$, occurring as reddish brown crystals, which is soluble in acids and alcohol and slightly soluble in water. It is used, usually as the hydrochloride, in the preparation of other dyes and as a component of basic fuchsin.

rosary (ro′zah-re) a structure resembling a string of beads. **rachitic r.,** rachitic beads; see under *bead.*

rose (rōz) [L. *rosa*] any plant or species of the genus *Rosa.* The flowers of *R. gallica, R. damascena, R. alba, R. centifolia,* and varieties of these species afford rose oil. **r. bengal,** a dye, the dichlor- or the tetrachlorerythrosin, $NaO\cdot(C_6HI_2\cdot O)_2C\cdot C_6H_2Cl_2\cdot COONa$.

Rose's position (ro′zez) [Frank Atcherly *Rose,* British surgeon] see under *position.*

Rose's test (ro′zez) [Joseph Constantin *Rose,* German physician, 1826–1893] see under *tests.*

Rose's tetanus (ro′zez) [Edmund *Rose,* German physician, 1836–1914] see *kofp-tetanus.*

rosein (ro′ze-in) fuchsin.

Rosenbach's sign, etc. (ro′zen-bahks) [Ottomar *Rosenbach,* physician in Berlin, 1851–1907] see under *sign, syndrome,* and *tests.*

Rosenbach's tuberculin (ro′zen-bahks) [F. J. R. *Rosenbach,* German physician, 1843–1923] see under *tuberculin.*

Rosenmüller's body (organ), gland (node), valve, recess (cavity, fossa) (ro′zen-mil″erz) [Johann Christian *Rosenmüller,* German anatomist, 1771–1820] see *epoophoron, nodi lymphatici inguinalis profundi, plica lacrimalis,* and *recessus pharyngeus.*

Rosenthal's canal (ro′zen-tahlz) [Isidor *Rosenthal,* German physiologist, 1836–1915] canalis spiralis modioli.

Rosenthal's test (ro′zen-thahlz) [Sanford Morris *Rosenthal,* American physician, born 1897] see under *tests.*

Rosenthal's vein (ro′zen-tahlz) [Friedrich Christian *Rosenthal,* German anatomist, 1779–1829] vena basalis.

roseola (ro-ze′o-lah, ro″ze-o′lah) [L.] any rose-colored rash, as in measles, syphilis, etc.; sometimes used alone to mean roseola infantum. **r. infan′tilis, r. infan′tum,** exanthema subitum. **syphilitic r.,** an eruption of rose-colored spots in early secondary syphilis; called also *syphilitic exanthem* and *macular syphilid.* **r. typho′sa,** rose spots.

Roser's sign (ro′zerz) [Wilhelm *Roser,* German surgeon, 1817–1888] see under *sign.*

roset (ro-zet′) rosette.

rosette (ro-zet′) [Fr.] any structure or formation resembling a rose, such as (*a*) the clusters of polymorphonuclear leukocytes around a globule of lysed nuclear material, as observed in the test for disseminated lupus erythematosus, or (*b*) a figure formed by the chromosomes in an early stage of mitosis. **malarial r.,** a stage in the asexual cycle of malarial plasmodia at which the parasites have attained full growth and are arranged around the periphery of the erythrocyte in the form of small bodies resembling a rosette and ready to break up into merozoites; seen especially in *Plasmodium malariae* and *P. ovale.*

rosin (roz′in) [L. *resina*] [NF] the solid resin obtained from *Pinus palustris* Mill. (Pinaceae) and other species of pine, occurring as sharply angular, translucent, amber-colored fragments, frequently covered with yellow dust. It contains about 90 per cent resin and 10 per cent neutral matter. Most of the resin acids are isomeric with abietic acid, $C_{44}H_{62}O_4$. It is used as a stiffening agent in the preparation of plasters and ointments. Formerly called *colophony.*

Rosin's test (ro′zenz) [Heinrich *Rosin,* Berlin physician, born 1855] see under *tests.*

Rosmarinus (ros″mah-ri′nus) [L. "sea-dew"] a genus of labiate plants. *R. officina′lis,* or common rosemary, affords the fragrant volatile oil of rosemary.

rosoxacin (ro-soks′ah-sin) chemical name: 1-ethyl-1,4-dihydro-4-oxo-7-(4-pyridinyl)-3-quinolinecarboxylic acid; an antibacterial, $C_{17}H_{14}N_2O_3$.

Ross's black spores, cycle (ros′ez) [Sir Ronald *Ross,* British physician and protozoologist, 1857–1932, noted for his demonstration of the life history of the malarial parasite and proof of its transmission by the bite of the female anopheline mosquito; winner of the Nobel prize for medicine in 1902] see under *spore* and *cycle.*

Ross's bodies (ros′ez) [Edward Halford *Ross,* English pathologist, born 1875] see under *body.*

Rossbach's disease (ros′bahks) [Michael Josef *Rossbach,* German physician, 1842–1894] hyperchlorhydria.

Rossel's test (ros-elz′) [Otto *Rossel,* Swiss physician, 1875–1911] see under *tests.*

Rossolimo's reflex (sign) (ros″o-le′mōz) [Gregorij Ivanovich *Rossolimo,* Russian neurologist, 1860–1928] see under *reflex.*

Rostan's asthma (ros-tahz′) [Louis Léon *Rostan,* Paris physician, 1790–1866] cardiac asthma.

rostellum (ros-tel′um), pl. *rostel′la* [L. "little beak"] a small protuberance or beak, especially the fleshy protuberance of the scolex of a tapeworm, which may or may not bear hooks.

rostrad (ros′trad) 1. toward a rostrum; situated nearer the rostrum in relation to a specific point of reference. 2. cephalad.

rostral (ros′tral) [L. *rostralis,* from *rostrum* beak] 1. pertaining to or resembling a rostrum; having a rostrum or beak. 2. situated toward a rostrum or toward the beak (oral and nasal region), which may mean superior (in relationships of areas of the spinal cord) or anterior or ventral (in relationships of brain areas).

rostralis (ros-tra′lis) [L.] rostral.

rostrate (ros′trāt) [L. *rostratus* beaked] having a beaklike process.

rostriform (ros′trĭ-form) [L. *rostrum* beak + *forma* form] shaped like a beak.

rostrum (ros′trum), pl. *ros′trums* or *ros′tra* [L. "beak"] a beaklike appendage or part; [NA] a general term for such a structure. **r. cor′poris callo′si** [NA], the anterior and lower end of the corpus callosum. **sphenoidal r., r. sphenoida′le** [NA], the prominent ridge on the inferior surface of the sphenoid bone that articulates with a deep depression between the wings of the vomer.

R.O.T. right occipitotransverse (position of the fetus).

Rot see *Roth.*

rot (rot) 1. decay. 2. a disease of sheep, and sometimes of man, caused by *Fasciola hepatica*. **Barcoo r.,** desert sore. **black r.,** a condition sometimes seen in storage eggs, even when kept in a refrigerator; it is caused by *Proteus melanovogenes*. **foot r.,** a disease of the feet of cattle and sheep, marked by decay of the hoof and an offensive discharge; it is caused by *Fusobacterium necrophorum* in cattle and *Bacteroides nodosus* in sheep, especially on soft, wet pasture. Called also *leg ill.* **liver r.,** a disease of sheep and cattle caused by the liver fluke, *Fasciola hepatica*. **pizzle r.,** enzootic balanoposthitis. **sheath r.,** enzootic balanoposthitis.

rotameter (ro-tam′ĕ-ter) a flow-rate meter of variable area with a rotating float in a tapered tube, used for measuring the gases in administering an anesthetic.

rotary (ro′ter-e) marked by or produced by rotation.

rotate (ro′tāt) to turn around an axis; to twist.

rotation (ro-ta′shun) [L. *rotatio, rotare* to turn] the process of turning around an axis; movement of a body about its axis, called the *axis of r.* In labor, the turning of the fetal head through 90 degrees so that the long diameter of the head corresponds with the long diameter of the pelvic outlet. It should occur naturally, but if it does not the rotation must be accomplished manually or instrumentally by the obstetrician. See also *maneuver.* In dentistry, the rotation of a malturned tooth in its central axis into a normal position; also malposition of a tooth due to turning around a longitudinal axis. **molecular r.,** the figure obtained by multiplying the specific rotation by the molecular weight and dividing by 100. **optical r.,** the quality of certain optically active substances whereby the plane of polarized light is changed, so that it is rotated in an arc the length of which is characteristic of the substance. **specific r.,** the arc through which a substance rotates the plane of polarization as observed in a polarimeter. **van Ness r.,** fusion of the knee joint and rotation of the ankle to function as the knee; done to correct a congenitally missing femur.

rotatory (ro″tah-to′re) occurring in or caused by rotation.

rotavirus (ro″tah-vi′rus) [L. *rota* wheel + *virus*] a group of doubled-stranded RNA viruses having a wheel-like appearance and responsible for acute infantile gastroenteritis and for diarrhea in mice, calves, and pigs.

Rotch's sign (roch′es) [Thomas Morgan *Rotch*, physician in Boston, 1849–1914] see under *sign*.

röteln (ret′eln) [Ger.] rubella.

rotenone (ro′tĕ-nōn) a poisonous compound, $C_{23}H_{22}O_6$, from derris root and other roots; used as an insecticide and as a scabicide.

rotexed (ro′tekst) rotated and bent to one side.

rotexion (ro-tek′shun) act of rotating and flexing; also the state of being rotated and flexed.

Roth's (Rot's) disease, syndrome (rōts) [Vladimir Karlovich *Roth*, Russian neurologist, 1848–1916] meralgia paraesthetica.

Roth's spots, vas aberrans (rōts) [Moritz *Roth*, Swiss physician, 1839–1915] see under *spot*, and see *ductuli aberrantes*.

Roth-Bernhardt disease, syndrome (rōt-bern′hart) [Vladimir K. *Roth*, Russian neurologist, 1848–1916; Martin *Bernhardt*, neurologist in Berlin, 1844–1915] meralgia paraesthetica.

rotifer (ro′tĭ-fer) any individual of the class Rotifera.

Rotifera (ro-tif′er-ah) [L. *rota* wheel + *ferre* to bear] a class of small, usually transparent, mostly free-living animals of the phylum Aschelminthes, the rotifers, which characteristically possess a corona of cilia around the anterior end, a cleft foot at the posterior end, and internal jaws. In some systems of classification, they are considered to be a separate phylum.

rotlauf (rot′lowf) [Ger.] swine erysipelas.

rotoxamine (ro-toks′ah-mēn) chemical name: (−)-2-[(4-chlorophenyl)(2-pyridinyl)methoxy]-*N,N*-dimethylethanamine. The *l*-isomer of carbinoxamine, $C_{16}H_{19}ClN_2O$, having antihistaminic potency about twice that of the racemic form. **r. tartrate,** the tartrate salt of rotoxamine, $C_{16}H_{19}ClN_2O \cdot C_4H_6O_6$, occurring as a white to creamy white, crystalline powder, having the same actions as the base; used in the treatment of allergic disorders, administered orally.

Rotter's test (rot′erz) [H. *Rotter*, physician in Budapest] see under *tests*.

rottlera (rot′ler-ah) kamala.

rottlerin (rot′ler-in) a powerful and toxic chromene derivative, $C_{30}H_{28}O_8$, obtained from *Kamala* or *Mallotus philippinensis* (Lam.) Muell.-Arg. (Euphorbiaceae); called also *mallotoxin*.

rotula (rot′u-lah) [L., dim. of *rota* wheel] 1. the patella. 2. any disklike bony process. 3. a troche or lozenge.

rotulad (rot′u-lad) toward the patella, or the patellar aspect.

rotular (rot′u-lar) pertaining to the patella.

rotz (rōts) [Ger.] glanders in horses.

rouge (roozh) a fine red powder composed of iron oxide (Fe_2O_3), usually in cake form but sometimes impregnated on paper or cloth; used in dentistry as a polishing agent for restorations of gold and precious metal alloys.

rouget du porc (roo-zha′ du pork′) [Fr.] the urticarial form of swine erysipelas.

Rouget's bulb (roo-zhāz′) [Antoine D. *Rouget*, French physiologist] bulb of the ovary.

Rouget's cells, muscle (roo-zhāz′) [Charles Marie Benjamin *Rouget*, French physiologist and anatomist, 1824–1904] see *pericyte*, and see under *cell*.

rough (ruf) not smooth; having an irregular, roughened surface.

roughage (ruf′ij) indigestible material such as fibers, cellulose, etc., in the diet.

Rougnon-Heberden disease (roon-yaw′-heb′er-den) [Nicholas François *Rougnon* de Magny, French physician, 1727–1799; William *Heberden*, Sr., English physician, 1710–1801] angina pectoris.

rouleau (roo-lo′), pl. *rouleaux′* [Fr. "roll"] a roll of red blood corpuscles like a pile of coins.

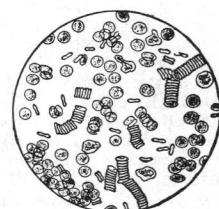

Human red blood cells arranged in rouleaux (Funke).

rouleaux (roo-lo′) [Fr.] plural of *rouleau*.

roundworm (rownd′wurm) any worm of the class Nematoda; a nematode.

Rous sarcoma, test (rows) [Francis Peyton *Rous*, American pathologist, born 1879; co-winner, with Charles B. Huggins, of the Nobel prize in medicine for 1966; for his discovery of tumor-inducing viruses] see under *sarcoma* and *tests*.

Roussel's law, sign (roo-selz′) [Theophile *Roussel*, French physician, 1816–1903] see under *law* and *sign*.

Roussy-Dejerine syndrome (roo-se′-deh″zher-ēn′) [Gustave *Roussy*, French pathologist, 1874–1948; Joseph Jules *Dejerine*, French neurologist, 1849–1917] thalamic syndrome.

Roussy-Lévy disease (roo-se′ la′ve) [Gustave *Roussy*] see under *disease*.

Roux's anastomosis (operation) (rooz) [César *Roux*, Swiss surgeon] see under *anastomosis*.

Roux's operation (rooz) [Philibert Joseph *Roux*, Paris surgeon, 1780–1854] see under *operation*.

Roux's serum (rooz) [Pierre Paul Emile *Roux*, French bacteriologist, 1853–1933] antidiphtheria serum (def. 2); see under *serum*.

Roux-en-Y see under *anastomosis*.

Rovighi's sign (ro-vig′ēz) [Alberto *Rovighi*, Bologna physician, 1856–1919] see under *sign*.

Rowntree-Geraghty test (roun′tre; ger′ah-te) [Leonard George *Rowntree*, American physician, born 1883; John Timothy *Geraghty*, Baltimore physician, 1876–1924] the phenolsulfonphthalein test.

RPF renal plasma flow.

R. Ph. abbreviation for Registered Pharmacist.

rpm revolutions per minute.

RPS renal pressor substance.

R.Q. respiratory quotient.

-rrhage, -rrhagia [Gr. *rhegnynai* to burst forth] word terminations denoting excessive flow.

-rrhea [Gr. *rhoia* flow] a word termination denoting flow or discharge.

R.R.L. Registered Record Librarian.

rRNA ribosomal RNA; see *ribonucleic acid*, under *acid*.

R.S.A. right sacroanterior (position of the fetus).

R.S.B. Regimental Stretcher Bearer.

R.Sc.A. right scapuloanterior (position of the fetus).

R.S.C.N. Registered Sick Children's Nurse.

R.Sc.P. right scapuloposterior (position of the fetus).

R.S.M. Royal Society of Medicine.

R.S.N.A. Radiological Society of North America.

R.S.P. right sacroposterior (position of the fetus).

R.S.T. right sacrotransverse (position of the fetus).

R.S.T.M.H. Royal Society of Tropical Medicine and Hygiene.

RSV Rous sarcoma virus.

R.T. reading test.

RTF resistance transfer factor; see *R factor*, under *factor*.

R.U. rat unit.

Ru chemical symbol for *ruthenium*.

rub (rub) an auscultatory sound caused by the rubbing together of two serous surfaces, as in pericardial rub; called also *friction r.* **friction r.,** see *rub.* **pericardial r.,** a scraping or grating noise heard with the heart beat, usually a to-and-fro sound, associated with an inflamed pericardium. **pleural r., pleuritic r.,** a rub produced by friction between the visceral and costal pleurae.

rubber-dam (rub′er-dam) a sheet of thin latex rubber used by dentists to isolate teeth from the fluids of the mouth during dental treatment.

rubefacient (roo″bĕ-fa′shent) [L. *ruber* red + *facere* to make] 1. reddening the skin. 2. an agent that reddens the skin by producing active or passive hyperemia.

rubella (roo-bel′ah) German measles: a mild viral infection characterized by a pink discrete and confluent macular exanthem. After an incubation period of 14 to 21 days, lymph node enlargement (postauricular, posterior cervical, and elsewhere) often precedes the appearance of a pink, macular eruption, occurring first on the face before spreading rapidly to involve the trunk and finally the extremities. No rash occurs in up to 40 per cent of those with the infection. Rhinorrhea, sore throat, bulbar and occasionally palpebral conjunctivitis precede or accompany the exanthem, which lasts little more than 3 to 4 days before fading. Arthralgia is common, and monoarticular arthritis occurs in 20 per cent of patients, more so in adults than children. Transplacental infection of the fetus in the first trimester produces developmental abnormalities of the heart, eyes, brain, bone, and ears in up to 40 per cent of cases without interrupting the pregnancy. See also under *syndrome.* In certain non–English-speaking countries, the disease is called *rubeola.*

rubeola (roo-be′o-lah, ru″be-o′lah) [L. *ruber* red] a synonym of measles in English and of German measles (see *rubella*) in French and Spanish.

rubeosis (roo″be-o′sis) redness. **r. i′ridis,** a condition characterized by a new formation of vessels and connective tissue on the surface of the iris, frequently seen in diabetics (*r. i′ridis diabet′ica*) and following occlusion of the central retinal vein or artery. It gives rise to severe intractable glaucoma. **r. ret′inae,** a name proposed for a condition characterized by formation of new vessels in front of the optic papilla in retinitis proliferans, seen in nondiabetics, as well as in diabetics (*r. ret′inae diabet′ica*), and usually leading to retinal detachment.

ruber (roo′ber) [L.] red.

rubescent (roo-bes′ent) [L. *rubescere* to become red] reddish; becoming red.

rubidiol (roo-bid′e-ol) a solution in oil of rubidium and potassium mercuric iodide, used externally as a resolvent.

rubidium (roo-bid′e-um) [L. *rubidus* red] a rare metallic alkaline element; atomic number, 37; atomic weight, 85.47; symbol, Rb. **r. and ammonium bromide,** a substance, $RbBr + 3NH_4Br$, used like potassium bromide.

rubidomycin (roo-bid′o-mi″sin) daunorubicin.

rubiginous, rubiginose (roo-bij′ĭ-nus; roo-bij′ĭ-nōs) [L. *rubigo* rust] having a rusty, brownish color; said of sputum.

rubin (roo′bin) fuchsin.

Rubin's test (roo′binz) [Isidor Clinton *Rubin,* New York physician, 1883–1958] see under *tests.*

Rubner's law, test (roob′nerz) [Max *Rubner,* German physiologist, 1854–1932] see under *law* and *tests.*

rubor (roo′bor) [L.] redness, one of the cardinal signs of inflammation.

rubriblast (roo′brĭ-blast) pronormoblast.

rubric (roo′brik) red; specifically, pertaining to the red nucleus.

rubricyte (roo′brĭ-sīt) [L. *rubrum* red + Gr. *kytos* cell] polychromatic normoblast.

rubrospinal (roo″bro-spi′nal) pertaining to the red nucleus and the spinal cord.

rubrothalamic (roo″bro-thah-lam′ik) pertaining to the red nucleus and the thalamus.

rubrum (roo′brum) [L.] red. **r. Con′go,** Congo red. **r. scarlati′num,** scarlet red.

Rubus (roo′bus) [L.] a genus of rosaceous plants, including the blackberries, raspberries, brambles, dewberries, and cloudberries. The root barks of several species of blackberry are tonic and astringent, and have been used in diarrhea. The fruits of *R. idae′us* L. and *R. strigo′sus* Michx. (Rosaceae), red raspberries, are used in pharmacy as vehicles for syrups, etc. See *raspberry juice,* under *juice.*

Ruck's watery extract tuberculin [Karl von *Ruck,* American physician, 1849–1922] see under *tuberculin.*

ructus (ruk′tus) [L.] the belching of wind; eructation. **r. hysteri′cus,** a hysterical condition in which wind is belched frequently and noisily.

Rudbeckia (rud-bek′e-ah) [O. *Rudbeck,* 1630–1702, and O. *Rudbeck,* Jr., 1660–1740] a genus of composite-flowered herbs of North America; the cone flower, *R. lacinia′ta,* thimble weed, is diuretic and tonic.

rudiment (roo′dĭ-ment) 1. primordium; the first indication of a

structure in the course of its development. 2. a structure that has remained undeveloped, or one with little or no function at present but which was functionally developed earlier either in the individual or in its phylogenetic ancestors. **lens r.,** a thickening of the ectoderm of the sides of the embryonic head, from which the crystalline lens develops. **r. of vaginal process,** vestigium processus vaginalis.

rudimentary (roo″dĭ-men′tah-re) 1. imperfectly developed. 2. vestigial.

rudimentum (roo″dĭ-men′tum), pl. *rudimen′ta* [L. "a first beginning"] 1. [NA] the first indication of a structure in the course of its development; a primordium. 2. a vestigial structure. **r. processus vaginalis,** vestigium processus vaginalis.

rue (roo) [L. *Ruta*] the rutaceous herb, *Ruta graveolens;* the volatile oil (*oleum rutae*) from the leaves is an irritant poison.

rufescine (roo′fe-sin) a substance obtained from a mollusk, *Haliotis rufescens,* which corresponds to the bile pigments in man.

Ruffini's brushes (organ), corpuscles (cylinders) (roo-fe′nēz) [Angelo *Ruffini,* Italian anatomist, 1864–1929] see under *brush* and *corpuscle.*

rufiopin (roo″fe-o′pin) a reddish yellow, crystalline substance, $C_{14}H_8O_4$, derivable from opianic acid, and isomeric with rufigallic acid.

rufous (roo′fus) [L. *rufus* red] 1. dull red. 2. having reddish hair and a ruddy complexion.

Rufus (roo′fus) **of Ephesus** (c. 100 A.D.) a physician and anatomist whose surviving writings are noteworthy, particularly those on anatomy, gout, the pulse, and clinical history taking.

ruga (roo′gah), pl. *ru′gae* [L.] a ridge, wrinkle, or fold, as of mucous membrane. **rugae gas′tricae,** rugae of stomach. **r. palati′na,** any one of the transverse ridges extending outward on both sides of the raphe of the palate. **rugae of stomach,** large folds of the mucous membrane of the stomach, occurring especially in the corpus, which are seen when the stomach is empty or undistended. **rugae of vagina, ru′gae vagina′les** [NA], small transverse folds of the mucous membrane of the vagina extending outward from the columns.

rugae (roo′je) [L.] plural of *ruga.*

Ruge-Phillipp test (roo″gah-fil′ip) [Reinhold *Ruge,* German hygienist, 1862–1936; Ernst *Phillipp,* German gynecologist, born 1893] see under *tests.*

rugine (roo-zhēn′) a raspatory.

rugitus (roo′jĭ-tus) [L. "roaring"] rumbling in the intestines caused by movement of flatus; see *borborygmus.*

rugoscopy (roo-gos′ko-pe) the study of the patterns of the grooves and ridges (rugae) of the palate to identify individual patterns.

rugose, rugous (roo′gōs, roo′gus) [L. *rugosus*] characterized by wrinkles.

rugosity (roo-gos′ĭ-te) [L. *rugositas*] 1. the condition of being wrinkled. 2. a fold, wrinkle, or ruga.

R.U.L. right upper lobe (of a lung).

rule (rōōl) [L. *regula*] a statement of conditions commonly observed in a given situation, or a statement of a prescribed course of action to obtain a result. **Abegg's r.** (*obs.*), all atoms have the same number of valences. **Allen's r.,** the extended body parts of warm-blooded species (tail, ears, and limbs) are relatively shorter in the colder regions of a species range than in the warmer. **Anstie's r.,** one used in connection with life insurance examination: the maximum amount of absolute alcohol which can be taken without injury by an adult is 1½ oz. daily. This is equivalent to about 3 oz. of whisky, brandy, gin, or rum; about 4 glasses of sherry or other strong wine; to 1 pint of claret, champagne, or other light wine; to 3 glasses of strong ale or porter; or 5 glasses of beer or light ale. **Arey's r.,** the total length of an embryo or fetus in inches, for the first five months, equals the numerical sum of the numbers of the previous lunar months since conception; for the last five lunar months, it equals the product of the number of the month multiplied by 2. **Bartholomews' r. of fourths,** if the uterine fundus is one-fourth of the way from the pubic symphysis to the umbilicus, the pregnancy is of two months duration; one-half of the way, three months duration; three-quarters of the way, four months duration; at the umbilicus, five months duration. The fundus then rises one-quarter of the way to the ensiform process each month until the ninth, when it sinks to the level it occupied at eight months. **Bastedo's r.,** the dose of a drug for a child is obtained by multiplying the adult dose by the child's age in years, adding 3 to the product, and dividing the sum by 30. **Bergmann's r.,** the body size of geographical races of warm-blooded species is smaller in the warmer parts of the species range than in the colder parts of the range. **Budin's r.,** a bottle-fed baby should not take more than ⅒ of its own weight of cow's milk per day. **Clark's r.,** the dose of a drug for a child is obtained by multiplying the adult dose by the weight of the child in pounds and dividing the result by 150. **Cowling's r.,** the dose of a drug for a child is obtained by multiplying the adult dose by the age of the child at his next birthday and dividing by 24. **delivery date r.,** Nägele's r. **dermatomal r.,** visceral pain is referred to the dermatomes supplied by the posterior roots through which the visceral afferent impulses reach the spinal cord. **Durham r.,** a court decision which states that the M'Naghten rule (q.v.) and irresistible impulse test (q.v.) are not compatible with modern psychiatric thought, and holds that "an accused is not criminally responsible if his unlawful act was the product of mental disease or mental defect." **Fried's r.,** the dose of a drug for an infant less than 2 years old is obtained by multiplying the child's age in months by the adult dose and dividing the result by 150. **Gibson's r.,** in pneumonia, if the pulse pressure in millimeters of mercury does not fall below the pulse rate, the prognosis is good; if it does, prognosis is bad. **Haase's r.,** the total length of an embryo or fetus in centimeters, for the first five months, equals the square of the number of lunar months since conception; for the last five months it equals the product of the number of the month multiplied by 5. **Hardy-Weinburg r.,** if mating is random with respect to genotype, and if p is the frequency of an allele A, and q the frequency of a, then the frequency of genotypes AA, Aa, and aa will be p^2, 2pq, and q^2, respectively. **Hudson's lactone r.,** molecular optical rotation of a carbohydrate or its derivatives is given as the sum of the rotation contributions at each asymmetric center. Certain other empirical conclusions may also be drawn from existing data. **Jackson's r.,** after epileptic attacks, simple nervous processes are more quickly recovered from than complex ones. **Liebermeister's r.,** in febrile tachycardia, the pulse beats increase at the rate of about eight to every degree centigrade of temperature. **Lossen's r.,** in hemophilia, only women transmit the condition, only men inherit it. **McDonald's r.,** the length in centimeters of the abdominal contour from the upper margin of the pubic symphysis to the fundus divided by 3.5 gives the duration of pregnancy in lunar months. **M'Naghten r.,** "to establish a defense on the ground of insanity, it must be clearly proved that at the time of committing the act the party accused was laboring under such a defect of reason from disease of the mind as not to know the nature and quality of the act he was doing, or, if he did know it, that he did not know he was doing what was wrong." **Nägele's r.** (for predicting day of labor), subtract three months from the first day of the last menstruation and add seven days. **octet r.,** when atoms combine to form molecules, they tend to share or transfer electrons until eight (four pairs) are in the valence shell of each atom. **phase r.,** a homogeneous chemical substance of n components is capable of $n + 1$ modifications of phase; e.g., the phases of H_2O are ice, water, and steam. A heterogeneous chemical system of p coexistent phases and c variable components has $p + 2 - c$ degrees of freedom or variations of phase, i.e., the sum of its coexistent phases and its possible changes of phase exceeds the number of its components by 2. **Quetelet's r.,** the body weight of an adult ought to be as many kilograms as his body length in centimeters exceeds 100. **Rolleston's r.,** the ideal systolic pressure for an adult is the figure represented by 100 plus half the age in years. **Schütz's r., Schütz-Borissov r.,** the amount of substrate decomposed in the same time interval by varying enzyme concentrations is not always proportional to the concentration of the enzyme, but is often proportional to the square root of this quantity. **van't Hoff's r.,** the velocity of chemical reactions is increased twofold or more for each rise of 10° C. in temperature; called also *van't Hoff's law.* Cf. *temperature coefficient,* under *coefficient.* **Weinberg's r.,** the total number of dizygotic twins in any population is twice the number of twins of different sex, and the sum of these subtracted from the total number of all twins gives the number of monozygotic twins. **Young's r.,** the dose of a drug for a child is obtained by multiplying the adult dose by the age in years and dividing the result by the sum of the child's age plus 12.

rumbatron (rum'bah-tron)   a high efficiency radio oscillator in which atoms are shattered and which employs electrons as the bombarding particles.

rumen (roo'men)   the first stomach of a ruminant, or cud-chewing animal; also called *paunch.*

rumenitis (roo"mĕ-ni'tis)   inflammation of the rumen.

rumenotomy (roo"mĕ-not'o-me) [*rumen* + Gr. *tomē* a cutting]   the operation of cutting into the rumen of an animal for the purpose of removing foreign bodies or impacted food or for evacuating gases.

ruminant (roo'mĭ-nant)   1. chewing the cud.   2. one of the order of animals which have a stomach with four complete cavities (1, rumen; 2, reticulum; 3, omasum; 4, abomasum), through which the food passes in digestion. The division includes oxen, sheep, goats, deer, and antelopes.

rumination (roo"mĭ-na'shun) [L. *ruminatio*]   1. the casting up of the food to be chewed a second time, as in cattle. In man, the regurgitation of food after almost every meal, part of it being vomited and the rest swallowed: a condition seen in infants. See *merycism.* 2. meditation.   **obsessive r.,** the constant preoccupation with certain thoughts, with inability to dismiss them from the mind.

ruminative (roo"mĭ-na'tiv)   characterized by rumination; constantly dwelling on certain topics or ideas.

Rummo's disease (room'ōz) [Gaetano *Rummo,* Italian physician, 1853–1917]   cardioptosis.

rump (rump)   the buttock or gluteal region.

Rumpel-Leede phenomenon (sign, test) (room'pel-la'dĕ) [Theodor *Rumpel,* German physician, 1862–1923; Stockbridge Carl *Leede,* German physician, born 1882]   see under *phenomenon.*

Rumpf's sign (symptom, reaction) (roompfs) [Heinrich Theodor Maria *Rumpf,* German physician, born 1851]   see under *sign.*

Runeberg's anemia (disease, type) formula (roo'nĕ-bergs) [Johan Wilhelm *Runeberg,* Finnish physician, 1843–1918]   see under *anemia* and *formula.*

Ruphos (roo'fos)   see *Rufus of Ephesus.*

rupia (roo'pe-ah) [Gr. *rhypos* filth]   thick, dark, raised, lamellated, adherent crusts on the skin somewhat resembling oyster shells, as in late recurrent secondary syphilis.

rupial (roo'pe-al)   pertaining to or resembling rupia.

rupioid (roo'pe-oid)   resembling rupia.

rupture (rup'chur)   1. forcible tearing or disruption of tissue.   2. a hernia.   **defense r.,** a breaking down of the body's defense against infection, such as is seen when silica particles inhaled by a worker break down the resistance against tuberculosis.

Rusconi's anus (roos-ko'nēz) [Mauro *Rusconi,* Italian biologist, 1776–1849]   the blastopore.

rush (rush)   a powerful wave of contractile activity which travels extremely long distances down the small intestine; it is caused by intense irritation or unusual distention. Called also *peristaltic r.*

Russell's bodies (rus'elz) [William *Russell,* physician in Edinburgh, 1852–1940]   see under *body.*

Russell effect (rus'el) [W. J. *Russell,* British physicist]   see under *effect.*

Russell's viper, viper venom (rus'elz) [Patrick *Russell,* Aleppo physician, 1727–1805]   see under *viper* and *venom.*

Russo's reaction (test) (roo'sōz) [Mario *Russo,* Italian physician, born 1866]   see under *reaction.*

rust (rust)   1. iron oxide or hydroxide, forming a reddish deposit on metallic iron where the latter has been exposed to moisture; also a similar deposit on other metals that have been exposed to dampness.   2. a fungal disease of plants characterized by the formation of rust-like spots on them.

Rust's disease, phenomenon (sign), syndrome (roosts) [Johann Nepomuk *Rust,* German surgeon, 1775–1840]   see under *disease, phenomenon,* and *syndrome.*

rut (rut) [L. *rugitus* roaring]   1. the period or season of heightened sexual activity in some male mammals that coincides with the season of estrus in the females.   2. estrus.

rutaecarpine (roo"te-kar'pin)   a crystalline alkaloid, $C_{18}H_{13}$-ON_3, from *Evodia rutaecarpa,* a small Asiatic shrub or tree.

ruthenium (roo-the'ne-um)   a rare, very hard metallic element; symbol, Ru; atomic weight, 101.07; atomic number, 44.

rutherford (ruth'er-ford) [Ernest *Rutherford,* British physicist, 1871–1937]   the unit representing one million disintegrations of radioactive matter per second. Abbreviated rd.

rutherfordium (ruth"er-ford'e-um) [named for Sir Ernest *Rutherford,* British physicist, 1871–1937]   a transuranic element, atomic number 104, atomic weight 261, symbol Rf, produced by an induced nuclear reaction.

rutidosis (roo"tĭ-do'sis)   rhytidosis.

rutilism (roo"tĭ-lizm) [L. *rutilis* red, inclining to golden yellow]   red-headedness.

rutin (roo'tin)   chemical name: 3,3',4',5,7-penta-hydroxyflavone-3-rutinoside. A bioflavonoid, $C_{27}H_{30}O_{16}$, occurring as a greenish yellow powder, obtained from buckwheat or other sources, which has been reported to reduce capillary fragility.

rutinose (roo'tĭ-nōs)   rhamnosidoglucose, a disaccharide occurring in rutin.

rutoside (roo'to-sīd)   rutin.

Ruysch's glomeruli, membrane (tunic), muscle, tube, veins (roish'ez) [Frederic *Ruysch,* Dutch anatomist, 1638–1731]   see *glomeruli renis, lamina choriocapillaris,* and *venae vorticosae,* and see under *muscle* and *tube.*

RV   residual volume.

R.V.H.   right ventricular hypertrophy.

rye (ri)   the cereal plant, *Secale cereale,* and its nutritious seed.   **spurred r.,** see *ergot,* def. 1.

Ryle tube (ril) [G. A. *Ryle,* British physician]   see under *tube.*

S

S chemical symbol for *sulfur.*

S. abbreviation for Latin *se'mis* half; *sacral* (in vertebral formulas); *siemens; sig'na* mark (see *prescription* and *signature,* def. 2); *smooth* (colony); *sinis'ter* left; *subject; supravergence;* and *Svedberg unit of sedimentation coefficient* (10^{-13} sec.).

Σ the capital of Greek sigma; symbol for summation.

σ sigma, the eighteenth letter of the Greek alphabet; symbol for one-thousandth part of a second and standard deviation.

S.A. abbreviation for L. *secun'dum ar'tem,* according to art.

Saathoff's test (saht'ofs) [Lübhard *Saathoff,* German physician, 1877–1929] see under *tests.*

S.A.B. Society of American Bacteriologists.

saber-legged (sa'ber-legd) having the angle of the hock more acute than normal, so that the hind feet stand well under the body; said of horses.

Sabin's vaccine (sa'binz) [Albert Bruce *Sabin,* American virologist, born 1906] live oral poliovirus vaccine; see under *vaccine.*

sabinism (sab'ĭ-nizm) poisoning by savin.

sabinol (sab'ĭ-nol) a terpene alcohol, $(CH_3)_2CH \cdot C_6H_6(OH):CH_2$, from the evergreen shrub, *Juniperus sabina* L., which is the chief constituent of savin oil; see *savin.*

Sabouraud's agar (sab'oo-rōz) [Raymond Jacques Adrien *Sabouraud,* French dermatologist, 1864–1938] see under *culture media.*

Sabouraudia (sab″oo-ro'de-ah) *Trichophyton.*

Sabouraudites (sab″oo-ro-di'tēz) *Microsporum.*

sabulous (sab'u-lus) [L. *sabulosus; sabulum* sand] gritty or sandy.

saburra (sah-bur'ah) [L.] foulness of the stomach, mouth, or teeth.

saburral (sah-bur'al) [L. *saburra* sand] pertaining to or of the nature of sordes, or of foulness of the stomach.

sac (sak) [L. *saccus;* Gr. *sakkos*] a pouch; a baglike organ or structure. **abdominal s.,** a serous sac in the embryo which develops into the abdominal cavity. **air s's,** alveoli pulmonis. **allantoic s.,** the dilated portion of the allantois which becomes a part of the placenta in many mammals. **alveolar s's,** sacculi alveolares. **amniotic s.,** amnion. **aneurysmal s.,** the chamber of a sacculated aneurysm. **aortic s.,** the homologue in mammalian embryos of the ventral aorta, from which arise the series of aortic arches. **chorionic s.,** the mammalian chorion. **conjunctival s.,** saccus conjunctivae. **dental s.,** the dense fibrous layer of mesenchyme surrounding the enamel organ and dental papilla. **dural s.,** the continuation of the dura mater below the caudal end of the spinal cord. **embryonic s.,** the blastocyst. **enamel s.,** the enamel organ during the stage in which its outer layer forms a sac enclosing the whole dental germ. **endolymphatic s.,** saccus endolymphaticus. **epiploic s.,** omental bursa. **gestation s.,** the extraembryonic membranes that envelop the embryo or fetus; in man, the fused amnion and chorion. **greater s. of peritoneum,** the peritoneum of the peritoneal cavity proper. **heart s.,** the pericardium. **hernial s.,** the pouch of peritoneum enclosing a hernia. **Hilton's s.,** sacculus laryngis. **lacrimal s.,** saccus lacrimalis. **laryngeal s.,** ventriculus laryngis. **lesser s. of peritoneal cavity,** omental bursa. **Lower's s's,** sacculated portions of the jugular vein at exit of the vein from the skull. **omental s.,** omental bursa. **pericardial s.,** pericardium. **pleural s.,** cavum pleurae. **serous s.,** the sac made up of the pleura, pericardium, and peritoneum. **splenic s.,** recessus lienalis. **tear s.,** saccus lacrimalis. **vitelline s.,** yolk s. **yolk s.,** the extraembryonic membrane that connects with the midgut; at the end of the fourth week of development it expands into a pear-shaped vesicle (*umbilical vesicle*) connected to the body of the embryo by a long narrow tube (*yolk stalk*). In marsupial and placental mammals, it produces a complete vitelline circulation in the early embryo and then undergoes regression; in oviparous vertebrates, it encloses the yolk mass, breaks down yolk, and makes it available to the developing organism.

sacbrood (sak'brōōd) an infectious disease of the larvae of bees, caused by a virus.

saccade (sah-kād') the series of involuntary, abrupt, rapid, small movements or jerks of both eyes simultaneously in changing the point of fixation.

saccadic (sah-kad'ik) [Fr. *saccader* to jerk] denoting the rapid involuntary small movements of both eyes simultaneously in changing the point of fixation on a visualized object, such as the series of jumps the eyes make in scanning a line of print.

saccate (sak'āt) [L. *saccatus*] 1. shaped like a sac. 2. contained in a sac.

saccharascope (sak'ah-rah-skōp) [Gr. *sakcharon* sugar + *skopein* to examine] a fermentation saccharimeter; see *saccharimeter.*

saccharase (sak'ah-rās) β-fructofuranosidase.

saccharate (sak'ah-rāt) a salt of saccharic acid.

saccharated (sak'ah-rāt″ed) [L. *saccharatus,* from *saccharum* sugar] charged with or containing sugar.

saccharephidrosis (sak″ar-ef″ĭ-dro'sis) [Gr. *sakcharon* sugar + *ephidrōsis* sweating] the discharge of sugar in the sweat.

saccharide (sak'ah-rid) one of a series of carbohydrates, including the sugars. The saccharides are divided into monosaccharides, disaccharides, trisaccharides, etc., or into oligosaccharides and polysaccharides, according to the number of saccharide groups ($C_nH_{2n}O_{n-1}$) composing them.

sacchariferous (sak″ah-rif'er-us) [L. *saccharum* sugar + *ferre* to bear] containing or yielding sugar.

saccharification (sak″ar-ĭ-fi-ka'shun) [L. *saccharum* sugar + *facere* to make] conversion into sugar.

saccharimeter (sak″ah-rim'ĕ-ter) [L. *saccharum* sugar + *metrum* measure] a device for estimating the proportion of sugar in a solution. It is either a polarimeter, indicating the proportion of sugar by the number of degrees through which it rotates the plane of polarization, or a hydrometer, indicating the proportion of sugar by the specific gravity of the solution. **Einhorn's s.,** a form of fermentation saccharimeter. **fermentation s.,** a saccharimeter in the form of a bent graduated tube and closed at one end. The amount of sugar in the urine is indicated by the gas which collects at the closed end when yeast is added to the urine. **Lohnstein's s.,** an instrument for performing a quantitative fermentation test of sugar in the urine.

saccharin (sak'ah-rin) [NF] chemical name: 1,2-benzisothiazolin-3-(2H)-one-1,1-dioxide. A white crystalline compound, C_7H_5-NO_3S, several hundred times sweeter than sucrose; used as a sweetening agent in pharmaceutical preparations. **s. calcium** [USP], a salt, $C_{14}H_8CaN_2O_2 \cdot 3\frac{1}{2}H_2O$, used as a non-nutritive sweetener when sugar is contraindicated. **s. sodium** [USP], a salt, $C_7H_4NNaO_3S \cdot 2H_2O$, used like the calcium salt.

saccharine (sak'ah-rin) [L. *saccharinus*] sugary; having a sweet taste.

saccharinol (sah-kar'ĭ-nol) saccharin.

saccharinum (sak″ah-ri'num) saccharin.

saccharo- (sak'ah-ro) [L. *saccharum;* Gr. *sakcharon* sugar] a combining form denoting relationship to sugar.

saccharobiose (sak″ah-ro-bi'ōs) a disaccharide.

saccharocoria (sak″ah-ro-ko're-ah) abhorrence of sugar.

saccharogalactorrhea (sak″ah-ro-gah-lak″to-re'ah) [*saccharo-* + Gr. *gala* milk + *rhoia* flow] the secretion of milk containing an excess of sugar.

saccharolytic (sak″ah-ro-lit'ik) [*saccharo-* + Gr. *lysis* dissolution] capable of chemically splitting up sugar.

saccharometabolic (sak″ah-ro-met″ah-bol'ik) pertaining to the metabolism of sugar.

saccharometabolism (sak″ah-ro-mĕ-tab'o-lizm) the metabolism of sugar.

saccharometer (sak″ah-rom'ĕ-ter) saccharimeter.

Saccharomyces (sak″ah-ro-mi'sēz) [*saccharo-* + Gr. *mykēs* fungus] a genus of ascomycetous fungi of the family Saccharomycetaceae, the yeasts. **S. al'bicans,** *Candida albicans.*

Saccharomyces (de Rivas).

S. an'ginae, *Candida albicans.* **S. apicula'tus,** *Kloekera apiculatus.* **S. baya'nus,** a species from fermenting wine and beer; called also *S. pastorianus.* **S. cant'liei,** a species reported from a tropical blastomycosis; it is now known to be *Pityrosporon ovale.* **S. capillit'ii,** a species from the scalp, with spherical cells, said to cause alopecia seborrheica; it is now known to be *Pityrosporon ovale.* **S. carlsbergen'sis,** a species used in microbiological assay in measuring vitamin B₆ in the urine, and in the brewing of beer. **S. cerevis'iae,** a species with oval or spherical cells, known as *brewers'* or *bakers' yeast;* it causes alcoholic fermentation, and is a very rare cause of lung disease. **S. dairen'sis,** a species with oval or elliptical cells that produces a fermentation in milk; called also *S. galacticolus.*

1165

S. ellipsoi′deus, a form from wine yeast, forming elliptical cells, solitary or in branching chains; it causes alcoholic fermentation in wines. **S. exig′uus,** a form in beer yeast, whose cells are elliptical and solitary, or in branching chains; it causes late fermentation in beer. **S. galact′olus,** *S. dairensis.* **S. glu′tinis,** *Rhodotorula glutinis.* **S. granulomato′sus,** *Cryptococcus neoformans.* **S. guttula′tus,** *Saccharomycopsis guttulatus.* **S. hansen′ii,** *Debaryomyces hansenii.* **S. hom′inis,** a species once isolated in chronic infectious pyemia; it is now known to be *Bacillus megatherium.* **S. lemonnie′ri,** a pathogenic fungus found in bronchitis; it was probably *Candida albicans.* **S. litho′genes,** a species from the lymph glands of an ox suffering from carcinoma of the liver; it is pathogenic to animals. It is now known to be *Cryptococcus neoformans.* **S. mesenter′icus,** *Candida mesenterica.* **S. mycoder′ma,** *Candida vini.* **S. neofor′mans,** *Cryptococcus neoformans.* **S. pastoria′nus,** *S. bayanus.* **S. ru′brum,** a Brazilian species reported to cause a parapsoriasic affection; it was probably the skin contaminant *Rhodotorula rubra.* **S. subcuta′neus tumefa′ciens,** a species, which is probably the same as *Cryptococcus neoformans,* once found in a myxoma of the thigh; it is pathogenic for animals. **S. tumefa′ciens al′bus,** a species discovered in certain cases of pharyngitis, pathogenic for mice, guinea pigs, and rabbits; it is now known to be *Candida albicans.*

saccharomyces (sak″ah-ro-mi′sēz), pl. *saccharomyce′tes.* An organism of the genus *Saccharomyces.* **Busse's s.,** *Cryptococcus neoformans.*

Saccharomycetacea (sak″ah-ro-mi-sĕ-ta′se-e) a family of ascomycetous fungi of the order Endomycetales, subclass Hemiascomycetidae, the members of which are usually unicellular yeasts and reproduce sexually by formation of ascospores; it includes the genus *Saccharomyces.*

saccharomycetes (sak″ah-ro-mi-se′tēz) plural of *saccharomyces.*

saccharomycetic (sak″ah-ro-mi-set′ik) pertaining to or due to the presence of yeastlike fungi.

saccharomycetolysis (sak″ah-ro-mi″sĕ-tol′ĭ-sis) [*saccharomyces* + Gr. *lysis* dissolution] the splitting up of saccharomyces.

Saccharomycopsis (sak″ah-ro-mi-kop′sis) a genus of perfect yeasts of the family Saccharomycetaceae. **S. guttula′tus,** a species found in the intestinal tract of herbivorous animals; formerly called *Saccharomyces guttulatus.*

saccharopine (sak′ah-ro-pēn″) an intermediate compound in the metabolism of lysine.

saccharorrhea (sak″ah-ro-re′ah) [*saccharo-* + Gr. *rhoia* flow] glycosuria.

saccharosan (sak′ah-ro-san) a form of anhydrosugar.

saccharose (sak′ah-ro-rōs) [*saccharo-* + *-ose*] sucrose.

saccharosuria (sak″ah-ro-su′re-ah) [*saccharose* + Gr. *ouron* urine + *-ia*] sucrosuria.

Saccharum (sak′ah-rum) a genus of graminaceous plants. *S. officina′rum* L., sugar cane, affords a large part of the commercial supply of sugar.

saccharum (sak′ah-rum) [L.; Gr. *sakcharon*] sugar, especially cane sugar, or sucrose. **s. acer′num, s. canaden′se,** maple sugar. **s. lac′tis,** sugar of milk; lactose. **s. us′tum,** caramel.

saccharuria (sak″ah-roo′re-ah) [*saccharo-* + Gr. *ouron* urine + *-ia*] glycosuria.

sacciform (sak′sĭ-form) [L. *saccus* sac + *forma* form] shaped like a sac or bag.

saccular (sak′u-lar) shaped like a sac.

sacculated (sak′u-lāt″ed) [L. *sacculatus*] characterized by sacculation or by the presence of saccules.

sacculation (sak″u-la′shun) 1. a sacculus, or pouch. 2. the quality of being sacculated, or pursed out with little pouches. **s's of colon,** haustra coli.

saccule (sak′ūl) [L. *sacculus*] 1. a little bag or sac. 2. see *sacculus.* **air s's, alveolar s's,** sacculi alveolares. **laryngeal s., s. of larynx,** sacculus laryngis.

sacculi (sak′u-li) [L.] plural of *sacculus.*

sacculocochlear (sak″u-lo-kok′le-ar) pertaining to the sacculus and cochlea.

sacculus (sak′u-lus), pl. *sac′culi* [L., dim. of *saccus*] a little bag or sac; applied in official anatomical nomenclature specifically to the smaller of the two divisions of the membranous labyrinth of the vestibule, which communicates with the cochlear duct by way of the ductus reuniens. Called also *s. proprius, s. rotundus, s. sphaericus, s. vestibularis,* and *saccule.* **sac′culi alveola′res** [NA], alveolar saccules: the spaces into which the alveolar ducts open distally, and with which the alveoli communicate; called also *alveolar sacs.* **s. commu′nis,** utriculus. **s. den′tis,** a fibrous sac in the jaw which encloses an unerupted tooth, being connected with the overlying gingiva by the gubernaculum dentis. **s. endolymphat′icus,** saccus endolymphaticus. **s. lacrima′lis,** saccus lacrimalis. **s. laryn′gis** [NA], laryngeal saccule: a diverticulum extending upward from the front of the laryngeal ventricle, between the vestibular fold medially and the thyroarytenoid muscle and thyroid cartilage laterally; called also

appendix ventriculi laryngis. **s. Morgag′nii,** ventriculus laryngis. **s. pro′prius, s. rotun′dus, s. sphae′ricus,** see *sacculus.* **s. ventricula′ris,** s. laryngis. **s. vestibula′ris,** see *sacculus.*

saccus (sak′kus), pl. *sac′ci* [L.; Gr. *sakkos*] a sac or pouch; [NA] a general term for a saclike structure. **s. conjuncti′vae** [NA], conjunctival sac: the potential space, lined by conjunctiva, between the eyelids and the eyeball. **s. endolymphat′icus** [NA], endolymphatic sac: the blind, flattened cerebral end of the endolymphatic duct. **s. lacrima′lis** [NA], lacrimal sac: the dilated upper end of the nasolacrimal duct.

Sachs' disease [Bernard (Barney) *Sachs,* New York neurologist, 1858–1944] see *amaurotic familial idiocy,* under *idiocy.*

Sachs-Georgi test (reaction) [Hans *Sachs,* German immunologist, 1877–1945; Walter *Georgi,* German bacteriologist, 1889–1920] see under *tests.*

Sachs-Witebsky test (reaction) (saks′ wĭ-teb′ske) [Hans *Sachs;* Ernest *Witebsky,* German-born immunologist in the United States, born 1901] see under *tests.*

Sachsse's test (zahk′sez) [Georg Robert *Sachsse,* German chemist, 1840–1895] see under *tests.*

sacrad (sa′krad) toward the sacrum, or sacral aspect.

sacral (sa′kral) [L. *sacralis*] pertaining to or situated near the sacrum.

sacralgia (sa-kral′je-ah) [*sacrum* + *-algia*] pain in the sacrum.

sacralization (sa″kral-i-za′shun) anomalous fusion of the fifth lumbar vertebra to the first segment of the sacrum, so that the sacrum consists of six segments.

sacrarthrogenic (sa″krar-thro-jen′ik) [*sacrum* + Gr. *arthron* joint + *gennan* to produce] resulting from disease of a sacral joint.

sacrectomy (sa-krek′to-me) [*sacrum* + Gr. *ektomē* excision] excision or resection of the sacrum.

sacro- (sa′kro) [L. *sacrum* sacred] a combining form denoting relationship to the sacrum.

sacroanterior (sa″kro-an-te′re-or) having the sacrum directed forward; see under *position.*

sacrococcygeal (sa″kro-kok-sij′e-al) pertaining to or located in the region of the sacrum and coccyx.

sacrococcyx (sa″kro-kok′siks) the sacrum and coccyx together.

sacrocoxalgia (sa″kro-kok-sal′je-ah) pain in the sacroiliac joint.

sacrocoxitis (sa″kro-kok-si′tis) [*sacro-* + L. *coxa* hip + *-itis*] inflammation of the sacroiliac joint.

sacrodynia (sa″kro-din′e-ah) [*sacro-* + Gr. *odynē* pain] pain in the sacral region.

sacroiliac (sa″kro-il′e-ak) pertaining to the sacrum and ilium; denoting the joint or articulation between the sacrum and ilium and the ligaments associated therewith.

sacroiliitis (sa″kro-il″e-i′tis) inflammation in the sacroiliac joint.

sacrolisthesis (sa″kro-lis-the′sis) the condition in which the sacrum lies anterior to the fifth lumbar vertebra.

sacrolumbar (sa″kro-lum′bar) [*sacro-* + L. *lumbus* loin] pertaining to the sacrum and the loin.

sacroperineal (sa″kro-per″ĭ-ne′al) pertaining to the sacrum and the perineum.

sacroposterior (sa″kro-pos-te′re-or) having the sacrum directed backward; see under *position.*

sacropromontory (sa″kro-prom′on-to-re) the promontory of the sacrum.

sacrosciatic (sa″kro-si-at′ik) pertaining to the sacrum and the ischium.

sacrospinal (sa″kro-spi′nal) [*sacro-* + L. *spina* spine] pertaining to the sacrum and the spine, or vertebral column.

sacrotomy (sa-krot′o-me) [*sacro-* + Gr. *temnein* to cut] the operation of cutting out the lower end of the sacrum.

sacrotransverse (sa″kro-trans-vers′) relating to the direction of the fetal sacrum in breech presentation; see under *position.*

sacrouterine (sa″kro-u′ter-in) pertaining to the sacrum and the uterus.

sacrovertebral (sa″kro-ver′tĕ-bral) pertaining to the sacrum and the vertebral column.

sacrum (sa′krum) [L. "sacred"] the triangular bone just below the lumbar vertebrae, formed usually by five fused vertebrae (sacral vertebrae) that are wedged dorsally between the two hip bones; called also *os sacrum* [NA]. See Plate accompanying *skeleton.* **assimilation s.,** see *assimilation pelvis,* under *pelvis.* **tilted s.,** a condition marked by separation of the sacroiliac joint and forward displacement of the sacrum.

sactosalpinx (sak″to-sal′pinks) [Gr. *saktos* stuffed + *salpinx* tube] dilatation of the inflamed uterine tube by retained secretions.

saddle (sad′l) a part or section of the base of a partial denture.

sadism (sad′izm) [Marquis de *Sade,* 1740–1814] sexual perversion in which satisfaction is derived from humiliating or hurting another. **anal s.,** in Freudian theory, the sadistic manifestations of anal erotism, such as aggressiveness, selfishness, and stinginess. **oral s.,** in Freudian theory, a sadistic form of oral erotism manifested by fantasies of chewing, biting, etc.

sadist (sad′ist) a practicer of sadism.

sadistic (să-dis′tik) pertaining to or characterized by sadism.

sadomasochism (sad″o-mas′o-kizm) a state characterized by both sadistic and masochistic tendencies.

sadomasochistic (sad″o-mas″o-kis′tik) characterized by both sadism and masochism.

Saemisch's operation (section), ulcer (sa′mish-ez) [Edwin Theodor *Saemisch*, ophthalmologist in Bonn, 1833–1909] see under *operation*, and see *ulcus serpens corneae*.

Saenger's macula (zeng′erz) [Max *Saenger*, gynecologist in Prague, 1853–1903] see *macula gonorrhoeica*.

Saenger's sign (reflex) (zeng′erz) [Alfred *Saenger*, German neurologist, 1861–1921] see under *sign*.

Saff (saf) trademark for a preparation of safflower oil.

Safflor (saf′flor) trademark for a preparation of safflower oil.

safrene (saf′rēn) a hydrocarbon, $C_{10}H_{16}$, obtained from sassafras oil.

safrol (saf′rol) an oily, volatile (melting point, 11° C.) substance, the methylene ether of 3,4-dihydroxyallylbenzene from sassafras oil; has been used as anodyne.

safrosin (saf′ro-sin) bluish eosin.

safu (sah′foo) Japanese name for leukopathia punctata reticularis symmetrica.

sagittal (saj′ĭ-tal) [L. *sagittalis; sagitta* arrow] 1. shaped like or resembling an arrow; straight. 2. situated in the direction of the sagittal suture; said of an anteroposterior plane or section parallel to the median plane of the body.

sagittalis (saj″ĭ-ta′lis) sagittal; [NA] a general term denoting a structure situated in the direction of the sagittal suture.

sago (sa′go) a starch mainly derived from the pith of various species of palm, chiefly of the genus *Sagus*.

Sahli's reaction, method, test (sah′lēz) [Herman *Sahli*, physician in Bern, 1856–1933] see *desmoid reaction*, under *reaction*, and see under *method* and *tests*.

S.A.L. abbreviation for L. *secun′dum ar′tis le′ges*, according to the rules of art.

sal (sal) [L.] salt. **s. ammoniac,** ammonium chloride. **s. diuret′icum,** potassium acetate. **s. so′da,** sodium carbonate. **s. volat′ile, volat′ilis,** ammonium carbonate.

Sala's cells (sal′ahz) [Luigi *Sala*, Italian zoologist, 1863–1930] see under *cell*.

salamander (sal″ah-man′der) [Gr. *salamandra* a kind of lizard] a tailed amphibian, many species of which are used in various types of experiments.

salamanderin (sal″ah-man′der-in) a poisonous base from the skin of a species of salamander.

salantel (sal′an-tel) chemical name: *N*-[3-chloro-4-(4-chlorobenzoyl)phenyl]-2-hydroxy-3,5-diiodobenzamide; a veterinary anthelmintic, $C_{20}H_{11}Cl_2I_2NO_3$.

salazosulfapyridine (sal″ah-zo-sul″fah-pir′ĭ-den) sulfasalazine.

salbutamol (sal-bu′tah-mol) albuterol.

salcolex (sal′ko-leks) chemical name: choline salicylate (salt) compound with magnesium sulfate (2:1); an analgesic, anti-inflammatory, and antipyretic, $[C_{12}H_{19}NO_4]_2 \cdot MgSO_4 \cdot 4H_2O$.

salethamide maleate (sal-eth′ah-mīd) chemical name: *N*-[2-(diethylamino)ethyl]salicylamide maleate (1:1) (salt); an analgesic, $C_{13}H_{20}N_2O_2 \cdot C_4H_4O_4$.

salicylaldehyde (sal″ĭ-sil-al′dĕ-hīd) salicylic aldehyde.

salicylamide (sal″ĭ-sil-am′id) chemical name: 2-hydroxybenzamide. An amide of salicylic acid, $C_7H_7NO_2$, occurring as a white, crystalline powder; used as an analgesic and antipyretic, administered orally.

salicylanilide (sal″ĭ-sil-an′ĭ-lid) chemical name: 2-hydroxy-*N*-phenylbenzamide. A compound usually prepared by the interaction of salicylic acid and aniline, $C_{13}H_{11}NO_2$, occurring as white or slightly pink crystals; used as a topical antifungal in the treatment of tinea capitis.

salicylase (sah-lis′ĭ-lās) an enzyme oxidizing salicylaldehyde into salicylic acid.

salicylate (sal′ĭ-sil″āt, sah-lis′ĭ-lāt) any salt of salicylic acid; the salicylates used as drugs include aspirin, choline salicylate, methyl salicylate, magnesium salicylate, sodium salicylate, and choline magnesium trisalicylate. **s. meglumine,** chemical name: 2-hydroxybenzoic acid compound with 1-deoxy-1-(methylamino)-D-glucitol; an antirheumatic and analgesic, $C_7H_{11}NO_5 \cdot C_7H_6O_3$.

salicylated (sal′ĭ-sil″āt-ed) containing or impregnated with salicylic acid.

salicylazosulfapyridine (sal″ĭ-sil″ah-zo-sul″fah-pir′ĭ-den) sulfasalazine.

salicylemia (sal″ĭ-sil-e′me-ah) [*salicylate* + Gr. *haima* blood + *-ia*] the presence of salicylate in the blood.

salicylic (sal″ĭ-sil′ik) pertaining to the radical salicyl; see under *acid*.

salicylism (sal″ĭ-sil′izm) a group of commonly occurring toxic effects of excessive dosage with salicylic acid or its salts, usually marked by tinnitus, nausea, and vomiting.

salicyltherapy (sal″ĭ-sil-ther′ah-pe) treatment by salicylic acid or salicylates.

salifiable (sal″ĭ-fi″ah-b'l) [L. *sal* salt + *fieri* to become] capable of combining with acids so as to form salts.

salify (sal′ĭ-fi) to convert into a salt.

salimeter (sah-lim′ĕ-ter) [L. *sal* salt + *metrum* measure] a hydrometer for ascertaining the concentration of saline solutions.

saline (sa′lēn, sa′līn) [L. *salinus; sal* salt] salty; of the nature of a salt; containing a salt or salts. **physiological s.,** an isotonic aqueous solution of NaCl for temporarily maintaining living cells.

salinigrin (sal″ĭ-ni′grin) a glycoside, $C_{13}H_{16}O_7$, from the bark of several species of *Salix* (willow) of the family Salicaceae, and from the needles and sprouts of certain coniferous trees.

salinometer (sal″ĭ-nom′ĕ-ter) an instrument (hydrometer) for direct reading of the salt content of a liquid.

saliva (sah-li′vah) [L.] the clear, alkaline, somewhat viscid secretion from the parotid, submaxillary, sublingual, and smaller mucous glands of the mouth. It serves to moisten and soften the food, keeps the mouth moist, and contains ptyalin, a digestive enzyme which converts starch into maltose. The saliva also contains mucin, serum albumin, globulin, leukocytes, epithelial debris, and potassium thiocyanate. Certain toxins frequently occur in it. **chorda s.,** submaxillary saliva produced in response to stimulation of the chorda tympani nerve, less viscid and turbid than that of the unstimulated gland. **ganglionic s.,** saliva obtained by irritating the submaxillary gland. **lingual s.,** the secretion of Ebner's glands and other serous glands of the tongue. **parotid s.,** saliva produced by the parotid gland; thinner and less viscid than the other varieties. **ropy s.,** saliva which is highly viscid. **sublingual s.,** that produced by the sublingual gland, the most viscid of all. **submaxillary s.,** that produced by the submaxillary gland. **sympathetic s.,** submaxillary saliva produced in response to stimulation of its sympathetic nerve supply; more viscid and turbid than that of the unstimulated gland.

salivant (sal′ĭ-vant) provoking a flow of saliva.

salivary (sal′ĭ-ver-e) [L. *salivarius*] pertaining to the saliva.

salivate (sal′ĭ-vāt) to produce an excessive flow of saliva.

salivation (sal″ĭ-va′shun) [L. *salivatio*] 1. the secretion of saliva. 2. ptyalism.

salivator (sal′ĭ-va″tor) an agent that causes salivation.

salivatory (sal′ĭ-vah-to″re) causing salivation.

salivin (sal′ĭ-vin) ptyalin.

salivolithiasis (sah-li″vo-lĭ-thi′ah-sis) sialolithiasis.

Salk vaccine (sahlk) [Jonas Edward *Salk*, American physician and virologist, born 1914] see under *vaccine*.

Salkowski's method, test (sal-kow′skēz) [Ernst Leopold *Salkowski*, physiologic chemist in Berlin, 1844–1923] see under *method* and *tests*.

salmiac (sal′me-ak) ammonium chloride.

salmin (sal′min) a toxic substance derived from the milt of salmon.

Salmonella (sal″mo-nel′ah) [Daniel Elmer *Salmon*, American pathologist, 1850–1914] a genus of microorganisms of tribe Salmonelleae, family Enterobacteriaceae, order Eubacteriales, made up of rod-shaped, gram-negative, usually but not invariably motile bacteria set apart from other enteric bacilli by failure to ferment lactose. It includes the typhoid-paratyphoid bacilli and bacteria usually pathogenic for lower animals which are often transmitted to man. The genus is separated into species or serotypes on the basis of O and H antigens, the latter occurring in two phases and identified by antigenic formulae taking the general form: O antigen: phase 1 ⇌ phase 2 in which the O antigens are designated by Roman numerals, the phase 1 antigens by lower case letters, and the phase 2 antigens by Arabic numerals. More than 1000 different serotypes have been described. **S. abor′tus e′qui,** a species causing infectious abortion in mares; not found in other animals. Called also *bacillus abortivus equinus*. **S. abor′tus o′vis,** a species isolated from cases of abortion in sheep. **S. aer′trycke,** S. typhimurium. **S. ana′tum,** a species causing keel in ducklings and intestinal disorder in man. **S. choleraesu′is,** a parasite of pigs and an important secondary invader in hog cholera. A member of the suipestifer group that also includes *S. paratyphi C* or Eastern type, the Kunzendorf variety or European type, and the Glässer-Voldagsen type that contains two species, *S. typhisuis* and *S. typhisuis var. Voldagsen*. Man is occasionally infected. The antigenic formula is VI,VII : (c) : 1,5. Formerly called *Bacterium cholerae*. **S. enterit′idis,** a widely distributed parasite of rodents occurring as a number of serotypes, namely, var. *Danysz*, var. *Chaco*, var. *Essen*, and var. *Jena*. It may produce epidemic diarrheal disease of rodents, and is a common cause of gastroenteritis in man. The antigenic formula is (I), IX, XII : g,m :—. Called also *Gärtner bacillus*, and formerly *Bacillus enteritis*. **S. gallina′rum,** the causative agent of fowl typhoid, with little or no pathogenicity for man; it has the antigenic formula (I),IX,XII : : — and is notable because only somatic O antigen is present. **S. hirschfel′dii,** *S. paratyphi C.* **S. mor′gani,** *Proteus morgani.* **S. paraty′phi,** *S. paratyphi A.* **S. paraty′phi A,** an etiologic agent of paratyphoid in man; usually found in man but occurring occasionally in lower animals. The antigenic formula is (I),II,XII : a:—. Called also *S. paratyphi.* **S. paraty′phi B,** an etiologic agent of paratyphoid in man, which also produces the acute syndrome of food-poisoning. Occurs in man and in lower animals. The antigenic formula is (I),IV,(V),XII : b:(1,2). **S. paraty′phi C,** an etiologic agent of paratyphoid in man in Asia, Africa, and southeastern Europe, and an important cause of death in British Guiana; closely related to strains of *S. choleraesuis.* **S. pullo′rum,** the causative agent of bacillary white diarrhea of chickens; serologically identical with *S. gallinarum.* **S. schottmül′leri,** *S. paratyphi B.* **S. sen′-dai,** a species causing paratyphoid in man. **S. suipes′tifer,** *S. choleraesuis.* **S. ty′phi,** *S. typhosa.* **S. typhimu′rium,** a parasite of rodents, especially mice, and the causative agent of mouse typhoid and of food poisoning in man. The antigenic formula is (I),IV,(V),XII : i:1,2,3. Called also *Nocard's bacillus* and *S. aertrycke.* **S. typhisu′is,** a species identical with *S. choleraesuis* except in minor cultural features. **S. typho′sa,** the etiologic agent of typhoid fever, occurring only in man. The antigenic formula is IX,XII(Vi): d—. Strains containing the Vi (virulence) antigen are designated V strains; those that have partially lost Vi antigen, V-W strains; and those that do not contain Vi antigen, W strains. The species is also subdivided into phage types on the basis of susceptibility to empirically numbered bacteriophages. Called also *S. typhi* and *typhoid bacillus.* Formerly called *Bacillus typhi, B. typhosa, Eberthella typhi,* and *Bacterium typhosum.*

salmonella (sal″mo-nel′ah), pl. *salmonel′lae.* Any microorganism of the genus *Salmonella.*

salmonellae (sal″mo-nel′e) plural of *salmonella.*

salmonellal (sal-mo-nel′al) caused by salmonellae.

Salmonelleae (sal″mo-nel′e-e) a tribe of the family Enterobacteriaceae, order Eubacteriales, made up of gram-negative, rod-shaped organisms which are usually but not invariably motile by means of peritrichous flagella. It includes two genera, *Salmonella* and *Shigella.*

salmonellosis (sal″mo-nel-lo′sis) infection with certain species of the genus *Salmonella,* usually caused by the ingestion of food containing the organisms or their products and marked by violent diarrhea attended by cramps and tenesmus and/or paratyphoid fever.

salocoll (sal′o-kol) phenocoll salicylate, $C_2H_5O \cdot C_6H_4 \cdot NH \cdot CO \cdot CH_2 \cdot NH_2 \cdot C_6H_4(OH)CO_2H$, a crystalline salt used as an antirheumatic.

salol (sa′lol) phenyl salicylate.

Salomon's test (sal′o-monz) [Hugo *Salomon,* German physician in Buenos Aires, 1872–1954] see under *tests.*

salpingectomy (sal″pin-jek′to-me) [*salpingo-* + Gr. *ektomē* excision] surgical removal of the uterine tube.

salpingemphraxis (sal″pin-jem-frak′sis) [*salpingo-* + Gr. *emphraxis* stoppage] obstruction of the auditory tube.

salpingian (sal-pin′je-an) pertaining to the auditory or to the uterine tube.

salpingion (sal-pin′je-on) a point at the apex of the petrous bone on its lower surface.

salpingitic (sal″pin-jit′ik) pertaining to or characterized by salpingitis.

salpingitis (sal″pin-ji′tis) [*salpingo-* + *-itis* inflammation] 1. inflammation of the uterine tube. 2. inflammation of the auditory tube. **chronic interstitial s.,** inflammation of the uterine tube associated with infiltration of connective tissue and muscle with lymphocytes and plasma cells. **chronic vegetating s.,** inflammation of the uterine tube, with marked hypertrophy of the mucosa. **eustachian s.,** inflammation of the auditory tube. **hemorrhagic s.,** inflammation of the uterine tube associated with rupture of a blood vessel and effusion of blood. **hypertrophic s.,** pachysalpingitis. **s. isth′mica nodo′sa,** a condition marked by nodular thickening of parts of both uterine tubes, most characteristically of the isthmic portion, pathogenically related to adenomyosis of the uterus. **mural s.,** pachysalpingitis. **nodular s.,** inflammation attended with formation of nodules in the wall and mucous lining of the uterine tube. **parenchymatous s.,** pachysalpingitis. **s. prof′luens,** inflammation of the uterine tube, with accumulation in its lumen of fluid that ultimately escapes. **pseudofollicular s.,** inflammation of the uterine tube characterized by agglutination of its walls, causing a formation of saccules. **purulent s.,** inflammation of the uterine tube attended with suppuration; called also *pyosalpingitis.* **tuberculous s.,** infection of the uterine tube by the tubercle bacillus, *Mycobacterium tuberculosis.*

salpingo- (sal-ping′go) [Gr. *salpinx* tube] a combining form denoting relationship to a tube, specifically to the uterine or to the auditory tube.

salpingocatheterism (sal-ping″go-kath′ĕ-ter-izm) catheterization of the auditory tube.

salpingocele (sal-ping′go-sēl) [*salpingo-* + Gr. *kēlē* hernia] hernial protrusion of a uterine tube.

salpingography (sal″ping-gog′rah-fe) [*salpingo-* + Gr. *graphein* to write] roentgenography of the uterine tubes after the injection of an opaque medium.

salpingolithiasis (sal-ping″go-lĭ-thi′ah-sis) the presence of calcareous deposits in the wall of the uterine tubes.

salpingolysis (sal″ping-gol′ĭ-sis) surgical separation of adhesions involving the uterine tubes.

salpingo-oophorectomy (sal-ping″go-o″of-o-rek′to-me) surgical removal of a uterine tube and ovary.

salpingo-oophoritis (sal-ping″go-o″of-o-ri′tis) inflammation of a uterine tube and ovary.

salpingo-oophorocele (sal-ping″go-o-of′or-o-sēl) hernia containing a uterine tube and ovary.

salpingo-oothecitis (sal-ping″go-o″o-the-si′tis) [*salpingo-* + Gr. *ōon* egg + *thēkē* case + *-itis*] salpingo-oophoritis.

salpingo-oothecocele (sal-ping″go-o″o-the′ko-sēl) [*salpingo-* + Gr. *ōon* egg + *thēkē* case + *kēlē* hernia] salpingo-oophorocele.

salpingo-ovariectomy (sal-ping″go-o-va″re-ek′to-me) salpingo-oophorectomy.

salpingo-ovariotomy (sal-ping″go-o-va″re-ot′o-me) salpingo-oophorectomy.

salpingoperitonitis (sal-ping″go-per″ĭ-to-ni′tis) inflammation of the peritoneum covering the uterine tube.

salpingopexy (sal-ping′go-pek″se) [*salpingo-* + Gr. *pēxis* fixation] the operation of fixing the uterine tube.

salpingopharyngeal (sal-ping″go-fah-rin′je-al) pertaining to the auditory tube and the pharynx.

salpingoplasty (sal-ping′go-plas″te) [*salpingo-* + Gr. *plassein* to form] plastic operation on the uterine tube. Called also *tuboplasty.*

salpingorrhaphy (sal″ping-gor′ah-fe) [*salpingo-* + Gr. *rhaphē* suture] the stitching of a uterine tube to the ipsilateral ovary after removal of part of the ovary.

salpingoscopy (sal″ping-gos′ko-pe) inspection of the auditory tube.

salpingostaphyline (sal-ping″go-staf′ĭ-lin) pertaining to the auditory tube and the uvula.

salpingostomatomy (sal-ping″go-sto-mat′o-me) [*salpingo-* + Gr. *stoma* mouth + *tomē* a cutting] surgical resection of a portion of the uterine tube, with creation of a new abdominal ostium.

salpingostomatoplasty (sal-ping″go-sto-mat′o-plas″te) salpingostomatomy.

salpingostomy (sal″ping-gos′to-me) [*salpingo-* + Gr. *stomoun* to provide with an opening or mouth] 1. formation of an opening or fistula into a uterine tube for the purpose of drainage. 2. surgical restoration of the patency of a uterine tube.

salpingotomy (sal″ping-got′o-me) [*salpingo-* + Gr. *tomē* a cutting] surgical incision of a uterine tube.

salpinx (sal′pinks) [Gr.] a tube. **s. auditi′va,** tuba auditiva. **s. uteri′na,** tuba uterina.

salsalate (sal′sah-lāt) chemical name: 2-hydroxybenzoic acid 2-carboxyphenyl ester; an analgesic and anti-inflammatory, $C_{14}H_{10}O_5$. Called also *salicylsalicylic acid.*

salt (sawlt) [L. *sal;* Gr. *hals*] 1. sodium chloride, or common salt. 2. any compound of a base and an acid; any compound of an acid some of whose replaceable hydrogen atoms have been substituted. 3. [pl.] a saline purgative. See *magnesium sulfate* (Epsom s.), *sodium sulfate* (Glauber's s.), and *potassium sodium tartrate* (Preston's, Rochelle, or Seignette's s.). **acid s.,** any salt in which the combining power of the acid is not completely exhausted. **baker's s.,** ammonium carbonate; sometimes used in leavening cakes. **basic s.,** any salt with more than the normal proportion of the basic elements. **bile s's,** glycocholate and taurocholate, the salts of bile acids synthesized by the liver and stored in and released by the gallbladder; they activate pancreatic lipase, facilitate the digestion of triglyceride fat, and stimulate the metabolism of intestinal mucosal cells. **bone s's,** the crystalline salts deposited in the organic matrix (principally collagen fibers) of bone, composed chiefly of calcium and phosphate. **buffer s.,** a salt, such as sodium bicarbonate and sodium phosphate, the anion of which functions as a conjugate base in a buffer system. **Carlsbad s.,** a mixture of sodium sulfate, potassium sulfate, sodium chloride, and sodium bicarbonate, used as a purgative. **common s.,** sodium chloride, NaCl. **diuretic s.,** potassium acetate. **double s.,** any salt in which the two hydrogen atoms of a dibasic acid have been replaced by two separate metals or basic radicals, as in potassium ammonium tartrate. **Epsom s.,** magnesium sulfate. **Everitt's s.,** potassium ferrous ferrocyanide, $K_2Fe[Fe(CN)_6]$. **Glauber's s.,** sodium sulfate. **halide s., haloid s.,** any binary compound of a metal or basic radical with a halogen—i.e., chlorine, iodine, bromine, fluorine. **Kissingen s's,** an aperient salt from the waters of a spring at Kissingen, Bavaria. **Monsel's s.,** iron subsulfate. **neutral s., normal s.,** any salt which is neither acidic nor basic in reaction. **pancreatic s.,** a mixture of the pancreatic ferments with common salt, used as a digestant. **peptic s.,** common salt mixed with pepsin, used as a digestant. **Plimmer's s.,** sodium antimony tartrate. **Preston's s., Rochelle s., Seignette's s.,** potassium sodium tartrate. **smelling s's,** aromatized ammonium carbonate: stimulant and restorative. **table s.,** sodium chloride, NaCl. **Wurster's s's,** the univalent oxidation products of the aromatic *p*-diamines. They are free radicals which may polymerize in a sufficiently concentrated solution and at low temperatures or in the solid state.

saltation (sal-ta′shun) [L. *saltatio* from *saltare* to jump] the action of leaping, especially (1) chorea, or the dancing which sometimes accompanies it; (2) conduction along myelinated nerves; (3) in genetics, an abrupt variation in species; a mutation.

saltatorial, saltatoric (sal″tah-to′re-al; sal″tah-to′rik) saltatory.

saltatory (sal′tah-to″re) pertaining to or characterized by saltation; see also under *evolution* and *spasm.*

Salter's incremental lines (sawl′terz) [Sir James A. *Salter,* English dentist of the nineteenth century] see under *line.*

salting-out (sawl′ting-owt) the separation of serum or plasma protein fractions in the serum or plasma by precipitation in increasing concentrations of neutral salts; the hydration of the salt progressively added removes water molecules so that each protein fraction becomes dehydrated and consequently less soluble at a different concentration of the salt.

saltpeter (sawlt-pe′ter) [L. *salpetra* or *sal petrae*] potassium nitrate, KNO₃. **Chile s.,** sodium nitrate.

salubrious (sah-lu′bre-us) [L. *salubris*] conducive to health; wholesome.

saluresis (sal″u-re′sis) [L. *sal* salt + Gr. *ourēsis* a making water] the excretion of sodium and chloride ions in the urine.

saluretic (sal″u-ret′ik) 1. pertaining to, characterized by, or promoting saluresis. 2. an agent that promotes saluresis.

Saluron (sal′u-ron) trademark for a preparation of hydroflumethiazide.

salutarium (sal″u-ta′re-um) [L. *salus* health] a resort for the preservation of health.

salutary (sal′u-ta″re) [L. *salutaris*] favorable to the preservation or restoration of health.

salvarsan (sal′var-san) see *arsphenamine.* **s. copper,** a yellowish-red powder, a combination of arsphenamine and copper, suggested by Ehrlich for use in protozoan infections. **silver s.,** silver arsphenamine. **sulfoxylate s.,** a modified arsphenamine.

salve (sav) a thick ointment or cerate; see *ointment.* **Dreuw's s.,** salicylic acid 10, chrysarobin 20, birch tar 20, green soap 25, petrolatum 25. **fetron s.,** a salve composed of from 3 to 5 per cent of the anilide of stearic acid with petrolatum. **scarlet s.,** a synthetic cell proliferant, toluylazo-toluyl-azo-beta-naphthol.

Salvia (sal′ve-ah) [L.] a genus of labiate plants. The leaves of *S. officinalis* L., sage, contain a volatile oil, and are sudorific, carminative, and astringent. The dried leaves are used as an antisecretory agent in hyperhidrosis, sialorrhea, pharyngitis, and bronchitis, and have been used to check excessive milk secretion. *S. reflexa* L., mint weed, sometimes causes poisoning in stock.

Salyrgan (sal′er-gan) trademark for a preparation of mersalyl.

Salzmann's nodular corneal dystrophy (salz′manz) [Maximilian *Salzmann,* German ophthalmologist, 1862–1954] see under *dystrophy.*

samaderin (sah-mad′er-in) a light-yellow, bitter, crystalline principle from the fruit and bark of *Samadera indica,* a tree of India, Ceylon, and Java; a decoction of the leaf is used as an emetic and purgative.

samandaridine (sam″an-dar′ĭ-din) an alkaloid, C₂₁H₃₁O₃N, from the skin of various salamanders; less poisonous than samandarine.

samandarine (sah-man′dah-rin) a poisonous alkaloid, C₁₉H₃₁O₂N, from the skin of various salamanders.

samarium (sah-ma′re-um) a very rare, metallic element; symbol, Sm; atomic number, 62; atomic weight, 150.35.

Sambucus (sam-bu′kus) [L. "the elder-tree"] a genus of caprifoliaceous trees and shrubs; elder. The dried flowers have been used as a carminative, stimulant, and diuretic; the berries (elder berries) were thought to possess some laxative principles.

sample (sam′p'l) [L. *exemplum* example] a representative part taken to typify the whole. **random s.,** a representative part so chosen that each item has an equal chance of being selected.

Sampson's cyst (samp′sunz) [John Albertson *Sampson,* American gynecologist, 1873–1946] chocolate cyst.

Sanarelli's serum (san″ah-rel′lēz) [Giuseppe *Sanarelli,* Rome physician, 1864–1940] see under *serum.*

sanative (san′ah-tiv) [L. *sanare* to heal] having a tendency to heal; curative.

sanatorium (san″ah-to′re-um) [L. *sanatorius* conferring health, from *sanare* to cure] 1. an establishment for the treatment of sick persons, especially a private hospital for convalescents or those who are not extremely ill. The term is now applied particularly to an establishment for the open-air treatment of tuberculous patients. 2. a health station; a health resort in a hot region.

sanatory (san′ah-to″re) [L. *sanatorius*] conducive to health; salubrious.

Sanctorius (sank-to′re-us) [It. Santorio Santorio, 1561–1636] an Italian physician, professor of medicine at Padua, who devised several instruments of precision (e.g., a clinical thermometer and a pulse clock), and made quantitative experiments on basal metabolism; a famous illustration in his most important book, *De statica medicina* (1614), depicts the author in a steel-yard chair, presumably about to weigh himself after a meal.

sand (sand) material occurring in small, gritty particles. **brain s.,** acervulus. **intestinal s.,** small gritty particles made up of oxides of calcium and phosphorus, bacteria, bile pigment, etc., formed in the intestine.

sandalwood (san′dal-wood) [L. *santalum*] 1. the fragrant wood of *Santalum album,* white or yellow sandal, and of other trees of the genera *Santalum* and *Fusanus.* See also *santal oil,* under *oil.* 2. the dried heart wood of the leguminous tree *Pterocarpus santalinus,* red sandal or santalum rubrum, used as a coloring agent.

sandarac (san′dah-rak) [Gr. *sandarakē*] a white, transparent resin from *Callitris quadrivalvis,* a tree of Africa, used in dentistry in an alcoholic solution as a separating fluid and as a preservative varnish for plastic casts. Sometimes, by extension, used also as a verb to denote treatment with the solution.

sand crack (sand krak) a crack starting at the bearing surface of a horse's hoof; it rarely causes lameness.

Sander's disease (san′derz) [Wilhelm *Sander,* German physician, 1838–1922] see under *disease.*

Sanders' disease [Murray *Sanders,* New York bacteriologist, born 1910] epidemic keratoconjunctivitis.

sandfly (sand′fli) a name applied to various two-winged flies of the families Heleidae, Simuliidae, and Psychodidae, but especially to flies of the latter family (of the genus *Phlebotomus*).

Sandril (san′dril) trademark for preparations of reserpine.

Sandström's bodies, glands (zant-strämz) [Ivar Victor *Sandström,* Swedish anatomist, 1852–1889] see *parathyroid glands,* under *gland,* and see *glandulae thyroideae accessoriae.*

Sandwith's bald tongue (sand′withs) [Fleming Mant *Sandwith,* British physician, 1853–1918] see under *tongue.*

sane (sān) [L. *sanus*] of sound mind; compos mentis.

Sänger see *Saenger.*

Sanger (Sang′er), Frederick. English biochemist, born 1918; winner of the Nobel prize in chemistry in 1958 for his work on the insulin molecule.

sangui- (sang′gwĭ) [L. *sanguis* blood] a combining form denoting relationship to blood.

sanguicolous (sang-gwik′o-lus) [sangui- + L. *colere* to dwell] inhabiting or living in the blood.

sanguifacient (sang″gwĭ-fa′shent) [sangui- + L. *facere* to make] hematopoietic.

sanguiferous (sang-gwif′er-us) [sangui- + L. *ferre* to bear] conveying or containing blood.

sanguification (sang″gwĭ-fi-ka′shun) [sangui- + L. *facere* to make] hematopoiesis.

sanguimotor, sanguimotory (sang″gwĭ-mo′tor; sang″wĭ-mo′tor-e) [sangui- + L. *motor* mover] pertaining to blood circulation.

sanguinaria (sang″gwĭ-na′re-ah) the dried rhizome and root of the bloodroot, *Sanguinaria canadensis,* a perennial herb, used as an ingredient of compound white pine syrup. It was formerly used as an expectorant and externally in the treatment of chronic eczema and cancer of the skin. It contains several alkaloids, e.g., sanguinarine.

sanguinarine (sang″gwĭ-na′rēn) an alkaloid, C₂₀H₁₅NO₅, obtained from sanguinaria and other species of the same family.

sanguine (sang′gwin) [L. *sanguineus; sanguis* blood] 1. abounding in blood. 2. ardent; hopeful.

sanguineous (sang-gwin′e-us) abounding in blood; pertaining to the blood.

sanguinolent (sang-gwin′o-lent) [L. *sanguinolentus*] of a bloody tinge.

sanguinopoietic (sang″gwĭ-no-poi-et′ik) hematopoietic.

sanguinopurulent (sang″gwĭ-no-pu′ru-lent) containing both blood and pus.

sanguinous (sang′gwĭ-nus) sanguineous.

sanguirenal (sang″gwĭ-re′nal) [sangui- + L. *ren* kidney] pertaining to the blood and the kidneys.

sanguis (sang′gwis) [L.] [NA]   the blood: the fluid that circulates through the heart, arteries, capillaries, and veins, carrying nutriment and oxygen to the body cells. See *blood.*

sanguivorous (sang-gwiv′o-rus) [*sangui*- + L. *vorare* to eat]   blood-eating; said of female mosquitoes which prefer blood to other nutrients.

sanicult (san′ĭ-kult)   a certain system of quack medicine.

sanies (sa′ne-ēz) [L.]   a fetid, ichorous discharge from a wound or ulcer, containing serum, pus, and blood.

saniopurulent (sa″ne-o-pu′roo-lent)   partly sanious and partly purulent.

sanioserous (sa″ne-o-se′rous)   partly sanious and partly serous.

sanious (sa′ne-us) [L. *saniosus*]   of the nature of sanies.

sanipractic (san″ĭ-prak′tik)   a system of medical practice based on applied prophylactic and therapeutic sanitation.

sanitarian (san″ĭ-ta′re-an)   a person who is expert in matters of sanitation and public health.

sanitarium (san″ĭ-ta′re-um) [L.]   an institution for the promotion of health. The word was originally coined to designate the institution established by the Seventh Day Adventists at Battle Creek, Michigan, to distinguish it from institutions providing care for mental or tuberculous patients.

sanitary (san′ĭ-ta″re) [L. *sanitarius*]   promoting or pertaining to health.

sanitation (san″ĭ-ta′shun) [L. *sanitas* health]   the establishment of environmental conditions favorable to health; assanation.

sanitization (san″ĭ-ti-za′shun)   the process of making or the quality of being made sanitary; see *sanitize.*

sanitize (san′ĭ-tīz)   to clean and sterilize, as eating or drinking utensils.

sanity (san′ĭ-te) [L. *sanitas* soundness]   soundness, especially soundness of mind.

Sanorex (san′o-reks)   trademark for a preparation of mazindol.

Sansert (san′sert)   trademark for a preparation of methysergide maleate.

Sansom's sign (san′somz) [Arthur Ernest *Sansom,* English physician, 1838–1907]   see under *sign.*

Sanson's images (san′sonz) [Louis Joseph *Sanson,* French physician, 1790–1841]   *Purkinje's images;* see under *image.*

santalum (san′tah-lum)   sandalwood. **s. ru′brum,** the dried heart wood of *Pterocarpus santalinus;* used as a coloring agent.

santonica (san-ton′ĭ-kah) [L.]   the dried unexpanded flower heads of *Artemisia maritima,* formerly used as an anthelmintic and stomachic; called also *semen contra.*

santonin (san′to-nin)   a lactone, $C_{15}H_{18}O_3$, which may be obtained from the unexpanded flower heads of *Artemisia maritima* and other species of *Artemisia;* used as an anthelmintic against *Ascaris lumbricoides.* Called also *santoninic acid.*

Santorini's cartilages, etc.   (sahn″to-re′nēz) [Giovanni Domenico *Santorini,* Italian anatomist, 1681–1737]   see under *cartilage, duct, fissure, ligament, muscle, papilla, plexus,* and *tubercle.*

sap (sap)   the natural juice of a living organism or tissue. **cell s.,** hyaloplasm, def. 1. **nuclear s.,** karyolymph.

saphena (sah-fe′nah) [L.; Gr. *saphēnēs* manifest]   either of two large superficial veins of the leg; see *vena saphena.*

saphenectomy (saf″ĕ-nek′to-me) [*saphena* + Gr. *ektomē* excision]   excision of a saphenous vein.

saphenous (sah-fe′nus)   pertaining to or associated with a saphena; applied to certain arteries, nerves, veins, etc.

sapid (sap′id) [L. *sapidus*]   having or imparting an agreeable taste.

sapin (sa′pin)   a nontoxic ptomaine, $C_5H_{14}N_2$, isomeric with cadaverine and neuridine.

sapo (sa′po) [L. "soap"]   1. soap; a compound of a fatty acid with a suitable base.   2. white castile soap made of soda and olive oil, used in pills, suppositories, plasters, and liniments: detergent. **s. anima′lis,** s. domesticus.   **s. cine′reus,** gray soap, or mercurial salve soap, a soap containing 50 per cent, by weight, of mercury and 5 per cent of benzoinated fat.   **s. domes′ticus,** a preparation of a soft soap made of animal fat and potash.   **s. du′rus,** soda soap.   **s. mol′lis,** soft soap.   **s. mol′lis medina′lis,** green soap.   **s. vir′idis,** green soap.

sapogenin (sah-poj′ĕ-nin)   a compound resulting from the decomposition of saponin, $C_{14}H_{22}O_2$.

saponaceous (sa″po-na′shus) [L. *sapo* soap]   of a soapy quality or nature.

Saponaria (sa″po-na′re-ah)   a genus of plants. The root of *S. officinalis,* or soapwort, has alterative properties and was formerly used in skin diseases. It contains saponin, saponarin, and sapotoxin.

saponarin (sa″po-na′rin)   a glycoside, $C_{27}H_{30}O_{16}$, from *Saponaria officinalis* L. (Caryophyllaceae).

saponatus (sa″po-na′tus) [L.]   charged or mixed with soap.

saponification (sa″po-pon″ĭ-fi-ka′shun) [L. *sapo* soap + *facere* to make]   the act or process of converting fats into soaps and glycerol by heating with alkalis. In chemistry, the term now denotes hydrolysis, of an ester by an alkali, resulting in the production of a free alcohol and an alkali salt of the ester acid.

saponin (sap′o-nin)   a group of glycosides, widely distributed in plants, such as *Quillaja saponaria* Molina (Rosaceae) and *Saponaria officinalis* L. (Caryophyllaceae), and characterized by (1) their property of forming a durable foam when their watery solutions are shaken, (2) by their ability to dissolve red blood cells even in high dilutions, and (3) by their having sapogenin as their aglycones.   **cholan s's,** a group of saponins that on hydrolysis yield sterol-like compounds.   **triterpenoid s's,** a group of saponins that on hydrolysis yield 1,2,7-trimethyl naphthalene.

sapophore (sap′o-for) [L. *sapor* taste + Gr. *phoros* bearing]   the group of atoms in the molecule of a compound that gives the substance its characteristic taste.

sapotalene (sap′o-tal″ēn)   a hydrocarbon, 1,2,7-trimethylnaphthalene, formed by the reduction of sapogenin.

sapotoxin (sa″po-tok′sin)   any of various toxic saponins found in such plants as *Quillaja saponaria* Molina (Rosaceae) and *Saponaria officinalis* L. (Caryophyllaceae).

Sappey's fibers, ligament, nucleus, veins (sahp-pāz′) [Marie Philibert Constant *Sappey,* French anatomist, 1810–1896]   see under *fiber* and *ligament,* and see *venae paraumbicales* and *nucleus ruber.*

sapphism (saf′izm) [*Sappho,* Greek poetess, about 600 B.C.]   homosexuality between women; lesbianism.

Sappinia diploidea (sah-pin′e-ah dĭ-ploi′de-ah)   a coprozoic ameba of the order Amoebida, class Rhizopoda, having a definite cuticle, two closely associated nuclei, and a few short lobopodia; found in the feces of various animals.

saprin (sa′prin) [Gr. *sapros* rotten]   a ptomaine, $C_5H_{14}N_2$, from decaying visceral substances; not poisonous.

sapro- (sap′ro) [Gr. *sapros* rotten]   a combining form meaning rotten or putrid, or designating relationship to decay or to decaying material.

saprobe (sah′prōb)   a name proposed for a vegetable organism living on dead or decaying organic matter.

saprobic (sah-prōb′ik)   of the nature of, or being a saprobe.

Saprolegnia (sap″ro-leg′ne-ah) [*sapro*- + Gr. *legnon* border]   a genus of partially saprophytic, phycomycetous water molds of the order Saprolegniales, subclass Oomycetes. *S. fe′rax* is destructive to salmon and to various water animals.

Saprolegniales (sap″ro-leg″ne-a′lēz)   an order of mostly saprophytic molds of the subclass Oomycetes, class Phycomycetes, which have an extensive mycelial thallus that has no cross walls, including the genera *Saprolegnia* and *Achlya.* These fungi are commonly called "water molds," although some inhabit soil.

saprophilous (sah-prof′ĭ-lus) [*sapro*- + Gr. *philein* to love]   saprophytic.

saprophyte (sap′ro-fīt) [*sapro*- + Gr. *phyton* plant]   any organism, such as a bacterium, living upon dead or decaying organic matter. Cf. *autophyte.*

saprophytic (sap′ro-fit′ik)   of the nature of or pertaining to a saprophyte; growing on dead or decomposing organic matter.

saprophytism (sap′ro-fi-tizm)   the condition of being a saprophyte.

Saprospira (sap″ro-spi′rah) [*sapro*- + Gr. *speira* coil]   a genus of microorganisms of the family Spirochaetaceae, order Spirochaetales, made up of actively motile cells containing spiral protoplasm without evident axial filament and with a definite periplast membrane found free-living in marine ooze. It contains three species, *S. gran′dis, S. lep′ta,* and *S. punc′tum,* the type species being *S. gran′dis.*

saprozoic (sap″ro-zo′ik) [*sapro*- + Gr. *zōon* animal]   living on dead or lifeless matter; said of animal organisms.

saprozoite (sap″ro-zo′īt)   an animal organism living upon dead or decaying animal matter.

saralasin acetate (sar-al′ah-sin)   chemical name: 1-(*N*-methylglycine)-5-L-valine-8-L-alaninangiotensin II acetate (salt) hydrate. An angiotensin-II antagonist, $C_{42}H_{65}N_{13}O_{10} \cdot xC_2H_4O_2 \cdot x$-$H_2O$, used as an antihypertensive in the treatment of severe hypertension and in the diagnosis of renin-dependent hypertension.

Sarbó's sign (sar′bōz) [Arthur von *Sarbó,* Budapest neurologist, born 1867]   see under *sign.*

Sarcina (sar-si′nah)   a genus of microorganisms of the family Micrococcaceae, order Eubacteriales, occurring as spherical, gram-positive cells in cubical packets of eight cells, found in soil and water as saprophytes and rarely observed in disease processes.

sarcina (sar′si-nah), pl. *sar′cinae* [L.]   1. a spherical bacterium occurring predominantly in cubical packets of eight cells as a consequence of failure of daughter cells to separate following cell division in three planes.   2. an organism of the genus *Sarcina.*

sarcinae (sar′si-ne) [L.]   plural of *sarcina.*

sarcitis (sar-si′tis) [*sarco*- + -*itis*]   myositis.

sarco- (sar′ko) [Gr. *sarx, sarkos* flesh] a combining form denoting relationship to flesh.

Sarcobiot (sar″ko-bi′ot) [*sarco-* + Gr. *bios* life] a species of fly which deposits its larvae in or near living animal tissue.

sarcoblast (sar′ko-blast) [*sarco-* + Gr. *blastos* germ] the primitive cell which develops into a muscle cell.

sarcocarcinoma (sar″ko-kar″sĭ-no′mah) sarcoma and carcinoma combined.

sarcocele (sar′ko-sēl) [*sarco-* + Gr. *kēlē* tumor] any fleshy swelling or tumor of the testis.

sarcocol (sar′ko-kol) [L. *sarcocolla; sarco-* + Gr. *kolla* glue] a nauseous gum-resin from various species of *Penaea*, a shrub of southern Africa.

sarcocyst (sar′ko-sist) [*sarco-* + Gr. *kystis* bladder] 1. an individual organism of the genus *Sarcocystis*. 2. a sarcosporidian cyst; one of the cylindrical cysts containing banana-shaped spores, found in the muscles of those infected with *Sarcocystis*.

sarcocystin (sar″ko-sis′tin) a toxin obtained from species of *Sarcocystis*.

Sarcocystis (sar″ko-sis′tis) [*sarco-* + Gr. *kystis* bladder] a genus of sporozoa of the order Sarcosporidia (considered to be of uncertain status by some authorities), which parasitize mammals, birds, and reptiles. Infection, which occurs following ingestion of the spores, is manifested by the formation of cysts (sarcosporidian cysts, or sarcocysts) containing the parasites in the host's muscles. Representative species include *S. lindemanni* in man, *S. tenella* in sheep, *S. miescheriana* in pigs, *S. bertrami* in horses, and *S. muris* in rats and mice.

sarcocyte (sar′ko-sīt) [*sarco-* + *-cyte*] the middle layer of ectoplasm of a protozoon lying between the epicyte and the myocyte.

sarcode (sar′kōd) [*sarco-* + Gr. *eidos* form] (*obs.*) the protoplasm of animal cells.

Sarcodina (sar″ko-di′nah) [Gr. *sarkōdēs* fleshlike] a subphylum of Protozoa, including all the amebae, both free-living and parasitic, characterized by the ability to produce pseudopodia during most of the life cycle; flagella, when present, develop only during the early stages. It includes the class Rhizopoda. Called also *Rhizopoda*.

sarcoenchondroma (sar″ko-en″kon-dro′mah) chondrosarcoma.

sarcogenic (sar″ko-jen′ik) [*sarco-* + Gr. *gennan* to produce] forming flesh.

sarcoglia (sar-kog′le-ah) [*sarco-* + Gr. *glia* glue] the substance which composes the eminences of Doyen at the entrance of nerves into muscle fibers.

sarcohydrocele (sar″ko-hi′dro-sēl) sarcocele combined with hydrocele.

sarcoid (sar′koid) [*sarco-* + Gr. *eidos* form] 1. tuberculoid; characterized by noncaseating epithelioid cell tubercles. 2. pertaining to or resembling sarcoidosis. 3. (*obs.*) resembling flesh; fleshy. **s. of Boeck,** sarcoidosis. **Darier-Roussy s.,** a form of sarcoidosis characterized by the large size of the nodules and their subcutaneous location. **multiple benign s.,** sarcoidosis. **Schaumann's s.,** sarcoidosis. **Spiegler-Fendt s.,** lymphadenosis benigna cutis.

sarcoidosis (sar″koi-do′sis) a chronic, progressive, generalized granulomatous reticulosis of unknown etiology, involving almost any organ or tissue, including the skin, lungs, lymph nodes, liver, spleen, eyes, and small bones of the hands and feet. It is characterized histologically by the presence in all affected organs or tissues of noncaseating epithelioid cell tubercles. Laboratory findings may include hypercalcemia and hypergammaglobinemia; there is usually diminished or absent reactivity to tuberculin, and, in most active cases, a positive Kveim reaction. The acute form has an abrupt onset and a high spontaneous remission rate, whereas the chronic form, insidious in onset, is progressive. Formerly called *Besnier-Boeck disease, Boeck's disease, benign lymphogranulomatosis*, and *sarcoid of Boeck*. **s. cor′dis,** involvement of the heart in sarcoidosis, with lesions ranging from a few asymptomatic, microscopic granulomas to widespread infiltration of the myocardium by large masses of sarcoid tissue. **muscular s.,** sarcoidosis involving the skeletal muscles, with sarcoid tubercles, interstitial inflammation with fibrosis, and disruption and atrophy of the muscle fibers.

sarcolactate (sar″ko-lak′tāt) any salt of sarcolactic acid.

sarcolemma (sar″ko-lem′ah) [*sarco-* + Gr. *lemma* husk] the delicate plasma membrane which invests every striated muscle fiber.

sarcolemmic (sar″ko-lem′ik) pertaining to or of the nature of sarcolemma.

sarcolemmous (sar″ko-lem′us) sarcolemmic.

sarcolysis (sar″ko-lol′ĭ-sis) [*sarco-* + Gr. *lysis* dissolution] disintegration of the soft tissues; disintegration of flesh.

sarcolyte (sar′ko-līt) 1. a cell concerned in the disintegration of the soft tissues. 2. a disintegrating muscle fiber.

sarcolytic (sar″ko-lit′ik) pertaining to, characterized by, or causing sarcolysis.

sarcoma (sar-ko′mah), pl. *sarcomas* or *sarco′mata* [*sarco-* + *-oma*] a tumor made up of a substance like the embryonic connective tissue; tissue composed of closely packed cells embedded in a fibrillar or homogeneous substance. Sarcomas are often highly malignant. See also *chondrosarcoma, fibrosarcoma, lymphosarcoma, melanosarcoma, myxosarcoma, osteosarcoma,* etc. **Abernethy's s.,** a variety of fatty tumor found principally on the trunk. **adipose s.,** liposarcoma. **alveolar soft part s.,** a variety having a reticulated fibrous stoma enclosing groups of sarcoma cells, which resemble epithelial cells and are inclosed in alveoli walled with connective tissue. **ameloblastic s.,** the malignant counterpart of ameloblastic fibroma. **botryoid s., s. botryoi′des,** a variety of embryonal rhabdomyosarcoma, arising in submucosal tissue, presenting grossly as a polypoid grape-like structure, and found most often in young children or infants in the upper vagina, cervix uteri, or neck of urinary bladder. **chicken s.,** a sarcoma of chickens which may be of several various cell types. **chloromatous s.,** chloroma. **chondroblastic s.,** see *osteogenic s.* **s. col′li u′teri hydro′picum papilla′re,** botryoid s. **deciduocellular s.,** choriocarcinoma. **embryonal s.,** Wilms' tumor. **endometrial stromal s.,** a pale, polypoid, fleshy, malignant tumor of the endometrial stroma, usually arising from the uterine fundus. **Ewing's s.,** see under *tumor*. **fascial s.,** a sarcoma arising in the fasciae about the joints, especially in the lower extremities. **fibroblastic s.,** see *osteogenic s.* **fowl s.,** chicken s. **giant cell s.,** a malignant form of giant cell tumor of bone; see under *tumor*. **granulocytic s.,** chloroma. **Hodgkin's s.,** Hodgkin's disease of the lymphocytic depletion type. **idiopathic multiple pigmented hemorrhagic s.,** Kaposi's s. **Jensen's s.,** a malignant tumor in mice transmissible to healthy mice by transplanting a small portion of the tumor. **Kaposi's s.,** a multifocal, metastasizing, malignant reticulosis with features resembling those of angiosarcoma, principally involving the skin, although visceral lesions may be present; it usually begins on the distal parts of the extremities, most often on the toes or feet, as reddish blue or brownish soft nodules and tumors. Called also *multiple idiopathic hemorrhagic s.* and *idiopathic multiple pigmented hemorrhagic s.* **Kupffer cell s.,** angiosarcoma of the liver in adults. **leukocytic s.,** leukosarcoma. **lymphatic s.,** lymphosarcoma. **melanotic s.,** malignant melanoma. **mixed cell s.,** malignant mesenchymoma. **multiple idiopathic hemorrhagic s.,** Kaposi's s. **osteoblastic s.,** see *osteogenic s.* **osteogenic s.,** a malignant primary tumor of bone composed of a malignant connective tissue stroma with evidence of malignant osteoid, bone, and/or cartilage formation. Depending on which component is dominant, three major subtypes are recognized: osteoblastic, fibroblastic, and chondroblastic. Called also *osteosarcoma, osteoid s.* and *osteolytic s.* **osteoid s.,** osteogenic s. **osteolytic s.,** osteogenic s. **parosteal s.,** a sarcoma situated close to the outer surface of a bone. **polymorphous s.,** malignant mesenchymoma. **reticulocytic s., reticuloendothelial s.,** reticulum cell s. **reticulum cell s.,** malignant lymphoma of the undifferentiated or histiocytic type, depending on the degree of differentiation of the malignant cells. **retothelial s.,** reticulum cell s. **Rous s.,** a peculiar sarcoma-like growth found in some fowls; from it can be obtained a filterable virus, the first known to cause tumors, which on inoculation into other fowls produces similar growths. **serocystic s.,** a proliferous cyst with intracystic growth. **synovial s.,** synoviosarcoma. **telangiectatic s.,** a sarcoma which develops such a rich vascular network that the endothelial cells are mistaken for the neoplastic element.

sarcomagenesis (sar″ko-mah-jen′ĕ-sis) the production of sarcoma.

sarcomagenic (sar″ko-mah-jen′ik) causing sarcoma.

sarcomata (sar-ko′mah-tah) plural of *sarcoma*.

sarcomatoid (sar-ko′mah-toid) resembling sarcoma.

sarcomatosis (sar″ko-mah-to′sis) a condition characterized by the formation of sarcomas. **s. cu′tis,** the development of sarcomatous growths on the skin. **general s.,** the occurrence of sarcomas in several parts of the body at the same time.

sarcomatous (sar-ko′mah-tus) pertaining to or of the nature of sarcoma.

sarcomere (sar′ko-mēr) [*sarco-* + Gr. *meros* part] the contractile unit of myofibrils; sarcomeres are repeating units, delimited by the Z bands along the length of the myofibril.

sarcomphalocele (sar″kom-fal′o-sēl) [*sarco-* + Gr. *omphalos* navel + *kēlē* tumor] a fleshy tumor of the umbilicus.

Sarcophaga (sar-kof′ah-gah) [*sarco-* + Gr. *phagein* to eat] a genus of flies of the family Sarcophagidae. The larvae of several

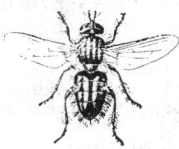

Sarcophaga carnaria.

species have been found in wounds, ulcers, the nasal passages, and sinuses. The most important species is *S. haemorrhoida'lis*. Other species are *S. carna'ria*, *S. fuscicau'da*, *S. dux*, *S. nificor'nis*, and *S. rubicor'nis*.

Sarcophagidae (sar″ko-faj'ĭ-de) a family of flies of the order Diptera, including the flesh flies; two genera *Sarcophaga* (type genus) and *Wohlfahrtia* produce myiasis in man and domestic animals.

sarcoplasm (sar'ko-plazm) [*sarco-* + Gr. *plasma* anything formed or molded] the interfibrillary matter of the striated muscles; the substance in which the fibrillae of the muscle fiber are embedded.

sarcoplasmic (sar″ko-plaz'mik) composed of or containing sarcoplasm; see also under *reticulum*.

sarcoplast (sar'ko-plast) [*sarco-* + Gr. *plastos* formed] an interstitial cell of a muscle, itself capable of being transformed into a muscle.

sarcopoietic (sar″ko-poi-et'ik) [*sarco-* + Gr. *poiein* to make] producing flesh or muscle.

Sarcopsylla (sar″kop-sil'ah) *Tunga*. **S. pen'etrans**, *Tunga penetrans*.

Sarcoptes (sar-kop'tēz) [*sarco-* + Gr. *koptein* to cut] a genus of acarids, including *S. scabie'i* (*Acarus scabiei*), the itch mite of humans, which produces scabies (q.v.). Varieties of *S. scabiei* cause mange of domestic animals, including pigs, horses, cows, and dogs.

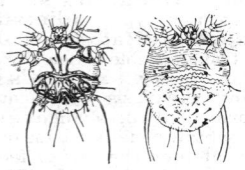

Sarcoptes scabiei, male and female.

sarcoptic (sar-kop'tic) of, relating to, or caused by *Sarcoptes*.

sarcoptidosis (sar-kop″tĭ-do'sis) infestation with *Sarcoptes*.

sarcosine (sar'ko-sēn) chemical name: *N*-methylglycine. An amino acid intermediate between glycine and dimethyl glycine in the one-carbon cycle, $C_3H_7NO_2$, found in shellfish, peanut protein, actinomycins, and, in low levels, in normal human blood.

sarcosis (sar-ko'sis) [*sarco-* + *-osis*] abnormal increase of flesh.

sarcosome (sar'ko-sōm) [*sarco-* + Gr. *sōma* body] former name for one of the mitochondria of a myofibril.

Sarcosporidia (sar″ko-spo-rid'e-ah) an order of sporozoan parasites found in the cardiac and striated muscles of vertebrates. It includes the genus *Sarcocystis*.

sarcosporidia (sar″ko-spo-rid'e-ah) plural of *sarcosporidium*.

sarcosporidiasis (sar″ko-spo″rĭ-di'ah-sis) sarcosporidiosis.

sarcosporidiosis (sar″ko-spo-rid'e-o'sis) the condition of being infected with the sporozoan *Sarcocystis*.

sarcosporidium (sar″ko-spo-rid'e-um), pl. *sarcosporid'ia*. An individual organism of the order Sarcosporidia.

sarcostosis (sar″kos-to'sis) [*sarco-* + Gr. *osteon* bone] ossification of fleshy tissues.

sarcostyle (sar'ko-stīl) [*sarco-* + Gr. *stylos* column] 1. a myofibril. 2. a bundle of myofibrils; called also *column of Kolliker* and *muscle column*.

sarcotherapeutics (sar″ko-ther″ah-pu'tiks) treatment of disease by the use of animal extracts.

sarcotherapy (sar″ko-ther'ah-pe) sarcotherapeutics.

sarcotic (sar-kot'ik) [Gr. *sarkōtikos*] promoting the growth of flesh.

sarcotubules (sar″ko-tu'būlz) membrane-limited structures that extend throughout the sarcoplasm and form a closely meshed canalicular network around each myofibril.

sarcous (sar'kus) pertaining to flesh or to muscular tissues.

sardonic (sar-don'ik) [L. *sardonicus*; Gr. *Sardonikos* Sardinian] denoting a kind of spasmodic or tetanic grin or involuntary smile, as *risus sardonicus*.

sarmentocymarin (sar-men″to-si'mah-rin) a cardiac glycoside, $C_{30}H_{46}O_8$, from the seeds of *Strophanthus sarmentosus*. On hydrolysis, it yields sarmentogenin and sarmentose.

sarmentogenin (sar″men-toj'ĕ-nin) an aglycone, $C_{23}H_{34}O_5$, from sarmentocymarin; it has been studied as a possible source of cortisone.

sarmentose (sar'men-tōs) a methyl ether of a 2-desoxyhexomethyl sugar from sarmentocymarin.

Sarothamnus (sa″ro-tham'nus) [Gr. *saron* broom + *thamnos* shrub] *Cytisus*.

sarpicillin (sar″pĭ-sil'in) chemical name: 6-(2,2-dimethyl-5-oxo-4-phenyl-1-imidazolidinyl)-3,3-dimethyl-7-oxo-4-thia-1-azabicyclo[3.2.0]heptane-2-carboxylic acid; an antibacterial, $C_{21}H_{27}N_3O_5S$.

Sarracenia (sar″ah-se'ne-ah) [Michel *Sarrazin*, Quebec physician

and naturalist, 1659–1734] a genus of polypetalous plants, known as *side-saddle flower* and *pitcher plant*, type of the order Sarraceniaceae. *S. purpu'rea* is the commonest of the pitcher plants of North America. The secretion of the pitcher of this plant is said to contain digestant enzymes. It is a stimulant, diuretic, and aperient.

sarsa (sar'sah), gen. *sar'sae* [L.; Sp. *sarça* briar] sarsaparilla.

sarsaparilla (sar″sap-ah-ril'ah) [L.; Sp. "briar vine"] the dried root of *Smilax aristolochiaefolia* Mill. (Liliaceae) and other related species; used as a flavoring agent in beverages, and in the treatment of psoriasis. It contains sarsasapogenin, a precursor in the manufacture of compounds in the pregnane series. Called also *sarsa*.

sarsasapogenin (sar″sah-sap″o-jen'in) a steroid sapogenin from sarsaparilla, used in the synthesis of hormones of the pregnane series.

Sassafras (sas'ah-fras) [L.] a genus of lauraceous trees. The root bark of *S. albi'dum* Nutt. (Lauraceae) (*S. variifo'lia*, *S. officina'le*), or sassafras, a tree of North America, is used as an aromatic and flavoring agent, and was formerly used as a sudorific. The volatile oil contains safrene and safrol. It is the source of the popular American beverage, root beer.

satellite (sat'ĕ-līt) [L. *satelles* companion] 1. a vein that closely accompanies an artery, such as the brachial. 2. a minor, or attendant, lesion situated near a larger one. 3. a globoid mass of chromatin attached at the secondary constriction to the ends of the short arms of acrocentric autosomes. 4. exhibiting satellitism. **bacterial s.,** satellite colony. **chromosomal s.,** see *satellite*. **nucleolar s.,** a small mass of chromatin found next to the nucleolar membrane in most nerve cells of the female; sex chromatin.

satellitism (sat'ĕ-li-tizm) the phenomenon in which certain bacterial species grow more vigorously in the immediate vicinity of colonies of other unrelated species (e.g., *Hemophilus influenzae* near a colony of streptococci), owing to the production of an essential metabolite by the latter species.

satellitosis (sat″ĕ-li-to'sis) accumulation of neuroglial cells about neurons; seen whenever neurons are damaged.

satiety (sah-ti'e-ty) [L. *satis* sufficient + *-ety* state or condition of] sufficiency, or satisfaction, as full gratification of appetite or thirst, with abolition of the desire to ingest food or liquids.

Satterthwaite's method (sat'er-thwāts) [Thomas Edward *Satterthwaite*, New York physician, 1843–1934] see under *method*.

Sattler's layer (sat'lerz) [Hubert *Sattler*, Austrian ophthalmologist, 1844–1928] see under *layer*.

saturated (sach'ĕ-rāt″ed) 1. having all the chemical affinities satisfied. 2. unable to hold in solution any more of a given substance. 3. denoting a fatty acid having only single bonds in its carbon chain.

saturation (sach'ĕ-ra″shun) [L. *saturatio*] 1. the act of saturating or condition of being saturated. 2. in radiotherapy, the delivery of a maximum tolerable tissue dose within a short time period and then maintaining this biologic effect for an extended period of time by additional smaller fractional doses. 3. an effervescing draft or potion. **oxygen s.,** a measure of the degree to which oxygen is bound to hemoglobin, given as a percentage calculated by dividing the maximum oxygen capacity into the actual oxygen content and multiplying by 100.

saturnine (sat'ur-nīn) [L. *saturninus; saturnus* lead] pertaining to or produced by lead; having the dull, heavy properties associated with lead.

saturnism (sat'ur-nizm) [L. *saturnus* lead] lead poisoning.

satyriasis (sat″ĭ-ri'ah-sis) [Gr. *satyros* satyr] excessive sexual desire in the male. Cf. *nymphomania*.

satyromania (sat″ĭ-ro-ma'ne-ah) [Gr. *satyros* satyr + *mania* madness] satyriasis.

saucer (saw'ser) a rounded, shallow depression. **auditory s.,** see under *placode*.

saucerization (saw″ser-i-za'shun) 1. the excavation of tissue to form a shallow shelving depression usually performed to facilitate drainage from infected areas of bone. 2. the shallow, saucer-like depression on the upper surface of a vertebra which has suffered a compression fracture.

Sauer's vaccine (sow'erz) [Louis W. *Sauer*, American pediatrician, born 1885] see under *vaccine*.

Sauerbruch's cabinet, prosthesis (sow'er-brooks) [Ernst Ferdinand *Sauerbruch*, surgeon in Berlin, 1875–1951] see under *cabinet* and *prosthesis*.

Saundby's test (sawnd'bēz) [Robert *Saundby*, English physician, 1849–1918] see under *tests*.

Saunders' disease, sign (sawn'derz) [Edward Watt *Saunders*, physician in St. Louis, 1854–1927] see under *disease* and *sign*.

sauroid (saw'roid) [Gr. *sauros* lizard + *eidos* form] resembling a reptile.

Saussure's hygrometer (so-sūrz') [Horace Bénédict de *Saussure*, Swiss physicist, 1740–1779] see under *hygrometer*.

savin (sav'in) [L. *sabina*] the evergreen shrub, *Juniperus sabina*

L. Cupressaceae. The fresh tops afford an acrid volatile oil which has been used in folk medicine for its emmenagogic, antirheumatic, and anthelmintic properties, and is used in perfumery. A preparation of the young twigs was formerly used as a diuretic.

saw (saw) a cutting instrument with a cutting or serrated edge. **Adams' s.,** a small straight saw with a long handle, for osteotomy. **amputating s.,** one for use in performing amputations. **bayonet s.,** a surgical bone saw used for the excision of the nasal dorsal hump. **Butcher's s.,** an amputating saw with a blade that can be set at various angles. **chain s.,** one in which the teeth are set upon links, the saw being moved by pulling upon one or the other handle. **crown s.,** a form of trephine. **Farabeuf's s.,** a saw the blade of which can be set at any desired angle. **Gigli's wire s.,** a flexible wire with saw teeth. **Hey's s.,** a

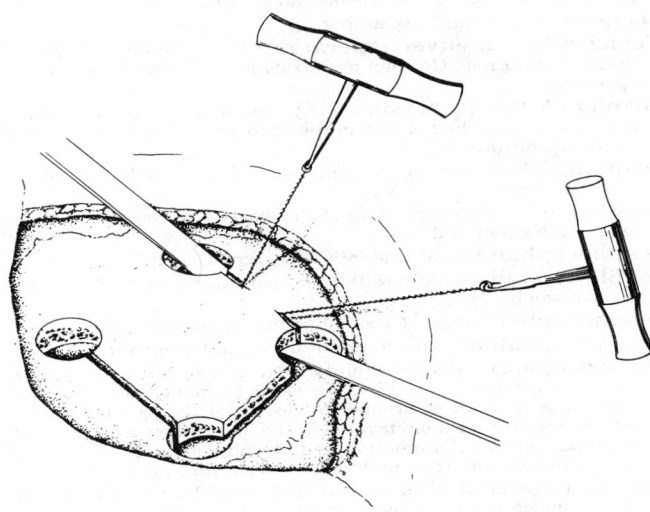

Gigli's wire saw as used in removing segment of the skull.

small saw for enlarging orifices in bones. **hole s.,** a trephine. **separating s.,** a saw for separating teeth. **Shrady's s., subcutaneous s.,** a saw for bone work operated through a fenestrated cannula which has been introduced alongside the bone by a trocar.

saxitoxin (sak″sĭ-tok′sin) a term used to designate the toxin obtained from poisonous mussels (*Mytilus*), clams (*Saxidomus*), and plankton (*Gonyaulax*), said to have the molecular formula $C_{10}H_{17}$-$N_7O_4 \cdot 2HCl$. The term is used interchangeably with paralytic shellfish poison or gonyaulax poison (q.v. under *poison*).

Sayre's apparatus, etc. (sa′erz) [Lewis Albert *Sayre*, American surgeon, 1820–1900] see under *apparatus, bandage, jacket,* and *operation.*

Sb chemical symbol for *antimony* (L. *stibium*).

SbCl₃ antimony trichloride.

Sb₂O₃ antimony trioxide.

Sb₂O₅ antimony pentoxide.

Sb₄O₆ antimony trioxide.

S.C. closure of the semilunar valves.

Sc chemical symbol for *scandium.*

scab (skab) 1. crust. 2. to become covered with a crust or scab. **foot s.,** sheep scab. **head s.,** any acariasis of the head, especially the sarcoptic scab of the head of sheep. **sheep s.,** a disease of sheep caused by the mite *Psoroptes ovis,* which infests the skin at the base of the hairs. A scab is formed which comes off, bringing the wool along with it.

scabetic (skah-bet′ik) scabietic.

scabicide (ska′bĭ-sīd) 1. destructive to *Sarcoptes scabiei;* used in the treatment of scabies. 2. an agent for destroying *Sarcoptes scabiei.*

scabies (ska′bēz) [L., from *scabere* scratch] a contagious skin disease due to the itch mite, *Sarcoptes scabiei,* which bores into the stratum corneum, forming cuniculi or burrows. The disease is attended with intense itching, together with the eczema caused by scratching. **bovine s.,** a disease of cattle resembling sheep scab, which is caused by *Psoroptes ovis.* **Norwegian s.,** a rare form associated with an immense number of mites and with marked scales and crusts.

scabietic (ska″be-et′ik) pertaining to or affected with scabies.

scala (ska′lah), pl. *sca′lae* [L. "staircase"] a stairlike structure; applied especially to various passages of the cochlea. **s. me′dia, s. of Löwenberg,** ductus cochlearis. **s. tym′pani** [NA], the perilymph-filled part of the cochlea that is continuous with the scala vestibuli at the helicotrema, is separated from other

cochlear structures by the spiral lamina and the cochlear duct, and ends blindly near the fenestra cochleae. Called also *tympanic canal of cochlea.* **s. vestib′uli** [NA], the perilymph-filled part of the cochlea that begins in the vestibule, is separated from other cochlear structures by the spiral lamina and the cochlear duct, and becomes continuous with the scala tympani at the helicotrema. Called also *vestibular canal.*

scalariform (skah-lar′ĭ-form) [L. *scalaris* like a ladder + *forma* shape] resembling the rungs of a ladder.

scald (skawld) 1. a burn caused by hot liquid or hot, moist vapor. 2. to burn with hot liquid or steam.

scale (skāl) 1. [Fr. *écale* shell, husk] a thin, compacted, platelike structure, as of cornified epithelial cells, on the surface of the body, or shed from the skin. 2. [L. *scala,* usually pl., *scalae,* a series of steps] a scheme or device by which some property may be evaluated or measured, such as a linear surface bearing marks at regular intervals, representing certain predetermined units. 3. to remove material from a body surface, as incrusted material from the surface of the teeth. **absolute s.,** a temperature scale with zero at the absolute zero of temperature. **Apgar s.,** see under *score.* **Baumé's s.,** a scale for expressing the specific gravity of fluids. **Bloch's s.,** a series of solutions of tincture of benzoin in glycerinated water, employed to determine, by comparison of turbidity, the amount of albumin precipitated in urine or other fluid by heat. **Brazelton behavioral s.,** a method for assessing infant behavior by its responses to environmental stimuli. **Cattell Infant Intelligence S.,** a test for evaluating the developmental status of infants in the first two years of life. **Celsius s.,** a temperature scale with the ice point at 0 and the normal boiling point of water at 100 degrees (100° C.). See Table. **centigrade s.,** one in which the interval

TABLE OF EQUIVALENTS OF CELSIUS (CENTIGRADE) AND
FAHRENHEIT TEMPERATURE SCALES

CELSIUS	FAHR.	CELSIUS	FAHR.	CELSIUS	FAHR.
Deg.	Deg.	Deg.	Deg.	Deg.	Deg.
−40	−40.0	9	48.2	57	134.6
−39	−38.2	10	50.0	58	136.4
−38	−36.4	11	51.8	59	138.2
−37	−34.6	12	53.6	60	140.0
−36	−32.8	13	55.4	61	141.8
−35	−31.0	14	57.2	62	143.6
−34	−29.2	15	59.0	63	145.4
−33	−27.4	16	60.8	64	147.2
−32	−25.6	17	62.6	65	149.0
−31	−23.8	18	64.4	66	150.8
−30	−22.0	19	66.2	67	152.6
−29	−20.2	20	68.0	68	154.4
−28	−18.4	21	69.8	69	156.2
−27	−16.6	22	71.6	70	158.0
−26	−14.8	23	73.4	71	159.8
−25	−13.0	24	75.2	72	161.6
−24	−11.2	25	77.0	73	163.4
−23	−9.4	26	78.8	74	165.2
−22	−7.6	27	80.6	75	167.0
−21	−5.8	28	82.4	76	168.8
−20	−4.0	29	84.2	77	170.6
−19	−2.2	30	86.0	78	172.4
−18	−0.4	31	87.8	79	174.2
−17	+1.4	32	89.6	80	176.0
−16	3.2	33	91.4	81	177.8
−15	5.0	34	93.2	82	179.6
−14	6.8	35	95.0	83	181.4
−13	8.6	36	96.8	84	183.2
−12	10.4	37	98.6	85	185.0
−11	12.2	38	100.4	86	186.8
−10	14.0	39	102.2	87	188.6
−9	15.8	40	104.0	88	190.4
−8	17.6	41	105.8	89	192.2
−7	19.4	42	107.6	90	194.0
−6	21.2	43	109.4	91	195.8
−5	23.0	44	111.2	92	197.6
−4	24.8	45	113.0	93	199.4
−3	26.6	46	114.8	94	201.2
−2	28.4	47	116.6	95	203.0
−1	30.2	48	118.4	96	204.8
0	32.0	49	120.2	97	206.6
+1	33.8	50	122.0	98	208.4
2	35.6	51	123.8	99	210.2
3	37.4	52	125.6	100	212.0
4	39.2	53	127.4	101	213.8
5	41.0	54	129.2	102	215.6
6	42.8	55	131.0	103	217.4
7	44.6	56	132.8	104	219.2
8	46.4				

between two established points is divided into 100 equal units, such as the Celsius scale. See Table. **Charrière s.,** a scale for grading the size of urethral sounds and catheters; see *French s.* **Clark's s.,** a scale used in denoting the hardness of water, based on the number of grains of calcium carbonate per imperial gallon. **Columbia Mental Maturity S.,** a test of specific kinds of mental function and general abilities, suitable for children (ages 3 to 12) with no speech or with limited physical capabilities, such as those with cerebral palsy. **Dunfermline s.,** a scheme used in denoting the nutritional status of children: 1, superior condition; 2, passable condition; 3, requiring supervision; 4, requiring medical treatment. **Fahrenheit s.,** a temperature scale with the ice point at 32 and the normal boiling point of water at

212 degrees (212° F.). See Table. **French s.,** a scale used for denoting the size of catheters, sounds, and other tubular instruments, each unit being roughly equivalent to 0.33 mm. in diameter, i.e., 18 French indicates a diameter of 6 mm. **Gaffky s.,** a scale used in denoting the prognosis in tuberculosis, based on the number of tubercle bacilli in the sputum. **gray s.,** see under *ultrasonography.* **hydrometer s.,** a scale used for expressing the specific gravity of liquids. **Kelvin s.,** an absolute scale on which the unit of measurement corresponds with that of the Celsius (centigrade) scale, but the ice point is at 273.15 degrees (273.15° K). **Kent Emergency S.,** a rapid screening test for determining the mental age of a child, consisting of a set of oral questions graded according to age. **Rankine s.,** an absolute scale on which the unit of measurement corresponds with that of the Fahrenheit scale, but the ice point is at 491.67 degrees (491.67° R). **Réaumur s.,** a temperature scale with the ice point at 0 and the normal boiling point of water at 80 degrees (80° R.). **Tallqvist's s.,** a series of lithographed colors formerly used to quantitate hemoglobin. **temperature s.,** a scale used for expressing the degree of heat, which is based on absolute zero as a reference point (absolute scale), or with a certain value arbitrarily assigned to such temperatures as the ice point and boiling point of water under certain stipulated conditions, the range between and beyond them being divided into a designated number of identical units. **Wechsler Adult Intelligence S. (W.A.I.S.)** a test consisting of verbal and performance elements, designed to measure adult intelligence. **Wechsler Intelligence S. for Children,** an intelligence test used to identify the retarded child.

scalene (ska'lēn) [Gr. *skalēnos* uneven] 1. unequally three sided. 2. pertaining to one of the scalene muscles.

scalenectomy (ska″lĕ-nek'to-me) [*scalenus* + Gr. *ektomē* excision] the operation of resecting a scalenus muscle.

scalenotomy (ska″lĕ-not'o-me) [*scalenus* + Gr. *tomē* a cutting] the operation of severing the scaleni muscles close to their insertion on the ribs to restrict respiratory activity of the upper part of the thorax and thus induce apical rest in pulmonary tuberculosis.

scalenus (ska-le'nus) [L.; Gr. *skalēnos*] uneven; a name given to various muscles of the neck. See *Table of Musculi.*

scaler (ska'ler) a dental instrument used in removing calculus from the surface of the teeth. **chisel s.,** a straight instrument which curves slightly as the blade extends from the shank, the straight cutting edge, at the end of the instrument, being beveled at a 45 degree angle. **deep s.,** a dental instrument designed for use in removal of subgingival calculus. **hoe s.,** one made with different angular relationships of shank and handle, but with the blade bent at a 99 degree angle, and the flattened termination surface beveled at an angle of 45 degrees. **sickle s.,** a node-shaped instrument, available in various sizes and shapes, designed for the removal of tenacious supragingival deposits of calculus. **superficial s.,** a dental instrument designed for use in removal of supragingival calculus. **wing s.,** a variation of the sickle scaler, consisting of a short curved blade with a flare at the very edge; used for the removal of supragingival calculus.

scaling (skāl'ing) removal of calculus material from the exposed tooth surfaces and that part of the teeth covered by the marginal gingiva.

scall (skawl) (*obs.*) 1. any scaly, or scabby, disease of the skin. 2. favus of animals. **honeycomb s.** (*obs.*), an eruption consisting of small ulcers separated by raised edges. **milk s.,** crusta lactea.

scalp (skalp) that part of the skin of the head, exclusive of the face and ears, which normally is covered with hair. **gyrate s.,** cutis verticis gyrata.

scalpel (skal'pel) [L. *scalpellum*] a small surgical knife with a straight handle and, usually, a blade with a convex edge.

scalpriform (skal'pri-form) shaped like a chisel.

scaly (ska'le) [L. *squamosus*] 1. scalelike. 2. characterized by scales.

scammonia (skah-mo'ne-ah) scammony.

scammony (skam'o-ne) [L. *scammonium, scammonia*] the plant *Convolvulus scammonia* L. (Convolvulaceae), of Asia Minor and Syria; the root affords a gummy and resinous exudate, which has anthelmintic and cathartic properties. **Mexican s.,** ipomea.

scan (skan) 1. shortened form of *scintiscan,* q.v.; variously designated, according to the organ under examination, as *brain scan, kidney scan, thyroid scan,* etc. 2. a visual display of ultrasonographic echoes. An *A-scan* is a display on a cathode ray tube in which one axis represents the time required for return of the echo and the other corresponds to the strength of the echo. In *B-scan,* the position of a bright dot on the tube corresponds to the time elapsed, and the brightness of the spot to the strength of the echo; movement of the transducer across the skin surface yields a two-dimensional cross-sectional display. **CAT s.,** computerized axial tomography; see under *tomography.*

scandium (skan'de-um) a very rare metallic element; symbol, Sc; atomic number, 21; atomic weight, 44.956.

scanner (skan'er) something that scans; a scintiscanner.

EMI s., an instrument for reconstructing tomographic images for display on a cathode ray tube; see *computerized axial tomography,* under *tomography.* **scintillation s.,** scintiscanner.

scanning (skan'ning) 1. the act of examining visually, as a small area or different isolated areas, in detail. 2. a manner of utterance characterized by somewhat regularly recurring pauses. **radioisotope s.,** the production of a two-dimensional picture (scintiscan, or scan), representing the gamma rays emitted by a radioactive isotope concentrated in a specific tissue of the body, such as the brain or thyroid gland.

scanography (skan-og'rah-fe) a method of making radiographs by the use of a narrow slit beneath the tube in such a manner that only a line or sheet of x-rays is employed and the x-ray tube moves over the object so that all the rays of the central beam pass through the part being radiographed at the same angle.

scansion (skan'shun) scanning.

Scanzoni's maneuver (operation) (skan-tso'nēz) [Friedrich Wilhelm *Scanzoni,* German obstetrician, 1821–1891] see under *operation.*

scapha (ska'fah) [L. "a skiff"] [NA] the long curved depression which separates the helix from the anthelix; called also *scaphoid fossa* and *fossa helicis.*

scaphion (ska'fe-on) [Gr. *skaphion* a small bowl or basin] basis cranii externa.

scapho- [Gr. *skaphē* skiff or light boat] a combining form meaning boat-shaped.

scaphocephalia (skaf″o-sĕ-fa'le-ah) scaphocephaly.

scaphocephalic (skaf″o-sĕ-fal'ik) pertaining to or characterized by scaphocephaly.

scaphocephalism (skaf″o-sef'ah-lizm) scaphocephaly.

scaphocephalous (skaf″o-sef'ah-lus) scaphocephalic.

scaphocephaly (skaf″o-sef'ah-le) [Gr. *skaphē* skiff + *kephalē* head] a condition in which the skull is abnormally long and narrow, as a result of premature closure of the sagittal suture, with heavy centers of ossification in the line of the suture; usually accompanied by inflammation and atrophy of the optic papillae and by mental retardation. Called also *sagittal synostosis.*

scaphohydrocephalus (skaf″o-hi″dro-sef'ah-lus) hydrocephalus in which the head assumes a boatlike shape.

scaphohydrocephaly (skaf″o-hi″dro-sef'ah-le) scaphohydrocephalus.

scaphoid (skaf'oid) [Gr. *skaphē* skiff + *eidos* form] shaped like a boat; navicular. Used especially in reference to the most lateral bone in the proximal row of carpal bones (os scaphoideum [NA]). See also *os naviculare.*

scaphoiditis (skaf″oi-di'tis) inflammation of the scaphoid bone. **tarsal s.,** inflammation involving the navicular (scaphoid) bone of the tarsus. See also *Köhler's bone disease* (def. 1), under *disease.*

Scaptocosa (skap″to-co'sah) a genus of wolf spiders. **S. rapto'ria,** a species of Brazil that has a powerful hemolytic venom that has been shown to cause necrotic arachnidism.

scapula (skap'u-lah), pl. *scap'ulae* [L.] [NA] the flat, triangular bone in the back of the shoulder; the shoulder blade. See illustration. **alar s., s. ala'ta,** winged s. **elevated ,s.,** Sprengel's deformity. **Graves' s.,** scaphoid s. **scaphoid s.,** a scapula in which the vertebral border is more or less concave. **winged s.,** a scapula having a prominent vertebral border.

scapulalgia (skap″u-lal'je-ah) pain in the scapular region.

scapular (skap'u-lar) of or pertaining to the scapula.

scapulary (skap'u-la're) a shoulder bandage, with the appearance of a pair of suspenders or braces, to hold in place a body bandage or girdle.

scapulectomy (skap″u-lek'to-me) [*scapula* + Gr. *ektomē* excision] the surgical removal of the scapula or a part of it (resection).

scapuloanterior (skap″u-lo-an-te're-or) denoting a position of the fetus in transverse lie, with the scapula directed anteriorly.

scapuloclavicular (skap″u-lo-klah-vik'u-lar) pertaining to the scapula and the clavicle.

scapulodynia (skap″u-lo-din'e-ah) [*scapula* + Gr. *odynē* pain + -*ia*] pain in the region of the shoulder.

scapulohumeral (skap″u-lo-hu'mer-al) pertaining to the scapula and the humerus.

scapulopexy (skap'u-lo-pek″se) [*scapula* + Gr. *pēxis* fixation] surgical fixation of the scapula.

scapuloposterior (skap″u-lo-pos-te're-or) denoting a position of the fetus in transverse lie, with the scapula directed posteriorly.

scapus (ska'pus), pl. *sca'pi* [L.] shaft; [NA] a general term for a shaftlike structure. **s. pe'nis,** corpus penis. **s. pi'li** [NA], hair shaft: the major portion of a hair, designating especially the portion that extends beyond the surface of the skin.

scar (skahr) [Gr. *eschara* the scab or eschar on a wound caused by burning] a mark remaining after the healing of a wound or other morbid process; a cicatrix. By extension applied to other visible manifestations of an earlier event. **hypertrophic s.,** one formed by exuberant cicatrization, giving it the appearance of a keloid but without the latter's tendency to progressive extension,

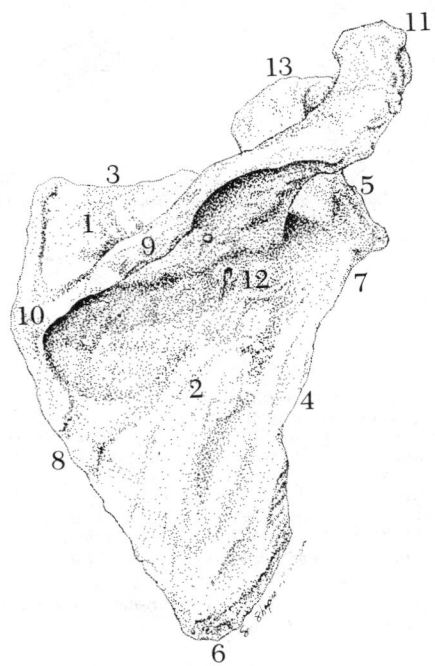

Right scapula, dorsal view: 1, supraspinous fossa. 2, infraspinous fossa. 3, superior margin. 4, lateral margin. 5, glenoid cavity. 6, inferior angle. 7, neck of scapula. 8, medial margin. 9, spine. 10, triangular commencement of spine, upon which the tendon of the trapezius muscle moves. 11, acromion. 12, arterial foramen. 13, coracoid process.

and recurrence after excision. **Reichert's s.,** an area over the implanting blastocyst of some species consisting of a fibrinous membrane in place of the decidual tissue. **white s. of ovary,** corpus albicans, def. 1.

scarf (skahrf) a broad strip of fabric. **Mayor's s.,** a triangular bandage for immobilizing the upper limbs.

scarification (skar″ĭ-fĭ-ka′shun) [L. *scarificatio,* Gr. *skariphismos* a scratching up] production in the skin of many small, superficial scratches or punctures, as for the introduction of smallpox vaccine. The term is sometimes used erroneously for scarring.

scarificator (skar′ĭ-fĭ-ka″tor) scarifier.

scarifier (skar′ĭ-fi″er) an instrument bearing many sharp points, used in scarification.

scarlatina (skahr″lah-te′nah) [L. "scarlet"] scarlet fever; see under *fever.* **s. angino′sa,** scarlet fever associated with painful pharyngitis, with tonsillar enlargement or peritonsillar abscess. Called also *Fothergill's disease.* **s. haemorrha′gica,** scarlet fever in which there is extravasation of the blood into skin and mucous membranes. **puerperal s.,** a scarlet rash sometimes seen in puerperal fever.

scarlatinal (skahr-lat′ĭ-nal) pertaining to or due to scarlatina (scarlet fever).

scarlatinella (skahr-lat″ĭ-nel′ah) Duke's disease.

scarlatiniform (skahr″lah-tin′ĭ-form) resembling scarlatina.

scarlatinoid (skahr-lat′ĭ-noid) scarlatiniform.

scarlet (skar′let) 1. bright red tinged with orange or yellow. 2. a scarlet dye. **Biebrich s., water-soluble,** an azo dye used as a plasma stain, $C_6H_4(SO_2 \cdot ONa) \cdot N{:}N \cdot C_6H_2(SO_2 \cdot ONa) \cdot N{:}N \cdot C_{10}H_3 \cdot OH.$ **s. G,** sudan III. **s. R,** scarlet red.

Scarpa's fascia, etc. (skar′pahz) [Anthony *Scarpa,* Italian anatomist and surgeon, 1747–1832] see under *fascia, fluid, foramen, ganglion, ligament, membrane, nerve, operation, sheath, shoe, staphyloma,* and *triangle.*

SCAT sheep cell agglutination test.

scatemia (skah-te′me-ah) [*scato-* + Gr. *haima* blood + *-ia*] alimentary toxemia in which the chemical poisons are absorbed through the intestine.

scato- (skat′o) [Gr. *skōr, skatos* dung] a combining form denoting relation to dung, or fecal matter; see also words beginning *skato-.*

scatol (ska′tōl) skatole.

scatologic (skat″o-loj′ik) pertaining to fecal matter, or to scatology.

scatology (skah-tol′o-je) [*scato-* + *-logy*] the study of the feces.

scatoma (skah-to′mah) [*scato-* + *-oma*] stercoroma.

scatophagy (skah-tof′ah-je) [*scato-* + Gr. *phagein* to eat] the eating of excrement.

scatophilia (skat″o-fil′e-ah) [*scato-* + Gr. *philein* to love] a perverted fondness for dung.

scatoscopy (skah-tos′ko-pe) [*scato-* + Gr. *skopein* to examine] inspection of the feces.

scatter (skat′er) the diffusion or deviation of roentgen rays produced by a medium through which the rays pass. Backward diffusion is called *backscatter.*

scattergram (skat′er-gram) a graph in which the values found in a statistical study are represented by separate, unconnected symbols (dots, crosses, hollow or solid circles, etc.).

scattering (skat′er-ing) in radiology, a change in direction of a photon or subatomic particle as the result of a collision or interaction.

scatula (skat′u-lah) [L. "parallelepiped"] an oblong paper box for powders or pills.

scavenger (skav′en-jer) a substance that influences the course of a chemical reaction by ready combination with free radicals, e.g., diphenylpicrylhydrazyl.

Sc.D. Doctor of Science.

Sc.D.A. abbreviation for L. *scapulodextra anterior* (right scapulo-lo-anterior, a presentation of the fetus).

Sc.D.P. abbreviation for L. *scapulodextra posterior* (right scapuloposterior, a presentation of the fetus).

Scedosporium (se-do-spo′re-um) *Monosporium.*

scelalgia (ske-lal′je-ah) [Gr. *skelos* leg + *algos* pain + *-ia*] pain in the leg.

Sceleth treatment (ske′leth) [Charles Edward *Sceleth,* Chicago physician, 1873–1942] see under *treatment.*

scelotyrbe (sel-o-ter′be) [Gr. *skelos* leg + *tyrbē* disorder] spastic paralysis of the legs.

Schacher's ganglion (shah′kerz) [Polycarp Gottlieb *Schacher,* German physician, 1674–1737] the ciliary ganglion.

Schachowa's spiral tubes (shah′ko-vahz) [Seraphina *Schachowa,* Russian histologist in Bern, born 1854] tubuli renales.

Schafer's method (sha′ferz) [Sir Edward Albert Sharpey-*Schafer,* English physiologist, 1850–1935] see under *respiration, artificial.*

Schäffer's reflex (shef′erz) [Max *Schäffer,* German neurologist, 1852–1923] see under *reflex.*

Schamberg's dermatosis (disease) (sham′bergz) [Jay Frank *Schamberg,* Philadelphia dermatologist, 1870–1934] progressive pigmentary dermatosis.

Schanz's disease, syndrome (shants′ez) [Alfred *Schanz,* German orthopedist, 1868–1931] see under *disease* and *syndrome.*

scharlach R (shar′lak) scarlet red.

Schaudinn's fluid (shaw-dinz′) [Fritz Richard *Schaudinn,* German bacteriologist, 1871–1906] see under *fluid.*

Schaumann's bodies, sarcoidosis (disease, lymphogranuloma, syndrome) (shaw′manz) [Jörgen *Schaumann,* Swedish dermatologist, 1879–1953] see under *body* and *sarcoidosis.*

Schauta's operation (shaw′tahz) [Friedrich *Schauta,* Vienna gynecologist, 1849–1919] see under *operation.*

Schauta-Wertheim operation (shaw′tah-ver′tīm) [Friedrich *Schauta;* Ernst *Wertheim,* Vienna gynecologist, 1864–1920] Wertheim-Schauta operation.

Schede's clot, operation (method, resection, treatment) (sha′dez) [Max *Schede,* surgeon in Bonn, 1844–1902] see under *clot* and *operation.*

Scheiner's experiment (shi′nerz) [Christoph *Scheiner,* German mathematician, 1575–1650] see under *experiment.*

schema (ske′mah) [Gr. *schēma* form, shape] a plan, outline, or arrangement. **Hamberger's s.,** the external intercostal and the intercartilaginous muscles are inspiratory muscles, the internal intercostal muscles are expiratory.

schematic (ske-mat′ik) [Gr. *schēma* form, shape] serving as a diagram or model; see *eye.*

Scherer's test (shār′erz) [Johann Joseph von *Scherer,* German physician, 1814–1869] see under *tests.*

scherlievo (skār-lya′vo) a contagious disorder formerly prevalent in Illyria and Dalmatia, supposed to have been syphilis.

scheroma (ske-ro′mah) xerophthalmia.

Scheuermann's disease, kyphosis (shoi′er-manz) [Holger Werfel *Scheuermann,* Danish surgeon, 1877–1960] osteochondrosis of the vertebrae; see *osteochondrosis.*

Schick's sign, test (reaction) (shiks) [Béla *Schick,* Hungarian pediatrician in the United States, born 1877] see under *sign* and *tests.*

Schiefferdecker's disk, symbiosis, theory (she-fer-dek′erz) [Paul *Schiefferdecker,* Bonn anatomist, 1849–1931] see under *disk, symbiosis,* and *theory.*

Schiff's biliary cycle (shifs) [Moritz *Schiff,* German physiologist, 1823–1896] see under *cycle.*

Schiff's reagent, test (shifs) [Hugo (Ugo) *Schiff,* German chemist in Florence, 1834–1915] see under *reagent* and *tests.*

Schilder's disease (encephalitis) (shil′derz) [Paul Ferdinand

Schilder, Austrian neurologist in the United States, 1886–1940] see under *disease*.

Schiller's test (shil′erz) [Walter *Schiller*, Austrian pathologist in the United States, 1887–1960] see under *tests*.

Schilling blood count (shil′ing) [Victor *Schilling*, German hematologist, 1883–1960] see under *count*.

Schilling test (shil′ing) [Robert Frederick *Schilling*, American hematologist, born 1919] see under *tests*.

Schimmelbusch's disease (shim′el-boosh″ez) [Curt *Schimmelbusch*, German surgeon, 1860–1895] cystic disease of the breast; see under *disease*.

schindylesis (skin″dĭ-le′sis) [Gr. *schindylēsis* a splintering] a form of articulation in which a thin plate of one bone is received into a cleft in another, as in the articulation of the perpendicular plate of the ethmoid bone with the vomer.

Schinus (ski′nus) [Gr. *schinos* mastic] a genus of anacardiaceous trees of warm regions. *S. mol′le*, L., of tropical America (pepper tree), affords a kind of American mastic, and is a mild purgative and aromatic.

Schiotz's tonometer (she-ets′) [Hjalmar *Schiotz*, Norwegian physician, 1850–1927] see under *tonometer*.

schistasis (skis′tah-sis) a splitting; specifically, a congenital defect consisting of a cleft or fissure of the body, as schistocormia, schistomelia, schistosomia.

schisto- [Gr. *schistos* split] a combining form meaning split or cleft.

schistocelia (shis″, skiz′to-se′le-ah) schistocoelia.

schistocephalus (shis″, skis″to-sef′ah-lus) [schisto- + Gr. *kephalē* head] a fetus born with a cleft head.

schistocoelia (shis″, skiz′to-se′le-ah) [schisto- + Gr. *koilia* belly] congenital fissure of the abdomen.

schistocormia (shis″, skiz′to-kor′me-ah) [schisto- + Gr. *kormos* trunk + *-ia*] a developmental anomaly characterized by a cleft condition of the trunk.

schistocormus (shis″, skiz′to-kor′mus) a fetus exhibiting schistocormia.

schistocystis (shis″to-sis′tis) [schisto- + Gr. *kystis* bladder] fissure of the bladder.

schistocyte (shis′, skis′to-sīt) a fragment of a red blood corpuscle, commonly observed in the blood in hemolytic anemias; called also *helmet cell*.

schistocytosis (shis″, skis″to-si-to′sis) the accumulation of schistocytes in the blood.

schistoglossia (shis″, skis″to-glos′e-ah) [schisto- + Gr. *glōssa* tongue + *-ia*] bifid tongue.

schistomelia (shis″, skis″to-me′le-ah) [schisto- + Gr. *melos* limb + *-ia*] a developmental anomaly characterized by a cleft condition of a limb.

schistomelus (shis-, skis-tom′e-lus) a fetus exhibiting schistomelia.

schistometer (shis-, skis-tom′ĕ-ter) [schisto- + Gr. *metron* measure] (*obs.*) an instrument for measuring the aperture between the vocal cords.

schistoprosopia (shis″, skis″to-pro-so′pe-ah) [schisto- + Gr. *prosōpon* face + *-ia*] a developmental anomaly characterized by fissure of the face; schizoprosopia.

schistoprosopus (shis″, skis″to-pros′o-pus) a fetus exhibiting schistoprosopia.

schistorachis (shis-, skis-tor′ah-kis) [schisto- + Gr. *rachis* spine] rachischisis.

schistosis (shis-, skis-to′sis) [Schist a form of slate + *-osis*] pneumoconiosis in slate workers.

Schistosoma (shis″, skis″to-so′mah) [schisto- + Gr. *sōma* body] a genus of trematode parasites or flukes; the blood flukes; sometimes called also *Bilharzia*. **S. bo′vis**, a species found in the portal system of sheep and oxen in Africa, Mesopotamia, Corsica, Sardinia, and Sicily. **S. haemato′bium**, a common parasite of Africa, especially Egypt, the Mediterranean littoral, and the Arabian peninsula. The adult worms are found in the veins, especially those of the vesical plexus, producing irritability of the bladder, hematuria, and dysentery. The parasites enter the body through the skin of persons coming in contact with infested waters, the invertebrate hosts being small snails of the genus *Bulinus*, including the subgenus *Physopsis*. Called also *Bilharzia haematobia* and, formerly, *Distoma haematobium* and *D. capense*. **S. in′dicum**, a species occurring in cattle, sheep, goats, etc., in India and Rhodesia. **S. intercala′tum**, a species found in West Central Africa, which causes schistosomiasis intercalatum by penetrating the skin of persons coming in contact with infested water; the proven transmitting hosts are certain snails of the genus *Bulinus*. **S. japon′icum**, a species found in Japan, China, the Philippines, Taiwan, the Celebes, and probably Laos and Cambodia, which causes schistosomiasis japonica by penetrating the skin of persons coming in contact with infested waters; the usual transmitting hosts are small snails of the genus *Oncomelania*. **S. manso′ni**, a species found in Egypt and elsewhere in Africa as well as in South America and the West Indies, including

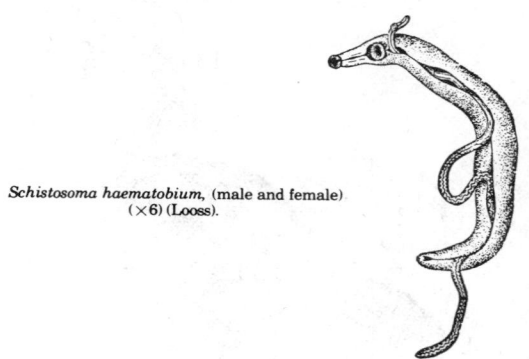

Schistosoma haematobium, (male and female) (×6) (Looss).

Puerto Rico, which causes schistosomiasis mansoni by penetrating the skin of persons coming in contact with infested waters; the transmitting hosts are planorbid snails, especially those of the genus *Biomphalaria*. **S. mat′thei**, a species found in the portal mesenteric vein of sheep, goats, game animals, monkeys, and rarely man in South Africa. **S. spinda′le**, a species parasitic in water buffalo, cattle, sheep, and goats in India, Malaya, Sumatra, Northern Rhodesia, and South Africa.

schistosomacidal (shis″, skis″to-so″mah-si′dal) schistosomicidal.

schistosomacide (shis″, skis″to-so′mah-sīd) schistosomicide.

schistosomal (shis″, skis″to-so′mal) pertaining to or caused by *Schistosoma*.

Schistosomatium (shis″, skis″to-so-ma′she-um) a genus of blood flukes allied to *Schistosoma*. *S. douthitti* is found in the hepatic portal veins of the meadow mouse.

schistosome (shis′, skis′to-sōm) an individual of the genus *Schistosoma*.

schistosomia (shis″, skis″to-so′me-ah) [schisto- + Gr. *soma* body + *-ia*] a developmental anomaly characterized by a fissure of the abdomen and lower extremities rudimentary or lacking.

schistosomiasis (shis″, skis″to-so-mi′ah-sis) the state of being infected with flukes of the genus *Schistosoma*; sometimes called *bilharziasis*. **cutaneous s.**, a condition resulting from invasion of the skin of bathers by the cercariae of schistosomes, marked by prickling sensation and intense itching; swimmer's itch. **eastern s.**, s. japonica. **s. haemato′bia**, urinary s. **hepatic s.**, schistosomiasis in which the ova of the parasites lodge in the hepatic portal venules, stimulating an inflammatory reaction with fibrosis; portal venous destruction leads to portal hypertension. **s. intercala′tum**, an endemic intestinal disease of West Central Africa due to infection by flukes of the species *Schistosoma intercalatum*, with abdominal pain, diarrhea in which the stools may contain blood and mucus, hyperplasia of the mucosa of the rectal valves, inflammation of the rectal walls, and sometimes polyposis. **intestinal s.**, Manson's s. **s. japon′ica**, infection by flukes of the species *Schistosoma japonicum*. The acute infection is marked by fever, allergic symptoms, and diarrhea. Chronic effects of infection, which may be very severe, are caused by fibrosis around the eggs deposited by the parasite in the liver, lungs, and central nervous system. Called also *Katayama disease*. **Manson's s.**, **s. manso′ni**, infection with flukes of the species *Schistosoma mansoni*, living principally in the inferior and superior mesenteric veins but migrating to deposit their eggs in venules, primarily of the large intestine. Eggs lodging in the liver may lead to peripheral fibrosis, hepatosplenomegaly, and ascites. **Oriental s.**, s. japonica. **pulmonary s.**, schistosomiasis in which migrating cercariae cause a type of pneumonia, and the ova, and sometimes the adult worms, cause embolization of pulmonary arterioles. Allergic pneumonia, allergic asthma, and emphysema may occur. **urinary s., vesical s.**, infection with *Schistosoma haematobium*, involving the urinary tract and causing cystitis and hematuria; called also *endemic hematuria*, *genitourinary schistosomiasis*, and *schistosomiasis haematobia*. **visceral s.**, infection with *Schistosoma mansoni* or *S. japonicum*, in contradistinction to urinary schistosomiasis caused by *S. haematobium*.

schistosomicidal (shis″, skis″to-so″mĭ-si′dal) destructive to schistosomes.

schistosomicide (shis″, skis″to-so′mĭ-sīd) an agent which destroys schistosomes.

Schistosomum (shis″, skis″to-so′mum) *Schistosoma*.

schistosomus (shis″, skis″to-so′mus) a monster exhibiting schistosomia.

schistosternia (shis″, skis″to-ster′ne-ah) [schisto- + *sternum*] schistothorax.

schistothorax (shis″, skis″to-tho′raks) [schisto- + Gr. *thōrax* chest] a developmental anomaly characterized by fissure of the chest.

schistotrachelus (shis″, skis″to-trah-ke′lus) [schisto- + trachēlos neck]   a fetus with fissure of the neck.

schizamnion (skiz-am′ne-on) [Gr. schizein to divide + amnion]   an amnion formed by cavitation over or in the inner cell mass, as occurs in human development.

schizaxon (skiz-ak′sŏn)   an axon which is divided into two equal, or nearly equal, branches.

schizencephalic (skiz″en-sĕ-fal′ik)   having abnormal clefts in the brain substance; see under porencephaly, def. 2.

schizencephaly (skiz″en-sef′ah-le) [Gr. schizein to divide + enkephalos brain]   schizencephalic porencephaly.

schizo- (skiz′o) [Gr. schizein to divide]   a combining form meaning divided, or denoting relationship to division.

Schizoblastosporion (skiz″o-blas″to-spo′re-on)   Geotrichum.

schizocephalia (skiz″o-sĕ-fa′le-ah)   a developmental anomaly characterized by a longitudinal fissure of the head.

schizocyte (skiz′o-sīt)   schistocyte.

schizocytosis (skiz″o-si-to′sis)   schistocytosis.

schizogenesis (skiz″o-jen′ĕ-sis) [schizo- + Gr. genesis production]   reproduction by fission.

schizogenous (skĭ-zoj′ĕ-nus)   reproducing by fission.

schizogony (skĭ-zog′o-ne) [schizo- + Gr. gonē seed]   the asexual cycle of sporozoa; particularly the life cycle of the malarial parasite (Plasmodium) in the blood corpuscle of man. Cf. sporogony.

schizogyria (skiz″o-ji′re-ah)   a condition in which the cerebral convolutions are marked by wedge-shaped cracks.

schizoid (skiz′oid, skit′soid)   1. resembling schizophrenia: a term applied by Bleuler to the shut-in, unsocial, introspective type of personality (see under personality) and by Kretschmer to the physical type resembling that of persons with dementia praecox, i.e., the asthenic dysplasic type. Cf. cycloid (def. 2.) and syntonic. 2. a person of schizoid personality.

schizoidism (skiz′oid-izm)   (obs.) the splitting of the psyche or the personality traits which are characteristic of schizophrenia.

schizokinesis (skiz″o-ki-ne′sis)   the condition in which, when an overt specific conditioned response has been extinguished, concomitant nonspecific responses continue to be elicited by the stimulus.

schizomycete (skiz″o-mi-sēt′)   any organism or species belonging to the Schizomycetes.

Schizomycetes (skiz″o-mi-se′tēz) [schizo- + Gr. mykēs fungus]   a taxonomic class comprising the bacteria; they are typically unicellular organisms, considered plants, which commonly multiply by cell division, and which may be free living, saprophytic, parasitic, or even pathogenic, the last causing disease in plants or animals. It includes 10 orders, Actinomycetales, Beggiatoales, Caryophanales, Chlamydobacteriales, Eubacteriales, Hyphomicrobiales, Mycoplasmatales, Myxobacterales, Pseudomonadales, and Spirochaetales.

schizont (skiz′ont) [schizo- + Gr. ōn, ontos being]   the stage in the development of the malarial parasite (Plasmodium) following the trophozoite whose nucleus divides into many smaller nuclei. This stage is followed by the segmenter, in which the cytoplasm divides to surround each nucleus or merozoite. Called also monont and agamont. Cf. sporont.

schizonticide (skĭ-zon′tĭ-sīd)   an agent that destroys schizonts.

schizonychia (skiz″o-nik′e-ah) [schizo- + Gr. onyx nail + -ia]   splitting of the nails.

schizophasia (skiz″o-fa′ze-ah)   the incomprehensible, disordered speech characteristic of schizophrenia.

schizophrenia (skiz″o-fre′ne-ah, skit″so-fre′ne-ah) [schizo- + Gr. phrēn mind + -ia]   any of a group of severe emotional disorders, usually of psychotic proportions, characterized by misinterpretation and retreat from reality, delusions, hallucinations, ambivalence, inappropriate affect, and withdrawn, bizarre, or regressive behavior. Popularly and erroneously called split personality. In the U.S., formerly called dementia praecox, a term still used in Europe for process schizophrenia. **ambulatory s.,** a term applied to the condition of schizophrenics who are nonhospitalized; the individuals in this group appear normal, but may suddenly commit aggressive, antisocial acts. **catatonic s.,** schizophrenia marked by excessive and sometimes violent motor activity and excitement, or by generalized inhibition; called also catatonia and Kahlbaum's disease. **childhood s.,** schizophrenia having the onset before puberty, characterized by autism, withdrawal, and atypical behavior. **chronic undifferentiated s.,** a condition manifested by schizophrenic symptoms that are of mixed or indefinite type which cannot be classified under other forms of schizophrenia. **hebephrenic s.,** a psychotic state characterized by shallow and inappropriate affect, giggling, silly behavior and mannerisms, regression, and hypochondriasis; called also hebephrenia. **latent s.,** a susceptibility to the development of schizophrenia, without a previous history of a psychotic schizophrenic episode. **paranoid s.,** a psychotic state characterized by delusions of grandeur or persecution, often accompanied by hallucinations; called also dementia paranoides and heboid paranoia. **process s.,** severe, progressive schizo-

phrenia seldom resulting in remission or recovery, believed by many to be caused by organic brain changes although definitive evidence is lacking; cf. reactive s. **pseudoneurotic s.,** schizophrenia in which the underlying psychosis is masked by pervasive symptoms of neurosis and anxiety. **reactive s.,** schizophrenia attributed chiefly to environmental conditions, with the expectation of a benign prognosis; cf. process s. **residual s.,** a condition manifested by individuals with symptoms of schizophrenia who, after a psychotic schizophrenic episode, are no longer psychotic. **schizo-affective s.,** a subtype of schizophrenia with prominent mood disorder, either manic or depressive. **simple s.,** a slow, insidiously progressive form of schizophrenia, marked by apathy, lack of initiative, indifference, and withdrawal.

schizophreniac (skiz″o-fre′ne-ak)   (obs.) schizophrenic, def. 2.

schizophrenic (skiz″o-fren′ik)   1. pertaining to or characterized by schizophrenia. 2. a person affected with schizophrenia.

schizophreniform (skiz″o-fren′ĭ-form)   resembling schizophrenia.

schizophrenosis (skiz″o-fre-no′sis)   Southard's term for any disease of the dementia praecox (schizophrenia) group.

Schizophyceae (skiz″o-fi′se-e) [schizo- + Gr. phykos seaweed]   Cyanophyceae.

schizoprosopia (skiz″o-pro-so′pe-ah)   ununited fissure of the face, as in harelip, cleft palate, etc.; schistoprosopia.

Schizosaccharomyces hominis (skiz″o-sak″ah-ro-mi′sēz hom′ĭ-nis)   Saccharomyces hominis.

Schizosiphon (skiz″o-si′fon)   a genus of nematogenous schizomycetes with flagelliform filaments, slender toward the extremity.

schizosis (skĭ-zo′sis)   (obs.) autism.

schizothorax (skiz″o-tho′raks)   a fetus with a fissure of the chest wall.

schizotonia (skiz″o-to′ne-ah) [schizo- + Gr. tonos tension + -ia]   division of the influx of tone to the muscles, so that, for instance, the flexor groups of the arm become hypertonic, while in the leg the extensors become hypertonic.

schizotrichia (skiz″o-trik′e-ah) [schizo- + Gr. thrix hair]   splitting of the hairs at the ends.

schizotropic (skiz″o-trop′ik)   having an affinity for schizonts.

schizotrypanosis, schizotrypanosomiasis (skiz″o-trip″ah-no′sis; skiz″o-trip″ah-no-so-mi′ah-sis)   Chagas' disease.

Schizotrypanum cruzi (skiz″o-trip′ah-num kroo′ze)   Trypanosoma cruzi.

schizozoite (skiz″o-zo′it) [schizo- + Gr. zōon animal]   merozoite.

schlafkrankheit (shlahf-kron′kīt) [Ger.]   African trypanosomiasis.

schlammfieber (shlahm′fe-ber) [Ger. "slime fever"]   a disease resembling leptospiral jaundice, due to Leptospira grippotyphosa, which prevailed among young persons who worked in the flooded districts near Breslau in the summer of 1891.

Schlatter's disease (sprain), operation (shlat′erz) [Carl Schlatter, surgeon in Zurich, 1864–1934]   see Osgood-Schlatter disease, under disease, and see under operation.

Schlatter-Osgood disease (shlat′er-oz′good) [Carl Schlatter; Robert Bayley Osgood, Boston orthopedist, born 1873]   Osgood-Schlatter disease.

Schlemm's canal, ligaments (shlemz) [Friedrich S. Schlemm, German anatomist, 1795–1858]   see sinus venosus sclerae, and under ligament.

Schlepper (shlep′er) [Ger. "tugboat"]   a substance that acts as a carrier for a nonimmunogenic or poorly immunogenic substance and induces a good immune response to the substance with which it has been chemically conjugated.

Schlesinger's sign (phenomenon) (shla′zing-erz) [Hermann Schlesinger, Austrian physician, 1866–1934]   see under sign.

Schlösser's treatment (injection, method) (shles′erz) [Carl Schlösser, German ophthalmologist, 1857–1925]   see under treatment.

schlusskoagulum (shluss″ko-ag′u-lum) [Ger.]   the clot that closes the gap made in the uterine lining by the implanting blastocyst; closing coagulum.

Schmidel's anastomosis (shme′delz) [Casimir Christoph Schmidel, German anatomist, 1718–1792]   see under anastomosis.

Schmidt's diet, syndrome, test (shmits) [Adolf Schmidt, physician in Bonn, 1865–1918]   see under diet, syndrome, and tests.

Schmidt's fibrinoplastin (shmits) [Eduard Oskar Schmidt, German anatomist, 1823–1886]   paraglobulin.

Schmidt-Lantermann incisures, segment (shmit′lahn″ter-mahn′) [Henry D. Schmidt, American anatomist, 1823–1888; A. J. Lantermann, American anatomist at Strassburg, 19th century]   see incisures of Lantermann, under incisure, and medullary segment, under segment.

Schmincke tumor (shmin′kĕ) [Alexander Schmincke, German pathologist, 1877–1953]   lymphoepithelioma.

Schmitz bacillus (shmits) [Karl Eitel Friedrich Schmitz, German physician, born 1889]   Shigella dysenteriae type 2.

Schmorl's body, disease, nodule (shmorlz) [Christian Georg

Schmorl, German pathologist, 1861–1932] see under *body, disease*, and *nodule*.

schmutzdecke (shmoots′dek-ĕ) [Ger.] the carpet-like layer of bacteria, algae, and other microorganisms which forms on the surface of a slow sand filter and which aids in purifying the water.

Schnabel's caverns (shnab′elz) [Isidor *Schnabel*, Vienna ophthalmologist, 1842–1908] see under *cavern*.

schnauzkrampf (shnowts′krampf) [Ger.] a facial grimace resembling pouting.

Schneider's carmine (shni′derz) [Franz Coelestin *Schneider*, German chemist, 1813–1897] see under *carmine*.

schneiderian membrane (shni-de′re-an) [Conrad Victor *Schneider*, German physician, 1614–1680] see under *membrane*.

Schoemaker's line (she′mah-kerz) [Jan *Schoemaker*, Dutch surgeon, 1871–1940] see under *line*.

Scholz's disease (shōlts′ez) [Willibald Oscar *Scholz*, German neurologist, born 1889] see under *disease*.

Schön's theory (shānz) [Wilhelm *Schön*, German ophthalmologist, 1848–1917] see under *theory*.

Schönbein's reaction, test (shān′bīnz) [Christian Friedrich *Schönbein*, German chemist, 1799–1868] see under *reaction* and *tests*.

Schönlein's purpura (disease) (shān′līnz) [Johann Lukas *Schönlein*, German physician, 1793–1864] purpura rheumatica.

Schönlein-Henoch purpura (disease, syndrome) (shān′-lin-hen′ōk) [J. L. *Schönlein*; Edouard Heinrich *Henoch*, German pediatrician, 1820–1910] see under *purpura*.

Schott's treatment (bath) (shots) [Theodor *Schott*, physician in Nauheim, 1850–1921] see under *treatment*.

Schottmüller's disease (shot′mil-erz) [Hugo *Schottmüller*, physician in Hamburg, 1867–1936] paratyphoid, def. 2.

schradan (schra′dan) octamethyl pyrophosphoramide.

Schreger's bands, lines, striae (shra′gerz) [Bernhard Gottlob *Schreger*, German anatomist, 1766–1825] see *bands of Hunter-Schreger*, under *band*.

Schreiber's maneuver (shri′berz) [Julius *Schreiber*, German physician, 1849–1932] see under *maneuver*.

Schridde's disease, granules (shrid′ez) [Hermann August *Schridde*, German pathologist, born 1875] see under the nouns.

Schroeder's disease (shra′derz) [Robert *Schroeder*, German gynecologist, 1884–1959] see under *disease*.

Schroeder's syndrome (shro′derz) [Henry Alfred *Schroeder*, St. Louis physician, born 1906] see under *syndrome*.

Schroeder's test (shra′derz) [Woldemar von *Schroeder*, German physician, 1850–1898] see under *tests*.

Schroetter see *Schrötter*.

Schrön's granule (shränz) [Otto von *Schrön*, German pathologist in Naples, 1837–1917] see under *granule*.

Schrön-Much granules (shrän-mook) [Otto von *Schrön*; Hans Christian *Much*, German physician, 1880–1932] Much's granules.

Schroth's treatment (shrōts) [Johann *Schroth*, German physician, 1800–1856] see under *treatment*.

Schrötter's catheter, chorea (shret′erz) [Leopold *Schrötter* von Kristelli, Viennese laryngologist, 1837–1908] see under *catheter*, and see *diaphragmatic chorea*, under *chorea*.

Schuchardt's incision (shoo′karts) [Karl August *Schuchardt*, German surgeon, 1856–1901] paravaginal incision.

Schüffner's dots (granules, punctuation, stippling) (shif′nerz) [Wilhelm August Paul *Schüffner*, German pathologist, 1867–1949] see under *dot*.

Schüle's sign (she′lez) [Heinrich *Schüle*, German psychiatrist, 1839–1916] omega melancholicum.

Schüller's disease (syndrome), phenomenon (shil′erz) [Artur *Schüller*, Vienna neurologist, born 1874] see *Hand-Schüller-Christian disease*, under *disease*, see *osteoporosis circumscripta cranii*, and see under *phenomenon*.

Schüller's method (shil′erz) [Karl Heinrich Anton Ludwig Max *Schüller*, surgeon in Berlin, 1843–1907] see under *method*.

Schüller-Christian disease (syndrome) (shil′er-kris′chan) [Artur *Schüller*; Henry A. *Christian*, American physician, 1876–1951] Hand-Schüller-Christian disease.

Schultz's angina (disease, syndrome) (shoolt′sez) [Werner *Schultz*, German internist, 1878–1947] agranulocytosis.

Schultz-Charlton reaction (phenomenon, test) (shoolts-charl′ton) [Werner *Schultz*; Willy *Charlton*, Berlin physician, born 1889] see under *reaction*.

Schultz-Dale reaction (shoolts-dāl) [Werner *Schultz*, German internist, 1878–1947; Sir Henry Hallett *Dale*, British physiologist and pharmacologist, born 1875] see under *reaction*.

Schultze's bundle (tract), cells (shoolt′sez) [Max Johann Sigismund *Schultze*, German biologist, 1825–1874] see *interfascicular fasciculus*, under *fasciculus*, and *olfactory cells*, under *cell*.

Schultze's fold (shoolt′sez) [Bernhard Sigismund *Schultze*, German gynecologist, 1827–1919] see under *fold*.

Schultze's sign, type (shoolt′sez) [Friedrich *Schultze*, German physician, 1848–1934] see *Chvostek's sign*, under *sign*, *tongue phenomenon*, under *phenomenon*, and see (for type) under *acroparesthesia*.

Schultze's test (shoolt′sez) [Ernst *Schultze*, Swiss chemist, 1860–1912] see under *tests*.

Schultze-Chvostek's sign (shoolt′se-vos′tek) [Friedrich *Schultze*; Franz *Chvostek*, Austrian surgeon, 1835–1884] Chvostek's sign.

Schumm's test (shoomz) [Otto *Schumm*, German chemist, born 1874] see under *tests*.

Schürmann's test (sher′manz) [Walter *Schürmann*, German serologist, born 1880] see under *tests*.

Schütz's micrococcus (shitz′ez) [Johann Wilhelm *Schütz*, German veterinarian, 1839–1920] *Streptococcus equi*.

Schwabach's test (shvah′baks) [Dagobert *Schwabach*, otologist in Berlin, 1846–1920] see under *tests*.

Schwalbe's corpuscles, etc. (shvahl′bez) [Gustav Albert *Schwalbe*, German anatomist, 1844–1917] see under *corpuscle, foramen, fissure, ring, sheath*, and *space*.

Schwann's cell, membrane (sheath), nucleus, substance (shvonz) [Theodor *Schwann*, German anatomist and physiologist, 1810–1882; professor of anatomy at Louvain, and the founder of the cell theory] see under *cell* and *nucleus*, and see *myelin* and *neurilemma*.

schwannitis (shwon-ni′tis) schwannosis.

schwannoglioma (shwon″o-gli-o′mah) schwannoma.

schwannoma (shwon-no′mah) a neoplasm originating from Schwann cells (of the myelin sheath) of neurons; schwannomas include neurofibromas and neurilemomas. **granular cell s.**, see under *tumor*.

schwannosis (shwon-no′sis) hypertrophy of the sheaths of Schwann.

Schwartz's test (shvarts′es) [Charles Edouard *Schwartz*, French surgeon, born 1852] see under *tests*.

Schwarz's test (shvarts′es) 1. [Karl Leonhard Heinrich *Schwarz*, German chemist, 1824–1890] see under *tests* (def. 1). 2. [Gottwald *Schwarz*, German roentgenologist, 1880–1959] see under *tests* (def. 2).

Schwediauer (shva′de-ow″er) see *Swediauer*.

Schweigger-Seidel sheath (shvi′ger-si′del) [Franz *Schweigger-Seidel*, Leipzig physiologist, 1834–1871] see under *sheath*.

schweinerotlauf (shvi″nĕ-rot′lowf) [Ger.] swine erysipelas.

schweineseuche (shvi″nĕ-zoi′ke) [Ger.] hemorrhagic septicemia of swine.

Schweitzer's reagent (shvīt′serz) [Matthias Eduard *Schweitzer*, German chemist, 1818–1860] see under *reagent*.

schwelle (shvel′ĕ) [Ger.] threshold, def. 1.

Schweninger's method (shven′in-gerz) [Ernst *Schweninger*, German physician, 1850–1924] see under *method*.

scia- for other words beginning thus, see also those beginning *skia-*.

sciage (se-azh′) [Fr.] a sawing movement in massage.

scialyscope (si-al′ĭ-skōp) an apparatus for throwing one image of an operative field into a darkened room separated from the operating room.

sciatic (si-at′ik) [L. *sciaticus*; Gr. *ischiadikos*] pertaining to or located near the ischium, as the sciatic nerve or vein.

sciatica (si-at′ĭ-kah) [L.] a syndrome characterized by pain radiating from the back into the buttock and into the lower extremity along its posterior or lateral aspect, and most commonly caused by prolapse of the intervertebral disk; the term is also used to refer to pain anywhere along the course of the sciatic nerve.

SCID severe combined immunodeficiency disease.

science (si′ens) [L. *scientia* knowledge] 1. the systematic observation of natural phenomena for the purpose of discovering laws governing those phenomena. 2. the body of knowledge accumulated by such means. **applied s.**, that concerned with the application of discovered laws to the matters of everyday living. **behavioral s.**, the interdisciplinary study of the behavior of man and lower animals for the purpose of understanding man as an individual and social being; it involves principally psychology, sociology, and anthropology, but also political science and other social sciences. **pure s.**, that concerned solely with the discovery of unknown laws relating to particular facts.

scientist (si′en-tist) one learned in science, especially one active in some particular field of investigation.

scieropia (si-er-o′pe-ah) [Gr. *skieros* shady + *ōps* eye + *-ia*] visual defect in which objects appear in a shadow.

scilla (sil′ah) [L.] squill.

scillabiose (sil″ah-bi′ōs) glucosidorhamnose, $C_{12}H_{22}O_{10}$, obtained by acid hydrolysis of scillaren A.

scillaren (sil′ah-ren) a mixture of cardioactive glycosides, scillaren A and B, from fresh squill.

scilliroside (sil'ir-o-sīd) a cardioactive glycoside from red squill that is poisonous to rodents.

scillism (sil'izm) poisoning from squill.

scillitic (sil'it-ik) pertaining to squill.

scintigram (sin'tĭ-gram) scintiscan.

scintigraphic (sin"tĭ-graf'ik) pertaining to scintigraphy.

scintigraphy (sin-tig'rah-fe) the production of two-dimensional images of the distribution of radioactivity in tissues after the internal administration of radionuclide, the images being obtained by a scintillation camera. **thyroidal lymph node s.**, radioisotopic thyroidolymphography.

scintillascope (sin-til'ah-skōp) [L. *scintilla* spark + Gr. *skopein* to examine] spinthariscope.

scintillation (sin"tĭ-la'shun) [L. *scintillatio*] 1. an emission of sparks. 2. a subjective visual sensation, as of seeing sparks. 3. a particle emitted in disintegration of a radioactive element; see also under *counter.*

scintiphotograph (sin"tĭ-fo'to-graf) a photograph made with a camera using scintillation energy sources.

scintiphotography (sin"tĭ-fo-tog'rah-fe) photography of the pattern of radioactivity of tissues after administration of radionuclides.

scintiscan (sin'tĭ-skan) a two-dimensional representation (map) of the gamma rays emitted by a radioisotope, revealing its varying concentration in a specific tissue of the body, such as the brain, kidney, or thyroid gland.

scintiscanner (sin"tĭ-skan'er) the system of equipment used in the making of a scintiscan.

sciopody (ski-op'o-de) unusually large feet, especially in children.

scirrho- (skir'o) [Gr. *skirrhos* hard] a combining form meaning hard, or denoting relationship to a hard cancer or scirrhous carcinoma.

scirrhoid (skir'oid) [*scirrho-* + Gr. *eidos* form] resembling scirrhous carcinoma.

scirrhoma (skir-ro'mah) [*scirrho-* + *-oma*] scirrhous carcinoma. **s. caminiano'rum,** chimney-sweeper's cancer, or soot cancer.

scirrhophthalmia (skir"of-thal'me-ah) [*scirrho-* + Gr. *ophthalmos* eye + *-ia*] scirrhous carcinoma of the eye.

scirrhous (skir'us) [L. *scirrhosus*] pertaining to or of the nature of a hard cancer; see also under *carcinoma.*

scirrhus (skir'us) [Gr. *skirrhos*] scirrhous carcinoma.

scission (sizh'un) [L. *scindere* to split] fission; splitting. In chemistry, the splitting of a molecule into two or more simpler molecules.

scissors (siz'erz) a cutting instrument with two opposed shearing blades. **canalicular s.,** delicate scissors with one of the blades probe pointed; used in slitting the lacrimal canal. **cannula s.,** scissors used in slitting a canal lengthwise. **craniotomy s.,** strong *f*-shaped shears for use in opening the fetal head. **de Wecker's s.,** small scissors for operations on the eyeball, in which the blades are operated by pressure on two springs joined at the end like a pair of tweezers. **Fox s.,** delicate, fine-pointed scissors designed for use in interproximal areas of the mouth. **Liston's s.,** scissors for cutting plaster-of-Paris bandages. **Smellie's s.,** short, strong-bladed scissors with external cutting edges, used in craniotomy.

scissors-bite (siz'erz-bīt') total lingual cross-bite of the mandible, with the mandibular teeth completely contained within the maxillary dental arch in habitual occlusion.

scissura (sĭ-su'rah), pl. *scissu'rae* [L.] an incisure; a splitting.

Sc.L.A. abbreviation for L. *scapulolaeva anterior* (left scapulo-anterior; a presentation of the fetus).

Sclavo's serum (sklah'vōz) [Achille *Sclavo,* Italian physician, 1861–1930] see under *serum.*

sclera (skle'rah), pl. *sclerae* [L.; Gr. *skleros* hard] [NA] the tough white outer coat of the eyeball, covering approximately the posterior five-sixths of its surface, and continuous anteriorly with the cornea and posteriorly with the external sheath of the optic nerve. **blue s.,** a condition of unusual blueness of the sclera; it is a prominent feature of osteogenesis imperfecta, and is seen in certain other abnormalities.

scleradenitis (skle"rad-ĕ-ni'tis) [*sclero-* + Gr. *adēn* gland + *-itis*] inflammation and hardening of a gland.

scleral (skle'ral) pertaining to the sclera.

scleratitis (skle"rah-ti'tis) scleritis.

scleratogenous (skle"rah-toj'ĕ-nus) sclerogenous.

sclerectasia (skle"rek-ta'ze-ah) [*sclero-* + Gr. *ektasis* extension + *-ia*] a bulging out of the sclera.

sclerectasis (skle-rek'tah-sis) sclerectasia.

sclerectoiridectomy (skle-rek"to-ir"ĭ-dek'to-me) the operation of excision of a portion of the sclera and of the iris for glaucoma; called also *Lagrange's operation.*

sclerectoiridodialysis (skle-rek"to-ir"ĭ-do-di-al'ĭ-sis) sclerectomy and iridodialysis.

sclerectome (skle-rek'tōm) an instrument for performing sclerectomy.

sclerectomy (skle-rek'to-me) [*sclero-* + Gr. *ektomē* excision] 1. excision of the sclera by scissors (Lagrange's operation), by punch (Holth's operation), or by trephining (Elliot's operation). 2. removal of the sclerosed parts of the middle ear after otitis media.

scleredema (skle"rĕ-de'mah) a chronic disorder of unknown etiology, occurring in both children and adults, characterized by progressive thickening and induration of the dermis, which is mainly a result of accumulation of metachromatic material in the ground substance between the collagen bundles; it typically begins on the nape and upper back and slowly extends downward and anteriorly. Although the disorder is not restricted to adults, it is also called *s. adultorum,* and sometimes, erroneously, *sclerema adultorum.* **s. adulto'rum, Buschke's s.,** scleredema. **s. neonato'rum,** sclerema.

sclerema (skle-re'mah) patchy or generalized progressive hardening of the subcutaneous fat, often with fatal outcome, occurring in infants predisposed by reason of prematurity, marasmus, hypothermia, gastrointestinal or respiratory infection, or gross malformations. The lesions are cold, yellowish, and boardlike. Called also *sclerema neonatorum,* and, erroneously, *scleredema neonatorum.* **s. adipo'sum,** sclerema. **s. adulto'rum,** scleredema. **s. neonato'rum,** sclerema.

sclerencephalia (skle"ren-sĕ-fa'le-ah) sclerencephaly.

sclerencephaly (skle"ren-sef'ah-le) [*sclero* + Gr. *enkephalos*] sclerosis of the brain.

sclerenchyma (skle-reng'kĭ-mah) [Gr. *sklēros* hard + *enchyma* infustion] supportive tissue occurring in many plant stems and roots, composed of thick-walled, usually dead cells impregnated with lignin. Cf. *collenchyma.*

sclerenchymatous (skle"reng-kim'ah-tus) of the nature of sclerenchyma.

sclererythrin (skle-rer'ĭ-thrin) [*sclerotium* + Gr. *erythros* red] a red coloring matter from ergot.

scleriasis (skle-ri'ah-sis) [Gr. *sklēriasis*] a hardened state of an eyelid.

scleriritomy (skle"rĭ-rit'o-me) [*sclera* + *iris* + Gr. *temnein* to cut] incision of the sclera and iris in anterior staphyloma.

scleritis (skle-ri'tis) [*sclera* + *-itis*] inflammation of the sclera; it may be superficial (*episcleritis*) or deep, the latter form causing bulging and thinning of the sclera. **annular s.,** scleritis occurring in a ring around the limbus of the cornea. **anterior s.,** inflammation of the sclera adjoining the limbus of the cornea. **brawny s.,** scleritis involving a thickening of the periphery of the cornea. **nodular s.,** that marked by localized dark blue patches in the anterior portion of the sclera, resulting from the choroid being visible through a translucent sclera. **posterior s.,** scleritis involving the sclera and the underlying retina and choroid.

sclero- (skle'ro) [Gr. *sklēros* hard] a combining form meaning hard, often used especially to denote relationship to the sclera.

scleroadipose (skle"ro-ad'ĭ-pōs) composed of fibrous and fatty tissue.

scleroblastema (skle"ro-blas-te'mah) [*sclero-* + *blastema*] the embryonic tissue which takes part in the formation of bone.

scleroblastemic (skle"ro-blas-tem'ik) pertaining to the scleroblastema.

sclerocataracta (skle"ro-kat"ah-rak'tah) [*sclero-* + Gr. *katarrhaktēs* waterfall] a hard cataract.

sclerochoroiditis (skle"ro-ko"roi-di'tis) inflammation of the sclera and the choroid coat, resulting in atrophy of both coats and protrusion of the former. **s. ante'rior,** a form involving the anterior portions of the sclera and causing anterior staphyloma. **s. poste'rior,** a condition seen in progressive myopia in which posterior staphyloma occurs in the region of the optic disk.

scleroconjunctival (skle"ro-kon"junk-ti'val) pertaining to the sclera and conjunctiva.

scleroconjunctivitis (skle"ro-kon-junk"tĭ-vi'tis) inflammation of the sclera and the conjunctiva.

sclerocornea (skle"ro-kor'ne-ah) the sclera and the cornea considered as forming a single coat or layer.

sclerocorneal (skle"ro-kor'ne-al) pertaining to the sclera and the cornea.

sclerodactylia (skle"ro-dak-til'e-ah) sclerodactyly.

sclerodactyly (skle"ro-dak'tĭ-le) [*sclero-* + Gr. *daktylos* finger] localized scleroderma of the digits, as in acrosclerosis.

scleroderma (skle"ro-der'mah) [*sclero-* + Gr. *derma* skin] chronic hardening and shrinking of the connective tissues of any part of the body, including the skin, heart, esophagus, kidney, and lung. The skin may be thickened, hard, and rigid, and pigmented patches may occur. It may be generalized (*systemic* or *diffuse s.*) limited to the distal parts of the extremities and face (*acrosclerosis*) or to the digits (*sclerodactyly*), or localized to oval or linear areas a few centimeters across (*morphea*). **circumscribed s., s. circumscrip'tum,** morphea. **diffuse s.,** systemic s. **generalized s.,** systemic s. **linear s.,** a form of morphea or circumscribed scleroderma in which the lesions occur in a line or band. A single sagittal linear lesion (*en coup de sabre*) may occur on the scalp and forehead; single or multiple ribbon-like lesions may occur on the extremities, where they extend from the hip to heel or shoulder to hand (*scleroderma en bande*). Called also *linear morphea* or *morphea linearis*. **localized s.**, morphea. **systemic s.**, a form involving large areas of the body surface and internal structures, marked by increase and swelling of collagen fibers, loss or fragmentation of elastic elements, atrophy of rete pegs, deposition of melanin in the basal cells, and retention of calcium; called also *diffuse* or *generalized s.*, *progressive systemic sclerosis*, *diffuse systemic sclerosis*, and *systemic sclerosis*. Cf. *morphea*.

sclerodermatous (skle″ro-der′mah-tous) pertaining to or characterized by scleroderma.

sclerodesmia (skle″ro-des′me-ah) [*sclero-* + Gr. *desmos* ligament + *-ia*] hardening of ligaments.

sclerogenic (skle″ro-jen′ik) sclerogenous.

sclerogenous (skle-roj′ĕ-nus) [*sclero-* + Gr. *gennan* to produce] producing sclerosis or sclerous tissue.

sclerogummatous (skle″ro-gum′ah-tus) composed of fibrous and gummatous tissue.

scleroid (skle′roid) [*sclero-* + Gr. *eidos* form] having a hard texture.

scleroiritis (skle″ro-i-ri′tis) inflammation of the sclera and of the iris.

sclerokeratitis (skle″ro-ker″ah-ti′tis) 1. inflammation of the sclera and of the cornea. 2. sclerosing keratitis.

sclerokeratoiritis (skle″ro-ker″ah-to-i-ri′tis) inflammation of the sclera, cornea, and iris.

sclerokeratosis (skle″ro-ker″ah-to′sis) sclerokeratitis.

scleroma (skle-ro′mah) [Gr. *sklērōma* induration] a hardened patch or induration, especially of the nasal or laryngeal tissues. **s. respirato′rium**, rhinoscleroma.

scleromalacia (skle″ro-mah-la′she-ah) [*sclero-* + Gr. *malakia* softness] 1. degeneration and thinning (softening) of the sclera, occurring in patients with rheumatoid arthritis; called also *scleromalacia perforans*. 2. Kienbock's name for osteitis deformans.

scleromeninx (skle″ro-me′ninks) [*sclero-* + Gr. *mēninx* membrane] the dura mater.

scleromere (skle′ro-mēr) [*sclero-* + Gr. *meros* part] 1. any segment or metamere of the skeletal system. 2. the caudal half of a sclerotome (def. 3).

sclerometer (skle-rom′ĕ-ter) [*sclero-* + Gr. *metron* measure] an instrument for determining the hardness of substances.

scleromucin (skle″ro-mu′sin) a slimy, active principle from ergot.

scleromyxedema (skle″ro-mik″sĕ-de′mah) a variant of lichen myxedematosus which is characterized not only by a generalized eruption of nodules but also by diffuse thickening of the skin.

scleronychia (skle″ro-nik′e-ah) [*sclero-* + Gr. *onyx* nail + *-ia*] a simultaneous thickening and dryness of the nails.

scleronyxis (skle″ro-nik′sis) [*sclero-* + Gr. *nyxis* puncture] surgical puncture of the sclera.

sclero-oophoritis (skle″ro-o-of″o-ri′tis) sclerosing inflammation of an ovary.

sclero-oothecitis (skle″ro-o″o-the-si′tis) sclero-oophoritis.

sclerophthalmia (skle″rof-thal′me-ah) [*sclero-* + Gr. *ophthalmos* eye + *-ia*] the condition in which, from imperfect differentiation of the sclera and cornea, the periphery of the cornea is opaque and only the central part remains clear.

scleroprotein (skle″ro-pro′te-in) [*sclero-* + *protein*] a simple protein which is characterized by its insolubility and fibrous structure, and which usually serves a supportive or protective function in the body; called also *albuminoid*.

sclerosal (skle-ro′sal) sclerous.

sclerosant (skle-ro′sant) a chemical irritant injected into a vein to produce inflammation and eventual fibrosis and obliteration of the lumen, used in the treatment of varicose veins.

sclerosarcoma (skle″ro-sar-ko′mah) [*sclero-* + Gr. *sarkōma* a fleshy excrescence.] a fibrosing sarcoma.

sclerose (skle-rōs′) to become sclerotic; to harden.

sclerosed (skle-rōst′) affected with sclerosis.

sclérose en plaques (skla-rōz″ aw-plak′) [Fr.] multiple sclerosis.

sclerosing (skle-rōs′ing) causing or undergoing sclerosis.

sclerosis (skle-ro′sis) [Gr. *sklērōsis* hardness] an induration, or hardening; especially hardening of a part from inflammation and in diseases of the interstitial substance. The term is used chiefly for such a hardening of the nervous system due to hyperplasia of the connective tissue or to designate hardening of the blood vessels. **Alzheimer's s.**, presenile dementia. **amyotrophic lateral s.**, a disease marked by progressive degeneration of the neurons that give rise to the corticospinal tract and of the motor cells of the brain stem and spinal cord, and resulting in a deficit of upper and lower motor neurons; it usually ends fatally

within two to three years. Called also *Charcot's syndrome* and *Dejerine type*. **annular s.**, sclerosis of the spinal cord, forming a band around it. **anterolateral s.**, sclerosis of the ventral and lateral columns of the spinal cord, leading to spastic paraplegia; called also *ventrolateral s.* **arterial s.**, **arteriocapillary s.**, arteriosclerosis. **arteriolar s.**, arteriolosclerosis. **bone s.**, eburnation. **combined s.**, subacute combined degeneration of the spinal cord; see under *degeneration*. **dentinal s.**, regressive alteration in tooth substance with calcification of the dentinal tubules, caused by caries or abrasion or occurring with age, and producing translucent zones (transparent dentin). **diaphyseal s.**, diaphyseal dysplasia. **diffuse s.**, a form affecting large areas of the brain and spinal cord. **diffuse systemic s.**, systemic scleroderma. **disseminated s.**, multiple sclerosis. **endocardial s.**, see under *fibroelastosis*. **Erb's s.**, primary lateral spinal sclerosis; see under *lateral s.* **familial centrolobar s.**, a familial form of leukoencephalopathy (q.v.) occurring in early life and running a slowly progressive course into adolescence or adulthood. It is marked by nystagmus, ataxia, tremor, choreoathetotic movements, parkinsonian facies, dysarthria, and mental deterioration. Pathologically, there is diffuse demyelination in the white substance of the brain, which may involve the brain stem, cerebellum, and spinal cord. Called also *aplasia axialis extracorticalis congenita*, *hereditary central leukodystrophy*, and *Pelizaeus-Merzbacher disease*. **focal s.**, multiple s. **gastric s.**, linitis plastica. **hyperplastic s.**, a form of arteriosclerosis seen in small arteries and arterioles as a subintimal thickening of the wall of the vessel. **insular s.**, multiple s. **lateral s.**, a degeneration of the lateral columns of the spinal cord. It may occur as a *primary* affection, resulting in spastic paraplegia, attended with rigidity of the limbs, increase of the tendon reflexes, and absence of nutritive and sensory disturbance; called also *Erb's sclerosis*. Or it may be *secondary* to myelitis, in which there is spastic paraplegia, with sensory and other disturbances; called also *spastic spinal paralysis*. **lobar s.**, presence of narrow, scar-distorted convolutions over a large area (lobe) of the surface of the cerebral hemispheres; seen frequently in cerebral palsy. **Marie's s.**, hereditary form of cerebellar sclerosis. **miliary s.**, sclerosis occurring in minute spots. **Mönckeberg's s.**, see under *arteriosclerosis*. **multiple s.**, a disease in which there are patches of demyelination throughout the white matter of the central nervous system, sometimes extending into the gray matter. Typically, the symptoms of lesions of the white matter are weakness, incoordination, paresthesias, speech disturbances, and visual complaints. The course of the disease is usually prolonged, with remissions and relapses over a period of many years. The etiology is unknown. Called also *disseminated s.* and *insular s.* **Pelizaeus-Merzbacher s.**, familial centrolobar s. **posterior s.**, tabes dorsalis. **posterolateral s.**, subacute combined degeneration of spinal cord; see under *degeneration*. **presenile s.**, presenile dementia. **progressive systemic s.**, systemic scleroderma. **s. re′dux**, chancre redux. **renal arteriolar s.**, arteriosclerosis involving chiefly the renal arterioles, resulting in contracted kidney. **subendocardial s.**, endocardial fibroelastosis. **systemic s.**, see under *scleroderma*. **s. tubero′sa**, **tuberous s.**, a congenital familial disease characterized pathologically by tumors on the surfaces of the lateral ventricles and sclerotic patches on the surface of the brain and marked clinically by progressive mental deterioration and epileptic convulsions. There may be adenoma sebaceum, congenital tumor of the eye (phakoma), and tumors of the viscera, especially the kidney and heart muscle. Called also *Bourneville's disease* and *epiloia*. **unicellular s.**, the development of bands of fibrous material between the cells of a gland. **vascular s.**, arteriosclerosis. **valvular s.**, fibrous thickening of a cardiac valve, especially the mitral valve. **venous s.**, phlebosclerosis. **ventrolateral s.**, anterolateral s.

scleroskeleton (skle″ro-skel′ĕ-ton) [*sclero-* + *skeleton*] those parts of the bony skeleton that are formed by the ossification of ligaments, tendons, or fasciae.

sclerostenosis (skle″ro-stĕ-no′sis) [Gr. *sklērōs* hard + *stenōsis* narrowing] induration or hardening combined with contraction.

Sclerostoma (skle-ros′to-mah) *Strongylus*. **S. duodena′le**, *Ancylostoma duodenale*. **S. syn′gamus**, *Syngamus trachea*.

sclerostomy (skle-ros′to-me) [*sclero-* + Gr. *stoma* opening] the surgical creation of an opening through the sclera; it is usually performed in the treatment of glaucoma.

sclerotherapy (skle″ro-ther′ah-pe) the injection of sclerosing solutions in the treatment of hemorrhoids or varicose veins.

sclerotic (skle-rot′ik) [L. *scleroticus*; Gr. *sklērōs* hard] 1. hard, or indurated; affected with sclerosis. 2. sclera.

sclerotica (skle-rot′ĭ-kah) [L.] sclera.

scleroticectomy (skle-rot″ĭ-sek′to-me) sclerectomy.

scleroticochoroiditis (skle-rot″ĭ-ko-ko″roid-i′tis) sclerochoroiditis.

scleroticonyxis (skle-rot″ĭ-ko-nik′sis) scleronyxis.

scleroticopuncture (skle-rot″ĭ-ko-punk′tūr) scleronyxis.

scleroticotomy (skle-rot″ĭ-kot′o-me) sclerotomy.

Sclerotinia (skle″ro-tin′ĭ-ah) a genus of ascomycetous fungi of the order Helotiales, family Sclerotiniaceae, which includes many pathogens of plants. Its imperfect (sexual) stage is *Monilia*.

Sclerotiniaceae (skle″ro-tin-i-a′she-e) a family of ascomycetes of the order Heleotiales, series Pyrenomycetes, including the genus *Sclerotina*.

sclerotitis (skle″ro-ti′tis) scleritis.

sclerotium (skle-ro′she-um) the hard, thick-walled, blackish mass formed by certain fungi, such as the ergot of rye or the sclerotic cells seen in chromomycosis.

sclerotome (skle′ro-tōm) 1. an instrument used in the incision of the sclera. 2. the area of a bone innervated from a single spinal segment. 3. one of the paired masses of mesenchymal tissue, separated from the ventromedial part of a somite, which develop into vertebrae and ribs.

sclerotomy (skle-rot′o-me) [*sclero-* + Gr. *tomē* a cutting] surgical incision of the sclera. **anterior s.**, the surgical opening of the anterior chamber of the eye, chiefly done for the relief of glaucoma. **posterior s.**, an opening made into the vitreous through the sclera, as for detached retina or the removal of a foreign body.

sclerous (skle′rus) hard; indurated.

sclerozone (skle′ro-zōn) [*sclero-* + Gr. *zōnē* zone] any surface on a bone giving attachment to the muscles from a given myotome.

Sc.L.P. abbreviation for L. scapulo-laeva posterior (left scapuloposterior; a presentation of the fetus).

S.C.M. State Certified Midwife.

scoleces (sko′lĕ-sēz) [L.] plural of *scolex*.

scoleciasis (sko-lĕ-si′ah-sis) [*scoleco-* + *-iasis*] the condition caused by the presence of larvae of moths or butterflies in the body.

scoleciform (sko-les′ĭ-form) resembling a scolex.

scoleco- (sko′lĕ-ko) [Gr. *skōlēx* worm] a combining form denoting relationship to a worm.

scolecoid (sko′lĕ-koid) [Gr. *skōlekoeidēs* vermiform] 1. resembling a worm. 2. resembling a scolex; hydatid.

scolecology (sko″lĕ-kol′o-je) [*scoleco-* + *-logy*] helminthology.

scolex (sko′leks), pl. *sco′leces* [Gr. *skōlēx* worm] the attachment (or holdfast) organ, of a tapeworm, generally considered the anterior, or cephalic end.

scolio- (sko′le-o) [Gr. *skolios* twisted] a combining form meaning twisted or crooked.

scoliokyphosis (sko″le-o-ki-fo′sis) [*scolio-* + *kyphosis*] combined lateral (scoliosis) and posterior (kyphosis) curvature of the spine.

scoliorachitic (sko″le-o-rah-kit′ik) affected with scoliosis and rickets.

scoliosiometry (sko″le-o-se-om′ĕ-tre) [*scoliosis* + Gr. *metron* measure] measurement of curvatures, especially those of the vertebral column.

scoliosis (sko″le-o′sis) [Gr. *skoliōsis* curvation] an appreciable lateral deviation in the normally straight vertical line of the spine. Cf. *kyphosis* and *lordosis*. **Brissaud's s.**, sciatic s. **cicatri-**

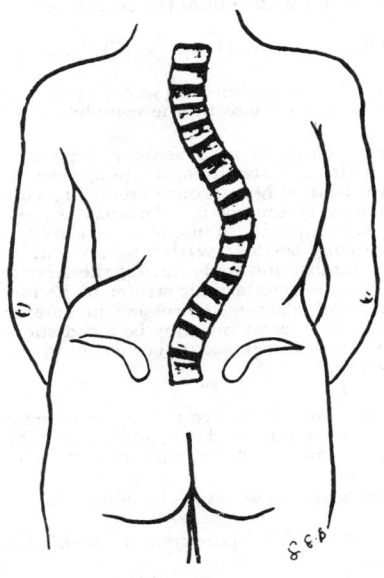

Scoliosis

cial s., that which is due to a cicatricial contraction following caries or necrosis. **coxitic s.**, scoliosis in the lumbar region caused by hip disease. **empyematic s.**, that which is caused

by empyema. **habit s.**, scoliosis due to improper posture. **inflammatory s.**, that which is due to vertebral disease. **ischiatic s.**, that which is due to hip disease. **myopathic s.**, paralytic s. **ocular s., ophthalmic s.**, scoliosis attributed to tilting of the head on account of astigmatism or muscle imbalance. **osteopathic s.**, that which is caused by disease of the vertebrae. **paralytic s.**, lateral curvature of the spinal column due to muscle paralysis; called also *myopathic s.* **rachitic s.**, spinal curvature due to rickets. **rheumatic s.**, that which is due to rheumatism of the dorsal muscles. **sciatic s.**, a list of the lumbar part of the spine away from the affected side in sciatica; called also *Brissaud's s.* **static s.**, that which is due to difference in the length of the legs.

scoliosometer (sko″le-o-som′ĕ-ter) an apparatus for measuring curves, especially those of the spinal column.

scoliotic (sko″le-ot′ik) [Gr. *skoliōtos* looking askew] pertaining to or characterized by scoliosis.

scoliotone (sko′le-o-tōn) an apparatus for the forcible correction of scoliosis.

Scolopendra (sko″lo-pen′drah) [Gr. *skolops* anything pointed] a genus of venomous centipedes of the class Chilopoda. The bite of some large species may produce a severe local inflammation attended with pain, glandular enlargement, vomiting, headache, vertigo, and fever. *S. he′ros* and *S. mor′sitans* are American species; *S. gigan′tea* is a tropical species.

scolopsia (sko-lop′se-ah) [Gr. *skolops* anything pointed] a suture between two bones that allows motion of one on the other.

scombrine (skom′brin) a protamine found in mackerel sperm.

scombroid (skom′broid) 1. of or pertaining to the suborder Scombroidea. 2. a fish of the suborder Scombroidea. See also under *poisoning*.

Scombroidea (skom-broi′de-ah) a suborder of larger, bony, marine fish having oily flesh, including tunas, bonitos, mackerels, albacores, and skipjacks. The flesh of these fish may contain a toxic histamine-like substance and, if ingested, can cause a condition known as *scombroid poisoning* (q.v.).

scombrone (skom′bron) a histone from spermatozoa of mackerel.

scombrotoxic (skom″bro-toks′ik) pertaining to or caused by the histamine-like toxin of scombroid fish; see *scombroid poisoning*, under *poisoning*.

scombrotoxin (skom″bro-toks′in) the histamine-like toxin formed in scombroid fish by bacterial action; it causes scombroid poisoning.

scoop (skōōp) a spoonlike instrument for evacuating cavities. **Mules's s.**, a form of curet used in eye operations.

scopafungin (sko-pah-fun′jin) an antibacterial with antifungal properties derived from a variant of *Streptomyces hygroscopicus*.

scoparin (sko-pa′rin) chemical name: 8-glycosyl-4′,5,7-trihydroxy-3′-methoxyflavone. A yellowish, crystalline active principle, $C_{22}H_{22}O_{11}$, from scoparius, the tops of *Cytisus scoparius*.

scoparius (sko-pa′re-us) the tops of *Cytisus scoparius*, (L.) Link. (Leguminosae), or broom, a leguminous shrub; they contain the alkaloid sparteine and the principle scoparin, and are diuretic, purgative, and emetic. Scoparius is also abused by being smoked for its euphoric properties.

-scope (skōp) [Gr. *skopein* to view, examine] a word termination meaning an instrument for examining or observing.

scopin (sko′pin) a substance formed by the gentle hydrolysis of scopolamine. It is $OH \cdot C_6H_8O \cdot N \cdot CH_3$, and readily changes into oscine.

scopola (sko-po′lah) the dried rhizome and larger roots of *Scopolia carniolica* Jacq. (Solanaceae). It contains the same constituents as belladonna, is used as an anticholinergic, and is a source of scopoletin.

scopolagnia (sko″po-lag′ne-ah) [Gr. *skopein* to view + *lagneia* lust] scopophilia.

scopolamine (sko-pol′ah-mēn) chemical name: α-(hydroxymethyl)benzeneacetic acid 9-methyl-3-oxa-9-azatricyclo[3.3.1.0²·⁴] non-7-yl ester. An anticholinergic alkaloid, $C_{17}H_{21}NO_4$, derived from several solanaceous plants, including *Atropa belladonna* L., *Hyoscyamus niger* L., *Datura* species, and *Scopolia* species. It has effects on the autonomic nervous system similar to those of atropine. Called also *hyoscine*. **s. hydrobromide** [USP], the trihydrate salt of scopolamine, $C_{17}H_{21}NO_4 \cdot HBr \cdot 3H_2O$, occurring as colorless or white crystals. It is used as a cerebral sedative, administered orally or subcutaneously, and as a cycloplegic and mydriatic, applied topically to the conjunctiva. **s. methylbromide**, methscopolamine bromide.

scopoletin (sko-pol′ĕ-tin) 7-hydroxy-5-methoxycoumarin, a growth factor in plants obtained from scopola.

Scopolia (sko-po′le-ah) [Johann-Antoni *Scopoli*, physician in Pavia, 1723–1788] a genus of solanaceous plants. *S. carniolica atropoi′des* of Europe, and *S. japon′ica* and *S. lu′rida*, of Asia, have properties like those of hyoscyamus and belladonna.

scopometer (sko-pom′ĕ-ter) [Gr. *skopein* to examine + *metron* measure] an instrument for measuring the turbidity of solutions, i.e., the density of a precipitate.

scopometry (sko-pom'ĕ-tre) measurement of the optical density of a precipitate to determine the amount of a substance in suspension.

scopophilia (sko-po-fil'e-ah) [Gr. *skopein* to view + *philein* to love] voyeurism; the derivation of sexual pleasure from looking at another's genital organs (*active s.*). 2. exhibitionism; a morbid desire to be seen (*passive s.*).

scopophobia (sko"po-fo'be-ah) [Gr. *skopein* to view + *phobein* to be affrighted by] a morbid dread of being seen.

scoptolagnia (skop"to-lag'ne-ah) scopophilia.

scoptophilia (skop"to-fil'e-ah) scopophilia.

scoptophobia (skop"to-fo'be-ah) scopophobia.

Scopulariopsis (skop"u-la"re-op'sis) a genus of imperfect fungi of the family Moniliaceae, order Moniliales. *S. brevicaulis* sometimes causes onychomycosis. Formerly called *Acaulium*.

scopulariopsosis (skop"u-la"re-op-so'sis) infection with a fungus of the genus *Scopulariopsis*.

-scopy (skop'e) [Gr. *skopein* to examine] word termination meaning the act of examining.

scorbutic (skor-bu'tik) [L. *scorbuticus*] pertaining to or affected with scurvy.

scorbutigenic (skor-bu"tĭ-jen'ik) causing scurvy.

scorbutus (skor-bu'tus) [L.] scurvy.

scordinema (skor"dĭ-ne'mah) [Gr. *skordinēma*] yawning and stretching with a feeling of lassitude, occurring as a preliminary symptom of some infectious disease.

score (skor) a rating, usually expressed numerically, based on achievement or the degree to which certain qualities are present. **Apgar s.**, a numerical expression of the condition of a newborn infant, usually determined at 60 seconds after birth, being the sum of points gained on assessment of the heart rate, respiratory effort, muscle tone, reflex irritability, and color. Cf. *recovery s.* **Bishop s.**, a score for estimating the prospects of induction of labor, arrived at by evaluating the extent of cervical dilatation, effacement, the station of the fetal head, consistency of the cervix, and the cervical position in relation to the vaginal axis. **recovery s.**, a number expressing the condition of an infant at various intervals, which should be stipulated, greater than 1 minute after birth, based on the same features assessed by the Apgar score at 60 seconds after birth.

scorings (skor'ingz) small transverse lines caused by increased density of bone, seen in roentgenograms at the metaphysis of growing bones, and due to temporary cessation of growth.

scorpion (skor'pe-on) an arthropod of warm countries, having a venomous sting. More important species are *Buthus quinquestriatus* of Egypt, *Centruroides suffusus* of Mexico, *Euscorpius italicus*, or black scorpion, of Europe and North Africa, and *Tityus serrulatus* of Brazil.

scorpionism (skor'pe-un-izm) poisoning by scorpion stings.

scoto- (sko'to) [Gr. *skotos* darkness] combining form denoting relationship to darkness.

scotochromogen (sko"to-kro'mo-jen) [*scoto-* + Gr. *chrōma* color + *gennan* to produce] a microorganism whose pigmentation develops in the dark as well as in the light; specifically, a member of Group II of the so-called "unclassified" mycobacteria, but applicable also to many other organisms.

scotochromogenic (sko"to-kro"mo-jen'ik) pertaining to or characterized by scotochromogenicity.

scotochromogenicity (sko"to-kro"mo-jĕ-nis'ĭ-te) the property of forming pigment in the dark, the coloration occurring irrespective of exposure to light.

scotodinia (sko"to-din'e-ah) [Gr. *skotos* darkness + *dinos* whirl] dizziness with blurring of vision and headache.

scotogram, scotograph (sko'to-gram; sko'to-graf) [Gr. *skotos* darkness + *graphein* to write] 1. roentgenogram. 2. the effect produced upon a photographic plate in the dark by certain substances.

scotographic (sko"to-graf'ik) affecting a photographic plate in the dark.

scotography (sko-tog'rah-fe) roentgenography.

scotoma (sko-to'mah), pl. *scoto'mata* [Gr. *skotōma*] 1. an area of depressed vision within the visual field, surrounded by an area of less depressed or of normal vision. 2. mental s. **absolute s.**, an area within the visual field in which perception of light is entirely lost. **annular s.**, a circular area of depressed vision in the visual field, surrounding the point of fixation. **arcuate s.**, an arc-shaped defect of vision arising in an area near the blind spot, and extending toward it. **aural s. au'ris**, loss of ability to perceive auditory stimuli coming from a certain direction. **Bjerrum's s.**, a further development of Seidel's scotoma, the sickle-shaped defect contiguous to the blind spot extending above and below the fixation point and encircling it more or less completely. **central s.**, an area of depressed vision corresponding with the point of fixation and interfering with or entirely abolishing central vision. **centrocecal s.**, a horizontal oval defect in the field of vision situated between and embracing both the point of fixation and the blind spot. **color**

s., an isolated area of depressed or defective vision for color in the visual field. **flittering s.**, teichopsia. **insular s.**, an isolated area of defective or absent vision in the visual field, surrounded on all sides by more nearly normal vision. **mental s.**, in psychiatry, a figurative blind spot in a person's psychological awareness, the patient being unable to gain insight into and to understand his mental problems; lack of insight. See also *scotomization*. **motile s's**, positive scotomas occurring as a result of opacities in the vitreous, muscae volitantes being an example of such a defect. **negative s.**, a scotoma which appears as a blank spot or hiatus in the visual field; a blind spot. **paracentral s.**, an area of depressed vision situated near the point of fixation. **peripapillary s.**, an area of depressed vision in the visual field near that corresponding with the optic disk. **peripheral s.**, an area of depressed vision distant from the point of fixation, toward the periphery of the visual field. **physiologic s.**, that area of the visual field corresponding with the optic disk, in which the photosensitive receptors are absent. **positive s.**, one which appears as a dark spot in the visual field. **relative s.**, an area of the visual field in which perception of light is only diminished, or the loss is restricted to light of certain wavelengths. **ring s.**, annular s. **scintillating s.**, teichopsia. **Seidel's s.**, a further development of an arcuate scotoma, which extends at either or both ends, the concavity of the prolongation always being directed toward the fixation point.

scotomagraph (sko-to'mah-graf) [*scotoma* + Gr. *graphein* to write] an instrument for recording a scotoma.

scotomata (sko-to'mah-tah) plural of *scotoma*.

scotomatous (sko-tom'ah-tus) pertaining to or affected with scotoma.

scotometer (sko-tom'ĕ-ter) [*scotoma* + Gr. *metron* measure] an instrument for diagnosing and measuring scotomata. **Bjerrum's s.**, campimeter.

scotometry (sko-tom'ĕ-tre) the measurement of isolated areas of depressed vision (scotomata) within the visual field.

scotomization (sko"tŏ-mi-za'shun) [*scotoma* + Gr. *-izein* to make into] the development of scotomata, or blind spots, especially the development of mental scotomata (mental "blind spots"), the patient attempting to deny existence of everything which conflicts with his ego.

scotophilia (sko"to-fil'e-ah) [*scoto-* + Gr. *philein* to love] love of darkness; abnormal preference for night over day.

scotophobia (sko"to-fo'be-ah) [*scoto-* + Gr. *phobein* to be affrighted by] morbid fear of darkness.

scotophobin (sko"to-fo'bin) [*scoto-* + Gr. *phobein* to be affrighted by] a peptide composed of 15 amino acids that has been isolated from the brain tissue of rats and mice conditioned to fear the dark; on injection into normal rodents, it is said to induce fear of dark.

scotopia (sko-to'pe-ah) [*scoto-* + Gr. *ōpē* sight + *-ia*] night vision; see also *dark adaptation*.

scotopic (sko-top'ik) pertaining to night vision; said of an eye which has become adapted to the dark. See *dark adaptation*, under *adaptation*.

scotopsin (sko-top'sin) the protein moiety in the rods of the retina that combines with retinal (11-*cis* retinal) to form rhodopsin.

scotoscopy (sko-tos'ko-pe) [*scoto-* + Gr. *skopein* to examine] skiascopy.

scototherapy (sko"to-ther'ah-pe) [*scoto-* + Gr. *therapeia* treatment] treatment of disease by the complete exclusion of light rays.

scours (skowrz) diarrhea or dysentery, especially in newborn animals; see *white s.* **black s.**, acute dysentery in cattle, accompanied by intestinal hemorrhage producing a dark color of the feces; the etiology is unknown. **bloody s.**, black scours in swine. **calf s.**, white scours in calves. **peat s.**, molybdenum poisoning in grazing cattle. **white s.**, an acute infectious disease of calves, lambs, and foals during the first few days after birth, caused by enteropathogenic strains of *Escherichia coli* and marked by fever, dehydration, depression, and diarrhea, with fetid feces that are light in color but may be blood-stained late in the disease. **winter s.**, black scours occurring in cattle when stabled for the winter.

scr. scruple.

scrapie (skra'pe) one of the transmissible spongiform viral encephalopathies occurring in sheep and goats, characterized by severe pruritus, debility, and muscular incoordination, and invariably ending fatally.

scratches (skrach'ez) eczematous inflammation of the feet of a horse.

screatus (skre-a'tus) [L.] paroxysmal hawking and snorting, due to neurosis.

screen (skrēn) 1. a structure resembling a curtain or partition, used as a protection or shield; such a structure used in fluoroscopy; or such a structure on which light rays are projected. 2. to examine by *fluoroscopy* (Great Britain). 3. an agent that affords defense against a deleterious influence, such as a substance applied to the skin (*skin s.*) to protect against the effects of the sun's rays (*solar s.*) or other noxious influences; called also *protectant* and *protective*. **Bjerrum s.,** tangent s. **fluorescent s.,** 1. a sheet of cardboard, paper, or glass coated with suitable material, which fluoresces visibly, as calcium tungstate, used as an intensifying screen in roentgenography; as the chief part of a fluoroscope; as a substitute for a fluoroscope in a darkened room. 2. a sheet of cardboard, paper, or glass coated with anthracene or other fluorescing materials to observe the ultraviolet radiations. **intensifying s.,** a thin sheet of celluloid or other substance coated with a finely divided substance which fluoresces under the influence of roentgen rays and intended to be used in close contact with the emulsion of a photographic plate or film for the purpose of reinforcing the image. **tangent s.,** a large square of black cloth, stretched on a frame, hung from a roller, and having a central mark for fixation; used with a campimeter to map the field of vision. Called also *Bjerrum screen*. **vestibular s.,** a screen made of acrylic resin that covers the labial or buccal surface of one or both dental arches, extending into the vestibule; it is used to treat oral habits and to stimulate tooth movement.

screening (skrēn′ing) 1. mass examination of the population to detect the existence of a particular disease, as diabetes or tuberculosis. 2. fluoroscopy (Great Britain). **multiphasic s., multiple s.,** the simultaneous use of multiple laboratory procedures for the detection of various diseases, or pathologic conditions, as anemia, diabetes, heart diseases, hypertension, syphilis, and tuberculosis and other pulmonary diseases.

screwworm (skru′werm) the larva of *Cochliomyia hominivorax*.

scribomania (skrib″o-ma′ne-ah) graphorrhea.

scrobiculate (skro-bik′u-lāt) [L. *scrobiculatus*] marked with pits or cavities.

scrobiculus (skro-bik′u-lus) [L. "little trench," "pit"] a small hollow, pit, or cavity. **s. cor′dis,** fossa epigastrica.

scrofula (skrof′u-lah) [L. "brood sow"] primary tuberculosis of the cervical lymph nodes; it may be accompanied by slowly suppurating abscesses and fistulous passages (scrofuloderma), the inflamed structures being subject to a cheesy degeneration. It is essentially a disease of early life. See also *tuberculous lymphadenitis*, under *lymphadenitis*.

scrofuloderma (skrof″u-lo-der′mah) [*scrofula* + Gr. *derma* skin] suppurating abscesses and fistulous passages opening on the skin, secondary to tuberculosis of lymph nodes, most commonly those of the neck (scrofula), and sometimes of bones and joint surfaces. It is essentially a disease of early life. Called also *tuberculosis cutis colliquativa*.

scrofulous (skrof′u-lus) pertaining to or characterized by scrofuloderma or scrofula.

scrotal (skro′tal) pertaining to the scrotum.

scrotectomy (skro-tek′to-me) [*scrotum* + Gr. *ektomē* excision] excision of a portion of the scrotum.

scrotitis (skro-ti′tis) inflammation of the scrotum.

scrotocele (skro′to-sēl) [*scrotum* + Gr. *kēlē* hernia] scrotal hernia.

scrotoplasty (skro′to-plas″te) [*scrotum* + Gr. *plassein* to form] plastic operation on the scrotum.

scrotum (skro′tum) [L. "bag"] [NA] the pouch which contains the testes and their accessory organs. It is composed of skin, the dartos, the spermatic, cremasteric, and infundibuliform fasciae, and the tunica vaginalis. **s. lapillo′sum,** calcareous atheroma of the scrotum. **lymph s.,** elephantiasis scroti. **watering-can s.,** a condition in which the under surface of the scrotum and the perineum are marked by multiple sinuses discharging urine; due to neglected stricture of the perineal urethra.

scruple (skroo′p'l) [L. *scrupulus*, dim. of *scrupus* a sharp stone, a worry or anxiety] 1. a fear of transgression. 2. a unit of mass (weight) of the apothecaries' system; being 20 grains, or the equivalent of 1.296 gm. Abbreviated scr.; symbol ℈.

scrupulosity (skroo″pu-los′ĭ-te) morbid sensitiveness in matters of conscience; preoccupation with transgressions of religious ritual as a manifestation of obsessive-compulsive disorder.

S.C.S. Society of Clinical Surgery.

scultetus (skul-te′tus) [named for Johann *Schultes* (Scultetus), German surgeon, 1595–1645] scultetus bandage, a many-tailed binder; see under *bandage*.

scurvy (skur′ve) [L. *scorbutus*] a condition due to deficiency of ascorbic acid (vitamin C) in the diet and marked by weakness, anemia, spongy gums, a tendency to mucocutaneous hemorrhages and a brawny induration of the muscles of the calves and legs. **hemorrhagic s.,** infantile scurvy. **infantile s.,** a nutritional disease of infants characterized by the same symptoms as scurvy in adults; called also *Barlow's disease*. **sea s.,** true scurvy; so called because it was most often seen in mariners.

scute (skūt) [L. *scutum* shield] 1. any squama or scalelike structure. 2. the tympanic scute. **tympanic s.,** the bony plate which divides the upper part of the tympanic cavity from the mastoid cells.

scutiform (sku′tĭ-form) [L. *scutum* shield + *forma* form] shaped like a shield; thyroid.

scutular (sku′tu-lar) marked by scutula, or small, saucer-shaped crusts.

scutulum (sku′tu-lum), pl. *scu′tula* [L.] one of the disklike or saucer-like crusts characteristic of favus.

scutum (sku′tum) [L. "shield"] 1. the tympanic scute. 2. the thyroid cartilage. 3. the patella. 4. a hard chitinous plate on the anterior portion of the dorsal surface of the Ixodidae, or hard-bodied ticks. **s. pec′toris,** the sternum.

scybala (sib′ah-lah) [Gr.] plural of *scybalum*.

scybalous (sib′ah-lus) of the nature of or composed of scybala.

scybalum (sib′ah-lum), pl. *scyb′ala* [Gr. *skybalon*] a dry, hard mass of fecal matter in the intestine.

scyllite (sil′īt) a hexose from the liver and kidneys of sharks, skates, etc.

scyllitol (sil′ĭ-tol) the 2-isomer of inositol isolated from the dog fish, *Scyllum canicula*, as well as from sharks and rays.

scymnol (sim′nol) a bile alcohol, $C_{27}H_{48}O_5$, with a 24:26-epoxy group, and a ring-system similar to that of cholic acid; found in the bile of *Scymnus borealis*, a marine fish of the shark family, and in other elasmobranchi.

scyphoid (si′foid) [Gr. *skyphos* cup + *eidos* form] shaped like a cup.

scythropasmus (si″thro-paz′mus) [Gr. *skythrōpasmos; skythōpazein* to look sullen] a dull, fatigued expression, regarded as a grave symptom in serious disease.

scytoblastema (si″to-blas-te′mah) [Gr. *skytos* skin + *blastēma* sprout] the rudimentary skin of the embryo.

Scytonema (si″to-ne′mah) [Gr. *skytos* skin + *nēma* thread] a genus of blue-green algae with cylindrical branching filaments.

S.D. skin dose; standard deviation.

S.D.A. abbreviation for L. *sacrodex′tra ante′rior* (right sacroanterior; a presentation of the fetus), and specific dynamic action.

S.D.E. specific dynamic effect (or action); see under *action*.

S.D.P. abbreviation for L. *sacrodex′tra poste′rior* (right sacroposterior; a presentation of the fetus). abbreviation for L. *sacrodextra transversa* (right sacrotransverse; a presentation of the fetus).

S.E. standard error.

SE sphenoethmoidal suture, a cephalometric landmark designating the junction of the sphenoid and ethmoid bones, in the anterior cranial base.

Se chemical symbol for *selenium*.

seal (sēl) something that effects a firm closure. **border s.,** the contact of the denture border with the underlying or adjacent tissues to prevent the passage of air or other substances. **double s.,** a seal consisting of gutta-percha underneath another material (e.g., temporary cement); used to close the coronal opening in a tooth during endodontic treatment. **posterior palatal s.,** the seal at the posterior border of a denture produced by displacing some of the soft tissue covering the palate by extra pressure developed in the impression or by scraping a depression in the cast. **velopharyngeal s.,** closure between the oral and nasopharyngeal cavities, accomplished by the action of the muscles of the soft palate and the superior constrictor muscle.

seam (sēm) a line of union. **pigment s.,** the portion of the pigmented epithelium of the iris which bends forward around the pupillary border.

searcher (surch′er) a sound used in searching for stone in the bladder; called also *stone searcher*.

seasickness (se′sik-nes) nausea and malaise caused by the motion of a ship at sea.

seat (sēt) a supporting structure. **basal s.,** oral tissues which support a complete or partial denture. **rest s.,** see under *area*.

seatworm (sēt′werm) any oxyurid, especially *Enterobius vermicularis*.

seaweed (se′wēd) a plant growing in the sea, especially one of the algae.

sebaceous (sĕ-ba′shus) [L. *sebaceus*] 1. pertaining to sebum. 2. secreting a greasy lubricating substance, sebum. See under *gland*.

sebiferous (sĕ-bif′er-us) [L. *sebiferus*, from *sebum* suet + *ferre* to bear] sebiparous.

Sebileau's bands, hollow (seb″ĭ-lōz′) [Pierre *Sebileau*, French surgeon, 1860–1953] see under *band* and *hollow*.

sebiparous (sĕ-bip′ah-rus) [L. *sebiparus; sebum* suet + *parere* to produce] producing a fatty secretion.

S.E.B.M. Society for Experimental Biology and Medicine.

sebolith (seb′o-lith) [*sebum* + Gr. *lithos* stone] a concretion formed in a sebaceous gland.

seborrhea (seb″o-re′ah) [L. *sebum* suet + Gr. *rhoia* flow] 1. excessive secretion of sebum; called also *hypersteatosis*. 2. seborrheic dermatitis. **s. adipo′sa,** that in which the secretion is oily, especially occurring about the nose and forehead; called also *s. oleo′sa*. **s. congesti′va,** lupus erythematosus. **s. oleo′sa,** seborrhea adiposa. **s. sic′ca,** dry, scaly seborrheic dermatitis.

seborrheal (seb″o-re′al) characterized by or pertaining to seborrhea.

seborrheic (seb″o-re′ik) affected with or of the nature of seborrhea.

seborrheid (seb″o-re′id) seborrheic dermatitis.

seborrhoea (seb″o-re′ah) seborrhea.

seborrhoic (seb″o-ro′ik) seborrheic.

sebotropic (seb″o-trop′ik) having an affinity for or a stimulating effect on sebaceous glands; promoting the excretion of sebum.

sebum (se′bum) [L.] 1. suet. 2. the secretion of the sebaceous glands; a thick, semifluid substance composed of fat and epithelial debris from the cells of the malpighian layer. **cutaneous s., s. cuta′neum,** the fatty secretion of the sebaceous glands. **s. palpebra′le,** the secretion of the tarsal glands.

Secale (se-ka′le) [L. "rye"] a genus of graminaceous plants. **S. cerea′le,** the common rye.

secale cornutum (se-ka′le kor-nu′tum) the name under which ergot was adopted in the first edition of the U.S.P.

secalin (sek′ah-lin) one of the active principles of ergot; said to be identical with trimethylamine, $N(CH_3)_3$.

secalintoxin (sek″ah-lin-tok′sin) a principle obtainable from ergot.

secalose (sek′ah-lōs) a carbohydrate obtainable from rye; when dried, it forms a white, hygroscopic powder, convertible by inversion into levulose.

Sechenoff's center (setsh′en-ofs) see *Setschenow.*

seclazone (sek′lah-zōn) chemical name: 7-chloro-3,3a-dihydro-2H,9H-isorazolo[3,2-b][1,3]benzoxazin-9-one; an anti-inflammatory with uricosuric properties, $C_{10}H_8ClNO_3$.

secobarbital (se″ko-bar′bǐ-tal) [USP] chemical name: 5-(1-methylbutyl)-5-(2-propenyl)-2,4,6(1H,3H,5H)pyrimidinetrione. A short-acting barbiturate, $C_{12}H_{18}N_2O_3$, occurring as a white, amorphous or crystalline powder; used as a hypnotic and sedative, administered orally. Called also *quinalbarbitone.* **s. sodium** [USP], the monosodium salt of secobarbital, $C_{12}H_{17}N_2NaO_3$, occurring as a white powder, having the actions and uses of the base; administered orally, intravenously, and intramuscularly.

secodont (se′ko-dont) [L. *secare* to cut + Gr. *odous* tooth] having teeth in which the tubercles of the molars are provided with cutting edges, as in many carnivorous mammals.

Seconal (sek′ō-nol) trademark for preparations of secobarbital.

second (sek′und) the unit of time equal to $\frac{1}{60}$ of a minute. **milliampere s's,** in radiographic exposure technique, the product of the milliamperes and the time in seconds.

secondary (sek′un-der″e) [L. *secundarius; secundus* second] second or inferior in order of time, place, or importance; derived from or consequent to a primary event or thing.

second intention (sek′und in-ten′shun) see under *healing.*

secreta (se-kre′tah) [L. pl.] secretion products.

secretagogue (se-krēt′ah-gog) [*secretion* + Gr. *agōgos* drawing] 1. stimulating secretion. 2. an agent that stimulates secretion.

secrete (se-krēt′) [L. *secernere, secretum* to separate] to separate or elaborate cell products.

secretin (se-kre′tin) a strongly basic polypeptide hormone secreted by the mucosa of the duodenum and jejunum when acid chyme enters the intestine. Carried by the blood, it stimulates the secretion of a watery pancreatic juice high in salt content but low in enzymes. It has a lesser stimulatory effect on bile and intestinal secretion. See also *S cells* (def. 2), under *cell.* **gastric s.,** former term for gastrin.

secretinase (se-kre′tǐ-nās) an enzymic substance in blood and other body fluids which inactivates secretin.

secretion (se-kre′shun) [L. *secretio,* from *secernere* to secrete] 1. the process of elaborating a specific product as a result of the activity of a gland; this activity may range from separating a specific substance of the blood to the elaboration of a new chemical substance. 2. any substance produced by secretion. **antilytic s.,** saliva secreted by the submaxillary gland with nerves intact, as distinguished from that secreted when the nerve is divided. **external s.,** one that is discharged upon an external or internal surface of the body; the glands of external secretion are the exocrine glands (q.v.). Cf. *internal s.* **internal s.,** any of the specific substances (hormones) that are not discharged by a duct from the body, but are given off into the blood and lymph, and effect a response distant from the site of origin. Such substances are secreted by the organs and structures of the endocrine system (q.v.). Cf. *external s.* **paralytic s.,** secretion from a gland after paralysis or division of its nerve.

secretogogue (se-kre′to-gog) secretagogue.

secretoinhibitory (se-kre″to-in-hib′ǐ-to″re) inhibiting secretion; antisecretory.

secretomotor (se-kre″to-mo′tor) exciting or stimulating secretion; said of nerves.

secretomotory (se-kre″to-mo′tor-e) secretomotor.

secretor (se-kre′tor) in genetics, an individual who secretes the ABH antigens of the ABO blood group in the saliva and other body fluids. Also, the gene that determines this trait.

secretory (se-kre′to-re) pertaining to secretion or affecting the secretions.

sectarian (sek-ta′re-an) a practitioner of medicine who "follows a dogma, tenet, or principle based on the authority of its promulgator to the exclusion of demonstration and practice" (Judicial Council A.M.A.).

sectile (sek′tīl) [L. *sectilis,* from *secare* to cut] 1. susceptible of being cut. 2. of several parts into which a whole is divided.

sectio (sek′she-o), pl. sectio′nes [L., from *secare* to cut] 1. an act of cutting. 2. a section; [NA] a general term for a segment or subdivision of an organ. **s. al′ta,** suprapubic cystotomy. **s. cadav′eris,** necropsy. **sectio′nes cerebel′li** [NA], the various internal anatomical subdivisions of the cerebellum. **sectio′nes corpo′rum quadrigemino′rum,** the anatomical divisions of the corpora quadrigemina. **sectio′nes hypothal′ami** [NA], the various internal anatomical subdivisions of the hypothalamus. **sectio′nes isth′mi,** see *sectiones mesencephali.* **s. latera′lis,** lateral lithotomy. **s. media′na,** median lithotomy. **sectio′nes medul′lae oblonga′tae** [NA], the various internal anatomical subdivisions of the medulla oblongata. **sectio′nes medul′lae spina′lis** [NA], the various internal anatomical subdivisions of the spinal cord. **sectio′nes mesence′phali** [NA], the various internal anatomical subdivisions of the mesencephalon. **sectio′nes pedun′culi cer′ebri,** sectiones mesencephali. **sectio′nes pon′tis** [NA], the various internal anatomical subdivisions of the pons. **sectio′nes telence′phali** [NA], the various internal anatomical subdivisions of the telencephalon. **sectio′nes thalamence′phali** [NA], the various internal anatomical subdivisions of the thalamencephalon.

section (sek′shun) [L. *sectio*] 1. an act of cutting. 2. a cut surface. 3. a segment or subdivision of an organ; called also *sectio* [NA]. **abdominal s.,** laparotomy. **celloidin s.,** a section cut by a microtome from tissue that has been embedded in celloidin. **cesarean s.,** incision through the abdominal and uterine walls for delivery of a fetus. The procedure was included (*lex cesarea*) in the codification of Roman law in 715 B.C., as a means of salvaging a fetus, if living, or of providing for its separate burial, in event of the mother's death. **cesarean s., cervical,** cesarean section in which the lower uterine segment is incised, either intraperitoneally or extraperitoneally. **cesarean s., classic, cesarean s., corporeal,** cesarean section in which the upper segment, or corpus, of the uterus is incised. **cesarean s., extraperitoneal,** cesarean section performed without incision of the peritoneum, the peritoneal fold being displaced upward and the bladder being displaced downward or to the midline, the uterus then being opened by an incision in its lower segment. **cesarean s., Latzko's,** extraperitoneal cesarean section with the incision made through one side of the lower segment of the uterus. **cesarean s., low,** cesarean s., cervical. **cesarean s., Porro** (*obs.*), cesarean s. **cesarean s., transperitoneal,** cesarean section performed with an incision through the uterovesical fold of peritoneum. **cesarean s., vaginal,** cesarean section performed through an incision through the anterior vaginal wall into the uterine cavity. **coronal s.,** frontal s. **frontal s.,** a section parallel with the long axis of the body and at right angles to a sagittal section; it divides the body into a dorsal and ventral part. Called also *coronal s.* **frozen s.,** a section cut by a microtome from tissue that has been frozen. **paraffin s.,** a section cut by a microtome from tissue which has been embedded in paraffin. **perineal s.,** external urethrotomy. **Pitres' s's,** a series of six coronal sections through the brain: a *prefrontal* section, through the prefrontal part of the frontal lobe; two *frontal* sections, the first being 2 cm. in front of the central sulcus (*pediculofrontal s.*), and the second being through the precentral gyrus; two *parietal* sections, one through the postcentral gyrus, and the other (*pediculoparietal s.*) 3 cm. behind the central sulcus; and an *occipital* section, through the middle of the occipital lobe. **Saemisch's s.,** Saemisch's operation. **sagittal s.,** a section that follows the sagittal suture and runs the entire length of the body, thus dividing the latter into more or less equal right and left halves. **serial s.,** histologic section made in a consecutive order and so arranged for the purpose of microscopical examination. **transverse s.,** one made at right angles to the long axis of a body or structure.

sectiones (sek″she-o′nēz) [L.] plural of *sectio.*

sector (sek′tor) [L. "cutter"] 1. the area of a circle included between an arc and the radii bounding it. 2. an area, zone, or part of something. 3. to divide into sectors.

sectorial (sek-to′re-al) [L. *sector* cutter] 1. pertaining or relating to a sector. 2. in genetics, pertaining to the presence of a sector of tissue which carries a somatic mutation and which is therefore different phenotypically from the tissues of the rest of the body; also, an individual having such a sector of tissue (a mosaic). 3. cutting or adapted for cutting, as the molar teeth of carnivores.

secundigravida (se-kun″dǐ-grav′ǐ-dah) [L. *secundus* second + *gravida* pregnant] a woman pregnant for the second time; written gravida II.

secundina (se″kun-di′nah), pl. *secundi′nae* [L., from *secundus* following] that which follows; see *secundines*. **s. oc′uli,** the middle coat of the choroid. **s. u′teri,** the chorion.

secundinae (se″kun-di′ne) [L.] plural of *secundina*; secundines.

secundines (se-kun′dīnz, se-kun-dēnz) [L. *secundinae*] the placenta and membranes expelled after childbirth; the afterbirth.

secundipara (se″kun-dip′ah-rah) [L. *secundus* second + *parere* to bring forth, produce] a woman who has had two pregnancies which resulted in viable offspring; written para II or II-para.

secundiparity (se-kun″dĭ-par′ĭ-te) the condition of being a secundipara.

secundiparous (se″kun-dip′ah-rus) having borne two viable offspring in separate pregnancies.

secundum artem (se-kun′dum ar′tem) [L.] in an approved or professional manner.

securinine (se-ku′rĭ-nēn) an alkaloid, $C_{13}H_{15}NO_2$, obtained from the leaves and roots of *Securinega suffruticosa* Rehder (Euphorbiaceae); its nitrate salt is used in neurasthenic states and cardiac insufficiency, and in the treatment of impotence.

S.E.D. skin erythema dose.

sedation (se-da′shun) [L. *sedatio*] the production of a sedative effect; the act or process of calming.

sedative (sed′ah-tiv) [L. *sedativus*] 1. allaying activity and excitement. 2. an agent that allays excitement. **Battley's s.,** a solution made up of extract of opium, boiling water, alcohol, and cold water. **cardiac s.,** one that abates the force of the heart's action. **cerebral s.,** one which principally affects the brain. **gastric s.,** one which soothes or lessens irritability of the stomach. **general s.,** one which affects all the organs and functions. **intestinal s.,** one which diminishes intestinal irritation; in general, they are also gastric sedatives. **nerve trunk s.,** one which acts upon the trunks of the nerves. **nervous s.,** a sedative which acts upon and through the nervous system; the cerebral, spinal, and nerve trunk sedatives belong to this class. **respiratory s.,** one which affects especially the respiratory centers and organs. **spinal s.,** any drug which abates the functional or abnormal activity of the spinal cord. **vascular s.,** one which affects the vasomotor activities.

sedentary (sed′en-ter″e) [L. *sedentarius*] 1. sitting habitually; of inactive habits. 2. pertaining to a sitting posture.

Sédillot's operation (sa-de-yōz′) [Charles Emmanuel *Sédillot,* French surgeon, 1804–1883] see under *operation*.

sediment (sed′ĭ-ment) [L. *sedimentum*] a precipitate, especially one that is formed spontaneously. **urinary s.,** the deposit of solid matter left after the urine has been allowed to stand for some time.

sedimentable (sed″ĭ-ment′ah-b′l) in microbiology, capable of forming sediment.

sedimentation (sed″ĭ-men-ta′shun) the act of causing the deposit of sediment, especially by the use of a centrifugal machine. **erythrocyte s.,** the sinking of red cells in a volume of drawn blood; see *erythrocyte sedimentation rate*, under *rate*. **formalin-ether s. (Ritchie),** a technique for detecting parasites in the feces, involving the centrifugation of diluted feces, the addition of formalin and ether to the sample, recentrifugation, and examining the final sediment as a wet mount.

sedimentator (sed″ĭ-men-ta′tor) a centrifugal machine for separating sediments from the urine.

sedopeptose (se″do-pep′tōs) a monosaccharide occurring in herbs of the genus *Sedum*.

seed (sēd) 1. the mature ovule of a flowering plant. 2. semen. 3. a small cylindrical shell of gold or other suitable material, used in application of radiation therapy. 4. to inoculate a culture medium with microorganisms. **cardamom s.** [NF], the dried ripe seed of *Elettaria cardamomum,* a perennial herb of the ginger family of tropical Asia; used as a flavoring agent. **celery s.,** see *Apium.* **larkspur s.,** see *Delphinium.* **plantago s.** [USP], **psyllium s.,** the cleaned dried, ripe seed of *Plantago psyllium, P. indica,* or *P. ovata,* used as a fecal softener. The mucilaginous portion of the seeds of *P. ovata* are used in preparing psyllium hydrophilic mucilloid. **radiogold (^{198}Au) s.,** a solid piece of radioactive gold wire about 2.5 mm. long and 0.8 mm. thick, used as a permanent interstitial radioactive implant in the treatment of cancer. **radon s.,** a small sealed container or tube for carrying radon, made of gold or glass for insertion into tissues for the treatment of certain malignant diseases; it is visible roentgenographically.

Seeligmüller's sign (za′lik-mil″erz) [Otto Ludovicus G. A. *Seeligmüller,* German neurologist, 1837–1912] see under *sign*.

Seessel's pouch (pocket) (za′selz) [Albert *Seessel,* American embryologist and anatomist, 1850–1910] see under *pouch*.

Séglas type (sa-glahz′) [Jules Ernest *Séglas,* French psychiatrist, 1856–1939] see under *type*.

segment (seg′ment) [L. *segmentum* a piece cut off] a portion of a larger body or structure, set off by natural or arbitrarily established boundaries. **bronchopulmonary s.,** one of the smaller subdivisions of the lobes of the lungs; see *segmenta bronchopulmonalia.* **cranial s's,** three segments into which the bones of the cranium may be divided; they are distinguished as the occipital, the parietal, and the frontal. **frontal s.,** the anterior of the three cranial segments. **hepatic s's,** segmenta hepatis. **interannular s.,** the portion of a nerve fiber between two consecutive nodes of Ranvier. **s's of kidney,** segmenta renalia. **s's of liver,** segmenta hepatis. **medullary s.,** a division of the medullary sheath of a nerve fiber between two Schmidt-Lanterman incisures. **mesoblastic s.,** a somite. **mesodermal s.,** a somite. **neural s.,** a neuromere. **occipital s.,** the posterior of the three cranial segments. **parietal s.,** the central of the three cranial segments. **primitive s., protovertebral s.,** somite. **pubic s. of the pelvis,** that portion of the floor of the pelvis which is between the symphysis pubis and the anterior wall of the vagina, which latter it includes. **Ranvier's s's,** the portions of the medullary substance of a nerve fiber between the nodes of Ranvier. **renal s's,** segmenta renalia. **rivinian s., s. of Rivinus.** an irregular notch at the upper border of the tympanic sulcus; called also *incisura tympanica* [*Rivini*]. **rod s.,** the two segments which make up one of the rods of the retina; the *outer rod s.* is the portion presenting a uniform diameter, while the *inner rod s.* has a slightly increased diameter. **sacral s.,** that portion of the floor of the pelvis which lies between the sacrum and the posterior vaginal wall. **Schmidt-Lanterman s.,** medullary s. **spinal s.,** a portion of the spinal cord to which a pair of spinal nerves is attached by dorsal and ventral roots. **uterine s.,** either of the portions into which the uterus becomes differentiated early in labor: the upper contractile portion (corpus uteri) becomes thicker as labor advances, and the lower noncontractile portion is thin-walled and passive in character.

segmenta (seg-men′tah) [L.] plural of *segmentum*.

segmental (seg-men′tal) pertaining to or forming a segment or a product of division, especially into serially arranged or nearly equal parts; undergoing segmentation.

segmentation (seg″men-ta′shun) 1. division into parts more or less similar, such as somites or metameres. 2. cleavage. **haustral s.,** the formation of pouches in the wall of the large intestine, by alternating contraction and relaxation of circular muscle fibers. It keeps the intestinal contents plastic and assists in propelling them toward the rectum.

segmenter (seg′ment-er) a malarial organism of the stage in which it divides into merozoites in the blood cell. See also *schizont*.

Segmentina (seg″men-ti′nah) a genus of fresh-water snails of the Orient; *S. hemisphaerula, S. trochoideus,* and *S. largillierti* are first intermediate hosts of the intestinal fluke *Fasciolopsis buski*.

segmentum (seg-men′tum), pl. *segmen′ta* [L.] a portion of a larger body or structure; [NA] a general term for a part of an organ or other structure set off by natural or arbitrarily established boundaries. **segmen′ta bronchopulmona′lia** [NA], bronchopulmonary segments: the smaller subdivisions of the lobes of the lungs, separated by connective tissue septa and supplied by branches of the respective lobar bronchi. Called also *lobuli pulmonum*. They include: RIGHT LUNG—(*superior lobe*) s. apicale, s. posterius, and s. anterius; (*middle lobe*) s. laterale and s. mediale; (*inferior lobe*) s. apicale (or superius), s. basale mediale (or cardiacum), s. basale anterius, s. basale laterale, and s. basale posterius; LEFT LUNG—(*superior lobe*) s. apicoposterius, s. anterius, s. lingulare superius, and s. lingulare inferius; (*inferior lobe*) s. apicale (or superius), s. subapicale (or subsuperius), s. basale mediale (or cardiacum), s. basale anterius, s. basale laterale, and s. basale posterius. See Plate accompanying *lung*. **segmen′ta hep′atis** [NA], hepatic segments: subdivisions of the hepatic lobes based on arterial and biliary supply and venous drainage; they are the *segmentum anterius* and *s. posterius* of the right lobe, and the *s. mediale* and *s. laterale* of the left lobe. **segmen′ta rena′lia** [NA], renal segments: subdivisions of the kidney that have independent blood supply from branches of the renal artery; they are: *segmentum superius, s. anterius superius, s. anterius inferius, s. inferius,* and *s. posterius.*

segregation (seg″re-ga′shun) 1. in genetics the separation of allelic genes during meiosis as homologous chromosomes begin to migrate toward the poles of the cell, so that eventually the members of each pair of allelic genes go to separate gametes. 2. the separation of different elements of a population. 3. the progressive restriction of potencies in the zygote to the various regions of the forming embryo.

segregator (seg′re-ga″tor) an instrument for securing the urine from each kidney separately. **Cathelin's s.,** an appliance inserted into the bladder, separating the cavity into two parts so that the urine from each ureter may be collected separately. **Harris' s.,** an instrument for collecting the urine from each kidney separately. **Luys' s.,** an instrument for collecting the urine from each kidney separately.

Séguin's signal symptom (sign) (sa-ganz′) [Edouard *Séguin,* French alienist, 1812–1880] see under *symptom*.

Sehrt's clamp (compressor) (sārts) [Ernst *Sehrt,* German surgeon, born 1879] see under *clamp*.

Seidel's scotoma (sign) (si′delz) [Erich *Seidel,* German ophthalmologist, 1882–1948] see under *scotoma*.

Seidelin bodies (si′dĕ-lin) [Harold *Seidelin*, British physician] see under *body*.

Seidlitz powder, powder test (sīd′litz) [named from a mineral spring in Bohemia] see under *powder* and *tests*.

Seignette's salt (sīn-yets′) [Pierre *Seignette*, apothecary in Rochelle, 1660–1719] potassium sodium tartrate.

seisesthesia (sīs″es-the′ze-ah) seismesthesia.

seismesthesia (sīs″mes-the′ze-ah) [Gr. *seismos* a shaking + *aisthēsis* perception + *-ia*] tactile perception of vibrations in a liquid or aerial medium.

seismocardiogram (sīz″mo-kar′de-o-gram″) the graphic record obtained by seismocardiography.

seismocardiography (sīz″mo-kar″de-og′rah-fe) [Gr. *seismos* a shaking, shock + *kardia* heart + *graphē* representation by means of lines] the selective recording of cardiac vibrations.

seismotherapy (sīz″mo-ther′ah-pe) [Gr. *seismos* a shaking + *therapy*] the treatment of disease by mechanical vibration.

seizure (se′zhur) 1. the sudden attack or recurrence of a disease. 2. an attack of epilepsy. See also *ictus*. **absence s.,** an epileptic seizure marked by a momentary break in the stream of thought and activity, accompanied by a symmetrical 3-c.p.s. spike and wave activity on the electroencephalogram; called also *petit mal epilepsy*. **audiogenic s.,** an epileptic seizure brought on by sound. **cerebral s.,** an attack of epilepsy. **febrile s.,** convulsions associated with high fever, occurring in infants and children. **jackknife s.,** a severe myoclonus appearing in the first 18 months of life and associated with general cerebral deterioration; it is marked by severe flexion spasms of the head, neck, and trunk and extension of the arms and legs. Called also *infantile massive spasms*. **photogenic s.,** an epileptic seizure brought on by light. **psychic s.,** psycholepsy. **psychomotor s.,** psychomotor epilepsy. **uncinate s.,** see under *epilepsy*.

sejunction (se-junk′shun) an interruption of the continuity of association complexes which leads to a breaking up of the personality (Wernicke).

sekisanine (sek-is′ah-nin) an alkaloid, $C_{16}H_{19}O_4N$, from *Lycoris radiata*.

selachian (sĕ-la′ke-an) one of a class of vertebrates which includes the sharks and rays.

selection (sĕ-lek′shun) the play of forces that determines the relative reproductive performance of the various genotypes in a population. **artificial s.,** the interference by man in the selection of the genotypes to produce succeeding generations of a given organism. **natural s.,** the survival in nature of those individuals and their progeny best equipped to adapt to environmental conditions. **sexual s.,** natural selection in which certain characteristics attract male or female members of a species, thus ensuring survival of those characteristics. **truncate s.,** in medical genetics, the selection of families in a population in such a way that one or more kinds of sibships are not ascertained, usually those sibships in which no member is affected with the trait under study.

selective (sĕ-lek′tiv) having a high degree of selectivity.

selectivity (sĕ-lek-tiv′ĭ-te) in pharmacology, the degree to which a dose of a drug produces the desired effect in relation to adverse effects.

selene (sĕ-le′ne) [L.; Gr. *selēnē* moon] a moon-shaped object or structure. **s. un′guium** ["moon of the nails"], lunula unguis.

selenide (sel′ĕ-nīd) a compound of selenium with another element or radical.

selenium (sĕ-le′ne-um) [Gr. *selēnē* moon] a nonmetallic element resembling sulfur; symbol, Se; atomic number, 34; atomic weight, 78.96. It is an essential mineral, being a constituent of the enzyme glutathione peroxidase, and believed to be closely associated with vitamin E in its functions, but it occurs in toxic levels in several kinds of plants growing in soil with high levels, causing disease in grazing animals (see *selenium poisoning*, under *poisoning*). **s. sulfide** [USP], the sulfide salt of selenium, SeS_2, occurring as a reddish brown to bright orange powder; used as a topical antifungal in the treatment of tinea versicolor, as a topical keratolytic, and applied topically to the scalp to control seborrheic dermatitis and dandruff.

selenodont (sĕ-le′no-dont) [Gr. *selēnē* moon + *odous* tooth] having posterior teeth on which the individual cusps assume a crescentic outline, as in many herbivorous mammals.

selenomethionine (sel″en-o-mĕ-thi′o-nēn) methionine in which selenium replaces the sulfur atom; the radioactive form (^{75}Se) is used in tests of tissue uptake of methionine.

Selenomonas (se″le-no-mo′nas) a genus of microorganisms of the family Spirillaceae, suborder Pseudomonadineae, order Pseudomonadales, made up of motile, kidney- to crescent-shaped cells with blunt ends. It includes three species, *S. pal′pitans, S. ruminan′tium,* and *S. sputi′gena*.

selenoplegia, selenoplexia (sĕ-le″no-ple′je-ah; sĕ-le″no-plek′se-ah) [Gr. *selēnē* moon + *plēxis* stroke] a morbid condition once believed to be due to the influence of the moon's rays.

selenosis (se″le-no′sis) selenium poisoning; see under *poisoning*.

self (self) an expression used by Burnet and Fenner to denote an animal's own antigenic constituents, in contrast to "not self," denoting foreign antigenic constituents. The "self" constituents are metabolized without antibody formation, whereas the antigens which are "not self" are eliminated through the immune response mechanism. It was postulated that there exists some mechanism of "self recognition" which enables the organism to distinguish between "self" and "not self."

self-differentiation (self″dif-er-en″she-a′shun) perseverance in a course of development by a part independently of outside influences or changed surroundings.

self-digestion (self″di-jes′chun) autodigestion; autolysis (def. 1).

self-fermentation (self″fer-men-ta′shun) autolysis; (def. 1); autodigestion.

self-fertilization (self″fer-tĭ-lĭ-za′shun) the fusion of male and female gametes from the same individual.

self-hypnosis (self″hip-no′sis) hypnosis by autosuggestion.

self-inductance (self″in-duk′tans) the property of an electric circuit which determines, for a given rate of change of current in the circuit, the electromotive force induced in the circuit itself.

self-infection (self″in-fek′shun) autoinfection.

selfing (self′ing) continuous cross-fertilization between different proglottids of the same tapeworm.

self-limited (self-lim′it-ed) limited by its own peculiarities, and not by outside influence; said of a disease that runs a definite limited course.

self-suspension (self″sus-pen′shun) the suspension of the body by the head and axillae (*axillocephalic s.*) or by the head (*cephalic s.*) for the purpose of stretching the vertebral column.

self-tolerance (self-tol′er-ans) immunological tolerance to self-antigens; called also *horror autotoxicus*. See also *clonal selection theory*, under *theory*.

selfwise (self′wīz) developing in a previously determined manner despite transplantation to a new and strange location; said of embryonic cells or tissue. Cf. *neighborwise*.

Selivanoff's (Seliwanow's) test (reaction) [Feodor Fedorowich *Selivanoff*, Russian chemist, born 1859] see under *tests*.

sella (sel′ah), pl. *sel′lae* [L.] a saddle-shaped depression. **s. tur′cica** [NA], a transverse depression crossing the midline on the superior surface of the body of the sphenoid bone, and containing the hypophysis.

sellae (sel′e) [L.] plural of *sella*.

sellanders (sel′an-derz) malanders.

sellar (sel′ar) pertaining to the sella turcica.

Sellards' test (sel′ardz) [Andrew Watson *Sellards*, American physician, born 1884] see under *tests*.

Selsun (sel′sun) trademark for a preparation of selenium sulfide. **S. Blue,** trademark for a preparation of selenium sulfide.

Selter's disease (sel′terz) [Paul *Selter*, German pediatrist, born 1866] acrodynia.

semantic (se-man′tik) pertaining to or affecting the meanings or significance of words.

semantics (se-man′tiks) [Gr. *sēmantikos* significant, from *sēma* a sign] the study of the meanings of words and the rules of their use; the study of the relationship between language and significance.

semasiology (se-ma″se-ol′o-je) semantics.

Semb's operation (sāmz) [Carl *Semb*, Oslo surgeon, born 1895] see under *operation*.

semeiography (se″mi-og′rah-fe) [Gr. *sēmeion* sign + *graphein* to write] a description of the signs or symptoms of disease.

semeiology (se″mi-ol′o-je) [Gr. *sēmeion* sign + *-logy*] symptomatology.

semeiotic (se″mi-ot′ik) [Gr. *semeiōtikos*] 1. pertaining to the signs or symptoms of disease. 2. pathognomonic.

semeiotics (se″mi-ot′iks) symptomatology.

semelincident (sem″el-in′sĭ-dent) [L. *semel* once + *incidens* falling upon] attacking only once, as an infectious disease which induces immunity thereafter.

semelparity (sem″el-par′ĭ-te) [L. *semel* once + *parere* to bear] the state, in an individual organism, of reproducing only once in a lifetime.

semelparous (sem-el′pah-rus) pertaining to or characterized by semelparity.

semen (se′men), gen. *sem′inis* [L. "seed"] 1. any seed or seedlike fruit. 2. the thick, whitish secretion of the reproductive organs in the male; composed of spermatozoa in their nutrient plasma, secretions from the prostate, seminal vesicles, and various other glands, epithelial cells, and minor constituents. **s. con′tra,** santonica.

semenologist (se″mĕ-nol′o-jist) seminologist.

semenology (se″mĕ-nol′o-je) seminology.

semenuria (se″mĕ-nu′re-ah) seminuria.

semi- (sem′e) [L. *semis* half] a prefix signifying one half, or partly.

semiantigen (sem″e-an′tĭ-jen) half antigen.

semiapochromat (sem″e-ap″o-kro′mat) [*semi-* + *apo-* + *chromatic* aberration] semiapochromatic objective.

semiapochromatic (sem″e-ap″o-kro-mat′ik) see under *objective.*

semicanal (sem″e-kah-nal′) a channel which is open on one side; called also *semicanalis*. **s. of auditory tube,** semicanalis tubae auditiva. **s. of humerus,** sulcus intertubercularis humeri. **s. of tensor tympani muscle,** semicanalis musculi tensoris tympani.

semicanales (sem″e-kah-na′lēz) [L.] plural of *semicanalis*.

semicanalis (sem″e-kah-na′lis), pl. *semicana′les* [L.] semicanal: a channel which is open on one side. **s. mus′culi tenso′ris tym′pani** [NA], semicanal of tensor tympani muscle: a small canal hidden in the temporal bone, constituting the superior part of the musculotubal canal, and lodging the tensor tympani muscle. **s. tu′bae auditi′vae** [NA], semicanal of auditory tube: a small canal in the temporal bone, opening on the inferior surface of the skull just posterior and superior to the foramen spinosum. It constitutes the inferior part of the musculotubal canal and lodges the auditory tube.

semicartilaginous (sem″e-kar″tĭ-laj′ĭ-nus) partially cartilaginous.

semicoma (sem″e-ko′mah) a stupor from which the patient may be aroused.

semicomatose (sem″e-ko′mah-tōs) in a condition of semicoma.

semicrista (sem″e-kris′tah), pl. *semicris′tae* [L.] a small or rudimentary crest. **s. incisi′va,** crista nasalis maxilla.

semidecussation (sem″e-de″kus-sa′shun) 1. an incomplete crossing of nerve fibers. 2. decussatio pyramidum.

semidiagrammatic (sem″e-di″ah-grah-mat′ik) partly diagrammatic; modified so as to illustrate a principle, rather than to serve as an exact copy of nature.

semiflexion (sem″e-flek′shun) 1. the position of a limb midway between flexion and extension. 2. the act of bringing to such a position.

semifluctuating (sem″e-fluk′chu-āt″ing) giving a somewhat fluctuating sensation on palpation.

semiglutin (sem″e-gloo′tin) a substance, $C_{55}H_{85}N_{17}O_{22}$, derived from gelatin and resembling a peptone.

Semih. abbreviation for L. *semiho′ra*, half an hour.

Semikon (sem′ĭ-kon) trademark for preparations of methapyrilene.

semilunar (sem″e-lu′nar) [L. *semilunaris; semi-* half + *luna* moon] resembling a crescent, or half-moon.

semilunare (sem″e-lu-na′re) [L.] the second bone of the first row of carpal bones, counting from the thumb side (os lunatum [NA]).

semiluxation (sem″e-luk-sa′shun) subluxation.

semimembranous (sem″e-mem′brah-nus) made up in part of membrane or fascia.

seminal (sem′ĭ-nal) [L. *seminalis*] pertaining to seed or to the semen.

seminarcosis (sem″e-nar-ko′sis) twilight sleep.

semination (sem″ĭ-na′shun) [L. *seminatio*] insemination.

seminiferous (se″mĭ-nif′er-us) [L. *semen* seed + *ferre* to bear] producing or conveying semen.

seminin (se′min-in) a proteolytic enzyme of human semen.

seminologist (se″mĭ-nol′o-jist) a specialist in the study of semen and spermatozoa.

seminology (se″mĭ-nol′o-je) the scientific study of the semen, in relation to the possible causes of infertility in the male.

seminoma (se″mĭ-no′mah) [*semen* + *-oma*] a radiosensitive, malignant neoplasm of the testis, thought to be derived from primordial germ cells of the sexually undifferentiated embryonic gonad, and occurring as a gray to yellow-white nodule or mass; three histologic variants are recognized: *classical* (typical), the most common type; *anaplastic;* and *spermatocytic.* The classical tumor is composed of fairly well-differentiated sheets or cords of uniform polygonal or round cells (seminoma cells), each cell having abundant clear cytoplasm, distinct cell membranes, a centrally placed round nucleus; and one or more nucleoli. In the female, a grossly and histologically identical neoplasm, known as *dysgerminoma,* occurs. **ovarian s.,** a dysgerminoma of an ovary.

seminormal (sem″e-nor′mal) of one-half the normal or standard strength.

seminose (sem′ĭ-nōs) mannose.

seminuria (se″mĭ-nu′re-ah) [L. *semen* seed + Gr. *ouron* urine + *-ia*] the presence of semen in the urine.

semiography (se″me-og′rah-fe) semeiography.

semiology (se″me-ol′o-je) symptomatology.

semiorbicular (sem″e-or-bik′u-lar) semicircular.

semiotic (se″mi-ot′ik) semeiotic.

semiparasite (sem″e-par′ah-sīt) an organism having potential pathogenicity, occurring both as a saprophyte and as a parasite.

semipenniform (sem″e-pen′ĭ-form) penniform on one side; said of a muscle the fibers of which are attached to one side of the tendon.

semipermeable (sem″e-per′me-ah-b'l) permitting the passage of certain molecules and hindering that of others; see under *membrane.*

semiplacenta (sem″e-plah-sen′tah) Strähl's term for a placenta in certain animals in which the fetal and maternal sections of the organ can be separated without tearing.

semiplegia (sem″e-ple′je-ah) hemiplegia.

semipronation (sem″e-pro-na′shun) 1. the act of bringing to a semiprone position. 2. a semiprone position.

semiprone (sem″e-prōn′) [L. *semis* half + *pronus* prone] partly prone; see *Sims's position,* under *position.*

semiquantitative (sem″ĭ-kwon″tĭ-ta′tiv) yielding an approximation of the quantity or amount of a substance; falling short of a quantitative result.

semiquinone (sem″e-kwin′ōn) a free radical derived from quinones or quinone imines by the addition of a single H atom to a molecule.

semirecumbent (sem″e-re-kum′bent) reclining but not completely recumbent.

semis (se′mis) [L.] half; abbreviated *ss.*

semisideratio (sem″e-sid″er-a′she-o) hemiplegia.

semisomnus (sem″e-som′nus) semicoma.

semisopor (sem″e-so′por) semicoma.

semispeculum (sem″e-spek′u-lum) a blunt gorget shaped like a half-speculum, used in lithotomy.

semistarvation (sem″e-star-va′shun) the so-called hunger cure.

semisulcus (sem″e-sul′kus) [L. *semis* half + *sulcus* furrow] a slight channel on the edge of a bone or other structure, which unites with a similar channel on a corresponding adjoining structure to form a complete sulcus.

semisupination (sem″e-su″pĭ-na′shun) 1. a position of partial or incomplete supination. 2. the act of bringing to such a position.

semisupine (sem″e-su′pīn) partly but not completely supine.

semisynthetic (sem″e-sin-thet′ik) produced by chemical manipulation of naturally occurring substances.

semitendinous (sem″e-ten′dĭ-nus) in part having a tendinous structure.

semivalent (sem-iv′ah-lent) (*obs.*) having one-half the power which is normal.

Semmelweis (sem′el-vīs), Ignaz Philipp (1818–1865). A Hungarian physician, who in Vienna (1847–1849) proved that puerperal fever is a form of septicemia, thus becoming the pioneer of antisepsis in obstetrics. The contagiousness of puerperal fever had been affirmed by Oliver Wendell Holmes of Boston in 1843, and important observations had been made even earlier by Alexander Gordon of Aberdeen and Charles White of Manchester.

Semon's law, sign (se′monz) [Sir Felix *Semon,* German laryngologist in London, 1849–1921] see under *law* and *sign.*

Semon-Hering hypothesis, theory (za′mon-ha′ring) [Richard Wolfgang *Semon,* German naturalist, 1859–1918; Ewald *Hering,* German physiologist, 1834–1918] see *mnemic theory,* under *theory.*

Semoxydrine (sem-ok′sĭ-drin) trademark for a preparation of methamphetamine hydrochloride.

Semple's treatment, vaccine (sem′p'lz) [Sir David *Semple,* British physician, 1856–1937] see under *treatment* and *vaccine.*

semustine (sĕ-mus′tēn) chemical name: *N-*(2-chloroethyl)-*N′-*(4-methylcyclohexyl)-*N*-nitrosourea; an antineoplastic, $C_{10}H_{18}ClN_3O_2$.

Senear-Usher syndrome (se-nēr′ush′er) [Francis Eugene *Senear,* Chicago dermatologist, 1889–1958; Barney *Usher,* Canadian dermatologist, born 1899] pemphigus erythematosus.

senecifolin (sen″ĕ-sif′o-lin) a poisonous alkaloid, $C_{18}H_{27}O_8N$, of *Senecio,* found in the vascular bundles of the young plant before flowering.

Senecio (sĕ-ne′she-o) [L. "old man"] a genus of composite-flowered plants. *S. aureus* L. (golden ragwort) and related species were once used as emmenagogues, but are now listed as poisonous to livestock; they contain senecine, senecifoline, and similar alkaloids. **S. jaco′bae** L. (Compositae), a species causing Pictou's disease in horses and cattle in Nova Scotia; also known as *Tansy ragwort.*

senega (sen′e-gah) [L.] the dried root of *Polygala senega* L. (Polygalaceae), seneca or senega snakeroot, a plant of North America, the main constituents of which are polygalic acid and senegenin; expectorant and emetic. It has been used in veterinary medicine as an expectorant.

senegenin (sen″ĕ-jen′in) a bitter saponin, $C_{30}H_{45}ClO_6$, which is an active principle of senega; called also *polygalin*.

senescence (se-nes′ens) [L. *senescere* to grow old] the process or condition of growing old, especially the condition resulting from the transitions and accumulations of the deleterious aging processes. Cf. *aging*. **dental s.,** deterioration of the teeth and other oral structures as a consequence of advancing age or of premature aging processes.

senescent (se-nes′ent) exhibiting senescence.

Sengstaken-Blakemore tube (sengz′ta-ken-blāk′mōre) [Robert William *Sengstaken*, American neurosurgeon, born 1923; Arthur H. *Blakemore*, American surgeon, born 1897] see under *tube*.

senile (se′nīl) [L. *senilis*] pertaining to or characteristic of old age; manifesting senility.

senilism (se′nil-izm) premature old age.

senility (sĕ-nil′ĭ-te) [L. *senilitas*] old age; the physical and mental deterioration associated with old age.

senium (se′ne-um) [L. "the weakness of old age"] old age; the period of life marked by the weaknesses and deterioration that may accompany advanced years.

Senn's bone plates, operation (senz) [Nicholas *Senn*, American surgeon, 1844–1908] see under *operation* and *plate;* see also *Kader-Senn operation*, under *operation*.

senna (sen′ah) [USP], the dried leaflets of *Cassia senna* L. (Alexandria senna) or of *C. angustifolia* Vahl. (India or Tinnevelly senna), (Leguminosae). They contain sennoside A and B, glycosides of rhein, and chrysophanic acid. Used chiefly as a cathartic.

sennoside (sen′o-sīd) either of two anthraquinone glucosides, sennoside A and B, found in senna. A mixture of *sennosides A and B* [USP] is used as a cathartic, administered orally.

senograph (se′no-graf) the apparatus used in senography; also, the resultant film.

senography (se-nog′rah-fe) a low voltage, constant-potential x-ray technique designed especially for mammography.

Senokot (sen′ŏh-kot) trademark for preparations of senna.

senopia (se-no′pe-ah) [L. *senium* old age + Gr. *ōpē* sight + *-ia*] an apparent decrease in presbyopia in the elderly, which is related to the development of nuclear sclerosis and resultant myopia.

sensation (sen-sa′shun) [L. *sensatio*] an impression conveyed by an afferent nerve to the sensorium. **articular s.,** the sensation produced by the contact of moving joint surfaces. **cincture s.,** zonesthesia. **common s.** (Gemeingefühl), the general feeling superinduced by the summation of all the bodily sensation (E. H. Weber, 1846). **concomitant s.,** a secondary sensation, developed, without special stimulation, along with a primary sensation. **cutaneous s.,** dermal s. **delayed s.,** a sensation which is not perceived until some time after the application of the stimulation. **dermal s.,** a sensation that arises from a receptor situated in the skin. **epigastric s.,** a peculiar, weak, sinking or anxious feeling localized in the stomach; a visceral sensation of undefined nature. **external s.,** the effect produced upon the mind by an external object through the medium of the senses. **general s.,** a sensation felt throughout the body. **girdle s.,** zonesthesia. **gnostic s's,** sensations that are perceived by the more recently developed senses, such as those of light touch and the epicritic sensibility to muscle, joint, and tendon vibrations; called also *new sensations*. **internal s.,** a sensation perceptible only to the subject himself, and not connected with any object external to his body. **joint s.,** articular s. **light s.,** the sensation produced when radiant energy of wavelength from 400 to 760 mμ enters a normal eye. **negative s.,** the condition produced by a stimulation below the threshold. **new s's,** gnostic s's. **objective s.,** external s. **palmesthetic s.,** pallesthesia. **primary s.,** a sensation which is the direct result of the reception of a stimulus. **referred s.,** **reflex s.,** a sensation felt at a place other than the point of application of the stimulus. **skin s.,** dermal s. **strain s.,** a sensation as of a strain or straining. **subjective s.,** internal s. **transferred s.,** referred s. **vascular s.,** the sensation felt when there is a change in vascular tone, as in blushing. **s. of warmth,** the comfortable sensation experienced when the environment is not too cold, also the sensation felt when moderate heat is imparted to the body by radiation or contact.

sense (sens) [L. *sensus*, from *sentire* to perceive, feel] a faculty by which the conditions or properties of things are perceived. Hunger, thirst, malaise, and pain are varieties of sense; a sense of equilibrium, of well being (euphoria), and other senses are also distinguished. **chemical s.,** a general sense which causes avoidance reactions in water creatures and residual reactions in man to various irritants, such as onion, pepper, snuff, ammonia, and war gases. **color s.,** the faculty by which various colors are perceived and distinguished. **equilibrium s.,** static s. **form s.,** the ability of the eye to recognize objects as solid. **internal s.,** any sense that is normally stimulated from within the body. **kinesthetic s.,** muscle s. **labyrinthine s.,** static s. **light s.,** the faculty by which different degrees of brilliancy are distinguished. **muscle s., muscular s.,** the faculty by which muscular movements are perceived. **pain s.,**

the sense by which pain is perceived. **posture s.,** a variety of muscular sense by which the position or attitudes of the body or its parts are perceived. **pressure s.,** the faculty by which pressure upon the surface of the body is perceived; called also *baresthesia.* **proprioceptive s.,** proprioceptive sensibility. **seventh s.,** visceral s. **sixth s.,** the general feeling of consciousness of the entire body; cenesthesia. **space s.,** that combination of the senses (chiefly of sight and touch) which gives information as to the relative positions and relations of objects in space. **special s.,** any one of the five senses of seeing, feeling, hearing, taste, and smell. **static s.,** the sense that enables man to maintain an upright position. **stereognostic s.,** the sense by which form and solidity are perceived. **temperature s.,** the faculty by which a person is able to appreciate differences of temperature. **time s.,** the ability to appreciate time intervals, especially in sound and in music. **tone s.,** the power of distinguishing one tone from another. **visceral s.,** the internal and subjective sensations supposed to appertain to the ganglionic portion of the nervous system.

Sensibamine (sen-sib′ah-mīn) trademark for an equimolar mixture of ergotamine and ergotamine.

sensibilatrice (sen″sĭ-be″lah-trēs′) (obs.) antibody.

sensibiligen (sen″sĭ-bil′ĭ-jen) anaphylactogen.

sensibilin (sen″sĭ-bil′in) anaphylactin.

sensibilisin (sen″sĭ-bil′ĭ-sin) anaphylactin.

sensibilisinogen (sen″sĭ-bil′ĭ-sin′o-jen) anaphylactinogen.

sensibility (sen″sĭ-bil′ĭ-te) [L. *sensibilitas*] susceptibility of feeling; ability to feel or perceive. **bone s.,** pallesthesia. **common s.,** cenesthesia. **cortical s.,** the sensibility controlled by the cerebral cortex which is concerned with the recognition and discrimination of sensory impressions. **deep s.,** the sensibility to pressure and movement which exists after the skin area is made completely anesthetic. **electromuscular s.,** sensibility of muscles to electric stimulation. **epicritic s.,** the sensibility to gentle stimulations which furnishes the means for making fine discriminations of touch and temperature; this sensibility exists in the skin only. **joint s.,** arthresthesia. **mesoblastic s.,** deep s. **pallesthetic s., palmesthetic s.,** pallesthesia. **proprioceptive s.,** the largely ignored and unconscious sense that gives us knowledge of the position and state of muscles, joints, limbs, and other parts; see *proprioceptor*. **protopathic s.,** the sensibility to stimulations of pain and temperature which is low in degree and poorly localized. Such sensibility exists in the skin and in the viscera, and acts as a defensive agency against pathologic changes in the tissues. **recurrent s.,** sensibility exhibited in the anterior root of a spinal nerve when the distal portion is stimulated after division. **somesthetic s.,** proprioceptive s. **splanchnesthetic s.,** the consciousness or sensibility dependent on the splanchnic receptors. **vibratory s.,** pallesthesia.

sensibilization (sen″sĭ-bil-i-za′shun) 1. the act of making more sensitive. 2. sensitization.

sensibilizer (sen′sĭ-bil-īz″er) obsolete term for antibody.

sensible (sen′sĭ-b′l) [L. *sensibilis*] capable of sensation; perceptible to the senses.

sensiferous (sen-sif′er-us) [L. *sensus* sense + *ferre* to carry] transmitting sensations.

sensigenous (sen-sij′ĕ-nus) [L. *sensus* sense + Gr. *gennan* to produce] producing sensory impulses.

sensimeter (sen-sim′ĕ-ter) an instrument for measuring the degree of sensitiveness of anesthetic and hyperesthetic areas on the body.

sensitin (sen′sĭ-tin) a name suggested for a nonantigenic substance, prepared from a pathogenic agent (virus, bacterium, or fungus), capable of revealing sensitivity of the delayed type evoked by the agent, such as coccidioidin, histoplasmin, and avian and human tuberculin.

sensitinogen (sen″sĭ-tin′o-jen) a general term including all the antigens which have a sensitizing effect on the body or which produce a hypersusceptible condition, such as anaphylactogen and allergen.

sensitive (sen′sĭ-tiv) [L. *sensitivus*] able to receive or respond to stimuli; often used to mean abnormally responsive to stimulation, or responding quickly and acutely.

sensitivity (sen″sĭ-tiv′ĭ-te) the state or quality of being sensitive; often used to denote a state of abnormal responsiveness to stimulation, or of responding quickly and acutely. **proportional s.,** the relationship in which a response bears some quantitative algebraic relationship to the intensity of the stimulus.

sensitization (sen″sĭ-ti-za′shun) 1. the initial exposure of an individual to a specific antigen, resulting in an immune response; subsequent exposure then induces a much stronger (secondary or anamnestic) immune response. Said especially of such exposure resulting in a hypersensitivity reaction. 2. the coating of cells with antibody, as in complement-fixation tests and the Schultz-Dale test, as a preparatory step in eliciting an immunological reaction. 3. the preparation of a tissue or organ by one hormone so that it will respond functionally to the action of another. **active s.,** the sensitization that results from the injection of antigen into an animal. **autoerythrocyte s.,** see under *syndrome*. **passive s.,** the sensitization which results when blood serum containing specific antibodies or immune lymphoid cells from a sensitized animal is injected into a normal animal. **photodynamic s.,** the increased lethal effects of light on microorganisms when certain dyes are present in the solution. **protein s.,** that bodily state in which the individual is sensitive or hypersusceptible to some foreign protein. **Rh s.,** the process or state of becoming sensitized to the Rh factor (i.e., Rh antigen(s), especially D antigen) as when an Rh-negative woman is pregnant with an Rh-positive fetus.

sensitized (sen′sĭ-tīzd) rendered sensitive.

sensitizer (sen′sĭ-tīz-er) obsolete term for antibody.

sensitizin (sen′sĭ-ti′zin) anaphylactogen.

sensitogen (sen′sĭ-to-jen) any antigen that elicits sensitizing antibody formation in an atopic individual.

sensitometer (sen″sĭ-tom′ĕ-ter) a set of sensitive photographic plates for testing the reaction of the eye to light rays.

sensomobile (sen″so-mo′bil) moving in response to a stimulus.

sensomobility (sen″so-mo-bil′ĭ-te) the capacity of man or animals for movement in response to a sensory stimulus.

sensomotor (sen″so-mo′tor) sensorimotor.

sensor (sen′sor) something that senses; a device specifically designed to respond to a physical stimulus (light, heat, pressure, etc.) by generating an impulse that can be measured or otherwise interpreted, or used as a control.

sensorial (sen-so′re-al) [L. *sensorialis*] pertaining to the sensorium.

sensoriglandular (sen″so-re-glan′du-lar) producing glandular activity as one of the consequences of stimulation of the sensory nerves.

sensorimetabolism (sen″so-re-mě-tab′o-lizm) the production of some metabolic action as a result of stimulation of the sensory nerves.

sensorimotor (sen″so-re-mo′tor) both sensory and motor.

sensorimuscular (sen″so-re-mus′ku-lar) producing reflex muscular action in response to a sensory impression.

sensorineural (sen″so-re-nu′ral) of or pertaining to a sensory nerve; pertaining to or affecting a sensory mechanism and/or a sensory nerve (see under *deafness* and *hearing loss*).

sensorium (sen-so′re-um) [L. *sentire* to experience, to feel the force of] 1. a sensory nerve center. 2. the seat of sensation, located in the brain (s. *commu′ne*); the term is often used to designate the condition of a subject relative to his consciousness or mental clarity.

sensorivascular (sen″so-re-vas′ku-lar) producing vascular changes as a result of stimulation applied through the sensory nerves.

sensorivasomotor (sen″so-re-vas″o-mo′tor) sensorivascular.

sensory (sen′so-re) [L. *sensorius*] pertaining to or subserving sensation.

sensualism (sen′shu-al-izm) [L. *sensus* sense] the condition of being dominated by bodily passions.

sentic (sen′tik) pertaining to the communication of emotions, or to sentics.

sentics (sen′tiks) the scientific study of the communication of emotions, including their expression, recognition, and generation.

sentient (sen′she-ent) [L. *sentiens*] able to feel; sensitive; having sensation or feeling.

sepal (se′pal) one of the divisions of leaves of the calyx of a flower.

sepaloid (sep′ah-loid) resembling or shaped like a sepal.

separator (sep′ah-ra″tor) [L.] a device for effecting a separation; in dentistry, an appliance for forcing adjoining teeth apart. **Harris' s.,** see under *segregator*. **Luys' s.,** see under *segregator*.

separatorium (sep″ah-rah-to′re-um) an instrument used in separating the pericranium from the subjacent bone.

sepazonium chloride (sep″ah-zo′ne-um) chemical name: 1-[2-(2,4-dichlorophenyl)-2-[2,4-dichlorophenyl)methoxy]ethyl]-3-(2-phenylethyl)-1*H*-imidazolium chloride; a topical anti-infective, $C_{26}H_{23}Cl_5N_2O$.

sepedogenesis (sep″ĕ-do-jen′ĕ-sis) sepedonogenesis.

sepedon (sep′ĕ-don′) [Gr. *sēpedōn* rottenness, putrefaction] a septic condition; putridity.

sepedonogenesis (sep″ĕ-do″no-jen′ĕ-sis) [*sepedon* + Gr. *genesis* production] the production of septic conditions.

seperidol hydrochloride (sě-per′ĭ-dōl) chemical name: 4-[4-(4-chloro-α,α,α-trifluoro-*m*-toyl)-4-hydroxypiperidino-4′-fluoro-butyrophenone; a tranquilizer, $C_{22}H_{22}ClF_4NO_2 \cdot HCl$.

Sephadex (sef′ah-deks) trademark for gel particles of cross-linked dextran, used in gel filtration; particle size is graded for separating substances of various atomic weights.

sepia (se′pe-ah) [L.; Gr. *sēpia* cuttlefish] a dark brown, inspissated inky juice secreted by cuttlefish (*Sepia*), squidlike cephalo-

pod marine mollusks; also, the dark brown colored pigment originally prepared from the juice.

sepium (se′pe-um) [L.; Gr. *sēpia* cuttlefish] the bone or internal shell of the cuttlefish; cuttlebone. It is used in preparing polishing agents and tooth powder, and is hung in bird cages for the purpose of supplying supplementary lime.

sepsin (sep′sin) [Gr. *sēpsis* decay] a poisonous crystallizable substance from decaying yeast and from animal matter.

sepsis (sep′sis) [Gr. *sēpsis* decay] the presence in the blood or other tissues of pathogenic microorganisms or their toxins; the condition associated with such presence. **s. agranulocyt′ica,** agranulocytosis. **catheter s.,** a complication of intravenous catheterization in which sepsis occurs with no known locus and which resolves on removal of the catheter. **incarcerated s.,** an infection which is latent after the primary lesion has apparently healed, but which may be stirred into activity by a slight trauma. **s. intestina′lis,** poisoning from the eating of contaminated food, such as canned meats, ice cream, sausages, or cheese. **s. len′ta,** a condition produced by infection with α-hemolytic streptococci, characterized by a febrile illness with endocarditis. **mouse s., murine s.,** see under *septicemia*. **oral s.,** a disease condition in the mouth or adjacent parts which may affect the general health through the dissemination of toxins. **puerperal s.,** sepsis occurring after childbirth, due to matter absorbed from the parturient canal.

Sepsis violacea (sep′sis vi″o-la′se-ah) the common dung fly, which may be found in houses.

Sept. abbreviation for L. *sep′tem*, seven.

septa (sep′tah) [L.] plural of *septum*.

septal (sep′tal) pertaining to a septum; see also under *area*.

septan (sep′tan) [L. *septem* seven] recurring every seventh (sixth) day, as a fever.

septanose (sep′tah-nōs) a monosaccharide having a seven-numbered ring structure.

septate (sep′tāt) divided by a septum.

septation (sep-ta′shun) division into parts by a septum.

septatome (sep′tah-tōm) septotome.

septavalent (sep″tah-va′lent) septivalent.

septectomy (sep-tek′to-me) [*septum* + Gr. *ektomē* excision] excision of a portion of the nasal septum.

septemia (sep-te′me-ah) septicemia.

septic (sep′tik) [L. *septicus*; Gr. *sēptikos*] produced by or due to decomposition by microorganisms; putrefactive.

septicemia (sep″tĭ-se′me-ah) [*septic* + Gr. *haima* blood + -*ia*] systemic disease associated with the presence and persistence of pathogenic microorganisms or their toxins in the blood. Called also *blood poisoning*. **bronchopulmonary s.,** septicemia resulting from the aspiration of infected wound secretions into the trachea in operations on the larynx. **Bruce's s.,** brucellosis. **cryptogenic s.,** septicemia in which the focus of infection is not evident during life. **fowl s.,** a disease of fowls resembling fowl cholera caused by *Vibrio metschnikovii*, marked by diarrhea, hyperemia of the alimentary canal, and the presence of a blood-tinged yellowish liquid in the small intestine. **hemorrhagic s., s. hemorrhagica,** any of a group of animal diseases caused by *Pasteurella multocida*, marked by the presence of pneumonia and some hemorrhagic areas in the subcutaneous tissues, serous membranes, muscles, lymph glands, and throughout the internal organs. It includes fowl cholera, swine plague, and bovine and swine pneumonias. **s. hemorrhag′ica bo′vum,** hemorrhagic septicemia of cattle. **s. hemorrhag′ica bubalo′rum,** pasteurellosis in the buffalo. **s. hemorrhag′ica o′vum,** hemorrhagic septicemia of sheep. **lymphovenous s.,** infection of the deep cellular planes of the body. **melitensis s.,** brucellosis. **metastasizing s.,** pyemia. **morphine injector's s.,** melioidosis in man. **mouse s.,** an infectious disease of mice, due to *Erysipelothrix insidiosa*. **phlebitic s.,** pyemia. **plague s.,** septicemic plague. **s. plurifor′mis,** hemorrhagic septicemia of sheep. **puerperal s.,** see under *fever*. **rabbit s.,** pasteurellosis in rabbits. **sputum s.,** a form produced by inoculation of certain of the microorganisms of the sputum. **typhoid s.,** general infection with typhoid bacillus.

septicemic (sep″tĭ-se′mik) pertaining to, or of the nature of, septicemia.

septicine (sep′tĭ-sin) a ptomaine, or compound of hexylamine and amylamine, from putrid flesh.

septicophlebitis (sep″tĭ-ko-fle-bi′tis) [*septic* + *phlebitis*] inflammation of the veins, due to septicemia.

septicopyemia (sep″tĭ-ko-pi-e′me-ah) septicemia and pyemia combined. **cryptogenic s.,** spontaneous septicopyemia. **metastatic s.,** a form marked by septic deposits in the lungs caused by embolism from putrid thrombi. **spontaneous s.,** a variety developing without obvious cause or from a slight wound of the skin; called also *cryptogenic s.*

septicopyemic (sep″tĭ-ko-pi-e′mik) pertaining to septicopyemia.

septicozymoid (sep″tĭ-ko-zi′moid) a hypothetical substance supposed by some to supply the necessary feeding ground for septic processes.

septigravida (sep″tĭ-grav′ĭ-dah) [L. *septem* seven + *gravida* pregnant] a woman pregnant for the seventh time; also written gravida VII.

septile (sep′tīl) of or pertaining to a septum.

septimetritis (sep″tĭ-mĕ-tri′tis) [*septic* + *metritis*] septic inflammation of the uterus.

septineuritis (sep″te-noo-ri′tis) neuritis due to sepsis. **Nicolau's s.,** a generalized, diffuse neuritis of the entire nervous system due to the multiplication and migration of viruses in nervous tissue, as occurs in rabies.

septipara (sep-tip′ah-rah) [L. *septem* seven + *parere* to bring forth, produce] a woman who has had seven pregnancies which resulted in viable offspring; also written para VII or VII-para.

septivalent (sep″tĭ-va′lent) [L. *septem* seven + *valens* able] able to combine with or to replace seven hydrogen atoms.

septomarginal (sep″to-mar′ji-nal) pertaining to the margin of a septum.

septonasal (sep-to-na′zal) pertaining to the nasal septum.

septoplasty (sep″to-plas′te) [*septum* + Gr. *plassein* to form or mold] surgical reconstruction of the nasal septum.

septostomy (sep-tos′to-me) [*septum* + Gr. *stomoun* to provide with an opening] surgical creation of an opening in a septum. **balloon atrial s.,** surgical creation of an opening in the interatrial septum of the heart by passage of a balloon catheter from the right atrium through the septum to the left atrium, at which point the balloon is inflated and the catheter is then withdrawn to create an interatrial septal defect; performed in transposition of the great vessels with an intact septum.

septotome (sep′to-tōm) an instrument for operating on the nasal septum.

septotomy (sep-tot′o-me) [*septum* + Gr. *tomē* a cutting] the operation of incising the nasal septum.

septula (sep′tu-lah) [L.] plural of *septulum*.

septulum (sep′tu-lum), pl. *sep′tula* [L., dim. of *septum*] a small separating wall or partition; used in anatomical nomenclature as a general term to designate such a structure. **sep′tula tes′tis** [NA], septa of testis: connective tissue lamellae from the inner surface of the tunica albuginea, which unite to form the mediastinum testis.

septum (sep′tum), pl. *sep′ta* [L.] a dividing wall or partition; [NA] a general term for such a structure. The term is often used alone to refer to the septal area (see under *area*) or to the septum pellucidum. **s. alve′oli,** see *interalveolar s.* and *interradicular s.* **s. atri′orum cor′dis,** s. interatriale cordis. **atrioventricular s. of heart, s. atrioventricula′re cor′dis** [NA], the portion of the membranous part of the interventricular septum between the right atrium and left ventricle. **s. of auditory tube, s. canalis musculotubarii. s. auricula′rum,** s. interatriale cordis. **Bigelow's s.,** a layer of hard, bony tissue in the neck of the femur. **bony s. of eustachian canal,** s. canalis musculotubarii. **bony s. of nose,** s. nasi osseum. **bronchial s., s. bronchia′le,** carina tracheae. **bulbar s.,** a septum, formed by fusion of the bulbar ridges, that divides the bulbus cordis into aortic and pulmonary trunks. **s. bul′bi ure′thrae,** the fibrous septum dividing the interior of the bulb of the urethra into two approximately equal parts. **s. cana′lis musculotuba′rii** [NA], septum of musculotubal canal: the thin lamella of bone that divides the musculotubal canal into the semicanals for the tensor tympani muscle and the auditory tube. **s. cartilagin′eum na′si,** pars cartilaginea septi nasi. **cervical s., intermediate, s. cervica′le interme′dium** [NA], a glial–pia mater septum which dips into the posterior intermediate sulcus of the posterior funiculus of the cervical and upper lumbar parts of the spinal cord; it separates the fasciculus gracilis and fasciculus cuneatus. **cloacal s.,** urorectal s. **s. of Cloquet,** s. femorale. **s. corpo′rum cavernoso′rum clitor′idis** [NA], an incomplete fibrous septum between the two lateral halves of the clitoris. **crural s.,** s. femorale. **Douglas' s.,** the septum formed by the union of Rathke's folds, forming the rectum of the fetus. **enamel s.,** enamel cord. **femoral s., s. femora′le** [NA], **s. femora′le [Cloque′ti],** the thin fibrous membrane that helps to close the anulus femoralis; it is derived from the fascia transversalis, is perforated for the passage of lymphatic vessels, and is embedded in fat. **s. of frontal sinuses,** s. sinuum frontalium. **gingival s.,** the part of the gingiva interposed between adjoining teeth. **s. glan′dis pe′nis** [NA], **s. of glans penis,** an incomplete fibrous septum in the median plane of the glans penis, especially below the urethra. **gum s.,** gingival s. **hemal s.,** a structure of lower animals which in man is represented by the linea alba and the transversalis, iliac, and rectovesical fasciae. **interalveolar s.,** one of the partitions of bone separating the alveoli of different teeth (*septa interalveolaria mandibulae* [NA], and *septa interalveolaria maxillae* [NA]). **sep′ta interalveola′ria mandib′ulae** [NA], interalveolar septa of mandible: the partitions between the tooth sockets in the alveolar part of the mandible. **sep′ta interalveola′ria maxil′lae** [NA], interalveolar septa

of maxilla: the partitions between the tooth sockets in the alveolar process of the maxilla. **interatrial s. of heart, s. interatria′le cor′dis** [NA], **interauricular s.,** the wall that separates the atria of the heart; called also *s. atriorum cordis.* **interdental s.,** interalveolar s. **intermuscular s. of arm, external,** s. intermusculare brachii laterale. **intermuscular s. of arm, internal,** s. intermusculare brachii mediale. **intermuscular s. of arm, lateral,** s. intermusculare brachii laterale. **intermuscular s. of arm, medial,** s. intermusculare brachii mediale. **intermuscular s. of leg, anterior,** s. intermusculare anterius cruris. **intermuscular s. of leg, posterior,** s. intermusculare posterius cruris. **intermuscular s. of thigh, external,** s. intermusculare femoris laterale. **intermuscular s. of thigh, lateral,** s. intermusculare femoris laterale. **intermuscular s. of thigh, medial,** s. intermusculare femoris mediale. **s. intermuscula′re ante′rius cru′ris** [NA], **s. intermuscula′re ante′rius fibula′re,** anterior intermuscular septum of leg: a fascial sheet in the leg extending between the extensor digitorum longus and peroneal muscles to the anterior fibular crest. **s. intermuscula′re bra′chii latera′le** [NA], lateral intermuscular septum of arm: the fascial sheet extending from the lateral border of the humerus to the under surface of the fascia investing the arm; called also *s. intermusculare humeri laterale.* **s. intermuscula′re bra′chii media′le** [NA], medial intermuscular septum of arm: the fascial sheet extending from the medial border of the humerus to the under surface of the fascia investing the arm; called also *s. intermusculare humeri mediale.* **s. intermuscula′re fem′oris latera′le** [NA], lateral intermuscular septum of thigh: the fascial sheet in the thigh separating the vastus lateralis muscle from the biceps femoris. **s. intermuscula′re fem′oris media′le** [NA], medial intermuscular septum of thigh: the fascial sheet in the thigh separating the vastus medialis from the adductor and the pectineus muscles. **s. intermuscula′re hu′meri latera′le,** s. intermusculare brachii laterale. **s. intermuscula′re hu′meri media′le,** s. intermusculare brachii mediale. **s. intermuscula′re poste′rius cru′ris** [NA], **s. intermuscula′re poste′rius fibula′re,** posterior intermuscular septum of leg: the fascial sheet extending between the peroneal muscles and soleus to the lateral fibular crest. **interradicular s., s. interradicula′re,** one of the thin bony partitions separating the crypts of a dental alveolus occupied by the separate roots of a multi-rooted tooth. **interventricular s. of heart, s. interventricula′re cor′dis** [NA], the partition that separates the left ventricle from the right ventricle, consisting of a muscular and a membranous part; called also *s. ventriculorum cordis.* **s. intra-alveola′rium,** interradicular s. **Körner's s.,** petrosquamosal lamina. **s. lin′guae** [NA], **lingual s.,** the median vertical fibrous part of the tongue. **s. lu′cidum,** septum pellucidum. **mediastinal s., s. mediastina′le,** mediastinum, def. 2. **s. membrana′ceum na′si,** pars membranacea septi nasi. **s. membrana′ceum ventriculo′rum cor′dis,** pars membranacea septi interventricularis cordis. **membranous s. of nose,** pars membranacea septi nasi. **s. mo′bile na′si,** mobile s. of nose, pars mobilis septi nasi. **s. muscula′re ventriculo′rum cor′dis,** pars muscularis septi interventricularis cordis. **s. of musculotubal canal,** s. canalis musculotubarii. **nasal s., s. na′si** [NA], the partition separating the two nasal cavities in the midplane, composed of cartilaginous, membranous, and bony parts. **s. na′si os′seum** [NA], osseous septum of nose: the bone of the skull interposed between the openings of the nose, consisting primarily of the vomer below and the perpendicular plate of the ethmoid bone above. Called also *bony s. of nose.* **neural s.,** a prolongation, chiefly in the lower vertebrates, of the general investing fascia, extending medially from the surface toward the skeleton; represented in man by the ligamentum nuchae and the supraspinous and interspinous ligaments. **orbital s., s. orbita′le** [NA], a fibrous membrane anchored to the periorbita along the entire margin of the orbit, extending to the levator palpebrae superioris muscle in the upper lid and to the tarsal plate in the lower lid; called also *tarsal membrane.* **osseous s. of nose,** s. nasi osseum. **parietal s.,** cuspis posterior valvae atrioventricularis sinistrae. **s. pectinifor′me,** s. penis. **pellucid s., s. pellu′cidum** [NA], a triangular double membrane separating the anterior horns of the lateral ventricles of the brain; situated in the median plane, it is bounded by the corpus callosum and the body and columns of the fornix. **s. pe′nis** [NA], the fibrous sheet between the two corpora cavernosa of the penis, formed by union of the tunicae albugineae of the two sides. **pharyngeal s.,** the transitory partition which separates the mouth cavity from the pharynx in the embryo; called also *buccopharyngeal membrane.* **placental s.,** tissue that divides the placenta into cotyledons. **s. pon′tis,** raphe pontis. **posterior median cervical s., s. pos′ticum,** a glial–pia mater septum which dips into the posterior median sulcus of the spinal cord and separates the two posterior funiculi. **s. pri′mum,** a septum in the embryonic heart, dividing the primitive atrium into right and left chambers. **rectovaginal s., s. rectovagina′le** [NA], the membranous partition between the rectum and the vagina. **rectovesical s., s. rectovesica′le** [NA], a membranous partition separating the rectum from the prostate and urinary bladder. **s. re′nis,** see *columnae renales.* **s. scro′ti** [NA], **s. of scrotum,** a fibromuscular partition in the median plane, dividing the scrotum into two nearly equal parts. **s. secun′dum,** a septum in the embryonic heart to the right of the septum primum; after birth it fuses with the septum primum to close the foramen ovale. **s. si′nuum fronta′lium** [NA], septum of frontal sinuses: a thin lamina of bone, in the lower front part of the frontal bone, that lies more or less in the median plane and separates the frontal sinuses. **s. si′nuum sphenoida′lium** [NA], **sphenoidal s., s. of sphenoidal sinuses,** a thin lamina of bone in the body of the sphenoid bone, lying more or less in the median plane and separating the sphenoidal sinuses. **spurious s., s. spu′rium,** a structure formed by union of the two folds, one on either side, guarding the opening of the sinus venosus into the dorsal wall of the right atrium of the heart in the early embryo. **subarachnoidal s.,** an incomplete fibrous sheath which lies in the median plane and which connects the arachnoid to the pia mater along the posterior median sulcus of the cervical and upper thoracic parts of the spinal cord. **septa of testis,** septula testis. **s. of tongue,** s. linguae. **tracheoesophageal s.,** the septum that, during the fourth week of embryonic development, separates the trachea from the ventral surface of the foregut. **transverse s. of ampulla,** crista ampullaris. **s. tu′bae,** processus cochleariformis. **urorectal s.,** the caudally and outwardly growing wedge of endoderm-covered mesoderm that divides the cloaca into urogenital sinus and rectum; called also *cloacal s.* **s. of ventricles of heart, s. ventriculo′rum cor′dis,** s. interventriculare cordis.

septuplet (sep′tu-plet, sep-tup′let, sep-too′plet) [L. *septuplum* a group of seven] one of seven offspring produced in one gestation period.

seq. luce. abbreviation for L. *sequen′ti lu′ce,* the following day.

sequel (se′kwel) sequela.

sequela (se-kwe′lah), pl. *seque′lae* [L.] any lesion or affection following or caused by an attack of disease.

sequelae (se-kwe′le) [L.] plural of *sequela.*

sequence (se′kwens) a connected series of things or events. **nearest neighbor s.,** in biochemistry, the relative frequency with which pairs of the four nucleotide bases occur next to one another.

sequester (se-kwes′ter) [L.; Fr. *sequestrer* to shut up illegally] to detach or separate abnormally a small portion from the whole; see *sequestration* and *sequestrum.*

sequestra (se-kwes′trah) [L.] plural of *sequestrum.*

sequestral (se-kwes′tral) pertaining to or of the nature of a sequestrum.

sequestrant (se-kwes′trant) a sequestering agent, as, for example, cholestyramine resin, which binds bile acids in the intestine, thus preventing their absorption.

sequestration (se″kwes-tra′shun) [L. *sequestratio*] 1. the formation of a sequestrum. 2. the isolation of a patient. 3. a net increase in the quantity of blood within a limited vascular area, occurring physiologically, with forward flow persisting or not, or produced artificially by the application of tourniquets. **pulmonary s.,** loss of connection of lung tissue with the bronchial tree and with the pulmonary veins, the tissue receiving its arterial supply from the systemic circulation. The mass may be completely separated anatomically and physiologically from normally connected lung (*extralobar pulmonary s.*) or be in anatomical contiguity with and partly surrounded by normal lung (*intralobar pulmonary s.*).

sequestrectomy (se″kwes-trek′to-me) [*sequestrum* + Gr. *ektomē* excision] the surgical removal of a sequestrum.

sequestrotomy (se″kwes-trot′o-me) [*sequestrum* + Gr. *tomē* a cutting] sequestrectomy.

sequestrum (se-kwes′trum), pl. *seques′tra* [L.] a piece of dead bone that has become separated during the process of necrosis from the sound bone. **primary s.,** a sequestrum that is en-

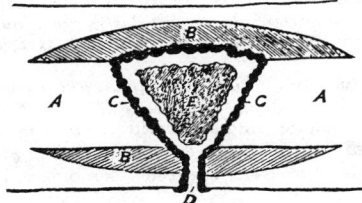

Illustrating the formation of a sequestrum: *A, A,* Sound bone; *B, B,* new bone; *C, C,* granulations lining involucrum; *D,* cloaca; *E,* sequestrum (DaCosta).

tirely detached. **secondary s.,** a sequestrum that is partially detached and may be pushed into place. **tertiary s.,** a sequestrum that is separated by only a slight dividing line and remains in its place.

sequoiosis (se″kwoi-o′sis) a form of allergic alveolitis due to in-

halation of and tissue reaction to dust from moldy redwood bark; species of *Graphium* provide the offending antigen.

Ser serine.

sera (se′rah) [L.] plural of *serum.*

seractide acetate (ser-ak′tīd) chemical name: 25-L-aspartic acid-26-L-alanine-27-glycine-30-L-glutamine-31-L-serine-α$^{1-39}$-corticotropin (pig); a synthetic adrenocorticotropic hormone, $C_{207}H_{308}N_{56}O_{58}S·(C_2H_4O_2)_x·xH_2O.$

seral (ser′al) of or pertaining or relating to a sere, as a seral stage.

seralbumin (se″ral-bu′min) serum albumin; the albumin of the blood.

serangitis (se″ran-ji′tis) [Gr. *sēranx* cavern + *-itis*] cavernitis.

serapheresis (se″rah-fĕ-re′sis) [*serum* + Gr. *aphairesis* removal] the production of serum by permitting the clotting of plasma derived by plasmapheresis.

Serapion (sĕ-ra′pe-on) **of Alexandria** (c. 280 B.C.) a Greek physician who is believed to have been one of the founders of the Empiric school of medicine.

Serax (ser′aks) trademark for a preparation of oxazepam.

sere (sēr) the entire sequence of ecological communities that successively occupy a given area, the transitory communities of which are called *seral stages,* or seral communities. The series finally lead to a stable, mature climax community.

serempion (se-rem′pe-on) a fatal form of measles occurring in the West Indies.

serendipity (ser″en-dip′ĭ-te) the discovery of some important scientific fact, by accident or sagacity, which was not the original objective of the quest.

Serenium (sĕ-re′ne-um) trademark for a preparation of ethoxazene hydrochloride.

Serenoa (ser″e-no′ah) [*Sereno* Watson] a genus of palms. *S. serrula′ta* is the saw palmetto or sabal of the southern United States. A fluidextract of the berries is diuretic, expectorant, and aphrodisiac, and has been used in diseases of the prostate and bladder.

Serentil (sĕ-ren′til) trademark for preparations of mesoridazine besylate.

seretin (ser′e-tin) carbon tetrachloride.

Serfin (ser′fin) trademark for a preparation of reserpine.

Sergent's white adrenal line (sār-zhawz′) [Emile *Sergent,* French physician, 1867–1943] see under *line.*

serglobulin (ser-glob′u-lin) paraglobulin.

serial (se′re-al) arranged in or forming a series.

serialograph (se″re-al′o-graf) an apparatus for making series of x-ray pictures.

sericin (ser′ĭ-sin) silk glue or silk gelatin; a protein, $C_{15}H_{25}N_5O_3,$ derivable from silk.

sericite (se′rĭ-sīt) a form of mica or muscovite, a complex silicate, causing pneumoconiosis.

Sericopelma (ser″ĭ-ko-pel′mah) a genus of huge hairy spiders of the family Theraphosidae. **S. commu′nis,** a large black species found in the Canal Zone whose venom is harmful to man.

series (sēr′ēz) [L. "row"] 1. a group or succession of objects or substances arranged in regular order or forming a kind of chain. In electricity, an arrangement of the parts of a circuit by connecting them successively to form a single path for the current. Parts thus arranged are in series. 2. a taxonomic category subordinate to a subclass and superior to an order, as the Basidiomycetes. **aliphatic s.,** the compounds having an open chain structure; see *open chain,* under *chain.* **aromatic s.,** the compounds derived from benzene. **erythrocyte s., erythrocytic s.,** the group of developing cells which sequentially and ultimately culminate in the mature erythrocytes. For immature forms in this series, see *normoblast.* **fatty s.,** methane and its derivatives and the homologous hydrocarbons. **granulocyte s., granulocytic s.,** the succession of developing cells that ultimately culminates in the mature granulocyte or granular leukocyte (*basophil, eosinophil,* or *neutrophil*); it begins with the myeloblast, which matures to form sequentially the promyelocyte, myelocyte, metamyelocyte, and mature segmented (polymorphonuclear) cell. Called also *myeloid, myelocytic,* or *leukocytic s.* See also *granular leukocytes,* under *leukocyte.* **Hofmeister s.,** the sequence of ions arranged with respect to their effects on the solubility of proteins, e.g., on their salting-out effects; called also *lyotropic s.* **homologous s.,** a series of compounds each member of which differs from the one preceding it by the radical $CH_2.$ **leukocytic s.,** granulocytic s. **lymphocyte s., lymphocytic s.,** the succession of developing cells that ultimately culminates in the lymphocyte; it begins with the lymphoblast which matures to form sequentially the lymphoblast, prolymphocyte, and mature lymphocyte. **lyotropic s.,** Hofmeister s. **monocyte s., monocytic s.,** the succession of developing cells that ultimately culminates in the monocyte; it begins with the monoblast, which matures to form sequentially the promonocyte and the mature cell. **myeloid s., myelocytic s.,** granulocytic s. **plasmacyte s., plasmacytic s.,** the succession of developing cells that ultimately culminates in the plasma cell; it begins with the plasmablast, which matures to form sequentially the proplasmacyte and the mature cell. **thrombocyte s., thrombocytic s.,** the succession of developing cells that ultimately culminates in the blood platelets (thrombocytes); it begins with the megakaryoblast, which matures to form sequentially the promegakaryocyte, megakaryocyte, and the mature cell.

seriflux (ser′ĭ-fluks) [L. *serum* whey + *fluxus* flow] a thin, watery discharge.

serifuge (se′rĭ-fūj) a small centrifuge for use with sera.

serine (ser′ēn) chemical name: 2-amino-3-hydroxypropionic acid. A naturally occurring, nonessential amino acid, $C_3H_7NO_3$. It may be synthesized from glycine, and is used as a dietary supplement and feed additive, in biological studies and tests, and in culture media.

serioscopy (se″re-os′ko-pe) roentgenographic visualization of the body in a series of parallel planes by means of multiple exposures. Two or more roentgenograms are taken from different directions. They are laid on each other and moved until the projections of the various planes of the object coincide consecutively.

seriscission (ser″ĭ-sizh′un) [L. *sericum* silk + *scindere* to cut] the division of soft tissues by an encircling silk ligature pulled tightly.

seroalbuminous (se″ro-al-bu′mĭ-nus) containing serum and albumin.

seroalbuminuria (se″ro-al-bu″mĭ-nu′re-ah) the presence in the urine of serum albumin.

seroanaphylaxis (se″ro-an″ah-fĭ-lak′sis) anaphylaxis produced by the use of blood serum.

serochrome (se′ro-krōm) [*serum* + Gr. *chrōma* color] the coloring matter of normal serum.

serocolitis (se″ro-ko-li′tis) inflammation of the serous surface of the colon.

seroconversion (se″ro-kon-ver′shun) the development of antibodies in response to infection or administration of a vaccine.

seroconvert (se″ro-kon-vert′) to develop antibodies in response to a vaccine.

seroculture (se′ro-kul-tūr) a bacterial culture on blood serum.

serocystic (se″ro-sis′tik) made up of serous cysts.

serodiagnosis (se″ro-di″ag-no′sis) diagnosis made by means of reactions taking place in the blood serum.

serodiagnostic (ser″ro-di″ag-nos′tik) pertaining to serodiagnosis.

seroenteritis (se″ro-en″tĕ-ri′tis) inflammation of the serous coat of the intestine.

seroenzyme (se″ro-en′zīm) an enzyme existing in the blood serum.

seroepidemiologic (se″ro-ep″ĭ-de″me-o-loj′ik) pertaining to serologic studies as used to delineate epidemiologic patterns of a disease.

seroepidemiology (se″ro-ep″i-de″me-ol′o-je) the study of disease in a human community by subjecting a portion of the population to a specific serologic test of immunity.

sero-fast (se′ro-fast′) serum-fast.

serofibrinous (se″ro-fib′rin-us) both serous and fibrinous.

serofibrous (se″ro-fi′brus) pertaining to serous and fibrous surfaces; as, *serofibrous* apposition.

seroflocculation (se″ro-flok″u-la′shun) flocculation produced in blood serum by an antigen. Cf. *Henry test,* under *tests.*

serofluid (se″ro-floo′id) a serous fluid.

serogastria (se″ro-gas′tre-ah) the presence of blood serum in the stomach; protein-losing gastropathy.

serogenesis (se″ro-jen′ĕ-sis) 1. the production of a serum. 2. the regular appearance of the natural antibodies during the life of an individual.

seroglobulin (se″ro-glob′u-lin) serum globulin; the globulin of the blood serum.

seroglycoid (se″ro-gli′koid) a glycoprotein found in serum albumin.

serohemorrhagic (se″ro-hem″o-raj′ik) characterized by serum and blood.

serohepatitis (se″ro-hep″ah-ti′tis) inflammation of the peritoneal coat which covers the liver; perihepatitis.

seroimmunity (se″ro-ĭ-mu′nĭ-te) immunity produced by antiserum; passive immunity.

serolactescent (se″ro-lak-tes′ent) resembling serum and milk.

serolemma (se″ro-lem′ah) [*serous* + Gr. *lemma* sheath] the membrane from which the serosa or chorion is developed.

serolipase (se″ro-li′pās) lipase from blood serum.

serologic, serological (se″ro-loj′ik; se″ro-loj′ĕ-kal) pertaining to serology.

serologist (se-rol′o-jist) one who is an expert in serology.

serology (se-rol′o-je) [*serum* + *-logy*] the study of antigen-antibody reactions in vitro. **diagnostic s.,** serodiagnosis.

serolysin (se-rol′ĭ-sin) a lysin present in the blood serum.

seroma (sēr-o′mah) a tumor-like collection of serum in the tissues.

seromembranous (se″ro-mem′brah-nus) both serous and membranous; composed of serous membrane.

seromucoid (se″ro-mu′koid) seromucous.

seromucous (se″ro-mu′kus) partly serous and partly mucous.

seromucus (se″ro-mu′kus) a secretion which is part serum and part mucus.

seromuscular (se″ro-mus′ku-lar) pertaining to the serous and muscular coats of the intestine.

Seromycin (ser′o-mi″sin) trademark for preparations of cycloserine.

seronegative (se″ro-neg′ah-tiv) serologically negative; showing negative results on serological examination; showing a lack of antibody.

seronegativity (se″ro-neg″ah-tiv′ĭ-te) the state of being seronegative, or of showing negative results on serological examination.

seroneutralization (se″ro-nu″tral-i-za′shun) neutralizing by use of serum.

seroperitoneum (se″ro-per″ĭ-to-ne′um) the presence of free fluid in the peritoneum; ascites.

seropheresis (se″ro-fĕ-re′sis) serapheresis.

serophysiology (se″ro-fiz″e-ol′o-je) the study of the physiologic mechanism of serum action.

seroplastic (se″ro-plas′tik) serofibrinous.

seropneumothorax (se″ro-nu″mo-tho′raks) pneumothorax with a serous effusion in the pleural cavity.

seropositive (se″ro-poz′ĭ-tiv) serologically positive; showing positive results on serological examination; showing a high level of antibody.

seropositivity (se″ro-poz″ĭ-tiv′ĭ-te) the state of being seropositive, or of showing positive results on serological examination.

seroprevention (se″ro-pre-ven′shun) a method of inducing passive immunity by the injection of immunoglobulins.

seroprognosis (se″ro-prog-no′sis) the prognosis of a disease based on study of its seroreactions.

seroprophylaxis (se″ro-pro″fĭ-lak′sis) the injection of immune serum or convalescent serum for protection purposes.

seropurulent (se″ro-pu′roo-lent) both serous and purulent.

seropus (se″ro-pus′) serum mingled with pus.

seroreaction (se″ro-re-ak′shun) a reaction occurring in a serum or as a result of the action of a serum. Cf. *fixation of the complement.*

serorelapse (se″ro-re-laps′) a definite rise in serological titer occurring after treatment.

seroresistant (se″ro-re-zis′tant) pertaining to seroresistance; showing a seropositive reaction to a pathogen after treatment.

seroresistance (se″ro-re-zis′tans) failure of the serological titer to fall satisfactorily after treatment.

seroreversal (se″ro-re-vers′al) a fall in serological titer after treatment.

serosa (se-ro′sah; se-ro′zah) 1. any serous membrane (tunica mucosa). 2. the tunica serosa. 3. the chorion.

serosal (se-ro′sal) pertaining to or composed of serosa.

serosamucin (se-ro″sah-mu′sin) a protein resembling mucin, found in inflammatory ascitic exudates.

serosanguineous (se″ro-sang-gwin′e-us) pertaining to or containing both serum and blood.

seroscopy (se-ros′ko-pe) [*serum* + Gr. *skopein* to examine] diagnostic examination of serum with the agglutinoscope.

serose (se′rōs) an albumose obtained from serum albumin.

seroserous (se″ro-se′rus) pertaining to two or more serous membranes.

serosites (se″ro-si′tĭ-dēz) plural of *serositis.*

serositis (se″ro-si′tis), pl. *serosites* [*serous membrane* + *-itis*] inflammation of a serous membrane. **multiple s.,** polyserositis.

serosity (se-ros′ĭ-te) the quality possessed by serous fluids.

serosurvey (se″ro-sur′va) a screening test of the serum of persons at risk to determine susceptibility to a particular disease.

serosynovial (se″ro-sĭ-no′ve-al) both serous and synovial.

serosynovitis (se″ro-sin″o-vi′tis) synovitis with effusion of serum.

serotherapeutical (se″ro-ther″ah-pu′tĭ-kal) pertaining to serotherapy.

serotherapist (se″ro-ther′ah-pist) one who treats disease by serotherapy.

serotherapy (se″ro-ther′ah-pe) [*serum* + Gr. *therapeia* treatment] the treatment of disease by the injection of blood serum from immune individuals, especially immunized animals.

serothorax (se″ro-tho′raks) hydrothorax.

serotonergic (se″ro-tōn-er′jik) serotoninergic.

serotonin (ser″o-to′nin) chemical name: 3-(2-aminoethyl)-5-indolol. A vasoconstictor, $C_{10}H_{12}N_2O$, found in various animals from coelenterates to vertebrates, in bacteria, and in many plants. In humans, it is released by the blood platelets and is found in high concentrations in many body tissues, including the intestinal mucosa, pineal body, and central nervous system. Produced enzymatically from tryptophan by hydroxylation and decarboxylation, serotonin has many physiologic properties; e.g., it inhibits gastric secretion, stimulates smooth muscle, serves as a central neurotransmitter, and is a precursor of melatonin. Called also *enteramine, thrombocytin, thrombotonin, 5-hydroxytryptamine,* and *5-HT.*

serotoninergic (ser″o-to′nin-er′gik) 1. containing or activated by serotonin, as the neurons of the raphe nuclei of the brain stem. 2. of or pertaining to neurons that secrete serotonin, which, in turn, stimulates release of pituitary hormones. Called also *serotonergic.*

serotoxin (se″ro-tok′sin) 1. a toxin formed in and from blood serum when the latter is treated with kaolin, barium sulfate, or in other ways. 2. anaphylatoxin, which is formed in the body and responsible for anaphylactic shock.

serotype (se′ro-tīp) 1. the type of a microorganism as determined by the kinds and combinations of constituent antigens present in the cell. 2. a taxonomic subdivision of bacteria based on the kinds and combinations of constituent antigens present in the cell, or a formula expressing the antigenic analysis on which such a subdivision is based. **heterologous s.,** a related but not identical serotype. **homologous s.,** an identical serotype.

serous (se′rus) [L. *serosus*] 1. pertaining to or resembling serum. 2. producing or containing serum, as a serous gland or cyst.

serovaccination (se″ro-vak″sĭ-na′shun) injection of serum combined with bacterial vaccination to produce passive immunity by the former and active immunity by the latter.

serozyme (se′ro-zīm) [L. *serum* + Gr. *zymē* yeast] (*obs.*) Bordet's name for the prothrombin present in the blood serum.

Serpasil (ser′pah-sil) trademark for preparations of reserpine.

serpentaria (ser″pen-ta′re-ah) [L. *serpens* snake] the dried rhizome and roots of *Aristolochia serpentaria,* Virginia snakeroot, and *A. reticulata,* or Texas snakeroot, herbs of North America. Serpentaria is an astringent bitter, the major bitter principle of which is aristolochic acid. Formerly used as an analgesic and in the treatment of snakebite.

Serpentes (ser′pen-tēz) *Ophidia.*

serpiginous (ser-pij′ĭ-nus) [L. *serpere* to creep] having a wavy or much indented margin, as a lesion in noduloulcerative cutaneous syphilis.

serrated (ser′āt-ed) [L. *serratus,* from *serra* saw] having a sawlike edge.

Serratia (sĕ-ra′she-ah) [named for Serafino *Serrati,* an Italian physicist of the 18th century] a genus of bacteria of the tribe Serratieae, family Enterobacteriaceae, order Eubacteriales. It is made up of small, motile, gram-negative rods which produce characteristic red pigments and are saprophytic on decaying plant or animal materials. The organisms are opportunistic pathogens, especially causing nosocomial infections. The type species is *S. marces′cens.* Formerly called *Erythrobacillus.*

Serratieae (ser″ah-ti′e-e) a tribe of the family Enterobacteriaceae, order Eubacteriales, made up of small, gram-negative rods which produce characteristic red pigments and are saprophytic on decaying plant or animal materials. It includes a single genus, *Serratia.*

serration (sĕ-ra′shun) [L. *serratio*] a structure or formation with teeth like those of a saw; the condition of being serrated.

serratus (ser-ra′tus) [L.] serrated.

serrefine (sār-fēn′) [Fr.] a small spring forceps for compressing bleeding vessels.

Serres' angle, glands (sārz) [Antoine Etienne Reynaud Augustin *Serres,* French physiologist, 1786–1868] see *metafacial angle,* under *angle,* and see under *gland.*

serrulate (ser′u-lāt) [L. *serrulatus*] marked or bordered with small serrations or projections.

Sertoli's cell, column (ser-to′lēz) [Enrico *Sertoli,* Italian histologist, 1842–1910] see under *cell* and *column.*

serum (se′rum), pl. *serums* or *se′ra* [L. "whey"] 1. the clear portion of any animal liquid separated from its more solid elements; especially the clear liquid (*blood s.*) which separates in the clotting of blood from the clot and the corpuscles. 2. blood serum from animals that have been inoculated with bacteria or their toxins. Such serum, when introduced into the body, produces passive immunization by virtue of the antibodies which it contains. 3. see *blood serum,* under B. **ACS s.,** antireticular cytotoxic s. **active s.,** a serum that contains complement. **allergenic s., allergic s.,** a serum which produces hypersensitiveness (anaphylaxis) to antigen injections. **anallergenic s., anallergic s.,** a serum which does not produce hypersensitiveness (anaphylaxis) to serum injections. **antibothropic s.,** serum used to produce immunization against the bites of rattlesnakes. **anti-**

cholera s., a serum made by injecting horses with killed and/or live cultures of *Vibrio cholerae,* or with toxins or other products of the germs. **anticomplementary s.,** a serum which interferes with or destroys the activity of complement. **anticrotalus s.,** an antivenomous serum which is protective against the poison of the rattlesnake. **antidiphtheric s.,** diphtheria antitoxin. **antihepatic s.,** serum of an animal into which has been injected liver matter from another animal; this serum is destructive to the liver of animals of the species from which the injected matter was taken. **antilymphocyte s., (ALS),** serum from animals immunized with lymphocytes from a different species; it is a powerful immunosuppressive agent that inhibits the humoral immune response and especially the cell-mediated immune response, its major effect being the destruction of the circulatory pool of lymphocytes. **antimeningococcus s.,** a polyvalent serum prepared by injecting first an autolysate of the strains and later living cultures (method of Flexner and Jobling); called also *Flexner's serum.* **antiophidic s.,** antivenomous s. **antipancreatic s.,** serum of an animal into which has been injected pancreatic extract from another animal; this serum is destructive to the pancreas of animals of the species from which the injected matter was taken. **antipertussis s.,** blood serum from patients convalescent from pertussis. **antipest s.,** antiplague s. **antiphagocytic s.,** a serum which destroys phagocytes. **antiplague s.,** a serum obtained from animals which have been repeatedly injected with killed or living plague microorganisms (*Pasteurella pestis*), or with both, or with some preparation of the microorganisms. **antiplatelet s.,** a serum that destroys blood platelets by lysis, agglutination, or by other mechanism. **antipneumococcus s. (horse),** a serum obtained from the blood of horses which have been injected with pneumococci of various types. **antipneumococcus s. (rabbit),** serum obtained from blood of rabbits immunized by cultures of pneumococci of any one of the several types. **antirabies s.** [USP], a sterile solution containing antiviral substances obtained from the blood serum or plasma of a healthy animal, usually the horse, that has been immunized against rabies by means of vaccine; used as a passive immunizing agent. **antireticular cytotoxic s.,** a serum made by inoculating horses with an extract of spleen and bone marrow; said to have, in small doses, a stimulating effect on the reticuloendothelial system, and in large doses a cytotoxic effect on that system. Abbreviated ACS. Called also *Bogomolets' s.* **antisarcomatous s.,** serum from an animal into which has been injected sarcoma tissue has been injected. **antiscarlatinal s.,** see *Dick's s.* and *Moser's s.* **anti-snakebite s.,** antivenomous s. **antispermotoxic s.,** antispermotoxin. **antistaphylococcus s.,** a serum raised by injection of a staphylococcus vaccine (e.g., autogenous vaccine) into a suitable animal. **antistreptococcus s.,** a serum obtained from the blood of animals which have been injected with killed or living streptococci or with both. **antitetanic s. (A.T.S.),** tetanus antitoxin. **antitoxic s.,** a serum which contains antitoxin. **antitubercle s.,** a serum prepared by injecting an animal with killed or with living tubercle bacilli (*Mycobacterium tuberculosis*) or with both or with a preparation of the microorganisms. **antitularense s.,** Foshay's s. **antityphoid s.,** serum containing antibody to the typhoid bacillus. **antivenomous s.,** a serum used as a remedy for snake bite, prepared from the blood of animals which have been immunized against the venom of serpents; called also *Calmette's s.* See also *antivenin.* **articular s.,** synovia. **bacteriolytic s.,** a serum which contains the bacteriolysin of a microorganism. **Banzhaf's s.,** a concentrated and purified antipneumococcus serum. **Bardel's s.** (*obs.*), a mixture of sodium chloride, phenol, sodium phosphate, sodium sulfate, and water. **Bargen's s.,** a serum prepared from cultures of an organism from the lesions of chronic ulcerative colitis. **blister s.,** the serous fluid found in a blister. **Blondel's s.,** the serum of fresh milk, prepared by filtration after coagulation and neutralization. **blood s.,** see *blood serum,* under B. **Bogomolets' s.,** antireticular cytotoxic s. **Calmette's s.,** antivenomous s. **Cattani's s.,** a mixture of sodium chloride, sodium carbonate, and boiled distilled water, for injection in infectious diseases. **Cheron's s.,** a mixture of crystalline phenol, sodium chloride, sodium phosphate, sodium sulfate, and boiled distilled water; formerly used for injection in infectious diseases. **chicken s.,** serum containing antibodies, prepared by the immunization of chickens. **convalescence s., convalescent s., convalescents' s.,** blood serum from a patient who is convalescent from an infectious disease; such a serum was once used as a prophylactic injection in such diseases as measles, scarlet fever, whooping cough, etc. **cytotropic s.,** a serum containing cytotropic antibodies. **despeciated s.,** serum which has lost its species-specific qualities. **Dick's s., Dochez's s.,** antitoxic serum once used for the treatment of scarlet fever, obtained by immunizing horses with the toxin of the streptococcus of scarlet fever. **Dopter's s.,** a serum effective against the parameningococcus. **Dorset-Niles s.,** a serum for immunizing against hog cholera. **Dunbar's s.,** an antitoxin from the pollen of ragweed, goldenrod, rye, etc.; used in the treatment of hay fever. **endotheliolytic s.,** serum which destroys endothelial cells; it is obtained from the blood of animals immunized with endothelial cells. **s. equi′num,** horse s. **Felix Vi s.,** a typhoid antiserum rich in Vi (virulence) antibodies. **Felton's s.,** a concentrated antipneumococcus horse serum. **Flexner's s.,** antimeningococcus s. **foreign s.,** serum from an animal to be injected into one of another species. **Foshay's s.,** a serum once used in the treatment of tularemia. **gastrotoxic s.,** a serum toxic to the gastric mucous membrane. **glycerin s.,** blood serum which contains 5 per cent of glycerin; used as a culture medium for tubercle bacilli. **heterologous s.,** 1. serum obtained from an animal belonging to a species different from that of the recipient. 2. serum prepared from an animal immunized by an organism differing from that against which it is to be used. **Hoffmann's s.,** epitheliolysin. **hog cholera s.,** serum obtained from hogs having some immunity, either following recovery from an attack of the disease or as a result of an injection of hog cholera serum, made hyperimmune by intravenous injection, at intervals of three to four weeks, of blood from a hog sick with hog cholera; once used in the prevention and in the cure of hog cholera. **homologous s.,** 1. serum obtained from an animal belonging to the same species as the recipient. 2. serum prepared from an animal immunized by the same organism against which it is to be used. **horse s.,** serum obtained from the blood of horses. **hyperimmune s.,** a serum unusually rich in antibody, obtained by a vigorous course of active immunization. **immune s.,** a serum containing one or more antibodies, especially one in which the antibody content has been increased by recovery from its specific infection or by injection with its specific antigen. **inactivated s.,** serum which has been heated to 56° C. for 30 minutes, to destroy the lytic activity of contained complement components. **leukocytolytic s.,** serum that destroys leukocytes; it is from the blood of animals immunized with leukocytes. **leukotoxic s.,** a serum that destroys leukocytes. **Löffler's s.,** see *Löffler's blood serum,* under *blood serum.* **lymphatolytic s.,** serum which destroys lymphatic tissues, such as the spleen and lymph glands. **Merz's s.,** a preparation containing hamamelis extract in tubes for use in hemorrhoids. **monovalent s.,** antiserum containing antibody to only one strain or species of microorganism or only one kind of antigen. **Moser's s.,** antistreptococcus serum produced by inoculating horses with several kinds of streptococci from the blood of scarlet fever patients. **motile s.,** an immune serum containing flagellar agglutinins. **multipartial s.,** polyvalent s. **muscle s.,** muscle plasma deprived of its myosin. **nephrolytic s., nephrotoxic s.,** a serum having a specific toxic effect on the kidney, produced by immunizing an animal with a brei or emulsion of kidney tissue. **neurolytic s., neurotoxic s.,** a serum having a specific toxic effect on the brain and spinal cord, produced by immunizing an animal with a brei or emulsion of nerve tissue. **normal s.,** serum from a normal untreated animal. **pericardial s.,** liquor pericardii. **petit s.,** a nonsensitizing, nontoxic, but vaccinating substance derived from serum by mixing with 2 parts of 90 per cent alcohol, treating the resulting precipitate with physiologic salt solution, and filtering. Cf. *Vaughan's split products,* under *product.* **plague s.,** antiplague s. **polyvalent s.,** antiserum containing antibody to more than one strain or species of microorganism or to more than one kind of antigen; it is produced by mixing monovalent sera or by immunizing the animal with multiple antigen. **pooled s.,** the mixed serum from a number of individuals. **pregnancy s.,** blood serum taken from pregnant women. **prophylactic s.,** a serum for immunizing against a disease. **Roux's s.,** diphtheria antitoxin. **salvarsanized s.,** blood serum taken from a patient after an intravenous injection of salvarsan; see *Swift-Ellis treatment,* under *treatment.* **Sanarelli's s.,** a serum used in protective inoculation against yellow fever. **specific s.,** antiserum containing antibody to a specific microorganism or antigen. **streptococcus s.,** antistreptococcus s. **thymotoxic s.,** a serum which has a specific toxic effect on thymus tissue. **thyrolytic s., thyrotoxic s.,** a serum having a specific destructive or toxic effect on thyroid tissue. **truth s.,** a misnomer for the drugs sometimes employed to facilitate interviews; especially applied to sodium amobarbital and sodium thiopental when used in criminal interrogation. The agent used is not a serum and its use does not guarantee truthfulness. **Yersin's s.,** antiplague s.

serumal (se-roo′mal) pertaining to or formed from serum.

serum-fast (se′rum-fast) resistant to the destructive effect of serum; said of bacteria.

serumuria (se″rum-u′re-ah) albuminuria.

Serv. abbreviation for L. *ser′va,* keep, preserve.

Servetus (ser-ve′tus), Michael (1511–1553). A Spanish theologian who also wrote, among other subjects, on geography, astrology, and medicine. His *Christianismi restitutio* (1553) contains the first printed description of the lesser circulation; Servetus was burned at the stake for heresy the same year, and only three copies of the book have survived.

servomechanism (ser″vo-mek′ah-nizm) a control system in which feedback is used to control errors in another system. The term is also applied to biological systems, such as the mechanism that controls the diameter of the pupil of the eye according to the amount of incident light.

sesame (ses′ah-me) [L. *sesamum;* Gr. *sēsamon*] the plant *Sesa-*

mum indicum L.; also its oil-bearing seeds. The oil, called oil of benne, is used as olive oil. The seeds are demulcent, and are used as a laxative. Currently also used in topical skin lotions, as an emollient, and as a parenteral vehicle for intramuscular injections.

sesamoid (ses′ah-moid) [L. *sesamoides;* Gr. *sēsamon* sesame + *eidos* form] 1. denoting a small nodular bone embedded in a tendon or joint capsule. 2. a sesamoid bone. See under *bone.*

sesamoiditis (ses″ah-moi-di′tis) inflammation of the sesamoid bones and surrounding structures of a horse's foot.

sesqui- [L. *sesqui* a half more] a prefix meaning one and a half.

sesquih. abbreviation for L. *sesquiho′ra,* an hour and a half.

sesquihora (ses″kwe-ho′rah) [L.] an hour and a half.

sesquioxide (ses″kwe-ok′sid) a compound of three parts of oxygen with two of another element.

sesquisulfate (ses″kwe-sul′fāt) a sulfate containing three parts of sulfuric acid united with two of another element.

sesquisulfide (ses″kwe-sul′fid) a sulfide containing three parts of sulfur united with two of another element.

sessile (ses′il) [L. *sessilis*] attached by a base; not pedunculated or stalked.

Sessinia (ses-sin′e-ah) a genus of blistering beetles, coconut beetles, of certain Pacific islands.

sesunc. abbreviation for L. *sesun′cia,* an ounce and a half.

set (set) 1. to align bones or bone fragments, as in reducing a fracture. 2. in psychology, a readiness to perceive or respond in a certain way because of past experience, requirements of a task, etc. **phalangeal s.,** a surgical office procedure for correction of deformities of the lesser toes, involving incision to reach the bony joint and manipulation for proper positioning.

seta (se′tah), pl. *se′tae* [L.] 1. bristle. 2. any bristle-like structure, such as the multicellular stalk of certain plants.

setaceous (se-ta′shus) [L. *setaceus; seta* bristle] slender and rigid, like a bristle.

Setaria (se-ta′re-ah) a genus of filarial nematodes. **S. cer′vi, S. cervi′na,** *S. labiatopapillosa.* **S. equi′na,** a species found in the abdominal cavity of the horse and related species, buffalo, cattle, and sometimes man. **S. labiatopapillo′sa,** a species found in the peritoneal cavity of cattle and various game animals in Africa.

Setchenow's centers (nuclei) (sech′ĕ-nofs) [Ivan Mikhailovich *Setchenow,* Russian neurologist, 1829– 1905, the father of Russian physiology and neurology] see under *center.*

setiferous (se-tif′er-us) [L. *seta* bristle + *ferre* to bear] bearing bristles; covered with bristles.

setigerous (se-tij′er-us) [L. *seta* bristle + *gerere* to carry] setiferous.

seton (se′ton) [Fr. *seton;* L. *seta* bristle] a thread of silk, linen, or other finely drawn material for passage through a sinus, fistula, or epithelial tract, often to serve as a guide for subsequent dilatation with instruments of larger diameter.

setup (set′up) the arrangement of teeth on a trial denture base. **diagnostic s.,** a procedure involving dissection of teeth from a plaster model and repositioning of the teeth in desired positions to aid in case analysis preliminary to constructing an appliance.

Seutin's bandage (su-tanz′) [Louis Joseph *Seutin,* Brussels surgeon, 1793–1862] see under *bandage.*

Sever's disease (se′verz) [James Warren *Sever,* Boston orthopedic surgeon, born 1878] see under *disease.*

sevoflurane (se-vo-floo′rān) chemical name: fluoromethyl-2,2,2-trifluoro-1-(trifluoromethyl)ethyl ether; an inhalation anesthetic, $C_4H_3F_7O$.

sevum (se′vum) [L.] suet.

sewage (su′ij) the matters found in sewers; it consists of the excreta of man and animals, and other waste material from homes and other structures inhabited by man. **activated s.,** sewage mixed with activated sludge. **domestic s.,** sewage from dwellings, business buildings, factories, or institutions. **septic s.,** sewage undergoing anaerobic putrefaction.

sex (seks) [L. *sexus*] 1. the fundamental distinction, found in most species of animals and plants, based on the type of gametes produced by the individual or the category into which the individual fits on the basis of that criterion; ova, or macrogametes, are produced by the female, and spermatozoa, or microgametes, are produced by the male, the union of these distinctive germ cells being the natural prerequisite for the production of a new individual in sexual reproduction. 2. to determine the sex of an organism. **chromosomal s.,** sex as determined by the presence of the XX (female) or the XY (male) genotype in somatic cells, and without regard to phenotypic manifestations; called also *genetic s.* **endocrinologic s.,** the phenotypic manifestations of sex determined by endocrine influences, such as breast development, etc. **genetic s.,** chromosomal s. **gonadal s.,** the sex as determined on the basis of the gonadal tissue present, whether ovarian or testicular. **morphological s.,** sex determined on the basis of the morphology of the external genitals. **nuclear s.,** the sex as determined on the basis of the presence or absence of sex chromatin in somatic cells, its presence normally indicating the XX (female) genotype, and its absence the XY (male) genotype.

psychological s., the self-image of the gender role of an individual. **social s.,** the complex of attitudes, expectations, etc., that a society attaches to the male and female roles.

sex-conditioned (seks″kon-dish′und) sex-influenced.

sexdigitate (seks-dij′ĭ-tāt) [L. *sex* six + *digitus* digit] having six fingers on the hand or six toes on the foot.

sexduction (seks-duk′shun) in bacterial genetics, the process whereby part of the bacterial chromosome is attached to the autonomous F factor (sex factor) and thus is transferred with high frequency from the donor (male) bacterium to the recipient (female); called also *F-duction.*

sex-influenced (seks-in′floo-enst) denoting an autosomal trait that is expressed differently, either in frequency or degree, in males and females, as for example, the trait of baldness; called also *sex-conditioned.*

sexivalent (sek-siv′ah-lent) [L. *sex* six + *valere* to have power] able to combine with or displace six atoms of hydrogen.

sex-limited (seks-lim′it-ed) denoting a genetic trait exhibited by one sex only, although not determined by an X-linked gene.

sex-linked (seks-linkt′) determined by a gene located on a sex chromosome. Although a trait may be X-linked or Y-linked, virtually all clinically significant sex-linked traits are transmitted by genes located on the X chromosome, and the terms sex-linked and X-linked are used synonymously.

sexology (seks-ol′o-je) that branch of science which deals with sex and sexual relations from the biological point of view.

sexopathy (seks-op′ah-the) abnormality or perversion of sexual expression.

sextan (seks′tan) [L. *sextanus* of the sixth] recurring every sixth day; said of fevers.

sextigravida (seks″tĭ-grav′ĭ-dah) [L. *sextus* sixth + *gravida* pregnant] a woman pregnant for the sixth time; also written gravida VI.

sextipara (seks-tip′ah-rah) [L. *sextus* sixth + *parere* to bring forth, produce] a woman who has had six pregnancies which resulted in viable offspring; also written para VI or VI-para.

sextuplet (seks′tu-plet) [L. *sextus* sixth] one of six offspring produced in one gestation period.

sexual (seks′u-al) [L. *sexualis*] 1. pertaining to sex. 2. a person considered in his sexual relations. **contrary s.,** a sexual invert.

sexuality (seks″u-al′ĭ-te) 1. the characteristic quality of the male and female reproductive elements. 2. the constitution of an individual in relation to sexual attitudes or activity. **pregenital s.,** the sexuality of early infantile life before object love and the genital zone have become dominant.

Seyderhelm's solution (si′der-helmz) [Richard *Seyderhelm,* Göttingen physician, 1888–1940] see under *solution.*

S.-G. Sachs-Georgi test.

S.G.O. Surgeon-General's Office.

SGOT serum glutamic-oxaloacetic transaminase; see *glutamic-oxaloacetic transaminase,* under *transaminase.*

SGPT serum glutamic-pyruvic transaminase; see *glutamic-pyruvic transaminase,* under *transaminase.*

SH serum hepatitis.

shadow (shad′o) 1. an attenuated image of an actual object, as a faded or colorless erythrocyte. 2. a figure or image created by the interruption of light or other rays, such as the representation on a roentgenogram of radiopaque structures. **bat's wing s.,** a roentgenographic shadow that radiates through both lungs from the hilar region toward the periphery, leaving a clear zone at the apices, periphery, and bases. **blood s.,** a phantom corpuscle. **heart s.,** the shadow of the heart on a roentgenogram. **Purkinje's s's,** see under *image.*

shadow-casting (shad″o-kast′ing) a technique for increasing the visibility of ultramicroscopic specimens under the microscope by applying a coating of chromium, gold, or other metal.

shadowgram, shadowgraph (shad′o-gram, shad′o-graf) roentgenogram.

shadowgraphy (shad′o-graf″e) roentgenography.

Shaffer's method (sha′ferz) [Philip Anderson *Shaffer,* American biochemist, born 1881] see under *method.*

shaft (shaft) a long slender part, such as the portion of a long bone between the wider ends or extremities; see also *diaphysis* [NA]. **s. of femur,** corpus femoris. **s. of fibula,** corpus fibulae. **hair s.,** scapus pili. **s. of humerus,** corpus humeri. **s. of metacarpal bone,** corpus ossis metacarpalis. **s. of metatarsal bone,** corpus ossis metatarsalis. **s. of penis,** corpus penis. **s. of phalanx of fingers,** corpus phalangis digitorum manus. **s. of phalanx of toes,** corpus phalangis digitorum pedis. **s. of radius,** corpus radii. **s. of rib,** corpus costae. **s. of tibia,** corpus tibiae. **s. of ulna,** corpus ulnae.

shakes (shāks) a vernacular term for the cold paroxysm of intermittent fever. **hatter's s.,** mercury poisoning among fur

hat workers. **kwaski s.,** a condition seen in children who, having been severely malnourished, suffer rhythmic twitches and shaking a week or two after introduction of a better diet. The "shakes" gradually disappear over a period of a few weeks. **spelter s.,** metal fume fever seen among brass-founders. **Teflon s.,** polymer fume fever.

shamanism, shamanismus (sham′ah-nizm; sham″ah-niz′mus) a state of excitement into which certain Dyaks and other people are able to throw themselves for religious purposes.

sham-feeding (sham-fēd′ing) sham feeding; see under *feeding.*

shank (shangk) a leg, or leglike part.

shaping (shāp′ing) a behavior therapy technique in which new behavior is produced by providing reinforcement for progressively closer approximations of the final desired behavior. Called also *successive approximation.*

Sharpey's fibers (shar′pēz) [William *Sharpey,* English anatomist and physiologist, 1802–1880] see under *fiber.*

shashitsu (shah-shit′soo) scrub typhus.

shear (shēr) an applied force that tends to cause an opposite but parallel sliding motion of the planes of an object. Also, the strain resulting from such force.

Shear's test (sherz) [Murray Jacob *Shear,* American chemist, born 1899] see under *tests.*

sheath (shēth) [L. *vagina;* Gr. *thēkē*] a tubular structure enclosing or surrounding some organ or part. **arachnoid s.,** the delicate membrane between the pial and dural sheaths of the optic nerve. **bulbar s.,** see *vagina bulbi.* **carotid s.,** a portion of the cervical fascia enclosing the carotid artery, the internal jugular vein, and the vagus nerve. **caudal s.,** a tubular cytoplasmic structure at the base of the nucleus in the early spermatid. **chordal s.,** notochordal s. **common s. of tendons of peroneal muscles,** vagina synovialis musculorum peroneorum communis. **common s. of testis and spermatic cord,** fascia spermatica interna. **connective tissue s. of Key and Retzius,** endoneurium, especially the delicate continuation around terminal branches of nerve fibers. **crural s.,** femoral s. **dentinal s.,** the layer of tissue forming the wall of a dentinal tubule. **dural s.,** the external investment of the optic nerve, overlying the arachnoid sheath. **enamel rod s's,** envelopes of organic tissue enclosing the enamel rods. **epithelial s. of Hertwig, epithelial root s. of Hertwig,** root s., def 1. **s. of eyeball,** vagina bulbi. **fascial s. of prostate,** the sheath, derived from the rectovesical fascia, which surrounds the prostate. **female s.,** vagina (def. 2). **femoral s.,** the fascial covering of the proximal portion of the femoral vessels, derived from the intra-abdominal fascia; the most medial portion of the sheath, separated by a septum, forms the canalis femoralis. Called also *crural s.* **fibrous s's of fingers,** vaginae fibrosae digitorum manus. **fibrous s. of optic nerve,** vagina externa nervi optici. **fibrous s. of spermatozoon,** the fibrous sheath surrounding the principal piece of the tail of a spermatozoon. **fibrous s. of tendon,** vagina fibrosa tendinis. **fibrous s's of toes,** vaginae fibrosae digitorum pedis. **s. of Henle,** connective tissue s. of Key and Retzius. **s. of Hertwig,** root s., def. 1. **s. of Key and Retzius,** connective tissue s. of Key and Retzius. **lamellar s.,** perineurium. **masculine s.,** utriculus prostaticus. **Mauthner's s.,** axolemma. **medullary s.,** myelin s. **mitochondrial s.,** the sheath of circumferentially oriented mitochondria arranged end to end, which surrounds the middle piece of a spermatozoon and is thought to control the movements of the tail. **mucous s's,** bursa synovialis and vaginal synoviales. **mucous s., intertubercular,** septum intermusculare anterius cruris. **mucous s. of tendon,** vagina synovialis tendinis. **mucous s's of tendons of fingers,** vaginae synoviales digitorum manus. **mucous s's of tendons of toes,** vaginae synoviales digitorum pedis. **myelin s.,** the sheath surrounding the axon of some (the myelinated) nerve cells, consisting of concentric layers of myelin, formed in the peripheral nervous system by the plasma membrane of Schwann cells, and in the central nervous system by oligodendrocytes. It is interrupted at intervals along the length of the axon by gaps known as nodes of Ranvier. Myelin is an electrical insulator that serves to speed the conduction of nerve impulses. **Neumann's s.,** dentinal s. **neurilemmal s.,** neurilemma. **notochordal s.,** an elastic sheath surrounding the notochord. **nucleated s.,** neurilemma. **s's of optic nerve,** vaginae nervi optici. **s. of optic nerve, external,** vagina externa nervi optici. **s. of optic nerve, internal,** vagina interna nervi optici. **perinephric s.,** the sheath of fascia investing the kidney. **perivascular s.,** a pia glial membrane which accompanies blood vessels into the brain. **pial s.,** the innermost of the three sheaths of the optic nerve, underlying the arachnoid sheath. **s. of plantar tendon of long peroneal muscle,** vagina tendinis musculi peronei longi plantaris. **primitive s.,** neurilemma. **prism s's,** enamel rod s's. **s. of rectus abdominis muscle,** vagina musculi recti abdominis. **root s.,** 1. an investment of epithelial cells around the unerupted tooth and inside the dental follicle which are derived by budding from the enamel organ; called also *s. of Hertwig.* 2. the epithelial portion of the hair follicle, divided into an *inner root sheath* (hair cuticle plus the layers of Huxley and

Henle) and an *outer root sheath* from which the sebaceous gland is derived. **Scarpa's s.,** fascia cremasterica. **Schwalbe's s.,** the thin envelope of an elastic fiber. **s. of Schwann,** neurilemma. **Schweigger-Seidel s.,** a spindle-shaped thickening in the walls of the second portion of the arterial branches forming the penicilli in the spleen. See *sheathed artery,* under *artery.* **spiral s.,** a heavily staining filament winding around the axial filament of the middle piece of a spermatozoon. **s. of styloid process,** vagina processus styloidei. **synovial s. of bicipital groove,** vagina synovialis intertubercularis. **synovial s. of intertubercular groove,** vagina synovialis intertubercularis. **synovial s. of tendon,** vagina synovialis tendinis. **synovial s. of tendons of foot,** vaginae synoviales digitales pedis. **tendinous s's of flexor muscles of fingers,** vaginae fibrosae digitorum manus. **tendinous s's of flexor muscles of toes,** vaginae fibrosae digitorum pedis. **tendinous s. of leg,** fascia cruris. **tendinous s. of long peroneal muscle, plantar,** vagina tendinis musculi peronei longi plantaris. **tendon s. of anterior tibial muscle,** vagina tendinis musculi tibialis anterioris. **tendon s's of long extensor muscles of toes,** vaginae tendinum musculi extensoris digitorum pedis longi. **tendon s's of long flexor muscles of toes,** vaginae tendinum musculi flexoris digitorum pedis longi. **tendon s. of posterior tibial muscle,** vagina synovialis tendinis musculi tibialis posterioris.

sheep-pox (shēp-poks) a highly infectious and sometimes fatal eruptive disease of sheep, spread by both direct and indirect contact, and caused by a virus closely related to the vaccinia virus. A form affecting man is known as *ecthyma contagiosum.* Called also *orf, ovinia,* and *ovine smallpox.*

sheet (shēt) a rectangular piece of cotton, linen, etc., for a bed covering. **draw s.,** a folded sheet placed under a patient in bed so that it may be withdrawn without lifting the patient. **drip s.,** a wet sheet from which the water is wrung out and which is then wrapped around a patient standing in a tub of water. **secretory s.,** the simplest form of multicellular gland, consisting of secreting cells alone, e.g., the surface epithelium of the mammalian gastric mucosa.

shelf (shelf) a shelflike structure, normal or abnormal, in the body. **buccal s.,** the surface of the mandible from the residual alveolar ridge or the alveolar ridge to the external oblique line in the region of the lower buccal vestibule; it is covered with cortical bone. **dental s.,** the shelflike epithelial invagination formed by the dental ridge, beneath which the dental papillae are formed. **mesocolic s.,** the transverse mesocolon and the great omentum taken together. **palatine s.,** see *lateral palatine process* and *median palatine process,* under *process.*

shell (shel) a covering or encasement, such as the calcareous, horny, or chitinous covering of an animal. **egg s.,** the thin, hard, brittle, outer covering of an egg; called also *testa ovi.*

shellac (shĕ-lak′) a product of lac from India, produced on various plants by an insect, *Laccifer lacca* Kerr (Coccidae); sometimes used in dentistry and surgery, and in coating confections and medicinal tablets.

Shenton's line (arch) (shen′tonz) [Thomas *Shenton,* English radiologist] see under *line.*

Shepherd's fracture (shep′ards) [Francis John *Shepherd,* Canadian surgeon, 1851–1929] see under *fracture.*

Sherman unit (shur′man) [Henry Clapp *Sherman,* American biochemist, 1875–1955] Sherman-Munsell unit.

Sherman-Bourquin unit (shur′man boor′kwin) [Henry C. *Sherman;* Ann *Bourquin,* American nutritionist, born 1897] see under *unit.*

Sherman-Munsell unit (shur′man-mun′sel) [Henry C. *Sherman;* Hazel E. *Munsell,* American nutritionist, born 1891] see under *unit.*

Sherrington's law (sher′ing-tonz) [Sir Charles Scott *Sherrington,* English physiologist, 1857–1952, noted for his work on physiology of the nervous system; co-winner, with Edward Douglas Adrian, of the Nobel prize for physiology and medicine in 1932] see under *law.*

shield (shēld) any protecting structure. **Buller's s.,** a watch glass fitted over the eye to guard it from infection. **embryonic s.,** the double-layered disk from which the embryo proper develops. **eye s.,** a covering for the eyes to protect them from light or injury. **lead s.,** in radiology, a lead barrier for protecting personnel from radiation. **nipple s.,** a cover to protect the nipple of a nursing woman. **oral s.,** a removable appliance used in orthodontic treatment, usually between the buccal mucosa and the teeth; see *vestibular screen,* under *screen.* **phallic s.,** a device for the antiseptic protection of the male genitals during surgical operations.

shift (shift) a change, as of position, status, etc. **chloride s.,** the exchange of chloride (Cl) and bicarbonate (HCO₃⁻) between the plasma and the red blood cells which takes place whenever HCO₃⁻ is generated or decomposed within the red cells. Called also *Hamburger's phenomenon.* **Doppler s.,** the magnitude of the change in frequency caused by the Doppler effect. **s. to the left,** Arneth's term for a preponderance of young neutrophils in the blood picture. **Purkinje s.,** shift of the region of maxi-

mum visual intensity in the spectrum from the yellow toward the violet as intensity of illumination diminishes. **regenerative blood s.,** the rapid outpouring of leukocytes of the juvenile and myelocyte type, occurring as the result of an acute stimulus to the bone marrow. **s. to the right,** Arneth's term for a preponderance of older neutrophils in the blood picture.

Shiga's bacillus, toxin (she′gahz) [Kiyoshi *Shiga,* Japanese physician, 1870–1957] see *Shigella dysenteriae* type 1, and see under *toxin.*

Shigella (shǐ-gel′ah) [Kiyoshi *Shiga*] a genus of microorganisms of tribe Salmonelleae, family Enterobacteriaceae, order Eubacteriales, made up of nonmotile, rod-shaped, gram-negative bacteria. These microorganisms, which cause dysentery and for that reason are called dysentery bacilli, are separated into the non-mannitol-fermenting and the mannitol-fermenting type; the former make up Group A, and the latter are subdivided into Groups B, C, and D, each group making up a species. See *S. boydii, S. dysenteriae, S. flexneri,* and *S. sonnei.* **S. alkales′cens,** a name given a serologically homogeneous group of microorganisms occasionally causing diarrheal disease in man; culturally and serologically distinct from other *Shigella* species, they are serologically related to coliform bacilli and are formally classified with them as *Escherichia alkalescens.* **S. ambig′ua,** *S. dysenteriae* type 2. **S. arabinotar′da type A,** a dysentery bacillus identical with *S. dysenteriae* type 3. **S. arabinotar′da type B,** a dysentery bacillus identical with *S. dysenteriae* type 4. **S. boy′dii,** the species name given to Group C dysentery bacilli, the cause of an acute diarrheal disease in man, especially in tropical regions; culturally identical with *S. flexneri* but serologically unrelated, the species includes 15 independent numbered serotypes. **S. ceylonen′sis,** a dysentery-like bacillus, occasionally associated with diarrheal disease in man, and classified with the coliform bacilli as *Escherichia dispar* var. *ceylonensis.* **S. dispar,** a slow lactose-fermenting dysentery bacillus of limited or doubtful pathogenicity; serologically heterogeneous but related to some types of *S. flexneri.* Now formally classified with the coliform bacilli as *Escherichia dispar.* **S. dysente′riae,** the species name given to Group A dysentery bacilli, and separated into numbered serotypes. TYPE 1, the classic Shiga bacillus, which is set apart from other dysentery bacilli by the production of a potent exotoxin, is more common in tropical regions and causes severe dysentery. TYPE 2, the Schmitz bacillus, is a non-mannitol-fermenting organism serologically related to *Escherichia coli* type 0112. Of limited pathogenicity, but occasionally the cause of epidemic diarrheal disease in man, the organism has been found in the chimpanzee but not in other lower animals. The other numbered types include the Large-Sachs group of parashiga bacilli (see *S. parashigae*). Formerly called *Bacillus dysenteriae* and *Bacterium dysenteriae.* **S. etou′sae,** *S. boydii* type 7, Lavington, type T, type 1296/7. **S. flexne′ri,** a species name given to Group B dysentery bacilli, one of the commonest causes of acute diarrheal disease in man, occurring as eight related serotypes, designated by numbers 1 to 6 and letters X and Y. Called also *S. paradysenteriae* and *Flexner's bacillus.* **S. madampen′sis,** a dysentery-like bacillus, occasionally associated with diarrheal disease in man, and classified with the coliform bacilli as *Escherichia dispar* var. *madampensis.* **S. new′castle,** *S. flexneri* type 6, Boyd 88. **S. paradysente′riae,** *S. flexneri.* **S. parashi′gae,** a name formerly given to a group of non-mannitol-fermenting dysentery bacilli serologically differentiable from the Shiga bacillus (now *S. dysenteriae* type 1); also known as the Large-Sachs group of parashiga bacilli, they are now known as *S. dysenteriae,* types 3 to 7, inclusive. **S. schmit′zii,** *S. dysenteriae* type 2. **S. shi′gae,** *S. dysenteriae* type 1. **S. son′nei,** a species name given to Group D dysentery bacilli, one of the commonest causes of bacillary dysentery in temperate climates; slow (5–14 days) lactose fermenters, the organisms are serologically homogeneous, but two antigens, designated I and II, occur in varying proportions. Called also *Sonne-Duval bacillus* and formerly *Bacterium sonnei.* **S. wake′field,** a species name given a paracolon bacillus.

shigella (shǐ-gel′ah), pl. *shigel′lae.* An individual organism of the genus *Shigella.*

shigellae (shǐ-gel′e) plural of *shigella.*

shigellosis (shǐ″gel-lo′sis) the condition produced by infection with organisms of the genus *Shigella.* See individual species under *Shigella,* and *bacillary dysentery,* under *dysentery.*

shikimene (shik′ǐ-mēn) sikimin.

shin (shin) 1. the crest or anterior edge of the tibia. 2. the anterior aspect of the leg below the knee. **bucked s's,** sore s's. **cucumber s.,** a tibia which is curved with the concavity anteriorly. **saber s.,** a tibia with a marked anterior convexity as seen in congenital syphilis, yaws, and osteitis deformans. Called also *Fournier's sign.* **sore s's,** periostitis of the large metacarpal or metatarsal bone of the horse.

shingles (shing′g′lz) [L. *cingulus*] herpes zoster.

shiver (shiv′er) 1. a slight chill or tremor. 2. to tremble, as from a chill.

shivering (shiv′er-ing) 1. involuntary trembling or quivering of the body caused by contraction or twitching of the muscles, a physiologic method of heat production in man and other mammals. 2. a disease of horses characterized by trembling or quivering of various muscles.

shock (shok)   1. a sudden disturbance of mental equilibrium.   2. a condition of acute peripheral circulatory failure due to derangement of circulatory control or loss of circulating fluid. It is marked by hypotension, coldness of the skin, usually tachycardia, and often anxiety. See also under *therapy*. **allergic s.**, anaphylactic s.   **anaphylactic s.**, a violent attack of symptoms produced by a second injection of serum or protein and due to anaphylaxis; see *anaphylaxis*. **anaphylactoid s.**, colloidoclasia. **anesthesia s.**, a shocklike condition caused by an overdose of anesthetic. **apoplectic s.**, apoplexy (def. 1). **asthmatic s.**, status asthmaticus. **bomb s.**, a condition of dread and loss of emotional equilibrium among children in the British Isles, as a result of repeated bombings. **break s.**, the shock produced by breaking the electric current as it is passing through the body. **burn s.**, shock resulting from the loss of plasma into a burn wound. **cardiac s.**, heart s. **cardiogenic s.**, shock resulting from diminution of cardiac output in heart disease, as in myocardial infarction. **cerebral s.**, a form of shock sometimes occurring in severe head injury affecting the centers of cardiovascular control. **colloid s.**, pseudoanaphylaxis. **colloidoclastic s.**, see *colloidoclasia*. **deferred s., delayed s.**, severe physical or mental disturbance, of which the symptoms occur a considerable time after the injury or mental impression is received. **diastolic s.**, the cardiac impulse which strikes the palpating hand in early diastole. **electric s.**, the effects produced by the passage of an electric current through any part of the body. When the current is intense, it may cause (*a*) reversible loss of consciousness or death, owing to effects on the nervous system or heart, (*b*) coagulation of tissue and resultant necrosis due to heat, and (*c*) violent tetanic muscular contractions which may lead to injury. See also *electroconvulsive therapy*, under *therapy*. **endotoxic s., endotoxin s.**, septic shock due to release of endotoxins by gram-negative bacteria. **epigastric s.**, the systemic effect of a sudden blow upon the epigastrium. **erethismic s.**, a form of shock in which the patient is excited and restless. **faradic s.**, the effect produced by faradization. **gravitation s.**, peripheral circulatory collapse on assumption of the erect position. **heart s.**, a sudden collapse of the functions of the heart. **hematogenic s.**, shock due to diminished blood volume; hypovolemic shock. **hemoclastic s.**, hemoclastic crisis. **hemorrhagic s.**, hematogenic shock resulting from hemorrhage. **histamine s.**, the reaction, resembling anaphylactic shock, which follows the injection of histamine. **hypnoclastic s.**, interruption of sleep by sudden awakening. **hypoglycemic s.**, insulin s. **hypovolemic s.**, hematogenic s. **insulin s.**, a condition of circulatory insufficiency resulting from overdosage with insulin which causes too sudden reduction of blood sugar. It is marked by tremor, sweating, vertigo, diplopia, convulsions, and collapse. See also *insulin coma therapy*, under *therapy*. **irreversible s.**, a condition in which the changes produced cannot be corrected by treatment, and death is inevitable. **liver s.**, a serious collapse which sometimes follows sudden relief of common bile duct obstruction of long duration. **micro s.**, the reaction produced by a preliminary injection of a small amount of a substance, as an antiserum, so that a therapeutic dose will not cause a serious reaction; see *skeptophylaxis*. **neurogenic s.**, shock due to action of the nervous system producing vasodilatation. **oligemic s.**, hematogenic s. **osmotic s.**, the destructive effect on certain phages of rapid reduction in osmotic pressure produced by dilution of the medium in which they have been suspended. **paralytic s.**, a sudden paralytic attack. **peptone s.**, protein s. **pleural s.**, a condition sometimes following thoracocentesis, and characterized by cyanosis, pallor, dilated pupils, and disturbance of pulse and respiration. **postoperative s.**, a state of shock following a surgical operation. **postpartum s.**, a condition of shock following childbirth. **protein s.**, a state of acute intoxication manifested by a chill with fever, spasm of the bronchi, acute emphysema, and vomiting and diarrhea, produced by the intravenous injection of peptone or other substance of protein nature, such as bacterial proteins, animal or vegetable proteins, organic extracts, and the like. **psychic s.**, a shocklike condition produced by strong emotion. **secondary s.**, shock appearing one or more hours after injury; delayed shock. **septic s.**, shock developing in the presence of severe infections, especially following bacteremia with gram-negative bacteria and release of endotoxins (*endotoxin s.*). **serum s.**, see *serum sickness*, under *sickness*, and see *anaphylactic s.* **shell s.**, a term in use during World War I to describe a condition of lost nervous control with numerous psychic symptoms, ranging from extreme fear to actual dementia, produced in soldiers under fire by the noise and concussion from bursting shells; it would now be classified as an adjustment reaction of adult life. **spinal s.**, the loss of spinal reflexes after injury of the spinal cord which affects the muscles innervated by the cord segments situated below the site of the lesion. **surgical s.**, shock that occurs during or after surgical operation. **testicular s.**, the effect of a sharp blow upon the testes. **thyroxin s.**, thyrotoxic symptoms produced by overdoses of thyroxin. **torpid s.**, shock in which the patient lies prostrate and immobile. **traumatic s.**,

any shock produced by trauma, whether psychic or physical. **vasogenic s.**, shock caused by marked vasodilatation.

shoe (shoo)   a covering or appliance for the foot.   **Charlier's s.**, a horse's shoe which allows the sole and the frog to come to the ground exactly as in the unshod foot.   **Scarpa's s.**, a metal brace used in treating talipes equinus by preventing plantar extension of the foot beyond a right angle.

Shope papilloma (shōp) [Richard Edwin *Shope*, American pathologist, born 1902]   rabbit papilloma.

shortsightedness (short-sīt'ed-nes)   myopia.

shot-compressor (shot'kom-pres"or)   see under *compressor*.

shot-silk   see under *retina*.

shotty (shot'e)   like shot; resembling the lead pellets used in shotgun cartridges.

shoulder (shōl'der)   the junction of the arm and trunk; also that part of the trunk which is bounded at the back by the scapula. **bull's-eye s.**, a horse's shoulder having on it a loose flabby disk of hyperplastic skin with a central denuded surface.   **drop s.**, depression of one shoulder below the level of the other.   **frozen s.**, adhesive capsulitis.   **knocked-down s.**, separation or dislocation of the shoulder at the acromioclavicular joint occurring in athletes. Called also *shoulder separation*.   **loose s.**, a condition seen in progressive muscular atrophy in which, when attempts to lift the patient by grasping the upper arms at their sides are made, the arms move up but the trunk remains behind.   **stubbed s.**, sprain of the shoulder joint occurring in athletes.

shoulder-blade (shōl'der-blād)   the scapula.

shoulder slip (shōl'der slip)   inflammation and atrophy of the shoulder muscles and tendons in the horse; called also *sweeny*.

show (sho)   the appearance of blood as a forerunner of labor or menstruation.

shower (show'er)   a sudden emission or appearance. **uric acid s.**, temporary increase in the uric acid contents of the urine; occurring in the course of a gouty attack.

Shrady's saw (shra'dēz) [George Frederick *Shrady*, New York surgeon, 1837–1907]   see under *saw*.

Shrapnell's membrane (shrap'nelz) [Henry Jones *Shrapnell*, English anatomist and Army surgeon, 19th century]   pars flaccida membranae tympani.

shunt (shunt)   1. to turn to one side; to divert; to bypass.   2. a passage or anastomosis between two natural channels, especially between blood vessels. Such structures may be formed physiologically (e.g., to bypass a thrombosis), or they may be structural anomalies (see *cardiovascular s.*).   3. a surgically created anastomosis; also, the operation of forming a shunt.   **arteriovenous**

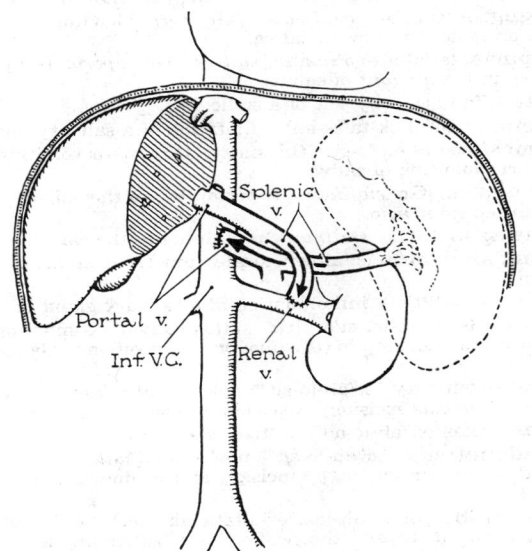

Portal shunts, showing two types of portal to systemic venous shunt. (Blakemore and Vorhees, Jr.)

(A-V) s., direct passage of blood from an artery to a vein. Also a U-shaped plastic tube inserted between an artery and a vein (usually between the radial artery and cephalic vein), bypassing the capillary network; commonly done to allow repeated access to the arterial system for the purpose of hemodialysis.   **cardiovascular s.**, an abnormality of blood flow between the sides of the heart or between the systemic and pulmonary circulation; see *left-to-right s.* and *right-to-left s.*   **hexose monophosphate s.**, pentose phosphate pathway.   **left-to-right s.**, diversion of blood from the left side of the heart to the right side or from the systemic to the pulmonary circulation through an anomalous opening such as a septal defect or patent ductus arteriosus. **LeVeen peritoneovenous s.,** the diversion of blood flow from the jugular vein through plastic tubing which passes through the peritoneal cavity and back to the venous circulation; a valve in the tubing permits absorption of fluid to relieve intractable ascites. **pentose s.,** pentose phosphate pathway. **peritoneovenous s.,** LeVeen peritoneovenous s. **portacaval s., postcaval s.,** surgical creation of an anastomosis between the portal vein and vena cava. **reversed s.,** right-to-left s. **right-to-left s.,** diversion of blood from the right side of the heart to the left side or from the pulmonary to the systemic circulation through an anomalous opening such as a septal defect or patent ductus arteriosus; called also *reversed s.* **ventriculoatrial s.,** the surgical creation of a communication between a cerebral ventricle and a cardiac atrium by means of a plastic tube, to permit drainage of cerebrospinal fluid for relief of hydrocephalus. **ventriculoperitoneal s.,** a communication between a cerebral ventricle and the peritoneum by means of plastic tubing; done for the relief of hydrocephalus.

Shwartzman's phenomenon (reaction) (shwarts'manz) [Gregory *Shwartzman*, Russian bacteriologist in the United States, 1896–1965] see under *phenomenon.*

SI Système International d'Unités, or International System of Units. See *SI unit,* under *unit.*

S.I. soluble insulin.

Si chemical symbol for *silicon.*

siagantritis, siagonantritis (si″ag-an-tri′tis; si″ag-on-an-tri′tis) [Gr. *siagōn* jaw bone + *antritis*] (*obs.*) inflammation of the maxillary sinus.

siagonagra (si″ag-o-nag′rah) [Gr. *siagōn* jaw bone + *agra* seizure] (*obs.*) pain in the maxilla.

sial- see *sialo-.*

sialaden (si-al′ah-den) [Gr. *sial-* + Gr. *adēn* gland] a salivary gland.

sialadenectomy (si″al-ad″ĕ-nek′to-me) sialoadenectomy.

sialadenitis (si″al-ad″ĕ-ni′tis) inflammation of a salivary gland. **chronic nonspecific s.,** an inflammatory disease of the major salivary glands characterized by intermittent swelling of the glands, which may progress to the development of fibrous masses; it is caused by obstruction of the salivary ducts with subsequent pyogenic bacterial infection.

sialadenography (si″al-ad″ĕ-nog′rah-fe) radiography of the salivary glands and ducts.

sialadenosis (si″al-ad″ĕ-no′sis) noninflammatory swelling of the salivary glands.

sialadenotomy (si″al-ad″ĕ-not′o-me) sialoadenotomy.

sialagogic (si″ah-lah-goj′ik) promoting the flow of saliva.

sialagogue (si-al′ah-gog) [sial- + Gr. *agōgos* leading] an agent that promotes the flow of saliva.

sialaporia (si″al-ah-po′re-ah) [sial- + Gr. *aporia* lack] deficiency in the amount of saliva.

sialate (si′ah-āt) any salt of a sialic acid.

sialectasia (si″al-ek-ta′se-ah) dilatation of a salivary duct.

sialemesis (si″al-em′ĕ-sis) [Gr. *sial-* + Gr. *emesis* vomiting] the hysteric vomiting of saliva.

sialic (si-al′ik) [Gr. *sialikos*] 1. pertaining to the saliva. 2. pertaining to sialic acid.

sialine (si′ah-lin) [L. *sialinus*] pertaining to the saliva.

sialism, sialismus (si′al-izm; si″al-iz′mus) [Gr. *sialismos*] ptyalism.

sialitis (si″ah-li′tis) inflammation of a salivary gland or duct.

sialo-, sial- (si′ah-lo, si′al) [Gr. *sialon* saliva] combining form denoting relationship to (*a*) saliva or to the salivary glands or (*b*) sialic acid.

sialoadenectomy (si″ah-lo-ad″ĕ-nek′to-me) [sialo- + Gr. *adēn* gland + *ektomē* excision] excision of a salivary gland.

sialoadenitis (si″ah-lo-ad″ĕ-ni′tis) sialadenitis.

sialoadenotomy (si″ah-lo-ad″ĕ-not′o-me) [sialo- + Gr. *adēn* gland + *tomē* a cutting] incision and drainage of a salivary gland.

sialoaerophagia (si″ah-lo-a″er-o-fa′je-ah) [sialo- + Gr. *aēr* air + *phagein* to eat + *-ia*] the swallowing of saliva and air.

sialoangiectasis (si″ah-lo-an″je-ek′tah-sis) [sialo- + Gr. *angeion* vessel + *ektasis* distention] dilatation of the salivary ducts.

sialoangiitis (si″ah-lo-an″je-i′tis) inflammation of the salivary ducts.

sialoangiography (si″ah-lo-an″je-og′rah-fe) radiography of the ducts of the salivary glands after injection of radiopaque material.

sialoangitis (si″ah-lo-an-ji′tis) sialoangiitis.

sialocele (si′ah-lo-sēl″) [sialo- + Gr. *kēlē* tumor] a salivary cyst or tumor.

sialodochitis (si″ah-lo-do-ki′tis) [sialo- + Gr. *dochos* receptacle + *-itis*] inflammation of the salivary ducts.

sialodochoplasty (si″ah-lo-do′ko-plas″te) [sialo- + Gr. *dochos* re-

ceptacle + *plassein* to form] plastic operation on the salivary ducts.

sialoductitis (si″ah-lo-duk-ti′tis) sialoangiitis.

sialogastrone (si″ah-lo-gas′trōn) a substance in saliva reputed to inhibit gastric secretion and motility.

sialogen (si′ah-lo-jen) an agent that induces salivation.

sialogenous (si″ah-loj′ĕ-nus) [sialo- + Gr. *gennan* to produce] producing saliva.

sialogogic (si″ah-lo-goj′ik) sialagogic.

sialogogue (si-al′o-gog) sialagogue.

sialogram (si-al′o-gram) [sialo- + Gr. *gramma* a mark] a radiograph produced by sialography.

sialograph (si-al′o-graf) sialogram.

sialography (si″ah-log′rah-fe) [sialo- + Gr. *graphein* to write] radiographic demonstration of the salivary ducts by means of the injection of substances opaque to x-radiation.

sialolith (si-al′o-lith) [sialo- + Gr. *lithos* stone] salivary calculus, def. 1.

sialolithiasis (si″ah-lo-lĭ-thi′ah-sis) [sialo- + Gr. *lithiasis* formation of a stone] the formation of salivary calculi or concretions within a salivary gland or duct.

sialolithotomy (si″ah-lo-lĭ-thot′o-me) [sialolith + Gr. *tomē* a cutting] incision of a salivary gland or duct for the removal of a calculus.

sialology (si″ah-lol′o-je) [sialo- + *-logy*] the study of the saliva.

sialoma (si″ah-lo′mah) a salivary tumor.

sialometaplasia (si″ah-lo-met″ah-pla′ze-ah) metaplasia of the salivary glands. **necrotizing s.,** a self-healing disease of the hard and soft palates marked by one or two deeply excavating ulcers; histologically, there is necrosis of the mucous cells of the minor salivary glands with partial replacement by squamous epithelium.

sialomucin (si″ah-lo-mu′sin) a component of the airway secretions of the lungs.

sialophagia (si″ah-lo-fa′je-ah) [sialo- + Gr. *phagein* to eat] the excessive swallowing of saliva.

sialorrhea (si″ah-lo-re′ah) [sialo- + Gr. *rhoia* flow] ptyalism. **s. pancreat′ica,** the expectoration of fluid resembling saliva or pancreatic juice, sometimes seen in disease of the pancreas.

sialoschesis (si″ah-los′kĕ-sis) [sialo- + Gr. *schesis* suppression] suppression of the salivary secretion.

sialosemeiology (si″ah-lo-se″mi-ol′o-je) [sialo- + *semeiology*] analysis of the saliva as a means of determining the physiologic status of the patient, especially in regard to metabolic processes.

sialosis (si″ah-lo′sis) [sial- + *-osis*] 1. the flow of saliva. 2. ptyalism.

sialostenosis (si″ah-lo-stĕ-no′sis) [sialo- + Gr. *stenos* narrow] stenosis, or narrowing, of a salivary duct.

sialosyrinx (si″ah-lo-si′rinks) [sialo- + Gr. *syrinx* pipe] 1. a salivary fistula. 2. a syringe for washing out the salivary ducts, or a drainage tube for the salivary ducts.

sialotic (si″ah-lot′ik) pertaining to or marked by the flow of saliva.

sib (sib) [Anglo-Saxon *sib* kin] 1. a blood relative; one of a group of persons all of whom are descendants of a common ancestor. 2. sibling.

sibbens (sib′enz) a form of treponematosis formerly prevalent in Scotland; considered to have been nonvenereal syphilis.

sibilant (sib′ĭ-lant) [L. *sibilans* hissing] of a shrill, hissing, or whistling character.

sibilus (sib′ĭ-lus) [L.] a whistling or sibilant rale.

sibling (sib′ling) [Anglo-Saxon *sib* kin + *ling* a diminutive] any of two or more offspring of the same parents; a brother or sister. Called also *sib.*

sibship (sib′ship) 1. relationship by blood. 2. a group of persons all of whom are descendants of a common ancestor, commonly used as the basis of study to determine genetic influences. 3. a group of siblings.

Sibson's aponeurosis (fascia), furrow, groove, notch, vestibule (sib′sunz) [Francis *Sibson,* English physician, 1814–1876] see under *furrow, groove,* and *notch,* and see *membrana suprapleuralis* and *vestibule of aorta.*

Sicard's syndrome (se-karz′) [Jean Athanase *Sicard,* Paris neurologist, 1872–1929] Collet's syndrome.

siccative (sik′ah-tiv) [L. *siccus* dry] drying; removing moisture from surrounding objects; xeransis.

sicchasia (sĭ-ka′ze-ah) [Gr. *sikchasia*] nausea.

siccolabile (sik″o-la′bĭl) altered or destroyed by drying.

siccostabile (sik″o-sta′bĭl) not altered by drying.

siccus (sik′us) [L.] dry.

sick (sik) 1. not in good health; afflicted by disease; ill. 2. affected with nausea.

sick bay (sik′ba) hospital and dispensary quarters on a naval vessel or station.

sicklemia (sik-le′me-ah) sickle cell anemia; see under *anemia*.

sicklemic (sik-le′mik) pertaining to or characterized by sicklemia.

sickling (sik′ling) the development of sickle cells in the blood, as in sickle cell anemia.

sickness (sik′nes) any condition or episode marked by pronounced deviation from the normal healthy state; illness. **aerial s.**, air s. **African horse s.**, an infectious pulmonary disease of horses and mules in South Africa, caused by a virus and marked by serous exudations. Called also *pestis equorum* and *equine plague*. **African sleeping s.**, African trypanosomiasis. **air s.**, sickness due to change in air pressure and to the movements experienced in an airplane, marked by nausea, salivation, and cold sweats. **altitude s.**, high-altitude s. **athletes′ s.**, weakness, blurred vision, nausea, and headache, following a short period of intense physical exercise. **aviation s.**, air s. **balloon s.**, a condition similar to mountain sickness occurring during balloon ascents. **bay s.**, Haff disease. **black s.**, kala-azar. **Borna s.**, Borna disease. **bush s.**, a disease similar to enzootic marasmus, occurring in New Zealand. **caisson s.**, decompression s. **car s.**, nausea and malaise produced by the motion of trains or automobiles or other vehicles. **cave s.**, a febrile disease of the lungs occurring in persons who were engaged in excavating in an abandoned mine, due to infection with *Histoplasma capsulatum* (histoplasmosis). **compressed-air s.**, decompression s. **decompression s.**, a disorder characterized by joint pains, respiratory manifestations, skin lesions, and neurologic signs, occurring in aviators flying at high altitudes and following rapid reduction of air pressure in persons who have been breathing compressed air in caissons and diving apparatus. **falling s.**, epilepsy. **gall s.**, see *gallsickness*. **Gambian horse s.**, a fatal infection of horses throughout central Africa caused by *Trypanosoma congolense*. See also *nagana*. **Gambian sleeping s.**, Gambian trypanosomiasis. **green s.**, chlorosis. **green tobacco s.**, a transient, recurrent occupational illness of tobacco harvesters, marked by headache, dizziness, vomiting, and prostration. **high-altitude s.**, the condition resulting from difficulty in adjusting to diminished oxygen pressure at high altitudes. It may take the form of mountain sickness (q.v.), high-altitude pulmonary edema, or cerebral edema. **Jamaican vomiting s.**, a disease occurring in Jamaica, marked by severe vomiting of acute onset, usually followed by convulsions, coma, and death, due to injestion of damaged or unripe fruit of akee (*Blighia sapida*). Called also *akee poisoning*. **lambing s.**, a condition of ewes almost identical with milk fever of cows. **laughing s.**, pseudobulbar paralysis. **milk s.**, 1. an acute, often fatal disease caused by the ingestion of milk, milk products, or the flesh of cattle or sheep which have a disease known as trembles. It is marked by weakness, anorexia, vomiting, constipation, and sometimes muscular tremors. Called also *lactimorbus*. 2. trembles. **morning s.**, the nausea of early pregnancy. **motion s.**, sickness caused by motion experienced in any kind of travel, such as sea sickness, train sickness, car sickness, and air sickness. **mountain s.**, a syndrome caused by exposure to altitude high enough to cause hypoxia, occurring as a result of decreased atmospheric pressure with consequent lowering of arterial oxygen content. The *acute* form (Acosta′s disease) may appear a few hours after exposure to high altitude, with manifestations that include fatigue, dizziness, breathlessness, headache, nausea, vomiting, insomnia, impairment of mental capacity and judgment, and prostration. The *chronic* form (Andes disease, Monge′s disease) is characterized by loss of tolerance to hypoxia in a previously acclimatized person, and by secondary polycythemia. It occurs in two types: an *emphysematasus* type, in which dyspnea is the dominant symptom and bronchitis and laryngitis are common, and cyanosis is present; and in an *erythremic* type, in which the prominent symptoms include an erythremic color that turns to cyanosis on mild exertion, fatigue, headache, episodic stupor, paresthesias, anorexia, nausea, vomiting, and diminution of visual acuity. The *subacute* form is milder than the chronic form and resembles the acute form clinically, but is persistent. Both the chronic and subacute forms can be cured by descent to a lower altitude or to sea level. **protein s.**, symptoms, such as eruptions, fever, edema, and pain in the joints, following the injection of foreign proteins into the body. **radiation s.**, a condition sometimes produced by exposure to sources of ionizing radiation; it is characterized by malaise, nausea, emesis, diarrhea, leukopenia, etc. **railroad s.**, transit tetany. **Rhodesian sleeping s.**, Rhodesian trypanosomiasis. **salt s.**, a disease similar to enzootic marasmus, occurring in Florida. **sea s.**, nausea and malaise caused by the motion of a ship. **serum s.**, a hypersensitivity reaction following the administration of foreign serum and other antigens, and marked by urticarial rashes, edema, adenitis, joint pains, high fever, and prostration. The *acute* reaction is attributable to the formation of antibodies against the foreign serum or antigens, which are usually present in antigen excess at initial antibody production. Soluble antigen-antibody complexes that mediate immunologic injury are deposited in the tissues. In the *chronic* form, the injury is due to repeated administration of antigen to immune animals with continuous formation of antigen-antibody complexes over a prolonged period. Serum sickness is a form of Type III hypersensitivity. Called also *immune-complex disease, serum disease,* and *serum intoxication*. See also *serum sickness syndrome*, under *syndrome*. **sleeping s.**, a disease characterized by increasing drowsiness and lethargy, caused by a protozoal infection, such as African trypanosomiasis, or by a viral infection, such as lethargic encephalitis, St. Louis encephalitis, or eastern or western encephalomyelitis. **stiff s.**, ephemeral fever of cattle. **sweating s.**, miliary fever. **talking s.**, epidemic encephalitis marked by extreme excitement, muscular twitching, and talkativeness. **three-day s.**, ephemeral fever of cattle. **veld s., veldt s.**, heartwater. **vomiting s.**, Jamaican vomiting s. **West African sleeping s.**, African trypanosomiasis. **x-ray s.**, radiation s. **Zambezi sleeping s.**, African trypanosomiasis as it occurs today in the Zambezi-Okovango basin.

S.I.D. Society for Investigative Dermatology.

side (sīd) the lateral (right or left) portion or aspect of the body or structure. **balancing s.**, the segment of a dentition or denture, on the side opposite to that toward which the mandible is moved. **working s.**, the segment of a denture or dentition on the same side as that toward which the mandible is moved.

side-bone (sīd′bōn) a condition of horses marked by ossification of the lateral cartilages of the third phalanx of the foot.

side effect (sīd′ef-fekt″) a consequence other than the one(s) for which an agent or measure is used, as the adverse effects produced by a drug, especially on a tissue or organ system other than the one sought to be benefited by its administration.

sideration (sid″er-a′shun) [L. *siderari* to be blasted by a constellation] 1. sudden destruction of vital forces. 2. therapeutic application of electric sparks.

siderinuria (sid″er-ĭ-nu′re-ah) [Gr. *sidēros* iron + *ouron* urine + *-ia*] excretion of iron in the urine.

siderism (sid′er-izm) metallotherapy.

sidero- (sid′er-o) [Gr. *sidēros* iron] a combining form denoting relationship to iron.

Siderobacter (sid″er-o-bak′ter) a genus of microorganisms of the family Siderocapsaceae, suborder Pseudomonadineae, order Pseudomonadales, occurring as bacilliform cells with rounded ends, singly, in pairs or short chains, or united to form colonies, with iron or manganese compounds in the membranes or on the surfaces of the cells. It includes five species, *S. bre′vis, S. du′plex, S. gra′cilis, S. la′tus,* and *S. linea′ris.*

sideroblast (sid′er-o-blast″) a nucleated red blood cell containing granules of iron in its cytoplasm.

Siderocapsa (sid″er-o-kap′sah) a genus of microorganisms of the family Siderocapsaceae, suborder Pseudomonadineae, order Pseudomonadales, occurring as one to many small, ellipsoidal cells embedded in a primary capsule, with iron stored on the surface. It includes six species, *S. botryoi′des, S. corona′ta, S. eusphae′ra, S. ma′jor, S. monoe′ca,* and *S. treu′bii.*

Siderocapsaceae (sid″er-o-kap-sa′se-e) a family of microorganisms (order Pseudomonadales, suborder Pseudomonadineae), occurring as spherical, ellipsoidal, or bacilliform cells, frequently embedded in a thick mucilaginous capsule in which there may be deposits of iron or manganese compounds. It includes ten genera, *Ferribacterium, Ferrobacillus, Naumanniella, Ochrobium, Siderobacter, Siderocapsa, Siderococcus, Sideromonas, Sideronema,* and *Siderosphaera.*

Siderococcus (sid″er-o-kok′us) a genus of microorganisms of the family Siderocapsaceae, order Pseudomonadales, suborder Pseudomonadineae, occurring as small coccoid cells without a gelatinous capsule. It includes two species, *S. commu′nis* and *S. limoni′ticus.*

siderocyte (sid′er-o-sīt″) an erythrocyte containing nonhemoglobin iron.

sideroderma (sid″er-o-der′mah) bronzed coloration of the skin from disorder of the metabolism of the iron from degenerated hemoglobin.

siderofibrosis (sid″er-o-fi-bro′sis) fibrosis of the spleen marked by iron-containing deposits.

siderogenous (sid″er-oj′ĕ-nus) [*sidero-* + Gr. *gennan* to produce] (*obs.*) producing or forming iron.

Sideromonas (sid″er-o-mo′nas) a genus of microorganisms of the family Siderocapsaceae, suborder Pseudomonadineae, order Pseudomonadales, occurring as short coccoid to rod-shaped cells embedded in a large capsule impregnated or completely encrusted with iron or manganese compounds. It includes four species, *S. conferva′rum, S. du′plex, S. ma′jor,* and *S. vulga′ris.*

Sideronema (sid″er-o-ne′mah) a genus of microorganisms of the family Siderocapsaceae, suborder Pseudomonadineae, order Pseudomonadales, occurring as coccoid cells in short chains, embedded in a gelatinous sheath. The type species is *S. globulife′rum.*

sideropenia (sid″er-o-pe′ne-ah) [*sidero-* + Gr. *penia* poverty] iron deficiency; deficiency of iron in the body.

sideropenic (sid″er-o-pe′nik) pertaining to or characterized by deficiency of iron.

Siderophacus (sid″er-o′fah-kus) [*sidero-* + Gr. *phakos* lentil] a genus of microorganisms of the family Caulobacteraceae, suborder Pseudomonadineae, order Pseudomonadales, occurring as biconcave or rodlike cells on horn-shaped stalks, in which ferric hydroxide accumulates. The type species is *S. corne'olus.*

siderophage (sid'er-o-fāj") a histiocyte laden with phagocytosed particles.

siderophil (sid'er-o-fil) 1. siderophilous. 2. a siderophilous tissue or structure.

siderophilin (si'der-of''ĭ-lin) transferrin.

siderophilous (sid"er-of'ĭ-lus) [*sidero-* + Gr. *philein* to love] having a tendency to absorb iron.

siderophone (sid'er-o-fōn) [*sidero-* + Gr. *phonē* voice] an instrument for detecting, by a telephone-like arrangement, the presence of iron splinters in the eyeball.

siderophore (sid'er-o-fōr") a macrophage containing hemosiderin.

sideroscope (sid'er-o-skōp) [*sidero-* + Gr. *skopein* to examine] a magnet or other appliance for determining the presence of metallic iron as a foreign body in the eye.

siderosilicosis (sid"er-o-sil"ĭ-ko'sis) pneumoconiosis due to the inhalation of iron-ore dust containing silica.

siderosis (sid"er-o'sis) 1. pneumoconiosis due to the inhalation of iron particles. 2. excess of iron in the blood. 3. the deposit of iron in a tissue. **s. bul'bi,** the deposit of an iron pigment within the eyeball. **s. conjuncti'vae,** a rust brown or yellowish discoloration of the conjunctiva due to the presence of an iron foreign body; the condition may also be seen in hemochromatosis. **hematogenous s.,** pigmentation with an iron compound derived from the blood. **hepatic s.,** the deposit of an abnormal quantity of iron in the liver; see also under *hemosiderosis.* **nutritional s.,** excessive iron in the blood due to a diet very high in iron and low in protein and calories. **pulmonary s.,** siderosis (def. 1). **urinary s.,** presence of hemosiderin granules in the urine. **xenogenous s.,** pigmentation with an iron oxide derived from a foreign body.

Siderosphaera (sid"er-o-sfe'rah) a genus of microorganisms of the family Siderocapsaceae, suborder Pseudomonadineae, order Pseudomonadales, occurring as small coccoid cells, in pairs and embedded in a primary capsule. The type species is *S. conglomera'ta.*

siderotic (sid"er-ot'ik) pertaining to or characterized by siderosis.

siderous (sid'er-us) containing iron.

SIDS sudden infant death syndrome; see under *syndrome.*

Siebold's operation (se'boltz) [Karl Kaspar von *Siebold,* German surgeon, 1736–1807] pubiotomy.

Siegert's sign (se'gertz) [Ferdinand *Siegert,* German pediatrician, born 1865] see under *sign.*

Siegle's otoscope (ze'gelz) [Emil *Siegle,* French aurist in Stuttgart, 1833–1900] see under *otoscope.*

siemens (se'menz) the SI unit of conductivity, measured by the quantity of electricity transferred across the unit area, per unit potential gradient per unit time. Called also *mho.* Abbreviated S.

Siemerling's nucleus (se'mer-lingz) [Ernst *Siemerling,* German neurologist and psychiatrist, 1857–1931] see under *nucleus.*

Sieur's test (sign) (se-erz') [Célestin *Sieur,* French surgeon, 1860–1955] see *coin test,* under *tests.*

sieve (siv) a device having pores or perforations of uniform size used for separating objects or particles of different sizes. **molecular s.,** a crystalline substance having uniform pores of molecular size that adsorbs smaller but not larger molecules; used in chemical separation.

Sig. abbreviation for L. *signe'tur,* let it be labeled.

sigh (si) [L. *suspirium*] an audible and prolonged inspiration, followed by an audible expiration.

sight (sīt) 1. the act or faculty of vision. 2. a thing seen. **day s.,** nyctalopia (def. 1), or night blindness. **far s., long s.,** hyperopia. **near s.,** myopia. **night s.,** hemeralopia, or day blindness. **old s.,** presbyopia. **second s.,** senopia. **short s.,** myopia.

sigma (sig'mah) the eighteenth letter of the Greek alphabet σ, ς, or Σ: used as the symbol for one thousandth of a second, standard deviation, and summation.

sigmasism (sig'mah-sizm) sigmatism.

sigmatism (sig'mah-tizm) the incorrect, difficult, or too frequent use of the *s* sound.

sigmoid (sig'moid) [L. *sigmoides;* Gr. *sigmoeidēs*] 1. shaped like the letter S or the letter C. 2. the sigmoid colon.

sigmoidectomy (sig"moi-dek'to-me) excision of the sigmoid flexure of the colon.

sigmoiditis (sig"moi-di'tis) inflammation of the sigmoid flexure.

sigmoidopexy (sig-moi'do-pek"se) [*sigmoid* + Gr. *pēxis* fixation] suspension of the sigmoid flexure, usually performed for treatment of rectal prolapse.

sigmoidoproctostomy (sig-moi"do-prok-tos'to-me) the cre-

ation of an artificial opening between the sigmoid flexure and the rectum; also, the opening so created.

sigmoidorectostomy (sig-moi"do-rek-tos'to-me) sigmoidoproctostomy.

sigmoidoscope (sig-moi'do-skōp) [*sigmoid* + Gr. *skopein* to examine] an endoscope with appropriate illumination for examining the sigmoid flexure.

sigmoidoscopy (sig"moi-dos'ko-pe) inspection of the sigmoid flexure through a sigmoidoscope.

sigmoidosigmoidostomy (sig-moi"do-sig-moi-dos'to-me) the operative formation of an anastomosis between two portions of the sigmoid; also, the opening so created.

sigmoidostomy (sig"moi-dos'to-me) [*sigmoid* + Gr. *stomoun* to provide with a mouth, or opening] the formation of an artificial opening from the surface of the body into the sigmoid flexure; also, the opening so produced.

sigmoidotomy (sig"moi-dot'o-me) operative incision into the sigmoid.

sigmoidovesical (sig-moi"do-ves'ĭ-kal) pertaining to or communicating with the sigmoid flexure and the urinary bladder, as a sigmoidovesical fistula.

Sigmund's glands (zig'moonts) [Karl Ludwig *Sigmund,* Austrian physician, 1810–1883] see under *gland.*

sign (sīn) [L. *signum*] an indication of the existence of something; any objective evidence of a disease, i.e., such evidence as is perceptible to the examining physician, as opposed to the subjective sensations (symptoms) of the patient. **Aaron's s.,** a sensation of pain or distress in the epigastric or precordial region on pressure over McBurney's point in appendicitis. **Abadie's s.,** 1. spasm of the levator palpebrae superioris muscle; a sign of Graves' disease. 2. insensibility of the Achilles tendon to pressure; seen in tabes dorsalis. **Abrahams' s.,** 1. a sound between dull and flat obtained on percussion over the acromion process in early tuberculosis of the apex of the lung. 2. acute pain produced in vesical lithiasis when pressure is applied midway between the umbilicus and the ninth right costal cartilage. **accessory s.,** any nonpathognomonic sign of disease. **air-cushion s.,** Klemm's s. **Allis' s.,** relaxation of the fascia between the crest of the ilium and the greater trochanter: a sign of fracture of the neck of the femur. **Amoss' s.,** in painful flexure of the spine, the patient, when rising to a sitting posture from lying in bed, does so by supporting himself with his hands placed far behind him in the bed. **Andral's s.,** see under *decubitus.* **André-Thomas s.,** if during the finger to nose test, the patient is directed to raise his arm over his head and is then suddenly ordered to let it fall to his head, the arm will rebound; seen in disease of the cerebellum. **Anghelescu's s.,** inability to bend the spine while lying on the back so as to rest on the head and heels alone, seen in tuberculosis of the vertebrae. **antecedent s.,** any precursory indication of an attack of disease. **anterior tibial s.,** involuntary contraction of the tibialis anterior muscle when the thigh is forcibly flexed on the abdomen; seen in spastic paraplegia. **anticus s.,** Piotrowski's s. **Argyll Robertson pupil s.,** see under *pupil.* **Arroyo's s.,** asthenocoria. **Aschner's s.,** oculocardiac reflex. **assident s.,** accessory s. **Auenbrugger's s.,** a bulging of the epigastrium, due to extensive pericardial effusion. **Aufrecht's s.,** noisy breathing heard just above the suprasternal notch, indicative of tracheal stenosis. **Babinski's s's,** 1. loss or lessening of the Achilles tendon reflex in sciatica: this distinguishes it from hysteric sciatica. 2. Babinski's reflex. 3. in hemiplegia, the contraction of the platysma muscle in the healthy side is more vigorous than on the affected side, as seen in opening the mouth, whistling, blowing, etc. 4. the patient lies supine on the floor, with arms crossed upon his chest, and then makes an effort to rise to the sitting posture. On the paralyzed side, the thigh is flexed upon the pelvis and the heel is lifted from the ground, while on the healthy side the limb does not move. This phenomenon is repeated when the patient resumes the lying posture. It is seen in organic hemiplegia, but not in hysterical hemiplegia. 5. when the paralyzed forearm is placed in supination, it turns over to pronation: seen in organic paralysis. Called also *pronation sign.* **Babinski's toe s.,** Babinski's reflex. **Baccelli's s.,** whisper heard over the chest in pleural effusion. **Baillarger's s.,** inequality of the pupils in paralytic dementia. **Ballance's s.,** resonance of right flank when the patient lies on the left side; said to be present in splenic rupture. **Ballet's s.,** ophthalmoplegia externa, with loss of all voluntary eye movements, the pupillary movements and reflex eye movements persisting; seen in Graves' disease and hysteria. **Bamberger's s.,** 1. allochiria. 2. presence of signs of consolidation at the angle of the scapula, which disappear when the patient leans forward; a sign of pericardial effusion. **Bárány's s.,** see under *symptom.* **Bard's s.,** in organic nystagmus the oscillations of the eye increase as the patient's attention follows the finger moved alternately from one side to the other; but in congenital nystagmus the oscillations disappear in like condition. **Barré's s.,** contraction of the iris is retarded in mental deterioration. **Barré's pyramidal s.,** the patient lies face down and the legs are flexed at the knee; he is unable to hold the legs in this vertical position if there is disease of the pyramidal tracts. **Baruch's s.,** resistance of the temperature in the rectum to a bath of 75° F. for fifteen minutes; a sign of typhoid fever. **Bastian-Bruns' s.**, see under *law*. **Battle's s.**, discoloration in the line of the posterior auricular artery, the ecchymosis first appearing near the tip of the mastoid process; seen in fracture of the base of the skull. **Becker's s.**, increase of pulsation in the retinal arteries in Graves' disease. **Béclard's s.**, a sign of the maturity of the fetus consisting of a center of ossification in the lower epiphysis of the femur. **Beevor's s.** 1. a sign of functional paralysis consisting in inability of the patient to inhibit the antagonistic muscles. 2. in paralysis of the lower parts of the recti abdominis muscles, there is upward excursion of the umbilicus. **Béhier-Hardy s.**, aphonia in the early stages of pulmonary gangrene. **Beisman's s.**, a bruit over the closed eye in thyrotoxicosis. **Bekhterev's s.** 1. in tabes dorsalis, anesthesia of the popliteal space. 2. Bekhterev's reflex. **Bell's s.**, see under *phenomenon*. **Berger's s.**, an irregularly shaped or elliptical pupil in the early stages of tabes dorsalis, paralytic dementia, and certain paralyses. **Bergman's s.**, in urologic radiography, (*a*) the ureter is dilated immediately below a neoplasm, rather than collapsed as below an obstructing stone and (*b*) the ureteral catheter tends to coil in this dilated portion of the ureter. **Bespaloff's s.**, in the early stage of measles, the tympanic membrane is red and there is nasopharyngeal catarrh. **Bethea's s.**, when the examiner, standing back of the patient, places his fingers so that the tips rest on the upper surfaces of corresponding ribs high up in the patient's axillae, unilateral impairment of chest expansion is indicated by the lessened degree of respiratory movement of the ribs on the side affected. **Bezold's s.**, an inflammatory swelling below the apex of the mastoid process; and evidence of mastoiditis. **Biederman's s.**, a dark red color (instead of the normal pink) of the anterior pillars of the throat, seen in some syphilitic patients. **Bieg's entotic s.**, (*obs.*) when sounds are heard by the patient only when spoken through an ear trumpet joined by a catheter to the eustachian tube, disease of the malleus or incus is indicated. **Biermer's s.**, the metallic resonance over hydropneumothorax varies in pitch with change of position of the patient; seen in pneumothorax. Called also *change of sound* and *Gerhardt's sign*. **Biernacki's s.**, analgesia of the ulnar nerve in paralytic dementia and tabes dorsalis. **Binda's s.**, a sudden movement of the shoulder when the head is passively and sharply turned toward the other side, an early sign of tuberculous meningitis. **Biot's s.**, see under *respiration*. **Bird's s.**, a definite zone of dullness with absence of the respiratory sounds in hydatid disease of the lung. **Bjerrum's s.**, see under *scotoma*. **Blatin's s.**, hydatid thrill. **Blumberg's s.**, pain on abrupt release of steady pressure (rebound tenderness) over the site of a suspected abdominal lesion indicates peritonitis. Repeated comparison of the pain felt on application and release has prognostic significance: a comparative increase in the release pain indicates advancing peritonitis. **Bonnet's s.**, pain on thigh adduction in sciatica. **Bordier-Fränkel s.**, an outward and upward rolling of the eye in peripheral facial paralysis. **Borsieri's s.**, when the fingernail is drawn along the skin in early stages of scarlet fever, a white line is left which quickly turns red; called also *Borsieri's line*. **Boston's s.**, in Graves' disease, when the eyeball is turned downward there is arrest of descent of the lid, spasm, and continued descent. **Bouchard's s.**, a few drops of Fehling's solution are added to the urine and the mixture is shaken; if pus from the kidney is present, fine bubbles will form which push to the surface the coagulum formed by heating. **Bouillaud's s.**, permanent retraction of the chest in the precordial region; a sign of adherent pericardium. **Boyce's s.**, a gurgling sound heard on pressure by the hand on the side of the neck, in diverticulum of the esophagus. **Bozzolo's s.**, a visible pulsation of the arteries within the nostrils; said to indicate aneurysm of the thoracic aorta. **Bragard's s.**, with the knee stiff, the lower extremity is flexed at the hip until the patient experiences pain; the foot is then dorsiflexed. Increase of pain points to disease of the nerve root. **Branham's s.**, bradycardia produced by digital closure of an artery proximal to an arteriovenous fistula. **Braunwald s.**, occurrence of a weak pulse instead of a strong one immediately after a premature ventricular contraction. **Braxton Hicks' s.**, Hicks' s. **Brickner's s.**, diminished oculoauricular associated movements seen in impairment of function of the facial nerve. **Brissaud-Marie s.**, see under *syndrome*. **Broadbent's s.**, a retraction seen on the left side of the back, near the eleventh and twelfth ribs, related to pericardial adhesion. **Broadbent's inverted s.**, pulsations synchronizing with ventricular systole on the posterior lateral wall of the chest in gross dilatation of the left atrium. **Brockenborough's s.**, occurrence of a weak pulse instead of a strong one immediately after a premature ventricular contraction. **Brodie's s.** 1. a black spot on the glans penis: a sign of urinary extravasation into the spongiosum. 2. Brodie's pain. **Brown-Séquard's s.**, see under *syndrome*. **Brudzinski's s.** 1. in meningitis, flexion of the neck usually results in flexion of the hip and knee. 2. in meningitis, when passive flexion of the lower limb on one side is made, a similar movement will be seen in the opposite limb; called also *contralateral sign*. **Brunati's s.**, the appearance of opacities in the cornea during the course of pneumonia or typhoid fever. **Bruns' s.**, see under *syndrome*. **Bryant's s.**, lowering of the

axillary folds in dislocation of the shoulder. **Bryson's s.**, lessened power of expansion of the thorax, sometimes noticed in Graves' disease. **Burger's s.**, Heryng's s. **Burghart's s.**, see under *symptom*. **Burton's s.**, lead line. **Cantelli's s.**, dissociation between the movements of the head and eyes: as the head is raised the eyes are lowered, and vice versa. Called also *doll's eye s.* **Capps' s.**, see under *reflex*. **Carabelli's s.**, see under *cusp*. **Cardarelli's s.**, transverse pulsation of the laryngotracheal tube in aneurysms and in dilatation of the arch of the aorta. **cardinal s's** (of inflammation), dolor, calor, rubor, tumor, and functio laesa; see *inflammation*. **cardiorespiratory s.**, a change in the normal pulse-respiration ratio from 4:1 to 2:1; seen in infantile scurvy. **Carman's s.**, meniscus s. **Carnett's s.**, the test for demonstrating parietal tenderness consists of palpation during a period in which the patient holds his anterior abdominal muscles as tense as possible. The tense abdominal muscles prevent the examiner's fingers from coming in contact with the underlying viscera and any tenderness that is elicited over them will be parietal in location. Tenderness elicited over relaxed muscles may be either parietal or intra-abdominal in origin. Tenderness present with relaxed muscles and absent with tense muscles is due to a subparietal lesion and its cause should be sought inside of the abdomen. Tenderness found both when the muscles are relaxed and when voluntarily tensed is due to an anterior parietal lesion and its cause should be sought outside the abdominal cavity. **Castellino's s.**, Cardarelli's s. **Cegka's s.**, invariability of the cardiac dullness during the different phases of respiration; a sign of adherent pericardium. **Chaddock's s.**, see under *reflex*. **Charcot's s.** 1. the raising of the eyebrow in peripheral facial paralysis, and the lowering of the same part in facial contraction. 2. intermittent limping in arteriosclerosis of the legs and feet. **Charcot-Vigouroux s.**, Vigouroux's s. **Cheyne-Stokes s.**, see under *respiration*. **chin-retraction s.**, a sign of the third stage of anesthesia: the chin and larynx move downward during inspiration. **Chvostek's s.**, **Chvostek-Weiss s.**, spasm of the facial muscles elicited by tapping the facial nerve in the region of the parotid gland; seen in tetany. **Claude's hyperkinesis s.**, reflex movements of paretic muscles elicited by painful stimuli. **clavicular s.**, a tumefaction at the inner third of the right clavicle; seen in congenital syphilis. Called also *Higouménakis's s.* **Cleeman's s.**, creasing of the skin just above the patella, indicative of fracture of the femur with overriding of fragments. **Cloquet's needle s.**, a clean needle is plunged into the biceps muscle; if life is not extinct, the needle oxidizes in 20–60 minutes. **Codman's s.**, in rupture of the supraspinatus tendon, the arm can be passively abducted without pain, but when support of the arm is removed and the deltoid contracts suddenly, pain occurs again. **cogwheel s.**, see under *phenomenon*. **coin s.**, see under *tests*. **Cole's s.**, deformity of the duodenal contour as seen in the roentgenogram, a sign of the presence of duodenal ulcer. **commemorative s.**, any sign of a previous disease. **Comolli's s.**, a sign of scapular fracture consisting in the appearance in the scapular region, shortly after the accident, of a triangular swelling reproducing the shape of the body of the scapula. **complementary opposition s.**, Grasset-Gaussel-Hoover s. **contralateral s.**, Brudzinski's s., def. 2. **Coopernail s.**, ecchymosis on the perineum and scrotum or labia: a sign of fracture of the pelvis. **Cope's s.**, tenderness over the appendix on stretching the psoas muscle by extending the thigh. **Corrigan's s.** 1. a purple line at the junction of the teeth with the gum in chronic copper poisoning. 2. a peculiar expanding pulsation indicative of aneurysm of the abdominal aorta; see also *Corrigan's pulse*, under *pulse*. 3. see under *respiration*. **coughing s.**, Huntington's s. **Courvoisier's s.**, see under *law*. **Cowen's s.**, jerky constriction of the contralateral pupil when light is shown into the pupil, a sign of Graves' disease. **Crichton-Browne's s.**, tremor of the outer angles of the eyes and of the labial commissures in the earlier stages of paralytic dementia. **Cruveilhier's s.**, a swelling in the groin is palpated when the patient coughs: in saphenous varix there is felt a tremor as of a jet of water entering and filling the pouch. **Cullen's s.**, a bluish discoloration of the skin around the umbilicus sometimes associated with intraperitoneal hemorrhage, especially following rupture of the uterine tube in ectopic pregnancy. A similar discoloration is seen in acute hemorrhagic pancreatitis. **Dalrymple's s.**, abnormal wideness of the palpebral opening in Graves' disease. **D'Amato's s.**, in pleural effusion, the location of dullness is altered from the vertebral area in the sitting position to the heart region when the patient assumes a lateral position on the side opposite the effusion. **Damoiseau's s.**, Ellis' line. **Darier's s.**, urtication and itching occurring on rubbing the lesions of urticaria pigmentosa. **Davidsohn's s.**, decrease of illumination of the pupil on transillumination with an electric light placed in the mouth; indicates tumor or fluid in the maxillary antrum. **Davis' s.**, an empty state and a yellowish or pale tint of the pulseless arteries; a sign of death. **Dawbarn's s.**, in acute subacromial bursitis, when the arm hangs by the side palpation over the bursa causes pain, but when the arm is abducted this pain disappears. **Dejerine's s.**, aggravation of symptoms of radiculitis produced by coughing, sneezing, and straining at stool. **de la Camp's s.**, relative dullness over and at each side of the fifth and sixth vertebrae in tuberculosis of the bronchial lymph nodes. **Delbet's s.,** in aneurysm of the main artery of a limb, if the nutrition of the part distal to the aneurysm is maintained, although the pulse may have disappeared, the collateral circulation is sufficient. **Delmege's s.,** deltoid flattening; said to be an early sign of tuberculosis. **Demarquay's s.,** fixation or lowering of the larynx during phonation and deglutition; a sign of syphilis of the trachea. **Demianoff's s.,** a sign that permits the differentiation of pain originating in the sacrolumbalis muscles from lumbar pain of any other origin. The sign is obtained by placing the patient in dorsal decubitus and lifting his extended leg. In the presence of lumbago this produces a pain in the lumbar region which prevents raising the leg high enough to form an angle of 10 degrees, or even less, with the table or bed on which the patient reposes. The pain is due to the stretching of the sacrolumbalis. **de Musset's s.,** Musset's s. **de Mussy's s.,** see under *point.* **Dennie's s.,** Morgan's line. **Desault's s.,** a sign of intracapsular fracture of the femur, consisting of alteration of the arc described by rotation of the great trochanter, which normally describes the segment of a circle, but in this fracture rotates only as the apex of the femur as it rotates about its own axis. **d'Espine's s.,** in the normal person, on auscultation over the spinous processes, pectoriloquy ceases at the bifurcation of the trachea, and in infants opposite the seventh cervical vertebra. If pectoriloquy is heard lower than this, it indicates enlargement of the bronchial lymph nodes. **Dew's s.,** in diaphragmatic hydatid abscess beneath the right cupola, the area of resonance moves caudally with the patient on hands and knees. **Dixon Mann's s.,** Mann's s. **doll's eye s.,** Cantelli's s. **Dorendorf's s.,** fullness of the supraclavicular groove on one side in aneurysm of the aortic arch. **Drummond's s.,** a whiff heard at the open mouth during respiration in cases of aortic aneurysm. **D.T.P. s.** (*distal tingling on percussion*), Tinel's s. **Du Bois' s.,** shortness of the little finger in congenital syphilis. **Duchenne's s.,** the sinking in of the epigastrium on inspiration in paralysis of the diaphragm or in certain cases of hydropericardium. **Duckworth's s.,** see under *phenomenon.* **duct s.,** a red spot seen at the orifice of the parotid duct in mumps. **Dugas' s.,** see under *tests.* **Duncan-Bird s.,** Bird's s. **Dunphy's s.,** injection anterior to the insertion of the lateral rectus in Graves' disease. **Dupuytren's s.,** 1. a crackling sensation on pressure over a sarcomatous bone. 2. in congenital dislocation of the head of the femur, there is a free up-and-down movement of the head of the bone. **Duroziez's s.,** see under *murmur.* **echo s.,** 1. a percussion sound resembling an echo which is heard over a hydatid cyst. 2. the repetition of the last word or clause of a sentence, seen in certain brain diseases; echolalia. **Elliot's s.,** 1. induration of the edge of a syphilitic skin lesion. 2. a scotoma extending from the blind spot and made up of numerous points or spots. **Ellis' s.,** the peculiar curved line of dullness discoverable during resorption of a pleuritic exudate. **Ely's s.,** see under *tests.* **Enroth's s.,** abnormal fullness of the eyelids in Graves' disease. **Erb's s.,** 1. increased electric irritability of motor nerves in cases of tetany. 2. dullness in percussion over the manubrium of the sternum in acromegaly. **Erben's s.,** see under *reflex.* **Erichsen's s.,** when the iliac bones are sharply pressed toward each other pain is felt in sacroiliac disease but not in hip disease. **Erni's s.,** the cavernous tympany developed over an apical cavity that has previously been filled with fluid. Sometimes gently rapping over such a filled cavity with a hard instrument will excite coughing, which will expel the secretion, and thus the cavernous signs are developed. **Escherich's s.,** in tetany, percussion of the inner surface of the lips or tongue produces contraction of the lips, tongue, and masseter muscles. **ether s.,** a sign of death: 1 or 2 ml. of ether is injected subcutaneously. If the ether spurts back when the needle is withdrawn, death has occurred. Its absorption indicates that life still persists. **Eustace Smith's s.,** Smith's s. **Ewart's s.,** 1. undue prominence of the sternal end of the first rib in certain cases of pericardial effusion. 2. bronchial breathing and dullness on percussion at the lower angle of the left scapula in pericardial effusion. **Ewing s.,** tenderness at the upper inner angle of the orbit: a sign of obstruction of the outlet of the frontal sinus. **external malleolar s.,** Chaddock's reflex. **extinction s.,** extinction of the eruption over an area of skin about the size of the palm when normal human serum is injected intracutaneously; see *Schultz-Charlton reaction,* under *reaction.* **fabere s.,** see *Patrick's test,* under *tests.* **facial s.,** Chvostek's s. **Faget's s.,** see under *law.* **Fajersztajn's crossed sciatic s.,** in sciatica, when the leg is flexed, the hip can also be flexed, but not when the leg is held straight; flexing the sound thigh with the leg held straight causes pain on the affected side. **fan s.,** spreading apart of the toes following the stroking of the sole of the foot; it forms part of the Babinski reflex. **Federici's s.,** on auscultation of the abdomen, the cardiac sounds can be heard in cases of intestinal perforation with gas in the peritoneal cavity. **Filipovitch's s.,** the yellow discoloration of prominent parts of the palms and soles in typhoid fever. **Fischer's s.,** 1. on auscultation over the manubrium with the patient's head bent backward, there is sometimes heard, in tuberculosis of the bronchial glands, a murmur due to pressure of the glands on the innominate veins. 2.

a presystolic murmur in certain cases of adherent pericardium. **flag s.,** dyspigmentation of the hair occurring as a band of light hair, seen in children who have recovered from kwashiorkor. **flush-tank s.,** the passage of a large amount of urine and the coincident temporary disappearance of a lumbar swelling; a sign of hydronephrosis. **forearm s.,** Leri's s. **formication s.,** Tinel's s. **Fournier's s.,** 1. the sharp delimitation characteristic of a syphilitic skin lesion. 2. saber shin. **Fränkel's s.,** excessive range of passive movement of the hip joint, indicating diminished tone of the surrounding musculature in tabes dorsalis. **Friedreich's s.,** 1. diastolic collapse of the cervical veins due to adherent pericardium. 2. lowering of the pitch of the percussion note over an area of cavitation during forced inspiration; called also *Friedreich's change of note.* **Froment's paper s.,** flexion of the distal phalanx of the thumb when a sheet of paper is held between the thumb and index finger; seen in affections of the ulnar nerve. **Fürbringer's s.,** in cases of subphrenic abscess, the respiratory movements will be transmitted to a needle inserted into the abscess, which is thus distinguished from abscess above the diaphragm. **Gaenslen's s.,** with the patient on his back on the operating table, the knee and hip of one leg are held in flexed position by the patient, while the other leg, hanging over the edge of the table, is pressed down by the examiner to produce hyperextension of the hip: pain occurs on the affected side in lumbosacral disease. **Galeazzi's s.,** in congenital dislocation of the hip, the dislocated side is shorter when both thighs are flexed 90 degrees. **Gangolphe's s.,** a serosanguineous abdominal effusion in strangulated hernia. **Garel's s.,** Heryng's s. **Gerhardt's s.,** Biermer's s. **Gianelli's s.,** Tournay's s. **Gifford's s.,** inability to evert the upper lid; seen in Graves' disease. **Gilbert's s.,** opsiuria indicative of hepatic cirrhosis. **Glasgow's s.,** a systolic sound in the brachial artery in latent aneurysm of the aorta. **Goggia's s.,** in health, the fibrillary contraction produced by striking and then pinching the brachial biceps extends throughout the whole muscle: in debilitating disease, such as typhoid fever, the contraction is local. **Goldstein's s.,** wide space of distance between the great toe and the adjoining toe seen in cretinism and Down's syndrome. **Goldthwait's s.,** the patient lying supine, his leg is raised by the examiner with one hand, the other hand being placed under the patient's lower back; leverage is then applied to the side of the pelvis. If pain is felt by the patient before the lumbar spine is moved, the lesion is a sprain of the sacroiliac joint. If pain does not appear until after the lumbar spine moves, the lesion is in the sacroiliac or lumbosacral articulation. **Golonbov's s.,** tenderness on percussion over the tibia in chlorosis. **Goodell's s.,** if the woman's cervix uteri is soft she is pregnant; if it is hard she is not. **Gordon's s.,** finger phenomenon (def. 1). **Gottron's s.,** bluish red plaques on the backs of the fingers, especially over the knuckles, seen in dermatomyositis, and sometimes preceding the onset of muscle weakness by weeks or as long as two to three years. **Gowers' s.,** abrupt intermittent oscillation of the iris under the influence of light; seen in certain stages of tabes dorsalis. **Graefe's s.,** failure of the upper lid to move downward promptly and evenly with the eyeball in looking downward, instead it moves tardily and jerkingly; seen in Graves' disease. **Grancher's s.,** equality of pitch between expiratory and inspiratory murmurs; a sign of obstruction to expiration. **Granger's s.,** if in the radiograph of an infant two years old or less, the anterior wall of the lateral sinus is visible, extensive destruction of the mastoid is indicated. **Grasset's s., Grassett-Bychowski s.,** Grasset's phenomenon. **Grasset-Gaussel-Hoover s.,** when the patient in a recumbent position attempts to lift the paretic limb, there is greater downward pressure on the examiner's hand with the sound limb than is observed in the test with a normal person. **Greene's s.,** outward displacement of the free cardiac border by the expiratory movement in pleuritic effusion; it is detected by percussion. **Grey Turner's s.,** Turner's s. **Griesinger's s.,** edematous swelling behind the mastoid process; seen in thrombosis of the transverse sinus. **Griffith's s.,** lower lid lag on upward gaze, a sign of Graves' disease. **Grisolle's s.,** if, on stretching an affected portion of the skin, the papule becomes impalpable to the touch, the eruption is caused by measles; if, on the contrary, the papule can still be felt, the eruption is one of smallpox. **Grocco's s.,** 1. a sign of pleural effusion consisting in the presence of a triangular area of dullness (*Grocco's, Korányi-Grocco, paravertebral,* or *Rauchfuss' triangle*) on the back, on the side opposite to that on which the effusion is present. Called also *Grocco's triangular dullness.* 2. acute dilatation of the heart produced by muscular effort in the early stages of Graves' disease. 3. extension of the liver dullness to the left of the midspinal line, indicating enlargement of the organ. **Grossman's s.,** dilatation of the heart as a sign of pulmonary tuberculosis. **Gubler's s.,** see under *tumor.* **Guilland's s.,** brisk flexion at the hip and knee joint when the contralateral quadriceps muscle is pinched; a sign of meningeal irritation. **Gunn's s.,** a raising of a ptosed eyelid on opening the mouth and moving the jaw toward the opposite side. **Gunn's crossing s.,** a crossing of an artery over a vein in the fundus of the eye, indicative of essential hypertension. **Gunn's pupillary s.,** swinging flashlight s. **Guttmann's s.,** a humming sound heard over the thyroid in Graves' disease.

Guye's s., aprosexia in children with adenoids. **Guyon's s.,** the ballottement and palpation of a floating kidney. **Hahn's s.,** persistent rotation of the head from side to side in cerebellar disease of childhood. **Hall's s.,** a tracheal diastolic shock felt in aneurysm of the aorta. **halo s.,** a halo effect produced in the roentgenogram of the fetal head between the subcutaneous fat and the cranium; said to be indicative of intrauterine death of the fetus. **Hamman's s.,** a loud crunching, clicking sound, synchronous with the heart beat, heard in mediastinal emphysema; it is pathognomonic for pneumopericardium. **harlequin s.,** reddening of the lower half of the laterally recumbent body and blanching of the upper half, due to temporary vasomotor disturbance in newborn infants. **Hatchcock's s.,** tenderness on running the finger toward the angle of the jaw in mumps. **Haudek's s.,** a projecting shadow in radiographs of penetrating gastric ulcer, due to settlement of bismuth in pathologic niches of the stomach wall; called also *Haudek's niche.* **Heberden's s's,** see under *node.* **Hefke-Turner s.,** a widening and change in contour of the normal obturator x-ray shadow, indicative of pathologic condition of the hip joint; called also *obturator s.* **Hegar's s.,** softening of the lower segment of the uterus, an indication of pregnancy. **Heilbronner's s.,** see under *thigh.* **Heim-Kreysig s.,** a depression of the intercostal spaces occurring along with the cardiac systole in adherent pericarditis. **Helbing's s.,** medialward curving of the Achilles tendon as viewed from behind; seen in flatfoot. **Hellat's s.** (*obs.*), in mastoid suppuration, a tuning fork placed on the diseased area is heard for a shorter time than when placed on any other part. **Hellendall's s.,** Cullen's s. **Hennebert's s.,** in the labyrinthitis of congenital syphilis, compression of the air in the external auditory canal produces a rotatory nystagmus to the diseased side; rarefaction of the air in the canal produces a nystagmus to the opposite side. Called also *pneumatic s.* or *test.* **Henning's s.,** an angular deformity of the angulus of the stomach, in which it assumes a Gothic arch shape; a sign of chronic gastric ulcer. Called also *Gothic arch formation.* **Heryng's s.,** an infraorbital shadow produced by fluid or by a hypertrophied, hyperplastic, or neoplastic membrane in the maxillary antrum and observable by electric illumination of the buccal cavity; seen in diseases of the antrum of Highmore (maxillary sinus). **Hicks' s.,** light, usually painless, irregular uterine contractions during pregnancy, gradually increasing in intensity and frequency and becoming more rhythmic during the third trimester. Called also *Braxton Hicks'* or *Hicks' contractions,* and *Braxton Hicks' s.* **Higouménakis' s.,** clavicular s. **Hill's s.,** disproportionate femoral systolic hypertension. **Hirschberg's s.,** adduction, inversion, and slight plantar flexion of the foot on stroking the inner aspect (not the sole) of the foot from the great toe to the heel; called also *adductor reflex of foot.* **Hochsinger's s.,** 1. indicanuria in the tuberculosis of childhood. 2. see under *phenomenon.* **Hoehne's s.,** absence of uterine contractions during delivery despite repeated injections of oxytocics, regarded as a sign of rupture of the uterus. **Hoffmann's s.,** 1. increased mechanical irritability of the sensory nerves in tetany; the ulnar nerve is usually tested. 2. a sudden nipping of the nail of the index, middle, or ring finger produces flexion of the terminal phalanx of the thumb and of the second and third phalanx of some other finger; called also *digital reflex, Hoffmann's reflex,* and *Trömmer's s.* **Holmes' s.,** rebound phenomenon. **Homans' s.,** discomfort behind the knee on forced dorsiflexion of the foot; a sign of thrombosis in the veins of the calf. **Hoover's s.,** 1. in the normal state or in genuine paralysis, if the patient, lying on a couch, is directed to press the leg against the couch, there will be a lifting movement seen in the other leg; this phenomenon is absent in hysteria and malingering. 2. movement of the costal margins toward the midline in inspiration, occurring bilaterally in pulmonary emphysema and unilaterally in conditions causing flattening of the diaphragm, such as pleural effusion and pneumothorax. **Hope's s.,** double heart beat in aortic aneurysm. **Horn's s.,** pain produced by traction on the right spermatic cord in acute appendicitis. **Horner's s.,** Spalding's s. **Horsley's s.,** if there is a difference in the temperature in the two axillae, the higher temperature will be on the paralyzed side. **Hoyne's s.,** a sign elicited in paralytic or nonparalytic poliomyelitis: with the patient in the supine position, his head falls back when his shoulders are elevated. **Huchard's s.,** paradoxical percussion resonance in pulmonary edema. **Hueter's s.,** the absence of the transmission of osseous vibration in cases of fracture with fibrous material interposed between the fragments. **Human's s.,** chin-retraction s. **Huntington's s.,** the patient is recumbent, with his legs hanging over the edge of a table, and is told to cough. If the coughing produces flexion of the thigh and extension of the leg in the paralyzed limb, it indicates that the paralysis is due to an upper motor neuron lesion. **Hutchinson's s.,** 1. interstitial keratitis and a dull-red discoloration of the cornea in inherited syphilis. 2. see under *tooth.* 3. see under *triad.* **hyperkinesis s.,** see *Claude's hyperkinesis s.* **interossei s.,** Souques's phenomenon. **Itard-Cholewa s.,** anesthesia of the tympanic membrane in otosclerosis. **Jaccoud's s.,** prominence of the aorta in the suprasternal notch. **Jackson's s.,** 1. [Chevalier Jackson] see *asthmatoid wheeze,* under *wheeze.* 2. [James Jackson, Jr.] prolongation of the expira-

tory sound over the affected area in pulmonary tuberculosis. **Jellinek's s.,** the pigmentation, usually brownish, occurring on the lid margins in many cases of hyperparathyroidism; called also *Rasin's s.* **Jendrassik's s.,** paralysis of the extraocular muscles in Graves' disease. **Joffroy's s.,** absence of forehead wrinkling in Graves' disease when the patient suddenly turns his eye upward. **jugular s.,** Queckenstedt's s. **Jürgensen's s.,** delicate crepitation sometimes heard in auscultation in acute pulmonary tuberculosis. **Kanavel's s.,** a point of maximum tenderness in the palm 1 inch proximal to the base of the little finger in infection of tendon sheath. **Kantor's s.,** a thin stringlike shadow in the roentgenogram of the colon through the filling defect; seen in colitis and regional ileitis. **Karplus' s.,** a modification of the vocal resonance, in which, on auscultation over a pleural effusion, the vowel *u* spoken by the patient is heard as *a.* **Kashida's s.,** spasm of muscles and hyperesthesia produced by applying heat or cold; seen in tetany. **Keen's s.,** increased diameter of the leg at the malleoli in Pott's fracture of the fibula. **Kehr's s.,** severe pain in the left shoulder in some cases of rupture of the spleen. **Kellock's s.,** increase of the vibration of the ribs on sharp percussion with the right hand, the left hand being placed firmly on the thorax under the nipple; a sign of pleural effusion. **Kelly's s.,** if the ureter is teased with an artery forceps, it will contract like a snake or worm. **Kerandel's s.,** deep hyperesthesia accompanied by pain, often retarded, after some slight blow upon a bony projection of the body; seen in African trypanosomiasis. **Kergaradec's s.,** uterine souffle. **Kernig's s.,** in dorsal decubitus, the patient can easily and completely extend the leg; in the sitting posture or when lying with the thigh flexed upon the abdomen the leg cannot be completely extended; it is a sign of meningitis. **Kerr's s.,** alteration of the texture of the skin below the somatic level in lesions of the spinal cord. **Kestenbaum's s.,** a decrease in number of arterioles traversing the optic disk margin as a criterion for optic atrophy. **Kleist's s.,** the fingers of the patient when gently elevated by the fingers of the examiner will hook into the examiner's fingers; indicative of frontal and thalamic lesions. **Klemm's s.,** in the roentgenogram in chronic appendicitis, there is often an indication of tympanites in the right lower quadrant. **Klippel-Feil s.,** flexion and adduction of the thumb when the patient's flexed fingers are quickly extended by the examiner; indicative of pyramidal tract disease. **Knie's s.,** unequal dilatation of the pupils in Graves' disease. **Kocher's s.,** a sign of Graves' disease: the examiner places his hand on a level with the patient's eyes and then lifts it higher; the patient's upper lid springs up more quickly than does his eyeball. **Koplik's s.,** see under *spot.* **Korányi's s.,** increase of resonance over the dorsal segment on percussion of the spinal processes of the thoracic vertebrae; a sign of pleural effusion. **Kreysig's s.,** Heim-Kreysig s. **Krisovski's (Krisowski's) s.,** cicatricial lines which radiate from the mouth in congenital syphilis. **Kussmaul's s.,** 1. distention of the jugular veins on inspiration, seen in constrictive pericarditis and mediastinal tumor. 2. convulsions and coma in stomach disease as a result of toxin absorption. 3. paradoxical pulse. **Küstner's s.,** a cystic tumor on the median line anterior to the uterus in cases of ovarian dermoids. **Laborde's s.,** Cloquet's needle s. **Ladin's s.,** a sign of pregnancy, consisting in a circular elastic area, which offers a sensation of fluctuation to the examining finger, situated in the median line of the anterior surface of the body of the uterus just above the junction of the body and the cervix. This area increases in size as pregnancy advances. **Laennec's s.,** the occurrence of rounded, gelatinous masses (Laennec's pearls) in the sputum of bronchial asthma. **Lafora's s.,** picking of the nose regarded as an early sign of cerebrospinal meningitis. **Langoria's s.,** relaxation of the extensor muscles of the thigh; a symptom of intracapsular fracture of the femur. **Larcher's s.,** grayish, cloudy discolorations of the conjunctivae that are speedily blackened; a sign of death. **Lasègue's s.,** in sciatica, flexion of the hip is painful when the knee is extended, but painless when the knee is flexed. This distinguishes the disorder from disease of the hip joint. **Laugier's s.,** a condition in which the styloid process of the radius and of the ulna are on the same level; seen in fracture of the lower part of the radius. **leg s.,** 1. Schlesinger's s. 2. Neri's s. **Leichtenstern's s.,** in cerebrospinal meningitis, tapping lightly any bone of the extremities causes the patient to wince suddenly. **Lennhoff's s.,** a furrow appearing on deep inspiration below the lowest rib and above an echinococcus cyst of the liver. **Leri's s.,** passive flexion of the hand and wrist of the affected side in hemiplegia shows no normal flexion at the elbow. **Leser-Trélat s.,** telangiectases, warts, and pigmented spots that appear suddenly and increase rapidly in number, and may indicate abdominal cancer in the elderly. It may take the form of acanthosis nigricans, dermatomyositis, amyloidosis, herpes zoster, or senile keratoses. **Leudet's s.,** see under *tinnitus.* **Levasseur's s.,** the failure of the scarificator and cupping-glass to draw blood; a sign of death. **Lhermitte's s.,** the development of sudden, transient, electric-like shocks spreading down the body when the patient flexes the head forward; seen mainly in multiple sclerosis but also in compression and other disorders of the cervical cord. **Libman's s.,** extreme tenderness, but without pain on pressure, of the tips of the mastoid bones.

Lichtheim's s., in subcortical aphasia, although the patient cannot speak, he is able to indicate with his fingers the number of syllables in the word he is thinking of. **ligature s.,** in hematuria, the development of ecchymoses in the distal part of a limb to which a ligature has been applied. **Linder's s.,** with the patient recumbent or sitting with outstretched legs, passive flexion of the head will cause pain in the leg or the lumbar region in sciatica. **Litten's s.,** see under *phenomenon.* **Livierato's s.,** vasoconstriction when the abdominal sympathetic nerve is irritated by striking the anterior abdomen along the xiphoumbilical line. **Lloyd's s.,** a symptom of renal calculus, consisting of pain in the loin on deep percussion over the kidney, even when pressure causes no pain. **Lombardi's s.,** the appearance of venous varicosities in the region of the spinous processes of the seventh cervical and first three thoracic vertebrae; seen in early pulmonary tuberculosis. **Lorenz's s.,** ankylotic rigidity of the spinal column, especially of the thoracic and lumbar segments; sometimes seen in incipient tuberculosis. **Lucas' s.,** distention of the abdomen in the early stages of rickets. **Lucatello's s.,** the external (axillary) temperature is higher than the oral by 0.2–0.3 degree in hyperthyroid patients. **Ludloff's s.,** swelling and ecchymosis at the base of Scarpa's triangle together with inability to raise the thigh when in a sitting posture, a sign of traumatic separation of the epiphysis of the greater trochanter. **Lust's s.,** see under *phenomenon.* **McBurney's s.,** tenderness at a point two-thirds the distance from the umbilicus to the anterior superior spine of the ilium; indicative of appendicitis. See also under *point.* **Macewen's s.,** on percussion of the skull behind the junction of the frontal, temporal, and parietal bones, there is a more resonant note than normal in internal hydrocephalus and cerebral abscess. **McGinn-White s.,** a Q wave and late inversion of the T wave in lead III, low S-T intervals and T waves in lead II, and inverted T waves in chest leads V_2 and V_3, the electrocardiographic evidence of right ventricular dilatation due to massive pulmonary embolism, plus the clinical signs of acute cor pulmonale. **McMurray s.,** occurrence of a cartilage click during manipulation of the knee; indicative of meniscal injury. **Magendie's s., Magendie-Hertwig s.,** skew deviation. **Magnan's s.,** see under *symptom.* **Mangus' s.,** after death, light ligation of a finger causes no visible change in its distal portion. **Mahler's s.,** a steady increase of pulse rate without corresponding elevation of temperature; seen in thrombosis. **Maisonneuve's s.,** marked hyperextensibility of the hand; a symptom of Colles' fracture. **Mann's s.,** 1. in Graves' disease the two eyes appear not to be on the same level. 2. lessened resistance of the scalp to a constant electric current; seen in certain traumatic neuroses. Called also *Dixon Mann's s.* **Mannkopf's s.,** increase in the frequency of the pulse on pressure over a painful spot; not present in simulated pain. **Marañón's s.,** a vasomotor reaction following stimulation of the skin over the throat; seen in Graves' disease. **Marcus Gunn's pupillary s.,** swinging flashlight s. **Marfan's s.,** a red triangle at the tip of a coated tongue indicates typhoid fever; a rarely observed phenomenon. **Marie's s.,** tremor of the body or extremities in Graves' disease. **Marie-Foix s.,** withdrawal of lower leg on transverse pressure of tarsus or forced flexion of toes, even when the leg is incapable of voluntary movement. **Marinesco's s.,** Marinesco's succulent hand; see under *hand.* **Masini's s.,** marked dorsal extension of the fingers and toes in mentally unstable children. **Mayo's s.,** relaxation of the muscles controlling the lower jaw, indicative of profound anesthesia. **Means' s.,** lag of the eyeball on upward gaze in Graves' disease. **Meltzer's s.,** loss of the normal second sound, heard on auscultation of the heart after swallowing; symptomatic of occlusion or contraction of the lower part of the esophagus. **Mendel-Bekhterev s.,** see under *reflex.* **meniscus s.,** the radioscopic appearance of a crescentic shadow made by the crater of a gastric ulcer: when the convexity of the crescent points outward the ulcer is on the lesser curvature; when the convexity points downward the ulcer is distal to the angular incisure. **Mennell's s.,** an examining thumb is placed over the posterosuperior spine of the sacrum and then made to slide, first outward and then inward. If on pressure over the former point tenderness is detected, it is due to a sensitive deposit in the structures of the gluteal aspect of the posterosuperior spine. If the tenderness is over the inner point, it is probable that the superior ligaments of the sacral iliac joint are strained and sensitive. If the tenderness is increased by pressure backward on the anterosuperior aspect of the ilium and decreased by pulling forward the crest from behind, this is positive proof that it is caused by the sensitive ligaments. **Meunier's s.,** daily loss of weight in measles, following the incubative stage and preceding the eruptive stage. **Meyer's s.,** formication of the hands and sometimes of the feet, experienced particularly after immersion of the extremities in water; once used to distinguish the eruptive stage of scarlet fever from other eruptions. **Michelson-Weiss s.** (*obs.*), in otitis media associated with tuberculosis of the lungs, the patient is able to hear his own respiratory sounds with his affected ear. **Milian's s.,** in subcutaneous inflammation of the head and face, the ears are not involved but in skin diseases they are. **Minor's s.,** the method of rising from a sitting position characteristic of the patient with sciatica; he supports himself on the healthy side,

placing one hand on the back, bending the affected leg and balancing on the healthy leg. **Mirchamp's s.,** when a sapid substance, such as vinegar, is applied to the mucous membrane of the tongue, a painful reflex secretion of saliva in the gland about to be affected is indicative of sialadenitis, e.g., mumps. **Möbius' s.,** inability to keep the eyeballs converged in Graves' disease; due to insufficiency of the internal recti muscles. **Moebius' s.,** Möbius' s. **Monteverde's s.,** failure of any response to the subcutaneous injection of ammonia; a sign of death. **Morquio's s.,** the patient lying supine resists all attempts to raise the trunk to a sitting posture until the legs are passively flexed; noticed in epidemic poliomyelitis. **Moschcowitz's s.,** see under *tests.* **Mosler's s.,** sternal tenderness in acute myeloblastic anemia. **moulage s.,** a waxy cast appearance of bowel segments, a roentgenographic sign of celiac disease. **Müller's s.,** a sign of aortic insufficiency consisting of pulsation of the uvula and redness of the tonsils and velum palati, occurring synchronously with the action of the heart. **Munson's s.,** abnormal bulging of the lower lid when the patient rolls his eyes downward, caused by abnormal curvature of the cornea (keratoconus). **Murat's s.,** in the tuberculous patient there is vibration of the affected side of the chest with a feeling of discomfort when speaking. **Murphy's s.,** a sign of gallbladder disease consisting of inability of the patient to take a deep inspiration when the physician's fingers are pressed deeply beneath the right costal arch, below the hepatic margin. **Musset's s.,** rhythmical jerking movement of the head; seen in cases of aortic aneurysm and aortic insufficiency. **Myerson's s.,** ready induction of blepharospasm when the frontalis muscle is tapped, a sign of Parkinson's disease. **neck s.,** Brudzinski's s., def. 1. **Negro s.,** cogwheel phenomenon. **Neri's s.,** 1. a sign of organic hemiplegia, consisting in the spontaneous bending of the knee of the affected side as the leg is passively lifted, the patient being in the dorsal position. 2. with the patient standing, forward bending of the trunk will cause flexion of the knee on the affected side in lumbosacral and iliosacral lesions. **niche s.,** Haudek's s. **Nicoladoni's s.,** Branham's s. **Nikolsky's s.,** easy separation of the outer portion of the epidermis from the basal layer on exertion of firm sliding pressure by the finger or thumb, as in pemphigus vulgaris and some other bullous diseases. **Ober's s.,** see under *tests.* **objective s.,** one that can be seen, heard, or felt by the diagnostician; called also *physical s.* **obturator s.,** 1. pain on outward pressure on the obturator foramen as a sign of inflammation in the sheath of the obturator nerve probably caused by appendicitis. 2. see *Hefke-Turner s.* **Oliver's s.,** tracheal tugging; see under *tugging.* **ophthalmoscopic s.,** as death approaches, the blood in the retinal vessels gradually ceases to move and the column of blood splits into fragments. **Oppenheim's s.,** dorsiflexion of the big toe on stroking downward the medial side of the tibia; seen in pyramidal tract disease. **orange-peel s.,** a sign for distinguishing lipoma: on compressing the tumor between the thumb and forefinger, it will be perceived that the skin overlying the mass is irregularly dimpled by the downward traction of the vertical trabeculae; called also *signe de peau d'orange.* **orbicularis s.,** in hemiplegia, inability to close the eye on the paralyzed side without closing the other. **Ortolani's s.,** see under *click.* **Osler's s.,** small, painful, erythematous swellings in the skin of the hands and feet in malignant endocarditis; Osler's nodes. **palmoplantar s.,** Filipovitch's s. **Parkinson's s.,** see under *facies.* **Parrot's s.,** 1. dilatation of the pupil on pinching the skin of the neck; seen in meningitis. 2. bony nodes on the outer table of the skull of infants with congenital syphilis, giving it a buttock shape. **Pastia's s.,** hemorrhagic lines appearing in body creases, as in the antecubital fossae, inguinal areas, and the wrists, during scarlet fever; they are visible at the onset of the rash and persist after its desquamation. **patent bronchus s.,** the radiologic finding of an unobstructed bronchus supplying a collapsed lung, lobe, or segment. **Patrick's s.,** see under *tests.* **Pende's s.,** André-Thomas s. **Perez's s.,** a friction sound heard over the sternum when the patient raises and drops his arms; a sign of mediastinal tumor or of aneurysm of the arch of the aorta. **peroneal s.,** dorsal flexion and abduction of the foot, a sign of latent tetany elicited by tapping the peroneal nerve just below the head of the fibula, while the knee is relaxed and slightly flexed. **Pfuhl's s.,** inspiration increases the force of flow in paracentesis in the case of subphrenic abscess, but lessens it in the case of pyopneumothorax. This distinction is lost when the diaphragm is paralyzed. **Pfuhl-Jaffé s.,** in pyopneumothorax the liquid issues from the exploratory puncture or incision with considerable force during inspiration; in true pneumothorax during expiration. **physical s.,** objective s. **Piltz's s.,** 1. attention reflex of pupil; see under *reflex.* 2. Westphal-Piltz phenomenon. **Pins' s.,** Ewart's s., def. 2. **Piotrowski's s.,** percussion of the anterior tibialis muscle produces dorsal flexion and supination of the foot. When this reflex is excessive it indicates organic disease of the central nervous system. Called also *anticus s.* or *reflex.* **Piskacek's s.,** asymmetrical enlargement of the corpus uteri, a sign of pregnancy. **Pitres' s.,** 1. hyperesthesia of the scrotum and testes in tabes dorsalis. 2. anterior deviation of the sternum in pleuritic effusion. **placental s.,** implantation bleeding. **plumb-line s.,** the estimation in sternal displacement by a plumb-line in the diagnosis of pleuritic effusion. **Plummer's s.**, inability to step up onto a chair or to walk up steps, in Graves' disease. **pneumatic s.**, Hennebert's s. **Pool-Schlesinger s.**, Schlesinger's s. **Porter's s.**, tracheal tugging; see under *tugging.* **Potain's s.**, 1. extension of percussion dullness over the arch of the aorta, in dilatation of the aorta, from the manubrium to the third costal cartilage on the right-hand side. 2. timbre métallique. **Pottenger's s.**, 1. intercostal muscle rigidity on palpation in pulmonary and pleural inflammatory conditions. 2. different degrees of resistance on light touch palpation, noted (1) over solid organs when compared with hollow organs; (2) over foci of disease in the lungs and pleura when compared with that over normal organs. **Prehn's s.**, elevation and support of the scrotum will relieve the pain in epididymo-orchitis, but not in torsion of the testicle. **Prévost's s.**, conjugate deviation of the head and eyes, the eyes looking toward the affected hemisphere and away from the palsied extremities; seen in hemiplegia. **pronation s.**, 1. Babinski's s. (def. 5). 2. Strümpell's s. (def. 3). **pseudo-Babinski's s.**, in poliomyelitis the Babinski reflex is modified so that only the big toe is extended, because all the foot muscles except the dorsiflexors of the big toe are paralyzed. **pseudo-Graefe's s.**, slow descent of the upper lid on looking down, and quick ascent on looking up; seen in conditions other than Graves' disease. **puddle s.**, in examination for ascites, a method for detecting free fluid in the abdominal cavity. The patient lies prone for five minutes, then rises to his hands and knees. While the examiner lightly flicks a finger against one flank, a Bowles stethoscope is moved slowly from the most dependent part of the abdomen to the flank. That part of the ventral abdomen containing the fluid "puddle" shows a loss of high-frequency vibration, which will be detected as soon as the edge of the fluid is reached, indicating the amount of fluid. **pyramid s., pyramidal s.**, any sign pointing to disease of the pyramidal tract. **Quant's s.**, a T-shaped depression in the occipital bone, sometimes seen in rickets. **Queckenstedt's s.**, when the veins in the neck are compressed on one or both sides, there is a rapid rise in the pressure of the cerebrospinal fluid of healthy persons, and this rise quickly disappears when pressure is taken off the neck. But when there is a block in the vertebral canal the pressure of the cerebrospinal fluid is little or not at all affected by this maneuver. **Quénu-Muret s.**, in aneurysm, the main artery of the limb is compressed and then a puncture is made at the periphery; if blood flows, the collateral circulation is probably established. **Quincke's s.**, see under *pulse.* **Quinquaud's s.**, trembling of the patient's fingers, felt when his fingers, spread apart, are placed vertically in the palm of the examiner's hand; said to be a sign of alcoholism. **radialis s.**, Strumpell's s., def. 2. **Radovici's s.**, palmchin reflex. **Raimiste's s.**, the patient's hand and arm are held upright by the examiner: if the hand is sound, it remains upright on being released; if paretic the hand flexes abruptly at the wrist. **Ramond's s.**, rigidity of the erector spinae muscle indicative of pleurisy with effusion; the rigidity relaxes when the effusion becomes purulent. **Rasin's s.**, Jellinek's s. **Raynaud's s.**, acrocyanosis. **Remak's s.**, see under *symptom.* **Revilliod's s.**, orbicularis s. **Richardson's s.**, the application of a tight fillet to the arm as a test of death: if life is present, the veins on the distal side of the fillet become more or less distended. **Riesman's s.**, 1. a bruit heard with the stethoscope over the closed eye in Graves' disease. 2. softening of the eyeball in diabetic coma. **Ripault's s.**, external pressure upon the eye during life causes only a temporary change in the normal roundness of the pupil; but after death the change so caused may be permanent. **Ritter-Rollet s.**, see under *phenomenon.* **Riviere's s.**, an area of change in percussion note denoting a band of increased density across the back at the plane of the spinous processes of the fifth, sixth, and seventh dorsal vertebrae: a sign of pulmonary tuberculosis. **Robertson's s.**, 1. fibrillary contraction of the pectoralis muscle over the cardiac area in approaching death from heart disease. 2. absence of pupillary dilatation on pressure over alleged painful areas in malingering. 3. in ascites, fullness and tension in the patient's flanks, felt by the examiner with the patient supine. **Roche's s.**, in torsion of the testis, the epididymis cannot be distinguished from the body of the testis, whereas in epididymitis the body of the testis can be felt in the enlarged crescent of the epididymis. **Rockley's s.**, two straight edges are placed vertically at the outer edges of the orbits from the prominence of the zygomatic bone: if depression fracture of the zygomatic arch exists, the difference in the two angles is obvious. **Romaña's s.**, unilateral ophthalmia with palpebral edema, conjunctivitis, and swelling of regional lymph glands as a sign of Chagas' disease. **Romberg's s.**, swaying of the body or falling when standing with the feet close together and the eyes closed; observed in tabes dorsalis. **Rommelaere's s.**, an abnormally small proportion of normal phosphates and of sodium chloride in the urine in cancerous cachexia. **rope s.**, acute angulation between chin and larynx, due to weakness of hyoid muscles, noted in bulbar poliomyelitis. **Rosenbach's s.**, 1. absence of the abdominal skin reflex in inflammatory disease of the intestines. 2. absence of the abdominal skin reflex in pinching the skin of the abdomen on the paralyzed side in hemiplegia. 3. a fine rapid tremor of the closed eyelids in Graves' disease. 4. inability to close the eyes

immediately on command; seen in neurasthenia. **Roser's s., Roser-Braun s.**, absence of dural pulsation, a sign of cerebral tumor or abscess. **Rossolimo's s.**, see under *reflex.* **Rotch's s.**, dullness on percussion of the right fifth intercostal space, a sign of pericardial effusion. **Rothschild's s.**, 1. preternatural flattening and mobility of the sternal angle; seen in tuberculosis. 2. rarefaction of the outer third of the eyebrows in thyroid inadequacy. **Roussel's s.**, sharp pain on light percussion on the subclavicular region, between the clavicle and fourth rib; a sign of incipient tuberculosis. **Rovighi's s.**, a fremitus felt on percussion and palpation of a superficial hepatic hydatid cyst. **Rovsing's s.**, pressure on the left side over the point corresponding to McBurney's point will elicit the typical pain at McBurney's point in appendicitis. **Ruggeri's s.**, see under *reflex.* **Rumpel-Leede s.**, see under *phenomenon.* **Rumpf's s.**, 1. alternating fibrillary and tonic contractions after the cessation of strong faradization; seen in traumatic neuroses. Called also *Rumpf's traumatic reaction.* 2. quickening of the pulse on pressure over a painful point; seen in neurasthenia. **Rust's s.**, see under *phenomenon.* **Saenger's s.**, a light reflex of the pupil that has ceased returns after a short stay in the dark; observed in cerebral syphilis but not in tabes dorsalis. **Salisbury and Melvin's s.**, ophthalmoscopic s. **Sansom's s.**, 1. marked increase of the area of dullness in the second and third intercostal spaces, due to pericardial effusion. 2. a rhythmical murmur heard with a stethoscope applied to the lips in aneurysm of the thoracic aorta. **Sarbó's s.**, analgesia of the peroneal nerve; sometimes noticed in tabes dorsalis. **Saunders' s.**, on wide opening of the mouth there take place in children associated movements of the hand consisting of opening of the hand and extension and separation of the fingers; called also *mouth-and-hand synkinesia.* **Schepelmann's s.**, in dry pleurisy, the pain is increased when the patient bends his body toward the normal side, whereas in intercostal neuralgia it is increased by bending toward the affected side. **Schick's s.**, stridor heard on expiration in an infant with tuberculosis of the bronchial glands. **Schlesinger's s.**, in tetany, if the patient's leg is held at the knee joint and flexed strongly at the hip joint, there will follow within a short time an extensor spasm at the knee joint, with extreme supination of the foot. Called also *Pool's phenomenon.* **Schüle's s.**, omega melancholium. **Schultze's s.**, 1. Chvostek's sign. 2. tongue phenomenon. **Schultze-Chvostek s.**, Chvostek's s. **Seeligmüller's s.**, mydriasis on the side of the face affected with neuralgia. **Séguin's s.**, see *Séguin's signal symptom,* under *symptom.* **Seidel's s.**, see under *scotoma.* **Seitz's s.**, bronchial inspiration which begins harshly and then becomes faint; indicative of a cavity in the lung. **Semon's s.**, impairment of the mobility of the vocal cords in malignant disease of the larynx. **setting-sun s.**, downward deviation of the eyes, so that each iris appears to "set" beneath the lower lid, with white sclera exposed between it and the upper lid; indicative of intracranial pressure (hemorrhage or meningoependymitis) or irritation of the brain stem (as in kernicterus). **Shibley's s.**, in the presence of consolidation of the lung or a collection of fluid in the pleural cavity, all spoken vowels are heard through the stethoscope as "ah." **Sicar's s.**, a metallic resonance on percussion with two coins on the front of the chest and auscultation at the back; observed in some cases of effusion within the pleura. **Siegert's s.**, in Down's syndrome, the little fingers are short and curved inward. **Sieur's s.**, see *coin test,* under *tests.* **Signorelli's s.**, extreme tenderness on pressure on the retromandibular point in meningitis. **Silex's s.**, furrows radiating from the mouth in congenital syphilis. **Simon's s.**, 1. [*C. E. Simon*] retraction or fixation of the umbilicus during inspiration. 2. [*J. Simon*] absence of the usual correlation between the movements of the diaphragm and thorax; seen in beginning meningitis. **Sisto's s.**, constant crying as a sign of congenital syphilis in infancy. **Skeer's s.**, a small circle in the iris, near the pupil, in both eyes; seen in tuberculous meningitis. **Skoda's s.**, a tympanitic sound heard on percussing the chest above a large pleural effusion or above a consolidation in pneumonia. **Smith's s.**, a murmur heard in cases of enlarged bronchial glands on auscultation over the manubrium with the patient's head thrown back. **Snellen's s.**, the bruit heard with a stethoscope over the closed eye in Graves' disease. **Somagyi's s.**, see under *reflex.* **Soto-Hall s.**, with the patient flat on his back, on flexion of the spine beginning at the neck and going downward, pain will be felt at the site of the lesion in back abnormalities. **Souques' s.**, 1. when the patient seated in a chair is suddenly thrown back, the lower extremities do not extend normally or otherwise attempt to counteract the loss of balance; it indicates advanced striatal disease. 2. Souques' phenomenon. **Spalding's s.**, in the x-ray film of the fetus in utero, overriding of the bones of the vault of the skull indicates death of the fetus. **spinal s.**, tonic contraction of the spinal muscles on the diseased side in pleurisy. **spine s.**, disinclination to flex the spine anteriorly on account of pain; seen in poliomyelitis. **Squire's s.**, alternate contraction and dilatation of the pupil, indicative of basilar meningitis. **stairs s.**, difficulty in descending a stairway in tabes dorsalis. **Stellwag's s.**, retraction of the upper eyelids producing apparent widening of the palpebral opening with which is associated infrequent and incomplete blinking; seen in Graves' disease. **Sterles' s.,** increased pulsation over the cardiac region in intrathoracic tumors. **Sterling-Okuniewski s.,** the patient is unable to put out his tongue when directed to do so; once considered to be symptomatic of louse-borne typhus fever. **Sternberg's s.,** sensitiveness to palpation of the muscles of the shoulder girdle in pleurisy. **Stewart-Holmes s.,** rebound phenomenon. **Stierlin's s.,** see under *symptom.* **Stiller's s.,** a floating tenth rib, suggestive of a tendency to neurasthenia. **Stimson's s.,** a transverse line of conjunctival inflammation, sharply demarcated along the eyelid margin, occurring in the prodromal stage of measles. **Stocker's s.,** in typhoid fever, if the bed clothes are pulled down, the patient takes no notice; but in tuberculous meningitis the patient resents the interference and immediately draws the clothes up again. **Strauss' s.,** increase of fat following the use of fatty foods in chylous ascites. **string s.,** 1. Kantor's s. 2. the stringing out of tubules, observed on pulling the tissues of an intact testis or one in which there is active spermatogenesis, a phenomenon which is prevented by the fibrosis and hyalinization about the tubules when the testis is atrophic. **Strümpell's s.,** 1. dorsal flexion of the foot when the thigh is drawn up toward the body; seen in spastic paralysis of the lower limb. Called also *tibialis s.* 2. inability to close the fist without marked dorsal extension of the wrist; called also *radialis s.* 3. pronation sign: passive flexion of the forearm caused by pronation; seen in hemiplegia. **Strunsky's s.,** a sign for detecting lesions of the anterior arch of the foot. The examiner grasps the toes and flexes them suddenly. This procedure is painless in the normal foot, but causes pain if there is inflammation of the anterior arch. **Suker's s.,** deficient complementary fixation in lateral eye rotation; seen in Graves' disease. **Sumner's s.,** on gentle palpation of the iliac fossa, a slight increase in tonus of the abdominal muscles indicates appendicitis, stone in the ureter or kidney, or a twisted pedicle of an ovarian cyst. **swinging flashlight s.,** with the patient's eyes fixed at a distance and a strong light shining before the intact eye, a crisp bilateral contraction of the pupil is noted. On moving the light to the affected eye, both pupils dilate for a short period. Then on return of the light to the intact eye, both pupils contract promptly and remain contracted. Indicative of minimal damage to the optic nerve. Called also *Marcus Gunn pupillary phenomenon* or *sign.* **Tay's s.,** see *cherry-red spot,* under *spot.* **Tellais' s.,** pigmentation of the eyelid in Graves' disease. **Testivin's s.,** the formation of a collodion-like pellicle on the urine after removing the albumin and treating with acid and then with one third of its volume of ether; said to occur during the incubation of infectious diseases. **Theimich's lip s.,** a protrusion or pouting of the lips elicited by tapping the orbicularis oris muscle. **thermic s.,** Kashida's s. **Thomas' s.,** 1. flexion of the hip joint can be compensated by lordosis. 2. pinching of the trapezius muscle causes goose flesh above the level of a spinal cord lesion. **Thomson's s.,** Pastia's s. **Thornton's s.,** severe pain in the region of the flanks in nephrolithiasis. **tibialis s.,** Strümpell's s., def. 1. **Tinel's s.,** a tingling sensation in the distal end of a limb when percussion is made over the site of a divided nerve. It indicates a partial lesion or the beginning regeneration of the nerve. Called also *formication s.* and *distal tingling on percussion* (D.T.P.). **toe s.,** Babinski's reflex. **Tommasi's s.,** alopecia on the posteroexternal aspect of the legs, found almost exclusively in men with gout. **Tournay's s.,** unilateral dilatation of the pupil of the abducting eye on extreme lateral fixation. **Traube's s.,** a faint double sound heard in auscultation over the femoral arteries in aortic regurgitation. **Trendelenburg's s.,** see under *tests.* **trepidation s.,** patellar clonus. **Tresilian's s.,** a reddish appearance in Stensen's duct in mumps. **Trimadeau's s.,** if the dilatation above an esophageal stricture is conic, the stricture is fibrous; if cup shaped, the stricture is malignant. **Troisier's s.,** enlargement of the lymph nodes above the clavicle; a sign of intra-abdominal malignant disease or of retrosternal tumor. **Trömner's s.,** Hoffmann's s., def. 2. **Trousseau's s.,** 1. see under *phenomenon.* 2. tache cérébrale. **Turner's s.,** discoloration (bruising) of the skin of the loin in acute hemorrhagic pancreatitis. **Turyn's s.,** in sciatica, if the patient's great toe is bent dorsally, pain will be felt in the gluteal region. **Uhthoff's s.,** nystagmus occurring in multiple cerebrospinal sclerosis. **Unschuld's s.,** a tendency to cramp in the calves of the legs; an early indication of diabetes. **Uriolla's s.,** the presence in the urine of malarial patients of minute black granules of blood pigment. **Vanzetti's s.,** in sciatica the pelvis is always horizontal in spite of scoliosis, but in other lesions with scoliosis the pelvis is inclined. **Vedder's s's** (*of beriberi*), slight pressure on muscles of calf causes pain; ascertain the presence of anesthesia with a pin over anterior surface of leg; note any changes in patellar reflexes; when patient squats upon heels, note the inability to rise without use of hands. **vein s.,** a bluish cord along the midaxillary line formed by the swollen junction of the thoracic and superficial epigastric vein; seen in tuberculosis of the bronchial glands and in superior vena cava obstruction. **Vigouroux's s.,** diminished electric resistance of the skin in Graves' disease. **vital s's,** the pulse, respiration, and temperature. **Voltolini's s.,** Heryng's s. **von Graefe's s.,** Graefe's s. **Wartenberg's s.,** 1. a sign of ulnar palsy, consisting of a position of

abduction assumed by the little finger. 2. reduction or absence of the pendulum movements of the arm in walking; seen in patients with cerebellar disease. **Weber's s.,** paralysis of the oculomotor nerve of one side and hemiplegia of the opposite side. See *syndrome of Weber.* **Wegner's s.,** a broadened, discolored appearance of the epiphyseal line in infants dying from hereditary syphilis. **Weill's s.,** absence of expansion in the subclavicular region of the affected side in infantile pneumonia. **Weiss's s.,** Chvostek's s. **Wernicke's s.,** hemiopic pupillary reaction. **Westermark's s.,** transient clearing (avascularity) of the normal radiologic shadow of pulmonary tissue distal to a pulmonary embolism. **Westphal's s.,** loss of the knee jerk in tabes dorsalis. **Widowitz's s.,** protrusion of the eyeballs and sluggish movements of the eyeballs and eyelids seen in diphtheritic paralysis. **Wilder's s.,** an early sign of Graves' disease consisting in a slight twitch of the eyeball when it changes its movement from adduction to abduction or vice versa. **Williams' s.,** a dull tympanitic resonance heard in the second intercostal space in severe pleural effusion. **Williamson's s.,** markedly diminished blood pressure in the leg as compared with that in the arm on the same side; seen in pneumothorax and pleural effusion. **Wimberger's s.,** erosion of the upper end of the tibia in early syphilis. **Winterbottom's s.,** enlargement of posterior cervical lymph nodes in African trypanosomiasis. **Wintrich's s.,** a change in the pitch of the percussion note when the mouth is opened and closed; it indicates a cavity in the lung. **Wood's s.,** relaxation of the orbicularis muscle, fixation of the eyeball, and divergent strabismus, indicative of profound anesthesia. **Wreden's s.,** presence of a gelatinous matter in the external auditory meatus in children who are born dead. **Zaufal's s.,** saddle nose.

signa (sig′nah) [L.]   mark, or write; abbreviated S. or sig. on prescriptions. See *prescription.*

signature (sig′nah-tūr) [L. *signatura*]   1. that part of a prescription which gives directions as to the taking of the medicine. See *prescription.* 2. any characteristic feature of a substance formerly regarded as an indication of its medicinal virtues: thus, the eyelike mark on the flower of the euphrasia was supposed to show its usefulness in eye diseases; the liver-like shape of the leaf of liverwort pointed to its use in hepatic diseases; the yellow color of saffron indicated its use in jaundice.

signaturist (sig′nah-tūr″ist)   one who believes in the doctrine of signatures.

signe (sēn) [Fr.]   sign.   **s. de journal** (sēn-dě-zhoor-nal′), Froment's paper sign.   **s. de peau d'orange** (sēn-dě-po-dor-anzh′), orange-peel sign.

significant (sig-nif′ĭ-kant)   in statistics, probably resulting from something other than chance.

Signorelli's sign (sēn-yor-el′ēz) [Angelo *Signorelli,* Italian physician, 1876–1952]   see under *sign.*

Sig. n. pro.   abbreviation for L. *sig′na nom′ine pro′prio,* label with the proper name.

siguatera (sig″wah-ta′rah) [Sp.]   ciguatera.

sikimi (sik′ĭ-me) [Japanese]   the plant *Illicium religiosum.*

sikimin (sik′ĭ-min)   a poisonous hydrocarbon, $C_{10}H_{16}$, found in the leaves of *Illicium religiosum.*

sikimitoxin (sik-im″ĭ-tok′sin)   a poisonous substance extracted from sikimi.

silafocon A (sil″ah-fo′kon)   chemical name: 3-[3,3,5,5,5-pentamethyl-1, 1-bis[(pentamethyldisiloxanyl)oxy]trisiloxanyl]propyl methacrylate polymer with methyl methacrylate, methacrylic acid, and tetraethylene glycol dimethacrylate. A hydrophilic contact lens material, $(C_{22}H_{56}O_8Si_7)_w(C_5H_8O_2)_x(C_4H_8O_2)_y(C_{16}H_{26}O_7)_z.$

Silain (si′lān)   trademark for preparations of simethicone.

silandrone (sĭ-lan′drōn)   chemical name: 17β-(trimethylsiloxy)-androst-4-en-3-one; an androgenic steroid, $C_{22}H_{36}O_2Si.$

Silastic (sĭ-las′tik)   trademark for polymeric silicone substances having the properties of rubber; it is biologically inert and used in surgical prostheses.

silent (si′lent)   producing no detectable signs or symptoms; noiseless.

silex (si′leks)   a noncrystalline form of silica, as precipitated silica, used in cements.

Silex's sign (se′leks-ez) [Paul *Silex,* German ophthalmologist, 1858–1929]   see under *sign.*

silica (sil′ĭ-kah) [L. *silex* flint]   silicon dioxide, $SiO_2,$ or silicic anhydride. It may occur in various allotropic forms, some of which are used in dental materials.

silicate (sil′ĭ-kāt) [L. *silicus*]   a salt of any of the many silicic acids.

silicatosis (sil″ĭ-kah-to′sis)   pneumoconiosis caused by the inhalation of the dust of silicates.

silicea (sĭ-lis′e-ah)   a homeopathic preparation of silica.

siliceous, silicious (sĭ-lish′us)   containing silica or a compound of silicon.

silicoanthracosis (sil″ĭ-ko-an″thrah-ko′sis)   silicosis combined with pneumoconiosis of coal workers.

silicofluoride (sil″ĭ-ko-floo′o-rīd) fluorosilicate.

silicol (sil′ĭ-kol) an organic silica compound, silicic oxide casein metaphosphate; used in the treatment of tuberculosis.

silicon (sil′ĭ-kon) [L. *silex* flint] a nonmetallic light element whose dioxide is silica; symbol, Si; atomic number, 14; atomic weight, 28.086. **s. carbide**, a compound produced by the reaction of silicon and carbon at extremely high temperature, used in dentistry as an abrasive agent. **s. dioxide**, silica. **s. dioxide, colloidal** [NF], a submicroscopic fumed silica prepared by the vapor-phase hydrolysis of a silicon compound; used as a tablet diluent and as a suspending and thickening agent. **s. fluoride**, SiF₄, a colorless gas sometimes fatal to workers in superphosphate factories.

silicone (sil′ĭ-kōn) any organic compound in which all or part of the carbon has been replaced by silicon.

silicosiderosis (sil″ĭ-ko-sid″er-o′sis) pneumoconiosis in which the inhaled dust is that of silica and iron.

silicosis (sil″ĭ-ko′sis) [L. *silex* flint] pneumoconiosis due to the inhalation of the dust of stone, sand, or flint containing silicon dioxide, with formation of generalized nodular fibrotic changes in both lungs. Called also *grinders' disease*. **infective s.**, silicotuberculosis.

Silicote (sil′ĭ-kōt) trademark for preparations of dimethicone.

silicotic (sil′ĭ-kot′ik) pertaining to or characterized by silicosis.

silicotuberculosis (sil″ĭ-ko-tu-ber″ku-lo′sis) tuberculous infection of the silicotic lung; infective silicosis.

siliqua (sil′ĭ-kwah) [L.] pod, or husk. **s. oli′vae** ["husk of the olive"], the fibers which appear to encircle superficially the inferior olive of the brain; their outer and inner portions are termed *funiculus lateralis medullae oblongatae*. Called also *amiculum olivae*.

siliquose (sil′ĭ-kwōs) pertaining to or resembling a pod or husk; see under *cataract*.

silkworm-gut (silk′werm-gut) a strand drawn from a silkworm which has been killed when ready to spin its cocoon; less pliable than catgut and nonabsorbable, it is used for retention sutures, which are later removed.

sillonneur (se-yon-nur′) [Fr.] (*obs.*) a three-bladed scalpel for operations on the eye.

Silvadene (sil′vah-dēn) trademark for a preparation of silver sulfadiazine.

silvatic (sil-vat′ik) [L. *silva* a wood or woods] pertaining to or occurring in the woods; as *silvatic plague*.

silver (sil′ver) [L. *argentum*] a white, soft, malleable, and ductile metal; symbol, Ag; atomic number, 47; atomic weight, 107.870. Its compounds are extensively used in medicine, and metallic silver is employed in surgery and in the manufacture of instruments. It is an important component in alloys used as filling materials in dentistry. **s. arsphenamine**, see under *arsphenamine*. **s. chloride**, an insoluble white salt, AgCl, that darkens in light; called *horn silver* in mineral form. **colloidal s.**, a silver preparation in which the silver exists as free ions to only a small extent. See *protein s., mild*, and *protein s., strong*. **s. cyanide**, a soluble salt, AgCN. **s. iodide**, an insoluble, light-yellowish binary, powdery compound, AgI, that turns black in the light; used in treatment of syphilis, nervous diseases, and conjunctivitis. **s. iodide, colloidal**, silver iodide in solution rendered stable by gelatin, an antiseptic for treating inflammations of mucous membranes. **s. nitrate** [USP], a powerful germicide, AgNO₃, occurring as colorless or white crystals; used as an antiseptic, applied topically to the conjunctiva as a prophylactic against ophthalmia neonatorum, and also used as an antiseptic and astringent, especially in infections of the skin and mucous membranes. It has also been used to purify drinking water. **s. nitrate, toughened** [USP], a compound prepared by fusing silver nitrate with hydrochloric acid, sodium chloride, or potassium nitrate, occurring as white crystalline masses molded into pencils or cones, and containing 94.5 per cent of silver nitrate; used as a caustic and applied topically after being dipped in water. Called also *lunar caustic, fused silver nitrate*, and *molded silver nitrate*. **s. orthophosphate**, an insoluble yellow powder, Ag₃PO₄. **s. oxide**, a heavy brownish-black powder, Ag₂O. **s. picrate**, yellow crystals, C₆H₂(NO₂)₃OAg·H₂O, used as a topical anti-infective, especially in infections of the skin and mucous membranes; it has been used in the treatment of vaginal trichomoniasis and candidiasis, administered by insufflation or in pessaries. **s. protein, mild**, a preparation containing 19–23 per cent of silver, rendered colloidal by the presence of, or combination with, protein; it occurs as dark brown or almost black scales or granules and is used as a topical anti-infective in various rectal, ocular, vaginal, urethral, otic, nasal, and pharyngeal infections. **s. protein, strong**, a pale yellowish orange to brownish black powdered compound of silver and protein containing 7.5–8.5 per cent of silver, an active germicide with a local irritant and astringent effect. It may cause argyria. **s. sulfadiazine**, the silver derivative of sulfadiazine, C₁₀H₉Ag N₄O₂S, having bactericidal activity against many gram-positive and gram-negative organisms, as well as being effective against yeasts; used as a topical anti-infective for the prevention and treatment of wound

sepsis in patients with second and third degree burns. **s. sulfate**, a moderately soluble colorless salt, Ag₂SO₄. **s. sulfide**, a black insoluble powder, Ag₂S.

Silverman's needle (sil′ver-manz) [Irving *Silverman*, Brooklyn surgeon, born 1904] see under *needle*.

silverskin (sil′ver-skin) the pericarp and germ of grains which are removed in processing, as in polished rice, but which contain the thiamine.

Silvester's method (sil-ves′terz) [Henry Robert *Silvester*, English physician, 1828–1908] see under *respiration, artificial*.

silvestrene (sil-ves′trēn) a hydrocarbon, C₁₀H₁₆, obtainable from European oil of turpentine.

Silvius (sil′ve-us) a genus of tabanid flies found abundantly in Australia.

Simaruba (sim″ah-roo′bah) a genus of tropical American trees, several species of which are medicinal. The root bark of *S. ama′ra* Aubl. (Simarubaceae) is a bitter tonic and astringent, and has been used in amebiasis. The active principle is simarubidin.

simarubidin (sim″ah-roo′-bĭ-din) the active principle, C₂₂H₃₂O₉, of the bark and wood of *Simaruba amara;* used experimentally in canine amebiasis.

simesthesia (sim″es-the′ze-ah) osseous sensibility.

simethicone (sĭ-meth′ĭ-kōn) [USP] a mixture of dimethicones and silicon dioxide, with a molecular weight between 14,000 and 21,000, occurring as a translucent, gray, viscous fluid. It is administered orally as an antifoaming agent in gastroscopy, and is also used as an antiflatulent and as a releasing agent in pharmaceutical preparations. Called also *dimethicone* or *activated dimethicone*. It is used in veterinary medicine in the treatment and prevention of bloat in cattle.

similia similibus curantur (sĭ-mil′e-ah sĭ-mil′ĭ-bus ku-ran′tur) [L. "likes are cured by likes"] the doctrine, or the brocard expressing it, which lies at the foundation of homeopathy; namely, that a disease is cured by those remedies which produce effects resembling the disease itself.

similimum (sĭ-mil′ĭ-mum) [L. "likest"] the homeopathic remedy which most exactly reproduces the symptoms of any disease.

Simmonds' disease (syndrome) (sim′ondz) [Morris *Simmonds*, physician in Hamburg, 1855–1925] see *panhypopituitarism*.

Simon's septic factor, sign (si′monz) [Charles Edmund *Simon*, Baltimore physician, 1866–1927] see under *factor* and under *sign*, def. 1.

Simon's sign (si′monz) [John *Simon*, English surgeon, 1824–1876] see under *sign*.

Simon's speculum (ze′monz) [Gustav *Simon*, German surgeon, 1824–1876] see under *speculum*.

Simonart's thread (band) (se″mo-narz′) [Pierre Joseph Cécilien *Simonart*, Belgian obstetrician, 1817–1847] see under *thread*.

Simonea folliculorum (sĭ-mo′ne-ah fŏ-lik″u-lo′rum) *Demodex folliculorum*.

Simonelli's test (si″mo-nel′ēz) [F. *Simonelli*, Italian physician] see under *tests*.

Simons' disease (si′monz) [Arthur *Simons*, Berlin physician, born 1877] *lipodystrophia progressiva*.

Simonsiella (si-mon″se-el′ah) a genus of blue-green algae isolated from the intestinal tracts of men and many animals; it was once thought to be a pathogen.

simple (sim′p'l) [L. *simplex*] 1. neither compound nor complex; single. 2. an old term for any herb with real or supposed medicinal virtues.

simpler (sim′pler) an herb doctor.

Simpson's forceps (simp′sunz) [Sir James Young *Simpson*, Scottish obstetrician, 1811–1870] see under *forceps*.

Simpson light (lamp) (simp′sun) [William Speirs *Simpson*, British civil engineer, died 1917] see under *light*.

Simpson's splint (simp′sunz) [William Kelly *Simpson*, laryngologist in New York, 1855–1914] see under *splint*.

Sims' position, etc. (simz) [James Marion *Sims*, New York gynecologist, 1813–1883] see under *depressor, position*, and *speculum*.

simul (sim′ul) [L.] at the same time as.

simulation (sim″u-la′shun) [L. *simulatio*] 1. the act of counterfeiting a disease; malingering. 2. the mimicking of one disease by another.

simulator (sim″u-la′tor) something that simulates, such as an apparatus that simulates conditions that will be encountered in real life. **electrocardiographic s.**, a device that produces simulations of electrocardiographic wave forms.

Simuliidae (si″mu-le′ĭ-de) a family of flies of the suborder Nematocerca, order Diptera, characterized by small size, a humped back, and short stubbed antennae of 10 or 11 segments. It contains approximately 600 species, known variously as black flies, buffalo gnats, or turkey gnats. The females of several species are vicious biters.

Simulium (si-mu′le-um) a genus of flies of the family Simuliidae. They are widely distributed and a great pest at times. *S.*

arc'ticum occurs in Alaska. *S. columbaczen'se,* a species in southern Europe which has been known to kill animals. *S. damno'sum* is an intermediate host of *Onchocerca volvulus* in Africa. *S. metal'licum* and *S. ochra'ceum* transmit *Onchocerca volvulus* in Mexico. *S. pecua'rium,* the buffalo gnat, a terrible scourge to horses and cattle. *S. venus'tum,* a species widely distributed in North America and Denmark.

simultanagnosia (si''mul-tān''ag-no'se-ah) the inability to comprehend more than one element of a visual scene at the same time or to integrate the parts as a whole.

sinal (si'nal) pertaining to a sinus; sinusal.

sinapism (sin'ah-pizm) [L. *sinapismus;* Gr. *sinapismos, sinapisma*] a plaster or paste of ground mustard seed; a mustard plaster.

Sinaxar (sin'aks-ar) trademark for a preparation of styramate.

sincalide (sin'kah-līd) chemical name: 1-de(5-oxo-L-proline)-2-de-L-glutamide-5-L-methioninecaerulin; a choleretic, $C_{49}H_{62}N_{10}$-$O_{16}S_3$.

sincipital (sin-sip'ĭ-tal) pertaining to the sinciput.

sinciput (sin'sĭ-put) [L.] [NA] the anterior and upper part of the head.

sinefungin (sin''ĕ-fun'jin) chemical name: 6,9-diamino-1-(6-amino-9*H*-purin-9-yl)-1,5,6,7,8,9-hexadeoxy-β-D-*ribo*-decofuranuronic acid; an antifungal antibiotic derived from *Streptomyces griseolus,* $C_{15}H_{23}N_7O_5$.

Sinequan (sin'ĕ-kwan) trademark for a preparation of doxepin hydrochloride.

sinew (sin'u) the tendon of a muscle. **back s.,** the large flexor tendon at the back of the cannon bone of quadrupeds. **weeping s.,** an encysted ganglion, chiefly on the back of the hand, containing synovial fluid.

sing. abbreviation of L. *singulo'rum,* of each.

Singoserp (sing'go-serp) trademark for preparations of syrosingopine.

singultation (sing''gul-ta'shun) a hiccup.

singultous (sing-gul'tus) affected with hiccup.

singultus (sing-gul'tus) [L.] hiccup. **s. gas'tricus ner-vo'sus,** hiccup due to a nervous condition of the stomach.

sinigrin (sin'ĭ-grin) potassium myronate, $CH_2:CH\cdot CH_2(S\cdot C_6\cdot H_{11}O_5)N\cdot CO\cdot SO_2\cdot OK$, a glycoside found in black mustard seed.

sinister (sin-is'ter) [L.] left; in official anatomical nomenclature, used to designate the left hand one of two similar structures, or the one situated on the left side of the body.

sinistrad (sin-is'trad) to or toward the left.

sinistral (sin'is-tral) [L. *sinistralis*] 1. pertaining to the left side. 2. a left-handed person.

sinistrality (sin''is-tral'ĭ-te) the preferential use, in voluntary motor acts, of the left member of the major paired organs of the body, as ear, eye, hand, and leg.

sinistraural (sin''is-traw'ral) [L. *sinister* + *auris* ear] hearing better with the left ear.

sinistro- (sin'is-tro) [L. *sinister* left] a combining form meaning left, or denoting relationship to the left side.

sinistrocardia (sin''is-tro-kar'de-ah) [*sinistro-* + Gr. *kardia* heart] location of the heart in left side of the thorax; levocardia.

sinistrocerebral (sin''is-tro-ser'ĕ-bral) pertaining to or situated in the left cerebral hemisphere.

sinistrocular (sin''is-trok'u-lar) [*sinistro-* + L. *oculus* eye] left eyed; having the left eye the dominant eye.

sinistrocularity (sin''is-trok''u-lar'ĭ-te) the state of having the left eye the dominant eye.

sinistrogyration (sin''is-tro-ji-ra'shun) [*sinistro-* + L. *gyrus* a turn] a turning to the left, as a movement of the eye or the plane of polarization.

sinistromanual (sin''is-tro-man'u-al) [*sinistro-* + L. *manus* hand] left handed.

sinistropedal (sin''is-trop'ĕ-dal) [*sinistro-* + L. *pes* foot] using the left foot in preference to the right.

sinistrorse (sin'is-trors) turned to the left.

sinistrose (sin'is-trōs) a levorotatory sugar sometimes found in the urine.

sinistrotorsion (sin''is-tro-tor'shun) [*sinistro-* + L. *torsio* twist] a twisting toward the left; said mainly of the eye.

sinkaline (sing'kah-lin) choline.

Sinkler's phenomenon (singk'lerz) [Wharton *Sinkler,* Philadelphia neurologist, 1847–1910] see under *phenomenon.*

sinoatrial (si''no-a'tre-al) pertaining to the sinus venosus and the atrium of the heart; see also under *node.*

sinoauricular (si''no-aw-rik'u-lar) sinoatrial.

sinobronchitis (si''no-brong-ki'tis) [*sino-* + Gr. *bronchos* bronchus + *-itis*] chronic paranasal sinusitis with recurrent episodes of bronchitis.

sinography (si-nog'rah-fe) [*sinus* + Gr. *graphein* to write] roentgenography of the sinuses.

sinomenine (si-nom'ĕ-nin) a crystalline alkaloid, $C_{19}H_{23}NO_4$, from *Sinomenium diversifolium,* a plant of eastern Asia.

Si non val. abbreviation for L. *si non va'leat,* if it is not enough.

sinopulmonary (si''no-pul'mo-ner''e) involving the paranasal sinuses and the lungs.

sinospiral (si''no-spi'ral) pertaining to the sinus venosus and having a spiral course; said of certain muscle fibers of the heart.

sinoventricular (si''no-ven-trik'u-lar) pertaining to the sinus venosus and the ventricle of the heart.

sinter (sin'ter) 1. the calcareous or silicious matter deposited by mineral springs. 2. [Ger.] to transform into a solid mass by heating without melting.

sintoc (sin'tok) the bark of *Cinnamomum sintoc,* of the East Indies; it resembles cinnamon.

Sintrom (sin'trom) trademark for a preparation of acenocoumarol.

sinuate (sin''u-āt) having a wavy margin.

sinuatrial (sin''u-a'tre-al) sinoatrial.

sinuauricular (sin''u-aw-rik'u-lar) sinoatrial.

sinuitis (sin''u-i'tis) sinusitis.

sinuotomy (si''nu-ot'o-me) sinusotomy.

sinuous (sin'u-us) [L. *sinuosus*] bending in and out; winding.

sinus (si'nus), pl. *si'nus* or sinuses [L. "a hollow"] 1. a cavity, or channel; [NA] a general term for such spaces as the dilated channels for venous blood in the cranium, or the air cavities in the cranial bones. 2. an abnormal channel or fistula permitting the escape of pus. **accessory s's of the nose,** s. paranasales. **air s.,** an air-containing space within the substance of a bone. **s. a'lae par'vae,** old term for s. sphenoparietalis. **anal s's, s. ana'les** [NA], furrows, with pouchlike recesses at the lower end, separating the rectal columns; called also *s. rectales* and *crypts of Morgagni.* **s. of anterior chamber,** the narrow space at the edge of the anterior chamber of the eye, between the border of the cornea and the root of the iris. **s. aor'tae** [NA], **s. aor'tae [Valsal'vae], aortic s.,** a dilatation between the aortic wall and each of the semilunar cusps of the aortic valve; from two of these sinuses the coronary arteries take origin. Called also *Petit's s., s. of Morgagni,* and *s. of Valsalva.* **Arlt's s.,** s. of Maier. **s. arte'riae pulmona'lis,** s. trunci pulmonalis. **articular s. of atlas,** fovea dentis atlantis. **articular s. of atlas, superior,** fovea articularis superior atlantis. **articular s. of axis, anterior,** facies articularis anterior axis. **arores vertebrarum. s. of atlas, anterior,** fovea dentis atlantis. **basilar s.,** plexus basilaris. **s. of Bochdalek,** hiatus pleuroperitonealis. **branchial s.,** an abnormal opening between a branchial groove and its corresponding pharyngeal pouch, homologous with an ancestral gill slit. **Breschet's s.,** s. sphenoparietalis. **s. carot'icus** [NA], **carotid s.,** the dilated portion of the internal carotid artery, situated above the division of the common carotid artery into its two main branches, or sometimes on the terminal portion of the common carotid artery, containing in its wall pressoreceptors that are stimulated by changes in blood pressure. Called also *bulbus caroticus.* **s. caverno'sus** [NA], **cavernous s.,** an irregularly shaped venous space in the dura mater at either side of the body of the sphenoid bone, extending from the medial end of the superior orbital fissure in front to the apex of the petrous temporal bone behind. It receives the superior ophthalmic vein, the superficial middle cerebral vein, and the sphenoparietal sinus, and communicates with the opposite cavernous sinus and with the transverse sinus and internal jugular vein by way of the petrosal sinuses. Commonly comprising one or more main venous channels, it contains the internal carotid artery and abducent nerve. **cerebral s.,** any of the ventricles of the brain. **cervical s.,** a temporary depression caudal to the embryonic hyoid arch, containing the succeeding branchial arches; it is overgrown by the hyoid arch and closes off as the cervical vesicle. **circular s., s. circula'ris,** the venous ring around the hypophysis formed by the two cavernous and the anterior and posterior intercavernous sinuses; called also *Ridley's s.* **s. circula'ris i'ridis,** s. venosus sclerae. **coccygeal s.,** a sinus or fistula situated just over or close to the tip of the coccyx, being the remains of the end of the neurenteric canal; see also *pilonidal s.* **s. coch'leae,** vena canaliculi cochleae. **s. condylo'rum fem'oris,** fossa intercondylaris femoris. **s. corona'rius** [NA], **coronary s.,** the terminal portion of the great cardiac vein, which lies in the coronary sulcus between the left atrium and ventricle, and empties into the right atrium. **cortical s's,** lymph sinuses in the cortex of a lymph node, which arise from the marginal sinuses and continue into the medullary sinuses; called also *intermediate s's.* **costal s's of sternum,** incisurae costales sterni. **costodiaphragmatic s.,** recessus costodiaphragmaticus pleurae. **costomediastinal s. of pleura, s. costomediastina'lis pleu'rae,** recessus costomediastinalis pleurae. **costophrenic s.,** recessus costodiaphragmaticus pleurae. **cranial s's,** see under *duct.* **Cuvier's s's,** see under *duct.* **dermal s.,** a congenital sinus tract extending from the surface of the body, between the bodies of two adjacent lumbar vertebrae, to the spinal canal. **s. du′rae ma′tris** [NA], large venous channels forming an anastomosing system between the layers of the dura mater encephali. They are devoid of valves, do not collapse when drained, and in some parts contain numerous trabeculae. They drain the cerebral veins and some diploic and meningeal veins into the veins of the neck. Those at the base of the skull also drain most of the blood from the orbit. In some places they communicate with superficial veins by small emissary vessels. Called also *cranial s's* and *venous s's of dura mater.* **s. epididym′idis** [NA], **s. of epididymis**, a long, slitlike serous pocket between the upper part of the testis and the overlying epididymis. **Eternod's s.**, a loop of vessels connecting the vessels of the chorion with those in the under side of the yolk sac. **ethmoidal s.**, **s. ethmoida′lis** [NA], one of the paranasal sinuses, located in the ethmoid bone, consisting of the cellulae ethmoidales collectively, and communicating with the ethmoidal infundibulum and bulla and with the superior and highest meatuses of the nasal cavity. **falcial s.**, **falciform s.**, old term for s. sagittalis inferior. **Forssell's s.**, a smooth space in the wall of the stomach surrounded by folds of the mucosa; seen on roentgen-ray examination. **frontal s.**, **bony**, s. frontalis osseus. **s. fronta′lis** [NA], frontal sinus: one of the paired paranasal sinuses located in the frontal bone, and communicating by way of the nasofrontal duct with the middle meatus of the nasal cavity on the same side. See also *s. frontalis osseus.* **s. fronta′lis os′seus** [NA], bony frontal sinus: an irregular air cavity situated in the frontal bone on either side, deep to the superciliary arch; separated from its fellow of the opposite side by a bony septum, and communicating with the middle meatus of the bony nasal cavity on the same side. **Guérin's s.**, a diverticulum behind Guérin's fold. **Huguier's s.**, a depression in the tympanum between the fenestra ovalis and the fenestra rotunda. **s. interarcua′lis**, fossa tonsillaris. **s. intercaverno′si** [NA], intercavernous sinuses: two venous channels that connect the two cavernous sinuses, one passing anterior and the other posterior to the infundibulum of the hypophysis. **s. intercaverno′sus ante′rior**, the anterior of the two spaces connecting the cavernous sinuses; see *s. intercavernosi.* **s. intercaverno′sus poste′rior**, the posterior of the two spaces connecting the cavernous sinuses; see *s. intercavernosi.* **intercavernous s's**, s. intercavernosi. **intermediate s's**, cortical s's. **s. of internal jugular vein, inferior**, bulbus venae jugularis inferior. **s. of internal jugular vein, superior**, bulbus venae jugularis superior. **s. of kidney**, s. renalis. **lacteal s's**, **s. lacteus**, **s. lactif′eri** [NA], **lactiferous s's**, enlargements in the lactiferous ducts just before they open onto the mammary papilla. **laryngeal s.**, **s. of larynx**, ventriculus laryngis. **lateral s.**, s. transversus durae matris. **s. lie′nis** [NA], sinuses of the spleen: dilated venous sinuses, not lined by ordinary endothelial cells, found in the splenic pulp. **longitudinal s.**, **inferior**, s. sagittalis inferior. **longitudinal s.**, **superior**, s. sagittalis superior. **lunate s. of radius**, incisura ulnaris radii. **lunate s. of ulna**, incisura radialis ulnae. **lymph s's**, **lymphatic s's**, irregular tortuous spaces within lymphoid tissue (nodes) through which a continuous stream of lymph passes, to enter the efferent lymphatic vessels. See also *cortical s's, marginal s's,* and *medullary s's.* **s. of Maier**, a slight diverticulum from the upper part of the lacrimal sac, into which the lacrimal canaliculi open, either together or separately; called also *Arlt's sinus.* **marginal s.**, 1. marginal lakes; see under *lake.* 2. bow-shaped lymph sinuses separating the capsule from the cortical parenchyma of a lymph node, and from which lymph flows into the cortical sinuses; called also *subcapsular s's.* **mastoid s.**, see *cellulae mastoideae.* **s. maxilla′ris** [NA], **s. maxilla′ris [Highmo′ri]**, maxillary sinus: one of the paired paranasal sinuses, located in the body of the maxilla on either side and communicating with the middle meatus of the nasal cavity on the same side. Called also *antrum of Highmore.* (See also *s. maxillaris osseus.*) **s. maxilla′ris os′seus** [NA], bony maxillary sinus: an air cavity of variable size and shape located in the body of each maxilla, communicating with the middle meatus of the bony nasal cavity on the same side. **maxillary s.**, s. maxillaris. **maxillary s.**, **bony**, s. maxillaris osseus. **medullary s's**, lymph sinuses in the medulla of a lymph node, which divide the lymphoid tissue into a number of medullary cords. **Meyer's s.**, **s. Mey′eri**, a small depression in the floor of the external auditory canal just in front of the tympanic membrane. **middle s. of atlas**, fovea dentis atlantis. **s. of Morgagni**, 1. see *sinus anales.* 2. sinus aortae. 3. ventriculus laryngis. **mucous s's of male urethra**, lacunae urethrales. **oblique s. of pericardium**, **s. obli′quus pericar′dii** [NA], a recess of serous pericardium that passes upward behind the left atrium and between the left and right pulmonary veins. **occipital s.**, **s. occipita′lis** [NA], a single venous sinus of the dura mater that begins in right and left branches, the marginal sinuses, and passes upward along the attached margin of the cerebellar falx to end in the confluence of the sinuses. **oral s.**, stomodeum. **paranasal s's**, **s. paranasa′les** [NA], the mucosa-lined air cavities in the cranial bones which communicate with the nasal cavity, including the ethmoidal, frontal, maxillary, and sphenoidal sinuses. **parasinoidal s.**, any one of several spaces in the dura mater opening

into one of the dural sinuses; called also *lacuna lateralis* or *lacus lateralis.* **s. pericar′dii**, s. transversus pericardii. **s. pericra′nii**, a soft fluctuating vascular tumor of the scalp which communicates directly with an intracranial sinus through a defect in the skull. **peroneal s. of tibia**, incisura fibularis tibiae. **Petit's s.**, s. aortae. **petrosal s., inferior**, s. petrosus inferior. **petrosal s., superior**, s. petrosus superior. **s. petro′sus infe′rior** [NA], inferior petrosal sinus: a venous sinus arising from the cavernous sinus and running along the line of the petrooccipital synchondrosis to the superior bulb of the internal jugular vein. **s. petro′sus supe′rior** [NA], superior petrosal sinus: a sinus arising at the cavernous sinus, passing along the attached margin of the cerebellar tentorium, and draining into the transverse sinus. **phrenicocostal s.**, **s. phrenicocosta′lis**, recessus costodiaphragmaticus pleurae. **pilonidal s.**, a suppurating sinus containing a tuft of hair, occurring chiefly in the coccygeal region, but also in other regions of the body. See also *coccygeal s.* **piriform s.**, recessus piriformis. **s. pleu′rae**, **pleural s.**, recessus pleurales. **pleuroperitoneal s.**, hiatus pleuroperitonealis. **s. pocula′ris**, utriculus prostaticus. **s. poste′rior ca′vi tym′pani** [NA], posterior sinus of tympanic cavity: a groove in the posterior wall of the tympanic cavity above the pyramidal eminence. **s. precervica′lis**, the depression at the side of the neck, produced in the developing embryo by the growth of the branchial arches. **prostatic s.**, **s. prostat′icus** [NA], the posterolateral recess between the seminal colliculus and the wall of the urethra. **s's of pulmonary trunk**, s. trunci pulmonalis. **pyriform s.**, recessus piriformis. **rectal s's**, **s. recta′les**, s. anales. **s. rec′tus** [NA], a venous sinus of the dura mater situated in the line of union of the cerebral falx and the cerebellar tentorium, formed by the junction of the great cerebral vein and the inferior sagittal sinus, and commonly ending in the opposite transverse sinus at the confluence of the sinuses. Called also *straight s.* **renal s.**, **s. rena′lis** [NA], a cavity within the substance of the kidney, occupied by the renal pelvis, calices, vessels, nerves, and fat. **s. reu′niens**, the sinus venosus of the embryonic heart into which empty all the veins that go to the heart. **rhomboid s.**, 1. fossa rhomboidea. 2. cavum septi pellucidi. **rhomboid s. of Henle**, ventriculus terminalis medullae spinalis. **s. rhomboi′deus cer′ebri**, cavum septi pellucidi. **Ridley's s.**, s. circularis. **Rokitansky-Aschoff s's**, small outpouchings of the mucosa of the gallbladder extending through the lamina propria and the muscular layer. **sacrococcygeal s.**, pilonidal s. **sagittal s., inferior**, s. sagittalis inferior. **sagittal s., superior**, s. sagittalis superior. **s. sagitta′lis infe′rior** [NA], inferior sagittal sinus: a small venous sinus of the dura mater, situated in the posterior half of the lower concave border of the cerebral falx and opening into the upper end of the straight sinus. **s. sagitta′lis supe′rior** [NA], superior sagittal sinus: a single venous sinus of the dura mater which begins in front of the crista galli and extends backward in the convex border of the falx cerebri. Near the internal occipital protuberance it ends in a variable way in the confluence of the sinuses. It receives the superior cerebral veins, communicates with the lateral lacunae of adjacent dura mater, and is partially invaginated by arachnoidal granulations. **semilunar s. of tibia**, incisura fibularis tibiae. **sigmoid s.**, **s. sigmoi′deus** [NA], either of two venous sinuses within the dura mater that are continuations of the transverse sinuses; each curves downward from the tentorium cerebelli to become continuous with the superior bulb of the internal jugular vein. **sphenoidal s.**, s. sphenoidalis. **sphenoidal s., bony**, s. sphenoidalis osseus. **s. sphenoida′lis** [NA], sphenoidal sinus: one of the paired paranasal sinuses, located in the anterior part of the body of the sphenoid bone and communicating with the highest meatus of the nasal cavity on the same side. See also *s. sphenoidalis osseus.* **s. sphenoida′lis os′seus** [NA], bony sphenoidal sinus: an air cavity of variable size and shape situated in the anterior part of the body of the sphenoid bone; separated from its fellow of the opposite side by a septum, and opening into the nasal cavity above the superior nasal concha on the same side. **sphenoparietal s.**, **s. sphenoparieta′lis** [NA], a dural venous sinus which begins at a meningeal vein next to the apex of the small wing of the sphenoid bone and which drains into the anterior part of the cavernous sinus. Called also *Breschet's s.* **s's of spleen**, s. lienis. **straight s.**, s. rectus. **subarachnoidal s's**, cisternae subarachnoideales. **subcapsular s's**, marginal s's (def. 2.) **subpetrosal s.**, s. petrosus inferior. **superpetrosal s.**, s. petrosus superior. **tarsal s.**, **s. tar′si** [NA], the space between the calcaneus and talus, containing the interosseous ligament; called also *tarsal canal.* **tentorial s.**, s. rectus. **terminal s.**, a vein which encircles the vascular area in the blastoderm. **tonsillar s.**, **s. tonsilla′ris**, fossa tonsillaris. **transverse s. of dura mater**, s. transversus durae matris. **transverse s. of pericardium**, s. transversus pericardii. **s. transver′sus du′rae ma′tris** [NA], transverse sinus of dura mater: either of two large venous sinuses of the dura mater that begin in a variable fashion at the confluence of the sinuses near the internal occipital protuberance. Each follows the attached margin of the tentorium cerebelli to the petrous temporal, where it becomes the sigmoid sinus. At their origin in the confluence, the right and left sinuses communicate with each other, and with the superior sagittal sinus and the straight sinus. **s. transver′sus pericar′dii** [NA], transverse sinus of pericardium: a passage behind the aorta and pulmonary trunk and in front of the atria; it is lined by serous pericardium. **traumatic s.**, a sinus due to trauma. **s. trun′ci pulmona′lis** [NA], sinuses of pulmonary trunk: slight dilatations in the wall of the pulmonary trunk immediately above the pulmonary valve. **s. tym′pani** [NA], **tympanic s.**, a deep fossa in the posterior part of the tympanic cavity; it is bounded superiorly by the eminentia pyramidalis, inferiorly by the subiculum promontorii, and it opens anteriorly into the fossula fenestrae cochleae. **s. of tympanic cavity, posterior,** s. posterior cavi tympani. **s. un′guis** [NA], the space underlying the advancing free edge of the fingernail or toenail. **urogenital s., s. urogenita′lis** [NA], an elongated sac formed by division of the cloaca in the early embryo, communicating with the mesonephric ducts and bladder, and forming the vestibule, urethra, and vagina in the female and some of the urethra in the male. **uterine s′s,** venous channels in the wall of the uterus in pregnancy. **s. of Valsalva,** s. aortae. **s. of venae cavae, s. vena′rum cava′rum** [NA], the portion of the right atrium bounded medially by the interatrial septum and laterally by the crista terminalis, and into which the superior and inferior venae cavae empty; it is often called the sinus venosus because it develops from that embryonic structure. **s. veno′sus,** 1. [NA] the common venous receptacle in the embryo midheart, attached to the posterior wall of the primitive atrium; it receives the umbilical and vitelline veins and the ducts of Cuvier. 2. s. venarum cavarum. **s. veno′sus scle′rae** [NA], venous sinus of sclera: a circular channel at the junction of the sclera and cornea, which is the main pathway for elimination of aqueous humor from the eye. Called also *Schlemm's canal*. **venous s.,** 1. a large vein or channel for the circulation of venous blood. 2. sinus venosus. **venous s′s of dura mater,** s. durae matris. **venous s. of sclera,** s. venosus sclerae. **s. ventric′uli,** Forssell's s. **s. vertebra′les longitudina′les,** old term for internal vertebral venous plexus.

sinusal (si′nus-al) pertaining to a sinus.

sinusitis (si″nŭ-si′tis) inflammation of a sinus. The condition may be purulent or nonpurulent, acute or chronic. Depending on the site of involvement it is known as ethmoid, frontal, maxillary, or sphenoid sinusitis. **infectious s. of turkeys,** a common, sometimes highly fatal respiratory disease of turkeys and game birds, caused by organisms of the pleuropneumonia-like group and marked by swelling below the eyes and sneezing; called also *airsac disease*.

sinusoid (si′nŭ-soid) [*sinus* + Gr. *eidos* form] 1. resembling a sinus. 2. a form of terminal blood channel consisting of a large, irregular anastomosing vessel, having a lining of reticuloendothelium but little or no adventitia. Sinusoids are found in the liver, suprarenals, heart, parathyroid, carotid gland, spleen, hemolymph glands, and pancreas; sinusoids in the anterior pituitary gland, adrenal cortex, and islets of Langerhans have a continuous basal lamina and a thin endothelium penetrated by pores closed by thin diaphragms (*fenestrated s′s*), and in many mammals the endothelial cells lining those of the liver meet and overlap in some areas, while there are gaps between the cells in other areas (*discontinuous s′s*). Called also *sinusoidal capillaries*. **myocardial s′s,** blood sinusoids that lie between the myocardial bundles or fibers.

sinusoidalization (si″nŭ-soi″dal-i-za′shun) the application of a sinusoidal current.

sinusotomy (si″nŭ-sot′o-me) [*sinus* + Gr. *tomē* a cutting] incision into a sinus.

sinuventricular (si″nu-ven-trik′u-lar) sinoventricular.

SiO₂ silicon dioxide (silica).

Si op. sit. abbreviation for L. *si o′pus sit*, if it is necessary.

siphon (si′fun) [Gr. *siphōn* tube] a bent tube with two arms of unequal length, used to transfer liquids from a higher to a lower level by the force of atmospheric pressure.

siphonage (si′fun-ij) the use of the siphon, as in gastric lavage or in draining the bladder.

Siphona irritans (si-fon′ah ir′ĭ-tans) *Haematobia irritans*.

Siphonaptera (si″fo-nap′ter-ah) [Gr. *siphon* tube + *apteros* wingless] an order of laterally compressed, highly chitinized and sclerotized small wingless blood-sucking ectoparasites of mammals and birds, commonly known as fleas. More than 800 species have been described, grouped in six or more families.

Siphunculata (si-fun″ku-la′tah) an order of insects including the lice.

Siphunculina (si-fun″ku-li′nah) a genus of dipterous insects of the family Chloropidae. **S. funic′ola,** the common "eye-fly" of India, where it spreads conjunctivitis; trachoma may also be transmitted by it.

Sippy diet, treatment (method) (sip′e) [Bertram Welton *Sippy*, American physician, 1866–1924] see under *diet* and *treatment*.

siqua (si′kwah) [coined from L. *sidentis altitudinis quadratio*, the square of the sitting height] Pirquet's unit for calculating the

area of the absorptive surface of the intestine; it is the square of the sitting height (in centimeters).

sirenomelus (si″ren-om′ĕ-lus) [Gr. *seirēn* siren + *melos* limb] a fetus with fused legs and no feet. Cf. *sympus*.

siriasis (sir-i′ah-sis) [Gr. *seiriasis* a disease produced by the heat of the sun] sunstroke.

sirikaya (sir″ĭ-ka′yah) the tree *Annona squamosa*, L. (Annonaceae), sugar apple or custard apple, whose fruit is edible and whose leaves are sudorific and bark purgative.

sirup (sir′up) syrup.

-sis a word termination of Greek origin, signifying state or condition. With a combining vowel it usually appears as *-asis, -esis, -iasis,* or *-osis*.

SISI short increment sensitivity index; see under *index*.

sismotherapy (sis″mo-ther′ah-pe) seismotherapy.

sisomicin (sis″o-mi′sin) chemical name: (2S-cis)-4-O-[3-amino-6-(aminomethyl)-3, 4-dihydro-2H-pyran-2-yl]-2-deoxy-6-O[3-deoxy-4-O-methyl-3-(methylamino)-β-L-arabinopyranosyl-D-streptamine. An aminoglycoside antibiotic derived from *Micromonospora inyoensis*, $C_{19}H_{37}N_5O_7$, closely related to C_{1a} component of the gentamicin complex; it is bactericidal for many gram-negative and some gram-positive organisms. **s. sulfate,** the sulfate salt of sisomicin, $(C_{19}H_{37}N_5O_7)_2 \cdot 5H_2SO_4$, having the antibacterial properties of the base.

sissorexia (sis″o-rek′se-ah) a tendency of the spleen to accumulate blood corpuscles.

sister (sis′ter) the nurse in charge of a hospital ward (Great Britain).

Sisto's sign (sēs′tōz) [Genero *Sisto*, Chilean pediatrician, died 1923] see under *sign*.

Sistrurus (sis-troo′rus) a genus of small rattlesnakes, the ground rattlesnakes, widely distributed throughout the United States, which have symmetrical plates covering the head. See table accompanying *snake*.

Sisyrinchium galaxioides (sis″ĭ-rin′ke-um gah-lak″se-oi′dēz) a South American iridaceous plant; its bulbs are purgative and diuretic.

site (sīt) a place, position, or locus. **active s.,** that subunit of an enzyme molecule which binds with the substrate molecule, inducing the conversion of the substrate into its reaction product; called also *catalytic s.* **allosteric s.,** that subunit of an enzyme molecule which binds with a nonsubstrate molecule, inducing a conformational change that results in inactivation of the enzyme for its substrate. **catalytic s.,** active s. **combining s.,** that portion of an antibody molecule that combines specifically with the antigenic determinant. **operator s.,** a site adjacent to the structural genes in the operon, believed to be the site on the DNA to which repressor molecules are bound, thereby inhibiting the synthesis of mRNA by the genes in the adjacent operon. **privileged s′s,** anatomical regions without lymphatic drainage where grafted tissues or organs can be situated without provoking an immune response. Examples include the anterior chamber of the eye and meninges of the brain.

sitfast (sit′fast) an inverted conical area of dry gangrene involving the skin and superficial fasciae of the neck in draft animals, caused by arrest of blood supply from pressure.

sitiology (sit″e-ol′o-je) sitology.

sitiomania (sit″e-o-ma′ne-ah) sitomania.

sito- (si′to) [Gr. *sitos* food] a combining form denoting relationship to food.

sitology (si-tol′o-je) the sum of knowledge regarding food, diet, and nutrition.

sitomania (si″to-ma′ne-ah) [*sito-* + Gr. *mania* madness] 1. excessive hunger, or morbid craving for food. 2. periodic bulimia.

sitosterol (si-tos′ter-ol) a generic term for a group of closely related natural plant sterols, the individual compounds being designated by Greek letters, and sometimes subscript numerals, as $\alpha_1, \alpha_2, \alpha_3, \beta$, and γ, on the basis of differing characteristics. A pharmaceutical preparation, called *sitosterols*, consisting of β-sitosterol and related sterols of plant origin, and containing not less than 95 per cent of total sterols and not less than 85 per cent of unsaturated sterols, calculated on the dried basis as β-sitosterol, is used as an oral anticholesterolemic agent.

β-sitosterolemia (si-tos″ter-ol-e′me-ah) the presence of excessive levels of plant sterols, especially β-sitosterol, in the blood. A rare form is associated with xanthomatosis, with tuberous and tendon xanthomas appearing in childhood.

sitotaxis (si″to-tak′sis) sitotropism.

sitotherapy (si″to-ther′ah-pe) [*sito-* + Gr. *therapeia* treatment] dietetic treatment.

sitotoxin (si″to-tok′sin) any basic food poison, especially that generated in a cereal food by a plant microorganism.

sitotoxism (si″to-tok′sizm) [*sito-* + Gr. *toxikon* poison] poisoning from ingested foods; food poisoning; alimentary toxicosis.

sitotropism (si-tot′ro-pizm) [*sito-* + Gr. *tropos* a turning] response of living cells to the presence of nutritive elements.

situation (sit″u-a′shun) the combination of factors with which an individual is confronted. In psychology, applied to the stimulus pattern, or the total sum, of all the factors affecting an individual at a given time.

situs (si′tus), pl. *si′tus* [L.] site, or position. **s. inver′sus vis′cerum,** lateral transposition of the viscera of the thorax and abdomen; a familial pattern and consanguineous parents have been reported. Complete transposition of the viscera in the absence of other defects is structurally sound, but see *dextrocardia, levocardia,* and *Kartagener's syndrome.* **s. perver′sus,** dislocation of any viscus. **s. sol′itus,** the normal position of the viscera. **s. transver′sus,** s. inversus viscerum.

Si vir. perm. abbreviation for L. *si vi′res permit′tant,* if the strength will permit.

606 (siks-o-siks) arsphenamine.

Sjögren's syndrome (disease) (sho′grenz) [Henrik Samuel Conrad *Sjögren,* Swedish ophthalmologist, born 1899] see under *syndrome.*

Sjöqvist's method (sho′kwistz) [John August *Sjöqvist,* Swedish physician, 1863–1934] see under *method.*

SK 1. streptokinase. 2. Sloan-Kettering. Used with numbers, as SK 1133, SK 1424, to designate various chemical compounds which have been used experimentally in the treatment of cancer at Sloan-Kettering Institute for Cancer Research.

skatole (skat′ōl) [Gr. *skōr, skatos* dung] chemical name: β-methylindole. A crystalline amine, with a strong characteristic odor, $C_6H_4 \cdot C(CH_3):CH \cdot NH$, from human feces. It is produced by the decomposition of proteins in the intestine and directly from the amino acid tryptophan by decarboxylation.

skatologic (skat″o-loj′ik) scatologic.

skatology (skah-tol′o-je) scatology.

skatophagy (skah-tof′ah-je) scatophagy.

skatosin (skah-to′sin) a base, $C_{10}H_{16}N_2O_2$, derived from certain proteins.

skatoxyl (skah-tok′sil) an oxidation product of skatole, $CH_3 \cdot C_8H_6NO$, found in the urine in certain cases of disease of the large intestine.

skein (skān) spireme. **Holmgren's s's, test s's,** skeins of colored worsted used in Holmgren's test of color perception.

skelalgia (ske-lal′je-ah) [Gr. *skelos* leg + *algos* pain + *-ia*] pain in the leg.

skelasthenia (ske″las-the′ne-ah) [Gr. *skelos* leg + *a* neg. + *sthenos* strength + *-ia*] weakness of the legs.

Skelaxin (skĕ-laks′in) trademark for a preparation of metaxalone.

skeletal (skel′ĕ-tal) pertaining to the skeleton.

skeletin (skel′ĕ-tin) any of a number of gelatinous substances occurring in invertebrate tissue, and including chitin, sericin, spongin, etc.

skeletization (skel″ĕ-ti-za′shun) 1. extreme emaciation. 2. the removal of the soft parts from the skeleton.

skeletogenous (skel″ĕ-toj′ĕ-nus) producing skeletal or bony structures.

skeletogeny (skel″ĕ-toj′ĕ-ne) the formation of the skeleton; the origin and development of the skeleton.

skeletography (skel″ĕ-tog′rah-fe) [*skeleton* + Gr. *graphein* to write] a description of the skeleton.

skeletology (skel″ĕ-tol′o-je) [*skeleton* + *-logy*] the sum of what is known regarding the skeleton.

skeleton (skel′ĕ-ton) [Gr. "a dried body, mummy"] the hard framework of the animal body, especially the bony framework of the body of higher vertebrate animals; the bones of the body collectively. See Plate XLIV. See *endoskeleton, exoskeleton,* and *splanchnoskeleton.* **appendicular s.,** the bones of the limbs; the *s. membri inferioris liberi* and *s. membri superioris liberi.* **axial s.,** the bones of the cranium, vertebral column, ribs, and sternum. **cardiac s.,** the connective tissue framework of the heart, which supports and gives attachment to the musculature; its main components are the pars membranacea septi interventricularis cordis and the anuli fibrosi cordis. **s. extremita′tis inferio′ris li′berae,** s. membri inferioris liberi. **s. extremita′tis superio′ris li′berae,** s. membri superioris liberi. **s. of heart,** cardiac s. **s. mem′bri inferio′ris li′beri** [NA], the bones of the thigh, leg, and foot; called also *s. extremitatis inferioris liberae.* **s. mem′bri superio′ris li′beri** [NA], the bones of the arm, forearm, and hand; called also *s. extremitatis superioris liberae.* **visceral s.,** that portion of the skeleton which protects the viscera, as the sternum, ribs, and os coxae.

skeletopia, skeletopy (skel″ĕ-to′pe-ah; skel′ĕ-to″pe) [*skeleton* + Gr. *topos* place] the position of an organ in relation to the skeleton.

Skene's catheter, glands (ducts, tubules) (skēnz) [Alexander Johnston Chalmers *Skene,* American gynecologist, 1838–1900] see under *catheter,* and see *ductus paraurethrales.*

skenitis (ske-ni′tis) inflammation of the ductus paraurethrales (Skene's glands).

skenoscope (ske′no-skōp) [*Skene's* glands + Gr. *skopein* to examine] an endoscope for examining Skene's glands.

skeocytosis (ske″o-si-to′sis) [Gr. *skaios* left + *kytos* hollow vessel + *-osis*] (*obs.*) presence of immature forms of white cells (neutrophils) in the blood; called also *shift to the left.*

skeptophylaxis (skep″to-fi-lak′sis) [Gr. *skēptein* to support + *phylaxis* a guarding] 1. a condition in which a minute dose of a substance poisonous to animals will produce immediate temporary immunity to the action of the poison, although the blood of the animal may be highly toxic during that period of immunity. 2. the method of allergic desensitization by the preliminary injection of a small amount of the allergen as is commonly done before the injection of an antiserum.

skew (sku) deviating from a straight line; see under *deviation.* In statistics, deviating from symmetry of frequency distribution.

skewfoot (sku′foot) a general term for any deformity of the foot in which its forepart deviates toward the midline; see *metatarsus varus* and *pes varus.*

skia- (ski′ah) [Gr. *skia* shadow] a combining form denoting reference to shadows, especially of internal structures as produced by roentgen rays.

skiagram (ski′ah-gram) [*skia-* + Gr. *gramma* a writing] a roentgenogram.

skiagraph (ski′ah-graf) a roentgenogram.

skiagraphy (ski-ag′rah-fe) roentgenography.

skiameter (ski-am′ĕ-ter) [*skia-* + Gr. *metron* measure] an instrument for measuring the intensity of the roentgen rays, and thus determining how long an exposure is needed.

skiametry (ski-am′ĕ-tre) retinoscopy.

skiascope (ski′ah-skōp) retinoscope.

skiascopy (ski-as′ko-pe) [*skia-* + Gr. *skopein* to examine] 1. retinoscopy. 2. examination of the body by the roentgen ray; fluoroscopy.

Skillern's fracture (skil′ernz) [Penn Gaskell *Skillern,* American surgeon, born 1882] see under *fracture.*

skimming (skim′ing) the removing of floating matter from a liquid. **plasma s.,** the action of red cells in flowing blood which leaves a zone near the wall of a vessel that is relatively free of cells.

skin (skin) the outer integument or covering of the body, consisting of the corium, or dermis, and the epidermis, and resting upon the subcutaneous tissues; called also *cutis* [NA]. See illustration on following page. **alligator s.,** ichthyosis sauroderma. **beaters' s.,** goldbeaters' s. **bronzed s.,** bronze colored skin, as seen in Addison's disease. **chamois s.,** a soft leather of sheep skin used in surgery. **collodion s.,** the covering membrane, somewhat resembling parchment or oiled silk, in lamellar exfoliation of the newborn; see under *exfoliation.* **crocodile s.,** ichthyosis sauroderma. **elastic s.,** Ehlers-Danlos syndrome. **farmers' s.,** sailors' s. **fish s.,** the appearance of the skin in ichthyosis vulgaris. **goldbeaters' s.,** a very thin, tough membrane prepared from ox's cecum and from the intestine of other animals; see *cobalt aurate membrane.* **India rubber s.,** Ehlers-Danlos syndrome. **lax s.,** cutis laxa. **marble s.,** cutis marmorata. **parchment s.,** a dry condition of the skin of cattle and sheep, especially such a condition accompanying verminous bronchitis. **piebald s.,** a term sometimes applied to the lesions of partial albinism. **porcupine s.,** ichthyosis hystrix. **sailors' s.,** skin rendered prematurely senile by excessive exposure to sunlight, with elastosis, atrophy, telangiectasia, and actinic keratoses, sometimes eventuating in carcinoma; seen especially in fair-skinned individuals. Called also *farmers' s.* **shagreen s.,** a form of connective tissue nevus in which the lesion—a soft skin-colored or yellowish plaque up to 10 cm. by 5 cm. in size and sometimes having a rough, pigmented surface—occurs during early childhood, usually in the lumbosacral region and occasionally on the trunk. The name is derived from the resemblance of the skin to shagreen, a leather (from shark skin) having a finely granular or knobbed surface.

Skinner box (skin′er) [Burrhus Frederic *Skinner,* American psychologist, born 1904] see under *box.*

Skiodan (ski′o-dan) trademark for preparations of methiodal sodium.

sklero- for words beginning thus, see those beginning *sclero-.*

Sklowsky's symptom (sklow′skēz) [E. L. *Sklowsky,* German physician] see under *symptom.*

Skoda's sign, tympany (sko′dahz) [Josef *Skoda,* Austrian physician, 1805–1881] see under *sign,* and see *skodaic resonance,* under *resonance.*

skodaic (sko-da′ik) named for Josef *Skoda;* see under *resonance.*

skole- for words beginning thus, see those beginning *scole-.*

skopometer (sko-pom′ĕ-ter) an instrument for measuring color, cloudiness, and other optical phenomena of liquids without using standards for comparison.

skoto- for words beginning thus, see those beginning *scoto-.*

SKSD an abbreviation for *streptokinase-streptodornase;* a

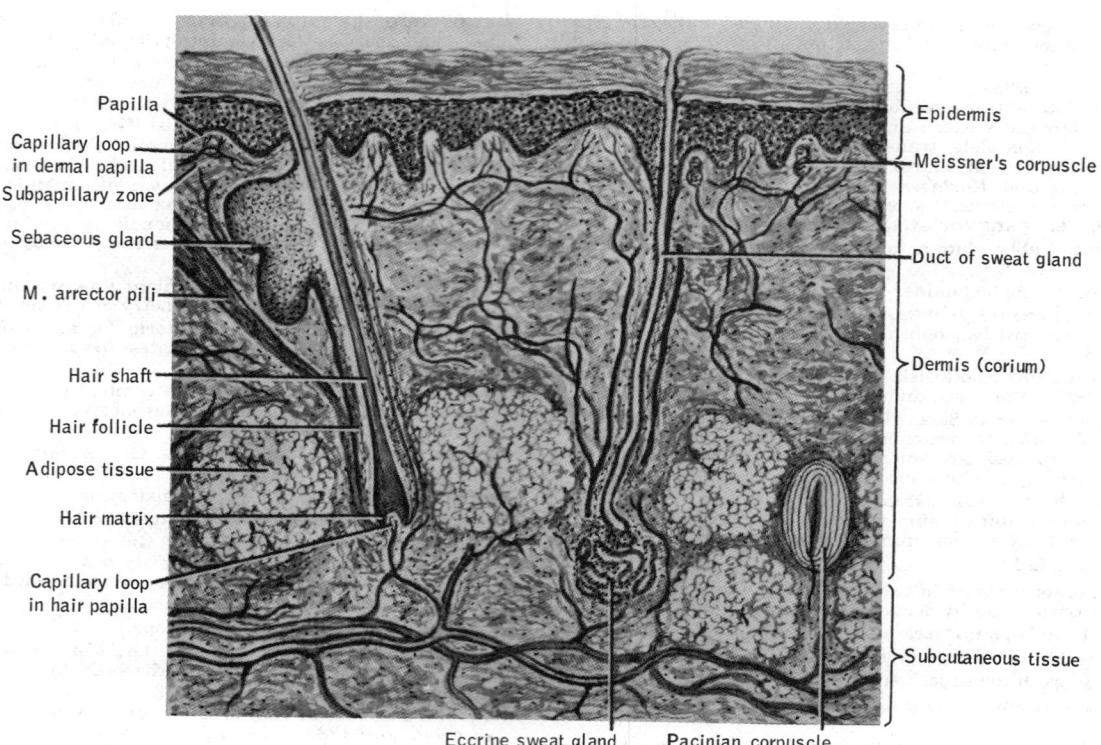

Papilla
Capillary loop in dermal papilla
Subpapillary zone
Sebaceous gland
M. arrector pili
Hair shaft
Hair follicle
Adipose tissue
Hair matrix
Capillary loop in hair papilla

Epidermis
Meissner's corpuscle
Duct of sweat gland
Dermis (corium)
Subcutaneous tissue

Eccrine sweat gland   Pacinian corpuscle

The skin and its appendages (Domonkos).

compound used in skin tests to determine either primary or secondary abnormalities of cell-mediated immunity.

skull (skul) the bony framework of the head, composed of the cranial bones and the bones of the face. It includes the ethmoid, frontal, hyoid, lacrimal, nasal, occipital, palatine, parietal, sphenoid, temporal, and zygomatic bones, and the inferior nasal conchae, mandible, maxillae, and vomer. Called also *cranium*. **cloverleaf s.**, kleeblattschädel. **hot cross bun s.**, see *Parrot's sign*, def. 2. **lacuna s.**, craniolacunia. **maplike s.**, a skull marked by irregular tracings resembling outlines on a map; seen in x-ray films of the cranial bones in Hand-Schüller-Christian disease. **natiform s.**, see *Parrot's sign*, def. 2. **steeple s., tower s.**, oxycephaly. **West's lacuna s., West-Engstler's s.**, a honeycomb appearance of the skull in roentgenograms, associated with spina bifida or meningocele and occasionally with encephalocele.

S.L.A. abbreviation for L. *sacrolaeva anterior* (left sacroanterior, a presentation of the fetus).

slant (slant) 1. a sloping surface of agar in a test tube. 2. a slant culture.

SLE systemic lupus erythematosus.

sleep (slēp) a period of rest for the body and mind, during which volition and consciousness are in partial or complete abeyance and the bodily functions partially suspended. Sleep has also been described as a behavioral state marked by a characteristic immobile posture and diminished but readily reversible sensitivity to external stimuli. Sleep is divisible into two stages: *NREM* (non-rapid eye movement) *sleep* and *REM* (rapid eye movement) *sleep*. **crescendo s.**, sleep which is marked by gradually increasing movements on the part of the sleeper. **deep s.**, NREM s. **desynchronized s.**, REM s. **dreaming s.**, REM s. **electric s.**, loss of voluntary movement and presence of general anesthesia induced by the application to the head of a rapidly interrupted electric current. **electrotherapeutic s.**, electrosleep. **fast s.**, REM s. **frozen s.**, treatment of cancer by local exposure of the tissues to a temperature of 40°–50° F. and a lowering of the general body temperature to 70°–90° F. **non–rapid eye movement s.**, NREM s. **NREM s.**, the deep, dreamless period of sleep during which the brain waves are slow and of high voltage, and autonomic activities, such as heart rate and blood pressure, are low and regular. Brief episodes of REM sleep occur at intervals during this type of sleep; in adults, about 80 per cent of sleep is NREM sleep. Called also *non–rapid eye movement s., orthodox s., slow wave s.*, and *synchronized s.* **orthodox s.**, NREM s. **paradoxical s.**, REM s. **paroxysmal s.**, narcolepsy. **prolonged s.**, treatment of neuroses by sustained and continuous sleep for several days under profound drug narcosis; called also *dauerschlaf* and *dauernarkose.*

rapid eye movement s., REM s. **REM s.**, the period of sleep during which the brain waves are fast and of low voltage, and autonomic activities, such as heart rate and respiration, are irregular. This type of sleep is associated with dreaming, mild involuntary muscle jerks, and rapid eye movements (REM). It usually occurs three to four times each night at intervals of 80 to 120 minutes, each occurrence lasting from 5 minutes to more than an hour. In adults, about 20 per cent of sleep is REM sleep and 80 per cent is NREM (non-rapid eye movement) sleep. Called also *desynchronized s., paradoxical s.*, and *rapid eye movement s.* See also *REM rebound*, under *rebound.* **slow wave s.**, NREM s. **synchronized s.**, NREM s. **temple s.**, incubation, def. 4. **twilight s.**, a condition of analgesia and amnesia, produced by hypodermic administration of morphine and scopolamine. In this state the patient, while responding to pain, does not retain it in her memory. Formerly widely used in obstetrics. Called also *twilight anesthesia, Freiburg method*, and *seminarcosis.*

slide (slīd) a glass plate on which objects are placed for microscopic examination. **Robinson-Cohen s.**, a modification of the astigmatic dial used in refraction of the eye.

slijmziekte (slim′zēk-te) a bacterial wilt disease of peanuts.

sling (sling) a bandage or suspensory for supporting all or a particular part of the body. **Glisson's s.**, a leather collar applied

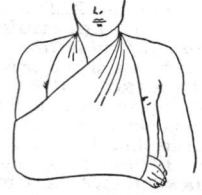

Sling (Christopher).

around the neck and under the chin to which is attached an extension apparatus over a pulley at the head of the patient's bed: for applying extension to the vertebral column. **Rauchfuss' s.**, an appliance for attaching to a bed for the purpose of supporting the spine in such a way that discharges from the diseased part may escape.

slit (slit) 1. a long narrow opening or incision. 2. to make a long narrow opening or incision. **filtration s's**, slit pores. **gill s.**, a long narrow opening from the pharynx to the exterior of the body of many aquatic animals, such as fishes and salamanders, through which water is drawn to bathe the gills.

slope (slōp) 1. an inclined plane; a surface which is neither horizontal nor vertical. 2. to deviate from the horizontal and from the vertical plane; said of a surface intersecting the horizontal at

Plate XLIV

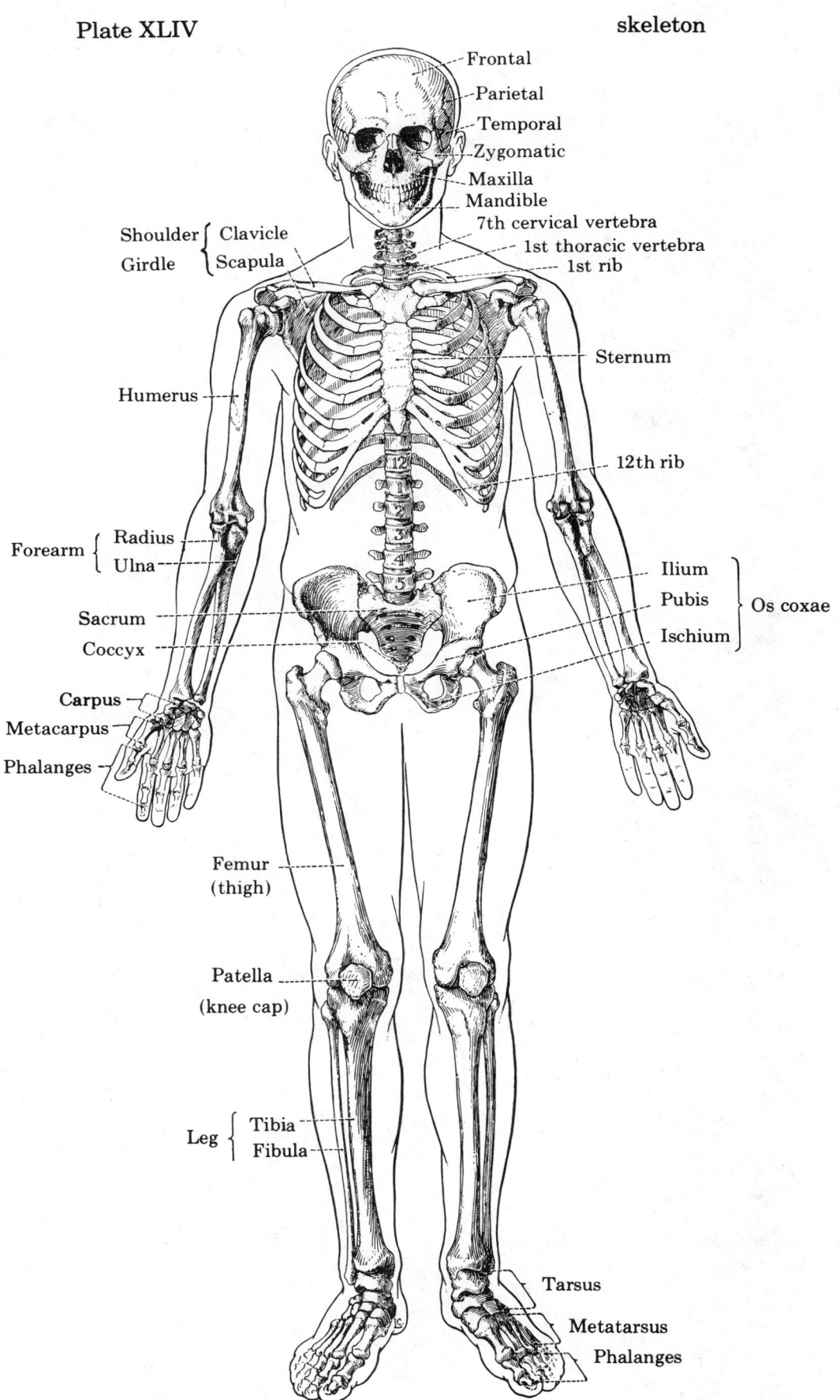

Frontal
Parietal
Temporal
Zygomatic
Maxilla
Mandible
7th cervical vertebra
Shoulder { Clavicle
Girdle { Scapula
1st thoracic vertebra
1st rib
Sternum
Humerus
12th rib
Forearm { Radius
Ulna
Ilium
Pubis } Os coxae
Ischium
Sacrum
Coccyx
Carpus
Metacarpus
Phalanges
Femur
(thigh)
Patella
(knee cap)
Leg { Tibia
Fibula
Tarsus
Metatarsus
Phalanges

ANTERIOR VIEW OF HUMAN SKELETON

(King and Showers)

an angle between 1 and 90 degrees. **lower ridge s.,** the slope of the mandibular residual ridge in the second and third molar region as seen from the buccal side.

slough (sluf) 1. necrotic tissue in the process of separating from viable portions of the body. 2. to shed or cast off.

sloughing (sluf'ing) the formation or separation of a slough.

slows (slōz) trembles.

S.L.P. abbreviation for L. *sacrolaeva posterior* (left sacroposterior, a presentation of the fetus).

S.L.T. abbreviation for L. *sacrolaeva transversa* (left sacrotransverse, a presentation of the fetus).

Sluder's neuralgia (syndrome), operation (method) (slu'derz) [Greenfield *Sluder,* American laryngologist, 1865–1928] see under *neuralgia* and *operation.*

sludge (sluj) a suspension of solid or semisolid particles in a fluid which itself may or may not be a truly viscous fluid. **activated s.,** sludge from well aerated sewage, which, being well supplied with oxidizing bacteria, ensures the presence of sufficient oxidizing organisms to activate the next tankful of sewage.

sludging (sluj'ing) the settling out of solid particles from solution. **s. of blood,** see *intravascular agglutination,* under *agglutination.*

slug (slug) a large group of terrestrial gastropods closely related to the snails but having a rudimentary or absent shell.

slurry (slur'e) a watery mixture or suspension of insoluble matter.

slyke (slīk) a unit of buffer value, named after D. D. Van Slyke, a pioneer in buffering analysis; abbreviated sl.

Sm chemical symbol for *samarium.*

smallpox (smawl'poks) variola; an acute infectious disease caused by a poxvirus. The incubation period is twelve days, followed by beginning of biphasic febrile course. The first phase lasts three to four days, during which there is fever and a transient red macular or petechial eruption on the trunk. It fades, the temperature recedes for a day, and then reappears when a papular eruption develops on the face, hands, and feet, vesiculates, and promptly become pustular. The lesions progress from distal points on palms, soles, arms, and legs toward the trunk. Each lesion is surrounded by others of exactly the same size and age, appearing primarily on exposed body areas, sparing the axillae and groin. The pustules umbilicate, crust, scab, and after 7 to 10 days fall off, leaving small depressed, depigmented scars. Other manifestations include pneumonia, arthritis, osteomyelitis (variole), and hemorrhage into cutaneous and oral mucosal lesions. Back pains, headache, and prostration are common accompaniments. **black s.,** hemorrhagic s. **bovine s.,** cowpox. **coherent s.,** a kind in which the pustules cohere at the edges, but do not become confluent. **confluent s.,** a severe form in which the pustules become more or less confluent. **discrete s.,** a form in which the pustules remain more or less distinct. **equine s.,** horsepox. **hemorrhagic s.,** a form in which hemorrhage occurs into the vesicles or from the mucous surfaces. **inoculation s.,** smallpox resulting from the direct, purposeful transfer of smallpox virus from a patient to a well person, which was widely practiced before the advent of vaccination. **malignant s.,** a severe and very fatal form of hemorrhagic smallpox. **mild s.,** variola minor. **modified s.,** varioloid. **ovine s.,** sheep-pox. **Sanaga s.,** variola minor.

smear (smēr) a specimen for microscopic study prepared by spreading the material across the glass slide. **Pap s., Papanicolaou s.,** see under *tests.*

Smee cell (sme) [Alfred *Smee,* English surgeon, 1818–1877] see under *cell.*

smegma (smeg'mah) [Gr. *smēgma* soap] the secretion of sebaceous glands, especially the cheesy secretion, consisting principally of desquamated epithelial cells, found chiefly beneath the prepuce. **s. embryo'num,** vernix caseosa.

smegmatic (smeg-mat'ik) pertaining to or composed of smegma.

smegmolith (smeg'mo-lith) [*smegma* + Gr. *lithos* stone] a calcareous concretion in the smegma.

smell-brain (smel'brān) rhinencephalon, def. 1.

Smellie's method, scissors (smel'ēz) [William *Smellie,* British obstetrician, 1697–1763] see under *method* and *scissors.*

smilacin (smi'lah-sin) [Gr. *smilakinos* pertaining to smilax] a poisonous glycoside, $C_{18}H_{36}O_6$, from sarsaparilla.

smilagenin (smi''lah-jen'in) a steroid precursor, $C_{27}H_{44}O_3$, from several species of *Smilax;* used in the manufacture of compounds of the pregnane series.

Smilax (smi'laks) [L., Gr. "bindweed"] a genus of climbing smilaceous plants, which are the source of sarsaparilla; the starchy root of several species was used as food by the Indians. Several species yield a steroid precursor, smilagenin. **S. aristolochiaefo'lia,** Mexican sarsaparilla, a species used as a beverage flavor and for digestive disorders, kidney ailments, skin diseases, and rheumatism in several tropical countries and Mexico.

Smith's disease, sign [Eustace *Smith,* London physician, 1835–1914] see *mucous colitis,* under *colitis,* and see under *sign.*

Smith's dislocation, fracture [Robert William *Smith,* Irish surgeon, 1807–1873] see under *dislocation* and *fracture.*

Smith's operation [Henry *Smith,* English surgeon in India, 1862–1948] see under *operation.*

Smith's phenomenon, reaction [Theobald *Smith,* American pathologist, 1859–1934] see *Theobald Smith phenomenon,* under *phenomenon,* and see *anaphylaxis.*

Smith's test [Walter George *Smith,* Irish physician, born 1844] see under *tests.*

Smith-Petersen nail [Marius Nygaard *Smith-Petersen,* American orthopedic surgeon, 1886–1953] see under *nail.*

S.M.O. Senior Medical Officer (in Navy); Medical Officer of Schools.

smog (smog) a mixture of smoke and fog; a colloid system in which the disperse phase consists of a mixture of gas and moisture and the dispersion medium is air.

smoke (smōk) a colloid system in which one or more solids is dispersed in a gas or vapor.

smudging (smuj'ing) a defect of speech in which the difficult consonants are omitted.

smut (smut) a disease of cereal grasses (wheat, oats, rye, Indian corn) caused by basidiomycetous fungi of the genera *Tilletia, Ustilago,* and *Urocystis.* See *Tilletia, Ustilago,* and *Urocystis.* **corn s.,** a smut of maize which is caused by *Ustilago maydis;* ingestion of the infected seeds cause ustilaginism, a condition similar to ergotism. **rye s.,** ergot formed by the ascomycete *Claviceps purpurea.*

Sn chemical symbol for *tin* [L. *stannum*].

S.N. abbreviation for L. *secun'dum natu'ram,* according to nature.

snail (snāl) a gastropod mollusk with a spiral shell. Certain fresh-water snails in tropical countries are intermediate hosts of parasitic trematodes; the miracidium of the fluke developing into a cercaria in the body of the snail.

snake (snāk) a limbless reptile of the suborder Ophidia, some of which are poisonous. See also *viper.* **brown s.,** a venomous elapid snake of Australia and New Guinea belonging to the genus *Demansia.* **cabbage s.,** see *Mermithidae.* **colubrid s.,** a snake of the family Colubridae, most of which are inoffensive, but the boomslang is venomous. **coral s.,** a venomous elapid snake, *Micrurus fulvius,* found in the southern United States and tropical America, whose body is marked with bright red, yellow, and black bands. **crotalid s.,** a snake of the family Crotalidae, a pit viper. **elapid s.,** any snake of the family Elapidae, including cobras, kraits, mambas, blacksnakes, brown snakes, copperheads, tiger snakes, death adder, and coral snakes. **hair s.,** see *Gordius.* **harlequin s.,** coral s. **poisonous s.,** any snake that contains a poison, either in venom glands or in other organs or tissues; commonly, a venomous snake. **sea s.,** a snake of the family Hydrophidae. **tiger s.,** a very venomous elapid snake, *Notechis scutatus,* of Australia, whose body is chiefly brown with dark bands. **venomous s.,** any snake that secretes substances (venoms) capable of producing a deleterious effect on the blood (hematoxins) or nervous system (neurotoxins), the venom being injected into the body of the victim by the snake's bite. Collectively, they are called the *thanatophidia* or *toxicophidia.* See table on following page. **viperine s.,** any snake of the family Viperidae, the true vipers, including European vipers, Russell's viper, sand vipers, puff adders, Gaboon vipers and rhinoceros vipers.

snap (snap) a short sharp sound. **opening s.,** a short sharp sound in early diastole caused by the movement of the mitral leaflet into the ventricle at the beginning of ventricular filling.

snare (snār) a wire loop or noose for removing polyps and tumors by encircling them at the base and closing the loop. **cold s.,** a snare that has not been heated. **hot s.,** a wire snare heated by a galvanic current, and used for simultaneous coagulation and removal of tumors. Called also *galvanocaustic s.*

sneeze (snēz) 1. to expel air forcibly and spasmodically through the nose and mouth. 2. an involuntary, sudden, violent, and audible expulsion of air through the mouth and nose.

Snell's law (snelz) [Simeon *Snell,* English ophthalmologist, 1851–1909] Descartes' law.

Snellen's chart, etc. (snel'enz) [Hermann *Snellen,* ophthalmologist in Utrecht, 1834–1908] see under *chart, eye, tests,* and *test type.*

Snider match test (sni'der) [Thomas H. *Snider,* American physician, born 1925] see under *test.*

snore (snor) 1. rough, noisy breathing during sleep, due to vibration of the uvula and soft palate; called also *stertor.* 2. to produce such sounds during sleep.

snow (sno) a freezing or frozen mixture consisting of discrete particles or crystals. **carbon dioxide s.,** Dry Ice: solid carbon dioxide, formed by rapid evaporation of liquid carbon dioxide; it gives a temperature of about 110 degrees below zero Fahrenheit (−79° C.); it has been used in cryotherapy to freeze the skin, thus

IMPORTANT VENOMOUS SNAKES OF THE WORLD*

FAMILY AND TYPE OF FANGS	COMMON NAMES	TYPE OF VENOM	DISTRIBUTION	REMARKS
COLUBRIDAE; rear, immovable, grooved	Colubrids	Mostly mild	Warm parts of both hemispheres	Over 1000 species, the few poisonous ones not dangerous
Example:	Boomslang	Hemorrhagin	South Africa	Arboreal, timid
ELAPIDAE; front, immovable, grooved	Elapids	Predominantly neurotoxin	Mostly in Old World	Over 150 species, very poisonous
Examples:	Cobras	Mostly neurotoxin	Africa, India, Asia, Philippines, Celebes	Spitting cobra in Africa aims at eyes
	Kraits	Strong neurotoxin	India, S.E. Asia, Indonesia	Sluggish, often buried in dust
	Mambas	Neurotoxin	Tropical W. Africa	Arboreal
	Blacksnake	Neurotoxin	Australia	Large snake, wet terrain
	Copperhead	Neurotoxin	Australia, Tasmania, Solomons	Damp environment
	Brown snake	Neurotoxin	Australia, New Guinea	Slender
	Tiger snake	Strong neurotoxin	Australia	Dry environment; aggressive; very dangerous
	Death adder	Neurotoxin	Australia, New Guinea	Sandy terrain
	Coral snakes	Neurotoxin	United States, tropical America	About 26 species, 2 in southern U. S. A.
HYDROPHIDAE; front, immovable, hollow	Sea snakes	Some mild; others very toxic	Tropical, Indian and Pacific Oceans	Gentle. Rudder-like tail. Over 50 species
VIPERIDAE; front, movable, hollow	True vipers; viperines; viperids	Predominantly hematoxin	Entirely in Old World	About 50 species
Examples:	European viper	Hematoxin	Europe (rare), N. Africa, Near East	Dry rocky country
	Russell's viper	Hematoxin	S.E. Asia, Java, Sumatra	Mostly open terrain; deadly
	Sand vipers	Hematoxin	N. Sahara	Buried in sand
	Puff adder	Hematoxin	Arabia, Africa	Open terrain; sluggish
	Gaboon viper	Neurotoxin and hematoxin	Tropical W. Africa	Forests; deadly
	Rhinoceros viper	Hematoxin	Tropical Africa	Wet forests
CROTALIDAE; front, movable, hollow	Pit vipers; crotalids; crotalines	Predominantly hematoxin	Old and New Worlds; none in Africa	Over 80 species; pit between eye and nostril
Examples:	Habu viper	Neurotoxin	Warmer parts of E. Asia; Ryukyu Islands	Caves and dry rocky country
	Rattlesnakes†	Predominantly hematoxin	N., Central and S. America	South American form neurotoxic
	Bushmaster	Hematoxin	Central and S. America	Large. In wet forests
	Fer-de-lance	Hematoxin	Central America, N. South America, few West Indies	Common on plantations
	Palm vipers	Hematoxin(?)	S. Mexico, Central and South America	Arboreal; small, greenish. Bite face
	Copperhead	Hematoxin	United States	Dry stony terrain
	Water moccasin	Hematoxin	Southeast U. S. A. to Texas	Swamps
	Asiatic pit vipers	Hematoxin	Southeast Asia, Taiwan	Most arboreal

*Manual of Tropical Medicine, Hunter, Frye, and Swartzwelder.
†All rattlesnakes are venomous.

producing local anesthesia and arrest of blood flow, and, in the form of a slush, as an escharotic to destroy certain skin lesions, such as warts, moles, etc.

snowblindness (sno'blīnd-nes) temporary loss of sight due to injury to superficial cells of the cornea caused by ultraviolet rays of the sun reinforced by those reflected by snow.

SNS Society of Neurological Surgeons; sympathetic nervous system.

snuff (snuf) a medicinal or errhine powder to be inhaled through the nose.

snuffles (snuf'f'lz) a catarrhal discharge from the nasal mucous membrane in infants, generally in congenital syphilis.

SO the spheno-occipital synchondrosis, a cephalometric landmark designating the most superior point at the junction of the sphenoid and occipital bones.

SO₂ sulfur dioxide.

SOAP a device for conceptualizing the process of recording the progress notes in the *problem-oriented record* (see under *record*): S indicates subjective data obtained from the patient and others close to him; O designates objective data obtained by observation, physical examination, diagnostic studies, etc.; A refers to assessment of the patient's status through analysis of the problem, possible interaction of the problems, and changes in the status of the problems; P designates the plan for patient care.

soap (sōp) [L. *sapo*] any compound of one or more fatty acids, or their equivalents, with an alkali. Soap is detergent and is much employed in liniments, enemas, and in making pills. It is also a mild aperient, antacid, and antiseptic. **animal s.,** sapo domesticus. **carbolic s.,** a disinfectant soap containing 10 per cent of phenol. **castile s.,** a hard soap, either white or mottled, prepared from olive oil and soda. See *sapo*, def. 2. **curd s.,** sapo domesticus. **green s.** [USP], a potassium soap made by the saponification of vegetable oils, excluding coconut oil and palm kernel oil, without the removal of glycerin. It is the chief ingredient of green soap tincture (q.v.). Called also *medicinal soft s., sapo mollis medicinalis,* and *soft s.* **hexachlorophene liquid s.** [USP], a solution of hexachlorophene in a 10 to 13 per cent solution of potassium soap, containing in each 100 gm., 225 to 260 mg. of hexachlorophene; used as a topical anti-infective and detergent. **guaiac s.,** a resin of guaiacum saponified with liquor potassae. **hard s.,** soda s. **McClintock's s.,** a disinfectant soap containing an active mercury salt. **medicinal soft s.,** green s. **potash s.,** green s. **soda s.,** soap made from soda and olive oil; called also *hard s.* **soft s.,** 1. a liquid soap made from potash and some oil; called also *potash s.* and *sapo mollis.* 2. green s. **Starkey's s.,** a soap made of potassium carbonate, turpentine oil, and Venice turpentine in equal parts. **superfatted s.,** a soap having an excess of fat over that necessary to neutralize all the alkali. **zinc s.,** a soap containing zinc oxide or zinc sulfate; for use as an ointment or plaster.

socaloin (so-kal'o-in) a variety of aloin, C₁₅H₁₆O₇, from Socotrine aloes.

socia (so'she-ah) [L. "a comrade, associate"] a detached part or exclave of an organ. **s. parot'idis,** accessory parotid gland.

socialization (so"shă-lĭ-za'shun) the process by which society integrates the individual, and the individual learns to behave in socially acceptable ways.

socioacusis (so"se-o-ah-ku'sis) the acceleration of the normal hearing loss associated with aging, which results from the noise encountered in modern civilization.

sociologic, sociological (so"se-o-bi"o-loj'ik; so"se-o-bi"o-loj'ĭ-kal) pertaining to sociobiology.

sociobiologist (so"se-o-bi-ol'o-jist) an individual trained in sociobiology.

sociobiology (so"se-o-bi-ol'o-je) the branch of theoretical biology which proposes that all animal (including human) behavior has a biological basis, which is controlled by the genes; the study of the biological basis of behavior.

sociogenic (so"se-o-jen'ik) arising from or imposed by society.

sociologist (so"se-ol'o-jist) an individual trained in sociology.

sociology (so"se-ol'o-je) [L. *socius* fellow + *-logy*] the science dealing with social relations and phenomena.

sociometry (so"se-om'ĕ-tre) [L. *socius* fellow + *metrum* a measure] the branch of sociology concerned with the measurement of human social behavior.

sociopath (so'se-o-path") a person with an antisocial (sociopathic) personality (q.v.).

sociopathic (so"se-o-path'ik) pertaining to a person with an antisocial personality (q.v.); antisocial.

sociopathy (so"se-op'ah-the) the condition of being antisocial (sociopathic).

sociotherapy (so"se-o-ther'ah-pe) any treatment emphasizing socioenvironmental and interpersonal rather than intrapsychic factors.

socket (sok'et) a hollow or depression, into which a corresponding part fits. **dry s.,** a condition sometimes occurring after tooth extraction, resulting in exposure of bone with localized osteomyelitis of an alveolar crypt, and symptoms of severe pain;

called also *alveolar osteitis, alveolitis sicca dolorosa,* and *localized alveolar osteitis.* **tooth s's,** the dental alveoli, the cavities in the maxilla and mandible in which the teeth are embedded; called also *alveoli dentales maxillae* and *alveoli dentales mandibulae.*

soda (so'dah) a term loosely applied to sodium bicarbonate (baking s.), sodium hydroxide (caustic s.), or sodium carbonate (washing s.). **baking s.,** sodium bicarbonate. **bicarbonate of s.,** sodium bicarbonate. **caustic s.,** sodium hydroxide. **chlorinated s.,** a mixture of sodium chloride and sodium hypochlorite. **s. cum cal'ce,** an escharotic preparation of equal parts of sodium hydroxide and lime. **s. lime,** [NF], hydroxide with sodium or potassium hydroxide, or both; used as adsorbent of carbon dioxide in equipment for metabolism tests, inhalant anesthesia, or oxygen therapy. **washing s.,** sodium carbonate.

sodiarsphenamine (so"di-ars-fen'ah-min) sodium arsphenamine; see under *arsphenamine.*

sodii (so'de-i) [L.] genitive of *sodium.*

sodiocitrate (so"de-o-sit'rāt) a compound containing sodium and a salt of citric acid.

sodiotartrate (so"de-o-tar'trāt) a compound containing sodium and a salt of tartaric acid.

sodium (so'de-um), gen. *so'dii* [L. *na'trium,* gen. *na'trii*] a soft, silver white, alkaline metallic element; symbol, Na; atomic number, 11; atomic weight, 22.990; specific gravity, 0.971. With a valence of 1, it has a strong affinity for oxygen and other nonmetallic elements. Sodium provides the chief cation of the extracellular body fluids. See also *sodium pump,* under *pump.* The salts of sodium are the most widely used salts in medicine. (NOTE: For sodium salts not listed below, see the name of the active ingredient.) **s. acetate** [USP], the trihydrate sodium salt of acetic acid, C₂H₃NaO₂·3H₂O, occurring as colorless, transparent crystals, or white, granular crystalline powder, or white flakes; used as a source of sodium ions in solutions for hemodialysis and peritoneal dialysis. It has also been used as a systemic and urinary alkalizer, diuretic, and expectorant. **s. acid phosphate,** s. biphosphate, NaH₂PO₄. **s. alginate** [NF], a purified carbohydrate product extracted from brown seaweeds with dilute alkali; used as a suspending agent. It is also used for its emulsifying, stabilizing, thickening, and water-binding qualities in foods, medicines, and cosmetics. **s. alizarinsulfonate,** chemical name: 9,10-dihydro-3,4-dihydroxy-9,10-dioxo-2-anthracenesulfonic acid sodium salt. A dye, C₁₄H₇O₂(OH)₂SO₃Na·H₂O, occurring as a yellow-brown or orange-yellow powder; used as a stain in microscopy, as a reagent for aluminum, as an acid-base indicator, and in the determination of fluorine. Called also *alizarin red S* and *alizarin water-soluble red.* **s. amylosulfate,** the sodium salt of the sulfurated form of amylopectin, derived from potatoes; an enzyme inhibitor, it has been used in the treatment of peptic ulcer. **s. antimony gluconate,** antimony sodium gluconate. **s. antimonyltartrate,** antimony sodium tartrate; see under *antimony.* **s. antimonylthioglycollate,** antimony sodium thioglycollate. **s. arsenate,** Na₂HAsO₄, an odorless, amorphous white powder used when effects of arsenic are desired. **s. ascorbate** [USP], the monosodium salt of ascorbic acid, C₆H₇NaO₆, occurring as white or very faintly yellow crystals or crystalline powder; used in the preparation of parenteral dosage forms of ascorbic acid. **s. aurothiomalate,** gold sodium thiomalate; see under *gold.* **s. aurothiosulfate,** gold sodium thiosulfate; see under *gold.* **s. benzoate** [NF], the sodium salt of benzoic acid, C₇H₅NaO₂, occurring as a white, granular or crystalline powder; used as an antifungal preservative in pharmaceutical preparations and foods. It may also be used as a test for liver function, administered orally or intravenously. **s. bicarbonate** [USP], a white, crystalline powder, NaHCO₃, chiefly used as a gastric antacid. It is also used to combat systemic acidosis and to alkalinize urine. In aqueous solution it is used locally for washing the nose, mouth, and vagina, and as a cleansing enema; in saturated solution it is used as a dressing for minor burns. Called also *baking soda* and *bicarbonate of soda.* **s. biphosphate** [USP], the monohydrate monosodium salt of phosphoric acid, NaH₂PO₄·H₂O, occurring as colorless crystals or white, crystalline powder. It is given orally with sodium phosphate as an antihypercalcemic; orally and rectally with sodium phosphate as a cathartic; and orally as a urinary acidifier. **s. bisulfite** [NF], a white or yellowish white granular powder or crystals, NaHSO₃, used as an antioxidant in various pharmaceutical preparations. **s. borate** [NF], the sodium salt of boric acid, Na₂B₄O₇, occurring as a white, crystalline powder, or as colorless transparent crystals; used as an alkalizing agent in pharmaceutical preparations. It has also been used for its weak antibacterial and mild astringent properties in lotions, gargles, and mouthwashes. Called also *borax, sodium pyroborate,* and *s. tetraborate.* **s. bromide,** a sedative, NaBr, occurring in white or colorless crystals; used occasionally in the management of grand mal seizures. See also *bromide* and *brominism.* **s. cacodylate,** an arsenical remedy, (CH₃)₂AsO·ONa·3H₂O, in the form of white crystals, or a white, granular powder, soluble in water; formerly used in tuberculosis, anemia, malaria, psoriasis, etc. **s. caprylate,** the sodium salt of caprylic acid; used in treatment of fungal infections of the skin. **s. carbonate** [NF], a compound, Na₂CO₃·H₂O, occurring as colorless crystals or as a white, crystalline powder, used as an alkalizing agent in pharmaceutic preparations. It has also been used as a lotion or bath in the treatment of scaly skin, and as a detergent. Called also *sal soda* and *washing soda*. **s. caseinate** casein-sodium. **s. chlorate,** a salt, $NaClO_3$, with properties similar to those of potassium chlorate, and occurring in colorless or white crystals or granules. It has been used as an antiseptic wash. **s. chloride,** common salt or table salt: a mineral, NaCl, soluble in water and occurring as colorless, cubic crystals or white, crystalline powder, found widely distributed over the earth, in sea water, etc., which is a necessary constituent of the body and consequently of the diet. It makes up over 90 per cent of the inorganic constituents of the blood serum and is the principal salt involved in maintaining osmotic tension of blood and tissues. It is used in medicine [USP] for many purposes, as in the preparation of isotonic and physiologic saline solutions; as a fluid and electrolyte replenisher, an isotonic vehicle for drugs, an antihypercalcemic, and an antidote to silver nitrate poisoning, administered by intravenous infusion; as a topical anti-inflammatory; to irrigate wounds and body cavities; as an enema to flush the colon and promote evacuation; as a mucolytic, administered by inhalation; and as a topical osmotic agent in ophthalmology. Also used widely as a food preservative and seasoning. **s. citrate** [USP], the trisodium of citric acid, $C_6H_5Na_3O_7$, occurring as colorless crystals, or white, crystalline powder; used as an anticoagulent for blood or plasma that is to be fractionated or for blood that is to be stored. It is also administered orally as a urinary alkalizer. **s. dimethylarsenate,** s. cacodylate. **s. fluoride** [USP], a white, odorless powder, NaF, used in the fluoridation of water, and also applied locally to the teeth, in 2 per cent solution, to reduce the incidence of dental caries. **s. fluosilicate,** s. silicofluoride. **s. folate,** chemical name: sodium *N*-[4-{[(2-amino-4-hydroxy-6-pteridyl)-methyl]amino}benzoyl]glutamate. A water-soluble compound, $C_{19}H_{18}N_7NaO_6$, used in various anemias and in sprue. **s. glutamate,** the monosodium salt of L-glutamic acid, COOH·-$CHNH_2 \cdot CH_2 \cdot CH_2 \cdot COONa$, occurring as a white or nearly white crystalline powder; used in treatment of encephalopathies associated with hepatic disease. It is also used to enhance the flavor of foods and tobacco. See also *Chinese restaurant syndrome*, under *syndrome*. **s. glycerophosphate,** a compound, $C_3H_5(OH)_2$-PO_4Na_2, formerly thought useful in various conditions of disordered metabolism. **s. glycocholate,** a yellowish white, bitter salt, $NaC_{26}H_{42}O_6N$, with a pH of 6.6; used as a laboratory reagent. **s. gold thiosulfate,** gold sodium thiosulfate; see under *gold*. **s. hydrate,** s. hydroxide. **s. hydroxide** [NF], a caustic alkali, NaOH, occurring as white, or nearly white, fused masses, in small pellets, flakes, sticks, and other forms; used as an alkalizing agent in pharmaceutical preparations. Called also *caustic soda* and *s. hydrate*. **s. hypochlorite,** the sodium salt of hypochlorous acid, NaClO, having germicidal and disinfectant properties. **s. hypophosphite,** a salt, $NaPH_2O_2 \cdot H_2O$, occurring in colorless, rectangular plates, or as a white, granular powder. **s. hyposulfite,** s. thiosulfate. **s. iodate,** a white crystalline powder, $NaIO_3$, which has been used as an antiseptic in diseases of the mucous membranes. **s. iodide** [USP], a binary haloid, NaI, occurring in colorless crystals or white crystalline powder, used in various conditions as a source of iodine. It is also used as an expectorant. **s. ipodate** [NF], chemical name: sodium 3-[[(dimethylamino)methylene]amino]-2,4,6-triiodohydrocinnamate. A white to off-white, odorless, fine crystalline powder, $C_{12}H_{12}I_3$-N_2NaO_2, used as a radiopaque medium in cholecystography. **s. lactate** [USP], $C_3H_5NaO_3$, the sodium salt of racemic or inactive lactic acid, $C_3H_5NaO_3$, used intravenously in one-sixth molar solution as a fluid and electrolyte replenisher to combat acidosis. **s. lauryl sulfate** [NF], an anionic surfactant, $CH_3(CH_2)_{10}CH_2$-OSO_3Na, occurring in white or light yellow crystals; used as a wetting agent, emulsifying aid, and detergent in various cosmetic and dermatologic preparations, and as an ingredient of tooth pastes. Called also *irium*. **s. metabisulfite** [NF], chemical name: disulfurous acid disodium salt. An antioxidant, $Na_2S_2O_5$, occurring as white crystals or as a white to yellowish crystalline powder; used in pharmaceutical preparations. **s. methylarsonate,** a crystalline powder, $CH_3AsO(ONa)_2 \cdot 5H_2O$, easily soluble in water and less soluble in alcohol, sometimes employed for its arsenical effects. **s. monofluorophosphate** [USP], chemical name: phosphorofluoridic acid disodium salt. A dental caries prophylactic, Na_2PFO_3, occurring as a white to slightly gray powder; applied topically to the teeth. **s. nitrate,** a compound, $NaNO_3$, occurring as colorless crystals or in white granules or powder; formerly used as a diuretic and in treatment of dysentery, but now used as a reagent and in certain industrial processes; called also *Chile saltpeter*. **s. nitrite** [USP], a compound, $NaNO_2$, occurring as a white to slightly yellow, granular powder or as white or nearly white, opaque fused masses or sticks, used as an antidote for cyanide poisoning. It is also used in the relief of the pain of angina pectoris, Raynaud's disease, asthma, and such conditions as lead colic and spastic colitis. **s. nitroferricyanide,** s. nitroprusside. **s. nitroprusside,** chemical name: (*OC*-6-22)-pentakis(cyano-*C*)nitrosylferrate(2–) disodium dihydrate. An antihypertensive, $Na_2[Fe(CN)_5NO] \cdot 2H_2O$, occurring as reddish brown crystals or powder; used in the treatment of hypertensive crisis and to produce controlled hypotension during surgery, administered by intravenous infusion. Sterile sodium nitroprusside conforms to USP specifications. It is also used as a reagent and testing solution. Called also *s. nitroferricyanide*. **s. oleate,** the sodium salt of oleic acid, C_{17}-$H_{33}COONa$, formerly considered useful in treatment of gallstones. **s. oxybate,** chemical name: sodium 4-hydroxybutyrate; a hypnotic agent, $C_4H_7NaO_3$, used as an adjunct in anesthesia. **s. para-aminosalicylate,** s. aminosalicylate. **s. perborate,** a compound, $NaBO_3 \cdot 4H_2O$, prepared by interaction of boric acid or sodium borate with sodium or hydrogen peroxide. It is an antiseptic compound, used in 2 per cent solution as a mouthwash and in a 10–20 per cent powder in dentrifices. **s. peroxide,** a white powder, Na_2O_2, soluble in water in which it liberates oxygen, which has been used externally in acne, and as a dental bleach. **s. phenolsulfonate,** chemical name: hydroxybenzenesulfonic acid sodium salt. An odorless, saline compound, $NaC_6H_5OSO_3 \cdot 2H_2O$, in colorless transparent prisms or crystalline granules; formerly used as an intestinal antiseptic. **s. phosphate** [USP], the heptahydrate monosodium salt of phosphoric acid, $Na_2HPO_4 \cdot 7H_2O$, occurring as a colorless or white, granular salt. It is given orally as a cathartic; orally and rectally with sodium biphosphate as a cathartic; and orally with sodium biphosphate as an antihypercalcemic. **s. phosphate, dried** [USP], the anhydrous salt, $NaHPO_4 \cdot xH_2O$, dried at 105° C. for four hours; used as an oral cathartic. **s. phosphate, effervescent** [USP], a dry granular mixture of citric acid, dried sodium phosphate, tartaric acid, and sodium bicarbonate; used as an oral cathartic. **s. phosphate, exsiccated,** dried s. phosphate. **s. phytate,** the sodium salt of phytic acid, $C_6H_9Na_9O_{24}P_6$; a calcium chelating agent. **s. polyphosphate,** disodium salt of polyphosphoric acid; a pharmaceutic aid, $(NaPO_3)_n$. **s. polystyrene sulfonate** [USP], a cation-exchange resin prepared in the sodium form, each gram of which exchanges 110 to 135 mg. of potassium, calculated on the anhydrous basis; used in the treatment of hyperpotassemia. **potassium s. tartrate,** see under *potassium*. **s. propionate** [NF], the sodium salt of propionic acid, CH_3CH_2COONa, occurring as colorless, transparent crystals or as a granular, crystalline powder, having antifungal properties; used alone or in combination with calcium propionate or other agents as a preservative to inhibit mold production in bakery and dairy products and other foods and in pharmaceuticals. It is also used as a topical antifungal in the treatment of various mycoses. **s. psylliate,** the sodium salt of the liquid fatty acids obtained by hydrolysis of the fixed oil of the seeds of *Plantago ovata;* used as a sclerosing agent. **s. pyroborate,** s. borate. **s. pyrophosphate,** a compound, $Na_4P_2O_7$, produced by heating sodium phosphate at a red heat; used in detergents. **radioactive s.,** radiosodium. **s. salicylate** [USP], the monosodium salt of salicylic acid, $C_7H_5NaO_3$, occurring as an amorphous or microcrystalline powder or as scales; used as an analgesic, antipyretic, and antirheumatic, administered orally. **s. santoninate,** a colorless crystalline compound, $C_{15}H_{19}NaO_4 \cdot 3\frac{1}{2}H_2O$, once used as a vermifuge. **s. silicate,** a compound of sodium, silicon, and oxygen in various ratios, formerly used as an antiseptic, and in tuberculosis, bronchial asthma, and arteriosclerosis. **s. silicofluoride,** a white, granular powder, Na_2SiF_6, which is toxic in high concentrations. It is sometimes added to water to produce 0.7 to 1 part per million of fluorine, to prevent dental caries and is sometimes used in insecticides. Called also *s. fluosilicate*. **s. stearate** [NF], a mixture of sodium stearate, sodium palmitate, and small amounts of the sodium salts of other fatty acids; used as a stiffening and emulsifying agent in pharmaceutical preparations. **s. stibocaptate,** stibocaptate. **s. stibogluconate,** antimony sodium gluconate. **s. succinate,** chemical name: succinic acid sodium salt. A compound, $C_4H_4Na_2O_4$, used as a respiratory stimulant, analeptic, urinary alkalizer, diuretic, and laxative. It has also been used as a hepatic stimulant. **s. sulfate** [USP], the decahydrate disodium salt of sulfuric acid, Na_2-$SO_4 \cdot 10H_2O$, occurring as large, colorless, transparent crystals, or a granular powder; used as an antihypercalcemic and antidote to barium poisoning, administered by intravenous infusion. It is also used orally as a cathartic or laxative and has been applied topically as a lymphagogue for infected wounds. Called also *Glauber's salt*. **s. sulfite,** a compound, $Na_2SO_3 \cdot 7H_2O$, occurring as colorless, efflorescent crystals; formerly used in treatment of dyspepsia, and externally in parasitic infections. **s. sulfite, anhydrous,** a fairly stable compound, Na_2SO_3, occurring as small white crystals or powder; used as a reagent. **s. sulfite, exsiccated,** s. sulfite, anhydrous. **s. sulfocarbolate,** s. phenolsulfonate. **s. tetraborate,** s. borate. **s. tetradecyl sulfate,** an anionic surfactant with sclerosing properties, $C_{14}H_{29}$-$NaSO_4$, occurring as a white, waxy solid; used as a wetting agent and in the treatment of varicose veins and hemorrhoids. **s. thiamylal,** chemical name: sodium 5-allyl-5-(1-methylbutyl)-2-thiobarbiturate; an ultrashort-acting barbiturate, $C_{12}H_{17}N_2Na$-O_2S. A sterile mixture of sodium thiamylal with anhydrous sodium carbonate (*s. thiamylal for injection* [NF]) is used intravenously as the sole anesthetic in relatively short surgical procedures, as a supplement to local anesthetics during regional and spinal anesthesia, and for induction prior to general anesthesia in prolonged surgical procedures. **s. thiosulfate** [USP], a compound, $Na_2S_2O_3 \cdot 5H_2O$, occurring as large colorless crystals or as a coarse crystalline powder, used intravenously as an antidote to cyanide poisoning. It is also used in solution as a foot bath to prevent ringworm infection at swimming pools and public shower-baths, topically in tinea versicolor, and in measuring the volume of extracellular body fluid and the renal glomerular filtration rate. It was formerly used in the treatment of arsenic poisoning. **s. trimetaphosphate**, the trisodium salt of metaphosphoric acid; a pharmaceutic aid, $Na_3P_3O_9$.

sodokosis (so″do-ko′sis) rat-bite fever.

sodoku (so′do-koo) [Japanese *so* rat + *doku* poison] the spirillary form of rat-bite fever (see under *fever*), caused by *Spirillum minor*.

sodomist (sod′o-mist) one who practices sodomy.

sodomite (sod′o-mīt) sodomist.

sodomy (sod′o-me) [after the city of *Sodom*] a form of paraphilia, variously defined by law to include sexual contact between humans and animals of other species, and mouth-genital or anal contact between humans; in medical usage, it is restricted to human-animal sexual contact and anal intercourse.

sodophthalyl (so″do-thal′il) disodoquinone phenolphthalein; used as a laxative.

Soemmering's foramen, gray substance (ganglion), spot (sem′er-ingz) [Samuel Thomas *Soemmering*, German anatomist, 1755–1830] see *fovea centralis retinae*, *macula retinae*, and *substantia nigra*.

softening (sof′en-ing) [Gr. *malakia*] the process of becoming soft; any morbid process of becoming soft, as of the brain or spinal cord, or of the vascular coats. **anemic s.**, disintegration of brain matter from deficient blood supply. **s. of the brain,** 1. a popular designation for paralytic dementia. 2. true softening of the brain substance; encephalomalacia. **colliquative s.**, softening in which the tissues become liquefied. **gray s.**, a stage in which the fat produced by degeneration has been more or less absorbed. **green s.**, a stage in which there is green pus present in the degenerated spot. **hemorrhagic s.**, softening of a part due to hemorrhage into it. **inflammatory s.**, a form of red softening due to inflammation. **mucoid s.**, myxomatous degeneration. **pyriform s.**, yellow s. **red s.**, softening of a patch or of patches of brain substance, with local redness due to congestion. **s. of the stomach**, gastromalacia; softening of the stomach walls due to an extremely acid condition of its contents, a condition usually seen after death. **white s.**, the stage next following yellow softening, in which the spot has become white from the presence of fatty deposit. **yellow s.**, the second of the three stages of the myelic process, characterized by fatty degeneration; the stage following red softening, in which the patch has become yellow as a result of degenerative changes in the brain substance.

soja bean (so′yah) soy bean.

sokosha (so-ko′shah) rat-bite fever.

Sol. solution.

sol (sol) 1. a colloid system in which the dispersion medium is liquid. 2. a contraction of *solution*. **metal s.**, a colloidal dispersion of a metal in a liquid. Such dispersions often have catalytic properties similar to those of enzymes, and are therefore sometimes called inorganic enzymes. **solid s.**, a colloidal system in which both the dispersed phase and the dispersion medium are solids.

Solanaceae (sōl″ah-na′se-e) a large family of widely distributed herbs, shrubs, and trees, having great economic importance, and including many poisonous species and numerous species that have medicinal properties. *Atropa, Capsicum, Datura, Duboisia, Hyoscyamus, Nicotiana, Scopolia,* and *Solanum* are some of the important genera.

solanaceous (sōl″ah-na′shus) of or pertaining to the family Solanaceae.

solandrine (so-lan′drin) pseudohyoscyamine.

solanine (so′lah-nēn) solatunine; a steroidal glycoalkaloid, $C_{45}H_{73}NO_{15}$, found in several species of *Solanum*; formerly used in bronchitis, epilepsy, and asthma. On hydrolysis, it yields solanidine and three sugars. Its aglycone portion is considered most toxic.

solanocyte (so-lah′no-sīt) flame cell.

solanoid (so′lah-noid) [L. *solanum* potato + Gr. *eidos* form] resembling a raw potato in texture.

solanoma (sō″lah-no′mah) (*obs.*) scirrhous carcinoma.

Solanum (so-la′num) [L. "nightshade"] a genus of solanaceous plants, including the potato, tomato, egg plant, several of the nightshades, and many poisonous and medicinal species. **S. carolinen′se** L. (Solanaceae), a plant of the United States. The fluidextracts of the root and berries were formerly used as anticonvulsive and sedative agents in epilepsy. The fruit is listed as poisonous to both animals and humans. Also known as *bull nettle, sand-brier, radical weed,* and *horse nettle.* **S. tubero′sum** L., the common potato.

solapsone (so-lap′sōn) chemical name: 1,1′-[sulfonylbis(*p*-phenyleneimino)]bis[3-phenyl-1,3-propanedisulfonic acid]tetrasodium salt. An antibacterial derivative of dapsone, $C_{30}H_{28}N_2Na_4$-

$O_{14}S_5$, having actions similar to those of the parent compound but less toxic; used as a leprostatic, administered orally and intramuscularly. Called also *solasulfone*.

solar (so′lar) [L. *solaris*] 1. pertaining to the sun. 2. denoting the great sympathetic plexus and its principal ganglia (especially the celiac); so called because of their radiating nerves.

solarium (so-la′re-um) [L.] a room especially designed to allow exposure to light of the sun or to artificial light.

solasulfone (so″lah-sul′fōn) solapsone.

solation (so-la′shun) the conversion of a gel into a sol.

Soldaini's test (reagent) (sol″dah-e′nēz) [Arturo *Soldaini*, Italian chemist] see under *tests*.

solder (sod′er) 1. a fusible alloy of metals used to unite the edges or surfaces of two pieces of metal. 2. to produce a union between two pieces of metal by use of a fusible alloy.

sole (sōl) [L. *solea; planta*] the bottom of the foot; called also *planta pedis* [NA]. **convex s., dropped s.**, pumiced foot.

soleno- (so′lĕ-no) [Gr. *sōlēn* a channel, gutter, pipe] a combining form denoting relationship to a pipe or gutter; tubular or grooved.

Solenoglypha (so″lĕ-nog′lĭ-fah) [*soleno-* + Gr. *glyphein* to cut out with a knife] a group of venomous snakes with fangs that are hollow like a hypodermic needle and that normally fold back against the roof of the mouth but can be erected for striking and piercing. Examples are the massasauga and the rattlesnakes.

solenoid (so′lĕ-noid) [Gr. *sōleno-eides* pipe-shaped, grooved] a coil of wire spaced equally between turns, which acts like a magnet when an electric current is passed through it.

solenoma (so″lĕ-no′mah) (*obs.*) endometrial carcinoma.

solenonychia (so″lĕ-no-nik′e-ah) [*soleno-* + Gr. *onyx, onychos* nail + *-ia*] dystrophia unguis mediana canaliformis.

Solenopotes (so″lĕ-no-po′tēz) [*soleno-* + Gr. *pōtēs* a drinker] a genus of lice of the order Anoplura. **S. capilla′tus,** a species of sucking lice occasionally found parasitic on cattle.

Solenopsis (so″lĕ-nop′sis) a genus of stinging ants, including the fire ants that attack man and inflict painful burning stings and may cause severe local and systemic reactions; *S. geminata* is indigenous to the United States; *S. saevissima richteri* is a viciously aggressive South American species that has been imported into the United States and gained a strong foothold.

solferino (sol″fer-e′no) fuchsin.

Solganal (sol′gah-nal) trademark for a preparation of aurothioglucose.

solid (sol′id) [L. *solidus*] 1. not fluid or gaseous; not hollow. 2. a substance or tissue not fluid or gaseous. **color s.**, a three-dimensional geometrical body, devised to show the relation of all hues and brightnesses, including black, white, and grays, in their various modes.

Solidago (sol″ĭ-da′go) [L.] a genus of composite-flowered plants: the golden-rods. *S. virgau′rea* L., of Europe and North America, is aromatic and diuretic. Some species are considered to be toxic to livestock.

solidism (sol′ĭ-dizm) [L. *solidus* solid] the obsolete doctrine that changes in the solids of the body, e.g., their expansion or contraction, are the causes of every disease.

solidist (sol′ĭ-dist) one who accepts the doctrine of solidism.

solidistic (sol″ĭ-dis′tik) pertaining to solidism or to the solidists.

solipsism (sōl′ip-sizm) [L. *solus* alone + *ipse* one's self] the belief that the world exists only in the mind of the individual, or that it consists solely of the individual himself and his own experiences.

solipsistic (sōl″ip-sis′tik) pertaining to or characterized by solipsism.

solitary (sol′ĭ-ter″e) [L. *solitarius*] placed alone; not grouped with others.

sol-lunar (sol-lu′nar) [L. *sol* sun + *luna* moon] pertaining to or caused by the sun and moon.

solpugid (sol-pu′jid) an individual of the order Solpugida.

Solpugida (sol″pu-jid′ah) the solpugids, a family of hairy, jointed spiders (class Arachnida) that are differentiated from true spiders by having a segmented abdomen, which is more broadly joined to the cephalothorax; solpugids are capable of inflicting deep painful bites and are found mainly in desert, tropical, and subtropical areas.

solubility (sol″u-bil′ĭ-te) the quality or fact of being soluble; susceptibility of being dissolved.

soluble (sol′u-b′l) [L. *solubilis*] susceptible of being dissolved.

Solu-Cortef (sol′u-kor′tef) trademark for a preparation of hydrocortisone sodium succinate.

solum (so′lum), pl. *so′la* [L.] [NA] the bottom or lowest part. **s. tym′pani,** paries jugularis cavi tympani.

solute (so′lūt) a substance dissolved in a solvent; a solution consists of a solute and a solvent.

solutio (so-lu′she-o) [L., from *solvere* to dissolve] solution.

solution (so-lu′shun) [L. *solutio*] 1. a homogeneous mixture of one or more substances (solutes) dispersed molecularly in a sufficient quantity of dissolving medium (solvent). The solute may be gas, liquid, or solid; the solvent is usually liquid, but may be solid, as in a solid solution of copper in silver (sterling silver). In pharmacology, a liquid preparation containing one or several soluble chemical substances usually dissolved in water and not, for various reasons, falling into another category. 2. the process of dissolving. 3. a loosening or separation. **A.C.D. s., acid citrate dextrose s.,** see *anticoagulant citrate dextrose s.* **acetylcysteine s.** [USP], a sterile solution of acetylcysteine in water, prepared with the aid of sodium hydroxide, containing 95 to 105 per cent of the labeled amount of acetylcysteine; administered by nebulization or installation for adjunct therapy in bronchopulmonary disorders when mucolysis is desired. **Albright's s.,** one consisting of 75 gm. of sodium citrate, 25 gm. of potassium citrate, 140 gm. of citric acid, and 1000 ml. of water; used in the treatment of renal tubular acidosis. **alcoholic s.,** a solution in which alcohol is used as the solvent. **Alsever's s.,** a solution for preserving sheep's red blood cells for use in complement fixation tests. **aluminum acetate topical s.** [USP], a preparation of aluminum subacetate solution, glacial acetic acid, and water, containing, in each 100 ml., 4.8–5.8 gm. of aluminum acetate, and used topically on the skin and mucous membranes, diluted with 10 to 40 parts of water, as an astringent. It is also used as a topical antiseptic and antipruritic in a wide variety of dermatologic conditions. Called also *Burow's s.* **aluminum subacetate topical s.** [USP], a solution containing aluminum sulfate, acetic acid, precipitated calcium carbonate, and water, yielding, from each 100 ml., 2.3–2.6 gm. aluminum oxide and 5.43–6.13 gm. acetic acid, and used topically on the skin and mucous membranes as an astringent. It is also used as a topical antiseptic and as a wet dressing in various skin diseases. **amaranth s.,** a clear, vivid red solution of amaranth in purified water containing, in each 100 ml., 0.9–1.1 gm. of amaranth; used as a coloring agent. **amaranth s., compound,** a solution composed of amaranth solution, caramel, alcohol, and purified water; used as a coloring agent. **aminoacetic acid sterile s.,** a sterile, aqueous solution containing 95 to 105 per cent of the labeled amount of aminoacetic acid; used as a nutrient. **aminobenzoic acid s.** [USP], a straw-colored solution containing 5 per cent aminobenzoic acid; applied topically to the skin as a sunscreening agent. **ammonia s., diluted,** a colorless, transparent liquid of alkaline reaction, containing, in each 100 ml., 9–10 gm. of ammonia; used as a pharmaceutic necessity. Called also *ammonia water* or *diluted ammonium hydroxide solution.* **ammonia s., strong** [NF], a colorless, transparent liquid, strongly alkaline in reaction, containing 27–30 per cent of ammonia; used as a solvent and a source of ammonia. **ammoniacal silver nitrate s.,** a mixture of silver nitrate, purified by water and strong ammonia solution; used as a dental protective. **ammonium acetate s.,** a clear, colorless liquid, containing ammonium acetate, which has been used as a diaphoretic and diuretic. Called also *spirit of Mindererus.* **ammonium citrate s., alkaline,** a preparation of dibasic ammonium citrate and strong ammonia solution; used in tests for zinc. **ammonium hydroxide s., diluted,** ammonia s., diluted. **ammonium hydroxide s., stronger,** ammonia s., strong. **anisotonic s.,** a solution having tonicity differing from that of the standard of reference. **antazoline phosphate ophthalmic s.,** a sterile, aqueous solution, containing 90 to 100 per cent of the labeled amount of antazoline phosphate; used topically in the eye as an antihistaminic. **anticoagulant citrate dextrose s.** [USP], a sterile solution used as an anticoagulant for storage of whole blood obtained for transfusion purposes, and consisting of dihydrous trisodium citrate, monohydrous citric acid, and dextrose. Formerly called *anticoagulant acid citrate dextrose s.* **anticoagulant citrate phosphate dextrose s.** [USP], a sterile solution used as an anticoagulant for storage of whole blood, and consisting of anhydrous citric acid, dihydrous sodium citrate, monohydrous sodium biphosphate, and monohydrous dextrose. **anticoagulant heparin s.** [USP], a sterile solution used as an anticoagulant, containing sodium heparin and sodium chloride in water for injection. **anticoagulant sodium citrate s.** [USP], an aqueous solution of sodium citrate containing 3.80–4.20 gm. of sodium citrate; used as an anticoagulant for plasma and for blood for fractionation. Formerly called *sodium citrate anticoagulant s.* **antipyrine and benzocaine s.** [NF], a solution of antipyrine and benzocaine in glycerin, containing 90 to 110 per cent of the labeled amount of antipyrine and benzocaine; instilled in the ear as a local anesthetic. **antiseptic s.,** a clear, colorless liquid, containing boric acid, thymol, chlorothymol, menthol, eucalyptol, methyl salicylate, thyme oil, alcohol, and purified water, used as an antibacterial for external and oral use. **aqueous s.,** a solution in which water is used as the solvent. **aromatic s., alkaline,** a preparation of glycerin, potassium bicarbonate, sodium borate, and other ingredients; used as a mouthwash. **arsenic chloride s.,** a partly hydrolyzed solution of antimony trichloride in water. **arsenical s.,** potassium arsenite s. **arsenious acid s.,** a clear, colorless, odorless liquid, with an acid reaction, containing arsenic trioxide. **atropine sulfate ophthalmic s.** [USP], a sterile, aqueous solution containing 93 to 107 per cent of the labeled amount of atropine sulfate; applied topically to the conjunctiva as an anticholinergic to produce mydriasis or cycloplegia. **Benedict's s.,** sodium citrate, sodium carbonate, and

copper sulfate water solution. Its normal blue color changes to yellow, orange, or red in the presence of a reducing sugar such as glucose. It is used in urinalysis. **benzalkonium chloride s.** [USP], a clear, colorless, aqueous solution, with an aromatic odor and a slightly bitter taste, which contains 95–105 per cent of the labeled amount of benzalkonium chloride in concentrations of 1 per cent or more, and 93–107 per cent of the labeled amount in concentrations of less than 1 per cent; used as a topical antiseptic, effective against gram-positive and gram-negative bacteria and certain viruses, fungi, yeasts and protozoa. It is also used as an antimicrobial preservative in ophthalmic solutions. **benzethonium chloride topical s.** [USP], a clear colorless liquid, without odor and with a slightly bitter taste, which contains 95–105 per cent of the labeled amount of benzethonium chloride; used as a local anti-infective, applied topically to the skin and nasal mucosa, and as a preservative in pharmaceutical preparations. **Bonain's s.,** an anesthetic and antiseptic solution used in operations on the tympanic membrane, consisting of equal parts of menthol, phenol, and cocaine hydrochloride. **boric acid s.,** a clear, colorless, odorless liquid, each 100 ml. of which contains at least 4.25 gm. of boric acid; used as an external anti-bacterial. **Bouin's s.,** see under *fluid.* **buffer s.,** a solution which resists appreciable change in its hydrogen ion concentration when acid or alkali is added to it. **Burnett's s.,** see under *fluid.* **Burow's s.,** aluminum acetate s. **butacaine sulfate s.** [USP], a sterile solution containing 95–105 per cent of the labeled amount of butacaine sulfate in water; used to produce topical anesthesia of the eye. **s. C3,** a solution resembling intracellular fluid used in perfusion of tissues or organs prior to freezing them for preservation, as of kidneys for transplantation; called also *Collins' s.* **calciferol s.,** ergocalciferol s. **calcium cyclamate and calcium saccharin s.,** a clear, colorless solution containing 90 to 110 per cent of the labeled amounts of calcium cyclamate and calcium saccharin; used as a non-nutritive sweetener. **calcium hydroxide topical s.** [USP], clear, colorless liquid with an alkaline reaction, each 100 ml., at 25° C., containing not less than 140 mg. of calcium hydroxide; used in preparing various astringent solutions and lotions. It has been added to infant formulas to decrease the curd size formed from cow's milk, and is used as an antacid in infants. Called also *aqua calcis* and *lime water.* **carbachol ophthalmic s.** [USP], a sterile solution of carbol in an isotonic, aqueous medium, containing 95 to 105 per cent of the labeled amount of carbol; used as a cholinergic applied topically to the conjunctiva in the treatment of glaucoma. **carbol-fuchsin topical s.** [USP], a dark purple solution containing, in each 1000 ml., basic fuchsin (3 gm.), phenol (45 gm.), resorcinol (100 gm.), acetone (50 ml.), alcohol (100 ml.), and purified water; used as a local antifungal in the treatment of dermatophytosis, tinea, and other skin infections. Called also *Castellani's paint.* **carmine s.,** a deep red, rather viscous liquid, compounded of carmine, diluted ammonia solution, glycerin, and water; used as a coloring agent. **Carnoy's s.,** an acid fixative used for studying the cell nucleus and chromosomes, composed of: 3 parts absolute ethanol, 1 part glacial acetic acid (or Bowin's fluid), 5 parts saturated picric acid, 5 parts 40 per cent formaldehyde (formalin), and 1 part glacial acetic acid. **carphenazine maleate s.** [USP], a solution containing 95–110 per cent of the labeled amount of carphenazine maleate; used as an antipsychotic in the treatment of acute and chronic schizophrenic reactions in hospitalized patients. **centinormal s.,** hundredth-normal s. **cetylpyridinium chloride s.** [USP], a clear solution containing 95 to 105 per cent of the labeled amount of cetylpyridinium chloride; used as a local anti-infective applied topically to the skin and mucous membranes, and as a preservative in pharmaceutical preparations. **chloramphenicol ophthalmic s.** [USP], a sterile, buffered solution, containing 90–130 per cent of the labeled amount of chloramphenicol; used as an antibacterial, applied topically to the conjunctiva. **chloramphenicol for ophthalmic s.** [USP], a sterile, dry mixture of chloramphenicol and suitable buffers, containing 90–120 per cent of the labeled amount of chloramphenicol; used as an antibacterial, applied topically to the conjunctiva. **chymotrypsin for ophthalmic s.** [USP], a sterile preparation containing 80–120 per cent of the labeled potency of chymotrypsin; used for enzymatic zonulolysis for intracapsular lens extraction, applied by irrigation to the posterior chamber of the eye, under the iris. **clindamycin palmitate hydrochloride for oral s.** [USP], a dry mixture containing clindamycin palmitate hydrochloride equivalent to 90–120 per cent of the labeled amount of clindamycin; used as an antibacterial, primarily in the treatment of penicillin-resistant gram-positive infections and in patients allergic to penicillin. **cloxacillin sodium for oral s.** [USP], a preparation containing 90–120 per cent of the labeled amount of cloxacillin; used as an oral antibacterial, primarily in the treatment of infections due to penicillinase-resistant staphylococci. **coal tar topical s.** [USP], a solution of coal tar and polysorbate 80 in alcohol, used, diluted, as a local antieczematic. **cochineal s.,** a dark, purplish red fluid with a slightly aromatic odor, compounded of cochineal, potassium carbonate, alum, potassium bitartrate, glycerin, and water; used as a coloring agent. **Cohn's s.,** a synthetic medium for growing yeast and molds, containing monopotassium acid phosphate, calcium phosphate, magnesium sulfate, and ammonium tartrate, in water. **Collins' s.**, s. C3. **colloid s., colloidal s.**, a preparation consisting of minute particles of matter suspended in a solvent, the solvent being called the continuous phase, and the suspended matter, the disperse phase. Called also *disperse system.* See *dispersoid* and *emulsoid.* **contrast s.**, a solution of a substance opaque to the roentgen ray, used to facilitate roentgen visualization of some organ or structure in the body. **cresol s., compound,** cresol s., saponated. **cresol s., saponated,** a mixture of cresol, vegetable oil, potassium hydroxide, alcohol, and water, and containing, in each 100 ml., 46–52 ml. of cresol; used as a disinfectant. Called also *compound cresol s.* **crystal violet s.**, methylrosaniline chloride s. **cyanocobalamin Co 57 s.** [USP], a clear colorless to pink solution, suitable for oral administration, containing cyanocobalamin in which a portion of the molecules contain radioactive cobalt (^{57}Co); used as a diagnostic aid in pernicious anemia. **cyanocobalamin Co 60 s.** [USP], a clear colorless to pink solution suitable for oral administration, containing cyanocobalamin in which a portion of the molecules contain radioactive cobalt (^{60}Co); used as a diagnostic aid in pernicious anemia. Formerly called *radiocyanocobalamin s.* **cyclopentamine hydrochloride s.** [USP], a solution of cyclopentamine hydrochloride in a suitable isotonic vehicle, containing 95 to 105 per cent of the labeled amount of cyclopentamine hydrochloride; applied intranasally as a vasoconstrictor to reduce nasal congestion. **cyclopentolate hydrochloride ophthalmic s.** [USP], a sterile solution of cyclopentolate hydrochloride in a buffer, isotonic, aqueous medium, containing 95 to 105 per cent of the labeled amount of cyclopentolate hydrochloride; applied topically to the conjunctiva as an anticholinergic. **Czapek-Dox s.**, a solution used for growing molds, containing glucose, sodium nitrate, monopotassium phosphate, potassium chloride, magnesium sulfate, iron sulfate, and water. **Dakin's s., Dakin's s., modified,** sodium hypochlorite s., diluted. **decimolar s.**, a solution having one-tenth the concentration of a molar solution. **decinormal s.**, tenth-normal s. **demecarium bromide ophthalmic s.** [USP], a sterile, aqueous solution containing 92 to 108 per cent of the labeled amount of demecarium bromide; applied topically to the conjunctiva as a cholinergic in treatment of glaucoma and convergent strabismus. **dexamethasone sodium phosphate ophthalmic s.** [NF], a sterile, aqueous solution containing 90 to 115 per cent of the labeled amount of dexamethasone phosphate; applied topically to the eye as an anti-inflammatory glucocorticoid. **diatrizoate sodium s.** [USP], a solution of diatrizoate sodium in purified water, or a solution of diatrizoic acid in purified water prepared with the aid of sodium hydroxide; used orally as a diagnostic radiopaque medium in radiography of the gastrointestinal tract. **diethyltoluamide topical s.** [USP], a solution of diethyltoluamide in alcohol or isopropyl alcohol, containing 92 to 108 per cent of the labeled amount of diethyltoluamide; applied to the skin and clothing to repel arthropods. **dioctyl calcium sulfosuccinate s.**, a clear solution containing 95 to 105 per cent of the labeled amount of dioctyl calcium sulfosuccinate; used as a wetting agent and as a nonlaxative fecal matter softener. **dioctyl sodium sulfosuccinate s.** docusate sodium s. **diphenoxylate hydrochloride and atropine sulfate oral s.** [USP], a solution containing 93 to 107 per cent of the labeled amount of diphenoxylate hydrochloride and 80 to 120 per cent of the labeled amount of atropine sulfate; used as an antiperistaltic in treatment of diarrhea. **disclosing s.**, a solution which is used for the purpose of making something apparent, such as one to be painted on the surface of a tooth in order to stain, and thus render visible, foreign matter or bacterial plaques. **Dobell's s.**, sodium borate s., compound. **docusate sodium s.** [USP], a solution containing 95 to 105 per cent of the labeled amount of docusate sodium; used as a fecal softener, administered rectally. Called also *dioctyl sodium sulfosuccinate s.* **double-normal s.**, a solution having double the strength of a normal solution: designated 2 N. **dyclonine hydrochloride topical s.** [USP], a sterile, aqueous solution containing 92 to 108 per cent of the labeled amount of dyclonine hydrochloride; used as a topical anesthetic. **echothiophate iodide for ophthalmic s.** [USP], a preparation containing 95–115 per cent of the labeled amount of echothiophate iodide; a cholinergic used as a miotic in the treatment of certain forms of glaucoma, applied topically to the conjunctiva. **dl-ephedrine hydrochloride s.**, racephedrine hydrochloride s. **ephedrine sulfate s.** [USP], a clear, colorless solution with a slightly camphoraceous odor and taste, and a neutral or acid reaction, used as a nasal vasoconstrictor. **epinephrine s.** [USP], a nearly colorless, slightly acid solution of epinephrine in purified water, prepared with the aid of hydrochloric acid, each 100 ml. containing 90–115 mg. of epinephrine; used as a vasoconstrictor. **epinephrine bitartrate ophthalmic s.** [USP], a buffered, aqueous solution, containing 90–115 per cent of the labeled amount of epinephrine bitartrate; used to reduce intraocular pressure in the management of simple chronic (open-angle) glaucoma, applied topically to the conjunctiva. **epinephryl borate ophthalmic s.** [USP], a sterile solution containing epinephryl borate equivalent to 90–115 per cent of the labeled amount of epinephrine; used as an adrenergic in ophthalmology, administered by instillation into the eye. **ergocalciferol**

oral s. [USP], a solution of ergocalciferol in an edible vegetable oil, in polysorbate 80, or in propylene glycol, containing, in each gram, not less than 0.25 mg. of ergocalciferol; used in the prophylaxis and treatment of vitamin D deficiency. Called also *calciferol s.* **erythrosine sodium topical s.** [USP], a preparation containing 90–110 per cent of the labeled amount of erythrosine sodium in purified water; applied topically to the teeth to disclose plaque. **ethereal s.**, a solution in which ether is used as the solvent. **Farrant's s.**, a mounting preparation used in bacteriological work, containing glycerin, water, arsenious acid solution, and gum arabic. **Fehling's s.**, dissolve 34.66 gm. of copper sulfate in water to make 500 ml., dissolve 173 gm. of crystallized potassium sodium tartrate and 50 gm. of sodium hydroxide in water to make 500 ml. Keep the two solutions in small well-stoppered bottles; for use, mix equal parts of the two solutions. **ferric chloride s.**, a yellowish orange liquid with a faint odor of hydrochloric acid and an acid reaction, containing 37.2–42.7 gm. of ferric chloride and 3.85–6.6 gm. of hydrochloric acid in each 100 ml.; formerly used as a hematinic in the treatment of iron deficiency anemias. **ferric subsulfate s.**, a reddish-brown, almost odorless, aqueous solution of basic ferric sulfate, used as an astringent. **ferrous sulfate oral s.** [USP], a solution containing 94–106 per cent of the labeled amount of ferrous sulfate; used as a hematinic in the treatment of iron deficiency anemia. **fiftieth-normal s.**, a solution having one-fiftieth the strength of a normal solution: designated N/50 or 0.02 N. **fixative s.**, see *fixative.* **Flemming's s.**, a solution for hardening histological specimens, consisting of chromium trioxide, osmium tetroxide, glacial acetic acid, and water. **fluocinolone acetonide topical s.** [USP], a solution containing 90–110 per cent of the labeled amount of fluocinolone acetonide; used as an anti-inflammatory in glucocorticoid-responsive dermatoses. **fluorouracil topical s.** [USP], a preparation containing 90–110 per cent of the labeled amount of fluorouracil; used as an antineoplastic in the treatment of actinic keratoses. **Fonio's s.**, a solution of magnesium sulfate in water, used as a diluent for blood platelets. **formaldehyde s.** [USP], a solution of formaldehyde in water, containing not less than 37 per cent of formaldehyde; used as a disinfectant. Called also *formalin* and *formol.* **formol-Zenker s.**, a fixing solution consisting of Zenker's solution and formaldehyde solution. **Fowler's s.**, potassium arsenite s. **gelatin s., special intravenous,** a 5 or 6 per cent sterile, pyrogen-free solution of gelatin in isotonic sodium chloride solution; used as a plasma volume expander. **gentian violet topical s.** [USP], a purple liquid with a slight odor of alcohol, containing gentian violet, alcohol, and purified water, each 100 ml. containing 0.95–1.05 gm. of gentian violet; used topically as an anti-infective. Called also *crystal violet s.* and *methylrosaniline chloride s.* **Gilson's s.**, a fixative solution consisting of mercuric chloride, nitric acid, glacial acetic acid, 70 per cent alcohol, and water. **glycerin oral s.** [USP], a preparation containing 95–105 per cent of the labeled amount of glycerin; used as a diuretic to reduce intraocular pressure in glaucoma and before cataract surgery. **gold s.**, any of a variety of gold compounds available for medicinal purposes with differences in their physical properties and clinical effectiveness, e.g., aurothioglucose, aurothioglycanide, gold sodium thiomalate, and gold sodium thiosulfate. See also *gold* ^{198}*Au s.* **gold** ^{198}**Au s.**, a sterile, pyrogen-free, cherry-red, colloidal solution of radiogold (^{198}Au) stabilized by the addition of gelatin and suitable reducing agents, used by intracavitary or interstitial injection in the treatment of certain types of cancer. Called also *radiogold s.* **Gowers' s.**, a solution of sodium sulfate, glacial acetic acid, and water, used for the dilution of blood prior to enumerating red blood cells microscopically with a hemocytometer. **Gram's s.**, see *Table of Stains and Staining Methods,* under *stain.* **gram molecular s.**, molar s. **half-normal s.**, a solution having half the strength of a normal solution; designated N/2. **haloperidol oral s.** [USP], a solution containing 90 to 110 per cent of the labeled amount of haloperidol; used as a tranquilizer, especially in the management of psychoses and for control of the manifestations of Gilles de la Tourette's syndrome. **Hamdi's s.**, a solution for preserving histological specimens, consisting of sodium sulfate, salt, glycerin, and water. **Harrington's s.**, a solution for hand disinfection, consisting of alcohol, hydrochloric acid, water, and corrosive mercuric chloride. **Hartman's s.**, a solution once used for dentin desensitization, consisting of thymol, 95 per cent ethyl alcohol, and sulfuric ether. **Hayem's s.**, a solution used in diluting blood prior to enumerating red blood cells microscopically with a hemocytometer, and consisting of mercury bichloride, sodium chloride, sodium sulfate, and water. **hexylcaine hydrochloride topical s.** [NF], a clear, colorless, aqueous solution containing 93 to 107 per cent of the labeled amount of hexylcaine hydrochloride; applied topically as a local anesthetic. **homatropine hydrobromide ophthalmic s.** [USP], a sterile, buffered, aqueous solution containing 95 to 105 per cent of the labeled amount of homatropine hydrobromide; applied topically to the conjunctiva to produce cycloplegia and mydriasis. **hundredth-normal s.**, a solution having one-hundredth the strength of a normal solution; designated N/100 or 0.01 N. **hydrogen dioxide s.**, hydrogen peroxide s. **hydrogen peroxide topical s.** [USP], a solution containing 2.5–3.5 gm. of hydrogen peroxide per 100 ml.; used as a topical anti-infective to the skin and mucous membrane. Called also *hydrogen dioxide solution.* **hydroxyamphetamine hydrobromide ophthalmic s.** [USP], a sterile, buffered, aqueous solution containing 0.95 to 1.05 per cent of hydroxyamphetamine hydrobromide; applied topically to the conjunctiva as a mydriatic. **hydroxypropyl methylcellulose ophthalmic s.** [USP], a sterile solution containing 85–115 per cent hydroxypropyl methylcellulose; applied topically to the conjunctiva to protect the cornea during certain ophthalmic procedures and to lubricate the cornea. **hyperbaric s.,** a solution having a greater specific gravity than a standard of reference, such as one used for spinal anesthesia having a specific gravity greater than that of the spinal fluid, causing it to migrate downward and produce anesthesia below the level of injection. **hypertonic s.,** see *hypertonic.* **hypobaric s.,** a solution having a specific gravity less than that of a standard of reference, such as one used for spinal anesthesia having a specific gravity less than that of the spinal fluid, causing it to migrate upward and produce anesthesia above the level of injection. **hypotonic s.,** see *hypotonic.* **idoxuridine ophthalmic s.,** [USP], a sterile, aqueous solution containing 0.09 to 0.11 per cent of idoxuridine; used as an antiviral agent in the treatment of herpes virus keratitis, applied topically to the conjunctiva. **iodine topical s.** [USP], a transparent, reddish brown liquid, with the odor of iodine, consisting of iodine and sodium iodide in purified water, each 100 ml. of which contains 1.8–2.2 gm. of iodine and 2.1–2.6 gm. of sodium iodide; used as a local anti-infective. **iodine s., compound,** iodine s. strong. **iodine s., strong** [USP], a transparent, deep brown liquid, with the odor of iodine, consisting of iodine and potassium iodide in purified water, each 100 ml. containing 4.5–5.5 gm. of iodine and 9.5–10.5 gm. of potassium iodide. It is used as a source of iodine. Called also *compound iodine s.* and *Lugol's s.* **iron and ammonium acetate s.,** a clear, reddish brown liquid, with an aromatic odor, compounded of ferric chloride tincture, diluted acetic acid, ammonium acetate solution, aromatic elixir, glycerin, and distilled water. Formerly used as a hematinic and as a diuretic. Called also *Basham's mixture.* **isobaric s.,** a solution having the same specific gravity as a standard of reference, such as one used for spinal anesthesia having a specific gravity same as that of the spinal fluid, causing it to remain and produce anesthesia at the level of injection. **isoflurophate ophthalmic s.,** a sterile solution containing 0.09–0.11 per cent of isoflurophate in a suitable vegetable oil; used as a cholinergic in the treatment of glaucoma, applied topically to the conjunctiva. **isotonic s.,** see *isotonic.* **Kaiserling s.,** 1. for *fixation:* formalin 400 ml., water 2,000 ml., potassium nitrate 30 gm., potassium acetate 60 gm. 2. *for restoring color:* alcohol 80 per cent. 3. *for preservation:* potassium acetate 200 gm., glycerol 400 ml., sodium arsenate 100 gm., water 2,000 ml. **Labarraque's s.** [NF], sodium hypochlorite solution, diluted with an equal volume of water. **Lang's s.,** see under *fluid.* **Lange's s.,** a solution of colloidal gold. **lead subacetate s.,** an aqueous solution of lead acetate and lead monoxide; used as an astringent and as a local sedative. **lead subacetate s., diluted,** a colorless, slightly turbid liquid, with a sweet, astringent taste, prepared by diluting lead subacetate solution with water. **lime s., sulfurated,** a solution of lime and sublimed sulfur in water; formerly much used as a keratolytic in acne vulgaris and seborrhea. Called also *Vleminckx's s.* **liver s.,** a brownish liquid prepared from mammalian livers and containing the soluble thermostable fraction which stimulates hematopoiesis in patients with pernicious anemia. Called also *liquid liver extract.* **Locke's s.,** a solution of sodium chloride, calcium chloride, potassium chloride, sodium bicarbonate, and dextrose; used in physiological experiments to keep the mammalian heart beating. **Locke's s., citrated,** a solution of sodium chloride, potassium chloride, calcium chloride, sodium citrate, and water, with pH adjusted to 7.4. **Locke-Ringer's s.,** a test solution containing sodium chloride, potassium chloride, calcium chloride, magnesium chloride, sodium bicarbonate, dextrose, and water. **Lugol's s.,** iodine s., strong. **Magendie's s.,** a solution for parenteral use containing morphine sulfate. **magnesium citrate oral s.** [USP], a colorless to slightly yellow, clear, effervescent liquid, with a sweet, acidulous taste and a lemon flavor, which consists of magnesium carbonate, anhydrous citric acid, syrup, talc, lemon oil, potassium bicarbonate, and purified water, each 100 ml. containing an amount of magnesium citrate equal to 1.55–1.9 gm. magnesium oxide. It is used as a cathartic. **malt extract s.,** a solution of malt extract in water; used as a bacteriological culture medium. **Massier's s.,** a solution used as a spray in laryngitis, consisting of resorcinol (1.5 gm.), menthol (0.1 gm.), 3.0 strong tincture of iodine, and glycerin (30 ml.). **Mencière's s.,** see under *mixture.* **merbromin s.,** a clear, red liquid with a yellow-green fluorescence, compounded of merbromin and water, each 100 ml. of which contains 1.8–2.2 gm. of merbromin; used as an antibacterial. **merbromin s., surgical,** a clear, red liquid with a yellow-green fluorescence, compounded of merbromin, water, acetone, and neutralized alcohol, the merbromin containing 24–26.7 per cent of mercury, and 18–21.3 per cent of bromine; used as an antibacterial. **methoxsalen topical s.** [USP], a preparation containing 9.2–10.8

mg. of methoxsalen per milliliter; used in conjunction with exposure to ultraviolet light to facilitate repigmentation in idiopathic vitiligo, and also as a suntan accelerator and sun protectant. **methylcellulose ophthalmic s.** [USP], a sterile solution containing 85–115 per cent of the labeled amount of methylcellulose; applied topically to protect the cornea during certain ophthalmic procedures and to lubricate the cornea. **methylrosaniline chloride s.,** gentian violet s. **molal s.,** a solution containing 1 mole of solute dissolved in 1,000 gm. of solvent. **molar s.,** a solution each liter of which contains 1 gram-molecule of the dissolved substance: designated M/1 or 1 M. The concentration of other solutions may be expressed in relation to that of molar solutions as tenth-molar (M/10 or 0.1 M), etc. **molecular disperse s.,** a solution in which the dispersed particles have a diameter of about 0.1 micromicron. **Monsel's s.,** ferric subsulfate s. **Naegeli's s.,** a synthetic culture medium containing dibasic potassium phosphate, magnesium sulfate, calcium chloride, and ammonium tartrate, in water; used for growing yeasts and molds. **nafcillin sodium for oral s.** [USP], a preparation containing nafcillin sodium equivalent to 90–120 per cent of the labeled amount of nafcillin; used as an antibacterial, chiefly in the treatment of resistant staphylococcal infections. **naphazoline hydrochloride nasal s.** [USP], a solution containing 90–110 per cent of the labeled amount of naphazoline hydrochloride in water; used as a vasoconstrictor, applied topically to the nasal mucosa. **naphazoline hydrochloride ophthalmic s.** [USP], a solution containing 90–110 per cent of the labeled amount of naphazoline hydrochloride in water; used as a vasoconstrictor, applied topically to the conjunctiva. **neomycin sulfate oral s.** [USP], a solution containing, in each 5 ml. of solution, an amount of neomycin sulfate equivalent to 90 to 125 per cent of the equivalent of 87.5 mg. of neomycin base; used as an antibacterial. **neomycin and polymyxin B sulfates and gramicidin ophthalmic s.** [USP], a sterile isotonic solution containing 90 to 130 per cent of the labeled amounts of neomycin base, polymyxin B sulfate, and gramicidin; applied topically to the eye as a local anti-infective. **Nessler's s.,** see under *reagent.* **nitrofurazone topical s.** [USP], a solution containing 95–105 per cent of the labeled amount of nitrofurazone; used as a local anti-infective against a wide variety of gram-negative and gram-positive bacteria in the treatment of many skin lesions, especially second and third degree burns and to aid healing and prevent infection of skin grafts, applied topically. **nitromersol topical s.** [USP], a clear, reddish orange liquid, compounded of nitromersol, sodium hydroxide, monohydrated sodium carbonate, and purified water, each 100 ml. of which yields 180–220 mg. of nitromersol; used as a topical anti-infective. **normal s.,** a solution each liter of which contains 1 gram equivalent weight of the dissolved substance: designated N/1 or 1 N. **normal saline s., normal salt s.,** physiological salt s. **normobaric s.,** isobaric s. **ophthalmic s.,** a sterile solution, essentially free from foreign particles and suitably compounded and dispensed, for instillation into the eye. **Orth's s.,** a solution for fixing histological specimens, consisting of Müller's fluid and formaldehyde solution. **oxacillin sodium for oral s.** [USP], a preparation containing 90–120 per cent of the labeled amount of oxacillin; used as an antibacterial, primarily in the treatment of infections due to penicillinase-resistant staphylococci. **oxymetazoline hydrochloride nasal s.** [USP], a solution of oxymetazoline hydrochloride in water adjusted to a suitable pH and tonicity, containing 95 to 115 per cent of the labeled amount of oxymetazoline hydrochloride; instilled into the nostrils as a vasoconstrictor. **paramethadione oral s.** [USP], a solution of paramethadione in dilute alcohol, containing, in each milliliter, 282 to 318 mg. of paramethadione; used as an anticonvulsant, especially in petit mal epilepsy. **parathyroid s.,** parathyroid injection. **Pasteur's s.,** a solution of ammonium tartrate, cane sugar, and ash from yeast, in water; used as a medium for growing yeasts and molds. **Perenyi's s.,** an embryological fixing solution, consisting of 10 per cent solution of nitric acid, alcohol, and 0.5 per cent solution of chromic acid. **phenylephrine hydrochloride nasal s.** [USP], a clear, colorless, or slightly yellow liquid, which contains 95–105 per cent of the labeled amount of phenylephrine hydrochloride; used as a nasal vasoconstrictor, applied topically. **phenylephrine hydrochloride ophthalmic s.** [USP], a sterile, buffered, aqueous solution containing 90 to 115 per cent of the labeled amount of phenylephrine hydrochloride; applied topically to the conjunctiva as a vasoconstrictor to produce mydriasis without cycloplegia. **physiological salt s., physiological sodium chloride s.,** an aqueous solution of sodium chloride having an osmolality similar to that of blood serum. **physostigmine salicylate ophthalmic s.** [USP], a sterile, aqueous solution containing 90–110 per cent of the labeled amount of physostigmine salicylate; used as a cholinergic to produce miosis and to decrease intraocular pressure in the treatment of glaucoma, applied topically to the conjunctiva. **Pickrell's s.,** a solution of sulfadiazine in ethanolamine, with sodium benzoate as a preservative. **pilocarpine hydrochloride ophthalmic s.** [USP], a sterile, buffered, aqueous solution containing 90 to 110 per cent of the labeled amount of pilocarpine hydrochloride; applied topically to the conjunctiva as a cholinergic. **pilocarpine nitrate ophthalmic s.** [USP], a sterile, buffered, aqueous solution containing 90 to 110 per cent of the labeled amount of pilocarpine nitrate; applied topically to the conjunctiva as a cholinergic. **Pitkin's s.**, a solution of procaine in a solvent having a specific gravity lower than that of the spinal fluid; used as a spinal anesthetic. **pituitary s., pituitary s., posterior,** posterior pituitary injection. **potassium arsenite s.**, a solution of arsenic trioxide, potassium bicarbonate, and alcohol in water. It has been used in the treatment of chronic myelogenous leukemia and chronic dermatitides. In veterinary medicine, it is used in the treatment of pulmonary emphysema, chronic nonparasitic dermatitides, chronic coughs, and general debility. Called also *arsenical s., Fowler's solution,* and *kali arsenicosum.* **potassium iodide oral s.** [USP], a solution containing 97–103 gm. of potassium iodide in each ml.; used as an expectorant, as a source of iodine in thyrotoxic crises and in the preparation of thyrotoxic patients for thyriodectomy, and as an antifungal in the treatment of lymphocutaneous sporotrichosis, administered orally. **povidone-iodine topical s.** [USP], a reddish brown, transparent solution of povidone-iodine and water, containing 85 to 120 per cent of the labeled amount of iodine; applied topically as an anti-infective. **prednisolone sodium phosphate ophthalmic s.** [USP], a sterile solution of prednisolone sodium phosphate in a buffered, aqueous medium, containing 90 to 115 per cent of the labeled amount of prednisolone phosphate, present as the disodium salt; used as an anti-inflammatory adrenocortical steroid. **prochlorperazine edisylate oral s.** [USP], a solution containing 92–108 per cent of the labeled amount of prochlorperazine; used as an antiemetic and tranquilizer, administered orally. **promazine hydrochloride oral s.** [USP], a solution containing 95–110 per cent of the labeled amount of promazine hydrochloride; used mainly as an antipsychotic agent, administered orally. **proparacaine hydrochloride ophthalmic s.** [USP], a sterile, aqueous solution containing 95 to 110 per cent of the labeled amount of proparacaine hydrochloride; applied topically to the conjunctiva as an anesthetic. **racephedrine hydrochloride s.**, a clear, colorless solution with a camphoraceous odor and taste, compounded of racephedrine hydrochloride, chlorobutanol, and Ringer's solution, each 100 ml. of which contains between 930 mg. and 1.07 gm. of racephedrine; used as an adrenergic. Called also *dl-ephedrine hydrochloride s.* **radiocyanocobalamin s.,** radioactive cyanocobalamin. **radiogold s.**, gold ^{198}Au s. **Randall's s.,** a solution consisting of the acetate, bicarbonate, and citrate salts of potassium; used especially in the treatment of potassium deficiency, administered orally. **Rees-Ecker s.,** see under *fluid.* **Ringer's s.,** see under irrigation. **Ruge's s.,** a solution of glacial acetic acid, 40 per cent formalin, and water; used as a stain. **saline s., salt s.,** a solution of sodium chloride, or common salt, in purified water. **saturated s.**, a solution in which the solvent has taken up all of the dissolved substance that it can hold in solution. **Schällibaum's s.,** a solution of celloidin and oil of cloves used in histological work to attach paraffin sections to slides. **sclerosing s.,** a solution of an irritant substance for injection into a vein to produce obliteration of the vein, or into a hernia to induce fibrous formation and obliteration of the sac. **scopolamine hydrobromide ophthalmic s.** [USP], a sterile, buffered, aqueous solution, containing 90 to 110 per cent of the labeled amount of scopolamine hydrobromide; used as a mydriatic and cycloplegic, applied topically to the conjunctiva. **seminormal s.,** half-normal s. **Seyderhelm's s.,** a colloidal mixture of Congo red and trypan blue, for staining urinary sediment. **Shohl's s.,** a solution containing 140 gm. citric acid and 98 gm. hydrated crystalline salt of sodium citrate, distilled water to make 1000 ml.; used to correct electrolyte imbalance in the treatment of renal tubular acidosis. **silver nitrate s., ammoniacal,** a clear, colorless, almost odorless liquid, compounded of silver nitrate, water, and strong ammonia solution, and containing, in each 100 ml., 28.5–30.5 gm. of silver, and 9.0–9.7 gm. of ammonia; used as a dental protective to fill minute crevices in teeth. **silver nitrate ophthalmic s.** [USP], a solution of silver nitrate in a buffered water medium, containing 0.95–1.05 per cent of $AgNO_3$; used as a local anti-infective applied topically to the conjunctiva as a prophylactic against ophthalmia neonatorum. **sodium borate s., compound,** a solution containing sodium borate, sodium bicarbonate, liquefied phenol, glycerin, and purified water; formerly used as a gargle or mouth wash. **sodium chloride s.,** see under *irrigation.* **sodium cyclamate and sodium saccharin s.,** a clear, colorless solution containing 90 to 110 per cent of the labeled amounts of sodium cyclamate and sodium saccharin; used as a non-nutritive sweetener. **sodium fluorescein ophthalmic s.** [USP], a sterile buffered solution containing, in each 100 ml., 1.86 to 2.10 gm. of sodium fluorescein, and a suitable antimicrobial agent; applied topically to the conjunctiva as a corneal trauma indicator. **sodium fluoride oral s.** [USP], a solution containing 95–105 per cent of the labeled amount of sodium fluoride; used as a dental caries prophylactic, used in the fluoridation of water and applied topically to the teeth. **sodium hypochlorite s.** [USP], a clear, pale, greenish yellow liquid with the odor of chlorine, containing 4–6 per cent of sodium hypochlorite; used as a disinfectant for utensils, etc., but not suitable for application to

wounds. It has also been used as a deodorant and bleaching agent. **sodium hypochlorite s., diluted,** a colorless to light yellow liquid with a faint odor of chlorine, compounded of sodium hypochlorite solution, sodium bicarbonate, and water, each 100 ml. containing 450–500 mg. of sodium hypochlorite; used as a topical anti-infective. It is also used for wound irrigation, and has been used to irrigate the urinary bladder. Called also *Dakin's antiseptic, Dakin's fluid, Dakin's s., Dakin's modified s.,* and *surgical s. of chlorinated soda.* See also *Carrel's treatment,* under *treatment.* **sodium iodide I 125 s.** [USP], a solution suitable for either oral or intravenous administration, containing radioiodine (^{125}I) as sodium iodide; used in the determination of thyroid function. **sodium iodide I 131 s.** [USP], a solution suitable for either oral or intravenous use, containing radioiodine (^{131}I) as sodium iodide; used for thryroid function determination and thyroid scans, as a thyroid inhibitor in the treatment of hyperthyroidism and cardiac diseases associated with hyperthyroidism, and for the palliation of thyroid cancer. **sodium phosphate s.,** a clear colorless liquid without odor and with a salty taste, the consistency of thick syrup, each 100 ml. of which contains the equivalent of 71–79 gm. of sodium phosphate; used as a mild saline cathartic. It was formerly administered orally or intravenously in the treatment of lead poisoning. **sodium phosphate P 32 s.** [USP], a solution suitable for either oral or intravenous administration, containing radiophosphorus (^{32}P) as sodium phosphate; used especially as an antipolycythemic and as a diagnostic aid for localization of tumors, e.g., intraocular and brain lesions, and has been used in the treatment of certain leukemias. Formerly called *sodium radiophosphate s.* **sodium phosphate and biphosphate oral s.** [USP], a solution of sodium phosphate and sodium biphosphate, or sodium phosphate and phosphoric acid, in purified water, containing in each 100 ml., 17.1–18.9 gm. of sodium phosphate and 45.6–50.4 gm of sodium biphosphate; used as a cathartic. **sodium radioiodide s.,** sodium iodide I 131 s. **sodium radiophosphate s.,** sodium phosphate P 32 s. **sorbitol s.** [USP], a clear, colorless, syrupy liquid with a sweet taste, containing in each 100 ml., 69–71 gm. of total solids consisting essentially of D-sorbitol with a small quantity of mannitol and other isomeric polyhydric alcohols; used as a flavored humectant in pharmaceutic preparations. **standard s.,** one which contains in each liter a definitely stated amount of reagent; usually expressed in terms of normality (equivalent weights of solute per liter of solution) or molarity (g.mol.wts. of solute per liter of solution). **sulfacetamide sodium ophthalmic s.** [USP], a sterile solution containing 95–105 per cent of the labeled amount of sulfacetamide sodium; used as an antibacterial in sulfonamide-responsive eye infections, applied topically to the conjunctiva. **sulfisoxazole diolamine ophthalmic s.,** [USP], a sterile solution containing sulfisoxazole diolamine equivalent to 90–115 per cent of the labeled amount of sulfisoxazole; used as an antibacterial in the treatment of sulfonamide-responsive eye infections. **supersaturated s.,** an unstable solution that contains more of the solute than it can permanently hold. **surgical s. of chlorinated soda,** see *sodium hypochlorite s., diluted.* **susa s.,** a decalcifying solution composed of corrosive sublimate, sodium chloride, trichloracetic acid, glacial acetic acid, formalin, and water. **tenth-normal s.,** one having one-tenth the strength of a normal solution: designated N/10 or 0.1 N. **test s's,** standard solutions (in purity and concentration) of specified chemical substances used in performing certain test procedures. **tetracaine hydrochloride ophthalmic s.** [USP], a sterile aqueous solution containing 90–110 per cent of the labeled amount of tetracaine hydrochloride; used as a topical anesthetic, applied to the conjunctiva. **tetracaine hydrochloride topical s.** [USP], an aqueous solution containing 95–105 per cent of tetracaine hydrochloride; used as a topical anesthetic, applied to the mucous membranes of the nose and throat. **tetrahydrozoline hydrochloride nasal s.** [USP], a solution of tetrahydrozoline hydrochloride in water adjusted to a suitable tonicity, containing 90 to 110 per cent of the labeled amount of tetrahydrozoline hydrochloride; a vasoconstrictor applied in 0.05 or 0.1 per cent solution as nasal drops or spray, or in 0.05 solution to the eye. **tetrahydrozoline hydrochloride ophthalmic s.** [USP], a sterile, aqueous solution containing 90 to 110 per cent of the labeled amount of tetrahydrozoline hydrochloride; a vasoconstrictor applied to the eye in 0.05 per cent solution. **thimerosal topical s.** [USP], a clear solution having a characteristic odor, compounded of thimerosal, ethylenediamine, monoethanolamine, sodium chloride, sodium borate, and purified water, each 100 ml. containing 95 to 105 mg. of thimerosal; applied topically as an anti-infective. **thioridazine hydrochloride oral s.** [USP], a solution containing, in each 100 ml., 2.70 to 3.30 gm. of thioridazine hydrochloride; used as a tranquilizer. **thousandth-normal s.,** a solution having one-thousandth the strength of a normal solution: designated N/1,000 or 0.001 N. **Toison's s.,** a fluid used in diluting blood for the counting of the erythrocytes, consisting of crystal violet, sodium chloride, sodium sulfate, glycerin, and water. **tolnaftate topical s.** [USP], a solution containing 90 to 115 per cent of the labeled amount of tolnaftate; used as a topical antifungal. **tribromoethanol s., tribromethyl alcohol s.,** a preparation containing in each 100 ml., 95–105 gm.

of tribromoethanol in amylene hydrate; used as a rectally administered basal anethestic, and has been used as an anticonvulsive. Called also *bromethol*. **tribromoethyl alcohol s.**, tribromoethanol s. [USP], a solution containing 94 to 106 per cent of the labeled amount of trimethadione; used as an oral anticonvulsant for control of petit mal seizures. **tropicamide ophthalmic s.** [USP], a sterile solution of tropicamide in a suitable buffered, aqueous medium, containing 95 to 105 per cent of tropicamide; applied topically to the conjunctiva as an anticholinergic. **tuaminoheptane sulfate nasal s.** [USP], a solution of tuaminoheptane sulfate, sodium hydroxide, phenylmercuric nitrate, monobasic potassium nitrate, sodium chloride, and purified water; used as an adrenergic applied topically to the nasal mucosa to relieve congestion. **Tyrode's s.**, a modified Locke's solution containing magnesium. **Vleminckx's s.**, lime s., sulfurated. **volumetric s.**, one which contains a specific quantity of solute per stated unit of volume; see also *standard s.* **xylometazoline hydrochloride nasal s.** [USP], a solution of xylometazoline hydrochloride in water adjusted to a suitable pH and tonicity, containing 90 to 110 per cent of the labeled amount of $C_{16}H_{24}N_2 \cdot HCl$; applied topically as a vasoconstrictor in nasal congestion. **Zenker's s.**, a fixative solution consisting of mercury bichloride, potassium dichromate, glacial acetic acid, and water. **Ziehl's s.**, see *Table of Stains and Staining Methods*. **zinc sulfate ophthalmic s.** [USP], a sterile solution of zinc sulfate in water rendered isotonic by the addition of suitable salts, containing 95 to 105 per cent of the labeled amount of zinc sulfate; applied topically to the conjunctiva as an astringent. Considered specific for conjunctivitis due to *Hemophilus duplex*.

solv. abbreviation for L. *sol've*, dissolve.

solvable (sol'vah-b'l) soluble.

solvate (sol'vāt) a compound of one or more molecules of a solvent with the ions or with the molecules of a dissolved substance.

solvation (sol-va'shun) chemical combination of a solvent with the solute.

solvent (sol'vent) [L. *solvens*] 1. dissolving; effecting a solution. 2. a liquid that dissolves or that is capable of dissolving; the component of a solution that is present in greater amount. Cf. *solute*.

solvolysis (sol-vol'ĭ-sis) a general term for double decomposition reactions of the type of hydrolysis, ammonolysis, and sulfolysis.

Soma (so'mah) trademark for preparations of carisoprodol.

soma (so'mah) [Gr. *sōma* body] 1. the body as distinguished from the mind. 2. the body tissue as distinguished from the germ cells. 3. the cell body.

somal (so'mal) somatic.

somalin (som'ah-lin) a cardioactive glycoside from plants of the genus *Adenium*.

somaplasm (so'mah-plazm) somatoplasm.

somasthenia (sōm''as-the'ne-ah) [*soma* + *a* neg. + Gr. *sthenos* strength + *-ia*] a condition of bodily weakness, poor appetite and sleep, and inability to maintain a normal active life without easy exhaustion.

somatalgia (so''mah-tal'je-ah) [*somato-* + Gr. *algos* pain + *-ia*] bodily pain.

somatasthenia (so''mat-as-the'ne-ah) somasthenia.

somatesthesia (so''mat-es-the'ze-ah) [*somato-* + Gr. *aisthēsis* perception + *-ia*] the consciousness of having a body.

somatesthetic (so''mat-es-thet'ik) pertaining to somatesthesia.

somatic (so-mat'ik) [Gr. *sōmatikos*] 1. pertaining to or characteristic of the soma or body. 2. pertaining to the body wall in contrast to the viscera.

somaticosplanchnic (so-mat''ĭ-ko-splank'nik) somaticovisceral.

somaticovisceral (so-mat''ĭ-ko-vis'er-al) pertaining to the body proper and viscera.

somatist (so'mah-tist) one who believes that neuroses and psychoses are of physical origin and are based on bodily lesions.

somatization (so''mah-ti-za'shun) in psychiatry, the conversion of mental experiences or states into bodily symptoms.

somato- (so'mah-to) [Gr. *sōma*, *sōmatos* body] a combining form denoting relationship to the body.

somatoceptor (so-mat'o-sep''tor) a receptor concerned in receiving stimuli of the skeletal and somatic musculature.

somatochrome (so-mat'o-krōm) [*somato-* + Gr. *chrōma* color] any nerve cell which has a well marked cell body completely surrounding the nucleus, its colorable protoplasm having a distinct contour; used also adjectively.

somatoderm (so-mat'o-derm) [*somato-* + Gr. *derma* skin] the somatic layer of mesoderm.

somatodidymus (so''mah-to-did'ĭ-mus) a double fetus exhibiting somatodymia.

somatodymia (so''mah-to-dim'e-ah) [*somato-* + Gr. *didymos* twin + *-ia*] a developmental anomaly resulting in the production of conjoined twins whose trunks are fused into one.

somatogenesis (so''mah-to-jen'ĕ-sis) [*somato-* + Gr. *genesis* production] the formation or emergence of bodily structure out of hereditary sources; the formation of somatoplasm out of germ plasm.

somatogenetic (so-mat''o-jĕ-net'ik) 1. pertaining to somatogenesis. 2. somatogenic.

somatogenic (so''mah-to-jen'ik) [*somato-* + Gr. *gennan* to produce] originating in the cells of the body, as a disease process; opposed to psychogenic.

somatogram (so-mat'o-gram) [*somato-* + Gr. *gramma* a writing] a roentgenogram of the body.

somatology (so''mah-tol'o-je) [*somato-* + *-logy*] the sum of what is known regarding the body; the study of the anatomy and physiology of the body.

somatome (so'mah-tōm) [*soma* + Gr. *temnein* to cut] 1. an appliance for cutting the body of the fetus. 2. a somite.

somatomedin (so''mah-to-me'din) any of a group of peptides formed in the liver (molecular weight, approximately 8000) and found in plasma which mediate the effect of growth hormone (somatotropin) on cartilage; they are responsible for uptake of sulfate and increased synthesis of collagen and other proteins by cartilage. Somatomedins also increase ribonucleic acid (RNA) synthesis and promote deoxyribonucleic acid (DNA) synthesis. Postulated as a "second messenger" in the somatotropic actions of growth hormone. Called also *sulfation factor*.

somatomegaly (so''mah-to-meg'ah-le) [*somato-* + Gr. *megaleios* stately + *-ia*] abnormal size of body; gigantism.

somatometry (so-mah-tom'ĕ-tre) [*somato-* + Gr. *metron* measure] measurement of the body.

somatomic (so''mah-tom'ik) pertaining to a somatome.

somatopagus (so''mah-top'ah-gus) [*somato-* + Gr. *pagos* thing fixed] a double fetus with trunks more or less merged.

somatopathic (so''mah-to-path'ik) [*somato-* + Gr. *pathos* disease] pertaining to or characterized by somatopathy.

somatopathy (so''mah-top'ah-the) a bodily disorder as distinguished from a mental one.

somatophrenia (so''mah-to-fre'ne-ah) [*somato-* + Gr. *phrēn* mind + *-ia*] a mental condition which exaggerates or imagines body ills.

somatoplasm (so-mat'o-plazm) [*somato-* + Gr. *plasma* anything formed or molded] the protoplasm of the body cells as distinguished from that of the germ cells. Cf. *germ plasm*.

somatopleural (so''mah-to-ploor'al) pertaining to the somatopleure.

somatopleure (so-mat'o-ploor) [*somato-* + Gr. *pleura* side] the embryonic body wall, formed by ectoderm and somatic mesoderm.

somatopsychic (so''mah-to-si'kik) [*somato-* + Gr. *psychē* soul] pertaining to both body and mind; denoting a physical disorder that produces mental symptoms.

somatopsychosis (so''mah-to-si-ko'sis) [*somato-* + *psychosis*] Southard's name for a mental disease symptomatic of bodily disease.

somatoschisis (so''mah-tos'kĭ-sis) [*somato-* + Gr. *schisis* fissure] a developmental anomaly characterized by a fissure of the trunk.

somatoscopy (so''mah-tos'ko-pe) [*somato-* + Gr. *skopein* to examine] viewing or examination of the body.

somatosexual (so''mah-to-seks'u-al) [*somato-* + L. *sexus* sex] pertaining to both physical and sex characteristics; pertaining to the physical manifestations of sexual development.

somatosplanchnopleuric (so''mah-to-splank''no-ploor'ik) pertaining to the somatopleure and the splanchnopleure.

somatostatin (so''mah-to-stat'in) a cyclic tetradecapeptide elaborated primarily by the median eminence of the hypothalamus and by the delta cells of the islets of Langerhans; it inhibits release of somatotropin, thyrotropin, and corticotropin by the adenohypophysis, of insulin and glucagon by the pancreas, or gastrin by the gastric mucosa, of secretin by the intestinal mucosa, and of renin by the kidney.

somatotherapy (so''mah-to-ther'ah-pe) [*somato-* + Gr. *therapeia* treatment] treatment aimed at curing the ills of the body.

somatotonia (so''mah-to-to'ne-ah) [*somato-* + Gr. *tonos* tension + *-ia*] a group of personality traits dominated by muscular activity and vigorous body assertiveness (Sheldon).

somatotopic (so''mah-to-top'ik) related to particular areas of the body; describing the organization of the motor area of the brain, control of the movement of different parts of the body being centered in specific regions of the cortex.

somatotridymus (so''mah-to-trid'ĭ-mus) [*somato-* + Gr. *tri-* three + *didymos* twin] a monster with three trunks.

somatotrope (so-mat'o-trōp) any of the acidophils (alpha cells) of the adenohypophysis that stain preferentially with orange G, and are thought to be responsible for the secretion of growth hormone. Called also *somatotropic cell*.

somatotroph (so-mat'o trōf) somatotrope.

somatotrophic (so''mah-to-trōf'ik) [*somato-* + Gr. *trophē* nourishment] having a stimulating effect on body nutrition and growth.

somatotrophin (so″mah-to-tro′fin) somatotropin.

somatotropic (so″mah-to-trop′ik) [somato- + Gr. tropos a turning] 1. having an affinity for or attacking the body or the body cells; also having an influence on the body. 2. having the properties of somatotropin.

somatotropin (so″mah-to-tro′pin) growth hormone; see under hormone.

somatotype (so-mat′o-tīp) [somato- + type] a particular category of body build, determined on the basis of certain physical characteristics. See ectomorph, endomorph, and mesomorph.

somatotyping (so-mat′o-tīp″ing) a method of studying objectively the physical types of individuals.

somatotypy (so-mat′o-ti″pe) the determination of the type of body build.

somatropin (so-mat′ro-pin) somatotropin.

Sombulex (som′bu-leks) trademark for a preparation of hexobarbital.

somesthesia (so″mes-the′ze-ah) somatesthesia.

somesthetic (so″mes-thet′ik) somatesthetic.

somite (so′mīt) one of the paired, blocklike masses of mesoderm, arranged segmentally alongside the neural tube of the embryo, forming the vertebral column and segmental musculature; called also mesoblastic or mesodermal segment.

somnambulance (som-nam′bu-lans) somnambulism.

somnambulation (som-nam″bu-la′shun) somnambulism.

somnambulism (som-nam′bu-lizm) [L. somnambulismus; somnus sleep + ambulare to walk] 1. sleep walking; habitual walking in the sleep. Called also noctambulation. 2. a hypnotic state in which the subject has the full possession of his senses but no subsequent recollection.

somnambulist (som-nam′bu-list) a person who walks in his sleep.

somni- (som′ne) [L. somnus sleep] a combining form denoting relationship to sleep.

somnifacient (som″nĭ-fa′shent) [somni- + L. facere to make] 1. causing sleep; hypnotic. 2. an agent that induces sleep.

somniferous (som-nif′er-us) [somni- + L. ferre to bring] inducing or causing sleep.

somnific (som-nif′ik) somniferous.

somniloquence (som-nil′o-kwens) somniloquism.

somniloquism (som-nil′o-kwizm) [somni- + L. loqui to speak] the habit of talking in one's sleep.

somniloquist (som-nil′o-kwist) one who talks in his sleep.

somniloquy (som-nil′o-kwe) somniloquism.

somnipathist (som-nip′ah-thist) [somni- + Gr. pathos disease] a person in or subject to hypnotic trance.

somnipathy (som-nip′ah-the) [somni- + Gr. pathos disease] any disorder of sleep; a condition of hypnotic trance.

somnocinematograph (som″no-sin″e-mat′o-graf) [somnus + cinematograph] an apparatus for recording movements made during sleep.

somnolence (som′no-lens) [L. somnolentia sleepiness] sleepiness; also unnatural drowsiness.

somnolent (som′no-lent) [L. somnolentus] affected with somnolence; sleepy.

somnolentia (som″no-len′she-ah) [L.] 1. drowsiness, or somnolence. 2. sleep drunkenness; a condition of incomplete sleep marked by loss of orientation and by excited or violent behavior.

somnolism (som′no-lizm) a state of hypnotic trance.

Somnos (som′nos) trademark for preparations of chloral hydrate.

somnus (som′nus) [L.] sleep.

somosphere (so′mo-sfēr) [Gr. sōma body + sphaira sphere] one of the elements of the archiplasm.

sonarography (so″nar-og′rah-fe) ultrasonic scanning that provides a two-dimensional image corresponding to clear sections of acoustic interfaces in tissues.

sonde (sond) [Fr.] sound. **s. coudé** (sond′koo-da′) [Fr. "bend sound"], a catheter with an elbow, or sharp, beaklike bend, near the end.

sone (sōn) a unit of loudness, being the loudness of a simple tone of 1,000 cycles per second, 40 decibels above a listener's threshold.

sonicate (son′ĭ-kāt) 1. to expose to sound waves; to disrupt bacteria by exposure to high-frequency sound waves. 2. the products of such disruption.

sonication (son″ĭ-ka′shun) exposure to sound waves; disruption of bacteria by exposure to high-frequency sound waves.

sonifer (son′ĭ-fer) [L. sonus sound + ferre to bear] a variety of ear trumpet.

Sonilyn (son′ĭ-lin) trademark for a preparation of sulfachlorpyridazine.

sonitus (son′ĭ-tus) [L. "sound"] a sounding or tinkling in the ears; tinnitus aurium.

Sonne dysentery (son′e) [Carl Olaf Sonne, Danish bacteriologist, 1882–1948] see under dysentery.

sonogram (so′no-gram) a record or display obtained by ultrasonic scanning.

sonographic (so′no-graf′ik) ultrasonographic.

sonography (so-nog′rah-fe) ultrasonography.

sonolucency (so′no-loo′sen-se) the property of being sonolucent.

sonolucent (so′no-loo′sent) in ultrasonography, permitting the passage of ultrasound waves without reflecting them back to their source (without giving off echoes).

sonorous (so-no′rus) [L. sonorus] resonant; sounding.

sophistication (so-fis″tĭ-ka′shun) [Gr. sophistikos deceitful] the adulteration of food or medicine.

sophomania (sof″o-ma′ne-ah) [Gr. sophos wise + mania madness] an irrational belief in one's own great wisdom.

Sophora (so-fo′ra) [Arabic sofara] a genus of leguminous trees and shrubs. The root and seed of S. tomentosa are used in India to arrest choleraic vomiting. Some species are poisonous; see loco.

sophoretin (sof″o-re′tin) quercetin.

sophorin (sof′o-rin) rutin.

sophorine (sof′o-rēn) cytisine.

sopor (so′por) [L.] sound, deep, or profound sleep.

soporiferous (so″po-rif′er-us) [L. sopor deep sleep + ferre to bring] inducing deep or profound slumber.

soporific (sop″o-rif′ik, so″po-rif′ik) [L. soporificus] 1. causing or inducing profound sleep. 2. a drug or other agent which induces sleep.

soporous (so′por-us) [L. soporus] associated or affected with coma or profound slumber.

S. op. s. abbreviation for L. si o′pus sit, if it is necessary.

Sorangiaceae (so-ran″je-a′se-e) a systematic family of Schizomycetes, order Myxobacterales, made up of saprophytic soil microorganisms, and comprising a single genus, Sorangium.

Sorangium (so-ran′je-um) a genus of Schizomycetes of the order Myxobacterales, family Sorangiaceae.

Soranus (so-ran′us) **of Ephesus** (2nd century A.D.) a celebrated Greek physician of the Methodist school, and the most renowned gynecologist and obstetrician of antiquity. He practiced in Alexandria and, later, in Rome. His surviving writings on obstetrics, gynecology, and pediatrics are outstanding.

sorb (sorb) to attract and retain substances by absorption or adsorption.

sorbefacient (sor″bĕ-fa′shent) [L. sorbere to suck + facere to make] 1. promoting absorption. 2. an agent that promotes absorption.

sorbent (sor′bent) an agent that sorbs.

sorbin (sor′bin) sorbose.

sorbinose (sor′bĭ-nōs) sorbose.

sorbitan (sor′bĭ-tan) a generic name for an anhydride of sorbitol, $C_6H_8O(OH)_4$, the fatty acids of which (s. monolaurate [NF], s. monooleate, s. monopalmitate [NF], s. monostearate [NF], s. sesquioleate, s. trioleate, s. tristearate) are surfactants; called also sorbitol anhydride. See also polysorbate.

sorbite (sor′bīt) sorbitol.

sorbitol (sor′bĭ-tol) a crystalline, hexahydric alcohol, $CH_2OH \cdot (CHOH)_4CH_2OH$, first found in ripe berries of the tree Sorbus aucuparia, and occurring in small quantities in other berries, cherries, plums, pears, etc. It is formed in mammals from glucose and is then converted to fructose; this process is responsible for fructose found in seminal plasma. It is also found in lens deposits in diabetes mellitus. A pharmaceutical preparation [NF] is obtained by catalytic hydrogenation of glucose and certain other sugars; it contains between 91 and 100.6 per cent sorbitol, calculated on the anhydrous basis; used as a sweetening agent and tablet excipient in pharmecutical preparations and, in a 50 per cent solution, as an intravenous osmotic diuretic.

Sorbitrate (sor′bĭ-trāt) trademark for a preparation of isosorbide dinitrate.

sorbose (sor′bōs) a ketohexose, $CH_2OH(CHOH)_3CO \cdot CH_2OH$, resembling levulose in its properties.

Sordariaciae (sor′dah-re-a′se-e) a family of fungi of the order Sphaeriales, series Pyrenomycetes, including the genus Neurospora.

sordes (sor′dēz) [L. "filth"] materia alba. **s. gas′tricae**, undigested food, mucus, etc., in the stomach.

sore (sōr) 1. a popular term for almost any lesion of the skin or mucous membranes. 2. painful. **bed s.**, decubitus ulcer. **canker s.**, aphthous stomatitis. **chrome s.**, chrome ulcer. **Cochin s.**, tropical ulcer. **Cochin China s.**, cutaneous leishmaniasis. **cold s.**, herpes febrilis, especially of the lips or face. **Delhi s.**, cutaneous leishmaniasis. **desert s.**, a form of tropical ulcer resembling varicose ulcer and appearing on the face, back of hands and lower extremities. It occurs in desert areas of Africa, Australia and the Near East. Called also *Gallipoli s.*, *Umballa s.*, *veldt s.* and *Barcoo rot.* **fungating s.,** see under *chancre.* **Gallipoli s.,** desert s. **hard s.,** chancre, def 1. **Kandahar s., Lahore s., Madagascar s.,** cutaneous leishmaniasis. **mixed s.,** see under *chancre.* **Moultan s.,** cutaneous leishmaniasis. **Naga s.,** a form of tropical ulcer occurring among workers in tea gardens in Assam; see *tropical ulcer* (def. 1), under *ulcer.* **Natal s., oriental s., Penjdeh s.,** cutaneous leishmaniasis. **pressure s.,** decubitus ulcer. **soft s.,** chancroid. **summer s's,** cutaneous habronemiasis. **tropical s.,** cutaneous leishmaniasis. **Umballa s.,** desert s. **veldt s.,** desert s. **venereal s.,** any sore that accompanies or manifests a venereal disease, especially a chancroid.

Sörensen's reagent (sor'en-senz) [Sören Peer Lauritz *Sörensen*, Danish biochemist, 1868–1939] see under *reagent.*

sore throat (sōr thrōt) see *laryngitis, pharyngitis,* and *tonsillitis.* **clergyman's s. t.,** dysphonia clericorum. **diphtheria s. t.,** diphtheria. **epidemic streptococcal s. t.,** septic s. t. **Fothergill's s. t.,** scarlatina angiosa. **hospital s. t.,** septic inflammation of the pharynx and fauces sometimes affecting nurses and interns in hospitals. **putrid s. t.,** gangrenous pharyngitis. **septic s. t.,** a severe type of sore throat occurring in epidemics, marked by intense local hyperemia with or without a grayish exudate and enlargement of the cervical lymph glands. It is usually caused by *Streptococcus pyogenes* and sometimes by *S. equisimilis.* The infection is probably largely spread by droplets or in air, but is also transmitted by direct contact and by food and milk. Called also *streptococcal sore throat* and *streptococcal tonsillitis.* **spotted s. t.,** follicular tonsillitis. **streptococcal s. t.,** septic s. t. **ulcerated s. t.,** gangrenous pharyngitis.

Soret band, effect (phenomenon) (so-ra') [C. *Soret,* French physicist, died 1931] see under *band* and *effect.*

soroche, sorroche (so-ro'cha) [Sp. "antimony"] mountain sickness of the Andes, incorrectly ascribed to metallic exhalations.

sororiation (so-ro″re-a'shun) [L. *sororiare* to increase together] increase in size of the breasts at puberty.

sorption (sorp'shun) [L. *sorbere* to suck in] the process or state of being sorbed; absorption or adsorption.

S.O.S. abbreviation for L. *si o'pus sit,* if it is necessary.

sotalol hydrochloride (so'tah-lōl) chemical name: *N*-[4-[1-hydroxy-2-[(1-methylethyl)amino]ethyl]phenyl]mathanesulfonamide monohydrochloride; a beta-adrenergic blocking agent, $C_{12}H_{20}N_2O_4 \cdot HCl$, having the same actions as propranolol (q.v.).

soterenol hydrochloride (so-ter'ĕ-nōl) chemical name: 2′-hydroxy-5′-[1-hydroxy-2-(isopropylamino)ethyl]methanesulfonanilide; an adrenergic with bronchodilator properties, $C_{12}H_{20}N_2O_4 \cdot$ S·HCl.

soteria (so-tēr'e-ah) [Gr. *sōtēria* a way or means of safety; a guarantee of safekeeping] *(obs.)* the experiencing of a feeling of security and protection, apparently out of proportion to the stimulus, derived from an external object, which becomes a neurotic object-source of comfort.

Soto-Hall sign (so'to-hawl) [Ralph *Soto-Hall,* San Francisco surgeon, born 1899] see under *sign.*

Sottas disease (sot'tahz) [Jules *Sottas,* French neurologist, born 1866] progressive hypertrophic interstitial neuropathy.

Sotteau's operation (so-tōz') [Augusté Joseph Henrí *Sotteau,* French surgeon, 1802–1851] see under *operation.*

soudan (soo-dan') Sudan.

souffle (soof'f'l) [Fr. "a puff"; L. *suffare* to blow] a soft, blowing, auscultatory sound; called also *bruit de soufflet* and *bellows murmur.* **cardiac s.,** any cardiac or vascular murmur of a blowing quality. **fetal s.,** a blowing sound sometimes heard in pregnancy; supposed to be due to compression of the umbilical vessels. **funic s., funicular s.,** a hissing souffle synchronous with the fetal heart sounds, and supposed to be produced in the umbilical cord. **placental s.,** a souffle supposed to be produced by the blood current in the placenta. **splenic s.,** a sound said to be sometimes audible over a diseased spleen. **umbilical s.,** funic s. **uterine s.,** a sound made by the blood within the arteries of the gravid uterus.

sound (sownd) [L. *sonus*] 1. the effect produced on the organ of hearing and its central connections by the vibrations of the air or other medium. 2. mechanical radiant energy, the motion of particles of the material medium through which it travels (air, water, or solids) being along the line of transmission (longitudinal); such energy, of frequency between 8 and 20,000 cycles per second, provides the stimulus for the subjective sensation of hearing. 3. an instrument to be introduced into a cavity to detect a foreign body or to dilate a stricture. 4. a noise, normal or abnormal, heard within the body; for other sounds see under *bruit, fremitus, murmur,* and *rale.* **auscultatory s.,** any sound heard on auscultation. **bandbox s.,** a highly resonant sound elicited by percussion over the chest in cases of emphysema of the lung. **Beatty-Bright friction s.,** the friction sound of pleurisy. **bell s.,** bruit d'airain. **Bellocq's s.,** see under *cannula.* **bellows s.,** a double murmur (systolic and diastolic) resembling the sound made by a bellows. **Béniqué's s.,** a lead or tin

sound, having a wide curve, for dilating urethral strictures. **bottle s.,** amphoric rale. **cardiac s's,** heart s's. **coin s.,** bruit d'airain. **cracked-pot s.,** a percussion sound indicative of a pulmonary cavity into which the breath may pass. **cracked-pot s., cranial,** a peculiar sound due to the separation of the cranial sutures; seen in children with raised intracranial pressure. **ejection s's,** high-pitched clicking sounds occurring very shortly after the first heart sound, attributed to sudden distention of a dilated pulmonary artery or aorta or to forceful opening of the pulmonic or aortic cusps; most often heard in septal defects or patent ductus associated with high pulmonary resistance and hypertension. Called also *ejection clicks.* **entotic s's,** sounds that originate within the ear, such as tinnitus. **esophageal s.,** a long, flexible sound for exploring the esophagus. **first s.,** see *heart s's.* **flapping s.,** the peculiar sound made by the closure of the heart valves. **fourth s.,** see *gallop rhythm,* under *rhythm.* **friction s.,** any sound produced by the rubbing of one surface over another. **heart s's,** the sounds heard over the cardiac region, which are produced by the functioning of the heart. The *first,* occurring at the beginning of ventricular systole, is dull, firm, and prolonged, and is heard as a "lubb" sound; the *second,* produced essentially by closure of the semilunar valves, is shorter and sharper than the first, and is heard as a "dupp" sound; the *third,* produced by vibrations of the ventricular walls when they are suddenly distended by the rush of blood from the atria, is weak, low-pitched, and dull, and is usually audible only in children and young adults; and the *fourth,* produced by atrial contraction and ventricular filling, is low-pitched and short, and is rarely audible in the normal heart. Called also *cardiac s's.* **hippocratic s.,** the succussion sound heard in pyopneumothorax or seropneumothorax. **Korotkoff s's,** sounds heard during auscultatory determination of blood pressure, produced by sudden distention of the artery, the walls of which were previously relaxed because of the proximally placed pneumatic cuff. **lacrimal s.,** a sound of small caliber for use in the lacrimal canal. **metallic s.,** a sound having a metallic quality heard especially over cavities in the chest. **muscle s.,** the sound heard over a muscle when in a condition of contraction. **peacock s.,** a quality of voice due to various defects and lesions of the air passages. **percussion s.,** any sound obtained by percussion. **physiological s's,** sounds heard when the auditory canals are plugged, caused by the rush of blood through blood vessels in or near the inner ear and by adjacent muscles in continuous low frequency vibration. **pistol-shot s.,** a sharp sound accompanying each pulsation heard with the stethoscope pressed over the femoral artery in aortic insufficiency. **respiratory s.,** any sound heard on auscultation over any portion of the respiratory tract. **second s.,** see *heart s's.* **second s., pulmonic,** the audible vibrations related to the closure of the pulmonary semilunar valve; abbreviated P_2. **shaking s.,** succussion s. **subjective s.,** 1. phonism. 2. the sound sometimes produced by the blood current in the examiner's ears during auscultation. **succussion s's,** splashing sounds heard on succussion over a distended stomach and in hydropneumothorax. **third s.,** see *heart s's.* **tick-tack s's,** heart sounds in which there is little or no difference in the quality of the first and second sounds. **to-and-fro s.,** a friction sound or murmur heard with both systole and diastole. **urethral s.,** a long, slim, slightly conical instrument of steel for exploring and dilating the urethra. **vesicular breath s's,** sounds heard on auscultation over the normal lung during respiration. **water-wheel s.,** bruit de moulin. **white s.,** that produced by a mixture of all frequencies of mechanical vibration perceptible as sound. **Winternitz's s.,** a double-current catheter. **xiphisternal crunching s.,** a peculiar sound, of unknown origin, frequently heard (20 per cent of healthy men) over the lower sternum and xiphoid process.

Souques's phenomenon, sign (soo'kez) [Alexandre Achille *Souques,* French neurologist, 1860–1944] see under *phenomenon* and *sign.*

Soxhlet's apparatus (soks'lets) [Franz Ritter von *Soxhlet,* German chemist, 1848–1926] see under *apparatus.*

soya (soi'ah) see *soy bean.*

soybean (soi'bēn) the bean of the leguminous plant, *Soja hispida* (*Glycine soja*) or Chinese bean. It contains little starch and is rich in protein. From it is prepared a meal which is used as a protein supplement. It also furnishes an enzyme, urease. See *urease.*

Soymida febrifuga (soi'mĭ-dah feb-rif'u-gah) a tree of southern Asia; the bark is bitter, astringent, and aromatic.

sp. abbreviation for L. *spir'itus,* spirit.

space (spās) 1. a delimited area. 2. an actual or potential cavity of the body; called also *spatium* [NA]. 3. the expanse of the universe beyond the earth and its atmosphere. **anatomical dead s.,** see *dead s.* **apical s.,** the region between the wall of the alveolus and the apex of the root of a tooth. **arachnoid s.,** see *cavum subarachnoideale* and *cavum subdurale.* **axillary s.,** axilla. **Blessig's s's,** see under *cyst.* **Bogros's s.,** a region bounded by the peritoneum above and the fascia transversalis below, in which the lower part of the external iliac artery can be found without cutting the peritoneum; called also *retroinguinal s.* **Bowman's s.,** capsular s. **bregmatic s.,** the anterior fontanel (fonticulus frontalis). **Burns' s.,** fossa jugularis, def. 1. **capsular s.,** a narrow chalice-shaped cavity between the glomerular and the capsular epithelium of the glomerular capsule of the kidney; called also *Bowman's space.* **cartilage s's,** the spaces in hyaline cartilage which contain the cartilage cells. **cathodal dark s.,** Crookes s. **cell s's,** the spaces in the ground substance of connective tissue enclosing the connective tissue corpuscles. **chyle s's,** the central lymphatic spaces of the villi of the intestine. **circumlental s.,** the space between the ciliary body and the equator of the lens. **Colles' s.,** a space under the perineal fascia containing the transversus perinei, ischiocavernosus, and bulbocavernosus muscles, the posterior scrotal or labial vessels and nerves, and the bulbous portion of the urethra. **complemental s.,** portions of the pleural cavity that are not occupied by lung tissue, such as the triangular spaces below the lower borders of the lungs and irregular spaces about the heart. **corneal s's,** the spaces between the lamellae of the substantia propria of the cornea which contain corneal cells and tissue fluid. **Cotunnius' s.,** the space within the membranous labyrinth. **Crookes s.,** a dark space at the cathode of a nearly exhausted roentgen-ray tube through which a current is being passed; called also *cathodal dark s.* **cupular s.,** pars cupularis recessus epitympanici. **Czermak's s's,** spatia interglobularia; see under *spatium.* **dead s.,** 1. space remaining after incomplete closure of surgical or other wounds, permitting the accumulation of blood or serum and resultant delay in healing. 2. in the respiratory tract: (*a*) *anatomical dead space,* those portions, from the nose and mouth to the terminal bronchioles, in which exchange of oxygen and carbon dioxide does not occur, and (*b*) *physiologic dead space,* which reflects nonuniformity of ventilation and perfusion in the lung, is the anatomical dead space plus the space in alveoli occupied by air that does not participate in oxygen–carbon dioxide exchange. **s's in dentin,** spatia interglobularia. **Disse's s's,** small spaces which separate the sinusoids of the liver from the liver cells and which carry the lymph of the liver. **Douglas' s.,** excavatio rectouterina. **epicerebral s.,** the potential space between the brain and the pia mater. **epidural s.,** cavum epidurale. **episcleral s.,** spatium episclerale. **epispinal s.,** the potential space between the substance of the spinal cord and the pia mater. **epitympanic s.,** recessus epitympanicus. **escapement s's,** spaces which permit the escape of material being comminuted between the occlusal surfaces of the teeth, provided by the cusps and ridges, sulci and developmental ridges of the teeth, and the embrasures between the teeth. **Faraday's dark s.,** the dark region separating the negative glow from the positive column in a Crookes tube. **s's of Fontana,** spaces beneath the pectinate ligament of the iridocorneal angle, present throughout life in lower animals and up to six months of gestation in the human eye; thereafter smaller rudimentary spaces in the human eye serve to drain the aqueous humor from the anterior chamber into the canal of Schlemm. Called also *spatia anguli iridocornealis* [NA]. **free way s.,** interocclusal distance (clearance). **globular s's of Czermak,** spatia interglobularia. **H. s.,** Holzknecht's s. **haversian s.,** haversian canal (canalis nutricius ossis [NA]). **Henke's s.,** a space containing connective tissue between the spinal column and the pharynx and esophagus. **His' perivascular s.,** the space between the adventitia of the blood vessels of the brain and spinal cord and the perivascular limiting membrane of glia tissue. **Holzknecht's s.,** the middle one of the three clear lung fields in the roentgenogram of the chest in oblique projection when the rays pass from the left posteriorly to the right anteriorly; called also *H. s., prevertebral s.,* and *retrocardiac s.* **iliocostal s.,** the area between the twelfth rib and the crest of the ilium. **interarytenoid s.,** pars intercartilaginea rimae glottidis. **intercostal s.,** spatium intercostale. **intercristal s.,** 1. all of the area within the inner membrane of a mitochondrion. 2. the clefts between the inward extensions of the mitochondrial membrane space. **intercrural s.,** a triangular space between the crura cerebri. **interfascial s.,** spatium intervaginale. **interglobular s's (of Owen),** spatia interglobularia. **interlamellar s's,** the spaces between the lamellae of the cornea. **interocclusal rest s.,** interocclusal distance (clearance). **interosseous s's of metacarpus,** spatia interossea metacarpi. **interosseous s's of metatarsus,** spatia interossea metatarsi. **interpeduncular s.,** fossa interpeduncularis. **interpleural s.,** mediastinum, def. 2. **interproximal s., interproximate s.,** the space between the proximal surfaces of adjoining teeth; sometimes used to designate especially the space between the proximal surfaces of adjoining teeth that is gingival to the area of contact (*septal s.*). Cf. *embrasure.* **interradicular s.,** the space between roots; in dentistry, the entire extent of the space between the roots of a tooth, from apex to base. **interseptal s.,** a space between the two folds uniting to form the spurious septum in the heart of the early embryo. **intervaginal s.,** spatium episclerale. **intervaginal s's of optic nerve,** spatia intervaginalia nervi optici. **intervillous s.,** the cavernous space of the placenta into which project the chorionic villi and through which maternal blood circulates. **s's of iridocorneal angle,** spatia anguli iridocornealis. **Kiernan's s's,** the triangular spaces bounded by invaginated Glisson's capsule between the liver lobules, containing the larger interlobular branches of the portal vein, hepatic artery, and hepatic duct. **Kiesselbach's s.,** see under *area.* **Kretschmann's s.,** a depressed area in the recessus epitympanicus, below Prussak's space. **Larrey's s's,** intervals between those parts of the diaphragm which are attached to the ribs and that which is attached to the sternum. **leeway s.,** see *Nance's leeway s.* **Lesgaft's s.,** a rhombus which in some persons exists between the external oblique muscle in front, the latissimus dorsi behind, the serratus posticus above, and the internal oblique below; frequently the site of pointing of an abscess, or occurrence of a hernia. Called also *Lesgaft's triangle* and *Grynfelt's triangle.* **lymph s.,** any space in tissue occupied by lymph. **Magendie's s's,** subarachnoid spaces between the pia and arachnoid, corresponding to the principal sulci of the brain. **Malacarne's s.,** substantia perforata posterior. **Marie's quadrilateral s.,** see *quadrilateral s. of Marie.* **marrow s.,** cavum medullare ossium. **Meckel's s.,** cavum trigeminale. **mediastinal s.,** mediastinum, def. 2. **medullary s.,** the central cavity and the intervals between the trabeculae of bone which contain the marrow. **midpalmar s.,** the palmar space lying between the middle metacarpal bone and the radial side of the hypothenar eminence. **mitochondrial membrane s.,** a narrow space between the inner and outer membranes of a mitochondrion, including its inward projections between the cristae. **Mohrenheim's s.,** a groove on the deltoid muscle for the cephalic vein and a branch of the acromiothoracic artery. **Nance's leeway s.,** the amount by which the space occupied by the deciduous canine and first and second deciduous molars exceeds that occupied by the canine and premolar teeth of the permanent dentition, usually averaging 1.7 mm. on each side of the dental arch. **Nuel's s's,** fluid-filled spaces in the organ of Corti between the outer hair cells, communicating with the inner tunnel through the spaces between the pillar cells. Called also *outer tunnel.* **Obersteiner-Redlich s.,** see under *area.* **palmar s.,** a large fascial space in the hand, divided by a fibrous septum into the midpalmar space and the thenar space. **parapharyngeal s.,** pharyngomaxillary s. **parasinoidal s's,** lateral lacunae in the dura mater, along the superior sagittal sinus, which receive meningeal and diploic veins. **Parona's s.,** a space between the pronator quadratus muscle and the deep flexor tendons in the forearm, about 5 cm. above the wrist, in direct continuity with the tendon sheaths and the midpalmar space. **perforated s., anterior,** substantia perforata anterior. **perforated s., posterior,** substantia perforata posterior. **periaxial s.,** a fluid-filled cavity surrounding the nuclear bag and myotubule regions of a muscle spindle. **perichorioidal s., perichoroidal s.,** spatium perichoroideale. **perilymphatic s.,** spatium perilymphaticum. **perineal s., deep,** spatium perinei profundum. **perineal s., superficial,** spatium perinei superficiale. **perineuronal s.,** the extracellular compartment surrounding nerve cells of the central nervous system; its histologic appearance as a space is an artefact. **perinuclear s.,** see under *cisterna.* **peripharyngeal s.,** retropharyngeal s. **periplasmic s.,** a zone between the plasma membrane and the outer membrane of the cell wall of gram-negative bacteria. **perisinusoidal s's,** Disse's s's. **perivascular s.,** a lymph space occurring within the walls of an artery. **perivitelline s.,** a space between the ovum and the zona pellucida; in the ovum of some animals, a fluid-filled space separating the fertilization membrane from the surface of the egg. **pharyngomaxillary s.,** the space included between the lateral wall of the pharynx, the internal pterygoid muscle, and the cervical vertebrae. **phrenocostal s.,** the space between the outer edge of the diaphragm and the costal surface. **physiologic dead s.,** see *dead s.* **pneumatic s.,** a portion of bone occupied by air-containing cells; applied especially to spaces in the bones of the head constituting the paranasal sinuses. **Poiseuille's s.,** that part of the lumen of a tube where no flow of liquid occurs, as next to the wall of a blood vessel, where the red cells are virtually motionless and constitute a layer over which the inner layers of liquid slide. **popliteal s.,** fossa poplitea. **postperforated s.,** substantia perforata posterior. **preperitoneal s.,** spatium retropubicum. **preputial s.,** the space between the prepuce and the glans penis. **prevertebral s.,** Holzknecht's s. **prevesical s.,** spatium retropubicum. **prezonular s.,** portion of the eyeball anterior to the zonula ciliaris, occupied by the aqueous humor. **proximal s., proximate s.,** interproximal s. **Prussak's s.,** recessus membranae tympani superior. **quadrilateral s. of Marie,** a space in the cerebral hemisphere bounded externally by the cortex, medially by the internal capsule, and anteriorly and posteriorly by the insula. **retrobulbar s.,** the space lying behind the fascia of the bulb of the eye, containing the eye muscles and the ocular vessels and nerves. **retrocardiac s.,** Holzknecht's s. **retroinguinal s.,** Bogros' s. **retromylohyoid s.,** the part of the alveololingual sulcus distal to the lingual tuberosity (the distal end of the mylohyoid ridge). **retro-ocular s.,** retrobulbar s. **retroperitoneal s.,** spatium retroperitoneale. **retropharyngeal s.,** the space behind the pharynx, containing areolar tissue. **retropubic s.,** Retzius' s. **Robin's s's,** minute lymph spaces in the external coat of an artery communicating with lymphatic vessels. **Schwalbe's s's,** spatia intervaginalia nervi optici. **semilunar s.,** see *Traube's semilunar s.* **septal s.,** that portion of the interproximal space gingival to the contact area of adjacent teeth in a dental arch. **subarachnoid s.,** cavum subarachnoideale. **subchorial s.,** see under *lake.* **subdural s.,** cavum subdurale. **subepicranial s.,** the potential space between the epicranius muscle and the pericranium; it is traversed by small arteries which supply the pericranium and by the emissary veins connecting the intracranial venous sinuses with the superficial veins of the scalp. **subgingival s.,** gingival crevice. **submaxillary s.,** trigonum submandibulare. **subphrenic s.,** the space between the diaphragm and subjacent organs. **subumbilical s.,** the somewhat triangular space within the body cavity just below the umbilicus. **suprasternal s.,** fossa jugularis, def. 1. **Tarin's s.,** recessus anterior fossae interpeduncularis [Tarini]. **Tenon's s.,** spatium episclerale. **thenar s.,** the palmar space lying between the middle metacarpal bone and the tendon of the flexor pollicis longus. **thiocyanate s.,** a quantitative expression of the space occupied by the extracellular fluid in the body, computed after intravenous injection of sodium thiocyanate. **thyrohyal s.,** the depressed space between the thyroid cartilage and hyoid bone in front. **Traube's semilunar s.,** an area on the left side and front of the lower part of the chest, over which the air in the stomach produces a vesiculotympanitic sound. **Tröltsch's s's,** see *recessus membranae tympani anterior* and *recessus membranae tympani posterior.* **urogenital s.,** rima pudendi. **Virchow-Robin s's,** potential spaces surrounding blood vessels for a short distance as they enter the brain, the inner wall being formed by a prolongation of a membrane like the arachnoid, and the outer wall by a continuation of the pia; the intervening channel communicates with the subarachnoid space. **Westberg's s.,** the space between the pericardium and the beginning of the aorta. **yolk s.,** the space formed by retraction of the vitellus of the ovum from the zona pellucida. **Zang's s.,** fossa supraclavicularis minor. **zonular s's,** spatia zonularia.

spadic (spa'dik) the native name in western South America for the leaves of the coca plant, used for chewing.

spagyric (spah-jir'ik) [Gr. *span* to draw + *ageirein* to bring together] pertaining to the obsolete paracelsian system of medicine.

spagyrist (spaj'ĭ-rist) a follower of the paracelsian system of medicine.

Spallanzani's law (spal"an-zan'ēz) [Lazaro *Spallanzani,* eminent Italian anatomist, 1729–1799] see under *law.*

spallation (spawl-la'shun) splintering; the process of breaking into small bits; see *spallation products,* under *product.*

span (span) 1. a measurement of reach or extent. 2. the distance in a fully extended hand between the tips of the thumb and little finger.

Spaniopsis (span"ĭ-op'sis) a genus of blood-sucking flies of the family Rhagionidae found in Australia.

Spanish windlass (span'ish wind'las) see *windlass.*

spano- (span'o) [Gr. *spanos* scarce] a combining form meaning scanty or scarce.

spanopnea (span"op-ne'ah) [*spano-* + Gr. *pnoia* breath] a nervous affection, with slow, deep breathing and a subjective feeling of dyspnea.

spar (spar) a nonmetallic, rather lustrous mineral. **Iceland s.,** a crystalline form of calcium carbonate, usually found in Iceland, and used in making Nicol prisms.

sparganosis (spar"gah-no'sis) infection with the migrating larvae (spargana) of any of several species of pseudophyllidean tapeworms, which invade the subcutaneous tissues, causing inflammation and fibrosis suggestive of cellulitis.

sparganum (spar-ga'num), pl. *sparga'na* [Gr. *sparganon* swaddling clothes] the larval stage (plerocercoid) of various pseudophyllidean cestodes, especially in the genera *Diphyllobothrium* and *Spirometra,* which may migrate in the subcutaneous tissues of man and other animals (see *sparganosis*). Also, a genus name applied to such larvae, usually when the adult stage is not known.

Sparine (spar'ēn) trademark for preparations of promazine hydrochloride.

spark (spark) a flash of light attended with a crackling sound, made by a discharge of electricity. **direct s.,** an electric spark which passes through the body from electrodes without the use of a Leyden jar.

sparteine (spar'te-in) [L. *spartium* broom] chemical name: dodecahydro-7,14-methano-2H,6H-dipyrido[1,2-*a*:1',2'-*e*][1,5]diazocine. An alkaloid $C_{15}H_{26}N_2$, obtained from the legumes *Cystius scoparius* (L.) Link. (broom), *Lupinus luteus* L. (yellow lupin bean), *L. niger* Hort. (black lupin bean), and *Anagyris foetida* L. (Mediterranean stinkbush). It is poisonous, and acts like digitalis. **s. sulfate,** the pentahydrate sulfate salt of sparteine, $C_{15}H_{26}N_2 \cdot H_2SO_4 \cdot 5H_2$, used as an oxytocic for the induction of labor and stimulation of hypotonic or subnormal uterine contractions. Formerly used as a substitute for digitalis.

spartium (spar'she-um) [Gr. *sparton*] scoparius.

spasm (spazm) [L. *spasmus;* Gr. *spasmos*] 1. a sudden, violent, involuntary contraction of a muscle or a group of muscles, attended by pain and interference with function, producing involuntary movement and distortion. 2. a sudden but transitory constriction of a passage, canal, or orifice. **s. of accommodation,** spasm of the ciliary muscles, producing excess of accommodation for near objects. **athetoid s.,** a spasm in which the affected member makes movements like those of athetosis. **Bell's s.,** convulsive tic. **bronchial s.,** spasmodic contraction of the muscular coat of the bronchial tubes, such as occurs in asthma. **cadaveric s.,** rigor mortis causing movements of the limbs. **canine s.,** risus sardonicus. **carpopedal s.,** spasm of the hand or foot, or of the thumbs and great toes, seen in tetany. **cerebral s.,** spasm due to a cerebral lesion. **clonic s.,** a spasm in which rigidity of the muscles is followed immediately by relaxation. **cynic s.,** risus sardonicus. **dancing s.,** saltatory s. **diffuse esophageal s.,** strong, incoordinated, nonpropulsive contractions of the esophagus evoked by deglutition, especially in the elderly; on barium radiography, the esophageal lumen appears as an irregular series of concentric narrowings, or a spiral coil (curling). Called also *esophageal dysrhythmia.* **esophageal s.,** diffuse esophageal s. **facial s.,** tonic spasm of the muscles supplied by the facial nerve, either involving the entire side of the face or confined to a limited region around the eye. **fixed s.,** permanent rigidity of a muscle or set of muscles. **functional s.,** occupation neurosis. **glottic s.,** laryngospasm. **habit s.,** tic. **handicraft s.,** occupation neurosis. **histrionic s.,** convulsion of the facial muscles analogous to writers' cramp. **infantile massive s's,** jackknife seizure. **inspiratory s.,** spasmodic contraction of the muscles of inspiration. **intention s.,** muscular spasm occurring on attempting voluntary movement. **lock s.,** a firm tonic spasm that seems to lock the fingers together, as in writers' cramp and in similar affections. **malleatory s.,** malleation. **massive s.,** a seizure characterized by contraction of most of the body musculature. **mixed s.,** a spasm in which there are both extensor and flexor movements. **mobile s.,** athetosis. **myopathic s.,** that which accompanies a disease of the muscles. **nictitating s.,** winking s. **nodding s.,** clonic spasm of the sternomastoid muscles, producing bowing motions; called also *salaam convulsions.* **occupation s.,** occupation neurosis. **perineal s.,** perineal vaginismus. **phonatory s.,** spasm of the tensors of the vocal bands. **professional s.,** occupation neurosis. **progressive torsion s.,** dystonia musculorum deformans. **respiratory s.,** spasm of the muscles of respiration. **retrocollic s.,** spasmodic retroflexion of the head. **Romberg's s.,** masticatory spasm of the muscles supplied by the fifth nerve. **rotatory s.,** intermittent spasm of the splenius muscle causing rotation of the head. **salaam s.,** nodding s. **saltatory s.,** clonic spasm of the muscles of the legs, producing a peculiar jumping or springing motion whenever the patient stands. Called also *Bamberger's disease, palmus,* and *saltatory tic.* **synclonic s.,** clonic spasm of more than one muscle. **tetanic s.,** 1. the muscular spasm occurring in tetanus. 2. tonic spasm. **tonic s.,** spasm in which rigidity persists for a considerable time. **tonoclonic s.,** a convulsive twitching of the muscles. **torsion s.,** spasm marked by a twisting or turning of the body, especially of the pelvis, as in dystonia musculorum deformans. **toxic s.,** that which is due to a poison. **winking s.,** spasmodic twitching of the orbicularis palpebrarum muscle and of the eyelid. **writers' s.,** writers' cramp.

spasmo- (spaz'mo) [L. *spasmus;* Gr. *spasmos*] a combining form denoting relationship to a spasm.

spasmodic (spaz-mod'ik) [Gr. *spasmōdēs*] of the nature of a spasm.

spasmogen (spaz'mo-jen) [*spasmo-* + Gr. *gennan* to produce] a substance that produces or causes spasms.

spasmogenic (spaz"mo-jen'ik) relating to the production of or causing spasms.

spasmology (spaz-mol'o-je) [*spasmo-* + *-logy*] the sum of what is known regarding spasms.

spasmolygmus (spaz"mo-lig'mus) [*spasmo-* + Gr. *lygmos* hiccup] hiccup.

spasmolysant (spaz-mol'ĭ-zant) 1. relieving or relaxing spasms. 2. an agent that relieves spasm.

spasmolysis (spaz-mol'ĭ-sis) the elimination or checking of spasm.

spasmolytic (spaz"mo-lit'ik) checking spasms; antispasmodic.

spasmophile (spaz'mo-fīl) spasmophilic.

spasmophilia (spaz"mo-fil'e-ah) [*spasmo-* + Gr. *philein* to love] spasmophilic diathesis; a condition in which the motor nerves show abnormal sensitiveness to mechanical or electric stimulation, and the patient shows a tendency to spasm, tetany, and convulsions.

spasmophilic (spaz"mo-fil'ik) marked by a tendency to spasms.

spasmotin (spaz'mo-tin) a poisonous ecbolic and acid principle, $C_{20}H_{21}O_9$, from ergot, which has oxytocic but not hallucinogenic properties.

spasmus (spaz′mus) [L.] spasm. **s. nu′tans**, nodding spasm.

spastic (spas′tik) [Gr. *spastikos*] 1. of the nature of or characterized by spasms. 2. hypertonic, so that the muscles are stiff and the movements awkward; see *cerebral palsy*, under *palsy*. 3. a person exhibiting spasticity, such as occurs in spastic paralysis or in cerebral palsy.

spasticity (spas-tis′ĭ-te) a state of hypertonicity, or increase over the normal tone of a muscle, with heightened deep tendon reflexes. **clasp-knife s.**, the phenomenon occurring when a hypertonic muscle is passively stretched: after initial increased resistance there is a sudden relaxation.

spatia (spa′she-ah) [L.] plural of *spatium*.

spatial (spa′shal) pertaining to space.

spatic (spa′tik) pertaining to a space, especially an interproximal space.

spatium (spa′she-um), pl. *spa′tia* [L.] a space or delimited area; [NA] a general term for an actual or potential open region. **spa′tia an′guli i′ridis [Fonta′nae], spa′tia an′guli iridocornea′lis** [NA], spaces of the iridocorneal angle: the spaces between the fibers of the pectinate ligament through which communication is effected between the anterior chamber and the canal of Schlemm. See also *Fontana's spaces*, under *space*. **s. episclera′le** [NA], episcleral space: the space between the bulbar fascia and the eyeball; called also *s. intervaginale, s. interfasciale [Tenoni], intervaginal space*, and *Tenon's space*. **s. intercosta′le** [NA], intercostal space: the space intervening between two adjacent ribs. **spa′tia intercosta′lia**, see *spatium intercostale*. **s. interfascia′le [Teno′ni]**, s. episclerale. **spa′tia interglobula′ria** [NA], interglobular spaces: numerous small irregular spaces in the deeper parts of the dentin of the crown of a tooth, representing areas of incompletely calcified dentin. Called also *interglobular spaces of Owen* and *interglobular dentin*. **spa′tia interos′sea metacar′pi** [NA], interosseous spaces of the metacarpus: the four spaces between the metacarpal bones. **spa′tia interos′sea metatar′si** [NA], interosseous spaces of metatarsus: the four spaces between the metatarsal bones. **s. intervagina′le**, former NA term for s. episclerale. **spa′tia intervagina′lia ner′vi op′tici** [NA], intervaginal spaces of optic nerve: the subdural and subarachnoid spaces between the internal and external sheaths of the optic nerve; called also *Schwalbe's spaces*. **s. perichorioidea′le, s. perichoroidea′le** [NA], perichoroidal space: any of the spaces between the laminae of the nonvascular layer of the choroid nearest the sclera. **s. perilymphat′icum** [NA], perilymphatic space: the fluid-filled space separating the membranous from the osseous labyrinth; called also *Retzius space*. **s. perine′i profun′dum** [NA], deep perineal space: the area between the superior and inferior fascia of the urogenital diaphragm. **s. perine′i superficia′le** [NA], superficial perineal space: the region between the inferior fascia of the urogenital diaphragm and the membranous layer of the superficial perineal fascia; it contains the root of the penis and associated muscles. **s. retroperitonea′le** [NA], retroperitoneal space: the space between the posterior parietal peritoneum and the posterior abdominal wall, containing the kidneys, suprarenal glands, ureters, duodenum, ascending and descending colon, pancreas, and the large vessels and nerves. **s. retropu′bicum** [NA], retropubic space: the extraperitoneal space between the inferior aspect of the apex of the bladder, and the transversalis fascia and the posterosuperior aspect of the pubic symphysis, extending along the sides of the bladder to the lateral ligaments and limited below by the puboprostatic ligaments. **spa′tia zonula′ria** [NA], zonular spaces: the lymph-filled interstices between the fibers of the zonula ciliaris, communicating with the posterior chamber of the eye; called also *Petit's canal*.

spatula (spach′u-lah) [L.] a flat, blunt, usually flexible instrument, used for spreading plasters or for mixing ointments and masses; a spatulate structure. **s. mal′lei**, the flat end of the handle of the malleus, attached to the membrana tympani.

spatular (spach′u-lar) spatulate.

spatulate (spach′u-lāt) 1. having a flat blunt end. 2. to mix or manipulate with a spatula.

spatulation (spach″u-la′shun) the mixing of combined materials to a homogeneous mass by repeatedly scraping them up and smoothing out the mass on a flat surface with a spatula.

spavin (spav′in) in general, an exostosis, usually medial, of the tarsus of equines, distal to the tibiotarsal articulation and often involving the metatarsals. **blood s.**, a dilatation of either or both of the medial metatarsal or of the saphenous veins, forming a soft enlargement on the dorsomedial surface of the tarsus in equines. **bog s.**, a distention of the synovial capsule of the tibiotarsal joint in equines. **bone s.**, osteoperiostitis or arthritis of the intertarsal or tarsometatarsal articulations in equines, commonly followed by exostosis and ankylosis. Classified as visible, occult, anterior, posterior and high. **Jack s.**, a very large exostotic spavin.

spavined (spav′ind) affected with spavin.

spay (spa) to castrate a female animal, usually by oophorohysterectomy.

SPCA serum prothrombin conversion accelerator (blood coagulation factor VII).

spearmint (spēr′mint) [NF] the dried leaf and flowering top of *Mentha spicata* (*M. viridis*), common spearmint, or of *Mentha caridiaca*, Scotch spearmint; used as a flavoring agent.

specialism (spesh′al-izm) limitation of practice or study to a particular branch of medicine or surgery.

specialist (spesh′al-ist) a physician whose practice is limited to a particular branch of medicine or surgery, especially one who, by virtue of advanced training, is certified by a specialty board as being qualified to so limit his practice. **clinical nurse s., nurse s.**, see under *nurse*.

specialization (spesh″al-i-za′shun) in medicine, medical practice limited to some special department of medicine or surgery.

specialty (spesh′al-te) the field of practice of a specialist.

speciation (spe″se-a′shun) the evolutionary formation of new species, or the process of such formation.

species (spe′shēz, spe′sēz) [L.] 1. a taxonomic category subordinate to a genus (or subgenus), and superior to a subspecies or variety, composed of individuals possessing common characters distinguishing them from other categories of individuals of the same taxonomic level. In taxonomic nomenclature, species are designated by the genus name followed by a Latin or latinized adjective or noun. 2. (*obs.*) a mixture of dried herbs, seeds, or barks, used chiefly as a decoction. **diovulatory s.**, a species of animal, the females of which ordinarily discharge two ova in one ovulatory cycle. **monovulatory s.**, a species of animal, the females of which usually discharge only one ovum in any one ovulatory cycle. **polyovulatory s.**, a species of animal, the females of which normally discharge several (3–16) ova at each ovulatory cycle. **type s.**, the original species from which a description of the genus of organisms is made.

species-specific (spe′sēz-spĕ-sif′ik) characteristic of a particular species; having a characteristic effect on, or interaction with, cells or tissues of members of a particular species; said of an antigen, drug, or infective agent.

specific (spĕ-sif′ik) [L. *specificus*] 1. pertaining to a species. 2. produced by a single kind of microorganism. 3. restricted in application, effect, etc., to a particular structure, function, etc. 4. a remedy specially indicated for any particular disease. 5. in immunology, pertaining to the special affinity of antigen for the corresponding antibody.

specificity (spes″ĭ-fis′ĭ-te) the quality or state of being specific. **neuronal s.**, the invariance of the locations, trajectories, and spatial arrangement of neurons in all members of the same species. **organ s.**, the state of being organ-specific. **species s.**, the state of being species-specific.

specificness (spe-sif′ik-nes) specificity.

specimen (spes′ĭ-men) 1. a sample or part of a thing, or of several things, taken to show or to determine the character of the whole, as a specimen of urine. 2. a preparation of tissue for pathological examination or of a normal tissue, organ, or organism for study of its structure. **corrosion s.**, a preparation of an organ, such as the liver, by injection of certain of its structures, as the arteries and veins, and chemical digestion of surrounding substance.

spectacles (spek′tah-k′lz) [L. *spectacula; spectare* to see] a pair of lenses in a frame to assist vision; see also *glasses* and *lens*. **compound s.**, spectacles fitted with extra colored glasses, or extra lenses, to be used as occasion requires. **decentered s.**, spectacles with lenses formed from eccentric portions of two convex lenses. **divided s.**, bifocal glasses. **Masselon's s.**, spectacles with an attachment for keeping the upper lid raised in cases of paralytic ptosis. **mica s.**, spectacles of sheet mica used to protect the eye from foreign bodies. **pantoscopic s.**, bifocal glasses. **periscopic s.**, spectacles with either menisci or concavoconvex lenses, with the concave surfaces toward the eyes; they allow the eyes considerable latitude of motion. **prismatic s.**, spectacles with prismatic lenses for correcting muscular defects. **pulpit s.**, spectacles containing the lenses in the lower segments of the glasses only. **stenopeic s.**, spectacles fitted with metal plates, having each a small central aperture. **tinted s.**, spectacles of a glass so colored as to protect the eyes from the effects of too bright light. **wire frame s.**, a kind of spectacles of wire gauze worn to protect the eye from the entrance of foreign bodies.

spectinomycin (spek″tĭ-no-mi′sin) chemical name: decahydro-4α,7,9-trihydroxy-2-methyl-6,8-bis(methylamino)-4*H*-pyrano[2,3-*b*][1,4]-benzodioxin-4-one. An antibiotic, $C_{14}H_{24}N_2O_7$, derived from *Streptomyces spectabilis*, that has moderate antibacterial activity against many gram-positive and gram-negative organisms, but is especially effective against *Neisseria gonorrhoeae*. It is also used in veterinary medicine in bacterial enteritis and coccidiosis of dogs. **s. hydrochloride**, the pentahydrate dehydrochloride salt of spectinomycin, $C_{14}H_{24}N_2O_7 \cdot 2HCl \cdot 5H_2O$, having the same actions as the base. A preparation suitable for intramuscular administration [USP] is used in the treatment of acute gonorrheal urethritis and proctitis in the male and acute gonorrheal cervicitis and proctitis in the female when due to susceptible strains of *Neisseria gonorrhoeae*.

spectra (spek′trah) plural of *spectrum.*

spectral (spek′tral) pertaining to a spectrum; performed by means of a spectrum.

spectrin (spek′trin) a contractile protein attached to glycophorin at the cytoplasmic surface of the cell membrane of erythrocytes, considered to be important in the determination of red-cell shape.

spectrochrome (spek′tro-krōm) [L. *spectrum* + Gr. *chrōma* color] a term applied to a method of treatment consisting of exposure of the part to be treated to light of various colors.

spectrocolorimeter (spek″tro-kul″or-im′ĕ-ter) an ophthalmospectroscope used in detecting color blindness for one color.

spectrofluorometer (spek″tro-floo″or-om′ĕ-ter) an optical instrument for analysis of fluorescence spectra.

spectrograph (spek′tro-graf) an instrument for photographing spectra on a sensitive photographic plate. **mass s.,** mass spectrometer.

spectrometer (spek-trom′ĕ-ter) 1. an instrument for measuring the index of refraction by measuring the external angle of a prism of the substance. 2. a spectroscope for measuring the wavelengths of rays of a spectrum. **mass s.,** an analytical instrument which identifies a substance by sorting a stream of electrified particles (ions) according to their mass; the sorting is most commonly done as follows: when the stream of charged particles enters a magnetic field, it is deflected into a semicircular path, ultimately striking a photographic plate or photomultiplier tube sensor. Called also *mass spectrograph.* **Mossbauer s.,** an instrument that detects small changes in interaction between an atomic nucleus and its environment caused by changes in temperature, pressure, and chemical state; used in chemical-physical research with applications in medicine.

spectrometry (spek-trom′ĕ-tre) [L. *spectrum* image + *metrum* measure] the determination of the places of the lines in a spectrum.

spectrophotofluorometer (spek″tro-fo″to-floo″or-om′ĕ-ter) an analytical instrument combining the techniques of spectrophotometry and fluorescence analysis.

spectrophotometer (spek″tro-fo-tom′ĕ-ter) [*spectrum* + *photometer*] 1. an apparatus for measuring the light sense by means of a spectrum. 2. an apparatus for estimating the quantity of coloring matter in solution by the quantity of light absorbed (as indicated by the spectrum) in passing through the solution. **absorption s.,** an analytical instrument for comparing the absorption of radiation of a given wavelength against a standard to identify a sample material.

spectrophotometry (spek″tro-fo-tom′ĕ-tre) the use of the spectrophotometer.

spectropolarimeter (spek″tro-po″lar-im′ĕ-ter) a combined spectroscope and polariscope for determining optical rotation.

spectropyrheliometer (spek″tro-pir-he″le-om′ĕ-ter) [*spectrum* + Gr. *pyr* fire + *hēlios* sun + *metrum* measure] an instrument for measuring the radiation from the sun.

spectroscope (spek′tro-skōp) [*spectrum* + Gr. *skopein* to examine] an instrument for developing and analyzing spectra.

spectroscopic (spek″tro-skop′ik) of, pertaining to, or performed by, the spectroscope.

spectroscopy (spek-tros′ko-pe) the propagation and analysis of spectra; examination by means of a spectroscope.

spectrum (spek′trum), pl. *spec′tra* [L. "apparition"] a charted band of wavelengths of electromagnetic vibrations obtained by refraction and diffraction. See *invisible s.* and *visible s.* By extension, a measurable range of activity, such as the range of bacteria affected by an antibiotic (antibacterial s.) or the complete range of manifestations of a disease. **absorption s.,** the spectrum afforded by light which has passed through various gaseous media, each gas absorbing those rays of which its own spectrum is composed. **action s.,** the range of wavelength of incident light producing a response in the material under study (e.g., the inactivation of an enzyme); also, a graph plotting the magnitude of the response as a function of the wavelength of the incident light. **broad-s.,** effective against a wide range of microorganisms; said of an antibiotic. **chemical s.,** that part of the spectrum which includes the ultraviolet or actinic rays. **chromatic s.,** that portion of the range of wavelengths of electromagnetic vibrations (from 7700 to 3900 A.U.) which gives rise to the sensation of color (red to violet) to the normally perceptive eye; coincident with the visible spectrum. **color s.,** chromatic s. **continuous s.,** one in which Fraunhofer's lines are not developed. **diffraction s.,** a spectrum formed by the passage of light through a diffraction grating. **electromagnetic s.,** the continuous range of electromagnetic energy from cosmic rays to electric waves, including gamma, x-, and ultraviolet rays, visible light, infrared waves, and radio waves. **fortification s.,** teichopsia. **gaseous s.,** one which is afforded by an incandescent gas. **invisible s.,** that made up of vibrations of wavelengths less than 3900 A.U. (ultraviolet, grenz rays, x-rays, and gamma rays) and between 7700 and 120,000 A.U. (infrared). **ocular s.,** after-image. **prismatic s.,** one produced by the passage of light through a prism. **solar s.,** that portion of the

range of wavelengths of electromagnetic vibrations emanating from the sun, including the visible (chromatic, or color) spectrum and small portions of the infrared and ultraviolet radiations at either extreme. **thermal s.,** that portion of the range of wavelengths of electromagnetic vibrations (> 7700 A.U.) containing the infrared or heat rays. **toxin s.,** a diagrammatic representation of the neutralizing power of an antitoxin. **visible s.,** that portion of the range of wavelengths of electromagnetic vibrations (from 7700 to 3900 A.U.) which is capable of stimulating specialized sense organs and is perceptible as light. **x-ray s.,** the spectrum of a heterogeneous beam of roentgen rays produced by a suitable grating, generally a crystal.

speculum (spek′u-lum), pl. *spec′ula* [L. "mirror"] 1. an instrument for exposing the interior of a passage or cavity of the body. 2. the septum pellucidum. **Bozeman's s.,** a bivalve speculum the blades of which remain parallel when separated. **Brinkerhoff's s.,** a rectal speculum consisting of a conical tube having a closed extremity, but provided with a sliding bar on the side which provides an opening. **Cook's s.,** a three-pronged rectal speculum. **duck-billed s.,** a form of two-valved vaginal speculum. **eye s.,** an appliance for keeping the eyelids apart. **Fergusson's s.,** a cylindrical vaginal speculum made of silvered glass. **Fränkel's s.,** a form of nasal speculum. **Gruber's s.,** a form of ear speculum. **Hartmann's s.,** a form of nasal speculum. **s. Helmon′tii,** centrum tendineum. **Kelly's s.,** a rectal speculum tubular in shape and fitted with an obturator; called also *Kelly's sphincteroscope.* **Martin's s., Martin and Davy s.,** a rectal speculum consisting of a conical cylinder with an obturator. **Mathews′ s.,** a four-pronged rectal speculum. **Politzer's s.,** a form of ear speculum. **Sims′ s.,** a double duck-billed vaginal speculum. **stop s.,** an eye speculum with an appliance for controlling the degree to which its branches spread. **wire bivalve s.,** a two-valved vaginal speculum made of heavy wire.

Spee's curve (spāz) [Ferdinand Graf von *Spee,* German embryologist, born 1855] see under *curve.*

speech (spēch) the utterance of vocal sounds conveying ideas. **clipped s.,** speech in which the words are slurred over and uncompleted; sometimes one of the features of dementia paralytica. **echo s.,** echolalia. **esophageal s.,** speech produced by vibration of the column of air in the esophagus against the contracting cricopharyngeal sphincter, after laryngectomy. **explosive s.,** loud, sudden enunciation, seen in certain brain diseases. **incoherent s.,** speech in which the consecutive ideas expressed are not related; due to disturbance of the train of thought. **jumbled s.,** anarthria. **mirror s.,** a speech abnormality in which the order of syllables in a sentence is reversed. **plateau s.,** speech which is characterized by a level, monotonous, unvaried pitch. **pressured s.,** a rapid, accelerated, frenzied speech, which may exceed the ability of the vocal musculature to articulate or may be incoherent to the listener. **scamping s.,** clipped s. **scanning s.,** speech in which the syllables are separated by pauses. **slurred s.,** clipped s. **staccato s.,** speech in which each syllable is uttered separately; seen in multiple sclerosis.

Spemann's induction [Hans *Spemann,* German zoologist, 1869–1941; noted for his researches on embryonic development, and winner of the Nobel prize for medicine and physiology in 1935] see under *induction.*

Spencer-Parker vaccine (spen′ser-par′ker) [Roscoe Roy *Spencer,* American physician, born 1888; Ralph Robinson *Parker,* American zoologist, 1888–1949] see under *vaccine.*

Spencer Wells facies see *Wells.*

Spengler's fragments, immune body, tuberculin (speng′lerz) [Carl *Spengler,* Swiss physician, 1860–1937] see under *fragment, body,* and *tuberculin.*

Spens' syndrome (spenz) [Thomas *Spens,* Scottish physician, 1764–1842] Adams-Stokes disease.

sperm (sperm) [Gr. *sperma* seed] 1. the semen or testicular secretion. 2. one of the mature germ cells of a male animal; see *spermatozoon.* **muzzled s.,** spermatozoa which are unable to adhere to the ovum.

sperma (sper′mah) semen.

spermaceti (sper″mah-set′e) [Gr. *sperma* seed + *kētos* whale] a waxy substance obtained from the head of the sperm whale, *Physeter macrocephalus,* occurring as white, somewhat translucent, slightly unctuous masses, having a crystalline fracture and a pearly luster; used in the preparation of ointment bases, such as cold cream and rose water ointment. **synthetic s.,** cetyl esters wax.

spermacrasia (sper″mah-kra′zhe-ah) [Gr. *sperma* seed + *akrasia* ill mixture] deficiency of spermatozoa in the semen.

spermagglutination (sperm″ah-gloo″tĭ-na′shun) the agglutination of spermatozoa.

spermalist (sper′mah-list) spermist.

spermase (sper′mās) an oxidizing enzyme found in barley.

spermateliosis (sper″mah-te″le-o′sis) spermiogenesis.

spermatemphraxis (sper″mat-em-frak′sis) [Gr. *sperma* seed + *emphraxis* stoppage] obstruction to the discharge of semen.

spermatic (sper-mat′ik) [L. *spermaticus;* Gr. *spermatikos*] pertaining to the semen; seminal.

spermaticide (sper-mat′ĭ-sīd) spermicide.

spermatid (sper′mah-tid) a cell derived from a secondary spermatocyte by fission, and developing into a spermatozoon; called also *spermatoblast.*

spermatin (sper′mah-tin) an albuminoid substance derived from the semen; it is related to mucin and to nucleoalbumin.

spermatism (sper′mah-tizm) [Gr. *spermatismos*] the production or discharge of semen.

spermatitis (sper′mah-ti′tis) inflammation of a vas deferens; deferentitis or funiculitis.

spermato-, spermo- (sper′mah-to, sper′mo) [Gr. *sperma, spermatos* seed] combining form denoting relationship to seed, specifically to the male generative element.

spermatoblast (sper′mah-to-blast″) [*spermato-* + Gr. *blastos* germ] a term originally applied to the supporting cells of Sertoli, but now used with the same meaning as *spermatid.*

spermatocele (sper′mah-to-sēl″) [*spermato-* + Gr. *kēlē* tumor] a cystic distention of the epididymis or the rete testis containing spermatozoa.

spermatocelectomy (sper-mat″o-sě-lek′to-me) [*spermatocele* + Gr. *ektomē* excision] operative excision of a lesion of the epididymis (spermatocele).

spermatocidal (sper″mah-to-si′dal) spermicidal.

spermatocyst (sper′mah-to-sist″) [*spermato-* + Gr. *kystis* sac, bladder] 1. a seminal vesicle. 2. a spermatocele.

spermatocystectomy (sper″mah-to-sis-tek′to-me) [*spermatocyst* + Gr. *ektomē* excision] excision of the seminal vesicles.

spermatocystitis (sper″mah-to-sis-ti′tis) seminal vesiculitis.

spermatocystotomy (sper″mah-to-sis-tot′o-me) [*spermatocyst* + Gr. *tomē* a cutting] the operation of making an incision into the seminal vesicles for the purpose of drainage.

spermatocytal (sper″mah-to-si′tal) pertaining to a spermatocyte.

spermatocyte (sper′mah-to-sīt″) [*spermato-* + *-cyte*] the parent cell of a spermatid. **primary s.,** a cell derived from a spermatogonium and dividing into two secondary spermatocytes; called also *spermiocyte.* **secondary s.,** one of the two cells into which a primary spermatocyte divides, and which in turn gives origin to spermatids; called also *prespermatid.*

spermatocytogenesis (sper″mah-to-si″to-jen′ě-sis) the first stage of formation of spermatozoa in which the spermatogonia develop into spermatocytes and then into spermatids.

spermatocytoma (sper″mah-to-si-to′mah) seminoma.

spermatogenesis (sper″mah-to-jen′ě-sis) [*spermato-* + Gr. *genesis* production] the process of formation of spermatozoa, including spermatocytogenesis and spermiogenesis.

spermatogenic (sper″mah-to-jen′ik) [*spermato-* + Gr. *gennan* to produce] producing semen or spermatozoa.

spermatogenous (sper″mah-toj′ě-nus) spermatogenic.

spermatogeny (sper″mah-toj′ě-ne) spermatogenesis.

spermatogone (sper′mah-to-gōn″) spermatogonium.

spermatogonia (sper″mah-to-go′ne-ah) plural of *spermatogonium.*

spermatogonium (sper″mah-to-go′ne-um), pl. *spermatogo′nia* [*spermato-* + Gr. *gonē* generation] an undifferentiated germ cell of a male, originating in a seminiferous tubule and dividing into two primary spermatocytes; called also *spermatophore, spermatospore,* and *spermospore.*

spermatoid (sper′mah-toid) [*spermato-* + Gr. *eidos* form] resembling semen.

spermatology (sper″mah-tol′o-je) [*spermato-* + *-logy*] the sum of what is known regarding the semen.

spermatolysin (sper″mah-tol′ĭ-sin) a substance causing spermatolysis.

spermatolysis (sper″mah-tol′ĭ-sis) [*spermato-* + Gr. *lysis* dissolution] destruction or solution of spermatozoa.

spermatolytic (sper″mah-to-lit′ik) pertaining to, characterized by, or causing spermatolysis.

spermatomere (sper″mah-to-mēr″) spermatomerite.

spermatomerite (sper″mah-to-me′rīt) [*spermato-* + Gr. *meros* part] one of the chromosomes into which the sperm nucleus resolves during fertilization of the ovum.

spermatomicron (sper″mah-to-mi′kron) a minute particle found in the semen of various animals; seen best with a dark-field microscope, when they show brownian motion.

spermatopathia (sper″mah-to-path′e-ah) [*spermato-* + Gr. *pathos* affection] a morbid condition of the semen.

spermatopathy (sper″mah-top′ah-the) spermatopathia.

spermatophore (sper′mah-to-fōr″) [*spermato-* + Gr. *phorein* to carry] 1. a capsule, containing several spermatozoa, extruded by some of the lower animals. 2. spermatogonium.

spermatopoietic (sper″mah-to-poi-et′ik) [*spermato-* + Gr.

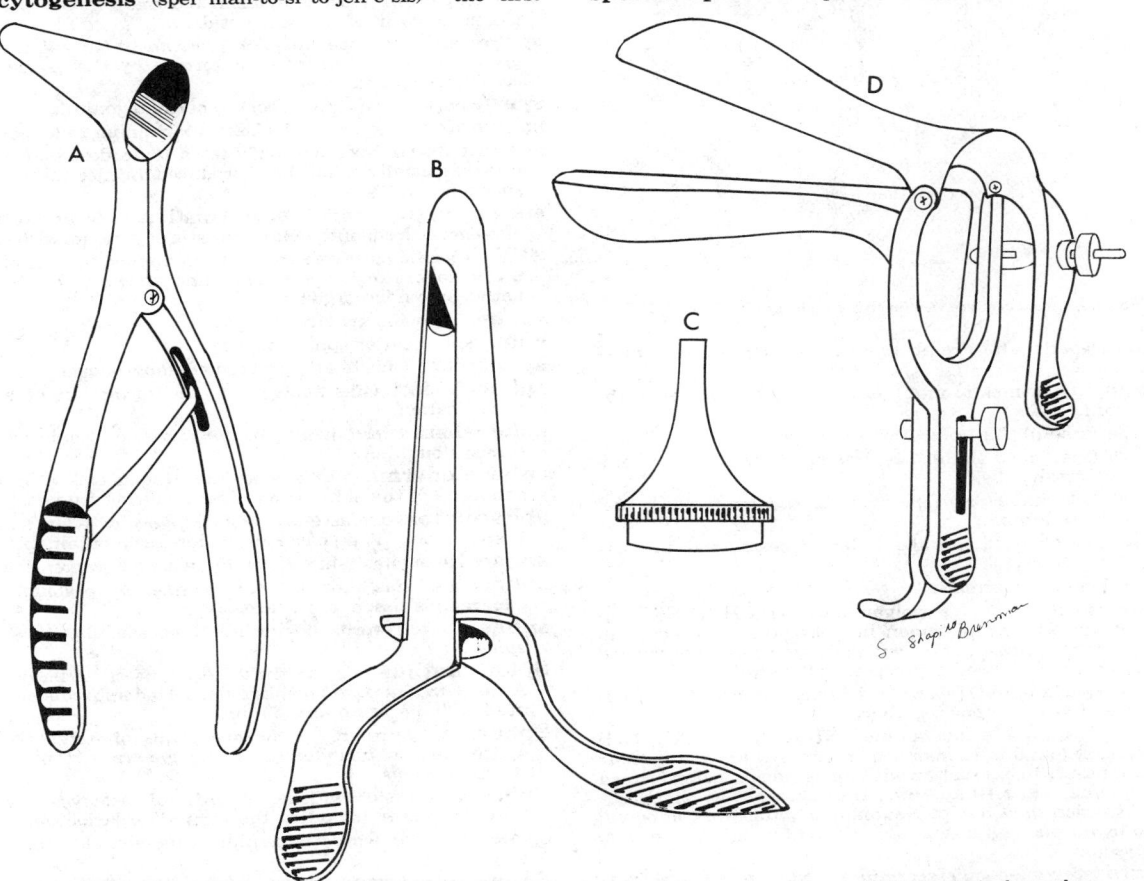

Specula: *A,* Vienna nasal speculum; *B,* Brinckerhoff rectal speculum; *C,* speculum for otoscope; *D,* Graves vaginal speculum.

poiētikos creative, productive] subserving or promoting the secretion of semen.

spermatorrhea (sper"mah-to-re'ah) [*spermato-* + Gr. *rhoia* flow] involuntary, too frequent, and excessive discharge of semen without copulation.

spermatoschesis (sper"mah-tos'kĕ-sis) [*spermato-* + Gr. *schesis* check] suppression of the secretion of semen.

spermatosome (sper-mat'o-sōm) spermatozoon.

spermatospore (sper-mat'o-spōr) [*spermato-* + Gr. *sporos* spore] a spermatogonium.

spermatotoxin (sper"mah-to-tok'sin) spermotoxin.

spermatovum (sper"mat-o'vum) [*spermato-* + L. *ovum* egg] a fertilized ovum.

spermatoxin (sper"mah-tok'sin) spermotoxin.

spermatozoa (sper"mah-to-zo'ah) [Gr.] plural of *spermatozoon*.

spermatozoal (sper"mah-to-zo'al) pertaining to spermatozoa.

spermatozoicide (sper"mah-to-zo'ĭ-sīd) spermicide.

spermatozoid (sper"mah-to-zoid) [*spermatozoon* + Gr. *eidos* form] 1. spermatozoon. 2. the male germ cell in plants.

spermatozoon (sper"mah-to-zo'on), pl. *spermatozo'a* [*spermato-* + Gr. *zōon* animal] a mature male germ cell, the specific output of the testes. It is the generative element of the semen which serves to fertilize the ovum. It consists of a head (or nucleus), a neck, a middle piece, and a tail with an end piece. Spermatozoa, formed in the seminiferous tubules, are derived from spermatogonia, which first develop into spermatocytes, which, in turn, undergo meiosis to produce spermatids; the spermatids then differentiate into spermatozoa.

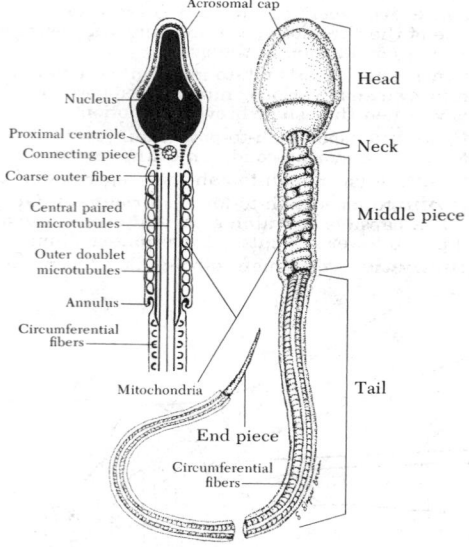

Human spermatozoon: side view (in cross-section) and flat view.

spermaturia (sper"mah-tu're-ah) [*spermato-* + Gr. *ouron* urine + *-ia*] seminuria.

spermectomy (sper-mek'to-me) excision of a portion of the spermatic cord.

spermia (sper'me-ah) [L.] plural of *spermium*.

spermiation (sper"me-a'shun) the freeing of mature spermatozoa from the Sertoli cells.

spermicidal (sper"mĭ-si'dal) [*sperm* + L. *caedere* to kill] destructive to spermatozoa.

spermicide (sper'mĭ-sīd) an agent that is destructive to spermatozoa.

spermid (sper'mid) spermatid.

spermidine (sper'mĭ-din) a polyamine, NH₂(CH₂)₃NH(CH₂)₄-NH₂, first found in human semen but now known to occur in almost all tissues, in association with nucleic acids; it is formed from putrescine and is itself a precursor of spermine.

spermiduct (sper'mĭ-dukt) [*sperm* + L. *ductus* duct] the ejaculatory duct and vas deferens together.

spermine (sper'min) a polyamine, NH₂(CH₂)₃NH(CH₂)₄NH-(CH₂)₃NH₂, first found in human semen but now known to occur in almost all tissues in association with nucleic acids, being formed from spermidine. **s. phosphate,** the substance, (C₂H₅N)₄H₄-Ca(PO₄)₂, of which the Charcot-Neumann crystals are composed; found also in various organs and secretions in leukemia, asthma, and emphysema.

spermiocyte (sper'me-o-sīt") [*spermia* + *-cyte*] a primary spermatocyte.

spermiogenesis (sper"me-o-jen'ĕ-sis) the second stage in the formation of spermatozoa in which the spermatids transform into spermatozoa.

spermiogonium (sper"me-o-go'ne-um) spermatogonium.

spermiogram (sper'me-o-gram) a diagram of the various cells formed during the development of the sperm.

spermioteleosis (sper"me-o-te"le-o'sis) [*spermio-* + Gr. *teleiōsis* perfection, completion] the progressive development of the spermatogonium through the successive changes necessary for becoming a mature spermatozoon.

spermioteleotic (sper"me-o-te"le-ot'ik) [*spermio-* + Gr. *teleiōtikos* perfective] pertaining to or characteristic of spermioteleosis.

spermist (sper'mist) a believer in the theory of preformation, which held that the spermatozoon was a complete miniature individual.

spermium (sper'me-um), pl. *sper'mia.* The mature spermatozoon.

spermo- see *spermato-*.

spermoblast (sper'mo-blast) [*spermo-* + Gr. *blastos* germ] a spermatid.

spermocytoma (sper"mo-si-to'mah) seminoma.

spermolith (sper'mo-lith) [*spermo-* + Gr. *lithos* stone] a calculus in the spermiduct.

spermoloropexis (sper"mo-lo"ro-pek'sis) spermoloropexy.

spermoloropexy (sper"mo-lo'ro-pek"se) [*spermo-* + Gr. *lōron* thong + *pēxis* fixation] fixation of the spermatic cord to the periosteum of the pubes in operation for undescended testicle.

spermolysin (sper-mol'ĭ-sin) spermotoxin.

spermolysis (sper-mol'ĭ-sis) spermatolysis.

spermolytic (sper"mo-lit'ik) spermatolytic.

spermoneuralgia (sper"mo-nu-ral'je-ah) [*spermo-* + Gr. *neuron* nerve + *-algia*] neuralgic pain in the spermatic cord.

Spermophilus (sper-mof'ĭ-lus) a genus of rodents which harbor organisms transmissible to man. *S. beech'eyi,* the ground squirrel of California, is extensively infected with plague, and, along with *S. mol'lis,* the ground squirrel of Utah, and *S. orego'nus* of Oregon, is a natural reservoir of *Francisella tularensis.*

spermophlebectasia (sper"mo-fle"bek-ta'ze-ah) [*spermo-* + Gr. *phelps* vein + *ektasis* distention + *-ia*] varicosity of the spermatic veins.

spermoplasm (sper'mo-plazm) [*spermo-* + Gr. *plasma* plasm] the protoplasm of the spermatids.

spermosphere (sper'mo-sfēr) [*spermo-* + Gr. *sphaira* sphere] a group or mass of spermatids formed by the segmentation of a secondary spermatocyte.

spermospore (sper'mo-spōr) spermatogonium.

spermotoxic (sper"mo-tok'sik) pertaining to a spermotoxin.

spermotoxin (sper"mo-tok'sin) a toxin destructive to spermatozoa; especially an antibody produced by injecting an animal with spermatozoa.

spes (spēs) [L.] hope. **s. phthis'ica,** a feeling of hopefulness of recovery frequently characteristic of patients with tuberculosis.

SPF specific-pathogen free, a term applied to animals reared for use in laboratory experiments, and known to be free of specific pathogenic microorganisms.

sp. gr. specific gravity.

sph. spherical or spherical lens.

sphacelate (sfas'ĕ-lāt) to become gangrenous.

sphacelation (sfas"ĕ-la'shun) the formation of a sphacelus; mortification.

sphacelism (sfas'ĕ-lizm) [Gr. *sphakelismos*] sphacelation or necrosis; sloughing.

sphaceloderma (sfas"ĕ-lo-der'mah) [*sphacelus* + Gr. *derma* skin] gangrene of the skin, or an ulcer resulting from it.

sphacelotoxin (sfas"ĕ-lo-tok'sin) [*sphacelus* + Gr. *toxikon* poison] 1. spasmotin. 2. a poisonous, yellow resin obtainable from ergot.

sphacelous (sfas'ĕ-lus) affected with gangrene; sloughing.

sphacelus (sfas'ĕ-lus) [L.; Gr. *sphakelos*] a slough or mass of gangrenous tissue; mortification.

sphaer- for words beginning thus, see also those beginning *spher-*.

Sphaeranthus (sfe-ran'thus) a genus of herbaceous plants of Asia. *S. indicus* L. furnishes a purported aphrodisiac oil. It is also used in India as an anthelmintic.

Sphaeria (sfe're-ah) a former genus of fungi, the species of which are now included in various genera. **S. sinen'sis,** *Cordyceps sinensis.*

Sphaeriales (sfe"re-a'lēz) an order of ascomycetes of the series Pyrenomycetes, including the family Sordariaceae.

sphaero- for words beginning thus, see also those beginning *sphero-*.

Sphaeroides maculatus (sfe'roi-dēz mak"u-la'tus) the Atlantic Coast puffer fish that contains a potent toxin concentrated in the gonads and viscera, which when eaten without special cooking preparation causes generalized paralysis and, in severe cases, unconsciousness and death.

Sphaerophorus (sfe-ro′fo-rus) *Bacteroides.* **S. necroph′orus,** *Fusobacterium necrophorum.*

Sphaerotilus (sfe-ro′tĭ-lus) a genus of microorganisms of the family Chlamydobacteriaceae, order Chlamydobacteriales, made up of attached or free-floating filaments, frequently showing false branching. It includes three species, *S. dicho′tomus, S. flu′itans,* and *S. na′tans.*

sphagiasmus (sfa″je-az′mus) [Gr. *sphagiasmos* a slaying, sacrificing] 1. contraction of the neck muscles in an epileptic attack. 2. petit mal; see *epilepsy.*

sphagitides (sfah-jit′ĭ-dēz) [Gr. *sphagitis* jugular; *sphage* throat] an old name for the so-called jugular vessels.

sphagitis (sfa-ji′tis) [Gr. *sphage* throat + *-itis*] any throat inflammation.

sphenethmoid (sfen-eth′moid) sphenoethmoid.

sphenion (sfe′ne-on), pl. *sphe′nia* [Gr. *sphen* wedge + *on* neuter ending] the cranial point at the sphenoid angle of the parietal bone.

spheno- (sfe′no) [Gr. *sphen* wedge] a combining form denoting relationship to the sphenoid bone or to a wedge, or meaning wedge-shaped.

sphenobasilar (sfe″no-bas′ĭ-lar) pertaining to the sphenoid bone and the basilar part of the occipital bone.

sphenoccipital (sfe″nok-sip′ĭ-tal) spheno-occipital.

sphenocephalus (sfe″no-sef′ah-lus) a fetus exhibiting sphenocephaly.

sphenocephaly (sfe″no-sef′ah-le) [*spheno-* + Gr. *kephale* head] a developmental anomaly characterized by a wedge-shaped appearance of the head.

sphenoethmoid (sfe″no-eth′moid) denoting the curved plate of bone in front of the lesser wing of the sphenoid bone.

sphenofrontal (sfe″no-frun′tal) pertaining to the sphenoid and frontal bones.

sphenoid (sfe′noid) [*spheno-* + Gr. *eidos* form] wedge-shaped; designating especially a very irregular wedge-shaped bone at the base of the skull (os sphenoidale, or sphenoid bone).

sphenoidal (sfe-noi′dal) pertaining to the sphenoid bone.

sphenoiditis (sfe″noi-di′tis) inflammation of the sphenoidal sinus.

sphenoidostomy (sfe″noi-dos′to-me) [*sphenoid* + Gr. *stomoun* to provide with an opening, or mouth] operative removal of the anterior wall of the sphenoidal sinus.

sphenoidotomy (sfe″noi-dot′o-me) incision into the sphenoidal sinus.

sphenomalar (sfe″no-ma′lar) sphenozygomatic.

sphenomaxillary (sfe″no-mak′sĭ-ler″e) pertaining to the sphenoid bone and the maxilla.

sphenometer (sfe-nom′ĕ-ter) [*spheno-* + Gr. *metron* measure] an instrument for measuring a wedge of bone removed in operations for correcting curvatures.

spheno-occipital (sfe″no-ok-sip′ĭ-tal) pertaining to the sphenoid and occipital bones.

sphenopagus (sfe″nop′ah-gus) [*spheno-* + Gr. *pagos* a thing fixed] symmetrical twins conjoined at the sphenoid bone at the base of the skull.

sphenopalatine (sfe″no-pal′ah-tin) pertaining to or in relation with the sphenoid and palatine bones.

sphenoparietal (sfe″no-pah-ri′ĕ-tal) pertaining to the sphenoid and parietal bones.

sphenopetrosal (sfe″no-pe-tro′sal) pertaining to the sphenoid bone and the petrosa.

sphenorbital (sfe-nor′bĭ-tal) pertaining to the sphenoid bone and the orbits.

sphenosquamosal (sfe″no-skwa-mo′sal) pertaining to the sphenoid bone and the squamous portion of the temporal bone.

sphenotemporal (sfe″no-tem′po-ral) pertaining to the sphenoid and temporal bones.

sphenotic (sfe-not′ik) [*spheno-* + Gr. *ous* ear] denoting a fetal bone which becomes that part of the sphenoid which is adjacent to the carotid groove.

sphenotresia (sfe″no-tre′ze-ah) [*spheno-* + Gr. *tresis* boring] boring of the skull in craniotomy.

sphenotribe (sfe′no-trīb) [*spheno-* + Gr. *tribein* to rub] an instrument for crushing the basal portion of the fetal skull.

sphenotripsy (sfe′no-trip″se) the crushing of the fetal head with the sphenotribe.

sphenoturbinal (sfe″no-tur′bĭ-nal) denoting a thin, curved bone in front of each of the lesser wings of the sphenoid, with which bone it becomes fused.

sphenovomerine (sfe″no-vo′mer-in) pertaining to the sphenoid and to the vomer.

sphenozygomatic (sfe″no-zi″go-mat′ik) pertaining to the sphenoid and zygomatic bones.

sphere (sfēr) [Gr. *sphaira* sphere] a ball, globe, or orb. **attraction s.,** centrosome. **embryotic s.,** the morula. **Morgagni's s's,** Morgagni's globules. **segmentation s.,** 1. the morula. 2. a blastomere. **vitelline s., yolk s.,** the morula.

spheresthesia (sfe″res-the′ze-ah) [Gr. *sphaira* sphere + *aisthesis* perception + *-ia*] a morbid sensation of a lump or ball in the throat; globus hystericus.

spherical (sfer′ĭ-kal) [Gr. *sphairikos*] pertaining to a sphere; sphere-shaped.

sphero- (sfe′ro) [Gr. *sphaira* a ball or globe] a combining form meaning round, or denoting relationship to a sphere.

spherocylinder (sfe″ro-sil′in-der) a combined spherical and cylindrical lens.

spherocyte (sfe′ro-sit) [*sphero-* + Gr. *kytos* cell] a small, globular, completely hemoglobinated erythrocyte without the usual central pallor, found characteristically in hereditary spherocytosis but also observed in acquired hemolytic anemia.

spherocytic (sfe″ro-sit′ik) characterized by the presence of spherocytes.

spherocytosis (sfe″ro-si-to′sis) the presence of spherocytes in the blood. **hereditary s.,** a congenital, familial form of hemolytic anemia characterized by spherocytosis, abnormal fragility of erythrocytes, jaundice, and splenomegaly. Called also *globe cell anemia, congenital hemolytic icterus, constitutional hemolytic anemia, chronic familial icterus, chronic acholuric jaundice,* and *acholuric jaundice.*

spheroid (sfe′roid) [*sphero-* + Gr. *eidos* form] a globular body, or one resembling a sphere.

spheroidal (sfe-roi′dal) having the form or shape of a sphere.

spheroidin (sfe-roi′din) [*Sphaeroides* (Gr. *sphaira* sphere) a puffer fish + *-in,* suffix denoting a chemical compound] a toxic fraction from tetrodotoxin, believed to have the empirical formula $C_{12}H_{17}O_{13}N_3$.

spherolith (sfe′ro-lith) [*sphero-* + Gr. *lithos* stone] any of the minute spherical deposits found in the kidney tissue of the newborn; they are probably uratic deposits.

spheroma (sfe-ro′mah) a globular tumor.

spherometer (sfe-rom′ĕ-ter) [*sphero-* + Gr. *metron* measure] an instrument for measuring the curvature of a surface.

Spherophorous (sfer-of′o-rus) *Sphaerophorus.*

spheroplast (sfer′o-plast) a spherical bacterial or plant cell, produced in hypertonic media under conditions that result in partial absence of the cell wall which no longer serves as a supporting structure. Cf. *protoplast,* def. 3.

spherospermia (sfe-ro-sper′me-ah) [*sphero-* + Gr. *sperma* seed] a round, tailless spermatozoon.

spherule (sfer′ūl) 1. a small sphere. 2. a spherical multinucleate cell of the parasitic stage of *Coccidioides immitis,* in which endospores are developed. **s's of Fulci,** numerous spherical red bodies seen in the spinal cord in inflammatory conditions of the cord. **rod s.,** the pear-shaped ending of a retinal rod cell, which synapses with the bipolar and horizontal cells in the outer plexiform layer.

sphincter (sfingk′ter) [L.; Gr. *sphinkter* that which binds tight] a ringlike band of muscle fibers that constricts a passage or closes a natural orifice; called also *musculus sphincter* [NA]. **s. a′ni,** see *musculus sphincter ani externus* and *musculus sphincter ani internus.* **s. of Boyden,** a superior choledochal sphincter encircling the common bile duct just proximal to the duodenum. **cardiac s., cardioesophageal s.,** muscle fibers about the opening of the esophagus into the stomach. **cornual s.,** tubal s. **s. of eye,** musculus orbicularis oculi. **gastroesophageal s.,** the terminal few centimeters of the esophagus, which prevents reflux of gastric contents into the esophagus. **Giordano's s.,** musculus sphincter ductus choledochi. **Henle's s.,** muscle fibers surrounding the prostatic urethra. **hepatic s.,** a thickened portion of the muscular coat of the hepatic veins near their entrance into the inferior vena cava. **s. of hepatopancreatic ampulla,** musculus sphincter ampullae hepatopancreaticae. **Hyrtl's s.,** an incomplete band or thickening of the muscle fibers in the rectum a few inches above the anus in the upper part of the rectal ampulla; called also *rectal s.* **inguinal s.,** a ring of muscle fibers around the spermatic cord at the internal opening of the inguinal canal. **s. i′ridis,** musculus sphincter pupillae. **Lütkens' s.,** a thickening of the muscle fibers in the neck of the gallbladder. **Nélaton's s.,** an occasional and often incomplete band of muscle fibers about the rectum at the level of the prostate. **O'Beirne's s.,** circular muscle fibers in the wall of the large intestine at the junction of the sigmoid colon and rectum. **s. oc′uli,** musculus orbicularis oculi. **Oddi's s.,** the sheath of muscle fibers investing the associated bile and pancreatic passages as they traverse the wall of the duodenum; called also *musculus sphincter ampullae hepatopancreaticae* [NA] and *Oddi's muscle.* **s. o′ris,** musculus orbicularis oris. **palatopharyngeal s.,** a transverse band of muscle fibers in the posterior wall of the pharynx, derived from the superior constrictor or palatopharyngeal muscle, which contracts during swallowing to form Passavant's bar; it also contracts during speech in persons with cleft palate. **pharyngoesoph-ageal s.,** a region of higher muscular tone at the junction of the pharynx and esophagus, which is involved in movements of swallowing. **precapillary s.,** a smooth muscle fiber encircling a true capillary where it originates from the arterial capillary, which can open and close the capillary entrance. **prepyloric s.,** a band of muscle fibers in the wall of the stomach proximal to the pyloric sphincter. **s. pupil′lae,** musculus sphincter pupillae. **pyloric s.,** a thickening of the circular muscle of the stomach around its opening into the duodenum; called also *musculus sphincter pylori* [NA]. **rectal s.,** Hyrtl's s. **tubal s.,** an encircling band of muscle fibers at the junction of the uterine tube and the uterus. **s. ure′thrae,** musculus sphincter urethrae. **s. vagi′nae,** the musculus bulbospongiosus in the female. **s. vesi′cae,** musculus sphincter vesicae urinariae.

sphincteral (sfingk′ter-al) pertaining to a sphincter.

sphincteralgia (sfingk″ter-al′je-ah) [*sphincter* + Gr. *algos* pain + *-ia*] pain in a sphincter muscle, as of the anus.

sphincterectomy (sfingk″ter-ek′to-me) [*sphincter* + Gr. *ektomē* excision] excision of any sphincter, such as the sphincter iridis.

sphincteric (sfingk-ter′ik) pertaining to a sphincter.

sphincterismus (sfingk″ter-iz′mus) spasm of the sphincter ani.

sphincteritis (sfingk″ter-i′tis) inflammation of a sphincter, particularly of the sphincter of Oddi.

sphincterolysis (sfingk″ter-ol′ĭ-sis) [*sphincter* + Gr. *lysis* dissolution] the operation of separating the iris from the cornea in anterior synechia.

sphincteroplasty (sfingk′ter-o-plas″te) [*sphincter* + Gr. *plassein* to mold] surgical repair of a defective sphincter.

sphincteroscope (sfingk′ter-o-skōp″) [*sphincter* + Gr. *skopein* to examine] a speculum for inspecting the anal sphincter. **Kelly's s.,** see under *speculum.*

sphincteroscopy (sfingk″ter-os′ko-pe) inspection of the anal sphincter.

sphincterotome (sfingk′ter-o-tōm″) an instrument for cutting a sphincter.

sphincterotomy (sfingk″ter-ot′o-me) [*sphincter* + Gr. *tomē* a cutting] division of a sphincter. **internal s.,** incision of the internal sphincter of the anus.

sphingo- [Gr. *sphingein* to bind fast] a combining form denoting relationship to sphingosine or a sphingolipid.

sphingogalactoside (sfing″go-gah-lak′to-sīd) a substance composing part of the material characteristic of the spleen in Gaucher's disease.

sphingoglycolipid (sfing″go-gli″ko-lip′id) any glycolipid that contains sphingosine, including the cerebrosides, globosides, hematosides, and gangliosides.

sphingoin (sfing′go-in) a leukomaine, $C_{17}H_{35}NO_2$, from the substance of the brain.

sphingol (sfing′gol) an alcohol, $C_9H_{18}O$, obtained from sphingomyelinic acid by hydrolysis.

sphingolipid (sfing″go-lip′id) [Gr. *sphingein* to bind tight + lipid] a lipid containing sphingosine; a fatty acid is attached to the nitrogen atom, and these *N*-acylsphingosines are called ceramides. Sphingolipids are combinations of different compounds with the hydroxyl group of ceramides, e.g., sphingomyelins (with phosphoryl choline), gangliosides (with branched-chain oligosaccharides), and cerebrosides (with glucose or galactose). They occur in membranes and in particularly high concentrations in brain and nerve tissue.

sphingolipidoses (sfing″go-lip″ĭ-do′sēz) [Gr.] plural of *sphingolipidosis.*

sphingolipidosis (sfing″go-lip″ĭ-do′sis), pl. *sphingolipidoses.* A general designation applied to diseases characterized by abnormal storage of sphingolipids, such as Gaucher's disease, Niemann-Pick disease, generalized gangliosidosis, and Tay-Sachs disease. **cerebral s.,** a group of hereditary disorders transmitted as an autosomal recessive trait and due to an inborn defect of lipid metabolism in which spingolipids accumulate in the brain. They are characterized by cerebromacular degeneration, progressive dementia, progressive loss of vision resulting in blindness, paralysis, and death, and are classified according to age of onset. The *infantile form* usually occurs between 4 and 6 months of age, chiefly affecting children of Jewish ancestry, and marked by a cherry-red spot with a gray-white border on both retinas; called also *Sachs'* or *Tay-Sachs disease.* The *late infantile form* occurs between 3 and 4 years of age, shows no racial predilection, and progresses more slowly than the infantile form. The cherry-red spot seen in the infantile form is frequently absent, but there are pigmentary changes of the retina. Called also *Bielschowsky's* or *Bielschowsky-Jansky disease.* The *juvenile form* shows no racial predilection, occurs between 5 and 10 years of age, and is marked by "salt and pepper" pigmentation of the retina; called also *Batten-Mayou, Spielmeyer-Vogt,* and *Vogt-Spielmeyer disease.* The *late juvenile,* or *adult, form* occurs between the ages of 15 and 26, and shows no racial predilection or ocular lesions; clinical findings

are those of cerebellar or basal ganglia disorders. Called also *Kufs' disease.*

sphingolipodystrophy (sfing″go-lip″o-dis′tro-fe) any of a group of disorders of sphingolipid metabolism, including Gaucher's disease, metachromatic leukodystrophy, Niemann-Pick disease, etc.

sphingomyelin (sfing″go-mi′ĕ-lin) a general designation of a group of phospholipids which on hydrolysis yield phosphoric acid, choline, sphingosine, and a fatty acid. They occur primarily in nervous tissue and generally in membranes.

sphingomyelinosis (sfing″go-mi″ĕ-lin-o′sis) Niemann-Pick disease.

sphingophospholipid (sfing″go-fos″fo-lip′id) a sphingolipid containing sphingosine or a related base and phosphorylcholine.

sphingosine (sfing″go-sin) a long-chain, mono-unsaturated aliphatic amino alcohol, $C_{18}H_{37}O_2N$, usually present in sphingomyelin.

sphygmic (sfig′mik) [Gr. *sphygmikos*] pertaining to the pulse; see *sphygmic period,* under *period.*

sphygmo- (sfig′mo) [Gr. *sphygmos* pulse] a combining form denoting relationship to the pulse.

sphygmobologram (sfig″mo-bo′lo-gram) a tracing made by the sphygmobolometer.

sphygmobolometer (sfig″mo-bo-lom′ĕ-ter) [*sphygmo-* + Gr. *bōlos* mass + *metron* measure] an instrument for measuring and recording the energy of the pulse wave, and so, indirectly, the strength of the systole.

sphygmobolometry (sfig″mo-bo-lom′ĕ-tre) the use of the sphygmobolometer.

sphygmocardiogram (sfig″mo-kar′de-o-gram) the tracing made by a sphygmocardiograph.

sphygmocardiograph (sfig″mo-kar′de-o-graf) [*sphygmo-* + Gr. *kardia* heart + *graphein* to write] an instrument for recording the pulse waves and heart beat at the same operation.

sphygmocardioscope (sfig″mo-kar′de-o-skōp) [*sphygmo-* + Gr. *kardia* heart + *skopein* to examine] an apparatus that records or displays the behavior of the pulse, heart action, and sounds.

sphygmochronograph (sfig″mo-kro′no-graf) [*sphygmo-* + Gr. *chronos* time + *graphein* to write] a form of self-registering sphygmograph.

sphygmodynamometer (sfig″mo-di″nah-mom′ĕ-ter) [*sphygmo-* + Gr. *dynamis* power + *metron* measure] an instrument for determining the force of the pulse.

sphygmogenin (sfig-moj′e-nin) [*sphygmo-* + Gr. *gennan* to produce] epinephrine.

sphygmogram (sfig′mo-gram) [*sphygmo-* + Gr. *gramma* a writing] a sphygmographic tracing; the record or tracing made by a sphygmograph. It consists of a curve having a sudden rise (*primary elevation*), followed by a sudden fall, after which there is a gradual descent marked by a number of secondary elevations.

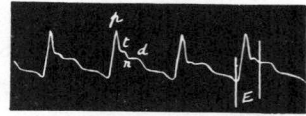

Radial sphygmogram from a healthy individual: *p,* The percussion wave; *t,* tidal or predicrotic wave; *n,* dicrotic or aortic notch; *d,* dicrotic wave; *E,* the sphygmic period during which the semilunar valves are open. (Hay.)

sphygmograph (sfig′mo-graf) [*sphygmo-* + Gr. *graphein* to write] an instrument for registering the movements, form, and force of the arterial pulse. Vierordt's sphygmograph (1835) and Marey's (1860) were the earliest. The latter, variously modified, is the kind principally used.

sphygmographic (sfig″mo-graf′ik) pertaining to the sphygmograph.

sphygmography (sfig-mog′rah-fe) the production of pulse tracings with the sphygmograph.

sphygmoid (sfig′moid) [*sphygmo-* + Gr. *eidos* form] resembling the pulse.

sphygmology (sfig-mol′o-je) [*sphygmo-* + *-logy*] the sum of what is known regarding the pulse.

sphygmomanometer (sfig″mo-mah-nom′ĕ-ter) an instrument for measuring blood pressure in the arteries. There are many forms of the instrument, each named for the person who devised it, as *Riva-Rocci s., Faught's s., Erlanger's s., Janeway's s., Mosso's s., Rogers' s., Staunton's s., Tycos s.*

sphygmometer (sfig-mom′ĕ-ter) [*sphygmo-* + Gr. *metron* measure] an instrument for measuring the force and frequency of the pulse.

sphygmometrograph (sfig″mo-met′ro-graf) an apparatus for recording the maximal and minimal arterial pressures.

sphygmometroscope (sfig″mo-met′ro-skōp) an instrument for taking the blood pressure by the auscultatory method.

sphygmo-oscillometer (sfig″mo-os″ĭ-lom′ĕ-ter) a form of

sphygmomanometer in which the disappearance and reappearance of the pulse are indicated by an oscillating needle.

sphygmopalpation (sfig″mo-pal-pa′shun) the act of palpating or feeling the pulse.

sphygmophone (sfig′mo-fōn) [*sphygmo-* + Gr. *phōnē* sound] an apparatus for rendering audible the vibrations of the pulse.

sphygmoplethysmograph (sfig″mo-plĕ-thiz′mo-graf) a plethysmograph which traces a record of the pulse, together with the curve of fluctuation of volume.

sphygmoscope (sfig′mo-skōp) [*sphygmo-* + Gr. *skopein* to examine] a device for rendering the pulse beat visible. **Bishop's s.,** an apparatus for measuring the blood pressure, especially the diastolic pressure.

sphygmoscopy (sfig-mos′ko-pe) examination of the pulse.

sphygmosystole (sfig″mo-sis′to-le) [*sphygmo-* + *systole*] that part of the sphygmogram that corresponds to the systole of the heart.

sphygmotonogram (sfig″mo-to′no-gram) (*obs.*) the graphic record produced by the sphygmotonograph.

sphygmotonograph (sfig″mo-to′no-graf) [*sphygmo-* + Gr. *tonos* tension + *graphein* to write] (*obs.*) an instrument for recording simultaneously the blood pressure, the carotid or jugular pulse, the brachial pulse, and the time in fifths of a second.

sphygmotonometer (sfig″mo-to-nom′ĕ-ter) [*sphygmo-* + Gr. *tonos* tension + *metron* measure] an instrument for measuring the elasticity of the arterial walls.

sphygmoviscosimetry (sfig″mo-vis″ko-sim′ĕ-tre) [*sphygmo-* + *viscosity* + Gr. *metron* measure] measurement of the blood pressure and the viscosity of the blood.

sphyrectomy (sfi-rek′to-me) [Gr. *sphyra* malleus + *ektomē* excision] surgical removal of the malleus.

sphyrotomy (sfi-rot′o-me) [Gr. *sphyra* malleus + *tomē* a cutting] surgical removal of a portion of the malleus.

spica (spi′kah) [L. "ear of wheat"] a figure-of-8 bandage with turns that cross one another usually at the shoulder or hip; see under *bandage*.

spicular (spik′u-lar) pertaining to a spicule.

spicule (spik′ūl) [L. *spiculum*] a sharp, needle-like body.

spiculum (spik′u-lum), pl. *spic′ula* [L.] spicule.

spider (spi′der) 1. an arthropod of the class Arachnida, some species of which have venomous bites. Cf. *arachnidism.* 2. a spider-like nevus; see *vascular s.* **arterial s.,** vascular s. **banana s.,** *Heteropoda venatoria.* **black widow s.,** see *Latrodectus.* **brown recluse s.,** *Loxosceles reclusa.* **cat-headed s.,** *Mastophora gasteracanthoides.* **comb-footed s.,** see *Theridiidae.* **European wolf s.,** European tarantula. **funnel-web s.,** see *Atrax.* **jointed s.,** see *Solpugida.* **lynx s.,** *Peucetia viridans.* **tree funnel-web s.,** *Atrax formidabilis.* **vascular s.,** a telangiectasis composed of small vessels a few millimeters long radiating from a central arteriole, the whole somewhat resembling the legs of a spider. They may occur singly or numerously, most often in children and pregnant women, but also in persons with liver disease. The upper chest and arms are most frequently affected, but they may occur anywhere. Called also *spider nevus, nevus araneus,* or *stellate angioma.* **wandering s.,** *Ctenus ferus.*

spider burst (spi′der burst) radiating lines of capillaries on the leg caused by venous dilatation but without distinct varicosity.

Spiegelberg's sign (spig′el-bergz) [Otto *Spiegelberg,* German gynecologist, 1830–1881] see under *sign.*

Spieghel's line (spig′elz) [Adriaan van der *Spieghel* (L. *Spigelius*), Flemish anatomist, 1578–1625] linea semilunaris.

Spiegler's test (reagent) (spe′glerz) [Eduard *Spiegler,* dermatologist of Vienna, 1860–1908] see under *tests.*

Spigelia (spi-je′le-ah) [Adriaan van der *Spieghel,* 1578–1625] a genus of loganiaceous plants; the rhizome and roots of *S. marilan′dica* L. (pinkroot) have been used as an anthelmintic.

spigelian (spi-je′le-an) named for Adriaan van der *Spieghel* (L. *Spigelius*), Flemish anatomist, 1578–1625, as *spigelian* line (linea semilunaris) or *spigelian* lobe (lobus caudatus).

spigeline (spi-je′lēn) an alkaloid resembling coniine and nicotine occurring in *Spigelia marilandica* L., a perennial herb of Eastern North America.

spignet (spig′net) *Aralia.*

spike (spīk) a sharp upward deflection in a curve, such as the main deflection of the oscillographic tracing of the action potential wave, the following smaller wave being called the *after-potential.* See also under *potential.*

spikenard (spīk′nard) [L. *nardus,* or *spica nardi*] the plant *Nardostachys jatamansi* and various fragrant valerianaceous and other plants; used now chiefly in oriental medicine for nervous disorders. **American s.,** *Aralia.* **false s.,** *Andropogon nardus,* an aromatic and stimulant East Indian grass; also *Smilacina racemosa,* a North American plant.

Spilanthes (spi-lan′thēz) [Gr. *spilos* spot + Gr. *anthos* flower] a genus of composite-flowered plants. *S. acmella* Murr., the Para

cress of tropical America and Asia, was formerly used as a remedy for toothache. It is also a powerful mosquito larvicide.

spillway (spil′wa) a channel or passageway through which food escapes from the occlusal surfaces of the teeth during mastication. The occlusal, developmental, and supplemental grooves, as well as the incisal, occlusal, labial, buccal, and lingual embrasures, become spillways during function.

spina (spi′nah), pl. *spi′nae* [L.] a spine: a thornlike process or projection; [NA] a general term for such a process. **s. angula′ris,** spina ossis sphenoidalis. **s. bif′ida,** a developmental anomaly characterized by defective closure of the bony encasement of the spinal cord, through which the cord and meninges may (s. bifida cystica) or may not (s. bifida occulta) protrude. **s. bif′ida ante′rior,** a defect of closure on the anterior surface of the bony spinal canal, often associated with defective development of the abdominal and thoracic viscera. **s. bif′ida aper′ta,** s. bifida cystica. **s. bif′ida cys′tica,** spina bifida in which there is protrusion through the defect of a cystic swelling involving the meninges (meningocele), spinal cord (myelocele), or both (meningomyelocele). **s. bif′ida manifes′ta,** s. bifida cystica. **s. bif′ida occul′ta,** spina bifida in which there is a defect of the bony spinal canal without protrusion of the cord or meninges. **s. bif′ida poste′rior,** a defect of closure on the posterior surface of the bony spinal canal. **s. fronta′lis,** s. nasalis ossis frontalis. **s. hel′icis** [NA], spine of helix: a small, forward-projecting cartilaginous process on the anterior portion of the helix at about the junction of the helix and its crus, just above the tragus. **s. ili′aca ante′rior infe′rior** [NA], anterior inferior iliac spine: a blunt bony process projecting forward from the lower part of the anterior margin of the ilium, just above the acetabulum. **s. ili′aca ante′rior supe′rior** [NA], anterior superior iliac spine: a blunt bony projection on the anterior border of the ilium, forming the anterior end of the iliac crest. **s. ili′aca poste′rior infe′rior** [NA], posterior inferior iliac spine: a blunt bony projection from the posterior border of the ilium, corresponding to the posterior lower extremity of the facies auricularis and the posterior upper extremity of the incisura ischiadica major. **s. ili′aca poste′rior supe′rior** [NA], posterior superior iliac spine: a blunt bony projection on the posterior border of the ilium, forming the posterior end of the iliac crest. **s. intercondyloi′dea,** eminentia intercondylaris. **s. ischiad′ica** [NA], ischial spine: a strong process of bone projecting backward and medialward from the posterior border of the ischium, on a level with the lower border of the acetabulum and serving to separate the major and minor ischiadic notches. **s. mea′tus,** s. suprameatum. **s. menta′lis** [NA], mental spine: any of the small bony projections (usually four in number) located on the internal surface of the mandible, near the lower end of the midline, serving for attachment of the genioglossal and geniohyoid muscles. Called also *genial apophysis.* **s. nasa′lis ante′rior maxil′lae** [NA], anterior nasal spine of maxilla: the sharp anterosuperior projection at the anterior extremity of the nasal crest of the maxilla. **s. nasa′lis os′sis fronta′lis** [NA], nasal spine of frontal bone: a rough and somewhat irregular process of bone projecting downward and forward from the front part of the inferior surface of the pars nasalis of the frontal bone and fitting between the nasal bones and the ethmoid bone; called also *spina frontalis.* **s. nasa′lis os′sis palati′ni** [NA], **s. nasa′lis poste′rior os′sis palati′ni,** nasal spine of palatine bone: a small, sharp, backward-projecting bony spine forming the medial posterior angle of the horizontal portion of the palatine bone; called also *posterior nasal spine.* **s. os′sis sphenoida′lis** [NA], spine of sphenoid bone: a small bony process projecting downward from the inferior aspect of the great wing of the sphenoid bone where the wing projects into the angle between the petrous and squamous portions of the temporal bone; it is just posterior to the foramen spinosum and serves for attachment of the sphenomandibular and pterygospinous ligaments. Called also *s. angularis.* **spi′nae palati′nae** [NA], palatine spines: ridges which are laterally placed on the inferior surface of the maxillary part of the hard palate, separating the palatine sulci. **s. scap′ulae** [NA], spine of scapula: a triangular plate of bone attached by one edge to the back of the scapula, its tip being at the vertebral border of the scapula; it passes laterally toward the shoulder joint and at its base bears the acromion. **s. su′prameat′um** [NA], suprameatal spine: a pointed process that sometimes projects from the temporal bone, just above and at the back of the external acoustic meatus. **s. tib′iae,** tuberositas tibiae. **s. trochlea′ris** [NA], trochlear spine: a spicule of bone on the anteromedial part of the orbital surface of the frontal bone for attachment of the trochlea of the superior oblique muscle; when absent, it is represented by the trochlear fovea. **s. tympan′ica ma′jor** [NA], greater tympanic spine: a spine of the temporal bone forming the anterior edge of the tympanic notch (deficient part of tympanic sulcus). **s. tympan′ica mi′nor** [NA], lesser tympanic spine: a spine of the temporal bone forming the posterior edge of the tympanic notch. **s. vento′sa,** a true dactylitis occurring mostly in infants and young children, characterized by enlargement of the fingers or toes, with caseation, sequestration, and sinus formation.

spinacin (spi′nah-sin) a protein obtained from the cytoplasm of the cells of spinach leaves. It is insoluble in water and in salt solutions, but soluble in very slight excess of either acid or alkali.

spinae (spi′ne) [L.] plural of *spina.*

spinal (spi′nal) [L. *spinalis*] pertaining to a spine or to the vertebral column. See also under *animal.*

spinalgia (spi-nal′je-ah) [*spine* + Gr. *algos* pain + *-ia*] pain in the spinal region. **Petruschky's s.,** tenderness in the interscapular region in tuberculosis of the bronchial lymph nodes.

spinalis (spi-na′lis) [L.] spinal.

spinant (spi′nant) any agent that acts directly upon the spinal cord, increasing its reflex activity.

spinate (spi′nāt) [L. *spinatus*] having thorns; shaped like a thorn.

spindle (spin′d'l) 1. the fusiform figure occurring in the cell nucleus during the metaphase of mitosis, composed of microtubules radiating from the centrioles and connecting the chromosomes at their centromeres. Called also *achromatic s., mitotic s.,* and *nuclear s.* 2. see *brain waves,* under *wave.* 3. muscle s. **aortic s.,** the dilated part of the aorta just below the isthmus. **Axenfeld-Krukenberg s.,** Krukenberg's s. **Bütschli's nuclear s.,** spindle, def. 1. **central s.,** the bundle of fibers in the axial part of the spindle of an amphiaster. **cleavage s.,** any spindle formed during cleavage of the ovum. **enamel s's,** spindle-shaped extensions of the dentinal tubules passing across the dentinoenamel junction into the enamel. **His' s.,** aortic s. **Krukenberg's s.,** a vertical spindle-shaped, brownish-red opacity on the posterior surface of the cornea. **Kühne's s.,** muscle s. **mitotic s.,** spindle, def. 1. **muscle s.,** a mechanoreceptor found between skeletal muscle fibers; the muscle spindles are arranged in parallel with muscle fibers, and respond to passive stretch of the muscle but cease to discharge if the muscle contracts isotonically, thus signaling muscle length. The muscle spindle is the receptor responsible for the stretch or myotatic reflex. **neuromuscular s.,** muscle s. **neurotendinal s.,** Golgi tendon organ. **nuclear s.,** see *spindle,* def. 1. **tendon s.,** Golgi tendon organ. **tigroid s's,** Nissl bodies. **urine s's,** spindle-shaped, urine-filled segments of the ureter due to incomplete occlusion of the ureter during peristalsis.

spine (spīn) 1. a thornlike process or projection; called also *spina* [NA]. 2. the spinal column (columna vertebralis [NA]). 3. the central ridge on the internal surface of a horse's hoof, between the branches of the frog; called also *frog stay.* **alar s., angular s.,** spina ossis sphenoidalis. **bamboo s.,** the ankylosed spine produced by rheumatoid spondylitis; so called because of the roentgenographic appearance caused by lipping of the vertebral margins. **basilar s.,** tuberculum pharyngeum. **Civinini's s.,** processus pterygospinosus. **cleft s.,** see *spina bifida.* **dendritic s.,** gemmule, def. 2. **dorsal s.,** columna vertebralis. **Erichsen's s.,** an obscure condition occurring as the result of alleged accidental injury to the vertebral column. **ethmoidal s. of Macalister,** crista sphenoidalis. **frontal s., external,** spina nasalis ossis frontalis. **s. of greater tubercle of humerus,** crista tuberculi majoris. **s. of helix,** spina helicis. **hemal s.,** a ventral projection from the hemal arch, which is attached to the underside of certain vertebral centra in lower vertebrates. **s. of Henle,** spina supra meatum. **hysterical s.,** simulated vertebral disease in neurotic patients. **iliac s., anterior inferior,** spina iliaca anterior inferior. **iliac s., anterior superior,** spina iliaca anterior superior. **iliac s., posterior inferior,** spina iliaca posterior inferior. **iliac s., posterior superior,** spina iliaca posterior superior. **iliopectineal s.,** eminentia iliopubica. **intercondyloid s.,** eminentia intercondylaris. **ischial s., s. of ischium,** spina ischiadica. **jugular s.,** processus jugularis ossis occipitalis. **kissing s's,** a condition in which the spinous processes of adjacent vertebra are in contact; called also *Baastrup's disease* or *syndrome.* **s. of lesser tubercle of humerus,** crista tuberculi minoris. **s. of maxilla,** spina nasalis anterior maxillae. **meatal s.,** spina suprameatum. **mental s.,** spina mentalis. **mental s., external,** protuberantia mentalis. **nasal s., anterior,** spina nasalis anterior maxillae. **nasal s., posterior,** spina nasalis ossis palatini. **nasal s. of frontal bone,** spina nasalis ossis frontalis. **nasal s. of maxilla, anterior,** spina nasalis anterior maxillae. **nasal s. of palatine bone,** spina nasalis ossis palatini. **neural s.,** processus spinosus vertebrarum. **obturator s.,** crista obturatoria. **occipital s., external,** protuberantia occipitalis externa. **occipital s., internal,** protuberantia occipitalis interna. **palatine s's,** spinae palatinae. **peroneal s. of os calcis,** trochlea peronealis calcanei. **pharyngeal s.,** tuberculum pharyngeum. **poker s.,** the ankylosed spine produced by rheumatoid spondylitis; so called because of its rigidity. **s. of pubic bone, s. of pubis,** tuberculum pubicum ossis pubis. **railway s.,** traumatic neurosis following spinal injury. **rigid s.,** poker s. **s. of scapula,** spina scapulae. **sciatic s.,** spina ischiadica. **s. of sphenoid bone, sphenoidal s.,** spina ossis sphenoidalis. **suprameatal s.,** spina suprameatum. **s. of tibia, tibial s.,** tuberositas tibiae. **trochanteric s., greater,** labium laterale lineae asperae femoris. **trochanteric s., lesser,** labium mediale lineae asperae femoris. **trochlear s.,** spina trochlearis. **tympanic s., anterior, tympanic s., greater,** spina

tympanica major. **tympanic s., lesser, tympanic s., posterior,** spina tympanica minor. **typhoid s.,** a painful condition of the spine due to osteomyelitis of the vertebrae following typhoid fever. **s. of vertebra,** processus spinosus vertebrarum.

Spinelli's operation (spe-nel′ēz) [Pier Giuseppe *Spinelli,* Italian gynecologist, 1862–1929] see under *operation.*

spinifugal (spi-nif′u-gal) [L. *spina* spine + *fugere* to flee] going, conducting, or moving away from the spinal cord.

spinipetal (spi-nip′e-tal) [L. *spina* spine + *petere* to seek] tending, conducting, or moving toward the spinal cord.

Spinitectus gracilis (spi″ne-tek′tus gras′ĭ-lis) a parasitic nematode in the intestines of fishes in the United States.

spinnbarkeit (spin′bahr-kīt) [Ger.] the formation of a thread by mucus from the cervix uteri when spread onto a glass slide and drawn out by a coverglass; the time at which it can be drawn to the maximum length usually precedes or coincides with the time of ovulation.

spinobulbar (spi″no-bul′bar) pertaining to the spinal cord and the medulla oblongata.

spinocellular (spi″no-sel′u-lar) containing, made up of, or marked by prickle cells.

spinocerebellar (spi″no-ser′e-bel′ar) pertaining to the spinal cord and the cerebellum.

spinocortical (spi″no-kor′tĭ-kal) corticospinal.

spinocostalis (spi″no-kos-ta′lis) the serratus posterior superior and inferior muscles together.

spinogalvanization (spi″no-gal″vah-ni-za′shun) galvanization of the spinal cord, performed by moving the anode slowly up and down the spine.

spinoglenoid (spi″no-gle′noid) pertaining to the spine of the scapula and the glenoid cavity.

spinogram (spi′no-gram) a roentgenogram of the spine or of the spinal cord.

spinopetal (spi-nop′e-tal) spinipetal.

spinose (spi′nōs) spinous.

spinotectal (spi″no-tek′tal) tectospinal.

spinous (spi′nus) [L. *spinosus*] 1. like a spine; acanthoid. 2. pertaining to a spine or to a spinelike process.

spinthariscope (spin-thar′ĭ-skōp) [Gr. *spintharis* spark + *skopein* to examine] an instrument for viewing the emanations of radium.

spintherism (spin′ther-izm) [Gr. *spinthērizein* to emit sparks] synchysis scintillans.

spintherometer (spin″ther-om′ĕ-ter) [Gr. *spinthēr* spark + *metron* measure] an apparatus for measuring the changes which occur in the vacuum of the roentgen-ray tube, and hence the penetrating power of the rays.

spintheropia (spin″ther-o′pe-ah) [Gr. *spinthēr* spark + *ōpē* sight + *-ia*] synchysis scintillans.

spintometer (spin-tom′ĕ-ter) spintherometer.

spiperone (spip′ĕ-rōn) chemical name: 8-[3-(*p*-fluorobenzoyl)-propyl]-1-phenyl-1,3,8-triazaspiro[4.5]-decan-4-one; a tranquilizer, $C_{23}H_{26}FN_3O_2$, used in treatment of schizophrenia.

spir. abbreviation for L. *spir′itus,* spirit.

spir- see *spiro.*

spiracle (spir′ah-k'l) [L. *spirare* to breathe] a breathing orifice of arthropods; an accessory opening for the intake of water in the respiratory system of cartilaginous fish.

spiradenoma (spi″rad-ĕ-no′mah) [Gr. *speira* coil + *adenoma*] adenoma sudoriparum. **cylindromatous s.,** cylindroma, def. 2. **eccrine s.,** a benign, solitary, deep-seated nodule arising from the coil portion of an eccrine gland; it is covered by normal appearing skin and may be accompanied by paroxysmal pain.

spiral (spi′ral) [L. *spiralis* from *spira;* Gr. *speira*] 1. winding about a center like a coil or the thread of a screw. 2. anything coiled or winding about a center. **Curschmann's s's,** coiled mucinous fibrils sometimes found in the sputum of bronchial asthma. **Golgi-Rezzonico s.,** see under *thread.* **Herxheimer's s's,** see under *fiber.* **Perroncito's s's,** see under *apparatus.* **tendon s.,** a spiral receptor connected with a tendon.

Spiranthes (spi-ran′thēz) [Gr. *speira* coil + *anthos* flower] a genus of orchidaceous plants. **S. autumna′lis,** a species reputed to be aphrodisiac. **S. diuret′ica,** a species of Chile, said to be a valuable diuretic.

spireme (spi′rēm) [Gr. *speirēma* coil] the threadlike, continuous or segmented figure formed by the chromosome material during the prophase of mitosis or meiosis. Called also *skein.*

spirilla (spi-ril′ah) [L.] plural of *spirillum.*

Spirillaceae (spi″ril-la′se-e) a family of Schizomycetes (order Pseudomonadales, suborder Pseudomonadineae), made up of gram-negative, simple curved or spirally twisted rods, frequently forming chains of spirally twisted cells. It includes 10 genera: *Cellfalcicula, Cellvibrio, Desulfovibrio, Methanobacterium, Micro-*

cyclus, Myconostoc, Paraspirillum, Selenomonas, Spirillum, and *Vibrio.*

spirillemia (spi″ril-e′me-ah) [*spirilla* + Gr. *haima* blood + *-ia*] the presence of spirilla in the blood.

spirillicidal (spi-ril″ĭ-si′dal) destroying spirilla.

spirillicide (spi-ril″ĭ-sīd) [*spirilla* + L. *caedere* to kill] 1. destroying spirilla. 2. an agent that destroys spirilla.

spirillicidin (spi-ril″ĭ-si′din) a substance formed in the blood of patients immunized against spirilla and capable of destroying spirilla.

spirillolysis (spi″rĭ-lol′ĭ-sis) [*spirilla* + Gr. *lysis* dissolution] the breaking up of or destruction of spirilla.

spirillosis (spi″rĭ-lo′sis) 1. any disease condition attended or marked by the presence of spirilla in the body. 2. fowl spirochetosis.

spirillotropic (spi″rĭ-lo-trop′ik) having an affinity for spirilla.

spirillotropism (spi″rĭ-lot′ro-pizm) [*spirilla* + Gr. *tropos* a turning] the property of having an affinity for spirilla.

Spirillum (spi-ril′um) a genus of microorganisms of the family Spirillaceae, suborder Pseudomonadineae, order Pseudomonadales, made up of cells which form long spirals, or portions of a turn. It includes nine species: *S. iterso′nii, S. kutsch′eri, S. lipo′ferum, S. mi′nus, S. ser′pens, S. ten′ue, S. un′dula, S. virginia′num,* and *S. vol′utans.* Many of the organisms placed in this genus in earlier taxonomic nomenclature have been reclassified in other genera. **S. mi′nor, S. mi′nus,** a species that is a normal parasite of the nasopharynx of rats and mice, which can assume a pathogenic role for the rodent host. It is the etiologic agent of the spirillary form of rat-bite fever.

spirillum (spi-ril′um), pl. *spiril′la* [L.] 1. a relatively rigid, spiral-shaped bacterium. 2. an organism of the genus *Spirillum.* **Deneke's s.,** *Vibrio tyrogenus.* **s. of Finkler and Prior,** *Vibrio proteus.* **s. of Vincent,** *Borrelia vincentii.*

spirit (spir′it) [L. *spiritus*] 1. any volatile or distilled liquid. 2. a solution of a volatile material in alcohol. **ammonia s.,** aromatic ammonia s. **ammonia s., aromatic** [USP], **s. of ammonia, aromatic,** a preparation compounded of ammonia, ammonium carbonate, strong ammonia solution, lemon oil, lavender oil, myristica oil, alcohol, and purified oil, and containing, in each 100 ml., 1.7–2.1 gm. ammonia and 3.5–4.5 gm. ammonium carbonate; used as a respiratory stimulant in syncope, weakness, or threatened faint. In veterinary medicine, it is used as a respiratory and circulatory stimulant, and sometimes as a carminative and antacid. Called also *ammonia s.* **anise s.,** a mixture of anise oil and alcohol; used as a carminative. **benzaldehyde s.,** a mixture of benzaldehyde, alcohol, and distilled water; used as a flavoring agent. **camphor s.** [USP], a solution of camphor and alcohol, each 100 ml. of which contains 9–11 gm. of camphor; used topically as a local irritant. It was formerly used for the treatment of diarrhea, and in hysteria and nervous excitement. **cardamom s., compound,** a preparation of cardamom oil, orange oil, cinnamon oil, clove oil, anethole, caraway oil, and alcohol, used as a flavoring vehicle. **cinnamon s.,** an alcoholic solution of cinnamon oil, each 100 ml. of which contains 9–11 ml. of the oil; used as a flavoring agent. **ether s.,** a transparent, colorless liquid with a burning sweetish taste and an ether odor, consisting of ethyl oxide and alcohol; formerly used as a carminative. Called also *Hoffmann's drops.* **ether s., compound,** a mixture of ethyl oxide, alcohol, and ethereal oil, which has been used as a carminative. In veterinary medicine, it is used as a stomachic and carminative. **ethyl nitrite s.,** an alcoholic solution containing 3.5–4.5 per cent of ethyl nitrite, which has been used as a diaphoretic and diuretic. Called also *s. of nitrous ether* and *sweet s. of nitre.* **glyceryl trinitrate s.,** nitroglycerin s. **lavender s.,** an alcoholic solution of lavender oil, each 100 ml. of which contains 4–6 ml. of lavender oil; used as a flavoring agent. **methylated s.,** denatured alcohol. **s. of Mindererus,** ammonium acetate solution. **nitroglycerin s.,** a clear, colorless liquid with the odor of alcohol, compounded of nitroglycerin 1–1.1 per cent in alcohol; used as a coronary vasodilator. Called also *glyceryl trinitrate s.* **s. of nitrous ether,** ethyl nitrite s. **orange s., compound** [USP], an alcoholic preparation containing orange, lemon, coriander, and anise oils; used as a flavoring agent. **peppermint s.** [USP], a preparation of peppermint, peppermint oil, and alcohol, used as a digestive aid and flavor. Called also *essence of peppermint.* **perfumed s.,** an aqueous solution of various fragrant oils, such as bergamot, lavender, lemon, orange flower, and rosemary, with alcohol, to which ethyl acetate has been added. **proof s.,** a product containing 50 per cent by volume of C_2H_2OH. **rectified s.,** alcohol. **spearmint s.,** an alcoholic solution of spearmint oil and powdered spearmint, each 100 ml. of which contains 9–11 ml. of spearmint oil. It has been used as a carminative. **sweet s. of nitre,** ethyl nitrite s. **s. of turpentine,** turpentine oil. **vanillin s., compound,** a preparation of vanillin and cardamom, cinnamon, and orange oils in alcohol; used as a flavoring agent. **s. of wine,** alcohol.

spirituous (spir′it-u-us) [L. *spirituosus*] alcoholic; containing a considerable proportion of alcohol.

spiro-, spir- 1. [Gr. *speira* coil] a combining form denoting relationship to a coil or spiral. 2. [L. *spirare* to breath] a combining form denoting relation to the breath or to breathing.

Spiro's test (spe′ro) [Karl *Spiro,* German chemist, 1867–1932] see under *tests.*

Spirocerca sanguinolenta (spi″ro-ser′kah sang″gwĭ-no-len′tah) a nematode of the family Spiruroidea, found in the walls of the aorta, esophagus, and stomach of dogs.

Spirochaeta (spi″ro-ke′tah) [Gr. *speira* coil + *chaitē* hair] a genus of microorganisms of the family Spirochaetaceae, order Spirochaetales, made up of flexible, undulating, spiral rods, found in fresh- or sea-water slime, especially when hydrogen sulfide is present. It includes five species: *S. daxen′sis, S. eurystrep′ta, S. mari′na, S. plica′tilis,* and *S. stenostrep′ta.* Most of the organisms placed in this genus in earlier taxonomic nomenclature have been reclassified in other genera. **S. grippotypho′sa,** *Leptospira grippotyphosa.* **S. pseudoicteroge′nes,** the name used in Germany to designate *Leptospira biflexa.*

Spirochaetaceae (spi″ro-ke-ta′se-e) a family of Schizomycetes (order Spirochaetales), made up of coarse spiral organisms, 30 to 5000 μ long, with definite protoplasmic structures, found in the intestinal tracts of bivalve mollusks and in stagnant fresh or salt water. It includes three genera: *Cristaspira, Saprospira,* and *Spirochaeta.*

Spirochaetales (spi″ro-ke-ta′lēz) an order of class Schizomycetes, made up of slender, undulating, motile organisms, 6 to 500μ long, in the form of spirals with at least one complete turn. It includes two families, Spirochaetaceae and Treponemataceae.

spirochetal (spi″ro-ke′tal) pertaining to or caused by spirochetes.

spirochete (spi′ro-kēt) 1. a spiral bacterium; a general term for any microorganism of the order Spirochaetales. 2. an organism of the genus *Spirochaeta.* **Dutton's s.,** *Borrelia duttonii.*

spirochetemia (spi″ro-ke-te′me-ah) [*spirochete* + Gr. *haima* blood + *-ia*] the presence of spirochetes in the blood.

spirocheticidal (spi″ro-ke″tĭ-si′dal) [*spirochete* + L. *caedere* to kill] destructive to spirochetes.

spirocheticide (spi″ro-ke″tĭ-sīd) an agent that causes the destruction of spirochetes.

spirochetogenous (spi″ro-ke-toj′ĕ-nus) caused by spirochetes.

spirochetolysin (spi″ro-ke-tol′ĭ-sin) a substance which causes lysis of spirochetes.

spirochetolysis (spi″ro-ke-tol′ĭ-sis) [*spirochete* + Gr. *lysis* dissolution] the destruction of spirochetes by lysis.

spirochetolytic (spi″ro-ke″to-lit′ik) pertaining to, characterized by, or causing spirochetolysis.

spirochetosis (spi″ro-ke-to′sis) infection with spirochetes. **s. arthrit′ica,** spirochetosis in which there is rheumatoid involvement of the joints. **bronchopulmonary s.,** bronchospirochetosis. **fowl s.,** a septicemic disease of fowls caused by the spirochete *Borrelia anserina,* and spread by the fowl tick *Argas persicus;* called also *spirillosis.* **icterogenic s., s. icterohaemorrhag′ica,** leptospiral jaundice.

spirocheturia (spi″ro-ke-tu′re-ah) [*spirochete* + Gr. *ouron* urine + *-ia*] the presence of spirochetes in the urine.

spirofibrilla (spi″ro-fi-bril′lah), pl. *spirofibril′lae* [*spiro-* (1) + L. *fibrilla*] Fayod's name for one of the hypothetical hollow, twisted fibrils forming the spirosparotae.

spirogram (spi′ro-gram) [L. *spirare* to breathe + Gr. *gramma* a writing] a tracing or graph of respiratory movements.

spirograph (spi′ro-graf) [L. *spirare* to breathe + Gr. *graphein* to write] an instrument for registering the respiratory movements.

spirographidin (spi″ro-graf′ĭ-din) (*obs.*) a hyalin derived from spirographin.

spirographin (spi-rog′rah-fin) a hyalogen derivable from the cartilage and skeletal structures of *Spirographis,* a marine worm.

spirography (spi-rog′rah-fe) the graphic measurement of breathing, including breathing movements and breathing capacity.

Spirogyra (spi″ro-ji′rah) a genus of fresh-water green algae having spiral chlorophyll bands and forming slimy masses in still waters and slow streams.

spiroid (spi′roid) resembling a spiral.

spiro-index (spi″ro-in′deks) [L. *spirare* to breathe + *index*] the value obtained by dividing the vital capacity by the height of the individual.

spirolactone (spi″ro-lak′tōn) a group of compounds bearing 17α-propionic acid as gamma-lactone with 17β-hydroxyl, capable of opposing the action of sodium-retaining steroids on renal transport of sodium and potassium. Three such compounds have been studied. The first contained angular methyl at C_{13} and C_{10}, and is 3-(3-keto-17β-hydroxy-4-androsten-17α-yl)-propionic acid-γ-lactone; the second, without angular methyl at C_{10}, is more potent, and the third (spironolactone), with a thioacetyl group at C_7, is highly active orally.

spiroma (spi-ro′mah) spiradenoma.

spirometer (spi-rom′ĕ-ter) [L. *spirare* to breathe + *metrum* measure] an instrument for measuring the air taken into and exhaled from the lungs.

Spirometra (spi″ro-met′rah) [*spiro-* (1) + Gr. *metra* womb, uterus] a genus of tapeworms of the family Diphyllobothriidae, order Pseudophyllidea, which are parasites of fish-eating cats, dogs, and birds. Infection in man is caused by eating inadequately cooked fish. **S. erinaceieuropa′ei**, a species parasitic in man, dogs, and cats. **S. mansonoi′des**, a species parasitic in dogs and cats, especially bobcats, which may cause diarrhea and anemia; infection with the larvae may cause sparganosis in man.

spirometric (spi″ro-met′rik) pertaining to spirometry or the spirometer.

spirometry (spi-rom′ĕ-tre) the measurement of the breathing capacity of the lungs. **bronchoscopic s.,** bronchospirometry.

Spironema (spi″ro-ne′mah) [Gr. *speira* coil + *nēma* thread] a name in Pribram's classification for a genus of spiral-shaped organisms, most of which are now included in the genus *Borrelia.*

spironolactone (spi-ro″no-lak′tōn) [USP] chemical name: 7α-(acetylthio)-17-hydroxy-3-oxo-pregn-4-ene-21-carboxylic acid γ-lactone acetate. A spirolactone, $C_{24}H_{32}O_4S$, occurring as a light-cream-colored to light tan, crystalline powder; it is an aldosterone antagonist, which increases urinary excretion of sodium and chloride, reduces excretion of potassium and ammonium and decreases the titratable acidity of urine. It is used in treatment of edema and ascites of hepatic cirrhosis, edema of congestive heart failure, and nephrotic syndrome.

spirophore (spi′ro-fōr) [L. *spirare* to breathe + Gr. *phorein* to bear] an apparatus to effect artificial respiration.

Spiroptera neoplastica (spi-rop′ter-ah ne″o-plas′tĭ-kah) a nematode which produces gastric carcinoma in certain species of rats.

Spiroschaudinnia (spi″ro-shaw-din′e-ah) a genus name proposed by Sambon (1907) for a group of spiral-shaped microorganisms found in the blood, most of which are now included in the genus *Borrelia.*

spiroscope (spi′ro-skōp) [L. *spirare* to breathe + Gr. *skopein* to examine] an apparatus for respiration exercises by which the patient can see the amount of water displaced in a given time and thus gauge his respiratory capacity.

spiroscopy (spi-ros′ko-pe) the use of the spiroscope.

spirosparta (spi″ro-spar′tah), pl. *spirospar′tae* [Gr. *speira* coil + *sparte* a rope] Fayod's name for one of the ropelike structures, formed by spirofibrillae, which constitute the protoplasm and nuclei of vegetable cells.

Spirotricha (spi″ro-trik′ah) [*spiro-* + Gr. *thrix* hair] an order of ciliate protozoa of the subclass Euciliata; it includes the suborder Hypotricha.

Spiruroidea (spi″roo-roi′de-ah) a superfamily of phasmid nematodes, including the genera *Gnathostoma, Gongylonema, Habronema, Physaloptera, Physocephalus, Spirocerca,* and *Thelazia.*

spissated (spis′āt-ed) [L. *spissatus*] inspissated: thickened by evaporation.

spissitude (spis′ĭ-tūd) [L. *spissitudo*] the state or quality of being inspissated.

Spitzka's nucleus, tract (spits′kahz) [Edward Charles *Spitzka,* New York neurologist, 1852–1914] see *Perlia's nucleus,* under *nucleus,* and see *tractus dorsolateralis.*

Spitzka-Lissauer tract (column) (spits′kah lis′ow-er) [E. C. *Spitzka;* Heinrich *Lissauer,* German neurologist, 1861–1891] tractus dorsolateralis.

Spivack's operation (spiv′aks) [Julius Leo *Spivack,* American surgeon, 1889–1956] see under *operation.*

splanchnapophyseal (splank″nap-o-fiz′e-al) pertaining to a splanchnapophysis.

splanchnapophysis (splank″nah-pof′ĭ-sis) [*splanchno-* + *apophysis*] a skeletal element, like the lower jaw, connected with the alimentary canal.

splanchnectopia (splank″nek-to′pe-ah) [*splanchno-* + Gr. *ektopos* out of place + *-ia*] displacement of a viscus.

splanchnesthesia (splank″nes-the′ze-ah) [*splanchno-* + Gr. *aisthēsis* perception + *-ia*] visceral sensation.

splanchnesthetic (splank″nes-thet′ik) pertaining to splanchnesthesia.

splanchnic (splank′nik) [Gr. *splanchnikos;* L. *splanchnicus*] pertaining to the viscera.

splanchnicectomy (splank″ne-sek′to-me) [*splanchnic* + Gr. *ektomē* excision] excision of a section (resection) of the greater splanchnic nerve; splanchnic neurectomy. This operation is combined with sympathectomy for the relief of essential hypertension.

splanchnicotomy (splank″ne-kot′o-me) [*splanchnic* + Gr. *tomē* a cutting] division of a splanchnic nerve.

splanchno- (splank′no) [Gr. *splanchnos* viscus] a combining form denoting relationship to a viscus, or to the splanchnic nerve.

splanchnoblast (splank′no-blast) [*splanchno-* + Gr. *blastos* germ] the rudiment or anlage of any viscus.

splanchnocele (splank′no-sēl) [*splanchno-* + Gr. *kēlē* hernia] hernial protrusion of a viscus.

splanchnocoele (splank′no-sēl) [*splanchno-* + Gr. *koilos* hollow] that portion of the embryonic body cavity, or coelom, from which are developed the abdominal, pericardial, and pleural cavities; called also *pleuroperitoneal cavity.*

splanchnocranium (splank″no-kra′ne-um) [*splanchno-* + *cranium*] those parts of the skull that are of branchial arch origin.

splanchnoderm (splank′no-derm) splanchnopleure.

splanchnodiastasis (splank″no-di-as′tah-sis) [*splanchno-* + Gr. *diastasis* separation] separation of a viscus; displacement of a viscus.

splanchnography (splank-nog′rah-fe) [*splanchno-* + Gr. *graphein* to write] the descriptive anatomy of the viscera.

splanchnolith (splank′no-lith) [*splanchno-* + Gr. *lithos* stone] an intestinal calculus or concretion.

splanchnologia (splank″no-lo′je-ah) splanchnology; in NA terminology *splanchnologia* encompasses the nomenclature relating to the viscera.

splanchnology (splank-nol′o-je) [*splanchno-* + Gr. *logos* treatise] the scientific study of the viscera of the body; applied also to the body of knowledge relating thereto.

splanchnomegalia (splank″no-mĕ-ga′le-ah) splanchnomegaly.

splanchnomegaly (splank″no-meg′ah-le) [*splanchno-* + Gr. *megas* large] enlargement of the viscera; visceromegaly.

splanchnomicria (splank″no-mik′re-ah) [*splanchno-* + Gr. *mikros* small] abnormal smallness of the viscera.

splanchnopathy (splank-nop′ah-the) [*splanchno-* + Gr. *pathos* disease] disease of the abdominal viscera.

splanchnopleural (splank″no-ploor′al) pertaining to the splanchnopleure.

splanchnopleure (splank′no-ploor) [*splanchno-* + Gr. *pleura* side] the layer formed by the union of the splanchnic mesoderm with entoderm; from it are developed the muscles and the connective tissue of the digestive tube.

splanchnoptosis (splank″no-to′sis) [*splanchno-* + Gr. *ptōsis* falling] the prolapse, or downward displacement, of the viscera; called also *visceroptosis.*

splanchnosclerosis (splank″no-skle-ro′sis) [*splanchno-* + Gr. *sklērōsis* hardening] induration of the viscera.

splanchnoscopy (splank-nos′ko-pe) [*splanchno-* + Gr. *skopein* to examine] inspection of the viscera by endoscopy.

splanchnoskeleton (splank″no-skel′e-ton) [*splanchno-* + Gr. *skeleton* a dried body, mummy] the totality of the skeletal structures connected with the viscera, especially the bony structure that forms within certain organs of animals, as in the gills, tongue, eye, penis, etc.

splanchnosomatic (splank″no-so-mat′ik) [*splanchno-* + Gr. *sōmatikos* of or for the body] pertaining to the viscera and the body proper.

splanchnotomy (splank-not′o-me) [*splanchno-* + Gr. *tomē* a cutting] the anatomy or dissection of the viscera.

splanchnotribe (splank′no-trīb) [*splanchno-* + Gr. *tribein* to crush] an instrument for crushing the intestine and so closing its lumen.

S-plasty in plastic surgery, a technique for distributing the contractile forces of wound healing in more than one direction by making an S-shaped incision, instead of a straight line, in areas where skin is loose.

splayfoot (spla′foot) flatfoot; talipes valgus.

spleen (splēn) [Gr. *splēn;* L. *splen*] a large glandlike but ductless organ situated in the upper part of the abdominal cavity on the left side and lateral to the cardiac end of the stomach. Called also *lien* [NA]. It is of a flattened oblong shape and about 125 mm. long, the largest structure in the lymphoid system; it has a purple color and a pliable consistency, and is distinguished by two types of tissue: red pulp and white pulp (see under *pulp*). It disintegrates the red blood cells and sets free the hemoglobin, which the liver converts into bilirubin; gives rise to new red blood cells during fetal life and in the newborn; serves as a reservoir of blood, produces lymphocytes and plasma cells, and has other important functions, the full scope of which is not entirely determined. **accessory s.,** a connected or detached outlying portion, or exclave, of the spleen; called also *lien accessorius.* **bacon s.,** a spleen with areas of amyloid degeneration, giving its cut surfaces the appearance of fried bacon. **cyanotic s.,** a contracted form of spleen due to passive congestion. **diffuse waxy s.,** amyloid degeneration of the spleen involving especially the coats of the venous sinuses and the reticulum of the organ. **enlarged s.,** splenomegaly. **flecked s. of Feitis,** multiple necroses of the spleen, characterized by nonembolic multiple areas of anemic necrosis. **floating s.,** a spleen displaced and preternaturally movable; called also *wandering s.* **Gandy-Gamna s.,** sideromegaly **hard-baked s.,** a condition of the spleen in Hodgkin's disease, marked by the presence of grayish areas resembling the diseased lymph nodes in structure. **lardaceous s.,** waxy s. **movable s.,** floating s. **porphyry s.,** a spleen which is the seat of nodular infiltration. **sago s.,** a spleen having on its cut surface the appearance of grains of sago; due to amyloid infiltration. **speckled s.,** flecked s. of Feitis. **wandering s.,** floating s. **waxy s.,** a spleen affected with amyloid degeneration; called also *lardaceous s.*

splen (splen) [Gr. *splēn*] spleen.

splen- see *spleno-*.

splenadenoma (splēn″ad-ĕ-no′mah) [splen- + Gr. *adēn* gland + *-oma*] hyperplasia of the spleen pulp.

splenalgia (sple-nal′je-ah) [splen- + Gr. *algos* pain + *-ia*] neuralgic pain in the spleen.

splenatrophy (splen-at′ro-fe) atrophy of the spleen.

splenauxe (sple-nawk′se) [splen- + Gr. *auxē* increase] splenomegaly.

splenceratosis (splen″ser-ah-to′sis) splenokeratosis.

splenculus (spleng′ku-lus) [L. "little spleen"] an accessory spleen, or splenic exclave.

splenectasis (sple-nek′tah-sis) [splen- + Gr. *ektasis* enlargement] splenomegaly.

splenectomize (sple-nek′to-mīz) to remove the spleen.

splenectomy (sple-nek′to-me) [splen- + Gr. *ektomē* excision] excision or extirpation of the spleen.

splenectopia (sple-nek-to′pe-ah) [splen- + Gr. *ek* out + *topos* place + *-ia*] displacement of the spleen; wandering or floating spleen.

splenectopy (sple-nek′to-pe) splenectopia.

splenelcosis (sple″nel-ko′sis) [splen- + Gr. *helkōsis* ulceration] ulceration of the spleen.

splenemia (sple-ne′me-ah) [splen- + Gr. *haima* blood + *-ia*] congestion of the spleen with blood.

splenemphraxis (sple″nem-frak′sis) [splen- + Gr. *emphraxis* stoppage] congestion of the spleen.

spleneolus (sple-ne′o-lus) accessory spleen.

splenetic (sple-net′ik) affected with splenic disorder; ill humored.

splenial (sple′ne-al) pertaining to the splenium or to the splenius muscle.

splenic (splen′ik) [Gr. *splēnikos;* L. *splenicus*] pertaining to the spleen; lienal.

splenicterus (splen-ik′ter-us) [splen- + Gr. *ikteros* jaundice] inflammation of the spleen associated with jaundice.

splenification (splen″ĭ-fi-ka′shun) splenization.

spleniform (splen′ĭ-form) resembling the spleen.

spleniserrate (splen″ĭ-ser′āt) pertaining to the splenius and the serratus muscles.

splenitis (sple-ni′tis) [splen- + *-itis*] inflammation of the spleen, a condition usually produced by pyemia. It is attended by enlargement of the organ with pus, and is marked by much local pain. **spodogenous s.,** that due to accumulation of foreign particles in the spleen.

splenium (sple′ne-um) [L.; Gr. *splēnion*] a bandlike structure; a bandage or compress. **s. cor′poris callo′si** [NA], the posterior rounded end of the corpus callosum.

splenization (splen″ĭ-za′shun) that condition of a part, especially the lung, in which it has the appearance of the tissue of the spleen, owing to engorgement and condensation. **hypostatic s.,** splenization produced by hypostatic pneumonia.

spleno-, splen- [Gr. *splēn* spleen] a combining form denoting relationship to the spleen.

splenoblast (sple′no-blast) the cell from which a splenocyte develops.

splenocele (sple′no-sēl) [spleno- + Gr. *kēlē* hernia] hernia of the spleen.

splenoceratosis (sple″no-ser″ah-to′sis) splenokeratosis.

splenocleisis (sple″no-kli′sis) [spleno- + Gr. *kleisis* closure] irritation of the surface of the spleen to induce the development of new fibrous tissue.

splenocolic (sple″no-kol′ik) [spleno- + Gr. *kolon* colon] pertaining to the spleen and colon.

splenocyte (splen′o-sīt) the monocyte characteristic of the spleen.

splenodynia (sple″no-din′e-ah) [spleno- + Gr. *odynē* pain + *-ia*] pain in the spleen.

splenogenous (sple-noj′ĕ-nus) arising in or formed by the spleen.

splenogram (sple′no-gram) 1. a roentgenogram of the spleen. 2. a differential count of the cells found in a stained preparation of material obtained by splenic puncture.

splenography (sple-nog′rah-fe) [spleno- + Gr. *graphein* to write] 1. roentgenography of the spleen. 2. a description of the spleen.

splenohepatomegalia (sple″no-hep″ah-to-me-ga′le-ah) splenohepatomegaly.

splenohepatomegaly (sple″no-hep″ah-to-meg′ah-le) [spleno- +

Gr. *hēpar* liver + *megas* large] enlargement of the spleen and liver.

splenoid (sple′noid) [spleno- + Gr. *eidos* form] resembling the spleen.

splenokeratosis (sple″no-ker″ah-to′sis) [spleno- + Gr. *keras* horn + *-osis*] hardening of the spleen.

splenolaparotomy (sple″no-lap″ah-rot′o-me) laparosplenotomy.

splenology (sple-nol′o-je) [spleno- + *-logy*] the sum of knowledge regarding the spleen, its functions and diseases.

splenolymphatic (sple″no-lim-fat′ik) pertaining to the spleen and lymph nodes.

splenolysin (sple-nol′ĭ-sin) [spleno- + Gr. *lyein* to dissolve] a lysin destructive to splenic tissue.

splenolysis (sple-nol′ĭ-sis) destruction of spleen tissue.

splenoma (sple-no′mah), pl. *splenomas* or *spleno′mata* [spleno- + *-oma*] a tumor of the spleen.

splenomalacia (sple″no-mah-la′she-ah) [spleno- + Gr. *malakia* softness] abnormal softness of the spleen; softening of the spleen.

splenomedullary (sple″no-med′u-ler″e) of or pertaining to the spleen and bone marrow.

splenomegalia (sple″no-me-ga′le-ah) splenomegaly.

splenomegaly (sple″no-meg′ah-le) [spleno- + Gr. *megas* large] enlargement of the spleen. **congestive s.,** enlargement of the spleen occurring secondary to portal hypertension, with ascites, anemia, thrombocytopenia, leukopenia, and episodic hemorrhage from the gastrointestinal tract. Called also *Banti's syndrome.* See also *Banti's disease,* under *disease.* **Egyptian s.,** that caused by *Schistosoma mansoni.* **Gaucher's s.,** see under *disease.* **hemolytic s.,** hemolytic anemia. **infective s., infectious s.,** splenomegaly associated with an infection. **myelophthisic s.,** enlargement of the spleen marked by decrease in myeloid tissue and by fibrosis. **Niemann's s.,** Niemann-Pick disease. **siderotic s.,** splenomegaly characterized by marked fibrosis with deposit of iron and calcium (Gamna nodules); called also *Gandy-Nanta disease.* **spodogenous s.,** enlargement of the spleen attributed to accumulation of erythrocytes in the organ. **thrombophlebitic s.,** Opitz's disease. **tropical s., febrile s.,** kala-azar.

splenometry (sple-nom′ĕ-tre) determination of the size of the spleen.

splenomyelogenous (sple″no-mi″ĕ-loj′ĕ-nus) formed in the spleen and bone marrow; splenomedullary.

splenomyelomalacia (sple″no-mi″ĕ-lo-mah-la′she-ah) [spleno- + Gr. *myelos* marrow + *malakia* softening] softening of the spleen and bone marrow.

splenoncus (sple-nong′kus) [spleno- + Gr. *onkos* bulk, mass] tumor of the spleen.

splenonephric (sple″no-nef′rik) pertaining to the spleen and the kidney.

splenonephroptosis (sple″no-nef″rop-to′sis) [spleno- + Gr. *nephros* kidney + *ptōsis* falling] downward displacement of the spleen and kidney on the same side.

splenopancreatic (sple″no-pan″kre-at′ik) pertaining to the spleen and the pancreas.

splenoparectasis (sple″no-pah-rek′tah-sis) [spleno- + Gr. *parektasis* extension] excessive enlargement of the spleen.

splenopathy (sple-nop′ah-the) [spleno- + Gr. *pathos* disease] any disease of the spleen.

splenopexia (sple″no-pek′se-ah) splenopexy.

splenopexis (sple′no-pek′sis) splenopexy.

splenopexy (sple′no-pek″se) [spleno- + Gr. *pexis* fixation] surgical fixation of a mobile spleen.

splenophrenic (splen-o-fren′ik) [spleno- + Gr. *phrēn* diaphragm] pertaining to the spleen and diaphragm.

splenopneumonia (splen″o-nu-mo′ne-ah) pneumonia attended with splenization of the lung.

splenoportography (sple″no-por-tog′rah-fe) splenic portography.

splenoptosia (sple″nop-to′se-ah) splenoptosis.

splenoptosis (sple″nop-to′sis) [spleno- + Gr. *ptōsis* falling] prolapse or downward displacement of the spleen.

splenorenal (sple″no-re′nal) pertaining to the spleen and kidney, or to splenic and renal veins.

splenorenopexy (sple″no-re′no-pek″se) nephrosplenopexy.

splenorrhagia (sple″no-ra′je-ah) [spleno- + Gr. *rhēgnynai* to burst forth] hemorrhage from the spleen.

splenorrhaphy (sple-nor′ah-fe) [spleno- + Gr. *rhaphē* suture] surgical repair of the spleen.

splenosis (sple-no′sis) a condition in which multiple implants of splenic tissue are present throughout the peritoneal cavity. **pericardial s.,** development between the heart and pericardium of splenic tissue deliberately introduced into the pericardial cavity as a means of increasing the blood supply to the heart muscle.

splenotomy (sple-not′o-me) [*spleno-* + Gr. *tome* a cutting] surgical incision of the spleen.

splenotoxin (sple″no-tok′sin) a toxin produced by or acting on the spleen.

splenulus (splen′u-lus) little spleen; an accessory spleen.

splenunculus (sple-nung′ku-lus) lienunculus.

splint (splint) 1. a rigid or flexible appliance for the fixation of displaced or movable parts. 2. [pl.] a condition characterized by development of exostoses on the rudimentary second or fourth metacarpal or metatarsal bone in the horse. **abutment s.**, adjacent tooth restorations that have been rigidly united at their proximal contact areas to form a multiple abutment. **Agnew's s.**, 1. one for fracture of the patella. 2. one used in fracture of the metacarpus. **airplane s.**, one which holds the arm in abduction; see illustration. **anchor s.**, a splint for fracture of the jaw, with metal loops fitting over the teeth and held together by a rod. **Anderson s.**, a splint for external internal fixation of fractures: two or more long screws, Kirschner wire, or nails are inserted through the tissues into the bone above and below the fracture; each group of screws, wires or nails is attached to an external plate and the plates are joined by an adjustable screw. **Angle's s.** a splint for fracture of the mandible; see illustration. **Asch's s.**, a tube splint for fracture of the nose. **Ashhurst's s.**, a bracketed splint of wire with a foot piece; made to cover the thigh and leg, and used after excision of the knee joint. **Balkan s.**, see under *frame*. **banjo traction s.**, a splint for the fingers constructed from a steel rod shaped like a banjo. **Bavarian s.**, a dressing formed by two pieces of flannel, folded once and sutured along the margin of the fold; between the layers of each fold, plaster cream is introduced, the seam serving as a hinge in the removal of the splint. **Böhler s.**, a piece of wood measuring 12 × 6 × 2 inches, rounded at the upper end to fit the axilla. **Bond's s.**, a form of splint for fracture of the lower end of the radius. **Bowlby's s.**, a splint for fracture of the shaft of the humerus. **bracketed s.**, a splint composed of two pieces of metal or wood joined by brackets. **Cabot's s.**, a posterior wire splint (see illustration). **cap s.**, a plastic or metallic fracture or stabilization appliance designed to cover the crowns of the teeth and usually cemented to them. **Carter's intranasal s.**, a fenestrated steel bridge, the wings of which are connected by a hinge; used in the bridge splint operation for depressed bridge of the nose. **Chandler felt collar s.**, see illustration. **Chatfield-Girdleston s.**, an apparatus for enabling a paralyzed poliomyelitis patient with bilateral deltoid paralysis to walk with crutches. **clavicular cross s.**, see illustration. **coaptation s's**, small splints adjusted about a fractured limb for the purpose of producing coaptation of fragments. **Cramer's s.**, a flexible wire splint consisting of parallel stout wires between which smaller wires are stretched like the rounds of a ladder. **Denis Browne s.**, a splint for the correction of talipes equinovarus. **drop foot s.**, see illustration. **Dupuytren's s.**, a splint to prevent eversion in Pott's fracture. **dynamic s.**, a support or protective apparatus for the hand or any other part of the body which also aids in initiating and performing motion of that part or adjacent parts and assists in dealing with the forces resulting from the action, thus assisting in those motions necessary to perform the activities of daily living. **Engelmann s.**, a big splint consisting of two strips of metal connecting at the top with a ring which fits over the thigh as high as it can be pushed up against the crotch. It is fastened at the lower end with a spike in each side which is driven into the shoe between the sole and upper, close to the heel. **Essig-type s.**, a stainless steel wire passed labially and lingually around a segment of the dental arch and held in position by individual ligature wires around the contact areas of the teeth; used to stabilize fractured or repositioned teeth. **Fox's s.**, an apparatus for fractured clavicle. **fracture s.**, any device fabricated of metal or plastic and used to fix segments in the treatment of fractures or facial deformities. Also, a plastic material contoured to the lingual and buccal-labial aspects of the teeth and fixed with wire or cement. **Frejka pillow s.**, one used for maintaining abduction and flexion of the femurs in congenital dislocation of the hip. **functional s.**, dynamic s. **Gibson's s.**, a form of Thomas splint. **Gilmer's s.**, a stainless steel wire fastening for holding the lower teeth to the upper ones in fracture of the mandible. **Gooch s.**, a flexible coaptation splint consisting of strips of wood arranged edge to edge and glued to cloth or leather. **Gordon's s.**, a side splint for the arm and hand in Colles' fracture. **Gunning's s.**, an interdental splint used in treating fractured mandible or maxilla. **Hodgen s.**, a wire splint for fracture of the femur below the upper third; see illustration. **interdental s.**, a plastic or metallic appliance for application to the dentition of the labial and/or lingual aspects to provide lugs for applying mandibular and/or maxillofacial traction or fixation. **Jones' nasal s.**, a splint for fracture of the nasal bones. **Kanavel's cock-up s.**, a splint for application to stiffened hands; see illustration. **Keller-Blake s.**, a hinged half-ring modification of the Thomas traction splint for fracture of the femur. **Kingsley s.**, a splint consisting of a base plate, precisely adapted to the upper dental arch, with steel metal arms that extend out through the mouth and then curve backward along the sides of the cheek to provide fixation to a head cap; used for fractures of the jaw. **Kirsch-**

ner wire s., a splint used to hold multiple metacarpophalangeal joints in flexion following excision of the collateral ligaments. **knee s.**, see illustration. **labial s.**, an appliance of plastic or metal, or both, made to conform to the outer aspect of the dental arch; used in the management of jaw and facial injuries. **Levis' s.**, a splint of perforated metal extending from below the elbow to the end of the palm. **lingual s.**, one similar to the labial splint, but conforming to the inner aspect of the dental arch. **Liston's s.**, a simple straight splint adapted to the side of the leg and body. **live s.**, dynamic s. **McIntire's s.**, a posterior splint for the leg and thigh, in the form of a double inclined plane. **Mason's s.**, a splint for the after-treatment of amputation at the elbow. **Middeldorpf's s.**, see under *triangle*. **plaster s.**, a splint composed of gauze impregnated with plaster of Paris. See illustration. **plastic s.**, an inflatable double-walled plastic tube for limb immobilization. **poroplastic s.**, a splint which can be softened with water and molded upon the limb. **Porzett s.**, a splint for controlling movement of the arms and of the head of the child after harelip operations. **Sayre's s.**, one of three varieties of splint: one for the ankle, one for the knee, and one for use in hip joint disease. **shin s's**, strain of the flexor digitorum longus muscle occurring in athletes, marked by pain along the shin bone. **Simpson's s.**, a shaped tampon of compressed cotton for inserting into the nasal fossa. **Stader s.**, a splint for external-internal fixation of fractures, consisting of a metal bar having a steel pin at each end for insertion into the bone on either side of the fracture so that the bar bridges the fracture; the ends of the fractured bone are drawn together by adjusting screws. **Stromeyer's s.**, a splint consisting of two hinged portions which can be fixed at any angle. **T s.**, a T-shaped splint made by tacking a transverse piece of splint board across the end of a vertical piece. **Taylor s.**, a steel support for the spine, used in disease or mechanical derangement of the spine; called also *Taylor's apparatus*. See illustration. **therapeutic s.**, dynamic s. **Thomas' knee s.**, a splint for removing the pressure of the weight of the body from the knee joint by transferring it to the ischium and perineum; see illustration. **Thomas' posterior s.**, a form of splint used in hip joint disease. **Tobruk s.**, an immobilizing split plaster cast applied from the foot to the groin, with skin traction tapes through openings in the plaster and connected with a Thomas splint. It was used in the North African campaign of World War II. **Toronto s.**, 1. a splint for poliomyelitis cases in which adjustable splints for the arms and legs are used with and attached to a Bradford frame. 2. a splinting catheter for use in the ureter after plastic operation. **Valentine's s.**, a splint for fracture of the clavicle. **Volkmann's s.**, a guttered splint with a foot piece and two lateral supports, for fracture of the lower extremity. **Wertheim s.**, a splint for fracture of a metacarpal bone.

splinter (splin′ter) 1. a small slender fragment, as a piece of fractured bone. 2. to break into small fragments.

splinting (splint′ing) 1. application of a splint, or treatment by use of a splint. 2. in dentistry, the application of a fixed restoration to join two or more teeth into a single rigid unit. 3. rigidity of muscles occurring as a means of avoiding pain caused by movement of the part.

splints (splintz) see *splint*, def. 2.

splitting (split′ing) division into fragments. In chemistry, the separation of a complex substance into two or more simpler substances. **s. of heart sounds**, the presence of two components in the first or second heart sound complexes; used chiefly to denote the separation of the elements of the second sound, which is related to closure of the aortic and pulmonary semilunar valves. **sagittal s. of mandible**, intraoral osteotomy of the ascending mandibular ramus and posterior body of the mandible in the sagittal plane for correction of prognathism, retrognathism, or open bite; an alternative procedure confines the split to the body of the mandible.

spodiomyelitis (spo″de-o-mi″ĕ-li′tis) [Gr. *spodios* ash colored + *myelos* marrow + *-itis*] acute anterior poliomyelitis.

spodo- (spod′o) [Gr. *spodos* ashes] a combining form denoting relation to waste materials.

spodogenous (spo-doj′ĕ-nus) [*spodo-* + Gr. *gennan* to produce] pertaining to or caused by waste materials in an organ.

spodogram (spod′o-gram) [*spodo-* + Gr. *gramma* a mark] the pattern created by the ash after incineration of a minute amount of tissue or other material; called also *ash picture*.

spodography (spo-dog′rah-fe) [*spodo-* + Gr. *graphein* to write] the incineration of a minute quantity of tissue and observation of the ashes (spodogram) under a dark-field microscope, as a means of studying the mineral constituents of the cells.

spondee (spon-de) any word (e.g., pancake) of two syllables having equal stress on each syllable; used in tests of speech reception threshold.

spondyl- (spon′dil) see *spondylo-*.

spondylalgia (spon″dĭ-lal′je-ah) pain in a vertebra.

spondylarthritis (spon″dil-ar-thri′tis) [*spondyl-* + Gr. *arthron* joint + *-itis*] arthritis of the spine. **s. ankylopoiet′ica**, rheumatoid s.

Plate XLV

splint

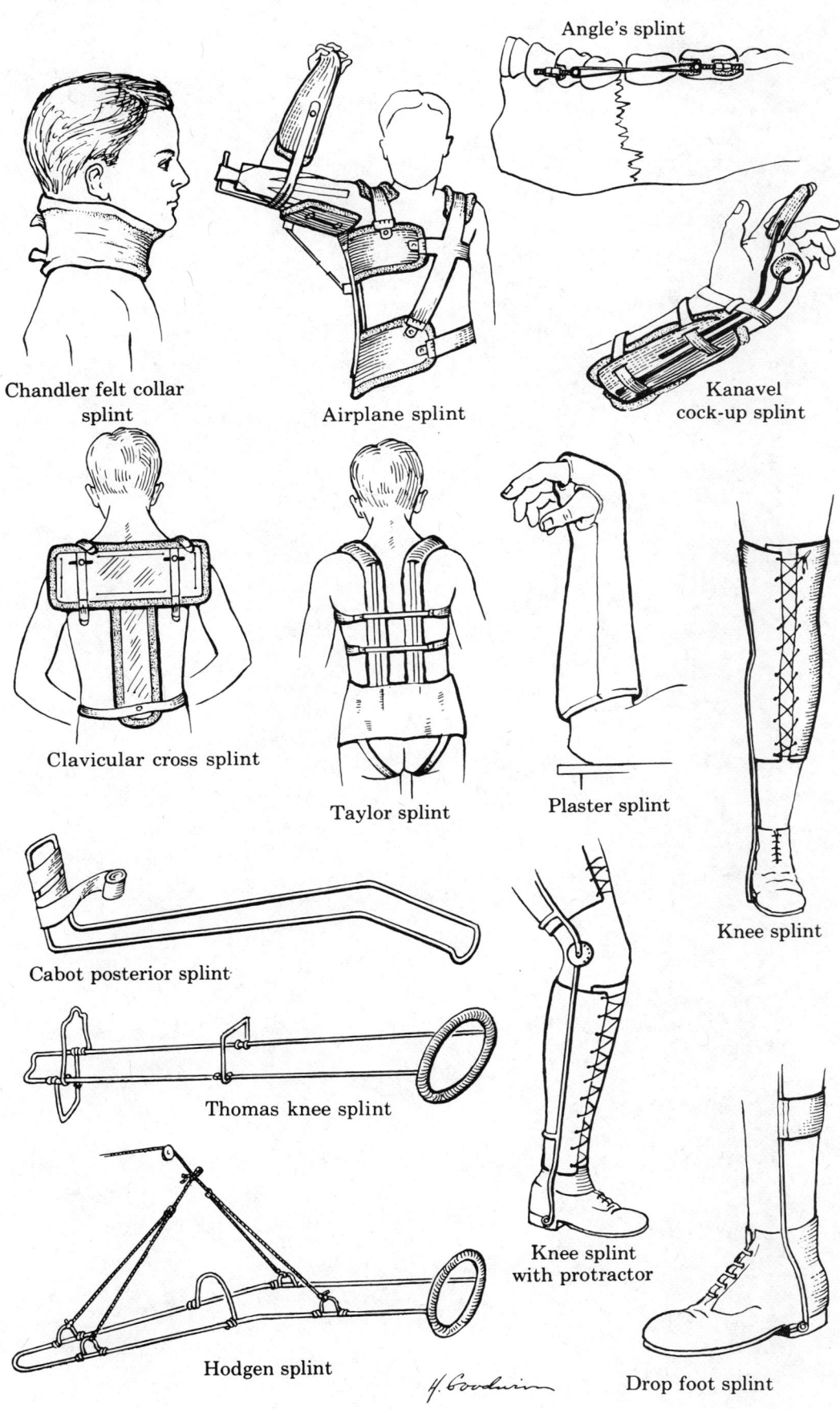

Angle's splint

Chandler felt collar
splint

Airplane splint

Kanavel
cock-up splint

Clavicular cross splint

Taylor splint

Plaster splint

Knee splint

Cabot posterior splint

Thomas knee splint

Hodgen splint

Knee splint
with protractor

Drop foot splint

VARIOUS TYPES OF SPLINT

spondylarthrocace (spon″dil-ar-throk′ah-se) [*spondyl-* + Gr. *arthron* joint + *kakē* badness] tuberculosis of the vertebrae.

spondyloarthropathy (spon″dĭ-lo-ar-throp′ah-the) disease of the joints of the spine.

spondylexarthrosis (spon″dil-eks″ar-thro′sis) [*spondyl-* + Gr. *exarthrōsis* dislocation] dislocation of a vertebra.

spondylitic (spon″dĭ-lit′ik) pertaining to or characterized by spondylitis.

spondylitis (spon″dĭ-li′tis) inflammation of the vertebrae. **s. ankylopoiet′ica, s. ankylo′sans, ankylosing s.,** rheumatoid s. **Bekhterev's s.,** rheumatoid s. **s. defor′mans,** rheumatoid s. **hypertrophic s.,** spondylitis with evidences of hypertrophic changes in the vertebrae. **s. infectio′sa,** inflammation of the vertebrae caused by a specific pathogen. **Kümmell's s.,** see under *disease*. **Marie-Strümpell s.,** rheumatoid s. **muscular s.,** a morbid condition of the spine resulting from muscular weakness and not a true inflammation. **post-traumatic s.,** Kümmell's disease. **rheumatoid s.,** the form of rheumatoid arthritis that affects the spine. It is a systemic illness of unknown etiology, affecting young males predominantly, and producing pain and stiffness as a result of inflammation of the sacroiliac, intervertebral, and costovertebral joints; paraspinal calcification, with ossification and ankylosis of the spinal joints, may cause complete rigidity of the spine and thorax. Called also *Bekhterev's disease* and *Marie-Strümpell disease.* **rhizomelic s., s. rhizome′lica, s. rhizomélique′,** rheumatoid s. **traumatic s.,** spondylitis occurring as a result of injury to the vertebrae. **s. tuberculo′sa, tuberculous s.,** tuberculosis of the spine. **s. typho′sa,** inflammation of the vertebrae following typhoid fever.

spondylizema (spon″dĭ-li-ze′mah) [*spondyl-* + Gr. *izēmia* depression] downward displacement of a vertebra in consequence of the destruction or softening of the one below it.

spondylo-, spondyl- [Gr. *spondylos* vertebra] combining form denoting relationship to a vertebra, or to the spinal column.

spondylocace (spon″dĭ-lok′ah-se) [*spondylo-* + Gr. *kakē* badness] tuberculosis of the vertebrae.

spondylodesis (spon″dĭ-lod′ĕ-sis) [*spondylo-* + Gr. *desis* binding] the operation of fusing the vertebrae by a short bone graft in cases of tuberculous spine.

spondylodidymia (spon″dĭ-lo-di-dim′e-ah) [*spondylo-* + Gr. *didymos* twin + *-ia*] teratic union of twins by the vertebrae.

spondylodymus (spon″dĭ-lod′ĭ-mus) twin fetuses united by the vertebrae.

spondylodynia (spon″dĭ-lo-din′e-ah) [*spondyl-* + Gr. *odynē* pain + *-ia*] pain in a vertebra.

spondylolisthesis (spon″dĭ-lo-lis′the-sis) [*spondyl-* + Gr. *olisthanein* to slip] forward displacement of one vertebra over another, usually of the fifth lumbar over the body of the sacrum, or of the fourth lumbar over the fifth, usually due to a developmental defect in the pars interarticularis.

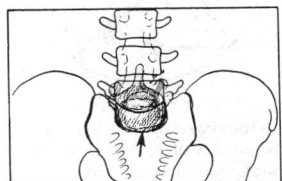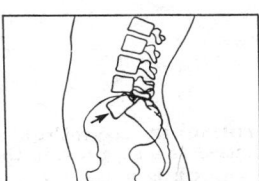

Spondylolisthesis of fifth lumbar vertebra over the sacrum (Meschan).

spondylolisthetic (spon″dĭ-lo-lis-thet′ik) pertaining to or caused by spondylolisthesis.

spondylolysis (spon″dĭ-lol′ĭ-sis) [*spondylo-* + Gr. *lysis* dissolution] dissolution of a vertebra; a condition marked by platyspondylia, aplasia of the vertebral arch, and separation of the pars interarticularis.

spondylomalacia (spon″dĭ-lo-mah-la′she-ah) softening of vertebrae. **s. traumat′ica,** Kümmell's disease.

spondylopathy (spon″dĭ-lop′ah-the) [*spondylo-* + Gr. *pathos* disease] any disorder of the vertebrae. **traumatic s.,** Kümmell's disease.

spondyloptosis (spon″dĭ-lo-to′sis) spondylolisthesis.

spondylopyosis (spon″dĭ-lo-pi-o′sis) [*spondylo-* + Gr. *pyōsis* suppuration] suppuration of a vertebra or of vertebrae.

spondyloschisis (spon″dĭ-los′kĭ-sis) [*spondylo-* + Gr. *schisis* fissure] congenital fissure of a vertebral arch.

spondylosis (spon″dĭ-lo′sis) ankylosis of a vertebral joint; also, a general term for degenerative changes due to osteoarthritis. **cervical s.,** degenerative joint disease affecting the cervical vertebrae, intervertebral disks, and surrounding ligaments and connective tissue, sometimes with pain or paresthesia radiating down the arms as a result of pressure on the nerve roots. **s. chron′ica ankylopoiet′ica, rhizomelic s.,** rheumatoid spondylitis. **lumbar s.,** degenerative joint disease affecting

the lumbar vertebrae and intervertebral disks, causing pain and stiffness, sometimes with sciatic radiation due to nerve root pressure by associated protruding disks or osteophytes. **s. uncovertebra′lis,** cervical spondylosis affecting the uncinate process of a vertebra.

spondylosyndesis (spon″dĭ-lo-sin′de-sis) [*spondylo-* + Gr. *syndesis* a binding together] operative immobilization or ankylosis of the spine; spinal fusion.

spondylotherapy (spon″dĭ-lo-ther′ah-pe) [*spondylo-* + Gr. *therapeia* treatment] treatment by physical methods applied to the spinal region; spinal therapeutics.

spondylotic (spon″dĭ-lot′ik) pertaining to or due to spondylosis.

spondylotomy (spon″dĭ-lot′o-me) [*spondylo-* + Gr. *temnein* to cut] rachitomy.

spondylous (spon′dĭ-lus) pertaining to a vertebra; vertebral.

spongarion (spon-ga′re-on) [Gr.] an ancient eye salve.

sponge (spunj) [L., Gr. *spongia*] 1. the elastic fibrous skeleton of certain marine animals; used mainly as an absorbent. 2. an absorbent pad of folded gauze or cotton. **Bernays' s.,** compressed disks of cotton which expand under moisture; used in checking epistaxis. **ear s.,** a small piece of sponge attached to a handle and used for washing the ear. **fibrin s.,** a spongy form of fibrin, used as a hemostatic. **gelatin s.,** a spongy form of denatured gelatin used as a hemostatic, especially when wet with thrombin. **gelatin s., absorbable** [USP], a sterile, absorbable, water-insoluble gelatin-base sponge; used as a local hemostatic.

spongeitis (spon″je-i′tis) spongiitis.

spongia (spon′je-ah) [L.; Gr.] sponge. **s. gelati′na absorben′da,** absorbable gelatin sponge.

spongiform (spon′jĭ-form) [L. *spongia* sponge + *forma* shape] resembling a sponge.

spongiitis (spon″je-i′tis) inflammation of the corpus spongiosum of the penis; periurethritis.

spongin (spon′jin) a horny, albuminoid material forming the basis of sponge.

spongio- [L., Gr. *spongia* sponge] a combining form meaning like a sponge, or denoting relationship to a sponge.

spongioblast (spon′je-o-blast″) [*spongio-* + Gr. *blastos* germ] 1. any of the embryonic epithelial cells, developed about the neural tube, which become transformed, some into neuroglial and some into ependymal cells. 2. amacrine (def. 2).

spongioblastoma (spun″je-o-blas-to′mah) a tumor containing spongioblasts; gliosarcoma or glioblastoma. **s. multifor′me,** one in which the cells are of various forms of arrangements; called also *glioma multiforme.* **s. unipola′re,** one in which the spongioblasts are mostly unipolar.

spongiocyte (spun′je-o-sīt″) 1. a neuroglial cell. 2. one of the cells with spongy vacuolated protoplasm in the cortex of the suprarenal gland.

spongiocytoma (spun″je-o-si-to′mah) spongioblastoma.

spongioid (spun′je-oid) [*spongio-* + Gr. *eidos* form] resembling a sponge in structure or appearance.

spongioplasm (spun′je-o-plazm) [*spongio-* + Gr. *plasma* anything formed or molded] 1. a substance which forms the network of fibrils pervading the cell substance and forming the reticulum of the fixed cell. 2. the granular material of an axon.

spongiosa (spun″je-o′sah) [L.] spongy; sometimes used alone to mean the substantia spongiosa ossium.

spongiosaplasty (spun″je-o″sah-plas′te) autoplasty of the substantia spongiosa ossium to potientiate formation of new bone or to cover bone defects.

spongiosis (spun″je-o′sis) intercellular edema of the spongy layer (malpighian layer) of the skin.

spongiositis (spun″je-o-si′tis) inflammation of the corpus spongiosum of the penis.

spongiotic (spun″je-ot′ik) pertaining to or characterized by spongiosis.

spongosterol (spon-gos′ter-ol) a mono-unsaturated sterol, 24α-methyl-22-cholestene-3β-ol, found in certain sponges.

spongy (spun′je) of a spongelike appearance or texture.

spontaneous (spon-ta′ne-us) [L. *spontaneus*] 1. voluntary; instinctive. 2. occurring without external influence.

Spontin (spon′tin) trademark for a lyophilized preparation of ristocetins A and B.

spool (spōōl) a tubular surgical instrument around which suture material is usually wound. **Carassini's s.,** a sectional spool made of aluminum for use in end-to-end intestinal anastomosis.

spoon (spōōn) a metallic instrument with an oval bowl to which a handle is attached. **Bunge's s.,** an instrument for eviscerating the eyeball. **Daviel's s.,** an instrument used in removing the crystalline lens from the eye. **excavator s.,** a spoon-shaped dental excavator. **marrow s.,** a gouge for removing marrow from bones. **sharp s.,** a spoon with a sharp-edged bowl; used for scraping away granulations, etc. **test s.,** a small spoon with a spatula-like handle for taking up small quantities of a powder, etc., in chemical experiments. **Volkmann's s.,** sharp s.

sporadic (spo-rad'ik) [Gr. *sporadikos* scattered; L. *sporadicus*] not widely diffused or epidemic; occurring only occasionally.

sporadin (spo'rah-din) trophozoite.

sporadoneure (spo-rad'o-nūr) [Gr. *sporadikos* sporadic + *neuron* nerve] an isolated nerve cell occurring in any of the tissues.

sporangia (spo-ran'je-ah) [L.; Gr.] plural of *sporangium.*

sporangial (spo-ran'je-al) pertaining to a sporangium.

sporangiophore (spo-ran'je-o-fōr) the threadlike stalk which bears at its tip the sporangium of phycomycetous molds.

sporangiospore (spo-ran'je-o-spōr) a spore contained in a sporangium.

sporangium (spo-ran'je-um), pl. *sporan'gia* [spore + Gr. *angeion* vessel] any encystment containing spores or sporelike bodies, as in certain of the fungi. See *spore.*

sporation (spo-ra'shun) sporulation.

spore (spōr) [L. *spora;* Gr. *sporos* seed] 1. a refractile, oval body formed within bacteria, especially *Bacillus* and *Clostridium,* which is regarded as a resting stage during the life history of the cell, and is characterized by its resistance to environmental changes. Called also *bacterial s.* 2. the reproductive element, produced sexually or asexually, of one of the lower organisms, such as protozoa, fungi, algae, etc. Spores arising as a result of a nonsexual process include: *conidia,* which are deciduous and develop from the hyphae by budding; *aleuriospores,* which are nondeciduous and also develop from the hyphae by budding; *endospores,* which are formed in the interior of special spore cases called *sporangia; zoospores,* which are flagellated motile spores formed in cases known as *zoosporangia;* and *chlamydospores,* which are resting spores, with thick walls, produced by enlargement of special cells. Those arising as a result of a sexual process include: *ascospores,* which are contained in special spore cases called *asci; basidiospores,* which are formed at the ends of club-shaped structures called *basidia; zygospores,* which are formed by conjugation between two morphologically identical cells, or from the fusion of like gametangia; and *oospores,* which are formed by heterogamous fertilization. See also *sporulation.* **asexual s.,** a spore produced by various methods, but not involv-

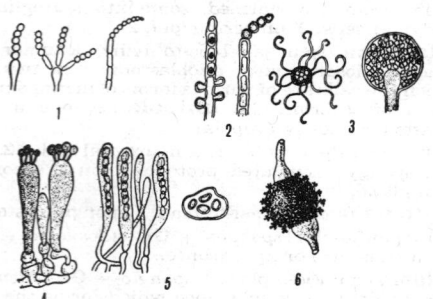

Various types of spores in fungi: 1, conidiospores; 2, chlamydospores; 3, sporangiospores; 4, basidiospores; 5, ascospores; 6, zygospores (de Rivas).

ing a sexual process. **bacterial s.,** see *spore,* def. 1. **black s's of Ross,** pigmented malarial oocysts in the stomach wall of a mosquito. **swarm s.,** a spore made up of numerous active motile individuals; a zoospore. **washed s's,** spores of bacteria which have been freed from their toxin by washing.

sporenrest (spo'ren-rest) [Ger.] residual body.

sporetia (spo-re'she-ah) that part of the extranuclear chromatin of a cell that is concerned in the reproductive function of the cell.

sporicidal (spo"ri-si'dal) [spore + L. *caedere* to kill] destroying spores.

sporicide (spo'ri-sīd) an agent that destroys spores.

sporidesmin (spōr"i-des'min) a poisonous substance isolated from the fungus *Pithomyces chartarum* (class Deuteromycetes), which causes facial eczema and liver damage in sheep and cattle in New Zealand and Australia.

sporiferous (spo-rif'er-us) [spore + L. *ferre* to bear] producing or bearing spores.

sporiparous (spo-rip'ah-rus) [spore + L. *parere* to produce] producing spores.

sporo- (spo'ro) [Gr. *sporos* seed] a combining form denoting relationship to a spore.

sporoagglutination (spo"ro-ah-gloo"ti-na'shun) agglutination of spores in the diagnosis of sporotrichosis.

sporoblast (spo'ro-blast) [sporo- + Gr. *blastos* germ] one of the bodies developed within the oocyst of the malarial parasite (*Plasmodium*) in the mosquito from which the sporozoite later

develops; also used to refer to similar stages in other sporozoa, e.g., *Isospora* and *Toxoplasma.*

sporocyst (spo'ro-sist) [sporo- + Gr. *kystis* sac, bladder] 1. any cyst or sac containing spores or reproductive cells, especially in lower eukaryotic organisms, e.g., protists. 2. a saclike organism which develops from a miracidium in the body of a snail host and contains germ cells which give rise to other sporocysts or to rediae in the life cycle of certain helminths. 3. the stage formed from a sporoblast, within the oocyst, in which sporozoites develop; it is differentiated from the sporoblast by the presence of a cyst wall.

Sporocytophaga (spo"ro-si-to'fah-gah) [Sporo- + Gr. *phagein* to eat] a genus of bacteria of the family Myxococcaceae.

sporoduct (spo'ro-dukt) a tubelike structure in the walls of certain sporocysts through which the spores are given off.

sporogenesis (spo"ro-jen'ĕ-sis) [sporo- + Gr. *genesis* production] the formation of spores; reproduction by spores.

sporogenic (spo"ro-jen'ik) capable of developing into or producing spores.

sporogenous (spo-roj'ĕ-nus) [sporo- + Gr. *gennan* to produce] reproduced by spores.

sporogeny (spo-roj'ĕ-ne) [sporo- + Gr. *gennan* to produce] the development of spores.

sporogony (spo-rog'o-ne) [sporo- + Gr. *goneia* generation] the sexual cycle of sporozoa, especially the life cycle of the malarial parasite (*Plasmodium*) in the stomach and body of the mosquito, in which the encysted zygote undergoes multiple divisions, giving rise to sporozoites. Cf. *schizogony.*

sporont (spo'ront) [sporo- + Gr. *ōn, ontos* being] a mature protozoon in its sexual cycle. Cf. *schizont.*

sporophore (spo'ro-fōr) [sporo- + Gr. *phorein* to bear] that part of an organism that supports the spores.

sporophyte (spo'ro-fīt) [sporo- + Gr. *phyton* plant] the diploid or asexual stage in the antithetic alternation of generation.

sporoplasm (spo'ro-plazm) [sporo- + Gr. *plasma* anything formed or molded] the protoplasm of spores.

sporoplasmic (spo"ro-plaz'mik) pertaining to or of the nature of sporoplasm.

Sporothrix (spo'ro-thriks) a genus of imperfect fungi of the family Moniliaceae, order Moniliales. *S. schenck'ii* (formerly called *Sporotrichum schenckii*) causes sporotrichosis, and many species, including *S. car'nis,* cause the formation of white mold on meat in cold storage.

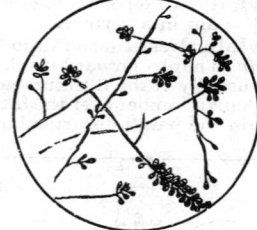

Sporothrix schenckii (de Rivas).

sporotrichin (spo-rot'ri-kin) a derivative of *Sporothrix schenkii* used as a skin test in the diagnosis of sporotrichosis.

sporotrichosis (spo"ro-tri-ko'sis) a chronic fungal infection caused by *Sporothrix schenckii,* occurring in three forms. The *cutaneous lymphatic form* is characterized by a single pustule, papule, or nodule at the site of invasion, followed by lymphatic spread and the development of multiple, painless, subcutaneous granulomas, which tend to break down and form indolent ulcers or cold abscesses. The *disseminated form* is marked by multiple, painless, cutaneous or subcutaneous nodules, which may form cold abscesses, ulcers, or fistulas; this form may involve the muscles, joints, bones, eyes, gastrointestinal system, mucous membranes, and nervous system. The *pulmonary form* results from the inhalation of spores and causes acute disease or chronic granulomas similar to those seen in other mycoses.

sporotrichotic (spo"ro-tri-kot'ik) 1. pertaining to or caused by fungi of the genus *Sporothrix.* 2. pertaining to sporotrichosis.

Sporotrichum (spo-rot'ri-kum) [sporo- + Gr. *thrix* hair] a genus of soil-inhabiting imperfect fungi of the family Moniliaceae, order Moniliales, which formerly included the etiologic agent of sporotrichosis. See *Sporothrix.*

Sporovibrio (spōr"o-vib'bre-o) a genus of hydrogen bacteria.

Sporozoa (spo"ro-zo'ah) [sporo- + Gr. *zōon* animal] a subphylum of diverse endoparasitic protozoa characterized by the lack of locomotor organs in the adult stages and by a complex life cycle usually involving an alternation of a sexual with an asexual generation. It includes the orders Gregarinida, Coccidia, Haemosporidia, Sarcosporidia, Microsporidia, and Myxosporidia.

sporozoa (spo"ro-zo'ah) [Gr.] plural of *sporozoon.*

sporozoan (spo"ro-zo'an) 1. pertaining to sporozoa. 2. a sporozoon.

sporozoite (spo″ro-zo′īt) [*sporo-* + Gr. *zōon* animal] A spore formed after fertilization; any of the elongated, nucleated cells formed by division of the encysted zygote (sporogony) of a sporozoon, which undergo multiple fission (schizogony) to give rise to merozoites. In malaria, the sporozoites are the forms of *Plasmodium* which are liberated from the oocysts in the mosquito, accumulate in the salivary glands, and are transferred to man when the mosquito bites. Called also *falciform body*. See illustration accompanying *Plasmodium*.

sporozooid (spo″ro-zo′oid) 1. resembling a sporozoon. 2. a falciform body resembling a sporozoon.

sporozoon (spo″ro-zo′on), pl. *sporozo′a*. Any organism or species belonging to the subphylum Sporozoa.

sporozoosis (spo″ro-zo-o′sis) infection with sporozoa.

sport (spōrt) a mutation; lusus naturae.

sporular (spōr′u-lar) pertaining to a spore.

sporulation (spōr″u-la′shun) the formation of spores. A form of reproduction seen in lower eukaryotic organisms, such as protozoa, fungi, most algae, etc., consisting of spontaneous division of the cell into four or more daughter elements, each with a part of the original cell nucleus. Also, in response to conditions no longer favorable for growth of the cell, the formation, by certain bacteria, of a resting spore, which is resistant to adverse environmental conditions; on restoration of a favorable environment, the cell becomes vegetative again. Called also *spore formation*. See also *spore*. **endogenous s.,** sporulation of a protozoon within its host. **exogenous s.,** sporulation of a protozoon to produce the infection of fresh hosts.

sporule (spor′ūl) a small spore.

spot (spot) a circumscribed area or place distinguished by its color; a loculus or macula; see also *tâche*. **acoustic s's,** the maculae sacculi and maculae utriculi. **Bitot's s's,** superficial, foamy gray, triangular spots on the conjunctiva, consisting of keratinized epithelium; they are associated with vitamin A deficiency. See also *xerosis conjunctivae*. **blind s.,** the area marking the site of entrance of the optic nerve on the retina (optic disk); so called because there are no sensory receptors in this region and hence no response to stimuli restricted to it. **blind s., mental,** mental scotoma. **blue s.,** 1. [pl.] maculae caeruleae. 2. mongolian spot. **Brushfield's s's,** small white spots on the periphery of the iris, usually crescentic, with the concavity outward, frequently but not exclusively seen in children with Down's syndrome. **café au lait s's** (kah-fa′o-la′) [Fr.], pigmented macules of a distinctive light brown color, like coffee with milk, as in neurofibromatosis and Albright's syndrome. **Carleton's s's,** sclerosed spots in the bones in gonorrheal disease. **Cayenne pepper s's,** minute, punctate telangiectases (cherry angiomas) lying within individual dermal papillae in lesions of angioma serpiginosum. **cherry-red s.,** a red circular area (the choroid) surrounded by gray-white retina, seen through the fovea centralis of the eye in the infantile and sometimes in the late infantile form of amaurotic familial idiocy; called also *Tay's sign* or *spot*. **Christopher's s's,** Maurer's dots; see under *dot*. **chromatin s.,** sex chromatin. **cold s.,** see *temperature s's*. **cotton-wool s's,** white or gray soft-edged opacities in the retina composed of cytoid bodies; seen in hypertensive retinopathy, lupus erythematosus, and numerous other conditions. Called also *cotton-wool exudates* or *patches*. **cribriform s's,** maculae cribrosae. **deaf s.,** deaf point. **De Morgan's s's,** cherry angiomas; see under *disk*. **epigastric s.,** a point of tenderness exactly over the xiphoid process. **eye s.,** 1. the rudiment of an eye in the embryo. 2. eyespot. 3. stigma (def. 5). **flame s's,** flame-shaped hemorrhages. **focal s.,** the part of the target of an x-ray tube which is bombarded by the focused electron stream when the tube is energized. **Fordyce's s's,** enlarged and ectopic sebaceous glands that appear as minute yellow papules on the oral mucosa; called also *Fordyce's disease* or *granules*. **Forschheimer s's,** a fleeting exanthem consisting of discrete rose spots on the soft palate, which may coalesce into a red blush and may extend over the fauces; sometimes seen in rubella just prior to the onset of the skin rash. **germinal s.,** the nucleolus of an ovum. **Graefe's s's,** spots over the vertebrae, pressure on which produces relaxation of blepharofacial spasm. **hot s.,** 1. see *temperature s's*. 2. the sensitive area of a neuroma. 3. an area of increased density on an x-ray or thermographic film. **hypnogenetic s.,** any superficial area the stimulation of which will bring on sleep. **Janeway's s's,** small nodular hemorrhagic spots on the palms and soles in cases of subacute bacterial endocarditis. **Koplik's s's,** small, irregular, bright red spots on the buccal and lingual mucosa, with a minute bluish white speck in the center of each; seen in the prodromal stage of measles. Called also *Koplik's sign*. **light s.,** cone of light; see under *cone*. **liver s.,** a lay term for brownish spots on the face, neck, or back of the hand in many older people. **Mariotte's s.,** blind s. **Maurer's s's,** see under *dot*. **Maxwell's s.,** macula retinae. **milk s's,** 1. whitish spots of fibrous thickening seen on the visceral layer of the pericardium in postmortem examination. 2. dense masses of macrophages in the omentum. **milky s's,** aggregations of macrophages in the subserous connective tissue of the pleura and peritoneum. **mongolian s.,** a flat, smooth, brown to grayish

blue nevus, 2 to 15 cm. in diameter, consisting of an excess of dermal melanocytes, typically found at birth in the sacral region in Orientals, Negroes, American Indians, and many southern European babies, and usually disappearing completely during childhood. Exceptionally, it may occur on almost any other part of the body. See *nevus of Ota* and *nevus of Ito*, under *nevus*. **pain s's,** spots on the skin where alone the sense of pain can be produced by a stimulus. **pelvic s's,** round or oval shadows often seen on fluoroscopic examination in the region of the inferior spine of the ilium and the horizontal ramus of the pubic bone. **plague s's,** ecchymotic or purpuric spots seen in some cases of bubonic plague. **rose s's,** an eruption of rose-colored spots, appearing on the abdomen and loins during the first seven days of typhoid fever; called also *typhoid spots*. **Roth's s's,** round or oval white spots sometimes seen in the retina early in the course of subacute bacterial endocarditis. **sacral s.,** mongolian s. **sacral bald s.,** sacrococcygeal dimple, a congenital abnormality in the sacrococcygeal region marked by the absence of hair follicles on the epidermis. **Soemmering's s.,** macula retinae. **soldier's s's,** milk s's, def. 1. **spongy s.,** zona vasculosa. **Stephen's s's,** Maurer's dots. **Tardieu's s's,** spots of ecchymosis under the pleura following death by suffocation. **Tay's s.,** cherry-red s. **temperature s's,** hot and cold spots: spots on the skin normally anesthetic to pain and pressure and sensitive respectively to heat and cold; they are arranged in lines, often somewhat curved, and show the peculiar arrangement of the end-organs with respect to the temperature sense. **tendinous s's,** maculae albidae. **Trousseau's s's,** tache cérébrale. **typhoid s's,** rose s's. **vital s's,** a name sometimes given to any of the major autonomic centers in the pons and medulla oblongata which are indispensable to life. **Wagner's s.,** the nucleolus of the human ovum. **warm s's,** minute areas in the skin that are peculiarly sensitive to temperatures above body temperature; see *temperature s's*. **Willner's s's,** efflorescent spots, soon becoming pustules, on the internal layer of the prepuce; seen in the early stages of smallpox. **yellow s.,** macula retinae.

sprain (sprān) a joint injury in which some of the fibers of a supporting ligament are ruptured but the continuity of the ligament remains intact. **riders' s.,** sprain of the adductor longus muscle of the thigh, resulting from strain in riding horseback. **Schlatter's s.,** Osgood-Schlatter disease.

spray (sprā) a liquid minutely divided or nebulized as by a jet of air or steam. **ether s.,** ether applied in a nebulized form to produce local anesthesia by chilling the part. **needle s.,** a water spray administered through a device having needle-sized jets. **Peet-Schultz s.** (*obs.*), a nasal spray for preventive application against poliomyelitis. **Pickrell's s.,** a solution of 3.5 per cent sulfathiazine in 6 per cent triethanolamine for spraying on burned areas; called also *Pickrell's method*. **Tucker's s.** (*obs.*), a nasal spray for asthma containing 1 per cent cocaine and 5 per cent potassium nitrate. **tyrothricin s.,** a solution of tyrothricin and water, made with suitable, harmless, solubilizing and wetting agents; it may contain a small proportion of alcohol and a suitable vasoconstrictor. It is used as a topical antibiotic.

spreader (spred′er) an instrument for distributing something over a broader area. **root canal s.,** a pointed instrument of variable diameter and taper, specifically designed for laterally condensing the root canal filling material.

Sprengel's deformity (spreng′elz) [Otto Gerhard Karl *Sprengel*, German surgeon, 1852–1915] see under *deformity*.

sprew (sproo) sprue.

spring (spring) an elastic wire attached to a denture or other appliance. **auxiliary s.,** a short piece of wire attached to an orthodontic appliance to serve as a lever to apply force to a tooth or teeth. **coil s.,** lengths of coil spring used as a part of orthodontic appliances to open or to close spaces between teeth. **Z s.,** a spring bent in the form of a Z with a coil loop at each end, used to move an individual tooth or groups of teeth buccally or labially.

sprue (sproo) 1. a chronic form of malabsorption syndrome occurring in both tropical and nontropical forms; called also *catarrhal dysentery*. 2. in dentistry, the hole through which metal or other material is poured or forced into a mold. **nontropical s.,** a malabsorption syndrome affecting both children and adults, precipitated by the ingestion of gluten-containing foods; its etiology is unknown, but a hereditary factor has been implicated. Pathologically, the proximal intestinal mucosa loses its villous structure, surface epithelial cells exhibit degenerative changes, and their absorptive function is severely impaired. It is characterized by diarrhea in which the stools are bulky, frothy, fatty (steatorrhea), and fetid (occasionally, malabsorption may be associated with the passage of a single bulky stool without diarrhea), and by abdominal distention, flatulence, weight loss, asthenia, deficiency of vitamins B, D, and K, and electrolyte depletion. Called also *celiac disease* and *gluten enteropathy*. In the *infantile form* the onset is insidious, and is marked by irritability, loss of appetite, weakness, extreme wasting, growth retardation, and celiac crisis; called also *infantile celiac disease*. The *adult form* is marked by extreme lassitude, fatigue, difficulty in breathing, clubbing of the fingers, bone pain, cramping of the muscles, tetany, abdominal distention during the day, megacolon, tympanitis, and skin pigmentation; called also *adult celiac disease*. **tropical s.,** a malabsorption syndrome occurring in the tropics and subtropics. Protein malnutrition is usually precipitated by the malabsorption, and anemia due to folic acid deficiency is particularly common. Administration of antibiotics (especially tetracycline) and folic acid usually results in remission. Called also *Ceylon sore mouth, Cochin-China diarrhea, psilosis stomatitis intertropica,* and *stomatitis tropica.*

Spt. abbreviation for L. *spir'itus,* spirit.

spur (sper) a projecting body, as from a bone. In dentistry, a piece of metal projecting from a plate, band, or other dental appliance. **calcaneal s.,** a bone excrescence on the lower surface of the calcaneus which frequently causes pain on walking. **Morand's s.,** calcar avis. **occipital s.,** an abnormal process of bone on the occipital bone behind the posterior process of the atlas. **olecranon s.,** an abnormal process of bone at the insertion of the triceps muscle.

spurious (spu're-us) [L. *spurius*] simulated; not genuine; false.

sputamentum (spu"tah-men'tum) [L.] sputum.

sputum (spu'tum) [L.] matter ejected from the lungs, bronchi, and trachea, through the mouth. **s. aerogino'sum,** green s. **albuminoid s.,** a yellowish, frothy sputum of persons from whom large amounts of pleural fluid have been withdrawn; believed to be due to pulmonary edema. **s. coc'tum,** the opaque mucopus of the later stages of bronchitis and laryngitis. **s. cru'dum,** the clear, tenacious mucus of the early stages of laryngitis and bronchitis. **s. cruen'tum,** bloody sputum. **globular s.,** sputum in yellow spherical lumps; said to be characteristic of the late stages of tuberculosis. **green s.,** sputum stained with a green pigment, as in certain cases of jaundice. **icteric s.,** sputum stained with a greenish or yellow tint by bile pigments, as in jaundice. **moss-agate s.,** a grayish, opalescent, gelatinous mottled sputum, usually projected from the mouth in a more or less globular form during coughing; characteristic of diseases of the trachea (Chevalier Jackson). **nummular s.,** sputum in rounded disks, shaped somewhat like coins. **prune juice s.,** dark, reddish brown, bloody sputum of certain forms of pneumonia, cancer of the lung, gangrene, etc. **rusty s.,** sputum stained with blood or blood pigments; seen in pneumonia, etc.

SQ abbreviation (symbol) for *subcutaneous.*

squalene (skwal'ēn) an unsaturated terpene hydrocarbon, $[(CH_3)_2C:CH(CH_2)_2C(CH_3):CH(CH_2)_2C(CH_3):CH \cdot CH_2]_2$, from the liver oil of sharks and certain other elasmobranch fishes; it is an intermediate in cholesterol biosynthesis (by way of lanosterol) in all animals examined. It is found in small amounts in human blood plasma and in increased amounts in viral influenza. A preparation [NF] is used as an oleaginous vehicle in pharmaceuticals.

squama (skwa'mah), pl. *squa'mae* [L.] a scale or platelike structure; [NA] a general term for such a structure. **s. alveola'ris,** a thin plate covering the bare areas of pulmonary alveoli. **frontal s., s. of frontal bone, s. fronta'lis** [NA], the broad, curved portion of the frontal bone, situated above the supraorbital margin and forming the forehead. **mental s., external,** protuberantia mentalis. **occipital s.,** s. occipitalis. **occipital s., superior,** os interparietale. **s. occipita'lis** [NA], occipital squama: the largest of the four parts of the occipital bone, extending from the posterior edge of the foramen magnum to the lambdoid suture, its external surface bearing the external occipital protuberance and nuchal lines. **perpendicular s.,** s. frontalis. **temporal s., s. of temporal bone, s. tempora'lis,** pars squamosa ossis temporalis.

squamae (skwa'me) [L.] plural of *squama.*

squamate (skwa'māt) [L. *squamatus,* from *squama* scale] scaly; having or resembling scales.

squamatization (skwa"mah-ti-za'shun) the transformation of cells of other types into squamous cells; squamous metaplasia.

squame (skwām) [L. *squama*] a scale or scalelike substance.

squamocellular (skwa"mo-sel'u-lar) [L. *squama* scale + *cellula* cell] having squamous cells.

squamofrontal (skwa"mo-fron'tal) pertaining to the squama frontalis.

squamomastoid (skwa"mo-mas'toid) pertaining to the squamous and mastoid portions of the temporal bone.

squamo-occipital (skwa"mo-ok-sip'ĭ-tal) pertaining to the squama occipitalis.

squamoparietal (skwa"mo-pah-ri'ĕ-tal) pertaining to the pars squamosa ossis temporalis and the parietal bone.

squamopetrosal (skwa"mo-pe-tro'sal) pertaining to the squamous and petrous portions of the temporal bone.

squamosa (skwa-mo'sah) [L.] scaly, or platelike; see *pars squamosa.*

squamosal (skwa-mo'sal) squamous.

squamosoparietal (skwa-mo"so-pah-ri'ĕ-tal) squamoparietal.

squamosphenoid (skwa"mo-sfe'noid) pertaining to the squamous portion of the temporal bone and to the sphenoid bone.

squamotemporal (skwa"mo-tem'po-ral) pertaining to the squamous portion of the temporal bone.

squamous (skwa'mus) [L. *squamosus* scaly] scaly, or platelike.

squamozygomatic (skwa"mo-zi"go-mat'ik) pertaining to the squamous portions of the temporal bone and the zygomatic bone.

squatting (skwot'ing) a position of flexion of the knees and hips, the buttocks being lowered to the level of the heels. It is sometimes adopted by the parturient at delivery. Children with certain types of cyanotic cardiac defects, particularly those with tetralogy of Fallot, frequently adopt the position.

squeeze (skwēz) subjection to pressure; compression. **tussive s.,** the compression of the lung in coughing, which is said to force material from the alveoli and smaller air passages into the bronchi.

squill (skwil) [L. *scilla;* Gr. *skilla*] the fleshy inner scales of the bulb of the white variety of *Urginea maritima* (L.) Baker (a liliaceous plant). It contains glucoscillaren A, scillaren A, proscillaridin A, other related cardioactive glycosides, and several other principles, and has been used as a diuretic, emetic, expectorant, and cardiotonic. The red variety is used as a rat poison. Called also *scilla.*

squillitic (skwil-lit'ik) [L. *scilliticus;* Gr. *skillitikos*] pertaining to or containing squill.

squint (skwint) strabismus; for types of squint not entered here, see under *strabismus.* **accommodative s.,** convergent strabismus. **comitant s., concomitant s.,** concomitant strabismus. **convergent s.,** esotropia. **divergent s.,** exotropia. **upward and downward s.,** hypertropia.

Squire's catheter (skwīrz) [Trumann Hoffman *Squire,* American surgeon, 1823–1889] vertebral catheter.

S.R. sedimentation rate (see *erythrocyte sedimentation rate,* under *rate*); sigma reaction.

Sr chemical symbol for *strontium.*

SRF somatotropin releasing factor; see *growth hormone releasing hormone,* under *hormone.*

SRH somatotropin releasing hormone; see *growth hormone releasing hormone,* under *hormone.*

S.R.N. State Registered Nurse (England and Wales).

sRNA soluble ribonucleic acid; see *ribonucleic acid,* under *acid.*

SRS-A slow reacting substance.

ss. abbreviation for L. *se'mis,* one half.

Ssabanejew-Frank operation (sab-an"ej-ef frank) [Ivan *Ssabanejew,* Russian surgeon, born 1856; Rudolf *Frank,* Vienna surgeon, 1862–1913] see *Frank's operation,* under *operation.*

S.S.D. source-skin distance.

SSS specific soluble substance (polysaccharide hapten).

s.s.s. abbreviation for L. *stra'tum su'per stra'tum,* layer upon layer.

S.S.V. abbreviation for L. *sub sig'no vene'ni,* under a poison label.

St. abbreviation for L. *stet,* let it stand; or *stent,* let them stand.

S. T. 37 trademark for a solution of hexylresorcinol.

stab (stab) see under *culture,* and see *staff cell,* under *cell.*

stabilarsan (sta-bil'ar-san) a double glycoside of arsphenamine, $C_6H_{11}O_5 \cdot NH(OH)C_6H_3As.$

stabilate (sta'bĭ-lāt) a population of organisms preserved in viable condition on a unique occasion; distinguished from a strain because of its assured stability.

stabile (sta'bil, sta'bīl) [L. *stabilis* stable, abiding] not moving; stationary; resistant to chemical change; opposed to *labile.* **heat s.,** thermostabile.

stability (stah-bil'ĭ-te) the quality of maintaining a constant character in the presence of forces which threaten to disturb it; resistance to change. **dimensional s.,** the resistance of a material to change in its shape or measurements.

stabilization (sta"bil-i-za'shun) the creation of a stable state.

stabilograph (sta'bil-o-graf") an instrument for measuring motor instability (sway patterns) during alcohol withdrawal.

stable (sta'b'l) not moving, fixed, firm; resistant to change.

staccato (stah-kah'to) [Ital. "detached"] denoting a manner of utterance in which the speech is delivered in a quick, jerky manner, with an interval between each two syllables.

stachydrine (stah-kid'rin) chemical name: *N*-methylproline-methylbetaine. An alkaloid, $C_7H_{13}NO_2,$ found in various plants, such as alfalfa, chrysanthemum, citrus, and species of hedge nettles.

stachyose (stak'e-ōs) an indigestible tetrasaccharide, $C_{24}H_{42}O_{21},$ from the tubers of the hedge nettle, *Stachys tubifera,* the seeds of various leguminous plants, and the roots and rhizomes of various labiate plants.

Stacke's operation (stak'ez) [Ludwig *Stacke,* German otologist, 1859–1918] see under *operation.*

stactometer (stak-tom'ĕ-ter) [Gr. *staktos* oozing out in drops + *metron* measure] an instrument for measuring drops.

Stader splint (sta'der) [Otto *Stader,* American veterinary surgeon] see under *splint.*

Staderini's nucleus (stad″er-e′nēz) [Rutilio *Staderini*, Italian anatomist] nucleus intercalatus.

stadium (sta′de-um), pl. *sta′dia* [L.; Gr. *stadion* course] a stage or period in a disease. See *stage*, def. 1. **s. ac′mes**, the height of a disease. **s. augmen′ti**, s. incrementi. **s. calo′ris**, the hot stage of a fever or disease. **s. decremen′ti**, the period of decrease of severity in a disease; the defervescence of fever. **s. defervescen′tiae**, s. decrementi. **s. fluorescen′tiae**, eruptive stage (of an exanthem). **s. frig′oris**, the cold stage of an intermittent fever. **s. incremen′ti**, the period of increase in the intensity of a disease; the stage of development of fever. **s. invasio′nis**, the incubative stage. **s. sudo′ris**, the sweating stage.

Staehelin's test (sta′ĕ-linz) [Rudolf *Staehelin*, Swiss internist, 1875–1943] see under *tests*.

staff (staf) 1. a wooden rod or rodlike structure. 2. a grooved director used as a guide for the knife in lithotomy. 3. the professional personnel of a hospital. 4. see under *cell*. **s. of Æsculapius**, a rod or staff with a snake entwined around it, which always appeared in the ancient representations of Æsculapius,

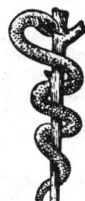

Staff of Æsculapius.

the god of medicine. It is the symbol of medicine and is the official insignia of the American Medical Association. **attending s.**, the corps of attending physicians and surgeons of a hospital. **consulting s.**, the corps of physicians and surgeons attached to a hospital who do not visit regularly, but may be consulted by members of the attending staff. **house s.**, the resident physicians and surgeons of a hospital. **s. of Wrisberg**, a slight mounding up of the mucosa over Wrisberg's cartilage (cartilago cuneiformis) seen in the normal larynx during examination with the laryngoscope.

stage (stāj) 1. a period or distinct phase in the course of a disease, the life history of an organism, or any biological process. See also *staging*. 2. the platform of a microscope on which a slide is placed for viewing of the specimen. **algid s.**, a condition characterized by a flickering pulse, subnormal temperature, and varied nervous symptoms. **amphibolic s.**, the stage which intervenes between the acme and the decline of an attack. **anal s.**, in psychoanalysis, the stage of psychosexual development from 12 months to as late as 36 months, characterized by libidinous experience of anal function; it follows the oral stage and precedes the phallic stage. **asphyxial s.**, the preliminary stage of an attack of epidemic cholera, marked by cramps, severe pain, and great thirst. **cold s.**, the chill or rigor of a malarial attack. **defervescent s.**, stadium decrementi. **eruptive s.**, that period during the course of an eruptive fever or exanthem when the rash is present. **expulsive s.**, the stage of labor during which the child is being expelled from the uterus; the second stage of labor. **s. of fervescence**, pyrogenetic s. **first s.** (of labor), the earliest stage of labor, ending with dilatation of the os uteri. **fourth s.** (of labor), a name sometimes applied to the immediate postpartum period. **genital s.**, in psychoanalysis, the psychosexual stage in which libidinous pleasure is associated with the genitals; the adult sexual stage, which follows the latent period. **hot s.**, the period of pyrexia in a malarial paroxysm. **incubative s.**, incubation period. **knäuel s.**, skein. **s. of latency**, 1. the incubation period of any infectious disorder. 2. the quiescent period following an active period in certain infectious diseases, during which the pathogen remains dormant for a variable length of time before again initiating signs of active disease. **mechanical s.**, a platform of a microscope by which the specimen being viewed can be moved in either of two mutually perpendicular directions. **oral s.**, in psychoanalysis, the first stage of the infantile period in psychosexual development, lasting from birth to 12 months, or even to 24 months of age, in which sensual or libidinous pleasure is associated with oral activities; it is followed by the anal stage. **phallic s.**, in psychoanalysis, the psychosexual stage from about two and a half to six years of age, during which sexual interest, curiosity, and pleasurable experience center about the penis in boys, and in girls, to a lesser extent, the clitoris; it follows the anal stage and precedes the latency period. **placental s.**, third s. **precystic s.**, the stage in the life cycle of an ameba in which it becomes nonmotile and secretes a wall about itself to become a cyst. **preeruptive s.**, the stage after infection and before eruption. **premenstrual s.**, the condition of the uterine mucosa after ovulation and the formation of a corpus luteum. **prodromal s.**, the period of early signs of disease, occurring at the end of the incubative stage of an infection and just before the appearance of its characteristic signs; it is typified by the preeruptive cough,

fever, and conjunctivitis of measles and the grippal symptoms that precede the meningeal and paralytic signs of poliomyelitis. **progestational s.**, the secretory stage of the endometrial cycle immediately preceding menstruation or implantation of the ovum. **proliferative s.**, the phase of the uterine mucosa following the first stage of rest: the mucosa shows hypertrophy of the glands and increase of the lining epithelium. **pyretogenic s.**, **pyrogenetic s.**, the stage of invasion of a febrile attack. **Ranke's s's**, the hypothesis that tuberculosis of the lungs develops in three stages: (1) the primary focus, (2) generalized spread of the tubercle bacillus, and (3) isolated organ tuberculosis, chiefly of the lungs. **rest s.**, the stage of the uterine mucosa immediately following the completion of menstruation. **resting s.**, the stage of a cell or its nucleus when no mitotic changes are going on; interphase. **ring s.**, see *signet ring*, under *ring*. **second s.** (of labor), period during which the infant is expelled from the uterus and vagina. **seral s.**, any of the individual transitional series of communities of an ecological sere, which finally leads to a stable, mature *climax community*. Called also *seral community*. **stepladder s.**, an early stage of enteric fever; so called from the peculiar form of the temperature curve. **sweating s.**, the final stage of a malarial paroxysm, marked by sweating. **third s.** (of labor), the period following expulsion of the infant and ending with expulsion of the placenta and membranes from the uterus. **transitional pulp s.**, a condition of the dental pulp tissue characterized by the presence of lymphocytes and macrophages; commonly found as a result of dental caries. **ugly duckling s.**, a dental development stage in the mixed dentition when the upper central and lateral incisors may be flared, before the maxillary canine teeth erupt. **vegetative s.**, resting s. **zooglea s.**, the stage in the life history of a microorganism in which it forms zooglea.

staggers (stag′erz) 1. gid. 2. a form of vertigo occurring in decompression sickness. **blind s.**, 1. gid. 2. an acute form of selenium poisoning in animals. **grass s.**, locoism. **sleepy s.**, **stomach s.**, a disease of horses, of unknown causation, but usually associated with the eating of moldy hay and grain; called also *forage poisoning*.

staging (sta′jing) 1. the determination of distinct phases or periods in the course of a disease, the life history of an organism, or any biological process. 2. the classification of neoplasms according to the extent of the tumor; see *TNM s*. **TNM s.**, staging of tumors according to three basic components: primary tumor (T), regional nodes (N), and metastasis (M). Subscripts are used to denote size and degree of involvement; for example, 0 indicates undetectable, and 1, 2, 3, and 4 a progressive increase in size or involvement. Thus a tumor may be described as $T_1N_2M_0$.

Stahl's ear (stahlz) [Friedrich Karl *Stahl*, German physician, 1811–1873] see under *ear*.

Stahr's gland (stahrz) [Hermann *Stahr*, German anatomist and pathologist, born 1868] see under *gland*.

stain (stān) 1. any dye, reagent, or other material used in producing coloration, such as a substance used in coloring tissues or microorganisms for microscopical study. See *Table of Stains and Staining Methods* and names of specific compounds. 2. a superficial discoloration, or an artificially colored spot in the skin. **acid s.**, a stain which is acid in reaction and more readily colors the protoplasm of cells. **after s.**, see *after-stain*. **basic s.**, a stain which is basic in reaction and shows an affinity for the nuclei of cells. **contrast s.**, material used to color an unstained portion of a tissue after another portion has been stained with another dye. **counter s.**, see *counterstain*. **differential s.**, one which facilitates differentiation of various elements in a specimen. **electron s's**, substances containing heavy atoms, such as osmic tetroxide, uranyl, and lead ions, which, under certain conditions, act as "electron stains," comparable to histologic stains, by combining selectively with certain regions of the specimen; used in the visualization of the ultrastructure. **heavy-metal s.**, any of the elements of high atomic weight often used as stains in electron microscopy. **lipoid s.**, a stain made from any fatlike, or lipid, substance, e.g., Sudan III. **metachromatic s.**, a stain that colors certain cell constituents a color different from that of the stain itself. **neutral s.**, a combination of an acid and a basic stain for staining neutrophil tissues. **nuclear s.**, a stain which has a special affinity for the nuclei of cells. **plasmatic s.**, **plasmic s.**, a stain which colors the tissue uniformly throughout. **port-wine s.**, nevus flammeus. **protoplasmic s.**, a stain which has a special affinity for the protoplasm of cells. **selective s.**, a stain which has a special affinity for a certain tissue element, staining it more vividly than, or to the exclusion of, other elements of the same specimen. **tumor s.**, an area of increased density in a radiograph due to collection of contrast material in distorted and abnormal vessels, prominent in the capillary and venous phase of arteriography, and presumed to indicate neoplasm.

staining (stān′ing) the artificial coloration of a substance, such as the introduction or application of material to facilitate examination of tissues, microorganisms, or other cells under the microscope. In dentistry, the modification of the color of a tooth or denture base. For various methods, see *Table of Stains and Staining Methods*. **bipolar s.**, staining at the two poles only, or staining differently at the two poles. **differential s.**, staining with a substance for which different bacteria or different elements of the bacteria or specimen being stained show varying affinities, resulting in their differentiation. **double s.,** staining with two different dyes which have an affinity for different tissue elements. **fluorescent s.,** the coloration of tissues with a fluorescent dye. **intravital s.,** vital s. **multiple s.,** staining with several different dyes to facilitate identification of different tissue elements. **negative s.,** staining of the background and not the organism, to facilitate the microscopical study of bacteria. **polar s.,** staining in which the ends of the rod stain deeply while the central portion of the organism is nearly or quite unstained, as in the pasteurellas. **postvital s.,** staining that occurs after death of a tissue which has been previously stained by vital methods. **preagonal s.,** vital s. **simple s.,** staining with a single substance, such as the staining of microorganisms with a single dye. **substantive s.,** the coloration of tissues by direct absorption of dyes in which they are immersed. **supravital s.,** staining of living tissue removed from the body, but before cessation of the chemical life of the cells. **triple s.,** staining with three different dyes to facilitate identification of the different elements. **vital s.,** staining of a tissue by a dye which is introduced into a living organism and which, by virtue of affinity for certain tissues, will stain those tissues; called also *intravital staining.*

TABLE OF STAINS AND STAINING METHODS

Listing some of the preparations and methods commonly employed in histologic and pathologic technique (*arranged alphabetically*). For other stains, see under *blue, red,* etc.

Achucárro's s., a silver-tannin stain for impregnating connective tissue.

acid-fast s., a staining procedure for demonstrating acid-fast microorganisms. After being stained with carbolfuchsin, either hot or by prolonged (16–24 hour) exposure, the microorganisms resist decolorization with dilute acid and do not show the counterstain (usually methylene blue) that is taken up by the decolorized, non–acid-fast microorganisms and tissue elements. Called also *Ziehl-Neelsen s.* or *method.*

acid fuchsin s., a diffuse stain containing acid fuchsin and diluted hydrochloric acid in purified water, for demonstrating axons.

Albert's diphtheria s., a stain containing toluidine blue and methyl (or malachite) green. Following treatment with iodine solution, the metachromatic granules appear black, the bars dark green to black, and the remainder of the diphtheria bacillus a light green.

alum-carmine s., a preparation of ordinary alum and carmine.

Alzheimer s., a methylene blue and eosin polychrome stain for demonstrating Negri bodies.

Anthony's capsule s., a method of staining the capsules of bacteria in which the microorganisms are heavily stained with acetic acid–crystal violet, followed by treatment with copper sulfate solution. The bacterial cells appear dark blue, and the capsules bluish violet.

azan s., Heidenhain's modification of Mallory's triple stain.

basic fuchsin s., a stain containing basic fuchsin in distilled water.

Benda's s., a method for demonstrating nerve tissue.

Bensley's neutral gentian orange G s., a preparation used for demonstrating secretion granules.

Best's carmine s., a stain for demonstrating glycogen.

Bethe's method, a method of fixing methylene blue stains of nerve fibers.

Bielschowsky's s., an ammoniacal silver stain for demonstrating axons and neurofibrils.

Bodian method, a method of staining nerve fibers and nerve endings with colloidal silver.

Bowie s., a stain used to demonstrate the slightly basophilic cytoplasm and the specific granules of juxtaglomerular cells.

C method, C-staining method, centric heterochromatin method.

Cajal method, a method of staining astrocytes by a gold chloride–mercuric chloride compound.

Cajal's double method, a method of demonstrating ganglion cells.

carbol-fuchsin s., a stain for microorganisms, containing basic fuchsin and dilute phenol as a mordant.

carbol-gentian violet s., a solution containing gentian violet and carbolic acid.

Castaneda's s., a method of demonstrating rickettsiae.

centric heterochromatin method, the DNA of chromosomes is denatured by alkali treatment, renatured, and then treated with Giemsa stain; bands of heavily stained regions (C bands) appear near the centromere of most chromosomes. Called also *constitutive* or *C method.*

Ciaccio's s., a stain for demonstrating lipoids.

constitutive heterochromatin method, centric heterochromatin method.

Cox's modification of Golgi's corrosive sublimate method, a method for staining ganglion cells.

Davenport's s., a stain for demonstrating various elements of nerve tissue, dependent upon the special affinity of nerve cells and their processes for silver.

Delafield's hematoxylin [USP], a preparation of hematoxylin, alcohol, ammonia alum, water, glycerin, and methanol, used as a nuclear stain.

Ehrlich's acid hematoxylin, a preparation of hematoxylin, used as a nuclear stain.

Ehrlich's neutral s., a mixture of methylene blue and acid fuchsin, used to stain blood corpuscles.

Ehrlich's triacid s., a stain containing acid fuchsin, orange G, and methyl green; used for demonstrating various formed elements in the blood.

F method, F-staining method, chromosomes are treated with phosphate buffer, rinsed and stored for 60–72 hours in saline citrate solution, then fixed in methanol-acetic acid, and stained by the Feulgen method; chromosomes display light and dark bands (F bands) at characteristic loci.

Feulgen s., a method of demonstrating chromatin and deoxyribonucleic acid (DNA).

Fontana's s., a method of staining spirochetes by silver impregnation, using ammoniacal silver nitrate solution.

G method, G-staining method, Giemsa method (for chromosomes).

Giemsa s., a solution containing azure II-eosin, azure II, glycerin, and methanol; used for staining protozoan parasites such as trypanosomes, *Leishmania*, etc., and *Leptospira, Borrelia,* viral inclusion bodies, and *Rickettsia.*

Giemsa method (*for chromosomes*), chromosomes stained with Giemsa stain at pH 9.0 show deeply stained bands (G bands) that are characteristic for each chromosome; called also *G method.*

Golgi's mixed method, a method of staining nerve cells and all of their processes; historically of very great importance.

Gomori's s's, stains used for histological demonstration of enzymes, especially phosphatases and lipases in sections; also methods for demonstration of connective tissue fibers and secretion granules. Called also *Gomori-Takamatsu s's.*

Gomori-Takamatsu s's, Gomori's s's.

Gomori-Wheatley s., trichrome s.

Goodpasture's s., a method for demonstrating the peroxidase reaction.

Gram's method, Gram's s., an empirical staining procedure devised by Gram in which microorganisms are stained with crystal violet, treated with 1:15 dilution of Lugol's iodine, decolorized with ethanol or ethanol-acetone, and counterstained with a contrasting dye, usually safranin. Those microorganisms that retain the crystal violet stain are said to be gram-positive, and those that lose the crystal violet stain by decolorization but stain with the counterstain are said to be gram-negative.

Hale's iron s., a stain used on substances with a high acid polysaccharide content because of the ability of polyanionic polysaccharides to bind polyvalent cations. Its main component is colloidal iron (Fe^{+++}).

Harris' hematoxylin, a nuclear stain.

Harris' method, a method for demonstrating Negri bodies.

Heidenhain's iron hematoxylin, an important cytological method for the demonstration of most cellular structures: nuclei, chromosomes, centrioles, fibrils, mitochondria, cilia, etc.

hemalum s., a nuclear stain containing hematoxylin and alum, widely used, especially in combination with eosin.

hematoxylin-eosin s., a mixture of hematoxylin in distilled water and aqueous eosin solution, employed also universally for routine examination of tissues; numerous variations are employed in execution of the stain.

hematoxylin-eosin-azure II, Maximow's method for the staining of blood-forming organs.

Hiss capsule s., a method of demonstrating bacterial capsules by mixing the bacterial suspension with India ink, drying and fixing, and staining with crystal violet or basic fuchsin. The bacterial cells are stained violet or red, and the capsules appear as unstained halos against the black background.

Hortega method, a method of demonstrating microglia, employing ammoniacal silver carbonate.

iron hematoxylin method, a staining procedure in which the sections are treated with an iron salt, stained with hematoxylin, and differentiated with the same iron salt.

Janus green B, a stain used supravitally for the demonstration of mitochondria.

Jenner's method, a method for demonstrating blood corpuscles.

Leishman's s., a mixture of methylene blue and eosin for staining blood cells and certain parasites.

Levaditi's method, a method for demonstrating *Treponema pallidum* in sections, employing reduced silver.

lithium-carmine s., a diffuse stain used intravitally for the demonstration of macrophages.

Löffler's alkaline methylene blue, methylene blue solution made slightly alkaline with potassium hydroxide.

Löffler's flagella s., a staining procedure for the demonstration of bacterial flagella; the smear is fixed in ferric chloride–tannic acid solution, and stained with methylene blue–aniline (or carbol-) fuchsin.

Lorrain Smith s., Nile blue sulfate staining fatty acids blue and neutral fat pink.

Macchiavello's s., a rickettsial stain in which the heat-fixed smear is stained with basic fuchsin, decolorized in citric acid, and counterstained with methylene blue. Rickettsiae are stained red, and tissue components blue. The stain may also be used for the elementary bodies of organisms of the psittacosis-lymphogranuloma venereum group (*Chlamydia*).

Mallory's acid fuchsin, orange G, and aniline blue s., a stain for demonstrating connective tissue and secretion granules. Called also *Mallory's triple stain.*

Mallory's phosphotungstic acid–hematoxylin s., a stain used for demonstrating nuclear and cytoplasmic detail and connective tissue fibers.

Mallory's triple s., Mallory's acid fuchsin, orange G, and aniline blue s.

Marchi's method, a method of demonstrating degenerated nerve fibers, the tissue first being fixed in a solution containing potassium bichromate, which prevents the normal myelinated fibers from staining with osmic acid.

Masson s., a trichrome stain for connective tissue.

Maximow's method, hematoxylin-eosin-azure II.

May's spore s., a method of staining the spores of bacteria in which they are treated with 5 per cent chromic acid, then with ammonia, stained with hot carbol-fuchsin, decolorized with dilute sulfuric acid, and counterstained with methylene blue. The spores appear red, the vegetative cells blue.

May-Grünwald s., an alcoholic neutral mixture of methylene blue and eosin.

Mayer's hemalum, an aqueous solution of hematein, alum, thymol, and 90 per cent alcohol.

Mayer's muchematein, a specific stain for mucus.

methyl green-pyronine s., Unna-Pappenheim s.

methyl violet s., an aniline dye used as a bacteriological stain.

methylene blue, an aniline dye much used as a staining agent; prepared in a saturated solution (7 per cent) in absolute alcohol, which is diluted for use.

Michaelis's., a mixture of alcoholic solution of methylene blue and a solution of eosin in acetone; used for demonstrating blood corpuscles.

Milligan's trichrome s., a differential stain for connective tissue and smooth muscle. Nuclei and muscle appear magenta; collagen appears green or blue, depending on whether fast green or aniline blue is used as a counterstain; and red blood cells appear orange to orange red.

N method, N-staining method, a method for staining exclusively the satellite regions of acrocentric autosomes by means of Giemse stain; distinct purplish red spots (N bands) are restricted to the satellite region.

neutral red, an important supravital stain for the demonstration of vacuoles in cells, and especially of the vacuome.

Nissl's method, a method employed in the study of nerve cell bodies.

Pal's modification of Weigert's myelin sheath s., a method for the study of myelinated nerves, the specimen being treated for several weeks in a solution containing potassium bichromate.

Papanicolaou's s., a method of staining smears of various body secretions, from the respiratory, digestive or genitourinary tract, for the examination of exfoliated cells, to detect the presence of a malignant process.

Pappenheim's s., a method for differentiating basophilic granules of erythrocytes and nuclear fragments.

PAS s., periodic acid–Schiff s.

Perdrau's method, a modification of Bielschowsky's method for staining collagen and reticulin.

periodic acid–Schiff (PAS) s., see under *reaction.*

Perls' s., see under *tests.*

peroxidase s., see Goodpasture's s.

phosphotungstic acid–hematoxylin s., see *Mallory's phosphotungstic acid–hematoxylin s.*

polychrome methylene blue, a stain for demonstrating plasma cells and mast cells, employing potassium carbonate and methylene blue.

Q method, Q-staining method, quinacrine fluorescent method.

quinacrine fluorescent method, chromosomes are exposed to quinacrine derivatives, after which they fluoresce, the degree of fluorescence varying from one chromosome segment to another; the resultant fluorescent patterns (Q bands) are characteristic for each chromosome. Called also *Q method.*

R method, R-staining method, reverse Giemsa method.

Ranson's pyridine silver s., a stain used for demonstrating nerve cells and their processes.

reverse Giemsa method, a method in which the reciprocal (R-bands) of the banding pattern seen in the Giemsa method for chromosomes is obtained; called also *R method.*

Romanovsky's (Romanowsky's) s., the prototype of the many eosin-methylene blue stains for blood smears and malarial parasites, including Giemsa stain, Leishman's stain, and Wright's stain.

Seller's s., a combination of alcoholic solutions of methylene blue and basic fuchsin which stains Negri bodies a bright red against a purplish-pink background; used in rapid diagnosis of rabies.

Shaeffer's spore s., a method of staining spores with hot malachite green, rinsing the stain out of the vegetative cells with water, and counterstaining with safranin. The spores appear bright green, and the vegetative cells pink.

spore s., a method of staining the spores of bacteria, usually with carbol-fuchsin or malachite green, heat being used to drive the stain into the spores, which later resist decolorization with ethanol or dilute acid. The preparation is usually counterstained with a dye of a contrasting color.

Sternheimer-Malbin s., a stain used in urinalysis which has ready affinity for hyaline casts, epithelial casts, red cells, bladder epithelial nuclei, nuclei of vaginal epithelium, and trichomonads, staining each a different color.

T method, T-staining method, a method for staining only the terminal ends of chromosomes by means of either Giemsa stain or acridine orange; it results in bands (T bands) of dark violet (Giemsa) or fiery orange (acridine orange).

tetrachrome s., a stain combining eosin Y, methylene blue, azur A, and methylene violet, in methyl alcohol.

trichrome s., a rapid staining method which adequately demonstrates structural details of the various intestinal protozoa. The solution is as follows: chromotrope 2R 0.6 gm., light green SF 0.3 gm., phosphotungstic acid 0.7 gm., acetic acid 1.00 ml., and distilled water 100.00 ml. Called also *Gomori-Wheatley s.*

Unna's alkaline methylene blue, a strongly alkaline solution of methylene blue which is valuable for staining plasma cells.

Unna-Pappenheim s., a stain for plasma cells, employing methyl green and pyronine; also widely used for demonstrating nucleoproteins.

van Gieson's solution of trinitrophenol and acid fuchsin, a stain for connective tissue, consisting of acid fuchsin and aqueous solution of trinitrophenol.

Verhoeff's s., a stain for demonstrating elastic tissue.

von Kossa's s., a silver nitrate stain for bone mineral.

Wade's method, a method of demonstrating *Mycobacterium leprae,* in which a drop of tissue pulp and lymph is obtained from a lepromatous lesion by inserting a scalpel or razor blade into a pinched-up fold of skin and then rotating the instrument so as to scrape the sides of the incision. The specimen is then dried and stained with carbolfuchsin.

Wade-Fite method, a method of demonstrating acid-fast bacilli, in which paraffin tissue sections are dewaxed by dipping in a mixture of rectified turpentine and heavy paraffin oil, stained in carbolfuchsin, decolorized in sulfuric acid, and stained in picric acid and acid fuchsin in water. Acid-fast bacilli stain deep blue or blue-black.

Wade-Fite-Faraco method, a method of demonstrating acid-fast bacilli, including *Mycobacterium leprae,* in which paraffin tissue sections are dewaxed by dipping in a mixture of paraffin oil and aviation gasoline or of paraffin oil and rectified turpentine, stained with carbolfuchsin, decolorized in hydrochloride and ethanol until the sections are pink, and counterstained with methylene blue. Acid-fast bacilli are stained red on a light blue background.

Weigert's fibrin s., a method, many variations of which have been used in both fixation and staining; stains gram-positive bacteria as well as fibrin.

Weigert's iron hematoxylin s., a simple method for staining most nuclear and cytoplasmic constituents.

Weigert's myelin sheath m., a method of demonstrating the myelin sheath of nerve cell processes.

Weigert's neuroglia fiber s., a complicated method for demonstrating fibrous glia, which works best on human material.

Weigert's resorcin-fuchsin s., a method for the demonstration of elastic fibers.

Weil's s., a method for staining myelin sheaths.

Wright's s., a mixture of eosin and methylene blue, used for demonstrating blood corpuscles and malarial parasites.

Ziehl's carbol-fuchsin s., see *carbolfuchsin s.*

Ziehl-Neelsen s., see *acid-fast s.*

Ziehl-Neelsen carbolfuchsin, a mixture of basic fuchsin, alcohol, liquefied phenol, and purified water.

stalactite (stah-lak'tīt) a long filamentous formation which hangs down from the surface of a broth culture of *Pasteurella pestis* into the liquid below.

stalagmometer (stal″ag-mom'ĕ-ter) [Gr. *stalagmos* dropping + *metron* measure] an instrument for measuring surface tension by determining the exact number of drops in a given quantity of a liquid. See *miostagmin reaction*, under *reaction*.

stalagmon (stah-lag'mon) a colloidal substance that changes the surface tension of a liquid containing it.

staling (stāl'ing) urination in cattle and horses.

stalk (stawk) an elongated, more or less slender anatomical structure resembling the stalk of a plant. **abdominal s.**, the umbilical cord. **allantoic s.**, the more slender tube interposed in most mammals between the urogenital sinus and the allantoic sac. It is the precursor of the umbilical cord. Called also *connecting s.* **belly s.**, the umbilical cord. **body s.**, a bridge of mesoderm connecting the caudal end of the young embryo with the chorion and eventually giving passage to the allantois with its important accompanying blood vessels; it is the precursor of the allantoic stalk. **cerebellar s.**, any of the cerebellar peduncles. **connecting s.**, allantoic s. **hypophyseal s.**, 1. pars infundibularis lobi anterioris hypophyseos. 2. infundibulum hypothalami. **infundibular s.**, infundibulum hypothalami. **neural s.**, infundibulum hypothalami. **optic s.**, a slender structure attaching the optic vesicle to the brain wall in the early embryo. **pituitary s.**, 1. pars infundibularis lobi anterioris hypophyseos. 2. infundibulum hypothalami. **yolk s.**, the narrow tube connecting the yolk sac (umbilical vesicle) with the midgut of the early embryo, which becomes incorporated into the embryo and usually undergoes complete obliteration, but occasionally persists in the embryo, and, rarely, is found in the adult as a diverticulum from the small intestine (*Meckel's diverticulum*). Called also *omphalomesenteric duct, umbilical duct*, and *vitelline duct*.

stallimycin hydrochloride (stal″ĭ-mi'sin) chemical name: *N*-[5-[[(3-amino-3-iminopropyl)amino]carbonyl]-1-methy-1*H*-pyrrol-3-yl]-4-[[[4-(formylamino)-1-methyl-1*H*-pyrrol-2-yl]carbonyl]amino]-1-methyl-1*H*-pyrrole-2-carboxamide monohydrochloride; an antibacterial, $C_{22}H_{27}N_9O_4 \cdot HCl$.

stamen (sta'men) the structure of a flower which bears the male gamete, or pollen.

stamina (stam'ĭ-nah) [L.] vigor or endurance.

stammering (stam'er-ing) a disorder of speech behavior marked by involuntary pauses in speech; sometimes used synonymously with stuttering, especially in Great Britain.

Stammler's reaction (stam'lerz) [D. *Stammler*, German surgeon] see under *reaction*.

Stamnosoma (stam″no-so'mah) [Gr. *stamnos* jar + *sōma* body] a genus of flukes. *S. arma'tum* and *S. formosa'num* are parasites of birds, but experimental human infections have been reported.

standard (stan'dard) something established as a measure or model to which other similar things should conform. **Pignet's s.**, see *Pignet's formula*, under *formula*.

standardization (stan″dard-i-za'shun) 1. the bringing of any preparation to a specified standard as to quality or ingredients. 2. the formulation of standards for a substance or for a procedure.

standardize (stan'dard-īz) to compare with or conform to a standard; to establish standards.

standstill (stand'stil) a quiet state resulting from the suspension of activity or movement, as cardiac standstill. **atrial s.**, cardiac arrhythmia in which there is a pause in atrial contraction secondary to sinus arrest or sinoatrial block, the ventricle continuing to respond to its own pacemaker. **auricular s.**, atrial s. **cardiac s.**, cessation of contraction of the myocardium; see also *cardioplegia*. **respiratory s.**, suspension of the movements of respiration; termed *expiratory s.* when it occurs at the end of an expiration, and *inspiratory s.* when it occurs at the end of an inspiration. **sinus s.**, see under *arrest*. **ventricular s.**, cardiac arrhythmia in which there is an absence of ventricular contraction.

Stanley (stan'le), Wendell Meredith. An American biochemist (born 1904), co-winner, with J. B. Sumner and J. H. Northrop, of the Nobel prize in chemistry for 1946 for pioneering work in crystallizing protein.

Stanley bacillus (stan'le) [*Stanley*, England] see under *bacillus*.

Stanley Kent see *Kent*.

stannate (stan'āt) any salt of stannic acid.

stannic (stan'ik) containing tin as a quadrivalent element. **s. chloride**, an irritant war smoke, $SnCl_4$.

stanniferous (stan-nif'er-us) [L. *stannum* tin + *ferre* to bear] containing tin.

stannosis (stan-o'sis) benign pneumoconiosis due to the inhalation of tin oxide; it is symptomless unless accompanied by silicosis.

stannous (stan'us) containing tin as a bivalent element. For stannous compounds, see under the salt, e.g., *chloride* and *fluoride*.

stannum (stan'um) [L.] tin (symbol Sn).

stanolone (stan'o-lōn) chemical name: 17β-hydroxy-5α-androstan-3-one. A semisynthetic androgen (dihydrotestosterone), $C_{19}H_{30}O_2$, occurring as a white crystalline powder, and having the same actions and uses as testosterone. It is used for its anabolic and antineoplastic actions in inoperable breast cancer and in postoperative metastatic breast cancer.

stanozolol (stan'o-zo-lol″) [USP] chemical name: 17-methyl-2′*H*-5α-androst-2-eno[3,2-*c*]-pyrazol-17β-ol. An androgenic anabolic steroid, $C_{21}H_{32}N_2O$, occurring as a white, crystalline powder; used orally, especially to increase hemoglobin levels in some patients with aplastic (congential and idiopathic) anemia.

stapedectomy (sta″pĕ-dek'to-me) [L. *stapes* stirrup + Gr. *ektomē* excision] excision of the stapes.

stapedial (stah-pe'de-al) pertaining to the stapes.

stapediolysis (stah-pe″de-ol'ĭ-sis) mobilization of the stapes in the surgical treatment of otosclerosis.

stapedioplasty (stah-pe″de-o-plas'te) replacement of the stapes with other material (wire, bone, plastic) in correction of defective hearing resulting from otosclerosis, the prosthesis serving to conduct the sound waves from the incus to the oval window (fenestra vestibuli).

stapediotenotomy (stah-pe″de-o-tĕ-not'o-me) the cutting of the tendon of the stapedius muscle.

stapediovestibular (stah-pe″de-o-ves-tib'u-lar) pertaining to the stapes and vestibule.

stapes (sta'pēz) [L. "stirrup"] [NA] the innermost of the auditory ossicles, shaped somewhat like a stirrup; it articulates by its head with the incus, and its base is inserted into the fenestra vestibuli. Called also *stirrup*.

Staphcillin (staf-sil'in) trademark for preparations of sodium methicillin.

staphisagria (staf″ĭ-sa'gre-ah) [Gr. *staphis* raisin + *agrios* wild] the poisonous seeds of *Delphinium staphisagria*, stavesacre, or lousewort. The plant and its seeds are poisonous and narcotic. The ripe seeds were formerly used externally as a parasiticide.

staphisagrine (staf″ĭ-sa'grin) a poisonous alkaloid, $C_{22}H_{33}NO_5$, from staphisagria.

staphyl- see *staphylo-*.

staphylagra (staf″ĭ-la'grah) [*staphyl-* + Gr. *agra* a way of catching] a forceps for holding the uvula.

staphylectomy (staf″ĭ-lek'to-me) [*staphyl-* + Gr. *ektomē* excision] uvulectomy; excision of the uvula.

staphyledema (staf″il-ĕ-de'mah) [*staphyl-* + Gr. *oidēma* swelling] an enlargement or swollen state of the uvula.

staphylematoma (staf″il-em″ah-to'mah) hemorrhage from the uvula (Pauli).

staphyline (staf'ĭ-līn) 1. shaped like a bunch of grapes. 2. pertaining to the uvula; uvular.

staphylinid (staf-ĭ-lin'id) 1. pertaining to or due to beetles of the family Staphylinidae. 2. a beetle of the family Staphylinidae.

Staphylinidae (staf″ĭ-lin'ĭ-de) a family of beetles (order Coleoptera), some members of which produce an irritating substance that causes blistering one or two days after contact.

staphylinus (staf″ĭ-li'nus) [L.] pertaining to the uvula.

staphylion (stah-fil'e-on) [Gr. "little grape"] 1. an encephalometric landmark on the posterior edge of the hard palate at the median line. 2. the uvula. 3. a nipple or teat.

staphylitis (staf″ĭ-li'tis) inflammation of the uvula; uvulitis.

staphylo-, staphyl- (staf'ĭ-lo, staf'il) [Gr. *staphylē* a bunch of grapes] combining form denoting resemblance to a bunch of grapes, used especially to denote relationship to the uvula or to staphylococci.

staphyloangina (staf″ĭ-lo-an'ji-nah) a mild form of sore throat, marked by a pseudomembranous deposit in the throat due to a staphylococcus.

staphylobacterin (staf″ĭ-lo-bak'ter-in) a bacterial vaccine prepared from staphylococci.

staphylocide (staf″ĭ-lo-sīd″) staphylococcide.

staphylocoagulase (staf″ĭ-lo-ko-ag'u-lās) a coagulase produced by staphylococci which may be important in the virulence of staphylococcic infections.

staphylococcal (staf″ĭ-lo-kok'al) pertaining to or caused by staphylococci.

staphylococcemia (staf″ĭ-lo-kok-se'me-ah) [*staphylococcus* + Gr. *haima* blood + *-ia*] a condition in which staphylococci are present in the blood; septicemia caused by staphylococci.

staphylococci (staf″ĭ-lo-kok'si) [L.; Gr.] plural of *staphylococcus*.

staphylococcic (staf″ĭ-lo-kok'sik) pertaining to or caused by staphylococci.

staphylococcide (staf″ĭ-lo-kok'sīd) an agent that is destructive to staphylococci.

staphylococcosis (staf″ĭ-lo-kok-o'sis) infection caused by staphylococci.

Staphylococcus (staf″ĭ-lo-kok'us) [Gr. *staphyl* bunch of grapes + *kokkus* berry] a genus of microorganisms of the family Micrococcaceae, order Eubacteriales, that are the commonest cause of localized suppurative infections. Slightly less than 1μ in diameter and spherical in shape, they tend to form masses of cells. **S. al'bus,** the white form of staphylococci, an occasional agent of staphylococcal pneumonia. Although not very pathogenic and rarely invasive, these bacteria are numerous in the sputum and readily obtained in pure culture. **S. au'reus,** a species comprising the pigmented, coagulase-positive, mannitol-fermenting pathogenic form. **S. epider'midis,** a species made up of non-pigmented, coagulase-negative, mannitol-negative nonpathogenic microorganisms commonly found on the skin. **S. pyog'enes var. al'bus,** the white staphylococci occasionally found in infectious processes.

staphylococcus (staf″ĭ-lo-kok′us), pl. *staphylococ'ci.* 1. a spherical bacterium occurring predominantly in irregular masses of cells as a consequence of failure of the daughter cells to separate following cell division in more than one plane. 2. an organism of the genus *Staphylococcus.*

staphyloderma (staf″ĭ-lo-der′ma) cutaneous pyogenic infection by staphylococci.

staphylodialysis (staf″ĭ-lo-di-al′ĭ-sis) [*staphylo-* + Gr. *dialysis* loosing] relaxation of the uvula.

staphyloedema (staf″ĭ-lo-ĕ-de′mah) staphyledema.

staphylokinase (staf″ĭ-lo-ki′nās) a bacterial kinase produced by certain strains of staphylococci, which is capable of activating plasminogen in the blood of various species of animals; see also *kinase* (def. 2).

staphyloleukocidin (staf″ĭ-lo-lu″ko-si′din) a toxin from staphylococcus cultures that is destructive to leukocytes.

staphylolysin (staf″ĭ-lol′ĭ-sin) a principle with hemolytic activity produced by staphylococci. **α s., alpha s.,** a hemolysin produced by pathogenic staphylococci which lyses both sheep and rabbit erythrocytes at 37° C. and has leukocidin activity. **β s., beta s.,** a hot-cold hemolysin produced by staphylococci which lyses sheep but not rabbit erythrocytes in the cold following preliminary incubation at 37° C. **δ s., delta s.,** a hemolysin produced by pyogenic staphylococci which lyses red cells from man and several other species; it differs immunologically from the α and β staphylolysins, and is both dermonecrotic and lethal. **ε s., epsilon s.,** a hemolysin formed almost exclusively by nonpathogenic, coagulase-negative strains of staphylococci. **γ s., gamma s.,** a hemolysin produced by staphylococci which is similar to, but serologically distinguishable from, the α staphylolysin.

staphyloma (staf″ĭ-lo′mah) [Gr. *staphylōma* a defect in the eye inside the cornea] protrusion of the cornea or sclera lined with uveal tissue, resulting from inflammation. **annular s.,** staphyloma of the sclera in the ciliary region, extending around the margin of the cornea. **anterior s.,** scleral or corneal staphyloma in the anterior part of the eye. **ciliary s.,** scleral staphyloma in the part covered by the ciliary body. **s. cor'neae, corneal s.,** 1. ectasia of the cornea with adherent uveal tissue; called also *prolapsus corneae* and *projecting staphyloma.* 2. staphyloma formed by an iris which has protruded through a wound in the cornea. **s. cor'neae racemo'sum,** staphyloma corneae (def. 2) in which there are a number of perforations from which small portions of iris protrude. **equatorial s.,** scleral staphyloma occurring in the equatorial region of the eye. **intercalary s.,** that which occurs in the rim of sclera anterior to the insertion of the ciliary body. **posterior s., s. posti'cum,** backward bulging of the sclera at the posterior pole of the eye; called also *Scarpa's s.* **projecting s.,** s. corneae. **retinal s.,** a forward bulging of the retina. **Scarpa's s.,** posterior s. **scleral s.,** protrusion of the contents of the eyeball at a point where the sclera has become too thin. **uveal s.,** protrusion of the uvea through a ruptured sclera.

staphylomatous (staf″ĭ-lom′ah-tus) pertaining to or resembling staphyloma.

staphyloncus (staf″ĭ-long′kus) [*staphylo-* + Gr. *onkos* mass] a tumor or swelling of the uvula.

staphylopharyngorrhaphy (staf″ĭ-lo-far″in-gor′ah-fe) [*staphylo-* + Gr. *pharynx* the throat + *rhaphē* suture] the stitching of the halves of the velum palatini to the posterior wall of the pharynx.

staphyloplasty (staf′ĭ-lo-plas″te) [*staphylo-* + Gr. *plassein* to mold] plastic repair of the soft palate and uvula.

staphyloptosia (staf″ĭ-lop-to′se-ah) [*staphylo-* + Gr. *ptōsis* falling + *-ia*] elongation of the uvula.

staphyloptosis (staf″ĭ-lop-to′sis) staphyloptosia; uvuloptosis.

staphylorrhaphy (staf″ĭ-lor′ah-fe) [*staphylo-* + Gr. *rhaphē* suture] surgical correction of a midline cleft in the uvula and soft palate; cf. *palatorrhaphy.*

staphyloschisis (staf″ĭ-los′kĭ-sis) [*staphylo-* + Gr. *schisis* splitting] fissure of the uvula and soft palate.

staphylotome (staf′ĭ-lo-tōm) [*staphylotomon*] a knife for cutting the uvula; uvulotome.

staphylotomy (staf″ĭ-lot′o-me) [*staphylo-* + Gr. *tomē* a cutting] 1. incision of the uvula. 2. the removal of a staphyloma by cutting.

staphylotoxin (staf″ĭ-lo-tok′sin) a toxin occurring in cultures of staphylococci.

staphylotropic (staf″ĭ-lo-trop′ik) having a selective affinity for staphylococci.

star (star) any structure with an appearance like that of a star. **daughter s.,** amphiaster. **dental s.,** a marking on the incisor teeth of horses, first appearing in the lower central incisors at about the age of eight years; used in judging a horse's age. **lens s's,** starlike lines formed within the lens of the eye by fibers which pass from the anterior to the posterior surface. **mother s.,** monaster. **polar s's,** the starlike figures of the amphiaster. **s's of Verheyen,** venulae stellatae renis. **Winslow's s's,** whorls of capillary vessels from which arise the vorticose veins of the choroid coat of the eye.

starch (starch) [L. *amylum*] 1. any of a group of polysaccharides of the general formula $(C_6H_{10}O_5)_n$, composed of a long-chain polymer of glucose in the form of amylose and amylopectin; it is the chief storage form of energy reserve (carbohydrates) in plants. 2. [NF] a preparation consisting of the granules separated from the mature grain of corn or wheat, or from potato tubers, occurring as irregular, angular, white masses or fine powder; used as a dusting powder and as a filler, binder, and disintegrant in pharmaceutical preparations. **animal s.,** glycogen. **cassava s.,** the starch from the roots of cassava (*Manihot utilissima* and *M. aipi*) which is the source of tapioca. **corn s.,** a starch from maize. **s. glycerite** [NF], a preparation of starch, benzoic acid, purified water, and glycerin; used as an emollient in pharmaceutical preparations intended for external use. **hydroxyethyl s.,** a starch product which has been suggested as a plasma substitute in man. **lichen s., moss s.,** lichenin. **pregelatinized s.,** [NF], starch chemically or mechanically processed to rupture all or part of the granules in the presence of water, and subsequently dried; it occurs as a moderately coarse to fine, white to off-white powder and is used as a tablet excipient in pharmaceutical preparations. **sago s.,** starch from the sago palm. **soluble s.,** amidulin.

stare (stār) a fixed, unblinking gaze. **postbasic s.,** a peculiar expression of the eyes in posterior basic meningitis due to downward rolling of the eyeball and retraction of the upper lid.

Starling's hypothesis, law (star′lingz) [Ernest Henry *Starling*, English physiologist, 1866–1927] see under *hypothesis* and *law.*

starter (star′ter) a culture of microorganisms used to initiate fermentation, as in dairy products.

starvation (star-va′shun) long-continued deprival of food.

stasimorphia (stas″ĭ-mor′fe-ah) stasimorphy.

stasimorphy (stas″ĭ-mor′fe) [Gr. *stasis* standing + *morphē* form] deformity or abnormality of shape in any organ, due to arrest of development.

stasis (sta′sis) [Gr. *stasis* a standing still] 1. a stoppage or diminution of the flow of blood or other body fluid in any part. 2. a state of equilibrium among opposing forces. **ileal s.,** abnormal delay in the passage of the intestinal contents through the ileum; it is usually associated with dilatation of the ileum. **intestinal s.,** any condition in which normal passage of intestinal content is impaired; it may be due to mechanical obstruction or impaired intestinal motility. **papillary s.,** papilledema. **pressure s.,** stoppage of the circulation caused by undue pressure on a part. **urinary s.,** stoppage of the flow or discharge of urine, which may occur at any level of the urinary tract. **venous s.,** cessation or impairment of venous flow.

-stasis (sta′sis) [Gr. "a standing still"] a word termination indicating the maintenance of (or maintaining) a constant level; preventing increase or multiplication.

Stas-Otto method (stahs-ot′o) [Jean Servais *Stas,* a Belgian chemist, 1813–1891] see under *method.*

stat. abbreviation for L. *sta'tim,* immediately.

state (stāt) [L. *status*] 1. condition or situation; status. 2. the crisis, or the turning point of an attack of disease. **alpha s.,** the state of relaxation and peaceful awakefulness, associated with prominent alpha brain wave activity. **anelectrotonic s.,** the condition which obtains in a nerve near the anode during the passage of a continuous current. **anxiety tension s. (A.T.S.),** neuromuscular hypertension. **anxious s.,** a state of fear with no particular object, as in panophobia. **borderline s.,** a diagnostic term used when it is difficult to determine whether symptoms are predominantly neurotic or psychotic. Symptoms often include acting out and behavior which is suggestive of schizophrenia. **carrier s.,** see carrier, def. 1. **catelectrotonic s.,** the condition of a nerve near the cathode during the passage of an electric current. **central excitatory s.,** a condition in which there is stored up in a reflex center of the spinal cord a number of stimuli which do not reveal themselves in reflex response. **constitutional psychopathic s.,** antisocial personality. **correlated s.,** dynamic equilibrium. **dream s.,** a state of defective consciousness in which the environment is imperfectly perceived. **epileptic s.,** status epilepticus. **excited s.,** the condition of a nucleus, atom, or molecule produced by the addition of energy to the system as the result of absorption of photons or of inelastic collisions with other particles or systems. **ground s.,** the condition of lowest energy of a nucleus, atom, or molecule, as opposed to the excited state. **hypnagogic s.,** that state of semiconsciousness which immediately precedes falling asleep. **hypnoidal s.,** a condition in which portions of unrecognized past experience come up into consciousness from the subconscious life. **hypnoidic s.,** a state in which more or less connected experiences of the past come up into consciousness from the subconscious state. **hypnoleptic s.,** a state occurring between two experiences of double personality. **hypnopompic s.,** that state of semiconsciousness which immediately precedes complete awakening from sleep. **local excitatory s.,** the condition of a nerve produced by an ineffectual stimulus. **marble s.,** status marmoratus. **metastable s.,** the condition of a system (nucleus, atom, or molecule) capable of undergoing quantum transition to a state of lower energy. **paranoid s.,** an emotional condition marked by paranoid trends or paranoid character defenses; it may be of short or long duration. **persistent vegetative s.,** a condition of profound nonresponsiveness in the wakeful state caused by brain damage at whatever level and characterized by a nonfunctioning cerebral cortex, the absence of any discernible adaptive response to the external environment, akinesia, mutism, and inability to signal; the electroencephalogram may be isoelectric or show abnormal activity. **plastic s., pluripotent s.,** the state of parts of the zygote or early embryo in which they may develop into any adult tissue or part. **refractory s.,** a condition of subnormal excitability of muscle and nerve following excitation. **resting s.,** the physiological condition achieved by complete bed rest for a period of at least one hour, a condition required in a number of different tests of various body functions. **steady s.,** dynamic equilibrium. **twilight s.,** a temporary absence of consciousness in which the patient may perform certain acts involuntarily and without remembrance of them afterward. **typhoid s.,** a condition of great muscular weakness and stupor, with dry, brown tongue, sordes on the teeth, muttering delirium, feeble pulse, and involuntary discharge of feces and urine; seen in certain wasting diseases, as typhoid and other fevers.

stathmokinesis (stath″mo-ki-ne′sis) a state of arrested mitosis, or pseudometaphase, as that induced by subjecting cells to the action of an agent such as colchicine, which destroys the fibrillar structure of cell spindles and thus permits the calculation of mitosis time.

static (stat′ik) [L. *staticus;* Gr. *statikos*] 1. at rest; in equilibrium; not in motion. 2. not dynamic.

statics (stat′iks) that phase of mechanics which deals with the action of forces and systems of forces on bodies at rest.

statim (sta′tim) [L.] immediately, at once. Abbreviated *stat.*

station (sta′shun) [L. *statio,* from *stare* to stand still] 1. the position assumed in standing; the manner of standing; in ataxic conditions it is sometimes pathognomonic. See *attitude.* 2. the location of the presenting part of the fetus in the birth canal, designated as −5 to −1 according to the number of centimeters the part is above a imaginary plane passing through the ischial spines, 0 when at the plane, and +1 to +5 according to the number of centimeters the part is below the plane. 3. a specified site to which the sick and wounded are brought. **Romberg s.,** the position assumed by the patient when the Romberg sign is being sought, i.e., standing upright with the feet close together.

stationary (sta′shun-er″e) [L. *stationarius*] not subject to variations or to changes of place.

statistics (stah-tis′tiks) numerical facts pertaining to a body of things; also the science which deals with the collection and tabulation of such facts. **vital s.,** that branch of biometry which deals with the data and laws of human mortality, morbidity, natality, and demography; called also *biostatistics.*

statoacoustic (stat″o-ah-koo′stik) pertaining to balance and hearing.

statoconia (stat″o-ko′ne-ah), pl. of statoconium [Gr. *statos* standing + *konos* dust] [NA] minute calciferous granules within the gelatinous statoconic membrane surmounting the acoustic maculae; called also *otoconia.*

statoconium (stat″o-ko′ne-um) singular of *statoconia;* called also *otoconium* and *otoconite.*

statocyst (stat′o-sist) [Gr. *statos* standing + *kystis* sac, bladder] one of the sacs of the labyrinth of the ear to which is attributed an influence in the maintenance of static equilibrium.

statolith (stat′o-lith) 1. one of the granules constituting the statoconia; called also *ear crystal, otolith, otolite,* and *otosteon.* 2. a solid or semisolid body occurring in the statocyst of animals.

statolon (stat′o-lon) an antiviral agent derived from *Penicillium stoloniferum,* which inhibits the multiplication of certain picornaviruses and arboviruses.

statometer (stah-tom′ĕ-ter) [Gr. *statos* standing + *metron* measure] an apparatus for measuring the degree of exophthalmos.

statosphere (stat′o-sfēr) centrosome.

statural (stat′u-ral) pertaining to stature.

stature (stat′ūr) [L. *statura*] the height or tallness of a person standing.

status (sta′tus) [L.] state or condition. **s. angino′sus,** angina which occurs at rest and is refractory to treatment; called also

preinfarction angina. **s. arthrit′icus,** the gouty diathesis; predisposition to gout. **s. asthmat′icus,** asthmatic crisis; asthmatic shock; a sudden intense and continuous aggravation of a state of asthma, marked by dyspnea to the point of exhaustion and collapse and not responding to the usual therapeutic efforts. **s. calcif′ames,** calcium hunger. **s. cholera′icus,** a state occurring in the algid stage of cholera, characterized by a dull countenance, weak pulse, and cold skin. **s. chore′icus,** a severe and persistent form of chorea. **s. convul′vus,** s. epilepticus. **s. criba′lis, s. cribro′sus,** a sievelike condition of the brain due to dilatation of the perivascular lymph spaces. **s. crit′icus,** a severe and persistent form of tabetic crises. **s. degenerati′vus,** a condition characterized by the presence of an unusual number of degenerative stigmata (developmental anomalies) in a single individual. **s. dysgraph′icus,** dysgraphia. **s. dysmyelina′tus, s. dysmyelinisa′tus,** Hallervorden-Spatz syndrome. **s. dysraph′icus,** faulty closure of the embryonic neural tube resulting in faulty formation of midline adult structures, such as the spine, sternum, breasts, and palate. **s. epilep′ticus,** a series of rapidly repeated epileptic convulsions without any periods of consciousness between them. **s. hemicra′nicus,** a state marked by constantly recurring attacks of migraine. **s. lacuna′ris, s. lacuno′sus,** a condition of the brain marked by numerous small infarcts or losses of substance. **s. lymphat′icus,** lymphatism, def. 2. **s. marmora′tus,** a condition marked by excessive myelinization of the nerve fibers of the corpus striatum, as in Vogt's syndrome; called also *état marbré* and *marble state.* **s. parathyreopri′vus,** a condition due to absence of parathyroid. **petit mal s.,** a state of mental confusion lasting for minutes or hours, and accompanied by nearly continuous 3-cps spike and wave discharges in the electroencephalogram. **s. prae′sens,** the condition of a patient at the time of observation. **s. rap′tus,** a condition of ecstasy. **s. spongio′sus,** extensive vacuolization of the cerebral cortex; called also *spongiform encephalopathy.* **s. thymicolymphat′icus,** a condition resembling lymphatism, with enlargement of the lymphadenoid tissue generally and with enlargement of the thymus as the special influencing factor. **s. thy′micus,** lymphatism, def. 2. **s. typho′sus,** the typhoid state. **s. verruco′sus,** a wartlike appearance of the cerebral cortex, produced by disorderly arrangement of the neuroblasts so that the formation of fissures and sulci is irregular and unpredictable. **s. vertigino′sus,** prolonged vertigo.

statuvolence (stat-u′vo-lens) [L. *status* state + *volens* willing] a voluntary, self-induced state of hypnotism.

statuvolent (stat-u′vo-lent) affected with or able to enter a condition of statuvolence.

statuvolic (stat″u-vol′ik) statuvolent.

statuvolism (stat-u′vo-lizm) statuvolence.

Staub-Traugott effect (test) (stawb-traw′got) [Hans *Staub,* Swiss (Basel) internist, born 1890; Carl *Traugott,* Frankfort internist, born 1885] see under *effect.*

staurion (staw′re-on) [Gr., dim. of *stauros* cross] a point at the crossing of the median and transverse palatine sutures.

stauroplegia (staw″ro-ple′je-ah) [Gr. *stauros* cross + *plēgē* stroke] alternate hemiplegia.

stavesacre (stāvz′a-ker) staphisagria.

staxis (stak′sis) [Gr. "a dripping"] hemorrhage.

stay (sta) a narrow structure that gives support, such as the bar of a horse's hoof. **s. of white line,** adminiculum lineae albae.

STD skin test dose.

steal (stēl) the diversion, as of blood flow, from its normal course, as in occlusive arterial disease. **subclavian s.,** in occlusive disease of the subclavian artery, a reversal of blood flow in the ipsilateral vertebral artery (which may deprive the brain of blood) from the basilar artery to the subclavian artery beyond the point of occlusion.

steapsin (ste-ap′sin) [Gr. *stear* fat + *pepsis* digestion] the lipase of the pancreatic juice.

steapsinogen (ste″ap-sin′o-jen) a pre-enzyme of steapsin.

stearaldehyde (ste″ah-ral′dĕ-hīd) a long-cain, aliphatic aldehyde of the class of free aldehydes with the formula $CH_3(CH_2)_{16}$-CHO; it is found in plasmalogens, which give the so-called plasmal reaction upon direct treatment of the tissue with Schiff's reagent.

stearate (ste′ah-rāt) octadecanoate: the ionic form of stearic acid, a naturally occurring fatty acid. Also, any compound of stearic acid.

steariform (ste-ar′ĭ-form) fatlike.

stearin (ste′ah-rin) tristearin.

Stearns' alcoholic amentia (sternz) [Albert Warren *Stearns,* American physician, 1885–1959] see under *amentia.*

stearo-, steato- (ste′ah-ro; ste′ah-to) [Gr. *stear, steatos* fat] combining forms denoting relationship to fat.

stearopten (ste″ah-rop′ten) [stearo- + Gr. *ptēnos* volatile] a camphor; the more solid substance which, combined with an eleopten, constitutes a typical volatile oil.

stearrhea (ste″ah-re′ah) [stearo- + Gr. *rhoia* flow] steatorrhea.

steatite (ste′ah-tīt) talc.

steatitis (ste″ah-ti′tis) [*steato-* + *-itis*] inflammation of adipose tissue.

steato- see *stearo-*.

steatocele (ste-at′o-sēl) [*steato-* + Gr. *kēlē* tumor] a fatty mass formed within the scrotum.

steatocystoma (ste″ah-to-sis-to′mah) an epithelial cyst. **s. mul′tiplex,** steatomatosis, a rare skin disorder with a high familial tendency, probably having an autosomal dominant mode of inheritance, affecting men more often than women, and characterized by the presence on the upper anterior trunk, proximal extremities, and scrotum of multiple cutaneous epithelial cysts containing an oily liquid, abortive hair follicles, and sebaceous glands.

steatogenous (ste″ah-toj′ĕ-nus) [*steato-* + Gr. *gennan* to produce] lipogenic.

steatolysis (ste″ah-tol′ĭ-sis) [*steato-* + Gr. *lysis* dissolution] the emulsifying process fats undergo preparatory to absorption.

steatolytic (ste″ah-to-lit′ik) pertaining to, characterized by, or promoting steatolysis.

steatoma (ste″ah-to′mah), pl. *steato′mata* or *steatomas.* 1. a lipoma. 2. a fatty mass retained within a sebaceous gland.

steatomatosis (ste″ah-to-mah-to′sis) 1. the presence of numerous steatomas. 2. steatocystoma multiplex.

steatomery (ste″ah-tom′er-e) [*steato-* + Gr. *mēros* thigh] a deposit of fat on the outer aspect of the thighs and buttocks.

steatonecrosis (ste″ah-to-nĕ-kro′sis) fat necrosis.

steatopygia (ste″ah-to-pij′e-ah) [*steato-* + Gr. *pygē* buttock + *-ia*] excessive fatness of the buttocks, usually seen in women. Sometimes called *Hottentot bustle* because it is commonly seen in the Hottentot people of southern Africa.

steatopygous (ste″ah-top′ĭ-gus) pertaining to or characterized by steatopygia.

steatorrhea (ste″ah-to-re′ah) [*steato-* + Gr. *rhoia* a flow] excessive amounts of fats in the feces, as in malabsorption syndromes. **idiopathic s.,** nontropical sprue.

steatosis (ste″ah-to′sis) fatty degeneration. **s. cardi′aca,** cardiomyoliposis.

stechiology (stek″e-ol′o-je) stoichiology.

stechiometry (stek″e-om′ĕ-tre) stoichiometry.

Steclin (stek′lin) trademark for preparations of tetracycline.

Steell's murmur (stēlz) [Graham *Steell,* English physician, 1851–1942] Graham Steell's murmur; see under *murmur.*

Steenbock unit (stēn′bok) [Harry *Steenbock,* American biochemist, 1886–1967] see under *unit.*

steffimycin (stef-ĭ-mi′sin) an antibacterial with antiviral properties, produced by *Streptomyces steffisburgensis* var. *steffisburgensis.*

stege (ste′je) [Gr. *stegos* roof] the internal layer of the rods of Corti.

stegnosis (steg-no′sis) [Gr. *stegnōsis* obstruction] constriction; stenosis.

stegnotic (steg-not′ik) pertaining to, characterized by, or promoting stegnosis; astringent.

Stegomyia (steg″o-mi′yah) [Gr. *stegos* roof + *myia* fly] a subgenus of mosquitoes. *S. argen′teus, S. cal′opus* and *S. fascia′tus* are old names for *Aedes aegypti.*

Stein's test (stīnz) [Stanislav Aleksandr Fyodorovich von *Stein,* Russian otologist, born 1855] see under *tests.*

Stein-Leventhal syndrome (stīn-lev′en-thal) [Irving F. *Stein,* Sr., American gynecologist, born 1887; Michael Leo *Leventhal,* American obstetrician and gynecologist, born 1901] see under *syndrome.*

Steinach's operation (method) (sti′nahks) [Eugen *Steinach,* Austrian physician, 1861–1944] see under *operation.*

Steiner's tumors (sti′nerz) [Gabriel *Steiner,* German neurologist, born 1883] Jeanselme's nodules.

Steinmann's pin (extension) (stīn′manz) [Fritz *Steinmann,* Bern surgeon, 1872–1932] see *nail extension,* under *extension.*

Stelangium (ste-lan′je-um) a genus of Schizomycetes of the order Myxobacterales, family Archangiaceae.

Stelazine (stel′ah-zēn) trademark for preparations of trifluoperazine hydrochloride.

stele (stēl) [Gr. *stechelo* stem] the cylindrical central core of vascular tissue of a plant, consisting of the pericycle and the tissues within it—xylem, phloem, and parenchyma.

stella (stel′ah), pl. *stel′lae* [L.] star. **s. len′tis hyaloi′dea,** the posterior pole of the crystalline lens. **s. len′tis irid′ica,** the anterior pole of the crystalline lens.

Stellaria (stel-la′re-ah) a genus of caryophyllaceous plants, the chickweeds. *S. holos′tea* and *S. me′dia* were formerly used as demulcent medicines.

stellate (stel′āt) [L. *stellatus*] shaped like a star; arranged in a roset, or in rosets.

stellectomy (stel-lek′to-me) removal of the stellate ganglion; done for the relief of pain.

stellite (stel′it) a very hard, noncorrosive alloy of cobalt, chromium, and tungsten, used for surgical instruments.

stellreflexe (stel″re-flek′sĕ) [Ger.] a postural reflex.

stellula (stel′u-lah), pl. *stel′lulae* [L., dim. of *stella*] little star. **stel′lulae vasculo′sae winslow′ii,** Winslow's stars. **stel′lulae of Verheyen,** venulae stellatae renis. **stel′lulae verhey′enii,** venulae stellatae renis.

stellulae (stel′u-le) [L.] plural of *stellula.*

Stellwag's sign (symptom) (stel′vagz) [Carl *Stellwag* von Carion, Austrian ophthalmologist, 1823–1904] see under *sign.*

stem (stem) a supporting structure comparable to the stalk or stem of a plant. **brain s.,** see under *B.* **infundibular s.,** infundibulum hypothalami.

Stender dish (sten′der) [Wilhelm P. *Stender,* manufacturer in Leipzig] see under *dish.*

Stenediol (sten′di-ol) trademark for preparations of methandriol.

stenion (sten′e-on), pl. *sten′ia* [Gr. *stenos* narrow + *-on* neuter ending] an encephalometric landmark, the craniometrical point situated at each end of the smallest transverse diameter of the head in the temporal region.

Steno (ste′no) see *Stensen.*

steno- (sten′o) [Gr. *stenos* narrow] a combining form meaning contracted or narrow.

stenobregmatic (sten″o-breg-mat′ik) [*steno-* + Gr. *bregma* the front part of the head] having the upper and anterior portion of the head narrowed.

stenocardia (sten″o-kar′de-ah) angina pectoris.

stenocephalia (sten″o-sĕ-fa′le-ah) stenocephaly.

stenocephalous (sten″o-sef′ah-lus) having a narrow head.

stenocephaly (sten″o-sef′ah-le) [*steno-* + Gr. *kephalē* head] excessive narrowness of the head.

stenochoria (sten″o-ko′re-ah) [*steno-* + Gr. *chōros* space] stenosis, or narrowing.

stenocoriasis (sten″o-ko-ri′ah-sis) [*steno-* + Gr. *korē* pupil] contraction of the pupil of the eye.

stenocrotaphia (sten″o-kro-ta′fe-ah) [*steno-* + Gr. *krotaphos* temple + *-ia*] narrowness of the temporal region.

stenocrotaphy (sten″o-krot′ah-fe) stenocrotaphia.

stenopeic (sten″o-pe′ik) [*steno-* + Gr. *opē* opening] having a narrow slit or opening, as stenopeic spectacles.

stenophotic (sten″o-fo′tik) [*steno-* + Gr. *phōs* light] able to see in a weak light.

stenosal (ste-no′sal) stenotic.

stenosed (stĕ-nōst′, stĕ-nōzd′) narrowed or constricted.

stenosis (stĕ-no′sis) [Gr. *stenōsis*] narrowing or stricture of a duct or canal. **aortic s.,** a narrowing of the aortic orifice of the heart or of the aorta itself. **buttonhole mitral s.,** mitral stenosis in which adhesion and shortening of the mitral cusps produces a diaphragmatic slit resembling a buttonhole; called also *buttonhole deformity* and *fishmouth mitral s.* **cardiac s.** (*obs.*), a narrowing or diminution of any heart passage or cavity. **caroticovertebral s.,** atherosclerotic stenosis of the cervical portions of the vertebral arteries, resulting in cerebral ischemia. **cicatricial s.,** stenosis caused by the contraction of a cicatrix. **fishmouth mitral s.,** buttonhole mitral s. **granulation s.,** stenosis or narrowing caused by the deposit of granulations or by their contraction. **idiopathic hypertrophic subaortic s.,** a cardiomyopathy of unknown cause, in which the left ventricle is hypertrophied (commonly with disproportionate involvement of the interventricular septum) and the cavity is small; it is marked by obstruction to left ventricular outflow. Called also *muscular subaortic s.* **infundibular s.,** stenosis below the pulmonary valve, within the infundibulum (conus arteriosus) of the right ventricle of the heart. **mitral s.,** a narrowing of the left atrioventricular orifice (mitral orifice). **muscular subaortic s.,** idiopathic hypertrophic subaortic s. **myocardial infundibular s.,** infundibular stenosis due to hypertrophy of the surrounding myocardium, resulting in a long narrow channel. **postdiphtheritic s.,** stenosis of the larynx or trachea following diphtheria. **pulmonary s.,** narrowing of the opening between the pulmonary artery and the right ventricle. **pyloric s.,** obstruction of the pyloric orifice of the stomach; it may be congenital as in hypertrophic pyloric stenosis, or acquired due to peptic ulceration or prepyloric carcinoma. **subaortic s., subvalvular aortic s.,** aortic stenosis due to an obstructive lesion in the left ventricle below the aortic valve, causing a pressure gradient across the obstruction within the ventricle. **supravalvular s.,** a rare form of aortic stenosis occurring above the aortic valve, usually caused by a complete circumferential fibrous ring of constricting tissue at the level of the sinus of Valsalva. **tricuspid s.,** narrowing or stricture of the tricuspid orifice of the heart. **valvular s.,** stenosis affecting any of the valves of the heart; see *aortic s., mitral s., pulmonary s.,* and *tricuspid s.*

stenostomia (sten″o-sto′me-ah) [*steno-* + Gr. *stoma* mouth + *-ia*] narrowing of the mouth.

stenothermal (sten″o-ther′mal) stenothermic.

stenothermic (sten″o-ther′mik) [*steno-* + Gr. *thermē* heat] a term applied to bacteria which can develop only within a narrow range of temperature.

stenothorax (sten″o-tho′raks) [*steno-* + Gr. *thōrax* chest] abnormal narrowness of the chest.

stenotic (stĕ-not′ik) [Gr. *stenotēs* narrowness] pertaining to or characterized by stenosis; abnormally narrowed.

Stensen's canal, duct, experiment, foramen, plexus (sten′senz) [Niels *Stensen*, Danish priest-physician, anatomist, physiologist, and theologian, 1638–1686] see under *experiment* and *plexus*, and see *canalis incisivum*, *ductus parotideus*, and *foramen incisivum*.

stent (stent) a mold for keeping a skin graft in place, made of Stent's mass or some acrylic or dental compound. By extension used to designate a device or mold of a suitable material, used to hold a skin graft in place or to provide support for tubular structures that are being anastomosed.

step (step) one of a series of footrests on different levels, or a structure resembling it. **Rönne's nasal s.,** a steplike defect in the nasal side of the visual field; seen in glaucoma.

stephanial (ste-fa′ne-al) pertaining to the stephanion.

stephanion (stĕ-fa′ne-on) [Gr. *stephanos* crown + *-on* neuter ending] the point on the side of the cranium at which the coronal suture meets the superior temporal line.

Stephanofilaria (stef″ah-no-fĭ-la′re-ah) a genus of filarial nematodes. **S. stile′si,** a species causing dermatitis in cattle in the United States.

stephanofilariasis (stef″ah-no-fil″ah-ri′ah-sis) a chronic skin disease of cattle in certain parts of the United States, due to infestation with the nematode *Stephanofilaria stilesi;* called also *verminous dermatitis.*

Stephanurus (stef″ah-nu′rus) a genus of nematode parasites of the family Syngamidae. **S. denta′tus,** a species parasitic in the urinary tract and occasionally in other tissues of swine.

steradian (ste-ra′de-an) [Gr. *ster-* solid + *radian*] the unit of measurement of solid angles, equivalent to the angle subtended at the center of a sphere by an area on its surface equal to the square of its radius.

Sterane (ster′ān) trademark for preparations of prednisolone.

sterco- (ster′ko) [L. *stercus* dung] a combining form denoting relation to feces.

stercobilin (ster″ko-bi′lin) [*sterco-* + *bilin*] a bile pigment derivative, $C_{33}H_{46}N_4O_6$, formed by air oxidation of stercobilinogen, which is in turn derived by reduction of bilirubin; it is a brown-orange-red pigmentation contributing to the color of feces and urine.

stercobilinogen (ster″ko-bi-lin′o-jen) a bilirubin metabolite and precursor of stercobilin, formed by reduction of urobilinogen.

stercolith (ster′ko-lith) [*sterco-* + Gr. *lithos* stone] a fecal concretion.

stercoporphyrin (ster″ko-por′fĭ-rin) coproporphyrin.

stercoraceous (ster″ko-ra′shus) [L. *stercoraceus*] consisting of or containing feces; fecal.

stercoral (ster′ko-ral) stercoraceous.

stercorin (ster′ko-rin) coprostanol.

stercorolith (ster′ko-ro-lith) stercolith.

stercoroma (ster″ko-ro′mah) a large accumulation of fecal matter forming a tumor-like mass in the rectum.

stercorous (ster′ko-rus) [L. *stercorosus*] of the nature of excrement.

Sterculia (ster-ku′le-ah) a genus of trees and shrubs, including many species, mostly tropical; some have edible seeds and others are medicinal, while still others afford a gummy exudation with cathartic and adhesive properties (see *karaya gum*, under *gum*). The hairs of *S. apetala* of Panama may be very irritating.

stercus (ster′kus), pl. *ster′cora* [L.] dung, or feces.

stere (stēr) [Gr. *stereos* solid] a cubic meter.

stereo- (ste′re-o) [Gr. *stereos* solid] a combining form meaning solid, having three dimensions, or firmly established.

stereoagnosis (ste″re-o-ag-no′sis) astereognosis.

stereoanesthesia (ste″re-o-an″es-the′ze-ah) reduced tactile ability to identify the form, size, weight, and texture of objects.

stereoarthrolysis (ste″re-o-ar-throl′ĭ-sis) [*stereo-* + Gr. *arthron* joint + *lysis* dissolution] operative formation of a movable new joint in cases of bony ankylosis.

stereoauscultation (ste″re-o-aws″kul-ta′shun) auscultation by means of two phonendoscopes each on different parts of the chest. One tube of each instrument is placed in the ears, the other tube of each being closed with the fingers.

stereoblastula (ste″re-o-blas′tu-lah) a solid blastula, all of whose cells reach the external surface.

stereocampimeter (ste″re-o-kam-pim′ĕ-ter) [*stereo-* + L. *campus*

field + *metrum* measure] an instrument for studying unilateral central scotomas and defects in the central retinal area.

stereochemical (ste″re-o-kem′e-kal) pertaining to stereochemistry, or to the space relations of the atoms of a molecule.

stereochemistry (ste″re-o-kem′is-tre) that chemical theory which supposes an arrangement of the atoms of certain molecules in three dimensional spaces; that branch of chemistry which treats of the space relations between atoms.

stereocilia (ste″re-o-sil′e-ah) [L.] plural of *stereocilium.*

stereocilium (ste″re-o-sil′e-um), pl. *stereocil′ia.* A nonmotile protoplasmic filament on the free surface of a cell. Cf. *kinocilium.*

stereocinefluorography (ste″re-o-sin″ĕ-floo″or-og′rah-fe) photographic recording by motion picture camera of x-ray images produced by stereofluoroscopy, affording three-dimensional visualization.

stereocognosy (ste″re-o-kog′no-se) stereognosis.

stereoencephalotome (ster″e-o-en-sef′ah-lo-tōm″) a guiding instrument used in stereoencephalotomy.

stereoencephalotomy (ster″e-o-en-sef″ah-lot′o-me) [*stereo-* + Gr. *enkephalos* brain + *tomē* a cutting] stereotaxic surgery.

stereofluoroscopy (ste″re-o-floo″o-ros′ko-pe) stereoscopic fluoroscopy.

stereognosis (ste″re-og-no′sis) [*stereo-* + Gr. *gnōsis* knowledge] 1. the faculty of perceiving and understanding the form and nature of objects by the sense of touch. 2. perception by the senses of the solidity of objects.

stereognostic (ste″re-og-nos′tik) pertaining to stereognosis.

stereogram (ste″re-o-gram) 1. a stereoscopic roentgenogram. 2. a stereoscopic drawing.

stereograph (ste″re-o-graf) stereogram.

stereoisomer (ste″re-o-i′so-mer) a compound exhibiting, or capable of exhibiting, stereoisomerism.

stereoisomeric (ster″e-o-i″so-mer′ik) pertaining to or exhibiting stereoisomerism.

stereoisomerism (ster″e-o-i-som′er-izm) [*stereo-* + *isomerism*] a type of isomerism in which two or more compounds possess the same molecular and structural formulas but different spatial or configurational formulas, the spatial relationships of the atoms being different, but not the linkages. Stereoisomerism is divided into two branches, *optical isomerism* (which includes enantiomorphism and diastereoisomerism), and *geometric isomerism.* See *structural isomerism* under *isomerism*, and see *mutarotation, racemization,* and *tautomerism.*

stereology (ste″re-ol′o-je) the study of the three-dimensional properties of objects usually seen in two dimensions.

stereometer (ste″re-om′ĕ-ter) [*stereo-* + Gr. *metron* measure] an instrument for performing stereometry.

stereometry (ste″re-om′ĕ-tre) the measurement of the cubic or solid contents of a solid body, or of the capacity of a hollow space.

stereo-ophthalmoscope (ste″re-o-of-thal′mo-skōp) an ophthalmoscope by which the fundus of the eye is viewed with both eyes through two eyepieces.

Stereo-orthopter (ste″re-o-thop′ter) trademark for a mirror-reflecting instrument used to correct strabismus.

stereophorometer (ste″re-o-fo-rom′ĕ-ter) a prism-refracting instrument for use in orthoptic training.

stereophoroscope (ste″re-o-for′o-skōp) [*stereo-* + Gr. *phoros* bearing + *skopein* to examine] a form of zoetrope, employed in the study of visual perception.

stereophotography (ste″re-o-fo-tog′rah-fe) stereoscopic photography.

stereophotomicrograph (ste″re-o-fo-to-mi′kro-graf) a stereoscopic photograph of a microscopical subject.

stereoplasm (ste′re-o-plazm″) [*stereo-* + Gr. *plasma* anything formed or molded] the more solid portions of protoplasm.

stereopsis (ste″re-op′sis) [*stereo-* + Gr. *opsis* vision] stereoscopic vision.

stereoradiography (ste″re-o-ra″de-og′rah-fe) stereoroentgenography.

stereoroentgenography (ste″re-o-rent″gen-og′rah-fe) the making of a roentgenogram giving an impression of depth as well as of width and height.

stereoroentgenometry (ste″re-o-rent″gen-om′ĕ-tre) measurement of the solid dimensions of a radiopaque object from its stereoscopic roentgenograms.

stereosalpingography (ste″re-o-sal″ping-gog′rah-fe) salpingography in which an impression of depth is achieved.

stereoscope (ste′re-o-skōp″) [*stereo-* + Gr. *skopein* to examine] an instrument for producing the appearance of solidity and relief by combining the images of two similar pictures of an object.

stereoscopic (ste″re-o-skop′ik) having the effect of a stereoscope; giving to objects seen a solid or three-dimensional appearance.

stereoskiagraphy (ste″re-o-ski-ag′rah-fe) stereoroentgenography.

stereospecific (ste″re-o-spĕ-sif′ik) exhibiting marked structural specificity in interacting with a substrate or a limited class of substrates; said of enzymes or of synthetic organic reactions.

stereotactic (ste″re-o-tak′tik) stereotaxic.

stereotaxic (ste″re-o-tak′sik) 1. pertaining to or characterized by precise positioning in space; said especially of discrete areas of the brain that control specific functions. See also under *surgery*. 2. pertaining to or exhibiting stereotaxis.

stereotaxis (ste″re-o-tak′sis) taxis in response to contact with a solid or rigid surface.

stereotaxy (ste″re-o-tak′se) stereotaxic surgery.

stereotropic (ste″re-o-trop′ik) pertaining to or characterized by stereotropism.

stereotropism (ste″re-ot′ro-pizm) [*stereo-* + Gr. *tropos* a turning] the movement of an organism in response to contact with a solid or with a rigid surface.

stereotypy (ste′re-o-ti″pe) [*stereo-* + Gr. *typos* type] the persistent repetition of senseless acts or words. It may be a persistent maintaining of a bodily attitude (*s. of attitude*), repetition of senseless movements (*s. of movement*, echopraxia), or constant repetition of certain words or phrases (*s. of speech*, echolalia, verbigeration).

Stereum (ste′re-um) a genus of basidiomycetous fungi of the order Polyporales, series Hymenomycetes, composed of the bracket fungi, and including some species causing tree and wood rot. *S. hirsu′tum* is the source of hirsutic acid.

steric (ste′rik) pertaining to the arrangement of atoms in space; pertaining to stereochemistry.

sterid (ster′id) steroid.

sterigma (ste-rig′mah), pl. *sterig′mata* [Gr. *stērigma* support] any of the flask-shaped structures projecting radially from the vesicle of fungi of the genus *Aspergillus*, from the tips of which conidia bud off consecutively; also any of the similar structures in *Penicillium* and other conidia-producing fungi.

Sterigmatocystis (ste-rig″mah-to-sis′tis) *Aspergillus*.

Sterigmocystis (ste-rig″mo-sis′tis) *Aspergillus*.

sterilant (ster′ĭ-lant) a sterilizing agent, i.e., an agent that destroys microorganisms.

sterile (ster′il) [L. *sterilis*] 1. unable to produce offspring; barren. 2. aseptic; not producing microorganisms; free from living microorganisms.

sterility (stĕ-ril′ĭ-te) [L. *sterilitas*] 1. the inability to produce offspring, i.e., the inability to conceive (*female s.*) or to induce conception (*male s.*). Cf. *infertility*. 2. the state of being aseptic, or free from microorganisms. **absolute s.**, complete and irremediable inability to produce offspring. **female s.**, inability of the female to conceive as a result of a structural or functional defect in the reproductive organs. **male s.**, inability of the male to fertilize the ovum as a result of failure to produce living spermatozoa (*aspermatogenic s.*), an abnormality in spermatozoa production (*dysspermatogenic s.*), or some cause other than inability to produce live, normal spermatozoa (*normospermatogenic s.*). **one-child s.**, inability to produce further offspring after having produced one. **primary s.**, 1. inability to produce offspring because of the absence of some factor essential for reproduction. 2. sterility in which no offspring has ever been produced. **relative s.**, infertility. **secondary s.**, 1. inability to produce further offspring after having conceived or induced conception. See *one-child s.* and *two-child s.* 2. inability to produce offspring resulting from a noncongenital defect. **two-child s.**, inability to produce further offspring after having produced two.

sterilization (ster″ĭ-li-za′shun) 1. the complete elimination of microbial viability. 2. any procedure by which an individual is made incapable of reproduction, as by castration, vasectomy, or salpingectomy. **chemical s.**, destruction of microbial viability by means of a chemical substance. **eugenic s.**, the process of rendering a person incapable of reproduction because the offspring would probably be undesirable types. **fractional s., intermittent s.**, destruction of microbial viability by successive application of the procedure at intervals, to allow spores to develop into vegetative forms, which are more easily destroyed. **mechanical s.**, the elimination of microorganisms by passing the fluid through a bacteria-proof filter.

sterilize (ster′ĭ-līz) 1. to render sterile; to free from microorganisms. 2. to render incapable of reproduction.

sterilizer (ster′ĭ-līz″er) an apparatus used for the destruction of microorganisms; see *sterilization*. **Arnold s.**, an apparatus for sterilizing objects by means of live steam at atmospheric pressure.

Sterisil (ster′ĭ-sil) trademark for a preparation of hexetidine.

Stern's position (sternz) [Heinrich *Stern*, American physician, 1868–1918] see under *position*.

Stern's test (sternz) [Margarete *Stern*, German scientist] see under *tests*.

sternad (ster′nad) toward the sternum, or sternal aspect.

sternal (ster′nal) [L. *sternalis*] pertaining to the sternum.

sternalgia (ster-nal′je-ah) [Gr. *sternon* sternum + *algos* pain + *-ia*] 1. pain in the sternum. 2. angina pectoris.

Sternberg's disease, giant cells (stern′bergz) [Carl *Sternberg*, Austrian pathologist, 1872–1935] see *Hodgkin's disease*, under *disease*, and *Sternberg-Reed cells*, under *cell*.

Sternberg-Reed cells (stern′berg-rēd) [Carl *Sternberg*; Dorothy *Reed*, American pathologist] see under *cell*.

sternebra (ster′ne-brah), pl. *ster′nebrae* [*sternum* + *vertebrae*] any of the segments of the sternum in early life, which later fuse to form the corpus sterni.

Sterneedle (stern′ne-d′l) trademark for a controlled depth, multiple puncture apparatus used in the diagnosis of tuberculosis. See *tuberculin test, Sterneedle*, under *tests*.

sternen (ster′nen) pertaining to the sternum alone.

sterno- (ster′no) [Gr. *sternon* breast] a combining form denoting relationship to the sternum.

sternoclavicular (ster″no-klah-vik′u-lar) pertaining to the sternum and clavicle.

sternoclavicularis (ster″no-klah-vik″u-la′ris) [L.] sternoclavicular.

sternocleidal (ster″no-kli′dal) [*sterno-* + Gr. *kleis* key] sternoclavicular.

sternocleidomastoid (ster″no-kli″do-mas′toid) pertaining to the sternum, clavicle, and mastoid process.

sternocostal (ster″no-kos′tal) [*sterno-* + L. *costa* rib] pertaining to the sternum and ribs.

sternodymia (ster″no-dim′e-ah) the union of two fetuses by the anterior wall of the chest.

sternodymus (ster-nod′ĭ-mus) [*sterno-* + Gr. *didymos* twin] a pair of twin fetuses united by the anterior wall of the chest.

sternodynia (ster″no-din′e-ah) sternalgia.

sternogoniometer (ster″no-go″ne-om′ĕ-ter) an instrument for measuring the sternal angle.

sternohyoid (ster″no-hi′oid) pertaining to the sternum and to the hyoid bone.

sternoid (ster′noid) resembling the sternum.

sternomastoid (ster″no-mas′toid) pertaining to the sternum and the mastoid process of the temporal bone.

sternopagia (ster″no-pa′je-ah) sternodymia.

sternopagus (ster-nop′ah-gus) [Gr. *sternon* sternum + *pagos* thing fixed] sternodymus.

sternopericardial (ster″no-per″ĭ-kar′de-al) pertaining to the sternum and the pericardium.

sternoscapular (ster″no-skap′u-lar) pertaining to the sternum and the scapula.

sternoschisis (ster-nos′kĭ-sis) [*sterno-* + Gr. *schisis* cleft] a developmental anomaly characterized by a fissure of the sternum.

sternothyreoideus (ster″no-thi″re-oi′de-us) [L.] sternothyroid.

sternothyroid (ster″no-thi′roid) pertaining to the sternum and to the thyroid cartilage or gland.

sternotomy (ster-not′o-me) [*sterno-* + Gr. *tome* a cutting] the operation of cutting through the sternum.

sternotracheal (ster″no-tra′ke-al) [*sterno-* + *trachea*] pertaining to the sternum and to the trachea.

sternotrypesis (ster″no-tri-pe′sis) [*sterno-* + Gr. *trypēsis* trephination] surgical perforation of the sternum.

sternovertebral (ster″no-ver′te-bral) pertaining to the sternum and vertebrae.

sternoxiphopagus (ster″no-zi-fop′ah-gus) [*sterno-* + *xiphoid* process + Gr. *pagus* thing fixed] a double fetus consisting of two similar components united in the frontal plane, in the region of the sternum and xiphoid process.

sternum (ster′num) [L.; Gr. *sternon*] [NA] a longitudinal unpaired plate of bone forming the middle of the anterior wall of the thorax, and articulating above with the clavicles and along the sides with the cartilages of the first seven ribs. It consists of three portions, the manubrium, the body, and the xiphoid process. **cleft s.**, a sternum which is longitudinally fissured.

sternutatio (ster″nu-ta′she-o) [L.] sternutation. **s. convulsi′va**, paroxysmal and convulsive sneezing.

sternutation (ster″nu-ta′shun) [L. *sternutatio*] the act of sneezing; a sneeze.

sternutator (ster′nu-ta″tor) a gas or other substance that causes sneezing.

sternutatory (ster-nu′tah-tor″e) [L. *sternutatorius*] 1. producing or causing sneezing. 2. an agent that causes sneezing.

sternzellen (stern′tsel-en) [Ger. "star cells"] Kupffer's cells.

steroid (ste′roid) a group name for lipids that contain a hydrogenated cyclopentenanthrene-ring system. Some of the substances included in this group are progesterone, adrenocortical hormones, the gonadal hormones, cardiac aglycones, bile acids, sterols (such as cholesterol), toad poisons, saponins, and some of the carcinogenic hydrocarbons. **anabolic s.**, any of a group of synthetic derivatives of testosterone, having pronounced anabolic properties and relatively weak androgenic properties, which are used clinically mainly to promote growth and repair of body tissues in senility, debilitating illness, and convalescence.

steroidogenesis (ste-roi″do-jen′ĕ-sis) the production of steroids, as by the adrenal glands.

steroidogenic (ste-roi″do-jen′ik) producing steroids; giving rise to steroids.

sterol (ste′rol) [Gr. *stereos* solid + *-ol* (L. *oleum* oil)] steroids with long (8–10 carbons) aliphatic side-chains at position 17 and at least one alcoholic hydroxyl group, usually at position 3. They have lipid-like solubility. Examples are cholesterol and ergosterol.

stertor (ster′tor) [L.] an act of snoring; stertorous or sonorous breathing. **hen-cluck s.**, a respiration sound like a hen's cluck in cases of postpharyngeal abscess.

stertorous (ster′to-rus) characterized by stertor.

steth- see *stetho-*.

stethacoustic (steth″ah-koo′stik) heard with the stethoscope.

stethalgia (steth-al′je-ah) pain in the chest or chest wall.

stethemia (steth-e′me-ah) [*steth-* + Gr. *haima* blood + *-ia*] congestion of the lungs.

stethendoscope (steth-en′do-skōp) [*steth-* + Gr. *endon* within + *skopein* to examine] a fluoroscope used in examination of the chest.

stetho-, steth- (steth′o, steth) [Gr. *stēthos* chest] combining form denoting relationship to the chest.

stethocyrtograph (steth″o-ser′to-graf) stethokyrtograph.

stethogoniometer (steth″o-go″ne-om′ĕ-ter) [*stetho-* + Gr. *gōnia* angle + *metron* measure] an apparatus for measuring the curvature of the chest.

stethograph (steth′o-graf) [*stetho-* + Gr. *graphein* to write] an instrument for recording movements of the chest.

stethography (steth-og′rah-fe) 1. use of the stethograph to record movements of the chest. 2. phonocardiography.

stethokyrtograph (steth″o-kir′to-graf) [*stetho-* + Gr. *kyrtos* bent + *graphein* to write] an instrument for recording and measuring the curves of the chest.

stethometer (steth-om′ĕ-ter) [*stetho-* + Gr. *metron* measure] an instrument for measuring the circular dimension or expansion of the chest.

Stethomyia (steth″o-mi′yah) a subgenus of anopheline mosquitoes.

stethomyitis (steth″o-mi-i′tis) stethomyositis.

stethomyositis (steth″o-mi″o-si′tis) [*stetho* + Gr. *myos* of muscle + *-itis*] inflammation of the muscles of the chest.

stethoparalysis (steth″o-pah-ral′ĭ-sis) paralysis of the chest muscles.

stethophone (steth′o-fōn) [*stetho-* + Gr. *phōnē* voice] 1. an instrument designed to transmit stethoscopic sounds so that many persons can hear them simultaneously. 2. a term proposed as a more accurate name for stethoscope.

stethophonometer (steth″o-fo-nom′ĕ-ter) [*stetho-* + Gr. *phōnē* voice + *metron* measure] an instrument for measuring the intensity of auscultatory sounds.

stethopolyscope (steth″o-pol′ĭ-skōp) [*stetho-* + Gr. *polys* many + *skopein* to examine] a stethoscope for the simultaneous use of several persons.

stethoscope (steth′o-skōp) [*stetho-* + Gr. *skopein* to examine] an instrument of various form, size, and material for performing mediate auscultation. By means of this instrument the respiratory, cardiac, pleural, arterial, venous, uterine, fetal, intestinal, and other sounds are conveyed to the ear of the observer. **binaural s.**, one with two adjustable branches, designed for use with both ears. **Cammann's s.**, a binaural stethoscope. **DeLee-Hillis obstetric s.**, a stethoscope worn on the head of the examiner, used for listening to the fetal heart. **differential s.**, one by means of which sounds at two different portions of the body may be compared. **electronic s.**, an electronic amplifier of sounds within the body; selective controls permit tuning for low or high frequency tones. An auxiliary output permits the recording or viewing of audio patterns. **esophageal s.**, one which is positioned within the esophagus to transmit heart and respiratory sounds. **Leff s.**, one for listening to the fetal heart.

stethoscopic (steth″o-skop′ik) pertaining to or performed by means of the stethoscope.

stethoscopy (steth-os′ko-pe) examination by means of the stethoscope.

stethospasm (steth′o-spazm) spasm of the chest muscles.

Stevens-Johnson syndrome (ste′venz-jon′son) [Albert Mason *Stevens*, 1884–1945, and Frank Chambliss *Johnson*, 1894–1934, American pediatricians] see under *syndrome*.

Stewart's purple (stu′artz) [Douglas Hunt *Stewart*, New York surgeon, 1860–1933] see under *purple*.

Stewart's test (stu′artz) [George Neil *Stewart*, Canadian-American scientist, 1860–1930] see under *tests*.

Stewart-Holmes sign (stu′art-hōmz) [Purves *Stewart*, London physician, 1869–1949; Gordon *Holmes*, British neurologist] rebound phenomenon.

STH somatotropic (growth) hormone.

sthenia (sthe′ne-ah) [Gr. *sthenos* + *-ia*] a condition of strength and activity.

sthenic (sthen′ik) active; strong.

stheno- (sthen′o) [Gr. *sthenos* strength] a combining form denoting relationship to strength.

sthenometer (sthen-om′ĕ-ter) an instrument for measuring the muscular strength of a part.

sthenometry (sthen-om′ĕ-tre) [*stheno-* + Gr. *metron* measure] the measurement of bodily strength.

sthenophotic (sthen″o-fo′tik) [*stheno-* + Gr. *phōs* light] able to see in a strong light.

sthenoplastic (sthen″o-plas′tik) [*stheno-* + Gr. *plastikos* formed] a term applied to the body form which resembles the long or dolichomorphic form.

stibamine (stib′ah-min) chemical name: sodium 4-aminobenzenestibonic acid. A brown, amorphous powder, $NH_2C_6H_5SbO(OH)_2$, formerly used in the treatment of leishmaniasis.

stibialism (stib′e-al-izm) [L. *stibium* antimony] poisoning with antimony.

stibiated (stib′e-āt″ed) containing antimony.

stibiation (stib″e-a′shun) [L. *stibium* antimony] administration of antimonials in large quantities; treatment by bringing the patient under the full influence of antimony.

stibium (stib′e-um) [L.] antimony.

stibocaptate (stib″o-kap′tāt) chemical name: 2,2′-(1,2-dicarboxy-1,2-ethanediyl)bis-1,3,2-dithiastibolane-4,5-dicarboxylic acid hexosodium salt. A trivalent antimony compound, $C_{12}H_8Na_6O_{12}Sb_2$, used as an antischistosomal, administered intramuscularly. Called also *antimony dimercaptossiccinate* and *antimony sodium dimercaptosuccinate*.

stibogluconate sodium (stib″o-glu′ko-nāt) antimony sodium gluconate.

stibonium (stĭ-bo′ne-um) the radical SbH_4.

stibophen (stib′o-fen) chemical name: bis[4,5-dihydroxy-1,3-benzenedisulfonato(4-)-O⁴,O⁵]antimonato(5-)pentasodium heptahydrate. A trivalent antimony compound, $C_{12}H_4Na_5O_{16}S_4$-Sb·7H₂O, occurring as a white or slightly yellow or pink, crystalline powder; used as an anthelmintic, chiefly in the treatment of schistosomiasis due to *Schistosoma mansoni*, *S. haematobium*, and *S. japonicum*. It is also effective in the treatment of granuloma inguinale, administered intramuscularly and intravenously. Called also *neoantimosan*.

stichochrome (stik′o-krōm) [Gr. *stichos* row + *chrōma* color] any nerve cell having the stainable substance (chromophilic bodies) arranged in more or less regular striae or layers. Cf. *arkyochrome*, *gyrochrome*, and *perichrome*.

Sticker's disease (stik′erz) [Georg *Sticker*, German physician, 1860–1960] erythema infectiosum.

Sticta (stik′tah) [Gr. *stiktos* punctured] a genus of lichens; lungwort.

Stieda's disease, fracture (ste′dahz) [Alfred *Stieda*, German surgeon, 1869–1945] see *Pellegrini's disease*, under *disease*, and see under *fracture*.

Stieda's process (ste′dahz) [L. *Stieda*, German anatomist, 1837–1918] processus posterior tali.

Stierlin's symptom (sign) (stēr′linz) [Eduard *Stierlin*, Munich surgeon, 1878–1919] see under *symptom*.

stifle (sti′f'l) the part of a horse's limb corresponding to the human knee.

stigma (stig′mah), pl. *stigmas* or *stig′mata* [Gr. "mark"] 1. any mental or physical mark or peculiarity which aids in the identification or in the diagnosis of a condition. 2. follicular stigma. 3. purpuric or hemmorhagic lesions of the hands and/or feet, which resemble crucifixion wounds. 4. in botany the uppermost part of a pistil, which secretes a moist, sticky substance to trap and hold the pollen that reach it. 5. a reddish or brownish red dot or short rod located in the anterior region of chromatophore-bearing protozoa and rarely in colorless forms; its exact nature is unknown. Called also *eyespot*. **costal s.**, Stiller's sign. **s. of degeneracy**, any of the developmental anomalies which are found in considerable number in status degenerativus. **follicular s.**, a spot on the surface of an ovary where the vesicular follicle will rupture and permit passage of the ovum during ovulation. Called also *macula folliculi*. **Giuffrida-Ruggieri s.**, abnormal shallowness of the glenoid fossa. **hysteric s.**, a bodily mark or sign characteristic of hysteria. **malpighian s's**, the points where the smaller veins enter into the larger veins of the spleen. **psychic s.**, mental conditions marked by susceptibility to suggestion. **somatic s.**, the bodily signs of certain nervous diseases.

stigmal (stig′mal) stigmatic.

stigmasterol (stig-mas′tĕ-rol) an unstaurated plant sterol, $C_{29}H_{48}O$, occurring in physostigma, cacao butter, rape oil, soybean oil, and elsewhere. An important starting material for industrial synthesis of steroid hormones.

stigmata (stig′mah-tah) [Gr.] plural of *stigma*.

stigmatic (stig-mat′ik) pertaining to a stigma.

stigmatism (stig′mah-tizm) 1. the condition due to or marked by stigmas. 2. the accurate rendition of points by a lens system.

stigmatization (stig″mah-ti-za′shun) 1. the formation of impressions on the skin. 2. the formation of bleeding points or of red lines upon the skin by hypnotic suggestion.

stigmatometer (stig″mah-tom′ĕ-ter) an instrument for testing the refraction of the eye by the objective method and for direct ophthalmoscopy.

stigmatoscope (stig-mat′o-skōp) the viewing instrument used in stigmatoscopy.

stigmatoscopy (stig″mah-tos′ko-pe) measurement of errors of refraction by having the patient observe a point of light (stigma) and describe the appearance under controlled conditions with different lenses.

stijfziekte (stēf-zēk′te) [Dutch] a phosphorus-deficiency disease of the joints of young cattle in South Africa, marked by retardation of growth, skeletal abnormalities, stiffness, and lameness.

stilalgin (stil-al′jin) mephenesin.

Stilbaceae (stil-ba′se-e) a family of imperfect fungi of the order Moniliales, including the genus *Dendrochium.*

stilbazium iodide (stil-baz′ĭ-um) chemical name: 1-ethyl-2,6-bis-(*p*-1-pyrrolidinylstyryl)pyridinium iodide; an anthelmintic, $C_{31}H_{36}IN_3$.

stilbene (stil′bēn) toluylene.

stilbestrol (stil-bes′trol) diethylstilbestrol.

stilet (sti-let′) [Fr. *stilette*] stylet.

stilette (sti-let′) [Fr.] stylet.

stili (sti′li) [L.] plural of *stilus.*

Still's disease (stilz) [Sir George Frederick *Still,* English physician, 1868–1941] see under *disease.*

Still-Chauffard syndrome (stil-sho-far′) [Sir G. F. *Still;* Anatole Marie Emile *Chauffard,* French physician, 1855–1932] Chauffard's syndrome.

stillbirth (stil′berth) the delivery of a dead child; see *fetal death,* under *death.*

stillborn (stil′born) born dead.

Stiller's rib, sign (stil′erz) [Berthold *Stiller,* physician in Budapest, 1837–1922] see under *rib* and *sign.*

stillicidium (stil″ĭ-sid′e-um) [L. *stilla* drop + *cadere* to fall] a dribbling or flowing by drops, as in epiphora. **s. lacrima′rum,** epiphora. **s. na′rium,** coryza. **s. uri′nae,** strangury.

Stilling's canal, column, fibers, fleece, nucleus (stil′ingz) [Benedict *Stilling,* German anatomist 1810–1879] see under the nouns.

Stillingia (stil-lin′je-ah) [Benjamin *Stillingfleet,* English botanist, 1702–1771] a genus of euphorbiaceous trees, shrubs, and herbs. The root of *S. sylvat′ica* L., a plant of North America, is sialagogue, diuretic, and laxative.

Stilphostrol (stil-fos′trōl) trademark for a preparation of diethylstilbestrol diphosphate.

stilus (sti′lus), pl. *sti′li* [L.] stylus.

stimulant (stim′u-lant) [L. *stimulans*] 1. producing stimulation; especially producing stimulation by causing tension on muscle fiber through the nervous tissue. 2. an agent or remedy that produces stimulation. **alcoholic s.,** one of which ethylic alcohol is the basis, such as wine, brandy, whisky, and malt liquors. **cardiac s.,** one which increases the heart's action. **central s.,** a stimulant of the central nervous system. **cerebral s.,** one which exalts the functional activities of the brain. **diffusable s.,** one which acts promptly and strongly, but transiently. **general s.,** one which acts upon the whole body. **genital s.,** an aphrodisiac. **hepatic s.,** one which stimulates the functions of the liver. **intestinal s.,** a cathartic agent. **local s.,** one which affects only, or mainly, that part to which it is applied. **nervous s.,** one which acts mainly upon the nerve centers; a cerebral or a spinal stimulant. **respiratory s.,** one which increases respiratory movements. **spinal s.,** one which acts upon and through the spinal cord. **stomachic s.,** one that promotes the digestion of food in the stomach. **topical s.,** local s. **uterine s.,** an agent which stimulates uterine contraction or menstruation. **vascular s., vasomotor s.,** one which affects the vasomotor centers.

stimulate (stim′u-lāt) to excite to functional activity.

stimulation (stim″u-la′shun) [L. *stimulatio,* from *stimulare* to goad] the act or process of stimulating; the condition of being stimulated. **areal s.,** stimulation of an extended portion of a sense organ. **audio-visual-tactile s.,** the simultaneous rhythmic excitation of the receptors for the senses of hearing, sight, and touch. **nonspecific s.,** stimulation of a sense organ by other than the specific exciting agent. **paradoxical s.,** application of a warm object to one of the cold spots of the body produces a sensation of cold. **paraspecific s.,** nonspecific s. **punctual s.,** excitation of a sense organ by stimulation at a single point.

stimulator (stim″u-la′tor) any agent that excites functional activity. **electronic s.,** a device for applying electronic pulses or signals to activate muscles, to identify nerves, to treat muscular

disorders, etc. **long-acting thyroid s.,** a substance found in the blood in Graves' disease which exerts a stimulating effect on the thyroid of longer duration than does thyrotropin; it also differs chemically and antigenically from thyrotropin and is not elaborated in the pituitary; rather it is associated with IgG immunoglobulin, and may function as an autoantibody. Abbreviated LATS.

stimuli (stim′u-li) plural of *stimulus.*

stimulin (stim′u-lin) a name given by Metchnikoff to an element in the blood serum that stimulates the action of phagocytes.

stimulon (stim′u-lon) a viral antigen postulated to have anti-interferon activity and which therefore promotes the multiplication of other viruses.

stimulus (stim′u-lus), pl. *stim′uli* [L. "goad"] any agent, act, or influence that produces functional or trophic reaction in a receptor or in an irritable tissue. **adequate s.,** a stimulus of the specific form of energy to which the receptor is most sensitive; called also *homologous s.* **aversive s.,** one which, when applied following the occurrence of a response, decreases the strength of that response on later occurrences. **chemical s.,** a chemical substance capable of exciting a response in an organism mediated through specialized nerve endings. **conditioned s.,** a neutral object or event which is psychologically related to a naturally stimulating object or event (unconditioned stimulus) and which induces a conditioned response. Abbreviated CS. **discriminative s.,** a stimulus associated with reinforcement, which exerts control over a particular form of behavior; the subject discriminates between closely related stimuli and responds positively only in the presence of that stimulus. **electric s.,** a galvanic, induced, or other electric current or shock as applied to a responsive tissue. **eliciting s.,** any stimulus, conditioned or unconditioned, which elicits a response. **heterologous s.,** one which produces an effect or sensation when applied to any part whatever of a nerve tract. **heterotopic s.,** a stimulus to heart contraction arising elsewhere than in the sinoatrial node, the normal pacemaker of the heart. **homologous s.,** adequate s. **liminal s.,** one near the threshold. **mechanical s.,** a stimulant application of mechanical force, as in friction or pinching. **nomotopic s.,** a stimulus to heart contraction arising in the sinoatrial node. **reinforcing s.,** any stimulus that follows a response and that increases the probability of eliciting that response. **structured s.,** a well-organized and unambiguous stimulus, the perception of which is influenced to a greater extent by the characteristics of the stimulus than by those of the perceiver. Called also *unambiguous s.* **subliminal s.,** one well below the threshold. **supraliminal s.,** one well above the threshold. **thermal s.,** application of heat. **threshold s.,** a stimulus that is just strong enough to elicit a response; see also *threshold* (def. 1 and 2). **unconditioned s.,** any stimulus capable of eliciting an unconditioned response. **unstructured s.,** an unclear or ambiguous stimulus, the perception of which is influenced to a greater extent by the characteristics of the perceiver than by those of the stimulus. Called also *ambiguous s.*

sting (sting) 1. an injury caused by the venom of a plant or animal (biotoxin) introduced into the individual or with which he has come in contact, together with the mechanical trauma caused by the organ responsible for its introduction. 2. the organ used to inflict such injury. **Irukandji s.,** a clinical syndrome observed in the vicinity of Cairns in Queensland, Australia, attributed to stinging by the carybdeid jellyfish *Carukia barnesi.*

Stintzing's tables (stint′zingz) [Roderich *Stintzing,* Jena internist, 1854–1933] see under *table.*

Stipa viridula (sti′pah vi-rid′u-lah) a grass of the southwestern United States, called *sleepygrass:* poisonous to cattle and horses; said to be a powerful narcotic, diuretic, sudorific, and cardiac poison.

stippling (stip′pling) a spotted condition or appearance, such as an appearance of the retina as if dotted with light and dark points, or the spotted appearance of red blood cells in basophilia. See *basophilia.* It may also be the result of irregular indentations or undulations in a surface, such as the adaptive specialization of normal gingivae which sometimes disappears in disease. **malarial s.,** the finely granular appearance often seen in stained red blood cells which harbor tertian malarial parasites; the granules are called *Schüffner's dots.* **Maurer's s.,** Maurer's dots. **Schüffner's s.,** malarial s.

stirofos (sti′ro-fos) chemical name: (*Z*)-2-chloro-1-(2,4,5-trichlorophenyl)ethenyl dimethyl ester phosphoric acid; a veterinary insecticide, $C_{10}H_9Cl_4O_4P$.

stirpicultural (ster″pĭ-kul′tu-ral) pertaining to stirpiculture.

stirpiculture (ster′pĭ-kul″tūr) [L. *stirps* stock + *cultura* culture] the systematic attempt at improving a stock or race by attention to the laws of breeding.

stirrup (stir′up) 1. a structure or device resembling the stirrup of a saddle, or the portion of an apparatus on which to rest the feet. 2. the stapes. **Finochietto's s.,** an apparatus for exerting skeletal traction in leg fractures, with a U-shaped steel band, passed over the posterior process of the calcaneous and fixed by a cross bar, from which traction is applied.

stitch (stich) 1. to pass lengths of material (thread, catgut, wire, etc.) through tissue by means of a needle, usually to approximate wound edges but also to fix or mobilize an organ or other structure. 2. a single suture. 3. a popular term for a severe pain, generally at the costal margin on one side.

stithe (stĭth) incus.

stizolobin (sti″zo-lo′bin) the globulin of the Chinese velvet bean.

stochastic (sto-kas′tik) [Gr. *stochastikos* skillful in aiming at, able to guess] able to conjecture skillfully; arrived at by skillful conjecturing; random.

stoechiology (stek″e-ol′o-je) stoichiology.

Stoerk's blennorrhea (sterks) [Carl *Stoerk*, Austrian laryngologist, 1832–1899] see under *blennorrhea*.

stoichiology (stoi″ke-ol′o-je) [Gr. *stoicheion* element + *-logy*] the science of elements, especially the physiology of the cellular elements of tissues.

stoichiometry (stoi″ke-om′ĕ-tre) [Gr. *stoicheion* element + *metron* measure] the study of the numerical relationships of chemical elements and compounds and the mathematical laws of chemical changes; the mathematics of chemistry.

stoke (stōk) a unit of kinematic viscosity, being that of fluid with a viscosity of 1 poise and a density of 1 gram per cubic centimeter.

Stokes' amputation (operation) [Sir William *Stokes*, Irish surgeon, 1839–1900] Gritti-Stokes amputation.

Stokes' disease, etc. (stōks) [William *Stokes*, Irish physician, 1804–1878] see under *collar, disease, expectorant, law, sign,* and *syndrome*.

Stokes' reagent (test) (stōks) [William Royal *Stokes*, American pathologist, born 1870] see under *reagent*.

Stokes-Adams disease (syndrome) [William *Stokes*, Irish physician, 1804–1878; Robert *Adams*, Irish physician, 1791–1875] see *Adams-Stokes disease*, under *disease*.

Stokvis' disease, test (stok′vis) [Barend Joseph E. *Stokvis*, Dutch physician, 1834–1902] see *enterogenous cyanosis*, under *cyanosis*, and see under *tests*.

Stokvis-Talma syndrome (stok′vis-tal′mah) [B.J.E. *Stokvis*; Sape *Talma*, Dutch physician, 1847–1918] enterogenous cyanosis.

stoma (sto′mah), pl. *sto′mas* or *sto′mata* [Gr. "mouth"] 1. any minute pore, orifice, or opening on a free surface. 2. the opening established in the abdominal wall by colostomy, ileostomy, etc.; also the opening between two portions of the intestine in an anastomosis.

stomacace (sto-mak′ah-se) [Gr. *stoma* mouth + *kakē* badness] ulcerative stomatitis.

stomach (stum′ak) [L. *stomachus*; Gr. *stomachos*] the musculomembranous expansion of the alimentary canal between the esophagus and the duodenum. Called also *ventriculus* [NA]. The proximal portion is the cardiac part; the portion above the entrance of the esophagus is the fundus; the distal portion is the pyloric part; and the body is between the fundus and the pyloric part. The upper concave surface or edge is the *lesser curvature;* the lower convex edge is the *greater curvature*. The coats of the stomach are four: an outer, peritoneal, or *serous* coat; a *muscular coat,* made up of longitudinal, oblique, and circular fibers; a *submucous* coat; and the *mucous* coat or membrane forming the inner lining. Gastric glands, which are in the mucous coat, secrete gastric juice containing hydrochloric acid, pepsin, and various other digestive enzymes into the cavity of the stomach. Food mixed with this secretion forms a semifluid substance (chyme) suitable for further digestion by the intestine. **aberrant umbilical s.,** an umbilical structure containing gastric mucosa. **aviator's s.,** aeroneurosis. **bilocular s.,** hourglass s. **cardiac s.,** the portion of the stomach close to the esophagus. **cascade s.,** an atypical form of hourglass stomach, characterized roentgenologically by a drawing up of the posterior wall; an opaque medium first fills the upper sac and then cascades into the lower sac. **cup-and-spill s.,** a roentgenographic finding in which the barium remains for a time in the gastric fundus, before spilling over into the main cavity of the stomach, as a result of pressure by a distended colon. **dumping s.,** a complication that sometimes follows gastroenterostomy, in which food is emptied rapidly from the stomach into the jejunum through the new opening, producing weakness, sweating, palpitation, and varying degrees of syncope. See *dumping syndrome,* under *syndrome*. **Holzknecht s.,** a stomach the roentgen picture of which shows it placed diagonally with the pylorus at the lower end of the diagonal. **hourglass s.,** a stomach more or less completely and permanently divided into two parts, so that it resembles an hour-glass in shape; the deformity is due to scarring which complicates chronic gastric ulcer. **leather bottle s.,** linitis plastica. **miniature s.,** Pavlov's s. **Pavlov's s.,** a portion of the stomach of a dog isolated from communication with the rest of the stomach and opening on to the abdominal wall through a fistula: used in studying gastric secretion. **powdered s.,** the dried and powdered defatted wall of the stomach of the hog, *Sus scrofa,* formerly used in the treatment of anemia. **sclerotic s.,** linitis plastica. **thoracic s.,** a stomach which is situated or drawn up above the

level of the diaphragm; i.e., that part of the stomach which has herniated through the diaphragmatic hiatus. **trifid s.,** a stomach with two constrictions, producing three pouches. **upside-down s.,** thoracic s. **waterfall s.,** cascade s. **water-trap s.,** a stomach with an extremely high pylorus, so that it does not readily empty itself.

stomachal (stum′ah-kal) pertaining to the stomach.

stomachalgia (stum″ah-kal′je-ah) pain in the stomach.

stomachic (sto-mak′ik) [L. *stomachicus;* Gr. *stomachikos*] 1. pertaining to the stomach. 2. a medicine which promotes the functional activity of the stomach; a stomachic tonic.

stomachodynia (stum″ah-ko-din′e-ah) [*stomach* + Gr. *odynē* pain + *-ia*] pain in the stomach.

stomachoscopy (sto″mah-kos′ko-pe) [*stomach* + Gr. *skopein* to examine] gastroscopy.

stomadeum (sto″mah-de′um) stomodeum.

stomal (sto′mal) pertaining to a stoma or stomata.

stomalgia (sto-mal′je-ah) stomatalgia.

stomata (sto′mah-tah) [Gr.] plural of *stoma*.

stomatal (sto′mah-tal) pertaining to stomata.

stomatalgia (sto″mah-tal′je-ah) pain in the mouth.

stomatic (sto-mat′ik) pertaining to the mouth.

stomatitides (sto″mah-tit′ĭ-dēz) plural of *stomatitis*. A general term applied collectively to inflammatory conditions of the oral mucosa.

stomatitis (sto-mah-ti′tis), pl. *stomatit′ides* [*stomato-* + *-itis*] inflammation of the oral mucosa, due to local or systemic factors, which may involve the buccal and labial mucosa, palate, tongue, floor of the mouth, and the gingivae. **allergic s.,** stomatitis venenata caused by exposure to allergens. **angular s.,** perlèche. **aphthobullous s.,** foot-and-mouth disease. **s. aphtho′sa, aphthous s.,** a disease of the oral mucosa characterized by small whitish ulcerative lesions surrounded by a red border (aphthae); its onset has been chiefly associated with mild local traumatic injury, allergic conditions, endocrine-associated conditions (such as menstruation), and emotional stress. The exact cause is unknown, but appears to be related to infection by a pleomorphic transitional L-form of α-hemolytic streptococcus, and an immunologic hypersensitivity reaction to the organism has been implicated. Herpes simplex viral infection, (*herpetic s., s. herpetica, vesicular s.*) has been eliminated as a possible factor. In the more severe form, it is known as *periadenitis mucosa necrotica recurrens* (q.v.). Called also *canker sore*. **s. arsenica′lis** stomatitis due to arsenical poisoning. **catarrhal s.,** a clinically and histologically nonspecific stomatitis that develops as a complication of a wide variety of conditions. **contact s.,** s. venenata. **epidemic s., epizootic s.,** foot-and-mouth disease. **erythematopultaceous s.,** stomatitis characterized by a reddened mucous membrane, covered with a layer of thick, sticky matter; seen in uremia. **s. exanthemat′ica,** stomatitis secondary to an exanthematous disease. **fusospirochetal s.,** necrotizing ulcerative gingivostomatitis. **s. gangreno′sa, gangrenous s.,** a form of noma; a severe fusospirochetal infection of grave prognosis, occurring in debilitated patients, with gangrene of the oral and facial tissues. Called also *cancrum oris*. **gonococcal s.,** a rare infection of the oral mucosa caused by *Neisseria gonorrhoeae,* occurring in newborn infants (infected from the birth canal) and in adults. **herpetic s., s. herpet′ica,** an acute infection of the oral mucosa with vesicle formation, caused by the virus of herpes simplex; called also *vesicular s*. **s. hyphomycet′ica,** thrush, def. 1. **infectious s.,** a general term for a usually mild infection of the oral mucosa, beginning with a circumscribed red, itchy area. **s. intertrop′ica,** stomatitis associated with tropical sprue. **lead s.,** the oral manifestations of lead poisoning, including a bluish line along the free gingival margin, pigmentation of the mucosa in contact with the teeth, metallic taste, excessive salivation, and swelling of the salivary glands. **s. medicamento′sa,** eruptive involvement of the oral mucosa resulting from an allergic reaction to some medication, such as antibiotics, arsenic, barbiturates, or salicylates. **membranous s.,** infection of the oral mucosa, accompanied by the formation of false membrane. **mercurial s.,** stomatitis due to mercurial poisoning. **s. mycetogenet′ica,** stomatitis resulting from a fungus infection. **mycotic s.,** thrush, def. 1. **necrotizing ulcerative s.,** necrotizing ulcerative gingivostomatitis. **s. nicoti′na,** irritation of the palate resulting from the coal tar products of tobacco, sometimes contributing to neoplasia. **nonspecific s.,** inflammation of the oral mucosa occurring in association with other conditions, such as menstruation, diabetes, or uremia. **s. scarlati′na,** the oral manifestations of scarlet fever (scarlatina), the most typical being strawberry tongue followed by raspberry tongue. **s. scorbu′tica,** stomatitis associated with vitamin C deficiency. **syphilitic s.,** stomatitis due to systemic syphilis. **s. traumat′ica,** stomatitis produced by some mechanical, thermal, or chemical cause. **tropical s.,** see under *sprue*. **ulcerative s. of sheep,** orf, def. 1. **uremic s.,** the oral manifestations of uremia, including varying degrees of erythema, exudation, ulceration, pseudomembrane formation, foul breath, and burning sensations. **s. venena′ta,** lesions of the oral mucosa resulting from contact with ordinarily innocuous substances such as denture bases, dentifrices, lipstick, food items, or flavoring in gum and candy. **vesicular s.,** 1. herpetic s. 2. a vesicular eruption on the oral mucosa of viral etiology, which affects swine, cattle, and horses. In swine, it is accompanied by vesicles on the snout and interdigital spaces, in cattle on the udder and teats, and in horses on the coronary band. It must be distinguished from foot-and-mouth disease. **Vincent's s.,** necrotizing ulcerative gingivostomatitis.

stomato- (sto′mah-to) [Gr. *stoma, stomatos* mouth] a combining form denoting relationship to the mouth or to the ostium uteri.

stomatocace (sto″mah-tok′ah-se) [stomato- + Gr. *kakē* badness] ulcerative stomatitis.

stomatocyte (sto′mah-to-sīt) a form of red blood cell in which a slit or mouthlike area replaces the normal circle of pallor, as seen in a rare form of hemolytic anemia and in liver disease.

stomatocytosis (sto″mah-to-si-to′sis) a rare congenital hemolytic anemia characterized by the presence of stomatocytes in the peripheral blood.

stomatodynia (sto″mah-to-din′e-ah) [stomato- + Gr. *odynē* pain + -ia] pain in the mouth.

stomatodysodia (sto″mah-to-dis-o′de-ah) [stomato- + Gr. *dysōdia* stench] a bad odor coming from the mouth.

stomatogastric (sto″mah-to-gas′trik) pertaining to the stomach and the mouth.

stomatoglossitis (sto″mah-to-glos-si′tis) inflammation involving the oral mucous membranes and the tongue, occurring in nutritional disorders such as pellagra, beriberi, vitamin B complex deficiency, and in infections, etc.

stomatognathic (sto″mah-tog-nath′ik) [stomato- + Gr. *gnathos* jaw] denoting the mouth and jaws collectively; see under *system.*

stomatography (sto″mah-tog′rah-fe) [stomato- + Gr. *graphein* to write] a description of the mouth.

stomatolalia (sto″mah-to-la′le-ah) speaking through the mouth with the nares closed.

stomatological (sto″mah-to-loj′e-kal) pertaining to stomatology.

stomatologist (sto″mah-tol′o-jist) an expert in stomatology.

stomatology (sto″mah-tol′o-je) that branch of medicine which treats of the mouth and its diseases. **forensic s.,** the application of the sum of knowledge regarding the mouth and its structures to questions of law.

stomatomalacia (sto″mah-to-mah-la′she-ah) [stomato- + Gr. *malakia* softness] softening of the structures of the mouth.

stomatomenia (sto″mah-to-me′ne-ah) [stomato- + Gr. *mēniaia* menses] bleeding from the mucous membrane of the mouth at the time of menstruation.

stomatomy (sto-mat′o-me) [stoma- + Gr. *tomē* a cutting] surgical incision of the ostium uteri.

stomatomycosis (sto″mah-to-mi-ko′sis) [stomato- + Gr. *mykēs* fungus] any oral disease due to a fungus.

stomatonecrosis (sto″mah-to-ne̅-kro′sis) stomatitis gangrenosa.

stomatonoma (sto″mah-to-no′mah) stomatitis gangrenosa.

stomatopathy (sto″mah-top′ah-the) [stomato- + Gr. *pathos* suffering] any disorder of the mouth.

stomatoplastic (sto″mah-to-plas′tik) pertaining to stomatoplasty.

stomatoplasty (sto′mah-to-plas″te) [stomato- + Gr. *plassein* to mold] plastic surgery of, or operative repair of, defects of the mouth or of the ostium uteri.

stomatorrhagia (sto″mah-to-ra′je-ah) [stomato- + Gr. *rhēgnynai* to burst forth] hemorrhage from the mouth. **s. gingiva′rum,** hemorrhage from the gingivae.

stomatoschisis (sto″mah-tos′kĭ-sis) [stomato- + Gr. *schisis* split] harelip.

stomatoscope (sto-mat′o-skōp) [stomato- + Gr. *skopein* to examine] an instrument used in inspecting the mouth.

stomatosis (sto″mah-to′sis) stomatopathy.

stomatotomy (sto″mah-tot′o-me) stomatomy.

stomatotyphus (sto″mah-to-ti′fus) typhus fever with severe lesions of the mouth.

stomencephalus (sto″men-sef′ah-lus) stomocephalus.

stomion (sto′me-on) [Gr. *stomion,* dim. of *stoma* mouth] an anthropometric landmark, being the central point in the oral fissure when the lips are closed.

stomocephalus (sto″mo-sef′ah-lus) [stomo- + Gr. *kephalē* head] a fetus with a rudimentary head and jaws, so that the skin hangs in folds about the mouth.

stomodeal (sto″mo-de′al) pertaining to the stomodeum.

stomodeum (sto″mo-de′um) [stomo- + Gr. *hodaios* pertaining to a way] an invagination of the ectoderm of the embryo at the point where later the mouth is formed.

stomoschisis (sto-mos′kĭ-sis) [stomo- + Gr. *schisis* a splitting] fissure of the mouth.

Stomoxys (sto-mok′sis) a genus of flies of the family Muscidae. **S. bouffar′di,** a species transmitting *Trypanosoma cazalboui,* a parasite of goats in French Guiana. **S. cal′citrans,** the common stable fly; it is annoying to man and beast, and is capable of transmitting anthrax, tetanus, *Trypanosoma evansi,* which causes surra in horses, and infectious anemia of horses. Called also *legsticker.*

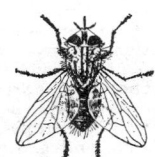

Stomoxys calcitrans.

-stomy (sto′me) [Gr. *stomoun* to provide with an opening, or mouth] a word termination denoting the surgical creation of an artificial opening into a hollow organ (colostomy, tracheostomy) or a new opening between two such structures (gastroenterostomy, pyeloureterostomy); also denoting the opening so created.

stone (stōn) 1. a mass of extremely hard and unyielding material, as a gallstone; a calculus. 2. a unit of weight recognized in Great Britain, being the equivalent of 14 pounds (avoirdupois), or about 6.34 kg. (metric). **artificial s.,** a specially calcined gypsum derivative used for making models or casts of oral structures; similar to plaster of Paris but with less porous grains, so that the product is stronger than one made of plaster of Paris. **bladder s.,** vesical calculus. **blue s.,** cupric sulfate. **chalk s.,** articular calculus. **dental s.,** 1. denticle (def. 2). 2. artificial stone. **eye s.,** the operculum of a small shell or other small calcareous object; used for removing foreign bodies from the eye. **kidney s.,** renal calculus. **lung s.,** lung calculus. **metabolic s.,** cholesterol calculus. **pulp s.,** denticle, def. 2. **rotten s.,** a siliceous mineral used as a polishing material. **salivary s.,** see under *calculus.* **s.-searcher,** a sound for exploring the bladder wherein a calculus is suspected. **skin s's,** calcareous nodules in the skin. **staghorn s.,** see under *calculus.* **struvite s.,** see under *calculus.* **tear s.,** dacryolith. **vein s.,** phlebolith. **womb s.,** uterine calculus.

Stookey's reflex (stook′ēz) [Byron Polk *Stookey,* New York neurologic surgeon, born 1887] see under *reflex.*

stool the fecal discharge from the bowels. **bilious s.,** the yellowish or brownish stools, turning darker on exposure, that are characteristic of bilious diarrhea. **caddy s.,** the stools seen in yellow fever; they look like dark, sandy mud. **fatty s.,** stools containing fat; seen in diseases of the pancreas and in malabsorption syndromes. **lienteric s.,** stool that contains much undigested food. **mucous s.,** stool containing a large amount of mucus; seen in intestinal inflammation or mucous colitis. **pea soup s.,** the characteristic liquid evacuation of typhoid fever. **pipe-stem s.,** stool resembling the shape of a pipe stem, seen in stricture of the lower rectum. **ribbon s.,** a long flattened stool seen in lower rectal stricture. **rice water s.,** the characteristic watery evacuations of cholera. **sago-grain s.,** stools of amebiasis in which the liquid feces contain small flecks of blood-stained mucus. **silver s.,** stools having the color of aluminum or silver paint, due to a mixture of melena and white fatty stools; it occurs in tropical sprue and in children with diarrhea who are given sulfonamides, and is indicative of carcinoma of the ampulla of Vater. **spinach s.,** dark-green stool resembling cooked spinach, resulting from the use of calomel in infants.

storax (sto′raks) [L. *storax, styrax;* Gr. *styrax* [USP] a balsam from the trunk of *Liquidambar orientalis* Mill (Levant s.), a tree of western Asia, or of *L. styraciflua* L. (American s.) of North America, occurring as a semiliquid, grayish brown, sticky, opaque mass which deposits on standing a heavy brown layer, or as a semisolid, sometimes solid mass, softened by warming; used as an ingredient of compound benzoin tincture (see under *tincture*). It has been used as an expectorant and topical parasiticide. Called also *styrax.*

storiform (stor′ĭ-form) [L. *storea, storia* a rush mat + *form*] denoting a matted, irregularly whorled pattern, somewhat resembling that of a straw mat; said of the microscopic appearance of fibrous histiocytomas.

storm (storm) an outburst; a temporary and sudden increase in symptoms. **thyroid s., thyrotoxic s.,** a sudden and dangerous increase of the symptoms of thyrotoxicosis (Graves' disease), especially after thyroidectomy.

Storm van Leeuwen chamber [William *Storm van Leeuwen,* a pharmacist in Leyden, 1882–1933] see under *chamber.*

stoss (stos) [Ger.] see *stosstherapy.*

stosstherapy (stos′ther-ah-pe) [Ger. *stoss* shock, stroke + *therapy*] treatment of a disease by a single massive dose of a therapeutic agent, or by short-term administration of unphysiologically large doses.

Stoxil (stok′sil) trademark for a preparation of idoxuridine.

STP popular designation for 2,5-dimethoxy-4-methylamphetamine.

strabismal (strah-biz′mal) strabismic.

strabismic (strah-biz′mik) pertaining to or of the nature of strabismus.

strabismology (strah″bis-mol′o-je) the study of strabismus.

strabismometer (strah-biz-mom′ĕ-ter) [strabismus + Gr. metron measure] an apparatus for measuring strabismus.

strabismus (strah-biz′mus) [Gr. strabismos a squinting] deviation of the eye which the patient cannot overcome. The visual axes assume a position relative to each other different from that required by the physiological conditions. The various forms of strabismus are spoken of as tropias, their direction being indicated by the appropriate prefix, as cyclotropia, esotropia, exotropia, hypertropia, and hypotropia. Called also cast, heterotropia, manifest deviation, and squint. **absolute s.,** that which occurs at all distances of the fixation point. **accommodative s.,** that which is due to excessive or deficient accommodative effort. **alternating s., bilateral s., binocular s.,** that which affects each eye alternately. **Braid's s.** (obs.), the turning of the eyes simultaneously upward and inward; a means sometimes adopted of inducing the hypnotic state. **comitant s.,** concomitant s. **concomitant s.,** that which is due to faulty insertion of the eye muscles, resulting in the same amount of deviation in whatever direction the eyes are looking, because the squinting eye follows the movements of the other eye; called also comitant s. and concomitant squint. **constant s.,** strabismus that is constantly present. **convergent s.,** esotropia. **cyclic s.,** intermittent strabismus that recurs at regular intervals. **s. deor′sum ver′gens,** that in which the visual axis of the squinting eye falls below the fixation point. **divergent s.,** exotropia. **dynamic s.,** the tendency to strabismus due to insufficiency of the ocular muscles, but which may be overcome by the effort of binocular vision. **external s.,** exotropia. **horizontal s.,** strabismus in which the deviation of the visual axis is in the horizontal plane; see esotropia and exotropia. **incomitant s.,** nonconcomitant s. **intermittent s.,** that which occurs only at intervals. **internal s.,** esotropia. **kinetic s.,** strabismus due to overactivity of the muscles controlling ocular movements. **latent s.,** that which occurs only when one eye is occluded. **manifest s.,** strabismus which occurs when vision by both eyes is possible. **mechanical s.,** that due to pressure or traction on the eye, as by a tumor, producing deflection. **monocular s., monolateral s.,** unilateral s. **muscular s.,** concomitant s. **noncomitant s.,** nonconcomitant s. **nonconcomitant s.,** that in which the amount of deviation of the squinting eye varies according to the direction in which the eyes are turned; called also incomitant or noncomitant s. **nonparalytic s.,** concomitant strabismus that is not due to paralysis of the extraocular muscles. **paralytic s.,** that which is due to paralysis of an eye muscle. **paralytic s., acute,** strabismus attended by dizziness and double vision. **periodic s.,** that occurring only during efforts at accommodation. **relative s.,** that which occurs for some and not for other distances of the fixation point. **spasmodic s.,** that which is due to spasm of the muscles of the eye. **suppressed s.,** heterophoria. **s. sur′sum ver′gens,** that in which the visual axis of the squinting eye lies above the fixation point. **unilateral s., uniocular s.,** strabismus affecting only one eye. **vertical s.,** strabismus in which the deviation of the visual axis is in the vertical plane; see hypertropia and hypotropia.

strabometer (strah-bom′ĕ-ter) strabismometer.

strabometry (strah-bom′ĕ-tre) measurement of the amount of strabismus.

strabotome (strab′o-tōm) a knife for performing strabotomy.

strabotomy (strah-bot′o-me) [Gr. strabos squinting + tomē cutting] the cutting of the tendon of a muscle of the eye in treatment of strabismus.

strain (strān) 1. to overexercise; to use to an extreme and harmful degree. 2. to filter or subject to colation. 3. an overstretching or overexertion of some part of the musculature. 4. excessive effort or undue exercise. 5. a group of organisms within a species or variety, characterized by some particular quality, as rough or smooth strains of bacteria. **cell s.,** cells derived from a primary culture or cell line by the selection and cloning of cells having specific properties. **heterologous s.,** a strain of microorganisms different from the strain originally isolated, tested, etc. **high-jumper's s.,** strain of the rotator muscles of the thigh occurring in high jumpers. **homologous s.,** a strain of microorganisms similar to the strain originally isolated, tested, etc. **resistant s.,** a strain of organisms that is resistant to the effects of the agents, such as antibiotics or insecticides, used to control them. **R s., rough s.,** the rough strain that results from bacterial dissociation; R colonies have a dull, uneven surface and irregular border, the growth in fluid media tends to flake out, no capsules are seen, and the culture tends to be less virulent. **S s., smooth s.,** the smooth strain that results from bacterial dissociation. The S colonies have a smooth surface and an unbroken border, growth in fluid media tends to be diffuse,

capsules, if present at all, are found in this strain, and the culture tends to be more virulent. **Vi s.,** a strain of Salmonella typhosa which contains the Vi (virulence) antigen of Felix.

strainer (strān′er) an apparatus for straining.

strait (strāt) a narrow passageway. **pelvic s., inferior,** the pelvic outlet. **pelvic s., superior,** the pelvic inlet.

straitjacket (strāt′jak″et) a contrivance for restraining the limbs, especially the arms, of a violently disturbed person; called also camisole.

stramonium (strah-mo′ne-um) the dried leaf and flowering or fruiting tops of Datura stramonium; used like belladonna and in the treatment of asthma. Called also thorn apple.

strand (strand) a thread or fiber. **Billroth's s's,** trabeculae lienis. **lateral enamel s.,** a structure in a developing tooth connecting the enamel organ with the dental lamina.

strangalesthesia (strang″g'l-es-the′ze-ah) [Gr. strangalizein to choke + aisthēsis perception + -ia] zonesthesia.

strangle (strang′g'l) [L. strangulare] to choke, or to be choked by compression or other obstruction of the windpipe.

strangles (strang′g'lz) 1. an infectious disease of horses, characterized by a mucopurulent inflammation of the respiratory mucous membrane, with lymph node abscesses, and caused by the Streptococcus equi. Called also colt distemper. 2. a condition in swine, characterized by infection of the lymph nodes, producing heavily encapsulated abscesses in the region of the pharynx.

strangulated (strang′gu-lāt″ed) [L. strangulatus] congested by reason of constriction or hernial stricture; see hernia.

strangulation (strang″gu-la′shun) [L. strangulatio] 1. choking or throttling arrest of respiration, due to occlusion of the air passage. 2. arrest of the circulation in a part, due to compression.

stranguria (strang-gu′re-ah) strangury.

strangury (strang′gu-re) [Gr. stranx drop + ouron urine] slow and painful discharge of the urine, due to spasm of the urethra and bladder.

strap (strap) 1. a band or slip, as of adhesive plaster, used in attaching parts to each other. 2. to bind down tightly. **crib s.,** a strap to be placed around the neck of a horse to prevent cribbing by compressing the windpipe. **Montgomery s's,** straps made of lengths of adhesive tape, used to secure dressings that must be changed frequently. Called also Montgomery's tapes. **Wyman's s's** (obs.), a set of straps for keeping a violently disturbed person in bed.

strapping (strap′ing) the application of strips of adhesive plaster, one overlapping the other, to cover and exert pressure upon an extremity or other area of the body; see Plate XLVI and see also bandaging. **Gibney's s.,** see under bandage.

Strasburger's cell plate (strahs-burg′erz) [Eduard Adolf Strasburger, German botanist, 1844–1912] midbody.

Strassburg's test (strahs′boorgz) [Gustav Adolf Strassburg, German physiologist, born 1848] see under tests.

strata (stra′tah) [L.] plural of stratum.

stratification (strat″ĭ-fi-ka′shun) [L. stratum layer + facere to make] disposal in layers.

stratified (strat′ĭ-fīd) disposed in layers.

stratiform (strat′ĭ-form) [L. stratum layer + forma form] having the form of strata.

stratigram (strat′ĭ-gram) a roentgenogram of a selected layer of the body made by body section roentgenography.

stratigraphy (strah-tig′rah-fe) [L. stratum layer + Gr. graphein to write] see body section roentgenography, under roentgenography.

stratum (stra′tum), pl. stra′ta [L.] a layer; [NA] a general term for a sheetlike mass of substance of nearly uniform thickness, particularly when the layer is one of several associated layers. **s. adamanti′num,** the enamel of a tooth (enamelum [NA]). **s. al′bum profun′dum cor′poris quadrigem′ini,** a layer of white matter between the corpora quadrigemina and the central gray layer of the cerebral aqueduct. **s. bacillo′rum,** s. neuroepitheliale retinae. **s. basa′le,** basal layer: the deepest layer of the endometrium, which contains the blind ends of the uterine glands; the cells of this layer undergo minimal change during the sexual cycle. **s. basa′le epider′midis** [NA], basal layer of epidermis: the deepest stratum of the epidermis, composed of a single layer of deeply basophilic cells; called also s. cylindricum epidermidis [NA alternative]. **cerebral s. of retina, s. cerebra′le ret′inae** [NA], the internal, transparent, light-sensitive layer of the optic part of the retina. **circular s. of muscular tunic of colon,** s. circulare tunicae muscularis coli. **circular s. of muscular tunic of rectum,** s. circulare tunicae muscularis recti. **circular s. of muscular tunic of small intestine,** s. circulare tunicae muscularis intestini tenuis. **circular s. of muscular tunic of stomach,** s. circulare tunicae muscularis ventriculi. **s. circula′re membra′nae tym′pani** [NA], circular layer of tympanic membrane: the layer of circularly coursing fibers deep to the mucous layer of the tympanic membrane; it is best developed near the periphery. **s. circula′re tu′nicae muscula′ris co′li**

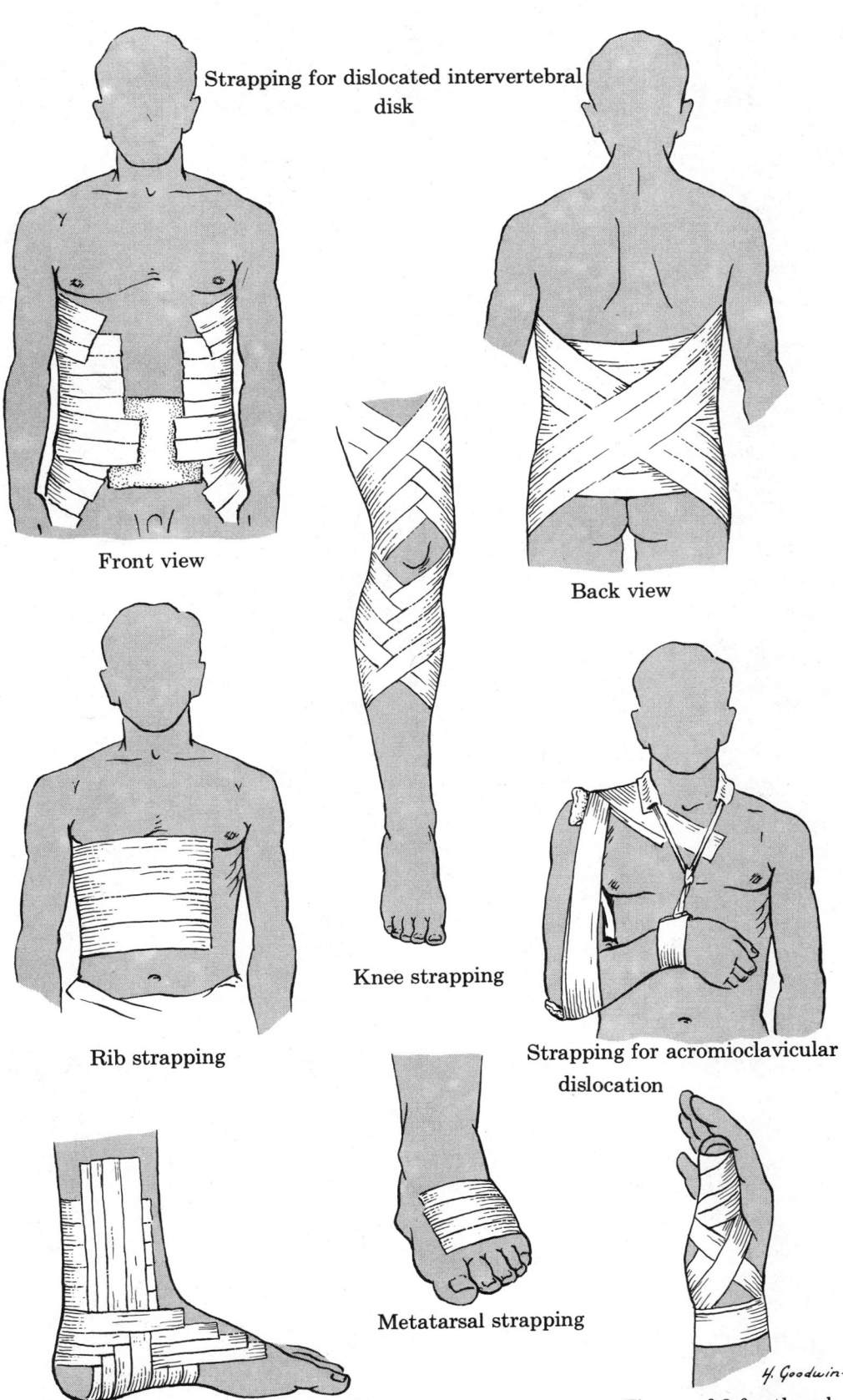

Plate XLVI

strapping

Strapping for dislocated intervertebral disk

Front view

Back view

Knee strapping

Rib strapping

Strapping for acromioclavicular dislocation

Metatarsal strapping

H. Goodwin-

Figure-of-8 for thumb

Basket weave for ankle

VARIOUS TYPES OF STRAPPING

[NA], circular layer of muscular tunic of colon: the inner layer of circularly coursing fibers in the muscular coat of the colon. **s. circula′re tu′nicae muscula′ris intesti′ni ten′uis** [NA], circular layer of muscular tunic of small intestine: the inner layer of circularly coursing fibers in the muscular coat of the small intestine. **s. circula′re tu′nicae muscula′ris rec′ti** [NA], circular layer of muscular tunic of rectum: the inner layer of circularly coursing fibers in the muscular coat of the rectum. **s. circula′re tu′nicae muscula′ris tu′bae uteri′nae,** the layer of circularly coursing fibers in the muscular coat of the uterus. **s. circula′re tu′nicae muscula′ris ure′thrae mulie′bris,** the layer of circularly coursing fibers in the muscular coat of the female urethra. **s. circula′re tu′nicae muscula′ris ventric′uli** [NA], circular layer of muscular tunic of stomach: the layer of circularly coursing fibers in the muscular coat of the stomach. **s. compac′tum,** compact layer: the layer of the endometrium nearest the surface, which contains the necks of the uterine glands; together with the stratum spongiosum, it forms the *stratum functionale* (q.v.). **connective tissue s. of mesentery,** lamina mesenterii propria. **s. cor′neum epider′midis** [NA], horny layer of epidermis: the outermost layer of the epidermis, consisting of cells that are dead and desquamating; the term once embraced also the layers now called *s. lucidum epidermidis* and *s. granulosum epidermidis.* **s. cor′neum un′guis** [NA], horny layer of nail: the outer, compact layer of the nail; called also *nail plate.* **s. cuta′neum membra′nae tym′pani** [NA], cutaneous layer of tympanic membrane: a very thin form of skin that constitutes the lateral layer of the tympanic membrane. **s. cylin′dricum epider′midis,** NA alternative for *s. basale epidermidis.* **s. denta′tum epider′midis,** s. germinativum epidermidis (Malpighii). **s. ebo′ris,** the dentin of a tooth (dentinum [NA]). **s. exter′num tu′nicae muscula′ris duc′tus deferen′tis,** the outer layer of fibers in the muscular coat of the ductus deferens. **s. exter′num tu′nicae muscula′ris ure′teris,** the outer layer of fibers in the muscular coat of the ureter. **s. exter′num tu′nicae muscula′ris ves′icae urina′riae,** the outer layer of fibers in the muscular coat of the urinary bladder. **s. fibro′sum cap′sulae articula′ris,** membrana fibrosa capsulae articularis. **s. functiona′le,** functional layer: the stratum compactum and stratum spongiosum considered together (i.e., all of the endometrium except for the stratum basale), the cells of which are cast off at menstruation and at parturition. It is known as the *decidua* during pregnancy. Called also *pars functionalis.* **s. gangliona′re ner′vi op′tici** [NA], ganglionic layer of optic nerve: the layer of the cerebral stratum of the retina that contains the multipolar neurons, the axons of which form the fibers of the optic nerve. **s. gangliona′re ret′inae** [NA], ganglionic layer of retina: the layer of the cerebral stratum of the retina that contains the bipolar cells. **ganglionic s. of optic nerve,** s. ganglionare nervi optici. **ganglionic s. of retina,** s. ganglionare retinae. **s. gangli-o′sum cerebel′li,** ganglionic layer of cerebellum: the thin middle gray layer of the cortex cerebelli, consisting of a single layer of Purkinje cells; called also *s. Purkinje.* **s. germinativum, s. germinati′vum epider′midis [Malpig′hii],** germinative layer of epidermis: the innermost layer of the epidermis. Called also malpighian layer and *s. malpighii.* Sometimes used to designate only the *stratum basale epidermidis.* **s. germinati′vum un′guis** [NA], germinative layer of nail: the lower layer of the nail, from which the nail grows; it is continuous with the stratum basale and stratum spinosum of the epidermis. **s. granulo′sum cerebel′li** [NA], granular layer of cerebellum: the deep layer of the cortex of the cerebellum; it contains many small neurons (granule cells) and is separated from the molecular layer by the Purkinje cells. **s. granulo′sum epider′midis** [NA], granular layer of epidermis: the layer of the epidermis between the stratum lucidum epidermidis and the stratum spinosum epidermidis. **s. granulo′sum follic′uli ooph′ori vesiculo′si,** s. granulosum folliculi ovarici vesiculosi. **s. granulo′sum follic′uli ova′rici vesiculo′si** [NA], **s. granulo′sum ova′rii,** granular layer of follicle of ovary: the layer of follicle cells lining the theca of a vesicular ovarian follicle. **s. gris′eum centra′le cer′ebri,** substantia grisea centralis cerebri. **s. gris′eum collic′uli superio′ris** [NA], gray layer of superior colliculus: a thick layer, containing few myelinated fibers, near the outer surface of the superior colliculus. **s. interme′dium,** the layer of cells of the enamel organ of a tooth just peripheral to the ameloblastic layer. **s. inter′num tu′nicae muscula′ris duc′tus deferen′tis,** the inner layer of fibers in the muscular coat of the ductus deferens. **s. inter′num tu′nicae muscula′ris ure′teris,** the inner layer of fibers in the muscular coat of the ureter. **s. inter′num tu′nicae muscula′ris ves′icae urina′riae,** the inner layer of fibers in the muscular coat of the urinary bladder. **s. interoliva′re lemnis′ci,** fibers from the nucleus gracilis and cuneatus that ascend between the olives to form the medial lemnisci. **s. lacuno′sum,** a subdivision of the superficial layer of cells of the hippocampus, lying deep to the stratum moleculare. **s. lemnis′ci,** s. interolivare lemnisci. **longitudinal s. of muscular tunic of colon,** s. longitudinale tunicae muscularis coli. **longitudinal s. of muscular tunic of**

rectum, s. longitudinale tunicae muscularis recti. **longitudinal s. of muscular tunic of small intestine,** s. longitudinale tunicae muscularis intestini tenuis. **longitudinal s. of muscular tunic of stomach,** s. longitudinale tunicae muscularis ventriculi. **s. longitudina′le tu′nicae muscula′ris co′li** [NA], longitudinal layer of muscular tunic of colon: the outer layer of the muscular coat of the colon, consisting of longitudinally coursing fibers; it is thick in the regions of the three teniae coli and very thin between them. **s. longitudina′le tu′nicae muscula′ris intesti′ni ten′uis** [NA], longitudinal layer of muscular tunic of small intestine: the outer layer of the muscular coat of the small intestine, consisting of longitudinally coursing fibers. **s. longitudina′le tu′nicae muscula′ris rec′ti** [NA], longitudinal layer of muscular tunic of rectum: the outer layer of the muscular coat of the rectum, consisting of longitudinally coursing fibers. **s. longitudina′le tu′nicae muscula′ris tu′bae uteri′nae,** the layer of longitudinally coursing fibers in the muscular coat of the uterus. **s. longitudina′le tu′nicae muscula′ris ure′thrae mulie′bris,** the layer of longitudinally coursing fibers in the muscular coat of the female urethra. **s. longitudina′le tu′nicae muscula′ris ventric′uli** [NA], longitudinal layer of muscular tunic of stomach: the layer of longitudinally coursing fibers in the muscular coat of the stomach. **s. lu′cidum epider′midis** [NA], clear layer of epidermis: the clear translucent layer of the epidermis, just beneath the stratum corneum epidermidis. **s. lu′cidum hippocam′pi,** the cellular (as opposed to dendritic) segment of the pyramidal cell layer of the hippocampus; cf. *s. radiatum.* **s. malpig′hii,** s. germinativum epidermidis (Malpighii). **s. me′dium tu′nicae muscula′ris duc′tus deferen′tis,** the middle layer of the muscular coat of the ductus deferens. **s. me′dium tu′nicae muscula′ris ure′teris,** the middle layer of the muscular coat of the ureter. **s. me′dium tu′nicae muscula′ris ves′icae urina′riae,** the middle layer of the muscular coat of the urinary bladder. **s. molecula′re cerebel′li** [NA], molecular layer of cerebellum: the superficial layer of the cortex of the cerebellum, containing a relatively small number of stellate neurons. **s. molecula′re hippocam′pi,** a subdivision of the superficial layer of cells of the hippocampus. **s. muco′sum membra′nae tym′pani** [NA], mucous layer of tympanic membrane: the inner layer of the tympanic membrane, continuous with the mucosa lining the tympanic cavity. **s. neuroepithelia′le ret′inae** [NA], neuroepithelial layer of retina: the outer layer of the cerebral stratum of the retina, which contains the rods and cones. **s. nuclea′re medul′lae oblonga′tae,** the column of gray substance in the medulla oblongata containing the nuclei of the lower cranial nerves. **s. op′ticum,** a layer of white fibers in the superior colliculus, just below the stratum griseum. **s. o′riens,** a layer of polymorphic cells of the hippocampus. **s. papilla′re cor′ii** [NA], **s. papilla′re cu′tis,** papillary layer of corium: the outer layer of the corium, characterized by ridges or papillae which protrude into the epidermis; called also *corpus papillare corii.* **s. perichorioi′deum,** lamina suprachoroidea. **s. pigmen′ti bul′bi oc′uli** [NA], pigmented layer of eyeball: a layer of pigmented epithelium, the outer of the two parts of the retina, extending from the entrance of the optic nerve to the pupillary margin of the iris, and comprising the stratum pigmenti retinae, stratum pigmenti corporis ciliaris, and stratum pigmenti iridis. **s. pigmen′ti cor′poris cilia′ris** [NA], pigmented layer of ciliary body: the part of the pigmented layer of the eyeball that rests on the ciliary body. **s. pigmen′ti i′ridis** [NA], pigmented layer of iris: the part of the pigmented layer of the eyeball that rests on the posterior surface of the iris. **s. pigmen′ti ret′inae** [NA], pigmented layer of retina: the part of the pigmented layer of the eyeball that forms the outer layer of the pars optica of the retina. **s. Purkin′je,** s. gangliosum cerebelli. **s. pyramida′le,** either of two layers of human cerebral cortex: the external pyramidal layer (layer III), or the internal pyramidal or ganglionic layer (layer V). **s. radia′tum,** the superficial part of the pyramidal cell layer of the hippocampus, containing numerous apical dendrites. **s. radia′tum membra′nae tym′pani** [NA], radiate layer of tympanic membrane: the layer of fibers beneath the cutaneous layer of the tympanic membrane, radiating outward from the manubrium of the malleus to pass into the fibrocartilaginous ring. **s. reticula′re cor′ii** [NA], **s. reticula′re cu′tis,** reticular layer of corium: the inner layer of the corium, consisting chiefly of dense fibrous tissue; called also *tunica propria corii* and *proper coat of corium.* **s. spino′sum epider′midis** [NA], spinous layer of epidermis: the layer of the skin between the stratum granulosum epidermidis and the stratum basale epidermidis characterized by the presence of prickle cells. Called also *prickle-cell layer* and *spinous layer of epidermis.* **s. spongio′-sum,** spongy layer: the middle layer of the endometrium, which contains the tortuous portions of the uterine glands; together with the stratum compactum, it forms the *stratum functionale* (q.v.). **s. submuco′sum,** the inner layer of the myometrium, which is in contact with the endometrium; called also *s. subvasculare.* **submucous s. of bladder,** tela submucosa vesicae urinariae. **submucous s. of colon,** tela submucosa coli. **submucous s. of rectum,** tela submucosa recti. **submucous s. of small intestine,** tela submucosa intestini tenuis. **submu-**

cous s. of stomach, tela submucosa ventriculi. **s. sub-sero'sum,** the outer layer of the myometrium, which is in contact with the serous coat of the uterus. **s. subvascula're,** s. submucosum. **s. supravascula're,** the layer of the myometrium that lies between the stratum vasculare and the stratum subserosum. **s. synovia'le cap'sulae articula'ris,** membrana synovialis capsulae articularis. **s. vascula're,** the middle layer of the myometrium, forming most of its bulk, and composed of circular and spiral fibers. **white s. of quadrigeminal body, deep,** s. album profundum corporis quadrigemini. **s. zona'le cor'poris quadrigem'ini** zonal layer of quadrigeminal body: a superficial layer of white fibers of the corpora quadrigemina. **s. zona'le thal'ami** [NA], zonal layer of thalamus: a layer of myelinated fibers covering the dorsal surface of the thalamus.

Straus' reaction (phenomenon, test) (strows') [Isidore *Straus,* French physician, 1854–1896] see under *reaction.*

Strauss' sign (strows') [Hermann *Strauss,* physician in Berlin, 1868–1944] see under *sign.*

streak (strēk) a line, stria, striation, or stripe. **angioid s's,** red to black irregular bands observed in the ocular fundus running outward from the region of the optic disk, which are seen in certain conditions, including pseudoxanthoma elasticum, osteitis deformans, and sickle-cell anemia. The lesions are thought to represent ruptures in Bruch's membrane. **germinal s.,** primitive s. **Knapp's s's,** lines resembling blood vessels seen occasionally in the retina after hemorrhage. **medullary s.,** the neural groove. **meningeal s.,** tache cérébrale. **primitive s.,** a faint white trace at the caudal end of the embryonic disc, formed by the movement of cells at the beginning of mesoderm formation; it provides the earliest evidence of the embryonic axis.

stream (strēm) a current or flow of water or other fluid. **axial s.,** the core of rapid flow in the center of a channel, as in the lumen of a blood vessel, bordered or surrounded by a zone in which the elements move less rapidly, or are motionless. **electron s.,** a stream of negatively charged particles (electrons) moving from cathode to anode across a potential difference in a low-pressure gas tube or a vacuum tube.

streblomicrodactyly (streb″lo-mi″kro-dak'tĭ-le) [Gr. *streblos* twisted + *mikros* small + *daktylos* finger] streptomicrodactyly.

stremma (strem'ah) [Gr. "a twist"] a sprain.

streph- see *strepho-.*

strephenopodia (stref″ĕ-no-po'de-ah) [*streph-* + Gr. *en* in + *pous* foot] talipes varus.

strephexopodia (stref″ek-so-po'de-ah) [*streph-* + Gr. *exō* out + *pous* foot] talipes valgus.

strepho-, streph- (stref'o; stref) [Gr. *strephein* to twist] combining form meaning twisted.

strephopodia (stref″o-po'de-ah) talipes equinus.

strephosymbolia (stref″o-sim-bo'le-ah) [*strepho-* + Gr. *symbolon* symbol + *-ia*] 1. a disorder of perception in which objects seem reversed as in a mirror. 2. a reading difficulty inconsistent with a child's general intelligence, beginning with confusion between similar but oppositely oriented letters (b-d, q-p) and a tendency to reverse direction in reading.

strepitus (strep'ĭ-tus) [L.] a noise; a sound heard on auscultation.

strepogenin (strep″o-gen'in) a factor present in casein and certain other proteins which is essential to optimal growth of animals; called also *chick growth factor.*

strepsinema (strep″sĭ-ne'mah) [Gr. *strepsis* a twist + *nēma* thread] the threads of chromatin in the strepsitene stage.

strepsitene (strep'sĭ-tēn) a stage of meiosis, after the diplotene stage, in which the threads become twisted about each other.

streptamine (strep-tam'in) chemical name: 1,3-diamino-2,4,5,6-tetrahydroxycyclohexane. One of the fractions derived from the degradation of streptomycin.

strepticemia (strep″tĭ-se'me-ah) streptococcemia.

streptidine (strep'tĭ-dīn) one of the fractions derived from degradation of streptomycin, the other fraction being streptobiosamine; it is 1,3-diguanido-2,4,5,6-tetrahydroxycyclohexane.

strepto- (strep'to) [Gr. *streptos* twisted] a combining form meaning twisted.

streptoangina (strep″to-an'jĭ-nah) a pseudomembranous deposit in the throat due to a streptococcal infection.

streptobacilli (strep″to-bah-sil'i) [L.] plural of *streptobacillus.*

Streptobacillus (strep″to-bah-sil'lus) a name given a genus of microorganisms of family Bacteroidaceae, order Eubacteriales, said to be made up of pleomorphic bacteria which vary from short rods to long interwoven filaments. **S. monilifor'mis,** the etiological agent of the bacillary form of rat-bite fever; formerly called *Haverhillia multiformis.*

streptobacillus (strep″to-bah-sil'us), pl. *streptobacil'li.* 1. a rod-shaped bacterium remaining loosely attached end-to-end in long chains as a consequence of failure of daughter cells to separate following cell division. 2. an organism of the genus *Streptobacillus.*

streptobacteria (strep″to-bak-te're-ah) (pl.) a group including those bacteria (*Actinomyces, Streptomyces, Nocardia,* etc.) which are linked together into twisted chains.

streptobacterin (strep″to-bak'ter-in) the vaccine prepared from streptococci.

streptobiosamine (strep″to-bi-o'sah-mēn) one of the fractions, $C_{13}H_{23}NO_9$, derived from the degradation of streptomycin, the other fraction being streptidine.

streptocerciasis (strep″to-ser-ki'ah-sis) infection with *Dipetalonema streptocerca,* whose microfilariae produce a pruritic rash resembling that in onchocerciasis; transmitted by midges of the genus *Culicoides,* it occurs in Central Africa.

Streptococcaceae (strep″to-kok-ka'se-e) a family of gram-positive, facultative anaerobic cocci, which are usually nonmotile, and occur in pairs, chains, or tetrads. It includes the genera *Aerococcus, Gemella, Leuconostoc, Pediococcus,* and *Streptococcus.*

streptococcal (strep″to-kok'al) pertaining to or caused by a streptococcus.

streptococcemia (strep″to-kok-se'me-ah) [*streptococcus* + Gr. *haima* blood + *-ia*] the presence of streptococci in the blood; streptococcal infection.

streptococci (strep″to-kok'si) [L.; Gr.] plural of *streptococcus.*

streptococcic (strep″to-kok'sik) streptococcal.

streptococcicide (strep″to-kok'sĭ-sīd) an agent that is destructive to streptococci.

streptococcolysin (strep″to-kok-kol'ĭ-sin) streptolysin.

Streptococcus (strep″to-kok'us) [*strepto-* + Gr. *kokkos* berry] a genus of gram-positive, facultatively anaerobic cocci occurring in pairs or chains, assigned to the family Streptococcaceae. The genus is separable into the pyogenic group, the viridans group, the enterococcus group, and the lactic group. The first group includes the β-hemolytic human and animal pathogens, the second and third include α-hemolytic parasitic forms occurring as normal flora in the upper respiratory tract and the intestinal tract, respectively, and the fourth is made up of saprophytic forms associated with the souring of milk. See also *hemolytic streptococcus* under *streptococcus.* **S. agalac'tiae,** β-hemolytic streptococci of group B, causing mastitis in cattle and seldom infecting man. **S. anaero'bius,** a microaerophilic or obligate anaerobe found in war wounds, gangrene, and puerperal infections. **S. anhemolyt'icus,** a former species name for anhemolytic streptococci. **S. bo'vis,** a serologically heterogeneous species of the enterococcus group, found in the bovine alimentary tract and sometimes in human feces; also sometimes associated with the subacute form of bacterial endocarditis. **S. bre'vis,** a former species name for a shorter-chained streptococcus thought to be less virulent than those occurring in longer chains. **S. cremo'ris,** an anhemolytic, nonpathogenic streptococcus of the lactis group, occurring in dairy products; its action on milk results in the production of buttermilk. **S. du'rans,** a β-hemolytic streptococcus of the enterococcus group, found in the human intestine. **S. epidem'icus,** former name for *S. pyogenes,* thought to be disease-specific for epidemic infection of the upper respiratory tract. **S. e'qui,** β-hemolytic streptococci of group C, the specific etiologic agent of strangles in horses; it is nonpathogenic for man. **S. equi'nus,** a species of the viridans group, found in the intestines of horses and in the feces in humans and cows. **S. equisim'ilis,** β-hemolytic streptococci of group C, producing about 5 per cent of human streptococcal disease, and known as "human C." **S. erysipel'atis,** former name for *S. pyogenes,* some strains of which were formerly thought to be disease-specific for erysipelas. **S. evolu'tus,** a microaerophilic or obligate anaerobe found in the mouth, respiratory tract, and vagina. **S. faeca'lis,** α-hemolytic streptococci of the enterococcus group, found as a normal inhabitant of the intestinal tract and a cause of subacute bacterial endocarditis. **S. foe'tidus,** a microaerophilic or obligate anaerobe found in gangrene and fetid suppurations. **S. hemolyt'icus,** former name for *S. pyogenes.* **S. interme'dius,** a microaerophilic or obligate anaerobe found in the vagina and in the respiratory and intestinal tracts. **S. lac'ticus, S. lac'tis,** an α-hemolytic or anhemolytic, nonpathogenic streptococcus of the lactis group, found in dairy products and commonly responsible for the souring of milk. **S. lanceola'tus,** *Diplococcus pneumoniae.* **S. liquefa'ciens,** an α-hemolytic streptococcus of the enterococcus group which hydrolyzes gelatin. **S. lon'gus,** former species name for a longer-chained streptococcus, thought to be more virulent than those occurring in shorter chains. **S. mastit'idis,** *S. agalactiae.* **S. mi'cros,** a microaerophilic or obligate anaerobe found in pulmonary gangrene and in puerperal infections. **S. mi'tis,** α-hemolytic streptococci of the viridans group, found in the normal upper respiratory tract and etiologically related to regional focal abscesses and the subacute form of bacterial endocarditis. **S. mu'tans,** a species implicated in the formation of dental caries. **S. pneumo'niae,** a facultative anaerobe that is the most common cause of lobar pneumonia; it also causes numerous other serious, acute pyogenic disorders, e.g., meningitis, septicemia, empyema, and peritonitis. These lanceolate bacteria occur in pairs, are heavily encapsulated in exudates, and are gram-positive. There are more than 80 serotypes (fewer if some are condensed as subtypes) on the basis of the specificity of the polysaccharide hapten making up the capsular substance. Called also *Diplococcus pneumoniae, pneumococcus,* and *S. lanceolatus.* See also Plate accompanying bacterium. **S. pyog′enes,** β-hemolytic, toxigenic pyogenic streptococci of group A, separable into numbered serotypes on the basis of the specificity and combination of the M and T antigens, and causing septic sore throat, scarlet fever, rheumatic fever, puerperal sepsis, acute glomerulonephritis, and other conditions in man. **S. saliva′rius,** α-hemolytic streptococci of the viridans group, making up a part of the normal flora of the upper respiratory tract, and occasionally associated with apical abscesses of the teeth and the subacute form of bacterial endocarditis. **S. scarlati′nae,** former species name for *S. pyogenes,* some strains of which were formerly thought to be disease-specific for scarlet fever. **S. thermoph′ilus,** a streptococcus of the viridans group, found in milk and milk products. **S. vir′idans,** a former species name for α-hemolytic streptococci, especially those strains found in human disease; see *hemolytic streptococcus,* under *streptococcus.* **S. zooepidem′icus,** β-hemolytic streptococci of group C, commonly causing pyogenic disease in lower animals and known as "animal pyogenes"; it is rarely found in man. **S. zymog′enes,** a β-hemolytic of the enterococcus group.

streptococcus (strep-to-kok′us), pl. *streptococ′ci.* 1. a spherical bacterium occurring predominantly in chains of cells often surrounded by continuous capsular material as a consequence of failure of daughter cells to separate following cell division in one plane. 2. an organism of the genus *Streptococcus.* **alpha s.,** see under *hemolytic s.* **anhemolytic s.,** a streptococcus which does not cause any change in the medium when cultured on blood-agar. **Bargen's s.,** *Streptococcus bovis.* **beta s.,** see under *hemolytic s.* **Fehleisen's s.,** *Streptococcus pyogenes.* **gamma s.,** anhemolytic s. **group A, B, C (etc.) streptococci,** a classification of β-hemolytic streptococci based on cell-wall carbohydrate antigens; see *Lancefield classification,* under *classification.* **hemolytic s.,** any streptococcus that is capable of hemolyzing red blood cells, or of producing a zone of hemolysis about the colonies on blood-agar. The great majority of streptococci found in pathologic processes belong to this type. The hemolytic streptococci have been classified as the *alpha* (α-hemolytic) or *viridans type,* which produces about the colony on blood-agar a zone of greenish discoloration considerably smaller than the clear zone produced by the beta type; and the *beta* (β-hemolytic) *type,* which produces a clear zone of hemolysis immediately surrounding the colony on blood-agar. On immunological grounds, the β-hemolytic streptococci may be divided into Group A (primarily pathogens of man), Group B (almost exclusively found in bovine mastitis), Group C (primarily pathogens of lower animals), Group D (found in cheese), Group E (found in milk), Group F, and so on. A further classification groups the hemolytic streptococci according to the presence of antigenic carbohydrates in the cell wall, and includes Groups A through O; see *Lancefield classification,* under *classification.* **indifferent s.,** anhemolytic s. **s. MG,** any of a strain of biochemically and antigenically homogeneous, anhemolytic streptococci isolated from the sputum in primary atypical pneumonia. **s. of Ostertag,** a species causing vaginitis verrucosa in cattle. **viridans s.,** α-hemolytic s.; see hemolytic s.

streptodornase (strep″to-dor′nās) [*streptococci* + *deoxyribonuclease*] a deoxyribonuclease produced by hemolytic streptococci. **streptokinase-s.,** see under *streptokinase.*

streptoduocin (strep″to-du′o-sin) an antibiotic compound consisting of approximately equal parts of dihydrostreptomycin sulfate and streptomycin sulfate.

streptogenin (strep″to-jen′in) a hypothetical substance in the proteins of milk and other foods, which are thought to be required for optimal growth in bacteria and laboratory animals.

streptohemolysin (strep″to-he-mol′ĭ-sin) streptolysin.

streptokinase (strep″to-ki′nās) [*streptococcus* + *kinase*] a proteolytic enzyme elaborated by hemolytic streptococci, which produces fibrinolysis by activating plasminogen to plasmin; it is used as a thrombolytic agent. See also *kinase,* def. 2. **s.-streptodornase,** a mixture of the proteolytic enzymes (streptokinase and streptodornase) produced by hemolytic streptococci; used topically on surface lesions and by instillation in closed body cavities to remove clotted blood or fibrinous or purulent accumulations.

streptoleukocidin (strep″to-lu″ko-si′din) a toxin from streptococcus cultures which is destructive to leukocytes.

streptolysin (strep-tol′ĭ-sin) [*streptococcus* + *hemolysin*] a filterable hemolysin produced by various streptococci. **s. O,** a hemolysin which is inactive in the oxidized state but is readily activated by treatment with mild reducing agents, such as sulfite. **s. S,** a hemolysin which is sensitive to treatment with heat or acid, but is not inactivated by oxygen.

streptomicrodactyly (strep″to-mi″kro-dak′tĭ-le) [*strepto* + Gr. *mikros* small + *daktylos* finger] camptodactyly in which the little fingers only are involved.

Streptomyces (strep″to-mi′sēz) [*strepto-* + Gr. *mykēs* fungus] a genus of microorganisms of the family Streptomycetaceae, order

Actinomycetales, separable into 150 different species, usually soil forms but occasionally parasitic on plants and animals, and notable as the source of various antibiotics, such as the tetracyclines; called also *Streptothrix.*

Streptomycetaceae (strep″to-mi″se-ta′se-e) a family of Schizomycetes, order Actinomycetales, made up of primarily soil forms, sometimes thermophilic in rotting manure, and some parasitic species. It includes three genera: *Micromonospora, Streptomyces,* and *Thermoactinomyces.*

streptomycin (strep′to-mi′sin) a bactericidal antibiotic of the aminoglycoside class, which is produced by the soil actinomycete, *Streptomyces griseus,* and is effective against most gram-negative and acid-fast bacteria and some gram-positive forms, but is used chiefly in the treatment of tuberculosis. It causes both inhibition and decreased fidelity in protein synthesis. **s. hydrochloride,** the trihydrochloride salt of streptomycin, $C_{21}H_{39}N_7O_{12} \cdot 3HCl$, having the same actions as the base; it has been used for the same purposes as the sulfate salt. **s. sulfate,** the sesquisulfate salt of streptomycin, $(C_{21}H_{39}N_7O_{12})_2 \cdot 3H_2SO_4$, occurring as a white or practically white powder, used primarily as a tuberculostatic, usually concomitantly with another tuberculostatic; it also may be used in certain cases in the treatment of nontuberculous infections due to susceptible organisms, such as plague, tularemia, brucellosis, klebsiella pneumonia, meningitis, and bacterial endocarditis. It is administered intramuscularly.

streptomycosis (strep″to-mi-ko′sis) infection with fungi of the genus *Streptomyces.*

streptonivicin (strep″to-ni′vĭ-sin) former name for novobiocin.

streptosepticemia (strep″to-sep″tĭ-se′me-ah) septicemia due to a streptococcus.

Streptosporangium (strep″to-spo-ran′je-um) [*strepto-* + Gr. *sporos* seed + *angeion* vessel] a genus of microorganisms of the family Actinoplanaceae, order Actinomycetales, made up of mycelium-forming saprophytic microorganisms found in soil and water.

streptothricin (strep″to-thri′sin) an antibiotic substance active against both gram-negative and gram-positive bacteria; it was the first antibiotic isolated, but was found to be too toxic for systemic use.

streptothricosis (strep″to-thri-ko′sis) streptotrichosis.

Streptothrix (strep′to-thriks) [*strepto-* + Gr. *thrix* hair] 1. a name formerly given a genus of microorganisms, species of which are now classified under *Actinomyces, Streptomyces, Nocardia,* and other genera. 2. a former name for *Dermatophilus.*

streptotrichal (strep-tot′rĭ-kal) pertaining to or caused by streptothrix.

streptotrichosis (strep″to-tri-ko′sis) 1. infection with organisms of the former genus *Streptothrix;* see *actinomycosis, nocardiosis* and *streptomycosis.* 2. a former name for dermatophilosis.

streptozocin (strep″to-zo′sin) chemical name: 2-deoxy-2-[[(methylnitrosoamino)carbonyl]amino]-D-glucopyranose. An antineoplastic antibiotic, $C_8H_{15}N_3O_7$, derived from *Streptomyces achromogenes* or produced by synthesis; used principally in the treatment of islet-cell tumors of the pancreas.

stress (stres) 1. forcibly exerted influence; pressure. In dentistry, the pressure of the upper teeth against the lower in mastication. 2. the sum of the biological reactions to any adverse stimulus, physical, mental, or emotional, internal or external, that tends to disturb the organism's homeostasis; should these compensating reactions be inadequate or inappropriate, they may lead to disorders. The term is also used to refer to the stimuli that elicit the reactions.

stress-breaker (stres′brāk-er) a device which abolishes or lessens the occlusal forces acting on abutment teeth.

stretcher (strech′er) a litter for carrying the sick or injured.

stria (stri′ah), pl. *stri′ae* [L. "a furrow, groove"] 1. a streak, or line. 2. a narrow bandlike structure; [NA] a general term for such longitudinal collections of nerve fibers in the brain. **acoustic striae,** striae medullares ventriculi quarti. **stri′ae albican′tes,** see *striae atrophicae.* **striae of Amici,** Z band; see under *band.* **stri′ae atro′phicae,** linear, depressed, atrophic, pinkish or purplish, scarlike lesions that later become white (*striae albicantes, lineae albicantes*), occurring on the abdomen, breasts, buttocks, and thighs. They are due to weakening of the elastic tissues, and are associated with pregnancy (*striae gravidarum*), excessive obesity, rapid growth during puberty and adolescence, Cushing's syndrome, or topical or prolonged treatment with corticosteroids. Called also *striae distensae* and *lineae atrophicae.* **auditory striae,** striae medullares ventriculi quarti. **striae of Baillarger,** Baillarger's lines. **stri′ae cilia′res,** slight dark ridges running parallel with each other from the teeth of the ora serrata of the retina to the valleys between the ciliary processes. **stri′ae disten′sae,** striae atrophicae. **s. for′nicis** (*obs.*), s. medullaris thalami. **s. of Gennari,** see *Baillarger's lines,* under *line.* **stri′ae gravida′rum,** see *striae atrophicae.* **habenular s.** (*obs.*), s. medullaris thalami. **s. interme′dia trigo′ni olfacto′rii, intermediate s. of olfactory trigone,** a more or less distinct branch of the posterior end of the olfactory tract, which spreads out in the olfactory trigone and the anterior perforated substance of the brain. **s. kaesbekhtere'vi,** Bekhterev's layer. **Knapp's striae,** see under *streak*. **s. lancis'ii,** s. longitudinalis medialis corporis callosi. **Langhans' s.,** cytotrophoblast. **Liesgang's striae,** see under *phenomenon*. **longitudinal s. of corpus callosum, lateral,** s. longitudinalis lateralis corporis callosi. **longitudinal s. of corpus callosum, medial,** s. longitudinalis medialis corporis callosi. **s. longitudina'lis latera'lis cor'poris callo'si** [NA], lateral longitudinal stria of corpus callosum: one of two slender bands of myelinated fibers which form longitudinal ridges in the indusium griseum on the superior aspect of each half of the corpus callosum. **s. longitudina'lis media'lis cor'poris callo'si** [NA], medial longitudinal stria of corpus callosum: one of two slender bands of myelinated fibers which form longitudinal ridges in the indusium griseum on the superior aspect of each half of the corpus callosum. **mallear s. of tympanic membrane, s. mallea'ris membra'nae tym'pani** [NA], **s. malleola'ris membra'nae tym'pani,** a nearly vertical radial band seen on the outer surface of the tympanic membrane; it extends from the umbo upward to the prominentia mallearis and is caused by the manubrium mallei. **s. media'lis trigo'ni olfacto'rii,** the portion of the posterior end of the olfactory tract that turns medialward to the area parolfactoria. **stri'ae medulla'res acus'ticae, stri'ae medulla'res fos'sae rhomboi'deae,** striae medullares ventriculi quarti. **s. medulla'ris thal'ami** [NA], medullary stria of thalamus: a fiber bundle that arises from the subcallosal and paraterminal gyri, the preoptic area, and amygdaloid area, and runs backward along the junction of the dorsal and medial surfaces of the thalamus to reach the habenular nucleus. **stri'ae medulla'res ventric'uli quar'ti** [NA], medullary striae of fourth ventricle: bundles of white fibers coursing transversely across the floor of the fourth ventricle; they arise from the arcuate nuclei, pass dorsally close to the midline, and after having reached the fourth ventricle finally enter the inferior cerebellar peduncle. Called also *striae medullares fossae rhomboideae*. **medullary striae of fourth ventricle, medullary striae of rhomboid fossa,** striae medullares ventriculi quarti. **medullary s. of thalamus,** 1. stria medullaris thalami. 2. see *laminae medullares thalami*. **meningitic s.,** tache cérébrale. **Nitabuch's s.,** see under *layer*. **striae olfacto'riae** [NA], **olfactory striae,** three bands of fibers diverging from the olfactory trigone: the medial olfactory stria becomes the medial olfactory gyrus, the lateral olfactory stria runs toward the insula, and the intermediate olfactory stria (only occasionally present) attaches to the anterior perforated substance. **s. pinea'lis** (*obs.*), s. medullaris thalami. **Retzius' parallel striae,** incremental lines. **Rohr's s.,** a layer of canalized fibrin in the developing placenta, within the intervillous space at the fetal-maternal junction. **Schreger's striae,** bands of Hunter-Schreger. **s. semicircula'ris,** s. terminalis. **s. termina'lis** [NA], a band of fibers along the lateral margin of the ventricular surface of the thalamus, covering the thalamostriate vein and, following the course of the vein, marking the line of separation between the thalamus and the caudate nucleus; it extends from the region of the interventricular foramen to the inferior horn of the lateral ventricle, carrying fibers from the amygdaloid nuclei to the septal, hypothalamic, and thalamic areas. **stri'ae transver'sae cor'poris callo'si,** transverse bands of fibers on the upper surface of the corpus callosum. **s. vascula'ris duc'tus cochlea'ris** [NA], a layer of fibrous vascular tissue covering the outer wall of the cochlear duct, which is thought to secrete the endolymph. **s. ventric'uli ter'tii** (*obs.*), s. medullaris thalami. **Wickham's striae,** pale grayish dots or lines forming a network on the surface of the papules, characteristic of lichen planus.

striae (stri'e) [L.] plural of *stria*.

striascope (stri'ah-skōp) an instrument for use in ophthalmologic refraction.

striatal (stri-a'tal) pertaining to the corpus striatum.

striate (stri'āt) striated.

striated (stri'āt-ed) [L. *striatus*] striped; marked by striae.

striation (stri-a'shun) 1. the quality of being marked by stripes or striae. 2. a streak or scratch. **Baillarger's s's,** see under *line*. **tabby cat s., tigroid s.,** a striation or marking on muscle tissue that has undergone marked fatty degeneration; seen especially in degenerated heart muscle.

striatonigral, strionigral (stri''ah-to-ni'gral; stri''o-ni'gral) projecting from the corpus striatum to the substantia nigra.

Striatran (stri'ah-tran) trademark for a preparation of emylcamate.

striatum (stri-a'tum) [L.] 1. striped, or grooved. 2. corpus striatum. 3. neostriatum.

stricture (strik'chur) [L. *strictura*] decrease in the caliber of a canal, duct, or other passage, as a result of cicatricial contraction or the deposition of abnormal tissue. **annular s.,** a stricture which encircles the lumen of a tubular structure. **bridle s.,** a fold of membrane stretched across a canal, and partially closing it. **cicatricial s.,** one which follows an operative or traumatic wound, particularly a wound which has been infected. **con-**

tractile s., one which may be mechanically dilated, but which soon returns to its contracted condition; called also *recurrent s.* **false s., functional s.,** spasmodic s. **Hunner's s.,** stricture of the ureter due to local inflammation of the wall of the ureter. **hysterical s.,** spasmodic stricture of the esophagus seen in hysterical subjects. **impassable s., impermeable s.,** one that does not permit the passage of an instrument. **irritable s.,** one through which the passage or attempted passage of an instrument produces pain. **organic s.,** a stricture due to a structural change in or about a canal. **permanent s.,** one which persists despite treatment. **recurrent s.,** contractile s. **spasmodic s., spastic s.,** one that is due to muscular spasm; called also *false s., functional s.,* and *temporary s.* **temporary s.,** spasmodic s.

stricturization (strik''chur-i-za'shun) the process of decreasing in caliber or of becoming constricted.

stricturotome (strik'chur-o-tōm'') a knife for cutting strictures.

stricturotomy (strik''chur-ot'o-me) incision of a stricture.

strident (stri'dent) stridulous.

stridor (stri'dor) [L.] a harsh, high-pitched respiratory sound such as the inspiratory sound often heard in acute laryngeal obstruction. Cf. *laryngismus stridulus*. **congenital laryngeal s.,** stridor and dyspnea of the newborn due to an indrawing or infolding of a congenitally flabby epiglottis and aryepiglottic folds (laryngomalacia) during inspiration; the condition is usually outgrown in two years. **s. den'tium** (*obs.*), bruxism. **laryngeal s.,** stridor due to laryngeal obstruction; see also *congenital laryngeal s.* **s. serrat'icus,** a sound like that made by filing a saw, caused by respiration through a tracheostomy tube.

stridulous (strid'u-lus) [L. *stridulus*] attended with stridor; shrill and harsh in sound.

string-halt (string'halt) myoclonus of the hind leg of a horse, causing a gait in which the leg is suddenly raised and then stamped on the ground.

striocellular (stri''o-sel'u-lar) [L. *stria* streak + *cellular*] composed of striated muscle fibers and cells.

striocerebellar (stri''o-ser''e-bel'ar) pertaining to or affecting both the corpus striatum and the cerebellum, as striocerebellar tremor.

striomotor (stri''o-mo'tor) pertaining to or affecting neurons supplying skeletal muscle.

striomuscular (stri''o-mus'ku-lar) pertaining to or composed of striated muscle.

strip (strip) 1. to press the contents from a canal, such as the urethra or a blood vessel, by running the finger along it. 2. to excise lengths of large veins and incompetent tributaries by subcutaneous dissection and the use of a stripper. 3. to remove tooth structure or restorative material from the mesial or distal surfaces of teeth utilizing abrasive strips; usually done to alleviate crowding.

stripe (strīp) a streak or stria. **Baillarger's s's, Gennari's s.,** see under *line*. **Hensen's s.,** a band near the middle of the under surface of the membrana tectoria of the ear. **Mees's s's,** diagonal white stripes on the fingernails in arsenic poisoning. **s's of Retzius,** incremental lines. **Vicq d'Azyr's s.,** the line of Kaes in the cerebral cortex.

stripper (strip'er) a surgical instrument for excision of veins, consisting of a flexible stainless steel cable with a stripping cup or disk at one end and a guide tip at the other; a rigid type of external stripper is also utilized.

strobila (stro-bi'lah), pl. *strobi'lae* [L.; Gr. *strobilos* anything twisted up] 1. the chain of proglottids constituting the bulk of the body of adult tapeworms; considered by some to include the entire body, including the head, neck, and proglottids. 2. The chain of individuals produced by strobilation, such as the series of buds produced at the oral end of the body of certain jellyfish, which during the process of formation somewhat resemble a pile of plates; each bud is released to form an immature, free-swimming jellyfish.

strobile (stro'bīl) strobila.

strobiloid (stro'bĭ-loid) resembling a row of tapeworm segments.

strobilus (stro-bi'lus) [L.; Gr. *strobilos* anything twisted up] strobila.

stroboscope (stro'bo-skōp) [Gr. *strobos* whirl + *skopein* to examine] an instrument by which the successive phases of animal movements may be studied; motion may appear to come to rest.

stroboscopic (stro''bo-skop'ik) pertaining to the stroboscope.

Stroganoff's (Stroganov's) treatment (stro-gan'ofs) [Vasilii Vasilovich *Stroganov*, Russian obstetrician, 1857–1938] see under *treatment*.

stroke (strōk) a sudden and severe attack; see *stroke syndrome*, under *syndrome*. **apoplectic s.,** apoplexy (def. 1). **back s.,** 1. the recoil of the ventricles at the time the blood is forced into the aorta. 2. the influence which a peripheral organ of response exerts back upon the nerve center from which the response was generated. **effective s.,** see *cilium* (def. 3). **heat s.,** a condition caused by exposure to excessive heat, natural or artificial, and marked by dry skin, vertigo, headache, thirst, nausea, and muscular cramps; body temperature may be dangerously elevated, contrasting with heat exhaustion in which the body temperature may be subnormal. Called also *heat apoplexy* and *thermoplegia*. Cf. *sunstroke*. **light s.**, a fatal narcosis produced in sensitized mice by exposure to light. **lightning s.**, loss of consciousness and shock with burns, frequently fatal, caused by lightning. **paralytic s.**, a sudden attack of paralysis from injury to the brain or spinal cord. **recovery s.**, see *cilium* (def. 3). **sun s.**, see *sunstroke*.

stroma (stro′mah), pl. *stro′mata* [Gr. *strōma* anything laid out for lying or sitting upon] the supporting tissue or matrix of an organ, as distinguished from its functional element, or parenchyma. **s. of cornea**, substantia propria corneae. **s. glan′dulae thyreoi′deae, s. glan′dulae thyroi′deae** [NA], stroma of thyroid gland: the tissue that forms the framework of the thyroid gland. **s. i′ridis** [NA], **s. of iris**, the soft mass of connective tissue fibers that make up the major portion of the iris. **s. ova′rii** [NA], **s. of ovary**, the fibrous tissue and smooth muscle composing the framework of the ovary. **Rollet′s s.**, that part of a red blood cell which remains after the hemoglobin has been removed. **s. of thyroid gland**, s. glandulae thyroideae. **vitreous s., s. vit′reum** [NA], the framework of firmer material making up the vitreous body of the eye, and enclosing within its meshes the more fluid portion (humor vitreus).

stromal (stro′mal) pertaining to or resembling stroma.

stromatic (stro-mat′ik) stromal.

stromatin (stro′mah-tin) a protein constituent of the stroma of erythrocytes.

stromatogenous (stro″mah-toj′ĕ-nus) [*stroma* + Gr. *gennan* to produce] originating in the stroma or connective tissue of an organ.

stromatolysis (stro″mah-tol′ĭ-sis) [*stroma* + Gr. *lysis* dissolution] destruction of the stroma of a cell, especially that of a red blood cell.

stromatosis (stro″mah-to′sis) adenomyosis in which the invading endometrial substance is stromal and not glandular; stromal adenomyosis.

Stromeyer′s cephalhematocele, splint (stro′mi-erz) [Georg Friedrich Ludwig *Stromeyer*, German surgeon, 1804–1876] see under *cephalhematocele* and *splint*.

stromuhr (strōm′oor) [Ger. "stream clock"] Ludwig′s instrument for measuring the velocity of the blood flow (1867).

Strong′s bacillus (strongz) [Richard Pearson *Strong*, American physician, 1872–1948] *Shigella flexneri*.

strongyli (stron′jĭ-li) plural of *strongylus*.

strongyliasis (stron″jĭ-li′ah-sis) strongylosis.

strongylid (stron′jĭ-lid) 1. of or pertaining to the superfamily Strongyloidea. 2. strongylus.

Strongylidae (stron-jil′ĭ-de) a family of nematodes of the superfamily Strongyloidea, including the genera *Strongylus* and *Œsophagostomum*.

Strongyloidea (stron″jĭ-loi′de-ah) a superfamily of phasmids, including the hookworms and related bursate nematodes. It comprises the families Ancylostomidae, Strongylidae, Trichostrongylidae, Metastrongylidae, and Syngamidae.

Strongyloides (stron″jĭ-loi′dēz) a genus of phasmids belonging to the superfamily Rhabditoidea, widely distributed as intestinal parasites of mammals. In some systems of classification, included in the superfamily Rhabdiasoidea. **S. intestina′lis**, *S. stercoralis*. **S. papillo′sus**, a species found in cows, pigs, sheep, goats, rabbits, and rats. **S. ranso′mi**, a species found in pigs. **S. rat′ti**, a species found in rats. **S. stercora′lis**, a roundworm occurring widely in tropical and subtropical countries. The female worm and her larvae inhabit the mucosa and submucosa of the small intestine, where they cause diarrhea and ulceration (intestinal strongyloidiasis or Cochin-China diarrhea). The larvae expelled from an infected person with his feces develop in the soil and penetrate the human skin on contact. They eventually are carried in the bloodstream to the lungs, where they cause hemorrhage (pulmonary strongyloidiasis) when they rupture into the alveoli; from the lungs they reach the intestine via the trachea and esophagus. Massive infections may be seen in patients treated with corticosteroids, immunosuppressive drugs, etc. An endogenous cycle of development may occur, allowing infections to persist for many years. Called also *Anguillula intestinalis, Anguillula stercoralis*, and *Strongyloides intestinalis*.

strongyloidiasis (stron″jĭ-loi-di′ah-sis) infection with *Strongyloides stercoralis* (see under *Strongyloides*).

strongyloidosis (stron″jĭ-loi-do′sis) strongyloidiasis.

strongylosis (stron″jĭ-lo′sis) infection with worms of the genus *Strongylus*.

Strongylus (stron′jĭ-lus) [Gr. *strongylos* round] a genus of parasitic nematode worms of the family Strongylidae. **S. edenta′tus**, a species found in horses. **S. equi′nus**, a worm parasitic in the intestines of horses; called also *palisade worm*. **S. fila′ria**, *Dictyocaulus filaria*. **S. gibso′ni**, *Mecistocirrhus*

digitatus. **S. gi′gas**, *Dioctophyma renale*. **S. longevagina′tus**, *Metastrongylus elongatus*. **S. micru′rus**, *Dictyocaulus viviparus*. **S. paradox′us**, *Metastrongylus elongatus*. **S. rena′lis**, *Dioctophyma renale*. **S. sub′tilis**, *Trichostrongylus colubriformis*. **S. vulga′ris**, a species found in horses.

strongylus (stron′jĭ-lus), pl. *stron′gyli*. An individual organism of the genus *Strongylus*.

strontia (stron′she-ah) strontium oxide.

strontium (stron′she-um) [*Strontian* in Scotland] a dark yellowish metal: symbol, Sr; atomic number, 38; atomic weight, 87.62. See also *radiostrontium*. **s. bromide**, a clear, colorless, crystalline substance, $SrBr_2 + 6H_2O$, used like other bromides. **s. hydroxide**, colorless crystals or white powder, $Sr(OH)_2 \cdot 8H_2O$, soluble in 50 parts water and in acids. **s. oxide**, a white, strongly basic substance, SrO, which reacts vigorously with water to give strontium hydroxide; called also *strontia*. **radioactive s.**, radiostrontium. **s. salicylate**, a salt, $(OH \cdot C_6H_4 \cdot CO \cdot O)_2Sr$, in white crystals, soluble in 40 parts of water and freely in alcohol.

strontiuresis (stron″she-u-re′sis) the elimination of strontium from the body by way of the urine.

strontiuretic (stron″she-u-ret′ik) pertaining to, characterized by, or promoting strontiuresis.

strophanthidin (stro-fan′thĭ-din) chemical name: 3β,5,14-trihydroxy-19-oxo-5β-card-20(22)-enolide. An aglycone, $C_{23}H_{32}O_6$, obtained by hydrolysis of glycosides from *Strophanthus kombé*.

strophanthin (stro-fan′thin) a glycoside or a mixture of steroidal glycosides obtained from *Strophanthus kombé*, occurring as a white or yellowish white powder. It is a cardioactive drug with actions similar to those of ouabain, and is used intravenously when a cardiotonic of rapid onset and short duration is desired. Called also *K-s* or *s.-K*. **G-s., s.-G**, ouabain.

Strophanthus (stro-fan′thus) [Gr. *strophos* a twisted band + *anthos* flower] a genus of shrubs, trees, and woody vines growing especially in tropical Africa, and including several poisonous species. *S. gratus* yields ouabain; *S. hispidus* yields pseudostrophanthin; *S. kombé* yields strophanthidin and strophanthin; and *S. sarmentosus* yields sarmentocymarin, sarmentogenin, and sarmentose.

strophocephalus (strof″o-sef′ah-lus) a fetus exhibiting strophocephaly.

strophocephaly (strof″o-sef′ah-le) [Gr. *strophos* a twisted band + *kephalē* head] a developmental anomaly characterized by distortion of the head and face.

strophosomus (strof″o-so′mus) [Gr. *strophos* a twisted band + *sōma* body] a celosomus, especially in chicks, in which the extremities are reflexed onto the back with the distal ends resting on the head.

strophulus (strof′u-lus) [L.] papular urticaria.

struck (struk) a usually fatal enterotoxemia of young calves, lambs, and piglets, caused by *Clostridium perfringens* type C, occurring chiefly in the winter and spring, apparently throughout the world; it is characterized by hemorrhagic enteritis and peritonitis. It was first reported as a disease of mature sheep in the Romney Marsh district of England. Called also *hemorrhagic enterotoxemia*.

structural (struk′tūr-al) pertaining to or affecting the structure.

structure (struk′chur) [L. *struere* to build] the components and their manner of arrangement in constituting a whole. **antigenic s.** (of microorganisms), the mosaic of individual antigens present in cells of a microorganism. **denture-supporting s′s**, the tissues, either the teeth or residual ridges, or both, which serve as the foundation for removable partial or complete dentures. **fine s.**, ultrastructure.

struma (stroo′mah) [L.] goiter. **s. aberran′ta**, goiter affecting an accessory thyroid gland. **adrenal s.**, suprarenal hyperplasia. **s. aneurysmat′ica**, vascular goiter in which the vessels are dilated. **s. basedowifica′ta**, Graves′ disease. **s. ba′seos lin′guae**, an accessory and ectopic portion of thyroid tissue at the base of the tongue. **s. calculo′sa**, a goiter that has undergone calcification. **cast iron s.**, Riedel′s s. **s. colloi′des**, distention of the follicles of the thyroid gland with colloid secretion. **s. colloi′des cys′tica**, a colloid goiter in which the walls of the follicles have broken down, forming cysts or cystlike cavities. **s. cys′tica os′sea**, a goiter in which bone has formed. **s. endothora′cica**, intrathoracic goiter. **s. fibro′sa**, thyroid enlargement caused by hyperplasia of the connective tissue. **s. follicula′ris**, parenchymatous goiter. **s. gelatino′sa**, colloid goiter. **Hashimoto′s s.**, s. lymphomatosa. **s. hyperplas′tica**, s. fibrosa. **ligneous s.**, Riedel′s s. **s. lipomato′des aberra′ta re′nis**, hypernephroma. **s. lymphat′ica**, lymphatism, def. 2. **s. lymphomato′sa**, a progressive disease of the thyroid gland, with extensive acidophilic degeneration of its epithelial elements and replacement by lymphoid and fibrous tissue; called also *Hashimoto′s disease* or *thyroiditis*. **s. malig′na**, cancer of the thyroid body. **s. mol′lis**, thyroid enlargement due to hyperplasia of the cellular and colloid elements. **s. nodo′sa**, adenoma of the thyroid gland. **s. ova′rii**, a rare teratoid tumor of the ovary composed almost entirely of thyroid tissue, with large follicles containing abundant colloid; occasionally there are symptoms of hyperthyroidism. **s. parenchymato'sa,** enlargement of the thyroid gland due to follicular hyperplasia. **s. pituita'ria,** permanent enlargement of the pituitary gland. **s. postbranchia'lis** (obs.), Hürthle cell tumor; see under *tumor.* **retrosternal s.,** substernal s. **Riedel's s.,** a chronic proliferating, fibrosing, inflammatory process involving usually one but sometimes both lobes of the thyroid gland, as well as the trachea and the muscles, fascia, nerves, and vessels in the vicinity of the gland. Called also *Riedel's disease* and *ligneous thyroiditis.* **substernal s.,** a goiter that extends down back of the sternum. **s. suprarena'lis,** a peculiar tumor of the suprarenal gland, consisting mainly of fatty tissue. **thymus s.,** persistence of the thymus gland beyond the time when it usually atrophies. **s. vasculo'sa,** vascular goiter.

strumectomy (stroo-mek'to-me) [L. *struma* goiter + Gr. *ektomē* excision] surgical removal of a goiter. **median s.,** excision of a median goiter or an enlarged isthmus of the thyroid.

strumiprival (stroo-mip'rĭ-val) strumiprivous.

strumiprivic (stroo"mĭ-priv'ik) strumiprivous.

strumiprivous (stroo"mĭ-pri'vus) [L. *strumiprivus; struma* goiter + *privus* deprived] caused by the removal of the thyroid gland.

strumitis (stroo-mi'tis) inflammation of the thyroid gland; thyroiditis. **eberthian s.,** thyroiditis due to infection with the typhoid bacillus.

Strümpell's disease, sign, type (strim'pelz) [Adolf von *Strümpell,* physician in Leipzig, 1853–1925] see under *disease, sign,* and *type.*

Strümpell-Leichtenstern disease (strim'pel-lik'ten-stern) [A. von *Strümpell;* Otto *Leichtenstern,* German physician, 1845–1900] hemorrhagic encephalitis.

Strümpell-Marie disease (strim'pel-mah-re') [A. von *Strümpell;* Pierre *Marie,* French physician, 1853–1940] rheumatoid spondylitis.

Strümpell-Westphal pseudosclerosis (strim'pel-vest'fawl) [A. von *Strümpell;* Carl Friedrich Otto *Westphal,* German neurologist, 1833–1890] hepatolenticular degeneration.

Strunsky's sign (strun'skēz) [Max *Strunsky,* New York orthopedic surgeon, born 1873] see under *sign.*

Struve's test (stroo'vez) [Heinrich *Struve,* physician in Petrograd] see under *tests.*

struvite (stroo'vīt) see under *calculus.*

strychnine (strik'nīn) an extremely poisonous alkaloid, $C_{21}H_{22}N_2O_2$, obtained chiefly from *Strychnos nux-vomica* and other species of *Strychnos,* which causes excitation of all portions of the central nervous system by blocking postsynaptic inhibition of neural impulses; it has been used as a central nervous system stimulant and was formerly used as a bitter tonic, circulatory stimulant, and with cathartic drugs. In veterinary medicine it is occasionally used as a tonic and stimulant. See also *strychninism.* **s. hydrochloride,** a crystalline salt, $C_{21}H_{22}N_2O_2 \cdot HCl + 2H_2O$. **s. nitrate,** a salt, $C_{21}H_{22}N_2O_2 \cdot HNO_3$, occurring as colorless odorless needles or as a white crystalline powder; its medical use is the same as that of strychnine, and its veterinary use is the same as that of strychnine sulfate. **s. phosphate,** a salt, $C_{21}H_{22}N_2O_2 \cdot H_3PO_4 \cdot 2H_2O$, occurring as colorless or white crystals or as a white powder; its medical use is the same as that of strychnine, and its veterinary use is the same as that of strychnine sulfate. It was formerly used in compounding iron, quinine, and strychnine phosphates elixir. **s. sulfate,** a salt, $(C_{21}H_{22}N_2O_2)_2 \cdot H_2SO_4 \cdot 5H_2O$, occurring as colorless or white crystals or as a white crystalline powder; used the same as strychnine. In veterinary medicine it is used in tonics, and in noninflammatory paraplegia, rumen, and intestinal impactions.

strychninism (strik'nin-izm) a toxic condition due to the misuse of strychnine; chronic strychnine poisoning. Symptoms include increased acuity of hearing, vision, touch, taste, and smell, followed by tonic convulsions and vomiting; in severe cases, it may culminate in respiratory paralysis and death.

strychninization (strik"nin-i-za'shun) the act of bringing under the influence of strychnine.

strychninomania (strik"nin-o-ma'ne-ah) [*strychnine* + Gr. *mania* madness] mental aberration due to strychnine poisoning.

strychnism (strik'nizm) poisoning by strychnine.

strychnize (strik'nīz) to put under the influence of strychnine.

Strychnos (strik'nos) [Gr. "nightshade"] a genus of loganiaceous tropical trees. *S. nux-vomica* affords strychnine, curare, brucine, and nux-vomica; *S. ignatii* affords ignatia and brucine.

S.T.S. serologic test for syphilis.

S.T.U. skin test unit; see under *unit.*

stump (stump) the distal end of the part of the limb left in amputation. **conical s.,** a cone-shaped amputation stump produced as a result of undue retraction of the muscles.

stun (stun) to knock senseless; to render unconscious by a blow or other force; to daze.

stunt (stunt) to retard the growth of. **bushy s.,** a viral disease of tomatoes marked by stunting and discoloration of the leaves.

stupe (stūp) [L. *stupa* tow] a cloth, sponge, or the like, for external application, charged with hot water, wrung out nearly dry, and then made irritant or otherwise medicated.

stupefacient (stu"pĕ-fa'shent) [L. *stupefacere* to make senseless] 1. inducing stupor. 2. an agent that induces stupor.

stupefactive (stu"pĕ-fak'tiv) producing narcosis or stupor.

stupor (stu'por) [L.] partial or nearly complete unconsciousness, manifested by responding only to vigorous stimulation. Also, in psychiatry, a disorder marked by reduced responsiveness. **anergic s.,** a form of dementia in which the patient is quiet, listless, and nonresistant. **benign s.,** a condition of stupor sometimes observed in the depressive phase of manic-depressive psychosis. **delusion s.,** stuporous psychosis or acute dementia. **epileptic s.,** stupor following an epileptic convulsion; called also *postconvulsive s.* **lethargic s.,** trance. **postconvulsive s.,** epileptic s.

stuporose (stu'por-ōs) stuporous.

stuporous (stu'por-us) affected with or characterized by stupor.

stupp (stup) a poisonous kind of soot which accumulates in the condensers of mercury smelters; it contains metallic mercury in a finely divided condition.

sturdy (stur'de) gid.

Sturge's disease, syndrome (ster'jez) [William Allen *Sturge,* British physician, 1850–1919] Sturge-Weber syndrome.

Sturge-Weber syndrome (sterj-web-er) [W. A. *Sturge;* Frederick Parkes *Weber,* British physician, 1863–1962] see under *syndrome.*

Sturm's conoid, interval (sturmz) [Johann Christoph *Sturm,* 1635–1703] see under *conoid,* and see *focal interval,* under *interval.*

stuttering (stut'er-ing) a problem of speech behavior involving three definitive factors: (1) speech disfluency, most significantly repetitions of parts of words and whole words, prolongations of sounds, interjections of sounds or words, and unduly prolonged pauses; (2) reactions of the listeners to the speaker's disfluency as evaluated by them as undesirable, abnormal, or unacceptable; and (3) the reactions of the speaker to the listeners' reactions, as well as to his own speech disfluency and to his conception of himself as a stutterer. Stuttering is usually distinguished from *stammering,* which is characterized by blocking or involuntary pauses in speech, sometimes with repetition of sounds. **labiochoreic s.,** labiochorea. **urinary s.,** interruption of the flow during urination.

sty (sti), pl. *sties* [L. *hordeolum*] stye.

stycosis (sti-ko'sis) the presence of calcium sulfate in the organs of the body, especially in the lymph nodes.

stye (sti), pl. *styes* [L. *hordeolum*] hordeolum. **meibomian s.,** one involving a meibomian gland, usually draining through the conjunctival surface of the lid. **zeisian s.,** one involving a zeisian gland, occurring on the surface of the skin at the edge of the lid.

style (stīl) stylet.

stylet (sti'let) [L. *stilus;* Gr. *stylos* pillar] 1. a wire run through a catheter or cannula to render it stiff or to remove debris from its lumen. 2. a slender probe.

styliform (sti'lĭ-form) [L. *stilus* stake, pole + *forma* shape] long and pointed; styloid.

styliscus (sti-lis'kus) [L.; Gr. *styliskos* pillar] a slender cylindrical tent.

stylo- (sti'lo) [L. *stilus* a stake, pole; Gr. *stylos* pillar] a combining form denoting resemblance to a stake or pole, used especially to denote relationship to the styloid process of the temporal bone.

stylohyal (sti"lo-hi'al) stylohyoid.

stylohyoid (sti"lo-hi'oid) pertaining to the styloid process and to the hyoid bone.

styloid (sti'loid) [Gr. *stylos* pillar + *eidos* form] resembling a pillar; long and pointed; styliform.

styloiditis (sti"loi-di'tis) inflammation of tissues about the styloid process.

stylomandibular (sti"lo-man-dib'u-lar) pertaining to the styloid process and the mandible.

stylomastoid (sti"lo-mas'toid) pertaining to the styloid and mastoid processes.

stylomaxillary (sti"lo-mak'sĭ-ler"e) pertaining to the styloid process and to the maxilla.

stylomyloid (sti"lo-mi'loid) [*stylo-* + Gr. *mylē* mill + *eidos* form] pertaining to the styloid process and to the region of the lower molar teeth.

stylopodium (sti"lo-po'de-um) see *limb.*

Stylosanthes (sti"lo-san'thēz) [*stylo-* + Gr. *anthos* flower] a genus of leguminous herbs, chiefly South American. *S. ela'tior,* the pencil-flower of North America, is a uterine sedative.

stylostaphyline (sti″lo-staf′ĭ-lin) pertaining to the styloid process of the temporal bone and the velum palatinum.

stylosteophyte (sti-los′te-o-fīt) a pillar-shaped exostosis.

stylostixis (sti″lo-stik′sis) [stylo- + Gr. stixis pricking] acupuncture.

stylus (sti′lus) [L. stilus] 1. a stylet. 2. a pencil-shaped medicinal preparation, as a stick of caustic.

stymatosis (sti″mah-to′sis) [Gr. styma priapism] priapism with a bloody discharge.

stypage (sti′pij, ste-pahzh′) [Fr.] the application of a stype to produce local anesthesia.

stype (stīp) [Gr. styppeion tow] a tampon or pledget.

stypsis (stip′sis) [Gr. stypsis contraction] 1. astringency; astringent action. 2. treatment by astringents.

styptic (stip′tik) [Gr. styptikos] 1. astringent; arresting hemorrhage by means of an astringent quality. 2. an astringent and hemostatic remedy. **Binelli's s.**, a solution of creosote, formerly used for arresting hemorrhage. **chemical s.,** one which arrests hemorrhage by causing coagulation through chemical action. **mechanical s.,** one which acts by causing coagulation mechanically, as a pledget of cotton. **vascular s.,** one which acts by producing contraction of injured or divided blood vessels of small caliber.

Stypven (stip′ven) trademark for a preparation of Russell's viper venom; used as a hemostatic agent. See also under *tests*.

styramate (stir′ah-māt) chemical name: carbamic acid β-hydroxyphenethyl ester. A crystalline substance, $C_9H_{11}NO_3$, used as a skeletal muscle relaxant.

Styrax (sti′raks) a genus of shrubs and trees of worldwide distribution but growing mainly in Java, Sumatra, and Thailand, various species of which are the source of benzoin (def. 1).

styrax (sti′raks) storax.

styrene (sti′rēn) a fragrant liquid or oil hydrocarbon, vinyl benzene, $C_6H_5CH:CH_2$, from storax; called also *cinnamene, cinnamol,* and *styrol.*

styrol (sti′rol) styrene.

styrolene (sti′ro-lēn) styrene.

styrone (sti′ron) cinnamyl alcohol.

su. abbreviation for L. *su′mat,* let him take.

sub- [L. *sub* under] a prefix signifying *under, near, almost,* or *moderately.*

subabdominal (sub″ab-dom′ĭ-nal) situated below the abdomen.

subabdominoperitoneal (sub″ab-dom″ĭ-no-per″ĭ-to-ne′al) subperitoneal.

subacetabular (sub″as-ĕ-tab′u-lar) situated below the acetabulum.

subacetate (sub-as′ĕ-tāt) any basic acetate.

subacid (sub-as′id) somewhat acid.

subacidity (sub″ah-sid′ĭ-te) deficient acidity.

subacromial (sub″ah-kro′me-al) situated below or beneath the acromion.

subacute (sub″ah-kūt′) somewhat acute; between acute and chronic.

subalimentation (sub″al-ĭ-men-ta′shun) insufficient nourishment.

subanal (sub-a′nal) situated below the anus.

subapical (sub-ap′ĕ-kal) situated below an apex.

subaponeurotic (sub″ap-o-nu-rot′ik) situated beneath an aponeurosis.

subarachnoid (sub″ah-rak′noid) situated or occurring between the arachnoid and the pia mater.

subarcuate (sub-ar′ku-āt) [sub- + L. arcuatus arched] somewhat arched or bent.

subareolar (sub″ah-re′o-lar) beneath the areola.

subastragalar (sub″as-trag′ah-lar) situated or occurring under the astragalus (talus).

subastringent (sub″ah-strin′jent) moderately astringent.

subatloidean (sub″at-loi′de-an) situated beneath the atlas.

subatomic (sub″ah-tom′ik) of or pertaining to the constituent parts of an atom as considered under the theory of the nuclear atom; occurring within an atom; smaller than an atom.

subaural (sub-aw′ral) situated beneath the ear.

subaurale (sub″aw-ra′le) an anthropometric landmark, the lowest point on the inferior border of the ear lobule when the subject is looking straight ahead.

subauricular (sub″aw-rik′u-lar) below the pinna (auricle) of the ear.

subaxial (sub-ak′se-al) below an axis.

subaxillary (sub-ak′sĭ-ler′e) below the axilla, or armpit.

subbasal (sub-ba′sal) below a base.

subbrachial (sub-bra′ke-al) relating to the brachium colliculi inferioris.

subbrachycephalic (sub″bra-ke-sĕ-fal′ik) somewhat brachycephalic; having a cephalic index of 78 to 79.

subcalcareous (sub″kal-ka′re-us) slightly calcareous.

subcalcarine (sub-kal′kar-īn) beneath the calcarine fissure.

subcalorism (sub-ka′lor-izm) frigorism.

subcapsular (sub-kap′su-lar) situated below a capsule.

subcapsuloperiosteal (sub-kap″su-lo-per″e-os′te-al) beneath the capsule and the periosteum of a joint.

subcarbonate (sub-kar′bo-nāt) any basic carbonate.

subcartilaginous (sub″kar-tĭ-laj′ĭ-nus) 1. situated beneath a cartilage. 2. partly cartilaginous.

subcentral (sub-sen′tral) located deep to the center.

subception (sub-sep′shun) perception below the level of awareness.

subchloride (sub-klo′rīd) that chloride of any series which contains the smallest proportion of chlorine.

subchondral (sub-kon′dral) beneath a cartilage.

subchordal (sub-kor′dal) situated below the notochord or below the vocal cords.

subchorionic (sub″ko-re-on′ik) situated beneath the chorion.

subchoroidal (sub″ko-roi′dal) beneath the choroid.

subchronic (sub-kron′ik) between chronic and subacute.

subclass (sub′klas) a taxonomic category sometimes established, subordinate to a class and superior to an order.

subclavian (sub-kla′ve-an) situated under the clavicle, as the subclavian artery.

subclavicular (sub″klah-vik′u-lar) situated under the clavicle.

subclinical (sub-klin′ĭ-kal) without clinical manifestations; said of the early stages, or a slight degree, of a disease.

subclone (sub′klōn) the progeny of a mutant cell arising in a clone.

subconjunctival (sub″kon-junk-ti′val) situated or occurring beneath the conjunctiva.

subconscious (sub-kon′shus) 1. imperfectly or partially conscious. 2. preconscious.

subconsciousness (sub-kon′shus-nes) the state of being partially conscious.

subcontinuous (sub″kon-tin′u-us) nearly continuous; remittent.

subcoracoid (sub-kor′ah-koid) situated beneath the coracoid process.

subcortex (sub-kor′teks) that part of the brain substance which underlies the cortex.

subcortical (sub-kor′tĭ-kal) situated beneath the cortex.

subcostal (sub-kos′tal) situated beneath a rib.

subcostalis (sub″kos-ta′lis), pl. *subcosta′les* [L.] subcostal.

subcranial (sub-kra′ne-al) beneath the cranium.

subcrepitant (sub-krep′ĭ-tant) pertaining to a rale that is slightly more coarse than a crepitant rale; see under *rale.*

subcrepitation (sub″krep-ĭ-ta′shun) the sound of subcrepitant rales; see under *rale.*

subculture (sub′kul-tūr) a culture of bacteria derived from another culture.

subcutaneous (sub″ku-ta′ne-us) beneath the skin.

subcuticular (sub″ku-tik′u-lar) situated beneath the epidermis; subepidermal.

subcutis (sub-ku′tis) [sub- + L. cutis skin] 1. panniculus adiposus. 2. subcutaneous tissue (tela subcutanea [NA]).

subdelirium (sub″de-lir′e-um) partial or mild delirium.

subdeltoid (sub-del′toid) beneath the deltoid muscle.

subdental (sub-den′tal) [sub- + L. dens tooth] beneath the teeth.

subdiaphragmatic (sub″di-ah-frag-mat′ik) situated under the diaphragm; subphrenic.

subdorsal (sub-dor′sal) situated below the dorsal region.

subduct (sub-dukt′) to depress or draw down; see *subduction.*

subduction (sub-duk′shun) a drawing downward; specifically the duction of the eyeball exerted by the inferior rectus muscle.

subdural (sub-du′ral) situated between the dura mater and the arachnoid.

subendocardial (sub″en-do-kar′de-al) beneath the endocardium.

subendothelial (sub″en-do-the′le-al) situated beneath an endothelium.

subendothelium (sub″en-do-the′le-um) Debove's membrane.

subendymal (sub-en′dĭ-mal) situated beneath the endyma (ependyma).

subependymal (sub″ep-en′dĭ-mal) situated beneath the ependyma.

subependymoma (sub″ep-en″dĭ-mo′mah) an ependymoma in which there is a diffuse proliferation of subependymal fibrillary astrocytes among the ependymal tumor cells.

subepidermal, subepidermic (sub″ep-ĭ-der′mal; sub″ep-ĭ-der′-mik) beneath the epidermis.

subepiglottic (sub″ep-ĭ-glot′ik) below the epiglottis.

subepithelial (sub″ep-ĭ-the′le-al) situated beneath an epithelium.

suberin (soo′ber-in) an insoluble variety of cellulose derived from cork.

suberitin (soo-ber′ĭ-tin) [*Suberites*, a marine sponge (from L. *suber* cork) + chemical suffix *-in*] a toxic substance derived from the marine sponge, *Suberites domunculus*, which, when injected into dogs, produces intestinal hemorrhages and respiratory distress.

suberosis (su″ber-o′sis) [L. *suber* cork + *-osis*] a form of allergic alveolitis due to inhalation of and tissue reaction to moldy cork dust; the offending antigen is from species of *Penicillium*.

subexcite (sub″ek-sīt′) to excite in a partial manner.

subextensibility (sub″eks-ten″sĭ-bil′ĭ-te) decreased extensibility.

subfamily (sub-fam′ĭ-le) a taxonomic category sometimes established, subordinate to a family and superior to a tribe.

subfascial (sub-fash′al) situated beneath a fascia.

subfertile (sub-fer′til) characterized by less than normal fertility.

subfertility (sub″fer-til′ĭ-te) the state of being less than normally fertile; relative sterility.

Sub fin. coct. abbreviation for L. *sub fi′nem coctio′nis*, toward the end of boiling.

subflavous (sub-fla′vus) [*sub-* + L. *flavus* yellow] yellowish.

subfoliar (sub-fo′le-ar) pertaining to a subfolium.

subfolium (sub-fo′le-um) [*sub-* + L. *folium* leaf] any of the elementary divisions of a cerebellar folium.

subgaleal (sub-ga′le-al) situated beneath the galea aponeurotica.

subgallate (sub-gal′āt) a basic gallate.

subgemmal (sub-jem′al) [*sub-* + L. *gemma* bud] situated under a taste bud or other bud.

subgenus (sub-je′nus) a taxonomic category between a genus and a species.

subgerminal (sub-jer′mĭ-nal) below or under the germ.

subgingival (sub-jin′jĭ-val) beneath the gingiva.

subglenoid (sub-gle′noid) situated under the glenoid fossa.

subglossal (sub-glos′al) sublingual.

subglossitis (sub″glos-si′tis) [*sub-* + L. *glossa* tongue + *-itis*] inflammation of the lower surface of the tongue.

subglottic (sub-glot′ik) beneath the glottis.

subgranular (sub-gran′u-lar) somewhat granular.

subgrondation (sub″gron-da′shun) [Fr.] the depression of one fragment of bone beneath another.

subgyrus (sub-ji′rus) any gyrus that is partly concealed or covered by another or by others.

subhepatic (sub″hĕ-pat′ik) situated beneath the liver.

subhumeral (sub-hu′mer-al) below or beneath the humerus.

subhyaloid (sub-hi′ah-loid) situated or occurring beneath the hyaloid membrane.

subhyoid (sub-hi′oid) situated below the hyoid.

subhyoidean (sub″hi-oi′de-an) subhyoid.

subicteric (sub″ik-ter′ik) somewhat jaundiced.

subicular (sŭ-bik′u-lar) of or pertaining to the uncinate gyrus.

subiculum (sŭ-bik′u-lum) [L., from *subicere* to raise, lift] an underlying or supporting structure. **s. cor′nu ammo′nis, s. hippocam′pi,** gyrus parahippocampalis. **s. promonto′rii ca′vi tym′pani** [NA], **s. of promontory of tympanic cavity,** a ridge of bone bounding the tympanic sinus posteriorly.

subiliac (sub-il′e-ak) below the ilium.

subilium (sub-il′e-um) the lowest portion of the ilium.

subimbibitional (sub″im-bĭ-bish′on-al) due to deficient intake of liquid.

subinflammation (sub″in-flah-ma′shun) a slight or mild inflammation.

subinflammatory (sub″in-flam′ah-tor″e) pertaining to or causing only mild inflammation.

subintimal (sub-in′tĭ-mal) beneath the intima (of a vessel).

subintrance (sub-in′trans) recurrence of a paroxysm after a shorter period than usual.

subintrant (sub-in′trant) [L. *subintrans* entering by stealth] 1. beginning before the completion of a previous cycle or paroxysm; anticipating. 2. characterized by recurrence at lessening intervals.

subinvolution (sub″in-vo-lu′shun) incomplete involution; failure of a part to return to its normal size and condition after enlargement due to functional activity, as subinvolution of the uterus after delivery of a baby. **chronic s. of uterus,** a diffuse, symmetrical uterine enlargement commonly associated with painless menorrhagia.

subiodide (sub-i′o-dīd) that iodide of any series which contains the smallest proportion of iodine.

subjacent (sub-ja′sent) [*sub-* + L. *jacere* to lie] lying just beneath or underneath.

subject¹ (sub-jekt′) [L. *subjectare* to throw under] to cause to undergo, or submit to; to render subservient.

subject² (sub′jekt) [L. *subjectus* cast under] 1. a person or animal which has been the object of treatment, observation, or experiment. 2. a body for dissection.

subjective (sub-jek′tiv) [L. *subjectivus*] pertaining to or perceived only by the affected individual; not perceptible to the senses of another person.

subjectoscope (sub-jek′to-skōp) [*subjective sensation* + Gr. *skopein* to examine] an instrument used in the study of subjective visual sensations.

subjee (sub′je) [Hind. *sabzī*, literally, "greenness"] the capsules and larger leaves of *Cannabis indica*.

subjugal (sub-ju′gal) situated below the zygomatic bone.

sublatio (sub-la′she-o) [L.] sublation. **s. ret′inae,** detachment of the retina.

sublation (sub-la′shun) [L. *sublatio*] a lifting up, or elevation.

sublesional (sub-le′shun-al) performed or occurring beneath a lesion.

sublethal (sub-le′thal) not quite fatal; insufficient to cause death.

sublimate (sub′lĭ-māt) [L. *sublimatum*] 1. a substance obtained or prepared by sublimation. 2. to divert consciously unacceptable instinctual drives into personally and socially acceptable channels through a mechanism operating outside of and beyond conscious awareness. **corrosive s.,** mercury bichloride.

sublimation (sub″lĭ-ma′shun) [L. *sublimatio*] 1. the direct change of state from solid to vapor. 2. Freud's term for the process of deviating sexual motive powers from sexual aims or objects to new aims or objects other than sexual.

Sublimaze (sub′lĭ-māz) trademark for a preparation of fentanyl citrate.

sublime (sub-līm′) [L. *sublimare*] to volatilize a solid body by heat and then to collect it in a purified form as a solid or powder.

subliminal (sub-lim′ĭ-nal) [*sub-* + L. *limen* threshold] below the limen, or threshold, of sensation.

sublimis (sub-li′mis) [L.] superficial.

sublingual (sub-ling′gwal) located beneath the tongue.

sublinguitis (sub″ling-gwi′tis) inflammation of the sublingual gland.

sublobe (sub′lōb) a division of a lobe; a lobule.

sublobular (sub-lob′u-lar) situated beneath a lobule.

subluxate (sub-luks′āt) to partially dislocate.

subluxation (sub″luk-sa′shun) [*sub-* + L. *luxatio* dislocation] an incomplete or partial dislocation. **s. of lens,** partial dislocation of lens of the eye. **Volkmann's s.,** a type of tuberculosis arthritis marked by flexion contracture of the knee, external rotation of the leg, valgus position of the knee, and bending of the upper third of the tibia.

sublymphemia (sub″lim-fe′me-ah) hypolymphemia.

submammary (sub-mam′ar-e) situated or occurring beneath a mammary gland.

submandibular (sub″man-dib′u-lar) below the mandible.

submania (sub-ma′ne-ah) hypomania.

submarginal (sub-mar′jĭ-nal) situated beneath a margin.

submaxilla (sub″mak-sil′ah) [*sub-* + L. *maxilla* jaw] the mandible.

submaxillaritis (sub-mak″sĭ-ler-i′tis) inflammation of the submaxillary gland.

submaxillary (sub-mak′sĭ-ler″e) situated beneath the maxilla.

submedial, submedian (sub-me′de-al; sub-me′de-an) beneath or near the middle.

submembranous (sub-mem′brah-nus) partly membranous.

submental (sub-men′tal) [*sub-* + L. *mentum* chin] situated below the chin.

submersion (sub-mer′shun) [*sub-* + L. *mergere* to dip] the act of placing or the condition of being under the surface of a liquid.

submetacentric (sub″met-ah-sen′trik) having the centromere more or less equidistant from the center of the chromosome and one end, so that one arm is shorter than the other. Cf. *acrocentric* and *metacentric*.

submicroscopic (sub-mi″kro-skop′ik) too small to be visible under the microscope.

submicroscopical (sub″mi-kro-skop′ĭ-kal) too small to be visible with the light microscope.

submorphous (sub-mor′fus) neither amorphous nor perfectly crystalline.

submucosa (sub″mu-ko′sah) the layer of areolar tissue situated beneath the mucous membrane; see under *tela* the terms beginning *t. submucosa*.

submucosal (sub″mu-ko′sal) pertaining to the submucosa, or situated beneath the mucous membrane.

submucous (sub-mu′kus) situated or performed beneath the mucous membrane.

subnarcotic (sub″nar-kot′ik) moderately narcotic.

subnasal (sub-na′zal) situated below the nose.

subnasale (sub″na-sa′le) an anthropometric landmark, the point at which the nasal septum merges, in the midsagittal plane, with the upper lip.

subnasion (sub-na′ze-on) subnasale.

subnatant (sub-na′tant) 1. situated below or at the bottom of something. 2. the liquid phase situated below a solid phase; it arises when a solid has a lower density than the liquid with which it is in contact.

subneural (sub-nu′ral) situated beneath a nerve, as a subneural apparatus.

subnitrate (sub-ni′trāt) a basic nitrate.

subnormal (sub-nor′mal) below or less than normal; characterized by qualities, such as intelligence, lower than the level usually observed.

subnormality (sub″nor-mal′ĭ-te) the state of being subnormal.

subnotochordal (sub″no-to-kor′dal) situated beneath the notochord.

subnucleus (sub-nu′kle-us) a partial or secondary nucleus into which a large nerve nucleus may be split up.

subnutrition (sub″nu-trish′un) defective nutrition.

suboccipital (sub″ok-sip′ĭ-tal) situated below the occiput.

suboptimal (sub-op′tĭ-mal) less than the optimum.

suboptimum (sub-op′tĭ-mum) a condition lower than that which is optimal or best.

suborbital (sub-or′bĭ-tal) situated beneath the orbit.

suborder (sub-or′der) a taxonomic category sometimes established, subordinate to an order and superior to a family.

suboxide (sub-ok′sīd) that oxide in any series which contains the smallest proportion of oxygen.

subpapillary (sub-pap′ĭ-lar-e) underlying the stratum papillare of the skin, as the subpapillary layer.

subpapular (sub-pap′u-lar) indistinctly papular.

subparalytic (sub″par-ah-lit′ik) partially paralytic.

subparietal (sub″pah-ri′ĕ-tal) situated below a parietal bone, lobe, etc.

subpatellar (sub″pah-tel′ar) situated below the patella.

subpectoral (sub-pek′tor-al) situated beneath or below the pectoral region or muscles.

subpelviperitoneal (sub-pel″ve-per″ĭ-to-ne′al) situated beneath the pelvic peritoneum.

subpericardial (sub″per-ĭ-kar′de-al) beneath the pericardium.

subperiosteal (sub″per-e-os′te-al) situated beneath the periosteum.

subperiosteocapsular (sub″per-e-os″te-o-kap′su-lar) subcapsuloperiosteal.

subperitoneal (sub″per-ĭ-to-ne′al) situated beneath or deep to the peritoneum, as a subperitoneal abscess.

subperitoneoabdominal (sub″per-ĭ-to-ne″o-ab-dom′ĭ-nal) subperitoneal.

subperitoneopelvic (sub″per-ĭ-to-ne″o-pel′vik) occurring beneath the peritoneum of the pelvis.

subpharyngeal (sub″fah-rin′je-al) situated below the pharynx.

subphrenic (sub-fren′ik) situated under the diaphragm; subdiaphragmatic.

subphyla (sub-fi′lah) plural of *subphylum.*

subphylum (sub-fi′lum), pl. *subphy′la.* A taxonomic category sometimes established, subordinate to a phylum and superior to a class.

subpial (sub-pi′al) situated beneath the pia mater.

subpituitarism (sub″pĭ-tu′ĭ-tar-izm) hypopituitarism.

subplacenta (sub″plah-sen′tah) the decidua basalis.

subpleural (sub-ploor′al) situated beneath the pleura.

subpreputial (sub″pre-pu′shal) situated beneath the prepuce.

subpubic (sub-pu′bik) situated or performed below the pubic arch.

subpulmonary (sub-pul′mo-ner″e) situated or occurring below the lung, between the lung and the diaphragm.

subpulpal (sub-pul′pal) below the dental pulp.

subpyramidal (sub″pi-ram′ĭ-dal) below a pyramid, as the subpyramidal fossa.

subrectal (sub-rek′tal) below the rectum.

subretinal (sub-ret′ĭ-nal) below the retina.

subscaphocephaly (sub″skaf-o-sef′ah-le) the condition of being moderately scaphocephalic.

subscapular (sub-skap′u-lar) situated below or under the scapula.

subscleral (sub-skle′ral) located or occurring beneath the sclera.

subsclerotic (sub-skle′rot-ik) 1. subscleral. 2. partly sclerosed.

subscription (sub-skrip′shun) that part of a prescription which gives the directions for compounding the ingredients; see *prescription.*

subserosa (sub″sĕ-ro′sah) a layer of tissue situated beneath a serous membrane.

subserous (sub-se′rus) situated beneath a serous membrane.

subsibilant (sub-sib′ĭ-lant) having a muffled, whistling sound.

subsonic (sub-son′ik) infrasonic.

subspecialty (sub-spesh′al-te) a branch of medicine subordinate to a specialty, as gastroenterology is a subspecialty of internal medicine.

subspecies (sub′spe-sēz) a taxonomic category subordinate to a species, whose members differ morphologically from other members of the species but remain capable of interbreeding with them; a variety or race.

subspinale (sub″spi-na′le) point A; see under *point.*

subspinous (sub-spi′nus) situated below a spinous process.

subsplenial (sub-sple′ne-al) beneath the splenium of the corpus callosum.

substage (sub′stāj) that part of the microscope which is situated beneath the stage.

substance (sub′stans) [L. *substantia*] the material constituting an organ or body; called also *substantia* [NA]. **accessory food s.,** vitamin. **ad s.,** a name given to the substance which effects transmission of a nerve impulse across a synapse. **adamantine s. of tooth,** enamel (enamelum [NA]). **agglutinable s.,** a substance existing in erythrocytes and bacteria, with which an agglutinin unites to produce specific agglutination. **agglutinating s.,** agglutinin. **α-s., alpha s.,** reticular s. **antidiuretic s.,** see under *hormone.* **anti-immune s.,** antiantibody. **arborescent white s. of cerebellum,** arbor vitae cerebelli. **autacoid s.,** autacoid. **β-s., beta s.,** see *Heinz-Ehrlich bodies.* **black s.,** substantia nigra. **blood group s's,** secreted soluble mucopolysaccharides in the body fluids having structures characteristic of red cells and some other body tissues and having the same blood group specificity as red cell isoantigens (e.g., the A, B, and H substances of the ABO blood group). **blood grouping specific s's** [USP], a sterile, isotonic solution of the polysaccharide-containing complexes that are capable of reducing the titer of the anti-A and the anti-B isoagglutinins of group O blood. Specific substance A is usually isolated from hog gastric mucin, and specific substance B usually from the glandular portion of horse gastric mucosa. **Blum s.,** katechin. **bony s. of tooth,** cementum. **cement s., cementing s.,** material which serves to hold together the different components of a tissue, as the intercellular substance in endothelium or the interprismatic substance in tooth enamel. **chromidial s.,** granular endoplasmic reticulum. **chromophil s.,** Nissl bodies. **colloid s.,** a jelly-like material formed in colloid degeneration. **compact s. of bones,** substantia compacta ossium. **contact s.,** catalyst. **controlled s.,** any of the drugs regulated under the Controlled Substances Act (see under C). **cortical s. of bone,** substantia corticalis ossium. **cortical s. of kidney,** cortex renis. **cortical s. of lens,** cortex lentis. **cortical s. of lymph nodes,** cortex nodi lymphatici. **cortical s. of suprarenal gland,** the adrenal cortex (cortex glandulae suprarenalis [NA]). **cytotoxin s.,** cytolysin. **depressor s.,** a substance that tends to decrease activity or blood pressure. **exophthalmos-producing s.,** a substance isolated from crude anterior pituitary extracts which produces exophthalmos in experimental animals. **external s. of suprarenal gland,** cortex glandulae suprarenalis. **fundamental s. of tooth,** dentin (dentinum [NA]). **gelatinous s. of gray substance,** substantia gelatinosa. **gelatinous s. of spinal cord,** substantia gelatinosa. **glandular s. of prostate,** substantia glandularis prostatae. **gray s.,** substantia grisea. **gray s. of cerebrum, central,** substantia grisea centrale cerebri. **gray s. of spinal cord,** substantia grisea medullae spinalis. **ground s.,** the amorphous gel-like material in which connective tissue cells and fibers are embedded. **H s.,** 1. a red cell isoantigen in individuals having blood group O of the ABO system; it also appears to be the precursor which, under the influence of A and B genes, is converted into antigens of the A and B blood groups. 2. released s. **hemolytic s.,** a substance that lyses erythrocytes. **I s.,** an inhibitory substance which appears in the synapses of the vertebrate central nervous system, which seems generally to act as a hypopolarizer of the postsynaptic junction. **interfibrillar s. of Flemming, interfilar s.,** hyaloplasm, def. 1. **intermediate s. of spinal cord, central,** substantia intermedia centralis medullae spinalis. **intermediate s. of spinal cord, lateral,** substantia intermedia lateralis. **intermediate s. of suprarenal gland, internal s. of suprarenal gland,** medulla glandulae suprarenalis. **interprismatic s.,** the ground substance in which the enamel rods are embedded. **interspongioplastic s.,** hyaloplasm, def. 1. **interstitial s.,** ground s. **intertubular s. of tooth, ivory s. of tooth,** dentin (dentinum [NA]).

s. of lens, substantia lentis. **medullary s.,** 1. the white matter of the central nervous system, consisting of axons and their myelin sheaths. 2. the soft, marrow-like substance of the interior of an organ; see under *medulla*. **medullary s. of bones,** medulla ossium. **medullary s. of bones, red,** medulla ossium rubra. **medullary s. of bones, yellow,** medulla ossium flava. **medullary s. of kidney,** medulla renis. **medullary s. of suprarenal gland,** medulla glandulae suprarenalis. **metachromatic s.,** fine particles seen in erythrocytes, especially after supravital staining. **molecular s.,** neuropil. **muscular s. of prostate,** substantia muscularis prostatae. **neurosecretory s.,** neurosecretion, def. 2. **s. of Nissl,** see *Nissl bodies.* **no-threshold s's,** those substances in the blood which are excreted into the urine in proportion to their absolute amount in the blood. Cf. *threshold s's.* **onychogenic s.,** the nail-forming substance which occurs in parallel fibrils in the nail matrix. **organ-forming s's,** specialized materials that become segregated in definite blastomeres, thus bringing about a mosaic type of development. **s. P,** a peptide composed of 11 amino acids, present in the intestine, where it serves to contract the intestine and dilate blood vessels; it is also present in a number of neuronal pathways in the brain and in primary sensory fibers of peripheral nerves and has been suggested to be a neurotransmitter associated with transmission of pain impulses. **P.-P. s., pellagra-preventing s.,** a dietary substance which will prevent or abolish pellagra. **perforated s., anterior,** substantia perforata anterior. **perforated s., posterior,** substantia perforata posterior. **periventricular gray s.,** diffuse collections of small cells immediately surrounding the ependymal lining of the third ventricle of the brain, around the cerebral aqueduct, and in the floor of the fourth ventricle. **prelipid s.,** degenerated nerve tissue which has not yet been converted into fat. **pressor s.,** any substance that tends to increase blood pressure. **preventive s.,** antibody. **proper s. of cornea,** substantia propria corneae. **proper s. of sclera,** substantia propria sclerae. **proper s. of tooth,** dentin (dentinum [NA]). **receptive s.,** a hypothetical substance supposed to exist in muscle tissue, especially near the motor end-plates of the nerves, and to conduct excitation. **red s. of spleen,** pulpa lienis. **Reichert's s.,** the posterior portion of the anterior perforated substance. **Reichstein's s. Fa,** cortisone. **Reichstein's s. M,** hydrocortisone, or cortisol. **released s.,** a histamine-like substance liberated at the site of inflammation and responsible for increased vascular permeability; called also *H s.* **reticular s.,** the netlike mass of threads seen in erythrocytes after vital staining; called also *reticular s.* and *filar mass.* **reticular s., white, of Arnold,** formatio reticularis pontis. **Rolando's gelatinous s.,** substantia gelatinosa. **Rollett's secondary s.,** the transparent material lying in narrow zones on each side of Krause's membranes. **sarcous s.,** the substance composing the sarcous element of muscle. **s. sensibilis'atrice, sensibilizing s., sensitizing s.,** antibody. **slow-reacting s., slow-reactive s.,** a substance released in the anaphylactic reaction that induces slow, prolonged contraction of certain smooth muscles; symbol SRS-A. **Soemmering's gray s.** (*obs.*), substantia nigra. **specific capsular s., specific soluble s.,** a polysaccharide from bacterial capsules having haptenic properties. **spongy s. of bones,** substantia spongiosa ossium. **threshold s's,** those substances in the blood, such as glucose, which are excreted into the urine only when their concentration in plasma exceeds a certain value. **thromboplastic s.,** a general term for any material with procoagulant activity. **tigroid s.,** see *Nissl bodies.* **transmitter s.,** neurotransmitter. **vitreous s. of tooth,** enamel (enamelum [NA]). **white s.,** substantia alba. **white s. of Schwann,** myelin, def. 1. **white s. of spinal cord,** substantia alba medullae spinalis. **zymoplastic s.,** thromboplastic s.

substandard (sub-stan′dard) falling short of the accepted or usual standard.

substantia (sub-stan′she-ah), pl. *substan′tiae* [L.] material of which a tissue, organ, or body is composed; used as a general term in nomenclature. Called also *substance.* **s. adamanti′na den′tis,** enamel (enamelum [NA]). **s. al′ba** [NA], white substance: the white nervous tissue, constituting the conducting portion of the brain and spinal cord, and composed mostly of myelinated nerve fibers. **s. al′ba medul′lae spina′lis** [NA], the white substance of the spinal cord, consisting of long myelinated nerve fibers arranged in parallel longitudinal bundles. **s. cine′rea,** s. grisea. **s. compac′ta os′sium** [NA], compact substance of bone: bone substance which is dense and hard; called also *compact bone.* **s. cortica′lis cerebel′li,** cortex cerebelli. **s. cortica′lis cer′ebri,** old term for cortex cerebri. **s. cortica′lis glan′dulae suprarena′lis,** the adrenal cortex (c. glandulae suprarenalis [NA]). **s. cortica′lis len′tis,** cortex lentis. **s. cortica′lis lymphoglan′dulae,** cortex nodi lymphatici. **s. cortica′lis os′sium** [NA], cortical substance of bone: the substance comprising the hard outer layer of a bone. **s. cortica′lis re′nis,** cortex renis. **s. denta′lis pro′pria,** dentin (dentinum [NA]). **s. ebur′nea den′tis,** dentin (dentinum [NA]). **s. ferrugin′ea,** locus ceruleus. **s. fundamenta′lis den′tis,** dentin (dentinum [NA]). **s. gelatino′sa cen-**

tra′lis, intermedia centralis. **s. gelatino′sa colum′nae posterio′ris,** s. gelatinosa. **s. gelatino′sa** [NA], **s. gelantio′sa (Rolan′di),** gelatinous substance of spinal cord: the gelatinous-appearing cap that forms the dorsal part of the posterior horn of the spinal cord. **s. glandula′ris pro′statae** [NA], glandular substance of prostate: tissue composed of branched tubuloalveolar glands, outgrowths of the tunica mucosa of the urethra, which terminate in excretory ducts opening into the male urethra; it is enclosed in muscular substance and permeated by muscular strands. Called also *corpus glandulare prostatae.* **s. gris′ea** [NA], gray substance: the gray nervous tissue composed of nerve cell bodies, unmyelinated nerve fibers, and supportive tissue. **s. gris′ea centra′lis cer′ebri** [NA], central gray substance of cerebrum: the gray substance in the brain surrounding the cerebral aqueduct; called also *stratum griseum centrale cerebri.* **s. gris′ea centra′lis medul′lae spina′lis,** see *s. intermedia centralis medullae spinalis* and *s. intermedia lateralis medullae spinalis.* **s. gris′ea medul′lae spina′lis** [NA], gray substance of the spinal cord: it contains fewer myelinated fibers but more nerve cell bodies, unmyelinated nerve fibers, and blood vessels than the white substance. **s. hyali′na,** the more fluid interstitial part of the protoplasm of a cell. Cf. *s. opaca.* **s. innomina′ta,** nerve tissue immediately caudad to the anterior perforated substance, and ventral to the globus pallidus and ansa lenticularis. Also known as the *s. innominata of Reichert* or *of Reil.* **s. innomina′ta of Reichert, s. innomina′ta of Reil,** s. innominata. **s. interme′dia centra′lis** [NA], central intermediate substance of spinal cord: the gray substance surrounding the central canal of the spinal cord. **s. interme′dia latera′lis** [NA], lateral intermediate substance of spinal cord: the gray substance of the spinal cord that intervenes between the central intermediate substance, the lateral column, and the anterior and posterior columns. **s. intertubula′ris den′tis,** dentin (dentinum [NA]). **s. len′tis** [NA], the fibrous material making up the bulk of the lens of the eye. **s. medulla′ris glan′dulae,** medulla glandulae suprarenalis. **s. medulla′ris lymphoglan′dulae,** medulla nodi lymphatici. **s. medulla′ris re′nis,** medulla renis. **s. metachromaticogranula′ris,** see *Heinz-Ehrlich bodies.* **s. muscula′ris pro′statae** [NA], muscular substance of prostate: the muscular stroma of the prostate, which is intimately blended with the fibrous capsule and permeates the glandular substance; called also *musculus prostaticus.* **s. ni′gra** [NA], black substance: the layer of gray substance that separates the tegmentum of the midbrain from the crus cerebri and which consists of two zones, a dorsal compact zone with melanin-containing cells and a ventral reticular zone whose cells lack melanin; called also *body of Vicq d'Azyr, ganglion of Soemmering,* and *locus niger.* **s. opa′ca,** the reticulum of the protoplasm of a cell. Cf. *s. hyalina.* **s. os′sea den′tis,** cementum. **s. perfora′ta ante′rior** [NA], anterior perforated substance: an area on the ventral surface of the brain bounded by the olfactory trigone and the optic tract; it is pierced by numerous small arteries. **s. perfora′ta poste′rior** [NA], posterior perforated substance: the floor of the interpeduncular fossa, between the cerebral peduncles; it is pierced by numerous branches of the posterior cerebral arteries. **s. pro′pria cor′neae** [NA], proper substance of cornea: the fibrous, tough, and transparent main part of the cornea, between the anterior and the posterior limiting lamina; called also *stroma of cornea.* **s. pro′pria den′tis,** dentin (dentinum [NA]). **s. pro′pria scle′rae** [NA], proper substance of sclera: the chief part of the sclera, lying between the lamina fusca and the episcleral lamina, composed of dense bands of fibrous tissue, mostly parallel with the surface, and crossing each other in all directions. It is structurally continuous with the substantia propria corneae. **s. reticula′ris al′ba of Arnold,** formatio reticularis pontis. **s. reticula′ris al′ba gy′ri fornica′ti [Arnol′di],** a name given to a reticular mixture of gray and white substance on the portion of the surface of the gyrus parahippocampalis that adjoins the gyrus dentatus. **s. reticula′ris al′ba medul′lae oblonga′tae,** white reticular formation: the white substance forming part of the formatio reticularis medullae oblongatae [NA]. **s. reticula′ris gris′ea medul′lae oblonga′tae,** gray reticular formation: the gray substance forming part of the formatio reticularis medullae oblongatae [NA]. **s. reticulofilamento′sa,** reticular substance. **s. Rolan′di,** s. gelatinosa. **s. spongio′sa medul′lae spina′lis,** see *s. intermedia centralis medullae spinalis, s. intermedia lateralis medullae spinalis,* and *columnae griseae.* **s. spongio′sa os′sium** [NA], spongy substance of bone: bone substance made up of thin intersecting lamellae, usually found internal to compact bone; called also *spongy,* or *cancellated bone.* **s. vit′rea den′tis,** enamel (enamelum [NA]).

substantiae (sub-stan′she-e) plural of *substantia.*

substernal (sub-ster′nal) situated beneath the sternum.

substernomastoid (sub″ster-no-mas′toid) beneath the sternomastoid muscle.

substituent (sub-stich′u-ent) 1. a substitute; especially an atom, radical, or group substituted for another in a compound. 2. of or pertaining to such an atom, radical, or group.

substitute (sub′sti-tūt) a material which may be used in place of another. **blood s., plasma s.,** a fluid which may be used instead of whole blood or plasma for replacement of circulating fluid in the body.

substitution (sub″stĭ-tu′shun) [L. *substitutio,* from *sub* under + *statuere* to place] 1. the act of putting one thing in the place of another, especially the chemical replacement of one element or radical by some other. 2. a defense mechanism, operating unconsciously, in which an unattainable or unacceptable goal, emotion, or object is replaced by one that is attainable or acceptable. **creeping s. of bone,** the formation of new bone on the surfaces of necrotic trabeculae by osteoblasts, occurring after the revascularization of an area that has been disrupted by fracture, as at the head of the femur after fracture of the neck has disrupted the blood supply to the head of the bone.

substitutive (sub′stĭ-tu″tive) effecting a change or substitution.

substrate (sub′strāt) [L. *sub* under + *stratum* layer] a substance upon which an enzyme acts.

substratum (sub-stra′tum) [L.] 1. a substrate. 2. a lower layer or stratum.

substructure (sub′struk-chur) the underlying or supporting portion of an organ or appliance; in dentistry, that portion of an implant denture which is embedded in the tissues of the jaw.

subsulcus (sub-sul′kus) a sulcus concealed by another.

subsulfate (sub-sul′fāt) a basic sulfate. **ferric s.,** reddish brown scales or powder, $Fe_4(OH)_2(SO_4)_5$, used in solution as a styptic; called also *iron subsulfate.*

subsultus (sub-sul′tus) [L. *subsilire* to spring up] a spasmodic movement. **s. ten′dinum,** a twisting movement of the muscles and tendons such as is observed in a typhoid state.

subsylvian (sub-sil′ve-an) situated deep in the lateral sulcus (fissure of Sylvius).

subtalar (sub-ta′lar) [*sub-* + L. *talus* ankle] beneath the talus, as the subtalar joint.

subtarsal (sub-tar′sal) situated below the tarsus.

subtelocentric (sub-tel″o-sen′trik) having the centromere almost, but not quite, at the telocentric position.

subtemporal (sub-tem′por-al) beneath the temple or any temporal structure or part; see also under *decompression.*

subtenial (sub-te′ne-al) situated beneath a tenia.

subtentorial (sub-ten′to-re-al) situated beneath the tentorium of the cerebellum.

subterminal (sub-ter′mĭ-nal) situated near an end or extremity.

subtetanic (sub″te-tan′ik) mildly tetanic.

subthalamic (sub″thah-lam′ik) situated below the thalamus; pertaining to the subthalamus.

subthalamus (sub-thal′ah-mus) the ventral thalamus or subthalamic tegmental region: a transitional region of the diencephalon interposed between the (dorsal) thalamus, the hypothalamus, and the tegmentum of the mesencephalon (midbrain); it includes the subthalamic nucleus, Forel's fields, and the zona incerta.

subthyroidism (sub-thi′roid-izm) hypothyroidism.

subtile (sut′'l) [L. *subtilis*] keen and acute.

subtilin (sub′til-in) an antibiotic substance isolated from strains of the soil bacteria *Bacillus subtilis,* which is chiefly effective against gram-positive bacteria and certain acid-fast bacilli.

subtilisin (sub-til′ĭ-sin) a proteolytic enzyme isolated from strains of the soil bacteria *Bacillus subtilis,* which catalyzes the hydrolysis of certain peptide bonds; analysis has shown it to be composed of 274 amino acid residues.

subtle (sut′'l) [L. *subtilis*] 1. very fine. 2. subtile.

subtotal (sub-to′tal) nearly but not quite total.

subtrapezial (sub″trah-pe′ze-al) situated beneath the trapezius muscle.

subtribe (sub′trīb) a taxonomic category sometimes established, subordinate to a tribe and superior to a genus.

subtrochanteric (sub″tro-kan-ter′ik) situated below a trochanter.

subtrochlear (sub-trok′le-ar) situated beneath the trochlea.

subtuberal (sub-tu′ber-al) situated under a tuber.

subtympanic (sub″tim-pan′ik) 1. below the tympanum. 2. having a somewhat tympanic quality.

subtypical (sub-tip′ĭ-kal) falling short of being typical.

subumbilical (sub″um-bil′e-kal) situated beneath the umbilicus.

subungual (sub-ung′gwal) [*sub-* + L. *unguis* nail] situated beneath a nail; hyponychial.

suburethral (sub″u-re′thral) situated or occurring beneath the urethra.

subvaginal (sub-vaj′ĭ-nal) situated under a sheath, or below the vagina.

subvertebral (sub-ver′te-bral) situated on the ventral side of the vertebral column.

subvirile (sub-vir′il) characterized by deficient virility.

subvitaminosis (sub-vi″tah-min-o′sis) a condition due to vitamin deficiency.

subvitrinal (sub-vit′rĭ-nal) situated beneath the vitreous.

subvolution (sub″vo-lu′shun) [*sub-* + L. *volvere* to turn] the operation of reversing a flap; especially the operation of dissecting and turning up a pterygium, so that the outer or cutaneous surface comes in contact with the raw surface of the dissection. It is done to prevent readhesion.

subwaking (sub-wāk′ing) intermediate between waking and sleeping.

subzonal (sub-zo′nal) situated beneath a zone, as below the zona pellucida.

subzygomatic (sub″zi-go-mat′ik) situated below the zygoma.

Sucaryl (su′kah-ril) trademark for a noncaloric sweetening agent (cyclamate calcium or cyclamate sodium) for use in restricted diets.

succagogue (suk′ah-gog) [L. *succus* juice + Gr. *agōgos* leading] 1. inducing glandular secretion. 2. an agent that stimulates glandular secretion.

succedaneous (suk″sĕ-da′ne-us) ensuing; in place of; of the nature of a succedaneum.

succedaneum (suk″sĕ-da′ne-um) [L. *succedaneus* taking another's place] a medicine or material that may be substituted for another of like properties.

succenturiate (suk″sen-tu′re-āt) [L. *succenturiare* to substitute] accessory; serving as a substitute.

succinate (suk′sĭ-nāt) any salt of succinic acid; in biochemistry, the term is used interchangeably with succinic acid (see under *acid*).

succinodehydrogenase (suk″sĭ-no-de-hi′dro-jen-ās) an enzyme that splits off hydrogen from succinic acid; it occurs in most tissues.

succinoresinol (suk″sĭ-no-rez′ĭ-nol) a resinol from amber, $C_{12}H_{20}O$.

succinous (suk′sĭ-nus) pertaining to amber.

succinum (suk′sĭ-num) [L.] amber.

succinyl (suk′sĭ-nil) a radical of succinic acid.

succinylcholine chloride (suk″sĭ-nil-ko′lēn) [USP] chemical name: 2,2′-[(1,4-dioxo-1,4-butanediyl)bis(oxy)]bis-[*N,N,N*-trimethylethanaminium]dichloride. A neuromuscular blocking agent, $C_{21}H_{22}H_2O_2$, occurring as a white, crystalline powder, which produces skeletal muscle relaxation by blocking transmission at the myoneural junction; used for its muscle relaxant action during shock therapy and such procedures as endotracheal intubation and endoscopy, and as an adjunct to surgical anesthesia, administered intravenously and intramuscularly.

succinyl-CoA (suk′sĭ-nil) a high-energy intermediate formed in the tricarboxylic acid (Krebs) cycle by the oxidation of α-ketoglutaric acid; it then undergoes deacylation to form succinic acid, a step which also involves formation of guanosine triphosphate.

succinylsulfathiazole (suk″sĭ-nil-sul″fah-thi′ah-zōl) chemical name: 4-oxo-4-[[4-[(2-thiazolylamino)sulfonyl]phenyl]amino]butanoic acid. A sulfonamide, $C_{13}H_{13}N_3O_5S_2 \cdot H_2O$, occurring as a white or yellowish, crystalline powder; used as an antibacterial in patients undergoing gastrointestinal surgery and in the treatment of gastrointestinal infections due to susceptible organisms, administered orally.

succorrhea (suk″o-re′ah) [L. *succus* juice + Gr. *rhoia* flow] an excessive flow of a juice or secretion, as in ptyalism.

succuba (suk′u-bah) [L.; from *succumbere* to lie under] an imaginary female monster, or demon.

succubus (suk′u-bus) [L.; from *succumbere* to lie under] an imaginary monster, or demon, formerly regarded as a cause of nightmare.

succus (suk′us) pl. *suc′ci* [L.] any fluid derived from living tissue; used in anatomical nomenclature as a general term for a bodily secretion or a fluid derived from body tissue; called also *juice.* **s. cera′si,** cherry juice. **s. enter′icus,** intestinal juice: the liquid secreted by the glands in the wall of the small intestine. **s. gas′tricus,** gastric juice: the liquid secretion of the glands of the stomach. **s. pancreat′icus,** pancreatic juice: the liquid secretion of the pancreas, which is discharged into the duodenum. **s. prostat′icus,** the secretion of the prostate gland, which contributes to formation of the semen. **s. ru′bi idae′i,** raspberry juice.

succussion (sŭ-kush′un) [L. *succussio* a shaking from beneath, earthquake] a procedure in which the body is shaken, a splashing sound being indicative of the presence of fluid and air in a body cavity. **hippocratic s.,** succussion to elicit a splashing sound in the chest, usually pathognomonic of pneumohydrothorax.

sucholoalbumin (su″ko-lo-al-bu′min) [L. *sus* pig + Gr. *cholē* bile + *albumin*] a poisonous protein characteristic of hog cholera, and obtained from cultures of the bacillus; it is injected for the purpose of giving immunity to the disease.

suckle (suk′'l) to derive or to provide nourishment by feeding at the breast.

Sucostrin (su-kos'trin) trademark for a preparation of succinylcholine.

Sucquet-Hoyer anastomosis (canal) (sik-a'oy-ār) [*Sucquet*; Henryk *Hoyer*, Polish anatomist, 1864–1947] see under *anastomosis*.

sucralfate (soo-kral'făt) chemical name: β-D-fructofuranosyl-glucopyranoside octakis (hydrogen sulfate) aluminum complex; a gastrointestinal antiulcerative, $C_{12}H_mAl_{16}O_nS_8$.

sucrase (su'krās) β-fructofuranosidase.

sucrate (su'krāt) a compound of a substance with sucrose.

sucre (su'k'r) [Fr.] sugar. **s. actuelle'**, actual sugar. **s. virtuelle'**, virtual sugar.

sucroclastic (su″kro-klas'tik) [Fr. *sucre* sugar + Gr. *klastos* broken] splitting of sugar.

sucrose (su'krōs) [L. *sucrosum*] a disaccharide $C_{12}H_{22}O_{11}$, obtained from sugar cane, sugar beet, or other sources, crystallizing in prisms, soluble in water, and turning the plane of polarization to the right. By boiling with acids and by the action of certain enzymes it is hydrolyzed and converted into dextrose and fructose. The official preparation conforms to NF specifications. It is extensively used as a food and as a sweetening agent, and is much employed in pharmacy, forming the basis of many pharmaceutical preparations. **s. octaacetate** [NF], a white, almost odorless, hygroscopic powder, having an intensely bitter taste; used as an alcohol denaturant.

sucrosemia (su″kro-se'me-ah) [*sucrose* + Gr. *haima* blood + -*ia*] the presence of sucrose in the blood.

sucrosum (su-kro'sum) [L.] sucrose.

sucrosuria (su″kro-su're-ah) [*sucrose* + Gr. *ouron* urine + -*ia*] the presence of sucrose in the urine.

suction (suk'shun) [L. *sugere* to suck] aspiration of gas or fluid by mechanical means. **post-tussive s.**, a sucking sound heard over a lung cavity just after a cough. **Wangensteen s.**, see under *tube*.

Suctoria (suk-to're-ah) a class of protozoa of the subphylum Ciliophora, characterized by the presence of cilia only during the larval stage, the mature organism having suctorial tentacles that serve as locomotor and food-acquiring mechanisms. Most are free-living, but some are parasitic on ciliates, while others are parasitic in other protozoa and in mammals.

suctorial (suk-to're-al) fitted for performing suction.

suctorian (suk-to're-an) 1. any individual of the class Suctoria. 2. of or pertaining to the class Suctoria.

sucuuba (soo″koo-oo'bah) the *Plumeria phagedenica*, a medicinal plant of South America.

Sudafed (soo'dah-fed) trademark for preparations of pseudoephedrine hydrochloride.

sudamen (su-da'men), pl. *sudam'ina* [L., from *sudare* to sweat] a whitish vesicle caused by the retention of sweat in the sudorific ducts or the layers of the epidermis. In the plural (*sudamina*), an eruption of such vesicles, known as *miliaria crystallina*.

sudamina (su-dam'ĭ-nah) [L.] plural of *sudamen*.

sudaminal (su-dam'ĭ-nal) pertaining to or resembling sudamina.

Sudan (su-dan') a group of azo compounds used as stains for fats. **S. G**, **S. III**. **S. I**, $C_6H_5 \cdot N{:}N \cdot C_{10}H_6 \cdot OH$. **S. II**, $(CH_3)_2$-$C_6H_3 \cdot N{:}N \cdot C_{10}H_6 \cdot OH$. **S. III**, chemical name: 1-(*p*-phenylazophenylazo)-2-naphthol. A red fat-soluble azo dye, $C_6H_5 \cdot N \cdot N \cdot C_6H_4 \cdot N{:}N \cdot C_{10}H_6 \cdot OH$, an important stain for the demonstration of neutral fats. **S. IV**, scarlet red. **S. yellow G**, a brown powder, $C_{12}H_{10}N_2O_2$, used as a stain for fats.

sudanophil (su-dan'o-fil) an element that stains readily with Sudan.

sudanophilia (su-dan″o-fil'e-ah) [*sudan* + Gr. *philein* to love] affinity for Sudan stain.

sudanophilic (su-dan″o-fil'ik) staining readily with Sudan.

sudanophilous (su″dan-of'ĭ-lus) sudanophilic.

sudarium (su-da're-um) [L.] a sweat bath.

sudarshan shurna (soo-dar'shan shoor'nah) a Hindu febrifuge containing fifty drugs.

sudation (su-da'shun) [L. *sudatio*] the excretion of sweat.

sudatoria (su″dah-to're-ah) [L.] plural of *sudatorium*.

sudatorium (su-dah-to're-um), pl. *sudato'ria* [L.] 1. a hot air bath. 2. a room for the administration of hot air baths.

Sudeck's atrophy (disease), point (soo'deks) [Paul Hermann Martin *Sudeck*, Hamburg surgeon, 1866–1938] see *post-traumatic osteoporosis*, under *osteoporosis*, and see under *point*.

Sudeck-Leriche syndrome (soo'dek-lĕ-rēsh') [P. H. M. *Sudeck*; René *Leriche*, French surgeon, 1879–1955] see under *syndrome*.

sudogram (su'do-gram) [L. *sudor* sweat + Gr. *gramma* a writing] a graphic representation of the areas of the body on which sweating is present.

sudomotor (su″do-mo'tor) [L. *sudor* sweat + *motor* move] stimulating the sweat glands.

sudor (su'dor) [L.] (*obs.*) sweat, or perspiration. **s. cruen'tus**, **s. sanguin'eus**, hematidrosis.

sudoresis (su″do-re'sis) diaphoresis.

sudoriferous (su″do-rif'er-us) [L. *sudor* sweat + *ferre* to bear] 1. conveying sweat. 2. sudoriparous.

sudorific (su″do-rif'ik) [L. *sudorificus*] 1. promoting the flow of sweat; diaphoretic. 2. an agent that causes sweating.

sudoriparous (su″do-rip'ah-rus) [L. *sudor* sweat + *parere* to produce] secreting or producing sweat.

sudoxicam (soo-dok'sĭ-kam) chemical name: 4-hydroxy-2-methyl-*N*-2-thiazolyl-1,2-benzothiazine-3-carboxamide; and anti-inflammatory, $C_{13}H_{11}N_3O_4S_2$.

suet (su'et) [L. *sevum*] the fat from the abdominal cavity of a ruminant animal, especially the sheep or ox; used in the preparation of cerates and ointments and as an emollient. The preparation employed in pharmacy is the internal fat of the abdomen of the sheep. **benzoinated s.**, prepared suet 1000, benzoin 30. **prepared s.**, the internal fat of the abdomen of the sheep purified by melting and straining.

sufentanil (su-fen'tah-nil) chemical name: *N*-[4-(methoxymethyl)-1-[2-(2-thienyl)ethyl]-4-piperidinyl]-*N*-phenylpropanamide; an analgesic, $C_{22}H_{30}N_2O_2S$.

suffocant (suf'o-kant) an agent that causes suffocation.

suffocation (suf″o-ka'shun) [L. *suffocatio*] asphyxiation; the stoppage of respiration, or the asphyxia that results from it.

suffraginis (suf-fraj'ĭ-nis) [L.] the large pastern bone or first phalanx of the horse.

suffusion (sŭ-fu'zhun) [L. *suffusio*] 1. the process of overspreading, or diffusion. 2. the condition of being moistened or of being permeated through, as by blood.

sugar (shoog'ar) [L. *saccharum*; Gr. *sakcharon*] a sweet carbohydrate of various kinds, and of both animal and vegetable origin. It is an aldehyde or ketone derivative of polyhydric alcohols. The two principal groups of sugars are the disaccharides, having the formula $C_{12}H_{22}O_{11}$, and the monosaccharides, $C_6H_{12}O_6$; all are white, crystallizable solids, soluble in water and dilute alcohol. The disaccharides are sucrose or saccharose, *beet s.*, *cane s.*, *maple s.*, *palm s.*, *malt s.* (maltose), *milk s.* (lactose), and others. The monosaccharides include ordinary dextrose (δ-glucose) (*diabetic s.*, *grape s.*, *liver s.*, *potato s.*, *starch s.*), fructose (*fruit s.*), inositol (*heart s.*, *muscle s.*). Besides these, a very considerable number of artificial and other sugars are known to chemistry. **actual s.**, (sucre actuelle of Lépine), the free glucose in the blood. **anhydrous s.**, anhydrosugar. **barley s.**, a clear hard form of sugar formed by heating ordinary granulated sugar (sucrose) to 160° F. **beechwood s.**, xylose. **beet s.**, sucrose derived from the root of the beet. **blood s.**, glucose, the form in which carbohydrate is carried in the blood, usually in a concentration of 70–100 mg. per 100 ml. **brain s.**, cerebrose. **burnt s.**, caramel. **cane s.**, sucrose obtained from sugar cane. **collagen s.**, aminoacetic acid. **compressible s.** [NF], a preparation which contains 95–98 per cent sucrose and which may contain starch, dextrin, and invert sugar; used as a sweetening agent and tablet excipient in pharmaceutical preparations. **confectioner's s.** [NF], sucrose ground together with corn starch to a fine powder, containing 95–97 per cent sucrose; used as a sweetening agent and tablet excipient in pharmaceutical preparations. **diabetic s.**, the dextrose found in the urine in diabetes mellitus. **fruit s.**, fructose. **gelatin s.**, aminoacetic acid. **grape s.**, dextrose. **heart s.**, inositol. **invert s.**, the mixture of dextrose and fructose obtained by hydrolysing sucrose; used in solution as a parenteral nutrient. Called also *invertose*. **larch s.**, melezitose. **s. of lead**, lead acetate. **Leo's s.**, laiose. **liver s.**, dextrose from the liver. **malt s.**, maltose. **maple s.**, sucrose from maple sap. **milk s.**, lactose. **muscle s.**, inositol. **oil s.**, eleosaccharum. **palm s.**, sucrose from palm sap. **potato s.**, dextrose from potatoes. **reducing s.**, a sugar which will reduce an alkaline copper tartrate solution. **simple s.**, a monosaccharide. **starch s.**, dextrin. **sulfur s.**, thioglucose. **threshold s.**, the lower limit of hyperglycemia at which dextrose appears in the urine. **virtual s.** (sucre virtuelle of Lépine), sugar in the blood in a colloidal state. **wood s.**, xylose.

sugarin (shoog'ar-in) chemical name: methylbenzoylsulfimide. A crystalline substance said to be 500 times as sweet as sugar.

suggestibility (sug-jes″tĭ-bil'ĭ-te) a condition of abnormal susceptibility to suggestion.

suggestible (sug-jes'tĭ-b'l) abnormally susceptible to suggestion.

suggestion (sug-jes'chun) [L. *suggestio*] 1. the impartation of an idea to a subject from without. 2. an idea introduced from without. **hypnotic s.**, a suggestion imparted to a person in the hypnotic state, by which he is led to believe certain things contrary to fact or is induced to perform certain actions. **post-hypnotic s.**, implantation in the mind of a subject during hypnosis of a suggestion to be acted upon after recovery from the hypnotic state.

suggillation (sug″jĭ-la'shun) [L. *suggillatio*] 1. a bruise or ecchymosis. 2. a mark of postmortem lividity.

suicide (soo'ĭ-sīd) [L. *sui* of himself + *caedere* to kill] the taking of one's own life. **psychic s.**, the termination of one's own life without employment of physical agents.

suint (swint) a fat-like substance derivable from sheep's wool, from which anhydrous lanolin is prepared. Called also *suint de laine.*

suit (sūt) an outer garment covering the entire body. **anti-blackout s., anti-g s., g s.**, a garment worn by pilots, designed to increase their ability to withstand without ill effects the accleratory forces experienced in certain aerial maneuvers.

sukkla pakla (sook′lah pak′lah) [Hind. "dry suppuration"] ainhum.

Sulamyd (sul′am-id) trademark for a preparation of sulfacetamide.

sulazepam (sul-ah′zĕ-pam) chemical name: 7-chloro-1,3-dihydro-1-methyl-5-phenyl-2*H*-1,4-benzodiazepine-2-thione; a minor tranquilizer, $C_{16}H_{13}ClN_2S$.

sulbenox (sul′ben-oks) chemical name: (4,5,6,7-tetrahydro-7-oxobenzo[*b*]thien-4-yl)urea; a veterinary growth stimulant, $C_9H_{10}N_2O_2S$.

sulcate (sul′kāt) [L. *sulcatus*] furrowed or marked with sulci.

sulcation (sul-ka′shun) the formation of sulci; the state of being marked by sulci.

sulci (sul′si) [L.] plural of *sulcus.*

sulciform (sul′sĭ-form) formed like a groove.

sulconazole nitrate (sul-kon′ah-zōl) chemical name: (+)-1-[2-[[(4-chlorophenyl)methyl]thio]-2-(2,4-dichlorophenyl)ethyl]-1*H*-imidazole mononitrate; an antifungal, $C_{18}H_{15}CL_3N_2S \cdot HNO_3$.

sulculi (sul′ku-li) plural of *sulculus.*

sulculus (sul′ku-lus), pl. *sul′culi* [L.] a small or minute sulcus.

sulcus (sul′kus), pl. *sul′ci* [L.] 1. a groove, trench, or furrow; [NA] a general term for such a depression, especially one of those on the surface of the brain, separating the gyri. Cf. *fissure.* 2. a linear depression or valley in the occlusal surface of a tooth, the sloping sides of which meet at an angle. **alveolabial s.,** the furrow between the dental arch and the lips. **alveolingual s.,** the depression between the dental arch and the tongue. **s. ampulla′ris** [NA], **ampullary s.**, a transverse groove on the membranous ampulla of each semicircular duct, for the ampullary branch of the pars vestibularis nervi octavi. **angular s.,** incisura angularis ventriculi. **s. anthel′icis transver′sus** [NA], transverse sulcus of anthelix: the depression on the medial surface of the pinna corresponding to the lower crus of the anthelix. **aortic s., s. aor′ticus,** a longitudinal groove on the median surface of the left lung corresponding to the thoracic aorta. **s. arte′riae occipita′lis** [NA], sulcus of occipital artery: the groove just medial to the mastoid notch on the temporal bone, lodging the occipital artery. **s. arte′riae subcla′viae** [NA], sulcus of subclavian artery: a transverse groove on the cranial surface of the first rib, just posterior to the anterior scalene tubercle; it lodges the subclavian artery; called also *s. subclavius.* **s. arte′riae tempora′lis me′diae** [NA], sulcus of middle temporal artery: a nearly vertical groove running just superior to the external acoustic meatus on the external surface of the squamous part of the temporal bone; it lodges the middle temporal artery. **s. arte′riae vertebra′lis atlan′tis** [NA], sulcus of vertebral artery of atlas: the groove on the cranial surface of the posterior arch of the atlas; it lodges the vertebral artery and the first spinal nerve. **arterial sulci, sul′ci arterio′si** [NA], grooves on the internal surfaces of the cranial bones for the meningeal arteries; called also *arterial grooves.* **atrioventricular s.,** s. coronarius cordis. **s. of auditory tube,** s. tubae auditivae. **s. of auricle, posterior, s. auric′ulae poste′rior** [NA], the slight depression on the pinna that separates the anthelix from the antitragus. **s. of auricular branch of vagus nerve,** s. canaliculi mastoidei. **basilar s. of occipital bone,** s. sinus petrosi inferioris ossis occipitalis. **basilar s. of pons, s. basila′ris pon′tis** [NA], the anteromedian groove in the pons, lodging the basilar artery. **bicipital s., lateral,** s. bicipitalis lateralis. **bicipital s., medial,** s. bicipitalis medialis. **s. bicipita′lis latera′lis** [NA], lateral bicipital sulcus: a longitudinal groove on the lateral side of the arm which marks the limit between the lateral border of the biceps muscle and the brachialis; called also *lateral bicipital groove.* **s. bicipita′lis media′lis** [NA], medial bicipital sulcus: a longitudinal groove on the medial side of the arm which marks the limit between the medial border of the biceps muscle and the brachialis; called also *medial bicipital groove.* **calcaneal s., s. calca′nei** [NA], a rough, deep groove on the upper surface of the calcaneus, between the medial and the posterior articular surfaces and giving attachment to the interosseous talocalcaneal ligament. **calcarine s., s. calcari′nus** [NA], a sulcus on the medial surface of the occipital lobe, separating the cuneus from the lingual gyrus; called also *fissura calcarina.* **callosal s.,** s. corporis callosi. **callosomarginal s.,** s. cinguli. **s. callo′sus,** s. corporis callosi. **s. canalic′uli mastoi′dei,** a small groove in the petrous portion of the temporal bone leading to the mastoid canaliculus. **s. cana′lis innomina′tus,** s. nervi petrosi minoris. **s. carot′icus os′sis sphenoida′lis** [NA], **carotid s.,** the groove on the side of the body of the sphenoid bone that lodges the internal carotid artery and the cavernous sinus. **carpal s., s.**

car′pi [NA], a broad deep groove on the volar surface of the carpal bones, which transmits the flexor tendons and the median nerve into the palm of the hand. **central s. of cerebrum,** s. centralis cerebri. **s. centra′lis cer′ebri** [NA], **s. centra′lis cere′bri [Rolan′di],** central sulcus of cerebrum: a relatively deep, nearly vertical sulcus on the cerebral hemisphere, which separates the frontal from the parietal lobe. **s. centra′lis in′sulae** [NA], a deep, oblique furrow which divides the insula into a larger anterior and a smaller posterior part. **sul′ci cerebel′li, sulci of cerebellum,** fissurae cerebelli. **cerebral s., lateral,** s. lateralis cerebri. **sul′ci cer′ebri** [NA], **sulci of cerebrum,** the furrows between the gyri of the cerebrum. **s. of chiasm, s. chias′matis** [NA], a furrow on the superior surface of the sphenoid bone located just anterior to the tuberculum sellae, and lodging the optic chiasm; called also *optic groove* or *sulcus.* **cingulate s., s. cin′guli** [NA], **s. of cingulum,** a long, irregularly shaped sulcus on the medial surface of a hemisphere, which separates the cingulate gyrus below from the medial frontal gyrus and the paracentral lobule above. It may be divided into frontal and marginal portions. **circular s. of insula, s. circula′ris in′sulae** [NA], **s. circula′ris [Rei′li],** a groove that separates the floor of the insula from the opercula. **collateral s., s. collatera′lis** [NA], a longitudinal sulcus on the inferior surface of the cerebral hemisphere between the fusiform gyrus and the parahippocampal gyrus; called also *fissura collateralis.* **s. col′li mandib′ulae,** the shallow groove between the ridge of the mandibular neck and the line of attachment of the sphenomandibular ligament. **s. corona′rius cor′dis** [NA], **coronary s. of heart,** a groove on the external surface of the heart, separating the atria from the ventricles; portions of it are occupied by the major arteries and veins of the heart; called also *atrioventricular groove.* **s. cor′poris callo′si** [NA], **s. of corpus callosum,** a sulcus encircling the convex aspect of the corpus callosum at the bottom of the longitudinal cerebral fissure. **s. cos′tae** [NA], **costal s.,** a sulcus that follows the inferior and internal surface of a rib anteriorly from the tubercle, gradually becoming less distinct; it lodges the intercostal vessels and nerves. **costal s., inferior,** s. costae. **s. cru′ris hel′icis** [NA], **s. of crus of helix,** a transverse sulcus on the medial surface of the pinna, corresponding to the crus helicis on the lateral surface. **cuboid, s.,** s. tendinum musculorum peroneorum calcanei. **sul′ci cu′tis** [NA], sulci of skin: the fine depressions on the surface of the skin between the ridges of the skin. **ethmoidal s. of Gegenbaur,** foramen ethmoidale anterius. **ethmoidal s. of nasal bone, s. ethmoida′lis os′sis nasa′lis** [NA], a groove that extends the entire length of the posteromedial surface of the nasal bone and lodges the external nasal branch of the anterior ethmoid nerve. **s. of eustachian tube,** s. tubae auditivae. **frontal s.,** 1. see *s. frontalis inferior* and *s. frontalis superior.* 2. sulcus sinus sagittalis superioris ossis frontalis. **frontal s., inferior,** s. frontalis inferior. **frontal s., superior,** s. frontalis superior. **s. fronta′lis infe′rior** [NA], inferior frontal sulcus: a short longitudinal sulcus that separates the inferior and middle frontal gyri. **s. fronta′lis supe′rior** [NA], superior frontal sulcus: a longitudinal sulcus that separates the middle and superior frontal gyri. **gingival s.,** a furrow surrounding a tooth, bounded internally by the surface of the tooth and externally by the epithelium lining the free gingiva. **gluteal s., s. glute′us** [NA], a curved transverse groove or fold on the back of the upper thigh, separating the upper part of the thigh from the nates. **greater palatine s. of maxilla,** s. palatinus major maxillae. **greater palatine s. of palatine bone,** s. palatinus major ossis palatini. **s. of greater petrosal nerve,** s. nervi petrosi majoris. **s. ham′uli pterygoi′dei** [NA], sulcus of pterygoid hamulus: a smooth groove on the lateral surface of the medial pterygoid plate of the sphenoid bone, in the angle at the base of the pterygoid hamulus; it lodges the tendon of the tensor veli palatini muscle. **Harrison′s s.,** see under *groove.* **hippocampal s., s. hippocam′pi** [NA], the sulcus that extends from the splenium of the corpus callosum almost to the tip of the temporal lobe, and forms the medial boundary of the parahippocampal gyrus; called also *fissura hippocampi* or *hippocampal fissure.* **s. horizonta′lis cerebel′li,** fissura horizontalis cerebelli. **hypothalamic s., s. hypothalam′icus** [NA], **s. hypothalam′icus [Monro′i],** a shallow curved sulcus on the wall of the third ventricle, extending from the interventricular foramen to the cerebral aqueduct. **s. of inferior petrosal sinus of occipital bone,** s. sinus petrosi inferioris ossis occipitalis. **s. of inferior petrosal sinus of temporal bone,** s. sinus petrosi inferioris ossis temporalis. **infraorbital s. of maxilla, s. infraorbita′lis maxil′lae** [NA], a groove in the orbital surface of the maxilla, commencing near the middle of the posterior edge of the surface and running anteriorly for a short distance to become continuous with the infraorbital canal. **infrapalpebral s., s. infrapalpebra′lis** [NA], the furrow below the lower eyelid. **s. of innominate canal,** s. nervi petrosi minoris. **interarticular s. of calcaneus,** s. calcanei. **interarticular s. of talus,** s. tali. **intermediate s. of spinal cord, anterior,** s. intermedius anterior medullae spinalis. **intermediate s. of spinal cord, posterior,** s. intermedius posterior medullae spinalis. **s. interme′dius gastri′cus,** a slight groove in the stomach about 2.5 cm. from the duodenopyloric junction. **s. interme′dius ante′rior medul′lae spina′lis**, anterior intermediate sulcus of spinal cord: an occasional furrow between the anterior median fissure and the anterior lateral sulcus of the spinal cord. **s. interme′dius poste′rior medul′lae spina′lis** [NA], posterior intermediate sulcus of spinal cord: a groove in the cervical and upper thoracic part of part of the spinal cord between the fasciculus gracilis and the fasciculus cuneatus. **interparietal s., s. interparieta′lis**, s. intraparietalis. **intertubercular s. of humerus, s. intertubercula′ris hu′meri** [NA], a longitudinal groove on the anterior surface of the humerus, lying between the tubercula above and between the cristae tuberculi farther down, and lodging the tendon of the long head of the biceps muscle. **interventricular s., anterior,** s. interventricularis anterior. **interventricular s., posterior,** s. interventricularis posterior. **interventricular s. of heart,** s. coronarius cordis. **s. interventricula′ris ante′rior** [NA], anterior interventricular sulcus: a groove on the sternocostal surface of the heart marking the position of the interventricular septum and the line of separation between the ventricles; called also *s. longitudinalis anterior cordis*. **s. interventricula′ris poste′rior** [NA], posterior interventricular sulcus: a groove on the diaphragmatic surface of the heart marking the position of the interventricular septum and the line of separation between the ventricles; called also *s. longitudinalis posterior cordis*. **intraparietal s., s. intraparieta′lis** [NA], an irregular sulcus on the convex surface of the parietal lobe of the cerebrum and between the inferior and superior parietal lobuli; called also *s. interparietalis* and *Pansch's fissure*. **Jacobson's s.,** 1. sulcus promontorii cavi tympani. 2. sulcus tympanicus ossis temporalis. **labiodental s.,** the arched groove in the embryo which separates off the anterior part of the mandibular process, thus helping to form the lower lip. **lacrimal s. of lacrimal bone,** s. lacrimalis ossis lacrimalis. **lacrimal s. of maxilla,** s. lacrimalis maxillae. **s. lacrima′lis maxil′lae** [NA], lacrimal sulcus of maxilla: a groove directed inferiorly and somewhat posteriorly on the nasal surface of the body of the maxilla, just anterior to the large opening into the maxillary sinus; it is converted into the nasolacrimal canal by the lacrimal bone and inferior nasal concha. **s. lacrima′lis os′sis lacrima′lis** [NA], lacrimal sulcus of lacrimal bone: a deep vertical groove on the anterior part of the lateral surface of the lacrimal bone, which with the maxilla forms the fossa for the lacrimal sac. **lateral s. for lateral sinus of occipital bone,** s. sinus transversi. **lateral s. for lateral sinus of parietal bone,** s. sinus sigmoidei ossis parietalis. **lateral s. of medulla oblongata, anterior,** s. lateralis anterior medullae oblongatae. **lateral s. of medulla oblongata, posterior,** s. lateralis posterior medullae oblongatae. **lateral s. for sigmoidal part of lateral sinus,** s. sinus sigmoidei ossis temporalis. **lateral s. of spinal cord, posterior,** s. lateralis posterior medullae spinalis. **s. latera′lis ante′rior medul′lae oblonga′tae** [NA], anterior lateral sulcus of medulla oblongata: a longitudinal sulcus on the surface of the medulla oblongata, lateral to the pyramid, from which emerge the fibers of the hypoglossal nerve. **s. latera′lis ante′rior medul′lae spina′lis**, the longitudinal groove on the anterolateral surface of the spinal cord from which the ventral nerve roots emerge; it separates the anterior and lateral funiculi. **s. latera′lis cer′ebri** [NA], lateral cerebral sulcus: a deep cleft beginning at the anterior perforated substance, extending laterally between the temporal and frontal lobes, and turning posteriorly between the temporal and parietal lobes. It divides into posterior, ascending, and anterior branches. Called also *fissura cerebri lateralis [Sylvii]*, *fissure* or *fossa of Sylvius*, and *sylvian fissure* or *fossa*. **s. latera′lis mesenceph′ali**, a longitudinal groove on the side of the mesencephalon, separating the crus cerebri from the tegmentum. **s. latera′lis pedun′culi cer′ebri**, s. lateralis mesencephali. **s. latera′lis poste′rior medul′lae oblonga′tae** [NA], posterior lateral sulcus of medulla oblongata: an upward extension of the posterolateral sulcus of the spinal cord; it gives attachment to the fibers of the glossopharyngeal, vagus, and accessory nerves. **s. latera′lis poste′rior medul′lae spina′lis** [NA], posterior lateral sulcus of spinal cord: a longitudinal sulcus on the posterolateral surface of the spinal cord; it gives entrance to the dorsal nerve roots and separates the lateral and posterior funiculi. **s. of lesser petrosal nerve,** s. nervi petrosi minoris. **s. lim′itans** [NA], a groove midway on the inner surface of each lateral wall of the neural tube, which separates it into a dorsal, alar plate and a ventral, basal plate; called also *s. limitans ventriculorum cerebri*. **s. lim′itans fos′sae rhomboi′deae** [NA], a longitudinal groove on the lateral side of the medial eminence, extending the entire length of the floor of the fourth ventricle. **s. lim′itans in′sulae,** s. circularis insulae. **s. lim′itans ventriculo′rum cer′ebri,** s. limitans. **longitudinal s. of frontal bone,** s. sinus sagittalis superioris ossis frontalis. **longitudinal s. of heart, anterior,** s. interventricularis anterior. **longitudinal s. of heart, posterior,** s. interventricularis posterior. **longitudinal s. of occipital bone,** s. sinus sagittalis superioris ossis occipitalis. **longitudinal s. of parietal bone,** s. sagittalis ossis parietalis. **s. lon-**

gitudina′lis ante′rior cor′dis, s. interventricularis anterior. **s. longitudina′lis os′sis occip′itis,** s. sinus sagittalis superioris ossis occipitalis. **s. longitudina′lis poste′rior cor′dis,** s. interventricularis posterior. **lunate s., s. luna′tus** [NA], a small semilunar furrow sometimes seen on the lateral surface of the occipital lobe of the cerebrum; this sulcus is conspicuous in the brain of certain apes and was called by Reidinger *Affenspalte* [Ger. "ape fissure"]. **malleolar s., s. malleola′ris tib′iae** [NA], a short longitudinal groove on the posterior surface of the medial malleolus of the tibia, which lodges the tendons of the posterior tibial muscle and the long flexor muscle of the toes. **mandibular s.,** s. colli mandibulae. **s. of mastoid canaliculus,** s. canaliculi mastoidei. **s. ma′tricis un′guis** [NA], s. of matrix of nail, the cutaneous fold in which the proximal part of the nail is embedded; called also *proximal nail fold*. **medial s. of crus cerebri, s. media′lis cru′ris cer′ebri** [NA], a longitudinal furrow on the medial surface of a cerebral peduncle, marking the separation of the crus cerebri from the tegmentum and lodging the root of the oculomotor nerve. Called also *s. nervi oculomotorii*. **s. media′lis mesenceph′ali,** s. medialis cruris cerebri. **median s. of fourth ventricle,** s. medianus ventriculi quarti. **median s. of medulla oblongata, posterior,** s. medianus posterior medullae oblongatae. **median s. of spinal cord, posterior,** s. medianus posterior medullae spinalis. **median s. of tongue, s. media′nus lin′guae** [NA], a shallow groove on the dorsal surface of the tongue in the midline. **s. media′nus poste′rior medul′lae oblonga′tae** [NA], posterior median sulcus of medulla oblongata: a narrow groove, existing only in the closed part of the medulla oblongata, which is the continuation of the posterior median sulcus of the spinal cord; it separates the two fasciculi gracili. Called also *fissura mediana posterior medullae oblongatae*. **s. media′nus poste′rior medul′lae spina′lis** [NA], posterior median sulcus of spinal cord: a shallow vertical groove on the posterior surface of the spinal cord in the median plane; it separates the two posterior funiculi. **s. media′nus ventric′uli quar′ti** [NA], median sulcus of fourth ventricle: a median groove in the floor of the fourth ventricle. **meningeal sulci,** sulci arteriosi. **mentolabial s., s. mentolabia′lis** [NA], the depression between the lower lip and the chin. **s. mesenceph′ali media′lis,** s. medialis cruris cerebri. **s. of middle temporal artery,** s. arteriae temporalis mediae. **s. of Monro,** s. hypothalamicus. **muscular s. of tympanic cavity,** semicanalis musculi tensoris tympani. **s. mus′culi flexo′ris hal′lucis lon′gi calca′nei,** s. tendinis musculi flexoris hallucis longi calcanei. **s. mus′culi flexo′ris hal′lucis lon′gi ta′li,** s. tendinis musculi flexoris hallucis longi tali. **s. mus′culi peronae′i calca′nei,** s. tendinum musculorum peroneorum calcanei. **s. mus′culi peronae′i os′sis cuboi′dei,** s. tendinis musculi peronei longi. **mylohyoid s. of mandible, s. mylohyoi′deus mandib′ulae** [NA], a groove on the medial surface of the ramus of the mandible, passing downward and forward from the foramen mandibulae and lodging the mylohyoid artery and nerve. **nasal s., posterior,** meatus nasopharyngeus. **s. of nasal process of maxilla,** s. lacrimalis maxillae. **nasolabial s., s. nasolabia′lis** [NA], the depression between the nose and the upper lip. **s. ner′vi oculomoto′rii,** s. medialis cruris cerebri. **s. ner′vi petro′si majo′ris** [NA], sulcus of greater petrosal nerve: a small groove in the floor of the middle cranial fossa, running anteromedially from the hiatus of the facial canal to the foramen lacerum, and lodging the greater petrosal nerve; called also *s. nervi petrosi superficialis majoris*. **s. ner′vi petro′si mino′ris** [NA], sulcus of lesser petrosal nerve: a small groove in the floor of the middle cranial fossa, running anteromedially just lateral to the sulcus of the greater petrosal nerve, and lodging the lesser petrosal nerve. Called also *s. nervi petrosi superficialis minoris*. **s. ner′vi petro′si superficia′lis majo′ris,** s. nervi petrosi majoris. **s. ner′vi petro′si superficia′lis mino′ris,** s. nervi petrosi minoris. **s. ner′vi radia′lis** [NA], sulcus of radial nerve: a broad oblique groove on the posterior surface of the humerus for the radial nerve and the deep brachial artery; called also *radial groove*. **s. ner′vi spina′lis** [NA], sulcus of spinal nerve: the groove on the upper surface of each transverse process of a cervical vertebra, extending from the foramen transversarium lateralward and separating the anterior and posterior tubercles. It lodges the ventral branch of a cervical nerve. **s. ner′vi ulna′ris** [NA], sulcus of ulnar nerve: a shallow vertical groove on the posterior surface of the medial epicondyle of the humerus for the ulnar nerve; called also *groove of ulnar nerve* or *ulnar groove*. **nymphocaruncular s., nymphohymeneal s.,** a groove between either labium minus and the carunculae hymenales. **obturator s. of pubis, s. obturato′rius os′sis pu′bis** [NA], a groove that obliquely crosses the inferior surface of the superior ramus of the pubis, giving passage to the obturator vessels and nerve. **occipital sulci, lateral,** sulci occipitales laterales. **occipital sulci, superior,** sulci occipitales superiores. **occipital s., transverse,** sulcus occipitalis transversus. **s. of occipital artery,** s. arteriae occipitalis. **s. occipita′lis ante′rior,** anterior occipital sulcus: a variable, vertically disposed furrow on the convex surface of the cerebrum, which by some is taken as the line of division between the parietal and the occipital lobes. **sul′ci occipita′les latera′les,** lateral occipital sulci: horizontal furrows that divide the lateral occipital gyri into upper and lower portions. **sul′ci occipita′les superio′res,** superior occipital sulci: irregular sulci associated with the superior occipital gyri. **s. occipita′lis transver′sus** [NA], transverse occipital sulcus: a vertical sulcus back of the gyrus angularis, which may help to form the anterior boundary of the occipital lobe or may lie within it. **s. occip′itis,** s. sinus sagittalis superioris ossis occipitalis. **occipitotemporal s., s. occipitotempora′lis** [NA], a longitudinal sulcus on the inferior surface of the temporal lobe that separates the inferior temporal gyrus from the lateral occipitotemporal gyrus; called also *s. temporalis inferior.* **s. oculomoto′rius,** s. medialis cruris cerebri. **s. olfacto′rius lo′bi fronta′lis** [NA], olfactory sulcus of frontal lobe: a straight parasagittal sulcus on the inferior surface of the frontal lobe, lodging the olfactory bulb and tract, and separating the gyrus rectus from the gyri orbitales. **s. olfacto′rius na′si** [NA], olfactory sulcus of nose: a shallow sulcus on the wall of the nasal cavity, passing upward from the level of the anterior end of the middle concha just above the agger nasi to the lamina cribrosa. **olfactory s. of frontal lobe,** s. olfactorius lobi frontalis. **olfactory s. of nose,** s. olfactorius nasi. **optic s.,** s. chiasmatis. **orbital sulci of frontal lobe, sul′ci orbita′les lo′bi fronta′lis** [NA], irregular sulci between the orbital gyri of the frontal lobe. **palatine sulci of maxilla, sul′ci palati′ni maxil′lae** [NA], the laterally placed furrows, between the palatine spines on the inferior surface of the hard palate, that lodge the palatine vessels and nerves. **palatinovaginal s., s. palatinovagina′lis** [NA], the groove on the vaginal process of the pterygoid process of the sphenoid bone that participates in formation of the palatinovaginal canal. **s. palati′nus ma′jor maxil′lae** [NA], greater palatine sulcus of maxilla: the sulcus on the nasal surface of the maxilla which, along with the corresponding one on the perpendicular plate of the palatine bone, forms the canal for the greater palatine nerve. **s. palati′nus ma′jor os′sis palati′ni** [NA], greater palatine sulcus of palatine bone: a vertical groove on the maxillary surface of the perpendicular plate of the palatine bone; it articulates with the maxilla to form the canal for the greater palatine nerve; called also *s. pterygopalatinus ossis palatini.* **paracolic sulci, sul′ci paracol′ici** [NA], small shallow and variable peritoneal pockets situated lateral to the descending colon; called also *recessus paracolici.* **paraglenoid sulci of hip bone, sul′ci paraglenoida′les os′sis cox′ae,** slight grooves, anterior and inferior to the auricular surface of the ilium, that serve for attachment of the ventral and interosseous sacroiliac ligaments. **parietooccipital s.,** 1. sulcus parietooccipitalis. 2. sulcus intraparietalis. **s. parietooccipita′lis** [NA], parietooccipital sulcus: a sulcus in the medial surface of each cerebral hemisphere, running upward from the calcarine sulcus and marking the boundary between the cuneus and precuneus, and also between the parietal and occipital lobes. Called also *fissura parietooccipitalis.* **s. parolfacto′rius ante′rior,** a sulcus on the medial surface of the cerebral hemisphere, between the area parolfactoria behind and the inferior frontal gyrus in front. **s. parolfacto′rius poste′rior,** a curved sulcus on the medial surface of the cerebral hemisphere, below the splenium of the corpus callosum and between the gyrus paraterminalis and the area parolfactoria. **petrobasilar s.,** s. sinus petrosi inferioris ossis temporalis. **petrosal s. of occipital bone, inferior,** s. sinus petrosi inferioris ossis occipitalis. **petrosal s. of temporal bone, inferior,** s. sinus petrosi inferioris ossis temporalis. **petrosal s. of temporal bone, posterior,** s. sinus petrosi inferioris ossis temporalis. **petrosal s. of temporal bone, superior,** s. sinus petrosi superioris. **s. petro′sus infe′rior os′sis occipita′lis,** s. sinus petrosi inferioris ossis occipitalis. **s. petro′sus infe′rior os′sis tempora′lis,** s. sinus petrosi inferioris ossis temporalis. **s. petro′sus supe′rior os′sis tempora′lis,** s. sinus petrosi superioris. **polar s.,** any of the small fissures which surround the posterior end of the calcarine sulcus. **pontobulbar s.,** the sulcus that separates the pons from the medulla oblongata. **pontopeduncular s.,** the sulcus that separates the pons from the mesencephalon (as represented by the cerebral peduncles). **postcentral s., s. postcentra′lis** [NA], a sulcus on the superolateral surface of the cerebrum, separating the postcentral gyrus from the remainder of the parietal lobe. **postclival s.,** a fissure of the cerebellum between the declive and the folium vermis. **postnodular s.,** a sulcus on the underside of the cerebellum between the nodule and the uvula. **postpyramidal s.,** a sulcus on the underside of the cerebellum between the pyramid and the tuber vermis. **s. praecentra′lis,** s. precentralis. **precentral s., s. precentra′lis** [NA], a vertical sulcus on the convex surface of a cerebral hemisphere, separating the precentral gyrus from the remainder of the frontal lobe. **preclival s.,** a fissure of the cerebellum between the culmen and the declive. **prepyramidal s.,** a sulcus on the inferior surface of the cerebellum between the uvula and the pyramid. **prerolandic s.,** s. precentralis. **s. promonto′rii ca′vi tym′pani** [NA], a groove in the surface of the promontory of the tympanic cavity, lodging the tympanic nerve. **s. of pterygoid hamulus,** s.

hamuli pterygoidei. **pterygoid s. of pterygoid process,** s. pterygopalatinus processus pterygoidei. **pterygopalatine s. of palatine bone,** s. palatinus major ossis palatini. **pterygopalatine s. of pterygoid process,** s. pterygopalatinus processus pterygoidei. **s. pterygopalati′nus os′sis palati′ni,** s. palatinus major ossis palatini. **s. pterygopalati′nus proces′sus pterygoi′dei** [NA], pterygopalatine sulcus of pterygoid process: a small groove on the inferior surface of the vaginal process of the medial pterygoid plate of the sphenoid bone, forming part of the wall of the vomerovaginal canal. **s. pulmona′lis thora′cis** [NA], **pulmonary s. of thorax,** a large vertical groove in the posterior part of the chest cavity, one on either side of the bodies of the vertebrae posterior to the level of their ventral surface, lodging the posterior, bulky portion of the lung. **radial s. of humerus, s. of radial nerve,** s. nervi radialis. **Reil's s.,** s. circularis insulae. **retrocentral s.,** s. postcentralis. **rhinal s., s. rhina′lis** [NA], a fissure on the inferior surface of the hemisphere, separating the anterior part of the parahippocampal gyrus from the rest of the temporal lobe. **sagittal s. of frontal bone,** s. sinus sagittalis superioris ossis frontalis. **sagittal s. of occipital bone,** s. sinus sagittalis superioris ossis occipitalis. **sagittal s. of parietal bone,** s. sagittalis ossis parietalis. **s. sagitta′lis os′sis fronta′lis,** s. sinus sagittalis superioris ossis frontalis. **s. sagitta′lis os′sis occipita′lis,** s. sinus sagittalis superioris ossis occipitalis. **s. sagitta′lis os′sis parieta′lis** [NA], sagittal sulcus of parietal bone: a shallow sulcus along the sagittal margin on the internal surface of the parietal bone; with its fellow of the opposite side it forms a groove for the middle portion of the superior sagittal sinus. **s. scle′rae** [NA], **scleral s., sclercorneal s.,** the groove at the junction of the sclera and cornea. **s. of semicanal of humerus,** s. intertubercularis humeri. **s. of semicanal of vidian nerve,** s. nervi petrosi majoris. **semilunar s. of radius,** incisura ulnaris radii. **sigmoid s., s. of sigmoid sinus,** s. sinus sigmoidei. **s. of sigmoid sinus of occipital bone,** s. sinus sigmoidei ossis occipitalis. **s. of sigmoid sinus of parietal bone,** s. sinus sigmoidei ossis parietalis. **s. of sigmoid sinus of temporal bone,** s. sinus sigmoidei ossis temporalis. **s. sigmoi′deus os′sis tempora′lis,** s. sinus sigmoidei ossis temporalis. **s. si′nus petro′si inferio′ris os′sis occipita′lis** [NA], sulcus of inferior petrosal sinus of occipital bone: the groove in the floor of the posterior cranial fossa at the line of junction between the basilar part of the occipital and the petrous portion of the temporal bone; it lodges the inferior petrosal sinus. Called also *s. petrosus inferior ossis occipitalis.* **s. si′nus petro′si inferio′ris os′sis tempora′lis** [NA], sulcus of inferior petrosal sinus of temporal bone: a groove on the posteromedial edge of the internal surface of the petrous portion of the temporal bone, which, with a corresponding groove on the adjacent basilar part of the occipital bone, lodges the inferior petrosal sinus. Called also *s. petrosus inferior ossis temporalis.* **s. si′nus petro′si superio′ris** [NA], sulcus of superior petrosal sinus: a small posterolaterally directed sulcus that runs along the internal surface of the petrous part of the temporal bone on the angle separating the posterior and middle cranial fossae; it lodges the superior petrosal sinus. Called also *s. petrosus superior ossis temporalis.* **s. si′nus sagitta′lis superio′ris os′sis fronta′lis** [NA], sulcus of superior sagittal sinus of frontal bone: a median groove on the cerebral surface of the squama of the frontal bone; in the upper part only, it is continuous with the sagittal sulcus of the parietal bone and lodges the anterior portion of the superior sagittal sinus. Called also *s. sagittalis ossis frontalis.* **s. si′nus sagitta′lis superio′ris os′sis occipita′lis** [NA], sulcus of superior sagittal sinus of occipital bone: a broad sulcus on the internal surface of the squama of the occipital bone, generally to the right of the superior division of the cruciform eminence; it lodges the posterior part of the superior sagittal sinus. Called also *s. sagittalis ossis occipitalis.* **s. si′nus sigmoi′dei** [NA], sulcus of sigmoid sinus: an S-shaped sulcus beginning on the internal surface of the posteroinferior edge of the parietal bone and continuous with the lateral end of the sulcus of the transverse sinus; it passes onto the internal surface of the mastoid part of the temporal bone, where it bends inferiorly and medially to continue onto the lateral portion of the occipital bone, ending at the jugular foramen. It lodges the sigmoid sinus. **s. si′nus sigmoi′dei os′sis occipita′lis** [NA], sulcus of sigmoid sinus of occipital bone: the portion of the sulcus of the sigmoid sinus found on the occipital bone. **s. si′nus sigmoi′dei os′sis parieta′lis** [NA], sulcus of sigmoid sinus of parietal bone: a short groove on the internal surface of the posteroinferior angle of the parietal bone, continuous with both the sulcus for the sigmoid sinus on the temporal bone and the sulcus for the transverse sinus on the occipital bone; it lodges the superior part of the sigmoid sinus. Called also *s. transversus ossis parietalis.* **s. si′nus sigmoi′dei os′sis tempora′lis,** sulcus of sigmoid sinus of temporal bone: the portion of the sulcus of the sigmoid sinus found on the temporal bone; called also *s. sigmoideus ossis temporalis.* **s. si′nus transver′si** [NA], sulcus of transverse sinus: a wide groove that passes horizontally, lateralward and forward from the internal occipital protuberance to the parietal bone, where it becomes continuous with the sulcus of the sigmoid sinus; it lodges the transverse sinus. Called also *s. transversus ossis occipitalis.* **sulci of skin,** sulci cutis. **s. of spinal nerve,** s. nervi spinalis. **spiral s., external,** s. spiralis externus. **spiral s., internal,** s. spiralis internus. **spiral s. of humerus,** s. nervi radialis. **s. spira'lis,** see *s. spiralis externus* and *s. spiralis internus.* **s. spira'lis exter'nus** [NA], external spiral sulcus: a concavity within the cochlear duct immediately above the basilar crest. **s. spira'lis inter'nus** [NA], internal spiral sulcus: the C-shaped concavity within the cochlear duct formed by the limbus laminae spiralis and its tympanic and vestibular labia along the edge of the osseous spiral lamina. **s. subcla'viae,** s. arteriae subclaviae. **subclavian s.,** s. arteriae subclaviae. **subclavian s. of lung,** s. subclavius pulmonis. **s. of subclavian artery,** s. arteriae subclaviae. **s. of subclavian vein,** s. venae subclaviae. **s. subcla'vius,** s. arteriae subclaviae. **s. subcla'vius pulmo'nis,** subclavian sulcus of lung: a broad, shallow, transverse groove across the top of the lung, lodging the subclavian artery. **subparietal s., s. subparieta'lis** [NA], a sulcus on the medial surface of a cerebral hemisphere, above the splenium of the corpus callosum, separating the precuneus from the cingulate gyrus. **s. of superior petrosal sinus,** s. sinus petrosi superioris. **s. of superior sagittal sinus of frontal bone,** s. sinus sagittalis superioris ossis frontalis. **s. of superior sagittal sinus of occipital bone,** s. sinus sagittalis superioris ossis occipitalis. **supraorbital s.,** foramen supraorbitalis. **suprasplenial s.,** s. subparietalis. **s. Syl'vii,** fossa lateralis cerebri. **s. ta'li** [NA], **s. of talus,** a transverse groove on the inferior surface of the talus, between the medial and the posterior articular surface, which helps to form the sinus tarsi. **temporal s., inferior, temporal s., middle,** s. temporalis inferior [NA]. **temporal s., superior,** s. temporalis superior. **temporal sulci, transverse,** sulci temporales transversi. **temporal s. of temporal bone,** s. arteriae temporalis mediae. **s. tempora'lis infe'rior,** 1. [NA] inferior temporal sulcus: a longitudinal sulcus on the lateral surface of the temporal lobe, separatiing the middle and the inferior temporal gyri. Formerly called *s. temporalis medius.* 2. sulcus occipitotemporalis. **s. tempora'lis me'dius,** s. temporalis inferior. **s. tempora'lis supe'rior** [NA], superior temporal sulcus: a longitudinal sulcus on the lateral surface of a cerebral hemisphere, passing downward and forward from the gyrus angularis to the temporal pole and separating the superior and the middle temporal gyri. **sul'ci tempora'les transver'si** [NA], transverse temporal sulci: irregularly vertical sulci in the part of the temporal lobe that lies within the lateral sulcus. **s. ten'dinis mus'culi flexo'ris hal'lucis lon'gi calca'nei** [NA], sulcus of tendon of flexor hallucis longus of calcaneus: a groove on the inferior surface of the sustentaculum tali of the calcaneus, lodging the tendon of the flexoris hallucis longus muscle; called also *s. musculi flexoris hallucis longi calcanei.* **s. ten'dinis mus'culi flexo'ris hal'lucis lon'gi ta'li** [NA], sulcus of tendon of flexor hallucis longus of talus: the sagittal groove on the posterior surface of the body of the talus that transmits the tendon of the flexor hallucis longus muscle; called also *s. musculi flexoris hallucis longi tali.* **s. ten'dinis mus'culi perone'i lon'gi** [NA], sulcus of tendon of peroneus longus muscle: a deep groove on the inferior surface of the cuboid bone, which in certain foot positions lodges the tendon of the peroneus longus muscle; called also *s. musculi peronaei ossis cuboidei.* **s. ten'dinum musculo'rum fibula'rium calca'nei,** NA alternative for *s. tendinum musculorum peroneorum calcanei.* **s. ten'dinum musculo'rum peroneo'rum calca'nei** [NA], sulcus of tendons of peroneus muscles: a slight groove on the inferior part of the lateral surface of the calcaneus, lodging the tendons of the peroneus longus and brevis muscles; called also *s. musculi peronaei calcanei.* **s. of tendon of flexor hallucis longus muscle of calcaneus,** s. tendinis musculi flexoris hallucis longi calcanei. **s. of tendon of flexor hallucis longus muscle of talus,** s. tendinis musculi flexoris hallucis longi tali. **s. of tendons of peroneus muscles,** s. tendinum musculorum peroneorum calcanei. **s. of tendon of peroneus longus muscle,** s. tendinis musculi peronei longi. **terminal s. of right atrium,** s. terminalis atrii dextri. **terminal s. of tongue,** s. terminalis linguae. **s. termina'lis a'trii dex'tri** [NA], terminal sulcus of right atrium: a shallow groove on the external surface of the right atrium of the heart between the superior and inferior venae cavae; it represents the junction of the sinus venosus with the primitive atrium in the embryo, and corresponds to a ridge on the internal surface, the crista terminalis. **s. termina'lis lin'guae** [NA], terminal sulcus of tongue: a more or less distinct groove on the tongue, extending from the foramen cecum forward and lateralward to the margin of the tongue on either side, and dividing the dorsum of the tongue from the root. It is marked by a row of vallate papillae. **s. of tongue,** see *s. medianus linguae* and *s. terminalis linguae.* **transverse s. of anthelix,** s. anthelicis transversus. **transverse s. of heart,** s. coronarius cordis. **transverse s. of occipital bone,** s. sinus transversi. **transverse s. of parietal bone,** s. sinus sigmoidei ossis parietalis. **s. of transverse sinus,** s. sinus transversi. **transverse s. of temporal bone,** s. sinus sigmoidei ossis temporalis. **s. transver'sus os'sis occipita'lis,** s. sinus transversi.

s. transver'sus os'sis parieta'lis, s. sinus sigmoidei ossis parietalis. **s. tu'bae auditi'vae** [NA], **s. tu'bae eusta'chii,** sulcus of auditory tube: a groove on the medial part of the base of the spine of the sphenoid bone; it lodges a portion of the cartilaginous part of the auditory tube. **Turner's s.,** s. intraparietalis. **tympanic s. of temporal bone, s. tympan'icus os'sis tempora'lis** [NA], a narrow groove in the medial part of the external acoustic meatus of the temporal bone, into which the tympanic membrane fits; it is deficient above. **s. of ulnar nerve,** s. nervi ulnaris. **s. of umbilical vein,** s. venae umbilicalis. **sulci for veins,** sulci venosi. **s. of vena cava, s. ve'nae ca'vae** [NA], a groove on the upper part of the posteroinferior surface of the liver, separating the right lobe from the caudate lobe and lodging the inferior vena cava; called also *fossa venae cavae.* **s. ve'nae subcla'viae** [NA], sulcus of subclavian vein: a transverse groove on the cranial surface of the first rib, just anterior to the anterior scalene tubercle; it lodges the subclavian vein. **s. ve'nae umbilica'lis** [NA], sulcus of umbilical vein: the impression on the visceral surface of the liver in the fetus, which lodges the umbilical vein. **sul'ci veno'si** [NA], **venous sulci,** grooves on the internal surfaces of the cranial bones for the meningeal veins; called also *venous grooves.* **s. ventra'lis medul'lae spina'lis,** fissura mediana anterior medullae spinalis. **vermicular s.,** a fissure between the vermis and the hemisphere of the cerebellum. **s. of vertebral artery of atlas,** s. arteriae vertebralis atlantis. **vertical s.,** s. precentralis. **vomerovaginal s., s. vomerovagina'lis** [NA], the groove on the vaginal process of the pterygoid process of the sphenoid bone that helps form the vomerovaginal canal. **Waldeyer's s.,** see *s. spiralis externus* and *s. spiralis internus.* **s. of wrist,** s. carpi.

sulfabenzamide (sul''fah-benz'ah-mīd) chemical name: *N*-sulfanilylbenzamide; an antibacterial, $C_{13}H_{12}N_2O_3S$.

sulfacetamide (sul''fah-set'ah-mīd) chemical name: *N*-sulfanilylacetamide. A sulfonamide $C_8H_{10}N_2O_3S$, occurring as a white crystalline powder, which has been used in the treatment of urinary tract infections. **sodium s.** [USP], the sodium salt of sulfacetamide, used topically in ointment or solution as an antibacterial in the management of various ophthalmic infections.

sulfacid (sulf-as'id) sulfonic acid.

sulfacytine (sul''fah-si'tēn) chemical name: 4-amino-*N*-(1-ethyl-1,2-dihydro-2-oxo-4-pyrimidinyl)benzenesulfonamide. A short-acting sulfonamide, $C_{12}H_{14}N_4O_3S$, used orally in the treatment of acute urinary tract infections when due to susceptible strains of *Escherichia coli; Klebsiella-Enterobacter* group, *Staphylococcus aureus, Proteus mirabilis,* and *P. vulgaris.*

sulfadiazine (sul''fah-di'ah-zēn) [USP] chemical name: 4-amino-*N*-2-pyrimidinylbenzenesulfonamide. A sulfonamide, $C_{10}H_{10}N_4O_2S$, occurring as a white or slightly yellow powder; frequently used in combination with other sulfonamides in the treatment of infections due to susceptible organisms, including meningitis caused by *Hemophilus influenzae,* chancroid, acute urinary tract infections, early manifestations of lymphogranuloma venereum, and falciparum malaria caused by chloroquine-resistant plasmodia. It is administered orally. **s. silver,** the silver derivative of sulfadiazine, $C_{10}H_9AgN_4O_2S$, used as a topical antibacterial to prevent wound sepsis in the treatment of second and third degree burns. **s. sodium** [USP], the monosodium salt of sulfadiazine, $C_{10}H_9N_4NaO_2S$, occurring as a white powder, having the same actions and uses as the base; administered subcutaneously and intravenously.

sulfadimethoxine (sul''fah-di''mĕ-thoks'ēn) chemical name: 4-amino-*N*-(2,6-dimethoxy-4-pyrimidinyl)benzenesulfonamide. A long-acting sulfonamide, $C_{12}H_{14}N_4O_4S$, occurring as an almost white, crystalline powder; used as an antibacterial in a variety of infections, administered orally.

sulfadimetine (sul''fah-di'mĕ-tēn) sulfisomidine.

sulfadimidine (sul''fah-di'mĭ-dēn) sulfamethazine.

sulfadoxine (sul'' fah-doks' ēn) chemical name: 4-amino-*N*-(5,6-dimethoxy-4-pyrimidinyl)benzenesulfonamide. A long-acting sulfonamide, $C_{12}H_{14}N_4O_4S$, which has been used in the treatment of leprosy and falciparum malaria.

sulfaethidole (sul''fah-eth'ĭ-dōl) chemical name: 4-amino-*N*-(5-ethyl-1,3,4-thiadiazol-2-yl)benzenesulfonamide. A short-acting sulfonamide, $C_{10}H_{12}N_4O_2S_2$, occurring as a white to yellowish white, crystalline powder; used principally as a urinary antiseptic, administered orally.

sulfafurazole (sul''fah-fu'rah-zōl) sulfisoxazole.

sulfaguanidine (sul''fah-gwan'ĭ-dēn) chemical name: *N*¹-amidinosulfanilamide. A sulfonamide, $C_7H_{10}N_4O_2S$, which is not well absorbed and occurs as a white needle-like crystalline powder, used as an antibacterial agent in infections of the gastrointestinal tract.

sulfalene (sul'fah-lēn) chemical name: 4-amino-*N*-(3-methoxypyrazinyl)-benzenesulfonamide. A long-acting sulfonamide, $C_{11}H_{12}N_4O_3S$, used as an antibacterial, especially in the treatment of urinary tract infections.

sulfamerazine (sul''fah-mer'ah-zēn) [USP] chemical name: *N*¹-(4-methyl-2-pyrimidinyl)sulfanilamide. A readily absorbed antibacterial substance, $C_{11}H_{12}N_4O_2S$, occurring as white or faintly yellowish white crystals or powder, usually used in combination with other sulfonamides. See *trisulfapyrimidines oral suspension*, under *suspension*. Called also *sulfamethyldiazine*.

sulfameter (sul″fah-me″ter) chemical name: 4-amino-*N*-(5-methoxy-2-pyrimidinyl)benzenesulfonamide. A long-acting sulfonamide, $C_{11}H_{12}N_4O_3S$, occurring as a fine, white to yellowish-white, powder; used as an antibacterial, especially in the treatment of acute and chronic urinary tract infections, administered orally.

sulfamethazine (sul″fah-meth′ah-zēn) [USP] chemical name: 4-amino-*N*-(4,6-dimethyl-2-pyrimidinyl)benzenesulfonamide. A sulfonamide, $C_{12}H_{14}N_4O_2S$, occurring as a white to yellowish white powder; used as an antibacterial in a variety of infections, usually, in the United States, in combination with other sulfonamides. It is administered orally. Called also *sulfadimidine*.

sulfamethizole (sul″fah-meth′ĭ-zōl) [USP] chemical name: N^1-(5-methyl-1,3,4-thiadiazol-2-yl)sulfanilamide. A compound, $C_9H_{10}N_4O_2S_2$, occurring as white crystals or powder, used as an antibacterial agent mainly in the treatment of infections of the urinary tract. Called also *sulfamethylthiadiazole*.

sulfamethoxazole (sul″fah-meth-oks′ah-zōl) [USP] chemical name: 4-amino-*N*-(5-methyl-3-isoxazolyl)benzenesulfonamide. A sulfonamide, $C_{10}H_{11}N_3O_3S$, occurring as a white to off-white, crystalline powder; used as an antibacterial, especially for the prophylaxis and treatment of acute urinary tract infections and of pyodermata and infections of wounds and soft tissues, administered orally.

sulfamethoxypyridazine (sul″fah-meth-ok′se-pi-rid′ah-zēn) chemical name: N^1-(6-methoxy-3-pyridazinyl)sulfanilamide. A compound, $C_{11}H_{12}N_4O_3S$, occurring as a white or yellowish white, crystalline powder, used as an antibacterial agent in the treatment of infections of the urinary tract and other infections.

sulfamethyldiazine (sul″fah-meth′il-di′ah-zēn) sulfamerazine.

sulfamethylthiadiazole (sul″fah-meth″il-thi″ah-di′ah-zōl) sulfamethizole.

Sulfamezathine (sul″fah-mez′ah-thēn) trademark for a preparation of sulfamethazine.

sulfamido (sul-fam′ĭ-do) one of a group of compounds containing an aminosulfone group $SO_2 \cdot NH_2$.

sulfamine (sul-fam′in) the univalent radical, —SO_2NH_2.

sulfamonomethoxine (sul″fah-mon″o-mĕ-thoks′ēn) chemical name: N^1-(6-methoxy-4-pyrimidinyl)sulfanilamide; an antibacterial, $C_{11}H_{12}N_4O_3S$.

sulfamoxole (sul″fah-moks′ōl) chemical name: N^1-(4,5-dimethyl-2-oxazolyl)sulfanilamide; an antibacterial, $C_{11}H_{13}N_3O_3S$.

Sulfamylon (sul″fah-mi′lon) trademark for preparations of mafenide.

sulfanilamide (sul″fah-nil′ah-mīd) chemical name: *p*-aminobenzenesulfonamide. A potent antibacterial compound, $NH_2 \cdot C_6H_4 \cdot SO_2NH_2$, the first of the sulfonamides discovered. Formerly used in the treatment of various infections, it has been replaced by more effective and less toxic derivatives, and by antibiotics. Called also *prontosil album*.

sulfanilate (sulf-an′ĭ-lāt) a salt of sulfanilic acid.

sulfanitran (sulf-ah-ni′tran) chemical name: 4′-[(*p*-nitrophenyl)sulfamoyl]acetanilide. A substance, $C_{14}H_{13}N_3O_5S$, used as an antibacterial and as a coccidiostatic agent in poultry.

sulfanuria (sulf″ah-nu′re-ah) anuria resulting from the use of sulfonamide drugs.

sulfapyridine (sul″fah-pir′ĭ-dēn) [USP] chemical name: N^1-2-pyridylsulfanilamide. An antibacterial compound, $C_{11}H_{11}N_3O_2S$, occurring as white or faintly yellowish white granules, crystals, or powder; used as an oral suppressant for dermatitis herpetiformis. It was formerly used in the treatment of pneumonia and streptococcal infections.

sulfaquinoxaline (sul″fah-kwin-ok′sah-lēn) chemical name: N^1-(2-quinoxalinyl)sulfanilamide. An antibacterial, $C_{14}H_{12}N_4O_2S$, used in veterinary medicine as a coccidiostat, and in the treatment of fowl cholera, fowl typhoid, infectious enteritis of swine, shipping dysentery of lambs, and foot rot of cattle.

sulfarsphenamine (sulf″ar-sfen′ah-min) the disodium salt of dihydroxy-diaminoarsenobenzenemonomethylene sulfonate, $NH_2(OH)C_6H_3 \cdot As:AsC_6H_3(OH)NH \cdot CH_2 \cdot SO_2 \cdot ONa$. It contains 18–20 per cent of arsenic and was formerly used in the treatment of syphilis. It differs from neoarsphenamine in having two side chains instead of one and in that the sulfur has a valence of four instead of two.

sulfasalazine (sul″fah-sal′ah-zēn) [USP] chemical name: 2-hydroxy-5-[[4-[(2-pyridinylamino)sulfonyl]phenyl]azo]benzoic acid. An antibacterial sulfonamide derivative, $C_{18}H_{14}N_4O_5S$, occurring as a bright yellow to brownish yellow powder; used orally in the treatment of mild to moderate ulcerative colitis and as adjunctive therapy in severe ulcerative colitis due to susceptible organisms, administered orally. Called also *salazosulfapyridine* and *salicylazosulfapyridine*.

Sulfasuxidine (sul″fah-suk′sĭ-dēn) trademark for preparations of succinylsulfathiazole.

sulfatase (sul′fah-tās) an enzyme that catalyzes the hydrolysis of various sulfuric acid esters into sulfuric acid and alchohol.

sulfate (sul′fāt) [L. *sulphas*] any salt of sulfuric acid. **acid s.,** one in which only one half of the hydrogen of the sulfuric acid is replaced; a bisulfate. **basic s.,** one in which the normal sulfate of the base is combined with a hydroxide of the same base; a subsulfate. **chondroitin s.,** see *chrondroitin*. **conjugated s's,** aromatic substances, such as phenol, scatoxyl, and indoxyl, which occur in the urine along with mineral sulfates. **cupric s.** [USP], the pentahydrate sulfate salt of copper, $CuSO_4 \cdot 5H_2O$, occurring as deep blue, triclinic crystals or as blue crystalline granules or powder, which is a powerful emetic; used orally as an antidote to phosphorus poisoning. Topical application of a 1 per cent solution is used in the treatment of phosphorus burns of the skin. It is also used as a catalyst with iron in the treatment of iron deficiency anemia. In 1:1,000,000 concentration it is used to prevent growth of algae in ponds, reservoirs, and swimming pools. Called also *blue vetriol*, *copper sulfate*, and *bluestone*. **dermatan s.,** chondroitin sulfate B; see *chondroitin*. **ethereal s's,** conjugated s's. **ferrous s.** [USP], pale bluish green odorless crystals or granules, $FeSO_4 \cdot 7H_2O$, used orally in treatment of iron deficiency anemia. Called also *copperas*, *green vitriol*, *iron protosulfate*, and *iron sulfate*. **ferrous s. dried** [USP], a grayish white powder, $FeSO_4 \cdot H_2O$, used as a hematinic. **mineral s's,** sulfates in the urine which are combinations of sulfuric acid with mineral substances such as sodium, potassium, calcium, and magnesium. **neutral s., normal s.,** one in which all the hydrogen of the sulfuric acid is replaced. **preformed s's,** mineral s's.

sulfatemia (sul″fāt-e′me-ah) the presence of sulfates in the blood.

Sulfathalidine (sul″fah-thal′ĭ-dēn) trademark for phthalylsulfathiazole.

sulfathiazole (sul″fah-thi′ah-zōl) chemical name: N^1-2-thiazolylsulfanilamide. A compound, $C_9H_9N_3O_2S_2$, once widely used as an antibacterial agent but replaced by less toxic sulfonamides and antibiotics. Called also *M & B 760*, *norsulfazole*.

sulfatide (sul′fah-tīd) one of a class of cerebroside sulfuric esters; they are found largely in the medullated nerve fibers, and may accumulate in the white matter of the brain in metachromatic leukodystrophy.

sulfazamet (sul-fah′zah-met) chemical name: N^1-(3-methyl-1-phenylpyrazol-5-yl)sulfanilamide; an antibacterial, $C_{16}H_{16}N_4O_2S$.

sulfhemoglobin (sulf″he-mo-glo′bin) sulfmethemoglobin.

sulfhemoglobinemia (sulf″he-mo-glo″bin-e′me-ah) the presence of sulfmethemoglobin in the blood.

sulfhydrate (sulf-hi′drāt) any compound of a base with sulfhydric acid or, more correctly, with the radical sulfhydryl, SH, or hydrogen sulfide.

sulfhydryl (sulf-hi′dril) the univalent radical, —SH.

sulfide (sul′fīd) any binary compound of sulfur; a compound of sulfur with another element or radical or base. **mercuric s.,** a brilliant scarlet powder, HgS, formerly used in the treatment of syphilis.

sulfindigotate (sul-fin′dĭ-go-tāt) any salt of sulfindigotic acid.

sulfinpyrazone (sul″fin-pi′rah-zōn) [USP] chemical name: 1,2-diphenyl-4-[2-(phenylsulfinyl)ethyl]3,5-pyrazolidinedione. A sulfoxide analogue of phenylbutazone, $C_{23}H_{20}N_2O_3S$, used as a uricosuric agent in treatment of gout.

sulfinyl (sul″fĭ-nil) the bivalent radical, —SO—.

sulfisomidine (sul-fĭ-som′ĭ-dēn) chemical name: N^1-(2,6-dimethyl-4-pyrimidinyl)sulfanilamide. A compound, $C_{12}H_{14}N_4O_2S$, closely related to sulfamethazine, occurring as a white or creamy-white powder, used as an antibacterial agent in the treatment of systemic and urinary tract infections. Called also *sulfadimetine*.

sulfisoxazole (sul″fĭ-sok′sah-zōl) [USP] chemical name: 4-amino-*N*-(3,4-dimethyl-5-isoxazolyl)benzenesulfonamide. A short-acting sulfonamide, $C_{11}H_{13}N_3O_3S$, occurring as a white to slightly yellowish, crystalline powder; used as an antibacterial in the treatment of a wide variety of infections, administered orally. Called also *sulfafurazole*. **acetyl s.** [USP], a tasteless derivative of sulfisoxazole, having the same actions as the base. **s. diethanolamine, s. diolamine** [USP], a soluble salt of sulfisoxazole, administered parenterally.

sulfite (sul′fīt) [L. *sulfis*] any salt of sulfurous acid. **s. oxidase,** an oxidoreductase that catalyzes the oxidation of sulfite (with O_2) to sulfate with release of H_2O_2; it is a hemoprotein containing molybdenum, occurring in the intermembrane space of mitochondria.

sulfmethemoglobin (sulf″met-he″mo-glo′bin) a greenish substance formed by treating blood with hydrogen sulfide or by the absorption of this gas from the intestinal tract; it is the cause of the greenish color seen in the abdominal walls and along the vessels of cadavers. Called also *sulfhemoglobin*.

sulfo- a prefix used in naming chemical compounds, indicating the presence of divalent sulfur or of the group SO_2OH.

sulfoacid (sul′fo-as′id) sulfonic acid.

sulfobromophthalein (sul″fo-bro″mo-thal′e-in) chemical name: 3,3′-(tetrabromophthalidylidene) bis[6-hydroxybenzenesulfonate]. Its disodium salt [USP], a white odorless crystalline powder, $C_{20}H_8Br_4Na_2O_{10}S_2$, is soluble in water and is used as a hepatic function determinant.

sulfoconjugation (sul″fo-kon″ju-ga′shun) the formation of conjugated sulfates.

sulfocyanate (sul″fo-si′ah-nāt) thiocyanate.

sulfogel (sul′fo-jel) a gel in which sulfuric acid is the medium instead of water.

sulfohydrate (sul″fo-hi′drāt) sulfhydrate.

sulfoichthyolate (sul″fo-ik′the-o-lāt) a salt of sulfoichthyolic acid; see *ichthammol*.

sulfolipid (sul″fo-lip′id) a lipid which on hydrolysis yields sulfuric acid.

sulfolysis (sul-fol′ĭ-sis) [*sulfo-* + Gr. *lysis* dissolution] a double decomposition, similar to hydrolysis, but in which sulfuric acid takes the place of water.

sulfomucin (sul″fo-mu′sin) a glucoprotein found in cartilage, cornea, and gastrointestinal mucosa, which contains sulfuric acid, uronic acid, and chondrosamine or glucosamine.

sulfonamide (sul-fon′ah-mīd) the chemical group SO_2NH_2. The sulfonamides, or sulfa drugs, are derivatives of sulfanilamide, which competitively inhibit folic acid synthesis in microorganisms, and are bacteriostatic against gram-positive cocci (streptococci and pneumococci), gram-negative cocci (meningococci and gonococci), gram-negative bacilli (*Escherichia coli* and shigellae), and a wide variety of other bacteria. Sulfonamides have been largely supplanted by more effective and less toxic antibiotics.

sulfonamidemia (sul″fōn-am″ĭ-de′me-ah) the presence of a sulfonamide compound in the blood.

sulfonamidocholia (sul″fōn-am″ĭ-do-ko′le-ah) the presence of a sulfonamide compound in the bile.

sulfonamidotherapy (sul″fōn-am″ĭ-do-ther′ah-pe) treatment with sulfonamide compounds.

sulfonamiduria (sul″fōn-am″ĭ-du′re-ah) the presence of a sulfonamide compound in the urine.

sulfone (sul′fōn) 1. the radical SO_2. 2. any compound containing two hydrocarbon radicals attached to the radical SO_2, especially dapsone (4,4′-sulfonylbisbenzenamine) and its derivatives, which are potent antibacterials effective against many gram-positive and gram-negative organisms, and are widely used as leprostatics. **Angeli's s.,** glucosulfone sodium.

sulfonethylmethane (sul″fōn-eth″il-meth′ān) chemical name: 2,2-bis(ethylsulfonyl)butane; a hypnotic, $C_8H_{18}O_4S_2$.

sulfonic (sul-fon′ik) indicating chemical compounds containing the monovalent $-SO_2OH$ or $-SO_3H$ radical.

sulfonmethane (sul″fōn-meth′ān) chemical name: 2,2-bis(ethylsulfonyl)propane. A white, crystalline compound, $(CH_3)_2C(SO_2\cdot C_2H_5)_2$, readily soluble in alcohol and slowly in 100 parts of water. It has moderate hypnotic properties, and was formerly used in insomnia of functional origin.

Sulfonsol (sul-fon′sol) trademark for trisulfapyrimidines oral suspension; see under *suspension*.

sulfonterol hydrochloride (sul-fon′ter-ōl) chemical name: α-[[(1,1-dimethylethyl)amino]methyl]-4-hydroxy-3-[(methylsulfonyl)methyl]benzenemethanol hydrochloride; a bronchodilator, $C_{14}H_{23}NO_4S\cdot HCl$.

sulfonyl (sul′fo-nil) the bivalent radical, $-SO_2-$.

sulfoprotein (sul″fo-pro′te-in) any of a series of albumins containing loosely combined sulfur.

sulfosalt (sul′fo-sawlt) a salt of sulfonic acid.

Sulfose (sul′fōs) trademark for preparations of trisulfapyrimidines.

sulfosol (sul′fo-sol) a sol in which sulfuric acid is the dispersion medium.

sulfotransferase (sul″fo-trans′fer-ās) an enzyme that catalyzes the transfer of sulfo groups, as from the phosphoadenylsulfates to form adenosine diphosphates.

sulfoxide (sul-fok′sīd) 1. the bivalent radical, $=SO$. 2. any member of a group of compounds intermediate between the sulfides and the sulfones.

sulfoxism (sul-fok′sizm) sulfuric acid poisoning.

sulfoxone sodium (sul-foks′on) [USP] chemical name: [sulfonylbis(1,4-phenyleneimino)]bismethanesulfinic acid disodium salt. An antibacterial derivative of dapsone, $C_{14}H_{14}N_2Na_2O_6S_3$, having actions similar to those of the parent compound, occurring as a white to pale yellow powder; used primarily as a leprostatic in the treatment of lepromatous and turberculoid leprosy, administered orally.

sulfur (sul′fur), gen. *sul′furis* [L.] a nonmetallic element existing in many allotropic forms; symbol, S; atomic number, 16; atomic weight, 32.064. It occurs in protein, being a constituent of the amino acids cysteine and methionine. Sulfur is a laxative and diaphoretic and is used in diseases of the skin and formerly in the treatment of a wide variety of diseases. **colloidal s.,** sulfur in a state of extremely fine division; milk of sulfur. **s. dioxide**

[NF], a colorless, nonflammable gas, SO_2, having a strong, suffocating odor; used as an antioxidant in pharmaceutical preparations. Dry sulfur dioxide is often used to kill fleas, mosquitoes, flies, rats, and other vermin. Called also *sulfurous anhydride*. **flower of s.,** sublimed s. **hepar-s.,** sulfurated potash. **s. hydride,** H_2S, a poisonous gas having the smell of rotten eggs. **s. iodide,** a binary compound, S_2I_2, which has been used externally in the treatment of various diseases of the skin, and, internally, in the treatment of human glanders. **lac s.,** precipitated s. **liver of s.,** sulfurated potash. **s. lo′tum,** washed s. **milk of s.,** sulfur in a state of extremely fine division; colloidal sulfur. **s. monochloride,** a lacrimating war gas, S_2Cl_2. **precipitated s.** [USP], a very fine, pale yellow, amorphous or microcrystalline powder, containing not less than 99.5 per cent sulfur, obtained by adding acid to a solution containing a polysulfide and a thiosulfate; used topically as a scabicide, and also used in various dermatologic formulations for its antiparasitic, antifungal, and keratolytic effects. Called also *lac sulfuris* and *milk of sulfur*. **radioactive s.,** radiosulfur. **roll s.,** sulfur melted and cast in the form of rods or cylinders. **sublimed s.** [USP], a fine yellow powder, containing not less than 99.5 per cent sulfur, obtained by subliming elemental sulfur and condensing the vapor. It is used topically as a scabicide and parasiticide. Called also *flores sulfuris* and *flowers of sulfur*. **s. vasogen,** an ointment containing sulfur and vasogen, either semisolid or fluid. **vegetable s.,** lycopodium. **washed s.,** sublimed sulfur purified by washing with water.

sulfuraria (sul″fu-ra′re-ah) a yellow powder, the sediment from certain springs in Italy, said to contain sulfur, calcium sulfide, strontium sulfate, silica, etc.; used in skin diseases.

sulfurated, sulfureted (sul′fu-rāt″ed; sul′fu-ret″ed) combined or charged with sulfur.

sulfurator (sul′fu-ra″tor) an apparatus for applying sulfur fumes, as in disinfecting.

sulfuret (sul′fu-ret) sulfide.

sulfurize (sul′fu-rīz) to cause to combine with sulfur.

sulfurtransferase (sul″fur-trans′fer-ās) an enzyme that catalyzes the transfer of a sulfur group, as from thiosulfate to cyanide to form thiocyanate.

sulfuryl (sul′fu-ril) the radical SO_2.

sulfydryl (sul-fi′dril) sulfhydryl.

sulindac (sul-in′dak) chemical name: (Z)-5-fluoro-2-methyl-1-[[4-(methylsulfinyl)phenyl]methylene]-1H-indene-3-acetic acid; a nonsteroidal anti-inflammatory, analgesic, and antipyretic, $C_{20}H_{17}FO_3S$, used in the treatment of rheumatic disorders.

sulisobenzone (sul″ĭ-so-ben′zōn) chemical name: 5-benzoyl-4-hydroxy-2-methoxybenzenesulfonic acid; an ultraviolet screen, $C_{14}H_{12}O_6S$.

Sulkowitch's test (sul′ko-wich″ez) [Hirsh Wolf *Sulkowitch*, American physician, born 1906] see under *tests*.

Sulla (sul′ah) trademark for a preparation of sulfameter.

sullage (sul′ij) sewage.

sulnidazole (sul-nĭd′ah-zōl) chemical name: [2-(2-ethyl-5-nitro-1H-imidazol-1-yl)ethyl]carbamothioic acid O-methyl ester; an antiprotozoal, $C_9H_{14}N_4O_3S$, effective against *Trichomonas*.

suloctidil (sul-ok′tĭ-dil) chemical name: (R*,S*)-4-[(1-methylethyl)thio]-α-[1-(octylamino)ethyl]benzenemethanol; a peripheral vasodilator, $C_{20}H_{35}NOS$.

suloxifen oxalate (sul-ok′sĭ-fen) chemical name: N-[2-(diethylamino)ethyl]-S,S-diphenylsulfoximine ethanedioate (1:1); a bronchodilator, $C_{18}H_{24}N_2OS\cdot C_2H_2O_4$.

sulph- for words beginning thus, see those beginning *sulf-*.

Sulphetrone (sul′fĕ-trōn) trademark for a preparation of solapsone.

sulpiride (sul′pĭ-rīd) chemical name: N-[(1-ethyl-2-pyrrolidinyl)methyl]-5-sulfamoyl-o-anisamide; an antidepressant, $C_{15}H_{23}N_3O_4S$.

sulprostone (sul-pros′tōn) chemical name: [1R-[1α(Z),2β(1E,3R*),3α]]-7-[3-hydroxy-2-(3-hydroxy-4-phenoxy-1-butenyl)-5-oxocyclopentyl]-N-(methylsulfonyl)-5-heptenamide; a prostaglandin, $C_{23}H_{31}NO_7S$.

Sul-Spansion (sul-span′shun) trademark for a preparation of sulfaethidole.

sulthiame (sul-thi′ām) chemical name: 4-(tetrahydro-2H-1,2-thiazin-2-yl)benzenesulfonamide S,S-dioxide. A carbonic anhydrase inhibitor, $C_{10}H_{14}N_2O_4S_2$, used as an anticonvulsant in the treatment of all forms of epilepsy except petit mal.

sum. abbreviation for L. *su′mat*, let him take; or *sumen′dum*, to be taken.

sumac (soo′mak) a name of various species of *Rhus*, applied principally to the nonpoisonous species. **poison s., swamp s.,** a species, *R. vernix*, usually found in swamps, which causes an itching rash on contact with the skin.

summation (sum-ma′shun) [L. *summa* total] the accumulative effects of a number of stimuli applied to a muscle, nerve, or reflex arc. **central s.,** the condition in which successive subliminal stimuli accumulate in a reflex center until they finally produce a reflex discharge.

summit (sum′it) [L. *summus,* superlative of *superus*] the highest point. **s. of bladder,** apex vesicae urinariae. **s. of nose,** radix nasi.

Sumner's method, reagent (sum′nerz) [James Batcheller *Sumner,* American biochemist, 1887–1955; co-winner, with W. M. Stanley and J. H. Northrop, of the Nobel prize in chemistry for 1946 for pioneering work in crystallizing proteins] see under *method* and *reagent.*

Sumner's sign (sum′nerz) [F.W. *Sumner,* British surgeon] see under *sign.*

Sumycin (soo-mi′sin) trademark for preparations of tetracycline hydrochloride.

sunburn (sun′bern) injury to the skin, with erythema, tenderness, and sometimes blistering, following excessive exposure to sunlight, and produced by ultraviolet rays, which are not filtered out by clouds or water.

suncillin sodium (sun-sil′in) chemical name: 3,3-dimethyl-7-oxo-6-[2-phenyl-D-2-(sulfoamino)acetamido]-4-thia-1-azabicyclo[3.2.0]heptane-2-carboxylic acid disodium salt; an antibacterial, $C_{16}H_{17}N_3Na_2O_7S_2$.

SunDare (sun′dār) trademark for preparations of cinoxate.

sunstroke (sun′strōk) insolation, or thermic fever; a condition produced by exposure to the sun, and marked by convulsions, coma, and a high temperature of the skin. Cf. *heat exhaustion* and *heat stroke.*

super- [L. *super* above] a prefix signifying above, or implying excess.

superabduction (soo″per-ab-duk′shun) extreme or excessive abduction.

superacid (soo″per-as′id) excessively acid.

superacidity (soo″per-ah-sid′ĭ-te) excessive acidity.

superacromial (soo″per-ah-kro′me-al) supra-acromial.

superactivity (soo″per-ak-tiv′ĭ-te) activity greater than normal; hyperactivity.

superacute (soo″per-ah-kūt′) extremely acute.

superalimentation (soo″per-al″ĭ-men-ta′shun) therapeutic treatment by excessive feeding beyond the requirements of the appetite: employed in wasting diseases; called also *gavage.*

superalkalinity (soo″per-al″kah-lin′ĭ-te) excessive alkalinity.

superaurale (soo″per-aw-ra′le) an anthropometric landmark, the highest point on the superior border of the helix of the ear.

supercarbonate (soo″per-kar′bon-āt) bicarbonate.

supercentral (soo″per-sen′tral) above a center.

supercilia (soo″per-sil′e-ah) [L., pl. of *supercilium*] [NA] the hairs growing on the transverse elevation at the junction of the forehead and the upper lid of either eye; called also *eyebrow.*

superciliary (soo″per-sil′e-a-re) [L. *superciliaris*] pertaining to the eyebrow.

supercilium (soo″per-sil′e-um), pl. *supercil′ia* [L.] [NA] the transverse elevation at the junction of the forehead and the upper eyelid; see *eyebrow* (def. 1), and see also *supercilia.*

superclass (soo′per-klas) a taxonomic category sometimes established, subordinate to a phylum and superior to a class.

supercoil (su′per-koil) a shape assumed by chromosomes when they have attained their maximum length during interphase, resembling a "zig-zag" pattern with broad turns.

superdistention (soo″per-dis-ten′shun) excessive distention.

superduct (soo″per-dukt′) [super- + L. *ducere* to draw] to carry up or elevate.

superego (soo″per-e′go) a part of the psyche with components derived from both the id and the ego, functioning largely in the unconscious zone, and acting as a monitor over the ego; the conscience.

superexcitation (soo″per-ek″si-ta′shun) [super- + L. *excitatio* excitement] extreme or excessive excitement.

superextended (soo″per-eks-tend′ed) extended beyond the normal.

superextension (soo″per-eks-ten′shun) excessive extension.

superfamily (soo″per-fam′ĭ-le) a taxonomic category sometimes established, subordinate to an order and superior to a family.

superfecundation (soo″per-fe″kun-da′shun) [super- + L. *fecundare* to fertilize] fertilization of two or more ova during the same ovulatory cycle by separate coital acts.

superfemale (soo″per-fe′māl) a female organism whose cells contain more than the ordinary number of sex-determining (X) chromosomes.

superfetation (soo″per-fe-ta′shun) [super- + *fetus*] the fertilization and subsequent development of an ovum when a fetus is already present in the uterus, a result of fertilization of ova during different ovulatory cycles and yielding fetuses of different ages.

superficial (soo″per-fish′al) [L. *superficialis*] pertaining to or situated near the surface.

superficialis (soo″per-fish″e-a′lis) superficial; [NA] a term used to designate a structure situated closer than another to the surface of the body.

superficies (soo″per-fish′e-ēz) [L.] an outer surface.

superflexion (soo″per-flek′shun) extreme or excessive flexion.

superfunction (soo″per-funk′shun) excessive activity of an organ or structure; hyperfunction.

supergenual (soo″per-jen′u-al) above the knee.

superimpregnation (soo″per-im″preg-na′shun) [super- + impregnation] superfetation.

superinduce (soo″per-in-dūs′) to induce or bring on in addition to some already existing condition.

superinfection (soo″per-in-fek′shun) a new infection complicating the course of antimicrobial therapy of an existing infectious process, and resulting from invasion by bacteria or fungi resistant to the drug(s) in use. It may occur at the site of the original infection or at a remote site.

superinvolution (soo″per-in″vo-lu′shun) prolonged involution of the uterus after delivery, to a size much smaller than the normal, occurring in nursing mothers. Called also *hyperinvolution.*

superior (soo-pe′re-or) [L. "upper"; neut. *superius*] situated above, or directed upward; [NA] a term used in reference to a structure occupying a position nearer the vertex.

superjacent (soo″per-ja′sent) located immediately above; overlying.

superlactation (soo″per-lak-ta′shun) hyperlactation.

superlethal (soo″per-le′thal) more than sufficient to cause death.

supermaxilla (soo″per-mak-sil′ah) the maxilla.

supermedial (soo″per-me′de-al) situated above the middle.

supermoron (soo″per-mo′ron) a person who is only slightly deficient mentally.

supermotility (soo″per-mo-til′ĭ-te) excessive motility.

supernatant (soo″per-na′tant) [super- + L. *natare* to swim] 1. situated above or on top of something. 2. the overlying liquid after precipitation of a solid component of a system.

supernate (soo′per-nāt) supernatant, def. 2.

supernormal (soo″per-nor′mal) more than normal.

supernumerary (soo″per-nu′mer-ar″e) [L. *supernumerarius*] in excess of the regular or normal number.

supernutrition (soo″per-nu-trish′un) excessive nutrition.

superoccipital (soo″per-ok-sip′ĭ-tal) supraoccipital.

superolateral (soo″per-o-lat′er-al) above and at the side.

superovulation (soo″per-ov″u-la′shun) extraordinary acceleration of ovulation.

superoxide (soo″per-oks′īd) any compound containing the highly reactive oxygen ion O_2^-, produced when molecular oxygen is reduced by (gains) a single electron; it is a common intermediate in numerous biological oxidations.

superparasite (soo″per-par′ah-sīt) 1. a parasite involved in superparasitism. 2. hyperparasite.

superparasitism (soo″per-par″ah-si″tizm) 1. infestation with more parasites of one species than the host can support or bring to maturity. 2. hyperparasitic.

superphosphate (soo″per-fos′fāt) any acid phosphate, especially calcium superphosphate (see *calcium phosphate, monobasic*).

super-regeneration (soo-per-re-jen″ĕ-ra′shun) the development of superfluous tissue, organs, or parts as a result of regeneration.

supersalt (soo′per-sawlt) any salt obtained by reaction with an excess of acid; a persalt or acid salt.

supersaturate (soo″per-sat′u-rāt) to add more of an ingredient than can be held in solution permanently.

superscription (soo″per-skrip′shun) [L. *superscriptio*] the sign ℞ before a prescription; see *prescription.*

supersecretion (soo″per-se-kre′shun) excessive secretion.

supersedent (soo″per-se′dent) a remedy which cures or prevents a disease in a part.

supersensitization (soo″per-sen″sĭ-ti-za′shun) hypersensitization.

supersoft (soo″per-soft′) extremely soft; applied to roentgen rays of extremely long wavelengths, large absorption coefficients, and low penetrating power.

supersonic (soo″per-son′ik) [super- + L. *sonus* sound] 1. having a speed greater than the velocity of sound, that is, faster than approximately one-fifth mile per second (or 720 miles an hour) in air. 2. ultrasonic.

supersonics (soo″per-son′iks) the general science relating to phenomena associated with speed greater than the velocity of sound (as in case of aircraft and projectiles traveling faster than sound).

supersphenoid (soo″per-sfe′noid) above the sphenoid bone.

superstructure (soo″per-struk′chur) the overlying or visible portion of an appliance. In dentistry, that portion of an implant denture which is outside the tissues of the mouth.

supertension (soo″per-ten′shun) extreme or excessive tension.

supervascularization (soo″per-vas″ku-lar-i-za′shun) in radiotherapy, the relative increase in vascularity that occurs when tumor cells are destroyed so that the remaining tumor cells are better supplied by the (uninjured) capillary stroma.

supervenosity (soo″per-ve-nos′ĭ-te) an abnormally diminished level of oxygen in venous blood.

supervention (soo″per-ven′shun) the development of some condition in addition to an already existing one.

supervirulent (soo″per-vir′u-lent) excessively virulent.

supervisor (soo″per-viz″er) an individual who oversees the activities of others, such as a nurse who oversees the nursing activities in a specific ward or department of a hospital.

supervitaminosis (soo″per-vi″tah-min-o′sis) hypervitaminosis.

supervoltage (soo′per-vol″tij) very high voltage. In x-ray therapy, it is generally considered to be voltage in the range of 500 kilovolts, as contrasted with orthovoltage (140 to 400 kilovolts) and with megavoltage (greater than 1 megavolt).

supinate (soo″pĭ-nāt) to assume or place in a supine position.

supination (soo″pĭ-na′shun) [L. *supinatio*] the act of assuming the supine position, or the state of being supine. Applied to the hand, the act of turning the palm forward (anteriorly) or upward, performed by lateral rotation of the forearm. Applied to the foot, it generally implies movements resulting in raising of the medial margin of the foot, hence of the longitudinal arch. Cf. *pronation*.

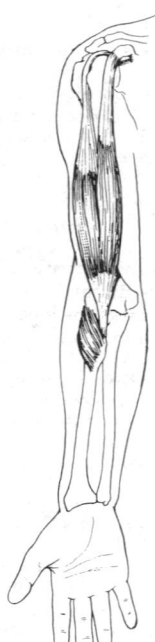

Supinators contracted; forearm, hand supinated. (King and Showers.)

supine (soo′pīn) [L. *supinus* lying on the back, face upward] lying with the face upward; see also *supination*.

suppedania (sup″ĕ-da′ne-ah) [L. *sub* under + *pes* foot] local applications to the soles of the feet.

supplemental (sup″lĕ-men′tal) serving as a supplement or addition.

support (sup-port′) 1. an appliance which helps maintain a part in position. 2. in dentistry, that location or point at which is placed one of the induced equilibrants to the applied loads.

suppositoria (sup-poz′ĭ-to″re-ah) [L.] plural of *suppositorium*.

suppositorium (sup-poz′ĭ-to″re-um), pl. *suppos′itoria* [L.] suppository.

suppository (sup-poz′ĭ-to-re) [L. *suppositorium*] a medicated mass adapted for introduction into the rectal, vaginal, or urethral orifice of the body; suppository bases are solid at room temperature but melt or dissolve at body temperature. Commonly used bases are cocoa butter, glycerinated gelatin, hydrogenated vegetable oils, polyethylene glycols of various molecular weights, and fatty acid esters of polyethylene glycol. **glycerin s.** [NF], a suppository made up of a mixture of glycerin and sodium stearate; used as a rectal evacuant.

suppressant (sŭ-pres′sant) 1. inducing suppression. 2. an agent that stops secretion, excretion, or normal discharge.

suppression (sŭ-presh′un) [L. *suppressio*] 1. the sudden stoppage of a secretion, excretion, or normal discharge. 2. in psychoanalysis, conscious inhibition as contrasted with repression, which is unconscious. 3. in genetics, the restoration of a lost function by a second mutation either in a gene other than that involved in the primary mutation (*intergenic s.*), or within the same gene (*intragenic s.*).

suppurant (sup′u-rant) [L. *suppurans*] 1. characterized by suppuration. 2. an agent that causes suppuration.

suppurantia (sup′u-ran′she-ah) substances that cause suppuration.

suppuration (sup′u-ra′shun) [L. *sub* under + *puris* pus] the formation of pus; the act of becoming converted into and discharging pus. **alveodental s.,** periodontitis with the formation of pus.

suppurative (sup′u-ra″tiv) producing pus, or associated with suppuration.

supra- [L. "above"] a prefix signifying above or over.

supra-acromial (soo″prah-ah-kro′me-al) situated above or over the acromion.

supra-anal (soo-prah-a′nal) situated above the anus.

supra-auricular (soo″prah-aw-rik′u-lar) situated above the ear.

supra-axillary (soo″prah-ak′sĭ-ler″e) situated above the axilla.

suprabuccal (soo″prah-buk′al) above the buccal region.

suprabulge (soo″prah-bulj) the surfaces of a tooth occlusal to the height of contour, or sloping occlusally. Cf. *infrabulge*.

suprachoroid (soo″prah-ko′roid) situated above or upon the choroid.

suprachoroidea (soo″prah-ko-roi′de-ah) lamina suprachoroidea.

supraciliary (soo″prah-sil′e-er″e) superciliary.

supraclavicular (soo″prah-klah-vik′u-lar) situated above the clavicle.

supraclavicularis (soo″prah-klah-vik″u-la′ris) [L.] supraclavicular.

supraclusion (soo″prah-kloo′zhun) the condition in which the occluding surface of a tooth extends beyond the normal occlusal plane.

supracondylar (soo″prah-kon′dĭ-lar) situated above a condyle or condyles.

supracondyloid (soo″prah-kon′dĭ-loid) supracondylar.

supracostal (soo″prah-kos′tal) situated above or upon a rib or ribs.

supracotyloid (soo″prah-kot′ĭ-loid) situated above the acetabulum.

supracranial (soo″prah-kra′ne-al) on the upper surface of the cranium.

supradiaphragmatic (soo″prah-di″ah-frag-mat′ik) situated above the diaphragm.

supraduction (soo″prah-duk′shun) [supra- + L. *ducere* to lead] sursumduction.

supraepicondylar (soo″prah-ep″ĭ-kon′dĭ-lar) situated above an epicondyle.

supraepitrochlear (soo″prah-ep″ĭ-trok′le-ar) situated above the medial epicondyle of the humerus.

supraglenoid (soo″prah-gle′noid) situated above the glenoid cavity.

supraglottic (soo″prah-glot′ik) situated above the glottis.

suprahepatic (soo″prah-he-pat′ik) situated above the liver.

suprahyoid (soo″prah-hi′oid) situated above the hyoid bone.

suprainguinal (soo″prah-in′gwĭ-nal) situated above the groin.

supraintestinal (soo″prah-in-tes′tĭ-nal) situated above the intestine.

supraliminal (soo″prah-lim′ĭ-nal) above the limen of sensation; more than just perceptible.

supralumbar (soo″prah-lum′bar) situated above the loin.

supramalleolar (soo″prah-mah-le′o-lar) situated above a malleolus.

supramammary (soo″prah-mam′ah-re) situated above a mammary gland.

supramandibular (soo″prah-man-dib′u-lar) situated above the mandible.

supramarginal (soo″prah-mar′jĭ-nal) situated above a margin.

supramastoid (soo″prah-mas′toid) situated above the mastoid portion of the temporal bone.

supramaxilla (soo″prah-mak-sil′ah) the maxilla.

supramaxillary (soo″prah-mak′sĭ-ler″e) 1. pertaining to the upper jaw. 2. situated above the maxilla.

supramaximal (soo″prah-mak′sĭ-mal) above the maximum.

suprameatal (soo″prah-me-a′tal) situated above a meatus.

supramental (soo″prah-men′tal) [supra- + L. *mentum* chin] situated above the chin.

supramentale (soo″prah-men-ta′le) point B; see under *point*.

supranasal (soo″prah-na′zal) above the nose.

supranormal (soo″prah-nor′mal) greater than normal; present or occurring in excess of normal amounts or values.

supranuclear (soo″prah-nu′kle-ar) situated or occurring above or on the cortical side or surface of a nucleus; see also under *paralysis*.

supraoccipital (soo″prah-ok-sip′ĭ-tal) situated above or in the upper portion of the occiput.

supraocclusion (soo″prah-ŏ-kloo′zhun) supraclusion.

supraocular (soo″prah-ok′u-lar) above the eye.

supraoptimal (soo″prah-op′tĭ-mal) greater than optimal.

supraoptimum (soo″prah-op′tĭ-mum) a condition or quantity exceeding the optimum.

supraorbital (soo″prah-or′bĭ-tal) situated above the orbit.

suprapatellar (soo″prah-pah-tel′ar) situated above the patella.

suprapelvic (soo″prah-pel′vik) situated above the pelvis.

suprapharmacologic (soo″prah-fahr″mah-ko-loj′ik) much greater than the usual therapeutic dose or pharmacologic concentration of a drug.

suprapontine (soo″prah-pon′tīn) situated above or in the upper part of the pons.

suprapubic (soo″prah-pu′bik) situated or performed above the pubic arch.

suprarenal (soo″prah-re′nal) [*supra-* + L. *ren* kidney] situated above a kidney; pertaining to the suprarenal (adrenal) gland.

suprarenalectomy (soo″prah-re″nal-ek′to-me) [*suprarenal* + Gr. *ektomē* excision] adrenalectomy; excision of the adrenal gland.

suprarenalemia (soo″prah-re″nal-e′me-ah) [*suprarenal* + Gr. *haima* blood + *-ia*] increase of adrenal secretion (epinephrine) in the blood.

suprarenalism (soo″prah-re′nal-izm) the condition produced by abnormal adrenal activity.

suprarenalopathy (soo″prah-re″nal-op′ah-the) [*suprarenal* + Gr. *pathos* disease] a disorder due to derangement of the adrenal gland.

suprarene (soo″prah-rēn′) [*supra* + L. *ren* kidney] an adrenal gland.

Suprarenin (soo″prah-ren′in) trademark for a preparation of epinephrine.

suprarenogenic (soo″prah-re″no-jen′ik) originating in the adrenal gland; due to abnormal adrenal activity.

suprarenoma (soo″prah-re-no′mah) a tumor derived from the adrenal tissue.

suprarenopathy (soo″prah-re-nop′ah-the) suprarenalopathy.

suprarenotropic (soo″prah-re″no-trop′ik) having an influence on the adrenal gland; adrenotropic.

suprarenotropism (soo″prah-re-not′ro-pizm) an endocrine make-up in which the adrenal hormone is dominant.

suprascapular (soo″prah-skap′u-lar) situated on the upper part of the scapula.

suprascleral (soo″prah-skle′ral) on the outer surface of the sclera.

suprasellar (soo″prah-sel′ar) above the sella turcica.

supraseptal (soo″prah-sep′tal) situated above a septum.

suprasonics (soo″prah-son′iks) ultrasonics.

supraspinal (soo″prah-spi′nal) situated upon or above a spine.

supraspinous (soo″prah-spi′nus) situated above a spine or a spinous process.

suprastapedial (soo″prah-stah-pe′de-al) situated above the stapes.

suprasternal (soo″prah-ster′nal) situated above the sternum.

suprasterol (soo″prah-ster′ol) an isomer of ergosterol.

suprasylvian (soo″prah-sil′ve-an) situated above the sylvian fissure.

supratemporal (soo″prah-tem′po-ral) situated above the temporal bone, fossa, or region.

supratentorial (soo″prah-ten-to′re-al) above the tentorium of the cerebellum.

suprathoracic (soo″prah-tho-ras′ik) situated above, or cephalad, of the thorax.

supratip (soo″prah-tip″) above the tip of the nose.

supratonsillar (soo″prah-ton′sĭ-lar) situated above a tonsil.

supratrochlear (soo″prah-trok′le-ar) situated above the trochlea.

supratympanic (soo″prah-tim-pan′ik) above the tympanum.

supraumbilical (soo″prah-um-bil′ĭ-kal) situated above the umbilicus.

supravaginal (soo″prah-vaj′ĭ-nal) situated above or outside of a sheath, specifically above the vagina.

supraventricular (soo″prah-ven-trik′u-lar) situated or occur-

ring above the ventricles, especially in an atrium or atrioventricular node.

supravergence (soo″prah-ver′jens) [*supra-* + L. *vergere* to turn] sursumvergence.

supraversion (soo″prah-ver′zhun) 1. the condition of a tooth when it is abnormally elongated from its socket. 2. sursumversion.

supravital (soo″prah-vi′tal) denoting a staining method in which the dye is added to a medium of cells already removed from the living organism.

supraxiphoid (soo″prah-zi′foid) above the xiphoid process.

suprofen (soo-pro′fen) chemical name: α-methyl-4-(2-thienyl-carbonyl)-benzeneacetic acid; a prostaglandin inhibitor, $C_{14}H_{12}O_3S$, having anti-inflammatory activity.

sura (su′rah) [L.] [NA] the muscular posterior portion of the leg; called also *calf*.

Suragina (su-rah-ji′nah) a genus of flies of the family Rhagionidae. *S. longipes* of Mexico is a vicious biter.

sural (su′ral) pertaining to the calf of the leg.

suralimentation (sur″al-ĭ-men-ta′shun) superalimentation.

suramin sodium (soo′rah-min) chemical name: 8,8′-[carbonyl-bis[imino-3,1-phenylenecarbonylimino(4-methyl-3,1-phenylene)-carbonylimino]]bis-1,3,5-naphthalenesulfonic acid hexasodium salt. An antitrypanosomal and antifilarial agent, $C_{51}H_{34}N_6Na_6O_{23}S_6$, occurring as a white or slightly pink powder; used in the treatment of African trypanosomiasis, especially that due to *Trypanosoma gambiense*, and of onchocerciasis, administered intravenously.

surdimute (sur′dĭ-mūt) [L. *surdus* deaf + *mutus* mute] 1. both deaf and mute. 2. a deaf-mute.

surdimutism (sur′dĭ-mu′tizm) deaf-mutism.

surdimutitas (sur′dĭ-mu′tĭ-tas) [L. *surdus* deaf + *mutus* unable to speak + *-tas* state] deaf-mutism.

surditas (sur′dĭ-tas) [L.] deafness. **s. congen′ita,** congenital deafness.

surdity (sur′dĭ-te) [L. *surditas*] deafness.

surexcitation (sur″ek-si-ta′shun) [L. *super* over + *excitation*] excessive excitation.

Surfacaine (sur′fah-kān) trademark for preparations of cyclomethycaine.

surface (sur′fis) the outer part or an external aspect of an object. For names included in official anatomical nomenclature, see under *facies*. **alveolar s. of maxilla,** arcus alveolaris maxillae. **anterior s.,** that surface which is toward the front of the body (on or nearest the ventral aspect) in man (*facies anterior* [NA]), or toward the head in quadrupeds; in dentistry, the proximal surface of any tooth that is closest to the midline of the dental arch. **anterior s. of manubrium and gladiolus,** planum sternale. **anterior s. of sacrum,** facies pelvina ossis sacri. **anterior s. of scapula,** facies costalis scapulae. **anterior s. of stomach,** paries anterior ventriculi. **approximal s.,** proximal s. **articular s.,** that surface of a bone or cartilage which forms a joint with another (*facies articularis* [NA]). **articular s. of acetabulum,** facies lunata acetabuli. **articular s. of sacral bone, lateral,** facies auricularis ossis sacri. **axial s.,** any surface parallel with an axis; in dentistry, any surface of a tooth which is parallel with its long axis, including the buccal, distal, labial, lingual, and medial surfaces. **basal s.,** that surface of a denture the detail of which is determined by the impression and which rests upon the supporting tissues of the mouth. **buccal s.,** the surface of a posterior tooth (or of a denture) which faces the cheek (*facies buccalis dentis*). **condyloid s. of tibia,** facies articularis superior tibiae. **contact s.,** the portion of the surface of a tooth which lies in contact with the next tooth in the same row; see also *proximal s.* **diaphragmatic s.,** the surface of an organ of the thoracic or abdominal cavity that is directed toward the diaphragm (*facies diaphragmatica* [NA]). **distal s.,** that surface of a structure which is farther from a point of reference; in dentistry, the proximal or contact surface of a tooth farthest from the midline of the dental arch (*lateral s.* or *posterior s.*). **dorsal s.,** the aspect of a structure that is toward the back of the body. In man, synonymous with posterior surface (*facies dorsalis, facies posterior* [NA]). **extensor s.,** the aspect of a joint of a limb (such as the knee or the elbow) on the side toward which the movement of extension is directed. **facial s.,** vestibular s. **flexor s.,** the aspect of a joint of a limb (such as the knee or the elbow) on the side toward which the movement of flexion is directed. **foundation s.,** basal s. **impression s.,** the surface of a denture that is determined by the impression made of the structures in the mouth. **incisal s.,** the surface of an anterior tooth which functions by incising food during the process of mastication. **inferior s.,** that surface which is lower (directed away from the head, in man) (*facies inferior* [NA]). **infratemporal s. of maxilla,** facies infratemporalis maxillae. **labial s.,** the surface of an anterior tooth (or of a denture) which faces the lip (*facies labialis dentis*). **lateral s.,** a surface nearer to or directed toward the side of the body (*facies lateralis* [NA]); in dentistry, the proximal surface of an incisor or canine tooth that is farthest from the midline of the dental arch. **lingual s.,** the surface of a tooth (or of a denture) which faces the tongue (*facies lingualis dentis* [NA]). **masticatory s.,** 1. facies occlusalis dentis. 2. facies masticatoria dentis. **medial s.,** a surface nearer to or directed toward the midline of the body (*facies medialis* [NA]); mesial s. **mesial s.,** in dentistry, the proximal or contact surface of the incisor or canine teeth that is closest to the midline of the dental arch; medial s. **morsal s's,** the occlusal surfaces of the mandibular and maxillary teeth which make contact in centric occlusion. **occlusal s.,** facies occlusalis dentis. **occlusal s., working,** facies masticatoria dentis. **polished s.,** one that is smoothed to a fine finish; in dentistry, that portion of the surface of a denture that is usually polished, including the palatal surface, and the buccal and lingual surfaces of the teeth. **posterior s.,** that surface which is toward the back of the body (on or nearest the dorsal aspect) in man (*facies posterior, facies dorsalis* [NA]), or toward the tail in quadrupeds; in dentistry, the surface of any tooth that is farthest from the midline of the dental arch. **posterior s. of sacrum,** facies dorsalis ossis sacri. **posterior s. of scapula,** facies dorsalis scapulae. **posterior s. of stomach,** paries posterior ventriculi. **proximal s.,** a surface that is nearer to a point of reference; used in dentistry to designate that surface of a tooth which faces an adjoining tooth in the same dental arch (*facies contactus dentis* [NA]). **proximate s.,** proximal s. **sacropelvic s. of the ilium,** facies sacropelvina ossis ilii. **suboccusal s.,** a portion of the surface of a tooth which is directed toward but does not make contact with the occlusal surface of its opposite number in the other jaw. **superior s.,** that surface which is upper or higher (toward the head, in man) (*facies superior* [NA]). **superior articular s. of atlas,** fovea articularis superior atlantis. **tentorial s.,** the portion of the cerebral surface that is in contact with the tentorium cerebelli. **ventral s.,** 1. the anterior surface, in man. 2. that surface which is lower, or on or nearest the abdominal aspect in quadrupeds. **vestibular s.,** the surface of a tooth that is directed outward toward the vestibule of the mouth, including the buccal and labial surfaces (*facies vestibularis dentis* [NA]); called also *facial s.*

surfactant (sur-fak′tant) a surface-active agent, such as soap or a synthetic detergent. In pulmonary physiology, a mixture of phospholipids (chiefly lecithin and sphingomyelin) secreted by the alveolar type II cells into the alveoli and respiratory air passages, which reduces the surface tension of pulmonary fluids and thus contributes to the elastic properties of pulmonary tissue.

Surfak (sur′fak) trademark for a preparation of docusate calcium.

surgeon (sur′jun) [L. *chirurgio;* Fr. *chirurgien*] 1. a physician who specializes in surgery. 2. the senior medical officer of a military unit. **acting assistant s.,** contract s. **barber s.,** formerly a barber who was authorized to practice surgery. **contract s.,** in the U.S. Army a physician or dentist engaged for temporary service in the medical department; called also *acting assistant surgeon.* **s. general,** 1. the chief of medical services in one of the armed forces. 2. the chief medical officer of the United States Bureau of Public Health, or of a state public health agency. 3. a member of the medical staff of the British Army. **house s.,** a surgeon resident in a hospital. **post s.,** the surgeon of an established army post.

surgery (sur′jer-e) [L. *chirurgia,* from Gr. *cheir* hand + *ergon* work] 1. that branch of medicine which treats diseases, injuries, and deformities by manual or operative methods. 2. the place in a hospital or doctor's or dentist's office where surgery is performed. 3. in Great Britain, a room or office where a doctor sees and treats patients. 4. the work performed by a surgeon. **abdominal s.,** surgery of the abdominal viscera. **antiseptic s.,** surgery conducted in accordance with antiseptic principles. **aseptic s.,** surgery performed in an environment so free from microorganisms that significant infection or suppuration does not supervene. **aural s.,** the surgical treatment of diseases of the ear. **bench s.,** surgery performed on an organ that has been removed from the body, after which it is reimplanted. **cardiac s.,** surgery of the heart. **cerebral s.,** that which deals with operations upon the brain. **cineplastic s.,** creation of a skin-lined tunnel through a muscle adjacent to the stump of an amputated limb, to permit use of the muscle in operating a prosthesis. **clinical s.,** the study of surgical disease by symptomatic analysis, examination, and observation. **conservative s.,** surgery designed to preserve, or to remove with minimal risk, diseased or injured organs, tissues, or extremities. Cf. *radical s.* **cosmetic s.,** that department of plastic surgery which deals with procedures designed to improve the patient's appearance by plastic restoration, correction, removal of blemishes, etc. **dental s.,** operative dentistry. **dentofacial s.,** that branch of the healing arts which deals with the surgical and adjunctive treatment of diseases, injuries, and defects involving the face and structures of the mouth. **general s.,** that which deals with surgical problems of all kinds. **ionic s.,** surgical ionization and electrolysis. **major s.,** surgery which involves the more important, difficult, and hazardous operations. **minor s.,** surgery restricted to the management of minor problems and injuries. **open heart s.,** surgery that involves incision into one or more chambers of the heart. **operative s.,** the operative or me-

chanical aspect of surgery; that which deals with manual and manipulative methods or procedures. **oral s.,** that branch of the healing arts which deals with the diagnosis and the surgical and adjunctive treatment of diseases, injuries, and defects of the mouth, the jaws, and associated structures. **orthopedic s.,** that branch of surgery which deals with the correction of deformities; orthopedics. **pelvic s.,** the surgery of the pelvis; chiefly in gynecological and obstetrical cases. **physiologic s.,** the indirect treatment of certain disorders by surgically altering normal physiologic functions. **plastic s.,** surgery concerned with the restoration, reconstruction, correction, or improvement in the shape and appearance of body structures that are defective, damaged or misshapened by injury, disease, or growth and development. **radical s.,** surgery designed to extirpate all areas of locally extensive disease and adjacent zones of lymphatic drainage; cf. *conservative s.* **reconstructive s.,** plastic s. **rectal s.,** the surgical treatment of diseases of the rectum. **sonic s.,** the use of focused ultrasonic waves to produce precisely circumscribed alterations within tissues at predetermined sites. **stereotactic s., stereotaxic s.,** a technique for the production of sharply circumscribed lesions in specific groups of cells in deep-seated brain structures after locating the discrete structure by means of three-dimensional coordinates; the lesions are made by such agents as heat, cold, x-ray or ultrasonic radiation, etc. Called also *stereoencephalotomy.* **structural s.,** surgery devoted to the correction of morphologic abnormalities. **veterinary s.,** the surgery of domestic animals.

surgibone (sur′jĭ-bōn) bone and cartilage obtained from bovine embryos and young calves, subjected to special processing to reduce antigenicity; it has been used as an internal bone splint in orthopedic and reconstructive surgery, but is used rarely now because of foreign body reaction.

surgical (sur′je-kal) of, pertaining to, or correctable by surgery.

Surgicel (sur′jĭ-sel) trademark for an absorbable knitted fabric prepared by controlled oxidation of cellulose, used as a hemostatic covering for surgical wounds to control hemorrhage when other conventional methods are impractical or ineffective.

surinamine (su-rin′ah-min) chemical name: paraoxyphenyl-alphamethylamino-propionic acid. A methyl tyrosine, $OH \cdot C_6H_4 \cdot CH_2 \cdot CH(COOH) \cdot NH \cdot CH_3$, found in many plants.

Surital (sur′ĭ-tal) trademark for preparations of sodium thiamylal.

surma (sur′mah) a lead sulfide (originally antimony sulfide) traditionally applied to the eyelids in India for cosmetic and medical purposes; it can be a source of lead poisoning.

surra (soor′ah) a disease of horses, camels, and other domestic animals in India, China, northern Africa, and the Philippine Islands, caused by an animal microparasite, the *Trypanosoma evansi.* It is marked by fever, petechia of mucous surfaces, edema, progressive anemia, and emaciation, ending in death. It is transmitted by the bite of gadflies or horseflies (Tabanidae) and probably also by fleas.

surrogate (sur′o-gāt) [L. *surrogatus* substituted] something used as a substitute for another. In psychoanalysis, an imagined person who conceals from conscious recognition the identity of that person, e.g., in dreams a king may represent the dreamer's father (*father s.*).

sursanure (sur-sān′ūr) an old name for a sore healed outwardly, but not inwardly.

sursumduction (sur″sum-duk′shun) [L. *sursum* upward + *ducere* to lead] the turning upward of a part, as of the eyes. Called also *supraduction.*

sursumvergence (sur″sum-ver′jens) [L. *sursum* upward + *vergere* to turn] an upward movement, especially of the eyes. Called also *supravergence.*

sursumversion (sur″sum-ver′zhun) [L. *sursum* upward + *vertere* to turn] an act of turning or directing upward; especially the simultaneous and equal upward turning of both eyes. Called also *supraversion.*

suruçucu (soo″roo-soo′koo) the bushmaster, *Lachesis muta,* a venomous snake of South America.

surveillance (sur-vāl′ans) in immunological theory, the constant monitoring of the body tissues by the immune (T-lymphocyte) system for abnormal cells.

susceptibility (sus-sep″tĭ-bil′ĭ-te) the state of being readily affected or acted upon. In immunology, the condition may be acquired, familial, individual, inherited, racial, etc., the same as is immunity. **differential s.,** nonhomogeneity in response by the various regions of an embryo when subjected to a diffusely applied injurious agent.

susceptible (sus-sep′tĭ-b'l) 1. capable of impression; readily acted on. 2. an individual who is not known to have become immune to an infectious disease by either natural or artificial means.

suscitate (sus′ĭ-tāt) to arouse to greater activity.

suscitation (sus″ĭ-ta′shun) [L. *suscitatio*] an arousal or excitation.

suspenopsia (sus″pen-op′se-ah) [L. *suspendere* to cause to waver + Gr. *opsis* vision + *-ia*] a condition of frequently occurring momentary suppression of attention in the visual cortex to impulses arising in the central retinal areas.

suspensiometer (sus-pen"se-om'ĕ-ter) nephelometer.

suspension (sus-pen'shun) [L. *suspensio*] 1. a condition of temporary cessation, as of animation, of pain, or of any vital process. 2. treatment, chiefly of spinal disorders, by suspending the patient by the chin and the shoulders. 3. a preparation of a finely divided drug intended to be incorporated (suspended) in some suitable liquid vehicle before it is used, or already incorporated in such a vehicle. **alumina and magnesia oral s.** [USP], a mixture of variable amounts of aluminum oxide, in the form of aluminum hydroxide and hydrated aluminum oxide, and magnesium hydroxide, which contains, on a weight/weight basis, the equivalent of 3.6 to 4 per cent aluminum oxide, 1.7 to 2.2 per cent magnesium hydroxide, and 5.3 to 6.2 per cent combined aluminum oxide and magnesium hydroxide; used as an antacid. **ampicillin for oral s.** [USP], a suspension containing 90 to 120 per cent of the labeled amount of ampicillin (anhydrous or as the trihydrate); used as an antibacterial against gram-negative bacteria. **betamethasone sodium phosphate and betamethasone acetate s., sterile** [USP], a sterile preparation of betamethasone sodium phosphate in solution and betamethasone acetate in suspension in water for injection, containing betamethasone sodium phosphate equivalent to 90 to 115 per cent of the labeled amount of betamethasone and 90 to 115 per cent of the labeled amount of betamethasone acetate; used as an anti-inflammatory glucocorticoid. **cephalic s.,** suspension of a patient by the head in order to make extension of the vertebral column. **chloramphenicol palmitate oral s.** [USP], a suspension containing 90 to 120 per cent of the labeled amount of chloramphenicol palmitate; used as an antibacterial and antirickettsial. **chlorothiazide oral s.** [USP], a suspension containing 90 to 110 per cent of the labeled amount of chlorothiazide; used as a diuretic and antihypertensive. **cholestyramine for oral s.** [USP], a mixture of cholestyramine resin, containing 85–115 per cent of the labeled amount of dried cholestyramine resin; used as an ion-exchange resin for bile salts for the relief of pruritus associated with cholestasis occurring in partial biliary obstruction and as adjunctive therapy to diet in the management of elevated cholesterol due to primary type II hyperlipoproteinemia (patients with pure hypercholesterolemia). **colistin sulfate for oral s.** [USP], a preparation containing colistin sulfate equivalent to 90–120 per cent of the labeled amount of colistin activity; used in the treatment of *Shigella* and intestinal *Pseudomonas* infections, and infant diarrhea due to *Escherichia coli* and susceptible gram-negative organisms. **colloid s.,** a suspension in which the suspended particles are very small. **corticotropin hydroxide s., sterile** [USP], a sterile suspension of corticotropin with prolonged action, adsorbed on zinc hydroxide; administered intramuscularly for diagnostic testing of adrenocortical function and to stimulate adrenal cortex activity. **cortisone acetate s., sterile** [USP], a sterile suspension of cortisone acetate in a suitable aqueous medium, containing 90 to 110 per cent of the labeled amount of total steroids, calculated as cortisone acetate; administered intramuscularly as an anti-inflammatory adrenocortical steroid. **cortisone acetate ophthalmic s.** [USP], a sterile suspension of cortisone acetate in an aqueous medium containing a suitable antimicrobial agent and 90 to 110 per cent of the labeled amount of total steroids, calculated as cortisone acetate; applied topically to the conjunctiva as an anti-inflammatory adrenocortical steroid. **demeclocycline oral s.** [USP], a suspension containing demeclocycline equivalent to not less than 85 per cent of the labeled amount of demeclocycline hydrochloride; used as an antibacterial. **desoxycorticosterone pivalate s., sterile** [USP], a sterile suspension containing 90 to 110 per cent of the labeled amount of desoxycorticosterone pivalate in an aqueous medium; used as a mineralocorticoid for replacement therapy in adrenocortical insufficiency in Addison's disease and in the treatment of salt-losing adrenogenital syndrome, administered intramuscularly. **dicloxacillin sodium for oral s.** [USP], a dry mixture containing the equivalent of 90–120 per cent of the labeled amount of dicloxacillin; used as an antibacterial, primarily in the treatment of penicillinase-resistant staphylococci. **diphenylhydantoin oral s.,** phenytoin oral s. **epinephrine oil s., sterile** [USP], a sterile suspension of epinephrine in a suitable vegetable oil, containing, in each milliliter, 1.8 to 2.4 mg. of epinephrine; an adrenergic as a bronchodilator. **estradiol s., sterile** [USP], a sterile suspension containing 90 to 110 per cent of the labeled amount of estradiol in water for injection; used as an estrogen. **hydrocortisone acetate s., sterile** [USP], a sterile suspension containing 90–100 per cent of total steroids, calculated as hydrocortisone acetate, in a suitable aqueous medium; used in various conditions responsive to the anti-inflammatory action of glucocorticoids, administered by intra-articular injection or soft-tissue infiltration. **hydrocortisone acetate ophthalmic s.** [USP], a sterile suspension of hydrocortisone acetate in an aqueous medium containing a suitable antimicrobial agent and 90 to 110 per cent of the labeled amount of total steroids, calculated as hydrocortisone acetate; applied topically to the conjunctiva as an anti-inflammatory adrenocortical hormone. **hydrocortisone cypionate oral s.** [NF], a preparation containing hydrocorti-

sone cypionate equivalent to 90–110 per cent of the labeled amount of hydrocortisone; used in the treatment of various conditions responsive to the anti-inflammatory action of glucocorticoids. **hydroxyzine pamoate oral s.** [USP], a suspension containing hydroxyzine pamoate equivalent to 90 to 110 per cent of the labeled amount of hydroxyzine hydrochloride; used as a minor tranquilizer. **insulin zinc s.** [USP], a sterile suspension of insulin modified by the addition of zinc chloride, so that the solid phase consists of approximately 7 parts of crystalline insulin and 3 parts of amorphous insulin, containing 40, 80, or 100 USP insulin units per ml., and having an intermediate action; administered subcutaneously in the treatment of diabetes mellitus. Called also *insulin lente.* **insulin zinc s., extended** [USP], a sterile suspension of insulin modified by the addition of zinc chloride, so that the solid phase is predominantly crystalline insulin, containing 40, 80, or 100 USP insulin units per ml., and having a prolonged action; administered subcutaneously in the treatment of diabetes mellitus. Called also *ultralente insulin.* **insulin zinc s., prompt** [USP], a sterile suspension of insulin modified by the addition of zinc chloride, so that the solid phase is amorphous, containing 40, 80, or 100 USP insulin units per ml., and having a rapid action; administered subcutaneously in the treatment of diabetes mellitus. Called also *semilente insulin.* **ipodate calcium for oral s.** [USP], a dry mixture of calcium ipodate and one or more suitable suspending, dispersing, or flavoring agents; used as a radiopaque medium in cholecystography. **isophane insulin s.** [USP], a sterile suspension made from zinc-insulin crystals modified by the addition of protamine in buffered water for injection, containing 40, 80, or 100 USP insulin units per ml., and having an intermediate action; administered subcutaneously in the treatment of diabetes mellitus. Called also *NPH insulin.* **levopropoxyphene napsylate oral s.** [USP], a preparation containing an amount of levopropoxyphene napsylate equivalent to 90–110 per cent of the labeled amount of levopropoxyphene; used as an antitussive. **magaldrate oral s.** [USP], a suspension containing the equivalent of 2.5 to 3.0 per cent (w/w) of magnesium oxide and the equivalent of 1.5 to 2.0 per cent (w/w) of aluminum oxide; used as an antacid. **magnesia and alumina oral s.** [USP], a mixture containing magnesium hydroxide, and variable amounts of aluminum oxide in the form of aluminum hydroxide and hydrated aluminum oxide; used as an antacid. **medroxyprogesterone acetate s., sterile** [USP], a sterile suspension in a suitable aqueous medium containing 90 to 110 per cent of the labeled amount of medroxyprogesterone acetate; used as a progestin in the treatment of endometriosis, uterine cancer, habitual and threatened abortion, and menstrual disorders, administered intramuscularly. **medrysone ophthalmic s.** [USP], a sterile suspension containing 90–115 per cent of the labeled amount of medrysone in a buffered aqueous medium; used as a topical anti-inflammatory in allergic and inflammatory eye conditions, such as episcleritis, allergic and vernal conjunctivitis, and epinephrine sensitivity. **meprobamate oral s.** [USP], a suspension containing 95 to 110 per cent of the labeled amount of meprobamate; used as a sedative. **methacycline hydrochloride oral s.** [USP], a suspension containing 90 to 125 per cent of the labeled amount of methacycline base and one or more suitable and harmless buffers, dispersants, colorings, flavorings, and preservatives; used as an antibacterial. **methenamine mandelate oral s.** [USP], a suspension of methenamine mandelate in vegetable oil, containing 90 to 110 per cent of the labeled amount of methenamine mandelate; used as a urinary antibacterial. **methylprednisolone acetate s., sterile** [USP], a sterile solution containing 90 to 110 per cent of the labeled amount of methylprednisolone acetate in a suitable aqueous medium; used as an anti-inflammatory glucocorticoid. **nitrofurantoin oral s.** [USP], a suspension of nitrofurantoin in a suitable aqueous vehicle, containing, in each 100 ml., 460 to 540 mg. of nitrofurantoin; used as a urinary antibacterial. **novobiocin calcium oral s.,** a suspension of novobiocin calcium in an aqueous vehicle, containing, in each 100 ml., novobiocin calcium equivalent to 2.25–3 gm. of novobiocin (as the free acid), one or more suitable suspending agents, colors, flavors, and preservatives; used as an antibacterial, chiefly in the treatment of infections in children due to staphylococci and other gram-positive organisms resistant to other antibiotics. **oxytetracycline calcium oral s.** [NF], a suspension containing 90–120 per cent of the labeled amount of oxytetracycline calcium in an aqueous vehicle containing one or more suitable suspending agents, flavors, colors, and preservatives; used as an antibacterial in various tetracycline-responsive conditions. **penicillin G benzathine s., sterile** [USP], a sterile suspension of penicillin G benzathine in water for injection with one or more suitable dispersing agents, buffers, and antimicrobial agents; used as an antibacterial in the treatment of infections due to penicillin G–susceptible organisms, administered intramuscularly. **penicillin G procaine s., sterile** [USP], a sterile suspension of procaine penicillin G in water for injection and one or more suitable suspending or dispersing agents and buffers; administered intramuscularly as an antibacterial in the treatment of infections due to penicillin G–susceptible organisms. **penicillin G procaine with aluminum stearate s., sterile** [USP], a sterile suspension of procaine penicillin G in refined peanut oil or sesame oil that has been gelled with 2 per cent of aluminum monostearate; used as an antibacterial in penicillin G–susceptible organisms, administered intramuscularly. **penicillin V benzathine oral s.** [USP], a preparation containing penicillin V benzathine equivalent to not less than 85 per cent of the labeled amount of penicillin V; used as an antibacterial in infections due to penicillin-susceptible organisms. **penicillin V hydrabamine oral s.** [USP], a preparation containing penicillin V hydrabamine equivalent to 90–125 per cent of the labeled amount of penicillin V; used as an antibacterial in the treatment of infections due to penicillin-susceptible organisms. **phensuximide oral s.** [USP], a suspension containing 90 to 110 per cent of the labeled amount of phensuximide; used as an anticonvulsant. **phenytoin oral s.** [USP], a suspension containing 90–110 per cent of the labeled amount of phenytoin in a suitable medium; used as an anticonvulsant in the treatment of all forms of epilepsy except petit mal. Called also *diphenylhydantoin oral s.* **prednisolone acetate s., sterile** [USP], a sterile suspension of prednisolone acetate in a suitable aqueous medium, containing 90 to 110 per cent of the labeled amount of prednisolone acetate; used as an anti-inflammatory in the treatment of various glucocorticoid-responsive conditions, administered intra-articularly or intramuscularly. **primidone oral s.** [USP], a suspension of primidone in a suitable aqueous vehicle, containing, in each 100 ml., 4.5 to 5.5 gm. of primidone; used as an anticonvulsant. **progesterone s., sterile** [USP], a sterile suspension containing 93 to 107 per cent of the labeled amount of progesterone in water for injection; used as a progestin in the treatment of functional uterine bleeding, menstrual disorders, and threatened abortion, administered intramuscularly. **propoxyphene napsylate oral s.** [USP], a preparation containing 90–110 per cent of the labeled amount of propoxyphene napsylate; used as an analgesic. **propyliodone s., sterile** [USP], a sterile suspension of propyliodone in water for injection, containing 47.5 to 52.5 per cent of propyliodone and a suitable suspending or dispersing agent; used as a radiopaque medium in bronchography. **propyliodone oil s., sterile**, a sterile suspension of propyliodone in peanut oil, containing 57 to 63 per cent of propyliodone; used as a radiopaque medium in bronchography. **protamine zinc insulin s.** [USP], a sterile suspension of insulin modified by the addition of zinc chloride and protamine, having a prolonged action; used as a hypoglycemic. Abbreviated PZI. **pyrantel pamoate oral s.** [USP], a suspension containing 90–110 per cent of the labeled amount of pyrantel in a suitable aqueous vehicle; used as an anthelmintic in the treatment of ascariasis and enterobiasis. **pyrvinium pamoate oral s.** [USP], a suspension containing, in each 100 ml., an amount of pyrvinium pamoate equivalent to 0.90 to 1.10 gm. of pyrvinium; used as an anthelmintic in the treatment of enterobiasis. **salicylamide oral s.**, a suspension containing 93 to 107 per cent of the labeled amount of salicylamide; used as an analgesic. **selenium sulfide detergent s.**, an aqueous, stabilized suspension of selenium sulfide containing a suitable dispersing agent, buffer, and detergent, and containing between 90 and 110 per cent selenium sulfide; used as an antiseborrheic shampoo to control seborrheic dermatitis and dandruff. **simethicone oral s.** [USP], a suspension containing 90–110 per cent of the labeled amount of dimethicone; used as an antiflatulent. **sitosterols s.**, a suspension containing 90 to 110 per cent of the labeled amount of sitosterols; used as an anticholesterolemic. **sulfacetamide, sulfadiazine, and sulfamerazine oral s.**, a suspension containing 90 to 110 per cent of the labeled amounts of sulfacetamide, sulfadiazine, and sulfamerazine; used as an antibacterial. **sulfadimethoxine oral s.** [USP], a suspension containing 93 to 107 per cent of the labeled amount of sulfadimethoxine; used as an antibacterial. **sulfamethizole oral s.** [USP], a buffered aqueous suspension containing 90 to 110 per cent of the labeled amount of sulfamethizole; used as an antibacterial. **sulfamethoxazole oral s.** [USP], a suspension containing 95 to 110 per cent of the labeled amount of sulfamethoxazole; used as an antibacterial. **sulfisoxazole acetyl oral s.** [USP], a suspension containing sulfisoxazole acetyl equivalent to 93 to 107 per cent of the labeled amount of sulfisoxazole; used as an antibacterial in a wide variety of infections due to sulfonamide-susceptible organisms, usually given to infants and children. **testolactone s., sterile** [USP], a suspension containing 90–110 per cent of the labeled amount of testolactone in a suitable aqueous medium; used as an antineoplastic agent for adjunctive therapy in the palliative treatment of advanced or disseminated breast cancer in postmenopausal women; administered orally or by intramuscular injection. **testosterone s., sterile** [USP], a suspension containing 90 to 110 per cent of the labeled amount of testosterone in an aqueous medium; used as an androgen chiefly in the treatment of male hypogonadism, cryptorchidism, and the symptoms of the male climacteric; administered intramuscularly. **tetracycline oral s.** [USP], tetracycline suspended in one or more suitable suspending and dispersing agents, containing 90 to 120 per cent of the labeled amount of tetracycline hydrochloride; used as an antiamebic, antibacterial, and antirickettsial. **thiabendazole oral s.** [USP], a suspension containing 90 to 110 per cent of the labeled amount of thiabendazole; used as an anthelmintic in the treatment of pinworm, threadworm, whipworm, roundworm,

and hookworm infections, and in cutaneous larva migrans. **triamcinolone acetonide s., sterile** [USP], a sterile suspension of triamcinolone acetonide in a suitable aqueous medium, containing 90 to 115 per cent of the labeled amount of triamcinolone acetonide; administered intra-articularly or intramuscularly as an anti-inflammatory adrenocortical steroid. **triamcinolone diacetate s., sterile** [USP], a sterile suspension containing 90 to 115 per cent of the labeled amount of triamcinolone diacetate in a suitable aqueous medium; used as an anti-inflammatory glucocorticoid. **triamcinolone hexacetonide s., sterile** [USP], a sterile suspension of triamcinolone hexacetonide in a suitable aqueous medium, containing 90–115 per cent of the labeled amount of triamcinolone hexacetonide; administered by intra-articular, intralesional, and sublesional injection in conditions responsive to the anti-inflammatory action of glucocorticoids. **trisulfapyrimidines oral s.** [USP], a suspension of sulfadiazine, sulfamerazine, and sulfamethazine, used as an antibacterial agent. **troleandomycin oral s.**, a suspension containing 90 to 120 per cent of the labeled amount of troleandomycin and one or more suitable suspending and dispersing agents, colors, flavors, buffers, and preservatives in an aqueous vehicle; used as an antibacterial, chiefly in the treatment of infections due to staphylococci and other gram-positive bacteria resistant to other systemic antibiotics.

suspensoid (sus-pen'soid) suspension colloid.

suspensorius (sus"pen-so're-us) [L.] suspensory.

suspensory (sus-pen'so-re) [L. *suspensorius*] 1. serving to hold up a part. 2. a ligament, bone, muscle, sling, or bandage which serves to hold up a part.

Sus-Phrine (sus'frin) trademark for a preparation of epinephrine.

suspirious (sus-pi're-us) breathing heavily; sighing.

sustentacular (sus"ten-tak'u-lar) [L. *sustentare* to support] pertaining to a sustentaculum; serving to support; see *supporting cells,* under cell, and see under *tissue.*

sustentaculum (sus"ten-tak'u-lum), pl. *sustentac'ula* [L.] a support. **s. lie'nis,** ligamentum phrenicolienale. **s. ta'li** [NA], **s. of talus,** a process of the calcaneus which supports the talus.

susto (soos'to) a mental disturbance seen chiefly in South America, consisting of panic reactions due to fear of the evil eye, black magic, and spirit possession.

susurrus (su-sur'us) [L.] murmur.

sutika (su'tik-ah) a disease of pregnant women of Bengal, marked by digestive troubles and fever during pregnancy, with progressive pernicious anemia occurring after delivery.

sutilains (soo'tĭ-lāns) [USP] a substance containing proteolytic enzymes derived from *Bacillus subtilis*, occurring as a cream-colored powder; used as a proteolytic agent for débridement of wounds.

Sutton's disease (sut'onz) [Richard L. *Sutton,* Jr., American dermatologist, born 1908] periadenitis mucosa necrotica recurrens.

Sutton's nevus (disease) (sut'onz) [Richard Lightburn *Sutton,* American dermatologist, 1878–1952] halo nevus.

sutura (su-tu'rah), pl. *sutu'rae* [L. "a seam"] [NA] a type of fibrous joint in which the apposed bony surfaces are so closely united by a very thin layer of fibrous connective tissue that no movement can occur; found only in the skull. Called also *suture, sutura vera,* and *true suture.* **s. corona'lis** [NA], coronal suture: the line of junction of the frontal bone with the two parietal bones. **sutu'rae cra'nii** [NA], cranial sutures: the sutures between the various bones of the skull, named generally for the specific components participating in their formation. **s. denta'ta,** s. serrata. **s. ethmoidomaxilla'ris** [NA], ethmoidomaxillary suture: the line of junction between the orbital lamina of the ethmoid bone and the orbital surface of the maxilla. **s. fronta'lis** [NA], frontal suture: the usually transient line of junction between the right and left halves of the frontal bone. The inferior part often persists in the adult; if the entire suture persists, it is called the metopic suture. **s. frontoethmoida'lis** [NA], frontoethmoidal suture: the line of junction in the anterior cranial fossa between the frontal bone and the cribriform plate of the ethmoid bone. **s. frontolacrima'lis** [NA], frontolacrimal suture: the line of junction between the upper edge of the lacrimal bone and the orbital part of the frontal bone. **s. frontomaxilla'ris** [NA], frontomaxillary suture: the line of junction between the frontal bone and the frontal process of the maxilla. **s. frontonasa'lis** [NA], frontonasal suture: the line of junction between the frontal and the two nasal bones; called also *s. nasofrontalis* or *nasofrontal suture.* **s. frontozygomat'ica** [NA], frontozygomatic suture: the line of junction between the zygomatic bone and the zygomatic process of the frontal bone; called also *s. zygomaticofrontalis,* or *zygomaticofrontal suture.* **s. harmo'nia,** s. plana. **s. incisi'va** [NA], incisive suture: an indistinct suture sometimes seen extending laterally from the incisive fossa to the space between the canine tooth and the lateral incisor, indicating the line of fusion between the premaxilla and the maxilla. **s. infraorbita'lis** [NA], infraorbital suture: a suture sometimes seen extending from the infraorbital foramen to the infraorbital groove. **s. intermaxilla′ris** [NA], intermaxillary suture: the line of junction between the maxillary bones of either side, just below the anterior nasal spine. **s. internasa′lis** [NA], internasal suture: the line of junction between the two nasal bones. **s. lacrimoconcha′lis** [NA], lacrimoconchal suture: the line of junction between the lacrimal bone and the inferior nasal concha. **s. lacrimomaxilla′ris** [NA], lacrimomaxillary suture: a suture on the inner wall of the orbit, between the lacrimal bone and the maxilla. **s. lambdoi′dea** [NA], lambdoid suture: the line of junction between the occipital and parietal bones, shaped like the Greek letter lambda. **s. limbo′sa**, a type of suture in which there is interlocking of the beveled surfaces the bones. **s. nasofronta′lis**, s. frontonasalis. **s. nasomaxilla′ris** [NA], nasomaxillary suture: the line of junction between the lateral edge of the nasal bone and the frontal process of the maxilla. **s. no′tha**, a type of suture formed by apposition of the roughened surfaces of the two participating bones. **s. occipitomastoi′dea** [NA], occipitomastoid suture: an extension of the lamboid suture between the occipital bone and the posterior edge of the mastoid portion of the temporal bone. **s. palati′na media′na** [NA], median palatine suture: the line of junction between the horizontal part of the palatine bones of either side. **s. palati′na transver′sa** [NA], transverse palatine suture. the line of junction between the palatine processes of the maxillae and the horizontal parts of the palatine bones. **s. palatoethmoida′lis** [NA], palatoethmoidal suture: the line of junction between the orbital process of the palatine bone and the orbital lamina of the ethmoid bone. **s. palatomaxilla′ris** [NA], palatomaxillary suture: the suture in the floor of the orbit, between the orbital processes of the palatine bone and the orbital portion of the maxilla. **s. parietomastoi′dea** [NA], parietomastoid suture: the line of junction between the posterior inferior angle of the parietal bone and the mastoid process of the temporal bone. **s. pla′na** [NA], flat suture: a type of suture in which there is simple apposition of the contiguous surfaces, with no interlocking of the edges of the participating bones. **s. sag′ittalis** [NA], sagittal suture: the line of junction between the two parietal bones. **s. serra′ta** [NA], serrated suture: a type of suture in which the participating bones are united by interlocking processes resembling the teeth of a saw. **s. sphenoethmoida′lis** [NA], sphenoethmoidal suture: the line of junction between the body of the sphenoid bone and the orbital lamina of the ethmoid bone. **s. sphenofronta′lis** [NA], sphenofrontal suture: a long suture joining the orbital part of the frontal bone to the greater and lesser wings of the sphenoid bone on either side of the skull. **s. sphenomaxilla′ris** [NA], sphenomaxillary suture: a suture occasionally seen between the pterygoid process of the sphenoid bone and the maxilla. **s. sphenoorbi′talis**, spheno-orbital suture: the line or junction between the orbital process of the palatine bone and the body of the sphenoid bone. **s. sphenoparieta′lis** [NA], sphenoparietal suture: the line of junction between the great wing of the sphenoid bone and the parietal bone. **s. sphenosquamo′sa** [NA], sphenosquamous suture: the line of junction between the great wing of the sphenoid bone and the squamous part of the temporal bone. **s. sphenozygomat′ica** [NA], sphenozygomatic suture: the line of junction between the great wing of the sphenoid bone and the zygomatic bone. **s. squamo′sa** [NA], squamous suture: a type of suture formed by overlapping of the broad beveled edges of the participating bones. **s. squamo′sa cra′nii** [NA], squamous suture of cranium: the suture between the squamous part of the temporal bone and the parietal bone. **s. squamosomastoi′dea** [NA], squamosomastoid suture: a suture existing early in life between the squamous and mastoid portions of the temporal bone. **s. temporozygomat′ica** [NA], temporozygomatic suture: the line of junction between the zygomatic process of the temporal bone and the temporal process of the zygomatic bone; called also *s. zygomaticotemporalis.* **s. ve′ra**, a true suture, in which no movement of the participating bones can occur. See *sutura.* **s. zygomaticofronta′lis**, s. frontozygomatica. **s. zygomaticomaxilla′ris** [NA], zygomaticomaxillary suture: the line of junction between the zygomatic bone and the zygomatic process of the maxilla. **s. zygomaticotempora′lis**, s. temporozygomatica.

suturae (su-tu′re) plural of *sutura.*

sutural (su″tu-ral) of or pertaining to a suture.

suturation (su″tu-ra′shun) the act or process of suturing.

suture (su′chur) [L. *sutura* a seam] 1. a type of fibrous joint in which the opposed surfaces are closely united, as in the skull; see *sutura.* 2. material used in closing a surgical or traumatic wound with stitches. 3. a stitch or series of stitches made to secure apposition of the edges of a surgical or accidental wound; used also as a verb to indicate the application of such stitches. 4. the act or process of uniting a wound by stitches. **absorbable s.,** a strand of material used for closing wounds which is subsequently dissolved by the tissue fluids. **absorbable surgical s.** [USP], a sterile strand prepared from collagen derived from healthy animals, which is available in various diameters and tensile strengths. It is capable of being absorbed by living mammalian tissue, but may be treated to modify its resistance to absorption. It may be impregnated with a suitable antimicrobial

agent, and may be colored by a color additive approved by the federal Food and Drug Administration. **Albert's s.,** a form of Czerny suture in which the first row of stitches is passed through the entire thickness of the intestine. **Appolito's s.,** Gély's s. **apposition s.,** a superficial suture used for the exact approximation of the cutaneous edges of a wound. **approximation s.,** a deep suture for securing apposition of the deep tissues of a wound. **arcuate s.,** sutura coronalis. **atraumatic s.,** a suture fused into the end of a small eyeless needle. **basilar s.,** fissura sphenooccipitalis. **bastard s.,** false s. **Bell's s.,** a form of lock-stitch in which the needle is passed from within outward alternately on the two edges of the wound. **biparietal s.,** sutura sagittalis. **bolster s.,** a suture the ends of which are tied over a tiny roll of gauze or a piece of rubber tubing, in order to lessen the pressure on the skin. **bony s.,** sutura. **bregmatomastoid s.,** sutura parietomastoidea. **buried s.,** one that is placed deep in the tissues and concealed by the skin. **button s.,** one in which the stitch is passed through a button-like disk to prevent the suture material from cutting through the skin. **catgut s.,** see *catgut.* **chain s.,** a continuous suture in which each loop of thread is caught by the next adjacent loop. **circular s.,** one that is applied to the entire circumference of a hollow viscus to secure closure, or to a portion of a visceral wall to achieve inversion of the enclosed circular area. **coaptation s.,** apposition s. **cobblers′ s.,** one made with suture material threaded through a needle at each end. **Connell s.,** a U-shaped continuous suture used in intestinal anastomosis, the stitches being placed parallel to and about 4 mm. from the edge of the wound, and passing through all the layers of the bowel. **continuous s.,** one in which a continuous, uninterrupted length of material is used to approximate the cut edges of one or more layers of tissues. **continuous running s.,** a suture with a knot at only the beginning and end of a sutured incision. **coronal s.,** sutura coronalis. **cranial s′s,** the lines of junction between the bones of the skull; see *suturae cranii* [NA]. **Cushing s.,** a continuous inverting suture used for closing the seromuscular layers in surgery of the gastrointestinal tract. **cutaneous s. of palate,** raphe palati. **Czerny's s.,** 1. an intestinal suture in which the thread is passed through the mucous membrane alone. 2. a method of uniting a ruptured tendon by splitting one of the ends and suturing the other end into the slit. **Czerny-Lembert s.,** a combination of Czerny and Lembert sutures in circular enterorrhaphy. **dentate s.,** sutura serrata. **double-button s.,** a form of stitch in which the suture material is passed deep across the edges of the wound, between two buttons placed on the surface of the skin, one on either side of the suture line. **Dupuytren's s.,** a continuous Lembert suture. **ethmoidomaxillary s.,** sutura ethmoidomaxillaris. **everting s.,** a method by which the approximated edges of a wound are everted; used in early blood vessel surgery to achieve apposition of the tunica intima of the divided segments. **everting interrupted s.,** an interrupted suture done by inserting the needle into the skin close to the incision line and diverging from the edge of the wound in order to encircle a larger amount of tissue in the lower depths of the skin than at the periphery. **false s.,** a line of junction between apposed surfaces, without fibrous union of the bones. **figure-of-eight s.,** one in which the thread follows the contours of the figure 8. **flat s.,** sutura plana. **frontal s.,** sutura frontalis. **frontoethmoidal s.,** sutura frontoethmoidalis. **frontolacrimal s.,** sutura frontolacrimalis. **frontomalar s.,** sutura frontozygomatica. **frontomaxillary s.,** sutura frontomaxillaris. **frontonasal s.,** sutura frontonasalis. **frontoparietal s.,** sutura coronalis. **frontosphenoid s.,** sutura sphenofrontalis. **frontozygomatic s.,** sutura frontozygomatica. **furrier's s.,** a method of stitching intestinal wounds by piercing first one margin of the incision and then the other from within outward; overlying sutures are placed through the seromuscular layers to reinforce the closure and prevent leakage. **Gaillard-Arlt s.,** a suture used in correction of entropion. **Gély's s.,** a continuous suture for repair of intestinal wounds, made by a thread with a needle at each end, and consisting of a series of cross-stitches closing the wound. **glovers′ s.,** lock-stitch s. **s. of Goethe,** sutura incisiva. **Gussenbauer's s.,** a figure-of-eight suture used in repairing a rent of the intestine. **Halsted s.,** a modification of the Lembert suture, consisting of a stitch parallel to the wound on one side, with the two free ends of the material emerging on the other side, where they are tied. **harelip s.,** a figure-of-eight suture used in the correction of harelip. **hemostatic s′s,** sutures used to control oozing of blood from raw areas. **incisive s.,** sutura incisiva. **infraorbital s.,** sutura infraorbitalis. **interdermal buried s.,** a suture with the knot placed downward in the lower layers of dermis. **interendognathic s.,** sutura palatina mediana. **intermaxillary s.,** sutura intermaxillaris. **internasal s.,** sutura internasalis. **interparietal s.,** sutura sagittalis. **interrupted s.,** a type of suture in which each stitch is made with a separate piece of material. **intradermal mattress s.,** a mattress suture below the level of the skin. **intradermic s.,** a suture applied parallel with the edges of the wound, but within the layers of the skin, usually a continuous stitch. **inverting s.,** a seromuscular stitch used in intestinal anastomosis to appose and invert the serosal surfaces of the two segments, as in the Cushing or Lembert suture. **jugal s.**, sutura sagittalis. **lacrimoconchal s.**, sutura lacrimoconchalis. **lacrimoethmoidal s.**, the vertical line of junction, on the medial wall of the orbit, between the lacrimal bone and the orbital plate of the ethmoid bone. **lacrimomaxillary s.**, sutura lacrimomaxillaris. **lacrimoturbinal s.**, sutura lacrimoconchalis. **lambdoid s.**, sutura lambdoidea. **Le Dentu's s.**, for a divided tendon: two stitches are passed on each side, right and left, and are tied in front; a third is taken from right to left above and below the cut, and is tied on one side. **Le Fort's s.**, for a divided tendon: a single loop is passed above the cut, entering at one side, coming out and going in in front; it is then passed below the cut at each side, coming out in front, and is there tied. **Lembert s.**, an inverting suture commonly used in gastrointestinal surgery: the needle is inserted about 2.5 mm. lateral to the incision, through the serous and muscular tunics but not the submucosa, and brought out near the edge of the incision, then inserted near the edge on the opposite side and brought out at the more distant point, without having entered the lumen of the gut. It may be either interrupted or continuous. **lock-stitch s.**, a continuous hemostatic suture used in intestinal surgery: the needle is passed through all layers of the bowel and the loop of suture material is made to fall over the point of emergence of the needle, which comes up through the loop, forming a self-locking stitch when the strand is pulled taut. **longitudinal s.**, sutura sagittalis. **longitudinal s. of palate**, sutura palatina mediana. **loop s.**, interrupted s. **malomaxillary s.**, sutura zygomaticomaxillaris. **mamillary s., mastoid s.**, sutura occipitomastoidea. **mattress s., horizontal,** a method in which the stitches are made parallel with the edges of the wound, the suture material crossing deeply from one side to the other. **mattress s., right-angle,** mattress s., vertical. **mattress s., vertical,** a method in which the stitches are made at right angles to the edges of the wound, taking both deep and superficial bites of tissue, the latter achieving more exact apposition of the cutaneous margins. **metopic s.**, a name given the frontal suture when it persists in the adult skull. **nasal s.**, sutura internasalis. **nasofrontal s.**, sutura frontonasalis. **nasomaxillary s.**, sutura nasomaxillaris. **nerve s.**, uniting a divided nerve by suturing; neurorrhaphy. **nonabsorbable s.**, material for closing wounds which is not absorbed in the body, e.g., silk, cotton, and stainless steel, or synthetic material such as nylon. **nonabsorbable surgical s.** [USP], a strand of material, either sterile or unsterilized, suitably resistant to the action of living mammalian tissue, which is available in various diameters and tensile strengths. It may be modified with respect to body or texture, or to reduce capillarity, impregnated or coated with a suitable antimicrobial agent, suitably bleached, and colored with a color additive approved by the federal Food and Drug Administration. **occipital s.**, sutura lambdoidea. **occipitomastoid s.**, sutura occipitomastoidea. **occipitoparietal s.**, sutura lambdoidea. **occipitosphenoidal s.**, fissura sphenooccipitalis. **over-and-over s.**, a method in which equal bites of tissue are taken on each side of the wound; it may be either interrupted or continuous. **overlapping s.**, a squamous suture (sutura squamosa), such as the sutura squamosa cranii. **palatine s., anterior,** sutura incisiva. **palatine s., median, palatine s., middle,** sutura palatina mediana. **palatine s., posterior, palatine s., transverse,** sutura palatina transversa. **palatoethmoidal s.**, sutura palatoethmoidalis. **palatomaxillary s.**, sutura palatomaxillaris. **Pancoast's s.**, a form of tongue-in-groove suture; see plastic s. **Paré's s.**, the use of strips of cloth applied along the edges of a wound, and then stitched together to bring the margins of the wound into apposition. **parietal s.**, sutura sagittalis. **parietomastoid s.**, sutura parietomastoidea. **parietooccipital s.**, sutura lambdoidea. **petrobasilar s., petrosphenobasilar s.**, synchondrosis petrooccipitalis. **petrosphenooccipital s. of Gruber,** fissura petrooccipitalis. **petrosquamous s.**, fissura petrosquamosa. **plastic s.**, a method in which a tongue is cut in one lip of the wound and a groove in the other, the tongue and groove then being stitched together, and the ends of the thread tied over a roll of adhesive plaster. **premaxillary s.**, sutura incisiva. **presection s.**, a stitch or series of stitches placed in the tissues before an incision is made. **primary s.**, prompt surgical closure of a wound. **pursestring s.**, a continuous, circular inverting suture commonly used to bury the stump of the appendix. **quilt s., quilted s.**, a continuous mattress suture. **relaxation s.**, any suture placed to close a wound but so formed that it may be loosened in order to relieve the tension should it become too great. **retention s.**, a reinforcing suture for abdominal wounds, utilizing exceptionally strong material like braided silk, stainless steel, or silkworm gut, and including a large amount of tissue in each stitch; intended to relieve pressure on the primary suture line and prevent postoperative disruption. **rhabdoid s.**, sutura sagittalis. **sagittal s.**, sutura sagittalis. **scaly s.**, sutura squamosa. **secondary s.**, 1. delayed closure of an operative or accidental wound, usually because of the presence or expectation of infection. 2. resuture of an operative wound following disruption. **seroserous s.**, a suture which apposes two serous surfaces. **serrated s.**, sutura serrata. **shotted s.**, one in which the two ends of the suture wire are passed through a split or perforated shot, which is then compressed. **silkworm gut s.**, material prepared from the entrails of the silkworm, for use in the closure of wounds, usually as nonabsorbable supporting sutures in large abdominal wounds. **Sims's s.**, a shotted suture. **s's of skull,** suturae cranii. **sphenoethmoidal s.**, sutura sphenoethmoidalis. **sphenofrontal s.**, sutura sphenofrontalis. **sphenomalar s.**, sutura sphenozygomatica. **sphenomaxillary s.**, sutura sphenomaxillaris. **sphenooccipital s.**, fissura sphenooccipitalis. **sphenoorbital s.**, sutura sphenoorbitalis. **sphenoparietal s.**, sutura sphenoparietalis. **sphenopetrosal s.**, synchondrosis petrooccipitalis. **sphenosquamous s., sphenotemporal s.**, sutura sphenosquamosa. **sphenozygomatic s.**, sutura sphenozygomatica. **squamosomastoid s.**, sutura squamosomastoidea. **squamosoparietal s.**, sutura squamosa cranii. **squamososphenoid s.**, sutura sphenosquamosa. **squamous s.**, sutura squamosa. **squamous s. of cranium,** sutura squamosa cranii. **subcuticular s.**, a method of skin closure involving placement of stitches in the subcuticular tissues parallel with the line of the wound; continuous or interrupted sutures may be used. **superficial s.**, one that is placed through the superficial fascia only. **temporal s.**, sutura squamosa cranii. **temporomalar s., temporozygomatic s.**, sutura temporozygomatica. **tongue-and-groove s.**, plastic s. **transverse s. of Krause,** sutura infraorbitalis. **true s.**, sutura vera. **uninterrupted s.**, continuous s. **uteroparietal s.**, stitching of the uterus to the inner surface of the abdominal wall at the incision line after cesarean section. **zygomaticofrontal s.**, sutura frontozygomatica. **zygomaticomaxillary s.**, sutura zygomaticomaxillaris. **zygomaticotemporal s.**, sutura temporozygomatica.

suxamethonium chloride (suk″sah-mĕ-tho′ne-um) succinylcholine chloride.

Sux-Cert (suks′sert) trademark for preparations of succinylcholine chloride.

suxemerid sulfate (suk-sem′ĕ-rid) chemical name: bis(1,2,-2,6,6-pentamethyl-4-piperidyl)succinate sulfate (1:2); an antitussive, $C_{24}H_{44}N_2O_4 \cdot 2H_2SO_4$.

Suzanne's gland (soo-zanz′) [Jean Georges Suzanne, French physician, born 1859] see under gland.

SV stroke volume; sinus venosus; simian virus.

SV40 simian virus 40; see vacuolating virus, under virus.

s.v. abbreviation for L. spir′itus vi′ni, alcoholic spirit.

s.v.r. abbreviation for L. spir′itus vi′ni rectifica′tus, rectified spirit of wine.

s.v.t. abbreviation for L. spir′itus vi′ni ten′uis, proof spirit.

swab (swahb) a wad of cotton or other absorbent material firmly attached to the end of a wire or stick, used for applying medication, removing material, collecting bacteriological material, etc.

swaddler (swahd′ler) a swaddling-suit for infants. **silver s.**, swaddling composed of polyester laminated on the inside surface with a thin layer of aluminum, used to prevent hypothermia in the newborn.

swage (swāj) 1. to shape metal by hammering or by adapting it to a die. 2. to fuse suture material to a needle, especially an eyeless needle. 3. a tool or form, often one of a pair, for shaping metal by pressure.

swager (swāj′er) an apparatus fitted with dies and counterdies for shaping wax patterns used in construction of crowns, inlays, etc., in dental work.

swallowing (swahl′o-ing) the taking in of a substance through the mouth and pharynx, past the cricopharyngeal constriction through the esophagus and into the stomach. The oral phase is a voluntary act, whereas the remainder is a reflex act mediated by an integrating swallowing center in the medulla oblongata.

swarming (sworm′ing) spreading in a swarm; a term applied to bacteria, especially Proteus species, which spread over the surface of the colony.

swayback (swa′bak) 1. abnormal downward curvature of the spinal column in the dorsal region in horses. 2. see lordosis. 3. enzootic ataxia.

sweat (swet) the perspiration; the liquid secreted by the sweat glands (glandulae sudoriferae), having a salty taste and a pH that varies from 4.5 to 7.5. Sweat produced by the eccrine sweat glands is clear with a faint characteristic odor, and contains water, sodium chloride, and traces of albumin, urea, and other compounds; its composition varies with many factors, e.g., fluid intake, external temperature and humidity, and some hormonal activity. Sweat produced by the larger, deeper, apocrine sweat glands of the axillae contains, in addition, organic material which on bacterial decomposition produces an offensive odor. **bloody s.**, hematidrosis. **blue s.**, chromhidrosis in which the sweat has a blue color; it may occur in copper workers. **fetid s.**, bromhidrosis. **green s.**, a greenish sweating seen among workers in copper. **night s.**, sweating during sleep, a symptom frequently occurring in tuberculosis. **phosphorescent s.**, phosphorescent perspiration, sometimes observed in miliaria and after the eating of phosphorescent fish.

Plate XLVII

Over-and-over suture

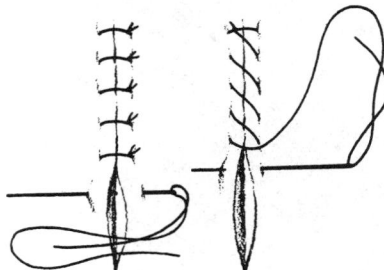

Vertical mattress suture

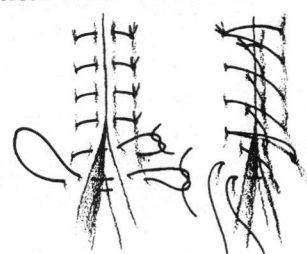

Horizontal mattress suture

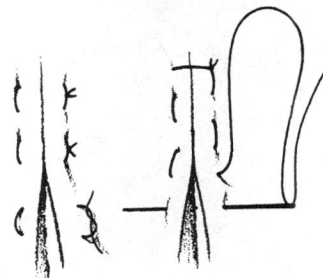

Lembert suture

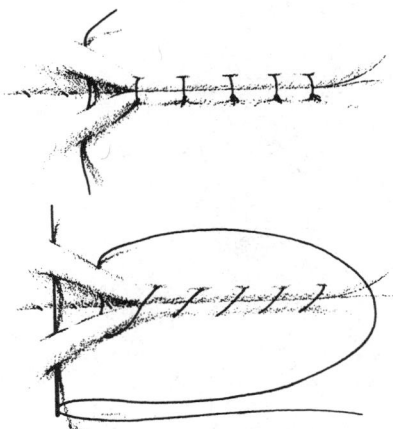

Lock-stitch suture

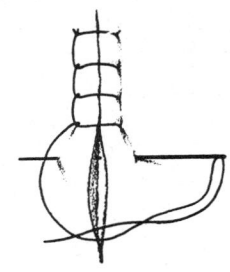

Connell suture

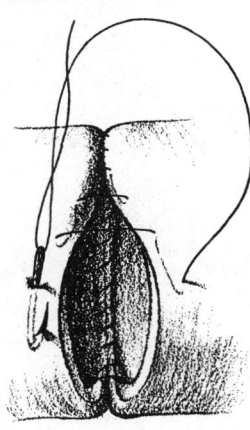

Purse-string suture

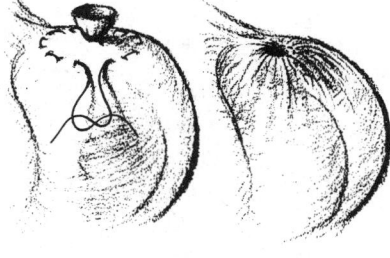

Halsted suture

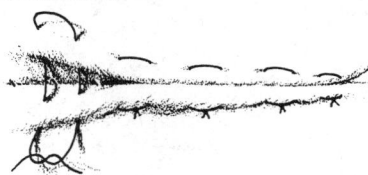

Cushing suture

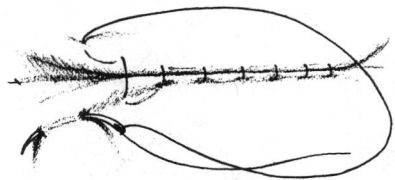

Everting sutures

Subcuticular suture

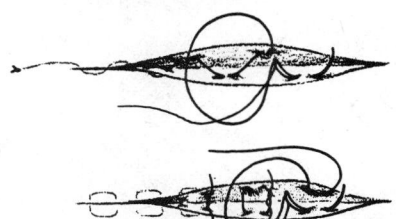

VARIOUS TYPES OF SUTURES AND KNOTS

(Nealon)

Swediaur's disease (swa″de-aw′erz) [François Xavier *Swediaur*, Austrian physician, 1748–1824] see under *disease*.

sweeny (swe′ne) shoulder slip.

swellhead (swel′hed) 1. lechuguilla fever. 2. swelled head.

swelling (swel′ing) 1. a transient abnormal enlargement or increase in volume of a body part or area not caused by proliferation of cells. 2. an eminence, or elevation. **albuminous s.,** cloudy s. **arytenoid s.,** an eminence on each side of the embryonic laryngeal orifice that presages the future larynx. **blennorrhagic s.,** swelling of the knee in gonorrheal synovitis. **Calabar s's,** edematous areas, up to several centimeters in diameter, appearing suddenly on various portions of the body, and lasting only 2 or 3 days; fever, pruritus, and urticaria may occur. It is caused by infection with *Loa loa.* Called also *ambulant edema* and *Calabar edema.* **capsular s.,** the development of a swollen appearance of capsulated pneumococci on exposure to type-specific antibody, due to the binding of antibody with capsular polysaccharide; called also *Neufeld's reaction.* **cloudy s.,** an early stage of toxic degenerative changes, especially in the protein constituents of organs in infectious diseases. The tissues appear swollen, parboiled and opaque but revert to normal when the cause is removed. At the cellular level, it is characterized by slight swelling of the cell and granularity and cloudiness of the cytoplasm. Called also *albuminous degeneration.* **fugitive s.,** an extremely short-lived swelling. **genital s.,** an elevation on each side of the embryonic phallus that becomes either a labial (labia majora) or a scrotal swelling. **giant s.,** angioneurotic edema. **glassy s.,** amyloid degeneration. **hunger s.,** edematous swellings in wet beriberi. **Kamerun s's,** Calabar s's. **labial s.,** the primordium of a labium majus. **labioscrotal s.,** genital s. **scrotal s.,** the primordium of one-half of the scrotum. **Soemmerring's crystalline s.,** annular edema of the lower portion of the lens capsule after the removal of a cataractous lens. **tropical s's,** Calabar s's. **tympanic s.,** intumescentia tympanica. **white s.,** former name for the swelling produced by tuberculous arthritis. Called also *tumor albus.*

Swift's disease (swifts) [H. *Swift*, Australian physician] acrodynia.

swinepox (swīn-poks) an acute infectious, eruptive disease of piglets, marked by lesions of the skin of the abdomen, flanks, head, and behind the ears, caused by a poxvirus; it usually runs a mild course but on occasion may be fatal.

swing (swing) a kind of suspensory cradle or sling.

swoon (swōōn) syncope.

sycephalus (si-sef′ah-lus) syncephalus.

sychnuria (sik-nu′re-ah) [Gr. *sychnos* frequent + *ouron* urine + *-ia*] pollakiuria.

sycosiform (si-ko′sĭ-form) resembling sycosis.

sycosis (si-ko′sis) [Gr. *sykōsis,* from *sykon* fig] 1. a disease marked by inflammation of the hair follicles, especially of the beard. 2. a kind of ulcer on the eyelids. **s. bar′bae,** 1. s. vulgaris. 2. pseudofolliculitis. **coccogenic s.,** s. vulgaris. **lupoid s.,** a chronic, scarring form of deep sycosis vulgaris, characterized by a persistent, slowly enlarging circinate patch with follicular papulopustules in the active, advancing border, and healing with scarring occurring in the central area. **parasitic s.,** tinea barbae. **s. staphylog′enes,** s. vulgaris. **s. tar′si,** blepharitis. **s. vulga′ris,** an inflammatory, papulopustular staphylococcal infection of the bearded region in which the primary lesion is a follicular, pin-head sized pustule pierced by a hair, which, if neglected, may become chronic. Called also *barber's itch* and *s. barbae.* See also *pseudofolliculitis.*

Sydenham's chorea, cough (sid′en-hams) [Thomas *Sydenham,* a celebrated English physician, sometimes called the "English Hippocrates," 1624–1689] see under *chorea* and *cough.*

syllabize (sil′ah-bīz) to divide speech sounds into syllables.

syllabus (sil′ah-bus) [L., a collection] an outline of a course of lectures.

syllepsiology (sĭ-lep″se-ol′o-je) [Gr. *syllēpsis* conception + *-logy*] the sum of knowledge regarding conception or pregnancy.

syllepsis (sil-lep′sis) conception, or pregnancy.

sylvan (sil′van) 1. a liguid obtained along with tetrol from distillation of pine wood. 2. sylvatic.

sylvatic (sil-vat′ik) sylvan; pertaining to, located in, or living in the woods. See under *plague.*

Sylvest's disease (sil-vests′) [Ejnar *Sylvest,* Norwegian physician, 1880–1931] epidemic pleurodynia.

sylvian (sil′ve-an) described by or named for Franciscus Sylvius de la Böe, 1614–1672, a Dutch anatomist, as the *sylvian artery* (arteria cerebri media), *fissure* (sulcus lateralis cerebri), *fossa* (fossa lateralis cerebri and sulcus lateralis cerebri), *line, point,* and *vein* (vena cerebri media superficialis); also *angle of Sylvius* and *valve of Sylvius* (valvula venae cavae inferioris). The name has also been ascribed to Jacobus *Sylvius* (Jacques Dubois), 1478–1555, a French anatomist who was a teacher of Vesalius, (*sylvian aqueduct* or *aqueduct of Sylvius* [aqueductus cerebri]).

symballophone (sim-bal′o-fōn) [Gr. *syn* together + *ballein* to throw + *phōnē* sound] a special type of double stethoscope making possible the comparison of sounds and detection of their direction.

symbiology (sim″bi-ol′o-je) the scientific study of symbiosis and symbiotic organisms.

symbion (sim′bi-on) symbiont.

symbionic (sim-bi-on′ik) pertaining to or characterized by symbiosis.

symbiont (sim′bi-ont, sim′be-ont) [Gr. *syn* together + *bioun* to live] an organism which lives in a state of symbiosis.

symbiosis (sim″bi-o′sis) [Gr. *symbiōsis*] 1. in parasitology, the living together or close association of two dissimilar organisms, each of the organisms being known as a *symbiont.* The association may be beneficial to both (mutualism), beneficial to one without effect on the other (commensalism), beneficial to one and detrimental to the other (parasitism), detrimental to one without effect on the other (amensalism), or detrimental to both (synnecrosis). 2. in psychiatry, a mutually reinforcing relationship between two persons who are dependent on each other; a normal characteristic of the relationship between the mother and infant child. 3. see *symbiotic psychosis,* under *psychosis.* **antagonistic s., antipathic s.,** an association between two organisms which is to the disadvantage of one of them; parasitism. **conjunctive s.,** association between two different organisms, with bodily union between them. **constructive s.,** an association between two organisms which is of benefit to the physiologic processes of one of them. **disjunctive s.,** symbiosis without actual union of the organisms.

symbiote (sim′bi-ōt) symbiont.

Symbiotes (sim″be-o′tēs) [Gr. *symbiōtēs* one who lives with] a genus of the tribe Wolbachieae, family Rickettsiaceae, order Rickettsiales, occurring as a single species, *S. lectula′rius,* which is parasitic on the bedbug.

symbiotic (sim″bi-ot′ik) associated in symbiosis; living together.

symblepharon (sim-blef′ah-ron) [Gr. *syn* together + *blepharon* eyelid] an adhesion between the tarsal conjunctiva and the bulbar conjunctiva. **anterior s.,** attachment of the lid to the eyeball by fibrous bands. **posterior s.,** adhesion between the lid and the eyeball extending into the fornix. **total s.,** adhesion of the entire conjunctival surfaces between the lid and the eyeball.

symblepharopterygium (sim-blef″ah-ro-ter-ij′e-um) a combination of symblepharon and pterygium; a form of symblepharon in which the lid is joined to the eyeball by a cicatricial band resembling a pterygium.

symbol (sim′bul) [Gr. *symbolon,* from *symballein* to interpret] a mark or character representing some quality or relation. In chemistry, a symbol is a letter or combination of letters representing an atom or a group of atoms. In psychiatry, an unconscious substitute which allows the libido to turn to an object not consciously concerned with sexuality. **phallic s.,** in psychoanalysis, any pointed or upright object which may represent the phallus or penis.

symbolia (sim-bo′le-ah) ability to recognize the nature of objects by the sense of touch.

symbolism (sim′bol-izm) 1. an abnormal mental condition in which every occurrence is conceived of as a symbol of the patient's own thoughts. 2. in psychoanalysis, a mechanism of unconscious thinking, usually of a sexual nature, whereby the real meaning becomes transformed so as not to be recognized as sexual by the super-ego.

symbolization (sim″bol-i-za′shun) a mental mechanism of the subconscious which consists in the representation of one object, idea, or quality by another.

symbrachydactylia (sim-brak″e-dak-til′e-ah) symbrachydactyly.

symbrachydactylism (sim-brak″e-dak′til-izm) symbrachydactyly.

symbrachydactyly (sim-brak″e-dak′tĭ-le) [Gr. *syn* together + *brachys* short + *daktylos* finger] a condition in which the fingers or toes are short and adherent; webbed fingers or toes.

symclosene (sim′klo-sēn) chemical name: 1,3,5-trichloro-*s*-triazine-2,4,6(1*H*,3*H*,5*H*)trione; a topical anti-infective, $C_3Cl_3O_3$.

Syme's amputation, operation (sīmz) [James *Syme,* Scottish surgeon, 1799–1870] see under *amputation* and *operation* (def. 2).

symelus (sim′ĕ-lus) symmelus.

Symington's body (si′ming-tonz) [Johnson *Symington,* Scottish anatomist, 1851–1924] the anococcygeal body; see under *body.*

symmelia (sim-me′le-ah) [Gr. *syn* together + *melos* limb + *-ia*] a developmental anomaly characterized by an apparent fusion of the lower limbs. There may be three feet (*tripodial s.*), two feet (*dipodial s.*), one foot (*monopodial s.*), or no feet (*apodial s.*).

symmelus (sim′e-lus) a fetus exhibiting symmelia.

Symmers' disease (sim′merz) [Douglas *Symmers,* American physician, 1879–1952] giant follicular lymphoma.

Symmetrel (sim'ĕ-trel) trademark for a preparation of amantadine hydrochloride.

symmetrical (sĭ-met're-kal) [Gr. *symmetrikos*] pertaining to or exhibiting symmetry; in chemistry, denoting compounds which contain atoms or groups at equal intervals in the molecule.

symmetry (sim'ĕ-tre) [Gr. *symmetria; syn* with + *metron* measure] the similar arrangement in form and relationships of parts around a common axis, or on each side of a plane of the body. **bilateral s.**, the configuration of an irregularly shaped body (as the human body or that of higher animals) which can be divided by a longitudinal plane into halves that are mirror images of each other. **inverse s.**, correspondence as between an object and its mirror image, in which one side of one object corresponds with the opposite side of another. **radial s.**, symmetry in which the body parts are arranged regularly around a central axis.

sympathectomize (sim"pah-thek'to-mīz) to subject to sympathectomy.

sympathectomy (sim"pah-thek'to-me) [*sympathetic* + Gr. *ektomē* excision] the transection, resection, or other interruption of some portion of the sympathetic nervous pathways. Operations may be named according to the topographic location of the nerve, ganglion, or plexus operation on, as *cervical, dorsal, lumbar,* or *thoracolumbar s.*, or in reference to the diaphragm, as *subdiaphragmatic, supradiaphragmatic,* or *transdiaphragmatic s.* **chemical s.**, suppression of the activity of the sympathetic nervous system by appropriate drugs. **periarterial s.**, surgical removal of the sheath of an artery containing the sympathetic nerve fibers; it produces temporary vasodilatation.

sympathetectomy (sim"pah-thĕ-tek'to-me) sympathectomy.

sympathetic (sim"pah-thet'ik) [Gr. *sympathētikos*] 1. pertaining to, caused by, or exhibiting sympathy. 2. a sympathetic nerve or the sympathetic nervous system; see under *system*.

sympatheticomimetic (sim"pah-thet"ĭ-ko-mi-met'ik) [*sympathetic* + Gr. *mimētikos* imitative] sympathomimetic.

sympatheticoparalytic (sim"pah-thet"ĭ-ko-par"ah-lit'ik) due to or affected with paralysis of the sympathetic nervous system.

sympatheticotonia (sim"pah-thet"ĭ-ko-to'ne-ah) a condition in which the sympathetic nervous system dominates the general functioning of the body organs, characterized by vascular spasm, heightened blood pressure, dermographic formation of goose flesh, and activity of the ciliospinal reflex.

sympatheticotonic (sim"pah-thet"ĭ-ko-ton'ik) [*sympathetic* + Gr. *tonos* tension] pertaining to or characterized by sympatheticotonia.

sympathetoblast (sim"pah-thet'o-blast) one of the embryonic nerve cells from the sympathetic system which develops into a sympathetic cell.

sympathic (sim-path'ik) sympathetic.

sympathicectomy (sim-path"ĭ-sek'to-me) sympathectomy.

sympathicoblast (sim-path"ĭ-ko-blast") the primitive pluripotential undifferentiated cell which develops into a sympathetic nerve cell.

sympathicoblastoma (sim-path"ĭ-ko-blas-to'mah) a malignant tumor containing sympathicoblasts; see *neuroblastoma*.

sympathicodiaphtheresis (sim-path"ĭ-ko-di"af-the-re'sis) Doppler's operation.

sympathicogonioma (sim-path"ĭ-ko-go"ne-o'mah) sympathicoblastoma.

sympathicolytic (sim-path"ĭ-ko-lit'ik) sympatholytic.

sympathicomimetic (sim-path"ĭ-ko-mi-met'ik) sympathomimetic.

sympathicopathy (sim-path"ĭ-kop'ah-the) any disease due to disorder of the sympathetic nervous system.

sympathicotherapy (sim-path"ĭ-ko-ther'ah-pe) treatment of certain diseases by stimulation or irritation of the turbinate bones and nasal septum, on the theory that such stimulation influences the sympathetic nerve.

sympathicotonia (sim-path"ĭ-ko-to'ne-ah) sympatheticotonia.

sympathicotonic (sim-path"ĭ-ko-ton'ik) sympatheticotonic.

sympathicotripsy (sim-path"ĭ-ko-trip'se) [*sympathetic ganglion* + Gr. *tribein* to crush] the surgical crushing of a nerve, ganglion, or plexus of the sympathetic nervous system.

sympathicotrope (sim-path'ĭ-ko-trōp) sympathicotropic.

sympathicotropic (sim-path"ĭ-ko-trop'ik) [*sympathetic* + Gr. *tropikos* turning] 1. having an affinity for the sympathetic nervous system. 2. an agent that has an affinity for or exerts its principal effect upon the sympathetic nervous system.

sympathicus (sim-path'ĭ-kus) the sympathetic nervous system.

sympathin (sim'pah-thin) a neurohormonal mediator of nerve impulses at sympathetic nerve synapses. The two most important mediators are epinephrine and norepinephrine, the term sympathin being used only when the nature of the mediator is unknown.

sympathism (sim'pah-thizm) susceptibility to hypnotic influence; suggestibility; the alleged transfer of feelings from one person to another.

sympathist (sim'pah-thist) one susceptible to sympathism.

sympathoadrenal (sim"path-o-ah-dre'nal) 1. pertaining to the sympathetic nervous system and the adrenal medulla. 2. involving the sympathetic nervous system and the adrenal glands, especially increased sympathetic activity that causes increased secretion of epinephrine by the adrenal medulla and of norepinephrine by the postganglionic sympathetic nerve endings.

sympathoblast (sim-path'o-blast) [*sympathetic* + Gr. *blastos* germ] sympathicoblast.

sympathoblastoma (sim"pah-tho-blas-to'mah) sympathicoblastoma.

sympathogone (sim"pah-tho-gōn') sympathogonium.

sympathogonia (sim"pah-tho-go'ne-ah) [pl., *sympathetic* + Gr. *gonē* seed] undifferentiated embryonic cells which develop into sympathetic cells.

sympathogonioma (sim"pah-tho-go"ne-o'mah) sympathicoblastoma.

sympathogonium (sim"pah-tho-go'ne-um) singular of *sympathogonia*.

sympatholytic (sim"pah-tho-lit'ik) [*sympathetic* + Gr. *lytikos* dissolving] 1. opposing the effects of impulses conveyed by adrenergic postganglionic fibers of the sympathetic nervous system. 2. an agent that opposes the effects of impulses conveyed by adrenergic postganglionic fibers of the sympathetic nervous system; called also *antiadrenergic*.

sympathomimetic (sim"pah-tho-mi-met'ik) [*sympathetic* + Gr. *mimētikos* imitative] 1. mimicking the effects of impulses conveyed by adrenergic postganglionic fibers of the sympathetic nervous system. 2. an agent that produces effects similar to those of impulses conveyed by adrenergic postganglionic fibers of the sympathetic nervous system. Called also *adrenergic*.

sympathy (sim'pah-the) [Gr. *sympatheia*] 1. an influence produced in any organ by disease or disorder in another part. 2. a relation which exists between the mind and the body, causing the one to be affected by the other. 3. the influence exerted by one individual upon another, or received by one from another, and the effects thus produced, as seen in hypnotism, in yawning, and in the transfer of hysterical symptoms.

sympectothiene (sim-pek"to-thi'ēn) ergothioneine.

sympectothion (sim-pek"to-thi'on) [Gr. *syn* together + *pexis* fixation + *theion* sulfur] ergothioneine.

sympexion (sim-pek'se-on), pl. *sympex'ia* [Gr. *sympēxis* condensation, coagulation + *on* neuter ending] a concretion.

symphalangia (sim"fah-lan'je-ah) [Gr. *syn* together + *phalanges* + *-ia*] congenital end-to-end fusion of contiguous phalanges of a digit, usually associated with other deformity of the hand or foot.

symphalangism (sim-fal'an-jizm) symphalangia.

symphoricarpus (sim"fōr-ĭ-kar'pus) [Gr. *symphorein* to bear together + *karpos* fruit] a homeopathic preparation of the fruit of *Symphoricarpos racemosus*, or snowberry, a shrub of North America.

Symphoromyia (sim"for-o-mi'yah) a genus of flies (snipe flies) of the family Rhagionidae, some of which are severe biters of man and animals.

symphyocephalus (sim"fe-o-sef'ah-lus) [Gr. *syn* together + *phyein* to grow + *kephalē* head] a twin fetus joined at the head.

symphyogenetic (sim"fe-o-jĕ-net'ik) [Gr. *syn* together + *phyein* to grow + *gennan* to produce] concerning the combined effects of hereditary determiners and environmental factors in producing the organism's structure and behavior.

symphyseal (sim-fiz'e-al) pertaining to a symphysis.

symphyseorrhaphy (sim-fiz"e-or'ah-fe) symphysiorrhaphy.

symphyses (sim'fĭ-sēz) [Gr.] plural of *symphysis*.

symphysial (sim-fiz'e-al) symphyseal.

symphysic (sim-fiz'ik) characterized by abnormal fusion of adjacent parts.

symphysiectomy (sim-fiz"e-ek'to-me) [*symphysis* + Gr. *ektomē* excision] resection of the symphysis pubis in order to facilitate impending and possible future deliveries.

symphysiolysis (sim-fiz"e-ol'ĭ-sis) [*symphysis* + Gr. *lysis* dissolution] separation or slipping of symphyses, especially the symphysis pubis.

symphysion (sim-fiz'e-on) [*symphysis* + Gr. *on* neuter ending] the middle point of the outer border of the alveolar process of the lower jaw.

symphysiorrhaphy (sim-fiz"e-or'ah-fe) [*symphysis* + Gr. *rhaphē* suture] suture of a divided symphysis.

symphysiotome (sim-fiz'e-o-tōm) a knife used in performing symphysiotomy.

symphysiotomy (sim-fiz"e-ot'o-me) [*symphysis* + Gr. *tomē* a cutting] the division of the fibrocartilage of the symphysis pubis, in order to facilitate delivery, by increasing the diameter of the pelvis.

symphysis (sim'fĭ-sis), pl. *sym'physes* [Gr. "a growing together, natural junction"] a site or line of union; used in official anatomical nomenclature to designate a type of cartilaginous joint in which the apposed bony surfaces are firmly united by a plate of fibrocartilage; called also *fibrocartilaginous joint.* **s. man-dib′ulae, s. men′ti,** the line of union, in the median plane, of the two halves of the fetal lower jaw. **s. os′sium pu′bis, pubic s.,** s. pubica. **s. pu′bica** [NA], **s. pu′bis,** the joint formed by union of the bodies of the pubic bones in the median plane by a thick mass of fibrocartilage; called also *s. ossium pubis* and *pubic s.* **s. sacrococcyg′ea, sacrococcygeal s.,** junctura sacrococcygea. **sacroiliac s.,** articulatio sacroiliaca.

symphysodactyly (sim″fĭ-so-dak′tĭ-le) [Gr. *symphysis* a growing together + *daktylos* finger] fusion of the fingers or toes.

Symphytum (sim′fĭ-tum) [L.; Gr. *symphyton*] a genus of boraginaceous plants; *S. officinale* L., common comfrey, is the comfrey of Europe and North America; its roots and leaves are demulcent and astringent.

symphytum (sim′fĭ-tum) a demulcent and astringent homeopathic preparation of *Symphytum officinale.*

symplasm (sim′plazm) tissue in which there is no cellular structure.

symplasmatic (sim″plaz-mat′ik) marked by union of protoplasm.

symplast (sim′plast) symplasm.

symplex (sim′pleks) a chemical compound in which a high molecular substance is bound by residual valencies; included are activators, adsorbents, hemoglobin, and toxin-antitoxin.

sympodia (sim-po′de-ah) [Gr. *syn* together + *pous* foot + *-ia*] fusion of the lower extremities. Cf. *sirenomelus* and *sympus.*

symport (sim′port) a mechanism of transporting two compounds simultaneously across a cell membrane in the same direction, one compound being transported down a concentration gradient, the other against a gradient.

symptom (simp′tum) [L. *symptoma*; Gr. *symptōma* anything that has befallen one] any subjective evidence of disease or of a patient's condition, i.e., such evidence as perceived by the patient; a change in a patient's condition indicative of some bodily or mental state. See also *sign.* **abstinence s′s,** withdrawal s′s. **accessory s.,** any symptom not pathognomonic. **Anton's s.,** denial of, and usually unawareness of, one's own blindness, with resort to confabulation, as seen in cortical blindness due to bilateral infarction of the occipital lobes; called also *Anton's syndrome.* **assident s.,** accessory s. **Bárány's s.,** 1. in disturbances of equilibrium of the vestibular apparatus, the direction of the fall is influenced by changing the position of the patient's head. 2. if the normal ear is irrigated with hot water (110–120° F.), a rotatory nystagmus is developed toward the side of the irrigated ear; if the ear is irrigated with cold water, a rotatory nystagmus is developed away from the irrigated side. There is no nystagmus if the labyrinth is diseased. Called also *caloric test.* **Baumés's s.,** see under *sign.* **Béhier-Hardy s.,** see under *sign.* **Bekhterev's s.,** paralysis of the facial muscles for automatic movements. **Berger's s.,** see under *sign.* **Bonhoeffer's s.,** loss of normal muscle tonus in chorea. **Brauch-Romberg s.,** see *Romberg's sign,* under *sign.* **Buerger's s.,** in thromboangiitis obliterans, the pain in the affected leg when the patient is lying down is relieved only by lying with the leg hung over the side of the bed. **Burghart's s.,** fine rales over the anterior inferior edge of the lung; an early sign of pulmonary tuberculosis. **Capgras s.,** the mental impression, but not an actual hallucination, of a person that the individual confronting him, though known to him, is a "double" or substitute for the real individual. **Cardarelli's s.,** see under *sign.* **cardinal s.,** 1. a symptom of greatest significance to the physician, establishing the identity of the illness. 2. [pl.] the symptoms shown in the pulse, temperature, and respiration. **Castellani-Low s.,** a fine tremor of the tongue seen in sleeping sickness. **characteristic s.,** a symptom that is almost universally associated with a particular disease or condition. **Chvostek's s.,** see under *sign.* **Colliver's s.,** a peculiar twitching, tremulous, or convulsive movement of the limbs, face, jaw, and sometimes of the entire body, seen in the preparalytic stage of poliomyelitis. **concomitant s.,** a symptom not essential to a disease, but which may have an accessory value in its diagnosis. **consecutive s.,** a symptom appearing during convalescence from a disease, but having no connection with the disease. **constitutional s.,** a symptom which is indicative of or due to disorder of the whole body. **crossbar s. of Fraenkel,** blocking of the peristaltic wave on the lesser curvature of the stomach at the site of an ulcer, on fluoroscopy of the stomach. **deficiency s.,** a symptom which is due to a deficiency of the secretion of some endocrine gland. **delayed s.,** one which does not appear for some time after the occurrence of the causes which produce it. **direct s.,** one which is directly caused by the disease. **dissociation s.,** anesthesia to pain and to heat and cold without loss of tactile sensibility; seen in syringomyelia. **endothelial s.,** see *Rumpel-Leede phenomenon,* under *phenomenon.* **Epstein's s.,** a symptom seen in nervous infants, consisting of failure of the upper lid to move downward, giving the child a frightened expression. **equivocal s.,** a symptom which may be produced by several different diseases. **esophagosalivary s.,** excessive flow of saliva in patients with cancer of the esophagus. **Fröschel's s.**

(obs.), if a child does not react to tickling at the opening of the auditory canal, yet is ticklish throughout the rest of his body, disease of the auditory apparatus is indicated. **Ganser's s.,** the giving of wrong or absurd answers to questions; seen in certain psychiatric conditions. See also *Ganser's syndrome,* under *syndrome.* **general s.,** constitutional s. **Goldthwait's s.,** see under *sign.* **Griesinger's s.,** see under *sign.* **guiding s.,** characteristic s. **Haenel's s.,** in tabes there is a lack of sensation on pressure over the eyeballs. **halo s.,** the seeing of colored rings around an individual light source; indicative of glaucoma. **Huchard's s.,** see under *sign.* **incarceration s.,** periodically recurring symptoms of displaced kidney, such as nephralgia, gastralgia, and severe collapse; called also *Dietl's crisis.* **indirect s.,** a symptom which points to a condition that may or may not be due to a particular disease or lesion. **induced s.,** one produced intentionally. **Jellinek's s.,** see under *sign.* **Jonas' s.,** spasm of the pylorus in rabies. **Kerandel's s.,** see under *sign.* **Kocher's s.,** see under *sign.* **Kussmaul's s.,** see under *sign* (def. 2). **labyrinthine s′s,** a group of symptoms indicating disease of the internal ear. **Lade s.,** a peculiar diarrhea or very soft stool occurring fourteen days prior to the eruption of chickenpox. **Liebreich's s.,** a symptom of red-green color blindness in which light effects appear red and shadows green. **local s.,** one due to local disease or to a particular lesion. **localizing s′s,** symptoms that indicate the location of a lesion. **Loewi's s.,** see under *tests.* **Magendie's s.,** skew deviation. **Magnan's s.,** a sensation as of a round body beneath the skin, sometimes experienced in chronic cocainism. **Mannkopf's s.,** see under *sign.* **neighborhood s.,** a symptom produced in an organ by disease in a neighboring organ, as by pressure of a tumor in one organ on an organ adjacent to it. **nostril s.,** dilatation of the nostrils during expiration and dropping during inspiration. **objective s.,** one that is obvious to the senses of the observer; see *sign.* **Oehler's s.,** coldness and pallor of the feet in intermittent claudication. **passive s.,** static s. **pathognomonic s.,** one that establishes with certainty the diagnosis of the disease. **Pel-Ebstein s.,** see under *fever.* **precursory s., premonitory s.,** signal s. **presenting s.,** the symptom or group of symptoms of which the patient complains the most or from which he seeks relief. **rainbow s.,** halo s. **rational s.,** subjective s. **reflex s.,** a symptom occurring in a part remote from that which is affected by the disease. **Remak's s.,** polyesthesia; also a prolongation of the lapse of time before a painful impression is perceived; both are noted in tabes dorsalis. **Roger's s.,** a temperature below the normal in the third stage of tuberculous meningitis. **Romberg-Howship s.,** see under *sign.* **Rumpf's s.,** see under *sign.* **Séguin's signal s.,** the involuntary contraction of the muscles just before an epileptic attack. **signal s.,** a sensation, aura, or other subjective experience that gives warning of the approach of an epileptic or other seizure. **Simon's s.,** polyuria seen in cancer of the breast, caused by metastasis of cancer to the pituitary gland. **Skeer's s.,** see under *sign.* **Sklowsky's s.,** when light pressure with the index finger is made upon the healthy skin near, and then over, a vesicle in varicella, the wall of the vesicle easily collapses and the contents are discharged. **static s.,** a condition indicative of the state of some particular organ independent of the rest of the body; called also *passive s.* **Stellwag's s.,** see under *sign.* **Stierlin's s.,** indurating and ulcerative processes, especially tuberculosis of the cecum and ascending colon, are shown in the roentgen plate by absence of the normal shadow following a contrast meal. **subjective s.,** one that is perceptible to the patient only. **sympathetic s.,** one due to sympathy, as when pain or other disorder affects a part when some other part is the seat of the disease proper. **Tar's s.,** in health the lower borders of the lungs are situated as deeply in the lying down position with moderate exhalation as in the upright position with deep inhalation; in infiltrating process of the lungs this is not the case. **Trendelenburg's s.,** a waddling gait due to paralysis of the gluteal muscles; see also *Trendelenburg's test,* def. 2, under *tests.* **Wanner's s.** (obs.), decrease of sound conduction through the bones of the head, without pain in the labyrinth, points to organic change in the skull. **Wartenberg's s.,** 1. itching of the nostrils and tip of the nose indicative of cerebral tumor. 2. flexion of the thumb occurring on flexion of the other fingers against resistance; seen in pyramidal lesions. **Weber's s.,** see under *sign.* **Wernicke's s.,** hemiopic pupillary reaction. **Westphal's s.,** see under *sign.* **Winterbottom's s.,** see under *sign.* **withdrawal s′s,** symptoms which follow sudden abstinence from a drug to which a person has become addicted.

symptomatic (simp″to-mat′ik) [Gr. *symptōmatikos*] 1. pertaining to or of the nature of a symptom. 2. indicative (of a particular disease or disorder). 3. exhibiting the symptoms of a particular disease but having a different cause. 4. directed at the allaying of symptoms, as symptomatic treatment.

symptomatology (simp″tom-ah-tol′o-je) 1. that branch of medicine which treats of symptoms; the systematic discussion of symptoms. 2. the combined symptoms of a disease.

symptomatolytic (simp″to-mah-to-lit′ik) [*symptom* + Gr. *lytikos* dissolving] causing the disappearance of symptoms.

symptome (samp-tōm′) [Fr.] symptom. **s's complice′** [Fr. "symptom complex"], a group of symptoms characteristic of a certain condition.

symptomolytic (simp″to-mo-lit′ik) symptomatolytic.

symptosis (simp-to′sis) [Gr. *syn* together + *ptōsis* fall] the gradual wasting of the whole body or of any organ.

sympus (sim′pus) [Gr. *syn* together + *pous* foot] a fetus exhibiting fusion of the lower limbs. Cf. *sirenomelus*. **s. a′pus,** sirenomelus. **s. di′pus,** a form in which both feet are present. **s. mo′nopus,** a form in which one foot is present.

Syms's tractor (simz′ez) [Parker *Syms*, American surgeon, 1860–1933] see under *tractor*.

syn- [Gr. *syn* with, together] a prefix signifying union or association.

synadelphus (sin″ah-del′fus) [*syn-* + Gr. *adelphos* brother] a monster with a single body and eight limbs.

synaetion (sin-e′te-on) [Gr. *synaitios* being a joint cause] the secondary or cooperative cause of a disease.

Synalar (sin′ah-lar) trademark for a preparation of fluocinolone acetonide.

synalbumin (sin″al-bu′min) a postulated competitive inhibitor of insulin, an insulin B chain bound to albumin.

synalgia (sin-al′je-ah) pain experienced in one place as the result of a lesion in another.

synalgic (sin-al′jik) affected with or of the nature of synalgia.

synanche (sin-an′ke) cynanche.

Synangium (sin-an′je-um) a genus of Schizomycetes of the order Myxobacterales, family Polyangiaceae.

synanthrin (sin-an′thrin) inulin.

synanthrose (sin-an′thrōs) levulin.

synaphymenitis (sin-af″ĭ-men-i′tis) conjunctivitis.

synapse (sin′aps) [Gr. *synapsis* a conjunction, connection] the site of functional apposition between neurons, at which an impulse is transmitted from one neuron to another by either electrical (see *ephapse*) or chemical means. In the typical synapse, the impulse is transmitted by a neurotransmitter (e.g., acetylcholine, norepinephrine, etc.) released by the axon terminal of the excited (presynaptic) cell, which diffuses across the synaptic cleft to bind with receptors on the postsynaptic cell membrane, and thereby effects electrical changes in the postsynaptic cell which result in depolarization (excitation) or hyperpolarization (inhibition). Synapses also occur at sites of apposition between nerve endings and effector organs (e.g., the neuromuscular junction). **axoaxonic s.,** one between the axon of one neuron and the axon of another neuron. **axodendritic s.,** one between the axon of one neuron and dendrites of another. **axodendrosomatic s.,** one between the axon of one neuron and the dendrites and body (soma) of another, as in motoneurons. **axosomatic s.,** one between the axon of one neuron and the body (soma) of another. **dendrodendritic s.,** one from a dendrite of one cell to a dendrite of another. **electrotonic s.,** see *gap junction*, under *junction*. **en passant s.,** synaptic contact characterized by a crossing of cells with similar fiber membranes lying alongside one another, as in coelenterates. **loop s.,** one having a relatively long area of contact of fiber membranes, as in many invertebrates.

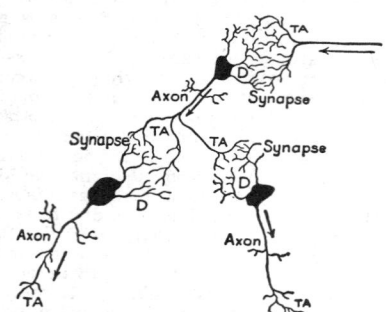

Diagram of three synapses. Nerve impulse is indicated by arrows, showing that the direction of passage is from terminal aborization (TA) or nerve endings of the axon of one neuron to the dendrites (D) of another neuron. (Williams.)

synapsis (sĭ-nap′sis) [Gr. "conjunction"] the pairing off in point-for-point association of homologous chromosomes from the male and female pronuclei during the early prophase of meiosis.

synaptase (sĭ-nap′tās) [Gr. *synaptos* joined] emulsin.

synaptene (sĭ-nap′tēn) amphitene.

synaptic (sĭ-nap′tik) pertaining to or affecting a synapse; pertaining to synopsis.

synaptology (sin″ap-tol′o-je) that branch of neurology which deals with the synaptic correlations of the nervous system.

synaptosome (sin-ap′to-sōm″) any of the membrane-bound sacs that break away from axon terminals at a synapse after brain

tissue has been homogenized in sugar solution; it contains synaptic vessels and mitochondria.

synarthrodia (sin″ar-thro′de-ah) [*syn-* + Gr. *arthrōdia* joint] synarthrosis.

synarthrodial (sin″ar-thro′de-al) pertaining to a synarthrosis.

synarthrophysis (sin″ar-thro-fi′sis) [*syn-* + Gr. *arthron* joint + *physis* growth] any ankylosing process; progressive ankylosis of joints.

synarthroses (sin″ar-thro′sēz) [Gr.] plural of *synarthrosis*.

synarthrosis (sin″ar-thro′sis), pl. *synarthro′ses* [*syn-* + Gr. *arthrōsis* joint] a form of articulation in which the bony elements are united by continuous intervening fibrous tissue. See *junctura fibrosa*.

synathresis (sin″ath-re′sis) synathroisis.

synathroisis (sin″ath-roi′sis) [*syn-* + Gr. *athroisis* collection] local hyperemia or congestion.

syncaine (sin-ka′in) procaine hydrochloride.

syncanthus (sin-kan′thus) [*syn-* + Gr. *kanthos* canthus] adhesion of the eyeball to the orbital structures.

syncaryon (sin-kar′e-on) [*syn-* + Gr. *karyon* nucleus] the nucleus formed by fusion of two pronuclei.

syncelom (sin-se′lom) the perivisceral cavities of the body considered as one structure, including the pleural, cardiac, and peritoneal cavities, and tunica vaginalis.

syncephalus (sin-sef′ah-lus) [*syn-* + Gr. *kephalē* head] a double monster with one head, there being a single face with four ears, two on the back of the head.

synchesis (sin′ke-sis) synchysis.

synchilia (sin-ki′le-ah) [*syn-* + Gr. *cheilos* lip + *-ia*] congenital adhesion of the lips.

synchiria (sin-ki′re-ah) [*syn-* + Gr. *cheir* hand + *-ia*] a condition in which the sensation produced by a stimulus applied to one side of the body is referred to both sides.

syncholia (sin-ko′le-ah) [*syn-* + Gr. *cholē* bile + *-ia*] the secretion of substances of exogenous origin in the bile.

synchondrectomy (sin″kon-drek′to-me) [*synchondrosis* + Gr. *ektomē* excision] surgical excision of a synchondrosis, especially of the symphysis of the pubic bone.

synchondroseotomy (sin″kon-dro″se-ot′o-me) [*synchondrosis* + Gr. *tomē* a cutting] an operation for exstrophy of the bladder done by cutting through the sacroiliac ligaments and forcibly drawing together the pelvic bones; called also *Trendelenburg's operation*.

synchondroses (sin″kon-dro′sēz) [Gr.] plural of *synchondrosis*.

synchondrosis (sin″kon-dro′sis), pl. *synchondro′ses* [Gr. *synchondrōsis* a growing into one cartilage] a type of cartilaginous joint that is usually temporary, the intervening hyaline cartilage ordinarily being converted into bone before adult life. **s. arycornicula′ta,** the cartilaginous union between the upper end of the arytenoid cartilage and the base of the corniculate cartilage. **costoclavicular s.,** ligamentum costoclaviculare. **synchondro′ses cra′nii** [NA], **synchondroses of cranium,** the cartilaginous junctions between certain bones of the cranium. **epiphyseal s., s. epiphy′seos,** cartilago epiphysialis. **intersphenoidal s., s. intersphenoida′lis,** the cartilaginous union of the two halves of the body of the sphenoid bone in the fetus. **intraoccipital s., anterior,** s. intraoccipitalis anterior. **intraoccipital s., posterior,** s. intraoccipitalis posterior. **s. intraoccipita′lis ante′rior** [NA], anterior intraoccipital synchondrosis: the cartilaginous union of the pars basilaris with the partes laterales of the occipital bone in the newborn. **s. intraoccipita′lis poste′rior** [NA], posterior intraoccipital synchondrosis: the cartilaginous union of the squama with the partes laterales of the occipital bone in the newborn. **petrooccipital s., s. petrooccipita′lis** [NA], the plate of cartilage in the petrooccipital fissure which helps to unite the basilar portion of the occipital bone and the petrous portion of the temporal bone. **pubic s., s. pu′bis,** symphysis pubica. **sacrococcygeal s.,** junctura sacrococcygea. **synchondroses of skull,** synchondroses cranii. **sphenobasilar s., spheno-occipital s.,** s. sphenooccipitalis. **s. sphenooccipita′lis** [NA], the cartilaginous union of the anterior end of the basilar portion of the occipital bone with the posterior surface of the body of the sphenoid bone. **s. sphenopetro′sa,** [NA], **sphenopetrosal s.,** the cartilaginous union of the lower border of the great wing of the sphenoid bone with the petrous portion of the temporal bone in the sphenopetrosal fissure. **sternal s., s. sterna′lis** [NA], the cartilaginous union between the manubrium and the body of the sternum.

synchondrotomy (sin″kon-drot′o-me) [*synchondrosis* + Gr. *tomē* a cutting] the division of the symphysis pubis or of any other synchondrosis.

synchorial (sin-ko′re-al) sharing a common placenta; said of multiple fetuses.

synchronia (sin-kro′ne-ah) 1. synchronism. 2. the formation of parts or tissues at the usual time. Cf. *heterochronia* (def. 1).

synchronism (sin′kro-nizm) occurrence at the same time; the quality of being synchronous.

synchronous (sin′kro-nus) [syn- + Gr. *chronos* time] occurring at the same time.

synchrotron (sin′kro-tron) a machine for generating high-speed electrons or protons. It combines features of the cyclotron and betatron and will produce 70 million volts.

synchysis (sin′kĭ-sis) [Gr. "a mixing together"] a softening or fluid condition of the vitreous body of the eye; synchysis corporis vitrei. **s. scintil′lans,** cholesterol crystals in the vitreous that develop as a degenerative change following inflammation or other ocular diseases.

syncinesis (sin″si-ne′sis) synkinesis.

synciput (sin′sĭ-put) sinciput.

synclinal (sin-kli′nal) [Gr. *synklinein* to lean together] bent or inclined together.

synclitic (sin-klit′ik) pertaining to or marked by synclitism.

synclitism, syncliticism (sin′klit-izm; sin-klit′ĭ-sizm) [Gr. *synklinein* to lean together] 1. parallelism between the planes of the fetal head and those of the pelvis. 2. normal, synchronous maturation of the nucleus and cytoplasm of blood cells. Cf. *asynclitism.*

synclonus (sin′klo-nus) [syn- + Gr. *klonos* turmoil] 1. muscular tremor, or the successive clonic contraction of various muscles together. 2. any disease characterized by muscular tremors. **s. beriber′ica,** muscular tremors associated with beriberi.

syncopal (sin′ko-pal) pertaining to or characterized by syncope.

syncope (sin′ko-pe) [Gr. *synkopē*] a temporary suspension of consciousness due to generalized cerebral ischemia; a faint or swoon. **Adams-Stokes s.,** see under *disease.* **s. angino′sa,** fainting with an episode of coronary insufficiency. **cardiac s.,** sudden loss of consciousness, with momentary or no premonitory symptoms, due to cerebral anemia caused by ventricular asystole, extreme bradycardia, or ventricular fibrillation. **carotid sinus s.,** carotid sinus syndrome. **cough s.,** tussive s. **digital s.,** a sudden temporary loss of strength in the fingers. **laryngeal s.,** tussive s. **micturition s.,** brief loss of consciousness during or immediately after micturition in certain men who arise from bed at night to urinate; it may be a form of orthostatic hypotension. **postural s.,** that resulting from orthostatic hypotension. **stretching s.,** syncope associated with stretching the arms upward with the spine extended. **swallow s.,** syncope associated with swallowing, a disorder of atrioventricular conduction mediated by the vagus nerve. **tussive s.,** brief loss of consciousness associated with vigorous and explosive paroxysms of coughing, usually seen in men; called also *cough s., laryngeal s.,* and *laryngeal vertigo.* **vasodepressor s.,** vasovagal attack. **vasovagal s.,** see under *attack.*

syncopic (sin-kop′ik) syncopal.

syncretio (sin-kre′she-o) [L.] a growing together or adhesion, as between inflamed serous surfaces in contact.

Syncryptidae (sin-krip′tĭ-de) a family of free-swimming flagellate protozoa of the order Chrysomonadina, class Phytomastigophora, including the genus *Synura.*

Syncurine (sin′ku-rēn) trademark for a preparation of decamethonium bromide.

syncytial (sin-sish′al) of, pertaining to, or producing a syncytium.

syncytiolysin (sin″sit-e-ol′ĭ-sin) a lysin destructive to the syncytium; formed in the blood of an animal into which matter from the placenta of another animal has been injected.

syncytioma (sin-sit″e-o′mah) syncytial endometritis. **s. malig′num,** choriocarcinoma.

syncytiotoxin (sin-sit″e-o-tok′sin) a toxin that has a specific action on the placenta.

syncytiotrophoblast (sin-sit″e-o-trof′o-blast) the outer syncytial layer of the trophoblast; called also *syntrophoblast.*

syncytium (sin-sish′e-um) a multinucleate mass of protoplasm produced by the merging of cells.

syncytoid (sin′sĭ-toid) resembling a syncytium.

syncytotoxin (sin″sĭ-to-tok′sin) a cytolytic serum produced by immunizing animals with placental cells.

syndactylia (sin″dak-til′e-ah) syndactyly.

syndactylism (sin-dak′tĭ-lizm) syndactyly.

syndactylous (sin-dak′tĭ-lus) pertaining to or characterized by syndactyly.

syndactylus (sin-dak′tĭ-lus) an individual exhibiting syndactyly.

syndactyly (sin-dak′tĭ-le) [Gr. *syn* with + *daktylos* finger] the most common congenital anomaly of the hand, marked by persistence of the webbing between adjacent digits, so they are more or less completely attached; generally considered an inherited condition, the anomaly may also occur in the foot. **complete s.,** syndactyly in which the connection extends from the base of the involved digits to the tip. **complicated s.,** syndactyly in which the bones or nails of the involved digits are fused. **double s.,** syndactyly involving three digits (two webs). **partial s.,** syndactyly in which the connecting web extends only part way up from the base of the involved digits. **simple s.,** syn-

dactyly in which the connecting web consists only of skin. **single s.,** syndactyly involving two digits (a single web). **triple s.,** syndactyly involving four digits (three webs).

syndectomy (sin-dek′to-me) [Gr. *syndesmos* band + *ektomē* excision] peritectomy.

syndelphus (sin-del′fus) synadelphus.

syndesis (sin′dĕ-sis, sin-de′sis) [syn- + Gr. *desis* binding] 1. arthrodesis. 2. synapsis.

syndesmectomy (sin″des-mek′to-me) [syndesmo- + Gr. *ektomē* excision] excision of a ligament or a portion of a ligament.

syndesmectopia (sin″des-mek-to′pe-ah) [syndesmo- + Gr. *ektopos* out of place + *-ia*] unusual situation of a ligament.

syndesmitis (sin″des-mi′tis) [syndesmo- + *-itis*] 1. inflammation of a ligament or ligaments. 2. conjunctivitis. **s. metatar′sea,** inflammation of the metatarsal ligaments occurring during strenuous marches; called also *march tumor.*

syndesmo- (sin-des′mo) [Gr. *syndesmos* band or ligament] a combining form denoting relationship to connective tissue or particularly the ligaments.

syndesmochorial (sin″des-mo-ko′re-al) a type of placentation, occurring in ruminants, characterized by limited destruction of the endometrial epithelium.

syndesmography (sin″des-mog′rah-fe) [syndesmo- + Gr. *graphein* to write] a description of the ligaments.

syndesmologia (sin″des-mo-lo′je-ah) syndesmology; in NA terminology *syndesmologia* encompasses the nomenclature relating to the articulations (joints) and ligaments.

syndesmology (sin″des-mol′o-je) [syndesmo- + Gr. *logos* treatise] the scientific study of ligaments, by extension including also study of the articulations and joints; applied also to the body of knowledge relating thereto.

syndesmoma (sin″des-mo′mah) a connective tissue tumor.

syndesmo-odontoid (sin-des″mo-o-don′toid) the posterior of the two atloaxoid articulations formed between the anterior surface of the transverse ligaments and the back of the odontoid process.

syndesmopexy (sin-des′mo-pek″se) [syndesmo- + Gr. *pēxis* fixation] the operative fixation of a dislocation by using the ligaments of the joint.

syndesmophyte (sin-des′mo-fīt) [syndesmo- + Gr. *phyton* plant] an osseous excrescence, or bony outgrowth, from a ligament.

syndesmoplasty (sin-des′mo-plas″te) [syndesmo- + Gr. *plassein* to form] plastic operation on a ligament.

syndesmorrhaphy (sin″des-mor′ah-fe) [syndesmo- + Gr. *rhaphē* suture] suture or repair of ligaments.

syndesmosis (sin″des-mo′sis), pl. *syndesmo′ses* [Gr. *syndesmos* band] [NA] a type of fibrous joint in which the intervening fibrous connective tissue forms an interosseous membrane or ligament. **tibiofibular s., s. tibiofibula′ris** [NA], a firm fibrous union formed at the distal end of the tibia and fibula between the fibular notch of the tibia and a roughened triangular surface on the fibula. **s. tympanostape′dia** [NA], **tympanostapedial s.,** the connection of the base of the stapes with the secondary membrane in the fenestra vestibuli.

syndesmotomy (sin″des-mot′o-me) [syndesmo- + Gr. *tomē* a cutting] the dissection or cutting of a ligament.

syndrome (sin′drōm) [Gr. *syndromē* concurrence] a set of symptoms which occur together; the sum of signs of any morbid state; a symptom complex. In genetics, a combination of phenotypic manifestations. **Aarskog's s.,** a hereditary syndrome, transmitted as an X-linked trait, characterized by ocular hypertelorism, anteverted nostrils, broad upper lip, peculiar scrotal "shawl" above the penis, and small hands. Called also *faciogenital dysplasia.* **Abercrombie's s.,** amyloid degeneration. **abstinence s.,** withdrawal symptoms. **abused-child s.,** battered-child s. **Achard-Thiers s.,** an association of diabetes and hirsutism in postmenopausal women; sometimes alleged to involve an increased incidence of uterine cancer. **acute organic brain s.,** severe mental symptoms arising suddenly in a person previously psychologically normal, caused by head injury, infections, endogenous and exogenous intoxications, nutritional deficiency, etc. It is characterized by a host of symptoms, including delirium, confusional states, disorientation for time and place, distractibility, restlessness, and excitement. Such disorders are reversible. **Adair-Dighton s.,** van der Hoeve's s. **Adams-Stokes s.,** see under *disease.* **addisonian s.,** the complex of symptoms resulting from adrenal insufficiency; see *Addison's disease,* under *disease.* **Adie's s.,** a syndrome consisting of a pathological pupil reaction (tonic pupil), the most important element of which is a myotonic condition on accommodation; the pupil on the affected side contracts on near vision more slowly than does the pupil on the opposite side, and it also dilates more slowly. The affected pupil does not usually react to direct or indirect light, but it may do so in an abnormal fashion. Certain tendon reflexes are absent or diminished, but there are no motor or sensory disturbances, nor demonstrable changes indicative of disease of the nervous system. **adiposogenital s.,** adiposogenital dystrophy. **adrenogenital s.,** hyperfunction of the adrenal cortex, with pseudohermaphroditism and virilism in the female, usually evident at birth, and precocious sexual development (macrogenitosomia precox) in the male, usually not appearing until three or four years after birth; the clinical findings are due to deficient production of cortisol and excessive production of androgen. Called also *congenital adrenal hyperplasia.* **adult respiratory distress s. (ARDS),** fulminant pulmonary interstitial and alveolar edema, which usually develops a few days after the initiating trauma, thought to result from a massive sympathetic discharge due to brain injury or hypoxia and from increased capillary permeability. Called also *shock lung.* **afferent loop s.,** chronic partial obstruction of the proximal loop (duodenum and jejunum) after gastrojejunostomy, resulting in duodenal distention, pain, and nausea following ingestion of food. **Ahumada-del Castillo s.,** a nonpuerperal triad consisting of galactorrhea, amenorrhea, and low gonadotropin secretion. **Albright's s., Albright-McCune-Sternberg s.,** fibrous dysplasia of bone, melanotic pigmentation of the skin, and sexual precocity in the female; called also *osteitis fibrosa disseminata.* **alcohol withdrawal s.,** the neurological effects in alcoholics of withdrawing from alcohol, characterized by agitation, disorientation, and hallucinosis, which may progress to convulsions and on to delirium tremens. **Aldrich's s.,** Wiskott-Aldrich s. **Alezzandrini's s.,** unilateral degenerative retinitis followed shortly by ipsilateral vitiligo and poliosis; deafness may occur. **Alport's s.,** a hereditary disorder characterized by progressive sensorineural hearing loss, progressive pyelonephritis or glomerulonephritis, and occasionally ocular defects. It is transmitted as an autosomal dominant trait. **Alstrom's s.,** a hereditary syndrome of retinitis pigmentosa with nystagmus and early loss of central vision, deafness, obesity, and diabetes mellitus. **amnestic s.,** Korsakoff's psychosis. **amniotic infection s. of Blane,** a syndrome in which fetal sepsis follows swallowing and at times aspiration of contaminated amniotic fluid. **amyostatic s.,** hepatolenticular degeneration. **Andersen's s.,** bronchiectasis, cystic fibrosis of the pancreas, and vitamin A deficiency. **Angelucci's s.,** excitable temperament, palpitation, and vasomotor disturbance in patients with vernal conjunctivitis. **anginal s., anginose s.,** the pain or other symptoms of coronary insufficiency. **anterior cord s.,** localized injury to the anterior portion of the spinal cord, characterized by complete paralysis and hypalgesia and hypesthesia to the level of the lesion, but with relative preservation of posterior column sensations of touch, position, and vibration. **anterior cornual s.,** muscular atrophy due to lesions of the anterior horns of the spinal cord. **anterior tibial compartment s.,** rapid swelling, increased tension, pain, and ischemic necrosis of the muscles of the anterior tibial compartment of the leg; the skin becomes glossy, erythematous, and edematous as the necrosis occurs. The cause is unknown, but usually there is a history of excessive exertion. **Anton's s.,** see under *symptom.* **anxiety s.,** the physical symptoms accompanying anxiety, such as palpitation of the heart, rapid and shallow respiration, sweating, pallor, and a feeling of panic. **aortic arch s.,** any of a group of disorders leading to occlusion of the arteries arising from the aortic arch; such occlusion may be caused by atherosclerosis, arterial embolism, syphilitic or tuberculous arteritis, etc. See also *pulseless disease,* under *disease.* **Apert's s.,** acrocephalosyndactyly. **argentaffinoma s.,** carcinoid s. **Arnold's nerve reflex cough s.,** a reflex cough due to irritation of the area supplied by Arnold's nerve (the auricular branch of the vagus nerve); this area is the posterior and inferior portion of the external auditory canal and the posterior half of the tympanic membrane. **Arnold-Chiari s.,** see under *deformity.* **Ascher's s.,** blepharochalasis occurring in association with goiter (adenoma of the thyroid) and redundancy of the mucous membrane and submucous tissue of the upper lip. **Asherman's s.,** persistent amenorrhea and secondary sterility due to intrauterine adhesions and synechiae, usually occurring as a result of uterine curettage. **asplenia s.,** Ivemark's s. **ataxia-telangiectasia s.,** see under *ataxia.* **auriculotemporal s.,** the appearance of a red area and of sweating on the cheek in connection with eating; seen in lesions of the parotid gland and due to some involvement of the auriculotemporal nerve. **autoerythrocyte sensitization s.,** a purpuric reaction occurring chiefly in young women, in which spontaneous, painful, recurrent single or multiple ecchymoses occur on any part of the body without trauma or after insufficient trauma. Sensitivity to a component of the erythrocytes' structural framework is responsible in many cases, but in some cases the leukocytes seem to be responsible. Emotional upsets are believed to be a precipitating factor. Called also *erythrocyte autosensitization syndrome, Gardner-Diamond syndrome,* and *painful bruising syndrome.* **Avellis' s.,** ipsilateral paralysis of vocal cord and soft palate, loss of pain and temperature sensibility in contralateral leg, trunk, arm, neck, and in the skin over the scalp; called also *ambiguospinothalamic paralysis.* **Axenfeld's s.,** a dominantly inherited syndrome consisting of posterior embryotoxon associated with adhesion of the base of the iris to Schwalbe's ring, defective development of the angular structures and trabecular region, and, frequently, glaucoma. Called also *Axenfeld's anomaly.* **Ayerza's s.,** pulmonary hypertension with dilatation of the pulmonary arteries,

related to disease of the lungs; formerly attributed to syphilis. **Baastrup's s.,** kissing spine. **Babinski's s.,** the association of cardiac and arterial disorders with chronic syphilitic meningitis, tabes dorsalis, paralytic dementia, and other late syphilitic manifestations. **Babinski-Fröhlich s.,** adiposogenital dystrophy. **s. of Babinski-Nageotte,** a syndrome due to multiple lesions affecting the pyramid and sensory tracts, the cerebellar peduncle, and the reticular formation, and marked by contralateral hemiplegia and hemianesthesia (usually only of the pain and temperature senses), ipsilateral hemiasynergia, hemiataxia, and Horner's syndrome. **Babinski-Vaquez s.,** Babinski's s. **Bäfverstedt's s.,** lymphadenosis benigna cutis. **Balint's s.,** cortical paralysis of visual fixation, optic ataxia, and disturbance of visual attention, with preservation of spontaneous and reflex eye movements. The parieto-occipital lesions are bilateral. **Banti's s.,** congestive splenomegaly. **Bardet-Biedl s.,** Laurence-Biedl s. **Barré-Guillain s.,** acute febrile polyneuritis. **Barrett's s.,** peptic ulcer of the lower esophagus, often with stricture, due to the presence of columnar-lined epithelium, which may contain functional mucous cells, parietal cells, or chief cells, in the esophagus instead of normal squamous cell epithelium. Called also *Barrett's esophagus.* **Bartter's s.,** hypertrophy and hyperplasia of the juxtaglomerular cells, producing hypokalemic alkalosis and hyperaldosteronism, characterized by absence of hypertension in the presence of markedly increased plasma renin concentrations, and by insensitivity to the pressor effects of angiotensin. It usually affects children and is perhaps hereditary, and may be associated with other anomalies, such as mental retardation and short stature. Called also *juxtaglomerular cell hyperplasia.* **basal cell nevus s.,** a hereditary disorder consisting of multiple basal cell carcinomas, jaw cysts, characteristic shallow pits of the skin of the hands and feet, multiple bony anomalies, and other defects; called also *nevoid basal cell carcinoma s., nevoid basalioma s., Gorlin's s.,* and *Gorlin-Goltz s.* **Bassen-Kornzweig s.,** abetalipoproteinemia. **battered child s.,** multiple traumatic lesions of the bones and soft tissues of young children, often accompanied by subdural hematomas; such lesions are usually willfully inflicted by an adult. Called also *abused child s.* **Beau's s.,** asystole. **Beckwith's s.,** a hereditary disorder marked by extreme cytomegaly of the fetal adrenal cortex, omphalocele, macroglossia, hyperplasia of the kidney and pancreas, Leydig-cell hyperplasia, and postnatal gigantism. **Beckwith-Wiedemann s.,** EMG s. **Behçet's s.,** severe uveitis and retinal vasculitis, optic atrophy, and aphtha-like lesions of the mouth and genitalia, often with other signs and symptoms suggesting a diffuse vasculitis; a rare disorder of unknown etiology, it most often affects young males. **s. of Benedikt,** a syndrome consisting of ipsilateral oculomotor paralysis, contralateral hyperkinesia, contralateral tremor and paresis of the arm and leg, and ipsilateral ataxia; caused by lesions that damage the third nerve and involve the nucleus ruber and corticospinal tract. **Bernard's s., Bernard-Horner s.,** Horner's s. **Bernard-Sergent s.,** diarrhea, vomiting, and collapse characteristic of Addison's disease. **Bernard-Soulier s.,** a hereditary coagulation disorder marked by mild thrombocytopenia, giant and morphologically abnormal platelets, hemorrhagic tendency, prolonged bleeding time, and abnormal prothrombin consumption. **Bernhardt-Rot s.,** meralgia paraesthetica. **Bernheim's s.,** right heart failure with absence of dyspnea or pulmonary congestion, in the presence of gross left ventricular hypertrophy, sometimes attributed to impairment of right ventricular capacity and filling. **Bertolotti's s.,** sacralization of the fifth lumbar vertebra together with sciatica and scoliosis. **Bianchi's s.,** a sensory aphasic syndrome with apraxia and alexia, seen in lesions of the left parietal lobe. **Biedl's s., Biemond's s.,** Laurence-Biedl s. **Björnstad's s.,** congenital cochlear deafness with pili torti. **Blatin's s.,** hydatid thrill. **blind loop s.,** a syndrome resulting from alterations in the anatomy of the small intestine, as by strictures or after surgery, in which a loop is disconnected from the main stream or when intestinal contents may gain access to it but not readily egress from it; it is associated with bacterial overgrowth, particularly anaerobic organisms, with resultant malabsorption of vitamin B_{12}, steatorrhea, and anemia. **Bloch-Sulzberger s.,** incontinentia pigmenti. **Bloom's s.,** dwarfism, photosensitivity, and butterfly telangiectatic erythema of the face, with numerous defects of skin pigmentation, keratinization, dentition, and development; it is transmitted as an autosomal recessive trait. **blue diaper s.,** a defect of tryptophan absorption in which, because of intestinal bacterial action on the tryptophan, the urine contains abnormal indoles, giving it a blue color. It is similar to Hartnup's disease. **Blum's s.,** hypochloremic azotemia. **body of Luys s.,** hemiballismus. **Boerhaave's s.,** spontaneous rupture of the esophagus. **Bonnevie-Ullrich s.,** a condition characterized by pterygium colli, lymphangiectatic edema of hands and feet, ocular hypertelorism, short stature, and other developmental anomalies. **Bonnier's s.,** a series of symptoms due to lesion of Deiters' nucleus or of the vestibular tracts related thereto; it consists of vertigo, pallor, and various aural and ocular disturbances. **Böök's s.,** PHC s. **Börjeson's s., Börjeson-Forssman-Lehmann s.,** a hereditary syndrome, transmitted as an X-linked recessive trait, characterized by severe mental retardation, epilepsy, hypogonadism, hypometabolism, marked obesity, swelling of the subcutaneous tissues of the face, and large ears. **Bouillaud's s.,** the coincidence of pericarditis and endocarditis in acute articular rheumatism. **Bouveret's s.,** paroxysmal tachycardia. **brachial s.,** a morbid condition resulting from compression or irritation of nerves of the brachial plexus. **Brachmann-de Lange s.,** de Lange's s. **bradycardia-tachycardia s.,** episodic or repetitive tachycardia of short duration followed by transient or protracted heart standstill, sometimes accentuated by quinidine. **brain s.,** see *acute brain s., chronic brain s.,* and *organic brain s.* **Brennemann's s.,** mesenteric and retroperitoneal lymphadenitis as a sequel of throat infections. **Briquet's s.,** shortness of breath and aphonia dependent on hysterical paralysis of the diaphragm. **Brissaud-Marie s.,** hysterical glossolabial hemispasm. **Brissaud-Sicard s.,** spasmodic hemiplegia caused by lesions of the pons. **Bristowe's s.,** a series of ingravescent symptoms characteristic of tumor of the corpus callosum: (1) gradual onset of hemiplegia; (2) association of hemiplegia on one side, vague hemiplegic symptoms on the other; (3) stupor and drowsiness, difficulty of swallowing, and speechlessness; (4) absence of direct implication of the cranial nerves; (5) death from coma. **brittle cornea s.,** an X-linked, recessively inherited syndrome, characterized by brittle cornea, blue sclerae, and red hair. **Brock s.,** middle lobe s. **Brown's vertical retraction s.,** adhesion of the muscles of the eye in the fetus. **Brown-Séquard s.,** a syndrome due to damage of one half of the spinal cord, resulting in ipsilateral paralysis and loss of discriminatory and joint sensation, and contralateral loss of pain and temperature sensation. Called also *Brown-Séquard's disease, paralysis,* or *sign.* **Bruns' s.,** intermittent headache, vertigo, vomiting, and visual disturbances on sudden movement of the head, characteristic of cysticercus infection of the fourth ventricle, lesion of the fourth ventricle, or tumors of the midline of the cerebellum and third or lateral ventricles; called also *Bruns' sign.* **Brunsting's s.,** a recurrent eruptive syndrome usually affecting middle-aged men, in which grouped, vesicular lesions occur about the head and neck, and result in scarring. **Brushfield-Wyatt s.,** a congenital syndrome consisting of extensive unilateral nevus flammeus, hemianopia affecting the right or left halves of the visual fields of both eyes, contralateral hemiplegia, cerebral angioma, and mental retardation; it is probably related to the Sturge-Weber syndrome. **Budd-Chiari s.,** symptomatic obstruction or occlusion of the hepatic veins, usually of unknown origin, but probably caused by a variety of circumstances, including neoplasms, strictures, liver disease, trauma, systemic infections, and hematologic disorders. It occurs in two forms: The *acute* form is characterized by abdominal and epigastric pain accompanied by rapid progressive enlargement and tenderness of the liver, massive ascites, and mild jaundice; the onset may be sudden and dramatic, with death occurring within a few hours or days, or it may be less dramatic with death occurring within 30 days. The *chronic* form is characterized by insidious onset, gradual enlargement of the liver, ascites, abdominal tenderness and pain of variable degree, vomiting, nausea, and edema of the lower extremities; death occurs after months or even years. Called also *Budd-Chiari disease, Chiari's disease* or *syndrome,* and *endophlebitis hepatica obliterans.* **bulbar s.,** Dejerine's syndrome, def. 2. **Bürger-Grütz s.,** hyperlipoproteinemia, type I. **Burnett's s.,** milk-alkali s. **burning feet s.,** Gopalan's s. **Buschke-Ollendorff s.,** dermatofibrosis lenticularis disseminata. **Bywaters' s.,** crush s. **Caffey's s., Caffey-Silverman s.,** infantile cortical hyperostosis. **callosal s.,** an association of symptoms thought to result from a lesion of the corpus callosum. **camptomelic s.,** osteochondrodysplasia associated with flat facies, bowed tibiae with skin dimpling, hypoplastic scapulae, and short vertebrae. **Canada-Cronkhite s.,** familial gastrointestinal polyposis with ectodermal defects, e.g., nail atrophy, alopecia, and excessive skin pigmentation, and sometimes with protein-losing enteropathy, malabsorption, and deficiency of blood calcium, potassium, and magnesium. **Capgras' s.,** a mental condition in which the patient cannot identify the person appearing before him. **Caplan's s.,** pneumoconiosis associated with rheumatoid arthritis. Radiographically, multiple spherical nodular lesions with clearly demarcated borders are found throughout both lungs. Called also *rheumatoid pneumoconiosis.* **capsular thrombosis s.,** hemiplegia due to thrombosis of a blood vessel supplying the internal capsule. **capsulothalamic s.,** hemiplegia, hemianopia, and perverted pain perception due to lesions of the thalamus and internal capsule. **carcinoid s.,** a symptom complex associated with carcinoid tumors (argentaffinoma) and characterized by attacks of severe cyanotic flushing of the skin lasting from minutes to days and by diarrheal watery stools, bronchoconstrictive attacks, sudden drops in blood pressure, edema, and ascites. Symptoms are caused by secretion by the tumor of serotonin, prostaglandins, and other biologically active substances. Called also *argentaffinoma s.* **cardiofacial s.,** a syndrome of congenital heart disease associated with unilateral partial lower facial paresis, the latter being transient or persistent. **carotid sinus s.,** syncope sometimes associated with convulsive seizures due to overactivity of the carotid sinus reflex when pressure is applied to one or both carotid

sinuses. **carpal tunnel s.,** a complex of symptoms resulting from compression of the median nerve in the carpal tunnel, with pain and burning or tingling paresthesias in the fingers and hand, sometimes extending to the elbow. **Carpenter's s.,** a hereditary disorder, transmitted as an autosomal recessive trait, characterized by acrocephalopolysyndactyly, brachydactyly, peculiar facies, obesity, mental retardation, hypogonadism, and other anomalies. Called also *acrocephalopolysyndactyly type II.* **cartilage–hair hypoplasia s.,** a hereditary syndrome transmitted as an autosomal recessive trait, consisting of short-limbed dwarfism with fine, sparse hair and deficient cellular immunity. **cat's cry s.,** cri du chat s. **cat-eye s., cat's eye s.,** an association of coloboma of the iris and anal atresia; there may also be many other anomalies, including preauricular skin tags or fistulas, hypertelorism, congenital heart disease, skeletal abnormalities, and renal malformations. It is associated with aneuploidy (an extra, acrocentric chromosome slightly smaller than the G-group chromosomes). **cauda equina s.,** dull aching pain of the perineum, bladder, and sacrum, generally radiating in a sciatic fashion, with associated paresthesias and areflexic paralysis, due to compression of the spinal nerve roots. **cavernous sinus s.,** edema of the conjunctiva, proptosis, edema of upper lid and root of the nose, together with paralysis of the third, fourth, and sixth nerves, due to thrombosis of the cavernous sinus. **celiac s.,** see under *disease.* **central cord s.,** injury to the central portion of the cervical spinal cord resulting in disproportionately more weakness or paralysis in the upper extremities than in the lower; pathological change is caused by hemorrhage or edema. **centroposterior s.,** syringomyelic dissociation of sensibility and vasomotor disorders, due to lesions of the centroposterior portion of the gray matter of the spinal cord. **cerebellar s.,** hereditary cerebellar ataxia. **cerebrocardiac s.,** Krishaber's disease. **cerebrohepatorenal s.,** a hereditary disorder, transmitted as an autosomal recessive trait, characterized by craniofacial abnormalities, hypotonia, hepatomegaly, polycystic kidneys, jaundice, and death in early infancy. **cervical s.,** a condition caused by irritation or compression of the cervical nerve roots, marked by pain in the neck radiating into the shoulder, arm, or forearm, depending on which nerve root is affected. **cervical rib s., cervicobrachial s.,** scalenus s. **Cestan's s., s. of Cestan-Chenais,** an association of contralateral hemiplegia, contralateral hemianesthesia, ipsilateral lateropulsion and hemiasynergia, Horner's syndrome, and ipsilateral laryngoplegia, due to scattered lesions of the pyramid, sensory tract, inferior cerebellar peduncle, nucleus ambiguus, and oculopupillary center. **Cestan-Raymond s.,** Raymond-Cestan s. **chancriform s.,** primary extrapulmonary coccidioidomycosis. **Charcot's s.,** 1. amyotrophic lateral sclerosis. 2. intermittent claudication. 3. intermittent hepatic fever, due to cholangitis. **Charcot-Weiss-Barker s.,** carotid sinus s. **Charlin's s.,** pain, iritis, corneitis, rhinorrhea, and tenderness along the nose in eye disturbance of nasal origin. **Chauffard's s., Chauffard-Still s.,** polyarthritis with fever and enlargement of the spleen and lymph nodes in persons infected with nonhuman tuberculosis. **Chédiak-Higashi s.,** a lethal, progressive, autosomal recessive, systemic disorder associated with oculocutaneous albinism, massive leukocyte inclusions (giant lysosomes), histiocytic infiltration of multiple body organs, development of pancytopenia, hepatosplenomegaly, recurrent or persistent bacterial infections, and a possible predisposition to development of malignant lymphoma. Called also *Béguez César disease* and *Chédiak-Higashi anomaly.* **Chiari's s.,** Budd-Chiari s. **Chiari-Arnold s.,** Arnold-Chiari deformity. **Chiari-Frommel s.,** a postparturient condition characterized by persistent lactation, amenorrhea, and atrophy of the uterus, ovaries, and vaginal tract, and low urinary levels of estrogen and gonadotropins; it may be due to pituitary or hypothalamic dysfunction. Called also *Frommel-Chiari s., Chiari-Frommel disease,* and *Frommel's disease.* **chiasma s., chiasmatic s.,** a syndrome indicative of lesion affecting the optic chiasma: impairment of vision, limitations of the field of vision, central scotoma, headache, vertigo, and syncope. **Chinese restaurant s. (CRS),** a transient syndrome associated with arterial dilatation, due to ingestion of monosodium glutamate, which is used liberally in seasoning Chinese food; it is characterized by throbbing of the head, lightheadedness, tightness of the jaw, neck, and shoulders, and backache. **Chotzen's s.,** a hereditary disorder, transmitted as an autosomal dominant trait, characterized by acrocephalosyndactyly in which the syndactyly is mild and by hypertelorism, ptosis, and sometimes mental retardation. Called also *acrocephalosyndactyly type III* and *Saethre-Chotzen s.* **Christian's s.,** Hand-Schüller-Christian disease. **Christ-Siemens s., Christ-Siemens-Touraine s.,** congenital ectodermal defect. **chronic brain s.,** a syndrome resulting from or associated with relatively permanent and more or less irreversible diffuse organic impairment of cerebral tissue function; disturbances of memory, orientation, comprehension, and affect of greater or lesser degree are characteristically present. It may occur in dementia paralytica, cerebral arteriosclerosis, brain trauma, Huntington's chorea, Pick's disease, brain tumor, etc. Abbreviated CBS. **Churg-Strauss s.,** allergic granulomatosis. **Citelli's s.,** mental backwardness, loss of power of concentration, drowsiness or insomnia; seen in persons with adenoids or sinus infection. **Clarke-Hadfield s.,** congenital pancreatic disease with infantilism; with enlarged liver, bulky fatty stools, and extensive atrophy of pancreas in undersized and underweight child. **Claude's s.,** paralysis of the third (oculomotor) nerve on one side and asynergia on the other side, together with dysarthria; called also *inferior s. of red nucleus* and *rubrospinal cerebellar peduncle s.* **Claude Bernard–Horner s.,** Horner's s. **Clérambault-Kandinsky s.,** see under *complex.* **click s.,** a left ventricular abnormality marked by apical midsystolic click and late murmur, with inversion of T waves. **closed head s.,** the complex of symptoms characteristic of cerebral injury without cranial penetration. **Clough and Richter's s.,** anemia in which the red corpuscles exhibit a severe degree of autoagglutination. **Clouston's s.,** hidrotic ectodermal dysplasia. **Cockayne's s.,** a hereditary syndrome transmitted as an autosomal recessive trait, consisting of dwarfism with retinal atrophy and deafness, associated with progeria, prognathism, mental retardation, and photosensitivity. **Cogan's s.,** nonsyphilitic keratitis with vestibuloauditory symptoms. **Collet's s., Collet-Sicard s.,** glossolaryngoscapulopharyngeal hemiplegia due to complete lesion of the ninth, tenth, eleventh and twelfth cranial nerves. **compression s.,** shock with hematuria and oliguria following long continued pressure on a limb, as in bombed buildings. **concussion s.,** encephalopathy due to trauma; see *postconcussional s.* **Conn's s.,** primary aldosteronism. **Conradi's s.,** chondrodystrophia calcificans congenita. **Cornelia de Lange's s.,** de Lange's s. **s. of corpus striatum,** Vogt's s. **Costen's s.,** temporomandibular joint s. **costoclavicular s.,** pain or other difficulties in the arm and/or hand, apparently due to pressure, stretching, or friction on the nerves or vessels at the cervicobrachial outlet. **Cotard's s.,** paranoia with delusions of negation, a suicidal tendency, and sensory disturbances. **Courvoisier-Terrier s.,** dilatation of the gallbladder, retention jaundice, and discoloration of the feces, indicating obstruction due to a tumor of the ampulla of Vater. **Creutzfeldt-Jakob s.,** a rare, usually fatal, transmissible spongiform viral encephalopathy, occurring in middle life in which there is partial degeneration of the pyramidal and extrapyramidal systems accompanied by progressive dementia and sometimes wasting of the muscles, tremor, athetosis, and spastic dysarthria. Called also *Creutzfeldt-Jakob disease, Jakob's disease, Jakob-Creutzfeldt disease,* and *spastic pseudoparalysis.* **cri du chat s.,** a hereditary congenital syndrome characterized by hypertelorism, microcephaly, severe mental deficiency, and a plaintive catlike cry, due to deletion of the short arm of chromosome 5. Called also *cat's cry s.* **Crigler-Najjar s.,** a congenital familial form of nonhemolytic jaundice, due to the absence of the hepatic enzyme glucuronide transferase, transmitted as an autosomal recessive trait. It is characterized by the presence in the blood of excessive amounts of unconjugated bilirubin and by kernicterus and severe disorders of the central nervous system. Called also *congenital hyperbilirubinemia* and *congenital nonhemolytic jaundice.* **s. of crocodile tears,** spontaneous lacrimation occurring parallel with the normal salivation of eating. It follows facial paralysis and seems to be due to straying of the regenerating nerve fibers, some of those destined for the salivary glands going to the lacrimal glands. **Cronkhite's s., Cronkhite-Canada s.,** Canada-Cronkhite s. **CRST s.,** diffuse progressive scleroderma in which calcinosis, Raynaud's phenomenon, sclerodactyly, and telangiectasia are prominent. **crush s.,** the edema, oliguria, and other symptoms of renal failure which follow the crushing of a part, especially a large muscle mass; see *lower nephron nephrosis,* under *nephrosis.* **Cruveilhier-Baumgarten s.,** cirrhosis of the liver with portal hypertension, associated with congenital patency of the umbilical or paraumbilical veins. It is characterized by hematemesis, ascites, splenomegaly, hypersplenism, esophageal varices, caput medusae, large tortuous veins in the abdominal wall, and a venous hum, often accompanied by a thrill, usually heard over the region of the xiphoid process. Called also *Cruveilhier-Baumgarten cirrhosis.* **cryptophthalmos s.,** an autosomal recessive abnormality, characterized by absence of the palpebral apertures, disorganization of one or both ocular globes, malformed ears, cleft palate, laryngeal stenosis, syndactyly, meningoencephalocele, imperforate anus, cardiac defects, and maldeveloped kidneys. **cubital tunnel s.,** a complex of symptoms resulting from injury or compression of the ulnar nerve at the elbow, with pain and numbness along the ulnar aspect of the hand and forearm, and weakness of the hand. **culture specific s.,** a form of disturbed behavior highly specific to certain cultural systems and that does not conform to Western nosologic entities; see also *hysterical psychosis,* under *psychosis.* **Curtius' s.,** hypertrophy of one side of the entire body or a portion of one side of the body, as of the face; called also *hemihypertrophy.* **Cushing's s.,** 1. a condition, more commonly seen in females, due to hyperadrenocorticism resulting from neoplasms of the adrenal cortex or the anterior lobe of the pituitary, or to prolonged excessive intake of glucocorticoids for therapeutic purposes (*Cushing's s. medicamentosus* or *iatrogenic Cushing's s.*). The symptoms and signs may include rapidly developing adiposity of the face, neck, and trunk, kyphosis caused by osteoporosis of the spine, hypertension, diabetes mellitus, amenorrhea, hypertrichosis (in females), impotence (in males),

dusky complexion with purple markings (striae), polycythemia, pain in the abdomen and back, and muscular wasting and weakness. When secondary to excessive pituitary secretion of adrenocorticotropin, it is known as Cushing's disease. Called also *Cushing's basophilism,* and *pituitary basophilism.* 2. in tumors of the cerebellopontine angle and acoustic tumors: subjective noises, impairment of hearing, ipsilateral cerebellar ataxia, and eventually ipsilateral impairment of the sixth and seventh nerve function together with elevated intracranial pressure. **Cushing's s. medicamentosus,** see *Cushing's s.,* def. 1. **Cyriax's s.,** a syndrome due to slipped rib cartilages pressing on the nerves at the interchondral joint, resulting in pain in the region of the cartilage, radiation of pain to the shoulder and arm, or pain similar to that of angina pectoris. **Da Costa's s.,** neurocirculatory asthenia. **Danbolt-Closs s.,** acrodermatitis enteropathica. **Dandy-Walker s.,** congenital hydrocephalus due to obstruction of the foramina of Magendie and Luschka; called also *Dandy-Walker deformity.* **Danlos' s.,** Ehlers-Danlos s. **Debré-Sémélaigne s.,** hereditary athyrotic cretinism associated with myotonia and muscular pseudohypertrophy, inherited as an autosomal recessive trait. Called also *Kocher-Debré-Sémélaigne s.* **defibrination s.,** diffuse intravascular coagulation; see under *coagulation.* **Degos' s.,** malignant papulosis. **Dejerine's s.,** 1. a syndrome in cortical sensory disturbances characterized by impairment of sensory discrimination (astereognosis), judgment of intensity and recognition of differences. 2. of bulbar lesions, those in the upper part of the bulb produce paralysis of the twelfth nerve of the side of the lesion and hemiplegia on the opposite side; lesions in the lower part of the bulb cause paralysis of the larynx and soft palate. 3. symptoms of radiculitis; namely, distribution of the pain, motor and sensory defects in the region of the radicular or segmental disturbance of the nerve roots rather than along the course of the peripheral nerve. 4. a syndrome resembling tabes dorsalis, with deep sensibility depressed but tactile sense normal. It is due to lesion of the long root fibers of the posterior column. **Dejerine-Klumpke s.,** Klumpke's paralysis. **s. of Dejerine-Roussy,** thalamic s. **Dejerine-Sottas s.,** progressive hypertrophic interstitial neuropathy. **de Lange's s.,** a congenital syndrome in which severe mental retardation is associated with many abnormalities, including short stature (Amsterdam dwarf), brachycephaly, low-set ears, webbed neck, carp mouth, depressed bridge of the nose with the end tilted up and forward-directed nostrils, bushy eyebrows meeting at the midline, unruly coarse hair growing low on the forehead and neck, and flat spadelike hands with short tapering fingers. Called also *Brachmann-de Lange s., Cornelia de Lange's s.,* and *typhus degenerativus amstelodamensis.* **Dennie-Marfan s.,** spastic paralysis and mental retardation in association with congenital syphilis. **depersonalization s.,** see under *neurosis.* **De Sanctis-Cacchione s.,** a hereditary syndrome, transmitted as an autosomal recessive trait, consisting of xeroderma pigmentosum associated with mental retardation, retarded growth, gonadal hypoplasia, and sometimes with neurologic complications and photosensitivity; called also *xerodermic idiocy.* **de Toni-Fanconi s.,** see *Fanconi's s.,* def. 2. **diencephalic s.,** failure to thrive, emaciation, and sometimes nevus unius lateralis. **DiGeorge's s.,** a congenital syndrome in which absence of the thymus and parathyroids due to defective development of the third and fourth embryonic pharyngeal pouches is associated with impairment of cell-mediated immunity and normal levels of immunoglobulins; it is characterized clinically by neonatal tetany, hypocalcemia, frequent viral and fungal infections, and, often, deformities of the ears, nose, mouth, and great vessels. Called also *thymic-parathyroid aplasia.* Cf. *Nezelof's s.* **Dighton-Adair s.,** van der Hoeve's s. **Di Guglielmo s.,** erythroleukemia. **Donohue's s.,** leprechaunism. **Down's s.,** a condition characterized by a small, anteroposteriorly flattened skull, short, flat-bridged nose, epicanthal fold, short phalanges, and widened space between the first and second digits of hands and feet, with moderate to severe mental retardation, and associated with a chromosomal abnormality, usually trisomy of chromosome 21 (Denver classification). Called also *mongolism* and *trisomy 21 s.* **Dresbach's s.,** elliptocytosis. **Dressler's s.,** postmyocardial infarction s. **Duane's s.,** a hereditary congenital syndrome in which the affected eye shows limitation or absence of abduction, restriction of adduction, retraction of the globe on adduction, narrowing of the palpebral fissure on adduction and widening on abduction, and deficient convergence. It is transmitted as an autosomal dominant trait. Called also *retraction s.* and *Stilling-Turk-Duane s.* **Dubin-Johnson s.,** a familial chronic form of nonhemolytic jaundice thought to be due to a defect in the excretion of conjugated bilirubin and certain other organic anions (e.g., sulfobromophthalein) by the liver. It is characterized by the presence of a brown, coarsely granular pigment in the hepatic cells, which is pathognomonic of the condition. **Dubin-Sprinz s.,** Dubin-Johnson s. **Dubreuil-Chambardel s.,** caries of the upper incisor teeth in persons between the ages of fourteen and seventeen followed after an interval by caries in the other teeth. **Duchenne's s.,** the collective signs of bulbar paralysis. **Duchenne-Erb s.,** see under *paralysis.* **dumping s.,** a complex reaction probably due to excessively rapid emptying of the gastric contents, manifested by nausea, weakness, sweating, palpitation, varying degrees of syncope, often a sensation of warmth, and sometimes diarrhea, occurring after ingestion of food by patients who have had partial gastrectomy and gastrojejunostomy. Called also *jejunal s.* and *postgastrectomy s.* **Duplay's s.,** (*obs.*), subacromial or subdeltoid bursitis; see *calcific tendinitis,* under *tendinitis.* **Dupré's s.,** meningism, def. 1. **Dyke-Davidoff s.,** a syndrome possibly due to injury to or severe disease affecting one side of the brain during the neonatal period, characterized by mental retardation, asymmetry of the face, and varying degrees of hemiplegia, neurological impairment, and atrophy of the side of the body contralateral to the lesion. **dysglandular s.,** the series of symptoms caused by an abnormality of the internal secretions (hormones). **dysplasia oculodentodigitalis s.,** oculodentodigital dysplasia. **Eaton-Lambert s.,** a myasthenia-like syndrome in which the weakness usually affects the limbs, and ocular and bulbar muscles are spared; there is reduced muscle action potential on stimulation of its nerve but with repetitive stimulation it becomes augmented. It is often associated with oat-cell carcinoma of the lung. Called also *myasthenic s.* **ectopic ACTH s.,** a condition in which tumors arising from nonendocrine tissue produce ACTH. Depending on its duration, the syndrome may resemble true Cushing's disease, but hypokalemic alkalosis and weakness are often the dominant manifestations. **Eddowes' s.,** blue scleras associated with osteogenesis imperfecta (q.v.). **Edwards' s.,** trisomy 18 s. **effort s.,** neurocirculatory asthenia. **egg-white s.,** biotin deficiency; see *biotin.* **Ehlers-Danlos s.,** a congenital hereditary syndrome characterized by hyperextensibility of the joints and hyperelasticity and fragility of the skin with poor healing of wounds, leaving scars resembling parchment, by capillary fragility, and by subcutaneous mucinous or fatty nodules following trauma. It occurs in many types with wide variability of expression, the classic type being inherited as an autosomal dominant trait. Called also *Danlos's s., cutis elastica, cutis hyperelastica, elastic skin,* and *India rubber skin.* **Eisenmenger's s.,** ventricular septal defect with pulmonary hypertension and cyanosis due to right-to-left (reversed) shunt of blood. Sometimes defined as pulmonary hypertension (pulmonary vascular disease) and cyanosis with the shunt being at the atrial, ventricular, or great vessel area. **Ekbom s.,** restless legs; see under *leg.* **Ellis-van Creveld s.,** chondroectodermal dysplasia. **EMG s.,** a congenital syndrome inherited as an autosomal recessive trait, characterized by exophthalmos, macroglossia, and gigantism, often associated with visceromegaly, adrenocortical cytomegaly, and dysplasia of the renal medulla. Called also *Beckwith-Wiedemann s.* and *exophthalmos-macroglossia-gigantism s.* **empty-sella s.,** a clinical syndrome in which the diaphragma sellae is vestigial, the sella turcica forms an extension of the subarachnoid space and is filled with cerebrospinal fluid, and the pituitary fossa appears to be empty, although the pituitary gland is present in a flattened form. **encephalotrigeminal vascular s.,** the combination of multiple angiomas of the brain and vascular nevi in the trigeminal region. **epiphyseal s.,** precocious development of external genitalia and sexual function, precocious abnormal growth of long bones, appearance of signs of internal hydrocephalus, absence of all other motor and sensory symptoms indicating lesion of the pineal body. Called also *Pellizzi's s., pineal s.,* and *macrogenitosomia precox.* **Epstein's s.,** nephrotic s. **Erb's s.,** the totality of signs of myasthenia gravis. **erythrocyte autosensitization s.,** autoerythrocyte sensitization s. **euthyroid sick s.,** the simulation of hypothyroidism as assessed by thyroid-function tests in a euthyroid patient suffering from systemic illness. **exophthalmos-macroglossia-gigantism s.,** EMG s. **extrapyramidal s.,** any of a group of clinical disorders characterized by abnormal involuntary movements, including parkinsonism, athetosis, and chorea. **Faber's s.,** hypochromic anemia. **Fabry's s.,** see under *disease.* **Fallot's s.,** tetralogy of Fallot. **Fanconi's s.,** 1. a rare hereditary disorder, transmitted in a recessive manner and having a poor prognosis, characterized by pancytopenia, hypoplasia of the bone marrow, and patchy brown discoloration of the skin due to the deposition of melanin, and associated with multiple congenital anomalies of the musculoskeletal and genitourinary systems. Called also *Fanconi's pancytopenia, pancytopenia-dysmelia s., congenital hypoplastic anemia, constitutional infantile panmyelopathy, Fanconi's anemia,* and *congenital pancytopenia.* 2. a general term for a group of diseases marked by dysfunction of the proximal renal tubules, with generalized hyperaminoaciduria, renal glycosuria, hyperphosphaturia, and bicarbonate and water loss; the most common cause is cystinosis (q.v.) but it is also associated with other genetic diseases and occurs in idiopathic and acquired forms. When unassociated with cystinosis, the disorder is also called *de Toni-Fanconi syndrome.* **Farber's s., Farber-Uzman s.,** a progressive form of lipidosis manifest at birth or within the first few months of life, transmitted as an autosomal recessive trait, and characterized by irritability, hoarse cry, nodular erythematous swellings with a predisposition for the extremities, cardiopulmonary and central nervous system involvement, and death occurring by two years of age. Called also *Farber's lipogranulomatosis.* **Favre-Racouchot s.,** nodular elastoidosis. **Felty's s.,** a combination of chronic (rheumatoid) arthritis, splenomegaly, leukopenia, pigmented spots on the skin

of the lower extremities, and other inconsistent evidence of hypersplenism, namely, anemia and thrombocytopenia. **feminizing testes s.,** testicular feminization s. **fertile eunuch s.,** a syndrome of eunuchoidism, with variable secondary sexual development, associated with normal spermatogenesis, normal levels of follicle-stimulating hormone, and variably low levels of luteinizing hormone. **fetal alcohol s.,** a syndrome of altered prenatal growth and morphogenesis occurring in infants born of women who were chronically alcoholic during pregnancy; it includes maxillary hypoplasia, prominence of the forehead and mandible, short palpebral fissures, microphthalmia, epicanthal folds, severe growth retardation, mental retardation, and microcephaly. **fetal face s.,** Robinow's s. **Fiessinger's s.,** Stevens-Johnson s. **Fiessinger-Leroy-Reiter s.,** Reiter's disease. **first arch s.,** malformations including macrostomia, hemignathia, and deformities of the external ear, resulting from an inhibitory process occurring toward the seventh week of embryonic life and affecting the facial bones derived from the first branchial arch. **Fitz's s.,** a series of symptoms indicative of acute pancreatitis, consisting of epigastric pain, vomiting, collapse, followed within twenty-four hours by a circumscribed swelling in the epigastrium or by tympanites. **Fitz-Hugh-Curtis s.,** perihepatitis occurring as a complication of gonorrhea in women, marked by fever, upper quadrant pain, tenderness and spasm of the abdominal wall, and occasionally by friction rub over the liver. **floppy infant s.,** a congenital myopathy of infants, characterized clinically by hypotonia and muscle weakness. The pathologic changes in skeletal muscle include numerous eosinophilic intranuclear crystals, characteristic crystal morphology, myofibrillar fragmentation, sarcoplasmic crystals, and expansion of the Z bands. **floppy valve s.,** mitral regurgitation due to myxomatous transformation of the leaflets of the mitral valve. **focal dermal hypoplasia s.,** a hereditary congenital syndrome of extensive ectodermal and mesodermal dysplasia, chiefly of skin and bones, with linear or serpiginous patches (especially on the buttocks and thighs), telangiectases, pigmentation, and orificial papillomas, often with syndactyly, oligodactyly, or adactyly. An X-linked dominant trait, lethal in the male, is believed responsible. Called also *Goltz's s.* and *Goltz-Gorlin s.* **Forbes-Albright s.,** spontaneous persistent nonpuerperal lactation, most often associated with a pituitary tumor. **Forssman's carotid s.,** neurologic disturbances following injection of a small dose of serum containing Forssman's antibodies into the carotid artery of a guinea pig, including disequilibrium, rotatory movement along the vertical and the longitudinal axes, forced deviation of the eyeballs, and nystagmus. **Foster Kennedy s.,** Kennedy's s. **four-day s.,** respiratory distress syndrome of newborn; so called because the infant usually recovers or dies within four days. **Foville's s.,** a syndrome similar to the Millard-Gubler syndrome (q.v.) except that, in addition to paralysis of the outward movement of the eye, there is paralysis of conjugate movement. **Franceschetti s.,** mandibulofacial dysostosis. **Franceschetti-Jadassohn s.,** Naegeli's s. **François' s.,** oculomandibulofacial s. **Freeman-Sheldon s.,** craniocarpotarsal dystrophy. **Frey's s.,** auriculotemporal s. **Friderichsen-Waterhouse s.,** Waterhouse-Friderichsen s. **Friedmann's vasomotor s.,** a train or cycle of symptoms due to a progressive subacute encephalitis of traumatic origin, including a sense of fullness in the head, headache, vertigo, irritability, insomnia, easy fatigability, and defect of memory. **Fröhlich's s.,** adiposogenital dystrophy. **Froin's s.,** a condition of the lumbar spinal fluid consisting of a transparent clear yellow color (xanthochromia), with the finding of large amounts of protein, rapid coagulation, and the absence of an increased number of cells. It is seen in certain organic nervous diseases in which the lumbar fluid is cut off from communication with the fluid in the ventricles. Called also *loculation s.* **Frommel-Chiari s.,** Chiari-Frommel s. **Fuchs's s.,** unilateral heterochromia, fine keratic precipitates, and secondary cataract. **G s.,** hypertelorism-hypospadias s. **Gaillard's s.,** dextrocardia from retraction of lungs and pleura to the right. **Gaisböck's s.,** stress polycythemia. **Ganser's s.,** amnesia, disturbance of consciousness, and hallucinations, generally of hysterical origin; the condition is marked by senseless answers to questions and by absurd acts. Called also *acute hallucinatory mania* and *nonsense s.* **Gardner's s.,** familial polyposis of the large bowel (with malignant potential), supernumerary teeth, fibrous dysplasia of the skull, osteomas, fibromas, and epithelial cysts. **Gardner-Diamond s.,** autoerythrocyte sensitization s. **Gasser's s.,** hemolytic-uremic s. **gastrocardiac s.,** a concept wherein disturbances of the circulatory system, particularly of the heart, are attributed to faulty function of the stomach. **Gee-Herter-Heubner s.,** the infantile form of nontropical sprue. **Gélineau's s.,** narcolepsy. **gender dysphoria s.,** a group of psychological problems associated with discrepancy between the physical sex assignment and the psychological gender identity. **general adaptation s.,** the total of all nonspecific systemic reactions of the body to long-continued exposure to systemic stress. **Gerhardt's s.,** bilateral abductor paralysis of the vocal cords causing inspiratory dyspnea. **Gerlier's s.,** Gerlier's disease. **Gerstmann's s.,** a combination of finger agnosia, right-left disorientation, agraphia, acalculia, and often constrictional apraxia, due to a lesion in the angular gyrus of the dominant hemisphere. **Gianotti-Crosti s.,** an acute transient dermatitis usually occurring in girls under the age of six, marked by the sudden appearance of nonpruritic asymmetrically distributed, red to purple, flat, dome-shaped, or pointed papules, which later assume a natural skin color, on the lower arms and thighs, the trunk, and sometimes the area around the front of the axillae; often accompanied by malaise, fever, respiratory or gastrointestinal symptoms, and lymphadenopathy. Called also *acrodermatitis papulosa infantum.* **Gilbert's s.,** see under *disease.* **Gilles de la Tourette's s.,** a syndrome of facial and vocal tics with onset in childhood, progressing to generalized jerking movements in any part of the body, with echolalia and coprolalia; once thought to have an unfavorable prognosis but recently shown to be responsive to treatment with butyrophenones. **glioma-polyposis s.,** Turcot s. **global s.,** a syndrome affecting infants between three and seven months of age who have been placed in a strange milieu; they are intensely preoccupied with scanning the new environment but are blankly unresponsive to the persons in it. Other symptoms include disturbances in eating and excessive sleepiness. **glomangiomatous-osseous malformation s.,** a congenital disorder, transmitted as an autosomal dominant trait, characterized by multiple glomus tumors with hypoplasia and osteoporosis of the bones of the affected extremity. **Goldenhar's s.,** oculoauriculovertebral dysplasia. **Goltz's s.,** Goltz-Gorlin s., focal dermal hypoplasia s. **Goodpasture's s.,** glomerulonephritis associated with hemoptysis, an uncommon, rapidly progressive, usually fatal condition affecting chiefly young men; it regularly begins with respiratory infection, variable pulmonary infiltrations, hemoptysis, and anemia, followed by a rapidly progressive renal disease in which hematuria, proteinuria, hypertension, and progressive azotemia are features. An antibody directed against the alveolar basement membrane of the lungs and the glomerular basement membrane of the kidneys has been implicated. **Gopalan's s.,** a symptom complex resulting from malnutrition, with signs suggestive of riboflavin deficiency, a burning sensation in the extremities, a feeling of "pins and needles" in the distal parts, and hyperhidrosis. **Gorlin's s.,** 1. basal cell nevus s. 2. Gorlin-Chaudhry-Moss s. **Gorlin-Chaudhry-Moss s.,** a syndrome consisting of craniofacial dysostosis, hypertrichosis, hypoplasia of labia majora, dental and eye abnormalities, and patent ductus arteriosus. Called also *Gorlin's s.* **Gorlin-Goltz s.,** basal cell nevus s. **Gorlin-Psaume s.,** orofaciodigital s. **Gougerot-Carteaud s.,** confluent and reticulated papillomatosis. **Gougerot-Nulock-Houwer s.,** Sjögren's s. **Gowers' s.,** vasovagal attack. **Gradenigo's s.,** palsy of the sixth nerve and unilateral headache in suppurative disease of the middle ear, caused by involvement of the abducens and trigeminal nerves by direct spread of the infection. **Graham Little s.,** lichen planus associated with acuminate follicular papules and alopecia. **gray s.,** a potentially fatal condition seen in neonates, particularly premature infants, due to a reaction to chloramphenicol, characterized by an ashen gray cyanosis, listlessness, weakness, and hypotension. **gray spinal s.,** muscular atrophy, syringomyelic disturbances of sensation, and vasomotor troubles, due to lesions of the gray matter of the spinal cord. **Greig's s.,** ocular hypertelorism. **Grönblad-Strandberg s.,** angioid streaks in the retina together with pseudoxanthoma elasticum of the skin. **Gruber's s.,** Meckel's s. **Guillain-Barré s.,** acute febrile polyneuritis. **Gunn's s.,** unilateral ptosis of the eyelid, with the association of movements of the affected upper eyelid with those of the jaw; called also *jaw-winking s.* **gustatory sweating s.,** auriculotemporal s. **Hadfield-Clark s.,** Clarke-Hadfield s. **Hakim's s.,** normal-pressure hydrocephalus. **Hallermann-Streiff s., Hallermann-Streiff-François s.,** oculomandibulofacial s. **Hallervorden-Spatz s.,** a hereditary disorder characterized by marked reduction in the number of the myelin sheaths of the globus pallidus and substantia nigra, with accumulations of iron pigment, progressive rigidity beginning in the legs, choreoathetoid movements, dysarthria, and progressive mental deterioration. Transmitted as an autosomal recessive trait, it usually begins in the first or second decade, with death usually occurring before the thirtieth year. Called also *Hallervorden-Spatz disease, status dysmyelinatus,* and *status dysmyelinisatus.* **Hallopeau-Siemens s.,** polydysplastic epidermolysis bullosa. **Hamman's s.,** see under *disease.* **Hamman-Rich s.,** see *idiopathic pulmonary fibrosis,* under *fibrosis.* **hand-foot-uterus s.,** a congenital syndrome consisting of small feet with unusually short great toes, abnormal thumbs, and, in females, duplication of the genital tract. **Hand's s., Hand-Schüller-Christian s.,** Hand-Schüller-Christian disease. **hand-shoulder s.,** reflex sympathetic dystrophy of the upper extremity; see under *dystrophy.* **Hanhart's s.,** a congenital syndrome characterized chiefly by severe micrognathia, high nose root, small eyelid fissures, low-set ears, and variable absence of digits or limbs, usually below the elbow or knee. **Hanot's s.,** 1. primary biliary cirrhosis. 2. secondary biliary cirrhosis. **Hanot-Chauffard s.,** hypertrophic cirrhosis with pigmentation and diabetes mellitus. **Harada's s.,** a syndrome, possibly caused by a virus, consisting of uveomeningitis associated with retinochoroidal detachment, temporary or permanent deafness

and blindness, and sometimes, though often transiently, alopecia, vitiligo, and poliosis; called also *Harada's disease.* **Hare's s.,** Pancoast's s., def. 1. **Harris' s.,** hyperinsulinism due to endogenous factors, such as functional disorders of the pancreas or insulinoma, manifested by hypoglycemia, weakness, perspiration, jitteriness, tachycardia, mental confusion, and disturbances of vision. **Hartnup s.,** a hereditary disease characterized by progressive mental deterioration, cerebellar ataxia, a pellagra-like condition of the skin, and aminoaciduria; it is due to a defect of intestinal and renal transport of certain alpha-amino acids and is transmitted as an autosomal recessive trait. **Hassin's s.,** protrusion of the ear on the side of the lesion combined with Horner's syndrome, in disease of the sympathetic nerve in the cervical region. **Hayem-Widal s.,** hemolytic anemia. **heart-hand s.,** Holt-Oram s. **Heerfordt's s.,** a rare manifestation of sarcoidosis, consisting of parotitis, uveitis, and cranial nerve paresis. **Heidenhain's s.,** a rapidly progressive degenerative disease manifested by cortical blindness, presenile dementia, dysarthria, ataxia, athetoid movements, and generalized rigidity. **hemangioma-thrombocytopenia s.,** Kasabach-Merritt s. **hemohistioblastic s.,** reticuloendotheliosis. **hemolytic-uremic s.,** a rare syndrome of unknown etiology occurring mainly in children under one year of age, characterized by renal failure, microangiopathic hemolytic anemia, and severe thrombocytopenia and purpura. Called also *Gasser's s.* **hemopleuropneumonic s.,** dyspnea, hemoptysis, tachycardia, and fever, with dullness at the base of the chest and tubular respiration over the middle zone of the chest; indicative of pneumonia and hydrothorax in puncture wounds of the chest. **hemorrhagic fever s.,** an acute, sometimes fatal syndrome of diverse viral etiologies, marked by severe hemorrhage and shock. In the Philippines and Southeast Asia, it is caused by dengue viruses, in Central and South America by Junin and Machupo viruses, in the U.S.S.R. by Omsk and Crimean hemorrhagic fever viruses, and in Korea by an unidentified virus. **Hench-Rosenberg s.,** palindromic rheumatism. **Henoch-Schönlein s.,** Schönlein-Henoch purpura. **hepatorenal s.,** functional renal failure, oliguria, and low urinary sodium concentration, without pathological renal changes, associated with cirrhosis and ascites or with obstructive jaundice. **hereditary benign intraepithelial dyskeratosis s.,** a syndrome characterized by plaques of the bulbar conjunctiva and by oral mucosal thickenings clinically similar to white-folded hypertrophy (white sponge nevus of Cannon); it is inherited as an autosomal dominant trait with a high degree of penetrance. **Hines-Bannick s.,** intermittent attacks of low temperature and disabling sweating. **Hoffmann-Werdnig s.,** Werdnig-Hoffmann paralysis. **Holmes-Adie s.,** Adie's s. **Holt-Oram s.,** hereditary heart disease, usually an atrial or ventricular septal defect, associated with skeletal malformation (hypoplastic thumb and short forearm); transmitted as an autosomal dominant trait. Called also *heart-hand s.* **Homén's s.,** a genetically determined disease of the nervous system with prominent abnormalities in the lenticular nucleus, marked by vertigo, ataxia, dysarthria, gradually increasing dementia, with rigidity of the body, especially the legs. **Horner's s., Horner-Bernard s.,** sinking in of the eyeball, ptosis of the upper eyelid, slight elevation of the lower lid, constriction of the pupil, narrowing of the palpebral fissure, anhidrosis and flushing of the affected side of the face; caused by paralysis of the cervical sympathetic nerves. Called also *Bernard's s., Bernard-Horner s.,* and *Horner's ptosis.* **Horton's s.,** 1. migrainous neuralgia. 2. temporal arteritis. **Hunt's s.,** Ramsay Hunt s. **Hunter's s., Hunter-Hurler s.,** a form of mucopolysaccharidosis clinically resembling Hurler's syndrome, but without gibbus and corneal clouding and with generally milder symptoms, although corneal opacities may develop later in life; other symptoms may include retinitis pigmentosa, nodular skin lesions, hypertrichosis, papilledema, optic atrophy, progressive deafness, and pulmonary hypertension. It is transmitted as an X-linked recessive trait. Called also *mucopolysaccharidosis II.* **Hurler's s.,** a hereditary disorder considered to be the prototypical form of the mucopolysaccharidoses, characterized by gargoyle-like facies with hypertelorism, depressed bridge of the nose, large prominent tongue, and widely spaced teeth; dwarf stature; severe somatic and skeletal changes, including short neck and trunk, scaphocephaly, and kyphosis with gibbus; short broad hands with short fingers; severe mental retardation after the first year of life; progressive opacities of the cornea; deafness; cardiovascular defects; hepatosplenomegaly; and joint contractures. It is due to deficiency of the enzyme α-L-iduronidase and is transmitted as an autosomal recessive trait. Called also *Hurler's disease, gargoylism, lipochondrodystrophy,* and *mucopolysaccharidosis I.* and *I-H.* See also *mucopolysaccharidosis.* **Hurler-Pfaundler s.,** Hurler's s. **Hutchinson's s.,** see under *triad.* **Hutchinson-Boeck s.,** sarcoidosis. **Hutchinson-Gilford s.,** progeria. **Hutchison s.,** see under *type.* **hyaline membrane s.,** see *respiratory distress s. of newborn.* **hydralazine lupus s.,** a drug-induced syndrome clinically and pathologically identical to systemic lupus erythematosus, occurring after therapy of long duration and high dosage of hydralazine; called also *hydralazine lupus* and *SLE-like s.* **17-hydroxylase deficiency s.,** congenital adrenal hyperplasia resulting from a deficiency of the enzyme 17-α-hydroxylase, leading to a deficiency of estrogen and androgen and consequent sexual infantilism; the compensatory increase in secretion of deoxycorticosterone and corticosterone results in hypokalemic alkalosis and hypertension. **hyperabduction s.,** thoracic outlet syndrome due to compression of the brachial plexus trunk roots and axillary vessels by the pectoralis minor muscle and the coracoid process when the arms are stretched above the head, as during sleep. **hypercalcemia s.,** milk-alkali s. **hypereosinophilic s.,** a massive increase in the number of eosinophils in the blood, mimicking leukemia, and characterized by eosinophilic infiltration of the heart, brain, liver, and lungs and by a progressively fatal course. **hyperkinetic s.,** a childhood disorder that usually abates during adolescence, characterized by hyperactivity, fidgetiness, excitability, impulsiveness, distractibility, short attention span, low tolerance for frustration, and difficulties in learning and perceptual motor function. Some cases are believed to be associated with brain damage and psychoses, but the specific causes of most cases has not been determined. Called also *hyperactivity* and *hyperkinesia.* **hyperkinetic heart s.,** increased cardiac output of unknown cause associated with slightly elevated systolic and pulse pressures, normal mean arterial pressure, and low systemic vascular resistance. **hyperlucent lung s.,** a syndrome simulating localized emphysema, but due to congenital absence or hypoplasia of pulmonary arteries; there may be lobar or segmental agenesis, and accessory lungs, lobes, or segments are not unusual. **hyperophthalmopathic s.,** proptosis, paresis of the external ocular muscles, swelling of the lids, edema of the conjunctiva, and retrobulbar pain. **hypersomnia-bulimia s.,** Kleine-Levin s. **hypertelorism-hypospadias s.,** a congenital condition consisting of hypertelorism associated with hypospadias and a neuromuscular abnormality of the esophagus and swallowing mechanism. Called also *G s.* **hyperventilation s.,** an emotional disorder in which rapid deep breathing caused by emotional tension, anxiety, or acute fear produces giddiness and clouding of consciousness, and sometimes apprehension, confusion, numbness of the hands and face, muscular cramps of the hands and feet, and a sense of air hunger. **hyperviscosity s.,** any syndrome associated with increased viscosity of the blood. In the *syndrome of serum hyperviscosity,* there is spontaneous bleeding and neurologic and ocular disorders. The *syndrome of polycythemic hyperviscosity,* in which increased viscosity is due to large numbers of red cells, is marked by retarded blood flow, organ congestion, reduced capillary perfusion, and increased cardiac effort. *Syndromes of sclerocythemic hyperviscosity* comprise those in which the deformability of erythrocytes is impaired, as in sickle cell anemia. **hypophyseal s.,** adiposogenital dystrophy. **hypoplastic left-heart s.,** a congenital malformation consisting of hypoplasia or atresia of the left ventricle and of the aorta or mitral valve or both, and characterized by respiratory distress and extreme cyanosis, with cardiac failure and death in early infancy. **inferior s. of red nucleus,** Claude's s. **inspissated bile s.,** biliary obstruction caused by plugging of the outflow tract. **intrauterine parabiotic s.,** placental transfusion s. **irritable bowel s., irritable colon s.,** see *mucous colitis,* under *colitis.* **Ivemark's s.,** congenital splenic agenesis, cardiac defects, and partial situs inversus viscerum; called also *asplenia s.* and *Polhemus-Schafer-Ivemark s.* **Jaccoud's s.,** chronic arthritis occurring after rheumatic fever, usually after repeated attacks, and characterized by fibrous changes in the joint capsules and tendons, leading to deformities that may resemble rheumatoid arthritis (especially ulnar deviation of fingers); the joints may be painful and rheumatic nodules are often present. **Jackson's s.,** paralysis of the tenth, eleventh, and twelfth cranial nerves, with paralysis of the soft palate, larynx, and one half of the tongue, associated with paralysis of the sternomastoid and trapezius muscles. **Jadassohn-Lewandowsky s.,** pachyonychia congenita. **Jaffe-Lichtenstein s.,** fibrous dysplasia. **Jahnke's s.,** a variant of the Sturge-Weber syndrome in which glaucoma is absent. **jaw-winking s.,** Gunn's s. **jejunal s.,** dumping syndrome. **Jervell and Lange-Nielsen s.,** a syndrome characterized by attacks of syncope and by sudden death in patients with congenital deafness and electrocardiographic anomalies, especially a prolonged Q-T interval. **Jeune's s.,** asphyxiating thoracic dystrophy. **Job's s.,** a variant of chronic granulomatous disease affecting girls with red hair and fair skin and marked by recurrent staphylococcal abscesses and eczema; it is associated with high levels of IgE in the serum. **jugular foramen s.,** Vernet's s. **Kallmann's s.,** the association of anosmia due to agenesis of the olfactory lobes, and secondary hypogonadism due to lack of gonadotropins. **Kanner's s.,** infantile autism. **Karroo s.,** a condition observed in youth among Afrikaners in the Karroo region, consisting of high fever, alimentary tract disturbance, and tenderness in the lymph glands of the neck. **Kartagener's s.,** a hereditary disorder involving a combination of dextrocardia (situs inversus), bronchiectasis, and sinusitis, transmitted as an autosomal recessive trait. **Kasabach-Merritt s.,** a syndrome occurring in infants, marked by giant hemangioma of the skin and spleen associated with thrombocytopenic purpura and afibrinogenemia. Called also *hemangioma-thrombocytopenia s.* **Kast's s.,** Maffucci's s. **Ken-**

nedy's s., retrobulbar optic neuritis, central scotoma, optic atrophy on the side of the lesion and papilledema on the opposite side, occurring in tumors of the frontal lobe of the brain which press downward. **Kiloh-Nevin s.,** ocular myopathy in patients with ptosis and progressive external ophthalmoplegia. **Kimmelstiel-Wilson s.,** intercapillary glomerulosclerosis. **kinky-hair s.,** Menkes' s. **Kinsbourne s.,** myoclonic encephalopathy of childhood; see under *encephalopathy.* **Klauder's s.,** ectodermosis erosiva pluriorificialis. **kleeblattschädel (cloverleaf skull) s.,** a congenital disorder, characterized by synostosis of multiple or all cranial sutures, hydrocephalus, and in some cases facial dysostosis and long bone anomalies. **Kleine-Levin s.,** the syndrome of periodic somnolence, morbid hunger, and motor unrest; it is sometimes associated with psychosis. **Klinefelter's s.,** a condition characterized by infertility, variable degrees of masculinization, the presence of small testes with fibrosis and hyalinization of seminiferous tubules, variable impairment of function and clumping of Leydig cells, and by an increase in urinary gonadotropins; patients tend to be of eunuchoid habitus, and about half have gynecomastia. It is associated typically with an XXY chromosome complement, although variants include XXYY, XXXY, XXXXY, and several mosaic patterns (XY/XXY, XXY, XXXY, etc.) **Klippel-Feil s.,** a condition characterized by shortness of the neck resulting from reduction in the number of cervical vertebrae or the fusion of multiple hemivertebrae into one osseous mass; the hairline is low and motion of the neck is limited. **Klippel-Trenaunay s., Klippel-Trenaunay-Weber s.,** a rare condition usually affecting one extremity, characterized by hypertrophy of the bone and related soft tissues, large cutaneous hemangiomas, nevus flammeus, and skin varices. **Klumpke-Dejerine s.,** Klumpke's paralysis. **Klüver-Bucy s.,** bizarre behavior disturbances following bilateral temporal lobectomy which destroys important limbic structures; it is characterized by a tendency to examine objects orally, depression of drive and emotional reactions, hypermetamorphosis, and lack of sexual inhibitions. **Kocher's s.** (*obs.*), leukopenia due to granulocytopenia with relative and absolute lymphocytosis and moderate eosinophilia occasionally accompanying thyrotoxicosis. **Kocher-Debré-Sémélaigne s.,** Debré-Sémélaigne s. **König's s.,** constipation alternating with diarrhea and attended with abdominal pain, meteorism, and gurgling sounds in the right iliac fossa. **Korsakoff's s.,** see under *psychosis.* **Kunkel's s.,** lupoid hepatitis. **Ladd's s.,** congenital obstruction of the duodenum due to peritoneal bands resulting from a malrotated cecum. **Landry's s.,** acute febrile polyneuritis. **Larsen's s.,** cleft palate, flattened facies, multiple congenital dislocations, and foot deformities. **Laubry-Soulle s.,** abnormal localized collections of gas in the colon (splenic flexure) and stomach following acute myocardial infarction. **Launois' s.,** gigantism due to excessive pituitary secretion, occurring before puberty and before the epiphyses close; it is most often caused by an eosinophilic adenoma, but sometimes results from a chromophobe adenoma. Called also *hyperpituitary* or *pituitary gigantism.* **Launois-Cléret's s.,** adiposogenital dystrophy. **Laurence-Biedl s., Laurence-Moon-Bardet-Biedl s., Laurence-Moon-Biedl s.,** a hereditary syndrome transmitted as an autosomal recessive trait, characterized by mental retardation, obesity, retinitis pigmentosa, hypogonadism, and polydactyly. **Läwen-Roth s.,** dwarfism with stippled epiphyses and thyroid deficiency; congenital hypothyroidism or cretinism. **Lawford's s.,** a variant of the Sturge-Weber syndrome in which there is glaucoma but without an increase in the size of the eye. **lazy leukocyte s.,** a syndrome occurring in children, marked by recurrent low-grade infections, associated with a defect in neutrophil chemotaxis and deficient random mobility of neutrophils. **Legg-Calvé-Perthes s.,** osteochondrosis of the capitular epiphysis. **Lennox s.,** a childhood epileptic encephalopathy characterized electroencephalographically by diffuse slow spike waves. **Lenz's s.,** a hereditary syndrome, transmitted as an X-linked trait, consisting of microphthalmia or anophthalmos, unilateral or bilateral, and digital anomalies; narrow shoulders, double thumbs, and other skeletal abnormalities; dental, urogenital, and cardiovascular defects may also occur. **leopard s.,** a hereditary syndrome transmitted as an autosomal dominant trait, consisting of multiple lentigines, asymptomatic cardiac defects, and typical coarse facies; it may also be associated with pulmonary stenosis, sensorineural deafness, skeletal changes, ocular hypertelorism, and abnormalities of the genitalia. Called also *multiple lentigines s.* **Leredde's s.,** severe dyspnea on exertion dating from early life, combined with advanced emphysema, recurrent attacks of acute febrile bronchitis; it is a remote sequel of syphilis, usually congenital. **Leriche's s.,** a syndrome caused by obstruction of the terminal aorta, usually occurring in males and characterized by fatigue in the hips, thighs, or calves on exercising, absence of pulsation in the femoral arteries and impotence, and often pallor and coldness of the lower extremities. **Lermoyez's s.,** tinnitus and hearing loss preceding an attack of vertigo and then subsiding after the vertigo has become established. **Lesch-Nyhan s.,** a rare disorder of purine metabolism due to deficiency of the enzyme hypoxanthine-guanine phosphoribosyltransferase, characterized by physical and mental retardation, compulsive self-mutilation of the fingers and lips by biting, choreoathetosis, spastic cerebral palsy, and impaired renal function, and by extremely excessive purine synthesis and consequently hyperuricemia and excessive urinary secretion of uric acid. It is transmitted as a sex-linked recessive trait. **levator s.,** episodic pain and a sensation of fullness and pressure in the rectum and sacrococcygeal area; attributed to spasm of the levator ani muscle. **Lévi's s.,** paroxysmal hyperthyroidism. **Lévy-Roussy s.,** Roussy-Lévy s. **Leyden-Moebius s.,** limb-girdle muscular dystrophy; see under *dystrophy.* **Lhermitte and McAlpine s.,** combined pyramidal and extrapyramidal system disease. **Libman-Sacks s.,** atypical verrucous endocarditis. **Lichtheim's s.,** subacute combined degeneration of the spinal cord; see under *degeneration.* **Lightwood's s.,** renal tubular acidosis. **Lignac's s., Lignac-Fanconi s.,** cystinosis. **liver-kidney s.,** hepatorenal s. **Lobstein's s.,** see *osteogenesis imperfecta.* **"locked-in" s.,** a condition of complete paralysis, except for some form of voluntary eye movement, due to bilateral lesions of motor pathways of the lower cranial nerves and limbs. **loculation s.,** Froin's s. **Löffler's s.,** a condition characterized by transient infiltrations of the lungs associated with an increase of the eosinophilic leukocytes in the blood; called also *Löffler's eosinophilia.* **Looser-Milkman s.,** Milkman s. **Louis-Bar s.,** ataxia-telangiectasia. **Lowe's s.,** oculocerebrorenal s. **Lowe-Terry-Machlachan s.,** oculocerebrorenal s. **lower radicular s.,** Klumpke's paralysis. **Lucey-Driscoll s.,** a syndrome of retention jaundice due to defective bilirubin conjugation, occurring in infants; apparently the result of an unidentified factor, presumably a steroid in maternal blood, transmitted to the infant. **Lutembacher's s.,** atrial septal defect associated with mitral stenosis. Called also *Lutembacher's disease* or *complex.* **Lyell's s.,** toxic epidermal necrolysis. **lymphoproliferative s.,** a general term applied to a group of diseases characterized by proliferation of lymphoid tissue, such as lymphocytic leukemia and malignant lymphoma. **McArdle s.,** see under *disease.* **McCune-Albright s.,** a syndrome of sexual precosity, polyostotic fibrous dysplasia, and patchy pigmentation of the skin. **Mackenzie's s.,** associated paralysis of the tongue, soft palate, and vocal cord on the same side. **Maffucci's s.,** enchondromatosis associated with multiple cutaneous or visceral hemangiomas. Called also *Kast's s.* **malabsorption s.,** a group of disorders in which there is subnormal absorption of dietary constituents, and thus excessive loss of nonabsorbed substances in the stool; the malabsorption may be due to an intraluminal (digestive) defect (e.g., pancreatic insufficiency), a mucosal abnormality (celiac disease or disaccharidase deficiency), or a lymphatic obstruction (intestinal lymphangiectasia). Unless there is a specific enzyme or transport defect, steatorrhea is usually present. Deficiency syndromes may result from excessive loss of vitamins, electrolytes, iron, calcium, etc. **Malin's s.,** anemia in which the red cells are ingested by the leukocytes; called also *autoerythrophagocytosis.* **Mallory-Weiss s.,** hematemesis or melena that follows typically upon many hours or days of severe vomiting and retching, traceable to one or several slitlike lacerations of the gastric mucosa, longitudinally placed at or slightly below the esophagogastric junction. **Marañón's s.,** a syndrome consisting of scoliosis and flatfoot, with ovarian insufficiency. **Marchesani's s.,** Weill-Marchesani s. **Marchiafava-Bignami s.,** see under *disease.* **Marchiafava-Micheli s.,** paroxysmal nocturnal hemoglobinuria; see under *hemoglobinuria.* **Marcus Gunn's s.,** Gunn's s. **Marfan's s.,** a congenital disorder of connective tissue characterized by abnormal length of the extremities, especially of fingers and toes, subluxation of the lens, cardiovascular abnormalities (commonly dilatation of the ascending aorta), and other deformities. It is inherited in an autosomal dominant manner with variable degree of expression. **Margolis s.,** sex-linked deaf-mutism with albinism. **Marie's s.,** 1. a complex of symptoms due to excessive secretion of the anterior pituitary, with acromegaly a prominent feature. 2. hypertrophic pulmonary osteoarthropathy. **Marie-Bamberger s.,** hypertrophic pulmonary osteoarthropathy. **Marie-Robinson s.,** melancholia, insomnia, and impotence in a form of levulosuria. **Marinesco-Sjögren's s.,** a hereditary syndrome transmitted as an autosomal recessive trait, consisting of cerebellar ataxia, mental and somatic growth retardation, congenital cataracts, inability to chew, thin brittle fingernails, and sparse, incompletely keratinized hair. **Maroteaux-Lamy s.,** a form of mucopolysaccharidosis transmitted as an autosomal recessive trait, closely resembling Hurler's syndrome (q.v.), except that the facial deformity is less marked, stiffness of the joints is minimal, and the intellect is not impaired; called also *mucopolysaccharidosis VI.* **Martorell's s.,** pulseless disease. **mast s.,** an inherited, early form of presenile dementia, transmitted as an autosomal recessive trait, having an onset in the late teens or twenties and a slow, progressive course with development of spastic paraparesis and basal ganglion disturbances; observed in an inbred Amish population. **maternal deprivation s.,** deprivation dwarfism. **Mauriac s.,** dwarfism, hepatomegaly, obesity, and retarded sexual maturation, in association with diabetes mellitus. **Mayer-Rokitansky-Kuster s.,** lack of müllerian development, congenital absence of the vagina and a rudimentary

uterus (typically bicornuate remnants), with normal uterine tubes, ovaries, and secondary female sex characteristics and normal growth. **Meckel's s., Meckel-Gruber s.,** a hereditary syndrome, transmitted as an autosomal recessive trait, most frequently characterized by sloping forehead, posterior meningo-encephalocele, polydactyly, and polycystic kidneys, with death occurring in the perinatal period. Called also *Gruber's s.* and *dysencephalia splanchnocystica.* **meconium plug s.,** a syndrome of intestinal obstruction caused by unusually thick or hard meconium in which neither enzymatic nor ganglion cell deficiency can be demonstrated. **megacystis-megaureter s.,** chronic ureteral dilatation (megaureter) associated with hypotonia and dilatation of the bladder (megacystis) and gaping of ureteral orifices, permitting vesicoureteral reflux of urine, and resulting in chronic pyelonephritis. **Meigs' s.,** ascites and hydrothorax associated with ovarian fibroma or other pelvic tumor. **Melkersson's s., Melkersson-Rosenthal s.,** a hereditary syndrome transmitted as an autosomal dominant trait, most often beginning in childhood or adolescence, and characterized chiefly by chronic noninflammatory facial swelling (usually confined to the lips), recurrent peripheral facial palsy, and sometimes fissured tongue. Associated ophthalmic symptoms may include lagophthalmos, burning sensation of the eyes, blepharochalasis, swelling of the eyelids, corneal opacities, retrobulbar neuritis, and bilateral recurrent exophthalmos. **Mengert's shock s.,** a condition resembling shock that sometimes occurs when pregnant women in the late antepartum period lie in the supine position; it is due to the pressure of the uterus on the vena cava. **Meniere's s.,** see under *disease.* **Menkes' s.,** a hereditary abnormality in copper absorption marked by severe cerebral degeneration and arterial changes resulting in death in infancy and by sparse, brittle scalp hair with a twisted appearance microscopically. It is transmitted as an X-linked recessive trait. Called also *Menkes' disease* and *kinky-* or *steely-hair s.* **metameric s.,** segmentary s. **methionine malabsorption s.,** Smith-Strang disease. **Meyer-Schwickerath and Weyers s.,** oculodentodigital dysplasia. **middle lobe s.,** atelectasis of the right middle pulmonary lobe, with chronic pneumonitis; called also *Brock's s.* **Mikulicz's s.,** a general term referring to bilateral enlargement of the salivary and lacrimal glands due to a variety of diseases, including leukemia, tuberculosis, and sarcoidosis. See also *Mikulicz's disease,* under *disease.* **milk-alkali s.,** a syndrome characterized by hypercalcemia without hypercalciuria or hypophosphatemia, with only mild alkalosis, normal serum phosphatase, severe renal insufficiency with hyperazotemia and calcinosis, attributed to ingestion of milk and absorbable alkali for long periods of time; called also *Burnett's s.* and *hypercalcemia s.* **Milkman's s.,** a generalized bone disease marked by multiple transparent stripes of absorption in the long and flat bones; called also *Looser-Milkman s.* **Millard-Gubler s.,** crossed paralysis, affecting the limbs on one side of the body and the face on the opposite side, together with paralysis of outward movement of the eye; it is due to infarction of the pons involving the sixth and seventh cranial nerves and the fibers of the corticospinal tract. Called also *Millard-Gubler paralysis.* Cf. *Foville's s.* **Minkowski-Chauffard s.,** hereditary spherocytosis. **Minot-von Willebrand s.,** von Willebrand's disease. **Möbius' s.,** agenesis or aplasia of the motor nuclei of the cranial nerves characterized by congenital bilateral facial palsy in various combinations, with unilateral or bilateral paralysis of the abductors of the eye, sometimes associated with involvement of the cranial nerves, particularly the oculomotor, trigeminal, and hypoglossal, and anomalies of the extremities. Called also *akinesia algera, congenital facial diplegia, nuclear agenesis* or *aplasia, congenital abducens-facial paralysis,* and *congenital oculofacial paralysis.* **Monakow's s.,** hemiplegia on the side opposite the lesion in occlusion of the anterior choroidal artery, sometimes with hemianesthesia and hemianopia. **Moore's s.,** abdominal epilepsy. **Morel's s.,** hyperostosis frontalis interna. **Morgagni's s.,** hyperostosis frontalis interna. **Morgagni-Adams-Stokes s.,** Adams-Stokes disease. **Morgagni-Stewart-Morel s.,** hyperostosis frontalis interna. **Morquio's s.,** a rare form of mucopolysaccharidosis which becomes evident when the affected infant starts to walk. The condition is marked by severe dwarfism, especially of the torso, short neck, prominent sternum, dorsolumbar kyphosis, genu valgum, flatfeet, and waddling gait. In contrast to Hurler's syndrome, the mental retardation is absent or slight, the facial deformities are less striking although marked by protruding mandible and short nose, the clouding of the cornea and deafness are mild, the muscles and ligaments are usually flaccid, and the cardiovascular changes are absent, except perhaps aortic valve disease. It is transmitted as an autosomal recessive trait. Called also *mucopolysaccharidosis IV, eccentro-osteochondrodysplasia, chondro-osteodystrophy, familial osteochondrodystrophy,* and *osteochondrodystrophia deformans.* **Morquio-Ullrich s.,** Morquio's s. **Morton's s.,** a congenital insufficiency of the first metatarsal segment of the foot, characterized by metatarsalgia due to shortening or relaxation of the part. **Morvan's s.,** edema and cyanosis, and sometimes recurring painless whitlows, usually symmetrically placed on the hands, though sometimes on the lower extremities, seen in cases of syringomyelia and occasionally in leprosy. **Mosse's s.,** polycythemia vera with cirrhosis of the liver. **Mucha-Habermann s.,** parapsoriasis lichenoides et varioliformis. **Muckle-Wells s.,** recurrent urticaria, deafness, and nephritis. **mucocutaneous lymph node s. (MLNS),** a syndrome of unknown etiology affecting most commonly infants and young children, and marked by fever, conjunctival injection, reddening of the lips and oral cavity, ulcerative gingivitis, enlarged cervical lymph nodes, and maculoerythematous skin eruption that becomes confluent and bright red in a glove-and-sock distribution, the skin becoming indurated and edematous and desquamating from the fingers and toes. It has been observed in Japan since 1967, but has recently been observed in the U.S. with some frequency. Called also *Kawasaki disease.* **multiple hamartoma s.,** Cowden's disease. **multiple lentigines s.,** leopard s. **Munchausen's s.,** a condition characterized by habitual presentation for hospital treatment of an apparent acute illness, the patient giving a plausible and dramatic history, all of which is false. Cf. *laparotomaphilia.* **Murchison-Sanderson s.,** Hodgkin's disease. **myasthenia gravis s.,** Erb's s. **myasthenic s.,** Eaton-Lambert s. **myelofibrosis-osteosclerosis s.,** a form of myeloproliferative disease characterized by fibrosis of the bone marrow, splenomegaly, extramedullary hematopoiesis, and leukoerythroblastosis. **myeloproliferative s.,** a general term applied to a group of diseases which may be related histogenetically and are characterized, at varying times and in varying degrees, by medullary and extramedullary proliferation of one or more lines of bone marrow constituents, including the myelocytic, erythrocytic, and megakaryocytic forms, in addition to the various cells derived from the reticulum and mesenchymal elements; the group includes acute and chronic myelocytic leukemia, polycythemia vera, agnogenic myeloid metaplasia with or without myelofibroma, essential hemorrhagic thrombocythemia, and erythremic myelosis (Di Guglielmo syndrome). **Naegeli's s.,** a hereditary disorder similar to incontinentia pigmenti, but differing in that it affects males and females with equal frequency (autosomal dominant inheritance) and involves plantar and palmar hypohidrosis and hypertrichosis; called also *Franceschetti-Jadassohn s.* **Naffziger's s.,** scalenus s. **nail-patella s.,** arthro-onychodysplasia. **Nelson's s.,** the development of an ACTH-producing pituitary tumor after bilateral adrenalectomy in Cushing's syndrome; it is characterized by aggressive growth of the tumor and hyperpigmentation of the skin. **neostriatal s.,** Hunt's striatal s., def. 2. **nephrotic s.,** a condition characterized by massive edema, heavy proteinura, hypoalbuminemia, and peculiar susceptibility to intercurrent infections; called also *Epstein's s.* **Netherton's s.,** a hereditary syndrome transmitted as an autosomal recessive trait, consisting of congenital ichthyosiform erythroderma and atopic dermatitis in association with trichorrhexis nodosa (bamboo hair). **neurocutaneous s.,** the formation of nevi and of deformities of the skeleton with symptoms of degeneration in the central nervous system. **nevoid basal cell carcinoma s., nevoid basalioma s.,** basal cell nevus s. **Nezelof's s.,** a hereditary syndrome transmitted as an autosomal recessive trait, in which thymic dysplasia is associated with normal levels of serum immunoglobulins and impaired cell-mediated immunity; it is characterized clinically by the early onset of severe recurrent infections, such as local and systemic candidiasis, disseminated varicella, plasma cell and bacterial pneumonia, and sepsis. Cf. *DiGeorge's s.* **nitritoid s.,** nitritoid crisis. **Noack's s.,** acrocephalopolysyndactyly (type I). **Nonne's s.,** hereditary cerebellar ataxia. **Nonne-Milroy-Meige s.,** Milroy's disease. **nonsense s.,** Ganser's s. **Noonan's s.,** the male phenotype of Turner's syndrome, with short stature, webbed neck, low nuchal hairline, low-set ears, and cubitus valgus; valvular pulmonary stenosis, rather than coarctation of the aorta, is often present. Called also *male Turner's s.* and *Ullrich-Turner s.* **Nothnagel's s.,** unilateral oculomotor paralysis combined with cerebellar ataxia, in lesions of the cerebral peduncles. **oculocerebrorenal s.,** a hereditary disorder characterized by vitamin D–refractory rickets, hydrophthalmia, congenital glaucoma and cataracts, mental retardation, and tubule reabsorption dysfunction as evidenced by hypophosphatemia, acidosis, and aminoaciduria. Seen only in males, it is transmitted as an X-linked recessive trait. Called also *Lowe's disease* or *syndrome.* **oculodento-osseous s.,** oculodentodigital dysplasia. **oculomandibulofacial s.,** a syndrome principally characterized by dyscephaly (usually brachycephaly), parrot nose, mandibular hypoplasia, proportionate nanism, hypotrichosis, bilateral congenital cataracts, and microphthalmia; called also *Hallermann-Streiff s., Hallermann-Streiff-François s., François' s.,* and *mandibulo-oculofacial dyscephaly.* **Ogilvie's s.,** a condition simulating colonic obstruction, with persistent contraction of intestinal musculature, but without evidence of organic disease of the colon, occurring as a result of a defect in the sympathetic nerve supply. Called also *false colonic obstruction.* **Oppenheim's s.,** see under *disease.* **organic brain s.,** any of the mental disorders caused by or associated with impairment of brain tissue function; they may be psychotic (e.g., senile dementia, alcoholic psychoses) or nonpsychotic, acute (reversible) or chronic (irreversible). Called also *organic psychosis.* See *acute* and *chronic organic brain s.* **orodigitofacial s.,** orofaciodigital syndrome. **orofaciodigital s.,** a condition occurring only in females, characterized by mental retardation and by anomalies of the mouth and tongue, the fingers, and frequently the face; called also *OFD s., orofacial-digital s.,* and *orodigitofacial dysostosis.* **Ostrum-Furst s.,** congenital synostosis of the neck, platybasia, and Sprengel's deformity. **outlet s.,** brachial s. **ovarian-remnant s.,** pelvic pain, sometimes cyclic, typically occurring several weeks or months after oophorectomy, usually associated with a pelvic mass, most frequently a corpus-luteum cyst, which sometimes leads to unilateral ureteral obstruction. It is due to survival of an ovarian fragment after the operation. **ovarian vein s.,** obstruction of the ureter due to compression by an enlarged or varicose ovarian vein; typically the vein becomes enlarged during pregnancy, the symptoms being those of obstruction or infection of the upper urinary tract. The right side is usually affected. **painful arc s.,** shoulder pain occurring at a particular portion of the arc described when the arm is abducted from the side to the fully raised position, as in inflammation of the tendons of the supraspinatus muscle. **painful bruising s.,** autoerythrocyte sensitization s. **paleostriatal s.,** juvenile paralysis agitans (of Hunt). **pallidal s.,** juvenile paralysis agitans (of Hunt). **pallidomesencephalic s.,** a syndrome made up of rigidity, poverty of movement, and bradykinesia, amounting to a parkinsonian state. **Pancoast's s.,** 1. roentgenographic shadow at apex of lung, neuritic pain in the arm, atrophy of the muscles of the arm and hand, and Horner's syndrome, observed in tumor near the apex of the lung and due to involvement of the brachial plexus. 2. osteolysis in the posterior part of one or more ribs and sometimes also involving the corresponding vertebra. **pancreaticohepatic s.,** extensive destruction of pancreatic tissue and fatty metamorphosis of the liver. **pancytopenia-dysmelia s.,** Fanconi's s., def. 1. **Papillon-Lefèvre s.,** a hereditary disorder transmitted as an autosomal recessive trait, characterized by hyperkeratosis palmaris et plantaris and periodontosis occurring in association with premature exfoliation of both the deciduous and the permanent teeth. **paraneoplastic s's,** a collective term for disorders arising from metabolic effects of cancer on tissues remote from the tumor; such disorders may, for example, appear as primary endocrine, hematologic, or neuromuscular disorders. **paratrigeminal s.,** paroxysmal neuralgic pain in the face associated with sympathetic palsy (Horner's syndrome). **Parinaud's s.,** 1. Parinaud's oculoglandular s. 2. see under *ophthalmoplegia.* **Parinaud's oculoglandular s.,** a general term applied to conjunctivitis, most often unilateral, usually of the follicular type, followed by tenderness and enlargement of the preauricular lymph nodes; it is often caused by infection with a leptothrix, or may be associated with other infections, such as cat-scratch fever, lymphogranuloma venereum, and tularemia. **parkinsonian s.,** a form of parkinsonism due to idiopathic degeneration of the corpus striatum or substantia nigra, frequently occurring as a sequel of lethargic encephalitis, although cerebral arteriosclerosis, toxins, neurosyphilis, and trauma have also been implicated. It is characterized by muscular rigidity, immobile facies (Parkinson's facies), slow involuntary tremor (present at rest but tending to disappear during sleep and on volitional movement), abolition of associated automatic movements, festinating gait, stooped posture, and salivation. Called also *postencephalitic parkinsonism.* See also *paralysis agitans.* **Parry-Romberg s.,** facial hemiatrophy. **Patau's s.,** trisomy 13 s. **Paterson's s.,** Plummer-Vinson s. **Paterson-Brown-Kelly s., Paterson-Kelly s.,** Plummer-Vinson s. **Pellegrini-Stieda s.,** calcification of the medial collateral ligament of the knee. **Pellizzi's s.,** epiphyseal s. **Pendred's s.,** a hereditary syndrome of congenital bilateral nerve deafness associated with development of goiter without hypothyroidism in middle childhood; the main biochemical feature is a partial inability to form organic iodine compounds. **pericolic-membrane s.,** symptoms resembling those of chronic appendicitis due to the pressure of pericolic membranes. **persistent müllerian duct s.,** the persistence, in otherwise normal males, of müllerian structures as well as male genital ducts, with undescended testes and bilateral uterine tubes, a uterus, and an upper vagina. There may be unilateral cryptorchidism with contralateral inguinal hernia containing a testis, uterus, and uterine tube (*hernia uteri inguinale*). The disorder is heritable; fertility has been described. **Peutz s.,** hereditary intestinal polyposis. **Peutz-Jeghers s.,** a hereditary syndrome characterized by gastrointestinal polyposis (usually hamartomas of the small bowel) associated with excessive melanin pigmentation of the skin and mucous membranes; gastrointestinal bleeding and intussusception are common complications. It is transmitted as an autosomal dominant trait. **Pfeiffer's s.,** a hereditary disorder, transmitted as an autosomal dominant trait, characterized by acroecephalosyndactyly associated with broad short thumbs and big toes. Called also *acrocephalosyndactyly type V.* **PHC s.,** a rare familial syndrome, marked by premolar aplasia, hyperhidrosis, and premature canities; it is transmitted as an autosomal dominant trait. Called also *Böök's s.* **Picchini's s.,** inflammation of the three serous membranes connected with the diaphragm, sometimes involving the meninges, synovial sheaths, and tunica vaginalis of the testicle; caused by a trypanosome. **Pick's s.,** 1. Pick's disease (def. 2). 2. (*obs.*) palpitation of the heart: a feeling of oppression on the chest, dyspnea, cyanosis, and dropsical phenomena; seen in certain heart diseases. **pickwickian s.,** the complex of obesity, somnolence, hypoventilation, and erythrocytosis. **Pierre Robin s.,** micrognathia in association with cleft palate and glossoptosis, and with absent gag reflex. **pineal s.,** epiphyseal s. **pituitary s.,** Marie's s., def. 1. **placental dysfunction s.,** malnutrition and hypoxia of the fetus due to degenerative changes in the placenta; in the full-blown condition the nails, skin, and vernix are stained a bright yellow and the umbilical cord a yellow-green. Called also *yellow vernix s.* **placental transfusion s.,** the birth of one anemic and one plethoric twin due to the forcing of blood of one fetal twin into the circulation of the other via interconnections between their blood vessels; called also *intrauterine parabiotic s.* **Plummer-Vinson s.,** dysphagia with glossitis, hypochromic anemia, splenomegaly, and atrophy in the mouth, pharynx, and upper end of the esophagus; called also *sideropenic dysphagia.* **pluriglandular s.,** polyglandular s. **Poland's s.,** unilateral absence of the sternocostal head of the pectoralis major muscle and ipsilateral syndactyly; called also *Poland's anomaly.* **Polhemus-Schafer-Ivemark s.,** Ivemark's s. **polycystic ovary s.,** Stein-Leventhal s. **polyglandular s.,** a series of symptoms believed to be due to pathologic action of several endocrine glands. **pontine s.,** Raymond-Cestan s. **popliteal pterygium s.,** a combination of popliteal pterygium, cleft lip and palate, lower lip pits, ankyloblepharon filiforme adnatum, and genital and digital anomalies; possibly transmitted as an autosomal dominant trait. **post-cardiotomy s.,** see *postcommissurotomy s.* and *postpericardiotomy s.* **postcholecystectomy s.,** the persistence or recurrence of abdominal pain or jaundice following cholecystectomy; it may be due to an incorrect preoperative diagnosis, a retained stone in the common bile duct, or to other physical or psychic abnormalities which are not apparent. **postcommissurotomy s.,** fever, chest pain, pleuritis, pericarditis, and pneumonitis, occurring frequently in patients who have undergone mitral commissurotomy, and sometimes related to cytomegalic inclusion disease. **postconcussional s.,** amnesia, headache, dizziness, tinnitus, irritability, fatigability, sweating, palpitations of the heart, insomnia, and difficulty in concentrating, occurring after concussion of the brain. **posterior cord s.,** sensory and ataxic phenomena derived from a lesion of the posterior columns of the spinal cord, as in locomotor ataxia. **posterolateral s.,** an ataxic and spasmodic condition due to lesion of the posterolateral elements of the spinal cord. **postgastrectomy s.,** dumping s. **postirradiation s.,** a symptom complex caused by massive irradiation, with hemorrhage, anemia, and malnutrition. **postmaturity s.,** placental dysfunction syndrome occurring in postmature fetuses. **postmyocardial infarction s.,** pericarditis with fever, leukocytosis, pleurisy, and pneumonia occurring after myocardial infarction; called also *Dressler's s.* **postperfusion s.,** an association of fever, hepatosplenomegaly, and atypical lymphocytes in the blood, often with abnormal liver-function tests. First found as a complication of open cardiac surgery with extracorporeal perfusion, it is now known to occur after simple transfusion. It is caused by a cytomegalovirus. Called also *post-transfusion s.* and *post-transfusion mononucleosis.* **postpericardiotomy s.,** delayed pericardial or pleural reaction following opening of the pericardium, characterized by fever, chest pain, and signs of pleural and/or pericardial inflammation. **postphlebitic s.,** post-thrombotic complications, including destruction of the valves of the deep veins and communicating veins of the leg, and obliteration of the thrombosed veins rather than recanalization, resulting in chronic venous insufficiency, marked by edema, stasis dermatitis, and ulceration of the leg. **post-transfusion s.,** postperfusion s. **post-traumatic brain s.,** a general term denoting all the symptoms occurring after a head injury; see *concussion of the brain, contusion of the brain,* and *postconcussional s.* **Potter's s.,** a rare condition combining a characteristic facial appearance with renal agenesis or hypoplasia and other defects. The face is flattened and features may include widely spaced eyes, epicanthal folds, a crease below the lower lids, large, low-set, floppy ears, micrognathia, and skin crease on the lower chin; skeletal abnormalities, such as clubbed feet and contracted joints, are frequent. Infants die shortly after birth. **Prader-Willi s.,** a congenital disorder characterized by rounded face, almond-shaped eyes, strabismus, low forehead, hypogonadism, and mental retardation. **preexcitation s.,** Wolff-Parkinson-White s. **premenstrual s.,** see under *tension.* **premotor s.,** the association of spastic hemiplegia with increased reflexes, disturbances of skilled movements, forced grasping and transient vasomotor disturbance; occurring in lesions of the premotor cortex. **Profichet's s.,** a gradual growth of calcareous nodules in the subcutaneous tissues (skin stones) especially about the larger joints, with a tendency to ulceration or cicatrization and attended by atrophic and nervous symptoms. **prune-belly s.,** a syndrome in which the lower part of the rectus abdominis muscle and the lower and medial parts of the oblique muscles are absent, the bladder and ureters are usually greatly dilated, the kidneys are small and dysplastic, with hydronephrosis, and the testes are undescended. The abdomen is protruding and thin-walled, with wrinkled skin, giving the syndrome its name. **pseudoclaudication s.,** a condition in which symptoms simi-

lar to those of intermittent claudication result from compression of the cauda equina owing to hypertrophic ridging or a herniated lumbar disk. **pulmonary dysmaturity s.,** Wilson-Mikity s. **Putnam-Dana s.,** subacute combined degeneration of spinal cord (see under *degeneration*). **radicular s.,** a syndrome due to lesion of the roots of the spinal nerves, consisting of restricted mobility of the spine and root pain. **Ramsay Hunt s.,** 1. facial paralysis accompanied by otalgia and a vesicular eruption involving the external canal of the ear, sometimes extending to the auricle caused by herpes zoster virus infection of the geniculate ganglion. Called also *geniculate neuralgia, herpes zoster oticus,* and *Hunt's disease* or *neuralgia.* 2. juvenile paralysis agitans (of Hunt). 3. dyssynergia cerebellaris progressiva. **Raymond-Cestan s.,** a syndrome due to obstruction of twigs of the basilar artery causing lesions of the pontine region; it is characterized by quadriplegia, anesthesia, and nystagmus. **Refsum's s.,** see under *disease.* **Reichmann's s.,** gastrosuccorrhea. **Reifenstein's s.,** a syndrome of familial male pseudohermaphrodism associated with hypospadias, primary hypogonadism, postpubertal testicular atrophy and azoospermia, signs of testosterone deficiency, and often gynecomastia. **Reiter's s.,** the triad of nongonococcal urethritis, conjunctivitis, and arthritis, frequently with mucocutaneous lesions; it is most commonly seen in males between the ages of 20 and 40 and rarely in women or children. Called also *Fiessinger-Leroy-Reiter s.* **Rendu-Osler-Weber s.,** hereditary hemorrhagic telangiectasia. **respiratory distress s. of newborn,** a condition of the newborn marked by dyspnea with cyanosis, heralded by such prodromal signs as dilatation of the alae nasi, expiratory grunt, and retraction of the suprasternal notch or costal margins, most frequently occurring in premature infants, children of diabetic mothers, and infants delivered by cesarean section, and sometimes with no apparent predisposing cause. The syndrome includes two patterns: (*a*) *hyaline membrane disease* or *syndrome,* in which affected infants frequently die of respiratory distress in the first few days of life and at autopsy have eosinophilic hyaline material lining the alveoli, alveolar ducts, and bronchioles, and (*b*) *idiopathic respiratory distress of newborn* in which the affected infants may live, but in those that die, only resorption atelectasis is seen and there is no formation of a hyaline membrane. Called also *congenital alveolar dysplasia* and *congenital aspiration pneumonia.* **restless legs s.,** see under *leg.* **retraction s.,** Duane's s. **s. of retroparotid space,** Villaret's s. **Reye's s.,** a rare, acute, and often fatal encephalopathy of childhood, marked by acute brain swelling associated with hypoglycemia, fatty infiltration of the liver, hepatomegaly, and disturbed consciousness and seizures. It most often occurs as a sequel of influenza and other viral infections of the upper respiratory tract. **Rh-null s.,** chronic hemolytic anemia affecting individuals who lack all Rh factors (Rh_{null}); it is marked by spherocytosis, stomatocytosis, and increased osmotic fragility. **Richards-Rundle s.,** a congenital syndrome consisting of ketoaciduria, mental retardation, underdevelopment of secondary sex characteristics, deafness, ataxia, and peripheral muscular wasting which progresses during childhood but eventually becomes static. **Rieger's s.,** a dominantly inherited syndrome consisting of posterior embryotoxon associated with mesodermal dysgenesis of the anterior segment of the eye, hypoplasia of the anterior stromal layer of the iris, adhesions between the iris and the trabecular network, and, frequently, glaucoma. It may be associated with various other abnormalities, such as dental defects, anal stenosis, hypertelorism, and agenesis of the facial bones. Called also *Rieger's anomaly.* **Riley-Day s.,** dysautonomia. **Riley-Smith s.,** macrocephaly without hydrocephalus, multiple hemangiomas, and pseudopapilledema. **Robert's s.,** a hereditary syndrome, transmitted as an autosomal recessive trait, consisting of imperfect development of the long bones of the limbs associated with cleft palate and lip and other anomalies. **Robin's s.,** Pierre Robin s. **Robinow's s.,** dwarfism associated with increased interorbital distance, malaligned teeth, bulging forehead, depressed nasal bridge, and short limbs. Called also *Robinow's dwarfism* and *fetal face s.* **Roger's s.,** a continuous excessive secretion of saliva as the result of cancer in the esophagus, or other esophageal irritation. **Rokitansky-Küster-Hauser s.,** Mayer-Rokitansky-Küster s. **rolandic vein s.,** hemiplegia resulting from interference with the cerebral venous circulation. **Romano-Ward s.,** an autosomal dominant disorder distinguished from the Jervell and Lange-Nielsen syndrome in that deafness does not occur in the Romano-Ward syndrome. **Rosenbach's s.,** paroxysmal tachycardia with gastric and respiratory complications. **Rosenthal s.,** a hereditary hemorrhagic diathesis clinically similar to hemophilia but due to deficiency of coagulation Factor XI. **Rosenthal-Kloepfer s.,** corneal leukomata, acromegaloid appearance, and cutis verticis gyrata. **Rosewater's s.,** a mild form of familial primary hypogonadism in the male of unknown pathogenesis, marked only by sterility and gynecomastia. **Rot's s.,** Rot-Bernhardt s.,** meralgia paresthetica. **Roth's s.,** Roth-Bernhardt s.,** meralgia paresthetica. **Rothmann-Makai s.,** idiopathic circumscribed panniculitis with fat cell necrosis, lipophagic granuloma, and cyst formation; it usually subsides spontaneously. **Rothmund-Thomson s.,** a hereditary syndrome transmitted as an autosomal recessive trait, characterized by poikiloderma and telangiectasia, and frequently associated with juvenile cataracts, saddle nose, congenital defects of the bones, and hypogonadism. Called also *poikiloderma congenita.* Cf. *Thomson's disease.* **Rotor's s.,** chronic familial nonhemolytic jaundice differing from Dubin-Johnson syndrome in the lack of liver pigmentation. **Roussy-Dejerine s.,** thalamic s. **Roussy-Lévy s.,** progressive neuropathic (peroneal) muscular atrophy with scoliosis and cerebellar ataxia. **Rovsing's s.,** horseshoe kidney with nausea, abdominal discomfort, and pain on hyperextension. **rubella s.,** a congenital syndrome due to intrauterine rubella infection (German measles), characterized most commonly by cataracts, cardiac anomalies (especially patent ductus arteriosus), deafness, microcephaly, and mental retardation. **Rubinstein's s., Rubinstein-Taybi s.,** a congenital condition characterized by mental and motor retardation, broad thumbs and great toes, short stature, characteristic facies, including high-arched palate and straight or beaked nose, various eye abnormalities, pulmonary stenosis, keloid formation in surgical scars, large foramen magnum, and abnormalities of the vertebra and sternum. **rubrospinal cerebellar peduncle s.,** Claude's s. **Rud's s.,** congenital syndrome consisting of ichthyosis simplex, mental deficiency, epilepsy, and infantilism. **runting s.,** graft-vs.-host reaction characterized by diarrhea, dermatitis, hepatosplenomegaly, hemolytic anemia, and pancytopenia. **Russell's s.,** a congenital syndrome consisting of low birth weight, short stature, a triangular face that appears small compared to the skull, disproportionately short arms, which may be associated with lateral asymmetry of the body, incurved fifth fingers, cryptorchidism, and various other abnormalities. Cf. *Silver's s.* **Rust's s.,** stiff neck, stiff carriage of the head, with the necessity of grasping the head with both hands in lying down or rising up from a horizontal posture, occurring in tuberculosis, cancer, fracture of the spine, rheumatic or arthritic processes, or syphilitic periostitis. **Sabin-Feldman s.,** chorioretinitis and cerebral calcifications, similar to the manifestations of toxoplasmosis, but having all tests for toxoplasmosis negative. **Saethre-Chotzen s.,** Chotzen's s. **salt-depletion s.,** salt-losing s. **salt-losing s.,** vomiting, dehydration, hypotension, and sudden death due to very large sodium losses from the body. It may be seen in abnormal losses of sodium into the urine (as in congenital adrenal hyperplasia, adrenocortical insufficiency, or one of the forms of salt-losing nephritis) or in large extrarenal sodium losses, usually from the gastrointestinal tract. Called also *salt-depletion crisis, salt-depletion syndrome, salt-losing crisis,* and *salt-losing defect.* **Sanfilippo's s.,** a form of mucopolysaccharidosis resembling Hurler's syndrome (q.v.), except that most of the somatic and skeletal changes are less severe, and corneal clouding and cardiovascular defects are absent; it is transmitted as an autosomal recessive trait. The syndrome occurs in two clinically indistinguishable types: type A, due to deficiency of heparan sulfate sulfamidase, and type B, due to deficiency of *N*-acetyl-α-D-glucosaminidase. Called also *mucopolysaccharidosis III* and *polydystrophic oligophrenia.* **scalded skin s.,** toxic epidermal necrolysis. **scalenus s., scalenus anticus s.,** pain over the shoulder, often extending down the arm (cervicobrachial s.) or radiating up the back of the neck due to compression of the nerves and vessels between a cervical rib and the scalenus anticus muscle; called also *Naffziger's s.* and *cervical rib s.* **scapulocostal s.,** pain in the superior or posterior aspect of the shoulder girdle, radiating to contiguous regions, as a result of long-standing alteration of the relationship of the scapula and the posterior thoracic wall. **Schafer's s.,** pachyonychia congenita associated with retardation of physical and mental development. **Schanz's s.,** a series of symptoms indicating spinal weakness, consisting of a sense of fatigue, pain on pressure over the spinous processes, pain on lying prone, and indications of spinal curvature. **Schaumann's s.,** sarcoidosis. **Scheie's s.,** a very rare type of mucopolysaccharidosis considered to be an atypical form of Hurler's syndrome (q.v.), in which the principal sign is marked progressive corneal clouding. Hirsutism, joint stiffness, mild deformities of the bones that may only affect the hands, disease of the aorta, and wide-mouthed facies occur, but there is no mental retardation. It is due to deficiency of α-L-iduronidase and is transmitted as an autosomal recessive trait. Called also *mucopolysaccharidosis I-S* and, formerly, *mucopolysaccharidosis V.* **Schirmer's s.,** a variant of the Sturge-Weber syndrome in which glaucoma occurs early in the course of the disease. **Schmidt's s.,** paralysis on one side, affecting the vocal cord, the velum palati, the trapezius muscle, and the sternocleidomastoid muscle, due to a lesion of the nucleus ambiguus and nucleus accessorius. **Schönlein-Henoch s.,** see under *purpura.* **Schroeder's s.,** high blood pressure with abnormal diminution of the salt content of the sweat, due to overactivity of the adrenal glands, and with notable gain in weight. **Schüller's s., Schüller-Christian s.,** Hand-Schüller-Christian disease. **Schultz s.,** agranulocytosis. **Schwachman s., Schwachman-Diamond s.,** primary pancreatic insufficiency and bone marrow failure, characterized by normal sweat chloride values, pancreatic insufficiency, and neutropenia; it may be associated with dwarfism and metaphyseal dysostosis of the hips. **scimitar s.,** complete or partial venous drainage of the right lung into the inferior vena cava, usually with hypoplasia of the right lung;

the name is derived from the convex shadow of the anomalous vein to the right of the lower border of the heart in the chest roentgenogram. **s. of sea-blue histiocyte,** a rare disorder characterized by the presence of a morphologically distinct, sea-blue, granulated histiocyte and by splenomegaly. Clinically, the disorder may range from a relatively benign course with mild purpura secondary to thrombocytopenia, to progressive hepatic cirrhosis, hepatic failure, and death. **Seabright bantam s.,** pseudohypoparathyroidism. **Seckel's s.,** see *bird-headed dwarf,* under *dwarf.* **segmentary s.,** a syndrome produced by a lesion of the gray matter of the spinal cord, and marked by weakness and wasting in the affected segment; called also *metameric s.* **Selye s.,** general adaptation s. **Senear-Usher s.,** pemphigus erythematosus. **Sertoli-cell-only s.,** congenital absence of the germinal epithelium of the testes, the seminiferous tubules containing only Sertoli cells, characterized by testes which are slightly smaller than normal, azoospermia, and elevated titers of follicle-stimulating hormone or of general gonadotropins. **serum sickness s.,** a serum sickness–like hypersensitivity reaction occurring after the administration of certain drugs. It is marked clinically by low-grade fever, urticaria, facial edema, pain and swelling of the joints, and lymphadenopathy, and occasionally may be associated with neuritis of the brachial plexus, Guillain-Barré syndrome, periarteritis nodosa, and nephritis. **Sézary s., Sézary reticulosis s.,** generalized exfoliative erythroderma produced by cutaneous infiltration of reticular lymphocytes and associated with intense pruritis, alopecia, edema, hyperkeratosis, and pigment and nail changes; although bone marrow and lymph nodes are normal, reticulemia may occur. Called also *Sézary erythroderma.* **Sheehan's s.,** postpartum pituitary necrosis. **short-bowel s., short-gut s.,** any of the malabsorption conditions resulting from massive resection of the small bowel, the degree and kind of malabsorption depending on the site and extent of the resection; it is characterized by diarrhea, steatorrhea, and malnutrition. **shoulder-hand s.,** a clinical disorder of the upper extremity, characterized by pain and stiffness in the shoulder, with puffy swelling and pain in the ipsilateral hand, sometimes occurring after myocardial infarction but also produced by other known or unknown causes. **Shy-Drager s.,** a progressive disorder of unknown cause that results in severe disability or death, beginning with symptoms of autonomic insufficiency including impotence (in males), constipation, urinary urgency or retention, anhidrosis, and most importantly, orthostatic hypotension, followed by signs of generalized neurologic dysfunction, such as parkinsonian-like disturbances, cerebellar incoordination, muscle wasting and fasciculations, and coarse tremors of the legs. **Sicard's s.,** Collet's s. **sicca s.,** Sjögren's s. **sick sinus s.,** a complex cardiac arrhythmia manifested as severe sinus bradycardia alone, sinus bradycardia alternating with tachycardia, or sinus bradycardia with atrioventricular block. **Silver's s.,** a congenital syndrome consisting of low birth weight despite normal duration of gestation, short stature, lateral asymmetry, slight to moderate increase in excretion of gonadotropins, which may be associated with incurved fifth fingers, café-au-lait spots, syndactyly, triangular-shaped face, turned down corners of the mouth, and precocious puberty. Cf. *Russell's s.* **Silverskiöld's s.,** a form of eccentro-osteochondrodysplasia in which the skeletal changes are chiefly in the extremities and which is inherited as a dominant character. **Silvestrini-Corda s.,** eunuchoid body type, absence of body hair, defective libido, atrophy of the testes, sterility, and gynecomastia: a syndrome indicative of abnormally high estrogenic activity, due to failure of the liver to inactivate the estrogens. **Simmonds' s.,** see *panhypopituitarism.* **Sipple's s.,** a hereditary association of pheochromocytoma, characteristically bilateral and multiple, medullary carcinoma of the thyroid, and a tendency to hyperparathyroidism due to hyperplasia or multiple parathyroid adenomas; associated abnormalities include mucosal neuromas, Marfan's syndrome, etc. It is transmitted as an autosomal dominant trait. **Sjögren's s.,** a symptom complex of unknown etiology, usually occurring in middle-aged or older women, marked by keratoconjunctivitis sicca, xerostomia, and enlargement of the parotid glands; it is often associated with rheumatoid arthritis and sometimes with systemic lupus erythematosus, scleroderma, or polymyositis. An abnormal immune response has been implicated. Called also *Gougerot-Nuloch-Houwer s., sicca s.,* and *Sjogren's disease.* **Sjögren-Larsson s.,** congenital oligophrenia, ichthyosis, and spastic pyramidal symptoms. **SLE-like s.,** hydralazine lupus s. **Sluder's s.,** see under *neuralgia.* **Smith-Lemli-Opitz s.,** a hereditary syndrome, transmitted as an autosomal recessive trait, characterized by multiple congenital anomalies, including microcephaly, mental retardation, hypotonia, incomplete development of male genitalia, short nose with anteverted nostrils, syndactyly of second and third toes, etc. **social breakdown s.,** a term used to express the concept that some of the mental patient's symptomatology, especially in large, understaffed institutions, is a result of treatment conditions and facilities and not part of the primary illness. **Sohval-Soffer s.,** a congenital syndrome consisting of male hypogonadism associated with multiple skeletal abnormalities of the cervical spine and ribs and mental retardation. **somnolence s.,** a transient condition of drowsiness, lethargy, anorexia, and irritability with electroencephalographic changes, occurring in children after irradiation of the head in acute leukemia or non-Hodgkin's lymphoma. **Sorsby's s.,** a congenital condition consisting of bilateral macular coloboma associated with apical dystrophy of the hands and feet, usually brachydactyly confined to the distal two phalanges. **Sotos' s., Sotos' s. of cerebral gigantism,** cerebral gigantism. **Spens's s.,** Adams-Stokes disease. **Speransky-Richen-Siegmund s.,** necrotizing perforation of the hard palate into the maxillary sinus, with detachment of the alveolar process. **spherophakia-brachymorphia s.,** Weill-Marchesani s. **splenic flexure s.,** discomfort in the left upper abdominal quadrant, which may give rise to pain in the precordium and left shoulder and arm, simulating angina. **split-brain s.,** an association of symptoms produced by disruption of or interference with the connection between the hemispheres of the brain. **Sprinz-Dubin s., Sprinz Nelson s.,** Dubin-Johnson s. **Spurway s.,** osteogenesis imperfecta associated with blue sclerae. **Steele-Richardson-Olszewski s.,** a progressive neurological disorder, having onset during the sixth decade, characterized by supranuclear ophthalmoplegia, especially paralysis of the downward gaze, pseudobulbar palsy, dysarthria, dystonic rigidity of the neck and trunk, and dementia. **steely-hair s.,** Menkes' s. **Stein-Leventhal s.,** a clinical symptom complex characterized by oligomenorrhea or amenorrhea, anovulation (hence infertility), and regularly associated with bilateral polycystic ovaries; excretion of follicle-stimulating hormone and 17-ketosteroids is essentially normal. Called also *polycystic ovary disease* or *syndrome*. **Steinbrocker's s.,** shoulder-hand s. **Steiner's s.,** Curtius' s. **Stevens-Johnson s.,** the severe form of erythema multiforme in which, in addition to other symptoms (see *erythema multiforme*), there is involvement of the oronasal and anogenital mucosa, the eyes, and viscera; constitutional symptoms include malaise, prostration, headache, fever, and arthralgia. It may be fatal. Called also *ectodermosis erosiva pluriorificialis, erythema multiforme exudativum,* and *Johnson-Stevens disease.* **Stewart-Morel s.,** hyperostosis frontalis interna. **Stewart-Treves s.,** lymphangiosarcoma which occurs as a late complication of severe lymphedema of the arm following excision of lymph nodes, usually associated with radical mastectomy. **"stiff heart" s.,** any cardiac disease characterized by restrictive hemodynamics; it may result from any pathologic process that renders the myocardial fibers abnormally rigid or that externally applies a constricting pressure and as a consequence impedes flow of blood into the ventricular cavities. **stiff-man s.,** a condition of unknown etiology characterized by progressive fluctuating rigidity of axial and limb muscles in the absence of signs of cerebral and spinal cord disease but with continuous electromyographic activity. **Still-Chauffard s.,** Chauffard's s. **Stilling s.,** Duane s. **Stilling-Turk-Duane s.,** Duane s. **Stokes's s., Stokes-Adams s.,** Adams-Stokes disease. **Stokvis-Talma s.,** enterogenous cyanosis. **straight back s.,** a skeletal deformity characterized by loss of the anterior concavity of the vertebral column in the upper thoracic region, with consequent reduction in the anteroposterior diameter of the thorax and compression of the heart between the dorsal spine and the sternum. **stroke s.,** a condition with sudden onset caused by acute vascular lesions of the brain, such as hemorrhage, embolism, thrombosis, or rupturing aneurysm, which may be marked by hemiplegia or hemiparesis, vertigo, numbness, aphasia, and dysarthria; it is often followed by permanent neurologic damage. Called also *cerebrovascular accident* and *stroke.* **Sturge's s., Sturge-Kalischer-Weber s.,** Sturge-Weber s. **Sturge-Weber s.,** a congenital syndrome consisting of nevus flammeus of the face, angiomas of the leptomeninges and choroid, and late glaucoma, frequently associated with intracranial calcification, mental retardation, contralateral hemiplegia, and epilepsy; called also *Sturge's s., Sturge-Kalischer-Weber s., Dimitri disease,* and various combinations of these names. **subclavian steal s.,** cerebral or brain stem ischemia resulting from diversion of blood flow from the basilar artery to the subclavian artery, in the presence of occlusive disease of the proximal portion of the subclavian artery. **sudden infant death s.,** the sudden and unexpected death of an apparently healthy infant, typically occurring between the ages of three weeks and five months, and not explained by careful postmortem studies; called also *crib* or *cot death.* Abbreviated SIDS. **Sudeck-Leriche s.,** post-traumatic osteoporosis associated with vasospasm. **Sulzberger-Garbe s.,** chronic exudative discoid and lichenoid dermatitis accompanied by severe nocturnal pruritus, occurring chiefly in middle-aged men of Jewish extraction; called also *oid-oid disease.* **superior caval s.,** venous engorgement, hepatic enlargement, and edema resembling that of right heart failure or constrictive pericarditis, resulting from lymphomatous, metastatic, or primary malignant neoplasms of the pericardium. **superior mesenteric artery s.,** compression of the third, or transverse, portion of the duodenum against the aorta by the superior mesenteric artery, resulting in chronic, intermittent, or acute, complete or partial obstruction; symptoms range from mild to nausea and vomiting, pain, and extreme distention of the stomach and duodenum. **superior sulcus tumor s.,** Pancoast's s., def. 1. **superior vena cava s.,** suffusion and brawny edema of the

face, neck, or upper arms due to increased venous pressure incident to compression of the superior vena cava, most commonly caused by metastatic mediastinal lymph node tumor in lung cancer. **suprarenogenic s.,** adrenal disorder characterized by adiposity, pigmentation, and hairiness. **supraspinatus s.,** tenderness over the supraspinatus tendon, a painful arc on movement of the arm, and a reversal of scapulohumeral rhythm. **sweat retention s.,** tropical anhidrotic asthenia. **Sweet's s.,** acute febrile neutrophilic dermatosis. **Takayasu's s.,** pulseless disease. **Tapia's s.,** unilateral paralysis of the tongue and larynx, the velum palati being unaffected. **tarsal tunnel s.,** a complex of symptoms resulting from compression of the posterior tibial nerve or of the plantar nerves in the tarsal tunnel, with pain, numbness, and tingling paresthesia of the sole of the foot. **Taussig-Bing s.,** a rare congenital malformation of the heart characterized by transposition of the great vessels and a ventricular septal defect straddled by a large pulmonary artery; hemodynamically it is characterized by pulmonary hypertension, pulmonary plethora, cyanosis, and greater O_2 saturation of blood in the pulmonary artery than in the aorta. **tegmental s.,** hemiplegia, alternating with disordered eye movements, indicative of lesions of the tegmentum. **temporomandibular joint s.,** dysfunction of the temporomandibular joint marked by a clicking or grinding sensation in the joint and often by pain in or about the ears, muscle tiredness and slight soreness upon waking, and stiffness of the jaw or actual trismus; it results from mandibular overclosure, condylar displacement, or stress, with deforming arthritis an occasional factor. **Terry's s.,** retrolental fibroplasia. **testicular feminization s.,** an extreme form of male pseudohermaphroditism, with female external development, including secondary sex characteristics, but with presence of testes and absence of uterus and tubes; it is due to end-organ resistance to the action of testosterone. **thalamic s.,** a combination of the following symptoms: (1) superficial persistent hemianesthesia; (2) mild hemiplegia; (3) mild hemiataxia and more or less complete astereognosis; (4) severe and persistent pains in the hemiplegic side; (5) choreoathetoid movements in the members of the paralyzed side. Called also *Dejerine-Roussy s.* and *thalamic hyperesthetic anesthesia.* **Thibierge-Weissenbach s.,** calcinosis. **Thiele s.,** tenderness and pain in the region of the lower portion of the sacrum and coccyx, or in contiguous soft tissues and muscles. **Thiemann's s.,** see under *disease.* **thoracic outlet s.,** compression of the brachial plexus nerve trunks, characterized by pain in arms, paresthesia of fingers, vasomotor symptoms (pallor, acrocyanosis, secondary Raynaud's phenomenon, etc.), and weakness and wasting of small muscles of the hand; it may be caused by drooping shoulder girdle, a cervical rib or fibrous band, an abnormal first rib, continual hyperabduction of the arm (see *hyperabduction s.*), or (rarely) compression of the edge of scalenus anterior muscle. **Thorn's s.,** see *salt-losing s.* **thrombocytopenia–absent radius (TAR) s.,** a hereditary syndrome, transmitted as an autosomal recessive trait, consisting of thrombocytopenia associated with absence of the radius and sometimes congenital heart disease and renal anomalies. **thromboembolic s.,** the association between the formation of thrombi in the deep veins of the leg and pulmonary embolism. **Tietze's s.,** 1. [Alexander *Tietze*] idiopathic painful nonsuppurative swellings of one or more costal cartilages, especially of the second rib; the anterior chest pain may mimic that of coronary artery disease. Called also *costal chondritis* and *Tietze's disease.* 2. albinism, except for normal eye pigment, deaf-mutism, and hypoplasia of the eyebrows. **Timme's s.,** ovarian and adrenal insufficiency with compensatory hypopituitarism. **tired housewife s.,** a form of mild hypothyroidism manifested in symptoms such as mild lassitude, fatigue, slight anemia, constipation, apathy, slight cold intolerance, menstrual irregularities, inability to conceive, dry skin, some loss of hair, and slight to moderate weight gain. **Tolosa-Hunt s.,** unilateral ophthalmoplegia associated with pain behind the orbit and in the area supplied by the first division of the trigeminal nerve; it is thought to be due to nonspecific inflammation and granulation tissue in the superior orbital fissure or cavernous sinus. **Tommaselli's s.,** see under *disease.* **Touraine-Solente-Golé s.,** pachydermoperiostosis. **toxic fat s.,** a condition occurring in 3- to 10-week old chickens that have been fed fat-supplemented diets, marked by edema of the pericardium and abdomen, waddling gait, and sudden death; called also *water belly.* **toxic shock s.,** a severe illness characterized by high fever of sudden onset, vomiting, diarrhea, and myalgia, followed by hypotension and, in severe cases, shock; a sunburn-like rash with peeling of the skin, especially of the palms and soles, occurs during the acute phase. The syndrome affects almost exclusively menstruating women using tampons, although a few women who do not use tampons and a few males have been affected. It is thought to be caused by infection with *Staphylococcus aureus.* **transfusion s.,** placental transfusion s. **Treacher Collins s.,** mandibulofacial dysostosis. **trichorhinophalangeal s.,** a hereditary syndrome, transmitted as an autosomal recessive trait, consisting of sparse, slowly growing hair, pear-shaped nose with high philtrum, and brachyphalangia with deformity of the fingers and wedge-shaped epiphyses. **triparanol s.,** alopecia, poliosis, ichthyosis, irreversible cataracts, and impotence, due to the use of triparanol, a drug formerly used to depress the synthesis of cholesterol. **trisomy C s.**, trisomy 8 s. **trisomy D s.**, trisomy 13 s. **trisomy E s.**, trisomy 18 s. **trisomy 8 s.**, a syndrome associated with an extra chromosome 8, usually mosaic (trisomy 8/normal, or trisomy C/normal), characterized by mild to severe mental retardation, prominent forehead, deep-set eyes, thick lips, prominent ears, and camptodactyly. Called also *trisomy C s.* **trisomy 13 s.**, holoprosencephaly due to an extra chromosome 13, in which central nervous system defects are associated with mental retardation, along with cleft lip and palate, polydactyly, dermal pattern anomalies, and abnormalities of the heart, viscera, and genitalia. Called also *Patau's s., trisomy D s.,* and *trisomy 13–15 s.* **trisomy 13–15 s.**, trisomy 13 s. **trisomy 16–18 s.**, trisomy 18 s. **trisomy 18 s.**, a condition characterized by mental retardation, scaphocephaly or other skull abnormality, micrognathia, blepharoptosis, low-set ears, corneal opacities, deafness, webbed neck, short digits, ventricular septal defects, Meckel's diverticulum, and other deformities. It is due to the presence of an extra chromosome 18. Called also *Edwards' s., trisomy E s.,* and *trisomy 16–18 s.* **trisomy 21 s.**, Down's s. **trisomy 22 s.**, a syndrome due to an extra chromosome 22, characterized typically by mental and growth retardation, microcephaly, low-set or malformed ears, micrognathia, long philtrum, preauricular skin tag or sinus, and congenital heart disease. In males, there is small penis and/or undescended testes. **Troisier's s.**, bronzed cachexia occurring in diabetes. **Trousseau's s.**, spontaneous venous thrombosis of upper and lower extremities occurring in association with visceral carcinoma. **Turcot s.**, familial polyposis of the colon associated with malignant tumors (gliomas) of the central nervous system. **Turner's s.**, a form of gonadal dysgenesis, marked by short stature, undifferentiated (streak) gonads, and variable abnormalities that may include webbing of the neck, low posterior hair line, increased carrying angle of the elbow, cubitus valgus, and cardiac defects; it is typically associated with absence of the second X chromosome (XO, or 45, X), although a defect of one X chromosome and mosaicism (X/XX or X/XXX) also occur. The phenotype is female; patients are invariably sterile. **Turner's s., male,** Noonan's s. **Ullrich-Feichtiger s.**, a condition of micrognathia, hexadactyly, and genital abnormalities, with depressed nose, small eyes, hypertelorism, and protuberant ears, along with other defects. **Ullrich-Turner s.**, Noonan's s. **Unverricht's s.**, myoclonus epilepsy. **urethral s.**, suprapubic aching and cramping, urinary frequency, and such bladder complaints as dysuria, urinary tenesmus, and low back pain, without evidence of urinary infection. **vagoaccessory s.**, Schmidt's s. **van Buchem's s.** hyperostosis corticalis generalisata. **van der Hoeve's s.**, a hereditary syndrome consisting of blue scleras, osteogenesis imperfecta, and otosclerotic deafness, usually transmitted as an autosomal dominant trait. Called also *Adair-Dighton s.* and *Dighton-Adair s.* See *osteogenesis imperfecta.* **Van der Woude's s.**, a hereditary syndrome, transmitted as an autosomal dominant trait, consisting of cleft lip and/or cleft palate occurring in association with cysts of the lower lip. **vanishing testes s.**, a disorder characterized by the absence of gonadal tissue, a small penis, and no adolescent virilization; the chromosome pattern is XY (male). **vascular s.**, any syndrome due to occlusion or stenosis of vessels supplying the nervous system. **Vernet's s.**, paralysis of the ninth, tenth, and eleventh cranial nerves due to a lesion in the region of the jugular foramen, and marked by paralysis of the superior constriction of the pharynx and difficulty in swallowing solids; paralysis of the soft palate and fauces with anesthesia of these parts and of the pharynx, and loss of taste in the posterior third of the tongue; paralysis of the vocal cords and anesthesia of the larynx; paralysis of the sternocleidomastoid and trapezius muscles. Called also *jugular foramen s.* **Villaret's s.**, unilateral paralysis of the ninth, tenth, eleventh, and twelfth cranial nerves and sometimes the seventh, due to a lesion in the retroparotid space, and characterized by paralysis of the superior constriction of the pharynx and difficulty in swallowing solids; paralysis of soft palate and fauces with anesthesia of these parts and of the pharynx; loss of taste in the posterior third of the tongue; paralysis of the vocal cords and anesthesia of the larynx; paralysis of the sternocleidomastoid and trapezius; and paralysis of the cervical sympathetic nerves (*Horner's syndrome*). Called also *s. of retroparotid space.* **Vinson's s.**, Plummer-Vinson s. **Vogt's s.**, a syndrome frequently associated with birth trauma, characterized by bilateral athetosis, walking difficulties, spasmodic outbursts of laughing or crying, speech disorders, excessive myelination of the nerve fibers of the corpus striatum, giving it a marbled appearance (*status marmoratus*), and sometimes mental deficiency. Called also *Vogt's disease* and *s. of corpus striatum.* **Vogt-Koyanagi s.**, uveomeningitis characterized by exudative iridocyclitis and choroiditis associated with patchy depigmentation of the skin and hair; the lashes and eyebrows also become whitened, and there may also be retinal detachment and associated deafness and tinnitus. **Volkmann's s.**, post-traumatic muscular hypertonia and degenerative neuritis; Volkmann's contracture. **Waardenburg's s.**, 1. a hereditary disorder, transmitted as an autosomal dominant trait, characterized by wide bridge of the nose due to lateral displacement of the inner canthi and puncta, pigmentary disturbances, including white forelock, heterochromia iridis, white eyelashes, leukoderma, and sometimes cochlear deafness. 2. a hereditary disorder, transmitted as an autosomal dominant trait, characterized by acrocephaly, orbital and facial deformities, and brachydactyly with mild soft tissue syndactyly; cleft palate, hydrophthalmos, cardiac malformation, and contractures of the elbows and knees may also be present. Called also *acrocephalosyndactyly type IV.* **Wallenberg's s.**, a syndrome due to occlusion of the posterior inferior cerebellar artery, marked by ipsilateral loss of temperature and pain sensations of the face and contralateral loss of these sensations of the extremities and trunk, ipsilateral ataxia, dysphagia, dysarthria, and nystagmus. **Waterhouse-Friderichsen s.**, the malignant or fulminating form of epidemic cerebrospinal meningitis, marked by sudden onset and short course, fever, coma, and collapse, cyanosis, petechial hemorrhages of the skin and mucous membranes, and bilateral adrenal hemorrhage. **s. of Weber,** paralysis of the oculomotor nerve on the same side as the lesion, producing ptosis, strabismus, and loss of light reflex and of accommodation; also spastic hemiplegia on the side opposite the lesion with increased reflexes and loss of superficial reflexes. Called also *alternating oculomotor hemiplegia* and *Weber's paralysis.* **Weber-Christian s.**, nodular nonsuppurative panniculitis. **Weber-Dubler s.**, s. of Weber. **Wegener's s.**, see under *granulomatosis.* **Weill-Marchesani s.**, a congenital disorder of connective tissue transmitted as an autosomal dominant or recessive trait, characterized by brachycephaly, brachydactyly, short stature with a broad chest and heavy musculature, reduced joint mobility, spherophakia, ectopia lentis, myopia, and glaucoma; called also *dystrophia mesodermalis congenita hyperplastica, Marchesani's s.,* and *spherophakia-brachymorphia s.* **Werdnig-Hoffmann s.**, see under *paralysis.* **Wermer's s.**, polyendocrine adenomatosis. **Werner's s.**, premature senility of an adult, characterized by early graying and some loss of hair, cataracts, hyperkeratinization, and scleroderma-like changes in the skin of the lower extremities, followed by chronic ulceration. **Wernicke's s.**, presbyophrenia. **Weyers' oligodactyly s.**, a congenital syndrome consisting of deficiency of the ulna and ulnar rays, antecubital pterygia, reduced sternal segments, malformations of the kidney and spleen, and cleft lip and palate. **Weyers-Thier s.**, oculovertebral dysplasia. **whistling face s.**, **whistling face–windmill vane hand s.**, craniocarpotarsal dystrophy. **Widal s.**, icteroanemia. **Willebrand's s.**, von Willebrand's disease. **Williams-Campbell s.**, congenital bronchomalacia due to absence of annular cartilage distal to the first division of the peripheral bronchi; it is marked by bronchiectasis. **Wilson's s.**, hepatolenticular degeneration. **Wilson-Mikity s.**, a rare form of pulmonary insufficiency in low-birth-weight infants, marked by hyperpnea and cyanosis of insidious onset during the first month of life and often resulting in death. Radiographically, there are multiple cystlike foci of hyperaeration throughout the lung with coarse thickening of the interstitial supporting structures. The disorder has been attributed to disparity of maturation of parenchymal elements, especially of alveoli proliferation, and hence has been called *pulmonary dysmaturity.* **Winter's s.**, a congenital syndrome consisting of renal hypoplasia or aplasia, anomalies of the internal genitalia, especially vaginal atresia, and anomaly of the ossicles of the middle ear. **Wiskott-Aldrich s.**, a condition characterized by chronic eczema, chronic suppurative otitis media, anemia, and thrombocytopenic purpura; it is an immunodeficiency syndrome transmitted as an X-linked recessive trait, in which there is poor antibody response to polysaccharide antigens and dysfunction of cell-mediated immunity. Called also *Aldrich's s.* **Wolf-Hirschhorn s.**, a syndrome associated with partial deletion of the short arm of chromosome 4, characterized by microcephaly, ocular hypertelorism, epicanthus, cleft palate, micrognathia, low-set ears simplified in form, cryptorchidism, and hypospadias. **Wolff-Parkinson-White s.**, the association of paroxysmal tachycardia (or atrial fibrillation) and preexcitation, in which the electrocardiogram displays a short P-R interval and a wide QRS complex which characteristically shows an early QRS vector (delta wave); called also *anomalous atrioventricular excitation.* **Wolfram's s.**, a hereditary association of diabetes mellitus, diabetes insipidus, optic atrophy, and neural deafness. **Wright's s.**, 1. (Irving S. Wright) a neurovascular syndrome caused by hyperabduction of the arm. Such hyperabduction may cause occlusion of the subclavian artery, leading to gangrene, or may produce sensory symptoms due to stretching of the brachial plexus. 2. a condition marked by multifocal areas of osteitis fibrosa, patchy cutaneous pigmentation, and precocious puberty. **XXY s.**, Klinefelter's s. **yellow nail s.**, a yellow or greenish discoloration of the nails preceded and accompanied by retardation of their growth, associated with lymphedema that is usually confined to the ankles but may involve other areas. **yellow vernix s.**, placental dysfunction s. **Young's s.**, amyotrophic lateral sclerosis of bulbar type associated with platybasia. **Zieve s.**, hypercholesterolemia, hepatosplenomegaly, fatty infiltration of the liver, hemolytic anemia, and hypertriglyceridemia following the ingestion of large amounts of ethanol. **Zollinger-Ellison s.**, a triad comprising (1) intractable, sometimes fulminating, and in many ways atypical peptic ulcers; (2) extreme gastric hyperacidity; and (3) gastrin-secreting, non–beta islet cell tumors of the pancreas, which may be single or multiple, small or large, benign or malignant. The gastrinoma sometimes occurs in sites (e.g., the duodenum) other than the pancreas. See also *polyendocrine adenomatosis,* under *adenomatosis.*

syndromic (sin-drom′ik) occurring as a syndrome.

syndromology (sin″drom-ol′o-je) the field concerned with the taxonomy, etiology, and patterns of congenital malformations.

Syndrox (sin′droks) trademark for preparations of methamphetamine hydrochloride.

synechia (sĭ-nek′e-ah), pl. *synech′iae* [Gr. *synecheia* continuity] adhesion of parts, especially adhesion of the iris to the cornea or to the lens. **annular s.,** adhesion of the whole rim of the iris to the lens. **anterior s.,** adhesion of the base of the iris to the cornea, producing occlusion of the chamber angle; it may be caused by glaucoma, cataract, intraocular tumors, or after perforation resulting from keratitis, iridocylitis, trauma, or surgery. **circular s.,** annular s. **s. pericar′dii,** concretio cordis. **posterior s.,** adhesion of the iris to the capsule of the lens or to the surface of the vitreous body, producing an irregularly shaped pupil. **total anterior s.,** adhesion of the entire surface of the iris to the cornea. **total posterior s.,** adhesion of the entire surface of the iris to the lens. **s. vul′vae,** fused vulva: a congenital condition in which the labia minora are sealed in the midline, with only a small opening below the clitoris through which urination and menstruation may occur.

synechiae (sĭ-nek′e-e) plural of *synechia.*

synechotome (sin-ek′o-tōm) a cutting instrument for use in synechotomy.

synechotomy (sin″ĕ-kot′o-me) [*synechia* + Gr. *tomē* a cutting] the operation of cutting a synechia.

synechtenterotomy (sin″ek-ten″ter-ot′o-me) [Gr. *synechēs* joined together + *enteron* bowel + *tomē* a cutting] division of an intestinal adhesion.

synecology (sin″ĕ-kol′o-je) the study of the environment of organisms in the mass, as distinguished from *autoecology.*

Synemol (sin′ĕ-mol) trademark for a preparation of fluocinolone acetonide.

synencephalocele (sin″en-sef′ah-lo-sēl″) [*syn-* + Gr. *enkephalos* brain + *kēlē* tumor] encephalocele with adhesions to the adjoining parts.

synencephalus (sin″en-sef′ah-lus) a monster exhibiting synencephaly.

synencephaly (sin″en-sef′ah-le) [*syn-* + Gr. *enkephalos* brain] a developmental anomaly in which there are two bodies and one head.

syneresis (sĭ-ner′ĕ-sis) [Gr. *synairesis* a taking or drawing together] a drawing together of the particles of the dispersed phase of a gel, with separation of some of the disperse medium and shrinkage of the gel, such as occurs in the clotting of blood.

synergenesis (sin″er-jen′ĕ-sis) the doctrine that every cell transmits its protoplasm to every generation of cells derived from it.

synergetic (sin″er-jet′ik) working together; said of muscles which cooperate in performing an action.

synergia (sin-er′je-ah) synergy.

synergic (sin-er′jik) acting together or in harmony.

synergism (sin′er-jizm) the joint action of agents so that their combined effect is greater than the algebraic sum of their individual effects.

synergist (sin′er-jist) 1. a medicine that aids or cooperates with another; an adjuvant. 2. an organ that acts in concert with another. **pituitary s.,** a substance occurring in extracts of the anterior pituitary which enhances the action of gonadotropic extracts of the urine of pregnant women or placenta.

synergistic (sin″er-jis′tik) acting together; enhancing the effect of another force or agent.

synergy (sin′er-je) [L. *synergia;* Gr. *syn* together + *ergon* work] correlated action or cooperation on the part of two or more structures or drugs. In neurology, the faculty by which movements are properly grouped for the performance of acts requiring special adjustments.

synesthesia (sin″es-the′ze-ah) [*syn-* + Gr. *aisthēsis* perception + *-ia*] a secondary sensation accompanying an actual perception; the experiencing of a sensation in one place, due to stimulation applied to another place; also the condition in which a stimulus of one sense is perceived as sensation of a different sense, as when a sound produces a sensation of color. **s. al′gica,** a painful synesthesia.

synesthesialgia (sin″es-the″ze-al′je-ah) a condition in which a stimulus produces pain on the affected side but no sensation or even a pleasant one on the normal side of the body.

synezesis (sin″e-ze′sis) synizesis.

Syngamidae (sin-gam′ĭ-de) a family of nematodes of the superfamily Strongyloidea, which includes the genera *Syngamus* and *Stephanurus.*

syngamous (sin′gah-mus) [*syn-* + Gr. *gamos* marriage] 1. pertaining to or characterized by syngamy. 2. having the sex of the individual determined at the time when the ovum is fertilized.

Syngamus (sin′gah-mus) a genus of nematode worms of the family Syngamidae that are parasitic in fowl and other birds. **S. tra′chea,** the gapeworm, a species of worms which are parasitic in chickens, pheasants, turkeys, and various wild birds, inhabiting the trachea and interfering with respiration when present in large numbers; it is the etiologic agent of gapes.

syngamy (sing′gah-me) [*syn-* + Gr. *gamos* marriage] 1. sexual reproduction. 2. the union of two gametes in fertilization to form a zygote.

syngeneic (sin″jĕ-ne′ik) in transplantation biology, denoting individuals or tissues that have identical genotypes, i.e., identical twins or animals of the same inbred strain, or their tissues. Called also *isogeneic.*

syngenesioplastic (sin″jĕ-ne″ze-o-plas′tik) [*syn-* + Gr. *genesis* origin + *plassein* to form] denoting transplantation of tissue from one individual to a related individual of the same species, as from a mother to her child, or from a brother to a sister.

syngenesiotransplantation (sin″jĕ-ne″ze-o-trans″plan-ta′shun) syngenesioplastic transplantation.

syngenesis (sin-jen′ĕ-sis) 1. the origin of an individual from a germ cell derived from both parents and not from either one alone, as occurs in mammals. 2. the state of having descended from a common ancestor.

syngnathia (sin-na′the-ah) [*syn-* + Gr. *gnathos* jaw + *-ia*] congenital bands or threads of mucous membrane extending between the jaws.

syngonic (sin-gon′ik) [*syn-* + Gr. *gonē* seed] having the sex of the individual determined at the time when the ovum is fertilized.

syngraft (sin′graft) isograft.

synizesis (sin″ĭ-ze′sis) [Gr. *synizēsis*] 1. occlusion. 2. a stage in mitosis in which the nuclear chromatin is massed. **s. pupil′lae,** occlusion of the pupil.

synkainogenesis (sin″ki-no-jen′ĕ-sis) [*syn-* + Gr. *kainos* new + *genesis* production] the process of developing a new formation simultaneously with another formation.

synkaryon (sin-kar′e-on) [*syn-* + Gr. *karyon* nucleus] the nucleus produced by the fusion of two pronuclei in karyogamy; the fertilization nucleus.

Synkayvite (sin′ka-vīt) trademark for preparations of menadiol sodium diphosphate.

synkinesia (sin″ki-ne′ze-ah) synkinesis.

synkinesis (sin″ki-ne′sis) [*syn-* + Gr. *kinēsis* movement] an associated movement; an unintentional movement accompanying a volitional movement. **imitative s.,** an involuntary movement on the healthy side accompanying an attempt at movement on the paralyzed side. **mouth-and-hand s.,** see *Saunders' sign,* under *sign.* **spasmodic s.,** a movement on the paralyzed side attending a voluntary movement on the healthy side.

synkinetic (sin″ki-net′ik) pertaining to or of the nature of synkinesis.

synnecrosis (sin″nĕ-kro′sis) [*syn-* + Gr. *nekrōsis* a state of death] a relationship between populations (or individuals) resulting in mutual depression or death.

synneurosis (sin″nu-ro′sis) [Gr. *synneurosis* union by sinews] syndesmosis.

synocha (sin′o-kah) [L.; Gr. *synochos* jointed together] a continued fever.

synochal (sin′o-kal) of or pertaining to synocha.

synochus (sin′o-kus) synocha.

synocytotoxin (sin″o-si″to-tok′sin) syncytotoxin.

synonychia (sin″o-nik′e-ah) [*syn-* + Gr. *onyx* nail + *-ia*] fusion of the nails of two or more digits in complicated syndactyly.

synophridia (sin″o-frid′e-ah) synophrys.

synophrys (sin-of′ris) [Gr. "with meeting eyebrows"] the condition in which the eyebrows grow together.

synophthalmia (sin″of-thal′me-ah) [*syn-* + Gr. *ophthalmos* eye + *-ia*] the usual form of cyclopia, in which the two eyes are more or less completely fused into one.

synophthalmus (sin″of-thal′mus) cyclops.

Synophylate (sin″o-fi′lāt) trademark for preparations of theophylline sodium glycinate.

synopsy (sin′op-se) [Gr. *syn* together + *opsis* vision] 1. a form of synesthesia in which certain colors are associated with certain tones. 2. the abnormal suggestion of types of the human face or figure by the various numerals.

synoptophore (sin-op′to-fōr) an instrument for diagnosing strabismus and for treating it by orthoptic methods.

synoptoscope (sin-op′to-skōp) [*syn-* + Gr. *optos* seen + *skopein* to examine] an instrument for examining the eye in strabismus.

synorchidism (sin-or′kĭ-dizm) synorchism.

synorchism (sin′or-kizm) [*syn-* + Gr. *orchis* testicle] fusion of the two testes into one mass, which may be located in the scrotum or in the abdomen.

synoscheos (sin-os′ke-os) [*syn-* + Gr. *oscheon* scrotum] adhesion between the penis and scrotum.

synosteology (sin″os-te-ol′o-je) [*syn-* + Gr. *osteon* bone + *-logy*] the sum of knowledge regarding the joints and articulations.

synosteosis (sin″os-te-o′sis) synostosis.

synosteotic (sin″os-te-ot′ik) pertaining to or marked by synosteosis.

synosteotomy (sin″os-te-ot′o-me) [*syn-* + Gr. *osteon* bone + *tomē* a cutting] the dissection of the joints.

synostosis (sin″os-to′sis), pl. *synosto′ses* [*syn-* + Gr. *osteon* bone] 1. [NA] a union between adjacent bones or parts of a single bone formed by osseous material, such as ossified connecting cartilage or fibrous tissue. 2. the osseous union of bones that are normally distinct. **radioulnar s.,** bony fusion of the proximal ends of the radius and ulna. **sagittal s.,** scaphocephaly. **tarsal s.,** fusion of various tarsal bones. **tribasilar s.,** fusion in infancy of the three bones at the base of the skull, producing mental retardation.

synostotic (sin″os-tot′ik) synosteotic.

synotia (si-no′she-ah) [*syn-* + Gr. *ous* ear] a developmental anomaly characterized by persistence of the ears in their horizontal position beneath the mandible.

synotus (si-no′tus) [*syn-* + Gr. *ous* ear] fetus exhibiting synotia.

synovectomy (sin″o-vek′to-me) [*synovia* + Gr. *ektomē* excision] excision of a synovial membrane, as of that lining the capsule of the knee joint, performed in treatment of rheumatoid arthritis of the knee, or of the synovial sheath of a tendon.

synovia (sĭ-no′ve-ah) [L.; Gr. *syn* with + *ōon* egg] [NA] a transparent alkaline viscid fluid, resembling the white of an egg, secreted by the synovial membrane, and contained in joint cavities, bursae, and tendon sheaths; called also *synovial fluid.*

synovial (sĭ-no′ve-al) [L. *synovialis*] of, pertaining to, or secreting synovia.

synovialis (sĭ-no″ve-a′lis) [L.] synovial.

synovialoma (sĭ-no″ve-ah-lo′mah) synovioma.

synovianalysis (sĭ-no″ve-ah-nal′ĭ-sis) the laboratory examination of joint fluid (synovia).

synovin (sin′o-vin) the mucin found in synovia.

synovioblast (sĭ-no′ve-o-blast) a fibroblast of synovial membrane.

synoviocyte (sĭ-no′ve-o-sīt) a cell of the synovial membrane.

synovioma (sĭ-no″ve-o′mah) a tumor of synovial membrane origin. **benign s.,** giant cell tumor of tendon sheath. **malignant s.,** synoviosarcoma.

synoviorthese (sin-o′ve-or-thēs″) [Fr.] irradiation of the synovium by intra-articular injection of radiocolloids to destroy inflamed synovial tissue.

synoviosarcoma (sĭ-no″ve-o-sar-ko′mah) a malignant neoplasm arising in the synovial membrane of the joints and also in synovial cells of tendons and bursae; called also *malignant synovioma* and *synovial sarcoma.*

synoviparous (sin″o-vip′ah-rus) [*synovia* + L. *parere* to produce] producing synovia.

synovitis (sin″o-vi′tis) inflammation of a synovial membrane. It is usually painful, particularly on motion, and is characterized by a fluctuating swelling, due to effusion within a synovial sac. Synovitis is qualified as *fibrinous, gonorrheal, hyperplastic, lipomatous, metritic, puerperal, rheumatic, scarlatinal, syphilitic, tuberculous, urethral,* etc. **bursal s.,** bursitis. **dendritic s.,** that in which villous growths are developed within the synovial sac. **dry s.,** synovitis with but little effusion. **fungous s.,** arthritis fungosa. **localized nodular s.,** lesions of the tendon sheaths that give histological evidence of evolution from a number of smaller nodules, or from villous structures. **pigmented villonodular s.,** synovial proliferation forming brown nodular masses, probably caused by hemangiomas of synovial membrane that become traumatized, resulting in synovial hyperplasia and inflammation; it is characterized by episodic monoarticular pain and swelling, with joint locking and hemorrhagic effusions. **purulent s.,** that in which there is an effusion of pus in a synovial sac. **serous s.,** synovitis with copious nonpurulent effusion. **s. sic′ca,** dry s. **simple s.,** that in which the effusion is clear or but slightly turbid. **tendinous s.,** inflammation of a tendon sheath. **vaginal s.,** tendinous s. **vibration s.,** synovitis produced by the passage of a missile through the tissues near a joint, but without actually wounding the joint. **villonodular s.,** proliferation of synovial tissue, especially of the knee joint, composed of synovial villi and fibrous nodules infiltrated by giant cells and by macrophages containing lipids and hemosiderin.

synovium (sĭ-no′ve-um) a synovial membrane.

synphalangism (sin-fal′an-jizm) symphalangia.

synpneumonic (sin″nu-mon′ik) occurring in association with pneumonia.

synprolan (sin′pro-lan) the name applied by Zondek to the synergistic principle in the anterior pituitary which enhances the action of the gonadotropic substance ("prolan") in the urine of pregnant women. See *pituitary synergist.*

synreflexia (sin″re-flek′se-ah) the association existing between various reflexes.

syntactic (sin-tak′tik) pertaining to or affecting syntax, or the proper arrangement of words in speech.

syntaxis (sin-tak′sis) [Gr. "a putting together in order"] articulation.

syntectic (sin-tek′tik) pertaining to or characterized by syntexis.

syntenic (sin-ten′ik) pertaining or relating to synteny.

syntenosis (sin″tě-no′sis) [*syn-* + Gr. *tenōn* tendon] a hinge joint surrounded by tendons.

synteny (sin′tě-ne) the presence together on the same chromosome of two or more gene loci whether or not in such proximity that they may be subject to linkage.

synteresis (sin″ter-e′sis) [*syn-* + Gr. *tērein* to watch over] preventive treatment; prophylaxis.

synteretic (sin″ter-et′ik) prophylactic.

syntexis (sin-tek′sis) [Gr. *syntēxis* colliquation] wasting or emaciation.

synthase (sin-thās) any enzyme, especially a lyase, which catalyzes a synthesis that does not involve the breakdown of a pyrophosphate bond, as opposed to *ligase.*

synthermal (sin-ther′mal) [*syn-* + Gr. *thermē* heat] having the same temperature.

synthescope (sin′thě-skōp) [Gr. *synthesis* placing together + *skopein* to examine] an instrument for observing the visible effect of placing two liquids in contact.

synthesis (sin′thě-sis) [Gr. "a putting together, composition"] 1. the artificial building up of a chemical compound, by the union of its elements or from other suitable starting materials. 2. the process of bringing back into consciousness activities or experiences that have become split off or dissociated. Cf. *dissociation* (3), and *subconscious.* **s. of continuity,** union of the edges of a wound or the ends of a fractured bone. **enzymatic s.,** synthesis brought about by enzymatic action. **inducible enzyme s.,** the formation of an enzyme within a cell only in the presence of its substrate or of a substance closely related to the substrate structurally. Called also *enzymatic adaptation.* **morphologic s.,** histogenesis.

synthesize (sin″thě-sīz′) to produce by means of synthesis.

synthetase (sin′thě-tās) ligase. **amide s.,** any ligase that catalyzes the linking together of an acid and an ammonia group, as in the formation of L-asparagine and L-glutamine. **glycogen s.,** an enzyme which acts during glycogen synthesis to catalyze the transfer of glucose residues in activated state from UDP-glucose to the nonreducing ends of a glycogen primer. **tryptophan s.,** the enzyme that catalyzes the union of indole and serine to form tryptophan.

synthetic (sin-thet′ik) [L. *syntheticus;* Gr. *synthetikos*] 1. pertaining to, of the nature of, or participating in synthesis. 2. produced by synthesis; artificial.

synthetism (sin′thě-tizm) [Gr. *synthetos* put together] the complete treatment of a fracture.

synthorax (sin-tho′raks) thoracopagus.

Synthroid (sin′throid) trademark for a preparation of levothyroxine sodium.

Syntocinon (sin-to′sĭ-non) trademark for a solution of synthetic oxytocin.

syntone (sin′tōn) a person of syntonic type.

syntonic (sin-ton′ik) [*syn-* + Gr. *tonos* tension] a term applied by Bleuler to the stable integrated type of personality which responds normally to the environment, as contrasted with the schizoid type.

syntonin (sin′to-nin) an acid metaprotein which precipitates from a gastric digestion mixture at or near the neutral point.

syntopie, syntopy (sin′to-pe) [*syn-* + Gr. *topos* place] the position of an organ in relation to neighboring organs.

syntripsis (sin-trip′sis) [*syn-* + Gr. *tribein* to rub] the comminution or crushing of a bone; comminuted fracture.

Syntropan (sin′tro-pan) trademark for a preparation of amprotropine phosphate.

syntrophism (sin′trōf-izm) [*syn-* + Gr. *trophē* nourishment] stimulation of the growth of a microorganism resulting from admixture with or nearness of another strain.

syntrophoblast (sin-trof′o-blast) syncytiotrophoblast.

syntrophus (sin′tro-fus) [Gr. *syntrophos* congenital] any congenital or inherited disease.

syntropic (sin-trop′ik) [*syn-* + Gr. *trepein* to turn] 1. turning or pointing in the same direction, as the ribs or the vertebral spines. 2. denoting the correlation of several factors, as the relation of one disease to the development or incidence of another disease. 3. Meyer's term for a well-balanced personality with a normal social outlook.

syntropy (sin′tro-pe) [syn- + Gr. *tropos* a turning]   the state of being syntropic.

synulosis (sin″u-lo′sis) [Gr. *synoulōsis*]   complete cicatrization.

synulotic (sin″u-lot′ik) [Gr. *synoulōtikos*]   1. promoting cicatrization.   2. an agent that promotes cicatrization.

Synura (sin-u′rah)   a genus of flagellate protozoa of the order Chrysomonadina, family Syncryptidae, which sometimes impart an unpleasant taste to drinking water.

synxenic (sin-zen′ik) [syn- + Gr. *xenos* a guest-friend, stranger]   associated with a known number of microbic species; applied to laboratory animals whose microfauna and microflora are known (gnotobiotes).

Syphacia (si-fa′se-ah)   a nematode parasite found in the intestines of rodents.   **S. obvela′ta,** a common cecal parasite of laboratory rats that has been reported occasionally in infants.

syphilid (sif′ĭ-lid)   a general term for the skin lesions of secondary syphilis, appearing (usually between six weeks and two years after infection) in a series of crops lasting a few days to a few months, and becoming progressively more severe and conspicuous, more persistent, and less widely generalized, in successive outbreaks. The serologic test for syphilis (STS) is invariably positive. Mucous membrane lesions in this stage are typically teeming with *Treponema pallidum* and are clinically the most contagious lesions of the disease. Syphilids are variously qualified by their shape (annular s.), site (plantar s.), and so on.   **macular s.,** syphilitic roseola.

syphilide (sif′ĭ-lĭd), pl. *syphil′ides* [Fr.]   syphilid.

syphiliphobia (sif″ĭ-lĭ-fo′be-ah)   syphilophobia.

syphilis (sif′ĭ-lis) [*Syphilus*, the name of a shepherd infected with the disease in the poem of Fracastorius (1530), in which the term first appears. Derived perhaps from Gr. *syn* together + *philein* to love, or from Gr. *siphlos* crippled, maimed]   a contagious venereal disease leading to many structural and cutaneous lesions, caused by the spirochete *Treponema pallidum* and transmitted by direct intimate contact or in utero. Its primary local seat is a hard or true chancre, whence it extends by means of the lymphatics to the skin, mucosa, and to nearly all the tissues of the body, even to the bones and periosteum. Syphilis is divided into primary, secondary, and tertiary stages or into early and late stages (see below). Called also *lues* and *venereal s.,* and formerly called *pox.* Cf. *nonvenereal s.*   **cerebrospinal s.,** Erb's spastic paraplegia.   **congenital s.,** syphilis acquired in utero, and manifested variously by any of several characteristic malformations of the teeth or bones known as stigmata and by active mucocutaneous syphilis at the time of birth or shortly afterward, ocular changes, such as interstitial keratitis, or by neurologic changes, such as deafness.   **s. d'emblée** (dawm-bla′), syphilis which develops without the formation of a chancre, or primary sore, as from blood transfusion.   **early s.,** the stage comprising primary, secondary, and early latent syphilis.   **early latent s.,** the stage following the primary stage (or *primary s.*) encompassing the first two years after infection, during which no signs or symptoms are present but relapse of the mucocutaneous lesion may occur.   **endemic s.,** nonvenereal s.   **equine s.,** dourine.   **s. heredita′ria tar′da,** congenital syphilis that manifests itself some time after birth.   **horse s.,** dourine.   **late s.,** the stage comprising late latent and tertiary syphilis.   **late latent s.,** the stage beginning two years after infection in the untreated patient, during which there is serologic or historical evidence of syphilis but no other signs or symptoms are detectable; it may last for many decades.   **latent s.,** syphilis manifested solely by serologic or historical evidence; see *early latent s.* and *late latent s.*   **meningovascular s.,** a form of neurosyphilis in which arteritis results in arterial thrombosis in the leptomeninges. It may involve the cranial nerves and nerve roots, and give rise to various neurological symptoms, as in Erb's spastic paraplegia (q.v.).   **nonvenereal s.,** a chronic treponemal infection that mainly affects children and occurs in many parts of the world, especially arid areas, including the Near East, Southeast Asia, Bechuanaland, Southern Rhodesia, Gambia, and Eastern Europe, especially Bosnia in Yugoslavia. Caused by an organism indistinguishable morphologically from *Treponema pallidum,* it is transmitted by direct nonsexual body contact and indirectly by the common use of table and drinking utensils. The first lesions are usually oral mucous patches; subsequent lesions are concentrated in the axillae, inguinal region, and rectum. A latent period usually follows the first stages, with the development of destructive lesions of the skin and bones appearing as late manifestations. It is called also *bejel, dichuchwa, njovera, frenga, siti,* and *endemic s.*   **primary s.,** syphilis in its first stage: the primary lesion (*chancre*) usually appears ten to forty days after infection, and is infectious and painless; the nearby lymph nodes become hard and swollen (satellite bubo), are painless, do not ulcerate, and slowly return to their normal condition. The spirochete can invariably be demonstrated by darkfield microscopy. The chancre heals spontaneously without leaving a scar.   **quaternary s.** (*obs.*), parasyphilis.   **rabbit s.,** a naturally occurring disease in rabbits caused by *Treponema cuniculi.*   **secondary s.,** syphilis in the second of its three stages: it begins after six weeks, usually within three months, and is attended with fever, copper-hued and multiform skin eruptions (see *syphilid*), iritis, alopecia, mucous patches, and severe pains in

the head, joints, and periosteum.   **tertiary s.,** late generalized syphilis, characterized by involvement of numerous organs and tissues, including the skin, bones, joints, the cardiovascular system, and the central nervous system (neurosyphilis). See *tabes dorsalis.*   **venereal s.,** syphilis.

syphilitic (sif″ĭ-lit′ik) [L. *syphiliticus*]   affected with, caused by, or pertaining to syphilis.

syphiloma (sif″ĭ-lo′mah)   a tumor of syphilitic origin; a gumma.

syphilomania (sif″ĭ-lo-ma′ne-ah) [*syphilis* + Gr. *mania* madness]   syphilophobia.

syphilophobia (sif″ĭ-lo-fo′be-ah) [*syphilis* + Gr. *phobein* to be affrighted by]   1. morbid fear of syphilis.   2. the delusion of being infected with syphilis.

syphilophobic (sif″ĭ-lo-fo′bik)   pertaining to or characterized by syphilophobia.

syphilophyma (sif″ĭ-lo-fi′mah) [*syphilis* + Gr. *phyma* growth]   any syphilitic growth or excrescence.

syphilopsychosis (sif″ĭ-lo-si-ko′sis)   any syphilitic mental disease.

syphilosis (sif″ĭ-lo′sis)   generalized syphilitic disease.

syphilous (sif′ĭ-lus)   syphilitic.

syphitoxin (sif″ĭ-tok′sin) [*syphilitis* + *toxin*]   an antisyphilitic serum.

Syr.   abbreviation for L. *syrupus*, syrup.

syrigmophonia (sir″ig-mo-fo′ne-ah) [Gr. *syrigmos* a shrill piping sound + *phōnē* voice + *-ia*]   a high, whistling sound of the voice.

syrigmus (sĭ-rig′mus) [Gr. *syrigmos* a shrill piping sound]   a ringing in the ears.

syringe (sĭ-rinj′, sir′inj) [L. *syrinxe*; Gr. *syrinx*]   an instrument for injecting liquids into or withdrawing them from any vessel or cavity.   **air s.,** chip s.   **Anel's s.,** a delicate syringe for the treatment of the lacrimal passages.   **chip s.,** a small, fine-nozzled syringe used to direct a current of air into a tooth cavity being excavated, to remove the small fragments detached from the tooth or to dry the cavity; called also *air s.*   **dental s.,** a small syringe into which is fitted a hermetically sealed cartridge which contains an anesthetic solution; used in operative dentistry.   **fountain s.,** an apparatus which injects a liquid by the action of gravity.   **hypodermic s.,** a syringe, usually of small caliber, by means of which drugs in solution or other liquids are injected through a hollow needle of small bore into the subcutaneous tissues.   **Luer's s., Luer-Lok s.,** a glass syringe for intravenous and hypodermic use, with a metallic tip and locking device to hold the needle firmly in place.   **Neisser's s.,** a urethral syringe for use in gonorrhea.   **probe s.,** a syringe whose point may be used also as a probe; used mostly in treating the lacrimal passages.

syringectomy (sir″in-jek′to-me) [*syringo-* + Gr. *ektomē* excision]   excision of the walls of a fistula.

syringin (sĭ-rin′jin)   chemical name: 4-(3-hydroxypropenyl)-2,6-dimethoxyphenyl D-glucoside. A white, crystalline glycoside, C_{17}-$H_{24}O_9$, soluble in hot water and in hot alcohol, from the bark of lilac, *Syringa vulgaris;* formerly used as an antiperiodic. Called also *ligustrin* and *lilacin.*

syringitis (sir″in-ji′tis)   inflammation of the auditory tube.

syringo- (sĭ-ring′go) [Gr. *syrinx* pipe, tube, fistula]   a combining form denoting relationship to a tube or a fistula.

syringoadenoma (sĭ-ring″go-ad″ĕ-no′mah)   syringocystadenoma.

syringobulbia (sĭ-ring″go-bul′be-ah) [*syringo-* + Gr. *bolbos* bulb + *-ia*]   the presence of cavities in the medulla oblongata; pontobulbia.

syringocarcinoma (sĭ-ring″go-kar″sĭ-no′mah)   carcinoma of a sweat gland.

syringocele (sĭ-ring′go-sēl)   a cavity-containing herniation of the spinal cord through the bony defect in spina bifida.

syringocoele (sĭ-ring′go-sēl) [*syringo-* + Gr. *koilia* hollow]   the central canal of the spinal cord (canalis centralis medullae spinalis [NA]).

syringocystadenoma (sĭ-ring″go-sis″tad-ĕ-no′mah) [*syringo-* + *cystadenoma*]   adenoma of the sweat glands; a skin disease marked by an eruption of small, hard papules; called also *hidradenoma* and *adenoma hidradenoides.*   **s. papillif′erum,** hamartoma of an apocrine sweat gland, the lesion being a circumscribed, firm, rose-red papule usually on the shoulder, axilla, genitals, inguinal region, or scalp.

syringocystoma (sĭ-ring″go-sis-to′mah) [*syringo-* + Gr. *kystis* cyst + *-oma*]   a cystic tumor of the sweat glands.

syringoencephalia (sĭ-ring″go-en″sĕ-fa′le-ah) [*syringo-* + Gr. *enkephalos* brain + *-ia*]   the formation of abnormal cavities in the brain substance.

syringoencephalomyelia (sĭ-ring″go-en-sef″ah-lo-mi-e′le-ah) [*syringo-* + Gr. *enkephalos* brain + *myelos* marrow + *-ia*]   the existence of cavities in the substance of the brain and spinal cord.

syringoid (sĭ-ring′goid) [L. *syringoides*, from Gr. *syrinx* pipe + *eidos* form]   resembling a pipe or tube; fistulous.

syringoma (sir″ing-go′mah) adenoma of sweat glands.

syringomeningocele (sĭ-ring″go-mĕ-nin′go-sēl) [*syringo-* + Gr. *mēninx* membrane + *kēlē* tumor] a meningocele resembling a syringomyelocele.

syringomyelia (sĭ-ring″go-mi-e′le-ah) [*syringo-* + Gr. *myelos* marrow + *-ia*] a condition marked by abnormal cavities filled with liquid in the substance of the spinal cord. **traumatic s.,** Kienböck's disease, def. 2.

syringomyelitis (sĭ-ring″go-mi″ĕ-li′tis) inflammation of the spinal cord, with the formation of cavities in its substance.

syringomyelocele (sĭ-ring″go-mi″ĕ-lo-sēl″) [*syringo-* + Gr. *myelos* marrow + *kēlē* tumor] hernial protrusion of the spinal cord through the bony defect in spina bifida, the mass containing a cavity connected with the central canal of the spinal cord.

syringomyelus (sĭ-ring″go-mi′ĕ-lus) dilatation of the central canal of the spinal cord, the gray matter being converted into connective tissue.

syringopontia (sĭ-ring″go-pon′she-ah) a condition in which cavities exist in the pons.

Syringospora (si″ring-gos′po-rah) former name of a genus of fungi now called *Candida.*

syringotome (sĭ-ring′go-tōm) a knife for cutting a fistula.

syringotomy (sir″in-got′o-me) [*syringo-* + Gr. *tomē* a cutting] incision of a fistula, particularly an anal fistula.

syrinx (sir′inks) [Gr. "a pipe"] 1. a tube or pipe; also a fistula. 2. the lower or posterior part of the trachea of birds in which vocal sounds are produced.

syrosingopine (si″ro-sing′go-pīn) chemical name: methyl carbethoxysyringoyl reserpate. A crystalline substance, $C_{35}H_{42}N_2O_{11}$, used as an antihypertensive agent.

Syrphidae (sir′phĭ-de) a family of flies, the hover flies, of the order Diptera, including the genera *Eristalis* and *Helophilus.*

syrup (sir′up) [L. *syrupus;* Arabic *sharāb*] a concentrated solution of a sugar, such as sucrose, in water or other aqueous liquid, sometimes with some medicinal substance added. The official preparation [NF] is a solution of sucrose in purified water, and is used as a flavored vehicle in pharmaceutical preparations. **acacia s.** [NF], a preparation of powdered acacia, sodium benzoate, vanilla tincture, sucrose, and water, used as a vehicle for drugs. **amantadine hydrochloride s.** [USP], a preparation containing 95 to 105 per cent of the labeled amount of amantadine hydrochloride; used as an antiviral agent for the prophylaxis of Asian (A_2) influenza. **aminocaproic acid s.** [USP], a preparation containing, in 5 ml., 1.25 gm. of aminocaproic acid; used as a hemostatic. **bromides s.,** a preparation containing potassium, sodium, ammonium, calcium, and lithium bromides, formerly used as a central nervous system depressant. **cacao s.,** cocoa s. **cherry s.,** a mixture of cherry juice, sucrose, alcohol, and purified water, used as a flavored vehicle for drugs. **chloral hydrate s.** [USP], a syrup containing 95 to 110 per cent chloral hydrate; used as a hypnotic and sedative. **chlorpheniramine maleate s.,** [USP], a preparation containing 36–44 mg. of chlorpheniramine maleate in each 100 ml., in a hydroalcoholic vehicle; used as an antihistaminic. Formerly called *chlorpheniramine maleate elixir.* **chlorpromazine hydrochloride s.** [USP], a liquid preparation containing between 190 and 210 mg. of chlorpromazine hydrochloride per 100 ml.; used as an antiemetic and tranquilizer. **citric acid s.,** a preparation of lemon tincture, hydrous citric acid, and purified water, in syrup, used as a flavored vehicle for drugs. **cocoa s.** [NF], a preparation of cocoa, sucrose, liquid glucose, glycerin, sodium chloride, vanillin, sodium benzoate, and purified water; used as a flavored vehicle for drugs. Called also *cacao s.* **cyprohetadine hydrochloride s.** [USP], a preparation containing 90 to 110 per cent of the labeled amount of cyprohetadine hydrochloride; used as an antihistaminic for relief of symptoms associated with allergy and as an antipruritic for relief of itching associated with skin disorders. **demethylchlortetracycline s.,** demeclocycline oral suspension. **dexchlorpheniramine maleate s.** [USP], a preparation containing 90 to 110 per cent of the labeled amount of dexchlorpheniramine maleate; used as an antihistaminic. **dextromethorphan hydrobromide s.** [USP], a preparation containing 95–105 per cent of the labeled amount of dextromethorphan hydrobromide; used as an antitussive. **dicyclomine hydrochloride s.** [USP], a preparation containing 95 to 105 per cent of the labeled amount of dicyclomine hydrochloride; used as an antispasmodic anticholinergic. **dihydrocodeinone bitartrate s.,** hydrocodone bitartrate s. **dimenhydrinate s.** [USP], a liquid preparation of dimenhydrinate, containing between 295 and 330 mg. of dimenhydrinate in each 100 ml.; used as an antiemetic. **dimethindene maleate s.,** a preparation containing 95 to 105 per cent of the labeled amount of dimethindene maleate; used as an antihistaminic. **dioctyl sodium sulfosuccinate s.,** docusate sodium s. **docusate sodium s.** [USP], a preparation containing 95 to 105 per cent of the labeled amount of dioctyl sodium sulfosuccinate; used as a fecal matter softener. Called also *dioctyl sodium sulfosuccinate s.* **doxylamine succinate s.** [USP], a preparation containing 90–110 per cent of the labeled amount of doxylamine succinate; used as an antihistaminic. **ephedrine sulfate s.** [USP], a preparation containing 360–440 mg. of ephedrine sulfate in each 100 ml.; used as a bronchodilator. **eriodictyon s., aromatic** [NF], a solution of eriodictyon fluidextract, potassium hydroxide solution, compound cardamom tincture, sassafras oil, lemon oil, clove oil, alcohol, sucrose, and magnesium carbonate, in purified water; used as a vehicle for drugs. **ferrous iodide s.,** a solution of iron, iodine, hypophosphorous acid, and sucrose, in purified water, used as a hematinic. **ferrous sulfate s.** [USP], a mixture of ferrous sulfate, hydrous citric acid, peppermint spirit, sucrose, and purified water, each 100 ml. of which contains 3.75–4.25 gm. of ferrous sulfate; used as an iron supplement. **glyceryl guaiacolate s.,** quaifenesin s. **glycyrrhiza s.,** a mixture of glycyrrhiza fluidextract, fennel and anise oil, and syrup, used as a flavored vehicle in compounding prescriptions. **guaifenesin s.** [USP], a preparation containing 95–105 per cent of the labeled amount of guaifenesin; used as an expectorant. Called also *glyceryl guaiacolate s.* **hydriodic acid s.,** a solution of diluted hydriodic acid and dextrose in purified water, each 100 ml. of which contains 1.3–1.5 gm. of HI; used as an expectorant. **hydrocodone bitartrate s.,** a preparation of hydrocodon bitartrate and cherry syrup in purified water, containing 90 to 110 per cent of hydrocodone bitartrate; used as an antitussive. **hydroxyzine hydrochloride s.** [USP], a preparation containing 90 to 110 per cent of the labeled amount of hydroxyzine hydrochloride; used as a tranquilizer and antihistamine. **ipecac s.** [USP], a mixture of ipecac fluidextract, glycerin, and syrup, used as an emetic. **isoniazid s.** [USP], a preparation, each 100 ml. of which contains 0.93 to 1.10 gm. of isoniazid; used as a tuberculostatic. **licorice s.,** glycyrrhiza s. **medicated s.,** one to which a medicinal substance has been added. **meperidine hydrochloride s.** [NF], a preparation containing 95 to 105 per cent of the labeled amount of meperidine hydrochloride; used as a narcotic analgesic. **methapyrilene fumarate s.** [USP], a preparation containing 90–110 per cent of the labeled amount of methapyrilene fumarate; used as an antihistaminic in the treatment of allergic manifestations, nausea and vomiting of pregnancy, and insomnia. **methdilazine hydrochloride s.** [USP], a preparation containing 93 to 107 per cent of the labeled amount of methdilazine hydrochloride; used as an antipruritic. **orange s.** [NF], a preparation of sweet orange peel tincture, citric acid, talc, and sucrose, in purified water, used as a flavored vehicle for pharmaceuticals. **phenindamine tartrate s.,** a syrup containing between 190 and 220 mg. of phenindamine tartrate in each 100 ml.; used as an antihistaminic. **piperazine citrate s.** [USP], a syrup containing between 10 and 12 gm. of anhydrous piperazine citrate in each 100 ml.; used as an anthelmintic. **prochlorperazine edisylate s.,** [USP], a syrup containing in each 100 ml. an amount of prochlorperazine edisylate equivalent to 95 to 105 mg. of prochlorperazine; used as an antiemetic and tranquilizer. **promazine hydrochloride s.** [USP], a preparation containing 95 to 110 per cent of the labeled amount of promazine hydrochloride; used mainly as an antipsychotic agent. **promethazine hydrochloride s.** [USP], a syrup containing in each 100 ml. between 112 and 138 mg. of promethazine hydrochloride; used as an antihistaminic. **pseudoephedrine hydrochloride s.** [USP], a preparation containing 90 to 110 per cent of the labeled amount of $C_{10}H_{15}NO·HCl$; used as a nasal decongestant and bronchodilator. **pyridostigmine bromide s.** [USP], a preparation, each 100 ml. of which contains 1.08 to 1.32 gm. of pyridostigmine bromide; used as an anticholinergic in the treatment of myasthenia gravis. **raspberry s.,** a syrup consisting of raspberry juice, sucrose, and alcohol, in purified water, used as a flavored vehicle for drugs. **sarsaparilla s., compound,** a solution of sarsaparilla and glycyrrhiza fluidextracts, sassafras and anise oils, methyl salicylate, alcohol, and syrup; used as a vehicle for drugs. **senna s.** [USP], a solution of senna fluidextract, coriander oil, sucrose, and purified water, used as a cathartic. **simple s.,** one compounded from purified water and sucrose. **s. of tolu,** tolu balsam s. **tolu balsam s.** [NF], a mixture of tolu balsam tincture, magnesium carbonate, sucrose, and purified water, used as a flavored vehicle for drugs. **triamcinolone diacetate s.** [USP], a preparation containing 90 to 110 per cent of the labeled amount of triamcinolone diacetate; used as an anti-inflammatory glucocorticoid. **trifluoperazine hydrochloride s.** [USP], a preparation containing trifluoperazine hydrochloride equivalent to 93–107 per cent of the labeled amount of trifluoperazine; used as an antipsychotic agent. **trimeprazine tartrate s.** [NF], a preparation containing trimeprazine tartrate equivalent to 90 to 110 per cent of the labeled amount of trimeprazine; used as an antipruritic. **triprolidine hydrochloride s.** [USP], a preparation containing 90–110 per cent of the labeled amount of triprolidine hydrochloride; used as an antihistaminic in the treatment of various allergic conditions and their manifestations. **white pine s., compound,** a solution containing coarsely powdered white pine, wild cherry, aralia, poplar bud, sanguinaria, and sassafras, combined with amaranth solution, chloroform, sucrose, glycerin, alcohol, and water; used as an antitussive and as a vehicle for other drugs. **white pine s., compound, with codeine,** compound white pine syrup combined with codeine phosphate dissolved in purified water, used as an antitussive. **wild cherry s.,** a mixture of a percolate of wild cherry, glycerin, sucrose, alcohol, and water; used as a flavored vehicle. **Yerba santa s., aromatic,** eriodictyon s., aromatic.

syrupus (sir′up-us) [L.] syrup. **s. auran′tii,** orange syrup. **s. cera′si,** cherry syrup. **s. cor′rigens,** aromatic eriodictyon syrup. **s. pi′ni al′bae compos′itus,** compound white pine syrup. **s. pi′ni al′bae compos′itus cum co′deina,** compound white pine syrup with codeine. **s. ru′bi ida′ei,** raspberry syrup. **s. sarsaparil′lae compos′itus,** compound sarsaparilla syrup.

syssarcosic (sis″sar-ko′sik) syssarcotic.

syssarcosis (sis″sar-ko′sis) [Gr. *syn* together + *sarkōsis* fleshy growth] the union or connection of bones by means of muscle, as the connection between the hyoid bone and the lower jaw, the scapula, and the breast bone.

syssarcotic (sis″sar-kot′ik) pertaining to or of the nature of a syssarcosis.

syssomus (sis-so′mus) [Gr. *syn* with + *sōma* body] a double monster with two heads and with the bodies united.

systaltic (sis-tal′tik) [Gr. *systaltikos* drawing together] alternately contracting and expanding; pulsating.

systatic (sis-tat′ik) affecting several of the sensory faculties at the same time.

system (sis′tem) [Gr. *systēma* a complex or organized whole] 1. a set or series of interconnected or interdependent parts or entities (objects, organs, or organisms) that function together in a common purpose or produce results impossible of achievement by one of them acting or operating alone. 2. a school or method of practice based on a specific set of principles, as the eclectic or galenic school. **absorbent s.,** lymphatic s. **accessory portal s. of Sappey,** small compensatory blood vessels formed around the liver and gallbladder in cases of cirrhosis of the liver. **adipose s.,** the fatty tissue of the body, considered collectively. **alimentary s.,** the organs concerned with the ingestion, digestion, and absorption of food or nutritional elements; see *apparatus digestorius.* **association s.,** the tracts of fibers in the brain by means of which perceptions are associated and thought rendered possible. **autonomic nervous s.,** the portion of the nervous system concerned with regulation of the activity of cardiac muscle, smooth muscle, and glands. See *systema nervosum autonomicum* [NA], and see Plate XLVIII. **biologic amplification s.,** a system of elements that augment the immune response, including the complement components and the kallikrein system. **biological s.,** a system composed of living material; such systems range from a collection of separate molecules to an assemblage of separate organisms. **blood group s.,** see *blood group.* **blood-vascular s.,** the blood vessels of the body. **brain cooling s.,** thermoregulated equipment for sensing and controlling brain temperature in neurophysiological and neuropsychological applications. **brunonian s.,** brunonianism. **buffer s.,** see *buffer.* **bulbospiral s.,** muscle bundles in the heart which arise in and are attached to the conus arteriosus and the root of the aorta. **cardiovascular s.,** the heart and blood vessels, by which blood is pumped and circulated through the body. **case s.,** a method of teaching based on the logical analysis of, and deductions formed from, reported cases of disease. **centimeter-gram-second s.,** see *C.G.S.* **central nervous s.,** that portion of the nervous system consisting of the brain and spinal cord (systema nervosum centrale [NA]). Abbreviated CNS. **centrencephalic s.,** the system of neurons located in the central core of the upper brain stem from the thalamus down to the medulla oblongata, and connecting the two hemispheres of the brain. **cerebrospinal s.,** central nervous s. **chemoreceptor s.,** the system of body structures, principally the carotid body, the aortic pulmonary bodies, and the glomus jugulare, that respond to variations in oxygen tension and carbon dioxide tension of the blood and may play a role in the regulation of respiration. **chromaffin s.,** the chromaffin cells of the body, which characteristically stain strongly with chromium salts, considered collectively; they occur along the sympathetic nerves, in the adrenal, carotid, and coccygeal glands, and in various other organs. **circulatory s.,** the channels through which the nutrient fluids of the body circulate; often restricted to the vessels conveying blood. **complement s.,** see *complement.* **conduction s., conductive s. (of the heart),** the system comprising the sinoatrial node, the atrioventricular node, the atrioventricular bundle, and the Purkinje fibers. **Conolly's s.,** a system of nonrestraint for treating the mentally and emotionally disturbed. **dentinal s.,** all the tubules radiating from a single pulp cavity. **dermal s., dermoid s.,** the skin and its appendages, including both the hair and the nails (integumentum commune [NA]). **digestive s.,** the organs associated with the ingestion, digestion, and absorption of food; see *apparatus digestorius* [NA]. **dioptric s.,** a system of lenses or of different media for refracting light. **disperse s., dispersion s.,** a colloid solution. **dosimetric s.,** a regular and determinate system of administration of a therapeutic agent. **ecological s.,** see *ecosystem.* **electron transmitter s.,** a system of enzymes localized within the substance of the mitochondrion in the mitochondrial membranes, which transfers electrons from foodstuff molecules to oxygen. **endocrine s.,** the system of glands and other structures that

elaborate internal secretions (hormones) which are released directly into the circulatory system and which influence metabolism and other body processes. Organs having endocrine function include the pituitary, thyroid, parathyroid, and adrenal glands, the pineal body, the gonads, the pancreas, and the paraganglia. The thymus is no longer considered to perform an endocrine function. See Plate accompanying *gland.* **endothelial s.,** see *reticuloendothelial s.* **exteroceptive nervous s.,** that portion of the afferent elements of the somatic nervous system which is sensitive to stimuli originating outside the body. **exterofective s.,** a little used term referring to the central nervous system, exclusive of the autonomic portion, as viewed in its function of maintaining homeostasis. Cf. *interofective s.* **extracorticospinal s.,** extrapyramidal tract. **extrapyramidal s.,** a functional, rather than anatomical, unit comprising the nuclei and fibers (excluding those of the pyramidal tract) involved in motor activities; they control and coordinate especially the postural, static, supporting, and locomotor mechanisms. It includes the corpus striatum, subthalamic nucleus, substantia nigra, and the red nucleus, along with their interconnections with the reticular formation, cerebellum, and cerebrum; some authorities include the cerebellum and the vestibular nuclei. Called also *extracorticospinal s.* or *tract* and *extrapyramidal tract.* **genitourinary s.,** the organs of reproduction, together with the organs concerned in the production and excretion of urine (apparatus urogenitalis or systema urogenitale [NA]). See Plate L. **glandular s.,** the glandular tissue of the body considered collectively. **Grancher s.,** the early removal of young children from contact with patients with tuberculosis, to save them from infection. **H-2 histocompatibility s.,** in the mouse, the major histocompatibility complex, where Ir (immune response) genes in addition to histocompatibility genes are located. Thus immune responsiveness as well as cell-surface antigens are determined by genes governed from this region. **haversian s.,** a haversian canal and its concentrically arranged lamellae, constituting the basic unit of structure of compact bone; see *osteon.* **hematopoietic s.,** the tissues concerned in production of the blood, including bone marrow and lymphatic tissue. **heterogeneous s.,** a system or structure made up of mechanically separable parts, as an emulsion. **homogeneous s.,** a system or structure made up of parts which cannot be mechanically separated, as a solution. **hormonopoietic s.,** endocrine s. **hypophyseoportal s.,** the venules connecting the capillaries (gomitoli) in the median eminence of the hypothalamus with the sinusoidal capillaries of the anterior lobe of the pituitary gland (hypophysis); called also *pituitary portal s.* **International S. of Units,** see *SI unit,* under *unit.* **interoceptive nervous s.,** that system which transmits afferent impulses from viscera by fibers which run centrally either in autonomic or somatic nerves. **interofective s.,** a seldom used term referring to the autonomic nervous system viewed in its role in maintaining homeostasis from within. Cf. *exterofective s.* **interrenal s.,** cortex glandulae suprarenalis. **interstitial s.,** see under *lamella.* **involuntary nervous s.,** Gaskill's name for the autonomic nervous system (systema nervosum autonomicum [NA]). **keratinizing s.,** the cells composing the bulk of the epithelium of the epidermis, which are of ectodermal origin and undergo keratinization and form the dead superficial layers of the skin; called also *malpighian s.* **kinesiodic s.,** a rarely used term for the efferent elements of the spinal cord, concerned in the transmission of motor impulses. **labyrinthine s.,** those parts of the vestibulocochlear organ concerned with the maintenance of equilibrium. **limbic s.,** a term loosely applied to a group of brain structures common to all mammals (including the hippocampus and dentate gyrus with their archicortex, the cingulate gyrus and septal areas, and the amygdala), associated with olfaction but of greater importance in other activities, such as autonomic functions and certain aspects of emotion and behavior; see also *rhinencephalon.* **lymphatic s.,** the lymphatic vessels and the lymphoid tissue, considered collectively (systema lymphaticum [NA]). **lymphoid s.,** the lymphoid tissue of the body, collectively; it consists of (a) a central component, including the bone marrow, thymus, and an unidentified portion called bursal equivalent tissue (see under *tissue*), and (b) a peripheral component of lymph nodes, spleen, and gut-associated lymphoid tissue (tonsils, Peyer's patches). **lymphoreticular s.,** the system consisting of the lymphoid tissues and the tissues of the reticuloendothelial system. **macrophage s.,** reticuloendothelial s. **malpighian s.,** keratinizing s. **masticatory s.,** the organs and structures which function primarily in mastication, including the jaws, the teeth with their supporting structures, the temporomandibular articulation, mandibular musculature, tongue, lips, cheeks, and oral mucosa. **melanocyte s.,** pigmentary s. **meter-kilogram-second s.,** see *M.K.S.* **metric s.,** a decimal system of weights and measures based on the meter. See also *SI unit,* under *unit;* see table accompanying *metric,* and see *Tables of Weights and Measures,* under *weight.* **mononuclear phagocyte s.,** the group of highly phagocytic cells considered to have a common origin from stem cells of the bone marrow and developing from promonocytes, to monocytes, to tissue macrophages, including those of connective tissue, the liver (Kupffer cells), lung, spleen, lymph nodes, etc. The term has been proposed to replace *reticulo-*

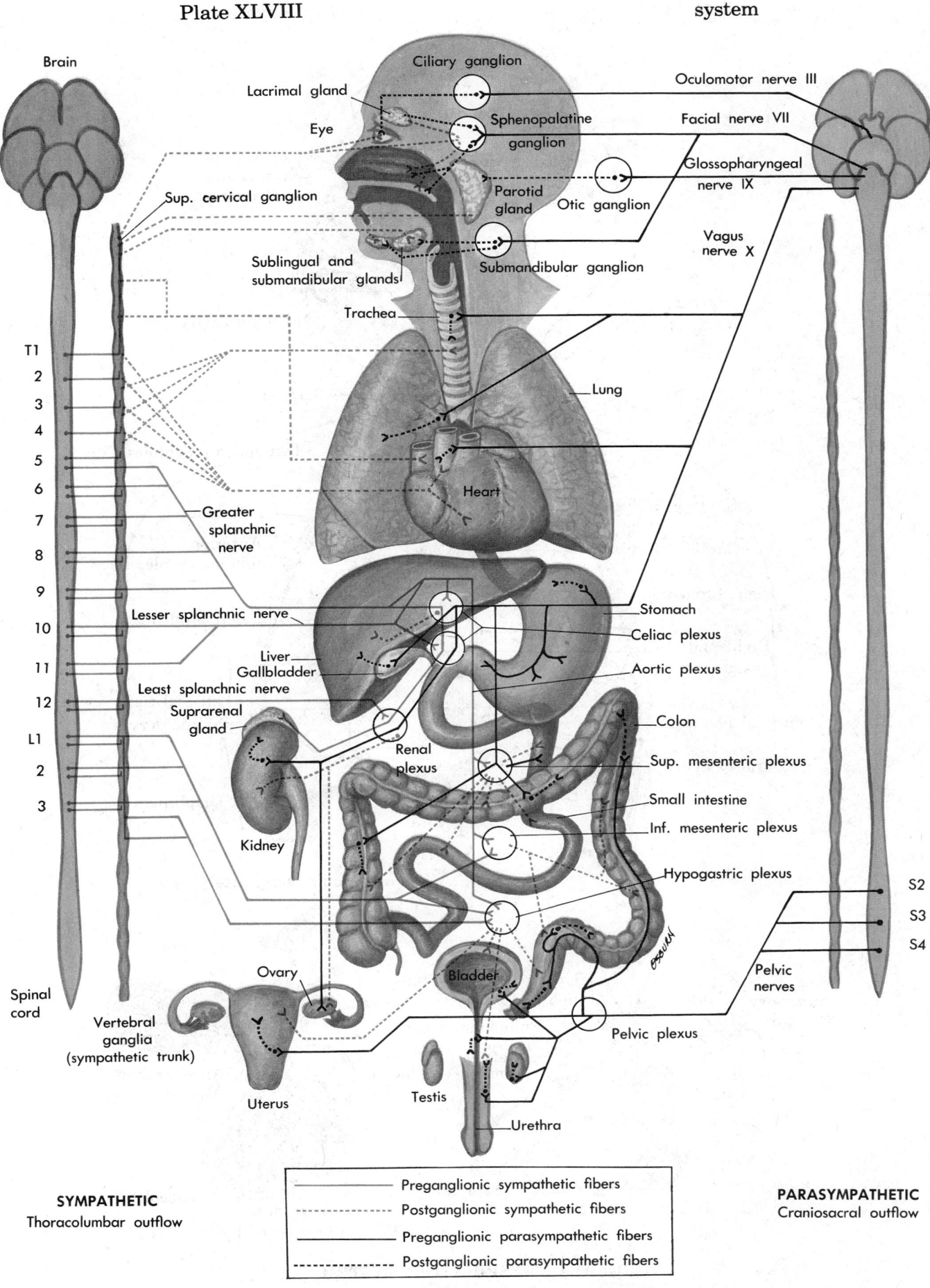

Plate XLVIII   system

Brain

Ciliary ganglion
Lacrimal gland
Eye
Sup. cervical ganglion

Oculomotor nerve III
Facial nerve VII
Sphenopalatine ganglion
Glossopharyngeal nerve IX
Parotid gland
Otic ganglion
Vagus nerve X
Sublingual and submandibular glands
Submandibular ganglion
Trachea

T1
2
3
4
5
6
7
8
9
10
11
12
L1
2
3

Lung

Heart

Greater splanchnic nerve
Lesser splanchnic nerve
Liver
Gallbladder
Least splanchnic nerve
Suprarenal gland
Renal plexus
Kidney

Stomach
Celiac plexus
Aortic plexus
Colon
Sup. mesenteric plexus
Small intestine
Inf. mesenteric plexus
Hypogastric plexus

S2
S3
S4
Pelvic nerves

Spinal cord
Vertebral ganglia (sympathetic trunk)
Ovary
Uterus
Bladder
Testis
Urethra
Pelvic plexus

SYMPATHETIC
Thoracolumbar outflow

PARASYMPATHETIC
Craniosacral outflow

Preganglionic sympathetic fibers
Postganglionic sympathetic fibers
Preganglionic parasympathetic fibers
Postganglionic parasympathetic fibers

AUTONOMIC NERVOUS SYSTEM

Plate XLIX   system

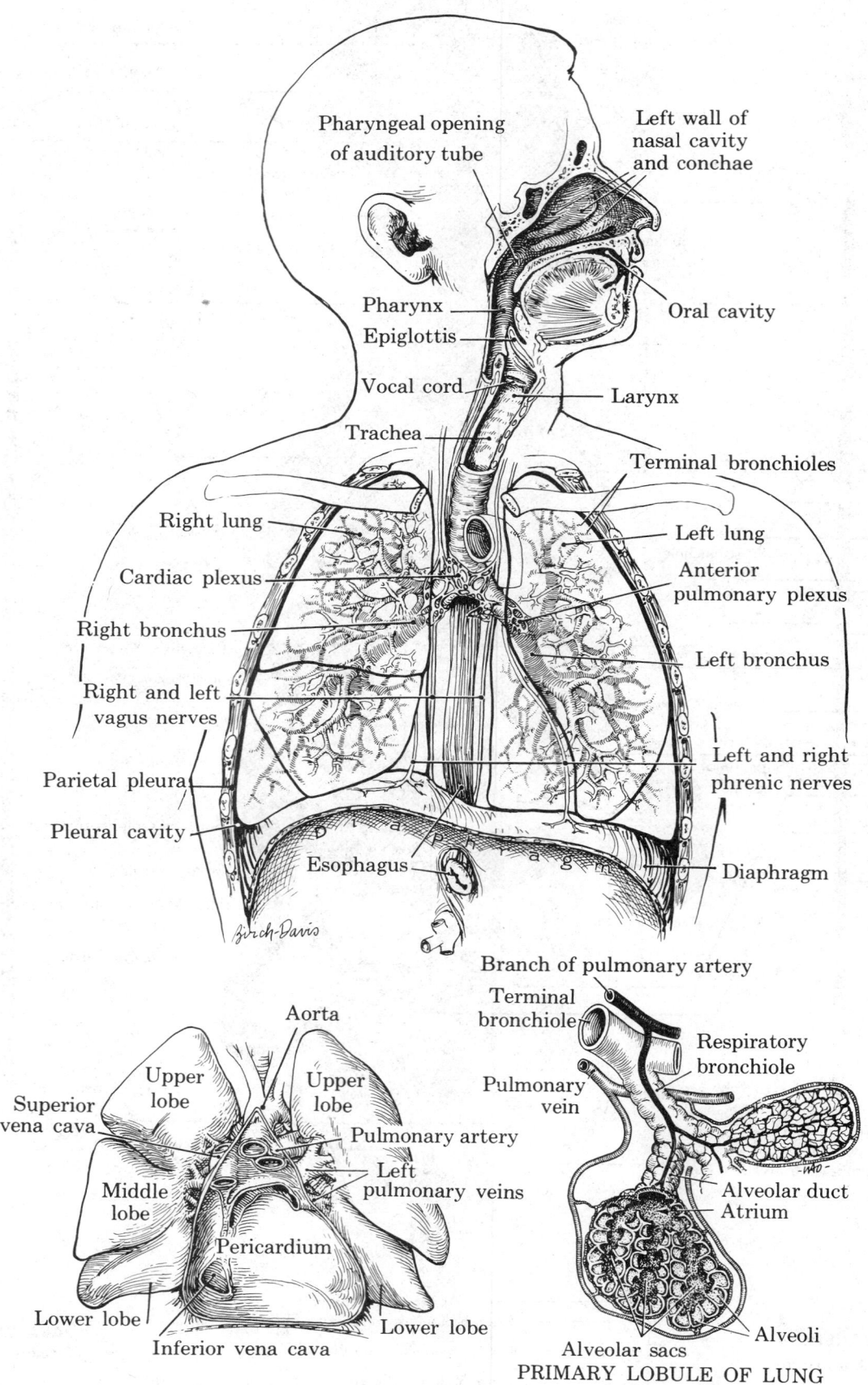

Pharyngeal opening
of auditory tube

Left wall of
nasal cavity
and conchae

Pharynx

Epiglottis

Oral cavity

Vocal cord

Larynx

Trachea

Terminal bronchioles

Right lung

Left lung

Cardiac plexus

Anterior
pulmonary plexus

Right bronchus

Left bronchus

Right and left
vagus nerves

Parietal pleura

Left and right
phrenic nerves

Pleural cavity

Esophagus

Diaphragm

Branch of pulmonary artery

Terminal
bronchiole

Aorta

Respiratory
bronchiole

Upper
lobe

Upper
lobe

Pulmonary
vein

Superior
vena cava

Pulmonary artery

Left
pulmonary veins

Middle
lobe

Alveolar duct
Atrium

Pericardium

Lower lobe

Lower lobe

Alveoli

Inferior vena cava

Alveolar sacs

PRIMARY LOBULE OF LUNG

ORGANS OF RESPIRATORY SYSTEM

Plate L system

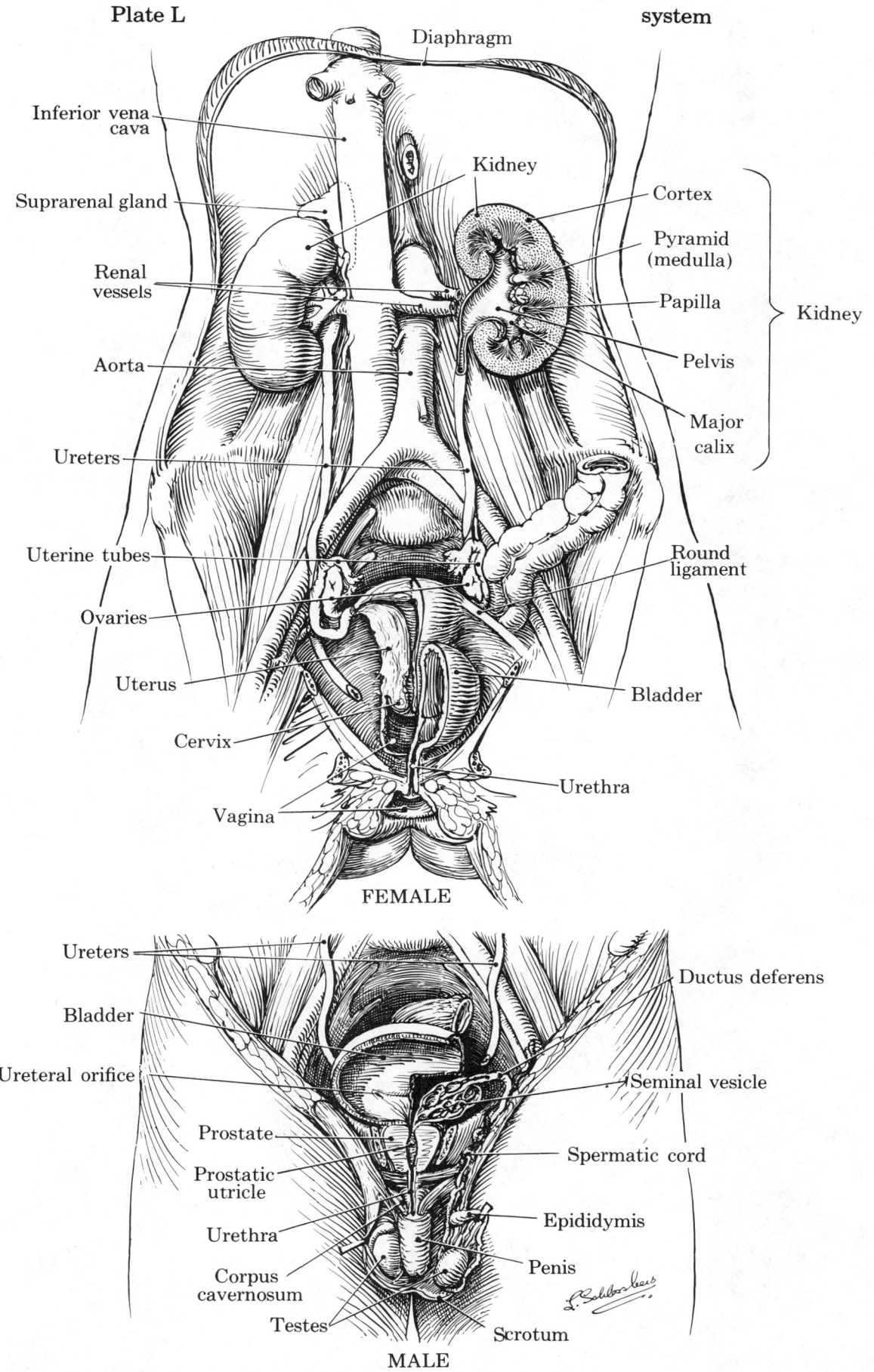

Diaphragm

Inferior vena cava

Kidney

Cortex

Suprarenal gland

Pyramid (medulla)

Renal vessels

Papilla

Kidney

Aorta

Pelvis

Ureters

Major calix

Uterine tubes

Round ligament

Ovaries

Uterus

Bladder

Cervix

Urethra

Vagina

FEMALE

Ureters

Ductus deferens

Bladder

Ureteral orifice

Seminal vesicle

Prostate

Spermatic cord

Prostatic utricle

Urethra

Epididymis

Corpus cavernosum

Penis

Testes

Scrotum

MALE

ORGANS OF THE UROGENITAL SYSTEM

endothelial s. **muscular s.,** all the muscles of the body considered collectively. **nervous s.,** the organ system which along with the endocrine system, correlates the adjustments and reactions of an organism to internal and environmental conditions. Called also *systema nervosum* [NA]. It comprises the central and peripheral nervous systems: the former is composed of the brain and spinal cord, and the latter includes all the other neural elements. See also *autonomic nervous s., parasympathetic nervous s.,* and *sympathetic nervous s.* **parasympathetic nervous s.,** the craniosacral portion of the autonomic nervous system (pars parasympathica systematis nervosi autonomici [NA]). See Plate XLVIII. **peripheral nervous s.,** that portion of the nervous system consisting of the nerves and ganglia outside the brain and spinal cord (systema nervosum periphericum [NA]). **periventricular s.,** collective name for the efferent pathways of the hypothalamus that arise mainly in the supraoptic, posterior, and tuberal nuclei and descend in the periventricular gray matter. **pigmentary s.,** the melanocytes, collectively. **Pinel's s.,** a method of management of the emotionally and mentally disturbed without the use of forcible restraint. **pituitary portal s.,** hypophyseoportal s. **plenum s.,** a system of ventilation based on the mechanical propulsion of air into the room. **portal s.,** an arrangement of vessels whereby blood collected from one set of capillaries passes through a large vessel or vessels and then through a second set of capillaries before it returns to the systemic circulation; such an arrangement occurs in the hypophysis and the liver. **proprioceptive nervous s.,** that portion of the afferent elements of the somatic nervous system which is sensitive to stimuli originating inside the body (from muscles, bones, joints, and ligaments). **Rademacher's s.,** the belief that there should be a specific remedy for every disease. **respiratory s.,** the tubular and cavernous organs and structures by means of which pulmonary ventilation and gas exchange between ambient air and the blood are brought about; called also *apparatus respiratorius* [NA]. See Plate XLIX. **reticular activating s.,** the system of cells of the reticular formation of the medulla oblongata that receive collaterals from the ascending sensory pathways and project to higher centers; they control the overall degree of central nervous system activity, including wakefulness, attentiveness, and sleep; abbreviated RAS. **reticuloendothelial s.,** a functional rather than anatomical system that serves as an important bodily defense mechanism, composed of highly phagocytic cells having both endothelial and reticular attributes and the ability to take up particles of colloidal dyes; these cells include macrophages lining the lymph sinuses and the blood sinuses of the liver (Kupffer's cells), spleen, and bone marrow, and the microglia, reticulum cells of lymphatic tissue, tissue macrophages, and circulating monocytes. Called also *macrophage s.* **SI s.,** see *SI unit,* under *unit.* **sinospiral s.,** muscle bundles in the heart which arise from and are inserted into the region of the sinus venosus. **somatic nervous s.,** the elements of the nervous system concerned with the transmission of impulses to and from the nonvisceral components of the body, such as the skeletal muscles, bones, joints, ligaments, skin, and eye and ear. **stomatognathic s.,** the structures of the mouth and jaws, considered collectively, as they subserve the functions of mastication, deglutition, respiration, and speech. **sympathetic nervous s.,** 1. the thoracolumbar portion of the autonomic nervous system (pars sympathica systematis nervosi autonomici [NA]). See Plate XLVIII. 2. the autonomic nervous system (formerly called *systema nervorum sympathica*). **T s.,** a system of transverse tubular invaginations (*T,* or *transverse, tubules*) of the sarcolemma, each of which penetrates deep into the muscle fiber. In mammalian skeletal muscle, they are located at the junction of the A band with the I band, and in mammalian cardiac muscle at the level of the Z band; the system plays a role in the excitation and relaxation of muscle and provides an important additional surface for the exchange of metabolites between muscle and the extracellular space. Called also *triad s.* See also *triad of skeletal muscle; terminal cisterns,* under *cistern;* and *T tubule,* and *tubule.* **triad s.,** T s. **urogenital s.,** the organs concerned in the production and excretion of urine, together with the organs of reproduction (apparatus urogenitalis or systema urogenitale [NA]). See Plate L. **uropoietic s.,** the organs concerned in secretion of urine (organa uropoëtica [NA]). **vascular s.,** the vessels of the body, especially the blood vessels. **vasomotor s.,** the part of the nervous system that controls the caliber of the blood vessels. **vegetative nervous s.,** an old term for the autonomic nervous system (systema nervosum autonomicum [NA]). **vestibular s.,** labyrinthine s. **visceral nervous s.,** autonomic nervous s. **Waring's s.,** see under *method.*

systema (sis-te'mah) [Gr. *systēma* a complex or organized whole] system: a series of interconnected or interdependent organs which together accomplish a specific function. **s. digesto'rium,** NA alternative for *apparatus digestorius.* **s. lymphat'icum** [NA], lymphatic system: the lymphatic vessels and the lymphoid tissue, considered collectively. **s. nervo'rum centra'le,** s. nervosum centrale. **s. nervo'rum peripher'icum,** s. nervosum periphericum. **s. nervo'rum sympath'icum,** s. nervosum autonomicum. **s. nervo'sum** [NA], the nervous system: the chief organ system that correlates the adjustments and reactions of the organism to internal and environmental conditions, composed of the central and the peripheral nervous system; the former comprises the brain and spinal cord, and the latter includes all other neural elements. **s. nervo'sum autonom'icum** [NA], the autonomic nervous system: the portion of the nervous system concerned with regulation of activity of cardiac muscle, smooth muscle, and glands; usually restricted to the two visceral efferent peripheral components, the pars sympathica systematis nervosi autonomici (thoracolumbar part, or sympathetic nervous system) and the pars parasympathica systematis nervosi autonomici (craniosacral part, or parasympathetic nervous system). Called also *s. nervorum sympathicum.* See Plate XLVIII. **s. nervo'sum centra'le** [NA], central nervous system: that portion of the nervous system consisting of the brain and spinal cord; called also *s. nervorum centrale.* **s. nervo'sum peripher'icum** [NA], peripheral nervous system: that portion of the nervous system consisting of the nerves and ganglia outside the brain and spinal cord; called also *s. nervorum periphericum.* **s. respirato'rium,** NA alternative for *apparatus respiratorius.* **s. urogenita'le,** NA alternative for *apparatus urogenitalis.* **s. vaso'rum,** the blood and lymph vessels of the body and all their ramifications, considered collectively.

systematic (sis"te-mat'ik) [Gr. *systēmatikos*] pertaining or according to a system.

systematization (sis-tem"ah-ti-za'shun) arrangement according to a system. In psychiatry, the arrangement of ideas into a logical sequence, or of delusions into a superficially coherent system.

systematized (sis'te-mah-tīzd) made systematic or arranged according to a system.

systematology (sis"tĕ-mah-tol'o-je) [Gr. *systēma* system + *-logy*] the doctrine or bibliography of systematic arrangements.

systemic (sis-tem'ik) pertaining to or affecting the body as a whole.

systemoid (sis'tĕ-moid) [Gr. *systēma* system + *eidos* form] 1. resembling a system. 2. denoting tumors made up of various kinds of tissue.

systogene (sis'to-jēn) tyramine.

systole (sis'to-le) [Gr. *systolē* a drawing together, contraction] the contraction, or period of contraction, of the heart, especially that of the ventricles; sometimes divided into components, as pre-ejection and ejection periods, or isovolumic, ejection, and relaxation periods. **aborted s.,** a systole, usually premature, not associated with pulsation of a peripheral artery. **atrial s.,** the contraction of the atria by which blood is propelled from them into the ventricles. **extra s.,** extrasystole. **frustrate s.,** aborted s. **hemic s.** (*obs.*), an independently occurring systole of a ventricle. **ventricular s.,** the contraction of the ventricles of the heart by which the blood is forced into the aorta and the pulmonary trunk.

systolic (sis-tol'ik) pertaining to or produced by the systole; occurring along with the ventricular systole.

systolometer (sis"to-lom'ĕ-ter) [Gr. *systolē* systole + *metron* measure] an instrument for determining the quality of the heart sounds.

systremma (sis-trem'ah) [Gr. "anything twisted up together"] a cramp in the muscles of the calf of the leg.

Sytobex (si'to-beks) trademark for preparations of cyanocobalamin.

syzygial (sĭ-zij'e-al) pertaining to syzygy.

syzygiology (sĭ-zij"e-ol'o-je) the study of the relationship of the whole as contrasted to that of isolated parts and functions.

Syzygium (sĭ-zij'e-um) a genus of tropical myrtaceous trees. S. *jambolanum,* the jambul tree of India, is astringent.

syzygium (sĭ-zij'e-um) syzygy.

syzygy (siz'ĭ-je) [Gr. *syzygia* a union of branches with the trunk] 1. the conjunction and fusion of organs without loss of identity. 2. the temporary adherence of male and female gregarines prior to encystment and the production of gametes.

Szabo's test (sah'bōz) [Dionys *Szabo,* Budapest physician, 1856–1918] see under *tests.*

Szent-Györgyi reaction (sent-jor'jĭ) [Albert *Szent-Györgyi,* Hungarian biochemist in America, born 1893, noted for his isolation of ascorbic acid and research in muscle contraction; winner of the Nobel prize for medicine and physiology in 1937] see under *reaction.*

T abbreviation for *temperature, tera, thoracic* (in vertebral formulas), and *intraocular tension*. Normal intraocular tension is indicated by the symbol Tn, while T + 1, T + 2, etc., indicate stages of increased tension, and T – 1, T – 2, etc., indicate stages of decreased tension.

T. tesla.

T$_m$ tubular maximum (of the kidneys); a notation used in reporting kidney function studies, with inferior letters representing the substance used in the test, as T$_{m_{PAH}}$ (tubular maximum for para-aminohippuric acid).

T$_3$ symbol for *triiodothyronine.*

T$_4$ symbol for *thyroxine.*

t in genetics, symbol for translocation.

t. abbreviation for *temporal.*

τ symbol for *life* (time).

τ$\frac{1}{2}$ symbol for *half-life* (time).

T-1824 Evans blue.

TA. alkaline tuberculin.

T.A. toxin-antitoxin.

Ta chemical symbol for *tantalum.*

tabacin (tab′ah-sin) a glycoside occurring in tobacco.

tabacism (tab′ah-sizm) tabacosis.

tabacosis (tab″ah-ko′sis) poisoning by tobacco, and chiefly by the inhalation of tobacco dust; also a form of pneumoconiosis attributed to tobacco dust (*t. pulmo′num*).

tabacum (tab′ah-kum) [L.] tobacco.

tabagism (tab′ah-jizm) the condition produced by excessive use of tobacco; nicotinism.

tabanid (tab′ah-nid) any gadfly of the family Tabanidae, of which the genus *Tabanus* is the type. Other genera are *Chrysops, Goniops, Silvius, Chrysozona,* and *Diachlorus.* Many of the species inflict painful bites upon men and aminals, and some species are mechanical vectors of diseases.

Tabanus (tah-ba′nus) [L. "gadfly"] a genus of bloodsucking biting flies; the horseflies or gadflies. They transmit trypanosomes and anthrax to various animals. **T. atra′tus,** the common black horsefly of North America. **T. bovi′nus,** the gadfly of cattle in Asia, Africa, and South America. **T. ditaenia′tus,**

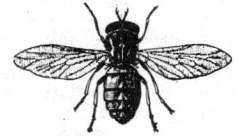

Tabanus bovinus.

T. fascia′tus, T. gra′tus, the Seroot flies of the Sudan, which are very troublesome to man and beast.

tabardillo (tab″ar-dēl′yo) [Sp.] murine typhus.

tabatière anatomique (tah-bah″te-ār′ ah-nah-to-mēk′) [Fr. "anatomical snuffbox"] the hollow on the back of the hand and at the base of the thumb, between the tendons of the extensor pollicis longus and extensor pollicis brevis muscles.

tabella (tah-bel′ah), pl. *tabel′lae* [L.] a medicated tablet or troche.

tabernanthine (tab″er-nan′thēn) an alkaloid, $C_{20}H_{26}N_2O$, isolated from the root of *Tabernanthe iboga* Baill. (Apocynaceae), which has both analgesic and serotonin antagonist properties. It is isomeric with ibogaine.

tabes (ta′bēz) [L. "wasting away, decay, melting"] 1. any wasting of the body; progressive atrophy of the body or a part of it. 2. tabes dorsalis. **abortive t.,** rudimentary t. **cerebral t.,** dementia paralytica. **cervical t.,** tabes dorsalis in which the upper extremities are first affected; called also *t. superior.* **diabetic t.,** a peripheral neuropathy occurring in diabetic patients with symptoms of tabes dorsalis. **t. dorsa′lis,** a degeneration of the dorsal columns of the spinal cord and of the sensory nerve trunks, with wasting, due to infection of the central nervous system with *Treponema pallidum.* The disease, the tertiary (or late) form of syphilis, is marked by paroxysms or crises of intense pain, incoordination, disturbances of sensation, loss of reflexes, paroxysms of functional disturbance of various organs, as the stomach, larynx, etc.; also by various trophic disturbances, especially of the bones and joints, incontinence or retention of urine, failure of sexual power, etc. The course of the disease is usually slow but progressive, and, although it may often be arrested, complete cure is very rare. The disease occurs mostly after middle life, and is more frequent in males. Called also *Duchenne's disease, locomotor ataxia,* and *syphilitic posterior spinal sclerosis.* **t. ergot′ica,** a condition resembling tabes dorsalis, due to ergotism. **Friedreich's t.,** Friedreich's ataxia. **t. infan′tum,** tabes as

seen in infants with congenital syphilis. **t. infe′rior,** tabes dorsalis affecting the lower extremities. **marantic t.,** tabes dorsalis marked by extreme emaciation. **t. mesenter′ica, t. mesara′ica,** tuberculosis of the mesenteric glands in children, resulting in digestive derangement and wasting of the body; called also *pedatrophia, pedatrophy,* and *atrophia mesenterica.* **monosymptomatic t.,** tabes dorsalis exhibiting a single symptom. **peripheral t.,** pseudotabes. **rudimentary t.,** tabes dorsalis with only a few symptoms, the condition remaining stationary for a long time; called also *abortive t.* **t. spina′lis,** t. dorsalis. **t. supe′rior,** cervical t. **vessel t.,** tabes due to an obliterative endarteritis occurring within a principal vessel supplying the posterior column of the spinal cord.

tabescent (tah-bes′ent) [L. *tabescere* to waste away] wasting away; shriveling.

tabetic (tah-bet′ik) pertaining to or affected with tabes.

tabetiform (tah-bet′ĭ-form) resembling tabes.

tabic (tab′ik) tabetic.

tabid (tab′id) [L. *tabidus* melting, dissolving] tabetic; wasting away.

tabification (tab″ĭ-fi-ka′shun) [L. *tabes* wasting away + *facere* to make] the process of wasting away.

tablature (tab′lah-chūr) the separation of the chief cranial bones into inner and outer tables, which are separated by a diploë.

table (ta′b'l) [L. *tabula*] a flat layer or surface. **Aub-Dubois t.,** a table of normal basal metabolic rates for persons of various ages. **Gaffky t.,** see under *scale.* **inner t. of bones of skull,** lamina interna ossium cranii. **inner t. of frontal bone,** facies interna ossis frontalis. **Mendeleev's t.,** periodic t. **outer t. of bones of skull,** lamina externa ossium cranii. **outer t. of frontal bone,** facies externa ossis frontalis. **periodic t.,** an ordering of all the known chemical elements in the form of a chart according to the periodic law, in which corresponding elements from the several periods form groups with similar properties; called also *Mendeleev's t.* **Reuss' t's,** see under *chart.* **Stintzing's t's,** tables showing the average value of the normal electric excitability of the muscles and nerves. **vitreous t.,** lamina interna ossium cranii. **water t.,** the upper surface of the impervious strata on which the ground water lies deep to the surface of the earth.

tablespoon (ta′b'l-spoon) a household unit of capacity, approximately equivalent to 4 fluid drams, or 15 milliliters.

tablet (tab′let) a solid dosage form of varying weight, size, and shape, which may be molded or compressed, and which contains a medicinal substance in pure or diluted form. Cf. *pill.* **buccal t.,** a small, flat, oval tablet to be held between the cheek and gum, permitting direct absorption through the oral mucosa of the medicinal substance contained therein. **dispensing t.,** a compressed or molded tablet containing a large quantity of a drug, used by dispensing pharmacists in compounding prescriptions. **enteric-coated t.,** one coated with material that delays release of the medication until after it leaves the stomach. **hypodermic t.,** one to be dissolved in water, containing a medicinal substance for hypodermic injection. **sublingual t.,** a small, flat, oval tablet to be held beneath the tongue, permitting direct absorption of the medicinal substance contained therein. **t. triturate,** a small, usually cylindrical, molded disk containing a medicinal substance diluted with a mixture of lactose and powdered sucrose, in varying proportions, with a moistening agent.

taboo (tah-boo′) any of the negative traditions and behaviors that are generally regarded as harmful to social welfare. Cf. *mores.*

taboparalysis (ta″bo-pah-ral′ĭ-sis) taboparesis.

taboparesis (ta″bo-pah-re′sis, ta″bo-par′e-sis) dementia paralytica occurring concomitantly with tabes dorsalis.

tabula (tab′u-lah), pl. *tab′ulae* [L.] table. **t. exter′na os′sis cra′nii,** lamina externa ossium cranii. **t. inter′na os′sis cra′nii, t. vit′rea,** lamina interna ossium cranii.

tabular (tab′u-lar) [L. *tabula* a board or table] resembling or shaped like a table.

tacahout (tak″ah-hoot′) [Arabic] a kind of gall from tamarisk trees; a source of gallic acid.

tacamahac (tak′ah-ma-hak″) a resin or gum derived from various trees, e.g., *Bursera gummifer* L. (Burseraceae) of tropical America; it is medicinally considered to be diaphoretic, diuretic, and purgative.

Tacaryl (tak′ah-ril) trademark for preparations of methdilazine.

TACE (tās) trademark for preparations of chlorotrianisene.

tache (tahsh) [Fr.] a spot or blemish. **t. blanche** (blahnsh) [Fr. "white spot"], a white spot on the liver in certain infectious diseases. **t's bleuâtres** (bleu-ahtr′) [Fr. "bluish spots"], maculae caeruleae. **t. cérébrale** (sa-ra-brahl′) [Fr. "cerebral spot"], a congested streak produced by drawing the nail across the skin: a concomitant of various nervous or cerebral diseases. Called also *t. méningéale.* **t's laiteuses** (la-tēz′) [Fr. "milky spots"], small spots, of a milky appearance in the omentum, made up of lymphoid cells and macrophages and especially prominent in the rabbit. **t. méningéale** (ma-nin-zha-al′) [Fr. "meningeal spot"], t. cérébrale. **t. motrice** (mo-trēs′) [Fr. "motor spot"], a kind of motor nerve ending in which the nerve fibril passes to a muscle cell, where it ends in a slight enlargement. **t. noire** (nwahr) [Fr. "black spot"], an ulcer covered with a black adherent crust, a characteristic local reaction occurring at the presumed site of the infective bite in certain tickborne rickettsioses, such as scrub typhus or boutonneuse fever. **t. spinale** (spe-nahl′) [Fr. "spinal spot"], a bulla resembling a burn, and due to a spinal cord disease.

tachistoscope (tah-kis′to-skōp) [Gr. *tachistos* swiftest + *skopein* to examine] a kind of stereoscope in which vision is interrupted by a movable diaphragm.

tacho- [Gr. *tachos* speed] a combining form denoting relationship to speed.

tachogram (tak′o-gram) [*tacho-* + Gr. *gramma* mark] a graphic record of the movement and velocity of the blood current.

tachography (tah-kog′rah-fe) [*tacho-* + Gr. *graphein* to write] the recording of the speed of the blood current.

tachy- (tak′e) [Gr. *tachys* swift] a combining form meaning swift or rapid.

tachyalimentation (tak″e-al″ĭ-men-ta′shun) [*tachy-* + *alimentation*] hypoglycemia occurring postprandially after gastric resection or gastroenterostomy, due to the accelerated passage of glucose into the small intestine, from which it enters the bloodstream at an increased rate, stimulating the production of insulin by the β-cells of the pancreas. It is a manifestation of the dumping syndrome.

tachyarrhythmia (tak″e-ah-rith′me-ah) [*tachy-* + *a* neg. + Gr. *rhythmos* rhythm] tachycardia associated with an irregularity in the normal heart rhythm.

tachyauxesis (tak″e-awk-ze′sis) [*tachy-* + Gr. *auxēsis* growth] heterauxesis in which the part grows more rapidly than the whole.

tachycardia (tak″e-kar′de-ah) [*tachy-* + Gr. *kardia* heart] excessive rapidity in the action of the heart; the term is usually applied to a heart rate above 100 per minute and may be qualified as atrial, junctional (nodal), or ventricular, and as paroxysmal. **atrial t.,** a rapid cardiac rate, usually between 160 and 190 per minute, originating from an atrial locus. **double t.,** the occurrence of two types of ectopic tachycardia, e.g., nodal and ventricular tachycardia, at the same time. **ectopic t.,** abnormally rapid heart action in response to impulses arising outside the sinoatrial node. **junctional t.,** that arising in response to impulses originating in the atrioventricular junction, i.e., in the atrioventricular node. **nodal t.,** tachycardia in response to impulses originating in or near the atrioventricular node; called also *atrioventricular nodal t.* **orthostatic t.,** disproportionate rapidity of the heart rate on rising from a reclining to a standing position. **paroxysmal t.,** a condition marked by attacks of rapid action of the heart having sudden onset and cessation; called also *Bouveret's disease* or *syndrome.* **reflex t.,** rapid action of the heart initiated through a relatively simple nerve pathway by an event occurring elsewhere in the body. **sinus t.,** simple tachycardia with origin in the sinus node. **t. strumo′sa exophthal′mica,** Graves' disease. **supraventricular t.,** a combination of junctional tachycardia and atrial tachycardia. **ventricular t.,** an abnormally rapid ventricular rhythm with aberrant ventricular excitation (wide QRS complexes), usually in excess of 150 per minute, which is generated within the ventricle and is most commonly associated with atrioventricular dissociation. Minor irregularities of rate may also occur. Evidence implicates a reentrant pathway as the usual cause.

tachycardiac (tak″e-kar′de-ak) 1. pertaining to, characterized by, or causing tachycardia. 2. an agent that acts to accelerate the pulse.

tachycardic (tak″e-kar′dik) tachycardiac.

tachygastria (tak″e-gas′tre-ah) the occurrence of a sequence of electric potentials at abnormally high frequencies in the gastric antrum.

tachygenesis (tak″e-jen′ĕ-sis) [*tachy-* + Gr. *genesis* production] the acceleration and compression of ancestral stages in embryonic development.

tachylalia (tak″e-la′le-ah) [*tachy-* + Gr. *lalein* to speak + *-ia*] rapidity of speech.

tachymeter (tah-kim′ĕ-ter) [*tachy-* + Gr. *metron* measure] any instrument for measuring rapidity of motion of any body.

tachyphagia (tak″e-fa′je-ah) [*tachy-* + Gr. *phagein* to eat + *-ia*] rapid or hasty eating.

tachyphasia (tak″e-fa′ze-ah) [*tachy-* + Gr. *phasis* speech + *-ia*] tachyphrasia.

tachyphemia (tak″e-fe′me-ah) [*tachy-* + Gr. *phēmē* speech + *-ia*] tachyphrasia.

tachyphrasia (tak″e-fra′ze-ah) [*tachy-* + Gr. *phrasis* speech + *-ia*] extreme volubility of speech; sometimes a sign of mental disorder.

tachyphrenia (tak″e-fre′ne-ah) [*tachy-* + Gr. *phrēn* mind + *-ia*] mental hyperactivity.

tachyphylaxis (tak″e-fi-lak′sis) [*tachy-* + Gr. *phylaxis* protection] 1. rapid immunization against the effect of toxic doses of an extract by previous injection of small doses of the same (Gley, 1911). 2. rapidly decreasing response to a drug or physiologically active agent after administration of a few doses.

tachypnea (tak″ip-ne′ah) [*tachy-* + Gr. *pnoia* breath] excessive rapidity of respiration; a respiratory neurosis marked by quick, shallow breathing.

tachypragia (tak″e-prag′e-ah) [*tachy-* + Gr. *prassein* to act] rapidity of action.

tachyrhythmia (tak″e-rith′me-ah) [*tachy-* + Gr. *rhythmos* rhythm + *-ia*] tachycardia, especially when the mechanism is obscure.

tachysterol (tak-is′te-rol) an isomer of ergosterol produced by irradiation.

tachysynthesis (tak″e-sin′thĕ-sis) tachyphylaxis.

tachytrophism (tak″e-tro′fizm) [*tachy-* + Gr. *trophē* nutrition] rapid metabolism.

taclamine hydrochloride (tah′klah-mēn) chemical name: 2,3,4,4a,8,9,13b,14 - octahydro -1*H*-benzo[6,7]cyclohepta[1,2,3 -*de*]-pyrido[2,1-α]isoquinoline; a minor tranquilizer, $C_{21}H_{23}N \cdot HCl$.

tactic (tak′tik) 1. exhibiting tacticity. 2. pertaining to or characterized by taxis.

tacticity (tak-tĭ′sĭ-te) the condition of having a regular chemical arrangement of the units making up the main chain of a polymer.

tactile (tak′til) [L. *tactilis*] pertaining to the touch.

tactilogical (tak″tĭ-loj′e-kal) pertaining to touch: tactual.

taction (tak′shun) [L. *tactio*] 1. a touch; an act of touching. 2. the sense of touch; perception by the touch.

tactometer (tak-tom′ĕ-ter) [L. *tactus* touch + *metrum* measure] an instrument for measuring the acuteness of the sense of touch; an esthesiometer.

tactor (tak′tor) a tactile end-organ.

tactual (tak′tu-al) [L. *tactus* touch] pertaining to or accomplished by the touch.

tactus (tak′tus) [L.] touch. **t. erudi′tus** [L. "trained touch"], delicacy of touch acquired by practice. **t. ex′pertus** [L. "experienced touch"], t. eruditus.

taedium (te′de-um) [L.] weariness; boredom. **t. vi′tae** [L. "weariness of life"], morbid disgust with life.

Taenia (te′ne-ah) [L. "a flat band," "bandage," "tape"] a genus of large tapeworms of the family Taeniidae. **T. africa′na,** *T. saginata.* **T. antarc′tica,** a species from dogs in Antarctic regions. **T. balan′iceps,** a species from dogs and bobcats in Nevada and New Mexico. **T. brachyso′ma,** a species infesting dogs in Italy. **T. brem′neri,** *T. confusa.* **T. cer′vi,** a species from dogs in Denmark. **T. confu′sa,** a species found in the Mississippi Valley and in East Africa, believed by some to be a variant of *T. saginata.* Called also *T. bremneri.* **T. cras′ciceps,** a cestode parasite of foxes in Alaska and Canada, found in rodents as an intermediate host. **T. crassicol′lis,** *T. taeniaeformis.* **T. cucurbiti′na,** *T. saginata.* **T. demararien′sis,** *Raillietina demarariensis.* **T. echinococ′cus,** *Echinococcus granulosus.* **T. ellip′tica,** *Dipylidium caninum.* **T. hydati′gena,** a tapeworm that is parasitic in dogs and wild carnivora; the larval stage (cysticercus) is found in the liver and abdominal cavity of various ruminants and rodents and occasionally in other animals, including man. Called also *T. marginata.* **T. krab′bei,** a cestode parasite found in the bobcat, dog, and wolf in the northern United States, Canada, Alaska, and Iceland. **T. madagascarien′sis,** *Raillietina madagascariensis.* **T. margina′ta,** *T. hydatigena.* **T. mediocanella′ta,** *T. saginata.* **T. na′na,** *Hymenolepis nana.* **T. o′vis,** a species parasitic in dogs; found in the musculature of sheep and goats as intermediate hosts. **T. philippi′na,** *T. saginata.* **T. pisifor′mis,** a tapeworm commonly found in dogs; parasitic in cats, foxes, wolves, and other animals; the cysticercus (larval stage) is found in the liver and peritoneal cavity of rabbits. **T. sagina′ta,** the commonest of the large tapeworms of man, a species 12 to 25 feet long, found in the adult form in the human intestine. The cysticerci (larval stage) develop in the muscles and other tissues of cattle and other ruminants. Human infection usually results from eating raw or rare beef. Called also *beef* or *unarmed tapeworm* and *T. africana.* **T. so′lium,** the pork tapeworm, a species 3 to 6 feet long found in the adult form in the human intestine; the cysticerci (larval stage) occur most often in the muscle and various tissues of the pig, but are also found in man, monkeys, camels, sheep, and dogs. It gains access to the human intestine through ingestion of inadequately cooked or measly pork (see *cysticerosis*). It is rare in the United States. Called also *armed* or *measly tapeworm.* **T. taeniaefor′mis,** a cestode parasite commonly found in cats, and more rarely in dogs, foxes, and other animals, having rats, mice, and other rodents as intermediate hosts. Called also *T. crassicollis.*

taenia (te′ne-ah), pl. *tae′niae* [L.] 1. tenia (def. 1). 2. an individual organism of the genus *Taenia.* **tae′niae acus′ticae,** striae medullares ventriculi quarti. **t. chorioi′dea,** tenia choroidea. **t. cine′rea,** a band of gray substance on the floor of the fourth ventricle outside the striae medullares ventriculi quarti. **tae′niae co′li,** teniae coli. **t. fim′briae,** the line of attachment of the choroid plexus to the lateral ventricle to the fimbria of the hippocampus; see *tenia fornicis* [NA]. **t. for′nicis,** tenia fornicis. **t. hippocam′pi,** fimbria hippocampi. **t. li′bera,** tenia libera. **t. medulla′ris thal′ami op′tici, medullary t. of thalamus,** tenia thalami. **t. mesocol′ica,** tenia mesocolica. **t. omenta′lis,** tenia omentalis. **t. pon′tis,** a bundle of fibers sometimes found on the cerebral peduncle along the rostral border of the pons, running an isolated course to the cerebellum between the superior and middle cerebellar peduncles. **tae′niae pylo′ri,** ligamenta pylori. **t. semicircula′ris cor′poris stria′ti,** stria terminalis. **t. tec′tae,** stria longitudinalis lateralis corporis callosi. **tae′niae tela′rum,** see *tenia telae* [NA]. **t. termina′lis,** 1. taenia fimbriae. 2. a slight ridge on the inner surface of the right atrium that marks the position of the sinoatrial node. **t. thal′ami,** tenia thalami. **t. tu′bae,** a thickened band of peritoneum along the upper border of the uterine tube. **taeniae of Valsalva,** teniae coli. **t. ventric′uli quar′ti,** tenia ventriculi quarti. **t. ventric′uli ter′tii,** tenia thalami.

taenia- for other words beginning thus, see also those beginning *tenia-.*

taeniacide (te′ne-ah-sīd″) [L. *taenia* tapeworm + *caedere* to kill] 1. destructive to tapeworms. 2. an agent that destroys tapeworms.

taeniae (te′ne-e) plural of *taenia.*

taeniafugal (te″ne-ah-fu′gal) expelling tapeworms.

taeniafuge (te′ne-ah-fūj″) [*taenia* + L. *fugare* to put to flight] an agent that expels tapeworms.

taenial (te′ne-al) 1. of or pertaining to tapeworms of the genus *Taenia.* 2. tenial (def. 1).

Taeniarhynchus (te″ne-ah-ring′kus) a genus name formerly given to beef tapeworms; see *Taenia confusa* and *T. saginata.*

taeniasis (te-ni′ah-sis) infection with any of the tapeworms of the genus *Taenia.*

taeniform (ten′ĭ-form) [*taenia* + L. *forma* shape] resembling the organism *Taenia,* or a tapeworm.

Taeniidae (te-ni′ĭ-de) a family of medium-sized or large tapeworms of the order Cyclophyllidea, subclass Cestoda, which are parasitic in mammals, including man; three medically important genera are *Taenia, Multiceps,* and *Echinococcus.*

taeniola (te-ni′o-lah) [L., dim of *taenia*] a slender bandlike structure. **t. cine′rea,** taenia cinerea. **t. cor′poris callo′si of Reil,** lamina rostralis.

Taeniorhynchus (te″ne-o-ring′kus) a genus of mosquitoes now called *Mansonia.*

T.A.F. 1. Tuberculin Albumose Frei (Ger.); see *albumose-free tuberculin,* under *tuberculin.* 2. toxoid-antitoxin floccules; see under *floccule.*

tag (tag) 1. a small appendage, flap, or polyp. 2. label. **auricular t′s,** rudimentary appendages of auricular tissue occurring on the face along the line of union of the first branchial arch. **cutaneous t.,** a small, flesh-colored or brown, pendulous outgrowth of the skin, such as an acrochordon, pendulous fibroma, or molluscum fibrosum; skin tags on the neck in middle life usually occur in pedunculated seborrheic keratosis. Called also *cutaneous papilloma* and *skin t.* **radioactive t.,** a radioisotope that has been incorporated within a biological chemical by metabolic or other processes. **skin t.,** cutaneous t.

Tagamet (tag′ah-met) trademark for preparations of cimetidine.

tagatose (tag′ah-tōs) a ketohexose, $CH_2OH(CHOH)_3 \cdot CO \cdot CH_2OH$, isomeric with fructose.

tagesrest (tah′gez-rest) [Ger.] day residue.

tagliacotian rhinoplasty or **operation** (tah″le-ah-ko′she-an) see under *rhinoplasty.*

tahaga (tah-hah′gah) a disease of camels in Algeria, similar to surra, caused by *Trypanosoma evansi.*

taiga (tī′ga) [Russian] the northern coniferous forest biome, found primarily in Canada, northern Europe, and Siberia.

tail (tāl) [L. *cauda;* Gr. *oura*] 1. any slender appendage; called also *cauda* [NA]. 2. the appendage that extends from the posterior trunk of animals. **t. of caudate nucleus,** cauda nuclei caudati. **t. of epididymis,** cauda epididymidis. **occult t.,** supernumerary segments of the coccyx, present in the buttock. **t. of pancreas,** cauda pancreatis. **t. of Spence,** the projection of mammary glandular tissue extending into the axillary region, sometimes forming a visible mass which may enlarge premenstrually or during lactation. **t. of spleen,** extremitas anterior lienis. **t. of spermatozoon,** the flagellum of a sper-

matozoon, which contains the axonema; it presents four regions: the *neck, middle piece, principal piece,* and *end piece.*

tailgut (tāl′gut) a prolongation of the hindgut into the tail of the early embryo.

Taillefer's valve (tah″u-fārs′) [Louis Auguste Horace Sydney Timeléon *Taillefer,* French physician, 1802–1868] see under *valve.*

Taka-diastase (tah′kah di′as-tās) [Jokichi *Takamine,* Japanese chemist in New York, 1854–1922] trademark for an amylolytic enzyme formed by the action of the spores of the fungus *Aspergillus oryzae* on the bran of wheat; used as a digestant.

Takata's reagent (tak-ah′tahz) [Maki *Takata,* Japanese pathologist, born 1892] see under *reagent.*

Takata-Ara test (tak-ah′tah ah′rah) [Maki *Takata;* Kiyoshi *Ara,* Japanese pathologist] see under *tests.*

Tal. abbreviation for L. *tal′is,* such a one.

talalgia (tal-al′je-ah) pain in the heel or ankle.

talampicillin hydrochloride (tal-amp″ĭ-sil′in) chemical name: [2*S*-[2α,5α,6β(*S**)]]-6-[(aminophenylacetyl)amino]-3,3-dimethyl-7-oxo-4-thia-1-azabicyclo[3.2.0]heptane-2-carboxylic acid 1,3-dihydro-3-oxo-1-isobenzofuranyl ester monohydrochloride. The monohydrochloride salt of the phthalidyl ester of ampicillin, $C_{24}H_{23}N_3O_6S \cdot HCl$, having the actions and uses of ampicillin (q.v.).

talantropia (tal″an-tro′pe-ah) [Gr. *talanton* balance + *tropos* a turning + *-ia*] nystagmus.

talar (ta′lar) of or pertaining to the talus.

Talauma elegans (tal-aw′mah el′e-gans) a plant of Java, valued as a stomachic, antispasmodic, and antihysteric remedy.

talbutal (tal′bu-tal) [USP] chemical name: 5-(1-methylpropyl)-5-(2-propenyl)-2,4-6(1*H,3H,5H*)-pyrimidinetrione. An intermediate-acting barbiturate, $C_{11}H_{16}N_2O_3$, occurring as a white, crystalline powder; used as a sedative and hypnotic, administered orally.

talc (talk) [USP] a native, hydrous magnesium silicate, sometimes containing a small proportion of aluminum silicate, used as a dusting powder; called also *purified talc.*

talcosis (tal-ko′sis) a morbid condition resulting from the inhalation or implantation in the body of talc. **pulmonary t.,** pneumoconiosis resulting from inhalation of particles of talc.

talcum (tal′kum) [L.] talc.

taleranol (tah-ler′ah-nōl) chemical name: [3*S*-(3*R**, 7*R**)]-3,4,5,6,7,8,9,10,11,12-decahydro-7,14,16-trihydroxy-3-methyl-1*H*-2-benzoxacyclotetradecin-1-one; an enzyme that inhibits gonadotropin, $C_{18}H_{26}O_5$.

tali (ta′li) plural of *talus.*

taliacotian (tal″e-ah-ko′shan) tagliacotian.

taliped (tal′ĭ-ped) 1. clubfooted. 2. a clubfooted person.

talipedic (tal″ĭ-pe′dik) clubfooted.

talipes (tal′ĭ-pēz) [L. "clubfoot"] a congenital deformity of the foot, which is twisted out of shape or position; called also *clubfoot.* See also under *pes.* **t. calcaneoval′gus,** a deformity of the

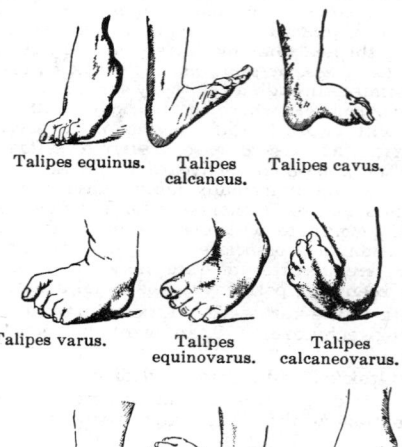

Talipes equinus. Talipes calcaneus. Talipes cavus.

Talipes varus. Talipes equinovarus. Talipes calcaneovarus.

Talipes valgus. Talipes calcaneovalgus. Talipes equinovalgus.

foot in which the heel is turned outward from the midline of the body and the anterior part of the foot is elevated. **t. calcaneova′rus,** a deformity of the foot in which the heel is turned toward the midline of the body and the anterior part is elevated. **t. calca′neus,** a deformity in which the foot is dorsiflexed. **t. cavoval′gus,** a deformity in which the longitudinal arch of the foot is abnormally high, and the heel is turned outward from the midline of the body. **t. ca′vus,** a deformity in which the longitudinal arch of the foot is abnormally high. **t.**

equinoval'gus, a deformity of the foot in which the heel is elevated and turned outward from the midline of the body. **t. equinova'rus,** a deformity of the foot in which the heel is turned inward from the midline of the leg and the foot is plantar flexed. This is associated with the raising of the inner border of the foot (supination) and displacement of the anterior part of the foot so that it lies medially to the vertical axis of the leg (adduction). With this type of foot the arch is higher (cavus) and the foot is in equinus (plantar flexion). This is a typical clubfoot. **t. equi'nus,** a deformity in which the foot is plantar flexed, causing the person to walk on the toes without touching the heel. **t. planoval'gus,** a deformity of the foot in which the heel is turned outward from the midline of the leg and the outer border of the anterior part of the foot is higher than the inner border. This results in a lowering of the longitudinal arch. The condition may be congenital and permanent, or it may be spasmodic as a result of reflex spasm of the muscles controlling the foot. **t. val'gus,** a deformity of the foot in which the heel is turned outward from the midline of the leg. **t. va'rus,** a deformity of the foot in which the heel is turned inward from the midline of the leg.

talipomanus (tal''ĭ-pom'ah-nus) [L. *talipes* clubfoot + *manus* hand] a deformity of the hand analogous with clubfoot, or talipes; i.e., the hand is twisted out of shape or position, usually in strong flexion and adduction; called also *clubhand.*

tallow (tal'o) suet.

Tallqvist's scale (tahl'kvists) [Theodor Waldemar *Tallqvist,* Finnish physician, 1871–1927] see under *scale.*

Talma's disease, operation (tal'mahz) [Sape *Talma,* physician in Utrecht, 1847–1918] see *myotonia acquisita,* and see under *operation.*

talocalcaneal (ta''lo-kal-ka'ne-al) pertaining to the talus and calcaneus.

talocalcanean (ta''lo-kal-ka'ne-an) talocalcaneal.

talocrural (ta''lo-kroo'ral) [L. *talus* ankle + *crus* leg] pertaining to the talus and the bones of the leg.

talofibular (ta''lo-fib'u-lar) pertaining to the talus and the fibula.

talon (tal'on) [L. "bird's claw"] the posterior portion of an upper molar. **t. noir** (nwahr) [F. "black claw"], a punctate pigmented dermatitis occurring on the heels, toes, or hands; thought to be related to trauma. Called also *basketball heels.*

talonavicular (ta''lo-nah-vik'u-lar) pertaining to the talus and the navicular bone.

talonid (tal'o-nid) the posterior portion of a lower molar.

talopram hydrochloride (tal'o-pram) chemical name: 1,3-dihydro-*N*,3,3-trimethyl-1-phenyl-1-isobenzofuran propanamine hydrochloride; a catecholamine potentiator, $C_{20}H_{25}NO \cdot HCl$.

taloscaphoid (ta''lo-skaf'oid) talonavicular.

talose (ta'lōs) an aldehyde hexose, $CH_2OH(CHOH)_4CHO$, an isomer of glucose.

talotibial (ta''lo-tib'e-al) pertaining to the talus and the tibia.

talus (ta'lus), pl. *ta'li* [L. "ankle"] 1. [NA] the highest of the tarsal bones and the one which articulates with the tibia and fibula to form the ankle joint; called also *ankle bone, astragalus, astragaloid bone,* and *os tarsi tibialis.* 2. the ankle (def. 1).

Talwin (tal'win) trademark for preparations of pentazocine.

T.A.M. toxoid-antitoxoid mixture.

tama (ta'mah) swelling of the feet and legs.

tambour (tam-boor') [Fr. "drum"] a drum-shaped appliance used in transmitting movements in a recording instrument. It consists of a cylinder having an elastic membrane stretched over it, from which passes a tube that transmits the changes in air pressure to a recording device.

tamoxifen citrate (tah-moks'ĭ-fen) chemical name: (*Z*)-2-[4-(1,2-diphenyl-1-butenyl)phenoxy]-*N,N*-dimethyl-2-hydroxy-1,2,3-propanetricarboxylate (1:1). A nonsteroidal oral antiestrogen, $C_{26}H_{29}NO \cdot C_6H_8O_7$, used in the palliative treatment of breast cancer in postmenopausal women and to stimulate ovulation in infertility.

tampan (tam'pan) see *Argas persicus* and *Ornithodorus moubata.*

tampicin (tam'pĭ-sin) a glycoside, $C_{34}H_{54}O_{14}$, from Tampico jalap, *Ipomoea simulans.*

tampon (tam'pon) [Fr. "stopper, plug"] a pack; a pad or plug made of cotton, sponge, or other material; variously used in surgery to plug the nose, vagina, etc., for the control of hemorrhage or the absorption of secretions. **Corner's t.,** a tampon composed of a segment of omentum for insertion into a gastric or intestinal wound. **tracheal t.,** an inflatable rubber bag surrounding a tracheotomy tube; used to prevent the entrance of blood into the trachea in operations on the mouth and nose. **Trendelenburg's t.,** see under *cannula.*

tamponade (tam''pon-ād') [Fr. *tamponner* to stop up] surgical use of the tampon; also pathologic compression of a part, as compression of the heart by pericardial fluid (see *cardiac t.*). **balloon t.,** esophagogastric tamponade by means of a device with a triple-lumen tube and two inflatable balloons, the third lumen providing for aspiration of blood clots. **cardiac t.,** acute compression of the heart which is due to effusion of the fluid into the pericardium or to the collection of blood in the pericardium from rupture of the heart or penetrating trauma. **chronic t.,** chronic compression of the heart caused by chronic pericardial effusion and pericardial thickening. **esophagogastric t.,** the exertion of pressure against bleeding esophageal varices by inflation of a sausage-shaped balloon introduced into the esophagus and a globular one into the stomach. **heart t.,** cardiac t.

tamponage (tam-po-nahzh') tamponade.

tamponing (tam'pon-ing) tamponade.

tamponment (tam-pon'ment) the act of plugging with a tampon.

Tamus (ta'mus) [L.] a genus of dioscoreaceous plants. *T. communis* L. is an old-world plant called black bryony, used homeopathically; the root is considered to be rubifacient and diuretic.

tan (tan) 1. to brown or become brown from exposure to sun or to ultraviolet light. 2. the brownish color of the skin acquired by such exposure, resulting from darkening of preformed melanin (Meirowsky phenomenon), accelerated formation of new melanin, and retention of melanin in the epidermis as a result of retardation of keratinization.

tandamine hydrochloride (tan'dah-mēn) chemical name: 9-ethyl-1,3,4,9-tetrahydro-*N,N,*1-trimethylthiopyrano[3,4-*b*]indole-1-ethanamine monohydrochloride; an antidepressant, $C_{18}H_{26}N_2S \cdot HCl$.

Tandearil (tan-de'ah-ril) trademark for a preparation of oxyphenbutazone.

tanghin (tan'gēn) the apocynaceous tree, *Cerbera tanghin,* of Madagascar, and its exceedingly poisonous seed; also an extract prepared from it, which is used as an arrow poison.

Tangier disease (tan-jēr') [*Tangier* Island, in Chesapeake Bay, where the disease was first discovered] see under *disease.*

tangoreceptor (tang''go-re-sep'tor) [L. *tangere* to touch + *receptor*] a sense organ that responds only to physical contact, such as touch.

tank (tank) an artificial receptacle for liquids. **activated sludge t.,** a tank through which sewage flows slowly or intermittently while compressed air is allowed to bubble up through it. **anaerobic t.,** septic t. **biological t.,** a modified septic tank. **digestion t.,** a deep septic tank in which sludge is separated and submitted to septic action without making the rest of the sewage offensive; called also *Emsher* or *Imhoff t.* **Dortmund t.,** a deep vertical flow settling tank for removing sludge from sewage. **Emsher t.,** digestion t. **Hubbard t.,** a tank in which a patient may be immersed for the purpose of permitting him to take underwater exercise. **hydrolytic t.,** septic t. **Imhoff t.,** digestion t. **septic t.,** a tank for the receipt of sewage, there to remain for a time in order that the solid matter may settle out and a certain amount of putrefaction occur from the action of the anaerobic bacteria present in the sewage; called also *anaerobic t.* and *hydrolytic t.* **settling t.,** a basin in which the rate of flow of the sewage is reduced and the sludge allowed to settle out.

tannal (tan'al) aluminum tannate. **insoluble t.,** basic aluminum tannate, a brown-yellow astringent powder, $Al_2(OH)_4(C_{14}H_9O_9)_2 + 10H_2O.$

tannalin (tan'al-in) a formaldehyde solution.

tannase (tan'ās) an esterase found in various tannin-bearing plants and produced in cultures by *Aspergillus niger* and *Penicillium glaucum,* which catalyzes the hydrolysis of various ester linkages in gallic acid compounds.

tannate (tan'āt) [L. *tannas*] any salt of tannic acid; all the tannates are astringent.

tannin (tan'in) tannic acid. **diacetyl t., t. diacetylate,** acetyltannic acid. **pathologic t.,** any tannin derived from galls, or vegetable excrescences due to a local disease of the plant. **physiologic t.,** any tannin normally produced by a healthy plant.

tanning (tan'ing) the treatment of burns with tannin.

Tanret's reagent, test (reaction) (tahn-rāz') [Charles *Tanret,* French chemist 1847–1917] see under *reagent* and *tests.*

Tansini's sign (tan-se'nēz) [Iginio *Tansini,* Italian surgeon, 1855–1943] see under *operation.*

tantalum (tan'tah-lum) a rare metallic element: symbol, Ta; atomic number, 73; atomic weight, 180.948. It is a noncorrosive and malleable metal which has been used for plates or disks to replace cranial defects, for wire sutures, and for making prosthetic appliances.

tantrum (tan'trum) a violent display of bad temper.

TAO (ta'o) trademark for preparations of troleandomycin.

taon (tah-on') infantile beriberi occurring in the Philippine Islands.

tap (tap) 1. a quick, light blow. 2. to drain off fluid by paracentesis. **bloody t.,** a lumbar puncture in which the fluid obtained is bloody or pinkish. **front t.,** a tap on the muscles of the front of the leg, producing contraction of the muscles of the calf in spinal irritability. **heel t.,** reflex movement of the toes on tapping the heel, occurring in pyramidal tract damage. **spinal t.,** lumbar puncture.

Tapazole (tap′ah-zol) trademark for a preparation of methimazole.

tape (tāp) a long, narrow strip of fabric or other flexible material. **adhesive t.** [USP], a strip of fabric and/or film evenly coated on one side with a pressure-sensitive, adhesive mixture, the whole having high tensile strength, used for the application of dressings and sometimes to produce immobilization; formerly called *adhesive plaster.* **adhesive t., sterile,** adhesive tape, the adhesive surface of which is covered by strips of a protective material of equal width, and which is sterilized after packaging; formerly called *sterile adhesive plaster.* **Montgomery's t's,** see under *strap.*

tapeinocephalic (tap″ĭ-no-sĕ-fal′ik) characterized by tapeinocephaly.

tapeinocephaly (tap″ĭ-no-sef′ah-le) [Gr. *tapeinos* low-lying + *kephalē* head] a low form of the skull, which is also flattened at front, having a vertical index below 72.

tapetal (tah-pe′tal) pertaining to a tapetum, especially to the tapetum lucidum.

tapetum (tah-pe′tum), pl. *tape′ta* [L.; Gr. *tapētion,* dim. of *tapēs* a carpet, rug] 1. a covering structure, or layer of cells. 2. a stratum in the human brain constituted by the fibers from the body and splenium of the corpus callosum sweeping outward over the lateral ventricle and forming the roof and lateral wall of its posterior horn, and the lateral wall of its inferior horn. **t. cellulo′sum,** a type of tapetum lucidum, being the more complex, more cellular type found in all but two species of the order Carnivora and in the seals. **t. choroi′deae,** t. lucidum. **t. cor′poris callo′si,** tapetum, def. 2. **t. fibro′sum,** a type of tapetum lucidum, being the simpler, fibrous type found almost exclusively in hoofed animals, in a few fish, and in marsupials, elephants, and whales. **t. lu′cidum,** the iridescent pigment epithelium of the choroid of animals which gives their eyes the properties of shining in the dark; called also *t. choroideae.* **t. ni′grum,** stratum pigmenti bulbi oculi. **t. oc′uli,** stratum pigmenti retinae. **t. ventric′uli,** fasciculus longitudinalis superior cerebri.

tapeworm (tāp′werm) a parasitic intestinal cestode worm having a flattened, bandlike form. Those infecting man are principally of the genera *Taenia, Diphyllobothrium, Hymenolepis, Echinococcus,* and *Dipylidium.* The eggs of tapeworms are ingested by the intermediate host, whence they make their way into the tissues, where the larval stages are produced (see *plerocercoid; cysticercus;* and *hydatid cyst,* under *cyst*). When the flesh of the intermediate host is eaten, the larvae develop within the alimentary canal of the definitive host into adult tapeworms, which consists of an attachment organ, or scolex, an undifferentiated neck, and a strobila made up of a variable number of separate segments, or proglottids, each of which is hermaphroditic and produces eggs. **African t.,** *Taenia saginata.* **armed t.,** *Taenia solium.* **beef t.,** *Taenia saginata.* **broad t.,** *Diphyllobothrium latum.* **dog t.,** 1. *Echinococcus granulosus.* 2. *Dipylidium caninum.* **double-pored dog t.,** *Dipylidium caninum.* **dwarf t.,** *Hymenolepis nana.* **fish t.,** *Diphyllobothrium latum.* **fringed t.,** *Thysanosoma actinioides.* **heart-headed t.,** *Diphyllobothrium cordatum.* **hydatid t.,** *Echinococcus granulosus.* **Madagascar t.,** *Raillietina madagascariensis.* **Manson's larval t.,** *Diphyllobothrium mansonoides.* **measly t.,** *Taenia solium.* **pork t.,** *Taenia solium.* **rat t.,** *Hymenolepis diminuta.* **Swiss t.,** *Diphyllobothrium latum.* **unarmed t.,** *Taenia saginata.*

Tapia's syndrome (tap′e-ahz) [Antonio Garcia *Tapia,* Spanish otolaryngologist, 1875–1950] see under *syndrome.*

tapinocephalic (tap″ĭ-no-se-fal′ik) tapeinocephalic.

tapinocephaly (tap″ĭ-no-sef′ah-le) tapeinocephaly.

tapioca (tap″e-o′kah) a fecula, or starch, derived from the root of *Jatropha manihot,* or manioc; used as a food.

tapiroid (ta′pĭ-roid) resembling the snout of a tapir.

tapotage (tah-po-tahzh′) coughing and expectoration following percussion in the supraclavicular region: a sign sometimes obtained in pulmonary tuberculosis.

tapotement (tah-pōt-maw′) [Fr.] a tapping or percussing movement in massage; it includes clapping, beating, and punctation.

tar (tahr) a dark-brown or black, viscid liquid, obtained by roasting the wood of various species of pine, or as a by-product of the destructive distillation of bituminous coal. It is a mixture of complex composition, and is the source of a number of substances, as cresol, creosol, guaiacol, naphthalene, paraffin, phenol, toluene, xylene, etc. Once used in chronic bronchitis, diarrhea, and diseases of the urinary organs, it now has only limited use in certain skin diseases, notably psoriasis and chronic eczematous disorders. **coal t.** [USP], tar obtained as a by-product of the destructive distillation of bituminous coal, used as a topical antieczematic and antipsoriatic. **gas t.,** a coal tar derived from the coal, rosin, petroleum, and other material used in gas works. **juniper t.** [USP], the volatile oil obtained from the woody portions of *Juniperus oxycedrus,* L. (Pinaceae), occurring as a thick brown liquid with a bitter taste; used as a pharmaceutic necessity, and for the topical therapy of dermatoses. Called also *cade oil, Haarlem oil, silver balsam,* and *oleum juniperi empyrheumaticum.* **pine t.** [USP], a viscid, blackish brown liquid obtained by destructive distillation of the wood of various pine trees; used as a local antieczematic and rubefacient, applied topically, and has been used as a stimulating expectorant incorporated in syrups.

Tar's symptom (tahrz) [Aloys *Tar,* Budapest physician, born 1886] see under *symptom.*

Taractan (tar-ak′tan) trademark for a preparation of chlorprothixene.

Taraktogenos kurzii King (tar″ak-toj′e-nos kur′ze-e) a tropical tree whose seeds are a source of chaulmoogra oil; called also *Hydnocarpus heterophyllus* Kurz.

tarantism (tar′an-tizm) a variety of dancing mania, popularly believed to be caused by the bite of a tarantula, and to be cured by dancing.

tarantula (tah-ran′tu-lah) a venomous spider whose bite causes local inflammation and pain, usually not to a severe extent. **American t.,** a large, dark, ferocious looking spider, *Eurypelma hentzii,* having a poisonous bite. **black t.,** a venomous spider of Panama, *Sericopelma communis.* **European t.,** the true tarantula, the large European wolf spider, *Lycosa tarentula,* the bite of which was believed to cause death.

Taraxacum (tah-rak′sah-kum) [L.] a genus of composite-flowered plants. The dried root of *T. officinale* Weber, the common dandelion or lion's tooth, contains taraxerol, choline, inulin, levulin, and pectin, and is a simple bitter.

taraxigen (tah-rak′sĭ-jen) see *taraxy.*

taraxin (tah-rak′sin) see *taraxy.*

taraxis (tah-rak′sis) an obsolete name for conjunctivitis.

taraxy (tah-rak′se) [Gr. *taraxis* disturbance] Novy's name for anaphylaxis, on the theory that the condition is due to a poisonous substance (*taraxin*) which is formed in the blood on the injection of an alien substance, as the result of a reaction with a substance which already exists in the blood serum (*taraxigen*).

tarbadillo (tahr″bah-dēl′yo) [Sp.] tabardillo.

tarbagan (tar′bah-gan) marmot.

Tardieu's spots, test (tar-dyuz′) [Auguste Ambroise *Tardieu,* French physician, 1818–1879] see under *spot* and *tests.*

tardive (tahr′div) [Fr. "tardy, late"] marked by lateness, late; said of a disease in which the characteristic lesion is late in appearing.

tare (tār) 1. the weight of the vessel in which a substance is weighed. 2. to take the weight of a vessel which is to contain a substance, in order to allow for it when the vessel and the substance are weighed together.

tarentism (tar′en-tizm) tarantism.

tarentula (tah-ren′tu-lah) tarantula.

target (tahr′get) 1. an object or area toward which something is directed, such as the metal or plate of a roentgen ray tube on which the electrons impinge and from which the roentgen rays are sent out. 2. denoting a cell or organ that is selectively affected by a particular agent, e.g., a hormone or drug. See also under *organ.*

tarichatoxin (tar″ik-ah-tok′sin) a neurotoxin from the newt (*Taricha*), identical with tetrodotoxin (q.v.).

Tarin, Tarini, Tarinus (tah-ră′, tah-ri′ni, tah-ri′nus), Pierre. A French anatomist and encyclopedist (1700–1761) who wrote a history of anatomy and described many anatomical structures, including the fossa interpeduncularis, gyrus dentatus, hiatus canalis nervi, petrosi majoris, horny band, recessus anterior fossae interpeduncularis, and velum medullare inferius.

Tarnier's forceps (tar-ne-āz′) [Etienne Stéphene *Tarnier,* French obstetrician, 1828–1897] see under *forceps.*

tarsadenitis (tahr″sad-ĕ-ni′tis) an inflammation of the tarsus of the eyelid and of the meibomian glands.

tarsal (tahr′sal) [L. *tarsalis*] 1. pertaining to the tarsus of an eyelid or to the instep. 2. any of the bones of the tarsus.

tarsalgia (tahr-sal′je-ah) pain in the ankle or foot.

tarsalia (tar-sa′le-ah) the bones of the tarsus.

tarsalis (tahr-sa′lis) [L.] tarsal.

tarsectomy (tahr-sek′to-me) [*tarso-* + Gr. *ektomē* excision] 1. excision of the tarsus, or a part of it. 2. excision of a tarsal cartilage.

tarsectopia (tahr″sek-to′pe-ah) [*tarso-* + Gr. *ektopos* out of place + *-ia*] dislocation of the tarsus.

tarsitis (tahr-si′tis) inflammation of the tarsus, or margin of an eyelid; blepharitis.

tarso- (tahr′so) [Gr. *tarsos* a broad flat surface] a combining form denoting relationship to the edge of the eyelid, or to the instep of the foot.

tarsocheiloplasty (tahr″so-ki′lo-plas″te) [*tarso-* + Gr. *cheilos* lip + *plassein* to mold] a plastic operation upon the edge of the eyelid, as in treatment of trichiasis.

tarsoclasis (tahr-sok′lah-sis) [*tarso-* + Gr. *klasis* breaking] the operation of fracturing the tarsus of the foot.

tarsomalacia (tahr″so-mah-la′she-ah) [*tarso-* + Gr. *malakia* softening] softening of the tarsus of an eyelid.

tarsomegaly (tahr″so-meg′ah-le) enlargement of the os calcis.

tarsometatarsal (tahr″so-met″ah-tahr′sal) pertaining to the tarsus and the metatarsus.

tarso-orbital (tahr″so-or′bĭ-tal) pertaining to the tarsus of the eyelid and to the orbit.

tarsophalangeal (tahr″so-fah-lan′je-al) pertaining to the tarsus and the phalanges of the toes.

tarsophyma (tahr″so-fi′mah) [*tarso-* + Gr. *phyma* growth] any tarsal tumor.

tarsoplasia (tahr″so-pla′se-ah) tarsoplasty.

tarsoplasty (tahr′so-plas″te) [*tarso-* + Gr. *plassein* to form] plastic surgery of the tarsus of an eyelid.

tarsoptosis (tahr″sop-to′sis) [*tarso-* + Gr. *ptōsis* falling] falling of the tarsus; flatfoot.

tarsorrhaphy (tahr-sor′ah-fe) [*tarso-* + Gr. *rhaphē* suture] the operation of suturing together a portion of (*partial t.*) or the entire (*total t.*) upper and lower eyelids for the purpose of shortening or closing entirely the palpebral fissure. The terms *external t.*, *median t.*, and *internal t.* are used to indicate the portion of the lids brought together in partial tarsorrhaphy. Called also *blepharorrhaphy*.

tarsotarsal (tahr″so-tahr′sal) pertaining to the articulation between the two rows of tarsal bones.

tarsotibial (tahr″so-tib′e-al) pertaining to the tarsus and the tibia.

tarsotomy (tahr-sot′o-me) [*tarso-* + Gr. *tomē* a cutting] the operation of incising the tarsus, or an eyelid; blepharotomy.

tarsus (tahr′sus) [L.; Gr. *tarsos* a frame of wickerwork; any broad flat surface] 1. [NA] the region of the articulation between the foot and the leg; see also *tarsus osseus.* 2. one of the plates of connective tissue forming the framework of an eyelid; see *t. inferior palpebrae* and *t. superior palpebrae.* **bony t.,** t. osseus. **t. infe′rior palpe′brae** [NA], the firm framework of connective tissue that gives shape to the inferior eyelid; called also *ciliary cartilage, palpebral cartilage,* and *tarsal cartilage.* **t. os′seus** [NA], the seven bones constituting the articulation between the foot and the leg: the talus, calcaneus, and navicular, in the proximal row; and the cuboid and the lateral, intermediate, and medial cuneiform bones, in the distal row. Called also *bony t.* **t. supe′rior palpe′brae** [NA], the firm framework of connective tissue that gives shape to the upper eyelid; called also *ciliary cartilage, palpebral cartilage,* and *tarsal cartilage.*

tartar (tahr′tahr) [L. *tartarum;* Gr. *tartaron*] 1. the lees, or sediment, of a wine cask; crude potassium bitartrate. 2. dental calculus. **borated t.,** a white powder prepared by evaporating a solution of 2 parts of sodium borate and 5 parts of potassium bitartrate. **cream of t.,** potassium bitartrate. **t. emetic,** antimony potassium tartrate; see under *antimony.* **serumal t.,** subgingival calculus. **vitriolated t.,** potassium sulfate.

tartarated (tahr′tahr-āt″ed) charged with tartaric acid.

tartarized (tahr′tahr-īzd) tartarated.

tartrate (tahr′trāt) [L. *tartras*] any salt of tartaric acid. **acid t.,** a bitartrate; any salt of tartaric acid in which one atom only of hydrogen is replaced by a base. **normal t.,** one in which two hydrogen atoms are replaced; various tartrates are employed as remedial agents.

tartrated (tahr′trāt-ed) [L. *tartratus*] containing tartar of tartaric acid.

tartrobismuthate (tahr″tro-biz′mu-thāt) bismuthotartrate.

tasikinesia (tas″ĭ-ki-ne′ze-ah) [Gr. *tasis* straining + *kinēsis* motion + *-ia*] a morbid inclination to get up and walk; inability to remain seated.

tastant (tās′tant) any substance, e.g., salt, capable of eliciting gustatory excitation, i.e., stimulating the sense of taste.

taste (tāst) [L. *gustus*] the peculiar sensation caused by the contact of soluble substances with the tongue; the sense effected by the tongue, the gustatory and other nerves, and the gustation center. Four qualities are distinguished by taste: sweet, sour, salty, and bitter. **color t.,** pseudogeusesthesia. **franklinic t.,** a sour taste produced by stimulating the tongue with static electricity.

taste-blindness (tāst-blīnd′nes) inability to taste certain substances, such as phenylthiocarbamide.

taster (tās′ter) an individual capable of tasting a particular test substance, such as phenylthiocarbamide, used in certain genetic studies.

TAT thematic apperception test.

T.A.T. toxin-antitoxin.

tätte melk (tet′ĕ melk) a food article in Sweden, prepared by inoculating milk with leaves of *Pinguicula vulgaris,* the butterwort, or bog violet.

tattooing (tah-too′ing) the insertion of permanent colors in the skin by introducing them through punctures. **t. of the cornea,** the permanent coloring of the cornea chiefly to conceal leukomatous spots.

Tatum (ta′tum), Edward Lawrie. United States biochemist, born 1909; co-winner, with George Wells Beadle and Joshua Lederberg, of the Nobel prize in medicine and physiology for 1958, for work in genetics and heredity.

taurine (taw′rin) a crystallizable acid, ethylamine sulfonic acid, $NH_2(CH_2)_2SO_2OH$, from the bile, produced by the hydrolysis of taurocholic acid. It is found also in small quantities in the tissues of the lungs and muscles. Its crystals are colorless and are readily soluble in water. It is a component of ox bile extract.

taurocholaneresis (taw″ro-ko″lan-er′ĕ-sis) [*taurocholic* acid + Gr. *hairesis* a taking] increase in the output or elimination of taurocholic acid in the bile. Cf. *cholaneresis.*

taurocholanopoiesis (taw″ro-ko-lan″o-poi-e′sis) synthesis of taurocholic acid by the liver.

taurocholate (taw″ro-ko′lāt) a salt of taurocholic acid; see *bile salts,* under *salt.*

taurocholemia (taw″ro-ko-le′me-ah) the presence of taurocholic acid in the blood.

taurodontism (taw″ro-don′tizm) [L. *taurus* bull + Gr. *odous* tooth + *-ism*] a variation in tooth form involving all or some of the primary and secondary molars, marked by elongation of the body of the tooth so that the pulp chambers are large apico-occlusally and the roots are reduced in size.

Taussig-Bing syndrome (taw′sig-bing) [Helen Brooke *Taussig,* American pediatrician, born 1898; Richard J. *Bing,* American surgeon, born 1909] see under *syndrome.*

tauto- [Gr. *tautos* from *to auto* the same] a combining form meaning the same.

tautomenial (taw″to-me′ne-al) [*tauto-* + Gr. *mēniaia* menses] pertaining to the same menstrual period.

tautomer (taw′to-mer) a chemical compound exhibiting, or capable of exhibiting, tautomerism.

tautomeral (taw-tom′er-al) [*tauto-* + Gr. *meros* part] pertaining to the same part, especially sending processes to help in the formation of the white matter in the same side of the spinal cord; said of certain neurons and neuroblasts. See *tautomeral cells,* under *cell.*

tautomerase (taw-tom′er-ās) an enzyme of the isomerase class which catalyzes tautomeric reactions. **phenylpyruvate t.,** an isomerase that catalyzes the interconversion of keto-phenylpyruvate to enol-phenylpyruvate.

tautomeric (taw″to-mer′ik) exhibiting, or capable of exhibiting, tautomerism.

tautomerism (taw-tom′er-izm) [*tauto-* + Gr. *meros* part] a form of stereoisomerism in which the compounds are mutually interconvertible, under normal conditions, forming a mixture which is in dynamic equilibrium. See *prototropy, anionotropy,* and *mutarotation.*

Tawara's node (tah-wah′rah) [Sunao *Tawara,* Japanese pathologist, born 1873] nodus atrioventricularis.

taxa (tak′sah) plural of *taxon.*

taxine (tak′sēn) an alkaloidal mixture obtainable from the yew, *Taxus baccata* L. (Taxaceae) and responsible for its poisonous properties.

taxis (tak′sis) [Gr. "a drawing up in rank and file"] 1. an orientation movement of a motile organism in response to an external stimulus. Such a response may be either positive (toward) or negative (away from the stimulus). Used also as a word termination, affixed to a stem denoting the nature of the stimulus (stereotaxis). 2. exertion of force in the manual replacement of a displaced or injured organ or structure, as in the reduction of a fracture or dislocation, or the replacement of a protruded intestine in hernia.

Taxodium distichum (L.) Rich. (Taxodiaceae) (taks-o′de-um dis′tik-um) the cypress, a timber tree of North America. The resin was formerly used in rheumatism.

taxology (taks-ol′o-je) taxonomy.

taxon (tak′son), pl. *tax′a* [Gr. *taxis* a drawing up in rank and file + *on* neuter ending] a particular group (category) into which related organisms are classified; the main categories are (in ascending order): species, genus, family, order, class, phylum, and kingdom.

taxonomic (tak″so-nom′ik) pertaining to taxonomy.

taxonomist (taks-on′o-mist) a specialist in taxonomy.

taxonomy (tak-son′o-me) [L. *taxinomia;* Gr. *taxis* a drawing up in rank and file + *nomos* law] the orderly classification of organisms into appropriate categories (taxa) on the basis of relationships among them, with the application of suitable and correct names. **numerical t.,** an arithmetic method of classifying larger numbers of bacterial strains on the basis of their overall similarity to one another, according to the number of phenotypic characters they share, each character being given equal weight. Called also *adansonian,* or *numerical, classification.*

Tay's choroiditis (disease), sign, spot (tāz) [Warren *Tay,* English physician, 1843–1927] see under *choroiditis,* and see *cherry-red spot,* under *spot.*

Tay-Sachs disease (ta saks′) [Warren *Tay;* Bernard (Barney)

Sachs, New York neurologist, 1858–1944] amaurotic family idiocy; see under *idiocy.*

Taylor splint (apparatus) (ta′ler) [Charles Fayette *Taylor,* orthopedic surgeon in New York, 1827–1899] see under *apparatus.*

tazettine (tāz′ĕ-tin) a crystalline alkaloid, $C_{18}H_{21}O_5N$, from the bulbs of daffodils, including *Lycoris radiata* and *Narcissus tazetta.* Called also *sekisanine.*

tazolol hydrochloride (ta′zo-lōl) chemical name: (±)-1-[(1-methylethyl)amino]-3-(2-thiazolyloxy)-2-propanol monohydrochloride. An adrenergic, $C_9H_{16}N_2O_2O_2S\cdot HCl$, having mainly beta$_1$-adrenergic activity; a cardiotonic.

TB see under *tuberculin.*

Tb chemical symbol for *terbium.*

T.b. abbreviation for *tubercle bacillus,* and, in speaking, for *tuberculosis.*

T.B.E. bacillen emulsion tuberculin; see under *tuberculin.*

TBN bacillus emulsions; see under *tuberculin.*

TBP bithionol.

T.C. tuberculin contagious; see under *tuberculin.*

Tc chemical symbol for *technetium.*

TCD$_{50}$ median tissue culture dose; see *TCID$_{50}$.*

TCID$_{50}$ abbreviation for *median tissue culture infective dose:* that quantity of a cytopathogenic agent (virus) that will produce a cytopathic effect in 50 per cent of the cultures inoculated.

TD$_{50}$ median toxic dose; a dose that produces a toxic effect in 50 per cent of a population.

t.d.s. abbreviation for L. *ter di′e sumen′dum,* to be taken three times a day.

Te 1. chemical symbol for *tellurium.* 2. tetanus.

TEA tetraethylammonium.

tea (te) [L. *thea*] 1. the dried leaves of *Camellia sinensis* (L.) Kuntze, containing caffeine, theophylline, tannic acid, and a pleasant volatile oil; also a decoction thereof, used as a stimulating beverage and soothing warm drink for various abdominal discomforts. 2. any decoction or infusion. **beef t.,** an infusion of lean beef. **pectoral t.,** an aqueous infusion of expectorant and demulcent herbs and aromatics.

TEAC tetraethylammonium chloride.

Teale's amputation (operation) (tēlz) [Thomas Pridgin *Teale,* Sr., English surgeon, 1801–1868] see under *amputation.*

tears (tērz) [L. *lacrimae;* Gr. *dakrya*] 1. the watery secretion of the lacrimal glands which serves to moisten the conjunctiva; the secretion is slightly alkaline and saline. 2. small, naturally formed, droplike masses of a gum or resin. **crocodile t.,** lacrimation on chewing and eating; see *syndrome of crocodile tears.*

teart (tert) 1. soil or plants that contain unusual amounts of molybdenum. 2. molybdenosis of farm animals caused by feeding on vegetation grown on soil that contains unusual amounts of molybdenum.

tease (tēz) to pull a tissue apart with needles for microscopical examination.

teaspoon (te′spōōn) a household unit of capacity, containing about 5 milliliters.

teat (tēt) the nipple of the mammary gland.

tebutate (teb′u-tāt) USAN contraction for tertiary butyl acetate.

technetium (tek-ne′she-um) the metallic, radioactive, synthetic chemical element of atomic number 43; its most stable isotope, technetium 99, has a half-life of 2×10^5 years; symbol, Tc. Formerly called *masurium.* **t. 99m,** a radioisotope of technetium having a half-life of 6.0 hours and emitting primarily gamma rays; used in preparations for scanning of the brain, lung, liver, kidney, etc. Symbol ^{99m}Tc. **t. Tc 99m aggregated albumin** [USP], a sterile, aqueous suspension of normal human serum that has been denatured to produce aggregates of controlled particle size that are labeled with ^{99m}Tc; used for lung scanning, administered intravenously. Called also *technetated (* ^{99m}Tc*) aggregated albumin (human).*

technic (tek′nik) technique.

technical (tek′nĭ-kal) pertaining to technique.

technician (tek-nish′an) a person trained in and expert in the performance of technical procedures.

technique (tek-nēk′) [Fr.] the method of procedure and the details of any mechanical process or surgical operation. See also under *method, treatment, maneuver, Table of Stains,* etc. **Begg t.,** a technique of light wire orthodontic therapy. **Coffey t.,** a method of correcting exstrophy of the bladder in which the ureters are transplanted between the coats of the colonic wall to achieve a valve-like function. **Conway t.,** a method of correcting severe macromastia, consisting in partial breast amputation and free transplantation of the nipples and areolae. **dilution-filtration t.,** a blood culture technique in which any culture inhibitors present in the blood are diluted out and red blood cells are removed before the sample is filtered and cultured, thereby permitting the identification of organisms in about 24 hours. **fluorescent antibody t.,** an immunofluorescence technique in which antigen in tissue sections is located by homologous antibody labeled with fluorochrome (the single-layer technique) or by treating the antigen with unlabeled antibody followed by a second layer of labeled antiglobulin which is reactive with the unlabeled antibody (double-layer technique). Variations include direct, indirect, inhibition, and complement staining techniques. **hanging drop t.,** a method of microscopic examination of organisms suspended in a drop on a special concave microscope slide. **Hartel's t.,** see under *treatment.* **Jerne plaque t.,** a hemolytic technique for detecting antibody-producing cells: a suspension of presensitized lymphocytes is mixed in an agar gel with erythrocytes; after a period of incubation, complement is added and a clear area of lysis of red cells can be seen around each of the antibody-producing cells. **Kleinschmidt t.,** rupture of the virion by osmotic shock so that viral DNA is exposed. **Krawitz's t.,** vaccination done by making multiple punctures at the same time. **Kristeller t.,** see under *method.* **Leboyer m.,** see under *method.* **Orr t.,** see under *treatment.* **Ouchterlony t.,** see under *test.* **Rebuck skin window t.,** a test of the inflammatory response: the skin is abraded and a cover slip or chamber is applied over the abraded area to permit direct observation of cell morphology. **scintillation counting t.,** a method of determining the amount of radioactivity by use of a scintillation crystal and appropriate electronic circuitry. **Seldinger t.,** a technique for percutaneous puncture of arteries or veins, used in angiography. **squash t.,** a method of preparing cells for chromosome study, suspending them in hypotonic solution, then incubating them and exposing them to colchicine for one hour; after fixing and staining, a drop of the stained material is placed on a glass slide and covered with a glass slip, which is then pressed against the slide with one thumb. **time diffusion t.,** a form of spinal anesthesia in which the anesthetic, of low specific gravity, is injected by lumbar puncture, with the patient in the sitting position. The anesthetic is allowed to flow upward for a measured number of seconds and then the patient is placed in the horizontal position. **Trueta t.,** see under *treatment.*

technocausis (tek″no-kaw′sis) [Gr. *technē* art + *kausis* burning] use of the actual cautery.

technologist (tek-nol′o-jist) technician.

technology (tek-nol′o-je) [Gr. *technē* art + *logos* treatise] scientific knowledge; the sum of the study of a technique.

technopsychology (tek″no-si-kol′o-je) [Gr. *technē* art + *psychology*] the psychology of the workman and his adaptation to his work.

teclozan (tek′lo-zan) chemical name: *N,N′-(* p-phenylenedimethylene) bis[2,2-dichloro-*N*-(2-ethoxyethyl)acetamide; an antiamebic, $C_{20}H_{28}Cl_4N_2O_4$.

tectocephalic (tek″to-sĕ-fal′ik) characterized by tectocephaly.

tectocephaly (tek″to-sef′ah-le) [L. *tectum* roof + Gr. *kephalē* head] scaphocephaly.

tectology (tek-tol′o-je) [Gr. *tektōn* builder + *-logy*] the science which treats of the building up of organisms from structured elements; the doctrine of structure, a division of morphology.

tectorial (tek-to′re-al) [L. *tectum* roof] of the nature of a roof or covering, as the tectorial membrane.

tectorium (tek-to′re-um), pl. *tecto′ria* [L. "roof"] membrana tectoria ductus cochlearis.

tectospinal (tek″to-spi′nal) extending from the tectum mesencephali to the spinal cord; see also under *tract.*

tectum (tek′tum) any rooflike structure. **t. mesenceph′ali** [NA], **t. of mesencephalon,** the roof of the mesencephalon: that part of the mesencephalon dorsal to the cerebral aqueduct, comprising the quadrigeminal plate and the superior and inferior colliculi.

T.E.D. threshold erythema dose.

teeth (tēth) see *tooth.*

teething (tēth′ing) the entire process which results in the eruption of the teeth.

Teflon (tef′lon) trademark for preparations of polytef (polytetrafluoroethylene). See also *polymer fume fever,* under *fever.*

teflurane (tef′loor-ān) chemical name: 2-bromo-1,1,1,2-tetrafluoroethane; an inhalation anesthetic, C_2HBrF_4.

tegmen (teg′men), pl. *teg′mina* [L. "cover"] any covering, or shelter; used in anatomical nomenclature as a general term to designate a covering structure or roof. **t. an′tri,** t. tympani. **t. cel′lulae,** t. mastoideum. **t. cra′nii,** calvaria. **t. cru′ris,** tegmentum, def. 2. **t. mastoideotympan′icum,** the tegmen mastoideum and tegmen tympani, which together roof over the mastoid cells. **t. mastoid′eum,** the bony roof of the mastoid cells. **t. tym′pani,** 1. [NA] the thin layer of translucent bone, on the petrous part of the temporal bone in the floor of the middle cranial fossa, separating the tympanic antrum from the cranial cavity; called also *roof of tympanum.* 2. paries tegmentalis cavi tympani. **t. ventric′uli quar′ti** [NA], the roof of the fourth ventricle, formed by the superior and inferior medullary vela.

tegmental (teg-men′tal) pertaining to or of the nature of a tegmen or tegmentum.

tegmentum (teg-men′tum), pl. *tegmen′ta* [L.] 1. a covering. 2. [NA] the part of the cerebral peduncle dorsal to the substantia nigra, consisting of an upward extension of the pontine tegmentum; it is made up of various nuclei, fiber tracts, and the reticular formation and is separated dorsally from the tectum by the cerebral aqueduct. **t. au′ris**, membrana tympani. **hypothalamic t.**, subthalamic t. **t. of pons, t. rhombenceph′ali** [NA], the dorsal half of the pons. **subthalamic t.**, the portion of the tegmentum of the cerebral peduncle extending beneath the thalamus.

Tegopen (teg′o-pen) trademark for preparations of cloxacillin sodium.

Tegretol (teg′rĕ-tol) trademark for preparations of carbamazepine.

Teichmann's crystals, test (tīk′mahnz) [Ludwig Carl *Teichmann*-Stawiarski, German histologist, 1825–1895] see under *crystal* and *tests*.

teichopsia (ti-kop′se-ah) [Gr. *teichos* wall + *opsis* vision + *-ia*] the sensation of a luminous appearance before the eyes, with a zigzag, wall-like outline; called also *fortification spectrum, flittering scotoma*, and *scintillating scotoma*.

T-1824 Evans blue.

teinodynia (ti″no-din′e-ah) tenodynia.

teknocyte (tek′no-sīt) [Gr. *teknon* that which is born + *kytos* cell] a young neutrophil leukocyte.

tektin (tek′tin) any of a group of insoluble structural protein having elastic properties.

tela (te′lah), pl. *te′lae* [L. "something woven," "web"] any weblike tissue; [NA] a general term for a thin membrane resembling a web. **t. ara′nea**, a spider web. **t. cellulo′sa**, t. conjunctiva. **t. choroi′dea ventric′uli latera′li**, the lateral extension of the tela choroidea ventriculi tertii into the choroid fissure of the lateral ventricle of the brain; from it, vascular folds invaginate the ventricular ependyma to form the choroid plexus of the lateral ventricle. **t. chorioi′dea ventric′uli quar′ti**, t. choroidea ventriculi quarti. **t. chorioi′dea ventric′uli ter′tii**, t. choroidea ventriculi tertii. **t. choroidea of fourth ventricle**, t. choroidea ventriculi quarti. **t. choroidea of third ventricle**, t. choroidea ventriculi tertii. **t. choroi′dea ventric′uli quar′ti** [NA], a double layer or fold of pia mater between the cerebellum and the lower part of the roof of the fourth ventricle; the anterior layer of the fold, together with the ventricular ependyma, contains vascular fringes which comprise the choroid plexus. **t. choroi′dea ventric′uli ter′tii** [NA], a double layer or fold of pia mater which, together with the ventricular ependyma, forms the roof of the third ventricle; from the lower fold two vascular fringes invaginate the roof to form the choroid plexuses. **t. conjuncti′va** [NA], a general term used to designate connective tissue. **t. elas′tica** [NA], a general term used to designate elastic tissue. **t. subcuta′nea** [NA], the layer of loose connective tissue situated directly beneath the skin; called also *hypodermis, subcutaneous fascia*, and *superficial fascia*. **t. submuco′sa** [NA], the layer of loose connective tissue between the lamina muscularis mucosae and the tunica muscularis in most parts of the digestive, respiratory, urinary, and genital tracts. **t. submuco′sa bronchio′rum** [NA], the layer of tissue underlying the tunica mucosa of the bronchi. **t. submuco′sa co′li** [NA], the layer of tissue underlying the tunica mucosa of the colon. **t. submuco′sa esoph′agi** [NA], the layer of tissue underlying the tunica mucosa of the esophagus. **t. submuco′sa intesti′ni ten′uis** [NA], the submucous layer of the wall of the small intestine. **t. submuco′sa pharyn′gis** [NA], the tissue underlying the tunica mucosa of the pharynx. **t. submuco′sa rec′ti** [NA], the submucous layer of the wall of the rectum. **t. submuco′sa tra′cheae** [NA], the tissue underlying the tunica mucosa of the trachea. **t. submuco′sa tu′bae uteri′nae**, the submucous layer of the wall of the uterus. **t. submuco′sa ventric′uli** [NA], the tissue underlying the tunica mucosa of the stomach. **t. submuco′sa vesi′cae urina′riae** [NA], the submucous layer of the wall of the urinary bladder. **t. subsero′sa** [NA], a layer of loose areolar tissue underlying the tunica serosa of various organs. **t. subsero′sa co′li** [NA], loose areolar tissue underlying the tunica serosa of the colon. **t. subsero′sa hep′atis** [NA], loose areolar tissue underlying the tunica serosa of the liver. **t. subsero′sa intesti′ni ten′uis** [NA], the subserous layer of the wall of the small intestine. **t. subsero′sa peritone′i** [NA], a web of loose areolar tissue underlying the tunica serosa of the peritoneum. **t. subsero′sa tu′bae uteri′nae** [NA], the subserous layer of the wall of the uterus; called also *tunica adventitia tubae uterinae*. **t. subsero′sa u′teri** [NA], the areolar tissue underlying the tunica serosa of the uterus. **t. subsero′sa ventric′uli** [NA], the tissue underlying the tunica serosa of the stomach. **t. subsero′sa vesi′cae fel′leae** [NA], the tissue underlying the tunica serosa of the gallbladder. **t. subsero′sa vesi′cae urina′riae** [NA], the subserous layer of the wall of the urinary bladder.

telae (te′le) [L.] plural of *tela*.

telalgia (tel-al′je-ah) pain occurring in a part distant from the lesion; referred pain.

telangiectasia (tel-an″je-ek-ta′ze-ah) [*tele-*(1) + Gr. *angeion* vessel + *ektasis* dilatation + *-ia*] a vascular lesion formed by dilatation of a group of small blood vessels, the basis for a variety of angiomas. **essential t.**, dilatations of small blood vessels. **hereditary hemorrhagic t.**, a hereditary disorder characterized by multiple small angiomas of the skin and mucous membranes, often with epistaxis or gastrointestinal bleeding and sometimes with pulmonary or hepatic arteriovenous fistula; called also *Rendu-Osler-Weber disease*. **t. lymphat′ica**, lymphangioma formed by dilatation of the lymph vessels. **t. macula′ris erupti′va per′stans**, a mild, chronic, adult form of urticaria pigmentosa, marked by unremitting macular lesions accompanied by telangiectasia and very little if any itching and redness; it may very rarely progress to systemic involvement. **spider t.**, vascular spider.

telangiectasis (tel-an″je-ek′tah-sis), pl. *telangiec′tases*. The spot formed, most commonly on the skin, by a dilated capillary or terminal artery; see *telangiectasia*. **spider t.**, a focal network of dilated capillaries, radiating from a central arteriole, seen chiefly in pregnancy and in hepatic cirrhosis.

telangiectatic (tel-an″je-ek-tat′ik) pertaining to or characterized by telangiectasia.

telangiectodes (tel-an″je-ek-to′dēz) marked by telangiectasia.

telangiitis (tel-an″je-i′tis) [*tele-*(1) + Gr. *angeion* vessel + *-itis*] inflammation of the capillaries.

telangion (tel-an′je-on) [*tele-*(1) + Gr. *angeion* vessel] a terminal artery.

telangiosis (tel″an-je-o′sis) [*tele-*(1) + Gr. *angeion* vessel + *-osis*] any disease of the capillary vessels.

telar (te′lar) pertaining to, affecting or resembling tela.

Teldrin (tel′drin) trademark for a preparation of chlorpheniramine maleate.

tele- 1. [Gr. *telos* end] a combining form denoting relation to the end. 2. [Gr. *tēle* far off, at a distance] a combining form meaning operating at a distance, or far away.

telebinocular (tel″ĕ-bi-nok′u-lar) a prism-refracting instrument for use in orthoptic training.

telecanthus (tel″e-kan′thus) [*tele-*(1) + L.; Gr. *kanthos* canthus] abnormally increased distance between the medial canthi of the eyelids.

telecardiogram (tel″ĕ-kar′de-o-gram) the tracing obtained by telecardiography.

telecardiography (tel″ĕ-kar′de-og′rah-fe) [*tele-*(2) + Gr. *kardia* heart + *graphein* to write] the recording of an electrocardiogram by transmission of impulses to a site at a distance from the patient.

telecardiophone (tel″ĕ-kar′de-o-fōn″) [*tele-*(2) + Gr. *kardia* heart + *phōnē* voice] an apparatus for rendering heart sounds audible to listeners at a distance from the patient.

teleceptive (tel″ĕ-sep″tiv) pertaining to a teleceptor.

teleceptor (tel″ĕ-sep″tor) [*tele-*(2) + *receptor*] a sensory nerve terminal which is sensitive to stimuli originating at a distance; such nerve endings exist in the eyes, ears, and nose.

telecinesia (tel″ĕ-si-ne′ze-ah) telekinesis.

telecinesis (tel″ĕ-si-ne′sis) telekinesis.

telecord (tel′ĕ-kord) an apparatus for attachment to an x-ray machine; by means of it each cardiac phase can be photographed in series.

telecurietherapy (tel″ĕ-ku″re-ther′ah-pe) [*tele-*(2) + *curietherapy*] treatment with a radioactive source, e.g., radium, located at a distance from the body.

teledactyl (tel″ĕ-dak′til) [*tele-*(2) + Gr. *daktylos* finger] an appliance for picking up objects from the ground without stooping; used in spinal diseases.

teledendrite, teledendron (tel″ĕ-den′drīt′, tel″ĕ-den′dron) telodendron.

telediagnosis (tel″ĕ-di″ag-no′sis) [*tele-*(1) + *diagnosis*] determination of the nature of a disease at a site remote from the patient on the basis of transmitted telemonitoring data or closed-circuit television consultation.

telefluoroscopy (tel″e-floo″or-os′ko-pe) [*tele-*(2) + *fluoroscopy*] television transmission of fluoroscopic images for observation and study at a distant location.

telegony (tĕ-leg′o-ne) [*tele-*(2) + Gr. *gonē* offspring] the alleged appearance in the offspring of one sire of characteristics derived from a previous sire to whom the dam has borne offspring.

telekinesis (tel″ĕ-ki-ne′sis) [*tele-*(2) + Gr. *kinēsis* movement] the power claimed by certain persons of moving objects without contact with the object moved; also motion produced without contact with a moving body.

telekinetic (tel″ĕ-ki-net′ik) pertaining to telekinesis.

telelectrocardiogram (tel″ĕ-lek″tro-kar′de-o-gram) telecardiogram.

telelectrocardiograph (tel″e-lek″tro-kar′de-o-graf) [*tele-*(2) +

electrocardiograph] a device for transmission and remote reception of electrocardiographic signals.

telemedicine (tel″e-med′ĭ-sin) [*tele-*(1) + *medicine*] the provision of consultant services by off-site physicians to health care professionals on the scene, as by means of closed-circuit television.

telemetry (tĕ-lem′e-tre) [*tele-*(2) + Gr. *metron* measure] the making of measurements at a distance from the subject, the measurable evidence of the phenomena under investigation being transmitted by radio signals. See *radioelectrocardiography* and *radioencephalography.*

telemnemonike (tel″ĕ-ne-mon′ĭ-ke) [*tele-*(2) + Gr. *mnēmonikos* pertaining to memory] the gaining of consciousness of things in the memory of another person.

telencephal (tel-en′sĕ-fal) telencephalon.

telencephalic (tel″en-sĕ-fal′ik) pertaining to the telencephalon.

telencephalization (tel″en-sef″al-i-za′shun) the transfer to the telencephalon, during the process of evolution, of the direction of the more complex nerve reactions.

telencephalon (tel″en-sef′ah-lon) [*tele-*(1) + Gr. *enkephalos* brain] 1. [NA] the paired cerebral vesicles, which are the anterolateral evaginations of the prosencephalon, together with the median, unpaired portion, the lamina terminalis; from it the cerebral hemispheres are derived. See Plate accompanying *brain.* 2. the anterior of the two vesicles formed by specialization of the prosencephalon in the developing embryo. Called also *endbrain.*

teleneurite (tel″ĕ-nu′rīt) the end expansion of an axon.

teleneuron (tel″ĕ-nu′ron) [*tele-*(1) + Gr. *neuron* nerve] a nerve ending.

teleological (te″le-o-loj′ĭ-kal) 1. pertaining to teleology. 2. serving an ultimate purpose in development.

teleology (tel″e-ol′o-je) [*tele-*(1) + Gr. *logos* treatise] the doctrine of final causes, or of adaptation to a definite purpose.

teleomitosis (tel″e-o-mi-to′sis) [*tele-*(1) + *mitosis*] completed mitosis.

teleonomic (tel″e-o-nom′ik) pertaining to or having evolutionary survival value.

teleonomy (tel″e-on′o-me) [*teleo-* + Gr. *nomos*, law] the doctrine that the existence of a structure or a function in an organism implies that it has had evolutionary survival value.

teleopsia (tel″e-op′se-ah) [*tele-* + Gr. *opsis* vision] a visual disturbance in which objects appear to be farther away than they actually are.

teleorganic (tel″e-or-gan′ik) necessary to life.

teleoroentgenogram (tel″e-o-rent-gen′o-gram) teleroentgenogram.

teleoroentgenography (tel″e-o-rent″gen-og′rah-fe) teleroentgenography.

teleost (tel′e-ost) a member of the Teleostei, comprising the higher bony fishes.

teleotherapeutics (tel″e-o-ther″ah-pu′tiks) [*tele-*(2) + *therapeutics*] (*obs.*) suggestive therapeutics.

Telepaque (tel′ĕ-pāk) trademark for a preparation of iopanoic acid.

telepathist (tĕ-lep′ah-thist) a professed mindreader.

telepathize (tĕ-lep′ah-thīz) to affect by sympathetic or other subtle means.

telepathy (tĕ-lep′ah-the) [*tele-*(2) + Gr. *pathos* feeling] extrasensory perception of the mental activity of another person. Cf. *clairvoyance.*

teleradiography (tel″ĕ-ra″de-og′rah-fe) radiography with the radiation source 6 to 7 feet from the subject.

teleradium (tel″ĕ-ra′de-um) [*tele-*(2) + *radium*] a radium source located at a distance from the body.

telergic (tel-er′jik) acting at a distance; pertaining to telergy.

telergy (tel′er-je) [*tele-*(2) + Gr. *ergon* work] 1. automatism. 2. a hypothetical action of one brain on another at a distance.

teleroentgenogram (tel″ĕ-rent-gen′o-gram) the picture or film obtained by teleroentgenography.

teleroentgenography (tel″ĕ-rent″gen-og′rah-fe) roentgenography with the x-ray tube 6½ to 7 feet away from the plate in order more nearly to secure parallelism of the rays.

teleroentgentherapy (tel″ĕ-rent″gen-ther′ah-pe) treatment with ionizing radiations from an x-ray source located at a distance from the body.

Telesphorus (tĕ-les′fo-rus) [Gr. *telesphoros* bringing to an end] the god of convalescence, a deity worshipped in company with Æsculapius, the god of healing, and Hygeia, the goddess of health.

telesthesia (tel″es-the′ze-ah) [*tele-*(2) + Gr. *aisthēsis* perception + *-ia*] telepathy; perception at a distance.

telesthetoscope (tel″es-thet′o-skōp) [*tele-*(2) + Gr. *aisthēsis* perception + *skopein* to examine] a combination of stethoscope and electrical amplification by which persons at a distance from the patient can hear the heart and lung sounds, as in demonstrating to a class or a medical audience.

telesyphilis (tel″ĕ-sif′ĭ-lis) metasyphilis, def. 1.

teletactor (tel″ĕ-tak′tor) [*tele-*(2) + L. *tangere* to touch] an instrument for communicating with the deaf by means of touch on a vibrating plate.

teletherapy (tel″ĕ-ther′ah-pe) [*tele-*(2) + Gr. *therapeia* treatment] treatment in which the source of the therapeutic agent, e.g., radiation, is at a distance from the body, as contrasted to contact therapy or brachytherapy.

telethermometer (tel″ĕ-ther-mom′ĕ-ter) an apparatus for determining temperature on which the reading is made at a distance from the object or subject being studied.

tellurate (tel′u-rāt) any salt of telluric acid.

telluric (tĕ-lu′rik) 1. pertaining to or originating from the earth. 2. pertaining to the element tellurium.

tellurism (tel′u-rizm) [L. *tellus* earth] the alleged production of disease by emanations from the earth or soil (telluric effluvium, or miasma).

tellurite (tel′u-rīt) any salt of tellurous acid.

tellurium (tĕ-lu′re-um) [L. *tellus* earth] a nonmetallic or metalloid element; symbol, Te; specific gravity, 6.24; atomic weight, 127.60; atomic number, 52.

Tellyesniczky's fluid (mixture) (tel″yets-nits′kēz) [Kálmár *Tellyesniczky*, Budapest anatomist, 1868–1932] see under *fluid.*

telo- [Gr. *telos* end] a combining form denoting relationship to an end.

telobiosis (tel″o-bi-o′sis) [*telo-* + Gr. *biōsis* way of life] the end-to-end union of embryos through operative procedures.

telocentric (tel″o-sen′trik) having the centromere at the extreme end of the replicating chromosome, so that the chromosome consists of only one arm.

telocinesia, telocinesis (tel″o-si-ne′se-ah; tel″o-si-ne′sis) telophase.

telocoele (tel′o-sēl) [*telo-* + Gr. *koilia* cavity] the cavity of the telencephalon.

telodendria (tel″o-den′dre-ah) plural of telodendrion.

telodendrion (tel″o-den′dre-on), pl. *teloden′dria.* Telodendron.

telodendron (tel″o-den′dron) [*telo-* + Gr. *dendron* tree] one of the many fine twiglike terminal branches of a neuron.

telogen (tel′o-jen) the quiescent, or resting, phase of the hair cycle, following catagen, the hair having become a club hair and not growing further.

teloglia (tel-og′lĭ-ah) terminal Schwann cells associated with the motor nerve endings.

telognosis (tel″og-no′sis) [*tele* + *otelephonic* dia*gnosis*] diagnosis based on interpretation of roentgenograms transmitted by telephonic or radio communication.

telokinesis (tel″o-ki-ne′sis) [*telo-* + Gr. *kinēsis* motion] telophase.

telolecithal (tel″o-les′ĭ-thal) [*telo-* + Gr. *lekithos* yolk] having the yolk concentrated toward one pole which, because of that concentration, is designated the vegetal pole. See under *ovum.* Cf. *eutelolecithal.*

telolemma (tel″o-lem′ah) [*telo-* + Gr. *lemma* rind] the twofold covering of a motor end-plate, made up of sarcolemma and an extension of Henle's sheath.

telomere (tel′o-mēr) [*telo-* + Gr. *meros* part] a term applied to each of the extremities of a chromosome, which possess special properties, among them a polarity which prevents their reunion with any fragment after a chromosome has been broken.

telophase (tel′o-fāz) [*telo-* + Gr. *phasis* phase] the last of the four stages of mitosis and of the two divisions of meiosis; it begins when the chromosomes arrive at the poles of the cell and the division of the cytoplasm starts. In plant cells the new cell wall that separates the daughter cells begins to form during this stage.

telophragma (tel″o-frag′mah) [*telo-* + Gr. *phragmos* a fencing in] a name given to the Z band; see also *inophragma.*

teloreceptor (te″lo-re-sep′tor) teleceptor.

telorism (tel′o-rizm) see *hypertelorism.*

telosynapsis (tel″o-sĭ-nap′sis) [*telo-* + Gr. *synapsis* conjunction] the union of chromosomes end to end during meiosis. Cf. *parasynapsis.*

telotaxis (tel″o-tak′sis) the tendency of an organism to maintain a constant angle to the source of a stimulus while it moves; observed in the behavior of social insects, such as bees and ants.

telotism (tel′o-tizm) 1. the complete performance of a function. 2. a complete erection of the penis.

telson (tel′son) an appendage on the terminal segment of some arthropods, especially the stinging organ of a scorpion.

TEM triethylenemelamine.

Temaril (tem′ah-ril) trademark for preparations of trimeprazine tartrate.

temazepam (tĕ-maz′ĕ-pam) chemical name: 7-chloro-1,3-dihydro-3-hydroxy-1-methyl-5-phenyl-2*H*-1,4-benzodiazepin-2-one; a minor tranquilizer, $C_{16}H_{13}ClN_2O_2$.

temefos (tem′ĕ-fos) chemical name: *O,O′-*(thiodi-4,1-phenylene)

O,O,O′,O′-trimethyl ester phosphorothioic acid; an organophosphorus insecticide, $C_{16}H_{20}O_6P_2S_3$, used as a veterinary ectoparasiticide.

Temin (te′min) Howard. American biologist, born 1935; co-winner, with David Baltimore and Renato Dulbecco, of the Nobel prize in medicine and physiology for 1975, for discoveries concerning the interaction between tumor viruses and the genetic material of host cells and the role of reverse transcriptase.

temodex (tem′o-deks) chemical name: 2-hydroxyethyl ester 3-methyl-2-quinoxalinecarboxylic acid 1,4-dioxide; a veterinary growth stimulant, $C_{12}H_{12}N_2O_5$.

temp. dext. abbreviation for L. *tem′pori dex′tro*, to the right temple.

temperament (tem′per-ah-ment) [L. *temperamentum* mixture] the peculiar physical character and mental cast of an individual. **atrabilious t.**, melancholic t. **bilious t.**, that characterized by a dark or sallow complexion, black hair, and a slow or moderate circulation of the blood. **choleric t.**, bilious t. **lymphatic t.**, one characterized by a fair but not ruddy complexion, light hair, and a general softness or laxity of the tissues. It results, according to the old physiologists, from the predominance of lymph or phlegm in the system. **melancholic t.**, one characterized by a predominance of *black bile* (which was supposed to be secreted by the spleen), rendering the disposition melancholic and morose, and, when in great excess, producing hypochondriasis. **nervous t.**, one characterized by the predominance of the nervous element, and by great activity or susceptibility of the great nervous center, the brain. **phlegmatic t.**, lymphatic t. **sanguine t., sanguineous t.**, one characterized by fair and ruddy complexion, yellow, red, or light auburn hair, a full, muscular development, large, full veins, and an active pulse, all indicating an abundant supply of blood.

temperantia (tem′per-an′she-ah) sedatives.

temperature (tem′per-ah-tūr) [L. *temperatura*] the degree of sensible heat or cold; the property of a system that determines whether or not the system is in thermal equilibrium with other systems; a measure of the escaping tendency of heat from a system. **absolute t.**, temperature reckoned from absolute zero (−273.15° C. or −459.67° F.), expressed on an absolute scale (Kelvin or Rankine). **body t.**, the temperature of the body: in cold-blooded animals it varies with environmental temperature; in warm-blooded animals it is usually constant within a narrow range. See *normal t.* **body t., basal,** the temperature of the body under conditions of absolute rest. Abbreviated B.B.T. **critical t.**, a temperature below which a gas may be liquefied by increased pressure. **maximum t.**, in bacteriology, the temperature above which growth does not take place. **mean t.**, the average temperature in a locality for a given period of time. **minimum t.**, in bacteriology, temperature below which growth does not take place. **normal t.**, that of the human body in health, about 98.6° F. or 37° C. when measured orally. This is maintained by the thermotaxic nerve mechanism, which maintains a balance between the thermogenetic, or heat-producing, and the thermolytic, or heat-dispelling, processes. **optimum t.**, the temperature promoting the most rapid growth of a given species of microorganism. **room t.**, the ordinary temperature of a room, 65°–80° F. **sub-normal t.**, temperature below the normal.

template (tem′plat) a pattern or mold. In dentistry, a curved or flat plate used as an aid in setting teeth for a denture. In theoretical immunology, an antigen that determines the configuration of combining (antigen-binding) sites of antibody molecules. In genetics, a strand of DNA which specifies the synthesis of a complementary strand of RNA (mRNA), which in turn serves as a template for the synthesis of nucleic acids or proteins. **surgical t.**, a thin plate of transparent resin shaped to duplicate the surface of an impression for an immediate denture and used as a guide in surgically shaping the alveolar process of the jaw to fit the prosthesis.

temple (tem′p'l) [L. *tempula*, dim. of *tempora*, pl. of *tempus*] the lateral region on either side of the upper part of the head; see *tempora*.

tempolabile (tem″po-la′bīl) [L. *tempus* time + *labilis* unstable] subject to change with the passage of time.

tempora (tem′po-rah) [L., pl. of *tempus*] [NA] the temples: the region on either side of the head, above the zygomatic arch.

temporal (tem′po-ral) [L. *temporalis*] 1. pertaining to the lateral region of the head, above the zygomatic arch. 2. pertaining to time; limited as to time; temporary.

temporalis (tem-po-ra′lis) [L.] pertaining to the lateral region of the head, above the zygomatic arch.

temporoauricular (tem″po-ro-aw-rik′u-lar) pertaining to the temporal and auricular regions.

temporofacial (tem″po-ro-fa′shal) pertaining to a temple and the face.

temporofrontal (tem″po-ro-fron′tal) pertaining to the temporal and frontal bones or regions.

temporohyoid (tem″po-ro-hi′oid) pertaining to the temporal and hyoid bones.

temporomalar (tem″po-ro-ma′lar) temporozygomatic.

temporomandibular (tem″po-ro-man-dib′u-lar) pertaining to the temporal bone and the mandible.

temporomaxillary (tem″po-ro-mak′sĭ-ler″e) pertaining to the temporal bone, or region, and the maxilla.

temporo-occipital (tem″po-ro-oks-ip′ĭ-tal) pertaining to the temporal and occipital bones or regions.

temporoparietal (tem″po-ro-pah-ri′ĕ-tal) pertaining to the temporal and parietal bones or regions.

temporopontile (tem″po-ro-pon′tĭl) pertaining to or connecting the temporal lobe and the pons.

temporospatial (tem″po-ro-spa′shal) [L. *tempus* time + *spatium* space] pertaining to both time and space.

temporosphenoid (tem″po-ro-sfe′noid) pertaining to the temporal and sphenoid bones.

temporozygomatic (tem″po-ro-zi″go-mat′ik) pertaining to the temporal and zygomatic bones, or to the region of the zygomatic arch.

tempostabile (tem″po-sta′bĭl) [L. *tempus* time + *stabilis* stable] not subject to change with the passage of time.

Tempra (tem′prah) trademark for preparations of acetaminophen.

temp. sinist. abbreviation for L. *tem′pori sinis′tro*, to the left temple.

temulence (tem′u-lens) [L. *temulentia*] drunkenness; intoxication.

temuline (tem′u-lēn) an alkaloid contained in seeds of darnel (*Lolium temulentum*) and at one time said to be toxic, though subsequent investigators have said the seeds are not toxic; the question is not yet settled.

tenacious (te-na′shus) [L. *tenax*] holding fast; adhesive.

tenacity (te-nas′ĭ-te) the quality of being tenacious; toughness; the condition of being tough. **cellular t.**, the inherent tendency of all cells to persist in a given form or direction of activity.

tenaculum (te-nak′u-lum) [L.] 1. a hooklike instrument for seizing and holding tissues. 2. any fibrous band for maintaining structures in place. **t. ten′dinum**, retinaculum tendinum.

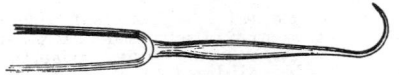

Tenaculum (Da Costa).

tenalgia (te-nal′je-ah) [Gr. *tenōn* tendon + *algos* pain + *-ia*] pain in a tendon.

tenderness (ten′der-nes) abnormal sensitiveness to touch or pressure. **pencil t.**, local tenderness on pressure with the rubber tip of a pencil. **rebound t.**, a sensation of pain felt on the release of pressure.

tendines (ten′dĭ-nēz) plural of *tendo*.

tendinitis (ten″dĭ-ni′tis) inflammation of tendons and of tendon-muscle attachments. **calcific t.**, inflammation and calcification of the subacromial or subdeltoid bursa, resulting in pain, tenderness, and limitation of motion in the shoulder. Called also *calcific bursitis* and *scapulohumeral bursitis*. **t. of horse**, inflammation of the flexor tendons, due to strain of wrenching, and causing great tenderness and lameness. **t. ossif′icans traumat′ica**, a condition in which areas of ossification develop in tendons as a result of trauma. **t. steno′sans, stenosing t.**, stenosing tendovaginitis of the flexor tendons of the finger.

tendinoplasty (ten′dĭ-no-plas″te) [L. *tendo* tendon + Gr. *plassein* to mold] the plastic surgery of the tendons.

tendinosuture (ten″dĭ-no-su′tūr) [L. *tendo* tendon + *sutura* sewing] the suturing of a tendon.

tendinous (ten′dĭ-nus) [L. *tendinosus*] pertaining to, resembling, or of the nature of a tendon.

tendo (ten′do), pl. *ten′dines* [L.] [NA] tendon: a fibrous cord of connective tissue in which the fibers of a muscle end and by which the muscle is attached to a bone or other structure. **t. Achil′lis**, NA alternative for *t. calcaneus*. **t. calca′neus** [NA], calcaneal tendon: a powerful tendon at the back of the heel which attaches the triceps surae muscle to the tuberosity of the calcaneus; called also *tendo Achillis* or *Achilles tendon*. **t. conjunc′vus**, NA alternative for *falx inguinalis*. **t. cordifor′mis**, centrum tendineum. **t. cricoesopha′geus** [NA], cricoesophageal tendon: the tendon giving origin to the longitudinal fibers of the esophagus that come from the upper part of the lamina of the cricoid cartilage. **t. oc′uli, t. palpebra′rum**, ligamentum palpebrale mediale.

tendolysis (ten-dol′ĭ-sis) [L. *tendo* tendon + Gr. *lysis* dissolution] tenolysis.

tendomucin (ten″do-mu′sin) a mucin derivable from tendons and closely related to submaxillary mucin.

tendon (ten′dun) [L. *tendo*; Gr. *tenōn*] a fibrous cord by which a muscle is attached; see *tendo*. **Achilles t.**, tendo calcaneus. **calcaneal t.**, tendo calcaneus. **central t. of diaphragm**, centrum tendineum. **central t. of perineum**, centrum tendineum perinei. **common t.**, a tendon that serves more than one muscle. **conjoined t.,** falx inguinalis. **cordiform t. of diaphragm,** centrum tendineum. **coronary t's,** two fibrous rings, one surrounding the cardiac orifice of the aorta and the other the pulmonary trunk orifice; see *anuli fibrosi cordis.* **cricoesophageal t.,** tendo cricoesophageus. **hamstring t.,** see *hamstring.* **t. of Hector, heel t.,** tendo calcaneus. **intermediate t. of diaphragm,** centrum tendineum. **kangaroo t.,** the prepared tendon from the tail of certain species of kangaroo, used as a material for sutures or ligatures. **membranaceous t.,** aponeurosis. **patellar t., anterior, patellar t., inferior,** ligamentum patellae. **pulled t.,** disruption of the fibers attaching a muscle to its point of origin, occurring as the result of unusual muscular effort. **riders' t.,** injury to the adductor tendons of the thigh incurred in horseback riding. **slipped t.,** perosis. **trefoil t.,** centrum tendineum. **t. of Zinn,** zonula ciliaris.

tendonitis (ten″do-ni′tis) tendinitis.

tendoplasty (ten′do-plas″te) [L. *tendo* tendon + Gr. *plassein* to mold] plastic surgery of the tendons.

tendosynovitis (ten″do-sin″o-vi′tis) tenosynovitis.

tendotome (ten′do-tōm) tenotome.

tendotomy (ten-dot′o-me) tenotomy.

tendovaginal (ten″do-vaj′ĭ-nal) [L. *tendo* tendon + *vagina* sheath] pertaining to a tendon and its sheath.

tendovaginitis (ten″do-vaj″ĭ-ni′tis) 1. inflammation of a tendon and its sheath. 2. tenosynovitis.

tenebrimycin (tĕ-neb″rĭ-mi′sin) tobramycin.

tenectomy (te-nek′to-me) [Gr. *tenōn* tendon + *ektomē* excision] excision of a lesion of a tendon or a tendon sheath.

tenemycin (ten″ĕ-mi′sin) tobramycin.

tenesmic (te-nez′mik) pertaining to or of the nature of tenesmus.

tenesmus (te-nez′mus) [L.; Gr. *teinesmos*] straining, especially ineffectual and painful straining at stool or in urination. **rectal t.,** painful, long-continued, and ineffective straining at stool. **vesical t.,** that which sometimes accompanies urination.

ten Horn see *Horn.*

tenia (te′ne-ah), pl. *te′niae* [L. "a flat band," "bandage," "tape"] 1. [NA] a flat band or strip of soft tissue; called also *taenia.* 2. taenia (def. 2). **te′niae acus′ticae,** striae medullares ventriculi quarti. **t. choroi′dea** [NA], the line of attachment of the lateral choroid plexus to the medial wall of the cerebral hemisphere; specifically, the line of attachment of the ependyma of the ventricle to the ependyma of the choroid plexus. **te′niae co′li** [NA], three thickened bands, about ⅓ inch wide and one-sixth shorter than the colon, formed by the longitudinal fibers in the muscular tunic of the large intestine and extending from the root of the vermiform appendix to the rectum, where the fibers spread out and form a continuous layer encircling the tube: they include the *t. libera, t. mesocolica,* and *t. omentalis.* **t. for′nicis** [NA], **t. of fornix,** the line of attachment of the choroid plexus of the lateral ventricle to the fornix, including the line of its attachment to the fimbria of the hippocampus (taenia fimbriae). **t. of fourth ventricle,** t. ventriculi quarti. **t. li′bera** [NA], the thickened band formed by anterior longitudinal muscle fibers of the large intestine, almost equidistant from the tenia mesocolica and the tenia omentalis. **t. mesocol′ica** [NA], the thickened band of longitudinal muscle fibers of the large intestine along the site of attachment of the mesocolon. **t. omenta′lis** [NA], the band of longitudinal muscle fibers of the large intestine along the site of attachment of the greater omentum. **t. plex′us choroi′dei ventric′uli quar′ti, t. si′nus rhomboi′deae,** t. ventriculi quarti. **t. te′lae** [NA], the line of attachment of the ependymal cells of the choroid plexus to various portions of the brain; called also *taenia telarum.* **t. thal′ami** [NA], **t. of thalamus,** the line of attachment of the ependymal cells of the roof of the third ventricle to the dorsal margin of the thalamus. **t. of third ventricle,** t. thalami. **t. ventric′uli quar′ti** [NA], tenia of fourth ventricle: the line of attachment of the ependymal cells of the choroid plexus to the ependyma along the edge of the caudal part of the fourth ventricle. **t. ventric′uli ter′tii,** t. thalami.

teniacide (te′ne-ah-sīd″) taeniacide.

teniae (te′ne-e) plural of *tenia.*

teniafugal (ten″e-ah-fu′gal) taeniafugal.

teniafuge (te′ne-ah-fūj″) taeniafuge.

tenial (te′ne-al) 1. pertaining to tenia of anatomical nomenclature. 2. taenial (def. 1).

teniamyotomy (te″ne-ah-mi-ot′o-me) an operation involving a series of transverse incisions of the teniae coli; done in diverticular disease.

teniasis (te-ni′ah-sis) taeniasis.

tenicide (ten′ĭ-sīd) taeniacide.

teniform (ten′ĭ-form) taeniform.

tenifugal (te-nif′u-gal) taeniafugal.

tenifuge (ten′ĭ-fūj) taeniafuge.

tenioid (te′ne-oid) taeniform.

teniola (te-ne′o-lah) [L. *taeniola*] a thin, grayish ridge which separates the striae of the floor of the fourth ventricle from the cochlear part of the acoustic nerve; called also *taeni′ola cine′rea.*

teniotoxin (te″ne-o-tok′sin) a poisonous principle occurring in tapeworms.

tennis thumb (ten′is) tendinitis of the tendon of the long flexor muscle of the thumb, with calcification.

teno-, tenonto- [Gr. *tenōn, tenontos* tendon] combining form denoting relationship to a tendon.

tenodesis (ten-od′ĕ-sis) [*teno-* + Gr. *desis* a binding together] tendon fixation; suturing of the end of a tendon to a bone.

tenodynia (ten″o-din′e-ah) [*teno-* + Gr. *odynē* pain] pain in a tendon.

tenofibril (ten′o-fi″bril) tonofibril.

tenolysis (ten-ol′ĭ-sis) [*teno-* + Gr. *lysis* dissolution] the operation of freeing a tendon from adhesions; called also *tendolysis.*

tenomyoplasty (ten″o-mi′o-plas″te) [*teno-* + Gr. *mys* muscle + *plassein* to form] a plastic operation involving tendon and muscle.

tenomyotomy (ten″o-mi-ot′o-me) [*teno-* + Gr. *mys* muscle + *tomē* a cutting] excision of a portion of tendon and muscle.

Tenon's capsule (fascia, membrane), space (te′nonz) [Jacques René *Tenon,* French surgeon, 1724–1816] see *vagina bulbi* and *spatium intervaginale.*

tenonectomy (ten″o-nek′to-me) [*teno-* + Gr. *ektomē* excision] excision of a part of a tendon for the purpose of shortening it.

tenonitis (ten″o-ni′tis) 1. tendinitis. 2. inflammation of Tenon's capsule.

tenonometer (ten″o-nom′ĕ-ter) [Gr. *teinein* to stretch + *metron* measure] an apparatus for measuring intraocular tension.

tenonostosis (ten″on-os-to′sis) tenostosis.

tenontagra (ten″on-ta′grah, ten-on′tag-rah) [*tenonto-* + Gr. *agra* seizure] a gouty affection of the tendons.

tenontitis (ten″on-ti′tis) inflammation of a tendon; tendinitis. **t. prolif′era calca′rea,** tendinitis.

tenonto- see *teno-.*

tenontodynia (ten″on-to-din′e-ah) [*tenonto-* + Gr. *odynē* pain + *-ia*] pain in the tendons.

tenontography (ten″on-tog′rah-fe) [*tenonto-* + Gr. *graphein* to write] a written description or delineation of the tendons.

tenontolemmitis (ten-on″to-lem-mi′tis) [*tenonto-* + Gr. *lemma* rind + *-itis*] tenosynovitis.

tenontology (ten″on-tol′o-je) the sum of what is known regarding the tendons.

tenontomyoplasty (ten-on″to-mi′o-plas″te) tenomyoplasty.

tenontomyotomy (ten-on″to-mi-ot′o-me) tenomyotomy.

tenontophyma (ten-on″to-fi′mah) [*tenonto-* + Gr. *phyma* growth] a tumorous growth in a tendon.

tenontoplasty (ten-on′to-plas″te) tenoplasty.

tenontothecitis (ten-on″to-the-si′tis) [*tenonto-* + Gr. *thēkē* sheath + *-itis*] inflammation of a tendon sheath.

tenontotomy (ten″on-tot′o-me) tenotomy.

tenophyte (ten′o-fīt) [*teno-* + Gr. *phyton* growth] a growth or concretion in a tendon.

tenoplastic (ten″o-plas′tik) of or relating to tenoplasty.

tenoplasty (ten′o-plas″te) [*teno-* + Gr. *plassein* to shape] plastic surgery of the tendons; operative repair of a defect in a tendon.

tenoreceptor (ten″o-re-sep′tor) [*teno-* + *receptor*] a proprioceptor situated in tendon; such receptors are stimulated by contraction.

tenorrhaphy (ten-or′ah-fe) [*teno-* + Gr. *rhaphē* suture] the union of a divided tendon by a suture.

tenositis (ten″o-si′tis) tendinitis.

tenostosis (ten″os-to′sis) [*teno-* + Gr. *osteon* bone + *-osis*] ossification of a tendon.

tenosuture (ten″o-su′tūr) [*teno-* + L. *sutura* suture] tenorrhaphy.

tenosynitis (ten″o-si-ni′tis) tendovaginitis.

tenosynovectomy (ten″o-sin″o-vek′to-me) excision or resection of a tendon sheath.

tenosynovitis (ten″o-sin″o-vi′tis) inflammation of a tendon sheath. **t. acu′ta purulen′ta,** tenosynovitis with pus formation. **adhesive t.,** tenosynovitis in which the tendons become bound in an inflammatory mass. **t. crep′itans,** a form accompanied by a crackling sound in the soft tissues on movement. **gonococcic t., gonorrheal t.,** tenosynovitis due to metastatic gonococcal infection. **t. granulo′sa,** tuberculosis of tendon sheaths, which become filled with granulation tissue. **t. hypertroph′ica,** a condition marked by swellings along the tendons and their sheaths. **nodular t.,** giant cell tumor of tendon sheath; see under *tumor.* **t. sero′sa chron′ica,** tenosynovitis with serous effusion. **t. steno′sans,** a painful condition of the wrist, marked by thickening and narrowing of the tendon sheath of the extensor brevis and abductor longus pollicis (De Quervain). **tuberculous t.,** chronic tuberculous infection of tendon sheaths and bursae. **villonodular t.,** a condition characterized by exaggerated proliferation of synovial membrane cells, producing a solid tumor-like mass, commonly occurring in periarticular soft tissues and less frequently in joints. **villous t.,** chronic infection of tendon sheaths and bursa, with proliferation of villous projections from the surface of the membranes.

tenotome (ten'o-tōm) a cutting instrument used in tenotomy.

tenotomize (ten-ot'o-mīz) to perform tenotomy.

tenotomy (ten-ot'o-me) [*teno-* + Gr. *tomē* a cutting] the cutting of a tendon as for strabismus or clubfoot. **curb t.,** the operation of cutting an eye muscle in squint and inserting it farther back on the globe of the eye. **graduated t.,** the incomplete division of a tendon.

tenovaginitis (ten"o-vaj"ĭ-ni'tis) inflammation of a tendon sheath; tenosynovitis.

tense (tens) drawn tight; rigid.

Tensilon (ten'sĭ-lon) trademark for a solution of edrophonium chloride.

tensio-active (ten"se-o-ak'tiv) having an effect on surface tension.

tensiometer (ten"se-om'ĕ-ter) [*tension* + Gr. *metron* measure] an apparatus for measuring the surface tension of liquids.

tension (ten'shun) [L. *tensio;* Gr. *tonos*] 1. the act of stretching. 2. the condition of being stretched or strained; the degree to which anything is stretched or strained. 3. voltage. 4. the partial pressure of a gas in a fluid, e.g., of oxygen in blood. **arterial t.,** blood pressure within an artery; intra-arterial pressure. **electric t.,** electromotive force. **interfacial surface t.,** the tension or resistance to separation possessed by the film of liquid between two well-adapted surfaces, as by the thin film of saliva between the denture base and the tissues. **intraocular t.,** see under *pressure.* **intravenous t.,** venous pressure. **muscular t.,** the condition of moderate contraction produced by stretching a muscle. **oxygen t.,** that concentration of dissolved oxygen at which its partial pressure is in equilibrium with the liquid (solvent). **premenstrual t.,** a syndrome sometimes occurring during the ten days preceding menstruation, marked by emotional instability, irritability, insomnia, and headache. There may also be pain in the breasts, abdominal distention, bearing-down pelvic discomfort, nausea, anorexia, constipation, urinary frequency, and general weakness. Called also *premenstrual syndrome.* **surface t.,** the tension or resistance which acts to preserve the integrity of a surface, such as the tension or resistance to rupture possessed by the surface film of a liquid, or the tension or strain upon the surface of a liquid in contact with another substance with which it does not mix. **tissue t.,** a state of equilibrium between tissues and cells which prevents overaction of any part. **wall t.,** the circumferential stretching force in a vessel wall, usually expressed as a function of intraluminal pressure and the radius according to the Laplace equation.

tensometer (tens-om'ĕ-ter) an apparatus by which the tensile strength of materials can be determined.

tensor (ten'sor) [L., "stretcher," "puller"] any muscle that stretches or makes tense.

tent (tent) [L. *tenta,* from *tendere* to stretch] 1. a covering of fabric designed to enclose an open space, especially such an arrangement over a patient's bed for the purpose of administering oxygen or vaporized medication by inhalation. 2. a conical and expansible plug of soft material, as lint, gauze, etc., for dilating an orifice or for keeping a wound open, so as to prevent its healing except at the bottom. **oxygen t.,** a tent erected over a bed into which a constant flow of oxygen can be maintained. **sponge t.,** a slender, cone-shaped piece of compressed sponge used for dilating the os uteri. **steam t.,** a tent erected over a bed into which steam is passed; used in certain respiratory conditions.

tentacle (ten'tah-k'l) a slender whiplike appendage in animals that may function in prehension and feeding or as a sense organ.

tentative (ten'tah-tiv) experimental and subject to change.

tenthmeter (tenth-me'ter) one ten-millionth of a meter.

tentoria (ten-to're-ah) plural of *tentorium.*

tentorial (ten-to're-al) pertaining to the tentorium of the cerebellum.

tentorium (ten-to're-um), pl. *tento'ria* [L. "tent"] an anatomical part resembling a tent or a covering. **t. cerebel'li** [NA], **t. of cerebellum,** the process of dura mater that supports the occipital lobes and covers the cerebellum. Its internal border is free and bounds the tentorial notch; its external border is attached to the skull and encloses the transverse sinus behind. **t. of hypophysis,** diaphragma sellae.

tentum (ten'tum) the penis.

Tenuate (ten'u-āt) trademark for preparations of diethylpropion hydrochloride.

tenulin (ten'u-lin) a crystalline principle, $C_{17}H_{22}O_5$, from the bitter weed, *Helenium tenuifolium,* and other species that is mildly sternutatory and poisonous to fish.

Tepanil (tep'ah-nil) trademark for preparations of diethylpropion hydrochloride.

tephromalacia (tef"ro-mah-la'she-ah) [Gr. *tephros* ash-colored + *malakia* softening] softening of the gray matter of the brain or cord.

tephromyelitis (tef"ro-mi"ĕ-li'tis) [Gr. *tephros* ash-colored + *myelos* marrow + *-itis*] inflammation of the gray substance of the spinal cord.

tephrosis (tef-ro'sis) [Gr. *tephrōsis*] incineration or cremation.

tephrylometer (tef"ril-om'ĕ-ter) [Gr. *tephros* ash-colored + *hylē* matter + *metron* measure] a graduated glass tube for measuring the thickness of the gray matter of the brain.

tepidarium (tep"ĭ-da're-um) [L., from *tepidus* lukewarm] a warm bath: more correctly, a place for a warm bath.

tepor (te'por) [L. "lukewarmness"] gentle heat.

teprotide (tep'ro-tīd) chemical name: 2-L-tryptophan-3-de-L-leucine-4-de-L-proline-8-L-glutamine-bradykinin potentiator B; a nonapeptide, $C_{53}H_{76}N_{14}O_{12}$, that inhibits the enzyme which converts angiotensin I to the active form (angiotensin II) and thus has antihypertensive properties.

ter- [L. *ter* thrice] a prefix meaning three, three-fold.

tera- [Gr. *teras* monster] a combining form used in naming units of measurement to indicate a quantity one trillion (10^{12}) times the unit specified by the root with which it is combined.

teracurie (ter"ah-ku're) a unit of radioactivity, being one trillion (10^{12}) curies.

teras (ter'as), pl. *ter'ata* [L.; Gr.] a monster. **ter'ata anadid'yma,** anadidymus; sometimes applied to a double monster with duplication of the cephalic pole and single toward the podalic pole. **ter'ata kata-anadid'yma,** anakatadidymus. **ter'ata katadid'yma,** katadidymus; sometimes applied to a double monster with duplication of the podalic pole and single toward the cephalic pole.

terata (ter'ah-tah) [Gr.] plural of *teras.*

teratic (ter-at'ik) [Gr. *teratikos*] monstrous; having the characters of a monster.

teratism (ter'ah-tizm) [Gr. *teratisma*] an anomaly of formation or development; the condition of a monster. See under *teras, monster,* and *monstrum,* and names of specific monsters.

terato- [Gr. *teras, teratos* monster] a combining form denoting relationship to a monster.

teratoblastoma (ter"ah-to-blas-to'mah) a neoplasm containing embryonic elements and differing from a teratoma in that its tissue does not represent all the germinal layers.

teratocarcinogenesis (ter"ah-to-kar"sĭ-no-jen'ĕ-sis) the production of teratomas.

teratocarcinoma (ter"ah-to-kar"sĭ-no'mah) a malignant neoplasm consisting of elements of teratoma with those of embryonal carcinoma or choriocarcinoma, or both; occurring most often in the testis.

teratogen (ter'ah-to-jen) an agent or factor that causes the production of physical defects in the developing embryo.

teratogenesis (ter"ah-to-jen'ĕ-sis) [*terato-* + Gr. *genesis* production] the production of physical defects in offspring in utero.

teratogenetic (ter"ah-to-jĕ-net'ik) pertaining to teratogenesis.

teratogenic (ter"ah-to-jen'ik) tending to produce anomalies of formation, or teratism.

teratogenous (ter"ah-toj'ĕ-nus) developed from fetal remains.

teratogeny (ter"ah-toj'ĕ-ne) teratogenesis.

teratoid (ter'ah-toid) [*terato-* + Gr. *eidos* form] resembling a monster.

teratologic, teratological (ter"ah-to-loj'ik; ter"ah-to-loj'ĭ-kal) pertaining to teratology.

teratology (ter"ah-tol'o-je) that division of embryology and pathology which deals with abnormal development and congenital malformations.

teratoma (ter"ah-to'mah), pl. *teratomas* or *terato'mata.* A true neoplasm made up of a number of different types of tissue, none of which is native to the area in which it occurs; most often found in the ovary or testis. **adult t.,** dermoid cyst. **benign cystic t., cystic t.,** dermoid cyst. **immature t.,** malignant t. **malignant t.,** a solid, malignant ovarian tumor resembling a dermoid cyst but composed of immature embryonal and/or extraembryonal elements derived from all three germ layers. Called also *immature t.* and *solid t.* **mature t.,** dermoid cyst. **solid t.,** malignant t.

teratomata (ter"ah-to'mah-tah) plural of *teratoma.*

teratomatous (ter"ah-to'mah-tus) pertaining to or of the nature of teratoma.

teratosis (ter"ah-to'sis) [Gr. *teras* monster + *-osis*] teratism.

teratospermia (ter"ah-to-sper'me-ah) the presence of malformed spermatozoa in the semen.

terbium (ter'be-um) a rare metallic element; symbol, Tb; atomic number, 65; atomic weight, 158.924.

terbutaline sulfate (ter-bu'tah-lēn) [USP] chemical name: 5-[2-[(1,1-dimethylethyl)amino]-1-hydroxyethyl]-1,3-benzenediol sulfate (2:1) salt. A β-adrenergic receptor antagonist, $(C_{12}H_{19}NO_3)_2 \cdot H_2SO_4$, used as a bronchodilator, administered orally, by aerosol inhalation, and subcutaneously.

terchloride (ter-klo′rīd) trichloride.

tere (te′re) rub.

terebene (ter′ĕ-bēn) [L. *terebenum*, from *terebinthus* turpentine] a thin, yellowish, fragrant mixture of terpene hydrocarbons, $C_{10}H_{16}$, obtained from oil of turpentine by the action of sulfuric acid. It is antiseptic and expectorant, and has been used in catarrh, bronchitis, cystitis, fermentative dyspepsia, genitourinary disease, and as an application to gangrenous wounds, etc.

terebenthene (ter″ĕ-ben′thēn) oil of turpentine.

terebinth (ter′ĕ-binth) [L. *terebinthus*] 1. the tree *Pistacia terebinthus*, L. (Anacardiaceae), formerly a source of turpentine. 2. turpentine; it also produces pistacia galls, a source of tannin.

terebinthina (ter″ĕ-bin′thĭ-nah) [L.] turpentine.

terebinthinate (ter″ĕ-bin′thĭ-nāt) resembling or containing turpentine.

terebinthinism (ter″ĕ-bin′thĭ-nizm) poisoning with oil of turpentine; symptoms include hemoglobinemia, pulmonary edema, convulsions, and damage to nervous system and kidneys.

terebrant, terebrating (ter′ĕ-brant; ter′ĕ-brāt″ing) [L. *terebrans* boring] of a boring or piercing quality.

terebration (ter′e-bra′shun) [L. *terebratio*] an act of boring or trephining; also a boring pain.

teres (te′rēz) [L.] long and round, as a muscle.

terfenadine (ter-fen′ah-dēn) chemical name: α-[4-(1,1-dimethylethyl)phenyl]-4-(hydroxydiphenylmethyl)-1-piperidine butanol; an antihistaminic, $C_{32}H_{41}NO_2$.

Terfonyl (ter′fo-nil) trademark for preparations of sulfamethazine, sulfadiazine, and sulfamerazine (trisulfapyrimidines). See *trisulfapyrimidines oral suspension*, under *suspension*.

tergal (ter′gal) [L. *tergum* back] pertaining to the back or the dorsal surface.

ter in die (ter in de′a) [L.] three times a day.

term (term) [L. *terminus*, from Gr. *terma*] 1. a word or combination of words commonly used to designate a specific entity. 2. a limit or boundary. 3. a definite period or specified time of duration, such as the culmination of pregnancy at the end of nine months. **ontogenetic t's,** termini ontogenetici.

terminad (ter′mĭ-nad) [L. *terminus* limit + *ad* to] toward the end or terminus.

terminal (ter′mĭ-nal) [L. *terminalis*] 1. forming or pertaining to an end; placed at the end. 2. a termination, end, or extremity; see *ending*. **C t.,** C-terminal. **N t.,** N-terminal.

terminatio (ter″mĭ-na′she-o), pl. *terminatio′nes* [L. "a limiting, bounding"] an ending; the site of discontinuation of a structure. **terminatio′nes nervo′rum li′berae** [NA], free nerve endings: those neural receptors having the simplest form, in which the peripheral nerve fiber divides into fine branches that terminate freely in connective tissue or epithelium.

termination (ter″mĭ-na′shun) [L. *terminatio*] a distal end; a cessation.

terminationes (ter″mĭ-na″she-o′nēz) [L.] plural of *terminatio*.

termini (ter′mĭ-ni) [L.] plural of *terminus*.

terminology (ter″mĭ-nol′o-je) [L. *terminus* term + -*logy*] 1. the vocabulary of an art or science. 2. the science which deals with the investigation, arrangement, and construction of terms.

terminus (ter′mĭ-nus), pl. *ter′mini* [L.] an ending. **ter′mini ad extremita′tes spectan′tes,** termini ad membra spectantes. **ter′mini ad mem′bra spectan′tes,** the NA category embracing terms relating to the upper and lower limbs; called also *termini ad extremitates spectantes*. **ter′mini genera′les,** the NA category embracing general terms (that is, terms not applied exclusively to one specific structure but to all structures belonging to the particular category or to which the term is applicable). **ter′mini ontogenet′ici** [NA], ontogenetic terms: terms relating to development, including those pertaining to the placenta and other fetal membranes or other structures. **ter′mini si′tum et directio′nem par′tium cor′poris indican′tes,** the NA category embracing terms indicating position and direction of parts of the body.

termolecular (ter″mo-lek′u-lar) involving three molecules.

ternary (ter′nah-re) [L. *ternarius*] 1. third in order. 2. made up of three distinct chemical elements.

ternitrate (ter-ni′trāt) a trinitrate.

terodiline hydrochloride (ter″-o-di′lēn) chemical name: *N*-(1,1-dimethylethyl)-α-methyl-γ-phenylbenzepropanamine hydrochloride; a coronary vasodilator, $C_{20}H_{27}N \cdot HCl$, used in the treatment of angina of effort.

teroxide (ter-ok′sīd) [L. *ter* three + *oxide*] trioxide.

terpene (ter′pēn) any hydrocarbon of the formula $C_{10}H_{16}$, derivable chiefly from essential oils, resins, and other vegetable aromatic products. They may be acyclic, bicyclic, or monocyclic, and differ somewhat in physical properties.

terpenism (ter′pen-izm) poisoning with a terpene, resulting in vomiting, convulsions, unconsciousness, pulmonary edema, and tachycardia.

terpin (ter′pin) [L. *terpinum*] a product, $(CH_3)_2C(OH)\cdot C_6H_9\cdot (OH)\cdot CH_3$, obtained by the action of nitric acid on oil of turpentine and alcohol. **t. hydrate** [USP], chemical name: 4-hydroxy-α,α,4-trimethylcyclohexanemethanol monohydrate. An expectorant, $C_{10}H_{20}O_2 \cdot H_2O$, occurring as colorless, lustrous crystals or as a white powder; administered orally.

terpineol (ter-pin′e-ol) chemical name: *p*-menth-1-en-8-ol. An alcohol, $(CH_3)_2 \cdot C(OH) \cdot C_6H_8 \cdot CH_3$, consisting of a mixture of several isomers occurring in many essential oils; formerly used as an antiseptic, but now used as a perfuming agent.

Terpinol (ter′pĭ-nol) trademark for terpin hydrate.

terra (ter′ah) [L.] earth. **t. al′ba,** white clay, used as an adsorbent. **t. lem′nia,** a yellowish, ferruginous clay. **t. mer′ita,** turmeric. **t. pondero′sa,** barium sulfate, or synthetic baryta. **t. sigilla′ta** [L. "sealed earth" of ancient Lemnos], Armenian bole, sold in masses stamped with a seal. **t. silic′ea purifica′ta,** purified silicious or infusorial earth; silicious earth, boiled, washed, and calcined; it is a fine gray powder and is used in certain pharmaceutical operations.

Terramycin (ter′ah-mi″sin) trademark for preparations of oxytetracycline.

terrein (ter′e-in) a cyclopentane compound, $C_8H_{10}O_2$, formed by the action of *Aspergillus terreus*.

Terridens (ter′rĭ-denz) a genus of nematode worms. **T. diminu′tus,** a parasite frequently present in monkeys and occasionally in man; called also *Triodontophorus diminutus*.

territoriality (ter′ĭ-tor″ĭ-al′ĭ-te) a pattern of behavior in which an individual organism or a group of organisms delineates a territory and vigorously defends it against intrusion by other members of the same or competing species.

terror (ter′er) intense fright. **day t's,** pavor diurnus. **night t's,** pavor nocturnus.

tersulfide (ter-sul′fīd) trisulfide.

tertian (ter′shun) [L. *tertianus*] recurring every third day, counting the day of occurrence as the first day; applied to the type of fever caused by certain forms of malarial parasites. **double t.,** an intermittent fever in which there are two sets of recurrences, each tertian.

tertiarism (ter′she-ah-rizm) former term for the combined symptoms of tertiary syphilis.

tertiary (ter′she-er-e) [L. *tertiarius*] third in order.

tertigravida (ter′she-grav′ĭ-dah) [L. *tertius* third + *gravida* pregnant] a woman pregnant for the third time; also written *gravida III*.

tertipara (ter-ship′ah-rah) [L. *tertius* third + *parere* to bring forth, produce] a woman who has had three pregnancies which resulted in viable offspring; also written *para III* or *III-para*.

tesicam (tes′ĭ-kam) chemical name: 4′-chloro-1,2,3,4-tetrahydro-1,3-dioxo-4-isoquinolinecarboxanilide; an anti-inflammatory, $C_{16}H_{11}ClN_2O_3$.

tesimide (tes′ĭ-mīd) chemical name: 5,6,7,8-tetrahydro-4-(phenylmethylene)isoquinolinedione; an anti-inflammatory, $C_{16}H_{15}NO_2$.

tesla (tes′lah) the SI unit of magnetic flux density, calculated as webers per square meter. It replaces the gauss. Abbreviated T.

Teslac (tes′lak) trademark for preparations of testolactone.

teslaization (tes″la-i-za′shun) [named for Nikola *Tesla*, a Serbian inventor in New York, 1856–1943] treatment by Tesla's currents; d'arsonvalism.

Tessalon (tes′sah-lon) trademark for a preparation of benzonatate.

tessellated (tes′el-lāt″ed) [L. *tessellatus; tessella* a square] divided into squares, like a checker board.

test (test) [L. *testum* crucible] 1. an examination or trial. 2. a significant chemical reaction. 3. a reagent. For specific tests, see *Table of Tests*. See also under *method, phenomenon, reaction, reagent, sign,* and *symptom*.

test card (test kard) a card printed with various letters or symbols, used in testing vision. **stigmometric t. c.,** a card with dots and squares arranged in groups, for testing vision (Fridenberg).

test letter (test let′er) see *test type*.

A TABLE OF TESTS

(See also under *method, phenomenon, reaction, reagent, sign,* and *symptom*.)

Abderhalden's t., see under *reaction*.

Abelin's t. (*for arsphenamine*), see under *reaction*.

abortus Bang ring (ABR) t.: a screening test for brucellosis in cattle; since *Brucella* agglutinins, as well as the organisms, are shed in the milk of infected cattle, a drop of hematoxylin-stained brucellae are mixed in a sample of pooled milk from the herd. After incubation, agglutinated bacteria rise to the surface to form a colored ring. Called also *milk-ring t.* and *ring t.*

ABR t., abortus Bang ring t.

Abrams' t. (*for lead in the urine*): add ammonium oxalate to urine (1:150) and introduce metallic magnesium (wire or rod). Lead is precipitated on the magnesium, and can be identified by warming with a fragment of iodine (yellow lead iodide), or dissolving in nitric acid and applying other reagents.

acetanilid t., see *Yvon's t.* (1).

acetic acid t. (*for albumin in urine*): a few drops of acetic acid are added to the boiled urine, when a white precipitate is formed.

acetic acid and potassium ferrocyanide t. (*for proteins*): acidify the unknown with acetic acid and add a few drops of potassium ferrocyanide; protein produces a white flocculent precipitate.

acetoacetic acid t., see specific tests, including *Arnold's t., Gerhardt's t.* (2), *Harding and Ruttan's t., Hurtley's t., Lindemann's t.,* and *Nobel's t.* (1). See also *acetoacetic acid, methods for,* under *method.*

acetone t.: a test for the presence of acetone in the urine made by adding a few drops of sodium nitroprusside, shaking, and pouring over the mixture stronger ammonia water: a magenta-colored line is formed over the area of contact if acetone is present. See specific tests, including *Bayer's t., Behre* and *Benedict's t., Braun's t., Chautard's t., Denigès' t.* (2), *Frommer's t., Gerhardt's t.* (1), *Gunning's t., Lange's t.* (2), *Legal's t.* (1), *Lieben's t., Lieben-Ralfe t., Malerba's t., Nobel's t.* (1), *Penzoldt's t.* (1), *Ralfe's t.* (1), *Rantzman's t., Reynold's t., Rothera's t., Stock t.,* and see *acetone, methods for,* under *method.*

acetonitrile t., see *Hunt's reaction,* under *reaction.*

Achard and Castaigne's t., see *methylene blue t.* (1).

acid elution t. (*for fetal hemoglobin*): air-dried blood smears on a glass slide are fixed in 80 per cent methanol and immersed in a buffer at pH 3.3 (citric acid and sodium phosphate); all hemoglobulins are eluted except fetal hemoglobulin, which remains fixed in the red cells and can be detected after staining.

acidity reduction t.: 250 ml. of 0.4 per cent hydrochloric acid is introduced into an empty stomach through a tube; samples are withdrawn at intervals of fifteen minutes and titrated for free acid.

acid-lability t.: a test to distinguish rhinoviruses from enteroviruses on the basis of their activity at various pH levels, rhinoviruses being inactivated by incubation at pH 3 to 5 for one to three hours.

acidosis t., see *Sabrazés t., Sellard's t.*

Acree-Rosenheim t. (*for proteins*): a few drops of formaldehyde solution (1:5000) are placed in a solution of the suspected matter. A little concentrated sulfuric acid is slowly placed in the test tube so that the solutions do not mix. At the line of contact a violet color appears if proteins are present.

acrolein t. (*for glycerol and fats*): heat the substance with an equal quantity of potassium acid sulfate and note the peculiar penetrating odor of acrolein.

Adamkiewicz's t. (*for proteins*): add the substance to a mixture of 1 volume of strong sulfuric acid and 2 volumes of glacial acetic acid and heat it; a reddish violet color shows the presence of proteins.

Adams' t. (*for fat in milk*): dry a known quantity of milk on filter paper, extract in Soxhlet's apparatus, dry to constant weight, and weigh.

Addis t.: after the patient is given a dry diet for 24 hours, the specific gravity of the urine is determined; called also *Addis method.*

Adler's t., see *benzidine t.*

Admiralty t.: a test for the efficiency of excremental disinfectants in which gelatin and starch are used as the organic test substances.

adrenalin t., see *epinephrine t.*

Adson's t. (*for thoracic outlet syndrome*): with the patient in a sitting position, his hands resting on thighs, the examiner palpates both radial pulses as the patient rapidly fills his lungs by deep inspiration and, holding his breath, hyperextends his neck and turns his head toward the affected side. If the radial pulse on that side is decidedly or completely obliterated, the result is considered positive. Called also *Adson's maneuver.*

agglutination t.: one of various specific and nonspecific tests the results of which depend on agglutination of bacteria or of other cells; used as an aid in diagnosis of certain bacterial or of viral and rickettsial diseases, and of rheumatoid arthritis. See also specific tests, such as *Bang t.* and *Bass-Watkin t.*

Agostini's t. (*for dextrose*): mix 5 drops of the urine with 5 drops of a 0.5 per cent solution of gold chloride and 3 drops of a 20 per cent solution of potassium hydroxide, and warm the mixture; dextrose will give a red tint.

air t., see *Franken's t.*

Albarrán's t. (*for renal inadequacy*): a test for the renal function based upon the principle that the greater the destruction of epithelium in the kidney, the less likely is that organ to respond by an increase in secretion after the administration of quantities of water. Called also *polyuria t.*

albumin t., see specific tests, including *acetic acid t., Almén's t.* (1), *Alper's t., ammonium sulfate t.* (2), *Axenfeld's t., Barral's t., Berzelius' t., Blum's t., Boedeker's t., Boston's t., Bychowski's t., Carrez's t., Castellani's t.* (1), *Cohen's t., Esbach's t., Exton's t., Fürbringer's t., Geissler's t., Heller's t.* (1), *Heynsius' t., Hindenlang's t., Ilimow's t., Johnson's t., MacWilliams' t., magnesionitric t., Méhu's t., Millard's t., Oliver's t.* (1), *Osgood-Haskin's t., oxyphenylsulfonic acid t., Parnum's t., Polacci's t., Posner's t.* (1), *Purdy's t.* (2), *Raabe's t., Rees' t., Riegler's t.* (1), *Roberts' t.* (1), *Spiegler's t., Suranyi's t., Tanret's t., Tidy's t.* (1), *Tretop's t., Tsuchiya's t., Ulrich's t., Zouchlos' t.* See also the tests listed under *protein t.,* and see *albumin in urine, methods for,* under *method.*

albumin A t., see *Kahn t.* (2).

alcohol t., see *Anstie's t., Berthelot's t.* (2), *chromic acid t., ethyl acetate t., iodoform t.* (2), *Woodbury's t.*

aldehyde t., see specific tests, including *formol-gel t., Napier's serum t.,* and *Tollens' t.* (1).

Aldrich-McClure t., see *McClure-Aldrich t.*

Alfraise's t. (*for iodine*): a reagent consisting of 1 drop of hydrochloric acid in 100 parts of water, 1 of starch, and 1 of potassium nitrate is boiled, and 1 drop of the reagent is added to the liquid being tested; a blue color will be produced if iodine is present.

alizarin t. (*for gastric secretion*): after a test drink containing alizarin the intensity of the coloration of the urine gives an indication of the degree of acidity of the urine.

alkali t., see specific tests, including *Bachmeier's t., Degener's t.*

alkali denaturation t.: a moderately sensitive spectrophotometric method for determining the concentration of fetal (F) hemoglobin, which depends on the resistance of the hemoglobin molecule to denaturation of its globin moiety when exposed to alkali.

alkali tolerance t.: 20 gm. of sodium bicarbonate given while fasting should raise the pH of the urine to 8 within two hours.

alkaloid t., see specific tests, including *Arnold's t.* (2), *Bouchardat's t., Erdman's t., Fröhde's t., Frohn's t., Mayer's t., Vitali's t.* (1) and (2), *Winckler's t.* (1), *Wormley's t.* (1) and (2), *Yvon's t.* (2).

allantoin t., see *Schiff's t.* (4).

Allen's t.: 1. (*for glucose in the urine*) add urine to boiling Fehling's solution, and allow it to cool; turbidity will be seen if dextrose is present. (Alfred Henry Allen.) 2. (*for phenol*) to 2 drops of the suspected liquid add 5 drops of hydrochloric acid and 1 of nitric acid. Phenol, if present, will produce a cherry-red color. (Alfred Henry Allen.) 3. (*for strychnine*) extract with ether, concentrate by letting drops fall into a warmed porcelain capsule, cool the residue, and treat with sulfuric acid and manganese dioxide. Strychnine gives a violet color. 4. (*obs.*) (*for tinea versicolor*) compound solution of iodine is applied to the suspected eruption; a dark mahogany stain will be produced if the eruption is tinea. (Charles Warren Allen.) 5. (*for occlusion of ulnar or radial arteries*) the patient makes a tight fist so as to express the blood from the skin of the palm and fingers; the examiner makes digital compression on either the radial or the ulnar artery. If on opening the hand blood fails to return to the palm and fingers, there is indicated obstruction to the blood flow in the artery that has not been compressed. (Edgar V. Allen.)

Allen-Doisy t. (*for estrogenic substance in laboratory animals*): a positive test is the presence in the vaginal secretion of cornified epithelial cells; a negative test shows only leukocytes in the secretion.

Allesandri-Guaceni t. (*for nitric acid; nitrates*): dissolve a few drops of phenol in hydrochloric acid by heating twelve hours on a water bath. Heat 10 drops of the reagent with the dry residue of suspected liquid on the water bath. Nitric acid or nitrates give an intense violet color, changed by ammonia to green.

Almén's t.: 1. (*for albumin in urine*) one part of Almén's reagent is added to 6 parts of the urine; a cloudiness is produced when albumin is present. 2. (*for blood or blood pigment*) shake the suspected liquid with a mixture of equal parts of tincture of guaiacum and oil of turpentine; blood pigment, if present, will turn the mixture blue. 3. (*for dextrose*) heat the liquid with bismuth subnitrate dissolved in sodium hydroxide solution and sodium potassium tartrate; dextrose will cause the mixture to become dark brown or nearly black, and to deposit a black precipitate.

aloin t., see *Rossel's aloin t.*

Alper's t. (*for albumin in the urine*): acidulate the urine with hydrochloric acid and add equal volumes of a 1 per cent mercury succinimide solution; a white cloudiness forms.

alpha t.: a psychological test designed to determine the mental capacity of persons able to read English.

alphanaphthol t., see specific tests, including *Molisch's t.* (2) and (3).

alternate cover t.: a test for determining the type of tropia and/or phoria done by alternately covering each eye and noting the movement of the uncovered eye.

Althausen t.: a test for the velocity of intestinal absorption by determining at intervals the concentration of galactose in the blood after the oral administration of sugar.

alum t., see *Bell's t.* (2).

Amann t. (*for indican in urine*): to 20 ml. of urine are added a few drops of pure sulfuric acid, 5 ml. of chloroform, and then 5 ml. of a 10 per cent solution of sodium pyrosulfate. They are mixed gently for several minutes. The chloroform is then allowed to settle and will be colored blue by the indigo.

Ames t. (*for carcinogenicity*): a strain of *Salmonella typhimurium* that lacks the enzyme necessary for histidine synthesis is mixed with rat-liver extract and is plated thinly on an agar medium; a disk of filter paper containing the suspected carcinogen is then placed on the bacteria. If the substance causes DNA damage resulting in mutations, some of the bacteria will regain the ability to synthesize histidine and will proliferate to form colonies. The ability to cause mutations indicates that the substance is carcinogenic.

amidopyrine t., see *aminopyrine t.*

amino acid t., see *Folin's t.* (4), and *Folin's method*, (3), under *method.*

amino-acid nitrogen t., see *triketohydrindene hydrate t.* See also *nitrogen, amino-acid, method for,* under *method.*

amino-nitrogen t., see *Van Slyke t.* (1).

aminopyrine t.: 1. (*for occult blood in feces*) a small portion of the feces is stirred up in 3 to 4 ml. of distilled water and filtered. To the filtrate add 3 or 4 ml. of a 90 per cent alcoholic solution of aminopyrine (Pyramidon) and several drops of a 30 per cent acetic acid with hydrogen peroxide. A violet-blue color indicates occult blood. 2. (*in urine*) to the urine add tincture of iodine; a yellow ring indicates aminopyrine (Pyramidon).

ammonia t., see specific tests, including *Brown's t.* (2), *Nessler's t., Ronchese's t., Spiro's t.* (1).

ammonium sulfate t. (*for spinal fluid*): 1. (*for globulin*) in a test tube place 2 ml. of a solution of 85 gm. of ammonium sulfate in 100 ml. of water. Overlay with spinal fluid. A clean-cut, grayish white ring appearing within five minutes indicates excess of globulin. 2. (*for albumin*) mix contents of tube, filter, add acetic acid and boil. A gray cloud indicates increase of albumin. A faint opalescence is normal.

Ammons quick t.: a rapid screening test for determining the mental age of a child. The subject indicates, by pointing, which of several printed drawings best illustrates the meaning of a given word.

amylase t.: 1. (*for kidney function*) the urine is tested for starch; a diminution below the normal starch content indicates a diminution of kidney function. 2. see *Hawk's t.*

amylopsin t.: add 0.5 ml. of duodenal contents to 50 ml. of a 3 per cent solution of soluble starch; incubate for one-half hour and test for reducing sugars.

Anderson's t. (*to distinguish pyridine chloroplatinate from quinoline chloroplatinate*): boil the salt in water; the pyridine salt becomes an insoluble double salt, and gives off hydrogen chloride, but the quinoline salt remains in solution.

Anderson and Goldberger's t. (*for typhus*): the patient's blood is injected into the peritoneal cavity of guinea-pigs; if the disease is typhus, a typical temperature curve will be obtained.

André's t. (*for quinine*): chlorine and ammonia produce a green color changing to blue on saturation with acid. Excess of acid changes the color to violet or bright red, but ammonia again turns it green.

Andreasch's t. (*for cysteine*): dissolve the substance in hydrochloric acid, and add a few drops of a dilute solution of ferric chloride and a little ammonia water; cysteine causes the liquid to assume a dark purplish tint.

Andrewes' t. (*for uremia*): to one volume of serum two volumes of alcohol are added. The mixture is centrifuged and the alcoholic supernatant layer removed. To four volumes of this alcoholic extract are added two volumes of alcohol and one volume of freshly prepared diazo reagent, as in van den Bergh's test. In uremia the mixture slowly develops a brown-buff color.

anemia t.: see specific tests, including *autohemolysis t., Ham t., Macht t., sickling t.*

Anstie's t. (*for alcohol in the urine*): a reagent consisting of a solution of potassium dichromate, 1, in concentrated sulfuric acid, 300, is added by drops; an emerald-green color signifies the presence of alcohol in toxic quantity.

antibody absorption t.: antiserum against one antigen is absorbed with a cross-reacting antigen, the titer of antibody against the original homologous antigen being determined both before and after absorption with the cross-reacting antigen.

antiglobulin t., Coombs' test.

antiglobulin consumption t., see *Coombs t.*

antimony t., see *Marsh's t.*

antipyrine t., see *Fieux's t.*

antithrombin t.: a test for typhoid based on the action of thrombin on the patient's serum.

antitrypsin t.: a test based on the power of the blood serum to inhibit the action of trypsin. The antitryptic power of the blood serum is increased in carcinoma, nephritis, pregnancy, etc. Called also *Bergmann-Meyer t., Fuld-Goss t.,* and *Müller-Jochmann t.*

Antonucci t.: a method for rapid cholecystography with tetraiodophenolphthalein.

anvil t.: the striking of a part with the closed fist used like a hammer: a blow so given on the sole of the foot with the leg extended produces pain in the hip in early hip-joint disease; such a blow given over the top of the head elicits pain in a diseased vertebra.

apomorphine t., see *Bedson's t.*

Apt t. (*for differentiating fetal from adult hemoglobin*): mix the infant's specimen (vomitus or stool) with 5 volumes of water,

centrifuge the mixture, and separate the clear pink supernatant. Add 1 ml. 1 per cent sodium hydroxide to 5 ml. of the supernatant. If hemoglobin F is present, the pink color persists for more than 2 minutes (indicating fetal blood). If hemoglobin A is present, it turns from pink to yellow within 2 minutes (indicating swallowed maternal blood).

aptitude t's: tests given to determine aptitude or ability to undertake study or training in a particular field.

Arakawa's t. (*for peroxidase in milk*), see under *reagent.*

Archetti's t. (*for caffeine*): heat a solution of potassium ferricyanide with half its volume of nitric acid to boiling, then dilute with water; the reagent gives a precipitate of Prussian blue with caffeine (uric acid does also).

arginine t., see *Sakaguchi t.*

Arloing-Courmont t.: the Widal test in tuberculosis.

Arnold's t.: 1. (*for aceto-acetic acid in urine*) a. Dissolve 1 gm. of para-amidoacetophenone in 80 to 100 ml. water by shaking and adding hydrochloric acid by drops, then add more concentrated acid until the solution is colorless. b. Dissolve 1 gm. sodium nitrite in 100 ml. distilled water. Just before using mix 2 parts a with 1 part b, add an equal volume of urine, and 2 or 3 drops concentrated ammonia water: an intense brownish red color develops. Now add 1 volume of this colored urine to 10 or 12 volumes of concentrated hydrochloric acid, 2 to 4 drops of ferric chloride, and 3 ml. of chloroform; a beautiful purplish violet color develops in the chloroform if acetoacetic acid is present. Strongly colored urine should first be decolorized with animal charcoal. 2. (*alkaloidal tests*) a. Some alkaloids heated on the water bath with syrupy phosphoric acid obtained by dissolving metaphosphoric acid or phosphoric acid anhydride in phosphoric acid yield characteristic color reactions: aconitine, violet; nicotine, yellow; coniine, green. b. Triturated with concentrated sulfuric acid, many alkaloids yield characteristic color reactions upon adding 30 to 40 per cent alcoholic (in some instances aqueous) potassium hydroxide solution.

Aron's t. (*for cancer*): a biopsy specimen of the adrenal cortex of a rabbit is taken; the animal is then injected with urinary extract from the patient. After two days the rabbit is killed and its adrenal cortex compared with the biopsy specimen.

arsenic t., see *Bettendorff's t., Fleitmann's t., Gutzeit's t., Marsh's t., Reinsch's t.* (1).

arsphenamine t., see *Abelin reaction,* under *reaction.*

Aschheim-Zondek t. (*for pregnancy*): the subcutaneous injection of the urine of pregnant women into immature female mice is followed by swelling, congestion, and hemorrhages of the ovaries and premature maturation of the ovarian follicles. Abbreviated AZT and A-Z t.

Aschner's t., Aschner-Danini t., see *Aschner's phenomenon,* under *phenomenon.*

Ascoli's t.: [Alberto *Ascoli*] the formation of a ring of precipitate at the junction of the two fluids when the extract of the infected tissue of an anthrax animal, after boiling with saline solution, is added to anthrax immune serum. 2. [Maurizio *Ascoli*] see *miostagmin reaction,* under *reaction.*

association t.: a test based on associative reaction. It is usually performed by mentioning words to a subject and noting what other words he will give as the ones called up in his mind. The reaction time is also noted.

Atkinson and Kendall's t. (*for blood*): a modified form of Teichmann's test.

atropine t., see *Dehio's t.* and *Reuss' t.*

attention-alertness t., see *Bourdon's t.*

Au t.: a test of donor blood for Australian (Au) antigen, an antigen associated with viral hepatitis.

augmented histamine t. (*of gastric function*): after a 12-hour fast, the residual gastric contents are aspirated. Basal gastric secretion is then collected for 1 hour in divided 15-minute aliquots. Thirty minutes before completion of collection, a suitable dose of antihistamine is given intramuscularly. At conclusion of basal secretion collection, histamine acid phosphate (0.04 mg. per kg. of body weight) is given subcutaneously, and gastric contents collected in 15-minute aliquots for 1 hour. Volume, pH, and titratable acidity are measured for each aliquot. When Histalog (1.7 mg. per kg. of body weight) is used in place of histamine, the antihistamine injection is omitted and 8 (rather than 4) 15-minute aliquots are taken after its injection.

Auricchio and Chieffi's t.: a test for leishmaniasis based on the fact that the serum of patients flocculates rapidly on the addition of a solution of iron peptonate.

autohemolysis t.: one performed in investigation of certain hemolytic states, particularly the congenital, nonspherocytic hemolytic anemias. Defibrinated blood is incubated at 37° C., under sterile conditions, for 24 and 48 hours, and the amount of spontaneous hemolysis is quantitated.

auto-urine t. (*former test for tuberculosis*): into the superficial layers of the patient's skin is injected 0.05 ml. of the patient's own urine. If the patient is actively tuberculous a local reaction develops which consists of a palpable lump of infiltration. Called also *Wildbolz's t.*

Axenfeld's t. (*for albumin in urine*): acidulate the urine with formic acid, and drop by drop add a 0.1 per cent solution of gold chloride. On warming, albumin, if present, will produce a red tint, which more of the gold chloride will turn to a blue. Many other substances will produce the blue tint, but not the red.

Ayer's t. (*for spinal block*): with a spinal manometer, the pressure in lumbar puncture and that in a cisterna magna puncture should be identical in the normal subject.

Ayer-Tobey t., see *Tobey-Ayer t.*

A-Z t., Aschheim-Zondek test.

Babcock's t. (*for fat in milk*): to 17.6 ml. of milk add 17.5 ml. sulfuric acid, specific gravity 1.82–1.83; centrifuge five minutes; bring level of liquid up to base of neck by adding hot water, at about 140° F.; centrifuge three minutes; add hot water to bring fat column well up into neck; centrifuge two minutes; read directly from scale on neck.

Babinski's t., see under *sign*.

Babinski-Weil t.: the patient, with his eyes shut, is made to walk forward and backward ten times in a clear space. A person with labyrinthine disease deviates from the straight path, bends to one side when walking forward and to the other side when walking backward.

Bachman t. (*for trichinosis*): an extract of powdered trichina larvae is injected intradermally; an immediate or delayed wheal-and-flare reaction denotes present or past infection; the immediate reaction is more reliable.

Bachmeier's t. (*for alkalis*): tannin solution produces a red to reddish brown color, changing to dirty green.

bactericidal t., see *Neisser and Wechsberg's t.,* and *Wright's method,* def. 2, under *method.*

bacteriolytic t., see *Pfeiffer's phenomenon,* under *phenomenon.*

Baermann t. (*for extraction of soil nematodes from earth and detecting larvae of Strongyloides stercoralis in feces*): a specimen of soil or feces is suspended over gauze or wire mesh in a water-filled funnel to which a piece of rubber tubing is attached; larval nematodes migrate from the specimen to the water, and collect in the rubber tubing.

Baeyer's t.: 1. (*for dextrose*) boil the liquid with orthonitrophenylpropiolic acid and sodium carbonate: if dextrose is present, indigo is formed; but an excess of dextrose will destroy the blue tint by forming white indigo. 2. (*for indole*) the suspected substance is dissolved in water, acidulated with 2 or 3 drops of fuming nitric acid; a 2 per cent solution added drop by drop produces a red color and then a red deposit of nitrosoindole nitrate.

balance t.: a functional test made by comparing the intake and output of a normal constituent, as of the urine.

Balfour's t.: the ascertainment of whether the heart is still active in cases of apparent death by inserting pins bearing paper streamers into the skin over the heart; movement of the heart muscles will be shown by movement of the papers.

ball t., see *Müller's test* (3).

Bang t.: abortus Bang ring t.

Bárány's t., see under *symptom,* def. 2.

Bárány's pointing t.: have the patient point at a fixed object alternately with the eyes open and closed; a constant error with the eyes closed indicates a brain lesion.

barbital t., see *Fabre's t.*

Bardach's t. (*for protein*): a test dependent on the fact that, in the presence of protein, acetone and potassium mercuric iodide and alkali react to yield canary-yellow needles instead of the usual hexagonal crystals of iodoform.

Bareggi's t. (*for typhoid fever*): the clot formed in the blood of typhoid patients after twenty-four hours is watery and soft, with only a small amount of separated serum.

Barfoed's t. (*for monosaccharides*): boil 5 ml. of Barfoed's reagent (dissolve 4.5 gm. of neutral crystallized copper acetate and 1.2 ml. of 50 per cent acetic acid in 100 ml. of water) and add the unknown slowly and with boiling. Monosaccharides reduce this mixture (formation of a red precipitate), while disaccharides do so only very slowly, if at all, and so can be distinguished from the former.

Barral's t. (*for albumin and biliary pigments*): overlay the urine with a 20 per cent solution of sozolic acid; a white ring develops at the contact point if albumin is present, a green ring if biliary pigments are present.

bar-reading t.: a test for binocular and stereoscopic vision, which consists of holding a ruler midway between the eyes and the printed page. It is also used as an exercise to develop stereoscopic vision.

Basham's t. (*for bile pigment*): the liquid is shaken with chloroform, evaporated, and a drop of nitric acid added; a play of bright colors is produced, finally becoming a fine red.

basophil t. (*for sensitivity*): a drop of the subject's blood is mixed with a small amount of solution of the substance being tested; disintegration of the basophils accompanies the release of histamine and is evidence of hypersensitivity to the substance.

basophil degranulation t. (*for hypersensitivity*): estimation of the amount of degranulation of basophil leukocytes following *in vitro* exposure to specific antigen, as compared to that in control preparations; the degranulation reaction is due to binding of the specific antigen by surface-bound IgE on the basophil membrane.

Bass-Watkins t. (*for agglutination*): a form of the Widal test so modified that it can be performed at the bedside in about five minutes. Place ¼ drop of the patient's blood on a glass slide, dissolve in 1 drop of water, add 1 drop of a rather heavy killed suspension of typhoid bacilli, and mix by tilting the slide from side to side. In a positive case small grayish clumps and a fine granular sediment form within two minutes.

Bauer's t.: 1. a modification of the Wassermann test by relying entirely on the antisheep amboceptor present in the patient's serum. 2. galactose tolerance test; test of carbohydrate tolerance of the liver, performed by administering 30 gm. of galactose, the urine being tested later for galactose by means of Fehling's solution: the elimination of more than 3 gm. indicates hepatic functional impairment. 3. (*for milk*) to 2 ml. of milk add 1 drop of 0.25 per cent aqueous solution of Nile-blue sulfate; the blue color can be extracted from human milk, but not from cow's milk by means of ether.

Baumann's t. (*for dextrose*): to a watery solution of the substance, add benzoyl chloride and an excess of sodium hydroxide, and shake until the odor of benzoyl chloride disappears and a precipitate of the benzoic acid ester of dextrose is formed.

Baumann and Goldmann's t. (*for cystine*): a solution containing the cystine is shaken with sodium hydroxide and benzoyl chloride; a voluminous precipitate is formed, composed of benzoyl cystine.

Bayer's t. (*for acetone in the urine*): equal volumes of urine and nitrobenzenaldehyde are mixed with alkaline water; acetone turns it to an indigo-blue tint.

Bayrac's t. (*for uric acid in urine*): evaporate 50 ml. of urine to dryness on the water bath, treat residue with hydrochloric acid (1:5), wash with alcohol, dissolve in 20 drops of sodium hydroxide solution heated to 90° or 100° C. on water bath, and decompose with sodium hypobromite in the apparatus for determining urea. Each 1 ml. of nitrogen at ordinary temperature equals 0.00357 gm. uric acid.

B. C. G. t., see *bicolor guaiac t.*

Becker's t.: 1. (*for picrotoxin*) Fehling's solution is added and the mixture is warmed; if the alkaloid is present, the solution is reduced. 2. (*for astigmatism*) the patient looks at a test card containing lines radiating in sets of three and points out which seem blurred.

Bekhterev's t.: the patient seated in bed is directed to stretch out both legs; in sciatica he cannot do this, but can stretch out each leg in turn.

Bedson's t. (*for apomorphine*): on boiling morphine solution containing apomorphine with potassium hydroxide, a brown color develops.

Behre and Benedict's t. (*for acetone bodies*): distill out the acetone bodies from acid solution, and determine colorimetrically with salicylic aldehyde and alkali. A red color is dihydroxy benzalacetone.

Bell's t.: 1. (*for percentage of free hydrochloric acid in stomach contents*) filter the contents, and to 4 ml. add drop by drop a solution of dimethyl-amido-azobenzol until the pink color ceases to grow darker. Compare with Bell's color scale for percentage. 2. (*for alum in flour or bread*) fresh 5 per cent logwood tincture in methylated spirit. Moisten 10 gm. flour with water, then add 1 ml. tincture and an equal quantity saturated ammonium carbonate solution. Sample, if pure, gives pinkish color, gradually fading to buff or brown. If alum is present, a lavender or bluish tint is formed, becoming more marked on drying.

belt t. (*for enteroptosis*): the lower abdomen of the patient is encircled by both hands and lifted up; the patient will experience a sensation of relief if enteroptosis is present.

Bender gestalt t., Bender visual-motor gestalt t.: a psychological test used for evaluating perceptual-motor coordination, for assessing personality dynamics, as a test of organic brain impairment, and for measuring neurological maturation. The subject is asked to make free-hand copies of nine simple geometric designs presented separately on cards or sometimes to reproduce the design from memory.

Bendien's t.: 1. a vanadic acid flocculation and spectrophotometric test for cancer. 2. a serum test for prognosis in tuberculosis.

Benedict's t.: 1. (*for dextrose*) 200 gm. of sodium or potassium citrate and 200 gm. crystallized sodium carbonate and 125 gm. of potassium sulfocyanate are dissolved in 800 ml. of boiling water. This is cooled and filtered and 18 gm. copper sulfate dissolved in 100 ml. of water are added and the whole diluted to make 1 liter. To 5 ml. of this reagent, in a test tube, 8 or 10 drops of the solution to be tested are added. Boil for one or two minutes and allow to cool slowly. If dextrose is present the solution will be filled with a precipitate red, yellow, or green in color. 2. (*for urea*) the urea is hydrolyzed to ammonium carbonate by $KHSO_4$ and $ZNSO_4$, made alkaline, and distilled as usual.

Benedict and Denis' t. (*for total sulfur in urine*), see under *method.*

Benedict and Murlin's t. (*for amino-acid nitrogen in urine*), see under *method.*

bentonite t.: a flocculation test for rheumatoid arthritis in which sensitized bentonite particles are added to inactivated serum; results are considered positive when half of the particles are clumped and half still remain in suspension.

benzidine t. (*for blood*): to a saturated solution of benzidine in glacial acetic acid add an equal volume of 3 per cent hydrogen peroxide and 1 ml. of the unknown; a blue color indicates blood.

benzidine peroxidase t. (*for raw milk*): to 10 ml. of the milk add 2 ml. of a 4 per cent alcoholic solution of benzidine and sufficient acetic acid to coagulate the milk. Mix and allow 2 ml. of a 3 per cent solution of hydrogen peroxide to flow slowly down the wall of the tube. An immediate blue color indicates raw milk (not heated to 78° C.).

benzoin t. (*for cerebrospinal syphilis*): when a colloidal solution of benzoin resin is added to syphilitic cerebrospinal fluid, flocculation or precipitation occurs.

Berenreuther t.: a test of interests and attitudes, consisting of 125 questions to be answered by yes or no.

Bergmann-Meyer t., see *antitrypsin t.*

Berthelot's t.: 1. (*for phenol*) an ammoniacal solution of phenol treated with solution of chlorinated soda takes on a fine blue color. 2. (*for alcohol*) shake with a few drops of benzyl chloride and an excess of sodium hydroxide until the irritating odor of benzyl chloride disappears; the aromatic odor of ethyl benzoate indicates alcohol.

Bertoni-Raymondi t. (*for nitrous acid in blood*): dialyze, evaporate the dialysate to dryness, take up with hot alcohol, and add starch paste and potassium iodide; a blue color develops.

Bertrand's t. (*for dextrose*): boil the unknown with an excess of Fehling's solution, filter out the cuprous oxide, dissolve in an acid solution of ferric sulfate, and titrate with potassium permanganate.

Berzelius's t. (*for albumin*): albumin is precipitated from solution by a fresh concentrated solution of metaphosphoric acid.

beta t.: a psychological test for intelligence to be used instead of the alpha test on persons unacquainted with English.

beta-oxybutyric acid t., see specific tests, including *Black's t., Hart's t., Kulz's t.* (1) (2), *Osterberg's t.*

Bettendorff's t. (*for arsenic*): the liquid to be tested is mixed with hydrochloric acid; a freshly prepared solution of stannous chloride is added, and a bit of tinfoil is put into it. A brown color or precipitate is formed.

Bettmann's t., see *Bettendorff's t.*

Bial's t. (*for pentose in urine*): make a reagent consisting of orcinol 1.5 gm., fuming hydrochloric acid 500 gm., and ferric chloride (10 per cent) 20–30 drops. Five ml. of this reagent are boiled in a test tube, and after removal from the flame, several drops of urine are added. A green color appearing at once indicates pentose.

bicarbonate tolerance t., see *Sellards' t.*

bicolor guaiac t.: a colloidal reaction in the cerebrospinal fluid: the reagents are a suspension of guaiac resin with two colored solutions, naphthol green and brilliant basic fuchsin; called also *B. C. G. t.*

bile acid t., see specific tests, including *Bischoff's t., Drechsel's t., Francis' t.* (1), *Hay's t., Mylius' t., Neukomm's t., Oliver's t.* (4), *Pettenkofer's t., Strassburg's t., Tyson's t., Udránsky's t.* (1).

bile pigment t., see specific tests, including *Barral's t., Basham's t., Bonanno's t., Brücke's t.* (1), *Capranica's t.* (1), *Cunisset's t., Dragendorff's t., Dumontpallier's t., Fleischl's t.,* foam *t., Gerhardt's t.* (3), *Gluzinski's t.* (1), *Gmelin's t., Hammarsten's t.* (2), *Huppert's t., Huppert-Cole t., Jolles' t.* (1), *Kapsinow's t., Krokiewicz's t., Maréchal's. t., Masset's t., Nakayami t., Nobel's t.* (2), *Quinlan's t., Rosenbach-Gmelin t., Salkowski and Schipper's t.,* sand *t., Schmidt's t.* (1), *Stokvis' t.* (1), *Torquay's t., Trousseau's t., Ultzmann's t., Vitali's t.* (3) (4). See also *bile pigments, methods for,* under *method.*

bile solubility t. (*for differentiation between pneumococci and streptococci*): the broth culture to be tested is divided into two parts in separate test tubes. Add 0.5 ml. of sterile ox bile to one tube and 0.5 ml. of salt solution to the other (control) tube. Pneumococci generally dissolve and the cultures become clear; cultures of streptococci remain cloudy.

bilirubin t., see specific tests, including *Fouchet's t., Harrison spot t., Schmidt's t.* (1), *van den Bergh's t.*

binaural distorted speech t's, tests of the capacity of the central nervous system to coordinate two incoming speech patterns, each of which is incomplete.

Binet's t.: a method of testing the mental capacity of children and youth by asking a series of questions adapted to, and standardized on, the capacity of normal children at various ages. According to the answers given the mental age of the subject is ascertained.

Binet-Simon t., see *Binet's t.*

Bing t.: a vibrating tuning fork is held to the mastoid process and the auditory meatus is alternately occluded and left open: an increase and decrease in loudness (positive Bing) is perceived by the normal ear and in sensorineural hearing impairment, but in conductive hearing impairment no difference in loudness is perceived (negative Bing).

Bing's entotic t.: when words are not audible through an ear trumpet as ordinarily applied, but may be heard when spoken into a trumpet joined to a catheter in the eustachian tube, it is probable that there is a lesion of the incus or malleus.

Binz's t. (*for quinine in urine*): the reagent consists of 2 parts iodine, 1 part potassium iodide, and 40 parts water.

Bio Lab t.: a modification of the Ide test for syphilis.

biological t., see *serum t.*

Birkhaug t.: a skin test for rheumatism: intracutaneous injection of 0.1 ml. of a 1 to 1000 dilution of the toxin of a streptococcus derived from a case of rheumatic fever.

Bischoff's t. (*for biliary acids*): heated with diluted sulfuric acid and cane sugar, these yield a red color.

bismuth t., see *Nylander's t.*

bitterling t. (*for pregnancy*): a small carplike fish of Japan (the bitterling) is placed in a quart of fresh water containing 2 teaspoonfuls of a woman's urine; if the woman is pregnant, there grows out from the belly of the bitterling its long tubular oviduct.

biuret t.: 1. (*for proteins*) to 2 ml. of unknown solution add 2 ml. of 2 N sodium hydroxide solution and then a few drops of 1 per cent copper sulfate solution. A pinkish-violet color indicates the presence of biuret or of a similar double —CO·NH— grouping. 2. (*for urea*) melt the substance in a dry test tube and gently heat it. Cool, and dissolve in 2 ml. of water. Add 2 ml. of 2 N sodium hydroxide solution, and mix drop by drop with a 1 per cent copper sulfate solution. A pink and finally a bluish color is produced.

Black's t. (*for beta-oxybutyric acid*): evaporate 50 ml. of urine in a small dish to about one-fourth; acidify with a few drops of hydrochloric acid and add plaster of paris to a thick paste. When the mass begins to harden, break it up into a meal, add 30 ml. of ether, and mix. Draw the clear ether into an evaporating dish; evaporate over a water bath and dissolve the residue in 10 ml. of water. Neutralize with an excess of dry barium carbonate; pour into a test tube, add a few drops of hydrogen peroxide and 5 drops of 10 per cent ferric chloride. A red color indicates beta-oxybutyric acid.

Blackberg and Wanger's t. (*for melanin*): concentrate the urine to one-third, add 1 per cent of potassium persulfate, and let it stand two hours. Precipitate the melanin with an equal volume of methyl alcohol. Filter, wash, and dry.

blanche t.: blanching of the tissues just lingual to the maxillary medial incisors after a tug on the upper lip indicates persistence of attachment of a heavy fibrous frenum which may well interfere with normal development closure of the spacing between the teeth.

blister t. (*for infectious disease*): a blister is raised on the skin and its contents examined. If the proportion of eosinophils present is less than 25 per cent, infectious disease is probable. Called also *Roger-Josué t.*

Block-Steiger t.: a test for simulated deafness based on the fact that if two tuning-forks, vibrating in unison, but one struck stronger than the other, are held before the two ears of a person with normal hearing, the louder fork only will be heard.

blood, tests for, see specific tests, including *Almén's t.* (2), *aminopyrine t., Atkinson* and *Kendall's t., benzidine t., Cowie's guaiac t., Day's t., Deen's t., Donogany's t., Fleig's t., Gannther's t., Gregerson and Boas' t.,* guaiac *t., Heller's t.* (2), *hematein t., hydrogen peroxide t., Klimow's t., Kobert's t., Ladendorff's t., Lechini's t., Lyle and Curtman's t., Meyer's t.* (3). *Nippe's t., phenolphthalein t.* (1), *Rose's t., Rosenthal's t.* (1), *Rossel's aloin t., Roussin's t., Ruttan and Hardisty's t.,* sand *t., Saundby's t., Schalfijew's t., Schönbein's t.* (1), serum *t., Stokes' t., Struve's t., Taylor's t., Teichmann's t., von Zeynek and Mencki's t., Weber's t.* (3), *Williamson's t.*

blood cholesterol t.: increase of the cholesterol content of the blood indicates deficiency of the cholaligenic power of the liver.

blood-urea clearance t.: a test for renal function based on the volume of blood which is cleared of its urea per minute.

Bloor's t.: 1. (*for fat*) the protein is precipitated, the fat is saponified, and the amount determined nephelometrically. 2. (*for cholesterol in blood*) extract the blood with a mixture of alcohol and ether and evaporate to dryness. Extract residue with chloroform and add acetic anhydride and sulfuric acid.

Bloxam's t. (*for urea*): if a nitrate is present, add a few drops of an ammonium chloride solution; if absent, acidulate with hydrochloric acid. Evaporate to dryness in a watch glass, and heat cautiously as long as thick, white fumes evolve. Dissolve the residue in a drop or two of ammonia, add a drop of barium chloride solution, and stir. If urea is present, a crystalline streak of barium cyanurate will form in the track of the rod.

Blum's t. (*for albumin*): dissolve 0.03 to 0.05 gm. manganous chloride in a little water; acidulate with hydrochloric acid, and treat with 100 ml. of 10 per cent solution sodium metaphosphate. Then add lead oxide a little at a time, let the liquid settle, and filter. Resulting pink solution of manganic metaphosphate detects albumin in urine. Place reagent in a test tube and filter urine into it.

Blumenau's t. (*for tuberculosis*): a drop of tuberculin is applied to the forearm and covered with adhesive plaster; an eruption develops if the patient has tuberculosis.

Blyth's t. (*for lead in drinking water*): a little alcoholic tincture of cochineal makes a precipitate with it.

Boas' t.: 1. (*for hydrochloric acid in the stomach contents*) dissolve 5 gm. of resorcinol and 3 gm. of sugar in 100 ml. of dilute alcohol. A thin layer of this reagent is warmed upon a porcelain dish. If a glass rod is dipped in this layer and touched to a drop of the filtered stomach juice, a scarlet streak is formed. Called also *resorcinol t.* 2. (*for free hydrochloric acid in the stomach contents*) resublimed resorcinol, 5 parts; cane sugar, 3 parts; 94 per cent alcohol, to make 100 parts; boil the fluid with the reagent: free hydrochloric acid will give a transient rose-red mirror. 3. (*for lactic acid*) test for lactic acid in gastric juice depends on oxidation of the acid to aldehyde and formic acid by action of sulfuric acid and manganese. The aldehyde is detected by addition of Nessler's reagent or by formation of iodoform when iodine solution is added. 4. chlorophyll t.

Bodal's t.: test of color perception by the use of colored blocks.

Boedeker's t. (*for albumin*): the liquid is treated with acetic acid, and potassium ferrocyanide in solution is added drop by drop; albumin will form a white precipitate.

Boerner-Lukens t.: a flocculation test for syphilis.

Bohmansson's t. (*for dextrose*): to 10 ml. of the urine add 2 ml. of 25 per cent hydrochloric acid and 5 ml. of bone black. Shake well, filter, and make Nylander's test on the filtrate.

Boltz's t. (*for diagnosis of schizophrenia*): place 1 ml. of fresh cerebrospinal fluid in a small glass test tube and to it add 0.3 ml. of acetic anhydride. Shake the mixture well and then add, drop by drop, 0.8 ml. of concentrated sulfuric acid. Shake the mixture gently once more. Then hold the test tube against a white background. The presence of a lilac tint indicates a positive reaction; a brownish-yellow, reddish-yellow, or clear fluid is noted if the reaction is a negative one.

Bonanno's t. (*for bile pigments*): to 5 ml. of the unknown add a few drops of concentrated hydrochloric acid containing 2 per cent of sodium nitrite; an emerald green color indicates bile pigments.

bone conduction t.: if a vibrating tuning-fork, when the handle is placed against the skull, is heard more distinctly than when held near the ear, it indicates loss in conduction through the middle ear.

borates and boric acid t.: dry the milk and ash the residue. Add 1 ml. of water and 2 drops of hydrochloric acid. Soak a strip of turmeric paper in the solution one minute and allow it to dry in the air. A deep red color which changes to green or blue on treatment with dilute alkali indicates boric acid.

Borchardt's t. (*for levulose in urine*): a few milliliters of a mixture of equal parts of water and concentrated hydrochloric acid are heated for one and one half minutes with an equal amount of urine and a few crystals of resorcin. The mixture is allowed to cool, made alkaline with sodium carbonate, then poured into a test tube and shaken with acetic ether; a yellow color in the ether indicates the presence of levulose.

Borden's t. (*for typhoid fever*): a modification of the Gruber-Widal reaction. The patient's blood serum is mixed with salt solution and then with a suspension of killed typhoid bacilli, so as to bring the dilution up to 1 to 50. The positive reaction consists of the sinking of the clump of bacteria to the bottom of the test tube, leaving a clear fluid above a small white mass of agglutinated bacilli.

Bordet's t., see *serum t.*

Boston's t.: a method of performing the ring tests for albumin in which the fluids are brought into contact in a glass pipet.

Botelho's t. (*for cancer*): to centrifugated suspect blood serum, dilute nitric acid and an iodine reagent are added in several small amounts at short intervals, the test tube being shaken after each addition. Normal serum remains clear, that of cancer patients continues clouded.

Böttger's t.: 1. [R. *Böttger*] (*for carbon monoxide*) paper moistened with palladium chloride solution (0.0002 gm. in 100 ml.) becomes darkened in the presence of carbon monoxide. 2. [W. C. *Böttger*] (*for dextrose in the urine*) the urine is treated with sodium hydroxide and then boiled with a very small amount of bismuth subnitrate; if dextrose is present the precipitate is black.

Bottu's t. (*for dextrose*): to 8 ml. of Bottu's reagent (3.5 gm. of orthonitrophenylpropiolic acid and 5 ml. of freshly prepared 10 per cent solution of sodium hydroxide per liter) in a test tube, add 1 ml. of the urine and mix. Boil the upper portion, add one more ml. of the mixture, and heat again. A blue color accompanied by the precipitation of small particles of indigo indicates dextrose.

Bouchardat's t. (*for alkaloids*): potassium tri-iodide as a test for alkaloids gives a brown precipitate, soluble in alcohol.

Bouin and Ancel t.: a test for the presence of progestin.

Bourdon's t. (*for mental alertness*): a test based on the accuracy and time required for a patient to strike out certain letters, numbers or words as required.

Bourget's t. (*for iodides in urine and saliva*): impregnate a filter paper with a 5 per cent starch solution, dry, and cut into squares 5 cm. each. Then drop 2 or 3 drops of a 5 per cent ammonium persulfate solution in the center of each square, and dry the pieces in the dark. Even with traces of iodine the prepared paper gives an intensely blue color.

Boveri's t. (*for excess of globulin in cerebrospinal fluid*): over 1 ml. of cerebrospinal fluid in a test tube is poured an equal quantity of a 1:1000 solution of potassium permanganate. If there is excess of globulin a yellow ring will form at the line of junction, and on shaking, the entire contents of the tube will become bright yellow.

Boyksen's t. (*for cancer*): serum from animals immunized with cancer material is injected intracutaneously; the resulting reaction is said to be more frequently positive in cancer patients than in controls.

Bozicevich's t.: a serologic test for the detection of trichinosis.

Brace t.: a method of testing the general motor ability of school-age children.

bracelet t.: the production of pain on moderate lateral compression of the lower ends of the radius and ulna; observed in rheumatoid arthritis.

Bram's t.: persons with Graves' disease are more tolerant of quinine hydrobromide than normal persons.

Brande's t. (*for quinine*): when a solution of quinine is treated with chlorine water and ammonia, a green color is produced.

Braun's t. (*for dextrose in urine*): the urine is alkalinized with sodium hydroxide and boiled with a solution of trinitrophenol; if dextrose is present, a deep-red color is produced. Acetone gives the same reaction, though less decidedly, whereas creatine will give it even in a cold solution.

Braun-Husler t.: to 1 ml. of cerebrospinal fluid add 5 ml. of 1:300 aqueous solution of hydrochloric acid; the mixture becomes cloudy if there is an excess of globulin in the cerebrospinal fluid.

Bremer's t. (*for diabetic blood*): the blood is prepared for staining, dried in a hot-air sterilizer, and stained with methylene blue and eosin. The red corpuscles of normal blood become brownish; but those of diabetic blood take on a greenish yellow tint.

Brenner's t., see under *formula*.

Brieger's t.: 1. (*for pyrocatechin*) add 1 drop of urine to 1 drop of very dilute ferric chloride solution on a watch glass—pyrocatechin causes an emerald-green color; on adding now a dilute solution of sodium bicarbonate or ammonium carbonate, the fluid becomes violet, changing back to green with acetic acid. 2. (*for strychnine*) pure chromic acid is added, and a violet color is produced. 3. see *cachexia reaction*, under *reaction*.

Broadbent's t. (*for cerebral dominance of language function*): different numbers (or words) are presented simultaneously to the two ears; right-handed persons tend to report first the words going into the right ear.

bromine t.: 1. (*for melanin*) see *Zeller's t.* (1). 2. (*for tryptophan*) see *tryptophan t.* (1). 3. (*for pregnancy*) a chemical test for the histamine found in the pituitary hormone excreted in the urine; in a test tube 2.5 ml. of urine are mixed with 1 ml. of bromine water, heating the solution to boiling. A positive reaction is indicated by a pink coloration.

Bromsulphalein t., see *sodium sulfobromophthalein.*

Brown's t.: 1. a modification of the Friedman test in which the patient's blood serum is used instead of urine. Called also *Brown's reaction*. [T. K. Brown.] 2. (*for quantitative estimation of ammonia in urine*) heat 60 ml. of urine with 3 gm. of basic lead acetate, stir well, let stand for a few minutes, and filter. This removes nitrogenous substances. Heat the filtrate with 2 gm. of neutral potassium oxalate, stir well, and filter. Take 10 ml. of the filtrate, add 50 ml. of water and 15 gm. of neutral potassium oxalate, and estimate the ammonia.

Brown fever t. (*for lesions of the sympathetic nervous system*): fever is induced with intravenous typhoid vaccine, and the increase of surface temperature is measured at half-hour intervals with a galvanometer.

brucellin t.: an allergic skin test made by the intradermal injection of melitin for the diagnosis of undulant fever (brucellosis).

Brücke's t.: 1. (*for bile pigments in urine*) it is made by shaking with nitric acid, and then slowly adding sulfuric acid; color reactions follow. 2. (*for proteins*) the suspected liquid is acidulated with hydrochloric acid and treated with potassic iodide; the proteins will be precipitated. 3. (*for urea*) the suspected liquid is heated with an alcoholic solution of fusel oil, filtered, and treated with a solution of oxalic acid in fusel oil; a crystalline deposit is formed.

Brugsch's t.: potassium ferrocyanide is injected intradermally as a test for iron in the skin: development of a blue stain at the site of injection denotes the presence of iron.

Bryce's t.: the determination of a degree of immunity against smallpox conferred by vaccination by repeating the inoculation after the lapse of several days; if the first is successful, the second will rapidly overtake it.

Bufano t. (*for liver function*): intravenous injection of 10 ml. of a 12 per cent solution of glycocoll is preceded and followed by measurement of the blood amino nitrogen. Normally there is a decrease in the amino acid after the injection.

Bühler's baby t.: a test for evaluating the development status of infants in the first two years of life.

Burchardt-Liebermann t., see *Liebermann's t.*

Bürger's t.: in persons without metabolic disturbance, there develops a hypercholesterolemia after the ingestion of cholesterol.

Burnam's t. (*for formaldehyde in urine*): to 10 ml. of urine in a test tube is added 3 drops of a 5 per cent solution of phenylhydrazine hydrochloride, 3 drops of a 5 per cent solution of sodium nitroprusside, and then a few drops of sodium hydroxide solution are poured down the side of the test tube. If formaldehyde is present, a deep purplish color is seen, changing to dark green, and then to pale yellow.

Buscaino's t.: three ml. of urine are mixed with 1.5 ml. of a 5 per cent solution of silver nitrate and the whole boiled for thirty minutes. The color of the precipitate indicates the reaction: a white precipitate is negative, a brown or black precipitate indicates disease of the brain.

butter t.: a test for pancreatic insufficiency based on the fact that in deficiency of the external secretion of the pancreas so much fat may be present in the stool after the ingestion of butter that the stool looks like butter.

butyric acid t., see *pineapple t.*, and *Noguchi reaction*, under *reaction.*

Bychowski's t. (*for albumin in urine*): two drops of urine are placed in a test tube of hot water and shaken; the water becomes cloudy if albumin is present.

caffeine t., see *Archetti's t.*, *Delff's t.*

Caillan's t. (*for dextrose in urine*): shake 2 parts of urine with 1 part of chloroform; on settling, dextrose will be present in the upper layer.

calcium t., see *Clark's t.* (2) and *Sulkowitch's t.* See also *calcium, methods for,* under *method.*

California mastitis t. (C.M.T.) (*for subclinical mastitis in cows*): equal amounts of milk, bromcresol purple, and an anionic surface-active substance are mixed in four separate cups within a plastic paddle by rapidly rotating the paddle horizontally; a positive reaction is indicated by various degrees of gel formation, according to the degree of abnormality of the milk. Called also *Schalm t.*

Callaway's t.: a test for dislocation of the humerus, consisting in the fact that the circumference of the affected shoulder, measured over the acromion and through the axilla, is greater than that on the unaffected side.

Calmette's t., see *ophthalmic reaction,* under *reaction.*

caloric t., see *Bárány's symptom* (def. 2), under *symptom.*

Calvert's t.: the patient takes his usual food, but no fluids from 12 noon. At 9 P.M. the bladder is emptied and 15 gm. of urea are drunk in 4 oz. of water; at 10 P.M. the bladder is again emptied and the urine discarded. The patient then goes to bed and all the night urine, together with that passed on rising—say 7 A.M.—is kept. A sample (*a*) of these mixed portions is analyzed for its urea content. The patient then drinks 30 oz. of weak tea or water and the urine passed up to the end of two hours—9 A.M.—is kept and a sample (*b*) again analyzed for its urea percentage. The two specimens *a* and *b* represent the maximum and minimum concentrations of urea in the urine and the difference between them represents the urea range.

Cammidge's t., pancreatic reaction.

Campani's t. (*for dextrose*): a mixture of a concentrated solution of lead subacetate and a dilute solution of copper acetate is productive of a yellow or red color.

Campbell's t.: the erythrocytes of pellagrous blood cause more rapid discoloration of iodine solutions than do other red corpuscles.

camphor t.: if 7½ grains of camphor are given by the mouth it should cause glycuronic acid to appear in the urine; this will not occur in liver disease.

cancer t., see specific tests including *antitrypsin t., Aron's t.,* (1), *Bolen's t., Botelho's t., Boyksen's t., Chrobak t., Clark t.* (1), *D'Amato's t., Fuchs' t., Gluzinski's t., glycyltryptophan t., Gröbly's t., Gross' t.,* (2), *Gruskin's t.* (1), *Haagensen t., Hirschfeldt's t., Huggins t., Kahn t.* (2), *Kelling's t.* (1), *Klein's t., Links' t., Lowy's t., Mendeléeff's t., miostagmin t., Pap t., Peret's t., Ringold t., Salomon's t., Schiller's t., Schubert-Dannmeyer t., Suranyi's t., tryptophan t.* (1), *Wolff-Junghans t.* See also *cancer reaction,* under *reaction.*

cane sugar t., see *Nicklés' t.*

Cannabis indica t., see *Gayer t.*

Cantani t. (*in syphilis*): Reagent A, 56 gm. of powdered ox heart, 300 ml. of 95 per cent ethyl alcohol, 150 ml. of 99.2 per cent ethyl alcohol and 2.5 gm. of cholesterol; reagent B, 20 gm. of egg lecithin, 370 ml. of 95 per cent ethyl alcohol and 3.75 ml. of pure phenol; reagent C, 225 ml. of 95 per cent ethyl alcohol, 25 ml. of pure phenol and 0.1 ml. of a 5 per cent solution of petrolatum in benzine. One part of reagent A, one part of reagent B and 0.5 part of reagent C are placed in a tube with two parts of a 3 per cent solution of sodium chloride. It is shaken for seven minutes before using. Eight times the original amount of sodium chloride solution is put in another tube, and after seven minutes the contents of the second tube are poured into the first tube and thoroughly mixed. Then 0.25 ml. of the mixture is poured into the tubes (generally five) containing the serum to be examined; the tubes are shaken at the rate of from 150 to 200 times per minute for four minutes, then left at rest for two minutes, and 2 ml. of an 0.85 per cent solution of sodium chloride is added to each tube. Negative serums show opalescence without flocculation; positive serums, clear flocculation; strongly positive serums, heavy flocculation with clarification of the liquid.

capillary fragility t., capillary resistance t.: apply blood pressure cuff for five minutes tightly enough to obstruct venous return only, or apply a cupping glass, and note the number of petechiae thus produced.

capon comb growth t.: a test for the presence of androgenic hormone based on the growth response of the comb of a capon following subcutaneous injection of the test material.

Cappagnoli's t. (*for dextrose*): a solution of cupric hydroxide and potassium hydroxide is added; a blue color is produced.

Capranica's t.: 1. (*for bile pigments*) shake the liquid with chloroform containing bromine; it turns green, blue, violet, yellowish red, and then becomes nearly colorless. 2. (*for guanine*) a warm solution of guanine hydrochloride gives a yellow precipitate in silky needles with a cold saturated solution of trinitrophenol. 3. (*for guanine*) mix the solution with a concentrated solution of potassium ferrocyanide: a yellowish-brown precipitate in prisms appears. 4. (*for guanine*) add to the suspected solution a concentrated solution of potassium dichromate; guanine will cause an orange-red precipitate in crystals.

carbohydrate t., see *Moore's t., Schiff's t.* (1).

carbohydrate tolerance t., see *Bauer's t.* (2) and *Killian's t.*

carbon clearance t., (*for activity of mononuclear phagocytes*): colloidal carbon particles are injected intravenously into an experimental animal; the amount of carbon remaining is then ascertained colorimetrically from lysed blood samples and the rate of carbon removed by phagocytosis is determined.

carbon monoxide t., see specific tests, including *Böttger's t.* (1), *Dejust's t., Hoppe-Seyler t.* (1), *Katayama's t., Preyer's t., Rubner's t.* (1), *Salkowski's t.* (1), *tannin t., Wetzel's t., Zaleski's t.*

carbon monoxide hemoglobin t., see *tannin t.*

Carnot's t. (*for atonic dilatation of the stomach*): the patient's stomach is emptied by the stomach pump and 500 ml. of water introduced. The patient remains in an erect posture for an hour, after which the water is withdrawn and measured. Then 500 ml. of water are introduced and the patient placed on his right side for an hour. In this position the stomach should be nearly empty in an hour.

carotid sinus t. (*for angina pectoris*): on slowing of the heart rate by massage over the right (or left) carotid sinus, the pain of an attack of angina pectoris will lessen or disappear.

carotinemia t.: to 2 ml. of serum add 2 ml. of 95 per cent alcohol and 2 ml. of petroleum ether; compare the color of the ether layer with a standard.

Carr-Price t.: a quantitative color test for vitamin A in oils.

Carrez's t. (*for albumin*): one gram of resorcinol is dissolved in 2 ml. of distilled water in a test tube and the urine is poured upon the surface; a white ring shows albumin.

Casamajor's t. (*for glucose*): the suspected liquid is shaken with methyl alcohol; glucose makes the mixture cloudy.

casein t., see *Leiner's t.* See also *casein, method for,* under *method.*

Casilli's t.: an adaptation of the Kahn antigen for slide agglutination.

Casoni's intradermal t. (*for hydatid disease*): injection into the skin of hydatid fluid followed by the immediate or delayed production of a wheal-and-flare reaction denotes hydatid infection.

Castellani's t.: 1. (*for albuminuria*) the filtered urine 5 ml., is placed in a test tube and 1.5 ml. of liquefied phenol is added by pouring it slowly down the sides of the tube by means of a pipet. The liquefied phenol will collect at the bottom of the tube. If within two minutes a definite white ring forms where the two liquids come in contact the test is considered positive; namely, the urine contains albumin. 2. an agglutination test for ascertaining the existence of a mixed infection with allied species of organisms.

catoptric t.: a test for cataract made by observing the reflections from the cornea and from the surfaces of the crystalline lens.

cellulose t., see *Cutola t., Schultze's t.* (1).

cephalin-cholesterol flocculation t., see *Hanger's t.*

Chapman's t. (*for acute abdominal conditions*): the patient is told to assume a supine position with his arms at his sides and then to raise himself by the abdominal muscles alone; when he fails to rise or feels great pain in doing so the test is positive.

Chautard's t. (*for acetone in the urine*): a drop of aqueous solution of magenta is dissolved with sulfurous acid and added to the urine; a violet color is produced.

Chediak's t. (*for syphilis*): a drop of blood is put on a slide, stirred for one minute and thus defibrinated, then exposed to the air and dried. To the dried drop 0.015 ml. of a solution containing 3.5 per cent of sodium chloride and 0.3 per cent of sodium carbonate is added. The blood is diluted with this solution and is placed in a paraffin ring (1.5 cm. in diameter) on another slide. Then 0.03 ml. of a dilution of the Meinicke clarification extract made with the aforementioned freshly prepared salt solution in a ratio of 1:10 is added. Before use, the extract and diluting fluid are heated separately for eight minutes in the water bath at 56° C. (132.8° F.), and, after being mixed, the solution remains two minutes longer in the water bath. The slide is shaken for three minutes and kept for thirty minutes in the moist chamber at room temperature. In negative tests the microscope reveals brown granules, but the positive reaction is indicated by black floccules and clots in the reddish-brown fluid.

Chick-Martin t.: a test for the efficiency of disinfectants in which dried human feces are used as the test material; see under *method.*

Chiene's t.: two strips of lead or tape are carried across the front of the body, the upper over the anterior superior spines, the lower over the great trochanters; convergence of these lines points to the side of upward displacement of the trochanter in fracture of the neck of the femur.

Chimani-Moos t.: a test for detecting simulated deafness.

chi-square t.: a statistical test in which the square of the difference between the expected frequency and the observed frequency is divided by the expected frequency, the sum of the quotients (for each category under test) being the chi-square (symbol X^2); the smaller the value of chi-square, the closer the agreement between the hypothetical and the actual frequency.

chloride balance t., see *balance t.*

chlorides t., see *Volhard's t.* (1).

chlorophyll t. (*for gastric motility*): on a fasting stomach the patient drinks 400 ml. of water which has been colored green by the addition of 20 drops of chlorophyll solution. After half an hour the residue is aspirated from the stomach, and the amount that has passed out of the stomach in one-half hour is ascertained.

cholera red t. (*for indole*): to the unknown add one tenth its volume of a 0.02 per cent solution of potassium nitrite and mix. Underlay with sulfuric acid. The purple color will change to bluish green on neutralization with potassium hydroxide.

cholesterol t., see *Bloor's t.* (2), *Bürger's t., Libermann-Burchardt's t., Obermüller's t., Salkowski's t.* (2), *Schiff's t.* (2), (3), *Schultze's t.* (2), and *Zwenger's t.* (1). See also *cholesterol, methods for,* under *method.*

Chopra's antimony t. (*for kala-azar*): see under *reaction.*

Chorine's t. (*for malaria*): dilute the serum with 10 parts of distilled water. Determine the optical density at once with the photometer of Vernes, Bricq, and Yvonne. Incubate three hours, allow to stand thirty minutes and take a second reading. The difference in the two readings in degrees represents the index of the serum.

Chovstek t. (for *hyperexcitability of muscles*): tap on the facial nerve just anterior to the ear; if positive, the muscles at the angle of the mouth on the same side contract.

Chrobak t.: if irritation of an eroded cervix by a sound causes bleeding and crumbling of the tissue, cancer should be suspected.

chromatin t. (for *determination of genetic sex*): examination of body cells for presence of the sex chromatin situated at the periphery of the nucleus in normal females but not in normal males.

chromic acid t. (for *alcohol*): warm with dilute sulfuric acid or hydrochloric acid and add 1 to 2 drops of very dilute potassium dichromate solution; the color will change from red to green and the odor of acetaldehyde will appear.

Ciamician and Magnanini's t. (for *skatole*): warm the solution with sulfuric acid; skatole produces a purplish-red tint.

Cipollina's t. (for *dextrose or levulose in urine*): four ml. of urine, 5 drops of pure phenylhydrazine, and 0.5 ml. of glacial acetic acid are boiled for one minute. Four or 5 drops of potassium hydroxide solution are added and the mixture boiled again for a few seconds. Cool and examine for crystals of phenyl-levulosazone or phenyl-dextrosazone.

cis-trans t.: in microbial genetics, a test to determine whether two mutations that have the same phenotypic effect (in a haploid cell or a cell with single phage infection) are located in the same gene (resulting in noncomplementation) or in different genes (resulting in complementation and hence in loss of the mutant defect). The test depends on the independent behavior of two alleles of a gene in a diploid cell or in a cell infected with two phages carrying different alleles.

citochol t., see *Sachs-Witebsky t.*

Clark's t.: 1. bleeding upon insertion into the interior of the uterus with a sound; usually indicative of cancer. 2. (for *calcium in blood*) precipitate the calcium with ammonium oxalate, remove excess of oxalate, dissolve precipitate in sulfuric acid, and titrate against potassium permanganate [Guy Wendell Clark].

Clauberg t.: a biological assay method for the standardization of corpus luteum preparations or progesterone. Immature rabbits are primed with estrogen before the material to be tested is administered. The degree of endometrial development is observed.

Clive's t.: an acetic anhydride method of testing the blood serum for syphilis.

C.M.T., see *California mastitis t.*

coagulase t.: a test for coagulase activity in which bacteria are added to citrated or oxalated (human or rabbit) blood plasma; in the presence of coagulase, the plasma gels within three hours. Coagulase activity is also demonstrable by mixing bacteria with blood plasma on a slide; if positive, clumping occurs, with fibrin formation.

coagulation t. (for *proteins in urine*): acidify the urine with acetic acid and boil; a white coagulum or a white precipitate or a cloudiness indicates protein.

cobra venom t., see *Weil's t.*

coccidioidin t.: an intracutaneous test for coccidioidomycosis; see *coccidioidin.*

cockscomb t.: a test for the activity of the ergot preparations, based on the fact that ergot, when administered to a cock, produces a blue coloration of its comb.

Cohen's t. (for *albumin*): to the acidulated solution add a solution of potassium bismuthic iodide and potassium iodide; albumin is precipitated.

Cohn's t.: a test for color perception by the use of variously colored embroidery patterns.

coin t.: a test for pneumothorax made by auscultating the chest while a coin laid against the chest is struck with another coin; a metallic, ringing sound is produced over a cavity containing air.

colchicin t., see *Zeisel's t.*

cold pressor t., see *Hines and Brown t.*

Cole's t.: 1. (for *dextrose*) add acetic acid to the urine and filter through blood charcoal to remove other reducing substances; then make a modified Fehling's test. 2. (for *lactose*) adsorb the lactose on to blood charcoal, extract it again with hot dilute acetic acid, and make an osazone test. 3. (for *uric acid*) add 2 drops of ammonium hydroxide to 5 ml. of urine and then saturate with ammonium chloride; pour off the supernatant fluid, filter, evaporate residue, and make murexid test.

collateral circulation t., see specific tests, including *Henle-Coenen t., Korotkoff's t., Pachon's t., tourniquet t.* (2), (3), *Tuffier's t., von Frisch t.*

colloidal benzoin t., see *benzoin t.*

colloidal gold t., (for *protein—globulin—in the cerebrospinal fluid, and thus for the diagnosis of certain central nervous system disorders, such as neurosyphilis, multiple sclerosis, poliomyelitis, and encephalitis*): progressive dilutions of cerebrospinal fluid are added to ten test tubes containing colloidal gold solution. The extent of precipitation is indicative of various diseases, and the results are interpreted according to the color changes that result. When no color change occurs the reaction is negative, i.e., the deep red colloidal gold color remains unchanged, and is recorded as 0. The appearance of the solution in the tube depends upon the amount of gold precipi-

tated and is scored as 1+ (reddish blue), 2+ (lilac to purple), 3+ (deep blue), 4+ (pale blue), and 5+ (colorless, due to complete precipitation of the gold). Called also *Lange's t.* or *Lange's colloidal gold t.*

color perception t.: see specific tests, including *Bodal's t., Cohn's t., Donders' t., Holmgren's t., Ishihara's t., Jenning's t., lantern t., Mauthner's t., Nagel's t.*

Comessatti's t. (for *epinephrine*): to 5 ml. of the unknown solution add an equal volume of 1 per cent sodium acetate solution and 1 ml. of 0.1 per cent mercuric chloride solution; a rose color indicates epinephrine.

complement fixation t., see under *fixation.*

concentration t. (for *renal function*): the patient is placed under conditions which cause the normal person to elaborate urine containing one or more constituents in high concentration and the results observed to see whether the patient is able to attain this concentration, as in the *urea concentration t., xylose concentration t.*

Congo red t. (for *amyloidosis*): Congo red is injected intravenously; if more than 60 per cent of the dye disappears after one hour, amyloidosis is indicated.

conjugate glycuronates t., see *Tollen's t.* (4).

conjunctival t.: 1. see *ophthalmic reaction,* under *reaction.* 2. the local reaction which occurs when a pollen or an extract of the pollen is instilled into the conjunctival sac of a person sensitive to that pollen.

connective tissue t., see *Schmidt's t.* (5).

consumption t.: a serological reaction in which antibody or antigen is removed from the reaction medium by its homologue. By comparing the quantity of reactant not removed with the amount originally present, the amount of reactant taken up during the reaction may be ascertained.

contact t., see *patch t.*

Contejean t.: dissolve freshly precipitated cobalt carbonate in specimen; a red color changing to blue on evaporation indicates free HCl.

Cooke's t. (for *purine bodies in urine*): in a centrifuge tube take 10 ml. urine and add 1 gm. sodium carbonate and 1 or 2 ml. strong ammonia. Shake until the sodium carbonate is dissolved; the earthy phosphates will be precipitated. Centrifuge and pour off clear fluid. Add 2 ml. ammonia and 2 ml. silver ammonionitrate solution; centrifuge again. Each 0.1 ml. of sediment represents 0.001176 gm. of purine bodies.

Coombs' t.: a test for detection of antibodies to red cells by means of antiglobulin. In the *direct* Coombs test, used to detect cell-bound antibody, the red cells are washed free of serum and unbound antibody, and antiglobulin is added. Agglutination indicates the presence of antibody. This method is used to detect sensitized red cells in erythroblastosis fetalis and autoimmune hemolytic anemia. In the *indirect* Coombs' test, used to detect circulating antibody, a sample of the subject's serum is incubated with donor red cells (or bacteria), the cells are washed, and the antiglobulin is added. If antibody has adsorbed to the cells, they will be agglutinated. Called also *antiglobulin t.*

Cope's t.: with the patient supine, the examiner flexes the right thigh and rotates the hip joint internally; an inflamed appendix will be irritated by this movement and pain will be felt in the hypogastrium.

copper t., see *Schönbein's t.* (2).

copper soap t. (for *lipase*): make up a hydrogel with 1 per cent of agar-agar, 2½ per cent of starch, and 2½ per cent of a neutral fat; pour into Petri dishes, cool, and place drops of the unknown on its surface. Incubate at 38° C. one hour and pour over the surface a saturated solution of cupric sulfate. Bluish green spots of copper soap where the drops were indicate lipase action.

Corner-Allen t.: a biological method of assay for progesterone or corpus luteum preparations containing it. The rabbits are mated, the ovaries removed eighteen hours later, and the material to be assayed injected. The results are read according to the intensity of the endometrial changes.

Costa t. (for *the activity of infections*): a test based on observing the rapidity with which precipitation is produced in blood serum by a procaine formaldehyde reagent.

cover t.: see *alternate cover t.* and *cover-uncover t.*

cover-uncover t.: a test for determining the type of phoria, by covering one eye and noting its movement as it is uncovered.

Cowie's guaiac t. (for *blood in feces*): add glacial acetic acid to the feces and extract with ether. To the filtrate add an equal volume of water, some powdered guaiac resin, and old turpentine or hydrogen peroxide. A blue color indicates blood.

Crafts' t.: in organic disease of the pyramidal tract, stroking with a blunt point upward over the dorsal surface of the ankle, the leg being extended and the muscles relaxed, produces dorsal extension of the great toe.

Craig's t.: 1. (for *tuberculosis*) a complement-fixation test for tuberculosis in which the antigen is made by growing several strains of bacilli on an alkaline bouillon containing a teaspoonful of aseptically removed egg white and egg yolk for each 250 ml. of bouillon. 2. a modification of the Wassermann test using a human hemolytic serum instead of a sheep hemolytic serum.

Cramer's t. (for *dextrose*): place 3 ml. of Cramer's "2.5 reagent" (0.4 gm. of mercuric oxide and 6 gm. of potassium iodide dissolved in 100 ml. of water and the reaction so adjusted that 10 ml. will be neutralized to phenolphthalein by 2.5 ml. of N/10 acid) in a test tube and boil. Add 3 ml. of the urine and again boil. If positive the mixture becomes turbid, darkens, and a precipitate of finely divided mercury settles out.

Crampton's t.: a test for physical resistance and condition based on the difference between the pulse and blood pressure in the recumbent position and in the standing position. A difference of 75 or more indicates good condition; one of 65 or less shows a poor condition.

creatinine t., see specific tests, including *balance t., Braun's t., Jaffé's t.* (1), *Kerner's t., Salkowski's t.* (5), *Thudichum's t., von Maschke's t., Weyl's t.* (1). See also *creatinine, methods for,* under *method.*

creatinine clearance t.: a test for renal function based on the rate at which ingested creatinine is filtered through the renal glomeruli.

Crismer's t. *(for dextrose)*: the solution is made alkaline, and is boiled with 1 part of safranine in 1000 parts of water: if dextrose is present, the mixture is decolorized or turned to a pale yellow.

Cronin Lowe t.: a precipitation test for malignancy.

cuff t.: a test for angina pectoris by producing ischemia in the left arm for five minutes by raising the pressure in a blood-pressure cuff on the arm to 50 mm. above the usual systolic pressure. This may produce an anginal attack in persons with coronary disease.

Cuignet's t. *(for simulated unilateral blindness)*: with the patient reading a book, the examiner inserts a pencil vertically between the eyes and the book. If patient continues to read uninterruptedly, he is seeing with both eyes.

Cunisset's t. *(for bile in the urine)*: the urine is shaken with chloroform; if biliary matter is present, a yellow color is produced.

currant t.: if, after a meal of currants, the seeds do not appear in the stools in twenty-four hours, there is defective motility.

Cutler-Power-Wilder t. *(for Addison's disease)*: the sodium chloride in the diet is restricted for a few days, and potassium citrate is administered; a marked rise in urinary chloride concentration on the third day indicates adrenal insufficiency.

Cutola t.: a 50 per cent hydriodic acid solution containing iodine colors cellulose blue.

Cutting's t. *(for spinal fluid)*: add a colloidal suspension of gum mastic to a series of dilutions of the spinal fluid; a heavy white precipitate is positive.

cysteine t., see specific tests, including *Andreasch's t., nitroprusside t.* (1), *Sullivan's t.*

cystine t., see specific tests, including *Baumann and Goldmann's t., Liebig's t., Müller's t.* (1).

cytopherometric t.: a method of assaying lymphocyte sensitization based on the principle that the interaction of sensitized lymphocytes with specific antigen results in liberation of a substance that slows electrophoretic migration of normal macrophages.

cytosine t., see *Wheeler and Johnson's t.*

cytotoxicity t.: any of a variety of tests of the ability to lyse cells, as when living cells are incubated with specific antibody and complement or with T-lymphocytes primed against cell surface antigens. Dead cells are then detected by staining, plaque formation, or other technique.

Daclin t.: shake 10 ml. of urine with 5 ml. of chloroform; allow this mixture to separate; decant the chloroform layer; evaporate this at a gentle heat; treat the residue with 2 drops of pure H_2SO_4. A violet color indicates santonine.

D'Amato's t.: in persons sensitized to the causative organism of a disease such as typhoid, paratyphoid, undulant fever, syphilis, the injection of the corresponding vaccine produces a hemoclastic reaction. In bearers of malignant tumors, the injection of neoplastic extracts produces a specific hemoclastic reaction.

dark-adaptation t. *(for vitamin A deficiency)*: a test based on the fact that with a deficient intake of vitamin A the ability to see a dimly illuminated object in a dark room is diminished.

darkroom t.: a test to determine the tendency to develop acute angle glaucoma: ocular pressure is measured by the applanation tonometer, the subject is placed in a darkroom for one hour, and applanation tonometry is then repeated.

Davidsohn's t. *(differential test for infectious mononucleosis)*: the determination of the agglutination of sheep erythrocytes by the patient's serum after absorption with Forssman antigen (guinea pig kidney or horse kidney) and beef antigen, respectively.

Davy's t. *(for phenol)*: to a drop or two of the suspected solution add 3 or 4 drops of a solution of 1 part of molybdic acid in 10 or 15 parts of concentrated sulfuric acid; if phenol is present, a pale yellow-brown tint is produced, changing to a reddish brown and then to a fine purple.

Day's t. *(for blood)*: the suspected substance is treated with fresh guaiacum tincture and then with hydrogen dioxide; if blood is present, a blue tint is produced.

Dedichen's t. *(for liver function)*: a test based on the assumption that urobilinuria is a sign of absolute liver insufficiency. Tincture of iodine is added to the urine, drop by drop, and then an equal amount of Schlesinger's reagent. The mixture is filtered. If urobilin is present, fluorescence takes place.

Deen's t. *(for blood in gastric juice)*: to the gastric juice is added 1 ml. of a fresh tincture of guaiac and 1 ml. of Hühnerfeld's solution (2 ml. of glacial acetic acid, 1 ml. of distilled water, and 100 ml. each

of oil of turpentine and alcohol). On shaking, the fluid turns blue if blood is present. Iron compounds give the same reaction as blood.

Degener's t. *(for alkalis)*: phenacetolin is turned red by alkalis.

Dehio's t.: if bradycardia is relieved by injections of atropine, the condition is caused by increased vagal tone; but if the bradycardia is not relieved, the cause is some affection of the heart muscle.

dehydrocholate t. *(for the speed of blood circulation)*: sodium dehydrocholate solution is injected intravenously; the usual time elapsing until a bitter taste in the mouth occurs is between 10 and 14 seconds.

Dejust's t. *(for carbon monoxide)*: if air containing carbon monoxide is passed through an ammoniacal silver solution, metallic silver will be deposited and the solution will take on a brown or black color.

Delff's t. *(for caffeine)*: a solution of red mercuric oxide and potassium iodide; it is used as a test for caffeine, which it throws down as a crystalline precipitate.

Denigès' t.: 1. *(for uric acid)* add nitric acid, which changes uric acid into alloxan, heat gently so as to drive off free nitric acid; add a few drops of sulfuric acid and of commercial benzol, which contains thiophen. This gives a blue color if alloxan has been formed. 2. *(for acetone in urine)* about 1 inch of the distillate in a test tube is mixed with an equal amount of a solution of the subsulfate of mercury (mercuric oxide 50, sulfuric acid 200, water up to 1000) and the mixture is allowed to simmer in a stoppered flask for about five minutes. A white crystalline precipitate occurs on cooling, which is very distinctive in appearance. If acetone is present in excess, the test is less distinct. If but a trace is present, a trace of sodium chloride will aid the precipitation. The precipitate is not soluble in dilute hydrochloric acid. 3. *(for morphine)* to 10 ml. of the unknown add 1 ml. of hydrogen peroxide, 1 ml. of ammonium hydroxide and 1 drop of 4 per cent solution of copper sulfate; a red color indicates morphine.

Dennis and Silverman's t. *(for the pH of stomach contents)*: a few drops of stomach contents are placed on test papers impregnated with Töpfer's reagent and with thymol blue. These are then matched up with similar test papers to which buffered solutions of known pH are applied.

Derrien's t. *(for alphadinitrophenol in the urine)*: to 10 ml. of urine add 1 ml. of 10 per cent H_2SO_4 and 1 ml. of 0.5 per cent $NaNO_2$. Shake and keep in the dark five minutes. Place 2 ml. of a fresh 0.5 per cent betanaphthol solution in ammonia water (22 B) in a 25 ml. capacity tube, and add the treated urine. Shake and after one minute add 10 ml. of sulfuric ether. Shake and cork. If the ether is violet, wine color, or orange-red the reaction is positive; if colorless or yellow, negative.

desmoid t., see under *reaction.*

dextrose t., see specific tests, including *Agostini's t., Allen's t.* (1), *Almén's t.* (3), *Baeyer's t.* (1), *Barfoed's t., Baumann's t., Benedict's t.* (1), *Bertrand's t., Bohmansson's t., Böttger's t.* (2), *Bottu's t., Braun's t., Caillan's t., Campani's t., Cappagnoli's t., Casamajor's t., Cipollina's t., Cole's t.* (1), *Cramer's t., Crismer's t., Donaldson's t.* (1), *Edlefsen's t., Fehling's t., fermentation t., Fischer's t., Folin's t.* (3), *Folin-McElroy t., Gawalowski's t., Gentele's t., Gerrard's t., Hager's t., Haines' t., Heller's t.* (3), *Horsley's t., hydroxylamine t., Jaffé's t.* (1), *Knapp's t.* (1), *Kowarsky's t.* (1), *Loewe's t., Löwenthal's t., Mathew's t., Maumené's t., Molisch's t.* (1), (2), *Moore's t., Mulder's t.* (1), *mycologic t., Nicklés' t., nitropropiol t., Nylander's t., Oliver's t.* (2), *Pavy's t., Pélouse-Moore t., Penzoldt's t.* (2), *Purdy's t.* (1), *Riegler's t.* (3), *Robert's t.* (2), *Rubner's t.* (2), *saccharimeter t., Sachsse's t., Salkowski's t.* (4), *Schmidt's t.* (2), *silver t., Soldaini's t., Tollen's t.* (2), *Trommer's t., von Jaksch's t.* (2), *Wender's t., Worm-Müller t.* See also *glucose (dextrose), methods for,* under *method.*

diabetes t.: see specific tests, including *Bremer's t., Hickey-Hare t., Kowarsky's t.* (2), *Loewi's t., Williamson's blood t.*

diacetic acid t., see *acetoacetic acid t.*

diacetyl t. *(for urea)*: the solution to be tested is mixed with concentrated hydrochloric acid and diacetyl monoxime; a yellow color develops on boiling if urea is present.

dialysis t., see *Abderhalden's reaction,* under *reaction.*

Diamond slide t.: a serologic test for Rh typing performed on open microscope slides.

diastase t., see *Wohlgemuth's t.*

diazo t., see *Ehrlich's diazo reaction,* under *reaction.*

Dick t. *(for susceptibility to scarlet fever)*: a small amount of erythrogenic toxin is injected intracutaneously; appearance within 24 to 48 hours of a small area of reddening of the skin indicates susceptibility of the subject.

Dicken's t. *(for salvarsan)*: to 10 ml. of urine add 3 drops of hydrochloric acid and 10 drops of a 0.5 per cent solution of sodium nitrite. Mix 5 ml. of 10 per cent resorcinol and 3 ml. of a 20 per cent solution of sodium carbonate. Stratify the two solutions; a rose-red ring indicates salvarsan, a yellow ring atoxyl.

differential t. for infectious mononucleosis: a test based on the fact that antisheep agglutinins in infectious mononucleosis are not absorbed by Forssman antigen (whereas as those in serum disease and of normal persons are), but are absorbed by beef cells (whereas those in conditions other than infectious mononucleosis may or may not be).

digitalin t., see *Grandeau's t.*

dilution t., see specific tests, including *Strauss' t.* (2), *Volhard t.,* and *water t.*

p-dimethylaminoazobenzene (*for free hydrochloric acid*): to a little of the filtered gastric juice in a test tube add a drop of 0.5 per cent alcoholic solution of *p*-dimethylaminoazobenzene; in the presence of free hydrochloric acid there will at once appear a cherry-red color.

diphtheria t.: see specific tests, including *Schick t.* and *tellurite t.*

dirt t. (*for milk*): filter a pint of milk through a little disk of absorbent cotton and note the stain produced.

Dold's t.: a flocculation test for syphilis.

Dolman's t. (*for ocular dominance*): the patient holds in both hands a card with a hole in it through which to sight at a light.

Donaldson's t.: 1. (*for sugar*) add to a suspected fluid a few drops of a solution of 5 parts of sodium carbonate, 5 of potassium hydroxide, 6 of potassium bitartrate, 4 of cupric sulfate, and 32 of water; heat it, and if sugar is present, a yellow-green color will be produced. 2. (*for amebic cysts*) add Donaldson's stain to a small amount of the feces; amebic cysts are stained yellow or brown.

Donath's t. (*for paroxysmal hemoglobinuria*), see under *phenomenon.*

Donath-Landsteiner t. (*for paroxysmal cold hemoglobinuria*): a test based on the fact that the blood of patients with this disease contains complement-dependent iso- and autohemolysin which unites with red cells only at low temperatures (2° to 10° C.), hemolysis occurring only after warming to 37° C.

Donders' t.: a color vision test performed by lanterns with sides of colored glass.

Donné's t. (*for pus in urine*): separate sediment from the urine, add to it a piece of solid potassium hydroxide, and stir. If pus is present the sediment will become slimy and tough, whereas mucus will pass into solution.

Donogany's t. (*for blood in urine*): one ml. of ammonium sulfide solution and 1 ml. of pyridine solution are added to 10 ml. of urine; an orange color appears if blood is present.

Dorn-Sugarman t.: a test for sex determination by observing the effect of urine from a pregnant woman on the testicles of rabbits.

double-blind t.: a study of the effects of a specific agent in which neither the administrator nor the recipient, at the time of administration and of recording of the effects, knows whether the active or an inert substance is being given.

double diffusion t.: a gel diffusion test in which solutions of antigen and antibody diffuse toward each other in a gel to form lines of precipitate. It may be in a single dimension as in a fine test tube, the antigen and antibody being separated by a layer of neutral agar, or in two dimensions, as in a Petri dish in which reagents are placed in opposing wells in a layer of agar (see *Ouchterlony t.*).

double glucagon t. (*for deficiency of amylo-1-6-glucosidase*): glucagon is administered after a twelve hour fast and again shortly after a meal; if the blood sugar fails to rise after the first administration but has a normal rise after the second, the test is positive.

Dragendorff's t. (*for bile pigments*): wet an unglazed porcelain plate with the suspected urine, which is soon absorbed; add a drop or more of nitric acid: if bile pigments are present, colored rings are formed.

Drechsel's t.: 1. (*for bile*) on heating the liquid on a water bath with phosphoric acid and cane sugar, a reddish brown color will be produced if bile is present. 2. (*for xanthine*) add cupric chloride to an ammoniacal solution of the substance; xanthine, if present, causes a muddy precipitate.

Dreyer's t.: an agglutination test for the differentiation of typhoid and paratyphoid infections from other infections in persons vaccinated against typhoid-paratyphoid infection.

drinking t. (*for glaucoma*): one quart of water is ingested as rapidly as possible before breakfast. The intraocular pressure is measured every fifteen minutes. A rise of from 8 to 15 mg. Hg in less than one-half hour indicates glaucoma.

Duane's t.: the employment of a candle blaze and prisms to measure the degree of ocular heterophoria.

Dugas' t.: a test for the existence of dislocation of the shoulder, made by placing the hand of the affected side on the opposite shoulder and bringing the elbow to the side of the chest. If this cannot be accomplished (Dugas' sign), dislocation of the shoulder exists.

Duke's t.: a test which measures bleeding time.

Dumontpallier's t. (*for bile pigments*): over the liquid to be tested carefully pour iodine tincture; if bile pigment is present, a green ring is seen between the two liquids.

Dungern's t., see *von Dungern's t.*

Dupont's t. (*for death*): the action of a drop of atropine in the pupil is observed.

dye exclusion t.: the determination of cell viability *in vitro.* Following exposure of a cell preparation to trypan blue or eosin, dead cells take up the dye from the medium whereas living cells remain unstained.

Eagle t. (*for syphilis*): an alcoholic beef heart antigen is prepared and is fortified by a combination of cholesterol and sitosterol to the point of oversaturation. One ml. of the fortified antigen is mixed with 1.3 ml. of a 4 per cent sodium chloride solution. This antigen-saline mixture is left at rest for thirty minutes, and 0.04 ml. is then placed into test tubes, followed by 0.4 ml. of the serum. The set is shaken in the Kahn shaker for two minutes, and the racks are incubated at

37° C. for four hours or longer. The tubes are then centrifugated for ten minutes. Physiologic solution of sodium chloride, 1.2 ml., is then run into each tube and the results are read.

early pregnancy t.: a do-it-yourself immunological test for pregnancy performed in the home as early as nine days after menstruation was expected (missed period). The test materials consist of a mixture of human chorionic gonadotropin (HCG) antiserum and HCG-coated red blood cells in a glass test tube, a vial of water, and a medical dropper. Three drops of urine are placed in the test tube and the vial of water is added. The tube is shaken for 10 seconds and placed in a holder for 2 hours. A brown ring of nonagglutinated red blood cells is positive (indicates pregnancy).

Ebbinghaus' t. (*for mental disease*): the examiner gives the patient sentences from which several words have been omitted, and asks him to complete them.

Edlefsen's t. (*for dextrose*), see under *reagent.*

Ehrlich's t.: 1. see *Ehrlich's diazo reaction,* under *reaction.* 2. the benzaldehyde test for urobilinogen; see *para-dimethylaminobenzaldehyde t.*

Ehrmann's t. (*for mydriatic substances*): the suspected substance is applied to an enucleated frog's eye, dilatation indicating the presence of a mydriatic substance.

Ehrmann's pancreatic t. (*for pancreatic efficiency*): after a test meal of hydrated fats and of chopped meat, the gastric contents and feces are examined for the fat-splitting of pancreatic lipase and for the presence of undigested muscle fibers which are characteristic for decrease of trypsin.

Eijkman's t.: (*for phenol*) add to the suspected solution a few drops of an alcoholic solution of ethylic ether and nitrous acid, each, 1 part, and concentrated sulfuric acid, 2 parts: a red color is produced.

Einhorn string t.: a test for determining whether the site of bleeding is in the low esophagus, stomach, or duodenum.

Eiselt's t. (*for melanin in the urine*): oxidizing agents like nitric and sulfuric acids or potassium dichromate render the urine dark colored if melanin is present.

Eitelberg's t. (*obs.*): large tuning-fork is held near the ear, at intervals, for twenty to thirty minutes. If the ear is normal the perception of the vibrations increases after each interval; if there is a lesion of the conducting apparatus, the perception decreases.

Ellermann and Erlandsen's t., see *tuberculin titer t.*

Elsberg's t.: a method of testing the sense of smell for determining the existence of brain tumor.

Ely's t.: with the patient prone, if flexion of the leg on the thigh causes the buttocks to arch away from the table and the leg to abduct at the hip joint, there is contracture of the lateral fascia of the thigh.

Emanuel-Cutting t., see *mastic t.*

emulsoid-gelatin t., see *gel t.*

epinephrine t.: 1. in persons with Graves' disease the injection of 1 mg. of epinephrine produces a lowering of blood pressure in vagotonic patients and an exaggerated rise of temperature in patients with sympathicotonia. 2. see *Goetsch's skin reaction,* under *reaction.* 3. see specific tests, including *Comessatti's t., Meyer's t.* (1), *Vulpian t.* See also *epinephrine, method for,* under *method.*

epiphanin t., see under *reaction.*

Erdmann's t. (*for alkaloids*), see under *reagent.*

ergot t., see specific tests, including *cockscomb t., Houghton's t.*

Erhard's t.: a test for detecting simulated deafness.

Erichsen t., see under *sign.*

erythrocyte sedimentation t., see under *rate.*

Esbach's t. (*for albumin*), see under *reagent.*

Escherich's t.: a modification of the von Pirquet reaction in which the tuberculin is injected subcutaneously.

Escudero's t. (*for gout*): after a meal containing a given quantity of purines, the quantity eliminated after a period of twenty-four to forty-eight hours is measured; if more than 50 per cent is eliminated gout is excluded.

ether t.: a small amount of a 25 per cent solution of sulfuric acid is added to urine in a test tube and a thin layer of ether is floated over it; the contents of the tube are shaken and allowed to stand. If the froth becomes sticky allergic asthma is indicated.

ethyl acetate t. (*for alcohol*): add an equal volume of concentrated sulfuric acid and a little sodium acetate and heat; the ethereal odor of ethyl acetate indicates alcohol.

ethyl butyrate t. (*for pancreatic lipase*): a neutral mixture of water, ethyl butyrate, and litmus turns red when acted on by lipase due to the liberation of butyric acid.

euglobulin lysis t.: a test for the presence of plasminogen activator, done by determining the time required to dissolve an incubated clot composed of precipitated plasma euglobulin and exogenous thrombin.

Ewald's t.: 1. (*for hydrochloric acid in stomach contents*) mix 2 ml. of a 10 per cent solution of potassium thiocyanate, 0.5 ml. of a neutral solution of iron acetate, and 7.5 ml. of water. This makes a ruby-red solution. A few drops are put into a porcelain dish and a drop or two of the suspected liquid are added. If HCl is present, a slight violet is seen; but on mixing the color becomes brown. 2. (*for motility of the stomach*) the injection of phenyl salicylate (salol) after a light meal. The phenyl salicylate passes into the intestine, where it is decomposed and salicyluric acid secreted in the urine. Normally the salicyluric acid should appear in from one to two hours, and may be detected by adding to the urine a weak solution of ferric chloride, when a purple color will appear. Called also *salol t.*

exercise t's, tests for detecting previously undetected coronary artery disease; they are graded tests of coronary fitness in which the subject performs exercise, as by walking a treadmill or pedaling a stationary bicycle, while under continuous electrocardiographic monitoring, usually by means by an oscilloscope, before, during, and after the exercise. Called also *stress t's.* See also *Master 2-step exercise t.*

extinction t.: Schultz-Charlton reaction.

Exton's t. (*for albumin in urine*): heat together equal volumes of Exton's reagent and urine; a precipitate indicates the presence of albumin.

Exton and Rose's glucose tolerance t.: 50 gm. of glucose are given and thirty minutes later another 50 gm.; the blood sugar level at sixty minutes should not be greater than at thirty minutes.

Fabre's t.: a test for barbital based on the formation of crystalline dicanthyl compounds developed in the presence of acetic acid.

Fahraeus' t.: erythrocyte sedimentation rate.

Falk and Tedesco's t.: a test for bronchial disease based on the fact that if salicylates are given to a patient in whom the bronchial mucosa is injured, salicylic acid will appear in the sputum.

Fantus t. (*for differentiating between predominant water or salt depletion*): place 10 drops of urine in a test tube with 1 drop of 20 per cent potassium chromate, then add 2.9 per cent silver nitrate 1 drop at a time, all the while agitating the tube, until there is a sudden color change from yellow to brick red. The number of drops of silver nitrate required to attain this change is the number of grams of chloride per liter in the urine; thus the addition of 4 drops to elicit the end point indicates a urine chloride concentration of 400 mg./100 ml. (4 gm./L.).

Farber's t.: presence of swallowed vernix cells in the meconium of a newborn baby indicates partial intestinal stenosis; their absence indicates intestinal atresia.

Farr t.: radioimmunoassay to measure the absolute amount of antibody.

fat t., see specific tests, including *acrolein t., Adams' t., Babcock's t., Bloor's t.* (1), *Leffmann-Beam t., Meigs's t., Saathoff's t., Valenta's t.*

fatigue t., see under *reaction.*

FE$_{Na}$ t.: excreted fraction of filtered sodium test, a measure of renal tubular reabsorption of sodium, calculated as follows: $(U/P)Na/(U/P)Cr \times 100$, where U and P represent concentrations of sodium and creatinine in urine and plasma, respectively.

Fearon's t. (*for vitamin A*): add 1 gm. of phosphorus pentoxide to 5 ml. of oil; a purple color indicates vitamin A.

Fehling's t. (*for dextrose in the urine*): mix the suspected liquid with freshly prepared Fehling's solution (q.v. under *solution*) and boil; a red precipitate of cuprous oxide shows the presence of dextrose.

femoral nerve stretch t. (*for lesions of third or fourth lumbar disk*): passive knee flexion in the prone position causes pain in the back or thighs.

fermentation t. (*for dextrose*): fill a graduated fermentation tube with the urine or unknown solution, add a small portion of compressed yeast, and incubate for twelve hours; the amount of gas that accumulates in the closed arm indicates the amount of dextrose present.

fern t. (*for estrogen*): the appearance of a fernlike pattern in dried smears of uterine cervical mucus indicates the presence of estrogen; the level of secretion is determined by the extent of ferning.

ferric chloride t.: 1. (*for thiocyanates in saliva*) add a few drops of dilute ferric chloride to saliva and acidify with hydrochloric acid; red ferric thiocyanate forms, which is decolorized by adding mercury bichloride. 2. (*for salicylic acid*) see *Remont's t.*

Feulgen's t.: 1. (*for animal nucleic acid*) hydrolyze with HCl solution and add a 1 per cent solution of decolorized rosaniline; a red color develops. 2. (*for deoxyribonucleic acid*) a microchemical test for the deoxyribose type of nucleic acid found in chromatin.

fibrinogen t. (*for liver function*): decrease in the amount of fibrinogen in the blood plasma below the normal amount points to liver injury. Whipple adds 1 ml. of a 2.5 per cent solution of calcium chloride to 1 ml. of plasma and judges the amount of fibrinogen by the toughness of the resulting clot. Rowntree heats the plasma on a water bath at 59° C. for twenty to thirty minutes, then washes, dries, and weighs the clot.

fibroderm bismuth capsule t., see *Schwarz's t.* (2).

Fieux's t. (*for antipyrine*): to the suspected liquid add 12 drops of sulfuric acid and 2.5 gm. of sodium metaphosphate; filter, and to the filtrate add a few drops of a solution of sodium nitrate. If antipyrine is present, a green color will be produced.

Finckh's t. (*for mental disease*): the patient is directed to explain the meaning of proverbs, such as "when the cat's away the mice wlll play," etc.

finger-to-finger t.: similar to finger-nose test, for testing coordinated movements of the extremities.

finger-nose t. (*for coordinated movements of the extremities*): with arm extended to one side the patient is asked to slowly try to touch the end of his nose with the point of his index finger.

Fischer's t. (*for dextrose*): the urine is boiled with phenylhydrazine and sodium acetate; if dextrose is present, yellow crystals of phenylglucosazone will be formed.

fish t., see *erythrophore reaction*, under *reaction.*

Fishberg concentration t. (*for renal function*): the patient is given supper with not more than 200 ml. of fluid and nothing thereafter. Urine voided during the night is discarded. The morning urine is saved, the patient kept in bed, and the urine of one hour later and of two hours later is saved. If the specific gravity of any of these three specimens is less than 1.024 there is impairment of renal function.

Fishberg and Friedfeld t., see *xylose concentration t.*

Fishman-Doublet t. (*for quick differential diagnosis of acute pancreatitis*): a minute amount of starch is incubated with serum for 5 minutes. A normal concentration of amylase will leave some of the starch undigested and give a blue color with iodine; a high serum amylase digests all the starch, and the addition of iodine will give only the yellow color of iodine. When the reaction color is yellow, the diagnosis of acute pancreatitis is strongly indicated. Called also *rapid serum amylase t.*

fistula t.: the air in the external auditory canal is compressed or rarefied: if there is erosion of the inner osseous wall of the tympanum exposing the membranous labyrinth, nystagmus will be produced, provided the labyrinth still functions. The site of the fistula is usually in the bony lateral semicircular canal.

fixation t., see *fixation of the complement*, under *fixation.*

Flack t. (*of physical efficiency*): after a full inspiration the subject blows as long as he can into a mercury manometer with a force of 40 mm. mercury.

Fleig's t. (*for blood in the urine*): a test based on the fact that fluorescein is easily reduced to fluorescin in the presence of oxygenated water and a catalytic agent, such as hemoglobin and its derivatives.

Fleischl's t. (*for bile pigments in urine*): heat the urine with a strong solution of sodium nitrate and add sulfuric acid with a pipet; the acid sinks to the bottom of the tube and forms colored layers.

Fleitmann's t. (*for arsenic compound*): in a tube containing the suspected fluid, hydrogen is generated from zinc and solution of potassium hydroxide. The mouth of the tube is closed by a piece of filter paper moistened with a solution of silver nitrate. On heating, if an inorganic arsenic compound is present, the filter paper will turn black.

flicker t.: see *flicker.*

flocculation t.: one in which a positive result depends on the degree of flocculent precipitation produced in the material being tested, as in the *Sachs-Georgi t., Sachs-Witebsky t.,* or *Vernes' t.*

Florence's t. (*for spermatic fluid*): to the suspected substance add a strong aqueous solution of iodine and potassium iodide; if spermatic fluid is present, brown plates or needles will be formed.

Fluhmann's t.: a modification of the Allen-Doisy test for estrogenic substance in the body, using mice in which a positive reaction is the mucinification of the vaginal mucosa.

fluorescent treponemal antibody absorption (FTA-ABS) t. (*for syphilis*): a specific serological test for syphilis using the *Treponema pallidum* (Nicols strain) as antigen. Syphilitic serum is bound to the surface of treponemes fixed onto a slide, and the antibody is made visible by utilizing fluorescein-tagged antiserum against human globulin.

foam t. (*for bile pigments*): shake the specimen of urine in a test tube; a brownish-yellow foam indicates bile pigments.

Focker's t.: to urine rendered alkaline with sodium hydroxide, add a solution of ammonium chloride; a precipitate of acid ammonium urate is formed.

Folin's t.: 1. (*for quantity of uric acid*) see *Folin-Shaffer method* (*for uric acid*), under *method.* 2. (*for uric acid*) to the unknown add a saturated solution of oxalic acid and evaporate to dryness; cool and extract phenols with 95 per cent alcohol; dissolve residue in water, add sodium carbonate and Folin's sodium phosphotungstate reagent. A blue color indicates uric acid. 3. (*for sugar in normal urine*) shake the urine with trinitrophenol and bone black to remove creatinin. Filter, add a small amount to Folin's sugar reagent, shake while boiling for one and a half minutes, and centrifugalize. A red layer of cuprous oxide in bottom of tube indicates sugar. 4. (*for amino acids*) amino acids develop a pink color in the presence of betanaphthaquinone sulfonic acid and alkali.

Folin and Denis' t. (*for tyrosine*): to 1 to 2 ml. of the unknown add an equal volume of the reagent (containing 10 per cent of sodium tungstate, 2 per cent of phosphomolybdic acid), and 3 to 10 ml. of a saturated solution of sodium carbonate. A blue color indicates tyrosine.

Folin and McEllroy's t. (*for dextrose*): (reagent: 100 gm. of sodium pyrophosphate, 30 gm. of disodium phosphate, and 50 gm. of dry sodium carbonate in 1 liter of water. Dissolve with heat and add 13 gm. of copper sulfate dissolved in 200 ml. of water.) To 5 ml. of the reagent add 5 to 8 drops of the urine and boil. In the presence of sugar the hot solution is filled with a colloidal greenish yellow or reddish precipitate.

Folin and Wu's t., see under *method.*

formaldehyde t., see specific tests, including *Burnam's t., Jorissen's t., Kentmann's t., Leach's t., Lebbin's t., Luebert's t., Schiff's t.* (6). See also *formalin t.*

formalin-gel t., formol-gel t. (*for kala-azar*): a drop of the patient's serum is placed on a slide, which is then inverted over a watch glass containing a few drops of formaldehyde solution; the serum from cases of kala-azar will solidify into a stiff opaque jelly.

Fornet's ring t., see *Fornet's reaction*, under *reaction*.

Foshay's t. *(for tularemia)*: a suspension of *Pasteurella tularensis* is injected into the skin; a positive reaction resembles that in a positive tuberculin test.

Fouchet's t. *(for bilirubin in blood)*: to a sample of the blood serum there is added an equal part of a reagent consisting of 5 gm. trichloracetic acid, 20 ml. water, and 2 ml. ferric chloride; a green color is produced if bilirubin is present.

Fournier t.: the patient is asked to rise on command from a sitting position; he is asked to rise and walk, then stop quickly on command; he is asked to walk and turn around quickly on command. The ataxic gait is thus brought out.

fragility t.: add 1 drop of blood to 25 ml. portions of salt solutions varying in concentration from 0.28 to 0.50 per cent. Shake and allow to stand two hours. Note concentration at which hemolysis begins to show a tinge of pink. Normal bloods begin at 0.42 to 0.44 and are complete at 0.36 to 0.32.

Francis' t.: 1. *(for bile acids in urine)* in a test tube is placed 2 gm. of dextrose in 15 gm. of sulfuric acid and the urine is placed on top of this; a purple color forms if bile acids are present. 2. an intracutaneous test in pneumonia for ascertaining the body response to the infection and whether the specific antibodies are present after treatment with antipneumococcus serum. The homologous pneumococcus polysaccharide is used in the skin test.

Fränkel's t.: examination of the nasal cavity with the patient's head bent down between his knees and rotated so that the side to be examined is turned upward. If pus is seen in the middle meatus, suppuration in some of the anterior accessory sinuses is indicated.

Franken's t. *(for completeness of placenta)*: the placenta held by the umbilical cord is put in a wash basin containing warm water; air is introduced through the umbilical vein. In this way defects in the placenta can be recognized.

Frei t.: sterile pus from the lesion is injected intracutaneously; the development of a raised red papule indicates venereal lymphogranuloma.

Friderichsen's t. *(for vitamin A deficiency)*: determination of the weakest light stimulus which will give rise to an oculomotor reflex. A variation from normal indicates vitamin A deficiency.

Friedman's t., Friedman-Lapham t. *(for pregnancy)*: the injection of the urine of a pregnant woman into female rabbits will cause the formation of corpora lutea and corpora haemorrhagica in the rabbits.

frog t., see *male frog t.*

Fröhde's t. *(for alkaloids)*: a 1 per cent solution of sodium molybdate in sulfuric acid.

Frohn's t.: the use of the double iodide of bismuth and potassium as a test for alkaloids.

Frommer's t. *(for acetone in urine)*: alkalinize about 10 ml. of the urine with 2 or 3 ml. of 40 per cent sodium hydroxide solution, add 10 or 12 drops of 10 per cent alcoholic solution of salicylous acid (salicylaldehyde), heat the upper portion to about 70°C. (it should not reach the boiling point), and keep at this temperature five minutes or longer. In the presence of acetone an orange color, changing to deep red, appears in the heated portion.

fructose t., see *levulose t.*

FTA-ABS t., fluorescent treponemal antibody absorption t.

Fuchs's t.: a test for cancer based on the observation that the serum of normal persons digests all fibrin except that of normal persons while the serum of cancer subjects digests all fibrin except that of cancer subjects.

Fuld's t. *(for antitryptic power of blood serum)*: three solutions are used: a 0.1 per cent solution of Grübler's dry trypsin in slightly alkaline normal saline, a 0.2 per cent neutral solution of casein, and an alcoholic solution of acetic acid. A series of test tubes are prepared containing definite amounts of casein solution and of diluted blood serum and increasing amounts of trypsin solution. After incubating, 1 or 2 drops of the acetic acid solution are added to each test tube. If any turbidity appears it indicates the presence of undigested casein. The amount of trypsin necessary to digest the casein completely in one-half hour can then be determined.

Fuld-Goss t., see *antitrypsin t.*

fundus reflex t., retinoscopy.

Funkenstein t.: an index of central autonomic reactivity, consisting of observing the response in systolic blood pressure after intramuscular injection of 10 mg. of acetylcholine.

Fürbringer's t. *(for albumin)*: in the urine are placed gelatin capsules opened at each end and containing mercuric chloride, sodium chloride, and citric acid; if albumin is present cloudiness or a flocculent precipitate is produced.

furfurol t. *(for proteins)*: heat the suspected substance with sulfuric acid; if proteins are present, furfurol is formed.

Gaenslen's t., see under *sign*.

Gairdner's coin t., see *coin t.*

galactose t., see *mucic acid t., phloroglucin t.*

galactose tolerance t., see *Bauer's t.* (2).

Galli Mainini t. *(for pregnancy)*: 10 ml. of urine from the patient is injected into a normal male batrachian (frog or toad); the presence of spermatozoa in a drop of the batrachian's urine indicates the existence of pregnancy.

Gallois' t. *(for inosite,* when proteins, tyrosine, and other sugars are present)*: evaporate a solution of the suspected substance to partial dryness, and moisten the residue with a solution of mercuric nitrate. On drying, it assumes a yellow color, which heating turns to a bright red and which disappears when the liquid cools.

Ganassini's t. *(for uric acid)*: precipitate the alkaline urate with $ZnCl_2$. In contact with the air the precipitate turns blue.

Gannther's t.: hydrogen dioxide, H_2O_2, liberates oxygen when brought into contact with blood.

Gardiner-Brown t. *(obs.)*: a vibrating tuning-fork is placed on the mastoid process of the patient: if the vibrations are heard longer than they can be felt by the examiner, or if they cease to be heard while they can still be felt by the examiner, there is disease of the middle ear.

Garriga's t.: a flocculation test for syphilis.

Garrod's t.: 1. *(for hematoporphyrin in urine)* to 100 ml. of urine, 20 ml. of a 10 per cent solution of sodium hydroxide is added, and the whole is filtered. The filtrate is washed in water-free alcohol and the precipitate dissolved in hydrochloric acid. The test is completed with the spectroscope, which gives two absorption bands indicative of hematoporphyrin (Sir A. E. Garrod). 2. *(for uric acid in the blood)* 30 ml. of blood serum are treated with 0.5 ml. of acetic acid. A fine thread is immersed in it, on which are formed crystals of uric acid (A. B. Garrod).

gastric function t., see specific tests, including *augmented histamine t., chlorophyll t., Ewald's t.* (2)*, pentagastrin t., Rehfuss t., Sahli's t., Sahli's glutoid t., saline load t., Schmidt's t.* (5)*, Schwarz's t.* (2).

Gault t. *(for simulated deafness)*: the patient's good ear is closed and a sound is made near the supposed bad ear; a winking motion of the lid on the tested side indicates hearing.

Gauran t.: a complement fixation test for the diagnosis of gonorrheal infection.

Gawalowski's t. *(for glycosuria)*: ammonium molybdate is added to suspected urine and heated to 100°C. If dextrose is present, the solution becomes blue.

Gay-Force t., see *typhoidin t.*

Gayer t. *(for Cannabis indica)*: the amount of the extract or pure drug which injected intravenously produces full anesthesia of the cornea in rabbits.

Geissler's t. *(for albumin in the urine)*: a test paper is dipped in citric acid and dried; another is dipped in a solution containing 3 per cent mercuric chloride and 14 per cent potassium iodide, and dried; the two papers are placed in the urine. If there is albumin present, a precipitate will be formed.

gel t.: differentiation of syphilitic serum by the opacity and rapid precipitation produced by addition of glacial acetic acid to small quantities of the serum (J. E. R. MacDonagh, 1916).

gel diffusion t., a precipitin test in which antigen and antibody are placed in a gel medium (e.g., agar) and one diffuses toward the other (single diffusion) or each diffuses toward the other (double diffusion) to form lines of precipitation.

Gellé's t.: a rubber tube is inserted in the ear and a tuning-fork is brought in contact with it; by means of a bulb on the tube, pressure is increased or decreased. If the change in pressure does not reduce the loudness, fixation of the ossicular chain is present.

Gentele's t. *(for dextrose or uric acid)*: add to the suspected liquid a solution of potassium ferrocyanide made alkaline with sodium hydroxide; on heating it becomes decolorized.

Georgi's t., Sachs-Georgi t.

Geraghty's t.: the phenolsulfonphthalein test.

Gerhardt's t.: 1. *(for acetone in the urine)* add a solution of ferric chloride and a red color is produced. This test is not reliable (Carl J. Gerhardt). 2. *(for acetoacetic acid in the urine)* filter, in order to remove the phosphates, and add a few drops of a solution of ferric chloride, which produces a deep red color, which disappears when sulfuric acid is added. 3. *(for bile pigments in the urine)* it is made by shaking with an equal measure of chloroform and soon after adding tincture of iodine and potassium hydroxide to the separated chloroform, when a yellow or yellowish brown color is produced (Charles Frédéric Gerhardt).

Gerrard's t. *(for dextrose in the urine)*: Fehling's solution is treated with a 5 per cent solution of potassium cyanide until the blue color begins to disappear. The suspected liquid is heated with this mixture, and if there is dextrose present, more or less discoloration takes place.

Gibbon and Landis t. *(for peripheral circulation)*: a pair of extremities (the hands, if the feet are to be tested; the feet, if the hands are to be tested) are immersed in a bath of 43°–45° C. If the temperature in the unimmersed extremities rises, the circulation is normal.

Gies' biuret t. *(for proteins)*: Gies uses the following reagent in making the test: mix 25 ml. of a 3 per cent solution of cupric sulfate and 975 ml. of a 10 per cent solution of potassium hydroxide.

globulin t., see specific tests, including *ammonium sulfate t.* (1)*, Boveri's t., Braun-Husler t., Gordon's t., Hammarsten's t.* (1)*, Kaplan's t., colloidal gold t., Mayerhofer's t., Noguchi's t.* (2)*, Nonne-Apelt t., Pandy's t., Pohl's t., Ross-Jones t., Weichbrodt's t.*

glucagon stimulation t. *(for deficiency of growth hormone)*: blood samples are taken immediately and at intervals of 1, 2, 2½, and 3 hours after subcutaneous or intramuscular injection of glucagon; radioimmunoassay of the serum is then done by enzyme partition.

glucose t., see *dextrose t.*

glucose tolerance t.: a metabolic test of carbohydrate tolerance; it measures active insulin, a hepatic function based on the power of the normal liver to absorb and store large quantities of glucose, and the effectiveness of intestinal absorption of glucose. Blood sugar should return to normal in two to two and one-half hours after ingesting 100 gm. of glucose into a fasting stomach. See also *Exton and Rose's glucose tolerance t.*

glutoid t., see *Sahli's glutoid t.*

Gluzinski's t.: 1. (*for bile pigments*) boil the solution with solution of formaldehyde until it becomes green; adding a little hydrochloric acid changes the tint to an amethyst violet. 2. (*for differentiation between ulcer and cancer of stomach*) examination of the gastric contents recovered from a fasting patient: (*a*) after a test breakfast consisting of the white of a boiled egg and 200 ml. of water, which is recovered after three quarters of an hour. (*b*) after a test dinner consisting of a beefsteak and 250 ml. of water, which is recovered after three and three-quarters hours. In ulcer, both the breakfast and the dinner give the reaction of free HCl. In beginning cancer, the first meal will give reaction of free HCl, whereas the second meal will show only a slight trace or none at all.

glycerol t., see specific tests, including *acrolein t.,* and *hypochlorite-orcinol t.*

glycerol-cholesterol t., see *Hinton's t.*

glycerophosphate t. (*for renal function*): 500 mg. of sodium glycerophosphate are injected intravenously, and then the free and total phosphorus in the urine collected during the following hour is determined.

glycosylated hemoglobin t.: measurement of the percentage of hemoglobin A molecules that have formed a stable ketoamine linkage between their terminal amino acid position of the β-chains and a glucose group; in normal persons this amounts to about 7 per cent of the total, in diabetics about 14.5 per cent.

glycuronates t., see specific tests, including *phloroglucin t., Tollens' t.* (4), *Tollens, Neuberg and Schwket's t.*

glycyltryptophan t. (*for carcinoma of stomach*): filtered gastric contents and glycyltryptophan are placed in a test tube and kept at body temperature for twenty-four hours; if on the addition of a few drops of bromine, a reddish violet color is formed, carcinoma is indicated.

glyoxylic acid t., see *Hopkins-Cole test.*

Gmelin's t. (*for bile pigments*): fuming nitric acid is so added to the suspected urine that it forms a layer under it. Near the junction of the two liquids, rings are formed—a green ring above, and under it a blue, violet-red, and reddish yellow. If the green and violet-red rings are absent, the reaction shows the probable presence of lutein.

Goetsch's t., see *Goetsch's skin reaction,* under *reaction.*

gold number t., see *colloidal gold t.*

Goldscheider's t. (*for cutaneous thermal sensibility*) (*obs.*): consists in touching the skin with the slightly pointed end of a metallic cylinder varyingly heated.

gold-sol t., see *colloidal gold t.*

Goodenough draw-a-man t., Goodenough draw-a-person t.: a method of testing the general intelligence of children by asking the subject to draw a picture of a man to the best of his ability.

Goodenough-Harris drawing t.: a revision of the Goodenough draw-a-man test, in which scoring emphasizes the presence or absence of body and clothing detail rather than artistic skill.

Gordon's t. (*for the presence of globulin-albumin in the spinal fluid*): one ml. of spinal fluid is placed in a small test tube and 0.1 ml. of 1 per cent solution of corrosive mercuric chloride in distilled water; the formation of a cloud or precipitate after standing an hour indicates a positive reaction.

Gordon's biological t. (*for Hodgkin's disease*): lymphadenomatous tissue injected intracerebrally into rabbits causes the development of a characteristic lesion in the rabbits' nervous tissues, accompanied by ataxia, spasm, and paralysis.

Göthlin's t.: a test for capillary fragility, done by testing the capillary resistance in the arm.

Graefe's t. (*for heterophoria*): on holding a prism of 10 degrees before one eye, base up or down, two images are formed; one of these images is displaced laterally in heterophoria.

Graham's t.: the intravenous or oral administration of tetra-iodophthalein sodium prior to roentgenologic examination of the gallbladder.

Grandeau's t. (*for digitalin*): the substance is dissolved in concentrated sulfuric acid, to which bromine is added; a rose color is formed if digitalin is present.

Gregerson and Boas' t. (*for blood*): a modification of the benzidine test to make it less sensitive for use in testing feces. Use a 0.5 per cent solution of benzidine instead of a saturated solution and barium peroxide instead of hydrogen peroxide.

Griess's t. (*for nitrites in the saliva*): mix it with 5 parts of water; add a few drops of dilute solution of sulfuric acid and a few drops of metadiamidobenzene; this produces a strong yellow color if nitrites are present.

Grigg's t. (*for proteins*): metaphosphoric acid precipitates all proteins except the peptones.

Grocco's t. (*obs.*): in slight cases of purpura and purpura rheumatica, if an elastic ligature is placed around the forearm, punctiform hemorrhages will appear in the bend of the elbow.

Gross' t.: 1. (*for trypsin in feces*) in a mortar, thoroughly rub up a portion of the fecal mass with three times its bulk of 0.1 per cent

sodium carbonate solution. Filter. Mix 10 ml. of the filtrate with 100 ml. of a fresh solution consisting of 0.5 gm. Grübler's pure casein, 1 gm. sodium carbonate, and 1000 ml. distilled water. Add a little toluol to prevent bacterial activity and place in an incubator at about 38° C. At intervals remove a few cubic centimeters and test for casein by adding a few drops of acetic acid of about 1 per cent strength. A white cloud appears as long as any casein remains undigested. With the patient upon a protein diet, there is normally a sufficient amount of trypsin to digest all the casein in from ten to fifteen hours. Delay or complete failure of digestion shows diminution or absence of trypsin. 2. a color reaction for the diagnosis of carcinoma.

group t.: a test of intelligence or aptitude given to a number of persons at one time.

Gruber's t. (*for the sensitivity of the ear to sounds*): (*obs.*) the end of the finger is inserted in the ear after the sound of a tuning-fork has ceased to be heard; the tuning-fork is then held against the finger, and the sound again becomes audible.

Gruber-Widal t. (*for typhoid fever*), Widal's t.

Gruskin's t.: 1. (*for malignancy*) inject intradermally a serum containing an alcoholic extract of embryonic tissue cells; a slight area of infiltration, with pseudopod formation, occurs in positive cases. 2. (*for tuberculosis*) a preparation of the fibrin from tuberculous guinea pigs is injected intracutaneously; the appearance of pseudopodia extending outward from the wheal within six minutes is positive.

guaiac t. (*for occult blood*): glacial acetic acid and a solution of gum guaiac are mixed with the specimen; on addition of hydrogen peroxide, the presence of blood is indicated by a blue tint.

guanine t., see *Capranica's t.* (2), (3), and (4).

Gunning's t. (*for acetone in urine*): to a few milliliters of urine or distillate in a test tube, add a few drops of tincture of iodine and of ammonia alternately until a heavy black cloud appears. This cloud will gradually clear up and, if acetone is present, iodoform, usually crystalline, will separate out. The iodoform can be recognized by its odor or by detection of the crystals microscopically. Iodoform crystals are yellowish six-pointed stars or six-sided plates.

Gunning-Lieben t., see *Gunning's t.*

Günzburg's t. (*for hydrochloric acid in the stomach contents*): dissolve 2 gm. of phloroglucin and 1 gm. of vanillin in 30 ml. of alcohol; of this mix 2 drops with 2 drops of filtered gastric juice; heat it slowly in a porcelain cell. Free HCl produces a bright-red color; it is not present if the color is brownish red or brown.

Gutzeit's t. (*for arsenic*): a paper is moistened with an acidulated silver nitrate solution and exposed to the fumes from the suspected liquid, which is mixed with zinc and dilute sulfuric acid. The formation of a yellow spot on the paper indicates the presence of inorganic arsenic compounds.

Haagensen t.: observation of the contour of the breasts when the patient leans forward as a means of detecting malignant changes in the mammae.

Hager's t. (*for dextrose*), see under *reagent.*

Haines' t. (*for dextrose*): copper sulfate, 30 grains; glycerin, $\frac{1}{2}$ fl.oz.; liquor potassae, 5 fl.oz.; water, sufficient to make 6 fl.oz. When boiled and a little urine added, and again boiled, a yellow or reddish yellow precipitate is produced.

Hallion's t., see *Tuffier's t.*

Ham t.: a test performed by incubating red cells in an acid environment for the diagnosis of paroxysmal nocturnal hemoglobinuria; a positive test may be obtained in other forms of anemia.

Hamburger's t.: a test made by injecting 0.1 ml. of a 1:10,000 dilution of tuberculin just below the skin; subcutaneous infiltration follows in twenty-four hours if the patient is tubercular.

Hamel's t. (*for slight jaundice*): a little blood is drawn by puncture from the lobe of the ear into a capillary tube and the tube is allowed to stand for a few hours; the serum which collects in the upper part of the tube will be yellow if jaundice is present.

Hamilton's t.: when the shoulder joint is luxated, a rule or straight rod applied to the humerus can be made to touch the outer condyle and the acromion at the same time.

Hammarsten's t.: 1. (*for globulin*) in a neutral solution suspected to contain globulin, dissolve magnesium sulfate to saturation; the globulin will be precipitated and may be filtered out. 2. (*for bile pigment*) to one volume of acid mixture (1 part HNO$_3$ and 19 parts HCl, each 25 per cent) add four volumes of alcohol, then a few drops of the unknown; a green color indicates biliverdin.

Hammer's t.: a complement fixation test for tuberculosis, in which the antigen is a mixture of Koch's old tuberculin and an extract of tuberculous granulation tissue.

Hammerschlag's t., see under *method.*

Hanganatziu-Deicher t. (*for infectious mononucleosis*): the serum of the patient is inactivated by a temperature of 58° C. Then a series of dilutions of serum with physiologic solution of sodium chloride is set up (1:4, 1:8, 1:16, and so on up to 1:4096). To each 0.5 ml. of serum dilution, 0.5 ml. of a 2 per cent suspension of washed corpuscles of sheep's blood and then 1 ml. of sodium chloride solution are added. The tubes are put in the incubator for two hours and then in the refrigerator over night. In infectious mononucleosis there is a thick clotted conglobation of the corpuscles of the sheep's blood up into the high dilutions; otherwise agglutination is either entirely absent or extremely weak in the 1:4, 1:8 and, in exceptional cases, the 1:16 tubes.

Hanger's t. (*for liver cell disease*): a test based on the flocculation of a cephalin-cholesterol emulsion by the patient's serum.

Hanke and Koessler's t. (*for phenols, hydroxyaromatic acids, and imidazoles*): to 5 ml. of 1.1 per cent sodium carbonate solution add 2 ml. of para-diazobenzene sulfonic acid reagent. Then add 1 ml. of solution to be tested.

hapten inhibition t.: serological characterization of an antigenic determinant by employing known haptens to mask the antigen binding site of antibody specific for it.

Harding and Ruttan's t. (*for acetoacetic acid*): acidify the urine with acetic acid, add 0.5 ml. of N/10 sodium nitroprusside, and then overlay the solution with concentrated aqueous NH_4OH; a violet ring is produced.

Harris and Ray t.: a microtitration for vitamin C in the urine.

Harrison spot t. (*for bilirubin in urine*): add to 10 ml. of urine 5 ml. of a 10 per cent solution of barium chloride, mix, and filter. Spread filter paper on dry filter paper. Add one to two drops of Fouchet's reagent (trichloroacetic acid 25 gm., water 100 ml., and 10 per cent solution of ferric chloride 10 ml.); a positive reaction gives a blue to green color (Godfried).

Hart's t. (*for oxybutyric acid in urine*): remove acetone and diacetic acid by diluting 20 ml. urine with 20 ml. of water, adding a few drops of acetic acid, and boiling down to 10 ml. To this add 10 ml. of water, mix, and divide between two test tubes. To one tube add 1 ml. of hydrogen peroxide, warm gently, and cool. This transforms β-hydroxybutyric acid to acetone. Now apply Lange's test for acetone to each tube. A positive reaction in the tube to which hydrogen peroxide has been added shows the presence of β-oxybutyric acid in the original sample of urine.

hatching t.: a test for the detection of schistosome eggs in urine or feces, dependent upon the eggs hatching to produce miracidia when placed in water; the miracidia are attracted to light and can readily be identified.

Hawk's t. (*for fecal amylase*): rub up and dilute the feces with seven volumes of a neutral mixture of Na_2HPO_4, NaH_2PO_4, and NaCl. Add varying amounts of this to tubes containing soluble starch and toluene and incubate for twenty-four hours. Test for digestion with iodine.

Hay's t. (*for bile salts*): a pinch of sublimated sulfur is dropped in the urine; the sulfur sinks if bile is present, but floats if it is absent.

Heaf t., see *tuberculin t., Sterneedle.*

Hecht's t. (*for syphilis*): a modification of Wassermann's reaction, based on the fact that normal human serum is capable of dissolving ten times its volume of a 2 per cent solution of sheep's blood.

Hecht-Weinberg t., see *Hecht's t.*

Hecht-Weinberg-Gradwohl t. (*for syphilis*): a modification of the Wassermann reaction using not only the natural antisheep amboceptor in human serum, but also the native hemolytic complement, the hemolytic index of the human serum being determined before the sheep corpuscles are added to the tube.

heel-knee t. (*for coordinated movements of the extremities*): the patient, lying on his back, is asked to touch the knee of one leg with the heel of the other and then to pass the heel slowly down the front of the shin to the ankle.

heel-tap t., see *heel tap,* under *tap.*

Heller's t.: 1. (*for albumin in urine*) stratify cold nitric acid below the urine in a test tube; albumin will form a white coagulum between the urine and the acid. 2. (*for blood in the urine*) add potassium hydroxide solution and heat; the earthy phosphates are precipitated, and if blood is present, they are stained red by hematin. 3. (*for dextrose in urine*) add a solution of potassium hydroxide; sugar will cause a brownish or reddish precipitate.

hemadsorption t.: an *in vitro* test for detecting hemagglutinating viruses based on the adherence of red blood cells to cells of the infected tissue in the presence of hemagglutinin.

hematein t. (*for blood*): to 5 ml. of the unknown add 5 ml. of sodium hydroxide, 2 drops of hematein solution, and 10 drops of hydrogen peroxide. If blood is present the contents will turn rapidly to violet red, then to clear brown, and then to pale yellow. Without blood these changes occur more slowly.

hematin t., see *Schumm's t.* (2).

hematoporphyrin t., see *Garrod's t.* (1).

heme t., see *Schumm's t.* (2).

hemin t. (*for blood*), see *Teichmann's t.*

hemoglobin t., see specific tests, including *alkali denaturation t., Almén's t.* (2), *Heller's t.* (2), *Katayama's t., Kobert's t., sand t., Stokes's t.* See also *hemoglobin, methods for,* under *method.*

hemosiderin t., see specific tests, including *Perl's t., Rous's t.*

Hench-Aldrich t. (*for the mercury-combining power of saliva*): titrate 5 ml. of saliva with a 5 per cent solution of bichloride of mercury until a drop gives a reddish brown color with a saturated solution of sodium carbonate.

Henle-Coenen t.: the amount of retrograde flow of blood which is obtained from the open end of the distal stump of a divided artery, while the proximal portion is being compressed with a clamp, is a measure (or index) of the adequacy of the collateral circulation.

Hennebert's t., see under *sign.*

Henry's t., Henry's melanoflocculation t. (*for malaria*): a seroflocculation test in which a formalized suspension of melanin from ox eyes is added to the suspected serum. It is a nonspecific test depending on increased levels of euglobin in the serum and precipitation of the melanin.

Henshaw t.: a test to aid in the selection of the appropriate homeopathic remedy in a given case of disease. A visible flocculation zone develops in the patient's blood serum when brought into contact with a potentized remedy homeopathically indicated in the case.

hepatic function t., see *liver function t.*

Hering's t.: the subject looks with both eyes through a tube blackened within and having a thread running vertically across the farther end, and a small round body is placed either before or behind the thread—if vision is binocular, the subject is able at once to tell whether the ball is nearer to him than the thread or farther off; but if vision is monocular, he cannot tell whether it is nearer or farther than the thread.

Herring's t., Herring-Binet t.: a modification of the Binet test for intelligence.

Herter's t.: 1. (*for indole*) to the unknown add 1 drop of a 2 per cent solution of beta-naphtha-quinone-sodium-mono-sulfonate, and then a drop of a 10 per cent solution of potassium hydroxide; a blue or bluish green color indicates indole. 2. (*for skatole*) to the unknown add 1 ml. of an acid solution of para-dimethyl-amino-benzaldehyde and heat to boiling. The purplish blue color is intensified by the addition of hydrochloric acid.

Herzberg's t. (*for free hydrochloric acid in the gastric juice*): moisten a paper with a solution of Congo red and dry it; free HCl colors it blue or bluish black.

Hess capillary t. (*for condition of the capillary walls*), see *tourniquet t.,* def. 1.

Heynsius' t. (*for albumin*): to a suspected liquid add enough acetic acid to render acidulous, and then boil with a saturated solution of sodium chloride; albumin will form a flocculent precipitate.

Hickey-Hare t. (*for diabetes insipidus*): intravenous infusion of hypertonic saline after establishment of water diuresis induces antidiuresis in normal subjects but not in patients with diabetes insipidus.

Hildebrandt's t. (*for urobilin in urine*): the reagent consists of an unfiltered solution of 10 parts of zinc acetate and 90 parts of absolute alcohol. The reagent is shaken before using, and equal parts of reagent and urine are mixed, the precipitate which forms being filtered off. With increase of urobilin the filtrate shows a distinct green fluorescence, either directly or after the addition of ammonia.

Hindenlang's t. (*for albumin*): to the liquid to be tested add solid metaphosphoric acid; albumin, if present, forms a precipitate.

Hines and Brown t.: cold pressor test; a test which measures the response of the blood pressure to the immersion of one hand in ice water: an excessive increase in pressure (hyperreaction) is said to identify a latent hypertensive state.

Hinton t. (*for syphilis*): (*a*) pipet into the first tube 0.1 ml. of serum, into the second, 0.2 ml., and into the third, 0.3 ml. with a 1 ml. pipet graduated in one tenths. (*b*) add 0.5 ml. of the glycerinated indicator to each tube with a 10 ml. pipet. (*c*) shake thoroughly the rack containing the tests by first inclining it at an angle of about 60 degrees to the body and then thrusting it quickly forward and backward. By repeating this ten times one obtains a quick but thorough mixture of the serum with the glycerinated indicator. The presence of distinct foam in each tube is the only safe criterion of adequate mixing. (*d*) place the rack containing the tubes in the Wassermann bath or incubator which registers a temperature continuously between 25° and 28° C. for from twelve to eighteen hours (overnight). At the end of six hours the difference between the positive and negative reactions is marked, but the final decision should not be made in less than twelve hours, and preferably only after eighteen hours.

hippuric acid t., see specific tests, including *Lücke's t., Quick's t.* (1), *Spiro's t.* (2). See also *hippuric acid, methods for,* under *method.*

Hirschfeldt's t. (*for cancer*): a complement fixation test for detecting in cancer patients antibodies for cancer lipoids.

Hirst t., Hirst and Hare t. (*for influenza*): heterophile antibodies, if present in the blood, agglutinate chicken erythrocytes.

Histalog t., see *augmented histamine t.*

histamine t.: 1. one ml. of a 0.1 per cent solution of histamine is injected subcutaneously as a stimulant of gastric secretion; see also *augmented histamine t.* 2. (*for lesions of the sympathetic nervous system*) a small area of skin on the wrist, ankle or knee is cleansed with alcohol, which is allowed to dry. A drop of 1:1000 solution of histamine phosphate is placed on it and introduced into the epidermis by multiple needle punctures in a manner similar to that used for cowpox vaccination. The excess histamine is gently removed. (*a*) A reddish purple spot appears as the result of local capillary dilatation. (*b*) A local wheal succeeds, because of transudation of serum from increased permeability of the capillaries. (*c*) A flare results as the effect of dilatation of the arteries by the reflex of a local axon. The flare being dependent on the integrity of the peripheral nerve, it therefore occurs in hysterical anesthesia and malingering but not in neural lesions. 3. (*for pheochromocytoma*) following rapid intravenous injection of histamine phosphate administered in a standardized dosage of 0.010 to 0.050 mg. of histamine base, normal individuals experience transient headache, flush, and a brief fall in blood pressure, but those with pheochromocytoma, after fall in blood pressure, experience a marked rise in blood pressure, fear, excitability, etc.

histamine flare t. (*for leprosy and postherpetic neuralgia*): a drop of 1:1000 histamine acid phosphate solution is placed on the skin and a needle puncture is made through it; the test is positive if there is no erythema flare when the puncture is made within the suspected lesion area, or if the flare stops at the border of the lesion when it is made slightly to the outside of it.

histidine loading t. (*for folic acid deficiency*): a loading dose of histidine is given, and the resultant urinary excretion of excess formiminoglutamic acid (FIGLU), secondary to decreased amounts of tetrahydrofolic acid, is measured. Called also *FIGLU excretion t.*

Hitzig t. (*for vestibular apparatus*): the positive electrode of a galvanic current is applied just in front of the ear being examined, while the negative electrode is held in the patient's hand, the patient standing with feet together and eyes closed. A current of 5 milliamperes causes a leaning toward the positive pole in normal persons.

hock t., spavin t.

Hoffmann's t. (*for tyrosine*): add mercuric nitrate to the suspected liquid and boil it; then add nitric acid with a little nitrous acid. A red color is produced if tyrosine is present, and a red precipitate is seen.

Hofmeister's t.: 1. (*for leucine*) warm the suspected liquid with mercurous nitrate; if leucine is present, metallic mercury is deposited. 2. (*for peptones*) mix phosphotungstic and hydrochloric acids; let the mixture stand twenty-four hours, and filter. With this reagent a solution containing peptones with no albumin will afford a precipitate.

Hogben t., see *Xenopus t.*

Holmgren's t.: the use of skeins of colored worsted as a test of the perception of colors; a skein is given to the subject of the test, and he is asked to match it out of a set of variously colored skeins.

Holten's t.: a creatinine clearance test for renal efficiency.

Hopkins' thiophene t. (*for lactic acid*): add a few drops of stomach contents to 5 ml. of concentrated sulfuric acid containing a little cupric sulfate and heat two minutes. Cool and add a very little thiophene. A cherry-red color indicates lactic acid.

Hopkins-Cole t. (*for protein*): glyoxylic acid is prepared by the action of sodium amalgam on a solution of oxalic acid. A few drops of this solution are added to the protein solution and strong sulfuric acid is poured down the side of the tube. A bluish violet color is produced at the junction of the two fluids due to the presence of tryptophan.

Hoppe-Seyler t.: 1. (*for carbon monoxide in the blood*) add to blood twice its volume of a solution of sodium hydroxide of 1.3 specific gravity: normal blood will form a dingy brown mass with a green shade if spread thin on a white surface; but if carbon monoxide is present, the mass is red, and so is the thin layer. 2. (*for xanthine*) add the substance to be tested to a mixture of chlorinated lime in a porcelain dish; a dark-green ring is formed at first.

hormone t., see specific tests, including *Aschheim-Zondek t.,* and *Siddall t.*

Horsley's t. (*for dextrose*): the solution is boiled with potassium hydroxide and potassium chromate; if dextrose is present a green color is produced.

Hotis t. (*for garget or mastitis in cows*): fresh milk containing bromcresol purple is incubated for twenty-four hours; a positive reaction is the formation of yellow flakes on the sides of the test tube.

Houghton's t.: ergot is given to a white leghorn cock; if the comb becomes darkened there is ergot activity and the result is positive.

Howard t. (*for renal function*): both ureters are catheterized and urine collected separately from each kidney; the quantity of urine in each collection and its sodium and creatinine concentrations are then determined. Called also *split-renal function t.*

Howell's t. (*for prothrombin*): a test for the amount of prothrombin in the blood depending on the clotting time of the oxalated plasma treated with calcium chloride and thromboplastin.

Huddleson's t.: an agglutination test for brucellosis in man.

Huggins t. (*for cancer*): a sample of patient's blood is treated with iodoacetate and is heated; the serum albumin clots more readily in healthy subjects than in subjects who have cancer.

Huhner t.: examination of the secretions aspirated from the vaginal fornix and the endocervical canal after coitus, to determine the number and condition of spermatozoa present and the extent to which they have penetrated the cervical mucus.

human erythrocyte agglutination t.: an adaptation of the sheep cell agglutination test, human Rh-positive cells coated with incomplete anti-Rh antibody being used instead of the sheep red blood cells sensitized with rabbit gamma globulin. The sera of some patients with rheumatoid arthritis will agglutinate these cells. The agglutination may be inhibited by some normal sera, and not others, and this test is the basis for the determination of the inherited gamma globulin groups (Gm system). Abbreviated HEAT.

Hunt's t., see under *reaction.*

Huppert's t. (*for bile pigments*): the suspected solution is treated with lime water or calcium chloride solution and then with a solution of ammonium or sodium carbonate. The precipitate of bile pigments may be removed by shaking with chloroform after washing with water and acidulating with acetic acid. Bilirubin colors the chloroform yellow and the acetic acid solution green.

Huppert-Cole t. (*for bile pigments*): to 50 ml. of the unknown add an excess of baryta water or lime water. To the precipitate add

5 ml. of 95 per cent alcohol, 2 drops of strong sulfuric acid, and 2 drops of a 5 per cent solution of potassium chlorate. Boil, and the supernatant liquid will be emerald or bluish green if bile is present.

Hurtley's t. (*for acetoacetic acid*): to 10 ml. of the unknown add 2 ml. of strong hydrochloric acid and 1 ml. of fresh 1 per cent sodium nitrite solution. Shake and add 15 ml. of concentrated ammonium hydroxide and 5 ml. of 10 per cent ferrous sulfate. A violet or purple color develops slowly if acetoacetic acid is present.

hydrobilirubin t., see *Schmidt's t.* (1).

hydrochloric acid t., see specific tests, including *Bell's t.* (1), *Boas' t.* (1), (2), *Contejean t., Dennis and Silverman's t., dimethyl-amino-azobenzene t., Ewald's t.* (1), *Günzburg's t., Herzberg's t., Leo's t., Lüttke's t., Maly's t.* (1), (2), *Mohr's t., Rabuteau's t.* (1), (2), *Riegler's t.* (2), *Scivoletto's t., Szabo's t., Töpfer's t., Uffelmann's t., von Jaksch's t.* (1), (2), *Winckler's t.* (2), *Witz's t.*

hydrogen peroxide t. (*for blood*): a 20 per cent solution of hydrogen peroxide is added to the suspected fluid; if blood is present even in minute proportion, bubbles will rise, forming foam on the surface of the fluid.

hydrostatic t.: floating of the lungs of a dead infant when placed in water indicates that the child was born alive; called also *Raygat's t.*

hydroxyaromatic acid t., see *Hanke and Koessler's t.*

hydroxylamine t. (*for dextrose*), see *Bang's method,* under *method.*

hyperemia t., see *Moschcowitz's t.*

hypochlorite-orcinol t. (*for glycerin*): to 3 ml. of the unknown add 3 drops of N/1 sodium hypochlorite solution and boil one minute to drive off chlorine. Then add an equal volume of strong hydrochloric acid and a little orcinol. Boil, and a violet or greenish blue color indicates glycerine or a sugar, or some substance that can be oxidized to a sugar.

hypoxanthine t., see *Kossel's t.*

icterus index t.: the comparison by dilution colorimetry of the blood serum with a standard solution of potassium bichromate.

Ide t. (*for syphilis*): one drop of blood, or serum, or cerebrospinal fluid, is mixed with saline on a hollow glass slide and the antigen is added. The slide is then shaken for four to five minutes and the result read under the low-power objective of a microscope or with a powerful lens. Positive reactions show purplish blue clumps, while in a negative reaction there is no sign of clumping. The preparation of the antigen: oxheart is extracted with alcohol, and then to the extract are added measured amounts of cholesterin, gum benzoin, and dyes (crystal violet and azure II).

Ilimow's t. (*for albumin*): acidulate with acid sodium phosphate, filter, and add a solution of phenol (1:20); a cloudy precipitate indicates albumin.

Ilosvay's t. (*for nitrites*), see under *reagent.*

imidazole t., see *Hanke and Koessler's t.*

immobilizaton t.: detection of antibody based on its ability to inhibit the motility of a bacterial cell or protozoon.

indican t., see specific tests, including *Amann's t., Jaffé's t.* (2), *Jolles' t.* (2), *MacMunn's t., Obermeyer's t., Porter's t.* (2), *Wang's t., Weber's t.* (2). See also *indican, methods for,* under *method.*

indigo carmine t. (*for renal permeability*): a solution of indigo carmine is injected intramuscularly and the time of its appearance in the urine is noted. Normally, it begins to appear in about five minutes. Delay beyond this points to defective renal adequacy.

indigo red t., see specific tests, including *Rosenbach's t.* and *Rosin's t.*

indole t., see specific tests, including *Baeyer's t.* (2), *cholera red t., Herter's t.* (1), *Kondo's t., Legal's t.* (2), *Nencki's t., nitroso-indole-nitrate t., pine wood t., Salkowski's t.* (3), *vanillin t.* See also *indole, methods for,* under *method.*

indophenol t. (*for the presence of oxidizing enzymes in cells and for detecting the presence of myeloblasts, etc.*): cover glass films of the cells are fixed in alcohol. Float for ten to twenty minutes, face down, upon a freshly prepared solution of equal parts of 1 per cent aqueous solutions of dimethyl paraphenylenediamine and of alphanaphthol (Nadi's reagent). Rinse and mount in glycerin. The cytoplasm of cells containing oxidase (myeloblasts, myelocytes, polymorphonuclears, and large mononuclears) will be colored blue by indophenol.

inkblot t., see *Rorschach t.*

inoculation t. (*for acute anterior poliomyelitis*): the cerebrospinal fluid of the suspected patient (i.e., before the appearance of paralytic symptoms) is injected into a monkey. Paralysis will appear in the monkey within seven days if the patient is affected.

inosite t., see specific tests, including *Gallois' t., Scherer's t.* (1), *Seidel's t.*

intelligence t., see specific tests, including *alpha t., beta t., Binet t., group t., Herring's t., Kuhlmann t., performance t., Pintner-Patterson t., Rorschach t., Stanford t., vocabulary t., Yerkes-Bridges t.*

intracutaneous t.: one which involves introduction of an antigen between the layers of the skin and evaluation of the reaction elicited by it.

intracutaneous tuberculin t., see *Mantoux t.*

intradermal salt solution t., McClure-Aldrich t.

inulin clearance t., see under *inulin.*

iodine t.: 1. (*for starch*) when a compound solution of iodine is added to starch, and especially to an acid or neutral solution of cooked starch paste, a deep-blue color is produced which disappears on heating and reappears on cooling. Erythrodextrin and glycogen give a red color with iodine. 2. see specific tests, including *Alfraise's t.*, *Bourget's t.*, *Lesser's t.*, *Winckler's t.* (3).

iodoform t.: 1. (*for acetone*) see *Gunning's t.* 2. (*for alcohol*) make the unknown alkaline, and add a few drops of iodine solution. Heat gently, and yellow iodoform crystals indicate alcohol or some similar body.

Iowa pressure articulation t.: a test of the ability to produce the consonant sounds in isolated words, particularly the pressure sounds.

iron t., see specific tests, including *Brugsch's t.*, and *Tizzoni's t.* See also *iron, methods for*, under *method*.

irresistible impulse t.: a court decision supplementing the M'Naghten rule, which stated that if it could be shown that a person accused of an unlawful act was impelled to commit the act by an urge which he could not resist, then he could not be held criminally responsible for such action. It is based on the assumption that mental illness produces sudden or spontaneous impulses to commit criminal acts. See also *M'Naghten rule*, under *rule*, and *Durham's decision*, under *decision*.

irrigation t.: the patient is examined with the bladder full. The anterior urethra is washed out with a warm solution of boric acid (3 per cent), the perineum being compressed to prevent the entrance of the fluid into the posterior urethra. When the washings are perfectly clear, the patient voids his urine and any turbidity must come from the posterior urethra.

Ishihara's t.: 1. a test for color vision made by the use of a series of plates composed of round dots of various sizes and colors. 2. a flocculation test for syphilis, using as antigen an alcoholic extract of the kidney of a pregnant rabbit.

Israelson's t.: the reagent consists of 1 part of alcoholic extract of dried brain of rabbit, guinea pig, or beef, 9 parts of physiologic solution of sodium chloride, and one or two drops of a 0.2 per cent solution of fuchsin for each milliliter of the reagent. To one drop of the suspected serum, placed on a microscopic slide, one drop of reagent is added and mixed with the aid of a glass rod. In positive reactions there are rosy, flaky shreds in transparent fluid. In negative reactions the appearance is uniformly rosy. In weakly positive reactions, the flocculent particles are very small but are plainly visible under the magnifying lens.

Ito-Reenstierna t.: intracutaneous injection of a vaccine of killed *Hemophilus ducreyi* elicits a positive skin reaction in persons who have been infected with chancroid.

Jacobsthal's t. (*for serodiagnosis of syphilis*): 1. the patient's serum is mixed with alcoholic extract of syphilitic liver in the proportion of 1 to 10, and the resulting precipitate is examined with the darkfield illuminator. A strong positive reaction appears as a clumpy precipitate, a weak positive reaction as a small conglomeration of little fat particles, while a negative reaction is shown as a thick emulsion of fine dancing particles: called also *optic serodiagnosis of syphilis*. 2. a modification of the Wassermann test in which complement fixation is done at a low temperature.

Jacoby's t. (*for pepsin*): the greatest dilution of gastric juice which will clarify an acid solution of ricin in three hours at 38° C. gives the number of peptic units in the juice.

Jacquemin's t. (*for phenol*): add to the suspected liquid an equal quantity of aniline and some sodium hypochlorite in solution; a blue color is produced.

Jadassohn's t., see *irrigation t.*

Jadassohn-Bloch t.: a skin test for allergic conditions made by holding the suspected substance in contact with the skin for a considerable time by binding it on.

Jaffé's t.: 1. (*for creatinine and dextrose*) to the liquid add trinitrophenol and then make alkaline with sodium hydroxide. A red color without heating indicates creatinine; a red color after heating indicates dextrose. 2. (*for indican*) to the suspected liquid are added an equal amount of concentrated hydrochloric acid, 1 ml. of chloroform, and a few drops of a strong solution of chlorinated soda. The chloroform is colored blue if indican is present.

Jaksch's t., see *von Jaksch's t.*

Janet's t. (*for differentiating between functional and organic anesthesia*): the patient is instructed to say "yes" or "no," according as he does or does not feel the examiner's touch. He may say "no" in functional anesthesia, but he will say nothing in cases of organic anesthesia.

Jansen's t. (*for osteoarthritis deformans of the hip*): the patient is told to cross his legs with a point just above the ankle resting on the opposite knee; this motion is impossible when the disease exists.

Javorski's t., Jaworski's t.: in hourglass stomach a splashing sound will be heard on succussion of the pyloric portion after siphonage.

Jendrasic's t. (*for water-soluble vitamin B*): prepare the reagent by mixing equal volumes of N/10 ferric chloride and N/10 potassium ferricyanide and use at once. To a concentrated aqueous solution of the substance add about 2 per cent of acetic acid, then add the reagent as long as the depth of the blue color increases. Stopper, let stand ten minutes, and read. One to five volumes of distilled water may be added to reduce the color. A distinct blue color or a bright blue precipitate is positive. A green color is negative.

Jenner-Kay t.: a test for serum phosphatase.

Jenning's t.: a modification of Holmgren's test for color perception. Small patches of colored worsted are placed so as to be protected

from light and dust. The person to be examined indicates his color selection by pricking the record sheet with a pointed pencil.

Jochmann's t., 1. Müller-Jochmann t. 2. antitrypsin t.

Johnson's t. (*for albumin*): put the urine in a test tube and carefully pour upon it a strong solution of trinitrophenol; a white coagulum of albumin appears at the junction of the liquids which heating augments.

Jolles's t.: 1. (*for bile pigments in urine*) the urine is shaken with barium chloride solution, chloroform, and a few drops of hydrochloric acid. The precipitate is removed and partially dried. Treatment with 2 drops of strong sulfuric acid will bring out the characteristic colors of the bile pigments. 2. (*for indican*) to the urine add a little alcoholic solution of thymol and fuming hydrochloric acid containing 0.5 per cent of ferric chloride; chloroform shaken with this mixture becomes violet in color.

Jones and Cantarow t., see *urea concentration t.*

Jorissen's t. (*for formaldehyde*): add 0.5 ml. of a 1 per cent solution of phloroglucinol in 10 per cent sodium hydroxide to 1 ml. of the urine; a bright red color indicates free formaldehyde.

Justus' t. (*for syphilis*): administration of mercury by inunction or subcutaneously; if syphilis is present, there will be a fall of hemoglobin of from 10 to 20 per cent.

Kabatschnik's t. (*for hearing*): (*obs.*) a tuning-fork is held near the open ear and removed the moment the sound ceases; it is then applied to the nail of the examiner's finger and this finger is placed so as to close the patient's external auditory meatus. In a normal ear the sound will be heard again, although the fork has not been struck a second time.

Kafka's t. for *cerebrospinal syphilis*): a modification of the mastic test, made with a solution of sodium bicarbonate, sodium chloride, mastic resin, and a stain.

Kahn t.: 1. [R. L. Kahn] a precipitation test for syphilis. The serum is inactivated as in the Wassermann test. To 0.3 ml. of serum in a test tube is added 0.05 ml. of diluted antigen. After shaking for three minutes the tube is incubated at 37° C. overnight. A positive reaction is shown by the presence of one or more lumps of precipitate. In the "presumptive" Kahn test a sensitized antigen is employed. 2. [Herbert Kahn] a test for the presence of cancer based on quantitative determination of a certain constituent of the patient's blood called albumin A.

Kantor and Gies' t. (*for proteins*): test papers, made by dipping them in Gies' reagent (see under *Gies' t.*), drying, and cutting into strips, are used in making biuret test.

Kaplan's t. (*for globulin-albumin in spinal fluid*): to 0.2 ml. of the fluid in a test tube is added 0.3 ml. of distilled water. This is boiled up twice. Three drops of a 5 per cent solution of butyric acid in physiologic salt solution are added and the mixture carefully underlaid with 0.5 ml. of a saturated aqueous solution of ammonium sulfate. After twenty minutes a definite ring will form at the point of contact if globulin-albumin is present.

Kapsinow's t. (*for bile pigments*): add Obermayer's reagent to the urine and heat; a green color indicates bile pigments.

Kashiwado's t. (*for pancreatic disease*): the patient swallows stained nuclei from a calf's thymus mixed with lycopodium grains; these later serve to indicate the portion of the feces which is to be examined.

Kastle's t. (*for raw milk*): to 5 ml. of the milk add 0.3 ml. of N/10 hydrogen peroxide solution and 1 ml. of a 1 per cent solution of tricresol; raw milk will give a slight yellow color, boiled milk will not.

Kastle-Meyer t., see *phenolphthalein t.*

Katayama's t. (*for carbonyl-hemoglobin*): to 5 drops of blood add 10 ml. of water, 5 drops of orange-colored ammonium sulfide, and enough acetic acid to make the mixture acid. CO causes a rose-red color; normal blood, a dirty greenish gray.

Kathrein's t., see *Maréchal's t.*

Kato t.: a technique for the quantitative estimation of the worm burden of an individual, based on estimation of a standard 50 mg. sample of fresh feces cleared with glycerine.

Kelling's t.: 1. (*for lactic acid in the stomach*) the stomach contents are diluted with water, and to them are added one or two drops of a 5 per cent watery solution of ferric chloride. A greenish yellow color is formed when lactic acid is present. 2. a test for the presence and location of an esophageal diverticulum by the sound of swallowing. 3. (*for gastric carcinoma*) a test based on the fact that the serum of cancer patients will dissolve the red corpuscles of the hen.

Kentmann's t. (*for formaldehyde*): dissolve in a test tube 0.1 gm. of morphine in 1 ml. of sulfuric acid; add, without mixing, an equal volume of the liquid to be tested: in a short time the latter will take on a reddish violet color if any formaldehyde is present.

Kerner's t. (*for creatinine*): acidify the suspected solution and add phosphomolybdic or phosphotungstic acid in solution; if creatinine is present, it will form a crystalline precipitate.

kidney function t., see specific tests, including *Albarran's t.*, *amylase t.* (1), *blood–urea clearance t.*, *concentration t.*, *creatinine clearance t.*, *Fishberg concentration t.*, *glycerophosphate t.*, *Holten's t.*, *Howard t.*, *indigo carmine t.*, *inulin clearance t.*, *lactose t.* (1), *methylene blue t.* (1), *Mosenthal's t.*, *Nyiri's t.*, *phenolsulfonphthalein t.*, *phlorhizin t.*, *potassium iodide t.*, *Pregl's t.*, *radioactive renogram t.*, *radioisotope renal excretion t.*, *Rehberg's t.*, *Simonelli's t.*, *Strauss's t.* (2), (4), *urea concentration t.*, *urine concentration t.*, *Volhard's t.* (2),

Wohlgemuth's t., xylose clearance or tolerance t., xylose concentration t.

Killian's t. *(for carbohydrate tolerance)*: two hours after a standard breakfast, give the patient 200 ml. of water. One hour later, give 1.75 gm. of dextrose per kilogram of body weight. Determine amount of dextrose in blood specimens taken at hourly intervals, and also in the twenty-four-hour specimen of urine.

Kinberg's t. *(for liver function)*: after a low nitrogen content diet for several days, 50 gm. of gelatin dissolved in hot chocolate is taken fasting; in liver disease there is an increase in the output of amino acids, except in congestion of the liver and catarrhal jaundice.

Kitzmiller t., see *antithrombin t.*

Kjeldahl's t. *(for nitrogen)*, see under *method.*

Klein t., see under *reaction.*

Klimow's t. *(for blood in urine)*: to a specimen of urine is added an equal quantity of H_2O_2 and a little powdered aloin; formation of a purple color indicates the presence of blood.

Kline t., Kline-Young t.: a microscope slide precipitation test for syphilis.

Knapp's t.: 1. *(for sugar in the urine)* ten gm. of mercuric cyanide are dissolved in 100 ml. of a solution of caustic soda and diluted; heated with diabetic urine, metallic mercury is precipitated. 2. *(for organic acids in stomach)* stomach contents are filtered and 1 ml. treated with 5 ml. of ether; the extract is floated on dilute iron solution in test tubes, and the various colored rings formed will indicate the presence of the various acids.

Knott t.: a test for microfilariae or worm larvae in the blood by lysis of the blood in a dilute (2 per cent) formalin solution, centrifugation, and examination of the stained sediment for microfilariae or larvae.

Kober t.: 1. *(for estrogens)* when estrogens are treated with a mixture of sulfuric acid and phenolsulfonic acid and then diluted with water, a clear pink color is formed. 2. *(for proteins in milk)* the proteins are precipitated with sulfosalicylic acid and the precipitate estimated nephelometrically.

Kobert's t. *(for hemoglobin)*: the suspected liquid is treated with zinc powder or a solution of zinc sulfate; the resulting precipitate is stained red by alkalis.

Kolmer's t.: 1. a modification of the Wassermann test for syphilis. 2. a specific complement-fixation test for various bacterial diseases.

Kondo's t. *(for indole or skatole)*: to 1 ml. of the unknown add 3 drops of solution of formaldehyde and 1 ml. of concentrated sulfuric acid; a violet-red color indicates indole, a yellow or brown color skatole.

Konew's t. *(for glanders)*: a test tube is filled to the depth of 3 cm. with mallease, and blood serum from the subject is introduced by means of a pipet at the bottom of the tube beneath the mallease. If the patient is affected with glanders a white cloudiness will appear along the line separating the two liquids. Called also *ring t.*

Korotkoff's t.: in aneurysm, if the blood pressure in the peripheral circulation remains fairly high while the artery above the aneurysm is compressed, the collateral circulation is good.

Kossel's t. *(for hypoxanthine)*: the liquid to be tested is treated with zinc and hydrochloric acid and with sodium hydroxide in excess; if hypoxanthine is present, a ruby-red color is produced.

Kottmann's t. *(for thyroid function)*: to 1 ml. of clear blood serum add 0.25 ml. of 0.5 per cent solution of KI and 0.3 ml. of 0.5 per cent solution of $AgNO_3$. Expose serum for five minutes to light of 500-watt Mazda lamp at 25 cm. distance. Then add 0.5 ml. of 0.25 per cent solution of hydrochinone. Normal serum turns brown in a short time; that of patients with hypothyroidism in a shorter time; that of patients with hyperthyroidism only after considerable delay.

Kowarsky's t.: 1. *(for dextrose in urine)* in a test tube place 5 drops of pure phenylhydrazine, 10 drops of glacial acetic acid, and 1 ml. of saturated solution of sodium chloride. To the mass which results add 2 or 3 ml. of urine; boil two minutes, and cool. If dextrose is present, crystals of phenylglucosazone will be seen with the microscope. 2. *(blood test for diabetes)* test of the patient's blood based on the reduction of a copper solution by the sugar in the blood to cuprous oxide, and the dissolving of the latter in an acid solution of ferrous sulphate, which causes the separation of an equal amount of ferrous oxide, which is measured by titration with potassium permanganate.

Krokiewicz' t. *(for bile pigment in urine)*: 1 ml. of a 1 per cent solution of sodium nitrate and 1 ml. of a 1 per cent solution of sulfanilic acid are mixed and added drop by drop to 0.5 ml. of urine. The amount added must not exceed 10 drops. The mixture becomes bright red, changing to amethyst on the addition of 1 or 2 drops of concentrated hydrochloric acid and a large amount of water.

Kuhlmann's t.: a modification of the Binet's test for intelligence so changed as to adapt it for use on infants.

Külz's t. *(for β-hydroxybutyric acid)*: 1. the fermented urine is evaporated to a syrupy consistence, strong sulfuric acid in equal volume is added, and the mixture is distilled. If hydroxybutyric acid is present, α-crotonic acid will be formed, which will crystallize. 2. if, after fermentation, the urine shows dextrorotatory properties, β-hydroxybutyric acid is present.

Kurzrok-Miller t.: an in vitro test of compatibility of cervical mucus and spermatozoa, involving observation, under the microscope, of the behavior of sperm placed beside a sample of mucus taken from the cervical canal at the time of ovulation.

Kveim t. *(for sarcoidosis)*: intracutaneous injection of an antigen prepared from human sarcoid tissue, usually lymph nodes or spleen; appearance in about a week of a red-purple papule which increases in size and on biopsy resembles the tuberculoid granulomas of sarcoidosis is considered positive for sarcoidosis.

Laborde's t. *(for death)*, see *Cloquet's needle sign,* under *sign.*

lactic acid t., see specific tests, including *Boas' t.* (3), *Hopkins' thiophene t., Kelling's t.* (1), *MacLean t., Strauss' t.* (1), *Uffelmann's t.* See also *lactic acid, methods for,* under *method.*

lactose t.: 1. *(for renal function)* twenty gm. of lactose dissolved in 20 ml. of distilled water are injected under aseptic precautions into a vein at the bend of the elbow. The urine is collected hourly and tested (Nylander's test) until the sugar reaction ceases to be positive. If lactose secretion continues for more than five hours, renal disease is indicated. 2. see specific tests, including *Cole's t.* (2), *Mathews' t., Meyer's t.* (2), *Moore's t., mucic acid t., Rubner's t.* (2).

Ladendorff's t. *(for blood)*: treat the suspected liquid with tincture of guaiacum, and afterward with eucalyptus oil; the upper stratum of the mixture is turned violet and the lower blue if blood is present.

Lancefield precipitation t.: a ring precipitation test used to classify and identify streptococci. Group specific antibody reacts *in vitro* with group specific polysaccharide to produce a ring of precipitation where the two reagents react at the interface.

Landau color t. *(for syphilis)*: to 0.2 ml. of clear serum from the patient add 0.01 ml. of a reagent consisting of a 1 per cent solution of iodine in carbon tetrachloride. Shake thoroughly until the iodine color has disappeared. Let stand for four or five hours. A positive reaction is shown by a clear, transparent, yellow color; a negative one by an opaque grayish color.

Lang's t. *(for taurine)*: the solution to be tested is boiled with freshly prepared mercuric oxide; taurine will cause a white precipitate to appear.

Lange's t., 1. see *colloidal gold t.* 2. *(for acetone in urine)* 15 ml. of urine are mixed with 0.5 to 1 ml. of acetic acid, and a few drops of a freshly prepared concentrated solution of sodium nitroprusside added. The mixture is overlaid with ammonia. At the point of junction a characteristic violet ring is formed.

lantern t.: a test for color blindness made with a set of specially devised lanterns.

latex agglutination t., latex fixation t.: a test in which soluble antigens are adsorbed to polystyrene latex, i.e., to very small spherical particles of the plastic in suspension. The antigen-coated latex particles agglutinate following the addition of specific antibody. This test has been used extensively for the detection of rheumatoid factor and of C-reactive protein.

Lautier's t. *(for tuberculosis)*: a few drops of a 1 per cent solution of Old Tuberculin are placed on the arm, covered with cotton, and left for forty-eight hours; if tuberculosis is present there will develop a patch of vesicles on an elevated reddened base.

LE t.: serum from patients with systemic lupus erythematosus is combined with normal leukocytes; following incubation at 37°C., polymorphonuclear leukocytes engulf nuclei or nuclear fragments of cells to form so-called LE cells.

Leach's t. *(for formaldehyde)*: to 10 ml. of milk add 10 ml. of concentrated hydrochloric acid containing 0.02 per cent of ferric chloride. Heat, and if formaldehyde is present a violet color will be produced.

lead t., see specific tests, including *Abrams' t.* and *Blyth's t.*

Lebbin's t. *(for formaldehyde in milk)*: a small amount of milk is boiled with a mixture of 0.05 gm. of resorcinol and the same quantity of a 5 per cent solution of sodium hydroxide. Change from a yellow to a red color indicates the presence of formaldehyde.

Lechini's t. *(for blood in urine)*: ten ml. of urine are treated with 1 drop of acetic acid and 3 ml. of chloroform; with blood the chloroform layer becomes red.

Lee's t. *(for rennin)*: add 5 drops of gastric juice to 5 ml. of milk; coagulation should take place in twenty minutes in the incubator.

Leffmann-Beam t.: a modification of the Babcock test used for determination of fat concentration in human breast milk.

Legal's t.: 1. *(for acetone)* render the urine acid with HCl and distill it. Solution of sodium hydroxide and sodium nitroprusside added to the distillate produce a ruby-red tint, which acetic acid changes to purple. Creatinine will also produce a red color, but this color disappears when acetic acid is put in. 2. *(for indole)* to the unknown add a few drops of sodium nitroprusside; make alkaline with potassium hydroxide. The violet color changes to blue on the addition of acetic acid.

Leiner's t. *(for casein or paracasein)*: a piece of feces is fixed by heat on a slide and stained with a solution of acid fuchsin and methyl green; a pale blue or violet color is formed.

leishmanin skin t., see *Montenegro t.*

Le Nobel's t., see *Nobel's t.*

lentochol t., see *Sachs-Georgi t.*

Leo's t. *(for free hydrochloric acid)*: calcium carbonate is added to the solution, which is neutralized if the acidity is due to free acid, but not if due to acid salts.

lepromin t. *(for leprosy)*: intradermal injection of lepromin is followed by development of an inflammatory papule, which may ulcerate, in persons with cellular immunity against *Mycobacterium leprae;* this includes well over half the normal adult population, and all patients with tuberculoid leprosy, but no patients with lepromatous leprosy. The test is read at three weeks. Called also *Mitsuda t.*

leprosy t., see specific tests, including *histamine flare t., lepromin t.*

Lesser's t.: any iodine-containing secretion turns yellow when treated with calomel.

leucine t., see specific tests, including *Hofmeister's t.* (1), *Scherer's t.* (2).

Levinson t. (*for tuberculous meningitis and other intracranial conditions*): one ml. of spinal fluid is placed in each of the two test tubes 8 mm. in diameter. To one is added 1 ml. of a 1 per cent solution of mercuric chloride and, to the other, 1 ml. of a 3 per cent solution of sulfosalicylic acid. The tubes are well shaken, stoppered, and allowed to stand at room temperature for forty-eight hours. At the end of twenty-four and forty-eight hours the column of precipitate in each tube is measured in millimeters. When the height of the precipitate in the first test tube is seen to be twice that of the precipitate in the second tube, the result of the test is positive.

levulose t., see *Borchardt's t., Cipollina's t., methylphenylhydrazine t., Rubner's t.* (2), *Selivanoff's t.*

levulose tolerance t.: a test of hepatic function based on the power of the liver to absorb and store large quantities of levulose.

Lewis and Pickering t.: the employment of a rapid rise of temperature to produce vasodilatation in the part to be tested for the state of the peripheral circulation.

Lichtheim t.: if a patient is able to indicate the number of syllables in a word which he cannot utter, it indicates that the cortex is less involved than the association fibers.

Lieben's t. (*for acetone in urine*): acidulate and distill it, and treat with ammonia and tincture of iodine; if acetone is present, a yellow precipitate of iodoform is produced.

Lieben-Ralfe t. (*for acetone*): boil 1.3 gm. of potassium iodide in 3.75 ml. of solution of potassium hydroxide; float the urine on the surface of the reagent in a test tube: a precipitate of phosphate is formed at the upper surface of the reagent, which, if acetone is present, will be rendered yellow by iodoform.

Liebermann's t. (*for proteins*): a precipitate is made from the urine with alcohol; wash this with ether and heat with strong hydrochloric acid: this produces a fine violet-blue color if proteins are present.

Liebermann-Burchardt t. (*for cholesterol*): dissolve the suspected substance in chloroform, add acetic anhydride, and treat with strong sulfuric acid; if cholesterol is present, a violet color is produced, which soon changes to green.

Liebig's t. (*for cystine*): boil the suspected substance with a sodium hydroxide solution and a little lead sulfide; if cystine is present, the lead sulfide will form a black precipitate.

Ligat's t. (*for cutaneous hyperesthesia in abdominal disease*): the skin is pinched between the thumb and forefinger and lifted up from the parts below.

Lignières' t.: a modification of the cutireaction consisting in shaving the skin and rubbing in a few drops of raw tuberculin; in tuberculous persons there appear papules whose color varies from pale pink to deep red.

limulus t.: an extract of blood cells from the horseshoe crab (*Limulus polyphemus*) is exposed to a blood sample from a patient; if gram-negative endotoxin is present in the sample, it will produce gelation of the extract of blood cells.

Lindemann's t. (*for acetoacetic acid in urine*): to about 10 ml. of urine add 5 drops of 30 per cent acetic acid, 5 drops Lugol's solution, and 2 or 3 ml. chloroform, and shake. The chloroform does not change color if diacetic acid is present, but becomes reddish violet in its absence. Uric acid also decolorizes iodine, and if much is present double the amount of Lugol's solution should be used.

Lindner's t., see under *sign*.

Links' t. (*for carcinoma*): a serum test for early carcinoma based on the relationship of the potassium and magnesium content of the serum to the erythrocyte count of the blood.

lipase t.: 1. (*for liver function*) a test based on the fact that lipase is present in the blood plasma of normal persons in a constant amount. Liver injury will cause a rise in the lipase of the blood plasma as measured by the power of the blood to split ethyl butyrate. 2. see specific tests, including *copper soap t., ethyl butyrate t., litmus milk t.*

Lipps's t., see *sand t.*

litmus milk t. (*for pancreatic lipase*): add pancreatic lipase to litmus milk, incubate, and note change of color; pancreatic lipase is indicated by a pink coloration.

liver function t., see specific tests, including *alkaline phosphate t., Bauer's t.*(2), *blood ammonia t., bromsulphalein excretion t., Bufano's t., camphor t., Dedichen's t., fibrinogen t., Hanger's t., Kinberg's t., levulose tolerance t., lipase t., Macdonald's t., nitrogen partition t., phenoltetrachlorophthalein t., Quick's t.* (1), *rose bengal t., Rosenthal's t.* (2), *santonin t., Strauss's t.* (3), *thymol turbidity t., Zappacosta's t.*

Loewe's t. (*for dextrose in urine*): treat the urine with a solution of sodium carbonate containing bismuth subnitrate and glycerine; sugar gives a dark precipitate.

Loewi's t.: three drops of epinephrine chloride solution 1:1000 are instilled into the conjunctival sac, followed in five minutes by 3 more drops. This causes dilatation of the pupil in pancreatic insufficiency, diabetes, and hyperthyroidism.

Lombard's t.: a test for simulated deafness using a noise apparatus.

loudness balance t's: tests for determining whether perception of loudness rises normally with progressive increases in intensity of a pure tone.

Löwenthal's t. (*for dextrose not in urine*): boil the suspected substance with a solution of ferric chloride, tartaric acid, and sodium carbonate; if dextrose is present, the liquid becomes dark, and iron oxide is freely precipitated.

Lowy's t.: a modified Abderhalden test for the diagnosis of cancer.

Lücke's t. (*for hippuric acid*): add boiling hot nitric acid, evaporate, and heat the dry residue; a strong odor of nitrobenzene proves the presence of hippuric acid.

Luebert's t. (*for formaldehyde in milk*): five gm. of coarsely powdered potassium sulfate are placed in a 100 ml. flask; 5 ml. of suspected milk are put over it by a pipet, and 10 ml. of sulfuric acid (specific gravity, 1.84) are run down the side of the flask. If formaldehyde is present, a violet coloration soon occurs; if none is present, the fluid becomes brown or black.

luetin t., see *Noguchi's luetin reaction,* under *reaction.*

lupus band t.: an immunofluoresence test to determine the presence and extent of immunoglobulin and complement deposits at the dermal-epidermal junction of skin specimens from patients with systemic lupus erythematosus.

lupus induction t.: serum from a patient suspected of having lupus erythematosus is mixed with normal blood and rotated in a vial with glass beads to induce the formation of the LE cell.

Lüttke's t. (*for free hydrochloric acid in gastric juice*): a quantitative determination in succession of the total chlorides, the chlorine in the fixed chlorides, and then the combined and free HCl.

Lyle and Curtman's t. (*for blood*): boil the stool with acetic acid, extract it with ether, and to the ethereal extract add a little guaiaconic acid in 95 per cent alcohol; a decided green, light-blue, or purple color indicates the presence of blood.

Lyon's t., Meltzer-Lyon t.

McClure-Aldrich t.: an 0.8 per cent solution of sodium chloride is injected intradermally; the rate with which it is absorbed (disappearance of wheal or Q. R. Z.) is decreased from the normal time in intoxications.

MacDonagh's t., see *gel t.*

Macdonald's t. (*for liver function*): inject 2 mg. per kilogram of sodium sulfobromophthalein (Bromsulphalein) and take blood specimens every five minutes for thirty minutes after the injection.

Machado t., Machado-Guerreiro t. (*for Chagas' disease*): a complement-fixation test, using as antigen an extract of the spleen of puppies severely infected with *Trypanosoma cruzi.*

Macht t.: the effect of blood sera on the growth of seedlings of *Lupinus albus;* the serum of pernicious anemia and other abnormal blood conditions delays the growth of the seedlings.

McKinnon's t. (*for smallpox*): material from the patient's lesion is inoculated intradermally into a normal rabbit and into a vaccinated rabbit; if the material contains smallpox virus the normal rabbit, but not the immunized one, will develop a local lesion.

Maclagan's t., see *thymol turbidity t.*

MacLean t. (*for lactic acid in gastric juice*): to 5 ml. of gastric juice add 5 drops of the following reagent: ferric chloride, 5 gm.; concentrated hydrochloric acid, 1.5 ml.; saturated solution of mercury bichloride, 100 ml. Lactic acid is indicated by a yellow coloration.

MacLean-de Wesselow t., see *urea concentration t.*

MacMunn's t. (*for indican*): boil the urine in an equal quantity of hydrochloric acid and a little nitric acid; cool, and shake with chloroform, which becomes violet, and shows one absorption band due to indigo blue and one due to indigo red.

McMurray's t. (*for torn meniscus*): as the patient lies supine with knee fully flexed, the examiner rotates the patient's foot fully outward and the knee is slowly extended; a painful "click" indicates a tear of the medial meniscus of the knee joint. If the click occurs when the foot is rotated inward, the tear is in the lateral meniscus.

MacQuarrie t.: a pencil and paper test for estimating general mechanical ability.

macrophage migration (inhibition) t.: migration inhibition t.

MacWilliams' t. (*for albumin*): take 20 ml. of urine and add 2 drops of a saturated solution of salicylsulfonic acid: if albumin is present, a cloudiness or precipitate will be seen; if albumoses or peptones are present, this precipitate will disappear on boiling, but appear again on cooling.

magnesionitric t. (*for albumin in urine*): mix 1 part of nitric acid and 1 part magnesium sulfate; turbidity indicates the presence of albumin.

Magpie's t. (*for salts of mercury*): stannous chloride is added to the suspected solution; a white and gray precipitate is formed, consisting of metallic mercury and mild mercurous chloride.

malaria t., see specific tests, including *Chorine's t., Henry's t., protein tyrosine t., Urriolla's t.*

male frog t., male toad t. (*for pregnancy*): urine or serum of a woman suspected of being pregnant is injected into the dorsal lymph sac of two male frogs (*Rana pipiens*) or male toads (*Bufo marinus*). The presence of spermatozoa in the cloacal fluid of both animals is positive; in one animal, inconclusive; in neither animal, negative.

Malerba's t. (*for acetone*): add a solution of dimethyl-paraphenylenediamine; a fine red or reddish color is seen.

mallein t., see *mallein*.

Malot's t.: a test for the quantitative determination of phosphoric acid in urine by the reaction with cochineal and a uranium salt.

maltose t., see *Rubner's t.* (2).

Maly's t.: 1. (*for free hydrochloric acid in the gastric juice*) a solution of methylene blue is added; the free acid will turn it from a violet to a green or blue tint. 2. (*for free hydrochloric acid in stomach contents*) filter into a glass dish and stain blue with ultramarine; place a piece of lead paper over it and cover; warm mixture. The free acid will turn the blue to brown and darken the lead paper.

Manson evaluation t.: a test for the psychometric differentiation of alcoholics and nonalcoholics.

Mantoux t. (*for tuberculosis*): give intracutaneous injection of 0.1 ml. of desired dilution of tuberculin and successive injections of gradually increasing concentration until a reaction occurs; called also *intracutaneous tuberculin t.*, *Mantoux reaction*, and *Mendel's t.*

Manzullo's t., see *tellurite t.*

Maréchal's t. (*for bile pigments in urine*): drop tincture of iodine carefully into the tube; when the drops touch the urine, a green color is seen.

Maréchal-Rosin t., see *Maréchal's t.*

Marie's three-paper t. (*of attention and recall*): three pieces of paper are given to the subject, who is told to cross the room, drop one piece into the waste basket, place another on the table, and return the third to the examiner.

Marlow's t. (*for heterophoria*): one eye is occluded by a bandage for some time; after the bandage is removed, measurements for heterophoria are made.

Marquardt's t. (*for fusel oil*): add a few drops of dilute potassium permanganate until the light pink color persists. Cork for twenty-four hours. Add more permanganate if necessary to keep the pink color. Note the sickening odor of valeric acid.

Marquis' t. (*for morphine*): evaporate the unknown to dryness on a white porcelain plate and touch with a mixture of 3 ml. of concentrated sulfuric acid and 2 drops of formalin. A purple-red color changing to violet and then to blue indicates morphine.

Marsh's t. (*for arsenic or antimony*): hydrogen obtained from zinc and dilute sulfuric acid is allowed to act on the suspected substance; if arsenic is present, hydrogen arsenide (AsH_3) is formed. Ignite this gas and hold a piece of porcelain in the jet of flame; metallic arsenic is deposited. For antimony the same test is serviceable, but the arsenical mirror is dissolved by sodium hypochlorite solution, while the antimonial mirror is not affected by it.

Marshall's t. (*for urea*): treat the specimen with urease and titrate the ammonia so formed; see under *method*.

Maschke's t., see *von Maschke's t.*

Masset's t. (*for bile pigments in urine*): add 2 or 3 drops of sulfuric acid and a crystal of potassium nitrite; a grass-green color shows the presence of bile pigments.

Master "2-step" exercise t. (*for coronary insufficiency*): an electrocardiographic test, the tracings being recorded while the subject repeatedly ascends and descends two steps, each 9 inches high, immediately after cessation of the climbs, and then 2 and 6 minutes later. The amount of work (number of trips) is standardized for age, weight, and sex.

mastic t. (*for cerebrospinal syphilis*): a test depending on the precipitation of a solution containing mastic in cases of syphilis; there is no change in the solution in negative cases. Called also *Emanuel-Cutting test*.

Matas' t., see *tourniquet t.*, def. 2.

match t.: a screening test of expiration in which a match is held 3 inches from the subject's wide open mouth and several attempts are made to blow it out. Failure after six attempts indicates a maximal breathing capacity below 40 liters per minute and a maximal midexpiratory flow rate below 0.6 liter per second.

Mátéfy t.: a serum test for the early diagnosis of pulmonary tuberculosis.

Mathews' t. (*for lactose and dextrose*): if both dextrose and lactose are suspected, make a total quantitative test by Benedict's method. Add yeast to the urine and ferment out the dextrose, then make a second quantitative determination. The second determination is or may be lactose; confirm with the osazone test. The difference between the two determinations is dextrose.

Maumené t. (*for dextrose*): heat the urine with a little stannous chloride; if sugar is present, a dark-brown precipitate will be formed.

Mauthner's t.: a method of testing color blindness by the use of small bottles filled with different pigments, some with one only and some with two, the latter containing either pseudoisochromatic or isochromatic solutions.

Mayer's t. (*for alkaloids*): mercuric chloride, 13$\frac{1}{2}$ gm., and potassium iodide, 50 gm., are dissolved in 1000 ml. of water: this is used as a test for alkaloid, with which it gives a white precipitate.

Mayerhofer's t.: the reduction of a decinormal solution of potassium permanganate solution by 1 ml. of spinal fluid in an acid medium as an index of the amount of protein substance present in

the fluid; used as an indication of the existence of tuberculous meningitis.

Mazzini t.: a flocculation test for the diagnosis of syphilis.

Méhu's t. (*for albumin in urine*): add a little nitric acid, and mix with 10 volumes of a solution of 2 parts of alcohol, 1 part of phenol, and 1 part of acetic acid; shake it and a white precipitate appears. This test is said not to be entirely trustworthy.

Meigs' t. (*for fat in milk*): to 10 ml. of milk in a special apparatus add 20 ml. of water, 20 ml. of ethyl ether, and shake. Then add 20 ml. of 95 per cent alcohol. Remove the ethereal layer, evaporate, and weigh.

Meinicke t. (*for syphilis*): 1. flocculation test: alcoholic extract of horse's heart diluted with water and a 2 per cent sodium chloride solution is added to the blood serum. After incubation for twenty-four hours flocculation is produced in syphilis. 2. turbidity test: the same solution, greatly diluted and containing balsam of tolu, gives a turbid mixture in syphilis. 3. clearing or clarification test: a milky dilution of alcoholic beef heart containing balsam of tolu will be cleared by the addition of syphilitic blood serum.

melanin t., see specific tests, including *Blackberg and Wagner's t.*, *Eiselt's t.*, *Thormählen's t.*, *von Jaksch's t.* (3), *Zeller's t.* (1).

Meltzer-Lyon t. (*for biliary disease*): a strong solution of magnesium sulfate is instilled into the duodenum by means of a tube, with the hope that this will paralyze the sphincter of Oddi, and that this paralysis will be followed by reflex contraction of the gallbladder, thus permitting the collection of separate specimens of bile from the common duct, the gallbladder, and the liver.

Mendel's t., see *Mantoux t.*

Mendeléeff's t.: a test for cancer based on the theory that there is a specific difference between the coagulating powers of leukocytic and erythrocytic extracts in cancerous and noncancerous subjects.

Mendelsohn's t.: a test for efficiency of the heart muscle based on the rapidity of the recovery of the pulse from its acceleration produced by exertion.

meningitis t.: see specific tests, including *Levinson's t.*, *Mayerhofer's t.*, *Takata-Ara t.*, *tryptophan t.* (2).

mercury t., see specific tests, including *Magpie's t.*, *Reinsch's t.* (2), *Vogel and Lee's t.*

Mester's t. (*for rheumatic disease*): blood is withdrawn from the middle finger of the right hand of a fasting patient before and again thirty and sixty minutes after administration of two or three intracutaneous injections of 0.2 ml. each of a sterile 0.1 per cent aqueous solution of salicylic acid, and the number of leukocytes is determined after each withdrawal. The injections are made at the flexor aspect of the right forearm at a distance of about 5 cm. from each other. They are followed by severe pain and burning sensation of short duration and by the formation, at the points of the injections, of wheals which disappear in a few hours. Positive results are shown by transient leukopenia within the first thirty minutes after administration of the injections.

methylene blue t.: 1. (*for renal permeability*) a solution of methylene blue is injected intramuscularly and the time of its appearance in the urine is noted. Normally, it appears in about thirty minutes. When delayed beyond this, renal permeability is reduced. Called also *Achard and Castaigne's t.* 2. (*for milk*) to 10 ml. of milk add 1 ml. of standard methylene blue solution, stopper, mix, and incubate at 37° C. in the dark. Mix each half hour. Good quality milk should not decolorize the mixture in less than six to eight hours.

methylphenylhydrazine t. (*for levulose*): add 4 gm. of methylphenylhydrazine to 10 ml. of unknown (containing about 2 gm. of levulose) and enough alcohol to clarify the solution; add 4 ml. of 50 per cent acetic acid and heat from five to ten minutes. Reddish yellow needles of methylphenyl-levulosazone indicate levulose.

Mett's t. (*for estimating pepsin*): tubes (Mett's tubes) of coagulated albumin are introduced into the unknown and into a standard pepsin HCl mixture and the amount of digestion occurring in a given time is noted.

Meyer's t.: 1. the blood vessel of a freshly killed ox is placed in the solution to be tested; if it contracts, epinephrine is assumed to be present. 2. (*for lactose*) precipitate the proteins of the milk with phosphotungstic acid and titrate the filtrate with Benedict's solution. 3. (*for blood*) see *Meyer's reagent*, under *reagent*.

Michailow's t. (*for proteins*): add ferrous sulfate to the solution, underlay it with strong sulfuric acid and a drop or so of nitric acid; a brown ring and red coloration indicate the presence of proteins.

microprecipitation t.: a precipitation test in which a minute quantity of the serum is employed.

Middlebrook-Dubos hemagglutination t.: a test for the detection of serum antibodies to certain components of *Mycobacterium tuberculosis*.

migration inhibition t.: an *in vitro* test for detection of cell-mediated immunity (or delayed hypersensitivity) in which peritoneal exudate cells (lymphocytes and macrophages) are packed in capillary tubes; if the medium contains an antigen to which the lymphocytes are primed, macrophage migration from the tubes is inhibited by lymphokines (macrophage inhibiting factor) released by the lymphocytes. Called also *macrophage migration (inhibition) t.*

milk t., see specific tests, including *Babcock's t.*, *Bauer's t.* (3), *benzidine peroxidase t.*, *dirt t.*, *Kastle's t.*, *Kober t.* (2), *methylene blue t.* (2), *phosphatase t.* (1), *Storck's t.*, *Wilkinson and Peter's t.*

milk-ring t., abortus Bang ring t.

Millard's t. (*for albumin*): make a reagent of 2 parts of liquefied carbolic acid, 6 parts of glacial acetic acid, and 22 parts of a solution of potassium hydroxide; this precipitates albumin.

Miller-Kurzrok t.: a laboratory procedure to test the ability of the sperm to penetrate the mucus plug in the woman's cervix.

40 millimeter t. (*for athletic efficiency*): the subject sits with nasal respiration occluded with a clamp, and by expiring through a mouthpiece, sustains a column of mercury at the height of 40 mm. as long as he can. The pulse rate is taken meanwhile, every five seconds. In a satisfactory test the pulse rate is unaltered for a minute or more.

Millon's t. (*for proteins and nitrogenous compounds*): a solution is made of 10 gm. of mercury and 20 gm. of nitric acid; this is diluted with an equal volume of water and decanted after standing twenty-four hours. This reagent gives a red color with proteins and other substances, such as tyrosine, phenol, and thymol, which contain the hydroxyphenyl group.

Mills's t. (*for tennis elbow*): with the wrist and fingers fully flexed and the forearm pronated, complete extension of the elbow is painful.

miostagmin t., see under *reaction.*

mirror t.: a mirror is held horizontally above the larynx and the patient instructed to cough. The mirror is thus sprayed with bronchial secretion. Small flecks of secretion on the mirror indicate the nature of the expectoration.

Mitscherlich's t. (*for phosphorus in the stomach*): the contents of the stomach are made acid and distilled in the dark. The condenser will contain a luminous ring. Small amounts of alcohol, ether, or turpentine will prevent the reaction.

Mitsuda t., lepromin t.

Mittelmeyer's t.: the patient is directed to take marching steps on one spot without progressing: in vestibular disorder he will turn to the side ipsilateral to vestibular loss, or contralateral to vestibular excitation.

mixed leukocyte culture t., mixed lymphocyte culture t., see *mixed leukocyte reaction,* under *reaction.*

Moerner-Sjöqvist t., Sjöqvist method.

Mohr's t. (*for hydrochloric acid in the stomach contents*): dilute to a light-yellow color a solution of iron acetate, free from alkaline acetates; add a few drops of a solution of potassium thiocyanate, and then the filtered contents of the stomach: if they contain the acid, a red coloring ensues, which is destroyed by sodium acetate.

Molisch's t.: 1. (*for dextrose in urine*) add 2 ml. of urine, 2 drops of a 15 per cent solution of thymol, and an equal volume of strong sulfuric acid; a deep-red color results. 2. (*for dextrose in urine*) to 1 ml. of urine add 2 or 3 drops of a 5 per cent solution of alphanaphthol in alcohol, then add 2 ml. of strong sulfuric acid; a deep-violet color is produced, and a violet precipitate follows if water is added. 3. (*for proteins*) the substance is treated with a 15 per cent alcoholic solution of alphanaphthol and then with concentrated sulfuric acid; a violet color is formed if proteins are present.

Moloney t. (*for delayed sensitivity to diphtheria toxoid*): 0.1 ml. of 1:10 dilution of fluid toxoid is injected intradermally on the flexor surface of the forearm; the appearance in 12 to 24 hours of an area of redness with induration of more than 12 mm. in diameter is a positive reaction. Called also *anatoxireaction, Moloney reaction,* and *Zeller's t.*

monaural distorted speech t's, tests to determine subtle unilateral disturbances in the central auditory pathways, in which various forms of distorted speech are used.

monosaccharide t., see *Barfoed's t.*

Montenegro t. (*for leishmaniasis*): an intradermal test of the delayed sensitivity type, using a killed suspension of leptomonads as antigen.

Montigne's t.: heat an alcoholic solution of a sterol with silicotungstic acid; a red-brown color appears.

Moore's t. (*for dextrose or any carbohydrate*): boil the suspected solution with sodium or potassium hydroxide; if dextrose or lactose is present, a yellow or brown color is produced.

Morelli's t. (*to differentiate between an exudate and a transudate*): add a few drops of the suspected fluid to a saturated solution of mercuric chloride in a test tube; a flaky precipitate indicates a transudate, a clot indicates an exudate.

Moretti's t. (*for typhoid fever*): twenty-five ml. of urine are saturated with 20 gm. of crystallized ammonium sulfate. After a quarter of an hour the urine is filtered and diluted to about one third. To 10 ml. of the filtrate one fifth of its volume of a 10 per cent solution of sodium hydroxide is added, and then a drop of 5 per cent tincture of iodine. The solution is shaken, and if the reaction is positive a persistent golden-yellow color is produced.

Moritz t., see *Rivalta's reaction,* under *reaction.*

Mörner's t.: 1. (*for tyrosine*) to a small quantity of the crystals in a test tube add a few milliliters of Mörner's reagent (solution of formaldehyde, 1 ml.; distilled water, 45 ml.; concentrated sulfuric acid, 55 ml.). Heat gently to the boiling point. A green color shows the presence of tyrosine. 2. see *nitroprusside t.* (1).

Moro's t., see under *reaction.*

morphine t., see specific tests, including *Denigès' t.* (3), *Marquis' t., Oliver's t.* (3), *Weppen's t.*

Morton's t.: in metatarsalgia, transverse pressure across the heads of the metatarsals causes a sharp pain, especially between the second and third metatarsals.

Moschcowitz t.: a test for arteriosclerosis made by rendering the lower limb bloodless by means of an Esmarch bandage. This is removed after five minutes have elapsed, when, in a normal limb, the color will return in a few seconds, but in one affected by arteriosclerosis the return of color takes place much more slowly. Called also *hyperemia t.*

Mosenthal's t. (*for kidney function*): with the patient on a prescribed general diet, take samples of urine in two-hour periods during the day and once at night. Examine them for volume, specific gravity, total nitrogen, and chlorides, and compare with normal.

Moynihan's t. (*for hourglass stomach*): the two parts of a Seidlitz powder are given separately; in hourglass stomach two separated protrusions on the abdominal wall can be observed.

mucic acid t. (*for galactose, lactose,* etc.): to the unknown add 20 per cent of its volume of nitric acid and evaporate on water bath to about 20 per cent of its original volume; a fine white precipitate of mucic acid indicates galactose or a carbohydrate containing galactose.

mucification t.: the vagina of a mouse is injected with blood serum; the extent of mucification of the mucosa developing in four days is noted.

Mulder's t.: 1. (*for dextrose*) alkalinize the solution with sodium carbonate; on adding a solution of indigo-carmine and heating, the mixture is decolorized, but becomes blue again when shaken with air. 2. (*for proteins*) treat the suspected substance with nitric acid: proteins are turned yellow by it; alkalinize the substance and it becomes an orange yellow, due to the presence of the phenyl group. Called also *xanthroproteic reaction.*

Müller's t.: 1. (*for cystine*) boil the substance with potassium hydroxide until dissolved; when cold, dilute it with water. A solution of sodium nitroprusside produces a violet coloration, which soon changes to a yellow [Edward Müller]. 2. a drop of pus is allowed to fall into a small vessel containing some Millon's reagent. Ordinary pus forms a little lump that soon disintegrates and colors the liquid bright red. Tuberculous pus forms a tough skin on the surface of the fluid, which, if pushed down, takes on a globular shape [Edward Müller]. 3. (*for syphilis*) a conglobation or clotting reaction for the diagnosis of syphilis, employing cholesterinized ox heart extract and an inactivated serum [Rudolf Müller]; called also *ball t., conglobation reaction,* and *Müller's reaction.*

Müller-Jochmann t.: 1. when a trace of pus is placed on some sterile coagulated blood serum, and the latter put in an incubator, no change takes place if the pus is tuberculous. Ordinary pus, on the other hand, will form a cup-shaped depression in the culture medium. 2. see *antitrypsin t.*

multiple-puncture t.: an intracutaneous test in which the material used (e.g., tuberculin) is introduced into the skin by pressure of several needles or pointed tines or prongs. See also *tine t.* and *tuberculin t., Sterneedle.*

Murata t.: a ring modification of the Sachs-Georgi test for syphilis.

murexide t., see *Weidel's t.* (1).

Murphy's t.: the patient sits with his arms folded in front of him; the examiner's thumb is placed under the twelfth rib and short jabbing movements are made. Thus deep-seated tenderness and muscular rigidity are determined. Called also *Murphy's kidney punch.*

mycobiologic t.: mycologic test.

mycologic t. (*for sugar in urine*): to the specimen of urine an equal quantity of 1 per cent peptone solution is added; this mixture is sown with some species of *Candida.* If sugar is present, gas is developed. Called also *mycobiologic t.*

mydriatic substances t., see *Ehrmann's t.*

Myers and Fine t. (*for amylolytic activity*): add decreasing amounts of stomach contents to constant amounts of starch solution and note by means of iodine the amount required to completely hydrolyze the starch.

Mylius' t. (*for bile acids*): to each milliliter of the solution of bile acids add 1 ml. of strong sulfuric acid and 1 drop of furfurol solution; if bile acids are present, a red color is produced, which turns to a bluish violet in the course of a day or so.

Naffziger's t. (*for nerve root compression*): increase or aggravation of pain or sensory disturbance over the distribution of the involved nerve root upon manual compression of the jugular veins bilaterally confirms the presence of an extruded intervertebral disk or other mass.

Nagel's t.: a test for color vision performed by means of cards with the colors printed in concentric circles.

Nagler's t., see under *reaction.*

Nakayama's t. (*for bile pigments*): add 5 ml. of acid urine to the same amount of 10 per cent barium chloride solution and centrifugalize. To the precipitate is added 2 ml. of a reagent consisting of 99 parts of 95 per cent alcohol, 1 part of fuming hydrochloric acid to a liter of which 4 gm. of ferric chloride has been added. The fluid is boiled; a green color is obtained, which, on the addition of yellow nitric acid, becomes violet or red.

Napier's serum t. (*for kala-azar*): add one drop of 40 per cent formaldehyde to 1 ml. of blood serum; if the serum becomes white and opalescent it indicates kala-azar.

Nathan's t. (*for tuberculosis*): a piece of gauze 1 cm. in diameter is moistened in Old Tuberculin and applied to healthy skin on the flexor surface of the forearm. The edges are secured to the skin by adhesive substance. The dressing is removed twenty-four hours later and the reaction is observed for the next five or six days. When positive, the reaction is characterized by the appearance of small vesicopapular lesions on a normal or somewhat hyperemic base.

NBT t., nitroblue tetrazolium dye t.

Neisser and Wechsberg's t. (*for bactericidal power of blood*): patient's serum is inactivated, mixed with fresh guinea-pig complement, and the bacteria incubated and then plated on agar.

Nencki's t. (*for indole*): treat the suspected material with nitric acid and a little nitrous acid; a red color follows, and in concentrated solution a red precipitate may appear.

Nessler's t. (*for free ammonia*), see under *reagent*.

Neubauer and Fischer's t.: the glycyltryptophan test.

Neufeld's t., see under *reaction*.

Neukomm's t. (*for bile acids*): a drop of the suspected substance is placed on a small white porcelain cover with a drop of dilute cane sugar solution and one of dilute sulfuric acid. The mixture is carefully evaporated over a flame, a violet stain being left if bile acids are present.

neutralization t.: a test for the power of an antiserum or other substance to antagonize the pathogenic properties of the virus or other organism concerned.

niacin t. (*for Mycobacterium tuberculosis*): in a chemical hood, add 0.1 ml. of heavy growth from a 10-day-old culture of organisms in Dubos' liquid Tween-albumin medium to 3 ml. of the same medium in a screw-cap tube. Add 1 ml. of 4 per cent aniline in 95 per cent ethanol and 1 ml. of 10 per cent aqueous cyanogen bromide. A distinct yellow color indicates the presence of niacin, a characteristic of human strains of *M. tuberculosis;* bovine strains are doubtful or negative; other strains are negative. Alternatively, add to the culture being tested, 0.5 to 0.1 ml. sterile saline or water, place the tube so that the fluid layers over the colonies, and allow to stand 15 minutes. Remove 0.5 ml. of the aqueous extract to a test tube. Add equal quantities of 4 per cent aniline in 95 per cent ethanol and 10 per cent aqueous cyanogen bromide. If niacin is present, a yellow color will appear.

Nickerson-Kveim t., see *Kveim t.*

Nicklés' t. (*for distinguishing cane sugar from dextrose*): heat the sugar with carbon tetrachloride to 100° C. This blackens cane sugar, but not dextrose.

Ninhydrin t., see *triketohydrindene hydrate t.*

Nippe's t. (*for blood*): a modified form of Teichmann's test.

nitrate reduction t., see *Ilosvay's reagent*, under *reagent*.

nitrates t., see *Allesandri-Guaceni t.*

nitric acid t.: 1. (*for albumin*) see *Heller's t.* (1). 2. see specific tests, including *Allesandri-Guaceni t.* and *Weyl's t.* (2).

nitric acid-magnesium sulfate t. (*for albumin*), see *Roberts' t.* (1).

nitrites t. (*in saliva*): to the saliva add 1 or 2 drops of H_2SO_4, a few drops of KI solution, and some starch paste; a blue color indicates nitrites. See also *Griess's t.*, *Ilosvay's t.*, *Schaffer's t.*

nitroblue tetrazolium (NBT) t.: a test of the phagocytic function of polymorphonuclear leukocytes based on the increased metabolic activity of phagocytes during particle uptake and digestion, as measured colorimetrically by the reduction of nitroblue tetrazolium to a dark blue formazan pigment.

nitrogenous compounds t., see *Millon's t.*

nitrogen partition t.: a test of hepatic function based on alterations in the distribution of nitrogen in the various nitrogenous bodies of the blood and urine.

nitropropiol t. (*for sugar in urine*): the urine is mixed with an alkali and heated with orthonitrophenylpropiolic acid; the indigo blue to green (blue and yellow) color reaction will be seen.

nitroprusside t.: 1. (*for cysteine*) if a protein containing cysteine is dissolved in water and 2 to 4 drops of a 4 or 5 per cent solution of sodium nitroprusside and then a few drops of ammonia are added, a deep purple-red color appears; called also *Morner's t.* 2. (*for acetone*) see *Legal's t.* (1). 3. (*for indole*) see *Legal's t.* (2). 4. (*for creatinine*) see *Weyl's t.* (1).

nitroso-indole-nitrate t. (*for indole and skatole*): acidify the unknown with nitric acid and add a few drops of potassium nitrite; a red color or a red precipitate indicates indole, a white turbidity indicates skatole.

nitrous acid t., see *Bertoni-Raymondi t.*

Nobel's t.: 1. (*for aceto-acetic acid and acetone*) stratify ammonium hydroxide on urine acidified with acetic acid and to which a little sodium nitroprusside has been added; a violet ring at the junction indicates acetoacetic acid or acetone. 2. (*for bile pigments*) add zinc chloride and a little of the tincture of iodine; a dichroic coloration follows.

Noguchi's t.: 1. see *Noguchi's reaction*, under *reaction*. 2. (*for globulin*) to 0.5 ml. of Noguchi's reagent add 0.1 ml. of spinal fluid; boil and add 0.1 ml. of N/1 sodium hydroxide. A flocculent precipitate indicates globulin.

Nonne's t., see *Ross-Jones t.*

Nonne-Apelt t., see under *reaction*.

nonverbal t.: a mental test in which language is not used.

nuclear t., nucleus t. (*for proteolytic pancreatic function*): a test based on the fact that cell nuclei are digested by the pancreatic juice, and not by the stomach.

nucleoalbumin t., see *Ott's t.*

Nyiri's t.: a concentration test for kidney function by the use of thiosulfate.

Nylander's t. (*for dextrose in urine*): dissolve 2 parts of bismuth subnitrate and 4 of sodium and potassium tartrate in 100 ml. of a 10 per cent solution of sodium hydroxide; of this add 1 part to 10 of the suspected urine and boil five minutes; a black coloration or black precipitate indicates a reducing sugar.

nystagmus t., see *Bárány's symptom*, under *symptom*.

Oakley-Fulthorpe t., a double diffusion test employing narrow tubes containing antibody in agar separated from antigen in solution by a layer of plain agar, into which both antigen and antibody diffuse to produce a precipitate.

Ober's t.: with the patient on his left side and his left leg and thigh flexed, the examiner holds the patient's right leg abducted and extended. If on the sudden withdrawal of the examiner's support the right leg holds up instead of dropping, there is contraction of the tensor fasciae femoris and the fascia lata.

Obermayer's t. (*for indican in urine*): precipitate the urine with a 1:5 lead acetate solution with care, lest an excess of the reagent be taken; filter and agitate the filtrate with an equal amount of fuming hydrochloric acid containing a little of the solution of ferric chloride; to this add chloroform, which is turned blue by indigo.

Obermüller's t. (*for cholesterin*): put the substance to be tested in a test tube and melt it with a drop or two of propionic anhydride over a small flame; on cooling, the mass becomes successively blue, green, orange, carmine, and copper colored.

obturator t., see *Cope's t.*

occult blood t., see tests listed under *blood t.*

Oliver's t.: 1. (*for albumin*) underlay the urine with a 1:4 solution of sodium tungstate and a 10:6 solution of citric acid; a white coagulum at the junction of the two layers shows the presence of albumin. 2. (*for sugar*) boil the suspected liquid with indigo carmine; sugar will change the blue to a red or yellow. 3. (*for morphine*) if, to a solution of morphine, a few milliliters of hydrogen peroxide is added and the mixture is stirred with a piece of copper wire, the solution takes on a deep port wine color, with the evolution of gas. 4. (*for bile acids*) to 5 ml. of the unknown add 2 to 3 drops of acetic acid and filter; an equal volume of 1 per cent solution of peptone will produce a precipitate insoluble in excess of acetic acid if bile acids are present.

one-stage prothrombin time t., see *Quick's t.* (2).

orcinol t. (*for pentose in urine*), see *Bial's t.*

organic acid t., see *Knapp's t.* (2).

orientation t.: see if patient can give correctly the time of day, the day of the week, month, and year, and the place.

orthotoluidine t. (*for blood*), see *Ruttan and Hardisty's t.*

osazone t. (*for sugars*), see *Kowarsky's t.* (1) and *von Jaksch's t.* (2).

Osgood-Haskins t. (*for albumin*): to 5 ml. of urine add 1 ml. of 50 per cent acetic acid; a precipitate at room temperature indicates bile salts, urates, or resin acids. Add 3 ml. of a saturated solution of sodium chloride; a precipitate suggests Bence Jones protein or globulin. The Bence Jones protein will redissolve on heating.

Osterberg's t. (*for beta-oxybutyric acid*): to 800 mg. of ammonium sulfate add 0.15 ml. of concentrated ammonium hydroxide solution, 2 drops of a 5 per cent solution of nitroprusside, and 1 ml. of the urine. Dilute to 50 ml. and compare with a standard.

Ott's t. (*for nucleoalbumin in urine*): to the urine is added an equal volume of saturated solution of sodium chloride, and then Almén's reagent (dissolve 5 gm. of tannic acid in 240 ml. of 50 per cent alcohol and add 10 ml. of 25 per cent acetic acid); a precipitate forms when nucleoalbumin is present.

Ouchterlony t.: a two-dimensional double diffusion test in which solutions of antigen and antibody are placed in separate wells in an agar plate and then diffuse radially to form lines of precipitate in any of three patterns (see *reaction of identity*, under *reaction*). Called also *Ouchterlony technique*. See also *double diffusion test*, under *test*.

Oudin t.: a single diffusion precipitin test in gel media. Antiserum incorporated into agar is placed in a narrow test tube and overlaid with antigen; precipitation rings form where the antigen diffuses into the agar and reacts with the antibody.

ovarian hyperemia t. (*for pregnancy*): the intraperitoneal injection of urine or blood serum of pregnant women into immature female mice produces a reddened appearance of the ovaries.

oxyphenylsulfonic acid t. (*for albumin in urine*): dissolve in 20 parts of water 3 parts of oxyphenylsulfonic acid and 1 part of salicylsulfonic acid; add to 1 ml. of urine a drop of the reagent: if albumin is present, a clear white precipitate appears.

Pachon's t.: measuring of the blood pressure for the purpose of determining the state of the collateral circulation in aneurysm.

Paget's t.: a solid tumor is most hard in its center, whereas a cyst is least hard in its center.

palmin t., palmitin t. (*for pancreatic efficiency*): after a test meal containing palmitin, the contents of the stomach are examined for the presence of fatty acids. They will be found in cases in which the pancreas is normal, for the presence of fat in the stomach causes the pylorus to open and admit the pancreatic juice, which splits palmitin into fatty acids.

pancreatic function t., see specific tests, including *butter t.*,

Ehrmann's pancreatic t., Kashiwado's t., litmus milk t., Loewi's t., nuclear t., palmin t., Sahli-Nencki t., secretin t.

Pándy's t.: a test for globulin in the cerebrospinal fluid. Mix 80 to 100 ml. pure phenol with distilled water, shake, and place in incubator several hours. After several days at room temperature pour off the top watery part, which serves as the reagent. With a Pasteur pipet a drop (0.01 ml.) of the fluid to be tested is deposited on the bottom of a watch crystal filled with the reagent. If no cloudy precipitate forms within five seconds the reaction is negative.

Pap t., Papanicolaou t.: an exfoliative cytological staining procedure for the detection and diagnosis of various conditions, particularly malignant and premalignant conditions of the female genital tract (cancer of the vagina, cervix, and endometrium), in which cells which have been desquamated from the genital epithelium are obtained by smears, fixed and stained, and examined under the microscope for evidence of pathologic changes. Cytologic findings have commonly been expressed in terms of histologic lesions classified as Class I to Class V, but preferably each examination should have an individual histological description. The test is also used in evaluating endocrine function, and in the diagnosis of malignancies of other organs, as of the respiratory tract and lungs, gastrointestinal tract, urinary tract, and breast. See also *Table of Stains.*

paracasein t., see *Leiner's t.*

paradimethylaminobenzaldehyde t. *(for urobilinogen)*: to the unknown add an equal volume of hydrochloric acid and boil; then add 2 drops of a 5 per cent solution of paradimethylaminobenzaldehyde in 10 per cent sulfuric acid. A red to violet color indicates urobilinogen. Called also *Ehrlich's t.*

Parnum's t. *(for albumin)*: filter the urine, add one-sixth volume of a saturated solution of magnesium or sodium sulfate, acidulate with acetic acid, and boil; if albumin is present, a white precipitate is formed.

partial thromboplastin time t.: a one-stage clotting test used clinically to detect deficiencies of the components of the intrinsic thromboplastin system; in reality prolonged clotting time may reflect deficiency or absence of coagulation factors I, II, V, and VIII through XII, separately or in combination.

passive cutaneous anaphylaxis t., see *passive cutaneous anaphylaxis.*

passive protection t.: a test in which antiserum is tested for protective antibody by parenteral inoculation of groups of animals with graded doses in constant volume.

passive transfer t., see *Prausnitz-Küstner reaction*, under *reaction.*

patch t.: a test for hypersensitiveness made by applying to the skin the substances in question by means of small pieces of linen or blotting paper impregnated with the substances; on removal of the patches the reactions of the skin are noted. The same method is used for applying tuberculin test for tuberculosis (*Vollmer's t.*).

Patrick's t.: with the patient supine, the thigh and knee are flexed and the external malleolus is placed over the patella of the opposite leg; the knee is depressed, and if pain is produced thereby arthritis of the hip is indicated. Patrick calls this test *fabere sign*, from the initial letters of movements that are necessary to elicit it, namely, flexion, abduction, external rotation, extension.

Patterson's t.: a chemical spot test for the diagnosis of uremia. A drop of Ehrlich's reagent is applied to a drop of blood placed on a white filter paper; if there is greatly increased blood urea, the spot on the filter paper turns a greenish color.

Paul's t.: pus from a suspected pustule is rubbed into the scarified eye of a rabbit; if the pus is variolous or vaccinial, a condition of epitheliosis develops in the rabbit in from thirty-six to forty-eight hours.

Paul-Bunnell t.: a method of testing for the presence of heterophil antibodies in the blood, used to confirm the clinical and hematologic diagnosis of infectious mononucleosis. The test is based on the agglutination of sheep red blood cells by the inactivated serum of patients with the disease. Called also *heterophil antibody reaction* and *Paul-Bunnell reaction.*

Paunz' t. *(for amyloidosis)*: inject intravenously 10 ml. per kg. of a 0.6 per cent solution of Congo red. After one hour withdraw some blood and to the serum add a little hydrochloric acid. No blue color in the coagulated proteins indicates amyloidosis.

Pavy's t. *(for dextrose in urine)*: prepare a reagent by mixing 120 ml. of Fehling's solution with 200 ml. of ammonia (specific gravity 0.88), 400 ml. of a solution of sodium hydroxide (specific gravity 1.14), and 1000 ml. of water; boil the suspected liquid with this solution: if dextrose is present, the reagent is decolorized.

PCA t., see *passive cutaneous anaphylaxis.*

Pélouse-Moore t. *(for sugar in urine)*: boil the urine with a solution of potassa, cool, and add 1 drop of concentrated sulfuric acid; the odor of burnt sugar will be given off.

pentose t., see *Bial's t., phloroglucin t.*

Penzoldt's t.: 1. *(for acetone)* to the suspected liquid add a warm saturated solution of orthonitrobenzaldehyde, and render it alkaline with sodium hydroxide: if acetone is present, the mixture becomes yellow and then green; thereafter a precipitate forms which, on shaking with chloroform, gives a blue color. 2. *(for dextrose in urine)* add sodium hydroxide solution and a slightly alkaline solution of sodium diazobenzosulfonate; shake the mixture until it foams: a red or yellow-red color is produced, the foam also being red.

Penzoldt-Fischer t. *(for phenol)*: alkalinize strongly the substance to be tested and dissolve in a solution of diazobenzolsulfonic acid; phenol, if present, produces a deep-red color.

peppermint t. *(for pulmonary perforation)*: the pneumothorax cavity is filled with the vapor of essence of peppermint; if there is a pulmonary perforation the patient will recognize the characteristic smell.

pepsin t., see specific tests, including *Jacoby's t.* and *Mett's t.*

peptide t., see *triketohydrindene hydrate t.*

peptone t., see specific tests, including *Hofmeister's t.* (2), *Ralfe's t.* (2), *Randolph's t., triketohydrindene hydrate t.*

perchloride t.: a port-wine colored reaction obtained by treating the urine of hyperemetic pregnant women with solution of ferric chloride; the intensity of the reaction indicates the gravity of the case.

percutaneous tuberculin t., see *Moro's reaction*, under *reaction.*

performance t.: an intelligence test such as the *Pinter-Patterson t.* or *Porteus maze t.*, in which the subject is required to do certain things rather than to answer questions.

Peria's t. *(for tyrosine)*, see *Piria's t.*

Perls' t.: a test for hemosiderin made by treating the substance with hydrochloric acid and potassium ferrocyanide; the Prussian blue reaction is produced if hemosiderin is present.

permanganate t., see *Weiss' t.*

peroxidase t., see *Arakawa's reagent*, under *reagent*, and *Goodpasture's stain*, under *stain.*

Perthes' t. *(for collateral circulation in varicose veins)*, see *tourniquet t.*, def. 3.

Peterman's t. *(for syphilis)*: 0.05 ml. of inactivated serum of the patient is stirred with 0.01 ml. of diluted beef heart antigen; this is inactivated between microscope slides at 37° C. for ten minutes and examined microscopically.

Petri's t. *(for proteins)*: add diazobenzolsulfonic acid and sodium hydroxide; an orange or brownish color is formed, and on shaking a red froth is produced.

Pettenkofer's t. *(for bile acids in urine)*: drop a solution of the suspected material into a mixture of sugar and sulfuric acid; a purplish crimson color is produced. This test is also given by aminomyelin, cephalin, lecithin, and myelin.

Petzetaki's t. *(for typhoid fever)*: 15 ml. of urine are placed in a test tube and to this is added a little 5 per cent alcoholic solution of iodine; if the upper part of the urine takes on a golden-yellow color, the test is positive.

phenacetin t. *(in urine)*: to the urine add a little concentrated hydrochloric acid, a little 1 per cent solution of sodium nitrate, and a little alkaline alphanaphthol solution; make alkaline and a red color indicates phenacetin.

phenol t., see specific tests, including *Allen's t.* (2), *Berthelot's t.* (1), *Davy's t., Eijkman's t.* (1), *Hanke and Koessler's t., Jacquemin's t., Penzoldt-Fischer's t., Plugge's t.* See also *phenol, methods for*, under *method.*

phenolphthalein t.: 1. *(for blood)* boil a thin fecal suspension, cool, and add it to half as much reagent (made by dissolving 1 to 2 gm. of phenolphthalein and 25 gm. of potassium hydroxide in water. Add 10 gm. of metallic zinc and heat until decolorized). A pink color indicates the presence of blood. 2. *(in urine)* make the urine alkaline; a red color indicates phenolphthalein.

phenolsulfonphthalein t. *(for kidney function)*: inject 1 ml. of 0.6 per cent solution of the monosodium salt of phenolsulfonphthalein intravenously or intramuscularly and collect the urine at hourly intervals. Make specimens alkaline with sodium hydroxide and match color in colorimeter with standard solution. Usually 60 to 75 per cent of the dye is excreted in two hours; 40 per cent or less indicates impaired function.

phenoltetrachlorophthalein t. *(for liver function)*: phenoltetrachlorophthalein is injected intravenously, and normally it appears in the feces, being excreted by the liver with the bile, and giving a bright color to the feces. A decrease in the normal excretion of this substance points to liver injury.

phenylhydrazine t., see specific tests, including *Kowarsky's t.* (1) and *von Jaksch's t.* (2).

phlorhizin t., phlorizin t. *(for renal insufficiency)*: the bladder is emptied and a hypodermic injection given of a mixture of 5 to 10 gm. each of sodium carbonate and phlorhizin. Sugar will appear in the urine within half an hour if the kidney is healthy. If only a small quantity of sugar appears, there is probably renal insufficiency; if none at all, then serious kidney disease probably exists.

phloroglucin t., phloroglucinol t., *(for galactose, pentose, and glycuronates in urine)*: a solution of phloroglucin in hydrochloric acid is added to the urine and warmed; a red color forms if suspected substances are present.

phosphatase t.: 1. *(for adequate pasteurization of milk)* Mycobacterium tuberculosis is killed more easily than milk phosphatase is destroyed by heat, so if there is no phosphatase in the milk, the pasteurization has been adequate. Add 2,6-dibromoquinonechloroimide and disodium phenyl phosphate to the sample of borax buffered milk. If phosphatase is present, the phenol will be set free and will undergo an indophenol reaction with the production of a blue color. 2. *(for serum phosphatase)* see *Jenner-Kay t.*

phosphoric acid t., see specific tests, including *Malot's t.* and *Mitscherlich's t.*

phthalein t., see *phenolsulfonphthalein t.*

phytotoxin t., see *Macht t.*

Piazza's t. (*for tuberculosis*): the patient's urine is mixed with the serum of a guinea pig or rabbit which has received an injection of Koch's old tuberculin; the formation of a precipitate is positive.

picrotoxin t., see *Becker's t.* (1).

Pincus t.: typical colors are produced on heating 17-ketosteroids with concentrated antimony trichloride in glacial acetic acid.

pineapple t. (*for butyric acid in stomach*): a few drops of sulfuric acid and alcohol are added to a dried ethereal extract of the gastric juice; if butyric acid is present, an odor of pineapple will be given off, caused by the formation of ethylbutyrate.

pine wood t. (*for indole*): a pine splinter moistened with concentrated hydrochloric acid is turned cherry red by a solution of indole.

Piotrowski's t., see *biuret t.* (1).

Piria's t. (*for tyrosine*): moisten the suspected material with strong sulfuric acid and warm it; then dilute and warm it again; neutralize it with barium carbonate, filter, and add ferric chloride in dilute solution: if tyrosine is present, a violet color is seen, which is destroyed by an excess of ferric chloride.

Pirquet's t., see under *reaction.*

P-K t., see under *reaction.*

plantar ischemia t.: a test for circulatory disturbances in the legs and feet, in which the plantar surface of the patient's foot is checked for blanching after he extends and flexes his inclined leg.

plasmacrit t.: a rapid but reasonably sensitive and specific screening test for syphilis, using plasma from microhematocrit tubes.

Plesch's t. (*for persistent ductus arteriosus*): determination of the amount of oxygen and of carbonic acid in the blood.

Plugge's t. (*for phenol*): a dilute solution containing phenol becomes red on mixture with a mercuric nitrate solution containing a trace of nitrous acid; mercury is also precipitated and the odor of salicylol is given off.

pneumatic t., Hennebert's sign.

Pohl's t. (*for globulins*): these substances are precipitated from solution by ammonium sulfate.

pointing t., see *Bárány's pointing t.*

Politzer's t. (*for deafness in one ear*): when a tuning-fork is placed in front of the nares, it is heard only by an unaffected ear during deglutition.

Pollacci's t. (*for albumin in urine*): dissolve in 100 ml. of water 1 gm. of tartaric acid, 5 gm. of mercuric chloride, and 10 gm. of sodium chloride, and add 5 ml. of solution of formaldehyde; this solution added to urine will cause coagulation of albumin in a white zone.

polyuria t., see *Albarran's t.*

Porges-Meier t. (*for syphilis*): a 1 per cent emulsion of lecithin in physiologic salt solution is mixed with an equal volume of blood serum and allowed to stand for five hours; when serum from the patient to be tested is added, the lecithin will be precipitated if the patient has syphilis.

Porges-Salomon t. (*for syphilis*): a 1 per cent sodium glycocholate solution is mixed with an equal volume of clear activated serum from the patient; if the serum is syphilitic, distinct flocculi will appear at the top of the fluid.

porphobilinogen t., see *Watson-Schwartz t.*

Porter's t.: 1. (*for excess of uric acid*) the upper portion of the urine is boiled in a test tube and a few drops of 4 per cent acetic acid added; in a few hours crystals of uric acid will form just below the surface. 2. (*for indican*) 10 ml. of urine is shaken with an equal amount of hydrochloric acid and 5 drops of a 0.5 per cent solution of potassium permanganate; add 5 ml. of chloroform and shake. A purple color with a deposit of blue matter indicates indican.

Porteus maze t.: a performance test in which the subject is required to trace with a pencil through printed mazes of increasing difficulty.

Posner's t.: 1. (*for the source of albumin in urine*) a twenty-four-hour sample of urine is preserved with solution of formaldehyde, shaken, and the leukocytes counted in the blood-counting chamber—100,000 leukocytes per 2 ml. of urine indicate 0.1 per cent of albumin. In this case the albumin is probably due solely to the pus. If albumin is present in greater proportion than this, it is probably due to Bright's disease. 2. (*for proteins*) Posner makes a ring biuret test by mixing the potassium hydroxide solution and the unknown and then stratifying very dilute copper sulfate solution on top of the mixture.

potassium iodide t. (*for renal function*): the patient receives 0.5 gm. of potassium iodide in solution by mouth, and the urine is tested every two hours for iodine; if iodine secretion is prolonged beyond sixty hours, excretion through the renal tubules is indicated.

Pratt's t.: a modification of Volhard's test combining the dilution and concentration tests.

Prausnitz-Küstner (P-K) t., see under *reaction.*

precipitation t., precipitin t.: any test in which the positive reaction consists in the formation and deposit of a precipitate in the fluid being tested.

Pregl's t. (*for kidney function*): determine the specific gravity of the urine obtained by catheterization of the ureters. Using Haeser's coefficient, estimate the amount of solid substances excreted, and compare it with the weight of ash. The diseased kidney may excrete the same volume of water, but less solid material. A predominance

of mineral substances (ash) over the organic also speaks for a lower function of the kidney.

pregnancy t., see specific tests, including *antitrypsin t., Aschheim-Zondek t., bitterling t., bromine t.* (3), *Brown's t.* (1), *early pregnancy t., Friedman's t., Galli Mainini t., male frog* or *male toad t., ovarian hyperemia t., pregnanediol t., Prostigmin t., Venning Browne t., Visscher-Bowman t., Xenopus t.*

Prendergast's t. (*for typhoid fever*): give an intradermal injection of 5 mg. of typhoid vaccine; in the nontyphoid patient there develops within twenty-four hours an area of redness about the site of the injection, while in the typhoid patient there is no reaction.

Preyer's t.: a spectroscopic test for carbon monoxide in the blood.

Proetz t. (*for acuity of sense of smell*): use of a series of substances each in 10 different concentrations in a liter of petroleum of specific gravity 0.880, to determine the least concentration at which the substance can be recognized; termed *olfactory coefficient* or *minimal identifiable odor.*

projective t., any of various tests in which an individual interprets ambiguous stimulus situations, e.g., a series of inkblots (Rorschach t.), according to his own unconscious dispositions, thus yielding information about his personality structure and its underlying dynamics.

Prostigmin t. (*for pregnancy*): administration of Prostigmin (neostigmine) to a woman who has missed her regular menstruation will bring on menstruation if she is not pregnant.

protection t., serum neutralization t.

protein t., see specific tests, including *acetic acid and potassium ferrocyanide t., Acree-Rosenheim t., Adamkiewicz's t., Bardach's t., biuret t.* (1), *Brücke's t.* (2), *coagulation t., colloidal gold t., Gies' biuret t., Grigg's t., Hopkins-Cole t., Kantor and Gies' t., Kober t.* (2), *Liebermann's t., Michaïlow's t., Millon's t., Molisch's t.* (3), *Mulder's t.* (2), *Petri's t., Posner's t.* (2), *Reichl's t., Schulte's t., Schultze's t.* (3), *Sicard-Cantelouble t., sulfur t., triketohydrindene hydrate t., von Aldor's t.* See also tests listed under *albumin t.*

protein tyrosin t. (*for malaria*): to 0.1 ml. of serum add 3 ml. of a 14 per cent solution of sodium sulfate, mix, and incubate for three hours. Centrifuge and wash the precipitate with fresh solution of sodium sulfate. Dissolve the precipitate in 1.75 ml. of water and add 0.1 ml. of a 5N solution of sodium hydroxide. Heat on water bath for ten minutes, add 0.15 ml. of Folin and Ciocalteu's phenol reagent, and compare with a standard.

proteose t.: proteose does not coagulate on boiling, but gives a ring test with trichloracetic acid. See also *von Aldor's t.*

prothrombin t.: a test for prothrombin based on clotting time; see under *time,* and see *Quick's t.* (2).

prothrombin consumption t.: a test used, for the most part, to measure the formation of intrinsic thromboplastin by determining the residual serum prothrombin after blood coagulation is complete. Because the test is made on whole blood, it also measures, indirectly, the thromboplastic function of platelets.

prothrombin-proconvertin t.: a test used in the control of coumarin-type anticoagulants similar to the Quick method, except that it employs a saline extract of brain as a thromboplastin and requires the presence of excess blood coagulation factor V, usually derived from deprothrombinized ox plasma.

protozoan t.: the use of protozoan protoplasm as a test for pathologic tissue change, by observing the rate of reproduction of cultures of paramecium bred on normal and pathologic tissue.

psychological t., any test to measure one's development, achievement, personality, intelligence, thought processes, etc.

psychometric t's, see *intelligence t.*

pulp t.: a diagnostic test to determine tooth pulp vitality or abnormality, usually by means of electric pulp testers or by application of a hot or cold stimulus.

Purdy's t. (*for albumin*): fill a test tube two thirds full of the clear urine, add one sixth of its volume of a saturated solution of sodium chloride and 5 to 10 drops of 50 per cent acetic acid. Gently heat the upper part of the tube and look for a cloud.

purine bodies t., see *Cooke's t.* See also *purine bodies, methods for,* under *method.*

pus t., see specific tests, including *Donné's t., Vitali's t.* (6), *Waterhouse pus t.*

Pyramidon t.: 1. (*for occult blood in feces*) see *aminopyrine t.* 2. (*in urine*) to the urine add tincture of iodine; a yellow ring indicates Pyramidon.

pyridine t., see *Anderson's t.*

pyrocatechin t., see *Brieger's t.* (1).

quadriceps t. (*for hyperthyroidism*): the patient sits well forward on the edge of a straight chair and holds the leg out at right angles to the body. Normal persons can hold this position for at least a minute; those with hyperthyroidism can maintain it for only a few seconds.

Queckenstedt's t., see under *sign.*

quellung t., see *Neufeld's reaction,* under *reaction.*

Quick's t.: 1. (*for liver function*) a test based on excretion of hippuric acid following the administration of sodium benzoate. 2. (*one-stage prothrombin time*) by adding an extrinsic thromboplastin such as dried rabbit brain and calcium to oxalated blood the integrity of the prothrombin complex, composed of factors II, V, VII, X, may be defined; used widely to control administration of coumarin-type anticoagulants.

Quick tourniquet t., see *tourniquet t.* (1).

quinine t., see specific tests, including *André's t., Binz's t., Brande's t., thalleioquin t.*

Quinlan's t. (*for bile*): a 3-mm. layer of the suspected liquid is examined by the spectroscope; if bile is present, some of the violet color of the spectrum will be absorbed.

Raabe's t. (*for albumin*): filter the urine into a test tube and drop a crystal of trichloracetic acid into it; albumin will form a white ring about the crystal; uric acid may form a similar ring, but it is not so well defined.

Rabuteau's t.: 1. (*for hydrochloric acid in urine*) add a little indigosulfonic acid to color the urine, and sulfurous acid to decompose what hydrochloric acid may be present; the urine will be decolorized. 2. (*for hydrochloric acid in stomach contents*) one gm. of potassium iodate and 0.5 gm. of potassium iodide are added to 50 ml. of starch mucilage; filtered stomach liquids are added to it; free hydrochloric acid will render the mixture blue.

radioactive renogram t.: an intravenous injection of radio-isotopic material is given and its uptake and excretion is monitored by an external scintillation counter over the kidneys.

radioallergosorbent t. (RAST): a radioimmunoassay assay test for the measurement of extremely small amounts of specific IgE antibody to a variety of allergens, in which antigen is fixed in a solid-phase matrix, the antibody-containing specimen is added to the matrix, and then a second, radiolabeled anti-gamma globulin is added.

radioimmunosorbent t. (RIST): a radioimmunoassay technique for measuring IgE immunoglobulins in serum; the serum sample is mixed with a standard amount of radiolabeled IgE and then exposed to Sephadex particles coated with anti-human IgE.

radioisotope renal excretion t. (*for study of renal function*): radioisotopic material diluted with saline is rapidly injected into a well-hydrated patient; urine collected by an indwelling urethral catheter or a ureteral catheter previously inserted into the kidney is collected at known intervals and the radioactivity of each specimen is determined and recorded.

Ralfe's t.: 1. (*for acetone in urine*) boil 4 ml. of solution of potassium hydroxide with 1.5 gm. of potassium iodide; overlay it with 4 ml. of urine; a yellow ring with specks of iodoform appears at the plane of contact. 2. (*for peptones in urine*) put 4 ml. of Fehling's solution in a test tube and overlay it with urine; a rose-colored ring shows the presence of peptones.

Ramon's flocculation t.: to a series of tubes containing a constant amount of toxin, e.g., diphtheria toxin, antitoxin is added in increasing amounts; when a zone of flocculation appears, the tube showing it contains a completely neutralized mixture of toxin and antitoxin. The first tube in which flocculation occurs is taken as the end-point.

Randolph's t. (*for peptones in urine*): add 2 drops of a saturated solution of potassium iodide and 3 drops of Millon's reagent to 5 ml. of cold and slightly acid urine; a yellow precipitate shows the presence of peptones.

Rantzman's t.: a modification of Lange's test for acetone, in which ammonium nitrate is used as a preservative.

rapid plasma reagin (RPR) t.: a group of screening flocculation tests for syphilis using a modified VDRL antigen containing choline chloride to check plasma or unheated serum; addition of charcoal particles to the antigen permits macroscopic identification of the flocculation.

rapid serum amylase t., Fishman-Doubilet t.

rash-extinction t., see *Schultz-Charlton reaction*, under *reaction*.

Raygat's t., see *hydrostatic t.*

Rebuck t., Rebuck skin window technique.

reckoning t.: a mental test consisting in requiring the patient to add in pairs a series of numbers. The total number of sums accomplished per minute indicates the patient's capacity for mental work, while their accuracy indicates the patient's fixed associations and power of attention.

red t., see *phenolsulfonphthalein t.*

Ree's t. (*for albumin*): small amounts of albumin are precipitated from solution by tannic acid in alcoholic solution.

Rehberg's t.: a test of kidney function based on the excretion of creatinine administered 2 gm. in 500 ml. of water.

Rehfuss' t. (*of gastric secretion*): by means of a specially devised tube (*Rehfuss tube*) inserted into the stomach immediately after an Ewald test meal, a specimen of the contents is drawn off at fifteen-minute intervals until the close of digestion. Each specimen is examined and the results are plotted in a graphic curve, the abscissa of which is the number of minutes at which the gastric contents were removed, and the ordinate the number of milliliters of decinormal sodium hydroxide solution necessary to titrate the free acidity and the total acidity of the gastric contents.

Reichl's t. (*for proteins*): add 2 or 3 drops of an alcoholic solution of benzaldehyde and a quantity of sulfuric acid previously diluted to twice its volume with water; then add a few drops of ferric sulfate solution. The mixture will sooner or later take on a deep-blue color if proteins are present.

Reid Hunt's t., see *Hunt's reaction*, under *reaction*.

Reinsch's t. (*for heavy metals, including arsenic, mercury, bismuth, antimony, and large amounts of selenium, tellurium, and sulfide*): insert a strip of clean copper into the suspected acidified liquid or finely ground tissue, and boil; if one or more heavy metals are present, a coating will form on the copper strip.

Remont's t. (*for salicylic acid*): make the milk acid with sulfuric acid, extract the salicylic acid with ether, and identify it by the purple or violet color produced on the addition of ferric chloride.

renal function t., see *kidney function t.*

rennin t., see individual tests, including *Lee's t.* and *Riegel's t.*

resorcinol t. (*for hydrochloric acid*), see *Boas's t.* (1).

resorcinol-hydrochloric acid t. (*for levulose*), see *Selivanoff's t.*

Reuss' t. (*for atropine*): the substance examined is treated with sulfuric acid and oxidizing agents; if atropine is present, an odor of roses and orange-flowers is given off.

Reynold's t. (*for acetone*): to the liquid to be examined add freshly prepared mercuric oxide, shake and filter, and overlay the filtrate with ammonium sulfide; the liquid turns black if acetone is present.

rheumatoid arthritis t., see specific tests, including *agglutination t., bentonite t., bracelet t., latex agglutination t., sheep cell agglutination t.*

rhubarb t. (*in urine*): make the urine alkaline; a red color indicates rhubarb.

Rieckenberg's t., see under *phenomenon*.

Riegel's t. (*for rennin*): to 10 ml. of milk add 5 ml. of neutral gastric juice and incubate for fifteen minutes; coagulation will occur if rennin is present.

Riegler's t.: 1. (*for albumin*) 10 gm. of betanaphtholsulfonic acid is dissolved in 200 ml. of distilled water and filtered; 5 ml. of urine is treated with 20 to 30 drops of solution. Turbidity shows the presence of albumin. 2. (*for hydrochloric acid in the gastric juice*) Congo red is changed to blue if hydrochloric acid is present. 3. (*for dextrose*) place in a test tube 0.1 gm. of phenyl-hydrazine-hydrochloride, 0.25 gm. of sodium acetate, and 20 drops of the urine. Heat to boiling. Add 10 ml. of a 3 per cent solution of potassium hydroxide and gently shake the tube. A red color indicates sugar.

Rimini's t., see *Burnam's t.*

ring t.: 1. (*for antibiotic activity*) the solution is placed in a ring resting on the surface of seeded agar and the size of the surrounding clear area of inhibition indicates the activity. 2. (*for glanders*) see *Konew's t.* 3. (*for protein*) see *Heller's t.* (1), *Posner's t.* (2), *Roberts' t.* (1).

Rinne t.: a hearing test made, with the opposite ear masked, with tuning forks of 256, 512, and 1024 Hz; by alternately placing the stem of the vibrating fork on the mastoid process of the temporal bone of the patient and holding it $\frac{1}{2}$ inch from the external auditory meatus until it is no longer heard at one of these positions. When air conduction is greater than bone conduction, it indicates normal hearing or sensorineural hearing loss. When bone conduction is greater than air conduction, it indicates conductive hearing loss.

Rivalta's t., see under *reaction*.

Roberts' t.: 1. (*for albumin*) underlay the urine with a mixture containing 5 parts of saturated solution of magnesium sulfate and 1 part of nitric acid; a white ring or layer forms at the plane of junction. 2. (*for dextrose*) determine the specific gravity of the urine at a certain temperature; add a little tartaric acid and some yeast; after twenty-four hours filter and again find the specific gravity. Each degree of density lost represents a grain of dextrose in a fluidounce of the urine.

Robinson-Kepler t. (*for adrenocortical insufficiency*): a test based on the fact that patients with adrenocortical insufficiency are unable to excrete a large water load at a normal rate, as opposed to normal subjects who will, for example, excrete 50 per cent of 1500 ml. of ingested water within four hours.

Robinson-Kepler-Power water t. (*for sprue*): a test based upon the fact that in sprue there is increased nocturnal elimination of urine, perhaps due to decreased absorption of water.

Roffo's t.: to 2 ml. of fresh centrifugalized blood serum are added 5 drops of a 5 per cent solution of neutral red; the normal yellow of the serum changes to red if the subject has cancer.

Roger's t., see *camphor t.*

Roger-Josué t., see *blister t.*

Romberg t. (*for differentiating between peripheral and cerebellar ataxia*): an increase in clumsiness in all movements and in the width and uncertainty of the gait when the patient's eyes are closed indicates peripheral ataxia; no change indicates the cerebellar type.

Römer's t.: intracutaneous injection of tuberculin into a tuberculous guinea-pig produces a papule with a hemorrhagic center; called also *cockade reaction* and *Römer's reaction.*

Ronchese t. (*for quantitative determination of ammonia in urine*): one based on the action of solution of formaldehyde on the ammonia salts. A 10 per cent solution of sodium carbonate is added, a drop at a time, to the urine until the reaction becomes neutral. The solution of formaldehyde (40 per cent) is neutralized with a one-fourth normal soda solution against phenolphthalein until a slight pink tint develops. Then 25 ml. of the neutral urine and 10 ml. of the neutral solution of formaldehyde are mixed and titrated against decinormal sodium carbonate solution until a deep pink develops. The calculation is simple: 1 ml. of the decinormal sodium carbonate solution for 100 ml. of urine corresponds to 0.017 gm. ammonia in 1000 ml. of urine.

Rorschach t.: a projective test (q.v.) which is sensitive to disorders of thought and emotion. It consists of a series of 10 ink blot designs, some black and some in colors. The patient is directed to look at the cards and tell what he sees. He is then asked to indicate which aspect of the blot and which location suggest the percept he reports.

Rose's t. (*for blood*): the scrapings from a blood stain are boiled in dilute caustic potash; when examined the liquid will show a greenish color in a thin layer and a red color in a thicker layer.

rose bengal t. (*for liver function*): rose bengal (1 per cent in sodium chloride solution) is injected into the blood stream. Normally it disappears from the blood rapidly; delay in the normal disappearance time points to diminished activity of the liver.

Rose-Waaler t. (*for rheumatoid factor*), see *sheep cell agglutination t.* (1).

Rosenbach's t.: 1. (*for indigo red*) boil with nitric acid; a blue color will be formed. 2. (*for circulating cold hemolysins*) immersion of the hands or feet in ice water will be followed by symptoms of paroxysmal cold hemoglobinuria if cold hemolysins are present.

Rosenbach-Gmelin t. (*for bile pigment*): filter the urine through a very small filter, and put a drop of nitric acid with a trace of nitrous acid on the inside of the filter; a pale-yellow spot will appear, surrounded with yellowish red, violet, blue, and green rings.

Rosenheim-Drummond t. (*for vitamin A*): dissolve 1 or 2 drops of cod liver oil in about 5 ml. of an anhydrous fat solvent. Add 1 drop of concentrated sulfuric acid. A temporary deep-violet color indicates vitamin A.

Rosenthal's t.: 1. (*for blood in urine*) add potassium hydroxide solution to the urine, remove the precipitate and dry it; place a small amount on a slide with a crystal of sodium chloride; apply a coverglass and cause a few drops of glacial acetic acid to flow under it; warm the plate. When it is cool hemin crystals will appear if blood is present. 2. (*for liver function*) a modification of the phenoltetrachlorophthalein test based on the amount of the dye which remains in the blood at definite periods after injection of 5 mg. per kilogram of body weight. The normal liver will remove most of the dye from the blood in fifteen minutes and all of it within an hour.

Rosin's t. (*for indigo red*): render the suspected liquid alkaline with sodium carbonate and extract with ether; this is colored red.

Ross-Jones t. (*for excess of globulin in cerebrospinal fluid*): 1 ml. of cerebrospinal fluid is floated over 2 ml. of concentrated ammonium sulfate solution; excess of globulin produces a fine white ring at the line of junction.

Rossel's aloin t. (*for blood in stools*): about 1 drachm of the feces is put in a test tube and extracted with 5 to 10 ml. of ether to remove the fat. After pouring off the ether the feces are thoroughly shaken up with 5 ml. of glacial acetic acid. The acid is then poured into another test tube and extracted with 5 to 10 ml. of ether. The test is then made with this ether. To that ether are added 20 to 30 drops of old oil of turpentine and 10 to 15 drops of a 1 to 4 per cent solution of Barbados aloin in 60 to 70 per cent alcohol. In the presence of blood the mixture takes on a light red color, turning to bright cherry red in about ten minutes.

Rothera's t. (*for acetone*): to 5 ml. of urine add a little solid ammonium sulfate and add 2 to 3 drops of a fresh 5 per cent solution of sodium nitroprusside and 1 to 2 ml. of ammonium hydroxide; a purple color forms if acetone is present.

Rotter's t. (*for ascorbic acid in the body*): cutaneous injection of 2,6-dichlorphenolindophenol produces colorization of the tissues; decolorization occurring in ten minutes indicates adequate ascorbic acid.

Rous t. (*for hemosiderin*): centrifuge the urine; to the sediment add 5 ml. of a 2 per cent solution of potassium ferrocyanide and 5 ml. of a 1 per cent solution of hydrochloric acid. Hemosiderin granules stain blue.

Roussin's t.: microscopic examination of suspected blood stains.

Rowntree and Geraghty's t., see *phenolsulfonphthalein t.*

RPR t., rapid plasma reagin t.

Rubin's t.: 1. a test for patency of the uterine tubes made by transuterine insufflation with carbon dioxide. If the tubes are patent the gas enters the peritoneal cavity and may be demonstrated by the fluoroscope or roentgenogram. This subphrenic pneumoperitoneum causes pain in one or both shoulders of the patient. If the manometer registers not over 100 mm. Hg the tubes are patent; if between 120 and 130, there may be stenosis or stricture, but not complete occlusion; if it rises to 200, the tubes are completely occluded. 2. a test to detect avian leukosis viruses in egg-culture vaccines; if the viruses are present, they induce a cellular resistance to Rous viruses subsequently inoculated (resistance-inducing factor).

Rubino's t., see under *reaction.*

Rubner's t.: 1. (*for carbon monoxide in blood*) shake the blood with 4 or 5 volumes of lead acetate in solution: if the blood contains CO, it will retain its bright color; if not, it becomes a chocolate brown. 2. (*for lactose, dextrose, maltose, and levulose in urine*) add lead acetate to the urine, boil, and then add an excess of ammonium hydroxide: lactose gives a brick-red color, dextrose a coffee-brown color, maltose a light-yellow color, and levulose no color at all.

Ruhemann's t. (*for uric acid in urine*), see under *method.*

ruler t., see *Hamilton's test.*

Rumpel-Leede t., see under *phenomenon.*

Russo's t., see under *reaction.*

Ruttan and Hardisty's t. (*for blood*): blood in the presence of a 4 per cent glacial acetic acid solution of orthotoluidine and hydrogen peroxide gives a bluish color.

Rytz t. (*for syphilis*): the test requires only one tube for each serum. In a tube 75 mm. by 10 mm., 0.15 ml. of serum is placed and heated in a water bath at 60° C. for three minutes; 0.05 ml. of half saturated ammonium sulfate is added and mixed by shaking. The antigen emulsion, 0.05 ml., is added, mixed by shaking, and 1 ml. of a 0.9 per cent solution of sodium chloride is added and rotated in such a manner that the antigen particles become evenly distributed. This is shaken in the Kahn shaker for three minutes, and then 2 ml. of a 0.9 per cent solution of sodium chloride is added and the tube is inverted slowly two or three times just before the reading is taken. A 1 plus reaction consists of tiny, densely scattered flocculation particles in a slightly opalescent fluid. Plus 2, 3, and 4 reactions show clumps of flocculation in a clear fluid, the clumps varying in size according to the positiveness of the serum. A negative test shows only minute antigen particles in a slightly hazy fluid without clumping.

Saathoff's t. (*for fat in stools*): rub up the feces with sudan and warm; fat droplets stain yellow to red.

Sabin-Feldman dye t.: a serologic test for the diagnosis of toxoplasmosis, based on the failure of living toxoplasmas, in the presence of specific antibody and accessory factor, to take up methylene blue dye.

saccharimeter t.: dextrose in solution rotates the plane of polarized light to the right, while levulose turns it to the left.

Sachs-Georgi t. (*for syphilis*): 1 ml. of a solution of cholesterinized alcoholic extract of human or beef heart (1 part) and 0.9 per cent sodium choride solution (9 parts), when added to 0.3 ml. of syphilitic serum, will cause a flocculent precipitation; called also *lentochol reaction.* Abbreviated S.-G. t.

Sachs-Witebsky t. (*for syphilis*): a quickly performed seroreaction for syphilis using a more concentrated cholesterinized extract of beef heart than that used in the Sachs-Georgi test; called also *citochol reaction* or *test,* and *Sachs-Witebsky reaction.*

Sachsse's t. (*for sugar in the urine*): a solution of 18 gm. of red mercuric iodide, 25 gm. of potassium iodide, 80 gm. of potassium hydroxide, in water enough to make a liter; sugar, if present, causes a black precipitate.

Sahli's t. (*for motive and digestive power of stomach*): the patient is fed a soup made of definite amounts of water, flour, butter, and salt, and in an hour the stomach contents are removed. The amount of fat present shows how much of the meal has been digested, and the acidity indicates how much the stomach has secreted.

Sahli's desmoid t., see *desmoid reaction,* under *reaction.*

Sahli's glutoid t. (*for digestive function*): a glutoid capsule containing 0.15 gm. of iodoform is taken with an Ewald breakfast. The capsule is not digested by the stomach fluid, but is readily digested by pancreatic juice. Appearance of iodine in the saliva and urine within four to six hours indicates normal gastric motility, normal intestinal digestion, and normal absorption. Glutoid capsules are prepared by soaking gelatin capsules in solution of formaldehyde.

Sahli-Nencki t. (*for lipolytic activity of the pancreas*): phenyl salicylate (salol) is administered: it is excreted as salicylic acid when pancreatic activity is normal.

Sakaguchi t. (*for arginine*): a reddish or wine color is produced in the presence of arginine when a tissue section is treated with an alkaline mixture of α-naphthol and sodium hypochlorite.

salicylaldehyde t. (*for acetone*), see *Frommer's t.*

salicylic acid t., see specific tests, including *Remont's t., Siebold and Bradbury's t.*

saline wheal t., see *McClure-Aldrich t.*

Salkowski's t.: 1. (*for CO in the blood*) add to the blood 20 volumes of water and sodium hydroxide in solution (specific gravity, 1.34). If CO is present, it becomes cloudy and then red; flakes of red afterward float on the surface. 2. (*for cholesterol*) dissolve in chloroform and add an equal volume of strong sulfuric acid: if cholesterol is present, the solution becomes bluish red, and slowly changes to a violet red, the sulfuric acid becomes red, with a green fluorescence. 3. (*for indole*) to the solution to be tested add a little nitric acid, and drop in slowly a solution of potassium nitrite (2 per cent): a red color shows that indole is present, and a red precipitate is afterward formed. 4. (*for dextrose*) a modified form of Trommer's t. 5. (*for creatinine*) to the yellow solution obtained in Weyl's test add an excess of acetic acid and heat; a green color results, which turns to blue.

Salkowski-Ludwig t. (*for uric acid*): a solution of silver ammonionitrate and ammonium and magnesium chlorides precipitates uric acid.

Salkowski and Schipper's t. (*for bile pigments*): to 10 ml. of the unknown add 5 drops of a 20 per cent solution of sodium carbonate and 10 drops of a 20 per cent solution of calcium chloride. To the precipitate add 3 ml. of alcohol containing 5 per cent of strong hydrochloric acid and a few drops of strong sodium nitrite. Heat. A green color indicates bile pigments.

salol t., see *Ewald's t.* (2) and *Sahli-Nencki t.*

Salomon's t.: test the stomach washing by means of Esbach's reagent, after twenty-four hours without protein food; the presence of albumin indicates ulcerative cancer.

salvarsan t., see *Dicken's t.*

sand t. (*for bile and hemoglobin in urine*): a layer of white sand is spread on a plate and on this is poured some of the urine; if the urine contains pigments, a spot is left on the sand, which is brown with hemoglobin and greenish with bile pigment. Called also *Lipp's t.*

Sandrock t. (*for thrombosis*): vigorous friction is applied to the part; the degree of hyperemia which follows is an indication of the condition of the circulation.

Sanford's t.: prepare a series of dilutions of salt from 0.28 to 0.5 per cent; add 1 drop of blood to each dilution, mix, allow to settle, and note the tubes which show hemolysis.

santonin t.: 1. (*for the antitoxic efficiency of the liver*) the patient is given 0.02 gm. of santonin on a fasting stomach; the urine is examined hourly for oxysantonin by treating it with a dilute sodium hydroxide solution which will produce a red color with oxysantonin. 2. see *Daclin t.*

Saundby's t. (*for blood in feces*): to a small quantity of feces in a test tube 10 drops of a saturated benzidine solution is added; to this is added 30 drops of hydrogen peroxide solution. A dark blue color will develop if blood is present.

scarification t., see *Pirquet reaction*, under *reaction*.

Schaffer's t. (*for nitrites in urine*): decolorize 4 ml. of urine with animal charcoal and add to it 4 ml. of 10 per cent acetic acid and 3 drops of 5 per cent solution of potassium ferrocyanide; an intense yellow color indicates nitrites.

Schalfijew's t. (*for blood*): treat defibrinated blood with excess of glacial acetic acid, heat to 80° C., cool, and examine for hemin crystals.

Schalm t., see *California mastitis t.*

Scherer's t.: 1. (*for inosite*) evaporate on platinum foil with nitric acid, add ammonia water and a single drop of calcium chloride in solution, and reevaporate to dryness; a rose-red coloration indicates the presence of inosite. 2. (*for pure leucine*) a small portion of leucine with a few drops of nitric acid are evaporated on platinum foil. The transparent residue turns a brownish color on the addition of a sodium hydroxide solution. When the mixture is concentrated an oil-like drop is obtained. 3. (*for tyrosine*) treat with nitric acid and dry with care on platinum foil; the formation of nitrotyrosine nitrate renders it yellow, and sodium hydroxide solution changes the color to reddish yellow.

Schick t.: intracutaneous injection of a quantity of diphtheria toxin equal to one fiftieth of the minimal lethal dose diluted in salt solution. If the patient has less than 0.03 unit of antitoxin per milliliter of blood, the toxin is not neutralized, and an area of inflammation is produced on the skin at the site of the injection. The test is a measure of immunity to diphtheria.

Schick t. control [USP], diagnostic diphtheria toxin that has been inactivated for use as control for the Schick test. Called also *inactivated diagnostic diphtheria toxin.*

Schiff's t.: 1. (*for carbohydrates in urine*) warm and add sulfuric acid; expose to the fumes of the urine a paper dipped in a mixture of equal volumes of xylidine and glacial acetic acid with alcohol and then dried: the paper becomes red if carbohydrates are present. 2. (*for cholesterol*) add a reagent composed of 2 parts of sulfuric acid with 1 part of a dilute solution of ferric chloride; evaporate to dryness and a violet color is produced. 3. (*for cholesterol*) evaporate with nitric acid and add ammonia water; a red color not changed by alkalis is produced. 4. (*for allantoin and urea*) add a solution of furfurol in hydrochloric acid; a yellow color appears, turning to purple and then to a brownish black. 5. (*for uric acid*) treat silver nitrate paper with an alkaline solution of the suspected substance; a brown stain shows the presence of uric acid. 6. (*for formaldehyde in milk*) the solution consists of an aqueous solution of magenta, 40 ml.; distilled water, 250 ml.; aqueous solution of sodium bisulfide, 10 ml.; pure concentrated sulfuric acid, 10 ml., which is allowed to stand until it is colorless; 2 ml. of this solution is added to a test tube two thirds full of milk. If formaldehyde is present, a pink or lilac color will appear in from thirty to sixty seconds.

Schiller's t. (*for cancer of cervix*): a test for early squamous cell cancer by treating the tissue with a solution of 1 gm. of pure iodine and 2 gm. of potassium iodide in 300 ml. of water: if the cervix is healthy, the surface turns brown; if there is cancer, the treated area turns white or yellow, because cancer cells do not contain glycogen and therefore do not stain with iodine.

Schilling t. (*for gastrointestinal absorption of vitamin B₁₂*): a measured amount of radioactive vitamin B₁₂ is given orally, followed by a parenteral flushing dose of the nonradioactive vitamin, and the percentage of radioactivity is determined in the urine excreted over a 24-hour period.

Schirmer's t. (*for keratoconjunctivitis sicca*): a test of tear production in which a piece of filter paper is inserted over the conjunctival sac of the lower lid, with the end of the paper hanging down on the outside. The range of normal wetting, determined by measuring the area of moisture on the projecting paper, depends on age and sex.

Schlesinger's t. (*for urobilin*): to about 5 ml. of the urine in a test tube, add a few drops of Lugol's solution to transform the chromogen into the pigment. Now add 4 or 5 ml. of a saturated solution of zinc chloride in absolute alcohol and filter. A greenish fluorescence, best seen when the tube is viewed against a black background and the light is concentrated upon it with a lens, shows the presence of urobilin. Bile pigment, if present, should be removed

by adding about one fifth volume of 10 per cent calcium chloride solution and filtering.

Schmidt's t.: 1. (*for bile*) particles of fresh feces are rubbed up with concentrated aqueous solution of corrosive mercuric chloride in a glass dish. After standing covered for twenty-four hours the matter is examined, bilirubin appearing as green particles, hydrobilirubin as red ones. 2. (*for sugar*) lead acetate is added and precipitated with ammonia water; on heating, the white precipitate remains unchanged if saccharose or milk sugar is present, but if dextrose is present, an orange tint is seen. 3. (*for proteolytic pancreatic function*) see *nuclear t.* 4. (*for intestinal indigestion*) the patient is placed upon a definite diet; after a few days the feces are examined for fermentation. If this occurs within forty-eight hours it points to the imperfect intestinal digestion of starch. 5. (*for digestive function of the stomach*) a test based upon the fact that when the gastric secretion is absent or greatly diminished, connective tissue masses appear in the stool after eating raw chopped meats.

Schönbein's t.: 1. (*for blood*) blue coloration obtained by adding solution of hydrogen peroxide to tincture of guaiac mixed with suspected blood. 2. (*for copper*) a solution containing a copper salt becomes blue if potassium cyanide and tincture of guaiac are added.

Schopfer's t. (*for urea*): minute amounts of vitamin B in the blood catalyze the mold *Phycomyces blaksleeanus.*

Schroeder's t. (*for urea*): add a crystal of the substance to a solution of bromine in chloroform; the urea will decompose and gas will be formed.

Schubert-Dannmeyer t.: a test for cancer based on the difference of certain electrical properties between a lipin extract of cancer serum and that from normal serum.

Schulte's t. (*for proteins*): remove all coagulable protein, precipitate with six volumes of absolute alcohol, dissolve the precipitate in water, and apply the biuret test.

Schultz-Charlton t., see under *reaction*.

Schultze's t.: 1. (*for cellulose*) iodine is dissolved to saturation in a zinc chloride solution (specific gravity, 1.8), and 6 parts of potassium iodide are added: this reagent colors cellulose blue. 2. (*for cholesterol*) evaporate with nitric acid, using a porcelain dish and water bath; if cholesterol is present, a yellow deposit is formed, which changes to yellowish red when ammonia is added. 3. (*for proteins*) to a suspected solution add a very little of a dilute solution of cane sugar and concentrated sulfuric acid; keep it at 60° C., and a bluish red coloration is produced.

Schultze's indophenol oxydase t., see *indophenol t.*

Schumm's t.: 1. see *benzidine t.* 2. (*for heme in plasma*) a given volume of plasma is covered with a layer of ether; one-tenth the volume of concentrated ammonium sulfide (analar) is then run in with a pipette and subsequently mixed by shaking. A positive reaction is indicated by the appearance of a hemochromogen with a sharply defined α band at 558 mμ in a depth up to 4 cm. of plasma.

Schürmann's t. (*for syphilis*): a color reaction proposed for the recognition of syphilitic blood serum.

Schwabach t.: a hearing test made, with the opposite ear masked, with tuning forks of 256, 512, 1024, and 2048 Hz, alternately placing the stem of the vibrating fork on the mastoid process of the temporal bone of the patient and that of the examiner (whose hearing should be normal) until it is no longer heard by one of them. The result is expressed as "Schwabach prolonged" if heard longer by the patient (indicative of conductive hearing impairment), as "Schwabach shortened or diminished" if heard longer by the examiner (indicative of sensorineural hearing impairment), and as "Schwabach normal" if heard for the same time by both.

Schwartz's t. (*for varicose veins*): the flats of the fingers are placed along the course of the supposed varicose saphenous vein in the thigh and some prominent part of the vessel below is tapped; a shock is transmitted to the fingers above if the vein is varicose.

Schwartz-McNeil t.: a complement fixation test for gonorrhea in which the antigen is an autolysate of a large number of strains of gonococci.

Schwarz's t.: 1. heat the substance with charcoal; the odor of mercaptan indicates the presence of sulfonmethane. (K. L. H. Schwarz.) 2. (*for digestive function of stomach*) with a test breakfast there is administered a capsule of goldbeaters' skin containing 4 gm. of bismuth carbonate and 0.25 gm. of neutral pepsin. The patient is then examined fluoroscopically. At first the capsule appears as a circular, sharply defined area, but if it is dissolved by the stomach juice the area becomes a broad band. If the shadow of the capsule remains unchanged after five hours, anacidity of the stomach is indicated. Called also *fibroderm bismuth capsule t.* (G. Schwarz.)

Scivoletto's t. (*for hydrochloric acid in urine*): dip filter paper in starch paste and dry; sprinkle it with urine and dry; hang it in a flask containing strontium acetate in solution: a blue color indicates the presence of the acid.

scratch t.: cutireaction.

screen t.: 1. alternate cover t. 2. cover-uncover t.

screening t., any test used to eliminate those who are definitely not affected by the disease in question, the remainder (those with positive reactions) being subjected to more refined diagnostic tests.

secretin t.: a test for pancreatic function done by examining the pancreatic secretion produced by the intravenous injection of secretin.

1343

sedimentation t.: 1. see *agglutination t.* 2. see *erythrocyte sedimentation rate,* under *rate.*

Seidel's t. (*for inosite*): evaporate in a platinum crucible with nitric acid, and treat with ammonia and strontium acetate in solution; inosite, if present, causes a green coloration and a violet precipitate.

Seidlitz powder t. (*for diaphragmatic hernia*): the stomach is distended by the administration of a Seidlitz powder, which will enable roentgen visualization of a herniated stomach loop.

Selivanoff's t., Seliwanow's t. (*for fructose in urine*): to the urine is added an equal volume of hydrochloric acid containing resorcinol in the following proportion: 5 mg. resorcinol, 5 ml. water, and 5 ml. 25 per cent concentrated hydrochloric acid. Formation of a burgundy-red color after boiling for 10 seconds indicates fructose.

Sellards' t. (*for acidosis*): the patient is given 5 gm. of sodium bicarbonate, dissolved in water, by mouth, every two or three hours until the urine, passed before each dose, becomes neutral or faintly alkaline. Tolerance of 20 to 30 gm. shows moderate acidosis; tolerance of from 75 to 100 gm. indicates distinct acidosis. Called also *bicarbonate tolerance t.*

semen t., see specific tests, including *Barberio's t., Florence t., Huhner t., serum t.*

senna t. (*in urine*): make the urine alkaline; a red color indicates senna.

sensitized sheep cell t., see *sheep cell agglutination t.* (1).

sero-enzyme t., see *Abderhalden's reaction,* under *reaction.*

serologic t.: any laboratory test on the blood serum of a patient.

serum t. (*for blood, meat, sperm, etc.*): the antigen, human blood serum, is injected several times, at intervals, into a rabbit. The suspected specimen is dissolved in physiologic salt solution and added to the serum of a rabbit treated in the way mentioned. The serum will become clouded if the suspected specimen is of the same species as the antigen used for immunizing the rabbit. Called also *biological t., Bordet's t.,* and *Uhlenhuth's t.*

serum neutralization t.: a test of the antimicrobial activity of a serum done by inoculating a mixture of the serum and the virus or other microorganism being tested into a susceptible animal; called also *protection t.*

shadow t.: retinoscopy.

Shear's t. (*for vitamin D*): to the oil add an equal volume of acid aniline (1 part concentrated HCl and 15 parts aniline). Mix and boil. A green color changing to red indicates vitamin D.

sheep cell agglutination t.: 1. (*for the presence of rheumatoid factor in serum*) sheep erythrocytes sensitized with rabbit antisheep erythrocyte immune globulin will agglutinate following the addition of human serum in which rheumatoid factor (IgM) is present. Called also *Rose-Waaler t., sensitized sheep cell t.,* and *Waaler-Rose t.* 2. (*for infectious mononucleosis*) when the antibody level of a person with infectious mononucleosis reaches a certain level, a sample of his blood will cause agglutination of sheep erythrocytes.

short increment sensitivity index (SISI) t., see under *index.*

Sia t. (*for macroglobulinemia*): a simple screening test performed by adding a drop of serum to 10 to 100 ml. of cold distilled water; a positive reaction is indicated by the formation of a heaving cloud of precipitate at the bottom of the container. It is not diagnostic, because it may be positive in other conditions, as in rheumatoid arthritis.

Sicard-Cantelouble t.: place 4 ml. of spinal fluid in a specially graduated tube, add 12 drops of a 33 per cent trichloracetic acid, mix, and read the amount of protein precipitated after twenty-four hours' sedimentation.

sickling t.: a method to demonstrate hemoglobin S and the sickling phenomenon in erythrocytes, particularly in the heterozygous state, performed by reducing the environmental oxygen to which the red cells are exposed. This may be done by simply sealing a drop of blood under a coverslip or, to hasten the morphologic change, by adding 2 per cent sodium metabisulfite or sodium dithionite to the preparation.

Siebold and Bradbury's t. (*for salicylic acid in urine*): alkalinize with potassium carbonate, add a solution of lead nitrate in excess, filter, and add a dilute solution of ferric chloride; a violet color will be produced.

Sieur's t., coin t.

sigma t., see under *reaction.*

silver t. (*for dextrose in the urine*): boil the urine with silver nitrate solution and an excess of ammonia; metallic silver will be deposited. Tartaric acid and aldehyde also produce this reaction.

Simonelli's t. (*for renal inadequacy*): iodine is administered and the urine and saliva tested for iodine; if iodine does not appear in the urine at the same time as in the saliva, the kidneys are diseased.

Sims' t.: a postcoital test for the ability of the spermatozoa to penetrate the cervical mucus.

skatole t., see specific tests, including *Ciamician and Magnanini's t., Herter's t.* (2), *Kondo's t., nitroso-indole-nitrate t.*

skin t., see *cutaneous reaction,* under *reaction,* and see *cutireaction.*

skin window t., Rebuck skin window technique.

slide t., see *Kline t.*

smear t., see *Papanicolaou's stain,* under *Table of Stains.*

Smith's t. (*for bile pigments*): overlay the suspected liquid with tincture of iodine diluted 1:10; a green ring or plane appears at the junction of the two liquids in the tube.

Snellen's t.: 1. (*for pretended blindness in one eye*) the patient is requested to look at alternate red and green letters; the admittedly sound eye is covered with a red glass and if the green letters are read, evidence of fraud is present. 2. determination of visual acuity by means of Snellen test types.

Snider match t. (*a screening test for pulmonary ventilation*): an ordinary book match which is burned nearly half way is held 6 inches from the mouth of the patient, who attempts to extinguish it by exhaling, after taking as deep a breath as possible, and without bringing the lips together.

sniff t.: when a patient sniffs, the paralyzed half of the diaphragm is seen to rise and the intact half to descend, as observed by fluoroscopy.

sodium chloride balance t., see *balance t.*

Soldaini's t. (*for glucose in the urine*): dissolve 15 gm. of copper carbonate and 416 gm. of potassium bicarbonate in 1400 ml. of water for a reagent; 2 parts of urine are boiled with 1 part of the reagent. A yellow precipitate of cupric oxide shows the presence of dextrose.

Solera's t. (*for thiocyanates*): saturate filter paper with 0.5 per cent starch paste containing 1 per cent of iodic acid; dry and preserve as test paper. A piece of this paper moistened with saliva will turn blue if thiocyanate is present.

solubility t. (*for pneumococcus*): reagent: sodium desoxycholate 10 gm., alcohol 10 ml., water 90 ml. Add 2 drops of the reagent to 1 ml. of a broth culture. Pneumococci dissolve within five minutes.

Sonnenschein's t. (*for strychnine*): the suspected substance is dissolved in a drop of sulfuric acid, some cerosoceric oxide is added, and stirred with a glass rod; a deep-blue color is formed, changing to violet, and finally to cherry red in the presence of strychnine.

soy bean t., see *urease t.*

spavin t.: a test for spavin in horses made by holding up the limb with the hock bent sharply; the horse is then started suddenly, and in cases of spavin the first steps are very lame. Called also *hock t.*

specific gravity t., see specific tests, including *Fishberg concentration t., urine concentration t., Volhard's t.* (2). See also *specific gravity, methods for,* under *method.*

sphenopalatine t.: the sphenopalatine ganglion is anesthetized with Novocain in order to determine whether the efferent current which is motivating a symptom is routed through either sphenopalatine ganglion, and if so, whether the left one or the right one.

Spiegler's t. (*for albumin*): acidulate with acetic acid and filter; prepare a reagent with 8 gm. of mercuric chloride, 10 gm. of sodium chloride, and 4 gm. of tartaric acid in 200 ml. of water and 20 ml. of glycerin; overlay the reagent with the filtrate. If albumin is present, a white ring appears at the junction of the liquids.

spinal t.: any laboratory serologic test of the spinal fluid.

Spiro's t.: 1. a test for the determination of ammonia and urea, embracing a combination of Folin's method for urea and the Sjöqvist method for urea. 2. (*for hippuric acid*) warm the unknown with acetic anhydride, anhydrous sodium acetate, and benzaldehyde. Cool, and crystals of phenylaminocinnamic acid—lactimide form.

split-renal function t., see *Howard t.*

sponge t.: a test performed by passing a hot sponge up and down the spine; if any lesion of the spine is present, pain is felt as the sponge passes over its locality.

Staehlin's t. (*for functional efficiency of myocardium*): the pulse rate after walking is more accelerated in impending heart failure than in health.

Stanford t.: a modified Binet test.

starch t., see *iodine t.* (1).

station t.: a test for disturbances of coordination, made by placing the patient in an erect posture, with the heels and toes of the two feet together; if the swaying of the body is beyond normal, coordination may be defective.

Staub-Traugott t., see under *effect.*

steapsin t., see *ethyl butyrate t.*

Stein's t.: inability to stand on one foot with the eyes shut; seen in disease of the labyrinth.

Steinle-Kahlenberg t.: heat a chloroform solution of a sterol with antimony pentachloride; the purple color changes to cobalt blue in the light.

Stenger t.: a test for detecting simulated unilateral hearing loss: a signal is presented at an intensity less than the admitted threshold to the affected ear and a less intense signal of the same frequency is presented simultaneously to the unaffected ear. If the subject is feigning a loss of hearing, the subject will not be able to detect the signal in the unaffected ear.

Stern's t.: a modification of the Wassermann test by using fresh active serum and the patient's complement, and overcoming nonspecific reactions by two fifths to one fifth of the usual dose of extract and three or four times the amboceptor unit.

Stock t. (*for acetone in urine*): the distillate of the urine is used; 50 to 100 ml. of urine is made acid by the addition of either acetic, hydrochloric, or sulfuric acid. The first 10 ml. of distillate will contain all the possible acetone. About 1 inch of the distillate is placed in a test tube; a drop or two of a 10 per cent solution of hydroxylamine hydrochloride is added, and sufficient sodium hydroxide or carbonate solution to render the solution alkaline to liberate hydroxylamine; the mixture is shaken and a couple of drops of pyridine is added and the mixture shaken; then 1 inch of ether is added and the mixture shaken. Bromine water is then added drop by drop, with mixing, until the ether layer becomes yellow; then a few drops of strong hydrogen peroxide is added; if acetone is present the ether will turn a distinctive green blue.

Stokes's t., see under *reagent.*

Stokvis' t. (*for bile pigment*): with 25 ml. of urine mix 8 ml. of a 1:5 zinc acetate solution; wash the precipitate in water on a filter, and dissolve in ammonia water. Filter again, and in a short time the filtrate shows a bluish green tint.

Stoll t.: a technique for the quantitative estimation of the worm burden of an individual based on collection of a 24-hour stool specimen and counting the number of ova present in an aliquot.

Storck's t. (*for human milk*): the ferment of human milk will decompose hydrogen dioxide.

Strange's t., see *Henderson's t.*

Strassburg's t. (*for bile acids in albumin-free urine*): add cane sugar to the urine; dip filter paper into it and dry; a drop of sulfuric acid on the paper will cause a red or violet spot if bile acids are present.

Straus's biological t. (*for glanders*), see *Straus' reaction,* under *reaction.*

Strauss's t.: 1. (*for lactic acid in stomach*) extract the lactic acid from the stomach contents by means of ether. To the ether add distilled water and a little ferric chloride solution; a green color indicates lactic acid. 2. a concentration test for kidney function by the ingestion of water. 3. a levulose tolerance test for hepatic function. 4. a urea balance test for renal function.

stress t's, exercise t's.

Struve's t. (*for blood in the urine*): alkalinize the urine and add tannic and acetic acids until the reaction becomes acid and a dark precipitate is formed. When this is dried, crystals of hemin may be obtained from it by adding ammonium chloride and glacial acetic acid.

strychnine t., see specific tests, including *Allen's t.* (3), *Brieger's t.* (2), *Sonnenschein's t., Wenzell's t.*

Stypven time t.: a test similar to the Quick one-stage prothrombin time test, but performed with Russell's viper venom (Stypven) as the thromboplastic agent; useful in defining deficiencies of blood coagulation factor X.

sugar t., see tests listed under *dextrose t., galactose t., levulose t.,* and *maltose t.*

sulfosalicylic acid t., same as *Exton's t.*

sulfur t. (*for protein*): the suspected liquid is heated with an excess of sodium hydroxide and a small quantity of acetate of lead; if proteins are present, a black precipitate of lead sulfide is formed.

Sulkowitch's t. (*for calcium in urine*): the precipitation of calcium in urine as an oxalate with use of a reagent consisting of 2.5 gm. of oxalic acid, 2.5 gm. of ammonium oxalate, and 5 ml. of glacial acetic acid dissolved in 150 ml. of distilled water.

Sullivan's t. (*for cysteine*): to 1 or 2 ml. of the unknown solution add 1 to 2 drops of a 0.5 per cent solution of 1,2-naphthoquinone-4-sodium sulfonate and then 5 ml. of a 20 per cent sodium thiosulfate made up in 0.25 normal sodium hydroxide. A brilliant red color indicates a free SH group, cysteine rather than cystine.

Suranyi's t.: an albumin reaction for the diagnosis of carcinoma.

syphilis t., see specific tests, including *Bauer's t.* (1), *benzoin t., Bio-Lab t., Boerner-Luken's t., Cantani t., Casilli's t., Chediak's t., Clive's t., colloidal gold t., Craig's t.* (2), *Dold's t., Eagle t., fluorescent treponemal antibody absorption t., Fornet's ring t., FTA t., Garriga's t., gel t., Hecht's t., Hecht-Weinberg-Gradwohl t., Hennebert's t., Hinton t., Ide t., Ishihara's t.* (2), *Jacobsthal's t.* (1), (2), *Justus' t., Kafka's t., Kahn t.* (1), *Kline t., Kolmer's t.* (1), *Landau color t., mastic t., Mazzini t., Meinicke t.* (1), (2), (3), *Müller's t.* (3), *Murata t., Peterman's t., plasmacrit t., Porges-Meier t., Porges-Salomon t., Rytz t., Sachs-Georgi t., Sachs-Witebsky t., Schürmann's t., Stern's t., Takata-Ara t., Targowla t., Treponema pallidum complement fixation t., Treponema pallidum cryolysis complement fixation t., treponemal hemagglutination t., Treponema pallidum immobilization t., Tschernogowbou's t., Venereal Disease Research Laboratory t., Wassermann t., Weil's t.* See also *syphilis reaction,* under *reaction.*

Szabo's t. (*for HCl in the stomach contents*): add to the suspected liquid a reagent containing equal parts of a 0.5 per cent solution of sodioferric tartrate and ammonium thiocyanate; if HCl is present, the reagent is changed from a pale yellow to a brownish red.

Takata-Ara t.: an obsolete, nonspecific test: by mixing a mercuric chloride solution with sodium carbonate in the presence of the normal spinal fluid, a colloidal solution of mercuric oxide is formed which turns a deep bluish violet by adding a solution of diamond-fuchsin. With pathologic spinal fluids the reaction is different. The abnormal protein content of the latter causes either a flocculation of the mercuric oxide with a discoloration of the fluid or color changes from bluish violet to pink with practically no precipitation. The first type of reaction, according to Takata and Ara, is typical of syphilis of the central nervous system while the change of the color occurs in bacterial meningitis.

tannic acid t. (*for nucleoalbumin*), see *Ott's t.*

tannin t. (*for carbon monoxide hemoglobin*): dilute the blood with 4 volumes of distilled water and add a little potassium ferricyanide to change the oxyhemoglobin into methemoglobin. Divide into two parts and thoroughly oxygenate one by shaking to decompose the carbon monoxide hemoglobin in it. Add to each part a little yellow ammonium sulfide and a little tannin solution. A bright red precipitate in the part not shaken indicates carbon monoxide hemoglobin. The methemoglobin in the other part gives a dirty, olive-green precipitate.

Tanret's t. (*for albumin*): Tanret's reagent gives a white precipitate with albumin. See under *reagent.*

Tardieu's t. (*for infanticide*): presence of air bubbles in gastric mucosa after establishment of fetal respiration.

Targowla's t., see under *reaction.*

taurine t., see *Lang's t.*

Taylor's t.: a modification of Schönbein's test for blood, the blue precipitate forming a deep sapphire blue solution when taken up by alcohol or ether.

Teichmann's t. (*for blood*): the suspected liquid is put under a coverglass with a crystal of sodium chloride and a little glacial acetic acid; heat carefully without boiling and then cool. If blood is present, rhombic crystals of hemin will appear.

tellurite t. (*for diphtheria*): a 2 per cent solution of potassium tellurite is applied to the membrane or exudate in the throat; any area affected with diphtheria will become blackened in from five to ten minutes (Manzullo, 1938).

Tensilon t. (*for myasthenia gravis*): after administration of Tensilon (edrophonium chloride), the patient's eye signs (ptosis and extraocular muscle abnormalities) markedly decrease.

Terman t.: the Stanford modification of the Binet test.

thalleioquin t. (*for quinine*): a neutralized solution of the suspected liquid is treated with chlorine, or bromine water, and then with an excess of ammonia; a green substance, thalleioquin, will be formed.

thematic apperception t. (TAT): a projective test in which the subject tells a story based on each of a series of standard ambiguous pictures, so that his responses reflect a projection of some aspect of his personality and current psychological preoccupations and conflicts.

thermoagglutination t.: a test to detect antigenic variants, in which slightly rough strains may be detected by their agglutination upon boiling saline for two hours.

thermoprecipitin t.: the finely divided organ or part is mixed with 5 to 10 parts of water, boiled, filtered, and stratified with a specific serum; a precipitate forming in five minutes is positive.

thiamine t., see *thiochrome t.*

thiochrome t. (*for thiamine*): oxidize the thiamine to thiochrome and then recognize the latter by its blue-violet fluorescence in ultraviolet radiation.

thiocyanate t., see *ferric chloride t.* (1), *Solera's t.*

Thomas t.: when one thigh is flexed on the abdomen to flatten lumbar lordosis, any flexion of the other thigh represents a fixed flexion contracture of that hip.

Thomas-Binetti t.: rapid decoloration of methylene blue by cancer serum in the presence of cancer extracts.

Thompson's t. (*for gonorrhea*), see *two-glass t.*

Thormählen's t. (*for melanin in urine*): treat urine with a solution of sodium nitroprusside, potassium hydroxide, and acetic acid; if melanin is present, a deep-blue color will form.

Thorn t.: a test of adrenal cortical response after injection of ACTH or of epinephrine.

thread t., see *Garrod's t.* (2).

three-glass t.: on arising in the morning the patient urinates successively into three glass receptacles labeled I, II, and III. In acute anterior urethritis the urine in I will be turbid from pus, while II and III will be clear; but in posterior urethritis the urine in all three glasses will be turbid. Blood in I comes only from the anterior urethra, but if it comes from the posterior urethra all three will contain blood. Shreds in glass III point to chronic prostatitis.

three-paper t., see *Marie's three-paper t.*

threshold tone decay t.: a test for abnormal auditory adaptation, in which continuous pure tones are presented at the threshold level to determine the amount of tone decay (auditory adaptation).

thromboplastin generation t.: a sensitive test for delineation of defects in formation of intrinsic thromboplastin (prothrombinase, intrinsic prothrombin-converting principle) and hence deficiencies of the factors involved. Patient plasma, serum, calcium chloride, and autologous platelets or platelet lipid substitute are incubated concurrently, and, at appropriate intervals, the clotting times of normal citrated plasma substrate, to which aliquots of the incubation mixture are added in sequential fashion, are determined.

Thudichum's t. (*for creatinine*): add to the suspected substance a dilute solution of ferric chloride; a dark-red color indicates the presence of creatinine.

thumb-nail t. (*for fractured patella*): the examiner's thumbnail is passed over the subcutaneous surface of the patella; a fracture will be felt as a sharp crevice.

thymol turbidity t. (*for disordered liver metabolism*): direct precipitation of a protein from the serum of a patient with hepatic insufficiency by means of a solution of thymol.

thyroid function t.: see specific tests, including *acetonitrile t., Kottmann's t., Loewi's t., quadriceps t.* See also *thyroid function reaction,* under *reaction,* and *thyroid activity, method for,* under *method.*

Tidy's t. (*for albumin in urine*): 1. add equal volumes of phenol and glacial acetic acids; albumin will form a white precipitate.

2. add 15 drops of alcohol and 15 drops of phenol; albumin will form a white precipitate.

tine t., tine tuberculin t. (Rosenthal): four tines or prongs 2 mm. long, attached to a plastic handle and coated with dip-dried Old tuberculin (O.T.) are pressed into the skin of the volar surface of the forearm, where they deposit a dose of the tuberculin in the outer layer. The skin is checked 48 to 72 hours later for the presence of palpable induration; if the induration around one or more of the puncture wounds is 2 mm. or more in diameter, the test is considered positive.

Tizzoni's t. (*for iron in tissues*): treat a section of tissue with a 2 per cent solution of potassium ferrocyanide, and then with a 0.5 per cent solution of HCl; the tissue will be stained a blue color if iron is present.

TNT t., see *Webster's t.*

toad t., 1. see *male frog* or *male toad t.* 2. see *Xenopus t.*

Tobey-Ayer t. (*in the diagnosis of lateral sinus thrombosis*): after spinal puncture a manometer is attached to the puncture needle: compression on both jugular veins causes the fluid to rise in the manometer; pressure on one jugular vein alone, causes a rise in spinal fluid pressure if the lateral sinus is normal, but little or no rise if there is thrombosis of the sinus on the same side as compression of the vein. The significance of the test is greater on the right side than on the left.

tolerance t.: 1. an exercise test to determine the efficiency of the circulation. 2. a test to determine the body's ability to metabolize a substance or to endure administration of a drug.

Tollens' t.: 1. (*for aldehyde*) treat the suspected solution with an ammoniacal solution of silver nitrate and potassium hydroxide; if aldehyde is present, a mirror of metallic silver appears. 2. (*for dextrose*) prepare a reagent by precipitating a silver nitrate solution with potassium hydroxide and dissolving with ammonia; this is reduced by dextrose. 3. (*for pentose*) see *phloroglucin t.* 4. (*for conjugate glycuronates*) to 5 ml. of the urine add 1 ml. of a 1 per cent solution of naphthoresorcinol in 95 per cent alcohol and 5 ml. of strong hydrochloric acid. Boil and cool. An ether extract of this mixture is violet red if glycuronates are present.

Tollens, Neuberg, and Schwket's t. (*for glycuronic acid*): extract the glycuronic acid from acidified urine with ether, add water, evaporate the ether, and make orcinol test.

tongue t., see under *phenomenon*.

Töpfer's t's: quantitative tests for hydrochloric acid in gastric contents. 1. (*for total acidity*) 1 per cent solution of phenolphthalein is used as the indicator. 2. (*for free HCl*) 0.5 per cent alcoholic solution of p-dimethylaminoazobenzene is used as the indicator. 3. (*for combined HCl*) 1 per cent aqueous solution of sodium alizarin sulfonate is used as the indicator.

Torquay's t. (*for bile*): a small amount of the suspected liquid is added to a test tube containing an aqueous solution of methyl violet, 1:2000. Bile will change the blue color to red.

tourniquet t.: 1. (*for capillary fragility*) after application of pressure midway between diastolic and systolic for 5 minutes by a manometer cuff, the petechiae are counted in a previously marked area, 2.5 cm. in diameter, on the inner aspect of the forearm, about 4 cm. below the crease of the elbow. A number between 10 and 20 is marginal, above 20, abnormal. Called also *Hess capillary t.* 2. (*for collateral circulation*) after hyperemia of the limb has been artificially produced by application of the tourniquet, the tourniquet is removed and the extent of collateral circulation is determined by compressing the main artery. Called also *Matas' t.* 3. (*for collateral circulation in patients with varicose veins*) a bandage is applied to the upper part of the leg below the knee and the patient walks around with it on; varicose veins of the leg will become evacuated from continuous compression if there is sufficient collateral circulation in the deep veins. Called also *Perthes' t.*

TPCF t., *Treponema pallidum* complement fixation t.
TPCP t., *Treponema pallidum* cryolysis complement fixation t.
TPHA t., treponemal hemagglutination t.
TPI t., *Treponema pallidum* immobilization t.

Trambusti t. (*for tuberculosis*), see under *reaction*.

trapeze t.: when the patient hangs from a trapeze, a spinal deformity will disappear if the deformity is postural but will remain if it is structural.

Trendelenburg's t.: 1. raise the leg above the level of the heart until the veins are empty, then lower it quickly. If the veins become distended at once, varicosity and incompetence of the valves are indicated. 2. the patient, standing erect, stripped, with back to the examiner, is told to lift one leg and then the other: when weight is supported by the affected limb, the pelvis on the sound side falls instead of rising; seen in disturbances of the gluteus medius mechanism, as in deformity of the femoral neck, dislocated hip joint, and weakness or paralysis of the gluteus medius muscle.

treponemal hemagglutination t. (TPHA) t. (*for syphilis*): a passive serological test for syphilis using as antigen disrupted *Treponema pallidum* coated onto tannin-treated sheep erythrocytes that are agglutinated in the presence of specific antibody.

Treponema pallidum complement fixation (TPCF) t. (*for syphilis*): a specific serological test for syphilis utilizing an antigen prepared from *Treponema pallidum* by making an extract of infected rabbit testicular tissue with citrate, acetone, and deoxycholate.

Treponema pallidum cryolysis complement fixation (TPCP) t. (*for syphilis*): a specific serological test for syphilis, utilizing an antigen obtained by differential centrifugation of *Treponema pallidum* from infected rabbit tissue, cryolysis, and ammonium sulfate precipitation.

Treponema pallidum immobilization (TPI) t. (*for syphilis*): a specific serological test for syphilis using living motile *Treponema pallidum* as antigen, immobilized by antibody in the presence of complement.

Treponema pallidum immune adherence (TPIA) t. (*for syphilis*): the spirochetes are mixed with complement, antiserum, and red cells, and the adherence of the red cells to the spirochetes is observed microscopically *in vitro*.

Tretop's t.: to fresh urine in a test tube a few drops of 40 per cent formalin are added; albumin in the urine is coagulated.

Triboulet's t. (*for tuberculous ulceration of the intestines*): a lump of feces as large as a walnut is dissolved in 20 ml. of distilled water and filtered; 3 ml. of the filtrate is diluted with 12 ml. of distilled water; 20 minims of Triboulet's reagent (sublimate 3.5, acetic acid 1, distilled water 100) are added. As a control the same solution is prepared without Triboulet's reagent. The test tubes containing the two solutions are well shaken, and are compared after five and twenty-four hours. A positive reaction is indicated by a cloudy gray or brown deposit.

trichophytin t. (*for trichophyton infection*): when filtrates of the fungus are injected into persons who have been infected with the disease, a reaction is produced somewhat resembling the tuberculin reaction.

tricresol peroxidase t. (*for raw milk*), see *Kastle's t.*

triketohydrindene hydrate t.: to 25 ml. of water add 10 mg. of aminoacetic acid. To 1 ml. of this solution add a solution of 50 mg. of sodium acid in 2 ml. of water, then add 0.2 ml. of a solution of 5 mg. of triketohydrindene hydrate (Ninhydrin) in 1 ml. of water. Add the suspected matter and boil for 1–2 minutes. A violet color indicates a free carboxyl and alpha-amino group in proteins, peptones, peptides, or amino acids.

Trommer's t. (*for dextrose in the urine*): to 2 parts of urine add 1 part of potassium or sodium hydroxide, then add a very dilute solution of copper sulfate drop by drop, and boil the whole. Sugar, if present, causes precipitation of an orange-red deposit.

Trousseau's t. (*for bile in urine*): tincture of iodine diluted with 10 parts of alcohol is added to urine in a test tube; a green ring is formed where the liquids touch if bilirubin is present.

trypsin t., see *antitrypsin t., Gross' t.* (1).

tryptophan t.: a test of the stomach contents for the presence of tryptophan, which indicates the presence of carcinoma of the stomach. The test is performed by adding to the suspected liquid a few drops of 3 per cent acetic acid, and then adding to this carefully, drop by drop, a few drops of bromine water. A reddish-violet color is formed if tryptophan is present. 2. see also *vanillin t.*

Tschernogowbou's t.: a modification of the Wassermann test, using the natural amboceptor and complement in the patient's serum against guinea-pig erythrocytes.

Tsuchiya's t. (*for albumin*): a modified test in which Tsuchiya's reagent is used instead of Esbach's reagent.

tuberculin t.: a test for the existence of tuberculosis, consisting in the subcutaneous injection of 5 mg. of tuberculin. In healthy persons it produces no appreciable effect, but in tuberculous patients it produces a moderate fever, which lasts for several hours, and also a swelling and redness in tuberculous lesions of the patient. The test does not differentiate between infection in a resistant individual without the disease and a person with clinical features of the disease. See also *ophthalmic reaction, Pirquet's reaction, Moro's reaction,* under *reaction,* and *Mantoux t.*

tuberculin t., Sterneedle: the needle points of the Sterneedle are dipped into 1 to 2 drops of tuberculin P.P.D. and then placed on the forearm, where the six needle points are caused to penetrate the skin (by means of a spring device in the handle), through the P.P.D. solution, to a depth of 1 mm., thus depositing tuberculin in the outer layer of the skin. Palpable, coalescing induration (edema) more than 5 mm. around the puncture wounds in three to seven days indicates a positive reaction. In England, it is known as the *Heaf test.*

tuberculin patch t.: a test made by applying to the skin a piece of surgical adhesive on which some Old tuberculin has been placed.

tuberculin titer t.: a test for the hypersensitivity of the organism to tuberculin by a graduated cutaneous tuberculin test with varying concentrations of the tuberculin; called also *Ellerman-Erlandsen's t.*

tuberculosis t., see specific tests, including *Arloing-Courmont t., Blumenau's t., Craig's t., Escherich's t., Gruskin's t.* (3), *Hamburger's t., Hammer's t., Imhof's t., Lautier's t., Lignières' t., Malmejde's t., Mantoux t., Mátéfy t., Merieux-Baillion t., mirror t., Müller's t.* (2), *Müller-Jochmann t., Nasso's t., Nathan's t., niacin t.* (1), (2), *Piazza's t., Römer's t., tine t., Triboulet's t., tuberculin t., tuberculin t., Sterneedle, tuberculin patch t., tuberculin titer t., urorosein t., Vollmer's t.* See also *tuberculosis reaction,* under *reaction.*

Tuffier's t.: in aneurysm, when the main artery and vein of a limb are compressed, swelling of the veins of the hand or foot will occur only if the collateral circulation is free.

two-glass t. (*for urethritis*): the patient collects his urine on rising, the first part in one glass and the second part in a separate glass. If he has anterior urethritis the first portion will be turbid and the second portion clear; if he has both anterior and posterior urethritis both portions will be turbid.

two-stage prothrombin t.: a method of quantitating prothrombin after tissue thromboplastin and excess Factor V have converted it to thrombin, by determining the clotting time of a standard fibrinogen solution to which the previously generated thrombin has been added.

typhoid fever t., see specific tests, including *antithrombin t., Bareggi's t., Borden's t., Dreyer's t., Ehrlich's t.* (1), *Marris' atropine t., miostagmin t., Moretti's t., Petzetaki's t., Prendergast's t., typhoidin t., urorosein t., Widal's t.* See also *typhoid fever reaction,* under *reaction.*

typhoidin t.: a cutaneous test for typhoid fever made by inoculating typhoidin into the skin of the forearm; a positive reaction consisting in the formation of an indurated and reddened area at the site of inoculation.

tyrosine t., see specific tests, including *Folin and Denis' t., Hoffmann's t., Mörner's t.* (1), *Piria's t., Scherer's t.* (3), *Udránszky's t.* (2), *Wurster's t.* (2).

Tyson's t. (*for bile acids in urine*): 180 to 240 ml. of urine are evaporated to dryness on the water bath. The residue is extracted with absolute alcohol, and to the extract 12 to 14 volumes of ether are added. The bile acids are precipitated, then are filtered off, dissolved in water, and the aqueous solution decolorized with animal charcoal.

Tzanck t.: examination of tissue from the floor of a lesion, in vesicular or bullous diseases, to discover the type of cell present as a means of diagnosing the disease. Certain cells are pathognomonic of varicella, herpes simplex, herpes zoster, or pemphigus.

Udránszky's t.: 1. (*for bile acids*) take 1 ml. of a solution of the suspected substance, add a drop of 0.1 per cent solution of furfurol in water, underlay with strong sulfuric acid, and cool; if bile is present, a bluish-red color is formed. 2. (*for tyrosine*) take 1 ml. of the suspected substance in solution, add a drop of 0.5 per cent aqueous solution of furfurol, and underlay with 1 ml. of concentrated sulfuric acid; a pink color shows the presence of tyrosine.

Uffelmann's t. (*for hydrochloric acid and lactic acid in the gastric contents*): to a quantity of material taken from the stomach add a few drops of a reagent containing 3 drops of a solution of ferric chloride, 3 drops of a concentrated solution of phenol, and 20 ml. of water; hydrochloric acid, if present, decolorizes this solution, while lactic acid turns it yellow.

Uhlenhuth's t., see *serum t.*

Ulrich's t. (*for albumin*): the reagent consists of saturated solution of common salt, 98 ml.; glacial acetic acid, 2 ml. It must be perfectly clear. Boil a few milliliters of this fluid in a test tube, and immediately overlay with the urine. Albumin and globulin give a white ring at the zone of contact.

Ultzmann's t. (*for bile pigments*): to 10 ml. of the urine to be tested add 3 or 4 ml. of a 1:3 solution of potassium hydroxide, and an excess of HCl; bile pigments will cause an emerald-green coloration.

Umber's t. (*for scarlet fever*): to a small quantity of urine add 2 drops of a solution made with 30 ml. concentrated hydrochloric acid, 2 gm. of paradimethylaminobenzaldehyde and 70 ml. of water; a red reaction indicates scarlet fever.

uracil t., see *Wheeler and Johnson's t.*

urea t., see specific tests, including *Benedict's t.* (2), *biuret t.* (2), *Bloxam's t., Brücke's t.* (3), *diacetyl t., Marshall's t., Schiff's t.* (4), *Schroeder's t., Spiro's t.* (1), *urease t., Van Slyke t.* (2). See also *urea, methods for,* under *method.*

urea clearance t., see *blood-urea clearance t.*

urea concentration t. (*for renal efficiency*): a test based on the fact that urea is absorbed rapidly from the stomach into the blood, and is excreted unaltered by the kidneys: 15 gm. of urea is given with 100 ml. of fluid, and the urine which is collected at the end of two hours is tested for urea concentration. Called also *MacLean-de Wesselow t.* and *Jones and Cantarow t.*

urease t.: a test for urea based on the conversion of urea into ammonium carbonate by the urease of soy bean; see *Marshall's method* and *urease, methods for,* under *method.*

Urecholine supersensitivity t. (*for neurogenic bladder*): administer 2.5 mg. of Urecholine (bethanechol) subcutaneously; the bladder is neurogenic if it exhibits a rise in intravesical pressure more than 15 cm. greater than that of a control.

uric acid t., see specific tests, including *Bayrac's t., Cole's t.* (3), *Denigès' t.* (1), *Folin's t.* (2), *Ganassini's t., Garrod's t.* (2), *Gentele's t., Porter's t.* (1), *Salkowski-Ludwig t., Schiff's t.* (5), *von Jaksch's t.* (4), *Weidel's t.* (1). See also *uric acid, methods for,* under *method.*

urine concentration t.: under a controlled diet the specific gravity of the urine should reach 1.18 or more at certain times.

urobilin t., see specific tests, including *Hildebrandt's t., paradimethylaminobenzaldehyde t., Schlesinger's t.* See also *urobilinogen, methods for,* under *method.*

urochromogen t., see *Weiss's t.*

urorosein t., urorrhodin t.: add to the urine half as much concentrated hydrochloric acid and a few drops of a 1 per cent solution of potassium nitrate; a red color indicates urorosein (urorrhodin); seen in typhoid fever, nephritis, pulmonary tuberculosis, and other diseases.

Urriolla's t.: the discovery of blood pigment in the urine is indicative of the existence of malaria.

Valenta's t. (*for foreign fats in butter*): the butter is heated with an equal amount of glacial acetic acid and then cooled. If opacity begins to show at 96° F., there is adulteration; if opacity is not observed until about 62° F., the butter is pure.

Valsalva's t. (*for pneumothorax*): after a deep inspiration, the mouth and nose are held tightly closed, and a strong attempt at expiration is made.

van Deen's t., see *Deen's t.*

van den Bergh's t.: a test for bilirubin in which diazotized serum or plasma is compared with a standard solution of diazotized bilirubin.

van den Velden's t., see *Maly's t.*

vanillin t. (*for indole and tryptophan*): to 5 ml. of the culture add 5 drops of 5 per cent vanillin solution in 95 per cent alcohol and 2 ml. of hydrochloric acid; indole gives an orange color, tryptophan a reddish violet color.

Van Slyke t.: 1. (*for amino-nitrogen*) nitrous acid acting on amino-nitrogen sets free nitrogen gas, which is collected and its volume determined. 2. (*for urea*) treat the sample with urease, pass the ammonia so formed into fiftieth normal acid, and titrate the excess of acid.

Van Slyke and Cullen's t., see under *method.*

Vaughan and Novy's t. (*for tyrotoxicon*): adding 2 or 3 drops each of sulfuric and carbolic acids and a few drops of an aqueous solution of the suspected substance to tyrotoxicon gives a yellow or orange-red color.

VDRL t.: a slide flocculation test for syphilis using VDRL antigen, which contains cardiolipin, cholesterol, and lecithin, to test serum or spinal fluid; the test was designed by the Venereal Disease Research Laboratory.

Venning Browne t.: the presence of pregnanediol in the urine indicates the presence of corpus luteum hormone in the body.

ventilation t.: measurement of the quantity of air expired by a person during a period of exercise.

Vernes' t.: either of two obsolete nonspecific tests. 1. (*for syphilis*) direct method: a test based on the degree of flocculation produced by various blood sera on a specially prepared extract of dried horse heart muscle, called perethynol. Indirect method: a test based on measuring the amount of flocculation produced in perethynol according to the degree of inhibition of hemolysis of sheep corpuscles by swine serum. The degree of flocculation by normal serum and that by syphilitic serum is noted during a course of time, and the various readings are plotted into curves (syphilimetry). Normal sera give a horizontal line, but with syphilitic sera the curve of flocculation oscillates up and down. 2. (*for tuberculosis*) the patient's blood is mixed with an equal amount of 1.25 per cent aqueous solution of resorcin. If the optic density of the mixture is below 15, the subject is free from tuberculosis; if it is above 30 the subject has tuberculosis.

Visscher-Bowman t. (*for pregnancy*): a chemical test for pregnancy, depending on the presence of anterior pituitary hormones in the urine.

Vitali's t.: 1. (*for alkaloids*) evaporate with fuming nitric acid and add a drop of potassium hydroxide; color reactions will occur. For atropine the color is violet, turning to red. 2. (*for alkaloids*) add sulfuric acid, potassium chlorate, and an alkaline sulfide; various color reactions will follow. 3. (*for bile pigments*) add a few drops of potassium nitrate in solution and dilute sulfuric acid. The color reactions are green, followed by blue or red and yellow. 4. (*for bile pigments*) add quinine bisulfate in solution and follow with ammonia water, sulfuric acid, a crystal of sugar, and alcohol; a violet color results. 5. (*for thymol*) distill, and pass the vapor through a mixture of chloroform and potassium hydroxide solution; a red color results. 6. (*for pus in the urine*) the urine is acidified with acetic acid and filtered. On the filter paper thus obtained a small quantity of guaiacum is dropped. The paper will turn a dark blue if pus is present.

vitality t., see *pulp t.*

vitamin t., see specific tests, including *Carr-Price t., Fearon's t., Gothlin's t., Harris and Ray t., Jendrasic's t., Rosenheim-Drummond t., Rotter's t., Schopfer's t., Shear's t., thiochrome t.*

vocabulary t.: a form of intelligence test based on the subject's knowledge of a selected list of words.

Voelcker and Joseph's t., see *indigo carmine t.*

Vogel and Lee's t. (*for mercury*): add 3 per cent of hydrochloric acid and concentrate the urine to one fifth its original volume. Add a piece of clean copper wire. A silvery film indicates mercury. To confirm, place the wire in a tube with a plug of gold foil and distill the mercury over onto the gold. Sublime a crystal of iodine onto the mercury and form the red iodide of mercury.

Voges-Proskauer t.: a test to detect the presence of acetyl-methyl carbinol and thus to distinguish between the colon group and the aerogenes group of bacteria.

Volhard's t.: 1. (*for chlorides*) the chlorides are precipitated by a known amount of $AgNO_3$. The excess of $AgNO_3$ is then titrated with KCNS. See under *method.* 2. (*specific gravity test for renal function*) the patient is given 1500 ml. of water to drink within three quarters of an hour in the early morning, and then nothing but a dry diet for the rest of the day. Following the ingestion of water, the specific gravity of the urine drops below 1.002 and the water taken is eliminated in about four hours. Later in the day, the specific gravity rises, passing 1.025 late in the afternoon.

Vollmer's t.: trademark for a tuberculin patch test done with an adhesive strip on which are two test squares and one control square of filter paper, the test squares saturated with concentrated Old Tuberculin and the control square with uninoculated broth.

von Aldor's t. (*for proteoses*): precipitate the urine with phosphotungstic acid, wash the precipitate with alcohol, bring into solution with potassium hydroxide, and apply the biuret test.

von Jaksch's t.: 1. (*for free HCl in gastric juice*) a test paper prepared with benzopurpurine B takes on a fine violet color is HCl is present. If present in considerable amount, it becomes dark blue. 2. (*for dextrose in urine*) add to the urine a mixture of 3 parts of sodium acetate and 2 parts of phenylhydrazine hydrochloride, warm it, and put the test tube in hot water for half an hour. On cooling, yellow needles of phenylglucosazone are seen as a precipitate. 3. (*for melanin*) add to the suspected liquid a few drops of a solution of ferric chloride. If melanin is present, a gray appearance is produced. After precipitation add more ferric chloride, and the precipitate will be redissolved. 4. (*for uric acid*) heat the powder slowly on a glass dish with a few drops of bromine water or chlorine water; the substance becomes red. After cooling, add ammonia, and it becomes purplish red.

von Maschke's t. (*for creatinine*): to the suspected solution add a few drops of Fehling's solution, after mixing with a cold solution of sodium carbonate; an amorphous, flocculent precipitate proves the presence of creatinine.

von Pirquet's t., see *Pirquet's reaction,* under *reaction.*

von Recklinghausen's t. (*of heart function*): a test based on the proposition that the product of the frequency of the pulse and the amplitude of the blood pressure is equal to the amount of blood expelled by the heart in a second, divided by the distensibility of the circulatory system.

von Zeynek and Mencki's t. (*for blood*): precipitate the urine with acetone, extract the precipitate with acidified acetone, and examine the colored extract under the microscope for small hemin crystals.

Vulpian t. (*for epinephrine*): add a few drops of ferric chloride solution, and a green color indicates epinephrine.

Waaler-Rose t. (*for rheumatoid factor*), see *sheep cell agglutination t.* (1).

Wada t. (*for cerebral dominance of language function*): amobarbital is injected into an internal carotid artery to produce transient hemiparesis of the contralateral limbs. Injection into the artery of the hemisphere dominant for language produces a transient aphasia, into that of the nondominant hemisphere does not interfere with language function.

Wagner's t. (*for occult blood*), see *benzidine t.*

Walter's bromide t.: a test based on the fact that in normal persons the ratio of the amount of bromide in the blood and cerebrospinal fluid is constant; in persons with mental disorder the ratio may vary.

Wang's t. (*quantitative test for indican*): the indican is converted into indigosulfuric acid and titrated by means of a potassium permanganate solution.

Warren's t., see *Trommer's t.*

Wassermann t., see under *reaction.*

water t. (*for Addison's disease*): the volume of urine excreted from 10:30 P.M. to 8:30 A.M. is measured. Twenty ml. of water per kilogram of body weight (9 ml. per pound) is administered without breakfast. The urine is collected at 9:30, 10:30, 11:30 A.M. and at 12:30 P.M. If the volume of any single specimen exceeds the volume of urine excreted during the night, Addison's disease is ruled out.

water-gurgle t. (*for stricture of the esophagus*): the swallowing of water causes a peculiar gurgle heard on auscultation.

water provocative t.: a test used in the early diagnosis of open-angle glaucoma. After the intraocular pressure is measured by applanation tonometry, the patient drinks a liter of water in 5 minutes. Forty-five to sixty minutes later the intraocular pressure is again measured; a pressure rise of 8 to 10 mm.Hg. is positive.

Watson-Schwartz t.: a simple qualitative procedure, depending upon the chloroform- and butanol-insolubility of porphobilinogen aldehyde, for differentiating porphobilinogen from urobilinogen and other Ehrlich reactors; it is of value in the diagnosis of acute porphyria.

Weber's t.: 1. (*for differentiating between hearing impairment of conductive or sensorineural origin*) the stem of a vibrating tuning fork is placed on the vertex or midline of the forehead; if the sound is heard best in the affected ear, the impairment is probably of the conductive type; if heard best in the normal ear, the impairment is probably of the sensorineural type. (Friedrich Eugen Weber.) 2. (*for indican*) boil 30 ml. of suspected urine with an equal volume of hydrochloric acid containing a little nitric acid; cool it, and shake with ether; if indican is present, the ether will become red or violet and the froth will be blue. (Ernest Heinrich Weber.) 3. (*for blood*) mix the blood with 30 per cent acetic acid and extract with ether; to the ethereal extract add an alcoholic solution of guaiac and hydrogen peroxide. A blue color indicates blood. (Ernest Heinrich Weber.)

Webster's t. (*for TNT in urine*): the urine is extracted with ether, then acidified with a mineral acid, and again extracted with ether. In the latter extract the presence of the azoxy-compound formed from TNT is shown by the development of a violet tint on the addition of alcoholic potash.

Weichbrodt's t. (*for globulin*): to 0.7 ml. of spinal fluid add 0.3 ml. of a 1 per cent solution of mercuric bichloride; a cloudiness or opalescence indicates globulin.

Weidel's t.: 1. (*for uric acid*) the substance tested is treated with nitric acid, evaporated, and moistened with ammonia water; if uric acid is present, murexide will be formed, and a purple color is produced. Called also *murexide t.* 2. (*for xanthine*) warm with freshly prepared chlorine water containing a trace of nitric acid until gas ceases to be produced; contact with gaseous ammonia develops a pink or purple color. 3. (*for xanthine bodies*) dissolve in warm chlorine water, evaporate, and treat with ammonia water, a pink or purple color will form, changing to violet on the addition of sodium or potassium hydroxide solution.

Weil's t. (*for syphilis*): a test for syphilis based on the fact that the erythrocytes of syphilitics are especially resistant to the hemolyzing power of cobra venom.

Weil-Felix t., see under *reaction.*

Weinberg's t.: a complement-fixation test for hydatid disease.

Weiss permanganate t., see *Weiss's t.*

Weiss's t. (*for urochromogen*): to 2 ml. of the urine add 4 ml. of distilled water and 3 drops of a 1:1000 solution of potassium permanganate; a canary yellow color indicates urochromogen.

Welland's t.: a vertical bar placed between the eyes and the letters to be read shows the degree of binocular fixation.

Wender's t. (*for dextrose*): make a reagent by dissolving 1 part of methylene blue in 300 parts of distilled water; alkalinize this with potassium hydroxide and heat with a suspected solution; dextrose, if present, will decolorize it.

Wenzell's t. (*for strychnine*): treat the suspected material with a solution of 1 part of potassium permanganate in 2000 parts of sulfuric acid; strychnine, even in very small proportion, will cause color reactions.

Weppen's t. (*for morphine*): treat with sugar, bromine, and sulfuric acid; a red color shows the presence of morphine.

Wernicke's t., see *hemiopic pupillary reaction,* under *reaction.*

Wetzel's t. (*for carbon monoxide in blood*): to the blood to be examined add 4 volumes of water and treat with 3 volumes of a 1 per cent tannin solution. If CO is present, the blood becomes carmine red; normal blood slowly assumes a grayish hue.

Weyl's t.: 1. (*for creatinine*) to the suspected solution add a little of a dilute solution of sodium nitroprusside, and then carefully put in a few drops of a weak solution of sodium hydroxide; a ruby-red color results, changing to blue on warming with acetic acid. 2. (*for nitric acid in the urine*) distill 200 ml. of urine with 0.2 part of sulfuric or hydrochloric acid, receiving the distillate in a potassium hydroxide solution. If metaphenyl-diamine is added, a yellow color will form; if there is added pyrogallic acid in aqueous solution with a little sulfuric acid, the color will be brown; but sulfanilic acid in solution, followed in ten minutes by naphthylamine hydrochlorate, produces a red tint.

Wheeler and Johnson's t. (*for uracil and cytosine*): to the unknown solution add bromine water until the color is permanent, but avoid excess. Now add an excess of barium hydroxide. A purple color indicates one of these substances.

Whipple's t., see *fibrinogen t.* (1), *lipase t.* (1), *phenoltetrachlorophthalein t.*

whisper t. (*obs.*): test for hearing in which the patient stands at one end of the room with the ear opposite to that being tested closed with the finger and with the eyes closed. The examiner, whispering as he goes, approaches the patient and notes at what point the whisper is perceived by the patient.

Whiteside t.: a test for the detection of subclinical mastitis in cows as indicated by an excessively high leukocyte count of the milk. Mix 2 ml. of a normal solution of sodium hydroxide with 10 ml. of milk; the development of a viscous mass is positive. A modified version consists in mixing 1 drop of milk with 5 drops of normal sodium hydroxide solution on a glass plate, and stirring for about 20 seconds with a glass rod. No changes in consistency—negative; threads, clumps, or flakes of coagulated material—positive; the development of a viscous mass with separation of a clear whey—strongly positive.

Widal's t., Widal's serum t. (*for typhoid fever*): agglutination of *Salmonella typhosa* by dilutions of the patient's serum.

Wideroe's t.: a test for the character of puncture fluids. A few drops of Millon's reagent is placed in a water glass, and 1 drop of the fluid to be tested is placed on the surface. A film of coagulated protein at once forms. If this film is coherent and can be lifted readily, the exudate is tuberculous; if less readily, it is inflammatory; if it breaks up so that it cannot be lifted at all, it is a transudate.

Widmark's t.: a blood test for the diagnosis of alcoholic intoxication.

Wijs' t.: an iodine number test which employs Wijs iodine solution; see *iodine number,* under *number.*

Wilbrand's prism t.: a small circle of white paper is placed upon a black surface, and the patient is seated before it with one eye bandaged. He is directed to look at the spot, and a strong prism is placed before the eye in such a way that the image of the spot is thrown upon the blind half of the retina. It is noticed if the eye at once moves to find the object again, and whether the movement is reversed when the prism is withdrawn. The presence of this reaction places the lesion in the cerebrum; the absence of the reaction locates it in the tract.

Wilkinson and Peter's t. (*for raw milk*): benzidine and hydrogen peroxide give a blue color in raw milk, but not in heated milk.

Williamson's blood t.: in a narrow test tube 4 ml. of water and 2 ml. of blood are placed; to this are added 1 ml. of methylene blue (1:6000) and 4 ml. of solution of potassium hydroxide. The tube is placed in a pot of boiling water. If the blood is from a diabetic patient, the blue soon disappears, but not otherwise.

Winckler t.: 1. (*for alkaloids*) a solution of mercuric chloride with an excess of potassium iodide is added; alkaloids will cause a white precipitate. 2. (*for free HCl in the gastric juice*) filter the juice into a porcelain cell with a few drops of the 5 per cent alcoholic solution of alphanaphthol containing 1 per cent or less of dextrose. Heat carefully, and a bluish-violet zone will appear, which rapidly grows darker. 3. (*for iodine*) sodium nitrate is mixed with a starch paste; iodine gives a blue color with it.

Winslow's t.: test for respiration in doubtful death by observing a vessel of water placed at the bottom of the chest.

Wishart t. (*for acetonemia*): a few drops of plasma are placed in a small test tube. Enough dry powdered ammonium sulfate is added to supersaturate, so that at the end of the test there will still be some of the solid sulfate in the bottom of the tube. A couple of drops of a fresh solution of sodium nitroprusside are next added and shaken, and finally 1 or 2 drops of ordinary ammonia water. On shaking, a purple color develops, a little more slowly than in the case of urine. The intensity of the color indicates the degree of acetonemia.

Witz's t. (*for hydrochloric acid in the gastric juice*): a 1:48 aqueous solution of methyl violet causes a violet color, changing to blue and then green.

Wohlgemuth's t. (*for renal inadequacy*): the urine is mixed with a solution of soluble starch, 1:1000, and is incubated to permit digestive reaction. The fluid is then tested with iodine to determine the amount of starch hydrolysis. The test is based on the fact that the normal kidney tissue secretes a diastatic enzyme which is diminished in proportion as the kidney parenchyma is diseased.

Woldman's t.: a test for gastrointestinal lesion based on the principle that free phenolphthalein may pass through a lesion in the gastrointestinal mucosa and appear in the urine.

Wolff-Eisner t., ophthalmic reaction.

Wolff-Junghans t. (*for gastric cancer*): quantitative estimation of the soluble albumin in the gastric extracts after giving a test meal; marked increase of dissolved albumin indicating malignant disease.

Woodbury's t. (*for alcohol in the urine*): to 2 ml. of urine 1 ml. of sulfuric acid is added, and a crystal of potassium dichromate; a green color will soon form.

Woods's t.: complement fixation with uveal pigment for sympathetic ophthalmitis.

Worm-Müller t. (*for dextrose in the urine*): a test made by boiling in a test tube 0.33 ml. of a 2.5 per cent solution of copper sulfate and 2.5 ml. of a solution of potassium hydroxide. Boil each and mix, and a yellowish or red precipitate will be formed.

Wormley's t. (*for alkaloids*): 1. made by treating with an alcoholic solution of picric acid; a yellow precipitate will be formed. 2. made by treating with a solution of 1 part of iodine and 2 parts of potassium iodide in 60 parts of water; a colored precipitate will be formed.

worsted t., see *Holmgren's t.*

Wurster's t.: 1. (*for hydrogen peroxide*) test paper is saturated with the solution of tetramethylparaphenylenediamine; hydrogen peroxide turns it to a blue-violet color. 2. (*for tyrosine*) the suspected material is dissolved in boiling water and a little quinone; a ruby-red color will form, changing slowly to brown.

X² t., chi-square t.

xanthemia t., see *carotinemia t.*

xanthine t., see specific tests, including *Drechsel's t.* (2), *Hoppe-Seyler t.* (2), *Weidel's t.* (2), (3).

xanthoproteic t., see *Mulder's t.* (2).

Xenopus t. (*for pregnancy*): a female African toad (*Xenopus laevis*) is injected with 2 ml. of urine, or 1 ml. of an extract, into the dorsal lymph sac; a deposit of 5–6 or more eggs within four to twelve hours indicates pregnancy.

xylidine t., see *Schiff's t.* (1).

xylose concentration t.: under uniform controlled conditions the ingestion of 50 gm. of xylose should result in a concentration of 2.5 per cent in the urine within two hours.

D-xylose absorption t., D-xylose tolerance t. (*for differential diagnosis in malabsorption syndromes*): after the oral administration of 25 gm. (sometimes 5 gm. is used) of D-xylose dissolved in 250 ml. of water, followed immediately by an additional 250 ml. of water, to a fasting adult, the amount excreted in the urine during a five-hour period is determined. Since poor renal function may also result in low xylose absorption, blood levels are also determined at two hours. Normally, more than 4.0 gm. of xylose should be excreted over the five-hour period; less than this amount suggests intestinal malabsorption. Blood values are normally more than 25 mg. xylose per 100 ml. of blood.

Yerkes-Bridges t.: a modified and improved form of the Binet test for intelligence.

Young's t. (*for cataract*): on a disk with a varied number of pinholes in different portions, the patient's ability to recognize the number of holes is a test of the integrity of macular function.

Yvon's t.: 1. (*for acetanilid in urine*) extract it with chloroform and heat the residue with mercurous nitrate; a green color will form. 2. (*for alkaloids*) add a solution of 3 gm. of bismuth subnitrate, made by boiling in 40 ml. of water, to which are added 14 gm. of potassium iodide and 40 drops of hydrochloric acid; a red color will show the presence of an alkaloid.

Zaleski's t. (*for carbon monoxide in blood*): to 2 ml. of blood add an equal volume of water and 3 drops of a one-third saturated solution of copper sulfate: if carbon monoxide is present, a brick-red deposit is thrown down; otherwise the precipitate is greenish brown.

Zangemeister t. (*for paternity*): a decrease in the light permeability (detected by the photometer) when the serum of the child is mixed with that of the father; when the serum of a man other than the father is added to a child's serum this decrease does not occur.

Zappacosta's t. (*for liver function*): glycocyamine is injected intravenously; if in one quarter of an hour after the injection the substance is still present in the blood, liver function is impaired.

Zeisel's t. (*for colchicine*): dissolve in hydrochloric acid, boil with ferric chloride, and shake with chloroform; a brown or dark-red layer will form at the bottom.

Zeller's t.: 1. (*for melanin in urine*) add bromine water; a yellow precipitate will form, changing slowly to black. 2. see *Moloney's t.*

Ziehen's t. (*for mental disease*): the patient is requested to explain the difference between such contrasted objects as ice and water, cat and dog, etc.

zinc fluorescence t. (*for urobilin*), see *Schlesinger's t.*

Zondek-Aschheim t., see *Aschheim-Zondek t.*

Zouchlos' t. (*for albumin in the urine*): 1. precipitate the urine with a mixture of 1 part of acetic acid and 6 parts of a 10 per cent solution of mercuric chloride. 2. prepare a reagent with 100 parts of a 10 per cent solution of potassium thiocyanate and 20 parts of acetic acid; drop it slowly into the urine until the albumin appears as a white cloudiness. 3. add equal parts of succinic acid and potassium thiocyanate; albumin, if present, will be precipitated.

Zsigmondy's gold number t., see *colloidal gold t.*

Zwenger's t.: 1. (*for cholesterol*) a crystal of cholesterol with 5 parts of sulfuric acid and 1 part water gives a red ring changing to violet. 2. see *Liebermann's t.*

---

test meal (test mēl)   a meal containing material given for the specific purpose for aiding diagnostic examination of the stomach, as by roentgenoscopy or by chemical analysis later of the stomach contents. See also *meal*. **Boas' t. m.,** a tablespoonful of oatmeal in a quart of water boiled down to a pint; once used to evaluate gastric secretion. **Boyden t. m.,** a motor meal for testing the evacuation of the gallbladder, containing three or four egg yolks combined with milk and seasoned with sugar, port wine, etc. **motor t. m.,** a meal or drink containing a radiopaque substance, permitting roentgenoscopic observation of its progress through the stomach, pylorus, and other portions of the gastrointestinal tract.

test type (test tīp)   printed letters of varying size, used in the testing of visual acuity; see also under *chart*. **Jaeger's t. t.,** ordinary printer's type of seven different sizes imprinted on a card; used in testing near vision. **Snellen's t. t.,** block letters used in testing visual acuity, so designed that the whole letter subtends, at the appropriate distance, a visual angle usually of 5 minutes, and each component part subtends an angle of 1 minute. See also *Snellen's chart.*

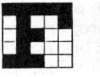

Two of Snellen's test types.

testa (tes'tah) [L.]   a shell; oyster shell. **t. o'vi,** egg shell.

testaceous (tes-ta'she-us) [L. *testa* shell]   of the nature of shell; having a shell.

testalgia (tes-tal'je-ah) [*testis* + *-algia*]   pain in the testicle.

Tes-Tape (tes'tāp)   trademark for a test strip impregnated with glucose oxidase, peroxidase, and orthotolidine; used for determining the approximate concentration of glucose in urine.

testectomy (tes-tek'to-me) [*testis* + Gr. *ektomē* excision]   orchiectomy.

testes (tes'tēz) [L.]   plural of *testis*.

testicle (tes'tĭ-k'l) [L. *testiculus*]   the testis.

testicond (tes'tĭ-kond) [*testis* + L. *condere* to hide]   having the testes retained within the abdominal cavity, as occurs normally in many mammals, such as the elephant and armadillo.

testicular (tes-tik′u-lar) pertaining to a testis.

testiculoma (tes-tik″u-lo′mah) a testicular tumor. **t. ova′rii,** arrhenoblastoma.

testiculus (tes-tik′u-lus) [L.] testis.

testis (tes′tis), pl. *tes′tes* [L.] [NA] the male gonad; either of the paired egg-shaped glands normally situated in the scrotum; each testis is surrounded by an outer mesothelial layer (tunica vaginalis) and an inner white capsule (tunica albuginea), and is composed of compartments (lobuli testis) which contain the seminiferous tubules, wherein the spermatozoa are produced. Specialized interstitial cells (Leydig cells) secrete testosterone. Called also *testicle.* **Cooper's irritable t.,** a testis affected with neuralgia. **ectopic t.,** a testis which has become lodged in some abnormal location. **inverted t.,** a testis whose position in the scrotum is reversed, the epididymis being attached to the anterior instead of the posterior surface. **t. mulie′bris,** an ovary. **obstructed t.,** a testis whose descent has been prevented by a fascial sheet at the entrance to the scrotum. **pulpy t.,** a testis affected with medullary sarcoma. **t. re′dux,** a testis which tends to be drawn to the upper part of the scrotum. **retained t.,** undescended t., see *cryptorchidism.* **undescended t.,** a testis which has failed to descend into the scrotum, but remains in the inguinal canal, and the condition so produced; called also *cryptorchism* or *cryptorchidism.*

testitis (tes-ti′tis) orchitis.

testitoxicosis (tes″ti-tok″si-ko′sis) [*testis* + Gr. *toxikon* poison] a condition of intoxication which sometimes follows double ligation of the vas deferens.

testoid (tes′toid) a term applied to testicular hormones and other natural or synthetic compounds having a similar effect.

testolactone (tes-to-lak′tōn) [USP] chemical name: D-homo-17α-oxaandrosta-1,4-diene-3,17-dione. An antineoplastic agent, $C_{19}H_{24}O_3$, occurring as a white to off-white, crystalline powder, which may be prepared from testosterone or progesterone. It is used as adjunctive therapy in the palliative treatment of advanced or disseminated breast cancer in postmenopausal women; administered orally or by intramuscular injection.

testopathy (tes-top′ah-the) [*testes* + Gr. *pathos* disease] any disease of the testes.

testosterone (tes-tos′tĕ-rōn) chemical name: 17β-hydroxy-androst-4-en-3-one. 1. the principal androgenic hormone, $C_{19}H_{28}O_2$, produced by the interstitial (Leydig) cells of the testes in response to stimulation by the luteinizing hormone of the anterior pituitary gland; it is thought to be responsible for regulation of gonadotropic secretion, spermatogenesis, and wolffian duct differentiation (formation of the epididymis, vas deferens, and seminal vesicle). It is also responsible for other male characteristics after its conversion to dihydrotestosterone (q.v.) by 5α-reductase in peripheral tissue. In addition, testosterone possesses protein anabolic properties, manifested by retention of nitrogen, calcium, phosphorus, and potassium, and is important in maintaining muscle mass and bone tissue in the adult male. It is also converted by aromatization to estradiol in peripheral tissue. See also *anabolic steroid,* under *steroid.* 2. [USP] the same principle prepared synthetically from cholesterol or isolated from bull testes, occurring as white or slightly creamy white crystals or crystalline powder; used in the treatment of male hypogonadism, cryptorchidism, and the symptoms of the male climacteric, and may be used for its anabolic properties; administered by subcutaneous implantation or intramuscular injection or buccally. **t. cyclopentylpropionate,** t. cypionate. **t. cypionate** [USP], an ester of testosterone, $C_{27}H_{40}O_3$, occurring as a white or creamy white, crystalline powder, having the same actions as the free alcohol but a prolonged duration of effect; used chiefly in the treatment of male hypogonadism, frigidity, and inoperable female breast cancer, to suppress lactation, and as an anabolic agent, administered by intramuscular injection. Called also *t. cyclopentylpropionate.* **t. enanthate** [USP], an ester of testosterone, $C_{26}H_{40}O_3$, occurring as a white or creamy white, crystalline powder, having the same actions as the free alcohol but a prolonged duration of effect; used chiefly in the treatment of male hypogonadism, oligospermia, and the symptoms of male climacteric, administered by intramuscular injection. Called also *t. heptanoate.* **ethinyl t.,** ethisterone. **t. heptanoate,** t. enanthate. **t. ketolaurate,** an ester of testosterone, having the same actions as the other esters. **methyl t.,** see *methyltestosterone.* **t. phenylacetate,** an ester of testosterone, $C_{28}H_{36}O_3$, occurring as a white to almost white, crystalline powder, having the same actions as the free alcohol but a prolonged duration of effect; administered by subcutaneous and intramuscular injection. **t. propionate** [USP], an ester of testosterone, $C_{22}H_{32}O_3$, occurring as white or creamy white crystals or crystalline powder, having the same actions as the free alcohol but with a relatively short duration of effect; used chiefly in the treatment of male hypogonadism, symptoms of male climacteric, postpubertal cryptorchidism, and inoperable female breast cancer, and to prevent postpartum breast engorgement; administered buccally or intramuscularly.

Testryl (tes′tril) trademark for a suspension of pure crystalline testosterone.

tetanal (tet′ah-nal) pertaining to or derived from tetanus.

tetania (tĕ-ta′ne-ah) [L.] tetany. **t. gravida′rum,** tetany in pregnant women. **t. parathyreopri′va,** tetany caused by removal of the parathyroids.

tetanic (tĕ-tan′ik) [Gr. *tetanikos*] 1. pertaining to or of the nature of tetanus. 2. producing tetanus.

tetaniform (tĕ-tan′ĭ-form) [*tetanus* + L. *forma* shape] like or resembling tetanus.

tetanigenous (tet″ah-nij′ĕ-nus) [*tetanus* + Gr. *gennan* to produce] producing tetanus or tetanic spasms.

tetanilla (tet″ah-nil′ah) 1. a form of tetany without rigidity, but attended by mental changes. 2. paramyoclonus multiplex.

tetanism (tet′ah-nizm) a form of more or less continuous muscular hypertonicity sometimes seen in young infants; a series of clinical conditions resembling those of tetanus, but dependent on infection with an organism other than the *Clostridium tetani.*

tetanization (tet″ah-ni-za′shun) the induction of tetanic convulsions or symptoms.

tetanize (tet′ah-nīz) to throw into a state or condition of tetanus or continuous spasm; to induce tetanic contractions in a muscle.

tetanocannabin (tet″ah-no-kan′ah-bin) a poisonous principle sometimes found in hemp; it resembles strychnine in its action.

tetanode (tet′ah-nōd) the unexcited stage of tetany.

tetanoid (tet′ah-noid) [*tetanus* + Gr. *eidos* form] like or resembling tetanus.

tetanolysin (tet″ah-nol′ĭ-sin) [*tetanus* + *lysin*] the hemolytic component of the exotoxin (tetanus toxin) produced by *Clostridium tetani,* which may or may not contribute to the pathogenesis of tetanus. See also *tetanospasmin.*

tetanometer (tet″ah-nom′ĕ-ter) [*tetanus* + Gr. *metron* measure] an apparatus for measurement and analysis of tetanus.

tetanospasmin (tet″ah-no-spaz′min) [*tetanus* + L. *spasmus* spasm + *-in* chemical suffix] the neurotoxic component of the exotoxin (tetanus toxin) produced by *Clostridium tetani,* which causes the typical muscle spasms of tetanus. See also *tetanolysin.*

tetanus (tet′ah-nus) [Gr. *tetanos,* from *teinein* to stretch] 1. an infectious disease in which tonic muscle spasm and hyperreflexia result in trismus ("lockjaw"), generalized muscle spasm, arching of the back (opisthotonus), glottal spasm, seizures, and respiratory spasms and paralysis; it is caused by the neurotoxin of anaerobically vegetating *Clostridium tetani,* with onset one to two weeks after inoculation of spore forms into a traumatized area of the body. 2. continuous tonic contraction of a muscle; steady contraction of a muscle without distinct twitching. **acoustic t.,** a series of induction shocks in a frog's nerve and muscle preparation; the speed is measured by the pitch of a vibrant rod. **anodal closure t.,** tetanic muscular contraction occurring at the anode when the electric circuit is closed. Abbreviated ACTe. **anodal opening t.,** tetanic muscular contraction occurring at the anode when the electric circuit is opened or broken. Abbreviated AOTe. **t. anti′cus,** tetanus in which the body is bowed forward. **apyretic t.,** tetany, def. 1. **artificial t.,** drug t. **cathodal closure t.,** tetanic muscular contraction occurring at the cathode when the electric circuit is closed. Abbreviated CCTe. **cathodal opening t.,** tetanic muscular contraction occurring at the cathode when the electric circuit is opened or broken. Abbreviated COTe. **cephalic t.,** a rare disease developing after injuries to the scalp, face, or neck, associated with palsies of cranial nerves 3, 4, 6, 7, 9, 10, 12, and invariably associated with some degree of trismus. **cerebral t.,** tetanus following a wound of the head, combining the generalized rigidity of the disease arising elsewhere and a cranial nerve palsy, especially of cranial nerve VII (the facial nerve); called also *cephalotetanus, kopf-tetanus, Janin's t.,* and *Klemm's t.* **chronic t.,** a form seen in man in which the onset is later, the progress of the disease is slower, and the prognosis more favorable than in the acute form. **cryptogenic t.,** tetanus which occurs without any wound or other ascertainable cause. **t. dorsa′lis,** t. posticus. **drug t.,** toxic spasm produced by some tetanic drug. **extensor t.,** that which affects especially the extensors. **flexor t.,** tonic spasm of flexor muscles. **head t., hydrophobic t.,** cerebral t. **idiopathic t.,** that which does not follow an obvious lesion. **imitative t.,** hysteria which simulates tetanus. **t. infan′tum,** t. neonatorum. **inoculation t.,** experimental tetanus produced by inoculation with a culture of *Clostridium tetani.* Called also *impf-tetanus.* **intermittent t.,** tetany, def. 1. **Janin's t., Klemm's t., kopf t.,** cerebral t. **t. latera′lis,** tetanus in which the body is bent sideways. **localized t.,** tetanic spasm of a single part. **modified t.,** localized t. **t. neonato′rum,** tetanus of very young infants, usually due to the infection of the umbilicus. **t. paradox′us,** cephalic tetanus in which trismus is combined with paralysis of the facial or other cranial nerve. **paralytic t.,** cerebral t. **partial t.,** tetany, def. 1. **t. posti′cus,** tetanus in which the body is bowed backward. **postserum t.,** tetanus which develops even after the administration of tetanus serum. **puerperal t.,** that which occurs in women after childbirth. **Ritter's t.,** tetanic contractions taking place at the opening of a constant current which has been passing for some time along a nerve; seen in tetany. **Rose's t.,** cerebral t. **splanchnic t.,** a form in which the muscles of deglutition and of respiration are severely involved and in which there is severe dysphagia. **toxic t.,** that produced by an overdose of nux vomica or strychnine. **traumatic t.,** that which follows wound infection with *Clostridium tetani.* **uterine t.,** puerperal t. **Wundt's t.,** tetanic contraction in a frog's muscle produced by electric current or injury.

tetany (tet'ah-ne) 1. a syndrome manifested by sharp flexion of the wrist and ankle joints (carpopedal spasm), muscle twitchings, cramps, and convulsions, sometimes with attacks of stridor. It is due to abnormal calcium metabolism and occurs in parathyroid hypofunction, vitamin D deficiency, alkalosis, and as a result of the ingestion of alkaline salts. 2. tetanus, def. 2. **duration t.,** a continuous tetanic contraction in response to a very strong continuous current; it occurs especially in degenerated muscles; abbreviated Dt. **gastric t.,** a severe form due to disease of the stomach, attended by difficult respiration and painful tonic spasms of the extremities. **grass t.,** an often fatal condition that may be produced in "fresh" cows that are turned out into lush pastures; it is apparently due to a deficiency of magnesium in the diet. **hyperventilation t.,** tetany produced by forced inspiration and expiration continued for a considerable time. **lactation t.,** grass tetany. **latent t.,** tetany elicited by the application of electrical and mechanical stimulation. **parathyroid t., parathyroprival t.,** tetany due to removal of the parathyroids. **transit t., transport t.,** a condition usually affecting well-fed cows and ewes in advanced pregnancy and in lactating mares that have been shipped long distances, which may result in paralysis, unconsciousness, and death unless treatment is begun early in the course of the disease. The etiology is unknown, but may be due to acute hypocalcium associated with improper care and feeding. Called also *railroad disease* or *sickness.*

tetarcone (tet'ar-kōn) tetartocone.

tetartanope (tet-ar'tah-nōp) an individual exhibiting tetartanopia.

tetartanopia (tet"ar-tah-no'pe-ah) [Gr. *tetartos* fourth + *an* neg. + *ōpē* sight + *-ia*] 1. quadrantanopia. 2. a rare problematic type of defective color vision, characterized by retention of the sensory mechanism for two hues only (red and green), and lacking that for blue and yellow, which are replaced in the spectrum by an achromatic (gray) band. Coined by G. E. Miller (1924), who conceded yellow as a fourth, "inner" primary. Cf. the correlative terms *protanopia, deuteranopia,* and *tritanopia,* in which the color vision deficiency is in the first, second, and third primary, respectively. Called also *blue-yellow blindness.*

tetartanopic (tet"ar-tah-nop'ik) pertaining to or characterized by tetartanopia.

tetartanopsia (tet"ar-tah-nop'se-ah) tetartanopia.

tetartocone (tet-ar'to-kōn) [Gr. *tetartos* fourth + *cone*] the posterior internal cusp of an upper premolar tooth.

tetartoconid (tet"ar-to-ko'nid) the posterior internal cusp of a lower premolar tooth.

tetia (te'te-ah) a native name for yaws on the Congo Coast.

tetiothalein sodium (te"she-o-thal'e-in so'de-um) iodophthalein sodium.

tetmil (tet'mil) ten millimeters taken as a unit of measurement.

tetra- [Gr. *tetra* four] a combining form meaning *four.*

tetra-amylose (tet"rah-am'ĭ-lōs) an anhydride obtained from dextrin; it consists of two units of diamylose, $[(C_6H_{10}O_5)_2]_2$.

tetrabasic (tet"rah-ba'sik) [*tetra-* + Gr. *basis* base] containing four atoms of replaceable hydrogen.

tetrablastic (tet"rah-blas'tik) having four germ layers.

tetrabrachius (tet"rah-bra'ke-us) [*tetra-* + Gr. *brachiōn* arm] a double monster having four arms.

tetrabromofluorescein (tet"rah-bro"mo-floo"o-res'e-in) eosin.

tetrabromophenolphthalein (tet"rah-bro"mo-fe"nol-thal'e-in) an indicator, $C_6H_4 \cdot CO \cdot O \cdot C(C_6H_2Br_2OH)_2$, which is colorless with acids and violet with alkalis.

tetrabromophthalein sodium (tet"rah-bro"mo-thal'e-in so'de-um) the sodium salt of tetrabromophenolphthalein, NaOOC·C₆H₄·C:C₆H₂Br₂O·C₆H₂Br₂ONa, used for roentgenological examination of the gallbladder, in which organ it appears after intravenous injection.

tetracaine (tet'rah-kān) [USP] chemical name: 4-(butylamino)-benzoic acid 2-(dimethylamino)ethyl ester. A local anesthetic, $C_{15}H_{24}N_2O_2$, occurring as a white or light yellow, waxy solid; applied topically to the eyeball and conjunctivia. **t. hydrochloride** [USP], a fine, white, crystalline powder, applied topically to the conjunctiva and eyeball, to the mucous membranes of the nose, throat, and respiratory tract, and to the skin to produce surface anesthesia and also used parenterally for conduction and infiltration anesthesia. Called also *amethocaine hydrochloride.*

tetracetate (tet-ras'ĕ-tāt) [*tetra-* + *acetate*] a compound of a base with four acetic acid molecules.

tetrachirus (tet"rah-ki'rus) [*tetra-* + Gr. *cheir* hand] a fetus having four hands.

tetrachlorethane (tet"rah-klōr-eth'ān) acetylene tetrachloride, $CHCl_2 \cdot CHCl_2$, formed by the action of chlorine on acetylene; it is anthelmintic, and is used as a solvent and in dry cleaning. Called also *cellon.*

tetrachloride (tet"rah-klo'rīd) a compound of a radical with four atoms of chlorine.

tetrachlormethane (tet"rah-klōr-meth'ān) carbon tetrachloride, CCl_4.

tetrachloroethylene (tet"rah-klo"ro-eth'ĭ-lēn) [USP] chemical name: perchloroethylene. An anthelmintic, C_2Cl_4, occurring as a clear, colorless, mobile liquid; used in the treatment of hookworm infections and certain trematode infections, administered orally.

tetrachlorphenoxide (tet"rah-klōr"fen-ok'sīd) a fungicide used for the preservation of lumber: it may cause a dermatitis in workmen.

tetrachromic (tet"rah-kro'mik) [*tetra-* + Gr. *chrōma* color] 1. pertaining to or exhibiting four colors. 2. able to distinguish only four of the seven colors of the spectrum.

tetracid (tet'ras-id) capable of replacing four atoms of hydrogen in an acid, or having four atoms of hydrogen replaceable by acid radicals.

tetracrotic (tet"rah-krot'ik) [*tetra-* + Gr. *krotos* beat] showing four elevations in the sphygmographic tracing of the pulse.

tetracycline (tet"rah-si'klēn) 1. any of a group of biosynthetic antibiotics isolated from certain species of *Streptomyces* or produced semisynthetically by catalytic hydrogenation of chlortetracycline or oxytetracycline. The tetracyclines, e.g., chlortetracycline (the first of the group to be discovered), oxytetracycline, tetracycline (see def. 2), demeclocycline, rolitetracycline, methacycline, doxycycline, and minocycline, are effective against a wide variety of organisms, including gram-positive and gram-negative bacteria, rickettsias, mycoplasmas, chlamydias, and certain viruses, protozoa, and actinomycetes. 2 [USP] chemical name: [4 S-(4α,4aα,5aα,6β,12aα)]-4-(dimethylamino)-1,4,4a,5,5a,6,11,12a-octahydro-3,6,10,12,12a-pentahydroxy-6-methyl-1,11-dioxa-2-naphthacenecarboxamide. A semisynthetic antibiotic, $C_{22}H_{24}N_2O_8$, occurring as a yellow, crystalline powder having the same wide spectrum of antimicrobial activity as the other tetracyclines (see def. 1), used as an antibacterial, antiamebic, and antirickettsial, administered orally. **t. hydrochloride** [USP], the monohydrochloride salt of tetracycline, $C_{22}H_{24}N_2O_8 \cdot HCl$, occurring as a yellow crystalline powder, having the same actions and uses as the base; administered orally, intramuscularly, or intravenously, or applied topically to the conjunctiva or eyelid. **t. phosphate complex** [NF], a phosphate complex salt of tetracycline, prepared by the addition of a solution of sodium metaphosphate to a solution of tetracycline or tetracycline hydrochloride; used as an antibacterial, administered orally; intramuscularly, or intravenously.

Tetracyn (tet'rah-sin) trademark for preparations of tetracycline.

tetrad (tet'rad) [Gr. *tetra-* four] a group of four similar or related entities, as (1) any element or radical having a valence, or combining power, of four; (2) a group of four chromosomal elements formed in the pachytene state in the first meiotic prophase; (3) a square of cells produced by the division into two planes of certain cocci (*Sarcina*). **Fallot's t.,** tetralogy of Fallot.

tetradactylous (tet"rah-dak'tĭ-lus) pertaining to or characterized by tetradactyly.

tetradactyly (tet"rah-dak'tĭ-le) [*tetra-* + Gr. *daktylos* finger] the condition of having four digits on the hand and foot.

tetradecanoate (tet"rah-dek"ah-no'āt) systemic name for myristate, denoting that it has fourteen (*tetra* four + *deca* ten) carbon atoms in a straight chain.

tetraerythrin (tet"rah-er'ĭ-thrin) crustaceorubin.

tetraethylammonium (tet"rah-eth"il-ah-mo'ne-um) the radical $(C_2H_5)_4N$; the bromide and chloride salts are short acting quaternary ammonium ganglion-blocking agents that have been used in the treatment of acute hypertension, peripheral vascular diseases, and other disorders of the peripheral circulation. They are now seldom employed, having been replaced by more effective drugs. Abbreviated TEA.

tetraethylthiuram disulfide (tet"rah-eth"il-thi'u-ram") disulfiram.

tetrafilcon A (tet"rah-fil'kon) chemical name: 2-hydroxyethyl methacrylate polymer with divinylbenzene methyl methacrylate and 1-vinyl-2-pyrrolidinone; a hydrophilic contact lens material, $(C_6H_{10}O_3)_w(C_{10}H_{10})_x(C_5H_8O_2)_y$.

tetragonum (tet"rah-go'num) [L.; Gr. *tetragōnon*] a square or quadrant; a quadrangular area or space. **t. lumba'le,** the quadrangular space bounded by the four lumbar muscles—by the serratus posterior inferior above, the internal oblique below, the erector spinae internally, and the external oblique externally.

tetragonus (tet"rah-go'nus) the platysma.

tetrahydric (tet″rah-hi′drik) containing four atoms of replaceable hydrogen: said of an acid or alcohol.

tetrahydrocannabinol (tet″rah-hi″dro-kah-nab′ĭ-nol) the active principle of cannabis, $C_{21}H_{30}O_2$, occurring in two isomeric forms: Δ^1-3,4-*trans* and Δ^6-3,4-*trans* tetrahydrocannabinol, both considered psychomimetically active. Abbreviated THC.

tetrahydrofolate (tet″rah-hi″dro-fo′lāt) an ester or dissociated form of tetrahydrofolic acid.

tetrahydropalmatine (tet″rah-hi″dro-pal′mah-tin) a crystalline, berberine type alkaloid, $C_{21}H_{25}NO_4$, from the roots of *Corydalis tuberosa* DC. (Fumariaceae).

tetrahydrozoline hydrochloride (tet″rah-hi-dro′zo-lēn) [USP] chemical name: 4,5-dihydro-2-(1,2,3,4-tetrahydro-1-naphthalenyl)-1*H*-imidazole monohydrochloride. An adrenergic, $C_{13}H_{16}N_2 \cdot HCl$, occurring as a white solid; applied topically to the nasal mucosa and to the conjunctiva to produce vasoconstriction.

Tetrahymena (tet″rah-hi′men-ah) a genus of ciliate protozoa of the subclass Euciliatia, which are normally free-living but are commonly found as facultative commensals in various vertebrates and invertebrates, and will become parasitic when experimentally injected into various hosts. **T. pyrifor′mis,** a species used extensively in experimental genetics.

tetraiodophenolphthalein (tet″rah-i″o-do-fe″nol-thal′e-in) chemical name: 3′,3″,5′,5″-tetraiodophenolphthalein. A dye, $C_6H_4 \cdot CO \cdot O \cdot C(C_6H_2I_2OH)_2$, which after intravenous injection is excreted in the bile in sufficient amount to make possible roentgenography of the gallbladder; it was once used in treating typhoid fever carriers.

tetraiodophthalein sodium (tet″rah-i″o-do-thal′e-in) iodophthalein sodium.

tetraiodothyronine (tet″rah-i″o-do-thi′ro-nēn) thyroxine; so called because it is formed by the conjugation of two molecules of diiodotyrosine.

tetralogy (tĕ-tral′o-je) a combination of four elements or factors, such as four concurrent symptoms or defects. **t. of Eisenmenger,** Eisenmenger's complex. **t. of Fallot,** a combination of congenital cardiac defects consisting of pulmonary stenosis, interventricular septal defect, dextroposition of the aorta so that it overrides the interventricular septum and receives venous as well as arterial blood, and right ventricular hypertrophy.

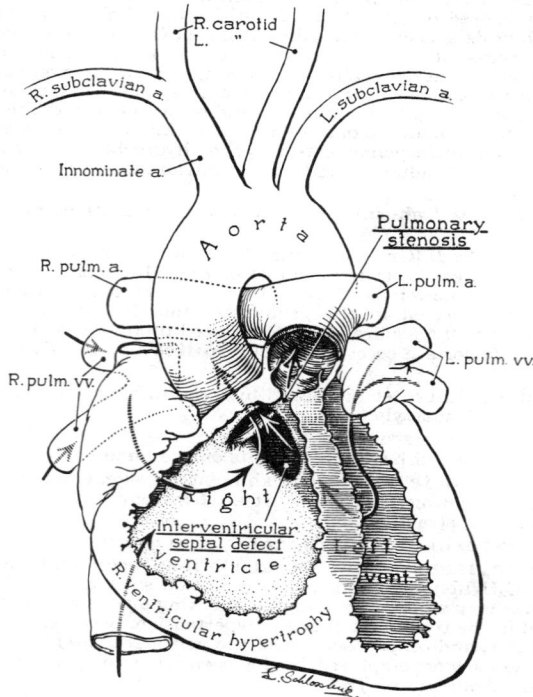

Tetralogy of Fallot. (Blalock and Taussig.)

tetramastigote (tet″rah-mas′tĭ-gōt) [*tetra-* + Gr. *mastix* lash] 1. having four flagella. 2. an organism having four flagella.

tetramazia (tet″rah-ma′ze-ah) [*tetra-* + Gr. *mazos* breast + *-ia*] the condition of having four mammary glands.

Tetrameres (tĕ-tram′er-ēz) a genus of nematode worms parasitic in the alimentary tract of chickens and other fowl. **T. america′na,** a parasite of the proventriculus of chickens and other birds.

tetrameric (tet″rah-mer′ik) having four parts.

tetramethyl (tet″rah-meth′il) a chemical compound each molecule of which contains four methyl groups.

tetramethylammonium hydroxide (tet″rah-meth″il-ah-mo′ne-um hi-drok′sīd) a toxic fraction, $N(CH_3)_4OH$, isolated from the sea anemone, *Actinia equina*, and from the salivary glands of whelks.

tetramethylenediamine (tet″rah-meth″il-ēn-di′am-in) putrescine.

tetramethylputrescine (tet″rah-meth″il-pu-tres′in) an extremely poisonous crystalline base, $N(CH_3)_2(CH_2)_4N(CH_3)_2$, derivable from putrescine; it produces symptoms like those of muscarine poisoning.

tetramine (tet′rah-mēn) tetramethylammonium hydroxide.

tetramisole hydrochloride (tĕ-tram′ĭ-sōl) chemical name: (+)-2,3,5,6-tetrahydro-6-phenylimidazo[2,1-*b*]-thiazol monohydrochloride; an anthelmintic, $C_{11}H_{12}N_2S \cdot HCl$, effective against roundworms, hookworms, and strongyloids.

Tetramitus mesnili (tĕ-tram′ĭ-tus mes-ni′le) *Chilomastix mesnili.*

tetramylose (tet-ram′ĭ-lōs) tetra-amylose.

tetranitrol (tet″rah-ni′trol) erythrityl tetranitrate.

tetranophthalmos (tet″ran-of-thal′mos) [*tetra-* + Gr. *ophthalmos* eye] a monster having four eyes.

tetranopsia (tet″ran-op′se-ah) quadrantanopia.

tetranucleotide (tet″rah-nu′kle-o-tīd) former name for nucleic acid, which was thought by Levene to be a polymer of four mononucleotides.

Tetranychus (tet-ran′ĭ-kus) [*tetra-* + Gr. *onyx* nail] a genus of mites. **T. autumna′lis,** *Trombicula autumnalis.* **T. molestis′simus,** an acarid attacking man and causing severe itching. **T. tela′rius,** the spider mite, which sometimes infests man.

Tetraodontoidea (tet-ra″o-don-toi′de-ah) a suborder of bony tropical marine fish, including puffers and sunfish; see also *tetrodotoxin* and *tetrodotoxism.*

tetraodontoxin (tet-ra″o-don-tok′sin) [*Tetraodon*, from Gr. *tetra* four + *odous* tooth, a puffer fish + *toxikon* poison] tetrodotoxin.

tetraodontoxism (tet-ra″o-don-tok′sizm) tetrodotoxism.

tetraotus (tet″rah-o′tus) [Gr. *tetraōtos* four-eared] a monster with two nearly separate heads, two faces, four eyes, and four ears.

tetraparesis (tet″rah-par′e-sis) muscular weakness affecting all four extremities.

tetrapeptide (tet″rah-pep′tid) a peptide which on hydrolysis yields four amino acids.

Tetraphyllidea (tet″rah-fil-lid′e-ah) an order of moderate-sized cestodes possessing four leaf-, trumpet-, or earlike sucking outgrowths on the scolex; the adults are intestinal parasites of elasmobranch fishes.

tetraplegia (tet″rah-ple′je-ah) [*tetra-* + Gr. *plēgē* stroke + *-ia*] paralysis of all four extremities; quadriplegia.

tetraploid (tet′rah-ploid) 1. pertaining to or characterized by tetraploidy. 2. an individual or cell having four sets of chromosomes.

tetraploidy (tet″rah-ploi″de) the state of having four sets of chromosomes (4n).

tetrapodisis (tet″rah-po-di′sis) locomotion on four feet; quadruped locomotion, as in young children.

tetrapus (tet′rah-pus) [*tetra-* + Gr. *pous* foot] a human fetus having four feet.

tetrasaccharide (tet″rah-sak′ah-rid) a carbohydrate composed of four monosaccharide groups, $C_{24}H_{42}O_{21}$.

tetrascelus (tet-ras′e-lus) [*tetra-* + Gr. *skelos* leg] a monster having four legs.

tetrasomic (tet″rah-so′mik) pertaining to or characterized by tetrasomy.

tetrasomy (tet′rah-so″me) [*tetra-* + Gr. *sōma* body] the presence of two additional chromosomes of one type in an otherwise diploid cell (2n + 2).

tetraspore (tet′rah-spōr) 1. a haploid asexual spore in the red algae, which is meiotically produced, usually in groups of four, from the carpospore. 2. in fungi, one of the spores of a four-spored basidium.

tetraster (tet-ras′ter) [*tetra-* + Gr. *astēr* star] a figure in abnormal mitosis characterized by four centrosomal centers or asters.

tetrastichiasis (tet″rah-stĭ-ki′ah-sis) [*tetra-* + Gr. *stichos* row + *-iasis*] an extremely rare condition in which there are four rows of eyelashes.

tetratomic (tet″rah-tom′ik) 1. consisting of four atoms. 2. having four replaceable atoms.

Tetratrichomonas buccalis (tet″rah-trik-om′o-nas buk-ka′lis) *Trichomonas tenax.*

tetravaccine (tet″rah-vak′sēn) a vaccine containing dead cultures of the bacteria of typhoid, paratyphoid A, paratyphoid B, and cholera.

tetravalent (tet-rav′ah-lent) having a chemical valence or combining power of four.

tetrodotoxin (tet″ro-do-tok′sin) a pure, crystalline, highly lethal neurotoxic substance, $C_{11}H_{17}N_3O_3$, present in numerous species of puffer fish of the suborder Tetraodontoidea and in newts of the genus *Taricha* (in which it is called tarichatoxin). Ingestion results, within minutes, in malaise, dizziness, and tingling about the mouth, which may be followed by ataxia, convulsions, respiratory paralysis, and death.

tetrodotoxism (tet″ro-do-tok′sizm) [*Tetraodon*, from Gr. *tetra* four + *odous* tooth, a puffer fish + *toxikon* poison] the most severe form of ichthyosarcotoxism, produced by ingestion of puffer fish which contain tetrodotoxin (q.v.).

tetronal (tet′ro-nal) diethylsulfondiethylmethane, $(C_2H_5)_2 \cdot C(SO_2C_2H_5)_2$, occurring in the form of colorless scales; it is hypnotic.

tetronerythrin (tet″ron-er′ĭ-thrin) a pigment from certain birds' feathers, mullets, and many invertebrates, e.g., lobsters.

tetrophthalmos (tet″rof-thal′mos) [*tetra-* + Gr. *ophthalmos* eye] a double-faced monster with two ears and four eyes.

tetrose (tet′rōs) a monosaccharide containing four carbon atoms in a molecule.

tetrotus (tet-ro′tus) tetraotus.

tetroxide (tĕ-trok′sīd) a compound of an element or a radical with four oxygen atoms, as osmium tetroxide.

tetrydamine (tet-tri′dah-mēn) chemical name: 4,5,6,7-tetrahydro-2*H*-methyl-3-(methylamino)-2*H*-indazole; an analgesic and anti-inflammatory, $C_9H_{15}N_3$.

tetryl (tet′ril) an organic explosive and expellant, tetra-nitromethyl-aniline, $(NO_2)_3C_6H_2N(NO)_2CH_3$, which may cause an industrial dermatitis.

tetter (tet′er) 1. a once popular name for various eczematous skin diseases. 2. a skin disease of animals communicable to man, and characterized by intense itching. **milky t.**, crusta lactea.

tetterwort (tet′ter-wort) *Sanguinaria canadensis* L. (Papaveraceae).

teucrin (tu′krin) a crystalline glycoside, $C_{21}H_{24}O_{11}$, from *Teucrium fruticans* L. (Labiatae).

Teucrium (tu′kre-um) [Gr. *teukrion* an herb of the germander kind] a genus of labiate plants called germander; generally used for their aromatic qualities.

teutlose (tūt′lōs) [Gr. *teutlon* beet] a kind of sugar found in beet root.

tewfikose (tu′fĭ-kōs) a sugar occurring in the milk of the Egyptian buffalo, *Bos bubalus*.

texis (tek′sis) [L.; Gr.] child-bearing.

textiform (teks′tĭ-form) [L. *textum* any material put together + *forma* form] formed like a tissue, network, or web.

textoblastic (teks″to-blas′tik) [L. *textum* any material put together + Gr. *blastos* germ] forming adult tissue; regenerative: said of cells.

textometer (teks″to-me′ter) [L. *textum* any material put together + Gr. *mētēr* mother] protoplasm regarded as the mother of tissues.

textural (teks′tu-ral) pertaining to the texture, or constitution, of the tissues.

texture (teks′tūr) [L. *textura*] the structure or organization of a tissue or organ.

textus (teks′tus) [L.] a tissue.

TF transfer factor.

T.F. tuberculin filtrate.

T-group training group; see *sensitivity group*, under *group*.

TGT thromboplastin generation test.

Th chemical symbol for *thorium*.

thalamectomy (thal″ah-mek′to-me) [*thalamus* + Gr. *tomē* cutting] a stereotaxic surgical technique for the discrete destruction of specific groups of cells with the thalamus, as for the relief of pain or for relief of tremor and rigidity in Parkinson's disease.

thalamencephalic (thal″ah-men″sĕ-fal′ik) pertaining to the thalamencephalon.

thalamencephalon (thal″ah-men-sef′ah-lon) [NA] the part of the diencephalon that comprises the thalamus, metathalamus, and epithalamus; called also *interbrain*.

thalami (thal′ah-mi) [L.] genitive singular and nominative plural of *thalamus*.

thalamic (thah-lam′ik) pertaining to the thalamus.

thalamocoele (thal′ah-mo-sēl″) [Gr. *thalamos* inner chamber + *koilia* hollow] the third ventricle of the brain (ventriculus tertius cerebri [NA]).

thalamocortical (thal″ah-mo-kor′tĭ-kal) pertaining to the thalamus and cerebral cortex.

thalamolenticular (thal″ah-mo-len-tik′u-lar) pertaining to the thalamus and the lenticular nucleus.

thalamomamillary (thal″ah-mo-mam′ĭ-ler″e) pertaining to the thalamus and mamillary bodies.

thalamotegmental (thal″ah-mo-teg-men′tal) pertaining to the thalamus and tegmentum.

thalamotomy (thal″ah-mot′o-me) [*thalamus* + Gr. *tomē* a cutting] a stereotaxic surgical technique for the discrete destruction of specific groups of cells within the thalamus, as for the relief of pain or for relief of tremor and rigidity in Parkinson's disease. **anterior t.**, production of lesions in the anterior nucleus of the thalamus. **dorsomedial t.**, production of lesions in the dorsomedial nucleus of the thalamus.

thalamus (thal′ah-mus), pl. *thal′ami* [L.; Gr. *thalamos* inner chamber] [NA] a constituent of the thalamencephalon, being the middle and larger portion of the diencephalon, which forms part of the lateral wall of the third ventricle and lies between the hypothalamus and the epithalamus. It comprises the medullary laminae and various nuclear groups, and is the main relay center for sensory impulses and cerebellar and basal ganglia projections to the cerebral cortex. Its nuclei include the anterior, central, intralaminar, lateral, medial, posterior, and reticular thalamic nuclei (see under *nucleus*). The lateral and medial geniculate bodies (the metathalamus) are also considered by many to be part of the thalamus. **optic t.**, corpus geniculatum laterale.

thalassanemia (thah-las″sah-ne′me-ah) thalassemia.

thalassemia (thal″ah-se′me-ah) [Gr. *thalassa* sea (because it was observed originally in persons of Mediterranean stock) + *haima* blood + *-ia*] a heterogeneous group of hereditary hemolytic anemias which have in common a decreased rate of synthesis of one or more hemoglobin polypeptide chains and are classified according to the chain involved (α, β, δ); the two major categories are α- and β-thalassemia. It is manifested in homozygotes by profound anemia or death in utero, and in heterozygotes by relatively mild red cell anomalies. **α-t.**, that caused by decreased rate of synthesis of the alpha chains of hemoglobin. The *homozygous* form is incompatible with life, the stillborn infant displaying severe hydrops fetalis. The *heterozygous* form may be asymptomatic or marked by mild anemia. **β-t.**, that caused by diminished synthesis of beta chains of hemoglobin. The *homozygous* form (Cooley's anemia; Mediterranean anemia; erythroblastic anemia of childhood; thalassemia major) in which hemoglobin A is completely absent and which appears in the newborn period, is a severe form marked by a hemolytic, hypochromic microcytic anemia, pronounced hepatosplenomegaly, skeletal deformation, mongoloid facies, and cardiac enlargement. The *heterozygous* form (thalassemia minor), in which hemoglobin A synthesis usually is retarded, is asymptomatic, but there is sometimes moderate anemia and splenomegaly. **δ-t.**, that involving suppression of the delta chains of hemoglobin, but having no clinical significance. **δ β-t.**, a form of heterozygous thalassemia in which synthesis of both delta and beta chains of hemoglobin is decreased; clinically it resembles β-thalassemia. **hemoglobin C-t.**, see under *disease*. **hemoglobin E-t.**, see under *disease*. **hemoglobin S-t.**, sickle cell–thalassemia disease. **t. interme′dia**, that which clinically appears to be intermediate between homozygous and heterozygous β-thalassemia. **t. major**, see *β-t.* **t. minor**, see *β-t.* **sickle cell–t.**, see under *disease*.

thalassin (thah-las′sin) a toxic substance derived from tentacles of the sea anemone, *Anemonia sulcata*, which, when injected into dogs, produces allergic symptoms.

thalassoposia (thah-las″so-po′ze-ah) [Gr. *thalassa* sea + *posis* drinking + *-ia*] the ingestion of sea water.

thalassotherapy (thah-las″so-ther′ah-pe) [Gr. *thalassa* sea + *therapeia* treatment] the treatment of disease by sea bathing, sea voyages, and sea air.

thalgrain (thal′grān) grain mixed with thallium sulfate; used as a poison for rodents.

thalidomide (thah-lid′o-mīd) chemical name: 2-(2,6-dioxo-3-piperidenyl)-1*H*-isoindole-1,3(2*H*)-dione. A sedative and hypnotic, $C_{13}H_{10}O_4$, commonly used in Europe in the late 1950's and early 1960's. Its use was discontinued because it was discovered to cause serious congenital anomalies in the fetus, notably amelia and phocomelia, when taken by a woman during early pregnancy. Thalidomide has been shown to be very effective in relieving severe pain associated with acute lepra reactions; it should not be used when pregnancy is possible.

thalleioquin (thal-i′o-kwin) a greenish, resinous substance, produced in a test for quinine; see under *tests*.

thallitoxicosis (thal″ĭ-tok″sĭ-ko′sis) poisoning by thallium or thallium-containing substances.

thallium (thal′e-um) [Gr. *thallos* green shoot] a heavy, soft, bluish white metal; symbol, Tl; atomic number, 81; atomic weight, 204.37; specific gravity, 11.85; its salts are active poisons. **t.-201**, a radioactive isotope of thallium having a half-life of 73.5 hours; used as a diagnostic aid in the form of thallous chloride (q.v.).

Thallophyta (tha-lof′ĭ-tah) [Gr. *thallos* green shoot + *phyton* plant] in former classifications, a taxonomic division of the plant kingdom comprising the fungi and algae, i.e., organisms possessing a thallus, and sometimes including bacteria and slime molds.

thallophyte (thal′o-fīt) [Gr. *thallos* green shoot + *phyton* plant] an individual of the Thallophyta.

thallospore (thal′o-spōr) a thallus modified to serve as an organ of reproduction.

thallotoxicosis (thal″o-tok″sĭ-ko′sis) thallitoxicosis.

thallous chloride Tl 201 (thal′us) the form in which thallium-201 in solution is injected intravenously as a diagnostic aid in scintillation scanning in myocardial disease. Called also *thallium chloride* (²⁰¹*TlCl*).

thallus (thal′us) 1. a simple plant body not differentiated into root, stem, and leaf, which is characteristic of mycelial fungi and some algae. 2. the actively growing vegetative organism as distinguished from reproductive or resting portions, as in fungi.

thalposis (thal-po′sis) [Gr. *thalpos* warmth] warmth sense; the sense which perceives warmth.

thalpotic (thal-pot′ik) pertaining to thalposis.

THAM tromethamine.

Thamnidium (tham-nid′e-um) [Gr. *thamnos* bush] a genus of molds of the family Mucoraceae, order Mucorales, which resembles *Mucor* and which is often found growing on meat in cold storage. It can grow at 28° F. and forms a profuse hairy growth. The species most frequently found are *T. elegans* and *T. chaetocladioides*.

thamuria (tham-u′re-ah) [Gr. *thamys* often + *ouron* urine + *-ia*] frequency of urination.

thanato- (than′ah-to) [Gr. *thanatos* death] a combining form denoting relationship to death.

thanatobiologic (than″ah-to-bi″o-loj′ik) [*thanato-* + Gr. *bios* life + *-logy*] pertaining to death and life.

thanatognomonic (than″ah-to-no-mon′ik) [*thanato-* + Gr. *gnōmonikos* decisive] indicating the approach of death.

thanatoid (than′ah-toid) [*thanato-* + Gr. *eidos* form] resembling death.

thanatology (than″ah-tol′o-je) the medicolegal study of death and conditions affecting dead bodies.

thanatometer (than″ah-tom′ĕ-ter) [*thanato-* + Gr. *metron* measure] a thermometer used to prove the occurrence of death by registering the reduction of the bodily temperature.

thanatophidia (than″ah-to-fid′e-ah) [*thanato-* + Gr. *ophis* snake] the venomous snakes collectively; toxicophidia.

thanatophidial (than″ah-to-fid′e-al) pertaining to venomous snakes.

thanatophoric (than″ah-to-fōr′ik) [*thanato-* + Gr. *pherein* to bear] deadly; lethal.

thanatopsia, thanatopsy (than″ah-top′se-ah; than′ah-top″se) [*thanato-* + Gr. *opsis* view] necropsy.

thanatosis (than″ah-to′sis) gangrene or necrosis.

Thane's method (thānz) [Sir George Dancer *Thane*, British anatomist, 1850–1930] see under *method.*

Thapsia (thap′se-ah) [L.; Gr. *thapsia;* named from the isle of *Thapsus*] a genus of umbelliferous plants. *T. garganica* L. (Umbelliferae), of Northern Africa, affords an irritant resin somewhat used in plasters; the plant is locally employed as a polychrest remedy.

thaumatropy (thaw-mat′ro-pe) [Gr. *thauma* wonder + *tropos* a turning] the transformation of an organ or structure into another organ or structure.

thaumaturgic (thaw″mah-ter′jik) [Gr. *thauma* wonder + *ergon* work] working wonders; magical; miraculous.

Thaysen's disease (thi′senz) [Thornwald Einar Hess *Thaysen,* Copenhagen physician, 1883–1936] nontropical sprue.

THC tetrahydrocannabinol.

thea (the′ah) [L.] tea.

theaism (the′ah-izm) a morbid condition resulting from ingestion of excessive quantities of tea.

thebaic (the-ba′ik) [L. *Thebaicus* Theban, named for Thebes, where opium was once prepared] pertaining to or derived from opium.

thebaine (the-ba′in) a crystalline, poisonous, and anodyne alkaloid from opium, $C_{19}H_{21}NO_3$, having properties similar to those of strychnine; called also *dimethyl morphine.*

thebesian (the-be′ze-an) named for or described by Adam Christian *Thebesius,* German physician, 1686–1732, as *thebesian foramen* (foramina venarum minimarum cordis), *thebesian valve* (valvula sinus coronarii), and *thebesian veins* (venae cordis minimae).

theca (the′kah), pl. *the′cae* [L.; Gr. *thēkē*] an enclosing case or sheath, as of an ovarian follicle or tendon. **t. cor′dis,** pericardium. **t. exter′na,** tunica externa thecae folliculi. **t. of follicle,** t. folliculi. **t. of follicle of von Baer,** tunica externa thecae folliculi. **t. follic′uli** [NA], an envelope of condensed connective tissue surrounding a vesicular ovarian follicle, comprising an internal vascular layer and an external fibrous layer. **t. inter′na,** tunica interna thecae folliculi. **t. medulla′re spina′lis,** dura mater of the spinal cord. **t. vertebra′lis,** dura mater of the spinal cord.

thecae (the′se) [L.] plural of *theca.*

thecal (the′kal) pertaining to a theca.

thecitis (the-si′tis) inflammation of the sheath of a tendon; tenosynovitis.

thecodont (the′ko-dont) [Gr. *thēkē* sheath + *odous* tooth] having the teeth inserted in sockets or alveoli.

thecoma (the-ko′mah) a theca cell tumor.

thecomatosis (the″ko-mah-to′sis) diffuse hyperplasia of the ovarian stroma.

thecostegnosis (the″ko-steg-no′sis) [Gr. *thēkē* sheath + *stegnōsis* narrowing] contraction of a tendon sheath.

Theden's bandage (ta′denz) [Johann Christian Anton *Theden,* German surgeon, 1714–1797] see under *bandage.*

Theelin (the′lin) trademark for preparations of estrone.

Theile's canal, glands (ti′lez) [Friedrich Wilhelm *Theile,* German anatomist, 1801–1879] see under *canal* and *gland.*

Theiler's disease, virus [Max *Theiler,* microbiologist and physician in U.S., born 1899 in South Africa; winner of the Nobel prize for medicine and physiology in 1951] see under *disease* and *virus.*

Theileria (thi-le′re-ah) [Sir Arnold *Theiler,* Swiss microbiologist, 1867–1936] a genus of minute intraerythrocytic protozoan parasites of the family Babesiidae, order Haemosporidia. **T. annula′ta,** *T. parva.* **T. dis′par,** *T. parva.* **T. hir′ci,** a species that causes a fatal disease in sheep and goats. **T. par′va,** a species causing a disease of cattle in Africa which is similar to Texas cattle fever and cattle anemia; called also *T. annulata* and *T. dispar.* See *East Coast fever,* under *fever.* **T. tsutsugamu′shi,** *Rickettsia tsutsugamushi.*

theileriasis (thi″lĕ-ri′ah-sis) infection with *Theileria.*

theine (the′in) the alkaloid of tea, isomeric with caffeine.

theinism (the′in-izm) theaism.

thelalgia (the-lal′je-ah) [Gr. *thēlē* nipple + *algos* pain + *-ia*] pain in the nipple.

thelarche (the-lar′ke) [Gr. *thēlē* nipple + *archē* beginning] the beginning of development of the breasts at puberty.

Thelazia (the-la′ze-ah) a genus of nematode worms of the superfamily Spiruroidea, which are allied to Filaria. Several species (*T. callipaeda, T. californiensis*) are parasitic in the eyes of animals.

thelaziasis (the″la-zi′ah-sis) infection of the eye with *Thelazia.*

theleplasty (the′le-plas″te) [Gr. *thēlē* nipple + *plassein* to form] a plastic operation upon the nipple.

thelerethism (thel-er′ĕ-thizm) [Gr. *thēlē* nipple + *erethisma* a stirring up] erection or protrusion of the nipple.

thelitis (the-li′tis) [Gr. *thēlē* nipple + *-itis*] inflammation of a nipple; mamillitis.

thelium (the′le-um), pl. *the′lia* [L.] 1. a papilla. 2. a nipple.

Thelohania (the″lo-ha′ne-ah) a genus of sporozoa of the order Microsporidia, which are parasitic in the larvae of the mosquito, *Culex pipiens.*

thelorrhagia (the″lo-ra′je-ah) hemorrhage from the nipple.

thelothism, thelotism (the′lo-thizm; the′lo-tizm) thelerethism.

thelyblast (thel′e-blast) [Gr. *thēlys* female + *blastos* germ] the female pronucleus.

thelyblastic (thel″e-blas′tik) pertaining to or of the nature of a thelyblast (female pronucleus).

thelygenic (the″le-jen′ik) [Gr. *thēlys* female + *gennan* to produce] producing only female offspring.

thelykinin (the″le-ki′nin) estrone.

thelytocia (thel′e-to′she-ah) [Gr. *thēlys* female + *tokos* birth] normal parthenogenesis producing females only.

thelytocous (the-lit′o-kus) pertaining to or characterized by thelytocia.

thelytoky (the-lit′o-ke) thelytocia.

Themison (them′ĭ-son) **of Laodicea** (1st century B.C.) a Greek physician who founded the Methodist school of medicine.

thenad (the′nad) toward the thenar eminence or toward the palm.

thenal (the′nal) pertaining to the palm or thenar.

thenar (the′nar) [Gr.] 1. [NA] the mound on the palm at the base of the thumb; called also *thenar eminence.* 2. pertaining to the palm.

thenium closylate (then′ĭ-um klo′sĭ-lāt) chemical name: dimethyl(2-phenoxyethyl)-2-thenylammonium *p*-chlorobenzenesulfonate; a veterinary anthelmintic, $C_{21}H_{24}ClNO_4S_2$.

thenyldiamine hydrochloride (then″il-di′ah-mēn) chemical name: *N,N*-dimethyl-*N*²-2-pyridinyl-*N*²-(3-thienylmethyl)-1,2-ethanediamine hydrochloride. An antihistamine, $C_{14}H_{19}N_3S \cdot HCl$, used for preoperative sedation, to control postoperative nausea, and to potentiate the action of analgesics.

Thenylene (then′ĭ-lĕn) trademark for a preparation of methapyrilene.

thenylpyramine (then″il-pir′ah-mēn) methapyrilene.

Theobaldia (the″o-bal′de-ah) [Frederic Vincent *Theobald,* British zoologist, 1868–1930] *Culiseta.*

Theobroma (the″o-bro′mah) [Gr. *theos* god + *brōma* food] a genus of sterculiaceous plants; the cacao. The seeds of *T. cacao* L. (called theobroma and cacao) contain the alkaloid theobromine, and are used in the preparation of cacao and chocolate.

theobromine (the″o-bro′min) chemical name: 3,7-dimethylxanthine. A white crystalline alkaloid, $C_7H_8N_4O_2$, prepared from the dried ripe seed of *Theobroma cacao*, or made synthetically from xanthine. It has physiologic properties similar to those of caffeine, and is used as a diuretic and smooth muscle relaxant and as a myocardial stimulant and vasodilator. Derivatives such as t. calcium salicylate, t. sodium acetate, t. sodium salicylate, t. sodium formate, and t. salicylate are available for use.

Theoglycinate (the″o-gli′sĭ-nāt) trademark for a preparation of theophylline sodium glycinate.

theolin (the′o-lin) a colorless, volatile liquid hydrocarbon, heptane, C_7H_{16}, obtainable from petroleum, etc.; it resembles benzine and has similar uses.

theophylline (the-of′ĭ-lin) [L. *thea* tea + Gr. *phyllon* leaf] [USP] chemical name: 3,7-dihydro-1,3-dimethyl-1*H*-purine-2,6-dione. A xanthine derivative, $C_7H_8N_4 \cdot H_2O$, found in tea leaves and prepared synthetically; it is a smooth muscle relaxant, used chiefly for its bronchodilator effect for the symptomatic treatment of chronic obstructive pulmonary emphysema, bronchial asthma, chronic bronchitis, and bronchospastic disorders; administered orally. It also may be used for its myocardial stimulant and coronary vasodilator actions, diuretic action, and respiratory center stimulant effect. **t. aminoisobutanol,** ambuphylline. **t. cholinate,** oxtriphylline. **t. ethanolamine,** t. olamine. **t. ethylenediamine,** aminophylline. **t. monoethanolamine,** t. olamine. **t. olamine** [USP], a compound containing theophylline (about 75 per cent) and monoethanolamine; used chiefly for its smooth muscle relaxant activity in the treatment of acute bronchial asthma and bronchospasm associated with chronic bronchitis and emphysema, administered rectally. Called also *t. ethanolamine* and *t. monoethanolamine.* **t. sodium acetate,** a hydrated mixture containing theophylline sodium and sodium acetate in approximately equimolecular proportions, and yielding 55 to 65 per cent of anhydrous theophylline; used as a smooth muscle relaxant and also as a diuretic. **t. sodium glycinate** [USP], an equilibrium mixture containing theophylline sodium and aminoacetic acid in approximately equal proportions, and yielding 49 to 52 per cent theophylline; used chiefly as a smooth muscle relaxant for the symptomatic treatment of bronchial asthma, administered orally.

Theorell (the″o-rel′), Axel Hugo Teodor. Swedish biochemist, born 1903; winner of the Nobel prize in medicine and physiology for 1955, for his discoveries concerning the nature and mode of action of oxidation enzymes.

theorem (the′o-rem) [Gr. *theorēma* a principle arrived at by speculation] a proposition capable of demonstration. **Gibbs's t.,** substances which lower the surface tension of the pure dispersion medium tend to collect on its surface. **Hazen's t.,** the proposition that for every death from typhoid fever avoided by the purification of public water supplies two or three deaths are avoided from other causes.

theory (the′o-re) [Gr. *theōria* speculation as opposed to practice] 1. the doctrine or the principles underlying an art as distinguished from the practice of that particular art. 2. a formulated hypothesis, or, loosely speaking, any hypothesis or opinion not based upon actual knowledge. **Adami's t.,** a hypothesis for the explanation of heredity, resembling Ehrlich's side-chain theory of immunity. **Adler's t.,** the theory that neuroses are developed as compensations for a social or physical inferiority. **aging t. of atherosclerosis,** a theory that atherosclerosis is an inevitable consequence of aging and therefore an irreversible process. **Altmann's t.,** a theory that protoplasm is made up of granular particles (bioblasts) grouped in masses and enclosed in indifferent matter. **apposition t.,** the theory that tissues grow by the deposit of cells from without. **Arrhenius' t.,** the theory of electrolytic dissociation. **atomic t.,** the theory that the molecules of a substance are made up of one or more atoms, each representing a definite amount of the element, which amount does not vary in the molecule, whatever combinations the molecule may enter. **avalanche t.,** the theory that nervous influence increases in force as it descends along an efferent nerve. **Bolk's retardation t.,** the theory that man, in his development, is at a stage which, in the higher primates, is still a fetal stage. **Bowman's t.** (*of urinary secretion*), the theory that water and inorganic salts are secreted by the glomeruli, whereas the urea and related bodies are secreted by the epithelial cells in the convoluted tubes. Cf. *Ludwig's t.* **brunonian t.,** brunonianism. **Buergi's t.,** two different substances causing identical therapeutic manifestations when combined are increased in their effects if they possess identical pharmacologic points of attack. **cell t.,** the doctrine that all living matter is composed of cells and that cell activity is the essential process of life. **cell-chain t.,** the theory that the nerve fiber consists of a chain of special cells which have only secondarily been brought into relation with the central cell. **chemicoparasitic t.,** the theory that dental caries is caused by combined chemical and microbial action. **cloaca t.,** in psychoanalysis, the fantasy of young children and some

schizophrenics that babies are expelled through the anal canal. **clonal-selection t. of immunity,** a selective theory of antibody formation proposed by Burnet, according to which a complement of clones of lymphoid cells capable of reacting with all possible antigenic determinants is present in the normal individual. During fetal life, those clones that react against self-antigens are suppressed on contact with antigen. By contrast, there occurs a change in the response to contact with antigen following birth, when the normal response is proliferation, antibody formation, and cell-mediated immunity. Thus, suppression of clones leads to the development of immunological tolerance. If suppressed clones against self-antigens again become active at some time later in life, autoimmune disease may result. **closed circulation t.,** one of the theories explaining how the blood in the spleen gets from the arteries to the venous sinuses; it holds that the capillaries empty directly into the venous sinuses. Cf. *open circulation t.* and *closed-open circulation t.* Called also *fast circulation t.* **closed-open circulation t.,** the theory that both an open and a closed circulation are present in the spleen; e.g., a closed circulation in a contracted spleen may become an open circulation when the organ is distended. Cf. *closed circulation t. and open circulation t.* **Cohnheim's t.,** 1. the theory that the emigration of leukocytes is the essential feature of inflammation. 2. the theory that tumors develop from embryonic rests which do not participate in the formation of normal surrounding tissue. **contractile ring t.,** a theory advanced to explain the formation of a furrow in a dividing cell. According to this theory, the gelated ring in the cortex of the dividing cell contracts (cortical gel contraction) like the nonmotile portion of an amoeba, and, therefore, decreases the surface area. Actually, however, before division the surface increases by about 26 per cent. **convergence-projection t.,** a theory advanced as an explanation for reference of pain, according to which some visceral afferent nerve fibers converge with cutaneous pain afferents to end upon the same neuron at some point in the sensory pathway. **core conductor t.,** a theory regarding the development of electrotonic potentials and their associated currents along nerve fibers, according to which the nerve fibers are considered to be core conductors, i.e., cylinders of conducting fluid material with a sheath of high electrical resistance, surrounded by a layer of conducting medium. **darwinian t.,** see *darwinism.* **De Vries' t.,** t. of mutations. **Dieulafoy's t.,** the theory that appendicitis is always due to the appendix becoming a closed cavity. **dimer t.,** the theory that the tooth organ of primates is composed of two halves, each of which is a representative of an independent tooth in the lower orders of animals. **dualistic t.,** the theory that the blood cells arise from two distinct types of primitive cells, the myeloblasts and lymphoblasts. Cf. *monophyletic t., polyphyletic t.,* and *trialistic t.* **ectopic focus t.,** a theory advanced by Rothberger, which states that atrial fibrillation arises as a result of rapid discharges from an ectopic focus. **Ehrlich's biochemical t.,** the theory that specific chemical affinity exists between the substance of specific living cells and specific chemical substances. **Ehrlich's side-chain t.,** a theory advanced regarding the phenomena concerned in immunity and cytolysis. According to this theory, the protoplasm of the body cells contains highly complex organic molecules, consisting of a tolerably stable central group, to which are attached less stable lateral chains (or side chains) of atoms or atomic groups. The ordinary chemical transformations in the protoplasm are carried on by means of these lateral chains (or *receptors*), the stable center of the molecule remaining unaffected. The lateral chains contain a group of atoms (*haptophore group*), which is capable of uniting with similar groups in toxins, bacterial cells, and foreign cells. See also *amboceptor* and *complement.* **electron t.,** all bodies are complex structures composed of small particles called atoms together with still smaller particles called electrons. **emergency t.,** Cannon's theory that the adrenal medulla is stimulated to secrete by activity on the part of the sympathetic nervous system in conditions of emotional excitement, pain, etc.; or, in other words, to meet bodily emergencies. **emigration t.,** Cohnheim's t., def. 1. **encrustation t.,** a theory advanced by Rokitansky, which states that fibrinous material derived from the blood is deposited on the inner surface of the intima of vessels and that fatty metamorphosis occurs secondarily in this deposit. **equilibrium t.,** a theory that the number of breeding species in a biome is a result of the rate of immigration of new species and the rate of extinction. **expanding surface t.,** a theory of cell division which postulates that a nuclear substance is liberated, probably from chromosomes, which causes expansion of the cellular membrane at the poles; as the polar areas expand, the equator contracts, leading to division. **fast circulation t.,** closed circulation t. **Flourens' t.,** the opinion that the entire cerebrum is concerned in each and every psychic operation or process, as opposed to the phrenologic views of Gall. **frequency t.,** a theory which postulates that the pattern of excitation of auditory nerve fibers is more important in perception of pitch than is the excitation of any of the fibers in any particular area of the cochlear basilar membrane. Cf. *place t.* **Frerichs' t.,** the theory that uremia is really a poisoning by ammonium carbonate formed by the action on urea of an enzyme contained in the blood. **gate t., gate-control t.,** neural impulses generated by noxious painful stimuli and transmitted to the spinal cord by small-diameter C-fibers and A-delta fibers are blocked at their synapses in the dorsal horn by the simultaneous stimulation of large-diameter myelinated A-fibers, thus inhibiting pain by preventing pain impulses from reaching higher levels of the central nervous system. Called also *gate hypothesis.* **germ t.,** the doctrine that infectious diseases are of microbic origin. **germ layer t.,** the teaching that the embryo develops three primary germ layers, each of which gives rise to definite organ derivatives. **gestalt t.,** see *gestaltism.* **Golgi's t.,** the theory that the neurons communicate by the axons of Golgi's cells and the collaterals of the axons of Deiters' cells. **Goltz's t.,** the theory that the function of the semicircular canals is to transmit sensations of position, and thus materially aid in the sense of equilibrium. **ground water t.,** Pettenkofer's t. **Helmholtz t.,** a theory of sound perception: each basilar fiber responds sympathetically to a definite tone and stimulates the hair cells of Corti's organ, which rest upon the fiber. The nerve impulse from this stimulation of the hair cells is carried to the brain. **Hering's t.,** the doctrine that color sensation depends on decomposition and restitution of the visual substance: disassimilation producing red, yellow, and white, and restitution producing blue, green, and black. **hit t.,** target t. **humoral t.,** the ancient theory that the body contains four humors—blood, phlegm, yellow bile, and black bile—health being the result of their proper adjustment, and disease resulting from their imbalance or irregular distribution. See also *humoralism.* **incasement t.,** the formerly advocated theory that all animals and plants develop from preexisting germs, and that they encase the germs of all future generations, one within another. **information t.,** a system for analyzing, chiefly by statistical methods, the characteristics of communicated messages and the systems that encode, transmit, distort, receive, and decode them. **ionic t.,** a theory that, on going into solution, the molecules of an electrolyte either completely or partially break up or dissociate into two or more portions, these portions being positively and negatively charged electrically, the positively charged portions being different chemically from those negatively charged. When an electric current is passed through the solution of an electrolyte the positively charged portions are attracted by the negative pole or electrode, and move toward it; the negatively charged portions are attracted by and migrate toward the positive electrode. From this property of moving toward one of the electrodes, these charged molecular fractions of electrolytes are called ions, from the Greek verb meaning "to move." **James-Lange t.,** the theory that emotion is the sensory awareness of response to the emotion-provoking stimulus, particularly autonomic response; e.g., we feel sad *because* we cry. **Kern plasma relation t.,** the theory that for each cell there exists a definite size relation of nuclear mass to cell mass. **Ladd-Franklin t.** (*of color vision*), that red, green, and blue stimulating substances are liberated in the nerve endings by suitable light waves from a complex photosensitive molecule. **Lamarck's t.,** the theory that acquired characteristics may be transmitted. **lateral-chain t.,** Ehrlich's side-chain t. **Liebig's t.,** the hydrocarbons which oxidize easily are the foods which produce animal heat. **local circuit t.,** in neurophysiology, the theory that current flows from the unstimulated, positively charged areas of the cell membrane of a neuron to the stimulated, depolarized or negative portion, and that as each new area becomes depolarized or negative, it in turn acts as the sink toward which the current flows from the adjacent area, which results in progressive depolarization, or reversal charge, along the neuron from the point of stimulation; the source of the current is the flow of Na^+ into the cell. **Ludwig's t.** (*of urinary secretion*), the theory that urine is formed by the simple process of filtration in the glomeruli and that reabsorption occurs in the urinary tubules by the process of diffusion. Cf. *Bowman's t.* **MacDougal's t.,** the hypothesis that many, if not all variations in nature are formed by chemical modifications of the germ cells. **t. of medicine,** the body of principles of the science and art of medicine as distinguished from the *practice of medicine,* or the application of those principles in actual practice. **membrane ionic t.,** the theory that the resting potential difference between the inside and outside of the cell is related to (1) the thin, electrically insulating membrane between the cytoplasm and the interstitial conducting medium, which is poorly and variably permeable to diverse ions; (2) the presence of a metabolic cellular pump that promotes the efflux of sodium ions from the cell interior to the outside against its electrochemical gradient and, coupled with this, the influx of potassium ions into the cell against its ionic concentration gradient. **mendelian t.,** see *Mendel's law,* under *law.* **metabolic t. of atherosclerosis,** a theory that atherosclerosis is caused by a disturbance in lipid metabolism, specifically cholesterol metabolism. **Metchnikoff's (Mechnikov's) t.,** the theory that bacteria and other harmful elements in the body are attached and destroyed by cells called phagocytes, and that the contest between such harmful elements and the phagocytes produces inflammation. **migration t.** (*obs.*), the theory that sympathetic ophthalmia is produced by migration of the pathogenic agent through the lymph channels of the optic nerve. **mnemic t.,** the theory that the cell has an inherited "memory" of the influences that are brought to bear upon it, and that consequently it tends to inherit acquired characteristics; called also *Semon-Hering hypothesis.* **Monakow's t.,** the theory of diaschisis; see *diaschisis.* **monophyletic t.,** the theory that all forms of blood cells, both red and white, have their origin in one and the same form of primordial blood cell (hemocytoblast), the several types of cells arising by a process of differentiation. Called also *unitarian t.* Cf. *dualistic t., polyphyletic t.,* and *trialistic t.* **t. of mutations,** the theory of heredity according to which the variability in the germ plasm is such that it may at times give rise not to fluctuating variations, but to marked and permanent variations, and these latter, if advantageous to the animal, are preserved by natural selection. Such permanent variations are called mutations or sports. Called also *De Vries' t.* **myogenic t.,** the theory that the muscle fibers of the heart possess in themselves the power of originating and maintaining the contraction of the heart. **neuron t.** (Waldeyer, 1801), the obsolete theory that the nervous system consists of innumerable neurons in contiguity, but not in continuity. See *neuron.* **open circulation t.,** one of the theories explaining how the blood in the spleen gets from the arteries to the venous sinuses; it holds that the capillaries open directly into the pulp reticulum, and that the blood gradually filters back into the venous sinuses. Called also *slow circulation t.* Cf. *closed circulation t.* and *closed-open circulation t.* **open-closed circulation t.,** see *closed-open circulation t.* **overproduction t.,** see *Weigert's law,* under *law.* **paralytic t.,** the doctrine that hyperemia is the most essential fact of inflammation, and is caused by paralysis of the vasomotor nerves. **Pasteur's t.,** the theory that the immunity secured by an attack of a disease is caused by the exhaustion of material needed for the growth of the organism of the disease; called also *t. of exhaustion of the medium.* **Pettenkofer's t.,** the theory that epidemics, as of typhoid fever, occur at the time when the ground water is at a low level; and that bacteria of the disease do not pass directly from the sick to the healthy, but pass into the soil, where they ripen when the soil is dry. **phlogiston t.,** see *phlogiston.* **pithecoid t.,** the theory that man is descended from apelike ancestors. **place t.,** a theory of pitch perception which postulates that excitation of specific areas of the basilar membrane of the cochlea determine the pitch that is perceived. Cf. *frequency t.* **Planck's t.,** quantum t. **point de repère t.,** the theory that there is always an external object, however small, to serve as a starting point for hallucination or for illusion (Binet). **polarization-membrane t.,** the theory that living, resting cells are surrounded by a semipermeable membrane lined by a series of electrical doublets, or dipoles, with negative charges on the inner and positive charges on the outer surface. When the membrane is electrically intact, its entire surface is surrounded by doublets, and is said to be polarized. **polyphyletic t.,** the theory that the various corpuscles and cells of the blood have their origin from two or more distinct varieties of primordial (mother) cells. Cf. *dualistic t., monophyletic t.,* and *trialistic t.* **P. O. U. t.,** Ishihara's theory of the placenta-ovary-uterus production of internal secretion. **preformation t.,** the outmoded theory that the individuals of successive generations are contained, completely formed, within the reproductive cell of one of the parents. **proteomorphic t.,** the theory that immunity against bacterial infection is handled by the hematopoietic system primarily, and secondarily by all the cells of the body, the waste products of the process being excreted by the liver. **quantum t.,** the theory that the radiation and absorption of energy take place in definite quantities called quanta (E) which vary in size and are defined by the equation $E = h\nu$, in which h is Planck's constant and ν is the frequency of the radiation. **recapitulation t.,** ontogeny recapitulates phylogeny; that is, an organism in the course of its development goes through the same successive stages as did the species in developing from the lower to the higher forms of animal life. Called also *biogenetic law* and *Haeckel's law.* **t. of reentry,** the theory that the sinus impulse preceding the premature beat activates the heart, but the activation wave is delayed in an area of diminished irritability; see *reentry.* **resonance t.,** 1. Helmholtz theory. 2. the theory of specificity which assumes that the surface forces of reacting substances must harmonize. **Ribbert's t.,** a tumor is formed from the development of cell rests owing to reduced tension in the surrounding tissues. **Schiefferdecker's symbiosis t.,** the theory that among the tissues of the body there is a sort of symbiosis, so that the products of metabolism in one tissue serve as a stimulus to the activities of other tissues. **Schön's t.,** the theory (of ocular accommodation) that the ciliary muscle exerts on the lens the same effect as is produced on a rubber ball held in both hands and compressed by the fingers. **Semon-Hering t.,** mnemic t. **side-chain t.,** Ehrlich's side-chain t. **single hit t.,** the theory that hemolysis results from a single complement-induced lesion of the erythrocyte surface, rather than that lesions at several sites are necessary. **sliding filament t.,** 1. a theory which postulates that the thin and thick filaments of a myofibril slide past each other, while maintaining their length, during muscle contraction. 2. a theory that postulates that contraction of cilia involves a sliding of filaments (microtubules) in a manner comparable to the sliding filament mechanism for the contraction of muscle (see def. 1). **slow circulation t.,** open circulation t. **spindle elongation t.,** the theory which suggests that the spindle and asters have a decisive role in cell division. The theory is based on the observation that the elongation of the cell at anaphase is accompanied by a shrinkage at the equator. The centers are believed to be pushed apart by the spindle tubules, since the spindles and asters appear to be rigid structures. **Spitzer's t.,** the formation of the septa in the heart are teleologically conditioned, phylogenetically brought about, and mechanically achieved by the appearance and development of the lungs through phylogeny. **target t.,** the theory advanced to explain some biological effects of radiation on the basis of ionization occurring in a very small sensitive region within the cell, which postulates that one or more ionizing events, or "hits," within the sensitive volume are necessary to bring about the biological end-effect; called also *hit t.* **thermostat t.,** a theory which suggests that the feeding and satiety centers of the brain, like the thermoregulatory centers, are sensitive to body temperature; a decrease in body temperature activates the feeding center and depresses the satiety center, whereas increased temperature acts on the centers in the opposite way. **Traube's resonance t.,** resonance t., def. 2. **trialistic t.,** the theory that the blood cells arise from three distinct types of primitive cells, the myeloblasts, lymphoblasts, and monocytes. Cf. *dualistic t., monophyletic t.,* and *polyphyletic t.* **undulatory t.,** wave t. **unitarian t.,** monophyletic t. **unitary t.,** the theory that disease is single in its nature and is not made up of separate and distinct morbid entities. **Villemin's t.,** the theory of the infectiousness and specificity of tuberculosis held before the discovery of the bacillus. **Wagner's t.,** migration t. **wave t.,** theory that light, heat, and electricity are transmitted through space in the form of waves. **Weismann's t.,** see *weismannism.* **Woods-Fildes t.,** the theory that the antibacterial activity of at least some chemotherapeutic drugs (especially the sulfonamides) is a consequence of a competitive inhibition of essential metabolic reactions of the microorganism. **Young-Helmholtz t.,** the doctrine that color vision depends on three sets of retinal fibers, corresponding to the colors red, green, and violet. **Zuntz's t.,** a theory of muscle contraction.

theotherapy (the″o-ther′ah-pe) [Gr. *theos* god + *therapeia* treatment] the treatment of disease by prayer and religious exercises.

Thephorin (thef′o-rin) trademark for preparations of phenindamine tartrate.

theque (tĕk) [Fr. a "box or small chest"] a round or oval collection, or nest, of melanin-containing nevus cells occurring at the dermoepidermal junction of the skin or in the dermis proper.

therapeusis (ther″ah-pu′sis) therapeutics.

therapeutic (ther″ah-pu′tik) [Gr. *therapeutikos* inclined to serve] 1. pertaining to therapeutics, or to the art of healing. 2. curative.

therapeutics (ther″ah-pu′tiks) 1. the science and art of healing. 2. a scientific account of the treatment of disease. **alimentary t.,** treatment by careful regulation of the diet. **cellular t.,** organotherapy. **dental t.,** that branch of dentistry which deals with the treatment of diseases of the teeth. **empiric t.,** treatment by remedies that experience has proved to be useful. **massive sterilizing t.,** therapia sterilisans magna. **mediate t.,** medication of a nursing child through its mother's milk, the remedy being administered to the mother. **mental t.,** treatment directed to influencing the mind, including hypnotic suggestion, etc. **rational t.,** treatment based upon a knowledge of the disease and of the action of the remedies employed. **ray t.,** therapy utilizing radiation from some part of the electromagnetic spectrum. **specific t.,** see under *therapy.* **stomatologic t.,** the treatment of diseases of the mouth. **testicular t.,** treatment by the hypodermic injection of testicular extract. **vibratory t.,** treatment by vibrations of various kinds, as by vibratory motions in massage.

therapeutist (ther″ah-pu′tist) therapist.

Theraphosidae (ther″ah-fo′sĭ-de) a family of very large hairy spiders (suborder Orthognatha) found in temperate and tropical areas. *Sericopelma communis* is the only species whose venom has a harmful effect on man, but some are capable of inflicting painful bites. The members of this family are sometimes improperly called tarantulas.

therapia (ther″ah-pi′ah) [L.; Gr.] therapy. **t. sterili′sans mag′na,** Ehrlich's procedure of treatment by the use of some chemical agent which will destroy the parasites in the body of a patient without being seriously toxic for the patient.

therapist (ther′ah-pist) [Gr. *therapeutēs* one who attends to the sick] a person skilled in the treatment of disease; often combined with a term indicating the specific type of disorder treated (as *speech therapist*) or a particular type of treatment rendered (as *physical therapist*). **physical t.,** a person skilled in the techniques of physical therapy and qualified to administer treatments prescribed by a physician and under his supervision; called also *physiotherapist.* **speech t.,** a person specially trained and qualified to assist patients in overcoming speech and language disorders.

therapy (ther′ah-pe) [Gr. *therapeia* service done to the sick] the treatment of disease; therapeutics. See also under *treatment.*

anticoagulant t., the use of drugs to render the blood sufficiently incoagulable to discourage thrombosis. **autoserum t.,** treatment of disease by the injection of the patient's own blood serum. **aversion t.,** therapy directed at associating an undesirable behavior pattern with unpleasant stimulation or at making the unpleasant stimulation a consequence of the undesirable behavior. **bacterial t.,** opsonic t. **beam t.,** 1. treatment by exposure to light from one of the colors of the spectrum. 2. treatment by radiation emitted from a source located at a distance from the body. **behavior t.,** a therapeutic approach in which the focus is on the patient's observable behavior, rather than on conflicts and unconscious processes presumed to underlie his maladaptive behavior. This is accomplished through systematic manipulation of the environmental and behavioral variables related to the specific behavior to be modified; operant conditioning, systematic desensitization, token economy, aversive control, flooding, and implosion are examples of techniques that may be used in behavior therapy. Called also *behavior modification* and *conditioning therapy.* **biological t.,** treatment of disease by the injection of the substances which produce a biological reaction in the organism. The term includes the use of sera, antitoxins, vaccines, and nonspecific proteins. **buffer t.,** intravenous injection of buffer substances, such as sodium bicarbonate, with the object of lowering the hydrogen ion concentration. **carbon dioxide t.,** a form of (rarely used) shock therapy employed to produce emotional abreactions and relieve anxiety, in which unconsciousness is induced by the administration of carbon dioxide gas by inhalation. **carbonic t.,** the administration of carbon dioxide for starting respiration in newborn infants and for resuscitating persons overcome by asphyxiating. **Chaoul t.,** short source-to-tissue distance, low-voltage roentgen therapy; see also under *tube.* **collapse t.,** treatment of pulmonary tuberculosis by operative collapse of the diseased lung; called also *collapsotherapy.* Cf. *artificial pneumothorax,* under *pneumothorax,* and *Forlanini's treatment,* under *treatment.* **conditioning t.,** behavior t. **convulsive shock t.,** electroconvulsive t. **corrective t.,** the planning and administration of progressive physical exercise and activities most effective in improving or maintaining general physical and emotional health, through individual or group participation. **Curie t.,** treatment with a radioactive source, e.g., radium. **deep roentgen-ray t.,** treatment by x-radiations generated by at least 150 kilovolts and capable of penetrating significantly below the skin level. **deleading t.,** the use of chelating agents in the mobilization and excretion from the body of heavy metals, such as lead, radium, etc. **diathermic t.,** treatment by thermopenetration; see *diathermy.* **duplex t.,** treatment by diathermic and galvanic currents in combination, both currents being passed through the body at the same time by way of the same two electrodes. **electric convulsive t.,** electroconvulsive t. **electroconvulsive t. (E.C.T.), electroshock t. (E.S.T.),** a form of shock therapy that is most effective in the treatment of depression, in which unconsciousness and/or convulsions are induced by the passage of an electric current through the brain; in contemporary practice, the convulsions are minimized by the administration of a muscle relaxant prior to treatment. **emanation t.,** treatment by ionizing radiations emitted by a radioactive source. **family t.,** group therapy in which the patient and his family are treated together. **fever t.,** treatment of disease by induction of high body temperature, accomplished by physical means or by injection of fever-producing vaccines. **Fleiss t.,** see under *treatment.* **gametocyte t.,** treatment aimed at destruction of the forms of the malarial parasites infective for mosquitoes. **grid t.,** therapeutic application of ionizing radiations through a metal grid having a pattern of small, evenly spaced perforations. **group t.,** psychotherapy carried out with a group of patients or the relatives of patients or both, which includes utilization of interactions of members of the group, under the guidance of a single therapist, who may be a psychiatrist, psychologist, psychoanalyst, social worker, clergyman, etc. Called also *group psychotherapy.* **heterovaccine t.,** bacterial vaccine therapy by the use of some infectious agent other than the specific one causing the disease. **high-voltage roentgen t.,** treatment by deeply penetrating x-rays generated by voltages of over 300 kilovolts. **humidification t.,** the use of air supersaturated with moisture in congestive conditions of the upper and lower respiratory tract. **hunger t.,** limotherapy. **hypoglycemic t.,** insulin coma t. **immunization t.,** treatment with antiserum and with actively antigenic substances, e.g., vaccines. **immunosuppressive t.,** treatment with agents, such as x-rays, corticosteroids, and cytotoxic chemicals, which suppress the immune response to antigen(s); it is used in various conditions, including autoimmune disease, allergy, multiple myeloma, chronic nephritis, and in organ transplantation. **Indoklon t.,** a form of shock therapy in which convulsions are induced by the inhalation of Indoklon (flurothyl). **inhalation t.,** treatment aimed at restoring toward normal any pathophysiologic alterations of gas exchange in the cardiopulmonary system, as by the use of respirators, aerosol-producing devices, and the therapeutic use of oxygen, helium-oxygen, and carbon dioxide mixtures. **insulin coma t., insulin shock t.,** a form of shock therapy, now rarely used, primarily employed in the treatment of schizophrenia, in which hypoglycemic coma is induced by the injection of insulin; called also *hypoglycemic t.* See also *subcoma insulin t.* **intraosseous t.,** the infusion of blood or other solutions into the circulation by injection through the bone marrow. **intravenous t.,** the introduction of therapeutic liquid agents directly into the venous circulation. **irritation t.,** stimulation t. **light t.,** the therapeutic application of radiation in the visible spectrum. **liquid air t.,** see *refrigeration.* **malarial t., malarization t.,** see *malariotherapy.* **metatrophic t.,** administration of a diet that acts as an adjunct to the drug taken. **Metrazol shock t.,** a form of shock therapy, now rarely used, in which convulsions are induced by intravenous injection of Metrazol (pentylenetetrazol). **milieu t.,** daily participation in group psychiatric therapy at a hospital, providing for observation and utilization of the patient's interpersonal relationships in a social setting, as well as occupational, physical, and individual psychotherapy. **Morita t.,** a school of psychotherapy originating in Japan, based on the essential elements of conduct in Zen Buddhism. It emphasizes the combating of egocentricity and the correction of alienation from nature. **myofunctional t.,** use of muscle exercises as an adjunct to mechanical correction of malocclusion. **narcosis t.,** treatment of certain intense anxiety reactions, exhaustion, and severe agitation by inducing prolonged sleep (18 to 20 hours a day for about two weeks) with drugs, usually barbiturates; called also *sleep t.* **nonspecific t.,** treatment of infections by the injection of nonspecific substances, such as proteins, proteoses, bacterial vaccines, etc., which produce a general and nonspecific effect on cellular activity. **occupational t.,** the use of any occupation for remedial purposes. **opsonic t.,** nonspecific therapy with bacterial vaccines to increase the opsonic index of the blood; called also *vaccine t.* **organic t.,** organotherapy. **orthomolecular t.,** treatment of disease, especially psychiatric disorders, based on the theory that restoration of optimal concentrations of substances normally present in the body will effect a cure. **oxygen t.,** treatment by means of oxygen inhalation. **paraspecific t.,** nonspecific t. **phage t.,** the use of bacteriophage in the treatment of bacterial infections. **physical t.,** the treatment of disease by physical agents and methods to assist in rehabilitation and restoration of normal bodily function after illness or injury, including the use of massage and manipulation, therapeutic exercises, hydrotherapy, and various forms of energy (electrotherapy, actinotherapy, and ultrasound). Called also *physiotherapy.* **play t.,** a method of psychotherapy used in treating emotional disorders in children, in which play is used to a considerable extent as a substitute for verbal communication between the patient and therapist. **primal t.,** psychotherapy in which the patient is encouraged to relive his early traumatic experiences. **protective t.,** sparing t. **protein t., protein-shock t.,** injection of foreign proteins by the parenteral route in inflammatory and venereal disease; nonspecific therapy. **pulp canal t.,** root canal t. **radium t.,** the treatment of disease by means of radium. **radium beam t.,** see *beam t.,* def. 2. **recurrence t.,** inoculation with *Treponema.* **reflex t.,** treatment by producing a reflex action. **replacement t.,** treatment to replace deficient formation or loss of body products by administration of the natural body products or synthetic substitutes. **root canal t.,** the treatment of diseases and injuries that affect the roots of the teeth and the pulp canals. **rotation t.,** in radiotherapy, circular movement of the patient or of the radiation source and beam around a fixed anatomical axis during a treatment exposure; it may entail complete, partial, or skip-field exposure. **serum t.,** see *serotherapy.* **shock t.,** the treatment of psychiatric illnesses, chiefly severe affective disorders, by convulsions induced by means of passing an electric current through the brain. Rarely convulsions are induced by the inhalation of Indoklon (flurothyl). Formerly comas were induced by the injection of insulin or the inhalation of carbon dioxide. Called also *shock treatment.* See also *electroconvulsive t.* **short wave t.,** short wave diathermy. **solar t.,** heliotherapy. **sparing t.,** treatment directed to the protecting and sparing of an organ by allowing it to rest as much as possible. Called also *protective t.* **specific t.,** treatment by a remedy which acts directly against the cause of the disease, as of malaria by quinine. **speech t.,** the use of special techniques for correction of speech and language disorders. **stimulation t.,** treatment by the parenteral injection of certain substances with the result that the nervous vascular systems of the body function more vigorously and the metabolism is increased: called also *irritation t.* **subcoma insulin t.,** the induction of a state of drowsiness or somnolence short of coma by the administration of insulin; used to relieve anxiety, stimulate appetite, and produce a feeling of well-being. See also *insulin coma t.* **substitution t.,** the administration of a hormone to compensate for deficiency of that gland. **substitutive t.,** see *substitutive medication,* under *medication.* **suggestion t.,** the treatment of disease by hypnotic suggestion. **thyroid t.,** treatment of various diseases with thyroid or with derivatives from it; it is used in various forms of hypothyroidism e.g., myxedema and cretinism. **vaccine t.,** active immunization against a disease by the injection of the infectious agents of the disease or their products directly into a patient. **zomo t.,** treatment by the administration of meat juice. **zone t.,** treatment of disorder by mechanical stimula-

tion of a body area located in the same longitudinal zone as the disorder; called also *Fitz Gerald method* or *treatment.*

Theria (the'rĭ-ah) [Gr. *thērion* beast, animal] in some systems of classification, a subclass of the Mammalia, including the infraclasses Eutheria and Metatheria, the members of which are viviparous.

theriac (ther'e-ak) theriaca.

theriaca (the-ri'ah-kah) [Gr. *thēriaka* antidotes to the poison of wild animals, from *thērion* wild animal] a mixture regarded as effective against bites by poisonous animals; it contained at one time 60 to 70 substances which were pulverized and made into an electuary with honey. **t. androm'achi,** a celebrated mixture of sixty-one drugs, formerly prescribed as an antidote for poisons, supposedly originated by Andromachus (the elder) of Crete.

theriatrics (the"re-at'riks) [Gr. *thērion* beast + *iatrikē* surgery, medicine] veterinary medicine.

Theridiidae (ther"ĭ-di'ĭ-de) a family of small, dark, comb-footed spiders (suborder Labidognatha), including the genus *Latrodectus,* whose venomous bite sometimes causes death in human beings.

theriogenologic (the"re-o"jen-o-loj'ik) pertaining or relating to theriogenology.

theriogenological (the"re-o-jen"o-loj'ĭ-kal) pertaining or relating to theriogenology; of or affecting the reproductive processes of animals.

theriogenologist (the"reo"jen-ol'o-jist) one who specializes in theriogenology.

theriogenology (the"re-o"jen-ol'o-je) [Gr. *thērion* beast + *gennan* to produce + *-logy*] that branch of veterinary medicine which deals with reproduction, including the physiology and pathology of male and female reproductive systems and the clinical practice of veterinary obstetrics, gynecology, and semenology.

theriotherapy (the"re-o-ther'ah-pe) [Gr. *thērion* beast + *therapeia* treatment] treatment of the diseases of lower animals.

therm (therm) [Gr. *thermē* heat] a unit of heat. The word has been used as equivalent to (*a*) large calorie; (*b*) small calorie; (*c*) 1000 large calories; (*d*) 100,000 British thermal units.

therm- see *thermo-.*

thermacogenesis (ther"mah-ko-jen'ĕ-sis) [Gr. *thermē* heat + *genesis* production] the action of a drug in elevating the body temperature.

thermae (ther'me) [L., pl.; Gr. *thermē* heat] 1. warm springs or warm baths. 2. establishments for the therapeutic use of warm medicinal springs.

thermaerotherapy (therm-a"er-o-ther'ah-pe) [*therm-* + Gr. *aēr* air + *therapeia* treatment] treatment by the application of hot air.

thermal (ther'mal) pertaining to or characterized by heat.

thermalgesia (ther"mal-je'ze-ah) [*therm-* + Gr. *algēsis* sense of pain + *-ia*] a condition in which the application of heat produces pain.

thermalgia (ther-mal'je-ah) [*therm-* + Gr. *algos* pain + *-ia*] a condition marked by sensations of intense burning pain; causalgia.

thermanalgesia (therm"an-al-je'se-ah) absence of pain on application of heat.

thermanesthesia (therm"an-es-the'ze-ah) [*therm-* + *an-* neg. + Gr. *aisthēsis* perception + *-ia*] inability to recognize sensations of heat and cold; absence of the heat sense.

thermatology (ther"mah-tol'o-je) the scientific study of heat as a therapeutic agent.

thermelometer (ther"mel-om'ĕ-ter) an electric thermometer.

thermesthesia (therm"es-the'ze-ah) [*therm-* + Gr. *aisthēsis* perception + *-ia*] ability to recognize heat and cold; the temperature sense.

thermesthesiometer (therm"es-the"ze-om'ĕ-ter) [*thermesthesia* + *metron* measure] an instrument for measuring sensibility to heat.

thermhyperesthesia (therm"hi-per-es-the'ze-ah) excessive sensitiveness to high temperatures.

thermhypesthesia (therm"hi-pes-the'ze-ah) [*therm-* + Gr. *hypo* under + *aisthēsis* perception + *-ia*] decrease in the normal sensitiveness to heat.

thermic (ther'mik) of or pertaining to heat.

thermion (ther'me-on) a particle containing an electric charge emitted by an incandescent substance; such as the electrons emitted from the cathode in a Coolidge tube.

thermionics (ther"me-on'iks) the science of the phenomena exhibited by thermions.

thermistor (ther-mis'tor) a thermometer whose impedance varies with the ambient temperature and so is able to measure extremely small changes in temperature.

thermo-, therm- [Gr. *thermē* heat] combining form denoting relationship to heat.

Thermoactinomyces (ther"mo-ak"tĭ-no-mi'sēz) [*thermo-* + Gr. *aktis, aktinos* a ray + *mykēs* fungus] a genus of microorganisms of the family Streptomycetaceae, order Actinomycetales, made up of saprophytic soil and water microorganisms distinguished by their ability to grow at high (50°–65° C.) temperatures.

thermoaesthesia (ther″mo-es-the′ze-ah) thermesthesia.

thermoalgesia (ther″mo-al-je′ze-ah) thermalgesia.

thermoanalgesia (ther″mo-an″al-je′ze-ah) thermanalgesia.

thermoanesthesia (ther″mo-an″es-the′ze-ah) thermanesthesia.

thermocauterectomy (ther″mo-kaw″ter-ek′to-me) [*thermocautery* + Gr. *ektomē* exision] excision of an organ by the thermocautery.

thermocautery (ther″mo-kaw′ter-e) cauterization by means of a hot wire or point.

thermochemistry (ther″mo-kem′is-tre) the aspect of physical chemistry dealing with heat changes that accompany chemical reactions.

thermochroic (ther″mo-kro′ik) [*thermo-* + Gr. *chroa* color] reflecting some of the heat rays and absorbing or transmitting others.

thermochroism, thermochrosis (ther-mok′ro-izm; ther″-mo-kro′sis) the state or condition of being thermochroic.

thermocoagulation (ther″mo-ko-ag″u-la′shun) coagulation of tissue by the action of high-frequency currents; used in removal of growths and also used to produce stereotactic lesions in the brain.

thermocouple (ther′mo-kup″l) a pair of dissimilar electrical conductors (such as platinum and platinum-rhodium, or copper and constantan), so joined that an electromotive force is developed by the thermoelectric effects when the junctions are at different temperatures; used for measuring temperature differences.

thermocurrent (ther″mo-kur′ent) a thermoelectric current.

thermodiffusion (ther″mo-dǐ-fu′zhun) diffusion under the influence of a temperature gradient.

thermodilution (ther″mo-di-lu′shun) a method of measuring ventricular blood volume and cardiac output in which a cold or cool indicator, such as a saline solution or distilled water, is injected and sampled by a thermistor.

thermoduric (ther″mo-du′rik) [*thermo-* + L. *durus* enduring] capable of withstanding high temperature.

thermodynamics (ther″mo-di-nam′iks) [*thermo-* + Gr. *dynamis* power] the branch of science which deals with heat, energy, and the interconversion of these, and with related problems. See also under *law*. **equilibrium t.,** that dealing with the application of the laws of thermodynamics to systems in equilibrium states, or undergoing transformations between two equilibrium states. **laws of t.,** see under *law*. **nonequilibrium t.,** that dealing with steady states and irreversible processes.

thermoelectric (ther″mo-e-lek′trik) pertaining to electricity generated by heat.

thermoelectricity (ther″mo-e″lek-tris′ǐ-te) electricity generated by heat.

thermoesthesia (ther″mo-es-the′ze-ah) thermesthesia.

thermoesthesiometer (ther″mo-es-the″ze-om′ĕ-ter) thermesthesiometer.

thermoexcitory (ther″mo-ek-si′tor-e) exciting or stimulating the production of heat in the body.

thermogenesis (ther″mo-jen′ĕ-sis) [*thermo-* + Gr. *genesis* production] the production of heat, especially within the animal body.

thermogenetic (ther″mo-jĕ-net′ik) pertaining to the production of heat.

thermogenic (ther″mo-jen′ik) producing heat.

thermogenics (ther″mo-jen′iks) the science relating to heat production.

thermogenous (ther-moj′ĕ-nus) caused by elevation of temperature, or by heat.

thermogram (ther′mo-gram) 1. a graphic record of variations in temperature (heat). 2. the visual record obtained by thermography.

thermograph (ther′mo-graf) 1. an instrument for recording variations in temperature (heat). 2. a thermogram (def. 2). 3. the apparatus or device employed in thermography. **continuous scan t.,** a thermograph that presents a continuous scan image of the thermal pattern (thermogram) of a patient or object on cathode ray tube.

thermographic (ther″mo-graf′ik) pertaining to a thermogram or to thermography.

thermography (ther-mog′rah-fe) [*thermo-* + Gr. *graphein* to write] a technique wherein an infrared camera is used to photographically portray the surface temperatures of the body, based on the self-emanating infrared radiation; sometimes employed as a means of diagnosing underlying pathologic processes, such as breast tumors.

thermogravimeter (ther″mo-grah-vim′ĕ-ter) an analytical instrument for measuring change in mass of a substance at changing temperature.

thermohyperalgesia (ther″mo-hi″per-al-je′ze-ah) a condition in which the application of moderate heat causes extreme pain.

thermohyperesthesia (ther″mo-hi″per-es-the′ze-ah) extreme sensitiveness to high temperatures.

thermohypesthesia (ther″mo-hi″pes-the′ze-ah) a state of diminished sensitiveness to high temperatures.

thermohypoesthesia (ther″mo-hi″po-es-the′ze-ah) thermohypesthesia.

thermoinactivation (ther″mo-in-ak″tǐ-va′shun) destruction of the power to act by exposure to heat.

thermoinhibitory (ther″mo-in-hib′ǐ-tor″e) inhibiting or retarding the production of bodily heat.

thermointegrator (ther″mo-in′te-gra″tor) an apparatus for recording environmental warmth.

thermolabile (ther″mo-la′bil) easily altered or decomposed by heat; called also *heat labile*.

thermolamp (ther″mo-lamp) [*thermo-* + Gr. *lampē* torch] a lamp for heating.

thermolaryngoscope (ther″mo-lah-ring′go-skōp) a laryngoscope heated by electricity so that the mirror does not become obscured by condensing moisture.

thermology (ther-mol′o-je) [*thermo-* + *-logy*] the science of heat.

thermoluminescence (ther″mo-lu-mǐ-nes′ens) the production of light by a substance when its temperature is increased.

thermolysis (ther-mol′ǐ-sis) [*thermo-* + Gr. *lysis* dissolution] 1. chemical dissociation by means of heat. 2. the dissipation of bodily heat by means of radiation, evaporation, etc.

thermolytic (ther″mo-lit′ik) [*thermo-* + Gr. *lytikos* dissolving] pertaining to, characterized by, or promoting thermolysis.

thermomassage (ther″mo-mah-sahzh′) massage with heat.

thermomastography (ther″mo-mas-tog′rah-fe) the use of thermography in the diagnosis of lesions of the breast.

thermometer (ther-mom′ĕ-ter) [*thermo-* + Gr. *metron* measure] an instrument for determining temperatures. In principle, it makes use of some substance with a physical property that varies in magnitude with temperature, to determine a value of temperature on some defined scale. See also under *scale*. **air t.,** one in which the expansible material is air. **alcohol t.,** a liquid-in-glass thermometer in which alcohol is the liquid used. **axilla t.,** a surface thermometer to be used in the axilla. **Beckmann t.,** a thermometer with a large bulb and fine bore stem for measurement of small differences in temperature. **bimetal t.,** one made of two metals of dissimilar temperature coefficients of expansion so bonded together that a change in temperature causes it to curl. **Celsius t.,** a thermometer employing the Celsius scale (q.v.). **centigrade t.,** one employing the Celsius scale (q.v.), that is, having the interval between the two established reference points divided into 100 units. **clinical t.,** one for use in determining temperature of the human body. **depth t.,** a thermometer whose sensitive element may be introduced into the tissues, for registering the actual temperature of a tissue. **differential t.,** one for measuring small differences in temperature. **Fahrenheit t.,** a thermometer employing the Fahrenheit scale (q.v.). **fever t.,** clinical t. **gas t.,** one in which the expansible material is a gas, such as air, carbon dioxide, helium, neon, nitrogen, or oxygen. **half-minute t.,** a clinical thermometer with a short time lag. **kata t.,** see *katathermometer*. **Kelvin t.,** a thermometer employing the Kelvin scale (q.v.). **liquid-in-glass t.,** the common type of thermometer, containing a liquid which expands with increase in temperature; most of the liquid is in a bulb, but its free surface is in a capillary tube graduated to indicate the degree of temperature causing expansion to each particular point. **maximum t.,** one which registers the highest temperature to which it has been exposed. **mercurial t.,** a liquid-in-glass thermometer in which mercury is the liquid used. **metallic t.,** one in which some solid metal is used as the expansible element. **metastatic t.,** one which indicates minute changes of temperature. **minimum t.,** one which registers the lowest temperature to which it has been exposed. **oral t.,** a clinical thermometer which is placed under the tongue, to record the temperature in the mouth; characteristically the bulb containing the mercury is elongated. **Rankine t.,** a thermometer employing the Rankine scale (q.v.). **Réaumur t.,** a thermometer employing the Réaumur scale (q.v.). **recording t.,** a temperature-sensitive instrument by which the temperature to which it has been exposed is continuously recorded on a specially designed chart. **rectal t.,** a clinical thermometer which is inserted in the rectum, for determining body temperature; characteristically the bulb containing the mercury is pear shaped. **resistance t.,** a thermometer which uses the electric resistance of metals for determining temperature; it consists of a resistance bulb of platinum or other metal wire, and uses a Wheatstone bridge. **self-registering t.,** recording t. **surface t.,** a clinical thermometer for determining the temperature on the surface of the body. **thermocouple t.,** a combination of a thermocouple with some device for measuring its electromotive force, such as a potentiometer; in use the thermocouple's reference junction is kept at a reference temperature (such as the ice point) and its measuring junction at the temperature being measured.

thermometric (ther″mo-met′rik) pertaining to a thermometer or to the measurement of degrees of temperature.

thermometry (ther-mom′ĕ-tre) the measurement of temperatures.

thermoneurosis (ther″mo-nu-ro′sis) pyrexia of vasomotor origin.

thermonuclear (ther″mo-nu′kle-or) of, pertaining to, or derived from nuclear reactions (e.g., the fusion of hydrogen nuclei) in which the energy required for the reaction is in the form of extraordinarily high temperatures.

thermopalpation (ther″mo-pal-pa′shun) palpation for the purpose of determining differences of temperature at different portions of the body.

thermopenetration (ther″mo-pen″ĕ-tra′shun) application of currents of low tension and high amperage, which produce warmth in the deeper parts of the body; medical diathermy.

thermophile (ther′mo-fīl) an organism which grows best at elevated temperatures.

thermophilic (ther″mo-fil′ik) [thermo- + Gr. philein to love] growing best at or having a fondness for high temperatures. Cf. mesophilic and psychrophilic.

thermophore (ther′mo-fōr) [thermo- + Gr. pherein to bear] 1. a device or apparatus for retaining heat. 2. an instrument for estimating heat sensibility.

thermopile (ther′mo-pīl) [thermo + L. pila pillar, pile] a number of thermocouples in series; used to increase the sensitivity for a temperature-measuring device, or for the direct conversion of heat into electric energy.

thermoplacentography (ther″mo-plas″en-tog′rah-fe) the use of thermography for determining the site of placental attachment.

thermoplastic (ther″mo-plas′tik) softening under heat and capable of being molded into shape with pressure, then hardening on cooling without undergoing chemical change.

thermoplegia (ther″mo-ple′je-ah) [thermo- + Gr. plēgē stroke + -ia] heat stroke or sunstroke (thermic fever).

thermopolypnea (ther″mo-pol″ip-ne′ah) [thermo- + Gr. polys many + pnoia breath] a quickening of the respiration due to great heat or high temperature.

thermopolypneic (ther″mo-pol″ip-ne′ik) pertaining to or characterized by the thermopolypnea.

thermoprecipitation (ther″mo-pre-sip″ĭ-ta′shun) precipitation by heat.

thermoprecipitin (ther″mo-pre-sip′ĭ-tin) a heated extract of a bacterium used for precipitin tests (a misleading term, since it does not describe a precipitin).

thermoprecipitinogen (ther″mo-pre-sip″ĭ-tin′o-jen) a heated precipitinogen; when injected into animals coctoprecipitins are produced.

thermoradiotherapy (ther″mo-ra″de-o-ther′ah-pe) application of ionizing radiation to an anatomical site whose tissue-temperature has been elevated by artificial means on the theory of increasing its radiosensitivity.

thermoreceptor (ther″mo-re-sep′tor) a nerve ending that is sensitive to stimulation by heat.

thermoregulation (ther″mo-reg′u-la″shun) heat regulation.

thermoregulator (ther″mo-reg′u-la″tor) 1. controlling or regulating heat. 2. thermostat.

thermoresistance (ther″mo-re-zis′tans) the quality of being little affected by heat.

thermoresistant (ther″mo-re-zis′tant) not greatly affected by heat.

thermoscope (ther′mo-skōp) [thermo- + Gr. skopein to examine] a differential thermometer.

thermostabile (ther″mo-sta′bil) unaffected by heat; able to withstand the effects of heat without undergoing change; called also heat stabile.

thermostability (ther″mo-stah-bil′ĭ-te) the quality of withstanding the effects of heat without undergoing change.

thermostasis (ther″mo-sta′sis) [thermo- + Gr. stasis a placing, setting] the maintenance of body temperature in warm-blooded animals.

thermostat (ther′mo-stat) [thermo- + Gr. histanai to halt] a device interposed in a heating system by which the temperature can be automatically maintained between certain levels.

thermosteresis (ther″mo-stĕ-re′sis) [thermo- + Gr. sterēsis deprivation] the deprivation of heat.

thermostromuhr (ther″mo-strōm′oor) an instrument for measuring the amount of blood flowing in a blood vessel.

thermosystaltic (ther″mo-sis-tal′tik) [thermo- + Gr. systellein to contract] contracting under the influence or stimulus of heat; pertaining to thermosystaltism.

thermosystaltism (ther″mo-sis′tal-tizm) [thermo- + Gr. systellein to contract] muscular contraction in response to temperature changes.

thermotactic (ther″mo-tak′tik) pertaining to thermotaxis.

thermotaxic (ther″mo-tak′sik) thermotactic.

thermotaxis (ther″mo-tak′sis) [thermo- + Gr. taxis arrangement] 1. the normal adjustment of the bodily temperature. 2. the movement of an organism in response to an increase in temperature.

thermotherapy (ther″mo-ther′ah-pe) [thermo- + Gr. therapeia treatment] treatment of disease by the application of heat.

thermotics (ther-mot′iks) the science of heat.

thermotolerant (ther″mo-tol′er-ant) enduring heat; said of bacteria whose activity is not checked by high temperature.

thermotonometer (ther″mo-to-nom′ĕ-ter) [thermo- + Gr. tonos tension + metron measure] an instrument for measuring the amount of muscular contraction caused by heat.

thermotracheotomy (ther″mo-tra″ke-ot′o-me) incision of the trachea by actual cautery.

thermotropic (ther″mo-tro′pik) pertaining to or exhibiting thermotropism; called also caloritropic.

thermotropism (ther-mot′ro-pizm) [thermo- + Gr. tropē turn] the orientation of a living cell in response to the stimulus of heat.

theroid (the′roid) [Gr. thēriōdēs beast-like] resembling an animal of a lower order.

theromorph (the′ro-morf) [Gr. thēr wild beast + morphē form] a morphologic part of an organism or individual with supernumerary, teratic, or absent parts, giving it a resemblance to a lower animal.

theromorphism (the″ro-mor′fizm) the abnormal resemblance of some part of the organism to the normal structure of the corresponding part of an animal of lower type.

Theromyzon (ther-o′mĭ-zon) a genus of leeches of the family Gnathobdellidae.

thesaurismosis (the-saw″riz-mo′sis) [Gr. thēsauros treasure] a metabolic disorder in which some substance accumulates or is stored in certain cells in unusually large amounts. The stored substances may be lipoids, proteins, carbohydrates, and other substances. See storage disease, under disease. **amyloid t.**, amyloidosis. **calcium t.**, calcinosis. **cholesterol t.**, Hand-Schüller-Christian disease. **glycogenic t.**, glycogen storage disease; see under disease. **kerasin t.**, Gaucher's disease. **lipoid t.**, lipoidosis. **melanin t.**, Addison's disease. **phosphatide t.**, Niemann-Pick disease. **urate t.**, gout. **water t.**, edema.

thesaurosis (the″saw-ro′sis) [Gr. thēsauros treasure + -osis] a condition resulting from the storing up in the body of unusual amounts of normal or foreign substance; see storage disease, under disease.

Thessalus (thes′sah-lus) **of Cos** (4th century B.C.) a Greek physician; the son of Hippocrates, he followed his father's teachings closely.

Thessalus (thes′sah-lus) **of Tralles** (1st century A.D.) a Greek physician of the Methodist school and a pupil of Themison.

thiabendazole (thi″ah-ben′dah-zol) [USP] chemical name: 2-(4-thiazolyl)-1H-benzimidazole. A broad-spectrum anthelmintic, $C_{10}H_7N_3S$, occurring as a white to almost white powder; used in the treatment of pinworm, threadworm, whipworm, roundworm, and hookworm infections, and in cutaneous larva migrans, administered orally.

thiacetazone (thi-ah-set′ah-zōn) chemical name: N-[4-[[(amino-thioxomethyl)hydrazono]methylene]phenyl]acetamide; an antibacterial, $C_{10}H_{12}N_3OS$, with tuberculostatic and antileprotic properties. Called also amithiozone.

thiadiazide, thiadiazine (thi″ah-di′ah-zīd; thi″ah-di′ah-zēn) thiazide.

thiamazole (thi-am′ah-zōl) methimazole.

thiamin (thi′ah-min) thiamine.

thiaminase (thi-am′ĭ-nās) an enzyme that catalyzes the splitting of thiamine into a pyrimidine derivative and a thiazole derivative; occurring in raw fish and certain bacteria and plants, e.g., bracken. **t. I**, a transferase that catalyzes the conversion of thiamine and pyridine to heteropyrithiamine and a methyl thiazole. **t. II**, a hydrolase that catalyzes the conversion of thiamine into pyrimidine and thiazole derivatives.

thiamine (thi′ah-min) 3-[(4-amino-2-methyl-5-pyrimidinyl)-methyl]-5-(2-hydroxyethy)-4-methylthiazolium. A water-soluble component of the B complex of vitamins, first isolated in 1926; present in beans, green vegetables, sweet corn, egg yolk, liver, corn meal, and brown rice, and found in blood plasma and cerebrospinal fluid in the free state. Its active form is thiamine pyrophosphate (q.v.). Deficiency of this vitamin results in beriberi. Called also vitamin B_1 and also written thiamin. See also phosphorylated t. **t. hydrochloride** [USP], the monohydrochloride salt of thiamine, $C_{12}H_{17}ClN_4OS \cdot HCl$, occurring as white crystals or crystalline powder; administered orally and intramuscularly for the prophylaxis and treatment of thiamine deficiency states. **t. mononitrate** [USP], the mononitrate salt of thiamine, $C_{12}H_{17}N_5O_4S$, occurring as white crystals or crystalline powder; used in the preparation of various multivitamin dosage forms. **phosphorylated t., t. pyrophosphate**, the active form of thiamine, which serves as a coenzyme in reactions involving oxidative decarboxylation of certain important intermediates in carbohydrate metabolism. Called also *cocarboxylase*.

thiamphenicol (thi-am-fen′ĭ-kōl)　chemical name: [R-(R^*,R^*)]-2,2-dichloro-N-[2-hydroxy-1-(hydroxymethyl)-2-[4-(methylsulfonyl)phenyl]ethyl]acetamide. A broad-spectrum antibacterial, $C_{12}H_{15}Cl_2NO_5S$, effective against a wide range of gram-positive and gram-negative organisms.

thiamylal sodium, (thi-am′ĭ-lal)　chemical name: dihydro-5-(1-methylbutyl)-5-(2-propenyl)-2-thioxo-4,6-(1H,5H)-pyrimidinedione monosodium salt. A very short-acting barbiturate, $C_{12}H_{17}N_2NaO_2S$. A preparation suitable for injection [NF] is administered intravenously to produce general anesthesia of brief duration, for induction of anesthesia, to supplement other anesthetics, or to induce hypnosis.

Thiara (thi-ah′rah)　a genus of widely distributed, fresh-water snails (family Meloniidae), species of which, such as *T. granifera* and *T. tuberculata*, act as the main snail hosts of various trematode parasites, including *Paragonimus*, *Metagonimus*, and *Haplorchis*.

thiasine (thi′ah-sin)　ergothioneine.

thiazide (thi′ah-zīd)　any of a group of benzothiadiazenesulfonamide derivatives, typified by chlorothiazide, that act as diuretics by inhibiting the reabsorption of sodium in the proximal renal tubule and stimulating chloride excretion, with resultant increase in excretion of water. Called also *benzothiadiazide*, *benzothiadiazine*, *thiadiazide*, and *thiadiazine*.

thiazole (thi′ah-zōl)　the chemical ring:

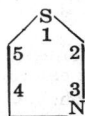

Thiele's syndrome (thēlz) [George Henry *Thiele*, American proctologist, born 1896]　see under *syndrome*.

thiemia (thi-e′me-ah) [Gr. *theion* sulfur + *haima* blood + *-ia*] an excess of sulfur in the blood.

Thiersch's graft operation (tērsh′ez) [Karl *Thiersch*, German surgeon, 1822–1895]　see *Ollier-Thiersch graft*, under *graft*, and see under *operation*.

thiethylperazine (thi-eth′il-per′ah-zēn)　chemical name: 2-(ethylthio)-10-[3-(4-methyl-1-piperazinyl)propyl]phenothiazine. A phenothiazine derivative, $C_{22}H_{29}N_3S_2$.　**t. malate** [USP], a slightly yellow, voluminous powder, having the same actions and uses as the maleate salt; administered by intramuscular injection. **t. maleate** [USP], the maleate salt of thiethylperazine, $C_{22}H_{29}N_3S_2 \cdot 2C_4H_4O_4$, occurring as a white to faintly yellow, crystalline powder; used as an antiemetic. It is useful in reducing nausea and vomiting associated with the use of general anesthesia and that following the use of radiation and mustard therapy and is possibly effective in the treatment of vertigo; administered orally or rectally.

thigh (thi)　the portion of the lower extremity situated between the hip above and the knee below; the femur (def. 2).　**cricket t.,** rupture of some of the fibers of the rectus femoris, which may occur in playing cricket or football; sometimes the tendon of the quadriceps or that of the patella is also ruptured.　**drivers′ t.,** sciatic neuralgia caused by pressure from the use of the accelerator in driving an automobile.　**Heilbronner's t.,** broadening and flattening of the thigh; seen in cases of organic paralysis when the patient lies on his back on a hard mattress; it does not appear in hysterical paralysis.

thigmesthesia (thig″mes-the′ze-ah) [Gr. *thigma* touch + *aisthēsis* perception + *-ia*]　tactile sensibility.

thigmotactic (thig″mo-tak′tik)　pertaining to, characterized by, or causing thigmotaxis.

thigmotaxis (thig″mo-tak′sis)　movement occurring in response to the stimulus of contact or touch, which may be toward (*positive t.*) or away from the stimulating object (*negative t.*).

thigmotropic (thig″mo-trop′ik)　pertaining to or exhibiting thigmotropism; responding to the stimulus of contact or touch.

thigmotropism (thig-mot′ro-pizm) [Gr. *thigma* touch + *tropē* turn]　the orientation of an organism in response to the stimulus of contact or touch.

thihexinol methylbromide (thi-hek′sĭ-nōl)　chemical name: α-[4-(diethylamino)cyclohexyl]-α-2-thienyl-2-thiophene methanol methyl bromide. An anticholinergic, $C_{18}H_{26}BrNOS_2$, claimed to inhibit intestinal hypermotility.

thimble (thim′b'l)　coping.

thimerosal (thi-mer′o-sal) [USP]　chemical name: ethyl(2-mercaptobenzoato-S)mercury sodium salt. An organomercurial antiseptic, $C_9H_9HgNaO_2S$, occurring as a light cream-colored, crystalline powder, which is actively antifungal and bacteriostatic for many nonsporulating bacteria; used as a topical anti-infective and as a preservative in pharmaceutical preparations. Called also *thiomersalate*.

thimethaphan camphorsulfonate (thi-meth′ah-fan)　trimethaphan camsylate.

thinking (thingk′ing)　the formulation of images or concepts in one's mind. **autistic t.,** autism. **dereistic t.,** see *dereism*.

thio- [Gr. *theion* sulfur]　a prefix signifying the presence of sulfur.

thio-acid (thi″o-as′id)　an organic compound produced by replacement of one of the oxygens of the carboxyl group by divalent sulfur.

thioalbumose (thi″o-al′bu-mōs)　an albumose that has a large sulfur content.

thioalcohol (thi″o-al′ko-hol)　mercaptan.

thioarsenite (thi″o-ar′se-nīt)　any compound of sulfur and arsenic of the type K_3AsS_3.

Thiobacillus (thi″o-bah-sil′us)　a genus of microorganisms of the family Thiobacteriaceae, suborder Pseudomonadineae, order Pseudomonadales, occurring as small, gram-negative, rod-shaped cells. It includes nine species, *T. concreti′vorus*, *T. coprolit′icus*, *T. denitri′ficans*, *T. ferroox′idans*, *T. neopolita′nus*, *T. novel′lus*, *T. thioox′idans*, *T. thio′parus*, and *T. trautwei′nii*.

Thiobacteriaceae (thi″o-bak-te″re-a′se-e)　a family of chemosynthetic microorganisms (order Pseudomonadales, suborder Pseudomonadineae) occurring as coccoid or straight or curved rod-shaped cells which oxidize sulfur compounds, usually depositing free sulfur granules inside or outside the cells. It includes four genera, *Thiobacillus*, *Thiobacterium*, *Thiospira*, and *Thiovulum*.

Thiobacterium (thi″o-bak-te″re-um)　a genus of microorganisms of the family Thiobacteriaceae, suborder Pseudomonadineae, order Pseudomonadales, occurring as rod-shaped sulfur bacteria in fresh or salt water or in the soil. It includes three species, *T. bovis′ta*, *T. crystallif′erum*, and *T. retifor′mans*.

thiobarbital (thi″o-bar′bĭ-tal)　chemical name: 5,5-diethyl-2-thio-barbituric acid. A salt of thiobarbituric acid, $C_8H_{12}N_2O_2S$, used as a thyroid depressant.

thiobarbiturate (thi″o-bar-bit′u-rāt)　a salt or derivative of thiobarbituric acid.

Thiocapsa (thi″o-kap′sah) [*thio-* + Gr. *kapsa* a case, casket]　a genus of microorganisms of the family Thiorhodaceae, suborder Rhodobacteriineae, order Pseudomonadales, occurring as spherical cells within a slime capsule. It includes two species, *T. florida′na* and *T. roseopersici′na*.

thiocarbamide (thi″o-kar′bah-mīd)　thiourea.

thiochrome (thi″o-krōm)　the fluorescent yellow coloring matter of yeast, $C_{12}H_{14}ON_4S$, resulting from the oxidation of thiamine.

thiocyanate (thi″o-si′ah-nat)　a salt analogous in composition to a cyanate, but containing sulfur instead of oxygen; called also *sulfocyanate*.

Thiocystis (thi″o-sis′tis) [*thio-* + Gr. *kystis* sac, bladder]　a genus of microorganisms of the family Thiorhodaceae, suborder Rhodobacteriineae, order Pseudomonadales, occurring as spherical to ovoid cells embedded in a common gelatinous capsule. It includes two species, *T. ru′fa* and *T. viola′cea*.

Thioderma (thi″o-der′mah) [*thio-* + Gr. *derma* skin]　a name formerly given a genus of sulfur bacteria.

Thiodictyon (thi″o-dik′te-on) [*thio-* + Gr. *diktyon* net]　a genus of microorganisms of the family Thiorhodaceae, suborder Rhodobacteriineae, order Pseudomonadales, occurring as rod-shaped cells arranged end to end in a netlike structure. The type species is *T. el′egans*.

thiodiphenylamine (thi″o-di-fen″il-am′in)　phenothiazine.

thiodotherapy (thi′o-do-ther′ah-pe) [*thio-* + *iodine* + *therapy*]　combined sulfur and iodine therapy.

thioether (thi″o-e′ther)　a sulfur ether; an ether in which sulfur replaces oxygen.

thioethylamine (thi″o-eth″il-am′in)　an amine, $SH(CH_2)_2NH_2$, formed from cysteine by the loss of CO_2.

thioflavine (thi″o-fla′vin) [*thio-* + *flavine*]　a yellow dye, methyl dehydrothio-p-toluidine sulfonate.

thiogenic (thi″o-jen′ik) [*thio-* + Gr. *gennan* to produce]　able to convert hydrogen sulfide into higher sulfur compounds.

thioglucose (thi″o-glu′kōs)　a synthetic glucose that contains a sulfhydryl group which replaces the oxygen in the aldehyde group.

thioglucosidase (thi″o-glu-ko′sĭ-dās)　an enzyme found in mustard seed that catalyzes the hydrolysis of thioglycoside to a thiol and a sugar; called also *myrosinase*.

thioguanine (thi″o-gwah′nēn) [USP]　chemical name: 2-amino-1,7-dihydro-6H-purine-6-thione. An antineoplastic derived from mercaptopurine, $C_5H_5N_5S \cdot xH_2O$, occurring as a pale yellow, crystalline powder; used in the treatment of acute leukemia and chronic granulocytic leukemia, administered orally.

thiokinase (thi″o-ki′nās)　any enzyme that catalyzes the joining of an acid and a thiol (—SH) group coupled with the release of inorganic phosphate from ATP or a similar triphosphate.

thiol (thi′ol)　1. sulfhydryl. 2. any organic compound containing the —SH group; the analogue of an alcohol, which contains the —OH group.

thiolase (thi′o-lās) acetyl-CoA acetyltransferase. **acetoacetyl t.,** acetyl-CoA acetyltransferase.

thiolhistidine (thi″ol-his′tĭ-din) the sulfur derivative of histidine occurring in the betaine form as ergothionine.

Thiomerin (thi-o′mer-in) trademark for a preparation of mercaptomerin sodium.

thiomersalate (thi″o-mer′sah-lāt) thimerosal.

thioneine (thi″o-ne′in) [Gr. *theion* sulfur + *neos* new] ergothioneine.

thionic (thi-on′ik) 1. pertaining to sulfur. 2. see under *acid*.

thionin (thi′o-nin) a dark-green powder, NH₂·C₆H₃(NS)·C₆H₃·· NH₂, giving a purple color in solution, and used as a metachromatic stain in microscopy. Called also *Lauth's violet*.

thionyl (thi′o-nil) the radical SO.

thiopectic (thi″o-pek′tik) fixing sulfur.

Thiopedia (thi″o-pe′de-ah) [*thio-* + Gr. *pedion* a plain] a genus of microorganisms of the family Thiorhodaceae, suborder Rhodobacteriineae, order Pseudomonadales, occurring as spherical to short rod-shaped cells. The type species is *T. ro′sea.*

thiopental sodium (thi″o-pen′tal) [USP] chemical name: 5-ethyldihydro-5-(1-methylbutyl)-2-thioxo-4,6(1*H*,5*H*)pyrimidine-dione monosodium salt. An ultra–short-acting barbiturate, C₁₁-H₁₇N₂NaO₂S, occurring as a white to off-white, crystalline powder, or yellowish, hygroscopic powder; administered intravenously to produce general anesthesia of brief duration, for induction of anesthesia prior to administration of other anesthetics, to supplement regional anesthesia, as an anticonvulsive, and for narcoanalysis and narcosynthesis in psychiatric disorders.

thiopentone (thi″o-pen′tōn) thiopental.

thiopexic (thi″o-pek′sik) thiopectic.

thiopexy (thi″o-pek′se) [*thio-* + Gr. *pēxis* fixation] the fixation of sulfur.

Thioploca (thi″o-plo′kah) a genus of Schizomycetes (order Beggiatoales, family Beggiatoaceae).

Thiopolycoccus (thi″o-pol″e-kok′us) a genus of microorganisms of the family Thiorhodaceae, suborder Rhodobacteriineae, order Pseudomonadales, occurring as spherical cells in irregularly shaped dense aggregates, held together by mucus. The type species is *T. ru′ber.*

thiopropazate hydrochloride (thi″o-pro′pah-zāt) chemical name: 4-[3-(2-chlorophenothiazine-10-yl)propyl]-1-piperazine-ethanol acetate dihydrochloride. A phenothiazine tranquilizer, C₂₃H₂₈ClN₃O₂·2HCl, occurring as a white, crystalline powder; used in the treatment of psychoses and to suppress involuntary muscular activity in Huntington's chorea, administered orally.

Thiorhodaceae (thi″o-ro-da′se-e) a family of Schizomycetes (order Pseudomonadales, suborder Rhodobacteriineae), occurring in environments containing sulfides, requiring light but little or no oxygen, and producing a pigment system composed of green bacteriochlorophyll and yellow and red carotenoids. It includes 13 genera: *Amoebobacter, Chromatium, Lamprocystis, Rhabdomonas, Rhodothece, Thiocapsa, Thiocystis, Thiodictyon, Thiopedia, Thiopolycoccus, Thiosarcina, Thiospirillum,* and *Thiothece.*

thioridazine hydrochloride (thi″o-rid′ah-zēn) [USP] chemical name: 10-[2-(1-methyl-2-piperidyl)ethyl]-2-(methylthio)phenothiazine monohydrochloride. A tranquilizer, with sedative and behavioral effects, C₂₁H₂₆N₂S₂·HCl, occurring as a white to slightly yellow, granular powder; administered orally.

Thiosarcina (thi″o-sar-si′nah) a genus of microorganisms of the family Thiorhodaceae, suborder Rhodobacteriineae, order Pseudomonadales, occurring as spherical cells in cubical packets. The type species is *T. ro′sea.*

thiosinamine (thi″o-sin′ah-min) a bitter, crystalline substance, (NH₂)CS·NHCH₂CH:CH₂, from oil of mustard and ammonia; it has been used to promote absorption of fibrous tissue. Called also *allyl thiocarbamide, allyl sulfocarbamide,* and *allyl thiourea.*

Thiospira (thi″o-spi′rah) a genus of microorganisms of the family Thiobacteriaceae, suborder Pseudomonadineae, order Pseudomonadales, occurring as colorless, slightly bent, large rods with a small number of polar flagella and containing sulfur granules within the cells. It includes two species, *T. bipuncta′ta* and *T. winograd′skyi.*

Thiospirillopsis (thi″o-spi″ril-lop′sis) a genus of Schizomycetes (order Beggiatoales, family Beggiatoaceae).

Thiospirillum (thi″o-spi-ril′lum) a genus of microorganisms of the family Thiorhodaceae, suborder Rhodobacteriineae, order Pseudomonadales, occurring singly as spirally wound cells. It includes five species, *T. jenen′se, T. rosenber′gii, T. ru′fum, T. sangui′neum,* and *T. viola′ceum.*

thiosulfate (thi″o-sul′fāt) any salt of thiosulfuric acid.

Thiosulfil (thi″o-sul′fil) trademark for preparations of sulfamethizole.

thiotepa (thi″o-te′pah) [USP] chemical name: 1,1′,1″-phosphino-thioylidynetris-aziridine. A cytotoxic alkylating agent, C₆H₁₂N₃-PS, occurring as fine, white, crystalline flakes; used as an antineoplastic, especially for the palliative treatment of certain malignant tumors as an adjunct to therapy, administered paren-

terally. Also written thio-*TEPA*. Called also *triethylenethiophosphoramide.*

Thiothece (thi″o-the′se) a genus of microorganisms of the family Thiorhodaceae, suborder Rhodobacteriineae, order Pseudomonadales, occurring as spherical to elongated cells embedded in a gelatinous capsule. The type species is *T. gelatino′sa.*

thiothixene (thi″o-thiks′ēn) [USP] chemical name: (*Z*)-*N*,*N*-dimethyl-9-[3-(4-methyl-1-piperazinyl)propylidene]-9*H*-thioxanthene-2-sulfonamide. An antipsychotic, C₂₃H₂₉N₃O₂S₂, occurring as white to tan crystals; administered orally. **t. hydrochloride** [USP], the dihydrate dihydrochloride salt of thiothixene, C₂₃H₂₉N₃O₂S₂·2HCl·2H₂O, occurring as a white, or nearly white, crystalline powder, having the same uses as the base; administered orally and intramuscularly.

Thiothrix (thi′o-thriks) a genus of Schizomycetes (order Beggiatoales, family Beggiatoaceae).

thiouracil (thi″o-u′rah-sil) chemical name: 2-mercapto-4-hydroxyprimidine. A thiourea derivative, C₄H₄N₂OS, which affects adversely the synthesis of the thyroid hormones. It has been used as an antithyroid agent in hyperthyroidism, and in angina pectoris and congestive heart failure.

thiourea (thi″o-u′re-ah) urea in which the oxygen is replaced by sulfur, H₂HCSNH₂; it inhibits the function of the thyroid gland, and was formerly used as an antithyroid agent. Called also *thiocarbamide.*

Thiovulum (thi-o′vu-lum) a genus of microorganisms of the family Thiobacteriaceae, suborder Pseudomonadineae, order Pseudomonadales, occurring as round to ovoid unicellular organisms, normally containing sulfur in the cytoplasm. The type species is *T. ma′jus.*

thioxanthene (thi″o-zan′thēn) a class of structurally related neuroleptic drugs, including chlorprothixene and thiothixene.

thiozine (thi′o-zin) ergothioneine.

thiphenamil hydrochloride (thi-fen′ah-mil) chemical name: α-phenylbenzene ethanethioic acid *S*-[2-(diethylamino)-ethyl]ester hydrochloride. An anticholinergic, C₂₀H₂₆ClNOS, having potent antispasmodic and smooth muscle relaxant properties; used to relieve pain and discomfort due to smooth muscle spasm associated with gastrointestinal disorders, administered orally.

thiram (thi′ram) chemical name: tetramethylthioperoxydicarbonic diamide; a topical antifungal, C₆H₁₂N₂S₄.

third intention see under *healing*.

thirst (therst) [L. *sitis*, Gr. *dipsa*] a sensation, often referred to the mouth and throat, associated with a craving for drink; ordinarily interpreted as a desire for water. **insensible t.,** subliminal t. **real t.,** true t. **subliminal t.,** a sensation of need for water which is insufficient to prompt the ingestion of water but is at times sufficient to maintain drinking once it is initiated. **true t.,** thirst which is associated with a bodily need for water and is satisfied by the ingestion of water. **twilight t.,** subliminal t.

Thiry's fistula (thi′rēz) [Ludwig *Thiry*, Austrian physiologist, 1817–1897] see under *fistula*.

thixolabile (thik″so-la′bil) easily affected by shaking or stirring.

thixotropic (thik″so-trop′ik) pertaining to or characterized by thixotropy.

thixotropism (thik-sot′ro-pizm) thixotropy.

thixotropy (thik-sot′ro-pe) [Gr. *thixis* a touch + *tropos* a turning] the property, exhibited by certain gels, of becoming fluid when shaken or stirred, and then becoming semisolid again.

thlipsencephalus (thlip″sen-sef′ah-lus) [Gr. *thlipsis* pressure + *enkephalos* brain] a monster with a deficient skull, or with the upper part of the skull lacking.

thoko (tho′ko) a Fijian word for yaws, which was once heavily endemic there.

Thoma's ampulla, fluid (to′mahz) [Richard *Thoma*, German histologist, 1847–1923] see under *ampulla* and *fluid*.

Thoma-Zeiss counting chamber (cell) (to′mah-zīs) [Richard *Thoma;* Carl *Zeiss,* German optician, 1816–1888] see under *chamber*.

Thomas' knee splint, posterior splint (tom′as) [Hugh Owen *Thomas,* orthopedic surgeon in Liverpool, 1834–1891] see under *splint*.

Thompson's test (tom′sonz) [Sir Henry *Thompson,* English surgeon, 1820–1904] two-glass test.

Thomsen's disease (tom′senz) [Asmus Julius Thomas *Thomsen,* Danish physician, 1815–1896] myotonia congenita.

Thomsen's phenomenon (tom′senz) [Oluf *Thomsen,* Danish physician, 1878–1940] Huebener-Thomsen-Friedenreich phenomenon.

Thomson's sign (tom′sunz) [Frederick Holland *Thomson,* British physician, 1867–1938] Pastia's sign; see under *sign*.

thomsonianism (tom-so′ne-an-izm) [Samuel *Thomson,* a New Hampshire farmer, 1769–1843] an empiric system of medical practice, chiefly based on use of plants as remedies.

thonzonium bromide (thon-zo′nĭ-um) chemical name: *N*-[2-

[[(4-methoxyphenyl)methyl]-2-pyrimidinylamino]ethyl]-*N*,*N*-dimethyl-1-hexadecanaminium bromide; a cationic detergent, $C_{32}H_{55}BrN_4O$.

thonzylamine hydrochloride (thon-zil′ah-mēn) chemical name: *N*-[(4-methoxyphenyl)methyl]-*N′*,*N′*-dimethyl-*N*-2-pyrimidinyl-1,2-ethanediamine monohydrochloride; an antihistaminic, $C_{16}H_{22}N_4O \cdot HCl$.

thoracal (tho′rah-kal) thoracic.

thoracalgia (tho″rah-kal′je-ah) pain in the chest wall.

thoracectomy (tho″rah-sek′to-me) [*thoraco-* + Gr. *ektomē* excision] thoracotomy with resection of a portion of a rib.

thoracentesis (tho″rah-sen-te′sis) [*thoraco-* + Gr. *kentēsis* puncture] surgical puncture of the chest wall into the parietal cavity for aspiration of fluids; called also *pleurocentesis* and *thoracocentesis*.

thoracic (tho-ras′ik) [L. *thoracicus;* Gr. *thōrakikos*] pertaining to or affecting the chest.

thoracicoabdominal (tho-ras″ĭ-ko-ab-dom′ĭ-nal) pertaining to the thorax and abdomen.

thoracicohumeral (tho-ras″ĭ-ko-hu′mer-al) pertaining to the thorax and the humerus.

thoracispinal (tho-ras″ĭ-spi′nal) pertaining to the thoracic portion of the spinal column.

thoraco- (tho′rah-ko) [Gr. *thōrax, thōrakos* chest] a combining form denoting relationship to the chest.

thoracoacromial (tho″rah-ko-ah-kro′me-al) pertaining to the chest and acromion.

thoracobronchotomy (tho″rah-ko-brong-kot′o-me) incision into the bronchus through the thoracic wall.

thoracoceloschisis (tho″rah-ko-se-los′kĭ-sis) [*thoraco-* + Gr. *koilia* belly + *schisis* fissure] congenital fissure of the thorax and abdomen.

thoracocentesis (tho″rah-ko-sen-te′sis) thoracentesis.

thoracocyllosis (tho″rah-ko-si-lo′sis) [*thoraco-* + Gr. *kyllōsis* crippling] deformity of the chest.

thoracocyrtosis (tho″rah-ko-sir-to′sis) [*thoraco-* + Gr. *kyrtōsis* a being humpbacked] abnormal curvature of the thorax, or unusual prominence of the chest.

thoracodelphus (tho″rah-ko-del′fus) [*thoraco-* + Gr. *adelphos* brother] a double monster with one head, two arms, and four legs, the bodies being joined above the navel.

thoracodidymus (tho″rah-ko-did′ĭ-mus) [*thoraco-* + Gr. *didymos* twin] conjoined twins united at the thorax.

thoracodynia (tho″rah-ko-din′e-ah) [*thoraco-* + Gr. *odynē* pain] pain in the chest.

thoracogastrodidymus (tho″rah-ko-gas″tro-did′ĭ-mus) [*thoraco-* + Gr. *gastēr* belly + *didymos* twin] conjoined twins united at the belly and chest.

thoracogastroschisis (tho″rah-ko-gas-tros′kĭ-sis) [*thoraco-* + Gr. *gastēr* belly + *schisis* fissure] fissure of the thorax and abdomen.

thoracograph (tho-rak′o-graf) [*thoraco-* + Gr. *graphein* to write] thoracopneumograph.

thoracolaparotomy (tho″rah-ko-lap″ah-rot′o-me) [*thoraco-* + Gr. *lapara* loin + *tomē* a cutting] incision through both the thorax and abdomen to gain access to the subphrenic space and adjoining regions.

thoracolumbar (tho″rah-ko-lum′bar) pertaining to the thoracic and lumbar parts of the spine.

thoracolysis (tho″rah-kol′ĭ-sis) [*thoraco-* + Gr. *lysis* dissolution] the freeing of adhesions of the chest wall.

thoracomelus (tho″rah-kom′e-lus) [*thoraco-* + Gr. *melos* limb] a monster with a supernumerary arm or leg attached to the thorax.

thoracometer (tho″rah-kom′ĕ-ter) [*thoraco-* + Gr. *metron* measure] stethometer.

thoracometry (tho″rah-kom′ĕ-tre) measurement of the thorax.

thoracomyodynia (tho″rah-ko-mi″o-din′e-ah) [*thoraco-* + Gr. *mys* muscle + *odynē* pain] pain in the muscles of the chest.

thoracopagus (tho″rah-kop′ah-gus) [*thoraco-* + Gr. *pagos* thing fixed] a double monster consisting of two nearly complete individuals joined in or near the sternal region, so the two components are face to face. **t. epigas′tricus,** an asymmetrical double monster in which the parasitic component is attached to the epigastric region of the autosite. **t. parasit′icus,** an asymmetrical double monster in which the parasitic component is attached to the thorax of the autosite.

thoracoparacephalus (tho″rah-ko-par″ah-sef′ah-lus) [*thoraco-* + Gr. *para* beside + *kephalē* head] asymmetrical conjoined twins, a parasite with rudimentary head being attached to the thorax of the autosite.

thoracopathy (tho″rah-kop′ah-the) [*thoraco-* + Gr. *pathos* disease] any disorder of the thorax or of the thoracic organs.

thoracoplasty (tho″rah-ko-plas′te) [*thoraco-* + Gr. *plassein* to mold] surgical removal of ribs, allowing the chest wall to move inward and collapse a diseased lung. **costoversion t.,** removal of several ribs and their replacement "inside out," occasionally with one rib placed vertically as a strut, providing a concave bony framework, to prevent paradoxical movement during the healing of the chest wall with the lung in the collapsed position.

thoracopneumograph (tho″rah-ko-nu′mo-graf) [*thoraco-* + Gr. *pneuma* breath + *graphein* to write] an instrument for recording the respiratory movements of the chest.

thoracoschisis (tho″rah-kos′kĭ-sis) [*thoraco-* + Gr. *schisis* fissure] congenital fissure of the chest, which may result in herniation of lung tissue.

thoracoscope (tho-ra′ko-skōp) 1. an endoscope for examining the pleural cavity; it is pushed into the cavity through an intercostal space. 2. a stethoscope.

thoracoscopy (tho″rah-kos′ko-pe) [*thoraco-* + Gr. *skopein* to examine] the diagnostic examination of the chest, specifically the direct examination of the pleural cavity by means of the endoscope; pleural endoscopy.

thoracostenosis (tho″rah-ko-stĕ-no′sis) [*thoraco-* + Gr. *stenōsis* contraction] abnormal contraction of the chest wall.

thoracostomy (tho″rah-kos′to-me) [*thoraco-* + Gr. *stomoun* to provide with an opening, or mouth] surgical creation of an opening in the wall of the chest for the purpose of drainage; also, the opening so created.

thoracotomy (tho″rah-kot′o-me) [*thoraco-* + Gr. *tomē* a cutting] surgical incision of the wall of the chest.

thoradelphus (tho″rah-del′fus) thoracodelphus.

thorax (tho′raks), pl. *tho′races* [Gr. *thōrax*] [NA] the part of the body between the neck and the respiratory diaphragm, encased by the ribs; the chest. **amazon t.,** a chest with only one mammary gland, or breast. **t. asthen′icus,** t. paralyticus. **barrel-shaped t.,** a malformed chest which is rounded like a barrel; seen in advanced pulmonary emphysema. **cholesterol t.,** accumulation in the pleural cavities of fluid with a high cholesterol content. **t. paralyt′icus,** the long flat thorax of patients with constitutional visceroptosis. **Peyrot's t.,** a chest that is obliquely oval; seen in large pleural effusions. **pyriform t.,** a pear-shaped thorax, large above, small below.

Thorazine (thor′ah-zēn) trademark for preparations of chlorpromazine hydrochloride.

Thorel's bundle (to′relz) [Christen *Thorel*, German physician, 1880–1935] see under *bundle*.

thoriagram (tho′re-ah-gram) [*thorium* + Gr. *gramma* mark] a photograph made with thorium.

thorium (tho′re-um) [*Thor*, a Norse deity] a rare, heavy gray metal, atomic number, 90; atomic weight, 232.038; symbol, Th. It is a radioactive metal with a half-life of the order of 10^{10} years, and the parent element of a radioactive disintegration series. Because of its radiopacity, various compounds of thorium have been used to facilitate visualization in roentgenography. **t. D,** the last element of the disintegration series derived from thorium, a stable isotope of lead with an atomic weight of 208. **t. dioxide,** ThO_2, used in roentgenography of the alimentary tract. **t. nitrate,** $Th(NO_3)_4 \cdot 4H_2O$, formerly used externally in parasitic skin diseases and internally in rheumatism. **radioactive t.,** radiothorium. **sodium t. tartrate,** used in roentgenography, especially the gastrointestinal tract. **t. X,** a radioactive element produced by disintegration of thorium, and an isotope of radium with a half-life of about $3\frac{2}{3}$ days; formerly used in treatment of superficial skin conditions, but replaced now by soft x-rays and grenz rays.

Thormählen's test (tor′ma-lenz) [Johann *Thormählen*, German physician] see under *tests*.

Thornton's sign (thorn′tonz) [Knowsley *Thornton*, British physician, 1845–1904] see under *sign*.

Thornwaldt see *Tornwaldt*.

thoron (tho′ron) thorium emanation.

thoroughpin (thur′o-pin) a distention of the synovial sheath of the flexor perforans tendon of the horse at the hock joint; also a similar distention on the carpal joint of the foreleg.

thozalinone (tho-zal′ĭ-nōn) chemical name: 2-(dimethylamino)-5-phenyl-2-oxazolin-4-one; an antidepressant, $C_{11}H_{12}N_2O_2$.

Thr threonine.

thread (thred) a long slender structure, such as a continuous filament of some substance used as suture material. **celluloid t.,** Pagenstecher's linen t. **t's of Golgi-Rezzonico,** threads of nerve tissue in the incisure of Lanterman surrounding the axon spiral arrangement. **Pagenstecher's linen t.,** ordinary linen thread which has been immersed in a solution of celluloid; used as a suture material. **Simonart's t.,** a band formed by the stretching of adhesions between the amnion and fetus when the amniotic cavity is distended with its proper fluid.

threadworm (thred′wurm) any long slender nematode, especially *Enterobius vermicularis*.

thremmatology (threm″ah-tol′o-je) [Gr. *thremma* nursling + *logos* treatise] the science of the laws of heredity and variation.

threonine (thre′o-nin) alpha-amino-beta-hydroxy butyric acid, $CH_3 \cdot CH(OH) \cdot CH(NH_2) \cdot COOH$; a natural amino acid essential for optimal growth in infants and for nitrogen equilibrium in adults.

threose (thre′ōs) a sugar, $C_4H_8O_4$, isomeric with erythrose.

threpsis (threp′sis) [Gr.] nutrition.

threpsology (threp-sol′o-je) [Gr. *threpsis* nutrition + *-logy*] the sum of what is known concerning nutrition; the science of nutrition.

threptic (threp′tik) pertaining to nutrition; pertaining to the nurturing of offspring by the parents, especially in certain insect species.

threshold (thresh′old) 1. that value at which a stimulus just produces a sensation, is just appreciable, or comes just within the limits of perception; see also *absolute t.* and *differential t.* 2. a hypothetical barrier that stimuli must pass to enter the mind. 3. that degree of concentration of a substance in the blood plasm above which the substance is excreted by the kidneys and below which it is not excreted; such a substance is called a *threshold substance.* 4. limen. **absolute t.,** the lowest possible limit of stimulation that is capable of producing sensation; called also *stimulus t.* **achromatic t.,** the least intensity of the spectrum that produces a sensation of color; reduction of intensity below this point produces a sensation of brightness only, without any color distinction. **auditory t.,** the *mini′mum audib′ile,* or slightest perceptible sound. **t. of consciousness,** the *mini′mum sensib′ile,* or lowest limit of sensibility; the point of consciousness at which a stimulus is barely perceived. **convulsant t.,** the minimum amount of electric current or drug required to produce a convulsion in shock treatment. **differential t.,** the lowest limit of discriminative sensibility; the ratio which the difference of two stimuli must bear to half their sum in order that their difference may be just perceptible. **displacement t.,** the threshold of perception of a break in the continuity of a contour or of a border; called also *Vernier acuity.* **double point t.,** the smallest distance apart at which two stimuli of touch are felt as distinct. **erythema t.,** the size of the radiation dose that is required to cause erythema of the skin. **flicker fusion t.,** the frequency at which a flickering light just appears to be continuous; see *flicker.* **galvanic t.,** rheobase. **neuron t.,** that degree of stimulation of a neuron which just suffices to call forth a fruitful excitation (sensation, movement, or the like) in a neuron. **t. of nose,** limen nasi. **parasite t.,** pyrogenic t. **pyrogenic t.,** the number of malarial parasites required to be in the blood to produce fever. **relational t.,** the ratio which two stimuli must have to each other in order that the difference between them may be just perceptible. **renal t.,** that concentration of a substance in plasma at which it begins to be excreted in the urine. **renal t. for glucose,** the point of sugar (glucose) concentration in the blood (180 mg. per ml. in the normal) at which the kidney will excrete sugar (glucosuria); called also *leak point.* **resolution t.,** t. of consciousness. **sensitivity t., stimulus t.,** absolute t. **swallowing t.,** the minimal stimulation necessary to elicit the reflex action that leads to swallowing. **t. of visual sensation,** the least possible amount of stimulus that gives rise to the sensation of sight.

thrill (thril) a sensation of vibration felt by the examiner on palpation of the body, as over an incompetent heart valve. **aneurysmal t.,** the vibratory sensation felt on the palpation of an aneurysm. **aortic t.,** a thrill perceptible over the aortic orifice in disease of its valves. **diastolic t.,** the vibratory sensation felt over the precordium in advanced aortic insufficiency. **fat t.,** a peculiar thrill sometimes felt in abdominal examinations due to excessive fatness of the parietes. **hydatid t.,** a tremulous impulse sometimes felt on palpation of the body surface over a hydatid cyst; called also *hydatid fremitus.* **presystolic t.,** a thrill felt just before the systole by the hand placed over the apex of the heart. **purring t.,** a thrill of a quality suggesting the purring of a cat. **systolic t.,** a thrill felt on systole over the precordium, as in aortic stenosis, pulmonary stenosis, and ventricular septal defect.

thrix (thriks) [Gr.] hair; used as a word termination denoting a resemblance or a relationship to hair.

-thrix [Gr. *thrix* hair] a word termination meaning hair.

throat (thrōt) 1. the pharynx. 2. the fauces. 3. the anterior part of the neck. **sore t.,** see *sore throat,* under S. **trench t.,** necrotizing ulcerative gingivitis.

throb (throb) a pulsating movement or sensation.

throbbing (throb′ing) beating; attended with a rhythmic beating sensation.

Throckmorton's reflex [Thomas Bentley *Throckmorton,* American neurologist, born 1885] see under *reflex.*

throe (thro) a severe pain or paroxysm.

thrombapheresis (throm″bah-fer′ĕ-sis) thrombocytapheresis.

thrombase (throm′bās) thrombin.

thrombasthenia (throm″bas-the′ne-ah) [*thrombocyte* + Gr. *astheneia* weakness] a platelet abnormality characterized by defective clot retraction, abnormal glass adhesion, impaired aggregation to ADP, collagen, and thrombin, and prolonged bleeding time; it is manifested clinically as Glanzmann's disease, with epistaxis, inappropriate bruising, and excessive bleeding, as during surgery. **Glanzmann's t.,** see *thrombasthenia.*

thrombectomy (throm-bek′to-me) [Gr. *thrombos* clot + *ektomē* excision] removal of a thrombus from a blood vessel; properly indicative of such removal by excision.

thrombembolia (throm″bem-bo′le-ah) thromboembolism.

thrombi (throm′bi) plural of *thrombus.*

thrombin (throm′bin) 1. the enzyme derived from prothrombin which converts fibrinogen to fibrin; called also *fibrinogenase* and *thrombase.* 2. [USP] a pharmaceutical preparation (*topical t.*), a sterile protein substance prepared from prothrombin of bovine origin through interaction with added thromboplastin in the presence of calcium is used therapeutically as a local hemostatic.

thrombinogen (throm-bin′o-jen) prothrombin.

thrombo- [Gr. *thrombos* clot] a combining form denoting relationship to a clot, or thrombus.

thromboangiitis (throm″bo-an″je-i′tis) [*thrombo-* + Gr. *angeion* vessel + *-itis*] inflammation of a blood vessel with thrombosis. **t. oblit′erans,** an inflammatory and obliterative disease of the blood vessels of the extremities, primarily the lower extremities, occurring chiefly in young men and leading to ischemia of the tissues and gangrene; called also *Buerger's disease.*

thromboarteritis (throm″bo-ar″ter-i′tis) thrombosis occurring in association with inflammation of an artery. **t. purulen′ta,** purulent softening of an arterial thrombosis, with infiltration of the artery walls.

thromboasthenia (throm″bo-as-the′ne-ah) thrombasthenia.

thromboclasis (throm-bok′lah-sis) [*thrombo-* + Gr. *klasis* a breaking] thrombolysis.

thromboclastic (throm″bo-klas′tik) thrombolytic.

thrombocyst (throm′bo-sist) [*thrombo-* + Gr. *kystis* cyst] the chronic sac which may form around a thrombus in a hematoma.

thrombocystis (throm″bo-sis′tis) thrombocyst.

thrombocytapheresis (throm″bo-sit″ah-fĕ-re′sis) [*thrombocyte* + Gr. *aphairesis* removal] the selective separation and removal of thrombocytes (platelets) from withdrawn blood, the remainder of the blood then being retransfused into the donor. Called also *plateletpheresis* and *thrombapheresis.*

thrombocyte (throm′bo-sīt) [*thrombo-* + Gr. *kytos* hollow vessel] a blood platelet.

thrombocythemia (throm″bo-sĭ-the′me-ah) [*thrombocyte* + Gr. *haima* blood + *-ia*] a fixed increase in the number of circulating blood platelets; called also *piastrinemia.* **essential t.,** hemorrhagic t. **hemorrhagic t.,** a clinical syndrome characterized by repeated spontaneous hemorrhages, either external or into the tissues, and a remarkable increase in the number of circulating platelets; regarded as one of the myeloproliferative syndromes. Called also *essential, idiopathic,* or *primary thrombocythemia,* and *megakaryocytic leukemia.* **idiopathic t., primary t.,** hemorrhagic t.

thrombocytic (throm″bo-sit′ik) 1. pertaining to, characterized by, or of the nature of a blood platelet (thrombocyte). 2. pertaining to the thrombocytic series.

thrombocytin (throm″bo-si′tin) serotonin.

thrombocytocrit (throm″bo-si′to-krit) [*thrombocyte* + Gr. *krinein* to separate] the volume of packed blood platelets in a given quantity of blood; the instrument used to measure the platelet volume.

thrombocytolysis (throm″bo-si-tol′ĭ-sis) destruction of blood platelets (thrombocytes).

thrombocytopathia (throm″bo-si″to-path′ĕ-ah) a heterogeneous hemorrhagic disorder characterized by platelets with defective clot-promoting (platelet factor 3) activity.

thrombocytopathic (throm″bo-si″to-path′ik) pertaining to or characterized by thrombocytopathy.

thrombocytopathy (throm″bo-si-top′ah-the) a general term applied to a qualitative disorder of the blood platelets, due mainly to deficiency of platelet factor 3, (PF-3). **constitutional t.,** Glanzmann's thrombasthenia.

thrombocytopenia (throm″bo-si″to-pe′ne-ah) [*thrombocyte* + Gr. *penia* poverty] decrease in the number of blood platelets. **essential t.,** idiopathic thrombocytopenic purpura. **immune t.,** that associated with the presence of anti-platelet antibodies (IgG). **malignant t.,** an old term for aleukia hemorrhagica.

thrombocytopoiesis (throm″bo-si″to-poi-e′sis) [*thrombocyte* + Gr. *poiēsis* a making, creation] the production of blood platelets.

thrombocytopoietic (throm″bo-si″to-poi-et′ik) concerned in the formation of blood platelets.

thrombocytosis (throm″bo-si-to′sis) increased numbers of platelets in the peripheral blood.

thromboelastogram (throm″bo-e-las′to-gram) the graphic record of the values determined by thromboelastography.

thromboelastograph (throm″bo-e-las′to-graf) an apparatus used in study of the rigidity of blood or plasma during coagulation.

thromboelastography (throm″bo-e″las-tog′rah-fe) determination of the rigidity of the blood or plasma during coagulation, by use of the thromboelastograph.

thromboembolia (throm″bo-em-bo′le-ah) thromboembolism.

thromboembolism (throm″bo-em′bo-lizm) obstruction of a blood vessel with thrombotic material carried by the blood stream from the site of origin to plug another vessel.

thromboendarterectomy (throm″bo-end″ar-ter-ek′to-me) [*thrombo-* + Gr. *endon* within + *artēria* artery + *ektomē* excision] removal of an obstructing thrombus together with the inner lining of an obstructed artery. **coronary t.,** excision of blood clot and the intima from an occluded coronary artery.

thromboendarteritis (throm″bo-end-ar″ter-i′tis) inflammation of the innermost coat of an artery, with thrombus formation.

thromboendocarditis (throm″bo-en″do-kar-di′tis) 1. formation of a thrombus on a heart valve which has previously been eroded. 2. an infectious disease of rabbits.

thrombogenesis (throm″bo-jen′ĕ-sis) the formation of blood clots.

thrombogenic (throm″bo-jen′ik) [*thrombo-* + Gr. *gennan* to produce] producing a clot, curd, or coagulum.

thromboid (throm′boid) [Gr. *thromboeidēs*] resembling a thrombus.

thrombokinase (throm″bo-kin′ās) activated Factor X; see *coagulation factors,* under *factor.*

thrombokinesis (throm″bo-ki-ne′sis) [*thrombo-* + Gr. *kinēsis* motion] the formation of a blood clot; clotting of blood.

thrombokinetics (throm″bo-ki-net′iks) the dynamics of blood coagulation.

thrombolymphangitis (throm″bo-lim″fan-ji′tis) inflammation of a lymph vessel due to a thrombus.

Thrombolysin (throm-bol′ĭ-sin) trademark for a preparation of fibrinolysin.

thrombolysis (throm-bol′ĭ-sis) [*thrombo-* + Gr. *lysis* dissolution] the phenomenon by which preformed thrombi are lysed by a complex series of events, the most important of which involves the local action of plasmin confined within the substance of the thrombus.

thrombolytic (throm″bo-lit′ik) 1. dissolving or splitting up a thrombus. 2. a thrombolytic agent.

thrombon (throm′bon) [*thrombo-* + Gr. *on* neuter ending] the element of the blood consisting of the platelets and their precursors; it is the counterpart of erythron and leukon.

thrombopathia (throm″bo-path′e-ah) a blood coagulation disorder due to failure of the platelets to release ADP in response to aggregating agents (collagen, epinephrine, thrombin).

thrombopathy (throm-bop′ah-the) see *thrombopathia.*

thrombopenia (throm″bo-pe′ne-ah) thrombocytopenia. **essential t.,** idiopathic thrombocytopenic purpura.

thrombopeny (throm″bo-pe′ne) thrombocytopenia.

thrombophilia (throm″bo-fil′e-ah) [*thrombo-* + Gr. *philein* to love] a tendency to the occurrence of thrombosis.

thrombophlebitis (throm″bo-fle-bi′tis) [*thrombo-* + Gr. *phleps* vein + *-itis*] inflammation of a vein associated with thrombus formation. Cf. *phlebothrombosis.* **iliofemoral t., postpartum,** thrombophlebitis of the iliofemoral vein following childbirth; called also *phlegmasia alba dolens puerperarum.* **t. mi′grans,** a recurring phlebitis usually affecting segments of superficial peripheral veins, and sometimes involving major and visceral veins; it may occur in multiple sites simultaneously or at intervals. **t. purulen′ta,** thrombophlebitis with purulent softening of the thrombus, and infiltration of the wall of the vessel.

thromboplastic (throm″bo-plas′tik) [*thrombo-* + Gr. *plassein* to form] causing or accelerating clot formation in the blood.

thromboplastid (throm″bo-plas′tid) a blood platelet.

thromboplastin (throm″bo-plas′tin) a substance having procoagulant properties or activity. **extrinsic t.,** the prothrombin activator formed as the result of interaction of coagulation Factors III, VII, and X which, with Factor IV, aids in the formation of thrombin: called *extrinsic* because not all of the components required for its production (e.g., Factor III, or tissue thromboplastin) are derived from intravascular sources. **intrinsic t.,** the prothrombin activator formed as the result of interaction of coagulation Factors V, VIII, IX, X, XI, and XII and platelet factor 3 (PF-3) which, with Factor IV, aids in the conversion of prothrombin to thrombin: called *intrinsic* because the components required for its production are derived from intravascular sources. **tissue t.,** Factor III; see *coagulation factors,* under *factor.* So called because it is released by or derived from extravascular tissues.

thromboplastinogen (throm″bo-plas-tin′o-jen) former term for Factor VIII; see *coagulation factors,* under *factor.*

thrombopoiesis (throm″bo-poi-e′sis) 1. thrombogenesis. 2. thrombocytopoiesis.

thrombopoietic (throm″bo-poi-et′ik) pertaining to or characterized by thrombopoiesis.

thrombopoietin (throm″bo-poi-e′tin) a hypothetical substance(s) believed to serve as the humoral regulator of the production of blood platelets.

thrombosed (throm′bōsd) affected with thrombosis.

thrombosinusitis (throm″bo-si″nu-si′tis) thrombosis of a sinus of the dura mater.

thrombosis (throm-bo′sis) [Gr. *thrombōsis*] the formation, development, or presence of a thrombus. **agonal t.,** clotting of blood in the heart and great vessels before death (Ribbert, 1916). **atrophic t.,** marasmic t. **cardiac t.,** thrombosis in the heart. **cavernous sinus t.,** thrombosis affecting the cavernous sinus. **cerebral t.,** thrombosis of a cerebral vessel, which may result in cerebral infarction. **coronary t.,** development of an obstructive thrombus in a coronary artery, often causing sudden death or a myocardial infarction. **creeping t.,** thrombosis gradually involving one portion of a vein after another. **dilatation t.,** thrombosis due to the slowing of circulation on account of dilatation of a vein. **infective t.,** that which is associated with a bacterial infection. **marantic t., marasmic t.,** thrombosis, chiefly of the longitudinal sinus, occurring in the wasting diseases of infancy and of old age; called also *atrophic t.* **mesenteric t.,** formation of a clot in an artery or arteriole of the mesentery. **placental t.,** 1. a normal formation of thrombi in the placenta. 2. an abnormal extension of the placental thrombus formation to the veins of the uterus. **plate t., platelet t.,** an aggregation of blood platelets forming the nidus of a thrombus; see also *white thrombus,* under *thrombus.* **propagating t.,** progressive clot formation upon an occlusive thrombus, producing an elongated mass sometimes extending into other blood vessels. **puerperal t.,** coagulation of blood in the veins (thrombophlebitis) occurring after childbirth. **Ribbert's t.,** agonal t. **sinus t.,** thrombosis of a venous sinus. **traumatic t.,** thrombosis following injury to a part. **venous t.,** the presence of a thrombus in a vein; phlebothrombosis.

thrombostasis (throm-bos′tah-sis) stasis of blood in a part, attended with the formation of a thrombus.

thrombosthenin (throm″bo-sthe′nin) [*thrombo-* + Gr. *sthenos* strength + *-in* chemical suffix] a contractile protein of platelets, active in clot retraction.

thrombotest (throm′bo-test) a test similar to the one-stage prothrombin test except that it is supposedly sensitive to depression of blood coagulation Factor IX and hence has an advantage over the one-stage test in controlling anticoagulant therapy; such superiority, however, has not been demonstrated.

thrombotic (throm-bot′ik) pertaining to or affected with thrombosis.

thrombotonin (throm″bo-to′nin) serotonin.

thromboxane (throm-boks′ān) an intermediate in the metabolic pathway of arachidonic acid, formed from prostaglandin endoperoxides and released from suitably stimulated platelets; the unstable form, thromboxane A_2, is a potent inducer of platelet aggregation and constrictor of arterial smooth muscle, but quickly breaks down to the inactive stable form, thromboxane B_2.

thrombus (throm′bus), pl. *throm′bi* [Gr. *thrombos* clot] an aggregation of blood factors, primarily platelets and fibrin with entrapment of cellular elements, frequently causing vascular obstruction at the point of its formation. Some authorities thus differentiate thrombus formation from simple coagulation or clot formation. Cf. *embolism.* **agonal t., agony t.,** a clot formed in the heart during the process of dying. **annular t.,** one which has an opening through its center, while the circumference is attached to the wall of the vessel. **antemortem t.,** a thrombus or a clot formed in the heart or in a large vessel before death. **ball t.,** a roughly spherical, organized thrombus which may obstruct an orifice (usually the mitral valve) intermittently like a ball valve. **bile t.,** a plug in one of the intrahepatic bile ducts, causing cholestasis. **blood plate t., blood platelet t.,** one formed by an abnormal accumulation of blood platelets. **calcified t.,** a phlebolith. **coral t.,** a red clot formed by coagulated fibrin enclosing red corpuscles. **currant jelly t.,** a soft, reddish, jelly-like clot. **fibrin t.,** a thrombus composed mainly of fibrin, and attached to the walls of a blood vessel. **hyaline t.,** a thrombus composed of erythrocytes which have lost their hemoglobin, forming a colorless translucent mass. **infective t.,** a thrombus associated with an infective agent. **laminated t.,** a thrombus whose substance is disposed in layers, suggesting different periods of formation. **lateral t.,** a clot attached to the side of a vessel, incompletely obstructing the blood current. **marantic t., marasmic t.,** a form associated with severe wasting diseases, often a terminal event; see also under *thrombosis.* **milk t.,** an accumulation of curdled milk in a lactiferous duct. **mixed t.,** laminated t. **mural t.,** a thrombus attached to the wall of the heart, the endocardium in the area being diseased. **obstructive t.,** one which plugs the lumen of the vessel at its site. **occluding t., occlusive t.,** one that occupies the entire lumen of a vessel and obstructs blood flow. **organized t.,** one which has been invaded by fibroblasts and thereby changed to loose fibrous tissue with varying degrees of vascularity. **pale t.,** a dull-white thrombus. **parasitic t.,** an accumulation of the pigmented bodies of free malarial parasites and their spores in the capillaries of the brain, and causing a condition known as *cerebral malaria*. **parietal t.,** one attached to the wall of a vessel. **phagocytic t.,** an accumulation of melaniferous leukocytes in the capillaries of the brain. **pigmentary t.,** an accumulation of free pigment in the capillaries of the brain. **plate t., platelet t.,** one formed by an abnormal accumulation of blood platelets. Called also *blood plate t.* or *blood platelet t.* **postmortem t.,** a thrombus or clot of blood formed in the heart or in a large vessel after death. **primary t.,** one which remains at the place of its origin. **propagated t.,** one which has grown beyond its original limits. **red t.,** a thrombus of a dark-red color formed by the coagulation of blood. **stratified t.,** one made up of layers of different colors. **traumatic t.,** one which results from an injury. **white t.,** 1. one which contains few or no red cells. 2. one composed chiefly of leukocytes. 3. one composed chiefly of platelets and fibrin, usually seen in arterial thrombosis.

thrush (thrush) 1. candidiasis of the mucous membranes of the mouth of infants (sometimes of adults), characterized by the formation of aphthae, or whitish spots in the mouth. It is due to infection by the fungus *Candida albicans*. The aphthae are followed by shallow ulcers. The disease is often accompanied by fever and gastrointestinal irritation. Such infection may spread to the groin, buttocks, and other parts of the body. Called also *mycotic stomatitis* and *white mouth.* 2. a disease of the horse's foot characterized by a fetid discharge. **sheep t.,** orf, def. 1.

thrust (thrust) a sudden forceful movement forward. **paraspinal t.,** the same as spinal thrust, except that the therapist's hands are placed on either side of the spinous processes, the fingers pointing toward the head. **spinal t.,** with the patient in the prone position on the examining table, the physician stands on the patient's right, facing him, places his right palm over the patient's lumbosacral joint perpendicular to the spinal axis, and using the left hand as reinforcement makes a series of short rapid thrusts downward and toward the head, progressing along each interspace to the midthoracic spine; done for relief of lumbosacral strain. **tongue t.,** the infantile pattern of the suckle-swallow in which the tongue is placed between the incisor teeth or alveolar ridges during the initial stages of deglutition, resulting sometimes in anterior open bite, deformation of the jaws, and abnormal function.

thrypsis (thrip′sis) [Gr. "a breaking in small pieces"] a comminuted fracture.

Thudichum's test (too′de-koomz) [John Lewis William *Thudichum*, London physician of German birth, 1829–1901] see under *tests.*

Thuja (thu′jah) [L.; Gr. *thyia*] a genus of coniferous trees, also called *arbor vitae;* secretions of the leafy twigs of *T. occidentalis* are poisonous to man on ingestion.

thuja (thu′jah) fresh tops of *Thuja occidentalis,* white cedar: diuretic, antipyretic, sudorific, and emmenagogue.

thujone (thu′jōn) an aromatic terpene ketone present in many essential oils. It is $CH_3 \cdot C_8H_6O \cdot CH(CH_3)_2$.

thulium (thu′le-um) [*Thule*, ancient name of Shetland] a very rare metallic element; symbol, Tm; atomic number, 69; atomic weight, 168.934.

thumb (thum) [L. *pollex, pollux*] the first digit of the hand, being the most preaxial of the five fingers, having only two phalanges, and being apposable to the four other fingers of the hand. Called also *pollex* [NA]. **bifid t.,** a deformed thumb in which the distal phalanx is divided or bifurcated. **tennis t.,** tendinitis with calcification in the flexor pollicis longus, resulting from repeated friction experienced in playing tennis.

thumbprint (thum′print) an imprint of the cutaneous ridges of the fleshy distal portion of the thumb. See also *thumbprinting*

thumbprinting (thum′print-ing) a roentgenographic sign appearing as smooth indentations on the barium-filled colon, as though made by depression with the thumb; seen in various disorders of the colon, especially ischemic colitis.

thumb-sucking (thum-suk′ing) an infantile oral habit that is normal quite early in the child's development but that may persist and cause deformation of supporting bony tissue and abnormal function.

thumps (thumps) 1. a disease of swine caused by *Ascaris* larvae in the lungs. 2. a kind of singultus, or hiccup, of horses, due to spasm of the diaphragm.

thylakoid (thi′lah-koid) [Gr. *thylakon* a small sac, a seed pouch + *eidos* form] any of the membranous sacs which are the widened portions of lamellae of chloroplasts and which are arranged in stacks to form grana; thylakoids contain the photosynthetic pigments of chloroplasts and the enzymes that catalyze light-dependent reactions.

thyme (tīm) [L. *thymus;* Gr. *thymos*] a plant of the genus *Thymus.* The *Thymus vulgaris* L. (Labiatae), or garden thyme, contains a volatile oil, which is aromatic and carminative. It also contains *thymol, thymene,* and *cumene.* **creeping t., wild t.,** *Thymus serpyllum,* which contains a volatile oil similar to that of *Thymus vulgaris* L.

thymectomize (thi-mek′to-mīz) to remove the thymus gland.

thymectomy (thi-mek′to-me) [Gr. *thymos* thymus + *ektomē* excision] surgical removal of the thymus gland.

thymelcosis (thi″mel-ko′sis) [Gr. *thymos* thymus + *helkōsis* ulceration] ulceration of the thymus.

thymene (thi′mēn) a clear, oily hydrocarbon, $C_{10}H_{16}$, from the oil of thyme.

thymergasia (thi″mer-ga′se-ah) see *thymergastic.*

thymergastic (thi″mer-gas′tik) [Gr. *thymos* mind + *ergon* work] Meyer's term for the affective psychoses (the manic-depressive group).

-thymia [Gr. *thymos* mind + *-ia*] a word termination denoting a condition of mind.

thymian (thim′e-an, tim′e-an) [Ger.] thyme.

thymiasis (thi-mi′ah-sis) yaws.

thymic (thi′mik) [L. *thymicus*] 1. pertaining to the thymus. 2. contained in or derived from thyme.

thymicolymphatic (thi″mi-ko-lim-fat′ik) pertaining to the thymus and the lymphatic glands.

thymidine (thi′mi-dēn) thymine deoxyriboside, a nucleoside isolable from deoxyribonucleotide.

thymidylate (thi″mi-dil′āt) a salt or ester of thymidylic acid, or thymidylic acid in dissociated form, which is important in the formation of DNA.

thymin (thi′min) a hormone-like substance secreted by the thymus that impairs postsynaptic neuromuscular transmission.

thymine (thi′min) a pyrimidine base, 5-methyl uracil, C_5H_6-N_2O, found in deoxyribonucleic acid.

thymion (thim′e-on) [Gr.] a cutaneous wart.

thymiosis (thim″e-o′sis) yaws.

thymitis (thi-mi′tis) inflammation of the thymus.

thymo- 1. [Gr. *thymos* thymus] a combining form denoting relationship to the thymus gland. 2. [Gr. *thymos* mind, spirit.] a combining form denoting relationship to the soul or emotions.

thymocrescin (thi″mo-kres′in) a hypothetical growth-promoting substance in extracts of the thymus gland.

thymocyte (thi′mo-sīt) [*thymo-*(1) + Gr. *kytos* hollow vessel] a lymphocyte arising in the thymus.

thymoform (thi′mo-form) a yellowish, antiseptic powder, thymoloform, $CH_2[C_6H_3(CH)_3(C_3H_7)O]_2$, prepared from formaldehyde and thymol.

thymogenic (thi″mo-jen′ik) [*thymo-*(2) + Gr. *gennan* to produce] of affective or hysterical origin.

thymohydroquinone (thi″mo-hi″dro-kwin-ōn′) chemical name: 2,5-dihydroxy-*p*-cymene. A compound, $CH_3 \cdot C_6H_2(OH)_2CH$-$(CH_3)_2$, occurring in the urine after the administration of thymol, and also found in various essential oils.

thymokesis (thi″mo-ke′sis) enlargement of the remnant of the thymus that is found in the adult.

thymokinetic (thi″mo-ki-net′ik) tending to stimulate the thymus.

thymol (thi′mol) [NF] chemical name: 5-methyl-2-(1-methylethyl)phenol. A phenol, $C_{10}H_{14}O$, occurring as colorless, often large, crystals, or white, crystalline powder, obtained from thyme oil or other volatile oils; used as a stabilizer in pharmaceutical preparations. It has been used for its antiseptic, antibacterial, and antifungal actions, and was formerly used as a vermifuge. **t. iodide,** a mixture of iodine derivatives of thymol, principally dithymol diiodide, $(C_6H_2 \cdot CH_3 \cdot C_3H_7 \cdot OI)_2$, occurring as a reddish brown or reddish yellow bulky powder, formerly used as an antifungal and antibacterial agent. **t. phthalein,** see *thymolphthalein.*

thymoleptic (thi″mo-lep′tik) [*thymo-* (2) + Gr. *lēpsis* a taking hold] any drug that favorably modifies mood in serious affective disorders such as depression or mania; the main categories of thymoleptics include the tricyclic antidepressants, monoamine oxidase inhibitors and lithium compounds. Also called antidepressants.

thymolize (thi′mo-līz) to treat with thymol.

thymolphthalein (thi″mol-thal′e-in) an indicator, $C_6H_4 \cdot CO$-$O \cdot C(C_6H_2 \cdot CH_3 \cdot C_3H_7 \cdot OH)_2$, with a pH range of 9.3 to 10.5, being colorless at 9.3 and blue at 10.5.

thymolysin (thi-mol′ĭ-sin) an antibody that damages or kills thymus cells.

thymolysis (thi-mol′ĭ-sis) [*thymo-*(1) + Gr. *lysis* dissolution] involution or dissolution of the thymus.

thymolytic (thi″mo-lit′ik) pertaining to, characterized by, or promoting thymolysis.

thymoma (thi-mo′mah) [*thymo-*(1) + *-oma*] a tumor derived from the epithelial or lymphoid elements of the thymus.

thymometastasis (thi″mo-mĕ-tas′tah-sis) a metastasis from the thymus.

thymopathic (thi″mo-path′ik) pertaining to, characterized by, or causing thymopathy.

thymopathy (thi-mop′ah-the) any disease of the thymus.

thymopoietin (thi″mo-poi′ĕ-tin) a polypeptide hormone secreted by the thymus, which induces differentiation of thymocytes and impairs postsynaptic neuromuscular transmission.

thymoprivic (thi″mo-priv′ik) thymoprivous.

thymoprivous (thi-mop′rĭ-vus) [thymo-(1) + L. privus without] pertaining to or caused by removal or atrophy of the thymus.

thymosin (thi′mo-sin) a humoral factor, believed to be a hormone, secreted by the thymus which promotes the maturation of T-lymphocytes and restores their function in thymus-deficient animals; called also *thymic hormone.*

thymotoxic (thi″mo-tok′sik) toxic for thymus tissue.

thymotoxin (thi″mo-tok′sin) an element that exerts a deleterious effect on the thymus.

thymotrophic (thi″mo-trōf′ik) having an influence on the thymus.

thymovidin (thi-mo′vĭ-din) a hormone which originates in the thymus of birds and stimulates the oviduct to the production of normal egg envelopes.

Thymus (thi′mus) a genus of herbs (family Labiatae) native to south central Europe and grown extensively in other countries. See *thyme.*

thymus (thi′mus) [L.; Gr. *thymos*] [NA] a lymphoid organ situated in the anterior superior mediastinum, which reaches its maximum weight at about puberty and then undergoes involution. It is necessary in early life for development and maturation of cell-mediated immunological functions. Of grayish red color, it originates as two separate primordia and develops into two lobes, which later become joined by connective tissue. The thymus is composed chiefly of epithelial cells (primarily in the medulla) and lymphocytes, or thymocytes (primarily in the cortex). Precursor cells migrate to the thymus, where they differentiate into lymphocytes, most of which are destroyed, but the remainder of which migrate to tissues to form T-lymphocytes. The thymus also secretes the hormone-like substances thymin, thymopoietin, and thymosin. **accessory t.,** a separated portion of the thymus gland which may be found occasionally. **persistent t., t. persis′tens hyperplas′tica,** a thymus which persists into adult life, sometimes even becoming hypertrophied.

thymus-dependent (thi′mus-de-pen′dent) depending on passage through or on being influenced by the thymus for the development of function; said of T-lymphocytes (see under *lymphocyte*). See also under *area.*

thymusectomy (thi″mus-ek′to-me) [thymus + Gr. *ektomē* excision] excision of the thymus.

thymus-independent (thi′mus-in-de-pen′dent) able to function without passing through or being influenced by the thymus; said of B-lymphocytes (see under *lymphocyte*). See also under *area.*

thynnin (thin′in) a protamine from the sperm of the tunny fish, *Thunnus thynnus.*

thypar (thi′pahr) deprived of the thyroid and parathyroid glands; lacking thyroid and parathyroid secretions.

Thyrar (thi′rar) trademark for a preparation of thyroid (def. 3).

thyratron (thi′rah-tron) a form of discharge tube containing mercury vapor and a multiplicity of electrodes, used as an electric valve to rectify alternating current.

thyremphraxis (thi″rem-frak′sis) [Gr. *thyreos* shield + *empharaxis* stoppage] obstruction of the thyroid gland.

thyreo- for other words beginning thus, see also those beginning *thyro-.*

thyreoitis (thi″re-o-i′tis) thyroiditis.

thyro- [Gr. *thyreos* shield] a combining form denoting relationship to the thyroid gland.

thyroactive (thi″ro-ak′tiv) having a metabolic effect similar to thyroid hormone.

thyroadenitis (thi″ro-ad″ĕ-ni′tis) [thyro- + Gr. *adēn* gland + -*itis*] inflammation of the thyroid gland.

thyroaplasia (thi″ro-ah-pla′ze-ah) [thyro- + *a* neg. + Gr. *plasis* molding + -*ia*] defective development of the thyroid gland with deficient activity of its secretion.

thyroarytenoid (thi″ro-ar″ĭ-te′noid) pertaining to the thyroid and arytenoid cartilages.

thyrocalcitonin (thi″ro-kal″sĭ-to′nin) calcitonin.

thyrocardiac (thi″ro-kar′de-ak) pertaining to the thyroid and the heart.

thyrocarditis (thi″ro-kar-di′tis) any affection of the heart muscle occurring in hyperthyroidism.

thyrocele (thi′ro-sēl) [thyro- + Gr. *kēlē* tumor] a tumor of the thyroid gland; goiter.

thyrochondrotomy (thi″ro-kon-drot′o-me) [thyro- + Gr. *chondros* cartilage + *tomē* a cutting] surgical incision of the thyroid cartilage.

thyrocolloid (thi″ro-kol′oid) the colloid matter of the thyroid gland.

thyrocricotomy (thi″ro-kri-kot′o-me) incision of the cricothyroid membrane.

thyrodesmic (thi″ro-dez′mik) [thyro- + Gr. *desmos* bond] thyrotropic.

thyroepiglottic (thi″ro-ep″ĭ-glot′ik) pertaining to the thyroid and to the epiglottis.

thyrofissure (thi″ro-fish′ur) the operation of making an opening through the thyroid cartilage for the purpose of gaining access to the interior of the larynx.

thyrogenic (thi″ro-jen′ik) thyrogenous.

thyrogenous (thi-roj′ĕ-nus) [thyro- + Gr. *gennan* to produce] originating in the thyroid gland.

thyroglobulin (thi-ro-glob′u-lin) 1. an iodine-containing glycoprotein of high molecular weight occurring in the colloid of the follicles of the thyroid gland; the iodinated tyrosine moieties of thyroglobulin form the active hormones thyroxine and triiodothyronine, which are released into the blood on proteolysis of thyroglobulin. 2. [USP] a substance obtained by fractionation of thyroid glands from the hog, *Sus scrofa* var. *domesticus,* containing not less than 0.7 per cent of total iodine, occurring as a cream to tan-colored, free-flowing powder; administered orally as a thyroid supplement in the treatment of hypothyroidism.

thyroglossal (thi″ro-glos′al) pertaining to the thyroid gland and the tongue.

thyrohyal (thi″ro-hi′al) 1. pertaining to the thyroid cartilage and the hyoid bone. 2. cornu majus ossis hyoidei.

thyrohyoid (thi″ro-hi′oid) pertaining to the thyroid gland or cartilage and the hyoid bone.

thyroid (thi′roid) [Gr. *thyreoeidēs; thyreos* shield + *eidos* form] 1. resembling a shield; scutiform. 2. the thyroid gland (glandula thyroidea [NA]); see under *gland.* 3. [USP] the cleaned, dried, and powdered thyroid gland previously deprived of connective tissue and fat, obtained from domesticated animals that are used for food by man, containing 0.17–0.23 per cent of iodine in thyroid combination, occurring as a yellowish to buff-colored amorphous powder; used as a source of thyroid hormones in the treatment of hypothyroidism. **aberrant t.,** a mass of thyroid tissue situated in an abnormal location. **accessory t.,** an exclave or detached portion of thyroid tissue. **intrathoracic t.,** a mass of thyroid tissue that is located within the thoracic cavity. **lingual t.,** thyroid tissue located at the base of the tongue, between the foramen cecum and the hyoid bone. It may project into the pharynx from the dorsum of the tongue, or be entirely within the tongue or located just beneath it; it may also be accessory to a normally located thyroid gland, or be the only thyroid tissue present. **retrosternal t., substernal t.,** a mass of thyroid tissue situated in the thorax behind the sternum.

thyroidea (thi-roi′de-ah) the thyroid gland. **t. accesso′ria, t. i′ma,** accessory thyroid.

thyroidectomize (thi″roi-dek′to-mīz) to deprive of the thyroid gland by surgical removal.

thyroidectomy (thi″roi-dek′to-me) [thyroid + Gr. *ektomē* excision] surgical removal of the thyroid. **medical t.,** diminution of thyroid function by the use of drugs.

thyroidism (thi′roid-izm) a morbid condition caused by overactivity of the thyroid gland (hyperthyroidism), or excessive doses of thyroid.

thyroiditis (thi″roi-di′tis) inflammation of the thyroid gland. **acute t.,** inflammation of the thyroid gland caused by staphylococcic, streptococcic, or other infection, with suppuration and abscess formation, and progressing to the subacute stage. **acute nonsuppurative t.,** granulomatous t. **chronic t., chronic fibrous t.,** Riedel's struma. **chronic lymphadenoid t., chronic lymphocytic t.,** struma lymphomatosa. **de Quervain's t.,** granulomatous t. **giant cell t., giant follicular t.,** granulomatous t. **granulomatous t.,** a condition characterized by fever, weakness, sore throat, and painful enlargement of the thyroid gland, with granulomas in the gland consisting of masses of colloid surrounded by giant cells and mononuclear cells, and a moderate amount of fibrosis. **Hashimoto's t.,** struma lymphomatosa. **invasive t., ligneous t.,** Riedel's struma. **lymphocytic t., lymphoid t.,** struma lymphomatosa. **t. parasita′ria, parasitic t.,** Chagas' disease. **pseudotuberculous t.,** granulomatous t. **Riedel's t.,** Riedel's struma. **subacute t., subacute diffuse t.,** granulomatous t. **woody t.,** Riedel's struma.

thyroidization (thi″roid-i-za′shun) 1. treatment with a preparation of the thyroid. 2. in histopathology, the thyroid-like appearance of a tissue.

thyroidomania (thi″roid-o-ma′ne-ah) mental disorder associated with hyperthyroidism.

thyroidotherapy (thi″roid-o-ther′ah-pe) thyrotherapy.

thyroidotomy (thi″roi-dot′o-me) [thyroid + Gr. *tomē* a cutting] surgical incision of the thyroid.

thyroidotoxin (thi″roid-o-tok′sin) a toxin specific for thyroid tissue.

thyroigenous (thi-roi′jĕ-nus) due to thyroid disorder.

thyrointoxication (thi″ro-in-tok″sĭ-ka′shun) thyroid poisoning; thyrotoxicosis.

Thyrolar (thi′ro-lar) trademark for a preparation of liotrix.

thyrolysin (thi-rol′ĭ-sin) a thyrolytic serum.

thyrolytic (thi″ro-lit′ik) [*thyroid* + Gr. *lysis* dissolution] destructive to thyroid tissue.

thyromegaly (thi″ro-meg′ah-le) [*thyro-* + Gr. *megaleia* bigness] enlargement of the thyroid gland; goiter.

thyromimetic (thi″ro-mi-met′ik) producing effects similar to those of thyroid hormones or the thyroid gland.

thyroncus (thi-rong′kus) [*thyroid* + Gr. *onkos* mass, tumor] goiter.

thyronucleoalbumin (thi″ro-nu″kle-o-al-bu′min) a nucleoalbumin present in the thyroid gland.

thyro-oxyindole (thi″ro-ok″se-in′dol) thyroxine.

thyroparathyroidectomy (thi″ro-par″ah-thi″roi-dek′to-me) [*thyroid* + *parathyroid* + Gr. *ektome* excision] excision of the thyroid and parathyroids.

thyroparathyroprivic (thi″ro-par″ah-thi″ro-priv′ik) lacking thyroid and parathyroid glands or secretions.

thyropathy (thi-rop′ah-the) [*thyroid* + Gr. *pathos* disease] any disease of the thyroid.

thyropenia (thi″ro-pe′ne-ah) [*thyroid* + Gr. *penia* poverty] deficiency of thyroid secretion.

thyrophyma (thi″ro-fi′mah) [*thyroid* + Gr. *phyma* tumor] thyrocele.

thyroprival (thi″ro-pri′val) [*thyroid* + L. *privus* without] pertaining to, characterized by, or resulting from deprivation or loss of thyroid function.

thyroprivia (thi″ro-priv′e-ah) [*thyroid* + L. *privus* without] hypothyroidism: the condition resulting from lack of thyroid hormone, as a consequence of removal of the thyroid gland or suppression of its functions.

thyroprivic, thyroprivous (thi″ro-priv′ik; thi-rop′rĭ-vus) thyroprival.

thyroptosis (thi″rop-to′sis) [*thyroid* + Gr. *ptosis* fall] downward displacement of the thyroid gland into the thorax.

thyrosis (thi-ro′sis), pl. *thyro′ses.* Any disease based on disordered thyroid action.

thyrotherapy (thi″ro-ther′ah-pe) treatment of disease by preparations of the thyroid glands of domestic animals used for food by man.

thyrotome (thi′ro-tōm) an instrument for cutting the thyroid cartilage.

thyrotomy (thi-rot′o-me) [*thyroid* + Gr. *tome* a cutting] 1. the surgical division of the thyroid cartilage. 2. the operation of cutting the thyroid gland.

thyrotoxemia (thi″ro-tok-se′me-ah) thyrotoxicosis.

thyrotoxia (thi″ro-tok′se-ah) thyrotoxicosis.

thyrotoxic (thi″ro-tok′sik) marked by toxic activity of the thyroid gland.

thyrotoxicosis (thi″ro-tok″sĭ-ko′sis) a morbid condition resulting from overactivity of the thyroid gland. See *Graves' disease,* under *disease.*

thyrotoxin (thi″ro-tok′sin) a toxic substance produced in the thyroid.

thyrotrope (thi′ro-trōp) any of the basophils (beta cells) of the adenohypophysis, the granules of which secrete thyrotropin; called also *beta basophil.*

thyrotroph (thi′ro-trōf) thyrotrope.

thyrotrophic (thi″ro-trōf′ik) thyrotropic.

thyrotrophin (thi″ro-trōf′in) thyrotropin.

thyrotropic (thi″ro-trop′ik) 1. pertaining to or marked by thyrotropism. 2. having an influence on the thyroid gland.

thyrotropin (thi-rot′ro-pin) a hormone of the anterior pituitary that has affinity for and specifically stimulates the thyroid gland.

thyrotropism (thi-rot′ro-pizm) [*thyroid* + Gr. *tropos* a turning] affinity for the thyroid.

thyroxin (thi-rok′sin) thyroxine.

thyroxine (thi-rok′sin) a crystalline iodine-containing hormone, 3,5,3′,5′-tetraiodothyronine, formed from thyroglobulin and secreted by the thyroid gland; its chief function is to increase the rate of cell metabolism. Thyroxine is deiodinated in peripheral tissues (liver, kidney, and heart) to form triiodothyronine, presumably the active "tissue" form of thyroid hormone, which is much more biologically active. Originally isolated by Kendall from the thyroid gland and later prepared synthetically, it is used in the treatment of hypothyroidism. Symbol T_4. **levo t.,** see *levothyroxine,* under L.

thyroxinemia (thi-rok″sin-e′me-ah) the presence of thyroxine in the blood.

thyroxinic (thi″rok-sin′ik) pertaining to thyroxine.

thyroxinsodium (thi-rok′sin-so′de-um) a preparation of thyroxine treated with sodium carbonate.

thyroxinum (thi-rok′sĭ-num) thyroxine.

thyrsus (thir′sus) [Gr. *thyrsos* Bacchic wand] the penis.

Thysanosoma (this″ah-no-so′mah) a genus of the family Anoplocephalidae. **T. actinioi′des,** the fringed tapeworm, found in the bile ducts and small intestine of sheep, cattle, antelope, and deer, in western and southwestern United States and in Africa.

Thytropar (thi′tro-par) trademark for a preparation of thyrotropin.

Ti chemical symbol for *titanium.*

tiacarana (te″ah-kar-an′yah) cutaneous leishmaniasis of the ulcerative type.

tiamenidine hydrochloride (ti″ah-men′ĭ-dēn) chemical name: *N*-(2-chloro-4-methyl-3-thienyl)-4,5-dihydro-1*H*-imidazol-2-amine monohydrochloride; an antihypertensive, $C_8H_{10}ClN_3S$·-HCl.

tiazuril (ti-az′ur-il) chemical name: 2-[4-[(4-chlorophenyl)thio]-3,5-dimethylphenyl]-1,2,4-triazine-3,5(2*H*,4*H*)-dione; a coccidiostat for poultry, $C_{17}H_{14}ClN_3O_2S$.

tibia (tib′e-ah) [L. "a pipe, flute"] [NA] the shin bone: the inner and larger bone of the leg below the knee; it articulates with the femur and head of the fibula above and with the talus below. See plate accompanying *skeleton.* **saber t., saber-shaped t.,** a tibia curved outward as a result of gummatous periostitis. **t. val′ga,** a bowing of the leg in which the angulation is away from the midline of the body. **t. va′ra,** osteochondrosis deformans tibiae.

tibiad (tib′e-ad) toward the tibial aspect.

tibial (tib′e-al) [L. *tibialis*] pertaining to the tibia.

tibiale (tib″e-a′le) a bone on the tibial side of the tarsus of the embryo, partly represented in the adult by the astragalus. **t. exter′num, t. posti′cum,** a sesamoid bone found in the tendon of the tibialis posterior muscle.

tibialgia (tib″e-al′je-ah) painful shin, with lymphocytosis and eosinophilia (von Schrötter, 1916).

tibialis (tib″e-a′lis) tibial; [NA] a term designating relationship to the tibia.

tibien (tib′e-en) pertaining to the tibia alone or in itself.

tibiocalcanean (tib″e-o-kal-ka′ne-an) pertaining to the tibia and the calcaneus.

tibiofemoral (tib″e-o-fem′or-al) pertaining to the tibia and the femur.

tibiofibular (tib″e-o-fib′u-lar) pertaining to the tibia and the fibula.

tibionavicular (tib″e-o-nah-vik′u-lar) pertaining to the tibia and the navicular bone.

tibioperoneal (tib″e-o-per′o-ne′al) tibiofibular.

tibioscaphoid (tib″e-o-skaf′oid) tibionavicular.

tibiotarsal (tib″e-o-tar′sal) pertaining to the tibia and the tarsus.

tibolone (tĭ′bo-lōn) chemical name: 17-hydroxy-7α-methyl-19-nor-17α-pregn-5(10)-en-20-yn-3-one; an anabolic steroid, $C_{21}H_{28}O_2$.

tic (tik) [Fr.] an involuntary, compulsive, repetitive, stereotyped movement, resembling a purposeful movement because it is coordinated and involves muscles in their normal synergistic relationships; tics usually involve the face and shoulders. **bowing t.,** nodding spasm. **convulsive t.,** spasm of those parts of the face supplied by the seventh nerve. **degenerative t.,** tic occurring in connection with degeneration of the central nervous system. **t. de pensée** (de pah-sa′), the habit of involuntarily expressing any thought that happens to come to mind. **diaphragmatic t.,** spasmodic twitching movements of the diaphragm; called also *respiratory t.* **t. douloureux** (doo-loo-roo′), trigeminal neuralgia. **facial t.,** spasm of the facial muscles. **gesticulatory t.,** that marked by spasmodic movements resembling the gestures of an orator or an actor. **t. de Guinon,** Gilles de la Tourette syndrome. **laryngeal t.,** that marked by a noisy expulsion of air through the glottis. **local t.,** a tic affecting only a limited locality, as the eye. **mimic t.,** facial tic. **motor t.,** a tic which is marked only by the spasmodic movement without mental disturbance; it includes facial spasm, rotatory spasm, blepharospasm, and diaphragmatic, laryngeal, and other varieties of tic. **t. nondouloureux,** myoclonus. **occupation t.,** occupation neurosis. **progressive choreic t.,** a chronic disease beginning in early life, marked by spasms which at first affect the neck muscles, but, as the disease advances, spread to the rest of the body. The disease ends fatally. **respiratory t.,** diaphragmatic t. **rotatory t.,** rotatory spasm. **saltatory t.,** saltatory spasm. **t. de sommeil,** an involuntary movement of the head during sleep. **spasmodic t.,** a condition marked by spasmodic movements of groups of muscles occurring at irregular intervals.

Ticar (ti′kar) trademark for a preparation of ticarcillin disodium.

ticarbodine (ti-kar′bo-dēn) chemical name: α,α,α-trifluoro-2,6-dimethylthio-1-piperidinecarboxy-*m*-toluidide; an anthelmintic, $C_{15}H_{19}F_3N_2S$.

ticarcillin (ti″kar-sil′in) chemical name: 6-[(carboxy-3-thienylacetyl)amino]-3,3-dimethyl-7-oxo-4-thia-1-azabicyclo[3.2.0]heptane-2-carboxylic acid. A semisynthetic penicillin bactericidal against both gram-negative and gram-positive organisms. **t. cresyl sodium,** a salt of ticarcillin, $C_{22}H_{21}N_2NaO_6S_2$. **t.**

disodium, t. sodium, the disodium salt of ticarcillin, $C_{15}H_{14}$-$N_2Na_2O_6S_2$, used primarily in the treatment of severe systemic infections and septicemia and infections of the genitourinary and respiratory tracts and of the soft tissues due to susceptible strains of *Pseudomonas aeruginosa, Proteus* species, and *Escherichia coli;* administered intramuscularly and intravenously. Sterile ticarcillin disodium conforms to USP specifications for antibiotics.

tick (tik) a blood-sucking acarid parasite of the suborder Ixodides, superfamily Ixodoidea. The ticks are larger than their relatives, the mites. There are two families: the Argasidae, or soft ticks, and the Ixodidae, or hard ticks. The former includes the genera *Antricola, Argas, Otobius,* and *Ornithodoros;* the latter the genera *Amblyomma, Anocenter, Aponomma, Boophilus, Dermacentor, Haemaphysalis, Hyalomma, Ixodes, Margaropus, Rhipicephalus,* and *Rhipicentor.* **adobe t.,** *Argas persicus.* **American dog t.,** *Dermacentor variabilis.* **bandicoot t.,** *Haemaphysalis humerosa.* **beady-legged winter horse t.,** *Margaropus winthemi.* **black pitted t.,** *Rhipicephalus simus.* **bont t.,** *Amblyomma hebraeum.* **British dog t.,** *Ixodes canisuga.* **brown dog t.,** *Rhipicephalus sanguineus.* **castor bean t.,** *Ixodes ricinus.* **cattle t.,** *Boophilus annulatus.* **dog t.,** 1. *Haemaphysalis leachi.* 2. *Dermacentor variabilis.* 3. *Rhipicephalus sanguineus.* **ear t.,** *Otobius megnini.* **Gulf Coast t.,** *Amblyomma maculatum.* **hard t., hard-bodied t.,** an individual of the family Ixodidae. **Kenya t.,** *Rhipicephalus appendiculatus.* **Lone Star t.,** *Amblyomma americanum.* **miana t.,** *Argas persicus.* **Pacific coast dog t.,** *Dermacentor occidentalis.* **pajaroello t.,** *Ornithodoros coriaceus.* **pigeon t.,** *Argas reflexus.* **rabbit t.,** *Haemaphysalis leporus-palustris.* **Rocky Mountain wood t.,** *Dermacentor andersoni.* **russet t.,** *Ixodes pilosus.* **scrub t.,** *Ixodes holocyclus.* **seed t.,** the young six-legged larva of a tick: after moulting it emerges as an eight-legged nymph. **sheep t.,** *Melophagus ovinus.* **soft t., soft-bodied t.,** an individual of the family Argasidae. **spinous t.,** *Otobius megnini.* **taiga t.,** *Ixodes persulcatus.* **tampan t.,** 1. *Ornithodoros moubata.* 2. *Argas persicus.* **winter t.,** *Dermacentor albipictus.* **wood t.,** *Dermacentor andersoni.*

tickling (tik′ling) light stimulation of a surface, and its reflex effect, such as involuntary laughter, etc.

ticlatone (tik′lah-tōn) chemical name: 6-chloro-1,2-benzisothiazolin-3(2*H*)-one; an antibacterial and antifungal, C_7H_4ClNOS.

ticlopidine hydrochloride (ti-klo′pĭ-dēn) chemical name: 5-[(2-chlorophenyl)methyl]-4,5,6,7-tetrahydrothieno[3,2-c] pyridine hydrochloride; a platelet inhibitor, $C_{14}H_{14}ClNS \cdot HCl$.

ticpolonga (tik″po-long′ah) an extremely venomous serpent of Ceylon and India, *Vipera russelli;* called also *Russell's viper* and *cobra-monil.*

ticrynafen (ti-krin′ah-fen) chemical name: [2,3-dichloro-4-(2-thienylcarbonyl)phenoxy]acetic acid; a diuretic, uricosuric, and antihypertensive, $C_{13}H_8Cl_2O_4S$. No longer used.

tictology (tik-tol′o-je) [Gr. *tiktein* to give birth + *logos* treatise] obstetrics.

t.i.d. abbreviation for L. *ter in di′e,* three times a day.

tide (tīd) a physiological variation or increase of a certain constituent in body fluids. **acid t.,** temporary increase in the acidity of the urine which sometimes follows fasting. **alkaline t.,** temporary increase in the alkalinity of the urine during gastric digestion. **fat t.,** the increase of fat in the lymph and blood following a meal.

Tidy's test (ti′dēz) [Charles Meymott *Tidy,* English physician, 1843–1892] see under *tests.*

Tiedemann's nerve (te′dĕ-manz) [Friedrich *Tiedemann,* German physician, 1781–1861] see under *nerve.*

Tietze's syndrome (disease) (tēt′sez) [Alexander *Tietze,* Breslau surgeon, 1864–1927] see under *syndrome.*

Tigan (ti′gan) trademark for preparations of trimethobenzamide hydrochloride.

tigestol (ti-jes′tōl) chemical name: 19-nor-17α-pregn-5(10)-en-20-yn-17-ol; a progestin, $C_{20}H_{28}O$.

tiglium (tig′le-um), gen. *tig′lii* [L.] the croton oil plant, *Croton tiglium* L. (Euphorbiaceae).

tigogenin (tig-oj′ĕ-nin) a complex aglycone, $C_{27}H_{44}O_3$, from tigonin.

tigonin (tig′o-nin) a saponin, $C_{56}H_{92}O_{27}$, from *Digitalis purpurea* L. and *D. lanata* Ehrh. (Scrophulariaceae). On hydrolysis, it yields tigogenin, glucose, galactose, and rhamnose.

tigretier (te-gret″e-a′) [Fr.] a form of hysterical dancing mania peculiar to Tigré, a region in Abyssinia.

tigroid (ti′groid) [Gr. *tigroeidēs* tiger-spotted] marked like a tiger; a term applied to Nissl bodies or masses of deeply staining substance in the protoplasm of neurons.

tigrolysis (ti-grol′ĭ-sis) chromatolysis, def. 2.

tikitiki (te″ke-te′ke) the Japanese name for rice polishings; see *polishing,* def. 2.

tiletamine hydrochloride (ti-let′ah-mēn) chemical name: 2-(ethylamino)-2-(2-thienyl)cyclohexanone hydrochloride; an anesthetic and anticonvulsant, $C_{12}H_{17}NOS \cdot HCl$.

tilidine hydrochloride (til′ĭ-dēn) chemical name: ($\pm$)-ethyl *trans-*2-(dimethylamino)-1-phenyl-3-cyclohexane-1-carboxylate hydrochloride; an analgesic, $C_{17}H_{23}NO_2 \cdot HCl$.

Tillaux's disease (te-yōz′) [Paul Jules *Tillaux,* French physician, 1834–1904] see under *disease.*

Tilletia (til-le′she-ah) a genus of basidiomycetous fungi of the order Ustilaginales, family Tilletiaceae, causing smut on cereals. *T. caries* causes stinking bunt of wheat.

Tilletiaceae (til-le″she-a′se-e) a family of basidiomycetous fungi of the subclass Heterobasidiomycetidae, order Ustilaginales, including the genera *Tilletia* and *Urocystis.*

tilmus (til′mus) [Gr. *tilmos* a plucking] carphology.

tilorone (til′or-ōn) a low-molecular-weight aromatic amine that stimulates the production of interferon in serum. **t. hydrochloride,** chemical name: 2,7-bis[2-(diethylamino)ethoxy]-9*H*-fluoren-9-one dihydrochloride; an antiviral agent, $C_{25}H_{34}N_2$-$O_3 \cdot 2HCl$.

tiltometer (til-tom′ĕ-ter) an instrument for measuring the degree of tilting of the operating table in spinal anesthesia and other procedures.

timbre (tim′ber, tam′br) [Fr.] a musical quality in a tone or sound. **t. métallique,** a high-pitched tympanic second sound heard in dilatation of the aorta. When heard in persons under fifty-five years of age it has been considered suggestive of syphilitic aortitis. Called also *Potain's sign* and *bruit de tabourka.*

time (tīm) [Gr. *chronos;* L. *tempus*] a measure of duration. **apex t.,** the interval at which the apex of the summated twitches of a muscle succeeds the second stimulus applied to the same muscle. **bleeding t.,** the period of duration of bleeding that follows controlled, standardized puncture of the earlobe (Duke method) or forearm (Ivy method); a relatively inconsistent measure of capillary and platelet function. **bleeding t., secondary,** the time required for the arrest of bleeding when the crust is removed from a traumatized area 24 hours after the original injury; this is generally prolonged in patients with Factor VIII deficiency (hemophilia) and with related hemophilioid states. **chromoscopy t.,** the time elapsing between the intramuscular injection of a dye and its appearance in the gastric secretion. **circulation t.,** the time required for blood to flow between two designated points, as arm-to-tongue time. **clot retraction t.,** the time required for 50 per cent of a blood clot (coagulum) to retract from the wall of the vessel containing it; a semiquantitative measure of this phenomenon is available. **clotting t.,** coagulation t. **coagulation t.,** the time required for blood to clot in a glass tube. **dextrinizing t.,** the time required for saliva to convert starch into sugar. **generation t.,** the time elapsing from one generation to the next, or in bacteria the time from one scission to the next. Also, the reciprocal of the growth rate, which is less than the doubling time since growth is exponential rather than linear. **inertia t.,** the time required to overcome the inertia of a muscle after the reception of a stimulus from a nerve. **prothrombin t.,** the time required for clot formation after thromboplastin (brain extract) and calcium have been added to blood plasma. **reaction t.,** the time elapsing between the application of a stimulus and the resulting reaction. **recalcification t.,** the interval required for clot formation when calcium ion is replaced in anticoagulated platelet-rich plasma; an insensitive measure of hemostasis. **sedimentation t.,** see *erythrocyte sedimentation rate,* under *rate.* **thermal death t.,** the duration of exposure required to kill a bacterium at a stated temperature.

timer (tīm′er) a clock mechanism which may be set to automatically signal the expiration of a given interval of time or to activate or cut off certain other apparatus at the desired time.

Timme's syndrome (tim′ez) [Walter *Timme,* American neurologist, 1874–1956] see under *syndrome.*

timolol maleate (ti′mo-lōl) chemical name: (*S*)-1-[(1,1-dimethylethyl)amino]-3-[[4-(4-morpholinyl)-1,2,5-thiadiazol-3-yl]oxy]-2-propanol (*Z*)-2-butanedioate (1:1) (salt). A beta-adrenergic blocking agent, $C_{13}H_{24}N_4O_3S \cdot C_4H_4O_4$, with antihypertensive and antiarrhythmic properties; it is used topically to lower intraocular pressure in glaucoma, by decreasing the formation of aqueous humor.

tin (tin) [L. *stannum*] a white, metallic element, atomic number, 50; atomic weight, 118.69; valence 2 or 4; symbol, Sn. Some of its salts are reagents, others are stains, while some of its compounds, particularly the oxide, have been tried in medicine. Its organic compounds exhibit moderate but variable toxicity. **t. chloride,** a compound, $SnCl_2 + 2H_2O$, or stannous chloride; used as a test reagent. **t. oxide,** a pure white powder, obtained from the product of a reaction between tin and concentrated nitric acid at a high temperature; used in dentistry as a polishing agent for teeth and metallic restorations in the mouth.

tina (te′nah) pinta.

Tinactin (tin-ak′tin) trademark for preparations of tolnaftate.

Tinbergen (tin′berg-en) Nikolaas. Dutch zoologist, born 1907; co-winner, with Karl von Frisch and Konrad Lorenz, of the Nobel prize in medicine and physiology for 1973, for his work on animal behavior.

tinct. abbreviation for *tincture*, or *tinctura*.

tinctable (tink′tah-b′l) stainable or tingible.

tinction (tink′shun) [L. *tingere* to dye] 1. the act of staining. 2. the addition of coloring or flavoring agents to a prescription.

tinctorial (tink-to′re-al) pertaining to dyeing or staining.

tinctura (tink-tu′rah), gen. and pl. *tinctu′rae* [L.] tincture.

tincturation (tink″tu-ra′shun) the preparation of a tincture; the treatment of a drug with a menstruum, such as alcohol or ether, for the purpose of preparing a tincture.

tincture (tink′tūr) [L. *tingere* to wet, to moisten] an alcoholic or hydroalcoholic solution prepared from animal or vegetable drugs or from chemical substances. **arnica t.**, a preparation of powdered arnica in equal parts of alcohol and water, formerly used as a local irritant. **belladonna t.** [USP], an alcoholic preparation of belladonna leaf, containing, in each 100 ml., 27–33 mg. of the alkaloids of belladonna leaf; used as an anticholinergic for the same purposes as atropine and hyoscyamine. **benzethonium chloride t.** [USP], a preparation containing 97–103 per cent of benzethonium chloride, calculated on a dried basis; used as a topical anti-infective. **benzoin t., compound** [USP], a preparation of benzoin, aloe, storax, and tolu balsam in alcohol, used as a topical protectant. Called also *friar's balsam*. **camphorated opium t.**, former name for paregoric. **capsicum t.**, a preparation of powdered capsicum in equal parts of alcohol and water; used as an irritant and carminative. **cardamom t., compound**, a preparation of powdered cardamom seed, cinnamon, caraway, and cochineal in glycerin and diluted alcohol; used as a flavoring agent. **digitalis t.**, finely powdered digitalis in a menstruum of alcohol and water, used as a cardiotonic. **ferric chloride t.**, a hydroalcoholic solution of ferric chloride, formerly used as a hematinic in the treatment of iron-deficiency anemias; it has also been used as a topical astringent and styptic. **ferric citrochloride t.**, a hydroalcoholic solution of ferric chloride and sodium citrate, used as a hematinic. **gentian t., compound**, a preparation of powdered gentian, bitter orange peel, and cardamom seed in a menstruum of glycerin, alcohol, and water; formerly used as a bitter. **green soap t.** [USP], a preparation of green soap, lavender oil, and alcohol used as a skin detergent; called also *medicinal soft soap liniment* and *linimentum saponis mollis*. **hyoscyamus t.**, a preparation of powdered hyoscyamus in alcohol and water; formerly used as an anticholinergic for the same purposes as atropine. **iodine t.** [USP], a preparation of iodine and sodium iodide in diluted alcohol, each 100 ml. of which contains 1.8–2.2 gm. of iodine and 2.1–2.6 gm. of sodium iodide; used as an anti-infective on the skin. **iodine t., strong**, an alcoholic solution of iodine and potassium iodide, each 100 ml. of which contains 6.8–7.5 gm. of iodine and 4.7–5.5 gm. of potassium iodide; used as an irritant, antibacterial, and antifungal agent. **lemon t.** [USP], **lemon peel t.**, a preparation of lemon peel in alcohol used as a flavoring agent. **myrrh t.**, a preparation of powdered myrrh in alcohol used as a protective. **nitromersol t.** [USP], a preparation of nitromersol, sodium hydroxide, and acetone, in alcohol and purified water; used as a local anti-infective, applied topically. **nux vomica t.**, a preparation of powdered nux vomica in equal parts of alcohol, hydrochloric acid, and water; used as a bitter. **opium t.** [USP], a preparation, obtained by percolation of granulated opium and concentration of the product, each 100 ml. of which yields 0.95–1.05 gm. of anhydrous morphine; used as an antiperistaltic. Called also *deodorized opium t.* **opium t., camphorated**, paregoric. **opium t., deodorized**, opium t. **rhubarb t., aromatic**, a preparation of powdered rhubarb, cinnamon, clove, and myristica in glycerin, alcohol, and water; used as a cathartic. **stramonium t.**, a hydroalcoholic solution of powdered stramonium formerly used as a parasympatholytic. **sweet orange peel t.** [USP], a preparation produced by the maceration in alcohol of the outer rind of the nonartificially colored fresh ripe fruit of *Citrus sinensis;* used as a flavoring agent. **thimerosal t.** [USP], a preparation of thimerosal, alcohol, acetone, ethylenediamine solution, and monoethanolamine in water; used as a local anti-infective, applied topically to the skin. **tolu balsam t.** [NF], a preparation of tolu balsam in alcohol; used as a flavor and as ingredient of *tolu balsam syrup*. **vanilla t.** [NF], a preparation of vanilla and sucrose in equal parts of diluted alcohol and water; used as a flavor and as an ingredient of *acacia syrup*.

Tindal (tin′dal) trademark for a preparation of acetophenazine maleate.

tinea (tin′e-ah) [L. "a grub, larva, worm"] a name applied to many different kinds of superficial fungal infection of the skin, the specific type (depending on characteristic appearance, etiologic agent, or site) usually being designated by a modifying term. Popularly called *ringworm*. **t. amianta′cea**, a nonfungal condition of the scalp, characterized by a dense concentration on its surface of silvery-white or gray scales which extend up on the hair shafts to form an asbestos-like encasement. **asbestoslike t.**, t. amiantacea. **t. axilla′ris**, trichomycosis axillaris. **t. bar′bae**, infection of the bearded area of the face and neck, caused by various species of fungi, the type depending on the organism involved: the inflammatory type, caused by *Trichophyton mentagrophytes* or *T. verrucosum* (see *t. kerion*); the ringworm type, caused by various species of fungi, with annular lesions

resembling those appearing on nonhairy skin; the sycosiform type, caused by *Trichophyton violaceum* or *T. rubrum* (see *t. sycosis*). **t. cap′itis**, fungal infection of the scalp, almost exclusively in children, caused by various species of *Microsporum* and *Trichophyton*, and characterized by irregular, patches of baldness, erythema, scaling, crusting, and black dots produced by breakage of infected hairs close to the scalp surface. Called also *ringworm of the scalp*. **t. cilio′rum**, fungal infection of the scalp, involving the eyelashes. **t. circina′ta**, fungal infection of glabrous skin, characterized by presence of the annular lesions responsible for the appellation "ringworm." **t. cor′poris**, fungal infection of glabrous skin, usually caused by various species of *Trichophyton* and *Microsporum*, sometimes acquired from animals or other infected persons and often named for some specific characteristic. See *t. circinata, trichophytic granuloma*, and *favus*. Called also *ringworm of the body*. **t. cru′ris**, a fungal infection common in males, starting in the crural or perineal folds, and extending onto the upper inner surfaces of the thighs; caused usually by *Epidermophyton floccosum* or species of *Trichophyton*. **t. favo′sa** (*obs.*), favus. **t. gal′li**, favus of fowl. **t. imbrica′ta**, a distinctive chronic type of tinea corporis, occurring in tropical countries, caused by *Trichophyton concentricum;* the early lesion is annular, with a circle of scales at the periphery, characteristically attached along one edge. New and larger concentric scaling rings form, sometimes reaching as many as 10 per lesion. **t. ke′rion**, kerion. **t. ni′gra**, a minor fungal infection, caused by *Cladosporium mansoni* or *C. wernecki*, producing strikingly dark lesions with the appearance of stains of spattered silver nitrate on the skin of the hands or, rarely, on other areas. **t. nodo′sa**, piedra. **t. pe′dis**, a chronic superficial fungal infection of the skin of the foot, especially of that between the toes and on the soles, caused by species of *Trichophyton* or by *Epidermophyton floccosum;* of different types and degrees of severity, it may be marked by maceration, cracking, and scaling of the skin, and by intense itching. Called also *athlete's foot*. **t. profun′da**, trichophytic granuloma. **t. syco′sis**, an inflammatory, deep type of tinea barbae. **t. tar′si**, blepharitis ulcerosa. **t. tonsu′rans**, a condition caused by *Trichophyton tonsurans*, which is similar to ordinary tinea capitis, except that the areas of baldness are smaller and the black dots are usually absent because there is less breakage of the infected hairs. **t. un′guium**, onychomycosis. **t. versic′olor**, a common chronic, noninflammatory and usually symptomless disorder, characterized only by occurrence of multiple macular patches, of all sizes and shapes, varying from whitish in pigmented skin to fawn-colored or brown in pale skin; seen most frequently in hot, humid tropical regions, and caused by *Pityrosporon orbiculare.*

Tinel's sign (tin-elz′) [Jules *Tinel*, French neurologist, 1879–1952] see under *sign*.

tingibility (tin″jĭ-bil′ĭ-te) the quality of being tingible.

tingible (tin′jĭ-b′l) [L. *tingere* to stain] susceptible of being tinged or stained.

tingling (ting′gling) a pricklike thrill, caused by cold or by striking a nerve, or as a result of various diseases of the central or peripheral nervous system. **distal t. on percussion**, see *Tinel's sign*, under *sign*.

tinidazole (ti-nid′ah-zōl) chemical name: 1-[2-(ethylsulfonyl)-ethyl]-2-methyl-5-nitroimidazole; an antiprotozoal, $C_8H_{13}N_3O_4S$, effective against *Trichomonas vaginalis, Entamoeba histolytica*, and *Giardia intestinalis*.

tinkle (ting′k′l) an auscultatory sound like the ringing of a small bell, sometimes heard over large pulmonary cavities and in pneumothorax. **metallic t.**, a ringing sound, as of a metallic object, sometimes heard in connection with other respiratory sounds.

tinnitus (tĭ-ni′tus) [L. "a ringing"] a noise in the ears, as ringing, buzzing, roaring, clicking, etc. Such sounds may at times be heard by others than the patient. **t. aurium**, a subjective sensation of noises in the ears. **clicking t.**, a clicking sound occurring in the ear in chronic catarrhal otitis media; it may be heard by others than the patient. **Leudet's t.**, a crackling sound in the ear, audible also to an observer, produced by involuntary contraction of an internal muscle, coinciding with a tic of some of the fibers of the mandibular division of the trigeminal (fifth cranial) nerve. **nervous t.**, that which arises from some disturbance of the otic nerve or its central connection. **nonvibratory t.**, tinnitus produced by biochemical changes occurring in the nerve mechanism of hearing. **objective t.**, abnormal or pathological sounds originating within the body of the patient, in the region of the ear, which are audible to others than the patient. **vibratory t.**, tinnitus resulting from transmission to the cochlea of vibrations originating in adjacent tissues of the body.

Tinospora (tin-os′po-rah) a genus of menispermaceous vines; the stalk and root of *T. cordifolia* Miers. are used in snakebite, indigestion, ulcers, and fevers.

tiodonium chloride (ti″o-do′ne-um) chemical name: (4-chlorophenyl)-2-thienyliodonium chloride; an antibacterial, $C_{10}H_7Cl_2$-IS.

tioperidone hydrochloride (ti″o-per′ĭ-dōn) chemical name:

3-[4-[4-[2-(propylthio)phenyl]-1-piperazinyl]butyl]-2,4(1H,3H)-quinazolinedione monohydrochloride; a tranquilizer, $C_{25}H_{32}N_4O_2S$·HCl.

tiopinac (ti-o′pĭ-nak) chemical name: 6,11-dihydro-11-oxodibenzo[b,e]thiepin-3-acetic acid; an anti-inflammatory, analgesic, and antipyretic, $C_{16}H_{12}O_3S$.

tioxidazole (ti″ok-si′dah-zōl) chemical name: (6-propoxy-2-benzothiazolyl)carbamic acid methyl ester; an anthelmintic, $C_{12}H_{14}N_2O_3S$.

tint B a color shown by the pastille in an x-ray–measuring instrument that denotes the amount of radiation which will cause depilation.

tintometer (tin-tom′ĕ-ter) [*tint* + Gr. *metron* measure] an instrument used in determining the relative proportion of coloring matter in a liquid.

tintometric (tin″to-met′rik) pertaining to tintometry.

tintometry (tin-tom′ĕ-tre) the use of the tintometer.

tip (tip) a pointed extremity of a body part; called also *apex*. **t. of nose,** apex nasi. **t. of sacral bone,** apex ossis sacri. **t. of tongue,** apex linguae. **Woolner's t.,** tuberculum auriculae.

tipping (tip′ing) a tooth movement in which its vertical position is altered.

tiprenolol hydrochloride (ti-pren′o-lōl) chemical name: (+)-1-(isopropylamino)-3-[*o*-(methylthio)phenoxy]-2-propanol hydrochloride; an antiadrenergic (β-receptor), $C_{13}H_{21}NO_2S$·HCl.

tiqueur (te-ker′) [Fr.] a person subject to a tic.

tiquinamide hydrochloride (ti-kwin′ah-mīd) chemical name: 5,6,7,8-tetrahydro-3-methyl-8-quinoline carbothioamide monohydrochloride; a gastric anticholinergic, $C_{11}H_{14}N_2S$·HCl.

tirebal (tēr-bahl′) [Fr.] an instrument resembling a corkscrew, for extracting bullets.

tirefond (tēr-fo′) [Fr.] an instrument like a corkscrew, for raising depressed portions of a bone.

tires (tīrz) trembles.

tiring (tīr′ing) the operation of passing a wire around a fractured patella, like a tire around a wheel; cerclage.

Tiselius apparatus (te-sa′le-us) [Arne Wilhelm Kaurin *Tiselius*, biochemist in Upsula, Sweden, born 1902; winner of the Nobel prize for chemistry in 1948] see under *apparatus*.

tisic (tiz′ik) phthisic.

tisis (tis′is) phthisis.

tissue (tish′u) [Fr. *tissu*] an aggregation of similarly specialized cells united in the performance of a particular function. **accidental t.,** a tissue growing in or upon a part to which it is foreign; it is either analogous or heterologous. **adenoid t.,** lymphoid t. **adipose t.,** fatty tissue; connective tissue made up of fat cells in a meshwork of areolar tissue. **adipose t., brown,** a thermogenic type of adipose tissue containing a dark pigment, and arising during embryonic life in certain specific areas in many mammals, including man; it is prominent in the newborn of all species in which it occurs and remains a distinct and conspicuous tissue in the adults of certain species, especially those that hibernate. Called also *brown fat*. Cf. *white adipose t.* **adipose t., white, adipose t., yellow,** the adipose tissue comprising the bulk of the body fat. Cf. *brown adipose t.* **adrenogenic t.,** the inner zone of the cortex of an adrenal gland which begins to involute shortly after birth, usually referred to as the fetal cortex. **analogous t.,** an accidental tissue similar to one found normally in other parts of the body. **areolar t.,** connective tissue made up largely of interlacing fibers. **areolar connective t.,** see *connective t.* **basement t.,** the substance of a basement membrane. **bony t.,** bone, whether normal or of a soft tissue, which has become ossified. **brown fat t.,** fatty tissue in various regions of the body of some mammals which contains a dark pigment. Called also *moruloid* or *mulberry fat*. The masses have been called interscapular gland, hibernating gland, and Bonnot's gland. **bursal equivalent t.,** an unidentified component of the lymphoid system, analogous to the bursa of Fabricius in birds, which is considered to be the primary site of the origin of B-lymphocytes and to consist of gut-associated lymphoid tissue, fetal liver, and bone marrow. **cancellous t.,** the loose spongy tissue of the interior and articular ends of bone. **cartilaginous t.,** the substance of the cartilages. **cavernous t.,** erectile t. **cellular t.,** loose connective tissue with large interspaces. **chondroid t.,** an embryonic form of cartilage composed of vesicular cells provided with elastic capsules and having collagenous fibers in its interstitial substance. **chordal t.,** the tissue of the notochord. **chromaffin t.,** a tissue composed largely of chromaffin cells, well supplied with nerves and vessels; it occurs in the adrenal medulla and also forms the paraganglia of the body. **cicatricial t.,** the dense fibrous tissue forming a scar or cicatrix and derived directly from granulation tissue; called also *scar t.* **compact t.,** the hard external portion of a bone. **connective t.,** the tissue which binds together and is the support of the various structures of the body. It is made up of fibroblasts, fibroglia, collagen fibrils, and elastic fibrils. It is derived from the mesoderm and in a broad sense includes the collagenous, elastic, mucous, reticular, osseous, and cartilaginous tissue. Some also

include the blood in this group of tissues. Cf. *fibroblast*. Connective tissue is classified according to concentration of fibers as loose (areolar) and dense, the latter having more abundant fibers than the former. **cribriform t.,** areolar t. **dartoid t.,** that which resembles the dartos in structure. **elastic t., elastic t., yellow,** connective tissue made up of yellow, elastic fibers, frequently massed into sheets. **endothelial t.,** endothelium. **episcleral t.,** the loose connective tissue over the sclera, between it and the conjunctiva. **epithelial t.,** epithelium. **epivaginal connective t.,** connective tissue surrounding the sheath of the optic nerve. **erectile t.,** tissue containing large venous spaces with which arteries communicate directly, as in the penis and clitoris. Another type formed of dilated venules occurs in the nasal mucosa. The smooth muscle of the nipples constitutes another erectile organ. **extracellular t.,** the total of tissues and body fluids outside the cells, including the plasma volume and all plasma components, the extracellular fluid volume and its components, plus the intercellular and extracellular tissue solids, most notably the collagen, cartilage, bone, elastin, and other connective tissues of the body framework and viscera. **fatty t.,** adipose t. **fibrohyaline t.,** chondroid t. **fibrous t.,** the ordinary connective tissue of the body, made up largely of yellow or white fibers. **fibrous t., white,** that which is composed almost wholly of collagenous fibers. **Gamgee t.,** a surgical dressing consisting of a thick layer of absorbent cotton between two layers of absorbent gauze. **gelatiginous t.,** that which yields gelatin on boiling with water. **gelatinous t.,** mucous tissue. **glandular t.,** an aggregation of epithelial cells that elaborate secretions. **granulation t.,** the newly formed vascular tissue normally produced in the healing of wounds of soft tissue and ultimately forming the cicatrix; it consists of small, translucent, red, nodular masses or granulations that have a velvety appearance. **gut-associated lymphoid t. (GALT),** lymphoid tissue associated with the gut, including the tonsils, Peyer's patches, lamina propria of the gastrointestinal tract, and appendix. **hematopoietic t.,** tissue that takes part in the production of the formed elements of the blood. **heterologous t.,** tissue unlike any other that is normal to the organism. **heterotopic t.,** choristoma. **homologous t.,** tissue identical with another tissue in structural type. **hylic t.,** Adami's term for embryonic tissues constituting the body of an organ, in contrast to lining (lepidic) tissue; see also *hylic*. **hyperplastic t.,** 1. tissue affected by hyperplasia. 2. in dentistry, an overgrowth of tissue about the maxilla or mandible that is excessively movable, or more readily displaced than is normal. **indifferent t.,** undifferentiated embryonic tissue. **interrenal t.,** the tissue composing the adrenal cortex. **interstitial t.,** the connective tissue between the cellular elements of a body; the stroma. **intertubular t.** (*obs.*), the dense tissue of dentin in which the dentinal tubes are embedded. **junctional t.,** the bridge between the atrium and ventricle of the heart formed by the atrioventricular node and the atrioventricular bundle. **Kuhnt's intermediary t.,** glial tissue surrounding the optic nerve and separating it from the retina. **lardaceous t.,** tissue charged with lardacein as a result of a degenerative process. **lepidic t.,** the lining membrane tissue of the embryo. Cf. *hylic t.* **loose connective t.,** see *connective t.* **lymphadenoid t.,** tissue resembling that of the lymph nodes, found in the spleen, bone marrow, tonsils, and other organs. **lymphatic t.,** lymphoid t. **lymphoid t.,** a lattice work of reticular tissue the interspaces of which contain lymphocytes; lymphoid tissue may be diffuse, or densely aggregated as in lymph nodules and nodes. **mesenchymal t.,** embryonic connective tissue composed of stellate cells and a ground substance of coagulable fluid; the mesenchyma. **metanephrogenic t.,** the more caudal nephrogenic tissue that gives rise to the nephrons of the permanent kidney. **mucous t.,** a jelly-like connective tissue, such as occurs in the umbilical cord. **muscular t.,** the substance of a muscle. **myeloid t.,** medulla ossis rubra. **nephrogenic t.,** tissue of the nephrotomes which furnishes the material out of which the three kidney types arise. **nerve t., nervous t.,** the substance of which the nerves and nerve centers are composed. **nodal t.,** tissue made up of nerve and muscle fibers, such as that composing the sinoatrial node of the heart. **osseous t.,** the specialized tissue forming the bones. **osteogenic t.,** that part of the periosteum adjacent to bone and concerned in the formation of osseous tissue; any tissue capable of generating bone. **osteoid t.,** uncalcified bone tissue. **parenchymatous t.,** parenchyma. **periodontal t.,** periodontium. **primitive pulp t.,** hylic t. **reticular t., reticulated t.,** connective tissue consisting of reticular cells and fibers. **rubber t.,** rubber in sheets for use in surgery. **scar t.,** cicatricial t. **sclerous t's,** the cartilaginous, fibrous, and osseous tissues. **shock t.,** that tissue in the animal body which bears the brunt of the antigen-antibody reaction in anaphylaxis. **skeletal t.,** the bony, ligamentous, fibrous, and cartilaginous tissue forming the skeleton and its attachments. **splenic t.,** red pulp. **subcutaneous t.,** the layer of loose connective tissue situated directly beneath the skin; called also *tela subcutanea* [NA]. **subcutaneous fatty t.,** panniculus adiposus. **sustentacular t.,** a non-nervous structure of the retina composed of the müllerian fibers of that organ. **symplastic t.,** symplasm. **target t.,** 1. tissue, either *in vivo* or *in vitro*, against which humoral or cell-mediated immunity is directed. 2. the tissue that responds specifically to a given hormone. **tuberculosis granulation t.,** the tissue that forms the characteristic tubercle in pulmonary productive tuberculosis, composed of epithelioid cells in concentric masses, lymphocytes, and often Langhans giant cells. **vesicular supporting t.,** chondroid t.

tissular (tish'u-lar)　pertaining to organic tissue.

titanium (ti-ta'ne-um) [L. *titan* the sun]　a dark-gray, metallic element of widespread distribution but occurring in small amounts; atomic number, 22; atomic weight, 47.90; symbol, Ti; specific gravity, 4.5; used for fixation of fractures. **t. dioxide** [USP], a white powder, TiO_2, used as a topical protectant against sunburn; it is also used in other protectant preparations and in dusting powders, and as a pigment in the manufacture of artificial teeth.

titer (ti'ter) [Fr. *titre* standard]　the quantity of a substance required to produce a reaction with a given volume of another substance, or the amount of one substance required to correspond with a given amount of another substance. **agglutination t.,** the highest dilution of a serum which causes clumping of microorganisms or other particulate antigens.

titillation (tit"ĭ-la'shun) [L. *titillatio*]　the act or sensation of tickling.

titrant (ti'trant)　the solution of known strength that is added in titration.

titrate (ti'trāt)　to determine by titration.

titration (ti-tra'shun) [Fr. *titre* standard]　determination of a given component in solution by addition of a liquid reagent of known strength until a given endpoint (e.g., change in color) is reached. **colorimetric t.,** a method of determining hydrogen ion concentration by adding an indicator to the unknown and then comparing the color with a set of tubes containing this same indicator in solutions of known hydrogen ion concentration. **complexometric t.,** titration of a substance (e.g., the calcium in clear serum) with a complexing agent (e.g., EDTA); the endpoint of the titration is generally observed as a change in color of the solution. **coulometric t.,** titration by determining the amount of electricity required to electrochemically generate a titrant which reacts with the substance in question. If the current is kept constant, as for chloride determination using the Cotlove titrator, the amount of electricity (coulombs) used is proportional to the elapsed time. **Dean and Webb t.,** a test for measuring antibody in which varying dilutions of antigen are mixed with a constant quantity of antiserum; antibody activity is determined by the dilution in which flocculation occurs most rapidly, i.e., the end point. In this dilution, antigen and antibody are together at a ratio of optimal proportions. **formol t.,** see *Sörensen's method,* under *method.* **potentiometric t.,** a method of determining hydrogen ion concentration by placing a hydrogen electrode in unknown solution and measuring the potential developed as compared with some standard electrode by means of a potentiometer.

titre (ti'ter) [Fr.]　titer.

titrimetric (tit"rĭ-met'rik)　pertaining to analysis by titration.

titrimetry (ti-trim'ĕ-tre) [*titration* + Gr. *metron* measure]　analysis by titration.

titubant (tit'u-bant)　a person who staggers.

titubation (tit"u-ba'shun) [L. *titubatio*]　the act of staggering or reeling; a staggering or stumbling gait with shaking of the trunk and head, commonly seen in cerebellar disease. **lingual t.,** stuttering or stammering.

Tityus serrulatus (tit'e-us ser"u-la'tus)　a scorpion of Brazil which inflicts a severe, sometimes fatal, sting.

tixanox (tiks'ah-noks)　chemical name: 7-(methylsulfinyl)-9-oxo-9*H*-xanthene-2-carboxylic acid; an antiallergic, $C_{15}H_{10}O_5S$.

Tizzoni's test (tid-zo'nez) [Guido *Tizzoni,* Italian physician, 1853–1932]　see under *tests.*

tjettek (tyet'ek)　a deadly poison prepared by the Javanese from the root of *Strychnos tieute.*

TKD　tokodynamometer.

TKG　tokodynagraph.

Tl　chemical symbol for *thallium.*

TLC　total lung capacity.

Tm　chemical symbol for *thulium.*

TMV　tobacco mosaic virus.

Tn　symbol for *normal intraocular tension (pressure).*

TNM　see under *staging.*

TNT　trinitrotoluene.

TO　abbreviation for *tinctura opii,* tincture of opium.

T.O.　original tuberculin; see *New tuberculin,* under *tuberculin.*

toadskin (tōd'skin)　phrynoderma.

toadstool (tōd'stul)　a popular name for a poisonous mushroom.

tobacco (to-bak'o) [L. *tabacum*]　the dried and prepared leaves of *Nicotiana tabacum* L. (Solenaceae), a solanaceous plant. Tobacco contains various alkaloids, the principal one being *nicotine,*

and unites the qualities of a sedative narcotic with those of an emetic and diuretic. It is also a heart depressant and antispasmodic. **mountain t.,** arnica. **poison t.,** hyoscyamus.

tobaccoism (to-bak'o-izm)　a morbid condition due to excessive use of tobacco; nicotinism.

Tobey-Ayer test (to'be a'er) [George Loring *Tobey,* Jr., Boston otolaryngologist, 1881–1947; James Bourne *Ayer,* Boston neurologist, born 1882]　see under *tests.*

tobramycin (to"brah-mi'sin) [USP]　chemical name: *O*-3-amino-3-deoxy-α-D-glucopyranosyl-(1 → 6)-*O*-[2,2-diamino-2,3,6-trideoxy-α-D-*ribo*-hexopyranosyl-(1 → 4)]-2-deoxy-D-streptamine. A purified fraction of an aminoglycoside antibiotic complex (see *nebramycin*) produced by *Streptomyces tenebrarius,* $C_{18}H_{37}N_5O_9$, bactericidal against many gram-negative and some gram-positive organisms. Administered intravenously or intramuscularly, as the sulfate salt, in the treatment of septicemia and neonatal sepsis, and in central nervous system, lower respiratory, gastrointestinal, skin, bone, and soft-tissue infections due to susceptible strains of *Pseudomonas aeruginosa, Escherichia coli,* indole-negative and indole-positive *Proteus, Providencia, Klebsiella-Enterobacter-Serratia* group, *Citrobacter,* and staphylococci, including coagulase-positive and coagulase-negative *S. aureus.* Called also *tenebrimycin* and *tenemycin.*

tocainide (to-ka'nīd)　chemical name: 2-amino-*N*-(2,6-dimethylphenyl)propanamide; a cardiac depressant (antiarrhythmic), $C_{11}H_{16}N_2O$.

tocamphyl (to-kam'fil)　chemical name: 1-(*p,α*-dimethylbenzyl)-camphorate compound with 2,2′-iminodiethanol (1:1); a choleretic obtained from tumeric, $C_{19}H_{26}O_4 \cdot C_4H_{11}NO_2$.

Toclase (to'klās)　trademark for preparations of carbetapentane citrate.

toco- [Gr. *tokos* childbirth]　a combining form denoting relationship to childbirth, or labor; see also words beginning *toko-.*

tocodynagraph (to"ko-di'nah-graf)　tokodynagraph.

tocodynamometer (to"ko-di"nah-mom'ĕ-ter)　tokodynamometer.

tocograph (tok'o-graf)　a recording tokodynamometer.

tocography (to-kog'rah-fe) [*toco-* + Gr. *graphein* to write]　the graphic recording of uterine contractions.

tocokinin (tok"o-kin'in) [*toco-* + Gr. *kinein* to move]　an extract from yeast and certain vegetables which has the properties of an estral hormone.

tocology (to-kol'o-je)　obstetrics.

tocometer (to-kom'ĕ-ter) [*toco-* + Gr. *metron* measure]　tokodynamometer.

tocopherol (to-kof'er-ol) [*toco-* + Gr. *pherein* to carry]　an alcohol which has the properties of vitamin E; isolated from the oil of the germ of wheat kernel, or produced synthetically. **α-t., alpha-t.,** vitamin E.

tocophobia (to"ko-fo'be-ah) [*toco-* + Gr. *phobein* to be affrighted by]　abnormal dread of childbirth.

tocus (to'kus) [L.; Gr. *tokos*]　labor; childbirth.

Todd bodies (tod) [John Launcelot *Todd,* Canadian physician, 1876–1949]　see under *body.*

Todd's cirrhosis, paralysis (palsy), process (todz) [Robert Bentley *Todd,* English physician, 1809–1860]　see under *paralysis,* see *primary biliary cirrhosis,* under *cirrhosis,* and see *fibrae intercrurales.*

Toddalia (to-dal'e-ah)　a genus of rutaceous shrubs. The root of *T. aculeata* Pers., of the East Indies, is an aromatic stomachic. The bark is used in India as a source of yellow dye. The rootbark is considered to be antimalarial, and possesses antiperiodic and antipyretic properties.

toddy (tod'e) [Hind. *tāre, tādi*]　1. the fermented sap of various palm trees. 2. a drink prepared from gin or whisky, sugar, and water.

toe (to)　any of the five digits of the foot. **curly t's,** a condition affecting chicks, in which the toes curl underneath the feet, due to a deficiency of riboflavin. **great t.,** the first digit of the foot; called also *hallux* [NA] and *digitus I* [NA alternative]. **hammer t.,** a condition in which the proximal phalanx of a toe—most often that of the second toe—is extended and the second and distal phalanges are flexed, causing a clawlike appearance. **little t.,** the fifth digit of the foot; called also *digitus minimus* [NA] and *digitus V* [NA alternative]. **mallet t.,** flexion contracture of the distal interphalangeal joint of any of the lesser toes. **Morton's t.,** a form of metatarsalgia due to compression of a branch of the plantar nerve by the metatarsal heads; chronic compression may lead to formation of a neuroma. Called also Morton's *disease, foot,* or *neuralgia.* **pigeon t.,** a permanent toeing-in position of the feet. **seedy t.,** a disease of horses' feet marked by a fungous growth of a horny, honeycombed texture between the coffin bone and the wall of the hoof. **tennis t.,** painful great toe associated with subungual hematoma, which, in the absence of treatment, may lead to subungual abscess; it usually develops after a vigorous tennis game, especially when tennis shoes with protective tips are worn. **webbed t's,** toes abnormally joined by strands of tissue at their base.

toenail (to′nāl) the nail on any of the digits of the foot. See *unguis* [NA]. **ingrown t.,** aberrant growth of a toenail, with one (usually the outer) margin or, less often, both lateral margins growing deeply into the nail groove and surrounding tissues. **ingrowing t.,** ingrown nail.

Toepfer (tep′fer) see *Töpfer.*

tofenacin hydrochloride (to-fen′ah-sin) chemical name: *N*-methyl-2-[(*o*-methyl-α-phenylbenzyl)oxy]ethylamine hydrochloride; an anticholinergic, $C_{17}H_{21}NO \cdot HCl$.

Tofranil (to-fra′nil) trademark for preparations of imipramine hydrochloride.

tofu (to′foo) a Japanese food preparation from the soy bean, in white tablets.

tofukasu (to-foo-kah′soo) a Japanese food prepared from soy beans.

togavirus (to″gah-vi′rus) a subgroup of arboviruses, including mosquito-borne and tickborne viruses that cause hemorrhagic fever; they are RNA viruses with envelopes (or "togas").

toilet (toi′let) the cleansing of an accidental wound and the surrounding skin, or of an obstetrical patient.

Toison's solution (fluid) (twah-zawz′) [J. *Toison*, French histologist, born 1858] see under *solution.*

tokelau (to-ke-lah′oo) [*Tokelau,* a South Pacific atoll] tinea imbricata.

toko- [Gr. *tokos* childbirth] for words beginning thus, see also those beginning *toco-.*

tokodynagraph (to″ko-di′nah-graf) [Gr. *tokos* childbirth + *graphein* to write] the record obtained with a tokodynamometer. Abbreviated TKG.

tokodynamometer (to″ko-di″nah-mom′ĕ-ter) [Gr. *tokos* childbirth + *dynamis* power + *metron* measure] an instrument for measuring the expulsive force of the uterine contractions in labor. Abbreviated TKD.

tolamolol (to-lah′mo-lōl) chemical name: 4-[2-[[2-hydroxy-3-(2-methylphenoxy)propyl]amino]ethoxy]benzamide. A beta-adrenergic blocking agent, $C_{19}H_{24}N_2O_4$, which has been used as a coronary vasodilator in the treatment of angina of effort and as a cardiac depressant in the treatment of arrhythmias.

tolazamide (tol-az′ah-mīd) [USP] chemical name: *N*-[[(hexahydro-1*H*-azepin-1-yl)amino]carbonyl]-4-methylbenzene sulfonamide. An orally effective hypoglycemic sulfonylurea, $C_{14}H_{21}N_3O_3S$, occurring as a white to off-white, crystalline powder; used in the treatment of diabetes mellitus.

tolazoline hydrochloride (tol-az′o-lēn) [USP] chemical name: 4,5-dihydro-2-(phenylmethyl)-1*H*-imidazole monohydrochloride. An adrenergic blocking agent and peripheral vasodilator, $C_{10}H_{12}N_2 \cdot HCl$, occurring as a white to off-white, crystalline powder; used in the treatment of peripheral vascular disorders due to vasospasm, administered orally.

tolbutamide (tol-bu′tah-mīd) [USP] chemical name: *N*-[(butylamino)carbonyl]-4-methylbenzenesulfonamide. An orally effective hypoglycemic sulfonylurea, $C_{12}H_{18}N_2O_3S$, occurring as a white, or practically white, crystalline powder; used in the treatment of diabetes mellitus. **t. sodium** [USP], the monosodium salt of tolbutamide, $C_{12}H_{17}N_2NaO_3S$, occurring as a white to off-white, crystalline powder, having the same actions as the base; used as a diagnostic test for diabetes mellitus, administered intravenously.

tolciclate (tōl-si′klāt) chemical name: *O*-1,2,3,4-tetrahydro-1,4-methanonaphthalen-6-yl)ester methyl(3-methylphenyl)carbamothioic acid; a topical antifungal, $C_{20}H_{23}NOS$.

Tolectin (tol′ek-tin) trademark for a preparation of tolmetin sodium.

tolerance (tol′er-ans) [L. *tolerantia*] the ability to endure without ill effect, unusually large doses of a drug, and to exhibit decreasing effect to continued use of the same dose of a drug. **acquired t.,** the increasing resistance to the usual effects of a drug due to continued use. **adoptive t.,** immunological tolerance induced by the passive transfer to an irradiated recipient animal of lymphoid cells from a donor rendered tolerant to an antigen. **alkali t.,** ability of the body to endure the administration of alkalis, measured by the amount of alkali that must be given to cause an alkaline urine; this forms a rough measure of the degree of acidosis. **crossed t.,** the lessened susceptibility which persons who have acquired a tolerance for one drug or poison may thereafter exhibit toward another drug. **drug t.,** progressive diminution of susceptibility to the effects of a drug, resulting from its continued administration. **glucose t.,** ability of the body to metabolize glucose; it is measured by the maximum amount of total glucose in a well-balanced diet, equally divided into three meals, which can be taken without having glucosuria at any time during the twenty-four hours. **high-zone t.,** acquired immunological tolerance due to the presence in very high concentrations of an antigen that would ordinarily stimulate lymphocytes to antibody production at intermediate concentrations. **immunologic t.,** an immunological response characterized by the development of specific nonreactivity of lymphoid tissues to a particular antigen capable under other conditions of inducing humoral or cell-mediated immunity. It may

be a consequence of contact with antigen in fetal or early postnatal life, or may occur in the presence of very high (*high-zone t.*) or very low (*low-zone t.*) doses of certain antigens to adults. The induction of tolerance to a given antigen does not affect immunological reactions to unrelated antigens. Called also *immunological paralysis.* **low-dose t.,** antigen-mediated specific immunosuppression induced in immunocompetent adult animals by successive minute doses of antigen. **low-zone t.,** immunological tolerance due to the continuous presence in extremely small concentrations (below the threshold required) of antigens that would ordinarily stimulate lymphocytes to antibody production at intermediate concentrations.

tolerant (tol′er-ant) able to endure, without effect, the action of any particular drug or other agent; exhibiting tolerance.

toleration (tol″er-a′shun) tolerance.

tolerogen (tol′er-o-jen) antigen in the animal body which induces a state of specific immunological unresponsiveness to subsequent challenging doses of the antigen.

tolerogenesis (tol″er-o-jen′ĕ-sis) induction of immunologic tolerance.

tolerogenic (tol″er-o-jen′ik) capable of inducing immunologic tolerance.

tolindate (to-lin′dāt) chemical name: *O*-2,3-dihydro-1*H*-inden-5-yl) ester carbamothioic acid; an antifungal, $C_{18}H_{19}NOS$.

Tolinase (tōl′in-ās) trademark for a preparation of tolazamide.

toliodium chloride (to-li′o-de-um) chemical name: bis(4-methylphenyl)iodonium chloride; a veterinary food additive, $C_{14}H_{14}ClI$.

Tollens' test (tol′enz) [Bernhard Christian Gottfried *Tollens,* German chemist, 1841–1918] see under *tests.*

tolmetin sodium (tol′met-in) chemical name: 1-methyl-5-(4-methylbenzoyl)-1*H*-pyrrole-2-acetic acid. An anti-inflammatory, analgesic, and antipyretic, $C_{15}H_{14}NNaO_3 \cdot 2H_2O$, used in the treatment of certain cases of rheumatoid arthritis, administered orally.

tolnaftate (tol-naf′tāt) [USP] chemical name: *O*-2-naphthalenyl ester carbamothioic acid. A synthetic antifungal, $C_{19}H_{17}NOS$, occurring as a white to creamy white, fine powder; used topically in the treatment of various forms of tinea of the skin.

tolonium chloride (to-lo′ne-um) chemical name: 3-amino-7-(dimethylamino)-2-methylphenothiazin-5-ium chloride. An antiheparin compound, $C_{15}H_{16}ClN_3S$, which has been used in the treatment of idiopathic functional uterine bleeding and menorrhagia, topically to detect and delineate oral and cervical neoplasia, and intravenously to stain the parathyroid glands. Called also *toluidine blue O.*

Tolserol (tol′ser-ol) trademark for preparations of mephenesin.

toluene (tol′u-ēn) the hydrocarbon methylbenzene, $C_6H_5 \cdot CH_3$; a colorless liquid obtainable from tolu and other resins and from coal tar. It is an organic solvent used in rubber and plastic cements, paint removers, etc. Poisoning may result from ingesting the solvent or inhaling its concentrated vapors. Called also *toluol* and *methyl benzene.*

toluidine (tol-u′ĭ-din) a compound, 2-amino-toluene, $CH_3 \cdot C_6H_4 \cdot NH_2$, made by reducing nitrotoluene. It is homologous with aniline. **t. blue O,** tolonium chloride.

toluol (tol′u-ol) toluene.

tolusafranine (tol″u-saf′rah-nin) a dibenzoparadiazine dye, $NH_2(CH_3) \cdot C_6H_3 \cdot N_2 \cdot (C_6H_5)Cl \cdot C_6H_3(CH_3) \cdot NH_2$, the chief constituent of safranin.

toluyl (tol′u-il) the univalent acid radical, $CH_3 \cdot C_6H_4$.

toluylene (tol-u′ĭ-lēn) the hydrocarbon, diphenyl ethylene, $C_6H_5 \cdot CH:CH \cdot C_6H_5$; called also *stilbene.*

tolyl (tol′il) the univalent radical, $CH_3 \cdot C_6H_4$, isomeric with benzyl. **t. hydroxide,** cresol.

tomatin (to-ma′tin) an antibiotic substance with antifungal properties, isolated from tomato plants affected with wilt.

-tome [Gr. *tomē* a cutting] a word termination signifying (*a*) an instrument for cutting or (*b*) a segment.

tomentum (to-men′tum) a little used term for a network of minute blood vessels of the pia mater and the cortex cerebri; called also *t. cerebri.*

Tomes' fibers (fibrils), layer, process (tōmz) [Sir John *Tomes,* English dentist, 1815–1895] see under *fiber* and *process,* and see *granular layer of Tomes,* under *layer.*

Tommaselli's disease (syndrome) (tom″ah-sel′ēz) [Salvatore *Tommaselli,* Italian physician, 1834–1906] see under *disease.*

Tommasi's sign (tom-mas′e) [L. *Tommasi,* Italian physician] see under *sign.*

tomo- [Gr. *tomē* a cutting] a combining form denoting relationship to a cutting, or to a designated layer, as might be achieved by cutting or slicing.

tomogram (to′mo-gram) a roentgenogram of a selected layer of the body made by tomography.

tomograph (to′mo-graf) an apparatus for moving an x-ray source in one direction as the film is moved in the opposite direction, thus showing in detail a predetermined plane of tissue while blurring or eliminating detail in other planes.

tomography (to-mog'rah-fe) [*tomo-* + Gr. *graphein* to write] the recording of internal body images at a predetermined plane by means of the tomograph; called also *body section roentgenography*. **computed t.,** computerized axial t. **computerized axial t. (CAT),** that in which the emergent x-ray beam is measured by a scintillation counter, the electronic impulses are recorded on a magnetic disk, and then are processed by a mini-computer for reconstruction display of the body in cross-section on a cathode ray tube. Called also *computed t.* and *CAT scan.* **ultrasonic t.,** the ultrasonographic visualization of a cross-section of a predetermined plane of the body by linear scanning with an ultrasonic probe across the desired site and displaying on a B-scan. **positron emission transaxial t. (PETT),** that accomplished by detection of gamma rays emitted from tissues after administration of a natural biochemical substance (e.g., glucose, fatty acids) into which positron-emitting isotopes have been incorporated The paths of the gamma rays, which result from collisions of positrons and electrons, are interpreted by a computer, and the resultant tomogram represents local concentrations of the isotope-containing substance.

-tomy [Gr. *tomē* a cutting] a word termination signifying the operation of cutting, or incision.

tonaphasia (ton"ah-fa'ze-ah) inability to recall a familiar tune; musical aphasia.

tone (tōn) [Gr. *tonos*; L. *tonus*] 1. the normal degree of vigor and tension; in muscle, the resistance to passive elongation or stretch. 2. a healthy state of a part; tonus. 3. a particular quality of sound or of voice. 4. to make permanent, or to change, the color of silver stain by chemical treatment, usually with a heavy metal. **feeling t.,** the condition or state of mind and feeling which accompanies every thought or act. **heart t's,** the sounds heard in the auscultation of the heart. **jecoral t.,** the sound produced by percussion over the liver. **plastic t.,** the posture-maintaining mechanism of muscle by virtue of which a limb passively placed in any position tends to maintain that position. **Traube's double t.,** a double heart sound heard in aortic regurgitation. **Williams' tracheal t.,** see under *sign,* def. 1.

tonga (tong'gah) a native name for yaws in New Caledonia and the Loyalty Islands.

tongs (tongs) an instrument for grasping and holding, consisting of two arms joined by a hinge or pivot. **skull t.,** tongs used to exert traction on the skull, as in surgery for fractures of cervical vertebrae; many forms are available, including Crutchfield t., Barton t., and Vinke t.

tongue (tung) [L. *lingua,* Gr. *glōssa*] 1. the movable, muscular organ on the floor of the mouth, subserving the special sense of taste and aiding in mastication, deglutition, and the articulation of sound. Called also *lingua* [NA]. 2. any structure or part having a shape similar to that of the oral organ of the same name. Called also *lingula* [NA]. **adherent t.,** a tongue that is abnor-

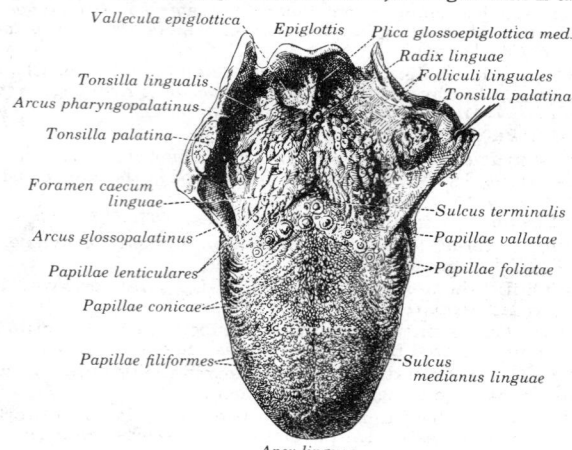

Vallecula epiglottica
Epiglottis
Plica glossoepiglottica med.
Tonsilla lingualis
Radix linguae
Folliculi linguales
Arcus pharyngopalatinus
Tonsilla palatina
Tonsilla palatina
Foramen caecum linguae
Sulcus terminalis
Arcus glossopalatinus
Papillae vallatae
Papillae lenticulares
Papillae foliatae
Papillae conicae
Papillae filiformes
Sulcus medianus linguae
Apex linguae

The tongue, showing principal structures (Eycleshymer and Jones).

mally attached by folds of connective tissue and mucous membrane to the sides and floor of the mouth. **amyloid t.,** enlargement of the tongue due to amyloidosis. **antibiotic t.,** glossitis caused by sensitivity to an antibiotic. **baked t.,** the dry, brown tongue of typhoid fever. **bald t.,** a tongue characterized by the absence of papillae, often seen in various nutritional disturbances. **beefy t.,** erythematous and/or atrophic glossitis, characterized by red, irregular ulcerations on the dorsal surface of the tongue. **bifid t.,** a tongue that is divided in its anterior part by a longitudinal fissure; called also *cleft t.* **black t., black hairy t.,** a condition characterized by the presence of a brown furlike patch on the dorsum of the tongue, composed of hypertrophied filiform papillae with microorganisms

and some pigment. Called also *anthracosis linguae, glossophytia, keratomycosis linguae, lingua villosa nigra, melanotrichia linguae,* and *nigrities linguae.* **blue t.,** a disease of sheep and cattle in South Africa, caused by a virus, and characterized by hyperemia, erosions, and edema of the lips, tongue, and oral mucosa. **burning t.,** glossopyrosis. **cardinal t.,** a tongue whose surface is denuded of epithelium, giving it a bright red appearance. **cerebriform t.,** fissured t. **choreic t.,** abrupt, snakelike protrusion and withdrawal of the tongue occurring in chorea. **cleft t.,** bifid t. **coated t.,** a tongue covered with a whitish or yellowish layer consisting of desquamated epithelium, debris, bacteria, fungi, etc. **cobble-stone t.,** a condition characterized by interstitial glossitis, with hypertrophy of the papillae and a verrucous white coating on the tongue. **crocodile t.,** fissured t. **dotted t.,** stippled t. **double t.,** bifid t. **earthy t.,** a tongue that is coated with a deposit of rough, calcareous matter. **encrusted t.,** a heavily coated tongue. **fern leaf t.,** a tongue with a central furrow having lateral branches. **filmy t.,** one marked with symmetrical whitish patches. **fissured t.,** a sometimes familial condition that may be congenital but whose incidence increases with age, characterized by uniformly arranged fissures radiating forward and outward from the median raphe of the tongue, without evidence of inflammation; seen in Melkersson-Rosenthal syndrome. Called also *lingua plicata.* **flat t.,** a condition in which the borders of the tongue cannot be rolled; it is due to paralysis of the transverse lingual muscles occurring as a result of congenital syphilis. **furred t.,** a tongue with papillae so changed as to give the mucous membrane the appearance of whitish fur. **furrowed t.,** fissured t. **geographic t.,** a tongue with denuded patches surrounded by thickened epithelium; called also *lingua geographica, erythema migrans, pityriasis linguae,* and *glossitis areata exfoliativa.* **grooved t.,** fissured t. **hairy t.,** a tongue the papillae of which have a hairlike appearance. **lobulated t.,** a tongue with a congenital second lobe lying on it. **magenta t.,** the magenta-colored tongue seen in cases of riboflavin deficiency. **mappy t.,** geographic t. **parrot t.,** the dry, horny tongue of low fever, which cannot be protruded. **plicated t.,** fissured t. **raspberry t.,** a red, uncoated tongue, with elevated papillae, as seen a few days after appearance of the rash in scarlet fever. **Sandwith's bald t.,** an extremely clean tongue sometimes seen in the late stages of pellagra. **scrotal t.,** fissured t. **smokers' t.,** leukoplakia of the tongue. **t. of sphenoid bone,** lingula sphenoidalis. **split t.,** bifid t. **stippled t.,** a tongue on which each papilla is covered with a separate white patch of epithelium; called also *dotted t.* **strawberry t.,** a coated tongue with enlarged, red, fungiform papillae, seen in the first 24 hours after appearance of the rash in scarlet fever. **sulcated t.,** fissured t. **timber t.,** wooden t. **trombone t.,** involuntary movement of the tongue, consisting of vigorous alternating protrusion and retraction. **white t.,** a condition in which all or part of the papillae and epithelium of the tongue have a dull white color. **wooden t.,** actinobacillosis of cattle in which hard tumor-like nodules form inside the tongue; called also *timber t.* **wrinkled t.,** fissured t.

tongue-tie (tung'ti) abnormal shortness of the frenum of the tongue, resulting in limitation of its motion; called also *ankyloglossia* and *lingua frenata.*

tonic (ton'ik) [Gr. *tonikos*] 1. producing and restoring the normal tone. 2. characterized by continuous tension. 3. a term formerly used for a class of medicinal preparations believed to have the power of restoring normal tone to tissue. **bitter t.,** a tonic of bitter taste, used for stimulating the appetite and improving digestion, such as quinine, quassia, and gentian. **cardiac t.,** one which strengthens the heart's action, such as digitalis, strophanthus, or strychnine. **digestive t.,** an intestinal or stomachic tonic. **general t.,** one which braces up the whole system; cold baths, electricity, and exercise are general tonics. **intestinal t.,** one that improves the tone of the intestinal tract. **stomachic t.,** one which aids the functions of the stomach; here are classed the alcoholic stimulants, vegetable bitters, hydrochloric and nitrohydrochloric acids. **vascular t.,** one which increases the tone of the blood vessels; among them are belladonna, digitalis, ergot, and strychnine.

tonicity (to-nis'i-te) the state of tissue tone or tension; in body fluid physiology, the effective osmotic pressure equivalent.

tonicize (ton'i-sīz) 1. to improve the tone of a part. 2. to induce tonic contraction of a muscle.

tonicoclonic (ton"i-ko-klon'ik) tonoclonic.

tonka bean (tong'kah bēn) the seed of *Dipteryx odorata* Willd. (Leguminosae), a North America tree; it affords coumarin, and has been used as a flavoring agent and to disguise odors in pharmaceutical and tobacco.

tono- [Gr. *tonos* tension] a combining form denoting relationship to tone or tension.

tonoclonic (ton"o-klon'ik) both tonic and clonic; said of a spasm consisting of a convulsive twitching of the muscles.

tonofibril (ton'o-fi"bril) a bundle of fine filaments (tonofilaments) in certain cells, especially epithelial cells, the individual strands of which transverse the cytoplasm in all directions and extend into the cell processes to converge and insert on the desmosomes; they are thought to have a supportive or cytoskeletal function and, in keratinizing epithelia, to be the principal precursor of keratin.

tonofilament (ton″o-fil′ah-ment) any of the fine filaments of a tonofibril.

tonogram (to′no-gram) the record produced by tonography.

tonograph (to′no-graf) [*tono-* + Gr. *graphein* to write] a recording tonometer.

tonography (to-nog′rah-fe) the recording of changes in intraocular pressure produced by the constant application of a known weight on the globe of the eye, reflecting the facility of outflow of the aqueous humor from the anterior chamber. **carotid compression t.,** a test for occlusion of the carotid artery by measuring ocular pressure and pulse before, during, and after the proximal portion of the carotid artery is compressed by the fingers.

tonometer (to-nom′ĕ-ter) [*tono-* + Gr. *metron* measure] an instrument for measuring tension or pressure; usually used specifically in reference to an instrument by which intraocular pressure is measured. **air-puff t.,** an instrument for measuring intraocular pressure; it does not touch the eye, but rather senses deflections of the cornea in reaction to a puff of pressurized air. **applanation t.,** an instrument that measures intraocular pressure by determination of the force necessary to flatten a corneal surface of constant size. **electronic t.,** one having an electronic readout. **Gärtner's t.,** an instrument for measuring blood pressure by means of a compressing ring applied to the finger. **Goldmann's applanation t.,** an instrument for measuring intraocular pressure which eliminates the effects of scleral resistance. **impression t.,** an instrument that measures direct pressure on the eyeball, such as the Schiøtz, McLean, or MacKay-Marg electronic tonometer. **MacKay-Marg electronic t.,** an electronic applanation tonometer equipped with a flat plunger which measures intraocular pressure by direct application to the cornea. **McLean t.,** an instrument that registers intraocular pressure, with a scale from which the pressure can be read directly. **Musken's t.,** an instrument for measuring the tonicity of the Achilles tendon. **Recklinghausen's t.,** an instrument for observing oscillatory blood pressure. **Schiøtz' t.,** an instrument that registers intraocular pressure by direct application to the cornea, the reading on the scale being translated into millimeters of mercury by means of a conversion table.

tonometry (to-nom′ĕ-tre) the measurement of tension or pressure, especially the indirect estimation of the intraocular pressure from determination of the resistance of the eyeball to indentation by an applied force. **applanation t.,** that done by means of the applanation tonometer. **digital t.,** estimation of the degree of intraocular pressure by pressure exerted on the eyeball by the finger of the examiner.

tonophant (ton′o-fant) [*tono-* + Gr. *phainein* to show] (*obs.*) an instrument for rendering acoustic vibrations visible.

tonoplast (ton′o-plast) [*tono-* + Gr. *plassein* to form] a small intracellular body which forms powerful osmotic substances within itself and thus swells up to form a small vacuole (De Vries, 1885). The term is now applied to the limiting membrane of an intracellular vacuole, the vacuole membrane.

tonoscope (ton′o-skop) [*tono-* + Gr. *skopein* to examine] (*obs.*) 1. an apparatus for rendering sound visible by registering the vibrations on a screen. 2. a device for examining the head or brain by means of sound. 3. tonometer.

tonotopic (ton″o-top′ik) having a spatial arrangement such that certain tone frequencies are transmitted along a particular portion of the structure, as in the cochlear nuclei.

tonotopicity (ton″o-top-is′ĭ-te) the property of being tonotopic.

tonsil (ton′sil) a small rounded mass of tissue, especially of lymphoid tissue. The term is often used without qualification to designate the palatine tonsil. Called also *tonsilla.* **buried t.,** submerged t. **t. of cerebellum,** tonsilla cerebelli. **eustachian t.,** see *noduli lymphatici tubarii tubae auditivae.* **faucial t.,** see *palatine t.* **Gerlach's t.,** see *noduli lymphatici tubarii tubae auditivae.* **intestinal t.,** see *folliculi lymphatici aggregati.* **lingual t.,** tonsilla lingualis. **Luschka's t.,** tonsilla pharyngea. **palatine t.,** a small, almond-shaped mass between the palatoglossal and palatopharyngeal arches on either side, composed mainly of lymphoid tissue, covered with mucous membrane, and containing various crypts and many lymph follicles; believed to act as sources for supply to the mouth and pharynx of phagocytes which destroy bacteria entering the mouth. Called also *tonsilla palatina* [NA]. **pharyngeal t.,** tonsilla pharyngea. **resected t.,** a palatine tonsil part of which has been excised. **submerged t.,** a palatine tonsil that is shrunken and atrophied and is partly or entirely hidden by the palatoglossal arch. **third t.,** tonsilla pharyngea. **t. of torus tubarius,** tonsilla tubaria. **tubal t's,** noduli lymphatici tubarii tubae auditivae.

tonsilla (ton-sil′ah), pl. *tonsil′lae* [L.] tonsil: [NA] a general term for a small rounded mass of tissue, especially of lymphoid tissue. **t. cerebel′li** [NA], **t. of cerebellum,** a rounded mass forming part of the cerebellum on its inferior surface, between the uvula and the biventral lobule; called also *amygdala*

of cerebellum. **t. intestina′lis,** see *folliculi lymphatici aggregati.* **t. lingua′lis** [NA], lingual tonsil: an aggregation of lymph follicles on the floor of the oropharyngeal passageway, at the root of the tongue. **t. palati′na** [NA], a small, almond-shaped mass between the palatoglossal and palatopharyngeal arches on either side; see *palatine tonsil.* **t. pharyn′gea** [NA], pharyngeal tonsil: the diffuse lymphoid tissue and follicles in the roof and posterior wall of the nasopharynx. See also *adenoid* (def. 2). **t. tuba′ria** [NA], lymphoid tissue associated with the opening of the auditory tube; called also *tonsil of torus tubarius.*

tonsillar (ton′sĭ-lar) [L. *tonsillaris*] of or pertaining to a tonsil; amygdaline.

tonsillectome (ton″sĭ-lek′tōm) an instrument for performing tonsillectomy.

tonsillectomy (ton″sĭ-lek′to-me) [L. *tonsilla* tonsil + Gr. *ektomē* excision] surgical removal of a tonsil or tonsils.

tonsillith (ton′sĭ-lith) tonsillolith.

tonsillitic (ton″sĭ-lit′ik) pertaining to or affected with tonsillitis.

tonsillitis (ton″sĭ-li′tis) [L. *tonsilla* tonsil + *-itis*] inflammation of the tonsils, especially the palatine tonsils. **caseous t.,** lacunar t. **catarrhal t., acute,** a form associated with acute catarrhal pharyngitis, in which the tonsils are red and swollen; called also *erythematous t.* **catarrhal t., chronic,** a form attended by permanent hypertrophy, and usually requiring tonsillectomy. **diphtherial t.,** see *diphtheria.* **erythematous t.,** catarrhal t., acute. **follicular t.,** that which especially affects the crypts (once referred to as follicles). **herpetic t.,** a local manifestation of herpes on the tonsil. **lacunar t.,** tonsillitis in which the crypts of the tonsils are filled with plugs of caseous matter; called also *caseous t.* **t. len′ta,** chronic inflammation of the tonsils producing a prolonged chronic sepsis. **lingual t.,** inflammation of a lymphoid mass at the base of the tongue. **mycotic t.,** a form due to fungi. **parenchymatous t., acute,** inflammation of the whole substance of the tonsil. **preglottic t.,** inflammation of the lingual tonsil. **pustular t.,** that which is characterized by the formation of pustules. **streptococcal t.,** see *septic sore throat,* under *sore throat.* **superficial t.,** inflammation of the mucous membrane over a tonsil. **suppurative t.,** parenchymatous t., acute. **Vincent's t.,** tonsillitis caused by Vincent's organism (*Fusobacterium plauti-vincenti*).

tonsilloadenoidectomy (ton″sil-o-ad″ĕ-noi-dek′to-me) excision of palatine tonsils and adenoids.

tonsillohemisporosis (ton″sĭ-lo-hem″ĭ-spo-ro′sis) infection of the tonsil with *Hemispora.*

tonsillolith (ton-sil′o-lith) [*tonsil* + Gr. *lithos* stone] a concretion or calculus in a tonsil.

tonsillomoniliasis (ton-sil″o-mo″nĭ-li′ah-sis) infection of the tonsil with *Monilia* (*Candida*).

tonsillomycosis (ton-sil″o-mi-ko′sis) any mycotic infection of the tonsils.

tonsillo-oidiosis (ton-sil″o-o-id″e-o′sis) infection of the tonsil with *Oidium* (*Candida*).

tonsillopathy (ton″sĭ-lop′ah-the) [*tonsil* + Gr. *pathos* disease] any disease of the tonsil.

tonsilloprive (ton′sĭ-lo-prīv) [*tonsil* + L. *privare* to deprive] having the tonsils removed; due to removal or absence of the tonsils.

tonsilloscopy (ton″sĭ-los′ko-pe) diagnostic inspection of the tonsils.

tonsillotome (ton-sil′o-tōm) a knife used in tonsillotomy.

thymopoietin (tri″mo-poi′ĕ-tin) a polypeptide hormone secreted by the thymus, which induces differentiation of thymocytes and impairs postsynaptic neuromuscular transmission.

tonsillotomy (ton″sĭ-lot′o-me) [L. *tonsilla* tonsil + Gr. *tomē* a cutting] incision of a tonsil; the surgical removal of a part of a tonsil.

tonsillotyphoid (ton″sĭ-lo-ti′foid) pharyngotyphoid.

tonsolith (ton′so-lith) tonsillolith.

tonus (to′nus) [L.; Gr. *tonos*] the slight, continuous contraction of muscle, which in skeletal muscles aids in the maintenance of posture and in the return of blood to the heart. See *tone.* **acerebral t.,** tonic contraction of muscles after removal of the cerebrum. **chemical t.,** the state of slight but continuous chemical activity in muscles when at rest. **myogenic t.,** tonic contraction of muscle dependent upon some property of the muscle itself or of its intrinsic nerve cells. **neurogenic t.,** tonic contraction of muscle due to stimulation received through the nervous system.

tooth (tōōth), pl. *teeth.* One of a set of small hard structures in the jaws used for mastication of food (dens, *pl.* dentes [NA]), or a similar structure in various organisms other than man in the animal or plant kingdom. In man, there are two sets of teeth; the *deciduous teeth* and the *permanent teeth.* Each tooth has two main sections, a *crown* and a *root* or roots; the two divisions are further divided into crown, cervix (or neck), root, and apex. Clinical landmarks include the coronal portion, the cervical portion, the

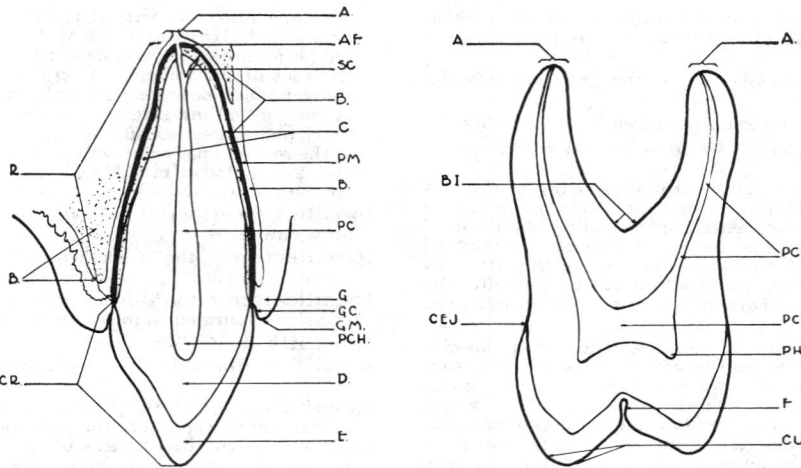

Schematic cross section of an anterior and a posterior tooth in upper jaw. **Left,** Anterior tooth: *A*, apex; *AF*, apical foramen; *SC*, supplementary canal; *C*, cementum; *PM*, periodontal membrane; *B*, bone; *PC*, pulp canal; *G*, gingiva; *GC*, gingival sulcus; *GM*, gingival margin; *PCH*, pulp chamber; *D*, dentin; *E*, enamel; *CR*, crown; *R*, root. **Right,** Posterior tooth: *A*, apices; *PC*, pulp canal; *PCH*, pulp chamber; *PH*, pulp horn; *F*, fissure; *CU*, cusp; *CEJ*, cemento-enamel junction; *BI*, bifurcation of roots. (Wheeler.)

radicular portion and the apical portion. The tooth is solid except for a *pulp cavity* centered within it. The major portion of the tooth is made up of *dentin* or ivory. A layer of *enamel,* a very hard inorganic substance, covers the crown portion of the tooth, mostly in evidence above the gum line, and a thin layer of *cementum* covers the root portion set in the jaw bones. Cementum (crusta petrosa) is true bone. The *pulp cavity* may be divided into two portions: the *pulp chamber,* mostly within the crown, and the *pulp canal* traversing the interior of the root, ending in a constricted opening at the root apex. There is at least one pulp canal in each root even when the tooth has multiple roots. The pulp cavity contains the *dental pulp,* a soft tissue containing connective tissue, blood vessels, and nerves. The *eruption* or "cutting" of the teeth follows generally an orderly schedule as follows: *Deciduous teeth*—first incisors, 6 to 8 months; second incisors, 7 to 9 months; first molars, 12 to 14 months; canines, 16 to 18 months; second molars, 20 to 24 months. *Permanent teeth*—first molars, 6 to 7 years; first incisors, 6 to 8 years; second incisors, 7 to 9 years; premolars, 10 to 12 years; canines, 9 to 12 years; second molars, 11 to 13 years; third molars, 17 to 21 years. **accessional teeth,** the permanent molars, so called because they do not supplant any deciduous predecessors in the dental arch. Cf. *succedaneous teeth.* **acrylic resin t.,** an artificial tooth made of acrylic resin. **anatomic teeth,** a term applied to artificial teeth in which the cusps and ridges of the natural teeth are reproduced on the occlusal surface. **ankylosed t.,** a primary tooth, with or without permanent successors, which remains submerged below the occlusal level of the dentition. **anterior teeth,** the three teeth on either side in each jaw situated closest to the midline of the dental arch, including the incisor and canine (cuspid) teeth. **artificial t.,** a tooth made of porcelain or other synthetic compound in imitation of a natural tooth; see also *denture.* **auditory teeth of Huschke,** dentes acustici. **t. of axis,** dens axis. **bicuspid teeth,** premolar teeth (dentes premolares [NA]). **brown opalescent teeth, hereditary,** see *amelogenesis imperfecta.* **buccal teeth,** posterior teeth. **canine teeth,** the four teeth, one on either side in each jaw, immediately lateral to the lateral, or second, incisors; they have a long conical crown and the longest, most powerful root of all the teeth. Called also *dentes canini* [NA]. **cheek teeth,** posterior teeth. **cheoplastic teeth,** artificial teeth attached to a cheoplastic base without pins. **connate t.,** geminate t. **corner t.,** the third incisor on either side of each jaw in the horse. **cross-bite teeth,** posterior teeth designed to permit positioning of the modified buccal cusps of the upper teeth in the fossae of the lower teeth. **cross-pin teeth,** artificial teeth in which the pins are inserted horizontally. **cuspid teeth,** canine teeth (dentes canini [NA]). **cuspless teeth,** artificial teeth designed without cusps on the occlusal surface. **deciduous teeth,** the teeth of the first dentition, which are shed and followed, in the dental arch, by the permanent teeth. The 20 deciduous teeth, 10 in each jaw, include 4 incisor, 2 canine, and 4 molar teeth. Called also *dentes decidui* [NA], and *milk,* or *primary,* or *temporary teeth.* **diatoric teeth,** artificial teeth with holes in their bases into which the denture base material flows and, when processed, attaches the teeth to the base. **dummy t.,** pontic. **embedded t.,** an un-erupted tooth, usually one completely covered by bone. **t. of epistropheus,** dens axis. **eye t.,** colloquial term for a canine tooth of the upper jaw. **Fournier teeth,** Moon's teeth.

fused teeth, the fusion, early in odontogenesis, of two normally separate tooth germs, the completeness of the fusion depending on the stage at which the union took place. **geminate t.,** a tooth with a single root and root canal, but with two completely or incompletely separated crowns, resulting from invagination of a single tooth germ, causing incomplete formation of two teeth. **Goslee t.,** an interchangeable tooth attached to a metal base. **hag teeth,** upper medial incisors that are widely separated. **hair teeth,** dentes acustici. **Horner's teeth,** incisor teeth that are horizontally grooved owing to a deficiency of enamel. **Hutchinson's teeth,** notched and narrow-edged permanent incisors; regarded as a sign of congenital syphilis, but not always of such origin. **impacted t.,** a tooth so placed in the jaw that it is unable to erupt, or unable to attain its normal position in occlusion. **incisor teeth,** the four front teeth, two on each side of the midline in each jaw; the cutting teeth, each with one long root. Called also *dentes incisivi* [NA]. See *incisor.* **labial teeth,** anterior teeth. **lion's t.** [Fr. *dent-de-lion* dandelion], *Taraxacum officinale* Weber. (Compositae). **malacotic teeth,** teeth that are soft in structure and are abnormally susceptible to caries. **malposed t.,** a tooth out of its normal position. **mandibular teeth,** the teeth of the mandible, or lower jaw. **maxillary teeth,** the teeth of the maxilla, or upper jaw. **metal insert teeth,** artificial teeth containing metal in the occlusal surface. **milk teeth,** deciduous teeth (dentes decidui [NA]). **molar teeth** [L. *molaris* to do with grinding], the most posterior teeth on either side in each jaw, totaling 8 in the

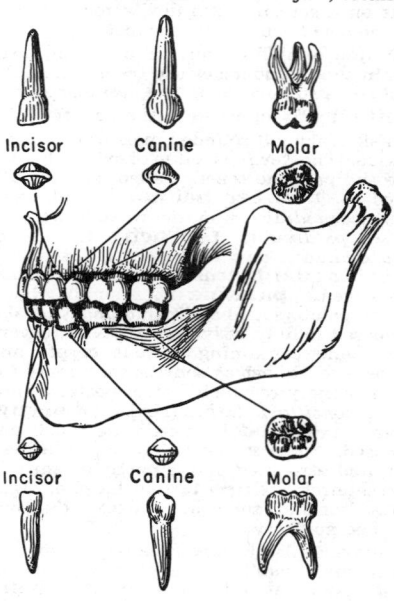

Typical Deciduous Teeth

deciduous dentition (2 on each side, upper and lower), and usually 12 in the permanent dentition (3 on each side, upper and lower). They are the grinding teeth, having large crowns with broad chewing surfaces. The upper molars characteristically have 4 major cusps and three roots. The lower first molars characteristically have 5 cusps, and the remaining lower molars 4 cusps. Normally all lower molars have two roots. The third molars ("widsom teeth") are often malformed, but when developed normally their crown and root form corresponds in general with neighboring molars in the same jaw. Called also *dentes molars* [NA]. **Moon's teeth,** small, domed first molars observed in patients with congenital syphilis. **morsal teeth** [L. *morsus* a seizing], anterior teeth. **mottled teeth,** teeth whose enamel is marked with discoloration. **mulberry t.,** mulberry molar. **natal t.,** a prematurely erupted deciduous tooth, visible in the jaw at birth. **neonatal t.,** a primary tooth that erupts during the neonatal period. **nonanatomic teeth,** a term applied to artificial teeth the occlusal surfaces of which are especially designed on the basis of engineering concepts, without regard to the features of natural teeth. **peg t.,** a tooth whose sides converge or taper together incisally, instead of being parallel or diverging mesially and distally; a condition frequently observed in the maxillary lateral incisor. **permanent teeth,** the teeth of the second dentition; the 32 permanent teeth, 16 in each jaw. They

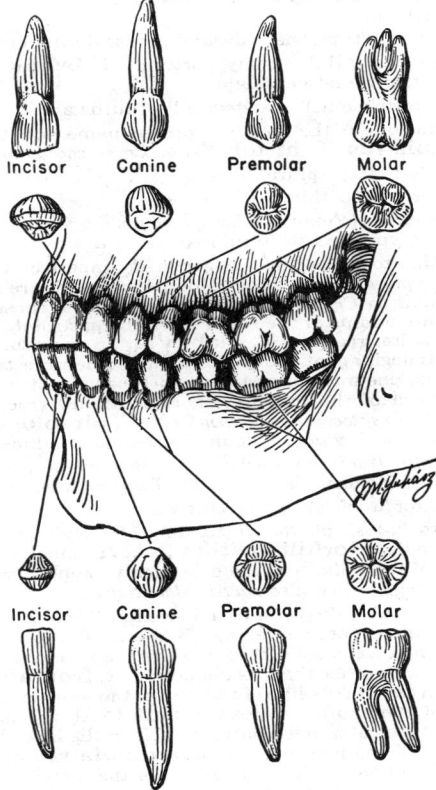

Typical Permanent Teeth

include 4 incisor, 2 canine, 4 premolar, and 6 molar teeth in each jaw. Called also *dentes permanentes* [NA]. **pink t. of Mummery,** internal resorption of a tooth, so called because of the pink color given the crown by the hyperplastic, vascular pulp filling the area formerly occupied by the resorbed dentin. **pinless teeth,** diatoric teeth. **plastic t.,** an artificial tooth made of synthetic resin. **posterior teeth,** the teeth on either side in each jaw, distal to the canine teeth, including the premolar (bicuspid) and molar teeth; called also *buccal* or *cheek teeth.* **predeciduous t.,** a term applied to a hornified epithelial structure, without roots, occurring on the gingiva over the crest of the ridge of the alveolar process before the eruption of deciduous teeth. **premilk t.,** 1. natal t. 2. neonatal t. **premolar teeth,** the eight permanent teeth, two on either side in each jaw, between the canine teeth and the molars; the upper premolars have two cusps (bicuspid), but the lower have from one to three. They are succedaneous to the deciduous molar teeth. Called also *dentes premolares* [NA], and *bicuspid teeth.* In zoology, those teeth which succeed the deciduous molars regardless of the number to be succeeded. **primary teeth,** deciduous teeth. **pulpless t.,** a tooth from which the pulp has been extirpated. **rake teeth,** teeth that are widely separated. **rootless teeth,** dentin dysplasia. **sclerotic teeth,** teeth that are hard in structure and resistant to caries. **screw-driver teeth,** Hutchinson's teeth.

shell t., a tooth in which the enamel appears essentially normal, the dentin is extremely thin, and the pulp chamber is enlarged. **snaggle t.,** a tooth out of proper line with the others. **stomach t.,** a canine tooth of the lower jaw, or mandible. **straight-pin teeth,** artificial teeth in which the pins are inserted vertically. **"submerged" t.,** a deciduous tooth, most commonly a mandibular second molar, which has undergone a variable degree of root resorption and then become ankylosed to the bone, preventing its exfoliation and subsequent replacement by a permanent tooth. It appears submerged in relation to the adjacent erupted permanent teeth. **succedaneous teeth, successional teeth,** the permanent teeth that have deciduous predecessors in the dental arch. Cf. *accessional teeth.* **superior teeth,** the teeth of the upper jaw, or maxilla. **supernumerary teeth, supplemental teeth** natural teeth in excess of the number normally present in the jaw. **temporary teeth,** deciduous teeth (dentes decidui [NA]). **tube teeth,** artificial teeth having a vertical, cylindrical aperture from the center of the base up into the body of the tooth, into which a pin may be placed or cast for attachment of the tooth to the denture base. **Turner's t.,** a permanent tooth, usually a mandibular premolar, with hypoplasia of enamel, resulting from spread to the tooth germ of periapical infection and inflammation involving a primary tooth. **vital teeth,** teeth to which the nerve and vascular supply is intact. **wandering t.,** a tooth that moves from its normal position in the dental arch. **wisdom t.,** the third molar tooth, the tooth most distal from the medial line on either side in each jaw, so called because it is the last of the permanent dentition to erupt, usually at the age of 17 to 21 years. Called also *dens serotinus* [NA]. **wolf t.,** a vestigial first premolar tooth sometimes present in the jaw of a horse. **zero degree teeth,** artificial teeth which have no cusp angles in relation to the horizontal on their occlusal surfaces.

Tooth's atrophy, disease, type (tooths) [Howard Henry *Tooth,* English physician, 1856–1925] progressive neuropathic (peroneal) muscular atrophy.

tooth-borne (tōōth'born) supported entirely by the teeth; said of a prosthesis or part of a prosthesis entirely supported by the abutment teeth.

topagnosia (top″ag-no′ze-ah) 1. loss of touch localization. 2. loss of ability to recognize familiar surroundings.

topagnosis (top″ag-no′sis) [Gr. *topos* place + *a* neg. + *gnōsis* recognition] loss of touch localization.

topalgia (to-pal′je-ah) [Gr. *topos* place + *algos* pain + *-ia*] fixed or localized pain; seen in neurasthenia.

topectomy (to-pek′to-me) [*topo-* + Gr. *ektomē* excision] ablation of a small and specific area of the frontal cortex in the treatment of mental illness.

topesthesia (top″es-the′ze-ah) [Gr. *topos* place + *aisthēsis* perception + *-ia*] the power of localizing a tactile sensation.

Töpfer's test (tep′ferz) [Alfred Edouard *Töpfer,* German physician, born 1858] see under *tests.*

tophaceous (to-fa′shus) [L. *tophaceus: tophus* porous stone] hard or gritty; of the nature of or characterized by tophi.

tophi (to′fi) [L.] plural of *tophus.*

topholipoma (tof″o-lĭ-po′mah) a lipoma containing tophi.

tophus (to′fus), pl. *to′phi* [L. "porous stone"] a chalky deposit of sodium urate occurring in gout; tophi form most often around joints in cartilage, bone, bursae, and subcutaneous tissue and in the external ear, producing a chronic, foreign-body inflammatory response. **auricular t.,** a tophus on the ear. **dental t.,** dental calculus. **t. syphilit′icus,** a syphilitic node.

topical (top′e-kal) [Gr. *topikos*] pertaining to a particular surface area, as a topical anti-infective applied to a certain area of the skin and affecting only the area to which it is applied.

Topicort (top′ĭ-kort) trademark for a preparation of desoximetasone.

Topicycline (top′ĭ-si′klēn) trademark for a topical preparation of tetracycline hydrochloride; used in treatment of acne.

Topinard's angle, line (top″e-nārz′) [Paul *Topinard,* French physician and anthropologist, 1830–1911] see *ophryospinal angle,* under *angle,* and see under *line.*

topo- (top′o) [Gr. *topos* place] a combining form meaning place.

topoalgia (top″o-al′je-ah) topalgia.

topoanesthesia (top″o-an″es-the′ze-ah) loss of power to localize a tactile sensation.

topochemistry (top″o-kem′is-tre) the chemical composition at specific sites of a structure, as at the surface membrane of a cell.

topodysesthesia (top″o-dis″es-the′ze-ah) localized dysesthesia.

topognosis (top″og-no′sis) [*topo-* + Gr. *gnōsis* recognition] topesthesia.

topographic (top″o-graf′ik) describing or pertaining to special regions.

topographical (top″o-graf′ĭ-kal) pertaining to topography.

topography (to-pog′rah-fe) [*topo-* + Gr. *graphein* to write] the description of an anatomical region or of a special part.

topology (to-pol'o-je) [topo- + -logy] the relation between the presenting part of the fetus and the birth canal.

toponarcosis (top"o-nar-ko'sis) [topo- + Gr. *narkōsis* benumbing] localized anesthesia.

toponym (top'o-nim) the name of a region as distinguished from an organ.

toponymy (to-pon'ĭ-me) [topo- + Gr. *onoma* name] terminology pertaining to the regions of the body.

topoparesthesia (top"o-par"es-the'ze-ah) localized paresthesia.

topophylaxis (top"o-fi-lak'sis) the application of a constricting band, intended to confine the protection following arsphenamine injections to the limb in which the injection is made.

topothermesthesiometer (top"o-therm"es-the-ze-om'ĕ-ter) [topo- + Gr. *thermē* heat + *aisthēsis* perception + *metron* measure] an apparatus for measuring the local temperature sense.

topovaccinotherapy (top"o-vak"sĭ-no-ther'ah-pe) artificial local immunization.

Topsyn (top'sin) trademark for a preparation of fluocinonide.

topterone (top'tĕ-rōn) chemical name: 17β-hydroxy-17-propyl-androst-4-en-one; an antiestrogen, $C_{22}H_{34}O_2$.

torcular (tor'ku-lar) [L. "wine-press"] a hollow, or expanded area. **t. Heroph'ili,** confluens sinuum.

Torecan (tor'ĕ-kān) trademark for preparations of thiethylperazine.

Torek operation (to'rek) [Franz J. A. *Torek*, New York surgeon (born in Breslau), 1861–1938] see under *operation.*

tori (to'ri) [L.] plural of *torus.*

toric (to'rik) pertaining to or resembling a torus.

tormina (tor'mĭ-nah) [L.] colic, def. 2.

torminal (tor'mĭ-nal) pertaining to or characterized by griping pain, or colic.

Tornwaldt's (Thornwaldt's) bursa, bursitis (disease) (torn'vahlts) [Gustav Ludwig *Tornwaldt,* 1843–1910] see *bursa pharyngea,* and see under *bursitis.*

torose, torous (to'rōs; to'rus) [L. *torosus* muscular, brawny] bulging or knobby.

torpent (tor'pent) [L. *torpere* to be sluggish] 1. inactive; in abeyance. 2. an agent that reduces irritation.

torpid (tor'pid) [L. *torpidus* numb, sluggish] not acting with normal vigor and facility.

torpidity (tor-pid'ĭ-te) sluggishness; inactivity, slowness.

torpor (tor'por) [L.] lack of response to normal or ordinary stimuli. **t. ret'inae,** a condition in which the retina is excited to action only by stimuli of considerable luminous power.

torque (tork) [L. *torquere* to twist] a rotary force; in dentistry, the rotation of a tooth on its long axis, especially the movement of the apical portions of the teeth by use of orthodontic appliances.

torquing (tork'ing) the twisting of a tooth into position, as in the correction of malposition.

torr (tor) [after Evangelista *Torr*icelli, Italian mathematician, 1608–1647] a unit of pressure equal to $\frac{1}{760}$ of normal atmospheric pressure, or to the pressure necessary to support a column of mercury 1 mm. high at 0° C. and standard gravity.

torrefaction (tor"ĕ-fak'shun) [L. *torrefactio*] the act of roasting or parching.

torrefy (tor'e-fi) [L. *torrefacere*] to parch, roast, or dry by the aid of heat.

torricellian (to"re-chel'e-an) named for Evangelista *Torricelli,* Italian mathematician, 1608–1647; see under *vacuum.*

torsiometer (tor"se-om'ĕ-ter) [L. *torsio* twist + *metrum* measure] a form of clinoscope for measuring the amount of rotation of the eyeball on the visual axis.

torsion (tor'shun) [L. *torsio; torquere* to twist] 1. the act of twisting; the condition of being twisted. In dentistry, the condition of a tooth when it is turned on its long axis. 2. in ophthalmology, any rotation of the vertical corneal meridians. **negative t.,** rotation in a counterclockwise direction. **positive t.,** rotation in a clockwise direction.

torsionometer (tor"shun-om'ĕ-ter) [torsion + Gr. *metron* measure] an apparatus for estimating the degree of rotation of the spinal column.

torsive (tor'siv) twisted.

torsiversion (tor"sĭ-ver'zhun) the turning or rotation of a tooth on its long axis out of its normal position.

torso (tor'so) the trunk without the head or extremities.

torsoclusion (tor"so-kloo'zhun) [L. *torquere* to twist + *cludere* to shut] 1. acupressure combined with pressure of the bleeding vessel. 2. torsiversion.

torso-occlusion (tor"so-ŏ-kloo'zhun) torsiversion.

torticollar (tor"tĭ-kol'ar) pertaining to or affected with torticollis.

torticollis (tor"tĭ-kol'is) [L. *tortus* twisted + *collum* neck] wryneck; a contracted state of the cervical muscles, producing twisting of the neck and an unnatural position of the head. **congenital t.,** torticollis due to injury to the sternocleidomastoid muscle on one side at the time of birth and its transformation into a fibrous cord which cannot lengthen with the growing neck. **dermatogenic t.,** torticollis caused by contraction of the skin of the neck. **fixed t.,** an unnatural position of the head due to actual and persistent organic muscular shortening. **hysteric t., hysterical t.,** torticollis due to hysteric contracture. **intermittent t.,** spasmodic t. **labyrinthine t.,** torticollis due to irritation of the semicircular canals on one side. **mental t.,** a form of tic, or habit spasm, in which there is spasmodic contraction of the neck muscles, producing deviation of the head. This deviation usually ceases on the patient lying down, or it may be controlled by slight pressure. **myogenic t.,** a transient condition due to muscular contraction in rheumatism, and to cold. **neurogenic t.,** torticollis due to pressure or irritation of the accessory nerve. **ocular t.,** torticollis due to a high degree of astigmatism or to ocular muscle palsy. **reflex t.,** torticollis caused by inflammation or suppuration in the neck, enlarged cervical lymph nodes, or tumor in the tonsil, neck, or pharynx. **rheumatoid t.,** that which is due to rheumatism, chiefly of the sternomastoid and adjacent muscles. **spasmodic t.,** that which is due to spasm of certain muscles, occurring intermittently. **spurious t.,** twisting or stiffness of the neck due to caries of the cervical vertebrae. **symptomatic t.,** stiffness of the neck due to rheumatism.

tortipelvis (tor"tĭ-pel'vis) dystonia musculorum deformans.

tortua (tor'tu-ah) [L.] agony; torture. **t. fa'cies,** Avicenna's name for trigeminal neuralgia.

tortuous (tor'choo-us) twisted; full of turns and twists.

Torula (tor'u-lah) [L. "roll"] former name for *Cryptococcus.* **T. capsula'tus, T. histolyt'ica,** *Cryptococcus neoformans.*

toruli (tor'u-li) [L.] plural of *torulus.*

torulin (tor'u-lin) thiamine.

toruloma (tor-u-lo'mah) a tumor or nodule which is one of the lesions of cryptococcosis (torulosis).

Torulopsis (tor"u-lop'sis) a genus of imperfect fungi of the family Cryptococcaceae, order Moniliales, which are morphologically similar to *Cryptococcus* but do not have a capsule, and are normal inhabitants of the respiratory and gastrointestinal tracts and urogenital region. **T. glabra'ta,** an opportunistic organism, an etiologic agent of torulopsosis and other infections, such as meningitis, pneumonia, cystitis, and fungemia; it is part of the normal flora of the mouth, gut, and urinary tract. **T. histolyt'ica,** *Cryptococcus neoformans.* **T. pintolope'sii,** a species similar to *T. glabrata,* found in the mouse alimentary tract.

torulopsosis (tor"u-lop'so-sis) an infection of the tissues resembling histoplasmosis, caused by *Torulopsis glabrata.*

torulosis (tor"u-lo'sis) cryptococcosis.

torulus (tor'u-lus), pl. *tor'uli* [L., dim. of *torus*] a small elevation; a papilla. **tor'uli tac'tiles** [NA], the small elevations on the skin of the palm and the sole, richly supplied with sensory nerve endings; called also *tactile elevations.*

torus (to'rus), pl. *to'ri* [L. "a round swelling," "protuberance"] 1. a bulging projection, a swelling; [NA] a general term for such a protuberance. 2. a solid developed by the revolution of a circle about any axis other than its diameter. **t. fronta'lis,** a protuberance in the middle line of the root of the nose, on the external surface of the skull. **t. levato'rius** [NA], the mucosal fold covering the levator veli palatini muscle in the lateral wall of the nasal part of the pharynx. **t. mandibula'ris,** an outgrowth of bone found on the lingual surface of the mandible, above the mylohyoid line and usually opposite the premolar tooth; commonly bilateral, and single or multiple in type. **t. occipita'lis,** a rounded edge occasionally seen on the occipital bone in the region of the superior nuchal line. **t. palati'nus** [NA], a bony protuberance sometimes found on the hard palate at the junction of the intermaxillary and transverse palatine sutures. **t. tuba'rius** [NA], the projecting posterior lip of the pharyngeal opening of the auditory tube. **t. ureter'icus,** interureteric ridge (plica interureterica [NA]).

tosifen (to'sĭ-fen) chemical name: (S)-4-methyl-N-[[(1-methyl-2-phenylethyl)amino]carbonyl]benzenesulfonamide; an antianginal, $C_{17}H_{20}N_2O_3S.$

tosylate (to'sĭ-lāt) USAN contraction for *p*-toluenesulfonate.

Totacillin (to"tah-sil'in) trademark for preparations of ampicillin.

Toti's operation (to'tēz) [Addeo *Toti,* Italian ophthalmologist, born 1861] dacryocystorhinostomy.

totipotency (to"te-po'ten-se) [L. *totus* all + *potentia* power] the ability of a part to develop in any manner, or of a cell to develop into any type of cell.

totipotent (to-tip'o-tent) totipotential.

totipotential (to"te-po-ten'shal) [L. *totus* all + *potentia* power] characterized by ability to develop in any direction; said of cells which can give rise to cells of all orders, i.e., to the complete individual. Cf. *unipotential.*

totipotentiality (to″tĭ-po-ten″she-al′ĭ-te) the ability to differentiate along any line or into any type of cell.

touch (tuch) [L. *tactus*] 1. the sense by which contact with objects gives evidence as to certain of their qualities. 2. palpation or exploration with the finger. **abdominal t.,** digital palpation of the abdomen. **double t.,** digital examination of the rectum and vagina at the same time. **rectal t.,** exploration of the rectum with the finger. **royal t.,** the touching or tapping of a person with scrofula; once practiced by the kings of England and France as a supposedly curative measure; called also *adenochirapsology*. **vaginal t.,** digital exploration of the vagina. **vesical t.,** digital examination of the bladder.

tour (toor) [Fr.] turn. **t. de maître** (dĕ mātr) [Fr. "master's turn"], a method of passing the sound or catheter into the male bladder or into the uterus. It is first introduced in a position with its stem parallel to the thighs and between them and its convexity upward, and then, by a sweep, is brought to the ordinary position and carried on into the bladder. The motion is reversed in the uterus.

Tourette's syndrome (disease) (too-retz′) see *Gilles de la Tourette* (for biographical note) and see *Gilles de la Tourette syndrome*, under *syndrome*.

tournesol (tur′nĕ-sol) litmus.

tourniquet (toor′nĭ-ket) [Fr.] an instrument for the compression of a blood vessel by application around an extremity to control the circulation and prevent the flow of blood to or from the distal area. Tourniquets are of various kinds, named chiefly for their inventors. **automatic rotating t.,** a system consisting of a motor, air compressor, and four blood pressure cuffs for application to the extremities; the cuffs are inflated and deflated in series and in sequence for treatment of acute pulmonary edema. **Esmarch's t.,** a tourniquet consisting of a piece of strong, flat rubber bandage, which, after the blood has been forced from the limb by gravity or compression, is wound about the proximal part of the limb to arrest the circulation. **garrote t.,** Spanish windlass. **pneumatic t.,** a narrow rubber bag to be wound around a limb, pressure being applied by pumping air into the inflatable cuff. **scalp t.,** a tourniquet placed around the scalp with enough pressure to occlude the superficial blood vessels and thereby to lessen the risk of drug-induced alopecia. **Spanish t., torcular t.,** Spanish windlass.

tousey (tow′ze) [Sinclair *Tousey*, New York radiologist, 1864–1937] a unit of roentgen-ray power; being the radiance which will produce on a photographic film an effect equal to that produced by a one-candlepower incandescent electric light.

Touton giant cell (toot′on) [Karl *Touton*, German dermatologist, born 1858] see under *cell*.

towelette (tow′el-et′) a small towel.

toxalbumic (tok″sal-bu′mik) (*obs.*) relating to or caused by toxalbumin.

toxalbumin (tok″sal-bu′min) (*obs.*) any poisonous albumin, including those found in plant juices (abrin, ricin, phallin), serpent venoms, etc. See *toxin*.

toxanemia (tok″sah-ne′me-ah) anemia due to a poison.

toxaphene (toks′ah-fēn) a chlorinated hydrocarbon, $C_{10}H_{10}Cl_8$, used as an agricultural insecticide.

Toxascaris (tok-sas′kah-ris) a genus of parasitic nematodes of the superfamily Ascaridoidea. **T. leoni′na,** a species found commonly in lions, tigers, and other large Felidae; found also in dogs and cats, but usually only in older animals. Its larvae differ from those of *Toxocara canis* and *Toxocara cati* by not passing through the lungs of the infected animal.

toxemia (tok-se′me-ah) [*toxin* + Gr. *haima* blood + *-ia*] 1. the condition resulting from the spread of bacterial products (toxins) by the bloodstream. 2. a condition resulting from metabolic disturbances, e.g., toxemia of pregnancy. **alimentary t.,** toxemia due to absorption from the alimentary canal of chemical poisons generated therein; a form of autointoxication. **eclamptic t., eclamptogenic t.,** t. of pregnancy. **hydatid t.,** toxemia with urticaria caused by hydatid fluid which has escaped into the peritoneal cavity. **preeclamptic t.,** see *preeclampsia*. **t. of pregnancy,** a group of pathologic conditions, essentially metabolic disturbances, occurring in pregnant women, and manifested by preeclampsia and fully developed eclampsia. **pregnancy t. in ewes,** an acute disorder leading to impaired nervous function, coma, and death, occurring during the last few weeks of pregnancy in ewes that are typically carrying twins, triplets, or a particularly large single lamb; the principal predisposing cause is undernutrition association with stress. Called also *pregnancy disease, twin-lamb disease,* and *lambing paralysis.*

toxemic (toks-e′mik) pertaining to or caused by toxemia.

toxenzyme (toks-en′zīm) any poisonous enzyme.

toxic (tok′sik) pertaining to, due to, or of the nature of a poison or toxin; manifesting the symptoms of severe infection.

toxicant (toks′ĭ-kant) [L. *toxicans* poisoning] 1. poisonous. 2. a poisonous agent.

toxication (tok″sĭ-ka′shun) poisoning.

toxicemia (toks″ĭ-se′me-ah) toxemia.

toxicide (tok′sĭ-sīd) [*toxin* + L. *caedere* to kill] a drug capable of overcoming toxic agents.

toxicity (tok-sis′ĭ-te) the quality of being poisonous, especially the degree of virulence of a toxic microbe or of a poison. **O₂ t., oxygen t.,** serious, sometimes irreversible, damage to the pulmonary capillary endothelium associated with breathing high partial pressures of oxygen for prolonged periods. Called also *O₂* or *oxygen poisoning.*

toxico- [Gr. *toxikon* poison] a combining form meaning poisonous or denoting relationship to poison.

toxicodendrol (tok″sĭ-ko-den′drol) a poisonous, nonvolatile oil found in certain plants of the genus *Rhus* (*Toxicodendron*).

Toxicodendron (tok″sĭ-ko-den′dron) [*toxico-* + Gr. *dendron* tree] *Rhus.*

toxicogenic (tok″sĭ-ko-jen′ik) [*toxico-* + Gr. *gennan* to produce] producing or elaborating toxins.

toxicohemia (tok″sĭ-ko-he′me-ah) toxemia.

toxicoid (tok″sĭ-koid) [*toxico-* + Gr. *eidos* form] resembling a poison.

toxicologic (tok″sĭ-ko-loj′ik) pertaining to toxicology.

toxicologist (tok″sĭ-kol′o-jist) an individual who specializes in toxicology.

toxicology (tok″sĭ-kol′o-je) the sum of what is known regarding poisons; the scientific study of poisons, their actions, their detection, and the treatment of the conditions produced by them.

toxicomania (tok″sĭ-ko-ma′ne-ah) [*toxico-* + Gr. *mania* madness] an intense desire for poisons, narcotic drugs, or intoxicants.

toxicomaniac (tok″sĭ-ko-ma′ne-ak) a person affected with toxicomania.

toxicopathic (tok″sĭ-ko-path′ik) pertaining to toxicopathy.

toxicopathy (tok″sĭ-kop′ah-the) [*toxico-* + Gr. *pathos* disease] any disease induced by a poison.

toxicopectic (tok″sĭ-ko-pek′tik) pertaining to, characterized by, or promoting toxicopexis.

toxicopexic (tok″sĭ-ko-pek′sik) toxicopectic.

toxicopexis (tok″sĭ-ko-pek′sis) [*toxico-* + Gr. *pēxis* fixation] the fixing or neutralizing of a poison in the body.

toxicopexy (tok′sĭ-ko-pek″se) toxicopexis.

toxicophidia (tok″sĭ-ko-fid′e-ah) [*toxico-* + Gr. *ophis* snake] thanatophidia.

toxicophobia (tok″sĭ-ko-fo′be-ah) [*toxico-* + Gr. *phobein* to be affrighted by] morbid dread of poisons.

toxicosis (tok″sĭ-ko′sis) [Gr. *toxikon* poison + *-osis*] any disease condition due to poisoning. **alimentary t.,** sitotoxism, or food poisoning. **endogenic t.,** autointoxication. **exogenic t.,** poisoning by the ingestion of toxic material, as in the food. See *food poisoning,* under *poisoning.* **gestational t.,** gestosis. **hemorrhagic capillary t.,** Frank's name for a hemorrhagic condition attributed to capillary weakening from some toxic action; see *Henoch's purpura,* under *purpura.* **proteinogenous t.,** an acute and fatal intoxication which appears in white mice which are fed an exclusive diet of various proteins. **retention t.,** that which is due to the nonexcretion of noxious waste products.

toxicosozin (tok″sĭ-ko-so′zin) a defensive protein which counteracts a toxin.

toxiferous (tok-sif′er-us) [*toxin* + L. *ferre* to bear] conveying or producing a poison.

toxigenic (tok″sĭ-jen′ik) toxicogenic.

toxigenicity (tok″sĭ-jĕ-nis′ĭ-te) the disease-producing virulence of a parasite which acts by virtue of a soluble toxin.

toxignomic (toks″ig-nom′ik) [*toxin* + Gr. *gnōmē* a means of knowing] characteristic of the toxic action of a poison.

toxin (tok′sin) [L. *toxicum* poison, from Gr. *toxikos* of or for the bow] a poison; frequently used to refer specifically to a protein produced by some higher plants, certain animals, and pathogenic bacteria, which is highly toxic for other living organisms. Such substances are differentiated from the simple chemical poisons and the vegetable alkaloids by their high molecular weight and antigenicity. **amanita t.,** a toxin from *Amanita phalloides.* **animal t.,** one produced by an animal; a zootoxin. **bacterial t's,** toxic substance produced by bacteria, including exotoxins, endotoxins, and toxic enzymes. **botulinus t.,** any of the six type-specific, immunologically differentiable exotoxins (types A to F, inclusive), produced by *Clostridium botulinum.* See *botulin.* **Coley's t.,** an unfiltered mixture of cultures of certain bacteria; once used in treatment of inoperable malignant growths. **dermonecrotic t.,** an exotoxin that produces extensive local necrosis on intradermal inoculation; produced primarily by coagulase-positive staphylococci and regarded as identical with δ staphylolysin. **Dick t.,** erythrogenic t. **diphtheria t.,** a protein exotoxin produced by *Corynebacterium diphtheriae* that is primarily responsible for the pathogenesis of diphtheritic infection; it is an enzyme that inactivates transferase II of the mammalian protein-synthesizing system. **diphtheria t., diagnostic** [USP], a sterile solution of the toxic products of *Corynebacterium diphtheriae*; used as a dermal reactivity indicator (Schick test). **diphtheria t., inactivated diagnostic**

[USP], a portion of a manufacturer's lot of diphtheria toxin, inactivated by heat, used simultaneously with the diagnostic toxin of the same lot as a control. **diptheria t. for Schick test** [USP], a sterile solution of the diluted, standardized toxic products of *Corynebacterium diptheriae;* used as a dermal reactivity indicator. Called also *diagnostic diphtheria t.* See also *Schick test,* under *tests.* **dysentery t.,** a toxin produced by various species of *Shigella.* That formed by *Shigella dysenteriae* type I (Shiga toxin) is a soluble protein. The toxins produced by other dysentery bacilli are endotoxins, immunologically distinct between species but with a closely similar pharmacological action. **erysipelas t.,** a toxin obtained from cultures of *Streptococcus pyogenes,* the causative agent of erysipelas, which was once used in treatment of malignant growths. **erythrogenic t.,** an exotoxin produced by many, but not all, strains of *Streptococcus pyogenes,* which produces a erythematous reaction on intradermal inoculation in man and to a lesser extent in the rabbit, and is responsible for the scarlatiniform rash of scarlet fever. **extracellular t.,** a toxin excreted by a bacterial cell; an exotoxin. **fatigue t.,** a toxin formed in the body as a result of muscular effort; a kenotoxin. **fugu t.,** tetrodotoxin. **fusarial t.,** any mycotoxin produced by molds of the genus *Fusarium.* **gonococcal t.,** an endotoxin present in the gonococcus, which is extractable in dilute alkali. **intracellular t.,** a toxin developed and retained within the bacterial cell; an endotoxin. **meningococcal t.,** an endotoxin present in the meningococcus, which is extractable in dilute alkali. **necrotizing t.,** dermonecrotic t. **plant t.,** one produced by a plant; a phytotoxin. **Prigge's t.,** a hemolytic, lethal, oxygen-labile, and thermolabile toxin from *Clostridium perfringens,* which probably produces necrosis in high concentrations. **scarlatinal t.,** erythrogenic t. **Shiga t.,** the exotoxin formed by *Shigella dysenteriae* type 1. **soluble t.,** exotoxin. **staphylococcal t.,** a mixture of exotoxins formed by coagulase-positive *Staphylococcus pyogenes* var. *aureus,* including two or more hemotoxins (α, β, and δ hemolysins) having leukocidin activity (α staphylolysin) and dermonecrotic activity (δ staphylolysin), staphylocoagulase, staphylokinase, and enterotoxin. **streptococcal t.,** a mixture of exotoxins formed by *Streptococcus pyogenes,* including the hemotoxins (streptolysin O and streptolysin S), streptokinase, hyaluronidase, and erythrogenic toxin. **tetanus t.,** the potent exotoxin produced by *Clostridium tetani,* consisting of two components, one a neurotoxin (*tetanospasmin*) and the other a hemolysin (*tetanolysin*). **true t.,** exotoxin.

toxin-antitoxin (tok″sin-an′tĭ-tok″sin)   a nearly neutral mixture of diphtheria toxin with its antitoxin. Such a mixture is used for immunization against diphtheria, the mixture being in such proportion that the diphtheria toxin has 85 per cent of its toxicity neutralized by the antitoxin. Called also *T. A. T.* and *T.-A. mixture.*

toxinemia (tok″sĭ-ne′me-ah) [*toxin* + Gr. *haima* blood + *-ia*] poisoning of the blood.

toxinology (tok″sin-ol′o-je)   the science dealing with the toxins produced by certain higher plants and animals and by pathogenic bacteria.

toxinosis (tok″sĭ-no′sis)   any disease condition due to the presence of a toxin.

toxinum (tok-si′num) [L.]   toxin.

toxipathy (tok-sip′ah-the)   toxicosis.

toxiphobia (tok″sĭ-fo′be-ah)   toxicophobia.

toxiphrenia (tok″sĭ-fre′ne-ah) [*toxin* + Gr. *phrēn* mind]   schizophrenia occurring with a toxic, delirious state.

toxiresin (tok″sĭ-rez′in)   a poisonous resinous substance obtainable from digitoxin.

toxisterol (tok-sis′ter-ol) [*toxin* + *sterol*]   a poisonous isomer of ergosterol, produced by ultraviolet radiation of the latter.

toxitabellae (tok″sĭ-tah-bel′e)   poison tablets.

toxo- [Gr. *toxikon;* L. *toxinum*]   a combining form denoting relationship to a toxin, or poison.

Toxocara (tok″so-ka′rah)   a genus of nematode worms of the superfamily Ascaridoidea. **T. ca′nis,** a nematode worm parasitic in the intestine of dogs; migrating larvae may cause lesions of the lung, liver, kidney, brain, and eye. In human infections, the larvae do not complete their cycle but cause visceral larva migrans (see under *larva*). **T. ca′ti,** a species closely related to *T. canis* but commonly found in cats; it has also been reported from man, both as an accidental intestinal parasite and as causing visceral larva migrans (see under *larva*). Called also *T. mystax.* **T. mys′tax,** *T. cati.*

toxocaral (tok″so-kār′al)   pertaining to or caused by *Toxocara.*

toxocariasis (tok″so-kār-i′ah-sis)   infection by roundworms of the genus *Toxocara.* **human t.,** visceral larva migrans (see under *larva*).

toxogen (tok′so-jen)   something that produces a poison.

toxogenin (toks-oj′e-nin) [*toxo-* + Gr. *gennan* to produce]   a substance supposed to develop in the blood under the influence of the action of an injected antigen, which, though itself inactive, on the injection of more antigen produces anaphylaxis.

toxoglobulin (tok″so-glob′u-lin)   a poisonous globulin.

toxoid (tok′soid) [*toxo-* + Gr. *eidos* form]   a modified bacterial exotoxin that has lost toxicity but retains the properties of

combining with, or stimulating the formation of, antitoxin. **adsorbed t.,** a bacterial toxoid adsorbed on aluminum hydroxide or aluminum phosphate, slowing its absorption in the body and providing a prolonged antigenic stimulus. **alum t.,** alum precipitated t. **alum precipitated t., (A.P.T.),** formol toxoid precipitated with potassium alum as an adjuvant and used as an active immunizing agent. **diphtheria t.** [USP], a sterile solution of formaldehyde-treated products of the growth of *Corynebacterium diphtheriae,* used as an active immunizing agent; called also *diphtheria vaccine, diphtheria anatoxin,* and *diphtherotoxin.* **diphtheria t. adsorbed** [USP], a sterile suspension of diphtheria toxoid precipitated or adsorbed by the addition of alum, aluminum hydroxide, or aluminum phosphate to a formaldehyde-treated solution of the products of growth of *Corynebacterium diphtheriae;* used as an active immunizing agent. **diphtheria and tetanus t's** [USP], a sterile solution prepared by mixing suitable quantities of fluid diphtheria toxoid and fluid tetanus toxoid. The potency and the proportions of the toxoids are such as to provide an active immunizing dose of each toxoid in the total dosage prescribed on the label. **diphtheria and tetanus t's adsorbed** [USP], a sterile suspension prepared by mixing suitable quantities of adsorbed diphtheria toxoid and adsorbed tetanus toxoid, each having been precipitated or adsorbed by the same precipitating or adsorbing agent (alum, aluminum hydroxide, or aluminum phosphate). The potency and the proportions of the toxoids are such as to provide an active immunizing dose of each toxoid in the total dosage prescribed on the label. **diphtheria and tetanus t's and pertussis vaccine** [NF], a sterile suspension of killed *Bordetella pertussis,* or a fraction of this organism, in a mixture of diphtheria toxoid and tetanus toxoid, the components being combined in such proportion as to yield a mixture that meets the antigenic and other requirements of each separate component; used as an immunizing agent, administered subcutaneously or intramuscularly. **diphtheria and tetanus t's and pertussis vaccine adsorbed** [USP], a sterile suspension of the precipitate obtained by treating a mixture of diphtheria and tetanus toxoids and pertussis vaccine with alum, aluminum hydroxide, or aluminum phosphate, the components being combined in such proportion as to yield a mixture containing an immunizing dose of each in the total dosage prescribed in the labeling; used as an active immunizing agent, administered intramuscularly. **fluid t.,** plain formol toxoid used as an active immunizing agent. **formol t.,** toxoid formed by the prolonged action of formaldehyde on toxins, usually bacterial exotoxins; called also *anatoxin.* **precipitated t.,** a toxoid which has been precipitated, usually by potassium alum, creating an insoluble precipitate which is more slowly absorbed in the body, providing a prolonged antigenic stimulus. **tetanus t.** [USP], a sterile solution of formaldehyde-treated products of the growth of *Clostridium tetani,* used as an active immunizing agent. **tetanus t. adsorbed** [USP], a sterile suspension of tetanus toxoid precipitated or adsorbed by the addition of alum, aluminum hydroxide, or aluminum phosphate to a formaldehyde-treated solution of the products of growth of *Clostridium tetani;* used as an active immunizing agent. **tetanus and diphtheria t's adsorbed** [USP], a sterile suspension of adsorbed tetanus toxoid and adsorbed diphtheria toxoid prepared by mixture in such proportions that each dose contains a specified quantity of tetanus toxoid and a specified smaller quantity of diphtheria toxoid; used as an active immunizing agent.

toxoid-antitoxoid (tok″soid-an′tĭ-tok″soid)   a toxoid mixed with an equivalent amount of antitoxic serum, the precipitate being suspended in saline.

toxolecithid (tok″so-les′ĭ-thid)   toxolecithin.

toxolecithin (tok″so-les′ĭ-thin)   a lecithin compounded with a toxin, as cobra venom.

toxolysin (toks-ol′ĭ-sin)   antitoxin.

toxonosis (tok″so-no′sis)   toxicosis.

toxopexic (tok″so-peks′ik) [*toxo-* + Gr. *pēxis* fixation]   toxicopectic.

toxophilic (tok″so-fil′ik) [*toxo-* + Gr. *philein* to love]   easily susceptible to a poison; having an affinity for toxins (like certain haptophore groups).

toxophilous (toks-of′ĭ-lus)   toxophilic.

toxophore (tok′so-fōr) [*toxo-* + Gr. *phoros* bearing]   the group of atoms in the molecule of a toxin which brings about its specific activity after the molecule has been properly anchored by the haptophore. See *Ehrlich's side-chain theory,* under *theory.*

toxophorous (tok-sof′o-rus)   carrying the toxin; see *toxophore.*

toxophylaxin (tok″so-fi-lak′sin)   any phylaxin which destroys or counteracts the poisons produced by bacteria.

Toxoplasma (toks″o-plaz′mah) [*toxo-* + Gr. *plasma* anything formed or molded]   a genus of sporozoa that are intracellular parasites of many organs and tissues of birds and mammals, including man. See *toxoplasmosis.* The only known complete hosts are cats and other Felidae, in which both asexual and sexual developmental cycles occur in the intestinal epithelium, culminating in the passage of oocysts in the feces. The intestinal stages do not occur in other hosts. **T. cunic′uli,** *T. gondii.* **T. gon′-**

dii, the etiologic agent of toxoplasmosis (q.v.); it also infects cats, swine, dogs, sheep, cattle, and rabbits.

toxoplasmin (tok″so-plas′min) an antigen prepared from mouse peritoneal fluids rich with *Toxoplasma gondii;* injected intracutaneously as a test for toxoplasmosis.

toxoplasmosis (tok″so-plaz-mo′sis) a protozoan disease of man caused by *Toxoplasma gondii. Congenital toxoplasmosis* is characterized by lesions of the central nervous system, which may lead to blindness, brain defects, and death. The acquired form is of two types: *lymphadenopathic toxoplasmosis,* which closely resembles mononucleosis, and *disseminated toxoplasmosis,* in which lesions involve chiefly the lungs, liver, heart, skin, muscle, brain, and meninges and which is characterized by pneumonitis, hepatitis, myocarditis, and meningoencephalitis in varying degrees. Chorioretinitis invariably accompanies the congenital form, and may occur in the acquired form.

toxoprotein (tok″so-pro′te-in) a toxic protein or a mixture of a toxin and a protein.

Toxothrix (tok′so-thriks) [Gr. *toxon* a bow + *thrix* hair] a genus of microorganisms of the family Chlamydobacteriaceae, order Chlamydobacteriales, made up of colorless, filamentous, cylindrical cells with a sheath originally thin but later thickened with impregnated iron oxide. It includes two species, *T. gelatino′sa,* and *T. trichog′enes.*

toxuria (toks-u′re-ah) uremia.

Toynbee's corpuscles, experiment, law, ligament, otoscope (toin′bēz) [Joseph *Toynbee,* English otologist, 1815–1866] see under *experiment, law,* and *otoscope,* see *corneal corpuscles,* under *corpuscle,* and see *musculus tensor tympani.*

TPN 1. total parenteral nutrition; see *parenteral hyperalimentation,* under *hyperalimentation.* 2. triphosphopyridine nucleotide; the former name for *nicotinamide-adenine dinucleotide phosphate.*

TPNH reduced triphosphopyridine nucleotide, the former name for the reduced form of nicotinamide-adenine dinucleotide phosphate.

T.R. tuberculin residue; see New tuberculin, under *tuberculin.*

trabecula (trah-bek′u-lah), pl. *trabec′ulae* [L., dim. of *trabs*] a little beam; [NA] a general term for a supporting or anchoring strand of connective tissue, as such a strand extending from a capsule into the substance of the enclosed organ. **arachnoid trabeculae,** delicate fibrous threads connecting the inner surface of the arachnoid to the pia mater. **trabeculae of bone,** anastomosing bony spicules in cancellous bone which form a meshwork of intercommunicating spaces that are filled with bone marrow. **trabec′ulae car′neae cor′dis** [NA], muscular ridges covering a great part of the interior of the walls of the ventricles of the heart; they may stand out in relief only, or be attached as bundles at both ends and free in the middle. **trabec′ulae cor′dis,** trabeculae carneae cordis. **trabeculae of corpora cavernosa of penis, trabec′ulae cor′porum cavernoso′rum pe′nis** [NA], numerous bands and cords of fibromuscular tissue traversing the interior of the corpora cavernosa of the penis, attached to the tunica albuginea and to the septum and creating the cavernous spaces that become filled with blood during erection. **trabeculae of corpus spongiosum of penis, trabec′ulae cor′poris spongio′si pe′nis** [NA], numerous bands and cords of fibromuscular tissue traversing the interior of the corpus spongiosum of the penis, creating the cavernous spaces that give the structure its spongy character. **trabec′ulae cra′nii,** a pair of longitudinal cranial bars of cartilage in the embryo, bounding the pituitary space that becomes the sella turcica. **fleshy trabeculae of heart,** trabeculae carneae cordis. **trabec′ulae lie′nis** [NA], trabeculae of spleen: fibrous bands that pass into the spleen from the tunica fibrosa and form the supporting framework of the organ. **Rathke's trabeculae,** trabeculae cranii. **septomarginal t., t. septomargina′lis** [NA], a bundle of muscle at the apical end of the right ventricle of the heart, connecting the base of the anterior papillary muscle to the interventricular septum; it usually contains a branch of the atrioventricular bundle. **trabeculae of spleen,** trabeculae lienis.

trabeculae (trah-bek′u-le) [L.] plural of *trabecula.*

trabecular (trah-bek′u-lar) pertaining to a trabecula.

trabecularism (trah-bek′u-lar-izm) the condition of having a trabecular structure.

trabeculate (trah-bek′u-lāt) [L. *trabecula* a small beam or bar] marked with cross bars or trabeculae.

trabeculation (trah-bek″u-la′shun) the formation of trabeculae in a part.

trabes (tra-bez) [L.] plural of *trabs.*

trabs (trabs), pl. *tra′bes* [L. "a beam"] a supporting or anchoring strand or structure. **tra′bes car′neae,** trabeculae carneae cordis.

tracer (trās′er) 1. a dissecting instrument for isolating vessels and nerves. 2. a mechanical device by which the outline of an object or the direction and extent of movement of a part may be graphically recorded; see also *tracing.* 3. a means or agent by which certain substances or structures can be identified or

followed, as a radioactive tracer. **needle-point t.,** a mechanical device used in recording jaw movements, in which the tracing is made on a horizontal plate by a weighted or a spring-loaded needle attached to the jaw. **radioactive t.,** a radioactive isotope replacing a stable chemical element in a compound introduced into the body, enabling the course of its metabolism, distribution, and elimination from the body to be traced by a Geiger-Müller counter or other type of counting instrument. **stylus t.,** a mechanical device used in recording jaw movements in which the element producing the tracing is a pointed instrument or stylus; see *needle-point t.*

trachea (tra′ke-ah) [L.; Gr. *tracheia artēria*] [NA] the cartilaginous and membranous tube descending from the larynx and branching into the right and left main bronchi. It is kept patent by a series of about twenty transverse horseshoe-shaped cartilages. **scabbard t.,** a trachea which is flattened by approximation of its lateral walls.

tracheaectasy (tra″ke-ah-ek′tah-se) dilatation of the trachea.

tracheal (tra′ke-al) [L. *trachealis*] pertaining to the trachea.

trachealgia (tra″ke-al′je-ah) [*trachea* + Gr. *algos* pain + *-ia*] pain in the trachea.

tracheid (tra′ke-id) [Gr. *tracheia* rough, rugged] any of the elongate, tapering conducting and supportive cells of the xylem of plant tissue, having thick, pitted walls without true perforations.

tracheitis (tra″ke-i′tis) inflammation of the trachea.

trachelagra (tra″ke-lag′rah, tra-kel′ah-grah) [Gr. *trachēlos* neck + *agra* seizure] gout in the neck.

trachelectomy (tra″ke-lek′to-me) [Gr. *trachēlos* neck + *ektomē* excision] cervicectomy.

trachelematoma (tra″ke-lem″ah-to′mah) a hematoma situated in the sternocleidomastoid muscle.

trachelism, trachelismus (tra′kĕ-lizm; tra″kĕ-liz′mus) [Gr. *trachēlismos*] spasm of the neck muscles; spasmodic retraction of the head in epilepsy.

trachelitis (tra″kĕ-li′tis) cervicitis.

trachelo- [Gr. *trachēlos* neck] a combining form denoting relationship to the neck or to a necklike structure.

trachelocele (trak′ĕ-lo-sēl) tracheocele.

trachelocyllosis (tra″kĕ-lo-si-lo′sis) [*trachelo-* + Gr. *kyllōsis* crooking] torticollis.

trachelocyrtosis (tra″kĕ-lo-sir-to′sis) [*trachelo-* + Gr. *kyrtos* curved + *-osis*] trachelokyphosis.

trachelocystitis (tra″kĕ-lo-sis-ti′tis) [*trachelo-* + Gr. *kystis* bladder + *-itis*] inflammation of the neck of the bladder.

trachelodynia (tra″kĕ-lo-din′e-ah) [*trachelo-* + Gr. *odynē* pain + *-ia*] pain in the neck.

trachelokyphosis (tra″kĕ-lo-ki-fo′sis) [*trachelo-* + Gr. *kyphōsis* a being hump backed] abnormal curvature of the cervical portion of the spine.

trachelologist (tra″ke-lol′o-jist) one skilled in trachelology.

trachelology (tra″kĕ-lol′o-je) [*trachelo-* + *-logy*] the study of the neck and its diseases and injuries.

trachelomyitis (tra″kĕ-lo-mi-i′tis) [*trachelo-* + Gr. *mys* muscle + *-itis*] inflammation of the muscles of the neck.

trachelopexia (tra″kĕ-lo-pek′se-ah) trachelopexy.

trachelopexy (tra′kĕ-lo-pek″se) [*trachelo-* + Gr. *pēxis* fixation] surgical fixation of the neck of the uterus to some other part.

tracheloplasty (tra′kĕ-lo-plas″te) [*trachelo-* + Gr. *plassein* to mold] the plastic surgery of the uterine neck; surgical repair of defects of the neck of the uterus.

trachelorrhaphy (tra″kĕ-lor′ah-fe) [*trachelo-* + Gr. *rhaphē* suture] suture of the lacerated cervix uteri.

tracheloschisis (tra″kĕ-los′kĭ-sis) [*trachelo-* + Gr. *schisis* fissure] congenital fissure of the neck.

trachelosyringorrhaphy (tra″kĕ-lo-sir″ing-gor′ah-fe) [*trachelo-* + Gr. *syrinx* pipe + *rhaphē* suture] trachelorrhaphy for fistula of the vagina.

trachelotomy (tra″kĕ-lot′o-me) [*trachelo-* + Gr. *tomē* a cutting] the surgical cutting of the uterine neck.

tracheo- a combining form denoting relationship to the trachea.

tracheoaerocele (tra″ke-o-a′er-o-sēl) [*tracheo-* + Gr. *aēr* air + *kēlē* hernia] a tracheal hernia containing air.

tracheobronchial (tra″ke-o-brong′ke-al) pertaining to the trachea and bronchi.

tracheobronchitis (tra″ke-o-brong-ki′tis) inflammation of the trachea and bronchi.

tracheobronchomegaly (tra″ke-o-brong″ko-meg′ah-le) a rare and probably congenital condition characterized by great enlargement of the lumen of the trachea and the larger bronchi.

tracheobronchoscopy (tra″ke-o-brong-kos′ko-pe) inspection of the interior of the trachea and bronchi.

tracheocele (tra′ke-o-sēl″) [*tracheo-* + Gr. *kēlē* hernia] hernial protrusion of the tracheal mucous membrane.

tracheoesophageal (tra″ke-o-e-sof′ah-je-al) pertaining to or communicating with both the trachea and esophagus.

tracheofissure (tra″ke-o-fish′er) the operation of splitting the trachea.

tracheofistulization (tra″ke-o-fis″tu-li-za′shun) 1. percutaneous puncture of the trachea for the introduction of medicinal agents. 2. an operation to create a permanent opening in the trachea communicating with the cervical skin.

tracheogenic (tra″ke-o-jen′ik) originating in the trachea.

tracheolaryngeal (tra″ke-o-lah-rin′je-al) pertaining to the trachea and larynx.

tracheolaryngotomy (tra″ke-o-lar″in-got′o-me) incision of the trachea and larynx.

tracheomalacia (tra″ke-o-mah-la′she-ah) softening of the tracheal cartilages.

tracheopathia (tra″ke-o-path′e-ah) [tracheo- + Gr. pathos disease] disease of the trachea. **t. osteoplas′tica,** a condition marked by the formation of a bony and cartilaginous deposit in the tracheal mucosa.

tracheopathy (tra″ke-op′ah-the) tracheopathia.

tracheopharyngeal (tra″ke-o-fah-rin′je-al) pertaining to the trachea and pharynx.

Tracheophilus cymbius (tra″ke-of′ĭ-lus sim′be-us) a trematode parasitic in the trachea of ducks in Europe and Asia.

tracheophonesis (tra″ke-o-fo-ne′sis) [tracheo- + Gr. phōnēsis sounding] auscultation of the heart at the sternal notch.

tracheophony (tra″ke-of′o-ne) [tracheo- + Gr. phōnē voice] a sound heard in auscultation over the trachea.

tracheophyte (tra′ke-o-fīt″) [tracheo- + Gr. phyton plant] a vascular plant containing both phloem and xylem.

tracheoplasty (tra′ke-o-plas″te) [tracheo- + Gr. plassein to mold] a plastic operation upon the trachea.

tracheopyosis (tra″ke-o-pi-o′sis) [tracheo- + Gr. pyon pus] purulent tracheitis.

tracheorrhagia (tra″ke-o-ra′je-ah) [tracheo- + Gr. rhēgnynai to burst forth] hemorrhage from the trachea.

tracheorrhaphy (tra″ke-or′ah-fe) [tracheo- + Gr. rhaphē suture] repair of an incised or wounded trachea.

tracheoschisis (tra″ke-os′kĭ-sis) [tracheo- + Gr. schisis fissure] fissure of the trachea.

tracheoscopic (tra″ke-o-skop′ik) pertaining to or of the character of tracheoscopy.

tracheoscopy (tra″ke-os′ko-pe) [tracheo- + Gr. skopein to examine] the inspection of the interior of the trachea. **percervical t.,** tracheoscopy through a previously made tracheotomy wound; low tracheoscopy. **peroral t.,** tracheoscopy by means of a tracheoscope passed through the mouth, between the vocal cords, and into the trachea; high tracheoscopy.

tracheostenosis (tra″ke-o-stĕ-no′sis) [tracheo- + Gr. stenōsis narrowing] contraction or narrowing of the trachea.

tracheostoma (tra″ke-os′to-mah) [tracheo- + Gr. stoma mouth] an opening into the trachea through the neck.

tracheostomize (tra″ke-os′to-mīz) to perform tracheostomy upon.

tracheostomy (tra″ke-os′to-me) [tracheo- + Gr. stomoun to furnish with an opening or mouth] the surgical creation of an opening into the trachea through the neck, with the tracheal mucosa being brought into continuity with the skin; also, the opening so created. The term is also used to refer to creation of an opening in the anterior trachea for insertion of a tube to relieve upper airway obstruction and to facilitate ventilation.

tracheotome (tra′ke-o-tōm) an instrument for use in incising the trachea.

tracheotomize (tra″ke-ot′o-mīz) to perform tracheotomy upon.

tracheotomy (tra″ke-ot′o-me) [tracheo- + Gr. tomē a cutting] incision of the trachea. **inferior t.,** incision of the trachea through the neck, below the isthmus of the thyroid. **superior t.,** incision of the trachea through the neck, above the isthmus of the thyroid.

trachitis (trah-ki′tis) tracheitis.

trachoma (trah-ko′mah), pl. trachomata [Gr. trachōma roughness] a chronic infectious disease of the conjunctiva and cornea, producing photophobia, pain, and lacrimation, caused by an organism once thought to be a virus but now classified as a strain of the bacteria Chlamydia trachomatis. Clinically, it can be divided into four stages (MacCallan): (1) mild infection marked by tiny follicles on the eyelid conjunctiva and subepithelial infiltration; (2) enlargement of the follicles and inflammatory changes forming hard red papillae, usually with vascular invasion of the cornea marking the onset of pannus; (3) severe scarring and contraction resulting in symblepharon, entropion, trichiasis, and corneal scarring which may result in blindness; (4) complete arrest with permanent scarring, entropion, and symblepharon. Called also Aret's t., Egyptian, granular, or trachomatous conjunctivitis, Egyptian ophthalmia, and granular lids. **Arlt's t.,** trachoma. **Türck's t.,** chronic catarrhal laryngitis. **t. of vocal bands,** development of nodular swellings on the vocal cords.

trachomata (trah-ko′mah-tah) [Gr.] plural of trachoma.

trachomatous (trah-ko′mah-tus) pertaining to, affected with, or of the nature of trachoma.

Trachybdella bistriata (tra″ke-del′ah bis″tre-ah′tah) a leech found in Brazil which attacks man and other animals.

trachychromatic (tra″ke-kro-mat′ik) [Gr. trachys rough + chrōma color] strongly or deeply staining.

trachyphonia (tra″ke-fo′ne-ah) [Gr. trachys rough + phōnē voice + -ia] roughness of the voice; hoarseness.

tracing (trās′ing) a graphic record produced by copying another, or scribed by an instrument capable of making a visual record of movements. In dentistry, the record of movements of the mandible produced by a tracer; the shape of the tracing depends on the relative location of the marking point and the tracing plate, and the apex of a properly made tracing is considered to indicate the most retruded unstrained position of the mandible in relation to the maxilla (centric jaw relation). In cephalometric roentgenography, the line drawing of structural outlines and landmarks on translucent paper to permit diagnostic assessment. **arrow point t.,** Gothic arch t. **cephalometric t.,** a tracing of the teeth, facial bones, and anthropometric landmarks made directly from a cephalometric radiograph and used to formulate a cephalometric analysis. **extraoral t.,** one made outside the oral cavity. **Gothic arch t.,** a tracing of the movements of the mandible that resembles the shape of an arrowhead, or a Gothic arch. **intraoral t.,** one made within the oral cavity.

track (trak) the path along which something moves, or the mark left by its movement. **fog t.,** the visible trail or track left when an electron or other particle passes through a supersaturated Wilson chamber. It consists of droplets of condensed moisture which can be photographed. **germ t.,** the lineage or continuity of germ cells which can be traced throughout innumerable generations of individuals.

tract (trakt) [L. tractus] a region, principally one of some length; specifically a collection or bundle of nerve fibers having the same origin, function, and termination (tractus [NA]), or a number of organs, arranged in series, subserving a common function. **alimentary t.,** canalis alimentarius. **ascending t.,** any bundle of nerve fibers that conveys impulses toward the brain. **Bekhterev's t.,** tractus tegmentalis centralis. **biliary t.,** the organs, ducts, etc., which participate in the secretion, storage, and delivery of bile into the duodenum. **Bruce's t.,** septomarginal t. **t. of Bruce and Muir,** septomarginal tract. **bulbar t.,** any of the bundles of nerve fibers of the medulla oblongata. **bulbospinal t.,** olivospinal t. **Burdach's t.,** fasciculus cuneatus medullae spinalis. **central t. of auditory nerve,** fibers that pass from the cochlear nuclei to the superior olive, to the lateral lemniscus on the same and the opposite side and then up through the brachium of the inferior colliculus into the medial geniculate body and from there to the cortex of the transverse temporal gyri. **central t. of cranial nerves,** fibers from several cranial nerves which pass upward to the thalamus closely associated with the medial lemniscus. **central t. of thymus,** tractus centralis thymi. **central t. of trigeminal nerve,** a more or less distinct bundle of fibers from the trigeminal nerve which passes upward to the thalamus on the dorsal side of the medial lemniscus. **cerebellar t., direct, of Flechsig,** tractus spinocerebellaris posterior. **cerebellorubral t.,** tractus cerebellorubralis. **cerebellorubrospinal t.,** fibers passing from one dentate nucleus of the cerebellum to the contralateral red nucleus, and thence to the spinal cord. **cerebellospinal t.,** uncinate fasciculus of the cerebellum, from the fastigial nucleus to the cervical cord. **cerebellotegmental t's of bulb,** fastigiobulbar t's. **cerebellothalamic t.,** tractus cerebellothalamicus. **cerebrospinal t., lateral,** former term for tractus pyramidalis lateralis. **comma t. of Schultze,** fasciculus interfascicularis. **conariohypophyseal t.,** a portion of the cavity of the embryonic brain connecting the pineal body and the pituitary gland. **cornucommissural t.,** fibers in the anterior part of the posterior column of the spinal cord, extending through the sacral and lumbar regions. **corticobulbar t.,** corticonuclear t. **corticocerebellar t's,** corticopontile t's. **corticohypothalamic t.,** tractus corticohypothalamicus. **corticonuclear t.,** former term for fibrae corticonucleares. **corticopontile t's, corticopontine t's,** tractus corticopontinus. **corticorubral t.,** fibers passing from the cerebral cortex to the red nucleus. **corticospinal t.,** pyramidal t. **corticospinal t., anterior,** tractus pyramidalis anterior. **corticospinal t., lateral,** tractus pyramidalis lateralis. **corticothalamic t.,** fibers uniting the cerebral cortex with the thalamus. **Deiters' t.,** tractus vestibulospinalis. **descending t.,** any bundle of nerve fibers that conveys impulses from the brain toward the periphery. **digestive t.,** canalis alimentarius. **direct cerebellar t. of Flechsig,** tractus spinocerebellaris posterior. **direct spinocerebellar t.,** tractus spinocerebellaris posterior. **dorsolateral t.,** tractus dorsolateralis. **extracorticospinal t.,** extrapyramidal system. **extrapyramidal t.,** see under system. **fastigiobulbar t's,** bundles of efferent fibers running from the nucleus fastigii to the medulla oblongata. **fiber t's of spinal cord,** distinct bundles in the white substance of the spinal cord, made up of fibers which have the same origin, termination, and function. **Flechsig's t.,** tractus spinocerebellaris posterior. **flow t. of the heart,** see *flow track,* under *F.* **foraminous spiral t.,** tractus spiralis foraminosus. **frontopontile t., frontopontine t.,** tractus frontopontinus. **gastrointestinal t.,** the stomach and intestines in continuity. **geniculocalcarine t.,** radiatio optica. **genitourinary t.,** apparatus urogenitalis. **Goll's t.,** fasciculus gracilis medullae spinalis. **Gowers' t.,** tractus spinocerebellaris anterior. **habenular t's,** a term for the habenulotectal, habenulodiencephalic, and habenulotegmental fibers, and the habenulopeduncular tract. **habenulopeduncular t.,** fasciculus retroflexus. **Helweg's t.,** olivospinal t. **hypothalamicohypophyseal t.,** one of the efferent pathways of the hypothalamus, as that leading from the supraoptic nuclei into the posterior lobe of the hypophysis. **iliopubic t.,** tractus iliopubicus. **iliotibial t.,** tractus iliotibialis. **intermediolateral t.,** columna lateralis medullae spinalis. **internuncial t.,** a fiber tract connecting two nuclei or centers. **intersegmental t., lateral,** see *fasciculi proprii.* **intestinal t.,** the small and large intestines in continuity. **Lissauer's t.,** tractus dorsolateralis. **Löwenthal's t.,** tractus tectospinalis. **Maissiat's t.,** tractus iliotibialis. **mamillopeduncular t.,** a fiber tract from the mamillary body to nuclei in the interpeduncular fossa. **mamillotegmental t.,** a branch from the mamillothalamic tract running caudally in the tegmentum of the mesencephalon. **mamillothalamic t.,** fasciculus mamillothalamicus. **Marchi's t.,** tractus tectospinalis. **marginal t., crossed,** tractus dorsolateralis. **mesencephalic t. of trigeminal nerve,** tractus mesencephalicus nervi trigemini. **t. of Meynert,** fasciculus retroflexus. **Monakow's t.,** tractus rubrospinalis. **motor t.,** any bundle of nerve fibers conveying motor impulses from the central nervous system to a muscle. **occipitopontine t.,** tractus occipitopontinus. **olfactory t.,** tractus olfactorius. **olivocerebellar t.,** tractus olivocerebellaris. **olivospinal t.,** a crossed tract descending from the olivary nucleus to the lower cervical or upper thoracic segments of the spinal cord; called also *bulbospinal t., Helweg's t., triangular t.,* and *Helweg's bundle.* **optic t.,** tractus opticus. **parietopontine t.,** tractus parietopontinus. **peduncular t., transverse,** a small band of fibers which passes from the brachium of the inferior colliculus to the sulcus medialis cruris cerebri. **t. of Philippe-Gombault,** Gombault-Philippe triangle. **predorsal t.** (*obs.*), tractus tectospinalis. **projection t.,** see under *fiber.* **pyramidal t.,** a term applied to two groups of fibers (corticonuclear and corticospinal) arising chiefly in the sensorimotor regions of the cerebral cortex and descending in the internal capsule, cerebral peduncle, and pons to the medulla oblongata, the corticonuclear fibers synapsing with motor nuclei throughout the brain stem. Most of the corticospinal fibers cross in the decussation of the pyramids and descend in the spinal cord as the lateral pyramidal (lateral corticospinal) tract; most of the uncrossed fibers form the anterior pyramidal (anterior corticospinal) tract; both end by synapsing with internuncial and motor neurons. The pyramidal tract is a phylogenetically new tract, most prominent in man, which provides for direct cortical control and initiation of skilled movements, especially those related to speech and involving the hand and fingers. Called also *tractus pyramidalis* [NA], *corticospinal t.,* and *pyramidal system.* **pyramidal t., anterior,** tractus pyramidalis anterior. **pyramidal t., crossed,** tractus pyramidalis lateralis. **pyramidal t., direct,** tractus pyramidalis anterior. **pyramidal t., lateral,** tractus pyramidalis lateralis. **pyramidoanterior t.,** former term for tractus pyramidalis anterior. **pyramidolateral t.,** former term for tractus pyramidalis lateralis. **respiratory t.,** apparatus respiratorius. **reticulospinal t.,** tractus reticulospinalis. **rubroreticular t.,** fibers from the red nucleus to the reticular formation of the pons and medulla oblongata. **rubrospinal t.,** tractus rubrospinalis. **Schultze's t., semilunar t.,** fasciculus interfascicularis. **sensory t.,** any bundle of nerve fibers conveying sensory impulses from a peripheral receptor to the central nervous system. **septomarginal t.,** a bundle of nerve fibers along the dorsal periphery of the posterior funiculus in the thoracic region, and along the septum in the lumbar region. Called also *Bruce's tract* and *tract of Bruce and Muir.* **solitary t. of medulla oblongata,** tractus solitarius medullae oblongatae. **spinal t. of trigeminal nerve,** tractus spinalis nervi trigemini. **spinocerebellar t., anterior,** tractus spinocerebellaris anterior. **spinocerebellar t., direct, spinocerebellar t., dorsal, spinocerebellar t., posterior,** tractus spinocerebellaris posterior. **spinocerebellar t., ventral,** tractus spinocerebellaris anterior. **spinocervicothalamic t.,** a tract ascending uncrossed in the dorsal part of the lateral funiculus to the lateral cervical nucleus, which relays to the thalamus by way of the opposite medial lemniscus. **spino-olivary t.,** an ascending tract of fibers arising from the posterior gray columns of the spinal cord and running to the olivary nucleus. **spinotectal t.,** tractus spinotectalis. **spinothalamic t., anterior,** tractus spinothalamicus anterior. **spinothalamic t., lateral,** tractus spinothalamicus lateralis. **spinothalamic t., ventral,** tractus spinothalamicus anterior. **spiral t., foraminous,** tractus spiralis foramino-

sus. **Spitzka's t., Spitzka-Lissauer t.,** tractus dorsolateralis. **strionigral t.,** a bundle of fibers from the corpus striatum to the substantia nigra. **sulcomarginal t.,** fasciculus sulcomarginalis. **supraopticohypophyseal t.,** tractus supraopticohypophysialis. **tectobulbar t.,** tractus tectobulbaris. **tectocerebellar t.,** a bundle of fibers from the tectum of the mesencephalon to the cerebellum. **tectospinal t.,** tractus tectospinalis. **tegmental t.,** a tract of fibers in the tegmentum, back of the nucleus posterior corporis trapezoidei, believed to connect the latter with the midbrain. **tegmental t., central,** tractus tegmentalis centralis. **tegmentospinal t.,** tractus reticulospinalis. **temporopontile t., temporopontine t.,** tractus temporopontinus. **thalamocortical t.,** fibers passing from the thalamus to the cerebral cortex. **thalamo-occipital t.,** radiatio optica. **thalamo-olivary t.,** a bundle of fibers descending from the thalamus to the olivary nucleus. **triangular t.,** olivospinal t. **triangular t. of Philippe-Gombault,** Gombault-Philippe triangle. **trigeminothalamic t.,** fibers from the trigeminal nerve to the thalamus. **tuberohypophyseal t.,** see *tractus supraopticohypophysialis.* **urinary t.,** the organs and ducts which participate in the secretion and elimination of the urine. **uveal t.,** the vascular tunic of the eye, comprising the choroid, ciliary body, and iris; called also *tunica vasculosa bulbi* [NA]. **vestibulocerebellar t.,** fibers of the pars vestibularis nervi octavi passing to the cortex of the cerebellum. **vestibulospinal t.,** tractus vestibulospinalis. **t. of Vicq d'Azyr,** fasciculus mamillothalamicus.

tractate (trak′tāt) to attract or to tend to come together.

tractellum (trak-tel′um), pl. *tractel′la* [L.] an anterior locomotive flagellum.

traction (trak′shun) [L. *tractio*] the act of drawing or exerting a pulling force, as along the long axis of a structure. **axis t.,** traction along an axis, as of the pelvis in obstetrics. **elastic t.,** traction by an elastic force or by means of an elastic appliance. **external t.,** traction applied by means of a fixed anchorage (as by a metal or plaster skull appliance) outside the oral cavity; used principally in the management of midfacial fractures. **halopelvic t.,** traction applied to the spine by means of two metal hoops, one (the halo) applied to the skull and the other to the pelvis, connected by four extension rods which can be lengthened by turn screws. **intermaxillary t.,** maxillomandibular t. **internal t.,** traction applied by using one of the cranial bones above the point of fracture for anchorage; used in the management of facial fractures. **maxillomandibular t.,** traction applied by means of elastic or wire ligatures and interdental wiring and/or splints. **Russell t.,** traction for the knee joint by means of a cuff applied just below the knee. **skeletal t.,** traction applied directly upon the long bones by means of pins, Kirschner's wire, etc. **skin t.,** traction on a body part maintained by an apparatus affixed by dressings to the body surface. **tongue t.,** 1. a remedial procedure which has been used as a cardiac stimulant. 2. the pulling forward of the tongue to improve the airway.

tractor (trak′tor) [L. "drawer"] an instrument for applying traction. **Perkins' t.** (*obs.*), a metallic appliance formerly drawn across the skin in the attempted cure of various disorders; see *perkinism.* **Syms' t.,** a tube with an inflatable rubber bag at the end; used to bring down a prostate into the perineal incision.

tractoration (trak″to-ra′shun) perkinism.

tractotomy (trak-tot′o-me) the operation of severing or incising a nerve tract. **mesencephalic t.,** surgical division of nerve tracts in the mesencephalon.

tractus (trak′tus), pl. *tractus* [L. "a track," "trail"] a tract: a region, principally one of some length; [NA] a general term, especially for a collection or bundle of nerve fibers having the same origin and termination, and serving the same function. **t. centra′lis thy′mi,** central tract of thymus: the medullary core of the thymus; an irregular fibrous bundle carrying the blood vessels and giving attachment to the lobules of the gland. **t. cerebellorubra′lis** [NA], cerebellorubral tract: fibers arising chiefly in the dentate nucleus of the cerebellum and projecting to the opposite red nucleus via the superior cerebellar peduncle; impulses are then relayed to the reticular formation and spinal cord. **t. cerebellothalam′icus** [NA], cerebellothalamic tract: fibers arising chiefly in the dentate nucleus of the cerebellum and projecting to the ventral lateral nucleus of the opposite thalamus via the superior cerebellar peduncle; impulses are then relayed to the frontal lobe. **t. corticopotham′icus** [NA], corticohypothalamic tract: a diffuse collection of fibers that arise from various parts of the frontal lobe and are distributed directly to the hypothalamus. **t. corticopon′tinus** [NA], corticopontine tract: a collective term for fibers arising in the frontal, temporal, parietal, and occipital lobes, which descend in the internal capsule and cerebral peduncle and are relayed to the opposite cerebellar hemisphere via the middle cerebellar peduncle. Formerly called *fibrae corticopontinae* or *corticopontine fibers.* **t. corticospina′lis ante′rior,** NA alternative for *t. pyramidalis anterior.* **t. corticospina′lis latera′lis,** NA alternative for *t. pyramidalis lateralis.* **t. dorsolatera′lis** [NA], dorsolateral tract: a group of nerve fibers in the lateral funiculus of the spinal cord dorsal to the posterior column, composed in part of primary pain and temperature fibers which enter the spinal cord, travel the distance of a few segments in the dorsolateral tract, and then synapse in the posterior column. Called also *dorsolateral fasciculus* and *Lissauer's marginal zone.* **t. fron-topon'tinus** [NA], frontopontine tract: the group of corticopontine fibers arising in the frontal lobe; see *t. corticopontinus.* **t. iliopu'bicus,** iliopubic tract: a thickened band of tissue that strengthens the lower part of the deep inguinal ring and forms the base of the internal spermatic fascia. **t. iliotibia'lis** [NA], **t. iliotibia'lis [Maissia'ti],** iliotibial tract: a thickened longitudinal band of fascia lata extending from the tensor muscle downward along the lateral side of the thigh to the lateral condyle of the tibia. **t. mesencephal'icus ner'vi trigem'ini** [NA], mesencephalic tract of trigeminal nerve: sensory fibers of the entering trigeminal nerve that continue rostrally along the medial aspect of the superior cerebellar peduncle, their cell bodies being located in the nucleus of the mesencephalic tract, which accompanies it. Called also *radix descendens[mesencephalica] nervi trigemini.* **t. occipitopon'tinus** [NA], occipitopontine tract: the group of corticopontine fibers arising in the occipital lobe; see *t. corticopontinus.* **t. olfacto'rius** [NA], olfactory tract: a narrow triangular band in the olfactory sulcus of the frontal lobe, which arises from the olfactory bulb and extends posteriorly, to end by dividing into medial and lateral olfactory striae, the latter ending in the primary olfactory cortex. **t. olivocerebella'-ris** [NA], olivocerebellar tract: a fiber tract that arises from the olive, crosses to the opposite side to pierce the other olive, and enters the cerebellum through its inferior peduncle; called also *fibrae cerebello-olivares.* **t. op'ticus** [NA], optic tract: the tract arising from the optic chiasma, proceeding backward, around the cerebral peduncle, and dividing into a lateral and a medial root; the roots end in the superior colliculus and lateral geniculate body, respectively. **t. parietopon'tinus** [NA], parietopontine tract: the group of corticopontine fibers arising in the parietal lobe; see *t. corticopontinus.* **t. pyramida'lis** [NA], pyramidal tract. **t. pyramida'lis ante'rior** [NA], anterior pyramidal tract: a group of nerve fibers in the anterior funiculus of the spinal cord, originating in the cerebral cortex; called also *t. corticospinalis anterior* [NA alternative]. See *pyramidal tract,* under *tract.* **t. pyramida'lis latera'lis** [NA], lateral pyramidal tract: a group of nerve fibers in the lateral funiculus of the spinal cord, originating in the cerebral cortex; called also *t. corticospinalis anterior* [NA alternative] and *fasciculus cerebrospinalis lateralis.* See *pyramidal tract,* under *tract.* **t. reticulospina'lis** [NA], reticulospinal tract: a system of fibers arising mostly from the medial parts of the reticular formation of the pons and medulla oblongata; chiefly homolateral, the fibers descend in the anterior and lateral funiculi to most levels of the spinal cord. **t. rubrospina'lis** [NA], rubrospinal tract: a group of nerve fibers in the lateral funiculus of the spinal cord, arising in the large cells of the red nucleus of the mesencephalon. **t. solita'rius medul'lae oblonga'tae** [NA], solitary tract of medulla oblongata: a descending tract in the medulla oblongata, ventrolateral to the caudal part of the fourth ventricle, near the dorsal nucleus of the vagus and glossopharyngeal nerves, and comprising primary visceral afferent fibers from the facial, glossopharyngeal, and vagus nerves. **t. spina'lis ner'vi trigem'ini** [NA], spinal tract of trigeminal nerve: a descending tract of the trigeminal nerve that extends from the level of entrance of the sensory root of the trigeminal nerves into the pons to the upper cervical segments of the spinal cord. Lying lateral to the nucleus of the spinal tract of the trigeminal nerve, in which its fibers synapse, this tract carries mainly pain and temperature impulses from the face. **t. spinocerebella'ris ante'rior** [NA], anterior spinocerebellar tract: a group of nerve fibers in the lateral funiculus of the spinal cord; arising mostly in the opposite gray matter, and activated by skin, muscle, tendon, and joint endings, they ascend to the cerebellum by way of the anterior part of the lateral funiculus and then the superior cerebellar peduncle. Called also *fasciculus anterolateralis superficialis [Gowersi].* **t. spinocerebella'ris poste'rior** [NA], posterior spinocerebellar tract: a group of nerve fibers in the lateral funiculus of the spinal cord; arising chiefly from the nucleus thoracicus and activated by skin, muscle, tendon, and joint endings, they ascend to the cerebellum by way of the dorsal part of the lateral funiculus and then the inferior cerebellar peduncle. Called also *fasciculus cerebellospinalis.* **t. spinotecta'lis** [NA], spinotectal tract: a group of nerve fibers in the lateral funiculus of the spinal cord, mostly crossed from their origin, which ascend to the superior and inferior colliculi, and carrying somatic sensory impulses. **t. spinothalam'icus ante'rior** [NA], anterior spinothalamic tract: a group of nerve fibers in the anterolateral funiculus of the spinal cord, which arise in the opposite gray matter; carrying impulses activated by light touch, they ascend to the thalamus, joining the medial lemniscus in the brain stem. **t. spinothalam'icus latera'lis** [NA], lateral spinothalamic tract: a group of nerve fibers in the lateral funiculus of the spinal cord, which arise in the opposite gray matter; carrying impulses activated by pain and temperature, they ascend to the thalamus, running with the lateral lemniscus in the brain stem. **t. spira'lis foramino'sus** [NA], foraminous spiral tract: a spiral area on the fundus of the internal acoustic meatus, below the

crista transversa and in front of the area vestibularis inferior; it corresponds to the base of the cochlea and is perforated with numerous holes for the passage of branches of the vestibulocochlear nerve. **t. subarcua'tus,** an area of small cell structure under the arch of the superior semicircular canal. **t. supraopticohypophysia'lis** [NA], supraopticohypophyseal tract: fibers arising in the supraoptic and paraventricular nuclei of the hypothalamus and descending to the neurohypophysis, where their neurosecretory material is stored as antidiuretic hormone and oxytocin. A portion of the tract arises in the tuber cinereum (tuberohypophyseal tract). **t. tectobulba'ris,** tectobulbar tract: fibers arising mostly in the superior colliculus; they descend to the lower border of the pons and end in the nuclei of the brain stem and in the reticular formation. **t. tecto-spina'lis** [NA], tectospinal tract: a group of nerve fibers, chiefly crossed, which arise mostly in the superior colliculus and descend to the cervical cord, where they lie in the anterior funiculus. **t. tegmenta'lis centra'lis** [NA], central tegmental tract: a composite nerve tract arising from the midbrain tegmentum, periaqueductal gray matter, and red nucleus; it descends in the tegmentum and reticular formation to end in the inferior olivary complex. The tract includes an ascending component from the reticular formation. Called also *Bekhterev's tract.* **t. temporopon'tinus** [NA], temporopontine tract: the group of corticopontine fibers arising in the temporal lobe; see *t. corticopontinus.* **t. triangula'ris,** olivospinal tract. **t. vestibulospina'lis** [NA], vestibulospinal tract: nerve fibers arising from the lateral vestibular nucleus which descend uncrossed, chiefly in the anterior part of the lateral funiculus, throughout most levels of the spinal cord. Some fibers to the caudal spinal segments lie in the anterior funiculus.

tragacanth (trag'ah-kanth) [NF] the dried gummy exudation from *Astragalus gummifer* or other species of *Astragalus;* used as a suspending agent for drugs. Called also *gum tragacanth.*

tragal (tra'gal) pertaining to the tragus.

tragi (tra'ji) [L., pl. of *tragus*] [NA] hair growing on the pinna of the external ear, especially on the cartilaginous projection anterior to the external opening (tragus).

Tragia (tra'je-ah) a genus of poisonous euphorbiaceous plants; several species (*T. urens,* etc.) are weeds of the southern United States.

tragion (traj'e-on) the anthropometric landmark located at the superior margin of the tragus of the ear.

tragomaschalia (trag"o-mas-kal'e-ah) [Gr. *tragos* goat + *maschalē* the armpit] odorous perspiration from the axilla.

tragophonia (trag"o-fo'ne-ah) egophony.

tragophony (trah-gof'o-ne) [Gr. *tragos* goat + *phōne* voice] egophony.

tragopodia (trag"o-po'de-ah) [Gr. *tragos* goat + *pous* foot] genu valgum.

tragus (tra'gus), pl. *tra'gi* [L.; Gr. *tragos* goat] [NA] the cartilaginous projection anterior to the external opening of the ear; see also *tragi.*

train (trān) 1. to prepare by instruction and practice for some definite occupation or pursuit. 2. a continuous succession of objects or of events, as of discharges of electric or magnetic energy.

trainable (tra'nah-b'l) capable of being trained; the term is used with special reference to persons with moderate mental retardation (I.Q. approximately 36–51) who are capable of achieving self-care, social adjustment at home, and economic usefulness under close supervision. Cf. *educable.*

training (trān'ing) a system of instruction or teaching; preparation by instruction and practice. **assertive t.,** a form of behavior therapy in which individuals are taught appropriate interpersonal responses, involving expression of their feelings, both negative and positive. Called also *expressive t.* **expressive t.,** assertive t.

trait (trāt) 1. any genetically determined characteristic; commonly used in medicine to designate the condition prevailing in the heterozygous state of a recessive disorder, as in sickle cell anemia. 2. a distinctive behavior pattern. **secretor t.,** the ability to secrete ABH antigens of the ABO blood group in the saliva, inherited in simple mendelian manner. **sickle cell t.,** the condition, usually asymptomatic, caused by heterozygosity for hemoglobin S.

trajector (trah-jek'tor) an instrument for locating a bullet in a wound.

Tral (tral) trademark for preparations of hexocyclium methylsulfate.

Trallianus, Alexander see *Alexander of Tralles.*

tralonide (tra'lo-nīd) chemical name: 9,11β-dichloro-6α,21-difluoro-16α,17-[(1-methylethylidene)bis(oxy)]pregna-1,4-diene-3,-20-dione; a glucocorticoid, $C_{24}H_{28}Cl_2F_2O_4$.

tramadol hydrochloride (trah'mah-dōl) chemical name: (±)-*trans*-2-[(dimethylamino)-methyl]-1-(*m*-methoxyphenyl)cyclohexanol hydrochloride; an analgesic, $C_{16}H_{25}NO_2 \cdot HCl$.

tramazoline hydrochloride (trah-maz'o-lēn) chemical name: 4,5-dihydro-*N*-(5,6,7,8-tetrahydro-1-naphthalenyl)-1*H*-imidazol-2-amine monohydrochloride; an adrenergic, $C_{13}H_{17}N_3 \cdot HCl$, with nasal decongestant properties.

Trambusti's reaction (test) (tram-boos′tēz) [Arnaldo *Trambusti*, Italian pathologist, born 1863]   see under *reaction*.

tramitis (tram-i′tis) [L. *trama* woof + *-itis*]   a condition of the pulmonary tissue in early tuberculosis seen in the roentgenogram as pleural adhesions, deviated mediastinum, sclerosed bands, calcified nodes, and areas of increased density.

trance (trans)   a profound or abnormal sleep, from which the patient cannot be aroused easily, and not due to organic disease. Voluntary movement is lost, though sensibility and consciousness may remain. It is usually due to hysteria, and may be induced by hypnotism.   **alcoholic t.,** a condition of automatism (dissociation of consciousness with complete forgetfulness) resulting from alcoholic indulgence.   **death t.,** that in which the patient appears to be dead.   **hypnotic t.,** an artificially induced trance.   **hysterical t.,** trance occurring as a symptom of hysteria.   **induced t.,** that which is mainly due to hysteria, but may be caused by hypnotism.

Trancopal (tran′ko-pal)   trademark for a preparation of chlormezanone.

tranquilizer (tran″kwĭ-līz′er) [L. *tranquillus* quiet, calm + *-ize* verb ending meaning to make + *-er* agent]   a large class of drugs used in the treatment of anxiety states, neuroses, and mental disorders. They are of two types; *major tranquilizers* (called also *antipsychotics* and *neuroleptics*) are used primarily for the treatment of psychoses and include the phenothiazines, thioxanthenes, and butyrophenones; *minor tranquilizers* (called also *anxiolytics*) are used primarily for the treatment of neuroses and anxiety states and include the benzodiazepines, certain barbiturates, and other drugs.

trans (tranz) [L., through]   in organic chemistry, having certain atoms or radicals on opposite sides; in genetics, having one of the two mutant genes of a pseudoallele on each homologous chromosome.

trans- [L. *trans* through]   1. a prefix meaning through, across, or beyond.   2. in organic chemistry, denoting the presence of certain atoms or radicals on opposite sides of the molecule. In genetics, having one of the two mutant genes of a pseudoallele on each homologous chromosome. Cf. *cis-*.

transabdominal (trans″ab-dom′ĭ-nal)   through the abdominal wall.

transacetylase (trans-as″ĕ-til-ās)   acetyltransferase.

transacetylation (trans-as″ĕ-til-a′shun)   a chemical reaction involving the transfer of the acetyl group CH_3—$\overset{\text{O}}{\underset{||}{C}}$—. It occurs in many metabolic reactions.

transacylase (trans-as′ĭ-lās)   an enzyme that catalyzes transacylation.

transacylation (trans-as″ĭ-la′shun)   a chemical reaction involving the transfer of the acyl radical between acetic and higher carboxylic acids.

transaldolase (trans-al′do-lās)   an enzyme (a transferase) that catalyzes the transfer of an aldehyde residue from sedoheptulose to form tetrose.

transamidinase (trans-am′ĭ-din-ās)   an enzyme (a transferase) that catalyzes the transfer of amidine, as from arginine to ornithine; called also *amidinotransferase*.

transaminase (trans-am′ĭ-nās)   an enzyme that catalyzes the reversible transfer of an amino group from an α-amino acid to an α-keto acid, usually α-ketoglutaric acid. Pyridoxal-5-phosphate and pyridoxamine phosphate act as coenzymes.   **glutamic-oxaloacetic t. (GOT),** an enzyme normally present in serum (SGOT) and in various body tissues, especially in the heart and liver; it is released into the serum as the result of tissue injury, hence the concentration in the serum may be increased in myocardial infarction or acute damage to hepatic cells.   **glutamic-pyruvic t. (GPT),** an enzyme normally present in serum (SGPT) and body tissues, especially in the liver; it is released into the serum as a result of tissue injury, hence the concentration in the serum may be increased in patients with acute damage to hepatic cells.

transamination (trans″am-i-na′shun)   the reversible transfer of an amino group from an amino acid to what was originally an α-keto acid, forming a new keto acid and a new amino acid, without the appearance of ammonia in the free state.

transanimation (trans-an″ĭ-ma′shun) [*trans-* + L. *anima* breath]   resuscitation by mouth-to-mouth breathing; see *mouth-to-mouth method of artificial respiration*, under *respiration*.

transaortic (trans″a-or′tik)   performed through the aorta; used especially in reference to surgical procedures on the aortic valve, performed through an incision in the wall of the aorta.

transappendageal (trans″ah-pen″dah-je′al)   across an appendage, as absorption across a hair follicle or other skin appendage.

transatrial (trans-a′tre-al)   performed through the atrium; used especially in reference to surgical procedures on a cardiac valve, performed through an incision in the wall of the atrium.

transaudient (trans-aw′de-ent)   permitting passage of the mechanical vibrations perceived as sound.

transaxial (trans-ak′se-al)   directed at right angles to the long axis of the body or a part.

transbasal (trans-ba′sal)   through the base, as a surgical approach through the base of the skull.

transcalent (trans-ka′lent) [*trans-* + L. *calere* to be hot]   permitting the passage of radiant heat.

transcalvarial (trans″kal-vār′e-al)   through or across the calvaria.

transcarbamoylase (trans-kar″bah-moi′lās)   carbamoyl-transferase.

transcarboxylase (trans″kar-bok′sĭ-lās)   carboxyltransferase.

transcatheter (trans-kath′ĕ-ter)   performed through the lumen of a catheter.

transcervical (trans-ser′vĭ-kal)   performed through the cervical opening of the uterus.

transclomiphene (trans-clo′mĭ-fēn)   zuclomiphene.

transcobalamin (trans″ko-bal′ah-min)   a group of proteins (of intestinal cells) that bind to cyanocobalamin (vitamin B_{12}) and transport it to other tissues.

transcondyloid (trans-kon′dĭ-loid)   through the condyles.

transcortical (trans-kor′tĭ-kal)   connecting two different parts of the cerebral cortex; also, dependent on disease of the tracts connecting different parts of the cerebral cortex.

transcortin (trans-kor′tin)   an α-globulin that binds and transports biologically active, unconjugated cortisol in plasma; called also *corticosteroid-binding globulin (CBG)*.

transcricothyroid (trans-kri″ko-thi′roid)   through or across the cricothyroid membrane.

transcriptase (trans-krip′tās)   RNA polymerase; an enzyme that catalyzes the synthesis (polymerization) of RNA from ribonucleoside triphosphates, with DNA serving as a template.   **reverse t.,** RNA-directed DNA polymerase; an enzyme of RNA viruses that catalyzes the transcription of RNA to DNA, which is then incorporated into the genome of the host cell.

transcription (trans-krip′shun)   the process by which genetic information contained in DNA produces a complementary sequence of bases in an RNA chain.

transducer (trans-du′ser)   a device that translates one form of energy to another, e.g., the pressure, temperature, or pulse to an electrical signal.   **neuroendocrine t.,** a neuron having the properties of both nerve and gland, such as a neurohypophyseal neuron, that on stimulation secretes a hormone, thereby translating neural information into hormonal information.

transduction (trans-duk′shun) [L. *transducere* to lead across]   a method of genetic recombination in bacteria, in which DNA from a lyzed bacterium is transferred to another bacterium by bacteriophage, thereby changing the genetic constitution of the second organism.

transdural (trans-du′ral)   through or across the dura mater.

transection (tran-sek′shun) [*trans-* + L. *sectio* a cut]   a section made across a long axis; a cross section; division by cutting transversely.

transepidermal (trans″ep-ĭ-der′mal)   occurring through or across the epidermis.

transepithelial (trans-ep″ĭ-thēl′e-al)   occurring through or across an epithelium.

transfaunation (trans″faw-na′shun)   the transfer of animal parasites from one host organism to another.

transfection (trans-fek′shun)   infection by naked viral nucleic acid.

transfer (trans′fer) [*trans-* + L. *ferre* to carry]   the conveyance of something from one place to another.   **group t.,** a chemical reaction involving the enzyme-induced transfer of a group (e.g., a phosphate group) to a substrate.   **linear energy t.,** see *LET*.   **passive t.,** the conference of immunity to a nonimmune host by injection of antibody or lymphocytes from an immune or sensitized donor.

transferase (trans′fer-ās)   any of a class of enzymes that catalyze the transfer, from one molecule to another, of a chemical group that does not exist in the free state during the transfer. **CoA-t.,** an enzyme that catalyzes the transfer of a CoA group, as from an acetyl group to propionate, oxalate, or malonate.

transference (trans-fer′ens)   1. the passage or conveyance of a symptom or affection from one part to another, a kind of metastasis.   2. in psychiatry, the shifting of an affect from one person to another or from one idea to another, especially the transfer by the patient to the analyst of emotional tones, either of affection or of hostility, based on unconscious identification. If the transfer is favorable it is *positive t.*, if unfavorable *negative t.*   **counter t.,** see *countertransference*.

transferrin (trans-fer′rin) [*trans-* + L. *ferrum* iron + *-in* chemical suffix]   serum β-globulin that binds and transports iron. Several types (e.g., C, B, D, and many others) have been distinguished on the basis of electrophoretic mobility and related as the products of corresponding dominant somatic genes, Tf^C, Tf^B, and Tf^D. Called also *siderophilin*.

transfix (trans'fiks) [*trans-* + L. *figere* to fix]   to pierce through and through.

transfixion (trans-fik'shun)   a cutting through from within outward, as in amputation.

transforation (trans″fo-ra'shun) [*trans-* + L. *forare* to pierce]   the perforation or piercing of the fetal skull.

transforator (trans'fo-ra″tor)   an instrument for making a transforation.

transformation (trans″for-ma'shun) [*trans-* + L. *formatio* formation]   change of form or structure; conversion from one form to another. In oncology, the change that a normal cell undergoes as it becomes malignant. **asbestos t.**, the deposition of extraneous fibers in hyaline cartilage, which gives it a silky, glossy appearance. **bacterial t.**, the process of intercellular transfer of genetic information in which a small portion of the total DNA of a lysed bacterium enters a related bacterium and is incorporated into its genetic constitution. **G-F t.**, globular-fibrous t., the reversible change of actin globules into long filaments, in the process of muscle contraction and relaxation. **lymphocyte t.**, the morphological and biochemical changes (increase in size, abundance of cytoplasm, visibility of nucleoli) in lymphocytes cultured in the presence of an antigen to which they were previously exposed, or in the presence of nonspecific stimulants such as plant mitogens, streptolysins, and anti-lymphocyte serum; these changes result in proliferation and differentiation.

transformiminase (trans″for-mim'ĭ-nās)   an enzyme that catalyzes the transfer of a formimino group, as from glutamate or glycine to tetrahydrofolate.

transfructosylase (trans-fruk″to-sil'ās)   fructosyltransferase.

transfusion (trans-fu'zhun) [L. *transfusio*]   the introduction of whole blood or blood component directly into the blood stream. Cf. *infusion.* **direct t.**, immediate t. **exchange t.**, repetitive withdrawal of small amounts of blood and replacement with donor blood, until a large proportion of the blood volume has been exchanged; used in newborn infants with erythroblastosis and in patients with severe uremia. **exsanguination t.**, exchange t. **fetomaternal t.**, transplacental passage of fetal blood into the circulation of the maternal organism. **immediate t.**, the transfer of blood from one person to another without use of an intermediate container or anticoagulant. **indirect t.**, transfer of blood from a donor to a flask or other container, and then to the recipient. **intraperitoneal t.**, infusion of blood into the peritoneal cavity; see *intrauterine t.* **intrauterine t.**, transfusion of Rh-negative blood into the peritoneal cavity of an unborn infant in the treatment of erythroblastosis fetalis *in utero.* **mediate t.**, indirect t. **placental t.**, return to the newborn, after birth, and through the umbilical vessels, of some of the blood contained in the fetal placenta. **replacement t., substitution t.**, exchange t.

transgenation (trans″jen-a'shun)   mutation.

transglucosylase (trans″glu-ko-sil'ās)   glucosyltransferase. **amylo-1,4 → 1,6-t.**, α-glucan-branching glycosyltransferase.

transglutaminase (tranz″gloo-tam'in-ās)   the activated form of protransglutaminase, which forms stabilizing covalent bonds within fibrin strands; called also *coagulation Factor XIIIa.*

transglycosidation (trans-gli″ko-sĭ-da'shun)   the formation of complex sugars by the transfer of monosaccharide units once glycosidic linkages are formed.

transglycosylase (trans″gli-ko′sil-ās)   glycosyltransferase.

transhexosylase (trans-hek″so-sil'ās)   hexosyltransferase.

transhiatal (trans″hi-a'tal)   across or through a hiatus.

transiliac (trans-il'e-ak)   across or between the two ilia.

transilient (tran-sil'e-ent) [*trans-* + L. *salire* to leap]   leaping or passing across.

transillumination (trans″ĭ-lu″mĭ-na'shun)   the passage of light through body tissues for the purpose of examination, the object or part under examination being interposed between the observer and the light source; diaphanoscopy.

transinsular (trans-in'su-lar)   across the insula; crossing the insula.

transischiac (trans-is'ke-ak)   between the two ischia.

transisthmian (trans-is'me-an)   across an isthmus, especially the isthmus of the gyrus fornicatus.

transistor (trans-is'tor)   a small wafer of semiconducting material having three electrodes, called the emitter, base, and collector, which perform functions similar to those of the cathode, grid, and plate of a vacuum tube.

transketolase (trans-ke'to-lās)   an enzyme that catalyzes the transfer of a ketonic residue to form a pentose.

translateral (trans-lat'er-al)   from side to side; in roentgenography, referring to the view obtained with the patient supine and the radiation directed horizontally.

translation (trans-la'shun) [*trans-* + L. *latus* borne]   a removal or change of place; in genetics, the formation of a polypeptide chain in the specific amino acid sequence directed by the genetic information carried by messenger RNA. See also *transcription.*

translocation (trans″lo-ka'shun) [*trans-* + L. *locus* place]   re-

moval to another place. In genetics, the shifting of a segment or fragment of one chromosome into another part of a homologous chromosome, or into a nonhomologous chromosome. Translocation between a chromosome of the D group and chromosome 21 sometimes results in Down's syndrome. Called also *interchange.* **balanced t.**, translocation which results in no more or no less than the normal diploid or haploid genetic material. **reciprocal t.**, the mutual exchange of fragments between two broken chromosomes, one part of one uniting with part of the other. **robertsonian t.**, that in which the breaks occur at the centromeres and entire chromosome arms are exchanged, usually involving two acrocentric chromosomes.

translucent (trans-lu'sent) [*trans-* + L. *lucens* shining]   transmitting light, but diffusing it so that objects beyond are not clearly distinguished.

transmethylase (trans-meth'ĭ-lās)   methyltransferase.

transmethylation (trans″meth-ĭ-la'shun)   the transfer of a methyl group (CH_3—) from the molecules of one compound to those of another.

transmigration (trans″mi-gra'shun) [*trans-* + L. *migratio* migration]   1. a wandering, especially a change of place from one side of the body to the other. 2. diapedesis. **external t.**, the passage of an ovum from one ovary to the uterine tube of the other side without going through its own oviduct. **internal t.**, the passage of an ovum from one oviduct to the other by way of the uterus.

transmissible (trans-mis'ĭ-b'l)   capable of being transmitted from one individual or one species to another.

transmission (trans-mish'un) [*trans-* + L. *missio* a sending]   a transfer, as of a disease or neural impulse; the communication of inheritable qualities to offspring. **duplex t.**, the transmission of neural impulses in two directions along a nerve. **ephaptic t.**, the conduction of a nerve impulse across an ephapse, as opposed to synaptic transmission. **horizontal t.**, the spread of an infectious agent from one individual to another, usually through contact with excreta, e.g., sputum, etc., containing the agent; cf. *vertical t.* **synaptic t.**, the transmission of a neural impulse across a synapse. **vertical t.**, transmission from one generation to another. The term is restricted by some to genetic transmission and extended by others to include also transmission of infection from one generation to the next, as by milk or through the placenta. Cf. *horizontal h.*

transmitter (trans-mit'er)   something that transmits; see also under *substance;* see also *neurotransmitter.*

transmural (trans-mu'ral) [*trans-* + L. *muralis,* from *murus* wall]   through the wall of an organ; extending through or affecting the entire thickness of the wall of an organ or cavity.

transmutation (trans″mu-ta'shun)   1. evolutionary change of one species into another. 2. the change of one chemical element into another; nucleonics, the changing of an atomic nucleus to one of a different atomic number by nuclear bombardment, causing rearrangement of the protons and neutrons.

transocular (trans-ok'u-lar) [*trans-* + L. *oculus* eye]   across the eye.

transonance (tran'so-nans) [*trans-* + L. *sonans* sounding]   transmission of a sound originating in one organ through the substance of another organ.

transorbital (trans-or'bĭ-tal)   performed through the bony socket of the eye.

transovarial (trans″o-va're-al)   through the ovary; referring to transmission of pathogens from the maternal organism, by invasion of the ovary and infection of eggs, to individuals of the next generation, as may occur in infections of arthropods, especially mites and ticks.

transovarian (trans″o-va're-an)   transovarial.

transoximinase (trans″oks-im'ĭ-nās)   oximinotransferase.

transpalatal (trans-pal'ah-tal)   performed through the roof of the mouth, or palate.

transparent (trans-par'ent) [*trans-* + L. *parere* to appear]   permitting the passage of rays of light, so that objects may be seen through the substance.

transparietal (trans″pah-ri'ĕ-tal) [*trans-* + L. *paries* wall]   through or across a wall, as through the intact body wall.

transpentosylase (trans-pen″to-sil'ās)   pentosyltransferase.

transpeptidase (trans-pep'tĭ-dās)   an enzyme that catalyzes the transfer of an amino group or a peptide group from one molecule to another.

transperitoneal (trans″per-ĭ-to-ne'al)   through or across the peritoneum.

transphosphorylase (trans″fos-for'ĭ-lās)   an enzyme that catalyzes the transfer of a phosphate group; see *kinase* (def. 1).

transphosphorylation (trans-fos″for-ĭ-la'shun)   the exchange of phosphate groups between organic phosphates, without their going through the stage of inorganic phosphate.

transpiration (tran″spĭ-ra'shun) [*trans-* + L. *spiratio* exhalation]   the discharge of air, sweat, or vapor through the skin; insensible perspiration. **pulmonary t.**, the exhalation of water vapor from the blood circulating through the lungs.

transplacental (trans″plah-sen′tal) through the placenta.

transplant 1. (trans-plant′) to transfer tissue from one part to another. 2. (trans′plant) an organ or tissue taken from the body for grafting into another area of the same body or into another individual. **Gallie t.,** strips of fascia lata employed as sutures in the repair of hernias.

transplantar (trans-plan′tar) [*trans-* + L. *planta* sole] across the sole.

transplantation (trans″plan-ta′shun) [*trans-* + L. *plantare* to plant] the grafting of tissues taken from the same body or from another. See also entries under *graft*. In dentistry, the insertion, into a prepared dental alveolus, of an autogenous or homologous tooth; it may be a developing tooth germ from the same mouth, or a frozen homologous transplant. **allogeneic t.,** transplantation of tissue between genetically dissimilar animals of the same species. **heterotopic t.,** transplantation of tissue typical of one area to a different recipient site. **homotopic t.,** orthotopic t. **orthotopic t.,** transplantation of tissue typical of one area to an identical recipient site. **syngeneic t.,** transplantation of tissues between animals in the same pure line, e.g., within an inbred strain. **syngenesioplastic t.,** transplantation of tissue from one individual to a related individual of the same species, as from a mother to her child, or from a brother to a sister. **tendon t.,** the operation of inserting the tendon of a sound muscle into the tendon of a paralyzed muscle or into bone.

transpleural (trans-ploor′al) through the pleura; by way of the pleural sac.

transport (trans′port) [L. *transportare* to carry across] the movement of materials in biological systems, particularly into and out of cells and across epithelial layers. **active t.,** the movement of materials across cell membranes and epithelial layers resulting directly from the expenditure of metabolic energy. **bulk t.,** the uptake by or extrusion from a cell of fluid and of particles too large to cross the cell membrane by diffusion or active transport, accomplished by invagination and vacuole formation (uptake) or by evagination (extrusion); it includes endocytosis, phagocytosis, pinocytosis, and exocytosis.

transposition (trans″po-zish′un) [*trans-* + L. *positio* placement] 1. displacement of a viscus to the opposite side. 2. the operation of carrying a tissue flap from one situation to another without severing its connection entirely until it is united at its new location. 3. the exchange of position of two atoms within a molecule. **corrected t. of great vessels,** a developmental cardiac anomaly characterized by transposition of the great vessels with inversion of the ventricles and atrioventricular valves; termed "corrected" because the inverted ventricles compensate for the transposition, producing a mirror-image blood flow in the heart. Called also *mixed levocardia*. **t. of great vessels,** a congenital cardiovascular malformation in which the aorta arises entirely from the right ventricle and the pulmonary artery from the left ventricle, so that the venous return from the peripheral circulation is recirculated by the right ventricle via the aorta to the systemic circulation without being oxygenated in the lungs. Life then depends on a crossflow of blood between blood in the right heart and that in the left heart, as through a ventricular septal defect or a patent duct arteriosus. Cyanosis is the chief symptom. **partial t. of great vessels,** Taussig-Bing syndrome.

transposon (tranz-po′zon) any discrete and characteristic genetic unit (DNA sequence) that may be transferred from one cell to another and be inserted into any of multiple sites in the recipient cell's plasmid- or chromosomal-DNA, with associated rearrangement of the recipient's DNA.

transpubic (trans-pu′bik) performed through the pubic bone after removal of a segment of the bone.

transsacral (trans-sa′kral) through or across the sacrum.

transsection (trans-sek′shun) transection.

transsegmental (trans″seg-men′tal) extending across a segment.

transseptal (trans-sep′tal) through or across a septum.

transsexual (trans-seks′u-al) 1. a person affected by transsexualism. 2. a person whose external anatomy has been changed to that of the opposite sex.

transsexualism (trans-seks′u-ah-lizm) a disturbance of gender identity in which the affected person has overwhelming desire to change anatomic sex stemming from the fixed conviction that he or she is a member of the opposite sex; such persons often seek hormonal and surgical treatment to bring their anatomy into conformity with their belief. Cf. *transvestism*.

transsphenoidal (trans″sfe-noi′dal) performed through the sphenoid bone.

transsternal (trans-ster′nal) through the sternum.

transtemporal (trans-tem′por-al) crossing the temporal lobe.

transthalamic (trans″thah-lam′ik) crossing the thalamus.

transthermia (trans-ther′me-ah) [*trans-* + Gr. *therme* heat] thermopenetration.

transthoracic (trans″tho-ras′ik) performed through the wall of the thorax, or through the thoracic cavity.

transtracheal (trans-tra′ke-al) performed by passage through the wall of the trachea.

transtympanic (trans″tim-pan′ik) across the tympanic membrane or the cavity of the middle ear.

transubstantiation (tran″sub-stan″she-a′shun) [*trans-* + L. *substantia* substance] the substitution of one tissue for another, as in surgical procedures.

transudate (trans″u-dāt) [*trans-* + L. *sudare* to sweat] a fluid substance which has passed through a membrane or been extruded from a tissue, sometimes as a result of inflammation. A transudate, in contrast to an exudate, is characterized by high fluidity and a low content of protein, cells, or of solid materials derived from cells.

transudation (trans″u-da′shun) 1. the passage of serum or other body fluid through a membrane or tissue surface, which may or may not be the result of inflammation. 2. transudate.

transuranium (trans″u-ra′ne-um) beyond uranium; see *transuranic elements*, under *element*.

transureteroureterostomy (trans″u-re″ter-o-u-re″ter-os′to-me) anastomosis of the distal and of the proximal portion of one ureter to the ureter of the opposite side.

transurethral (trans″u-re′thral) performed through the urethra.

transvaginal (trans-vaj′ĭ-nal) performed through the vagina.

transvaterian (trans″vah-te′re-an) through the papilla of Vater.

transvector (trans-vek′tor) an organism that conveys or transmits a poison which is not generated in its own body but is obtained from another source, such as the mussel, *Mytilus*, which serves as a transvector of paralytic shellfish poison derived from the dinoflagellate, *Gonyaulax*.

transventricular (trans″ven-trik′u-lar) performed through the ventricle; used especially in reference to surgical procedures on cardiac valves, performed through an incision in the wall of a ventricle.

transversalis (trans″ver-sa′lis) [*trans-* + L. *vertere, versum* to turn] transverse; [NA] a term designating a structure situated at a right angle to the long axis of the body or of an organ.

transverse (trans-vers′) [L. *transversus*] placed crosswise; situated at right angles to the long axis of a part.

transversectomy (trans″ver-sek′to-me) [*transverse* + Gr. *ektome* excision] surgical removal of the transverse process of a vertebra.

transversion (trans-ver′zhun) displacement of a tooth from its proper numerical position in the jaw.

transversocostal (trans-ver″so-kos′tal) costotransverse.

transversotomy (trans″ver-sot′o-me) [*transverse* + Gr. *tome* a cutting] the operation of cutting the transverse process of a vertebra.

transversourethralis (trans-ver″so-u″re-thra′lis) the transverse fibers of the sphincter urethrae muscle.

transversus (trans-ver′sus) transverse; [NA] a general term designating a position at right angles to a long axis.

transvesical (trans-ves′ĭ-kal) through the bladder.

transvestism (trans-ves′tizm) [*trans-* + L. *vestitus* clothed] a sexual deviation characterized by overwhelming desire to assume the attire, and be accepted as a member, of the opposite sex; called also *cross dressing* and *eonism*. Cf. *transsexualism*.

transvestite (trans-ves′tīt) an individual exhibiting transvestism.

transvestitism (trans-ves′tĭ-tizm) transvestism.

Trantas' dots (trans′tas) [Alexios *Trantas*, Greek ophthalmologist, born 1867] see under *dot*.

Tranxene (tran′zēn) trademark for a preparation of clorazepate dipotassium.

tranylcypromine sulfate (tran″il-si′pro-mēn) [USP] chemical name: (±)-*trans*-2-phenylcyclopropylamine sulfate. A monoamine oxidase inhibitor, $(C_9H_{11}N)_2 \cdot H_2SO_4$, occurring as a white crystalline powder; used as an antidepressant, administered orally.

trapezial (trah-pe′ze-al) pertaining to a trapezium.

trapeziform (trah-pez′ĭ-form) trapezoid.

trapeziometacarpal (trah-pe″ze-o-met″ah-kar′pal) pertaining to or connecting the trapezium and the metacarpus.

trapezium (trah-pe′ze-um) [L.; Gr. *trapezion*] an irregular four-sided figure; see os *trapezium*.

trapezoid (trap′e-zoid) [L. *trapezoides*; Gr. *trapezoeidēs* table shaped] 1. having the shape of a four-sided plane, with two sides parallel and two diverging. 2. the os trapezoideum.

Trapp's formula (coefficient) (traps) [Julius *Trapp*, Russian pharmacist, 1814–1908] see under *formula*.

Trasentine (tras′en-tin) trademark for preparations of adiphenine hydrochloride.

Traube's curves, etc. (trow′bez) [Ludwig *Traube*, German physician, 1818–1876] see under *curve, dyspnea, heart, membrane,* and *space,* and see *gallop rhythm,* under *rhythm.*

Traube-Hering curves, waves (trow′be-her′ing) [Ludwig *Traube*; Ewald *Hering*, physiologist in Leipzig, 1834–1918] see Traube's *curve*, under *curve*, and see under *wave*.

trauma (traw′mah), pl. *traumas* or *trau′mata* [L.; Gr.] a wound or injury, whether physical or psychic. **birth t.**, an injury to the infant received in or due to the process of being born. In some psychiatric theories, the psychic shock produced in an infant by the experience of being born. **occlusal t.**, pathologic changes in a tooth and its surrounding structures produced by abnormal occlusal stresses. **potential t.**, in dentistry, an alteration in tissue that may occur at any time as a result of an existing dental disharmony. **psychic t.**, an emotional shock that makes a lasting impression on the mind, especially upon the subconscious mind.

traumasthenia (traw″mas-the′ne-ah) [*trauma* + *a* neg. + Gr. *sthenos* strength + *-ia*] traumatic neurasthenia.

traumata (traw′mah-tah) [Gr.] plural of *trauma*.

traumatherapy (traw″mah-ther′ah-pe) [*trauma* + Gr. *therapeia* treatment] that branch of surgery which deals with the treatment of wounds and injuries.

traumatic (traw-mat′ik) [Gr. *traumatikos*] pertaining to, occurring as the result of, or causing trauma.

traumatin (traw′mah-tin) a substance which stimulates the growth of plant tissues; it may be identical with wound hormone.

traumatism (traw′mah-tizm) [Gr. *traumatismos*] 1. the physical or psychic state resulting from an injury or wound. 2. a wound.

traumato- (traw′mah-to) [Gr. *trauma, traumatos* wound] a combining form denoting relationship to trauma, or to a wound or injury.

traumatogenic (traw″mah-to-jen′ik) [*traumato-* + Gr. *gennan* to produce] 1. caused by or due to a wound or wounds. 2. capable of causing trauma.

traumatologist (traw″mah-tol′o-jist) a surgeon experienced in treating accidental injuries.

traumatology (traw″mah-tol′o-je) [*traumato-* + *-logy*] the branch of surgery which deals with wounds and disability from injuries.

traumatonesis (traw″mah-to-ne′sis) suture of a wound.

traumatopathy (traw″mah-top′ah-the) [*traumato-* + Gr. *pathos* disease] any pathological condition due to wound or injury.

traumatophilia (traw″mah-to-fil′e-ah) [*traumato-* + Gr. *philein* to love] a condition in which the patient takes a subconscious delight in injuries or surgical operations.

traumatopnea (traw″mah-top-ne′ah) [*traumato-* + Gr. *pnoia* breath] a condition of partial asphyxia with collapse caused by traumatic opening of the pleural space (open pneumothorax).

traumatopyra (traw″mah-to-pi′rah) [*traumato-* + Gr. *pyr* fever] traumatic fever.

traumatosis (traw″mah-to′sis) traumatism.

traumatotherapy (traw″mah-to-ther′ah-pe) treatment of wounds and other injuries.

traumatropism (traw-mat′ro-pizm) [*trauma* + Gr. *tropos* a turning] the growth or movement of organisms in relation to injury.

travail (trav′āl) childbirth; see *labor*.

Travasol (trav′ah-sol) trademark for a crystalline amino acid solution for intravenous administration, containing a mixture of essential and nonessential amino acids but no peptides.

tray (tra) a flat-surfaced utensil for the conveyance of various objects or material. **acrylic resin t.**, an impression tray made of acrylic resin. **impression t.**, in dentistry, a contoured metal or plastic container to hold the material with which an impression of the jaw or teeth is being made.

trazodone hydrochloride (tra′zo-dōn) chemical name: 2-[3-[4-(3-chlorophenyl)-1-piperazinyl]propyl]-1,2,4-triazolo[4,3-*a*]pyridin-3-(2*H*)-one monohydrochloride; an antidepressant, tranquilizer, and hypnotic, $C_{19}H_{22}ClN_5O \cdot HCl$.

TRBF total renal blood flow; see under *flow*.

treacle (tre′k'l) [Gr. *thēriaka*] a syrupy substance or mixture; molasses. **Venice t.**, theriaca andromachi.

tread (tred) injury of the coronet of a horse's hoof, due to striking with the shoe of the opposite side.

treatment (trēt′ment) the management and care of a patient for the purpose of combating disease or disorder. See also under *maneuver, method, technique, tests,* and *therapy.* **active t.**, that which is directed immediately to the cure of a disease or injury. **Albertini's t.**, complete rest and abstinence from food in aneurysm of the aorta. **Allen's t.**, treatment by certain days of fasting, followed by a restricted diet and attended by a careful determination of the quantity of food which the patient can consume without producing glycosuria and glycemia. Called also *starvation t.* **antigen t.**, the production of active immunity by the injection of antigens, including bacteriotherapy, and the use of vaccine and tuberculins. **Ascoli t.**, injection of epinephrine in malaria, with resultant contraction of the spleen which forces its contents, including the malaria parasites, into the circulation, facilitating diagnosis. **autoserous t.**, treatment of an infectious disease by inoculating the patient with his own serum. **Balfour's t.**, treatment of aneurysm by potassium iodide. **Banting's t.**, treatment of obesity by a diet low in carbohydrate, but rich in nitrogenous matters. **Baunscheidt's t.**, baunscheidtism. **Beard's t.**, treatment of cancer by trypsin. **Bell t.**, treatment of cancer by injections of a preparation of colloidal lead. **Bergonié's t.**, the application of general faradization for the reduction of corpulence. **Bier's t.**, see under *hyperemia.* **Bier's combined t.**, treatment of surgical tuberculosis by artifical hyperemia, heliotherapy, and iodides. **Bird's t.**, treatment of decubitus ulcer by mild galvanic currents. **Blanchard's t.**, the plugging of tuberculotic bone cavities with a mixture of white wax and petrolatum. **Bluemel's t.**, a method of treating the morphine habit, with complete withdrawal of morphine, a liquid diet, cathartics, intravenous sodium chloride solution, and chloral to insure sleep the first few nights. **Bouchardat's t.**, treatment of diabetes by use of a diet that excludes substances rich in carbohydrates. **Brandt t.** (obs.), see under *method.* **Brehmer's t.**, treatment of pulmonary tuberculosis by the use of dietetic and physical measures. **Brown-Séquard t.**, organotherapy. **Calot's t.**, treatment of tuberculosis of the spine (Pott's disease) by plaster jackets having an opening over the kyphos on which pressure is made by means of pads. **Cantani's t.**, former method of treating cholera by the repeated injection into the bowel of a large quantity of water containing tannic acid and tincture of opium at a temperature of from 100° to 104° F. **carbon dioxide t.**, see under *therapy.* **Carrel's t., Carrel-Dakin t.**, treatment of wounds, based on thorough exposure of the wound, removal of all foreign material and divitalized tissue, meticulous cleansing, and repeated irrigation with a dilute sodium hypochlorite solution. The adjacent skin is protected with petrolatum gauze. **Castellani's t.**, treatment of elephantiasis by complete rest in bed, bandaging with a flannel or rubber bandage, and daily injections of fibrolysin. **causal t.**, treatment that is directed against the cause of a disease. **Chervin's t.**, a method of treatment for stuttering; called also *Chervin's method.* **choline t.**, treatment of cancer by the intravenous injection of borate of choline in connection with the use of radioactive substances. **Coffey-Humber t.**, treatment of cancer by injection of an extract of adrenal cortex of sheep. **conservative t.**, treatment designed to avoid radical medical therapeutic measures or operative procedures; often reserved for elderly or debilitated patients. **Cox's t.**, treatment of cholera by intravenous isotonic saline. **curative t.**, active treatment designed to cure an existing disease, as opposed to *palliative t.* **Dancel's t.**, treatment of obesity by a diet containing as little water as possible. **Debove's t.**, treatment of tuberculosis by a special form of forced feeding. **denture t.**, a dental prosthesis used for the purpose of treating or conditioning the tissues which are to support and retain a denture base. **dietetic t.**, treatment of disease by regulation of the diet. **drug t.**, treatment with drugs, as distinguished from treatment with physical means, such as diet, exercise, electricity, etc. **Dubois' t.**, see under *method.* **Ebstein's t.**, see under *diet.* **Ehrlich-Hata t.**, see *arsphenamine.* **electroconvulsive t., electroshock t.**, see under *therapy.* **empiric t.**, treatment by means which experience has proved to be beneficial. **Etappen t.**, treatment of bowlegs and knock knee by plaster of Paris bandage and corrective wedging. **eventration t.**, application of ionizing irradiation to internal anatomical tissues through an open laparotomy wound. **expectant t.**, treatment designed only to relieve untoward symptoms, leaving the cure mainly to nature. **fever t.**, pyretotherapy. **Fichera's t.**, treatment of cancer by hypodermic injection of autolyzed human fetal tissue. **Finikoff's t.** (obs.), treatment for bone tuberculosis: iodized peanut oil is injected intramuscularly every five to eight days and 10 per cent calcium solution intravenously three times a week. **Finsen t.** (obs.), treatment of lupus vulgaris by direct application of rays of sunlight or artifical ultraviolet light. **Fitz Gerald t.**, zone therapy. **Fliess' t.**, anesthetization of the nasal conchae for the relief of pain in dysmenorrhea and in nervous stomach pains. **foam t.**, treatment with the foam produced by blowing a current of air through water containing saponin solution. **Fournier's t.**, former method of treating syphilis by administering mercury for two months, then stopping the mercury for a month or more. This is followed by a period of alternate administration and stopping of the mercury. **Fowler-Murphy t.**, Murphy's t., def. 2. **Fränkel's t.**, the use of strophanthin in cardiac failure. **Frenkel's t.**, see under *movement.* **Girard's t.**, treatment of seasickness by hypodermic or oral administration of atropine sulfate and strychnine sulfate. **gland t.**, gonadotherapy. **Goeckerman t.**, treatment of psoriasis by applying ointments of tar followed by irradiation with ultraviolet light. **Guinard's t.**, application of calcium carbide to ulcerating tumors. **Hartel's t.**, alcoholic injection for trigeminal neuralgia in which the needle is passed through the mouth into the region of the foramen ovale of the sphenoid bone. **high-frequency t.**, diathermy. **Högyes' t.**, former method of treating rabies, by the subcutaneous injection of a 1 per cent suspension of rabies virus diluted 1:100 or 1:1000. **hygienic t.**, that directed to the restoration or maintenance of hygienic conditions. **hypo-**

glycemic shock t., insulin coma therapy. **Indoklon t.,** see under *therapy*. **insulin coma t., insulin shock t.,** see under *therapy*. **Jacquet's biokinetic t.,** active gymnastics of the hand and fingers. **Jarotzky's (Jarotsky's) t.,** treatment of gastric ulcer by a diet of whites of eggs, fresh butter with bread, and milk or noodles. **Karell t.,** treatment of heart and kidney disease by keeping the patient in bed and giving only 800 ml. of milk daily for four or five days, the diet then being gradually increased until, on the thirteenth day, the regular diet is resumed. **Keating-Hart's t.,** see under *fulguration*. **Kenny's t.,** treatment of infantile paralysis by wrapping the patient's back and limbs in woolen cloths wrung out of hot water; after pain has subsided passive exercise is given and the patient taught to exercise his muscles by himself. **Killgren t.,** a system of medical gymnastics combined with passive exercise, friction, and vibrations, and laying special emphasis on the mechanical treatment of the nerves. **Kittel's t.,** massage and manipulation for the dispersion of the uratic deposits in gouty joints. **Klapp's creeping t.,** treatment of scoliosis by having the patient creep about on the floor, with exaggerated movements of the spine. **Koga t.,** treatment of thromboangiitis obliterans by diluting the blood by hypodermoclysis with normal salt solution. **Korányi's t.,** former method of treating leukemia by the use of benzol (benzene). **Kromayer's t.,** former method of treating syphilis by the inhalation of very finely divided mercury. **Lambert's t.,** a method of treating opium addiction based on gradual reduction of opium and increasing doses of codeine, which is continued for about a week after the opium is withdrawn. **Lambotte's t.,** a method of extension in fractures of the extremities by means of an extensible steel frame fastened to the bone by steel pegs. **La Porte t.,** treatment of chronic osteomyelitis by application over the infected areas of aluminum potassium nitrate in an oatmeal poultice. **Larat's t.,** treatment of diphtheritic paralysis of the palate by faradism. **Lerich's t.** (*of strains*), infiltration of the periarticular tissues with a 0.5–2 per cent solution of procaine. **light t.,** phototherapy. **McPheeters' t.,** treatment of varicose ulcer by bandaging a rubber sponge over the ulcerated area and directing the patient to walk as much as possible; called *venous heart treatment*. **Maisler's t.,** gaseous dilation, once used in the treatment of gonorrhea. **malarial t.,** malariotherapy. **Matas' t.,** treatment of neuralgia by the injection of alcohol under the nerve ganglions at the base of the skull. **medicinal t.,** that in which the treatment is mainly accomplished by the use of remedies. **Metrazol shock t.,** see under *therapy*. **Minot-Murphy t.,** the treatment of pernicious anemia by the addition to the diet of raw liver or liver extract. **Mitchell t.,** see *Weir Mitchell t.* **Muirhead's t.,** treatment of Addison's disease by epinephrine given to the point of tolerance and the administration of adrenal cortex by mouth. **Murphy's t.,** 1. treatment of pulmonary tuberculosis by injecting nitrogen gas into the pleural cavity in order to cause collapse of the lung and consequent obliteration of cavities. 2. treatment of peritonitis by placing the patient in the Fowler position to favor drainage into the pelvis from the abdomen, and then irrigating the colon with physiologic salt solution administered slowly. **Nägeli's t.,** see under *maneuver*. **Nauheim t.,** Schott's t. **Neuber's t.,** treatment of tuberculosis of bones and joints by excising the carious tissue and filling the cavity with an emulsion of iodoform in glycerin. **Neuendorf t.,** treatment of rheumatoid arthritis by the mud baths of Neuendorf, Germany. **Noorden t.,** oatmeal t. **Nordach t.,** treatment of pulmonary tuberculosis by fresh air, rest, and an abundance of nourishing food. **oatmeal t.,** treatment of diabetes by restricting the protein of the diet and limiting the carbohydrates to oatmeal. **Ochsner t.,** treatment of appendicitis by securing peristaltic rest so that peritoneal adhesions may form; this is achieved by abstention from food by mouth, gastric suction, and an inlying rectal tube to facilitate the escape of gas. **Oertel's t.,** treatment of heart disease, circulatory diseases, obesity, etc., by regulation of diet, diminution of fluid elements in the food, mountain climbing and other systematic exercises, and by massage and Swedish movements. **organ t.,** organotherapy. **Orr t.,** treatment of compound fractures and osteomyelitis by débridement of the wound, alignment of fracture, drainage with petrolatum gauze, and immobilization of limb in a plaster cast which is left on until the wound discharge has softened the plaster. **palliative t.,** treatment which is designed to relieve pain and distress, but which does not attempt a cure. **Paul's t.,** the therapeutic use of lymph for cutaneous therapy of chronic rheumatism. **Petrén's t.,** see under *diet*. **Playfair's t.,** treatment by rest and feeding. **Politzer's t.,** treatment of disease of the middle ear by blowing air into the nostril while the patient goes through the movements of swallowing. **Potter t.,** treatment of intestinal fistulas by administration of tenth normal solution of hydrochloric acid to neutralize the alkalinity of the pancreatic juice, thus preventing tryptic activity. **preventive t., prophylactic t.,** that in which the aim is to prevent the occurrence of the disease; prophylaxis. **Proetz t.,** the instillation of fluid into the paranasal sinuses by means of intermittent negative pressure for the treatment of sinus infection. **rational t.,** treatment based upon a knowledge of disease and the action of the remedies employed. **Retan's t.,** treatment of in-

tussusception by distending the colon with a barium mixture, followed by manipulations. **Ricord's t.,** former method of treating syphilis by administration of mercury for six months, followed by administration of potassium iodide for three months. **Roeder's t.,** removal of pus and debris from an inflamed tonsil by suction. **Rollier t.,** treatment of surgical tuberculosis by systematic exposure of the part to the rays of the sun. **salicyl t.,** treatment of rheumatism with salicylic acid or its derivatives. **sand t.,** treatment with sand baths. **Schede's t.,** see *Schede's operation* (def. 3), under *operation*. **Schlösser's t.,** treatment of facial neuralgia by injections of 80 per cent alcohol (Schlösser's injection) into the foramen from which the nerve emerges. **Schott's t.,** treatment of heart disease by use of warm saline baths of Nauheim and systematically conducted exercise. **Schroth's t.** (*obs.*), treatment of obesity by the exclusion of water in any form as far as possible. **Semple's t.,** the prevention of rabies by injection of Semple vaccine. **sewage t.,** the processing of sewage to remove or so alter some of its constituents as to render it less offensive or dangerous and more fit to discharge into a public water course. **shock t.,** see under *therapy*. **Sippy t.,** a regimen of treatment of peptic ulcer based on neutralization of hydrochloric acid by frequent feedings and the use of alkalies in carefully regulated but adequate quantities. See under *diet*. **slush t.,** the treatment of acne by the application of a mixture of carbon dioxide snow, acetone, and sulfur. **solar t.,** heliotherapy. **specific t.,** treatment that is particularly adapted to the special disease being treated. **starvation t.,** Allen t. **Stoker's t.,** treatment in bronchiectasis by continuous inhalation of oxygen. **string method t.,** treatment of esophageal stricture by passing a string through the mouth and through a gastric fistula, and then, by pulling the string up and down, cutting through the stricture so that a bougie may easily be passed. Called also *Abbe's string method*. **Stroganoff's (Stroganov's) t.** (*obs.*), treatment of puerperal eclampsia by morphine, chloral hydrate, and chloroform, according to a definite scheme. **subcoma insulin t.,** see under *therapy*. **supporting t.,** that which is mainly directed to sustaining the strength of the patient. **surgical t.,** that in which surgical methods are those chiefly employed. **symptomatic t.,** expectant t. **Tallerman t.,** the localized application of superheated dry air in rheumatism, gout, sprains, neuritis, eczema, etc. See also under *apparatus*. **teleradium t.,** treatment by a radium source located at a distance from the body. **terrain t.,** treatment of weak heart, neurasthenia, corpulence, etc., by regular exercise, mountain climbing, regulation of diet, etc. **three-dye t.,** treatment of burns by the application of 6 per cent gentian violet, 1 per cent brilliant green, and 0.1 per cent acriflavin base. **thymus t.,** treatment of progressive muscular atrophy by extracts from the thymus gland. **thyroid t.,** treatment of disease by preparations of the thyroid gland of domestic animals used for food by man. **tonic t.,** 1. treatment with tonics. 2. treatment of syphilis with small doses of mercury continued for a long period. **Trueta t.,** immediate treatment of fractures as follows: (1) adopt surgical treatment as soon as possible; (2) thoroughly wash wound and entire limb with water, soap, and a nail brush, shave hair, paint surrounding skin with weak alcoholic solution of iodine, avoiding the wound; (3) débride wound; (4) open neighboring cellular spaces and remove hematomas; (5) remove completely denuded or displaced bone fragments and all foreign matter; (6) reduce fracture; (7) dress wound with sterile gauze and immobilize with plaster, including two adjacent joints if possible; (8) give injection of tetanus antitoxin. **Tschmarke's t.,** treatment of a cutaneous burn by thorough washing with soap, water, and alcohol under general anesthesia. **Tuffnell's t.,** treatment of aneurysm by absolute rest and starvation diet. **underwater t.,** treatment of poliomyelitis patients by permitting active movements in the water of a bath or pool. **venous heart t.,** McPheeters' t. **Wagner-Jauregg t.,** treatment of dementia paralytica by infection of the patient with malaria. **Weir Mitchell t.,** a method of treating neurasthenia, hysteria, etc., by absolute rest in bed, frequent and abundant feeding, and the systematic use of massage and electricity. **Woodbridge t.,** treatment of typhoid fever with small doses of calomel, podophyllin, and intestinal antiseptics. **Yeo's t.,** treatment of obesity by giving large amounts of hot drinks and withholding carbohydrates.

trebenzomine hydochloride (trĕ-ben′zo-mēn) chemical name: (*cis* or *trans*)-(±)-3,4-dihydro-*N,N,*2-trimethyl-2*H*-1-benzopyran-3-amine hydrochloride; an antidepressant, $C_{12}H_{17}NO \cdot HCl$.

Trechona (trĕ-kon′ah) a genus of spiders (family Dipluridae), which is harmful to man.

tree (tre) 1. a perennial of the plant kingdom characterized by having a main stem or trunk and numerous branches. 2. an anatomical structure with branches resembling a tree. **bronchial t.,** the bronchi and their branching structures. **tracheobronchial t.,** the trachea, bronchi, and their branching structures.

trehala (tre-ha′lah) a mannitol-like substance deposited by an insect (*Larinus maculatus*) upon an Asiatic plant of the genus *Echinops*.

trehalase (tre-ha′lās) an enzyme of the intestinal mucosa that catalyzes the hydrolysis of trehalose to form 2 D-glucose.

trehalose (tre-ha′lōs) a disaccharide, $C_{12}H_{22}O_{11}$, from the cocoons of certain beetles (*Trehala manna*) and yeast; it is not digestible, but yields glucose when hydrolyzed with acids.

Treitz's arch, fossa, hernia, muscle (ligament) (trīts) [Wenzel *Treitz*, Austrian physician, 1819–1872] see under *arch* and *hernia*, see *musculus suspensorius duodeni*, and see *recessus duodenalis superior*.

treloxinate (trĕ-loks′ĭ-nāt) chemical name: methyl 2,10-dichloro-12*H*-dibenzo[*d,g*] [1,3]dioxocin-6-carbolate; an anticholesteremic, $C_{16}H_{12}Cl_2O_4$.

Trematoda (trem″ah-to′dah) [Gr. *trēmatōdēs* pierced] a class of the Platyhelminthes which includes the flukes. The trematodes or flukes are parasitic in man and animals, infection generally resulting from the ingestion of uncooked or insufficiently cooked fish, crustaceans, and vegatation. All flukes require a mollusk as their first intermediate host, in which a complex developmental cycle takes place. The larval stage, which escapes from the mollusk, may then enter a second intermediate host (fish, crustacean, or another mollusk), encyst on vegetation, or penetrate directly into the skin of the definitive host. The important trematodes of man belong to the genera (1) BLOOD: *Schistosoma*. (2) INTESTINE: *Echinostoma, Fasciolopsis, Gastrodiscoides, Heterophyes, Metagonimus*. (3) LIVER: *Clonorchis, Fasciola, Dicrocoelium, Opisthorchis*. (4) LUNG: *Paragonimus*.

trematode (trem′ah-tōd) any parasitic animal organism belonging to the class Trematoda.

trematodiasis (trem″ah-to-di′ah-sis) infection with trematodes.

trembles (trem′b'lz) poisoning in cattle and sheep that feed on the white snakeroot (*Eupatorium rugosum*), in which the animal has muscular tremors and becomes weak and may suddenly stumble and fall. Persons made ill by milk, milk products, or flesh from an animal so affected are said to have milk sickness (q.v.), which may be fatal. A similar condition is caused by *Haplopappus*.

tremelloid, tremellose (trem′ĕ-loid; trem′ĕ-lōs) like jelly.

tremetol (trem′ĕ-tol) chemical name: 2-isopropenyl-2,3-dihydro-5-acetylbenzofuran. A toxin, $C_{13}H_{14}O_2$, in the white snakeroot, *Eupatorium rugosum* (*E. urticaefolium*), which causes trembles in cattle and sheep and milk sickness in man. Called also *tremetone*.

tremetone (trem′ĕ-tōn) tremetol.

Tremin (trem′in) trademark for a preparation of trihexyphenidyl hydrochloride.

tremogram (tre′mo-gram) [*tremor* + Gr. *gramma* mark] the tracing or record made by a tremograph; a graphic tracing of a tremor. See *ataxiameter*.

tremograph (tre′mo-graf) [*tremor* + Gr. *graphein* to write] an instrument for recording tremors.

tremolabile (trem″mo-la′bil) [*tremor* + L. *labilis* unstable] susceptible to shaking; easily inactivated by shaking; said of a ferment.

tremor (trem′or, tre′mor) [L., from *tremere* to shake] an involuntary trembling or quivering. **action t.,** rhythmic, oscillatory, involuntary movements of the outstretched upper limb, as when writing or lifting a cup; it may also affect the voice and other parts. **arsenic t.,** a tremor resulting from arsenic poisoning. **coarse t.,** a tremor in which the vibrations are slow. **continuous t.,** a persistent tremor resembling that of paralysis agitans. **t. cor′dis,** palpitation of the heart. **darkness t.,** involuntary movements of the eyes, resembling nystagmus, which occur in young animals kept in the dark. **epidemic t.,** avian encephalomyelitis. **epileptoid t.,** intermitting clonic spasm with tremor. **essential t.,** a familial tremor with onset at varying ages, usually at about 50 years of age, beginning with a fine rapid tremor (as distinct from that of parkinsonism) of the hands, followed by tremor of the arms, tongue, heads, legs, and trunk; it is aggravated by emotional factors, is accentuated by volitional movement, and is temporarily improved by alcohol. Called also *familial t., heredofamilial t.,* and *hereditary essential t.* **familial t.,** essential t. **fibrillary t.,** a fine rhythmical trembling due to alternate contraction of the different fibrils of a muscle; fibrillation. **fine t.,** a tremor in which the vibrations are rapid. **flapping t.,** asterixis. **forced t.,** a movement persisting after voluntary motion, due to intermittent stimulation of the nerve centers. **hereditary essential t.,** essential t. **heredofamilial t.,** essential t. **Hunt's t.,** the tremor attending every voluntary movement which is characteristic of cerebellar lesions. **hysterical t.,** tremor seen in hysteria dependent upon uncertain nervous impulse. **intention t.,** tremor which arises or which is intensified when a voluntary, coordinated movement is attempted; seen in hemiplegia or when attempts at voluntary movement are made. **kinetic t.,** a tremor occurring in a limb during active movement. **t. lin′guae,** trembling of the tongue, as seen in alcoholism, typhoid fever, and paretic dementia. **t. mercuria′lis,** tremor due to mercurial poisoning. **metallic t.,** tremor seen in various metallic poisonings. **motofacient t.,** a tremor in muscles which participate in an action. **t. opio-**

phago′rum, the tremor of opium users. **passive t.,** a tremor occurring only when the patient is at rest. **persistent t.,** a tremor occurring whether the patient is at rest or in motion. **t. potato′rum** ["trembling of drinkers"], delirium tremens. **purring t.,** a thrill, like the purring of a cat, felt by the hand placed over the heart. **Rendu's t.,** a hysterical intention tremor. **rest t.,** tremor occurring in a relaxed and supported limb, as in parkinsonism. **senile t.,** a tremor resulting from the infirmities of age. **static t.,** a tremor occurring on effort to hold one of the limbs in a definite position. **striocerebellar t.,** a combined form of tremor with both striatal and cerebellar components, usually due to diffuse degeneration of the central nervous system. **t. ten′dinum** ["trembling of the tendons"], subsultus tendinum. **toxic t.,** a tremor seen in states of chronic poisoning. **trombone t. of tongue,** Magnan's movement. **volitional t.,** a trembling of the entire body during voluntary effort; seen in multiple sclerosis.

tremorgram (trem′or-gram) tremogram.

tremulor (trem′u-lor) a machine for the administration of vibratory treatment.

tremulous (trem′u-lus) [L. *tremulus*] shaking, trembling, or quivering.

trend (trend) inclination in a particular direction or course.

Trendelenburg cannula, etc. (tren-del′en-berg) [Friedrich *Trendelenburg*, surgeon in Leipzig, 1844–1924] see under *cannula, operation, position, symptom,* and *tests*.

trendscriber (trend′skrīb-er) the apparatus used in trendscription.

trendscription (trend′skrip″shun) a programmed method of continuous electrocardiographic monitoring, wherein the tracing is condensed on a rotating drum recorder and the program permits selective sampling of rhythm data.

trepan (trĕ-pan′) [Gr. *trypanon* auger] 1. an obsolete form of the trephine, resembling a carpenter's bit and brace. 2. to trepan.

trepanation (trep″ah-na′shun) [L. *trepanatio*] an operation with the trepan; trephination. **corneal t.,** excision of a disk of cornea in treatment of staphyloma.

trepanner (tre-pan′er) one who performs a trepanation; trephiner.

trephination (tref″ĭ-na′shun) the operation of trephining. **dental t.,** surgical formation of an opening through the gum and bone to the apical end of a tooth.

trephine (trĕ-fīn′, trĕ-fēn′) [L. *trephina*] 1. a crown saw for removing a circular disk of bone, chiefly from the skull. 2. an instrument for removing a circular area of cornea, as in corneal transplant operations. 3. to operate upon with the trephine. **Horsley's t.,** a trephine that may be taken apart and cleaned.

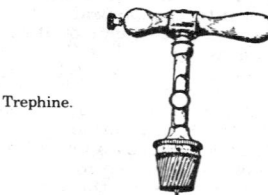

Trephine.

trephinement (tre-fīn′ment) the act or process of trephining.

trephiner (tre-fīn′er) one who performs the operation of trephining.

trephocyte (tref′o-sīt) [Gr. *trephein* to feed + *kytos* cell] a cell that furnishes nutrition to other cells, as a Sertoli cell.

trepidant (trep′ĭ-dant) [L. *trepidans* trembling] characterized by tremor.

trepidatio (trep″ĭ-da′she-o) [L.] trepidation. **t. cor′dis,** palpitation of the heart.

trepidation (trep″ĭ-da′shun) [L. *trepidatio*] 1. a trembling or oscillatory movement. 2. nervous anxiety and fear.

Treponema (trep″o-ne′mah) [Gr. *trepein* to turn + *nema* thread] a genus of microorganisms of the family Treponemataceae, order Spirochaetales, made up of cells 3 to 18 μ long, in acute, regular or irregular spirals, some of them being pathogenic and parasitic for man and other animals. **T. calligy′rum,** a parasitic microorganism found in smegma and in lesions of the pudenda; it is thought to be nonpathogenic. **T. carate′um,** the causative agent of pinta (carate). **T. cunic′uli,** the causative agent of rabbit syphilis; not pathogenic for man. **T. genita′lis,** a parasitic, nonpathogenic microorganism found on human genitalia. **T. herrejo′ni,** a spirochete which causes pinta. **T. macroden′tium,** an apparently nonpathogenic species which has been found in the mouth. **T. microden′tium,** a parasitic spiral microorganism found in the normal human mouth; nonpathogenic. **T. muco′sum,** a parasitic microorganism found in pyorrhea alveolaris; pathogenicity uncertain. **T. pal′lidum,** the causative agent of venereal syphilis in man; some authorities believe that it is also the etiologic agent of nonvenereal syphilis. **T. perten′ue,** the causative agent of yaws (frambesia tropica) in man. **T. recurren'tis,** the relapsing fever spirochete, called also *Borrelia recurrentis.*

treponema (trep''o-ne'mah) an organism of the genus *Treponema.*

treponemal (trep''o-ne'mal) of, pertaining to, or caused by treponemas.

Treponemataceae (trep''o-ne''mah-ta'se-e) a family of Schizomycetes (order Spirochaetales), made up of coarse or slender spirals, 4 to 16 μ long, sometimes showing terminal filaments and sometimes visible only with dark-field illumination. They commonly occur as parasites in vertebrates, and some of them cause disease. The family includes three genera, *Borrelia, Leptospira,* and *Treponema.*

treponematosis (trep''o-ne-mah-to'sis) an infection with treponema.

treponeme (trep'o-nēm) an organism of the genus *Treponema.*

treponemiasis (trep''o-ne-mi'ah-sis) infection with treponema; syphilis.

treponemicidal (trep''o-ne''mĭ-si'dal) destroying treponema.

trepopnea (tre''pop-ne'ah) [Gr. *trepein* to turn + *pnoia* breath] a condition in which breathing is most comfortable with the patient turned in a definite recumbent position.

treppe (trep'ĕ) [Ger. "staircase"] the phenomenon of gradual increase in the extent of muscular contraction following rapidly repeated stimulation (H. P. Bowditch, 1871). Also called *staircase phenomenon.*

Tresilian's sign (tre-sil'e-anz) [Frederick James *Tresilian,* English physician, 1862–1926] see under *sign.*

tresis (tre'sis) [Gr. *trēsis*] perforation.

Trest (trest) trademark for a preparation of methixene hydrochloride.

trestolone acetate (tres'to-lōn) chemical name: 17β-hydroxy-7α-methylestr-4-en-3-one acetate; an antineoplastic and androgenic steroid, $C_{21}H_{30}O_3$.

tretinoin (tret'ĭ-noin) [USP] the *all-trans* stereoisomer of retinoic acid, $C_{20}H_{28}O_2$, occurring as a yellow to light-orange, crystalline powder; used as a topical keratolytic, especially in the treatment of certain cases of acne vulgaris. Called also *retinoic acid* and *vitamin A acid.*

Treves' fold, operation (trēvs) [Sir Frederick *Treves,* English surgeon, 1853–1923] see *plica ileocecalis,* and see under *operation.*

TRF thyrotropin releasing factor; see *protirelin.*

TRH thyrotropin releasing hormone; see *protirelin.*

tri- [Gr. *treis;* L. *tres* three] a prefix meaning *three* or *thrice.*

triacetate (tri-as'ĕ-tāt) an acetate which contains three molecules of the acetic acid radical.

triacetin (tri-as'ĕ-tin) [USP] chemical name: 1,2,3-propanetriol. An antifungal agent, $C_9H_4O_6$, occurring as a colorless or pale straw-colored liquid; used topically in the treatment of superficial fungal infections of the skin. Called also *glyceryl triacetate.*

triacetyloleandomycin (tri-as''ĕ-til-o''le-an''do-mi'sin) troleandomycin.

triacid (tri-as'id) a base capable of neutralizing three equivalents of monobasic acid.

triacylglycerol (tri-as''il-glis'er-ol) a term proposed to replace triglyceride.

triad (tri'ad) [L. *trias;* Gr. *trias* group of three] 1. any trivalent element. 2. a group of three entities or objects, as an association of three symptoms. **acute compression t.,** Beck's t. **adrenomedullary t.,** the symptoms produced by activation of the adrenal medulla: tachycardia, vasoconstriction, and sweating. **Andersen's t.,** see under *syndrome.* **Basedow's t.,** Merseburg t. **Beck's t.,** three symptoms characteristic of cardiac compression: (1) a high venous pressure, (2) a low arterial pressure, and (3) a small quiet heart. **Bezold's t.,** prolonged bone conduction and lessened perception of low tones, indicating otosclerosis. **Charcot's t.,** nystagmus, intention tremor, and staccato speech, often seen in multiple sclerosis. **Dieulafoy's t.,** hypersensitiveness of the skin, reflex muscular contraction, and tenderness at McBurney's point in appendicitis. **Falta's t.,** the three organs cooperating in production of diabetes mellitus: the pancreas, liver, and thyroid. **Grancher's t.,** lessened vesicular quality of breathing, skodaic resonance, and increased vocal fremitus; seen in early pulmonary tuberculosis. **hepatic t's,** the grouping of the tributaries of the hepatic artery, vein, and bile duct at the angles of the lobules of the liver. **t. of Herz,** neurocirculatory asthenia. **Hutchinson's t.,** diffuse interstitial keratitis, labyrinthine disease, and Hutchinson teeth, seen in inherited syphilis. **Kartagener's t.,** see under *syndrome.* **t. of Luciani,** asthenia, atonia, and astasia, the three major symptoms of cerebellar disease. **Merseburg t., Merseburger t.,** goiter, exophthalmos, and tachycardia, the three cardinal symptoms of Graves' (Basedow's) disease; named after Merseburg, the home of Basedow. **Osler's t.,** telangiectasis, capillary fragility, and hereditary hemorrhagic diathesis. **portal t's,** hepatic t's. **Saint's t.,** hiatus hernia, colonic diverticula, and cholelithiasis, occurring concomitantly. **t. of retinal**

cone, the tip of two horizontal cell dendrites and one midget cell dendrite, enclosed in a synaptic invagination of a retinal cone pedicle. **t. of Schultz,** jaundice, gangrenous stomatitis, and leukopenia. **t. of skeletal muscle,** a pair of terminal cisterns in close apposition to the T tubule, running transversely across a myofibril of skeletal muscle; in mammalian muscle there are two triads to each sarcomere, situated at the A band–I band junction. See also *T system,* under *system* and *T tubule,* under *tubule.* **Whipple's t.,** the essential clinical features of insulin-producing tumors: (1) spontaneous hypoglycemia, (blood sugar levels below 50 mg. per 100 ml.), (2) accompanied by central nervous or vasomotor system symptoms, and (3) relief of symptoms by the oral or intravenous administration of glucose.

triaditis (tri''ad-i'tis) inflammation of three elements taken as a unit. **portal t.,** inflammation of the connective tissue around the hepatic artery, portal vein, and bile duct of the portal tract.

triafungin (tri''ah-fun'jin) chemical name: 3-(phenylmethyl)-pyrido[3,4-*e*]-1,2,4-triazine; an antifungal, $C_{13}H_{10}N_4$.

triage (tre-ahzh') [Fr. "sorting"] the sorting out and classification of casualties of war or other disaster, to determine priority of need and proper place of treatment.

trialism (tri'al-izm) trialistic theory; see under *theory.*

triallylamine (tri'al-il-am'in) a volatile, oily, liquid amine, $(CH_2:CH \cdot CH_2)_3N.$

triamcinolone (tri''am-sin'o-lōn) [USP] chemical name: 9-fluoro-11β,16α,17,21-tetrahydroxypregna-1,4-diene-3,20-dione. A potent synthetic glucocorticoid, $C_{21}H_{27}FO_6$, occurring as a white or almost white, crystalline powder, having practically no mineralocorticoid activity; used in the treatment of various conditions responsive to the anti-inflammatory action of glucocorticoids, administered orally. **t. acetonide** [USP], the acetonide ester of triamcinolone, $C_{24}H_{31}FO_6$, occurring as a white to cream-colored, crystalline powder; applied topically to the skin and oral mucosa or administered by intra-articular, intrabursal, intramuscular, and intradermal injection. **t. acetonide sodium phosphate,** the 21-disodium phosphate salt of triamcinolone acetonide, $C_{24}H_{30}FNa_2O_9P$, having anti-inflammatory actions similar to those of the base. **t. diacetate** [USP], the diacetate ester of triamcinolone, $C_{25}H_{31}FO_8$, occurring as a fine, white to off-white, crystalline powder; administered orally and by intramuscular, intra-articular, and soft tissue injection. **t. hexacetonide** [USP], the hexacetonide ester of triamcinolone, $C_{30}H_{41}FO_7$, occurring as a white to cream-colored powder; it is administered by intra-articular or by intralesional or sublesional injection for treatment of arthritis or of inflammatory skin lesions, respectively.

triamine (tri-am'in) a compound containing three amino (—NH_2) groups.

triamterene (tri-am'ter-ēn) [USP] chemical name: 6-phenyl-2,4,7-triamino-6-phenylpteridine. An orally effective diuretic, $C_{12}H_{11}N_7$, occurring as a yellow, odorless, crystalline powder, which increases sodium and chloride secretion but not potassium secretion.

triamylose (tri-am'ĭ-lōs) a polymerized anhydride of glucose, $(C_6H_{10}O_5)_3$, isolable from the amylopectin of starch.

triangle (tri'ang-g'l) [L. *triangulum; tres* three + *angulus* angle] a three-cornered area, figure, or object; see also *trigone* and *trigonum.* **Alsberg's t.,** an equilateral triangle with its apex upward, formed by a line passing through the long axis of the femur, a second line passing through the long axis of the neck of the femur, and a third line on a plane passing through the base of the head of the femur. The angle at the apex is known as *Alsberg's angle,* or *angle of elevation.* **Assézat's t.,** facial t. **auditory t.,** area vestibularis. **auricular t.,** one bounded by lines drawn from the tip of the auricle and the two ends of its base of insertion. **t. of auscultation,** the area limited by the lower edge of the trapezius muscle, the latissimus dorsi, and the medial margin of the scapula. **axillary t.,** the triangular area formed by the inner aspect of the arm, the axilla, and the pectoral region. **Béclard's t.,** the area lying between the posterior edge of the hyoglossal muscle, the posterior belly of the digastric muscle, and the greater cornu of the hyoid bone. **Bolton t.,** the triangle formed by drawing a line from the nasion to the sella turcica to the Bolton point. **Bonwill t.,** an equilateral triangle said by Bonwill to be formed by a line connecting the centers of the mandibular condyles and lines connecting either center with the mesial contact area of the mandibular medial incisors, each side being approximately 4 inches long. **brachial t.,** axillary t. **Burger's scalene t.,** a triangle providing a reference frame to represent the quantitative relationships between the electromotive forces of the heart and the extremity leads of the electrocardiograph. As compared to Einthoven's triangle, the lines representing leads I and II are considerably shortened. **Calot's t.,** the triangle formed by the cystic artery superiorly, the cystic duct inferiorly, and the hepatic duct medially; called also *cystohepatic t.* **cardiohepatic t.,** the triangular region in the fifth intercostal space of the right side, separating the heart from the upper edge of the liver. **carotid t., inferior,** the part of the trigonum caroticum medial to the omohyoid muscle; called also *t. of necessity.* **carotid t., superior,** the part of the trigonum caroticum lateral to the omohyoid muscle; called also *t. of election.* **cephalic t.,** one on the anteroposterior plane of the skull, between the lines from the occiput to the forehead and to the chin, and a third line extending from the chin to the forehead. **cervical t's,** see *t's of neck, anterior,* and *posterior.* **Codman's t.,** a triangular area visible roentgenographically where the periosteum, elevated by a bone tumor, rejoins the cortex of normal bone. **color t.,** a plane figure with red, green, and blue located at the three apices, and gray at the center, with lines drawn from side to side, as a guide to the color mixing equation needed to produce any intermediate hue. **crural t.,** the triangular area formed by the inner aspect of the thigh and the lower abdominal, inguinal, and genital regions. **cystohepatic t.,** Calot's t. **digastric t.,** trigonum submandibulare. **Dunham's t's,** see under *fan.* **Einthoven's t.,** an equilateral triangle used as a mathematical model of the standard electrocardiographic limb leads, in which the instantaneous heart vector in the frontal plane may be projected on the sides of the triangle thereby demonstrating that the algebraic sum of the potential differences as recorded in electrocardiographic leads I and III will equal that potential difference recorded in lead II. See *Einthoven's formula,* under *formula.* **t. of elbow,** a triangular area on the front of the elbow, having the brachioradialis muscle on the outside and the pronator teres inside, the base being toward the humerus. **t. of election,** superior carotid t. **extravesical t.,** Pawlik's t. **facial t.,** a triangular area whose points are the basion, the alveolar point, and the nasion; called also *Assézat's triangle.* **Farabeuf's t.,** one on the upper part of the neck, its sides being formed by the internal jugular vein and the facial vein, and its base by the hypoglossal nerve. **femoral t.,** trigonum femorale. **fetal t.,** a triangular space made by the side of the fetal trunk, the thigh above, and the arm below. **frontal t.,** one bounded by the maximum frontal diameter and lines from either end of this diameter to the glabella. **Garland's t.,** a triangular area of relative resonance in the lower back, close to the spine on the diseased side; seen in pleurisy with effusion. **Gerhardt's t.,** a triangular area of dullness to percussion above the third left rib, an inconstant sign in patent ductus arteriosus. **Gombault-Philippe t.,** a triangular field formed in the conus medullaris by the fibers of the septomarginal tract. **Grocco's t.,** see *Grocco's sign* (def. 1), under *sign.* **Grynfelt's t., t. of Grynfelt and Lesgaft,** Lesgaft's space. **Henke's t.,** a triangular area between the descending portion of the inguinal fold, the lateral portion of the inguinal fold, and the lateral border of the rectus muscle. **Hesselbach's t.,** trigonum inguinale. **hypoglossohyoid t.,** the triangular space in the subhyoid region, bounded above by the hypoglossal nerve, in front by the posterior border of the mylohyoid muscle, and behind and below by the tendon of the digastric muscle. Called also *Pinaud's t.* and *Pirogoff's t.* **iliofemoral t.,** a triangular area bounded by Nélaton's line, a line through the superior iliac spine, and one extending from this spine to the great trochanter. **infraclavicular t.,** trigonum deltoideopectorale. **inguinal t.,** 1. trigonum inguinale. 2. trigonum femorale. **Jackson's safety t.,** a triangular space bounded above by the lower end of the thyroid cartilage, its apex in the suprasternal notch, and its sides the inner edges of the sternocleidomastoid muscle; so called because it marks the limits of the area through which the trachea may safely be incised in tracheostomy. **Kanavel's t.,** a triangular area in the middle of the palm beneath which lies the common tendon sheath of the digital flexor tendons. **Korányi-Grocco t.,** see *Grocco's sign* (def. 1), under *sign.* **Labbé's t.,** one included between a horizontal line along the lower border of the cartilage of the ninth rib, the line of the false ribs, and the line of the liver, being the area where the stomach lies in contact with the anterior abdominal wall. **Langenbeck's t.,** one having its apex at the anterior superior spine of the ilium, its base along the anatomical neck of the femur, and its external side by the external face of the great trochanter. **Lesgaft's t.,** see under *space.* **Lesser's t.,** one bounded by the hypoglossal nerve above and the two bellies of the digastricus muscle on the other two sides. **Lieutaud's t.,** trigonum vesicae. **Livingston's t.,** a triangular area bounded by lines from the umbilicus to the crest of the ilium, from the latter to the right pubic spine, and from there to the umbilicus, marking an area which is hypersensitive to palpation in appendicitis. **lumbocostoabdominal t.,** a space between the obliquus externus abdominis muscle, the serratus posterior inferior, the erector spinae, and the obliquus internus abdominis. **lymphoid t.,** see *Waldeyer's tonsillar ring,* under *ring.* **Macewen's t.,** mastoid fossa of temporal bone. **Malgaigne's t.,** superior carotid t. **mesenteric t.,** a triangular space between the two layers of the mesentery as they diverge to enclose the intestine. **Middeldorpf's t.,** a padded triangular splint for supporting the upper arm in partial extension in fracture of the humerus. **Minor's t.,** an angular defect posterior to the anus, produced by attachment of the superficial portion of the external sphincter to the coccyx. **t. of necessity,** inferior carotid t. **t's of neck, anterior,** the inferior and superior carotid triangles, and the submandibular triangle. **t's of neck, posterior,** the occipital and subclavian triangles. **occipital t.,** the area bounded by the sterno-

cleidomastoid muscle anteriorly, the trapezius muscle posteriorly, and the omohyoid muscle inferiorly. **occipital t., inferior,** a triangular area having a line between the two mastoid processes as its base and the inion as its apex. **palatal t.,** one limited by the greatest transverse diameter of the palate and lines from either end of this diameter to the alveolar point. **paravertebral t.,** see *Grocco's sign* (def. 1), under *sign.* **Pawlik's t.,** one within the vagina corresponding exactly with the trigonum vesicae, and bounded laterally by Pawlik's folds. **Petit's t.,** trigonum lumbale. **Pinaud's t., Pirogoff's t.,** hypoglossohyoid t. **popliteal t. of femur,** facies poplitea femoris. **pubourethral t.,** one in the perineum bounded externally by the ischiocavernosus muscle, internally by the bulbocavernosus, and posteriorly by the transversus perinei superficialis. **Rauchfuss' t.,** see *Grocco's sign* (def. 1), under *sign.* **Reil's t.,** trigonum lemnisci. **retromandibular t.,** a shallow triangular fossa on the mandibular bone posterior to the third molar. **sacral t.,** a shallow triangular depression overlying the sacrum. **t. of safety,** the fifth or sixth left intercostal space, considered a safe site for pericardial aspiration. **Scarpa's t.,** trigonum femorale. **sternocostal t.,** trigonum sternocostale. **subclavian t.,** trigonum omoclaviculare. **subinguinal t.,** 1. hiatus saphenus. 2. trigonum femorale. **submandibular t.,** **submaxillary t.,** trigonum submandibulare. **submental t.,** a triangle bounded on either side by the anterior belly of the digastric muscle and below by the hyoid bone. **suboccipital t.,** a triangular area lying between the rectus capitis posterior major and the obliquus capitis superior and obliquus capitis inferior muscles. **suprameatal t.,** mastoid fossa of temporal bone. **surgical t.,** any triangular area or region in which certain nerves, vessels, or organs are located; established for reference in surgical operations. **Trautmann's t.,** a space with its anterior angle at the prominence containing the labyrinth, bounded posteriorly by the transverse sinus and superiorly by the inferior temporal line. When the bone is removed, the superior petrosal sinus will be encountered at the superior posterior angle of this triangle. **Tweed t.,** a mathematical triangle defined by facial and dental landmarks on a lateral cephalometric film, using the Frankfort horizontal plane as a base and intended for use as a guide in the evaluation and planning of orthodontic treatment. **umbilicomammillary t.,** one having its base formed by the line joining the nipples and its apex at the umbilicus. **urogenital t.,** diaphragma urogenitale. **vaginal t.,** Pawlik's t. **vesical t.,** trigonum vesicae. **von Weber's t.,** one on the sole of the foot formed by lines connecting the head of the first metatarsal, the head of the fifth metatarsal, and the center of the under surface of the heel. **Ward's t.,** the space formed by the angle of the trabeculae in the neck of the femur; a vulnerable point for fracture. **Wernicke's t.,** the area within the posterior limb on the internal capsule in which the optic radiation, having just left the lateral geniculate body, comes into close proximity to the auditory and somesthetic radiations.

triangular (tri-ang′gu-lar) [L. *triangularis*] having three angles or corners.

triangularis (tri-ang″gu-la′ris) [L.] triangular.

triantebrachia (tri″an-te-bra′ke-ah) [*tri-* + *antebrachium* + *-ia*] a developmental anomaly characterized by tripling of the forearm.

Triatoma (tri-at′o-mah) a genus of bugs of the family Reduviidae, called the cone-nosed bugs, important in medicine as vectors of *Trypanosoma cruzi,* the etiologic agent of Chagas' disease. **T. megis′ta,** former name for *Panstrongylus megistus.* **T. sanguisu′ga,** the blood-sucking cone-nose or Mexican bedbug of the southern United States. Its bite is painful and causes irritation, swelling, and nausea. Other species which are vectors of *Trypanosoma cruzi* are: *T. dimidia′ta,* of Central America; *T. genicula′ta (Panstrongylus geniculatus),* which inhabits the burrows of the armadillo; *T. gerstaeck′eri* of Texas; *T. (Panstrongylus) infes′tans,* the unchuca or great black bug of the Argentine and Paraguay; *T. mexica′na,* found in Mexico; *T. nigrova′rius,* widely distributed in South America; *T. protrac′ta,* of the southern United States; *T. recur′va* and *T. rubi′da* of Arizona; *T. (Entriatoma) sor′dida* of São Paulo; and *T. vit′ticeps,* of Rio de Janeiro.

triatomic (tri″ah-tom′ik) made up of three atoms.

triazol 156 (tri′ah-zol) a compound, 4-cyclohexyl 3-ethyl 1-2-4-triazol, once used as a convulsant in the treatment of schizophrenia.

triazolam (tri-a′zo-lam) chemical name: 8-chloro-6-(2-chlorophenyl)-1-methyl-4*H*-[1,2,4]triazolo[4,3-*a*][1,4]benzodiazepine; a tranquilizer, $C_{17}H_{12}Cl_2N_4$.

tribadism (trib′ah-dizm) [Gr. *tribein* to rub] 1. lesbianism in which heterosexual intercourse is simulated; sometimes used to refer to the use of an artificial penis. 2. mutual friction of the genitals between women.

tribady (trib′ah-de) tribadism.

tribasic (tri-ba′sik) [*tri-* + L. *basis* base] having three replaceable hydrogen atoms.

tribe (trīb) a taxonomic category subordinate to a family (or subfamily) and superior to a genus (or subtribe).

tribenoside (tri-ben′o-sīd) chemical name: ethyl-3,5,6-tri-*O*-

benzyl-D-glucofuranoside; a sclerosing agent, $C_{29}H_{34}O_8$, which has been used in inflammatory and varicose disorders of the veins.

Tribolium (tri-bo′le-um) a genus of small beetles that live in and are very destructive to flour and other cereal products. The two most common species, *T. confu′sum* and *T. casta′neum*, are reddish brown in color and 3.5 mm. in length.

tribology (trĭ-bol′o-je) [Gr. *tribē* a rubbing + *-logy*] the study of the lubrication, friction, and wear of the joints.

triboluminescence (tri″bo-lu″mĭ-nes′ens) [Gr. *tribein* to rub + *luminescence*] luminescence produced by mechanical energy, as by the grinding, rubbing, or breaking of certain crystals.

tribrachia (tri-bra′ke-ah) [*tri-* + Gr. *brachion* arm + *-ia*] a developmental anomaly characterized by tripling of an arm.

tribrachius (tri-bra′ke-us) 1. a monster exhibiting tribrachia. 2. a monster consisting of conjoined twins having only three arms.

tribromaloin (tri″brŏm-al′o-in) a yellow, crystalline compound, $C_{17}H_{15}Br_3O_7$, or bromine and barbaloin.

tribromethanol (tri″brŏm-eth′ah-nol) tribromoethanol.

tribromide (tri-bro′mīd) a bromine compound containing three atoms of bromine to one of the base.

tribromoethanol (tri-bro″mo-eth′ah-nol) chemical name: tribromoethyl alcohol. An anesthetic, $C_2H_3Br_3O$, occurring as a white, crystalline powder; administered by inhalation. Called also *ethobrom*. See also under *solution*.

tribromsalan (tri-brom′sah-lan) chemical name: 3,5-dibromo-*N*-(4-bromophenyl)-2-hydroxybenzamide. A disinfectant with antibacterial and antifungal activities, $C_{13}H_8Br_3NO_2$, used mainly in medicated soaps.

tribulosis (trib″u-lo′sis) poisoning in sheep in South Africa, caused by wilted plants of the species *Tribulus terrestris.*

Triburon (trib′u-ron) trademark for preparations of triclobisonium chloride.

tributyrin (tri-bu′tir-in) a colorless fat, $C_3H_5(OCOCH_2CH_2CH_3)_3$, found in cows' milk.

tributyrinase (tri″bu-tir′ĭ-nās) an enzyme in the saliva which cleaves tributyrin.

TRIC (trik) acronym for *trachoma inclusion conjunctivitis* (group of organisms); see *Chlamydia.*

tricalcic (tri-kal′sik) containing three atoms of calcium.

tricellular (tri-sel′u-lar) three celled.

tricephalus (tri-sef′ah-lus) [*tri-* + Gr. *kephalē* head] a monster having three heads.

triceps (tri′seps) [L.] having three heads, as a triceps muscle. **t. su′rae,** see *Table of Musculi.*

triceptor (tri-sep′tor) an intermediary having three combining groups.

Tricercomonas (tri″ser-kom′o-nas) *Enteromonas.*

tricheiria (tri-ki′re-ah) [*tri-* + Gr. *cheir* hand + *-ia*] a developmental anomaly characterized by tripling of a hand.

trichesthesia (trik″es-the′ze-ah) trichoesthesia.

trichiasis (trĭ-ki′ah-sis) [Gr.] 1. a condition of ingrowing hairs about an orifice, or of ingrowing eyelashes. 2. the appearance of hairlike filaments in the urine.

trichilemmal (trik″ĭ-lem′al) pertaining to the outer root sheath of a hair.

trichilemmoma (trik″ĭ-lem-o′mah) a benign neoplasm of the lower outer root sheath of the hair.

Trichina (trĭ-ki′nah) *Trichinella.*

trichina (trĭ-ki′nah), pl. *trichi′nae.* an individual organism of the genus *Trichinella.*

trichinae (trĭ-ki′ne) plural of *trichina.*

Trichinella (trik″ĭ-nel′ah) [Gr. *trichinos* of hair] a genus of nematode parasites of the superfamily Trichuroidea. **T. spira′lis,** the etiologic agent of trichinosis, one of the smallest of the parasitic nematodes, being only about 1.5 mm. in length. It is found coiled in a cyst in the muscles of the bear, rat, pig, and man. When infected meat is eaten without proper cooking the cyst dissolves, the parasite matures, deposits its larvae in the deep mucosa, whence they enter the lymphatics, are carried to all parts of the body, and again encyst. An extract of *Trichinella* larvae is used in an intradermal skin test for trichinosis. Called also *pork worm.*

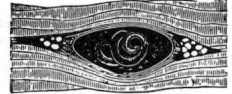

Trichinella spiralis encapsulated in muscle.

trichinelliasis (trik″ĭ-nel-li′ah-sis) trichinosis.
trichinellosis (trik″ĭ-nel-lo′sis) trichinosis.
trichiniasis (trik″ĭ-ni′ah-sis) trichinosis.
trichiniferous (trik″ĭ-nif′er-us) [*trichina* + L. *ferre* to bear] containing trichinae.

trichinization (trik″ĭ-ni-za′shun) infection with *Trichinella spiralis;* trichinosis.

trichinosis (trik″ĭ-no′sis) a disease due to infection with trichinae. It is produced by eating undercooked meat containing *Trichinella spiralis.* It is attended in the early stages by diarrhea, nausea, colic, and fever, and later by stiffness, pain, swelling of the muscles, fever, eosinophilia, circumorbital edema, splinter hemorrhages, sweating, and insomnia.

trichinous (trik′ĭ-nus) affected with or containing trichinae.

trichion (trik′e-on), pl. *trich′ia* [Gr.] an anthropometric landmark, the point at which the midsagittal plane of the head intersects the hairline.

trichite (tri′kīt) 1. A. Meyer's name for one of the radially arranged needle-shaped crystals composing a starch grain. 2. one of the needle-shaped plastids which may serve a supportive function in certain protozoa.

trichlorfon (tri-klōr′fon) metrifonate.

trichlorphon (tri-klōr′fon) metrifonate.

trichloride (tri-klo′rīd) any combination of three atoms of chlorine with one of another element.

trichlormethane (tri″klōr-meth′ān) chloroform.

trichlormethiazide (tri-klōr″mĕ-thi′ah-zīd) [USP] chemical name: 6-chloro-3-(dichloromethyl)-3,4-dihydro-2*H*-1,2,4-benzothiadiazine-7-sulfonamide 1,1-dioxide. A white or practically white, crystalline powder, $C_8H_8Cl_3N_3O_4S_2$, used as a diuretic and antihypertensive, administered orally.

trichloroacetaldehyde (tri-klo″ro-as″et-al′de-hīd) chloral.

trichloroethylene (tri″klo-ro-eth′ĭ-lēn) chemical name: trichloroethene. A clear, colorless, or blue, mobile liquid, C_2HCl_3, used as an inhalation anesthetic for short operative procedures. It is widely used as an industrial solvent, and exposure to its vapor in high concentrations has caused some poisonings, some of which were fatal. Called also *ethinyl trichloride.*

trichloromethylchloroformate (tri-klo″ro-meth″il-klo″ro-for′māt) a chlorine-containing gas which is irritating to lung tissue.

trichloromonofluoromethane (tri-klo″ro-mon″o-floor-o-meth′ān) [NF] chemical name: trichlorofluoromethane. A clear, colorless gas having a faint, ethereal odor, CCl_3F, used as an aerosol propellant.

trichlorophenol (tri″klor-o-fe′nol) a disinfectant and external antiseptic.

trichlorotrivinylarsine (tri-klo″ro-tri-vi″nil-ar′sin) a sternutatory war gas $(CHCl:CH)_3As.$

tricho- [Gr. *thrix, trichos,* hair] a prefix denoting relationship to hair.

trichoaesthesia (trik″o-es-the′ze-ah) trichoesthesia.

trichoanesthesia (trik″o-an″es-the′ze-ah) loss of hair sensibility.

trichobacteria (trik″o-bak-te′re-ah) [*tricho-* + Gr. *baktērion* rod] 1. a group of bacteria including those forms which possess flagella. 2. the filamentous or threadlike bacteria.

trichobasalioma hyalinicum (trik″o-ba-sal″e-o′mah) cylindroma, def. 2.

trichobezoar (trik″o-be′zor) [*tricho-* + *bezoar*] a hairball; a concretion within the stomach or intestines formed of hairs.

Trichobilharzia (trik″o-bil-har′ze-ah) a genus of flukes. **T. ocella′ta,** a blood fluke parasitic in European ducks.

trichocardia (trik″o-kar′de-ah) [*tricho-* + Gr. *kardia* heart] cor villosum, or hairy heart.

trichocephaliasis (trik″o-sef″ah-li′ah-sis) trichuriasis.

trichocephalosis (trik″o-sef″ah-lo′sis) trichuriasis.

Trichocephalus (trik″o-sef′ah-lus) [*tricho-* + Gr. *kephalē* head] former name for a genus of nematodes now called *Trichuris.*

trichoclasia (trik″o-kla′se-ah) trichorrhexis nodosa.

trichoclasis (trik-ok′lah-sis) [*tricho-* + Gr. *klasis* fracture] trichorrhexis nodosa.

trichocyst (trik′o-sist) [*tricho-* + Gr. *kystis* bladder] a cell structure derived from the cytoplasm.

Trichodectes (trik″o-dek′tēz) [*tricho-* + Gr. *dēktēs* biter] a genus of parasitic insects of the order Mallophaga, the biting lice. **T. can′is,** a biting louse that parasitizes dogs and is an intermediate host of *Dipylidium caninum.* **T. cli′max,** *Damalinia caprae.* **T. e′qui,** *Damalinia equi.* **T. herm′si,** *Damalinia hermsi.* **T. la′tus,** the dog louse, found on dogs, especially puppies. **T. pilo′sus,** *Damalinia pilosus.* **T. retu′sis,** a biting louse that infests ranch-raised mink. **T. sphaeroceph′alus,** the red-headed sheep louse, found in the wool of sheep in Europe and America.

Trichoderma (trik-o-der′mah) [*tricho* + *derma* skin] a genus of soil fungi (family Moniliaceae, order Moniliales), some species of which cause alimentary toxic aleukia.

Trichodina (trik-od′ĭ-nah) [*tricho-* + Gr. *dinos* whirling] a genus of the ciliate protoza of the order Peritrichida, species of which live on hydras and the gills of fish and salamanders.

trichoepithelioma (trik″o-ep″ĭ-the-le-o′mah) a benign skin tumor whose cell growth starts in the follicles of the lanugo; it may occur as a dominantly inherited condition characterized by multiple tumors (sometimes called *trichoepithelioma papillosum multiplex*) or as a solitary lesion. **t. papillo′sum mul′tiplex,** hereditary multiple trichoepithelioma; see *trichoepithelioma*. Called also *epithelioma adenoides cysticum*.

trichoesthesia (trik″o-es-the′ze-ah) [*tricho-* + Gr. *aisthēsis* perception + -*ia*] the sense by which one perceives when one of the hairs of the skin has been touched; hair sensibility.

trichoesthesiometer (trik″o-es-the″ze-om′ĕ-ter) [*tricho-* + Gr. *aisthēsis* perception + *metron* measure] an electric apparatus for measuring the hair sensibility, or the sensitiveness of the scalp by means of the hairs.

trichofibroacanthoma (trik″o-fi″bro-ak″an-tho′mah) trichoepithelioma.

trichofibroepithelioma (trik″o-fi″bro-ep″ĭ-the″le-o′mah) trichoepithelioma.

trichoglossia (trik″o-glos′e-ah) [*tricho-* + Gr. *glōssa* tongue + -*ia*] a hairy state of the tongue due to a thickening of the papillae.

trichographism (tri-kog′rah-fizm) pilomotor reflex.

trichohyalin (trik″o-hi′ah-lin) [*tricho-* + *hyalin*] a keratohyaline-like substance occurring in granules in the cytoplasm of the cells of Huxley's layer of a hair follicle.

trichoid (trik′oid) [*tricho-* + Gr. *eidos* form] like or resembling a hair, or the hair.

tricholabion (tri-ko-la′be-on) [Gr.] (*obs.*) epilating forceps.

tricholeukocyte (trik″o-lu′ko-sīt) hairy cell.

tricholith (trik′o-lith) [*tricho-* + Gr. *lithos* stone] a hairy concretion.

trichologia (trik″o-lo′je-ah) [*tricho-* + Gr. *legein* to pick out + -*ia*] the pulling out of the hair by delirious patients; trichotillomania.

trichology (tri-kol′o-je) the study of hair, or the sum of what is known about the hair.

trichoma (tri-ko′mah) entropion.

trichomadesis (trik″o-mah-de′sis) abnormally rapid or premature loss of hair from the scalp; called also *lipsotrichia* and *trichorrhea*.

trichomania (trik″o-ma′ne-ah) trichotillomania.

trichomatous (trĭ-kom′ah-tus) affected with, of the nature of, or pertaining to trichoma (entropion).

trichome (tri′kōm) [Gr. *trichōma* a growth of hair, hair generally] 1. a filamentous or hairlike structure. 2. a colony of filamentous blue-green algae in which the member cells grow end-to-end to form a chain-like structure.

trichomegaly (trik″o-meg′ah-le) [*tricho-* + Gr. *megalē* large] a congenital syndrome consisting of excessive growth of the eyelashes and brow hair associated with dwarfism, mental retardation, and pigmentary degeneration of the retina.

trichomonacidal (trik″o-mo′nah-si′dal) destructive to trichomonads.

trichomonacide (trik″o-mo′nah-sīd) an agent destructive to trichomonads.

trichomonad (trik″o-mo′nad, trik″o-mon′ad, trĭ-kom′o-nad) a parasite of the genus Trichomonas.

trichomonadicidal (trik″o-mo-nad″ĭ-si′dal) trichomonacidal.

trichomonal (trik″o-mo′nal, trik″o-mon′al, trĭ-kom′o-nal) pertaining to or caused by trichomonads.

Trichomonas (trik″o-mo′nas, trik″o-mon′as, trĭ-kom′o-nas) [*tricho-* + Gr. *monas* unit] a genus of parasitic flagellate protozoa of the order Polymastigida, class Zoomastigophora, occurring in the form of pear-shaped cells having four flagella in front, an undulating membrane, and a trailing flagellum. They cause rather serious disease in animals and birds and urogenital infection in man; called also *Pentatrichomonas* and *Tritrichomonas*. **T. bucca′lis,** *T. tenax.* **T. colum′bae, T.**

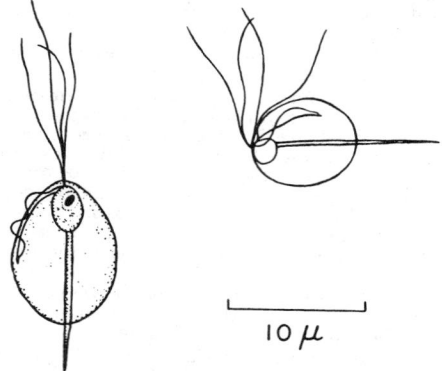

Trichomonas vaginalis; permanently stained preparation (Markell and Voge).

10 μ

columba′rum, *T. gallinae.* **T. elonga′ta,** *T. tenax.* **T. foe′tus,** a species parasitic in the genital tract of cattle, which causes abortion in infected animals. **T. gal′linae,** a species causing lesions in the upper digestive tract, liver, and pancreas of various birds, especially pigeons; sometimes fatal to the host. Called also *T. columbae* and *T. columbarum.* **T. gallina′rum,** a species found in the lower digestive tract, particularly the liver and cecum, of galliform birds, especially turkeys, producing drowsiness and liquid yellow droppings; it is often fatal to young turkeys. **T. homi′nis,** a common parasite in the intestine of man, which is not thought to be pathogenic; formerly called *Cercomonas hominis.* **T. intestina′lis,** *T. hominis.* **T. mu′ris,** a species found in the cecum of the rat. **T. pulmona′lis,** a name given to *T. tenax* isolated from pulmonary abscesses. **T. te′nax,** a nonpathogenic form found in the human mouth, especially about the tartar of the teeth; called also *T. buccalis, T. elongata,* and *Tetratrichomonas buccalis.* **T. vagina′lis,** a species found in the vagina, which produces a refractory vaginal discharge; it has also been found in the bladder and urethra of the male.

trichomoniasis (trik″o-mo-ni′ah-sis) infection with Trichomonas.

Trichomycetes (trik″o-mi-se′tēs) [*tricho-* + Gr. *mykēs* fungus] a group of organisms with a simple or branched thallus attached by a basal cell to the digestive tract or external cuticle of living arthropods. In some classifications, they are included in the Phycomycetes, and are also called *Microsiphonales.*

trichomycosis (trik″o-mi-ko′sis) [*tricho-* + Gr. *mykēs* fungus] any disease of the hair due to infection by a fungus. **t. axilla′ris, t. chromat′ica,** a minor infection of the axillary and sometimes of the pubic hairs, caused by *Corynebacterium tenuis* and not a fungus, as originally thought, which led to the name; occurring commonly in the tropics, it is characterized by development of dense colonies of bacteria on the hairs, appearing as yellow, red, or black nodules. **t. favo′sa,** favus. **t. nodo′sa, t. palmelli′na** (*obs.*), t. axillaris. **t. ru′bra** (*obs.*), t. axillaris characterized by red nodules.

trichon (trik′on) an autolyzed preparation of the fungi of the genus Trichophyton.

trichonodosis (trik″o-no-do′sis) a rare condition characterized by apparent or actual knotting of the hair, thought to be the result of inability of new hairs to grow freely from their follicles, because of toughness of the surrounding tissues.

trichopathic (trik″o-path′ik) pertaining to disease of the hair.

trichopathy (trĭ-kop′ah-the) [*tricho-* + Gr. *pathos* disease] disease of the hair.

trichophagy (tri-kof′ah-je) [*tricho-* + Gr. *phagein* to eat] the practice or habit of eating hair.

trichophytic (trik″o-fit′ik) pertaining to trichophytosis.

trichophytid (trĭ-kof′ĭ-tid) a secondary skin eruption that is the expression of an allergic reaction to a trichophyton infection occurring in an area far from the site of infection.

trichophytin (trĭ-kof′ĭ-tin) the soluble broth culture products of various species of *Trichophyton;* used in the trichophytin test.

trichophytobezoar (trik″o-fi″to-be′zōr) [*tricho-* + Gr. *phyton* plant + *bezoar*] a bezoar composed of animal hair and vegetable fibers.

Trichophyton (tri-kof′ĭ-ton) [*tricho-* + Gr. *phyton* plant] a genus of imperfect fungi of the order Moniliales, family Moniliaceae, consisting of flat, branched filaments and various types of spores. Species of *Trichophyton* attack the skin, nails, and hair (dermatophytes). As the perfect (sexual) stages are identified they are classified in the genus *Arthroderma.* The common species include *T. mentagrophy′tes, T. ru′brum, T. ton′surans, T. schoenlei′ni, T. concen′tricum, T. ferrugin′eum, T. viola′ceum, T. galli′nae,* and *T. sim′ii.*

trichophytosis (trik″o-fi-to′sis) a fungal infection caused by species of *Trichophyton.*

Trichoptera (tri-kop′ter-ah) [*tricho-* + Gr. *pteron* wing] an order of flies, the caddis flies. The hair and scales from the wings may produce allergic symptoms in susceptible persons.

trichoptilosis (trik″o-tĭ-lo′sis) [*tricho-* + Gr. *ptilon* feather + -*osis*] the condition in which the hairs are split and feather-like.

trichorrhea (trik″o-re′ah) [*tricho-* + Gr. *rhoia* flow] trichomadesis.

trichorrhexis (trik″o-rek′sis) [*tricho-* + Gr. *rhēxis* fracture] a condition in which the hairs break. **t. nodo′sa,** a condition characterized by what appear to be white nodes on the hairs but are actually sites where the cortex of the shaft has fractured and split into strands, weakening the hairs so they break at these nodes. Called also *bamboo hair.*

trichoschisis (trik-os′kĭ-sis) [*tricho-* + Gr. *schisis* fissure] splitting of the hairs.

trichoscopy (trĭ-kos′ko-pe) [*tricho-* + Gr. *skopein* to examine] examination of the hair.

trichosiderin (trik″o-sid′er-in) [*tricho-* + Gr. *sidēros* iron] an iron-containing brown pigment found in normal human red hair.

trichosis (tri-ko′sis) [Gr. *trichōsis*] any disease or abnormal growth of the hair. **t. carun′culae,** abnormal development of the hair on the lacrimal caruncle.

Trichosoma (trik″o-so′mah) [*tricho-* + Gr. *sōma* body] *Capillaria.* **T. contor′tum,** *Capillaria contorta.*

Trichosomoides (trik″o-so-moi′dēz) a genus of nematode parasites. **T. crassicau′da,** a nematode parasite of rats; the male is much smaller than the female, and is parasitic in the rat vagina or uterus.

Trichosporon (tri-kos′po-ron) [*tricho-* + Gr. *sporos* seed] a genus of imperfect fungi of the family Cryptococcaceae, order Moniliales, which are normal flora of the respiratory and digestive tract of man and animals, and may infect the hair. **T. beigel′ii,** *T. cutaneum.* **T. cuta′neum,** the etiologic agent of white piedra. It is a normal inhabitant of the skin and the respiratory and intestinal tracts, and rarely an opportunistic agent in debilitated patients, causing a fatal systemic infection. Called also *T. biegelii* and *T. giganteum.* **T. gigan′teum,** *T. cutaneum.* **T. pedrosia′num,** *Fonsecaea pedrosoi.*

trichosporosis (trik″o-spo-ro′sis) infestation with *Trichosporon;* see *piedra.* **t. in′dica, t. nodo′sa, t. trop′ica,** piedra.

Trichosporum (tri-kos′po-rum) *Trichosporon.*

trichostasis spinulosa (trī-kos′tah-sis spin″u-lo′sa) [*tricho-* + Gr. *stasis* a standing] a disorder in which the hair follicles appear to be obstructed with a spinulous dark plug, consisting of numerous lanugo hairs in a horny mass. The skin of the alae nasi and other areas of the face, or of the arms, chest, abdomen, or interscapular area may be affected.

trichostrongyliasis (trik″o-stron″jĭ-li′ah-sis) infection by nematodes of the genus *Trichostrongylus,* whose eggs are often mistaken for those of the hookworm. It is usually asymptomatic, but diarrhea may occur.

Trichostrongylidae (trik″o-stron-jil′ĭ-de) a family of nematodes of the superfamily Strongyloidea, including the genera *Trichostrongylus, Haemonchus, Nippostrongylus,* and *Nematodirus.*

trichostrongylosis (trik″o-stron″jĭ-lo′sis) infestation with *Trichostrongylus.*

Trichostrongylus (trik″o-stron′jĭ-lus) a genus of nematode worms (family Trichostrongylidae), comprising some of the species formerly included in the genus *Strongylus.* Adult worms are small and embed their heads in the mucosa of the small intestine; their eggs are often mistaken for those of the hookworm. Infection is usually asymptomatic. **T. caprico′la,** a species commonly found in ruminants. **T. colubriform′is,** a species frequently present in sheep and goats and occasionally in man; called also *Strongylus subtilis* and *T. instabilis.* **T. insta′bilis,** *T. colubriformis.* **T. orienta′lis,** a species found in man in Asia. **T. probolu′rus,** a species found in sheep, mountain goats, dromedaries, gazelles, and occasionally man in Europe, Africa, and North America. **T. vitri′nus,** a species found in sheep, goats, dromedaries, and occasionally in man.

Trichothecium (trik″o-the′se-um) [*tricho-* + Gr. *thēkē* case] a genus of imperfect fungi of the order Moniliales, family Moniliaceae. **T. ro′seum,** a species causing pinkrot of apples, lumber, etc., and very rarely recovered from otitis externa and mycotic keratitis.

trichotillomania (trik″o-til″o-ma′ne-ah) [*tricho-* + Gr. *tillein* to pull + *mania* madness] a morbid impulse to pull out one's own hair; trichologia.

trichotomous (tri-kot′o-mus) [Gr. *tricha* three-fold + *tomē* a cutting] divided into three parts.

trichotoxin (tri″ko-tok′sin) an antibody that has a toxic action on epithelial cells.

trichroic (tri-kro′ik) pertaining to or characterized by trichroism.

trichroism (tri′kro-izm) [*tri-* + Gr. *chroa* color] the exhibition of three different colors in three different aspects.

trichromat (tri′kro-mat) a person who has normal color vision.

trichromatic (tri″kro-mat′ik) trichromic.

trichromatism (tri-kro′mah-tizm) trichroism.

trichromatopsia (tri″kro-mah-top′se-ah) [*trichroic* + Gr. *opsis* vision + *-ia*] ability to see all three primary colors; normal color vision (Hering).

trichromic (tri-kro′mik) [*tri-* + Gr. *chrōma* color] 1. pertaining to or exhibiting three colors. 2. able to distinguish only three of the seven colors of the spectrum.

trichterbrust (trich′ter-broost) [Ger.] funnel chest.

trichuriasis (trik″u-ri′ah-sis) the state of being infected with nematodes of the genus *Trichuris.*

Trichuris (trik-u′ris) [*tricho-* + Gr. *oura* a tail] a genus of intestinal nematode parasites of the superfamily Trichuroidea. **T. trichiu′ra,** the species that principally infects man. It is about 2 inches in length, the front portion of its body, the esophageal zone, being hairlike in slimness. It inhabits the large intestine, and may cause diarrhea, vomiting, and rectal prolapse

in children heavily infected, although it usually produces no symptoms. Also known as *whipworm.*

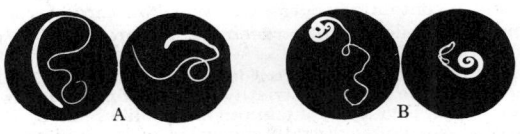

Trichuris trichiura: A, females; B, males. The posterior portion of the male is usually coiled as shown in B. Photographs of mounted specimens; natural size (Todd).

Trichuroidea (trik″u-roi′de-ah) a superfamily of aphasmid nematodes including the genera *Capillaria, Trichinella,* and *Trichuris.*

tricipital (tri-sip′ĭ-tal) [L. *tricipitis*] 1. pertaining to the triceps muscle. 2. having three heads.

triclobisonium chloride (tri″klo-bĭ-so′ne-um) chemical name: *N,N,N′,N′*-trimethyl-*N,N′*-bis[1-methyl-3-(2,2,6-trimethyl-cyclohexyl)propyl]-1,6-hexanediaminium dichloride. A quaternary ammonium compound, $C_{36}H_{74}Cl_2N_2$, occurring as a white, crystalline powder; used as a local anti-infective, primarily in the treatment of vulvitis, vaginitis, and other gynecological conditions due to *Trichomonas vaginalis, Candida albicans,* and *Hemophilus vaginalis* or to staphylococci and streptococci, administered intravaginally.

triclocarban (tri″klo-kar′ban) chemical name: *N*-(4-chloro-phenyl)-*N′*-(3,4-dichlorophenyl)urea. A disinfectant, $C_{13}H_9Cl_3N_2O$, effective against gram-positive bacteria and to a lesser extent against gram-negative bacteria and against fungi; used in the preparation of soaps and other cleansing products and dermatological compositions to control skin infections.

triclofenol piperazine (tri-klo′fen-ōl) chemical name: 2,4,5-trichlorophenol compound with piperazine (2:1); an anthelmintic, $C_4H_{10}N_2 \cdot 2C_6H_3Cl_3O$, effective against roundworms and hookworms.

triclofos sodium (tri′klo-fōs) chemical name: 2,2,2-trichloro-ethanol dihydrogen phosphate monosodium salt; an oral hypnotic and sedative, $C_2H_3Cl_3NaO_4P$, used especially to induce sleep in the treatment of insomnia. It may also be used as premedication for sleep induction in electroencephalography.

triclonide (tri-klo′nid) chemical name: 9,11β,21-trichloro-6α-fluoro-16α,17-[(1-methylethylidene)bis(oxy)]pregna-1,4-diene-3,-20-dione; an anti-inflammatory, $C_{24}H_{28}Cl_3FO_4$.

Triclos (tri′klōs) trademark for a preparation of triclofos sodium.

triclosan (tri-klo′san) chemical name: 5-chloro-2-(2,4-dichloro-phenoxy)phenol. An antibacterial, $C_{12}H_7Cl_3O_2$, effective against gram-positive and most gram-negative organisms and exhibiting slight activity against yeasts and fungi; used as a detergent in surgical scrubs, soaps, and deodorants.

Tricofuron (tri′ko-fu′ron) trademark for preparations of furazolidone.

Tricoloid (tri′ko-loid) trademark for a preparation of tricyclamol chloride.

tricorn (tri′korn) [*tri-* + L. *cornu* horn] a lateral ventricle of the brain.

tricornute (tri-kor′nūt) [*tri-* + L. *cornutus* horned] having three horns, cornua, or processes.

tricresol (tri-kre′sol) cresol.

tricrotic (tri-krot′ik) [Gr. *trikrotos* rowed with a triple stroke; triple beating] pertaining to or characterized by tricrotism.

tricrotism (tri′kro-tizm) the quality of having three sphygmographic waves or elevations to one beat of the pulse.

tricuspid (tri-kus′pid) [L. *tricuspis*] 1. having three points or cusps. 2. pertaining to the tricuspid valves of the heart.

tricyclamol chloride (tri-si′klah-mol) chemical name: 1-(3-cyclohexyl-3-hydroxy-3-phenylpropyl)-1-methyl pyrrolidinium chloride. A quaternary ammonium anticholinergic derived from procyclidine, $C_{20}H_{32}ClNO$, which inhibits gastrointestinal hypermotility and reduces secretion of gastric juices; it has been used in the treatment of peptic ulcer and as a gastrointestinal antispasmodic.

tricyclic (tri-sik′lik) containing three fused rings or closed chains in the molecular structure; see also under *antidepressant.*

Trid. abbreviation for L. *trid′uum,* three days.

tridactylism (tri-dak′tĭ-lizm) [*tri-* + Gr. *daktylos* finger] the condition of having only three digits on one hand or foot.

tridactylous (tri-dak′tĭ-lus) pertaining to or characterized by tridactylism.

trident, tridentate (tri′dent; tri-den′tāt) three pronged.

tridermic (tri-der′mik) [*tri-* + Gr. *derma* skin] derived from the ectoderm, endoderm, and mesoderm.

tridermogenesis (tri″der-mo-jen′ĕ-sis) [*tri-* + Gr. *derma* skin + *genesis* production] the formation of the three germ layers and, by extension, the stage in embryonic development during which it occurs.

tridermoma (tri″der-mo′mah) [*tri-* + Gr. *derma* skin + *-oma*] a teratoma containing representatives of all three germ layers.

Tridesilon (tri-des′ĭ-lon)   trademark for preparations of desonide.

tridihexethyl chloride (tri″di-heks-eth′il) [USP]   chemical name: γ-cyclohexyl-*N,N,N*-triethyl-γ-hydroxybenzenepropanaminium. A quaternary ammonium anticholinergic, $C_{21}H_{36}ClNO$, occurring as a white, crystalline powder, which inhibits gastrointestinal hypermotility and spasms and reduces secretion of gastric juices; used as adjunctive therapy in the treatment of peptic ulcer and in the irritable bowel syndrome, administered orally and parenterally.

Tridione (tri-di′ōn)   trademark for preparations of trimethadione.

tridymite (trid′ĭ-mīt)   a rare crystalline form of silica, SiO_2, obtainable from quartz by heating.

triencephalus (tri″en-sef′ah-lus) [*tri-* + Gr. *enkephalos* brain] a monster having no organs of sight, hearing, or smell.

-triene (tri′ēn)   a chemical suffix indicating the presence of three double bonds.

triester (tri′es-ter)   a compound containing three ester groups.

triethanolamine (tri″eth-ah-nōl′ah-mēn)   1. an alkanolamine produced by ammonolysis of ethylene oxide. 2. trolamine.

triethylamine (tri″eth-il-am′in)   a somewhat poisonous, oily liquid ptomaine, $N(C_2H_5)_3$, with an ammoniacal smell, derived from decaying fish.

triethylenemelamine (tri-eth″ĭ-lēn-mel′ah-mēn)   chemical name: 2,4,6-tris(1-aziridinyl)-1,3,5-triazine. A cytotoxic alkylating agent, $C_9H_{12}N_6$, occurring as a white, crystalline powder; used as an antineoplastic in the palliative treatment of certain cancers of the lymphatic and hematopoietic systems, such as Hodgkin's disease, leukemia, retinoblastoma, and lymphosarcoma, administered orally. Called also *TEM*.

triethylenethiophosphoramide (tri-eth″ĭ-lēn-thi″o-fos-fōr′-ah-mīd)   thiotepa.

trifacial (tri-fa′shal) [L. *trifacialis*]   designating the fifth cranial nerve (nervus trigeminus [NA]).

trifid (tri′fid) [L. *trifidus,* from *tres* three + *findere* to split]   split into three parts.

triflocin (tri-flo′sin)   chemical name: 4-(α,α,α-trifluoro-*m*-toluidino)nicotinic acid; a diuretic, $C_{13}H_9F_3N_2O$.

triflumidate (tri-floo′mĭ-dāt)   chemical name: ethyl *m*-benzoyl-*N*-(trifluoromethyl)sulfonyl]carbanilate; an anti-inflammatory, $C_{17}H_{14}F_3NO_5S$.

trifluoperazine hydrochloride (tri″floo-o-pār′ah-zēn) [USP]   chemical name: 10-[3-(4-methyl-1-piperazinyl)propyl]-2-(trifluoromethyl)-10*H*-phenothiazine dihydrochloride. An antipsychotic agent, $C_{21}H_{24}F_3N_3S \cdot 2HCl$, occurring as a white to pale yellow, crystalline powder; administered orally and intramuscularly.

trifluperidol (tri-flu-per′ĭ-dol)   chemical name: 4′-fluoro-4-[4-hydroxy-4-(α,α,α-trifluoro-*m*-tolyl)piperidino]butyrophenone; a tranquilizer, $C_{22}H_{23}F_4NO_2$, which has been used in the treatment of mania and schizophrenia.

triflupromazine (tri″floo-pro′mah-zēn) [USP]   chemical name: *N,N*-dimethyl-2-(trifluoromethyl)-10*H*-phenothiazine-10-propanamine. An antipsycotic agent, $C_{18}H_{19}F_3N_2S \cdot HCl$, occurring as a viscous, light amber-colored, oily liquid, which crystalizes on long standing to large irregular crystals; administered orally. **t. hydrochloride** [USP], the monohydrochloride salt of triflupromazine, $C_{18}H_{19}F_3N_2S \cdot HCl$, occurring as a white to pale tan, crystalline powder; administered orally and intramuscularly.

trifluridine (tri-floor′ĭ-den)   chemical name: α,α,α-trifluorothymidine; an antiviral for use in ophthalmology, $C_{10}H_{11}F_3N_2O_5$.

trifluromethylthiazide (tri-floor″o-meth″il-thi′ah-zīd)   flumethiazide.

trifoliosis (tri″fo-le-o′sis)   a disease of horses marked by irritation of the skin and of the mucous membrane of the mouth and by general disturbance; attributed to the eating of hybrid clover.

trifurcation (tri″fur-ka′shun) [*tri-* + L. *furca* fork]   division into three branches.

trigastric (tri-gas′trik) [*tri-* + Gr. *gastēr* belly]   having three bellies; said of a muscle.

trigeminal (tri-jem′ĭ-nal) [*tri-* + L. *geminus* twin]   1. triple. 2. pertaining to the fifth cranial nerve (nervus trigeminus [NA]).

trigeminus (tri-jem′ĭ-nus) [L.]   triple; see *nervus trigeminus.*

trigeminy (tri-jem′ĭ-ne)   the condition of occurring in threes, especially the occurrence of three pulse beats in rapid succession; see *trigeminal pulse,* under *pulse.*

trigenic (tri-jen′ik)   possessing three different alleles at any particular locus on the chromosome.

triglyceride (tri-glis′er-īd)   a compound consisting of three molecules of fatty acid esterified to glycerol; it is a neutral fat synthesized from carbohydrates for storage in animal adipose cells. On enzymatic hydrolysis, it releases free fatty acids in the blood.

trigocephalus (tri″go-sef′ah-lus)   trigonocephalus.

trigona (tri-go′nah) [L.]   plural of *trigonum.*

trigonal (tri′go-nal)   triangular; pertaining to a trigone.

trigone (tri′gōn)   1. a triangular area (trigonum [NA]); see also *triangle.* 2. the first three cusps of an upper molar tooth; see *hypocone, paracone,* and *protocone.* **t. of bladder,** trigonum vesicae. **carotid t.,** trigonum caroticum. **cerebral t.,** fornix cerebri. **collateral t.,** trigonum collaterale. **collateral t. of fourth ventricle,** trigonum nervi vagi. **femoral t.,** trigonum femorale. **fibrous t's of heart,** trigona fibrosa cordis. **t. of habenula, habenular t.,** trigonum habenulae. **Henke's t.,** Henke's triangle. **t. of hypoglossal nerve,** trigonum nervi hypoglossi. **iliopectineal t.,** fossa iliopectinea. **inguinal t.,** trigonum inguinale. **interpeduncular t.,** fossa interpeduncularis. **lumbar t.,** trigonum lumbale. **olfactory t.,** trigonum olfactorium. **omoclavicular t.,** trigonum omoclaviculare. **Pawlik's t.,** Pawlik's triangle. **t. of Reil,** trigonum lemnisci. **submandibular t.,** trigonum submandibulare. **urogenital t.,** diaphragma urogenitale. **t. of vagus nerve,** trigonum nervi vagi. **vesical t.,** trigonum vesicae.

trigonectomy (tri″gōn-ek′to-me) [*trigone* + Gr. *ektomē* excision]   excision of the base of the bladder (trigonum vesicae).

trigonelline (trig″o-nel′in)   an alkaloid, $C_7H_7NO_2$, found in fenugreek, cannabis, strophanthus, and various other plants, in sea urchins and jellyfish, and also in the urine after administration of nicotinic acid. It is a betaine of methyl nicotinic acid.

trigonid (tri-gon′id)   the first three cusps of a lower molar tooth. See *hypoconid, paraconid,* and *protoconid.*

trigonitis (trig″o-ni′tis) [*trigone* + *-itis*]   inflammation or localized hyperemia of the trigone of the bladder.

trigonocephalia (trig″o-no-sĕ-fa′le-ah)   trigonocephaly.

trigonocephalic (trig″o-no-sĕ-fal′ik)   pertaining to or characterized by trigonocephaly.

trigonocephalus (trig″o-no-sef′ah-lus)   an individual exhibiting trigonocephaly.

trigonocephaly (trig-go″no-sef′ah-le) [Gr. *trigonos* triangular + *kephalē* head]   a deformity of the head characterized by sharp angulation ventrad of the squamous portion of the frontal bones at the site of the suture between them.

trigonotome (tri-go″no-tōm)   an instrument for cutting the trigone of the bladder.

trigonum (tri-go′num), pl. *trigo′na* [L.; Gr. *trigōnon* triangle]   a three-cornered area; [NA] a general term for a triangular area. Called also *triangle* and *trigone.* **t. acus′tici,** area vestibularis. **t. carot′icum** [NA], carotid trigone: the triangular region bounded by the posterior belly of the digastric muscle, the sternocleidomastoid muscle, and the anterior midline of the neck; called also *fossa carotica.* **t. cerebra′le,** fornix cerebri. **t. cervica′le,** 1. t. caroticum. 2. t. omoclaviculare. **t. collatera′le** [NA], collateral trigone: the triangular area in the floor of the lateral ventricle between the diverging inferior and posterior horns. **t. collatera′le ventric′uli quar′ti,** t. nervi vagi. **t. col′li latera′le,** regio colli lateralis. **t. coracoacromia′le,** a triangle bounded by the coracoid process, the apex of the acromion, and the concave border of the clavicle. **t. deltoideopectora′le,** the deeper part of the infraclavicular region which is exposed by dissection. **t. femora′le** [NA], femoral trigone: a triangular area bounded superiorly by the inguinal ligament, laterally by the sartorius muscle, and medially by the adductor longus muscle; called also *Scarpa's triangle.* **trigo′na fibro′sa cor′dis** [NA], fibrous trigones of heart: two thickened and irregularly triangular portions of the fibrous skeleton of the base of the heart, one located between the right and left atrioventricular fibrous rings, posterior to the aortic orifice, and the other between the left atrioventricular fibrous ring and the left posterior margin of the aortic fibrous ring. **t. haben′ulae** [NA], trigone of habenula: the small, depressed triangular area on the dorsomedial aspect of the posterior part of the thalamus which contains the habenular nuclei and marks the habenular commissure. **t. inguina′le** [NA], inguinal trigone: the area on the inferoanterior abdominal wall bounded by the rectus abdominis muscle, the inguinal ligament, and the inferior epigastric vessels: the site in which a direct inguinal hernia begins. **t. interpeduncula′re,** fossa interpeduncularis. **t. lemnis′ci,** a small, more or less distinct triangular area on the side of the isthmus just lateral to the inferior colliculus, bounded below by the superior cerebellar peduncle, dorsomedially by the brachium colliculi inferioris, and anterolaterally by the sulcus lateralis mesencephali. **t. lumba′le** [NA], **t. lumba′le [Peti′ti],** lumbar trigone: a small triangular interval between the inferolateral margin of the latissimus dorsi muscle and the external oblique muscle of the abdomen, just above the ilium; called also *Petit's triangle.* **t. lumbocosta′le,** a triangular opening of variable size between the lateral lumbocostal arch and the pars costalis diaphragmatis. **t. ner′vi hypoglos′si** [NA], trigone of hypoglossal nerve: the tapering lower end of the medial eminence of the rhomboid fossa just superficial to the position of the hypoglossal nucleus. **t. ner′vi va′gi** [NA], trigone of vagus nerve: an area in the floor of the fourth ventricle immediately lateral to the trigonum nerve hypoglossi; beneath it lies the dorsal nucleus of the vagus nerve. Called also *ala cinerea.* **t. olfacto′rium** [NA], olfactory trigone: the area of the anterior perforated substance between the diverging lateral and medial olfactory striae, and bounded posteriorly by the diagonal band. **t. omoclavicula′re** [NA], omoclavicular trigone: a deep region of the neck, corresponding to the fossa supraclavicularis major on the surface, in which the brachial plexus may be palpated, and by downward pressure the subclavian artery can be compressed against the first rib; called also *subclavian triangle.* **t. sternocosta′le,** sternocostal triangle: a triangular opening between the pars costalis and the pars sternalis diaphragmatis; beyond this point the internal thoracic vessels become the superior epigastric vessels. Called also *Larrey′s cleft.* **t. submandibula′re** [NA], submandibular trigone: the triangular region of the neck bounded by the mandible, the stylohyoid muscle and posterior belly of the digastric muscle, and the anterior belly of the digastric muscle; called also *regio submaxillaris.* **t. urogenita′le,** diaphragma urogenitale. **t. va′gi,** t. nervi vagi. **t. ventric′uli latera′lis,** t. collaterale. **t. vesi′cae** [NA], **t. vesi′cae [Lieutau′di],** trigone of bladder: a smooth triangular portion of the mucous membrane at the base of the bladder; it is bounded behind by the interureteric fold and ends in front in the uvula of the bladder.

trihexyphenidyl hydrochloride (tri-hek″se-fen′ĭ-dil) [USP] chemical name: α-cyclohexyl-α-phenyl-1-piperidinepropanol hydrochloride. An anticholinergic, $C_{20}H_{31}NO \cdot HCl$, occurring as a white or slightly off-white crystalline powder, having atropine-like actions; used as an oral antiparkinsonian agent.

trihybrid (tri-hi′brid) a hybrid offspring of parents differing in three mendelian characters.

trihydrate (tri-hi′drāt) trihydroxide; a compound containing three hydroxyl groups.

trihydric (tri-hi′drik) containing three hydrogen atoms that are replaceable by bases.

trihydrol (tri-hi′drol) the associated water or ice molecule, $(H_2O)_3$.

trihydroxide (tri″hi-drok′sīd) trihydrate.

trihydroxyestrin (tri″hi-drok″se-es′trin) estriol.

tri-iniodymus (tri″in-e-od′ĭ-mus) [*tri-* + Gr. *inion* nape of the neck + *didymos* twin] a monster with a single body and three heads united posteriorly.

triiodide (tri-i′o-dīd) a compound containing three atoms of iodine to one of another element.

triiodomethane (tri-i″o-do-meth′ān) iodoform.

triiodothyronine (tri″i-o″do-thi′ro-nēn) one of the thyroid hormones: an organic iodine-containing compound liberated from thyroglobulin by hydrolysis, and thought to be formed by the conjugation of one molecule each of monoiodotyrosine and diiodotyrosine, or by the partial deiodination of thyroxine. It has several times the biological activity of thyroxine. Symbol T_3.

triketohydrindene hydrate (tri-ke″to-hi-drin′dēn) chemical name: 1,2,3-indantrione monohydrate. A compound, $C_9H_4O_3 \cdot H_2O$, occurring as white to brownish white crystals or crystalline powder, used as a reagent. See under *tests.*

triketopurine (tri″ke-to-pu′rin) uric acid.

trilabe (tri′lāb) [*tri-* + Gr. *labē* a handle] a three-pronged instrument for taking calculi from the bladder.

Trilafon (tri′lah-fon) trademark for preparations of perphenazine.

trilaminar (tri-lam′ĭ-nar) consisting of three layers.

trilateral (tri-lat′er-al) [*tri-* + L. *latus* side] having or pertaining to three sides.

trilaurin (tri-law′rin) a crystalline glyceride, $C_3H_5(OC_{12}H_{23}O)_3$, forming the principal constituent of coconut oil, and found in bayberry oil and palm nut oil.

Trilene (tri′lēn) trademark for a preparation of trichloroethylene.

trilinolein (tri″lin-o′le-in) a glyceride, $C_3H_5(OC_{18}H_{32}O)_3$, found in linseed oil, hempseed oil, sunflower oil, etc.

Trilisate (tril′ĭ-sāt) trademark for choline magnesium trisalicylate.

trilliin (tril′e-in) a concentration prepared from *Trillium erectum* L. (Liliaceae), a North American plant.

Trillium (tril′e-um) a genus of liliaceous plants. **T. erec′tum** L., wake-robin; the rhizome contains trilliin.

trilobate (tri-lo′bāt) [*tri-* + L. *lobus* lobe] having three lobes.

trilobectomy (tri″lo-bek′to-me) excision of three pulmonary lobes, two from one lung and one from the other.

trilobed (tri′lōbd) trilobate.

trilocular (tri-lok′u-lar) [*tri-* + L. *loculus* cell] having three compartments or cells.

trilogy (tril′o-je) a combination of three elements, such as three concurrent defects or symptoms. **t. of Fallot,** a term sometimes applied to the combination of pulmonic stenosis, atrial septal defect, and right ventricular hypertrophy.

trilostane (tri′lo-stān) chemical name: 4α,5-epoxy-17β-hydroxy-3-oxo-5α-androstane-2α-carbonitrile; an adrenocortical suppressant, $C_{20}H_{27}NO_3$.

trimanual (tri-man′u-al) [*tri-* + L. *manus* hand] accomplished by the use of three hands.

Trimastigamoeba (tri-mas″tĭg-ah-me′bah) a genus of amebae of the order Amoebida, class Rhizopoda, found in stagnant water, and having both an ameboid and a flagellate stage during its life history; in the latter stage it possesses three equal flagella. *T. philippen′sis* has been obtained in culture from city water.

trimastigote (tri-mas′tĭ-gōt) 1. having three flagella. 2. a cell having three flagella.

trimazosin hydrochloride (tri-ma′zo-sin) chemical name: 4-(4-amino-6,7,8-trimethoxy-2-quinazolinyl)-1-piperazine carboxylic acid 2-hydroxy-2-methylpropyl ester monohydrochloride monohydrate; an antihypertensive, $C_{20}H_{29}N_5O_6 \cdot HCl \cdot H_2O$.

trimenon (tri-me′non) [*tri-* + Gr. *mēn* month + *on* neuter ending] trimester.

trimensual (tri-men′su-al) occurring every three months.

trimeprazine tartrate (tri-mep′rah-zēn) [USP] chemical name: N,N,β-trimethyl-10H-phenothiazine-10-propanamine [R-(R*,R*)]-2,3-dihydroxybutanedioate (2:1). A phenothiazine derivative, $(C_{18}H_{22}N_2S)_2 \cdot C_4H_6O_6$, occurring as a white to off-white, crystalline powder, having mild central nervous system depressant, moderate antiemetic and anticonvulsant properties, and powerful antihistaminic actions; used as an antipruritic, administered orally.

trimer (tri′mer) 1. a compound formed by combination of three identical simpler molecules. 2. a capsomere having three structural units.

trimercuric (tri″mer-ku′rik) containing three atoms of bivalent mercury.

Trimeresurus (trim″ĕ-rē-su′rus) a genus of venomous pit vipers of East and Southeast Asia, which are usually green and possess a prehensile tail. *T. flavorvi′ridis* is the habu.

trimeric (tri′mer-ik) exhibiting the characteristics of a trimer.

trimester (tri-mes′ter) a period of three months.

trimetaphosphatase (tri″met-ah-fos′fah-tās) an enzyme occurring in the liver and kidneys that catalyzes the hydrolysis of trimetaphosphate to triphosphate.

trimethadione (tri″meth-ah-di′ōn) [USP] chemical name: 3,5,5-trimethyl-2,4-oxazolidinedione. An anticonvulsant with analgesic properties, $C_8H_9NO_3$, occurring as white, crystalline granules; used for the control of petit mal seizures, administered orally. In veterinary medicine, used as an anticonvulsant-analgesic for cats. Called also *troxidone.*

trimethaphan camsylate (tri-meth′ah-fan) [USP] chemical name: decahydro-2-oxo-1,3-bis(phenylmethyl)thieno[1′,2′:1,2]thieno[3,4]imidazol-5-ium salt with (+)-7-7-dimethyl-2-oxobicyclo-[2.2.1]heptane-1-methanesulfonic acid (1:1). A short-acting ganglionic blocking agent with direct vasodilator action, $C_{32}H_{40}N_2O_5S_2$, occurring as white crystals or white, crystalline powder; used as an antihypertensive to produce controlled hypotension during surgery and for the emergency treatment of hypertensive crises and pulmonary edema due to hypertension, administered by intravenous infusion. Called also *t. camphorsulfonate.*

trimethidinium methosulfate (tri-meth′ĭ-din′e-um) chemical name: 1,3,8,8-tetramethyl-3-[3-(trimethylammonio)propyl]-3-azoniabicyclo[3.2.1]octane bis(methyl sulfate). A quaternary ammonium ganglion blocking agent, $C_{19}H_{46}N_2O_8S_2$, occurring as a white, hygroscopic powder, used as an oral antihypertensive in the treatment of moderate to severe hypertension in certain patients.

trimethobenzamide hydrochloride (tri-meth″o-ben′zah-mīd) [USP] chemical name: N-[[4-[2-(dimethylamino)ethoxy]phenyl]methyl]-3,4,5-trimethoxybenzamide monohydrochloride. An antiemetic, $C_{21}H_{28}N_2O_5 \cdot HCl$, occurring as a white, crystalline powder; administered orally, intramuscularly, or rectally.

trimethoprim (tri-meth′o-prim) [USP] chemical name: 5-[3,4,5-trimethoxyphenyl)methyl]-2,4-pyrimidinediamine. An antibacterial, $C_{14}H_{18}N_4O_3$, closely related to the antimalarial pyrimethamine; administered orally, in combination with a sulfonamide because the two drugs markedly potentiate each other, in the treatment of urinary tract infections due to *Escherichia coli, Klebsiella-Enterobacter* group, *Proteus vulgaris, P. mirabilis,* and *P. morganii,* and in *Pneumocystic carinii* pneumonitis in children with reduced host defenses. In certain countries, it is used alone as an antimalarial.

trimethylamine (tri″meth-il-am′in) a colorless gaseous (boiling point 3.2°–3.8° C.) tertiary amine, $(CH_3)_3N$, with an ammoniacal, fishy odor, from beet sugar residue and herring brine. In the body it probably results from the decomposition of choline; it has been reported in menstrual blood.

trimethylene (tri-meth′ĭ-lēn) cyclopropane.

trimethylxanthine (tri-meth″il-zan′thin) caffeine.

trimetozine (tri-met′o-zēn) chemical name: 4-(3,4,5-trimethoxybenzoyl)morpholine; a sedative, $C_{14}H_{19}NO_5$.

trimipramine (tri-mip′rah-mēn) chemical name: 10,11-dihydro-N,N,β-trimethyl-5H-dibenz[b,f]azepine-5-propanamine; a tricyclic antidepressant, $C_{20}H_{26}N_2$. **t. maleate,** the maleate salt of trimipramine, $C_{20}H_{26}N_2 \cdot C_4H_4O_4$, having the same actions as the base.

trimorphous (tri-mor′fus) [*tri-* + Gr. *morphē* form]   existing in three different forms.

trimopam maleate (tri′mo-pam)   chemical name: (+)-2,3,4,5-tetrahydro-7,8-dimethoxy-3-methyl-1-phenyl-1*H*-3-benzazepine (*Z*)-2-butenedioate (1:1); a tranquilizer, $C_{19}H_{23}NO_2 \cdot C_4H_4O_4$.

trinegative (tri-neg′ah-tiv)   having three negative valencies or charges.

trineural (tri-nu′ral)   pertaining to three nerves.

trineuric (tri-nu′rik)   pertaining to or having three neurons.

trinitrate (tri-ni′trāt)   a nitrate which contains three radicals of nitric acid, as glycerol trinitrate.

trinitrin (tri-ni′trin)   nitroglycerin.

trinitrocellulose (tri″ni-tro-sel′u-lōs)   pyroxylin.

trinitrocresol (tri″ni-tro-kre′sol)   an antiseptic and highly explosive compound, $(NO_2)_3C_6H(CH_3)OH$, formed by the action of concentrated nitric acid on coal tar cresol.

trinitroglycerin (tri-ni″tro-glis′er-in)   nitroglycerin.

trinitroglycerol (tri-ni″tro-glis′er-ol)   nitroglycerin.

trinitrophenol (tri″ni-tro-fe′nol)   a yellow, crystalline, bitter-tasting substance, $C_6H_2(NO_2)_3OH$, sparingly soluble in water; it is used as a dye and a tissue fixative and as an antiseptic, astringent, and stimulant of epithelialization. It can be detonated by percussion or heating above 300° C. Called also *carbazotic, nitroxanthic, picric,* and *picronitric acid.*

trinitrotoluene (tri″ni-tro-tol′u-ēn)   a high explosive, C_6H_2-$(NO_2)_3CH_3$, obtained by nitrating toluene; called also TNT.

trinomial (tri-no′me-al) [*tri-* + L. *nomen* name]   composed of three names or terms.

trinucleate (tri-nu′kle-āt)   having three nuclei.

trinucleotide (tri-nu′kle-o-tīd)   a polymer made up of three mononucleotides.

triocephalus (tri″o-sef′ah-lus) [*tri-* + Gr. *kephalē* head]   a monster in which the structures of the mouth, nose, and eyes are wanting, the head being nearly a shapeless mass.

Triodontophorus diminutus (tri″o-don-tof′o-rus dim-ĭ-nu′tus)   *Territans diminutus.*

triolein (tri-o′le-in)   olein.

triolism (tri′o-lizm)   sexual interests or practices involving three persons, two of one sex and one of the opposite sex.

trionym (tri′o-nim) [*tri-* + Gr. *onyma* name]   a name made up of three terms.

triophthalmos (tri″of-thal′mos) [*tri-* + Gr. *ophthalmos* eye]   a double-faced monster with three eyes.

triopodymus (tri″o-pod′ĭ-mus) [*tri-* + Gr. *ops* face + *didymos* twin]   a monster having a fused head with three faces.

triorchid (tri-or′kid) [*tri-* + Gr. *orchis* testis]   an individual with three testes.

triorchidism (tri-or′kĭ-dizm)   the condition of having three testes.

triorchis (tri-or′kis)   triorchid.

triorchism (tri-or′kizm)   triorchidism.

triose (tri′ōs)   a monosaccharide containing three carbon atoms in a molecule.

triotus (tri-o′tus) [*tri-* + Gr. *ous* ear]   an individual with a supernumerary ear.

trioxide (tri-ok′sīd)   a compound containing three atoms of oxygen to one of another element.

trioxsalen (tri-ok′sah-len) [USP]   chemical name: 2,5,9-trimethyl-7*H*-furo[3.2-*g*][1]benzopyran-7-one. A synthetic psoralen, $C_{14}H_{12}O_3$, occurring as a white or grayish, crystalline solid; used orally in conjunction with exposure to ultraviolet light to facilitate repigmentation in vitiligo, and also as a suntan accelerator and sun protectant.

trioxypurine (tri″ok-se-pu′rin)   uric acid.

tripalmitin (tri-pal′mĭ-tin)   palmitin.

tripara (trip′ah-rah) [*tri-* + L. *parere* to bring forth, produce]   a woman who has had three pregnancies which resulted in viable offspring; also written para III.

triparanol (tri-par′ah-nol)   chemical name: 1-[*p*-(2-diethyl-aminoethoxy)phenyl]-1-(*p*-tolyl)-2-(*p*-chlorophenyl)ethanol. A crystalline substance, $C_{27}H_{32}ClNO_2$, formerly used as a cholesterol biosynthesis inhibitor but withdrawn from the market because of association with irreversible cataracts, baldness, and impotence.

tripartite (tri-par′tīt)   having three parts.

tripelennamine (tri″pĕ-len′ah-min)   chemical name: *N,N*-dimethyl-N′-(phenylmethyl)-N′-2-pyridinyl-1,2-ethanediamine. A histamine antagonist, $C_{16}H_{21}N_3$. **t. citrate** [USP], the citrate salt of tripelennamine, $C_{16}H_{21}N_3 \cdot C_6H_8O_7$, occurring as a white, crystalline powder; used as antihistaminic in the symptomatic treatment of allergic disorders, administered orally. **t. hydrochloride** [USP], the monohydrochloride salt of tripelennamine,

$C_{16}H_{21}N_3 \cdot HCl$, have the same appearance, actions, and uses as the citrate salt; administered orally, parenterally, and topically.

tripeptide (tri-pep′tid)   a peptide which on hydrolysis yields three amino acids.

Triperidol (tri-per′ĭ-dol)   trademark for a preparation of trifluperidol.

triphalangeal (tri″fah-lan′je-al)   pertaining to or characterized by triphalangia.

triphalangia (tri″fah-lan′je-ah)   triphalangism.

triphalangism (tri-fal′an-jizm)   the presence of three phalanges in the longitudinal axis of a digit normally composed of only two.

triphasic (tri-fa′zik) [*tri-* + Gr. *phasis* phase]   triply varied or triply phasic; used in describing the electromotive actions of muscles. Cf. *diphasic* and *monophasic.*

triphenylethylene (tri-fen″il-eth′ĭ-lēn)   a synthetic estrogen, $C_{20}H_{16}$ (*alpha*-phenyl-stilbene), not related to naturally occurring estrogens with the phenanthrene nucleus.

triphenylmethane (tri-fen″il-meth′ān)   a substance from coal tar, $(C_6H_5)_3CH$, the basis of various dyes and stains, including aurin, rosaniline, basic fuchsin, and gentian violet.

triphosphate (tri-fos′fāt)   a salt containing three phosphate radicals.

triphosphopyridine nucleotide (tri-fos″fo-pir′ĭ-dēn)   TPN; former name for nicotinamide-adenine dinucleotide phosphate (NADP).

triphthemia (trif-the′me-ah) [Gr. *tribein* to wear out + *haima* blood + *-ia*]   the retention of waste products in the blood.

Tripier's amputation (trip′e-āz) [Léon *Tripier,* French surgeon, 1842–1891]   see under *amputation.*

triple-angle (trip′l ang′g′l)   having three angles; Black's term for a dental instrument having three angulations in the shank connecting the handle, or shaft, with the working portion of the instrument, known as the blade, or nib.

triplegia (tri-ple′je-ah) [*tri-* + Gr. *plēgē* stroke]   paralysis of three of the extremities.

triplet (trip′let)   1. one of three individuals having coextensive gestation periods and produced at the same birth. 2. a combination of three objects or entities occurring or acting together, as three lenses constituting a microscope eyepiece or objective. 3. in molecular genetics, a unit of three successive bases in DNA or RNA, which codes for a specific amino acid.

triplex (tri′pleks) [Gr. *triploos* triple]   triple or three-fold.

triploblastic (trip″lo-blas′tik) [Gr. *triploos* triple + *blastos* germ]   having three germ layers or blastodermic membranes; said of an embryo.

triploid (trip′loid)   1. pertaining to or characterized by triploidy. 2. an individual or cell having three sets of chromosomes.

triploidy (trip′loi-de)   the presence in humans of 69 chromosomes, or three full sets, a frequent finding in abortuses.

triplokoria (trip″lo-ko′re-ah) [Gr. *triploos* triple + *korē* pupil + *-ia*]   the presence of three pupils in one eye.

triplopia (trip-lo′pe-ah) [Gr. *triploos* triple + *ōpē* sight + *-ia*]   the perception of three images of a single object; triple vision.

tripod (tri′pod) [Gr. *treis* three + *pous* foot]   anything having three feet or supports. **t. of the Empirics,** the three principles on which the Empirics based their theory of medicine: (1) their own chance observations; (2) learning obtained from contemporaries and predecessors; and, in case of a disease not previously encountered, (3) conclusions based on other diseases which it might resemble. **Haller's t.,** truncus celiacus. **t. of life, vital t.,** the brain, heart, and lungs regarded as the triple support of life.

tripodia (tri-po′de-ah) [Gr. *treis* three + *pous* foot]   a type of symmelia characterized by the presence of three feet.

tripoding (tri′pod-ing)   the use of three points of support, as adopted by paralyzed patients when changing from a sitting or standing position. See also *tripod position,* under *position.*

tripoli (trip′o-le)   a mild abrasive and polishing agent, used in dentistry, derived from certain porous rocks first found near Tripoli.

tripositive (tri-pos′ĭ-tiv)   having three positive valencies or charges.

triprolidine hydrochloride (tri-pro′lĭ-dēn) [USP]   chemical name: (*E*)-2-[1-(4-methylphenyl)-3-(1-pyrrolidinyl)-1-propenyl]-pyridine monohydrochloride monohydrate. An antihistaminic, $C_{19}H_{22}N_2 \cdot HCl \cdot H_2O$, occurring as a white, crystalline powder; used in the treatment of various allergic conditions and their manifestations, administered orally.

triprosopus (tri″pro-so′pus) [Gr. *treis* three + *prosōpon* face]   a monster having a triple face.

tripsis (trip′sis) [Gr. *tripsis* rubbing]   1. a trituration; the process of trituration. 2. the act of shampooing or of massage.

-tripsy (trip′se) [Gr. *tripsis* a rubbing, friction]   a word termination designating a surgical procedure in which a structure is intentionally crushed.

triptokoria (trip″to-ko′re-ah) triplokoria.

tripus (tri′pus) [Gr. *treis* three + *pous* foot] 1. a tripod. 2. a conjoined twin monster having three feet. **t. hal′leri,** truncus celiacus.

triquetrous (tri-kwe′trus) [L. *triquetrus*] triangular; three cornered.

triquetrum (tri-kwe′trum) [L.] three cornered; see os *triquetrum.*

triradial, triradiate (tri-ra′de-al; tri-ra′de-āt) [*tri-* + L. *radiatus* rayed] having three rays; radiating in three directions.

triradiation (tri″ra-de-a′shun) radiation in three directions.

triradius (tri-ra′de-us) in dermatoglyphics, a point from which the dermal ridges course in three directions at angles of approximately 120 degrees.

TRIS tris(hydroxymethyl)aminomethane; see *tromethamine.*

trisaccharidase (tri-sak′ah-rĭ-dās) an enzyme that catalyzes the hydrolysis of trisaccharides.

trisaccharide (tri-sak′ah-rid) a carbohydrate, $C_{18}H_{32}O_{16}$, composed of three saccharide groups.

tris(hydroxymethyl)aminomethane (tris″hi-drok″se-meth″il-am″ĭ-no-meth′ān) tromethamine.

trismic (triz′mik) of the nature of or pertaining to trismus.

trismoid (triz′moid) [*trismus* + Gr. *eidos* form] a variety of trismus nascentium, said to be due to pressure on the occiput during birth.

trismus (triz′mus) [Gr. *trismos* grating, grinding] motor disturbance of the trigeminal nerve, especially spasm of the masticatory muscles, with difficulty in opening the mouth (lockjaw); a characteristic early symptom of tetanus. **t. nascen′tium,** inability to open the jaws sometimes observed in an infant at birth. **t. neonato′rum,** tetanus of young infants due to infection of the navel.

trisnitrate (tris-ni′trāt) trinitrate.

trisomia (tri-so′me-ah) trisomy.

trisomic (tri-so′mik) pertaining to or characterized by trisomy.

trisomy (tri′so-me) [*tri* + Gr. *sōma* body] the presence of an additional (third) chromosome of one type in an otherwise diploid cell (2n +1): trisomy 8 (trisomy C) results in trisomy 8 syndrome; trisomy 13 (trisomy D or 13–15) results in Patau's syndrome; trisomy 18 (trisomy E or 16–18) results in trisomy 18 syndrome; trisomy 21 results in Down's syndrome; and trisomy 22 results in trisomy 22 syndrome. See these anomalies under *syndrome.*

Trisoralen (tri-sor′ah-len) trademark for a preparation of trioxsalen.

trisplanchnic (tri-splangk′nik) [Gr. *treis* three + *splanchna* viscera] pertaining to or supplying the three great body cavities and their viscera.

tristearin (tri-ste′ah-rin) a white, crystalline fat, glyceryl tristearate, $C_3H_5(C_{18}H_{35}O_2)_3$, found in the harder fats, such as tallow; called also *stearin.*

tristichia (tri-stik′e-ah) [Gr. *treis* three + *stichos* row] the existence of three rows of eyelashes.

tristimania (tris″tĭ-ma′ne-ah) [L. *tristis* sad + Gr. *mania* madness] melancholia.

trisubstituted (tri-sub′stĭ-tūt″ed) having three molecules or atoms replaced by three other molecules or atoms.

trisulcate (tri-sul′kāt) having three furrows.

trisulfapyrimidines (tri-sul″fah-pi-rim′ĭ-dēnz) preparations containing a mixture of the sulfonamides sulfadiazine, sulfamerazine, and sulfamethazine.

trisulfate (tri-sul′fāt) a binary compound containing three sulfate (SO_4) groups in the molecule.

trisulfide (tri-sul′fid) a sulfur compound containing three atoms of sulfur to one of the base.

Trit. abbreviation for L. *tri′tura,* triturate.

tritanomaly (tri″tah-nom-ah′le) tritanomalopia.

tritanomalous (tri″tah-nom′ah-lus) pertaining to or characterized by tritanomalopia.

tritanomalopia (tri″tah-nom″ah-lo-pe-ah) [Gr. *tritos* third + *anōmalos* irregular + *ōpē* sight + *-ia*] a rare form of defective color vision, similar to but milder than tritanopia, in which there is decreased sensitivity of, rather than absence of, blue-sensitive visual pigment. Cf. the correlative terms *deuteranomalopia* and *protanomalopia.*

tritanope (tri′tah-nōp″) an individual exhibiting tritanopia.

tritanopia (tri″tah-no′pe-ah) [Gr. *tritos* third + *an-* neg. + *ōpē* sight + *-ia*] a rare and obscure type of defective color vision, characterized by retention of the sensory mechanism for two hues only (red and green) of the normal 4-primary quota, and lacking blue and yellow, with loss of luminance and shift of brightness and hue curves toward the long-wave end of the spectrum. Often associated with drug administration, retinal detachment, or diseases of the nervous system. Formerly called "blue blindness." Cf. the correlative terms *protanopia, deuteranopia,* and *tetartanopia,* in which the color vision deficiency is in the first, second, and fourth primary, respectively.

tritanopic (tri″tah-nop′ik) pertaining to or characterized by tritanopia.

tritanopsia (tri″tah-nop′se-ah) tritanopia.

tritiate (trit′e-āt) to treat with tritium.

triticeous (tri-tish′us) [L. *triticeus*] resembling a grain of wheat.

triticeum (tri-tis′e-um) [L.] cartilago triticea.

triticin (trit′ĭ-sin) a fructose polysaccharide, $(C_6H_{10}O_5)_n$, which occurs in the rhizome of couch grass, *Agropyron repens* (L.) Beauv. (Gramineae).

Triticum (trit′ĭ-kum) [L.] a genus of grasses, including wheat. T. (*Agropyron*) *repens* (L.) Beauv., or couch grass, is diuretic; formerly used in the treatment of cystitis and as a nutritive agent in the form of a decoction.

triticum (trit′ĭ-kum) the dried rhizome and roots of couch grass, *Agropyron* (*Triticum*) *repens* (L.) Beauv. (Gramineae), which has diuretic properties, and was formerly used in the treatment of cystitis; it was also used as a nutritive agent in the form of a decoction. Called also *agropyrum.*

tritium (trit′e-um, trish′e-um) [Gr. *tritos* third] the mass three isotope of hydrogen, ³H, a radioactive gas obtained by bombardment of beryllium in the cyclotron with deuterium ions. It has a half-life of about 31 years and is used as an indicator or tracer in metabolic studies. Cf. *deuterium* and *protium.*

tritocone (tri′to-kōn) [Gr. *tritos* third + *kōnos* cone] the distobuccal cusp of a mammalian upper premolar tooth.

tritoconid (tri″to-ko′nid) the distobuccal cusp of a mammalian lower premolar tooth.

tritol (tri′tol) any emulsion of the extract of filix mas with the diastasic extract of malt.

triton (tri′ton) trinitrotoluene.

tritotoxin (tri″to-tok′sin) (*obs.*) a toxin which unites less easily with the antitoxin than the prototoxin and deuterotoxin. See *deuterotoxin, hemotoxin, heterotoxin, prototoxin.*

Tritrichomonas (tri-trik″o-mo′nas) *Trichomonas.*

triturable (trich′er-ah-bel) susceptible of being triturated.

triturate (trich′ĕ-rāt) 1. to rub to a powder. 2. a triturated substance.

trituration (trich′ĕ-ra′shun) [L. *tritura* the treading out of corn] 1. the reduction of solid bodies to a powder by continuous rubbing. 2. a triturated drug, especially one rubbed up with milk sugar. 3. the creation of a homogeneous whole by mixing, as the combining of particles of an alloy with mercury to form dental amalgam; called also *amalgamation.*

triturator (trit′u-ra′tor) an apparatus in which substances can be continuously rubbed, as in the process of amalgamating an alloy with mercury.

trivalence (triv′ah-lens) the condition or quality of being trivalent.

trivalent (triv′ah-lent) [*tri-* + L. *valens* powerful] uniting with or replacing three hydrogen atoms.

trivalve (tri′valv) having three valves or three blades, as a speculum.

trizonal (tri-zo′nal) arranged in three zones.

tRNA transfer-RNA; see *ribonucleic acid,* under *acid.*

Trobicin (tro-bi′sin) trademark for a preparation of spectinomycin hydrochloride.

trocar (tro′kar) [Fr. *trois quarts* three quarters] a sharp-pointed instrument equipped with a cannula, used to puncture the wall of a body cavity and withdraw fluid. **Duchenne's t.,** an instrument for removing small portions of tissues from deep parts for microscopical study. **Durham's t., piloting t.,** a trocar for introducing a jointed tracheostomy tube. **rectal t.,** a curved trocar for tapping the bladder through the rectum.

troch. trochiscus.

trochanter (tro-kan′ter) [L.; Gr. *trochantēr*] either of the two processes below the neck of the femur. **greater t.,** t. major. **lesser t.,** t. minor. **t. ma′jor** [NA], greater trochanter: a broad, flat process at the upper end of the lateral surface of the femur, to which several muscles are attached. **t. mi′nor** [NA], lesser trochanter: a short conical process projecting medially from the lower part of the posterior border of the base of the neck of the femur. **rudimentary t.,** t. tertius. **small t.,** t. minor. **t. ter′tius** [NA], **third t.,** a term applied to the gluteal tuberosity of the femur when it is unusually prominent.

trochanterian (tro″kan-ter′e-an) trochanteric.

trochanteric (tro″kan-ter′ik) pertaining to a trochanter.

trochanterplasty (tro-kan′ter-plas″te) surgical excision of a ridge of bone to form a new femoral neck.

trochantin (tro-kan′tin) trochanter minor.

trochantinian (tro″kan-tin′e-an) pertaining to the lesser trochanter.

troche (tro′ke) [Gr. *trochos* a round cake] a small circular or oblong tablet usually for solution in the mouth, especially for medication of the throat, consisting of an active ingredient incorporated in a mass made up of sugar and mucilage or fruit base, and air dried. Called also *lozenge, morsulus, rotula,* and *trochiscus.*

trochin (tro′kin) [L. *trochinus*] tuberculum minus humeri.

trochiscus (tro-kis′kus), pl. *trochis′chi* [L.; Gr. *trochiskos,* dim. of *trochos,* a small wheel or disk] a medicated tablet; a troche.

trochiter (trok′ĭ-ter) 1. trochanter major. 2. tuberculum majus humeri.

trochiterian (trok″ĭ-te′re-an) pertaining to the trochiter.

trochlea (trok′le-ah), pl. *troch′leae* [L.; Gr. *trochilia* pulley] a pulley-shaped part or structure; [NA] a general term for such a structure. **t. fibula′ris calca′nei,** NA alternative for *t. peronealis calcanei.* **t. hu′meri** [NA], **t. of humerus,** the pulley-like medial portion of the distal end of the humerus for articulation with the semilunar notch of the ulna; called also *trochlear eminence.* **t. labyrin′thi,** cochlea, def. 2. **muscular t., t. muscula′ris** [NA], an anatomical part that serves to change the direction of pull of a tendon; it may be fibrous or bony. **t. mus′culi obli′qui superio′ris bul′bi** [NA], **t. mus′culi obli′qui superio′ris oc′uli,** the fibrocartilaginous pulley near the internal angular process of the frontal bone, through which the tendon of the superior oblique muscle of the eyeball passes; called also *t. of superior oblique muscle.* **peroneal t. of calcaneus, t. peronea′lis calca′nei** [NA], a small eminence on the lateral surface of the calcaneus, separating the tendons of the peroneus brevis and longus muscles; called also *processus trochlearis calcanei* and *t. fibularis calcanei* [NA alternative]. **t. phalan′gis digito′rum ma′nus,** caput phalangis digitorum manus. **t. phalan′gis digito′rum pe′dis,** caput phalangis digitorum pedis. **t. of superior oblique muscle,** t. musculi obliqui superioris bulbi. **t. ta′li** [NA], **t. of talus,** the surface of the talus for articulation with the tibia and fibula.

trochlear (trok′le-ar) [L. *trochlearis*] 1. of the nature of or resembling a pulley. 2. pertaining to a trochlea.

trochleariform (trok″le-ar′ĭ-form) pulley-shaped.

trochlearis (trok″le-a′ris) [L.] trochlear.

trochocephalia (tro″ko-sĕ-fa′le-ah) trochocephaly.

trochocephaly (tro″ko-sef′ah-le) [Gr. *trochos* wheel + *kephalē* head] a rounded appearance of the head caused by synostosis of the frontal and parietal bones.

trochoid (tro′koid) [Gr. *trochos* wheel + *eidos* form] resembling a pivot or a pulley.

trochoides (tro-koi′dēz) [Gr. *trochoeidēs,* from *trochos* wheel + *eidos* form] articulatio trochoidea.

trochophore (tro′ko-fōr) [Gr. *trochos* wheel + *phoros* bearing] the pear- or top-shaped larva of certain mollusks and annelids that bears a girdle of cilia (prototroch).

Trocinate (tro′sĭ-nāt) trademark for a preparation of thiphenamil hydrochloride.

Troglodytella (trog″lo-di-tel′ah) a genus of ciliate protozoa, species of which occur in the gorilla and chimpanzee.

Troglotrema (trog″lo-tre′mah) a genus of flukes. **T. sal-min′cola,** a parasite found in the kidney and under the skin of various fish, especially salmon and trout, and which serves as a vector of *Neorickettsia helminthoeca,* the etiologic agent of salmon poisoning (q.v.). It is transmitted to man, dogs, cats, foxes, bears, mink, hogs, and other animals by the ingestion of raw, infected fish. Called also *Nanophyetus salmincola.*

troilism (troi′lizm) [Fr. *trois* three] paraphilia practiced by three persons, by two women and a man, or by two men and a woman.

Troisier's ganglion, node, sign, syndrome (trwah-ze-āz′) [Charles Emile *Troisier,* French physician, 1844–1919] see under *ganglion, sign,* and *syndrome,* and see *sentinel node,* under *node.*

trolamine (tro′lah-mēn) 1. [NF] chemical name: 2,2′,2″-nitrilotrisethanal. A mixture of alkanolamines, $C_8H_{15}NO_3$, consisting largely of triethanolamine and containing some di- and monoethanolamine; used as an alkalizing agent in pharmaceutical preparations. Called also *triethanolamine.* 2. USAN contraction for triethanolamine.

troland (tro′land) the retinal illuminance produced by the image of an object the luminance of which is 1 lumen per square meter for an area of the entrance pupil of 1 square millimeter.

Trolard's plexus (net), vein (tro-lardz′) [Paulin *Trolard,* French anatomist, 1842–1910] see *plexus venosus canalis* and *vena anastomotica inferior.*

troleandomycin (tro″le-an-do-mi′sin) the triacetyl ester of oleandomycin, $C_{41}H_{67}NO_{14}$, occurring as a white, odorless powder; used as an antibacterial, chiefly in the treatment of infections due to staphylococci and other gram-positive bacteria resistant to other systemic antibiotics, administered orally. Called also *triacetyloleandomycin.*

trolnitrate phosphate (trol-ni′trāt) chemical name: 2,2′2″-nitrilotrisethanol trinitrate (ester) phosphate (1:2) (salt). An organic nitrate, $C_6H_{12}N_4O_9$, occurring as a white, crystalline powder, having vasodilating actions; used to reduce the frequency and severity of anginal attacks, administered orally.

Tröltsch's corpuscles, recesses (spaces) (trel′ches) [Anton Friedrich von *Tröltsch,* German otologist, 1829–1890] see under *corpuscle,* and see *recessus membranae tympani anterior* and *recessus membranae tympani posterior.*

Trombicula (trom-bik′u-lah) a genus of acarine mites of the family Trombiculidae. **T. akamu′shi,** the kedani mite, whose larvae (chiggers) transmit *Rickettsia tsutsugamushi,* the

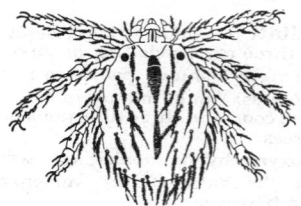

Trombicula akamushi (Tanaka).

etiologic agent of scrub typhus; it is the chief vector in Japan. Called also *Microtrombidium akamushi.* **T. alfredduge′si,** *Eutrombicula alfreddugèsi;* see also under *chigger.* **T. autumna′lis,** the autumnal chigger of Europe whose larvae cause lesions of the skin in man and animals; formerly called *Leptus autumnalis.* **T. delien′sis,** a species whose larvae transmit *Rickettsia tsutsugamushi,* the etiologic agent of scrub typhus; it is believed to be the chief vector outside of Japan. **T. fletch′eri,** a carrier of *Rickettsia tsutsugamushi,* the causative agent of scrub typhus. **T. holoseri′ceum,** *T. autumnalis.* **T. interme′dia,** a carrier of *Rickettsia tsutsugamushi,* the causative agent of scrub typhus. **T. ir′ritans,** *Eutrombicula alfreddugèsi.* **T. mus′cae domes′ticae,** a red acarid parasite on the housefly. **T. musca′rum,** *T. muscae domesticae.* **T. pal′lida,** a carrier of *Rickettsia tsutsugamushi,* the causative agent of scrub typhus. **T. scutella′ris,** a carrier of *Rickettsia tsutsugamushi,* the causative agent of scrub typhus. **T. tsalsahua′tl,** *Eutrombicula alfreddugèsi.*

trombiculiasis (trom-bik″u-li′ah-sis) infestation with *Trombicula.*

Trombiculidae (trom-bik′u-li″de) a family of mites which is cosmopolitan in distribution, ranging from Alaska and Labrador to New Zealand, and from sea level to an altitude of more than 16,000 feet in the Andes. The parasitic larvae of the mites infest vertebrates. The single genus of medical significance is *Trombicula,* with subgenera *Eutrombicula* and *Leptotrombidium.*

trombidiiasis (trom-bid″e-i′ah-sis) trombiculiasis.

trombidiosis (trom-bid″e-o′sis) trombiculiasis.

Trombidium (trom-bid′e-um) a name formerly given a genus of mites, now included in the genus *Trombicula.*

tromethamine (tro-meth′ah-mēn) [USP] chemical name: 2-amino-2-(hydromethyl)-1,3-propanediol. An amine base, $C_4H_{11}NO_3$, occurring as a white crystalline powder; used intravenously as an alkalizer for the correction of metabolic acidosis. Called also *THAM, TRIS* and *tris(hydroxymethyl)aminomethane.*

Trommer's test (trom′erz) [Karl August *Trommer,* German chemist, 1806–1879] see under *tests.*

Trömner's sign [Ernest L. O. *Trömner,* German neurologist, born 1868] Hoffmann's sign, def. 2.

tromomania (trom″o-ma′ne-ah) [Gr. *tromos* trembling + Gr. *mania* madness] delirium tremens.

tromophonia (trom″o-fo′ne-ah) a form of dysphonia characterized by a tremulous voice.

trona (tro′nah) [possible anagram of *natron*] a crude sodium salt.

tronchado (tron-kah′do) a name in Central America and Mexico for a fatal paralytic disease in cattle.

Tronothane (tron′o-thān) trademark for preparations of pramoxine.

tropate (tro′pāt) a salt of tropic acid.

tropesis (tro-pe′sis) [Gr. *tropos* a turning] Haekel's term for the tendency to action shown by every substance.

trophectoderm (trof-ek′to-derm) [*tropho-* + *ectoderm*] the outer layer of cells of the early blastodermic vesicle; the earliest trophoblast.

trophedema (trof″ĕ-de′mah) [*tropho-* + *edema*] a disease marked by permanent edema of the feet or legs. **congenital t., hereditary t.,** Milroy's disease.

trophesial, trophesic (tro-fe′ze-al; tro-fe′sik) pertaining to or characterized by trophesy.

trophesy (trof′ĕ-se) defective nutrition due to disorder of the trophic nerves.

trophic (trof′ik) [Gr. *trophikos*] of or pertaining to nutrition.

-trophic, -trophin [Gr. *trophikos* nourishing] word terminations denoting relationship to nutrition.

trophicity (tro-fis′ĭ-te) a trophic function or relation.

-trophin see *-tropin.*

trophism (trof'izm)   direct trophic influence.

tropho- (trof'o) [Gr. *trophē* nutrition]   a combining form denoting relationship to food or nourishment.

trophoblast (trof'o-blast) [*tropho-* + Gr. *blastos* germ]   a layer of extraembryonic ectodermal tissue on the outside of the blastocyst. It attaches the ovum to the uterine wall and supplies nutrition to the embryo. From it are derived the chorion and amnion. The inner cellular layer of the trophoblast covering a chorionic villus is called *cytotrophoblast* and its outer syncytial layer *syncytiotrophoblast*. The mesoblast, once thought to be trophoblastic, is now traced, in primates, to the caudal end of the primitive streak.

trophoblastic (trof'o-blas'tik)   pertaining to the trophoblast.

trophoblastoma (trof'o-blas-to'mah)   choriocarcinoma.

trophochromatin (trof'o-kro'mah-tin)   trophochromidia.

trophochromidia (trof'o-kro-mid'e-ah)   chromatin concerned with the nutrition of the cell rather than with reproduction. Cf. *idiochromidia*.

trophocyte (trof'o-sīt)   a lower type of cell which furnishes nourishment to a higher type of cell of a tissue. Cf. *trophospongium* (def. 1).

trophoderm (trof'o-derm) [*tropho-* + Gr. *derma* skin]   trophoblast.

trophodermatoneurosis (trof'o-der″mah-to-nu-ro'sis)   acrodynia.

trophodynamics (trof'o-di-nam'iks)   the study of the forces engaged in nutrition.

trophoedema (trof″o-ĕ-de'mah)   trophedema.

tropholecithal (trof'o-les'ĭ-thal)   pertaining to the tropholecithus.

tropholecithus (trof'o-les'ĭ-thus) [*tropho-* + Gr. *lekithos* yolk]   the food yolk of a meroblastic egg.

trophology (tro-fol'o-je)   the science of nutrition of the body.

trophon (trof'on)   the nutritive non-neural element of the neuron.

trophoneurosis (trof″o-nu-ro'sis)   any functional nervous disease due to the failure of nutrition from defective nerve influence. **facial t.**, facial hemiatrophy. **lingual t.**, progressive hemiatrophy of the tongue. **muscular t.**, trophic alteration of muscular tissue, dependent on nervous derangement. **t. of Romberg**, facial hemiatrophy.

trophoneurotic (trof'o-nu-rot'ik)   pertaining to or of the nature of a trophoneurosis.

trophonosis (trof″o-no'sis) [*tropho-* + Gr. *nosos* disease]   any disease or disorder due to nutritional causes.

trophonucleus (trof″o-nu'kle-us)   macronucleus.

trophopathia (trof″o-path'e-ah)   trophopathy.

trophopathy (tro-fop'ah-the) [*tropho-* + Gr. *pathos* disease]   any derangement of the nutrition.

trophoplasm (trof'o-plasm) [*tropho-* + Gr. *plasma* something formed]   (*obs.*) Strasburger's name for the material thought to constitute the main mass of a cell and to be the site of nutritive processes; cf. *kinoplasm*.

trophoplast (trof'o-plast) [*tropho-* + Gr. *plastos* formed]   a granular protoplasmic body; a plastid.

trophospongia (trof″o-spon'je-ah) [L.; Gr.]   plural of *trophospongium*.

trophospongium (trof″o-spon'je-um), pl. *trophospon'gia* [*tropho-* + Gr. *spongion* sponge]   1. a canalicular network in the cytoplasm of certain cells which was once believed to be instrumental in the circulation of nutritive material. 2. (*pl.*) the vascular endometrium between the myometrium and the trophoblast.

trophotaxis (trof″o-tak'sis) [*tropho-* + Gr. *taxis* a drawing up in rank and file]   an orientation movement of a motile organism in response to the stimulus provided by nutritive materials.

trophotherapy (trof″o-ther'ah-pe)   treatment of disease by dietetic measures.

trophozoite (trof″o-zo'īt) [*tropho-* + Gr. *zōon* animal]   the active, motile, feeding stage of a protozoan organism, as contrasted with the nonmotile encysted stage. In the malarial parasite, the stage of schizogony between the signet ring stage and the schizont.

-trophy [Gr. *trophē* nutrition]   a word termination indicating food or nutrition.

tropia (tro'pe-ah) [Gr. *tropē* a turning]   a manifest deviation of an eye from the normal position when both eyes are open and uncovered; strabismus, or squint. See *cyclotropia, esotropia, exotropia, hypertropia,* and *hypotropia*.

-tropic [Gr. *tropikos* turning]   a word termination denoting turning toward, changing, or tending to turn or change; see *tropism*.

tropical (trop'e-kal) [Gr. *tropikos* turning]   pertaining to the regions of the earth bounded by the parallels of latitude 23° 27' north and south of the equator.

tropicamide (tro-pik'ah-mīd) [USP]   chemical name: *N*-ethyl-α-(hydroxymethyl)-*N*-(4-pyridenylmethyl)benzene acetamide. An anticholinergic, $C_{17}H_{20}N_2O_2$, occurring as a white to practically white, crystalline powder, applied topically to the conjunctiva to produce mydriasis and cycloplegia.

tropicopolitan (trop″ĭ-ko-pol'ĭ-tan) [*tropical* + Gr. *polis* a city or a country]   1. occurring in all tropical areas. 2. an organism occurring in all tropical regions.

tropidine (trop'ĭ-din)   an oily, liquid base, $CH_3 \cdot N:C_8H_9:CH$, with an odor like that of coniine, formed by the dehydration of tropine.

tropin (tro'pin)   opsonin.

-tropin [Gr. *tropos* a turning]   a word termination meaning having an affinity for the structure or thing denoted by the stem to which it is affixed, as gonadotropin.

tropine (tro'pin)   a crystalline alkaloid, $C_8H_{15}NO$, with a smell like tobacco, derivable from atropine and from various plants.

tropism (tro'pizm) [Gr. *tropē* a turn, turning]   a growth response in a motile organism, elicited by an external stimulus. Such response may be either positive (toward) or negative (away from the stimulus). By extension, used as a word termination affixed to a stem denoting the nature of the stimulus (phototropism) or the material or entity for which an organism or substance shows a special affinity (neurotropism).

tropochrome (tro'po-krōm″) [*tropo-* + Gr. *chrōma* color]   refusing to stain with mucin stains after formol-bichromate fixation, as applied to certain serous cells of the salivary glands. Cf. *homeochrome*.

tropocollagen (tro″po-kol'ah-jen) [Gr. *tropē* a turning + *collagen*]   the molecular unit of collagen fibrils, about 1.4 nm. wide and 280 nm. long. It is a helical structure consisting of three polypeptide chains, each chain composed of about a thousand amino acids coiled around each other to form a spiral; tropocollagen is rich in glycine, proline, and hydroxyproline and hydroxylysine, all types of collagen being formed by interaction of these units.

tropoelastin (tro″po-e-las'tin)   the precursor of elastin.

tropometer (tro-pom'ĕ-ter) [Gr. *tropē* a turning + *metron* measure]   1. an instrument for measuring the rotation of the eyeball. 2. an instrument for measuring the twist or torsion of a long bone.

tropomyosin (tro″po-mi'o-sin)   muscle protein of the I band that inhibits contraction unless its position is modified by troponin so that the myosin molecules can make contact with the actin molecules. **t. A**, paramyosin.

tropon (trop'on)   a brownish powder prepared from vegetable and animal albumins; nutrient.

troponin (tro'po-nin)   a complex of globular muscle proteins of the I band that inhibits contraction by blocking the interaction of actin and myosin; when combined with Ca^{++}, it so modifies the position of the tropomyosin molecules that interaction takes place.

trotyl (tro'til)   trinitrotoluene.

trough (trof)   a shallow longitudinal depression or channel. **gingival t.**, gingival sulcus. **synaptic t's**, primary synaptic clefts. **vestibular t.**, the sulcus formed by reflection of the mucous membrane from the inner surface of the cheeks or lips onto the tissues overlying the alveoli of the teeth.

Trousseau's phenomenon, sign, spot, twitching (troo-sōz') [Armand *Trousseau*, French physician, 1801–1867]   see under *phenomenon, sign,* and *twitching,* and see *tache cérébrale*.

troxidone (trok'sĭ-dōn)   trimethadione.

troy (troi)   a system of weights commonly used in England and the United States for expressing quantities of gold and silver; for equivalents see *tables of weights and measures*.

Trp   tryptophan.

TRU   see under *unit*.

true (troo)   actually existing; not false; real; meeting all the criteria establishing its identity.

Trueta treatment (method, technique) (troo-a'tah) [José *Trueta,* Spanish surgeon in England, born 1897]   see under *treatment*.

truncal (trun'kal)   pertaining to the trunk.

truncate (trun'kāt) [L. *truncare, truncatus*]   1. to amputate; to deprive of limbs. 2. having the end cut squarely off.

trunci (trun'si) [L.]   plural of *truncus*.

truncus (trun'kus), pl. *trun'ci* [L. "trunk"]   the main part, a stem; [NA] a general term for the main part of the body, to which the head and limbs are attached, or a major, undivided and usually short, portion of a nerve or of a blood or lymphatic vessel or other duct. **t. arterio'sus**, an arterial trunk, especially the artery connected with the fetal heart, which gives off the aortic arches and develops into the aortic and pulmonary arteries. **t. arterio'sus, persistent**, a congenital anomaly, characterized by a single arterial trunk arising from the heart, receiving blood from both ventricles and supplying blood to the coronary, pulmonary, and systemic circulations; sometimes classified according to the arrangement of the arteries supplying the lungs. **t. brachiocephal'icus** [NA], brachiocephalic trunk: the first branch of the arch of the aorta, which behind the right sternoclavicular joint divides into the right common carotid and right subclavian arteries, with distribution to the right side of the head and neck and to the right arm; the lowest thyroid artery may arise from this trunk. Called also *arteria anonyma* or *innominate artery.* **t. bronchomediastina′lis** [NA], bronchomediastinal trunk: either of the two lymphatic vessels draining the pulmonary, bronchopulmonary, tracheobronchial, tracheal, and parasternal lymph nodes: that on the right side into the right lymphatic duct or subclavian vein, and that on the left into the thoracic duct or the subclavian vein. **t. bronchomediastina′lis dex′ter,** the truncus bronchomediastinalis on the right side. **t. celi′acus** [NA], celiac trunk: the arterial trunk that arises from the abdominal aorta, gives off the left gastric, common hepatic, and splenic arteries, and supplies the esophagus, stomach, duodenum, spleen, pancreas, liver, and gallbladder. Called also *arteria coeliaca* or *celiac artery.* **t. cor′poris callo′si** [NA], trunk of corpus callosum: the main central portion of the corpus callosum as distinguished from the rostrum and the splenium. **t. costocervica′lis** [NA], costocervical trunk: an artery that arises from the back of the subclavian artery, arches backward, and at the neck of the first rib divides into the deep cervical and highest intercostal arteries, thus supplying blood to the structures of the first two intercostal spaces, the vertebral column, the muscles of the back, and the deep neck muscles. **t. fascic′uli atrioventricula′ris** [NA], the undivided portion of the atrioventricular bundle, from its origin at the atrioventricular node to the point of division into right and left branches at the superior end of the muscular part of the interventricular septum. **t. infe′rior plex′us brachia′lis** [NA], inferior trunk of brachial plexus: the trunk of the brachial plexus that is formed by the ventral branches of the eighth cervical and first thoracic nerves; medial pectoral nerves may arise from it. Its anterior division becomes the medial cord of the plexus, and its posterior division helps form the posterior cord; modality, general sensory and motor. **trun′ci intestina′les** [NA], intestinal lymphatic trunks: short lymphatic vessels which leave the gastrointestinal tract and participate in formation of the thoracic duct. **t. jugula′ris** [NA], jugular trunk: either of the two vessels draining the deep cervical lymph nodes: on the right side, into the right lymphatic duct or subclavian vein, and on the left side, into the thoracic duct or subclavian vein. **t. linguofacia′lis** [NA], linguofacial trunk: the common trunk by which the facial and lingual arteries often arise from the external carotid artery. **trun′ci lumba′les [dex′ter et sinis′ter]** [NA], lumbar trunks: lymphatic vessels, one on either side, that drain lymph upward from the lumbar lymph nodes and help form the thoracic duct. **t. lumbosacra′lis** [NA], lumbosacral trunk: a trunk formed by union of the lower division of the ventral branch of the fourth lumbar nerve with the ventral branch of the fifth lumbar nerve. **t. me′dius plex′us brachia′lis** [NA], middle trunk of brachial plexus: the trunk of the brachial plexus that is formed by the ventral branch of the seventh cervical nerve. Its anterior division, from which lateral pectoral nerves may arise, helps form the lateral cord of the plexus, and its posterior division helps form the posterior cord; modality, general sensory and motor. **trun′ci plex′us brachia′lis** [NA], trunks of brachial plexus: the three trunks of the brachial plexus, arising from the ventral branches of the lower four cervical nerves and the first thoracic nerve near the lateral border of the scalenus anterior muscle; they continue laterally and downward, above and behind the subclavian artery, and near the clavicle form the lateral, medial, and posterior fasciculi or cords of the plexus. See *t. inferior plexus brachialis, t. medius plexus brachialis,* and *t. superior plexus brachialis.* **t. pulmona′lis** [NA], pulmonary trunk: the vessel arising from the conus arteriosus of the right ventricle, extending upward obliquely to divide into the right and left pulmonary arteries beneath the arch of the aorta, and conveying unaerated blood toward the lungs. Called also *arteria pulmonalis* or *pulmonary artery.* **t. subcla′vius** [NA], subclavian trunk: either of two lymphatic vessels draining the axillary lymph nodes; that on the right into the right lymphatic duct or subclavian vein, that on the left into the thoracic duct or the subclavian vein. **t. supe′rior plex′us brachia′lis** [NA], superior trunk of brachial plexus: the trunk of the brachial plexus that is formed by the ventral branches of the fifth and sixth cervical nerves. Its anterior division helps form the lateral cord of the plexus, its posterior division helps form the posterior cord, and it gives rise directly to the suprascapular and subclavian nerves; modality, general sensory and motor. **t. sympath′icus** [NA], sympathetic trunk: two long nerve strands, one on each side of the vertebral column, extending from the base of the skull to the coccyx. Interconnected by nerve strands, each has cervical, thoracic, lumbar, and sacral sympathetic ganglia. These receive preganglionic fibers from thoracic and upper lumbar ventral roots by way of rami communicantes, send postganglionic fibers to ventral roots by rami communicantes, and give branches to prevertebral plexuses and adjacent viscera and blood vessels. **t. thyreocervica′lis, t. thyrocervica′lis** [NA], thyrocervical trunk: a short artery that arises from the convex side of the subclavian artery just medial to the anterior scalene muscle and at once divides into the inferior thyroid, transverse cervical, and suprascapular arteries, supplying thyroid, neck, and scapular regions. **t. vaga′lis ante′rior** [NA], anterior vagal trunk: a nerve trunk (or trunks) formed by fibers from both left and right vagus nerves, collected from the anterior part

of the esophageal plexus; it descends through the esophageal opening of the diaphragm to supply branches to the anterior surface of the stomach. **t. vaga′lis poste′rior** [NA], posterior vagal trunk: a nerve trunk or trunks formed by fibers from both left and right vagus nerves, collected from the posterior part of the esophageal plexus; it descends through the esophageal opening of the diaphragm to supply branches to the posterior surface of the stomach.

trunk (trunk) [L. *truncus* the stem or trunk of a tree] 1. the main part of the body, to which head and limbs are attached. 2. a major, undivided and usually short, portion of a nerve or of a blood or lymphatic vessel, or other duct. See also *truncus.* **t. of atrioventricular bundle,** truncus fasciculi atrioventricularis. **basilar t.,** arteria basilaris. **t. of brachial plexus,** trunci plexus brachialis. **brachiocephalic t.,** truncus brachiocephalicus. **bronchomediastinal t.,** truncus bronchomediastinalis. **celiac t.,** truncus celiacus. **t. of corpus callosum,** truncus corporis callosi. **costocervical t.,** truncus costocervicalis. **inferior t. of brachial plexus,** truncus inferior plexus brachialis. **intestinal lymphatic t's,** trunci intestinales. **jugular t.,** truncus jugularis. **linguofacial t.,** truncus linguofacialis. **lumbar t's,** trunci lumbales [dexter et sinister]. **lumbosacral t.,** truncus lumbosacralis. **middle t. of brachial plexus,** truncus medius plexus brachialis. **pulmonary t.,** truncus pulmonalis. **subclavian t.,** truncus subclavius. **superior t. of brachial plexus,** truncus superior plexus brachialis. **sympathetic t.,** truncus sympathicus. **thyrocervical t.,** truncus thyrocervicalis. **vagal t., anterior,** truncus vagalis anterior. **vagal t., posterior,** truncus vagalis posterior.

trusion (troo′zhun) [L. *trudere* to shove] malposition of a tooth. **bimaxillary t.,** malposition of the teeth of both the upper and the lower jaw. **bodily t.,** malposition of the entire tooth, crown and root. **coronal t.,** malposition of the crown of a tooth, the root being normally placed. **mandibular t.,** malposition of the mandibular teeth. **maxillary t.,** malposition of the maxillary teeth.

truss (trus) an elastic, canvas, or metallic device for retaining a reduced hernia within the abdominal cavity. **nasal t.,** a trusslike support for fractured nasal bones. **yarn t.,** a trusslike bandage of worsted yarn for the support of inguinal hernia in infants.

truxilline (truks′ĭ-lin) an amorphous alkaloid prepared from coca leaves or made synthetically.

try-in (tri′in) a preliminary insertion of a dental restoration or prosthesis to determine its fit and suitability.

trypaflavine (trip″ah-fla′vin) acriflavine hydrochloride.

trypanblau (tri′pan-blaw″) [Ger.] trypan blue; see under *blue.*

trypanid (tri′pan-id) an eruption occurring in trypanosomiasis.

trypanocidal (tri-pan″o-si′dal) trypanosomicidal.

trypanocide (tri-pan′o-sīd) trypanosomicide.

trypanolysis (tri″pan-ol′ĭ-sis) the destruction of trypanosomes.

trypanolytic (tri″pan-o-lit′ik) destructive to trypanosomes.

Trypanoplasma (tri″pan-o-plaz′mah) [Gr. *trypanon* borer + *plasma* anything formed or molded] *Crystobia.*

Trypanosoma (tri″pan-o-so′mah) [Gr. *trypanon* borer + *sōma* body] a genus of protozoan parasites of the family Trypanosomatidae, order Protomastigida, found in the blood and lymph of invertebrates and vertebrates, including man. Typically, the adult body is elongate with a whiplike flagellum arising from the posterior end and attached to the cell by a delicate undulating membrane that runs the entire length of the body. Most species live part of their life cycle in the intestines of insects and other invertebrates, where they undergo remarkable transformations. The typical adult stage or stages occur only in the vertebrate host. Called also *Trypanosomonas* and *Trypanozoon.* **T. america′num,** a species infecting cattle in the United States. **T. a′riari,** *T. rangeli.* **T. a′vium,** a parasite 20–70μ long found in the blood of birds, but apparently not pathogenic. **T. ber′berum,** *T. evansi.* **T. bru′cei,** a widely distributed species found in horses, cattle, pigs, camels, and other domestic animals of Africa, transmitted by tsetse flies (*Glossina* spp.), and producing the disease nagana; it also causes a benign infection in wild animals, especially antelopes. Called also *T. pecaudi.* **T. calmet′ii,** a species found in the blood of a domestic fowl in Tonkin. **T. cap′rae,** *T. vivax.* **T. castella′ni,** *T. gambiense.* **T. cazal′boui,** *T. vivax.* **T. confu′sum,** *T. congolense.* **T. congolen′se,** a species found in cattle, horses, sheep, and other domestic animals in Central Africa, transmitted by flies of the genus *Glossina,* and causing nagana. Called also *T. dimorphon, T. montgomeryi,* and *T. nanum.* **T. cru′zi,** a species infecting man, armadillos, bats, cats, guinea pigs, and various other animals in Central and South America and as far north as the southwestern United States. It is commonly transmitted by *Panstrongylus megistus* and other reduviid bugs, and is the etiologic agent of Chagas' disease. Called also *Schizotrypanum cruzi.* **T. dimor′phon,** *T. congolense.* **T. equi′num,** a species now considered to be identical with *T. evansi,* found in horses, mules, and dogs in South America, transmitted by tabanid flies and by vampire bats (*Desmodus rotundus*), and causing the acute disease mal de caderas. **T. equiper′dum,** a widely distributed species found in horses, donkeys, and cattle; it is the cause of the disease dourine. Called also *T. rougeti.* **T. esco′mili,** *T. rangeli.* **T. evan′si,** a species found in elephants and in horses, mules, camels, and other domestic animals; it is the etiologic agent of surra, tahaga, and El debab. Called also *T. berberum, T. macrocanum,* and *T. soudanense.* **T. gambien′se,** a species found in domestic and wild animals, including antelopes, pigs, and buffaloes, of central Africa, transmitted to man by the bite of *Glossina palpalis* and other species of *Glossina,* and causing Gambian trypanosomiasis; called also *Castellanella gambiense, T. castellani, T. hominis, T. nigeriense,* and *T. ugandense.* See also *African trypanosomiasis,* under *trypanosomiasis.* **T. granulo′sum,** a species parasitic in the eel; its intermediate host is the leech, *Hemiclepsis marginata.* **T. guatemalen′sis,** *T. rangeli.* **T. guyanen′se,** *T. vivax.* **T. hip′picum,** a species now considered to be identical with *T. evansi,* found in horses and mules in Panama, transmitted by flies of the genus *Glossina* and by vampire bats (*Desmodus rotundus*), and causing murrina. Called also *T. venezuelense.* **T. hom′inis,** *T. gambiense.* **T. inopina′tum,** a species parasitic in the frog and transmitted by a leech, *Helobdella algira.* **T. lew′isi,** a species found in the blood of the rat, and transmitted by a second host, the rat flea, *Nosopsyllus fasciatus.* **T. lu′is,** *Treponema pallidum.* **T. macroca′num,** *T. evansi.* **T. melopha′gium,** a nonpathogenic species occurring in sheep. **T. montgom′eryi,** *T. congolense.* **T. na′num,** *T. congolense.* **T. neoto′mae,** a species found in woodrats in California, possibly identical with *T. cruzi.* **T. nigerien′se,** *T. gambiense.* **T. noc′tuae,** a species found in the blood of the little owl, and seminated by the gnat, *Culex pipiens.* **T. pecau′di,** *T. brucei.* **T. rangel′i,** a species of Venezuela, Colombia, and Guatemala, transmitted by the reduviid bug *Rhodnius prolixus,* and causing an asymptomatic infection in man; called also *T. ariari, T. guatemalensis, T. escomili.* **T. rhodesien′se,** a species found in wild and domestic animals and wild game of southeastern Africa, transmitted to man by the bite of *Glossina morsitans* and other species of *Glossina,* and causing Rhodesian trypanosomiasis; called also *Castellanella castellani.* See also *African trypanosomiasis,* under *trypanosomiasis.* **T. rotato′rium,** the type species of the genus, and found in the blood of several species of frogs. **T. rouge′ti,** *T. equiperdum.* **T. sim′iae,** a species infecting monkeys, pigs, sheep, goats, and camels, transmitted by flies of the genus *Glossina.* It causes a rapidly fatal disease in pigs and camels and a chronic disease in monkeys. **T. soudanen′se,** *T. evansi.* **T. thei′leri,** a nonpathogenic species found in cattle in South Africa. **T. tria′tomae,** a form very similar to *T. cruzi,* found in rodents in California, probably identical with *T. neotomae.* **T. uganden′se,** *T. gambiense.* **T. unifor′me,** *T. vivax.* **T. venezuelen′se,** *T. hippicum.* **T. vi′vax,** a species found in ruminants and equines and causing nagana in cattle, sheep, and goats throughout tropical Africa; it is also found in South America. It is transmitted by flies of the genus *Glossina.* Called also *T. uniforme, T. caprae, T. cazalboui,* and *T. guyanense.*

trypanosomal (tri-pan″o-so′mal) 1. pertaining to or caused by trypanosomes. 2. denoting a morphologic stage in the development of certain hemoflagellates; see *trypomastigote.*

trypanosomatic (tri-pan″o-so-mat′ik) pertaining to or caused by trypanosomes.

Trypanosomatidae (tri″pan-o-so-mat′ĭ-de) a family of monoflagellate, typically elongate protozoan parasites of the order Protomastigida, class Zoomastigophora, found in the blood and tissues of man and various animals; their life cycle includes at least two of the following morphologic stages: *amastigote* (leishmanial stage), *epimastigote* (crithidial stage), *promastigote* (leptomonad stage), trypomastigote (trypanosomal stage). It includes the genera *Trypanosoma, Leishmania, Crithidia, Leptomonas, Herpetomonas,* and *Phytomonas.*

trypanosomatosis (tri-pan″o-so″mah-to′sis) trypanosomiasis.

trypanosomatotropic (tri-pan″o-so″mah-to-trop′ik) having a selective affinity for trypanosomes.

trypanosome (tri-pan′o-sōm) 1. any organism of the genus *Trypanosoma.* 2. any individual of the family Trypanosomatidae when exhibiting the typical trypanosomal form (trypomastigote) during its life cycle.

trypanosomiasis (tri-pan″o-so-mi′ah-sis) the state of being infected with protozoa of the genus *Trypanosoma.* Trypanosomal infections of man include the Gambian and Rhodesian forms of African trypanosomiasis, and Chagas' disease. **African t.,** a disease common among natives of tropical Africa, due to infection with *Trypanosoma gambiense* (*Gambian t.*) or *T. rhodesiense* (*Rhodesian t.*), transmitted by the bite of various species of the genus *Glossina.* The early stage of the disease (known as trypanosome fever) is ushered in by fever, chills, headache, and vomiting. There are then alternating periods of fever and apyrexia lasting for several months. This is followed by pains in the extremities, enlargement of the lymph glands, and anemia. Later the central nervous system becomes involved, producing *sleeping sickness,* when the patients become depressed, tremulous, lethargic, and somnolent, until finally they sleep all the time, become emaciated, and eventually die. The disease may last for years, but it is always

fatal after the nervous system has become involved. It is also known as *African sleeping sickness, African lethargy,* and *Congo t.* **American t., Brazilian t.,** Chagas' disease. **Congo t.,** African t. **Cruz t.,** Chagas' disease. **Gambian t.,** a form of African trypanosomiasis prevalent in central Africa, caused by *Trypanosoma gambiense* and transmitted to man by the bite of the tsetse fly *Glossina palpalis* and other species of *Glossina;* called also *Gambian sleeping sickness.* **Rhodesian t.,** a virulent form of African trypanosomiasis prevalent in southeastern Africa, which is caused by *Trypanosoma rhodesiense* and transmitted to man by the bite of the tsetse fly *Glossina morsitans* and other species of *Glossina.* Called also *kaodzera* and *Rhodesian sleeping sickness.* **South American t.,** Chagas' disease.

trypanosomic (tri-pan″o-so′mik) pertaining to or infected with trypanosomes.

trypanosomicidal (tri-pan″o-so″mĭ-si′dal) destructive to trypanosomes.

trypanosomicide (tri-pan″o-so′mĭ-sīd) [*trypanosome* + L. *caedere* to kill] 1. destructive to trypanosomes. 2. a substance which destroys trypanosomes.

trypanosomid (tri-pan′o-so-mid) a skin eruption occurring in trypanosomiasis.

trypanosomosis (tri-pan″o-so-mo′sis) trypanosomiasis.

Trypanozoon (tri-pan″o-zo′on) a subgenus of *Trypanosoma.*

trypanroth (tri′pan-roth) [Ger.] trypan red.

tryparosan (tri-par′o-san) a preparation formed by introducing a halogen radical (e.g., chlorine) into the parafuchsin molecule; used by injection in trypanosomiasis.

tryparsamide (trip-ar′sah-mīd) chemical name: monosodium *N*-(carbamoylmethyl) arsanilate. An antitrypanosomal agent, $C_8H_{10}AsN_2NaO_4 \cdot \frac{1}{2}H_2O$, occurring as a white crystalline powder, used in the treatment of African trypanosomiasis. Called also *tryponarsyl* and *trypotan.*

trypasafrol (tri″pah-saf′rol) one of the safranine group of aniline dyes; believed to be useful in trypanosomiasis.

trypesis (tri-pe′sis) [Gr. *trypēsis*] trephination.

trypochete (tri′po-kēt) a name given to Döhle's inclusion bodies; see under *body.*

trypomastigote (tri″po-mas′tĭ-gōt) [Gr. *trypanon* borer + *mastix* whip] the morphologic stage in the development of certain hemoflagellates of vertebrate hosts, resembling the typical adult form of *Trypanosoma* and characterized by having a flagellum arising from a posteriorly situated blepharoplast and running forward to form the outer edge of the undulating membrane; it may be free at the anterior end of the body. Called also *trypanosomal stage* or *form.* Cf. *amastigote, promastigote,* and *epimastigote.*

tryponarsyl (tri″po-nar′sil) tryparsamide.

trypotan (tri′po-tan) tryparsamide.

trypsase (trip′sās) trypsin.

trypsin (trip′sin) [Gr. *tryein* to rub + pe*psin*] a proteolytic enzyme formed in the intestine by the action of enterokinase on trypsinogen, so named by Willy Kühne, in 1874. It is an endoproteinase, acting on peptide linkages containing the carboxyl group of either lysine or arginine. **crystallized t.** [USP], a purified, crystallized preparation from an extract of the pancreas of the ox, *Bos taurus,* occurring as a white to yellowish white, crystalline or amorphous powder; used topically for its proteolytic effect in the debridement of necrotic wounds and ulcers, abscesses, fistulas, and sinuses, and in the treatment of empyema.

trypsinize (trip′sĭ-nīz) to subject to the action of trypsin.

trypsinogen (trip-sin′o-jen) [*trypsin* + Gr. *gennan* to produce] the crystallizable pre-enzyme occurring in the pancreas, from which trypsin is formed when it comes into contact with enterokinase.

trypsogen (trip′so-jen) trypsinogen.

Tryptar (trip′tar) trademark for a preparation of crystallized trypsin.

tryptase (trip′tās) any of a class of enzymes which split native proteins to peptides in neutral or near neutral solutions.

tryptic (trip″tik) relating to or produced as a result of digestion by trypsin.

tryptolysis (trip-tol′ĭ-sis) [*tryptone* + Gr. *lysis* dissolution] cleavage of tryptone.

tryptolytic (trip″to-lit′ik) pertaining to the proteolytic properties of trypsin; splitting up of tryptone.

tryptone (trip′tōn) a peptone produced by proteolytic digestion with trypsin.

tryptophan (trip′to-fān) an amino acid, $C_8H_6N \cdot CH_2 \cdot CH \cdot NH_2 \cdot COOH$, or α-amino-β-3-indole propionic acid, existing in proteins, from which it is set free by tryptic digestion; essential for optimal growth in infants and for nitrogen equilibrium in human adults. It is a precursor of serotonin. Adequate levels of tryptophan in the diet may compensate deficiencies of niacin and thus mitigate pellagra. Before the name tryptophan was accepted, *proteinochromagen* was also suggested, both names being derived from the color produced in tests.

tryptophanase (trip′to-fān-ās) an enzyme that catalyzes the cleavage of tryptophan into indole, pyruvic acid, and ammonia.

tryptophane (trip′to-fān) an earlier spelling of tryptophan.

tryptophanuria (trip″to-fān-u′re-ah) the presence of excessive amounts of tryptophan in the urine; the symptoms resemble those of pellagra.

T.S. test solution.

TSA tumor-specific antigen.

Tsa (sah) denoting a virus mutant that can effect abortive malignant transformation of a cell but not stable transformation.

tsalsahuatl (tsal″sa-whaht′l) *Eutrombicula alfreddugèsi.*

tsetse (tset′se) an African fly of the genus *Glossina.*

TSH thyroid-stimulating hormone; see *thyrotropin.*

TSH-RF thyroid-stimulating hormone releasing factor; see *thyrotropin releasing factor,* under *factor.*

TSTA tumor-specific transplantation antigen.

Tsuga (tsoo′gah) a genus of coniferous trees. **T. canaden′sis** (L.) Carr. (Pinaceae), the eastern hemlock tree, affords Canada pitch, oil of spruce, and an astringent extract.

tsutsugamushi (soot″soo-gah-moosh′e) [Japanese "dangerous bug"] scrub typhus.

T.U. toxic unit; *tuberculin unit.* See under *unit.*

Tuamine (too′ah-min) trademark for preparations of tuaminoheptane.

tuaminoheptane (too-am′ĭ-no-hep′tān) [USP] chemical name: 2-heptanamine. An adrenergic, $C_7H_{17}N$, occurring as a volatile, colorless to pale yellow liquid; administered by inhalation to produce vasoconstriction of the nasal mucosa for relief of congestion. **t. sulfate** [USP], the sulfate of tuaminoheptane, $(C_7H_{17}N)_2 \cdot H_2SO_4$, occurring as a white, odorless powder, having the same actions and uses as the base; applied topically to the nasal mucosa.

tuba (too′bah), pl. *tu′bae* [L. "trumpet"] a tube: an elongated hollow cylindrical organ; [NA] a general term for such a structure. **t. acus′tica**, t. auditiva. **t. auditi′va** [NA], **t. auditi′va [Eusta′chii]**, auditory tube: a channel, about 36 mm. long, lined with mucous membrane, that establishes communication between the tympanic cavity and the nasopharynx and serves to adjust the pressure of air in the cavity to the external pressure. It comprises a pars ossea, located in the temporal bone, and a pars cartilaginea, ending in the nasopharynx. Called also *eustachian tube.* **t. uteri′na** [NA], **t. uteri′na [Fallop′pii]**, uterine tube: a long slender tube that extends from the upper lateral angle of the uterus to the region of the ovary of the same side; it is attached to the broad ligament by the mesosalpinx, and consists of an ampulla, an infundibulum, an isthmus, two ostia, and a pars uterina. Called also *fallopian tube.*

Tubadil (too′bah-dil) trademark for a preparation of tubocurarine chloride.

tubae (too′be) plural of *tuba.*

tubal (too′bal) pertaining to or occurring in a tube, as a tubal pregnancy.

Tubarine (too′bah-rin) trademark for a preparation of tubocurarine chloride.

tubatorsion (tu″bah-tor′shun) torsion or twisting of the uterine tube.

tubba, tubboe (tub′ah; tub′o) yaws attacking the soles and palms.

tube (tūb) [L. *tubus*] an elongated hollow cylindrical organ or instrument. **Abbott-Miller t.**, Miller-Abbott t. **Abbott-Rawson t.**, a double barrelled tube through which fluid may be both injected and aspirated; it may be used for lavage or decompression of the stomach. **air t.**, any tubular passage of the respiratory apparatus. **auditory t.**, the channel that establishes communication between the tympanic cavity and the nasopharynx; see *tuba auditiva* [NA]. **Bouchut's t's**, a set of tubes for use in the intubation of the larynx. **Bowman's t's**, tubes formed artificially between the lamellae of the cornea in the process of injection; called also *corneal t's.* **buccal t.**, see *end t.* **Cantor t.**, a mercury-weighted tube for intestinal intubation. **Carrel t.**, a small-bore rubber tube ligated at its distal end, with multiple holes proximal thereto, so designed as to convey antiseptic solution to the entire surface of the wound in Carrel's treatment. **cathode-ray t.**, a vacuum tube in which the cathode rays are accelerated as a beam to form luminous spots on a fluorescent screen. **Celestin's t.**, a plastic tube used to keep the esophagus open in inoperable esophageal carcinoma. **cerebromedullary t.**, neural t. **Chaoul t.**, a low voltage x-ray tube so designed as to permit the anode to be located at 2 cm. from the body, thus permitting intense but very superficial tissue penetration of the ionizing radiation beam. **collecting t's**, tubuli renales recti. **Coolidge t.**, a vacuum tube for the generation of roentgen rays in which the cathode consists of a spiral filament of incandescent tungsten, and the anode (the target) of massive tungsten. **corneal t.**, a tubelike passage sometimes seen between the layers of the cornea. **corneal t's**, Bowman's t's. **Crookes' t.**, an early form of vacuum tube by the use of which the roentgen rays were discovered. **Devine's t.**, a diag-

nostic aid in the study of the small intestine, a tube-within-a-tube arrangement to prevent the obstruction phenomenon caused by a vacuum, by the application of an air vent. **Diamond's t.**, a double-lumen tube used in the study of the small intestine; similar to the Abbot-Rawson tube. **digestive t.**, canalis alimentarius. **discharge t.**, a vessel of insulating material (usually glass) provided with metal electrodes which is exhausted to a low gas pressure and permits the passage of electricity through the residual gas when a moderately high voltage is applied to the electrodes. **drainage t.**, a tube used in surgery to facilitate the escape of fluids. **dressed t.**, a rubber drainage tube with a gauze strip wound around it, the whole covered with gutta-percha. **duodenal t.**, a tube intended to be passed into the duodenum. **Durham's t.**, 1. [Arthur Edward *Durham*] a jointed tracheostomy tube. 2. [Herbert Edward *Durham*] a small inverted test tube used in determining bacterial gas production. **empyema t.**, a rubber tube for draining pus in thoracic empyema. **end t.**, an attachment on the buccal surface of a terminal banded molar; often referred to as *buccal tube.* **endobronchial t.**, a double-lumen tube inserted into the bronchus of one lung and permitting the complete deflation of other lung; used in anesthesia and thoracic surgery. **endotracheal t.**, an airway catheter inserted in the trachea in endotracheal intubation. **Esmarch's t's**, tubes used in making roll cultures of bacteria. **esophageal t.**, a soft, flexible tube for lavage of the stomach and artificial forced feeding. **eustachian t.**, tuba auditiva. **Ewald t.**, a tube of large bore used to evacuate the stomach. **fallopian t.**, tuba uterina. **feeding t.**, a tube for introducing fluids of high caloric value into the stomach. **fermentation t.**, a U-shaped tube with one arm closed for determining gas production by bacteria. **Ferrein's t's**, the convoluted uriniferous tubules. **fusion t's**, the pair of tubes used in observing and cultivating the power of fusion in eyes affected with heterophoria. **gas t.**, a roentgen-ray tube which depends for its action on the presence of residual gas; the cathode is not heated and the target is usually connected electrically to the anode. **Geissler's t.**, Geissler-Pluecker t., a discharge tube for showing the luminous effects of discharges through rarefied gases. **granulation t.**, a laryngeal intubation tube with a large head which covers any granulations that may have been formed about the wound. **Guisez's t.**, a self-retaining rubber tube for use in cancer of the esophagus. **Harris t.**, a single-lumen tube utilizing mercury as a weight, used as a diagnostic aid in the study of the small intestine; the construction of the head is exactly the same as in the Miller-Abbott tube. **Hittorf t.**, Crookes' t. **horizontal t.**, a metal tube attachment placed in a horizontal position on the buccal surface of each anchor molar tooth to allow for the insertion of the labial arch wire. **hot-cathode t.**, a vacuum tube in which the cathode is electrically heated to incandescence and in which the stream of electrons depends on the temperature of the cathode. **intubation t.**, a breathing tube introduced in the air passage after tracheostomy or laryngostomy. **Killian's t's**, tubes for use in removing foreign bodies from the trachea and esophagus. **Kobelt's t's**, the remains of the tubules of the mesonephros in the paroophoron. **Kuhn's t.**, a flexible tube of metal for use in intratracheal anesthesia. **Leonard t.**, cathode-ray t. **Levin t.**, a gastroduodenal catheter of sufficiently small caliber to permit transnasal passage. **McCollum t.**, an apparatus for keeping a patient dry when there is a large amount of drainage from a sinus. **medullary t.**, neural t. **Mett's t's**, small glass tubes filled with coagulated egg white for testing peptic activity; see under *tests.* **Miescher's t's**, sarcosporidian cysts. **Miller-Abbott t.**, a double-channel intestinal tube with an inflatable balloon at its distal end, for use in the treatment of obstruction of the small intestine; occasionally useful also as a diagnostic aid. **multiple-lumen t.**, a tube containing more than two lumina, used primarily for experimental purposes. Perforations are made into the separate lumina at different levels depending on the location and number of segments of the intestine to be studied **nasogastric t.**, a tube of soft rubber or plastic inserted through a nostril and into the stomach, for instilling liquid foods or other substances, or for withdrawing gastric contents. **nephrostomy t.**, a tube inserted through the abdominal wall into the pelvis of the kidney, for direct drainage of the urine. **Neuber's t's**, drainage tubes of bone. **neural t.**, the epithelial tube developed from the neural plate and forming the central nervous system of the embryo; called also *medullary t.* and *cerebromedullary t.* **O'Dwyer's t.**, an intubation tube. **Olshevsky t.**, a roentgen-ray tube constructed to use only the stronger rays which pass through the target and armoring the rest of the tube. **otopharyngeal t.**, tuba auditiva. **ovarian t's**, groups of cells which grow down and are cut off from the much thickened surface layer of the ovary; they differentiate into primary oocytes, each with a follicular layer. Called also *Pflüger's t's* or *Pflüger's cords.* **Paul-Mixter t.**, a large-calibered, flanged drainage tube of glass used for temporary intestinal decompression. **Pflüger's t's**, the ovarian tubes. **pharyngotympanic t.**, tuba auditiva. **photomultiplier t.**, a vacuum tube that converts electromagnetic radiation signals into electrical pulses, consisting of a light-sensitive surface that emits electrons when light is incident on it, the electrons then passing through successive stages with electron multiplication at each stage. **pus t.**, pyosalpinx. **Rainey's t's**, sarcosporidian cysts. **Rehfuss' t.**, a specially designed stomach tube used in making the Rehfuss test. **Roida's t.**, a tube designed for the separation of motile from nonmotile bacteria; the motile organisms make their way through sand, glass-wool and other obstructions. **roll t.**, a test tube in which liquid agar culture medium is placed, the tube then being tilted and rotated so that the inside of the tube becomes coated with the culture medium. **Ruysch's t.**, a very small tubular opening on the nasal septum, just anterior and inferior to the nasopalatine foramen: it is a relic of the fetal Jacobson's organ. **Ryle's t.**, a thin rubber tube with an olive-shaped end used in giving a test meal. **salivary t's**, the interlobular ducts of the salivary glands. **Schachowa's spiral t's**, tubuli renales. **Sengstaken-Blakemore t.**, a device used for the tamponade of bleeding esophageal varices, consisting of three tubes: one leading to a balloon which is inflated in the stomach, to retain the instrument in place, and to compress the vessels around the cardia; another leading to a long narrow balloon by which pressure is exerted against the wall of the esophagus; and the third attached to a suction apparatus for aspirating contents of the stomach. **Shiner's t.**, a flexible plastic radiopaque tube for obtaining biopsy material from the jejunum under fluoroscopic control; the jejunal mucosa is drawn by suction into a small aperture in the knife cylinder head at the end of the tube, and a portion is excised. **sieve t.**, the conductive element of phloem. **Souttar's t.**, a metal tube used to keep the esophagus open in inoperable esophageal carcinoma. **sputum t.**, a graduated capillary tube for containing sputum to be rotated in the centrifuge. **stomach t.**, a tube for feeding or for irrigation of the stomach. **T t.**, a self-retaining drainage tube in the shape of a T. **tampon t.**, a piece of stout rubber tubing wound with iodoform gauze, used in plugging the rectum to control oozing and at the same time to allow the escape of gas. **test t.**, a tube of thin glass closed at one end, used for various procedures in chemistry and for observing the growth of bacterial cultures. **thoracostomy t.**, a tube inserted through an opening in the chest wall, for application of suction to the pleural cavity often used to facilitate reexpansion of the lung in spontaneous pneumothorax. **Thunberg t.**, a laboratory tube used extensively in studies of dehydrogenases. **tracheostomy t.**, a curved tube to be inserted into the trachea through the opening made in tracheostomy. **uterine t.**, tuba uterina. **vacuum t.**, a glass tube from which the air has been exhausted to a high degree of vacuum; see *Crookes's t.* and *Geissler's t.* **valve t.**, a vacuum tube used to rectify an alternating current. **Veillon t.**, a piece of glass tubing with a rubber cork at one end and a plug of cotton at the other, used in bacterial culture work. **vertical t.**, an orthodontic attachment usually placed on the lingual surface of the anchor band to allow for the insertion of the lingual arch wire. **Voltolini's t.**, a tube for keeping open an incision in the tympanic membrane. **Wangensteen t.**, a small tube passed through the nose into the stomach and connected with a special suction apparatus to maintain gastric and duodenal decompression; called also *Wangensteen's apparatus.* **x-ray t.**, a glass vacuum bulb containing two electrodes. Electrons are obtained either from gas in the tube or from a heated cathode. When suitable potential is applied, electrons travel at high velocity from cathode to anode, where they are suddenly arrested, giving rise to x-rays.

tubectomy (too-bek′to-me) excision of a portion of the uterine tube.

tuber (too′ber), pl. *tubers* or *tu′bera* [L.] 1. a swelling, protuberance; [NA] a general term for such a structure. See also *tubercle, tuberculum, tuberositas,* and *tuberosity.* 2. a thickened underground plant stem adapted for food storage, such as is found in the potato. **t. ante′rius hypothal′ami**, t. cinereum. **t. calca′nei** [NA], the posteroinferior projection of the calcaneus that forms the heel; called also *tuberosity of calcaneus.* **t. cine′reum** [NA], a layer of gray matter which is part of the hypothalamus; forming a part of the floor of the third ventricle, it lies in front of and between the corpora mamillaria and merges anteriorly into the infundibulum. Called also *tuberculum cinereum* and *gray tubercle.* **t. coch′leae**, promontorium tympani. **eustachian t.**, an eminence on the medial wall of the tympanum, below the vestibular window. **external t. of Henle**, tuberculum mentale mandibulae. **frontal t., t. fronta′le** [NA], one of the slight rounded prominences on the frontal bone on either side above the eyes, forming the most prominent portions of the forehead; called also *frontal eminence.* **iliopubic t.**, eminentia iliopubica. **t. ischiad′icum** [NA], **t. is′chii**, ischial tuberosity: a large elongated mass on the inferior part of the posterior margin of the body of the ischium, to which several muscles are attached. **t. maxil′lae** [NA], **t. maxilla′re**, maxillary t., a rounded eminence at the posteroinferior angle of the infratemporal surface of the maxilla; called also *tuberosity of maxilla.* **mental t.**, tuberculum mentale mandibulae. **omental t. of liver**, t. omentale hepatis. **omental t. of pancreas**, t. omentale pancreatis. **t. omenta′le hep′atis** [NA], omental tuber of liver: the rounded prominence on the posteroinferior surface of the left lobe of the liver, just cranial to the lesser curvature of the stomach. **t. omenta′le pancrea′tis** [NA], omental tuber of pancreas: a rounded prominence chiefly on the anterior surface of the neck of the pancreas. **papillary t. of liver**, processus papillaris hepatis. **parietal t., t. parieta′le** [NA], the somewhat laterally bulging prominence just superior to the superior temporal line on the external surface of the parietal bone. **t. ra′dii, t. of radius**, tuberositas radii. **sciatic t.**, t. ischiadicum. **t. val′vulae cerebel′li**, t. vermis. **t. ver′mis** [NA], the part of the vermis of the cerebellum between the folium vermis and the pyramid; called also *commissura brevis loborum posteriorum inferiorum cerebelli.* **t. zygomat′icum**, tuberculum articulare ossis temporalis.

tubera (too′ber-ah) [L.] plural of *tuber.*

tubercle (too′ber-k'l) 1. any of the small, rounded, granulomatous lesions produced by infection with *Mycobacterium tuberculosis;* it is the characteristic lesion of tuberculosis, and consists of a translucent mass, gray in color, made up of a collection of modified macrophages resembling epithelial cells (*epithelioid cells*), surrounded by a rim of mononuclear cells, principally lymphocytes, and sometimes a center of giant multinucleate cells (*Langhans' giant cells*). Called also *gray t.* 2. a nodule, or small eminence, such as a rough, rounded eminence on a bone; called also *tuberculum* [NA]. 3. (*obs.*) a nodule, especially a solid elevation of the skin, larger in size than a papule. 4. dental t. See also *tuber, tuberositas,* and *tuberosity.* **acoustic t.**, area vestibularis. **adductor t. of femur**, tuberculum adductorium femoris. **amygdaloid t. of Schwalbe**, area vestibularis. **anatomical t.**, tuberculosis verrucosa. **t. of anterior scalene muscle**, tuberculum musculi scaleni anterioris. **articular t. of temporal bone**, tuberculum articulare ossis temporalis. **t. of atlas, anterior**, tuberculum anterius atlantis. **t. of atlas, posterior**, tuberculum posterius atlantis. **auricular t.**, tuberculum auriculae. **Babès' t's**, cellular aggregations around degenerated neurons in the medulla oblongata and the spinal ganglia in cases of rabies and other types of encephalitis. **brachial t. of humerus**, processus supracondylaris humeri. **calcaneal t.**, processus lateralis tuberis calcanei. **Carabelli t.**, see under *cusp.* **carotid t. of sixth cervical vertebra**, tuberculum caroticum vertebrae cervicalis VI. **caseous t.**, a yellowish mass of cheesy material, thought to represent a typical lesion of tuberculosis that has undergone degeneration. **caudal t. of liver**, processus caudatus hepatis. **cervical t's**, two small eminences on the femur, a *superior* on the upper and anterior part of the neck at its junction with the greater trochanter, and an *inferior* at the junction with the lesser trochanter. **t. of cervical vertebrae, anterior**, tuberculum anterius vertebrarum cervicalium. **t. of cervical vertebrae, posterior**, tuberculum posterius vertebrarum cervicalium. **Chassaignac's t.**, tuberculum caroticum vertebrae cervicalis VI. **condyloid t.**, an eminence on the condylar process of the mandible for attachment of the lateral ligament of the temporomandibular articulation. **conglomerate t.**, a mass made up of an aggregation of many smaller nodules. **conoid t.**, tuberculum conoideum. **corniculate t.**, tuberculum corniculatum. **t. of crown of tooth**, dental t. **crude t.**, caseous t. **cuneiform t.**, tuberculum cuneiforme. **darwinian t.**, tuberculum auriculae. **deltoid t.**, 1. a prominence on the clavicle for attachment of the deltoid muscle. 2. tuberositas deltoidea humeri. **dental t.**, 1. a small elevation of indiscriminate size on some portion of the tooth crown, produced by extra formation of enamel. 2. tuberculum coronae dentis. **dorsal t. of radius**, an easily palpable prominence on the distal, dorsal aspect of the radius, which is grooved by the tendon of the extensor pollicis longus muscle; called also *Lister's t.* **epiglottic t.**, tuberculum epiglotticum. **Farre's t's**, masses beneath the capsule of the liver, felt on palpation in certain cases of hepatic cancer. **fibrous t.**, a tubercle of bacillary origin which contains connective tissue elements. **t. of fibula, posterior**, apex capitis fibulae. **genial t.**, tuberculum mentale mandibulae. **genital t.**, an eminence in front of the cloaca in the early embryo, which becomes the penis or the clitoris. **Ghon t.**, see under *focus.* **gracile t.**, tuberculum nuclei gracilis. **gray t.**, 1. the typical lesion of tuberculosis; see *tubercle* (def. 2). 2. tuberculum cinereum. 3. tuber cinereum. **greater t. of calcaneus**, processus medialis tuberis calcanei. **t. of greater multangular bone**, tuberculum ossis trapezii. **hippocampal t.**, an expansion of the hippocampus at its lower end, separating the fimbria from the gyrus dentatus. **His' t.**, a small prominence on the posteroinferior part of the pinna. **t. of humerus**, capitulum humeri. **t. of humerus, anterior, of Meckel**, tuberculum majus humeri. **t. of humerus, anterior, of Weber**, tuberculum minus humeri. **t. of humerus, external**, tuberculum majus humeri. **t. of humerus, greater**, tuberculum majus humeri. **t. of humerus, internal**, tuberculum minus humeri. **t. of humerus, lesser**, tuberculum minus humeri. **t. of humerus, posterior**, tuberculum majus humeri. **iliopectineal t.**, iliopubic t., eminentia iliopubica. **inferior t. of Humphrey**, processus accessorius vertebrarum lumbalium. **infraglenoid t.**, tuberculum infraglenoidale. **intercondylar t.**, eminentia intercondylaris. **intercondylar t., lateral**, tuberculum intercondylare laterale. **intercondylar t., medial**, tuberculum intercondylare mediale. **intervenous t.**, tuberculum intervenosum. **intravascular t.**, a tubercle in the intima of a blood vessel. **jugular t. of occipital bone,** tuberculum jugulare ossis occipitalis. **labial t.,** tuberculum labii superioris. **lacrimal t.,** papilla lacrimalis. *lateral or-***bital t.,** Whitnall's t. **lateral palpebral t.,** Whitnall's t. **lesser t. of calcaneus,** processus lateralis tuberis calcanei. **Lisfranc's t.,** tuberculum musculi scaleni anterioris. **Lister's t.,** dorsal t. of radius. **Lower's t.,** tuberculum inter-venosum. **Luschka's t.,** carina urethralis vaginae. **lymphoid t.,** a lesion of tuberculosis consisting of lymphoid cells. **mamillary t. of hypothalamus,** corpus mamillare. **mamillary t. of vertebrae,** processus mamillaris vertebra-rum. **marginal t. of zygomatic bone,** tuberculum marginale ossis zygomatici. **mental t.,** tuberculum mentale man-dibulae. **mental t., external,** protuberantia mentalis. **mental t. of mandible,** tuberculum mentale mandibulae. **miliary t.,** one of the many minute tubercles formed in many organs in acute miliary tuberculosis. **Montgomery's t's,** greatly enlarged sebaceous glands (Morgagni's tubercles) observed on the surface of the areola of the mammary gland during pregnancy. **Morgagni's t.,** 1. bulbus olfactorius. 2. one of the small nodules on the surface of the areola of the mammary gland produced by the superficially situated large sebaceous glands. **Müller's t.,** a protrusion into the urogenital sinus caused by the downward-growing mesonephric and paramesonephric ducts. **muscular t. of atlas,** tuberculum anterius atlantis. **naked t.,** an aggregation of large, pale-staining epithelioid cells with few or no intermingling small round cells, a characteristic finding in sarcoidosis. **t. of navicular bone,** tuberculum ossis scaphoidei. **necrogenic t's,** the papules of tuberculosis verrucosa cutis. **nuchal t.,** the prominence formed by the spinous process of the seventh cervical vertebra. **t. of nucleus cuneatus,** tuberculum nuclei cuneati. **t. of nucleus gracilis,** tuberculum nuclei gracilis. **obturator t., anterior,** tuberculum obturatorium anterius. **obturator t., posterior,** tuberculum obturatorium posterius. **olfactory t.,** bulbus olfactorius. **papillary t.,** processus papillaris hepatis. **pharyngeal t.,** tuberculum pharyngeum. **plantar t.,** tuberositas ossis metatarsalis I. **t. of posterior process of talus, lateral,** tuberculum laterale processus posterioris tali. **t. of posterior process of talus, medial,** tuberculum mediale processus posterioris tali. **pterygoid t.,** tuberositas pterygoidea mandibulae. **pubic t. of pubic bone,** tuberculum pubicum ossis pubis. **rabic t's,** Babès' t's. **t. of rib,** tuberculum costae. **t. of Rolando,** tuberculum cinereum, def. 1. **t. of root of zygoma,** tuberculum articulare ossis temporalis. **t. of Santorini,** tuberculum corniculatum. **scalene t.,** tuberculum musculi scaleni anterioris. **t. of scaphoid bone,** tuberculum ossis scaphoidei. **t. of sella turcica,** tuberculum sellae turcicae. **superior t. of Henle,** tuberculum obturatorium posterius. **superior t. of Humphrey,** processus mamillaris vertebrarum. **supraglenoid t.,** tuberculum supraglenoidalis. **supratragic t.,** tuberculum supratragicum. **t. of thalamus, anterior,** tuberculum anterius thalami. **t. of thalamus, posterior,** pulvinar. **thyroid t., inferior,** tuberculum thyroideum inferius. **thyroid t., superior,** tuberculum thyroideum superius. **t. of tibia,** eminentia intercondylaris. **transverse t. of fourth tarsal bone,** tuberositas ossis cuboidei. **t. of trapezium,** tuberculum ossis trapezii. **trochlear t.,** spina trochlearis. **t. of ulna,** tuberositas ulnae. **t. of upper lip,** tuberculum labii superioris. **t's of vertebra,** three elevations (*superior, inferior,* and *external*) upon the transverse process of the last thoracic vertebra, and represented on the lumbar vertebrae by more or less rudimentary structures. **Whitnall's t.,** a small eminence on the internal aspect of the middle of the orbital surface of the zygomatic bone; called also *lateral orbital* or *palpebral t.* **Wrisberg's t.,** tuberculum cuneiforme. **yellow t.,** caseous t. **t. of zygoma, zygomatic t.,** tuberculum articulare ossis temporalis.

tubercula (too-ber′ku-lah) [L.] plural of *tuberculum.*

tubercular (too-ber′ku-lar) of, pertaining to, or resembling tubercles or nodules. Cf. *tuberculous.*

Tuberculariaceae (too-ber″ku-lar″ĭ-a′se-e) a family of Fungi Imperfecti of the order Moniliales, including the genus *Fusarium.*

tuberculase (too-ber′ku-lās) an extract of tubercle bacilli once used for protective inoculation against tuberculosis.

tuberculate, tuberculated (too-ber′ku-lāt″; too-ber′ku-lāt″ed) covered with tubercles; affected with tubercle.

tuberculation (too-ber″ku-la′shun) the development of tubercles; the becoming affected with tubercles.

tuberculid (too-ber′ku-lid) a papular skin eruption usually attributed to a state of allergy to tuberculosis. **papulonecrotic t., rosacea-like t.,** a grouped, symmetric eruption appearing in successive crops in children and young adults with tuberculosis, and consisting of small papules or nodules which undergo necrosis and heal with scarring; called also *tuberculosis papulonecrotica.*

tuberculigenous (too-ber″ku-lij′ĕ-nus) [*tubercle* + Gr. *gennan* to produce] causing tuberculosis.

tuberculin (too-ber′ku-lin) a sterile liquid containing the growth products of, or specific substances extracted from, the tubercle bacillus. The form first prepared (Old tuberculin) by

boiling, filtering, and concentrating a bouillon culture of tubercle bacilli, was put forth as a cure for tuberculosis by Koch in 1890 (Koch's lymph paratoloid, paratoloidin). In various forms tuberculin is used in the diagnosis of tuberculosis infection, especially in children and cattle, and formerly also in the treatment of tuberculosis. The tuberculin test, as commonly applied, consists in the injection of tuberculin under or into the skin; the injection has no effect in nontuberculous subjects, but causes inflammation at the site of the injection in tuberculous subjects. See *tuberculin test,* under *tests.* **albumose-free (A.F.) t.,** tuberculin free from albumose, used for the subcutaneous tuberculin test. Called also *Tuberculin Albumose Frei (T.A.F.).* **T. Albumose Frei (T.A.F.),** albumose-free t. **alkaline t.,** a preparation obtained from tubercle bacilli by extracting with $\frac{1}{10}$ normal soda solution; much the same as the original tuberculin. **autogenous t.,** autotuberculin. **bacillary emulsion (B.E.) t. (T.B.E.),** tubercle cultures are dried, ground, and suspended (1 gm.) in equal parts of water and glycerol (200 ml.). It differs from New tuberculin in that the tubercle bacilli are not washed nor is the supernatant fluid from the first centrifugalization discarded. **Behring's t.,** 1. tuberculase. 2. tulase. **Béraneck's t.,** cultures of tubercle bacilli grown on a nonpeptonized, 5 per cent glycerin bouillon are filtered and the microorganisms are extracted in 1 per cent orthophosphoric acid by long-continued shaking. This extract (basiotoxin) is mixed with an equal volume of the filtrate (acidotoxin) for use. **t. bouillon filtrate (B.F.),** the clear glycerin bouillon in which tubercle cultures have been grown and from which they have been filtered out. It is not heated or concentrated. Called also *Denys' tuberculin.* **Calmette's t.,** purified tuberculin, prepared by precipitating Old tuberculin with alcohol, washing, dissolving in water, and filtering. When instilled in the conjunctiva of persons affected with tuberculosis or typhoid fever it produces a severe local reaction. Called also *tuberculin precipitation (T.P.).* See also *ophthalmic reaction,* under *reaction.* **t. contagious (T.C.),** von Behring's name for tuberculin which is said to be taken up by the cells of the body and there transformed into an integral part of those cells; in this form it is called *TX.* **Denys' t.,** t. bouillon filtrate. **Dixon's t.,** a tuberculin prepared by treating living tubercle cultures with ether and extracting in salt solution. **t. filtrate (T.F.),** a tuberculin preparation made by precipitating and filtering the dissolved precipitate separately. **Hirschfelder's t.,** oxytuberculin. **Klebs' t.,** tuberculocidin. **Klemperer's t.,** a tuberculin prepared from cultures of bovine tuberculosis. **Koch's t.,** see *New t., Old t.* **Maragliano's t.,** a tuberculin containing all the extracts of the tubercle bacillus that are soluble in water. **Maréchal's t.,** a mixture of Old tuberculin and guaiacol. **Moro's t.,** diagnostic t. **New t.,** a suspension of the fragments of tubercle bacilli, freed from all soluble materials and with glycerin added: tubercle bacilli are triturated to a fine consistency and suspended in distilled water or physiological salt solution. Centrifugation results in separation into a translucent supernatant (TO, *tuberculin ober*) and a muddy sediment (TR, *tuberculin rest*). This sediment is dried, again triturated, and suspended and centrifuged. The process is repeated until only an opalescent fluid is obtained. The addition of a sufficient quantity of glycerin to make a 20 per cent solution renders the preparation ready for use. Called also *Koch's t., original t.* (T.O.), *residue t.,* and *t. residue* (T.R.). **Old t. (O.T.)** [USP], a sterile solution of concentrated, soluble products of the growth of tubercle bacilli, adjusted to standard potency by addition of glycerin and isotonic sodium chloride solution, final glycerin content being about 50 per cent. It is used as a dermal reactivity indication in the diagnosis of tuberculosis. Called also *Koch's t.* and *tuberculinum pristinum.* **original t. (T.O.),** New t. **perlsucht t.,** Perlsucht T. Original (P.T.O.), Spengler's t. **Perlsucht T. Rest (P.T.R.),** a tuberculin prepared from bacilli of bovine tuberculosis in the same manner as New tuberculin. **t. precipitation (T.P.),** Calmette's t. **purified t.,** Calmette's t. **purified protein derivative (P.P.D.) of t.** [USP], a sterile, soluble partially purified product of growth of the tubercle bacillus prepared in a special liquid medium free from protein. It is used as a dermal reactivity indicator in the diagnosis of tuberculosis. **residual t., t. residue (T.R.),** New t. **Rosenbach's t.,** tuberculin prepared from cultures which have been infected with *Trichophyton holosericum-album,* which reduces the toxicity of the tubercle bacilli. **Ruck's watery extract t.,** tubercle cultures are concentrated in vacuo at 55° C. to one tenth volume and filtered. The filtrate is precipitated with an acid solution of sodium bismuth iodide. Filter, neutralize the filtrate, and filter again. Precipitate the filtrate with enough absolute alcohol to make 90 per cent alcohol, filter, and make a 1 per cent aqueous solution of the dry precipitate. **Seibert's t.,** 1. purified protein derivative of t. 2. a purified tuberculin used intradermally as a test for tuberculosis. **Selter's t.,** vital t. **Spengler's t.,** a preparation from the bacilli of bovine tuberculosis; called also *perlsucht t.* and *Perlsucht Tuberculin Original (P.T.O.).* **Thamm's t.,** tuberculoalbumin. **vacuum t. (V.T.),** Old tuberculin reduced in a vacuum to much less than its original volume. **Vaudremer's t.,** tuberculin prepared by macerating it in the ground up mycelia of *Aspergillus fumigatus,* which renders the tuberculin nearly free from toxicity. **vital t.,** a tuberculin prepared by triturating moist attenuated human tubercle bacilli; the preparation contains a few living tubercle bacilli of very slight virulence. **t. zymoplastiche (TZ),** the dried residue of the portions of the tubercle bacillus which are soluble in alcohol.

tuberculination (too-ber″ku-lin-a′shun) tuberculinization.

tuberculinization (too-ber″ku-lin″i-za′shun) treatment by use of tuberculin or the application of the tuberculin test.

tuberculinose (too-ber′ku-lin″ōs) a modified form of tuberculin.

tuberculinotherapy (too-ber″ku-lin″o-ther′ah-pe) the therapeutic use of tuberculin.

tuberculinum (too-ber″ku-li′num) [L.] tuberculin. **t. pristi′num,** Old tuberculin.

tuberculitis (too″ber-ku-li′tis) [*tubercle* + *-itis*] inflammation of or near a tubercle.

tuberculization (too-ber″ku-li-za′shun) 1. treatment with tuberculin or its modifications. 2. the formation of or conversion into tubercles.

tuberculoalbumin (too-ber″ku-lo-al-bu′min) (*obs.*) a preparation very much like tuberculase, but extracted by a different method.

tuberculocele (too-ber′ku-lo-sēl″) [*tubercle* + Gr. *kēlē* tumor] tuberculous disease of the testis.

tuberculocidal (too-ber′ku-lo-si′dal) lethal to *Mycobacterium tuberculosis.*

tuberculocide (too-ber′ku-lo-sīd″) an agent that is lethal to *Mycobacterium tuberculosis.*

tuberculocidin (too-ber″ku-lo-si′din) an albumose derived from tuberculin by treating it with platinum chloride. It is used like tuberculin, but is said to be free from the objectionable characters of the latter.

tuberculoderm (too-ber′ku-lo-derm) any tuberculous condition or disease of the skin.

tuberculofibroid (too-ber″ku-lo-fi′broid) characterized by a tubercle that has undergone a fibroid degeneration.

tuberculofibrosis (too-ber″ku-lo-fi-bro′sis) fibroid phthisis.

tuberculoid (too-ber′ku-loid) resembling a tubercle or tuberculosis.

tuberculoidin (too-ber″ku-loi′din) a form of modified tuberculin cleared of its bacilli by treatment with alcohol.

tuberculoma (too-ber″ku-lo′mah) a tumor-like mass resulting from enlargement of a caseous tubercle. **t. en plaque,** a flat plaque on the surface of the frontoparietal cortex in tuberculous meningoencephalitis, producing the symptoms of brain tumor.

tuberculomyces (too-ber″ku-lom′ĭ-sēz) [*tuberculosis* + Gr. *mykēs* fungus] a name for the group of bacteria including the *Mycobacterium tuberculosis* and similar bacteria.

tuberculo-opsonic (too-ber″ku-lo-op-son′ik) pertaining to the opsonin capable of sensitizing tubercle bacilli.

tuberculoprotein (too-ber″ku-lo-pro′te-in) protein derived from the bodies of tubercle bacilli.

tuberculosarium (too-ber″ku-lo-sa′re-um) a sanatorium for the tuberculous.

tuberculosilicosis (too-ber″ku-lo-sil″ĭ-ko′sis) silicosis complicated by pulmonary tuberculosis.

tuberculosis (too-ber″ku-lo′sis) any of the infectious diseases of man and animals caused by species of *Mycobacterium* and characterized by the formation of tubercles and caseous necrosis in the tissues. The common causative species are *M. tuberculosis, M. bovis,* and *M. avium,* but the disease is also caused by several atypical mycobacteria, including *M. kansasii* and others as yet unclassified. Atypical infections, which are clinically and morphologically indistinguishable from the typical disease, do not appear to be directly transmissible from man to man. Tuberculosis varies widely in its manifestations and has a tendency to great chronicity. Any organ may be affected, although in man the lung is the major seat of the disease and the usual portal through which the infection reaches other organs. **acute miliary t.,** an acute form of tuberculosis in which minute tubercles are formed in a number of organs of the body, due to dissemination of the bacilli throughout the body by the blood stream. **adrenal t.,** Addison's disease. **adult t.,** see *postprimary t.* and *primary t.* **aerogenic t.,** inhalation t. **anthracotic t.,** tuberculosis associated with pneumoconiosis of coal workers. **atypical t.,** mycobacteriosis. **avian t.,** a variety of tuberculosis affecting various birds, including chickens and ducks, caused by *Mycobacterium avium,* and characterized by tubercles consisting principally of epithelioid cells. It may be communicated to other animals and man. **basal t.,** tuberculosis situated in the lower part of the affected lung. **t. of bones and joints,** tuberculosis involving the bones and joints, producing strumous arthritis, or white swelling, and cold abscess. **bovine t.,** an infection of cattle caused by *Mycobacterium bovis,* transmissible to man and other animals. **cerebral t.,** tuberculous meningitis. **cestodic t.,** a disease simulating tuberculosis, but due to excessive infestation with cestode parasites. **chicken t.,** avian tuberculosis occurring in chickens. **childhood t.,** primary t. **t. col-**

liquati′va, scrofuloderma. **t. cu′tis,** tuberculosis of the skin, including lupus vulgaris, tuberculosis verrucosa cutis, scrofuloderma, tuberculosis cutis orificialis, papulonecrotic tuberculid, etc. **t. cu′tis colliquati′va,** scrofuloderma. **t. cu′tis indurati′va,** former name for *erythema induratum.* **t. cu′tis lichenoi′des,** lichen scrofulosorum. **t. cu′tis orificia′lis,** a condition occurring in patients with systemic tuberculosis, characterized by the development, about the mucocutaneous junctions and on the skin contiguous to the body orifices, of indolent, round, shallow granulating ulcers covered with thin crusts. **disseminated t.,** acute miliary t. **exudative t.,** the simplest form of pulmonary tuberculosis, frequently the earliest reaction to infection, in which the alveolar spaces and the smaller bronchi become filled with a cellular exudate consisting mainly of large mononuclear cells; called also *tuberculous pneumonia.* **fowl t.,** avian tuberculosis occurring in fowl. **genital t.,** tuberculosis of the genital tract, e.g., tuberculous endometritis. **genitourinary t.,** tuberculosis involving the genitourinary tract, often the result of hemic dissemination of pulmonary tuberculosis. **hematogenous t.,** infection with *Mycobacterium tuberculosis* carried through the blood stream to other organs from the primary site of infection. **hilus t.,** tuberculosis involving the hilus of the lung. **t. indurati′va,** former name for *erythema induratum.* **inhalation t.,** tuberculosis caused by aspiration of the tubercle bacilli into the lungs. **t. of intestines,** tuberculosis involving the intestines, marked by formation of spreading ulcers, especially of the lymphoid tissue; attended by diarrhea, and sometimes resulting in cicatricial stricture. **t. of kidney,** renal t. **t. of larynx,** tuberculosis involving the larynx, producing ulceration of the vocal cords and elsewhere on the mucosa, and commonly attended by hoarseness, cough, pain on swallowing, and hemoptysis. **t. lichenoi′des,** lichen scrofulosorum. **t. of lungs,** infection of the lungs caused by *Mycobacterium tuberculosis.* Characteristically, the course of the untreated disease is as follows: tuberculous pneumonia, formation of tuberculous granulation tissue, caseous necrosis, calcification, and cavity formation. It may spread to other lung segments via the bronchi, or to other organs via the blood or lymph vessels. Symptoms may include weight loss, lassitude and fatigue, night sweats, and wasting, with purulent sputum, hemoptysis, and chest pain. **t. lupo′sa,** lupus vulgaris. **t. of lymph nodes, lymphoid t.,** scrofula. **miliary t.,** see *acute miliary t.* **open t.,** 1. tuberculosis in which there are lesions from which the tubercle bacilli are being discharged out of the body. 2. tuberculosis of the lungs with cavitation. **t. orificia′lis,** t. cutis orificialis. **t. papulonecrot′ica,** papulonecrotic tuberculid. **postprimary t.,** pulmonary tuberculosis, formerly known as the adult type, that is typical of a fresh infection (a reinfection) of the lungs of a person who has had an earlier and probably subclinical attack of tuberculosis; it is distinguished by caseation and cavitation and by healing that results in fibrosis. Called also *reinfection t.* **primary t.,** tuberculosis of the lungs, formerly known as the childhood type, occurring when the individual is first infected with the disease. In children, it results in tuberculous pneumonia and is characterized by the formation of a primary complex, consisting of a parenchymal pulmonary lesion with a corresponding lymph node focus. In adults, it is more likely to be marked by a small subapical focus. **productive t.,** pulmonary tuberculosis in which a new type of tissue—tuberculous granulation tissue, consisting of epithelioid cells in concentric masses, lymphocytes, and often Langhans giant cells—appears at the site of infection. **pulmonary t.,** t. of lungs. **reinfection t.,** postprimary t. **t. of serous membranes,** tuberculosis involving the pleura, peritoneum, pericardium, and cerebral meninges, producing inflammation of those structures. **t. of skin,** t. cutis. **spinal t., t. of spine,** osteitis or caries of the vertebrae, usually occurring as a complication of tuberculosis of the lungs; it is marked by stiffness of the vertebral column, pain on motion, tenderness on pressure, prominence of certain of the vertebral spines, and occasionally abdominal pain, abscess formation, and paralysis. Called also *David's disease, dorsal phthisis, Pott's disease, spondylitis tuberculosa,* and *tuberculous spondylitis.* **surgical t.,** tuberculosis which is amenable to treatment by surgical means. **tracheobronchial t.,** productive tuberculous involvement of the bronchi, characterized by wheezing, mucosal redness and edema, granulation tissue, and sometimes ulceration and bronchial stricture due to cicatrization. **t. ulcero′sa,** t. cutis orificialis. **uveoparotid t.,** uveoparotid fever. **t. verruco′sa, t. verruco′sa cu′tis,** a condition usually resulting from external inoculation of the tubercle bacilli into the skin, but sometimes initiated by systemic infection, with wartlike papules coalescing to form distinctly verrucous patches with an inflammatory, erythematous border; called also *verruca necrogenica* and *warty tuberculosis.* **warty t.,** t. verrucosa.

tuberculostatic (too-ber″ku-lo-stat′ik) 1. inhibiting the growth of *Mycobacterium tuberculosis.* 2. an agent that inhibits the growth of *Mycobacterium tuberculosis.*

tuberculotic (too-ber″ku-lot′ik) pertaining to or affected with tuberculosis.

tuberculous (too-ber′ku-lus) pertaining to or affected with tuberculosis: tuberculotic; caused by the *Mycobacterium tuberculosis.* Cf. *tubercular.*

tuberculum (too-ber′ku-lum), pl. *tuber′cula* [L., dim. of *tuber*] a tubercle, nodule, or small eminence; [NA] general term for such a structure. See also *tubercle, tuber, tuberositas,* and *tuberosity.* **t. acus′ticum,** area vestibularis. **t. adducto′rium fem′oris** [NA], adductor tubercle of femur: a small projection from the upper part of the medial epicondyle of the femur, to which the tendon of the adductor magnus muscle is attached. **t. ante′rius atlan′tis** [NA], anterior tubercle of atlas: the conical eminence on the front of the anterior arch of the atlas. **t. ante′rius thal′ami** [NA], anterior tubercle of thalamus: a distinct enlargement on the dorsal surface of the most rostral part of the thalamus; it contains the anterior nuclear group. **t. ante′rius vertebra′rum cervica′lium** [NA], anterior tubercle of cervical vertebrae: a tubercle on the anterior part of the extremity of each transverse process of the cervical vertebrae. **t. arthrit′icum,** a gouty concretion in a joint. **t. articula′re os′sis tempora′lis** [NA], articular tubercle of temporal bone: an enlargement of the inferior border of the zygomatic process of the temporal bone, forming the anterior boundary of the mandibular fossa and part of the anterior root of the zygoma; it gives attachment to the lateral ligament of the temporomandibular articulation. Called also *tubercle of root of zygoma.* **t. auric′ulae** [NA], **t. auric′ulae [Darwin′i],** auricular tubercle: a small projection sometimes found on the edge of the helix, and conjectured by some to be a relic of a simioid ancestry. **t. carot′icum ver′tebrae cervica′lis VI** [NA], carotid tubercle of sixth cervical vertebra: either of the large anterior tubercles of the sixth cervical vertebra. **t. cine′reum,** 1. an elevation of the upper end of the lateral funiculus of the medulla oblongata, produced by the spinal tract of the trigeminal nerve and the inferior cerebellar peduncle. Called also *tubercle of Rolando, gray tubercle,* and *eminentia trigemina.* 2. Tuber cinereum. **t. conoi′deum** [NA], conoid tubercle: a prominent elevation on the inferior aspect of the lateral part of the clavicle, to which the conoid part of the coracoclavicular ligament is attached. **t. cornicula′tum** [NA], **t. cornicula′tum [Santorin′i],** corniculate tubercle: a rounded eminence near the posterior end of the aryepiglottic fold, posterior to the cuneiform tubercle, corresponding to the corniculate cartilage. **t. coro′nae den′tis** [NA], tubercle of crown of tooth: any of the projections on the crown of a tooth; called also *dental cusp* and *dental tubercle.* **t. cos′tae** [NA], tubercle of rib: a small eminence on the posterior surface of a rib where the neck and body join; it protrudes inferiorly and posteriorly, and bears on its medial part a surface that articulates with the transverse process of the corresponding vertebra. **t. cunea′tum,** t. nuclei cuneati. **t. cuneifor′me** [NA], **t. cuneifor′me [Wrisber′gi],** cuneiform tubercle: a rounded eminence in the posterior portion of the aryepiglottic fold, anterior to the corniculate tubercle, corresponding to the cuneiform cartilage; called also *Wrisberg's tubercle.* **t. doloro′sum,** a painful nodule or tubercle, such as one situated in the subcutaneous tissue near a joint, produced by enlargement of the end of a sensory nerve. **t. epiglot′ticum** [NA], epiglottic tubercle: a posterior projection on the inferior part of the posterior surface of the epiglottic cartilage. **t. genia′le** t. mentale mandibulae. **t. hypoglos′si,** trigonum nervi hypoglossi. **t. im′par,** a small tubercle in the midline on the floor of the pharynx of the embryo, between the ends of the mandibular and hyoid arches, which is the primordium of the tongue. **t. infraglenoida′le** [NA], infraglenoid tubercle: a roughened area, just below the glenoid cavity of the scapula, that gives origin to the long head of the triceps muscle; called also *tuberositas infraglenoidalis* or *infraglenoid tuberosity.* **t. intercondyla′re latera′le** [NA], lateral intercondylar tubercle: a lateral spur projecting upward from the intercondylar eminence at the proximal end of the tibia; called also *t. intercondyloideum laterale.* **t. intercondyla′re media′le** [NA], medial intercondylar tubercle: a medial spur projecting upward from the intercondylar eminence at the proximal end of the tibia; called also *t. intercondyloideum mediale.* **t. intercondyloi′deum,** eminentia intercondylaris. **t. intercondyloi′deum latera′le,** t. intercondylare laterale. **t. intercondyloi′deum media′le,** t. intercondylare mediale. **t. interveno′sum** [NA], **t. interveno′sum [Low′eri],** intervenous tubercle: a more or less distinct ridge across the inner surface of the right atrium between the openings of the venae cavae. **t. jugula′re os′sis occipita′lis** [NA], jugular tubercle of occipital bone: a smooth eminence overlying the hypoglossal canal on the superior surface of the lateral part of the occipital bone. **t. la′bii superio′ris** [NA], the central prominence of the upper border between the skin and the mucous membrane of the upper lip, marking the distal termination of the philtrum. Called also *procheilon, tubercle of upper lip,* and *labial tubercle.* **t. latera′le proces′sus posterio′ris ta′li** [NA], the lateral tubercle or eminence of the posterior process of the talus. **t. Low′eri,** t. intervenosum. **t. ma′jus hu′meri** [NA], greater tubercle of humerus: a large flattened prominence at the upper end of the lateral surface of the humerus, just lateral to the highest part of the anatomical neck, giving attachment to the infraspinatus, the supraspinatus, and the teres minor muscles. **t. margina′le os′sis zygomat′ici** [NA], marginal tubercle of zygomatic bone: a process on the superior part of the temporal border of the zygomatic bone to which a strong slip of the temporal

fascia is attached; called also *processus marginalis ossis zygomatici.* **t. media′le proces′sus posterio′ris ta′li** [NA], the medial tubercle or eminence of the posterior process of the talus. **t. menta′le mandib′ulae** [NA], mental tubercle of mandible: a more or less distinct prominence on the inferior border of either side of the mental protuberance of the mandible. **t. mi′nus hu′meri** [NA], lesser tubercle of humerus: a distinct prominence at the proximal end of the anterior surface of the humerus, just lateral to the anatomical neck; it gives insertion to the subscapular muscle. **t. mus′culi scale′ni anterio′ris** [NA], tubercle of anterior scalene muscle: the tubercle on the cranial surface of the first rib for the insertion of the anterior scalene muscle; called also *t. scaleni* [Lisfranci]. **t. nu′clei cunea′ti** [NA], tubercle of nucleus cuneatus: an enlargement of the fasciculus cuneatus in the medulla oblongata just lateral to the tubercle of the nucleus gracilis, produced by the underlying nucleus cuneatus. **t. nu′clei gra′cilis** [NA], tubercle of nucleus gracilis: an enlargement of the fasciculus gracilis in the medulla oblongata, forming the lower lateral border of the posterior part of the fourth ventricle, produced by the underlying nucleus gracilis. Called also *clava.* **t. obturato′rium ante′rius** [NA], anterior obturator tubercle: a small spur sometimes present on the margin of the obturator foramen, projecting from the superior ramus of the pubis. **t. obturato′rium poste′rius** [NA], posterior obturator tubercle: a small protuberance often present on the margin of the obturator foramen, projecting from the free edge of the acetabular fossa near the junction of the pubis and ischium. **t. os′sis multan′guli majo′ris,** t. ossis trapezii. **t. os′sis navicula′ris,** t. ossis scaphoidei. **t. os′sis scaphoi′dei** [NA], tubercle of scaphoid bone: a projection on the volar surface of the scaphoid bone of the wrist, giving attachment to the transverse carpal ligament; called also *t. ossis navicularis.* **t. os′sis trape′zii** [NA], tubercle of trapezium: a prominent ridge on the volar surface of the trapezium bone, forming the lateral margin of the groove that transmits the tendon of the flexor carpi radialis muscle; called also *t. ossis multanguli.* **t. pharyn′geum** [NA], pharyngeal tubercle: a midline eminence on the inferior surface of the basilar part of the occipital bone, for attachment of the pharynx (superior constrictor and pharyngeal raphe). **t. poste′rius atlan′tis** [NA], posterior tubercle of atlas: a variable prominence on the posterior surface of the posterior arch of the atlas, which represents a spinous process and gives attachment to the rectus capitis posterior minor muscle. **t. poste′rius thal′ami,** pulvinar. **t. poste′rius vertebra′rum cervica′lium** [NA], posterior tubercle of cervical vertebrae: a tubercle on the posterior part of the extremity of a transverse process of a cervical vertebra. **t. pu′bicum os′sis pu′bis** [NA], pubic tubercle of pubic bone: a prominent tubercle situated at the lateral end of the pubic crest and at the medial end of the superior border of the superior ramus of the pubic bone; it is the anterior medial terminal of the obturator crest and of the pecten of the pubic bone. **t. retroloba′re,** His' tubercle. **t. Santori′ni,** t. corniculatum. **t. scale′ni [Lisfran′ci],** t. musculi scaleni anterioris. **t. sel′lae os′sis sphenoida′lis,** t. sellae turcicae. **t. sel′lae tur′cicae** [NA], tubercle of sella turcica: a transverse ridge on the upper surface of the body of the sphenoid bone; it is in front of the sella turcica, back of the sulcus chiasmatis, and between the anterior clinoid processes. **t. sep′ti,** a tubercle or prominence on the superior anterior part of the nasal septum. **t. supraglenoida′le** [NA], supraglenoid tubercle: a raised roughened area, just superior to the glenoid cavity of the scapula, that gives attachment to the long head of the biceps muscle of the arm; called also *tuberositas supraglenoidalis scapulae.* **t. supratra′gicum** [NA], supratragic tubercle: a small tubercle sometimes seen on the pinna just superior to the tragus. **t. thyreoi′deum infe′rius,** t. thyroideum inferius. **t. thyreoi′deum supe′rius,** t. thyroideum superius. **t. thyroi′deum infe′rius** [NA], inferior thyroid tubercle: a more or less distinct tubercle at the inferior end of the oblique line of the thyroid cartilage; called also *t. thyreoideum inferius.* **t. thyroi′deum supe′rius** [NA], superior thyroid tubercle: a more or less distinct tubercle at the superior extremity of the oblique line of the thyroid cartilage; called also *t. thyreoideum superius.*

tuberin (too′ber-in) a simple globulin from potatoes.

tuberosis (too″ber-o′sis) a condition characterized by the development of nodules.

tuberositas (too″bĕ-ros′ĭ-tas), pl. *tuberosita′tes* [L.] tuberosity: an elevation or protuberance; [NA] a general term for such a structure. See also *tuber, tubercle,* and *tuberculum.* **t. coracoi′dea,** see *tuberculum conoideum* and *linea trapezoidea.* **t. cos′tae II,** t. musculi serrati anterioris. **t. costa′lis clavic′ulae,** impressio ligamenti costoclavicularis. **t. deltoi′dea hu′meri** deltoid tuberosity of humerus: a rough, triangular elevation, about the middle of the anterolateral border of the shaft of the humerus, for attachment of the deltoid muscle. **t. fem′oris exter′na,** epicondylus lateralis femoris. **t. fem′oris inter′na,** epicondylus medialis femoris. **t. glu′tea fem′oris** [NA], gluteal tuberosity of femur: an elevation on the upper part of the shaft of the femur for attachment of the gluteus maximus muscle. **t. ili′aca** [NA], iliac tuberosity: a roughened area on the sacropelvic surface of the ilium, between the iliac crest and the auricular surface, for the attachment of muscles and ligaments. **t. infraglenoida′lis,** tuberculum infraglenoidale. **t. masseter′ica** [NA], masseteric tuberosity: an elongated, raised and roughened area on the lateral side of the angle of the mandible, for the insertion of tendinous bundles of the masseter muscles. **t. mus′culi serra′ti anterio′ris** [NA], tuberosity for serratus anterior muscle: a roughened, raised area on the second rib that gives attachment to a slip of the anterior serratus muscle; called also *t. costae II.* **t. os′sis cuboi′dei** [NA], tuberosity of cuboid bone: a transverse ridge on the lower surface of the cuboid bone over which the tendon of the peroneus longus muscle plays. **t. os′sis metatarsa′lis I** [NA], tuberosity of first metatarsal bone: a blunt process projecting downward and laterally from the lower surface of the base of the first metatarsal bone, to which the tendon of the peroneus longus muscle is attached. **t. os′sis metatarsa′lis V** [NA], tuberosity of fifth metatarsal bone: a large conical protuberance projecting backward and laterally from the base of the fifth metatarsal bone, to which the tendon of the peroneus brevis muscle is attached. **t. os′sis navicula′ris** [NA], tuberosity of navicular bone: a rough protuberance on the navicular bone of the foot, projecting downward and medially, and giving attachment to the tendon of the posterior tibial muscle. **t. patella′ris,** t. tibiae. **t. phalan′gis dista′lis ma′nus** [NA], distal tuberosity of fingers: a roughened, raised bony mass on the palmar surface of the tip of a distal phalanx of the hand; called also *t. unguicularis manus.* **t. phalan′gis dista′lis pe′dis** [NA], distal tuberosity of toes: a roughened, raised bony mass on the plantar surface of the tip of a distal phalanx of the foot; called also t. unguicularis pedis. **t. pterygoi′dea mandib′ulae** [NA], pterygoid tuberosity of mandible: a roughened area on the inner side of the angle of the mandible for the insertion of the internal pterygoid muscle; called also *pterygoid tubercle.* **t. ra′dii** [NA], radial tuberosity: the tuberosity on the anterior inner surface of the neck of the radius, for the insertion of the tendon of the biceps muscle. **t. sacra′lis** [NA], sacral tuberosity: a roughened area on the pars lateralis of the sacrum, on the dorsal surface between the lateral sacral crest and the auricular surface, which gives attachment to the sacroiliac ligaments. **t. supraglenoida′lis scapulae,** tuberculum supraglenoidale. **t. tib′iae** [NA], tuberosity of tibia: a longitudinally elongated, raised and roughened area on the anterior crest of the tibia, located just distal to the intercondylar eminence, and giving attachment to the patellar ligament. **t. tib′iae exter′na,** condylus lateralis tibiae. **t. tib′iae inter′na,** condylus medialis tibiae. **t. ul′nae** [NA], tuberosity of ulna: a large roughened area on the volar surface of the ulna, located just distal to the coronoid process, and giving attachment to the brachialis muscle. **t. unguicula′ris ma′nus,** t. phalangis distalis manus. **t. unguicula′ris pe′dis,** t. phalangis distalis pedis.

tuberositates (too″ber-os′ĭ-tah′tēs) [L.] plural of *tuberositas.*

tuberosity (too″bĕ-ros′ĭ-te) an elevation or protuberance; called also *tuberositas.* **t. for anterior serratus muscle,** tuberositas musculi serrati anterioris. **bicipital t.,** tuberositas radii. **t. of calcaneus,** tuber calcanei. **t. of clavicle,** impressio ligamenti costoclavicularis. **coracoid t.,** see *tuberculum conoideum* and *linea trapezoidea.* **costal t. of clavicle,** impressio ligamenti costoclavicularis. **t. of cuboid bone,** tuberositas ossis cuboidei. **deltoid t. of humerus,** tuberositas deltoidea humeri. **distal t. of fingers,** tuberositas phalangis distalis manus. **distal t. of toes,** tuberositas phalangis distalis pedis. **t. of femur, external,** epicondylus lateralis femoris. **t. of femur, internal,** epicondylus medialis femoris. **t. of femur, lateral,** epicondylus lateralis femoris. **t. of femur, medial,** epicondylus medialis femoris. **t. of fifth metatarsal bone,** tuberositas ossis metatarsalis V. **t. of first carpal bone,** tuberculum ossis scaphoidei. **t. of first metatarsal bone,** tuberositas ossis metatarsalis I. **t. of fourth tarsal bone,** tuberositas ossis cuboidei. **gluteal t. of femur,** tuberositas glutea femoris. **greater t. of humerus,** tuberculum majus humeri. **t. of greater multangular bone,** tuberculum ossis trapezii. **t′s of humerus,** the three elevations on the humerus; see *tuberculum majus humeri, tuberculum minus humeri,* and *tuberositas deltoidea humeri.* **iliac t.,** tuberositas iliaca. **infraglenoid t.,** tuberculum infraglenoidale. **ischial t., t. of ischium,** tuber ischiadicum. **lesser t. of humerus,** tuberculum minus humeri. **malar t.,** the prominence of the zygomatic bone. **masseteric t.,** tuberositas masseterica. **t. of maxilla,** tuber maxillae. **t. of navicular bone,** tuberositas ossis navicularis. **patellar t.,** tuberositas tibiae. **pterygoid t. of mandible,** tuberositas pterygoidea mandibulae. **t. of pubic bone,** tuberculum pubicum ossis pubis. **pyramidal t. of palatine bone,** processus pyramidalis ossis palatini. **radial t., t of radius,** tuberositas radii. **sacral t.,** tuberositas sacralis. **t. of scaphoid bone,** 1. tuberculum ossis scaphoidei. 2. tuberositas ossis navicularis. **scapular t. of Henle,** processus coracoideus scapulae. **t. of second rib, t. for serratus anterior muscle,** tuberositas musculi serrati anterioris. **supraglenoid t.,** tuberculum supraglenoidale. **t. of tibia,** tuberositas tibiae. **t. of tibia, external,** condylus lateralis tibiae. **t. of tibia, internal,** condylus medialis tibiae. **t. of trapezium,** tuber-

culum ossis trapezii. **t. of ulna,** tuberositas ulnae. **ungual t., unguicular t.,** see *tuberositas phalangis distalis manus* and *tuberositas phalangis distalis pedis.*

tuberous (too′ber-us) covered with tubers; knobby. See also under *sclerosis.*

Tubifera (too-bif′er-ah) *Eristalis.*

tubiferous (too-bif′er-us) [L. *tuber* + *ferre* to bear] having tubers; tuberous.

tuboabdominal (too″bo-ab-dom′ĭ-nal) pertaining to the oviduct and the abdomen.

tuboadnexopexy (too″bo-ad-nek′so-pek″se) the operation of suturing the uterine adnexa in a fixed position.

tubocurarine (too″bo-ku-rah′rin) an alkaloid isolated from the bark and stems of *Chondodendron tomentosum* R. & P. (Menispermaceae); it is the active principle of curare (q.v.). **t. chloride** [USP], chemical name: 7′,12′-dihydroxy-6,6′-dimethoxy-2,2′,2′-trimethyltubocuraranium chloride hydrochloride pentahydrate. A neuromuscular blocking agent, $C_{37}H_{41}ClN_2O_6 \cdot HCl \cdot 5H_2O$, occurring as a white or yellowish white to grayish white, crystalline powder; administered intravenously to relax skeletal muscles in surgery, tetanus, and shock therapy, and may be used for diagnosis of myasthenia gravis in certain cases. **dimethyl t. iodide,** metocurine iodide.

tuboligamentous (too″bo-lig″ah-men′tus) pertaining to a uterine tube and a broad ligament.

tubo-ovarian (too″bo-o-va′re-an) of or pertaining to a uterine tube and ovary.

tubo-ovariotomy (too″bo-o-va″re-ot′o-me) salpingo-oophorectomy.

tubo-ovaritis (too″bo-o″vah-ri′tis) salpingo-oophoritis.

tuboperitoneal (too″bo-per″ĭ-to-ne′al) pertaining to a uterine tube and the peritoneum.

tuboplasty (too′bo-plas″te) 1. salpingoplasty. 2. plastic repair of a tube, such as the eustachian tube. **eustachian t.,** plastic repair of the eustachian tube.

tuborrhea (too″bo-re′ah) [*tube* + Gr. *rhoia* flow] a condition marked by a discharge from the auditory tube.

tubotorsion (too″bo-tor′shun) a twisting of a tube, especially of the auditory tube.

tubotympanal (too″bo-tim′pah-nal) pertaining to the auditory tube and the tympanic cavity.

tubotympanum (too″bo-tim′pah-num) the auditory tube and tympanic cavity considered together.

tubouterine (too″bo-u′ter-ĭn) pertaining to a uterine tube and the uterus.

tubovaginal (too″bo-vaj′ĭ-nal) pertaining to a uterine tube and the vagina.

tubular (too′bu-lar) [L. *tubularis*] shaped like a tube; of or pertaining to a tubule.

tubulature (too′bu-lah-tūr) [L. *tuba* tube] the tube of a receiver or retort.

tubule (too′būl) a small tube; called also *tubulus.* **Albarrán's t's,** small branching tubules in the cervical part of the prostate gland. **Bellini's t's,** tubuli renales recti. **biliferous t.,** any small channel conveying bile. **caroticotympanic t's,** canaliculi caroticotympanici. **collecting t's,** channels through which fluids pass from the secreting cells; see *tubuli renales recti.* **connecting t's,** channels connecting other tubules, such as the arching portion of a renal tubule that connects the distal convoluted tubule with the straight tubule. **convoluted t's,** channels which follow a tortuous course; see *tubuli renales contorti* and *tubuli seminiferi contorti.* **convoluted t., distal,** see *tubuli renales contorti.* **convoluted t., proximal,** see *tubuli renales contorti.* **dental t's, dentinal t's,** canaliculi dentales. **discharging t's,** channels by which a fluid is discharged from the substance of the gland or organ in which it is secreted; see *tubuli renales recti.* **Ferrein's t's,** the portions of the renal tubules making up the pars radiata of the lobules of the renal cortex. **galactophorous t's,** ductus lactiferi. **Henle's t's,** the straight ascending and descending portions of a renal tubule forming Henle's loop; called also *straight tubules.* **Kobelt's t's,** 1. the outer series of tubules in the epoophoron. 2. a similar series of tubules in the paradidymis of the male. **lactiferous t's,** ductus lactiferi. **mesonephric t's,** the tubules comprising the mesonephros, or temporary kidney of amniotes. **metanephric t's,** the tubules comprising the permanent kidney of amniotes. **Miescher's t's,** sarcosporidian cyst. **paraurethral t's,** ductus paraurethrales. **pronephric t's,** the tubules comprising the primitive kidney of vertebrates, rudimentary in amniotes. **Rainey's t's,** sarcosporidian cysts. **renal t's,** tubuli renales. **renal t's, convoluted,** tubuli renales contorti. **renal t's, straight,** 1. tubuli renales recti. 2. see *Henle's t's.* **segmental t's,** the tubules of the mesonephros. **seminiferous t's,** channels in the testis in which the spermatozoa develop and through which they leave the gland; see *tubuli seminiferi contorti* and *tubuli seminiferi recti.* **seminiferous t's, convoluted,** tubuli seminiferi contorti. **seminiferous t's, straight,** tubuli seminiferi recti.

Skene's t's, ductus paraurethrales. **spiral t's,** channels which follow a spiral course; see *tubuli renales contorti.* **straight t's,** channels which follow a comparatively straight course; see *tubuli renales recti* and *tubuli seminiferi recti.* **subtracheal t.,** ductus thyroglossus. **T t's,** the transverse intracellular tubules invaginating from the cell membrane and surrounding the myofibrils of the T system of skeletal and cardiac muscle, serving as a pathway for the spread of electrical excitation within a muscle cell, enabling the nearly simultaneous activation of all myofibrils; in skeletal muscle, a T tubule is the intermediate element of a triad of tubular structures, the other elements being a pair of terminal cisterns. See also *T system,* under *system; terminal cistern,* under *cistern;* and *triad of skeletal muscle.* **transverse t.,** T t. **uriniferous t's, uriniparous t's,** channels for the passage of urine; see *tubuli renales.* **vertical t's,** the inner set of tubules in the epoophoron.

tubuli (too′bu-li) [L.] plural of *tubulus.*

tubulin (too′bu-lin) the constituent protein of microtubules; thought to be involved in phagocyte motility.

tubulization (too″bu-li-za′shun) Foramitti's method of treating injured nerves by isolating the nerve stump in an absorbable cylinder which serves as a guide for new growth.

tubuloacinar (too″bu-lo-as′ĭ-nar) composed of tubular acini, as a tubuloacinar gland.

tubulocyst (too′bu-lo-sist) any cystic dilatation of a vestigial canal or functionless duct.

tubuloracemose (too″bu-lo-ras′ĕ-mōs) both tubular and racemose.

tubulorrhexis (too″bu-lo-rek′sis) [*tubule* + Gr. *rhēxis* a breaking] disruption of continuity of kidney tubules, the basement membrane being suddenly interrupted, or disintegrated into fibrils.

tubulosaccular (too″bu-lo-sak′u-lar) both tubular and saccular.

tubulous (too′bu-lus) containing tubules.

tubulus (too′bu-lus), pl. *tu′buli* [L., dim. of *tubus*] a tubule or a small tube; [NA] a general term for such a structure. **t. bilif′erus,** a channel for conveying bile; see *ductus cysticus.* **tu′buli contor′ti,** convoluted tubules; see *tubuli renales contorti* and *tubuli seminiferi contorti.* **tu′buli rec′ti,** straight tubules; see *tubuli renales recti* and *tubuli seminiferi recti.* **tu′buli rena′les** [NA], renal tubules: the minute, reabsorptive, secretory, and collecting canals, made up of basement membrane lined with epithelium, that form the substance of the kidneys. See also *nephron.* See plate accompanying *kidney.* **tu′buli rena′les contor′ti** [NA], convoluted renal tubules: the convoluted reabsorptive and secretory portions of the renal tubules, found in the renal cortex. The *proximal convoluted tubule* begins at the renal corpuscle and is continuous with the descending portion of Henle's loop; after passing back near the point of origin of the tubule, the ascending portion of the loop is continuous with the *distal convoluted tubule.* **tu′buli rena′les rec′ti** [NA], straight renal tubules: the excretory or collecting portions of the renal tubules, each of which descends from the distal convoluted tubule through the medulla, joining with others to form a common duct that opens at the apex of a renal papilla. **tu′buli seminif′eri contor′ti** [NA], convoluted seminiferous tubules: the numerous delicate, contorted canals within each lobule of the testis, from whose epithelial linings the spermatozoa are formed. **tu′buli seminif′eri rec′ti** [NA], straight seminiferous tubules: the straight terminal portions of the seminiferous tubules, which form the rete testis.

tubus (too′bus), pl. *tu′bi* [L.] tube; used as a general term in anatomical nomenclature. **t. digesto′rius,** canalis alimentarius.

Tuerck see *Türck.*

Tuffier's method, test (te′fe-āz) [Marin Théodore *Tuffier,* surgeon in Paris, 1857–1929] see under *method* and *tests.*

Tuffnell's treatment (tuf′nelz) [Thomas Joliffe *Tuffnell,* English surgeon, 1819–1885] see under *treatment.*

tuft (tuft) a small clump or cluster; a coil. **enamel t's,** groups or bunches of poorly calcified enamel rods extending from the dentoenamel junction through about one third the thickness of the enamel. **hair t's,** groups of several hairs from one follicle, consisting of one main hair and some secondary hairs. **malpighian t's, renal t's,** glomeruli renis. **synovial t's,** villi synoviales.

tuftsin (tuft′sin) a basic tetrapeptide, L-threonyl-L-bysyl-L-propyl-L-arginine, produced in the spleen that stimulates phagocytosis in polymorphonuclear leukocytes and in macrophages.

tugging (tug′ing) a pulling sensation. **tracheal t.,** a pulling sensation in the trachea, due to aneurysm of the arch of the aorta; it is most apparent when the head is extended and a finger is placed on the thyroid cartilage. Called also *Oliver's* or *Porter's sign.*

tularemia (too″lah-re′me-ah) [*Tulare* a district in California, where the disease was first described] a disease of rodents, resembling plague, which is transmitted by the bites of flies, fleas, ticks, and lice, and may be acquired by man through handling of contaminated animal products (leather) or infected animals, or the bites of fleas, ticks, and the deer fly. Caused by *Francisella*

tularensis, the disease is of three types: *ulceroglandular,* in which the primary lesion affects the skin, with associated regional lymph node enlargement; *oculoglandular,* marked by conjunctivitis and preauricular node inflammation; and *pneumonic,* marked by severe pulmonary infection due to inhalation or blood stream dissemination. Meningitis is an uncommon manifestation. All forms exhibit the constitutional signs of fever, chill, headache, and myalgia, which vary greatly in intensity. Called also *deer fly fever, Pahvant Valley plague, rabbit fever, alkali disease,* and *Francis' disease.*

tularine (too′lah-rēn) the antigen used in the Foshay skin test for tularemia.

tulase (too′lās) Von Behring's fluid, used by him in the treatment of tuberculosis.

tulle gras (tool-grah′) [Fr. "fatty tulle"] a close-meshed net cut into squares and impregnated with soft paraffin, Peruvian balsam, and vegetable oil; used in treating raw surfaces.

Tulpius' valve (tul′pe-us) [Nikolaas *Tulpius* (Nicolas *Tulp*), Dutch physician, 1593–1674] valva ileocecalis.

tumefacient (too″me-fa′shent) [L. *tumefaciens*] tending to cause or causing a swelling.

tumefaction (too″me-fak′shun) [L. *tumefactio*] a swelling; the state of being swollen, or the act of swelling; puffiness; edema.

tumentia (too-men′she-ah) [L.] swelling. **vasomotor t.,** irregular partial swelling of the lower limbs, and sometimes of the arms associated with vasomotor changes.

tumescence (too-mes′ens) 1. the condition of being tumid or swollen. 2. a swelling.

tumeur (too-mer′) [Fr.] tumor. **t. perlée** (too-mer′ per-la′) [Fr. "pearly tumor"], cholesteatoma. **t. pileuse** (too-mer′ peluz′) [Fr. "hairy tumor"], trichobezoar.

tumid (too′mid) [L. *tumidus*] swollen or edematous.

tumor (too′mor) [L., from *tumere* to swell] 1. swelling, one of the cardinal signs of inflammation; morbid enlargement. 2. a new growth of tissue in which the multiplication of cells is uncontrolled and progressive; called also *neoplasm.* **Abrikosov's t.,** myoblastoma. **acoustic nerve t.,** a tumor growing from the sheath of the acoustic nerve at the cerebellopontine angle. Called also *acoustic neuroma, acoustic neurilemoma, schwannoma,* and *acoustic neurinoma.* **acute splenic t.,** a swelling resulting from acute splenitis. **adenoid t.,** adenoma. **adenomatoid t.,** a small, circumscribed, benign tumor of the genital tract (the epididymis, tunic of testis, uterine corpus, or uterine tube), composed of small glandlike spaces lined by flattened or cuboidal mesothelium-like cells. **adipose t.,** lipoma. **adrenal rest t.,** lipoid cell t. of ovary. **t. al′bus,** "white swelling"; tuberculosis of a bone or joint. **t. al′bus pyo′genes,** a chronic inflammation of gunshot injuries of the bones and joints marked by great swelling of the capsule of the joint and surrounding soft parts, which become converted into a gelatinous, edematous granulation tissue (A. Tietze). **aniline t.,** cancer appearing in workers in the synthetic aniline dye industry. **benign t.,** one that lacks the properties of invasion and metastasis and that is usually surrounded by a fibrous capsule; its cells also show a lesser degree of anaplasia than those of malignant tumors. **blood t.,** 1. hematoma. 2. aneurysm. **Brenner t.,** a tumor of the ovary whose structure consists of groups of epithelial cells lying in a fibrous connecting tissue stroma. When small the tumor may be solid, resembling fibroma; when large it may appear like a cystadenoma with nodular masses of the tumor (Brenner nodules) in the cyst wall. Called also *oophoroma folliculare.* **Brooke's t.,** trichoepithelioma. **brown t.,** a giant-cell granuloma produced in and replacing bone, occurring in osteitis fibrosa cystica and due to hyperparathyroidism. **Brown-Pearce t.,** a transplantable anaplastic carcinoma that forms a soft, friable, necrotic, hemorrhagic lesion at the site of inoculation. **Burkitt's t.,** see under *lymphoma.* **Buschke-Löwenstein t.,** a large cauliflower-like mass of warts occurring on the prepuce, especially in uncircumcized males, and also in the perianal region; it tends to penetrate and destroy adjacent tissue. Called also *giant condyloma acuminatum.* **butyroid t.,** a collection of material in the mammary gland closely resembling butter. **carcinoid t. of bronchus,** a highly vascular tumor of the bronchus similar to carcinoid (argentaffinoma) of the gastrointestinal tract. **carotid body t.,** an invariably benign, encapsulated, firm round mass at the bifurcation of the common carotid artery, with nests of large polyhedral cells in alveolar or organoid arrangement; usually asymptomatic, but sometimes causing dizziness and nausea or vomiting. It is a form of chemodectoma. **cartilaginous t.,** a chondroma or an enchondroma. **cavernous t.,** angioma cavernosum. **cellular t.,** a tumor made up chiefly of cells in a homogeneous stroma. **chromaffin-cell t.,** pheochromocytoma. **Codman's t.,** chondroblastoma. **t. col′li,** a tumor in the neck. **colloid t.,** myxoma. **connective-tissue t.,** any tumor developed from some structure of the connective tissue, such as a lipoma, fibroma, glioma, chondroma, or sarcoma. **craniopharyngeal duct t.,** craniopharyngioma. **cystic t.,** one not solid, but more or less hollow. **dermoid t.,** a teratoma which contains fatty cutaneous elements, and sometimes hair, nails, etc.; such tumors are usually benign, but solid dermoids are more often malignant than cystic ones (dermoid cysts). Called also *teratoid t.* **desmoid t.,** desmoid. **dumb-bell t.,** hourglass t. **eiloid t.,** a skin tumor having the look of a coil of intestine. **embryonal t.,** embryoma. **embryoplastic t.,** one due to the growth of persistent embryo cells. **encysted t.,** a tumor enclosed in a membranous sac. **epithelial t.,** a tumor containing epithelium; an organized tumor. **erectile t.,** hemangioma cavernosum. **Ewing's t.,** a malignant tumor of the bone which always arises in medullary tissue, occurring more often in cylindrical bones, with pain, fever, and leukocytosis as prominent symptoms; called also *Ewing's sarcoma.* **false t.,** one due to extravasations, exudation, echinococcus, or retained sebaceous matter. **fatty t.,** lipoma. **fecal t.,** stercoroma. **fibrocellular t.,** fibroma. **fibroid t.,** fibroma. **fibroplastic t.,** a fibroma or a fibrosarcoma. **fluid t.,** lymphangioma cysticum. **fungating t.,** a tumor with exuberant granulation. **gelatinous t.,** myxoma. **germinal t.,** a tumor of germ cell origin. **giant cell t. of bone,** a bone tumor composed of cellular spindle cell stroma containing scattered multinucleated giant cells resembling osteoclasts; symptoms may include local pain and tenderness, functional disability, and, occasionally, pathologic fractures. The tumors range from benign to frankly malignant lesions. **giant cell t. of tendon sheath,** a benign tumor-like lesion of tendon sheath origin forming a small, yellow, discrete nodule, most commonly of the wrist and fingers, or ankle and toes; the tissue is laden with lipophages and contains multinucleated giant cells. Called also *benign synovioma* and *nodular tenosynovitis.* **glomus t.,** glomangioma. **glomus jugulare t.,** a chemodectoma arising from the chemoreceptors of the glomus jugulare. **granular cell t.,** a benign circumscribed tumor-like lesion of soft tissue, particularly of the tongue, skin, and muscle, composed of large cells having a prominent granular cytoplasm and considered by some to be derived from myoblasts (myoblastoma) and by others from neurogenic elements (granular cell schwannoma); still others regard it as a manifestation of lipid storage cell disease. **granulation t.,** a granuloma. **granulosa t., granulosa cell t.,** an ovarian tumor originating in the cells of the primordial membrana granulosa; it may be associated with excessive production of estrin inducing endometrial hyperplasia with menorrhagia. Called also *folliculoma* and *granulosa cell carcinoma.* **granulosa-theca cell t.,** an ovarian tumor predominantly composed of either granulosa cells (follicular cells) or theca cells, and often associated with excessive production of estrogen, with hyperplasia of the breast and endometrium, and carcinoma of the endometrium. When luteinized, i.e., having cells resembling those of the corpus luteum, it is known as luteoma. **Grawitz's t's,** hypernephroma; the tumors formerly known as adenomas of the kidney, but which Grawitz thought to be an overgrowth of fetal inclusion in the midst of the kidney substance of particles of suprarenal glandular tissue: now considered carcinoma of the renal parenchyma. **Gubler's t.,** a tumor on the back of the wrist, with paralysis of the extensors of the hand, in cases of lead poisoning. **gummy t.,** gumma. **heterologous t.,** one made up of tissue which differs from that in which it grows. **heterotypic t.,** heterologous t. **hilar cell t.,** a rare benign neoplasm of the hilus of the ovary, histologically resembling Leydig cell tumor of the testis; it may cause virilization. **histioid t.,** one which is formed of a single tissue resembling that of the surrounding parts. **homoiotypic t., homologous t.,** a tumor which resembles the surrounding parts in its structure. **Hortega cell t.,** a cellular tumor of the lymphoreticular system arising in the central nervous system. **hourglass t.,** a spinal tumor made up of intradural and extradural masses joined by a narrow pedicle passing through an enlarged intervertebral foramen. **Hürthle cell t.,** a new growth of the thyroid gland composed wholly or predominantly of large cells (Hürthle cells) having abundant granular, eosinophilic cytoplasm. Such tumors are usually benign (Hürthle cell adenoma) but on occasion may be locally invasive or may rarely metastasize (Hürthle cell carcinoma, or malignant Hürthle cell tumor). **infiltrating t.,** a tumor which is not clearly marked off from the surrounding tissue. **innocent t.,** benign t. **iron-hard t.,** Riedel's struma. **islet cell t.,** a tumor of the islets of Langerhans; such tumors may result in hyperinsulinism or in Zollinger-Ellison syndrome. **ivory-like t.,** osteoma durum. **Jensen's t.,** see under *sarcoma.* **Krompecher's t.,** rodent ulcer. **Krukenberg's t.,** a special type of carcinoma of the ovary, usually metastatic from cancer of the gastrointestinal tract, especially of the stomach. It is characterized by areas of mucoid degeneration and the presence of signet-ring–like cells. Called also *carcinoma mucocellulare.* **lacteal t.,** 1. mammary abscess. 2. galactocele. **Leydig cell t.,** the most common nongerminal tumor of the testis, derived from the Leydig cells of the testis; such tumors are rarely malignant. **t. lie′nis,** enlargement of the spleen less in degree than splenomegaly. **lipoid cell t. of ovary,** a rare, usually benign, ovarian tumor composed of eosinophilic cells or cells with lipoid vacuoles, arising from ovarian cells or embryonic rest cells of the adrenals; it causes masculinization. Called also *adrenal rest t.* and *masculinovoblastoma.* **luteinized granulosa-theca cell t.,** luteoma. **Malherbe t.,** pilomatricoma. **malignant t.,** one that has the properties of invasion and metastasis and that

shows a greater degree of anaplasia than do benign tumors. **march t.,** syndesmitis metatarsea. **margaroid t.,** a cholesteatoma. **mast cell t.,** a benign, local aggregation of mast cells forming a nodulous tumor. **melanotic neuroectodermal t.,** a benign, rapidly growing, deeply pigmented tumor of the jaw and occasionally of other sites, consisting of an infiltrating mass of cells arranged in an alveolar pattern, and occurring almost exclusively in infants. Its source of origin is in dispute, the various theories giving rise to its several names. Called also *melanoameloblastoma, melanotic ameloblastoma, pigmented ameloblastoma, melanotic progonoma,* and *retinal anlage tumor.* **migrated t., migratory t.,** a tumor arising from a portion of a primary tumor which has become detached from its original location and fixed in some other place or lies free in a cavity. **mixed t.,** a tumor composed of more than one type of neoplastic tissue; especially "a complex embryonal tumor of local origin, which reproduces the normal development of the tissues and organs of the affected part" (Ewing). **mucous t.,** a myxoma. **muscular t.,** a myoma. **Nélaton's t.,** a dermoid tumor of the wall of the abdomen. **neuroepithelial t.,** a highly malignant tumor of peripheral nerves, developed from elements derived from the neural crest and resembling tumors of the central nervous system. **oozing t.,** a rare disease, consisting of a large, flat tumor on one or both labia majora, divided with deep fissures, and discharging a large amount of acrid, offensive fluid. **organoid t.,** a teratoma. **oxyphil cell t.,** Hürthle cell t. **Pancoast's t.,** pulmonary sulcus t. **papillary t.,** a papilloma. **pearl t., pearly t.,** cholesteatoma. **Perlmann's t.,** a benign multiloculated cystic tumor of the kidney, surrounded by a dense fibrous capsule and showing a yellow-blue-gray color on its cut surface. **phantom t.,** an abdominal swelling not due to a structural change, but to a neurosis; it is generally due to gaseous distention of the bowels. **plasma cell t.,** plasmacytoma. **potato t.,** chemodectoma of the carotid body. **pregnancy t.,** a bright red or purplish red, smooth, mushroom-like mass on the gingiva, usually occurring after the third month of pregnancy, and due to a chronic inflammatory response to local irritation. Histopathologically and clinically, it resembles pyogenic granuloma; lesions clinically and histologically identical are also seen in men and nonpregnant women. **premalignant fibroepithelial t.,** premalignant fibroepithelioma. **pseudointraligamentous t.,** a kind of ovarian tumor simulating intraligamentous tumors, but in reality adherent to the posterior surface of the broad ligament. **pulmonary sulcus t.,** one at the apex of the lung, extending outward to destroy the ribs and vertebrae and invading the brachial plexus; called also *Pancoast's t.* **ranine t.,** ranula. **Rathke's t., Rathke's pouch t.,** craniopharyngioma. **Recklinghausen's t.,** adenoleiomyofibroma of the posterior uterine wall or of the wall of an oviduct. **retinal anlage t.,** melanotic neuroectodermal tumor. **sacrococcygeal t.,** a form of spina bifida containing teratomatous tissue. **sand t.,** psammoma. **Schmincke t.,** lymphoepithelioma. **Schwanncell t.,** a neoplasm of a nerve sheath (Schwann's sheath); schwannoma. **Sertoli cell t.,** androblastoma, def. 1. **Sertoli-Leydig cell t.,** arrhenoblastoma. **sheath t.,** a tumor of the sheaths of the brain or peripheral nerves, including meningioma, acoustic nerve tumor, and schwannoma. **Steiner's t's,** Jeanselme's nodules. **stercoral t.,** stercoroma. **superior sulcus t.,** pulmonary sulcus t. **teratoid t.,** teratoma. **theca cell t.,** a fibroid-like tumor of the ovary containing yellow areas of lipoid material derived from theca cells. It may be associated with excessive production of estrogen and have a tendency to cystic degeneration. The tumor is rarely composed entirely of theca cells; commonly both theca and follicular cells (granulosa cells) are found. Called also *thecoma* and *fibroma thecocellulare xanthomatodes.* See also *granulosa-theca cell t.* **transition t.,** one which recurs after removal and then shows malignant characters. **tridermic t.,** a teratoma. **true t.,** a neoplasm. **turban t.,** multiple cutaneous cylindromas of the scalp grouped together so as to cover the entire scalp like a turban. **varicose t.,** a swelling, composed of dilated veins. **vascular t.,** 1. a tumor of blood vessel elements; an angioma. 2. any tumor with a copious blood supply. **villous t.,** papilloma. **Warthin's t.,** papillary adenocystoma lymphomatosum. **warty cicatricial t.,** a neoplasm which appears as warty growths in parallel lines on the surface of a scar; it often breaks down and becomes what is known as Marjolin's ulcer. **white t.,** chronic tuberculous arthritis. **Wilms' t.,** a rapidly developing malignant mixed tumor of the kidneys, made up of embryonal elements; it usually affects children before the fifth year, but may occur in the fetus and rarely in later life. Called also *embryonal adenomyosarcoma, carcinosarcoma,* or *nephroma,* and *nephroblastoma.* **yolk sac t.,** mesonephroma (type 2).

tumoraffin (too″mor-af′in) [*tumor* + L. *affinis* related] having a special affinity for tumor cells; oncotropic.

tumoricidal (too″mor-ĭ-si′dal) destructive to cancer cells.

tumorigenesis (too″mor-ĭ-jen′ĕ-sis) the production of tumors.

tumorigenic (too″mor-ĭ-jen′ik) giving rise to tumors; said especially of a cell or group of cells capable of producing a tumor. Cf. *oncogenic.*

tumorous (too′mor-us) of the nature of a tumor.

tumultus (too-mul′tus) [L.] excessive organic action or motility.

Tunga (tung′gah) a genus of fleas of the family Hectopsyllidae. **T. pen′etrans,** a species widely distributed in the tropical and subtropical regions of America and Africa; called *Dermatophilus penetrans.* See *chigoe.*

tungiasis (tung-gi′ah-sis) infestation of the skin with *Tunga penetrans.* See *chigoe.*

tungstate (tung′stāt) a salt of tungstic acid.

tungsten (tung′sten) [Swed. "heavy stone"] the chemical element of atomic number 74, symbol W, and atomic weight 183.85; used in electric light filaments and in steel alloys to secure hardness.

tunic (too′nik) a covering or coat; see *tunica.* **Bichat's t.,** tunica intima vasorum. **Brücke's t.,** tunica nervea of Brücke. **fibrous t.,** tunica fibrosa. **fibrous t. of eyeball,** tunica fibrosa bulbi. **fibrous t. of liver,** tunica fibrosa hepatis. **mucous t.,** tunica mucosa. **muscular t.,** tunica muscularis. **pharyngeal t.,** pharyngobasilar t., fascia pharyngobasilaris. **proper t.,** tunica propria. **Ruysch's t.,** lamina choriocapillaris. **serous t.,** tunica serosa. **t's of spermatic cord and testis,** tunicae funiculi spermatici et testis.

tunica (too′nĭ-kah), pl. *tu′nicae* [L.] a covering or coat; [NA] a general term for a membrane or other structure covering or lining a body part or organ. Called also *tunic.* **t. abdomina′lis,** the aponeurosis of the abdominal muscles in certain quadrupeds, as the horse. **t. adna′ta oc′uli,** tunica conjunctiva; sometimes applied specifically to the tunica conjunctiva bulbi. **t. adna′ta tes′tis,** lamina parietalis tunicae vaginalis testis. **t. adventi′tia** [NA], the outer coat of various tubular structures, made up of connective tissue and elastic fibers. **t. adventi′tia duc′tus deferen′tis** [NA], the adventitious coat of the ductus deferens. **t. adventi′tia esoph′agi** [NA], the adventitious coat of the esophagus. **t. adventi′tia tu′bae uteri′nae,** tela subserosa tubae uterinae. **t. adventi′tia ure′teris** [NA], the adventitious coat of the ureter. **t. adventi′tia vaso′rum,** t. externa vasorum. **t. adventi′tia vesic′ulae semina′lis** [NA], the adventitious coat of the seminal vesicle. **t. albugin′ea** [NA], a dense, white, fibrous sheath enclosing a part or organ. **t. albugin′ea cor′poris spongio′si** [NA], the dense, white, fibroelastic sheath that encloses the corpus spongiosum of the penis. **t. albugin′ea corpo′rum caverno′rum** [NA], the dense, white, fibroelastic sheath that encloses the corpora cavernosi penis. Its superficial, longitudinal fibers form a tunic surrounding both corpora, and the deep circularly coursing fibers surround them separately, uniting medially to form the septum of the penis. **t. albugin′ea lie′nis,** t. fibrosa lienis. **t. albugin′ea tes′tis** [NA], the dense, white, inelastic tissue immediately covering the testis, beneath the visceral layer of the tunica vaginalis. **t. conjuncti′va** [NA], the thin, transparent mucous membrane lining the eyelids and covering the front surface of the eyeball; called also *conjunctiva.* It comprises the tunica conjunctiva bulbi and the tunica conjunctiva palpebrarum. **t. conjuncti′va bul′bi** [NA], **t. conjuncti′va bul′bi oc′uli,** bulbar conjunctiva: the portion of the tunica conjunctiva covering the cornea and front part of the sclera, appearing white because of the sclera behind it. **t. conjuncti′va palpebra′rum** [NA], palpebral conjunctiva: the portion of the tunica conjunctiva lining the eyelids, appearing red because of its great vascularity. **t. dar′tos** [NA], a layer of smooth muscle fibers situated in the superficial fascia of the scrotum; the deeper fibers help to form the septum of the scrotum; also called *dartos.* **t. elas′tica inter′na,** t. intima vasorum. **t. ex′terna the′cae follic′uli** [NA], the external, fibrous layer of the theca folliculi. **t. exter′na vaso′rum** [NA], **t. exter′na vaso′rum [adventi′tia],** the outer, fibroelastic coat of a blood vessel. **t. fibro′sa** [NA], fibrous tunic or coat: an enveloping fibrous membrane. **t. fibro′sa bul′bi** [NA], fibrous tunic of eyeball: the outer of the three tunics of the eye, comprising the cornea and the sclera; called also *t. fibrosa oculi.* **t. fibro′sa hep′atis** [NA], fibrous tunic of liver: the fibroelastic layer that surrounds the liver beneath the peritoneum; it is continuous at the hepatic portal with the perivascular fibrous capsule. **t. fibro′sa lie′nis** [NA], the fibroelastic coat of the spleen; called also *t. albuginea lienis.* **t. fibro′sa oc′uli,** t. fibrosa bulbi. **t. fibro′sa re′nis,** capsula fibrosa renis. **tu′nicae funic′uli spermat′ici** [NA], the coverings of the spermatic cord; see *tunicae funiculi spermatici et testis.* **tu′nicae funic′uli spermat′ici et tes′tis,** tunics of spermatic cord and testis: the coverings of the spermatic cord and testis, comprising the external spermatic fascia, the cremasteric muscle and fascia, the internal spermatic fascia, and the tunica vaginalis testis. **t. inter′na bul′bi** [NA], the internal nervous tunic of the eye; see *retina.* **t. inter′na the′cae follic′uli** [NA], the inner, vascular layer of secretory cells of the theca folliculi; called also *theca interna* and *internal coat of capsule of graafian follicle.* **t. in′tima vaso′rum** [NA], the inner coat of the blood vessels, made up of endothelial cells surrounded by longitudinal elastic fibers and connective tissue. **t. me′dia vaso′rum** [NA], the middle coat of the blood vessels, made up of transverse elastic and muscle fibers. **t. muco′sa** [NA], mu-

cous tunic or coat: the mucous membrane lining of various tubular structures, comprising the epithelium, basement membrane, lamina propria mucosae, and lamina muscularis mucosae. **t. muco′sa bronchio′rum** [NA], the mucous membrane lining the bronchi. **t. muco′sa ca′vi tym′pani** [NA], the mucous membrane covering the walls and much of the contents of the tympanic cavity; called also *t. mucosa tympanica* and *mucous coat of tympanic cavity.* **t. muco′sa co′li** [NA], the mucous coat of the colon. **t. muco′sa duc′tus deferen′tis** [NA], the mucous coat of the ductus deferens. **t. muco′sa esoph′agi** [NA], the mucous coat of the esophagus. **t. muco′sa intesti′ni rec′ti,** t. mucosa recti. **t. muco′sa intesti′ni ten′uis** [NA], the mucous coat of the small intestine. **t. muco′sa laryn′gis** [NA], the mucous coat of the larynx. **t. muco′sa lin′guae** [NA], the mucous membrane covering the tongue. **t. muco′sa na′si** [NA], the mucous membrane lining the nasal cavity; called also *membrana mucosa nasi.* See also *regio olfactoria* and *regio respiratoria.* **t. muco′sa o′ris** [NA], the tunica mucosa of the mouth. **t. muco′sa pharyn′gis** [NA], the mucous coat of the pharynx. **t. muco′sa rec′ti** [NA], the mucous coat of the rectum; called also *t. mucosa intestini recti.* **t. muco′sa tra′cheae** [NA], the mucous coat of the trachea. **t. muco′sa tu′bae auditi′vae** [NA], the mucous membrane lining the auditory tube. **t. muco′sa tu′bae uteri′nae** [NA], the mucous coat of the uterine tube. **t. muco′sa tympan′ica,** t. mucosa cavi tympani. **t. muco′sa ure′teris** [NA], the mucous coat of the ureter. **t. muco′sa ure′thrae femini′nae** [NA], **t. muco′sa ure′thrae mulie′bris,** the mucous coat of the female urethra. **t. muco′sa u′teri** [NA], the mucous membrane lining the uterus, the thickness and structure of which vary with the phase of the menstrual cycle; called also *endometrium* [NA alternative]. **t. muco′sa vagi′nae** [NA], the mucous coat of the vagina. **t. muco′sa ventric′uli** [NA], the mucous coat of the stomach. **t. muco′sa vesi′cae fel′leae** [NA], the mucous coat of the gallbladder. **t. muco′sa vesi′cae urina′riae** [NA], the mucous coat of the urinary bladder. **t. muco′sa vesic′ulae semina′lis** [NA], the mucous coat of the seminal vesicle. **t. muscula′ris** [NA], muscular tunic or coat: the muscular coat or layer surrounding the tela submucosa in most portions of the digestive, respiratory, urinary, and genital tracts. **t. muscula′ris bronchio′rum** [NA], the muscular coat of the bronchi. **t. muscula′ris cer′vicis u′teri,** the muscular coat of the cervix of the uterus. **t. muscula′ris coli** [NA], the muscular coat of the colon, consisting of layers of longitudinally and circularly coursing fibers. **t. muscula′ris duc′tus deferen′tis** [NA], the muscular coat of the ductus deferens. **t. muscula′ris esoph′agi** [NA], the muscular coat of the esophagus. **t. muscula′ris intesti′ni rec′ti,** t. muscularis recti. **t. muscula′ris intesti′ni ten′uis** [NA], the muscular coat of the small intestine, consisting of an inner circular and an outer longitudinal layer. **t. muscula′ris pharyn′gis** [NA], the muscular coat of the pharynx, consisting primarily of the pharyngeal constrictor muscles. **t. muscula′ris rec′ti** [NA], the muscular coat of the rectum, consisting of an outer longitudinal and an inner circular layer; called also *t. muscularis intestini recti.* **t. muscula′ris tra′cheae** [NA], the muscular coat of the trachea. **t. muscula′ris tu′bae uteri′nae** [NA], the muscular coat of the uterine tube. **t. muscula′ris ure′teris** [NA], the muscular coat of the ureter. **t. muscula′ris ure′thrae femini′nae** [NA], **t. muscula′ris ure′thrae mulie′bris,** the muscular coat of the female urethra. **t. muscula′ris u′teri** [NA], the smooth muscle coat of the uterus, which forms the mass of the organ; called also *myometrium* [NA alternative] and *mesometrium.* **t. muscula′ris vagi′nae** [NA], the muscular coat of the vagina. **t. muscula′ris ventric′uli** [NA], the muscular coat of the stomach, composed of longitudinal, circular, and oblique fibers. **t. muscula′ris vesi′cae fel′leae** [NA], the muscular coat of the gallbladder. **t. muscula′ris vesi′cae urina′riae** [NA], the smooth muscle coat of the urinary bladder. **t. muscula′ris vesic′ulae semina′lis** [NA], the muscular coat of the seminal vesicle. **t. ner′vea of Brücke,** the cerebral layer of the retina, exclusive of the rod and cone layer with its fibers and nuclei. **t. pro′pria** [NA], proper tunic: a general term in anatomical nomenclature for the proper coat or layer of a part, as distinguished from an investing membrane. **t. pro′pria co′rii,** stratum reticulare corii. **t. pro′pria tu′buli tes′tis,** the proper coat of the seminiferous tubules. **t. ruyschia′na,** lamina choriocapillaris. **t. sero′sa** [NA], the membrane lining the external walls of the body cavities and reflected over the surfaces of protruding organs; it consists of mesothelium lying upon a connective tissue layer, and it secretes a watery exudate; called also *serous coat, membrane,* or *coat.* **t. sero′sa co′li** [NA], the serous coat of the colon. **t. sero′sa hep′atis** [NA], the serous coat of the liver. **t. sero′sa intesti′ni ten′uis** [NA], the serous coat of the small intestine. **t. sero′sa lie′nis** [NA], the serous coat of the spleen. **t. sero′sa peritone′i** [NA], the serous coat of the peritoneum. **t. sero′sa tes′tis,** lamina visceralis tunicae vaginalis testis. **t. sero′sa tu′bae uteri′nae** [NA], the serous coat of the uterine tube. **t. sero′sa u′teri** [NA], the serous coat of the uterus; called also *perimetrium* [NA alternative]. **t. sero′sa ventric′uli** [NA], the serous coat of the stomach. **t. sero′sa vesi′cae fel′leae** [NA], the serous coat of the gallbladder. **t. sero′sa vesi′cae urina′riae** [NA], the serous coat of the urinary bladder. **t. submuco′sa ure′thrae mulie′bris**, the submucous coat of the female urethra. **tu′nicae tes′tis** [NA], the coverings of the testis; see *tunicae funiculi spermatici et testis*. **t. u′vea**, t. vasculosa bulbi. **t. vagina′lis commu′nis** [tes′tis et funic′uli spermat′ici], fascia spermatica interna. **t. vagina′lis pro′pria tes′tis**, t. vaginalis testis. **t. vagina′lis tes′tis** [NA], the serous membrane covering the front and sides of the testis and epididymis, composed of a visceral and a parietal layer. **t. vasculo′sa**, a vascular coat, or a layer well supplied with blood vessels. **t. vasculo′sa bul′bi** [NA], vascular tunic of the eye: the middle, pigmented, vascular coat of the eyeball, comprising the choroid, the ciliary body, and the iris; called also *uvea* and *uveal tract*. **t. vasculo′sa len′tis**, the vascular envelope which encloses and nourishes the developing lens of the fetus; it consists of the *pupillary membrane* in the region of the pupil, the *capsulopupillary membrane* around the edge of the lens, and the *capsular membrane* at the back of the lens. **t. vasculo′sa oc′uli**, t. vasculosa bulbi.

tunicary (too′nĭ-ker″e) pertaining to or possessing a tunic or enveloping membrane.

Tunicata (too″nĭ-ka′tah) [L. "clothed with a tunic"] Urochordata.

tunicate (too′nĭ-kāt) an animal belonging to the Urochordata (Tunicata); a urochordate.

tunicin (too′nĭ-sin) a substance resembling cellulose occurring in the body covering of some of the lowest vertebrates, such as the tunicates or ascidians; animal cellulose.

tuning fork (toon′ing fork) a two-tined forklike instrument of steel or aluminum, the tines of which when struck give off a musical note.

tunnel (tun′el) a passageway of varying length, through a solid body, completely enclosed except for the open ends, permitting entrance and exit. **aortico-left ventricular t.**, a congenital communication between the ascending aorta just above the coronary arteries, and the left ventricle. **carpal t.**, the osseofibrous passage for the median nerve and the flexor tendons, formed by the flexor retinaculum and the carpal bones. Called also *canalis carpi* [NA]. **cervical t′s**, small tubular canals which are extensions of the clefts in the uterine endocervical mucosa. **Corti's t.**, inner t. **cubital t.**, the opening between the two heads of the flexor carpi ulnaris muscle through which the ulnar nerve enters the forearm. **flexor t.**, carpal t. **inner t.**, a canal extending the length of the cochlea, formed by the pillar cells of the organ of Corti; called also *canal of Corti* and *Corti's t*. **outer t.**, Nuel's space. **tarsal t.**, the osseofibrous passage for the posterior tibial vessels, tibial nerve, and flexor tendons, formed by the flexor retinaculum and tarsal bones.

turacin (too′rah-sin) a red or crimson pigment, a copper salt of uroporphyrin.

turacoporphyrin (too″rah-ko-por″fĭ-rin) a derivative from turacin; nearly identical with hematoporphyrin.

turanose (too′rah-nōs) a reducing disaccharide, $C_{12}H_{22}O_{11}$, obtained by partially hydrolyzing melazitose.

Turbatrix (tur-ba′triks) a genus of nematodes. **T. aceti**, a minute nematode found in vinegar, where it helps form "mother of vinegar"; it sometimes occurs in the urine of patients who have used vinegar douches. It may also occur in sour paste and fermenting vegetable substances. Formerly called *Anguillula aceti*.

Turbellaria (tur″be-la′re-ah) a class of platyhelminths, usually found in fresh or salt water, although some are terrestrial.

turbid (tur′bid) [L. *turba* a tumult] cloudy; showing turbidity.

turbidimeter (tur″bĭ-dim′ĕ-ter) an instrument for measuring turbidity.

turbidimetric (tur″bid-ĭ-met′rik) performed by the turbidimeter.

turbidimetry (tur″bĭ-dim′ĕ-tre) the measurement of the tubidity of a fluid.

turbidity (tur-bid′ĭ-te) cloudiness; disturbance of solids (sediment) in a solution, so it is not clear.

turbinal (tur′bĭ-nal) [L. *turbinalis*, from *turbo* a child's top] 1. shaped like a top; turbinate. 2. a turbinate bone.

turbinate (tur′bĭ-nāt) [L. *turbineus*] 1. shaped like a top. 2. a turbinate bone (concha nasalis). **sphenoid t.**, concha sphenoidalis.

turbinated (tur′bĭ-nāt″ed) shaped like a top.

turbinectomy (tur″bĭ-nek′to-me) [*turbinate* + Gr. *ektomē* excision] the surgical removal of a turbinate bone.

turbinotome (tur-bin′o-tōm) a cutting instrument for use in the removal or cutting of a turbinate bone.

turbinotomy (tur″bĭ-not′o-me) [*turbinate* + Gr. *tomē* a cutting] the surgical cutting of a turbinate bone.

Türck's bundle, cell, column, degeneration, fasciculus (column), trachoma (tĕrks) [Ludwig *Türck*, neurologist and laryngologist in Vienna, 1810–1868] see under the nouns.

Turck's zone (turks) [Fenton Benedict *Turck*, New York physician, 1857–1932] see *zona transformans*.

turgescence (tur-jes′ens) [L. *turgescens* swelling] the distention or swelling of a part.

turgescent (tur-jes′ent) [L. *turgescens*] swelling or beginning to swell.

turgid (tur′jid) [L. *turgidus*] swollen and congested.

turgidization (tur″jid-i-za′shun) the creation of turgor in a tissue by the injection of fluid.

turgometer (tur-gom′ĕ-ter) [L. *turgor* swelling + *metrum* measure] an instrument for measuring the amount of turgescence.

turgor (tur′gor) [L.] the condition of being turgid; normal or other fullness. **t. vita′lis**, the normal consistency of living tissue.

turista (tu-rēs′tah) [Sp.] Mexican name for traveler's diarrhea.

Türk's cell (irradiation leukocyte) (tĕrks) [Wilhelm *Türk*, Austrian physician, 1871–1916] see under *cell*.

turmeric (tur′mer-ik) the rhizome of *Curcuma longa* L. (Zingiberaceae), a plant of India, China, and East Indies. It contains curcumin, an orange-yellow coloring principle, and several aromatic principles that give it a pepper-like and bitter taste; used as a coloring agent, chemical indicator, and condiment (as curry powder).

turmschadel (torm′sha-del) [Gr.] a developmental anomaly in which the skull is high and rounded, due to early synostosis of the three major sutures of the skull.

Turner's sign (tur′nerz) [George Grey *Turner*, English surgeon, 1877–1951] see under *sign*.

Turner's sulcus (tur′nerz) [William Aldren *Turner*, British neurologist, born 1864] sulcus intraparietalis.

Turner's syndrome (tur′nerz) [Henry Hubert *Turner*, American endocrinologist, born 1892] see under *syndrome*.

Turner tooth (hypoplasia) (tur′ner) [Joseph George *Turner*, British dentist, died 1955] see under *tooth*.

turnera (tur′ner-ah) damiana.

turnsick, turnsickness (turn′sik, turn′sik-nes) gid.

turnsol (turn′sol) litmus.

turpentine (tur′pen-tin) [L. *terebinthina*] the concrete oleoresin obtained from *Pinus palustris* Mill. (Pinaceae) and other species of *Pinus*. It contains a volatile oil, to which its properties are due, and in which form it is generally used; see under *oil*.

turricephaly (tur″ĭ-sef′ah-le) oxycephaly.

turunda (tu-run′dah) [L.] 1. a surgeon's tent. 2. a suppository.

Turyn's sign (too′rinz) [Felix *Turyn*, Warsaw physician, born 1899] see under *sign*.

tus. abbreviation for L. *tus′sis*, a cough.

tusk (tusk) an extremely large tooth projecting beyond the lips.

tussal (tus′al) [L. *tussis* cough] pertaining to a cough.

tussicula (tŭ-sik′u-lah) [L., dim. of *tussis* cough] a slight cough.

tussicular (tŭ-sik′u-lar) [L. *tussicula*] of or relating to a cough.

tussiculation (tŭ-sik″u-la′shun) a short, hacking cough.

tussigenic (tus″ĭ-jen′ik) [L. *tussis* cough + Gr. *gennan* to produce] causing cough.

tussis (tus′is) [L.] cough. **t. convul′siva**, pertussis.

tussive (tus′iv) pertaining to or due to a cough.

tutamen (tu-ta′men), pl. tutam′ina [L.] a protective covering or structure. **tutam′ina oc′uli** ["defenses of the eye"], the appendages of the eye: the eyelids, lashes, etc. (organa oculi accessoria [NA]).

tutamina (tu-tam′ĭ-nah) [L.] plural of *tutamen*.

Tuttle's proctoscope (tut′l'z) [Edward Gerry *Tuttle*, surgeon in New York, 1862–1913] see under *proctoscope*.

Tween (twēn) trademark for preparations of polysorbates, used with a numerical suffix; e.g., *Tween 80* is a trademark for polysorbate 80.

tween-brain (twēn′brān) diencephalon.

twig in anatomy, a final ramification, as of branches of nerves or blood vessels.

twin (twin) one of two offspring produced in the same pregnancy and developed from one ovum (monozygotic) or from two ova (dizygotic) fertilized at the same time. **acardiac t.**, acardius. **allantoidoangiopagous t's**, twins joined by the vessels of the umbilical cord only; called also *omphaloangiopagous t's*. **binovular t's**, dizygotic t's. **conjoined t's**, monozygotic twins ranging from two well-developed individuals joined by a superficial connection of varying extent, usually in the frontal, transverse, or sagittal body plane (*symmetrical* or *equal conjoined t's*) to those in which only a small part of the body is duplicated or one small and incompletely developed component, the parasite, is attached to a much larger and more fully developed one, the autosite (*asymmetrical* or *unequal t's*). Called also *Siamese t's*. **conjoined t's, asymmetrical**, see *conjoined t's*. **conjoined t's, equal**, see *conjoined t's*. **conjoined t's, symmetrical**, see *conjoined t's*. **conjoined t's, unequal**, see *conjoined t's*. **dichorial t's, dichorionic t's**, dizygotic t's.

dissimilar t's, dizygotic t's. **dizygotic t's,** two offspring developed from two separate ova fertilized at the same time; they may be of the same or different sex, and they have different genomes. Called also *binovular, dichorial, dichorionic, dissimilar, false, fraternal, heterologous, hetero-ovular, two-egg,* and *unlike t's.* **enzygotic t's,** monozygotic t's. **false t's,** dizygotic t's. **fraternal t's,** dizygotic t's. **heterologous t's,** dizygotic t's. **hetero-ovular t's,** dizygotic t's. **identical t's,** monozygotic t's. **impacted t's,** twins so situated during delivery that the pressure of one against the other prevents simultaneous engagement of both. **monoamniotic t's,** twins developing within a single amniotic cavity; they are always monozygotic. **monochorial t's, monochorionic t's,** monozygotic t's. **monoovular t's, monovular t's,** monozygotic t's. **monozygotic t's,** two offspring developed from one zygote or fertilized ovum, and therefore having identical genomes. Called also *enzygotic, identical, monochorial, monochorionic, mono-ovular, similar, true,* and *uniovular t's.* **omphaloangiopagous t's,** allantoidoangiopagous t's. **one-egg t's,** monozygotic t's. **Siamese t's,** conjoined t's. **similar t's,** monozygotic t's. **true t's,** monozygotic t's. **two-egg t's,** dizygotic t's. **unequal t's,** twins of which one is incompletely developed. **uniovular t's,** monozygotic t's. **unlike t's,** dizygotic t's.

twinge (twinj) a short, sharp pain.

twinning (twin′ing) 1. the simultaneous production of two (or more) offspring. 2. the production of symmetrical structures or parts by division. **experimental t.,** embryonic duplication produced by purposeful external intervention. **spontaneous t.,** embryonic duplication without external intervention, as occurs in nature.

twinship (twin′ship) the state of being a twin.

Twiston (twis′ton) trademark for preparations of rotoxamine tartrate.

twitch (twich) 1. a brief contractile response of a skeletal muscle elicited by a single maximal volley of impulses in the motor neurons supplying it. 2. a noose passed through a perforation in a board, used for compressing a part, as the lip of a horse, during slight operations.

twitching (twich′ing) the occurrence of a single contraction or a series of contractions of a muscle; see *twitch.* **fascicular t.,** repetitive brief contraction of large groups of bundles of muscle fibers. **fibrillar t.,** repetitive brief contraction of single bundles of muscle fibers. **Trousseau's t.,** repetitive brief contraction involving muscles of the face.

Twort-d'Herelle phenomenon (twort-dĕ-rel′) [Frederick William *Twort,* British bacteriologist, 1877–1950; Felix Hubert d'Herelle of the Pasteur Institute, Paris, 1873–1949] see under *phenomenon.*

TX a symbol for a derivative of contagious tuberculin (TC.); see under *tuberculin.*

tybamate (ti′bah-māt) chemical name: butylcarbamic acid 2-[[(aminocarbonyl)oxy]methyl]-2-methylpentyl ester. A minor tranquilizer, $C_{13}H_{26}N_2O_4$, occurring as a clear, viscous liquid; administered orally.

tychastics (ti-kas′tiks) [Gr. *tychē* chance, accident] the science of industrial accidents.

tylectomy (ti-lek′to-me) [Gr. *tylos* knot + *ektomē* excision] resection of the local lesion only, in carcinoma of the breast; partial mastectomy.

Tylenol (ti′lĕ-nol) trademark for preparations of acetaminophen.

tylion (til′e-on) [Gr. *tyleion* cushion] the point on the anterior edge of the optic groove in the median line.

tyloma (ti-lo′mah) [Gr. *tylōma*] a callus or callosity.

Tylophora asthmatica Wight et Arn. (ti-lof′o-rah az-mat′ĭ-kah) [Gr. *tylos* knot + *pherein* to bear] an asclepiadaceous plant of South Asia; it is the source of tylophorine.

tylophorine (ti-lof′o-rin) chemical name: 9,11,12,13,13a,14-hexahydro-2,3,6,7-tetramethoxydibenzo[*f,h*]pyrrolo[1,2-*b*]isoquinoline. A crystalline alkaloid, $C_{24}H_{27}O_4N$, from *Tylophora asthmatica* Wight et Arn. (Asclepiadaceae); it is emetic, and is useful in dysentery and asthma.

tylosis (ti-lo′sis) [Gr. *tylōs* a knob or callus] the formation of a callus or callosity. **t. cilia′ris,** thickening of the eyelids. **t. lin′guae,** leukoplakia buccalis. **t. palma′ris et planta′ris,** keratosis palmaris et plantaris.

tylotic (ti-lot′ik) pertaining to or affected with tylosis.

tyloxapol (ti-loks′ah-pōl) [USP] chemical name: 4-(1,1,3,3-tetramethylbutyl)phenol polymer with formaldehyde and oxirane. A nonionic liquid polymer of the alkyl aryl polyether alcohol type; used as a surfactant to aid liquefaction and removal of mucopurulent bronchopulmonary secretions, administered by inhalation through a nebulizer or with a stream of oxygen.

tympanal (tim′pah-nal) pertaining to the tympanic cavity or to the tympanic membrane.

tympanectomy (tim″pah-nek′to-me) [*tympanum* + Gr. *ektomē* excision] excision of the tympanic membrane.

tympania (tim-pan′e-ah) tympanites.

tympanic (tim-pan′ik) [L. *tympanicus*] 1. of or pertaining to the tympanum of the tympanic membrane. 2. bell-like; resonant.

tympanicity (tim″pah-nis′ĭ-te) a tympanic quality.

tympanion (tim-pan′e-on) [Gr.] a point at either end of the vertical diameter of the anulus tympanicus. **lower t.,** the lowest point on the anulus tympanicus. **upper t.,** the highest point on the anulus tympanicus.

tympanism (tim′pah-nizm) [Gr. *tympanon* drum] distention with gas; tympanites.

tympanites (tim″pah-ni′tēz) [Gr. *tympanitēs,* from *tympanon* drum] distention of the abdomen, due to the presence of gas or air in the intestine or in the peritoneal cavity, as in peritonitis and typhoid fever. **false t.,** pseudotympanites. **uterine t.,** physometra.

tympanitic (tim″pah-nit′ik) 1. pertaining to or affected with tympanites. 2. bell-like, or tympanic.

tympanitis (tim″pah-ni′tis) otitis media.

tympanoacryloplasty (tim″pah-no-ah-kril′o-plas″te) surgical obliteration of the mastoid cavity by instillation of an acrylic compound.

tympanocentesis (tim″pah-no-sen-te′sis) surgical puncture of the tympanic membrane (drumhead) or tympanum (middle ear).

tympanoeustachian (tim″pah-no-u-sta′ke-an) pertaining to the tympanic cavity and auditory tube.

tympanogenic (tim″pah-no-jen′ik) [*tympanum* + Gr. *gennan* to produce] arising from the tympanum or middle ear.

tympanogram (tim-pan′o-gram″) [*tympanum* + Gr. *metron* measure] a graphic representation of the relative compliance and impedance of the tympanic membrane and ossicles of the middle ear obtained by tympanometry.

tympanohyal (tim″pah-no-hi′al) 1. pertaining to the tympanum and the hyoid arch. 2. a small bone or cartilage at the base of the styloid process; in early life it becomes a part of the temporal bone.

tympanolabyrinthopexy (tim″pah-no-lab″ĭ-rin′tho-pek″se) Sourdille's operation of uniting a neotympanic system to a labyrinthine fistula for the cure of progressive hearing loss from otosclerosis.

tympanomalleal (tim″pah-no-mal′e-al) pertaining to the tympanic membrane and the malleus.

tympanomandibular (tim″pah-no-man-dib′u-lar) pertaining to the middle ear and the mandible.

tympanomastoiditis (tim″pah-no-mas″toi-di′tis) inflammation of the middle ear and the pneumatic cells of the mastoid process.

tympanometric (tim″pan-o-met′rik) pertaining to tympanometry.

tympanometry (tim″pah-nom′ĕ-tre) indirect measurement of the compliance (mobility) and impedance of the tympanic membrane and ossicles of the middle ear; it is done by subjecting the external acoustic meatus to positive, normal, and negative air pressure and monitoring the resultant sound energy flow.

tympanoplastic (tim″pah-no-plas′tik) relating to tympanoplasty.

tympanoplasty (tim″pah-no-plas′te) [*tympanum* + Gr. *plassein* to form] surgical reconstruction of the hearing mechanism of the middle ear, with restoration of the drum membrane to protect the round window from sound pressure, and establishment of ossicular continuity between the tympanic membrane and the oval window. See *myringoplasty.*

tympanosclerosis (tim″pah-no-sklĕ-ro′sis) a condition characterized by the presence of masses of hard, dense connective tissue around the auditory ossicles in the tympanic cavity.

tympanosquamosal (tim″pah-no-skwah-mo′sal) pertaining to the pars tympanica and pars squamosa of the temporal bone.

tympanostapedial (tim″pah-no-stă-pe′de-al) pertaining to the tympanum and the stapes.

tympanosympathectomy (tim″pah-no-sim″pah-thek′to-me) the operation of excising the tympanic plexus for the relief of tinnitus aurium.

tympanotemporal (tim″pah-no-tem′po-ral) pertaining to the tympanum and the region over the temporal bone or region.

tympanotomy (tim″pah-not′o-me) [*tympanum* + Gr. *tomē* a cutting] surgical puncture of the membrana tympani; myringotomy.

tympanous (tim′pah-nus) pertaining to or marked by tympanites; distended with gas.

tympanum (tim′pah-num) [L.; Gr. *tympanon* drum] the cavity of the middle ear, located just medial to the tympanic membrane, and containing the auditory ossicles and connecting with the mastoid cells and auditory tube. Called also *auris media* [NA].

tympany (tim′pah-ne) [Gr. *tympanias*] 1. tympanites. 2. a tympanic, or bell-like, percussion note. **bell t.,** a modified tympanitic note heard on percussion of the chest in some cases of pneumothorax. **Skoda's t., skodaic t.,** skodaic resonance. **t. of the stomach,** a kind of indigestion in cattle and sheep, marked by an abnormal collection of gas in the first stomach; called also *bloat*.

Tyndall light, phenomenon (effect) (tin′dal) [John *Tyndall*, British physicist, 1820–1893] see under *light* and *phenomenon*.

tyndallization (tyn″dal-i-za′shun) [John *Tyndall*] fractional sterilization.

type (tīp) [L. *typus*; Gr. *typos* mark] the general or prevailing character of any particular case of disease, person, substance, etc. See also under *habit* and *habitus*. Cf. *constitution* and *diathesis*. **allotropic t.**, a personality which tends to be preoccupied with what others do or think or mean. **amyostatic-kinetic t.**, a type of epidemic encephalitis marked by apathy, rigidity, akinesis, slowing of movement and sometimes tremor. **apoplectic t.**, see *habitus apoplecticus*. **asthenic t.**, a type of physical constitution: slender, flat in front, long chested, poor muscular development. **athletic t.**, a type of physical constitution, marked by broad shoulders, deep chest, flat abdomen, thick neck, and good muscular development. **Aztec t., bird's head t.**, see *microcephalic idiocy*, under *idiocy*. **blood t's**, see *blood group*, under B. **body t.**, the general character of the body structure or constitution. See *Kretschmer's types* and *ectomorphy*, *endomorphy*, and *mesomorphy*. **buffalo t.**, obesity confined to the neck, head, and trunk; seen in Cushing's syndrome (def. 1). **Charcot-Marie t., Charcot-Marie-Tooth t.**, see *progressive neuropathic (peroneal) muscular atrophy*, under *atrophy*. **cycloid t.**, see *syntonic*. **Dejerine t.**, amyotrophic lateral sclerosis. **Dejerine-Landouzy t.**, Landouzy-Dejerine dystrophy. **Duchenne's t.**, pseudohypertrophic muscular dystrophy. **Duchenne-Aran t.**, spinal muscular atrophy. **Duchenne-Landouzy t.**, Landouzy-Dejerine dystrophy. **dysplastic t.**, any body type which differs from the asthenic, the athletic, and the pyknic types. **Eichhorst's t.**, see under *atrophy*. **Erb-Zimmerlin t.**, the juvenile scapular type of primary muscular dystrophy. **Fazio-Londe t.**, the bulbofacial type of familial infantile progressive spinal muscular atrophy. **Hutchison t.**, neuroblastoma with cranial metastases. **Kalmuck t., Kalmuk t.**, Down's syndrome. **koinotropic t.**, the socially adjusted type; the "good mixer." **Kretschmer t's**, types of physique related to personality: the *asthenic* (leptosome) is schizoid; the *pyknic* is syntonic. **Landouzy's t., Landouzy-Dejerine t.**, Landouzy-Dejerine dystrophy. **leg t.**, progressive hereditary muscular atrophy. **Leichtenstern's t.**, hemorrhagic encephalitis. **leptosome t.**, asthenic t. **Levi-Lorain t.**, hypophyseal infantilism. **Leyden-Möbius t.**, limb-girdle muscular dystrophy. **Lorain t.**, arrested physical development (infantilism) of pituitary causation. **Nothnagel's t.**, see under *acroparesthesia*. **organic reaction t.**, a type of psychosis due to organic disease of the brain. **overactive t.**, a mental make-up characterized by mental and physical aggressiveness and activity, talkativeness and a tendency to exaltation. **Pepper's t.**, see under *syndrome*. **phage t.**, an intraspecies type of bacterium demonstrated by phage typing (see under *typing*); called also *lysotype* and *phagotype*. **phthinoid t.**, a body type characterized by a flat, narrow chest. **phthisic t.**, habitus phthisicus. **Putnam's t.**, subacute combined degeneration of spinal cord; see under *degeneration*. **pyknic t.**, a physical type marked by rounded body, large chest, thick shoulders, broad head, and short neck. **Raymond's t. of apoplexy**, see under *apoplexy*. **Remak's t.**, see under *paralysis*. **Runeberg's t.**, see under *anemia*. **scapulohumeral t.**, progressive spinal muscular atrophy beginning in the shoulder. **schizoid t.**, see *schizoid*, def. 1. **Schultze's t.**, see under *acroparesthesia*. **seclusive t.**, a mental make-up characterized by quietness, reserve, shyness, secretiveness, and aversion to social contacts. **Séglas t.**, the psychomotor type of paranoia. **Simmerlin t.**, Leyden-Möbius dystrophy. **sthenic t.**, a type of physical constitution characterized by muscular strength. **Strümpell's t.**, see under *disease*, def. 1. **suspicious t.**, a mental make-up characterized by abnormal mistrustfulness and suspicion. **sympatheticotonic t.**, a type of physical constitution characterized by sympathicotonia. **syntonic t.**, see *syntonic*. **test t.**, see *test type*. **Tooth's t.**, progressive neuropathic (peroneal) muscular atrophy. **unstable t.**, a mental make-up characterized by emotional changeableness. **vagotonic t.**, a physical type characteristic of deficient suprarenal activity: there are slow pulse, low blood pressure, localized sweating, high sugar tolerance, and oculocardiac reflex. **vesanic t.**, psychosis due to primary psychiatric disorder and not to any external cause, as injury, poisoning, or disease of some other organ; it includes mania, melancholia, etc. **visual t.**, an individual who depends mainly on sight and whose imagery is mostly visual. **Werdnig-Hoffmann t.**, see under *paralysis*. **Wernicke-Mann t.**, see under *hemiplegia*. **wild t.**, in genetics, the standard phenotype for any experimental organism; also a gene that determines a standard phenotypic trait. **Zimmerlin's t.**, see under *atrophy*.

typembryo (tīp-em′bre-o) an embryo in that stage of development at which the characteristics of the type to which it belongs may be seen.

Typhaceae (ti-fa′se-e) a name once proposed for the family including the causative organism of typhoid fever (*Salmonella typhosa*) and related forms.

typhemia (ti-fe′me-ah) [*typhus* + Gr. *haima* blood + *-ia*] the presence of typhoid bacilli in the blood.

typhia (tif′e-ah) typhoid fever.

typhic (ti′fik) pertaining to typhus or to typhoid fever.

typhlectasis (tif-lek′tah-sis) [Gr. *typhlon* cecum + *ektasis* distention] distention of the cecum.

typhlectomy (tif-lek′to-me) cecectomy.

typhlenteritis (tif″len-ter-i′tis) [Gr. *typhlon* cecum + Gr. *enteron* intestine] cecitis.

typhlitis (tif-li′tis) [Gr. *typhlon* cecum + *-itis*] inflammation of the cecum; the term was formerly used for the condition now called *appendicitis*.

typhlo- 1. [Gr. *typhlon* cecum] a combining form denoting relationship to the cecum. 2. [Gr. *typhlos* blind] a combining form denoting relationship to blindness.

typhlocele (tif′lo-sēl) cecocele.

Typhlocoelum (tif″lo-se′lum) a genus of trematode parasites. **T. cucumeri′num**, a trematode parasitic in the trachea, esophagus, and thoracic cavity of chicks in Brazil and certain ducks and wild aquatic birds in Madagascar.

typhlocolitis (tif″lo-ko-li′tis) [*typhlo*-(1) + *colitis*] colitis in the region of the cecum.

typhlodicliditis (tif″lo-dik″lĭ-di′tis) [*typhlo*-(1) + Gr. *diklis* door + *-itis*] inflammation of the ileocecal valve.

typhloempyema (tif″lo-em″pi-e′mah) [*typhlo*-(1) + *empyema*] appendicular abscess.

typhloenteritis (tif″lo-en″ter-i′tis) cecitis.

typhlohepatitis (tif″lo-hep″ah-ti′tis) histomoniasis of turkeys.

typhlolexia (tif″lo-lek′se-ah) [*typhlo*-(2) + Gr. *lexis* speech + *-ia*] alexia.

typhlolithiasis (tif″lo-lĭ-thi′ah-sis) [*typhlo*-(1) + Gr. *lithos* stone + *-ia*] the presence of calculi in the cecum.

typhlology (tif-lol′o-je) [*typhlo*-(2) + *-logy*] the sum of what is known in regard to blindness.

typhlomegaly (tif″lo-meg′ah-le) [*typhlo*-(1) + Gr. *megas* large] abnormal enlargement of the cecum.

typhlon (tif′lon) [Gr.] the cecum.

typhlopexia (tif″lo-pek′se-ah) typhlopexy.

typhlopexy (tif′lo-pek″se) [*typhlo*-(1) + Gr. *pēxis* fixation] operative suspension and fixation of the cecum.

typhloptosis (tif″lo-to′sis) [*typhlo*-(1) + Gr. *ptōsis* falling] cecoptosis.

typhlorrhaphy (tif-lor′ah-fe) cecorrhaphy.

typhlosis (tif-lo′sis) [Gr. *typhlōsis* a making blind] blindness.

typhlostenosis (tif″lo-stĕ-no′sis) [*typhlo*-(1) + Gr. *stenōsis* narrowing] contraction of the cecum.

typhlostomy (tif-los′to-me) [*typhlo*-(1) + Gr. *stomoun* to provide with an opening, or mouth] cecostomy.

typhloteritis (tif″lo-ter-i′tis) cecitis.

typhlotomy (tif-lot′o-me) [*typhlo*-(1) + Gr. *tomē* a cutting] cecotomy.

typhloureterostomy (tif″lo-u-re″ter-os′to-me) [*typhlo*-(1) + Gr. *ourētēr* ureter + *stomoun* to provide with an opening, or mouth] anastomosis of the ureter to the cecum.

typhobacillosis (ti″fo-bas″ĭ-lo′sis) [*typhus* + *bacillus* + *-osis*] a term formerly used to designate the symptoms due to poisoning by the toxins of *Salmonella typhosa*. **t. tuberculo′sa**, a condition due to tuberculous infection and exhibiting the symptoms of typhoid fever.

typhobacterin (ti″fo-bak′ter-in) typhoid vaccine.

typhoid (ti′foid) [Gr. *typhōdes* like smoke; delirious] 1. resembling typhus. 2. typhoid fever. **bilious t.**, leptospiral jaundice. **fowl t.**, an acute infectious disease of fowl caused by *Salmonella gallinarum*, marked by drowsiness, anorexia, extreme weakness, and usually diarrhea, finally ending in death in four days to two weeks after onset. Called also *Klein's disease*. **Manchurian t.**, a disease seen in Manchuria during the Russo-Japanese War, distinct from typhoid, and resembling in its symptoms Brill's disease. **pellagra t.**, pellagra marked by moderate fever with mild delirium. **provocation t.**, the systemic reaction to the endotoxin of killed typhoid bacilli in typhoid vaccine. **subcontinuous t.**, a form of malarial disease simulating typhoid fever, as typhomalarial fever.

typhoidal (ti-foid′al) resembling typhoid fever.

typhoidin (ti′foi-din) a ten-day culture of a single strain of *Salmonella typhosa* on glycerin broth evaporated to one-tenth volume (Gay and Force, 1914). It is also used in the cutaneous reaction for typhoid fever. See *typhoidin test*, under *tests*.

typhomalarial (ti″fo-mah-la′re-al) of malarial origin, but with typhoid symptoms; see under *fever*.

Typhonium trilobatum (L.) Schott. (Araceae) (ti-fo′ne-um tri″lo-ba′tum) [L.] an Asiatic plant, highly valued in oriental practice as a polychrest remedy.

typhopaludism (ti″fo-pal′u-dizm) typhomalarial fever.

typhopneumonia (ti″fo-nu-mo′ne-ah) pulmonary involvement during the course of infection with *Salmonella typhosa*.

typhous (ti′fus) pertaining to or resembling typhus.

typhus (ti′fus) [Gr. *typhos* stupor arising from fever] any of a group of related arthropod-borne infectious diseases caused by species of *Rickettsia* and marked by malaise, severe headache, sustained high fever, and a macular or maculopapular eruption which appears from the third to the seventh day. Called also *typhus fever*. In English-speaking countries, often used alone to refer to epidemic t., whereas in several European languages, it refers to typhoid fever. **Austra-lian tick t.,** North Queensland tick t. **amarillic t.,** yellow fever. **benign t.,** Brill's disease. **canine t.,** Stuttgart disease. **classic t.,** epidemic t. **collapsing t.,** an infectious typhoid fever occurring in Korea. **endemic t.,** murine t. **epidemic t.,** the classic form of typhus, caused by *Rickettsia prowazekii*, which is transmitted from man to man by the louse *Pediculus humanus*. After an incubation of 10 days to 2 weeks, the onset is usually abrupt, with severe headache, generalized aches and pains, and shaking chills. After a few days there is fever, lasting 10 to 14 days. A macular or maculopapular rash that becomes petechial appears about the fifth day, beginning on the back and covering the body except the face, palms, and soles; it fades with the fever. In the second week there may be delirium and stupor, progressing to coma and ending in death in 20 per cent of untreated cases. **European t.,** epidemic t. **exanthematic t.,** epidemic t. **exanthematic t. of São Paulo,** Rocky Mountain spotted fever. **t. exan-themat′icus, t. exanthematique′, exanthematous t.,** epidemic t. **flea t., flea-borne t.,** murine t. **Gubler-Robin t.,** the renal form of typhus. **Indian tick t.,** a rickettsial disease of India believed to be identical with boutonneuse fever. **K T t.,** rural t. **Kenya t.,** a rickettsial disease occurring in Kenya, believed to be identical with boutonneuse fever, except that tache noir is absent; it is transmitted by *Rhipicephalus sanguineus, R. simus, Haemaphysalis haebreum*, and the larvae of *Amblyomma leachi*. Called also *Kenya fever*. **louse t., louse-borne t.,** epidemic t. **Manchurian t.,** murine t. **Mexican t.,** murine t. **mite-borne t.,** scrub t. **Moscow t.,** murine t. **mouse t.,** an epizootic disease of mice caused by *Salmonella typhimurium*. **murine t.,** an infectious disease clinically similar to epidemic typhus, but caused by *Rickettsia typhi*, which is transmitted from rat to man by the rat flea, *Xenopsylla cheopis*, and by the rat louse, *Polyplax spinulosa;* called also *endemic, fleaborne*, or *rat t*. It is also known by various names according to the region in which it occurs, e.g., *Mexican t., Manchurian t., Moscow t., Congolian red fever*, etc. **North Asian tick t.,** Siberian tick t. **North Queensland tick t.,** a nonfatal febrile disease occurring in Australia, caused by *Rickettsia australis*, and characterized by headache, conjunctival injection, and an initial lesion somewhat resembling a cigarette burn; the vector may be the tick *Ixodes holocyclus*. Called also *Australian tick t.* and *Queensland tick t.* **petechial t.,** epidemic t. **Queensland tick t.,** North Queensland tick t. **rat t.,** murine t. **recrudescent t.,** Brill's disease. **rural t.,** a form of scrub typhus seen mostly in outdoor workers in Malaya. **São Paulo t.,** Rocky Mountain spotted fever. **scrub t.,** a self-limited, febrile disease of two weeks' duration, caused by *Rickettsia tsutsugamushi,* transmitted by larval mites of the genus *Trombicula*, especially *T. akamushi* (in Japan) and *T. deliensis* (outside Japan); it is characterized by sudden onset of fever with a primary skin lesion (tache noir, or eschar), and development of a rash about the fifth day. Called also *mite-borne t.* and *tsutsuga-mushi disease*. Known also by various names according to the region in which it is found, e.g., *Kedani fever* and *Japanese flood fever* in Japan, *Sumatran mite fever* in Sumatra, and *rural t.* in Malaya. **shop t.,** urban t. **Siberian tick t.,** a relatively mild, acutely febrile, spotted fever, characterized by headache, malaise, conjunctival injection, a maculopapular rash, and a primary ulcerative lesion at the site of the tick bite; it occurs in north, central, and east Asia. The causative agent is *Rickettsia siberica*, which is transmitted by ticks of the genera *Dermacentor* and *Haemaphysalis*. Called also *North Asian tick t.* **tick t.,** **tickborne t.,** Rocky Mountain spotted fever; also, any tickborne infectious disease (see *tick fever*, under *fever*). **Toulon t.,** murine t. **tropical t.,** scrub t. **urban t.,** a mild form of murine typhus, usually observed in indoor workers in Malaya and the Mediterranean regions; called also *shop t*.

typical (tip′ĭ-kal) [Gr. *typikos*] presenting the distinctive features of any type.

typing (tīp′ing) in transplantation immunology, a method of measuring the degree of organ, solid tissue, or blood compatibility between two individuals, in which specific histocompatibility antigens (e.g., those present on leukocytes or erythrocytes) are detected by means of suitable isoimmune antisera. **t. of blood,** classification of the blood with reference to various erythrocytic membrane antigens. See *blood type*. **phage t.,** characterization of bacteria, extending to strain differences, by demonstration of susceptibility to one or more (a spectrum) races of bacteriophage; widely applied to staphylococci, typhoid bacilli, etc., for epidemiological purposes. **tissue t.,** see *typing*.

typodont (ti′po-dont) a model of a tooth.

typology (ti-pol′o-je) the study of types; the science of classifying, as bacteria according to type.

typoscope (ti′po-skōp) [Gr. *typos* type + *skopein* to examine] an instrument to aid amblyopia and cataract patients in reading.

typus (ti′pus) [L.] type. **t. degenerati′vus amstelo-damen′sis,** de Lange's syndrome.

Tyr tyrosine.

tyramine (ti′rah-mēn) a decarboxylation product of tyrosine, which may be converted to cresol and phenol; closely related structurally to epinephrine and norepinephrine, it has a similar but weaker action. It is found in decayed animal tissue, ripe cheese, and ergot.

tyrannism (tir′ah-nizm) [Gr. *tyrrhanos* tyrant] morbid cruelty.

tyrein (ti′re-in) the coagulated casein of milk.

tyresin (ti-re′sin) a principle derivable from the venom of serpents and from the juice of mushrooms; it was thought to be an antidote for snake poisoning.

tyro- (ti′ro) [Gr. *tyros* cheese] a combining form denoting relationship to cheese.

tyrocidin (ti″ro-si′din) tyrocidine.

tyrocidine (ti″ro-si′din) a crystalline polypeptide antibiotic substance which is the major component of tyrothricin.

Tyrode's solution (ti′rōdz) [Maurice Vejux *Tyrode*, American pharmacologist, 1878–1930] see under *solution*.

tyrogenous (ti-roj′ĕ-nus) [*tyro-* + Gr. *gennan* to produce] originating in cheese.

Tyroglyphus (ti-rog′lĭ-fus) [*tyro-* + Gr. *glyphein* to carve] *Tyrophagus*. **T. castella′ni,** *Tyrophagus castellani*. **T. fari′nae,** *Tyrophagus farinae*. **T. lon′gior,** *Tyrophagus longior*. **T. si′ro,** *Acarus siro*.

tyroid (ti′roid) [*tyro-* + Gr. *eidos* form] caseous; resembling cheese.

tyroma (ti-ro′mah) a caseous tumor; a new growth or nodule of cheesy material.

tyromatosis (ti″ro-mah-to′sis) a condition characterized by caseous degeneration.

tyropanoate sodium (ti″ro-pah-no′āt) chemical name: α-ethyl-2,4,6-triiodo-3-[(1-oxobutyl)amino]benzene propanoic acid monosodium salt; a diagnostic radiopaque medium for use in cholecystography, $C_{15}H_{17}I_3NNaO_3$.

Tyrophagus (ti-rof′ah-gus) a genus of pale, soft-bodied mites, the meal mites; called also *Tyroglyphus*. **T. castella′ni,** the copra mite, the species that causes copra itch. **T. fari′nae,** the flour mite, found in flour mills and granaries. **T. lon′gior,** the cheese mite, which has been reported from both the urinary and digestive tracts and may be found in the stools. **T. si′ro,** *Acarus siro*.

tyrosamine (ti-rōs′ah-mēn) tyramine.

tyrosinase (ti-ro′sin-ās) an oxidizing enzyme in animal and plant tissues which catalyzes the oxidation of tyrosine and other phenolic compounds into black pigments.

tyrosine (ti-ro′sin) a crystallizable amino acid, *p*-hydroxy-phenylalanine, $C_9H_{11}O_3N$, found in most proteins and synthesized metabolically from phenylalanine; it is a precursor of thyroid hormones, catecholamines, and melanin. Sometimes called *oxy-phenylaminopropionic acid*.

tyrosinemia (ti″ro-sĭ-ne′me-ah) a disorder of tyrosine metabolism marked by an excess of tyrosine in the blood and by tyrosyluria. It occurs in two forms: *transient* or *neonatal tyrosinemia*, a benign condition of the newborn, especially of the premature, which responds to ascorbic acid, and *hereditary tyrosinemia*, which results in liver failure or severe nodular cirrhosis, with renal tubular involvement similar to Fanconi's syndrome, hypoglycemia, rickets, darkening of the skin, and slight mental retardation; it is transmitted as an autosomal recessive trait.

tyrosinosis (ti″ro-sĭ-no′sis) a condition characterized by a faulty metabolism of tyrosine in which an intermediate product, parahydroxyphenyl pyruvic acid, appears in the urine and gives it an abnormal reducing power.

tyrosinuria (ti″ro-sĭ-nu′re-ah) [*tyrosine* + Gr. *ouron* urine + *-ia*] the presence of tyrosine in urine, as in tyrosinemia.

tyrosis (ti-ro′sis) caseation, def. 2.

tyrosyluria (ti″ro-sil-u′re-ah) the increased urinary excretion of para-hydroxyphenyl compounds derived from tyrosine, as in tyrosinemia.

tyrothricin (ti″ro-thri′sin) [NF] an antibiotic substance isolated from the soil bacillus *Bacillus brevis*, occurring as a white, grayish white, or brownish white powder, consisting principally of two polypeptides: gramicidin and tyrocidine. It is used as a topical antibacterial.

Tyrothrix (ti′ro-thriks) [*tyro-* + Gr. *thrix* hair] a genus name once given to certain microorganisms later included in the genera *Lactobacillus, Bacillus,* or *Clostridium*.

tyrotoxicon (ti″ro-tok′sĭ-kon) chemical name: benzenediazonium hydroxide. A poisonous crystalline compound, C_6H_5N-(:N)OH, sometimes occurring in stale milk, cheese, and ice cream.

tyrotoxicosis (ti″ro-tok″sĭ-ko′sis) a morbid condition resulting from ingestion of tyrotoxicon; marked by vertigo, headache, vomiting, chills, muscular cramps, purging, prostration, and death. Called also *cheese poisoning*.

tyrotoxism (ti″ro-toks′izm) poisoning resulting from ingestion of contaminated cheese; see *tyrotoxicosis*.

Tyrrell's fascia, hook (tir′elz) [Frederick *Tyrrell*, English anatomist, 1793–1843] see *septum rectovesicale*, and see under *hook*.

Tyson's crypts, glands (ti′sunz) [Edward *Tyson*, English physician and anatomist, 1650–1708] glandulae preputiales.

tysonian (ti-so′ne-an) named for Edward *Tyson*.

tysonitis (ti″son-i′tis) inflammation of Tyson's glands.

tyvelose (ti′vel-ōs) an unusual sugar found to be a polysaccharide somatic antigen of *Salmonella* species.

Tyzine (ti′zēn) trademark for preparations of tetrahydrozoline hydrochloride.

Tyzzeria (ti-ze′re-ah) a genus of coccidia the oocysts of which contain eight naked sporozoites. *T. pernicio′sa* is highly pathogenic in the domestic duck, being parasitic in the small intestine.

TZ tuberculin zymoplastiche; see under *tuberculin*.

Tzanck cell, test (tsank) [Arnault *Tzanck*, Russian dermatologist in Paris, 1886–1954] see under *cell* and *tests*.

tzetze (set′se) tsetse. **Metrazol shock t.,** see under *therapy*.

U

U chemical symbol for *uranium*.

U. unit.

²³⁵U an isotope of uranium of mass number 235.

uarthritis (u″ar-thri′tis) gout due to excess of uric acid in the system.

uberous (u′ber-us) prolific.

uberty (u′ber-te) [L. *ubertas* fruitfulness] fertility.

ubiquinol (u-bik′wĭ-nol) the form of ubiquinone when reduced by two electrons.

ubiquinone (u-bik′wĭ-nōn) coenzyme Q.

udder (ud′er) the mammary organ of cattle and certain other mammals; within the large baglike envelope are two or more glands, each having a teat.

UDP uridine diphosphate.

UDPG uridine diphosphoglucose.

UDP-galactose uridine diphosphogalactose.

UDP-glucose uridine diphosphoglucose.

UDP-glucuronate uridine diphosphoglucuronate.

Udránszky's test (oo-dran′skēz) [László *Udránszky*, Budapest physiologist, 1862–1914] see under *tests*.

udruj (ud′ruj) an East Indian medicinal gum.

UFA unesterified fatty acids.

Uffelmann's test (reagent) (oof′el-mahnz) [Jules *Uffelmann*, German physician, 1837–1894] see under *tests*.

Uhlenhuth's test (oo′len-hootz) [Paul Theodore *Uhlenhuth*, German bacteriologist, 1870–1957] serum test.

Uhthoff's sign (oot′hofs) [Wilhelm *Uhthoff*, ophthalmologist in Breslau, 1853–1927] see under *sign*.

uixi (wik′se) the *Myristica platysperma*, a medicinal plant of South America.

Ulacort (u′lah-kort) trademark for preparations of prednisolone.

ulaganactesis (u-lag″an-ak-te′sis) [Gr. *oulon* gum + *anganaktēsis* irritation] irritation or itching of the gums.

ulalgia (u-lal′je-ah) [Gr. *oulon* gum + *algos* pain + *-ia*] gingivalgia.

ulatrophia (u″lah-tro′fe-ah) ulatrophy.

ulatrophy (u-lat′ro-fe) [Gr. *oulon* gum + *atrophy*] shrinkage of the gums; gum recession; a form of pericementoclasia marked by a decrease in the bulk of the marginal and cemental gingiva with exposure of the cementum. **afunctional u.,** ulatrophy due to congenital malocclusion. **atrophic u.,** ischemic u. **calcic u.,** ulatrophy that is caused by the presence of salivary concretions. **ischemic u.,** ulatrophy due to atrophy of the gum from deficient vascular nourishment. **traumatic u.,** ulatrophy due to excessive strain, as from nail biting, etc.

ulcer (ul′ser) [L. *ulcus*; Gr. *helkōsis*] a local defect, or excavation, of the surface of an organ or tissue, which is produced by the sloughing of inflammatory necrotic tissue. **Aden u.,** a form of cutaneous leishmaniasis. **Allingham's u.,** fissure in ano. **amebic u.,** the ulcerous lesion of amebiasis cutis. **amputating u.,** ulceration which encircles a part and destroys the tissues to the bone. **anastomotic u.,** ulcer at the anastomotic site occurring as a complication after gastroenterostomy performed for duodenal ulcer. **Annam u., annamite u.,** an obstinate endemic sore of Indochina, probably cutaneous leishmaniasis; called also *Cochin-China u.* **annular u.,** ring u. **aphthous u.,** the ulcerative lesion of aphthous stomatitis. **atheromatous u.,** a loss of intima over an atheroma, often giving rise to thrombus formation and/or emboli. **atonic u.,** a chronic ulcer with unhealthy granulations. **Barrett's u.,** chronic peptic ulcer of the esophagus, usually associated with heterotopic gastric mucosa and stricture formation; it is usually a late complication of peptic esophagitis. **Bouveret's u.,** an ulcer occurring in typhoid fever in the fauces just above and to the outer side of the tonsil.

Buruli u. [named for the *Buruli* district of Uganda], necrotizing ulcer of the skin and subcutaneous tissue affecting especially the extremities, caused by *Mycobacterium ulcerans;* it occurs in Australia, Africa, and Mexico. Called also *mycobacterial u.* **catarrhal corneal u.,** an ulcer near the corneal limbus occurring in catarrhal conjunctivitis. **chancroidal u.,** chancroid. **chicle u., chiclero u.,** an endemic, zoonotic forest disease, a form of cutaneous leishmaniasis of the New World, found chiefly in Central America and Yucatan, affecting forest workers, e.g., chicle workers, and caused by *Leishmania mexicana*, transmitted by *Lutzomyia flaviscutellala*. It is characterized by a pruriginous papule that ulcerates after one or two months and usually heals within six months, with the exception of ulcers on the pinna of the ear, which may last many years and destroy the cartilage. Called also *Mexican cutaneous leishmaniasis*. **chrome u.,** an ulcer produced by chromium or its salts; seen in tanners and others working in chromium. **Cochin-China u.,** annamite u. **concealed u.,** destructive inflammation affecting some internal tissue. **corrosive u.,** gangrenous stomatitis. **Crombie's u.,** ulcer of the gum in sprue. **Cruveilhier's u.,** simple gastric ulcer. **Curling's u.,** acute ulceration of the stomach or duodenum following a severe burn upon the surface of the body. **Cushing's u.,** a peptic ulcer associated with manifest or occult lesions of the central nervous system. **Cushing-Rokitansky u.,** Rokitansky-Cushing u. **cystoscopic u.,** ulcer of the bladder due to injury by the cystoscope. **decubital u., decubitus u.,** an ulceration caused by prolonged pressure in a patient allowed to lie too still in bed for a long period of time; called also *decubitus, bed sore,* and *pressure sore.* **dendriform u., dendritic u.,** ulcer of the cornea branching in various directions, usually caused by herpes simplex infection. **dental u.,** a lesion on the oral mucosa, resulting from trauma inflicted by the teeth, as by biting, or from irritation by a sharp or broken tooth. **diabetic u.,** an ulcer, usually of the lower extremities, associated with diabetes mellitus. **diphtheritic u.,** one the surface of which is partly or entirely covered by a dirty grayish membrane; it is sometimes, but not always, produced by diphtheria of the skin. **duodenal u.,** a peptic ulcer situated in the duodenum. **elusive u.,** Hunner's u. **endemic u.,** any form of ulcer prevailing in special districts or regions, as those of cutaneous leishmaniasis. **Fenwick-Hunner u.,** Hunner's u. **fistulous u.,** the ulcerated superficial end of a fistula. **flask u.,** an ulcer of the intestine in amebic dysentery. **follicular u.,** a small ulcer on the mucous membrane having its origin in a lymph follicle. **Gaboon u.,** a variety of cutaneous leishmaniasis occurring in the Republic of Congo, Africa. **gastric u.,** an ulcer of the gastric mucosa. **giant peptic u's,** very large, uncommon, peptic ulcers with characteristic clinical and radiological manifestations. **girdle u.,** a tuberculous ulcer that spreads along the wall of the intestine in an encircling manner. **gouty u.,** a superficial ulcer occurring over a gouty joint. **gummatous u.,** a broken-down superficial gumma. **gwaliar u.,** cutaneous leishmaniasis. **Hunner's u.,** a lesion occurring in chronic interstitial cystitis, involving all the layers of the bladder wall, and appearing as a small brownish red patch on the mucosa; it tends to heal superficially and is notoriously difficult to detect. **hypopyon u.,** a corneal ulcer accompanied by hypopyon. **Jacob's u.,** rodent ulcer, especially that of an eyelid. **Jeddah u.,** cutaneous leishmaniasis. **jejunal u.,** an ulcer of the jejunum; such an ulcer developing after gastroenterostomy is called *secondary jejunal u.* **kissing u's,** ulcers on directly opposing surfaces of the stomach, as on opposite sides of the lesser curvature. **Kocher's dilatation u.,** ulceration occurring in a greatly distended intestine or in the course of ileus. **Lahore u.,** tropical u. **Lipschütz u.,** ulcus vulvae acutum. **lupoid u.,** a skin ulcer that simulates or resembles lupus. **Malabar u.,** tropical u., def. 1. **Mann-Williamson u.,** progressive peptic ulcer produced in experimental animals by the performance of gastric resection or gastroenterostomy. **marginal u.,** a gastric ulcer in the jejunal mucosa near the site of a gastrojejunal anastomosis; called also *stoma u.* **Marjolin's u.,** an ulcer seated upon an old cicatrix; it may degenerate into a squamous cell carcinoma with a propensity for metastasis. **Meleney's u's,** deep, undermining, extremely painful, spreading ulcers associated with wounds, caused by microaerophilic nonhemolytic streptococci; they have an outer, bright red zone, a middle, dusky purple zone, and a central gangrenous zone. **Mooren's u.,** chronic serpiginous ulceration, usually bilateral, of the marginal cornea, seen in elderly individuals; it is of unknown etiology. **Mozambique u.,** an endemic ulcer of East Africa, apparently a form of cutaneous leishmaniasis. **mycobacterial u.,** Buruli u. **mycotic u.,** a noduloulcerative lesion due to a fungal infection. **neurogenic u., neurotrophic u.,** an ulcer caused by nervous disease or by psychic factors. **Parrot's u.,** the ulceration seen in thrush. **Pendinski u.,** cutaneous leishmaniasis. **penetrating u.,** an ulcerative lesion which involves also the wall or substance of an adjacent organ. **Penjdeh u.,** cutaneous leishmaniasis. **peptic u.,** an ulceration of the mucous membrane of the esophagus, stomach, or duodenum, caused by the action of the acid gastric juice. **perambulating u.,** phagedenic u. **perforating u.,** an ulcer which involves the entire thickness of an organ, as the foot, or the wall of the stomach or intestine, creating an opening on both surfaces. **Persian u.,** cutaneous leishmaniasis. **phagedenic u.,** one which spreads rapidly and destructively, eating away the tissues, and marked by sloughing particles in the discharge; called also *perambulating u.* and *sloughing u.* **Plaut's u.,** necrotizing ulcerative gingivitis. **pneumococcus u.,** ulcus serpens corneae. **pudendal u.,** granuloma inguinale. **ring u.,** fusion of foci of ulceration in the cornea to form a peripheral ring of ulceration. **rodent u.,** ulcerating basal cell carcinoma of the skin. **Rokitansky-Cushing u's,** an occasional ulcerative accompaniment of severe lesions of the central nervous system, affecting the lower third of the esophagus, the fundus of the stomach, or the duodenum. **round u.,** a peptic ulcer of the stomach. **Saemisch's u.,** ulcus serpens corneae. **scorbutic u.,** one due to scurvy. **sea anemone u.,** an intestinal ulcer in amebiasis, with a deep crater and partly necrotic undermined edges which are raised above the level of the surrounding mucosa. **secondary jejunal u.,** see *jejunal u.* **serpiginous corneal u.,** ulcus serpens corneae. **simple u.,** a mild form of ulcer which is neither of septic origin nor the expression of a general disease. **sloughing u.,** phagedenic u. **soft u.,** chancroid. **stasis u.,** ulceration on the ankle due to venous stasis or insufficiency. **stercoraceous u.,** stercoral u. **stercoral u.,** an ulcer caused by the pressure of impacted feces; also a fistulous ulcer through which fecal matter escapes. **stoma u., stomal u.,** marginal u. **stress u.,** peptic ulcer, usually gastric, resulting from stress; possible predisposing factors include changes in the microcirculation of the gastric mucosa, increased permeability of the gastric mucosa barrier to H^+, and impaired cell proliferation. **sublingual u.,** an ulcer on the frenum of the tongue, caused by irritation of the lower incisor teeth; also, an ulcer on the ventral surface of the tongue or floor of the mouth. **submucous u.,** Hunner's u.; so called because of the tendency of the lesion to heal superficially. **symptomatic u.,** an ulcer that indicates some general disease. **Syriac u.,** diphtheria. **Syrian u.,** 1. diphtheria. 2. Aleppo boil, or cutaneous leishmaniasis. **tanner's u.,** chrome u. **Tashkent u.,** one of the crusted ulcers that are developed in sartian disease, an endemic affection occurring in Tashkent, a city in the southwestern part of the Siberia. **traumatic u.,** one due to a local injury. **trophic u.,** an ulcer due to imperfect nutrition of the part. **trophoneurotic u.,** ulcer due to denervation. **tropical u.,** a chronic sloughing ulcer, usually on the lower extremities, of unknown causation, occurring in tropical regions. Spirochetes and fusiform bacilli are often present in the developing lesion. Protein and vitamin deficiency, with lowered resistance, may be important in the etiology. Called also *ulcus tropicum, Malabar ulcer, Cochin sore,* and *Naga sore.* Many other terms of only geographical significance have been applied to tropical ulcer. **Turkestan u.,** sartian disease; probably cutaneous leishmaniasis. **varicose u.,** one that is due to varicose veins, as a stasis ulcer. **venereal u.,** a disease marked by the formation of ulcers about the vulvae of women who have not been exposed to veneral disease; the ulcers resemble chancre or chancroid. **Yemen u.,** cutaneous leishmaniasis. **Zambesi u.,** an ulcer endemic among laborers of the Zambesi valley; it occurs on the leg or foot and is not attended with constitutional symptoms. It is caused by the larva of a dipterous fly which burrows into the subcutaneous tissue.

ulcera (ul'ser-ah) [L.] plural of *ulcus.*

ulcerate (ul'sĕ-rāt) [L. *ulcerare, ulceratus*] to become affected with ulceration.

ulceration (ul″sĕ-ra'shun) [L. *ulceratio*] 1. the formation or development of an ulcer. 2. an ulcer. **u. of Daguet,** ulceration of the uvula and other parts of the throat, seen in typhoid fever.

ulcerative (ul'ser-a″tiv) pertaining to or characterized by ulceration.

ulcerogangrenous (ul″ser-o-gang'grĕ-nus) characterized by both ulceration and gangrene; pertaining to a gangrenous ulcer.

ulcerogenic (ul″ser-o-jen'ik) causing ulceration; leading to the production of ulcers.

ulcerogranuloma (ul″ser-o-gran″u-lo'mah) a granuloma developing on an ulcer.

ulceromembranous (ul″ser-o-mem'brah-nus) characterized by ulceration and by a membranous exudation.

ulcerous (ul'ser-us) [L. *ulcerosus*] 1. of the nature of an ulcer. 2. affected with ulceration.

ulcus (ul'kus), pl. *ul'cera* [L.] ulcer. **u. am'bulans,** phagedenic ulcer. **u. cancro'sum,** rodent ulcer. **u. ex'edens,** rodent ulcer. **u. interdigita'le,** keratolysis of the horny layer of the skin between the toes, a disease similar to cracked heel. **u. mol'le, u. mol'le cu'tis** (obs.), chancroid. **u. pen'etrans,** one that penetrates not into the peritoneal cavity but into an abutting organ. **u. ro'dens,** rodent ulcer. **u. scorbu'ticum** (obs.), scorbutic ulcer. **u. ser'pens cor'neae,** an ulcer of the cornea; a creeping central suppurative ulcer of the cornea due usually to pneumococcus. Called also *pneumococcus ulcer.* **u. sim'plex vesi'cae,** Hunner's ulcer. **u. tro'picum,** tropical ulcer, def. 1. **u. ventric'uli,** gastric ulcer. **u. vul'vae acu'tum,** a nonvenereal rapidly growing lesion of the vulva. The etiology is uncertain, but *Bacillus crassus,* a normally nonpathogenic species sometimes found in vaginal cultures, has been implicated. Called also *Lipschütz disease* or *ulcer.*

uldazepam (ul-da'zah-pam) chemical name: 7-chloro-5-(2-chlorophenyl)-*N*-(2-propenyloxy)-3*H*-1,4-benzodiazepam-2-amine; a tranquilizer, $C_{18}H_{15}Cl_2N_3O.$

ule- see *ulo-.*

ulectomy (u-lek'to-me) 1. [Gr. *oulē* scar + Gr. *ektomē* excision] excision of scar tissue, i.e., in secondary iridectomy. 2. [Gr. *oulon* gum + *ektomē* excision] excision of the gingiva; gingivectomy.

ulegyria (u″le-ji're-ah) [Gr. *oulē* scar + *gyrus* + *-ia*] a condition in which the cerebral gyri are narrow and distorted by scars, resulting from lesions existing in fetal life or early infancy.

ulemorrhagia (u″lem-o-ra'je-ah) [Gr. *oulon* gum + *rhegnynai* to burst forth] bleeding or hemorrhage from the gingiva.

ulerythema (u″ler-ĭ-the'mah) [Gr. *oulē* scar + *erythēma* redness] an erythematous disease of the skin characterized by the formation of cicatrices and by atrophy. **u. ophryo'genes,** keratosis pilaris affecting the follicles of the eyebrow hairs of young men, associated with erythema, and leading to scarring and atrophy; it is transmitted as an autosomal dominant trait.

Ulex europaeus L. (Leguminosae) (u'leks u-ro'pe-us) a leguminous shrub, common gorse or furze, which is a source of cytisine (ulexine).

ulexine (u-leks'ēn) cytisine.

uliginous (u-lij'ĭ-nus) [L. *uliginosus* moist] muddy or slimy.

ulitis (u-li'tis) [Gr. *oulon* gum + *-itis*] inflammation of the gums; gingivitis. **aphthous u.,** ulitis combined with aphthae. **fungus u.,** ulitis due to presence of a fungus. **interstitial u.,** inflammation of the connective tissue of the gums around the teeth. **mercurial u.,** ulitis due to mercurialism. **scorbutic u.,** ulitis due to scurvy. **ulcerative u.,** ulitis with ulceration.

ullem (ul'em) a kind of dyspepsia occurring in Lapland.

Ullmann's line (ul'manz) [Emerich *Ullmann,* Hungarian surgeon, 1861–1937] see under *line.*

Ulmus (ul'mus) [L. "elm"] a genus of ulmaceous trees; the elms. **U. ful'va Michx.,** the slippery elm, the inner bark of which is mucilaginous and demulcent.

ulna (ul'nah), pl. *ul'nae* [L. "the arm"] [NA] the inner and larger bone of the forearm, on the side opposite that of the thumb; it articulates with the humerus and with the head of the radius at its proximal end; with the radius and bones of the carpus at the distal end. See Plate XLIV.

ulnad (ul'nad) toward the ulna.

ulnar (ul'nar) [L. *ulnaris*] pertaining to the ulna or to the ulnar (medial) aspect of the arm as compared to the radial (lateral) aspect.

ulnare (ul-na're) [L.] os triquetrum.

ulnaris (ul-na'ris) ulnar; in official anatomical nomenclature, designating relationship to the ulna.

ulnen (ul'nen) pertaining to the ulna alone.

ulnocarpal (ul″no-kar'pal) pertaining to the ulna and carpus.

ulnoradial (ul″no-ra'de-al) pertaining to the ulna and radius.

ULO trademark for a preparation of chlophedianol hydrochloride.

ulo- 1. [Gr. *oulē* scar] a combining form denoting relationship to a scar, or cicatrix. 2. [Gr. *oulon* gum] a combining form denoting relationship to the gingivae.

ulocace (u-lok'ah-se) [*ulo-*(2) + Gr. *kakē* badness] ulceration of the gingivae.

ulocarcinoma (u″lo-kar″sĭ-no'mah) [*ulo-*(2) + *carcinoma*] carcinoma of the gums.

uloglossitis (u″lo-glos-si'tis) [*ulo-*(2) + Gr. *glōssa* tongue + *-itis*] inflammation of the gums and the tongue.

uloncus (u-long'kus) [*ulo-*(2) + Gr. *onkos* mass, tumor] a swelling or tumor of the gums.

ulorrhagia (u″lo-ra′je-ah) [*ulo*-(2) + Gr. *rhēgnynai* to burst forth] a sudden or free discharge of blood from the gums.

ulorrhea (u″lo-re′ah) [*ulo*-(2) + Gr. *rhoia* flow] an oozing of blood from the gums.

ulotomy (u-lot′o-me) 1. [Gr. *oulē* scar + *tomē* a cutting] the cutting or division of scar tissue. 2. [Gr. *oulon* gum + *tomē* a cutting] incision of the gingivae.

ulotripsis (u″lo-trip′sis) [*ulo*-(2) + Gr. *tripsis* rubbing] gum revitalization by massage.

ultimate (ul′tĭ-māt) [L. *ultimus* last] the last or farthest; final or most remote.

ultimisternal (ul″tĭ-mĭ-ster′nal) pertaining to the xiphoid process.

ultimum moriens (ul′tĭ-mum mo′re-enz) [L. "last to die"] 1. the right atrium; said to be the last part of the body to cease moving in death. 2. the upper part of the trapezius muscle.

ult. praes. abbreviation for L. *ul′timum praescriptus*, last prescribed.

ultra- [L. "beyond"] a prefix denoting excess, or beyond.

ultrabrachycephalic (ul″trah-brak″e-sĕ-fal′ik) having a cephalic index of more than 90.

ultracentrifugation (ul″trah-sen-trif″u-ga′shun) subjection to the action of an ultracentrifuge.

ultracentrifuge (ul″trah-sen′trĭ-fūj) a centrifuge with an exceedingly high rate of rotation which will separate and sediment the molecules of a substance.

ultradian (ul-tra′de-an) [*ultra*- +L. *dies* day] pertaining to a period of less than 24 hours; applied to the rhythmic repetition of certain phenomena in living organisms occurring in cycles of less than a day (*ultradian rhythm*). Cf. *circadian* and *infradian.*

ultradolichocephalic (ul″trah-dol″ĭ-ko-sĕ-fal′ik) extremely dolichocephalic; having a cephalic index of not more than 64.

ultrafilter (ul″trah-fil′ter) an apparatus for performing ultrafiltration; a semipermeable membrane.

ultrafiltrate (ul″trah-fil′trāt) the liquid that has passed through an ultrafilter.

ultrafiltration (ul″trah-fil-tra′shun) filtration through filters with minute pores, thus allowing the separation of extremely minute particles. Ultrafiltration occurs naturally, as in the filtration of plasma at the capillary membrane, and it is performed in the laboratory, especially to separate a substance in colloidal solution from its dispersion medium, and usually under pressure in order to accelerate the process.

ultragaseous (ul″trah-gas′e-us) having the properties of gas at one millionth of atmospheric pressure; see *radiant matter,* under *matter.*

ultramicrochemistry (ul″trah-mi″kro-kem′is-tre) the chemical study of materials in extremely minute quantities.

ultramicron (ul″trah-mi′kron) an individual element of the dispersed phase of a colloid.

ultramicropipet (ul″trah-mi″kro-pi-pet′) a pipet designed to handle extremely small quantities of liquid (0.002 to 0.005 ml.).

ultramicroscope (ul″trah-mi′kro-skōp) a special darkfield microscope for the examination of particles of colloidal size. See *darkfield illumination,* under *illumination,* and *darkfield microscope,* under *microscope.*

ultramicroscopic (ul″trah-mi″kro-skop′ik) 1. pertaining to the ultramicroscope. 2. too small to be seen with an ordinary microscope.

ultramicroscopy (ul″trah-mi-kros′ko-pe) the employment of the ultramicroscope.

ultramicrotome (ul″trah-mi′kro-tōm) an instrument for making very thin tissue sections for electron microscopy.

Ultran (ul′tran) trademark for preparations of phenaglycodol.

ultraphagocytosis (ul″trah-fag″o-si-to′sis) ingestion of particles of submicroscopic dimensions.

ultraprophylaxis (ul″trah-pro″fĭ-lak′sis) prophylaxis directed toward the prevention of diseased or abnormal children by regulation of the marriage of the unfit.

ultraquinine (ul″trah-kwin′in) an alkaloid from cuprea bark.

ultra-red (ul″trah-red′) infrared.

ultrasonic (ul″trah-son′ik) [*ultra*- + L. *sonus* sound] pertaining to mechanical radiant energy having a frequency beyond the upper limit of perception by the human ear, that is, beyond about 20,000 Hz (cycles per second); see *ultrasonics.*

ultrasonics (ul″trah-son′iks) that part of the science of acoustics dealing with the frequency range beyond the upper limit of perception by the human ear (beyond 20 kilocycles per second), but usually restricted to frequencies above 500 kilocycles per second. Ultrasonic radiation is injurious to tissues because of its thermal effects when absorbed by living matter, but in controlled doses it is used therapeutically to selectively break down pathologic tissues, as in treatment of arthritis and lesions of the nervous system, and also as a diagnostic aid by visually displaying echoes received from irradiated tissues, as in echocardiography and echoencephalography.

ultrasonogram (ul″trah-son′o-gram) the record obtained by ultrasonography.

ultrasonographic (ul″trah-son″o-graf′ik) pertaining to or accomplished by ultrasonography; called also *sonographic.*

ultrasonography (ul″trah-son-og′rah-fe) the visualization of deep structures of the body by recording the reflections of (echoes of) pulses of ultrasonic waves directed into the tissues. Diagnostic ultrasonography, as in echocardiography and echoencephalography, utilizes a frequency range of 1 million to 10 million hertz (cycles per second), or 1 to 10 MHz. Such sound waves are transmissible only in liquids and solids. Called also *echography* and *sonography.* **Doppler u.,** that in which measurement and a visual record are made of the shift in frequency of a continuous ultrasonic wave proportional to the blood-flow velocity in underlying vessels; used in diagnosis of extracranial occlusive vascular disease. It is also used in detection of the fetal heart beat or of the velocity of movement of a structure such as the beating heart. **gray-scale u.,** a B-scan technique in which a television video-scan converter amplifies and processes echoes according to their strength into a visual display ranging from white for the strongest echoes to varying shades of gray.

ultrasonometry (ul″trah-so-nom′ĕ-tre) the measurement of certain physical properties of biologic fluids by means of ultrasound.

ultrasound (ul′trah-sownd) mechanical radiant energy (see *sound*), with a frequency greater than 20,000 cycles per second; see *ultrasonics.*

ultrastructure (ul′trah-struk″chur) the arrangement of the smallest elements making up a body; the structure beyond the resolution power of the light microscope, i.e., the structure visible only under the ultramicroscope and electron microscope. Called also *fine structure.*

ultratoxon (ul″trah-tok′son) a toxon of the lowest degree of toxicity.

ultraviolet (ul″trah-vi′o-let) beyond the violet end of the spectrum; said of electromagnetic rays or radiation between the violet rays and the roentgen rays, that is, with wavelengths between 4 and 400 nm. These rays have powerful actinic and chemical properties, inducing sunburn and tanning of the skin and producing ergocalciferol (vitamin D₂) by their action or ergosterol in the skin. **far u.,** ultraviolet radiation of shortest wavelength, between 200 and 300 nm. **near u.,** that portion of the ultraviolet near the visible spectrum, that is, with wavelengths between 300 and 400 nm.

ultravirus (ul″trah-vi′rus) (*obs.*) an extremely small pathogenic agent; see *filterable virus,* under *virus.*

ultravisible (ul″trah-viz′ĭ-b′l) ultramicroscopic.

ultromotivity (ul″tro-mo-tiv′ĭ-te) ability to move spontaneously.

Ultzmann's test (ooltz′mahnz) [Robert *Ultzmann,* German urologist, 1842–1889] see under *tests.*

ululation (ul″u-la′shun) [L. *ululare* to howl] the loud crying or wailing of hysterical patients.

umbauzonen (um″bou-zo′nen) [Ger., "rebuilding zones"] Looser's transformation zones; see under *zone.*

umbelliferone (um″bel-lif′er-ōn) 7-hydroxycoumarin, a substance present in many plants, particularly those of the Umbelliferae family; used to absorb ultraviolet rays in sunscreen creams and lotions.

umber (um′ber) a natural earth containing chiefly manganese, iron oxide, and silica; used as a pigment.

Umber's test (um′berz) [Friedrich *Umber,* German physician, 1871–1946] see under *tests.*

umbilectomy (um″bĭ-lek′to-me) [*umbilicus* + Gr. *ektomē* exicision] excision of the umbilicus.

umbilical (um-bil′ĭ-kal) [L. *umbilicalis*] pertaining to the umbilicus.

umbilicate (um-bil′ĭ-kāt) [L. *umbilicatus*] shaped like or resembling the umbilicus.

umbilicated (um-bil′ĭ-kāt″ed) marked by depressed areas resembling the umbilicus.

umbilication (um″bil-ĭ-ka′shun) a pit or depression resembling the umbilicus.

umbilicus (um-bil′ĭ-kus, um″bĭ-li′kus) [L.] [NA] the navel: the cicatrix marking the site of attachment of the umbilical cord in the fetus. **amniotic u.,** the oval aperture formed by converging amnion folds. **decidual u.,** a small cicatricial mark over the human blastocyst shortly after its migration through the uterine epithelium into the stroma, marking the place of the closure of the decidua capsularis. **posterior u.,** pilonidal sinus.

umbo (um′bo), pl. *umbo′nes* [L. "a boss"] a round projection; the projecting center of any rounded surface. **u. membra′nae tym′pani** [NA], **u. of tympanic membrane,** the slight projection at the center of the outer surface of the tympanic membrane, corresponding to the point of attachment of the tip of the manubrium of the malleus.

umbonate (um′bo-nāt) [L. *umbo* a knob] knoblike; button-like; having a button-like, raised center.

umbrascopy (um-bras′ko-pe) [L. *umbra* shade + Gr. *skopein* to examine] skiascopy.

UMP uridine monophosphate.

unazotized (un-a′zo-tīzd) containing no nitrogen.

unbalance (un-bal′ans) lack or loss of normal balance.

uncal (ung′kal) of or pertaining to the uncus.

Uncaria (un-ka′re-ah) [L.] a genus of rubiaceous shrubs native to Asia. **U. gam′bier, U. gam′bir** [Hunter] Roxb., Rubiaceae, a species of southeastern Asia, which is the source of gambir and catechin.

uncarthrosis (unk″ar-thro′sis) bone disease involving the uncinate processes of vertebrae.

uncia (un′se-ah) [L.] 1. ounce. 2. inch.

unciform (un′sĭ-form) [L. *uncus* hook + *forma* form] shaped like a hook, as the unciform bone.

unciforme (un″sĭ-for′me) [L.] hooked; see *os hamatum.*

uncinal (un′sĭ-nal) uncinate.

Uncinaria (un″sĭ-na′re-ah) [L. *uncus* hook] a genus of nematode worms of the family Ancylostomidae. **U. america′na,** *Necator americanus.* **U. duodena′lis,** *Ancylostoma duodenale.* **U. stenoceph′ala,** a hookworm commonly causing hookworm disease in dogs; also parasitic in foxes, cats, and other carnivores.

uncinariasis (un″sin-ah-ri′ah-sis) the state of being infected with worms of the genus *Uncinaria.* See *hookworm disease,* under *disease.*

uncinariatic (un″sĭ-na″re-at′ik) pertaining to or exhibiting uncinariasis (hookworm disease).

uncinate (un′sĭ-nāt) 1. hooked or barbed, as the uncinate bone. 2. relating to or affecting the uncinate gyrus, as in uncinate epilepsy.

uncinatum (un″sĭ-na′tum) [L.] hooked; see *os hamatum.*

uncipressure (un′sĭ-presh″ur) [L. *uncus* hook + *pressura* pressure] pressure with a hook to control hemorrhage.

uncomplemented (un-kom′ple-ment″ed) not joined with complement, and therefore not active.

unconscious (un-kon′shus) 1. insensible; incapable of responding to sensory stimuli and of having subjective experiences. 2. in freudian terminology, that part of mental activity which includes primitive or repressed wishes. Since these are concealed from consciousness by the psychic censor, the subject cannot know of them unless they are revealed to him through some psychotherapeutic procedure or as a result of severe emotional strain. Cf. *dissociation.* **collective u.,** in jungian psychology, the elements of the unconscious that are theoretically common to all mankind.

unco-ossified (un″ko-os′ĭ-fīd) not united into one bone.

uncotomy (ung-kot′o-me) [*uncus* + Gr. *tomē* a cutting] the production of a circumscribed lesion in the uncus in the treatment of psychotic states.

uncovertebral (un″ko-ver′tĕ-bral) pertaining to or affecting the uncinate processes of a vertebra.

unction (ungk′shun) [L. *unctio*] 1. an ointment. 2. the application of an ointment or salve; inunction.

unctuous (ungk′chu-us) greasy or oily; oleaginous.

uncus (ung′kus) [L. "hook"] [NA] the medially curved anterior end of the parahippocampal gyrus; called also *u. gyri fornicati. u. gyri hippocampi,* and *u. gyri parahippocampalis.* **u. of hamate bone,** hamulus ossis hamati.

undecane (un′de-kān) a colorless petroleum hydrocarbon, CH_3-$(CH_2)_9CH_3$.

undercut (un′der-kut) 1. that portion of a tooth which lies between the survey line (height of contour) and the gingivae. 2. the contour of a cross-section of a residual ridge or dental arch which would prevent the insertion of a denture. 3. the contour of flasking stone which interlocks in such a way as to prevent the separation of the parts.

underhorn (un′der-horn) cornu inferius ventriculi lateralis.

undernutrition (un″der-nu-trish′un) improper nutrition due to inadequate food supply or to failure to ingest, assimilate, or utilize any or all of the necessary food elements.

understain (un″der-stān) to stain less deeply than usual.

undertoe (un′der-to) a condition in which the great toe is displaced under the others.

Underwood's disease (un′der-woodz) [Michael *Underwood,* London obstetrician and pediatrician, 1737–1820] sclerema.

undifferentiation (un″dif-er-en″she-a′shun) absence of normal differentiation; anaplasia.

undine (un′dīn) a small glass flask for irrigating the eye.

undinism (un′din-izm) [*Undine* a water nymph, from L. *unda* wave] the association of sexual ideas with water, including urine and urination.

undulant (un′du-lant) [L. *unda* wave] characterized by wavelike fluctuations; see also under *fever.*

undulation (un″du-la′shun) [L. *undulatio*] a wavelike motion

in any medium; a vibration. **jugular u.,** venous pulse. **respiratory u.,** the variation of the blood pressure curve due to respiration.

ung. abbreviation for L. *unguen′tum,* ointment.

ungual (ung′gwal) [L. *unguis* nail] pertaining to the nails.

unguent (ung′gwent) [L. *unguentum*] an ointment, salve, or cerate.

unguentum (ung-gwen′tum) [L.] ointment. **u. ac′idi bo′rici,** boric acid ointment. **u. ac′idi undecylen′ici compos′itum,** compound undecylenic acid ointment. **u. aeth′ylis aminobenzoa′tis,** benzocaine ointment. **u. al′bum,** white ointment. **u. a′quae ro′sae,** rose water ointment. **u. a′quae ro′sae petrola′tum,** petrolatum rose water ointment. **u. belladon′nae,** belladonna ointment. **u. calami′nae,** calamine ointment. **u. epinephri′nae bitartra′tis ophthal′micum,** epinephrine bitartrate ophthalmic ointment. **u. fla′vum,** yellow ointment. **u. glycol′is polyethyle′ni,** polyethylene glycol ointment. **u. hydrar′gyri biochlo′ridi,** mercury bichloride ointment. **u. hydrar′gyri chlori′di mi′tis,** calomel ointment. **u. hydrar′gyri mi′te,** mild mercurial ointment. **u. hydrar′gyri ox′idi fla′vi,** yellow mercuric oxide ophthalmic ointment. **u. hydrophil′icum,** hydrophilic ointment. **u. ichthammol′lis,** ichthammol ointment. **u. menthol′is compos′itum,** compound menthol ointment. **u. nitrofurazo′ni,** nitrofurazone ointment. **u. pi′cis carbo′nis,** coal tar ointment. **u. pi′cis pi′ni,** pine tar ointment. **u. resorcinol′is compos′itum,** compound resorcinol ointment. **u. sulfacetami′di so′dici,** sodium sulfacetamide ointment. **u. sulfu′ris,** sulfur ointment. **u. zin′ci ox′idi,** zinc oxide ointment.

unguiculate (ung-gwik′u-lāt) provided with claws or nails; resembling a claw.

unguiculus (ung-gwik′u-lus) [L., dim. of *unguis*] a small nail or claw.

unguis (ung′gwis), pl. *un′gues* [L.] 1. [NA] the horny cutaneous plate on the dorsal surface of the distal end of the terminal phalanx of a finger or toe, made up of flattened epithelial scales developed from the stratum lucidum of the skin. Called also *nail* (q.v.). 2. a collection of pus in the cornea; an onyx. 3. a nail-like part or structure. **u. incarna′tus,** ingrown nail; see under *nail.* **u. ventric′uli latera′lis cer′ebri,** calcar avis.

ungula (ung′gu-lah) [L. "hoof," "claw," "talon"] the hoof of an animal.

ungulate (ung′gu-lāt) [L. *ungula* hoof] a hoofed mammal.

unguligrade (ung′gu-lĭ-grād″) [L. *ungula* hoof + *gradi* to walk] walking or running on the tips of one or two digits of each limb, a characteristic of certain quadrupeds known as ungulates.

uni- [L. *unus* one] a prefix meaning *one.*

uniarticular (u″ne-ar-tik′u-lar) [*uni-* + L. *articulus* joint] pertaining to a single joint.

uniaural (u″ne-aw′ral) monaural.

uniaxial (u″ne-ak′se-al) [*uni-* + L. *axis* axis] 1. having but one axis. 2. developing in an axial direction only, as, *uniaxial* organism.

unibasal (u″nĭ-ba′sal) [*uni-* + L. *basis* base] having only one base.

unicameral (u″nĭ-kam′er-al) [*uni-* + L. *camera* chamber] having only one cavity or compartment.

unicellular (u″nĭ-sel′u-lar) [*uni-* + L. *cellula* cell] made up of but a single cell, as the bacteria.

unicentral (u″nĭ-sen′tral) [*uni-* + L. *centrum* center] pertaining to or having a single center.

unicentric (u″nĭ-sen′trik) unicentral.

uniceps (u″nĭ-seps) [*uni-* + L. *caput* head] having one head or origin; said of a muscle.

uniceptor (u′nĭ-sep″tor) a ceptor with a single combining group; see *Ehrlich's side-chain theory,* under *theory.*

unicism (u′nĭ-sizm) [L. *unicus* single] the obsolete opinion that there is but one kind of venereal virus.

unicornous (u″nĭ-kor′nus) [L. *unicornis*] having only one horn or cornu.

unicuspid (u″nĭ-kus′pid) a tooth with only one cusp.

unicuspidate (u″nĭ-kus′pĭ-dāt) having only one cusp.

unidirectional (u″nĭ-di-rek′shun-al) flowing in only one direction.

uniflagellate (u″nĭ-flaj′ĕ-lāt) having one flagellum.

unifocal (u″nĭ-fo′kal) arising from or pertaining to a single focus.

uniforate (u″nĭ-fo′rāt) [*uni-* + L. *foratus* pierced] having only one opening.

unigeminal (u″nĭ-jem′ĭ-nal) [*uni-* + L. *geminus* twin] pertaining to or affecting one twin of a pair.

unigerminal (u″nĭ-jer′mĭ-nal) 1. pertaining to a single germ or ovum. 2. monozygotic.

uniglandular (u″nĭ-glan′du-lar) pertaining to or affecting only one gland.

unigravida (u″nĭ-grav′ĭ-dah) primigravida.

unilaminar (u″nĭ-lam′ĭ-nar) having only one layer or lamina.

unilateral (u″nĭ-lat′er-al) [uni- + L. latus side] affecting but one side.

unilobar (u″nĭ-lo′bar) having only one lobe; consisting of a single lobe.

unilocular (u″nĭ-lok′u-lar) [uni- + L. loculus] having but one loculus or compartment.

unimodal (u″nĭ-mo′dal) having only one mode.

uninephrectomized (u-ne-nĕ-frek′to-mīzd) having one kidney removed by excision.

uninuclear (u″nĭ-nu′kle-ar) pertaining to a single nucleus; mononuclear.

uninucleated (u″nĭ-nu′kle-āt″ed) having but one nucleus; mononuclear; mononucleate.

uniocular (u″ne-ok′u-lar) [uni- + L. oculus eye] pertaining to or affecting but one eye.

union (ūn′yun) [L. unio] the process of healing; the renewal of continuity in a broken bone or between the edges of a wound. See healing. **faulty u.,** an unfaithful fracture. **primary u.,** healing by first intention. **vicious u.,** union of the ends of a fractured bone so as to produce deformity.

uniovular (u″ne-ov′u-lar) [uni- + L. ovum egg] monozygotic; monovular.

unipara (u-nip′ah-rah) primipara.

uniparental (u″nĭ-pah-ren′tal) pertaining to one of the parents only.

uniparous (u-nip′ah-rus) [uni- + L. parere to bring forth, produce] 1. producing only one ovum or offspring at one time. 2. primiparous.

Unipen (u′nĭ-pen) trademark for preparations of nafcillin sodium.

unipolar (u″nĭ-po′lar) [uni- + L. polus pole] having but a single pole or process, as a nerve cell.

unipotency (u″nĭ-po′ten-se) [L. unus one + potentia power] the ability of a part to develop in one manner only, or of a cell to develop into only one type of cell.

unipotent (u-nip′o-tent) unipotential.

unipotential (u″nĭ-po-ten′shal) [uni- + L. potens able] capable in one way only; said of cells which have had their fates determined and can give rise to cells of one order only. Cf. totipotential.

unirritable (un-ir′ĭ-tah-b′l) not irritable; not capable of being stimulated.

uniseptate (u″ne-sep′tāt) having only one septum.

unisexual (u″nĭ-seks′u-al) [uni- + L. sexus sex] of only one sex; having the sexual organs of one sex only.

unit (u′nit) [L. unus one] 1. a single thing. 2. a quantity assumed as a standard of measurement. 3. a gene. **alexinic u.,** the smallest quantity of alexinic serum required to lyse a given amount of red blood cells in the presence of an excess of hemolytic serum. **Allen-Doisy u.,** see mouse u. and rat u. **amboceptor u.,** the least quantity of amboceptor with which a definite amount of red blood cells will be lysed by an excess of complement. **American Drug Manufacturers' Association u.,** one tenth of the Steenbock unit. **Angström u.,** the unit of wavelength of electromagnetic and corpuscular radiations, equal to 10^{-7} mm. Called also angstrom u., A., or A.U. **Ansbacher u.,** a unit of vitamin K dosage. **antigen u.,** the least quantity of antigen which will fix one unit of complement so as to prevent hemolysis. **antitoxic u.,** a unit for expressing the strength of an antitoxin. The unit of diphtheria antitoxin is approximately the amount of antitoxin which will preserve the life of a guinea pig weighing 250 gm. for at least four days after it is injected subcutaneously with a mixture of 100 times the minimum lethal dose of diphtheria toxin. Practically, it is the equivalent of a standard unit preserved in Washington. The unit of tetanus antitoxin is approximately ten times the amount of tetanus antitoxin which will preserve the life of a guinea pig weighing 350 gm. for at least ninety-six hours after injection of a mixture with 100 minimum lethal doses of tetanus toxin. The U.S. Public Health Service unit for scarlet fever antitoxin neutralizes 50 skin test doses of scarlet fever toxin. Abbreviated A.E. (Ger. antitoxineinheit). **atomic mass u.,** the unit mass equal to $\frac{1}{12}$ the mass of the nuclide of carbon-12, equivalent to 1.657×10^{-24} gm.; abbreviated amu. Called also atomic weight u. and dalton. **atomic weight u.,** atomic mass u. **avena u.,** the amount of auxin which applied to one side of the tip of an oat sprout will cause a curvature of 10 degrees. **Behnken's u.,** a unit of roentgen-ray exposure, being that quantity which, when applied in 1 cc. of air at 18° C. and 760 mm. Hg of pressure, engenders sufficient electric conductivity to equal one electrostatic unit, as measured by the saturation current. **Bodansky u.,** the quantity of phosphatase in 100 ml. of serum required to liberate 1 mg. of phosphorus as phosphate ion from sodium β-glycerophosphate in 1 hour at 37° C. and under other standardized conditions.

British thermal u., the amount of heat necessary to raise the temperature of 1 pound of water from 39° F. to 40° F., abbreviated B.T.U. **cat u.,** that amount of digitalis calculated per kilogram of weight of a cat which is just sufficient to kill when slowly and continuously injected into the vein (Hatcher). **C. G. S. u.,** any unit in the centimeter-gram-second system. **Clauberg's u.,** a unit of progestin which is essentially one half of a Corner-Allen unit. **clinical u.,** a unit of estrogenic activity equal to approximately one sixth of the international unit. **Collip u.,** a unit of dosage of parathyroid extract: it is one one-hundredth of the amount required to increase by 5 mg. the quantity of calcium in 100 ml. of blood at the end of fifteen hours in a dog of 20 kg. weight. **complement u.,** the least quantity of complement which will hemolyze a definite amount of red blood cells in the presence of an amboceptor unit. **Corner-Allen u.,** a unit of progestin dosage. **coronary care u.,** a specially designed and equipped hospital area containing a small number of private rooms, with all facilities necessary for constant observation and possible emergency treatment of patients with severe heart disease. **u. of current,** see ampere. **dental u.,** 1. a single tooth. 2. a piece of dental equipment providing several services (electrical, air, gas, etc.). **digitalis u.,** any of several units once used in bioassay of digitalis preparations and named according to the animal in which it was determined, as cat unit, etc. **electromagnetic u's,** that system of units based on the fundamental definition of a unit magnetic pole as one which will repel an exactly similar pole with a force of one dyne when the poles are 1 cm. apart. **electrostatic u's,** that system of units based on the fundamental definition of a unit charge as one which will repel an equal and like charge with a force of one dyne when the two charges are 1 cm. apart in a vacuum. Abbreviated E.S.E. (Ger., elektrostatische einheit) and e.s.u. **enzyme u.,** that amount of an enzyme which will catalyze the transformation of 1 micromole of substrate (or of 1 microequivalent of the substrate group when more than one bond is attacked, as in polysaccharides) per minute under standard conditions of temperature (30° C.), optimal pH, and optimal substrate concentration. **Felton's u.,** a mouse protective unit of antipneumococcic serum; it is that quantity of antibody capable of protecting a white Swiss mouse against one million fatal doses of a standard pneumococcus culture of the corresponding type. Frequently, it is considered to be the equivalent of the National Institutes of Health control serum (P-11). **Florey u.** (obs.), Oxford u. **u. of force,** see dyne. **Hampson u.,** a unit of roentgen-ray exposure; it is one quarter of the erythema dose. **Hanson u.,** a unit of parathyroid extract, being one one-hundredth of the amount required to increase by 1 mg. the amount of calcium in the blood serum of a parathyroidectomized dog weighing 15 kg. **u. of heat,** the quantity of heat required to raise the temperature of a kilogram of water 1° C. See calorie and British thermal u. **hemolytic u.,** the amount of inactivated immune serum which, in the presence of complement, will completely hemolyze 1 ml. of a 5 per cent suspension of washed red blood cells. **hemorrhagin u.,** the amount of snake venom necessary to produce hemorrhages in the vascular network of a three-day-old chick embryo. **Holzknecht u.,** a unit of roentgen-ray exposure equal to one-fifth of the erythema dose. Abbreviated H. **intensive care u.,** a hospital unit in which are concentrated special equipment and skilled personnel for the care of seriously ill patients requiring immediate and continuous attention; abbreviated ICU. **International u.,** a unit of biological material, as of enzymes, hormones, vitamins, etc., established by the International Conference for the Unification of Formulas. **international u. of estrogenic activity,** the estrus-producing activity represented in 0.1 microgram of the international standard estrone. **international u. of gonadotrophic activity,** the specific gonadotrophic activity of 0.1 mg. of the standard material preserved at and distributed from the National Institute for Medical Research, Hampstead, London. It is derived from pregnancy urine and it is approximately the amount required to produce cornification of the vaginal epithelium of the immature rat. **international insulin u.,** one twenty-second of a milligram of the pure crystalline product now adopted as the standard. **international u. of male hormone,** the androgenic activity represented in 0.1 mg. of crystalline androsterone. **international u. of penicillin,** the specific penicillin activity contained in 0.6 microgram of the international standard sodium salt of II or G penicillin. **international u. of vitamin A,** activity equivalent to 0.6 micrograms of pure beta-carotene. **international u. of vitamin D,** the activity of 1 mg. of the international standard solution of irradiated ergosterol (1 mg. in 10 ml. of olive oil). One mg. given daily to rachitic rats for eight consecutive days should produce a wide calcium line. **Kienböck u.,** a unit of roentgen-ray exposure equal to 0.1 erythema dose; symbol X. **King u., King-Armstrong u.,** the amount of phosphatase which, when allowed to act upon an excess of disodium phenylphosphate at a pH of 9 for 30 minutes at 37.5° C., will liberate 1 mg. of phenol. **Lf u.,** that amount of diphtheria toxin or toxoid which gives the most rapid flocculation with one standard unit of diphtheria antitoxin when mixed and incubated in vitro. **light u.,** see footcandle. **Mache u.,** a German unit for expressing the concentration of radium emanation in solution; it is equivalent to 3.64 eman. Abbreviated M.u.

map u., the relative distance between loci on a chromosome as determined by the recombination frequency; called also *map distance.* **morgan u.,** see *morgan.* **motor u.,** the unit of motor activity formed by a motor nerve cell and its many innervated muscle fibers. **mouse u.,** the least amount of estrus-producing hormone (estrogen) which will cause in a spayed mouse a characteristic change in the vaginal epithelium. Abbreviated m.u. **Noon pollen u.,** the activity present in the saline extract from one millionth of a grain of pollen. **Oxford u.,** that amount of penicillin which, when dissolved in 50 ml. of meat extract broth, just inhibits completely a test strain of *Staphylococcus aureus.* **pepsin u.,** a unit for measuring the proportion of pepsin in the gastric juice. **peripheral resistance u.,** the unit of resistance to blood flow in a vessel, being the resistance encountered when the pressure gradient between two points in a vessel is 1 mm. Hg and the blood flow is 1 ml. per second. **physiologic u.,** see *micelle.* **pilosebaceous u.,** the hair follicle and the associated apocrine gland. **quantum u.,** see *Planck's constant,* under *constant.* **rat u.,** the highest dilution of an estrus-producing hormone (estrogen) which when given to a mature spayed rat in three injections at four-hour intervals during the first day will produce cornification and desquamation of the vaginal epithelium. Abbreviated R.U. **u. of resistance,** see *ohm.* **Sherman u.** (for vitamin A), see *Sherman-Munsell u. of vitamin A.* **Sherman-Bourquin u. of vitamin B₂,** that amount of riboflavin which fed daily to a standard test rat for eight weeks will give a gain of 3 gm. a week. **Sherman-Munsell u. of vitamin A,** that amount of vitamin A which when fed daily just suffices to support a rate of gain of 3 gm. per week for eight weeks in a standard rat previously depleted of vitamin A. **SI u.,** any of the units of the Système International d'Unités, or International System of Units, adopted in 1960 at the Eleventh General Conference of Weights and Measures. SI units comprise the basic units *meter* (length), *kilogram* (mass), *second* (time), *ampere* (electric current), *kelvin* (temperature [absolute]), *candela* (luminous intensity), and *mole* (amount of substance); supplementary units *radian* (plane angle) and *steradian* (solid angle); and derived units, which are stated in terms of the basic units, *newton* (force), *pascal* (pressure), *joule* (energy), *watt* (power), *volt* (electric potential), *coulomb* (electric charge), *farad* (capacitance), *ohm* (electric resistance), *siemens* (electric conductance), *weber* (magnetic flux), *tesla* (magnetic flux density), *henry* (inductance), *hertz* (frequency), and *degree Celsius* (temperature). For multiples and submultiples of these units formed by the use of prefixes, see table under *metric* and *Tables of Weights and Measures,* under *weight.* **skin test u.,** that amount of scarlet fever toxin which when injected intradermally gives a positive reaction in susceptible persons and no reaction in unsusceptible or immune persons. A positive reaction is a faint to bright red area measuring as much as 10 mm. in one diameter. Abbreviated S.T.U. **Somogyi u.,** that amount of amylase which will destroy 1.5 mg. of starch in 8 minutes at 37° C. The normal range of the value in blood serum is considered by some to be between 80 and 200 units per 100 ml. **specific smell u.,** the smallest amount in substance in grams per liter which can be detected by smell. **spermatocyte u.,** the smallest amount of tuberculin which will destroy spermatogenesis when injected into the testicle of a guinea pig. **Steenbock u. of vitamin D,** the total amount of vitamin D which will produce a narrow line of calcium deposit in the rachitic metaphyses of the distal ends of the radii and ulnae of standard rachitic rats within ten days. **sudanophobic u.,** the smallest amount of corticotropic hormone which will cause the disappearance of the sudanophobic zone in at least two or three hypophysectomized rats when they are injected morning and evening on eight consecutive days. **Svedberg u.,** a unit of time (10⁻¹³ seconds) and velocity used in measuring the sedimentation constant of a colloid solution. **Thayer-Doisy u.,** a unit of vitamin K activity, being equivalent to the activity of 1 μg. of pure vitamin K₁. **toxic u., toxin u.,** the smallest dose of toxin which will kill a guinea pig weighing about 250 gm. in three to four days. **tuberculin u.,** 0.00002 mg. of purified protein derivative (P.P.D.) in 0.1 ml. of tuberculin solution, corresponding in potency to a 1:10,000 solution of Old tuberculin. **turbidity reducing u.,** the amount of hyaluronidase which is just sufficient to reduce the turbidity produced by 0.2 mg. of hyaluronate to that produced by 0.1 mg. after addition of acidified horse serum. **uranium u.,** a unit for measuring radioactivity, the activity of uranium being considered as 1. **urotoxic u.,** the smallest quantity of urotoxin which will kill an animal weighing 1 gm. **U.S.P. u.,** one used in the United States Pharmacopeia in expressing the potency of antibiotic, pharmacodynamic, and endocrine preparations, as well as most of the sera, toxins, vaccines, and related products, corresponding to units established internationally, by the Food and Drug Administration, or by the National Institutes of Health. **vitamin A u.,** see *international u. of vitamin A,* and *Sherman-Munsell u. of vitamin A.* **u. of vitamin B₁,** the antineuritic activity of 3 micrograms of the international standard preparation deposited at the National Institute for Medical Research, Hampstead. **vitamin D u.,** see *international u. of vitamin D, Steenbock u. of vitamin D* and *American Drug Manufacturers' Association u. of vitamin D.* **vitamin G u.,** see *Sherman-Bourquin u. of vitamin B₂.* **Voegtlin u.,** the amount of contraction produced in the isolated guinea-pig uterus by 0.5 mg. of the standard powdered preparation of the posterior pituitary. **x-ray u.,** Kienböck u.

unitage (u′nit-ij) a statement of the unit quantity in any system of measurement.

unitary (u′nĭ-ter″e) [L. *unitas* oneness] composed of or pertaining to a single unit.

United States Pharmacopeia see *U.S.P.*

Unitensen (u″nĭ-ten′sen) trademark for a preparation of cryptenamine acetates or cryptenamine tannates.

uniterminal (u″nĭ-ter″mĭ-nal) monoterminal.

univalence (u″nĭ-va′lens) the state or condition of being univalent.

univalent (u″nĭ-va′lent) [uni- + L. *valere* to be strong] having a valence of one; replacing or combining with one atom of hydrogen or its equivalent.

univitelline (u″nĭ-vi-tel′in) pertaining to or derived from a single ovum.

unmedullated (un-med′u-lāt″ed) not possessing a medulla or myelin sheath; said of a nerve fiber.

unmyelinated (un-mi′ĕ-lĭ-nāt″ed) not possessing a myelin sheath; said of a nerve fiber.

Unna's boot, etc. (oo′nahz) [Paul Gerson *Unna,* dermatologist in Hamburg, 1850–1929] see under *boot, cell, dermatosis, layer,* and *Table of Stains.*

Unna-Pappenheim stain (oo′nah-pahp′en-him) [Paul Gerson *Unna;* Artur *Pappenheim,* German physician, 1870–1916] see *Table of Stains.*

unorganized (un-or′gan-izd) not developed into an organic structure; not having organs.

unorientation (un″o-re-en-tā′shun) extreme disorder of memory in which the person loses the ideas of place and time; disorientation.

unphysiologic (un″fiz-e-o-loj′ik) not physiologic in character.

unrest (un-rest′) a state of uneasiness, or restlessness. **peristaltic u.,** a state of disturbed peristalsis of the stomach or intestine.

unsaturated (un-sat′u-rāt″ed) not saturated; applied to (1) a chemical compound in which two or more atoms are united by double or triple bonds. These bonds have two or three pairs of shared electrons characterized by pi-electrons (π-electrons) with orbital overlap. Such compounds may still add atoms or groups to the unsaturated bonding atoms up to a limit of bonding power or saturation. Most commonly refers to carbon-carbon bonds, as in unsaturated fatty acids. (2) a solution in which more solute may still be dissolved under stated conditions.

Unschuld's sign (oon′shooldz) [Paul *Unschuld,* German internist, born 1835] see under *sign.*

unsex (un-seks′) to deprive of the sex glands, or gonads.

unstriated (un-stri′āt-ed) having no striations or striae; see under *muscle.*

Unverricht's disease (syndrome) (oon′fer-ikts) [Heinrich *Unverricht,* German physician, 1853–1912] myoclonus epilepsy.

upsiloid (up′sĭ-loid) [Gr. υ + *eidos* form] shaped like the Greek upsilon (υ or Υ); see *hyoid* (def. 1) and *hypsiloid.*

uptake (up′tāk) absorption and incorporation of a substance by living tissue, as of iodine by the thyroid gland.

ur- see *uro-.*

urachal (u′rah-kal) pertaining to the urachus.

urachovesical (u″rah-ko-ves′ĭ-kal) pertaining to the urachus and the bladder.

urachus (u′rah-kus) [Gr. *ourachos*] [NA] a canal in the fetus that connects the bladder with the allantois; it persists throughout life as a cord (the median umbilical ligament) into which a patent canal may extend for part of the distance to the umbilicus.

uracil (u′rah-sil) a pyrimidine component, ($C_4H_4O_2N_2$), found in nucleic acid. **5-methyl u.,** see *thymine.*

uracrasia (u″rah-kra′se-ah) [ur- + Gr. *akrasia* bad mixture] a disordered state of the urine.

uracratia (u″rah-kra′she-ah) [ur- + Gr. *akrateia* lack of self control] urinary incontinence.

uragogue (u′rah-gog) [ur- + Gr. *agōgos* leading] 1. increasing urinary volume flow; diuretic. 2. an agent that increases production of urine.

uramil (u′rah-mil) a white crystalline pyrimidine derivative, $CO(NH \cdot CO)_2CH \cdot NH_2$, dialuramide, or 5-aminobarbituric acid, obtainable from uric acid, alloxantin, and other substances.

uranianism (u-ra′ne-an-izm) uranism.

uranidin (u-ran′ĭ-din) any one of a group of yellow animal pigments found in sponges, corals, medusae, and worms.

uranin (u′rah-nin) the sodium or potassium salt of fluorescein; see *sodium fluorescein.*

uranisco- [Gr. *ouraniskos,* the roof of the mouth] a combining form denoting relationship to the palate; see also *urano-.*

uraniscochasma (u″rah-nis″ko-kaz′mah) [*uranisco-* + Gr. *chasma* cleft] cleft palate.

uraniscolalia (u″rah-nis″ko-la′le-ah) [*uranisco-* + Gr. *lalia* talking] a speech defect due to cleft palate.

uraniscoplasty (u″rah-nis′ko-plas″te) palatoplasty.

uraniscorrhaphy (u″rah-nis-kor′ah-fe) [*uranisco-* + Gr. *rhaphē* seam] staphylorrhaphy.

uraniscus (u″rah-nis′kus) [Gr. *ouraniskos*, dim. of *ouranos*] the palate.

uranism (u′rah-nizm) [Gr. *ourania* the heavenly one, one of the epithets of Aphrodite, or Venus, as the patroness of homosexuals] homosexuality.

uranium (u-ra′ne-um) [L. *Uranus* a planet] a hard and heavy radioactive metallic element; symbol, U; atomic number, 92; atomic weight, 238.03; specific gravity, 18.68. Some of its compounds are medicinal. Naturally occurring uranium is composed of three isotopes of mass numbers 234, 235, and 238, respectively. Uranium 235 separated from U 238 undergoes fission with slow neutrons, giving up neutrons which can join the nucleus of U 238 to form neptunium, which in turn decays by beta particle emission to form plutonium. Cf. *neptunium* and *plutonium.*

urano- [Gr. *ouranos* the roof of the mouth, also the vault of heaven, or sky] a combining form denoting relationship to the palate; sometimes used in reference to the sky, or heaven.

uranoplastic (u″rah-no-plas′tik) pertaining to uranoplasty (palatoplasty).

uranoplasty (u′rah-no-plas″te) [*urano-* + Gr. *plassein* to mold] palatoplasty.

uranoplegia (u″rah-no-ple′je-ah) [*urano-* + Gr. *plēge* stroke + *-ia*] palatoplegia.

uranorrhaphy (u″rah-nor′ah-fe) [*urano-* + Gr. *rhaphē* seam] staphylorrhaphy.

uranoschisis (u″rah-nos′kĭ-sis) [*urano-* + Gr. *schisis* fissure] fissure of the palate; cleft palate.

uranoschism (u-ran′o-skizm) [*urano-* + Gr. *schisma* cleft] fissure of the palate; cleft palate.

uranostaphyloplasty (u″rah-no-staf″ĭ-lo-plas″te) an operation for repairing a defect of both the soft and hard palates; palatoplasty.

uranostaphylorrhaphy (u″rah-no-staf″ĭ-lor′ah-fe) [*urano-* + Gr. *staphylē* uvula + *rhaphē* suture] surgical palatorrhaphy.

uranostaphyloschisis (u″rah-no-staf″ĭ-los′kĭ-sis) fissure of both the hard and the soft palate.

uranosteoplasty (u″rah-nos′te-o-plas″te) palatoplasty.

Uranotaenia (u″rah-no-te′ne-ah) a genus of culicine mosquitoes. **U. sappari′nus,** a species occurring in the eastern United States.

uranyl (u′rah-nil) the UO++ ion, as in uranyl sulfate, UO₂SO₄. **u. acetate,** a yellow crystalline compound, UO₂(C₂H₃O₂)₂·2H₂O, used in coryza.

urapostema (u″rah-pos-te′mah) [*ur-* + Gr. *apostēma* abscess] an abscess which contains urine.

urarthritis (u″rar-thri′tis) gouty arthritis.

urase (u′rās) urease.

urasin (u-ras′in) an enzyme derivable from urea by the action of various bacteria.

urate (u′rāt) [L. *uras*] any salt of uric acid. Urates, especially that of sodium, are constituents of the urine, the blood, and of tophi, or calcareous concretions. **monosodium u.,** the urate ion form in which uric acid usually exists (in the serum) at the normal pH of body fluids.

uratemia (u″rah-te′me-ah) [*urate* + Gr. *haima* blood + *-ia*] the presence of urates in the blood.

uratic (u-rat′ik) pertaining to urates or to gout.

uratohistechia (u″rah-to-his-tek′e-ah) [*urate* + Gr. *histos* tissue + *echein* to hold] the presence of an excessive amount of urate, urea, or uric acid in a tissue.

uratoma (u″rah-to′mah) a tophus or concretion made up of urates.

uratosis (u″rah-to′sis) the deposition of crystalline urates in the tissues.

uraturia (u″rah-tu′re-ah) [*urate* + Gr. *ouron* urine + *-ia*] the presence of an excess of urates in the urine; lithuria.

urazin, urazine (u′rah-zin) diurea.

urazole (u′rah-zōl) a crystalline compound, 1,2,4-triazolidine-3,5-dione, (NH·CO)₂NH, formed by heating urea or biuret with hydrazine sulfate.

Urbach-Oppenheim disease (ur″bak op′en-hīm) [Erich *Urbach,* Philadelphia dermatologist, 1893–1946; Maurice *Oppenheim,* Chicago dermatologist, 1876–1949] necrobiosis lipoidica diabeticorum.

urceiform (ur-se′ĭ-form) [L. *urceus* pitcher + *forma* shape] pitcher-shaped.

urceolate (ur-se′o-lāt) urceiform.

ur-defense (ur″de-fens′) [Ger. *Ur* ultimate, transcendent + *de-*

fense] a belief essential to the psychological integrity of the individual. Such beliefs include faith in personal survival, in religious, philosophic, or scientific systems, and in human succorance.

urea (u-re′ah) 1. the diamide of carbonic acid, NH₂CO·NH₂; a white, crystallizable substance found in the urine, blood, and lymph. It is the chief nitrogenous constituent of the urine, and the chief nitrogenous end-product of the metabolism of proteins. It is formed in the liver from amino acids and from compounds of ammonia. See also *carbamide,* and see *urea cycle,* under *cycle.* 2. [USP] a preparation containing between 99.0 and 100.5 per cent of the labeled amount of urea, occurring as colorless to white, prismatic crystals or white, crystalline powder, used as an osmotic diuretic mainly to reduce intracranial and intraocular pressure, administered by intravenous infusion. Urea is also used in topical preparations, containing 2 or 10 per cent urea, to moisturize, soften, and smooth dry, rough skin. **diethyl malonyl u.,** barbital. **malonyl u.,** barbituric acid. **mesoxalyl u.,** alloxan. **u. nitrogen,** the nitrogen component of urea. The concentration of urea nitrogen in the blood (*blood urea nitrogen,* BUN) is measured in the determination of kidney function; elevated levels of blood urea nitrogen indicate a disorder of kidney function. **u. quinate, u. salicylate,** urea compounds once used in gouty conditions. **u. stibamine,** a mixture of different antimony compounds, used as an antileishmanial, administered intravenously.

ureagenetic (u-re″ah-jĕ-net′ik) [*urea* + Gr. *gennan* to produce] forming or producing urea.

ureal (u′re-al) pertaining to urea.

ureametry (u″re-am′ĕ-tre) the measurement of the urea present in the urine.

Ureaphil (u-re′ah-fil) trademark for a preparation of urea.

Ureaplasma urealyticum (u-re′ah-plaz″mah u-re″ah-lit′ĭ-kum) a species of nonmotile pleomorphic, gram-negative bacteria, lacking a cell wall, and forming very small granular colonies, 15–25 μm. in diameter; they are associated with nonspecific urethritis in males and genital tract infections in females. Called also *T-mycoplasma.*

ureapoiesis (u-re″ah-poi-e′sis) [*urea* + Gr. *poiein* to make] the formation of urea.

urease (u′re-ās) a colorless, crystalline globulin first extracted by Takeuchi from soy bean. It is also found in mucous urine passed during inflammation of the bladder. It is an enzyme elaborated by various microorganisms, and is capable of causing the change of urea into carbon dioxide and ammonia and of hippuric acid into benzoic acid and glycocoll. It was the first enzyme prepared in the crystalline state (Jesse Sumner). Called also *urea enzyme.*

urecchysis (u-rek′ĭ-sis) [*uro-* + Gr. *ekchysis* a pouring out] the effusion of urine into the cellular tissue.

Urechites (u-rek′ĭ-tēz) a genus of plants. **U. suberec′ta,** Savannah flower, an apocynaceous plant of tropical America with poisonous and antipyretic leaves.

urechitin (u-rek′ĭ-tin) a poisonous glycoside, C₂₈H₄₂O₈ + xH₂O, from *Urechites suberecta.*

urechitoxin (u-rek″ĭ-tok′sin) a poisonous glycoside, C₁₃H₂₀O₅, from *Urechites suberecta.*

Urecholine (u″re-ko′lin) trademark for a preparation of bethanechol chloride.

uredema (u″rĕ-de′mah) [*uro-* + Gr. *oidēma* swelling] a puffy condition of the tissues caused by infiltration of extravasated urine.

uredofos (u-re′do-fos) chemical name: [[[2-[[[[(4-methylphenyl)-sulfonyl]amino]carbonyl]amino]phenyl]amino]thioxomethyl]phosphoramidic acid diethyl ester; a veterinary antihelmintic, C₁₉H₂₅-N₄O₆PS₂.

ureide (u′re-id) a compound of urea and an acid or aldehyde formed by the elimination of water. Those from one molecule of urea, as alloxan, are monoureides; those derived from two, as uric acid, are diureides.

urein (u-re′in) a yellowish, oily substance isolated from the urine, and said to be the principal organic constituent and the true cause of uremia. It has a specific gravity of 1.27, and mixes freely with water and alcohol.

urelcosis (u″rel-ko′sis) [*uro-* + Gr. *helkōsis* ulceration] 1. ulceration of the urinary passages. 2. an ulcer due to derangement of the urinary apparatus.

uremia (u-re′me-ah) [Gr. *ouron* urine + *haima* blood + *-ia*] the retention of excessive by-products of protein metabolism in the blood, and the toxic condition produced thereby. It is marked by nausea, vomiting, headache, vertigo, dimness of vision, coma or convulsions, and an azotemic odor of the breath. It is due to nephron function inadequate to excrete urea and other products of protein metabolism. **azotemic u.,** retention u. **convulsive u.,** uremia in which the symptoms are due to spasm of the cerebral arteries or to increase of intracranial tension. **eclamptic u.,** convulsive u. **extrarenal u., prerenal u.,** uremia due to inhibition of renal function by disorders not related to the urinary tract. **puerperal u.,** uremic poisoning following childbirth. **retention u.,** uremia due to the retention of urinary nitrogenous substances in the blood.

uremic (u-re′mik) pertaining to or characterized by uremia.

uremigenic (u-re″mĭ-jen′ik) 1. caused by or due to uremia. 2. causing uremia.

ureo- for other words beginning thus, see those beginning *urea-*.

ureolysis (u″re-ol′ĭ-sis) [*urea* + Gr. *lysis* a loosing, setting free] the decomposition of urea to carbon dioxide and ammonia.

ureolytic (u″re-o-lit′ik) pertaining to, characterized by, or promoting ureolysis.

ureometry (u″re-om′ĕ-tre) ureametry.

ureotelic (u″re-o-tel′ik) [*urea* + Gr. *telikos* belonging to the completion, or end] having urea as the chief excretory product of nitrogen metabolism.

uresiesthesis (u-re″se-es-the′sis) [*uresis* + Gr. *aisthēsis* perception + *-ia*] the normal impulse to pass the urine.

uresis (u-re′sis) [Gr. *ourēsis*] the passage of urine; urination. Sometimes used as a word termination denoting excretion in the urine of the substance indicated by the stem to which it is affixed, as chloruresis, cupruresis, saluresis.

uret (u′ret) the chemical group CH₂NO.

uretal (u-re′tal) ureteral.

ureter (u-re′ter) [Gr. *ourētēr*] [NA] the fibromuscular tube which conveys the urine from the kidney to the bladder. It begins with the pelvis of the kidney, a funnel-like dilatation, and empties into the base of the bladder, being 16 to 18 inches long. It is divided into a pars abdominalis and a pars pelvina. See Plate accompanying *urogenital system*, under *system*. **circumcaval u.,** postcaval u. **ectopic u.,** a ureter which opens elsewhere than in the bladder wall, usually arising from the upper segment of a double kidney, and, in the female, opening in the vestibule, terminal urethra, vagina, cervix, or uterine cavity; in the male it invariably enters the genital or urinary tract above the level of the external sphincter. **postcaval u.,** a congenital anomaly in which the right ureter passes behind the inferior vena cava and curves round this vessel to regain its anterior position as it descends to the bladder; called also *circumcaval u.* and *retrocaval u.* **retrocaval u.,** postcaval u. **retroiliac u.,** a congenital anomaly in which a ureter passes behind the iliac artery.

ureteral (u-re′ter-al) pertaining to or used upon the ureter.

ureteralgia (u″re-ter-al′je-ah) pain in the ureter; neuralgia of the ureter.

ureterectasia (u-re″ter-ek-ta′se-ah) ureterectasis.

ureterectasis (u-re″ter-ek′tah-sis) [*ureter* + Gr. *ektasis* distention] distention of the ureter.

ureterectomy (u″re-ter-ek′to-me) [*ureter* + Gr. *ektomē* excision] the surgical removal of a ureter or of a part of it.

ureteric (u″rĕ-ter′ik) ureteral.

ureteritis (u″re-ter-i′tis) inflammation of a ureter. **u. cys′tica,** ureteritis characterized by the formation of multiple submucosal cysts. **u. glandula′ris,** ureteritis characterized by the conversion of transitional mucosal into cylindrical epithelium, with formation of glandular acini.

uretero- [Gr. *ourētēr* the duct which conveys urine from the kidney to the bladder] a combining form denoting relationship to the ureter.

ureterocele (u-re′ter-o-sēl″) [*uretero-* + Gr. *kēlē* hernia] sacculation of the terminal portion of the ureter into the bladder, as a result of stenosis of the ureteral meatus. **ectopic u.,** one which is located distal to the trigone of the bladder and which may extend into the urethra.

ureterocelectomy (u-re″ter-o-se-lek′to-me) excision of a ureterocele.

ureterocervical (u-re″ter-o-ser′vĭ-kal) pertaining to a ureter and to the cervix uteri.

ureterocolostomy (u-re″ter-o-ko-los′to-me) [*uretero-* + Gr. *kōlon* colon + *stomoun* to provide with an opening, or mouth] transplantation of the bladder end of a ureter into the colon.

ureterocutaneostomy (u-re″ter-o-ku-ta″ne-os′to-me) surgical creation of an opening of the ureter on the skin, permitting drainage of urine directly to the exterior of the body.

ureterocystanastomosis (u-re″ter-o-sis″tah-nas″to-mo′sis) ureteroneocystostomy.

ureterocystoneostomy (u-re″ter-o-sis″to-ne-os′to-me) [*uretero-* + Gr. *kystis* bladder + *neos* new + *stomoun* to provide with an opening, or mouth] ureteroneocystostomy.

ureterocystoscope (u-re″ter-o-sis′to-skōp) [*uretero-* + *cystoscope*] a cystoscope with an arrangement for catheterizing the ureters.

ureterocystostomy (u-re″ter-o-sis-tos′to-me) [*uretero-* + Gr. *kystis* bladder + *stomoun* to provide with an opening, or mouth] ureteroneocystostomy.

ureterodialysis (u-re″ter-o-di-al′ĭ-sis) [*uretero-* + Gr. *dialysis* separation] rupture of a ureter.

ureteroduodenal (u-re″ter-o-du″o-de′nal) pertaining to or communicating with a ureter and the duodenum, as a ureteroduodenal fistula.

ureteroenteric (u-re″ter-o-en-ter′ik) pertaining to or connecting the ureter and the intestine.

ureteroenteroanastomosis (u-re″ter-o-en″ter-o-ah-nas″to-mo′sis) ureteroenterostomy.

ureteroenterostomy (u-re″ter-o-en″ter-os′to-me) [*uretero-* + Gr. *enteron* bowel + *stomoun* to provide with an opening, or mouth] the operation of forming an anastomosis between a ureter and the intestine.

ureterogram (u-re′ter-o-gram) a radiograph of the ureter.

ureterography (u-re″ter-og′rah-fe) [*uretero-* + Gr. *graphein* to write] radiography of the ureter after injection of an opaque medium into the ureter.

ureteroheminephrectomy (u-re″ter-o-hem″ĭ-nĕ-frek′to-me) excision of the diseased portion of a reduplicated kidney and its ureter.

ureteroileostomy (u-re″ter-o-il″e-os′to-me) anastomosis of the ureters to an isolated loop of the ileum, drained through a stoma on the abdominal wall.

ureterointestinal (u-re″ter-o-in-tes′tĭ-nal) pertaining to or connecting the ureter and intestine.

ureterolith (u-re′ter-o-lith″) [*uretero-* + Gr. *lithos* stone] a calculus lodged or formed in a ureter.

ureterolithiasis (u-re″ter-o-lĭ-thi′ah-sis) the formation of a calculus in the ureter.

ureterolithotomy (u-re″ter-o-lĭ-thot′o-me) [*uretero-* + Gr. *lithos* stone + *tomē* a cutting] the removal of a calculus from the ureter by incision.

ureterolysis (u-re″ter-ol′ĭ-sis) [*uretero-* + Gr. *lysis* dissolution] 1. rupture of the ureter. 2. paralysis of the ureter. 3. the operation of freeing the ureter from adhesions.

ureteromeatotomy (u-re″ter-o-me″ah-tot′o-me) incision of the opening of the ureter in the bladder wall.

ureteroneocystostomy (u-re″ter-o-ne″o-sis-tos′to-me) [*uretero-* + Gr. *neos* new + *kystis* bladder + *stomoun* to provide with an opening, or mouth] surgical transplantation of the ureter to a different site in the bladder.

ureteroneopyelostomy (u-re″ter-o-ne″o-pi″ĕ-los′to-me) [*uretero-* + Gr. *neos* new + *pyelos* pelvis + *stomoun* to provide with an opening, or mouth] an operation for cutting out a stricture of the ureter and inserting the upper end of the lower segment of the ureter through a new aperture into the pelvis of the kidney.

ureteronephrectomy (u-re″ter-o-nĕ-frek′to-me) [*uretero-* + Gr. *nephros* kidney + *ektomē* excision] extirpation of a kidney and its ureter.

ureteropathy (u-re″ter-op′ah-the) [*uretero-* + Gr. *pathos* disease] any disease of the ureter.

ureteropelvic (u-re″ter-o-pel′vik) pertaining to or affecting the ureter and the renal pelvis.

ureteropelvioneostomy (u-re″ter-o-pel″ve-o-ne-os′to-me) ureteroneopyelostomy.

ureteropelvioplasty (u-re″ter-o-pel′ve-o-plas″te) surgical reconstruction of the junction of the ureter and renal pelvis. **Culp u.,** ureteropelvioplasty in which a spiral pelvic flap is turned down and incorporated into the adjacent ureter. **Foley Y-type u.,** an operation for correction of obstructive, congenital high insertion of the ureter into the renal pelvis. **Scardino u.,** ureteropelvioplasty in which a vertical pelvic flap is turned down and incorporated into the adjacent ureter.

ureterophlegma (u-re″ter-o-fleg′mah) [*uretero-* + Gr. *phlegma* phlegm] the presence of mucus in the ureter.

ureteroplasty (u-re′ter-o-plas″te) [*uretero-* + Gr. *plassein* to form] plastic operation upon the ureter for widening a stricture.

ureteroproctostomy (u-re″ter-o-prok-tos′to-me) [*uretero-* + Gr. *prōktos* anus + *stomoun* to provide with an opening, or mouth] the operation of forming an anastomosis between the ureter and the lower rectum.

ureteropyelitis (u-re″ter-o-pi-ĕ-li′tis) [*uretero-* + Gr. *pyelos* pelvis] inflammation of a ureter and of the pelvis of a kidney.

ureteropyelography (u-re″ter-o-pi-ĕ-log′rah-fe) roentgenography of the ureter and pelvis of the kidney.

ureteropyeloneostomy (u-re″ter-o-pi″ĕ-lo-ne-os′to-me) [*uretero-* + Gr. *pyelos* pelvis + *neos* new + *stomoun* to provide with an opening, or mouth] surgical formation of a new passage from the pelvis of a kidney to the ureter.

ureteropyelonephritis (u-re″ter-o-pi″ĕ-lo-nĕ-fri′tis) [*uretero-* + Gr. *pyelos* pelvis + *nephros* kidney + *-itis*] inflammation of the ureter and the pelvis of the kidney.

ureteropyelonephrostomy (u-re″ter-o-pi″ĕ-lo-nĕ-fros′to-me) operative anastomosis of the ureter and the pelvis of the kidney.

ureteropyeloplasty (u-re″ter-o-pi′ĕ-lo-plas″te) any plastic operation on the ureter and renal pelvis.

ureteropyelostomy (u-re″ter-o-pi″ĕ-los′to-me) ureteropyeloneostomy.

ureteropyosis (u-re″ter-o-pi-o′sis) [*uretero-* + Gr. *pyon* pus + *-osis*] suppurative inflammation of the ureter.

ureterorectal (u-re″ter-o-rek′tal) pertaining to or communicating with a ureter and the rectum, as a ureterorectal fistula.

ureterorectoneostomy (u-re″ter-o-rek″to-ne-os′to-me) ureteroproctostomy.

ureterorectostomy (u-re″ter-o-rek-tos′to-me) ureteroproctostomy.

ureterorenoscope (u-re″ter-o-re′no-skōp) a fiberoptic endoscope used in uterorenoscopy.

ureterorenoscopy (u-re″ter-o-re-nos′ko-pe) visual inspection of the interior of the ureter and kidney by means of a fiberoptic endoscope for such purposes as biopsy, removal or crushing of stones, etc.

ureterorrhagia (u-re″ter-o-ra′je-ah) [uretero- + Gr. rhēgnynai to burst forth] a discharge of blood from the ureter.

ureterorrhaphy (u″re-ter-or′ah-fe) [uretero- + Gr. rhaphē suture] the operation of suturing the ureter for fistula.

ureterosigmoidostomy (u-re″ter-o-sig″moi-dos′to-me) the operation of implanting the ureter into the sigmoid flexure.

ureterostegnosis (u-re″ter-o-steg-no′sis) [uretero- + Gr. stegnōsis contraction] ureterostenosis.

ureterostenoma (u-re″ter-o-stě-no′mah) [uretero- + Gr. stenōma stricture] ureterostenosis.

ureterostenosis (u-re″ter-o-stě-no′sis) [uretero- + Gr. stenōsis narrowing] stricture of the ureter.

ureterostoma (u″re-ter-os′to-mah) [uretero- + Gr. stoma mouth] 1. the vesical orifice of the ureter (ostium ureteris [NA]). 2. a ureteral fistula.

ureterostomosis (u-re″ter-o-sto-mo′sis) ureterostomy.

ureterostomy (u″re-ter-os′to-me) [uretero- + Gr. stomoun to provide with an opening, or mouth] surgical formation of a permanent fistula through which a ureter may discharge its contents. **cutaneous u.,** the operation of bringing the ureter to the skin through an incision in the iliac region; ureterocutaneostomy.

ureterotomy (u″re-ter-ot′o-me) [uretero- + Gr. tomē a cutting] surgical incision of a ureter.

ureterotrigonoenterostomy (u-re″ter-o-tri-go″no-en″ter-os′-to-me) implantation into the intestine of the ureter with the part of the bladder wall surrounding its termination.

ureterotrigonosigmoidostomy (u-re″ter-o-tri-go″no-sig″moi-dos′to-me) implantation into the sigmoid flexure of the ureter with the part of the bladder wall surrounding its termination.

ureteroureteral (u-re″ter-o-u-re′ter-al) connecting two parts of the ureter.

ureteroureterostomy (u-re″ter-o-u-re″ter-os′to-me) end-to-end anastomosis of the two portions of a transected ureter; see also transureteroureterostomy.

ureterouterine (u-re″ter-o-u′ter-in) pertaining to or communicating with a ureter and the uterus.

ureterovaginal (u-re″ter-o-vaj′ĭ-nal) pertaining to or communicating with a ureter and the vagina.

ureterovesical (u-re″ter-o-ves′ĭ-kal) pertaining to a ureter and the bladder.

ureterovesicoplasty (u-re″ter-o-ves″ĭ-ko-plas′te) plastic repair of the ureterovesical junction for correction of ureterovesical reflux or obstruction.

ureterovesicostomy (u-re″ter-o-ves″ĭ-kos′to-me) the operation of reimplanting the ureter at a different site in the bladder wall.

urethan (u′rě-than) [NF] chemical name: carbamic acid ethyl ester. An antineoplastic, $C_3H_7NO_2$, occurring as white crystals or white, granular powder; it has been used in the treatment of myeloid and lymphatic leukemia and plasma cell myeloma, but has been replaced largely by superior drugs.

urethane (u′rě-thān) urethan.

urethra (u-re′thrah) [Gr. ourēthra] the membranous canal conveying urine from the bladder to the exterior of the body. See Plate accompanying urogenital system, under system. **anterior u.,** the portion of the male urethra extending from the bulb to the meatus on the summit of the glans penis, tunneling the corpus spongiosum; it consists of three parts, the bulbous, the pendulous, and the most distal, glandular part. **double u.,** congenital complete or partial reduplication of the urethra; the urethral openings may be side by side or one above the other. **female u., u. femini′na** [NA], a canal, about 3.7 cm. long, extending from the neck of the bladder, running above the anterior vaginal wall and piercing the urogenital diaphragm, to reach the urinary meatus; called also u. muliebris. **male u., u. masculi′na** [NA], a canal extending from the neck of the bladder to the urinary meatus, measuring about 20 cm. in length, and presenting a double curve when the penis is flaccid; it is divided into a pars prostatica, pars membranacea, and pars spongiosa. Called also u. virilis. **u. mulie′bris,** u. feminina. **posterior u.,** the portion of the male urethra, extending from the bladder to the bulb, and consisting of the membranous and prostatic parts. **u. viri′lis,** u. masculina.

urethral (u-re′thral) pertaining to the urethra.

urethralgia (u″rě-thral′je-ah) pain in the urethra.

urethrascope (u-re′thrah-skōp) urethroscope.

urethratresia (u-re″thrah-tre′ze-ah) imperforation of the urethra.

urethrectomy (u″rě-threk′to-me) [urethra + Gr. ektomē excision] the surgical removal of the urethra or a part of it.

urethremphraxis (u″rě-threm-frak′sis) [urethra + Gr. emphraxis stoppage] obstruction of the urethra.

urethreurynter (u-rēth″roo-rin′ter) [urethra + Gr. eurynein to make wide] an instrument for dilating the urethra.

urethrism (u′rě-thrizm) [L. urethrismus] irritability or chronic spasm of the urethra.

urethritis (u″rě-thri′tis) inflammation of the urethra. **u. cys′tica,** inflammation of the urethra, with the formation of multiple submucosal cysts. **u. glandula′ris,** inflammation of the urethra, with conversion of transitional mucosal into cylindrical epithelium, with formation of glandular acini. **gonococcal u., gonorrheal u.,** gonorrhea in the male. **gouty u.,** urethritis due to gout. **u. granulo′sa,** urethritis in which the anterior urethra is filled with granulations. **nongonococcal u., nonspecific u.,** urethritis without evidence of gonococcal infection, as, for example, that caused by Chlamydia trachomatis; called also simple u. **u. orifi′cii exter′ni,** inflammation and ulceration of the external urethral meatus. **u. petri′ficans,** urethritis with the formation of calcareous matter in the urethral wall. **prophylactic u.,** a mild urethritis that sometimes follows irrigations used to prevent venereal infections. **simple u.,** nongonococcal u. **specific u.,** that due to infection with the gonococcus. **u. vene′rea,** gonorrhea.

urethro- [Gr. ourēthra the tube by which urine is discharged from the bladder] a combining form denoting relationship to the urethra.

urethroblennorrhea (u-re″thro-blen″o-re′ah) a purulent discharge from the urethra.

urethrobulbar (u-re″thro-bul′bar) pertaining to the urethra and the bulbus penis.

urethrocele (u-re″thro-sēl) [urethro- + Gr. kēlē tumor] 1. prolapse of the female urethra through the meatus urinarius. 2. a diverticulum of the urethral walls encroaching upon the vaginal canal.

urethrocystitis (u-re″thro-sis-ti′tis) inflammation of the urethra and bladder.

urethrocystogram (u-re″thro-sis′to-gram) a roentgenogram of the urethra and bladder.

urethrocystography (u-re″thro-sis-tog′rah-fe) [urethro- + Gr. kystis bladder + graphein to write] roentgenography of the urethra and bladder after the injection of a contrast medium.

urethrocystopexy (u-re″thro-sis″to-pek′se) [urethro- + Gr. kystis bladder + pēxis fixation] surgical fixation of the urethrovesical junction, and the area of the bladder just above it, to the back of the pubic bones, for relief of stress incontinence.

urethrodynia (u-re″thro-din′e-ah) [urethro- + Gr. odynē pain] pain in the urethra; urethralgia.

urethrograph (u-re′thro-graf) an instrument for recording graphically the caliber of the urethra.

urethrography (u″rě-throg′rah-fe) roentgenography of the urethra after the injection of an opaque medium.

urethrometer (u″rě-throm′ě-ter) [urethro- + Gr. metron measure] an instrument for measuring the urethra.

urethrometry (u″rě-throm′ě-tre) 1. determination of the resistance of various segments of the urethra to retrograde flow of fluid. 2. measurement of the urethra.

urethropenile (u-re″thro-pe′nīl) pertaining to the urethra and the penis.

urethroperineal (u-re″thro-per″ĭ-ne′al) pertaining to or communicating with the urethra and the perineum.

urethroperineoscrotal (u-re″thro-per-in″e-o-skro′tal) pertaining to the urethra, perineum, and scrotum.

urethropexy (u-re″thro-pek′se) [urethro- + Gr. pēxis fixation] surgical fixation of the urethra to the overlying symphysis pubis and fascia of the rectus abdominis muscle, in correction of stress incontinence in the female.

urethrophraxis (u-re″thro-frak′sis) [urethro- + Gr. phrassein to stop up] obstruction of the urethra.

urethrophyma (u-re″thro-fi′mah) [urethro- + Gr. phyma growth] a tumor or growth in the urethra.

urethroplasty (u-re″thro-plas″te) [urethro- + Gr. plassein to form] plastic surgery of the urethra; operative repair of a wound or defect in the urethra.

urethroprostatic (u-re″thro-pros-tat′ik) pertaining to the urethra and the prostate.

urethrorectal (u-re″thro-rek′tal) pertaining to or communicating with the urethra and the rectum.

urethrorrhagia (u-re″thro-ra′je-ah) [urethro- + Gr. rhēgnynai to burst forth] a flow of blood from the urethra.

urethrorrhaphy (u″rě-thror′ah-fe) [urethro- + Gr. rhaphē seam] suturation of the urethra; the closing of a urethral fistula by suture.

urethrorrhea (u-re″thro-re′ah) [*urethro-* + Gr. *rhoia* flow] an abnormal discharge from the urethra.

urethroscope (u-re′thro-skōp) [*urethro-* + Gr. *skopein* to examine] an instrument for viewing the interior of the urethra.

urethroscopic (u-re″thro-skop′ik) pertaining to the urethroscope or urethroscopy.

urethroscopy (u″re-thros′ko-pe) [*urethro-* + Gr. *skopein* to examine] visual inspection of the interior of the urethra.

urethroscrotal (u-re″thro-skro′tal) pertaining to or communicating with the urethra and scrotum, as a urethroscrotal fistula.

urethrospasm (u-re′thro-spazm) [*urethro-* + Gr. *spasmos* spasm] spasm of the muscular tissue of the urethra.

urethrostaxis (u-re″thro-stak′sis) [*urethro-* + Gr. *staxis* dropping] oozing of blood from the urethra.

urethrostenosis (u-re″thro-stĕ-no′sis) [*urethro-* + Gr. *stenōsis* stricture] stricture or stenosis of the urethra.

urethrostomy (u″rĕ-thros′to-me) [*urethro-* + Gr. *stomoun* to provide with an opening, or mouth] surgical formation of a permanent opening of the urethra at the perineal surface.

urethrotome (u-re′thro-tōm) an instrument for cutting a urethral stricture. **Maisonneuve's u.,** a urethrotome in which the knife is concealed until it reaches the stricture, when the knife may be exposed.

urethrotomy (u″rĕ-throt′o-me) [*urethro-* + Gr. *tomē* a cutting] a cutting operation for curing a stricture of the urethra. It may be performed either externally or internally. *External urethrotomy* (perineal section) consists in opening the urethra from the outside. *Internal urethrotomy* may be performed in two ways, viz.: Incising from before backward, as with the instrument of Maisonneuve; incising from behind forward, as with the urethrotome of S. W. Gross.

urethrotrigonitis (u-re″thro-tri″go-ni′tis) inflammation of the urethra and trigone of the bladder.

urethrovaginal (u-re″thro-vaj′ĭ-nal) pertaining to or communicating with the urethra and the vagina.

urethrovesical (u-re″thro-ves′ĭ-kal) pertaining to or communicating with the urethra and the bladder.

uretic (u-ret′ik) [L. *ureticus;* Gr. *ourētikos*] 1. pertaining to the urine. 2. diuretic.

Urevert (u′re-vert) trademark for a preparation of urea.

Urex (u′reks) trademark for a preparation of methenamine hippurate.

urgency (ur′jen-se) the sudden compelling urge to urinate.

Urginea (ur-jin′e-ah) [L.] a genus of liliaceous plants. *U. marit′ima* (L.) Baker, the Mediterranean or white variety, and *U. indica* Kunth., the Indian variety, afford squill (q.v.).

urhidrosis (ur″hid-ro′sis) [*ur-* + Gr. *hidrōs* sweat] the presence in the sweat of urinous materials, such as uric acid, urea, etc. **u. crystal′lina,** a form in which crystals of uric acid are deposited upon the skin.

-uria [Gr. *ouron* urine + *-ia* state] a word termination denoting a characteristic or constituent of the urine, indicated by the stem to which it is affixed, as oliguria, proteinuria.

urian (u′re-an) urochrome.

uric (u′rik) [Gr. *ourikos*] of or pertaining to the urine; see also under *acid.*

uricacidemia (u″rik-as″ĭ-de′me-ah) [*uric* acid + Gr. *haima* blood + *-ia*] the accumulation of uric acid in the blood; see *lithemia.*

uricaciduria (u″rik-as″ĭ-du′re-ah) [*uric* acid + Gr. *ouron* urine + *-ia*] presence in the urine of an excess of uric acid, and the morbid state produced thereby; see *lithuria.*

uricase (u′rĭ-kās) an enzyme found in most mammals except man, which catalyzes the complicated transformation of uric acid into allantoin.

uricemia (u″rĭ-se′me-ah) uricacidemia.

uricocholia (u″rĭ-ko-ko′le-ah) [*uric* acid + Gr. *cholē* bile] the presence of uric acid in the bile.

uricolysis (u″rĭ-kol′ĭ-sis) [*uric* acid + Gr. *lysis* dissolution] the cleavage of uric acid or of urates.

uricolytic (u″rĭ-ko-lit′ik) pertaining to, characterized by, or promoting uricolysis.

uricometer (u″rĭ-kom′ĕ-ter) [*uric* acid + Gr. *metron* measure] an instrument for measuring the amount of uric acid in the urine. **Ruhemann's u.,** one based on the principle that uric acid will absorb iodine.

uricopoiesis (u″rĭ-ko-poi-e′sis) the formation of uric acid.

uricosuria (u″rĭ-ko-su′re-ah) the excretion of uric acid in the urine.

uricosuric (u″rĭ-ko-su′rik) 1. pertaining to, characterized by, or promoting uricosuria. 2. an agent that promotes uricosuria.

uricotelic (u″rĭ-ko-tel′ik) [*uric* acid + Gr. *telikos* belonging to the completion, or end] having uric acid as the chief excretory product of nitrogen metabolism, as in reptiles and birds.

uricotelism (u″rĭ-ko-te′lizm) the excretion of uric acid as the end product of nitrogen metabolism, as in reptiles and birds.

uricoxidase (u″rĭ-kok′si-dās) an enzyme that oxidizes uric acid.

Uricult (u′rĭ-kult) trademark for a bacterial culture device, consisting of a glass slide in a sterile plastic container. On one face of the slide a 13 sq. cm. area is coated with MacConkey's medium, on the other a similar area is coated with nutrient agar. The slide is dipped into freshly voided urine, removed, and replaced in the container, where growth takes place.

uridine (u′rĭ-dēn, u′rĭ-din) a nucleoside (pentoside) from nucleic acid; on hydrolysis it yields uracil and ribose. **u. diphosphate,** a nucleotide containing uridine, which participates in glycogen metabolism and in some processes of nucleic acid synthesis; abbreviated UDP. **u. diphosphate galactose, u. diphosphogalactose,** a nucleotide derivative of galactose formed from galactose-1-phosphate and UTP; abbreviated UDP-galactose. **u. diphosphate glucose, u. diphosphoglucose,** a nucleotide derivative of glucose, formed from glucose-1-phosphate; it is an intermediate in the formation of glycogen and galactose and a source of several precursors of heteropolysaccharides. Abbreviated UDP-glucose. **u. diphosphoglucuronate,** a nucleotide formed by the oxidation of UDP-glucose; it serves in the synthesis of mucopolysaccharides. Abbreviated UDP-glucuronate. **u. monophosphate (UMP),** uridylic acid. **u. triphosphate,** a triphosphate which reacts with glucose-1-phosphate to form UDP-glucose and inorganic pyrophosphate, a step in tissue glycogen storage; abbreviated UTP.

uridrosis (u″rĭ-dro′sis) urhidrosis.

uriesthesis (u″re-es′the-sis) uresiesthesis.

urina (u-ri′nah) [L.] urine. **u. chy′li, u. ci′bi** ["urine of food"], the urine secreted after a full meal. **u. cruen′ta,** bloody urine; see *hematuria.* **u. galacto′des,** milky urine. **u. jumento′sa,** cloudy urine. **u. po′tus** ["urine of drink"], urine secreted after copious drinking. **u. san′guinis** ["urine of the blood"], urine passed after a night's rest, and so not influenced by food or drink.

urinable (u′rin-ah-b'l) capable of being excreted in the urine.

urinaccelerator (u″rin-ak-sel′er-a″tor) musculus bulbospongiosus.

urinacidometer (u″rin-as″ĭ-dom′ĕ-ter) an instrument for estimating the pH of urine.

urinaemia (u″rĭ-ne′me-ah) uremia.

urinal (u′rĭ-nal) [L. *urinalis* urinary] a vessel or other receptacle for urine.

urinalysis (u″rĭ-nal′ĭ-sis) physical, chemical, or microscopic analysis or examination of urine.

urinary (u′rĭ-ner″e) pertaining to the urine; containing or secreting urine.

urinate (u′rĭ-nāt) to void or discharge urine.

urination (u″rĭ-na′shun) the discharge or passage of urine. **precipitant u.,** a sudden and strong desire to urinate. **stuttering u.,** an intermittent flow of urine, due to vesical spasm.

urinative (u′rĭ-na″tiv) diuretic.

urine (u′rin) [L. *urina;* Gr. *ouron*] the fluid excreted by the kidneys, passed through the ureters, stored in the bladder, and discharged through the urethra. Urine, in health, has an amber color, a slight acid reaction, a peculiar odor, and a bitter, saline taste. The average quantity excreted under ordinary dietary conditions in twenty-four hours is about 1000 to 2000 ml. Specific gravity, about 1.024, varying from 1.005 to 1.030. One thousand parts of healthy urine contain about 960 parts of water and 40 parts of solutes, which consist chiefly of urea, 23 parts; sodium chloride, 11 parts; phosphoric acid, 2.3 parts; sulfuric acid, 1.3 parts; uric acid, 0.5 part; also hippuric acid, leukomaines, urobilin, and certain organic salts. The abnormal matters found in the urine in various conditions include ketone bodies, proteins, proteoses, bile, blood, cystine, glucose, hemoglobin, fat, pus, spermatozoa, epithelial cells, mucous casts, and crystals of sulfanilamide derivatives (crystalluria). **Bence Jones u.,** see *Bence Jones protein,* under *protein.* **black u.,** urine colored black by melanin (melanuria), or by derivatives of homogentisic acid (ochronosis). **chylous u.,** urine of a milky color from the presence of chyle or fat; chyluria. **cloudy u.,** urine having a cloudy appearance, usually due to phosphaturia or uraturia, but may be caused by pyuria; called also *nebulous u.* and *urina jumentosa.* **crude u.,** light-colored, watery urine, which deposits little sediment. **diabetic u.,** that which contains an excess of glucose. **dyspeptic u.,** the urine in dyspepsia, frequently containing calcium oxalate crystals. **febrile u.,** strong, odorous, high-colored, concentrated urine, such as is secreted in fever. **gouty u.,** scanty, high-colored urine containing large quantities of urates. **milky u.,** urine having a milky appearance, which may be due to chyluria or pyuria; called also *urina galactodes.* **nebulous u.,** cloudy u. **residual u.,** the urine that remains in the bladder after urination in disease of the bladder and hypertrophy of the prostate.

urinemia (u″rĭ-ne′me-ah) [*urine* + Gr. *haima* blood + *-ia*] uremia.

urine-mucoid (u″rin-mu′koid) a mucin-like substance found in the urine.

urinidrosis (u″rin-ĭ-dro′sis) urhidrosis.

uriniferous (u″rĭ-nif′er-us) [*urine* + L. *ferre* to bear] transporting or conveying the urine.

urinific (u″rĭ-nif′ik) uriniparous.

uriniparous (u″rĭ-nip′ah-rus) [*urine* + L. *parere* to produce] producing or elaborating urine.

urino- [L. *urina*] a combining form denoting relationship to urine; see also *uro-*.

urinocryoscopy (u-ri″no-kri-os′ko-pe) cryoscopy of the urine.

urinogenital (u″rĭ-no-jen′ĭ-tal) genitourinary; urogenital.

urinogenous (u″rĭ-noj′ĕ-nus) of urinary origin.

urinoglucosometer (u″rĭ-no-gloo″ko-som′ĕ-ter) an instrument for measuring the glucose in the urine.

urinologist (u″rĭ-nol′o-jist) urologist.

urinology (u″rĭ-nol′o-je) urology.

urinoma (u″rĭ-no′mah) a cyst containing urine.

urinometer (u″rĭ-nom′ĕ-ter) [*urino-* + Gr. *metron* measure] an instrument for determining the specific gravity of the urine.

urinometry (u″rĭ-nom′ĕ-tre) the ascertainment of the specific gravity of the urine.

urinophilous (u″rĭ-nof′ĭ-lus) [*urino-* + Gr. *philein* to love] having an affinity for urine, as a microorganism which grows best in urine, or an organism (such as a certain South American fish) which invades the urinary meatus of bathers.

urinoscopy (u″rĭ-nos′ko-pe) uroscopy.

urinosexual (u″rĭ-no-seks′u-al) genitourinary; urogenital.

urinous (u′rĭ-nus) pertaining to the urine; containing elements commonly excreted in the urine.

uriposia (u″rĭ-po′ze-ah) [*urine* + Gr. *posis* drinking + *-ia*] the drinking of urine.

urishiol (u-rish′e-ol) an extremely allergenically active mixture of catechol derivatives forming the major constituent of the irritant resin of poison ivy and other members of Anacardiaceae.

Urispas (u′rĭ-spaz) trademark for a preparation of flavoxate hydrochloride.

Uritone (u′rĭ-tōn) trademark for preparations of methenamine.

urningism (oor′ning-izm) uranism (homosexuality).

urnism (oorn′izm) uranism (homosexuality).

uro-, ur-, urono- [Gr. *ouron* urine] combining forms denoting relationship to urine, the urinary tract, or urination.

uroacidimeter (u″ro-as″ĭ-dim′ĕ-ter) an instrument for measuring the acidity of the urine.

uroammoniac (u″ro-ah-mo′ne-ak) containing uric acid and ammonia.

uroanthelone (u″ro-an′thĕ-lōn) urogastrone.

uroazotometer (u″ro-az″o-tom′ĕ-ter) an apparatus for measuring the nitrogenous matter of the urine.

urobilin (u″ro-bi′lin) [*uro-* + L. *bilis* bile] an amorphous, brownish pigment, $C_{35}H_{44}O_8N_4$, an oxidized form of urobilinogen, found in the feces and sometimes in urine left standing in the air.

urobilinemia (u″ro-bil″ĭ-ne′me-ah) [*urobilin* + Gr. *haima* blood + *-ia*] the presence of urobilin in the blood.

urobilinogen (u″ro-bi-lin′o-jen) [*urobilin* + Gr. *gennan* to produce] a colorless compound formed in the intestines by the reduction of bilirubin. Some is excreted in the feces, where by oxidation it becomes urobilin; some is reabsorbed, and re-excreted in the bile as bilirubin, or at times in the urine, where it may be later oxidized to urobilin.

urobilinogenemia (u″ro-bi-lin″o-jĕ-ne′me-ah) the presence of urobilinogen in the blood.

urobilinogenuria (u″ro-bi-lin″o-jĕ-nu′re-ah) the presence of urobilinogen in the urine.

urobilinoid (u″ro-bil′ĭ-noid) resembling urobilin.

urobilinoiden (u″ro-bil″ĭ-noi′din) a reduction product of hematin, resembling urobilin, sometimes found in the urine.

urobilinuria (u″ro-bil″ĭ-nu′re-ah) [*urobilin* + Gr. *ouron* urine + *-ia*] the presence of an excess of urobilin in the urine, as in cirrhosis of the liver.

urocanase (u″ro-ka′nās) an enzyme that catalyzes the conversion of urocanate to imidazolone propionate in the metabolism of histidine.

urocanate (u″ro-kan′āt) the dissociated form of urocanic acid, an intermediate product in histidine metabolism.

urocele (u′ro-sēl) [*uro-* + Gr. *kēlē* hernia] distention of the scrotum with extravasated urine.

urocheras (u-rok′er-as) [*uro-* + Gr. *cheras* gravel] uropsammus.

urochezia (u″ro-ke′ze-ah) [*uro-* + Gr. *chezein* to defecate + *-ia*] the discharge of urine in the feces.

Urochordata (u″ro-kor′da-tah) [Gr. *oura* tail + L. *chorda* string] a subphylum of chordates intermediate between the invertebrates and true vertebrates, including the sea squirts and their allies, the members of which have a saclike body and a leathery tunic; the notochord is present only during the larval stage. Called also *Tunicata*.

urochordate (u-ro-kor′dāt) any member of the Urochordata; a tunicate.

urochrome (u′ro-krōm) [*uro-* + Gr. *chrōma* color] a yellow, amorphous pigment of the urine, which gives the urine its yellow color.

urochromogen (u″ro-kro′mo-gen) a low oxidation product found in the urine, which on further oxidation becomes urochrome.

urocinetic (u″ro-si-net′ik) urokinetic.

uroclepsia (u″ro-klep′se-ah) [*uro-* + Gr. *kleptein* to steal] the unconscious escape of urine.

urocoproporphyria (u″ro-kop″ro-por-fir′e-ah) porphyria cutanea tarda symptomatica.

urocrisia (u″ro-kriz′e-ah) [*uro-* + Gr. *krinein* to judge] diagnosis by observing or examining the urine.

urocriterion (u″ro-kri-te′re-on) [*uro-* + Gr. *kritērion* test] an indication of disease observed in examination of the urine.

urocyanin (u-ro-si′ah-nin) [*uro-* + Gr. *kyanos* blue] uroglaucin.

urocyanogen (u″ro-si-an′o-jen) [*uro-* + Gr. *kyanos* blue + *gennan* to produce] a blue pigment of the urine, especially of that of cholera patients.

urocyanosis (u″ro-si″ah-no′sis) [*uro-* + Gr. *kyanos* blue] indicanuria.

urocyst (u′ro-sist) [*uro-* + Gr. *kystis* bladder] the urinary bladder (vesica urinaria [NA]).

urocystic (u″ro-sis′tik) pertaining to the urinary bladder.

Urocystis (u″ro-sis′tis) a genus of basidiomycetous fungi of the order Ustilaginales, family Tilletiaceae. **U. trit′ici**, a fungus which causes flag smut of wheat in Australia, China, and southern Asia.

urocystis (u″ro-sis′tis) [L.] the urinary bladder.

urocystitis (u″ro-sis-ti′tis) inflammation of the urinary bladder.

urodeum (u″ro-de′um) [*uro-* + Gr. *hodaios* on the way] the portion of the cloaca into which the ureters and genital ducts empty.

urodialysis (u″ro-di-al′ĭ-sis) [*uro-* + Gr. *dialysis* cessation] partial or complete suppression of the urine.

urodochium (u″ro-do′ke-um, u″ro-do-ki′um) [*uro-* + Gr. *docheion* holder] a urinal.

urodynamic (u″ro-di-nam′ik) pertaining to the flow and motion of liquids in the urinary tract.

urodynamics (u″ro-di-nam′iks) the dynamics of the propulsion and flow of urine in the urinary tract.

urodynia (u″ro-din′e-ah) [*uro-* + Gr. *odynē* pain + *-ia*] pain accompanying urination.

uroedema (u″ro-ĕ-de′mah″) edema due to infiltration of urine.

uroenterone (u″ro-en′ter-ōn) urogastrone.

uroerythrin (u″ro-er′ĭ-thrin) [*uro-* + Gr. *erythros* red] a dark reddish coloring matter found in the urine; it gives the red color seen in deposits of urates. Called also *purpurin*.

uroflavin (u″ro-fla′vin) a fluorescent compound closely related to riboflavin, excreted in the urine.

uroflometer, uroflowmeter (u″ro-flo′me-ter) a device for the continuous recording of urine flow in milliliters per second, consisting of a cylinder placed on a transducer that weighs the urine entering the cylinder and records it on a time scale.

urofuscin (u″ro-fus′in) [*uro-* + L. *fuscus* tawny] a pigment of the urine which is the precursor of hematoporphyrin.

urofuscohematin (u″ro-fus″ko-hem′ah-tin) a red-brown pigment from the urine in certain diseases.

urogaster (u″ro-gas′ter) [*uro-* + Gr. *gastēr* stomach] the urinary intestine; a part of the allantoic cavity of the embryo.

urogastrone (u″ro-gas′trōn) a polypeptide secreted by the salivary glands and by Brunner's glands, which is a potent inhibitor of gastric acid secretion; it is obtainable from the normal and pregnancy urine of man and other mammals; called also *anthelone U*.

urogenital (u″ro-jen′ĭ-tal) pertaining to the urinary and genital apparatus; genitourinary. See under *system*.

urogenous (u-roj′ĕ-nus) [*uro-* + Gr. *gennan* to produce] producing urine; also produced from or in the urine.

uroglaucin (u″ro-glaw′sin) [*uro-* + Gr. *glaukos* green] indigo blue occurring in the urine; it is due to oxidation of a colorless chromogen in the urine, and is seen in conditions such as scarlet fever.

Uroglena (u″ro-gle′nah) a genus of free-swimming, colonial, flagellate protozoa, of the order Chrysomonadina, family Ochromonadidae, which sometimes impart a fishy odor to a water supply.

Uroglenopsis (u″ro-gle-nop′sis) a genus of free-swimming, colonial, flagellate protozoa of the order Chrysomonadina, family Ochromonadidae, similar to *Uroglena* but without the connecting processes between individuals seen in the latter genus.

urogram (u′ro-gram) a roentgenogram of part of the urinary tract.

urography (u-rog′rah-fe) roentgenography of a part of the urinary tract which has been rendered opaque by some opaque medium. **ascending u.,** retrograde u. **cystoscopic u.,** retrograde u. **descending u., excretion u., excretory u., intravenous u.,** roentgen examination of the urinary tract after the intravenous injection of an opaque medium that is rapidly excreted in the urine. **oral u.,** urography in which the opaque medium is given by the mouth. **retrograde u.,** urography in which the contrast medium is injected into the bladder through the urethra.

urogravimeter (u″ro-grah-vim′ĕ-ter) [*uro-* + L. *gravis* heavy + *metrum* measure] urinometer.

urohematin (u″ro-hem′ah-tin) the coloring matter or pigments of the urine; regarded as identical with heme.

urohematonephrosis (u″ro-hem″ah-to-ne-fro′sis) distention of the kidney with urine and blood.

urohematoporphyrin (u″ro-hem″ah-to-por′fĭ-rin) hematoporphyrin derived from the urine.

urohypertensin (u″ro-hi-per-ten′sin) a mixture of bases obtained from the urine which acts as a pressor substance.

urokinase (u″ro-ki′nās) an enzyme found in the urine of mammals, including man, and of other vertebrates; it is elaborated by the parenchymal cells of the human kidney and functions as a plasminogen activator. It is used as a thrombolytic (fibrinolytic) agent.

urokinetic (u″ro-ki-net′ik) [*uro-* + Gr. *kinēsis* movement] caused by a reflex from the urinary organs; said of a form of dyspepsia.

urokymography (u″ro-ki-mog′rah-fe) kymography applied to study of the urogenital system.

urolagnia (u″ro-lag′ne-ah) [*uro-* + Gr. *lagneia* lust] a form of paraphilia in which sexual excitement is associated with the sight or thought of urine or urination.

urolith (u′ro-lith) [*uro-* + Gr. *lithos* stone] a urinary calculus or stone.

urolithiasis (u″ro-lĭ-thi′ah-sis) 1. the formation of urinary calculi. 2. the diseased condition associated with the presence of urinary calculi.

urolithic (u″ro-lith′ik) pertaining to urinary calculi.

urolithology (u″ro-lĭ-thol′o-je) the sum of knowledge regarding urinary calculi.

urologic, urological (u″ro-loj′ik; u″ro-loj′ĭ-kal) pertaining to urology.

urologist (u-rol′o-jist) a physician who specializes in urology.

urology (u-rol′o-je) that branch of medicine which concerns itself with the urinary tract in both male and female, and with the genital organs in the male.

urolutein (u″ro-lu′te-in) [*uro-* + L. *luteus* yellow] a yellow pigment of the urine.

uromancy (u′ro-man″se) [*uro-* + Gr. *manteia* a divination] prognosis based on examination of urine.

uromantia (u″ro-man′she-ah) uromancy.

uromelanin (u″ro-mel′ah-nin) [*uro-* + Gr. *melas* black] a black pigment, $C_{18}H_{43}N_7O_{10}$, sometimes found in urine; it results from the decomposition of urochrome.

uromelus (u-rom′e-lus) [Gr. *oura* tail + *melos* limb] a monster with fused legs and a single foot.

urometer (u-rom′ĕ-ter) [*uro-* + Gr. *metron* measure] urinometer.

urometric (u″ro-met′rik) pertaining to urometry.

urometry (u-rom′ĕ-tre) the measurement and recording of pressure changes caused by contraction of the ureter during ureteral peristalsis.

uromucoid (u″ro-mu′koid) an insoluble mucoprotein found in urine.

uronate (u′ro-nāt) a sugar in which the terminal alcohol group is oxidized to a carboxylate group.

uroncus (u-rong′kus) [*uro-* + Gr. *onkos* mass] a swelling containing urine.

Uronema caudatum (u″ro-ne′mah kaw-da′tum) a species of ciliate protozoa found in the feces; it is believed to be a free-living coprozoic contaminant.

uronephrosis (u″ro-ne-fro′sis) abnormal distention of the pelvis and tubules of the kidney with urine.

urono- see *uro-*.

uronology (u″ro-nol′o-je) urology.

urononcometry (u″ron-on-kom′ĕ-tre) [*urono-* + Gr. *onkos* mass

+ *metron* measure] the measurement of the quantity of urine excreted in twenty-four hours.

uronophile (u-ron′o-fīl) [*urono-* + Gr. *philein* to love] growing in a medium containing urine; said of a microorganism.

uronoscopy (u″ro-nos′ko-pe) examination of the urine.

uropathogen (u″ro-path′o-jen) a microorganism which causes diseases of the urinary tract.

uropathy (u-rop′ah-the) [*uro-* + Gr. *pathos* disease] any pathologic change in the urinary tract. **obstructive u.,** any pathologic change in the urinary tract due to obstruction.

uropenia (u″ro-pe′ne-ah) [*uro-* + Gr. *penia* poverty] deficiency of urine or urinary secretion.

uropepsin (u″ro-pep′sin) a pepsin-like enzyme occurring in the urine.

uropepsinogen (u″ro-pep-sin′o-jen) pepsinogen occurring in the urine.

urophanic (u″ro-fan′ik) [*uro-* + Gr. *phainein* to show] appearing in the urine.

urophein (u″ro-fe′in) [*uro-* + Gr. *phaios* gray] an odoriferous gray pigment of the urine.

urophobia (u″ro-fo′be-ah) fear of passing the urine.

urophosphometer (u″ro-fos-fom′ĕ-ter) an instrument for measuring the quantity of phosphorus in the urine.

uropittin (u″ro-pit′in) [*uro-* + Gr. *pitta* pitch] a resinous product, $C_9H_{10}N_2O_3$, of the decomposition of urochrome.

uroplania (u″ro-pla′ne-ah) [*uro-* + Gr. *planē* wandering + *-ia*] the presence of urine in, or its discharge from, organs not of the urogenital tract.

uropoiesis (u″ro-poi-e′sis) [*uro-* + Gr. *poiein* to make] the production of the urine.

uropoietic (u″ro-poi-et′ik) pertaining to or concerned in the production of the urine.

uroporphyria (u″ro-por-fir′e-ah) porphyria in which there is excessive excretion of uroporphyrin. **erythropoietic u.,** congenital erythropoietic porphyria.

uroporphyrin (u″ro-por′fĭ-rin) one of a group of porphyrins, $C_{40}H_{38}O_{16}N_4$, produced during biosynthesis of natural porphyrins. Their pyrrole groups, linked by methyne bridges, each have an acetate and propionate side chain. Urinary levels, normally low, are increased in porphyria. Uroporphyrin I differs from uroporphyrin III in having the acetate and propionate side chains interchanged at one of the pyrrole rings.

uroporphyrinogen (u″ro-por″fĭ-rin′o-jen) one of a group of porphyrins, precursors of uroporphyrins and of coproporphyrinogens. They are formed by the enzymatically catalyzed condensation of four porphobilinogen molecules, uroporphyrinogen I differing from uroporphyrinogen III in having one of the porphobilinogen residues reversed. Uroporphyrinogen III is also an intermediate in the biosynthesis of heme.

uropsammus (u″ro-sam′us) [*uro-* + Gr. *psammos* sand] sediment or gravel in the urine.

uropterin (u-rop′ter-in) a pigment, identical with xanthopterin, isolated from human urine; see *pterin*.

uropyonephrosis (u″ro-pi″o-nĕ-fro′sis) the presence of urine and pus in the pelvis of the kidney.

uropyoureter (u″ro-pi″o-u-re′ter) [*uro-* + Gr. *pyon* pus + *oureter* ureter] a collection of urine and pus in the ureter.

uroradiology (u″ro-ra″de-ol′o-je) radiology of the urinary tract.

urorhythmography (u″ro-rith-mog′rah-fe) [*uro-* + Gr. *rhythmos* rhythm + *graphein* to write] graphic registration of the ejaculation of the urine from the ureteral orifices.

urorosein (u″ro-ro′ze-in) urorrhodin.

uroroseinogen (u″ro-ro′se-in′o-jen) urorrhodinogen.

urorrhagia (u″ro-ra′je-ah) [*uro-* + Gr. *rhēgnynai* to burst forth] an excessive flow of urine; diabetes.

urorrhea (u″ro-re′ah) [*uro-* + Gr. *rhoia* flow] an involuntary discharge of urine; enuresis.

urorrhodin (u″ro-ro′din) [*uro-* + Gr. *rhodon* rose] a rose-colored pigment found in the urine in typhoid fever, nephritis, pulmonary tuberculosis, and other diseases. See under *tests*.

urorrhodinogen (u″ro-ro-din′o-jen) [urorrhodin + Gr. *gennan* to produce] a chromogen in the urine which, on decomposition, yields urorrhodin.

urorubin (u″ro-roo′bin) [*uro-* + L. *ruber* red] a red pigment derivable from the urine by the action of hydrochloric acid.

urorubinogen (u″ro-roo-bin′o-jen) a chromogen from which urorubin is derived.

urorubrohematin (u″ro-roo″bro-hem′ah-tin) [*uro-* + L. *ruber* red + *hematin*] a red pigment rarely found in the urine in certain constitutional diseases, as leprosy.

urosaccharometry (u″ro-sak″ah-rom′ĕ-tre) the measurement or estimation of sugar in the urine.

urosacin (u-ro′sa-sin) urorrhodin.

uroscheocele (u-ros′ke-o-sēl″) [*uro-* + Gr. *oscheon* scrotum + *kēlē* tumor] urocele.

uroschesis (u-ros′kĕ-sis) [*uro-* + Gr. *schesis* holding] retention of the urine.

uroscopic (u″ro-skop′ik) pertaining to uroscopy.

uroscopy (u-ros′ko-pe) [*uro-* + Gr. *skopein* to examine] diagnostic examination of the urine.

urosemiology (u″ro-se″me-ol′o-je) diagnostic study of the urine.

urosepsin (u″ro-sep′sin) a septic poison arising from urine in the tissues.

urosepsis (u″ro-sep′sis) [*uro-* + Gr. *sēpsis* decay] septic poisoning from the absorption and decomposition of urinary substances in the tissues.

uroseptic (u″ro-sep′tik) pertaining to or marked by urosepsis.

urosis (u-ro′sis) any disease of the urinary apparatus.

urospectrin (u″ro-spek′trin) [*uro-* + L. *spectrum* image] one of the pigments of normal urine; a substance obtainable from certain specimens of urine, allied to hematoporphyrin.

urostalagmometry (u″ro-stal″ag-mom′ĕ-tre) the use of the stalagmometer in the study of the urine.

urostealith (u″ro-ste′ah-lith) [*uro-* + Gr. *stear* fat + *lithos* stone] a fatty constituent of certain urinary calculi; a urinary calculus having fatty constituents.

urothelial (u″ro-the′le-al) pertaining to the urothelium.

urothelium (u″ro-the′le-um) the epithelium of the urinary bladder.

urotoxia (u″ro-tok′se-ah) [*uro-* + Gr. *toxikon* poison] 1. the toxicity of the urine. 2. the toxic substances of the urine. 3. the unit of the toxicity of the urine or a quantity sufficient to kill 1 kg. of living substance.

urotoxic (u″ro-tok′sik) pertaining to the toxic materials of the urine.

urotoxicity (u″ro-toks-is′ĭ-te) the toxic quality of the urine.

urotoxin (u″ro-tok′sin) the toxic or poisonous constituents of the urine.

urotoxy (u′ro-tok″se) urotoxia.

Urotropin (u-rot′ro-pin) trademark for a preparation of methenamine.

uroureter (u″ro-u-re′ter) distention of the ureter with urine.

uroxanthin (u″ro-zan′thin) [*uro-* + Gr. *xanthos* yellow] a yellow pigment of normal urine convertible into indigo blue.

uroxin (u-rok′sin) alloxantin.

urrhodin (u-ro′din) urorrhodin.

ursone (ur′sōn) ursolic acid; a crystallizable triterpene, $C_{30}H_{48}O_3$, from waxlike coatings of fruits (e.g., apples and pears) and leaves (e.g., rhododendron and uva ursi).

Urtica (ur-ti′kah) [L.] a genus of plants, including the true or typical nettles; plants covered with stinging hairs and secreting a poisonous fluid. **U. dio′ica,** a stinging nettle of temperate regions having stimulant, diuretic, and hemostatic properties.

urtica (ur-ti′kah), pl. *urti′cae* [L., "a stinging nettle"] (*obs.*) a wheal or pomphus.

urticant (ur′tĭ-kant) causing an itching or stinging sensation, or creating a wheal, or both.

urticaria (ur″tĭ-ka′re-ah) [L. *urtica* stinging nettle + *-ia*] a vascular reaction of the skin marked by the transient appearance of smooth, slightly elevated patches (wheals) which are redder or paler than the surrounding skin and often attended by severe itching. The eruption rarely lasts longer than two days, but may exist in a chronic form. Certain foods (e.g., shellfish), drugs (e.g., penicillin), infection, or emotional stress may be the exciting cause. Called also *hives*. **acute u.,** the sudden appearance of extensive wheals of relatively brief duration, as after insect bites or administration of drugs. **u. bullo′sa,** a rare form of urticaria characterized by the appearance of bullae. **cholinergic u.,** urticaria often associated with sweating, characterized by minute, pruritic, pale, punctate papules surrounded by areas of erythema, and produced by the action of acetylcholine or mast cells; it occurs in susceptible persons under conditions of exertion, emotional stress, or in increased environmental heat. **chronic u.,** urticaria in recurrent episodes over weeks or months; called also *recurrent u.* **cold u.,** edema and whealing of body areas exposed to the cold, a hypersensitivity reaction mediated by histamine. **endemic u., u. endem′ica,** a very rare variety caused by certain species of caterpillar, and occurring as an endemic. **epidemic u., u. epidem′ica,** a severe and very rare form ascribed to caterpillar poisoning. **u. facti′tia** (*obs.*), dermatographism. **giant u., u. gigan′tea,** angioneurotic edema. **heat u.,** generalized urticaria associated with cramps, weakness, flushing, and collapse, probably mediated by acetylcholine. **u. hemorrhag′ica,** purpura with urticaria. **heredofamilial u.,** urticaria associated with chills and fever during adolescence, followed years later by deafness, arthralgia, and nephropathy. **u. medicamento′sa,** urticaria caused by the use of a drug. **u. multifor′mis endem′ica,** harara. **papular u., u. papulo′sa,** a condition occurring in temperate parts of the world, usually seen in children, caused by the bites of fleas, bedbugs, and other insects, and representing a stage in the development of hypersensitization to them. **peptone u.,** urticaria attributed to overeating; the peptones, being absorbed before they are sufficiently digested, affect capillary permeability, producing hives. **u. photogen′ica,** solar u. **u. pigmento′sa,** mastocytosis manifested as persistent pink to brown macules or soft plaques of various size, the irritation of which results in localized pruritus and urtication (Darier's sign). **u. pigmento′sa, juvenile,** urticaria pigmentosa present at birth or occurring in the first few weeks of life. It may take the form of a single tumor or nodule (solitary mastocytoma), often on the back of the hand, or it may appear as a disseminated eruption of yellowish brown to yellowish red macules, plaques, or bullae. It usually disappears before puberty but may, rarely, continue into adulthood. **pressure u.,** that caused by prolonged pressure on the skin, as in sitting on a hard chair, but appearing after a latent period of many hours. **recurrent u.,** chronic u. **solar u., u. sola′ris,** a rare form of urticaria produced by exposure to sunlight; called also *photogenic u.* **u. subcuta′nea, subcutaneous u.,** a form manifested as subcutaneous edema instead of surface wheals; see also *angioneurotic edema,* under *edema.*

urticarial (ur″tĭ-ka′re-al) pertaining to, characterized by, or of the nature of urticaria.

urticariogenic (ur″tĭ-ka′re-o-jen′ik) causing urticaria.

urticarious (ur″tĭ-ka′re-us) urticarial.

urticate (ur′tĭ-kāt) 1. marked by the presence of wheals. 2. to perform urtication.

urtication (ur″tĭ-ka′shun) [L. *urtica* a stinging nettle] 1. the development or formation of urticaria. 2. a burning sensation as of stinging with nettles. 3. (*obs.*) the flogging of a part with green nettles for their revulsive or stimulant effect.

urushiol (u-roo′she-ol) the chief constituent of the irritant oil of *Rhus* (*Toxicodendron*) *radicans* L. (poison ivy), *R. diversiloba* L. (poison oak), *R. vernix* L., and related plants, consisting of a mixture of several oleoresins.

USAN (u′san) acronym for *United States Adopted Names,* a nonproprietary designation for any compound used as a drug, established by negotiation between the manufacturer of the compound and a nomenclature committee known as the USAN Council, which is sponsored jointly by the American Medical Association, the American Pharmaceutical Association, and The United States Pharmacopeial Convention. A liaison representative of the United States Food and Drug Administration sits on the USAN Council. The term is currently limited to names adopted by the Council since June, 1961. These names will appear as the monograph titles in the official compendia, U.S.P. and N.F., when and if the respective drugs are admitted to either compendium.

Uschinsky's culture medium (us-chin′skēz) [Nikolaus *Uschinsky,* Leningrad bacteriologist, 1863–1934] see *asparagin culture medium* (def. 2) and *protein-free culture medium,* under *culture medium.*

U.S.M.H. United States Marine Hospital.

Usnea barbata (us′ne-ah bar-ba′tah) a large lichen growing on forest trees; also its homeopathic preparation. The active ingredients include usnic acid (usnein), $C_{18}H_{16}O_7$, which has antibacterial activity. The crude plant is used as a dressing for wounds.

usnein (us′ne-in) usnic acid.

U.S.P. the United States Pharmacopeia, a legally recognized compendium of standards for drugs, published by The United States Pharmacopeial Convention, Inc., and revised periodically. It includes also assays and tests for the determination of strength, quality, and purity.

U.S.P.H.S. United States Public Health Service.

Ustilaginales (us″tĭ-laj′ĭ-na′lēz) an order of basidiomycetous fungi of the subclass Heterobasidiomycetidae, which includes the family Tilletiaceae.

ustilaginism (us″tĭ-laj′ĭ-nizm) a condition resembling ergotism caused by eating maize containing *Ustilago maydis.*

Ustilago (us″tĭ-la′go) [L.] a genus of basidiomycetous fungi of the order Ustilaginales, family Ustilaginaceae, called smuts, parasitic on plants. **U. hypody′tes,** a smut fungus on various grasses thought to be a cause of friente. **U. may′dis,** a fungus causing corn smut; the ingestion of infected seeds causes ustilaginism, a condition similar to ergotism.

ustion (us′chun) [L. *ustio*] burning with the actual cautery.

ustulation (us″tu-la′shun) [L. *ustulare* to scorch] the drying of a moist drug by heat.

ustus (us′tus) [L.] burnt; calcined.

usustatus (u-su′sta-tus) [L. *usus* use + *status* position] the ordinary erect or standing posture usual to an animal.

uta (oo′tah) a form of cutaneous leishmaniasis of the New World occurring in the Peruvian Andes, caused by *Leishmania peruviana* (considered by some to be a subspecies of *L. brasiliensis*), transmitted by *Lutzomyia verrucarum* and *L. peruensis,* and characterized by single or few skin lesions.

Ut dict. abbreviation for L. *ut dic′tum,* as directed.

Utend. abbreviation for L. *uten'dus*, to be used.

uteralgia (u″ter-al'je-ah) metralgia or metrodynia.

uteri (u'ter-i) [L.] plural and genitive of *uterus*.

uterine (u'ter-in) [L. *uterinus*] of or pertaining to the uterus.

uteroabdominal (u″ter-o-ab-dom'ĭ-nal) pertaining to the uterus and the abdomen.

uterocervical (u″ter-o-ser'vĭ-kal) pertaining to the uterus and the cervix uteri.

uterodynia (u″ter-o-din'e-ah) metralgia or metrodynia.

uterofixation (u″ter-o-fik-sa'shun) hysteropexy.

uterogenic (u″ter-o-jen'ik) formed in the uterus.

uterogestation (u″ter-o-jes-ta'shun) [*uterus* + L. *gestatio* a carrying] 1. uterine pregnancy; any pregnancy which is not extrauterine. 2. the full period of time of normal pregnancy.

uteroglobulin (u″ter-o-glob'u-lin) blastokinin.

uterography (u″ter-og'rah-fe) hysterography.

uterolith (u'ter-o-lith″) [*uterus* + Gr. *lithos* stone] a hysterolith.

uterometer (u″ter-om'ĕ-ter) an instrument for measuring the uterus.

uterometry (u″ter-om'ĕ-tre) measurement of the uterus.

utero-ovarian (u″ter-o-o-va're-an) pertaining to the uterus and ovary.

uteropexy (u'ter-o-pek″se) hysteropexy.

uteroplacental (u″ter-o-plah-sen'tal) pertaining to the uterus and the placenta.

uteroplasty (u'ter-o-plas″te) any plastic operation on the uterus.

uterorectal (u″ter-o-rek'tal) pertaining to the uterus and rectum, or communicating with the uterine cavity and rectum, as a uterorectal fistula.

uterosacral (u″ter-o-sa'kral) pertaining to the uterus and the sacrum.

uterosalpingography (u″ter-o-sal″ping-gog'rah-fe) hysterosalpingography.

uterosclerosis (u″ter-o-sklĕ-ro'sis) sclerosis of the uterus.

uteroscope (u'ter-o-skōp″) [*uterus* + Gr. *skopein* to examine] hysteroscope.

uterothermometry (u″ter-o-ther-mom'ĕ-tre) the measurement of the temperature in the uterus.

uterotomy (u″ter-ot'o-me) hysterotomy.

uterotonic (u″ter-o-ton'ik) 1. giving muscular tone to the uterus. 2. an agent that increases the tonus of the uterine muscle.

uterotropic (u″ter-o-trop'ik) having a special affinity for or exerting its principal influence upon the uterus.

uterotubal (u″ter-o-tu'bal) pertaining to the uterus and the oviducts.

uterotubography (u″ter-o-tu-bog'rah-fe) hysterosalpingography.

uterovaginal (u″ter-o-vaj'ĭ-nal) pertaining to the uterus and the vagina.

uteroventral (u″ter-o-ven'tral) pertaining to the uterus and the cavity of the abdomen.

uteroverdin (u″ter-o-ver'din) a term once applied to biliverdin when occurring in the placenta or in the eggs of some birds.

uterovesical (u″ter-o-ves'ĭ-kal) pertaining to the uterus and the bladder.

uterus (u'ter-us), pl. *u'teri* [L.; Gr. *hystera*] the hollow muscular organ in female mammals in which the fertilized ovum normally becomes embedded and in which the developing embryo and fetus is nourished. In the nongravid human [NA], it is a pear-shaped structure, about 3 inches in length, consisting of a body, fundus, isthmus, and cervix. Its cavity opens into the vagina below, and into the uterine tube on either side above. It is supported by direct attachment to the vagina and by indirect attachment to various other nearby pelvic structures. **u. acol'lis,** a uterus in which the vaginal portion is absent. **u. arcua'tus,** a uterus with a depressed fundus. **u. bicamera'tus vetula'rum,** a uterus in which the cervical orifices are closed by adhesions, resulting in distention of the cervix and corpus uteri. **u. bicor'nis,** a uterus which has two horns, or cornua. **u. bicor'nis bicol'lis,** a uterus with two horns and two cervices. **u. bicor'nis unicol'lis,** a uterus with two horns and a single cervix. **u. bif'oris,** a uterus in which the external os is divided by a septum. **u. bilocula'ris,** a uterus the cavity of which is divided into two parts by a partition. **u. biparti'tus,** u. bilocularis. **cochleate u.,** a small adult uterus with a conical cervix and body which is small, globular, and acutely flexed. **u. cordifor'mis,** a heart-shaped uterus. **Couvelaire u.,** see *uteroplacental apoplexy,* under *apoplexy.* **u. didel'phys,** either of two distinct uteri occurring side by side in the same individual. **duplex u., u. du'plex,** a double uterus; normal in marsupial mammals, and rarely seen in the human subject. **fetal u.,** a uterus in which the cervical canal is longer than the cavity of the corpus. **gravid u.,** the pregnant uterus. **u. incudifor'mis,** a uterus

bicornis which is broad between the two horns. **infantile u.,** pubescent u. **u. masculi'nus,** utriculus prostaticus. **u. parvicol'lis,** a uterus in which the cervical portion is very small, but the corpus is of normal size. **u. planifunda'lis,** u. incudiformis. **pubescent u.,** one which is adult in type but is undeveloped; called also *infantile u.* **ribbon u.,** an aplastic uterus found as a transverse ribbon of fibromuscular tissue between the blind ends of the uterine tubes and the bladder. **u. rudimenta'rius,** a hypoplastic uterus measuring 1 to 3 cm. in length; affected women are amenorrheic and sterile. **saddle-shaped u.,** u. arcuatus. **u. sep'tus,** u. bilocularis. **u. simplex,** one that is single throughout its length, as in the human. **u. subsep'tus,** u. bicornis. **u. triangula'ris,** u. incudiformis. **u. unicor'nis,** one with only one cornu, one lateral half being undeveloped or imperfectly developed.

Utibid (u'tĭ-bid) trademark for a preparation of oxolinic acid.

Uticillin VK (u″tĭ-sil'in) trademark for a preparation of penicillin V potassium.

UTP uridine triphosphate.

utricle (u'tre-k'l) [L. *utriculus*] 1. any small sac. 2. the larger of the two divisions of the membranous labyrinth; see *utriculus,* def. 2. **prostatic u., urethral u.,** utriculus prostaticus.

utricular (u-trik'u-lar) 1. pertaining to a utricle. 2. resembling a bladder.

utriculi (u-trik'u-li) [L.] plural of *utriculus*.

utriculitis (u-trik″u-li'tis) inflammation of the prostatic utricle or of the utricle of the ear.

utriculosaccular (u-trik″u-lo-sak'u-lar) pertaining to the utricle and saccule of the labyrinth.

utriculus (u-trik'u-lus), pl. *utric'uli* [L., dim. of *uter*] 1. a small sac. 2. [NA] the larger of the two divisions of the membranous labyrinth, located in the posterosuperior region of the vestibule. It is the major organ of the vestibular system, which gives information about position and movements of the head. Called also *utricle* and *utriculus vestibuli.* **u. masculi'nus,** u. prostaticus. **u. prostat'icus** [NA], prostatic utricle: the remains of the lower part of the paramesonephric duct in the male; it is a small blind pouch arising in the prostatic substance and opening onto the seminal colliculus. **u. vestib'uli,** utriculus (def. 2).

utriform (u'trĭ-form) having the shape of a bottle.

uva (u'vah), pl. *u'vae* [L. "grape"] the raisin; the dried fruit of *Vitis vinifera* L. (Vitaceae), grape vine. **u. ur'si** L. (Ericaceae) [L. "bear's grapes"], the leaves of *Arctostaphylos uva-ursi,* or bearberry, a trailing ericaceous shrub; used medicinally as astringent, diuretic tea.

Uval (u'val) trademark for preparations of sulisobenzone.

uvea (u've-ah) the vascular middle coat of the eye, comprising the iris, ciliary body, and choroid (tunica vasculosa bulbi [NA]).

uveal (u've-al) pertaining to the uvea.

uveitic (u″ve-it'ik) pertaining to uveitis.

uveitis (u″ve-i'tis) [*uvea* + *-itis*] inflammation of the uvea. **anterior u.,** uveitis involving the structures of the iris and/or ciliary body; iridocyclitis. **Förster's u.,** syphilitic involvement of the entire uvea. **granulomatous u.,** uveitis of any part of the uveal tract but particularly the posterior portion, characterized by nodular collections of epithelioid cells and giant cells surrounded by lymphocytes. **heterochromic u.,** see under *iridocyclitis.* **lens-induced u.,** an acute intraocular inflammation resulting from the escape of lens matter through an opening in the lens capsule; called also *phacogenic u.* See also *phacolytic u.* **nongranulomatous u.,** inflammation of the anterior portion of the uveal tract (iris and ciliary body). **phacolytic u.,** uveitis secondary to leakage of lens material into the aqueous from a hypermature cataract. **phacotoxic u.,** lens-induced u. **posterior u.,** uveitis involving the posterior segment of the eye, including choroiditis and chorioretinitis. **sympathetic u.,** see under *ophthalmia.* **toxoplasmic u.,** chorioretinitis as a complication of toxoplasmosis. **tuberculous u.,** granulomatous uveitis due to infection with the tubercle bacillus, usually a severe caseating granulomatous chorioretinitis.

uveolabyrinthitis (u″ve-o-lah″bĭ-rin-thi'tis) uveitis associated with labyrinthitis.

uveomeningitis (u've-o-men″in-ji'tis) a disorder characterized by lesions of the uvea accompanied by meningeal signs; see *Harada's disease* and *Vogt-Koyanagi syndrome.*

uveoneuraxitis (u″ve-o-nu″raks-i'tis) uveitis associated with involvement of the optic nerve.

uveoparotid (u″ve-o-pah-rot'id) affecting the uvea and the parotid gland; see under *fever.*

uveoparotitis (u″ve-o-par″o-ti'tis) uveoparotid fever.

uveoscleritis (u″ve-o-skle-ri'tis) scleritis resulting from an extension of the inflammation from the uvea to the sclera.

uviform (u'vĭ-form) [L. *uva* grape + *forma* form] having the form of a grape.

uviofast (u've-o-fast″) uvioresistant.

uviolize (u've-o-līz) to subject to the action of ultraviolet rays.

uviometer (u″ve-om′ĕ-ter) an instrument for measuring ultraviolet emanation.

uvioresistant (u″ve-o-re-zis′tant) resistant to or not affected by ultraviolet rays.

uviosensitive (u″ve-o-sen′sĭ-tiv) sensitive to ultraviolet rays.

uvula (u′vu-lah), pl. *u′vulae* [L. "little grape"] a pendent, fleshy mass; used as a general term in anatomical terminology. Usually used alone to designate the *uvula palatina*. **bifid u.**, a split uvula. **u. of bladder,** u. vesicae. **u. cerebel′li, u. of cerebellum,** u. vermis. **u. fis′sa,** a forked or split uvula. **Lieutaud's u.,** u. vesicae. **u. palati′na** [NA], **palatine u.,** the small, fleshy mass hanging from the soft palate above the root of the tongue, composed of the levator and tensor palati muscles and the muscle of the uvula, connective tissue, and mucous membrane. **u. ver′mis** [NA], the part of the vermis of the cerebellum between the pyramis and the nodulus; called also *u. of cerebellum.* **u. vesi′cae** [NA], a rounded elevation at the neck of the bladder, formed by convergence of many fibers of the trigonal muscle as they pass through the encircling musculus sphincter vesicae to terminate in the urethra. Called also *u. of bladder.*

uvulaptosis (u″vu-lap-to′sis) uvuloptosis.

uvular (u′vu-lar) pertaining to the uvula; staphyline.

uvularis (u″vu-la′ris) [L.] uvular.

uvulatome (u′vu-lah-tōm) uvulotome.

uvulatomy (u″vu-lat′o-me) uvulotomy.

uvulectomy (u″vu-lek′to-me) [*uvula* + Gr. *ektomē* excision] excision of the uvula; cionectomy.

uvulitis (u″vu-li′tis) [*uvula* + *-itis*] inflammation of the uvula; staphylitis.

uvuloptosis (u″vu-lop-to′sis) [*uvula* + Gr. *ptōsis* falling] falling of the palate: a relaxed and pendulous condition of the palate; staphyloptosia.

uvulotome (u′vu-lo-tōm) an instrument for cutting the uvula; staphylotome.

uvulotomy (u″vu-lot′o-me) [*uvula* + Gr. *tomē* a cutting] the operation of cutting off the uvula or a part of it.

uzara (u-zah′rah) the dried root of a species of *Gomphocarpus* (Asclepiadaceae), an African plant; used by certain natives in diarrhea and dysentery. It is the source of uzarin.

uzarin (u-zar′in) a constituent of uzara, $C_{35}H_{54}O_{14}$, which has antidiarrheal properties.

V

V chemical symbol for *vanadium.*

V. *Vibrio;* vision; visual acuity.

v. abbreviation for L. *vena* vein, and for *volt.*

V_T symbol for *tidal volume* (in pulmonary ventilation).

VA visual acuity.

V.A. Veterans Administration.

vaccigenous (vak-sij′ĕ-nus) [*vaccine* + Gr. *gennan* to produce] producing vaccine.

vaccin (vak′sin) vaccine.

vaccina (vak-si′nah) vaccinia.

vaccinable (vak-sin′ah-b'l) susceptible of being successfully vaccinated.

vaccinal (vak′sĭ-nal) [L. *vaccinus*] 1. pertaining to vaccinia, to vaccine, or to vaccination. 2. having protective qualities when used by way of inoculation.

vaccinate (vak′sĭ-nāt) to inoculate with vaccine for the purpose of producing immunity.

vaccination (vak″sĭ-na′shun) [L. *vacca* cow] the introduction of vaccine into the body for the purpose of inducing immunity. Coined originally to apply to the injection of smallpox vaccine, the term has come to mean any immunizing procedure in which vaccine is injected. **smallpox v.,** the application of smallpox vaccine upon the denuded or scarified skin, to produce immunity to smallpox.

vaccinationist (vak″sĭ-na′shun-ist) one who defends the practice of vaccination.

vaccinator (vak′sĭ-na″tor) 1. one who vaccinates. 2. an instrument for use in vaccination.

vaccine (vak′sēn) [L. *vaccinus*] a suspension of attenuated or killed microorganisms (bacteria, viruses, or rickettsiae), administered for the prevention, amelioration, or treatment of infectious diseases. **anthrax v.,** anthrax cultures attenuated by growing them at 42° C. for varying lengths of time and injected into horses, cattle, sheep, and goats to protect them against anthrax. It is a triple vaccine: No. 1 is the weakest and is given first; Nos. 2 and 3 are progressively stronger and are given after intervals of twelve days. **antirabic v.,** rabies v. **antityphoid v.,** typhoid v. **attenuated v.,** a vaccine prepared from live microorganisms or viruses cultured under adverse conditions leading to loss of their virulence but retention of their ability to induce protective immunity. **autogenous v.,** a vaccine prepared from microorganisms which have been freshly isolated from the lesion of the patient who is to be treated with it. **avian embryo v.,** a vaccine prepared from embryonate avian eggs infected with inactivated fixed virus. **bacterial v.,** a standardized suspension of attenuated or killed bacteria which is injected subcutaneously, intramuscularly or intradermally, to increase the patient's immunity to the organisms injected, or sometimes for pyrogenetic effects in treatment of certain noninfectious diseases. **BCG v.** (bacille Calmette-Guérin) [USP], a preparation used as an active immunizing agent against tuberculosis, consisting of a dried, living culture of the Calmette-Guérin strain of *Mycobacterium bovis,* which is grown on a suitable medium from a seed strain of known history that has been maintained to preserve its capacity for conferring immunity. It is usually administered intradermally, but may also be given by multiple punctures with a special instrument, or by scarification through a suspension, applied to the skin. Called also *Calmette's v.* and *tuberculosis v.* **brucellosis v.,** a vaccine made from an avirulent variant of

Brucella abortus, said to reduce the incidence of bovine brucellosis. **Calmette's v.,** BCG v. **caprinized v.,** a vaccine prepared from microorganisms that have been attenuated by passage in goats. **cholera v.** [USP], a sterile suspension, in isotonic sodium chloride solution or other suitable diluent, of killed cholera vibrios (*Vibrio cholerae*), prepared from equal portions of suspensions of cholera vibrios of the Inaba and Ogawa strains, and containing, at the time of manufacture, 8 billion cholera vibrios in each milliliter. Used as an active immunizing agent against cholera, it is administered subcutaneously or intramuscularly. **Cox v.,** typhus v. **crystal violet v.,** a vaccine prepared from the virus of hog cholera in pig's blood, attenuated by exposure to the dyestuff crystal violet; used for immunizing young pigs against hog cholera. **diphtheria v.,** see under *toxoid.* **diphtheria and tetanus toxoids and pertussis v.** [USP], a sterile suspension of killed *Bordetella pertussis* in a mixture of diphtheria toxoid and tetanus toxoid, the components being combined in such proportions as to yield a mixture that meets the antigenic and other requirements of each separate component; used as an active immunizing agent, administered subcutaneously. **diphtheria and tetanus toxoids and pertussis v. adsorbed** [USP], a sterile suspension of the precipitate obtained by treating a mixture of diphtheria toxoid, tetanus toxoid, and pertussis vaccine with alum, aluminum hydroxide, or aluminum phosphate, the components being combined in such proportions as to yield a mixture containing an immunizing dose of each in the total dosage prescribed on the label; used as an active immunizing agent, administered intramuscularly. **duck embryo v.,** vaccine prepared from embryonate duck eggs infected with inactivated fixed virus. **glycerinated v.,** vaccine material purified by treatment with glycerin. **heterologous v.,** a vaccine that confers protective immunity against a pathogen not present in the vaccine, because it contains microorganisms that possess cross-reacting antigens which they share in common with that pathogen. For example, vaccinia virus protects against smallpox. Called also *heterotypic v.* **heterotypic v.,** heterologous v. **hydrophobia v.,** rabies v. **inactivated v.,** a vaccine containing nonreplicating microorganisms or viruses which are noninfectious but which retain their protective antigens. Viral vaccines are usually inactivated by agents such as formalin, phenol, or β-propiolactone; bacterial vaccines by heat, acetone, ultraviolet rays, formaldehyde, or phenol. **influenza virus v.** [USP], a sterile, aqueous suspension of suitably inactivated influenza virus prepared from the extraembryonic fluid of influenza virus–infected chick embryo; it may contain an adsorbent, such as aluminum phosphate or protamine. It is an active immunizing agent, administered intramuscularly or subcutaneously. **live v.,** a vaccine prepared from live microorganisms or viruses that have been attenuated but that retain their immunogenic properties. **measles virus v., inactivated,** an aqueous suspension of suitable measles virus grown on either chicken embryo or monkey renal tissue cultures and inactivated by a suitable method; it has been administered intramuscularly as an active immunizing agent but the live attenuated measles virus vaccine is usually preferred. **measles virus v., live attenuated** [USP], a bacterially sterile preparation of live virus derived from a strain of measles virus suitable for human immunization, grown on cultures of either chicken embryo or canine renal tissue cultures; used as an active immunizing agent, administered subcutaneously. **measles and rubella virus v., live** [USP], a bacterially sterile preparation of a combination of live measles and rubella viruses found suitable for human immunization; the measles virus is grown on cultures of chicken embryo tissue and the rubella virus on cultures of duck embryo tissue. Used as an active immunizing agent, administered subcutaneously. **measles, mumps, and rubella virus v., live** [USP], a bacterially sterile preparation of a combination of the live measles, mumps, and rubella vaccines found suitable for human immunization, grown on cultures of either chicken or duck embryo tissue; used as an active immunizing agent, administered subcutaneously. **mixed v.,** polyvalent v. **mumps virus v., inactivated** [NF], a sterile suspension of killed mumps virus, prepared from the extraembryonic fluid of the virus-infected chick embryo tissue and concentrated and purified by differential centrifugation; used as an immunizing agent, administered subcutaneously. **mumps virus v., live** [USP], a bacterially sterile preparation of live virus derived from a strain of mumps virus suitable for human immunization, grown on chicken-embryo tissue culture; used as an active immunizing agent, administered subcutaneously. **pertussis v.** [USP], a sterile bacterial fraction or suspension, in an isotonic sodium chloride solution or other suitable diluent, of killed pertussis bacilli (*Bordetella pertussis*) of a strain or strains selected for high antigenic efficiency; used as an active immunizing agent, administered subcutaneously. **pertussis v. adsorbed** [USP], a sterile bacterial fraction or suspension, in a suitable diluent, of killed pertussis bacilli (*Bordetella pertussis*) of a strain or strains selected for high antigenic efficiency and precipitated or adsorbed by the addition of aluminum hydroxide or aluminum phosphate, and resuspended; used as an active immunizing agent, administered intramuscularly. **plague v.** [USP], a sterile suspension, in an isotonic sodium chloride solution or other suitable diluent, of killed plague bacilli (*Pasteurella pestis*) of a strain selected for high antigenic efficiency, and containing approximately 2 billion plague bacilli in each milliliter; used as an active immunizing agent, administered subcutaneously. Called also *vaccinum pestis*. **poliomyelitis v., polymyelitis v. inactivated** [USP], a sterile suspension of inactivated poliovirus of Types 1, 2, and 3, which are grown separately in primary cultures of monkey kidney tissue, and after inactivation are combined in suitable proportions; used as an active immunizing agent, administered intramuscularly and subcutaneously. Called also *Salk v.* See also *poliovirus v. live oral.* **poliovirus v. live oral** [USP], a preparation of one or a combination of the three types of live, attenuated polioviruses, grown separately in primary cultures of monkey kidney tissue; used as an active immunizing agent against poliomyelitis, it is administered orally. Called also *Sabin oral v.* **polyvalent v.,** a vaccine prepared from cultures or antigens of more than one strain or species. **rabies v.** [USP], a sterile preparation, in liquid or in dried form, of killed fixed virus of rabies, obtained from brain tissue of rabbits or from duck embryos, which have been infected with fixed rabies virus. It is used as an active immunizing agent in patients infected or contaminated with rabies virus, being administered subcutaneously daily for a minimum of 14 days. Called also *antirabies v.* and *hydrophobia v.* See also *Semple v.* **replicative v.,** any vaccine containing organisms that are able to reproduce, including live and attenuated viruses and bacteria. **Rocky Mountain spotted fever v.** [USP], a sterile, aqueous suspension of inactivated *Rickettsia rickettsii*, prepared by growing the virus in the embryonic tissues of the domestic fowl, *Gallus domesticus;* used as an active immunizing agent, administered subcutaneously. **rubella virus v., live** [USP], a bacterially sterile preparation of live rubella virus found suitable for human immunization, grown on cultures of either duck embryo tissue or rabbit kidney tissue; used as an active immunizing agent, administered subcutaneously. **rubella and mumps virus v., live** [USP], a bacterially sterile preparation of a combination of live rubella and mumps viruses found suitable for human immunization; the rubella virus is grown on cultures of duck embryo tissue, and the mumps virus on chicken embryo tissue. Used as an active immunizing agent, administered subcutaneously. **Sabin's oral v.,** see *poliovirus v. live oral.* **Salk v.,** poliomyelitis v. inactivated. **Sauer's v.,** a pertussis vaccine prepared from freshly isolated strains of *Bordetella pertussis;* used in immunizing children against whooping cough. **Semple v.,** an antirabies vaccine prepared from 4 per cent inoculated rabbit brain treated with 0.5 per cent phenol. **sensitized v.,** a vaccine consisting of bacteria which have been immersed in their specific immune serum. Such a vaccine is believed to cause no negative phase, but only a slight local reaction and to facilitate the antibody formation. **smallpox v.** [USP], the living virus of vaccinia (cowpox) that has been grown in the skin of a vaccinated bovine calf or in the membranes of the chick embryo, and is available in liquid or dried form. It is used as an active immunizing agent against smallpox, being administered by multiple punctures, with a special instrument, through a suspension applied to the skin. Called also *vaccinum vacciniae* and *vaccinum variolae.* **Sobernheim's v.,** a vaccine consisting of virulent *Bacillus anthracis* mixed with antiserum; used for immunization of cattle against anthrax. **Spencer-Parker v.,** a vaccine for Rocky Mountain spotted fever, prepared from ground infected ticks. **staphylococcus v.,** a bacterial vaccine prepared from one or more strains of staphylococci. **streptococcus v.,** a bacterial vaccine made from cultures of streptococci. **TAB v.,** typhoid and paraty-

phoid v. **triple v.,** a vaccine prepared from the cultures of three different species of organisms. **tuberculosis v.,** BCG v. **typhoid v.** [USP], a sterile suspension, in buffered isotonic sodium chloride solution or other suitable diluent, of killed typhoid bacilli (*Salmonella typhosa*) of a strain selected for high antigenic efficiency, and containing approximately 1 billion typhoid bacilli in each milliliter; used as an active immunizing agent, administered subcutaneously. Called also *antityphoid v., typhobacterin, vaccinum antityphicum,* and *vaccinum typhosum.* **typhoid and paratyphoid v.,** a sterile suspension in buffered, isotonic sodium chloride solution or other suitable diluent, of killed typhoid bacilli (*Salmonella typhosa*) of a strain selected for high antigenic efficiency, killed paratyphoid A bacilli (*S. paratyphi A*), and killed paratyphoid B bacilli (*S. paratyphi B*), which contains, in each milliliter, approximately 1 billion typhoid bacilli and 250 million of each type of the paratyphoid bacilli. It is an active immunizing agent against typhoid fever and paratyphoid fevers, administered subcutaneously. Called also *TAB v., typhoparatyphoid v., typhosum et paratyphosum,* and *vaccinium.* **typhoparatyphoid v.,** typhoid and paratyphoid v. **typhus v.** [USP], a sterile suspension of the killed rickettsial organisms of a strain or strains of epidemic typhus rickettsiae (*Rickettsia prowazeki*) selected for antigenic efficiency, consisting of refined material derived from an aqueous suspension of infected yolk sac membrane of chick embryos, and rickettsiae killed by a chemical agent; used as an active immunizing agent, administered subcutaneously. Called also *Cox v.* **univalent v.,** a vaccine containing only one variety of organism in pure culture. **Weigl v.,** a typhus fever vaccine prepared by inoculating lice per rectum with rickettsiae and then emulsifying the intestines of the lice in phenolized solution of sodium chloride. **yellow fever v.** [USP], an attenuated strain of living yellow fever virus selected for high antigenic activity and safety. It is prepared by culturing of the virus in the live chick embryo, from which a suspension is prepared, processed, dried from the frozen state, and sealed under dry nitrogen; used as an active immunizing agent, administered subcutaneously.

vaccinia (vak-sin′e-ah) [L., from *vacca* cow] a viral disease of cattle; see *cowpox.* In humans, a localized pustular eruption produced by inoculation of the vaccinia virus, used to produce antibody against smallpox. It is also transmissible by contact with a vaccinated person or with infected cows. It is occasionally associated with local and systemic complications due to the virus, to secondary infection by bacteria, and to postinfectious meningoencephalitis. **v. gangreno′sa,** generalized vaccinia characterized by failure to develop antibodies against the virus (due to agammaglobulinemia), as a result of which there is spreading necrosis at the inoculation site and metastasis of lesions throughout the body; called also *progressive v.* **generalized v.,** a benign systemic infection sometimes occurring after smallpox vaccination, not to be confused with eczema vaccinatum, with appearance of the virus in the blood and a widespread papular rash, which later vesiculates but leaves no scars; called also *vaccinid* and *vacciniola.* See also *v. gangrenosa.* **progressive v.,** v. gangrenosa.

vaccinial (vak-sin′e-al) pertaining to or characteristic of vaccinia (cowpox).

vacciniculturist (vak″sĭ-nĭ-kul′tūr-ist) one who raises heifers and uses them for the production of vaccine.

vaccinid (vak′sĭ-nid) generalized vaccinia.

vaccinifer (vak-sin′ĭ-fer) [*vaccine* + L. *ferre* to carry] the source (individual organism) from which smallpox vaccine is derived.

vacciniform (vak-sin′ĭ-form) resembling vaccinia (cowpox).

vaccinin (vak′sĭ-nin) the inoculable principle by which vaccinia is transmitted.

vacciniola (vak″sĭ-ne-o′lah) [L., dim. of *vaccinia*] generalized vaccinia.

vaccinization (vak″sin-i-za′shun) vaccination persistently repeated until the virus has no perceptible effect.

vaccinogen (vak-sin′o-jen) a source from which vaccine is derived.

vaccinogenous (vak″sĭ-noj′ĕ-nus) producing vaccine.

vaccinostyle (vak-sin′o-stil) a small lance used in vaccination.

vaccinotherapy (vak″sĭ-no-ther′ah-pe) therapeutic use of vaccines.

vaccinum (vak-si′num) [L.] vaccine. **v. antityph′icum,** typhoid vaccine. **v. pertus′sis,** pertussis vaccine. **v. pes′tis,** plague vaccine. **v. typho′sum,** typhoid vaccine. **v. typho′sum et paratypho′sum,** typhoid and paratyphoid vaccine. **v. vaccin′iae, v. vari′olae,** smallpox vaccine.

VACTERL an acronym for *v*ertebral, *a*nal, *c*ardiac, *t*racheal, *e*sophageal, *r*enal, and *l*imb; used to designate a pattern of congenital anomalies.

vacuolar (vak′u-o″lar) pertaining to a vacuole; characterized by the presence of vacuoles.

vacuolate (vak′u-o-lāt″) to form small spaces, or vacuoles.

vacuolated (vak′u-o-lāt″ed) pertaining to or characterized by vacuoles.

vacuolation (vak″u-o-la′shun) the process of forming vacuoles; the condition of being vacuolated.

vacuole (vak′u-ōl) [L. *vacuus* empty + *-ole* diminutive ending] any small space or cavity formed in the protoplasm of a cell. **autophagic v.**, autoplasmosome. **condensing v's**, membrane-bound spherical vacuoles in the Golgi complex of secretory cells, which contain secretory product in varying degrees of condensation and which mature, pass to the cell surface as secretory granules or droplets, and discharge their contents. **contractile v.**, a small cavity containing watery fluid, seen in the protoplasm of certain unicellular organisms; it gradually increases in size and then collapses. Its function is thought to be respiratory or excretory. **digestive v.**, secondary lysosome. **food v.**, a small cavity in protozoa containing ingested food particles. **heterophagic v.**, heterophagosome. **plasmocrine v.**, a small cavity containing crystalloids in a secretory cell. **rhagiocrine v.**, a small cavity containing colloids in a secretory cell. **water v.**, a small drop of water within the protoplasm of a cell.

vacuolization (vak″u-o-li-za′shun) vacuolation.

vacuome (vak′u-ōm) the system of vacuoles in a cell which stain with neutral red.

vacuum (vak′u-um) [L.] a space devoid of air or of other gas; a space from which the air has been exhausted. **high v.**, a vacuum in which the attenuation is extreme. **torricellian v.**, the vacuum in a barometric tube.

vadum (va′dum) [L. "a shallow"] an occasional elevation from the bottom of a cerebral sulcus, rendering the sulcus more or less shallow.

vagal (va′gal) pertaining to the vagus nerve.

vagi (va′ji) [L.] plural of *vagus*.

vagina (vah-ji′nah), pl. *vagi′nae* [L.] 1. a sheath, or sheathlike structure; used as a general term in anatomical nomenclature. 2. [NA] the canal in the female, extending from the vulva to the cervix uteri, which receives the penis in copulation. **v. bul′bi** [NA], connective tissue that forms the capsule enclosing the posterior part of the eyeball, extending anteriorly to the conjunctival fornix, and continuous with the muscular fascia of the eye; called also *fascia bulbi* [*Tenoni*], *bulbar fascia*, *sheath of eyeball*, and *Tenon's capsule*. **v. carot′ica fas′ciae cervica′lis** [NA], the portion of the cervical fascia that encloses the carotid vessels and vagus nerve. **v. cor′dis**, pericardium. **v. exter′na ner′vi op′tici** [NA], the thick outer sheath of the optic nerve, continuous with the dura mater and connecting it with the sclera; called also *external* or *fibrous sheath of optic nerve*. **v. fem′oris**, fascia lata femoris. **vagi′nae fibro′sae digito′rum ma′nus** [NA], strong fibrous, semicylindrical sheaths investing the grooved palmar surface of the proximal and middle phalanges of the fingers; called also *ligamenta vaginalia digitorum manus* and *fibrous sheaths of fingers*. **vagi′nae fibro′sae digito′rum pe′dis** [NA], more or less complete fascial sheaths surrounding the phalanges of the toes, for attachment of the tendons and their synovial membranes; called also *ligamenta vaginalia digitorum pedis* and *fibrous sheaths of toes*. **v. fibro′sa ten′dinis** [NA], the fibrous sheath of a tendon, usually confining it to an osseous groove. **v. inter′na ner′vi op′tici** [NA], the inner sheath of the optic nerve, continuous with the pia mater; called also *internal sheath of optic nerve*. **v. mas′culi′na**, utriculus prostaticus. **vagi′nae muco′sae**, vaginae synoviales. **v. muco′sa intertubercula′ris**, v. synovialis intertubercularis. **v. muco′sa ten′dinis**, v. synovialis tendinis. **vagi′nae muco′sae ten′dinum digito′rum pe′dis**, vaginae synoviales digitorum pedis. **vagi′nae muco′sae ten′dinum flexo′rum ma′nus**, vaginae synoviales digitorum manus. **v. mulie′bris**, the organ of copulation in the female; see *vagina*, def. 2. **v. mus′culi rec′ti abdo′minis** [NA], a sheath formed by the aponeuroses of other abdominal muscles, within which the rectus abdominis can move. **vagi′nae ner′vi op′tici**, the internal and external meningeal sheaths of the optic nerve within the orbit, continuous with the meninges of the brain. See *v. externa nervi optici* and *v. interna nervi optici*. Called also *sheaths of optic nerve*. **v. oc′uli**, *v. bulbi*. **v. pi′li**, folliculus pili. **v. proces′sus styloi′dei**, a ridge on the lower surface of the temporal bone, partly enclosing the base of the styloid process; called also *sheath of styloid process*. **vagi′nae synovia′les** [NA], double-layered, fluid-filled sheaths such as those that usually surround tendons running in osseofibrous tunnels. **v. synovia′lis commu′nis muscu-lo′rum flexo′rum** [NA], the common synovial sheath for the flexor tendons as they pass through osteofibrous canals of the fingers; called also *v. tendinum musculorum flexorum communium manus*. **vagi′nae synovia′les digito′rum ma′nus** [NA], the synovial sheaths of the tendons of the fingers; called also *vaginae mucosae tendinum flexorum manus*. **v. synovia′lis intertubercula′ris** [NA], the synovial membrane that surrounds the long head of the biceps brachii muscle as it passes through the intertubercular sulcus; called also *v. mucosa intertubercularis* and *synovial sheath of intertubercular groove*. **v. synovia′lis musculo′rum fibula′rium commu′nis**, NA alternative for *v. synovialis musculorum peroneorum communis*. **v. synovia′lis mus′culi obli′qui superio′ris** [NA],

the synovial sheath of the superior oblique muscle, particularly where its tendon passes through the trochlea; called also *bursa musculi trochlearis*. **v. synovia′lis musculo′rum peroneo′rum commu′nis** [NA], the double tendon sheath for the peroneus longus and peroneus brevis muscles; called also *v. tendinum musculorum peronaeorum communis*. **v. synovia′lis ten′dinis** [NA], a double-layered, fibrous sheath usually found surrounding a tendon running in an osteofibrous canal, with synovial fluid present between the layers; called also *v. mucosa tendinis* and *synovial sheath of tendon*. **vagi′nae synovia′les ten′dinum digito′rum ma′nus** [NA], the tendon sheaths of the long and short flexors of the fingers; called also *vaginae tendinum digitales manus*. **vagi′nae synovia′les ten′dinum digito′rum pe′dis** [NA], the synovial sheaths of the tendons of the toes; called also *vaginae mucosae tendinum digitorum pedis*. **v. synovia′lis ten′dinis mus′culi flexo′ris car′pi radia′lis** [NA], the tendon sheath of the flexor carpi radialis muscle; called also *bursa musculi flexoris carpi radialis*. **v. synovia′lis ten′dinis mus′culi flexo′ris hal′lucis lon′gi** [NA], the tendon sheath of the flexor hallucis longus muscle, extending from the medial malleolus to where it crosses the tendon of the flexor digitorum longus; called also *v. tendinis musculi flexoris hallucis longi*. **v. synovia′lis ten′dinis mus′culi tibia′lis posterio′ris** [NA], the tendon sheath of the tibialis posterior muscle, beginning at the medial malleolus and extending into the foot; called also *v. tendinis musculi tibialis posterioris*. **v. synovia′lis troch′leae**, bursa synovialis trochlearis. **vagi′nae ten′dinum digita′les ma′nus**, vaginae synoviales tendinum digitorum manus. **vagi′nae ten′dinum digito′rum pe′dis** [NA], the tendon sheaths of the long and short flexor muscles of the toes, beginning at the heads of the metatarsal bones. **v. ten′dinum musculo′rum abducto′ris lon′gi et extenso′ris bre′vis pol′licis** [NA], the tendon sheath of the long abductor and short extensor muscles of the thumb. **v. ten′dinum musculo′rum extenso′rum car′pi radia′lium** [NA], the tendon sheath of the short and long extensor carpi radialis muscles. **v. ten′dinis mus′culi extenso′ris car′pi ulna′ris** [NA], the tendon sheath of the extensor carpi ulnaris muscle. **v. ten′dinum musculo′rum extenso′ris digito′rum commu′nis et extenso′ris in′dicis**, v. tendinum musculorum extensoris digitorum et extensoris indicis. **v. ten′dinum musculo′rum extenso′ris digito′rum et extenso′ris in′dicis** [NA], the tendon sheath of the extensor digitorum and extensor indicis muscles. **v. ten′dinis mus′culi extenso′ris dig′iti min′imi** [NA], the tendon sheath of the extensor digiti minimi muscle. **vagi′nae ten′dinum mus′culi extenso′ris digito′rum pe′dis lon′gi** [NA], the tendon sheaths of the extensor digitorum longus muscle, running from the cruciate ligament to the intermediate cuneiform bone. **v. ten′dinis mus′culi extenso′ris hal′lucis lon′gi** [NA], the tendon sheath of the extensor hallucis longus muscle, extending from the cruciate ligament to the dorsal fascia of the foot. **v. ten′dinis mus′culi extenso′ris pol′licis lon′gi** [NA], the sheath of the extensor pollicis longus tendon. **v. ten′dinis mus′culi fibula′ris lon′gi planta′ris**, NA alternative for *v. tendinis musculi peronei longi plantaris*. **v. ten′dinum musculo′rum flexo′rum commu′nium ma′nus**, v. synovialis communis musculorum flexorum. **vagi′nae ten′dinum mus′culi flexo′ris digito′rum pe′dis lon′gi** [NA], the tendon sheaths of the flexor digitorum longus muscle, extending from the medial malleolus to below the navicular bone. **v. ten′dinis mus′culi flexo′ris hal′lucis lon′gi**, v. synovialis tendinis musculi flexoris hallucis longi. **v. ten′dinis mus′culi flexo′ris pol′licis lon′gi** [NA], the tendon sheath for the long flexor muscle of the thumb in the wrist and palm. **v. ten′dinum musculo′rum peronaeo′rum commu′nis**, v. synovialis musculorum peroneorum communis. **v. ten′dinis mus′culi perone′i lon′gi planta′ris** [NA], the tendon sheath of the peroneus longus muscle, beginning in the peroneal groove of the cuboid bone. **v. ten′dinis mus′culi tibia′lis anterio′ris** [NA], the tendon sheath of the tibialis anterior muscle, extending from the transverse crural ligament to the talonavicular joint. **v. ten′dinis mus′culi tibia′lis posterio′ris**, v. synovialis tendinis musculi tibialis posterioris. **v. vaso′rum** [NA], a fibrous sheath that encloses certain arteries, sometimes along with their veins and nerves.

vaginae (vah-ji′ne) plural of *vagina*.

vaginal (vaj′ĭ-nal) 1. of the nature of a sheath; ensheathing. 2. pertaining to the vagina. 3. pertaining to the tunica vaginalis testis.

vaginalectomy (vaj″ĭ-nah-lek′to-me) vaginectomy.

vaginalitis (vaj″ĭ-nah-li′tis) inflammation of the tunica vaginalis testis. **plastic v.**, pachyvaginalitis.

vaginapexy (vaj″ĭ-nah-pek′se) colpopexy.

vaginate (vaj′ĭ-nāt) [L. *vaginatus* sheathed] provided with a sheath.

vaginectomy (vaj″ĭ-nek′to-me) 1. resection of the tunica vaginalis testis. 2. excision of the vagina.

vaginiperineotomy (vaj″ĭ-nĭ-per″ĭ-ne-ot′o-me) paravaginal incision.

vaginismus (vaj″ĭ-niz′mus) [L.] painful spasm of the vagina due to local hyperesthesia; it is distinguished as *superficial* and *deep*, according as the seat is at the entrance of the vagina, or probably in the bulbocavernosus muscle, or in the levator ani muscle. **mental v.,** extreme aversion to coitus on the part of a woman, attended with contraction of the muscles when the act is attempted. **perineal v.,** spasm of the perineal muscles. **posterior v.,** vaginismus caused by spasm of the levator ani muscle. **vulvar v.,** vaginismus caused by spasm of the constrictor vaginae muscle.

vaginitis (vaj″ĭ-ni′tis) 1. inflammation of the vagina; it is marked by pain and by a purulent discharge. See also *colpitis.* 2. inflammation of a sheath. **v. adhaesi′va, adhesive v.,** see *atrophic v.* **atrophic v.,** vaginitis occurring in postmenopausal women and associated with estrogen deficiency. The common types are: *senile vulvovaginitis,* in which there is intense itching around the vagina, often with burning, almost complete lack of vaginal secretions, and evidence of tissue atrophy; and *senile vaginitis* or *adhesive vaginitis,* marked by the formation of superficial erosions, which often adhere to opposed surfaces, sometimes causing obliteration of the vaginal canal. **desquamative inflammatory v.,** vaginitis of unknown etiology, resembling atrophic vaginitis clinically and microscopically, but occurring in the absence of estrogen deficency, and characterized chiefly by recrudescent reddened superficial ulcerations. **diphtheritic v.,** diphtheritic inflammation of the vagina. **v. emphysemato′sa, emphysematous v.,** inflammation of the vagina and adjacent cervix, characterized by numerous, asymptomatic, gas-filled cystlike lesions; the gas filling the lesions has been shown to have a carbon dioxide content. **granular v.,** the most common variety, in which the papillae are enlarged and infiltrated with small cells. **senile v.,** see *atrophic v.* **v. tes′tis,** perididymitis. **trichomonas v.,** vaginitis produced by *Trichomonas.*

vaginoabdominal (vaj″ĭ-no-ab-dom′ĭ-nal) pertaining to the vagina and the abdomen.

vaginocele (vaj′ĭ-no-sēl″) [L. *vagina* sheath + Gr. *kēlē* tumor] 1. colpocele (def. 1). 2. colpoptosis.

vaginocutaneous (vaj″ĭ-no-ku-ta′ne-us) pertaining to the vagina and skin, or communicating with the vagina and the cutaneous surface of the body, as a vaginocutaneous fistula.

vaginodynia (vaj″ĭ-no-din′e-ah) [L. *vagina* sheath + Gr. *odynē* pain + *-ia*] pain in the vagina; colpodynia.

vaginofixation (vaj″ĭ-no-fiks-a′shun) colpopexy; suturing of the fundus of the uterus to the abdominal wall in cases of retroflexion. Called also *vaginal hysteropexy.*

vaginogram (vah-ji′no-gram) a roentgenogram of the vagina.

vaginography (vaj″ĭ-nog′rah-fe) roentgenography of the vagina.

vaginolabial (vaj″ĭ-no-la′be-al) pertaining to the vagina and the labia.

vaginometer (vaj″ĭ-nom′ĕ-ter) [*vagina* + Gr. *metron* measure] an instrument for measuring the length and diameter of the vagina.

vaginomycosis (vaj″ĭ-no-mi-ko′sis) [*vagina* + Gr. *mykēs* fungus] fungal disease of the vagina.

vaginopathy (vaj″ĭ-nop′ah-the) [*vagina* + Gr. *pathos* disease] any disease of the vagina.

vaginoperineal (vaj″ĭ-no-per″ĭ-ne′al) pertaining to the vagina and perineum.

vaginoperineorrhaphy (vaj″ĭ-no-per″ĭ-ne-or′ah-fe) colpoperineorrhaphy.

vaginoperineotomy (vaj′ĭ-no-per″ĭ-ne-ot′o-me) paravaginal incision.

vaginoperitoneal (vaj″ĭ-no-per″ĭ-to-ne′al) pertaining to the vagina and peritoneum.

vaginopexy (vah-ji′no-pek″se) [*vagina* + Gr. *pēxis* fixation] the operation of suturing the vagina to the abdominal wall in cases of vaginal relaxation.

vaginoplasty (vah-ji′no-plas″te) [*vagina* + Gr. *plassein* to form] colpoplasty.

vaginoscope (vaj′ĭ-no-skōp) [*vagina* + Gr. *skopein* to examine] a vaginal speculum; colposcope.

vaginoscopy (vaj″ĭ-nos′ko-pe) [*vagina* + Gr. *skopein* to examine] inspection of the vagina; colposcopy.

vaginotomy (vaj″ĭ-not′o-me) [*vagina* + Gr. *tomē* a cutting] colpotomy.

vaginovesical (vaj″ĭ-no-ves′ĭ-kal) pertaining to the vagina and bladder.

vaginovulvar (vaj″ĭ-no-vul′var) vulvovaginal.

vagitus (vah-ji′tus) [L.] the cry of an infant. **v. uteri′nus,** the crying of a child in the uterus. **v. vagina′lis,** the crying of a child while its head is still within the vagina.

vagoaccessorius (va″go-ak″ses-so′re-us) [L.] the vagus nerve and the cranial root of the accessory nerves regarded as together forming one nerve.

vagoglossopharyngeal (va″go-glos″o-fah-rin′je-al) pertaining to the vagus and glossopharyngeal nerves.

vagogram (va′go-gram) [*vagus* + Gr. *gramma* mark] a tracing showing the electrical variations of the vagus nerve; called also *electrovagogram.*

vagolysis (va-gol′ĭ-sis) [*vagus* + Gr. *lysis* dissolution] surgical lysis of the vagus nerve.

vagolytic (va″go-lit′ik) having an effect resembling that produced by interruption of impulses transmitted by the vagus nerve; parasympatholytic.

vagomimetic (va″go-mi-met′ik) having an effect which resembles that produced by vagal stimulation.

vagosplanchnic (va″go-splank′nik) vagosympathetic.

vagosympathetic (va″go-sim″pah-thet′ik) pertaining to both the vagus and sympathetic innervation.

vagotomy (va-got′o-me) [*vagus* + Gr. *tomē* a cutting] interruption of the impulses carried by the vagus nerve or nerves; so called because it was first performed by surgical methods. **bilateral v.,** transection of the right and left vagus nerves. **complete v.,** transection of all vagal secretory fibers sufficient to prevent increased flow or acidity of gastric secretion in insulin hypoglycemia. **highly selective v.,** division of only those vagal fibers supplying the acid-secreting glands of the stomach, with preservation of those supplying the antrum as well as the hepatic and celiac branches. **medical v.,** interruption of the impulses carried by the vagus nerve by administration of suitable drugs; vagus block. **parietal cell v.,** selective severing of the vagus nerve fibers supplying the proximal two-thirds (parietal area) of the stomach; done for duodenal ulcer. **selective v.,** division of the vagal fibers to the stomach with preservation of the hepatic and celiac branches. **surgical v.,** transection of the vagus nerve by surgical means. **truncal v.,** surgical division of the two main trunks of the abdominal vagus nerve.

vagotonia (va″go-to′ne-ah) [*vagus* + Gr. *tonos* tension + *-ia*] hyperexcitability of the vagus nerve; a condition in which the vagus nerve dominates in the general functioning of the body organs. It is marked by vasomotor instability, constipation, sweating, and involuntary motor spasms with pain.

vagotonic (va″go-ton′ik) pertaining to or characterized by vagotonia.

vagotonin (va-got′o-nin) a preparation of hormone from the pancreas which increases vagal tone, slows the heart, and increases the store of glycogen in the liver.

vagotony (va-got′o-ne) vagotonia.

vagotrope (va′go-trōp) vagotropic.

vagotropic (va″go-trop′ik) having an effect on the vagus nerve.

vagotropism (va-got′ro-pizm) [*vagus* + Gr. *tropos* a turning] affinity of a drug or poison for the vagus nerve.

vagovagal (va″go-va′gal) arising as a result of afferent and efferent impulses which are both mediated through the vagus nerve.

vagrant (va′grant) [L. *vagrans,* from *vagare* to wander] 1. wandering; moving from one place to another. 2. a vagabond.

vagus (va′gus), pl. *va′gi* [L. "wandering"] designating the tenth cranial nerve; see *nervus vagus.*

vagusstoff (va′gus-stof) [*vagus* + Ger. *Stoff* stuff, substance] a substance liberated by the vagus nerve endings that inhibits cardiac activity; it is identical to acetylcholine.

Vahlkampfia (vahl-kamp′fe-ah) a genus of amebae of the order Amoebida, class Rhizopodia, having a single nucleus and one broad psuedopodium. *V. limax* is found in fresh water, *V. patuxent* in the alimentary canal of oysters.

Val valine.

Valadol (val′ah-dol) trademark for preparations of acetaminophen.

valamin (val′ah-min) the valerian ester of amylene hydrate, $(CH_3)_2 \cdot C_2H_5 \cdot CO \cdot O \cdot C_5H_9$, formerly used as a hypnotic and sedative.

valence (va′lens) [L. *valentia* strength] the numerical measure of the capacity to combine. In chemistry it is an expression of the number of atoms of hydrogen (or its equivalent) which one atom of a chemical element can hold in combination, if negative, or displace in a reaction, if positive. An element is characterized as univalent or monovalent, bivalent or divalent, tervalent or trivalent, multivalent or polyvalent, according to its valence—one, two, three, many, etc. Valence is determined by the number of electrons in the outer (or valence) shell of an atom. In immunology, it is an expression of the number of antigenic determinants with which one molecule of a given antibody can combine. Most antibody molecules possess two combining sites (i.e., two antigen-binding sites) and are said to be divalent, i.e., those belonging to the IgG, IgA, and IgE immunoglobulin classes. The valence of the IgM molecule is frequently found to be 5, although theoretically it should possess 10 combining sites. In like manner, the valence of an antigen may be expressed as the number of antibody combining sites (i.e., antigen-binding sites) with which it can unite. Most large antigen molecules are multivalent, or polyvalent. Also an expression of the number of different organisms or antigens in a vaccine. **biologic v.,** the combining power of molecules of homologous antigen and antibody; see *valence*.

valency (va'len-se) [L. *valentia*] 1. strength; ability. 2. valence.

Valentin's corpuscles, ganglion (pseudoganglion) (val'-en-tēnz) [Gabriel Gustav *Valentin*, German physician, 1810–1883] see under *corpuscle*, and see *intumescentia tympanica*.

Valentine's position (val'en-tīnz) [Ferdinand C. *Valentine*, surgeon in New York, 1851–1909] see under *position*.

***n*-valeraldehyde** (vah-ler-al'dĕ-hīd) an aldehyde, $C_5H_{10}O$, which has narcotic properties and is a mild irritant; called also *amylic aldehyde* and *valeric aldehyde*.

valerian (va-le're-an) [L. *valeriana*] any plant of the genus *Valeriana*. The dried roots and rhizome of *V. officinalis* L. (Valerianaceae) of Europe are antispasmodic and nerve stimulant and have been used in nervousness and hysteria. **Greek v.,** the European plant *Polemonium caeruleum* L. (Polemoniaceae), or Jacob's ladder, used as a topical application to ulcers.

valethamate bromide (val-eth'ah-māt) chemical name: *N, N*-diethyl-*N*-methyl-2-[(3-phenyl-1-oxo-2-phenylpentyl)oxy]-ethanaminium bromide. A quaternary ammonium anticholinergic, $C_{19}H_{32}BrNO_2$, occurring as a white, crystalline powder; used as an antispasmodic in the treatment of hypermotility and spasm of the gastrointestinal, genitourinary, and biliary tracts, administered orally, intramuscularly, or intravenously.

valetudinarian (val″e-tu″dĭ-na're-an) [L. *valetudinarius* sickly] an invalid; a feeble person.

valetudinarianism (val″e-tu″dĭ-na're-an-izm) an infirm or feeble habit of body.

valgus (val'gus) [L.] bent outward, twisted; denoting a deformity in which the angulation of the part is away from the midline of the body, as in *talipes valgus*. The term valgus is an adjective and should be used only in connection with the noun it describes, as talipes valgus, genu valgum, coxa valga, etc. Cf. *varus*.

valine (val'in) an essential amino acid, alpha-aminoisovalerianic acid, $(CH_3)_2 \cdot CH \cdot CH(NH_2) \cdot COOH$, produced by the digestion or hydrolytic decomposition of proteins; it is essential for optimal growth in infants and for nitrogen equilibrium in human adults. Called also *2-aminoisovaleric acid* and *isopropyl-aminoacetic acid*.

valinemia (val″ĭ-ne'me-ah) hypervalinemia.

Valisone (val'ĭ-sōn) trademark for preparations of betamethasone valerate.

Valium (val'e-um) trademark for a preparation of diazepam.

vallate (val'āt) [L. *vallatus* walled] having a wall or rim; cup-shaped.

vallecula (vah-lek'u-lah), pl. *vallec'ulae* [dim. of L. *valles* a hollow] a depression or furrow; used as a general term in anatomical nomenclature. Sometimes used alone to designate the *vallecula epiglottica*. **v. cerebel'li** [NA], the longitudinal hollow on the inferior surface of the cerebellum, between the hemispheres, in which the medulla oblongata rests. **v. epiglot'tica,** a depression between the lateral and median glossoepiglottic folds on each side. **v. ova'ta,** fossa vesicae felleae. **v. for petrosal ganglion,** fossula petrosa. **v. syl'vii,** fossa lateralis cerebri. **v. un'guis,** sulcus matricis unguis.

vallecular (vah-lek'u-lar) pertaining to or affecting a vallecula.

Valleix's points (vahl-lāz') [François Louis Isidore *Valleix*, French physician, 1807–1855] see under *point*.

Vallestril (val-les'tril) trademark for a preparation of methallenestril.

valley (val'e) a small hollow. **v. of cerebellum,** vallecula cerebelli.

Valli-Ritter law (val″e-rit'er) [Eusebio *Valli*, Italian physiologist, 1755–1816; Johann Wilhelm *Ritter*, German physicist, 1776–1810] see *Ritter-Valli law*, under *law*.

vallicepobufagin (vah-lis″ĕ-po-bu'fah-jin) a cardiac poison, $C_{26}H_{38}O_5$, from the skin glands of the toad, *Bufo valliceps*.

vallis (val'is) [L. "valley"] vallecula cerebelli.

vallum (val'um), pl. *val'la* [L. "a fortification"] a mound, or wall. **v. un'guis** [NA], the fold of skin overlapping the sides and the proximal end of a nail; called also *wall of nail*.

Valmid (val'mid) trademark for a preparation of ethinamate.

valnoctamide (val-nok'tah-mīd) chemical name: 2-ethyl-3-methylvaleramide; a tranquilizer, $C_8H_{17}NO$.

Valpin (val'pin) trademark for preparations of anisotropine methylbromide.

valproate sodium (val-pro'āt) chemical name: 2-propylpentanoic acid sodium salt. It is the sodium salt, $C_8H_{15}NaO_2$, of valproic acid, a simple eight-carbon branched-chain fatty acid and is used as an antiepileptic especially for control of absence seizures.

Valsalva's ligaments, maneuver (experiment), sinus, zone (val-sal'vahz) [Antonio Maria *Valsalva*, an Italian anatomist, 1666–1723] see under *maneuver*, and see *ligamenta auricularia, lamina basilaris ductus cochlearis*, and *sinus aortae*.

Valsuani's disease (val″su-an'ēz) [Emilio *Valsuani*, Italian gynecologist of 19th Century] see under *disease*.

value (val'u) a measure of worth or efficiency; a quantitative measurement of the activity, concentration, etc., of specific substances (see *normal v's*). **acetyl v.,** acetyl number. **acid v.,** acid number. **buffer v.,** a numerical expression of the degree of change in pH of a solution in response to the addition of acid or alkali. **cryocrit v.,** the per cent volume of sedimented cryoglobulin after cold centrifugation of serum kept at 4° to 5° C. **fuel v.,** the potential heat energy of the food. **Hehner's v.,** the percentage of insoluble (nonvolatile) fatty acids that are yielded by a saponified fat. **liminal v.,** that intensity of a stimulus which produces a just noticeable impression. **mean clinical v.,** see *MCV*. **normal v's,** the range in concentration of specific substances found in normal healthy tissues, secretions, etc. **saponification v.,** saponification number. **threshold v.,** liminal v. **valence v.,** the number obtained by multiplying the lowering of the freezing point in degrees by the amount of urine in milliliters.

valva (val'vah), pl. *val'vae* [sing. of L. *valvae* folding doors] [NA] a valve: a membranous fold in a canal or passage, which prevents the reflux of the contents passing through it. **v. aor'tae** [NA], aortic valve: a valve composed of three semilunar cusps or segments (posterior, right, and left), guarding the aortic orifice in the left ventricle of the heart; it prevents backflow into the left ventricle. Called also *valvulae semilunares aortae* and *semilunar valve*. **v. atrioventricula'ris dex'tra** [NA], right atrioventricular valve: the valve between the right atrium and right ventricle of the heart; it usually has three cusps (anterior, posterior, and septal), but additional small cusps may be present. Called also *valvula tricuspidalis* or *tricuspid valve*. **v. atrioventricula'ris sinis'tra** [NA], left atrioventricular valve: the valve between the left atrium and left ventricle of the heart; it usually has two cusps (anterior and posterior), but additional small cusps may be present. Called also *valvula bicuspidalis [mitralis]* and *bicuspid* or *mitral valve*. **v. ileoceca'lis** [NA], ileocecal valve: a functional valve at junction of the ileum and cecum, consisting of circular muscle of the terminal ileum. The ileocecal opening has two folds, one above and one below, which project into the cecum. Called also *valvula coli*. **v. mitra'lis,** NA alternative for *v. atrioventricularis sinistra*. **v. tricuspida'lis,** NA alternative for *v. atrioventricularis dextra*. **v. trun'ci pulmona'lis** [NA], valve of pulmonary trunk: a valve composed of three semilunar segments (anterior, right, and left), guarding the pulmonary orifice in the right ventricle of the heart; it prevents backflow of blood into the right ventricle. Called also *pulmonary valve, semilunar valve*, and *valvulae semilunares arteriae pulmonalis*.

valval, valvar (val'val; val'var) pertaining to a valve.

valvate (val'vāt) pertaining to or having valves.

valve (valv) a membranous fold in a canal or passage, which prevents the reflux of the contents passing through it; see also *valva* and *valvula*. **anal v's,** valvulae anales. **v. of aorta, aortic v.,** valva aortae. **artificial v.,** a man-made cardiac valve. **atrioventricular v., left,** valva atrioventricularis sinistra. **atrioventricular v., right,** valva atrioventricularis dextra. **auriculoventricular v., left,** valva atrioventricularis sinistra. **auriculoventricular v., right,** valva atrioventricularis dextra. **Ball's v's,** valvulae anales. **ball-type v.,** an artificial cardiac valve that contains a small free-floating ball that prevents the reflux of blood during diastole; for various types, see under *prosthesis*. **Bauer v.,** a piece of unglazed porcelain fused into the wall of a gas tube by means of which air can be admitted as needed. **Bauhin's v.,** valva ileocecalis. **Béraud's v.,** a fold of mucous membrane sometimes found at the junction of the lacrimal sac and the nasolacrimal duct; called also *Arnold's fold* and *Krause's valve*. **Bianchi's v.,** the lower termination of the nasolacrimal duct. **bicuspid v.,** valva atrioventricularis sinistra. **Bochdalek's v.,** a fold within the lacrimal duct near the punctum lacrimale. **cardiac v's,** valves that control the flow of blood through and from the heart; they are the atrioventricular, aortic, and pulmonary trunk valves. **cardiac v's, artificial,** see under *prosthesis*. **caval v.,** valvula venae cavae inferioris. **v. of colon,** valva ileocecalis. **coronary v., v. of coronary sinus,** valvula sinus coronarii. **eustachian v.,** valvula venae cavae inferioris. **fallopian v.,** valva ileocecalis. **flair v.,** a cardiac valve having a cusp that has lost its normal support (as in ruptured chordae tendinae) and flutters in the blood stream. **Foltz's v.,** a fold of membrane in the lacrimal canaliculus. **v. of foramen ovale,** 1. valvula foraminis ovalis. 2. the septum primum of the fetal heart. **Gerlach's v.,** valvula processus vermiformis. **Guérin's v.,** valvula fossae navicularis. **Hasner's v.,** plica lacrimalis. **heart v's,** cardiac v's. **heart v., artificial,** see under *prosthesis*. **Heister's v.,** plica spiralis. **Hoboken's v's,** foldlike thickenings of the media of the umbilical arteries which protrude into the lumen of the arteries. **Houston's v's,** plicae transversales recti. **Huschke's v.,** plica lacrimalis. **hymenal v. of male urethra,** valvula fossae navicularis. **ileocecal v., ileocolic v.,** valva ileocecalis. **v. of inferior vena cava,** valvula venae cavae inferioris. **interauricular v.,** 1. limbus fossae ovalis. 2. valvula foraminis ovalis (def. 1). **Kerckring's v's,** plicae circulares. **Kohlrausch's v's,** plicae transversales recti. **Krause's v.,** Béraud's v.

lymphatic v., valvula lymphaticum. **v. of Macalister,** valva ileocecalis. **Mercier's v.,** interureteric ridge (plica interureterica [NA]). **mitral v.,** valva atrioventricularis sinistra. **Morgagni's v's,** valvulae anales. **v. of navicular fossa,** valvula fossae navicularis. **O'Beirne's v.,** see under *sphincter.* **pulmonary v., pulmonary trunk v., v. of pulmonary trunk,** valva trunci pulmonalis. **pyloric v.,** valvula pylori. **Rosenmüller's v.,** plica lacrimalis. **semilunar v.,** a valve having semilunar cusps, i.e., the aortic valve and the pulmonary valve. The term is sometimes used to designate the semilunar cusps composing these valves; see entries beginning *valvula semilunaris.* **semilunar v's of colon,** plicae semilunares coli. **semilunar v's of Morgagni,** sinus anales. **sigmoid v's of colon,** plicae semilunares coli. **spiral v. of cystic duct, spiral v. of Heister,** plica spiralis. **v. of Sylvius,** valvula venae cavae inferioris. **Taillefer's v.,** a fold of the mucous membrane of the nasolacrimal duct near the middle of its course. **Tarinus' v.,** velum medullare inferius. **thebesian v.,** valvula sinus coronarii. **tricuspid v.,** valva atrioventricularis dextra. **v. of Tulpius,** valva ileocecalis. **ureteral v.,** a congenital transverse fold across the lumen of the ureter, composed of redundant mucosa prominent by circular muscle fibers; it usually disappears in time but may rarely cause urinary obstruction. Pathological valves or kinks also occur. **v. of Varolius,** valva ileocecalis. **v. of veins,** valvula venosa. **v. of vermiform appendix,** valvula processus vermiformis. **v. of Vieussens, Willis' v.,** velum medullare superius.

valved (valvd) having valves; opening by valves.

valviform (val'vĭ-form) [L. *valva* valve + *forma* shape] shaped like a valve.

valvotome (val'vo-tōm) a surgical instrument for incising a heart valve.

valvotomy (val-vot'o-me) [L. *valva* valve + Gr. *tomē* a cutting] incision of a valve, such as a valve of the heart. **mitral v.,** dilation of the left atrioventricular (mitral) valve, the commissures being split and extended with the finger, with or without the aid of a knife or a mechanical dilator. **pulmonary v.,** transventricular closed v. **transventricular closed v.,** incision into the ventricle with a valvotome and dilation of the pulmonary valve, performed to avoid total extracorporeal circulation in young infants with pulmonary stenosis; called also *Brock's operation.*

valvula (val'vu-lah), pl. *val'vulae* [L., dim of *valva*] a small valve; once used in official nomenclature as a general term to designate a valve, such as in the heart, but in NA restricted to designation of a cusp of the aortic valve or of the valve of the pulmonary trunk, or the valves of the anus, foramen ovale, navicular fossa, coronary sinus, inferior vena cava, or of the lymphatic vessels and veins. **val'vulae ana'les** [NA], anal valves: archlike folds of mucous membrane connecting the caudal ends of the anal columns. **v. biscuspida'lis [mitra'lis],** valva atrioventricularis sinistra. **v. co'li,** valva ileocecalis. **val'vulae conniven'tes** [L. "closing valves"], plicae circulares. **v. fora'minis ova'lis,** 1. [NA] valve of foramen ovale: in the adult, a crescentic ridge on the left side of the interatrial septum, representing the edge of what was the septum primum before fusion of the septum; called also *falx septi* [NA alternative]. 2. the septum primum of the fetal heart. **v. fos'sae navicula'ris** [NA], valve of navicular fossa: a fold of mucous membrane occasionally occurring in the roof of the fossa navicularis of the urethra. **v. ileocol'ica,** valva ileocecalis. **v. lymphat'icum** [NA], a lymphatic valve: any of the usually doubled cusps in the collecting lymphatic vessels, serving to ensure flow in only one direction. **v. mitra'lis,** valva atrioventricularis sinistra. **v. proces'sus vermifor'mis,** an inconstant fold of mucous membrane at the opening into the cecum of the canal of the vermiform appendix. **v. pylo'ri,** pyloric valve: a prominent circular fold of mucous membrane at the pyloric orifice of the stomach; called also *Haller's circle.* **v. semiluna'ris,** a semilunar cusp. **v. semiluna'ris ante'rior arte'riae pulmona'lis,** v. semilunaris anterior trunci pulmonalis. **v. semiluna'ris ante'rior trun'ci pulmona'lis** [NA], the anterior cusp of the valve of the pulmonary trunk. **val'vulae semiluna'res aor'tae,** valva aortae. **val'vulae semiluna'res arte'riae pulmona'lis,** valva trunci pulmonalis. **v. semiluna'ris dex'tra aor'tae** [NA], the right cusp of the aortic valve. **v. semiluna'ris dex'tra arte'riae pulmona'lis,** v. semilunaris dextra trunci pulmonalis. **v. semiluna'ris dex'tra trun'ci pulmona'lis** [NA], the right cusp of the valve of the pulmonary trunk. **v. semiluna'ris poste'rior aor'tae** [NA], the posterior cusp of the aortic valve. **v. semiluna'ris sinis'tra aor'tae** [NA], the left cusp of the aortic valve. **v. semiluna'ris sinis'tra arte'riae pulmona'lis,** v. semilunaris sinistra trunci pulmonalis. **v. semiluna'ris sinis'tra trun'ci pulmona'lis** [NA], the left cusp of the valve of the pulmonary trunk. **v. si'nus corona'rii** [NA], **v. si'nus corona'rii [Thebe'sii],** valve of coronary sinus: a fold of endocardium along the right margin of the opening of the coronary sinus into the right atrium of the heart. **v. spira'lis [Heis'teri],** plica spiralis. **v. tricuspida'lis,** valva atrioventricularis dextra. **v. ve'nae ca'vae**

inferio'ris [NA], **v. ve'nae ca'vae inferio'ris [Eusta'chii],** valve of inferior vena cava: the variably-sized crescentic fold of endocardial and subendocardial tissue that is attached to the anterior margin of the opening of the inferior vena cava into the right atrium of the heart. **v. veno'sa** [NA], valve of veins: any of the small cusps or fold of the tunica intima found in many veins, serving to prevent the backflow of blood. **v. vestib'uli,** either of the two thin folds bordering the opening of the sinus reuniens into the right atrium of the embryonic heart; they develop into the valves of the inferior vena cava and coronary sinus.

valvulae (val'vu-le) [L.] plural of *valvula.*

valvular (val'vu-lar) pertaining to, affecting, or of the nature of a valve.

valvulitis (val"vu-li'tis) inflammation of a valve or valvula, especially a valve of the heart. **rheumatic v.,** involvement of a cardiac valve by the rheumatic process; endocarditis.

valvuloplasty (val'vu-lo-plas"te) plastic operation on a valve.

valvulotome (val'vu-lo-tōm") an instrument for cutting a valve.

valvulotomy (val"vu-lot'o-me) valvotomy.

valylene (val'ĭ-lēn) a hydrocarbon, C_5H_6.

vampire (vam'pīr) a neotropical bat belonging to the genera *Desmodus, Diaemus,* or *Diphylla.*

vanadate (van'ah-dāt) any salt of vanadic acid.

vanadium (vah-na'de-um) [*Vanadis,* a Norse deity] a rare, gray, metallic element; symbol, V; atomic number, 23; atomic weight, 50.942. Its salts have been used in treating various diseases. See also *vanadiumism.*

vanadiumism (vah-na'de-um-izm") a chronic intoxication caused by absorption of vanadium compounds, usually via the lungs; symptoms include irritation of the respiratory tract, pneumonitis, conjunctivitis, and anemia.

van Buren's disease (van-bu'renz) [William Holme *van Buren,* American surgeon, 1819–1883] Peyronie's disease.

Vancocin (van'ko-sin) trademark for a preparation of vancomycin hydrochloride.

vancomycin hydrochloride (van'ko-mi"sin) [USP] an antibiotic produced by the soil bacillus *Streptomyces orientalis,* which is highly effective against cocci, especially staphylococci, and other gram-positive bacteria, occurring as a tan to brown, free-flowing powder; used in the treatment of severe staphylococcal infections resistant to other antibiotics, administered intravenously or by intravenous infusion.

van Deen's test (van dēnz) [Izaak Abramson *van Deen,* Dutch physician, 1804–1869] see *Deen's test,* under *tests.*

Van de Graaff machine (van de grahf) [Robert Jemison *Van de Graaff,* American physicist, 1901–1967] see under *machine.*

van den Bergh's disease, test (van den bergz') [A. A. Hijmans (Hymans) *van den Bergh,* Dutch physician, 1869–1943] see *enterogenous cyanosis,* under *cyanosis,* and see under *tests.*

van der Velden's test (van der vel'denz) [Reinhardt *van der Velden,* German physician, 1851–1903] *Maly's test.*

van Gehuchten's cells, method (van-ga-hook'tenz) [Arthur *van Gehuchten,* Belgian anatomist, 1861–1914] see *Golgi type II neurons,* under *neuron,* and see under *method.*

Vanghetti's prosthesis (vahn-get'ēz) [Giuliano *Vanghetti,* Italian surgeon, 1861–1940] see under *prosthesis.*

van Gieson's stain (van-ge'sonz) [Ira *van Gieson,* New York neuropathologist, 1865–1913] see *Table of Stains.*

van Helmont's mirror (van hel'monts) [Johannes Baptista *van Helmont,* Belgian physician, 1577–1644] the central tendon of the diaphragm (centrum tendineum [NA]).

van Hook's operation (van hooks') [Weller *van Hook,* Chicago surgeon, 1862–1933] ureteroureterostomy.

van Hoorne's canal (van hornz) [Jean *van Hoorne,* Dutch anatomist, 1621–1670] the thoracic duct (ductus thoracicus [NA]).

Vanilla (vah-nil'ah) [L.] a genus of climbing orchidaceous plants of hot climates. The fruit of *V. planifolia* Andr. (Orchidaceae), of Mexico, are the vanilla beans, which contain vanilla and are used as a flavor and a mild stimulant; said to be aphrodisiac.

vanilla (vah-nil'ah) [NF] the cured, full-grown, unripe fruit of *Vanilla planifolia* Andr. (Mexican or Bourbon v.) or of *V. tahitensis* Moor. (Tahiti v.), used in medicine as a flavoring agent, usually in the form of a tincture.

vanillal (vah-nil'lal) ethyl vanillin.

vanillin (van'ĭ-lin, vah-nil'in) [NF] chemical name: 4-hydroxy-3-methoxybenzaldehyde. A constituent of vanilla and other plants, which also may be prepared synthetically, $C_8H_8O_3$, occurring as fine fluffy white to yellow crystals, usually needle-like; used as a flavor in pharmaceutical preparations. **ethyl v.** [NF], chemical name: 3-ethoxy-4-hydroxybenzaldehyde. Fine white or slightly yellowish crystals, $C_9H_{10}O_3$; used as a flavor in pharmaceutical preparations.

vanillism (vah-nil′izm) symptoms of dermatitis, coryza, and malaise seen in those handling raw vanilla and caused by the mite *Acarus siro.*

Vanogel (van′o-jel) trademark for an aqueous suspension of aluminum hydroxide gel.

Van Slyke's formula, etc. (van-slīks′) [Donald Dexter *Van Slyke,* American biochemist, born 1883] see under *formula, method,* and *tests.*

Van Slyke-Cullen method (test) (van-slik′-kul′en) [Donald D. *Van Slyke;* Glenn Ernest *Cullen,* American biochemist, born 1890] see under *method.*

Van Slyke-Fitz method (van-slik′fitz) [Donald D. *Van Slyke;* Reginald *Fitz,* American physician, 1885–1953] see under *method.*

van't Hoff's law, rule (vant hofs) [Jacobus Hendricus *van't Hoff,* Dutch chemist, 1852–1911; winner of the Nobel prize for chemistry in 1901] see under *law* and *rule.*

Vanzetti's sign (vahn-tset′ēz) [Tito *Vanzetti,* Italian surgeon, 1809–1888] see under *sign.*

vapocauterization (va″po-kaw″ter-i-za′shun) cauterization by means of steam or other hot vapor.

vapor (va′por), pl. *vapo′res, va′pors* [L.] steam, gas, or exhalation.

vaporarium (va″po-rār′e-um) [L.] an establishment or apparatus for treating certain diseases by the use of vapors.

vaporium (va-po′re-um) [L.] vaporarium.

vaporization (va″por-i-za′shun) 1. the conversion of a solid or liquid into a vapor without chemical change; distillation. 2. treatment by vapors.

vaporize (va′por-īz) to convert into vapor or to be transformed into vapor.

vaporizer (va″por-i′zer) a device for producing an aerosol or mist, as from a solution containing a medication to ease breathing.

vapors (va′porz) an old term for hypochondriasis or hysterical depression.

vapotherapy (va″po-ther′ah-pe) the therapeutic use of vapor, steam, or spray.

Vaquez's disease (vak-āz′) [Louis Henri *Vaquez,* French physician, 1860–1936] polycythemia vera.

var. variety.

variability (var″e-ah-bil′ĭ-te) the state of being variable.

variable (va′re-ah-b'l) [L. *variare* to change] 1. changing from time to time. 2. a quantity or value subject to change; in statistics, one of the separate numerical values from which a curve of variability can be constructed.

variant (vār′e-ant) 1. something that differs in some characteristic from the class to which it belongs, as a variant of a disease, trait, species, etc. 2. exhibiting such variation. **L-phase v.,** a bacterial variant that has a defective cell wall but can multiply on hypertonic medium; called also *L-form.*

variate (va′re-āt) variable.

variation (va″re-a′shun) in genetics, deviation in characters in an individual from those typical of the group to which it belongs; also, deviation in characters of the offspring from those of its parents. **continuous v.,** a series of small variations. **impressed v.,** a variation which occurs in response to a particular environmental stimulus. **inborn v.,** one which arises from changes in the germ cells and not from the somatic cells. **isotypic v.,** in immunology, the variability in the structure of antigens present in all members of a single species, e.g., antigenic differences in classes of immunoglobulins. **meristic v.,** variation in the number of parts in the offspring. **quasicontinuous v.,** variation in which the underlying distribution of variability is continuous but a threshold effect makes it appear discontinuous.

varication (var″ĭ-ka′shun) 1. the formation of a varix. 2. a varicose condition; a varicosity.

variceal (var″ĭ-se′al) pertaining to or caused by a varix.

varicella (var″ĭ-sel′ah) [L.] chickenpox. **v. gangreno′sa,** a rare form of chickenpox in which the eruption leads to a gangrenous ulceration, occurring mainly in children with leukemia or other severe underlying disease. **v. inocula′ta,** the inoculation of children with a virus from a fresh clear vesicle of chickenpox; usually no general symptoms develop. **pustular v., v. pustulo′sa,** chickenpox in which the eruption develops into furuncles. **vaccination v.,** v. inoculata.

varicellation (var″ĭ-sel-la′shun) prophylactic inoculation with the virus of varicella.

varicelliform (var″ĭ-sel′ĭ-form) resembling varicella.

varicellization (var″ĭ-sel-i-za′shun) varicellation.

varicelloid (var″ĭ-sel′oid) [*varicella* + Gr. *eidos* form] resembling varicella.

varices (vār′ĭ-sēz) [L.] plural of *varix.*

variciform (var-is′ĭ-form) [*varix* + L. *forma* form] resembling a varix; varicose.

varico- [L. *varix* a varicose vein] a combining form denoting relationship to a varix, or meaning twisted and swollen.

varicoblepharon (var″ĭ-ko-blef′ah-ron) [*varico-* + Gr. *blepharon* eyelid] a varicose swelling of the eyelid.

varicocele (var″ĭ-ko-sēl″) [*varico-* + Gr. *kēlē* tumor] a varicose condition of the veins of the pampiniform plexus, forming a swelling that feels like a "bag of worms," appearing bluish through the skin of the scrotum, and accompanied by a constant pulling, dragging, or dull pain in the scrotum. **ovarian v., pelvic v.,** a varicose condition of the veins of the broad ligament. **utero-ovarian v.,** a varicose condition of the veins of the pampiniform plexus of the female.

varicocelectomy (var″ĭ-ko-sĕ-lek′to-me) [*varicocele* + Gr. *ektomē* excision] the excision of a part of the scrotum and the enlarged veins for varicocele.

varicography (var″ĭ-kog′rah-fe) [*varico-* + Gr. *graphein* to write] roentgenological visualization of varicose veins.

varicoid (var′ĭ-koid) [*varico-* + Gr. *eidos* form] resembling a varix.

varicole (var′ĭ-kōl) varicocele.

varicomphalus (var″ĭ-kom′fah-lus) [*varico-* + Gr. *omphalos* navel] a varicose tumor at the umbilicus.

varicophlebitis (var″ĭ-ko-fle-bi′tis) varicose veins with inflammation.

varicose (var′ĭ-kōs) [L. *varicosus*] of the nature of or pertaining to a varix; unnaturally and permanently distended: said of a vein; variciform.

varicosis (var″ĭ-ko′sis) [L.] a varicose condition of the veins of any part.

varicosity (var″ĭ-kos′ĭ-te) 1. a varicose condition; the quality or fact of being varicose; varication. 2. a varix or varicose vein.

varicotomy (var″ĭ-kot′o-me) [*varico-* + Gr. *tomē* a cutting] the excision of a varix or of a varicose vein.

varicula (vah-rik′u-lah) [L.] a varix of the conjunctiva.

Varidase (var′ĭ-dās) trademark for preparations of streptokinase-streptodornase.

variety (vah-ri′ĕ-te) in taxonomy, a subcategory of a species.

variola (vah-ri′o-lah) [L.] smallpox. **v. capri′na,** goatpox. **v. crystal′lina,** chickenpox. **v. hemorrha′gica,** hemorrhagic smallpox. **v. inser′ta,** smallpox acquired by inoculation. **v. ma′jor,** a severe form of smallpox, such as hemorrhagic smallpox or malignant smallpox, characterized by a case fatality rate of 25 to 40 per cent. **v. milia′ris,** smallpox with an eruption of small vesicles. **v. mi′nor,** a mild form of smallpox, caused by a virus slightly less virulent for the chick embryo than the virus causing variola major, and distinguished from the latter condition by its much lower fatality rate. **v. mitiga′ta,** v. minor. **v. pemphigo′sa,** smallpox with an eruption of large blebs. **v. siliquo′sa,** smallpox in which the contents of the pustules become absorbed, leaving the walls empty. **v. ve′ra,** simple and unmodified smallpox. **v. verruco′sa,** a variety of smallpox in which the eruption does not pass beyond the papular stage.

variolar (vah-ri′o-lar) pertaining to smallpox.

Variolaria amara (va″re-o-la′re-ah ah-ma′rah) a febrifugal and anthelmintic lichen of the Old World, which is a source of litmus.

variolate (va′re-o-lāt) 1. having the nature or appearance of smallpox. 2. to inoculate with smallpox virus.

variolation (va″re-o-la′shun) deliberate inoculation with the virus of unmodified smallpox to produce immunity to the naturally occurring disease. As practiced in the Orient in ancient times, the dried crusts of smallpox lesions were applied to the skin or nasal mucous membranes, or were ingested. The method employed in Europe in the eighteenth century consisted in subcutaneous injection of material from the lesions. Variolation is now used only experimentally in animals. **bovine v.,** inoculation of a calf with smallpox.

variolic (var″e-ol′ik) variolar.

varioliform (va″re-o′lĭ-form) resembling smallpox.

variolization (va″re-o-li-za′shun) variolation.

varioloid (va′re-o-loid″) a modified and mild form of smallpox occurring in a patient who has had a previous attack or has been vaccinated.

variolous (vah-ri′o-lus) pertaining to or of the nature of smallpox.

variolovaccine (vah-ri″o-lo-vak′sēn) 1. pertaining to vaccine or bovine variola. 2. a virus obtained by vaccinating the heifer with the virus of smallpox.

variolovaccinia (vah-ri″o-lo-vak-sin′e-ah) cowpox in the heifer caused by inoculation with smallpox.

varistor (va-ris′tor) a voltage-variable resistor; a resistor, usually a semiconductor, designed to change its resistance with the voltage applied across it.

varix (vār′iks), pl. *var′ices* [L.] an enlarged and tortuous vein, artery, or lymphatic vessel. **anastomotic v.,** a varix composed of intercommunicating channels. **aneurysmal v., an-**

eurysmoid v., a markedly dilated tortuous vessel; sometimes used to denote a form of arteriovenous aneurysm in which the blood flows directly into a neighboring vein without the intervention of a connecting sac. Called also *Pott's aneurysm.* **arterial v.,** a racemose aneurysm or varicose artery. **cirsoid v.,** racemose aneurysm. **esophageal v.,** varicosities of the branches of the azygos vein which anastomose with tributaries of the portal vein in the lower esophagus, occurring in patients with portal hypertension. **lymph v., v. lymphat′icus,** a soft, lobulated swelling of a lymph node, resulting from obstruction and dilatation of the lymphatic vessels. **papillary varices,** Cayenne pepper spots.

varnish (var′nish) a solution of rosin, of resin, or of several resins in a suitable solvent or solvents, applied in a thin layer to form a hard, smooth surface; sometimes used in dentistry as a protective film for the dental pulp.

varolian (vah-ro′le-an) 1. described by or named for Costanzo Varolius (*Varoli, Varolio*), Italian anatomist and surgeon, 1543–1575. 2. pertaining to the pons.

Varolius′ bridge, valve (vah-ro′le-us) [Costanzo *Varolius* (*Varoli, Varolio*), Italian anatomist, 1543–1575] see *pons* (def. 2) and *valva ileocecalis.*

varus (va′rus) [L.] bent inward; denoting a deformity in which the angulation of the part is toward the midline of the body, as talipes varus. The term varus is an adjective and should be used only in connection with the noun it describes, as talipes varus, genu varum, coxa vara, etc. Cf. *valgus.*

vas (vas), pl. *va′sa* [L.] a vessel: any canal for carrying a fluid; [NA] a general term for such channels, especially those carrying blood, lymph, or spermatozoa. **v. aber′rans, 1.** a blind tubule sometimes connected with the epididymis; it is a vestigial mesonephric tubule. **2.** any anomalous or unusual vessel. **v. aber′rans of Roth,** see *ductuli aberrantes.* **va′sa aber′ran′tis hep′atis,** numerous vessels found in the inconstant fibrous appendix and in the capsule of the liver. **v. af′ferens glomer′uli** [NA], afferent vessel (or arteriole) of glomerulus: a branch of an interlobular artery that goes to a renal glomerulus. **va′sa afferen′tia,** vessels that convey fluid to a structure or part. **va′sa afferen′tia lymphoglan′dulae,** vasa afferentia nodi lymphatici. **va′sa afferen′tia no′di lymphat′ici** [NA], afferent vessels of lymph node: lymphatic vessels that carry lymph to a lymph node, entering through the capsule. **v. anastomot′icum** [NA], anastomotic vessel: a vessel that serves to interconnect other vessels; such communications are present in the palm of the hand, sole of the foot, base of the brain, and other regions. **va′sa au′ris inter′nae** [NA], vessels of the internal ear. **va′sa bre′via,** arteriae gastricae breves. **v. capilla′re** [NA], a capillary: any of the minute vessels connecting the arterioles and the venules, forming networks found in nearly all parts of the body. Their walls act as semipermeable membranes for the interchange of various substances between the blood and tissue fluid. See also *continuous capillaries* and *fenestrated capillaries,* under *capillary.* **v. collatera′le** [NA], collateral vessel: a vessel that parallels another vessel, nerve, or other structure. **v. def′erens,** ductus deferens. **v. ef′ferens glomer′uli** [NA], efferent vessel (or arteriole) of glomerulus: an arteriole that arises from a renal glomerulus, breaking up into capillaries to supply renal tubules. **va′sa efferen′tia,** efferent vessels: vessels that convey fluid away from a structure or part; see *vasa efferentia nodi lymphatici* and *ductuli efferentes testis.* **va′sa efferen′tia lymphoglan′dulae,** vasa efferentia nodi lymphatici. **va′sa efferen′tia no′di lymphat′ici** [NA], efferent vessels of lymph node: lymphatic vessels that carry lymph away from a lymph node, emerging at the hilus. **v. epididym′idis,** ductus epididymidis. **va′sa intesti′ni ten′uis,** arteriae intestinales. **v. lymphat′icum** [NA], a vessel that conveys lymph; pl. **va′sa lymphat′ica** [NA], lymphatic vessels: the capillaries, collecting vessels, and trunks which collect lymph from the tissues and through which the lymph passes to reach the blood stream. **va′sa lymphat′ica profun′da** [NA], deep lymphatic vessels: lymphatic vessels that accompany the deeply placed blood vessels. **va′sa lymphat′ica superficia′lia** [NA], superficial lymphatic vessels: lymphatic vessels located under the skin and superficial fascia, in the submucous areolar tissue of the digestive, respiratory, and genitourinary tracts, and in the subserous tissue of the walls of the abdomen and thorax. **va′sa nervo′rum,** blood vessels supplying the nerves. **va′sa nutri′tia,** see *vasa vasorum.* **va′sa prae′via,** presentation, in front of the fetal head during labor, of the blood vessels of the umbilical cord where they enter the placenta. **v. prom′inens duc′tus cochlea′ris** [NA], a small vessel often seen deep to the spiral prominence in the cochlear duct. **va′sa pro′pria of Jungbluth,** vessels situated beneath the amnion of the early embryo. **va′sa rec′ta** [L. "straight vessels"], arteriolae rectae renis. **va′sa sanguin′ea integumen′ti commu′nis,** the blood vessels of the skin, or common integument. **va′sa sanguin′ea ret′inae** [NA], the blood vessels of the retina, including all the arterioles, derived from the central artery of the retina, and the venules, which return blood to the central vein. **v. spira′le** [NA], a prominent vessel in the basilar membrane near the osseous spiral

lamina. **va′sa vaso′rum** [NA], the small nutrient arteries and the veins in the walls of the larger blood vessels. **va′sa vortico′sa,** venae vorticosae.

vasa (va′sah) [L.] plural of *vas.*

Vasal (vas′al) trademark for a preparation of papaverine hydrochloride.

vasal (va′sal) pertaining to a vas or to a vessel.

vasalgia (vah-sal′je-ah) pain in vessels.

vasalium (vah-sa′le-um) true vascular tissue, such as is found in closed or vascular organs.

vascular (vas′ku-lar) pertaining to blood vessels or indicative of a copious blood supply.

vascularity (vas″ku-lar′ĭ-te) the condition of being vascular.

vascularization (vas″ku-lar-i-za′shun) the process of becoming vascular, or the natural or surgically induced development of vessels in a tissue.

vascularize (vas′ku-lar″īz) to supply with vessels.

vasculature (vas′ku-lah-tūr) the vascular system of the body or any part of it.

vasculitic (vas′ku-lit′ik) pertaining to vasculitis.

vasculitis (vas″ku-li′tis) [L. *vasculum* vessel + *-itis*] inflammation of a vessel; angiitis. **allergic cutaneous v.,** see under *angiitis.* **livedo v.,** segmented hyalinizing v. **necrotizing v.,** polyarteritis. **nodular v.,** allergic cutaneous angiitis. **segmented hyalinizing v.,** chronic relapsing vasculitis of the lower legs, the lesions being nodular or purpuric, or both, at the onset and later becoming superficially ulcerated, resulting in scars; histologically, endothelial proliferations, hyaline degeneration, and thrombosis are seen in the mid and lower dermis. It usually affects middle-aged persons with circulatory difficulties. Called also *livedo v.*

vasculogenesis (vas″ku-lo-jen′ĕ-sis) [L. *vasculum* vessel + Gr. *genesis* production] the development of the vascular system.

vasculogenic (vas″ku-lo-jen′ik) inducing vascularization.

vasculolymphatic (vas″ku-lo-lim-fat′ik) pertaining to blood or lymph vessels.

vasculomotor (vas″ku-lo-mo′tor) vasomotor.

vasculopathy (vas″ku-lop′ah-the) any disorder of blood vessels.

vasculotoxic (vas″ku-lo-tok′sik) pertaining to or characterized by a deleterious or toxic effect on the vessels of the body.

vasculum (vas′ku-lum), pl. *vas′cula* [L., dim. of *vas*] a small vessel. **v. aber′rans,** vas aberrans.

vasectomized (vas-ek′to-mīzd) deprived of the ductus deferentes (vasa deferentia) by surgical means.

vasectomy (vah-sek′to-me) [*vas* + Gr. *ektomē* excision] surgical removal of the ductus (vas) deferens, or of a portion of it; done in association with prostatectomy, or to induce infertility. **cross-over v.,** vasectomy in which the right and the left vas deferens are transected, the lower portion of each (the portions still attached to the epididymis) then being tied together. The technique prevents recanalization while allowing surgical reconstruction.

vasifactive (vas″ĭ-fak′tiv) [*vas* + L. *facere* to make] vasoformative.

vasiform (vas′ĭ-form) [*vas* + L. *forma* form] having the appearance of a vessel.

vasitis (vah-si′tis) inflammation of the ductus (vas) deferens.

vaso- (vas′o) [L. *vas* vessel] a combining form denoting relationship to a vessel or to a duct.

vasoactive (vas″o-ak′tiv) exerting an effect upon the caliber of blood vessels.

vasoconstriction (vas″o-kon-strik′shun) the diminution of the caliber of vessels, especially constriction of arterioles leading to decreased blood flow to a part.

vasoconstrictive (vas″o-kon-strik′tiv) pertaining to, characterized by, or producing vasoconstriction.

vasoconstrictor (vas″o-kon-strik′tor) 1. causing constriction of the blood vessels. 2. an agent (motor nerve or chemical compound) that causes constriction of the blood vessels.

vasocorona (vas″o-ko-ro′nah) [*vaso-* + L. *corona* crown] the arterial vessels which pass radially from the spinal cord to its periphery.

vasodentin (vas″o-den′tin) [*vaso-* + L. *dens* tooth] dentin provided with blood vessels, as in the teeth of some fishes.

vasodepression (vas″o-de-presh′un) decrease in vascular resistance with hypotension.

vasodepressor (vas″o-de-pres′sor) 1. having the effect of lowering the blood pressure through reduction in peripheral resistance. 2. an agent that causes vasodepression.

Vasodilan (vas″o-di′lan) trademark for preparations of isoxsuprine hydrochloride.

vasodilatation (vas″o-di-lah-ta′shun) a state of increased caliber of the blood vessels.

vasodilatin (vas″o-di-la′tin) (*obs.*) a substance obtained from tissue extracts, causing vasodilation and stimulating gastric secretion; possibly identical with *histamine.*

vasodilation (vas″o-di-la′shun) dilation of a vessel, especially dilation of arterioles leading to increased blood flow to a part. **reflex v.,** vasodilation occurring as a reflex response to stimuli applied elsewhere, or subsequent to an initial vasoconstrictive response.

vasodilative (vas″o-di′la-tiv) pertaining to, characterized by, or producing vasodilatation.

vasodilator (vas″o-di-lāt′or) 1. causing dilation of the blood vessels. 2. an agent (motor nerve or chemical compound) that causes dilation of the blood vessels.

vasoepididymography (vas″o-ep″ĭ-did″ĭ-mog′rah-fe) radiography of the vas deferens and epididymis after injection of a contrast medium.

vasoepididymostomy (vas″o-ep″ĭ-did-ĭ-mos′to-me) operative formation of a communication between the ductus (vas) deferens and the epididymis.

vasofactive (vas″o-fak′tiv) vasoformative.

vasoformative (vas″o-for′mah-tiv) pertaining to or promoting the formation of blood vessels.

vasoganglion (vas″o-gang′gle-on) any vascular ganglion or rete.

vasography (vah-sog′rah-fe) [*vaso-* + Gr. *graphein* to write] roentgenography of the blood vessels.

vasohypertonic (vas″o-hi″per-ton′ik) vasoconstrictor.

vasohypotonic (vas″o-hi″po-ton′ik) vasodilator.

vasoinert (vas″o-in-ert′) exerting no effect on the caliber of blood vessels.

vasoinhibitor (vas″o-in-hib′ĭ-tor) an agent that inhibits the action of the vasomotor nerves.

vasoinhibitory (vas″o-in-hib′ĭ-tor-e) hindering the action of the vasomotor nerves.

vasoligation (vas″o-li-ga′shun) ligation of the ductus (vas) deferens.

vasoligature (vas″o-lig′ah-tūr) vasoligation.

vasomotion (vas″o-mo′shun) [*vaso-* + L. *motio* movement] change in the caliber of a vessel, especially of a blood vessel.

vasomotor (vas-o-mo′tor) [*vaso-* + L. *motor* mover] 1. affecting the caliber of a vessel, especially of a blood vessel. 2. any element or agent that affects the caliber of a blood vessel.

vasomotorial (vas″o-mo-to′re-al) 1. pertaining to the vasomotorium. 2. pertaining to the change in caliber of a blood vessel.

vasomotoricity (vas″o-mo-tor-is′ĭ-te) the power of producing change in the caliber of blood vessels.

vasomotorium (vas″o-mo-to′re-um) the vasomotor system of the body, i.e., the part of the nervous system that controls the caliber of blood vessels.

vasomotory (vas″o-mo′tor-e) affecting the caliber of a vessel, especially a blood vessel.

vasoneuropathy (vas″o-nu-rop′ah-the) a combined vascular and neurologic defect, the lesions being caused by simultaneous action of both the vascular and the nervous system, or by the interaction of the two systems.

vasoneurosis (vas″o-nu-ro′sis) angioneuropathy.

vaso-orchidostomy (vas″o-or″kid-os′to-me) the operation of suturing tubules of the epididymis to the ductus (vas) deferens.

vasoparesis (vas″o-pah-re′sis) [*vaso-* + Gr. *paresis* relaxation] partial paralysis of vasomotor nerves.

vasopermeability (vas″o-per″me-ah-bil′ĭ-te) the permeability of a blood vessel; the extent to which a blood vessel is permeable.

vasopressin (vas″o-pres′in) 1. one of two octapeptide hormones formed by the neuronal cells of the hypothalamic nuclei and stored in the posterior lobe of the pituitary gland (neurohypophysis), the other being oxytocin. It stimulates the contraction of the muscular tissue of the capillaries and arterioles, raising the blood pressure. It stimulates contraction of the intestinal musculature and increases peristalsis, and also exerts some influence on the uterus. It also has a specific effect on the epithelial cells of the distal portion of the uriniferous tubule, stimulating resorption of water independently of solutes, resulting in concentration of urine. Its rate of secretion is regulated chiefly by the osmolarity of the plasma. 2. [USP], a pharmaceutical preparation of the same principle, prepared synthetically or obtained from the posterior pituitary of healthy domestic animals used for food by man; used mainly as an antidiuretic in the treatment of acute or chronic diabetes insipidus, administered intramuscularly or subcutaneously or by nasal inhalation or topical application to the nasal mucosa. It is also administered intramuscularly as a test of renal function, and may be used to stimulate smooth muscle tissue, especially to induce vasoconstriction in the presence of hemorrhage. Called also *antidiuretic hormone (ADH)* and *beta-hypophamine.*

vasopressor (vas″o-pres′or) 1. stimulating contraction of the muscular tissue of the capillaries and arteries. 2. an agent that stimulates contraction of the muscular tissue of the capillaries and arteries.

vasopuncture (vas′o-punk″tūr) puncture of the ductus (vas) deferens.

vasoreflex (vas″o-re′flex) a reflex of a blood vessel.

vasorelaxation (vas″o-re-lak-sa′shun) decrease of vascular pressure.

vasoresection (vas″o-re-sek′shun) resection of the ductus (vas) deferens.

vasorrhaphy (vas-or′ah-fe) suture of the ductus (vas) deferens.

vasosection (vas″o-sek′shun) [*vaso-* + L. *sectio* a cutting] the severing of a vessel or vessels, especially of the ductus deferentes (vasa deferentia).

vasosensory (vas″o-sen′so-re) supplying sensory filaments to the vessels.

vasospasm (vas′o-spazm) spasm of the blood vessels, resulting in decrease in their caliber.

vasospasmolytic (vas″o-spaz″mo-lit′ik) arresting spasm of the vessels.

vasospastic (vas″o-spas′tik) producing or affected by vagospasm.

vasostimulant (vas″o-stim′u-lant) stimulating or arousing vasomotor action.

vasostomy (vah-sos′to-me) [*vas* deferens + Gr. *stomoun* to provide with an opening, or mouth] the operation of forming an opening into the ductus (vas) deferens.

vasotocin (vas″o-to′sin) a nonapeptide hormone having the properties of both vasopressin and oxytocin, occurring in birds, amphibians, and fishes.

vasotomy (vah-sot′o-me) [*vaso-* + Gr. *tomē* a cutting] incision into or cutting of the ductus (vas) deferens; called also *Belfield's operation.*

vasotonia (vas″o-to′ne-ah) [*vaso-* + Gr. *tonos* tone + *-ia*] tone or tension of the vessels; called also *angiotonia.*

vasotonic (vas″o-ton′ic) pertaining to, characterized by, or promoting vasotonia.

vasotribe (vas′o-trīb) angiotribe.

vasotripsy (vas′o-trip″se) angiotripsy.

vasotrophic (vas″o-trof′ik) [*vaso-* + Gr. *trophē* nutrition] affecting nutrition through the alteration of the caliber of the blood vessels.

vasotropic (vas″o-trop′ik) tending to act on blood vessels.

vasovagal (vas″o-va′gal) vascular and vagal; see *vasovagal attack,* under *attack.*

vasovasostomy (vas″o-vah-sos′to-me) anastomosis of the ends of the severed ductus (vas) deferens; done to restore fertility in vasectomized males.

vasovesiculectomy (vas″o-ve-sik″u-lek′to-me) excision of the ductus (vas) deferens and seminal vesicles.

vasovesiculitis (vas″o-ve-sik″u-li′tis) inflammation of the ductus deferentes (vasa deferentia) and seminal vesicles.

Vasoxyl (vas-ok′sil) trademark for preparations of methoxamine hydrochloride.

vastus (vas′tus) [L.] great or vast; description of muscles, as musculus vastus lateralis.

VATER an acronym for *v*ertebral defects, imperforate *a*nus, *t*racheoesophageal fistula, and *r*adial and *r*enal dysplasia, which together form a nonrandom association of congenital defects.

Vater's ampulla, corpuscles, papilla (fah′terz) [Abraham *Vater,* German anatomist, 1684–1751] see *ampulla hepatopancreatica, corpuscula lamellosa,* and *papilla duodeni major.*

Vater-Pacini corpuscles (fah′ter-pa-se′ne) [Abraham *Vater:* Filippo *Pacini,* Italian anatomist, 1812–1883] corpuscula lamellosa.

Vateria (vah-te′re-ah) [named for A. *Vater*] a genus of Asian trees of the family Dipterocarpaceae. **V. in′dica** L., an East Indian tree which affords Indian copal, piny varnish, white dammar, or Indian anime; used as a varnish, candle-stuff, and medicine.

Vaughan-Novy's test [Victor Clarence *Vaughan,* American pathologist, 1851–1929; Frederick George *Novy,* American bacteriologist, 1864–1957] see under *tests.*

vault (vawlt) a domelike or archlike structure. In dentistry, the longest palatal border obtainable through a coronal section of the maxilla; the shape of the palatal arch posteriorly. **v. of pharynx,** fornix pharyngis.

VC vital capacity.

VCG vectorcardiogram.

V-Cillin (ve-sil′in) trademark for preparations of penicillin V.

V.D. venereal disease.

VDEL Venereal Disease Experimental Laboratory.

V.D.G. venereal disease—gonorrhea.

V.D.H. valvular disease of the heart.

VDRL Venereal Disease Research Laboratories; see also under *antigen* and *test.*

V.D.S. venereal disease—syphilis.

vecordia (ve-kor′de-ah) [L. *vecors* without reason] an old term for a concept of partial insanity. Cf. *vesania*.

vection (vek′shun) [L. *vectio* a carrying] the carrying of disease germs from an infected person to a well person. It is *circumferential, indirect,* or *mediate* when pathogens are carried by an intermediate host; *direct, immediate,* and *radial* when transferred directly from one person to another.

vectis (vek′tis) [L. from *vehere* to carry] a curved lever for making traction upon the fetal head in labor.

vector (vek′tor) [L. "one who carries," from *vehere* to carry] 1. a carrier, especially the animal (usually an arthropod) which transfers an infective agent from one host to another. 2. a quantity possessing magnitude, direction, and sense (positivity or negativity), and commonly represented by a straight line resembling an arrow: the length of the line denotes magnitude, the arrowhead denotes sense, and the position of the line with respect to an axis of reference denotes direction. **biological v.,** an anthropod vector in whose body the infecting organism develops or multiplies before becoming infective to the recipient individual. **mechanical v.,** an arthropod vector which transmits an infective organism from one host to another but which is not essential to the life cycle of the parasite. **spatial v.,** one representing a three-dimensional force; see *vectorcardiography*.

vectorcardiogram (vek″tor-kar′de-o-gram″) the record, usually a photograph, of the loop formed on the oscilloscope in vectorcardiography, the inscribed loop representing the ends of the instantaneous vectors.

vectorcardiograph (vek″tor-kar′de-o-graf) the instrument used in vectocardiography.

vectorcardiography (vek″tor-kar′de-og′rah-fe) the registration, usually by formation of a loop display on an oscilloscope, of the direction and magnitude (vector) of the moment-to-moment electromotive forces of the heart during one complete cycle, as transmitted by electrocardiographic leads. **spatial v.,** that in which the potential vectors of cardiac excitation are projected upon three mutually perpendicular coordinates, which are usually designated X, Y, and Z, where X is the transverse (right or left), Y the vertical (up or down), and Z the sagittal (anterior or posterior).

vectorial (vek-to′re-al) pertaining to a vector.

vectorscope (vek′tor-skōp) a device utilized in viewing vectorcardiograms.

Vectrin (vek′trin) trademark for preparations of minocycline hydrochloride.

Vedder's culture medium (agar), sign (ved′erz) [Col. Edward Bright *Vedder*, U.S. Army Surgeon, retired, 1878–1952] see under *culture medium*, and see under *sign*.

VEE Venezuelan equine encephalomyelitis.

Veetids (ve′tidz) trademark for a preparation of penicillin V potassium.

vegan (vej′an) an extreme vegetarian who excludes all animal protein from his diet.

veganism (vej′ah-nizm) strict limitation to a vegetable diet, with exclusion of all protein of animal origin.

vegetable (vej′e-tah-b'l) [L. *vegetabilis* quickening] 1. pertaining to or derived from plants. 2. any plant or species of plant, especially one cultivated as a source of food.

vegetal (vej′e-tal) 1. pertaining to plants or to a plant. 2. vegetative.

vegetality (vej″e-tal′ĭ-te) the aggregate of phenomena that are common to plants.

vegetarian (vej″e-tār′e-an) one whose food is exclusively of vegetable origin.

vegetarianism (vej″e-tār′e-ah-nizm″) restriction of the diet to food substances of vegetable origin.

vegetation (vej″e-ta′shun) [L. *vegetatio*] any plantlike fungoid neoplasm or growth; a luxuriant fungus-like growth of pathologic tissue. **adenoid v.,** fungus-like growths of lymphoid tissue in the nasopharynx. **bacterial v's,** irregular excrescences on the cardiac valves or endocardium formed by bacteria. **dendritic v.,** 1. the shaggy appearance of a villous cancer. 2. the arachnoidal tufts and villous neoplasms on the pleura and other serous membranes. **verrucous v's,** small irregular excrescences on the cardiac valves.

vegetative (vej′e-ta″tiv) 1. concerned with growth and with nutrition. 2. functioning involuntarily or unconsciously, as the vegetative nervous system; see under *system*. 3. resting; denoting the portion of a cell cycle during which the cell is not involved in replication. 4. of, pertaining to, or characteristic of plants. 5. of or pertaining to asexual reproduction, as by budding or fission.

vegetoanimal (vej″e-to-an′ĭ-mal) common to plants and animals.

vehicle (ve′ĭ-k'l) [L. *vehiculum*] 1. an excipient. 2. any medium through which an impulse is propagated.

veil (vāl) 1. a covering structure; see *velum*. 2. a caul or piece of the amniotic sac occasionally covering the face of a newborn child. 3. a slight huskiness in the voice of a singer. **Fick's v.,** see under *phenomenon*. **Hottentot v.,** see under *apron*. **Jackson's v.,** see under *membrane*. **posterior v. of soft palate,** palatum molle. **Sattler's v.,** see *Fick's phenomenon*.

Veillon tube (va-yaw′) [Adrien *Veillon*, Paris bacteriologist, 1864–1931] see under *tube*.

Veillonella (va″yon-el′ah) [Adrien *Veillon*] a genus of microorganisms of the family Neisseriaceae, order Eubacteriales, made up of minute (0.3–0.4 μ) obligate anaerobic cocci, found as nonpathogenic parasites in the mouth, intestines, and urogenital and respiratory tracts of man and other animals. Six species have been named, *V. alcales′cens, V. discoi′des, V. orbic′ulus, V. par′vula, V. renifor′mis,* and *V. vulvovaginit′idis*.

vein (vān) [L. *vena*] a vessel through which blood passes from various organs or parts back to the heart. Called also *vena* [NA]. All veins except the pulmonary veins carry blood low in oxygen. Veins, like arteries, have three coats, an *inner, middle,* and *outer,* but the coats are not so thick, and they collapse when the vessel is cut. Many veins have *valves* formed of reduplications of their lining membrane, which prevent the backward flow of blood away from the heart. See Plates accompanying the *Table of Venae,* under *vena*. **accompanying v.,** vena comitans. **accom-**

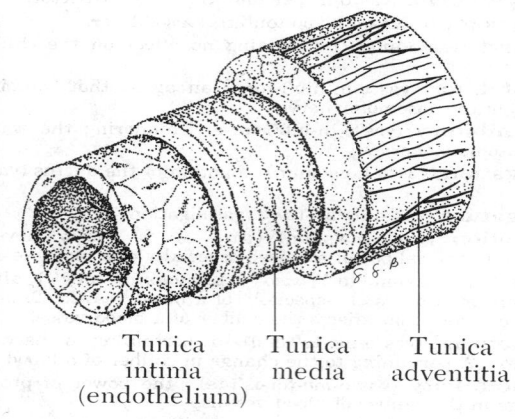

Tunica intima (endothelium)   Tunica media   Tunica adventitia

The three coats of a vein.

panying v. of hypoglossal nerve, vena comitans nervi hypoglossi. **adrenal v's,** venae suprarenales. **afferent v's,** veins that carry blood to an organ. **allantoic v's,** paired vessels that accompany the allantois, growing out from the primitive hindgut and entering the body stalk of the early embryo; they fuse later into one vessel, the umbilical vein. **anastomotic v., inferior,** vena anastomotica inferior. **anastomotic v., superior,** vena anastomotica superior. **angular v.,** vena angularis. **anonymous v's,** venae brachiocephalicae [dextra et sinistra]. **antebrachial v., median,** vena mediana antebrachii. **appendicular v.,** vena appendicularis. **v. of aqueduct of vestibule,** vena aqueductus vestibuli. **aqueous v's,** microscopic, blood vessel–like pathways on the surface of the eye, containing aqueous humor or diluted blood and connecting the sinus venosus sclerae (Schlemm's canal) with conjunctival or subconjunctival veins. Called also *Ascher's v's*. **arciform v's, arcuate v's of kidney,** venae arcuatae renis. **arterial v.,** truncus pulmonalis. **arterial v. of Soemmering,** vena portae. **ascending v's of Rosenthal,** venae cerebri inferiores. **Ascher's v's,** aqueous v's. **auditory v's, internal,** venae labyrinthi. **auricular v's, anterior,** venae auriculares anteriores. **auricular v., posterior,** vena auricularis posterior. **axillary v.,** vena axillaris. **azygos v.,** vena azygos. **azygos v., left,** vena hemiazygos. **azygos v., lesser superior,** vena hemiazygos accessoria. **basal v.,** vena basilis. **basilic v.,** vena basilica. **basilic v., median,** vena mediana basilica. **basivertebral v's,** venae basivertebrales. **brachial v's,** venae brachiales. **brachiocephalic v's,** venae brachiocephalicae [dextra et sinistra]. **Breschet's v's,** venae diploicae. **bronchial v's,** venae bronchiales. **Browning's v.,** the upper portion of the inferior anastomotic vein. **v. of bulb of penis,** vena bulbi penis. **v. of bulb of vestibule,** vena bulbi vestibuli. **Burow's v.,** a vessel formed by the two inferior epigastric veins and a branch from the bladder; it joins the portal vein. **v. of canaliculus of cochlea,** vena canaliculi cochleae. **cardiac v's,** venae cordis. **cardiac v's, anterior,** venae cordis anteriores. **cardiac v., great,** vena cordis magna. **cardiac v., middle,** vena cordis media.

Plate LI   veins

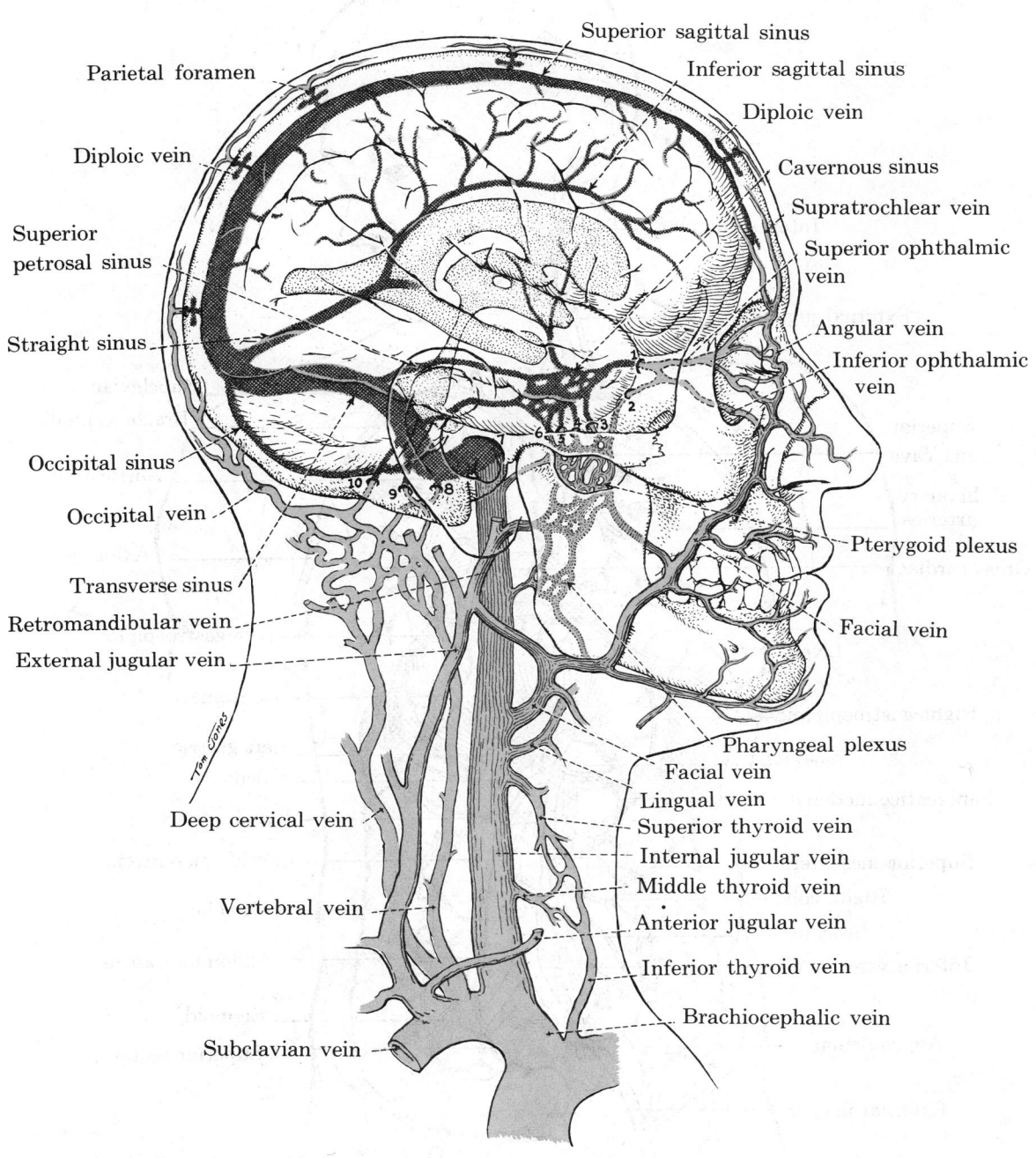

Parietal foramen

Diploic vein

Superior
petrosal sinus

Straight sinus

Occipital sinus

Occipital vein

Transverse sinus

Retromandibular vein

External jugular vein

Deep cervical vein

Vertebral vein

Subclavian vein

Superior sagittal sinus

Inferior sagittal sinus

Diploic vein

Cavernous sinus

Supratrochlear vein

Superior ophthalmic
vein

Angular vein

Inferior ophthalmic
vein

Pterygoid plexus

Facial vein

Pharyngeal plexus

Facial vein

Lingual vein

Superior thyroid vein

Internal jugular vein

Middle thyroid vein

Anterior jugular vein

Inferior thyroid vein

Brachiocephalic vein

VEINS OF THE HEAD AND NECK
(Modified from Jones and Shepard)

Plate LII   veins

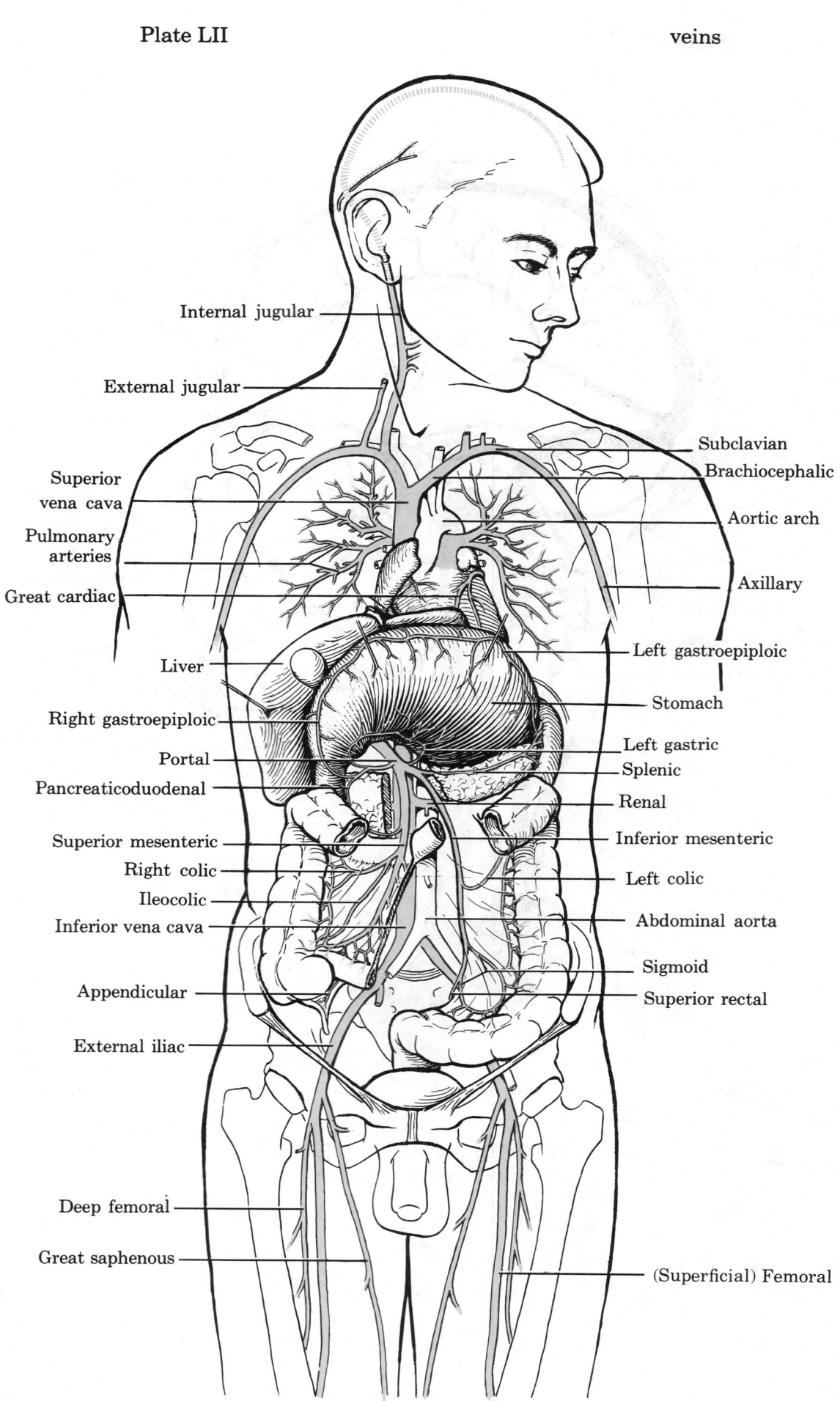

Internal jugular

External jugular

Superior
vena cava

Pulmonary
arteries

Great cardiac

Liver

Right gastroepiploic

Portal

Pancreaticoduodenal

Superior mesenteric

Right colic

Ileocolic

Inferior vena cava

Appendicular

External iliac

Deep femoral

Great saphenous

Subclavian

Brachiocephalic

Aortic arch

Axillary

Left gastroepiploic

Stomach

Left gastric

Splenic

Renal

Inferior mesenteric

Left colic

Abdominal aorta

Sigmoid

Superior rectal

(Superficial) Femoral

PRINCIPAL VEINS OF THE BODY

Plate LIII   veins

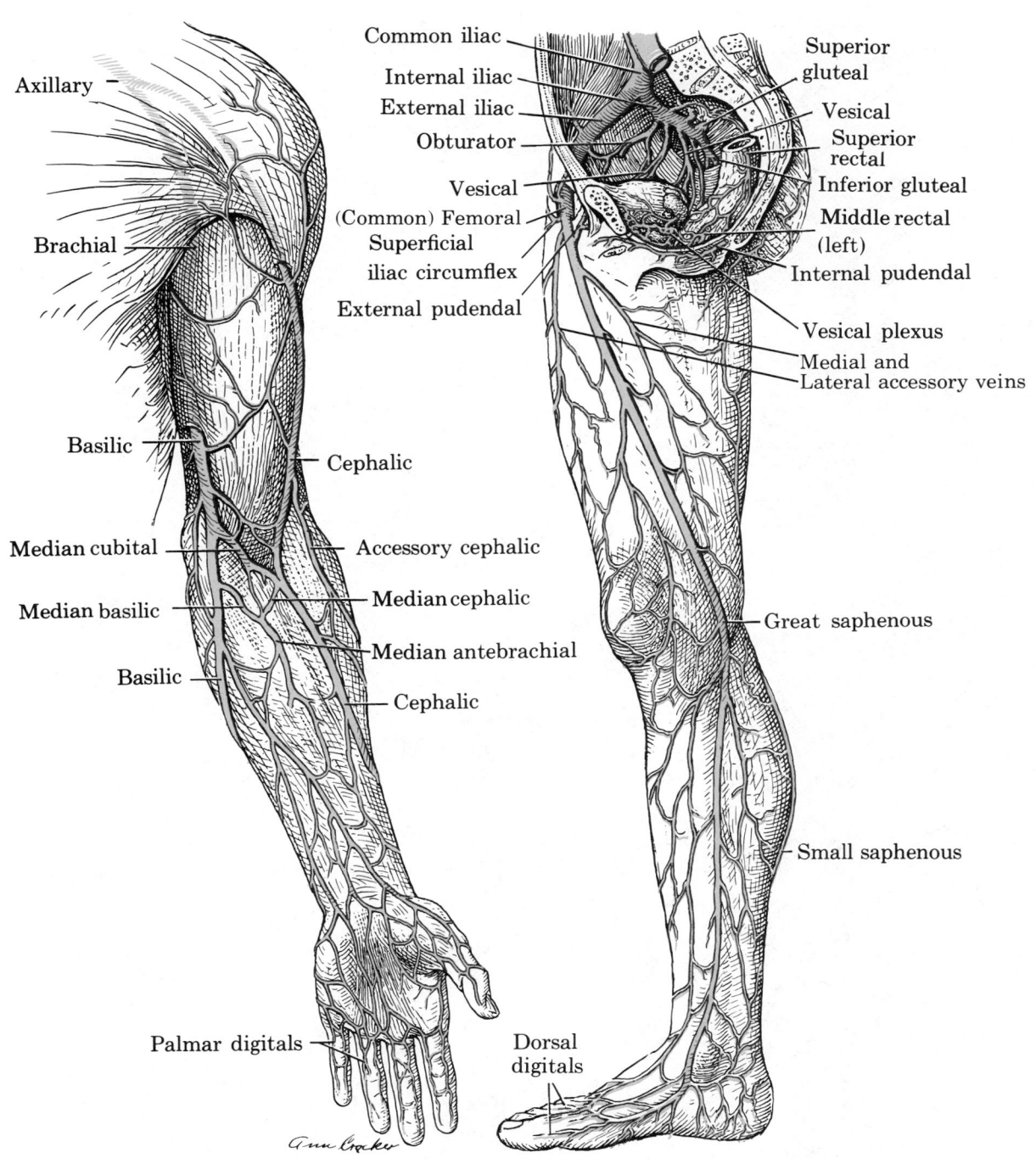

Axillary

Brachial

Basilic

Median cubital

Median basilic

Basilic

Palmar digitals

Common iliac

Internal iliac

External iliac

Obturator

Vesical

(Common) Femoral

Superficial
iliac circumflex

External pudendal

Cephalic

Accessory cephalic

Median cephalic

Median antebrachial

Cephalic

Dorsal
digitals

Superior
gluteal

Vesical

Superior
rectal

Inferior gluteal

Middle rectal

(left)

Internal pudendal

Vesical plexus

Medial and
Lateral accessory veins

Great saphenous

Small saphenous

SUPERFICIAL VEINS OF THE EXTREMITIES

cardiac v., small, vena cordis parva. **cardiac v's, smallest**, venae cordis minimae. **cardinal v's**, embryonic vessels that include the precardinal and postcardinal veins and the ducts of Cuvier (common cardinal veins). **carotid v., external**, vena retromandibularis. **cavernous v's of penis**, venae cavernosae penis. **central v.**, a vein that occupies the axis of an organ. **central v's of hepatic lobules, central v's of liver**, venae centrales hepatis. **central v. of retina**, vena centralis retinae. **central v. of suprarenal gland**, vena centralis glandulae suprarenalis. **cephalic v.**, vena cephalica. **cephalic v., accessory**, vena cephalica accessoria. **cephalic v., median**, vena mediana cephalica. **cerebellar v's, inferior**, venae cerebelli inferiores. **cerebellar v's, superior**, venae cerebelli superiores. **cerebral v's**, venae cerebri. **cerebral v., anterior**, vena cerebri anterior. **cerebral v., great**, vena cerebri magna. **cerebral v's, inferior**, venae cerebri inferiores. **cerebral v's, internal**, venae cerebri internae. **cerebral v., middle, deep**, vena cerebri media profunda. **cerebral v., middle, superficial**, vena cerebri media superficialis. **cerebral v's, superior**, venae cerebri superiores. **cervical v., deep**, vena cervicalis profunda. **cervical v's, transverse**, venae transversae colli. **choroid v.**, vena choroidea. **ciliary v's**, venae ciliares. **circumflex femoral v's, lateral**, venae circumflexae femoris laterales. **circumflex femoral v's, medial**, venae circumflexae femoris mediales. **circumflex iliac v., deep**, vena circumflexa ilium profunda. **circumflex iliac v., superficial**, vena circumflexa ilium superficialis. **v. of cochlear canal**, vena canaliculi cochleae. **colic v., left**, vena colica sinistra. **colic v., middle**, vena colica media. **colic v., right**, vena colica dextra. **conjunctival v's**, venae conjunctivales. **coronary v., left**, vena cordis magna. **costoaxillary v's**, venae costoaxillares. **cubital v., median**, vena mediana cubiti. **cutaneous v.**, vena cutanea. **cutaneous v., ulnar**, vena basilica. **cystic v.**, vena cystica. **deep v's of clitoris**, venae profundae clitoridis. **deep v's of penis**, venae profundae penis. **deep v. of thigh**, vena profunda femoris. **deep v. of tongue**, vena profunda linguae. **digital v's, palmar**, venae digitales palmares. **digital v's, plantar**, venae digitales plantares. **digital v's of foot, common**, venae digitales communes pedis. **digital v's of foot, dorsal**, venae digitales dorsales pedis. **diploic v's**, venae diploicae. **diploic v., frontal**, vena diploica frontalis. **diploic v., occipital**, vena diploica occipitalis. **diploic v., temporal, anterior**, vena diploica temporalis anterior. **diploic v., temporal, posterior**, vena diploica temporalis posterior. **dorsal v. of clitoris, deep**, vena dorsalis clitoridis. **dorsal v's of clitoris, superficial**, venae dorsales clitoridis superficiales. **dorsal v. of penis, deep**, vena dorsalis penis. **dorsal v's of penis, superficial**, venae dorsales penis superficiales. **dorsal v's of tongue**, venae dorsales linguae. **dorsispinal v's**, see *plexus venosi vertebrales externi* [*anterior et posterior*]. **duodenal v's**, venae duodenales. **emissary v.**, one passing through a foramen of the skull and draining blood from a cerebral sinus into a vessel outside the skull; called also *vena emissaria* [NA]. **emissary v., condylar**, vena emissaria condylaris. **emissary v., mastoid**, vena emissaria mastoidea. **emissary v., occipital**, vena emissaria occipitalis. **emissary v., parietal**, vena emissaria parietalis. **emulgent v.**, the portion of the left spermatic vein near its termination in the left renal vein. **epigastric v., inferior**, vena epigastrica inferior. **epigastric v., superficial**, vena epigastrica superficialis. **epigastric v's, superior**, venae epigastricae superiores. **episcleral v's**, venae episclerales. **esophageal v's**, venae esophageae. **ethmoidal v's**, venae ethmoidales. **facial v.**, vena facialis. **facial v., anterior**, see *vena facialis*. **facial v., common**, see *vena facialis*. **facial v., deep**, vena faciei profunda. **facial v., posterior**, vena retromandibularis. **facial v., transverse**, vena transversa faciei. **femoral v.**, vena femoralis. **femoral v., deep**, vena profunda femoris. **femoropopliteal v.**, vena femoropoplitea. **fibular v's**, venae peroneae. **frontal v's**, venae supratrochleares. **Galen's v's**, 1. venae cerebri internae. 2. vena cerebri magna. **gastric v., left**, vena gastrica sinistra. **gastric v., right**, vena gastrica dextra. **gastric v's, short**, venae gastricae breves. **gastroepiploic v., left**, vena gastroepiploica sinistra. **gastroepiploic v., right**, vena gastroepiploica dextra. **genicular v's**, venae genus. **gluteal v's, inferior**, venae gluteae inferiores. **gluteal v's, superior**, venae gluteae superiores. **hemiazygos v.**, vena hemiazygos. **hemiazygos v., accessory**, vena hemiazygos accessoria. **hemorrhoidal v's, inferior**, venae rectales inferiores. **hemorrhoidal v's, middle**, venae rectales mediae. **hemorrhoidal v., superior**, vena rectalis superior. **hepatic v's**, venae hepaticae. **hypogastric v.**, vena iliaca interna. **hypophyseoportal v's**, a system of venules connecting capillaries in the hypothalamus with sinusoidal capillaries in the anterior lobe of the hypophysis. **ileal v's**, veins draining blood from the ileum; see *venae jejunales et ilei*. **ileocolic v.**, vena ileocolica. **iliac v., common**, vena iliaca communis. **iliac v., external**, vena iliaca externa. **iliac v., internal**, vena iliaca interna. **iliolumbar v.**, vena iliolumbalis. **innomi-**

nate v's, venae brachiocephalicae [dextra et sinistra]. **intercapital v's**, venae intercapitales. **intercapitular v's of foot**, venae intercapitulares pedis. **intercapitular v's of hand**, venae intercapitales. **intercostal v's, anterior**, venae intercostales anteriores. **intercostal v., highest**, vena intercostalis suprema. **intercostal v's, posterior, IV–XI**, venae intercostales posteriores [IV–XI]. **intercostal v., superior, left**, vena intercostalis superior sinistra. **intercostal v., superior, right**, vena intercostalis superior dextra. **interlobar v's of kidney**, venae interlobares renis. **interlobular v's of kidney**, venae interlobulares renis. **interlobular v's of liver**, venae interlobulares hepatis. **interosseous v's of foot, dorsal**, venae metatarseae dorsales. **interosseous metacarpal v's, dorsal**, venae metacarpeae dorsales. **intervertebral v.**, vena intervertebralis. **jejunal v's**, veins that drain blood from the jejunum; see *venae jejunales et ilei*. **jugular v., anterior**, vena jugularis anterior. **jugular v., anterior horizontal**, arcus venosus juguli. **jugular v., external**, vena jugularis externa. **jugular v., internal**, vena jugularis interna. **v's of kidney**, venae renis. **Kohlrausch v's**, superficial veins passing from the under surface of the penis to the dorsal vein. **Krukenberg's v's**, venae centrales hepatis. **Kuhnt's postcentral v.**, a vein branching from the vena centralis retina, extending posteriorly from the center of the optic nerve, and draining into the canalis opticus. **Labbé's v.**, vena anastomotica inferior. **labial v's, anterior**, venae labiales anteriores. **labial v's, inferior**, venae labiales inferiores. **labial v's, posterior**, venae labiales posteriores. **labial v., superior**, vena labialis superior. **v's of labyrinth**, venae labyrinthi. **lacrimal v.**, vena lacrimalis. **laryngeal v., inferior**, vena laryngea inferior. **laryngeal v., superior**, vena laryngea superior. **lingual v.**, vena lingualis. **lingual v., deep**, vena profunda linguae. **lingual v's, dorsal**, venae dorsales linguae. **lumbar v's I and II**, venae lumbales [I et II], **lumbar v's III and IV**, venae lumbales [III et IV], **lumbar v., ascending**, vena lumbalis ascendens. **mammary v's, external**, venae costoaxillares. **mammary v., internal**, see *venae thoracicae internae*. **v. of Marshall, Marshall's oblique v.**, vena obliqua atrii sinistri. **masseteric v's**, venae massetericae. **maxillary v's**, venae maxillares. **median v. of elbow**, vena mediana cubiti. **median v. of forearm**, vena mediana antebrachii. **median v. of neck**, vena mediana colli. **mediastinal v's**, venae mediastinales. **meningeal v's**, venae meningeae. **meningeal v's, middle**, venae meningeae mediae. **mesenteric v., inferior**, vena mesenterica inferior. **mesenteric v., superior**, vena mesenterica superior. **metacarpal v's, dorsal**, venae metacarpeae dorsales. **metacarpal v's, palmar**, venae metacarpeae palmares. **metatarsal v's, dorsal**, venae metatarseae dorsales. **metatarsal v's, plantar**, venae metatarseae plantares. **muscular v's**, venae musculares. **musculophrenic v's**, venae musculophrenicae. **nasal v's, external**, venae nasales externae. **nasofrontal v.**, vena nasofrontalis. **oblique v. of left atrium**, vena obliqua atrii sinistri. **obturator v's**, venae obturatoriae. **occipital v.**, vena occipitalis. **oesophageal v's**, venae esophageae. **omphalomesenteric v's**, vitelline v's. **ophthalmic v., inferior**, vena ophthalmica inferior. **ophthalmic v., superior**, vena ophthalmica superior. **ophthalmomeningeal v.**, vena ophthalmomeningea. **ovarian v., left**, vena ovarica sinistra. **ovarian v., right**, vena ovarica dextra. **palatine v., external**, vena palatina externa. **palpebral v's**, venae palpebrales. **palpebral v's, inferior**, venae palpebrales inferiores. **palpebral v's, superior**, venae palpebrales superiores. **pancreatic v's**, venae pancreaticae. **pancreaticoduodenal v's**, venae pancreaticoduodenales. **paraumbilical v's**, venae paraumbilicales. **parietal v. of Santorini**, vena emissaria parietalis. **parotid v's**, venae parotideae. **parotid v's, anterior**, rami parotidei venae facialis. **parotid v's, posterior**, venae parotideae. **parumbilical v's**, venae paraumbilicales. **perforating v's**, venae perforantes. **pericardiac v's**, venae pericardiacae. **pericardiacophrenic v's**, venae pericardiacophrenicae. **peroneal v's**, venae peroneae. **pharyngeal v's**, venae pharyngeae. **phrenic v's, inferior**, venae phrenicae inferiores. **phrenic v's, superior**, venae pericardiacophrenicae. **popliteal v.**, vena poplitea. **portal v.**, vena portae. **postcardinal v's**, paired vessels in the embryo caudal to the heart. **posterior v. of left ventricle**, vena posterior ventriculi sinistri cordis. **precardinal v's**, paired venous trunks in the embryo cranial to the heart. **prepyloric v.**, vena prepylorica. **primary head v's**, vessels alongside the embryonic brain that continue into the precardinal veins. **v. of pterygoid canal**, vena canalis pterygoidei. **pudendal v's, external**, venae pudendae externae. **pudendal v., internal**, vena pudenda interna. **pulmonary v's**, venae pulmonales. **pulmonary v., inferior, left**, vena pulmonalis inferior sinistra. **pulmonary v., inferior, right**, vena pulmonalis inferior dextra. **pulmonary v., superior, left**, vena pulmonalis superior sinistra. **pulmonary v., superior, right**, vena pulmonalis superior dextra. **pulp v's**, vessels draining the venous sinuses of the spleen. **pyloric** v., vena gastrica dextra. **radial v's,** venae radiales. **radial v., external, of Soemmering,** vena cephalica accessoria. **ranine v.,** vena sublingualis. **rectal v's, inferior,** venae rectales inferiores. **rectal v's, middle,** venae rectales mediae. **rectal v., superior,** vena rectalis superior. **renal v's,** venae renales. **retromandibular v.,** vena retromandibularis. **Retzius's v's,** veins from the walls of the intestine to the branches of the inferior vena cava. **Rosenthal's v.,** vena basalis. **Ruysch's v's,** venae vorticosae. **sacral v's, lateral,** venae sacrales laterales. **sacral v., middle,** vena sacralis mediana. **salvatella v.,** a small vein of the little finger and dorsum of the hand. **saphenous v., accessory,** vena saphena accessoria. **saphenous v., great,** vena saphena magna. **saphenous v., small,** vena saphena parva. **v's of Sappey,** venae paraumbilicales. **scrotal v's, anterior,** venae scrotales anteriores. **scrotal v's, posterior,** venae scrotales posteriores. **v. of septum pellucidum,** vena septi pellucidi. **sigmoid v's,** venae sigmoideae. **small v. of heart,** vena cordis parva. **spermatic v.,** vena spermatica. **spinal v's,** venae spinales. **spiral v. of modiolus,** vena spiralis modioli. **splenic v.,** vena lienalis. **stellate v's of kidney,** venulae stellatae renis. **Stensen's v's,** venae vorticosae. **sternocleidomastoid v.,** vena sternocleidomastoidea. **striate v.,** vena striata. **stylomastoid v.,** vena stylomastoidea. **subcardinal v's,** paired vessels in the embryo, replacing the postcardinal veins and persisting to some degree as definitive vessels. **subclavian v.,** vena subclavia. **subcostal v.,** vena subcostalis. **subcutaneous v's of abdomen,** venae subcutaneae abdominis. **sublingual v.,** vena sublingualis. **sublobular v's,** tributaries of the hepatic veins that receive the central veins of hepatic lobules. **submental v.,** vena submentalis. **supracardinal v's,** paired vessels in the embryo, developing later than the subcardinal veins and persisting chiefly as the lower segment of the inferior vena cava. **supraorbital v.,** vena supraorbitalis. **suprarenal v., left,** vena suprarenalis sinistra. **suprarenal v., right,** vena suprarenalis dextra. **suprascapular v.,** vena suprascapularis. **supratrochlear v's,** venae supratrochleares. **sylvian v., v. of sylvian fossa,** vena cerebri media superficialis. **temporal v's, deep,** venae temporales profundae. **temporal v., middle,** vena temporalis media. **temporal v's, superficial,** venae temporales superficiales. **temporomandibular articular v's,** venae articulares temporomandibulares. **terminal v.,** vena thalamostriata. **testicular v., left,** vena testicularis sinistra. **testicular v., right,** vena testicularis dextra. **thalamostriata v.,** vena thalamostriata. **thebesian v's, v's of Thebesius,** venae cordis minimae. **thoracic v's, internal,** venae thoracicae internae. **thoracic v., lateral,** vena thoracica lateralis. **thoracoacromial v.,** vena thoracoacromialis. **thoracoepigastric v's,** venae thoracoepigastricae. **thymic v's,** venae thymicae. **thyroid v., inferior,** vena thyroidea inferior. **thyroid v's, middle,** venae thyroideae mediae. **thyroid v., superior,** vena thyroidea superior. **tibial v's, anterior,** venae tibiales anteriores. **tibial v's, posterior,** venae tibiales posteriores. **trabecular v's,** vessels coursing in splenic trabeculae, formed by tributary pulp veins. **tracheal v's,** venae tracheales. **transverse v. of face,** vena transversa faciei. **transverse v's of neck,** venae transversae colli. **Trolard's v.,** vena anastomotica superior. **tympanic v's,** venae tympanicae. **ulnar v's,** venae ulnares. **umbilical v.,** vena umbilicalis. **umbilical v., left,** vena umbilicalis sinistra. **uterine v's,** venae uterinae. **varicose v.,** a dilated tortuous vein, usually in the subcutaneous tissues of the leg; incompetency of the venous valves is associated. **vertebral v.,** vena vertebralis. **vertebral v., accessory,** vena vertebralis accessoria. **vertebral v., anterior,** vena vertebralis anterior. **vertebral v's, superficial, v's of vertebral column, external,** see *plexus venosi vertebrales externi* [*anterior et posterior*]. **vesalian v.,** an emissary vein connecting the cavernous sinus with the pterygoid venous plexus, sometimes passing through an opening in the great wing of the sphenoid bone. **vesical v's,** venae vesicales. **vestibular v's,** venae vestibulares. **vidian v's,** venae canalis pterygoidei. **v's of Vieussens,** venae cordis anteriores. **vitelline v's,** veins that return the blood from the yolk sac to the primitive heart of the early embryo. **vorticose v's,** venae vorticosae.

Veinamine (vān'ah-mēn) trademark for a crystalline amino acid solution for intravenous administration, containing a mixture of essential and nonessential amino acids but no peptides.

vela (ve'lah) [L.] plural of *velum.*

Velacycline (vel"ah-si'klēn) trademark for preparations of rolitetracycline.

velamen (ve-la'men), pl. *vela'mina* [L. "a covering"] a membrane, velum, meninx, or tegument. **v. vul'vae,** Hottentot apron.

velamenta (vel"ah-men'tah) [L.] plural of *velamentum.*

velamentous (vel"ah-men'tus) [L. *velamen* veil] membranous and pendent; like a veil.

velamentum (vel"ah-men'tum), pl. *velamen'ta* [L.] any covering, velum, or envelope. **velamen'ta cer'ebri,** the meninges.

velar (ve'lar) pertaining to a velum, especially to the velum palatinum (palatum molle).

Velban (vel'ban) trademark for a preparation of vinblastine sulfate.

veliform (vel'ĭ-form) velamentous.

Vella's fistula (ve'lahz) [Luigi *Vella,* Italian physiologist, 1825–1886] see under *fistula.*

vellosine (vel-lo'sin) a poisonous alkaloid occurring in yellow crystals, $C_{23}H_{28}N_2O_4$, from the bark of *Geissospermum laeve* (*vellosii*).

vellus (vel'us) [L. "fleece"] the fine hair which succeeds the lanugo over most of the body. **v. oli'vae,** a narrow band of tangential fibers surrounding the olive.

velonoskiascopy (ve"lo-no-ski-as'ko-pe) skiascopy of shadows made by the movement of a needle held before the patient's pupil.

velopharyngeal (vel"o-fah-rin'je-al) pertaining to the soft palate (velum palatinum) and pharynx; see also under *insufficiency* and *portal.*

Velosef (vel'o-sef) trademark for preparations of cephradine.

velosynthesis (vel"o-sin'thĕ-sis) [L. *velum* veil + Gr. *synthesis* a putting together] staphylorrhaphy.

Velpeau's bandage, deformity, hernia (vel-pōz') [Alfred Armand Louis Marie *Velpeau,* surgeon in Paris, 1795–1867] see under *bandage* and *hernia,* and see *silver fork fracture,* under *fracture.*

velum (ve'lum), pl. *ve'la* [L.] a covering; [NA] a general term for a veil or veil-like structure. **artificial v.,** a prosthetic appliance used in correction of a cleft of the soft palate. **Baker's v.,** an obturator used in cleft palate. **v. interpos'itum cer'ebri,** tela choroidea ventriculi tertii. **v. interpos'itum rhombenceph'ali,** v. medullare superius. **v. medulla're ante'rius,** v. medullare superius. **v. medulla're infe'rius** [NA], **v. medulla're poste'rius,** inferior medullary velum: a thin layer of white substance that forms part of the roof of the fourth ventricle below the fastigium; it is continuous above with the nodulus, on the sides with the pedunculus flocculi and the teniae, and ventrally it is fused with the choroid plexus. **v. medulla're supe'rius** [NA], superior medullary velum: a thin layer of white substance that forms the anterior portion of the roof of the fourth ventricle, extending from the tectal lamina in front to the fastigium behind, and between the superior cerebellar peduncles on the sides; called also *v. medullare anterius.* **medullary v., anterior,** v. medullare superius. **medullary v., inferior,** medullary v., **posterior,** v. medullare inferius. **medullary v., superior,** v. medullare superius. **nursing v.,** a suitable piece of soft rubber, attached to a handle, that may be held in an infant's mouth to enable it to nurse in spite of a cleft palate. **v. pala'ti,** palatum molle. **v. palati'num,** NA alternative for *palatum molle.* **v. pen'dulum pala'ti,** palatum palati. **v. semiluna're,** v. medullare inferius. **v. of Tarinus,** v. medullare inferius. **v. transver'sum,** a transverse fold of the tela choroidea marking the boundary between the diencephalon and the telencephalon in the embryonic brain.

vena (ve'nah), pl. *ve'nae* [L.] [NA] vein: a vessel that conveys blood to or toward the heart, or from the heart itself to the right atrium. See *vein.* For names and description of specific veins, see *Table of Venae* and accompanying Plates.

TABLE OF VENAE

Descriptions of veins are given on NA terms, and include anglicized names of specific veins.

ve'nae advehen'tes, channels in the early embryo that convey blood to the sinusoids of the liver and later become the portal vein.
v. anastomot'ica infe'rior [NA], inferior anastomotic vein: a vein that interconnects the superficial middle cerebral vein and the transverse sinus.
v. anastomot'ica supe'rior [NA], superior anastomotic vein: a vein that interconnects the superficial middle cerebral vein and the superior sagittal sinus.

v. angula'ris [NA], angular vein: a short vein between the eye and the root of the nose; it is formed by union of the supratrochlear and supraorbital veins and continues inferiorly as the facial vein.
ve'nae anon'ymae [dex'tra et sinis'tra], venae brachiocephalicae [dextra et sinistra].
v. appendicula'ris [NA], appendicular vein: the vena comitans of the appendicular artery; it unites with the anterior and posterior cecal veins to form the ileocolic vein.

v. aqueduc′tus vestib′uli [NA], vein of aqueduct of vestibule: a small vein from the internal ear that passes through the aqueduct of the vestibule and empties into the superior petrosal sinus.

ve′nae arcifor′mes re′nis, venae arcuatae renis.

ve′nae arcua′tae re′nis [NA], arcuate veins of kidney: a series of complete arches across the bases of the pyramids of the kidneys; they are formed by union of the interlobular veins and the venulae rectae and drain into the interlobar veins. Called also *venae arciformes renis.*

ve′nae articula′res mandib′ulae, venae articulares temporomandibulares.

ve′nae articula′res temporomandibula′res [NA], temporomandibular articular veins: small vessels that drain the plexus around the temporomandibular articulation in the retromandibular vein; called also *venae articulares mandibulae.*

ve′nae auditi′vae inter′nae, venae labyrinthi.

ve′nae auricula′res anterio′res [NA], anterior auricular veins: branches from the anterior part of the pinna that enter the superficial temporal vein.

v. auricula′ris poste′rior [NA], posterior auricular vein: a vein that begins in a plexus on the side of the head, passes down behind the pinna, and joins with the retromandibular vein to form the external jugular vein.

v. axilla′ris [NA], axillary vein; the venous trunk of the upper member; it begins at the lower border of the teres major muscle by junction of the basilic and brachial veins, and at the lateral border of the first rib is continuous with the subclavian vein.

v. az′ygos [NA], azygos vein: an intercepting trunk for the right intercostal veins as well as a connecting branch between the superior and inferior venae cavae: it arises from the ascending lumbar vein, passes up in front of and on the right side of the vertebrae, and empties into the superior vena cava.

v. basa′lis [NA], basal vein: a vein that arises at the anterior perforated substance, passes backward and around the cerebral peduncle, and empties into the internal cerebral vein; called also *v. basalis [Rosenthali].*

v. basa′lis [Rosentha′li], v. basalis.

v. basil′ica [NA], basilic vein: the superficial vein that arises from the ulnar side of the dorsal rete of the hand, passes up the forearm, and joins with the brachial veins to form the axillary vein.

ve′nae basivertebra′les [NA], basivertebral veins: venous sinuses in the cancellous tissue of the bodies of the vertebrae, which communicate with the plexus of veins on the anterior surface of the vertebrae and with the anterior internal vertebral plexus.

ve′nae brachia′les [NA], brachial veins: the venae comitantes of the brachial artery, which join with the basilic vein to form the axillary vein.

ve′nae brachiocephal′icae [dex′tra et sinis′tra] [NA], brachiocephalic veins: the two veins that drain blood from the head, neck, and upper extremities, and unite to form the superior vena cava. Each is formed at the root of the neck by union of the ipsilateral internal jugular and subclavian veins. The right vein (*v. brachiocephalica dextra*) passes almost vertically downward in front of the brachiocephalic artery, and the left vein (*v. brachiocephalica sinistra*) passes from left to right behind the upper part of the sternum. Each vein receives the vertebral, deep cervical, deep thyroid, and internal thoracic veins. The left vein also receives intercostal, thymic, tracheal, esophageal, phrenic, mediastinal, and pericardiac branches, as well as the thoracic duct. Called also *venae anonymae[dextra et sinistra].*

ve′nae bronchia′les [NA], bronchial veins: vessels that drain blood from the larger subdivisions of the bronchi into the azygos vein on the left, and into the hemiazygos or the superior intercostal vein on the right.

ve′nae bronchia′les anterio′res, ve′nae bronchia′les posterio′res, see *venae bronchiales.*

v. bul′bi pe′nis [NA], vein of bulb of penis: a vein draining blood from the bulb of the penis into the internal pudendal vein.

v. bul′bi vestib′uli [NA], vein of bulb of vestibule: a vein draining blood from the bulb of the vestibule of the vagina into the internal pudendal vein.

v. canalic′uli coch′leae [NA], vein of cochlear canal: a vein that arises in the cochlea and empties into the superior bulb of the internal jugular vein.

v. cana′lis pterygoi′dei [NA], vein of pterygoid canal: one of the veins that pass through the pterygoid canal and empty into the pterygoid plexus; called also *v. canalis pterygoidei [Vidii].*

v. cana′lis pterygoi′dei [Vid′ii], v. canalis pterygoidei.

ve′nae ca′vae, the vena cava inferior and superior.

v. ca′va infe′rior [NA], inferior vena cava: the venous trunk for the lower extremities and for the pelvic and abdominal viscera; it begins at the level of the fifth lumbar vertebra by union of the common iliac veins, passes upward on the right of the aorta, and empties into the right atrium of the heart.

v. ca′va supe′rior [NA], superior vena cava: the venous trunk draining blood from the head, neck, upper extremities, and chest; it begins by union of the two brachiocephalic veins, passes directly downward, and empties into the right atrium of the heart.

v. cava superior, persistent left, a developmental anomaly in which the left superior vena cava persists into postnatal life, usually draining into the left atrium; it is due to failure of the upper part of the left anterior cardinal vein to become obliterated. It may be an isolated anomaly or accompany other cardiovascular defects, such as tetralogy of Fallot.

ve′nae caverno′sae pe′nis [NA], cavernous veins of penis: veins that return the blood from the corpora cavernosa to the deep veins and the dorsal vein of the penis.

v. centra′lis glan′dulae suprarena′lis [NA], central vein of suprarenal gland: the large single vein into which the various veins within the substance of the gland empty, and which continues at the hilus as the suprarenal vein.

ve′nae centra′les hep′atis [NA], central veins of liver: veins in the middle of the hepatic lobules, draining into the hepatic vein.

v. centra′lis ret′inae [NA], central vein of retina: the vein that is formed by union of the retinal veins; it passes out of the eyeball in the optic nerve to empty into the superior ophthalmic vein.

v. cephal′ica [NA], cephalic vein: the superficial vein that arises from the radial side of the dorsal rete of the hand, and winds anteriorly to pass along the anterior border of the brachioradialis muscle; above the elbow it ascends along the lateral border of the biceps muscle and the pectoral border of the deltoid muscle, and opens into the axillary vein.

v. cephal′ica accesso′ria [NA], accessory cephalic vein: a vein arising from the dorsal rete of the hand, passing up the forearm to join the cephalic vein just above the elbow.

ve′nae cerebel′li inferio′res [NA], inferior cerebellar veins: rather large veins from the inferior surface of the cerebellum which empty into the transverse, sigmoid, and inferior petrosal sinuses, or into the occipital sinus.

ve′nae cerebel′li superio′res [NA], superior cerebellar veins: veins from the upper surface of the cerebellum, emptying into the straight sinus and the great cerebral vein, or into the transverse and superior petrosal sinuses.

ve′nae cer′ebri [NA], cerebral veins: veins that drain blood from the brain.

v. cer′ebri ante′rior [NA], anterior cerebral vein: the vein that accompanies the anterior cerebral artery and joins the basal vein.

ve′nae cer′ebri inferio′res [NA], inferior cerebral veins: veins that ramify on the base and the inferolateral surface of the brain. Those on the inferior surface of the frontal lobe drain into the inferior sagittal sinus and the cavernous sinus; those on the temporal lobe, into the superior petrosal sinus and the transverse sinus; those on the occipital lobe, into the straight sinus.

ve′nae cer′ebri inter′nae [NA], internal cerebral veins: two veins that arise at the interventricular foramen by the union of the thalamostriate and the choroid veins; they pass backward through the tela choroidea, collecting blood from the basal nuclei, and unite at the splenium of the corpus callosum to form the great cerebral vein.

v. cer′ebri mag′na [NA], great cerebral vein: a short median trunk, formed by union of the two internal cerebral veins, which curves around the splenium of the corpus callosum and empties into, or is continued as, the straight sinus; called also *v. cerebri magna [Galeni].*

v. cer′ebri mag′na [Gale′ni], v. cerebri magna.

v. cer′ebri me′dia, v. cerebri media superficialis.

v. cer′ebri me′dia profun′da [NA], deep middle cerebral vein: the vein that accompanies the middle cerebral artery in the floor of the lateral sulcus, and joins the basal vein.

v. cer′ebri me′dia superficia′lis [NA], superficial middle cerebral vein: a vein that drains the lateral surface of the cerebrum, follows the lateral cerebral fissure, and empties into the cavernous sinus; called also *v. cerebri media.*

ve′nae cer′ebri superio′res [NA], superior cerebral veins: about twelve veins that drain the superior, lateral, and medial surfaces of the cerebrum toward the longitudinal cerebral fissure, where they open into the superior sagittal sinus.

v. cervica′lis profun′da [NA], deep cervical vein: a vein that arises from a plexus in the suboccipital triangle, follows the deep cervical artery down the neck, and empties into the vertebral or the brachiocephalic vein.

v. chorioi′dea, v. choroidea.

v. choroi′dea [NA], choroid vein: the vein that runs along the whole length of the choroid plexus, draining it and the hippocampus, fornix, and corpus callosum; it unites with the thalamostriate vein to form the internal cerebral vein. Called also *v. chorioidea.*

ve′nae choroi′deae oc′uli, NA alternative for *venae vorticosae.*

ve′nae cilia′res [NA], ciliary veins: veins that arise inside the eyeball by branches from the ciliary muscle and drain into the superior ophthalmic vein. The *anterior ciliary veins* follow the anterior ciliary arteries, and receive branches from the sinus venosus, sclerae, the episcleral veins, and the tunica conjunctiva bulbi. The *posterior ciliary veins* follow the posterior ciliary arteries and empty also into the inferior ophthalmic vein.

ve′nae cilia′res anterio′res, ve′nae cilia′res posterio′res, see *venae ciliares.*

ve′nae circumflex′ae fem′oris latera′les [NA], lateral circumflex femoral veins: venae comitantes of the lateral circumflex femoral artery, emptying into the femoral or the deep femoral vein.

ve′nae circumflex′ae fem′oris media′les [NA], medial circumflex femoral veins: venae comitantes of the medial circumflex femoral artery, emptying into the femoral or the deep femoral vein.

1443

v. circumflex'a il'ium profun'da [NA], deep circumflex iliac vein: a common trunk formed from the venae comitantes of the homonymous artery and emptying into the external iliac vein.

v. circumflex'a il'ium superficia'lis [NA], superficial circumflex iliac vein: a vein that follows the homonymous artery and empties into the great saphenous vein.

v. col'ica dex'tra [NA], right colic vein: a vein that follows the distribution of the right colic artery and empties into the superior mesenteric vein.

v. col'ica me'dia [NA], middle colic vein: a vein that follows the distribution of the middle colic artery and empties into the superior mesenteric vein.

v. col'ica sinis'tra [NA], left colic vein: a vein that follows the left colic artery and opens into the inferior mesenteric vein.

v. com'itans [NA], an accompanying vein: such veins (venae comitantes), usually two in number, closely accompany their homonymous artery and are found especially in the extremities.

ve'nae comitan'tes arte'riae femora'lis, accompanying veins of the femoral artery, which empty into the external iliac vein.

v. com'itans ner'vi hypoglos'si [NA], accompanying vein of hypoglossal nerve: a vessel, formed by union of the vena profunda linguae and the vena sublingualis, that accompanies the hypoglossal nerve; it empties into the facial, lingual, or internal jugular vein.

ve'nae conjunctiva'les [NA], conjunctival veins: small veins that drain blood from the conjunctiva to the superior ophthalmic vein.

ve'nae conjunctiva'les anterio'res, ve'nae conjunctiva'les posterio'res, see *venae conjunctivales.*

ve'nae cor'dis [NA], cardiac veins: the veins of the heart, which drain blood from the various tissues making up the organ.

ve'nae cor'dis anterio'res [NA], anterior cardiac veins: small vessels from the anterior wall of the right ventricle that empty into the right atrium or join the lesser cardiac vein.

v. cor'dis mag'na [NA], great cardiac vein: a vein that collects blood from the anterior surface of the ventricles, follows the anterior longitudinal sulcus, and empties into the coronary sinus.

v. cor'dis me'dia [NA], middle cardiac vein: a vein that collects blood from the diaphragmatic surface of the ventricles, follows the posterior longitudinal sulcus, and empties into the coronary sinus.

ve'nae cor'dis min'imae [NA], smallest cardiac veins: numerous small veins arising in the muscular walls and draining independently into the cavities of the heart, and most readily seen in the atria.

v. cor'dis par'va [NA], small cardiac vein: a vein that collects blood from both parts of the right heart, follows the coronary sulcus to the left, and opens into the coronary sinus.

v. corona'ria ventric'uli, see *v. gastrica dextra, v. gastrica sinistra,* and *v. prepylorica.*

ve'nae costoaxilla'res, costoaxillary veins: veins that arise from the areolar venous plexus, anastomose with the upper six or seven posterior intercostal veins, and empty into the axillary vein.

v. cuta'nea [NA], cutaneous vein: one of the small veins that begin in the papillae of the skin, form subpapillary plexuses, and open into the subcutaneous veins.

v. cys'tica [NA], cystic vein: a small vein that returns the blood from the gallbladder to the right branch of the portal vein, within the substance of the liver.

ve'nae digita'les commu'nes pe'dis, common digital veins of foot: short veins formed by union of the dorsal digital and the intercapitular veins of the foot.

ve'nae digita'les dorsa'les pe'dis [NA], dorsal digital veins of foot: the veins on the dorsal surfaces of the toes that unite in pairs around each cleft to form the dorsal metatarsal veins; called also *venae digitales pedis dorsales.*

ve'nae digita'les palma'res [NA], palmar digital veins: the venae comitantes of the proper and common palmar digital arteries, which join the superficial palmar venous arch.

ve'nae digita'les pe'dis dorsa'les, venae digitales dorsales pedis.

ve'nae digita'les planta'res [NA], plantar digital veins: veins from the plantar surfaces of the toes which unite at the clefts to form the plantar metatarsal veins of the foot.

ve'nae digita'les vola'res commu'nes, see *venae digitales palmares.*

ve'nae digita'les vola'res pro'priae, see *venae digitales palmares.*

ve'nae diplo'icae [NA], diploic veins: veins of the skull, including the frontal, occipital, anterior temporal, and posterior temporal diploic veins, which form sinuses in the cancellous tissue between the laminae of the cranial bones. They send branches to the external and the internal lamina, the periosteum, and the dura mater, and empty in part inside and in part outside the skull.

v. diplo'ica fronta'lis [NA], frontal diploic vein: a vein that drains the frontal bone, emptying externally into the supraorbital vein or internally into the superior sagittal sinus.

v. diplo'ica occipita'lis [NA], occipital diploic vein: the largest of the diploic veins, which drains blood from the occipital bone and empties into the occipital vein or the transverse sinus.

v. diplo'ica tempora'lis ante'rior [NA], anterior temporal diploic vein: a vein that drains the lateral portion of the frontal and the anterior part of the parietal bone, opening internally into the sphenoparietal sinus and externally into a deep temporal vein.

v. diplo'ica tempora'lis poste'rior [NA], posterior temporal diploic vein: a vein that drains the parietal bone and empties into the transverse sinus.

v. dorsa'lis clitor'idis profun'da [NA], deep dorsal vein of clitoris: a vein that follows the course of its homonymous artery and opens into the vesical plexus.

ve'nae dorsa'les clitor'idis superficia'les [NA], superficial dorsal veins of clitoris: veins that collect blood subcutaneously from the clitoris and drain into the external pudendal vein.

ve'nae dorsa'les lin'guae [NA], dorsal lingual veins: veins that unite with a small vena comitans of the lingual artery and join the main lingual trunk.

v. dorsa'lis pe'nis profun'da [NA], deep dorsal vein of penis: the single vein lying subfascially in the midline of the penis between the dorsal arteries; it begins in small veins around the corona glandis, is joined by the deep veins of the penis as it passes proximally, and passes between the arcuate pubic and transverse perineal ligaments, where it divides into a left and right vein to join the prostatic plexus.

ve'nae dorsa'les pe'nis subcuta'neae, venae dorsales penis superficiales.

ve'nae dorsa'les pe'nis superficia'les [NA], superficial dorsal veins of penis: veins that collect blood subcutaneously from the penis and drain into the external pudendal vein; called also *venae dorsales penis subcutaneae.*

ve'nae duodena'les, duodenal veins: veins draining blood from the duodenum.

v. emissa'ria [NA], emissary vein: one of the small, valveless veins that pass through foramina of the skull, connecting the dural venous sinuses with scalp veins or with deep veins below the base of the skull; called also *emissarium.*

v. emissa'ria condyla'ris [NA], condylar emissary vein: a small vein running through the condylar canal of the skull, connecting the sigmoid sinus with the vertebral or the internal jugular vein; called also *emissarium condyloideum.*

v. emissa'ria mastoi'dea [NA], mastoid emissary vein: a small vein passing through the mastoid foramen of the skull and connecting the sigmoid sinus with the occipital or the posterior auricular vein; called also *emissarium mastoideum.*

v. emissa'ria occipita'lis [NA], occipital emissary vein: an occasional small vein running through a minute foramen in the occipital protuberance of the skull and connecting the confluence of the sinuses with the occipital vein; called also *emissarium occipitale.*

v. emissa'ria parieta'lis [NA], parietal emissary vein: a small vein passing through the parietal foramen of the skull and connecting the superior sagittal sinus with the superficial temporal veins; called also *emissarium parietale.*

v. epigas'trica infe'rior [NA], inferior epigastric vein: a vein that accompanies the inferior epigastric artery and opens into the external iliac vein.

v. epigas'trica superficia'lis [NA], superficial epigastric vein: a vein that follows its homonymous artery and opens into the great saphenous or the femoral vein.

ve'nae epigas'tricae superio'res [NA], superior epigastric veins: the venae comitantes of the superior epigastric artery, which open into the internal thoracic vein.

ve'nae episclera'les [NA], episcleral veins: the veins that ring the cornea and drain into the vorticose and ciliary veins.

ve'nae esopha'geae [NA], esophageal veins: small vessels that drain blood from the esophagus into the hemiazygos and azygos veins, or into the left brachiocephalic vein.

ve'nae ethmoida'les [NA], ethmoidal veins: veins that follow the anterior and posterior ethmoidal arteries, emerge from the ethmoidal foramina, and empty into the superior ophthalmic vein.

v. ethmoida'lis ante'rior, v. ethmoida'lis poste'rior, see *venae ethmoidales.*

v. facia'lis [NA], facial vein; the vein that begins at the medial angle of the eye as the angular vein, descends behind the facial artery, and usually ends in the internal jugular vein; formerly called the *anterior facial vein* or *vena facialis anterior,* this vessel sometimes joins the retromandibular vein to form a common trunk previously known as the *common facial vein* or *vena facialis communis.*

v. facia'lis ante'rior, v. facia'lis commu'nis, see *v. facialis.*

v. facia'lis poste'rior, v. retromandibularis

v. facie'i profun'da [NA], deep facial vein: a vein draining from the pterygoid plexus to the facial vein.

v. femora'lis [NA], femoral vein: a vein that lies in the proximal two-thirds of the thigh; it is a direct continuation of the popliteal vein, follows the course of the femoral artery, and at the inguinal ligament becomes the external iliac vein. NOTE: Vascular surgeons refer to the portion of the femoral vein proximal to the branching of the deep femoral vein as the *common femoral vein,* and to its continuation distal to the branching as the *superficial femoral vein.*

v. femoropoplite'a, femoropopliteal vein: a superficial descending vein draining the lower and back part of the thigh and opening into the small saphenous vein just before it perforates the deep fascia.

ve'nae fibula'res, NA alternative for *venae peroneae.*

ve'nae fronta'les, venae supratrochleares.

ve'nae gas'tricae bre'ves [NA], short gastric veins: small vessels draining the left portion of the greater curvature of the stomach and emptying into the splenic vein.

v. gas'trica dex'tra [NA], right gastric vein: the vena comitans of the right gastric artery, emptying into the portal vein.

v. gas'trica sinis'tra [NA], left gastric vein: the vena comitans of the left gastric artery, emptying into the portal vein.

v. gastroepiplo'ica dex'tra [NA], right gastroepiploic vein: a vein that follows the distribution of its homonymous artery and empties into the superior mesenteric vein.

v. gastroepiplo'ica sinis'tra [NA], left gastroepiploic vein: a vein that follows the distribution of its homonymous artery and empties into the splenic vein.

ve'nae ge'nus [NA], genicular veins: veins accompanying the genicular arteries and draining into the popliteal vein.

ve'nae gluta'eae inferio'res, venae gluteae inferiores.

ve'nae gluta'eae superio'res, venae gluteae superiores.

ve'nae glute'ae inferio'res [NA], inferior gluteal veins: venae comitantes of the inferior gluteal artery; they drain the subcutaneous tissue of the back of the thigh and the muscles of the buttock, unite into a single vein after passing through the greater sciatic foramen, and empty into the internal iliac vein.

ve'nae glute'ae superio'res [NA], superior gluteal veins: venae comitantes of the superior gluteal artery; they drain the muscles of the buttock, pass through the greater sciatic foramen, and empty into the internal iliac vein.

ve'nae haemorrhoida'les inferio'res, venae rectales inferiores.

v. haemorrhoida'lis me'dia, see *venae rectales mediae.*

v. haemorrhoida'lis supe'rior, v. rectalis superior.

v. hemiaz'ygos [NA], hemiazygos vein: an intercepting trunk for the lower left posterior intercostal veins; it arises from the ascending lumbar vein, passes up on the left side of the vertebrae to the eighth thoracic vertebra, where it may receive the accessory branch, and crosses over the vertebral column to open into the azygos vein.

v. hemiaz'ygos accesso'ria [NA], accessory hemiazygos vein: the descending intercepting trunk for the upper, often the fourth through the eighth, left posterior intercostal veins. It lies on the left side and at the eighth thoracic vertebra joins the hemiazygos vein or crosses to the right side to join the azygos vein directly; above, it may communicate with the left superior intercostal vein.

ve'nae hepat'icae [NA], hepatic veins: several veins that receive blood from the central veins of the liver; two or three large vessels in an upper group and six to twenty small veins in a lower group form successively larger vessels which ultimately open into the inferior vena cava on the posterior aspect of the liver.

ve'nae hepat'icae dex'trae [NA], the right hepatic veins that drain into the vena cava inferior.

ve'nae hepat'icae me'diae [NA], the middle hepatic veins that drain into the vena cava inferior.

ve'nae hepat'icae sinis'trae [NA], the left hepatic veins that drain into the vena cava inferior.

v. hypogas'trica, v. iliaca interna.

v. ileocol'ica [NA], ileocolic vein: a vein that follows the distribution of its homonymous artery and empties into the vena mesenterica superior.

v. ili'aca commu'nis [NA], common iliac vein: a vein that arises at the sacroiliac articulation by union of the external iliac and the internal iliac vein, and passes upward to the right side of the fifth lumbar vertebra where the two unite to form the inferior vena cava.

v. ili'aca exter'na [NA], external iliac vein: the continuation of the femoral vein from the inguinal ligament to the sacroiliac articulation, where it joins with the internal iliac vein to form the common iliac vein.

v. ili'aca inter'na [NA], internal iliac vein: a short trunk formed by union of parietal branches; it extends from the greater sciatic notch to the brim of the pelvis, where it joins the external iliac vein to form the common iliac vein; called also *v. hypogastrica.*

v. iliolumba'lis [NA], iliolumbar vein: a vein that follows the distribution of the iliolumbar artery and opens into the internal iliac or the common iliac vein, or it may divide to end in both.

inferior v. cava, v. cava inferior.

ve'nae intercapita'les [NA], intercapital veins: veins at the clefts of the fingers which pass between the heads of the metacarpal bones and establish communication between the dorsal and the palmar venous system of the hand; called also *venae intercapitulares manus.*

ve'nae intercapit'ulares ma'nus, venae intercapitales.

ve'nae intercapitula'res pe'dis, intercapitular veins of foot: veins at the clefts of the toes which pass between the heads of the metatarsal bones and establish communication between the dorsal and the plantar venous system.

ve'nae intercosta'les, veins that accompany the intercostal arteries; see *venae intercostales anteriores, venae intercostales posteriores, v. intercostalis superior dextra, v. intercostalis superior sinistra,* and *v. intercostalis suprema.*

ve'nae intercosta'les anterio'res [NA], anterior intercostal veins: the twelve paired venae comitantes of the anterior thoracic arteries, which drain into the internal thoracic vein.

ve'nae intercosta'les posterio'res IV–XI [NA], posterior intercostal veins IV–XI: venae comitantes of posterior intercostal

arteries IV to XI, draining on the right side into the azygos vein and on the left side into the hemiazygos or accessory hemiazygos vein.

v. intercosta'lis supe'rior dex'tra [NA], right superior intercostal vein: a common trunk formed by union of the second, third, and sometimes fourth posterior intercostal veins, which drains into the azygos vein.

v. intercosta'lis supe'rior sinis'tra [NA], left superior intercostal vein: the common trunk formed by union of the second, third, and sometimes fourth posterior intercostal veins, which crosses the arch of the aorta and joins the left brachiocephalic vein.

v. intercosta'lis supre'ma [NA], highest intercostal vein: the first posterior intercostal vein of either side, which passes over the apex of the lung and ends in the brachiocephalic, vertebral, or superior intercostal vein.

ve'nae interloba'res re'nis [NA], interlobar veins of kidney: veins that drain the venous arcades of the kidney, pass down between the pyramids, and unite to form the renal vein.

ve'nae interlobula'res hep'atis [NA], interlobular veins of liver: the veins that arise as tributaries of the portal vein between the hepatic lobules.

ve'nae interlobula'res re'nis [NA], interlobular veins of kidney: veins that collect blood from the capillary network of the cortex and empty into the venous arcades of the kidney.

ve'na intervertebra'lis [NA], intervertebral vein: any one of the veins that drain the vertebral plexuses, passing out through the intervertebral foramina and emptying into the regional veins: in the neck, into the vertebral; in the thorax, the intercostal; in the abdomen, the lumbar; and in the pelvis, the lateral sacral veins.

ve'nae intestina'les, the veins draining blood from the small intestines (venae jejunales et ilei [NA]).

ve'nae jejuna'les et il'ei [NA], jejunal and ileal veins: veins draining blood from the jejunum and the ileum into the superior mesenteric vein; called also *venae intestinales.*

v. jugula'ris ante'rior [NA], anterior jugular vein: a vein that arises under the chin, passes down the neck, and opens into the external jugular or the subclavian vein or into jugular venous arch.

v. jugula'ris exter'na [NA], external jugular vein: the vein that begins in the parotid gland behind the angle of the jaw by union of the retromandibular and the posterior auricular vein, passes down the neck, and opens into the subclavian, the internal jugular, or the brachiocephalic vein.

v. jugula'ris inter'na [NA], internal jugular vein: the vein that begins as the superior bulb in the jugular fossa, draining much of the head and neck; it descends with first the internal carotid and then the common carotid artery in the neck, and joins with the subclavian vein to form the brachiocephalic vein.

ve'nae labia'les anterio'res [NA], anterior labial veins: veins that collect blood from the anterior aspect of the labia and drain into the external pudendal vein; they are homologues of the anterior scrotal veins in the male.

ve'nae labia'les inferio'res [NA], inferior labial veins: veins that drain the region of the lower lip into the facial vein.

ve'nae labia'les posterio'res [NA], posterior labial veins: small branches from the labia which open into the vesical venus plexus; they are homologues of the posterior scrotal veins in the male.

v. labia'lis supe'rior [NA], superior labial vein: the vein that drains blood from the region of the upper lip into the facial vein.

ve'nae labyrin'thi [NA], veins of labyrinth: several small veins that pass through the internal acoustic meatus from the cochlea into the inferior petrosal or the transverse sinus; called also *venae auditivae internae.*

v. lacrima'lis [NA], lacrimal vein: the vein that drains blood from the lacrimal gland into the superior ophthalmic vein.

v. laryn'gea infe'rior [NA], inferior laryngeal vein: a vein draining blood from the larynx into the inferior thyroid vein.

v. laryn'gea supe'rior [NA], superior laryngeal vein: a vein that drains blood from the larynx into the superior thyroid vein.

v. liena'lis [NA], splenic vein: the vein formed by union of several branches at the hilus of the spleen, passing from left to right to the neck of the pancreas, where it joins the superior mesenteric vein to form the portal vein.

v. lingua'lis [NA], lingual vein: the deep vein that follows the distribution of the lingual artery and empties into the internal jugular vein.

ve'nae lumba'les, see *venae lumbales* [I et II] and *venae lumbales* [III et IV].

ve'nae lumba'les [I et II] [NA], lumbar veins I and II: venae comitantes of the first and second lumbar arteries, which drain into the ascending lumbar vein and thence into the azygos or hemiazygos vein.

ve'nae lumba'les [III et IV] [NA], lumbar veins III and IV: venae comitantes of the third and fourth lumbar arteries, which usually drain into the inferior vena cava.

v. lumba'lis ascen'dens [NA], ascending lumbar vein: an ascending intercepting vein for the lumbar veins of either side; it begins in the lateral sacral veins and passes up the spine to the first lumbar vertebra, where by union with the subcostal vein it becomes on the right side the azygos vein, and on the left side, the hemiazygos vein.

v. mamma'ria inter'na, see *venae thoracicae internae.*

ve′nae masseter′icae, masseteric veins: veins from the masseter muscle that empty into the facial vein.

ve′nae maxilla′res [NA], maxillary veins: veins from the pterygoid plexus, usually forming a single short trunk, passing back and uniting with the superficial temporal vein in the parotid gland to form the retromandibular vein.

v. media′na antebra′chii [NA], median antebrachial vein: a vein that arises from a palmar venous plexus and passes up the forearm between the cephalic and the basilic veins to the elbow, where it either joins one of these, bifurcates to join both, or joins the median cubital vein. Called also *v. mediana antibrachii.*

v. media′na antibra′chii, v. mediana antebrachii.

v. media′na basil′ica [NA], median basilic vein: a vein sometimes present as the medial branch, ending in the basilic vein, of a bifurcation of the median antebrachial vein.

v. media′na cephal′ica [NA], median cephalic vein: a vein sometimes present as the lateral branch, ending in the cephalic vein, formed by bifurcation of the median antebrachial vein.

v. media′na col′li, median vein of neck: a vein formed when the anterior jugular veins unite as they pass down the neck.

v. media′na cu′biti [NA], median cubital vein: the large connecting branch that arises from the cephalic vein below the elbow and passes obliquely upward over the cubital fossa to join the basilic vein.

ve′nae mediastina′les [NA], mediastinal veins: numerous small branches that drain blood from the anterior mediastinum into the brachiocephalic vein, azygos vein, or the superior vena cava; called also *venae mediastinales anteriores.*

ve′nae mediastina′les anterio′res, venae mediastinales.

ve′nae menin′geae [NA], meningeal veins: the venae comitantes of the meningeal arteries, which drain the dura mater, communicate with the lateral lacunae, and empty into the regional sinuses and veins.

ve′nae menin′geae me′diae [NA], middle meningeal veins: the venae comitantes of the middle meningeal artery, which end in the pterygoid venous plexus.

v. mesenter′ica infe′rior [NA], inferior mesenteric vein: a vein that follows the distribution of its homonymous artery and empties into the splenic vein.

v. mesenter′ica supe′rior [NA], superior mesenteric vein: a vein that follows the distribution of its homonymous artery and joins with the splenic vein to form the portal vein.

ve′nae metacar′peae dorsa′les [NA], dorsal metacarpal veins: veins that arise from the union of dorsal veins of adjacent fingers and pass proximally to join in forming the dorsal venous rete of the hand.

ve′nae metacar′peae palma′res [NA], palmar metacarpal veins: the venae comitantes of the palmar metacarpal arteries, which open into the deep palmar venous arch; called also *venae metacarpeae volares.*

ve′nae metacar′peae vola′res, venae metacarpeae palmares.

ve′nae metatar′seae dorsa′les [NA], dorsal metatarsal veins: veins that are formed by the dorsal digital veins of the toes at the clefts of the toes, joining the dorsal venous arch.

ve′nae metatar′seae planta′res [NA], plantar metatarsal veins: deep veins of the foot that arise from the plantar digital veins at the clefts of the toes and pass back to open into the plantar venous arch.

ve′nae muscula′res, muscular veins: veins that drain blood from the levator palpebrae, superior rectus, superior oblique, and medial rectus muscles into the superior ophthalmic vein.

ve′nae musculophren′icae [NA], musculophrenic veins: the venae comitantes of the musculophrenic artery, draining blood from parts of the diaphragm and from the wall of the thorax and abdomen.

ve′nae nasa′les exter′nae [NA], external nasal veins: small ascending branches from the nose that open into the angular and facial veins.

v. nasofronta′lis [NA], nasofrontal vein: a vein that begins at the supraorbital vein, enters the orbit, and joins the superior ophthalmic vein.

v. obli′qua a′trii sinis′tri [NA], oblique vein of left atrium: a small vein from the left atrium that opens into the coronary sinus; called also *v. obliqua atrii sinistri* [*Marshalli*].

v. obli′qua a′trii sinis′tri [**Marshal′li**], v. obliqua atrii sinistri.

ve′nae obturato′riae [NA], obturator veins: veins that drain the hip joint and the regional muscles, enter the pelvis through the obturator canal, and empty into the internal iliac or the inferior epigastric vein, or both.

v. occipita′lis [NA], occipital vein: a vein in the scalp that follows the distribution of the occipital artery and opens under the trapezius muscle into the suboccipital venous plexus; it may continue with the occipital artery and end in the internal jugular vein.

ve′nae oesopha′geae, venae esophageae.

v. ophthal′mica infe′rior [NA], inferior ophthalmic vein: a vein formed by confluence of muscular and ciliary branches, and running backward either to join the superior ophthalmic vein or to open directly into the cavernous sinus; it sends a communicating branch through the inferior orbital fissure to join the pterygoid venous plexus.

v. ophthal′mica supe′rior [NA], superior ophthalmic vein: the vein that begins at the medial angle of the eyelid, where it communicates with the frontal, supraorbital, and angular veins; it follows the distribution of the ophthalmic artery, and may be joined by the inferior ophthalmic vein at the superior orbital fissure before opening into the cavernous sinus.

v. ophthalmomenin′gea, ophthalmomeningeal vein: a small inferior meningeal vein that opens usually into the superior ophthalmic vein, or occasionally into the superior petrosal sinus.

v. ova′rica, see *v. ovarica dextra* and *v. ovarica sinistra.*

v. ova′rica dex′tra [NA], right ovarian vein: a vein that drains the pampiniform plexus of the broad ligament on the right into the inferior vena cava.

v. ova′rica sinis′tra [NA], left ovarian vein: a vein that drains the pampiniform plexus of the broad ligament on the left into the left renal vein.

v. palati′na, v. palatina externa.

v. palati′na exter′na [NA], external palatine vein: the vein that drains blood from the tonsils and the soft palate into the facial vein; called also *v. palatina.*

ve′nae palpebra′les [NA], palpebral veins: small branches from the eyelids that open into the superior ophthalmic vein.

ve′nae palpebra′les inferio′res [NA], inferior palpebral veins: branches that drain the blood from the lower eyelid into the facial vein.

ve′nae palpebra′les superio′res [NA], superior palpebral veins: branches that drain the blood from the upper eyelid to the angular vein.

ve′nae pancreat′icae [NA], pancreatic veins: numerous branches from the pancreas which open into the splenic and the superior mesenteric vein.

ve′nae pancreaticoduodena′les [NA], pancreaticoduodenal veins: four veins that drain blood from the pancreas and duodenum, closely following the homonymous arteries. A superior and an inferior vein originate from both an anterior and a posterior venous arcade. The anterior superior vein joins the right gastroepiploic vein; the posterior superior vein joins the portal vein. The anterior and posterior inferior veins join, sometimes as one trunk, the uppermost jejunal vein or the superior mesenteric vein.

ve′nae paraumbilica′les [NA], paraumbilical veins: veins that communicate with the portal vein and anastomose with the superior and inferior epigastric and the superior vesical veins in the region of the umbilicus. They form a part of the collateral circulation of the portal vein in event of hepatic obstruction. Called also *venae parumbilicales* [*Sappeyi*].

ve′nae paroti′deae [NA], parotid veins: small veins from the parotid gland that open into the superficial temporal vein; called also *venae parotideae posteriores.*

ve′nae paroti′deae anterio′res, rami parotidei venae facialis.

ve′nae paroti′deae posterio′res, venae parotideae.

ve′nae parumbilica′les [**Sap′peyi**], venae paraumbilicales.

ve′nae pectora′les [NA], collective term for branches of the subclavian vein that drain the pectoral region.

ve′nae perforan′tes [NA], perforating veins: the venae comitantes for the perforating arteries of the thigh, which empty into the deep femoral vein; called also *venae perforantes femoris.*

ve′nae perforan′tes fem′oris, venae perforantes.

ve′nae pericardi′acae [NA], pericardiac veins: numerous small branches that drain blood from the pericardium into the brachiocephalic, inferior thyroid, and azygos veins, and the superior vena cava.

ve′nae pericardiacophren′icae [NA], pericardiacophrenic veins: small veins that drain blood from the pericardium and diaphragm into the left brachiocephalic vein; called also *venae phrenicae superiores.*

ve′nae perone′ae [NA], peroneal veins: the venae comitantes of the peroneal artery, emptying into the posterior tibial vein; called also *venae fibulares* [NA alternative] or *fibular veins.*

ve′nae pharyn′geae [NA], pharyngeal veins: veins that drain the pharyngeal plexus and empty into the internal jugular vein.

ve′nae phren′icae inferio′res [NA], inferior phrenic veins: veins that follow the homonymous arteries, the one on the right entering the inferior vena cava, and the one on the left entering the left suprarenal or renal vein or the inferior vena cava.

ve′nae phren′icae superio′res, venae pericardiacophrenicae.

v. poplite′a [NA], popliteal vein: a vein following the popliteal artery, and formed by union of the venae comitantes of the anterior and posterior tibial arteries; at the adductor hiatus it becomes continuous with the femoral vein.

v. por′tae [NA], portal vein: a short thick trunk formed by union of the superior mesenteric and the splenic vein behind the neck of the pancreas; it passes upward to the right end of the porta hepatis, where it divides into successively smaller branches, following the branches of the hepatic artery, until it forms a capillary-like system of sinusoids that permeates the entire substance of the liver.

v. poste′rior ventric′uli sinis′tri cor′dis [NA], posterior vein of left ventricle: the vein that drains blood from the posterior surface of the left ventricle into the coronary sinus.

v. prepylo'rica [NA], prepyloric vein: a vein that accompanies the prepyloric artery, passing upward over the anterior surface of the junction between the pylorus and the duodenum and emptying into the right gastric vein.

ve'nae profun'dae, deeply situated veins, including *v. profunda femoris, v. profunda linguae,* and *v. profunda penis.*

ve'nae profun'dae clitor'idis [NA], deep veins of clitoris: small veins of the clitoris that drain into the vesical venous plexus.

v. profun'da fem'oris [NA], deep femoral vein: a vein that follows the distribution of the deep femoral artery and opens into the femoral vein.

v. profun'da lin'guae [NA], deep lingual vein: a vein that drains blood from the deep aspect of the tongue and joins the sublingual vein to form the vena comitans of the hypoglossal nerve.

ve'nae profun'dae pe'nis [NA], deep veins of penis: veins that follow the distribution of the homonymous artery and empty into the dorsal vein of the penis.

ve'nae puden'dae exter'nae [NA], external pudendal veins: veins that follow the distribution of the external pudendal artery and open into the great saphenous vein.

v. puden'da inter'na [NA], internal pudendal vein: a vein that follows the course of the internal pudendal artery, and drains into the internal iliac vein.

ve'nae pulmona'les [NA], pulmonary veins: the four veins, the right and left superior and inferior pulmonary veins, that return aerated blood from the lungs to the left atrium of the heart.

ve'nae pulmona'les dex'trae, see *v. pulmonalis inferior dextra* and *v. pulmonalis superior dextra.*

v. pulmona'lis infe'rior dex'tra [NA], right inferior pulmonary vein: the vein that returns blood from the lower lobe of the right lung (from the apical branch and from the common, superior, and inferior basal veins) to the left atrium of the heart.

v. pulmona'lis infe'rior sinis'tra [NA], left inferior pulmonary vein: the vein that returns blood from the lower lobe of the left lung (from the superior apical branch and the common basal vein) to the left atrium of the heart.

ve'nae pulmona'les sinis'trae, see *v. pulmonalis inferior sinistra* and *v. pulmonalis superior sinistra.*

v. pulmona'lis supe'rior dex'tra [NA], right superior pulmonary vein: the vein that returns blood from the upper and middle lobes of the right lung (from the apical, anterior, and posterior branches and the middle lobar branch) to the left atrium of the heart.

v. pulmona'lis supe'rior sinis'tra [NA], left superior pulmonary vein: the vein that returns blood from the upper lobe of the left lung (from the apicoposterior, anterior, and lingular branches) to the left atrium of the heart.

ve'nae radia'les [NA], radial veins: the venae comitantes of the radial artery, which open into the brachial veins.

ve'nae recta'les inferio'res [NA], inferior rectal veins: veins that drain the rectal plexus into the internal pudendal vein; called also *venae haemorrhoidales inferiores.*

ve'nae recta'les me'diae [NA], middle rectal veins: veins that drain the rectal plexus and empty into the internal iliac and superior rectal veins.

v. recta'lis supe'rior [NA], superior rectal vein: the vein that drains the upper part of the rectal plexus into the inferior mesenteric vein and thus establishes connection between the portal and the systemic system; called also *v. haemorrhoidalis superior.*

ve'nae rena'les [NA], renal veins: short thick trunks, the one on the left longer than that on the right, that pass from the kidneys to the inferior vena cava.

ve'nae re'nis [NA], the veins within the kidney, including the *venae interlobares renis, venae arcuatae renis, venae interlobulares renis, venulae rectae renis,* and *venulae stellatae renis.*

v. retromandibula'ris [NA], retromandibular vein: the vein that is formed in the upper part of the parotid gland behind the neck of the mandible by union of the maxillary and superficial temporal veins; it passes downward through the gland, communicates with the facial vein, and emerging from the gland joins with the posterior auricular vein to form the external jugular vein. Called also *v. facialis posterior.*

ve'nae revehen'tes, channels in the early embryo that convey blood from the sinusoids of the liver to the sinus venosus and later become the hepatic veins.

ve'nae sacra'les latera'les [NA], lateral sacral veins: veins that follow the homonymous arteries, help to form the lateral sacral plexus, and empty into the internal iliac vein or the superior gluteal veins.

v. sacra'lis me'dia, v. sacralis mediana.

v. sacra'lis media'na [NA], middle sacral vein: a vein that follows the middle sacral artery and opens into the common iliac vein; called also *v. sacralis media.*

v. saphe'na accesso'ria [NA], accessory saphenous vein: a vein that, when present, drains the medial and posterior superficial parts of the thigh and opens into the great saphenous vein.

v. saphe'na mag'na [NA], great saphenous vein: the longest vein in the body, extending from the dorsum of the foot to just below the inguinal ligament, where it opens into the femoral vein.

v. saphe'na par'va [NA], small saphenous vein: the vein that continues the marginal vein from behind the malleolus and passes up the back of the leg to the knee joint, where it opens into the popliteal vein.

v. scapula'ris dorsa'lis [NA], a branch of the subclavian vein.

ve'nae scrota'les anterio'res [NA], anterior scrotal veins: veins that collect blood from the anterior aspect of the scrotum and drain into the external pudendal vein.

ve'nae scrota'les posterio'res [NA], posterior scrotal veins: small branches from the scrotum that open into the vesical venous plexus.

v. sep'ti pellu'cidi [NA], vein of septum pellucidum: a vein from the septum pellucidum that empties into the thalamostriate vein.

ve'nae sigmoi'deae [NA], sigmoid veins: veins from the sigmoid colon that empty into the inferior mesenteric vein.

v. spermat'ica, spermatic vein: the vein that drains blood from the testis and epididymis, forms the pampiniform plexus of the spermatic cord, and accompanies the internal spermatic artery. The vein on the right enters the inferior vena cava; that on the left enters the left renal vein.

ve'nae spina'les [NA], spinal veins: anastomosing networks of small veins that drain blood from the spinal cord and its pia mater into the internal vertebral venous plexuses.

ve'nae spina'les exter'nae anterio'res, small longitudinal veins draining blood from the anterior part of the pia mater of the spinal cord; see *venae spinales.*

ve'nae spina'les exter'nae posterio'res, small longitudinal veins draining blood from the posterior part of the pia mater of the spinal cord; see *venae spinales.*

ve'nae spina'les inter'nae, minute veins draining blood from the substance of the spinal cord; see *venae spinales.*

v. spira'lis modi'oli [NA], spiral vein of modiolus: a small vein in the spiral modiolus, a tributary of the labyrinthine veins.

ve'nae stella'tae re'nis, venulae stellatae renis.

v. sternocleidomastoi'dea [NA], sternocleidomastoid vein: a vein that follows the course of the homonymous artery and opens into the internal jugular vein.

v. stria'ta [NA], striate vein: the vein that arises from the anterior perforated substance of the brain and joins the basal vein.

v. stylomastoi'dea [NA], stylomastoid vein: a vein following the stylomastoid artery and emptying into the retromandibular vein.

v. subcla'via [NA], subclavian vein: the vein that continues the axillary as the main venous stem of the upper member, follows the subclavian artery, and joins with the internal jugular vein to form the brachiocephalic vein.

v. subcosta'lis [NA], subcostal vein: the vena comitans of the subcostal artery, which joins the ascending lumbar vein to form the azygos or hemiazygos vein, on the right or left side respectively.

ve'nae subcuta'neae abdom'inis [NA], subcutaneous veins of abdomen: the superficial veins of the abdominal wall.

v. sublingua'lis [NA], sublingual vein: a vein that follows the sublingual artery and opens into the lingual vein.

v. submenta'lis [NA], submental vein: a vein that follows the submental artery and opens into the facial vein.

superior v. cava, v. cava superior.

v. supraorbita'lis [NA], supraorbital vein: the vein that passes down the forehead lateral to the supratrochlear vein, joining it at the root of the nose to form the angular vein.

ve'nae suprarena'les, see *v. suprarenalis dextra* and *v. suprarenalis sinistra.*

v. suprarena'lis dex'tra [NA], right suprarenal vein: a vein that drains the right suprarenal gland into the inferior vena cava.

v. suprarena'lis sinis'tra [NA], left suprarenal vein: the vein that returns blood from the left suprarenal gland to the left renal vein.

v. suprascapula'ris [NA], suprascapular vein: the vein that accompanies the homonymous artery (sometimes as two veins that unite), opening usually into the external jugular, or occasionally into the subclavian vein; called also *v. transversa scapulae.*

ve'nae supratrochlea'res [NA], supratrochlear veins: two veins, each beginning in a venous plexus high up on the forehead and descending to the root of the nose, where it joins with the supraorbital to form the angular vein; called also *venae frontales.*

v. tempora'lis me'dia [NA], middle temporal vein: the vein that arises in the substance of the temporal muscle and passes down under the fascia to the zygoma, where it breaks through to join the superficial temporal vein.

ve'nae tempora'les profun'dae [NA], deep temporal veins: veins that drain the deep portions of the temporal muscle and empty into the pterygoid plexus.

ve'nae tempora'les superficia'les [NA], superficial temporal veins: veins that drain the lateral part of the scalp in the frontal and parietal regions, the tributaries forming a single superficial temporal vein in front of the ear, just above the zygoma. This descending vein receives the middle temporal and transverse facial veins and, entering the parotid gland, unites with the maxillary vein deep to the neck of the mandible to form the retromandibular vein.

v. termina'lis, v. thalamostriata.

v. testicula'ris, see *v. testicularis dextra* and *v. testicularis sinistra.*

v. testicula'ris dex'tra [NA], right testicular vein: a vein that drains the right pampiniform plexus into the inferior vena cava.

v. testicula'ris sinis'tra [NA], left testicular vein: a vein that drains the left pampiniform plexus into the left renal vein.

v. thalamostria'ta [NA], thalamostriate vein: a vein that collects blood from the corpus striatum and thalamus, and joins with the choroid vein to form the internal cerebral veins; called also *v. terminalis.*

v. thoraca'lis latera'lis, v. thoracica lateralis.

ve'nae thora'cicae inter'nae [NA], internal thoracic veins: two veins formed by junction of the venae comitantes of the internal thoracic artery of either side; each continues along the artery to open into the brachiocephalic vein; called also (sing.) *v. mammaria interna.*

v. thora'cica latera'lis [NA], lateral thoracic vein: a large vein accompanying the lateral thoracic artery and draining into the axillary vein; called also *v. thoracalis lateralis.*

v. thoracoacromia'lis [NA], thoracoacromial vein: the vein that follows the homonymous artery and opens into the subclavian vein.

ve'nae thoracoepigas'tricae [NA], thoracoepigastric veins: long, longitudinal, superficial veins in the anterolateral subcutaneous tissue of the torso, which empty superiorly into the lateral thoracic and inferiorly into the femoral vein.

ve'nae thy'micae [NA], thymic veins: small branches from the thymus gland that open into the left brachiocephalic vein.

v. thyreoi'dea i'ma, an occasional vein formed by high junction of the right and left inferior thyroid veins, and emptying usually into the left brachiocephalic vein.

ve'nae thyreoi'deae inferio'res, see *v. thyroidea inferior.*

ve'nae thyreoi'deae superio'res, 1. see *vena thyroidea superior.* 2. veins draining blood from the upper portion of the thyroid gland into the posterior facial vein.

v. thyroi'dea infe'rior [NA], inferior thyroid vein: either of two veins, left and right, that drain the thyroid plexus into the left and right brachiocephalic veins; occasionally they may unite into a common trunk to empty, usually, into the left brachiocephalic vein.

ve'nae thyroi'deae me'diae [NA], middle thyroid veins: veins that drain blood from the thyroid gland into the internal jugular vein.

v. thyroi'dea supe'rior [NA], superior thyroid vein: a vein arising from the upper part of the thyroid gland on either side, opening into the internal jugular vein, occasionally in common with the facial vein.

ve'nae tibia'les anterio'res [NA], anterior tibial veins: venae comitantes of the anterior tibial artery, which unite with the posterior tibial veins to form the popliteal vein.

ve'nae tibia'les posterio'res [NA], posterior tibial veins: venae comitantes of the posterior tibial artery, which unite with the anterior tibial veins to form the popliteal vein.

ve'nae trachea'les [NA], tracheal veins: small branches that drain blood from the trachea into the brachiocephalic vein.

ve'nae transver'sae col'li [NA], transverse cervical veins: veins that follow the transverse artery of the neck and open into the subclavian vein.

v. transver'sa facie'i [NA], transverse facial vein: a vein that passes backward with the transverse facial artery just below the zygomatic arch to join the retromandibular vein.

v. transver'sa scap'ulae, v. suprascapularis.

ve'nae tympan'icae [NA], tympanic veins: small veins from the tympanic cavity that pass through the petrotympanic fissure, open into the plexus around the temporomandibular articulation, and finally drain into the retromandibular vein.

ve'nae ulna'res [NA], ulnar veins: the venae comitantes of the ulnar artery, which unite with the radial veins at the elbow to form the brachial veins.

v. umbilica'lis, umbilical vein: former NA term for either of the paired veins that carry blood from the chorion to the sinus venosus and heart in the early embryo; they later fuse and a single vessel persisting in the umbilical cord carries all the blood from the placenta to the ductus venosus of the fetus. See *v. umbilicalis sinistra.*

v. umbilica'lis sinis'tra [NA], left umbilical vein of the fetus, the vein formed by fusion of the atrophied right umbilical vein with the left umbilical vein, which carries all the blood from the placenta to the ductus venosus.

ve'nae uteri'nae [NA], uterine veins: veins that drain the uterine plexus into the internal iliac veins.

ve'nae vaso'rum, small veins that return blood from the tissues making up the walls of the blood vessels themselves.

v. vertebra'lis [NA], vertebral vein: a vein that arises from the suboccipital venous plexus, passes with the vertebral artery through the foramina of the transverse processes of the upper six cervical vertebrae, and opens into the brachiocephalic vein.

v. vertebra'lis acces'soria [NA], accessory vertebral vein: a vein that sometimes arises from a plexus formed around the vertebral artery by the vertebral vein, descends with the vertebral vein, and emerges through the transverse foramen of the seventh cervical vertebra to empty into the brachiocephalic vein.

v. vertebra'lis ante'rior [NA], anterior vertebral vein: a small vein arising from the venous plexus around the transverse processes of the upper cervical vertebrae, and descending to end in the vertebral vein.

ve'nae vesica'les [NA], vesical veins: veins passing from the vesical plexus to the internal iliac veins.

ve'nae vestibula'res [NA], vestibular veins: branches draining blood from the vestibule into the labyrinthine veins.

ve'nae vortico'sae [NA], vorticose veins: four veins that pierce the sclera and carry blood from the choroid to the superior ophthalmic vein; called also *venae choroideae oculi* [NA alternative].

---

venacavogram (ve″nak-ka′vo-gram) the film obtained by venacavography.

venacavography (ve″nah-ka-vog′rah-fe) radiography of a vena cava, usually of the inferior vena cava.

venae (ve′ne) [L.] plural of *vena.*

Vena medinensis (ve′nah med″ĭ-nen′sis) *Dracunculus medinensis.*

venation (ve-na′shun) [L. *vena* vein] the manner of distribution of the veins of a part.

venectasia (ve″nek-ta′ze-ah) phlebectasia; varicosity.

venectomy (ve-nek′to-me) phlebectomy.

veneer (vĕ-nēr′) in the construction of crowns or pontics, a layer of tooth-colored material, usually porcelain or acrylic resin, attached to the surface by direct fusion, cementation, or mechanical retention.

venenation (ven″ĕ-na′shun) [L. *venenum* poison] poisoning; a condition of being poisoned.

veneniferous (ven″ĕ-nif′er-us) [L. *venenum* poison + *ferre* to bear] carrying poison.

venenific (ven″ĕ-nif′ik) [L. *venenum* poison + *facere* to make] forming poison.

Venenosa (ven″ĕ-no′sah) [pl., L. *venenosus* poisonous] a term once used to designate venomous snakes collectively; thanatophidia.

venenosalivary (ven″ĕ-no-sal′ĭ-ver″e) venomosalivary.

venenosity (ven″ĕ-nos′ĭ-te) the condition of being venomous.

venenous (ven″ĕ-nus) [L. *venenosus*] venomous.

venenum (ve-ne′num), pl. *vene′na* [L.] a poison.

venepuncture (ven′e-punk″tūr) venipuncture.

venereal (ve-ne′re-al) [L. *venereus*] due to or propagated by sexual contact; see under *disease.*

venereologist (ve-ne″re-ol′o-jist) a practitioner who specializes in venereal disease.

venereology (ve-ne″re-ol′o-je) the branch of medicine which deals with venereal disease.

venerology (ven″er-ol′o-je) venereology.

venerupin (ven″er-oo′pin) [*Venerupis* (L. *veneris*) the Venus shell + *-in,* suffix for chemical compounds] a toxic substance, believed to be an amine, found in certain Japanese pelecypods which were formerly placed in the genus *Venerupis;* this toxin, the exact chemical nature of which is unknown, is entirely distinct from the paralytic shellfish poison found in other bivalves.

venery (ven′er-e) [L. *venereus* pertaining to Venus] coitus; sexual intercourse.

venesection (ven″ĕ-sek′shun) [L. *vena* vein + *sectio* cutting] phlebotomy.

venesuture (ven″ĕ-su′tūr) phleborrhaphy.

veniplex (ven′ĭ-pleks) [L. *vena* vein + *plexus* plexus] a venous plexus.

venipuncture (ven′ĭ-punk″tūr) puncture of a vein.

venisection (ven′ĭ-sek′shun) phlebotomy.

venisuture (ven′ĭ-su′tūr) [L. *vena* vein + *sutura* stitch] phleborrhaphy.

veno- (ve′no) [L. *vena* vein] a combining form denoting relationship to a vein. See also words beginning *phlebo-.*

venoatrial (ve″no-a′tre-al) pertaining to the vena cava and the right atrium.

venoauricular (ve″no-aw-rik′u-lar) venoatrial.

venoclysis (ve-nok′lĭ-sis) [*vena* + Gr. *klysis* injection] phleboclysis.

venofibrosis (ve″no-fi-bro′sis) a disease of the veins characterized by hyperplasia of the fibrous connective tissue of the median coat of the vein.

venogram (ve′no-gram) 1. phlebogram. 2. a venous-pulse tracing.

venography (ve-nog′rah-fe) phlebography. **intraosseous v.,** roentgenography of the veins after injection of the contrast medium into bone marrow at an appropriate site, such as the iliac crest, ischium, pubic bones, greater trochanter, spinous processes of the vertebrae, or sternum. **portal v.,** portography. **splenic v.,** splenic portography.

venom (ven'um) [L. *venenum* poison] a poison; specifically, a toxic substance normally secreted by a serpent, insect, or other animal. **Russell's viper v.,** the venom of Russell's viper, *Vipera russelli,* which acts *in vitro* as an intrinsic thromboplastin and is useful in defining deficiencies of blood coagulation Factor X. **snake v.,** the poisonous secretion of snakes, containing hemotoxins, hemagglutinins, neurotoxins, leukotoxins, or endotheliotoxins. The venoms of various species have been used as hemostatics. See also *antivenomous serum,* under *serum.* **spider v.,** the venom of a spider such as *Latrodectus, Atrax, Ctenus,* and *Lycosa.*

venomization (ven"um-i-za'shun) treatment of a substance with snake venom.

venomosalivary (ven"o-mo-sal'ĭ-ver"e) secreting a poisonous saliva.

venomotor (ve"no-mo'tor) pertaining to or producing constriction or dilatation of the veins.

venomous (ven'o-mus) secreting venom; poisonous.

veno-occlusive (ve"no-ŏ-kloo'siv) pertaining to or characterized by obstruction of the veins.

venoperitoneostomy (ve"no-per"ĭ-to"ne-os'to-me) [*veno-* + *peritoneum* + Gr. *stomoun* to provide with an opening, or mouth] anastomosis of the saphenous vein with the peritoneum for permanent drainage of the peritoneal cavity in ascites.

venopressor (ve-no-pres"or) 1. pertaining to venous blood pressure. 2. an agent that causes venous constriction.

venosclerosis (ve"no-sklĕ-ro'sis) phlebosclerosis.

venose (ve'nōs) provided with veins.

venosinal (ve"no-si'nal) pertaining to the venae cavae and the right atrium of the heart.

venosity (ve-nos'ĭ-te) 1. excess of venous blood in a part. 2. a plentiful supply of blood vessels or of venous blood.

venostasis (ve"no-sta'sis) [*veno-* + Gr. *stasis* stopping] retardation of venous outflow from a part, as from the leg on standing when venous valves are incompetent; see *phlebostasis.*

venotomy (ve-not'o-me) phlebotomy.

venous (ve'nus) [L. *venosus*] of or pertaining to the veins.

venovenostomy (ve"no-ve-nos'to-me) phlebophlebostomy.

vent (vent) [Fr. *fente* slit] 1. any opening or outlet; especially the anus. 2. an opening that discharges pus. **pulmonic alveolar v's,** interalveolar pores.

Ventaire (ventār) trademark for a preparation of protokylol hydrochloride.

venter (ven'ter), pl. *ven'tres* [L. "belly"] 1. any belly-shaped part; [NA] a general term for a fleshy contractile part of a muscle. 2. the abdomen or stomach. 3. any hollowed part or cavity. **v. ante'rior mus'culi digas'trici** [NA], anterior belly of digastric muscle: the shorter belly of the digastric muscle, arising from the digastric fossa on the mandible and extending backward to join the posterior belly through an intermediate tendon attached to the hyoid bone. **v. fronta'lis mus'culi occipitofronta'lis** [NA], the frontal belly of the occipitofrontal muscle, originating from the galea aponeurotica and inserting into the skin of the eyebrows and the root of the nose. Called also *musculus frontalis.* **v. il'ii,** the free (pelvic) portion of the sacropelvic surface of the ilium. **v. i'mus,** the lowermost of the great body cavities, the abdominal cavity (cavum abdominis). **v. infe'rior mus'culi omohyoi'dei** [NA], the lowermost belly of the omohyoid muscle. **v. me'dius,** the middle of the great body cavities, the thoracic cavity (cavum thoracis). **v. mus'culi** [NA], belly of muscle: the fleshy contractile part of a muscle. **v. occipita'lis mus'culi occipitofronta'lis** [NA], the occipital belly of the occipitofrontal muscle, originating from the highest nuchal line of the occipital bone and inserting into the galea aponeurotica; called also *musculus occipitalis.* **v. poste'rior mus'culi digas'trici** [NA], posterior belly of digastric muscle: the longer belly of the digastric muscle, arising from the mastoid notch of the temporal bone and extending forward to join the anterior belly through an intermediate tendon attached to the hyoid bone. **v. propen'dens,** pendulous abdomen. **v. scap'ulae,** fossa subscapularis. **v. supe'rior mus'culi omohyoi'dei** [NA], the uppermost belly of the omohyoid muscle. **v. supre'mus,** the uppermost of the great body cavities, the cranial cavity.

ventilation (ven"tĭ-la'shun) [L. *ventilatio*] 1. the process or act of supplying a house or room continuously with fresh air. 2. in respiratory physiology, the process of exchange of air between the lungs and the ambient air. *Pulmonary ventilation* (usually measured in liters per minute) refers to the total exchange, whereas *alveolar ventilation* refers to the effective ventilation of the alveoli, in which gas exchange with the blood takes place. 3. in psychiatry, the open discussion of grievances. **alveolar v.,** the amount of gas expelled from the alveoli to the outside of the body per minute. **downward v.,** that in which the outlets have places lower than those of the inlets. **exhausting v.,** ventilation by means of the exhausting fan or by some other

process which withdraws the foul air. **mechanical v.,** ventilation accomplished by extrinsic means as under positive end-expiratory pressure. **minute v.,** the total amount of gas (in liters) expelled from the lungs per minute. Called also *total ventilation.* **natural v.,** ventilation effected without any special appliance to render it certain. **plenum v.,** the supply of fresh air to a building by fan blowers. **upward v.,** that which introduces air below the place of its withdrawal. **vacuum v.,** that which is effected by the forced extraction of air.

ventilator (ven'tĭ-la'tor) an apparatus designed to qualify the air that is breathed through it or to assist or control pulmonary ventilation, either intermittently or continuously.

ventouse (vaw-tooz') [Fr.] a cupping glass.

ventrad (ven'trad) [L. *venter* belly + *ad* to] toward a belly, venter, or ventral aspect.

ventral (ven'tral) [L. *ventralis*] 1. pertaining to the belly or to any venter. 2. denoting a position more toward the belly surface than some other object of reference; same as *anterior* in human anatomy.

ventralis (ven-tra'lis) ventral; [NA] a general term used to designate a position closer to the belly surface. Cf. *anterior.*

ventralward (ven'tral-ward) ventrad.

ventri- see *ventro-.*

ventricle (ven'trĭ-k'l) a small cavity, such as one of the several cavities of the brain, or one of the lower chambers of the heart; called also *ventriculus.* **aortic v. of heart,** ventriculus sinister cordis. **v. of Arantius,** the fossa rhomboidea, especially its lower end; the eponym is also sometimes applied to the cavum septi pellucidi. **auxiliary v.,** an implanted pumping mechanism designed to assist the left ventricle of the heart in maintaining normal output, rate, and blood pressure; called also *booster heart.* **v's of the brain,** the cavities within the brain which are filled with cerebrospinal fluid, including the two lateral, the third, and the fourth ventricles. They are lined by ependyma which, in certain regions, is invaginated by vascular fringes of pia mater to form the choroid plexuses. The cavum septi pellucidi, to which the term ventricle is sometimes applied, is not a true ventricle. **v. of cord,** canalis centralis medullae spinalis. **double-outlet right v.,** incomplete transposition of the great vessels in which both the aorta and the pulmonary artery arise from the right ventricle, associated with a subaortic ventricular septal defect. In type I, the septal defect is posteroinferior to the crista supraventricularis and remote from the pulmonary valve. In type II, it is anterosuperior to the crista and close to the valve. **Duncan's v., fifth v.,** cavum septi pellucidi. **first v. of cerebrum,** ventriculus lateralis cerebri. **fourth v. of cerebrum,** an irregularly shaped cavity in the rhombencephalon; see *ventriculus quartus cerebri* [NA]. **Galen's v.,** ventriculus laryngis. **v. of heart,** one of a pair of cavities, with thick muscular walls, that make up the bulk of the heart; see *ventriculus dexter cordis* and *ventriculus sinister cordis.* Called also *ventriculus cordis* [NA]. **v. of larynx,** ventriculus laryngis. **lateral v. of cerebrum,** the cavity in each hemisphere, derived (developed) from the cavity of the embryonic neural tube; see *ventriculus lateralis cerebri.* **left v. of heart,** ventriculus sinister cordis. **Morgagni's v.,** ventriculus laryngis. **pineal v.,** recessus pinealis. **right v. of heart,** ventriculus dexter cordis. **second v. of cerebrum,** ventriculus lateralis cerebri. **single v.,** cor triloculare biatriatum. **sixth v.,** Verga's v. **v. of Sylvius,** cavum septi pellucidi. **terminal v. of spinal cord,** ventriculus terminalis medullae spinalis. **third v. of cerebrum,** ventriculus tertius cerebri. **Verga's v.,** an occasional space between the corpus callosum and the fornix; called also *sixth v.* **Vieussen's v.,** cavum septi pellucidi.

ventricornu (ven"trĭ-kor'nu) [*ventri-* + L. *cornu* horn] cornu anterius medullae spinalis.

ventricornual (ven"trĭ-kor'nu-al) pertaining to the ventricornu.

ventricose (ven'trĭ-kōs) having an expansion or belly on one side.

ventricular (ven-trik'u-lar) pertaining to a ventricle.

ventriculi (ven-trik'u-li) [L.] plural of *ventriculus.*

ventriculitis (ven-trik"u-li'tis) inflammation of a ventricle, especially of a ventricle of the brain.

ventriculo- (ven-trik'u-lo) [L. *ventriculus,* dim. of *venter* belly] a combining form denoting relationship to a ventricle, of the heart or brain.

ventriculoatriostomy (ven-trik"u-lo-a"tre-os'to-me) surgical creation of a passage, by means of subcutaneously placed catheters with a one-way valve, permitting drainage of cerebrospinal fluid from a cerebral ventricle to the right atrium by way of the jugular vein; performed for relief of hydrocephalus.

ventriculocisternostomy (ven-trik"u-lo-sis"ter-nos'to-me) surgical establishment of a communication between the third ventricle and the cisterna interpeduncularis; see *ventriculostomy.*

ventriculocordectomy (ven-trik"u-lo-kor-dek'to-me) Chevalier Jackson operation for laryngeal stenosis with bilateral recurrent paralysis, done by excising with the punch forceps the entire ventricular floor anterior to the vocal process and anteroexternal surface of the arytenoid.

ventriculogram (ven-trik′u-lo-gram) a roentgenogram of the cerebral ventricles.

ventriculography (ven-trik″u-log′rah-fe) [*ventriculo* + Gr. *graphein* to write] 1. roentgenography of the head following removal of cerebrospinal fluid from the cerebral ventricles and its replacement by air or other contrast medium. 2. roentgenography of a ventricle of the heart after injection of a contrast medium.

ventriculometry (ven-trik″u-lom′ĕ-tre) [*ventriculo-* + Gr. *metron* measure] the measurement of the intraventricular (intracranial) pressure.

ventriculomyotomy (ven-trik″u-lo-mi-ot′o-me) incision of the obstructing muscular band in treatment of subaortic stenosis.

ventriculonector (ven-trik″u-lo-nek′ter) [*ventriculo-* + L. *nector* joiner] bundle of His.

ventriculopuncture (ven-trik′u-lo-punk″tūr) puncture of a lateral ventricle of the brain by the insertion of a needle.

ventriculoscope (ven-trik′u-lo-skōp) an endoscope for examining the cerebral ventricles and for cauterizing the choroid plexus.

ventriculoscopy (ven-trik″u-los′ko-pe) [*ventriculo-* + Gr. *skopein* to examine] direct examination of the cerebral ventricles by means of an endoscope or cystoscope.

ventriculostium (ven-trik″u-los′tĭ-um) [*ventriculo-* + L. *ostium* mouth] the development of an opening between one of the cerebral ventricles and the external surface of the brain.

ventriculostomy (ven-trik″u-los′to-me) [*ventriculo-* + Gr. *stomoun* to provide with an opening, or mouth] the operation of establishing a free communication between the floor of the third ventricle and the underlying cisterna interpeduncularis; for the treatment of hydrocephalus.

ventriculosubarachnoid (ven-trik″u-lo-sub″ah-rak-′noid) pertaining to the cerebral ventricles and the subarachnoid spaces.

ventriculotomy (ven-trik″u-lot′o-me) [*ventriculo-* + Gr. *tomē* a cutting] incision of a ventricle of the heart.

ventriculovenostomy (ven-trik″u-lo-vĕ-nos′to-me) creation of a communication from a cerebral ventricle to the internal jugular vein, for the treatment of hydrocephalus.

ventriculovenous (ven-trik″u-lo-ve′nus) pertaining to or communicating with a cerebral ventricle and a vein.

ventriculus (ven-trik′u-lus), pl. *ventric′uli* [L., dim. of *venter* belly] [NA] 1. the stomach: the musculomembranous expansion of the alimentary canal between esophagus and duodenum. See also *stomach.* 2. a small cavity in an organ; called also *ventricle.* **v. cor′dis** [NA], ventricle of heart: one of the pair of cavities, with thick muscular walls, that make up the bulk of the heart. See *v. dexter cordis* and *v. sinister cordis.* **v. dex′ter cer′ebri,** the ventriculus lateralis cerebri of the right cerebral hemisphere. **v. dex′ter cor′dis** [NA], right ventricle of heart: the cavity of the heart that propels the blood through the pulmonary trunk and arteries into the lungs. See Plate XX. **v. laryn′gis** [NA], **v. laryn′gis [Morgag′nii],** ventricle of larynx: a lateral evagination of mucous membrane between the vocal and vestibular folds, reaching nearly to the angle of the thyroid cartilage. **v. latera′lis cer′ebri** [NA], lateral ventricle of cerebrum: the cavity in each cerebral hemisphere, derived (developed) from the cavity of the embryonic neural tube; it consists of a pars centralis and three horns—anterior, inferior, and posterior in the frontal, temporal, and occipital lobes respectively. Each lateral ventricle communicates with the third ventricle by an interventricular foramen through which also the choroid plexuses of the lateral ventricles become continuous with that of the third ventricle. Cerebrospinal fluid formed in the lateral ventricle flows into the third ventricle through the interventricular foramina. **v. quar′tus cer′ebri** [NA], fourth ventricle of cerebrum: an irregularly shaped cavity in the rhombencephalon, between the medulla oblongata, the pons, and the isthmus in front, and the cerebellum behind; it is continuous with the central canal of the cord below and with the cerebral aqueduct above, and through its lateral and median apertures it communicates with the subarachnoid space. **v. sinis′ter cer′ebri,** the ventriculus lateralis cerebri of the left cerebral hemisphere. **v. sinis′ter cor′dis** [NA], left ventricle of heart: the cavity of the heart that propels the blood out through the aorta into the systemic arteries. See Plate XX. **v. termina′lis medul′lae spina′lis** [NA], terminal ventricle of spinal cord: a saclike expansion of the central canal of the spinal cord within the conus medullaris. **v. ter′tius cer′ebri** [NA], third ventricle of cerebrum: a narrow cleft below the corpus callosum, within the diencephalon between the two thalami. Its floor is formed by the hypothalamus, its anterior wall by the lamina terminalis, and its roof by ependyma. It communicates with the lateral ventricles by the interventricular foramina, and with the fourth ventricle by the cerebral aqueduct.

ventricumbent (ven″trĭ-kum′bent) [*ventri-* + L. *cumbere* to lie] lying upon the belly; prone.

ventriduct (ven′trĭ-dukt) [*ventri-* + L. *ducere* to draw] to bring or carry ventrad.

ventriduction (ven″trĭ-duk′shun) the act of drawing a part ventrad.

ventriflexion (ven″trĭ-flek′shun) [*ventri-* + *flexion*] flexion toward the belly or ventral surface.

ventrimesal (ven″trĭ-me′sal) pertaining to the ventrimeson.

ventrimeson (ven-trim′e-son) [*ventri-* + Gr. *meson* middle] the middle line on the ventral surface.

ventro-, ventri- [L. *venter* belly or abdomen] combining form denoting relationship to the belly, or to the front (anterior) aspect of the body.

ventrocystorrhaphy (ven″tro-sis-tor′ah-fe) the stitching of a cyst, or of the bladder, to the abdominal wall.

ventrodorsad (ven″tro-dor′sad) from the ventral toward the dorsal aspect.

ventrodorsal (ven″tro-dor′sal) pertaining to the ventral and dorsal surfaces.

ventrofixation (ven″tro-fiks-a′shun) [*ventro-* + L. *fixare* to fix] the operation of suspending the retroplaced uterus to the abdominal wall. Cf. *hysteropexy.*

ventrohysteropexy (ven″tro-his′ter-o-pek″se) ventrofixation of the uterus.

ventroinguinal (ven″tro-ing′gwĭ-nal) pertaining to the abdomen and the inguinal region.

ventrolateral (ven″tro-lat′er-al) both ventral and lateral.

ventromedian (ven″tro-me′de-an) both ventral and median.

ventroposterior (ven″tro-pos-te′re-or) both ventral and posterior (caudal).

ventroptosia (ven″trop-to′se-ah) [*ventro-* + Gr. *ptōsis* falling + *-ia*] gastroptosis.

ventroptosis (ven″trop-to′sis) gastroptosis.

ventroscopy (ven-tros′ko-pe) [*ventro-* + Gr. *skopein* to examine] illumination of the abdominal cavity for the purpose of examination.

ventrose (ven′trōs) [L. *ventrosus*] having a belly-like expansion.

ventrosuspension (ven″tro-sus-pen′shun) ventrofixation.

ventrotomy (ven-trot′o-me) [*ventro-* + Gr. *tomē* a cutting] celiotomy.

ventrovesicofixation (ven″tro-ves″ĭ-ko-fiks-a′shun) [*ventro-* + L. *vesica* bladder + *fixatio* fastening] (*obs.*) the operation of suturing the uterus to the bladder and the abdominal wall. Cf. *hysteropexy* and *ventrohysteropexy.*

venturimeter (ven″tu-rim′ĕ-ter) [G. B. *Venturi* (Italian physicist, 1746–1822) + Gr. *metron* measure] an instrument for measuring the flow of liquids, as of the blood in vessels, by relating difference of pressures between a constricted and a nonconstricted portion of a tube through which fluid is flowing.

venula (ven′u-lah), pl. *ven′ulae* [L., dim. of *vena*] [NA] venule: any of the small vessels that collect blood from the capillary plexuses and join to form veins. **v. macula′ris infe′rior** [NA], inferior macular venule: the inferior venule draining blood from the macula retinae. **v. macula′ris supe′rior** [NA], superior macular venule: the superior venule draining blood from the macula retinae. **v. media′lis ret′inae** [NA], medial venule of retina: a small branch draining blood from the central region of the retina to the central retinal vein; called also *v. retinae medialis.* **v. nasa′lis ret′inae infe′rior** [NA], inferior nasal venule of retina: a small vein returning blood from the inferior nasal region of the retina to the central vein. **v. nasa′lis ret′inae supe′rior** [NA], superior nasal venule of retina: a small vein returning blood from the superior nasal region of the retina to the central vein. **ven′ulae rec′tae re′nis** [NA], straight venules of kidney: straight veins from the papillary part of the kidney, emptying into the arcuate veins. **v. ret′inae media′lis,** v. medialis retinae. **ven′ulae stella′tae re′nis** [NA], stellate venules of kidney: veins on the surface of the kidney that collect blood from the superficial parts of the cortex and empty into the interlobular veins; called also *venae stellatae renis.* **v. tempora′lis ret′inae infe′rior** [NA], inferior temporal venule of retina: a small vein returning blood from the inferior temporal region of the retina to the central vein. **v. tempora′lis ret′inae supe′rior** [NA], superior temporal venule of retina: a small vein returning blood from the superior temporal region of the retina to the central vein.

venulae (ven′u-le) [L.] plural of *venula.*

venular (ven′u-lar) pertaining to, composed of, or affecting venules.

venule (ven′ūl) any of the small vessels that collect blood from the capillary plexuses and join to form veins; called also *venula* [NA]. **macular v., inferior,** venula macularis inferior. **macular v., superior,** venula macularis superior. **medial v. of retina,** venula medialis retinae. **nasal v. of retina, inferior,** venula nasalis retinae inferior. **nasal v. of retina, superior,** venula nasalis retinae superior. **postcapillary v.,** a venous capillary. **stellate v's of kidney,** venulae stellatae renis. **straight v's of kidney,** venulae rectae renis. **temporal v. of retina, inferior,** venula temporalis retinae inferior. **temporal v. of retina, superior,** venula temporalis retinae superior.

Veracillin (ver″ah-sil′in) trademark for a preparation of dicloxacillin sodium.

Veraguth's fold (va′rah-goots) [Otto *Veraguth,* Zurich neurologist, 1870–1940] see under *fold.*

Veralba (ver-al′bah) trademark for a mixture of protoveratrines A and B.

verapamil (ver-ap′ah-mil) chemical name: α-[3-[[2-(3,4-dimethoxyphenyl) ethyl] methylamino] propyl] - 3, 4 - dimethoxy - α - (1-methylethyl)benzeneacetonitrile; a coronary vasodilator, $C_{27}H_{38}$-N_2O_4, used in the treatment and prophylaxis of angina of effort.

veratroidine (ver″ah-troi′din) a crystallizable base, $C_{32}H_{53}$-NO_9, from the liliacious plants *Veratrum album* L. and *V. viride* Aiton, a powerful nerve stimulant and cardiac inhibitor.

Veratrum (ve-ra′trum) [L.] a genus of poisonous liliaceous plants, including *V. album* L., or European white hellebore, and *V. viride* Aiton, or American or green hellebore, both of which are the source of antihypertensive alkaloids.

verbal (ver′bal) [L. *verbum*] consisting of words; pertaining to words or speech.

verbenol (ver-be′nol) a terpene alcohol, $(CH_3)_2C{:}C_6H_6(OH)$-CH_3, from *Boswellia carterii* Birdw. (Burseraceae), a tree of southern Europe, Arabia, and Somali; a source of the biblical frankincense.

verbenone (ver-be′nōn) a terpene ketone, $(CH_3)_2C{:}C_6H_5O{\cdot}CH_3$, from *Verbena triphylla,* an American herb.

verbigeration (ver-bij″er-a′shun) [L. *verbigerare* to chatter] the repetition of meaningless words and sentences; called also *catalogia.* Cf. *polyphrasia.*

verbomania (ver″bo-ma′ne-ah) [L. *verba* word + Gr. *mania* madness] morbid talkativeness.

Vercyte (ver′sīt) trademark for a preparation of pipobroman.

verdigris (ver′dĭ-gris) [Fr., from *vert de Grèce* green of Greece] a blue, hydrated, basic copper acetate, $(CH_3{\cdot}COO)_2{\cdot}Cu{\cdot}Cu(OH)_2$; astringent.

verdohemin (ver″do-he′min) a compound analogous to hemin, in which one porphyrin ring is open.

verdohemochromogen (ver″do-he″mo-kro′mo-jen) a compound analogous to hemochromogen, in which one porphyrin ring is open.

verdohemoglobin (ver″do-he″mo-glo′bin) a compound analogous to hemoglobin, in which one porphyrin ring is open.

verdoperoxidase (ver″do-per-ok′sĭ-dās) [Fr. *vert* green + *peroxidase*] an enzyme (peroxidase) occurring in leukocytes and having a greenish color.

verdunization (ver″dun-i-za′shun) [*Verdun,* a French city besieged during World War I] (*obs.*) the addition of small amounts of chlorine and potassium permanganate to water for the purpose of sterilizing it.

Verga's lacrimal groove, ventricle (ver′gahz) [Andrea *Verga,* Italian neurologist, 1811–1895] see under *groove* and *ventricle.*

verge (verj) a circumference, or ring. **anal v.,** the external or distal boundary of the anal canal; the line where the walls of the anus come in contact during the normal state of apposition.

vergence (ver′jens) [L. *vergere* to be inclined] disjunctive movement of the eyes in opposite directions, as in convergence and divergence, that is, in adjusting from far to near or from near to far vision.

vergency (ver′jen-se) vergence.

Verheyen's stars (ver-hi′enz) [Philippe *Verheyen,* Flemish anatomist, 1648–1710] venulae stellatae renis.

Verhoeff's operation, stain (ver′hefz) [Frederick Herman *Verhoeff,* American ophthalmologist, born 1874] see under *operation* and *Table of Stains.*

Veriloid (ver′ĭ-loid) trademark for a preparation of alkavervir.

Vermale's operation (ver-malz′) [Raymond de *Vermale,* French surgeon of the 18th century] see under *operation.*

Vermes (ver′mēz) obsolete term for the group of invertebrates called worms.

vermetoid (ver′mĕ-toid) wormlike.

vermian (ver′me-an) pertaining to the vermis of the cerebellum.

Vermicella (ver″mĭ-sel′ah) [L.] a genus of mildly venomous Australian serpents.

vermicidal (ver″mĭ-si′dal) destructive to worms.

vermicide (ver′mĭ-sīd) [*vermis* + L. *caedere* to kill] an anthelmintic drug or medicine destructive to intestinal animal parasites.

vermicular (ver-mik′u-lar) [L. *vermicularis,* from *vermis* worm] wormlike in shape or appearance.

vermiculation (ver-mik″u-la′shun) [L. *vermiculatio,* from *vermis* worm] peristaltic or wormlike movements, as of the intestine; peristalsis.

vermicule (ver′mĭ-kūl) a wormlike structure; see also *ookinete.* **traveling v.,** ookinete.

vermiculose (ver-mik′u-lōs) vermiculous.

vermiculous (ver-mik′u-lus) 1. wormlike. 2. infected with worms.

vermiform (ver′mĭ-form) [L. *vermiformis,* from *vermis* worm + *forma* shape] shaped like a worm.

vermifugal (ver-mif′u-gal) [*vermis* + L. *fugare* to put to flight] expelling worms or intestinal animal parasites.

vermifuge (ver′mĭ-fūj) an agent that expels worms or intestinal animal parasites; an anthelmintic.

vermilion (ver-mil′yun) cinnabar, or mercuric sulfide, HgS, a red pigment; see also under *border.*

vermilionectomy (ver-mil″yon-ek′to-me) excision of the vermilion border of the lip, the surgically created defect being resurfaced by advancement of the undermined labial mucosa.

vermin (ver′min) [L. *vermis* worm] an external animal parasite; animal ectoparasites collectively.

verminal (ver′mĭ-nal) pertaining to or due to worms; pertaining to or due to vermin.

vermination (ver″mĭ-na′shun) [L. *verminatio*] infection with worms; infestation with vermin.

verminosis (ver″mĭ-no′sis) vermination.

verminotic (ver″mĭ-not′ik) pertaining to or caused by infection with worms; pertaining to or caused by infestation with vermin.

verminous (ver′mĭ-nus) [L. *verminosus*] pertaining to, due to, or abounding in worms; pertaining to, due to, or abounding in vermin.

vermis (ver′mis) [L.] a worm or wormlike structure; often used alone to designate the vermis cerebelli. **v. cerebel′li** [NA], the median part of the cerebellum, between the two hemispheres; it comprises the lingula, lobulus centralis, culmen, declive, folium vermis, tuber vermis, pyramis vermis, uvula vermis, and nodulus. Called also *cauda cerebelli* and *vermiform process of cerebellum.* **inferior v.,** the inferior aspect of the vermis cerebelli, from the tuber vermis to the nodulus. **superior v.,** the superior aspect of the vermis cerebelli, from the lingula to the folium vermis.

vermix (ver′miks) appendix vermiformis.

vermography (ver-mog′rah-fe) roentgenography of the vermiform appendix.

vernal (ver′nal) [L. *vernalis* of the spring] pertaining to or occurring in the spring.

Vernes' test (vārnz) [Arthur *Veres,* French physician, born 1879] see under *tests.*

Vernet's syndrome (ver-nāz′) [Maurice *Vernet,* French neurologist, born 1887] see under *syndrome.*

Verneuil's canals, etc. (ver-na′ēz) [Aristide August Stanislaus *Verneuil,* French surgeon, 1823–1895] see under *canal, disease,* and *neuroma.*

vernier (ver′ne-er) [Pierre *Vernier,* French physicist, 1580–1637] a finely graduated scale accessory to a more coarsely graduated one for measuring fractions of the divisions of the latter.

vernin (ver′nin) a pentoside of adenine found in *Vicia* seedlings.

vernix (ver′niks) [L.] varnish. **v. caseo′sa** [“cheesy varnish”], an unctuous substance composed of sebum and desquamated epithelial cells, which covers the skin of the fetus.

Vernonia anthelmintica Willd. (ver-no′ne-ah an″thel-min′-tĭ-kah) a plant called *somraj* in India; it is anthelmintic. Also used there for skin diseases and leprosy and as an abortifacient.

Verocay bodies (ver′o-ka) [José *Verocay,* Prague pathologist, 1876–1927] see under *body.*

vérole (va-rōl′) [Fr.] syphilis. **v. nerveuse** neurosyphilis.

Veronicella (ve-ron″ĭ-sel′lah) a genus of slugs. **V. leydig′i,** an intermediate host of *Angiostrongylus cantonensis* in the Pacific, especially in Tahiti and Hawaii.

verruca (vĕ-roo′kah), pl. *verru′cae* [L.] 1. an epidermal tumor caused by a papillomavirus; the term is also loosely applied to any of various benign, epidermal proliferations of nonviral etiology, as verruca senilis (seborrheic keratosis). Called also *wart,* or *common wart.* 2. one of the wartlike elevations developing on the endocardium in various types of endocarditis. **v. acumina′ta,** condyloma acuminatum. **v. digita′ta,** a wart with finger-like excrescences growing from its surface. **v. filifor′mis,** a wart with soft, thin, threadlike projections on its surface. **v. gla′-bra** (*obs.*), a wart with a smooth surface. **v. necrogen′ica,** tuberculosis verrucosa. **v. perua′na, v. peruvia′na,** verruga peruana. **v. pla′na, v. pla′na juveni′lis,** a small, smooth, usually skin colored or light brown, slightly raised wart sometimes occurring in great numbers, on the face, neck, back of the hands, wrists, and knees; seen most frequently in children but also in adults. Called also *flat wart.* See also *epidermodysplasia verruciformis.* **v. planta′ris,** plantar wart: a viral epidermal tumor on the sole. **v. seborrhe′ica,** seborrheic keratosis. **v. seni′lis,** seborrheic keratosis. **v. vulga′ris,** former name for *verruca,* or *common wart.*

verrucae (vĕ-roo′se) [L.] plural of *verruca.*

verruciform (vĕ-roo′sĭ-form) [L. *verruca* wart + *forma* form] resembling or shaped like a verruca, or wart.

verrucose (ver'oo-kōs) [L. *verrucosus*] verrucous.

verrucosis (ver"oo-ko'sis) a condition marked by the presence of multiple warts, or verrucae.

verrucous (ver'oo-kus) rough; warty.

verruga (vĕ-roo'gah) [Sp.] verruca. **v. perua'na,** one of the characteristic hemangioma-like tumors or nodules which are sometimes the first manifestations of Carrión's disease (bartonellosis).

Versapen (ver'sah-pen) trademark for preparations of hetacillin.

versicolor (ver-sik'o-lor) [L. *vertere* to turn + *color* color] variegated; changing color.

version (ver-zhun) [L. *versio*] change of direction. In obstetrics, change of the polarity of the fetus with reference to the body of the mother, in order to convert an abnormal or relatively abnormal relation into a normal or relatively normal relation. **abdominal v.,** external v. **bimanual v.,** version done by combined external and internal manipulation, the cervix being open enough to admit the hand; called also *combined v.* **bipolar v.,** version done by purely external manipulation or by combined internal and external manipulation. **cephalic v.,** version in which the fetal head is brought down into the maternal pelvis. **combined v.,** bimanual v. **Denman's spontaneous v.,** see under *evolution.* **external v.,** manipulation of the fetal body applied through the abdominal wall of the mother. **internal v.,** turning of the fetus effected by the hand or fingers inserted through the dilated cervix. **pelvic v.,** version done by manipulating the buttocks of the fetus. **podalic v.,** version in which one or both legs of the fetus are brought down into the maternal pelvis. **Potter v.,** podalic version in head presentation when the cervix is fully effaced and dilated. **spontaneous v.,** conversion of an abnormal position of the fetus into a normal or relatively normal one, occurring without the aid of manipulation. **Wigand's v.,** external conversion of a transverse lie into a cephalic presentation, accomplished by pushing the fetal head down with one hand and its buttocks up with the other; called also *Wigand's maneuver.*

vertebra (ver'tĕ-brah), pl. *ver'tebrae* [L.] any of the thirty-three bones of the spinal column (columna vertebralis), comprising the seven *cervical,* twelve *thoracic,* five *lumbar,* five *sacral,* and four *coccygeal* vertebrae. **abdominal vertebrae,** vertebrae lumbales. **basilar v.,** the lowest or last of the lumbar vertebrae. **caudal vertebrae, caudate vertebrae,** vertebrae coccygeae. **cervical vertebrae, ver'tebrae cervica'les** [NA], the upper seven vertebrae, constituting the skeleton of the neck. **ver'tebrae coccyg'eae** [NA], **coccygeal vertebrae,** the lowest segments of the vertebral column, comprising three to five rudimentary vertebrae which form the coccyx. **ver'tebrae col'li,** vertebrae cervicales. **cranial v.,** the segments of the skull and facial bones, by some regarded as modified vertebrae. **v. denta'ta,** the second cervical vertebra (axis [NA]). **dorsal vertebrae,** vertebrae thoracicae. **false vertebrae,** the vertebrae that become fused, i.e., the sacral and coccygeal vertebrae. **ver'tebrae lumba'les** [NA], **lumbar vertebrae,** the five vertebrae between the thoracic vertebrae and the sacrum. **v. mag'num,** os sacrum. **odontoid v.,** the second cervical vertebra (axis [NA]). **v. pla'na,** a condition of spondylitis in which the body of the vertebra is reduced to a sclerotic disk; often due to eosinophilic granuloma. **v. prom'inens** [NA], **prominent v.,** the seventh cervical vertebra; so called because of the length of its spinous process. **sacral vertebrae, ver'tebrae sacra'les** [NA], the vertebrae below the lumbar vertebrae (usually five in number), which normally fuse to form the sacrum. **sternal v.,** sternebra. **terminal v., great,** os sacrum. **ver'tebrae thoraca'les, thoracic vertebrae,** vertebrae thoracicae. **ver'tebrae thora'cicae** [NA], thoracic vertebrae: the vertebrae, usually twelve in number, situated between

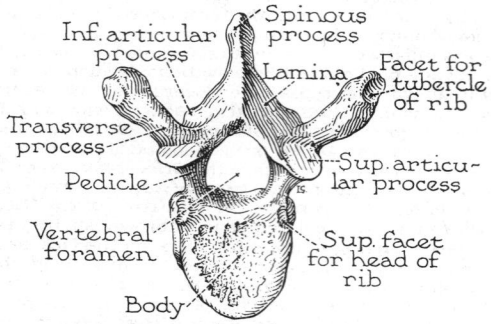

Typical (sixth) thoracic vertebra viewed from above (King & Showers).

the cervical and the lumbar vertebrae, giving attachment to the ribs and forming part of the posterior wall of the thorax; called also *vertebrae thoracales.* **tricuspid v.,** the sixth cervical vertebra

of quadrupeds. **true vertebrae,** the vertebrae that normally remain unfused throughout life, i.e., the cervical, thoracic, and lumbar vertebrae.

vertebrae (ver'tĕ-bre) [L.] plural of *vertebra.*

vertebral (ver'te-bral) [L. *vertebralis*] of or pertaining to a vertebra.

vertebrarium (ver"tĕ-bra're-um) [L.] the vertebral column.

vertebrarterial (ver"tĕ-brar-te're-al) pertaining to the vertebral artery.

Vertebrata (ver"tĕ-bra'tah) a subphylum of the Chordata comprising all animals that have a vertebral column, including mammals, birds, reptiles, amphibians, and fishes.

vertebrate (ver'tĕ-brāt) [L. *vertebratus*] 1. having a vertebral column. 2. an animal having a vertebral column; any member of the Vertebrata.

vertebrated (ver'tĕ-brāt"ed) made up of joints resembling the vertebrae.

vertebrectomy (ver"tĕ-brek'to-me) [*vertebro-* + Gr. *ektomē* excision] excision of a vertebra.

vertebro- [L. *vertebra,* from *vertere* to turn] a combining form denoting relationship to a vertebra, or to the vertebral column.

vertebroarterial (ver"tĕ-bro-ar-te're-al) vertebrarterial.

vertebrobasilar (ver"tĕ-bro-bas'ĭ-lar) pertaining to or involving the vertebral and basilar arteries.

vertebrochondral (ver"tĕ-bro-kon'dral) pertaining to a vertebra and a costal cartilage.

vertebrocostal (ver"tĕ-bro-kos'tal) [*vertebro-* + L. *costa* rib] pertaining to a vertebra and a rib.

vertebrodidymus (ver"tĕ-bro-did'ĭ-mus) [*vertebro-* + Gr. *didymos* twin] a twin monster united in the region of the spinal column.

vertebrodymus (ver"tĕ-brod'ĭ-mus) vertebrodidymus.

vertebrofemoral (ver"tĕ-bro-fem'or-al) relating to the vertebrae and the femur.

vertebrogenic (ver"tĕ-bro-jen'ik) arising in a vertebra or in the vertebral column.

vertebroiliac (ver"tĕ-bro-il'e-ak) pertaining to the vertebrae and the ilium.

vertebromammary (ver"tĕ-bro-mam'er-e) pertaining to or extending between the vertebral column and the pectoral region.

vertebrosacral (ver"tĕ-bro-sa'kral) pertaining to the vertebrae and the sacrum.

vertebrosternal (ver"tĕ-bro-ster'nal) pertaining to the vertebrae and the sternum.

vertex (ver'teks), pl. *ver'tices* [L.] a summit or top; used as a general term in anatomical nomenclature. Sometimes used alone to designate the top of the head (*vertex cranii*). **v. of bony cranium,** v. cranii ossei. **v. cor'dis,** vortex cordis. **v. of cornea, v. cor'neae** [NA], the central, thinner portion of the cornea. **v. cra'nii** [NA], the top or crown of the head. **v. cra'nii os'sei** [NA], vertex of bony cranium: the highest point of the skull; although its position varies somewhat in different skulls, it is generally located on the sagittal suture, usually near the midpoint of the suture. **v. of urinary bladder, v. vesi'cae urina'riae,** apex vesicae urinariae.

vertical (ver-tĭ-kal) 1. perpendicular to the plane of the horizon. 2. relating to the vertex.

verticalis (ver"tĭ-ka'lis) [L.] vertical, or perpendicular to the plane of the horizon; [NA] a general term used in reference to structures with the body in the anatomical, that is, upright, position.

verticillate (ver-tis'ĭ-lāt) [L. *vertex* a whorl] arranged in the form of a whorl.

Verticillium (ver"tĭ-sil'e-um) a genus of imperfect fungi of the order Moniliales, family Moniliaceae, some species of which cause apple wilt. **V. gra'phii,** a species of uncertain identity, which is considered by some to be a species of *Trichosporon,* sometimes reported in otitis externa and mycotic keratitis.

verticine (ver'tĭ-sin) a crystalline alkaloid, $C_{27}H_{45}NO_3$, from *Fritillaria verticillata* Willd. (Liliaceae), a bulbous herb.

verticomental (ver"tĭ-ko-men'tal) pertaining to the vertex and the chin.

vertiginous (ver-tij'ĭ-nus) [L. *vertiginosus*] pertaining to or affected with vertigo.

vertigo (ver'tĭ-go, ver-ti'go) [L. *vertigo*] an illusion of movement; a sensation as if the external world were revolving around the patient (*objective vertigo*) or as if he himself were revolving in space (*subjective vertigo*). The term is sometimes erroneously used to mean any form of dizziness. Vertigo may result from diseases of the inner ear or may be due to disturbances of the vestibular centers or pathways in the central nervous system. **v. ab au're lae'so,** Meniere's disease. **v. ab stom'acho lae'so,** stomachal v. **alternobaric v.,** a transient, true, whirling vertigo sometimes affecting those (caisson workers, air crew members, etc.) subjected to large, rapid variations in barometric pressure; called also *pressure v.* **angiopathic v.,** vertigo due to arteriosclerosis of the cerebral vessels. **apoplectic v.,** scotodinia. **arteriosclerotic v.,** angiopathic v. **auditory v., aural v.,** Meniere's disease. **benign paroxysmal positional (or postural) v.,** recurrent vertigo and nystagmus occurring when the head is placed in certain positions, usually not associated with lesions of the central nervous system. **cardiac v.,** vertigo due to some chronic disease of the heart. **cardiovascular v.,** vertigo due to sclerosis of the blood vessels and heart. **central v.,** vertigo due to disease of the central nervous system. **cerebral v.,** that which is due to some brain disease. **encephalic v.,** a sensation of movement of tissues within the skull, as of the brain turning over and over, or round and round. **endemic paralytic v.,** Gerlier's disease. **epidemic v.,** an epidemic condition characterized chiefly by vertigo but with some nausea and vomiting. See *epidemic nausea,* under *nausea.* Cf. *nausea epidemica.* **epileptic v.,** that which attends or follows an epileptic attack. **essential v.,** a vertigo, often severe, but of no discoverable cause; probably due to some disease or lesion in a brain center. **galvanic v.,** voltanic v. **gastric v.,** a form associated with disease or disorder of the stomach. **height v.,** dizziness (not a true vertigo) felt on looking down from a high location. **horizontal v.,** that which comes on when a person lies down. **hysterical v.,** vertigo associated with hysterical symptoms, often of a bizarre form. **labyrinthine v.,** a form associated with disease of the labyrinth of the ear. See *Meniere's disease,* under *disease.* **laryngeal v.,** tussive syncope. **lateral v.,** that which is caused by rapidly passing a row of similar objects, as a fence or series of pillars. **lithemic v.,** that which is associated with gout and lithemia. **mechanical v.,** vertigo due to long-continued turning or vibration of the body, as in seasickness. **neurasthenic v.,** a subjective form of vertiginous sensation associated with neurasthenia. **nocturnal v.,** a sensation of falling occurring as the subject is going to sleep. **objective v.,** a form in which the objects seen by the patient seem to be moving around him. **ocular v.,** a form due to eye disease, especially to paralysis of or lack of balance in the eye muscles. **organic v.,** vertigo due to vestibular brain disease or to tabes dorsalis. **paralyzing v.,** Gerlier's disease. **peripheral v.,** vestibular v. **pilot's v.,** spatial disorientation. **positional v.,** postural v. **postural v.,** vertigo associated with a specific position of the head in space or changes in the position of the head in space; called also *positional v.* **pressure v.,** alternobaric v. **primary v.,** vertigo resulting from a stimulus, e.g., an active disease process, within the vestibular system of the ear, and independent of body movement. **residual v.,** vertigo associated with motion, resulting from hypofunction or absence of vestibular sensory or neural elements; when it occurs only in one plane of movement, it is called *postural v.* **riders' v.,** motion sickness. **rotary v., rotatory v.,** vertigo in which there is a definite feeling of rotation. **sham-movement v.,** vertigo attended by a sensation as if objects were circling around the body. **special sense v.,** aural (Meniere's disease) or ocular v. **stomachal v.,** vertigo associated with a disorder of the digestive system. **subjective v.,** that in which the patient seems to himself to be turning round and round. **systematic v.,** rotary v. **tenebric v.,** scotodinia. **toxemic v., toxic v.,** a form of vertigo which results from poisoning, alcoholism, uremia, or lithemia. **vertical v.,** that which is caused by looking up or down at a distant object. **vestibular v.,** vertigo due to disturbances of the vestibular centers or pathways in the central nervous system; called also *peripheral v.* **villous v.,** that which is caused by a functional derangement of the liver. **voltaic v.,** an inclination of the head toward the shoulder on the side of the positive pole when a galvanic current is applied to the vestibular fibers of the eighth nerve.

vertigraphy (ver-tig′rah-fe) [L. *vertigo* a whirling + Gr. *graphein* to write] see *body section roentgenography,* under *roentgenography.*

verumontanitis (ve″ru-mon″tah-ni′tis) inflammation of the verumontanum (colliculus seminalis).

verumontanum (ve″ru-mon-ta′num) [L. "mountain ridge"] colliculus seminalis.

vesalian (ve-sa′le-an) named in honor of Andreas *Vesalius,* as the vesalian bone (os vesalianum) or vein.

vesalianum (ve-sa″le-a′num) [Andreas *Vesalius*] a name applied to several sesamoid bones: one on the outer border of the foot between the cuboid and fifth metatarsal bone, and one (sometimes more) in the tendon of origin of the gastrocnemius muscle.

Vesalius (ve-sa′le-us), Andreas (1514–1564) a Flemish anatomist and physician, the most eminent anatomist of the 16th century. His great work on anatomy (1543), entitled *De humani corporis fabrica libri septem* (Seven Books on the Structure of the Human Body), is said to be "one of the most remarkable known to science," and "one of the most noble and magnificent volumes in the history of printing" (Saunders & O'Malley). See also under *foramen* and *ligament.*

vesania (ve-sa′ne-ah) [L.] an old term for full-fledged mental disorder, marked by the four stages of mania, melancholia, paranoia, and dementia. Cf. *vecordia.*

vesanic (ve-san′ik) pertaining to or exhibiting vesania.

Vesic. abbreviation for L. *vesic′ula, vesicato′rium,* a blister.

vesica (ve̅-si′kah), pl. *vesi′cae* [L.] a membranous sac or receptacle for a secretion; [NA] a general term for such a structure. Called also *bladder.* **v. fel′lea** [NA], the gallbladder: the pear-shaped reservoir for the bile on the posteroinferior surface of the liver between the right and quadrate lobes. **v. prostat′ica,** utriculus prostaticus. **v. urina′ria** [NA], urinary bladder: the musculomembranous sac, situated in the anterior part of the pelvic cavity, that serves as a reservoir for urine; it receives the excretory products of the kidneys through the ureters, and expels them through the urethra.

vesicae (ve-si′se) [L.] plural of *vesica.*

vesical (ves′ĭ-kal) pertaining to the bladder.

vesicant (ves′ĭ-kant) [L. *vesica* blister] 1. causing blisters; blistering. 2. a blistering drug or agent.

vesication (ves″ĭ-ka′shun) 1. the process of blistering. 2. a blistered spot or surface.

vesicatory (ves′ĭ-kah-tor″e) [L. *vesicare* to blister] vesicant.

vesicle (ves′ĭ-k'l) [L. *vesicula,* dim. of *vesica* bladder] 1. a small bladder or sac containing liquid; see also *vesicula.* 2. a small (less than 1 cm. in diameter) blister; a small circumscribed elevation of the epidermis containing a serous liquid. Cf. *bulla* and *bleb.* 3. the swollen end of a conidiophore from which sterigmata are produced. **acoustic v.,** auditory v. **acrosomal v.,** a membrane-bounded vacuole-like structure containing the enlarging acrosomal granule, which undergoes collapse and spreads over the upper two thirds of the head (acrosome) of a spermatozoon to form a head cap. **allantoic v.,** see under *diverticulum.* **amniocardiac v's,** fissures in the mesoderm of the early embryo representing the paired primordia of the pericardial sac and the heart. **archoplasmic v.,** a sac developed from the attraction sphere of a spermatid and growing into the sheath of the tail of the spermatozoon. **Ascherson's v's,** small vesicles formed by shaking together oil and liquid albumin; they consist of drops of oil enclosed in a layer of albumin. **auditory v.,** a detached ovoid sac formed by closure of the auditory pit, in embryonic development of the internal ear. **Baer's v.,** the vesicular ovarian follicle (graafian follicle) of the ovary with its contained ovum. **blastodermic v.,** the blastocyst. **brain v's,** the five divisions of the closed neural tube in the developing embryo, including, in craniocaudal sequence, the telencephalon, diencephalon, mesencephalon, metencephalon, and myelencephalon. **brain v's, primary,** the three earliest subdivisions of the embryonic neural tube, including the prosencephalon, mesencephalon, and rhombencephalon. **brain v's, secondary,** the four brain vesicles formed by specialization of the prosencelphalon (the telencephalon and diencephalon) and of the rhombencephalon (the metencephalon and myelencephalon) in later embryonic development. **cephalic v's, cerebral v's,** brain v's. **cervical v.,** a temporary sac in the cervical region of the embryo formed by the closing off of the cervical sinus. **chorionic v.,** the mammalian chorion. **compound v.,** multilocular v. **concentrating v's,** condensing vacuoles. **encephalic v's,** brain v's. **germinal v.,** the fluid-filled nucleus of an oocyte toward the end of prophase of its meiotic division. **graafian v's,** folliculi ovarici vesiculosi. **intermediate v's,** transfer v's. **kerionic v.,** multilocular v. **lens v.,** a vesicle formed from the lens pit of the embryo and developing into the crystalline lens; called also *lens sac.* **Malpighi's v's,** alveoli pulmonis. **matrix v's,** small membrane-limited structures at sites of calcification of the cartilage matrix. **multilocular v.,** a vesicle having multiple chambers or compartments, usually by reason of intraepidermal origin, as from spongiosis, rather than of subepidermal origin; called also *compound v.* and *kerionic v.* **Naboth's v's,** nabothian follicles. **ocular v.,** vesicula ophthalmica. **olfactory v.,** 1. the vesicle in the embryo which later develops into the olfactory bulb and tract. 2. a bulbous expansion at the distal end of an olfactory cell, from which the olfactory hairs project. **ophthalmic v., optic v.,** vesicula ophthalmica. **otic v.,** auditory v. **phagocytotic v.,** phagosome. **pinocytotic v.,** pinosome. **pituitary v.,** Rathke's pouch. **plasmalemmal v.,** caveola. **prostatic v.,** utriculus prostaticus. **Purkinje's v.,** germinal v. **secretory v's,** condensing vacuoles. **seminal v.,** vesicula seminalis. **sense v.,** the vesicular primordium of a sense organ in the embryo. **simple v.,** a vesicle on the skin having a single chamber or compartment. **spermatic v., false,** utriculus prostaticus. **synaptic v's,** a profusion of small round structures in the end-feet of neurons, believed to contain protein-bound humoral transmitter substance. **transfer v's, transitional v's, transport v's,** small vesicles formed by budding off the granular endoplasmic reticulum, in which secretory material is transferred to the Golgi complex, where it is concentrated in condensing vacuoles (q.v.). Called also *intermediate v's.* **umbilical v.,** the pear-shaped expansion of the yolk sac growing out into the cavity of the chorion at the end of the fourth week of development, and joined to the midgut of the embryo by the yolk stalk. **Unna's v.** (obs.), the teardrop vesicle, containing a clear serum, which is characteristic of chickenpox and herpes zoster.

vesico- [L. *vesica* bladder] a combining form denoting relationship to the bladder, or to a blister.

vesicoabdominal (ves″ĭ-ko-ab-dom′ĭ-nal) pertaining to the urinary bladder and abdomen, or communicating with the bladder and an abdominal viscus, as a vesicoabdominal fistula.

vesicocavernous (ves″ĭ-ko-kav′er-nus) both vesicular and cavernous.

vesicocele (ves′ĭ-ko-sēl″) [*vesico-* + Gr. *kēlē* hernia] hernial protrusion of the bladder.

vesicocervical (ves″ĭ-ko-ser′vĭ-kal) [*vesico-* + L. *cervix* neck] pertaining to the urinary bladder and the cervix uteri, or communicating with the bladder and the cervical canal, as a vesicocervical fistula.

vesicoclysis (ves″ĭ-kok′lĭ-sis) [*vesico-* + Gr. *klysis* washing] the injection of a fluid into the urinary bladder.

vesicocolic (ves″ĭ-ko-kol′ik) vesicocolonic.

vesicocolonic (ves″ĭ-ko-ko-lon′ik) pertaining to or communicating with the urinary bladder and colon, as a vesicocolonic fistula. Called also *vesicocolic*.

vesicoenteric (ves″ĭ-ko-en-ter′ik) vesicointestinal.

vesicofixation (ves″ĭ-ko-fiks-a′shun) 1. the stitching of the uterus to the urinary bladder. 2. the surgical fixation of the urinary bladder; cystopexy.

vesicointestinal (ves″ĭ-ko-in-tes′tĭ-nal) pertaining to or communicating with the urinary bladder and intestine, as a vesicointestinal fistula.

vesicoperineal (ves″ĭ-ko-per′ĭ-ne′al) pertaining to or communicating with the urinary bladder and perineum, as a vesicoperineal fistula.

vesicoprostatic (ves″ĭ-ko-pros-tat′ik) pertaining to the urinary bladder and the prostate.

vesicopubic (ves″ĭ-ko-pu′bik) pertaining to the urinary bladder and the pubes.

vesicopustule (ves″ĭ-ko-pus′tūl) a vesicle which is developing into a pustule by entry of leukocytes into its contents.

vesicorectal (ves″ĭ-ko-rek′tal) pertaining to the urinary bladder and the rectum.

vesicorenal (ves″ĭ-ko-re′nal) pertaining to the urinary bladder and the kidney.

vesicosigmoid (ves″ĭ-ko-sig′moid) pertaining to the urinary bladder and sigmoid flexure.

vesicosigmoidostomy (ves″ĭ-ko-sig″moi-dos′to-me) [L. *vesica* bladder + *sigmoid* + Gr. *stomoun* to provide with an opening or mouth] the operation of making a permanent communication between the urinary bladder and sigmoid flexure.

vesicospinal (ves″ĭ-ko-spi′nal) pertaining to the urinary bladder and the spine.

vesicostomy (ves″ĭ-kos′to-me) the formation of an opening into the bladder; cystostomy. **cutaneous v.,** surgical anastomosis of the bladder mucosa to an opening in the skin below tne umbilicus, creating a stoma for bladder drainage.

vesicotomy (ves″ĭ-kot′o-me) [L. *vesica* bladder + Gr. *tomē* a cutting] incision of the urinary bladder; cystotomy.

vesicoumbilical (ves″ĭ-ko-um-bil′ĭ-kal) pertaining to the umbilicus and the urinary bladder.

vesicourachal (ves″ĭ-ko-u′rah-kal) pertaining to the urinary bladder and the urachus.

vesicoureteral, vesicoureteric (ves″ĭ-ko-u-re′ter-al; ves″ĭ-ko-u″rĕ-ter′ik) pertaining to or communicating with the urinary bladder and the ureter.

vesicourethral (ves″ĭ-ko-u-re′thral) pertaining to or communicating with the urinary bladder and the urethra.

vesicouterine (ves″ĭ-ko-u′ter-īn) pertaining to or communicating with the urinary bladder and the uterus.

vesicouterovaginal (ves″ĭ-ko-u″ter-o-vaj′ĭ-nal) pertaining to or communicating with the urinary bladder, uterus, and vagina.

vesicovaginal (ves″ĭ-ko-vaj′ĭ-nal) pertaining to or communicating with the urinary bladder and vagina.

vesicovaginorectal (ves″ĭ-ko-vaj″ĭ-no-rek′tal) pertaining to or communicating with the urinary bladder, vagina, and rectum.

vesicula (vĕ-sik′u-lah) pl. *vesic′ulae* [L., dim. of *vesica*] a vesicle: a small bladder or sac containing liquid; used as a general term in anatomical nomenclature. **v. bi′lis, v. fel′lea,** vesica felea. **v. germinati′va,** germinal vesicle. **vesic′ulae graafia′nae,** folliculi ovarici vesiculosi. **vesic′ulae nabo′thi,** Naboth's follicles. **v. ophthal′mica** [NA], optic vesicle: an evagination developing on either side of the forebrain of the early embryo, from which the percipient parts of the eye are formed. **v. prostat′ica,** utriculus prostaticus. **v. semina′lis** [NA], seminal vesicle: either of the paired, sacculated pouches attached to the posterior part of the urinary bladder; the duct of each joins the ipsilateral ductus deferens to form the ejaculatory duct. **v. sero′sa,** chorion.

vesiculae (vĕ-sik′u-le) [L.] plural of *vesicula*.

vesicular (vĕ-sik′u-lar) [L. *vesicula* a little bladder] 1. composed of or relating to small, saclike bodies. 2. pertaining to or made up of vesicles on the skin.

vesiculase (vĕ-sik′u-lās) a ferment from the prostate gland which coagulates semen.

vesiculated (vĕ-sik′u-lāt″ed) marked by the presence of vesicles.

vesiculation (vĕ-sik′u-la′shun) the presence or formation of vesicles.

vesiculectomy (vĕ-sik″u-lek′to-me) [*vesicle* + Gr. *ektomē* excision] excision of a vesicle, especially the seminal vesicle.

vesiculiform (vĕ-sik′u-lĭ-form″) [*vesicle* + L. *forma* form] shaped like a vesicle.

vesiculitis (vĕ-sik″u-li′tis) inflammation of a vesicle, especially of a seminal vesicle. **seminal v.,** inflammation of a seminal vesicle.

vesiculobronchial (vĕ-sik″u-lo-brong′ke-al) both vesicular and bronchial; bronchovesicular.

vesiculocavernous (vĕ-sik″u-lo-kav′er-nus) both vesicular and cavernous.

vesiculogram (vĕ-sik′u-lo-gram″) a roentgenogram of the seminal vesicles.

vesiculography (vĕ-sik″u-log′rah-fe) roentgenography of the seminal vesicles.

vesiculopapular (vĕ-sik″u-lo-pap′u-lar) pertaining to or characterized by vesicles and papules.

vesiculopustular (vĕ-sik″u-lo-pus′tu-lar) consisting of or pertaining to vesicles and pustules.

vesiculotomy (vĕ-sik″u-lot′o-me) [*vesicle* + Gr. *tomē* a cutting] incision of a vesicle. **seminal v.,** the operation of exposing and opening the seminal vesicles.

vesiculotubular (vĕ-sik″u-lo-tu′bu-lar) having both a vesicular and a tubular quality; said of auscultatory sounds.

vesiculotympanic (ve-sik″u-lo-tim-pan′ik) having both a vesicular and tympanic quality; said of percussion sounds.

vesperal (ves′per-al) [L. *vespera* evening] pertaining to or occurring in the evening.

Vesprin (ves′prin) trademark for preparations of triflupromazine.

vessel (ves′el) any channel for carrying a fluid, such as the blood or lymph, see also *vas*. **absorbent v's,** lymphatic vessels. **afferent v. of glomerulus,** vas afferens glomeruli. **afferent v's of lymph node,** vasa afferentia nodi lymphatici. **anastomotic v.,** vas anastomoticum. **arterioluminal v's,** small branches of coronary arterioles that lie near the endocardium, and after a short course open directly into the lumen of the heart. **arteriosinusoidal v's,** small branches of coronary arterioles that soon break up into sinusoids that lie between bundles or individual muscle fibers of the heart. **bile v.,** one of the vessels in the liver which conduct bile; called also *ductuli biliferi* [NA]. **blood v.,** any of the vessels conveying the blood, and comprising the arteries, arterioles, capillaries, venules, and veins. **chyliferous v's,** lacteal v's. **collateral v.,** 1. a vessel that parallels another vessel, nerve, or other structure (vas collaterale [NA]). 2. a vessel important in establishing and maintaining a collateral circulation; see under *circulation*. **efferent v. of glomerulus,** vas efferens glomeruli. **efferent v's of lymph node,** vasa efferentia nodi lymphatici. **great v's,** the large vessels entering the heart, including the aorta, the pulmonary arteries and veins, and the venae cavae. **hemorrhoidal v's,** veins of the rectum which have become dilated and swollen; see *hemorrhoid*. **Jungbluth's v's,** vasa propria of Jungbluth. **lacteal v's,** any of the intestinal lymphatic vessels that transport chyle (q.v.); so called because during absorption they are white from absorbed fat. Called also *chyliferous v's* and *lacteals*. **lymphatic v's,** the capillaries, collecting vessels, and trunks that collect lymph from the tissues and carry it to the blood stream; called also *vasa lymphatica* [NA]. **lymphatic v's, deep,** vasa lymphatica profunda. **lymphatic v's, superficial,** vasa lymphatica superficialia. **nutrient v's,** vessels that supply nutritive elements to special tissues, such as arteries entering the substance of bone, or supplying walls of the blood vessels themselves.

vessicnon, vessignon (ves′ik-non, ves″ēn-yaw) [Fr.] windgall.

vestibula (ves-tib′u-lah) [L.] plural of *vestibulum*.

vestibular (ves-tib′u-lar) pertaining to a vestibule.

vestibule (ves′tĭ-būl) a space or cavity at the entrance to a canal; called also *vestibulum* [NA]. **v. of aorta,** a space within the left ventricle at the root of the aorta. **buccal v.,** that portion of the vestibule of the mouth which lies between the cheeks and the teeth and gingivae, or the residual alveolar ridges. **v. of ear,** an oval cavity in the middle of the bony larynth; see *vestibulum auris* [NA]. **Gibson's v.,** v. of aorta. **labial v.,** that portion of the vestibule of the mouth which lies between the lips and the teeth and gingivae, or residual alveolar ridges. **v. of larynx,** vestibulum laryngis. **v. of mouth,** that portion of the oral cavity bounded on the one side by the teeth and gingivae, or the residual alveolar ridges, and on the other side by the lips (*labial v.*) and cheeks (*buccal v.*); called also *vestibulum oris*

[NA]. **v. of nose,** vestibulum nasi. **v. of omental bursa,** vestibulum bursae omentalis. **v. of pharynx,** 1. fauces. 2. oropharynx. **Sibson's v.,** v. of aorta. **v. of vagina, v. of vulva,** vestibulum vaginae.

vestibulogenic (ves-tib″u-lo-jen′ik)   arising in a vestibule, as that of the ear.

vestibulo-ocular (ves-tib″u-lo-ok′u-lar)   pertaining to the vestibular and oculomotor nerves; or to the maintenance of visual stability during head movements.

vestibuloplasty (ves-tib′u-lo-plas″te)   the surgical modification of the gingival–mucous membrane relationships in the vestibule of the mouth, including deepening of the vestibular trough, repositioning of the frenum or muscle attachments, and broadening of the zone of attached gingiva, after periodontal treatment.

vestibulotomy (ves-tib″u-lot′o-me) [*vestibule* + Gr. *tomē* a cutting]   surgical opening of the vestibule of the inner ear.

vestibulourethral (ves-tib″u-lc-u-re′thral)   pertaining to the vestibulum vaginae and to the urethra.

vestibulum (ves-tib′u-lum), pl. *vestib′ula* [L.]   a vestibule: a space or cavity at the entrance to a canal; [NA] a general term for such a structure. **v. au′ris** [NA], vestibule of ear: an oval cavity in the middle of the bony labyrinth, communicating anteriorly with the cochlea and posteriorly with the semicircular canals, and containing the sacculus and utriculus. **v. bur′sae omenta′lis** [NA], vestibule of omental bursa: that part of the omental bursa dorsal to the lesser omentum and adjacent to the epiploic foramen. **v. glot′tidis,** v. laryngis. **v. laryn′gis** [NA], vestibule of larynx: the portion of the laryngeal cavity above the vestibular folds. **v. na′si** [NA], vestibule of nose: the anterior part of the nasal cavity situated just inferior to the nares and limited posteriorly by the limen nasi. **v. o′ris** [NA], the part of the oral cavity exterior to the teeth; see *vestibule of mouth*. **v. vagi′nae** [NA], vestibule of vagina: the space between the labia minora into which the urethra and vagina open.

vestige (ves′tij)   the remnant of a structure which functioned in a previous stage of species or individual development; called also *vestigium*. **coccygeal v.,** the remnant of the caudal end of the neural tube. **v. of vaginal process,** vestigium processus vaginalis.

vestigia (ves-tij′e-ah) [L.]   plural of *vestigium*.

vestigial (ves-tij′e-al)   of the nature of a vestige, trace, or relic; rudimentary.

vestigium (ves-tij′e-um), pl. *vestig′ia* [L. "a trace"]   a vestige: the remnant of a structure which functioned in a previous stage of species or individual development; used in NA to designate the degenerating remains of any structure which served as a functioning entity in the embryo or fetus. **v. proces′sus vagina′lis** [NA], vestige of vaginal process: a band of connective tissue in the spermatic cord which is that vestige of the processus vaginalis; called also *rudimentum processus vaginalis*.

vesuvin (ve-su′vin)   aniline brown.

veta (va′tah) [Sp.]   mountain sickness of the Andes; see under *sickness*.

veterinarian (vet″er-ĭ-nār′e-an)   a person trained and authorized to practice veterinary medicine and surgery; a doctor of veterinary medicine.

veterinary (vet′er-ĭ-ner″e) [L. *veterinarius*]   pertaining to domestic animals and their diseases.

V.F.   vocal fremitus.

V.f.   field of vision.

VIA   virus inactivating agent; see under *agent*.

via (vi′ah), pl. *vi′ae* [L.]   a way or passage. **vi′ae natura′les,** the natural passages of the body. **pri′mae vi′ae,** canalis alimentarius.

viability (vi″ah-bil′ĭ-te)   ability to live after birth.

viable (vi′ah-b'l)   capable of living; especially said of a fetus that has reached such a stage of development that it can live outside of the uterus.

Viadril (vi′ah-dril)   trademark for a preparation of hydroxydione sodium.

viae (vi′e) [L.]   plural of *via*.

vial (vi′al) [Gr. *phialē*]   a small bottle.

vibesate (vi′bĕ-sāt)   a modified polyvinyl plastic applied topically as a spray, to form an occlusive dressing for surgical wounds and other surface lesions.

vibex (vi′beks), pl. *vibi′ces* [L. *vibix* mark of a blow]   a narrow linear mark or streak; a linear subcutaneous effusion of blood.

vibices (vĭ-bi′sēz) [L.]   plural of *vibex*.

Vibramycin (vi-brah-mi′sin)   trademark for a preparation of doxycycline.

vibratile (vi′brah-tīl) [L. *vibratilis*]   having an oscillatory motion; swaying or moving to and fro.

vibration (vi-bra′shun) [L. *vibratio*, form *vibrare* to shake]   1. a rapid movement to and fro; oscillation. 2. the shaking of the body as a therapeutic measure. 3. a form of massage. **photoelectric v.,** a change in the position of the visual cells, and a series of photoelectric movements in the rods and cones under the influence of light.

vibrative (vib′rah-tiv)   a conconantal sound like that or *r*, produced by so forcing the breath that the margins of a narrow portion of the respiratory canal are made to vibrate, the nasal cavity being shut off.

vibratode (vi′brah-tōd)   the instrument or appliance at the end of a vibratory appliance by which the vibrations are applied to the body.

vibrator (vi′bra-tor)   an instrument used in the mechanical treatment of disease.

vibratory (vi′brah-tor″e) [L. *vibratorius*]   vibrating or causing vibration.

Vibrio (vib′re-o)   a genus of microorganisms of the family Spirallaceae, suborder Pseudomonadineae, order Pseudomonadales, made up of short, slighly curved, actively motile gram-negative rods, occurring singly and occasionally found end-to-end. The 34 species described include the cholera and El Tor vibrios pathogenic for man, agents of specific disease in lower animals, and paracholera or cholera-like water vibrios (nonagglutinating, or NAG, vibrios). See also *vibrio*. **V. chol′erae, V. chol′eraeasiat′icae,** the etiologic agent of Asiatic cholera in man; characterized as nonhemolytic (Greig test) and the somatic antigen of vibrio O group I. It may occur in one of three serological types, the distribution of which has no epidemiological significance. Called also *V. comma*. **V. co′li,** the etiologic agent of swine dysentery. **V. com′ma,** V. cholerae. **V. danu′bicus,** see *paracholera vibrios*. **V. el′tor,** 1. a biotype of *V. cholerae* that may or may not be hemolytic, the etiologic agent of the seventh pandemic of cholera. 2. a member of the El Tor group of vibrios, first isolated at the El Tor Quarantine Station on the Sinai Peninsula, some strains of which are immunologically related to *V. cholerae*. **V. fe′tus,** *Campylobacter fetus*. **V. fink′leri,** *V. proteus*. **V. ghin′da,** see *paracholera vibrios*. **V. je-ju′ni,** the etiologic agent of a diarrheal disease in cows and calves. **V. leonar′dii,** a species causing disease in insects, such as the wax moth and the European corn borer. **V. massau′ah,** see *paracholera vibrios*. **V. mestchniko′vii,** a species morphologically and physiologically similar to the cholera vibrio, and highly pathogenic for pigeons and guinea pigs. In fowls, it produces an epidemic disease resembling fowl cholera. See *fowl septicemia*, under *septicemia*. **V. ni′ger,** an anaerobic species found frequently in man in certain pathologic conditions, such as purulent otitis, mastoiditis, or pulmonary gangrene. **V. parahaemolyt′icus,** the causative agent of a foodborne illness associated with eating contaminated raw or cooked fish, shellfish, salad, meat, and vegetables, and characterized by headache, chills, stomach pain, diarrhea, fever, and vomiting. **V. phosphores′cens,** a phosphorescent microorganism isolated from the intestinal contents of patients with cholera and other gastrointestinal infections. **V. pis′cium,** the etiologic agent of an epidemic disease of carp and other fish. **V. pro′teus,** a microorganism isolated from the feces of patients with a mild diarrheal disease. **V. sep′ticus,** *Clostridium septicum*. **V. tyrog′enus,** a curved, rod-shaped organism, somewhat smaller and more slender than *V. cholerae*, isolated from cheese.

vibrio (vib′re-o), pl. *vib′rios* or *vibrio′nes*.   An organism of the genus *Vibrio*, or other spiral motile organism. **Celebes v.,** the pathogenic El Tor biotype of *V. cholerae*, isolated in Celebes (Suluwasi); see *Vibrio eltor*, def. 1. **cholera v.,** the etiologic agent of classic (Asiatic) cholera, *Vibrio cholerae*. **El Tor v.,** see *Vibrio eltor*, def. 2. **NAG v's, nonagglutinating v's,** nonpathogenic paracholera vibrios, unrelated to the cholera vibrio O antigenic group. **paracholera v's,** microorganisms closely similar to *Vibrio cholerae*, but differing from it immunologically and having variable pathogenic properties. Many such organisms isolated from water and from the feces of individuals with mild diarrheal disease have been designated by the name of the place of their discovery, as *V. danu′bicus, V. ghin′da,* and *V. massau′ah*.

vibriocidal (vib″re-o-si′dal)   destructive to organisms of the genus *Vibrio*, especially *V. cholerae*.

vibrion (ve″bre-on′) [Fr.]   a vibrio, or spiral motile organism. **v. septique** (ve″bre-on′sep-tēk′), *Clostridium septicum*.

vibriones (vib″re-o′nēz)   plural of *vibrio*.

vibriosis (vib″re-o′sis)   infection with organisms of the genus *Vibrio*, especially infectious abortion of cattle, sheep, and goats caused by *Vibrio fetus* (it is a venereal disease of cattle and goats but is apparently spread by ingestion in sheep). A few human infections, resembling brucellosis, have been reported.

vibrissa (vi-bris′ah), pl. *vibris′sae* [L.]   a long coarse hair, such as those occurring about the nose (muzzle) of an animal, as of the dog or cat. See also *vibrissae*.

vibrissae (vi-bris′e) [L. pl. of *vibrissa*] [NA]   the hairs growing in the vestibular region of the nasal cavity.

vibrocardiogram (vi″bro-kar′de-o-gram″)   the graphic record produced by vibrocardiography.

vibrocardiography (vi″bro-kar′de-og′rah-fe)   the graphic recording of vibrations produced by the heart, usually those in the nonaudible low-frequency range.

vibrolode (vi'bro-lōd) vibratode.

vibromasseur (vib"ro-mah-sūr') [Fr.] (obs.) an instrument used in vibratory massage of the ear.

vibrometer (vi-brom'ĕ-ter) [L. *vibrare* to quiver + *metrum* measure] (obs.) a device used in the treatment of deafness due to deposits of plastic material or inspissated mucus; it acts by producing vibrations which tend to break up adhesions.

vibrophone (vib'ro-fōn) [L. *vibrare* to quiver + Gr. *phōne* sound] (obs.) an instrument similar to a vibrometer, and used for the same purpose.

vibrophonocardiograph (vi"bro-fo"no-kar'de-o-graf") an instrument for recording heart vibrations and sounds.

vibrotherapeutics (vi"bro-ther"ah-pu'tiks) [L. *vibrare* to shake + *therapeutics*] the therapeutic use of vibratory appliances.

Viburnum (vi-bur'num) [L.] a genus of caprifoliaceous trees and shrubs. **V. op'ulus**, the high bush or cranberry tree, the dried bark (cramp bark) of which has been used as an antispasmodic, uterine sedative, and antiscorbutic. **V. prunifo'lium** L., black haw, the dried bark of the root or stem of which has been used as a uterine sedative.

vicarious (vi-kar'e-us) [L. *vicarius*] acting in the place of another or of something else; occurring at an abnormal site, as vicarious menstruation.

vice (vīs) [L. *vitium*] 1. a blemish, defect, or imperfection. 2. depravity; immorality.

vicho (ve'cho) a vernacular Peruvian name for dysentery, the protrusion of the rectum being attributed to the presence of an insect (vicho).

Vicia (vish'e-ah) a genus of herbs including the vetch and broad bean. **V. fa'ba (fa'va),** a species whose beans or pollen contain a component that is capable of causing a condition known as *favism* in susceptible individuals; called also *fava*, *fava bean*, and *broad bean.*

vicianose (vīs'e-ah-nōs) a disaccharide, $C_{11}H_{20}O_{10}$, which on hydrolysis yields glucose and arabinose; obtained from the seeds of *Vicia angustifolia.*

vicilin (vi'sĭ-lin) a globulin from lentils and other legumes.

vicine (vi'sin) a white crystalline glycoside, $C_{10}H_{16}N_4O_8$, found in *Vicia sativa* and other species of vetch; it is a mononucleoside and on hydrolysis yields dextrose.

vicious (vish'us) [L. *vitio'sus*] 1. faulty or defective; malformed. 2. depraved; refractory or unruly.

Vicum album (vis'kum al'bum) European mistletoe.

Vicq d'Azyr's band, etc. (vēk dah-zērz') [Félix *Vicq d'Azyr,* French anatomist, 1748–1794] see under *band, body, fasciculus, foramen,* and *stripe.*

Vidal's disease (ve-dahlz') [Jean Baptiste Émile *Vidal,* dermatologist in Paris, 1825–1893] see *lichen chronicus simplex.*

Vidal's operation (ve-dahlz') [Auguste Théodore *Vidal* de Cassis, French surgeon, 1803–1856] see under *operation.*

vidarabine (vi-dār'ah-bēn) chemical name: 9-β-D-arabinofuranosyl-9H-purin-6-amine monohydrate. A purine analogue that inhibits DNA synthesis, $C_{10}H_{13}N_5O_4H_2O$, used as a topical antiviral agent in the treatment of herpes simplex keratitis and intravenously in the treatment of herpes simplex encephalitis. Sterile vidarabine conforms to USP specifications. Called also *adenine arabinoside* or *ara-A.*

videognosis (vid"e-og-no'sis) [*video-,* from L. *videre* to see + diagnosis] diagnosis based on the interpretation of roentgenograms transmitted by television techniques to a radiologic center.

vidian artery, canal, nerve (vid'e-an) [Guido Guidi (L. *Vidius*), Italian physician, 1500–1569] see *arteria canalis pterygoidei, canalis pterygoideus, nervus canalis pterygoidei,* and *nervus petrosus profundus.*

Vieussens' ansa, etc. (ve-uh-sahz') [Raymond de *Vieussens,* French anatomist, 1641–1715] see under *ansa, foramen, limbus, valve, vein,* and *ventricle.*

vigilambulism (vij"il-am'bu-lizm) a state resembling somnambulism, but not occurring in sleep; double or multiple personality.

vigilance (vij'ĭ-lans) [L. *vigilantia*] wakefulness; watchfulness; arousal.

vigintinormal (vi-jin"tĭ-nor'mal) [L. *viginti* twenty + *norma* rule] having one twentieth the strength of normal, as a solution.

Vignal's cells (vēn-yahlz') [Guillaume *Vignal,* French physiologist, 1852–1893] see under *cell.*

vignin (vig'nin) a protein from the cow pea.

vigor (vig'or) [L. *vigere* to flourish] a combination of attributes of living organisms which expresses itself in rapid growth, high fertility and fecundity, large size, and long life. **hybrid v.,** heterosis.

Vigouroux's sign (vēg"oo-rōōz') [Auguste *Vigouroux,* a French neurologist of the 19th century] see under *sign.*

Villard's button (ve-larz') [Eugêne *Villard,* surgeon in Lyons, born 1868] see under *button.*

Villaret's syndrome (ve-lar-āz') [Maurice *Villaret,* French neurologist, 1877–1946] see under *syndrome.*

Villarsia nymphaeoides (vil-lar"ze-ah nim"fe-oi'dēz) an old world gentianaceous plant having antiscorbutic properties.

Villemin's theory (vēl-maz') [Jean Antoine *Villemin,* French surgeon, 1827–1892] see under *theory.*

villi (vil'i) [L.] plural of *villus.*

villiferous (vil-lif'er-us) having or bearing villi.

villikinin (vil"ĭ-ki'nin) [*villi* + Gr. *kinein* to move] a hypothetical hormone said to stimulate villus movement and to be released by action of hydrochloric acid on the mucous membrane of the duodenum.

villioma (vil"e-o'mah) villoma.

villitis (vĭ-li'tis) [*villi* + -*itis*] inflammation of the villous tissue of the coronet and of the plantar substance of a horse's foot.

villoma (vĭ-lo'mah) a papilloma, chiefly of the rectum.

villonodular (vil"o-nod'u-lar) characterized by villous and nodular thickening; said of a proliferative disorder of the synovial tissue.

villose (vil-lōs') [L. *villosus*] shaggy with soft hairs; covered with villi.

villositis (vil"o-si'tis) a bacterial disease characterized by alterations in the villi of the placenta.

villosity (vĭ-los'ĭ-te) 1. the condition of being covered with villi. 2. a villus.

villous (vil'us) villose.

villus (vil'lus), pl. *vil'li* [L. "tuft of hair"] a small vascular process or protrusion, especially such a protrusion from the free surface of a membrane; [NA] a general term for such a structure. **amniotic v.,** one of the irregular, flat, opaque areas of imperfect skin on the amnion near the distal end of the umbilical cord. **anchoring v.,** a chorionic villus that attaches to the decidua basalis. **arachnoid villi,** 1. granulationes arachnoideales. 2. numerous microscopic projections of the arachnoid into some of the venous sinuses, which are thought by some to enlarge in man with advancing age to become the granulationes arachnoideales (q.v.). **chorionic v.,** one of the threadlike projections growing in tufts on the external surface of the chorion; see *primary, secondary,* and *tertiary v.* **free v.,** a chorionic villus that projects into the intervillous space. **intestinal villi, vil'li intestina'les** [NA], the multitudinous threadlike projections that cover the surface of the mucosa of the small intestine and

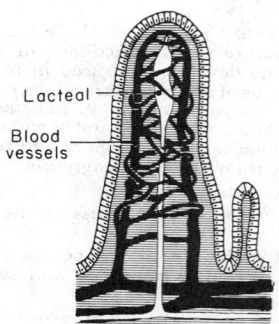

Intestinal villus (Routh).

serve as the sites of absorption (by active transport and diffusion) of fluids and nutrients. **lingual villi,** papillae filiformes. **pericardial v.,** one of the threadlike projections on the free surface of the pericardium. **pleural villi, vil'li pleura'les,** the shaggy appendages on the surface of the pleura near the costomediastinal sinus. **primary v.,** one of the earliest chorionic villi, composed of trophoblast only. **secondary v.,** an intermediate stage of chorionic villi, having a core of connective tissue (mesoblast) covered with trophoblast. **villi of small intestine,** villi intestinales. **synovial villi, vil'li synovia'les** [NA], slender projections of the synovial membrane from its free inner surface into the joint cavity. **tertiary v.,** one of the definitive type of chorionic villi, having trophoblastic cover, connective tissue (mesoblastic) core, and blood vessels.

villusectomy (vil"us-ek'to-me) synovectomy; excision of a synovial villus.

viloxazine hydrochloride (vĭ-loks'ah-zēn) chemical name: 2-[(2-ethoxyphenyl)methyl]morpholine hydrochloride; an antidepressant, $C_{13}H_{19}NO_3 \cdot HCl.$

Vinactane (vin-ak'tān) trademark for a preparation of viomycin.

vinbarbital (vin-bar'bĭ-tal) chemical name: 5-ethyl-5-(1-methyl-1-butenyl)-2,4,6(1H,3H,5H)-pyrimidinetrione. An intermediate-acting barbiturate, $C_{11}H_{16}N_2O_3$, it has been used as a hypnotic and sedative, administered orally. **v. sodium,** the sodium salt of vinbarbital, $C_{11}H_{15}N_2NaO_3$, having the same actions and uses as the base; administered orally and parenterally.

vinblastine sulfate (vin-blas'tēn) [USP] chemical name: vincaleukoblastine sulfate (1:1) (salt). The sulfate salt of an alkaloid extracted from *Vinca rosea* L. (Apocynaceae), $C_{46}H_{58}N_4O_9 \cdot H_2SO_4$, occurring as a white or slightly yellow, crystalline powder. It is used as an antineoplastic in the palliative treatment of lymphomas, including generalized Hodgkin's disease, lymphosarcoma, reticulum-cell sarcoma, and advanced mycosis fungoides, and of neuroblastoma, Letterer-Siwe disease, choriocarcinoma resistant to other agents, breast carcinoma resistant to other agents, and embryonal carcinoma of the testis. Administered intravenously.

Vinca (vin′kah) a genus of apocynaceous woody herbs, including the periwinkles. *V. minor* L. is the common, or lesser, periwinkle. *V. rosea* L. (*Catharanthus roseus* G. Don), the Madagascar periwinkle, contains many alkaloids, including vinblastine and vincristine.

vincamine (vin′kah-mēn) a major alkaloid, $C_{21}H_{26}N_2O_3$, obtained from *Vinca minor* L. (Apocynaceae); used to help improve intellectual capacity in patients with cerebrovascular disorders.

Vincent's angina, etc. (vin′sents) [Henri *Vincent*, physician in Paris, 1862–1950] see under *angina, spirillium, stomatitis,* and *tonsillitis.*

vincofos (vin′ko-fos) chemical name: phosphoric acid 2,3-dichloroethenyl methyl octyl ester; an anthelmintic, $C_{11}H_{21}Cl_2O_4P$.

vincristine sulfate (vin-kris′tēn) [USP] chemical name: 22-oxovincaleukoblastine sulfate (1:1) (salt). The sulfate salt of an alkaloid extracted from *Vinca rosea* L. (Apocynaceae), $C_{46}H_{56}N_4O_{10} \cdot H_2SO_4$, occurring as a white to slightly yellow, amorphous or crystalline powder; used as an antineoplastic, especially in the treatment of acute leukemia, administered intravenously.

vincula (ving′ku-lah) [L.] plural of *vinculum.*

vinculum (ving′ku-lum), pl. *vin′cula* [L.] a band or bandlike structure; [NA] a general term for such a structure. **v. bre′ve** [NA], either of two fan-shaped expansions near the ends of the flexor tendons of a finger, one connecting the superficial tendon to the proximal interphalangeal joint and the other connecting the deep tendon to the intermediate interphalangeal joint. **v. lin′-guae,** frenulum linguae. **vin′cula lin′gulae cerebel′li,** lateral prolongations of the lingula of the cerebellum. **v. lon′-gum** [NA], either of two independent pairs of slender bands in each finger, one connecting the deep flexor tendon to the superficial tendon after the latter becomes subjacent, and the other connecting the superficial tendon to the proximal phalanx. **vin′cula ten′dinum digito′rum ma′nus** [NA], vincula of tendons of fingers: small vascular bands that connect the tendons of the flexor digitorum profundus and flexor digitorum superficialis muscles to the phalanges and interphalangeal articulations of the hand. The tendon blood supply is also carried in them. See *v. breve* and *v. longum.* **vin′cula ten′dinum digito′rum pe′dis** [NA], vincula of tendons of toes: bands connecting the tendons of the flexor digitorum longus and flexor digitorum brevis muscles to the phalanges and interphalangeal articulations of the foot. They are similar to the vincula found in the hand. **vincula of tendons of fingers,** vincula tendinum digitorum manus. **vincula of tendons of toes,** vincula tendinum digitorum pedis.

vindesine (vin′dĕ-sēn) chemical name: 23-amino-O^4-deacetyl-23-demethoxyvincaleukoblastine; an antineoplastic, $C_{43}H_{55}N_5O_7$.

vinegar (vin′e-gar) [Fr. *vinaigre* sour wine] 1. a weak and impure dilution of acetic acid; especially a sour liquid consisting chiefly of acetic acid, formed by the fermentation of cider, wine, etc., or by the distillation of wood. 2. a medicinal solution of a drug in dilute acetic acid.

vinegaroon (vin″e-gah-rōōn′) the whip-scorpion, *Mastigoproctus giganteus,* so called because it produces an irritating excretion which has an odor resembling that of vinegar.

Vinethene (vin′ĕ-thēn) trademark for vinyl ether; see under *ether.*

vinic (vi′nik) [L. *vinum* wine] pertaining to wine.

vinometer (vi-nom′ĕ-ter) [L. *vinum* wine + L. *metrum* measure] an instrument for estimating the percentage of alcohol in wine.

vinous (vi′nus) [L. *vinosus,* from *vinum* wine] pertaining to or containing wine.

Vinson's syndrome [Porter Paisley *Vinson,* American surgeon, 1890–1959] see *Plummer-Vinson syndrome,* under *syndrome.*

vinum (vi′num), gen. *vi′ni* [L.] wine.

vinyl (vi′nil) the univalent group $CH_2{:}CH{-}$. **v. acetate,** a vinyl group to which the monovalent radical $CH_3COO{-}$ is attached, the monomer which polymerizes to polyvinyl acetate. **v. chloride,** a vinyl group to which an atom of chlorine is attached, $CH_2 \cdot CHCl$, the monomer which polymerizes to polyvinyl chloride.

viocid (vi′o-sid) gentian violet.

Viocin (vi′o-sin) trademark for a preparation of viomycin sulfate.

Vioform (vi′o-form) trademark for preparations of iodochlorhydroxyquin.

Viokase (vi′o-kās) trademark for a preparation of pancreatin.

Viola (vi′o-lah) [L.] a genus of plants (family Violaceae), the vio-

lets and pansies. **V. odora′ta** L., a sweet-scented violet of Europe and Asia; mainly used in perfumery as a source of oil. **V. tri′color** L., a species with emetic properties; it has been used in skin diseases and as an expectorant in cough preparations.

violacein (vi″o-la′se-in) a bacterial pigment showing antibiotic activity, from *Chromobacter violaceum.*

Violaquercitrin (vi-o″lah-kwer′sĭ-trin) rutin.

violescent (vi″o-les′ent) somewhat violet in color.

violet (vi′o-let) 1. the hue seen in the most refracted end of the spectrum. 2. a violet-colored dye. **amethyst v.,** a tetraethylphenosafranine used in triple staining, $(C_2H_5)_2N \cdot C_6H_3 \cdot N_2Cl(C_6H_5) \cdot C_6H_3 \cdot N(C_2H_5)_2$. Called also *heliotrope B.* and *iris v.* **ammonium oxalate crystal v.,** a type of Gram stain prepared by mixing 2 gm. of crystal violet (90 per cent dye content) and 20 ml. of ethyl alcohol (95 per cent) with 0.8 gm. of ammonium oxalate and 80 ml. of distilled water. **v. 7 B or C,** gentian v.; see under G. **chrome v.,** a tricarboxyl derivative of pararosolic acid, $COONa \cdot C_6H_3(O)C[C_6H_3(OH)COONa]_2$. **cresyl v., cresylecht v.,** a dye used in pathologic staining. **crystal v.,** gentian v.; see under G. **v. G,** gentian v.; see under G. **gentian v.** see under G. **hexamethyl v.,** gentian v. **Hofmann's v.,** iodine v., dahlia. **iris v.,** amethyst v. **Lauth's v.,** thionine. **methyl v.,** gentian v.; see under G. **methylene v.,** one of the constituents of polychrome methylene blue, $(CH_3)_2N \cdot C_6H_3(SN)CH_3{:}O$. **neutral v.,** a dye that resembles neutral red, but is more violet in color, $(CH_3)_2N \cdot C_6H_3 \cdot N_2 \cdot C_6H_2 \cdot (NH_2 \cdot HCl) \cdot NH \cdot C_6H_4 \cdot N(CH_3)_2$. **Paris v., pentamethyl v.,** gentian v.; see under G. **visual v.,** iodopsin.

viomycin sulfate (vi′o-mi″sin) the sulfate salt of an antibacterial antibiotic produced by *Streptomyces puniceus, S. floridae,* and *Actinomyces vinaceus,* or by other means, $C_{25}H_{43}N_{13}O_{10} \cdot xH_2SO_4$, occurring as a white to slightly yellow, crystalline powder; used as a tuberculostatic, administered intramuscularly.

viosterol (vi-os′ter-ol) ergocalciferol.

viper (vi′per) any venomous snake, especially any member of the families Viperidae and Crotalidae. See table accompanying *snake.* **European v.,** a venomous viperine snake, *Vipera berus,* native to Europe, North Africa, and the Near East; it may be red, brown, or gray with dark markings, or black; called also *adder.* **Gaboon v.,** a very deadly, brightly marked, viperine snake, *Bitis gabonica,* of tropical West Africa. **nose-horned v.,** sand v. **palm v.,** any of various small, greenish, arboreal pit vipers of the genera *Bothrops* and *Trimeresurus,* which have prehensile tails that enable them to move from tree to tree. **pit v.,** any of the venomous snakes of the family Crotalidae, having a depression or pit between the nostril and the eye. They include the habu, rattlesnake, copperhead, bushmaster, fer-de-lance, palm viper, and water moccasin. **rhinoceros v.,** a venomous, brightly colored, viperine snake, *Bitis nasicornis,* of tropical Africa, characterized by the presence on the snout of a pair of hornlike growths. **Russell's v.,** the daboia (*Vipera russelli*), an extremely venomous, brightly colored, viperine snake of southeastern Asia, Java, and Sumatra. **sand v.,** a snake, *Vipera ammodytes,* found from southern Europe to Asia Minor, which possesses a hornlike protuberance on the snout for burrowing; called also *nose-horned v.* **true v.,** any one of the snakes of the family Viperidae.

Vipera (vi′per-ah) a genus of venomous snakes of the family Viperidae, including *V. ammodytes,* the sand viper, *V. berus,* the adder or European viper, and *V. russelli,* Russell's viper.

viperid (vi′per-id) viperine.

Viperidae (vi-per′ĭ-de) a family of venomous snakes, the true or Old World vipers, characterized by front, movable, hollow fangs. It includes the European viper, Russell's viper, sand viper, puff adder, Gaboon viper, and rhinoceros viper. Cf. *Crotalidae.*

viperine (vi′per-in, vi′per-īn) 1. any snake of the family Viperidae; a true viper. 2. of or pertaining to the family Viperidae.

viraginity (vi″rah-jin′ĭ-te) [L. *virago* a manlike woman] a condition in which a woman has the sexual feelings and mentality of a man.

viral (vi′ral) pertaining to, caused by, or of the nature of virus.

Virales (vi-ra′lēz) the taxonomic order comprising the viruses; further classification under this taxon has been abandoned. See *virus.*

Virchow's angle, etc. (vēr′kōz) [Rudolf Ludwig Karl *Virchow,* German pathologist, 1821–1902] see under *angle, cell, corpuscle, crystal, degeneration, granulation, line,* and *node,* and see *psammoma.*

Virchow-Robin spaces (vēr′ko-ro-ba′) [Rudolf *Virchow;* Charles Philippe *Robin,* French anatomist, 1821–1885] see under *space.*

viremia (vi-re′me-ah) the presence of viruses in the blood, usually characterized by malaise, fever, and aching of the back and extremities.

virgin (vir′jin) [L. *virgo*] a woman or girl who has not had sexual intercourse.

virginal (vir′jĭ-nal) pertaining to a virgin or to virginity.

virginiamycin (ver-jin″yah-mi′sin) an antibiotic produced by

Streptomyces virginiae or by other means, consisting chiefly of two components, virginiamycin M$_1$ (factor M$_1$) and virginiamycin S$_1$ (factor S); used in animal feedstuffs and feed supplements and in infections due to sensitive organisms, especially gram-positive cocci.

virginity (vir-jin′ĭ-te) [L. *virginitas*] maidenhood; the condition of being a virgin.

virginium (vir-jin′e-um) a former name of the element francium.

viricidal (vir″ĭ-si′dal) virucidal.

viricide (vir′ĭ-sīd) virucide.

viridin (vi-rid′in) 1. an oily principle, C$_{12}$H$_{19}$N, distilled from bone oil and from coal tar. 2. an antifungal antibiotic, C$_{20}$H$_{16}$O$_6$, isolated from *Gliocladium virens*.

viridobufagin (vir″ĭ-do-bu′fah-jin) a cardiac poison, C$_{23}$H$_{34}$O$_5$, from the skin glands of the toad, *Bufo viridis*.

virile (vīr′il) [L. *virilis*] 1. peculiar to men or the male sex. 2. possessing masculine traits, especially copulative power.

virilescence (vir′ĭ-les′ens) the development of male secondary sex characters in the female; virilization.

virilia (vi-ril′e-ah) [L.] the male genital organs (organa genitalia masculina [NA]).

viriligenic (vir′ĭ-li-jen′ik) promoting virility or promoting male characteristics.

virilism (vir′ĭ-lizm) [L. *virilis* masculine] masculinity; the development of masculine physical and mental traits in the female (see virilization). **adrenal v.,** virilism due to inappropiate adrenal androgen production; in it the body changes toward the masculine type. **prosopopilary v.,** virilism marked by growth of hair on the face.

virility (vi″-ril′ĭ-te) [L. *virilitas*, from *vir* man] possession of the normal primary sex characters in one of the male sex.

virilization (vir″ĭ-li-za′shun) the induction or development of male secondary sex characters, especially the induction of such changes in the female, including enlargement of the clitoris, growth of facial and body hair, development of a hairline typical of the male forehead, stimulation of secretion and proliferation of the sebaceous glands (often with acne), and deepening of the voice. Called also *masculinization*.

virion (vi′re-on) the complete viral particle, found extracellularly and capable of surviving in crystalline form and infecting a living cell; it comprises the nucleoid (genetic material) and the capsid. Called also *viral particle*.

viripotent (vi-rip′o-tent) [L. *viripotens*; *vir* man + *potens* able] 1. sexually mature; said of a male. 2. marriageable or nubile; said of the female.

virogene (vi′ro-jēn) [*virus* + *gene*] in theoretical genetics, an RNA tumor virus assembled by the normal genetic complement of a cell.

virogenetic (vi″ro-jĕ-net′ik) having a viral origin; caused by a virus.

viroid (vi′roid) 1. a general term for any biological specific used in immunization. 2. a portion of a strand of infectious viral RNA.

virolactia (vi″ro-lak′she-ah) secretion of viruses in the milk.

virologist (vi-rol′o-jist) a microbiologist specializing in virology.

virology (vi-rol′o-je) that branch of microbiology which is concerned with viruses and viral diseases.

viromicrosome (vi′ro-mi′kro-sōm) a name sometimes applied to an incomplete virus particle released by premature disruption of the host cell.

viropexis (vi″ro-pek′sis) [*virus* + Gr. *pēxis* fixation] the fixation of virus to the membrane of an animal cell and its subsequent engulfment by the cell.

viroplasm (vi′ro-plazm) plaques of very fine granular substance that appear in cells before virions are observed and which correspond to the DNA material, as in poxvirus infections.

virose (vi′rōs) [L. *virosus*, from *virus* poison] having poisonous qualities.

virosis (vi-ro′sis), pl. *viro′ses*. a disease caused by a virus.

virostatic (vi″ro-stat′ik) 1. inhibiting the replication of viruses. 2. an agent that inhibits the replication of viruses.

virous (vi′rus) virose.

virtual (vir′tu-al) [L., *virtus* strength] see under *focus*.

virucidal (vi″ru-si′dal) capable of neutralizing or destroying a virus.

virucide (vi′ru-sīd) an agent that neutralizes or destroys a virus.

virulence (vir′u-lens) [L. *virulen′tia*, from *virus* poison] the degree of pathogenicity of a microorganism as indicated by case fatality rates and/or its ability to invade the tissues of the host. It is measured experimentally by the median lethal dose (LD$_{50}$) or median effective dose (ED$_{50}$). By extension, the competence of any infectious agent to produce pathologic effects.

virulent (vir′u-lent) [L. *virulentus*, form *virus* poison] pertain-

ing to or characterized by virulence; exceedingly pathogenic, noxious, or deleterious.

virulicidal (vir″u-lis′ĭ-dal) destructive of virulence; capable of destroying the deleterious potency of a virus or other noxious agent.

viruliferous (vir″u-lif′er-us) [L. *virus* poison + *ferre* to bear] conveying or producing a virus or other noxious agent.

viruria (vīr-u′re-ah) the presence of viruses in the urine.

virus (vi′rus) [L.] one of a group of minute infectious agents, with certain exceptions (e.g., poxviruses) not resolved in the light microscope, and characterized by a lack of independent metabolism and by the ability to replicate only within living host cells. Like living organisms, they are able to reproduce with genetic continuity and the possibility of mutation. They range from 200–300 nm. to 15 nm. in size and are morphologically heterogeneous, occurring as rod-shaped, spherical, or polyhedral, and tadpole-shaped forms; masses of the spherical or polyhedral forms may be made up of orderly arrays, to give a crystalline structure. The individual particle, or virion, consists of nucleic acid (the nucleoid), DNA or RNA (but not both) and a protein shell, or capsid, which contains and protects the nucleic acid and which may be multilayered. Viruses are customarily separated into three subgroups on the basis of host specificity, namely bacterial viruses, animal viruses, and plant viruses. They are also classified as to their origin (e.g., reoviruses), mode of transmission (arboviruses, tickborne viruses), or the manifestations they produce (polioviruses, polyomaviruses, poxviruses). They are sometimes named for the geographical location in which they were first isolated (e.g., coxsackievirus). **acute laryngotracheobronchitis v.,** parainfluenza 2 v.; see *parainfluenza v.* **adeno-associated v.,** a parvovirus that apparently cannot replicate unless associated with an adenovirus. **Amapari v.,** an arenavirus isolated from rodents in Brazil. **animal v's,** viruses that produce diseases of man and other animals. **v. anima′tum,** a living animal poison. **arbor v's** (arthropod-*borne*), former name for *arbovirus*. **Argentinian hemorrhagic fever v.,** Junin v. **attenuated v.,** one whose pathogenicity has been reduced by serial animal passage or by other means. **Australian X disease v.,** see under *disease*. **avian leukosis v.,** any of a complex of leukoviruses causing erythroblastosis, granulomatosis, lymphomatosis, and myelocytomatosis in chickens; see *avian leukosis,* under *leukosis*. **B v.,** a herpesvirus causing a mild disease in monkeys, the natural host, but a severe and usually fatal disease in humans accidentally infected by exposure to infected monkeys. **bacterial v.,** a virus capable of producing transmissible lysis of bacteria; the virus particle attaches to the bacterial cell wall and viral nucleoprotein enters the cell, resulting in the synthesis of virus and its liberation on physical disruption of the cell. Bacterial viruses are usually specific for bacterial species, but they may be strain-specific or may infect more than one species of bacteria. Called also *bacteriophage* or *phage*. See *Twort-d'Herelle phenomenon*, under *phenomenon*. **Bittner v.,** mouse mammary tumor v. **Bolivian hemorrhagic fever v.,** Machupo v. **Brunhilde v.,** the prototype strain of poliovirus type 1. **Bunyamwera v.,** an arbovirus isolated from *Aedes* mosquitoes in an uninhabited part of the Semliki Forest in western Uganda; it causes a mild febrile disease. **bushy stunt v.,** a small spherical plant virus, which causes bushy stunt of tomatoes. **Bwamba fever v.,** an arbovirus, originally isolated from the blood of natives in Bwamba county in Uganda, which causes a mild febrile disease. **C v.,** coxsackievirus. **CA v.** (croup-associated), parainfluenza 2 virus. **Cache Valley v.,** an arbovirus, related to the Bunyamwera virus, first isolated from *Culiseta inornata* in the Cache Valley in northern Utah. It has also been found in Brazil, and was isolated from *Aedes scapularis* in Trinidad. **California v.,** a virus isolated in California in 1943 from species of mosquitoes, capable of causing disease in laboratory animals and the probable cause of fatal encephalitis in an infant. **cancer-inducing v.,** a virus that causes uncontrolled proliferation of infected cells, including both RNA and DNA viruses. **Catu v.,** an arbovirus closely related to Guama virus. **CCA v. (chimpanzee coryza agent),** respiratory syncytial v. **CELO (chicken-embryo-*lethal* orphan) v.,** an enteric orphan virus which is lethal for chicken embryos and induces tumors in newborn and weanling hamsters. **Chagres v.,** an arbovirus causing fever associated with malaise, headache, and pains of localized and generalized distribution, in Panama. **Chenuda v.,** an arbovirus closely related to Quaranfil virus. **chikungunya v.,** an arbovirus found in the Newala district of Tanzania as the etiologic agent of an epidemic dengue-like disease known as chikungunya. It is closely related to Semliki Forest virus. **Coe v.,** coxsackievirus type A21. **Colorado tick fever v.,** the etiologic agent of a febrile disease occurring in regions of the Rocky Mountains where the tick vector, *Dermacentor andersoni*, is prevalent. **Columbia SK v.,** an encephalomyocarditis virus originally isolated in 1940 from a monkey which had previously been inoculated with the Yale SK strain of poliovirus. **common cold v's,** a subgroup of rhinoviruses considered to cause the common cold. **coryza v.,** rhinovirus. **Coxsackie v.,** coxsackievirus. **Crimean hemorrhagic fever v.,** an arbovirus, transmitted by the tick *Hyalomma marginatum*, which causes hemorrhagic fever in the

Crimea and the Lower Don and Volga River Valleys of the U.S.S.R. **croup-associated v.,** parainfluenza 2 virus. **cytomegalic inclusion disease v.,** see *cytomegalovirus*. **defective v.,** one that cannot be completely replicated or cannot form a protein coat; in some cases replication can proceed if missing gene functions are supplied by other (helper) viruses; see *helper v.* **dengue v.,** the etiologic agent of dengue, existing as two immunological types, designated 1 and 2, and related to other arboviruses. **EB v.,** Epstein-Barr v. **Ebola v.,** an RNA virus almost identical to the Marburg virus but serologically distinct; it causes a highly fatal hemorrhagic fever closely resembling Marburg virus disease; outbreaks of the disease have occurred in Central Africa. **ECBO v.,** ecbovirus. **ECDO v.,** ecdovirus. **ECHO v.,** echovirus. **ECHO 28 v.,** echovirus 28. **ECMO v.,** ecmovirus. **ECSO v.,** ecsovirus. **EEE v.,** eastern equine encephalomyelitis v.; see *equine encephalomyelitis v.* **EMC v.,** encephalomyocarditis v. **encephalomyocarditis v.,** an enterovirus found in Africa, South America, and elsewhere, which causes mild aseptic meningitis and encephalomyocarditis; it is represented by four strains which appear to be substantially identical in immunological and other respects. It includes the Columbia SK, Mengo, and MM viruses. **enteric v.,** enterovirus. **enteric orphan v's,** viruses isolated from the intestinal tract of man and various other animals, called orphan viruses because they are often not specifically associated with illness; they include such viruses isolated from cattle (ecboviruses), dogs (ecdoviruses), man (echoviruses), monkeys (ecmoviruses), and swine (ecsoviruses). **epidemic keratoconjunctivitis v.,** adenovirus type 8. **Epstein-Barr v. (EB v.; EBV),** a herpes-like virus that cause infectious mononucleosis and is associated with Burkitt's lymphoma and nasopharyngeal carcinoma. **equine encephalomyelitis v.,** a group of arboviruses causing encephalomyelitis in horses, mules, and man, with a reservoir of infection in birds, and transmitted by mosquitoes. The group includes *eastern equine encephalomyelitis virus (EEE v.),* the cause of equine encephalomyelitis in a region extending from New Hampshire to Texas, and as far west as Wisconsin in the United States, and also in Canada, the Caribbean, Mexico, and parts of Central and South America; *Venezuelan equine encephalomyelitis virus (VEE v.),* the cause of equine encephalomyelitis in Venezuela and other South American countries, and Mexico and Florida; and *western equine encephalomyelitis virus (WEE v.),* the cause of equine encephalomyelitis in the United States west of the Mississippi (with evidence suggesting its presence also in the Atlantic and Gulf Coast states), transmitted primarily by *Culex tarsalis.* **exanthematous disease v.,** any of a group of dermotropic viruses, including poxviruses, causing exanthematous disease in man and lower animals. **FA v.,** a strain of virus causing encephalomyelitis of mice. **filterable v., filtrable v.,** a pathogenic agent capable of passing through fine filters of diatomite or unglazed porcelain; ultravirus. **v. fixé, fixed v.,** rabies virus whose virulence and incubation period have been stabilized by serial passage and remain fixed during further transmission; used for inoculating animals from which rabies vaccine is prepared. **fowl plague v.,** a virus causing a disease of fowl in northern Italy, Germany, and France. **Friend v.,** a murine leukemia virus causing malignant reticulopathy in mice. **Germistan v.,** an arbovirus of the Bunyamwera group, causing a mild febrile disease in South Africa. **Graffi v.,** a murine leukemia virus which causes chloroleukemia in mice. **granulosis v.,** baculovirus. **Gross v.,** a virus resembling the Rous sarcoma virus, which causes many kinds of leukemia in newborn mice and rats. **Guama v.,** an arbovirus isolated in the Belem region of Brazil from foresters suffering from hyperthermia, headache, muscular and articular pains, and occasionally nausea and vertigo. **Guaroa v.,** an arbovirus isolated in Colombia from the blood of patients with a febrile disease; a member of the Bunyamwera group of viruses. **helper v.,** a virus (e.g., the Rous-associated virus) that aids the development of a defective virus by supplying or restoring the activity of a viral gene or enabling a defective virus (e.g., the Rous virus) to form a protein coat. **hemadsorption v., type 1 (HA1),** parainfluenza 3 virus. **hemadsorption v., type 2 (HA2),** a parainfluenza 1 virus isolated from children with febrile respiratory disease. **hemagglutinating v. of Japan,** Sendai v. **hepatitis v.,** the etiologic agent of viral hepatitis. Three types are recognized: *hepatitis virus A (hepatitis virus IH),* the agent causing infectious hepatitis, acquired by parenteral inoculation or by ingestion, and *hepatitis virus B (hepatitis virus SH),* the agent causing serum hepatitis, transmitted by inadequately sterilized syringes and needles, or through infectious blood plasma, or certain blood products, and *non-A, non-B hepatitis virus,* which closely resembles hepatitis virus B and causes a similar disease. **herpangina v.,** one of the viruses of the coxsackievirus A group, causing a febrile disease, usually of children, characterized by small herpes-like lesions on the soft palate or in the faucial area. **herpes v.,** see *herpesvirus.* **Ilheus v.,** an arbovirus first isolated from species of *Aedes* and *Psorophora* in Brazil; and also found in Panama, where birds may be hosts. It is related to St. Louis encephalitis virus, Japanese B encephalitis virus, and West Nile virus. **infectious porcine encephalomyelitis v.,** Teschen v. **infectious wart v.,** a papil-lomavirus that causes warts in man. **influenza v.,** any of a group of myxoviruses that cause influenza, including at least three serotypes (A, B, and C) and several antigenic variations, classified on the basis of their surface antigens (hemagglutinin and neuraminidase) as H_1N_1, H_2N_2, etc. Serotype A viruses are subject to major antigenic changes (antigenic shifts) as well as minor gradual antigenic changes (antigenic drift) and cause the major pandemics. Serotype B viruses appear to undergo only minor antigenic changes (antigenic drift) and cause more localized epidemics. Serotype C viruses appear to be antigenically stable and cause only sporadic disease. **insect v's,** viruses capable of causing disease in insects. **iridescent v.,** iridovirus. **Japanese B encephalitis v.,** the causative agent of Japanese B encephalitis, closely similar to the various agents causing the different types of equine encephalomyelitis and St. Louis encephalitis, but having a wider range of pathogenicity for experimental animals. **JH v.,** echovirus 28. **Junin v.,** an arenavirus first isolated in 1958 during an epidemic of hemorrhagic fever; it is serologically related to the Machupo virus. See *Argentinian hemorrhagic fever,* under *fever.* **K v.,** a nononcogenic polyomavirus that produces fatal pneumonia on inoculation into newborn mice. **Kemerova v.,** an arbovirus (tickborne) responsible for a benign febrile disease in western Siberia. **Kumba v.,** a virus isolated from mosquitoes in the Kumba region of the British Cameroons in West Africa; antigenically identical with the Semliki Forest virus. **Kyasanur Forest disease v.,** a tick-borne virus found in native monkeys in the Kyasanur Forest in Mysore, India, and the cause of a highly fatal disease in man; closely related to the Russian spring-summer encephalitis virus. **Langat v.,** a tickborne arbovirus that causes encephalitis in man and in mice. **Lansing v.,** the prototype strain of poliovirus type 2. **Lassa fever v.,** an extremely virulent arenavirus, originally isolated in Lassa, Nigeria, in 1969, which causes an acute, febrile disease with high fatality rate; it morphologically resembles the viruses of lymphocytic choriomeningitis and the Tacaribe-Junin-Machupo group. **latent v.,** masked v. **Latino v.,** an arenavirus isolated from rodents in Bolivia. **LCM v.,** lymphocytic choriomeningitis v. **Leon v.,** the prototype strain of poliovirus type 3. **louping ill v.,** a virus transmitted by the tick, *Ixodes ricinus;* it causes louping ill of sheep, is transmissible to man, and is closely related to Russian spring-summer encephalitis virus. **Lunyo v.,** a neurotropic variant of Rift Valley fever virus. **lymphocytic choriomeningitis (LCM) v.,** an arenavirus, the etiologic agent of lymphocytic choriomeningitis that occurs naturally in mice, dogs, and monkeys. **lytic v.,** one that is replicated in the host cell and causes death and lysis of the cell. **M-25 v.,** a virus with the properties of a myxovirus, although antigenically unrelated; isolated from a person with upper respiratory illness. **Machupo v.,** an arenavirus first isolated during an epidemic of hemorrhagic fever in Bolivia in 1959, indistinguishable from the Junin virus by complement fixation, but distinct by the neutralization test. See *Bolivian hemorrhagic fever,* under *fever.* **Makonde v.,** an arbovirus isolated along with the chikungunya virus in the region of the Makonde plateau in Tanzania. **mammary tumor v.,** mouse mammary tumor v. **Marburg v.,** an RNA virus occurring in Africa, transmitted by insect bite and causing Marburg disease. **masked v.,** a virus which ordinarily occurs in a noninfective state and is demonstrable by indirect methods which activate it, as by blind passage in experimental animals. **Mayaro v.,** an arbovirus found in Mayaro county, Trinidad, and in the region of the Guama River in Brazil as an etiologic agent of febrile disease; closely related to and possibly identical with Semliki Forest virus. **measles v.,** a paramyxovirus, the etiologic agent of measles. **Mengo v.,** an encephalomyocarditis virus isolated originally in 1948 from a captive monkey in Uganda and later from mosquitoes and a mongoose of the same area; identified also as the cause of an epizootic disease of swine in Panama. **MM v.,** an encephalomyocarditis virus originally isolated in 1943 from the brain of a hamster that was previously inoculated with material from a human case of paralytic disease. **molluscum contagiosum v.,** a poxvirus that causes molluscum contagiosum. **Moloney v.,** a murine leukemia virus which causes lymphoid leukemia in mice. **Mossuril v.,** a mosquito-borne arbovirus. **mouse mammary tumor v.,** a virus causing mammary adenocarcinoma in mice of certain genotype and influenced by estrogenic stimulation; it is usually transmitted from the mother to her offspring through the milk. Called also *Bittner agent, Bittner v., mammary tumor agent, milk agent* or *factor.* **mumps v.,** a paramyxovirus that causes mumps and, in some cases, tenderness and swelling of the testes, pancreas, ovaries, or other organs. **murine leukemia v.,** any of a group of leukoviruses causing leukemia and solid tumors in rats, mice, hamsters, and other animals; the group includes the Gross, Rauscher, Friend, Moloney, and Graffi viruses. **Murray Valley encephalitis v.,** a virus closely resembling the Japanese B encephalitis virus; see under *encephalitis.* **Nakiwogo v.,** Semunya v. **neurotropic v.,** one that has a predilection for and causes infection in nervous tissues, e.g., the rabies virus. **newborn pneumonitis v.,** Sendai v. **Newcastle disease v.,** a virus causing disease in chickens and occasionally in man; related to the influenza viruses. Abbreviated NDV. **nononcogenic v.,** one that does not cause cancer. **Ntaya v.,** a virus originally isolated in 1943 from various species of mosquitoes, including *Culex* and *Aedes,* in the Ntaya Swamp in western Uganda; it is fatal to mice infected by intracerebral inoculation. **Omsk hemorrhagic fever v.,** an arbovirus, closely related to the Kyasanur Forest disease virus, originally isolated in the Omsk region of the U.S.S.R., which causes a severe febrile illness in man. **oncogenic v.,** a cancer-inducing virus. **O'nyong-nyong v.,** an arbovirus found in Uganda and Kenya as the etiologic agent of an epidemic febrile, dengue-like disease. **Oropouche v.,** an arbovirus isolated from a patient with febrile disease in Trinidad; related to the Simbu virus. **orphan v's,** viruses which when isolated originally in tissue culture showed no specific association with disease, such as the enteric orphan viruses; some have since been found to occur in association with human disease. **papilloma v.,** papillomavirus. **pappataci fever v.,** the etiological agent of phlebotomus (pappataci) fever, transmitted by *Phlebotomus,* and occurring as two serotypes, the Naples and Sicilian types. **parainfluenza v.,** a group of viruses isolated from patients with upper respiratory tract disease of varying severity. Parainfluenza viruses are classified as: *Parainfluenza 1 v.,* comprising two immunologically related but not identical viruses, *Sendai virus* and *hemadsorption type 2 (HA2) virus; Parainfluenza 2 v.,* a virus isolated from patients with acute laryngotracheobronchitis; called also *CA v.* or *croup-associated v.; Parainfluenza 3 v.,* a virus causing bronchitis and pneumonia, especially in children; called also *hemadsorption v., type 1 (HAI v.); Parainfluenza 4 v.,* a virus associated with respiratory disease in children. **Parana v.,** an arenavirus isolated from rodents in Paraguay. **pharyngoconjunctival fever v.,** adenovirus type 3. **Pichinde v.,** an arenavirus infecting rodents in Colombia, and isolated from human subclinical infections. **Piry v.,** an arbovirus isolated from East African patients with an acute febrile syndrome. **plant v's,** viruses that replicate in and may produce diseases of higher plants. **poliomyelitis v.,** see *poliovirus.* **polyoma v.,** polyomavirus. **Pongola v.,** an arbovirus causing a febrile disease in Africa. **Powassan v.,** a tickborne virus isolated from a fatal case of encephalitis in Ontario, Canada; closely related to Russian spring-summer encephalitis virus. **pox v.,** see *poxvirus.* **Quaranfil v.,** an arbovirus found in Egypt, where it was isolated from the blood of children with febrile disease, from the blood of young egrets, and from ticks (*Argas arboreus* and *A. hermanni*). **rabbit fibroma v.,** a poxvirus closely related to the rabbit myxoma virus, which causes rabbit fibroma. **rabbit myxoma v.,** a poxvirus, closely related to the rabbit fibroma virus, which causes infectious myxomatosis in rabbits. **rabbit papilloma v.,** a papillomavirus, morphologically the same as the infectious wart virus, which causes rabbit papilloma. **rabies v.,** the etiologic agent of rabies, one of the most neurotropic of the viruses. **Rauscher leukemia v.,** a murine leukemia virus that causes lymphoid leukemia in mice. **respiratory syncytial v.,** a paramyxovirus resembling the influenza virus; it is the cause of an epidemic acute respiratory disease that is more serious in children, in whom it causes bronchopneumonia and bronchiolitis. In tissue cultures, the virus causes syncytium formation. First isolated from chimpanzees with symptoms of respiratory disease. Called also *chimpanzee coryza agent (CCA),* and *RS v.* **Rift Valley fever v.,** the etiologic agent of a febrile disease first seen in the Rift Valley of Kenya, South Africa, but now widespread in East and South Africa, transmitted by mosquitoes of the species *Aedes, Culex,* and *Erethmapodites.* **Rous-associated v. (RAV),** a helper virus in whose presence a defective Rous sarcoma virus is able to form a protein coat. **Rous sarcoma v.,** a leukovirus producing fibrosarcoma in fowl, especially chickens; some strains have been shown to produce tumors in other animals. See *Rous sarcoma,* under *sarcoma.* **RS v.,** respiratory syncytial v. **Russian spring-summer encephalitis v.,** a tickborne virus which causes spring-summer encephalitis in Russia and Central Europe. **SA v.,** a virus isolated from the hamster brain following inoculation with a chick embryo allantoic culture of nasal washings from a person with acute upper respiratory infection. **St. Louis encephalitis v.,** the etiologic agent of St. Louis encephalitis, with a distribution similar to that of western equine encephalomyelitis virus, but differing from it immunologically. **salivary gland v.,** cytomegalovirus. **satellite v.,** a strain of virus unable to replicate except in the presence of helper virus; considered to be deficient in coding for capsid formation. **Schwartz leukemia v.,** a virus that causes lymphoid leukemia in Swiss mice. **Semliki Forest v.,** an arbovirus isolated from mosquitoes of the Semliki Forest of western Uganda; it is pathogenic for laboratory animals and man. **Semunya v.,** an arbovirus isolated from East African patients with an acute febrile syndrome; called also *Nakiwogo v.* **Sendai v.,** a parainfluenza 1 virus, which seems to have been the etiologic agent of a highly fatal epidemic pneumonitis of newborn infants in Japan, and has been found in infants in Germany and Russia. It is related to the mumps virus. **sigma v.,** a virus that induces carbon dioxide sensitivity in *Drosophila melanogaster* and other fruit flies. **Simbu v.,** a virus isolated from a species of mosquitoes (*Aedes circumluteolis*) in Africa. **simian v's,** viruses that have been recovered from monkeys; they belong to many different groups, including adenoviruses,

enteroviruses, herpesviruses, and reoviruses. **simian v. 40 (SV40),** vacuolating v. **Sindbis v.,** an arbovirus first isolated from *Culex univittatus* and once from a hooded crow in the Sindbis district of northern Egypt, capable of causing infection in experimental animals. **slow v.,** any virus causing a disease characterized by a very long preclinical course and very gradual progression once the symptoms appear; slow viruses include etiologic agents of kuru, scrapie, and Aleutian disease of mink. **Spondweni v.,** an arbovirus originally isolated in 1955 from South African mosquitoes, which may cause a short-term febrile illness in man. **street v.,** rabies virus from a naturally infected animal, as opposed to a laboratory-adapted strain of the virus. **Tacaribe v.,** an arenavirus, isolated from bats in Trinidad, which is immunologically related to the Junin and Machupo viruses. **Tahyna v.,** a virus serologically related to the California virus, isolated in various European countries; it is suspected of causing human and animal disease. **Tamiami v.,** an arenavirus isolated from rodents in Florida. **temperate v.,** see under *bacteriophage.* **Teschen v.,** the etiologic agent of infectious porcine encephalomyelitis (Teschen disease). **Theiler's v.,** the etiologic agent of a spontaneous encephalomyelitis of mice (Theiler's disease); it resembles human poliovirus but is immunologically distinct from them. **tickborne v's,** viruses that are transmitted by ticks. **tobacco mosaic v.,** a plant virus containing RNA which causes mosaic disease of tobacco. **tumor v.,** a cancer-inducing v. **Turlock v.,** a mosquitoborne virus isolated from *Culex tarsalis* in California; it is unrelated to other arthropod-borne viruses and is not known to cause human disease. **2060 v.,** echovirus 28. **U v.,** a virus resembling the parainfluenza 2 virus but of uncertain status, found in children with subglottic laryngitis; called also *Uppsala v.* **Uganda S v.,** an arbovirus first isolated from species of *Aedes* in Bwamba county in Uganda. It causes mild febrile disease in certain areas in Africa, especially in Nigeria. **Uppsala v.,** U v. **Uruma v.,** an arbovirus causing epidemic febrile disease in Colombia. **vaccinia v., v. vaccin'icum,** the virus of cowpox, used in inoculating against smallpox. See also *poxvirus.* **vacuolating v.,** a polyomavirus isolated from *Rhesus* monkey kidney tissue, which produces malignancy in human and newborn hamster kidney cell cultures and tumors on inoculation into newborn hamsters; called also *simian v. 40.* **VEE v.,** Venezuelan equine encephalomyelitis v.; see *equine encephalomyelitis v.* **vesicular stomatitis v.,** a rhabdovirus, the etiologic agent of vesicular stomatitis of swine, cattle, and horses. **wart v.,** see *infectious wart v.* **WEE v.,** western equine encephalomyelitis v.; see *equine encephalomyelitis v.* **Wesselsbron v.,** an arbovirus repeatedly isolated in South Africa from mosquitoes and from sheep and man, in whom it causes a mild febrile disease. **West Nile v.,** an arbovirus related to Japanese encephalitis B virus and St. Louis encephalitis virus, which causes a mild disease in humans; it was first isolated in Uganda, but is widespread in Africa and has been observed in Israel. *Culex uvivittatus* is the most probable vector. **Wyeomyia v.,** a virus of the Bunyamwera group originally isolated in Colombia from the mosquito *Wyeomyia melanocephala* and later from man in Panama; it produces encephalitis in the infant mouse after intracerebral inoculation. **Yaba v.,** a virus that produces superficial benign tumors in the monkey. **Yale SK v.,** a strain of poliovirus. **Zika v.,** an arbovirus originally isolated in 1947 from monkeys in the Zika Forest, Uganda, and later found to infect *Aedes africanus;* human infection also occurs. **Zimmermann v.,** a neurotropic arbovirus of the tickborne encephalitis group.

virusemia (vi"rus-e'me-ah) viremia.

virustatic (vir"u-stat'ik) [*virus* + Gr. *statikos* bringing to a standstill] inhibiting the replication of viruses.

vis (vis), pl. *vi'res* [L.] force; energy. **v. a ter'go,** the factor of pressure transmitted through the capillaries to the veins by the blood pumped into the arteries by the heart. **v. conserva'trix,** the natural power of the organism to resist injury and disease. **v. formati'va,** energy manifesting itself in the formation of new tissue to replace that which has been destroyed. **v. in si'tu,** power or force inherent in a particular tissue. **v. medica'trix natu'rae,** the healing power of nature; the natural curative power inherent in the organism. **v. vi'tae, v. vita'lis,** the vital, or life, force.

viscera (vis'er-ah) [L.] plural of *viscus.*

viscerad (vis'er-ad) toward the viscera.

visceral (vis'er-al) [L. *visceralis,* from *viscus* a viscus] pertaining to a viscus.

visceralgia (vis"er-al'je-ah) [L. *viscus* viscus + Gr. *algos* pain + *-ia*] pain in the viscera or in any bodily organ.

visceralism (vis'er-al-izm) the opinion that the viscera are the principal seats of disease.

viscerimotor (vis"er-ĭ-mo'tor) [L. *viscus* viscus + *motor* mover] conveying motor impulses to a viscus.

viscero- [L. *viscus,* pl. *viscera*] a combining form denoting relationship to the organs (viscera) of the body.

viscerocranium (vis"er-o-kra'ne-um) that part of the skull which is derived from the branchial arches.

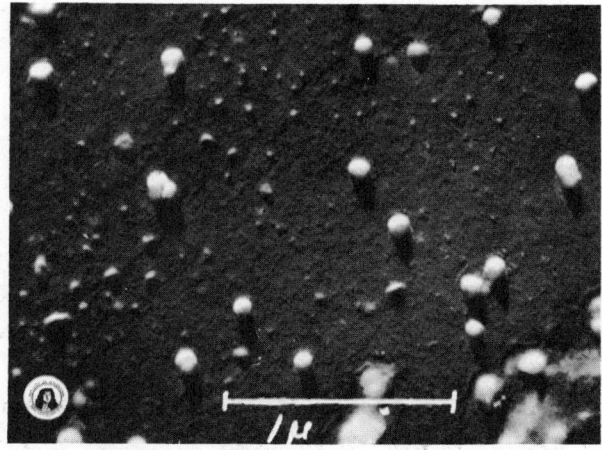

Influenza virus. (Williams and Wyckoff, S.A.B. LS-136.)

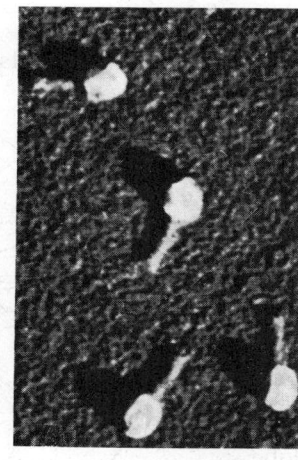

Bacteriophage (T₂) of *Escherichia coli.*
(Williams and Frazer, Virology, vol. 2.)

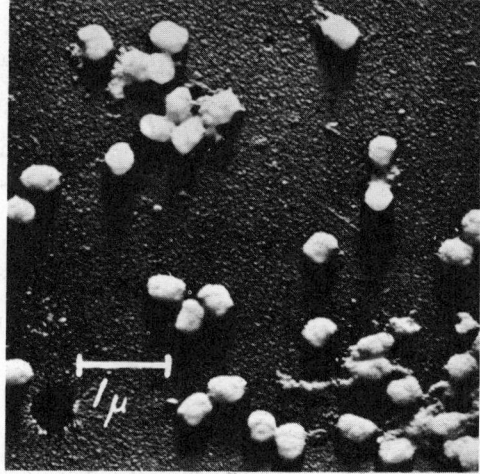

Vaccinia virus. (G. G. Sharp, S.A.B. LS-142.)

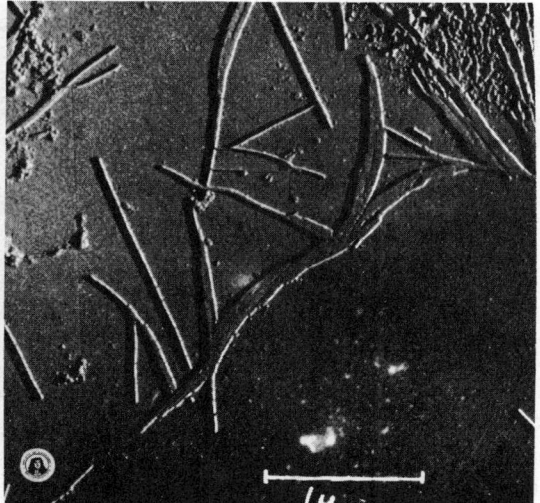

Tobacco mosaic virus. (Williams and Wyckoff, S.A.B.
LS-135.)

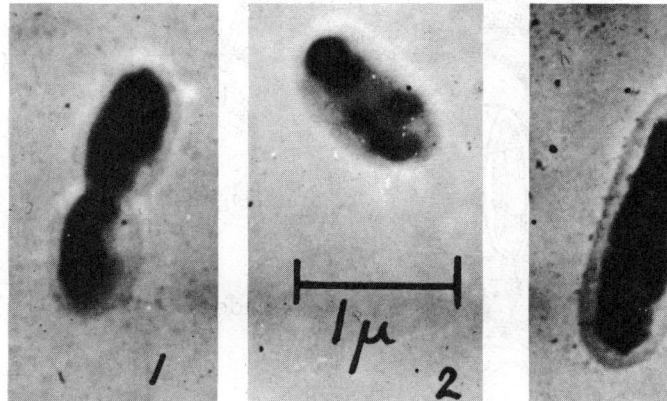
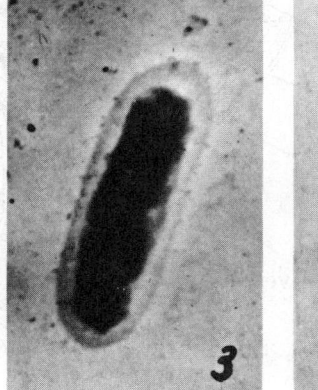
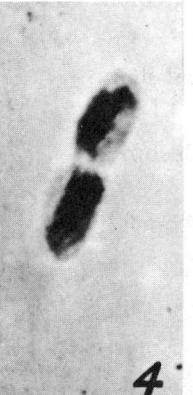

Rickettsiae: *1,* epidemic typhus fever; *2,* endemic typhus fever; *3,* Rocky Mountain spotted fever;
4, American Q fever. (Plotz, Smadel, Anderson, and Chambers, S.A.B. LS-25.)

ELECTRON MICROGRAPHS OF VIRUSES AND RICKETTSIAE

Plate LV

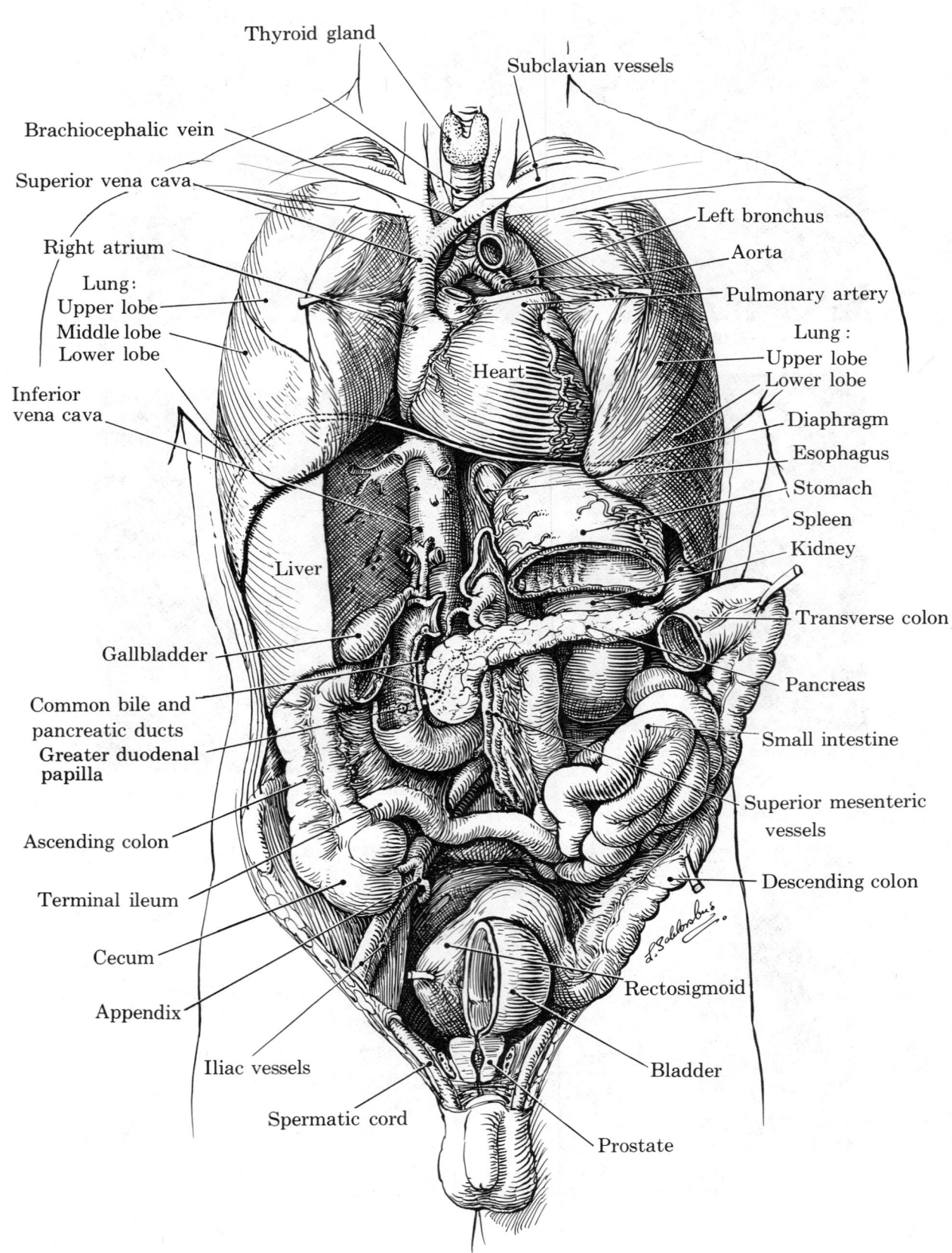

Thyroid gland

Subclavian vessels

Brachiocephalic vein

Superior vena cava

Left bronchus

Aorta

Right atrium

Pulmonary artery

Lung:
Upper lobe
Middle lobe
Lower lobe

Heart

Lung:
Upper lobe
Lower lobe

Inferior
vena cava

Diaphragm

Esophagus

Stomach

Spleen

Kidney

Liver

Transverse colon

Gallbladder

Pancreas

Common bile and
pancreatic ducts
Greater duodenal
papilla

Small intestine

Superior mesenteric
vessels

Ascending colon

Descending colon

Terminal ileum

Cecum

Appendix

Rectosigmoid

Iliac vessels

Bladder

Spermatic cord

Prostate

THORACIC AND ABDOMINAL VISCERA

viscerography (vis″er-og′rah-fe) roentgenography of the viscera.

visceroinhibitory (vis″er-o-in-hib′ĭ-tor″e) inhibiting the essential movements of any viscus or organ.

visceromegaly (vis″er-o-meg′ah-le) [*viscero-* + Gr. *megas* large] enlargement of the viscera; organomegaly.

visceromotor (vis″er-o-mo′tor) concerned in the essential movements of the viscera.

visceroparietal (vis″er-o-pah-ri′ĕ-tal) pertaining to the viscera and the abdominal wall.

visceroperitoneal (vis″er-o-per″ĭ-to-ne′al) pertaining to the viscera and the peritoneum.

visceropleural (vis″er-o-ploor′al) pertaining to both the viscera and the pleura.

visceroptosis (vis″er-op-to′sis) [L. *viscus* viscus + Gr. *ptōsis* fall] splanchnoptosis.

viscerosensory (vis″er-o-sen′so-re) pertaining to sensation in the viscera.

visceroskeletal (vis″er-o-skel′e-tal) pertaining to the visceral skeleton.

viscerosomatic (vis″er-o-so-mat′ik) pertaining to the viscera and body.

viscerotome (vis′er-o-tōm) 1. an instrument designed for obtaining specimens of liver tissue from cadavers by simple puncture. 2. an area on an abdominal viscus which is supplied with afferent nerve fibers by a single posterior root.

viscerotomy (vis″er-ot′o-me) [*viscero-* + Gr. *tomē* a cutting] incision of an organ, especially postmortem excision of a portion of the liver.

viscerotonia (vis″er-o-to′ne-ah) a group of traits characterized by general relaxation; love of comfort, sociability, and conviviality; and gluttony for food, people, and affection.

viscerotrophic (vis″er-o-trof′ik) trophic and dependent upon the viscera.

viscerotropic (vis″er-o-trop′ik) [*viscero-* + Gr. *tropos* a turning] primarily acting on the viscera; having a predilection for the abdominal or thoracic viscera.

viscid (vis′id) [L. *viscidus*] glutinous or sticky.

viscidity (vĭ-sid′ĭ-te) the quality of being viscid.

viscin (vis′in) [L. *viscum* mistletoe] a glutinous principle obtainable from mistletoe.

viscogel (vis′ko-jel) a gel which on melting gives a sol of high viscosity. Cf. *liquogel.*

viscometer (vis-kom′ĕ-ter) viscosimeter.

viscometry (vis-kom′ĕ-tre) viscosimetry.

viscosaccharase (vis″ko-sak′ah-rās) an enzyme that catalyzes the synthesis of dextran and levan from sucrose.

viscose (vis′kōs) 1. a glutinous product of the viscous fermentation of dextrose or of invertin. 2. viscous. 3. a form of cellulose acetate, used in dialysis membranes, etc.

viscosimeter (vis″ko-sim′ĕ-ter) an apparatus used in determination of the viscosity of a substance. **Ostwald v.,** one which measures relative viscosity by comparing the time required for the meniscus of the solution under study to move a fixed distance with the time required for a meniscus of water to move the same distance. **Stormer v.,** an apparatus for determining viscosity by measurement of the time required, under controlled conditions, for a definite number of revolutions of a rotating cylinder immersed in the substance to be tested.

viscosimetry (vis″ko-sim′ĕ-tre) the measurement of the viscosity of a substance.

viscosity (vis-kos′ĭ-te) a physical property of a substance that is dependent on the friction of its component molecules as they slide by one another.

viscous (vis′kus) [L. *viscosus*] characterized by a high degree of friction between component molecules as they slide by each other.

viscus (vis′kus), pl. *vis′cera* [L.] any large interior organ in any one of the three great cavities of the body, especially in the abdomen; see Plate LV.

visibility (viz″ĭ-bil′ĭ-te) [L. *visibilitas*] the quality of being visible.

visible (viz′ĭ-b'l) [L. *visibilis*] capable of being seen; perceptible by the sight.

visile (viz′il) pertaining to vision; recalling most readily impression of vision; a term applied to a type of individual who uses chiefly the sense of sight.

Visine (vi′sēn) trademark for a preparation of tetrahydrozoline hydrochloride.

vision (vizh′un) [L. *visio, videre* to see] 1. the act or faculty of seeing; sight. 2. an apparition; a subjective sensation of vision not elicited by actual visual stimuli. 3. visual acuity; symbol V. **achromatic v.,** a condition in which the entire solar spectrum is seen as colorless, that is, in bands of grays; it occurs in two types, cone and rod, with and without loss of central foveal function. **binocular v.,** the use of both eyes together without diplopia. **central v.,** that which is elicited by stimuli impinging directly on the macula retinae. **chromatic v.,** 1. color v. 2. chromatopsia. **color v.,** perception of the different colors making up the spectrum of visible light; it is mediated by the cones of the retina. **day v.,** visual perception in the daylight, or under conditions of bright illumination; see also *light adaptation.* **dichromatic v.,** a condition in which color perception is restricted to a pair of primaries, either blue and yellow or (rarely) red and green, the entire visible spectrum appearing either in various degrees of vividness and brightness of the effective color pair or the missing colors appearing as grays. The 150 hues discriminable in normal vision are reduced to two, with slight differences in saturation and brilliance doing duty for the varied hues. **direct v.,** central v. **double v.,** diplopia. **facial v.,** the power of judging of the distance, direction, etc., of objects in one's environment by the sensation felt in the skin of the face. **false v.,** pseudoblepsia. **finger v.,** the alleged ability to perceive colors and receive other sensations ordinarily elicited by visual stimuli, as a result of stimuli received through the skin of the fingertips. **foveal v.,** central v. **half v.,** hemianopia. **halo v.,** perception of a colored halo about a light source, one of the symptoms of glaucoma. **haploscopic v.,** stereoscopic v. **indirect v.,** peripheral v. **iridescent v.,** halo v. **low v.,** impairment of vision such that there is significant visual handicap but also significant usable residual vision; such impairment may involve visual acuity, visual fields, or ocular motility. **monocular v.,** vision with one eye. **multiple v.,** polyopia. **night v.,** visual perception in the darkness of night, or under conditions of reduced illumination; see also *dark adaptation.* **v. nul,** the existence of scotomas in the field of vision of which the patient is not aware. **v. obscure,** the existence of scotomas in the field of vision of which the patient is aware. **oscillating v.,** oscillopsia. **peripheral v.,** that which is elicited by stimuli falling on areas of the retina distant from the macula. **photopic v.,** day v. **Pick's v.,** a visual condition in which objects lose their normal horizontal-vertical alignment and converge toward or diverge from one another. **pseudoscopic v.,** the reverse of stereoscopic vision, an object appearing not as a solid body, but as a hollow one. **rainbow v.,** halo v. **rod v.,** vision in which the cones of the retina play little or no part, as in scotopic vision. **scoterythrous v.,** a form of anomalous color vision in which there is failure of perception of wavelengths at the red end of the spectrum. **scotopic v.,** night v. **shaft v.,** tunnel v. **solid v.,** stereoscopic v. **stereoscopic v.,** perception of the relief of objects or of their depth; vision in which objects are perceived as having three dimensions, and not merely as two-dimensional pictures. **triple v.,** the perception of three images of a single object; triplopia. **tunnel v.,** a condition characterized by great reduction in the visual field, as though the subject were looking through a long tunnel. **twilight v.,** night v. **violet v.,** ianthinopsia. **word v.,** the ability to perceive printed or written words.

visna (vis′nah) a viral disease of sheep affecting primarily the central nervous system, characterized by insidious onset and paresis of the hind limbs which progresses to total paralysis and death.

Vistaril (vis′tah-ril) trademark for preparations of hydroxyzine.

visual (vizh′u-al) [L. *visualis,* from *videre* to see] 1. pertaining to vision or sight. 2. a person in whom the visual centers are predominant in memory and learning.

visualization (vizh″u-al-i-za′shun) the act of viewing, or of achieving a complete visual impression of an object, as by roentgenography. **double contrast v.,** see *mucosal relief roentgenography,* under *roentgenography.*

visualize (vizh′u-al-īz) 1. to achieve a complete view of; to become visible. 2. to picture in the mind.

visuoauditory (vizh″u-o-aw′dĭ-tor″e) audiovisual.

visuognosis (vizh″u-og-no′sis) [L. *visus* sight + Gr. *gnōsis* knowledge] the recognition and interpretation of visual impressions.

visuolexic (vizh″u-o-lek′sik) [L. *visus* sight + Gr. *lexis* speech, word] pertaining to the visual aspects of language, as in perception of written language.

visuometer (vizh″u-om′ĕ-ter) [L. *visus* sight + *metrum* measure] an instrument for measuring the range of vision.

visuopsychic (vizh″u-o-si′kik) visual and psychic; a term applied to that area of the cerebral cortex concerned in the judgment of visual sensations.

visuosensory (vizh″u-o-sen′sor-e) pertaining to the perception of stimuli giving rise to visual impressions.

visuospatial (vizh″u-o-spa′shal) pertaining to visual perception of spatial relationships.

vitagonist (vi-tag′o-nist) a vitamin antagonist; a substance that produces deficiency of a given vitamin.

vital (vi′tal) [L. *vitalis,* from *vita* life] 1. necessary to or pertaining to life. 2. (pl.) the parts and organs necessary to life.

Vitali's test (ve-tal′ēz) [Dioscoride *Vitali,* Italian physician, 1832–1917] see under *tests.*

vitalism (vi′tah-lizm) [L. *vita* life] the theory that biological activities are directed by a supernatural force; opposed to mechanism (def. 3).

vitalist (vi′tal-ist) a believer in vitalism.

vitalistic (vi″tal-is′tik) pertaining to vitalism.

vitality (vi-tal′ĭ-te) 1. the life principle. 2. the condition of being alive.

vitalize (vi′tal-iz) to give life to.

Vitallium (vi-tal′e-um) trademark for a cobalt-chromium alloy used in dentures and in surgical appliances, prostheses, and instruments.

vitamer (vi′tah-mer) any of a number of compounds that possess a given vitamin activity, i.e., that act to overcome a given vitamin deficiency in one or another organism, plant or animal. Thus, there are biotin vitamers, niacin vitamers, thiamine vitamers, pyridoxin vitamers, A vitamers, D vitamers, K vitamers, etc. (Dean Burk).

vitameter (vi-tam′ĕ-ter) an intrument for assaying vitamins.

vitamin (vi′tah-min) [L. *vita* life + *amine*] a general term for a number of unrelated organic substances that occur in many foods in small amounts and that are necessary in trace amounts for the normal metabolic functioning of the body. They may be water-soluble or fat-soluble. See *Table of Vitamins*. **anticanitic v.**, a substance that counteracts or prevents graying of the hair; see *para-aminobenzoic acid*. **antihemorrhagic v.**, a substance that counteracts a hemorrhagic tendency; see *vitamin K* in *Table of Vitamins*. **anti-infection v.**, one that is useful in preventing infection; see *vitamin A* in *Table of Vitamins*. **antineuritic v.**, thiamine. **antipellagra v.**, niacin. **antiscorbutic v.**, ascorbic acid. **antisterility v.**, a substance that promotes fertility; see *vitamin E* in *Table of Vitamins*. **antixerophthalmic v.**, a substance that counteracts xerophthalmia; see *vitamin A* in *Table of Vitamins*. **fat-soluble v's**, those (vitamins A, D, E, and K) that are soluble in fat solvents and are absorbed along with dietary fats; they are not normally excreted in the urine and tend to be stored in the body in moderate amounts. **permeability v.**, a substance necessary to insure integrity of the capillary walls. **water-soluble v's**, all the vitamins soluble in water (i.e., all but vitamins A, D, E, and K); they are excreted in the urine and are not stored in the body in appreciable quantities.

vitaminogenic (vi-tam″ĭ-no-jen′ik) caused by or due to a vitamin.

vitaminoid (vi′tah-min-oid) 1. resembling a vitamin. 2. a substance having vitamin-like activity, e.g., a bioflavonoid.

vitaminology (vi″tah-min-ol′o-je) the study of vitamins.

vitaminoscope (vi″tah-min′o-skōp) [*vitamin* + Gr. *skopein* to examine] an instrument for measuring the time required for recovery from glare as an indication of the vitamin A reserve of the body.

vitanition (vi″tan-ish′un) nutritional disorder due to vitamin deficiency.

vitellarium (vit″ĕ-lār′e-um) an accessory genital gland found in flukes and tapeworms which secretes the yolk and shell for the fertilized egg; called also *vitelline gland*.

vitellary (vit′ĕ-lār″e) pertaining to the vitellus, or yolk.

vitellicle (vi-tel′ĭ-k'l) [L. *vitellus* yolk] the yolk sac.

vitellin (vi-tel′in) [L. *vitellus* yolk] a phosphoprotein found in the yolk of eggs.

vitelline (vi-tel′in) [L. *vitellus* yolk] resembling or pertaining to the yolk of an egg or ovum.

vitellogenesis (vi″tel-o-jen′ĕ-sis) production of yolk.

vitellolutein (vi″tel-o-lu′te-in) [L. *vitellus* yolk + *luteus* yellow] a yellow pigment obtainable from lutein.

vitellorubin (vi″tel-o-ru′bin) [L. *vitellus* yolk + *ruber* red] 1. a reddish pigment obtainable from lutein. 2. crustaceorubin.

vitellose (vi-tel′ōs) a form of proteose derived from vitellin.

vitellus (vi-tel′us) [L.] the yolk of an egg, or of an ovum.

vitiatin (vi-ti′ah-tin) a compound sometimes occurring in the urine along with creatine and creatinine; it is a homologue of choline.

vitiation (vish″e-a′shun) [L. *vitiatio*] impairment of efficiency; the perversion of any process so as to render it faulty or ineffective.

vitiligines (vit″ĭ-lij′ĭ-nēz) [pl. of *vitiligo*] depigmented areas of the skin, as those occurring in vitiligo, or the whitened lines of striae atrophicae.

vitiliginous (vit″ĭ-lij′ĭ-nus) relating to or affected with vitiligo.

vitiligo (vit″ĭ-li′go) [L.] an idiopathic, probably autoimmune, condition characterized by destruction of melanocytes in small or large circumscribed areas of the skin, resulting in patches of depigmentation often having a hyperpigmented border, and often enlarging slowly. Cf. *piebald skin* and *leukoderma*. **Cazenave's v.**, alopecia areata. **circumscribed v.**, halo nevus. **v. i′ridis**, depigmentation of the iris. **perinevic v.**, halo nevus.

Vitis (vi′tis) [L.] a genus of plants of the family Vitaceae, including various species of grape or grape vine. **V. vinif′era**, L., a species affording most of the more valuable varieties of cultivated and wine-producing grapes. Various preparations of the fruit have numerous medicinal uses by the laity.

vitium (vish′e-um), pl. *vit′ia* [L.] fault, defect. **v. conformatio′nis**, a defect in shape; a malformation. **v. cor′dis**, an

---

TABLE OF VITAMINS

Individual vitamins are listed here under their different designations (letters and subscript numbers or letters), with description or cross reference to the name of the specific compound.

v. A, a fat-soluble vitamin occurring in nature in two forms: retinol and dehydroretinol. Deficiency in the diet causes (*a*) inadequate production and regeneration of the visual purple of the retina with resulting night blindness and (*b*) disturbances in epithelial tissue resulting in keratomalacia, xerophthalmia, and lessened resistance to infections through the epithelial surfaces. Vitamin A is present in the liver oils of the cod and other fish, in butter, egg yolk, cheese, and liver as well as in tomatoes and many other vegetable foods in most of which it exists in precursor form as carotene. Vitamin A is toxic when taken in excess; see *hypervitaminosis A*. The term vitamin A is used sometimes to mean retinol alone. See *retinol* and *dehydroretinol*.

v. A$_1$, retinol.

v. A$_2$, dehydroretinol.

v. B, a member of the vitamin B complex.

v. B complex, a group of water-soluble substances including thiamine, riboflavin, niacin (nicotinic acid), niacinamide (nicotinamide), the vitamin B$_6$ group (including pyridoxine, pyridoxal, pyridoxamine), biotin, pantothenic acid, folic acid, possibly para-aminobenzoic acid, inositol, vitamin B$_{12}$, and possibly choline. Niacin and niancinamide are also known, together, as the pellagra-preventing factor, P.-P. factor, or antipellagra factor.

v. B$_1$, thiamine.

v. B$_2$, riboflavin.

v. B$_6$, water-soluble substances (including pyridoxine, pyridoxal, and pyridoxamine) found in most foods, especially meats, liver, vegetables, whole grain cereals, and egg yolk, and concerned in the metabolism of amino acids, in the degradation of tryptophan, and in the breakdown of glycogen to glucose-1-phosphate.

v. B$_{12}$, cyanocobalamin.

v. B$_{12b}$, hydroxocobalamine.

v. B$_c$, folic acid.

v. B$_c$ conjugate, folic acid.

v. C, ascorbic acid.

v. D, any one of several fat-soluble compounds, including chole-calciferol and ergocalciferol, which have antirachitic properties. Known collectively as *calciferol*, they may be produced artificially by the irradiation of ergosterol and a few related sterols. See *ergosterol*. Deficiency of vitamin D tends to cause rickets in children and osteomalacia and osteoporosis in adults. It is present in the liver oils of various fish, in butter and egg yolk, and is produced in the body on exposure to sunlight. Ingestion of excess amounts of vitamin D leads to hypercalcemia, weakness, loss of weight and other symptoms.

v. D$_2$, ergocalciferol.

v. D$_3$, cholecalciferol.

v. E, a fat-soluble vitamin necessary in the diet of many species for normal reproduction, normal development of muscles, normal resistance of erythrocytes to hemolysis, and various other biochemical functions. Chemically it is alpha-tocopherol, one of the three tocopherols (alpha, beta, and gamma) occurring in wheat germ oil, cereals, egg yolk, and beef liver. It is also prepared synthetically. Tocopherols act as antioxidants.

v. G, riboflavin.

v. H, biotin.

v. K, a group of fat-soluble vitamins (see *v. K$_1$, v. K$_2$, v. K$_3$*) which promote clotting of the blood by increasing the synthesis of prothrombin by the liver. They occur naturally in alfalfa, spinach, cabbage, putrefied fish meal, hog-liver fat, egg yolk, hempseed. Vitamin K and its synthetic analogues have an antihemorrhagic activity with a specific effect on prothrombin deficiency. They are used in obstructive jaundice, in hemorrhagic states associated with intestinal diseases and with disease of the liver, in the hypoprothrombinemia of the newborn, administered parenterally to the infant or to the mother during labor.

v. K$_1$, phytonadione.

v. K$_2$, menaquinone.

v. K$_3$, menadione.

v. L, a factor necessary for lactation in rats, L$_1$ is found in beef-liver extract, L$_2$ in yeast.

v. M, folic acid.

organic heart defect. **v. pri′mae formatio′nis**, a developmental anomaly.

vitochemical (vi″to-kem′ĭ-kal) organic; pertaining to organic chemistry.

vitodynamics (vi″to-di-nam′iks) biodynamics.

vit. ov. sol. abbreviation for L. *vitel′lo o′vi solu′tus*, dissolved in yolk of egg.

vitrectomy (vĭ-trek′to-me) [L. *vitreus* glassy + Gr. *ektomē* excision] surgical extraction via the pars plana of the contents of the vitreous chamber of the eye and their replacement by a physiological solution; done in diabetic retinopathy with vitreous hemorrhage.

vitreocapsulitis (vit″re-o-kap″su-li′tis) [L. *vitreus* glassy + *capsula* capsule + *-itis*] inflammation of the capsule enclosing the vitreous; hyalitis.

vitreodentin (vit″re-o-den′tin) [L. *vitreus* glassy + *dentin*] an unusually hard and glasslike form of dentin.

vitreoretinal (vit″re-o-ret′ĭ-nal) of or pertaining to the vitreous and retina.

Vitreoscilla (vit″re-os-sil′ah) a genus of schizomycetes of the family Vitreoscillaceae.

Vitreoscillaceae (vit″re-os″sil-la′se-e) a family of Schizomycetes (order Beggiatoales), made up of saprophytic microorganisms, found in decaying organic matter, occurring in colorless trichomes of varying flexibility, which show a gliding motion when attached to a substrate. It includes three genera, *Bactoscil′la*, *Microscil′la*, and *Vitreoscil′la*.

vitreous (vit′re-us) [L. *vitreus* glassy] glasslike or hyaline; often used alone to designate the vitreous body of the eye (corpus vitreum [NA]). **detached v.**, vitreous separated from its attachments, as from the retina. **primary v.**, the earliest vitreous in the embryo, formed from a mass of ectodermal and mesodermal fibrils and vascularized by the proliferating hyaloid system. It ceases to be formed when the hyaline capsule of the lens is formed, and is then enveloped by secondary vitreous. **primary persistent hyperplastic v.**, a congenital anomaly, usually unilateral, due to persistence of embryonic remnants of the fibromuscular tunic of the eye and part of the hyaloid vascular system. Clinically, there is a white pupil, elongated ciliary processes, and often microphthalmia; the lens, although clear initially, may become completely opaque. **secondary v.**, embryonic vitreous composed of densely packed fine fibrils formed around the primary vitreous by the inner layer of the optic cup. **tertiary v.**, embryonic zonular fibers derived from the primary vitreous and the basement membrane of the nonpigmented epithelium of the ciliary body; the fibers eventually attach to the lens capsule, giving rise to the zonule of Zinn.

vitreum (vit′re-um) the vitreous body of the eye (corpus vitreum [NA]).

vitrina (vĭ-tri′nah) [L. *vitrum* glass] a translucent or glassy material. **v. audito′ria, v. au′ris**, endolympha. **v. ocula′ris, v. oc′uli**, corpus vitreum.

vitriol (vit′re-ol) [L. *vitriolum*] any crystalline sulfate. **blue v.**, the pentahydrate form of cupric sulfate. **elixir of v.**, aromatic sulfuric acid. **green v.**, ferrous sulfate. **oil of v.**, sulfuric acid. **white v., zinc v.**, zinc sulfate.

vitriolated (vit′re-o-lāt″ed) containing vitriol; containing sulfuric acid.

vitrum (vit′rum) [L.] glass.

Vivactil (vi-vak′til) trademark for a preparation of protriptyline hydrochloride.

vivi- [L. *vivus* alive] a combining form meaning alive or denoting relationship to life.

vividialysis (viv″ĭ-di-al′ĭ-sis) removal by dialysis through a living membrane (the peritoneum). Cf. *peritoneal lavage*, under *lavage*.

vividiffusion (viv″ĭ-dĭ-fu′zhun) removal of diffusible substances from the circulating blood of living subjects by dialysis, performed by the continuous passage of the blood from an artery through a system of tubes made of celloidin immersed in saline solution, and its return to a vein, thus yielding by dialysis certain of its constituents to the fluid surrounding the tubes.

vivification (viv″ĭ-fi-ka′shun) [L. *vivificatio*, from *vivus* living + *facere* to make] the conversion of lifeless into living protein matter in the process of assimilation.

viviparity (viv″ĭ-par′ĭ-te) the quality of being viviparous.

viviparous (vi-vip′ah-rus) [*vivi-* + L. *parere* to bring forth, produce] bearing living young which derive nutrition directly from the maternal organism.

Viviparus (vi-vip′ah-rus) a genus of fresh-water snails. **V. javan′icus**, a second intermediate host of the fluke *Echinostoma ilocanum* in Java.

vivipation (viv″ĭ-pa′shun) the form of reproduction in which the embryo develops within and derives nutrition directly from the maternal organism.

viviperception (viv″ĭ-per-sep′shun) the study of the vital processes of the living organism.

vivisection (viv″ĭ-sek′shun) the performance of surgical procedures upon living animals for purposes of research.

vivisectionist (viv″ĭ-sek′shun-ist) one who practices or defends vivisection.

vivosphere (vi′vo-sfēr) [L. *vivus* alive + *atmosphere*] the region between the atmosphere above and the petrosphere below, in which life is found most abundantly; biosphere.

VLDL very low-density lipoprotein.

Vleminckx solution (vlem′inks) [Jean François *Vleminckx*, Belgian physician, 1800–1876] sulfurated lime solution.

V.M.D. Doctor of Veterinary Medicine [L. *Veterinariae Medicinae Doctor*].

vocal (vo′kal) [L. *vocalis*, from *vox* voice] pertaining to the voice.

Voegtlin's unit (vegt′lin) [Carl *Voegtlin*, American pharmacologist, born in Basel, 1879–1960] see under *unit*.

Voges-Proskauer test (reaction) [O. *Voges*, German physician; Bernhard *Proskauer*, German hygienist, 1851–1915] see under *tests*.

Vogt's angle (fōgts) [Karl *Vogt*, German naturalist and physiologist, 1817–1895] see under *angle*.

Vogt's point (fōgts) [Paul Frederick Emmanuel *Vogt*, surgeon in Greifswald, 1844–1885] see under *point*.

Vogt's syndrome (disease) (fōgts) [Oskar *Vogt*, German neurologist, 1870–1959] see under *syndrome*.

Vogt-Hueter point (fōgt-he′ter) [P. F. E. *Vogt*; Karl *Hueter*, German surgeon, 1838–1882] see Vogt's *point*, under *point*.

voice (vois) [L. *vox* voice] a sound produced by the larynx and modified by the vocal tract. **amphoric v.**, cavernous v. **cavernous v.**, a hollow sound heard on auscultation when the patient speaks; it indicates a cavity in the lung. **double v.**, diphonia. **eunuchoid v.**, a high falsetto voice in a man, resembling that of a eunuch or a woman. **whispered v.**, the transmission of a whisper to the auscultating ear, heard in pulmonary consolidation.

void (void) to cast out as waste matter.

Voigt's boundary lines (voits) [Christian August *Voigt*, Austrian anatomist, 1809–1890] see under *line*.

Voillemier's point (vwal-me-āz′) [Léon Clémont *Voillemier*, French urologist] see under *point*.

Voit's nucleus (foits) [Carl von *Voit*, physiologist in Munich, 1831–1908] see under *nucleus*.

voix (vwah) [Fr.] voice. **v. de polichinelle** (vwah″dĕ-pol″ish-ĭ-nel′) [Fr. "voice of Punch"], a variety of egophony.

vola (vo′lah) [L.] a concave or hollow surface. **v. ma′nus**, the hollow of the hand (palma manus [NA]). **v. pe′dis**, the hollow of the foot (planta pedis [NA]).

volar (vo′lar) pertaining to the palm or sole; indicating the flexor surface of the forearm, wrist, or hand.

volardorsal (vo″lar-dor′sal) from the volar to the dorsal surface.

volaris (vo-la′ris) palmar; designating relationship to the palm of the hand.

volatile (vol′ah-til) [L. *volatilis*, from *volare* to fly] tending to evaporate rapidly.

volatilization (vol″ah-til-i-za′shun) the conversion into vapor or gas without chemical change.

volatilize (vol′ah-til-īz) to convert into vapor.

volatilizer (vol′ah-til-īz″er) an apparatus for producing volatilization.

vole (vōl) a mouselike rodent of the genus *Microtus*. The field vole of Great Britain is affected by a disease resembling tuberculosis, being caused by *Mycobacterium microti*, formerly called the vole bacillus. From this organism has been prepared a vaccine for use in tuberculosis of man and cattle.

Volhard's test (fōl′harts) [Franz *Volhard*, German internist, 1872–1905] see under *tests*.

volition (vo-lish′un) [L. *velle* to will] the act or power of willing.

volitional (vo-lish′un-al) pertaining to the will.

Volkmann's canal, membrane (fōlk′mahnz) [Alfred Wilhelm *Volkmann*, German physiologist, 1800–1877] see under *canal* and *membrane*.

Volkmann's contracture, etc. (flōk′mahnz) [Richard von *Volkmann*, German surgeon, 1830–1889] see under *contracture, disease, operation, splint, paralysis*, and *spoon*.

volley (vol′e) a rhythmical succession of muscular twitches artificially induced; the aggregate of nerve impulses set up by a single stimulus. **antidromic v.**, the backfire excitation traveling centrad through the anterior root during the reflex arc.

volsella (vol-sel′ah) [L.] vulsella.

volt (vōlt) [Alessandro *Volta*, Italian physiologist and physicist, 1745–1827] the unit of electromotive force in the M.K.S. system of measurement, being the force necessary to cause one ampere of current to flow against one ohm of resistance. **electron v.**, the energy acquired by an electron when accelerated by a potential of one volt, being equivalent to 3.82×10^{-20} small calories, or 1.6×10^{-12} ergs; usually expressed in million electron-volts, or Mev.

voltage (vōl′tij) electromotive force measured in volts.

voltaic (vol-ta′ik) galvanic (def. 2).

voltaism (vol′tah-izm) galvanism.

voltammeter (vōlt-am′me-ter) an instrument for measuring both volts and amperes.

voltampere (vōlt-am′pēr) the product of multiplying a volt by a milliampere.

voltmeter (vōlt′me-ter) an instrument for measuring electromotive force in volts.

Voltolini's disease, tube (vol″to-le′nēz) [Frederic Edward Rudolf *Voltolini*, rhinologist and otologist in Breslau, 1819–1889] see under *disease* and *tube*.

volume (vol′ūm) the measure of the quantity or capacity of a substance. **atomic v.,** the value obtained by dividing the atomic weight of an element by its specific gravity in the solid condition. **blood v.,** the total quantity of blood in the body, usually expressed in liters or in liters per kilogram of body weight. **circulation v., v. of circulation,** the amount of blood pumped through the lungs and out to all the organs of the body by the heart, expressed in liters of blood flow per minute. **v. of distribution,** a dilution method for determining the volume of fluids, e.g., plasma, in a body fluid compartment. A solute (e.g., inulin) is injected into the compartment and, after it is equally distributed, a sample is taken. Then the quantity of solute removed (as by metabolism, excretion, etc.) is subtracted from the quantity administered, and the result is divided by the concentration per milliliter in the sample. **end-diastolic v.,** the volume of blood in each ventricle at the end of diastole, usually about 120–130 ml. but sometimes reaching 200–250 ml. in the normal heart. **end-systolic v.,** the volume of blood remaining in each ventricle at the end of systole, usually about 50–60 ml. but sometimes as little as 10–30 ml. in the normal heart. **expiratory reserve v.,** the maximal amount of gas that can be expired from the resting end-expiratory level. Abbreviated ERV. See illustration accompanying *capacity*. **inspiratory reserve v.,** the maximal amount of gas that can be inspired from the end-inspiratory position. Abbreviated IRV. **mean corpuscular v.,** see *MCV*, def. 1. **minute v.,** the quantity of gas expelled from the lungs per minute. Abbreviated MV. **packed-cell v.,** the number of packed red cells in milliliters per 100 ml. of centrifuged blood. Abbreviated PCV. **residual v.,** the amount of gas remaining in the lung at the end of a maximal expiration. Abbreviated RV. See illustration accompanying *capacity*. **stroke v.,** the amount of blood ejected from a ventricle at each beat of the heart. **tidal v.,** the amount of gas that is inspired and expired (i.e., ventilation) during one respiratory cycle. Abbreviated V_T. See illustration accompanying *capacity*.

volumenometer (vol″ūm-nom′ĕ-ter) volumometer.

volumetric (vol″u-met′rik) [*volume* + *metric*] pertaining to or accomplished by measurement in volumes.

volumette (vol″u-met′) an instrument for delivering repeatedly quantities of fluid in accurate predetermined amounts.

volumination (vol″u-mĭ-na′shun) the swelling of the bodies of bacteria produced by blood serum; normal serum produces a certain amount of swelling, but immune serum produces much more.

volumometer (vol″u-mom′ĕ-ter) [*volume* + Gr. *metron* measure] an instrument for measuring volume or changes in volume.

voluntary (vol′un-tār″e) [L. *voluntas* will] accomplished in accordance with the will.

voluntomotory (vo″lun-to-mo′tor-e) [L. *voluntas* will + *motor* mover] subject to voluntary motor influence.

volute (vo-lūt′) rolled up.

volutin (vo-lu′tin) bacterial polymetaphosphate occurring as cytoplasmic granules (metachromatic granules) having a marked affinity for basic dyes.

volvulate (vol′vu-lāt) [L. *volvere* to twist round] to twist or form a knot (volvulus).

volvulosis (vol″vu-lo′sis) onchocerciasis caused by *Onchocerca volvulus* (q.v.).

volvulus (vol′vu-lus) [L. *volvere* to twist round] intestinal obstruction due to a knotting and twisting of the bowel. **v. neonato′rum,** volvulus occurring in the newborn.

vomer (vo′mer) [L. "plowshare"] [NA] the unpaired flat bone that forms the inferior and posterior part of the nasal septum.

vomerine (vo′mer-īn) of or pertaining to the vomer.

vomerobasilar (vo″mer-o-bas′ĭ-lar) pertaining to the vomer and to the basilar portion of the cranium.

vomeronasal (vo″mer-o-na′sal) pertaining to the vomer and the nasal bone.

vomica (vom′ĭ-kah), pl. *vom′icae* [L. "abscess"] 1. the profuse and sudden expectoration of pus and putrescent matter. 2. an abnormal cavity in an organ, especially in the lung, caused by suppuration and the breaking down of tissue.

vomicose (vom′ĭ-kōs) full of ulcers; ulcerous.

vomit (vom′it) [L. *vomitare*] 1. to cast up from the stomach by the mouth. 2. matter cast up from the stomach; vomited matter. 3. an emetic. **Barcoo v.,** vomiting and nausea, with bulimia, occurring in southern Australia. **bilious v.,** vomited matter stained with bile. **black v.,** blackish matter consisting of blood which has been acted upon by the gastric juice, cast up from the stomach in yellow fever and other conditions in which blood collects in the stomach. **coffee-ground v.,** vomit containing dark altered blood mixed with stomach contents; see *black v.*

vomiting (vom′it-ing) the forcible expulsion of the contents of the stomach through the mouth. **cerebral v.,** spontaneous vomiting without nausea, frequently seen in intracranial disease. **cyclic v.,** vomiting recurring at irregular intervals, especially in children; called also *periodic v.* and *recurrent v.* **dry v.,** nausea with attempts at vomiting, but with the ejection of nothing but gas. **fecal v.,** stercoraceous v. **hysterical v.,** vomiting accompanying an attack of hysteria. **nervous v.,** vomiting as a symptom of gastric neurosis. **periodic v.,** cyclic v. **pernicious v.,** vomiting in pregnancy, so severe as to threaten the life of the mother. **v. of pregnancy,** vomiting occurring in pregnancy, especially the early morning vomiting common in that condition. **projectile v.,** vomiting in which the vomitus is ejected with force. **recurrent v.,** cyclic v. **stercoraceous v.,** the vomiting of fecal matter; it is seen in intestinal obstruction, appendicitis, etc., when bacterial overgrowth in the upper intestine has modified the intestinal contents.

vomitive (vom′ĭ-tiv) emetic.

vomito (vom′ĭ-to) [Sp.] vomit. **v. negro** (vom′ĭ-to na′gro) [Sp.], 1. black vomit. 2. yellow fever.

vomitory (vom′ĭ-tor″e) an emetic.

vomiturition (vom″it-u-rish′un) repeated ineffectual attempts at vomiting.

vomitus (vom′ĭ-tus) [L.] 1. vomiting. 2. matter vomited. **v. cruen′tus,** bloody vomit. **v. matuti′nus,** the morning vomiting of chronic gastric catarrh.

von Behring see *Behring.*

von Bekhterev see *Bekhterev.*

von Bergmann see *Bergmann.*

von Bezold see *Bezold.*

von Economo see *Economo.*

von Frisch (von frish), Karl Ritter. Austrian-born German zoologist, born 1886; co-winner, with Konrad Lorenz and Nikolaas Tinbergen, of the Nobel prize in medicine and physiology for 1973, for his work on the behavior of bees.

von Gierke see *Gierke.*

von Graefe see *Graefe.*

von Haller see *Haller.*

von Hippel see *Hippel.*

von Jaksch see *Jaksch.*

von Kossa see *Kossa.*

von Langenbeck see *Langenbeck.*

von Leyden see *Leyden.*

von Mikulicz see *Mikulicz.*

von Monakow see *Monakow.*

von Pirquet see *Pirquet.*

von Recklinghausen see *Recklinghausen.*

von Ruck see *Ruck.*

von Wahl see *Wahl.*

von Zenker see *Zenker.*

Vontrol (von-trōl′) trademark for preparations of diphenidol.

Voorhees' bag (voor′ēz) [James Ditmars *Voorhees*, obstetrician in New York, 1869–1929] see under *bag.*

Voranil (vor′ah-nil) trademark for a preparation of clortermine hydrochloride.

Voronoff's operation (vo′ro-nofs) [Serge *Voronoff*, Russian physician in Paris, 1866–1951] see under *operation.*

vortex (vor′teks), pl. *vor′tices* [L. "whirl"] a whorled arrangement, design, or pattern, as of muscle fibers, or of the ridges or hairs on the skin; [NA] a general term for a structure having a whorled arrangement, design, or pattern. **coccygeal v., v. coccyg′eus,** a spiral arrangement of hairs over the region of the coccyx. **v. cor′dis** [NA], **v. of heart,** the whorled arrangement of muscle fibers at the apex, in the left ventricle of the heart, through which the more superficial fibers pass to the interior of the left ventricle toward the base. **Fleischer's v.,** a rare congenital opacity characterized by ochre-colored whorls which radiate from the center of the cornea at the level of Bowman's membrane; called also *cornea verticillata.* **v. len′tis,** a spiral figure on the surface of the lens of the eye produced by the concentric arrangement of the fibers composing it; called also *nuclear arc* or *zone.* **vor′tices pilo′rum** [NA], whorled patterns of hair growth on the body, as that on the crown of the head.

Vorticella (vor″tĭ-sel′ah) a genus of ciliate protozoa of the order Peritrichida, found attached to aquatic plants and animals.

vortices (vor′tĭ-sēz) [L.] plural of *vortex*.

v. o. s. abbreviation for L. *vitel′lo o′vi solu′tus,* dissolved in yolk of egg.

Vossius lenticular ring (vos′e-us) [Adolf *Vossius,* German ophthalmologist, 1855–1925] see under *ring*.

vox (voks), pl. *vo′ces* [L.] voice. **v. choler′ica,** the peculiar suppressed voice of true cholera.

voyeur (voi-yer′) a person who practices voyeurism.

voyeurism (voi′yer-izm) a form of paraphilia in which sexual gratification is derived from watching or looking at others, particularly the genitals, or from observing sexual objects or acts.

V.R. vocal resonance.

V.S. volumetric solution.

v.s. vibration seconds (the unit of measurement of sound waves.)

V.T. vacuum tuberculin.

vuerometer (vu″er-om′ĕ-ter) [Fr. *vue* sight + Gr. *metron* measure] an instrument for measuring the distance between the eyes.

vulcanite (vul′kan-īt) vulcanized caoutchouc or India rubber, formerly used as a base for artificial dentures.

vulcanize (vul′kah-nīz) to subject caoutchouc, in the presence of sulfur, to heat and high steam pressure, producing a flexible or hard rubber, as desired.

vulgaris (vul-ga′ris) [L.] ordinary; common. See *acne vulgaris, lupus vulgaris,* etc.

vulnerability (vul″ner-ah-bil′ĭ-te) susceptibility to injury or to contagion.

vulnerant (vul′ner-ant) 1. inflicting injury or causing a wound. 2. an agent that causes injury.

vulnerary (vul′ner-er″e) [L. *vulnerarius,* from *vulnus* wound] 1. pertaining to wounds or the healing of wounds. 2. an agent that promotes the healing of wounds.

vulnerate (vul′ner-āt) [L. *vulnerare*] to wound.

vulnus (vul′nus), pl. *vul′nera* [L.] a wound.

Vulpian's atrophy, law, test (vul′pe-anz) [Edme Felix Alfred *Vulpian,* French physician, 1826–1887] see under *atrophy, law,* and *tests*.

vulsella, vulsellum (vul-sel′ah, vul-sel′um) [L.] a forceps with clawlike hooks at the extremity of each blade.

vulva (vul′vah) [L.] the region of the external genital organs of the female, including the labia majora, labia minora, mons pubis, bulb of the vestibule, vestibule of the vagina, greater and lesser vestibular glands, and vaginal orifice. See *pudendum femininum* [NA]. **fused v.,** synechia vulvae.

vulval, vulvar (vul′val; vul′var) pertaining to the vulva.

vulvectomy (vul-vek′to-me) excision of the vulva.

vulvismus (vul-viz′mus) vaginismus.

vulvitis (vul-vi′tis) [*vulva* + *-itis*] inflammation of the vulva. **diabetic v.,** vulvitis occurring in diabetes. **eczematiform v.,** vulvitis marked by the formation of vesicular pustules. **leukoplakic v.,** kraurosis vulvae. **phlegmonous v.,** see *noma.* **plasma cell v.,** Zoon's erythroplasia. **pseudoleukoplakic v.,** vulvitis in which the mucosa is whitish and opaque, resembling leukoplakia. **ulcerative v.,** a form with ulceration, pain, and lymphangitis.

vulvocrural (vul-vo-kroo′ral) pertaining to the vulva and the thigh.

vulvopathy (vul-vop′ah-the) [*vulva* + Gr. *pathos* disease] any disease of the vulva.

vulvorectal (vul″vo-rek′tal) pertaining to or communicating with the vulva and rectum, as a vulvorectal fistula.

vulvouterine (vul″vo-u′ter-in) pertaining to the vulva and uterus.

vulvovaginal (vul″vo-vaj′ĭ-nal) pertaining to the vulva and vagina.

vulvovaginitis (vul″vo-vaj″ĭ-ni′tis) inflammation of the vulva and vagina, or of the vulvovaginal glands. **infectious pustular v.,** an acute contagious nonvenereal viral disease of cattle characterized by inflammation, necrosis, and pustule formation of varying degree in the vulva and vagina; in the male, similar lesions occur on the skin of the penis. **senile v.,** see *atrophic vaginitis.*

vv. abbreviation for L. *ve′nae* (veins).

v/v volume (of solute) per volume (of solvent).

V.W. vessel wall.

W

W chemical symbol for *tungsten*.

W. wehnelt (a unit of hardness of roentgen rays).

w. watt.

Ω symbol for *ohm*.

Wachendorf's membrane (vahk′en-dorfs) [Eberhard Jacob *Wachendorf,* German anatomist of the 18th century] see under *membrane*.

wagaga (wah-gag′ah) Fiji name for filariasis.

Wagner's corpuscles, spot (vahg′nerz) [Rudolf *Wagner,* German physiologist, 1805–1864] see *corpuscula tactus,* and see under *spot*.

Wagner's disease (vahg′nerz) [Ernst Leberecht *Wagner,* Leipzig pathologist, 1829–1888] colloid milium.

Wagner's hammer (vahg′nerz) [Johann Philip *Wagner,* German physicist, 1799–1879] Neef's hammer.

Wagner's operation (vahg′nerz) [Wilhelm *Wagner,* German surgeon, 1848–1900] see under *operation*.

Wagner's theory (vahg′nerz) [Moritz *Wagner,* German zoologist, 1813–1887] see *migration theory,* under *theory*.

Wagner-Jauregg treatment (vahg′ner-yow′reg) [Julius *Wagner von Jauregg,* Austrian neuropsychiatrist, 1857–1940, noted for his research on cretinism and for treatment of dementia paralytica by malarial infection; winner of the Nobel prize for medicine in 1927] see under *treatment*.

Wagstaffe's fracture (wag′stafs) [William Warwick *Wagstaffe,* English surgeon, 1843–1910] see under *fracture*.

waist (wāst) the portion of the body between the thorax and the hips.

wakamba (wa-kam′bah) an African arrow poison.

wakefulness (wāk′ful-nes) a state marked by indisposition to sleep; sleeplessness; arousal.

Waksman (waks′man), Selman A. A Russian microbiologist in the United States, born 1888, noted for his research in the field of antibiotics; winner of the Nobel prize for medicine and physiology in 1952.

Walcheren fever (vahl′ka-ren) [*Walcheren,* a region in Holland] see under *fever*.

Waldenburg's apparatus (vahl′den-boorgz) [Louis *Waldenburg,* German physician, 1837–1881] see under *apparatus*.

Waldenström's disease (vahl′den-stremz) [Johan Henning *Waldenström,* orthopedic surgeon in Stockholm, born 1877] see *osteochondrosis.*

Waldenström's macroglobulinemia (vahl′den-stremz) [Jan *Waldenström,* Swedish biochemist, born 1906] see under *macroglobulinemia.*

Waldeyer's fluid, etc. (vahl′di-erz) [Heinrich Wilhelm Gottfried von *Waldeyer,* anatomist in Berlin, 1836–1921] see under *fluid, fossa, gland, layer, ring,* and *sulcus.*

walk (wok) 1. to move on foot. 2. the manner in which one moves on foot; see also *gait* and *walking.*

walking (wok′ing) progressing on foot, or the manner in which one moves on foot. **heel w.,** a gait marked by walking on the heels to avoid the pain of pressure upon the hyperalgesic soles of the feet in cases of peripheral neuritis. **sleep w.,** somnambulism, def. 1.

wall (wawl) the limiting structure of a space, as of the chest, abdomen, or hollow organ, or of a definitive mass of material. For official names of specific walls of various anatomical structures, see under *paries.* **axial w.,** in a cavity involving an axial surface of a tooth, that wall which lies nearest the pulp (parallel with the long axis of the tooth). **cavity w.,** a plane surface of a tooth cavity prepared to receive a restoration, being named for the surface which it faces, or most closely approximates, as buccal, distal, incisal, labial, lingual, mesial, occlusal; depending on the situation of the cavity there are also axial, gingival, pulpal, and subpulpal walls. **cell w.,** a rigid structure that lies just outside of and is joined to the plasma membrane of plant cells and most prokaryotic cells; it protects the cell and maintains its shape. **germ w.,** a ringlike thickening around the blastoderm of the bird, consisting of the advancing boundary zone at its margin. **gingival w.,** in a cavity involving an axial surface of a tooth, that wall which is nearest the gingiva. **nail w., w. of nail,** vallum unguis. **parietal w.,** somatopleure. **periotic w.,** the wall of the otic vesicle. **pulpal w.,** in a cavity involving the occlusal or incisal surface of a tooth, that wall which overlies the pulp. **splanchnic w.,** splanchnopleure. **subpulpal w.,** the exposed inner surface of the pulp chamber of a tooth after the pulp has been removed.

Wallenberg's syndrome (vahl′en-bergz) [Adolf *Wallenberg,* German physician, 1862–1949] see under *syndrome.*

wallerian degeneration, law (wahl-le′re-an) [Augustus Volney *Waller*, English physician, 1816–1870] see under *degeneration* and *law*.

walleye (wahl′i) 1. leukoma of the cornea. 2. exotropia.

Wallhauser-Whitehead method [A. *Wallhauser*; J. M. *Whitehead*, American physicians] see under *method*.

wall-plate (wahl′plāt) an electrical apparatus for giving off a current of low tension and low voltage.

Walter's bromide test (vahl′terz) [Friedrich Karl *Walter*, Bremen neurologist, born 1881] see under *tests*.

Walthard's islets (cell rests, inclusions) [Max *Walthard*, Swiss gynecologist, 1867–1933] see under *islet*.

Walther's ducts, ganglion, oblique ligament, (vahl′terz) [August Friedrich *Walther*, German anatomist, 1688–1746] see *ductus sublinguales minores, glomus coccygeum,* and *ligamentum talofibulare posterius*.

wambles (wahm′b′lz) milk sickness.

wandering (wahn′der-ing) moving about freely, as a wandering cell; abnormally movable; too loosely attached. **mind w.,** reverie, day dreaming, and similar states. **w. of a tooth,** displacement of a tooth due to destruction of the periodontal membrane by resorption or to absence of an adjacent tooth in the dental arch.

Wang's test (wangz) [*Wang* Chung Tik, Chinese physician, 1888–1931] see under *tests*.

wanganga (wan-gang′gah) a term applied to elephantoid fever in Fiji.

Wangensteen drainage, tube (apparatus, suction) (wan′-gen-stēn) [Owen Harding *Wangensteen*, American surgeon, born 1898] see under *drainage* and *tube*.

Wanner's symptom (vahn′erz) [Friedrich *Wanner*, Munich otologist, born 1870] see under *symptom*.

Wanscher's mask (vahn′sherz) [Oscar *Wanscher*, Danish physician, 1846–1906] see under *mask*.

warbles (war′b′lz) see *Hypoderma*. **ox w.,** larvae of flies of the genus *Hypoderma* (*H. bovis* and *H. lineatum*) which infest cattle of the Northern Hemisphere.

Warburg's coenzyme (war′boorgs) [Otto Heinrich *Warburg*, German physiological chemist, born 1883, noted for his research on the chemistry of respiration and on enzymes; winner of the Nobel prize for medicine and physiology in 1931] see *nicotinamide-adenine dinucleotide phosphate,* under *dinucleotide*.

ward (ward) a large room in a hospital for the accommodation of several patients. **isolation w.,** a hospital ward for the isolation of persons having or suspected of having infectious disease. **psychopathic w.,** a ward in a general hospital for temporary reception of psychiatric patients.

warfarin (war′fah-rin) [named for *Wisconsin Alumni Research Foundation*] chemical name: 4-hydroxy-3-oxo-1-phenylbutyl-2*H*-1-benzopyran-2-one. One of the synthetic coumarin anticoagulants, $C_{19}H_{16}O_4$. **w. potassium** [USP], the potassium salt of warfarin, $C_{19}H_{15}KO_4$, occurring as a white crystalline powder, having anticoagulant actions and uses similar to those of the sodium salt; administered orally. **sodium w.** [USP], the sodium salt of warfarin, $C_{19}H_{15}NaO_4$, occurring as a white, amorphous or crystalline powder, the anticoagulant action of which is of intermediate duration and cumulative; administered orally, intravenously, or intramuscularly. It is also used as a rodenticide.

Waring's method (system) (wār′ings) [George Edward *Waring*, American sanitarian, 1833–1898] see under *method*.

Warren's fat columns, incision (war′enz) [John Collins *Warren*, Boston surgeon, 1778–1856] see *fat columns,* under *column,* and see under *incision*.

wart (wort) [L. *verruca*] an epidermal tumor caused by a papillomavirus; the term is also loosely applied to any of various benign, wartlike, epidermal proliferations of nonviral etiology, as a senile wart (seborrheic keratosis); called also *verruca*. **acuminate w.,** condyloma acuminatum. **anatomical w.,** the wart in tuberculosis verrucosa. **cattle w.,** a condition of viral origin in cattle, characterized by development of nodular tumors, usually in the skin of the head, neck, and shoulders, and often on the udder. **common w.,** verruca (def. 1). **digitate w.,** verruca digitata. **flat w.,** verruca plana. **filiform w.,** verruca filiformis. **fugitive w.** (obs.), verruca plana. **Hassall-Henle w's,** hyaline excrescences in the periphery of Descemet's membrane (lamina limitans posterior corneae) occurring with advancing age. **juvenile w.,** verruca plana. **moist w.,** condyloma latum. **mosaic w.,** an irregularly shaped lesion on the sole of the foot, with a granular surface, formed by an aggregation of contiguous plantar warts. **mother w.,** a solitary wart that, after long period of slow growth, appears to give rise to eruption of many new warts. **mucocutaneous w.,** a variant of the common wart, found in the mucocutaneous junctional areas of the genitalia and anus, and occasionally of the nostrils and mouth. **necrogenic w.,** a warty lesion of tuberculosis verrucosa. **periungual w.,** a common wart occurring around the nails, where it is likely to become fissured and tender. **peruvian w.,** verruga peruana. **pitch w's,** precancerous, keratotic, epidermal tumors occurring in individuals who work in gas, tar, pitch, or various oils derived

from coal. **plane w.,** verruca plana. **plantar w.,** verruca plantaris. **pointed w.,** condyloma acuminatum. **postmortem w., prosector's w.,** tuberculosis verrucosa. **seborrheic w.,** seborrheic keratosis. **seed w.,** verruca or common wart; so called because of the minute black specks or "seeds" within it, which are actually thrombosed elongated capillary loops extending up into the substance of the wart. **senile w.,** seborrheic keratosis. **soot w.,** chimney-sweeps' cancer. **telangiectatic w.,** a misnomer for the verrucous papule of angiokeratoma. **tuberculous w.,** tuberculosis verrucosa. **venereal w.,** condyloma acuminatum.

Wartenberg's disease, etc. (wor′ten-bergz) [Robert *Wartenberg*, American neurologist, 1887–1956] see under *disease, sign,* and *symptom*.

wash (wosh) a solution used for cleansing or bathing a part, as an eye or the mouth. **eye w.,** collyrium. **mouth w.,** see *mouthwash*.

Wasielewskia (was″e-el-u′ske-ah) *Naegleria*.

Waskia (was′ke-ah) *Retortamonas*.

wasp (wosp) [L. *vespa*] any stinging hymenopterous insect of the family Vespidae, of which the genus *Vespa* is the type. Its venom contains histamine, 5-hydroxytryptamine, etc.

wasserhelle (vos′er-hel″le) [Ger. "water-clear"] see *water-clear cells,* under *cell*.

Wassermann reaction (test) (wos′er-man) [August Paul von *Wassermann*, bacteriologist in Berlin, 1866–1925] see under *reaction*.

Wassermann-fast (wos′er-man fast″) showing a persistent positive Wassermann reaction despite antisyphilitic treatment.

Wassilieff's disease (was-sil′e-efs) [Nikolai Porfiryevich *Wassilieff*, Russian physician, born 1861] leptospiral jaundice.

waste (wāst) 1. gradual loss, decay, or diminution of bulk. 2. useless and effete material, unfit for further use within the organism. 3. to pine away or dwindle. **phonetic w. of the breath,** a too rapid expiratory act, due to paralysis of a lateral cricoarytenoid muscle.

water (wah′ter) 1. a tasteless, odorless, colorless liquid, $(H_2O)_n$, used as the standard of specific gravity and of specific heat. It freezes at 32° F. (0° C.) and boils at 212° F. (100° C.). It is present in all organic tissues and in many other substances, and is the most universal of the solvents. 2. aromatic water. 3. purified water. **ammonia w.,** diluted ammonia solution. **ammonia w., stronger,** strong ammonia solution. **aromatic w.,** a solution, usually saturated, of a volatile oil or other aromatic or volatile substance in purified water, prepared by distillation or solution; called also *aqua aromatica*. **bound w.,** water in the tissues of the body bound to macromolecules or organelles. **capillary w.,** the water contained in the soil above the water table of the ground water. **carbon dioxide-free w.,** purified water which has been boiled vigorously for 5 minutes or more and protected from absorption of carbon dioxide from the atmosphere while it is cooling. **chlorine w.,** a saturated solution of chlorine in water. **cinnamon w.,** a clear, saturated solution of cinnamon oil in purified water, used as a flavored vehicle in pharmaceutical preparations; called also *aqua cinnamomi*. **w. of combustion,** metabolic w. **w. of crystallization,** that which is an ingredient of many salts, forming a structural part of the crystal. **distilled w.,** water which has been purified by distillation; called also *aqua distillata*. **egg w.,** 1. water that has bathed eggs of various invertebrates and acquired one or another substance detectable by a physiological reaction; e.g., oyster egg water may stimulate spawning of male oysters. 2. water containing fertilizin exuded from the ripe eggs of sea urchins and other aquatic animals, by which the spermatozoa are agglutinated. **free w.,** that portion of the water in body tissues which is not bound by macromolecules or organelles. **Goulard's w.,** diluted lead subacetate solution. **ground w.,** the water which lies in the depth of soils, being carried along under ground over impervious strata. **hamamelis w.,** an astringent solution prepared by maceration in water of cut dormant twigs of *Hamamelis virginiana;* called also *aqua hamamelidis* and *witch-hazel water*. **hard w.,** water that contains salts of calcium or magnesium, which resist the action of soap, so that it does not readily form lather. **heavy w.,** a compound analogous to water, but containing deuterium, the mass two isotope of hydrogen, the formula being D_2O or ^2H_2O. It differs from ordinary water in having a higher freezing point (3.8° C.) and boiling point (101.4° C.), and in the fact that it is incapable of supporting life. It is the stable isotope used as a moderator in nuclear reactors. Called also *deuterium oxide*. **Hiss' serum w.,** see *serum w.* **w. for injection** [USP], water for parenteral use, prepared by distillation, and meeting certain standards as to sterility and clarity. **w. for injection, bacteriostatic** [USP], sterile water for injection, containing one or more suitable antimicrobial agents. **w. for injection, sterile** [USP], water for injection that has been sterilized and suitably packaged. **lead w.,** diluted lead subacetate solution. **lime w.,** calcium hydroxide solution. **metabolic w.,** water in the body derived from metabolism of a food element such as starch, glucose, or fat; called also *w. of combustion*. **mineral w.,** water containing mineral salts in solution in sufficient quantity to give it special properties and taste. **orange flower w.** [NF], a saturated solution of the odoriferous principles of the flowers of *Citrus aurantium* Linné, used as a vehicle, flavor, and perfume in pharmaceutical preparations; called also *aqua aurantii florum.* **peppermint w.** [NF], a clear, saturated solution of peppermint oil in purified water; used as a vehicle in pharmaceutical preparations; called also *aqua menthae piperitae.* **peptone w.**, a solution of peptone, usually 1 per cent, used as a culture medium, especially as an enrichment medium for the isolation of the cholera vibrio. Called also *peptone water culture medium.* **potable w.**, water that is suitable for drinking purposes. **purified w.** [USP], water obtained by distillation or de-ionization, used for pharmaceutical or other purposes requiring mineral-free water. **rose w.**, a solution prepared by diluting stronger rose water with an equal volume of purified water; used as a perfuming agent in pharmaceutical preparations. **rose w., stronger** [NF], a saturated solution of the odoriferous principles of the flowers of *Rosa centifolia* Linné, used as a perfuming agent in pharmaceutical preparations; called also *aqua rosae fortior.* **saline w.**, water which contains neutral salts. **serum w.**, a mixture of blood serum and distilled water, with sugar and indicator added, used in preparing bacteriological culture mediums; called also *serum culture medium* and *Hiss' serum w.* **soft w.**, water that contains little or no mineral matter. **witch-hazel w.**, hamamelis w.

water brash (wah′ter brash′) hearburn with regurgitation of sour fluid or almost tasteless saliva into the mouth.

waterpox (wah′ter-poks) (obs.) ground itch.

water-bite (wah′ter-bīt″) see *trench foot,* under *foot.*

water-borne (wah′ter-born″) propagated by contaminated drinking water; said of diseases.

Waterhouse-Friderichsen syndrome (wah′ter-hous frid″er-ik′sen) [Rupert *Waterhouse,* British physician, 1873–1958; Carl *Friderichsen,* Danish physician, born 1886] see under *syndrome.*

watermelon (wah″ter-mel′on) the edible fruit of the plant *Citrullus vulgaris* (Curcurbitaceae), whose seeds are the source of cucurbitol and cucurbocitrin.

waters (wah′terz) a popular name for the amniotic fluid.

watershed (wah′ter-shed) a ridge which directs drainage toward either side. **abdominal w's**, the ridges formed in the supine position by the forward projection of the lumbar vertebrae and the projecting brim of the pelvis, causing free effusions to gravitate into the lumbar fossae and pelvis.

Watkins' operation (wot′kinz) [Thomas James *Watkins,* gynecologist in Chicago, 1863–1925] see under *operation.*

Watson (wot′son), James Dewey. United States biochemist, born 1928; co-winner, with Maurice Wilkins and Francis Crick, of the Nobel prize in medicine and physiology for 1962, for the discovery of the molecular structure of deoxyribonucleic acid.

Watson-Crick helix (wat′son-krik) [James Dewey *Watson;* Francis Harry Compton *Crick,* English biochemist, born 1916] see under *helix.*

Watson-Schwartz test (wot′son-shwarts) [Cecil James *Watson,* American physician, born 1901; Samuel *Schwartz,* American physician, born 1916] see under *tests.*

Watsonius watsoni (wot-so′ne-us wot-so′ni) [Malcolm *Watson,* British physician, 1873–1955] a pear-shaped amphistome trematode found in the intestines of man and monkeys in Africa; called also *Amphistoma watsoni.*

watt (wot) [after James *Watt,* 1736–1819] a unit of electric power, being the work done at the rate of 1 joule per second. It is equivalent to a current of 1 ampere under a pressure of 1 volt.

wattage (wot′ij) the power output or consumption of an electrical device expressed in watts.

watt-hour (wot′our) a unit of electrical work or energy, equal to the wattage multiplied by the time in hours.

wattmeter (wot′me-ter) an instrument for measuring electric activity in watts.

wave (wāv) a uniformly advancing disturbance in which the parts moved undergo a double oscillation; any wavelike pattern. **a w.**, see *phlebogram.* **alpha w's**, brain waves in the electroencephalogram which have a frequency of 8 to 13 per second; they are typical of the normal person awake and in a quiet resting state, and occur principally in the occipital region. **anacrotic w., anadicrotic w.**, see under *pulse.* **beta w's**, brain waves in the electroencephalogram, which have a frequency of 18 to 30 per second; they are typical during periods of intense activity of the nervous system, and occur principally in the parietal and frontal regions. **brain w's**, the fluctuations of electrical potential in the brain, as recorded by electroencephalography. See *alpha, beta, delta,* and *theta w's.* Some observers distinguish three types of waves: (1) *trains,* which correspond to alpha waves; (2) *spindles,* short series with a frequency of 14 per second; and (3) *random w's,* irregular changes of potential with no fixed frequency which appear at the beginning of sleep. **c w.**, see *phlebogram.* **catacrotic w., catadicrotic w.**, see under *pulse.* **contraction w.**, the wave of progression of the contraction in a muscle from the point of stimulation; also the graphic representation of

a contracting muscle. **delta w's**, 1. waves in the electroencephalogram which have a frequency below 3½ per second; they are typical in deep sleep, in infancy, and in serious brain disorders. 2. an early QRS vector in the electrocardiogram characteristic of Wolff- Parkinson-White syndrome. **dicrotic w.**, 1. the second portion of the arterial pulse or arterial pressure recording after the dicrotic notch and aortic valve closure. 2. recoil wave. **electroencephalographic w's**, see *brain w's.* **electromagnetic w's**, the entire series of ethereal waves which are similar in character, and which move with the velocity of light, but which vary enormously in wavelength. The unbroken series is known from the hertzian waves used in radio transmission which may be miles in length (one mile equals 1.6×10^5 cm.) through heat and light, the ultraviolet, roentgen rays, and the gamma rays of radium to the cosmic rays, the wavelength of which may be as short as 0.0004 of an Angström unit (4×10^{-12} cm.). **Erb's w's**, undulations in a muscle stimulated by a moderately powerful constant current; sometimes seen in myotonia congenita. **excitation w.**, an electric wave flowing from a muscle just previous to its contraction. **F w's**, a series of rapid minute waves in the venous pulse in atrial flutter. **fibrillary w's**, small irregular deflections in the electrocardiogram in atrial fibrillation. **h w.**, see *phlebogram.* **hertzian w's**, electromagnetic waves resembling light waves, but having greater wavelength; they are used in wireless telegraphy. **Liesegang's w's**, see under *phenomenon.* **light w's**, the electromagnetic waves that produce sensations in the retina; see *light.* **longitudinal w.**, one in which the oscillatory motion is parallel to the direction of propagation of the wave. **P w.**, a deflection in the electrocardiogram produced by excitation of the atria; see *electrocardiogram.* **papillary w., percussion w.**, the chief ascending portion of a sphygmographic tracing. **phrenic w.**, see *diaphragm phenomenon,* under *phenomenon.* **pulse w.**, the elevation of the pulse felt by the finger or shown graphically in a recording of pulse or pressure. **Q w.**, in the QRS complex, the initial downward (negative) deflection, related to the initial phase of depolarization (excitation) of the ventricular myocardium; see *electrocardiogram.* **R w.**, the initial upward deflection of the QRS complex, following the Q wave in the normal electrocardiogram. See *electrocardiogram.* **radio w's**, electromagnetic radiation of wavelength between 10^{-1} and 10^6 cm. and frequency of about 10^{11} to 10^4 cps. **random w's**, see *brain w's.* **recoil w.**, the second of the two principal waves of a dicrotic pulse, attributed to the reflected impulse of the closure of the aortic valves. **S w.**, a downward deflection of the QRS complex following the R wave in the normal electrocardiogram. See *electrocardiogram.* **short w.**, a wave having a wavelength of 60 meters or less. **sine w.**, the wave form of an alternating current characterized by a rise from zero to maximum positive potential, descending back through zero to its maximum negative value, and then rising back to zero. **sonic w's**, audible sound waves. **stimulus w.**, the wave which passes along a muscle as a result of a stimulus applied at a certain point. **supersonic w's**, a term applied to waves similar to ordinary sound waves but of frequencies from 200,000 to 1,500,000 cycles per second; they are highly destructive to some organisms and some chemical substances. **T w.**, the second major deflection of the normal electrocardiogram, reflecting the potential variations occurring with repolarization of the ventricles; see *electrocardiogram.* **theta w's**, brain waves in the electroencephalogram which have a frequency of 4 to 7 per second; they occur mainly in children but also in adults during periods of emotional stress. **tidal w.**, the sphygmographic wave next after the percussion wave; the second elevation of the sphygmographic tracing between the percussion wave and the dicrotic elevation. **transverse w.**, one in which the oscillatory motion is perpendicular to the direction of propagation of the wave. **Traube-Hering w's**, rhythmical rises and falls in the arterial pressure, attributed to rhythmical activity of the vasoconstrictor center. **tricrotic w.**, a third wave in the sphygmographic curve in addition to the tidal and dicrotic waves, occurring during systole. **U w.**, see *electrocardiogram.* **ultrashort w.**, an electromagnetic wave of wavelength of less than 10 meters; called also *microwave.* **ultrasonic w's**, waves similar to sound waves but of such high frequency that the human ear does not perceive them as sound; see *ultrasonics.* **v w.**, see *phlebogram.* **ventricular w.**, the part of the tracing of the venous pulse occurring during ventricular systole. **x w.**, see *phlebogram.* **y w.**, see *phlebogram.*

wavelength (wāv′length) the distance between the top of one wave and the identical phase of the succeeding one. **effective w., equivalent w.**, in radiology, the wavelength of monochromatic x-rays which would undergo the same percentage attenuation in a specified absorber as the heterogeneous beam under consideration. **minimum w.**, the shortest wavelength in an x-ray spectrum.

wax (waks) [L. *cera*] a plastic substance deposited by insects or obtained from plants. Waxes are esters of various fatty acids with higher, usually monohydric alcohols. The wax of pharmacy is principally yellow wax (beeswax), the material of which honeycomb is made. It consists chiefly of cerotic acid and myricin and is used in making ointments, cerates, etc. When yellow wax is bleached it becomes white (*white w.*). **bone w.**, see *Mosetig-*

Moorhof bone w. **boxing w.,** wax used for boxing impressions for dental prostheses. **candelilla w.,** a wax obtained from the plant *Euphorbia antisyphilitica* Zucc. (Euphorbiaceae), and used as a substitute for beeswax. **carnauba w.** [NF], a wax obtained from the leaves of *Copernic'ia cerif'era* Mart., a palm of South America; used as a tablet coating agent. **casting w.,** a compound of various waxes, having controlled properties of thermal expansion and contraction, which is used in making patterns for metal castings for dental prostheses. **cetyl esters w.** [NF], a mixture consisting primarily of esters of saturated fatty alcohols and saturated fatty acids; used as a stiffening agent in pharmaceutical preparations. Called also *synthetic spermaceti.* **Chinese w.,** a hard white wax deposited by certain insects on trees, such as the Chinese ash, *Fraxinus chinensis;* also a similar wax from the plant *Ligustrum madra.* **ear w.,** cerumen. **emulsifying w.** [NF], a waxy solid prepared from cetostearyl alcohol, containing a poloxyethylene derivative of a fatty acid ester of sorbitan; used as an emulsifying and stiffening agent in pharmaceutical preparations. **grave w.,** adipocere. **Horsley's w.,** a mixture of wax, petrolatum, and phenol, used for packing small bone cavities, as in the bones of the skull, and for controlling bleeding from them. **inlay w.,** wax used in preparation of the pattern from which a dental inlay is cast, the main ingredient generally being paraffin, with other natural sources from mineral or vegetable sources. **Japan w.,** a fat from the fruit of *Myri'ca cerif'era* L. (Myricaceae) and other species of the same genus. **Mosetig-Moorhof bone w.,** a preparation for filling sterile bone cavities; it consists of equal parts of spermaceti and oil of sesame, which are sterilized in a water bath. To 60 parts of this is added 40 parts of iodoform. **palm w.,** 1. carnauba wax. 2. a wax from *Cerox'ylon andic'ola,* a South American palm. **tubercle bacillus w.,** a complex phosphatide extracted from *Mycobacterium tuberculosis.* **vegetable w.,** a waxy substance, resembling beeswax, derived from various vegetable sources. **white w.** [NF], the bleached, purified wax from the honeycomb of the bee, *Apis mellifera,* used as an ingredient in several ointments. **yellow w.** [NF], the purified wax from the honeycomb of the bee *Apis mellifera;* used as a stiffening agent in pharmaceutical preparations and as an ingredient of yellow ointment. It was formerly used internally, in the treatment of diarrhea. Called also *beeswax* and *cera flava.*

waxing (wak'sing) the shaping of a wax pattern or the wax base of a trial denture into the contours desired; spoken of also as *waxing up.*

Wb weber.

W.B.C. white blood cell; white blood [cell] count (see *blood count,* under *count*).

wean (wēn) to discontinue the breast feeding of an infant, with substitution of other feeding habits.

weanling (wēn'ling) 1. newly changed to nourishment other than breast feeding. 2. an animal newly changed to other forms of nourishment than breast feeding.

weasand (we'zand) the trachea.

web (web) a tissue or membrane. **esophageal w.,** a congenital, soft, weblike stricture of the esophagus, usually of the lower portion, resulting in dysphagia. **laryngeal w.,** the most common congenital malformation of the larynx, it may be a thin, translucent diaphragm or thicker and more fibrotic; it is spread between the vocal folds near the anterior commissure and may cause obstruction, hoarseness, aphonia, etc. **subsynaptic w.,** a system of filaments or fine canaliculi which have been observed to penetrate at a varying distance into the postsynaptic cell. **terminal w.,** a feltwork of fine filaments in the cytoplasm immediately beneath the free surface of certain epithelial cells, especially those with a brush border of microvilli, such as the absorptive cells of the intestines and the hair cells of the inner ear; it is thought to have a supportive or cytoskeletal function.

webbed (webd) connected by a membrane.

weber (web'er) a unit of magnetic flux which, linking a circuit of one turn, produces in it an electromotive force of one volt as it is reduced to zero at a uniform rate in one second. In SI, it replaces the maxwell. Abbreviated Wb.

Weber's corpuscle (organ), glands, zone (va'berz) [Moritz Ignatz *Weber,* German anatomist, 1795–1875] see under *gland,* and see *utriculus prostaticus* and *zona orbicularis articulationis coxae.*

Weber's disease (web'erz) [Frederick Parkes *Weber,* British physician, 1863–1962] 1. localized epidermolysis bullosa. 2. Sturge-Weber syndrome.

Weber's douche (va'berz) [Theodor *Weber,* German physician, 1829–1914] see under *douche.*

Weber's law, paradox, test (va'berz) [Ernest Heinrich *Weber,* German anatomist and physiologist, 1795–1878] see under *law, paradox,* and *tests* (def. 1 and 2).

Weber's sign (symptom), syndrome (paralysis) (web'erz) [Sir Hermann David *Weber,* London physician, 1823–1918] see under *sign* and *syndrome.*

Weber's test (va'berz) [Friedrich Eugen *Weber,* German otologist, 1832–1891] see under *tests.*

Weber-Christian disease (panniculitis, syndrome) (web'er-kris'chan) [F. P. *Weber;* Henry Asbury *Christian,* American physician, 1876–1951] relapsing febrile nodular nonsuppurative panniculitis.

Weber-Fechner law (va'ber-fek'ner) [Ernest Heinrich *Weber;* Gustav Theodor *Fechner,* Prussian natural philosopher, 1801–1887] see under *law.*

Webster's operation (web'sterz) [John Clarence *Webster,* American gynecologist, 1863–1950] see under *operation.*

Webster's test (web'sterz) [John *Webster,* London chemist, 1878–1927] see under *tests.*

WEE western equine encephalomyelitis.

Weeks' bacillus (wēks) [John Elmer *Weeks,* New York ophthalmologist, 1853–1949] *Hemophilus aegyptius.*

weep (wēp) to slowly exude clear serum.

Wegner's disease, sign (veg'nerz) [Friedrich Rudolf Georg *Wegner,* German pathologist, born 1843] see under *disease* and *sign.*

wehnelt (va'nelt) the unit of hardness or penetrating ability of roentgen rays. Abbreviated W.

Weichardt's antikenotoxin (vi'karts) [Wolfgang *Weichardt,* German pathologist, 1875–1945] see *antikenotoxin.*

Weichbrodt's reaction, test (vīk'brōts) [Raphael *Weichbrodt,* Frankfurt neurologist, born 1886] see under *reaction* and *tests.*

Weidel's test (vi'delz) [Hugo *Weidel,* Austrian chemist, 1849–1899] see under *tests.*

Weigert's law, stain (method) (vi'gerts) [Karl *Weigert,* German pathologist, 1845–1904] see under *law,* and *Table of Stains.*

weight (wāt) heaviness; the degree to which a body is drawn toward the earth by gravity. See accompanying tables of weights and measures. **apothecaries' w.,** a system of weights used in compounding prescriptions based on the grain (equivalent 64.8 mg.). Its units are the scruple (20 grains), dram (3 scruples), ounce (8 drams), and pound (12 ounces). **atomic w.,** the weight of an atom of a substance as compared with the weight of an atom of carbon-12 isotope, which is taken as 12.00000; see also *mass.* Abbreviated At. wt. **avoirdupois w.,** the system of weight commonly used for ordinary commodities in English-speaking countries; its units are the dram (27.344 grains), ounce (16 drams), and pound (16 ounces). **combining w.,** the relative weight, compared with that of hydrogen (which is considered as 1), of an element that enters into combination with other elements. **equivalent w.,** the weight in grams of a substance which is equivalent in a chemical reaction to 1.008 gm. of hydrogen. **gram molecular w.,** a quantity of a substance which has a weight in grams numerically equivalent to its molecular weight. See *mole,* def. 3. **molecular w.,** the weight of a molecule of a substance as compared with that of an atom of carbon-12; it is equal to the sum of the atomic weights of its constituent atoms. Abbreviated Mol. wt. **troy w.,** a system of weights used by jewelers for gold and precious stones.

weights and measures see *Tables of Weights and Measures.*

Weil's basal layer (zone) (vīlz) [L. A. *Weil,* German dentist of the 19th century] see under *layer.*

Weil's disease (vīlz) [Adolf *Weil,* physician in Wiesbaden, 1848–1916] leptospiral jaundice.

Weil's stain (wīlz) [Arthur *Weil,* American neuropathologist, born 1887] see *Table of Stains.*

Weil's test (wīlz) [Richard *Weil,* New York physician, 1876–1917] see under *tests.*

Weil-Felix reaction (test) (vīl-fa'liks) [Edmund *Weil,* German physician in Prague, 1880–1922; Arthur *Felix,* Prague bacteriologist, 1887–1956] see under *reaction.*

Weill's sign (vēlz) [Edmond *Weill,* French pediatrician, 1858–1924] see under *sign.*

Weinberg's test (reaction) (vīn'bergz) [Michel *Weinberg,* French pathologist, 1868–1940] see under *tests.*

Weinmannia (wīn-man'e-ah) a genus of saxifragaceous plants with an astringent medicinal bark.

Weir's operation (wērz) [Robert Fulton *Weir,* New York surgeon, 1838–1927] appendicostomy.

Weir Mitchell treatment (wēr-mich'el) see *Mitchell,* and under *treatment.*

Weisbach's angle (vīs'bahks) [Albin *Weisbach,* Austrian anthropologist of the 19th century] see under *angle.*

Weismann's theory (vīs'manz) [August Friedrich Leopold *Weismann,* German biologist, 1834–1914] weismannism.

weismannism (wīs'man-izm) [named for August *Weismann*] the doctrine of the noninheritance of acquired characters.

Weiss' reflex (vīs') [Leopold *Weiss,* Austrian oculist, 1848–1901] see under *reflex.*

Weiss' sign (vīs') [Nathan *Weiss,* physician in Vienna, 1851–1883] Chvostek's sign.

Weiss' test (vīs') [Moriz *Weiss,* Vienna physician] see under *tests.*

Weitbrecht's cord (ligament), foramen (vīt'brekts) [Josias

TABLES OF WEIGHTS AND MEASURES

MEASURES OF MASS
AVOIRDUPOIS WEIGHT

GRAINS	DRAMS	OUNCES	POUNDS	METRIC EQUIVALENTS, GRAMS
1	0.0366	0.0023	0.00014	0.0647989
27.34	1	0.0625	0.0039	1.772
437.5	16	1	0.0625	28.350
7000	256	16	1	453.5924277

APOTHECARIES' WEIGHT

GRAINS	SCRUPLES (℈)	DRAMS (ʒ)	OUNCES (℥)	POUNDS (℔)	METRIC EQUIVALENTS, GRAMS
1	0.05	0.0167	0.0021	0.00017	0.0647989
20	1	0.333	0.042	0.0035	1.296
60	3	1	0.125	0.0104	3.888
480	24	8	1	0.0833	31.103
5760	288	96	12	1	373.24177

METRIC WEIGHT

MICRO-GRAM	MILLI-GRAM	CENTI-GRAM	DECI-GRAM	GRAM	DECA-GRAM	HECTO-GRAM	KILO-GRAM	METRIC TON	EQUIVALENTS	
									Avoirdupois	Apothecaries'
1	...	...	...	...	...	...	...	...	0.000015 grains	
10^3	1	...	...	...	...	...	...	...	0.015432 grains	
10^4	10	1	...	...	...	...	...	...	0.154323 grains	
10^5	100	10	1	...	...	...	...	...	1.543235 grains	
10^6	1000	100	10	1	...	...	...	...	15.432356 grains	
10^7	10^4	1000	100	10	1	...	...	...	5.6438 dr.	7.7162 scr.
10^8	10^5	10^4	1000	100	10	1	...	...	3.527 oz.	3.215 oz.
10^9	10^6	10^5	10^4	1000	100	10	1	...	2.2046 lb.	2.6792 lb.
10^{12}	10^9	10^8	10^7	10^6	10^5	10^4	1000	1	2204.6223 lb.	2679.2285 lb.

TROY WEIGHT

GRAINS	PENNYWEIGHTS	OUNCES	POUNDS	METRIC EQUIVALENTS, GRAMS
1	0.042	0.002	0.00017	0.0647989
24	1	0.05	0.0042	1.555
480	20	1	0.083	31.103
5760	240	12	1	373.24177

MEASURES OF CAPACITY
APOTHECARIES' (WINE) MEASURE

MINIMS	FLUID DRAMS	FLUID OUNCES	GILLS	PINTS	QUARTS	GALLONS	EQUIVALENTS		
							CUBIC INCHES	MILLILITERS	CUBIC CENTIMETERS
1	0.0166	0.002	0.0005	0.00013	.....	.....	0.00376	0.06161	0.06161
60	1	0.125	0.0312	0.0078	0.0039	.....	0.22558	3.6967	3.6967
480	8	1	0.25	0.0625	0.0312	0.0078	1.80468	29.5737	29.5737
1920	32	4	1	0.25	0.125	0.0312	7.21875	118.2948	118.2948
7680	128	16	4	1	0.5	0.125	28.875	473.179	473.179
15360	256	32	8	2	1	0.25	57.75	946.358	946.358
61440	1024	128	32	8	4	1	231	3785.434	3785.434

TABLES OF WEIGHTS AND MEASURES (*Continued*)

METRIC MEASURE

MICRO-LITER	MILLI-LITER	CENTI-LITER	DECI-LITER	LITER	DEKA-LITER	HECTO-LITER	KILO-LITER	MEGA-LITER	EQUIVALENTS (APOTHECARIES' FLUID)
1	...	...	...	...	...	...	...	...	0.01623108 min.
10^3	1	...	...	...	...	...	...	...	16.23 min.
10^4	10	1	...	...	...	...	...	...	2.7 fl.dr.
10^5	100	10	1	...	...	...	...	...	3.38 fl.oz.
10^6	10^3	100	10	1	...	...	...	...	2.11 pts.
10^7	10^4	10^3	100	10	1	...	...	...	2.64 gal.
10^8	10^5	10^4	10^3	100	10	1	...	...	26.418 gals.
10^9	10^6	10^5	10^4	10^3	100	10	1	...	264.18 gals.
10^{12}	10^9	10^8	10^7	10^6	10^5	10^4	10^3	1	26418 gals.

1 liter = 2.113363738 pints (Apothecaries).

MEASURES OF LENGTH
METRIC MEASURE

MI-CRON	MILLI-METER	CENTI-METER	DECI-METER	METER	DEKA-METER	HECTO-METER	KILO-METER	MEGA-METER	EQUIVALENTS	
1	0.001	10^{-4}	...	...	...	...	...	...	0.000039	inch
10^3	1	10^{-1}	...	...	...	...	...	...	0.03937	inch
10^4	10	1	...	...	...	...	...	...	0.3937	inch
10^5	100	10	1	...	...	...	...	...	3.937	inch
10^6	1000	100	10	1	...	...	...	...	39.37	inch
10^7	10^4	1000	100	10	1	...	...	...	10.9361	yards
10^8	10^5	10^4	1000	100	10	1	...	...	109.3612	yards
10^9	10^6	10^5	10^4	1000	1000	10	1	...	1093.6121	yards
10^{10}	10^7	10^6	10^5	10^4	1000	100	10	...	6.2137	miles
10^{12}	10^9	10^8	10^7	10^6	10^5	10^4	1000	1	621.370	miles

CONVERSION TABLES
AVOIRDUPOIS—METRIC WEIGHT

OUNCES	GRAMS	OUNCES	GRAMS	POUNDS	GRAMS	KILOGRAMS
1/16	1.772	7	198.447	1 (16 oz.)	453.59	
1/8	3.544	8	226.796	2	907.18	
1/4	7.088	9	255.146	3	1360.78	1.36
1/2	14.175	10	283.495	4	1814.37	1.81
1	28.350	11	311.845	5	2267.96	2.27
2	56.699	12	340.194	6	2721.55	2.72
3	85.049	13	368.544	7	3175.15	3.18
4	113.398	14	396.893	8	3628.74	3.63
5	141.748	15	425.243	9	4082.33	4.08
6	170.097	16 (1 lb.)	453.59	10	4535.92	4.54

METRIC—AVOIRDUPOIS WEIGHT

GRAMS	OUNCES	GRAMS	OUNCES	GRAMS	POUNDS
0.001 (1 mg.)	0.000035274	1	0.035274	1000 (1 kg.)	2.2046

APOTHECARIES'—METRIC WEIGHT

GRAINS	GRAMS	GRAINS	GRAMS	SCRUPLES	GRAMS
1/150	0.0004	2/5	0.03	1	1.296(1.3)
1/120	0.0005	1/2	0.032	2	2.592(2.6)
1/100	0.0006	3/5	0.04	3 (1 ℈)	3.888(3.9)
1/90	0.0007	2/3	0.043		
1/80	0.0008	3/4	0.05	DRAMS	GRAMS
1/64	0.001	7/8	0.057		
1/60	0.0011	1	0.065	1	3.888
1/50	0.0013	1 1/2	0.097(0.1)	2	7.776
1/48	0.0014	2	0.12	3	11.664
1/40	0.0016	3	0.20	4	15.552
1/36	0.0018	4	0.24	5	19.440
1/32	0.002	5	0.30	6	23.328
1/30	0.0022	6	0.40	7	27.216
1/25	0.0026	7	0.45	8 (1 ℨ)	31.103
1/20	0.003	8	0.50		
1/16	0.004	9	0.60	OUNCES	GRAMS
1/12	0.005	10	0.65		
1/10	0.006	15	1.00	1	31.103
1/9	0.007	20 (1 ℈)	1.30	2	62.207
1/8	0.008	30	2.00	3	93.310
1/7	0.009			4	124.414
1/6	0.01			5	155.517
1/5	0.013			6	186.621
1/4	0.016			7	217.724
1/3	0.02			8	248.828
				9	279.931
				10	311.035
				11	342.138
				12 (1 lb.)	373.242

METRIC—APOTHECARIES' WEIGHT

MILLIGRAMS	GRAINS	GRAMS	GRAINS	GRAMS	EQUIVALENTS
1	0.015432	0.1	1.5432	10	2.572 drams
2	0.030864	0.2	3.0864	15	3.858 "
3	0.046296	0.3	4.6296	20	5.144 "
4	0.061728	0.4	6.1728	25	6.430 "
5	0.077160	0.5	7.7160	30	7.716 "
6	0.092592	0.6	9.2592	40	1.286 oz.
7	0.108024	0.7	10.8024	45	1.447 "
8	0.123456	0.8	12.3456	50	1.607 "
9	0.138888	0.9	13.8888	100	3.215 "
10	0.154320	1.0	15.4320	200	6.430 "
15	0.231480	1.5	23.1480	300	9.644 "
20	0.308640	2.0	30.8640	400	12.859 "
25	0.385800	2.5	38.5800	500	1.34 lb.
30	0.462960	3.0	46.2960	600	1.61 "
35	0.540120	3.5	54.0120	700	1.88 "
40	0.617280	4.0	61.728	800	2.14 "
45	0.694440	4.5	69.444	900	2.41 "
50	0.771600	5.0	77.162	1000	2.68 "
100	1.543240	10.0	154.324		

APOTHECARIES'—METRIC LIQUID MEASURE

MINIMS	MILLILITERS	FLUID DRAMS	MILLILITERS	FLUID OUNCES	MILLILITERS
1	0.06	1	3.70	1	29.57
2	0.12	2	7.39	2	59.15
3	0.19	3	11.09	3	88.72
4	0.25	4	14.79	4	118.29
5	0.31	5	18.48	5	147.87
10	0.62	6	22.18	6	177.44
15	0.92	7	25.88	7	207.01
20	1.23	8 (1 fl.oz.)	29.57	8	236.58
25	1.54			9	266.16
30	1.85			10	295.73
35	2.16			11	325.30
40	2.46			12	354.88
45	2.77			13	384.45
50	3.08			14	414.02
55	3.39			15	443.59
60 (1 fl.dr.)	3.70			16 (1 pt.)	473.17
				32 (1 qt.)	946.33
				128 (1 gal.)	3785.32

METRIC—APOTHECARIES' LIQUID MEASURE

MILLILITERS	MINIMS	MILLILITERS	FLUID DRAMS	MILLILITERS	FLUID OUNCES
1	16.231	5	1.35	30	1.01
2	32.5	10	2.71	40	1.35
3	48.7	15	4.06	50	1.69
4	64.9	20	5.4	500	16.91
5	81.1	25	6.76	1000 (1 L.)	33.815
		30	7.1		

TABLE OF METRIC DOSES WITH APPROXIMATE APOTHECARY EQUIVALENTS

These *approximate* dose equivalents represent the quantities usually prescribed, under identical conditions, by physicians using, respectively, the metric system or the apothecary system of weights and measures. In labeling dosage forms in both the metric and the apothecary systems, if one is the approximate equivalent of the other, the approximate figure shall be enclosed in parentheses.

When prepared dosage forms such as tablets, capsules, pills, etc., are prescribed in the metric system, the pharmacist may dispense the corresponding *approximate* equivalent in the apothecary system, and vice versa, as indicated in the following table.

For the conversion of specific quantities in converting pharmaceutical formulas, exact equivalents must be used. In the compounding of prescriptions, the exact equivalents, rounded to three significant figures, should be used.

LIQUID MEASURE		LIQUID MEASURE	
METRIC	APPROXIMATE APOTHE-CARY EQUIVALENTS	METRIC	APPROXIMATE APOTHE-CARY EQUIVALENTS
1000 ml.	1 quart	3 ml.	45 minims
750 ml.	1 1/2 pints	2 ml.	30 minims
500 ml.	1 pint	1 ml.	15 minims
250 ml.	8 fluid ounces	0.75 ml.	12 minims
200 ml.	7 fluid ounces	0.6 ml.	10 minims
100 ml.	3 1/2 fluid ounces	0.5 ml.	8 minims
50 ml.	1 3/4 fluid ounces	0.3 ml.	5 minims
30 ml.	1 fluid ounce	0.25 ml.	4 minims
15 ml.	4 fluid drams	0.2 ml.	3 minims
10 ml.	2 1/2 fluid drams	0.1 ml.	1 1/2 minims
8 ml.	2 fluid drams	0.06 ml.	1 minim
5 ml.	1 1/4 fluid drams	0.05 ml.	3/4 minim
4 ml.	1 fluid dram	0.03 ml.	1/2 minim

WEIGHT		WEIGHT	
METRIC	APPROXIMATE APOTHE-CARY EQUIVALENTS	METRIC	APPROXIMATE APOTHE-CARY EQUIVALENTS
30 Gm.	1 ounce	30 mg.	1/2 grain
15 Gm.	4 drams	25 mg.	3/8 grain
10 Gm.	2 1/2 drams	20 mg.	1/3 grain
7.5 Gm.	2 drams	15 mg.	1/4 grain
6 Gm.	90 grains	12 mg.	1/5 grain
5 Gm.	75 grains	10 mg.	1/6 grain
4 Gm.	60 grains (1 dram)	8 mg.	1/8 grain
3 Gm.	45 grains	6 mg.	1/10 grain
2 Gm.	30 grains (1/2 dram)	5 mg.	1/12 grain
1.5 Gm.	22 grains	4 mg.	1/15 grain
1 Gm.	15 grains	3 mg.	1/20 grain
0.75 Gm.	12 grains	2 mg.	1/30 grain
0.6 Gm.	10 grains	1.5 mg.	1/40 grain
0.5 Gm.	7 1/2 grains	1.2 mg.	1/50 grain
0.4 Gm.	6 grains	1 mg.	1/60 grain
0.3 Gm.	5 grains	0.8 mg.	1/80 grain
0.25 Gm.	4 grains	0.6 mg.	1/100 grain
0.2 Gm.	3 grains	0.5 mg.	1/120 grain
0.15 Gm.	2 1/2 grains	0.4 mg.	1/150 grain
0.12 Gm.	2 grains	0.3 mg.	1/200 grain
0.1 Gm.	1 1/2 grains	0.25 mg.	1/250 grain
75 mg.	1 1/4 grains	0.2 mg.	1/300 grain
60 mg.	1 grain	0.15 mg.	1/400 grain
50 mg.	3/4 grain	0.12 mg.	1/500 grain
40 mg.	2/3 grain	0.1 mg.	1/600 grain

NOTE—A milliliter (ml.) is the equivalent of a cubic centimeter (cc.).

The above *approximate* dose equivalents have been adopted by the Pharmacopeia, National Formulary and New and Nonofficial Drugs, and these dose equivalents have the approval of the federal Food and Drug Administration.

Weitbrecht, German anatomist in Petrograd, 1702–1747] see *chorda obliqua membranae interosseae antebrachii*, and see under *foramen*.

Welch's bacillus (welch'ez) [William Henry *Welch*, pathologist in Baltimore, 1850–1934] *Clostridium perfringens*.

Welcker's method (vel'kerz) [Hermann *Welcker*, German physician, 1822–1897] see under *method*.

well (wel) a vessel or space for containing fluid. **atrial w.**, an adjuvant device used during surgical repair of atrial septal defects. Attached to the right atrial wall, it permits blood to rise within it while the surgeon explores and repairs the defect below the surface of the blood.

Weller (wel'ler), Thomas H. United States physician and parasitologist, born 1915; co-winner, with John F. Enders and Frederick C. Robbins, of the Nobel prize in medicine and physiology for 1954, for the discovery that poliomyelitis viruses multiply in human tissue.

weltmerism (welt'mer-izm) [Sidney A. *Weltmer*] an obsolete system of treatment based on suggestion and aiming to bring the mind and body into harmony; it was devised by Sidney Weltmer, who coined such words as *neropathy* and *manual gerocomia* to denote the laying on of hands.

wen (wen) 1. epidermal cyst. 2. pilar cyst.

Wenckebach's disease, period (ven'kĕ-bahks) [Karel Frederik *Wenckebach*, Dutch internist in Vienna, 1864–1940] see *cardioptosis*, and see under *period*.

Wender's test (ven'derz) [Neumann *Wender*, Austrian chemist] see under *tests*.

Wenzell's test (wen'zelz) [William Theodore *Wenzell*, American physician, born 1829] see under *tests*.

Werdnig-Hoffmann paralysis (atrophy, disease, syndrome, type) (verd'nig-hof'man) [Guido *Werdnig*, Austrian neurologist; Ernst *Hoffmann*, German neurologist, born 1868] see under *paralysis*.

Werlhof's disease (verl'hofs) [Paul Gottlieb *Werlhof*, German physician, 1699–1767] idiopathic thrombocytopenic purpura.

Werner-His disease (ver'ner-his') [Heinrich *Werner*, German physician, born 1874; William *His*, Jr., German physician, 1863–1934] trench fever.

Wernicke's aphasia, etc. (ver'nĭ-kez) [Karl *Wernicke*, German neurologist, 1848–1905] see under *aphasia, area, disease, fissure, reaction syndrome*, and *triangle*.

Wernicke-Mann hemiplegia (type) (ver'nĭ-kĕ-mahn) [Karl *Wernicke*; Ludwig *Mann*, German neurologist, 1866–1936] see under *hemiplegia*.

Wertheim's ointment (ver'tīmz) [Gustav *Wertheim*, physician in Vienna, 1822–1888] see under *ointment*.

Wertheim's operation (ver'tīmz) [Ernst *Wertheim*, gynecologist in Vienna, 1864–1920] see under *operation*.

Wertheim-Schauta operation (ver'tīm-show'tah) [Ernst *Wertheim*; Friedrich *Schauta*, Vienna gynecologist; 1849–1919] see under *operation*.

Westberg's space (vest'bergz) [Friedrich *Westberg*, German physician of the 19th century] see under *space*.

Westergren method (west'er-gren) [Alf *Westergren*, Swedish physician] see under *method*.

Westphal's nucleus, sign (phenomenon, symptom) (vest'fahls) [Carl Friedrich Otto *Westphal*, German neurologist, 1833–1890] see under *sign*, and see *nucleus accessorius*.

Westphal's phenomenon, pupillary reflex (vest'fahlz) [Alexander Karl Otto *Westphal*, Austrian neurologist, 1863–1941] see *Westphal-Piltz phenomenon*, under *phenomenon*, and see under *reflex*.

Westphal-Piltz phenomenon, reflex (vest'fahl-pilts') [A. K. O. *Westphal*; Jan *Piltz*, Austrian neurologist, 1871–1930] see under *phenomenon* and *reflex*.

Westphal-Strümpell disease, pseudosclerosis (vest'fahl-strim'p'l) [C. F. O. *Westphal*; Ernst Adolf Gustav Gottfried von *Strümpell*, physician in Leipzig, 1853–1925] hepatolenticular degeneration.

wet-nurse (wet'nurs) a woman who nurses the child of another at her own breast.

wetpox (wet'poks) a disease resembling fowlpox, with lesions occurring in the mouth and frequently causing death by suffocation.

wet-scald (wet'skahld) eczema in sheep.

Wetzel's grid (wet'selz) [Norman Carl *Wetzel*, Cleveland pediatrician, born 1897] see under *grid*.

Wetzel's test (vet'selz) [Georg *Wetzel*, German anatomist, born 1871] see under *tests*.

Weyl's test (vīlz) [Theodor *Weyl*, German chemist 1851–1913] see under *tests*.

Wharton's duct, jelly (gelatin) (hwar'tunz) [Thomas *Wharton*, English physician and anatomist, 1614–1673] see *ductus submandibularis*, and see under *jelly*.

wheal (hwēl, wēl) a smooth, slightly elevated area on the body surface, which is redder or paler than the surrounding skin; it is often attended with severe itching, and is usually evanescent, changing its size or shape, or disappearing, within a few hours. It is the typical lesion of urticaria, the dermal evidence of allergy, and in sensitive persons may be provoked by mechanical irritation of the skin.

wheat (hwēt) the plant *Triticum vulgare* and its cereal grain. The grain is a source of energy and of protein which is of lower biological value than animal protein; the bran and germ of the grain contain iron, phosphorus, and vitamins of the B complex, which are lost when wheat is highly milled.

wheatmeal (hwēt'mēl) eighty-five per cent extracted wheat flour. **National w.** (British), wheatmeal to which calcium carbonate has been added at the rate of 14 ounces to every 280 pounds of flour.

Wheatstone's bridge (hwēt'stōnz) [Sir Charles *Wheatstone*, English physicist, 1802–1875] see under *bridge*.

Wheelhouse's operation (hwēl-hows-ez) [Claudius Galen *Wheelhouse*, English surgeon, 1826–1909] see under *operation*.

wheeze (hwēz) a whistling sound made in breathing. **asthmatoid w.**, a sound similar to the wheezing heard when the ear is placed close to the mouth of an asthmatic; heard in cases of foreign body in the trachea or bronchus. Called also *Jackson's sign*.

whelp (hwelp) 1. an unweaned puppy. 2. to give birth to; said of the female dog.

whey (hwa) the thin serum of milk remaining after the curd and cream have been removed. **alum w.**, a whey prepared by boiling milk with a piece of alum and removing the curd by straining. **litmus w., Petruschky's litmus w.**, whey colored with litmus to a deep purplish-red color, and used as a culture medium. **wine w.**, a preparation of milk coagulated with white wine, strained from the curd, and sweetened with sugar.

whiplash (hwip'lash) a popular term for an acute cervical sprain; acceleration extension injury of the cervical spine.

Whipple's disease, tests (hwip'elz) [George Hoyt *Whipple*, American pathologist, born 1878; co-winner, with George R. Minot and William P. Murphy, of the Nobel prize in medicine and physiology for 1934] see *intestinal lipodystrophy*, under *lipodystrophy*, and see under *tests*.

Whipple's operation (hwip'elz) [Allen O. *Whipple*, American surgeon, 1881–1963] see under *operation*.

whipworm (hwip'werm) *Trichuris trichiura*.

whirlbone (hwirl'bōn) 1. the patella. 2. the head of the femur (caput femoris [NA]).

whisper (hwis'per) a soft, low, sibilant breathing sound produced by the unvoiced passage of the breath through the glottis.

whistle (hwis'el) 1. a shrill musical sound produced by the forcing of air or steam against a thin edge or into a cavity. 2. a device or apparatus which produces a whistling sound. **Edelmann-Galton w.**, a modification of Galton's whistle once used for testing acuity of hearing. **Galton's w.**, a metallic whistle once used in testing the sense of hearing.

White (hwīt), Charles (1728–1813). English surgeon and obstetrician, whose *Treatise on the Management of Pregnant and Lying-in Women* (1773) antedated the work of Semmelweis in its appeal for surgical cleanliness to combat puerperal fever.

white (hwīt) reflecting all the rays of the spectrum; the opposite of black. **Spanish w.**, bismuth subnitrate. **visual w.**, leukopsin.

White's operation (hwīts) [J. William *White*, Philadelphia surgeon, 1850–1916] see under *operation*.

whitecomb (hwīt'kōm) favus of fowl.

whitehead (hwīt'hed) milium.

Whitehead's operation (hwīt'hedz) [Walter *Whitehead*, English surgeon, 1840–1913] see under *operation*.

Whitehorn's method (hwīt'hornz) [John Clare *Whitehorn*, American biochemist, born 1894] see under *method*.

whiteleg (hwīt'leg) phlegmasia alba dolens.

whitepox (hwīt'poks) variola minor.

Whitfield's ointment (hwit'fēldz) [Arthur *Whitfield*, British dermatologist, 1868–1946] benzoic and salicylic acid ointment.

whitlow (hwit'lo) a felon. **melanotic w.**, a malignant tumor of the nail bed characterized by the formation of melanotic tissue about the nail border and under the nail. **thecal w.**, suppurative tenosynovitis of the terminal phalanx of a finger.

Whitman's operation (hwit'mahnz) [Royal *Whitman*, New York orthopedic surgeon, 1857–1946] see under *operation*.

Whitmore's bacillus, disease (fever) (hwit'mōrz) [Major Alfred *Whitmore*, of the Indian Medical Service] see *Pseudomonas pseudomallei* and *melioidosis*.

W.H.O. World Health Organization, an international agency associated with the United Nations and based in Geneva.

whoop (hōōp) the sonorous and convulsive inspiration of whooping cough.

whooping cough (hōōp'ing kawf) an infectious disease caused by *Bordetella pertussis* and characterized by catarrh of the respiratory tract and peculiar paroxysms of cough, ending in a prolonged crowing or whooping respiration. After an incubation period of about two weeks the *catarrhal stage* begins, with slight fever, sneezing, running at the nose, and a dry cough. In a week or two the *paroxysmal stage* begins, with the characteristic paroxysmal cough. This consists of a deep inspiration, followed by a series of quick, short coughs, continuing until the air is expelled from the lungs. During the paroxysm the face becomes cyanosed, the eyes injected, and the veins distended. The cough frequently induces vomiting, and, in severe cases, epistaxis or other hemorrhage. The close of the paroxysm is marked by a long-drawn, shrill, whooping inspiration, due to spasmodic closure of the glottis. The number of paroxysms varies from ten or twelve to forty or fifty in twenty-four hours. This stage lasts from three to four weeks, after which the paroxysms grow less frequent and less violent, and finally cease. The disease is most frequently met in children, is much more prevalent in cold weather, and is very contagious. Called also *pertussis*.

whorl (hwerl) a spiral turn or twist, such as one of the turns of the cochlea of the ear, the arrangement of muscle fibers in the heart (*vortex*), or a spiral arrangement of the ridges apparent in a finger print. **bone w.,** an enostosis. **lens w.,** the peculiar bowed appearance presented by the marginal portion of the lens in meridional sections.

Whytt's disease (hwits) [Robert *Whytt,* Scottish physician, 1714–1766] see under *disease.*

Wichmann's asthma (vik'mahnz) [Johann Ernst *Wichmann,* German physician, 1740–1802] laryngismus stridulus.

Wickersheimer's fluid (medium) (vik'er-shi"merz) [J. *Wickersheimer,* anatomist in Berlin, 1832–1896] see under *fluid.*

Wickham's striae (wik'amz) [Louis-Frédéric *Wickham,* Paris dermatologist, 1861–1913] see under *stria.*

Widal's syndrome, test (reaction, serum test) (ve-dahl') [Georges Fernand Isidore *Widal,* French physician, 1862–1929] see *icteroanemia,* and see under *tests.*

Widal-Abrami disease (ve-dahl'-ah-brahm'e) [G. F. I. *Widal;* Pierre *Abrami,* French physician, 1879–1943] acquired hemolytic anemia.

Wigand's version (maneuver) (ve'gants) [Justus Heinrich *Wigand,* German gynecologist, 1769–1817] see under *version.*

Wilbur-Addis test (wil'ber-ad'is) [Ray Lyman *Wilbur,* San Francisco physician, 1875–1949; Thomas *Addis,* San Francisco physician, 1881–1949] Schneider's test, def. 2.

Wildbolz test (reaction) (vilt'bōlts) [Hans *Wildbolz,* Swiss urologist, 1873–1940] autourine test.

Wilde's cords, incision, etc. (wīldz) [Sir William Robert Wills *Wilde,* Irish surgeon, 1815–1876] see *striae transversae corporis callosi,* and see under *incision.*

Wilder's diet (wil'derz) [Russell Morse *Wilder,* Sr., American physician, 1885–1959] see under *diet.*

Wilder's law of initial value (wil'derz) [Joseph *Wilder,* neuropsychiatrist in New York, born 1895] see under *law.*

Wilder's sign (wīl'derz) [William Hamlin *Wilder,* ophthalmologist in Chicago, 1860–1935] see under *sign.*

Wildermuth's ear (vil'der-moots) [Hermann A. *Wildermuth,* alienist in Stuttgart, 1852–1907] see under *ear.*

Wilkins (wil'kinz), Maurice Hugh Frederick. English biochemist, born 1916; co-winner, with Francis Crick and James Dewey Watson, of the Nobel prize in medicine and physiology for 1962, for the discovery of the molecular structure of deoxyribonucleic acid.

Willan's lepra (wil'anz) [Robert *Willan,* English physician, 1757–1812] psoriasis.

Willett forceps (wil'et) [J. Abernethy *Willett,* London obstetrician, died 1932] see under *forceps.*

Willia (wil'e-ah) former name for *Hansenula.*

Williams' sign (tracheal tone) (wil'yamz) [Charles J. B. *Williams,* English physician, 1805–1889] see under *sign,* def. 1.

Williamson's blood test (wil'yam-sunz) [Richard Thomas *Williamson,* English physician] see under *tests.*

Williamson's sign (wil'yam-sunz) [Oliver K. *Williamson,* London physician] see under *sign.*

Willis' antrum, circle, cords, nerve, paracusis (wil'is) [Thomas *Willis,* English anatomist and physician, 1621–1675] see *antrum pyloricum, circulus arteriosus cerebri,* and *nervus accessorius,* and see under *cord* and *paracusis.*

Wilms' tumor (vilmz) [Max *Wilms,* German surgeon, 1867–1918] see under *tumor.*

Wilson's degeneration (disease, syndrome) (wil'sunz) [Samuel Alexander Kinnier *Wilson,* English neurologist, 1878–1936] hepatolenticular degeneration.

Wilson's disease (wil'sunz) [William James Erasmus *Wilson,* English dermatologist, 1809–1884] dermatitis exfoliativa.

Wilson's muscle (wil'sunz) [James *Wilson,* English surgeon, 1765–1821] musculus sphincter urethrae.

wilt (wilt) a disease of plants characterized by plugging of the conducting tissues by a fungus, resulting in wilting; potato wilt is caused by *Fusarium solanae,* banana wilt by *Fusarium oxysporum,* and apple wilt by species of *Verticillium.*

Wimshurst machine (wimz'hurst) [James *Wimshurst,* English engineer, 1832–1903] see under *machine.*

Winckel's disease (ving'kelz) [Franz Karl Ludwig Wilhelm von *Winckel,* gynecologist in Munich, 1837–1911] see under *disease.*

windburn (wind'burn) chapping of the skin caused by excessive exposure to wind.

windchill (wind'chil) loss of heat from bodies subjected to wind.

windgall (wind'gawl) a distention of the joint capsule, or of a tendon sheath in the region of the fetlock of a horse.

windigo (wind'dĭ-go) [Ojibwa] a cannibalistic monster of the mythology of Eskimos and certain American Indians; also, a psychosis involving delusions of being possessed by the windigo, with fears of becoming cannabalistic, sometimes actual cannabilistic behavior, and agitated depression. Called also *witigo.*

windlass, Spanish (wind'las) an improvised tourniquet consisting of a handkerchief tied around a part and twisted by a stick passed under it.

window (win'do) [L. *fenestra*] a circumscribed opening in a plane surface. **aortic w.,** a transparent region below the aortic arch formed by the bifurcation of the trachea, visible in the left anterior oblique roentgenogram of the heart and adjacent vessels. **aorticopulmonary w.,** aortic septal defect. **oval w.,** fenestra vestibuli. **round w.,** fenestra cochleae. **skin w.,** see under *technique.*

windowing (win'do-ing) surgical creation of an opening in the cortex of a bone.

windpipe (wind'pīp) the trachea.

windpuff (wind'puf) a swelling just below the fetlock joint of a horse, caused by a collection of synovial fluid between the tendons of the leg.

wind-sucking (wind'suk-ing) cribbing.

wineglass (wīn'glas) a measure approximately equal to 2 fluid ounces.

wing (wing) [L. *ala*] 1. either of the anterior appendages of birds, which are modified for flight. 2. a structure or part resembling the wing of a bird; called also *ala.* **ash-like w.,** trigonum nervi vagi. **great w. of sphenoid bone, greater w. of sphenoid bone,** ala major ossis sphenoidalis. **w. of ilium,** ala ossis ilii. **w's of Ingrassias,** w's of sphenoid bone. **lateral w. of sacrum,** pars lateralis ossis sacri. **lateral w. of sphenoid bone,** ala major ossis sphenoidalis. **lesser w. of sphenoid bone,** ala minor ossis sphenoidalis. **major w. of sphenoid bone,** ala major ossis sphenoidalis. **minor w. of sphenoid bone,** ala minor ossis sphenoidalis. **w. of nose,** ala nasi. **orbital w. of sphenoid bone, small w. of sphenoid bone,** ala minor ossis sphenoidalis. **w's of sphenoid bone,** the laterally projecting processes of the sphenoid bone; see *ala major ossis sphenoidalis* and *ala minor ossis sphenoidalis.* **superior w. of sphenoid bone,** ala minor ossis sphenoidalis. **temporal w. of sphenoid bone,** ala major ossis sphenoidalis. **w. of vomer,** ala vomeris.

WinGel (win'jel) trademark for a preparation of alumina and magnesia.

Winiwarter's operation (vin'ĭ-var"terz) [Alexander von *Winiwarter,* German surgeon, 1848–1916] cholecystenterostomy.

winking (wingk'ing) quick closing and opening of the eyelids. **jaw w.,** involuntary closing movements of the eyelid occasionally associated with movements of the jaw; see *Gunn's syndrome,* under *syndrome.*

Winkler's disease (vink'lerz) [Max *Winkler,* Swiss physician, 1875–1952] chondrodermatitis nodularis chronica helicis.

Winslow's foramen, etc. (winz'lōz) [Jacob Benignus *Winslow,* anatomist in Paris, 1669–1760] see under *foramen, ligament, pancreas,* and *star.*

Winstrol (win'strol) trademark for a preparation of stanozolol.

Winterbottom's sign (symptom) (win'ter-bot"umz) [Thomas Masterman *Winterbottom,* English physician, 1765–1859] see under *sign.*

wintergreen (win'ter-grēn) *Gaultheria procumbens.*

Winternitz's sound (vin'ter-nits"ez) [Wilhelm *Winternitz,* physician in Vienna, 1835–1917] see under *sound.*

Wintrich's sign (vin'triks) [Anton *Wintrich,* German physician, 1812–1882] see under *sign.*

wire (wīr) 1. a long, slender, flexible structure of metal, used in surgery and dentistry. 2. to insert wires into a body structure, as into a broken bone to immobilize the fragments, or into an aneurysm to promote the formation of clots. **arch w.,** wire applied around the dental arch; used in correcting irregularities of the teeth. **ideal arch w.,** the configuration of an arch wire that conforms as closely as possible to the desired ultimate shape of the arch for a particular individual. **Kirschner w.,** a steel wire for skeletal transfixion of fractured bones and for obtaining skeletal traction in fractures; it is inserted through the soft parts and the bone and held tight in a clamp. **ligature w.,** a soft thin wire used to tie an arch wire to band attachments or brackets. **separating w.,** wire used in orthodontics to create space between the teeth prior to banding.

wireworm (wīr'werm) *Haemonchus contortus.*

wiring (wīr'ing) the fixing into position by means of wire, as of segments of fractured bone. **circumferential w.,** a technique for fixation of mandibular fractures in which wires are passed around a section of bone with the ends exiting into the oral cavity and then around a fixed intraoral splint. **continuous loop w.,** wiring of the teeth for the reduction and fixation of fractures, by using a single length of wire to form wire loops on both the maxillary and mandibular teeth, over which intermaxillary elastics can be placed; called also *Stout w.* **craniofacial suspension w.,** wiring of noncontiguous areas of bone (piriform aperture, zygomatic arch, zygomatic process of the frontal bone) for the support of fractured jaw segments. **Gilmer w.,** a method of intermaxillary fixation in which single opposing teeth are wired circumferentially and the wires twisted together. **Ivy loop w.,** wiring of adjacent teeth in groups of two to provide an attachment for intermaxillary elastics. **perialveolar w.,** the fixing of a splint to the maxillary arch by passing a wire through the alveolar process from the buccal plate to the palate. **piriform aperture w.,** wiring through the nasal bones at the piriform aperture for the stabilization of fractures of the jaws. **Stout w.,** continuous loop w.

Wirsung's canal, duct (vēr'soongz) [Johann Georg *Wirsung,* German physician, 1600–1643] ductus pancreaticus.

Wishart test (wish'art) [Mary B. *Wishart*] see under *tests.*

withdrawal (with-draw'al) 1. a pathological retreat from external reality. 2. abstention from drugs to which one is habituated or addicted. Also, denoting the symptoms occasioned by such withdrawal.

withers (with'erz) the top of the shoulders of the horse. **fistulous w.,** a name applied to a condition occurring in horses after a dual infection of the supraspinous bursa by *Brucella* and *Actinomyces,* leading to distention and sometimes to rupture of the bursa, with suppuration.

witigo (wĭ-ti'go) windigo.

witkop (wit'kop) favus in South African Bantus; called also *dikwakwadi.*

Witzel's operation (vit'selz) [Friedrich Oskar *Witzel,* German surgeon, 1856–1925] see under *operation.*

witzelsucht (vit'sel-zōōkt) [Ger.] a mental condition characteristic of frontal lobe lesions and marked by the making of poor jokes and puns and the telling of pointless stories, at which the patient himself is intensely amused.

Wladimiroff's operation (vlad''ĭ-mer'ofs) [Russian surgeon, 1837–1903] Mikulicz operation, def. 3.

WMA World Medical Association.

wobbles (wob'b'lz) posterior incoordination in the horse, beginning with a slight swaying action of the hindquarters, or stumbling, with worsening of the condition until the animal cannot trot without rolling from side to side and falling; it is usually associated with spinal cord malacia but the cause is unknown.

Wohlfahrtia (vōl-fahr'te-ah) a genus of flies of the family Sarcophagidae. **W. magnif'ica,** a very common flesh fly of the Old World; its larvae may produce wound myiasis in man and animals. **W. o'paca,** a North American species; its larvae cause cutaneous myiasis in man and animals, especially foxes and mink. **W. vig'il,** a North American species; its larvae may produce cutaneous myiasis in man and animals.

Wohlgemuth's test (vōl'ge-moots) [Julius *Wohlgemuth,* German physician, born 1874] see under *tests.*

Wolbachia (wol-bak'e-ah) [Simeon Burt *Wolbach,* American physician, 1880–1954] a genus of microorganisms of the tribe Wolbachieae, family Rickettsiaceae, order Rickettsiales; nine species of these rickettsia-like microorganisms have been described, none of which is pathogenic for mammals.

Wolbachieae (wol''bah-ki'e-e) [S. B. *Wolbach*] a tribe of the family Rickettsiaceae, order Rickettsiales, class Microtatobiotes, made up of rickettsia-like organisms occurring symbiotically or parasitically within the cells of arthropod hosts. Many organisms previously classified in the genus Rickettsia have been assigned to this tribe, which includes three genera, *Rickettsiella, Symbiotes,* and *Wolbachia.*

Woldman's test (wold'manz) [Edward Elbert *Woldman,* American physician, born 1897] see under *tests.*

Wolfe's graft (woolfs) [John Reissberg *Wolfe,* Scottish ophthalmologist, 1824–1904] Krause-Wolfe graft.

Wolfe-Krause graft (wolfe-krowz) [J. R. *Wolfe;* Fedor *Krause,* German surgeon, 1857–1937] Krause-Wolfe graft.

Wolfenden's position (wol'fen-denz) [Richard Norris *Wolfenden,* British laryngologist of the 19th century] see under *position.*

Wolff's law (volfs) [Julius *Wolff,* German anatomist, 1836–1902] see under *law.*

Wolff-Eisner reaction (test) (volf īz'ner) [Alfred *Wolff-Eisner,*

German serologist, 1877–1948] see *ophthalmic reaction,* under *reaction.*

Wolff-Parkinson-White syndrome [Louis *Wolff,* American cardiologist, born 1898; Sir John *Parkinson,* British physician, born 1885; Paul Dudley *White,* American cardiologist, 1886–1973] see under *syndrome.*

wolffian (woolf'e-an) described by Kaspar Friedrich *Wolff,* German anatomist and embryologist, 1733–1794, as wolffian body (mesonephros), cyst, duct (ductus mesonephricus), and ridge (mesonephric ridge).

Wölfler's operation (vel'flerz) [Anton *Wölfler,* surgeon in Prague, 1850–1917] see under *operation.*

wolfram (wool'fram) tungsten.

wolframium (wolf-ra'me-um) [L. "wolfram"] (*obs.*) tungsten.

Wolfring's glands (vōlf'ringz) [Emilij Franzevic von *Wolfring,* Polish ophthalmologist, 1832–1906] see under *gland.*

wolfsbane (wolfs'bān) 1. *Arnica.* 2. *Aconitum napellus.*

Wollaston's doublet (wool'as-tonz) [William Hyde *Wollaston,* English physician, 1766–1828] see under *doublet.*

womb (wōōm) the uterus.

Wong's method (wongz) [San Yin *Wong,* Chinese biochemist, born 1894] see under *method.*

Wood's light (filter, glass) (woodz) [Robert Williams *Wood,* American physicist, 1868–1953] see under *light.*

Wood's operation (woodz) [John *Wood,* English surgeon, 1825–1891] see under *operation.*

Woodbridge treatment (wood'brij) [John Eliot *Woodbridge,* American physician, 1845–1901] see under *treatment.*

wool (wool) [L. *lana*] the hair of sheep and lambs; by extension applied to any material existing as fine threads. **collodion w.,** pyroxylin. **gut w.,** catgut shredded into fine fibers. **lumpy w.,** dermatophilosis of sheep, characterized by erythematous, exudative, scaling lesions of the skin which develop into pyramidal scabby masses; called also *wool rot.* **styptic w.,** wool impregnated with ferric chloride. **synthetic w.,** thin fibers spun from a synthetic material, such as the precipitate of milk casein.

Woolner's tip (wool'nerz) [Thomas *Woolner,* English sculptor and poet, 1826–1892] tuberculum auriculae.

word salad (werd sal'ad) a mixture of words and phrases which lack any comprehensive meaning or logical coherence to the listener.

work-up (werk'up) the procedures done to arrive at a diagnosis, including history taking, laboratory tests, x-rays, and so on.

worm (werm) [L. *vermis*] 1. any of the soft-bodied, naked, elongated invertebrates of the phyla Platyhelminthes, Annelida, Acanthocephala, and Aschelminthes. Formerly classified as Vermes. 2. any anatomical structure resembling a worm; see *vermis.* 3. the spiral tube of a distilling apparatus. **bilharzia w.,** *Schistosoma.* **bladder w.,** a cysticercus; bladder worms exist in various parenchymatous tissues of a host; being then transferred to the stomach of another host, they develop into tapeworms. **blinding w.,** *Onchocerca volvulus.* **case w.,** *Echinococcus.* **cayor w.,** the larva of *Cordylobia anthropophaga.* **w. of cerebellum,** vermis cerebelli. **dragon w.,** *Dracunculus medinensis.* **eel w.,** *Ascaris.* **eye w.,** *Loa loa.* **flat w.,** any member of the Platyhelminthes. **fluke w.,** see *fluke.* **guinea w.,** *Dracunculus medinensis.* **heart w.,** *Dirofilaria immitis.* **horsehair w.,** *Gordius.* **kidney w.,** *Dioctophyma renale.* **lung w.,** see *lungworm.* **maw w.,** *Ascaris.* **meal w.,** *Asopia farinalis, Tenebrio molitor,* and other grain beetles. **Medina w.,** *Dracunculus medinensis.* **palisade w.,** *Strongylus equinus.* **pork w.,** *Trichinella spiralis.* **ribbon w.,** see *Rhynchocoela.* **screw w.,** see *screwworm.* **serpent w.,** *Dracunculus medinensis.* **spinyheaded w.,** Acanthocephala. **stomach w.,** *Haemonchus contortus.* **thorny-headed w.,** Acanthocephala. **tongue w.,** Pentastomida. **trichina w.,** *Trichinella.*

Worm-Müller's test (vorm-mil'erz) [Jacob *Worm-Müller,* Norwegian physician, 1834–1889] see under *tests.*

wormian bones (wer'me-an) [Olaus *Worm,* Danish anatomist, 1588–1654] ossa suturarum.

Wormley's test (worm'lēz) [Theodore George *Wormley,* Philadelphia chemist, 1826–1897] see under *tests.*

wormseed (werm'sēd) 1. santonica. 2. *Chenopodium.*

wormwood (werm'wood) absinthium.

Woulfe's bottle (woolfs) [Peter *Woulfe,* English chemist, 1727–1803] see under *bottle.*

wound (wōōnd) [L. *vulnus*] a bodily injury caused by physical means, with disruption of the normal continuity of structures. **aseptic w.,** one which is not infected with pathogens. **blowing w.,** open pneumothorax. **contused w.,** a wound in which the skin is unbroken. **incised w.,** one made by a cutting instrument. **lacerated w.,** one in which the tissues are torn or mangled by a dull or blunt instrument. **nonpenetrating w.,** one in which there is no disruption of the skin but there is injury to underlying structures. **open w.,** one that communicates with the atmosphere by direct exposure. **penetrating w.,** one caused by a sharp, usually slender object, such as a nail or ice pick, which passes through the skin into the underlying tissues. **perforating w.,** a penetrating wound which extends into a viscus or bodily cavity. **poisoned w.,** one into which septic matter has been introduced. **puncture w.,** one made by a pointed instrument; penetrating wound. **septic w.,** one that is infected with pathogens. **seton w.,** one which enters and exits on the same side of the injured part. **subcutaneous w.,** one which involves only the skin and subcutaneous tissue. **sucking w.,** a penetrating wound of the chest through which air is drawn in and out. **summer w's,** see *esponja* and *habronemiasis*, and *summer sores*, under *sore*. **tangential w.,** an oblique glancing wound which results in one edge being undercut. **traumatopneic w.,** sucking w.

W-plasty a technique in plastic surgery used mainly in the repair of straight scars that require the redistribution of tension. It consists in excising a series of consecutive small triangular areas of tissue on each side of the wound or scar, and imbricating the resultant triangular flaps.

W.R. Wassermann reaction.

wreath (rēth) an encircling structure, resembling a circlet of flowers or leaves such as may be worn about the head. **daughter w.,** the amphiaster as viewed from its surface. **hippocratic w.,** the sparse peripheral rim of scalp hair which is the ultimate stage of male pattern alopecia.

Wreden's sign (vra′denz) [Robert Robertovich *Wreden*, otologist in Petrograd, 1837–1893] see under *sign*.

Wright's method, stain (rītz) [James Homer *Wright*, Boston pathologist, 1871–1928] see under *method* and *Table of Stains*.

Wright's syndrome (rītz) [Irving Sherwood *Wright*, New York physician, born 1901] see under *syndrome*.

Wrisberg's cartilage, etc. (ris′bergz) [Heinrich August *Wrisberg*, German anatomist, 1739–1808] see under *cartilage, ganglion, ligament, line, nerve,* and *tubercle*.

wrist (rist) the region of the articulation between the forearm and hand, which is made up of eight bones. See *ossa carpi* and names of specific bones. The term is also applied to the corresponding part in the thoracic limb of quadrupeds. Called also *carpus*. **tennis w.,** tenovaginitis of the tendons of the wrist in tennis players.

wristdrop (rist′drop) a condition resulting from paralysis of the extensor muscles of the hand and fingers. Called also

carpoptosis and *drop hand*.

writing (rīt′ing) the inscription of letters or other symbols, and of words, phrases, and sentences, so that they may be perceived by the eyes or, by the blind, through the fingertips. **mirror w., specular w.,** writing in which the right and left relationships of letters and words are reversed, as if seen in a mirror.

wryneck (ri′neck) torticollis.

wt. weight.

Wuchereria (voo″ker-e′re-ah) [Otto *Wucherer*, German physician in Brazil, 1820–1873] a genus of filarial nematodes (roundworms) indigenous in various countries of warmer regions of the world. **W. bancrof′ti,** a white threadlike worm which causes elephantiasis, lymphangitis, and chyluria by interfering with the lymphatic circulation. The immature forms, or microfilariae (*microfilaria bancrofti*), are found in the circulating blood, especially at night, and are carried by *Culex* and other mosquitoes. In the Pacific form of *W. bancrofti,* sometimes called *W. bancrofti* var. *pacifica*, the microfilariae do not show the nocturnal periodicity seen elsewhere. **W. ma′layi,** *Brugia malayi*.

wuchereriasis (voo-ker″e-ri′ah-sis) infection with worms of the genus *Wuchereria*.

Wunderlich's curve (voon′der-liks) [Carl Reinhold August *Wunderlich*, German physician, 1815–1877] see under *curve*.

Wundt's tetanus (voonts) [Wilhelm *Wundt*, German physiologist, 1832–1920] see under *tetanus*.

Wurster's test (vurs′terz) [Casimir *Wurster*, Dresden physiologist, 1856–1913] see under *tests*.

Wützer's operation (vet′zerz) [Karl Wilhelm *Wützer*, German surgeon, 1789–1863] see under *operation*.

w./v. weight (of solute) per volume (of solvent).

Wyamine (wi′ah-min) trademark for preparations of mephentermine.

Wycillin (wi-sil′lin) trademark for preparations of penicillin G procaine.

Wydase (wi′dās) trademark for preparations of hyaluronidase for injection.

Wyeomyia (we″o-mi′yah) a genus of culicine mosquitoes.

Wyeth's operation (wi′eths) [John Allan *Wyeth*, surgeon in New York, 1845–1922] see under *operation*.

Wylie's drain, operation (wi′lēz) [Walker Gill *Wylie*, gynecologist in New York, 1848–1923] see under *drain* and *operation*.

X

X symbol for *Kienbock's unit* of x-ray exposure.

xanchromatic (zan″kro-mat′ik) xanthochromic.

xanoxate sodium (zah-noks′āt) chemical name: 7-(1-methylethoxy)-9-oxo-9H-xanthene-2-carboxylic acid sodium salt; a bronchodilator, $C_{17}H_{13}$ NaO₅.

xanthate (zan′thāt) any salt of xanthic acid.

xanthelasma (zan″thel-az′mah) [*xantho-* + Gr. *elasma* plate] the commonest form of xanthoma affecting the eyelids and characterized by soft yellowish spots or plaques; called also *xanthelasma palpebrarum*. See *plane xanthoma,* under *xanthoma*. **generalized x.,** see *plane xanthoma,* under *xanthoma*.

xanthelasmatosis (zan″thel-az″mah-to′sis) the generalized form of plane xanthoma (q.v.).

xanthematin (zan-them′ah-tin) an ill-defined yellow substance derivable from hematin, sometimes by the action of nitric acid.

xanthemia (zan-the′me-ah) [*xantho-* + Gr. *haima* blood + *-ia*] presence of yellow coloring matter in the blood; carotenemia.

xanthene (zan′thēn) the compound, $(C_6H_4)_2(O)CH_2$, or dibenzpyran, from which the xanthene dyes and indicators are derived.

xanthic (zan′thik) 1. yellow. 2. pertaining to xanthine.

xanthin (zan′thin) any of the yellow pigments obtained from yellow flowers and other plants, probably consisting of oxygen-containing carotenoids.

xanthine (zan′thēn) [Gr. *xanthos* yellow: named from the yellow color of its nitrate] a white, amorphous base, 2,6-dioxypurine, $C_5H_4N_4O_2$, from most of the body tissues and fluids, urinary calculi, and certain plants. It is formed by the oxidation of hypoxanthine and may be oxidized to uric acid. It is insoluble in cold water, but freely soluble in dilute acid and alkaline solutions. It possesses stimulant properties to muscle tissue, especially that of the heart. The three derivatives of xanthine most used in medicine are caffeine, theobromine, and theophylline and their derivatives. **dimethyl x.,** theobromine. **trimethyl x.,** caffeine.

xanthinin (zan′thĭ-nin) 1. a white, crystalline substance, C_4H_3-

N_3O_2, formed by heating ammonium thionurate. 2. a keto-lactone from leaves of *Xanthium pennsylvanicum*, or cocklebur.

xanthinoxidase (zan″thin-ok′sĭ-dās) an enzyme that oxidizes xanthine and hypoxanthine into uric acid.

xanthinuria (zan″thin-u′re-ah) [*xanthine* + Gr. *ouron* urine] a rare hereditary disorder of purine metabolism due to deficiency of the enzyme xanthine oxidase, which results in excessive urinary secretion of xanthine and hypoxanthine, in place of uric acid, and may lead to the formation of xanthine calculi in the urinary tract.

xanthinuric (zan″thin-u′-rik) pertaining to or resulting from xanthinuria.

xanthiuria (zan″the-u′re-ah) xanthinuria.

xantho- (zan′tho) [Gr. *xanthos* yellow] a combining form meaning yellow.

xanthochromatic (zan″tho-kro-mat′ik) xanthochromic.

xanthochromia (zan″tho-kro′me-ah) [*xantho-* + Gr. *chrōma* color + *-ia*] any yellowish discoloration, as of the skin or of the spinal fluid.

xanthochromic (zan″tho-kro′mik) having a yellow color; applied almost exclusively to cerebrospinal fluid.

xanthocyanopsia (zan″tho-si″ah-nop′se-ah) [*xantho-* + Gr. *kyanos* blue + *opsis* vision + *-ia*] ability to discern yellow and blue tints, but not red or green.

xanthocystine (zan″tho-sis′tin) a substance found in tubercles from a dead body.

xanthocyte (zan′tho-sīt) a cell that contains yellow pigment.

xanthodontous (zan″tho-don′tus) [*xantho-* + Gr. *odous* tooth] having yellowish teeth.

xanthoerythrodermia (zan″tho-ĕ-rith″ro-der′me-ah) a yellowish red coloration of the skin. **x. per′stans,** parapsoriasis en plaques.

xanthofibroma thecocellulare (zan″tho-fi-bro′mah the″ko-sel″u-lah′re) dermatofibroma.

xanthogranuloma (zan″tho-gran″u-lo′mah) a tumor having the histologic characteristics of both granuloma and xanthoma. **juvenile x.,** a dermatosis, typically beginning in infancy or early childhood, in which groups of yellow, yellow-brown, reddish yellow, or brown papules or nodules occur on the extensor surfaces of the extremities; the eyeball, meninges, and testes may also be involved. Spontaneous remission of the lesions usually occurs in one to three years. Formerly called *nevoxanthoendothelioma.*

xanthokyanopy (zan″tho-ki-an′o-pe)   xanthocyanopsia.

xanthoma (zan-tho′mah)   a papule, nodule, or plaque of a yellow color in the skin, due to deposits of lipids. Microscopically the lesions show light cells with foamy protoplasm (foam cells, or xanthoma cells). See also *xanthomatosis.* **craniohypophyseal x.,** deposits of cholesterol esters in bones around the hypophysis in Hand-Schüller-Christian disease. **diabetic x., x. diabetico′rum,** an eruptive xanthoma associated with diabetes mellitus; when the diabetes is brought under control, the skin lesions disappear. **x. dissemina′tum,** a chronic, benign, normolipoproteinemic xanthomatosis characterized by small, yellowish red to brown papules and nodules chiefly affecting the flexural and intertriginous surfaces and the mucous membranes of the oropharynx, larynx, and bronchi. Diabetes insipidus has been reported in a large percentage of patients. Called also *x. multiplex.* **eruptive x., x. erupti′vum,** xanthomatosis characterized by clusters of small yellow or yellowish-brown papules over the entire body; the lesions may be encircled by an erythematous halo. **generalized plane x.,** see *plane x.* **x. mul′tiplex,** x. disseminatum. **x. palpebra′rum,** xanthelasma. **planar x., plane x., x. planum,** xanthomatosis characterized by flat macules or slightly elevated plaques of yellowish to orange color, which may be localized to the eyelids (*xanthelasma, xanthelasma palpebralis*) or distributed over large areas of the skin (*generalized plane x., generalized xanthelasma, xanthelasmatosis*). It is usually associated with reticuloendothelial disorders, especially multiple myeloma. **x. stria′tum palma′re,** xanthoma planum affecting only the palms. **x. tendino′sum,** a hereditary lipid storage disease marked by formation of papules or nodules in the tendons, especially the extensor tendons of the hands and feet and the Achilles tendon. **x. tubero′sum, x. tubero′sum mul′tiplex, tuberous x.,** a hereditary lipid storage disease characterized by groups of flat, or elevated and rounded, yellowish or orangish nodules on the skin over joints, especially the elbows and knees. It may be associated with types I and II hyperlipoproteinemia, biliary cirrhosis, and myxedema.

xanthomatosis (zan″tho-mah-to′sis)   an accumulation of an excess of lipids in the body due to disturbance of lipid metabolism and marked by the formation of foam cells in skin lesions. See also entries under *xanthoma.* **biliary hypercholesterolemic x.,** widespread xanthomatosis resulting from hypercholesterolemia due to biliary tract obstruction. **x. bul′bi,** fatty degeneration of the cornea. **cerebrotendinous x.,** a lipid storage disease characterized by xanthomas of the tendons and the white matter of brain and by spasticity, ataxia, mental retardation, and early cataracts. The lesions contain cholesterol and dehydrocholesterol. **chronic idiopathic x.,** Hand-Schüller-Christian disease. **x. generalisa′ta os′sium,** lipid granulomatosis of the bones. **x. i′ridis,** the formation of yellow patches in the discolored iris of an eye blinded as the result of protracted iritis or glaucoma. **primary familial x.,** Wolman's disease. **Wolman's x.,** Wolman's disease.

xanthomatous (zan-tho′mah-tus)   pertaining to or of the nature of xanthoma.

Xanthomonas (zan″tho-mo′nas)   a genus of microorganisms of the family Pseudomonadaceae, suborder Pseudomonadineae, order Pseudomonadales, occurring as monotrichous cells producing a yellow pigment, the type species being *X. hyacin′thi.* Most of the 60 described species, as well as many of the 14 species provisionally included, are pathogenic for plants.

xanthone (zan′thōn)   xanthene ketone, CO:(C₆H₄)₂:O, a derivative of xanthine.

xanthophane (zan′tho-fān)   a yellow pigment from the retina.

xanthophore (zan′tho-fōr) [*xantho-* + Gr. *phoros* bearing]   a chromatophore of cold-blooded animals containing granules of yellow-red pigment.

xanthophose (zan′tho-fōz) [*xantho-* + Gr. *phōs* light]   any yellow or yellowish phose.

xanthophylase (zan″tho-fi′lās)   an enzyme discovered in the rabbit that determines the presence of its yellow fat.

xanthophyll (zan′tho-fil) [*xantho-* + Gr. *phyllon* leaf]   a yellow coloring matter of plants, one of a group of oxygenated carotenoids, e.g., 3,3-dihydroxy alpha-carotene, C₄₀H₅₆O₂, occurring along with carotene in green leaves, grass, and other vegetable matter.

xanthopia (zan-tho′pe-ah)   xanthopsia.

xanthoproteic (zan″tho-pro-te′ik)   pertaining to xanthoprotein.

xanthoprotein (zan″tho-pro′te-in)   an orange pigment produced by heating proteins with nitric acid.

xanthopsia (zan-thop′se-ah) [*xantho-* + Gr. *opsis* vision + *-ia*]   a form of chromatopsia in which objects looked at appear yellow.

xanthopsin (zan-thop′sin)   all-*trans* retinal; see *retinal.*

xanthopsis (zan-thop′sis) [*xantho-* + Gr. *opsis* appearance]   a yellow pigment or pigmentation in cancers.

xanthopterin (zan-thop′ter-in) [*xanto-* + Gr. *pteron* wing]   chemical name: 2-amino-4,6-pteridinediol. A yellow pigment, C₆H₅N₅O₂, from the integument of wasps and hornets and from butterfly wings, which has some hematopoietic activity in anemic animals. It is an inhibitor of xanthine oxidase. See *pterin.*

xanthopuccine (zan″tho-puk′sin) [*xantho-* + *puccoon,* Algonquin name for plants used as pigments]   an alkaloid from *Hydrastis canadensis* L. (Ranunculaceae), the goldenseal.

xanthorhammin (zan″tho-ram′nin)   chemical name: 3,3′,4′,5-tetrahydroxy-7-methoxyflavone-3-rhamninoside. A yellow glycoside, C₃₄H₄₂O₂₀, from the fruit of several species of *Rhamnus.*

xanthorubin (zan″tho-ru′bin)   xantorubin.

xanthosarcoma (zan″tho-sar-ko′mah)   giant cell tumor of the tendon sheath; see under *tumor.*

xanthosine (zan′tho-sēn)   a nucleoside, xanthine-9-ribofuranoside, C₁₀H₁₂O₆N₄, which on hydrolysis yields xanthine and ribose.

xanthosis (zan-tho′sis)   a yellowish discoloration; degeneration with yellowish pigmentation. **x. of septum nasi,** yellow pigmentation of the mucous membrane of the nose, due to degeneration of the blood after hemorrhage.

xanthotoxin (zan″tho-tok′sin)   methoxsalen.

xanthous (zan′thus)   yellow or yellowish.

xanthuria (zan-thu′re-ah) [*xanthine* + Gr. *ouron* urine + *-ia*]   xanthinuria.

xanthyl (zan′thil)   the monovalent radical C₁₃H₉O.

xanthylic (zan-thil′ik)   pertaining to xanthine.

xantorubin (zan″to-roo′bin)   a yellow pigment found in the blood serum after hepatectomy.

Xe   chemical symbol for *xenon.*

xenembole (zen-em′bo-le) [*xeno-* + Gr. *embolē* insertion]   the introduction of foreign substances into the system.

xenenthesis (zen″en-the′sis) [*xeno-* + Gr. *enthesis* putting in]   xenembole.

xenia (ze′ne-ah) [Gr. "a friendly relation between two foreigners"]   the appearance in the endosperm (seed) resulting from cross-pollination of dominant characters inherited from the male (pollen) plant.

xeno- [Gr. *xenos* a guest-friend; any stranger or foreigner]   a combining form meaning strange, or denoting relationship to foreign material.

xenobiotic (zen″o-bi-ot′ik)   a chemical foreign to the biologic system.

xenocytophilic (zen″o-si″to-fil′ik) [*xeno-* + Gr. *kytos* hollow vessel + *philein* to love]   having an affinity for cells derived from a different species.

xenodiagnosis (zen″o-di-ag-no′sis) [*xeno-* + *diagnosis*]   1. diagnosis by means of finding, in the feces of clean laboratory-bred bugs fed on the patient, the infective forms of the organism causing the disease; used in the early stages of Chagas' disease. 2. diagnosis of trichinosis by means of feeding laboratory-bred rats or mice on meat suspected of being infected with *Trichinella,* and then examining the animals for the parasite.

xenodiagnostic (zen″o-di″ag-nos′tik)   pertaining to xenodiagnosis.

xenodochia (zen″o-do′ke-ah)   medieval hospital for poor and infirm pilgrims.

xenogeneic (zen″o-jen-a′ik) [*xeno-* + *gennan* to produce]   in transplantation biology, denoting individuals or tissues from individuals of different species and hence of disparate cell type; called also *heterologous.* See *allogeneic.*

xenogenesis (zen″o-jen′ĕ-sis)   1. alternation of generation; heterogenesis. 2. the production of offspring unlike either parent.

xenogenous (zen-oj′ĕ-nus) [*xeno-* + Gr. *gennan* to produce]   caused by a foreign body, or originating outside the organism.

xenograft (zen′o-graft)   a graft of tissue transplanted between animals of different species. Called also *heterograft, heterologous graft,* and *heteroplastic graft.*

xenology (ze-nol′o-je)   the science of the relations of parasites to their hosts.

xenomenia (zen″o-me′ne-ah) [*xeno-* + Gr. *mēniaia* menses]   vicarious menstruation.

xenon (ze′non) [Gr. *xenos* stranger]   a chemically unreactive gaseous element found in the atmosphere; atomic number, 54; atomic weight, 131.30; symbol, Xe.

xenoparasite (zen″o-par′ah-sīt)   an organism not usually parasitic on the host, but which becomes so because of a weakened condition of the host.

xenophobia (zen″o-fo′be-ah) [*xeno-* + Gr. *phobein* to be affrighted by + *-ia*]   morbid dread of strangers.

xenophonia (zen″o-fo′ne-ah) [*xeno-* + Gr. *phōnē* voice + *-ia*]   alteration of the accent and intonation of a person's speech.

xenophthalmia (zen″of-thal′me-ah) [*xeno-* + Gr. *ophthalmia* ophthalmia]   ophthalmia caused by a foreign body in the eye.

Xenopsylla (zen″op-sil′ah) [*xeno-* + Gr. *psylla* flea] a genus of fleas, including more than 30 species, many of which transmit disease-producing microorganisms. **X. as′tia,** a rat flea of parts of Ceylon and India that has been implicated in the transmission of plague. **X. brasilien′sis,** a rat flea of Africa, Brazil, and India, a transmitter of plague. **X. che′opis,** a rat flea of worldwide distribution, which transmits plague and murine typhus; called also *Pulex cheopis* and *Asiatic rat flea.* **X. hawaiien′sis,** *X. vexabilis.* **X. vexabil′is,** a species infesting field rats in the Hawaiian islands; called also *X. hawaiiensis.*

Xenopus (zen′o-pus) a genus of amphibians. **X. lae′vis,** the South African clawed toad; see *Xenopus test,* under *tests.*

xenorexia (zen″o-rek′se-ah) [*xeno-* + *orexis* appetite + *-ia*] perversion of appetite leading to the repeated swallowing of foreign bodies not ordinarily ingested.

xenyl (zen′il) the univalent chemical group, $C_6H_5 \cdot C_6H_4$—.

xerantic (ze-ran′tik) causing dryness; siccative.

xeraphium (ze-raf′e-um) a drying powder.

xero- [Gr. *xēros* dry] a combining form meaning dry, or denoting relationship to dryness.

xerocheilia (ze″ro-ki′le-ah) [*xero-* + Gr. *cheilos* lip + *-ia*] dryness of the lips, a form of simple cheilitis.

xerocollyrium (ze″ro-ko-lir′e-um) [*xero-* + Gr. *kollyrion* collyrium] a dry collyrium; an eye salve.

xeroderma (ze″ro-der′mah) [*xero-* + Gr. *derma* skin] a mild form of ichthyosis, marked by a dry, rough, discolored state of the skin, with the formation of a scaly desquamation. **follicular x.** (*obs.*), keratosis pilaris. **x. of Kaposi** (*obs.*), x. pigmentosum. **x. pigmento′sum,** a rare and frequently fatal pigmentary and atrophic disease in which the skin and eyes are extremely sensitive to light. It begins in childhood and progresses to early development of ephelides, telangiectases, keratoses, papillomas, carcinoma, and melanoma. Ocular symptoms include photophobia, lacrimation, keratitis, opacities, and tumors of the lid and cornea. The disease is inherited as an autosomal recessive trait involving a defect in the enzymes active in the excision and repair of DNA damaged by ultraviolet irradiation. Total protection from sunlight prevents development of lesions completely.

xerodermatic (ze″ro-der-mat′ik) pertaining to or of the nature of xeroderma.

xerodermia (ze″ro-der′me-ah) xeroderma.

xerogel (ze′ro-jel) a gel containing little liquid. Cf. *lyogel.*

xerography (ze-rog′rah-fe) xeroradiography.

xeroma (ze-ro′mah) an abnormally dry condition of the conjunctiva; xerophthalmia.

xeromammography (ze″ro-mam-mog′rah-fe) xeroradiography of the breast.

xeromenia (ze″ro-me′ne-ah) [*xero-* + Gr. *mēniaia* menses] a condition in which the bodily symptoms of menstruation occur without any bloody flow.

xeromycteria (ze″ro-mik-te′re-ah) [*xero-* + Gr. *myktēr* nose] dryness of the nasal mucous membrane.

xerophagia (ze″ro-fa′je-ah) [*xero-* + Gr. *phagein* to eat] the eating of dry food.

xerophagy (ze-rof′ah-je) xerophagia.

xerophobia (ze″ro-fo′be-ah) inhibition of saliva flow because of fear, anger, or excitement.

xerophthalmia (ze″rof-thal′me-ah) [*xero-* + Gr. *ophthalmos* eye + *-ia*] dryness of the conjunctiva and cornea due to vitamin A deficiency. The condition begins with night blindness and conjunctival xerosis and progresses to corneal xerosis and, in the late stages, to keratomalacia.

xerophthalmus (ze″rof-thal′mus) xerophthalmia.

xeroradiography (ze″ro-ra″de-og′rah-fe) a dry, totally photoelectric process for recording x-ray images, using metal plates coated with a semiconductor, such as selenium.

xerosialography (ze″ro-si″ah-log′rah-fe) sialography in which the images are recorded by xerography.

xerosis (ze-ro′sis) [Gr. *xērosis*] abnormal dryness, as of the eye, skin, or mouth. **x. conjuncti′vae, conjunctival x.,** dryness of the conjunctiva. When associated with Bitot's spots, it is due to vitamin A deficiency and may progress to xerophthalmia and keratomalacia. **x. cor′neae, corneal x.,** dryness of the cornea, giving it a hazy or milky appearance; see *xerophthalmia.* **x. cu′tis,** asteatosis cutis. **x. parenchymato′sus,** xerophthalmia due to trachoma. **x. superficia′lis,** xerophthalmia due to abnormal exposure of the eyeball to the air.

xerostomia (ze″ro-sto′me-ah) [*xero-* + Gr. *stoma* mouth + *-ia*] dryness of the mouth from lack of the normal secretion, as in Sjögren's syndrome.

xerotes (zer′o-tēz) [Gr. *xērotēs*] dryness.

xerotic (ze-rot′ik) characterized by xerosis or dryness.

xerotomography (ze″ro-to-mog′rah-fe) tomography in which the images are recorded by xeroradiography.

xerotripsis (ze″ro-trip′sis) [*xero-* + Gr. *tripsis* friction] dry friction.

xilobam (zi′lo-bam) chemical name: *N*-(2,6-dimethylphenyl)-*N*′-(1-methyl-2-pyrrolidinylidene)urea; a muscle relaxant, $C_{14}H_{19}$-N_3O.

Ximenia (zi-me′ne-ah) a genus of African olacineous trees; the drupes of some species are edible and aromatic.

xipamide (zip′ah-mīd) chemical name: 5-(aminosulfonyl)-4-chloro-N-(2,6-dimethylphenyl)-2-hydroxybenzamide; a diuretic and antihypertensive, $C_{15}H_{15}ClN_2O_4S$.

xiphi- see *xipho-.*

xiphin (zif′in) a protamine from the sperm of the sword fish, *Xiphias gladius.*

xiphisternal (zif″ĭ-ster′nal) pertaining to the xiphisternum.

xiphisternum (zif″ĭ-ster′num) [*xiphi-* + Gr. *sternon* sternum] the xiphoid process (processus xiphoideus [NA]).

xipho-, xiphi- [Gr. *xiphos* sword] a combining form denoting relationship to the xiphoid process.

xiphocostal (zif″o-kos′tal) [*xipho-* + L. *costa* rib] pertaining to the xiphoid process and the ribs.

xiphodidymus (zif″o-did′ĭ-mus) [*xipho-* + Gr. *didymos* twin] xiphopagus.

xiphodymus (zi-fod′ĭ-mus) xiphopagus.

xiphodynia (zif″o-din′e-ah) [*xipho-* + Gr. *odynē* pain + *-ia*] pain in the xiphoid process.

xiphoid (zif′oid) [*xipho-* + Gr. *eidos* form] 1. shaped like a sword. 2. the xiphoid process (processus xiphoideus [NA]).

xiphoiditis (zif″oi-di′tis) inflammation of the xiphoid process.

xiphopagotomy (zi-fop″ah-got′o-me) surgical separation of conjoined twins fused in the region of the xiphoid process.

xiphopagus (zi-fop″ah-gus) [*xipho-* + Gr. *pagos* thing fixed] symmetrical conjoined twins fused in the region of the xiphoid process.

X-linked (eks′linkt) transmitted by genes on the X chromosome; sex-linked.

XO symbol for the presence of only one sex chromosome, the other X or the Y chromosome being absent.

X-Prep (eks′prep) trademark for a preparation of senna.

x-ray (eks′ra) roentgen ray; see under *ray.* **spark x-r's,** brush discharge.

xylanthrax (zi-lan′thraks) charcoal.

xylazine hydrochloride (zi′lah-zēn) chemical name: *N*-(2,6-dimethylphenyl)-5,6-dihydro-4*H*-1,3-thiazin-2-amine monohydrochloride; an analgesic, sedative, and muscle relaxant, $C_{12}H_{16}N_2S \cdot HCl$, used in veterinary medicine.

xylem (zi′lem) [Gr. *xylon* wood] the tissue in woody plants which conducts water and dissolved salts up from the roots, characterized by the presence of tracheids. In bulk it forms wood. Cf. *phloem.*

xylene (zi′lēn) 1. dimethylbenzene; an antiseptic hydrocarbon, $C_6H_4(CH_3)_2$, from methyl alcohol or coal tar; used in microscopy as a solvent and clarifier. 2. a group of hydrocarbons of the benzene series.

xylenol (zi′lĕ-nol) any of a series of colorless, crystalline substances, $(CH_3)_2C_6H_3OH$, resembling phenol. **x. salicylate,** a white antirheumatic powder, $OH \cdot C_6H_4 \cdot CO \cdot O \cdot C_6H_3(CH_3)_2$.

xylidine (zi′li-din) a compound, dimethylaniline $(CH_3)_2C_6H_3 \cdot NH_2$, used as a dyestuff intermediate and for blending gasoline.

xylitol (zi′li-tol) an alcohol, $CH_2OH(CHOH):CH_2OH$, from xylose.

xylitone (zi′li-tōn) an oil, $C_{12}H_{18}O$, formed by treating acetone with hydrochloric acid.

xylo- [Gr. *xylon* wood] a combining form denoting relationship to wood.

Xylocaine (zi′lo-kān) trademark for preparations of lidocaine.

xylogen (zi′lo-jen) lignin.

xyloidin (zi-loid′in) [*xylo-* + Gr. *eidos* form] a white, explosive substance, $C_6H_9(NO_2)O_5$, prepared from starch by the action of nitric acid.

xyloketose (zi″lo-ke′tōs) xylulose.

xyloketosuria (zi″lo-ke″to-su′re-ah) essential pentosuria.

xylol (zi′lol) [Gr. *xylon* wood] xylene.

xyloma (zi-lo′mah) a woody tumor on a tree or plant.

xylometazoline hydrochloride (zi″lo-met″ah-zo′lēn) [USP] chemical name: 2-(4-tert-butyl-2,6-dimethylbenzyl)-2-imidazoline monohydrochloride. An adrenergic, $C_{16}H_{24}N_2 \cdot HCl$, occurring as a white, crystalline powder; used topically as a vasoconstrictor to reduce swelling and congestion of the nasal mucosa.

xylonite (zi′lo-nīt) a substance which resembles celluloid manufactured from pyroxylin.

xylopyranose (zi″lo-pi′rah-nōs) xylose in the cyclic pyranose form.

xylosazone (zi-lo′sa-zōn) the phenyl-osazone of xylose.

xylose (zi′lōs) a pentose, $CH_2OH(CHOH)_3CHO$, in a pyranose form, occurring in mucopolysaccharides of connective tissue and sometimes in the urine (see *xylosuria*); also obtained from vegetable gums, beechwood, and jute. The official preparation is used as a diagnostic aid in determining intestinal function.

xyloside (zi-lo-sīd) a glycoside of xylose.

xylosidoglucose (zi″lo-sid″o-gloo′kōs) primaverose.

xylosuria (zi″lo-su′re-ah) presence of xylose in the urine. A form of alimentary pentosuria reportedly occurring after ingestion of certain fruits, e.g., cherries, plums, and grapes; the identity of the urinary pentose(s) has not been crisply established. It is to be distinguished from essential pentosuria, which results from a genetic defect.

xylotherapy (zi″lo-ther′ah-pe) [*xylo-* + Gr. *therapeia* treatment] medical treatment by the application of certain woods to the body.

xylulose (zi′lu-lōs) a pentose sugar, $CH_2OH(CHOH)_2CO \cdot CH_2$-OH, occurring in two forms: L-xylulose, one of the few L sugars found in nature and sometimes excreted in the urine (see *pentosuria*), and D-xylulose.

L-xylulosuria (zi″lu-lo-su′re-a) a pentosuria.

xylyl (zi′lil) the hydrocarbon radical, $CH_3C_6H_4CH_2$.

xyphoid (zi′foid) xiphoid.

xysma (zis′mah) [Gr. "that which is scraped or shaved off"] a material, like bits of membrane, seen in the stools of diarrhea.

xyster (zis′ter) [Gr. *xystēr* a scraper] a surgeon's file or raspatory.

Y

Y chemical symbol for *yttrium*.

yahourth (yah′oort) yogurt.

yard (yard) a unit of linear measure, 3 feet, or 36 inches, being the equivalent of 86.44 cm.

yatobyo (yah″to-bi′yo) [Japanese *ya* wild, or field + *to* rabbit, or hare + *byo* disease] tularemia.

yaw (yaw) a lesion of yaws (q.v.). **guinea corn y.,** a lesion of yaws which resembles a grain of maize. **mother y.,** the initial cutaneous lesion of yaws. **ringworm y.,** a circular or ring-shaped lesion of yaws.

yawey (yaw′e) affected with yaws.

yawning (yawn′ing) a deep, involuntary inspiration with the mouth open, often accompanied by the act of stretching. Cf. *pandiculation.*

yaws (yawz) a usually nonvenereal, systemic, infectious disease, caused by the spirochete *Treponema pertenue,* and most commonly occurring in children in tropical regions, such as Equatorial Africa, West Indies, and tropical areas of America and the Far East. It is divided into three stages: a *primary stage,* in which a granulomatous initial lesion, the mother yaw, appears at the site of implantation of the spirochete, usually the lower leg or foot, and increases in size, becomes crusted, and spontaneously disappears, leaving a scar; a *secondary stage,* which occurs weeks or months after the appearance of the primary lesion, and is marked by successive crops of granulomatous papules distributed over the body, especially the face, extremities, and anogenital area; and, rarely, a *tertiary stage,* in which gummatous lesions of the skin similar to those of syphilis and destructive lesions of the bones occur after an interval of several years. Called also *Breda's* or *Charlouis' disease.* Also known by numerous local names, e.g., *frambesia, pian, parangi,* and *bouba.* **crab y.,** yaws characterized by hyperkeratosis with fissuring and ulceration of the soles of the feet, and less commonly involving the palms of the hands. **forest y.,** pian bois.

Ya Yan Tzu the Chinese species of the simaroubaceous plant of the genus *Brucea,* e.g., *B. antidysenterica* J.F. Mill., the seeds of which are used in treating amebic dysentery.

Yb chemical symbol for *ytterbium*.

yd. yard.

yeast (yēst) a general term including single-celled, usually rounded fungi that produce by budding (blastospore formation). Some yeasts transform to a mycelial (mold) stage under certain environmental conditions, while others always remain single-celled. The perfect yeasts are included in the class Ascomycetes, subclass Hemiascomycetes, order Endomycetales, and the imperfect yeasts in the class Deuteromycetes, order Moniliales, family Cryptococcaceae. A few are pathogenic for man. **bakers' y., brewers' y.,** *Saccharomyces cerevisiae,* used in brewing beer, making alcoholic liquors, and baking bread. **dried y.,** the dry cells of any suitable strain of *Saccharomyces cerevisiae,* usually a by-product of the brewing industry; used as a natural source of protein and B-complex vitamins. **imperfect y.,** one whose perfect (sexual) stage is unknown. **perfect y.,** one whose perfect (sexual) stage is known.

yeki (ya′ke) [Japanese] bubonic plague.

yellow (yel′o) 1. one of the primary colors of wavelength of 571.5 to 578.5 millimicrons. 2. a dye or stain that produces a yellow color. **acid y.,** fast y. **alizarin y.,** an indicator used in the determination of hydrogen ion concentration with a pH range of 10.1–12.1. **brilliant y.,** an indicator used in determining hydrogen ion concentration of 6–8. **butter y.,** *p*-dimethylaminoazobenzene. **chrome y.,** lead chromate, $PbCrO_4$, used in paints and injection masses. **corallin y.,** yellow corallin. **fast y.,** a yellow, acid azo dye, $(N \cdot C_6H_4 \cdot SO_2ONa)_2 \cdot NH_2$, used in staining bone. **imperial y.,** aurantia. **Manchester y., Martius y.,** a poisonous, yellow, azo dye, $C_6H_5(NO_2)_2OH$, used as a stain and in the preparation of light filters. **metanil y., metaniline y. (extra),** an indicator used in the determination of hydrogen ion concentration, with a pH range of

1.2–2.3. **naphthol y.,** Manchester y. **Philadelphia y.,** phosphine, def. 2. **visual y.,** all-*trans* retinal; see *retinal.*

yellows (yel′ōz) 1. a form of canine leptospirosis resembling leptospiral jaundice in man, caused by *Leptospira icterohaemorrhagiae.* 2. a disease affecting sheep and cattle in Scotland during June and July; it is marked by photosensitization and jaundice after ingestion of clover or alfalfa followed by exposure to sunlight; called also *headgrit.*

Yeo's treatment (ye′ōz) [Isaac Burney *Yeo,* London physician, 1835–1914] see under *treatment.*

yerba (yer′bah) [Sp.] herb. **y. santa** (yer′bah sahn′tah) [Sp. "sacred herb"], *Eriodictyon.*

yerbine (yer′bin) an alkaloid resembling caffeine, obtained from *Ilex paraguayensis,* a holly tree of Brazil, Argentina, and Paraguay.

Yerkes-Bridges test (yer′kēz-brij′ez) [Robert M. *Yerkes,* Boston psychiatrist, 1876–1956; James W. *Bridges,* Canadian psychiatrist, born 1885] see under *tests.*

yerli (yer′le) a fine quality of Turkish opium.

Yersin's serum (yer′sinz) [Alexandre Emil Jean *Yersin,* Swiss bacteriologist in Paris, 1863–1943] antiplague serum.

Yersinia (yer-sin′e-ah) [A.J.E. *Yersin*] a genus made up of nonmotile, ovoid or rod-shaped, nonencapsulated, gram-negative bacteria of the family Enterobacteriaceae. **y. enterocolit′ica,** a ubiquitous species isolated from the feces and lymph nodes of animals and man; it is nonpathogenic for laboratory animals. **Y. pes′tis,** the etiologic agent of plague in man and rats, ground squirrels, and other rodents, transmitted from rat to rat and from rat to man by the rat flea, and from man to man by the human body louse; pathogenic for mice, guinea pigs, and rabbits. Formerly called *Pasteurella pestis.* **Y. pseudotuberculos′sis,** a gram-negative, polymorphic, coccoid or ovoid, motile species of bacteria which is a common pathogen of rodents and birds. It causes mesenteric lymphadenitis in man and pseudotuberculosis in guinea pigs, rabbits, and, rarely, in other animals. Formerly called *Pasteurella pseudotuberculosis.*

-yl [Gr. *hylē* matter of substance] a chemical suffix signifying a radical, particularly a univalent hydrocarbon radical.

ylang-ylang (e″lahng-e′lahng) a tree of the Malayan Islands, *Cananga odorata* Hook and Thoms. (Anonaceae); its flowers afford a fragrant volatile oil used in perfumes.

-ylene a suffix used in chemistry to denote a bivalent hydrocarbon radical.

yochubio (yo-chu′be-o) scrub typhus.

Yodoxin (yo-dok′sin) trademark for preparations of iodoquinol.

yogurt (yo′goort) a form of curdled milk, produced by fermentation with organisms of the genus *Lactobacillus.*

yohimbine (yo-him′bēn) an alkaloid, $C_{21}H_{26}N_2O_3$, from *Corynanthe johimbe* K. Schum. (Rubiaceae) and from *Rauwolfia serpentina* L. Benth. (Apocynaceae). It possesses adrenergic blocking properties and is used in arteriosclerosis and angina pectoris, and formerly as a local anesthetic and mydriatic and for its purported aphrodisiac properties.

yoke (yōk) a connecting structure; a depression or ridge connecting two structures. Called also *jugum.* **aleolar y's of mandible,** juga alveolaria mandibulae. **alveolar y's of maxilla,** juga alveolaria maxillae. **cerebral y's of bone of cranium,** juga cerebralia ossium cranii. **sphenoidal y.,** jugum sphenoidale.

yolk (yōk) [L. *vitellus*] 1. the stored nutrient of the ovum. 2. crude wool fat or suint. **accessory y.,** the part of the yolk that serves for the nutrition of the formative portion. **egg y.,** the yellow portion of the egg of a bird. **formative y.,** that part of the ovum from which the embryo is developed. **nutritive y.,** accessory y.

Young's operation (yungz) [Hugh Hampton *Young,* Baltimore urologist, 1870–1945] see under *operation.*

Young's rule (yungz) [Thomas *Young,* English physician, physicist, mathematician, and philologist, 1773–1829, the "father of physiologic optics"] see under *rule*.

Young-Helmholtz theory (yung-helm′hōlts) [Thomas *Young;* H. L. F. von *Helmholtz,* German physician, 1821–1894] see under *theory*.

yperite (i′per-īt) dichlorodiethyl sulfide.

ypsiliform (ip-sil′ĭ-form) upsiloid.

ypsiloid (ip′sĭ-loid) upsiloid.

y.s. yellow spot (of the retina); see *macula retinae*.

ytterbium (ĭ-ter′be-um) [from *Ytterby,* in Sweden] a very rare metal; symbol, Yb; atomic number, 70; atomic weight, 173.04.

yttrium (ĭ′tre-um) [from *Ytterby,* in Sweden] a very rare metal, allied to cerium; symbol Y; atomic number, 39, atomic weight, 88.905.

yukon (u′kon) [*Yukawa,* Japanese physicist] see *barytron*.

Yvon's coefficient, test (e′vonz) [Paul *Yvon,* French physician, 1848–1913] see under *coefficient* and *tests*.

Z

Z symbol for *atomic number*.

Z. abbreviation for Ger. *Zuckung,* contraction.

zacatilla (zak″ah-tēl′yah) [Sp.] the choicest quality of cochineal.

Zactane (zak′tān) trademark for a preparation of ethoheptazine citrate.

Zahn's lines (ribs) (zahnz) [Friedrich Wilhelm *Zahn,* Swiss pathologist, 1845–1904] see under *line*.

zaire (zi′ra) an epidemic form of cholera occurring in Portugal.

Zander apparatus (zan′der) [Jonas Gustaf Wilhelm *Zander,* Swedish physician, 1835–1917] see under *apparatus*.

Zang's space (zangz) [Christoph Bonifacius *Zang,* German surgeon, 1772–1835] fossa supraclavicularis minor.

Zangemeister's test (zan″gĕ-mīs′terz) [Wilhelm *Zangemeister,* German gynecologist, 1871–1930] see under *tests*.

Zappert's chamber (tsap′ertz) [Julius *Zappert,* physician in Vienna, born 1867] see under *chamber*.

zaranthan (zah-ran′than) [Heb.] a hardening of the breast.

Zarontin (zah-ron′tin) trademark for a preparation of ethosuximide.

Zaroxolyn (zah-roks′o-lin) trademark for a preparation of metolazone.

Zaufal's sign (tsow′fahlz) [Emanuel *Zaufal,* Prague rhinologist, 1833–1910] saddle nose.

Zea (ze′ah) 1. maize. 2. corn-silk, the fresh styles and stigmas of the flowers of American corn, *Zea mays* L. (Gramineae). Formerly used in the treatment of cystitis and urethritis.

zeatin (ze′ă-tin) [from *Zea mays,* the generic name for corn] a cytokinin, or growth-stimulating factor of plants, 6-(4-hydroxy-3-methyl-*trans*-2-butenytamino)purine, first isolated from young kernels of sweetcorn but now known to occur in peas and spinach as well.

zeaxanthin (ze″ah-zan′thin) [*zea* + Gr. *xanthos* yellow] a carotinoid, $C_{40}H_{56}O_2$, from yellow corn, egg yolk, and *Fucus vesiculosus,* a seaweed of the North Atlantic Ocean.

zedoary (zed′o-a″re) [L. *zedoaria*] the rhizome of *Curcuma zedoaria,* a plant of India, which resembles ginger; used medicinally as an aromatic stimulant and carminative.

Zeeman effect (tse′man) [Pieter *Zeeman,* Dutch physicist, 1865–1943] see under *effect*.

zein (ze′in) a yellowish prolamin obtainable from corn; molecular weight is about 40,000. It does not contain tryptophan or lysine.

zeinolysis (ze″in-ol′ĭ-sis) [*zein* + Gr. *lysis* dissolution] the decomposition or splitting up of zein.

zeinolytic (ze″in-o-lit′ik) pertaining to, characterized by, or promoting zeinolysis.

zeiosis (zi-o′sis) [Gr. *zeiein* to boil, seethe + -*osis*] bubbling or blebbing activity, giving the appearance of boiling in slow motion, observed at the periphery of cells cultured in artificial media.

zeisian gland, stye (zi′se-an) [Edourd *Zeis,* Dresden ophthalmologist, 1807–1868] see *glandulae sebaceae conjunctivales,* and see *external hordeolum,* under *hordeolum*.

zeism (ze′izm) [L. *zea* maize] any condition attributed to excessive use of maize in the diet, principally pellagra.

zeismus (ze-is′mus) zeism.

zeistic (ze-is′tik) pertaining to maize.

Zeller's test (zel′erz) [O. *Zeller,* German physician] see under *tests*.

Zenker's crystals, degeneration (necrosis), diverticulum (zeng′kerz) [Friedrich Albert von *Zenker,* German pathologist, 1825–1898] see *Charcot-Leyden crystals* under *crystal,* and see under *degeneration* and *diverticulum*.

Zenker's fixative (fluid, solution) (zeng′kerz) [Konrad *Zenker,* German histologist, died 1894] see under *fixative*.

zenkerism (zeng′ker-izm) [F. A. *Zenker*] Zenker's degeneration; see under *degeneration*.

zenkerize (zeng′ker-īs) [K. *Zenker*] to treat with Zenker's fixative.

zeolite (ze′o-lit) a hydrated double silicate with ion-exchange properties; probably the active constituent in permutit.

zeoscope (ze′o-skōp) [Gr. *zeein* to boil, seethe + *skopein* to examine] an apparatus for determining the alcoholic strength of a liquid by means of its boiling point.

Zephiran (zef′ĭ-ran) trademark for preparations of benzalkonium.

zeranol (zer′ah-nōl) chemical name: (3*S*,7 *X*)-3, 4, 5, 6, 7, 8, 9, 10, -11, 12-decahydro-7,14,16-trihydroxy-3-methyl-1 *H*-2-benzoxacyclotetradecin-1-one; an anabolic-estrogenic agent, $C_{18}H_{26}O_5$, which has been used for estrogen replacement in human subjects, but is used chiefly in veterinary medicine.

zero (ze′ro) [Ital. "naught"] the point on a thermometer scale at which the graduation begins. The zero of the Celsius (centigrade) and Réamur temperature scales is the ice point; that of the Fahrenheit scale is 32 degrees below the ice point. **absolute z.,** the lowest possible temperature, designated as 0 on the Kelvin or Rankine scale; by definition this is equivalent to –273.15° C. or –459.67° F. **limes z.,** see under *dose*. **physiologic z.,** the temperature at which a thermal stimulus ceases to cause a sensation.

Zero family see under *family*.

zerumbet (ze-rum′bet) [East Indian] a spice or drug, the dried rhizome of a species of ginger, *Zingiber zerumbet* (L.) Smith (Zingiberaceae), now little used.

zestocausis (zes″to-kaw′sis) [Gr. *zestos* boiling hot + *kausis* burning] the therapeutic application of a tube containing superheated steam.

zestocautery (zes″to-kaw′ter-e) a tube or appliance used in zestocausis.

zeugopodium (zu″go-po′de-um) zygopodium (see *limb*).

zidometacin (zi″do-met′ah-sin) chemical name: 1-4(4-azidobenzoyl)-5-methoxy-2-methyl-1 *H*-indole-3-acetic acid; an anti-inflammatory, $C_{19}H_{16}N_4O_4$.

ziega (ze-a′gah) a kind of curd made by treating milk with rennet and afterward with acetic acid.

Ziegler's operation (zēg′lerz) [Samuel Louis *Ziegler,* ophthalmologist in Philadelphia, 1861–1926] see under *operation*.

Ziehen's test (ze′henz) [Georg Theodor *Ziehen,* German neurologist, born 1862] see under *tests*.

Ziehen-Oppenheim disease (ze′hen-op′en-hīm) [Georg Theodor *Ziehen;* Herman *Oppenheim,* German neurologist, 1858–1919] dystonia musculorum deformans.

Ziehl's carbolfuchsin stain, solution (zēlz) [Franz *Ziehl,* German bacteriologist, 1857–1926] carbolfuchsin stain; see *Table of Stains*.

Ziehl-Neelsen's carbolfuchsin method, stain (zēl-nēl′senz) [Franz *Ziehl;* German bacteriologist, 1857–1926; Friederich Karl Adolf *Neelsen,* 1854–1894] see *acid-fast stain* and *carbolfuchsin stain* in *Table of Stains*.

Ziemssen's motor points (zēm′senz) [Hugo Wilhelm von *Ziemssen,* physician in Munich, 1829–1902] see under *point*.

Ziffern's test (zif′ernz) [Sidney Edward *Ziffern,* Iowa City pathologist, born 1912] see under *tests*.

zigzagplasty (zig′zag-plas″te) the surgical technique of minimizing the visual impact of a long linear scar by breaking it up into short irregular segments at right or acute angles to each another.

zilantel (zil-an′tel) chemical name: (diethoxyphosphinyl)carbonimidodithioic acid 1,2-ethanediyl bis(phenylmethyl)ester; an anthelmintic, $C_{26}H_{38}N_2O_6P_2S_4$.

zimelidine hydrochloride (zĭ-mel′ĭ-dēn) chemical name: (*Z*)-3-(4-bromophenyl)- *N, N*-dimethyl-3-(3-pyridinyl-2-propen-1-amine dihydrochloride monohydrate; an antidepressant, $C_{16}H_{17}Br-N_2 \cdot 2HCl \cdot H_2O$.

Zimmerlin's atrophy (type) (zim′er-linz) [Franz *Zimmerlin,* Swiss physician, 1858–1932] see under *atrophy*.

Zimmermann's arch, corpuscle (zim′er-mahnz) [Karl Wilhelm *Zimmermann,* German histologist, 1861–1935] see under *arch,* and see *achromocyte*.

zinc (zingk) [L. *zincum*] a blue-white metal, many of whose salts are used in medicine: symbol, Zn; atomic number, 30; atomic weight, 65.37. Zinc is necessary in trace amounts in the body (and hence in the diet); it forms an essential part of many enzymes (e.g., carbonic anhydrase, important in carbon dioxide metabolism), and plays an important role in protein synthesis and in cell division. Deficiency in zinc is associated with anemia, short stature, hypogonadism, impaired wound healing, and geophagia. Zinc salts are often poisonous when absorbed by the system, producing a chronic poisoning resembling that caused by lead. **z. acetate,** [USP], a salt $Zn(C_2H_3O_2)_2 \cdot 2H_2O$, produced by the reaction of zinc oxide with acetic acid, used as a pharmaceutic necessity for zinc-eugenol cement and as an astringent, styptic, and formerly as an emetic. **z. carbonate,** a salt, $2ZnCO_3 \cdot 3Zn(OH)_2$, used as a dusting powder or in the form of a cerate. **z. chloride** [USP], a white, or nearly white, odorless crystalline powder, $ZnCl_2$, used topically as an astringent and desensitizer for dentin. It is also used topically as a caustic antiseptic, and deodorant. **z. hydroxide,** a white powder, $Zn(OH)_2$, an ingredient of medicinal zinc peroxide. **z. iodide,** a white, granular powder, ZnI_2, which has been used as a topical antiseptic and astringent. **z. oxide** [USP], a very fine, odorless, amorphous, white or yellowish white powder, ZnO, used topically as an astringent and protectant in various cutaneous conditions. Called also *white z.* **z. permanganate,** a salt, $Zn(MnO_4)_2 \cdot 6H_2O$, in violet crystals, formerly used in solution as an astringent and antiseptic in the treatment of urethritis. **z. peroxide,** a white to yellowish white odorless powder, ZnO_2, used in pharmaceuticals. **z. peroxide, medicinal,** a mixture of zinc peroxide, zinc carbonate, and zinc hydroxide, used topically in a 40 per cent solution as a local anti-infective and oxidant. It is also used as an astringent and deodorant. **z. phenolsulfonate,** chemical name: *p*-hydroxybenzenesulfonic acid zinc salt. A colorless, crystalline salt, $(HO \cdot \cdot C_6H_4 \cdot SO_3)_2Zn \cdot 8H_2O$, formerly used as an antiseptic and astringent, and in the manufacture of insecticides. Called also *z. sulfocarbolate.* **z. pyrithione,** chemical name: bis[1-hydroxy-2(1*H*)-pyridinethionato]zinc. A compound, $C_{10}H_8N_2O_2S_2Zn$, used as an antibacterial, topical antifungal, and antiseborrheic. **z. salicylate,** a salt in colorless crystals, $(C_7H_5O_3)_2Zn \cdot 3H_2O$, which has been used as an antiseptic and astringent. **z. stearate** [USP], a compound of zinc with variable proportions of stearic acid and palmitic acid, containing 12.5 to 14.0 per cent of zinc oxide; used as a dusting powder. **z. sulfanilate,** chemical name: zinc sulfanilate tetrahydrate; an antibacterial, $C_{12}H_{12}N_2O_6S_2Zn \cdot 4H_2O$. **z. sulfate** [USP], the heptahydrate zinc salt of sulfuric acid, $ZnSO_4 7H_2O$, occurring as colorless, transparent prisms, or small needles; used as an astringent for the mucous membranes, especially for those of the eye, being considered specific for conjunctivitis due to *Hemophilus duplex.* It has also been used in various dermatological preparations, and internally as an antiemetic, especially in the treatment of poisoning. Called also *white vitriol* and *z. vitriol.* **z. sulfocarbolate,** z. phenolsulfonate. **z. undecylenate** [USP], the zinc salt of undecylenic acid, $C_{22}H_{38}O_4Zn$, occurring as a fine, white powder; used in combination with undecylenic acid as a topical antifungal. **z. vitriol,** z. sulfate. **white z.,** z. oxide.

zincalism (zingk'al-izm) zinc poisoning; symptoms include fever, chills, myalgia, vomiting, headache, and pneumonitis.

zincative (zingk'ah-tiv) electrically negative, i.e., like the zinc in a Daniell cell.

zinciferous (zing-kif'er-us) containing zinc.

zincoid (zing'koid) [L. *zincum* + Gr. *eidos* form] pertaining to or resembling zinc.

zincum (zing'kum), gen. *zin'ci* [L.] zinc.

Zinn's artery, etc. (zinz) [Johann Gottfried *Zinn*, German anatomist, 1727–1759] see under *aponeurosis, artery, cap, circle, ligament,* and *zone.*

Zinsser inconsistency (zin'ser) [Hans *Zinsser,* American bacteriologist, 1878–1940] lack of parallelism between local and systemic anaphylactic symptomatology.

zinterol hydrochloride (zin'tĕ-rōl) chemical name: *N*-[5-[2-[(1,1-dimethyl-2-phenylethyl) amino]-1-hydroxyethyl]-2-hydroxyphenyl]methanesulfonamide monohydrochloride; a bronchodilator, $C_{19}H_{26}N_2O_4S \cdot HCl$.

zipp (zip) a paste made by grinding together 1 part of zinc oxide, 2 parts of iodoform, and 2 to 3 parts of liquid paraffin; it is applied to wounds in veterinary surgery.

zirconium (zir-ko'ne-um) a rather rare metallic element; symbol Zr; atomic number, 40; atomic weight, 91.22; chiefly obtained from a mineral called zircon. **z. dioxide, z. oxide,** a heavy white powder, ZrO_2, formerly used as a radiopaque medium in roentgenography of the digestive tract, and once employed in an ointment for treating poison ivy dermatitis.

zisp (zisp) a modified form of zipp in which zinc peroxide is used in place of zinc oxide.

Zn chemical symbol for zinc.

ZnSO₄ zinc sulfate.

zoacanthosis (zo″ak-an-tho'sis) any dermatitis caused by the retention of animal structures, such as bristles, stings, hairs, etc.

zoamylin (zo-am'ĭ-lin) (obs.) glycogen.

zoanthropic (zo″an-throp'ik) pertaining to or characterized by zoanthropy.

zoanthropy (zo-an'thro-pe) [Gr. *zōon* animal + *anthrōpos* man] the abnormal belief of a patient that he has become a beast.

zoescope (zo'ĕ-skōp) [Gr. *zōē* life + *skopein* to examine] stroboscope.

zoetic (zo-et'ik) [Gr. *zōē* life] pertaining to life.

zoetrope (zo'ĕ-trōp) [Gr. *zōē* life + *trepein* to turn] an apparatus which affords pictures of objects apparently moving as in life.

zoic (zo'ik) [Gr. *zōikos* of or proper to animals] pertaining to or characterized by animal life.

zolamine hydrochloride (zo'lah-mēn) chemical name: *N*-[(4-methoxyphenyl)methyl]-*N'*,*N'*-dimethyl-*N*-2-thiazolyl-1,2-ethanediamine monohydrochloride. An antihistaminic with local anesthetic action, $C_{15}H_{21}N_3OS \cdot HCl$, which has been used as a topical anesthetic in the treatment of earache associated with otitis media and in the treatment of hemorrhoids.

Zollinger-Ellison syndrome (zol'lin-jer-el'lĭ-son) [Robert Milton *Zollinger,* American physician, born 1903; Edwin H. *Ellison,* American physician, born 1918] see under *syndrome.*

Zöllner's lines (figures) (zel'nerz) [Johann Carl Friedrich *Zöllner,* German physicist, 1834–1882] see under *line.*

zomepirac sodium (zo″mĕ-pēr'ak) chemical name: 5-(4-chlorobenzoyl)-1,4-dimethyl-1*H*-pyrrole-2-acetic acid sodium salt dihydrate; an analgesic and anti-inflammatory, $C_{15}H_{13}ClNNaO_3 \cdot 2H_2O$.

zometapine (zo-met'ah-pēn) chemical name: 4-(3-chlorophenyl)-1,6,7,8-tetrahydro-1,3-dimethylpyrazolo[3,4-*e*][1,4]diazepine; an antidepressant, $C_{14}H_{15}ClN_4$.

zomidin (zo'mĭ-din) [Gr. *zōmos* broth] a constituent of meat extract.

zomotherapy (zo″mo-ther'ah-pe) [Gr. *zōmos* broth + *therapeia* service done to the sick] the treatment of disease by muscle plasma, meat juice, or by meat diet.

zona (zo'nah), pl. *zo'nae* [L. "a girdle"] 1. a zone: an encircling region or area; [NA] a general term for an area with a specific boundary or characteristics. 2. herpes zoster. **z. arcua'ta,** canal of Corti. **z. cartilagin'ea,** limbus laminae spiralis osseae. **z. cilia'ris,** ciliary zone. **z. denticula'ta,** denticulate zone: the inner zone of the lamina basilaris ductus cochlearis with the limbus of the osseous spiral lamina. **z. dermat'ica,** an elevation of thick skin around the protruding mass in spina bifida. **z. epitheliosero'sa,** an area of membranous tissue inside the zona dermatica. **z. fascicula'ta,** fascicular zone: the thick middle layer of the cortex of the suprarenal gland. **z. ganglio'naris,** a mass of ganglion tissue on the pars cochlearis nervi octavi. **z. glomerulo'sa,** glomerular zone: the thin outer layer of the cortex of the suprarenal gland, which is contiguous with the capsule. **z. granulo'sa,** the peripheral stratified cuboidal epithelium of the ovarian follicle. **z. hemorrhoida'lis** [NA], hemorrhoidal zone: that part of the anal canal extending from the anal valves to the anus and containing the rectal venous plexus; called also *annulus haemorrhoidalis.* **z. incer'ta** [NA], a narrow band of gray matter between the subthalamic nucleus and the fasciculus thalamicus. **z. ophthal'mica,** herpetic infection of the cornea. **z. orbicula'ris articulatio'nis cox'ae** [NA], orbicular zone of hip joint: circular fibers of the articular capsule of the hip joint which form a ring around the neck of the femur; they are especially prominent at the inferior and posterior part of the capsule. **z. pectina'ta,** pectinate zone: the outer part of the lamina basilaris ductus cochlearis running from the rods of Corti to the spiral ligament. **z. pellu'cida,** 1. pellucid zone: a thick, transparent, noncellular layer or envelope of uniform thickness surrounding an oocyte; called also *oolemma.* Under the light microscope, it appears as a radially striated layer, which can be seen to be microvillous under the electron microscope, and is therefore called *zona radiata, zona striata,* or *striated membrane.* 2. area pellucida. **z. perfora'ta,** the inner portion of the lamina basilaris ductus cochlearis. **z. radia'ta,** see *z. pellucida,* def. 1. **z. reticula'ris,** reticular zone: the inner layer of the cortex of the suprarenal gland, consisting of cells arranged as clearly anastomosing cords, and abutting on the medulla. **z. rolan'dica,** the motor area of the cerebral cortex. **z. spongio'sa,** apex cornus posterioris medullae spinalis. **z. stria'ta,** see *z. pellucida,* def. 1. **z. tec'ta,** canal of Corti. **zo'nae tendino'sae cor'dis,** anuli fibrosi cordis. **z. transfor'mans,** transformation zone: the connective tissue layer of the intestinal wall where bacteria penetrating from the intestine are destroyed; called also *Turck's zone.* **z. Valsal'vae,** lamina basilaris ductus cochlearis. **z. vasculo'sa,** vascular zone: a region in the supramastoid fossa containing many foramina for the passage of blood vessels. **z. Web'eri,** z. orbicularis articulationis coxae.

zonae (zo'ne) [L.] plural of *zona.*

zonal (zo'nal) [L. *zona'lis*] of the nature of a zone.

zonary (zo'ner-e) zonal.

Zondek-Aschheim test (tson'dek-ash'hīm) [Bernhardt *Zondek,* German gynecologist, born 1891; Selmar *Aschheim,* German gynecologist, 1878–1965] Aschheim-Zondek test.

zone (zōn) [Gr. *zōnē* a belt, girdle] an encircling region or area; by extension any area with specific characteristics or boundary;

called also *zona.* **abdominal z's,** three zones into which the surface of the abdomen is divided by transverse lines. These zones are the *subcostal* or *epigastric*—that above the subcostal line; the *mesogastric*—that between the subcostal and intertubercular lines; and the *hypogastric*—that below the intertubercular line. **androgenic z.,** the provisional cortex of the embryonic suprarenal gland, which is possessed of certain testicular hormonal functions. **anelectrotonic z.,** polar z. **apical z.,** a narrow area along the mucous membrane over the apexes of the roots of the teeth. **arcuate z.,** canal of Corti. **biokinetic z.,** the range of temperatures within which the living cell carries on its life activities, lying approximately between 10° and 45° C. **border z.,** a zone at the boundary of two contiguous structures, as that where the trophoblast and the endometrium meet. **cervical z.,** that third of the coronal zone which is nearest the cervix of the tooth, marked by the cementoenamel junction of crown and root. **Charcot's z.,** hysterogenic z. **ciliary z.,** the outer of the two regions into which the anterior surface of the iris is divided by the angular line. Cf. *pupillary z.* **comfort z.,** an environmental temperature between 13° and 21° C. (55°–70° F.) with a humidity of 30 to 55 per cent. **contact area z.,** the zone which includes the contact area of adjoining teeth; usually it is in the middle third of the coronal zone between the occlusal and the cervical zone. **cornuradicular z.,** the outer part of the fasciculus cuneatus medullae spinalis. **coronal z.,** the entire enamel area of the tooth crown above the cementoenamel junction, the demarcation between crown and root. The coronal zone is subdivided horizontally into three areas; the occlusal zone, the contact area zone, and the cervical zone. These divisions are also spoken of as the occlusal third, the middle third, and the cervical third. **Cozzolino's z.,** fissula ante fenestram. **denticulate z.,** zona denticulata. **dentofacial z.,** the entire lower part of the face; the region of the face overlying the teeth and the alveolar processes of the jaws. **z's of discontinuity,** zones of varying optic density, seen with the slit lamp, in the lens of the eye; these zones are formed at particular periods in the prenatal development of the lens. **dolorogenic z.,** an area stimulation of which produces pain, or excites an attack of neuralgia. **dorsal z. of His,** the smaller upper thickening of the dorsal portion of the embryonic spinal cord projecting into the central canal. **entry z.,** the area of the spinal cord where the dorsal roots enter. **ependymal z.,** see under *layer.* **epigastric z.,** see *abdominal z's.* **epileptogenic z., epileptogenous z.,** an area stimulation of which may bring on an epileptic attack. **equivalence z.,** see *zone phenomenon,* under *phenomenon.* **erogenous z., erotogenic z.,** a portion of the body stimulation of which produces erotic excitation; such are the genitals, urethra, lips, anus, and breasts. **z. of exclusion** area of the cytoplasm devoid of all cytoplasmic components except the Golgi complex. **extravisual z.,** that part of the dioptric surfaces and media outside the visual zone, which is practically incapable of accurately focusing light. **fascicular z.,** zona fasciculata. **Flechsig's primordial z's,** the cortex of the ascending frontal gyrus and the ascending parietal gyrus of the brain. **glomerular z.,** zona glomerulosa. **Golgi z.,** the intracellular zone close to the nucleus and containing the Golgi complex; in most secretory cells, it is between the nucleus and the apical surface through which expulsion of the secretion occurs. **Head's z's,** areas of cutaneous sensitiveness associated with diseases of the viscera; called also *z's of hyperalgesia.* **hemorrhoidal z.,** zona hemorrhoidalis. **His's z's,** four thickenings which run the entire length of the embryonic spinal cord. **z's of hyperalgesia,** Head's z's. **hyperesthetic z.,** a region of the body surface marked by abnormal sensibility. **hypnogenic z., hypnogenous z.,** an area of the body on which pressure will characteristically induce sleep in particularly suggestible subjects. **hypogastric z.,** see *abdominal z's.* **hysterogenic z., hysterogenous z.,** a region of the body on which pressure may elicit a hysterial attack; called also *Charcot's z.* **inhibition z.,** see prozone. **intermediate z.,** that portion of the field of vision which lies between the fifteenth and forty-fifth concentric circles. **interpalpebral z.,** the part of the cornea not covered by the eyelids when the eye is open. **keratogenous z.,** the zone immediately above the dome of the dermal papilla, in which the cellular components of a hair follicle undergo keratinization and form the hair shaft. **language z.,** a general term referring to all cortical areas concerned with language mechanisms; usually in the dominant hemisphere. **Lissauer's marginal z.,** tractus dorsolateralis. **Looser's transformation z's,** dark lines seen on roentgenograms of bones, thought to represent pathological healing phases of fatigue fractures occurring in certain bone diseases. **mantle z.,** see under *layer.* **marginal z.,** 1. border zone. 2. marginal layer. **median root z.,** oval fasciculus. **mesogastric z.,** see *abdominal z's.* **motor z.,** an area of the cortex of the brain which, when electrically stimulated, causes contraction of voluntary muscles. **nephrogenic z.,** the subcapsular layer of the kidney. **neutral z.,** the potential space between the lips and cheeks on one side and the tongue on the other, natural or artificial teeth in this zone being subject to balancing forces from the surrounding musculature. **neutral z. of His,** a thickening of the dorsal portion of the embryonic spinal cord projecting

into the central canal. **Nitabuch z.,** see under *layer.* **nuclear z.,** vortex lentis. **Obersteiner-Redlich z.,** see under *area.* **occlusal z.,** that third of the coronal zone of the teeth which is nearest the occlusal plane. **orbicular z. of hip joint,** zona orbicularis articulationis coxae. **z. of oval nuclei,** a narrow band of sustentacular cells with oval nuclei in the olfactory mucosa. **pectinate z.,** zona pectinata. **pellucid z.,** zona pellucida. **peripolar z.,** the region surrounding a polar zone. **placental z.,** the area of the uterus to which the placenta is attached. **polar z.,** the region immediately around an electrode applied to the body. **proagglutinoid z.,** prozone. **pupillary z.,** the inner of the two regions into which the anterior surface of the iris is divided by the angular line. Cf. *ciliary z.* **reticular z.,** zona reticularis. **Rolando's z.,** the motor area of the cerebral cortex. **root z.,** those parts of the spinal cord to which dorsal and ventral roots are attached. **z. of round nuclei,** a broad band of olfactory cells with round nuclei in the olfactory mucosa. **rugae z.,** see under *area.* **segmental z.,** a zone of undifferentiated mesoderm between somites already formed and the primitive knot, from which additional somites will be produced. **subcostal z.,** see *abdominal z's.* **sudanophobic z.,** a broad zone of cells which appears in the adrenal cortex of rats following hypophysectomy, and which does not stain with Sudan. **tendinous z's of heart,** anuli fibrosi cordis. **transformation z.,** zona transformans. **transition z., transitional z.,** the circle in the equator of the lens of the eye in which epithelial fibers are developed into lens fibers. **transparent z.,** see *transparent dentin,* under *dentin.* **trigger z.,** dolorogenic z. **Turck's z.,** zona transformans. **umbau z's** [Ger.], Looser's transformation z's. **Valsalva's z.,** lamina basilaris ductus cochlearis. **vascular z.,** zona vasculosa. **visual z.,** that part of the dioptric surfaces and mediums around an optic axis in which there is practically no aberration of light rays. **Weber's z.,** zona orbicularis articulationis coxae. **Weil's basal z.,** see under *layer.* **Wernicke's z.,** see under *area.* **Westphal's z.,** a zone of the posterior gray column of the spinal cord in the lumbar region; it is said to contain the exodic fibers concerned in the patellar reflex. **X z.,** androgenic z. **z. of Zinn,** zonula ciliaris.

zonesthesia (zo″nes-the′ze-ah) [Gr. *zōnē* girdle + *aisthēsis* perception + *-ia*] a sensation of constriction, as by a girdle.

zonifugal (zo-nif′u-gal) [L. *zona* zone + *fugere* to flee from] passing outward from any area or region.

zoning (zōn′ing) the occurrence of a stronger fixation of complement in a lesser amount of suspected serum.

zonipetal (zo-nip′ĕ-tal) [L. *zona* zone + *petere* to seek] passing from outside into any area or region.

Zonomune (zo″no-mūn′) trademark for a preparation of influenza virus vaccine.

zonoskeleton (zōn″o-skel′ĕ-ton) see *limb.*

zonula (zōn′u-lah), pl. *zon′ulae* [L., dim. of zona] a small zone, or zonule. **z. adher′ens,** that portion of the junctional complex of columnar epithelial cells, just deep to the zonula occludens, where the cell membranes diverge to form an intercellular space 150 to 200 A wide and are supported on their inner aspect by moderately dense filamentous material forming a continuous band parallel to the zonula occludens. **z. cilia′ris** [NA], **z. cilia′ris [Zin′nii],** ciliary zonule: a system of fibers extending between the ciliary body and the equator of the lens, holding the lens in place; called also *Zinn's membrane* or *zonule.* **z. occlu′dens,** that portion of the junctional complex of columnar epithelial cells, just beneath the free surface, where the intercellular space is obliterated; it extends completely around the cell perimeter, above the zonula adherens. Called also *tight junction.*

zonulae (zon′u-le) [L.] plural of *zonula.*

zonular (zon′u-lar) pertaining to a zonule.

zonule (zōn′ul) a small zone; called also *zonula.* **ciliary z.,** zonula ciliaris. **lens z.,** zonula ciliaris. **z. of Zinn,** zonula ciliaris.

zonulitis (zōn″u-li′tis) inflammation of the ciliary zonule.

zonulolysis (zon″u-lol′ĭ-sis) [*zonule* + Gr. *lysis* dissolution] dissolution of the zonule of Zinn (zonula ciliaris) in surgery by means of enzymes such as alpha-chymotrypsin.

zonulotomy (zon″u-lot′o-me) [*zonule* + Gr. *tomē* a cutting] incision of the ciliary zonule.

zonulysis (zon″u-li′sis) zonulolysis.

zoo- [Gr. *zōon* animal] a combining form denoting relationship to an animal.

zoo-agglutinin (zo″o-ah-gloo′tĭ-nin) a substance in animal poisons having the power of agglutinating red blood cells.

zooamylon (zo″o-am′ĭ-lon) [*zoo-* + Gr. *amylon* starch] (*obs.*) glycogen.

zoo-anaphylactogen (zo″o-an″ah-fi-lak′to-jen) a protein substance of animal origin capable of producing anaphylaxis; called also *zoosensitinogen.*

zoobiology (zo″o-bi-ol′o-je) [*zoo-* + Gr. *bios* life + *-logy*] the biology of animals.

zoobiotism (zo″o-bi′o-tizm) biotics.

zooblast (zo'o-blast) [zoo- + Gr. *blastos* germ] an animal cell.

zoochemical (zo''o-kem'ĭ-kal) pertaining to zoochemistry.

zoochemistry (zo''o-kem'is-tre) the study of the chemical reactions occurring in animal tissues.

zoodermic (zo''o-der'mik) [zoo- + Gr. *derma* skin] performed with the skin of an animal; said of skin grafting in which the grafts are from the skin of an animal.

zoodetritus (zo''o-de-tri'tus) biodetritus produced by the disintegration and decomposition of animal organisms. Cf. *phytodetritus.*

zoodynamic (zo''o-di-nam'ik) pertaining to zoodynamics (animal physiology).

zoodynamics (zo''o-di-nam'iks) [zoo- + Gr. *dynamis* power] animal physiology.

zooerastia (zo''o-e-ras''te-ah) [zoo- + Gr. *erastēs* lover] bestiality.

zoofulvin (zo''o-ful'vin) a yellow pigment from the feathers of certain birds.

zoogenesis (zo''o-jen'ĕ-sis) zoogeny.

zoogenous (zo-oj'ĕ-nus) 1. acquired from animals. 2. viviparous.

zoogeny (zo-oj'ĕ-ne) [zoo- + Gr. *gennan* to produce] the development and evolution of animals.

zoogeography (zo''o-je-og'rah-fe) the study of the distribution of animal life on the earth.

zooglea (zo''o-gle'ah) [zoo- + Gr. *gloios* gum] a colony of bacteria embedded in a gelatinous matrix.

zoogleic (zo''o-gle'ik) pertaining to or characterized by the presence of zooglea.

Zoogloea (zo''o-gle'ah) a genus of microorganisms of the family Pseudomonadaceae, suborder Pseudomonadineae, order Pseudomonadales, occurring as rod-shaped cells embedded in a gelatinous matrix. It includes two species, *Z. filipen'dula* and *Z. rami'gera.*

zoogloea (zo''o-gle'ah) zooglea.

zoogloeic (zo''o-gle'ik) zoogleic.

zoogonous (zo-og'o-nus) viviparous.

zoogony (zo-og'o-ne) [zoo- + Gr. *gonē* offspring] the production of living young from within the body.

zoografting (zo''o-graft''ing) the grafting of animal tissue.

zoography (zo-og'rah-fe) [zoo- + Gr. *graphein* to write] a treatise on animals.

zoohormone (zo''o-hor'mōn) an animal hormone.

zooid (zo'oid) [zoo- + Gr. *eidos* form] 1. resembling an animal. 2. an object or form which resembles an animal. 3. one of the individuals in a united colony of animals.

zookinase (zo''o-kin'ās) a naturally occurring activator of autolytic activity in a cell.

zoolagnia (zo''o-lag'ne-ah) [zoo- + Gr. *lagneia* lust] sexual attraction toward animals.

zoology (zo-ol'o-je) [zoo- + Gr. *logos* treatise] the biology of animals; the sum of what is known regarding animals. **experimental z.,** the study of animals by means of experiments performed upon them.

zoomania (zo''o-ma'ne-ah) [zoo- + Gr. *mania* madness] a morbid love of animals.

Zoomastigophora (zo''o-mas''tĭ-gof'o-rah) a class of protozoa of the subphylum Mastigophora, including all the flagellates that parasitize higher animals; they are characterized by the absence of chromatophores and most have one nucleus, usually of the vesicular type. It includes the orders Rhizomastigida, Protomastigida, Protomonadina, Polymastigida, and Hypermastigida.

zoonerythrin (zo''on-er'ĭ-thrin) [zoo- + Gr. *erythros* red] crustaceorubin.

zoonite (zo'o-nīt) a cerebrospinal metamere.

zoonomy (zo-on'o-me) [zoo- + Gr. *nomos* law] zoobiology.

zoonoses (zo''o-no'sēz) plural of *zoonosis.*

zoonosis (zo''o-no'sis), pl. *zoono'ses* [zoo- + Gr. *nosos* disease] a disease of animals that may be transmitted to man under natural conditions (e.g., brucellosis, rabies).

zoonosology (zo''o-no-sol'o-je) [zoo- + Gr. *nosos* disease + *logos* treatise] the classification of diseases of animals.

zoonotic (zo''o-not'ik) transmissible from animals to man under natural conditions; pertaining to or constituting a zoonosis.

zooparasite (zo''o-par'ah-sīt) any parasitic animal organism or species; see *animal parasite,* under *parasite.*

zooparasitic (zo''o-par''ah-sit'ik) pertaining to or produced by zooparasites.

zoopathology (zo''o-pah-thol'o-je) animal pathology; the study of the diseases of animals.

zooperal (zo-op'er-al) pertaining to zoopery.

zoopery (zo-op'er-e) [zoo- + Gr. *peiran* to experiment] the performing of experiments on animals.

zoophagous (zo-of'ah-gus) [zoo- + Gr. *phagein* to eat] subsisting upon animal food.

zoopharmacology (zo''o-fahr''mah-kol'o-je) veterinary pharmacology.

zoopharmacy (zo-o-fahr'mah-se) veterinary pharmacy.

zoophile (zo'o-fīl) [zoo- + Gr. *philein* to love] 1. zoophilic. 2. an antivivisectionist.

zoophilia (zo''o-fil'e-ah) abnormal fondness for animals.

zoophilic (zo''o-fil'ik) preferring animals to man; said of certain mosquitoes. Cf. *anthropophilic* and *anthropozoophilic.*

zoophilism (zo-of'ĭ-lizm) 1. fondness for animals; antivivisection. 2. the state of being zoophilic. **erotic z.,** sexual pleasure experienced in the fondling of animals.

zoophilous (zo-of'ĭ-lus) zoophilic.

zoophobia (zo''o-fo'be-ah) [zoo- + Gr. *phobein* to be affrighted by] abnormal dread of animals.

zoophysiology (zo''o-fiz''e-ol'o-je) animal physiology.

zoophyte (zo'o-fīt) [zoo- + Gr. *phyton* plant] any plantlike animal, such as sponges or hydroids.

zooplankton (zo''o-plank'ton) [zoo- + Gr. *planktos* wandering] the minute animal organisms which, with those of the vegetable kingdom (phytoplankton), make up the plankton of natural waters.

zooplasty (zo'o-plast''te) [zoo- + Gr. *plassein* to form] zoografting.

zooprecipitin (zo''o-pre-sip'ĭ-tin) a precipitin obtained by injections of protein substances of animal origin.

zooprophylaxis (zo''o-pro''fĭ-lak'sis) 1. prophylaxis applied to animals; veterinary prophylaxis. 2. the prevention or amelioration of disease (e.g., smallpox) in man as a result of previous exposure to heterologous infection of animal origin (e.g., cowpox). 3. protecting man from bites of mosquitoes by providing cattle or other animals for the mosquitoes to feed on.

zoopsia (zo-op'se-ah) [zoo- + Gr. *opsis* vision + *-ia*] a hallucination in which the patient thinks he sees animals.

zoopsychology (zo''o-si-kol'o-je) animal psychology.

zoosadism (zo''o-sa'dizm) sadism directed toward animals.

zooscopy (zo-os'ko-pe) [zoo- + Gr. *skopein* to view] 1. zoopsia. 2. the scientific study or observation of animals.

zoosensitinogen (zo''o-sen''sĭ-tin'o-jen) zoo-anaphylactogen.

zoosis (zo-o'sis) [zoo- + *-osis*] any disease due to animal agents.

zoosperm (zo'o-sperm) [zoo- + Gr. *sperma* seed] spermatozoon.

zoospermia (zo''o-sper'me-ah) the presence of live spermatozoa in the ejaculated semen.

zoosporangia (zo''o-spo-ran'je-ah) plural of *zoosporangium.*

zoosporangium (zo''o-spo-ran'je-um), pl. *zoosporan'gia* [zoo- + Gr. *angeion* vessel] the structure in which zoospores are developed. See *spore.*

zoospore (zo'o-spōr) [zoo- + *spore*] a motile mitospore; a motile, flagellated, asexual spore, as produced by certain algae and fungi. Called also *flagellospore, flagellula,* and *swarm spore.* See *spore.*

zoosteroid (zo''o-ste'roid) any steroid of animal origin.

zoosterol (zo''o-ste'rol) any sterol of animal origin.

zootechnics (zo''o-tek'niks) [zoo- + Gr. *technē* art] the art of breeding, keeping, and handling animals in domestication or captivity.

zootic (zo-ot'ik) pertaining to the lower animals. Cf. *demic.*

zootomist (zo-ot'o-mist) a comparative anatomist.

zootomy (zo-ot'o-me) [zoo- + Gr. *tomē* a cutting] 1. the dissection of animals. 2. the anatomy of animals.

zootoxin (zo''o-tok'sin) [zoo- + Gr. *toxikon* poison] a toxic substance of animal origin, such as the venoms of snakes, spiders, and scorpions.

zootrophic (zo''o-trof'ik) [zoo- + Gr. *trophē* nutrition] pertaining to the nutrition of animals.

zootrophotoxism (zo''o-trof''o-tok'sizm) [zoo- + Gr. *trophē* nutrition + *toxikon* poison] poisoning with animal foods.

Zopfius (zop'fe-us) a former genus of bacteria, now named *Kurthia.*

zorbamycin (zor-bah-mi'sin) an antibacterial antibiotic derived from a variant of *Streptomyces bikiniensis.*

zorubicin hydrochloride (zo-ru'bĭ-sin) chemical name: (2S-cis)-benzoic acid[1-[4-[(3-amino-2,3,6-trideoxy-α-L-*lyxo*-hexopyranosyl)oxy]-1,2,3,4,6,11-hexahydro-2,5,12-trihydroxy-7-methoxy-6,11-dioxo-2-naphthacenyl]ethylidene]hydrazide; an antineoplastic, $C_{34}H_{35}N_3O_{10} \cdot HCl.$

zoster (zos'ter) [Gr. *zōstēr*] a girdle, or encircling structure or pattern; see *herpes zoster.*

Zostera marina (zos'ter-ah mah-ri'nah) seawrack or eelgrass, a marine plant.

zosteriform (zos-ter'ĭ-form) resembling herpes zoster.

zosteroid (zos'ter-oid) resembling herpes zoster.

zoxazolamine (zok''sah-zol'ah-mēn) chemical name: 2-amino-5-chlorobenzoxazole. A plate-like substance, $C_7H_{15}ClN_2O,$ occasionally used as a skeletal muscle relaxant and uricosuric agent in gout.

Z-plasty (ze-plas'te) a plastic operation for the relaxation of contractures, in which a Z-shaped incision is made, the middle bar of the Z being over the contracted scar, and the triangular flaps rotated so that their apices cross the line of contracture.

Zr chemical symbol for *zirconium*.

Zsigmondy's gold number method, test (sig-mon'dēz) [Richard Adolf *Zsigmondy*, German chemist, 1865–1929; winner of the Nobel prize in chemistry for 1925, for his work on colloids; inventor of the ultramicroscope in 1903] colloidal gold test.

Zuberella (zu"ber-el'ah) a genus of gram-negative anaerobic bacteria.

zuckergussdarm (tsook'er-goos"darm) [Ger. "sugar-ice skin"] peritonitis chronica fibrosa encapsulans.

zuckergussleber (tsook'er-goos"la-ber) [Ger. "sugar-ice liver"] perihepatitis chronica hyperplastica.

Zuckerkandl's body, convolution, gland, organs (tsook'-er-kan"d'lz) [Emil *Zuckerkandl*, German anatomist, 1849–1910] see under *body, gland,* and *organ,* and see *gyrus paraterminalis*.

zuclomiphene (zoo-klo'mĭ-fēn) chemical name: (Z)-2-[4-(2-chloro-1,2-diphenylethenyl) phenoxy]- N, N-diethylethanamine; the *trans*-isomer of the gonad-stimulating principle clomiphene citrate (q.v.), $C_{26}H_{28}ClNO$. Called also *transclomiphene*. Cf. *enclomiphene*.

Zuntz's theory (zoont'zes) [Nathan *Zuntz*, Berlin physician, 1847–1920] see under *theory*.

zwieback (tsve'bak) pieces of bread made of rich dough and heated in the oven until they are deep yellow in color.

Zwischenferment (tsvish"en-fer'ment) [Ger.] glucose 6-phosphate dehydrogenase.

Zwischenkörper (tsvish'en-ker"per) [Ger.] amboceptor; antibody.

zwischenscheibe (tsvish'en-shi"bě) [Ger.] Z band; see under *band*.

zwitterion (tsvit'er-i"on) a dipolar ion, i.e., an ion that has both positive and negative regions of charge; amino acids, for example, occur as zwitterions in neutral solution, and the pH value at which the zwitterion state is at a maximum is the isoelectric point.

zwölffingerdarm (tsvelf-fing'ger-darm) [Ger. *zwölf* twelve + *finger* finger + *darm* bowel] the duodenum.

zygadenine (zi-gad'ě-nin) a crystalline alkaloid, $C_{39}H_{63}NO_{10}$, from the plant *Zygadenus intermedius*.

zygal (zi'gal) [Gr. *zygon* yoke] shaped like a yoke.

zygapophyseal (zi"gah-po-fiz'e-al) pertaining to a zygapophysis.

zygapophysis (zi"gah-pof'ĭ-sis), pl. *zygapoph'yses.* An articular process of a vertebra; see *processus articularis inferior vertebrarum* and *processus articularis superior vertebrarum*.

zygia (zij'e-ah) plural of *zygion*.

zygion (zij'e-on), pl. *zyg'ia* [Gr.] an anthropometric landmark, being the most laterally situated point on either zygomatic arch.

zygo- [Gr. *zygon* yoke] a combining form meaning yoked or joined, or denoting relationship to a junction.

Zygocotyle lunatum (zi"go-ko'tĭ-le lu-na'tum) a trematode parasitic in the intestine of a variety of hosts, including rats, cattle, and ducks in North America.

zygocyte (zi'go-sīt) see *zygote*.

zygodactyly (zi"go-dak'tĭ-le) [*zygo-* + Gr. *daktylos* finger] a term sometimes used to designate simple syndactyly, as distinguished from syndactyly in which there is bony fusion between the phalanges of the digits involved; usually occurring in the hand between the third and fourth digits, and in the foot between the fourth and fifth.

zygoite (zi'go-īt) an organism formed by zygosis; a zygote.

zygoma (zi-go'mah) [Gr. *zygōma* bolt or bar] 1. processus zygomaticus temporalis. 2. arcus zygomaticus. 3. a term sometimes applied to os zygomaticum.

zygomatic (zi"go-mat'ik) pertaining to the zygoma.

zygomaticofacial (zi"go-mat"ĭ-ko-fa'shal) pertaining to the zygoma and the face.

zygomaticofrontal (zi"go-mat"ĭ-ko-fron'tal) pertaining to the zygoma and the frontal bone.

zygomaticomaxillary (zi"go-mat"ĭ-ko-mak'sĭ-ler"e) pertaining to the zygoma and the maxilla.

zygomatico-orbital (zi"go-mat"ĭ-ko-or'bĭ-tal) pertaining to the zygoma and the orbit.

zygomaticosphenoid (zi"go-mat"ĭ-ko-sfe'noid) pertaining to the zygoma and the sphenoid bone.

zygomaticotemporal (zi"go-mat"ĭ-ko-tem'por-al) pertaining to the zygoma and the temporal bone.

zygomaxillare (zi"go-mak'sĭ-la"re) [L.] a craniometric point at the lower end of the zygomatic suture.

zygomaxillary (zi"go-mak'sĭ-ler"e) pertaining to the zygoma and the maxilla.

Zygomycetes (zi"go-mi-se'tēz) a subclass of phycomycetous fungi, including the orders Mucorales and Entomophthorales.

zygon (zi'gon) [Gr.] the bar or stem connecting the two branches of a zygal fissure.

zygoplast (zi'go-plast) [*zygo-* + Gr. *plassein* to form] rhizoplast.

zygopodium (zi"go-po'de-um) see *limb*.

zygosis (zi-go'sis) [Gr. *zygōsis* a balancing] the sexual union of two unicellular organisms.

zygosity (zi-gos'ĭ-te) [Gr. *zygon* yoke + *-ity* state or condition] the condition relating to conjugation, or to the zygote, as (*a*) the state of a cell or individual in regard to the alleles determining a specific character, whether identical (homozygosity) or different (heterozygosity); or (*b*), in the case of twins, whether developing from one zygote (monozygosity) or two (dizygosity). Often used as a word termination affixed to a root descriptive of the condition.

zygosperm (zi'go-sperm) zygospore.

zygosphere (zi'go-sfēr) a gamete arising from a zygophore which unites with another to form a zygospore.

zygospore (zi'go-spōr) a spore formed by the conjugation of two cells (isogametes) which are morphologically identical, or in the Zygomycetes, from the fusion of like gametangia. See *spore*.

zygostyle (zi'go-stīl) the last coccygeal vertebra.

zygote (zi'gōt) [Gr. *zygōtos* yoked together] the cell resulting from union of a male and a female gamete, until it divides; the fertilized ovum. More precisely, the cell after synapsis at the completion of fertilization until first cleavage. Also, used loosely to refer to the fertilized ovum and derivatives for an indefinite period, extending even to birth. Cf. *conceptus.* **duplex z.,** one possessing two identical genes for a given dominant character. **multiplex z.,** one possessing no gene for a given dominant character. **simplex z.,** one possessing only one gene for a given dominant character.

zygotene (zi'go-tēn) [Gr. *zygōtos* yolked together] the synaptic stage of the first meiotic prophase in which the two leptotene chromosomes undergo pairing by the formation of synaptonemal complexes to form a bivalent structure. See also *diplotene, leptotene,* and *pachytene.* Called also *amphitene*.

zygotic (zi-got'ik) pertaining to a zygote.

zygotoblast (zi-go'to-blast) [*zygote* + Gr. *blastos* germ] sporozoite.

zygotomere (zi-go'to-mēr) [*zygote* + Gr. *meros* part] sporoblast.

zylonite (zi'lo-nīt) [Gr. *xylon* wood] xylonite.

Zyloprim (zi'lo-prim) trademark for a preparation of allopurinol.

zymase (zi'mās) [Gr. *zymē* leaven + *-ase*] 1. an enzyme. 2. the intracellular enzyme of yeast by which alcoholic fermentation is produced; called also *Buchner's z*.

zymasis (zi'mah-sis) the excretion of the active substance of yeast by hydraulic pressure.

zyme (zīm) [Gr. *zymē* leaven] 1. enzyme. 2. any pathogenic agent that produces a zymotic disease.

zymic (zi'mik) pertaining to enzymes.

zymin (zi'min) 1. a pancreatic extract prepared for therapeutic use. 2. zyme.

zymo- [Gr. *zymē* leaven] a combining form denoting relationship to an enzyme, or to fermentation.

Zymobacterium (zi"mo-bak-te're-um) [Gr. *zymē* leaven + *baktērion* little rod] a genus of microorganisms of the family Propionibacteriaceae, order Eubacteriales, non–spore-forming, anaerobic to microaerophilic, gram-positive bacilli, nonpathogenic but occurring as parasites in the intestinal tract.

zymochemistry (zi"mo-kem'is-tre) the chemistry of fermentation.

zymoexcitator (zi"mo-ek'si-ta"tor) any substance which serves to convert zymogens into their enzymes. Cf. *kinase*, def. 2.

zymoexciter (zi"mo-ek-si'ter) zymoexcitator.

zymogen (zi'mo-jen) [*zymo-* + Gr. *gennan* to produce] an inactive precursor that is converted to active enzyme by the action of acid, another enzyme, or by other means. Called also *pre-enzyme* or *proenzyme.* **lab z.,** an enzyme in the stomach that is transformed into rennin by acids of the gastric juice.

zymogenesis (zi"mo-jen'ě-sis) the formation of an enzyme from a zymogen.

zymogenic (zi"mo-jen'ik) 1. causing a fermentation. 2. pertaining to a fermentation.

zymogenous (zi-moj'ě-nus) zymogenic.

zymogic (zi-moj'ik) zymogenic.

zymogram (zi'mo-gram) a graphic representation of enzymatically active components separated electrophoretically.

zymohexase (zi"mo-hek'sās) an enzyme that catalyzes the splitting of fructose 1,6-diphosphate into dihydroxy acetone phosphate and phosphoglyceric aldehyde; said to be increased in tumor-bearing animals.

zymohydrolysis (zi"mo-hi-drol'ĭ-sis) zymolysis.

zymoid (zi'moid) [*zymo-* + Gr. *eidos* form] 1. resembling an enzyme. 2. any poison derived from a decaying tissue that has lost its power of decomposing the substratum, but not its power of uniting with it.

zymolysis (zi-mol'ĭ-sis) [*zymo-* + Gr. *lysis* dissolution] fermentation or digestion by means of an enzyme.

zymolytic (zi''mo-lit'ik) pertaining to, characterized by, or promoting zymolysis.

Zymomonas (zi''mo-mo'nas) a genus of microorganisms of the family Pseudomonadaceae, suborder Pseudomonadineae, order Pseudomonadales, occurring as rod-shaped or ellipsoidal cells in fermenting beverages. It includes two species, *Z. anaero'bia* and *Z. mo'bilis.*

Zymonema (zi''mo-ne'mah) [*zymo-* + Gr. *nēma* thread] a name formerly given a genus of fungi. **Z. al'bicans,** *Candida albicans.* **Z. capsula'tum, Z. dermatit'idis, Z. gilchris'ti,** *Blastomyces dermatitidis.* **Z. farcimino'sum,** *Histoplasma farciminosus.*

zymophore (zi'mo-fōr) [*zymo-* + Gr. *phoros* bearing] the group of atoms in the molecule of an enzyme which is responsible for its specific effect; the active site of an enzyme.

zymophorous (zi-mof'o-rus) pertaining to the zymophore; responsible for the specific action of an enzyme.

zymophosphate (zi''mo-fos'fāt) hexosephosphoric acid occurring in yeast; it may accumulate in large amounts.

zymoprotein (zi''mo-pro'te-in) any of a class of proteins having catalytic powers. They include catalase, chymase, papain, pepsin, peroxidase, and urease.

zymosan (zi'mo-san) a mixture of polysaccharides, proteins, and ash, of variable concentration, derived from the cell walls, or the entire cell, of yeast, commonly *Saccharomyces cerevisiae.* It is anticomplementary, absorbing the C3 component of complement, and is used in assaying properdin.

zymoscope (zi'mo-skōp) [*zymo-* + Gr. *skopein* to examine] an apparatus for determining the zymotic (fermentative) power of yeast.

zymose (zi'mōs) invertin.

zymosis (zi-mo'sis) [Gr. *zymōsis* fermentation] 1. fermentation. 2. the development of any zymotic disease; the propagation and development of an infectious disease, known by the growth of bacteria and their products. 3. any infectious or contagious disease. **z. gas'trica,** a condition marked by the formation of organic acids in the stomach, due to the action of yeasts.

zymosterol (zi-mos'ter-ol) mycosterol; a sterol, $C_{27}H_{44}O$, occurring in fungi and molds, which is second to ergosterol in abundance in yeast fat.

zymosthenic (zi''mos-then'ik) [*zymo-* + Gr. *sthenos* strength] increasing the activity of an enzyme.

zymotic (zi-mot'ik) 1. caused by or pertaining to zymosis. 2. a zymotic disease.

zymurgy (zi'mer-je) [Gr. *zymē* leaven + *ergon* work] (*obs.*) the art of brewing, distilling, and winemaking; the branch of chemistry that deals with the commercial application of fermentation.

zytase (zi'tās) an enzyme that changes xylan to xylose.

Zz. abbreviation for L. *zin'giber,* ginger.

Z.Z.'Z.'' increasing degrees of contraction.